Laboratory Parameter	SI	Conventional (C)	Conversion Factor (CF) CF × C = SI
Glucose, plasma			
Overnight fast, normal	4.2–6.4 mmol/L	75–115 mg/dL	0.05551
Overnight fast, diabetes mellitus			
National Diabetes Data Group	>7.8 mmol/L	>140 mg/dL	0.05551
American Diabetes Association	>7.0 mmol/L	>126 mg/dL	0.05551
72-h fast, normal men	>2.8 mmol/L	>50 mg/dL	0.05551
72-h fast, normal women	>2.2 mmol/L	>40 mg/dL	0.05551
Glucose Tolerance Test, 2-h postprandial plasma glucose			
Normal	<7.8 mmol/L	<140 mg/dL	0.05551
Impaired glucose tolerance	7.8–11.1 mmol/L	140–200 mg/dL	0.05551
Diabetes mellitus	>11.1 mmol/L	>200 mg/dL	0.05551
Gonadal Steroids, plasma			
Androstenedione			
Women	3.5–7.0 nmol/L	1–2 ng/mL	3.492
Men	3.0–5.0 nmol/L	0.8–1.3 ng/mL	3.492
Dihydrotestosterone			
Women	0.17–1 nmol/L	0.05–3 ng/mL	3.467
Men	0.87–2.6 nmol/L	0.25–0.75 ng/mL	3.467
Estradiol			
Women, basal	70–220 pmol/L	20–60 pg/mL	3.671
Women, ovulatory surge	>740 pmol/L	>200 pg/mL	3.671
Men	<180 pmol/L	<50 pg/mL	3.671
Progesterone			
Women, luteal phase	6–64 nmol/L	2–20 ng/mL	3.180
Women, follicular phase	<6 nmol/L	<2 ng/mL	3.180
Men	<6 nmol/L	<2 ng/mL	3.180
Testosterone			
Women	<3.5 nmol/L	<1 ng/mL	3.467
Men	10–35 nmol/L	3–10 ng/mL	3.467
Gonadotropins, plasma			
Follicle-Stimulating Hormone (FSH)			
Women, basal	1.4–9.6 IU/L	1.4–9.6 mIU/mL	—
Women, ovulatory surge	2.3–21 IU/L	2.3–21 mIU/mL	—
Women, postmenopausal	34–96 IU/L	34–96 mIU/mL	—
Men	0.9–15 IU/L	0.9–15 mIU/mL	—
Luteinizing Hormone (LH)			
Women, basal	0.8–26 IU/L	0.8–26 mIU/mL	—
Women, ovulatory surge	25–57 IU/L	25–57 mIU/mL	—
Women, postmenopausal	40–104 IU/L	40–104 mIU/mL	—
Men	1.3–13 IU/L	1.3–13 mIU/mL	—
Growth Hormone (GH), plasma			
After 100 g glucose orally	<2 μg/L	<2 ng/mL	—
After insulin-induced hypoglycemia	>9 μg/L	>9 ng/mL	—
Human Chorionic Gonadotropin β Subunit (β-hCG), plasma			
Men and nonpregnant women	<3 IU/L	<3 mIU/mL	—
β-Hydroxybutyrate, plasma	<300 μmol/L	<3 mg/dL	96.05
Insulin, plasma			
Fasting	35–145 pmol/L	5–20 uU/mL	7.175
During hypoglycemia (plasma glucose <2.8 nmol/L <50 mg/mL)	<35 pmol/L	<5 uU/mL	7.175
Insulin C Peptide, plasma	0.5–2 μg/L	0.5–2 pg/mL	—
Insulin-Like Growth Factor I (IGF-I, Somatomedin-C)			
Women	0.45–2.2 kU/L	0.45–2.2 U/mL	—
Men	0.34–1.9 kU/L	0.34–1.9 U/mL	—
Lactate, plasma	0.56–2.2 mmol/L	5–20 mg/dL	0.111
Magnesium, serum	0.8–1.30 mmol/L	1.8–3.0 mg/dL	0.4114
Osmolality, plasma	285–295 mmol/kg	285–295 mOsmol/L	—
Oxytocin, plasma			
Random	1–4 pmol/L	1.25–5 ng/L	0.80
Women, ovulatory surge	4–8 pmol/L	5–10 ng/L	0.80
Parathyroid Hormone, serum (**Intact PTH** using IRMA assay)	10–65 ng/L	10–65 pg/mL	—
Phosphorus, inorganic, serum	1–1.5 mmol/L	3.0–4.5 mg/dL	0.3229
Prolactin, serum			
Nonpregnant women and men	2–15 μg/L	2–15 ng/mL	—
Pyruvate, plasma	39–102 μmol/L	0.3–0.9 mg/dL	0.01129
Renin Activity, plasma, normal-sodium intake			
Supine	3.2 ± 1 μg/L/h	3.2 ± 1 ng/mL/h	—
Standing	9.3 ± 4.3 μg/L/h	9.3 ± 4.3 ng/mL/h	—
Sodium, serum	136–145 mmol/L	136–145 mEq/L	—
Thyroid Function Tests			
Free thyroxine estimate	9–26 pmol/L	0.7–2.0 ng/dL	12.87
Radioactive iodine uptake, 24 h	0.05–0.30	5–30%	—
Resin T_3 uptake, serum	0.25–0.35	25–35%	—
Reverse triiodothyronine (rT_3), serum	0.15–0.61 nmol/L	10–40 ng/dL	0.01536
Thyroid hormone-binding ratio (THBR)	0.85–1.10	85–110%	—
Thyrotropin (TSH), serum	0.5–5 mU/L	0.5–5 μU/mL	—
Thyroxine (T_4), serum	64–154 nmol/L	5–12 μg/dL	12.87
Triiodothyronine (T_3), serum	1.1–2.9 nmol/L	70–190 ng/dL	0.01536
Triglycerides, plasma	<1.80 mmol/L	<160 mg/dL	0.01129
Vitamin D, see **Calciferols**			

Williams Textbook of

Endocrinology

TENTH EDITION

P. Reed Larsen, MD, FACP, FRCP
Professor of Medicine
Harvard Medical School
Chief, Division of Endocrinology, Diabetes and Hypertension
Brigham and Women's Hospital
Boston, Massachusetts

Henry M. Kronenberg, MD
Professor of Medicine
Harvard Medical School
Chief, Endocrine Unit
Massachusetts General Hospital
Boston, Massachusetts

Shlomo Melmed, MD
Senior Vice President, Academic Affairs
Cedars Sinai Research Institute
Professor of Medicine and Associate Dean
University of California, Los Angeles, School of Medicine
Los Angeles, California

Kenneth S. Polonsky, MD
Adolphus Busch Professor and Chairman
Department of Medicine
Professor, Department of Cell Biology and Physiology
Washington University School of Medicine
St. Louis, Missouri

SAUNDERS
An Imprint of Elsevier Science

SAUNDERS
An Imprint of Elsevier Science

The Curtis Center
Independence Square West
Philadelphia, Pennsylvania 19106

WILLIAMS TEXTBOOK OF ENDOCRINOLOGY ISBN 0-7216-9184-6

Notice

Medicine is an ever-changing field. Standard safety precautions must be followed, but as new research and clinical experience broaden our knowledge, changes in treatment and drug therapy may become necessary or appropriate. Readers are advised to check the most current product information provided by the manufacturer of each drug to be administered to verify the recommended dose, the method and duration of administration, and contraindications. It is the responsibility of the treating physician, relying on experience and knowledge of the patient, to determine dosages and the best treatment for each individual patient. Neither the publisher nor the editor assumes any liability for any injury and/or damage to persons or property arising from this publication.

THE PUBLISHER

Library of Congress Cataloging-in-Publication Data

Williams textbook of endocrinology/P. Reed Larsen . . . [et al.].—10th ed.
p. ; cm.
ISBN 0-7216-9184-6
1. Endocrinology. 2. Endocrine glands—Diseases. I. Williams, Robert Hardin. II. Larsen, P. Reed.
RC648 .T48 2002
616.4—dc21
DNLM/DLC 2002019193

Acquisitions Editor: Catherine Carroll
Senior Developmental Editor: Faith Voit
Project Manager: Norman Stellander
Designer: Steven Stave

PIT/MVB

Printed in the United States of America.

Last digit is the print number: 9 8 7 6 5 4 3 2 1

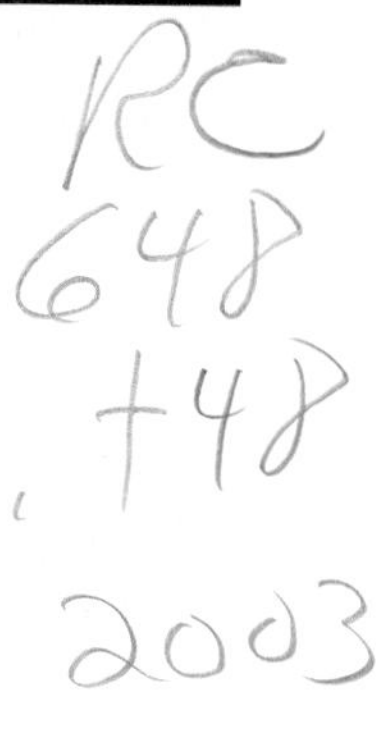

CONTRIBUTORS

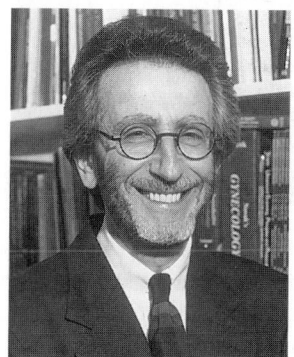

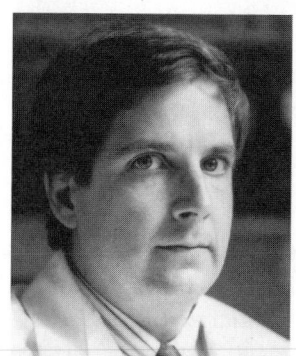

Eli Y. Adashi

Presidential Professor of Obstetrics and Gynecology and John A. Dixon Professor and Chair, Department of Obstetrics and Gynecology, University of Utah Health Sciences Center, Salt Lake City, Utah

The Physiology and Pathology of the Female Reproductive Axis; Fertility Control: Current Approaches and Global Aspects

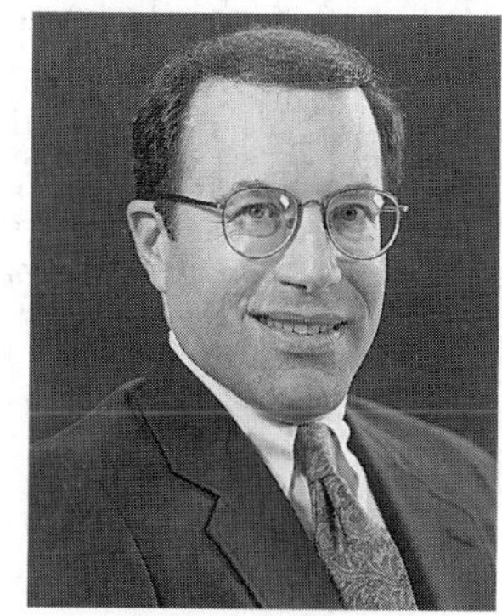

Andrew Arnold

Murray-Heilig Chair in Molecular Medicine and Professor of Medicine and Genetics, University of Connecticut School of Medicine; Director, Center for Molecular Medicine, and Chief, Division of Endocrinology and Metabolism, University of Connecticut, Farmington, Connecticut

Pathogenesis of Endocrine Tumors

Lloyd P. Aiello

Associate Professor of Ophthalmology, Harvard Medical School; Assistant Director, Beetham Eye Institute; Investigator and Head, Section of Eye Research, Joslin Diabetes Center, Boston, Massachusetts

Complications of Diabetes Mellitus

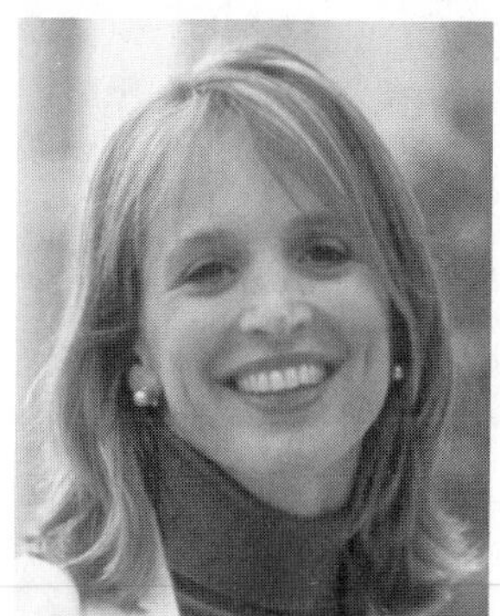

Jennifer Berman

Assistant Professor, Department of Urology, David Geffen School of Medicine at University of California, Los Angeles; Attending Surgeon, UCLA Medical Center; Co-Director, Female Sexual Medicine Center at UCLA, Los Angeles, California

Sexual Dysfunction in Men and Women

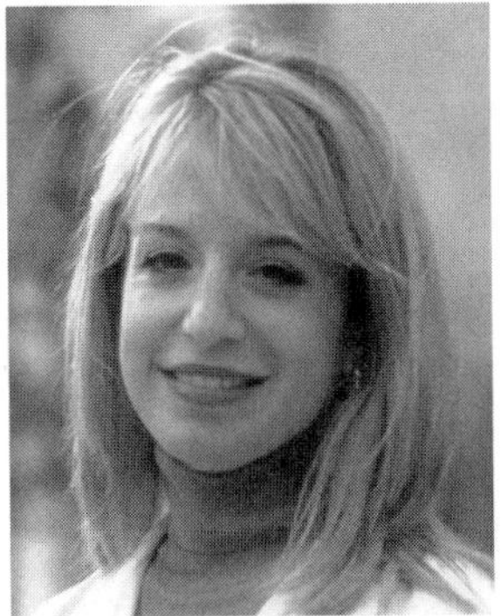

Laura Berman
Assistant Professor, Department of Urology, David Geffen School of Medicine at University of California, Los Angeles; Co-Director, Female Sexual Medicine Center at UCLA, Los Angeles, California
Sexual Dysfunction in Men and Women

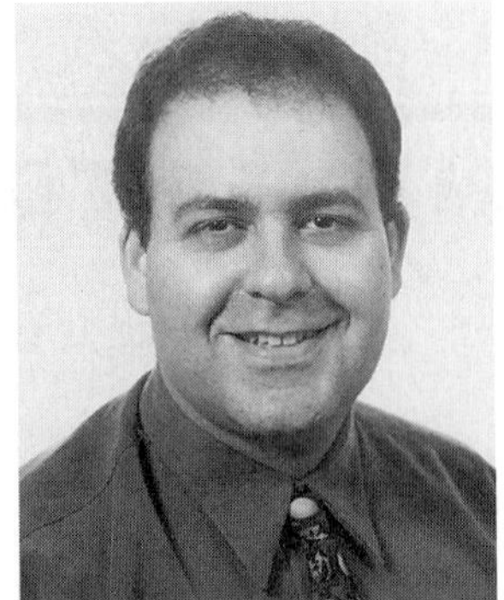

Robin P. Boushey
General Surgery Resident, Department of Surgery, University of Toronto, Toronto, Ontario, Canada
Gastrointestinal Hormones and Gut Endocrine Tumors

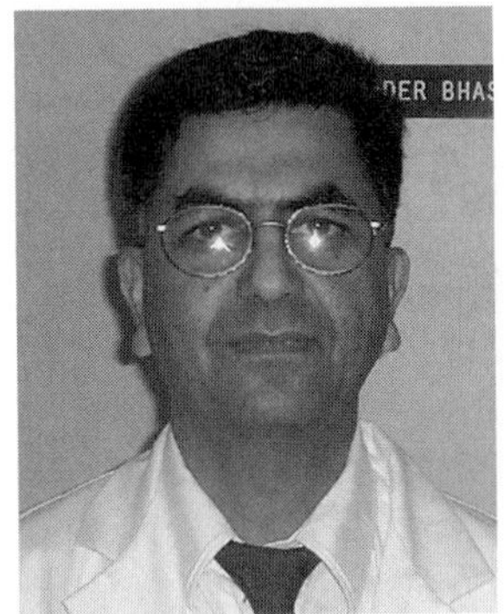

Shalender Bhasin
Professor of Medicine, University of California, Los Angeles, School of Medicine; Chief, Division of Endocrinology, Metabolism, and Molecular Medicine, Charles Drew University and King-Drew Medical Center, Los Angeles, California
Sexual Dysfunction in Men and Women

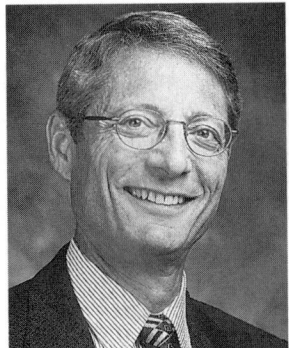

Glenn D. Braunstein
Professor of Medicine, University of California, Los Angeles, School of Medicine; Chairman, Department of Medicine, The James R. Klinenberg, MD, Chair in Medicine, Cedars-Sinai Medical Center, Los Angeles, California
Endocrine Changes in Pregnancy

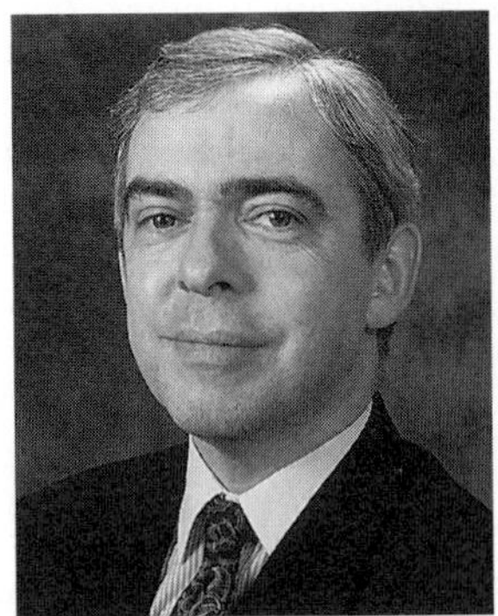

Andrew J. M. Boulton
Professor of Medicine, University of Manchester; Consultant Physician, Manchester Royal Infirmary, Manchester, United Kingdom
Complications of Diabetes Mellitus

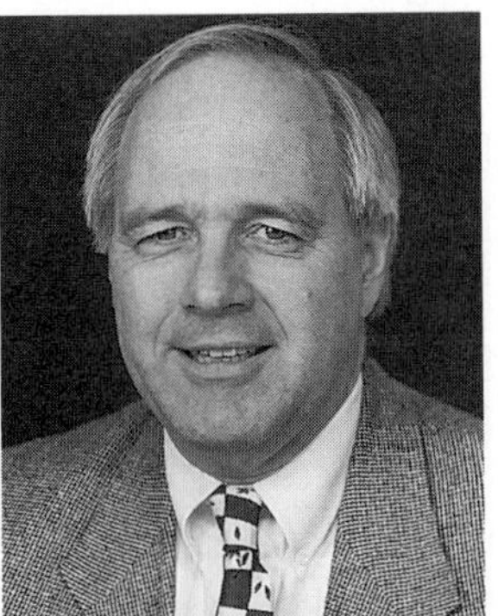

F. Richard Bringhurst
Associate Professor of Medicine, Harvard Medical School; Physician, Massachusetts General Hospital, Boston, Massachusetts
Hormones and Disorders of Mineral Metabolism

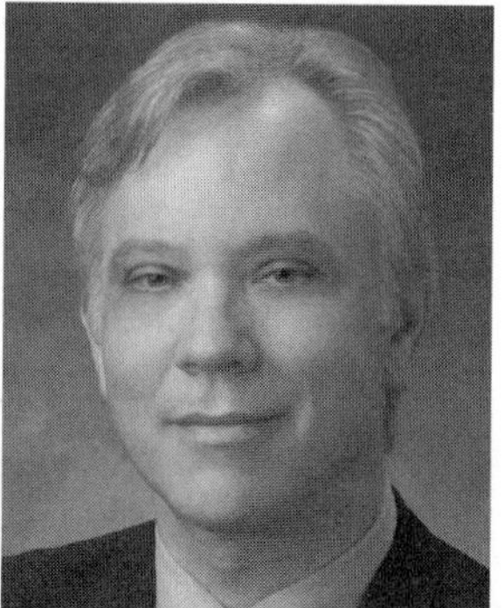

Michael Brownlee
Anita and Jack Saltz Professor of Diabetes Research and Professor of Medicine and Pathology, Albert Einstein College of Medicine, Bronx, New York
Complications of Diabetes Mellitus

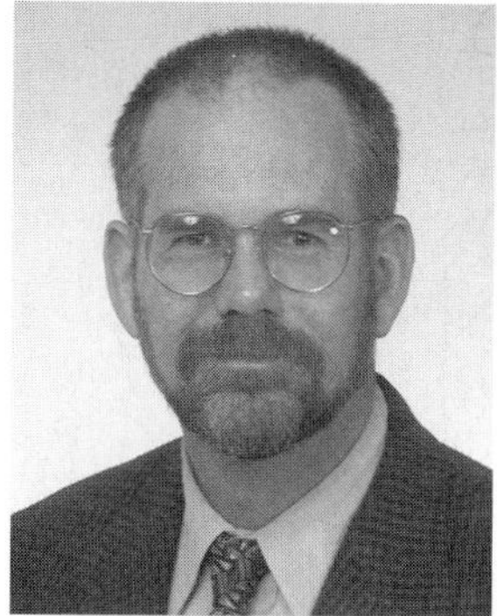

John B. Buse
Associate Professor of Medicine; Chief, Division of General Medicine and Clinical Epidemiology; Director, Diabetes Care Center, University of North Carolina School of Medicine, Chapel Hill, North Carolina
Type 2 Diabetes Mellitus; Type 1 Diabetes Mellitus

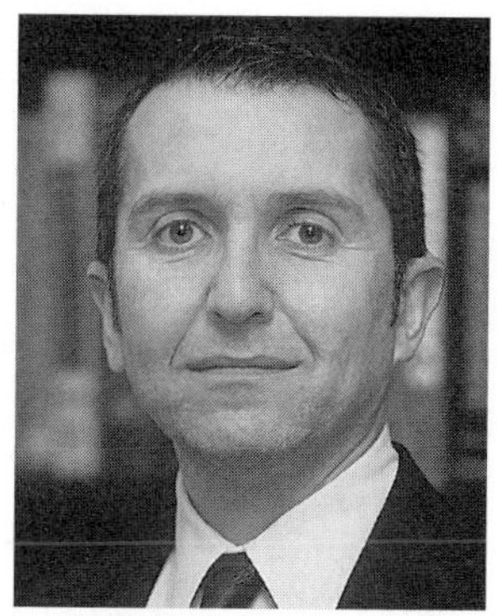

Serdar E. Bulun
Associate Professor of Obstetrics-Gynecology and Molecular Genetics; Director, Division of Reproductive Endocrinology and Infertility, University of Illinois, Chicago, Illinois
The Physiology and Pathology of the Female Reproductive Axis

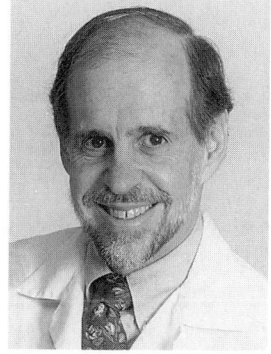

David A. Bushinsky
Professor of Medicine and of Pharmacology and Physiology, University of Rochester School of Medicine and Dentistry; Chief, Nephrology Unit, Strong Memorial Hospital, Rochester, New York
Kidney Stones

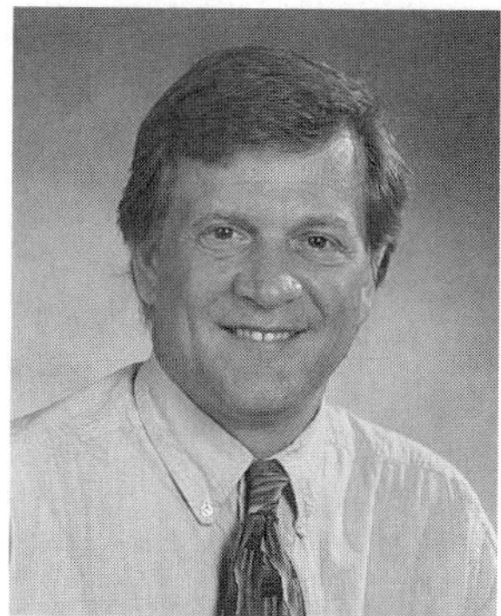

Charles F. Burant
Associate Professor, Department of Internal Medicine, University of Michigan; Attending Physician, University of Michigan Hospitals, Ann Arbor, Michigan
Type 2 Diabetes Mellitus

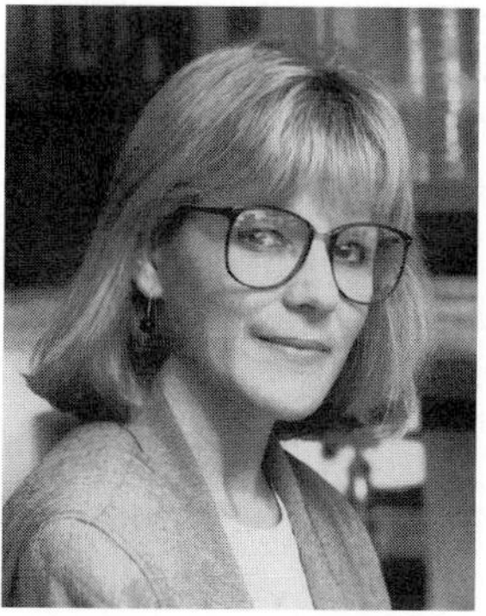

Judy L. Cameron
Associate Professor, Department of Psychiatry, University of Pittsburgh, Pittsburgh, Pennsylvania; Associate Scientist, Oregon National Primate Research Center, Oregon Health and Science University, Portland, Oregon
Neuroendocrinology

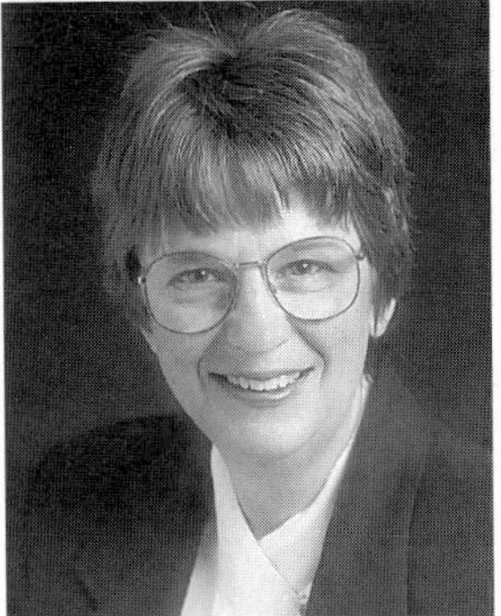

Christin Carter-Su

Professor of Physiology; Associate Director, Michigan Diabetes Research and Training Center, University of Michigan Medical School, Ann Arbor, Michigan

Mechanism of Action of Hormones That Act at the Cell Surface

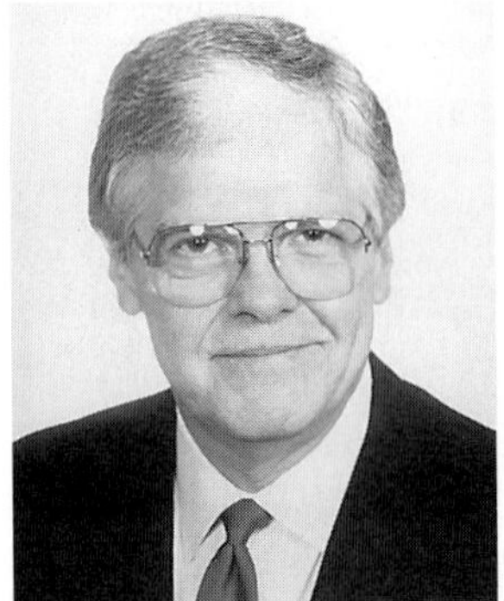

Philip E. Cryer

Irene E. and Michael M. Karl Professor of Endocrinology and Metabolism in Medicine, Washington University School of Medicine; Chief of Endocrinology, Diabetes, and Metabolism, Barnes-Jewish Hospital, St. Louis, Missouri

Glucose Homeostasis and Hypoglycemia

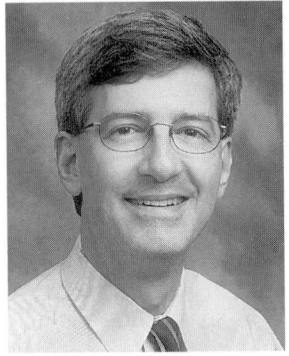

Roger D. Cone

Senior Scientist, Vollum Institute; Associate Professor, Department of Cell and Developmental Biology, Oregon Health and Science University, Portland, Oregon

Neuroendocrinology

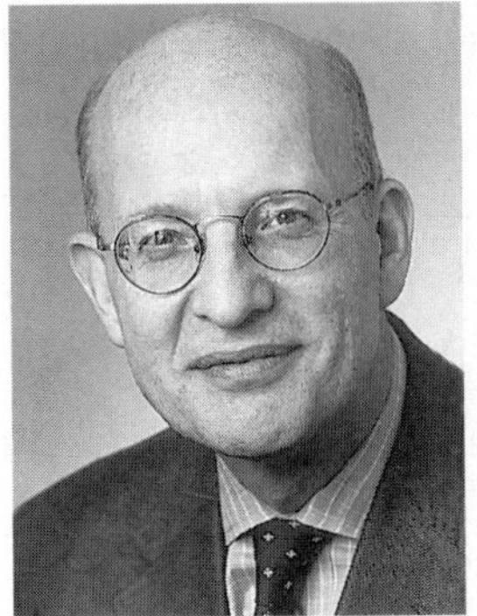

Terry F. Davies

Professor of Medicine and Director, Division of Endocrinology, Diabetes and Bone Diseases, Mount Sinai School of Medicine; Attending Physician, Mount Sinai Hospital, New York, New York

Thyroid Physiology and Diagnostic Evaluation of Patients with Thyroid Disorders; Thyrotoxicosis; Hypothyroidism and Thyroiditis

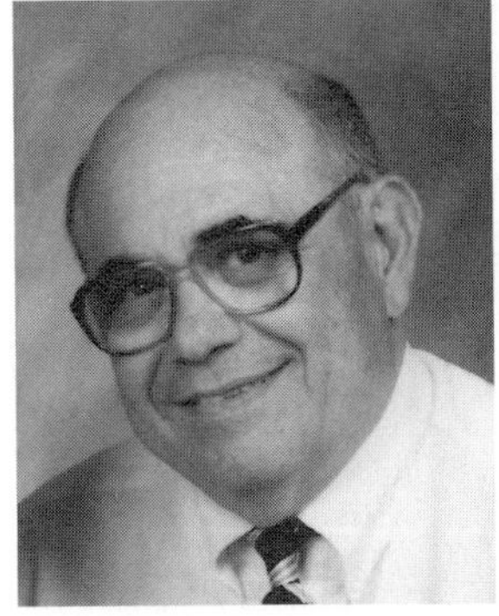

Felix A. Conte

Professor of Pediatrics, Department of Pediatrics, University of California, San Francisco, School of Medicine, San Francisco, California

Disorders of Sex Differentiation

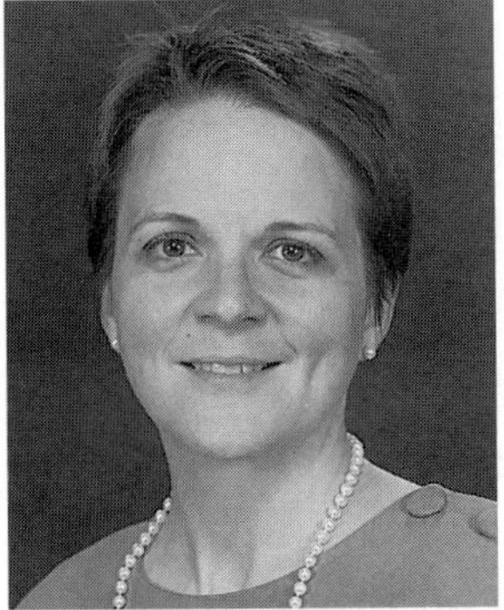

Marie B. Demay

Associate Professor of Medicine, Harvard Medical School; Associate Physician, Massachusetts General Hospital, Boston, Massachusetts

Hormones and Disorders of Mineral Metabolism

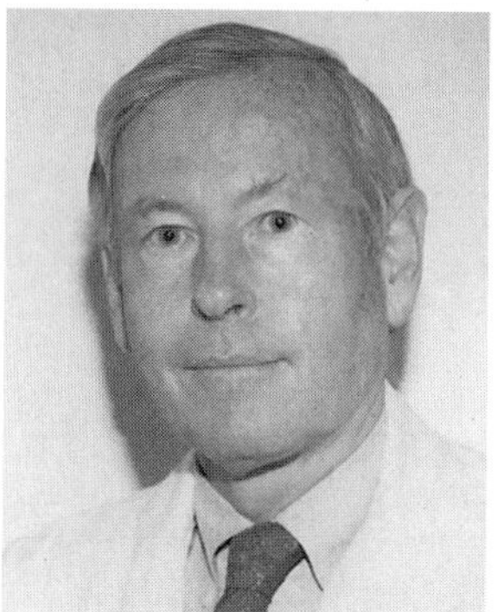

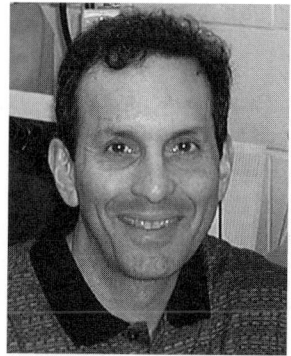

Robert G. Dluhy
Professor of Medicine, Harvard Medical School; Clinical Chief, Division of Endocrinology, Diabetes and Hypertension, Brigham and Women's Hospital, Boston, Massachusetts
Endocrine Hypertension

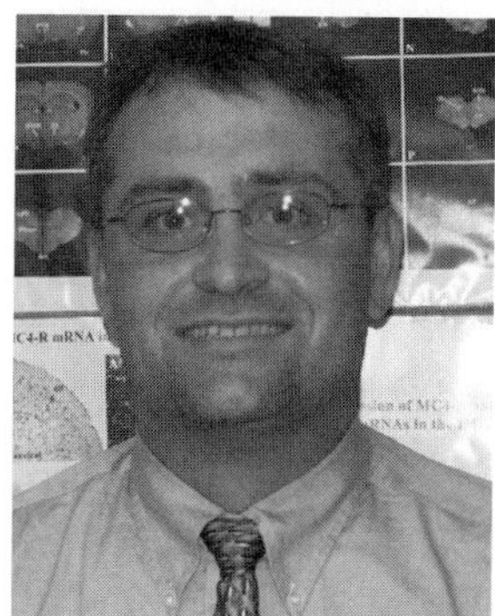

Joel K. Elmquist
Associate Professor of Medicine and Neurology, Harvard Medical School, Division of Endocrinology, Beth Israel Deaconess Medical Center, Boston, Massachusetts
Neuroendocrinology

Daniel J. Drucker
Professor of Medicine, University of Toronto Faculty of Medicine; Director, Banting and Best Diabetes Centre, Toronto General Hospital, Toronto, Ontario, Canada
Gastrointestinal Hormones and Gut Endocrine Tumors

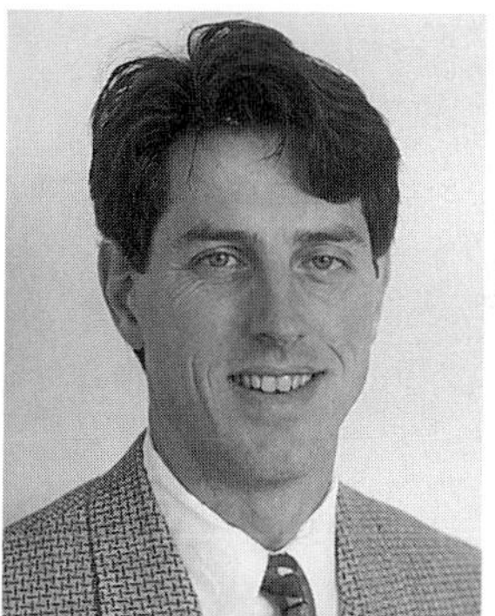

Robert V. Farese, Jr.
Professor of Medicine, University of California, San Francisco; Senior Investigator, Gladstone Institute of Cardiovascular Disease, San Francisco, California
Disorders of Lipid Metabolism

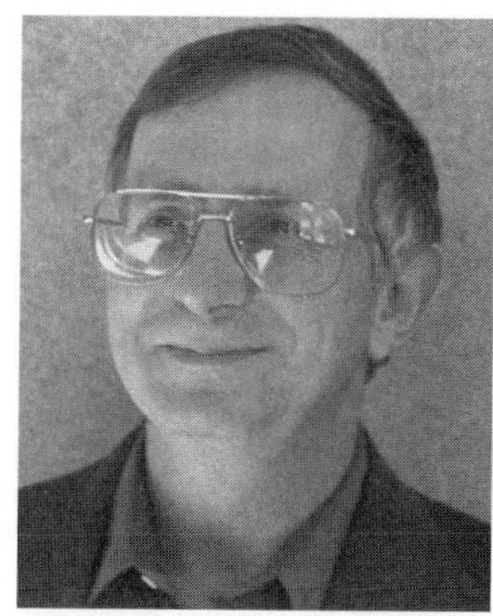

George S. Eisenbarth
Professor of Pediatrics, Medicine, and Immunology, University of Colorado School of Medicine; Executive Director, Barbara Davis Center for Childhood Diabetes, Denver, Colorado
Type 1 Diabetes Mellitus; The Immunoendocrinopathy Syndromes

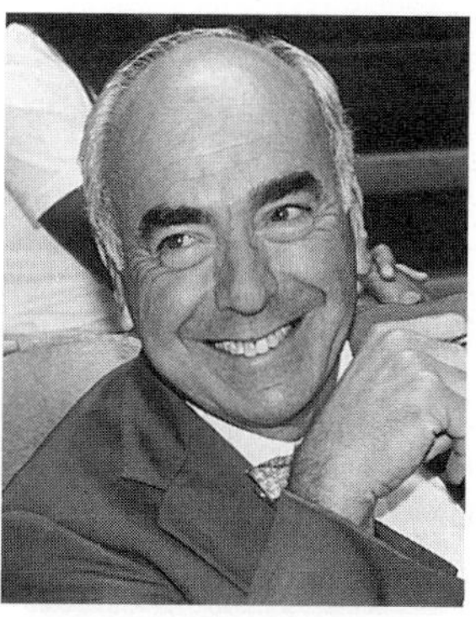

Daniel D. Federman
Carl W. Walter Distinguished Professor of Medicine and Medical Education, Harvard Medical School; Senior Physician, Brigham and Women's Hospital and Massachusetts General Hospital, Boston, Massachusetts
The Endocrine Patient

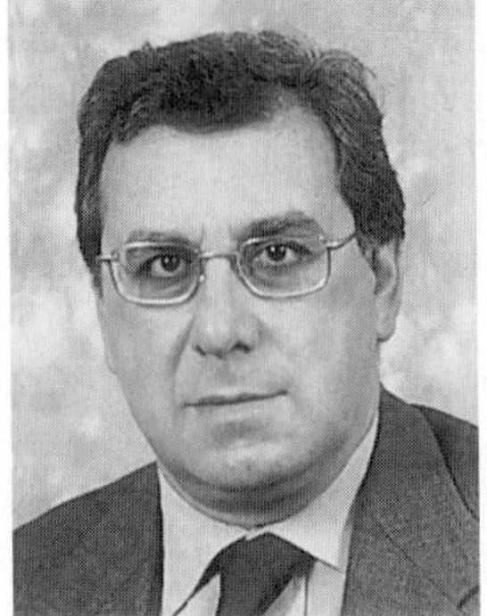

Sebastiano Filetti

Professor of Medicine, Department of Internal Medicine, University of Sapienza, and Chairman of Internal Medicine, and Policlinico Umberto I, Rome, Italy

Nontoxic Goiter and Thyroid Neoplasia

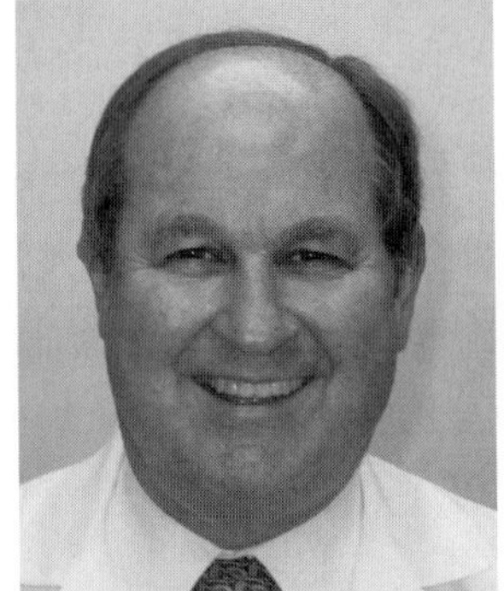

Robert F. Gagel

Professor of Medicine, Division of Internal Medicine, University of Texas/M.D. Anderson Cancer Center; Adjunct Professor of Medicine, Internal Medicine, and Cell Biology, Baylor College of Medicine, Houston, Texas

Multiple Endocrine Neoplasia

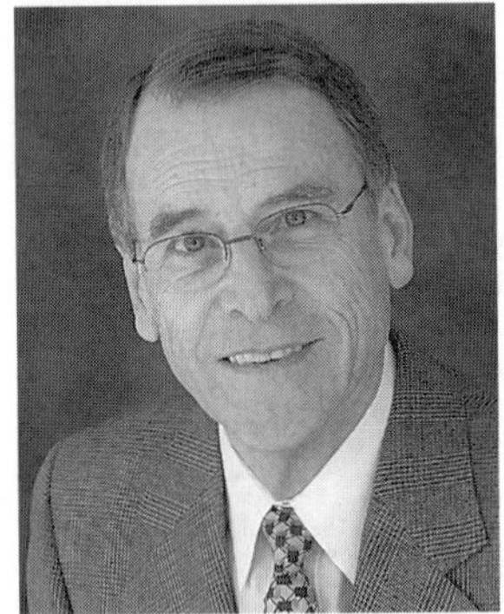

Delbert A. Fisher

Professor of Pediatrics and Medicine Emeritus, University of California, Los Angeles, School of Medicine; Vice President, Science and Innovation, Quest Diagnostics Inc., Nichols Institute, San Juan Capistrano, California

Endocrinology of Fetal Development

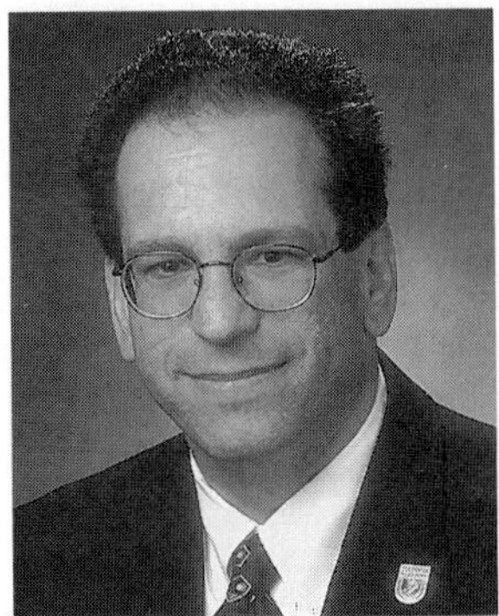

Peter A. Gottlieb

Assistant Professor of Pediatrics and Medicine, Barbara Davis Center for Childhood Diabetes, University of Colorado Health Sciences Center, Denver, Colorado

The Immunoendocrinopathy Syndromes

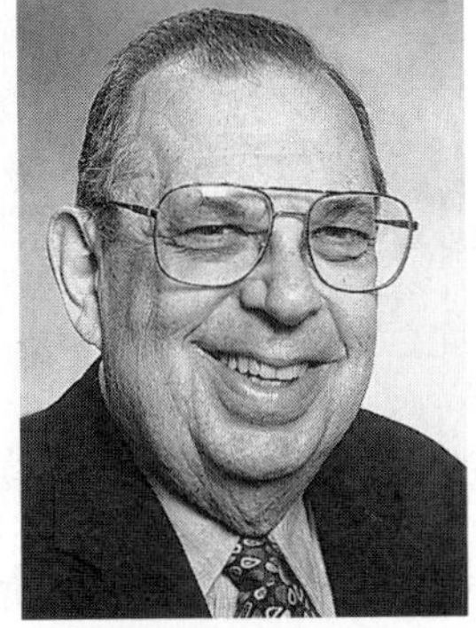

Eli Friedman

Distinguished Teaching Professor of Medicine, State University of New York; Chief, Division of Renal Disease, Department of Medicine, Downstate Medical Center; Attending Physician, University Hospital of Brooklyn and Kings County Hospital, Brooklyn, New York

Complications of Diabetes Mellitus

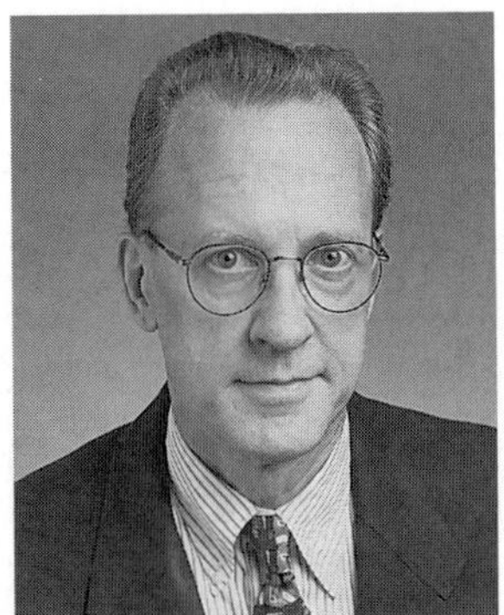

James E. Griffin

Professor of Internal Medicine and Diana and Richard C. Strauss Professor in Biomedical Research, The University of Texas Southwestern Medical Center, Dallas, Texas

Disorders of the Testes and Male Reproductive Tract

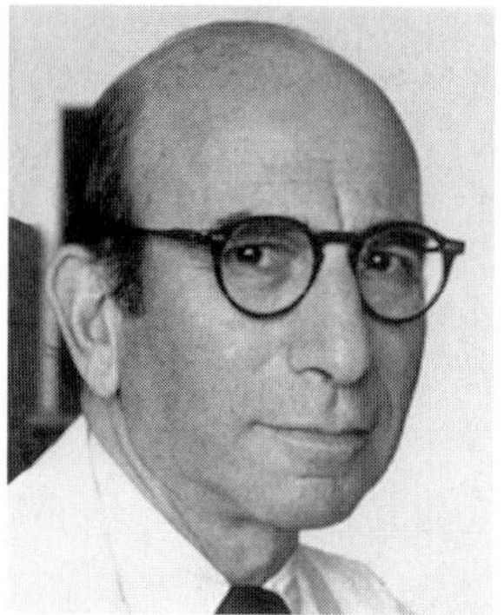

Melvin M. Grumbach
Edward B. Shaw Emeritus Professor of Pediatrics and Emeritus Chairman, Department of Pediatrics, University of California, San Francisco, San Francisco, California
Disorders of Sex Differentiation; Puberty: Ontogeny, Neuroendocrinology, Physiology, and Disorders

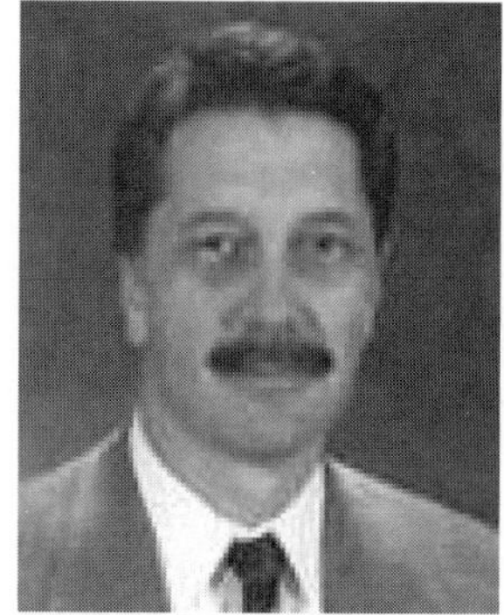

Wayne J. G. Hellstrom
Professor of Urology and Chief, Section of Andrology and Male Dysfunction, Tulane University Health Sciences Center, New Orleans, Louisiana
Sexual Dysfunction in Men and Women

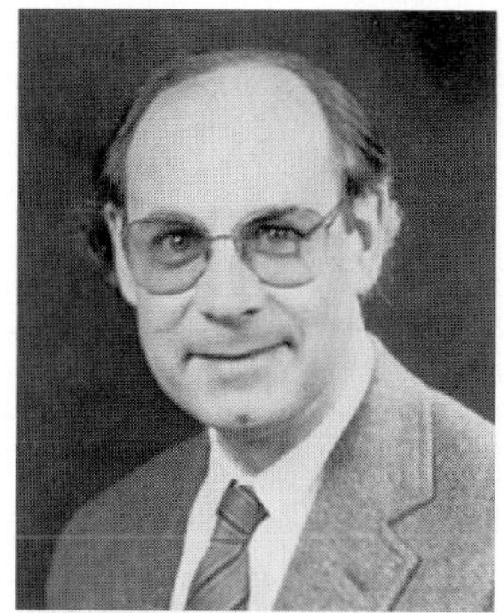

Joel F. Habener
Professor of Medicine, Harvard Medical School; Associate Physician and Chief, Laboratory of Molecular Endocrinology, Massachusetts General Hospital; Investigator, Howard Hughes Medical Institute, Boston, Massachusetts
Genetic Control of Peptide Hormone Formation

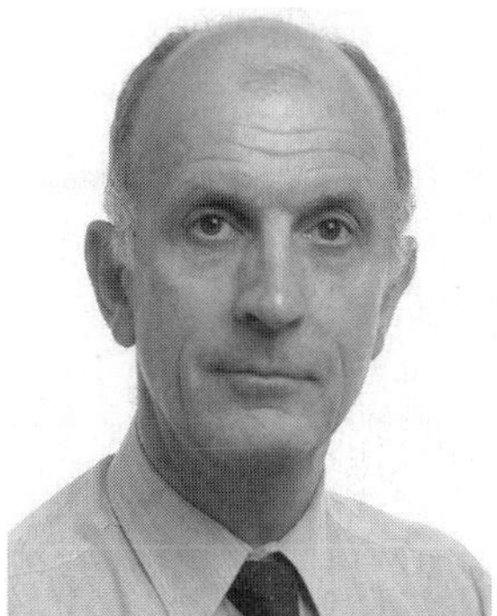

Ieuan A. Hughes
Professor of Paediatrics and Head, Department of Paediatrics, University of Cambridge; Honorary Consultant, Paediatric Endocrinology, Addenbrooke Hospital, Cambridge, United Kingdom
Disorders of Sex Differentiation

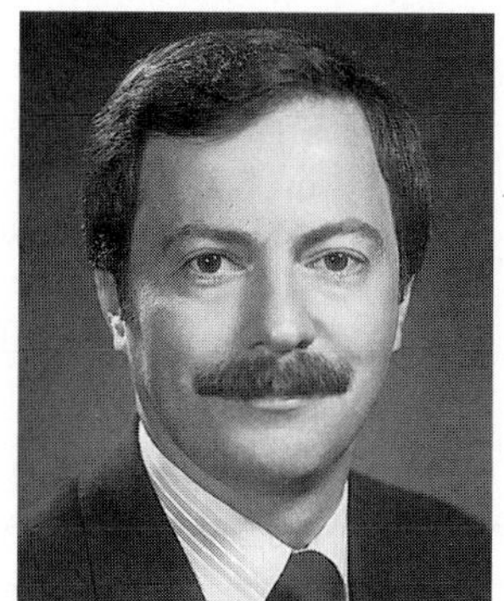

Ian D. Hay
Professor of Medicine, Mayo Medical School; Consultant in Endocrinology and Internal Medicine, Mayo Clinic, Rochester, Minnesota
Thyroid Physiology and Diagnostic Evaluation of Patients with Thyroid Disorders; Nontoxic Goiter and Thyroid Neoplasia

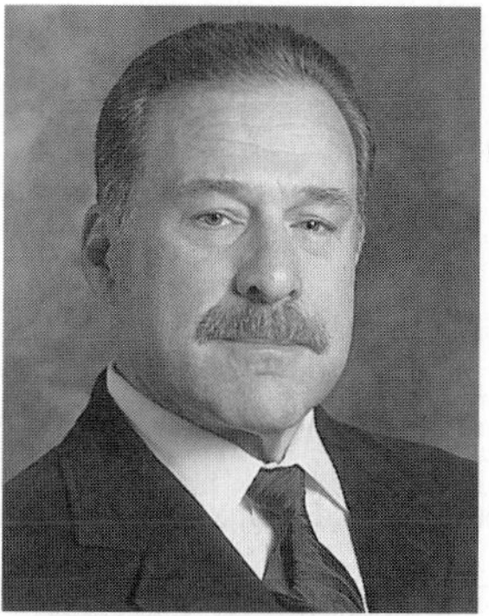

Michael Kafrissen
Adjunct Professor, Maternal and Child Health, University of North Carolina School of Medicine, Chapel Hill, North Carolina; Vice President, Ortho-McNeil Pharmaceutical Co., Raritan, New Jersey
Fertility Control: Current Approaches and Global Aspects

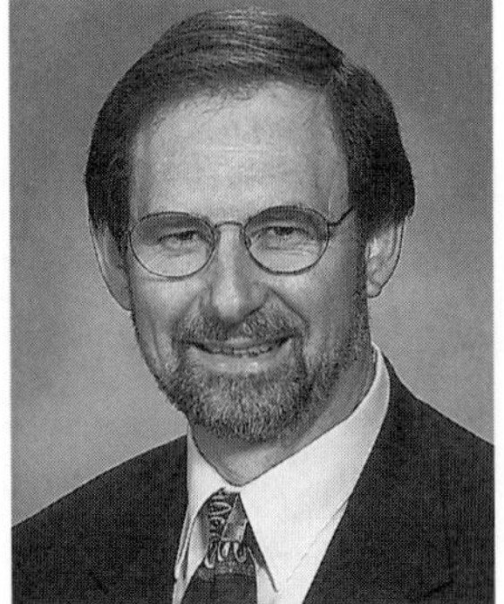

George G. Klee

Professor of Laboratory Medicine, Department of Laboratory Medicine, Mayo Medical School; Consultant in Clinical Pathology, Department of Laboratory Medicine and Pathology, Mayo Clinical Hospitals, Rochester, Minnesota

Laboratory Techniques for Recognition of Endocrine Disorders

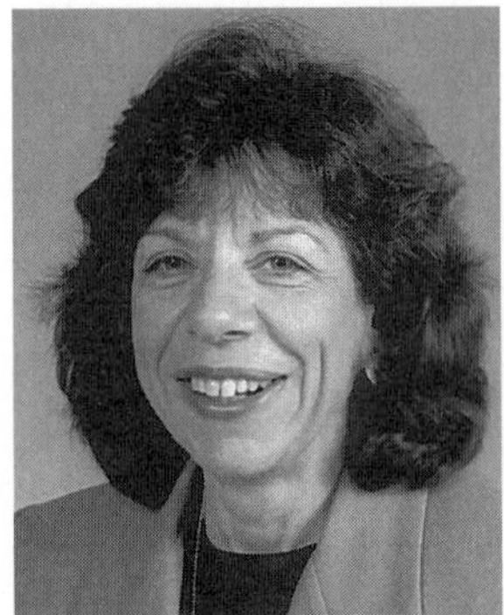

Barbara E. Kream

Professor, Departments of Medicine and Genetics and Developmental Biology, University of Connecticut Health Center, Farmington, Connecticut

Metabolic Bone Disease

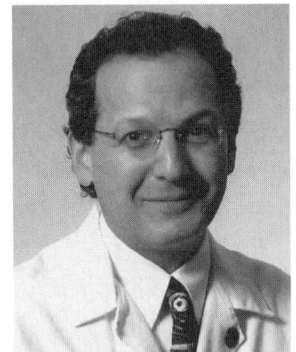

Samuel Klein

Danforth Professor of Medicine, Department of Medicine, Washington University School of Medicine, St. Louis, Missouri

Obesity

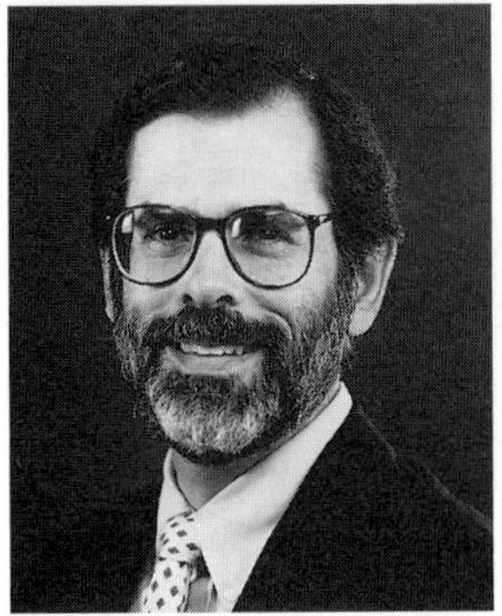

Henry M. Kronenberg

Professor of Medicine, Harvard Medical School; Chief, Endocrine Unit, Massachusetts General Hospital, Boston, Massachusetts

Principles of Endocrinology; Hormones and Disorders of Mineral Metabolism

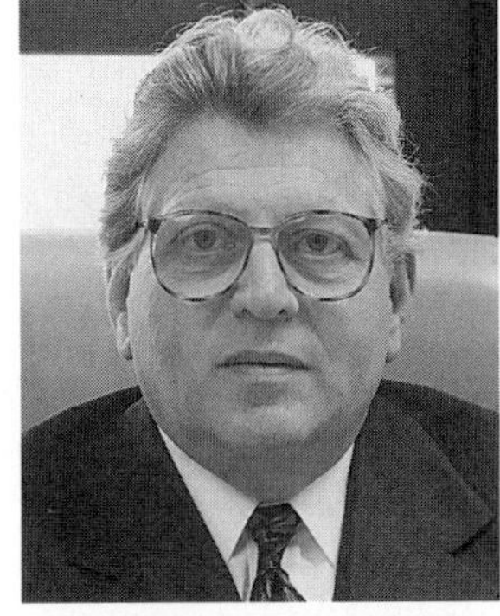

David L. Kleinberg

Professor of Medicine and Director, Neuroendocrine Research Medicine, New York University School of Medicine; Attending, Medicine, New York University Medical Center; Consultant in Medicine, New York Harbor Healthcare Veterans Administration Hospital, New York, New York

Anterior Pituitary

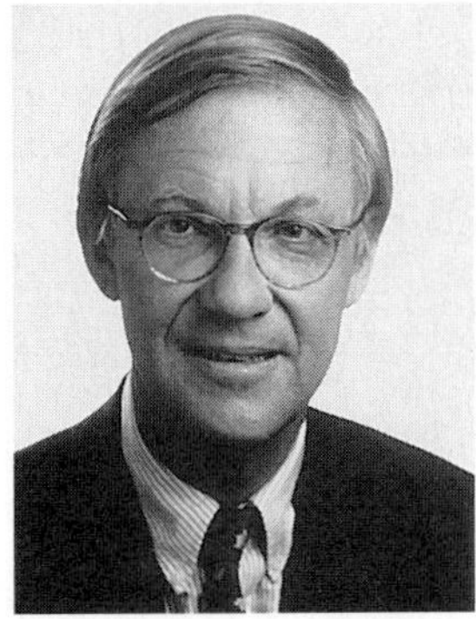

Steven W. J. Lamberts

Professor of Medicine, Erasmus University Rotterdam, Rotterdam, The Netherlands

Endocrinology and Aging

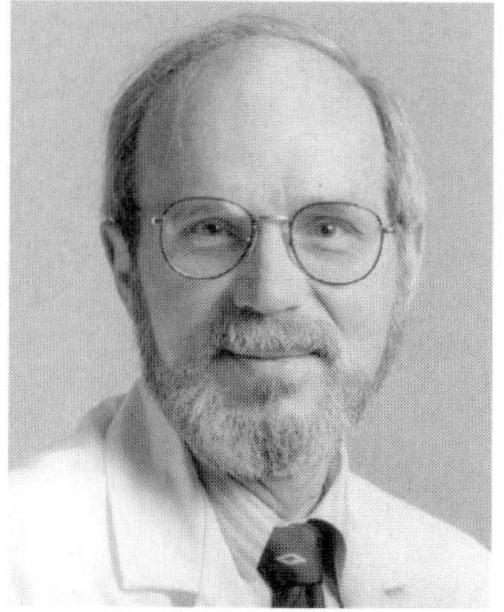

P. Reed Larsen

Professor of Medicine, Harvard Medical School; Chief, Division of Endocrinology, Diabetes and Hypertension, and Senior Physician, Brigham and Women's Hospital, Boston, Massachusetts

Principles of Endocrinology; Thyroid Physiology and Diagnostic Evaluation of Patients with Thyroid Disorders; Thyrotoxicosis; Hypothyroidism and Thyroiditis

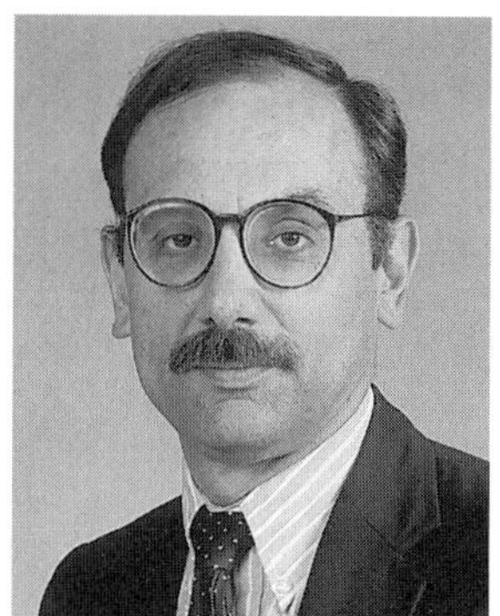

Joseph A. Lorenzo

Professor of Medicine, University of Connecticut School of Medicine; Attending Physician, John Dempsey Hospital/University of Connecticut Health Center, Farmington, Connecticut

Metabolic Bone Disease

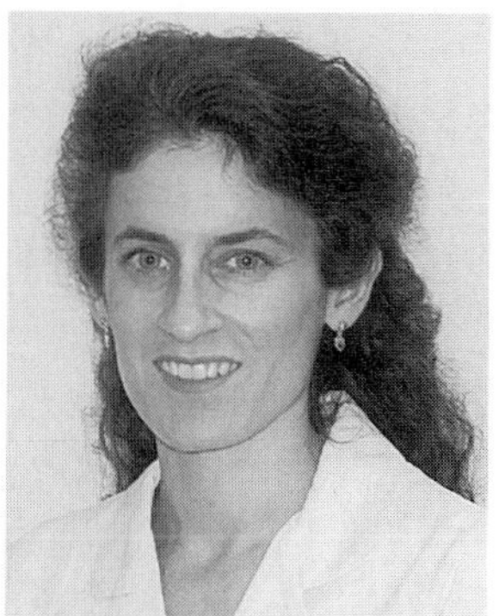

Jennifer E. Lawrence

Director, South Georgia Medical Center Diabetes Center; Chief, Division of Endocrinology, South Georgia Medical Center, Valdosta, Georgia

Endocrine Hypertension

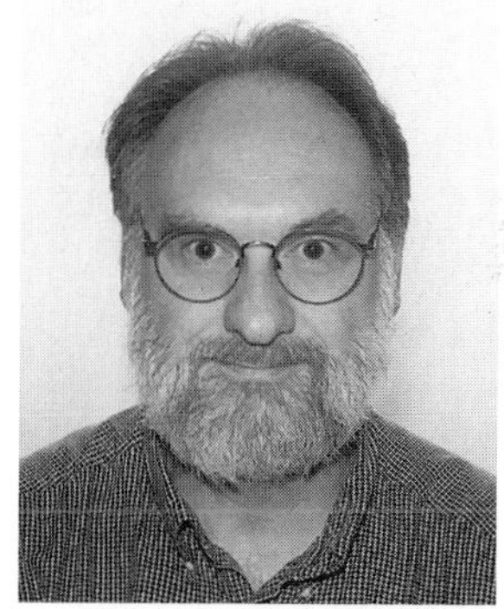

Malcolm J. Low

Professor, Department of Behavioral Neuroscience, Oregon Health and Science University; Scientist, Vollum Institute, Oregon Health and Science University, Portland, Oregon

Neuroendocrinology

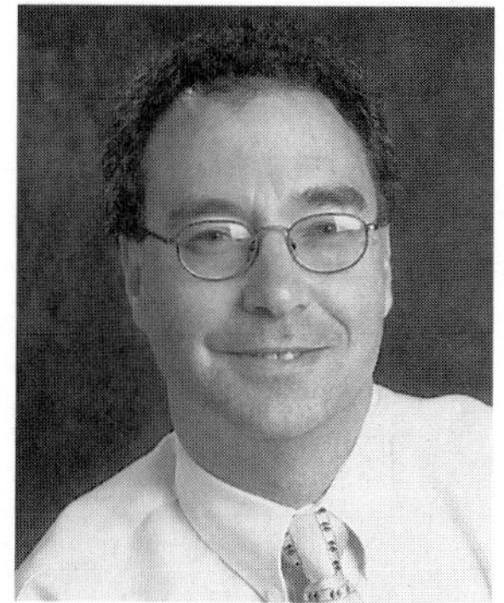

Mitchell A. Lazar

Sylvan H. Eisman Professor of Medicine and Genetics and Director, Penn Diabetes Center, University of Pennsylvania School of Medicine; Chief, Division of Endocrinology, Diabetes, and Metabolism, Hospital of The University of Pennsylvania, Philadelphia, Pennsylvania

Mechanism of Action of Hormones That Act on Nuclear Receptors

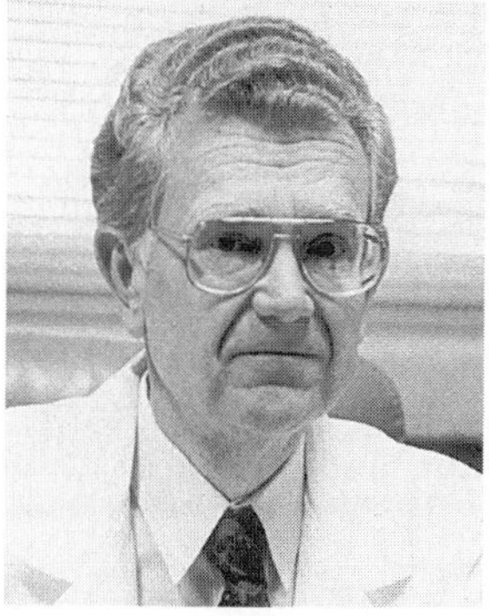

Robert W. Mahley

Professor of Pathology and Medicine, University of California, San Francisco; Director, Gladstone Institute of Cardiovascular Disease, San Francisco, California

Disorders of Lipid Metabolism

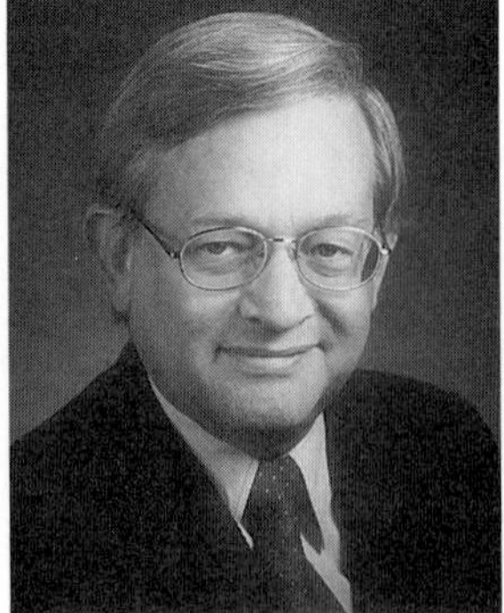

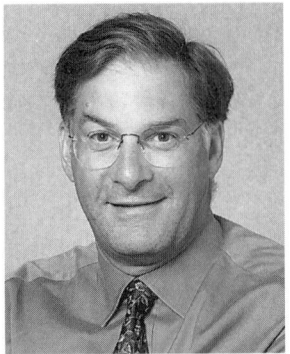

Stephen J. Marx
Chief, Metabolic Diseases Branch, and Chief, Genetics and Endocrinology Section, National Institute of Diabetes and Digestive and Kidney Diseases, National Institutes of Health, Bethesda, Maryland
Multiple Endocrine Neoplasia

Richard W. Nesto
Associate Professor of Medicine, Harvard Medical School, Boston; Chairman, Department of Cardiovascular Medicine, Lahey Clinic Medical Center, Burlington, Massachusetts
Complications of Diabetes Mellitus

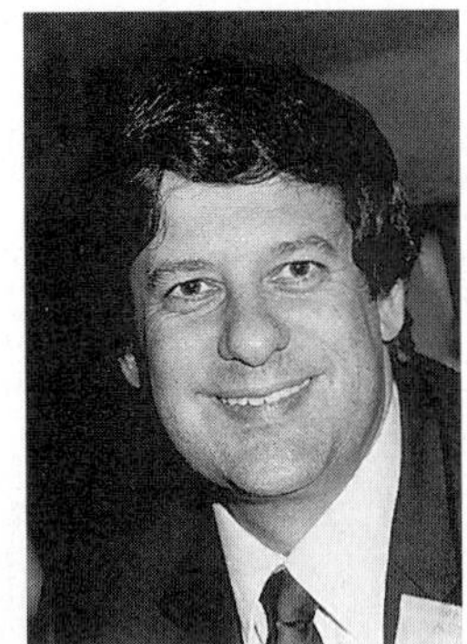

Shlomo Melmed
Senior Vice President, Academic Affairs, Cedars Sinai Medical Center; Professor of Medicine and Associate Dean, University of California, Los Angeles, School of Medicine, Los Angeles, California
Principles of Endocrinology; Anterior Pituitary

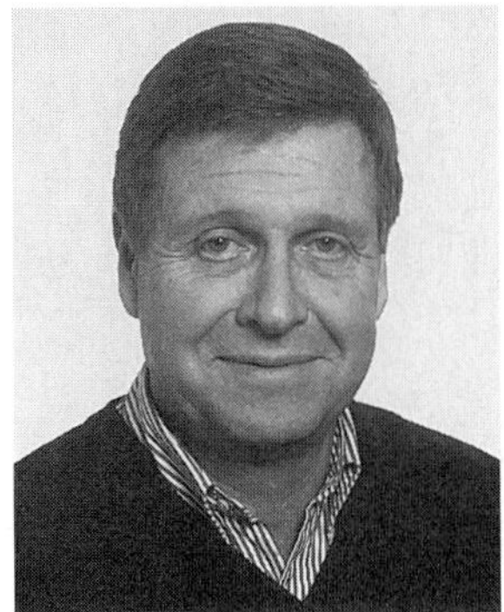

Kjell E. Öberg
Chairman, Department of Medical Sciences, Medical Faculty, Uppsala University; Professor of Endocrine Oncology, University Hospital, Uppsala, Sweden
Carcinoid Tumors, Carcinoid Syndrome, and Related Disorders

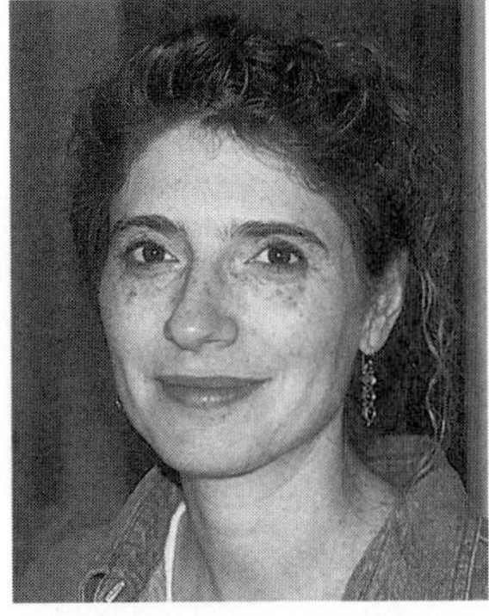

Rebeca D. Monk
Assistant Professor of Medicine, University of Rochester School of Medicine and Dentistry; Head, Urolithiasis Clinic, Strong Memorial Hospital, Rochester, New York
Kidney Stones

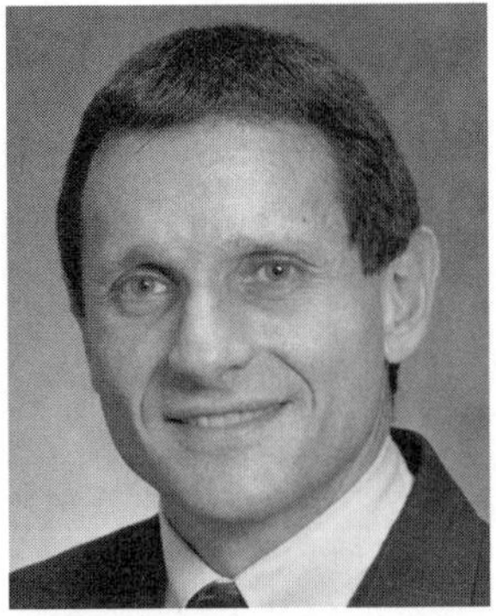

Kenneth S. Polonsky
Adolphus Busch Professor and Chairman, Department of Medicine, and Professor, Department of Cell Biology and Physiology, Washington University School of Medicine, St. Louis, Missouri
Principles of Endocrinology; Type 2 Diabetes Mellitus; Type 1 Diabetes Mellitus

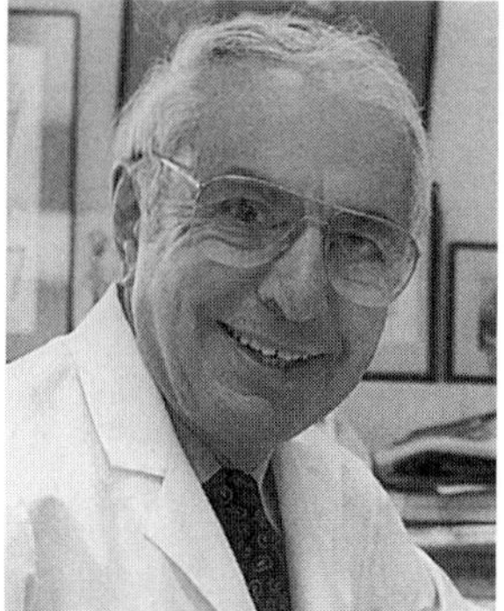

Lawrence G. Raisz
Professor of Medicine, University of Connecticut School of Medicine and Health Center, Farmington; Physician, Hartford Hospital and St. Francis Medical Center, Hartford, Connecticut
Metabolic Bone Disease

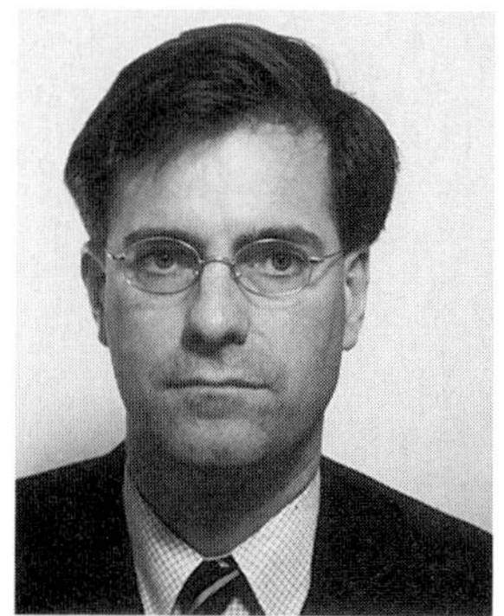

Johannes A. Romijn
Professor of Medicine and Endocrinology, Department of Endocrinology, Leiden University School of Medicine and Medical Center, Leiden, The Netherlands
Obesity

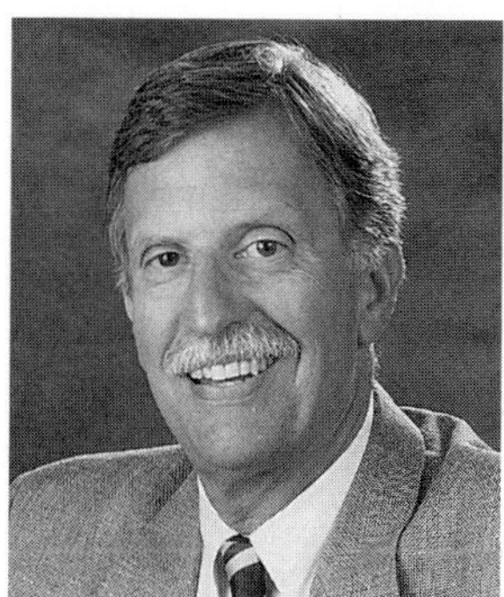

Edward O. Reiter
Professor of Pediatrics, Tufts University School of Medicine, Boston; Chairman, Department of Pediatrics, Baystate Medical Center, Children's Hospital, Springfield, Massachusetts
Normal and Aberrant Growth

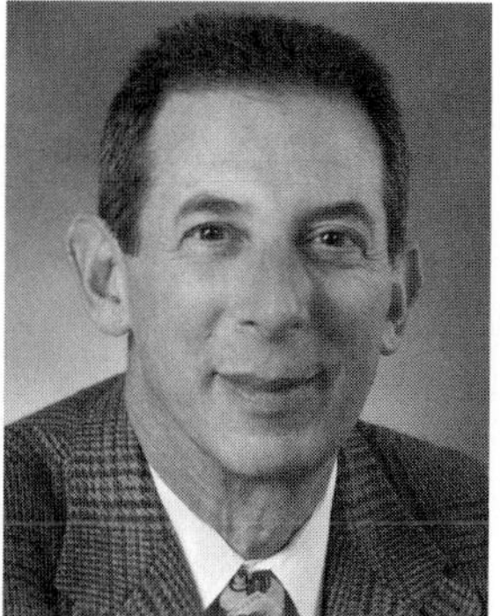

Ron G. Rosenfeld
Credit Union Endowment Professor and Chairman, Department of Pediatrics, and Professor, Cell and Developmental Biology, Oregon Health and Science University; Physician-in-Chief, Doermbecher Children's Hospital, Portland, Oregon
Normal and Aberrant Growth

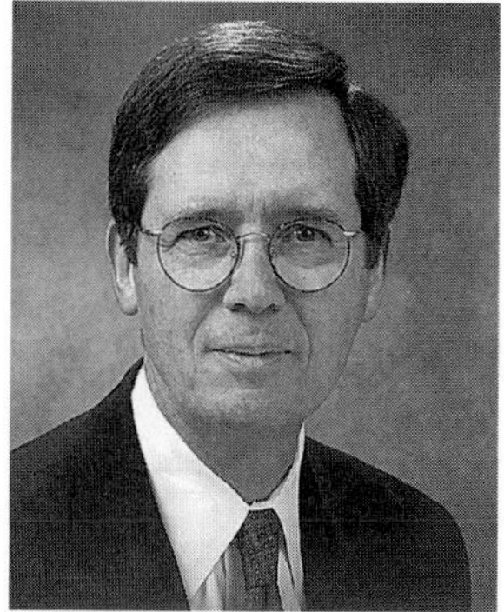

Alan G. Robinson
Vice Provost, Medical Sciences, and Executive Associate Dean and Professor of Medicine, University of California, Los Angeles, School of Medicine, Los Angeles, California
Posterior Pituitary Gland

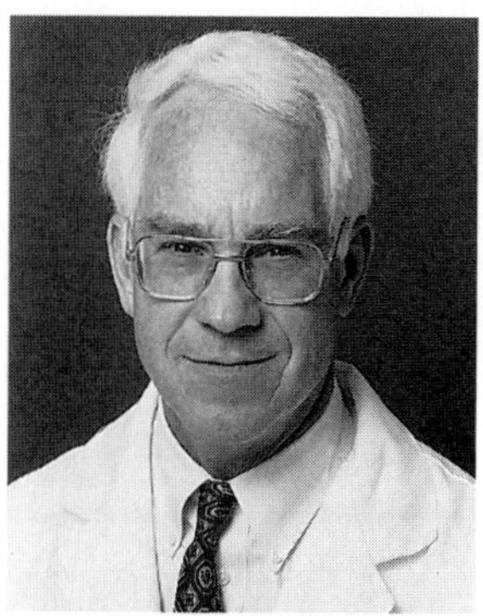

Richard Santen
Professor of Medicine, University of Virginia School of Medicine; Member, Division of Endocrinology, Department of Internal Medicine, University of Virginia Health System, Charlottesville, Virginia
Endocrine-Responsive Cancer

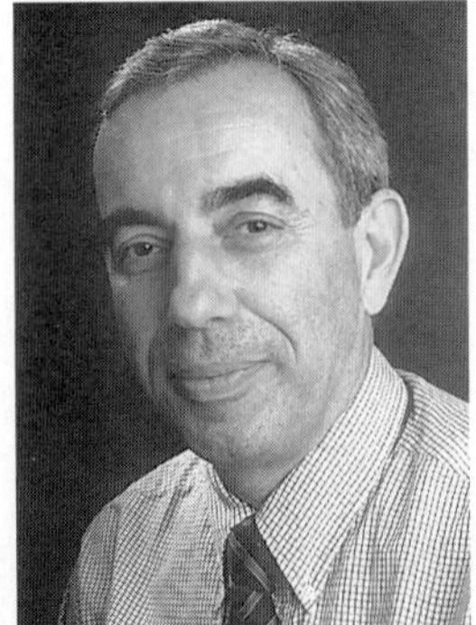

Martin-Jean Schlumberger

Professor, University of Paris, Sud; Chief, Department of Nuclear Medicine and Endocrine Tumors, Institute Gustave Roussy, Villejuif, France

Thyroid Physiology and Diagnostic Evaluation of Patients with Thyroid Disorders; Nontoxic Goiter and Thyroid Neoplasia

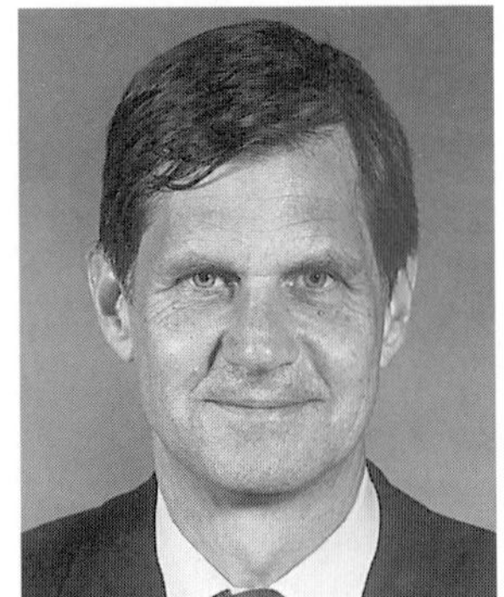

Gordon J. Strewler

Professor of Medicine and Master, Walter Bradford Cannon Society, Harvard Medical School; Physician, Beth Israel Deaconess Medical Center, Boston, Massachusetts

Humoral Manifestations of Malignancy

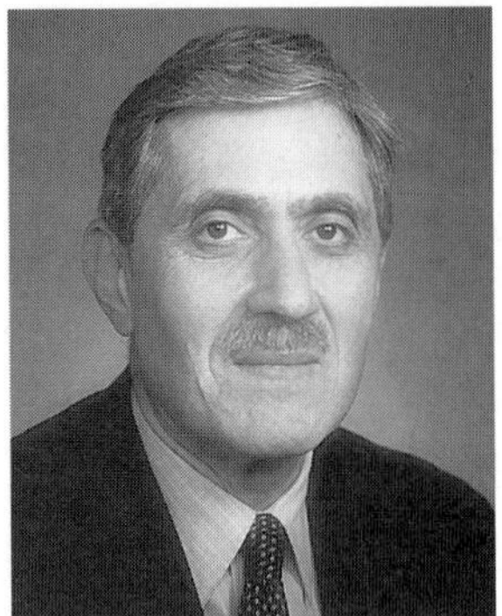

Allen Spiegel

Director, National Institute of Diabetes and Digestive and Kidney Diseases, National Institutes of Health, Bethesda, Maryland

Mechanism of Action of Hormones That Act at the Cell Surface

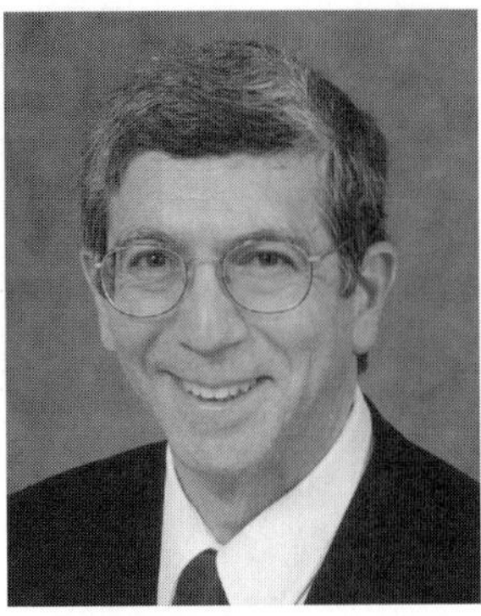

Dennis M. Styne

Professor and Chief, Pediatric Endocrinology, University of California, Davis, School of Medicine, Sacramento, California

Puberty: Ontogeny, Neuroendocrinology, Physiology, and Disorders

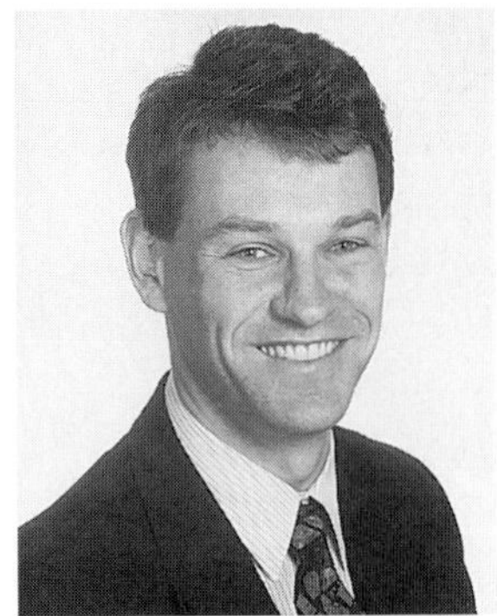

Paul M. Stewart

Professor of Medicine, School of Medicine, University of Birmingham; Consultant Physician, Queen Elizabeth Hospital, Birmingham, United Kingdom

The Adrenal Cortex

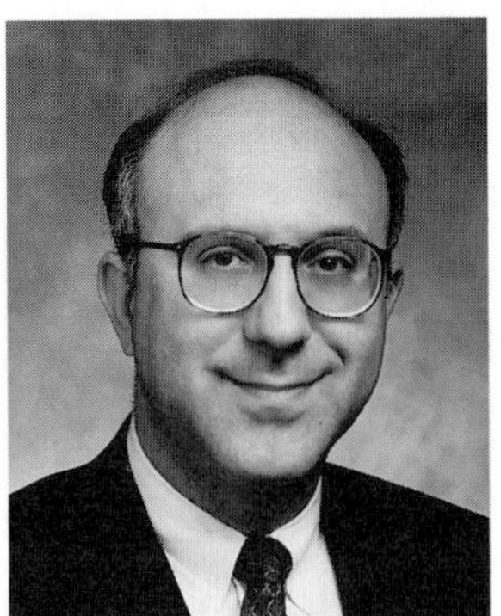

Simeon I. Taylor

Vice President, Discovery Biology, Bristol-Myers Squibb, Hopewell, New Jersey

Mechanism of Action of Hormones That Act at the Cell Surface

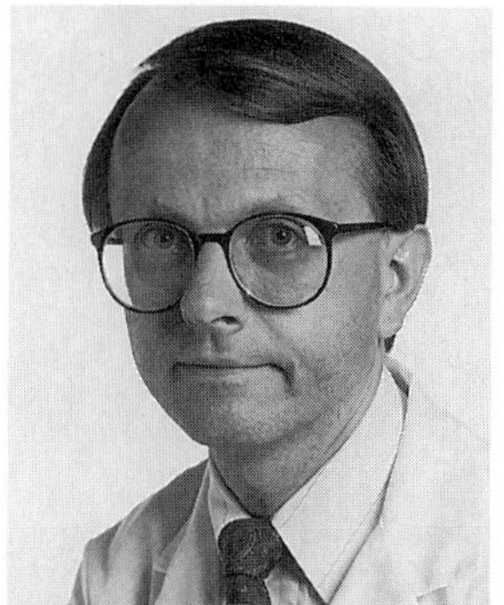

Joseph G. Verbalis
Professor of Medicine, Department of Medicine, Georgetown University School of Medicine; Chief, Division of Endocrinology and Metabolism, Georgetown University Medical Center, Washington, D.C.
Posterior Pituitary Gland

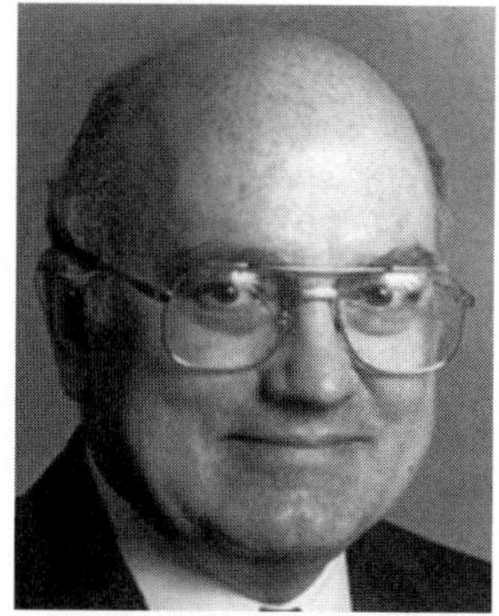

Gordon H. Williams
Professor of Medicine and Director of Scholars in Clinical Science Program, Harvard Medical School; Director, General Clinical Research Center and Center for Clinical Investigation, Brigham and Women's Hospital, Boston, Massachusetts
Endocrine Hypertension

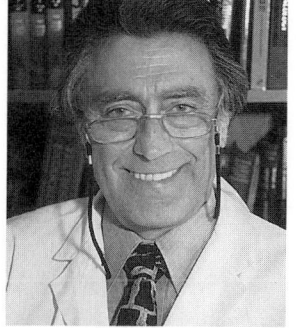

Aaron I. Vinik
Professor, Internal Medicine, Pathology, and Neurobiology, Eastern Virginia Medical School; Director, Strelitz Diabetes Research Institute, Norfolk, Virginia
Complications of Diabetes Mellitus

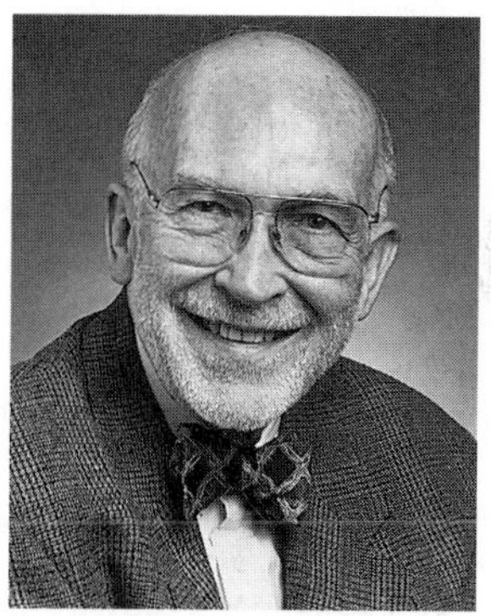

Jean D. Wilson
Charles Cameron Sprague Distinguished Chair in Biomedical Research, The University of Texas Southwestern Medical Center, Dallas, Texas
Disorders of the Testes and the Male Reproductive Tract

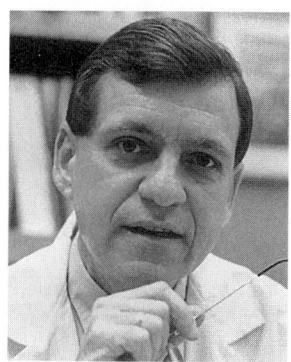

Karl H. Weisgraber
Professor of Pathology, University of California, San Francisco, School of Medicine; Deputy Director and Senior Investigator, Gladstone Institute of Cardiovascular Disease, San Francisco, California
Disorders of Lipid Metabolism

FOREWORD

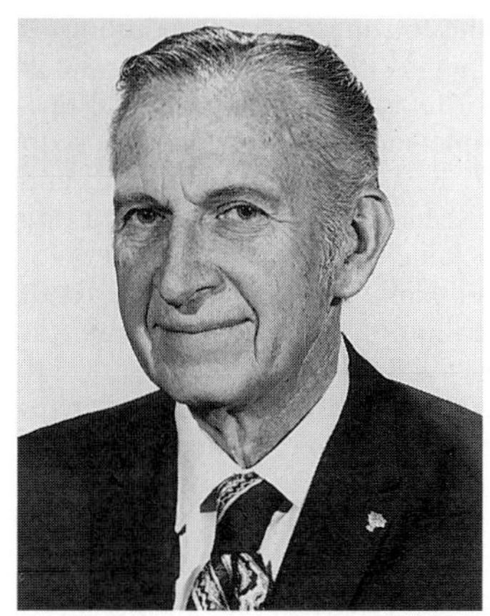
Robert H. Williams

The publication of the tenth edition comes 52 years after the first edition of Williams' *Textbook of Endocrinology.* There had been other large textbooks of endocrinology, such as Biedl's *Innere Sekretion* in 1916[1] and Rolleston's *The Endocrine Organs in Health and Disease* in 1936,[2] but only a handful of physicians could be identified as endocrinologists by the middle of the twentieth century. Consequently, Robert H. Williams exercised "powerful persuasion" to overcome the reluctance of the sales staff of the W. B. Saunders Company to publish a book that had no visible audience.[3] In fact, however, Williams was correct in predicting a large readership, because its publication coincided with an explosive increase in basic endocrine science and in the application of this basic information to patients, and with the evolution of endocrinology into a recognized subspecialty of several branches of medicine. Indeed, the book has had a profound impact on endocrine science and on the development of the clinical discipline, and it is appropriate at this time to remember Robert Williams and his contributions to the field and to *Textbook of Endocrinology.*

Williams described in a memoir the training and the background that led to his development of the textbook.[4] After his graduation from Washington and Lee University, he obtained the M.D. degree at Johns Hopkins University Medical School in 1934. His house staff training was spread between the Mallory Institute of Pathology at the Boston City Hospital, the Department of Medicine at Vanderbilt (where he did research with Tinsley R. Harrison), and the Department of Medicine at Johns Hopkins (where he worked with Warren Longcope). He finished his training at the Massachusetts General Hospital as an endocrine fellow at a time when there were "many quacks in this area throughout the world."[4] He and his mentor, Fuller Albright, became good friends and maintained close contact over the years.

In 1940, Williams was appointed to the staff of the Endocrine Unit of the Thorndike Laboratory in the Harvard Medical Unit at the Boston City Hospital. In 1942, he became head of the Unit, where his research focused principally on the biochemistry and physiology of thyroid disease, including pioneering work on the treatment of thyrotoxicosis with thionamide drugs and with radioactive iodine. In addition, he described the syndrome of biotin deficiency and published papers on adrenal physiology, obesity, and nephrogenic diabetes insipidus.

To attract students and fellows into the field, he developed the concept that "endocrinology is the backbone of metabolism and metabolism is the interstitium of medicine." His students and trainees included at least three future contributors to his textbook, Sidney Ingbar, Peter Forsham, and William H. Daughaday. Daughaday describes Williams as a man of extraordinary exuberance and enthusiasm who took great pleasure in lecturing and in bedside teaching and whose motto was "B(bright) and E(early) and on the B(ball)."[5]

Williams considered himself first and foremost an educator, and in 1948 he moved to the University of Washington as Chairman of the Department of Medicine, where his extraverted and outgoing personality made him a superb teacher, recruiter, administrator, and institution builder. The Endocrine Division in Seattle was very broad and encompassed diabetes mellitus, clinical nutrition, and metabolism, as well as endocrinology. Williams served as President of the Endocrine Society, the American Society for Clinical Investigation, and the Association of American Physicians, and he was the founder of the Association of the Professors of Medicine. In brief, he was an academic giant of twentieth century medicine.

The founding of the *Textbook of Endocrinology* evolved from his interest in education: "In view of the rapid progress in endocrinology and metabolism, and the fact that our unit at Boston City Hospital had registered very high in undergraduate, graduate, and postgraduate teaching, I decided that there was a great need for a new textbook in endocrinology."[4] The arrangements for the textbook were completed before Williams left Boston, and the aims were clearly described in the preface to the first edition:

> *The rapidity and extent of advances in endocrinology have made it increasingly difficult for the student and physician to take full advantage of information available for understanding, diagnosis and treatment of clinical disorders. It is the realization of these difficulties that prompted the writing of this book. The main*

objective is to provide a condensed and authoritative discussion of the management of clinical endocrinopathies, based upon the application of fundamental information obtained from chemical and physiologic investigations.

The product was a book that over the years has served as an effective bridge between clinical medicine and the science of endocrinology. There may be no other arena of medicine in which the basic and clinical sciences are so tightly interwoven into one discipline. On the one hand, the clinical discipline profits immensely from scientific advances; on the other hand, clinical observations often raise important questions for investigation and on occasion provide answers that have an impact on basic science. By reflecting advances in both areas, the *Williams Textbook* was designed to convey the intellectual excitement of a rapidly changing scientific base and, at the same time, to promote the integration of a spectrum of disciplines ranging from molecular genetics to patient care into a unified discipline. The achievement of this aim was possible because, from the initial edition, Williams chose contributors who were at the forefront of the field, thereby ensuring the freshness of each edition.

Now, of course, there are several textbooks of endocrinology, but Williams' pioneering book continues to enjoy a growing readership of both the English and the foreign language editions. Williams edited the first five editions, and Edwin L. Bierman completed the editing of the sixth edition after Williams' death in 1979. Jean D. Wilson and Daniel W. Foster edited the seventh and eighth editions and were joined by Henry M. Kronenberg and P. Reed Larsen as editors for the ninth edition. For the tenth edition, Larsen and Kronenberg are joined by editors Kenneth S. Polonsky and Shlomo Melmed, and continuing the tradition set by Williams, the editors of the tenth edition have enlisted an outstanding group of new and former contributors. Saunders continues as publisher.

Endocrinology has changed in many ways during the past 50 years, and the editorial challenges likewise change with each edition. On one level, these challenges reflect scientific advances, such as the explosion of knowledge about hormone action, the development of new and improved diagnostic techniques and imaging modalities, and the application of molecular genetics to biology. On another level, the concept that the discipline of endocrinology was defined by the concept of humoral control mechanisms has become blurred by recognition that the endocrine, immune, and neurologic signaling systems constitute a single integrated system rather than separate control mechanisms. The most significant challenge now, however, is the same as that faced by all textbooks at a time when the volume of published information is rapidly increasing, namely the dilemma of how to take full advantage of developments in electronic publishing and the evolving revolution in information retrieval systems to devise effective learning systems for the near and remote futures. The fundamental educational issues are the same that Williams faced in 1948, namely the need to integrate rapidly evolving basic and clinical science in a cohesive format appropriate for undergraduate, graduate, and continuing medical education. Now, however, the prose text can be enhanced by multimedia additions, and updating can be done in a continuum. How these tools will be utilized to create new types of teaching materials by academicians faced with multiple demands on their time is not entirely clear, but the response to this challenge will determine whether *Williams Textbook of Endocrinology* will continue to have the same impact over the next 50 years.

JEAN D. WILSON

References

1. Biedl A. Innere Sekretion. Ihre Physiologischen Grundlagen und Ihre Bedeutung für die Pathologie. Berlin: Urban & Schwarzenberg, 1916.
2. Rolleston HD. The Endocrine Organs in Health and Disease with an Historical Review. Oxford, Oxford University Press, 1936.
3. Dusseau JL. An Informal History of W. B. Saunders Company. Philadelphia: W. B. Saunders Company, 1988, pp 98–99.
4. Williams RH. My experiences in endocrinology: 1940–1948. In Finland M (ed). The Harvard Medical Unit at Boston City Hospital, Vol I. Boston, Harvard Medical School, 1982, pp 455–481.
5. Daughaday WH. Personal communication.

PREFACE

This tenth edition of *Williams Textbook of Endocrinology* is a milestone in many respects. A tenth edition *per se* is testimony to the enduring accomplishments of our predecessors, who have consistently created a product that remains the most popular textbook in this field. It is also now a half century since the publication of the first edition of *Williams*, a landmark suitably celebrated in a foreword by our coauthor and former editor, Dr. Jean Wilson. Two internationally renowned endocrinologists, Drs. Shlomo Melmed and Kenneth Polonsky, have joined Drs. Reed Larsen and Henry Kronenberg to formulate, co-edit, and assemble this volume. We will strive to meet the high standards maintained by Drs. Wilson and Daniel Foster during their editorial leadership.

Our goal for this first edition of the new millennium was to emulate the achievements of our predecessors by producing a definitive and fresh approach to the presentation of the essentials of clinical endocrinology. Accordingly, we invited a number of new authors, including several European colleagues, to prepare 23 of the 41 chapters. Our challenge to them and to those updating their material was to distill the burgeoning molecular and physiological knowledge into a complete, but relevant, scholarly presentation. Where appropriate, this would include a practical experienced guide as to how the author uses this information in the diagnosis and management of his or her own patients. Achieving such relevance, thoroughness, and practicality requires a unique combination of scientific knowledge and total clinical familiarity best encapsulated in the term "physician-scientist." We believe that our physician-scientist authors have again met Robert Williams' stipulation that this text should provide "a condensed and authoritative discussion of the management of clinical endocrinopathies based upon the application of fundamental information obtained from chemical and physiologic investigation." We hope our readers will agree.

Both new and revised chapters are replete with tables and figures. Highlights of this edition include a new and expanded diabetes section, new chapters on many old and new topics including endocrinology and aging, female reproduction and fertility control, sexual function and dysfunction, kidney stones, the adrenal cortex, endocrine hypertension, endocrine-responsive tumors, and non-insulin-secreting tumors of the gastroenteropancreatic system. A largely new, concise introductory section includes several new chapters discussing mechanisms of hormone action and the clinical approach to the endocrine patient, as well as a thorough guide to the intricacies of the rapidly changing laboratory techniques. The entire section containing chapters on the hypothalamus and both anterior and posterior pituitary disorders is original, and the thyroid section has been thoroughly revised and divided into expanded disorder-based presentations.

Stylistic innovations include page numbers in the introductory outlines for each chapter, which we hope will permit the reader ready access to specific topics. We have also introduced algorithms and clinical guidelines for diagnostic and treatment strategies to crystallize recommendations for each disease. Readers will also note that this edition is published only five years following its predecessor, reflecting the all-too-familiar rapidity with which new knowledge is accumulating in the biomedical disciplines. Its timely appearance despite so much new material reflects the diligent efforts of our editorial staff and especially the new authors.

We would like to express our deep gratitude to the coworkers in our offices, Anita Nichols, Debra Hession, Lynn Moulton, Grace Labrado, Linda Walker, Louise Ishibashi, and Sherri Turner, without whose dedication this project could not have been completed. We also wish to thank our colleagues at Elsevier, Richard Zorab and Cathy Carroll, and our tireless and effective developmental editors, Faith Voit and Joanne Husovski. Their painstaking attention to every detail is a major contribution to this new edition.

P. Reed Larsen
Henry M. Kronenberg
Shlomo Melmed
Kenneth S. Polonsky

CONTENTS

SECTION EIGHT

DISORDERS OF CARBOHYDRATE AND LIPID METABOLISM

SECTION NINE

POLYENDOCRINE DISORDERS

SECTION TEN

PARAENDOCRINE AND NEOPLASTIC SYNDROMES

SECTION ONE

HORMONES AND HORMONE ACTION

1 Principles of Endocrinology

Henry Kronenberg, Shlomo Melmed,
P. Reed Larsen, and Kenneth Polonsky

INTRODUCTION

Roughly a hundred years ago, Starling coined the term *hormone* to describe secretin, a substance secreted by the small intestine into the blood stream to stimulate pancreatic secretion. In his Croonian Lectures, Starling considered the endocrine and nervous systems as two distinct mechanisms for coordination and control of organ function. Thus, endocrinology found its first home in the discipline of mammalian physiology.

Work over the next several decades by biochemists, physiologists, and clinical investigators led to the characterization of many hormones secreted into the blood stream from discrete glands or other organs. These investigators showed for the first time that diseases such as hypothyroidism and diabetes could be treated successfully by replacing specific hormones. These initial triumphs formed the foundation of the clinical specialty of endocrinology.

Advances in cell biology, molecular biology, and genetics over the ensuing years began to help explain the mechanisms of endocrine diseases and of hormone secretion and action. Although these advances have embedded endocrinology into the framework of molecular cell biology, they have not changed the essential subject of endocrinology—the signaling that coordinates and controls the functions of multiple organs and processes. Here we would like to survey the general themes and principles that underpin the diverse approaches used by clinicians, physiologists, biochemists, cell biologists, and geneticists to understand the endocrine system.

THE EVOLUTIONARY PERSPECTIVE

Hormones can be defined as chemical signals secreted into the blood stream that act on distant tissues, usually in a regulatory fashion. Hormonal signaling represents a special case of the more general process of signaling between cells. Even unicellular organisms such as baker's yeast, *Saccharomyces cerevisiae*, secrete short peptide mating factors that act on receptors of other yeast cells to trigger mating between the two cells. These receptors resemble the ubiquitous family of mammalian 7-transmembrane spanning receptors that respond to ligands as diverse as photons and glycoprotein hormones. Because these yeast receptors trigger activation of heterotrimeric G proteins just as mammalian receptors do, this conserved signaling pathway must have been present in the common ancestor of yeast and humans.

Signals from one cell to adjacent cells, so-called paracrine signals, often trigger cellular responses that use the same molecular pathways used by hormonal signals. For example, the sevenless receptor controls the differentiation of retinal cells in the Drosophila eye by responding to a membrane-anchored signal from an adjacent cell. Sevenless is a membrane-spanning receptor with an intracellular tyrosine kinase domain that signals in a way that closely resembles the signaling by hormone receptors such as the insulin receptor tyrosine kinase. Since paracrine factors and hormones can share signaling mechanisms it is not surprising that hormones can, in some settings, act as paracrine factors. Testosterone, for example, is secreted into the blood stream but also acts locally in the testes to control spermatogenesis. Insulin-like growth factor I (IGF-I) is a hormone secreted into the blood stream from the liver and other tissues, but it is also a paracrine factor made locally in most tissues to control cell proliferation. Further, one receptor can mediate the actions of a hormone, such as parathyroid hormone, and of a paracrine factor, such as parathyroid hormone–related protein.

Target cells respond similarly to signals that reach them from the blood stream (hormones) or from the cell next door (paracrine factors); the cellular response machinery does not distinguish the sites of origin of signals. The shared final common pathways used by hormonal and paracrine signals should not, however, obscure important differences between hormonal and paracrine signaling system (Fig. 1–1). Paracrine signals do not travel very far; consequently, the specific site of origin of a paracrine factor determines where it will act and provides specificity to that action. When the paracrine factor BMP4 is secreted by cells in the developing kidney, it regulates the differentiation of renal cells; when BMP4 is secreted by cells in bone, it regulates bone formation. Thus, the site of origin

Regulation of signaling: endocrine

Source: gland
- No contribution to specificity of target
- Synthesis/secretion

Distribution: blood stream
- Universal—almost
  - Importance of dilution

Non-target organ
- Metabolism

Target cell
- Receptor: source of specificity
- Responsiveness:
  Number of receptors
  Downstream pathways
  Other ligands
  Metabolism of ligand/receptor
  All often regulated by ligand

A

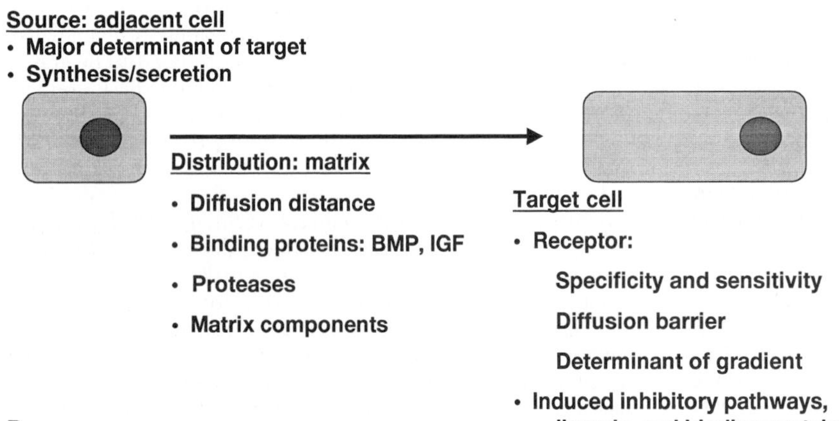

Figure 1–1. Comparison of determinants of endocrine (*A*) and paracrine (*B*) signaling.

of BMP4 determines its physiologic role. In contrast, since hormones are secreted into the blood stream, their sites of origin are often divorced from their functions. We know nothing about thyroid hormone function, for example, that requires that the thyroid gland to be in the neck.

Because the specificity of action of paracrine factors is so dependent on their precise site of origin, elaborate mechanisms have evolved to regulate and constrain the diffusion of paracrine factors. Paracrine factors of the hedgehog family, for example, are covalently bound to cholesterol to constrain the diffusion of these molecules in the extracellular milieu. Most paracrine factors interact with binding proteins that block their action and control their diffusion. Chordin, noggin, and many other distinct proteins all bind to various members of the BMP family to regulate their action, for example. Proteases such as tolloid then destroy the binding proteins at specific sites to liberate BMPs so that the BMPs can act on appropriate target cells.

Hormones have rather different constraints. Because they diffuse throughout the body, they must be synthesized in enormous amounts relative to the amounts of paracrine factors needed at specific locations. This synthesis usually occurs in specialized cells designed for that specific purpose. Hormones must then be able to travel in the blood stream and diffuse in effective concentrations into tissues. Therefore, for example, lipophilic hormones bind to soluble proteins that allow them to travel in the aqueous media of blood at relatively high concentrations. The ability of hormones to diffuse through the extracellular space means that the local concentration of hormone at target sites will rapidly decrease when glandular secretion of the hormone stops. Because hormones diffuse throughout extracellular fluid quickly, hormonal metabolism can occur in specialized organs such as the liver and kidney in a way that determines the effective concentration of the hormones in other tissues.

Paracrine factors and hormones thus use several distinct strategies to control their biosynthesis, sites of action, transport, and metabolism. These differing strategies may partly explain why a hormone such as IGF-I, unlike its close relative insulin, has multiple binding proteins that control its action in tissues. As noted earlier, IGF-I has a double life as both a hormone and a paracrine factor. Presumably, the local actions of IGF-I mandate an elaborate binding protein apparatus.

All the major hormonal signaling programs—G protein–

coupled receptors, tyrosine kinase receptors, serine/threonine kinase receptors, ion channels, cytokine receptors, nuclear receptors—are also used by paracrine factors. In contrast, several paracrine signaling programs are used only by paracrine factors and are probably not used by hormones. For example, Notch receptors respond to membrane-based ligands to control cell fate, but no bloodborne ligands use Notch-type signaling (at least none is currently known). Perhaps the intracellular strategy used by Notch, which involves cleavage of the receptor and subsequent nuclear actions of the receptor's cytoplasmic portion, is too inflexible to serve the purposes of hormones.

The analyses of the complete genomes of multiple bacterial species, the yeast *Saccharomyces cerevisiae*, the fruit fly *Drosophila melanogaster*, the worm *Caenorhabitis elegans*, the plant *Aradopsis thaliana*, and humans have allowed a comprehensive view of the signaling machinery used by various forms of life. As noted already, *S. cerevisiae* uses G protein–linked receptors; this organism, however, lacks tyrosine kinase receptors and nuclear receptors that resemble the estrogen/thyroid receptor family. In contrast, the worm and fly share with humans the use of each of these signaling pathways, although with substantial variation in numbers of genes committed to each pathway. For example, the *Drosophila* genome encodes 20 nuclear receptors, the *C. elegans* genome encodes 270, and the human genome encodes (tentatively) more than 50. These patterns suggest that ancient multicellular animals must have already established the signaling systems that are the foundation of the endocrine system as we know it in mammals.

Even before the sequencing of the human genome, sequence analyses had made clear that many receptor genes are found in mammalian genomes for which no clear ligand or function was known. The analyses of these "orphan" receptors has succeeded in broadening the current understanding of hormonal signaling. For example, the liver X receptor (LXR) was one such orphan receptor found when searching for unknown nuclear receptors. Subsequent experiments showed that oxygenated derivatives of cholesterol are the ligands for LXR, which regulates genes involved in cholesterol and fatty acid metabolism.[1] The example of LXR and many others raise the question of what constitutes a hormone. The classical view of hormones is that they are synthesized in discrete glands and have no function other than activating receptors on cell membranes or in the nucleus. In contrast, cholesterol, which is converted in cells to oxygenated derivatives that activate the LXR, uses a hormonal strategy to regulate its own metabolism. Other orphan nuclear receptors respond similarly to ligands, such as bile acids and fatty acids. These "hormones" have important metabolic roles quite separate from their signaling properties, although the hormone-like signaling serves to allow regulation of the metabolic function. The calcium-sensing receptor is an example from the G protein–linked receptor family of receptors that responds to a nonclassical ligand, ionic calcium. Calcium is released into the blood stream from bone, kidney, and intestine and acts on the calcium-sensing receptor in parathyroid cells, renal tubular cells, and other cells to coordinate cellular responses to calcium. Thus, many important metabolic factors have taken on hormonal properties as part of a regulatory strategy.

ENDOCRINE GLANDS

Hormone formation may occur either in localized collections of specific cells, in the endocrine glands, or in cells that have additional roles. Many protein hormones, such as growth hormone, parathyroid hormone, prolactin, insulin, and glucagon, are produced in dedicated cells by standard protein synthetic mechanisms common to all cells. These secretory cells usually contain specialized secretory granules designed to store large amounts of hormone and to release the hormone in response to specific signals. Formation of small hormone molecules initiates with commonly found precursors, usually in specific glands such as the adrenals, gonads, or thyroid. In the case of the steroid hormones, the precursor is cholesterol, which is modified by various hydroxylations, methylations, and demethylations to form the glucocorticoids, androgens, and estrogens, and their biologically active derivatives. In contrast, the precursor of vitamin D, 7-dehydrocholesterol, is produced in skin keratinocytes, again from cholesterol, by a photochemical reaction. Leptin, which regulates appetite and energy expenditure, is formed in adipocytes, thus providing a specific signal reflecting the organism's nutritional state to the central nervous system.

Thyroid hormone synthesis occurs via a unique pathway. The thyroid cell synthesizes a 660,000-kd homodimer, thyroglobulin, which is then iodinated at specific iodotyrosines. Certain of these "couple" to form the iodothyronine molecule within thyroglobulin, which is then stored in the lumen of the thyroid follicle. In order for this to occur, the thyroid cell must concentrate the trace quantities of iodide from the blood and oxidize it via a specific peroxidase. Release of thyroxine (T_4) from the thyroglobulin requires its phagocytosis and cathepsin-catalyzed digestion by the same cells.

Hormones are synthesized in response to biochemical signals generated by various modulating systems. Many of these systems are specific to the effects of the hormone product; for example, parathyroid hormone synthesis is regulated by the concentration of ionized calcium, whereas gonadal, adrenal, and thyroid hormone synthesis is achieved by the hormonostatic function of the hypothalamic–pituitary axis. Cells in the hypothalamus and pituitary monitor the circulating hormone concentration and secrete trophic hormones that activate specific pathways for hormone synthesis and release. Typical examples are luteinizing (LH) follicle-stimulating (FSH), thyroid-stimulating (TSH), and adrenocorticotrophic (ACTH) hormones.

These trophic hormones increase rates of hormone synthesis and secretion and also may induce target cell division, thus causing enlargement of the various target glands. For example, in hypothyroid individuals living in iodine-deficient areas of the world, TSH secretion causes a marked hyperplasia of thyroid cells. In such regions, the thyroid gland may be 20- to 50-fold its normal size. Adrenal hyperplasia occurs in patients with genetic deficiencies in cortisol formation. Hypertrophy and hyperplasia of parathyroid cells, in this case initiated by an intrinsic response to the stress of hypocalcemia, occur in patients with renal insufficiency or calcium malabsorption.

Hormones may be fully active when released into the blood stream (e.g., growth hormone or insulin) or may require activation in specific cells to produce their biological effects. These activation steps are often highly regulated. For example, the T_4 released from the thyroid cell is a prohormone that must undergo a specific deiodination to form the active 3,5,3′ triiodothyronine (T_3). This deiodination reaction can occur in target tissues, such as in the central nervous system; in the thyrotrophs, where T_3 provides feedback regulation of TSH production; or in hepatic and renal cells, from which T_3 is released into the circulation for uptake by all tissues. A similar post secretory activation step catalyzed by a 5α-reductase causes tissue-specific activation of testosterone to dihydrotestosterone in target tissues, including the male urogenital tract and genital skin, as well as in the liver. Vitamin D undergoes hydroxylation at the 25 position in the liver and in the 1 position in the kidney. Both hydroxylations must occur to produce the active hormone 1,25$(OH)_2$ vitamin D. The activity of the 1α-hydroxylase, but not that of the 25-hydroxylase, is stimulated by parathyroid hormone and reduced plasma phosphate but is inhibited by calcium and $1,25(OH)_2$ vitamin D.

Hormones are synthesized as required on a daily, hourly, or minute-to-minute basis with minimal storage, but there are significant exceptions. One such exception is the thyroid gland, which contains enough stored hormone to last for about two months. This permits a constant supply of this hormone despite significant variations in the availability of iodine. If iodine deficiency is prolonged, however, the normal reservoirs of thyroxine can be depleted.

The various feedback signaling systems exemplified above provide the hormonal *homeostasis* characteristic of virtually all endocrine systems. Regulation may include the central nervous system or local signal recognition mechanisms in the glandular cells, such as the calcium-sensing receptor of the parathyroid cell. Superimposed, centrally programmed increases and decreases in hormone secretion or activation through neuroendocrine pathways also occur. Examples include the circadian variation in the secretion of ACTH directing the synthesis and release of cortisol. The monthly menstrual cycle exemplifies a system with much longer periodicity that requires a complex synergism between central and peripheral axes of the endocrine glands. Disruption of hormonal homeostasis due to glandular or central regulatory system dysfunction has both clinical and laboratory consequences. Recognition and correction of these are the essence of clinical endocrinology.

TRANSPORT OF HORMONES IN BLOOD

Protein hormones and some small molecules such as the catecholamines are water-soluble and readily transported by the circulatory system. Others are nearly insoluble in water (e.g., the steroid and thyroid hormones), and their distribution presents special problems. Such molecules are bound to 50 to 60-kd carrier plasma glycoproteins such as thyroxine-binding globulin (TBG), sex hormone–binding globulin (SHBG), and corticosteroid-binding globulin (CBG), as well as to albumin. These ligand–protein complexes serve as reservoirs of these hormones, ensure ubiquitous distribution of their water-insoluble ligands, and protect the small molecules from rapid inactivation or excretion in the urine or bile. Without these proteins, it is unlikely that hydrophobic molecules would be transported much beyond the veins draining the glands in which they are formed. The protein-bound hormones exist in rapid equilibrium with the often minute quantities of hormone in the aqueous plasma. It is this "free" fraction of the circulating hormone that is taken up by the cell. It has been shown, for example, that if tracer thyroid hormone is injected into the portal vein in a protein-free solution, it is bound to hepatocytes at the periphery of the hepatic sinusoid. When the same experiment is repeated with a protein-containing solution, there is a uniform distribution of the tracer hormone throughout the hepatic lobule.[2] Despite the very high affinity of some of the binding proteins for their ligands, one specific protein may not be essential for hormone distribution. For example, in humans with a congenital deficiency of TBG, other proteins, transthyretin and albumin, subsume its role. Because the affinity of these secondary thyroid hormone transport proteins is several orders of magnitude lower than that of TBG, it is possible for the hypothalamic–pituitary feedback system to maintain free thyroid hormone in the normal range at a much lower total hormone concentration. The fact that the "free" hormone concentration is normal in subjects with TBG deficiency indicates that it is this free moeity that is defended by the hypothalamic–pituitary axis and is the active hormone.[3]

The availability of gene-targeting techniques has allowed specific tests of the physiologic role of several hormone-binding proteins. For example, mice with targeted inactivation of the vitamin D–binding protein (DBP) have been generated.[4] Although the absence of DBP markedly reduces the circulating concentration of vitamin D, the mice are otherwise normal. However, they show enhanced susceptibility to a vitamin D–deficient diet because of the reduced reservoir of this sterol. In addition, the absence of DBP markedly reduces the half-life of $25(OH)D_2$ by accelerating its hepatic uptake, making the mice less susceptible to vitamin D intoxication.

In rodents, transthyretin (TTR) carries retinol-binding protein and is also the principal thyroid hormone–binding protein. This protein is synthesized in the liver and in the choroid plexus. It is the major thyroid hormone–binding protein in the cerebrospinal fluid of both rodents and humans and was thought to perhaps serve an important role in thyroid hormone transport into the central nervous system. This hypothesis has been disproven by the fact that mice without TTR have normal concentrations of T_4 in the brain as well as of free T_4 in the plasma.[5, 6] To be sure, the serum concentrations of vitamin A and total T_4 are decreased, but the knockout mice have no signs of vitamin A deficiency or hypothyroidism. Such studies suggest that these proteins primarily serve distributive/reservoir functions.

Protein hormones and some small ligands (e.g., catecholamines) produce their effects by interacting with cell surface receptors. Others, such as the steroid and thyroid hormones, must enter the cell to bind to cytosolic or nuclear receptors. In the past, it has been thought that much of the transmembrane transport of hormones was passive. Evidence is now in hand that there are specific organic anion transporters involved in cellular uptake of thyroid hormone (see reference 7). This may be found to be the case for other small ligands as well, revealing yet another mechanism for ensuring the distribution of a hormone to its site of action.

TARGET CELLS AS ACTIVE PARTICIPANTS

Hormones determine cellular target actions by binding with high specificity to receptor proteins. Whether a peripheral cell is hormonally responsive depends to a large extent on the presence and function of specific and selective hormone receptors. Receptor expression thus determines which cells will respond, as well as the nature of the intracellular effector pathways activated by the hormone signal. Receptor proteins may be localized to the cell membrane, cytoplasm, and nucleus. Broadly, polypeptide hormone receptors are cell-membrane associated, whereas soluble intracellular proteins selectively bind to steroid hormones (Fig. 1–2). This idea of selective localization has recently been challenged, however, because related sequences can be found in multiple cellular compartments.

Membrane-associated receptor proteins usually consist of extracellular sequences that recognize and bind ligand, transmembrane anchoring hydrophobic sequences, and intracellular sequences, which initiate intracellular signaling. Intracellular signaling is mediated by soluble second messengers (e.g., cyclic AMP) or by activation of intracellular signaling molecules (e.g., signal transduces and activates of transcription [STAT] proteins). Receptor-dependent activation of heterotrimeric G-proteins, comprising α, β, and γ subunits, may either induce or suppress effector enzymes or ion channels.

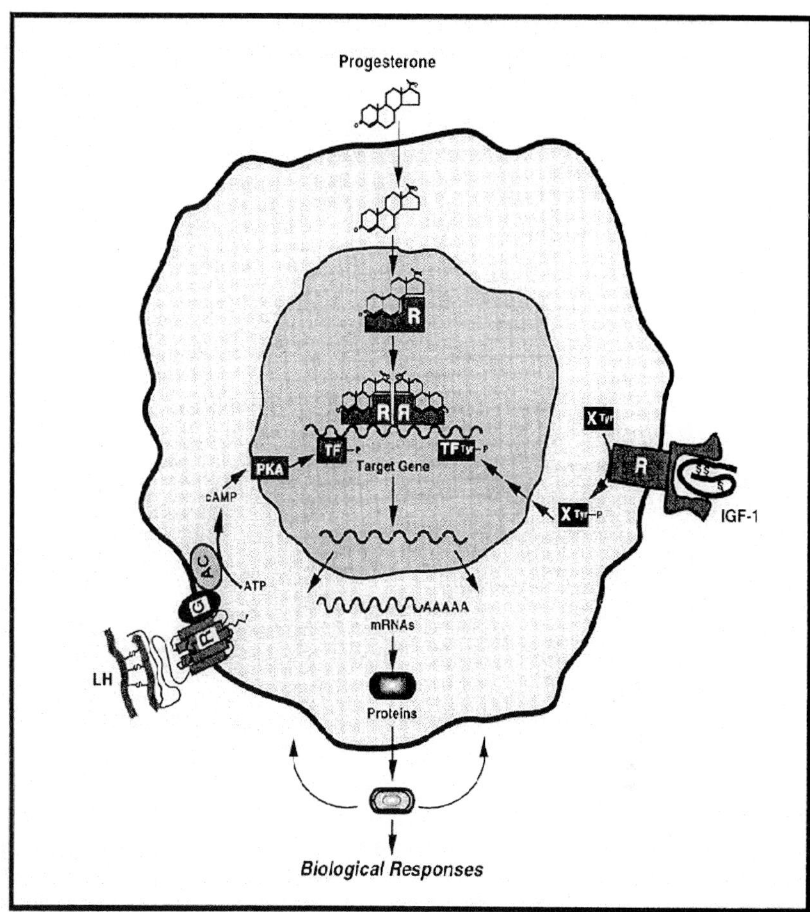

Figure 1–2. Hormonal signaling by cell-surface and intracellular receptors. The receptors for the water-soluble polypeptide hormones, LH, and IGF-I; are integral membrane proteins located at the cell surface. They bind the hormone-utilizing extracellular sequences and transduce a signal by the generation of second messengers, cAMP for the LH receptor, and tyrosine-phosphorylated substrates for the IGF-I receptor. Although effects on gene expression are indicated, direct effects on cellular proteins, for example, ion channels, are also observed. In contrast, the receptor for the lipophilic steroid hormone progesterone resides in the cell nucleus. It binds the hormone and becomes activated and capable of directly modulating target gene transcription. (Tf = transcription factor; R = receptor molecule.) (Reproduced from Mayo K. In Conn PM, Melmed S (eds). Endocrinology: Basic and Clinical Principles. Totowa, NJ, Humana Press, 1997, p. 11.)

Several growth factors and hormone receptors (e.g., for insulin) behave as intrinsic tyrosine kinases or activate intracellular protein tyrosine kinases. Ligand activation may cause receptor dimerization (e.g., growth hormone [GH]) or heterodimerization (e.g., interleukin-6 [IL-6]), followed by activation of intracellular phosphorylation cascades. These activated proteins ultimately determine specific nuclear gene expression.

Both the number of receptors expressed per cell and their responses are also regulated, thus providing a further level of control for hormone action. Several mechanisms account for altered receptor function. Receptor endocytosis causes internalization of cell surface receptors; the hormone–receptor complex is subsequently dissociated, resulting in abrogation of the hormone signal. Receptor trafficking may then result in recycling back to the cell surface (e.g., as for insulin), or the internalized receptor may undergo lysosomal degradation. Both these mechanisms triggered by activation of receptors effectively lead to impaired hormone signaling by down-regulation of these receptors. The hormone signaling pathway may also be down-regulated by receptor desensitization (e.g., as for epinephrine); ligand-mediated receptor phosphorylation leads to a reversible deactivation of the receptor. Desensitization mechanisms can be activated by a receptor's ligand (homologous desensitization) or by another signal (heterologous desensitization), thereby attenuating receptor signaling in the continued presence of ligand. Receptor function may also be limited by the action of specific phosphatases (e.g., Src homology 2 domain-containing protein tyrosine phosphatase [SHP]) or by intracellular negative regulation of the signaling cascade (e.g., suppressor of cytokine signaling [SOCS] proteins inhibiting Janus kinase [JAK]-STAT signaling).

Mutational changes in receptor structure can also determine hormone action. Constitutive receptor activation may be induced by activating mutations (e.g., TSH receptor), leading to endocrine organ hyperfunction, even in the absence of hormone. Conversely, inactivating receptor mutations may lead to endocrine hypofunction (e.g., testosterone or vasopressin receptors). These syndromes are now well characterized and are well described in this volume (Fig. 1–3).

The functional diversity of receptor signaling also results in overlapping or redundant intracellular pathways. For example, both GH as well as cytokines activate JAK-STAT signaling, whereas the distal effects of these stimuli clearly differ. Thus, despite common signaling pathways, hormones elicit highly specific cellular effects. Tissue or cell-type genetic programs or receptor–receptor interactions at the cell surface (e.g., dopamine D2 with somatostatin receptor hetero-oligonization) may also confer specific cellular response to a hormone and provide an additive cellular effect.[8]

CONTROL OF HORMONE SECRETION

Anatomically distinct endocrine glands are composed of highly differentiated cells that synthesize, store, and secrete hormones. Circulating hormone concentrations are a function of glandular secretory patterns and hormone clearance rates. Hormone secretion is tightly regulated to attain circulating levels that are most conducive to elicit the appropriate target tissue response. For example, longitudinal bone growth is initi-

Diseases Caused by Mutations in G Protein-Coupled Receptors

Condition	Receptor	Inheritance	Δ Function
Retinitis Pigmentosa	Rhodopsin	AD/AR	Loss
Nephrogenic Diabetes Insipidus	Vasopressin V2	X-linked	Loss
Isolated Glucocorticoid Deficiency	ACTH	AR	Loss
Color Blindness	Red/Green Opsins	X-linked	Loss
Familial Precocious Puberty	LH	AD (male)	Gain
Familial Hypercalcemia	Ca^{2+} Sensing	AD	Loss
Neonatal Severe Parathyroidism	Ca^{2+} Sensing	AR	Loss
Dominant Form Hypocalcemia	Ca^{2+} Sensing	AD	Gain
Congenital Hyperthyroidism	TSH	AD	Gain
Resistance to Thyroid Hormone	TSH	AR (comp het)	Loss
Hyperfunctioning Thyroid Adenoma	TSH	Somatic	Gain
Metaphyseal Chondrodysplasia	PTH-PTHrP	Somatic	Gain
Hirschsprung's Disease	Endothelin-B	Multigenic	Loss
Coat Color Alteration (*E* locus, mice)	MSH	AD/AR	Loss & Gain
Dwarfism (*little* locus, mice)	GHRH	AR	Loss

Figure 1–3. Diseases caused by mutations in G-protein-coupled receptors. All are human conditions with the exception of the final two entries, which refer to the mouse. (AD = autosomal dominant; AR = autosomal recessive inheritance.) Loss of function refers to inactivating mutations of the receptor, and gain of function to activating mutations. Abbreviations for G-protein-coupled receptors: ACTH = adrenocorticotropic hormone; LH = luteinizing hormone; TSH = thyroid-stimulating hormone; PTH-PTHrP = parathyroid hormone and parathyroid hormone-related peptide; MSH = melanocyte-stimulating hormone; GHRH = growth hormone-releasing hormone; FSH = follicle-stimulating hormone. (Reproduced from Mayo K. In Conn PM, Melmed S (eds), Endocrinology: Basic and Clinical Principles. Totowa, NJ, Humana Press, 1997, page 27.)

ated and maintained by exquisitely regulated levels of circulating GH, whereas mild GH hypersecretion results in gigantism and GH deficiency causes growth retardation. Ambient circulating hormone concentrations are not uniform, and secretion patterns determine appropriate physiologic function. Thus, insulin secretion occurs in short pulses elicited by nutrient and other signals and gonadotrophin secretion is episodic, determined by a hypothalamic pulse generator, whereas prolactin secretion appears to be relatively continuous, with secretory peaks elicited during suckling.

Hormone secretion also adheres to rhythmic patterns. Circadian rhythms serve as adaptive responses to environmental signals and are controlled by a circadian timing mechanism.[9] Light is the major environmental cue adjusting the endogenous clock. The retinohypothalamic tract entrains circadian pulse generators situated within hypothalamic suprachiasmatic nuclei. These signals subserve timing mechanisms for the sleep–wake cycle and determine patterns of hormone secretion and action. Disturbed circadian timing results in hormonal dysfunction and may also be reflective of entrainment or pulse generator lesions. For example, adult GH deficiency due to a damaged hypothalamus or pituitary is associated with elevations in integrated 24-hour leptin concentrations, decreased leptin pulsatility, and yet preserved circadian rhythm of leptin. GH replacement restores leptin pulsatility, followed by loss of body fat mass.[10] Sleep is also an important cue regulating hormone pulsatility. About 70% of overall GH secretion occurs during slow-wave sleep, and increasing age is associated with declining slow-wave sleep and concomitant decline in GH and elevation of cortisol secretion.[11] Most pituitary hormones are secreted in a circadian (day–night) rhythm, best exemplified by ACTH peaks before 9 AM, whereas ovarian steroids follow a 28-day menstrual rhythm. Disrupted episodic rhythms are often a hallmark of endocrine dysfunction. Thus, loss of circadian ACTH secretion with high midnight cortisol levels is a feature of Cushing's disease.

Hormone secretion is induced by multiple specific biochemical and neural signals. Integration of these stimuli results in the net temporal and quantitative secretion of the hormone (Fig. 1–4). Thus, signals elicited by hypothalamic hormones (GHRH, somatostatin), peripheral hormones (IGF-I, sex steroids, thyroid hormone), nutrients, adrenergic pathways, stress, and other neuropeptides, all converge on the somatotroph cell, resulting in the ultimate pattern and quantity of GH secretion. Networks of reciprocal interactions allow for dynamic adaptation and shifts in environmental signals. These regulatory systems embrace the hypothalamic, pituitary, and target endocrine glands, as well as the adipocyte and lymphocyte. Peripheral inflammation and stress elicit cytokine signals, which interface with the neuroendocrine system, resulting in hypothalamic–pituitary axis activation. The parathyroid and pancreatic secreting cells are less tightly controlled by the hypothalamus, but their functions are tightly regulated by the effects they elicit. Thus, parathyroid hormone (PTH) secretion is induced when serum calcium levels fall, and the signal for sustained PTH secretion is abrogated by rising calcium levels.

Several tiers of control subserve the ultimate net glandular secretion. First, central nervous system signals including stress, afferent stimuli, and neuropeptides signal the synthesis and secretion of hypothalamic hormones and neuropeptide (Fig. 1–5). Four hypothalamic releasing hormones (GHRH, corticotropin-releasing hormone [CRH], TRH, and gonadotrophin releasing hormone [GnRH]) traverse the hypothalamic portal vessels and impinge on their respective transmembrane trophic hormone-secreting cell receptors. These distinct cells express GH, ACTH, TSH, and gonadotrophins. In contrast, hypothalamic somatostatin and dopamine suppress GH, prolactin (PRL), or TSH secretion. Trophic hormones also maintain the structural–functional integrity of endocrine organs, including the thyroid and adrenal glands, and the gonads. Target hormones, in turn, serve as powerful negative feedback regulators of their respective trophic hormone and often also suppress secretion of hypothalamic releasing hormones. In certain circumstances, for example during puberty, peripheral sex steroids may positively induce the hypothalamic–pituitary–target gland axis. Thus, luteinizing hormone (LH) induces ovarian estrogen

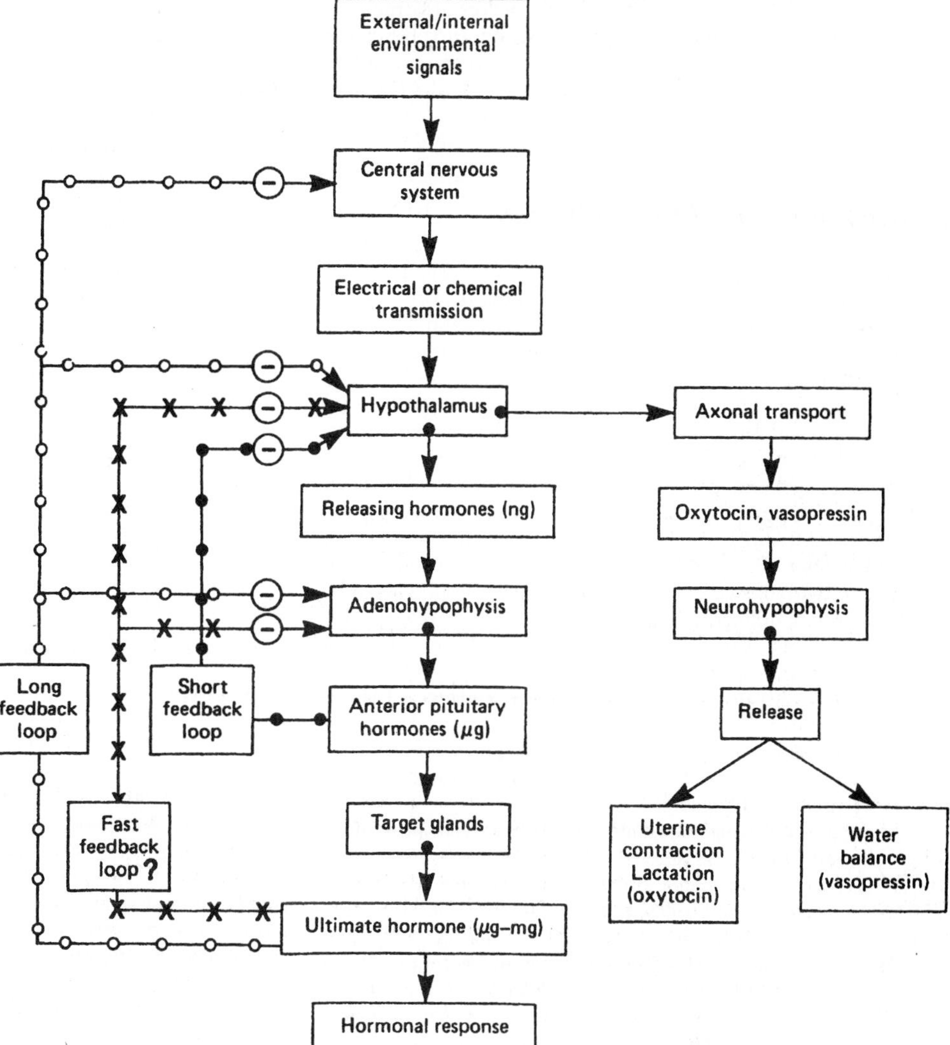

Figure 1–4. Peripheral feedback mechanism and a million-fold amplifying cascade of hormonal signals. Environmental signals are transmitted to the central nervous system, which innervates the hypothalamus, which responds by secreting nanogram amounts of a specific hormone. Releasing hormones are transported down a closed portal system, pass the blood–brain barrier at either end through fenestrations, and bind to specific anterior pituitary cell membrane receptors to elicit secretion of micrograms of specific anterior pituitary hormones. These enter the venous circulation through fenestrated local capillaries, bind to specific target gland receptors, trigger release of micrograms to milligrams of daily hormone amounts, and elicit responses by binding to receptors in distal target tissues. Peripheral hormone receptors enable widespread cell signaling by a single initiating environmental signal, thus facilitating intimate homeostatic association with the external environment. Arrows with a black dot at their origin indicate a secretory process. (Reproduced from Normal AW, Litwack G. Hormones, 2nd edn. New York, Academic Press, 1997, p 14.)

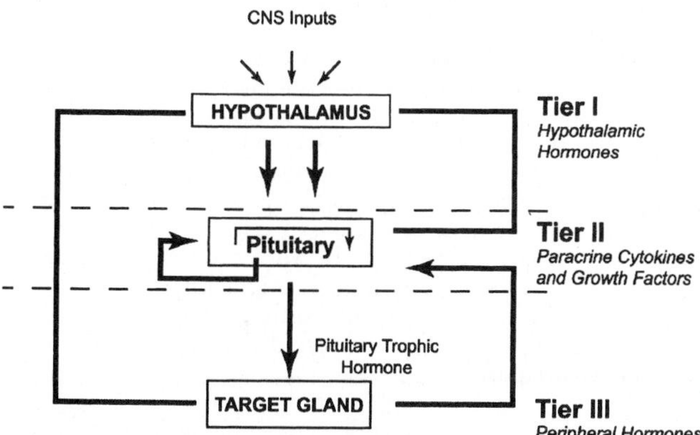

Figure 1–5. Model for regulation of anterior pituitary hormone secretion by three tiers of control. Hypothalamic hormones impinge directly on their respective target cells. Intrapituitary cytokines and growth factors regulate tropic cell function by paracrine (and autocrine) control. Peripheral hormones exert negative feedback inhibition of respective pituitary trophic hormone synthesis and secretion. (Reproduced with permission from Ray D, Melmed S. Pituitary cytokine and growth factor expression and action. Endocrin Rev 1997; 18:206–228.)

secretion, which feeds back positively to induce further LH release. Pituitary hormones themselves, in a short feedback loop, may also regulate their own respective hypothalamic controlling hormone. Hypothalamic releasing hormones are secreted in nanogram amounts and have short half-lives of a few minutes. Anterior pituitary hormones are produced in microgram amounts and have longer half-lives, whereas peripheral hormones can be produced in up to milligram amounts daily, with much longer half-lives.

A further level of secretion control occurs within the gland itself. Thus, intraglandular paracrine or autocrine growth peptides serve to autoregulate pituitary hormone secretion, as exemplified by epidermal growth factor (EGF) control of prolactin or IGF-I control of GH secretion. Molecules within the endocrine cell may also subserve an intracellular feedback loop. Thus, corticotrope SOCS-3 induction by gp 130-linked cytokines serves to abrogate the ligand-induced JAK-STAT cascade and to block pro-opiomelanocortin gene transcription and ACTH secretion. This rapid on–off regulation of ACTH secretion provides a plastic endocrine response to changes in environmental signaling and serves to maintain homeostatic integrity.[12]

In addition to the central–neuroendocrine interface mediated by hypothalamic chemical signal transduction, the CNS directly controls several hormonal secretory processes. Posterior pituitary hormone secretion occurs as direct efferent neural extensions. Postganglionic sympathetic nerves also regulate rapid changes in renin, insulin, and glucagon secretion, and preganglionic sympathetic nerves signal to adrenal medullary cells, eliciting adrenaline release.

HORMONE MEASUREMENT

Endocrine function can be assessed by measuring levels of basal circulating hormone, evoked or suppressed hormone, or hormone-binding proteins. Alternatively, peripheral hormone receptor function can be assessed. Meaningful strategies for timing hormonal measurements vary from system to system. In some cases, circulating hormone concentrations can be measured in randomly collected serum samples. This measurement, when standardized for fasting, environmental stress, age, and gender, is reflective of true hormone concentrations only when levels do not fluctuate appreciably. For example, thyroid hormone, prolactin, and IGF-I levels can be accurately assessed in fasting morning serum samples. On the other hand, when hormone secretion is clearly episodic, timed samples may be required over a defined time course to reflect hormone bioavailability. Thus, early morning and late evening cortisol measurements are most appropriate. Although 24-hour sampling for GH measurements, with samples collected every 2, 10, or 20 minutes, are expensive and cumbersome, they may yield valuable diagnostic information. Random sampling may also reflect secretion peaks or nadirs, thus confounding adequate interpretation of results.

In general, confirmation of failed glandular function is made by attempting to evoke hormone secretion by recognized stimuli. Thus, testing of pituitary hormone reserve may be accomplished by injecting appropriate hypothalamic releasing hormones. Injection of trophic hormones, including TSH and ACTH, evokes specific target gland hormone secretion. Pharmacologic stimuli, for example metoclopromide for induction of prolactin secretion, may also be useful tests of hormone reserve. In contrast, hormone hypersecretion can be diagnosed by suppressing glandular function. Thus, failure to appropriately suppress GH levels after a standardized glucose load implies inappropriate GH hypersecretion.

Radioimmunoassays utilize highly specific antibodies unique to the hormone, or a hormone fragment, to quantify hormone levels. Enzyme-linked immunoabsorbent assays (ELISA) employ enzymes instead of radioactive hormone markers, and enzyme activity is reflective of hormone concentration. This sensitive technique has allowed ultrasensitive measurements of physiologic hormone concentrations. Hormone-specific receptors may be employed in place of the antibody in a radioreceptor assay.

ENDOCRINE DISEASES

Endocrine diseases fall into four broad categories: (1) hormone overproduction; (2) hormone underproduction; (3) altered tissue responses to hormones; and (4) tumors of endocrine glands.

Hormone Overproduction

Occasionally, hormones are secreted in increased amounts because of genetic abnormalities that cause abnormal regulation of hormone synthesis or release. In glucocorticoid-remediable hyperaldosteronism, for example, an abnormal chromosomal crossing-over event puts the aldosterone synthetase gene under the control of the ACTH-regulated 11 β-hydroxylase gene. More often, diseases of hormone overproduction are associated with an increase in the total number of hormone-producing cells. For example, the hyperthyroidism of Graves' disease, in which antibodies mimic TSH and activate the TSH receptors on thyroid cells, is associated with dramatic increase in thyroid cell proliferation, as well as with increased synthesis and release of thyroid hormone from each thyroid cell. In this example, the increase in thyroid cell number represents a polyclonal expansion of thyroid cells, in which large numbers of thyroid cells proliferate in response to an abnormal stimulus. Most endocrine tumors are not polyclonal expansions, however, but instead represent monoclonal expansions of one mutated cell. Pituitary and parathyroid tumors, for example, are usually monoclonal expansions in which somatic mutations occur in multiple tumor suppressor genes and proto-oncogenes. These mutations lead to an increase in proliferation and/or survival of the mutant cells. Sometimes this proliferation is associated with abnormal secretion of hormone from each tumor cell as well. For example, mutant G_α proteins in somatotrophs can lead to both increased cellular proliferation and increased secretion of growth hormone from each tumor cell.

Hormone Underproduction

Underproduction of hormone can result from a wide variety of processes, ranging from surgical removal of parathyroid glands during neck surgery, to tuberculous destruction of adrenal glands, or to iron deposition in β-cells in hemochromatosis. A frequent cause of destruction of hormone-producing cells is autoimmunity. Autoimmune destruction of beta cells in type 1 diabetes mellitus and autoimmune destruction of thyroid cells in Hashimoto's thyroiditis are two of the most common disorders treated by endocrinologists. More uncommonly, a host of genetic abnormalities can also lead to decreased hormone production. These disorders can result from abnormal development of hormone-producing cells (e.g., hypogonadotrophic hypogonadism caused by KAL gene mutations), from abnormal synthesis of hormones (e.g., deletion of the growth hormone gene), or from abnormal regulation of hormone secretion (e.g., the hypoparathyroidism associated with activating mutations of the parathyroid cell's calcium-sensing receptor).

Altered Tissue Responses

Resistance to hormones can be caused by a variety of genetic disorders. Examples include mutations in the growth hormone receptor in Laron dwarfism and mutations in the G_α gene in the hypoparathyroidism of pseudohypoparathyroidism, type 1a. The insulin resistance in muscle and liver central to the etiology of type 2 diabetes mellitus appears to be polygenic in origin. Type 2 diabetes is also an example of a disease in which end organ insensitivity is worsened by signals from other organs, in this case by signals originating in fat cells. In other cases, the target organ of hormone action is more directly abnormal, as in the parathyroid hormone (PTH) resistance of renal failure.

Increased end organ function can be caused by mutations in signal reception and propagation. For example, activating mutations in TSH, LH, and PTH receptors can cause increased activity of thyroid cells, Leydig cells, and osteoblasts, even in the absence of ligand. Similarly, activating mutations in the G_s α protein can cause precocious puberty, hyperthyroidism, and acromegaly in McCune-Albright syndrome.

Tumors of Endocrine Glands

Tumors of endocrine glands, as noted above, often result in hormone overproduction. Some tumors of endocrine glands produce little if any hormone but cause disease by their local compressive symptoms or by metastatic spread. Examples include so-called nonfunctioning pituitary tumors, which are usually benign but can cause a variety of symptoms due to compression on adjacent structures, and thyroid cancer, which can spread throughout the body without causing hyperthyroidism.

THERAPEUTIC STRATEGIES

In general, hormones are employed pharmacologically for both their replacement and their suppressive effects. Hormones may also be used for diagnostic stimulatory effects (e.g., hypothalamic hormones) to evoke target organ responses or to diagnose endocrine hyperfunction by suppressing hormone hypersecretion (e.g., T_3). Ablation of endocrine gland function due to genetic or acquired causes can be restored by hormone replacement therapy. In general, steroid and thyroid hormones are replaced orally, where as peptide hormones (e.g., insulin, DH) require injection. Gastrointestinal absorption and first-pass kinetics determine oral hormone dosage and availability. Physiologic replacement can achieve both appropriate hormone levels (e.g., thyroid), as well as approximate hormone secretory patterns (e.g., GnRH delivered intermittently via a pump). Hormones can also be used to treat diseases associated with glandular hyperfunction. Long-acting depot preparations of somatostatin analogs suppress GH hypersecretion in acromegaly or 5-HIAA hypersecretion in carcinoid syndrome. Estrogen receptor antagonists (e.g., tarmoxilen) are useful for some patients with breast cancer, and GnRH analogs may downregulate the gonadotrophin axis and benefit patients with prostate cancer.

Novel formulations of receptor-specific hormone ligands are now being clinically developed (e.g., estrogen agonists/antagonists, somatostatin receptor subtype ligands), resulting in more selective therapeutic targeting. Modes of hormone injection (e.g., for PTH) may also determine therapeutic specificity and efficacy. Improved hormone delivery systems, including computerized minipumps, intranasal sprays (e.g., for 1-desamino-8-D-arginine vasopression [DDAVP]), pulmonary inhalations, and depot intramuscular injections, will also allow added patient compliance and ease of administration.

Despite this tremendous progress, some therapies, such as insulin delivery to rigorously control blood sugar, still require tremendous patient involvement and await innovative approaches.

References

1. Chawla A, Repa, JJ, Evans RM et al. Nuclear receptors and lipid physiology: Opening the X-files. Science 2001; 294: 1866–1870.
2. Mendel CM, Weisiger RA, Jones AL, et al. Thyroid hormone-binding proteins in plasma facilitate uniform distribution of thyroxine within tissues: A perfused rat liver study. Endocrinology 1987; 120:1742–1749.
3. Mendel CM. The free hormone hypothesis: A physiologically based mathematical model. Endocr Rev 1989; 10(3):232–274.
4. Safadi FF, Thornton P, Magiera H, et al. Osteopathy and resistance to vitamin D toxicity in mice null for vitamin D binding protein. J Clin Invest 1999; 103:239–251.
5. Palha JA, Fernandes R, de Escobar GM, et al. Transthyretin regulates thyroid hormone levels in the choroid plexus, but not in the brain parenchyma: Study in a transthyretin-null mouse model. Endocrinology 2000; 141:3267–3272.
6. Palha JA, Episkopou V, Maeda S, et al. Thyroid hormone metabolism in a transthyretin-null mouse strain. J Biol Chem 1994; 269: 33135–33139.
7. Hennemann G, Docter R, Friesema ECH, et al. Plasma membrane transport of thyroid hormones and its role in thyroid hormone metabolism and bioavailability. Endocr Rev 2001; 22:451–476.
8. Rochevill M, Lange DC, Kumar U, et al. Receptors for dopamine and somatostatin: formation of hetero-oligomers with enhanced functional activity. Science 2000; 288:154–157.
9. Moore RY. Circadian rhythms: Basic neurobiology and clinical applications. Ann Rev Med 1997; 48:253–266.
10. Aftab MA, Guzder R, Wallace AM, et al. Circadian and ultradian rhythm and leptin pulsitility in adult GH deficiency: Effects of GH replacement. J Clin Endocr Metab 2001; 86:3499–3506.
11. Cauter EV, Leproult R, Plat L. Age-related changes in slow wave sleep and REM sleep and relationship with growth hormone and cortisol levels in healthy men. JAMA 2000; 284:861–868.
12. Melmed S: The immuno-neuroendocrine interface. J Clin Invest 2001; 108:1563–1566.

2 The Endocrine Patient

Daniel D. Federman

A textbook of medicine is inevitably about disease, but the practice of medicine deals with illness, that is, a person experiencing a disease. It is for that reason that the present chapter has been entitled "The Endocrine Patient." It is my intention to lay out the general issues and approaches applicable to caring for patients with endocrine disorders. The topics to be discussed include initial evaluation and the nature of referral, the fact finding required in clinical evaluation, the use of the laboratory and imaging, the formulation of a differential diagnosis, decision making, and management. In each case, the steps are portrayed from the patient's point of view.

It is worth noting that, except for acute adrenal insufficiency, endocrine disorders are seldom life-threatening. They have enormous effect on the quality of life, however, and successful intervention can be extremely important to both patient and family.

GENERAL CONSIDERATIONS

Many features of being an endocrine patient are common to all experiences of illness. Most often, a perceived change in bodily function, a symptom, gets one to the doctor. Although generations of medical students have described new patients as being "in no acute distress," most patients are, in fact, worried and anxious when they see a physician, the more so when the physician is not known to them. A few minutes spent in getting to know the patient can pay enormous dividends in the accuracy of the history obtained and in setting the stage for further cooperation with testing and treatment.

Inasmuch as most endocrine consultation is elective rather than emergent, I favor asking a few simple questions, such as "Where are you from?" "What do you do?" "How did you come to us?" "Were you referred?" and so on. Almost always, some common experience or acquaintance is discovered that provides the basis for a rapport that does not emerge from formal medical questioning. This step also immediately conveys that you are interested in the patient as a person and not just as a disease.

SPECIAL FEATURES OF ENDOCRINE ILLNESS

Discovery through Screening

Numerous special features of endocrine disease make patient presentation quite different from that seen in general medicine. One is the discovery of abnormality through screening of asymptomatic individuals, for example, a high serum calcium level discovered through multiphasic screening or a high blood glucose level discovered in a shopping mall kiosk. The very absence of symptoms lends an unreality to the moment and should become an explicit topic of the patient-doctor interaction. In this circumstance, it is worth emphasizing the value of early discovery and prevention of greater morbidity.

Quantitative Rather Than Qualitative Abnormalities

A second special feature of endocrine disorders is that they are all quantitative, rather than qualitative, departures from normal. No endocrine disorder is due to a novel hormone. Everyone has cortisol circulating as a determining feature of his or her life. Hypercorticism and adrenal insufficiency represent just more or less of the hormone. Similarly, all hormones found in excess or in deficiency in disease are physiologic determinants of stature, weight, complexion, hairiness, temperament, and behavior. In contrast, no one has a little pneumonia or a little inflammatory bowel disease as a constitutive status. In addition, most endocrine glands have both a basal and a stimulable or reserve function. It is common to have partial diminution of capacity in which the basal function is adequate but a reserve called upon during part of each day—or, more dramatically, in emergencies—is not available.

Overlap with Other Diseases

The symptoms of endocrine disorders overlap a great range of normal characteristics, including body contour, facial configurations, weight distributions, skin and hair coloring, and muscular capacity. They also overlap with other conditions that are far more common, including depression and normal aging. The added adipose tissue of hyperadrenocorticism is more difficult to recognize in a person who is already obese. The nervousness associated with hyperthyroidism is less apparent in a thin, hyperkinetic man than in a person of moderate body weight. The effects of an androgen-producing adrenal tumor are less likely to be noticed in a family of swarthy, hirsute individuals.

Finally, most endocrine disorders evolve gradually over months to years instead of appearing suddenly, such as a heart attack or an acute infection. This combination of varied host background and slow evolution of disease leads to considerable delay in diagnosis: both the patient and primary care physician adapt to the changes as part of the person, and definitive evaluation, now relatively easy for most disorders, is not undertaken. Hypothyroidism and acromegaly are good examples of this phenomenon. All series show a remarkable delay in diagnosis despite sometimes disabling symptoms.

Hormones have more distant effects than local effects. This, of course, reflects their messenger status. Unlike an abscess, a myocardial infarction, or an esophageal cancer, endocrine disorders seldom produce symptoms near the gland of origin. (Subacute thyroiditis and large pituitary tumors, of course, are exceptions.) But because in most endocrinopathies the excess or missing hormone works on several or many systems, the resulting syndrome can be enigmatic.

Several endocrine disorders are important not because of their incidence but because of their curability: Cushing's disease, acromegaly, and pheochromocytoma are cases in point. Although these disorders enter the differential diagnosis of common problems such as diabetes, their occurrence is so rare that the primary care physician does not easily think of them.

Unique Features of Reproductive Disorders

Reproductive disorders have symptoms and signs that have no parallel in other areas. This is the one system in which sexual dimorphism is inherent rather than epiphenomenal; it is also the one with the greatest span of developmental change. Once the heart starts beating in the embryo, it goes on doing so until the last moment of life; but puberty, adult sexual functioning, and menopause establish time lines against which all symptoms are to be assessed. Thus, vaginal bleeding has entirely different meanings whether it occurs on the first day of life, as a natural appearance at age 12, between menstrual periods at age 25 years, as a harbinger of menopause at age 46 years, or as a highly probable symptom of cancer at age 66 years.

Physical appearance and function are important features of self-image. Thus, hirsutism, thinness, obesity, sexual arousal, and erectile capacity bear considerable psychological import to the endocrine patient. The clinician should be constantly aware of both spoken and unspoken thoughts that may be troubling the patient.

The Couple as a Clinical Unit

The ultimate goal of reproductive capacity is, of course, a fertile union. This means that the couple, rather than the individual, is the unit of clinical concern. It is thus the principal area in medicine whereby two people and their interaction, rather than a single person and her capacities, are studied and treated. In addition, there are dimensions of successful sexual function that are important at other times than when fertility is sought. Sex drive, erotic responsiveness, affection, and tenderness are all important aspects of life whether or not fertility is an issue. These areas are notoriously difficult to evaluate in a society that treats sexual function as such a special topic, particularly enshrouded in personal issues of such importance.

EVALUATION OF PATIENTS WITH ENDOCRINE DISORDERS

I have emphasized previously the belief that establishing an interested and warm relationship is the beginning of excellence in any elective medical interaction. In addition to its affective power, the relationship elicits a more informative history, establishes better cooperation in both testing and treatment, and provides a platform for informed decision making by the patient.

History

As in most areas of medicine, precision of diagnosis and economy of investigation begin with a carefully wrought history. An open-ended question, combined with an attentive silence, allows the patient to provide the background for the clinical moment. After the patient has spoken spontaneously, the physician provides a guided expansion of the information. Details of timing, sequence, changes of diet or activity, relationship to the menstrual cycle, changes in weight or size, and alterations in mood or sleep pattern—all of these may provide clues to underlying endocrine abnormality.

A good example of the power of the history is the interpretation of irregular periods in a woman of reproductive age. The simple statement, "I've never been regular," points to a presumptive diagnosis of polycystic ovary syndrome in a way that a very convoluted sequence of questions might actually fail to do. That statement is to be contrasted with this one: "I used to be regular, but in the last year or so, I never know when my period is going to come." If the presenting symptom is irregular periods, the simple invitation, "Tell me about your periods," is likely to be the key to the diagnosis.

Careful questioning about use of complementary and alternative medicines is an important and, occasionally, a very revealing step.

A thorough family history has become increasingly important as the genetic basis for more and more endocrine diseases becomes established. For practical purposes, I favor diagramming a pedigree of the first-order relatives—parents, siblings, children—of all patients, not just those for whom a genetic disorder is already suspected. Known disorders are readily revealed this way, and unknown conjunctions of clinical and genetic factors may also be disclosed (Fig. 2–1).

Physical Examination

General Examination

It is said that the history is 80% or more of clinical diagnosis, and that is no less true in endocrine disorders than in general medicine. Yet the physical examination is a critical element in the process of arriving at a diagnosis, and here I want to call particular attention to the first impression.

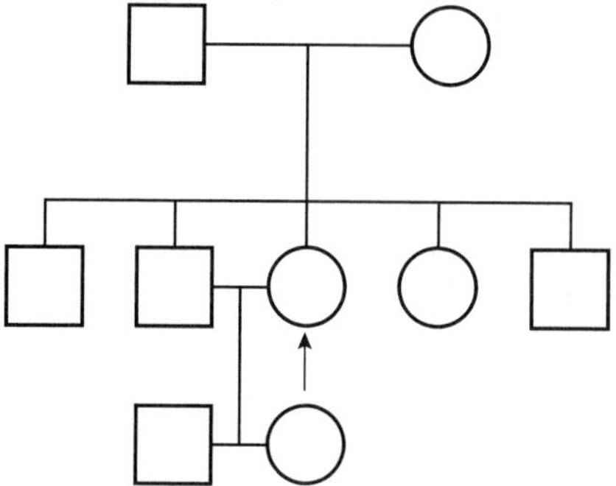

Figure 2–1. Simple pedigree of the propositi *(arrow)* and first-order relatives should be the standard family history in a new patient work-up. If the patient has children, their health status should be included as well.

The possibility of Cushing's syndrome, Addison's disease, hyperthyroidism and hypothyroidism, acromegaly, polycystic ovary syndrome, hypogonadism, and Turner's syndrome—these and other endocrine disorders should be considered from the first moment one encounters a new patient. Otherwise, one risks accepting that the appearance of the patient is just that and no more. In other words, as soon as one accepts that the initial impression is what the person looks like naturally, the quantitative departure from normal that is the essence of endocrine disease fails to impress one. This, incidentally, is why both families and primary care physicians often miss a diagnosis that seems obvious to the consultant endocrinologist.

A quantification of this last point may be helpful. If the signs of hypothyroidism or acromegaly, for example, take 3 years to become striking, the person living with the patient is exposed to 1/1095th of fractional change per day—well below the threshold of just noticeable difference. Similarly, a primary care physician seeing the patient perhaps four times a year for a general checkup and management of hypertension is exposed to 91/1095 fractional change. This can sometimes lead to a diagnosis but often does not. When one sees the patient for the first time, however, the imprint of the disease catches attention and the constitutional appearance is in the background.

Although a consultant participates because of a special area of interest and expertise, he or she is a general physician first and should be alert to all dimensions of the physical examination:

What is the height/weight ratio?
What is the basic degree of muscularity?
Is there evidence of heart disease to explain the chest pain and dyspnea one has heard about in the history?
What is the degree of hirsutism?
Are there signs of liver disease, malnutrition, or poor or excellent physical training?
What is the blood pressure with the patient standing as well as lying or sitting?

These and many other points of a general examination begin to modify the thinking one has undertaken on the basis of history.

Targeted Examination

The targeted physical examination of any consultant is an interesting interplay of general and specific goals. Theoretically, any experienced clinician should undertake a general examination and come to all the findings pertinent to an underlying endocrine disorder. In fact, however, the physical examination is greatly influenced by the hypotheses generated in the history. Let us look at a few examples.

If a patient reports weight loss despite a good appetite, there is only a very restricted differential diagnosis, principally malabsorption or hypermetabolism. In doing a physical examination, therefore, I would pay particular attention to signs of malabsorption (muscular wasting, vitamin deficiencies, purpura) and to signs of thyroid disease with its generalized hypermetabolism and localized autoimmune phenomena, including ophthalmopathy.

Similarly, if a patient complains of hirsutism or other signs of androgen excess, one is immediately thrust into a consideration of ethnic hair distribution and quality. Is there temporal recession of the hairline? Does the hair on the abdomen come up over the umbilicus? Is hair present on the back (rare without marked hyperandrogenism)? How much acne is there? At the extreme, is there evidence of clitoral enlargement?

Finally, and most important, does the patient look like or unlike the other women in her family?

Direct Assessment of Endocrine Glands

Three endocrine glands are palpable—the thyroid, the testis, and the ovary. Specific attention should be given to each of these.

The thyroid gland should be approached first by inspection—while the patient swallows—for size, symmetry, or localized enlargement. Many thyroid nodules are visible, and inspection often calls attention to lesions that would be missed on palpation. The thyroid should then be felt while the patient swallows, from the front with your thumbs or from behind the patient with the index and third fingers. It is crucial to keep your own fingers from moving while the patient is swallowing. The principal observation is whether there is diffuse enlargement of the thyroid gland (most often Graves' diffuse hyperplasia or Hashimoto's thyroiditis) or one or more nodules. Although the consistency of the gland is to be noted, in fact it is often not concordant with the pathology.

Functioning tumors of the testis may be too small to be felt with the fingers, and most internists and general physicians are not skilled in palpation of the ovaries. For this reason, ultrasound and other forms of imaging have become key features of gonadal evaluation and are discussed later.

The size of one other endocrine gland, the pituitary, can be inferred from physical examination for what Cushing called "neighborhood signs." As a pituitary tumor or diffuse enlargement proceeds, it pushes up on the optic chiasm from below, producing a bitemporal hemianopsia first manifested in the upper quadrants, often to a blinking or flashing red light. This finding is too subtle for the generalist's confidence, however, and pituitary assessment depends on formal visual fields and imaging.

Indirect Assessment of Endocrine Status

Many consequences of hormone action can be detected on physical examination; the results combine with the history to produce a highly reliable differential diagnosis and thus an informed basis for laboratory evaluation and imaging. Among the things to be looked for are the eye signs and dermopathy of Graves' disease, acanthosis nigricans as a clue to insulin resistance, muscular wasting and tremor, changes in the voice due to hypothyroidism or acromegaly, and a general impression of nutrition and its adequacy or excess. Each of these findings is described in more detail with the specific disorder in subsequent chapters.

that year, and endocrine testing in patients at risk can justify surgical thyroidectomy before the first birthday. Hereditary predispositions will certainly emerge for other endocrine disorders and will make it crucial for the clinician to take a revealing family history and follow up even minor clues.

The Internet

Never in history has so much medical information been available to patients. I therefore now routinely ask patients what they already know about their condition or their symptoms. A bit sheepishly in some cases, many patients admit to looking up topics on the World Wide Web and are about to compare what I tell them with what they have already read. Much of that information is accurate, but some is nonsense, and it requires patience and clear explanation before such patients go away satisfied.

Electronic Mail

Although opinions differ widely, I find e-mail an extremely useful advance in communicating with patients who have computers. They have access to you between appointments and on a time frame of mutual convenience. The computer thus reduces anxiety on the patient's part, particularly regarding questions or findings for which they might otherwise hesitate to make an appointment. Reporting laboratory test results is expedited, and accompanying the report with a few sentences of interpretation can be as useful as a telephone call.

It is wise to keep copies of e-mails so that a clear record of the exchange is available. There are, however, several important caveats. Never let an e-mail exchange substitute for a true evaluation, including history and physical examination. I believe that one should not prescribe for a patient whom one has not seen, and one should not provide much interpretation of history or laboratory tests without very fundamental disclaimers. On the whole, however, e-mail can be used to initiate a new relationship and can certainly support an ongoing one.

Managed Care

The effort to control health care costs by limiting reimbursement for physician services, laboratory testing, and imaging has had a profound impact throughout medicine. Without taking on the whole issue, I want to comment on several practical consequences.

"Curbsiding"—the request by a physician for patient guidance without being asked to see the patient—has increased strikingly. Consultants can provide some general help to primary care physicians without seeing the patient; however, much hinges on the history and physical examination done by the primary care physician. The failure to realize that hyperthyroidism is due to a hot nodule, for example, totally distorts the picture and will lead to an erroneous recommendation for treatment. The failure to distinguish a recent onset of amenorrhea and virilization from a polycystic ovary–like syndrome may hide the presence of a readily curable virilizing tumor. The failure to recognize hypoglycemic unresponsiveness may perpetuate a dangerous degree of overinsulinization and elicit inappropriate advice from the consultant. Thus, the consultant must set bounds and at some point indicate that it is important for a formal consultation to take place.

Costs

Some endocrine work-ups can be expensive and invite challenge from third-party insurers. The best approach to this concern is a careful history and physical examination, clear establishment of the prior probabilities of certain diagnoses, and then effective use of screening tests before embarking on an unnecessarily extensive evaluation.

For example, in a patient with suspected Cushing's syndrome, it is mandatory to establish the presence of hypercorticism before embarking on a search for its cause. Once this lethal but curable disorder has been properly diagnosed, however, no cost should deter one from finding the cause and correcting it. One argument I make is that expensive tests and imaging should be amortized rather than considered an extravagant or unnecessary expense. If a young woman age 30, with a life expectancy of 80 years or more, has a husband and two children to whom her life matters, the $3000 evaluation breaks down to $20 per loved one per year of life expectancy. Any plan manager has to see that this is an appropriate cost.

MANAGEMENT

There are few more gratifying experiences in medicine than recognizing and correcting an endocrine disorder. Patients feel that they have been rescued from a mysterious overtaking of their identity. Body contour, facial appearance, temperament, and well-being are restored to the patient's constitutive status. Deterioration attributed to aging or depression or chronic disease is reversed. In brief, something almost miraculous takes place. Even when these goals cannot be achieved, as in diabetes, a major impact on mortality and morbidity can be.

Of course, these optimal outcomes require accuracy of diagnosis—but that is only the beginning. A true sharing by patient and physician, based on a sound knowledge of normal physiology, provides the best foundation for choice of therapy and maintenance of a continuing program. The result can be, simply put, wonderful.

3 Genetic Control of Peptide Hormone Formation

Joel F. Habener

Advances in the fields of molecular and cellular biology have provided new insights into the mechanistic workings of cells. Recombinant deoxyribonucleic acid (DNA) technology and the sequencing (decoding) of the entire human and mouse genomes now make it possible to analyze the precise structure and function of DNA, the genetic substance that is the basis for life. The discovery of the unique biochemical and structural properties of DNA provided the conceptual framework with which to begin a systematic investigation of the origins, development, and organization of life forms.[1]

The near completion of the entire sequences of the human and mouse genomes was accomplished in the years 2000 and 2001, 5 years ahead of the originally anticipated schedule. The availability of a complete blueprint of the structure and organization of all expressed genes now provides profound insights into the basis of genetically determined diseases. Within the next decades, genotyping of individuals shortly after birth will be possible. Therapeutic approaches for the correction of genetic defects by techniques of gene replacement are likely to become a reality.

The polypeptide hormones constitute a critically important and diverse set of regulatory molecules encoded by the genome whose functions are to convey specific information among cells and organs. This type of molecular communication arose early in the development of life and evolved into a complex system for the control of growth, development, and reproduction and for the maintenance of metabolic homeostasis. These hormones consist of approximately 400 or more small proteins ranging from as few as three amino acids (thyrotropin-releasing hormone, TRH) to 192 amino acids (growth hormone). In a broader sense, these polypeptides function both as hormones, whose actions on distant organs are mediated by way of their transport through the blood stream, and as local cell-to-cell communicators (Fig. 3–1). The latter function of the polypeptide hormones is exemplified by their elaboration and secretion within neurons of the central, autonomic, and peripheral nervous systems, where they act as neurotransmitters. These multiple modes of expression of the polypeptide hormone genes have aroused great interest in the specific functions of these peptides and the mechanisms of their synthesis and release.

This chapter reviews the diverse structures of genes encoding peptide hormones and the multiple mechanisms that govern their expression. The synthesis of nonpeptide hormones (e.g., catecholamines, thyroid hormones, steroid hormones) involves the action of multiple enzymes—and hence the expression of multiple genes—and is discussed in the individual chapters devoted to such hormones.

EVOLUTION OF PEPTIDE HORMONES AND THEIR FUNCTIONS

Peptide hormones arose early in the evolution of life. Indeed, polypeptides that are structurally similar to mammalian peptides are present in lower vertebrates, insects, yeasts, and bacteria.[2] An example of the early evolution of regulatory peptides is the α factor (mating pheromone) of yeast, which is similar in structure to mammalian luteinizing hormone–releasing hormone (also called gonadotropin-releasing hormone [GnRH]).[3] The oldest member of the cholecystokinin-gastrin family of peptides appeared at least 500 million years ago in the protochordate *Ciona intestinalis*.[4]

Thus, the genes encoding polypeptide hormones, and particularly regulatory peptides, evolved early in the development of life and initially fulfilled the function of cell-to-cell communication to cope with problems concerning nourishment, growth, development, and reproduction. As specialized organs connected by a circulatory system developed during evolution, similar, if not identical, gene products became hormones for purposes of organ-to-organ communication.

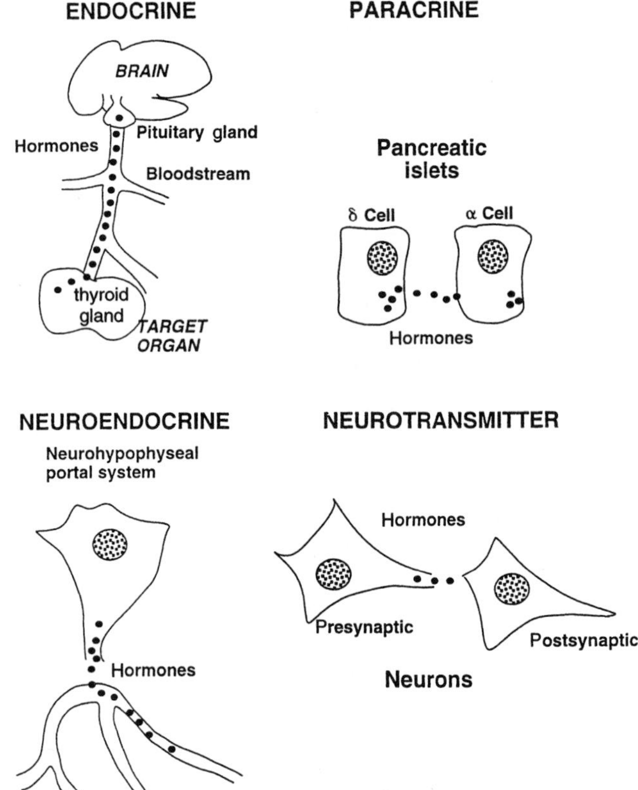

Figure 3–1. Different modes of utilization of polypeptide hormones in expression of their biologic actions. The peptide hormones are expressed in at least four ways in fulfilling their functions as cellular messenger molecules: (1) endocrine mode, for purposes of communication among organs (e.g., pituitary-thyroid axis); (2) paracrine mode, for communication among adjacent cells, often located within endocrine organs; (3) neuroendocrine mode, for synthesis and release of peptides from specialized peptidergic neurons for action on distant organs through the blood stream (e.g., neuroendocrine peptides of hypothalamus); and (4) neurotransmitter mode, for action of peptides in concert with classical amino acid–derived aminergic transmitters in the neuronal communication network. Identical polypeptides are often utilized in the nervous system both as neuroendocrine hormones and as neurotransmitters. In some instances, the same gene product is used in all four modes of expression.

STEPS IN EXPRESSION OF A PROTEIN-ENCODING GENE

The steps involved in transfer of information encoded in the polynucleotide language of DNA to the poly–amino acid language of biologically active proteins involve gene transcription, post-transcriptional processing of ribonucleic acids (RNAs), translation, and post-translational processing of the proteins. The expression of genes and protein synthesis can be considered in terms of several major processes, any one or more of which may serve as specific control points in the regulation of gene expression (Fig. 3–2):

1. *Rearrangements and transpositions of DNA segments.* These processes occur over many years (eons) in evolution, with the exception of uncommon mechanisms of somatic gene rearrangements such as the rearrangements in the immunoglobulin genes during the lifetime of an individual.
2. *Transcription.* Synthesis of RNA results in the formation of RNA copies of the two gene alleles and is catalyzed by the basal RNA polymerase II–associated transcription factors.
3. *Post-transcriptional processing.* Specific modifications of the RNA include the formation of messenger RNA (mRNA) from the precursor RNA by way of excision and rejoining of RNA segments (introns and exons) and modifications of the 3′ end of the RNA by polyadenylation and of the 5′ end by addition of 7-methylguanine "caps."
4. *Translation.* Amino acids are assembled by base pairing of the nucleotide triplets (anticodons) of the specific "carrier" aminoacylated transfer RNAs to the corresponding codons of the mRNA bound to polyribosomes and are polymerized into the polypeptide chains.
5. *Post-translational processing and modification.* Final steps in protein synthesis may involve one or more cleavages of peptide bonds, which result in the conversion of biosynthetic precursors (prohormones), to intermediate or final forms of the protein; derivatization of amino acids (e.g., glycosylation, phosphorylation, acetylation, myristoylation); and the folding of the processed polypeptide chain into its native conformation.

Each of the specific steps of gene expression requires the integration of precise enzymatic and other biochemical reactions. These processes have developed to provide high fidelity in the reproduction of the encoded information and to provide control points for the expression of the specific phenotype of cells.

The post-translational processing of proteins creates diversity in gene expression through modifications of the protein. Although the functional information contained in a protein is ultimately encoded in the primary amino acid sequence, the specific biologic activities are a consequence of the higher order secondary, tertiary, and quaternary structures of the polypeptide. Given the wide range of possible specific modifications of the amino acids, such as glycosylation, phosphorylation, acetylation, and sulfation,[5] any one of which may affect the conformation or function of the protein, a single gene may ultimately encode a wide variety of specific proteins as a result of post-translational processes.

Polypeptide hormones are synthesized in the form of larger precursors that appear to fulfill several functions in biologic systems (Fig. 3–3), including (1) intracellular trafficking, by which the cell distinguishes among specific classes of proteins and directs them to their sites of action, and (2) the generation of multiple biologic activities from a common genetically encoded protein by regulated or cell-specific variations in the post-translational modifications (Fig. 3–4).

All the peptide hormones and regulatory peptides studied thus far contain signal or leader sequences at the amino termini; these hydrophobic sequences recognize specific sites on the membranes of the rough endoplasmic reticulum, which results in the transport of nascent polypeptides into the secretory pathway of the cell (see Figs. 3–2 and 3–3).[6] The consequence of the specialized signal sequences of the precursor proteins is that proteins destined for secretion are selected from a great many other cellular proteins for sequestration and subsequent packaging into secretory granules and export from the cell. In addition, most, if not all, of the smaller hormones and regulatory peptides are produced as a consequence of post-translational cleavages of the precursors within the Golgi complex of secretory cells.

SUBCELLULAR STRUCTURE OF CELLS THAT SECRETE PROTEIN HORMONES

Cells whose principal functions are the synthesis and export of proteins contain highly developed, specialized subcellular organelles for the translocation of secreted proteins and their

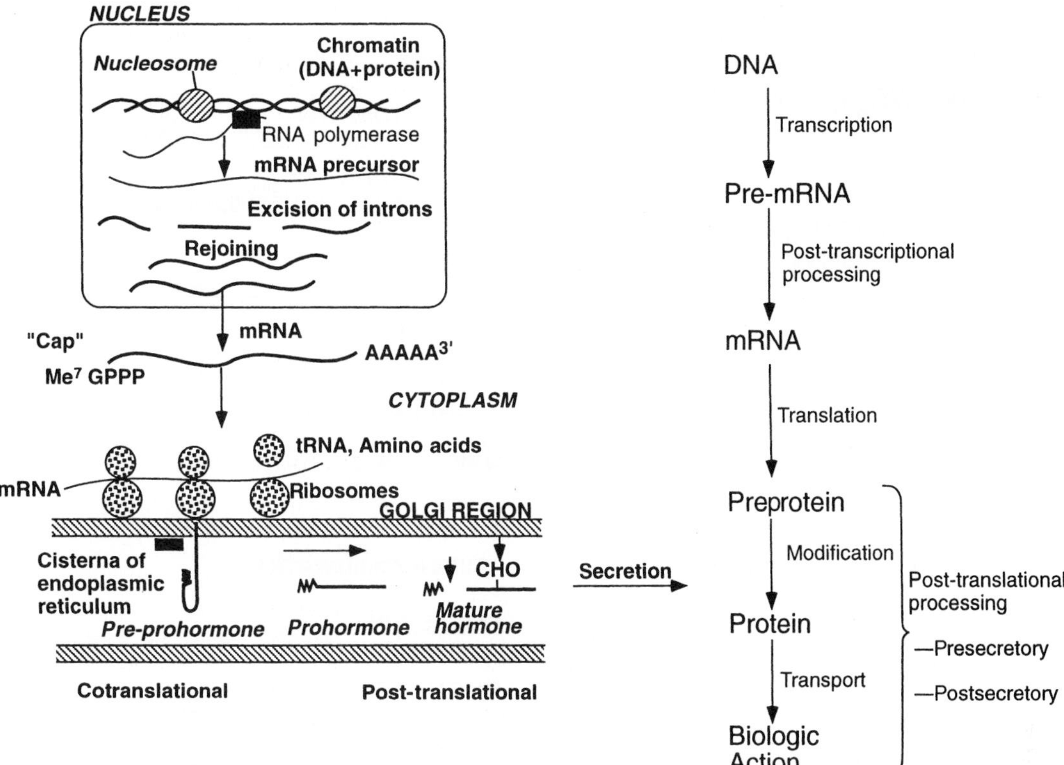

Figure 3–2. Steps in the cellular synthesis of polypeptide hormones. Steps that take place within the nucleus include transcription of genetic information into a messenger ribonucleic acid (mRNA) precursor (pre-mRNA) followed by post-transcriptional processing, which includes RNA cleavage, excision of introns, and rejoining of exons, resulting in formation of mRNA. Ends of mRNA are modified by addition of methylguanosine caps at the 5′ end and addition of poly(A) tracts at the 3′ ends. The cytoplasmic mRNA is assembled with ribosomes. Amino acids, carried by aminoacylated transfer RNAs (tRNAs), are then polymerized into a polypeptide chain. The final step in protein synthesis is that of post-translational processing. These processes take place both during growth of the nascent polypeptide chain (cotranslational) and after release of the completed chain (post-translational), and they include proteolytic cleavages of polypeptide chain (conversion of pre-prohormones or prohormones to hormones), derivatizations of amino acids (e.g., glycosylation, phosphorylation), and cross-linking and assembly of the polypeptide chain into its conformed structure. The diagram depicts post-translational synthesis and processing of a typical secreted polypeptide, which requires vectorial, or unidirectional, transport of the polypeptide chain across the membrane bilayer of the endoplasmic reticulum, thus resulting in sequestration of the polypeptide in the cisterna of the endoplasmic reticulum, a first step in the export of proteins destined for secretion from the cell (see Fig. 3–6). Most translational processing occurs within the cell as depicted (presecretory) and in some instances outside the cell, when further proteolytic cleavages or modifications of the protein may take place (postsecretory). CHO, carbohydrate.

packaging into secretory granules. The subcellular pathways utilized in protein secretion have been elucidated largely through the early efforts of Palade[7] and colleagues (reviewed by Jamieson[8]). Secretory cells contain an abundance of endoplasmic reticulum, Golgi complexes, and secretory granules (Fig. 3–5). The proteins that are to be secreted from the cells are transferred during their synthesis into these subcellular organelles, which transport the proteins to the plasma membrane.

Protein secretion begins with translation of the mRNA encoding the precursor of the protein on the rough endoplasmic reticulum, which consists of polyribosomes attached to elaborate membranous saccules that contain cavities (cisternae). The newly synthesized, nascent proteins are discharged into the cisternae by transport across the lipid bilayer of the membrane. Within the cisternae of the endoplasmic reticulum, proteins are carried to the Golgi complex by mechanisms that are incompletely understood. The proteins gain access to the Golgi complex either by direct transfer from the cisternae, which are in continuity with the membranous channels of the Golgi complex, or by way of shuttling vesicles known as transition elements (see Fig. 3–5).

Within the Golgi complex, the proteins are packaged into secretory vesicles or secretory granules by their budding from the Golgi stacks in the form of immature granules. Immature granules undergo maturation through condensation of the proteinaceous material and application of a specific coat around the initial Golgi membrane. On receiving the appropriate extracellular stimuli (regulated pathway of secretion), the granules migrate to the cell surface and fuse to become continuous with the plasma membrane, which results in the release of proteins into the extracellular space, a process known as exocytosis.

The second pathway of intracellular transport and secretion involves the transport of proteins contained within secretory vesicles and immature secretory granules (see Fig. 3–5). Although the use of this alternative vesicle-mediated transport pathway remains to be demonstrated conclusively (it is generally considered to be a constitutive, or unregulated, pathway), different extracellular stimuli may modulate hormone secretion differently, depending on the pathway of secretion. For example, in the parathyroid gland and in the pituitary cell line derived from corticotropic cells (AtT-20), newly synthesized hormone is released more rapidly than hormone synthesized

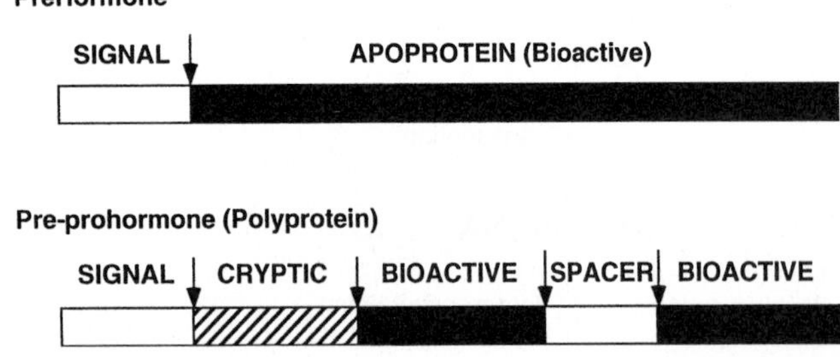

Figure 3–3. Diagrammatic depiction of two configurations of precursors of polypeptide hormones. Diagrams represent polypeptide backbones of protein sequences encoded in mRNA. One form of precursor consists of the NH_2-terminal signal, or presequence, followed by the apoprotein portion of the polypeptide that needs no further proteolytic processing for activity. A second form of precursor is a pre-prohormone that consists of the NH_2-terminal signal sequence followed by a polyprotein, or prohormone, sequence consisting of two or more peptide domains linked together that are subsequently liberated by cleavages during post-translational processing of the prohormone. The reason for synthesis of polypeptide hormones in the form of precursors is only partly understood. Clearly, NH_2-terminal signal sequences function in the early stages of transport of polypeptide into the secretory pathway. Prohormones, or polyproteins, often serve to provide a source of multiple bioactive peptides (see Fig. 3–4). However, many prohormones contain peptide sequences that are removed by cleavage and have no known biologic activity, and they are referred to as cryptic peptides. Other peptides may serve as spacer sequences between two bioactive peptides (e.g., the C peptide of proinsulin). In instances in which a bioactive peptide is located at the COOH terminus of the prohormone, the NH_2-terminal prohormone sequence may simply facilitate cotranslational translocation of polypeptide in endoplasmic reticulum (see Fig. 3–6).

earlier. These findings suggest that the newly synthesized hormone may be transported by way of a vesicle-mediated pathway without incorporation into mature storage granules.

INTRACELLULAR SEGREGATION AND TRANSPORT OF POLYPEPTIDE HORMONES

Specific amino acid sequences encoded in the proteins serve as directional signals in the sorting of proteins within subcellular organelles.[6, 9, 10] A typical eucaryotic cell synthesizes an estimated 5000 different proteins during its life span. These different proteins are synthesized by a common pool of polyribosomes. However, each of the different proteins is directed to a specific location within the cell, where its biologic function is expressed. For example, specific groups of proteins are transported into mitochondria, into membranes, into the nucleus, or into other subcellular organelles, where they serve as regulatory proteins, enzymes, or structural proteins. A subset of proteins is specifically designed for export from the cell (e.g., immunoglobulins, serum albumin, blood coagulation factors, and protein and polypeptide hormones).

This process of directional transport of proteins involves sophisticated informational signals. Because the information for these translocation processes must reside either wholly or in part within the primary structure or in the conformational properties of the protein, sequential post-translational modifications may be crucial for determining the specificity of protein function.

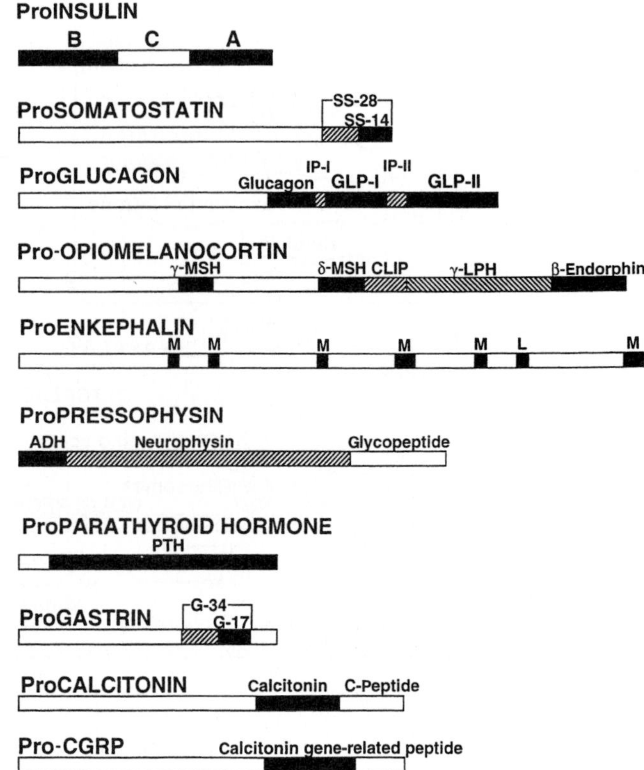

Figure 3–4. Diagrammatic illustration of primary structures of several prohormones. The *darkly shaded areas* of prohormones denote regions of sequence that constitute known biologically active peptides after their post-translational cleavage from prohormones. Sequences indicated by hatching denote regions of precursor that alter the biologic specificity of that region of precursor. For example, the precursor contains the sequence of γ-melanocyte-stimulating hormone (γ-MSH), but when the latter is covalently attached to the clip peptide, it constitutes adrenocorticotropic hormone (corticotropin, ACTH). Somatostatin-28 (SS-28) is an NH_2-terminally extended form of somatostatin-14 (SS-14) that has higher potency than somatostatin-14 on certain receptors. The neurophysin sequence linked to the COOH terminus of vasopressin (ADH) functions as a carrier protein for hormone during its transport down the axon of neurons in which it is synthesized. Precursor proenkephalin represents a polyprotein that contains multiple similar peptides within its sequence, either met-enkephalin (M) or leu-enkephalin (L). Procalcitonin and procalcitonin gene–related product (CGRP) share identical NH_2-terminal sequences but differ in their COOH-terminal regions as a result of alternative splicing during the post-transcriptional processing of the RNA precursor. γ-LPH, γ-lipotropin; GLP, glucagon-like peptide; IP, intervening peptide.

Signal Sequences in Peptide Prohormone Processing and Secretion

The early processes of protein secretion that result in the specific transport of exported proteins into the secretory pathway are now becoming better understood.[6, 10–12] Initial clues to this process came from determinations of the amino acid sequences of the proteins programmed by the cell-free translation of mRNAs encoding secreted polypeptides.[13] Secreted proteins are synthesized as precursors that are extended at their NH_2 termini by sequences of 15 to 30 amino acids, called *signal* or *leader sequences*. Signal sequence extensions, or their functional equivalents, are required for targeting the ribosomal or nascent protein to specific membranes and for the vectorial transport of the protein across the membrane of the endoplasmic reticulum. On emergence of the signal sequence

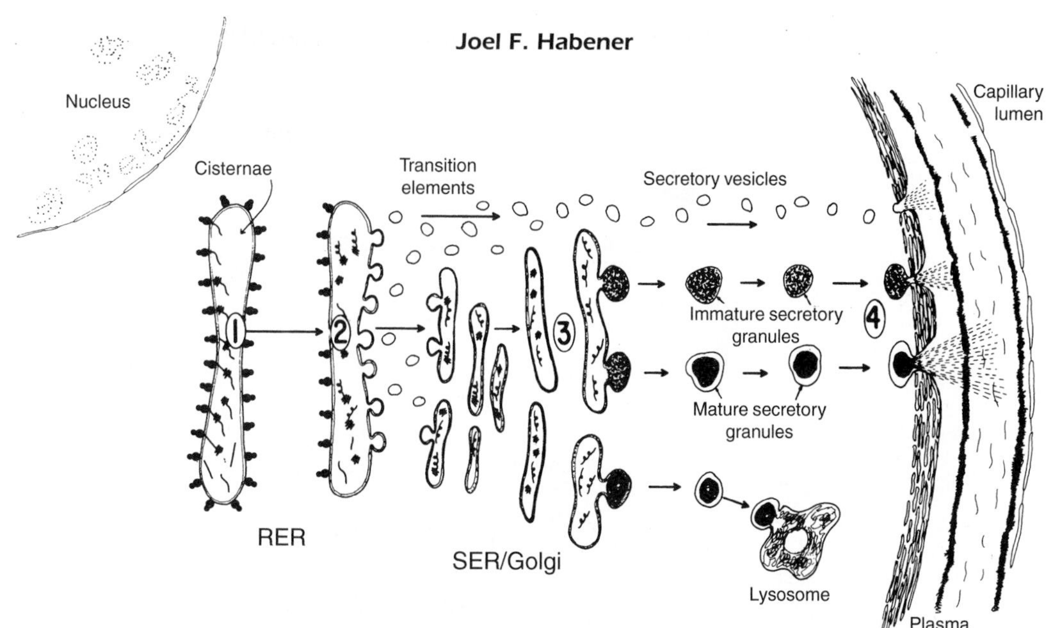

Figure 3–5. Schematic representation of subcellular organelles involved in transport and secretion of polypeptide hormones or other secreted proteins within a protein-secreting cell. (1) Synthesis of proteins on polyribosomes attached to endoplasmic reticulum (RER) and vectorial discharge of proteins through the membrane into the cisterna. (2) Formation of shuttling vesicles (transition elements) from endoplasmic reticulum followed by their transport to and incorporation by the Golgi complex. (3) Formation of secretory granules in the Golgi complex. (4) Transport of secretory granules to the plasma membrane, fusion with the plasma membrane, and exocytosis resulting in the release of granule contents into the extracellular space. Note that secretion may occur by transport of secretory vesicles and immature granules as well as mature granules. Some granules are taken up and hydrolyzed by lysosomes (crinophagy). Golgi, Golgi complex; RER, rough endoplasmic reticulum; SER, smooth endoplasmic reticulum. (From Habener JF. Hormone biosynthesis and secretion. In Felig P, Baxter JD, Broadus AE, et al. [eds]. Endocrinology and Metabolism. New York, McGraw-Hill, 1981, pp 29–59. Copyright © 1981 by McGraw-Hill, Inc. Used by permission of McGraw-Hill Book Company.)

from the large ribosomal subunit, the ribosomal complex specifically makes contact with the membrane, which results in translocation of the nascent polypeptide across the endoplasmic reticulum membrane into the cisterna as the first step in the transport of the polypeptide within the secretory pathway. These observations initially left unanswered the question of how specific polyribosomes that translate mRNAs encoding secretory proteins recognize and attach to the endoplasmic reticulum (Fig. 3–6).

Because microsomal membranes in vitro reproduce the processing activity of intact cells, it was possible to identify macromolecules responsible for processing of the precursor and for translocation activities.[14] The endoplasmic reticulum and the cytoplasm contain an aggregate of molecules, called a *signal recognition particle complex*, that consists of at least 16 different proteins, including three guanosine triphosphatases to generate energy[15] and a 7S RNA.[6, 10, 16] This complex, or particle, binds to the polyribosomes involved in the translation of mRNAs encoding secretory polypeptides when the NH_2-terminal signal sequence first emerges from the large subunit of the ribosome.

The specific interaction of the signal recognition particle with the nascent signal sequence and the polyribosome arrests further translation of mRNA. The nascent protein remains in a state of arrested translation until it finds a high-affinity binding protein on the endoplasmic reticulum, the signal recognition particle receptor, or docking protein.[6] On interaction with the specific docking protein, the translational block is released and protein synthesis resumes. The protein is then transferred across the membrane of the endoplasmic reticulum through a proteinaceous tunnel.

At some point, near the termination of synthesis of the polypeptide chain, the NH_2-terminal signal sequence is cleaved from the polypeptide by a specific signal peptidase located on the cisternal surface of the endoplasmic reticulum membrane. The removal of the hydrophobic signal sequence frees the protein (prohormone or hormone) so that it may assume its characteristic secondary structure during transport through the endoplasmic reticulum and the Golgi apparatus. Interestingly, after its cleavage from the protein by signal peptidase, the signal peptide may sometimes be further cleaved in the endoplasmic reticulum membrane to produce a biologically active peptide. The signal sequence of preprolactin of 30 amino acids, for example, is cleaved by a signal peptide peptidase to give a charged peptide of 20 amino acids that is released into the cytosol, where it binds to calmodulin and inhibits Ca^{2+}-calmodulin–dependent phosphodiesterase.[17]

This sequence in the directional transport of specific polypeptides ensures optimal cotranslational processing of secretory proteins, even when synthesis commences on free ribosomes. The presence of a cytoplasmic form of the signal recognition particle complex that blocks translation guarantees that the synthesis of the presecretory proteins is not completed in the cytoplasm; the efficient transfer of proteins occurs only after contact has been made with the specific receptor or docking protein on the membrane. Although the identification of the signal recognition particle and the docking protein explains the specificity of the binding of ribosomes containing mRNAs encoding the secretory proteins, it does not explain the mode of translocation of the nascent polypeptide chain across the membrane bilayer. Further dissection and analysis of the membrane have identified other macromolecules that are responsible for the transport process.[6]

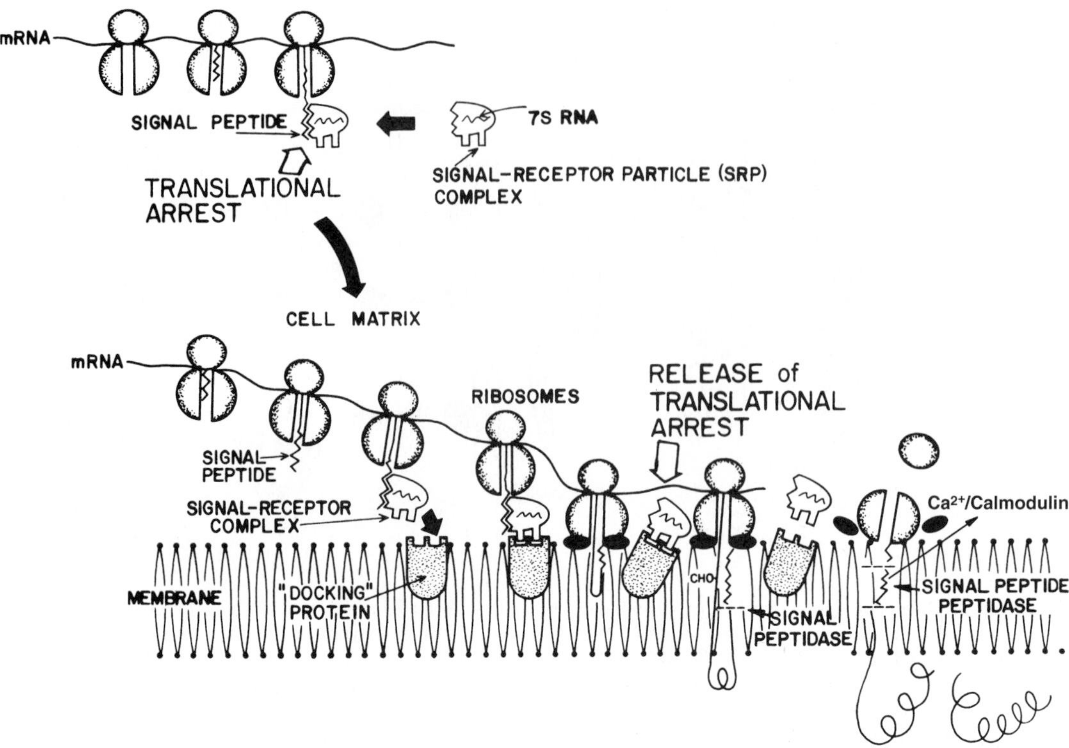

Figure 3–6. Diagram depicting cellular events in initial stages of synthesis of a polypeptide hormone according to the signal hypothesis. In this schema, a signal recognition particle, consisting of a complex of six proteins and an RNA (7S RNA), interacts with the NH_2-terminal signal peptide of the nascent polypeptide chain after approximately 70 amino acids are polymerized, which results in the arrest of further growth of the polypeptide chain. The complex of the signal recognition particle and the polyribosome nascent chain remains in a state of translational arrest until it recognizes and binds to a docking protein, which is a receptor protein located on the cytoplasmic face of the endoplasmic reticular membrane. This interaction of the signal recognition particle complex with docking protein releases the translational block, and protein synthesis resumes. The nascent polypeptide chain is discharged across the membrane bilayer into the cisterna of the endoplasmic reticulum and is released from the signal peptide by cleavage with a signal peptidase located in the cisternal face of the membrane. In this model, the signal peptide is cleaved from the polypeptide chain by signal peptidase before the chain is completed (cotranslational cleavage). The configuration of the polypeptide during transport across the membrane and the forces and mechanisms responsible for its translocation are unknown. The loop, or hairpin, configuration of the chain that is shown is an arbitrary model; other models are equally possible.

Cellular Processing of Prohormones

The signal sequences of prehormones and pre-prohormones are involved in the transport of these molecules, but the function of the intermediate hormone precursors (prohormones) is not fully understood. The conversion of prohormones to their final products begins in the Golgi apparatus. For example, the time that elapses between the synthesis of pre-proparathyroid hormone and the first appearance of parathyroid hormone correlates closely with the time required for radioautographic grains to reach the Golgi apparatus.[18] Similarly, the conversion of proinsulin to insulin takes place about an hour after the synthesis of proinsulin is complete, and processing of proinsulin to insulin and C peptide takes place during the transport within the secretory granule.[19] The conversion of prohormones to hormones can also be blocked by inhibitors of cellular energy production such as antimycin A and dinitrophenol[20] and by drugs that interfere with the functions of microtubules (vinblastine, colchicine).[21] Thus, the translocation of the prohormone from the rough endoplasmic reticulum to the Golgi complex depends on metabolic energy and probably involves microtubules.

There is no evidence that sequences that are specific to the prohormone contribute to or are chemically involved in transport of the newly synthesized protein from the rough endoplasmic reticulum to the Golgi apparatus or that they are involved in the packaging of the hormone in the vesicles or granules. Analyses of the structures of the primary products of translation of mRNAs encoding secretory proteins indicate that many of these are not synthesized in the form of prohormone intermediates (see Fig. 3–3). It remains puzzling that some secretory proteins (e.g., parathyroid hormone, insulin, serum albumin) are formed by way of intermediate precursors, whereas others (e.g., growth hormone, prolactin, albumin) are not.

Size constraints may be placed on the length of a secretory polypeptide. When the bioactivity of peptides resides at the COOH termini of the precursors (e.g., somatostatin, calcitonin, gastrin), NH_2-terminal extensions may be required to provide a sufficient "spacer" sequence to allow the signal sequence on the growing nascent polypeptide chain to emerge from the large ribosome subunit for interaction with the signal recognition particle and to provide adequate polypeptide length to span the large ribosomal subunit and the membrane of the endoplasmic reticulum during vectorial transport of the nascent polypeptide across the membrane (see Fig. 3–6). When the final hormonal product is 100 amino acids long or longer (e.g., growth hormone, prolactin, or the α and β subunits of the glycoprotein hormones), there may be no requirement for a prohormone intermediate.

Although the exact functions of prohormones remain unknown, certain details of their cleavages have been established.

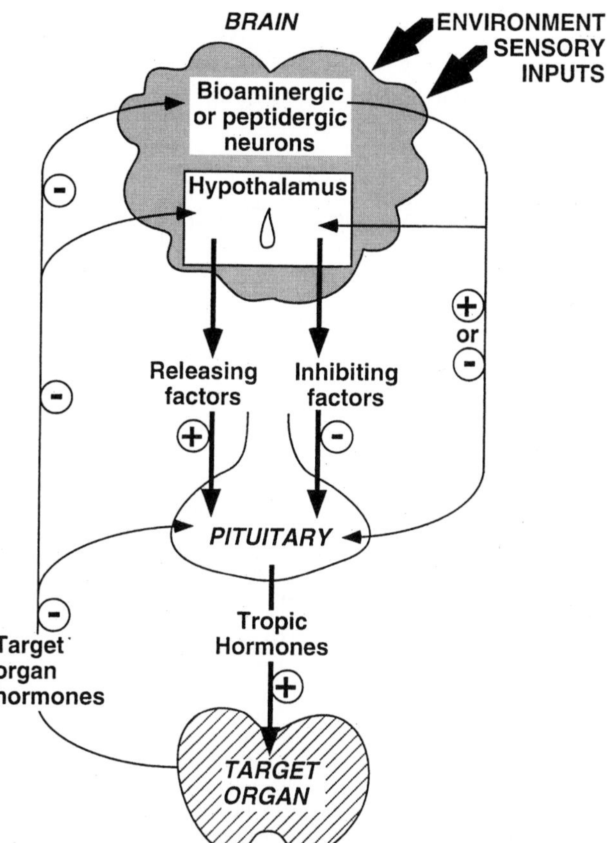

Figure 3–7. Regulatory feedback loops of the hypothalamic–pituitary–target organ axis. Being a combination of both stimulatory and inhibitory factors, hormones often act in concert to maintain homeostatic balance in the presence of physiologic or pathophysiologic perturbations. The concerted actions of hormones typically establish closed feedback loops by stimulatory and inhibitory effects coupled to maintain homeostasis.

Unlike the situation with prehormones, in which the amino acids at the cleavage site between the signal sequence and the remainder of the molecule (hormone or prohormone) vary from one hormone to the next, the cleavage sites of the prohormone intermediates consist of the basic amino acid lysine or arginine, or both, usually two to three in tandem. This sequence is preferentially cleaved by endopeptidases with trypsin-like activities.

Specific *prohormone-converting enzymes* (PCs) consist of a family of at least eight such enzymes.[22–24] The most studied of the isozymes are PC2 and PC1/3, which are responsible for the cleavages of proinsulin between the A chain/C peptide and B chain/C peptide, respectively. A rare patient missing PC1 presented with childhood obesity, hypogonadotropic hypogonadism, and hypercortisolism and was found to have elevated proinsulin levels and presumably widespread abnormalities in neuropeptide modification.[25] Targeted disruption of the PC2 gene in mice resulted in incomplete processing of proinsulin, leaving the A chain and C peptide intact.[26] Notably, proglucagon in the pancreas remains completely unprocessed, indicating that PC2 is required for the formation of glucagon. As a consequence of defective PC2 activity and low levels of glucagon, the mice have severe chronic hypoglycemia.

After endopeptidase cleavage, the remaining basic residues are selectively removed by exopeptidases with activity resembling that of carboxypeptidase B. In the instances in which the COOH-terminal residue of the peptide hormone is amidated, a process that appears to enhance the stability of a peptide by conferring resistance to carboxypeptidase, specific amidation enzymes in the Golgi complex work in concert with the cleavage enzymes for modification of the COOH terminal of the bioactive peptides.[27, 28]

All proproteins and prohormones are cleaved by PC enzymatic processes within the Golgi complex of cells of diverse origins. The significance of specific cleavages of specific prohormones remains incompletely understood, as does the reason for the existence of prohormone intermediates in some but not all secretory proteins. As indicated earlier, precursor peptides removed from the prohormones may have intrinsic biologic activities that are as yet unrecognized.

PROCESSES OF HORMONE SECRETION

Specific extracellular stimuli control the secretion of polypeptide hormones. The stimuli consist of changes in homeostatic balance; the hormonal products released in response to the stimuli act on the respective target organs to reestablish homeostasis (Fig. 3–7). Endocrine systems typically consist of closed-loop feedback mechanisms such that, if hormones from organ A stimulate organ B, organ B in turn secretes hormones that inhibit the secretion of hormones from organ A. The concerted actions of both positive and negative hormonal influences thereby maintain homeostasis. For example, an increase in the concentration of plasma electrolytes as a consequence of dehydration stimulates the release of arginine vasopressin (also called antidiuretic hormone [ADH]) in the neural lobe of the pituitary gland, and vasopressin in turn acts on the kidney to increase the reabsorption of water from the renal tubule, thereby readjusting serum electrolyte concentrations toward normal levels.

These regulatory processes commonly include inhibitory feedback loops in which the products elaborated by the target organs in response to the actions of a hormone inhibit further endocrine secretion. An example of such negative feedback regulation is the control of the secretion of adrenocorticotropic hormone (ACTH) by the anterior pituitary gland. Increased ACTH stimulates the adrenal cortex to produce and secrete cortisol, which in turn feeds back to suppress further pituitary secretion of ACTH.

In many instances, endocrine regulation is complex and involves the responses of several endocrine glands and their respective target organs. After a meal, the release of a dozen or more hormones is triggered as a result of gastric distention, variations in the pH of the contents of the stomach and duodenum, and increased concentrations of glucose, fatty acids, and amino acids in the blood. The rise in plasma glucose and amino acid levels stimulates the release of insulin and the incretin hormones glucagon-like peptide 1 and glucose-dependent insulinotropic peptide and suppresses the release of glucagon from the pancreas. Both effects promote the net uptake of glucose by the liver; insulin increases cellular transport and uptake of glucose, and the lower blood levels of glucagon decrease the outflow of glucose because of diminished rates of glycogenolysis and gluconeogenesis.

STRUCTURE OF A GENE ENCODING A POLYPEPTIDE HORMONE

Structural analyses of gene sequences have resulted in at least three major discoveries that are important for under-

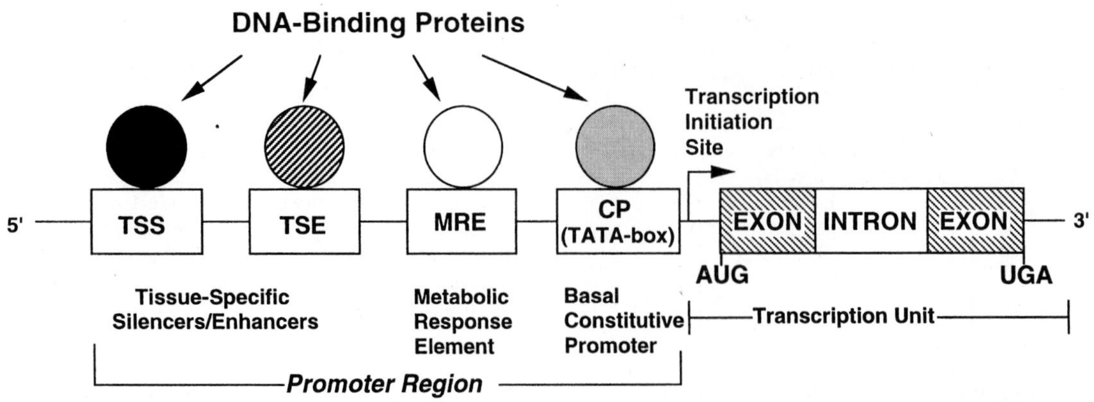

Figure 3–8. Diagrammatic structure of a "consensus" gene encoding a prototypical polypeptide hormone. Such a gene typically consists of a promoter region and a transcription unit. The transcription unit is the region of deoxyribonucleic acid (DNA) composed of exons and introns that is transcribed into a messenger ribonucleic acid (mRNA) precursor. Transcription begins at the cap site sequence in DNA and extends several hundred bases beyond the poly(A) addition site in the 3′ region. During post-transcriptional processing of the RNA precursor, the 5′ end of mRNA is capped by addition of methylguanosine residues. The transcript is then cleaved at the poly(A) addition site approximately 20 bases 3′ to the AATAAA signal sequence, and the poly(A) tract is added to the 3′ end of the RNA. Introns are cleaved from the RNA precursor, and exons are joined together. Dinucleotides GT and AG are invariably found at the 5′ and 3′ ends of introns. Translation of mRNA invariably starts with the codon ATG for methionine. Translation is terminated when the polyribosome reaches the stop codon TGA, TAA, or TAG. The promoter region of the gene located 5′ to the cap site contains numerous short regulatory DNA sequences that are targets for interactions with specific DNA-binding proteins. These sequences consist of the basal constitutive promoter (TATA box), metabolic response elements that modulate transcription (e.g., in response to cAMP, steroid hormone receptors, and thyroid hormone receptors), and tissue-specific enhancers and silencers that permit or prevent transcription of the gene, respectively. The enhancer and silencer elements direct expression of specific subsets of genes to cells of a given phenotype. Whether a gene is or is not expressed in a particular cellular phenotype depends on complex interactions of the various DNA-binding proteins among themselves and, most important, with the TATA box proteins of the basal constitutive promoter.

standing the expression of peptide-encoding genes. First, sequences of almost all the known biologically active hormonal peptides are contained within larger precursors that often encode other peptides, many of which are of unknown biologic activity. Second, the transcribed regions of genes (exons) are interrupted by sequences (introns) that are transcribed but subsequently cleaved from the initial RNA transcripts during their nuclear processing and assembly into specific mRNAs. Third, specific regulatory sequences reside in the regions of DNA flanking the 5′ ends of structural genes, and these DNA sequences constitute specific targets for the interactions of DNA-binding proteins that determine the level of expression of the gene.

The DNA of higher organisms is wound into a tightly and regularly packed chromosomal structure in association with a number of different proteins organized into elements called *nucleosomes*.[29, 30] Nucleosomes are composed of four or five different histone subunits that form a core structure about which approximately 140 base pairs of genomic DNA are wound. The nucleosomes are arranged similarly to beads on a string, and coils of nucleosomes form the fundamental organizational units of the eucaryotic chromosome.

The nucleosomal structure serves several purposes. For example, nucleosomes enable the large amount of DNA ($\sim 2 \times 10^9$ pairs) of the genome to be compacted into a small volume. Nucleosomes are involved in the replication of DNA and gene transcription. In addition to histones, other proteins are associated with DNA, and the complex nucleoprotein structure provides specific recognition sites for regulatory proteins and enzymes involved in DNA replication, rearrangements of DNA segments, and gene expression. The acetylation and deacetylation of histone-rich chromatin is involved in the regulation of gene transcription.

The topography of a typical protein-encoding gene consists of two functional units (Fig. 3–8):

- A transcriptional region
- A promoter or regulatory region

Transcriptional Regions

The transcriptional unit is the segment of the gene that is transcribed into an mRNA precursor. The sequences corresponding to the mature mRNA consist of the exon sequences that are spliced from the primary transcript during the post-transcriptional processing of the precursor RNA; these exons contain the code for the mRNA sequence that is translated into protein and for untranslated sequences at the 5′- and 3′-flanking regions. The 5′ sequence typically begins with a methylated guanine residue known as the cap site. The 3′-untranslated region contains within it a short sequence, AATAAA, that signals the site of cleavage of the 3′ end of the RNA and the addition of a poly(A) tract of 100 to 200 nucleotides located approximately 20 bases from the AATAAA sequence. Although the functions of these modifications of the ends of mRNAs are not completely understood, they appear to provide signals for leaving the nucleus; enhance stability, perhaps through providing resistance to degradation by exonucleases; and stimulate initiation of mRNA translation. The protein-coding sequence of the mRNA begins with the codon AUG for methionine and ends with the codon immediately preceding one of the three nonsense, or stop, codons (UGA, UAA, and UAG).

The nature of the enzymatic splicing mechanisms that result in the excision of intron-coded sequences and the rejoining of exon-coded sequences is incompletely understood. Short "consensus" sequences of nucleotides reside at the splice junctions—for example, the bases GT and AG at the 5′ and 3′ ends of the introns, respectively, are invariant—and a polypyrimidine stretch is found near the AG.[31] Splicing involves a series of cleavage and ligation steps that remove the introns as a lariat structure with its 5′ end ligated near the 3′ end of the introns and ligate the two adjacent exons together. An elaborate machinery (the spliceosome) consisting of five *small nuclear RNAs* (snRNAs) and roughly 50 proteins direct these steps, guided by base pairing between three of the snRNAs and the mRNA precursor.

Regulatory Regions

The regulation of the expression of genes that encode polypeptides is beginning to be understood in some detail. As a result of experiments involving the deletion of 5′ sequences upstream from structural genes, followed by analyses of the expression of the genes after introduction into cell lines, several insights have been obtained. These regulatory sequences, termed *promoters* and *enhancers*, consist of short polynucleotide sequences (see Fig. 3–8). They can be divided into at least four groups with respect to their functions and distances from the transcriptional initiation site.

First, the sequence *TATAA* (TATA, or Goldberg-Hogness, box) is usually present in the more proximal promoter within 25 to 30 nucleotides upstream from the point of transcriptional initiation. The TATA sequence is required to ensure the accuracy of initiation of transcription at a particular site. The TATA box directs the binding of a complex of several proteins, including RNA polymerase II. The proteins, referred to as *TATA box transcription factors* (TFs), number six or more basal factors (IIA, IIB, IID, IIE, IIF, IIH) and, along with RNA polymerase II, form the general or basal transcriptional machinery required for the initiation of RNA synthesis.[32]

The other three groups of regulatory sequences consist of *tissue-specific silencers* (TSSs), which function by binding repressor proteins; *tissue-specific enhancers* (TSEs), which are activated by the binding of transcriptional activator proteins; and *metabolic response elements* (MREs), which are regulated by the binding of specialized proteins whose transcriptional activities (repressor or activator) are regulated by metabolic signaling, often involving changes in their phosphorylation.

Introns and Exons

Genes encoding proteins and ribosomal RNAs in eukaryotes are interrupted by intervening DNA sequences (introns) that separate them into coding blocks (exons).[33] In bacterial genes the nucleotide sequences of the chromosomal genes match precisely the corresponding sequences in the mRNAs. Interruption of the continuity of genetic information appears to be unique to nucleated cells. The reasons for such interruption are not completely understood, but introns appear to separate exons into functional domains with respect to the proteins that they encode. An example is the gene for proglucagon, a precursor of glucagon in which five introns separate six exons, three of which encode glucagon and the two glucagon-related peptides contained within the precursor (Fig. 3–9).[34] A second example is the growth hormone gene, which is divided into five exons by four introns that separate the promoter region of the gene from the protein-coding region and the latter into three partly homologous repeated segments, two coding for the growth-promoting activity of the hormone and the third for its carbohydrate metabolic functions.[35] As a rule, the genes for the precursors of hormones and regulatory peptides contain introns at or about the region where the signal peptides join the apoproteins or prohormones, thus separating the signal sequences from the components of the precursor that are exported from the cell as hormones or peptides.

There are exceptions to the *one exon, one function theory* in mammalian cells. The genes of several precursors of peptide hormones are not interrupted by introns in a manner that corresponds to the separation of the functional components of the precursor. Notable in this regard is the precursor pro-opiomelanocortin, from which the peptides ACTH, α-melanocyte-stimulating hormone, and β-endorphin are cleaved during the post-translational processing of the precursor. The protein-coding region of the pro-opiomelanocortin gene is devoid of introns. Likewise, no introns interrupt the protein-coding re-

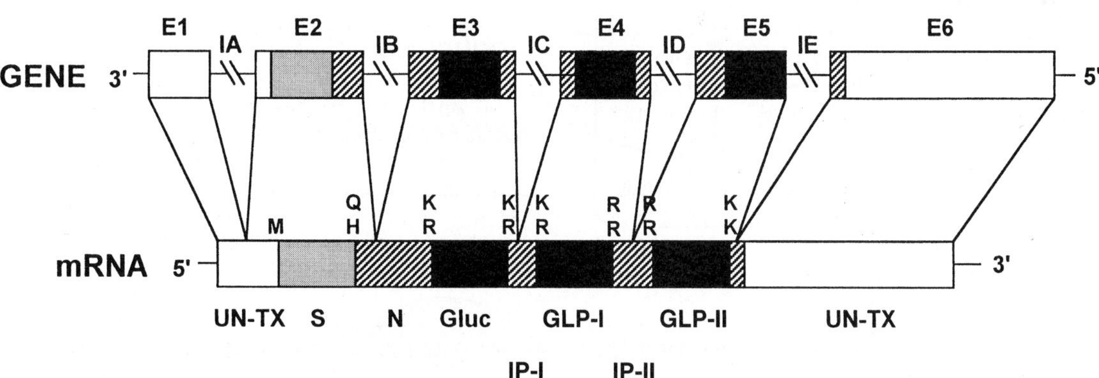

Figure 3–9. Diagram of the pancreatic glucagon gene and its encoded messenger RNA (mRNA) (complementary DNA). The glucagon gene is an example of a gene in which exons precisely encode separate functional domains. The gene consists of six exons (E1 to E6) and five introns (1A to 1E). The mRNA encoding pre-proglucagon, the protein precursor of glucagon, consists of 10 specific regions: from left to right, a 5′-untranslated sequence (UN-TX, *unshaded*), a signal sequence (S, *stippled*), an NH_2-terminal extension sequence (N, *hatched*), glucagon (Gluc, *shaded*), a first intervening peptide (IP-I, *hatched*), a first glucagon-like peptide (GLP-I, *shaded*), a second intervening peptide (IP-II, *hatched*), a second glucagon-like peptide (GLP-II, *shaded*), a dilysyl dipeptide *(hatched)* after the glucagon-like peptide II sequence, and an untranslated region (UN-TX, *unshaded*). Exons from left to right encode the 5′-untranslated region, signal sequence, glucagon, glucagon-like peptide I, glucagon-like peptide II, and 3′-untranslated sequence. Letters shown above the mRNA denote amino acids located at positions in pre-proglucagon that are cleaved during cellular processing of precursor. The amino acid methionine (M) marks the initiation of translation of mRNA into pre-proglucagon. H, histidine; K, lysine; Q, glutamine; R, arginine.

gion of the gene for the proenkephalin precursor, which contains seven copies of the enkephalin sequences. It is possible that, in the past, introns separated each of these coding domains and were lost during the course of evolution.

A precedent for the selective loss of introns appears to be exemplified by the rat insulin genes. The rat genome harbors two nonallelic insulin genes: one containing two introns and the other containing a single intron. The most likely explanation is that an ancestral gene containing two introns was transcribed into RNA and spliced; then that RNA was copied back into DNA by a cellular reverse transcriptase and inserted back into the genome at a new site.

REGULATION OF GENE EXPRESSION

The regulation of expression of genes encoding polypeptide hormones can take place at one or more levels in the pathway of hormone biosynthesis (Fig. 3–10)[36, 37]:

- DNA synthesis (cell growth and division)
- Transcription
- Post-transcriptional processing of mRNA
- Translation
- Post-translational processing

In different endocrine cells, one or more levels may serve as specific control points for regulation of production of a hormone (see also Generation of Biologic Diversification later).

Levels of Gene Control

Newly synthesized prolactin transcripts are formed within minutes after exposure of a prolactin-secreting cell line to TRH.[38] Cortisol stimulates growth hormone synthesis in both somatotropic cell lines and pituitary slices through increases in rates of gene transcription and enhancement of the stability of mRNA.[39, 40] The time required for cortisol to enhance transcription of the growth hormone gene is 1 to 2 hours, which is considerably longer than the time required for the action of TRH on prolactin gene transcription. Regulation of proinsulin biosynthesis appears to take place primarily at the level of translation.[41, 42] Within minutes after raising the plasma glucose level, the rate of proinsulin biosynthesis increases fivefold to 10-fold. Glucose acts either directly or indirectly to enhance the efficiency of initiation of translation of proinsulin mRNA.

Rapid metabolic regulation at the level of post-transcriptional processing of mRNA precursors is not yet clearly established. However, alternative exon splicing plays a major role in the regulation of the formation of mRNAs during development (see next section in chapter on Generation of Biologic Diversification). For example, the primary RNA transcripts derived from the calcitonin gene are alternatively spliced to provide two or more tissue-specific mRNAs that encode chimeric protein precursors with both common and different amino acid sequences, suggesting that regulation might take place at the level of processing of the calcitonin gene transcripts.

In many instances, the level of gene expression under regulatory control is optimal for meeting the secretory and biosynthetic demands of the endocrine organ. For example, after a meal there is an immediate requirement for the release of large amounts of insulin. This release depletes insulin stores of

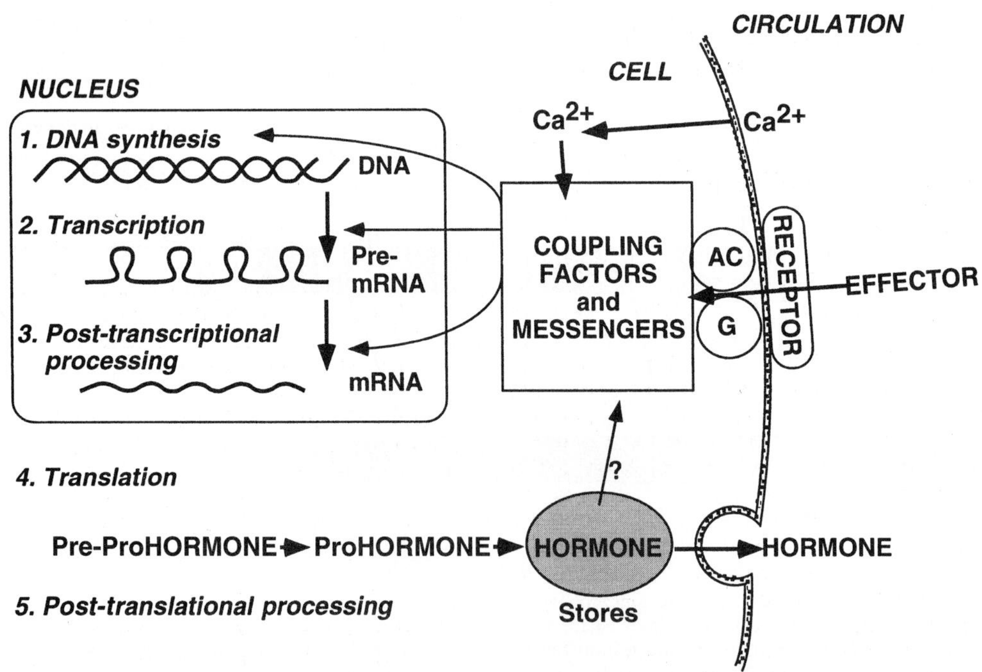

Figure 3–10. Diagram of an endocrine cell showing potential control points for regulation of gene expression in hormone production. Specific effector substances bind either to plasma membrane receptors (peptide effectors) or to cytosolic or nuclear receptors (steroids), which leads to initiation of a series of events that couple the effector signal with gene expression. In the illustration shown, peptide effector-receptor complex interactions act initially through activation of adenylate cyclase (AC) coupled with a guanosine triphosphate–binding protein (G). Coupling factors and substances such as glucose, cyclic adenosine monophosphate, and cations activate protein kinases, resulting in a series of phosphorylations of macromolecules. As discussed in the text, specific effectors for various endocrine cells appear to act at one or more of the indicated five levels of gene expression, with the possible exception of post-translational processing of prohormones, for which no definite examples of metabolic regulation have yet been found.

the pancreatic beta cells within a few minutes, and increasing the translational efficiency of preformed proinsulin mRNA provides additional hormone rapidly.

Tissue-Specific Gene Expression

Differentiated cells have a remarkable capacity for selective expression of specific genes. In one cell type, a single gene may account for a large fraction of the total gene expression, and in another cell type the same gene may be expressed at undetectable levels.

When a gene can be expressed in a particular cell type, the associated chromatin is loosely arranged; when the same gene is never expressed in a particular cell type, the chromatin organization is more compact. Thus, the DNA within the chromatin of expressed genes is more susceptible to cleavage by deoxyribonuclease than is the DNA in tissues in which the genes are quiescent.[43–45] This looseness may facilitate access of RNA polymerase to the gene for purposes of transcription. In addition, inactive genes appear to have a higher content of methylated cytosine residues than the same genes in tissues in which they are expressed.[46, 47]

Determinants for the tissue-specific transcriptional expression of genes exist in control sequences usually residing within 1000 base pairs of the 5′-flanking region of the transcriptional sequence. Enhancer sequences in animal cell genes were first described for immunoglobulin genes, a finding that extended the earlier observations of enhancer control elements in viral genomes.[48] However, the first clear demonstrations of these elements directing transcription to cells of distinct phenotypes came from studies of the comparative expression of two model genes, insulin and chymotrypsin, in the endocrine and exocrine pancreas, respectively.[49] The restricted expression of genes in a cell-specific manner is determined by the assembly of specific combinations of DNA-binding proteins on a predetermined array of control elements of the promoter regions of genes to create a transcriptionally active complex of proteins that includes the components of the general or basal transcriptional apparatus.

Transcription Factors in Developmental Organogenesis of Endocrine Systems

Certain families of transcription factors are critical for organogenesis and the development of the body plan. Among these factors are the homeodomain proteins[50] and the nuclear receptor proteins.[51–53] The family of homeotic selector, or homeodomain, proteins are highly conserved throughout the animal kingdom from flies to humans. The orchestrated spatial and temporal expression of these proteins and the target genes that they activate determine the orderly development of the body plan of specific tissues, limbs, and organs. Similarly, the actions of families of nuclear receptors (steroid and thyroid hormones, retinoic acid, and others) are critical for normal development to occur. Inactivating mutations in the genes encoding these essential transcription factors predictably result in loss or impairment of the development of the specific organ whose development they direct.

Three examples are described of impaired organogenesis attributable to mutations in essential transcription factors:

- Partial anterior pituitary agenesis (Pit-1)
- Adrenal and gonadal agenesis (SF-1, DAX-1)
- Pancreatic agenesis (IDX-1)

Partial Pituitary Agenesis

The transcription factor Pit-1 is a member of a family of pou-homeodomain proteins, which is a specialized subfamily of the larger family of homeodomain proteins.[54] Pit-1 is a key transcriptional activator of the promoters of the growth hormone, prolactin, and thyroid-stimulating hormone β genes, produced in the anterior pituitary somatotrophs, lactotrophs, and thyrotrophs, respectively. Pit-1 is also the major enhancer activating factor for the promoter of the growth hormone–releasing factor receptor gene.[55] Mutations in Pit-1 that impair its DNA-binding and transcriptional activation functions are responsible for the phenotype of the Jackson and Snell dwarf mice.[54]

Mutations in the gene encoding Pit-1 have been found in patients with combined pituitary hormone deficiency in which there is no production of growth hormone, prolactin, or thyroid-stimulating hormone, resulting in growth impairment and mental deficiency.[56] Notably, the production of the other two of the five hormones secreted by the anterior pituitary gland, adrenocorticotropin and the gonadotropins luteinizing hormone (LH) and follicle-stimulating hormone (FSH), is unaffected.[56] In these human Pit-1 mutations, Pit-1 can bind to its cognate DNA control elements but is defective in *trans*-activating gene transcription. Furthermore, the mutated Pit-1 acts as a dominant negative inhibitor of Pit-1 actions on the unaffected allele.

Pancreatic Agenesis

The homeodomain protein islet duodenum homeobox 1 or IDX-1 (somatostatin transcription factor 1 [STF-1], insulin promoter factor 1 [IPF-1]) appears to be responsible for the development and growth of the pancreas. Targeted disruption of the IDX-1 gene in mice resulted in a phenotype of pancreatic agenesis.[57] A child born without a pancreas was shown to be homozygous for inactivating mutations in the IDX-1 gene.[58] Notably, the parents and their ancestors who are heterozygous for the affected allele have a high incidence of maturity-onset (type 2) diabetes mellitus, suggesting that a decrease in gene dosage of IDX-1 may predispose to the development of diabetes. The possibility that a mutated IDX-1 allele may be one of several "diabetes genes" is supported by the observation that IDX-1 and the helix-loop-helix transcription factors E47 and beta-2 appear to be key up-regulators of the transcription of the insulin gene.[59]

Agenesis of the Adrenal Gland and Gonads

Two nuclear receptor transcription factors have been identified as critical for the development of the adrenal gland, gonads, pituitary gonadotrophs, and the ventral medial hypothalamus. These nuclear receptors are SF-1 (steroidogenic factor 1)[60] and DAX-1 (dosage-sensitive sex reversal, adrenal hypoplasia congenita, X chromosome).[61] SF-1 binds to half-sites of estrogen response elements that bind estrogen receptors in the promoters of genes. DAX-1 binds to retinoic acid receptor (RAR) binding sites in promoters and inhibits RAR actions. Targeted disruption of SF-1 in mice results in a phenotype of adrenal and gonadal agenesis. In addition, pituitary gonadotrophs are absent and the ventral medial hypothalamus is severely underdeveloped.

X-linked adrenal hypoplasia congenita is an X-linked, developmental disorder of the human adrenal gland that is lethal if untreated. The gene responsible for adrenal hypoplasia congenita has been identified by positional cloning and encodes DAX-1, a member of the nuclear receptor proteins related to RAR.[61] Several inactivating mutations identified in the DAX-1 gene result in the syndrome of adrenal hypoplasia congenita and hypogonadotropic hypogonadism. Thus, genetically defined and transmitted defects in the genes encoding the transcription factors SF-1 and DAX-1 result in profound arrest in the development of the target organs regulated by the hypo-

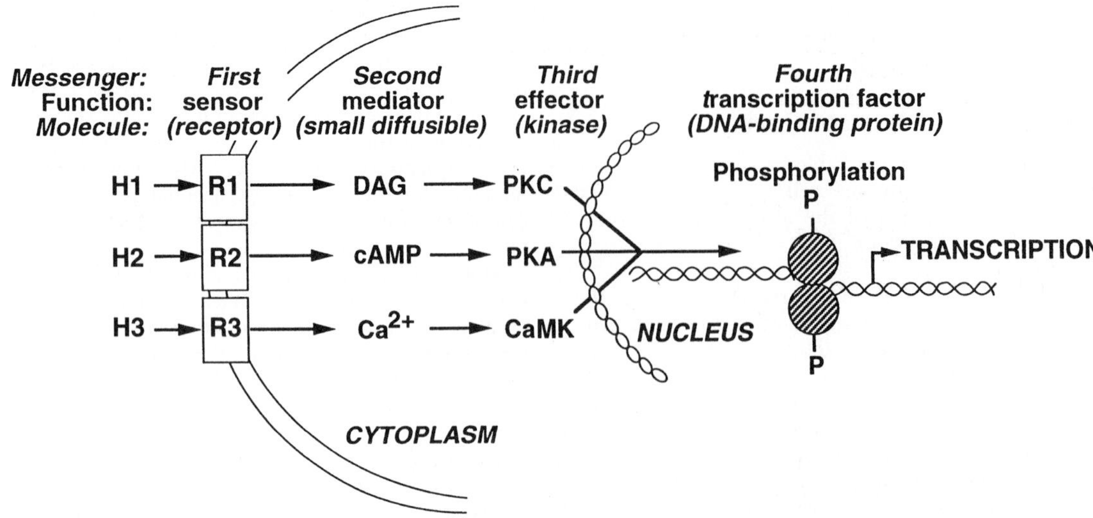

Figure 3–11. Diagram showing three cell-surface receptor–coupled signal transduction pathways involved in the activation of a superfamily of nuclear transcription factors. Peptide hormone molecules (H1, H2, and H3) interact with sensor receptors (R1, R2, and R3) coupled to the diacylglycerol (DAG)–protein kinase C (PKC), the cyclic adenosine monophosphate (cAMP)–protein kinase A (PKA), and the calcium-calmodulin pathways in which small diffusible second messenger molecules are generated (DAG, cAMP, Ca^{2+}). The third messengers or effector protein kinases are generated and phosphorylate transcription factors such as members of the CREB/ATF and jun/AP-1 families of DNA-binding proteins to modulate DNA-binding affinities or transcriptional activation, or both. The various proteins bind as dimers determined by a poorly understood code that is not promiscuous in as much as only certain homodimer or heterodimer combinations are permissible. AP-1, activator protein 1; ATF, activating transcription factor; CaMK, calcium/calmodulin-dependent protein kinase; CREB, cAMP response element-binding protein.

thalamic-pituitary-adrenal axis involved in steroidogenesis—the adrenal gland (glucocorticoids, mineral corticoids) and the gonads (estrogens and androgens).

Coupling of Effector Action to Cellular Response

Another mode of gene control consists of the induction and suppression of genes that are normally expressed in a specific tissue. These processes are at work in the minute-to-minute and day-to-day regulation of rates of production of the specific proteins produced by the cells (e.g., production of polypeptide hormones in response to extracellular stimuli).

At least two classes of signaling pathways—protein phosphorylation and activation of steroid hormone receptors by hormone binding—appear to be involved in the physiologic regulation of hormone gene expression. These two pathways mediate the actions of peptide and steroid hormones, respectively. Peptide ligands bind to receptor complexes on the plasma membrane, which results in enzyme activation, mobilization of calcium, formation of phosphorylated nucleotide intermediates, activation of protein kinases, and phosphorylation of specific regulatory proteins such as transcription factors (see Chapter 5).[62, 63]

Steroidal compounds, because of their hydrophobic composition, readily diffuse through the plasma membrane, bind to specific receptor proteins, and interact with other macromolecules in the nucleus, including specific domains on the chromatin located in and around the gene that is activated (see Chapter 4).[51–53] Phosphorylated nucleotides such as cyclic adenosine monophosphate (cAMP), adenosine triphosphate, and guanosine triphosphate, as well as calcium, appear to have important functions in secretory processes. In particular, fluxes of calcium from the extracellular fluid into the cell and from intracellular organelles (e.g., endoplasmic reticulum) into the cytosol are closely coupled to secretion.[64, 65]

The cellular signaling pathways that involve protein phosphorylations are multiple and complex. They typically consist of sequential phosphorylations and dephosphorylations of molecules referred to as *protein kinase* or *phosphatase cascades.*[66] These cascades are initiated by hormones, sensor molecules known as ligands, that bind to and activate receptors located on the surface of cells, resulting in the generation of small second messenger molecules such as cAMP, diacylglycerol, or calcium ions. These second messengers then activate protein kinases that phosphorylate and thereby activate key target proteins (Fig. 3–11). The final step in the signaling pathways is the phosphorylation and activation of important transcription factors, resulting in gene expression (or repression).

Insight has been gained into the identities of some of the phosphoproteins. As discussed earlier, a specific group of transcription factors, DNA-binding proteins, interacts with cAMP-responsive and phorbol ester–responsive DNA elements to stimulate gene transcription mediated by the cAMP–protein kinase A, diacylglycerol–protein kinase C, and calcium-calmodulin signal transduction pathways (see Fig. 3–11). These proteins are encoded by a complex family of genes and bind to the DNA elements in the form of heterodimers or homodimers through a coiled coil helical structure known as a leucine zipper motif.[67] There is evidence that phosphorylation of these proteins modulates dimerization, DNA recognition and binding, and transcriptional *trans*-activation activities. Phosphorylation of the protein substrates might change their conformations and activate the proteins, which, in turn, interact with coactivator proteins such as the cAMP response element–binding protein (CREB) and the protein components of the basal transcriptional machinery, thereby allowing RNA polymerase to initiate gene transcription.[68]

Generally, the second messengers activate serine/threonine kinases, which phosphorylate serine or threonine residues, or both, on proteins, whereas the receptor kinases are tyrosine-specific kinases that phosphorylate tyrosine residues.[66, 69] Examples of receptor tyrosine kinases are growth factor receptors such as those for insulin, insulin-like growth factor (IGF),

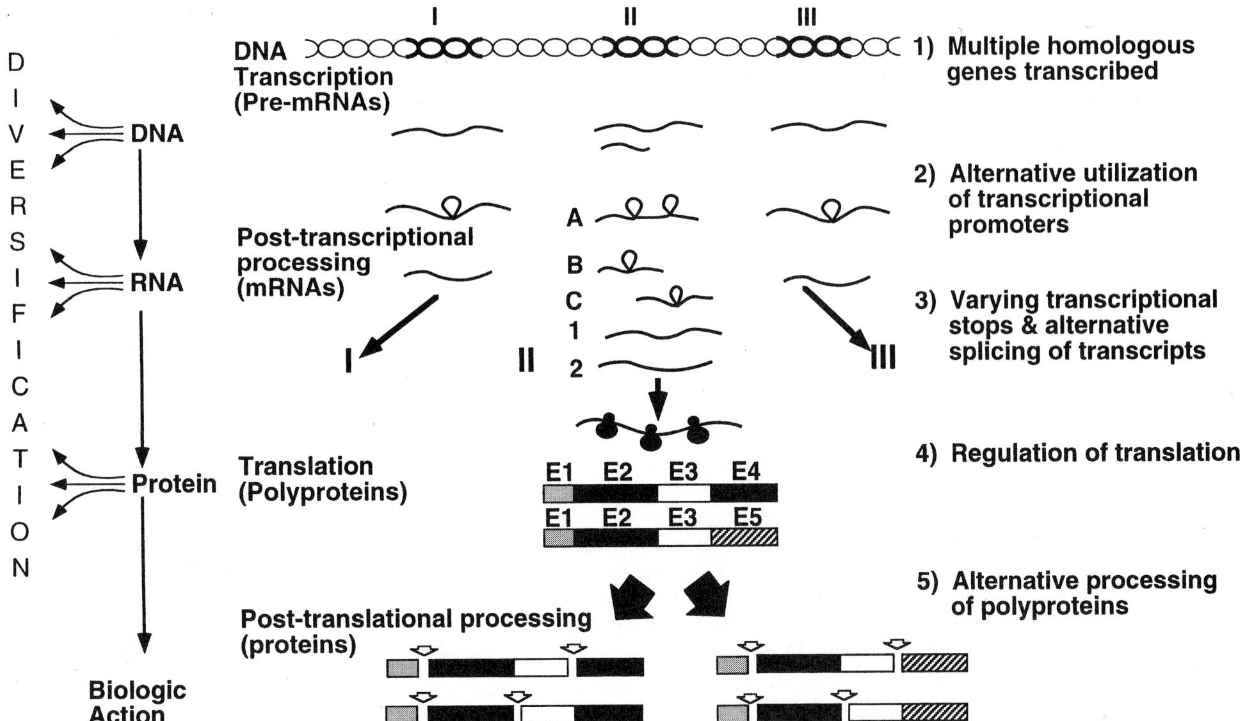

Figure 3–12. Schema indicating levels in expression of genetic information at which diversification of information encoded in a gene may take place. The three major levels of genetic diversification are (1) gene duplication, a process that occurs in terms of evolutionary time; (2) variation in the processing of ribonucleic acid (RNA) precursors, which results in formation of two or more messenger RNAs (mRNAs) by way of alternative pathways of splicing of transcript (see Figs. 3–13 and 3–14); and (3) use of alternative patterns in processing of protein biosynthetic precursors (polyproteins, or prohormones). These three levels in gene expression provide a means for diversification of gene expression at levels of deoxyribonucleic acid (DNA), RNA, or protein. One or a combination of these processes leads to formation of the final biologically active peptide or hormone. In the diagram, loops depicted in transcripts denote introns; in diagrammatic structures of proteins, the *stippled*, *shaded*, and *unshaded areas* denote exons. See text for details.

epidermal growth factor, and platelet-derived growth factor. Receptors in the cytokine receptor family, which include leptin, growth hormone, and prolactin, activate associated tyrosine kinases in a variation on the theme.

The different types of signal transduction pathways are described as more or less distinct pathways for semantic purposes. In reality, there is considerable cross-talk among the different pathways that occur developmentally and in cell type–specific settings. An active area of research in endocrine systems is attempting to understand these complex interactions among different signal transduction pathways. Although the growth factor and cytokine receptors are similar in some respects, they differ in other respects. For example, growth factor receptor tyrosine kinases activate transcription factors through cascades that involve both tyrosine phosphorylation and serine/threonine kinases such as mitogen-activated protein kinases, whereas the Janus kinases (JAKs) activated by cytokine receptors directly tyrosine phosphorylate the signal transducer and activator of transcription (STAT) factors.[69, 70]

GENERATION OF BIOLOGIC DIVERSIFICATION

In addition to providing control points for the regulation of gene expression, the various steps involved in transfer of information encoded in the DNA of the gene to the final bioactive protein are a means for diversification of information stored in the gene (Fig. 3–12). Five steps in gene expression can be arbitrarily described: (1) gene duplication and copy number, (2) transcription, (3) post-transcriptional RNA processing, (4) translation, and (5) post-translational processing.

Gene Duplications

At the level of DNA, diversification of genetic information comes about by way of gene duplication and amplification. Many of the polypeptide hormones are derived from families of multiple, structurally related genes. Examples include the growth hormone family, consisting of growth hormone, prolactin, and placental lactogen; the glucagon family, consisting of glucagon, vasoactive intestinal peptide, secretin, gastric inhibitory peptide, and growth hormone–releasing hormone; and the glycoprotein hormone family, thyrotropin, luteinizing hormone, follicle-stimulating hormone, and chorionic gonadotropin.

A remarkable example of diversification at the level of gene amplifications is the extraordinarily large number of genes encoding the pheromone and odorant receptors.[71] It is estimated that as many as 1000 such receptor genes may exist in mouse and rat genomes, each receptive to a particular odorant ligand. Over the course of evolution, an ancestral gene encoding a prototypic polypeptide representative of each of these families was duplicated one or more times and, through mutation and selection, the progeny proteins of the ancestral gene assumed different biologic functions. The exonic-intronic structural organization of the genomes of higher animals lends itself to gene recombination and RNA copying of genetic sequences with subsequent reintegration of DNA reverse-transcribed sequences back into the genome, resulting in rearrangement of transcriptional units and regulatory sequences.[72, 73]

Transcription

In addition to duplication of genes and their promoters, another way to create diversity in expression is at the level of gene transcription by providing genes with alternative promoters[74] and by utilizing a large array of *cis*-regulatory elements in the promoters regulated by complex combinations of transcription factors.

Alternative Promoters

Many of the genes encoding hormones and their receptors utilize more than one promoter during development or when expressed in different tissue types. The employment of alternative promoters results in the formation of multiple transcripts that differ at their 5′ ends (Fig. 3–13). It is presumed that some genes have multiple promoters because they provide flexibility in the control of expression of the genes. For example, in some cases, expression of genes in more than one tissue or developmental stage may require distinct combinations of tissue-specific transcription factors. This flexibility enables genes in different cell types to respond to the same signal transduction pathways or genes in the same cell type to respond to different signal transduction pathways. A single promoter may not be adequate to respond to a complex array of transcription factors and a changing environment of cellular signals.

The organization of alternative promoters in genes is manifested in several patterns within exons or introns in the 5′ noncoding sequence or the coding sequence (see Fig. 3–13). The most common occurrence of alternative promoters is within the 5′ noncoding or leader exons. The utilization of different promoters in the 5′ untranslated region of a gene, often accompanied by alternative exon splicing, results in the formation of mRNAs with different 5′ sequences. The alternative usage of promoters in 5′ leader exons can affect gene expression and generate diversity in several different ways. These include the developmental stage–specific and temporal expression of genes, the tissue-type specificity of expression, the levels of expression, the responsivity of gene expression to specific metabolic signals conveyed through signal transduction pathways, the stability of the mRNAs, the efficiencies of translation, and the structures of the amino termini of proteins encoded by the genes.[74]

Examples of genes that use alternative 5′ leader promoters during development are those encoding IGF-I, IGF-II, the retinoic acid receptors, and glucokinase, all of which are regulated by multiple promoters that are active in a variety of embryonic and adult tissues and are subject to developmental and tissue-specific regulation.[74] During fetal development, promoters P2, P3, and P4 of the IGF-II gene are active in the liver. These promoters are shut off after birth, at which time the P1 promoter is activated. The P1 and P2 promoters of the IGF-I gene are differentially responsive to growth hormone: P2 expressed in liver is responsive to growth hormone, whereas P1 expressed in muscle is not.

The retinoic acid receptor exists in three isoforms (RARα, RARβ, and RARγ) encoded by separate genes that give rise to at least 17 different mRNAs generated by a combination of multiple promoters and alternative splicing.[75] The RAR isoforms appear to differ in their specificity for retinoic acid–responsive promoters, in their affinities for ligand isoforms, and in *trans*-activating capabilities. The different RAR isoforms are expressed at different times in different tissues during development. It has been proposed that the different RAR isoforms provide a means of achieving a diverse set of cellular responses to a single, simple ligand, retinoic acid.[75]

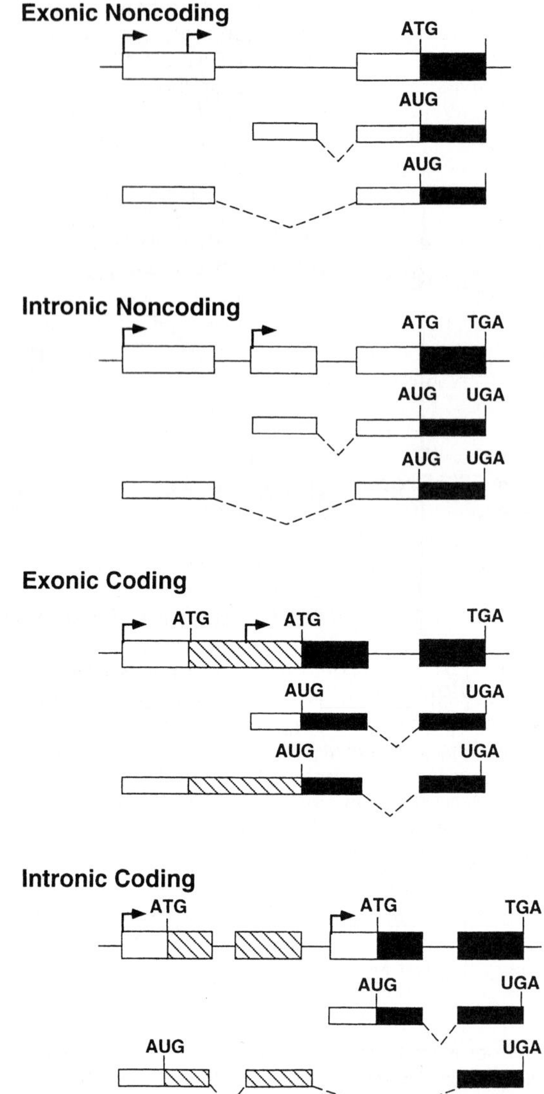

Figure 3–13. Utilization of alternative promoters in the expression of genes as a means to generate biologic diversification of gene expression. The use of alternative promoters allows a gene to be expressed in a variety of unique contexts that alter the properties of the messenger ribonucleic acid (mRNA) that is expressed. Such alternative promoter usage may render the mRNA more or less stable, affect translational efficiencies, or switch the translation of one protein isoform to another. The use of alternative promoters in genes characteristically occurs during development, or after development is completed, to designate tissue-specific patterns of expression of the gene. Exons are shown as boxes whose protein-coding regions are *shaded*. Introns are designated by horizontal lines. *Dashed lines* indicate introns that are spliced out. (Adapted from Ayoubi TAY, Van De Ven WJM. Regulation of gene expression by alternative promoters. FASEB J 1996; 10:453–460.)

Glucokinase is an example of the alternative use of 5′ leader promoters that have different metabolic responsiveness.[76] Expression of glucokinase in pancreatic beta cells and some other neuroendocrine cells utilizes an upstream promoter (1β), whereas in liver a promoter (IL) 26 kb downstream of the 1β promoter is used exclusively. In beta cells, expression of the glucokinase gene is apparently not responsive to hormones. In contrast, in liver expression mediated by the IL promoter is intensely up-regulated by insulin and down-regulated by glucagon.

The α-amylase gene provides an example in which two alternative promoters in the 5′ noncoding exons expressed in two different tissues have dramatically different strengths of expression.[74] A strong upstream promoter directs expression within the parotid gland, contrasting with weak expression directed by an alternative downstream promoter in liver.

Examples of the alternative usage of promoters in the coding regions of genes are the progesterone receptor (PR) and the transcription factor cAMP response element modulator (CREM). In both of these examples, different protein isoforms are produced that have markedly different functional activities. The genes encoding the chicken and human progesterone receptors express two isoforms of the receptor (isoforms A and B).[77] Isoform A initiates translation at a methionine residue located 164 amino acids downstream from the methionine that initiates the translation of the longer form B. Analyses of the mechanisms responsible for the synthesis of two different isoforms revealed that two promoters exist in the human PR gene: one upstream of the 5′ leader exon and the other in the first protein coding exon. The two isoforms of the human PR differ markedly in their capabilities to *trans*-activate transcription from different progesterone responsive elements (PRE). Both human PR isoforms equivalently activate a canonical PRE. Isoform B is much more efficient than A at activating the PRE in the mouse mammary tumor virus promoter, whereas isoform A, but not B, activates transcription from the ovalbumin promoter.[77]

The utilization of an alternative intronic promoter within the protein coding sequence of a gene is exemplified by the CREM gene.[78] The CREM gene employs a constitutively active, unregulated promoter (P1) that encodes predominantly activator forms of CREM and an internal promoter (P2) located in the fourth intron that is regulated by cAMP signaling and encodes a repressor isoform, ICER (inducible cAMP early response). The remarkable complexity of the alternative mechanisms of expression of the CREM and CREB genes is discussed subsequently.

Diversity of Transcription Factors

Another mechanism to create diversity at the level of gene transcription is that of the interplay of multiple transcription factors on multiple *cis*-regulatory sequences. The promoters of typical genes may contain 20 or 30 or more *cis*-acting control elements, either enhancers or silencers. These control elements may respond to ubiquitous transcription factors found in all cell types and to cell type–specific factors.

Unique patterns of control of gene expression can be affected by several different mechanisms acting in concert. The spacing, relative locations, and juxtapositioning of control elements with respect to each other and to the basal transcriptional machinery can influence levels of expression. Transcription factors often act in the form of dimers or higher oligomers among factors of the same or different classes. A given transcription factor may act as either an activator or a repressor as a consequence of the existing circumstances. The ambient concentrations of transcription factors within the nucleus in conjunction with their relative DNA-binding affinities and *trans*-activation potencies may determine the levels of expression of genes.

Post-transcriptional Processing (Alternative Exon Splicing)

Identification of the mosaic structure of transcriptional units encoding polypeptide hormones and other proteins that consist of exons and introns raised the possibility that the use of alternative pathways in RNA splicing could provide informationally distinct molecules. Different proteins could arise either by inclusion or exclusion of specific exonic segments or by utilization of parts of introns in one mRNA as exons in another mRNA. In addition, differences in the splice sites would result in expression of new translational reading frames. Alternative splicing utilizes two distinct mechanisms (Fig. 3–14). One is that of exon skipping or switching in or out of exons. The other mechanism, known as intron slippage, is to include part of an intron in an exon, to splice out part of an exon along with the intron, or to include a "coding" intron.

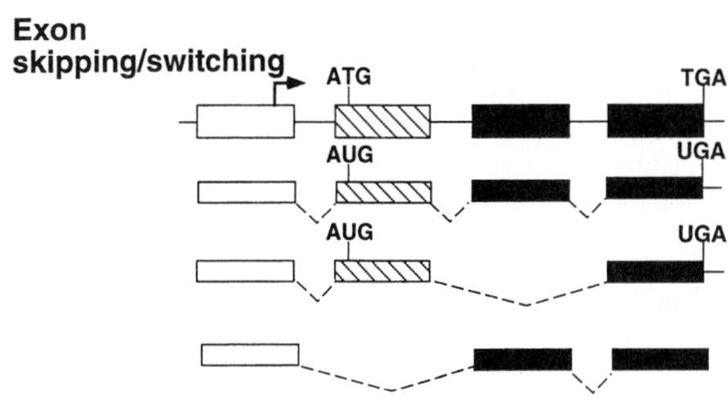

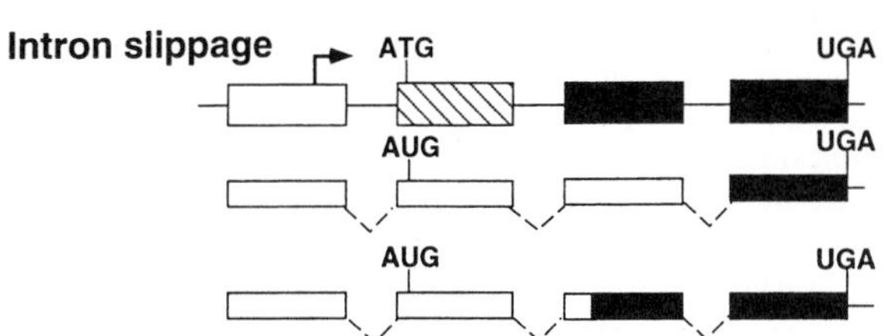

Figure 3–14. Alternative exon splicing provides a means to generate biologic diversification of gene expression. Mechanisms of exon skipping or switching and intron slippage are frequently utilized in the alternative processing of pre–messenger ribonucleic acids (mRNAs) to provide unique mRNAs and encoded proteins during development and in a tissue-specific pattern of expression in the fully differentiated tissues or organs. Exons are shown as boxes with protein-coding regions *shaded* to designate origin of protein isoforms. Introns are depicted as horizontal lines. *Dashed lines* denote spliced-out introns.

There are many examples of both mechanisms used to generate diversity in endocrine systems. Included among the genes encoding prohormones in which the pre-mRNAs are alternatively spliced by exon skipping or switching are those for procalcitonin/calcitonin gene-related peptide, prosubstance P/K, and the prokininogens. Alternative processing of the RNA transcribed from the calcitonin gene results in production of an mRNA in neural tissues that is distinct from that formed in the C cells of the thyroid gland.[79] The thyroid mRNA encodes a precursor to calcitonin, whereas the mRNA in the neural tissues generates a neuropeptide known as calcitonin gene–related peptide. Immunocytochemical analyses of the distribution of the peptide in brain and other tissues suggest functions for the peptide in perception of pain, ingestive behavior, and modulation of the autonomic and endocrine systems.

The splicing of the RNA precursor that encodes substance P can take place in at least two ways.[80] One splicing pattern results in the mRNA that encodes substance P and another peptide, called *substance K*, in a common protein precursor. Other mRNAs are apparently spliced so as to exclude the coding sequence for substance K. An alternative RNA splicing pattern also occurs in the processing of transcripts arising from the gene encoding bradykinin.[81] The high-molecular-weight and low-molecular-weight kininogens are translated from mRNAs that differ by the alternative use of 3′-end exons encoding the COOH termini of the prohormones, a situation similar to that found in the transcription of the calcitonin gene.

Other examples of genetic diversification arise from the programmed flexibility in the choice of splice acceptor sites within coding regions (intron slippage), which allows an array of coding sequences (exons) to be put together in a number of useful combinations. For example, the coding sequences of the growth hormone, lutropin-choriogonadotropin,[82] and leptin receptors[83] can be brought together in two different ways, one to include, the other to exclude, an exonic coding sequence specifying the transmembrane spanning domains of the polypeptide chains that anchor the receptors to the surface of cells. If mRNA splicing excludes the anchor's peptide sequence, a secreted rather than a surface protein is produced.

Translation

The process of translation provides a fourth level for the creation of diversity of gene expression. As discussed earlier in the section of the chapter on Regulation of Gene Expression, the rate of translational initiation can be regulated as typified by the proinsulin and prohormone convertase mRNAs, in which translation is augmented by glucose and cAMP. Molecular diversity of translation, however, is generated by the developmentally regulated utilization of alternative translation initiation (start) codons (methionine codons, AUGs). The mechanism of translation initiation involves the assembly of the 40S ribosome subunit on the 5′ methyl guanosine cap of the mRNA.[84] The ribosome subunit then scans 5′ to 3′ along the mRNA until it encounters an AUG sequence in a context of surrounding nucleotides favorable for the initiation of protein synthesis. Upon encountering such a favorable AUG, the subunit pauses and recruits the 60S subunit plus a number of other essential translation initiation factors, allowing the polymerization of amino acids.

The use of an alternative downstream start codon for translation can occur by mechanisms of loose scanning and reinitiation (Fig. 3–15).[85] Loose scanning is believed to occur when the most 5′ AUG codon is not in a strongly favorable context and allows the 40S ribosomal subunit to continue scanning until it encounters a more favorable AUG downstream. Thus, in the loose scanning mechanism, both translational start codons are used. In contrast, the mechanism of translational reinitiation involves the termination of translation followed by the reinitiation of translation at a downstream start codon. Thus, two proteins are encoded from the same mRNA by a start and stop mechanism.

This process of translational reinitiation can occur either by continued scanning of the 40S ribosomal subunit after termination of translation followed by reinitiation, as in loose scanning, or by complete dissociation of the ribosomal subunits at the time of termination followed by complete reassembly at a downstream start codon, referred to as an *internal ribosomal entry site* (IRES). Such utilization of alternative translation start codons occurs in mRNAs encoding certain classes of transcription factors illustrated by the basic leucine zipper (bZIP) proteins CREB, CREM, and certain of the CCAAT/enhancer binding proteins (C/EBPs), the C/EBPα and C/EBPβ isoforms. In all four of these DNA-binding proteins, the alternative use of internal start codons results in a switch from activators to repressors.

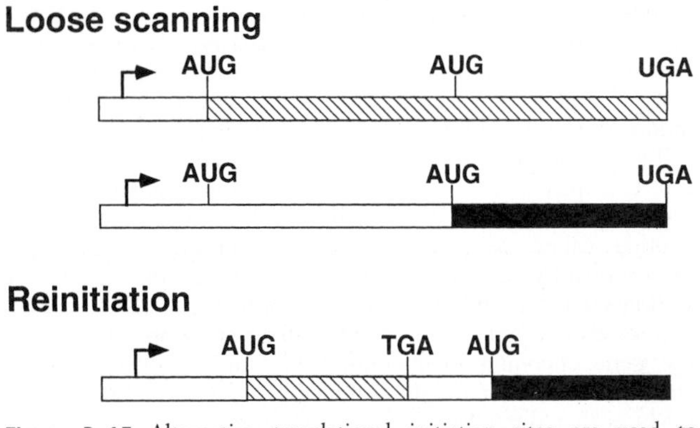

Loose scanning

Reinitiation

Figure 3–15. Alternative translational initiation sites are used to change the coding sequences of messenger ribonucleic acids to encode different protein isoforms. The two mechanisms illustrated involve loose scanning and reinitiation of translation. See text.

The CREB gene uses translational reinitiation by the somewhat novel mechanism of alternative exon switching that occurs during spermatogenesis.[86] At developmental stages IV and V of the seminiferous tubule of the rat, an exon (exon W) is spliced into the CREB mRNA. Exon W introduces an in-frame stop codon, thereby terminating translation approximately 40 amino acids upstream of the DNA-binding domain.[87, 88] The termination of translation then permits reinitiation of translation at each of two downstream start codons, resulting in the synthesis of two repressor or inhibitor isoforms of CREB known as I-CREBs that are powerful dominant negative inhibitors of activator forms of CREB and CREM because they consist of the DNA-binding domain devoid of any *trans*-activation domains.[86–88] The function, if any, of the amino-terminal truncated protein consisting of the activation domains devoid of the DNA-binding domain is unknown. It has been postulated that the role of the alternative splicing of exon W in the CREB pre-mRNA is to interrupt a forward positive feedback loop during spermatogenesis.

CREM, C/EBPα, and C/EBPβ mRNAs utilize alternative downstream start codons to synthesize repressors during development. Like the I-CREBs, these repressors consist of the DNA-binding domains and lack *trans*-activation domains. The CREM repressor (S-CREM) is expressed during brain development.[78] The C/EBPα-30 and C/EBPα-20 isoforms are expressed during the differentiation of adipoblasts to adipocytes, and the C/EBP repressor liver inhibitory protein (LIP) is expressed during the development of the liver.[78]

Post-translational Processing

A fifth level of gene expression at which diversification of biologic information can take place is that of post-translational processing. Many precursors of polypeptide hormones, particularly those encoding small peptides, contain multiple peptides that are cleaved during post-translational processing of the prohormones.[89] Certain polyprotein precursors, however, contain several copies of the peptide. Examples of prohormones that contain multiple identical peptides are the precursors encoding TRH[90] and the α mating factor of yeast,[91] each of which contains four copies of the respective peptide. Polyproteins that contain several distinct peptides include proenkephalins,[92] pro-opiomelanocortin,[93] and proglucagon.[94]

In many instances, biologic diversification at the level of post-translational processing occurs in a tissue-specific manner. The processing of pro-opiomelanocortin differs markedly in the anterior compared with the intermediate lobe of the pituitary gland. In the anterior pituitary the primary peptide products are ACTH and β-endorphin, whereas in the intermediate lobe of the pituitary one of the primary products is α-melanocyte-stimulating hormone. The smaller peptides produced are extensively modified by acetylation and phosphorylation of amino acid residues.

The processing of proglucagon in the pancreatic A cells and that in the intestinal L cells are also different (see Fig. 3–15).[34] In the pancreatic A cells, the predominant bioactive product of the processing of proglucagon is glucagon itself; the two glucagon-like peptides are not processed efficiently from proglucagon in the A cells and are biologically inactive by virtue of having NH_2-terminal and COOH-terminal extensions. On the other hand, in the intestinal L cell the glucagon immunoreactive product is a molecule, called *glicentin*, that consists of the NH_2-terminal extension of the proglucagon plus glucagon and the small COOH-terminal peptide known as intervening peptide I.

Glicentin has no glucagon-like biologic activity, and therefore the bioactive peptide (or peptides) in the intestinal L cells must be one or both of the glucagon-like peptides. In fact, glucagon-like peptide I in its shortened form of 31 amino acids, GLP-I (7–37), is a potent insulinotropic hormone in its actions of stimulating insulin release from pancreatic beta cells.[95] This peptide is released from the intestines into the blood stream in response to oral nutrients and appears to be a potent intestinal incretin factor implicated in the augmented release of insulin in response to oral compared with systemic (intravenous) nutrients. This potential for diversification of biologic information provided by the alternative pathways of gene expression is impressive when one considers that these pathways can occur in multiple combinations.

Unexpectedly Low Numbers of Expressed Genes in Genomes of Mammals (Humans and Mice)

A somewhat surprising initial conclusion, heralded in the lay press when the results of the sequencing of the human and mouse genomes were revealed, was that the number of genes in the human and mouse was approximately 30,000. This number was viewed as remarkably low because the number of genes in yeast *(Saccharomyces cerevisiae)*, worm *(Caenorhabditis elegans)*, and fly *(Drosophila melanogaster)* is about 20,000. However, it seems quite clear from the complexities of the mRNAs expressed in humans and mice, as exemplified by the growing database of expressed sequence tags, that tissue-specific alternative exon splicing and alternative promoter usage occur much more frequently in humans and mice than in yeast, worms, and flies. Considering the as yet incomplete database of expressed genes at the mRNA level, it seems reasonable to extrapolate that the human genome may actually express as many as 100,000 to 200,000 mRNAs that encode proteins with distinct, specific functions. This extrapolation is based on the observation that alternative exon splicing and promoter usage appear to be on the order of 5 to 10 times more frequent in higher vertebrate mammals than in yeasts and flies.

Acknowledgments

I am indebted to the members of the laboratory whose forbearance and helpful discussions of this chapter were invaluable. I thank Townley Budde for help in the preparation of the manuscript. J. F. H. is an Investigator with the Howard Hughes Medical Institute.

References

1. Watson JD, Crick FHC. Molecular structure of nucleic acids. Nature 1953; 171:737–738.
2. Roth J, LeRoith D, Shiloach J, et al. The evolutionary origins of hormones, neurotransmitters, and other extracellular chemical messengers. N Engl J Med 1982; 306:523–527.
3. Loumaye E, Thorner J, Catt KJ. Yeast mating pheromone activates mammalian gonadotrophs: evolutionary conservation of a reproductive hormone? Science 1982; 218:1323–1325.
4. Johnsen AH. Phylogeny of the cholecystokinin/gastrin family. Front Neuroendocrinol 1998; 19:73–99.
5. Uy R, Wold F. Post-translational covalent modification of proteins. Science 1977; 198:890–896.
6. Martoglio B, Dobberstein B. Signal sequences: more than just greasy peptides. Trends Cell Biol 1998; 8:410–415.
7. Palade G. Intracellular aspects of the process of protein synthesis. Science 1975; 189:347–358.
8. Jamieson JD. The Golgi complex: perspectives and prospectives. Biochim Biophys Acta 1998; 1404:3–7.
9. Blobel G. Intracellular protein topogenesis. Proc Natl Acad Sci USA 1980; 77:1496–1500.
10. Hegde RS, Lingappa VR. Regulation of protein biogenesis at the endoplasmic reticulum membrane. Trends Cell Biol 1999; 9:132–137.
11. Nelson DL, Cox MM. Lehninger's Principles of Biochemistry, 3rd ed. New York, Worth, 2000.
12. Agarraberes FA, Dice JF. Protein translocation across membranes. Biochim Biophys Acta 2001; 1513:1–24.
13. Blobel G, Dobberstein B. Transfer to proteins across membranes. II. Reconstitution of functional rough microsomes from heterologous components. J Cell Biol 1975; 67:852–862.
14. Walter P, Blobel F. Signal recognition particle contains a 7S RNA essential for protein translocation across the endoplasmic reticulum. Nature 1982; 299:691–698.
15. Bacher G, Pool M, Dobberstein B. The ribosome regulates the GTPase of the beta-subunit of the signal recognition particle receptor. J Cell Biol 1999; 146:723–730.
16. Wang L, Dobberstein B. Oligomeric complexes involved in translocation of proteins across the membrane of the endoplasmic reticulum. FEBS Lett 1999; 457:316–322.
17. Martoglio B, Graf R, Dobberstein B. Signal peptide fragments of preprolactin and NIV-1 p-gp160 interact with calmodulin. EMBO J 1997; 16:6636–6645.
18. Habener JF, Amgerdt M, Ravazzola M, et al. Parathyroid hormone biosynthesis. J Cell Biol 1979; 80:715–731.
19. Steiner DF, Docherty K, Carroll R. Golgi/granule processing of peptide hormone and neuropeptide precursors: a minireview. J Cell Biochem 1984; 24:121–130.
20. Chu LLH, MacGregor RR, Cohn DV. Energy-dependent intracellular translocation of proparathormone. J Cell Biol 1977; 72: 1–10.
21. Kemper B, Habener JF, Rich A, et al. Microtubules and the intracellular conversion of proparathyroid hormone to parathyroid hormone. Endocrinology 1975; 96:902–912.
22. Steiner DF. The proprotein convertases. Curr Opin Chem Biol 1998; 2:31–39.
23. Muller L, Lindberg I. The cell biology of the prohormone convertases PC1 and PC2. Prog Nucleic Acid Res Mol Biol 1999; 63: 69–108.
24. Seidah NG, Chretien M. Proprotein and prohormone convertases: a family of subtilases generating diverse bioactive polypeptides. Brain Res 1999; 848:45–62.
25. Jackson RS, Creemers JW, Ohagi S, et al. Obesity and impaired prohormone processing associated with mutations in the human prohormone convertase 1 gene. Nat Genet 1997; 16:303–306.
26. Furuta M, Yano H, Zhou A, et al. Defective prohormone processing and altered pancreatic islet morphology in mice lacking active SPC2. Proc Natl Acad Sci USA 1997; 94:6646–6651.
27. Bradbury AF, Smyth DG. Peptide amidation. Trends Biochem Sci 1991; 16:112–115.
28. Prigge ST, Mains RE, Eipper BA, et al. New insights into copper monooxygenases and peptide amidation: structure, mechanism and function. Cell Mol Life Sci 2000; 57:1236–1259.
29. Kornberg RD. Eukaryotic transcriptional control. Trends Cell Biol 1999; 9:M46–M49.
30. Wolffe AP, Kurumizaka H. The nucleosome: a powerful regulator of transcription. Prog Nucleic Acid Res Mol Biol 1998; 61:379–422.
31. Sharp PA. Split genes and RNA splicing. Cell 1994; 77:805–815.
32. Albright SR, Tjian R. TAFs revisited: more data reveal new twists and confirm old ideas. Gene 2000; 242:1–13.
33. Crick F. Split genes and RNA splicing. Science 1979; 204:264–271.
34. Mojsov S, Heinrich G, Wilson IB, et al. Preproglucagon gene expression in pancreas and intestine diversifies at the level of post-translational processing. J Biol Chem 1986; 261:11880–11889.
35. Miller W, Eberhardt NL. Structure and evolution of the growth hormone gene family. Endocr Rev 1983; 4:97–130.
36. Brown DD. Gene expression in eukaryotes. Science 1981; 211: 667–674.
37. Darnell JE. Variety in the level of gene control in eukaryotic cells. Nature 1982; 297:365–371.

38. Murdoch GH, Franco R, Evans RM, et al. Polypeptide hormone regulation of gene expression. J Biol Chem 1983; 258:15329–15335.
39. Baxter JD, Ivarie RD. Regulation of gene expression by glucocorticoid hormones: studies of receptors and responses in cultured cells. Receptors Horm Action 1978; 2:251–284.
40. Wegnez M, Schachter BS, Baxter JD, et al. Hormonal regulation of growth hormone mRNA. DNA 1982; 1:145–153.
41. Itoh N, Okamoto H. Translational control of proinsulin synthesis by glucose. Nature 1980; 283:100–102.
42. Skelly RH, Schuppin GT, Ishihara H, et al. Glucose-regulated translational control of proinsulin biosynthesis with that of the proinsulin endopeptidases PC2 and PC3 in the insulin-producing MIN6 cell line. Diabetes 1996; 45:37–43.
43. Wu C, Gilbert W. Tissue-specific exposure of chromatin structure at the 5′ terminus of the preproinsulin II gene. Proc Natl Acad Sci USA 1981; 78:1577–1580.
44. Barton MC, Crowe AJ. Chromatin alteration, transcription and replication: what's the opening line to the story? Oncogene 2001; 20:3094–3099.
45. Feil R, Khosla S. Genomic imprinting in mammals: an interplay between chromatin and DNA methylation? Trends Genet 1999; 15:431–435.
46. Stallcup MR. Role of protein methylation in chromatin remodeling and transcriptional regulation. Oncogene 2001; 20:3014–3020.
47. Wade PA. Methyl CpG binding proteins: coupling chromatin architecture to gene regulation. Oncogene 2001; 20:3166–3173.
48. Marx JL. Immunoglobulin genes have enhancers. Science 1983; 221:735–757.
49. Walker MD, Edlund T, Boulet AM, Rutter WJ. Cell-specific expression controlled by the 5′-flanking region of insulin and chymotrypsin genes. Nature 1983; 306:557–561.
50. Krumlauf R. Hox genes in vertebrate development. Cell 1994; 78: 191–201.
51. Beato M, Klug J. Steroid hormone receptors: an update. Hum Reprod Update 2000; 6:225–236.
52. McKenna NJ, Lanz RB, O'Malley BW. Nuclear receptor coregulators: cellular and molecular biology. Endocr Rev 1999; 20:321–344.
53. Rosenfeld MG, Glass CK. Coregulator codes of transcriptional regulation by nuclear receptors. J Biol Chem 2001; 276:36865–36868.
54. Rosenfeld MG. POU-domain transcription factors: pou-er-ful developmental regulators. Genes Dev 1991; 5:897–907.
55. Lin C, Lin S-C, Chang C-P, et al. Pit-1–dependent expression of the receptor for growth hormone releasing factor mediates pituitary cell growth. Nature 1992; 360:765–768.
56. Latchman DS. Transcription-factor mutations and disease. N Engl J Med 1996; 334:28–33.
57. Jonsson J, Carlsson L, Edlund T, et al. Insulin-promoter-factor 1 is required for pancreas development in mice. Nature 1994; 371: 606–609.
58. Stoffers DA, Zinkin NT, Stonojevic V, et al. Pancreatic agenesis attributable to a single nucleotide deletion in the human *IPF1* gene coding sequence. Nat Genet 1996; 15:106-110.
59. Peers B, Leonard J, Sharma S, et al. Insulin expression in pancreatic islet cells relies on cooperative interactions between the helix loop helix factor E47 and the homeobox factor STF-1. Mol Endocrinol 1994; 8:1798–1806.
60. Luo X, Ikeda Y, Parker KL. A cell-specific nuclear receptor is essential for adrenal and gonadal development and sexual differentiation. Cell 1994; 77:481–490.
61. Zanaria E, Muscatelli F, Bardoni B, et al. An unusual member of the nuclear hormone receptor superfamily responsible for X-linked adrenal hypoplasia congenita. Nature 1994; 372:635–641.
62. Cohen P. Signal integration at the level of protein kinases, protein phosphatases and their substrates. Trends Biochem Sci 1992; 17: 408–413.
63. Krebs EG, Graves JD. Interactions between protein kinases and proteases in cellular signaling and regulation. Adv Enzyme Regul 2000; 40:441–470.
64. Berridge MJ. Elementary and global aspects of calcium signalling. J Physiol (Lond) 1997; 499:291–306.
65. Bootman MD, Collins TJ, Peppiatt CM, et al. Calcium signalling: an overview. Semin Cell Dev Biol 2001; 12:3–10.
66. Hill CS, Treisman R. Transcriptional regulation by extracellular signals: mechanisms and specificity. Cell 1995; 80:199–211.
67. Habener JF, Miller CP, Vallejo M. Cyclic AMP–dependent regulation of gene transcription by CREB and CREM. Vitam Horm 1995; 51:1–57.
68. Janknecht R, Hunter T. A growing coactivator network. Nature 1996; 383:22–23.
69. Cobb MH, Goldsmith EJ. How MAP kinases are regulated. J Biol Chem 1995; 270:14843–14846.
70. Schindler C, Darnell JE Jr. Transcriptional responses to polypeptide ligands: the JAK-STAT pathway. Annu Rev Biochem 1995; 64:621–651.
71. Axel R. The molecular logic of smell. Sci Am 1995; 273(4):154–159.
72. Dover G. Molecular drive: a cohesive mode of species evolution. Nature 1982; 299:111–117.
73. Reanney D. Genetic noise in evolution. Nature 1984; 307:318–319.
74. Ayoubi TAY, Van De Ven WJM. Regulation of gene expression by alternative promoters. FASEB J 1996; 10:453–460.
75. Leid M, Kastner P, Chambon P. Multiplicity generates diversity in the retinoic acid signaling pathways. Trends Biochem Sci 1992; 117:427–433.
76. Davidson EH, Jacobs HT, Britten RJ. Very short repeats and coordinate induction of genes. Nature 1983; 301:468–470.
77. Kastner P, Krust A, Turcotte B, et al. Two distinct estrogen-regulated promoters generate transcripts encoding the two functionally different human progesterone receptor forms A and B. EMBO J 1990; 9:1603–1614.
78. Foulkes NS, Sassone-Corsi P. More is better: activators and repressors from the same gene. Cell 1992; 68:411–414.
79. Rosenfeld MG, Mermod JJ, Amara SG, et al. Production of a novel neuropeptide encoded by the calcitonin gene via tissue-specific RNA processing. Nature 1983; 304:129–135.
80. Nawa H, Hirose T, Takashima H, et al. Nucleotide sequences of cloned cDNAs for two types of bovine brain substance P precursor. Nature 1983; 306:32–36.
81. Kitamura N, Takagaki Y, Furuto S, et al. A single gene for bovine high molecular weight and low molecular weight kininogens. Nature 1983; 305:545–549.
82. Segaloff DL, Ascoli M. The lutropin/choriogonadotropin receptor . . . 4 years later. Endocr Rev 1993; 14:324–347.
83. Lee G-H, Proenca R, Montez JM, et al. Abnormal splicing of the leptin receptor in diabetic mice. Nature 1996; 379:632–635.
84. Dreyfuss G, Hentze M, Lamond AI, et al. From transcript to protein. Cell 1996; 85:963–972.
85. Kozak M. The scanning model for translation: an update. J Cell Biol 1989; 108:229–241.
86. Walker WH, Sanborn BM, Habener JF. An isoform of transcription factor CREM expressed during spermatogenesis lacks the phosphorylation domain and represses cAMP-induced transcription. Proc Natl Acad Sci USA 1994; 91:12423–12427.
87. Walker WH, Girardet C, Habener JF. An alternatively spliced, polycistronic mRNA controls a switch from activator to repressor isoforms of transcription factor CREB during spermatogenesis. J Biol Chem 1996; 271:20145–20158.
88. Walker WH, Habener JF. Role of transcription factors CREB and CREM in cAMP-induced regulation of transcription during spermatogenesis. Trends Endocrinol Metab 1996; 4:133–138.
89. Neurath H. Proteolytic processing and regulation. Enzyme 1991; 45:239–243.
90. Lechan RM, Wu P, Jackson IME, et al. Thyrotropin-releasing hormone precursor: characterization in rat brain. Science 1986; 231:159–161.
91. Kurjan J, Herskowitz I. Structure of a yeast pheromone gene (MF): a putative factor precursor contains four tandem copies of mature factor. Cell 1982; 30:933–943.
92. Noda M, Teranishi Y, Yakahashi T, et al. Isolation and structural organization of the human preproenkephalin gene. Nature 1982; 297:431–434.
93. Nakanishi S, Inoue A, Kita T, et al. Nucleotide sequence of cloned cDNA for bovine corticotropin-β-lipotropin precursor. Nature 1979; 278:423–427.
94. Heinrich G, Gros P, Lund PK, et al. Pre-proglucagon messenger RNA: nucleotide and encoded amino acid sequences of the rat pancreatic cDNA. Endocrinology 1984; 115:2176–2181.
95. Mojsov S, Weir GC, Habener JF. Insulinotropin: glucagon-like peptide I (7–37) coencoded in the glucagon gene is a potent stimulator of insulin release in perfused rat pancreas. J Clin Invest 1987; 79:616–619.

4 Mechanism of Action of Hormones That Act on Nuclear Receptors

Mitchell A. Lazar

Hormones can be divided into two groups on the basis of where they function in a target cell. The first group includes hormones *that do not enter cells;* instead, they signal via second messengers generated by interacting with receptors at the cell surface. All polypeptide hormones, as well as monoamines and prostaglandins, utilize cell surface receptors (see Chapter 5, "Mechanism of Action of Hormones That Act at the Cell Surface"). The second group, the focus of this chapter, includes hormones *that can enter cells.* These hormones bind to intracellular receptors that function in the nucleus of the target cell to regulate gene expression. Classical hormones that utilize intracellular receptors include thyroid and steroid hormones.

Hormones serve as a major form of communication between different organs and tissues that allows specialized cells in complex organisms to respond in a coordinated manner to changes in the internal and external environments. Classical endocrine hormones, such as thyroid and steroid hormones, are secreted by ductless glands and are distributed throughout the body via the blood stream. These hormones were discovered by purifying the biologically active substances from clearly definable glands.

It is now recognized that numerous other signaling molecules share with thyroid and steroid hormones the ability to function in the nucleus to convey intercellular and environmental signals. Not all of these molecules are produced in glandular tissues. Further, whereas some of these signaling molecules arrive at target tissues via the blood stream like classical endocrine hormones, others have *paracrine* functions (i.e., they act on adjacent cells) or *autocrine* functions (i.e., they act on the cell of origin).

Lipophilic signaling molecules that utilize nuclear receptors include the following:

- Derivatives of vitamins A and D
- Endogenous metabolites such as oxysterols and bile acids
- Non-natural chemicals encountered in the environment (*xenobiotics*)

These molecules are referred to generically as *ligands* for nuclear receptors. The nuclear receptors for all of these signaling molecules are structurally related and collectively referred to as the *nuclear receptor superfamily*.

LIGANDS THAT ACT VIA NUCLEAR RECEPTORS

General Features of Nuclear Receptor Ligands

Unlike polypeptide hormones that function via cell surface receptors, no ligands for nuclear receptors are directly encoded in the genome. To the contrary, all nuclear receptor ligands are small (molecular weight < 1000 daltons [d]) and lipophilic, enabling them to enter cells. Cellular uptake of nuclear receptor ligands may be a passive process, but in some cases a membrane transport protein is involved. For example, the oatp3 organic anion transporter mediates thyroid hormone entry into cells.[1] The lipophilicity of nuclear receptor ligands also allows them to be absorbed from the gastrointestinal tract, thus facilitating their use in replacement or pharmacologic therapies of disease states.

Another common feature of nuclear receptor ligands is that all are derived from dietary, environmental, and metabolic precursors. In this sense, the function of these ligands and their receptors is to translate cues from the external and internal environments into changes in gene expression. Their critical role in maintaining homeostasis in multicellular organisms is highlighted by the fact that nuclear receptors are found in all vertebrates as well as insects but not in single-cell organisms such as yeast.[2]

Subclasses of Nuclear Receptor Ligands

One classification of nuclear receptor ligands is outlined in Table 4–1 and is described next.

Classical Hormones

The classical hormones that utilize nuclear receptors for signaling are thyroid hormone and steroid hormones. Steroid hormones include receptors for cortisol, aldosterone, estrogen, progesterone, and testosterone. In some cases (e.g., thyroid hormone receptor [TR] α and β genes, estrogen receptor [ER] α and β), there are multiple receptor genes, encoding multiple receptors. Multiple receptors for the same hormone can also derive from a single gene either by alternative promoter usage or alternative splicing (e.g., TR $\beta 1$ and $\beta 2$).

Finally, some receptors can mediate the signal of multiple hormones. For example, the mineralocorticoid (aldosterone) receptor (MR) has equal affinity for cortisol and probably functions as a glucocorticoid receptor in some tissues, such as the brain.[3] The androgen receptor (AR) binds and responds to both testosterone and dihydrotestosterone (DHT).

Vitamins

Vitamins were discovered as essential constituents of a healthful diet. Two fat-soluble vitamins, A and D, are precursors of important signaling molecules that function as ligands for nuclear receptors.

Table 4–1. Nuclear Receptor Ligands and Their Receptors

Classical Hormones
Thyroid hormone: thyroid hormone receptor (TR), subtypes α, β
Estrogen: estrogen receptor (ER), subtypes α, β
Testosterone: androgen receptor (AR)
Progesterone: progesterone receptor (PR)
Aldosterone: mineralocorticoid receptor (MR)
Cortisol: glucocorticoid receptor (GR)
Vitamins
1,25-$(OH)_2$-vitamin D_3: vitamin D receptor (VDR)
All-*trans*-retinoic acid: retinoic acid receptor, subtypes α, β, γ
9-*cis*-retinoic acid: retinoid X receptor (RXR), subtypes α, β, γ
Metabolic Intermediates and Products
Oxysterols: liver X receptor (LXR), subtypes α, β
Bile acids: bile acid receptor (BAR)
Fatty acids: peroxisome proliferator–activated receptor (PPAR), subtypes α, β, γ
Xenobiotics
Pregnane X receptor (PXR), constitutive androstane receptor (CAR)

Precursors of vitamin D are synthesized and stored in skin and activated by ultraviolet light; vitamin D can also be derived from dietary sources. Vitamin D is then converted in the liver to 25(OH) vitamin D and in the kidney to 1,25-$(OH)_2$-vitamin D_3, the most potent natural ligand of the *vitamin D receptor* (VDR). 1,25-$(OH)_2$-vitamin D_3 acts as a circulating endocrine hormone.

Vitamin A is stored in the liver and is activated by metabolism to all-*trans*-retinoic acid, which is a high affinity ligand for retinoic acid receptors (RARs). Retinoic acid is likely to function as a signaling molecule in paracrine as well as endocrine pathways. Retinoic acid is also converted to its 9-*cis*-isomer, which is a ligand for another nuclear receptor called the *retinoid X receptor* (RXR).[4] These retinoids and their receptors are essential for normal life and development of multiple organs and tissues.[5] They also have pharmaceutical utility for conditions ranging from skin diseases to leukemia.[6]

Metabolic Intermediates and Products

Certain nuclear receptors have been discovered to respond to naturally occurring, endogenous metabolic products. One, called *liver X receptor* (LXR), is activated by oxysterol intermediates in cholesterol biosynthesis. Mice lacking LXR-α have dramatically impaired ability to metabolize cholesterol.[7]

Another "orphan receptor," *bile acid receptor* (BAR) also known as FXR, or "Farnesyl X receptor", is thus likely to play a role in regulation of bile synthesis and circulation in normal as well as disease states.[8]

The *peroxisome proliferator–activated receptors* (PPARs) constitute another subfamily of nuclear receptors.[9] There are three subtypes, and all are activated by polyunsaturated fatty acids. No single fatty acid has particularly high affinity for any PPAR, and it is possible that these receptors may function as integrators of the concentration of a number of fatty acids.

PPARα is expressed primarily in liver; to date, the natural ligand with highest affinity for PPARα is an eicosanoid, 8(S)-hydroxyeicosatetraenoic acid. The most potent PPARα ligands are the *fibrate class* of lipid-lowering pharmaceuticals. The name PPAR derives from the fact that compounds such as fibrates induce proliferation of hepatic peroxisomes, organelles involved in β-oxidation of fatty acids.

The other PPARs (δ and γ) are structurally related but are not activated by peroxisome proliferators. PPAR-δ is ubiquitous, and its ligands—other than fatty acids—are not well characterized. PPARγ is expressed primarily in fat cells (adipocytes) and is necessary for differentiation along the adipocyte lineage.[10, 11] PPARγ is also expressed in other cell types, including colonocytes, macrophages, and vascular endothelial cells, where it may play physiologic as well as pathologic roles. The natural ligand for PPARγ is not known, although prostaglandin J derivatives have the highest affinity (in the micromolar range). It is exciting news that PPARγ appears to be the target of thiazolidinedione antidiabetic drugs that improve insulin sensitivity.[12, 13] These pharmaceutical agents bind to PPARγ with nanomolar affinities, and non-thiazolidinedione PPARγ ligands are also insulin sensitizers, further implicating PPARγ in this physiologic role.

Xenobiotics

Other nuclear receptors appear to function as integrators of exogenous environmental signals, including natural *endobiotics* (e.g., medicinals and toxins found in plants) and *xenobiotics* (compounds that are not naturally occurring).[14] In these cases, the role of the activated nuclear receptor is to induce cytochrome P450 enzymes that facilitate detoxification of potentially dangerous compounds in the liver. Receptors in this class include:

- SXR, or *sterol and xenobiotic receptor*[15]
- CAR, or *constitutive androstane receptor*[16]
- PPARα, which is also activated by certain environmental chemicals

Unlike other nuclear receptors that have high affinity for very specific ligands, xenobiotic receptors have low affinity for a large number of ligands, reflecting their function in defense from a varied and challenging environment. Although these xenobiotic compounds are clearly not "hormones" in the classical sense, the function of these nuclear receptors is consistent with the general theme of helping the organism to cope with environmental challenges.

Orphan Receptors

The nuclear receptor superfamily is one of the largest families of transcription factors. The hormones and vitamins just described account for the functions of only a fraction of the total number of nuclear receptors. The remainder have been designated as *orphan receptors* because their putative ligands are not known.[17, 18]

From analyses of mice and humans with mutations in various orphan receptors, it is clear that many of these receptors are required for life or development of specific organs ranging from brain nuclei to endocrine glands. Some orphan receptors appear to be active in the absence of any ligand ("constitutively active") and may not respond to a natural ligand. Nevertheless, all of the receptors now known to respond to metabolites and environmental compounds were originally discovered as orphans. Thus, it is likely that future research will find that additional orphan receptors function as receptors for physiologic, pharmacologic, or environmental ligands.

Variant Receptors

As to be discussed later, the carboxyl (C-) terminus of the nuclear receptors is responsible for hormone binding. In the case of a few nuclear receptors, including TRα and the glucocorticoid receptor, alternative splicing leads to the production of variant receptors with unique C-termini that do not bind ligand.[19, 20] These variant receptors are normally expressed, but their biologic relevance is uncertain. It has been speculated that they modulate the action of the classical receptor to which they are related by inhibiting its function.

Another type of normally occurring variant nuclear receptors lacks a classical deoxyribonucleic acid (DNA) binding domain (see later). These include DAX-1, which is mutated in human disease,[21] and SHP-1.[22] Their ligands, if any, are not known, and it is likely that DAX-1 and SHP-1 bind to and repress the actions of other receptors.

Rare, naturally occurring mutations of hormone receptors can cause hormone resistance in affected patients, for instance:

1. Inheritance of the hormone resistance phenotype can be *dominant* if the mutant receptor inhibits the action of the normal receptor, as with generalized resistance to thyroid hormone.[23]
2. Inheritance is *recessive* if the mutation results in a complete loss of receptor function, as with the syndrome of hereditary 1,25-dihydroxyvitamin D-resistant rickets.[24]
3. Inheritance can be X-linked, as with the mutated androgen receptor in androgen insensitivity syndromes, including testicular feminization.[25]

Regulation of Ligand Levels

Ligand levels can be regulated in a number of ways (Table 4–2). A dietary precursor may not be available in required amounts, as occurs in hypothyroidism due to iodine deficiency. Pituitary hormones (e.g., thyroid-stimulating hormone) regulate the synthesis and secretion of classical thyroid and steroid hormones. When the glands that synthesize these hormones fail, hormone deficiency can occur.

Many of the nuclear receptor ligands are enzymatically converted from inactive *prohormones* to the biologically active hormone (e.g., 5′ deiodination of thyroxine [T_4] to triiodothyronine [T_3]). In other cases, one hormone is precursor for another (e.g., aromatization of testosterone to estradiol). Biotransformation may occur in a specific tissue that is not the main target of the hormone (e.g., renal 1-hydroxylation of vitamin D) or may occur primarily in target tissues (e.g., 5α-reduction of testosterone to DHT). Deficiency or pharmacologic inhibition of such an enzyme can also reduce hormone levels.

Hormones can be inactivated by standard hepatic or renal clearance mechanisms or by more specific enzymatic processes. In the latter case, reduction in enzyme activity due to gene mutations or pharmacologic agents can result in hormone excess syndromes, for example, the renal deactivation of cortisol by 11-β-hydroxysteroid dehydrogenase (11β-OHSD). Since, as noted earlier, cortisol can activate the mineralocorticoid receptor, insufficient 11β-OHSD activity due to licorice ingestion, gene mutation, or extremely high cortisol levels causes syndromes of apparent mineralocorticoid excess.[26]

NUCLEAR RECEPTOR SIGNALING MECHANISMS

Nuclear receptors are multifunctional proteins that transduce the signals of their cognate ligands. General features of nuclear receptor signaling are illustrated in Figure 4–1.

First and foremost, the ligand and the nuclear receptor must get to the nucleus. The nuclear receptor must also bind its ligand with high affinity. Because a major function of the receptor is to selectively regulate target gene transcription, it must recognize and bind to promoter elements in appropriate target genes. One discriminatory mechanism is dimerization of a receptor with a second copy of itself or with another nuclear receptor. The DNA-bound receptor must also work in the context of chromatin to signal the basal transcription machinery to increase or decrease transcription of the target gene.

Table 4–2. Regulation of Nuclear Receptor Ligand Levels

Precursor availability
Synthesis
Secretion
Activation (prohormone → active hormone)
Deactivation (active hormone → inactive hormone)
Elimination (hepatic, renal clearance)

Throughout the following discussion on the mechanisms and regulation of signaling by nuclear receptors, it should be kept in mind that some basic mechanisms are generally used by many or all members of the nuclear receptor superfamily, whereas other mechanisms impart the specificity that is crucial to the vastly different biologic effects of the many hormones and ligands that utilize these related receptors.

Domain Structure of Nuclear Receptors

The nuclear receptors are proteins whose molecular weights are generally between 50,000 and 100,000 d. They all share a common series of domains, referred to as A to F (Fig. 4–2). This linear depiction of the receptors is useful for describing and comparing the receptors, but it does not capture the role of protein folding and tertiary structure in mediating the various receptor functions. As of this writing, no full-length nuclear hormone receptor has been crystallized, but structures of individual domains have been extremely revealing, as will be clear from the discussions of specific receptor functions that follow.

Nuclear Localization

The nuclear receptors, like all cellular proteins, are synthesized on ribosomes that reside outside the nucleus. Import of

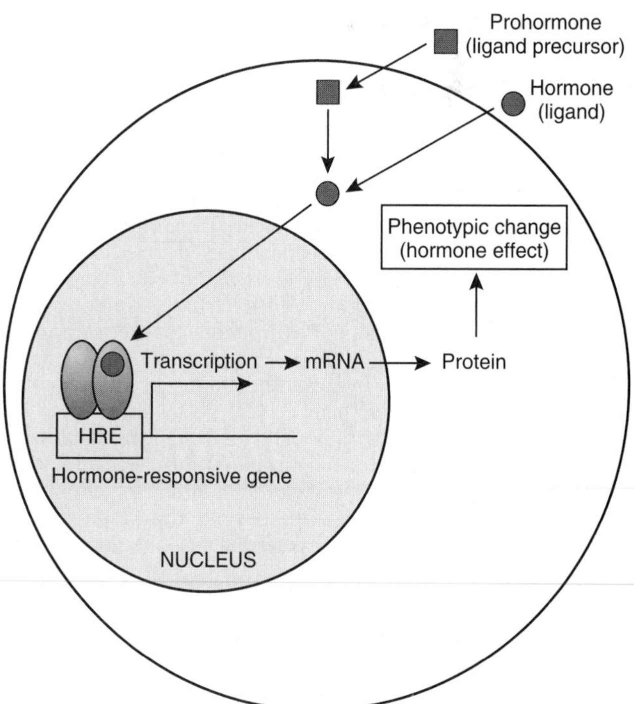

Figure 4–1. Signal transduction by hormones and other ligands that act via nuclear receptors. HRE, hormone response element; mRNA, messenger ribonucleic acid.

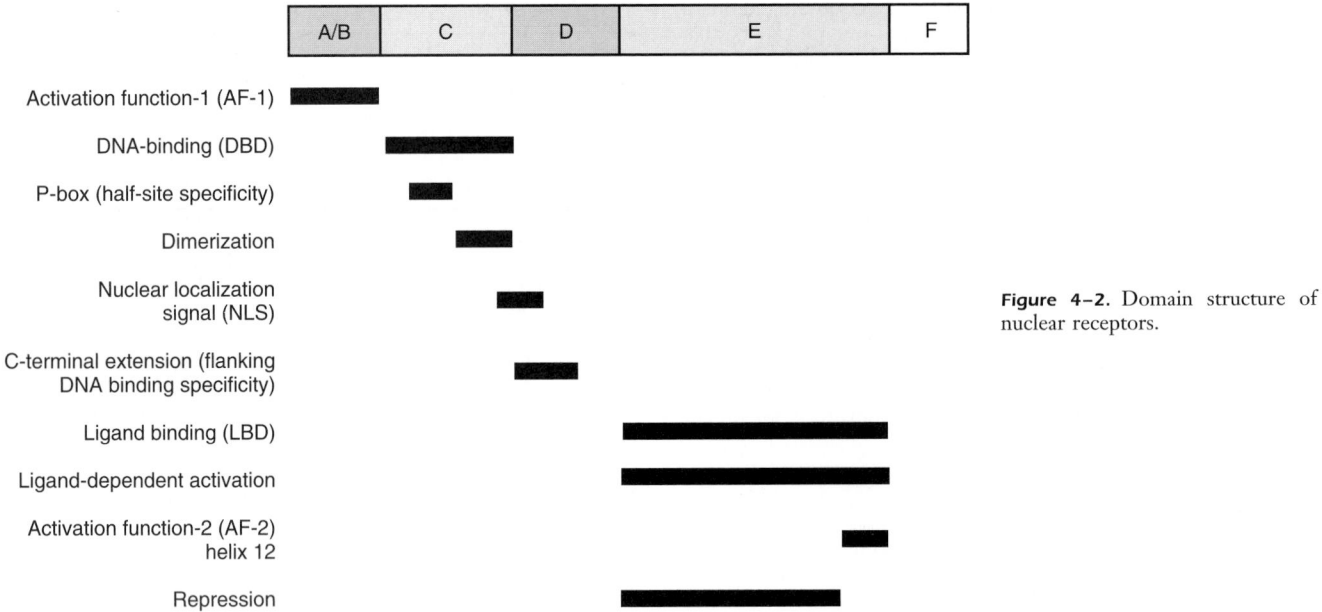

Figure 4–2. Domain structure of nuclear receptors.

the nuclear receptors into the nucleus requires the *nuclear localization signal* (NLS), located near the border of the C and D domains (see Fig. 4–2). As a result of their nuclear localization signals, most of the nuclear receptors reside in the nucleus in the absence, as well as in presence, of ligand. A major exception is the glucocorticoid receptor (GR), which, in the absence of hormone, is tethered in the cytoplasm to a complex of chaperone molecules, including *heat shock proteins* (hsps). Hormone binding to GR induces a conformational change that results in dissociation of the chaperone complex, thereby allowing the hormone-activated GR to translocate to the nucleus via its nuclear localization signal.

Hormone Binding

High-affinity binding of a lipophilic ligand is a shared characteristic of many nuclear receptors. This defining function of the receptor is mediated by the C-terminal *ligand-binding domain* (LBD), domains D and E in Figure 4–2. This region of the receptor also has many other functions, including dimerization and transcriptional regulation (see "Receptor Dimerization" and "Receptor Regulation of Gene Transcription" below).

The structure of the LBD has been solved for a number of receptors. All share a similar overall structure consisting of 12 α-helical segments in a highly folded tertiary structure (Fig. 4–3). The ligand binds within a hydrophobic pocket composed of amino acids in helix 3 (H3), H4, and H5. The major structural change induced by ligand binding is an internal folding of the most C-terminal helix (H12), which forms a cap on the ligand-binding pocket. Although the overall mechanism of ligand binding is similar for all receptors, the details are crucial in determining ligand specificity.[27, 28] Although the molecular details of ligand binding are beyond the scope of this chapter, this is the most critical determinant of receptor specificity.

Target Gene Recognition by Receptors

Another crucial specificity factor for nuclear receptors is their ability to recognize and bind to the subset of genes that are to be regulated by their cognate ligand. Target genes contain specific DNA sequences that are called *hormone response elements* (HREs). Binding to the HRE is mediated by the central C domain of the nuclear receptors (see Fig. 4–2). This region is typically composed of 66 to 68 amino acids, including two subdomains called *zinc fingers* because the structure of each subdomain is maintained by four cysteine residues that coordinate with a zinc atom.

The first of these zinc-ordered modules contains basic amino acids that contact DNA; as with the LBD, the overall structure of the DNA-binding domain (DBD) is very similar for all members of the nuclear receptor superfamily. The specificity of DNA binding is determined by multiple factors (Table 4–3). All steroid hormone receptors, except for the *estrogen receptor* (ER), bind to the double-stranded DNA sequence AG*AA*CA (Fig. 4–4).

By convention, the double-stranded sequence is described by the sequence of one of the complementary strands, with the bases ordered from the 5′ to the 3′ end. Other nuclear receptors recognize the sequence AG*GT*CA. The primary determinant of this specificity is a group of amino acids residues in the so-called P-box of the DBD (see Fig. 4–4). These hexamer DNA sequences are referred to as *half-sites*. The only two differences between these hexameric half-sites are the central two base pairs (underlined). For some nuclear receptors, the C-terminal extension of the DBD contributes specificity for extended half-sites containing additional, highly specific DNA sequences 5′ to the hexamer (see Fig. 4–2).[29]

Another source of specificity for target genes is the spacing and orientation of these half-sites, which in most cases are bound by receptor dimers.

Receptor Dimerization

As noted earlier, the nuclear receptor DBD has affinity for the hexameric half-site, or extended half-sites; many HREs, however, are composed of *repeats* of the half-site sequence, and most nuclear receptors bind such HREs as dimers. Steroid receptors, including ER, function primarily as homodimers, which preferentially bind to two half-sites oriented toward each other *(inverted repeats)* with three base pairs in between (IR3) (Fig. 4–4*A*). The major dimerization domain in steroid receptors is within the C-domain, although the LBD contributes. Ligand-binding facilitates dimerization and DNA binding of steroid hormone receptors. Most other receptors, including

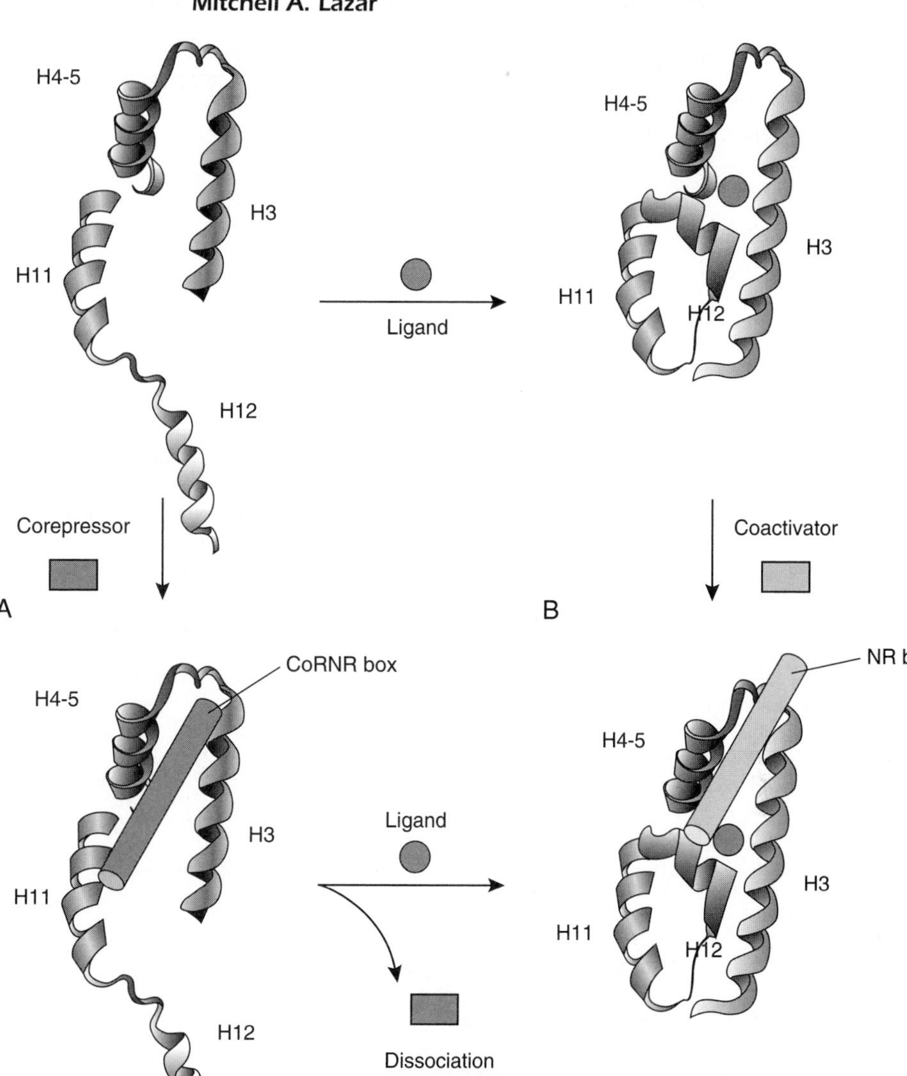

Figure 4–3. Structural basis of nuclear receptor ligand binding and cofactor recruitment.

TR, RAR, VDR, PPAR, LXR, and VDR, bind to DNA as heterodimers with RXR (Fig. 4–4*B*).

Heterodimerization is mediated by two distinct interactions. The receptor LBD mediates the strongest interaction, which occurs even in the absence of DNA. These receptor heterodimers bind to two half-sites arranged as *direct repeats* (DRs) with variable numbers of base pairs in between.

The spacing of the half-sites is a major determinant of target gene specificity. This is due to the second receptor-receptor interaction, which involves the DBDs and is highly sensitive to the spacing of the half-sites. For example, VDR/RXR heterodimers bind preferentially to direct repeats separated by three bases (DR3 sites), TR/RXR binds DR4, and RAR/RXR binds DR5 with highest affinity.[30]

The structural basis of this restriction on DNA binding is related to the fact that the RXR binds to the upstream half-site (farthest from the start of transcription). As a result of the periodicity of the DNA helix, each base pair separating the half-sites leads to a rotation of about 36° of one half-site relative to the other. Subtle differences in the structure of the receptor LBDs make the DBD interactions more or less favorable at the different degrees of rotation.[31]

Receptor Regulation of Gene Transcription

Nuclear receptors mediate a variety of effects on gene transcription. The most common modes of regulation (Table 4–4) are:

- Ligand-dependent gene activation
- Ligand-independent repression of transcription
- Ligand-dependent negative regulation of transcription

The remainder of this chapter describes these mechanisms.

Ligand-Dependent Activation

Ligand-dependent activation is the most well-understood function of nuclear receptors and their ligands. In this case, the ligand-bound receptor increases transcription of a target gene to which it is bound. The DBD serves to bring the receptor domains that mediate transcriptional activation to a specific gene. Transcriptional activation itself is mediated primarily by the LBD, which can function in the same way even when it is transferred to a DNA-binding protein that is not

Table 4–3. Determinants of Target Gene Specificity Of Nuclear Receptors

Specificity	Region of Receptor
1. Binding to DNA	1. DNA-binding domain (DBD, C domain)
2. Binding to specific hexamer (AGGTCA vs. AGAACA)	2. P-box in C-domain
3. Binding to sequences 5′ to hexamer	3. C-terminal extension of DBD
4. Binding to hexamer repeats	4. Dimerization domain (C domain for steroid receptors, D-E-F for others)
5. Recognition of hexamer spacing	5. Heterodimerization with retinoid X receptor (RXR) (nonsteroid receptors, C domain)

related to nuclear receptors. The *activation function* (AF) of the LBD is referred to as AF-2 (see Fig. 4–2).

Gene transcription is mediated by a large complex of factors that ultimately regulate the activity of ribonucleic acid (RNA) polymerase, the enzyme that uses the chromosomal DNA template to direct the synthesis of messenger RNA. Most mammalian genes are transcribed by RNA polymerase II, utilizing a large set of cofactor proteins, including *basal transcription factors*, and associated factors collectively referred to here as *general transcription factors* (GTFs). Details about GTFs are of fundamental importance and are available elsewhere.[32, 33]

Table 4–4. Regulation of Gene Transcription By Nuclear Receptors

1. Ligand-dependent gene activation: DNA binding and recruitment of coactivators
2. Ligand-independent gene repression: DNA binding and recruitment of corepressors
3. Ligand-dependent negative regulation of gene expression: DNA binding and recruitment of corepressors *or* recruitment of coactivators off DNA

The ligand-bound nuclear receptor communicates stimulatory signals to GTFs on the gene to which it is bound. This process involves recruiting positively acting cofactors, called *coactivators*.[34] These coactivators bind to the nuclear receptor on DNA only when hormone or ligand is bound. Thus, these coactivators specifically recognize the ligand-bound conformation of the LBD.

The most important determinant of coactivator binding is the position of H12, which changes dramatically when ligands bind receptors (see Fig. 4–3). Along with H3, H4, and H5, H12 forms a hydrophobic cleft that is bound by short polypeptide regions of the coactivator molecules.[35–37] These polypeptides, called *NR boxes*, have characteristic sequences of LxxLL, where L is leucine and xx can be any two amino acids.[38] A number of coactivator proteins containing LxxLL

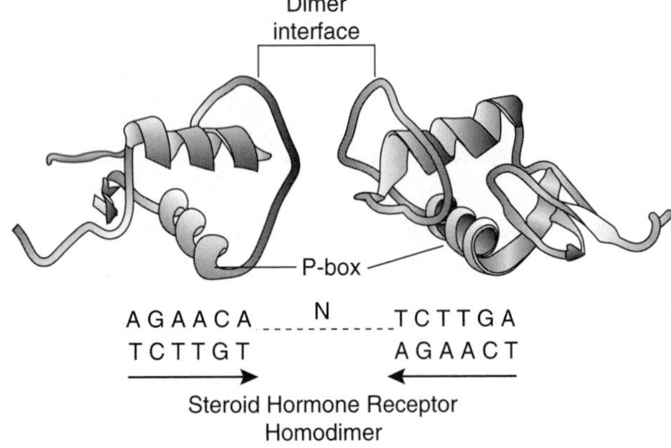

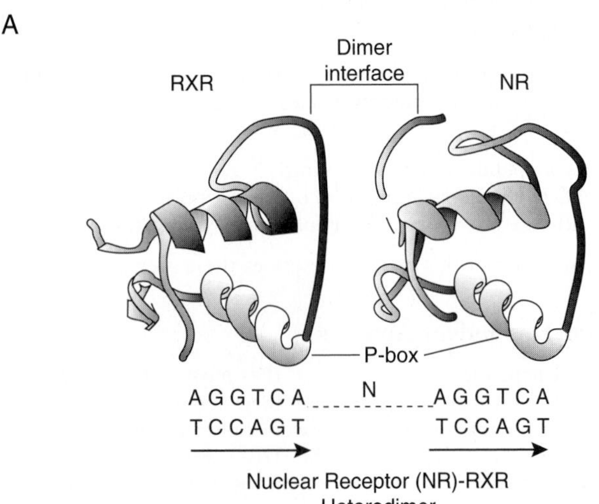

Figure 4–4. Structural basis of nuclear receptor (NR) DNA binding specificity. Ribbon diagrams of receptor DNA-binding domains (DBDs) are shown. *A*, Steroid hormone receptor binding as homodimer to inverted repeat (*arrows*) of AGAACA half-site. *B*, RXR-NR heterodimer binding to direct repeat of AGGTCA. The position of the P-box, the region of the DBD that makes direct contact with DNA, is shown. N, number of base pairs between the two half-sites; RXR, retinoid X receptor.

Table 4–5. Nuclear Receptor Coactivators and Corepressors

Coactivators
1. Chromatin remodeling
Swi/Snf complex
2. Histone acetyl transferase
p160 family (SRC-1, GRIP-1, pCIP)
p300/CBP
pCAF (p300/CBP–associated factor)
3. Activation
TRAP/DRIP (thyroid receptor–associated proteins/D receptor interacting proteins)
Corepressors
N-CoR (nuclear receptor corepressor)
SMRT (silencing mediator for retinoid and thyroid hormone receptors)

CBP, calcium-binding protein; SRC-1, steroid receptor coactivator 1; GRIP-1, glucocorticoid receptor interacting protein-1; pCIP, CBP interacting protein.

motifs that bind to liganded nuclear receptors have been described (Table 4–5).[34, 39]

Coactivators increase the rate of gene transcription. This is accomplished by enzymatic functions, including DNA unwinding activity as well as histone acetyltransferase (HAT) activity.[40] HAT activity is critically important for activation because chromosomal DNA is tightly wrapped around nucleosomal units composed of core histone proteins. Acetylation of lysine tails on histones "opens up" this chromatin structure.[41]

The best understood class of coactivator proteins is the so-called p160 family, whose name is based on their size (~160 kd).[42] There are at least three such molecules, each with numerous names (see Table 4–5).[34, 43] These factors possess HAT activity and also recruit other coactivators (CBP and p300), which are also HATs.[44] A third HAT, called p300/CBP–associated factor (pCAF), is also recruited by liganded receptors.[45] Together these HATs along with a complex of molecules called Swi/Snf, which directs adenosine triphosphate (ATP)–dependent DNA unwinding, create a chromatin structure that favors transcription (Fig. 4–5).

It is possible that the recruitment of multiple HATs reflects different specificities for core histones and potentially other, nonhistone proteins. Some HATs also interact directly with GTFs and further enhance their activities. An important complex that also links nuclear receptors to GTFs is the TRAP (TR-associated proteins) or DRIP (D receptor–associated proteins) complex.[46, 47]

Repression of Gene Expression by Unliganded Receptor

Although DNA binding is ligand-dependent for steroid hormone receptors, other nuclear receptors are bound to DNA even in the absence of their cognate ligand. The unliganded DNA-bound receptor is not passively waiting for hormone; instead, it actively represses transcription of the target gene. This repression both "turns off" the target gene and amplifies the magnitude of the subsequent activation by hormone or ligand. For instance, if the level of gene transcription in the repressed state is 10% of the basal level in the absence of receptor, a hormone-activation to 10-fold above that basal level represents a 100-fold difference of transcription rate between hormone-deficient (repressed) genes and hormone-activated genes (Fig. 4–6).[48]

In many ways, the molecular mechanism of repression is the mirror image of ligand-dependent activation. The unliganded nuclear receptor recruits negatively acting factors *(corepressors)* to the target gene. The two major corepressors are large (~270 kd) proteins[49, 50]:

- Nuclear receptor corepressor (N-CoR)
- Silencing mediator for retinoid and thyroid receptors (SMRT)

N-CoR and SMRT specifically recognize the unliganded conformation of nuclear receptors and use an amphipathic helical sequence similar to the NR box of coactivators to bind to a hydrophobic pocket in the receptor.

For corepressors, the peptide responsible for receptor binding is called the *CoRNR box* and contains the sequence (I or L) xx (I or V)I (where I is isoleucine, L is leucine, V is valine, and xx represents any two amino acids).[51] The receptor utilizes helices 3 to 5 to form the hydrophobic pocket, as in coactivator binding, but H12 does not promote and even hinders corepressor binding. This negative role of H12 highlights the role of the ligand-dependent change in the position of H12 as the switch that determines repression and activation by nuclear receptors (see Fig. 4–5).[52]

The transcriptional functions of N-CoR and SMRT are the opposite of those of the coactivators. The corepressors themselves do not possess enzyme activity but do recruit multiple histone deacetylases (HDAC) to the target gene, thereby reversing the effects of histone acetylation described earlier and leading to a compact, repressed state of chromatin. The corepressors also interact directly with GTFs to inhibit their transcriptional activities.

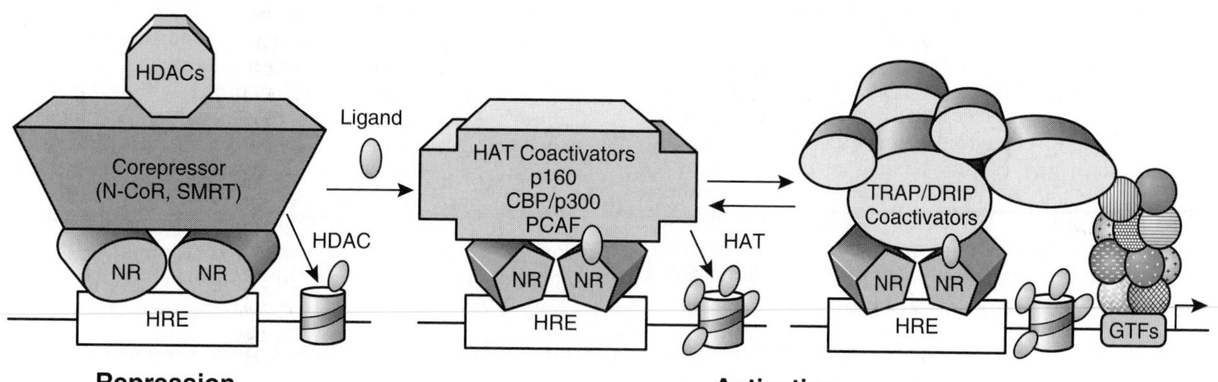

Figure 4–5. Coactivators and corepressors in transcriptional regulation by nuclear receptors. CBP, calcium-binding protein; DRIP, D receptor–interacting protein; HRE, hormone response element; HAT, histone acetyltransferase; HDAC, histone deacylase; N-CoR, nuclear receptor corepressor; NR, nuclear receptor; PCAF, p300/CBP–associated factor; SMRT, silencing mediator of retinoid and thyroid receptors; TRAP, thyroid hormone receptor–associated protein.

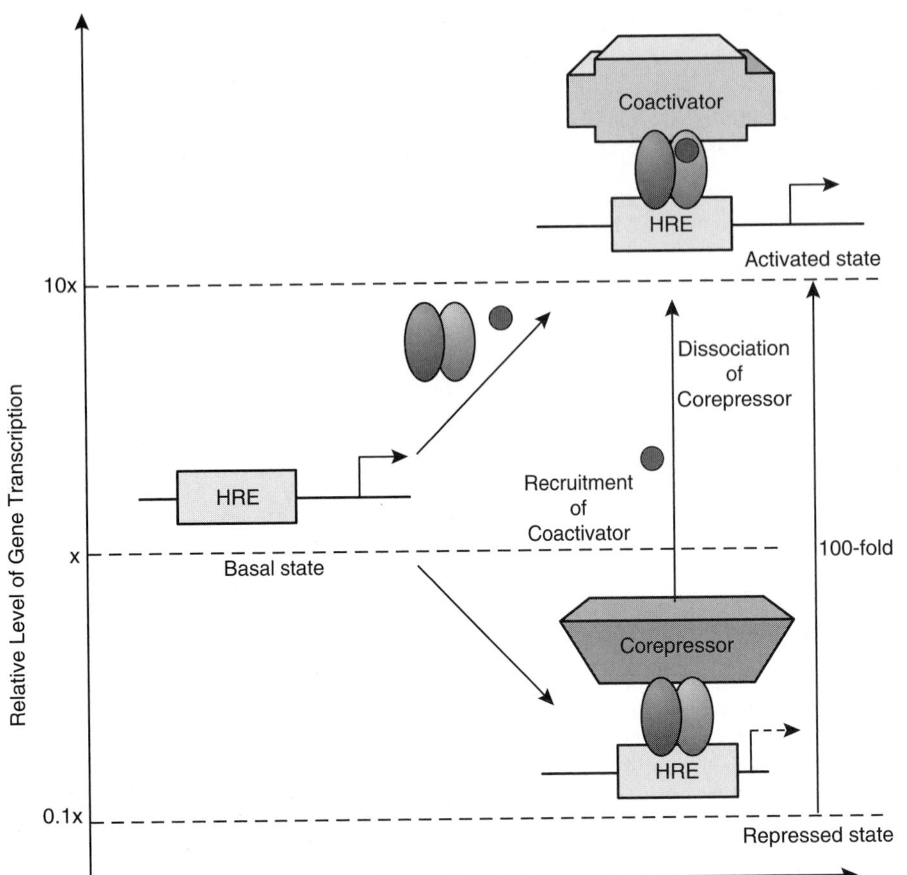

Figure 4–6. Repression and activation functions augmenting the dynamic range of transcriptional regulation by nuclear receptors. HRE, hormone response element.

Ligand-Dependent Negative Regulation of Gene Expression (Transrepression)

The ligand-dependent switch between the repressed and activated receptor conformations explains how hormones activate gene expression. However, many of the most important gene targets of hormones are turned off in the presence of the ligand. This is referred to as ligand-dependent negative regulation of transcription, or *transrepression*, to distinguish it from the repression of basal transcription by unliganded receptors.

The mechanism of negative regulation is less well understood than ligand-dependent activation, and, indeed, there may be more than one mechanism. One mechanism involves nuclear receptor binding to DNA binding sites that reverse the paradigm of ligand-dependent activation (*negative response elements*). Ligand-bound receptors recruit corepressors and HDAC activity to such binding sites.[53] For example, when the unliganded TR binds to the negative response element of the gene for the β subunit of thyroid-stimulating hormone (TSH), transcription is activated. Ligand binding recruits corepressors and HDAC to the TR and leads to suppression of transcription.[54] In other cases, it has been postulated that negative regulation may result from ligand binding to nuclear receptors that bind to other transcription factors without binding DNA. This interaction leads to removal of coactivators such as p300 and CBP from the other transcription factors that positively regulate the gene.[55] In this model, inhibition of the activity of the positively acting factors results in the observed negative regulation.

Table 4–6. Factors Modulating Receptor Activity in Different Tissues

Receptor concentration
Ligand concentration
Ligand function (agonist, partial agonist, antagonist)
Concentrations and types of coactivators and corepressors
Phosphorylation state of nuclear receptor

Role of Other Nuclear Receptor Domains

The N-terminal A/B domain of the nuclear receptors is the most variable region among all members of the superfamily in terms of length and amino acid sequence. Even subtypes of the same receptor often have completely different A/B domains. The function of this domain is least well defined. It is not required for unliganded repression or ligand-dependent activation. In many receptors, the A/B domain contains a positive transcriptional activity, often referred to as AF-1 (see Fig. 4–2), that is ligand-independent but probably interacts with coactivators[56] and may influence the magnitude of activation by agonists or partial agonists (see later). This activation function is tissue-specific and tends to be more important for steroid hormone receptors, whose A/B domains are notably longer than those of other members of the superfamily. The F domain of the nuclear receptors is hypervariable in length and sequence, and its function is not known.

Cross-talk with Other Signaling Pathways

Hormones and cytokines that signal via cell surface receptors also regulate gene transcription, often by activating protein kinases that phosphorylate transcription factors such as *cAMP-response element–binding protein* (CREB). Such signals can also lead to phosphorylation of nuclear receptors. Multiple signal-dependent kinases can phosphorylate nuclear receptors, leading to conformational changes that regulate function.[57] Phosphorylation can lead to changes in DNA binding, ligand binding, or coactivator binding; these variable consequences depend on the specific kinase, receptor, and domain of the receptor that is phosphorylated. The properties of coactivators and corepressor molecules are also regulated by phosphorylation.

Receptor Antagonists

Certain ligands function as receptor antagonists by competing with agonists for the ligand-binding site. In the case of steroid hormone receptors, the position of H12 in antagonist-bound conformation is not identical to that in the unliganded receptor or the agonist-bound receptor. H12, which itself has a sequence that resembles the NR box, binds to the coactivator-binding pocket and thereby prevents coactivator binding.[37, 58] This antagonist-bound conformation also favors corepressor binding to steroid hormone receptors.

Tissue-Selective Ligands

Some ligands function as antagonists in some tissues but as full or partial agonists in others. These *selective receptor modulators* include compounds such as tamoxifen, a selective estrogen receptor modulator (SERM). SERMs are estrogen receptor antagonists with respect to the functions of AF-2, including coactivator binding, and require the AF-1 function for their agonist activity.[59] Such agonism, like AF-1 activity, tends to be tissue-specific and therefore has great therapeutic utility.

In addition to drugs, certain endogenous ligands (e.g., testosterone, DHT) also mediate tissue-specific effects. The molecular basis of tissue-specific activity is not well understood but is probably due to the expression or activity of transcriptional cofactors that differentiate between receptors bound to different ligands. Table 4–6 summarizes factors contributing to tissue-specificity of receptor activity.

References

Nuclear Receptors and Ligands

1. Abe T, Kakyo M, Sakagami H, et al. Molecular characterization and tissue distribution of a new organic anion transporter subtype (oatp3) that transports thyroid hormones and taurocholate and comparison with oatp2. J Biol Chem 1998; 273:22395–22401.
2. Escriva H, Delaunay F, Laudet V. Ligand binding and nuclear receptor evolution. Bioessays 2000; 22:717–727.
3. Arriza JL, Weinberger C, Cerelli G, et al. Cloning of human mineralocorticoid receptor complementary cDNA: structure and functional kinship with the glucocorticoid receptor. Science 1987; 237:268–275.
4. Mangelsdorf DJ, Evans RM. The RXR heterodimers and orphan receptors. Cell 1995; 83:841–850.
5. Chambon P. A decade of molecular biology of retinoic acid receptors. FASEB J 1996; 10:940–954.
6. Nagpal S, Chandraratna RA. Recent developments in receptor-selective retinoids. Curr Pharm Des 2000; 6:919–931.
7. Peet DJ, Janowski BA, Mangelsdorf DJ. The LXRs: a new class of oxysterol receptors. Curr Opin Genet Dev 1998; 8:571–575.
8. Repa JJ, Mangelsdorf DJ. Nuclear receptor regulation of cholesterol and bile acid metabolism. Curr Opin Biotech 1999; 10:557–563.
9. Desvergne B, Wahli W. Peroxisome proliferator-activated receptors: nuclear control of metabolism. Endocr Rev 1999; 20:649–688.
10. Rosen ED, Spiegelman BM. Transcriptional regulation of adipogenesis. Genes Dev 2000; 14:1293–1307.
11. Rangwala SM, Lazar MA. Transcriptional control of adipogenesis. Ann Rev Nutr 2000; 8:535–559.
12. Lehmann JM, Moore LB, Smith-Oliver TA, et al. An antidiabetic thiazolidinedione is a high affinity ligand for the nuclear peroxisome proliferator-activated receptor g (PPARg). J Biol Chem 1995; 270:12953–12956.
13. Reginato MJ, Lazar MA. Mechanisms by which thiazolidinediones potentiate insulin action. Trends Endocrinol Metab 1999; 10:9–13.
14. Waxman DJ. P450 gene induction by structurally diverse xenochemicals: central role of nuclear receptors CAR, PXR, and PPAR. Arch Biochem Biophys 1999; 369:11–23.
15. Xie W, Barwick JL, Downes M, et al. Xenoregulation of cytochrome P450 gene by nuclear receptor PXR/SXR. Nature 2000; 406:435–439.
16. Wei P, Zhang J, Egan-Hafley M, et al. The nuclear receptor CAR mediates specific xenobiotic induction of drug metabolism. Nature 2000; 407:920–923.
17. Enmark E, Gustafsson J-A. Orphan nuclear receptors—the first eight years. Mol Endocrinol 1996; 10:1293–1307.
18. Giguere V. Orphan nuclear receptors: from gene to function. Endocr Rev 1999; 20:689–725.
19. Webster JC, Cidlowski JA. Mechanisms of glucocorticoid-receptor-mediated repression of gene expression. Trends Endocrinol Metab 1999; 10:396–402.
20. Zhang J, Lazar MA. The mechanism of action of thyroid hormone receptors. Ann Rev Physiol 2000; 62:439–466.
21. Achermann JC, Jameson JL. Fertility and infertility: genetic contributions from the hypothalamic-pituitary-gonadal axis. Mol Endocrinol 1999; 13:812–818.
22. Seol W, Choi HS, Moore DD. An orphan nuclear hormone receptor that lacks a DNA binding domain and heterodimerizes with other receptors. Science 1996; 272:1336–1339.

Nuclear Receptor Mutations

23. Weiss RE, Refetoff S. Thyroid hormone resistance. Ann Rev Med 1992; 43:363–375.
24. Haussler MR, Haussler CA, Jurutka PW, et al. The vitamin D hormone and its nuclear receptor: molecular actions and disease states. J Endocrinol 1997; 154:S57–S73.
25. McPhaul MJ, Marcelli M, Zoppi S, et al. Genetic basis of endocrine disease. 4. The spectrum of mutations in the androgen receptor gene that causes androgen resistance. J Clin Endocrinol Metab 1993; 76:17–23.
26. Stewart PM, Krozowski ZS. 11 beta-hydroxysteroid dehydrogenase. Vitam Horm 1999; 57:249–324.

Structure and Function of Nuclear Receptors

27. Moras D, Gronemeyer H. The nuclear receptor ligand-binding domain: structure and function. Curr Opin Cell Biol 1998; 10:384–391.
28. Weatherman RV, Fletterick RJ, Scanlan TS. Nuclear receptor ligands and ligand-binding domains. Ann Rev Biochem 1999; 68:559–581.
29. Zhao Q, Khorasanizadeh S, Miyoshi Y, et al. Structural elements of an orphan nuclear receptor-DNA complex. Mol Cell 1998; 1:849–861.
30. Umesono K, Murakami KK, Thompson CC, et al. Direct repeats as selective response elements for the thyroid hormone, retinoic acid, and vitamin D3 receptors. Cell 1991; 65:1255–1266.
31. Rastinejad F, Perlmann T, Evans RM, et al. Structural determinants of nuclear receptor assembly on DNA direct repeats. Nature 1995; 375:203–211.
32. Roeder RG. Role of general and gene-specific cofactors in the regulation of eukaryotic transcription. Cold Spring Harb Symp Quant Biol 1998; 63:201–218.
33. Reinberg D, Orphanides G, Ebright R, et al. The RNA polymerase II general transcription factors: past, present, and future. Cold Spring Harb Symp Quant Biol 1998; 63:83–103.
34. McKenna NJ, Lanz RB, O'Malley BW. Nuclear receptor coregulators: cellular and molecular biology. Endocr Rev 1999; 20:321–44.
35. Feng W, Ribeiro RCJ, Wagner RL, et al. Hormone-dependent coactivator binding to a hydrophobic cleft on nuclear receptors. Science 1998; 280:1747–1749.
36. Nolte RT, Wisely GB, Westin S, et al. Ligand binding and co-activator assembly of the peroxisome prolierator-activated receptor-g. Nature 1998; 395:137–143.

37. Shiau AK, Barstad D, Loria PM, et al. The structural basis of estrogen receptor/coactivator recognition and the antagonism of this interaction by tamoxifen. Cell 1998; 95:927–937.
38. Heery DM, Kalkhoven E, Hoare S, et al. A signature motif in transcriptional co-activators mediates binding to nuclear receptors. Nature 1997; 387:733–736.
39. Freedman LP. Increasing the complexity of coactivation in nuclear receptor signaling. Cell 1999; 97:5–8.
40. Belotserkovskaya R, Berger SL. Interplay between chromatin modifying and remodeling complexes in transcriptional regulation. Crit Rev Eukaryot Gene Expr 1999; 9:221–230.
41. Kuo MH, Allis CD. Roles of histone acetyltransferases and deacetylases in gene regulation. Bioessays 1998; 20:615–626.
42. Halachmi S, Marden E, Martin G, et al. Estrogen receptor–associated proteins: possible mediators of hormone-induced transcription. Science 1994; 264:1455–1458.
43. Glass CK, Rose DW, Rosenfeld MG. Nuclear receptor coactivators. Curr Opin Cell Biol 1997; 9:222–232.
44. Chrivia JC, Kwok RP, Lamb N, et al. Phosphorylated CREB binds specifically to the nuclear protein CBP. Nature 1993; 365: 855–859.
45. Blanco JC, Minucci S, Lu J, et al. The histone acetylase PCAF is a nuclear receptor coactivator. Genes Dev 1998; 12:1638–1651.
46. Rachez C, Suldan Z, Ward J, et al. A novel protein complex that interacts with the vitamin D3 receptor in a ligand-dependent manner and enhances VDR transactivation in a cell-free system. Genes Dev 1998; 12:1787–1800.
47. Ito M, Yuan CX, Malik S, et al. Identity between TRAP and SMCC complexes indicates novel pathways for the function of nuclear receptors and diverse mammalian activators. Mol Cell 1999; 3:361–370.
48. Hu X, Lazar MA. Transcriptional repression by nuclear hormone receptors. Trends Endocrinol Metab 2000; 11:6–10.
49. Horlein AJ, Naar AM, Heinzel T, et al. Ligand-independent repression by the thyroid hormone receptor mediated by a nuclear receptor co-repressor. Nature 1995; 377:397–404.
50. Chen JD, Evans RM. A transcriptional co-repressor that interacts with nuclear hormone receptors. Nature 1995; 377:454–457.
51. Hu X, Lazar MA. The CoRNR motif contols the recruitment of corepressors to nuclear hormone receptors. Nature 1999; 402:93–936.
52. Glass CK, Rosenfeld MG. The coregulator exchange in transcriptional functions of nuclear receptors. Genes Dev 2000; 14:121–141.
53. Sasaki S, Lesoon-Wood LA, Dey A, et al. Ligand-induced recruitment of a histone deacetylase in the negative-feedback regulation of thyrotropin beta gene. EMBO J 1999; 18:5389–5398.
54. Steinfelder HJ, Wondisford FE. Thyrotropin (TSH) beta-subunit gene expression: an example for the complex regulation of pituitary hormone genes. Exp Clin Endocrinol Diabetes 1997; 105: 196–203.
55. Kamei Y, Xu L, Heinzel T, et al. A CBP integrator complex mediates transcriptional activation and AP-1 inhibition by nuclear receptors. Cell 1996; 85:403–414.
56. McInerney EM, Tsai MJ, O'Malley BW, et al. Analysis of estrogen receptor transcriptional enhancement by a nuclear hormone receptor coactivator. Proc Natl Acad Sci U S A 1996; 93:10069–10073.
57. Shao D, Lazar MA. Modulating nuclear receptor function: may the phos be with you. J Clin Invest 1999; 103:1617–1618.
58. Brzozowski AM, Pike AC, Dauter Z, et al. Molecular basis of agonism and antagonism in the oestrogen receptor. Nature 1997; 389:753–758.
59. Osborne CK, Zaho H, Fuqua SA. Selective estrogen receptor modulators: structure, function, and clinical use. J Clin Oncol 2000; 18:3172–3186.

5 Mechanism of Action of Hormones That Act at the Cell Surface

Allen Spiegel, Christin Carter-Su, and
Simeon Taylor

Hormones are secreted into the blood and act upon target cells at a distance from the secretory gland. In order to respond to a hormone, a target cell must contain the essential components of a signaling pathway. First, there must be a receptor to bind the hormone. Second, there must be an effector—for example, an enzymatic activity—that is regulated when the hormone binds to its receptor. Finally, there must be appropriate downstream signaling pathways to mediate the physiologic responses to the hormone. In fact, this type of mechanism involving receptors, effectors, and downstream signaling pathways is quite general and also functions in nonendocrine systems such as neurotransmitters, cytokines, and paracrine and autocrine factors. This chapter reviews several examples of endocrine signaling pathways, with particular attention to the molecular mechanisms that function in normal physiology and to the molecular pathology causing disease.

RECEPTORS

Definition and Classification

There are two essential functions that define hormone receptors: (1) the ability to bind the hormone and (2) the ability to couple hormone binding to hormone action. Both components of the definition are essential; for example, many hormones bind to binding proteins, which are distinct from receptors because the binding proteins do not trigger the signaling pathways that mediate hormone action.

Many classes of receptors are of interest in endocrinology. Some receptors are located within the cell and function as transcription factors (e.g., receptors for steroid and thyroid hormones). Other receptors are located on the cell surface and function primarily to transport their ligands into the cell by a process referred to as receptor-mediated endocytosis (e.g., low-density lipoprotein receptors). In this chapter, we focus upon cell-surface receptors that trigger intracellular signaling pathways. These cell-surface receptors can be classified according to the molecular mechanisms by which they accomplish their signaling function:

1. Ligand-gated ion channels (e.g., nicotinic acetylcholine receptor).
2. Receptor tyrosine kinases (e.g., receptors for insulin and insulin-like growth factor I).
3. Receptor serine/threonine kinases (e.g., receptors for activins and inhibins).
4. Receptor guanylate cyclase (e.g., atrial natriuretic factor receptor).
5. G protein–coupled receptors (e.g., receptors for adrenergic agents, muscarinic cholinergic agents, glycoprotein hormones, glucagon, and parathyroid hormone).
6. Cytokine receptors (e.g., receptors for growth hormone, prolactin, and leptin).

The receptors belonging to classes 1 to 4 are bifunctional molecules that can bind hormone and also serve as effectors by functioning either as ion channels or as enzymes. In contrast, the receptors belonging to classes 5 and 6 have the ability to bind the hormone but must recruit a separate molecule to catalyze the effector function. For example, as the name implies, G protein–coupled receptors utilize G proteins to regulate downstream effector molecules. Similarly, cytokine receptors recruit cytosolic tyrosine kinases (e.g., Janus family tyrosine kinases, JAKs) as effectors to trigger downstream signaling pathways.

Hormone Binding

As predicted by the fact that hormones circulate in relatively low concentrations in the plasma, the binding interaction between a hormone and its receptor is characterized by high binding affinity. Furthermore, hormone binding has a high degree of specificity. Generally, the receptor binds its cognate hormone more tightly than it binds other hormones. However, some receptors may bind structurally related hormones with lower affinity. For example, the insulin receptor binds insulin-like growth factors (IGFs) with approximately 100-fold lower affinity than it binds insulin. Similarly, the thyrotropin receptor binds human chorionic gonadotropin with lower affinity than it binds thyrotropin. This phenomenon has been referred to as *specificity spillover* and provides an explanation of several pathologic conditions, such as hypoglycemia caused by tumors secreting IGF-II and hyperthyroidism associated with choriocarcinoma.[1]

Binding of a hormone (H) to its receptor (R) can be described mathematically as an equilibrium reaction:

$$\mathrm{H} + \mathrm{R} \leftrightarrows \mathrm{HR}$$

At equilibrium, $K_a = (RH)/(H)(R)$, where K_a is the association constant for the formation of the hormone receptor complex (HR). As originally shown by Scatchard, it is possible to rearrange this equation in terms of the total concentration of receptor binding sites, $R_0 = (R) + (RH)$, as follows:

$$K_a = (RH)/\{[R_o - (RH)](H)\}$$

$$(RH) = K_a[R_o - (RH)](H)$$

$$(RH)/(H) = K_aR_o - K_a(RH)$$

A straight line is obtained when (RH)/(H) (i.e., the ratio of bound to free hormone) is plotted as a function of (RH) (the concentration of bound hormone). The slope of the line is $-K_a$, and the line intercepts the horizontal axis at the point where $(HR) = R_0 =$ the total number of binding sites. This type of plot is referred to as a Scatchard plot and has been used as a graphic method to estimate the affinity with which a receptor binds its hormone. Although the binding properties of some receptors are described more or less accurately by these simple equations, other receptors exhibit more complex properties. This simple algebraic derivation of the Scatchard equation implicitly assumes that there is only one class of receptors and that the binding sites on the receptors do not interact with one another. If these assumptions do not apply to the interaction of a particular hormone with its receptor, the Scatchard plot may not be linear.

Several molecular mechanisms may contribute to nonlinearity of the Scatchard plot. For example, there may be more than one type of receptor that binds the hormone (e.g., a high-affinity, low-capacity site and a low-affinity, high-capacity site). Alternatively, some receptors have more than one binding site, and there may be cooperative interactions among the binding sites (e.g., the insulin receptor). In addition, the interaction between a G protein and a G protein–coupled receptor may affect the affinity with which the receptor binds its ligand; moreover, the effect on binding affinity depends on whether guanosine diphosphate (GDP) or guanosine triphosphate (GTP) is bound to the G protein. However, a detailed discussion of these complexities is beyond the scope of this chapter.

REGULATION OF HORMONE SENSITIVITY

Early in the history of endocrinology, attention was focused on the regulation of hormone secretion as the most important mechanism for regulating physiology. However, it has become apparent that the target cell is not passive. Rather, there are many influences that can alter the sensitivity of the target cell's response to a given concentration of hormone. For example, the number of receptors can be regulated. All things being equal, hormone sensitivity is directly related to the number of hormone receptors expressed on the cell surface. In addition, post-translational modifications of the receptor can modify either the affinity of hormone binding or the efficiency of coupling to downstream signaling pathways. Moreover, all of the downstream components in the hormone action pathway are subject to similar types of regulatory influences, which can have a significant impact on the ability of the target cell to respond to hormone.

Just as hormone sensitivity is subject to normal physiologic regulation, pathologic influences can cause disease by targeting components of the hormone action pathway. Multiple etiologic factors can impair the hormone action pathway, such as genetic, autoimmune, and exogenous toxins. For example, disease mechanisms can alter the functions of cell-surface receptors, effectors such as G proteins, and other components of the downstream signaling pathways. This chapter describes several examples illustrating these principles.

RECEPTOR TYROSINE KINASES

Receptor tyrosine kinases have several structural features in common: an extracellular domain containing the ligand-binding site, a single transmembrane domain, and an intracellular portion that includes the tyrosine kinase catalytic domain (Fig. 5–1). Analysis of the sequence of the human genome suggests that there are approximately 100 receptor tyrosine kinases. The tyrosine kinase domain is the most highly conserved sequence among all the receptors in this family. In contrast, there is considerable variation among the sequences of the extracellular domains. Indeed, the family of receptor tyrosine kinases can be classified into 16 subfamilies, primarily on the basis of the differences in the structure of the extracellular domain.[2] Furthermore, receptor tyrosine kinases mediate the biologic actions of a wide variety of ligands, including insulin, epidermal growth factor (EGF), platelet-derived growth factor (PDGF), and vascular endothelial cell–derived growth factor. The variation in the sequences of the extracellular domains enables the receptors to bind this structurally diverse collection of ligands.

The EGF receptor was the first cell-surface receptor demonstrated to possess tyrosine kinase activity[3] and also the first receptor tyrosine kinase to be cloned.[4] Like most receptor tyrosine kinases, the EGF receptor exists primarily as a monomer in the absence of ligand. However, binding of ligand induces receptor dimerization. As discussed later in this chapter, ligand-induced dimerization is central to the mechanism whereby the receptor mediates the biologic activity of EGF. In addition to the ability to form homodimers, the EGF receptor can form heterodimers with other members of the same subfamily of receptor tyrosine kinases. Because a small number of receptors can combine in a large number of pairings, heterodi-

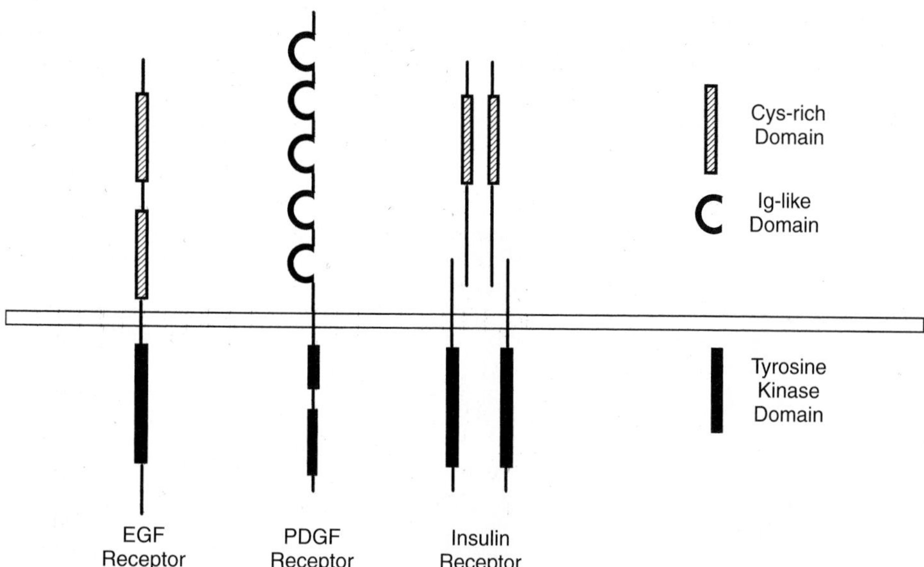

Figure 5–1. Receptor tyrosine kinases. This diagram illustrates 3 of the 16 families of receptor tyrosine kinases.[2, 99] All receptor tyrosine kinases possess an extracellular domain containing the ligand-binding site, a single transmembrane domain, and an intracellular domain containing the tyrosine kinase domain. Several structural motifs (i.e., cysteine-rich domain, immunoglobulin-like domain, tyrosine kinase domain) in these receptor tyrosine kinases are indicated on the right side of the figure. Cys, cysteine; EGF, epidermal growth factor; Ig, immunoglobulin; PDGF, platelet-derived growth factor.

mer formation has the potential to fine-tune the specificity of receptors with respect to both ligand binding and downstream signaling.

The insulin receptor is of special interest to endocrinologists because diabetes is among the most common diseases of the endocrine system. Furthermore, the insulin receptor closely resembles the type 1 receptor for IGFs.[5] This is the receptor that mediates the biologic actions of IGF-I and therefore also plays an important role in the physiology of growth hormone (GH) in vivo. Although the kinase domains of receptors for insulin and IGF-I closely resemble other receptor tyrosine kinases, at least two distinctive features set them apart. First, the receptors are synthesized as proreceptors that undergo proteolytic cleavage into two subunits (α and β). The α subunit contains the ligand-binding site; the β subunit includes the transmembrane and tyrosine kinase domains. Second, both receptors exist as $\alpha_2\beta_2$ heterotetramers that are stabilized by intersubunit disulfide bonds. In contrast to other receptor tyrosine kinases, which are thought to dimerize in response to ligand binding, the insulin receptor exists as a dimer of $\alpha\beta$ monomers even in the absence of ligand. The remainder of this section reviews the molecular mechanisms whereby receptor tyrosine kinases mediate biologic action, with special emphasis on the insulin receptor as an illustrative example.

Receptor Activation: Role of Receptor Dimerization

Dimerization plays a central role in the mechanism whereby most receptor tyrosine kinases are activated by their cognate ligands.[2, 6] Although receptor dimerization is a common theme, the detailed molecular mechanisms differ from receptor to receptor. The following are three examples of the mechanisms of receptor dimerization (Fig. 5–2):

Dimeric Ligand

PDGF and vascular endothelial cell–derived growth factor are examples of dimeric ligands (see Fig. 5–2).[70–9] Because each subunit of ligand can bind one receptor molecule, simul-

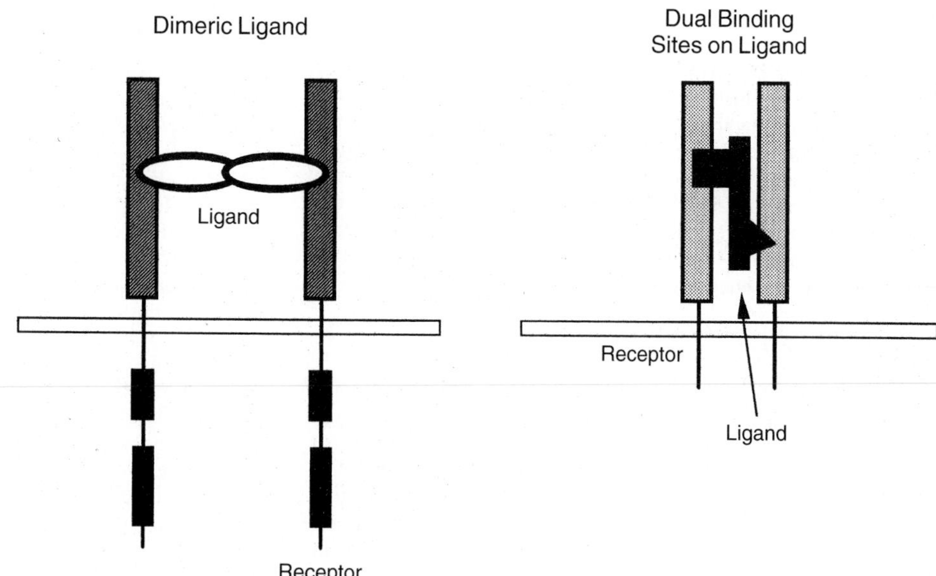

Figure 5–2. Ligand-induced dimerization of receptors. Two molecular mechanisms of ligand-induced receptor dimerization are illustrated. In the case of the platelet-derived growth factor, the ligand is dimeric and therefore contains two receptor binding sites.[7, 8] In the case of growth hormone, a single ligand molecule contains two binding sites so that it can bind simultaneously to two receptor molecules.[10–12]

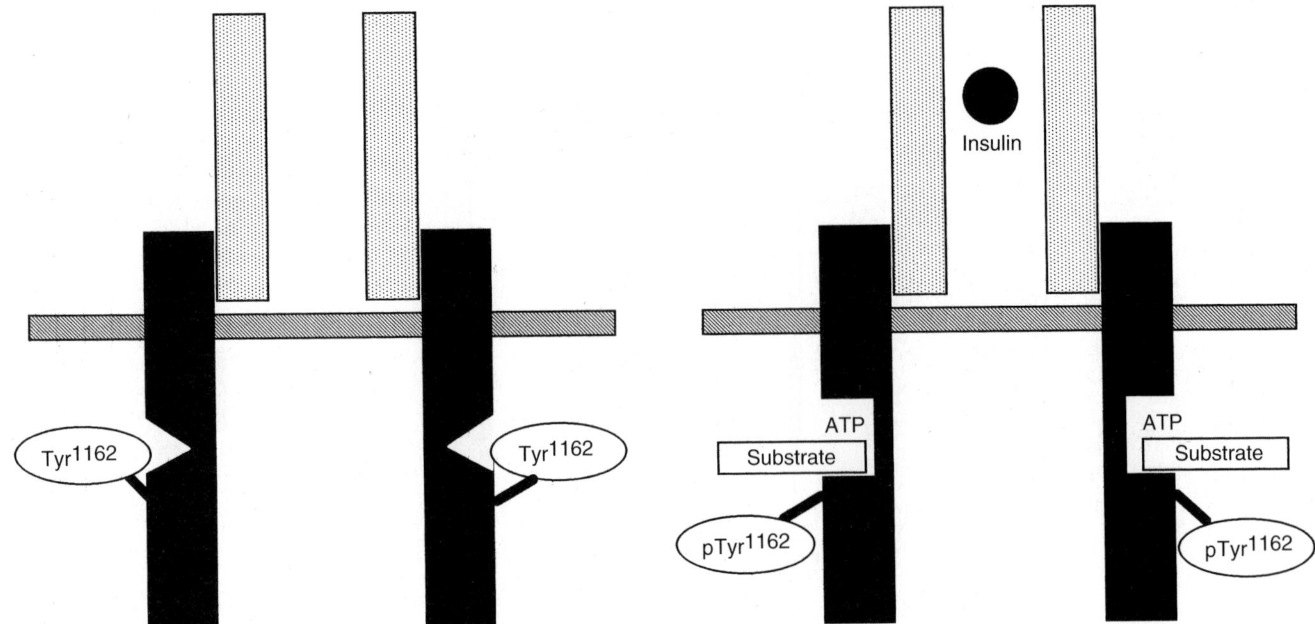

Figure 5–3. Phosphorylation of tyrosine residues in the activation loop leads to activation of the insulin receptor tyrosine kinase. A hypothetical mechanism for ligand-stimulated activation of the insulin receptor tyrosine kinase is illustrated. The model is based on the three-dimensional structure of the isolated insulin receptor tyrosine kinase as determined by x-ray crystallography.[18, 19, 22] In the inactive insulin receptor kinase *(left)*, Tyr1162 blocks the active site so that substrates cannot bind. In contrast, when the tyrosine residues in the activation loop (including Tyr1162) become phosphorylated *(right)*, Tyr1162 moves out of the way, and there is a conformational change that allows binding of adenosine triphosphate (ATP) and protein substrate so that the kinase reaction can proceed.

taneous binding of two receptor molecules drives receptor dimerization. Direct support for this type of mechanism is provided by the crystal structure of vascular endothelial cell–derived growth factor bound to its receptor (Flt-1).[9]

Two Receptor Binding Sites on a Monomeric Ligand

Although this mechanism is important for many receptor tyrosine kinases, it was first shown rigorously for the GH receptor, which is not a member of the receptor tyrosine kinase family (see Fig. 5–2).[10–12] As illustrated by the crystal structure of GH bound to its receptor, one molecule of ligand can bind two molecules of receptor. In fact, there are two distinct receptor-binding sites on each GH molecule, and this enables the ligand to promote receptor dimerization. This observation has an important implication for pharmacology. By abolishing one of the two receptor-binding sites, it is possible to design mutant ligands that lack the ability to promote receptor dimerization and therefore lack the ability to trigger hormone action. Nevertheless, by binding to receptors, the mutant ligand acquires the ability to inhibit the action of the endogenous hormone. Such mutant GH molecules are being evaluated as potential therapeutic agents, for example, in conditions such as acromegaly.

Preexisting Receptor Dimers

The insulin receptor represents a paradox. The insulin receptor exists as a dimer even in the absence of ligand. (Actually, it is an $\alpha_2\beta_2$ heterotetramer, which is a *dimer* of $\alpha\beta$ monomers.) If the receptor is already dimerized, why is it not active? Although the molecular details remain to be elucidated, it seems likely that the two halves of the insulin receptor are not oriented in an optimal way to permit receptor activation in the absence of ligand. Perhaps, insulin binding triggers a conformational change that somehow mimics the effects of dimerization in other receptor tyrosine kinases. In any case, several studies have demonstrated that receptor dimerization is necessary for the ability of insulin to activate its receptor. For example, $\alpha\beta$ monomers retain the ability to bind insulin but are not activated in response to insulin binding.[13, 14] Furthermore, indirect evidence suggests that a single insulin molecule binds simultaneously to both α subunits of the insulin receptor[15, 16]; the ability to bind simultaneously to both halves of the dimeric receptor appears to be essential to the ability of insulin to activate its receptor.

Receptor Activation: Conformational Changes in the Kinase Domain

When ligand binds to the extracellular domain, it stimulates the tyrosine kinase activity of the intracellular domain. Although the detailed mechanisms of transmembrane signaling are not completely understood, considerable progress has been made in elucidating the molecular mechanisms of receptor activation. Investigations of the three-dimensional structure of the insulin receptor tyrosine kinase domain help to explain why the receptor is maintained in a low-activity state in the absence of insulin (Fig. 5–3).[17–19] In the inactive form of the insulin receptor kinase, Tyr1162 is located in a position so that it blocks protein substrates from binding to the active site. Furthermore, in the inactive state of the tyrosine kinase domain, the active site assumes a conformation that does not accommodate magnesium adenosine triphosphate (ATP). Thus, the tyrosine kinase is inactive because the active site cannot bind either of its substrates. How does insulin activate the receptor? Insulin binding triggers autophosphorylation of three tyrosine residues (Tyr1158, Tyr1162, and Tyr1163) in the "activation loop." When the three tyrosine residues in the activation loop become phosphorylated, an important conformational change occurs. As a result of the movement of the activation loop, the active site acquires the ability to bind both ATP and protein substrates. Thus, the conformational change induced by autophosphorylation activates the receptor to phosphorylate other substrates.[20, 21]

It remains unclear how this process is initiated. Because the inactive state of the tyrosine kinase cannot bind ATP, it seems unlikely that phosphorylation of Tyr1162 proceeds by a true *auto*phosphorylation mechanism. Rather, it is likely that Tyr1162 in one β subunit is transphosphorylated by the second β subunit in the $\alpha_2\beta_2$ heterotetramer molecule.[2, 22] However, this proposed mechanism poses a "chicken and egg" problem. It requires that at least one of the β subunits is active before the Tyr residues in the activation loop become phosphorylated. Perhaps the activation loop is somewhat mobile so that some molecules of unphosphorylated tyrosine kinase can assume an active conformation and initiate a chain reaction of transphosphorylation and receptor activation.

Receptor Tyrosine Kinases Phosphorylate Other Intracellular Proteins

Once activated, tyrosine kinases are capable of phosphorylating other protein substrates. Several factors determine which proteins are phosphorylated under physiologic conditions within the cell.

Amino Acid Sequence Context of Tyr Residue

Tyrosine kinases do not exhibit strict specificity with respect to the amino acid sequence of the phosphorylation site. Nevertheless, most tyrosine phosphorylation sites are located in the vicinity of acidic amino acid residues (i.e., Glu or Asp).[2]

Binding to the Tyrosine Kinase

Some protein substrates bind directly to the intracellular domain of the receptor. The binding interaction brings the substrate into close proximity to the kinase, thereby promoting phosphorylation of the substrate. For example, the insulin receptor substrate (IRS) proteins are characterized by a highly conserved phosphotyrosine-binding (PTB) domain that binds to a conserved motif (Asn-Pro-Xaa-pTyr) in the juxtamembrane domain of the insulin receptor.[23–25] Binding of the PTB domain to the insulin receptor requires phosphorylation of the Tyr residue in the Asn-Pro-Xaa-pTyr motif. This provides another mechanism (in addition to activation of the intrinsic receptor tyrosine kinase) whereby autophosphorylation of the receptor enhances phosphorylation of IRS proteins. Similarly, substrates for some tyrosine kinases contain Src homology 2 (SH2) domains, highly conserved domains that bind phosphotyrosine residues (see later). For example, the activated PDGF receptor contains a phosphotyrosine residue near its C-terminus that binds the SH2 domain of phospholipase Cγ. This enables the PDGF receptor to phosphorylate and activate phospholipase Cγ.[2, 26]

Subcellular Localization

Because receptor tyrosine kinases are located in the plasma membrane, they are in close proximity to other plasma membrane proteins. This colocalization has the potential to promote phosphorylation. For example, the insulin receptor has been reported to phosphorylate pp120/hepatocyte antigen-4 (HA4).[27, 28] Like the insulin receptor, pp120/HA4 is an integral membrane glycoprotein associated with the plasma membrane of hepatocytes. Similarly, FGF receptor substrate-2 (FRS2), a substrate of the fibroblast-derived growth factor receptor, is targeted to the plasma membrane by an N-terminal myristoylation site.[29]

Functional Significance of Tyrosine Phosphorylation

There are at least two distinct mechanisms whereby tyrosine phosphorylation regulates protein function. First, tyrosine phosphorylation can induce a conformational change in a protein, thereby altering its function. For example, as discussed earlier, phosphorylation of the three Tyr residues in the activation loop of the insulin receptor changes the conformation of the active site, thereby facilitating binding of substrates and activating the receptor tyrosine kinase.[17–19] However, most of the effects of tyrosine phosphorylation on protein function are mediated indirectly by regulating protein-protein interactions. In order to understand how tyrosine phosphorylation regulates protein-protein interactions, it is useful to review the biochemistry of c-src, the prototype of a nonreceptor tyrosine kinase. When the amino acid sequence of c-src is analyzed, it is apparent that there are three highly conserved domains in the molecule: the kinase catalytic domain and two noncatalytic domains that are referred to as src homology domains 2 and 3 (SH2 and SH3, respectively).

SH2 Domains

SH2 domains consist of conserved sequences (approximately 100 amino acid residues) that are present in many proteins that function in signaling pathways. From a functional point of view, SH2 domains share the ability to bind pTyr residues. However, individual SH2 domains vary with respect to their binding specificity. The binding affinity of an SH2 is determined by the three amino acid residues downstream from the pTyr residue. For example, the SH2 domains of phosphatidylinositol (PI) 3-kinase exhibit a preference for pTyr-(Met/Xaa)-Xaa-Met, whereas the SH2 domain of growth factor receptor binding protein 2 (Grb-2) prefers to bind pTyr-Xaa-Asn-Xaa. Thus, a given SH2 domain binds to a tyrosine-phosphorylated protein if and only if the pTyr residue is located in a context that corresponds to the binding specificity of the SH2 domain.

SH3 Domains

SH3 domains consist of conserved sequences (approximately 50 amino acid residues) that bind to proline-rich sequences. Like SH2 domains, SH3 domains are found in many proteins that function in signaling pathways.

Downstream Signaling Pathways

Receptor tyrosine kinases mediate the action of a wide variety of ligands in a wide variety of cell types. The bewildering complexity of the downstream signaling pathways corresponds to the huge number of physiologic processes that are regulated by receptor tyrosine kinases. Although it is beyond the scope of this chapter to attempt an encyclopedic review of all the downstream signaling pathways, we have selected examples to illustrate general principles.

As discussed earlier, the activated insulin receptor phosphorylates multiple substrates including IRS-1, IRS-2, IRS-3, and IRS-4.[30] Each of these substrates contains multiple tyrosine phosphorylation sites, many of which correspond to consensus sequences for SH2 domains in important signaling molecules. Thus, IRS proteins serve as docking proteins that bind SH2 domain–containing proteins. Among these, two of the most important are PI 3-kinase and Grb-2. As discussed subsequently, binding of SH2 domains triggers multiple downstream signaling pathways.

Phosphatidylinositol 3-Kinase

The catalytic subunit of PI 3-kinase (p110; molecular mass approximately 110,000) is bound to a regulatory subunit. The classical isoforms of the regulatory subunit (p85; molecular mass approximately 85,000) contain two SH2 domains, both of which bind to pTyr in the context of pTyr-(Met/Xaa)-Xaa-Met motifs. Binding of pTyr residues to both SH2 domains of p85 leads to maximal activation of PI 3-kinase catalytic activity. (Submaximal activation can be achieved with occupancy of a single SH2 domain in p85.) Because all four IRS molecules (IRS-1, IRS-2, IRS-3, and IRS-4) contain multiple tyrosine phosphorylation sites that conform to the Tyr-(Met/Xaa)-Xaa-Met consensus sequence, insulin-stimulated phosphorylation promotes binding of IRS proteins to the SH2 domains in the regulatory subunit PI 3-kinase, thereby increasing the enzymatic activity of the catalytic subunit.[31–34] Activation of PI 3-kinase triggers activation of a cascade of downstream kinases, beginning with phosphoinositide-dependent kinases 1 and 2. These phosphoinositide-dependent kinases phosphorylate and activate multiple downstream protein kinases including protein kinase B and atypical isoforms of protein kinase C.[35–41]

A large body of evidence demonstrates that the pathways downstream from PI 3-kinase mediate the metabolic activities of insulin (e.g., activation of glucose transport into skeletal muscle, activation of glycogen synthesis, and inhibition of transcription of the phosphoenolpyruvate carboxykinase gene). Among other lines of evidence, PI 3-kinase inhibitors (e.g., LY294002 and wortmannin) block the metabolic actions of insulin.[42] Similarly, overexpression of dominant negative mutants of the p85 regulatory subunit of PI 3-kinase also inhibits the metabolic actions of insulin.[35] Although it is generally agreed that activation of PI 3-kinase is necessary, it is controversial whether it is sufficient to trigger the metabolic actions of insulin. For example, a second parallel pathway may also be required. The latter pathway involves tyrosine phosphorylation of Cbl, another protein that can be phosphorylated by the insulin receptor in some cell types.[43–45]

Grb-2 and the Activation of Ras

Grb-2 is a short adaptor molecule that contains an SH2 domain[46] capable of binding to pTyr residues in several signaling molecules, for example, IRS-1 and Shc, another PTB domain–containing protein that is phosphorylated by several receptor tyrosine kinases including the insulin receptor.[47, 48] The SH2 domain of Grb-2 is flanked by two SH3 domains[46] which bind to proline-containing sequences in mSos (the mammalian homologue of *Drosophila* son-of-sevenless).[49] mSos is capable of activating Ras, a small G protein that plays an important role in intracellular signaling pathways. mSos activates Ras by catalyzing the exchange of GTP for GDP in the guanine nucleotide–binding site of Ras. This, in turn, triggers the activation of a cascade of serine/threonine-specific protein kinases including Raf, mitogen-activated protein/extracellular signal–regulated kinase (MEK), and mitogen-activated protein (MAP) kinase. These pathways downstream from Ras contribute to the ability of tyrosine kinases to promote cell growth and regulate the expression of various genes.

We have focused on the signaling pathways downstream from the insulin receptor because of the importance of insulin and IGF-I in endocrinology (Fig. 5–4). In many ways, the molecular mechanisms closely resemble those downstream from other receptor tyrosine kinases. However, the insulin signaling pathway is atypical in at least one respect. The insulin receptor phosphorylates docking proteins (e.g., IRS-1), which bind SH2 domain–containing proteins (e.g., PI 3-kinase and Grb-2). In contrast, the intracellular domains of most receptor tyrosine kinases contain binding sites for SH2 domains. For example, the SH2 domain of Grb-2 binds to pTyr716 in the activated PDGF receptor.[2] Similarly, the PDGF receptor contains two Tyr-(Met/Xaa)-Xaa-Met motifs in the kinase insert domain that bind to the two SH2 domains in the p85 subunit of PI 3-kinase.[2, 50] It is not clear why some tyrosine kinases (e.g., the PDGF receptor) activate PI 3-kinase through a direct binding interaction, whereas others (e.g., the insulin receptor) utilize an indirect mechanism involving docking proteins. However, in contrast to PDGF receptors, which are associated with the plasma membrane, IRS proteins appear to be associated with the cytoskeleton.[51] Perhaps this differential subcellular localization contributes to signaling specificity. In other words, if insulin and PDGF receptors trigger translocation of PI 3-kinase to different locations within the cell, this compartmentation may permit two different receptors to elicit different biologic responses even though both responses are mediated by the same signaling molecule (i.e., PI 3-kinase).

Off Signals: Termination of Hormone Action

Just as there are complex biochemical pathways that mediate hormone action, there are also mechanisms to terminate the biologic response. The necessity for these mechanisms is illustrated by the following example. After we eat a meal, the concentration of plasma glucose increases. This elicits an increase in insulin secretion, which in turn leads to a decrease in plasma glucose levels. If these processes went on unchecked, the level of glucose in the plasma would eventually fall so low that it would lead to symptomatic hypoglycemia. How is insulin action terminated? The answers to this question are not yet entirely clear, but several mechanisms contribute to turning off the insulin signaling pathway.

Receptor-Mediated Endocytosis

Insulin binding to its receptor triggers endocytosis of the receptor. Although most of the internalized receptors are recycled to the plasma membrane, some receptors are transported to lysosomes, where they are degraded.[52, 53] As a result, insulin binding accelerates the rate of receptor degradation, thereby down-regulating the number of receptors on the cell surface. Furthermore, endosomes contain proton pumps, which acidify the lumen; the acidic pH within the endosome promotes dissociation of insulin from its receptor. Ultimately, insulin is transported to the lysosome for degradation. In fact, receptor-mediated endocytosis is the principal mechanism whereby insulin is cleared from the plasma.[54] Binding of ligands to other receptor tyrosine kinases also triggers receptor-mediated endocytosis by similar mechanisms.

Protein Tyrosine Phosphatases

Protein phosphorylation is a dynamic process. Tyrosine kinases catalyze the phosphorylation of tyrosine residues, but there are also protein tyrosine phosphatases (PTPases) to remove the phosphates.[2] Thus, PTPases antagonize the action of tyrosine kinases. Studies with knockout mice have demonstrated that the absence of PTPase-1B is associated with increased insulin sensitivity and also protects against weight gain.[55, 56] Nevertheless, the human genome encodes a large number of PTPases, and it is an important goal of research to elucidate their physiologic functions. If one could develop selective inhibitors of the PTPases that oppose the effects of the insulin receptor tyrosine kinase, it is possible that these inhibitors would provide novel therapies for diabetes.

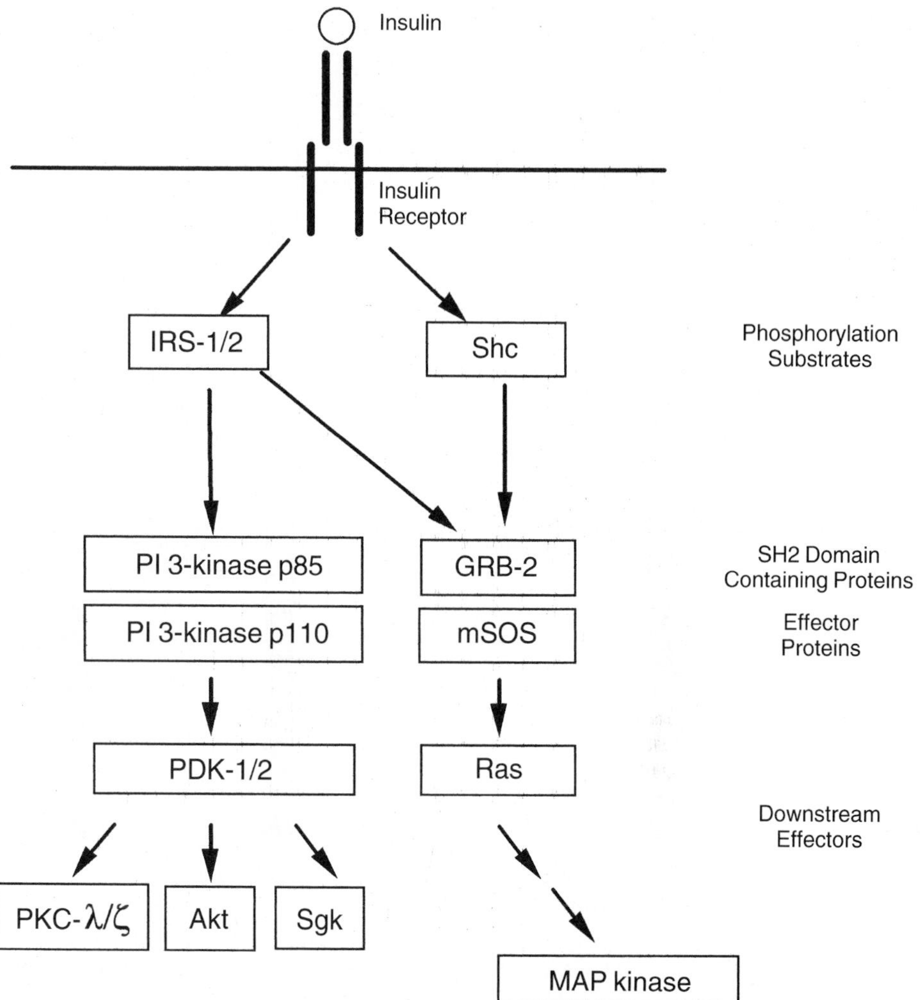

Figure 5–4. Simplified model of signaling pathways downstream from the insulin receptor. Insulin binds to the insulin receptor, thereby activating the receptor tyrosine kinase to phosphorylate tyrosine residues on insulin receptor substrates (IRSs) including IRS-1 and IRS-2.[30] Consequently, phosphotyrosine residues in IRS molecules bind to Src homology 2 (SH2) domains in molecules such as growth factor receptor–binding protein 2 (Grb-2) and the p85 regulatory subunit of phosphatidylinositol (PI) 3-kinase. These SH2 domain–containing proteins initiate two distinct branches of the signaling pathway. Activation of PI 3-kinase leads to activation of phosphoinositide-dependent kinases (PDKs) 1 and 2, which activates multiple protein kinases including Akt/protein kinase B, atypical protein kinase C (PKC) isoforms, and serum/glucocorticoid-activated protein kinases (Sgk).[100] Grb-2 interacts with m-SOS, a guanine nucleotide exchange factor that activates Ras.[101] Activation of Ras triggers a cascade of protein kinases leading to the activation of mitogen-activated protein (MAP) kinase.

Serine/Threonine Kinases

Most receptor tyrosine kinases, including the insulin receptor, are substrates for phosphorylation by Ser/Thr-specific protein kinases. Interestingly, the Ser/Thr phosphorylation appears to inhibit the action of the tyrosine kinase. Similarly, other phosphotyrosine-containing proteins are subject to inhibitory influences of Ser/Thr phosphorylation resistance. For example, it has been reported that Ser/Thr phosphorylation of IRS-1 may inhibit insulin action, thereby causing insulin resistance.[57–61]

Mechanisms of Disease

The simplest forms of endocrine disease are caused by either a deficiency or an excess of a hormone. However, hormone resistance syndromes resulting from defects in the signaling pathways can masquerade as hormone deficiency states. Similarly, diseases associated with constitutively activated receptors can mimic a state of hormone excess. In some cases, the abnormality in hormone action is genetic in origin, resulting from a mutation in a gene encoding one of the proteins in the signaling pathway. Similar syndromes can also be caused by other mechanisms; for example, there are autoimmune syndromes caused by autoantibodies directed against cell-surface receptors. These clinical syndromes illustrate the principle that understanding the biochemical pathways of hormone action can provide important insights into the pathophysiology of human disease.

Genetic Defects in Receptor Function

At least two distinct major types of genetic defects can cause hormone resistance.[62] First, mutations can lead to a decrease in the number of receptors. For example, in the case of the insulin receptor, mutations have been identified that decrease receptor number by at least three mechanisms: (1) impairing receptor biosynthesis, (2) inhibiting the transport of receptors to their normal location in the plasma membrane, and (3) accelerating the rate of receptor degradation. Second, mutations can impair the intrinsic activities of the receptor. In the case of the insulin receptor, mutations have been reported that decrease the affinity of insulin binding or inhibit receptor tyrosine kinase activity.

Receptor dimerization is known to play a central role in the mechanisms whereby ligands activate many cell-surface receptors. This role has been shown most convincingly in the case of the GH receptor (a member of the family of cytokine receptors) but has also been postulated for receptor tyrosine kinases. The syndromes of multiple endocrine neoplasia types 2A and 2B and familial medullary carcinoma of the thyroid are caused by mutations in the gene encoding the ret tyrosine kinase (a subunit of the receptor for glial cell–derived growth factor).[63] Ordinarily, there are cysteine residues in the extracel-

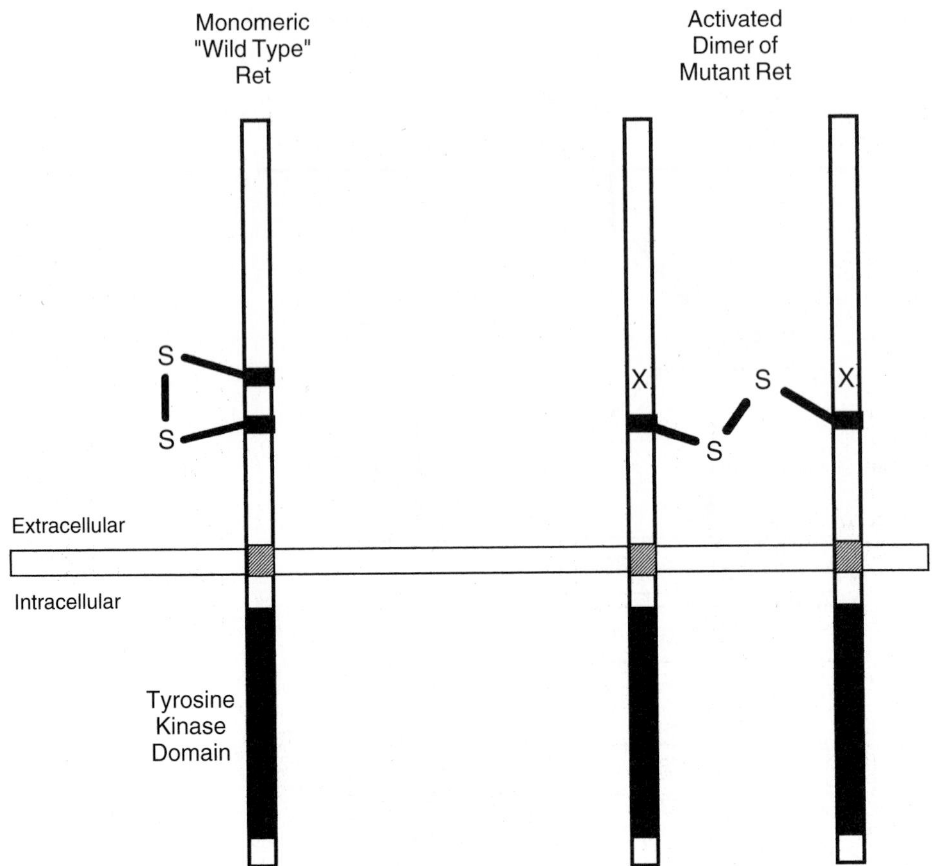

Figure 5–5. Mutations leading to constitutive activation of Ret. "Wild-type" Ret has intramolecular disulfide bonds formed by two cysteine residues in the same receptor molecule *(left)*. When one of the two cysteine residues is mutated, the unpaired cysteine residue is available to form an intermolecular disulfide bond with a cysteine residue on another receptor molecule. This leads to receptor dimerization *(right)*, which in turn leads to constitutive activation of the receptor tyrosine kinase.[63, 102, 103] This type of mutation has been identified in patients with multiple endocrine neoplasia type 2.

lular domain of Ret that participate in the formation of intramolecular disulfide bonds. Mutation of one of the cysteine residues leaves an unpaired cysteine residue that promotes dimerization of Ret molecules, thereby activating the Ret receptor tyrosine kinase (Fig. 5–5). Activation of the Ret tyrosine kinase through this germ line mutation converts Ret into an oncogene.

Autoantibodies Directed against Cell-Surface Receptors

Inhibitory antireceptor autoantibodies were first identified in myasthenia gravis.[64] In this neurologic disease, antibodies to the nicotinic acetylcholine receptor impair neuromuscular transmission, apparently by accelerating receptor degradation. Subsequently, autoantibodies to the insulin receptor were demonstrated to block insulin action in the syndrome of type B extreme insulin resistance.[65] Insulin resistance is caused by at least two mechanisms: (1) the antireceptor antibodies inhibit insulin binding to the receptor,[66] and (2) the antibodies accelerate receptor degradation.[67]

Graves' disease provided the first example of stimulatory antireceptor autoantibodies.[68] In Graves' disease, there are autoantibodies directed against the thyroid-stimulating hormone (TSH) receptor. These antireceptor antibodies activate the TSH receptor, thereby stimulating growth of the thyroid gland as well as hypersecretion of thyroid hormone. This "experiment of nature" demonstrates that the receptor can be activated by ligands other than the physiologic ligand and that the normal spectrum of biologic actions can be triggered by this unphysiologic ligand (i.e., the antireceptor antibody). Similarly, antibodies to the insulin receptor have been demonstrated to activate the insulin receptor by mimicking insulin action. Although it is more common for a patient with anti-insulin receptor autoantibodies to present with insulin resistance, patients with anti-insulin receptor autoantibodies have also been reported to experience fasting hypoglycemia.[69–71]

RECEPTORS THAT SIGNAL THROUGH ASSOCIATED TYROSINE KINASES

Overview

Members of the cytokine family of receptors resemble receptor tyrosine kinases in their mechanism of action, with one important difference. Instead of the tyrosine kinase being intrinsic to the receptor, enzymatic activity resides in a protein that associates with the cytokine receptor. As with receptor tyrosine kinases, ligand binding to the cytokine receptor activates the associated kinase. The more than 25 known ligands that bind to members of the cytokine receptor family have diverse functions. Three of the ligands are hormones: GH, which is vital for normal body height; prolactin (PRL), which is required for reproduction and lactation; and leptin, which is a potent appetite suppressant and a regulator of rates of metabolism. Other ligands of cytokine receptors, for example, erythropoietin, most interleukins, and interferons α, β, and γ, regulate hematopoiesis or the immune response. A number of genetic diseases can be traced to defects in cytokine receptors. For example, Laron dwarfism is caused by autosomal recessive mutations of the GH receptor[72] and autosomal recessive mutations of the leptin receptor can cause morbid obesity.[73]

Cytokine Receptors Are Composed of Multiple Subunits

Members of the cytokine family of receptors share homology in both the extracellular and cytoplasmic domains. Some cytokine receptors, including the receptors for GH, PRL, and leptin, are thought to be composed of dimers of a single receptor subunit (Fig. 5–6). One ligand is thought to bind to both receptor subunits, as discussed earlier for the GH receptor. However, most cytokine receptors are composed of two or more different subunits, with as many as six subunits constituting a single receptor.[74, 75] Some of these receptors are thought to bind ligand dimers. One or more of these receptor subunits is shared by receptors for other cytokines.

This phenomenon of "mixing and matching" receptor subunits is an efficient way for the cell to fine-tune its cellular responses and increase the number of ligands a group of receptor subunits can bind. For example, a receptor composed of gp130 and leukemia inhibitory factor receptor β subunit binds leukemia inhibitory factor, a pleiotropic cytokine with multiple functions that appears to serve as a molecular interface between the neuroimmune and endocrine systems.[76] The same receptor subunits, when combined with a ciliary neurotrophic factor receptor subunit, show a preference for ciliary neurotrophic factor, a trophic factor for motor neurons in the ciliary ganglion and spinal cord and a potent appetite suppressor.[77] Combine two gp130 subunits with an interleukin-6 (IL-6) receptor subunit, and the new receptor shows a preference for IL-6, an inducer of the acute phase response with additional anti-inflammatory properties.[78]

Cytokine Receptors Activate Members of the Janus Family of Tyrosine Kinases

Members of the cytokine family of receptors do not themselves exhibit enzymatic activity. Rather, they bind members of the Janus family of tyrosine kinases (JAKs) through a proline-rich region (see Fig. 5–6). There are four known JAKs, designated JAK1, JAK2, JAK3, and TYK2. As do the cytokine receptors, the JAKs mix and match in that some receptors show a strong preference for a single JAK, some require two different JAKs, and others appear to activate multiple JAK family members. For example, GH, PRL, and leptin preferentially activate JAK2. Interferon-γ activates JAK1 and JAK2, and IL-2 activates JAK1 and JAK3.[74, 79]

Binding of ligand to a cytokine receptor activates the appropriate JAK family member or members. In some cases (e.g., PRL), the JAKs appear to be constitutively associated with the cytokine receptor and ligand binding increases their activity.[80] In other cases (e.g., the GH receptor), ligand binding increases both the affinity of JAKs for the cytokine receptor and the activity of the associated JAKs.[81] Activation of JAKs requires receptor oligomerization, presumably to bring two or more JAKs into sufficiently close proximity to transphosphorylate each other on the activating tyrosine in the kinase domain, as described previously in the chapter for the receptor tyrosine kinases. Although receptor dimerization appears to be required for receptor activation, a conformational change in receptor may also be required.[82, 83] Transphosphorylation is believed to cause a conformational change that exposes the ATP- or substrate-binding site, or both. Once the JAKs are activated, they phosphorylate themselves and their associated receptor subunits on multiple tyrosines. JAKs appear to be vital for normal human function. Mutations in the JAK3 gene have been linked to an autosomal recessive form of severe combined immunodeficiency disease.[84] Targeted disruption of the JAK2 gene in mice is embryonic lethal.[85]

Signaling Pathways Initiated by Cytokine Receptor–JAK Complexes

Phosphorylated tyrosines within the cytokine receptor subunits and their associated JAKs form binding sites for various signaling proteins containing phosphotyrosine binding domains, such as SH2 and PTB domains. Each cytokine receptor–JAK complex would be expected to have some tyrosine-containing motifs shared with many other cytokine receptor–JAK complexes (e.g., tyrosines within JAKs) and some specific tyrosine-containing motifs (e.g., tyrosines within a specific combination of receptor subunits). Thus, ligand binding to cytokine receptors would be expected to initiate some signaling pathways that are shared by many cytokines and some that are more specialized to a particular cytokine receptor. The signaling proteins known to be recruited to subsets of cytokine receptor–JAK complexes are generally the same as those recruited to receptor tyrosine kinases. Examples include the IRS proteins, the adapter proteins Shc and Grb-2 that lead to activation of the Ras-MAP kinase pathway, phospholipase Cγ, and PI 3-kinase. However, there is one family of signaling proteins that appears to be particularly important for the function of cytokines—signal transducers and activators of transcription (STATs) (Fig. 5–7).

STAT proteins are latent cytoplasmic transcription factors. STATs bind, through their SH2 domains, to one or more phosphorylated tyrosines in activated receptor-JAK complexes. Once bound, they themselves are tyrosyl phosphorylated, presumably by the receptor-associated JAKs. STATs then dissociate from the receptor-JAK complexes, homodimerize or heterodimerize with other STAT proteins, move to the nucleus, and bind to gamma-activated sequence–like elements in the promoters of cytokine-responsive genes.[86] The transcriptional response depends on how many STAT binding sites exist in the receptor-JAK complex, with which of the seven known STATs a particular STAT heterodimerizes, to what other proteins a particular STAT binds, the degree of serine or threonine phosphorylation of the STAT, and what other transcription factors are also activated. For example, leukemia inhibitory factor, whose receptor contains seven STAT3 binding motifs (YXXQ, where Y = tyrosine, X = any amino acid, and Q = glutamine) is a particularly potent activator of STAT3.[87] The transcriptional activity of STAT5 is enhanced by its forming a complex with the glucocorticoid receptor.[88]

Precise Regulation of the Cytokine Receptors Is Required for Normal Function

Ligand binding to cytokine receptors normally activates JAKs rapidly and transiently. Conversely, constitutively activated JAKs and STATs are associated with cellular transformation. For example, in cells transformed by the Abl oncoprotein v-Abl, JAK1 is constitutively activated and inhibition of JAK1 blocks the ability of v-Abl to transform bone marrow cells.[89] Constitutively active JAKs and STATs are a common characteristic of leukemias,[90] and both JAK2 and STAT5b have been identified as fusion partners in translocations in leukemias. The Tel-JAK2 fusion protein is constitutively active, leading to constitutively active STAT proteins. Thus, an understanding of what turns off cytokine receptor signaling is of utmost importance in understanding normal signaling through cytokine receptors.

As with the receptor tyrosine kinases, several steps have been hypothesized to serve as points of signal termination for cytokine signaling. These include receptor degradation (e.g., through a ubiquitination-proteosome pathway) and dephospho-

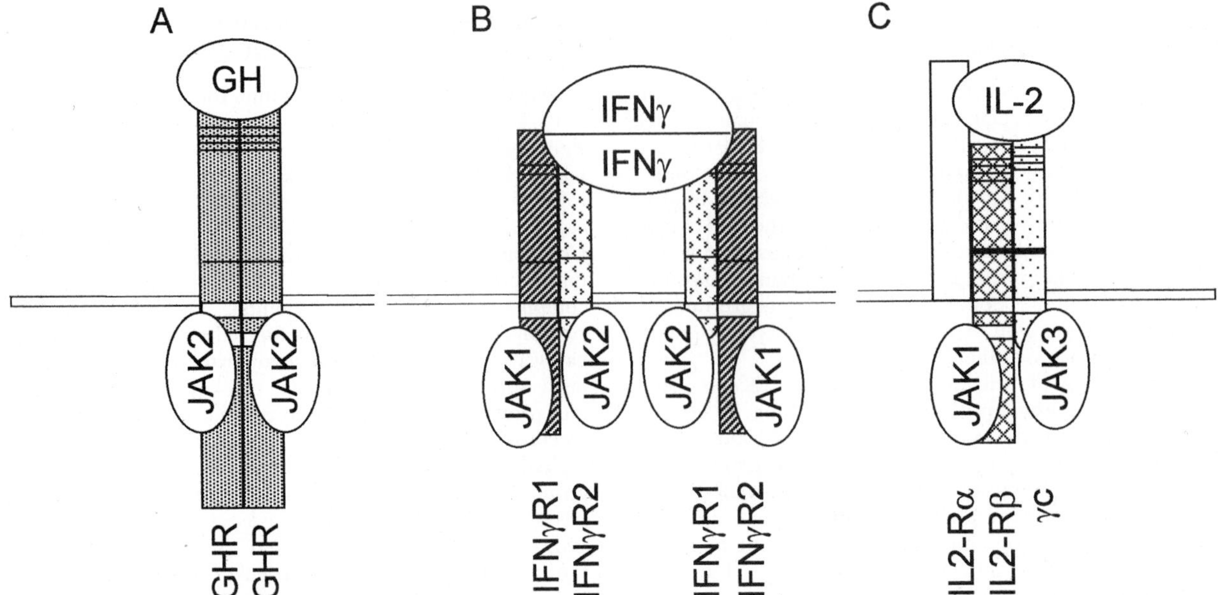

Figure 5–6. Cytokine receptors are composed of multiple subunits and bind to one or more members of the Janus kinase (JAK) family of tyrosine kinases. *A*, Growth hormone (GH), like prolactin and leptin, binds to receptor homodimers and activates JAK2. *B*, Interferon γ (IFNγ) homodimers bind to their ligand-binding γR1 subunits. The γR2 subunits are then recruited, leading to activation of JAK1, which binds to γR1 subunit, and JAK2, which binds to γR2 subunit. Both subunits and both JAKs are necessary for responses to IFNγ. *C*, Interleukin-2 (IL-2) binds to receptors composed of three subunits: a γc subunit shared with receptors for ILs 4, 7, 9, and 15; an IL-2Rβ subunit shared with the IL-15 receptor; and a noncytokine receptor subunit, IL-2Rα subunit. IL-2 activates both JAK3, bound to the γc subunit, and JAK1, bound to IL2-Rβ. Extracellular regions of homology are indicated by the *black lines and patterns*. Intracellular regions of homology are indicated by the *white boxes*.

rylation of tyrosines within JAK or receptor (e.g., by an SH2 domain containing tyrosine phosphatase recruited to receptor-JAK complexes). The suppressors of cytokine-signaling (SOCSs) are thought to be particularly important players in the termination or suppression of cytokine-signaling pathways. SOCS proteins are an excellent example of an effective negative feedback loop. They are generally synthesized in response to cytokines. The newly synthesized SOCS proteins in turn bind, through their SH2 domain, to phosphorylated tyrosines within the cytokine receptor–JAK complex and inhibit further cytokine signaling. In some cases (i.e., SOCS1), SOCS proteins are thought to bind to phosphotyrosines in the kinase domain of JAK and inhibit kinase activity.[91, 92] In other cases (i.e., SOCS 3), SOCS proteins bind to phosphorylated tyrosines in the receptor and inhibit JAK activity.[93] Finally, in some cases (i.e., cytokine-inducible SH2 protein [CIS]), SOCS proteins bind to phosphorylated tyrosines in the receptor and block STAT binding and activation.[94] SOCS proteins can also be synthesized in response to noncytokine receptors, suggesting a mechanism whereby prior exposure to one ligand suppresses subsequent responses to another. For example, SOCS proteins have been implicated in the well-known ability of endotoxin to cause resistance to GH.[95]

Summary

Hormones, growth factors, and cytokines that bind to members of the cytokine family of receptors activate JAK family tyrosine kinases. The activated kinases in turn phosphorylate tyrosines in themselves and associated receptors. The phosphorylated tyrosines form binding sites for other signaling proteins, including STAT proteins and a variety of other phosphotyrosine-binding proteins. STAT proteins promote the regulation of cytokine-sensitive genes, including SOCS proteins that serve a negative feedback function of terminating ligand activation of JAKs or STATs, or both.

Although this gives the general picture, it should be recognized that the picture is becoming much more complex every day. For example, there are reports that members of the Src family of tyrosine kinases can also be activated by some cytokine receptors (e.g., PRL receptor),[96] that some JAK-binding proteins (e.g., SH2-B) are potent activators of JAK2,[97] and that other proteins contribute to the down-regulation of cytokine-signaling pathways, including protein inhibitors of activated STAT (PIAS), that bind and inhibit specific STATs.[98]

G PROTEIN–COUPLED RECEPTORS

Overview

G protein–coupled receptors (GPCRs) are an evolutionarily conserved gene superfamily with members in all eucaryotes from yeast to mammals. They transduce a wide variety of extracellular signals including photons of light; chemical odorants; divalent cations; monoamine, amino acid, and nucleoside neurotransmitters; lipids; and peptide and protein hormones.[104] All members of the GPCR superfamily share a common structural feature, seven membrane-spanning helices, but various subfamilies diverge in primary amino acid sequence and in the domains that serve in ligand binding, G protein coupling, and interaction with other effector proteins (Fig. 5–8).

All GPCRs act as guanine nucleotide exchange factors. In their activated (agonist-bound) conformation, they catalyze exchange of GDP tightly bound to the α subunit of heterotrimeric G proteins for GTP (Fig. 5–9). This in turn leads to activation of the α subunit and its dissociation from the G protein βγ dimer. Both G protein subunits are capable of regulating effector activity.[105] Identified G protein–regulated

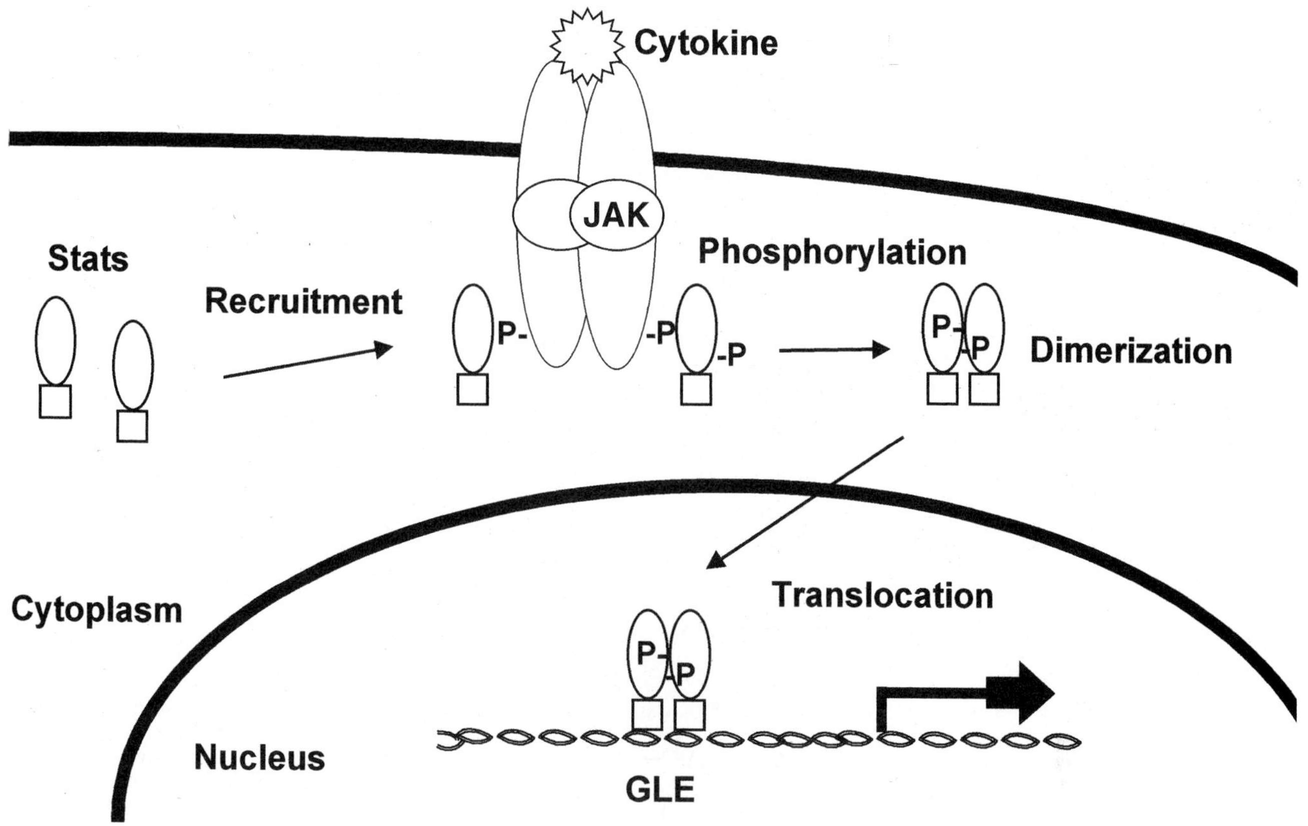

Figure 5–7. Cytokines activate signal transducers and activators of transcription (STATs). STAT proteins are latent cytoplasmic transcription factors. STATs bind, through their Src homology 2 (SH2) domains, to one or more phosphorylated tyrosines in activated receptor-JAK complexes. Once bound, they themselves are tyrosyl phosphorylated, presumably by the receptor-associated JAKs. STATs then dissociate from the receptor-JAK complexes, homodimerize or heterodimerize with other STAT proteins, move to the nucleus, and bind to gamma-activated sequence–like elements (GLEs) in the promoters of cytokine-responsive genes. (Adapted from figure by J. Herrington, with permission.)

effectors include enzymes of second messenger metabolism such as adenylyl cyclase and phospholipase C-β and a variety of ion channels. Agonist binding to GPCRs thus alters intracellular second messenger and ion concentrations with resultant rapid effects on hormone secretion, muscle contraction, and a variety of other physiologic functions. Long-term changes in gene expression are also seen as a result of second messenger–stimulated phosphorylation of transcription factors.

The G protein subunits are encoded by three distinct genes. The α subunit binds guanine nucleotides with high affinity and specificity and has intrinsic guanosine triphosphatase (GTPase) activity. The β and γ polypeptides are tightly but noncovalently associated in a functional dimer subunit. The three-dimensional structures of the individual and associated subunits have been determined.[105–107] There is considerable diversity in G protein subunits, with multiple genes encoding all three subunits and alternative gene splicing resulting in additional polypeptide products. There are at least 16 distinct α subunit genes in mammals. These vary widely in range of expression. Some such as Gs-α, which couples many GPCRs to stimulation of adenylyl cyclase, are ubiquitous; others such as Gtl-α, which couples the GPCR rhodopsin to cyclic guanosine monophosphate phosphodiesterase in retinal rod photoreceptor cells, are highly localized.

Because multiple distinct GPCRs, G proteins, and effectors are expressed within any given cell, the degree and basis for specificity in G protein coupling to GPCRs and to effectors are major subjects of investigation with implications for drug action and disease mechanisms.[108] Since the pioneering work of Rodbell[109] in discovering G proteins and showing that G protein–mediated signal transduction involves three separable components (receptor, G protein, and effector), additional complexity has emerged.

A large new gene family termed RGS (for regulators of G protein signaling) has been identified. RGS proteins bind to a transition state of the GTP-activated G protein α subunit and accelerate its GTPase activity, thus helping deactivate the α subunit. RGS domains have also been found in modular proteins with additional functions, in certain cases linking heterotrimeric G protein signaling with the function of low-molecular-weight GTP-binding proteins in the ras superfamily.[110] Lefkowitz[111] has shown that a family of GPCR kinases and of arrestin proteins is involved in GPCR desensitization after agonist binding. In addition, it is now clear that GPCRs interact directly with a number of other proteins in addition to G proteins. Not only are GPCRs important targets for treatment of many diseases, but also mutations in genes encoding GPCRs have been identified as the cause of a number of endocrine as well as nonendocrine disorders.

G Protein–Coupled Receptor Structure and Function

Structure

Hydropathy analysis of the primary sequence of all GPCRs predicts seven membrane-spanning α helices connected by three intracellular loops and three extracellular loops with an

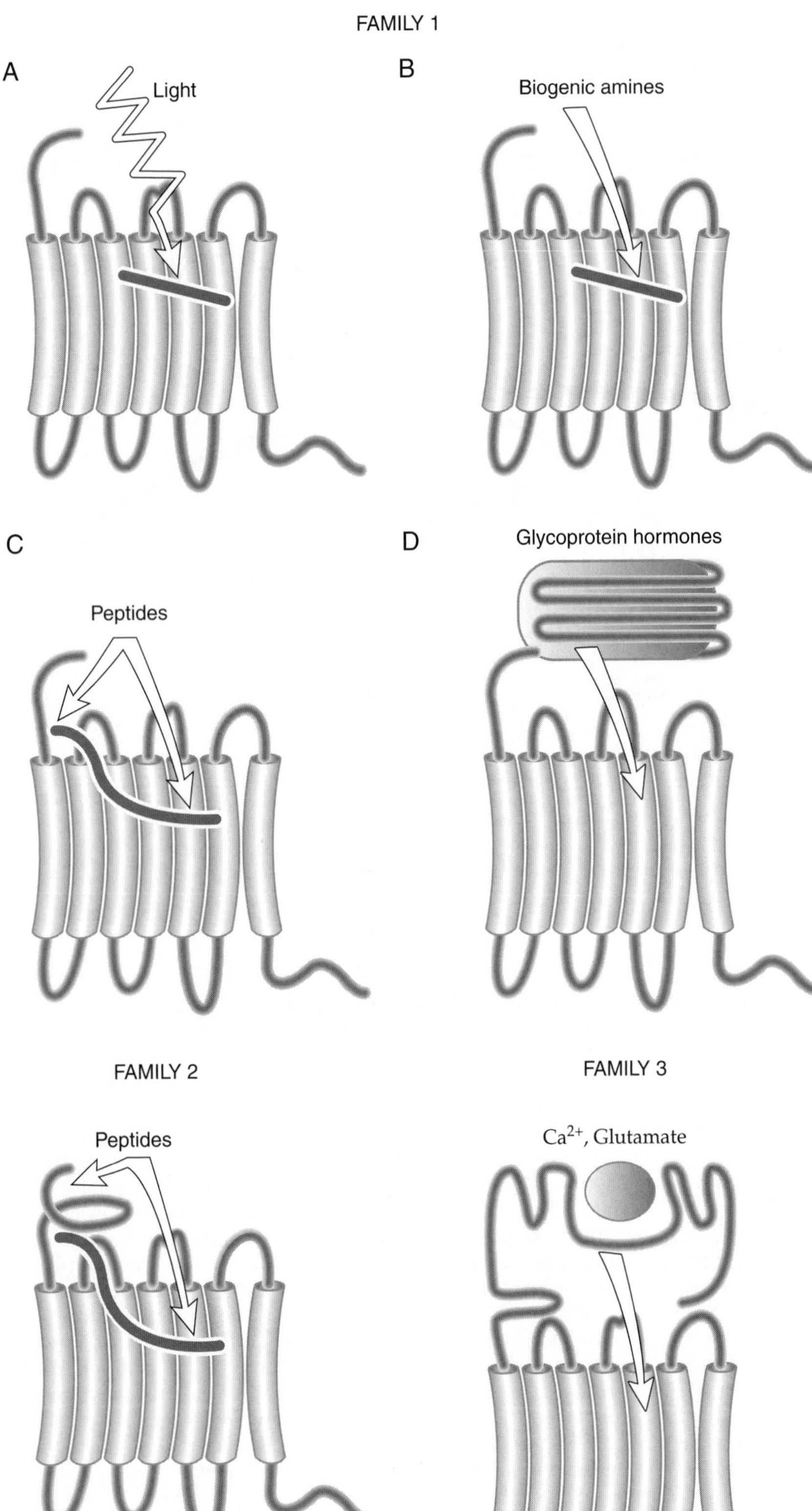

Figure 5–8. The G protein–coupled receptor (GPCR) superfamily: diversity in ligand binding and structure. Each panel depicts various members of the GPCR superfamily in cartoon form. The seven membrane-spanning α helices are shown as cylinders with the extracellular amino terminus and three extracellular loops above and the intracellular carboxyl terminus and three intracellular loops below. The superfamily can be divided into three subfamilies on the basis of amino acid sequence conservation within the transmembrane helices. Family 1 includes *(A)* the opsins, in which light *(jagged arrow)* causes isomerization of retinal covalently bound within the pocket created by the transmembrane helices *(bar)*; *(B)* monoamine receptors, in which agonists *(arrow)* bind noncovalently within the pocket created by the transmembrane helices *(bar)*; *(C)* receptors for peptides such as vasopressin, in which agonist binding *(arrow)* may involve parts of the extracellular amino terminus and loops as well as the transmembrane helices *(bar)*; and *(D)* glycoprotein hormone receptors, in which agonists *(oval)* bind to the large extracellular amino terminus, thereby activating the receptor through as yet undefined interactions with the extracellular loops or transmembrane helices *(arrow)*. Family 2 includes receptors for peptide hormones such as parathyroid hormone (PTH) and secretin. Agonists *(arrow)* may bind to residues in the extracellular amino terminus and loops as well as transmembrane helices *(bar)*. Family 3 includes the extracellular Ca^{2+} sensing receptor and metabotropic glutamate receptors. Agonists *(sphere)* bind in a cleft of the Venus flytrap–like domain in the large extracellular amino terminus, thereby activating the receptor through as yet undefined interactions with the extracellular loops or transmembrane helices *(arrow)*.

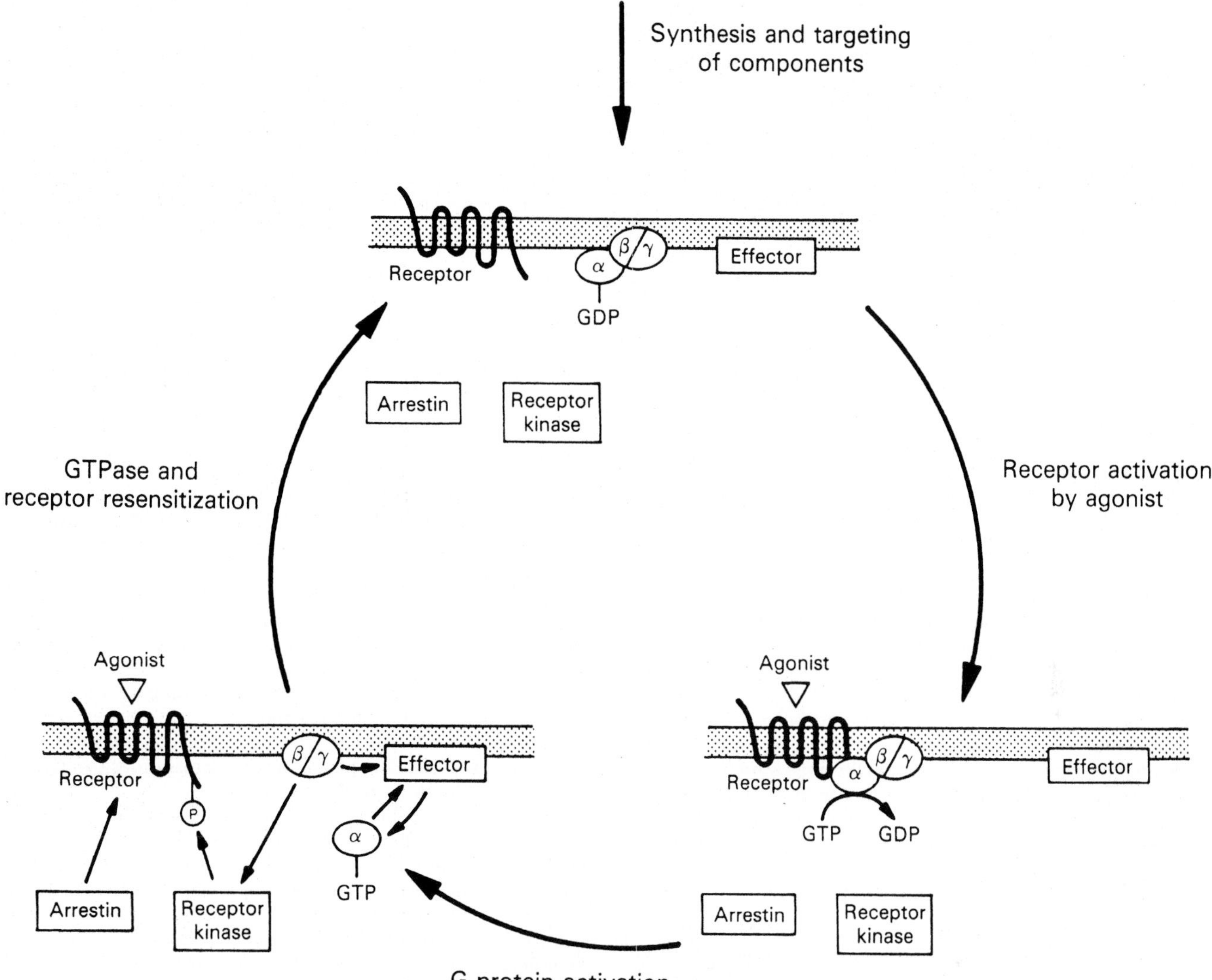

Figure 5–9. The G protein guanosine triphosphatase (GTPase) and G protein–coupled receptor (GPCR) desensitization-resensitization cycle. In each panel, the *stippled region* denotes the plasma membrane with extracellular above and intracellular below. In the basal state, the G protein is a heterotrimer with guanosine diphosphate (GDP) tightly bound to the α subunit. The agonist-activated GPCR catalyzes release of GDP, which permits guanosine triphosphate (GTP) to bind. The GTP-bound α subunit dissociates from the $\beta\gamma$ dimer. *Arrows* from α subunit to effector and from $\beta\gamma$ dimer to effector indicate regulation of effector activity by the respective subunits. *Arrow* from effector to α subunit indicates regulation of its GTPase activity by effector interaction. Under physiologic conditions, effector regulation by G protein subunits is transient and is terminated by the GTPase activity of the α subunit. The latter converts bound GTP to GDP, thus returning the α subunit to its inactivated state with high affinity for the $\beta\gamma$ dimer, which reassociates to form the heterotrimer in the basal state. In the basal state, the receptor kinase and arrestin are shown as cytosolic proteins. Dissociation of the GTP-bound α subunit from the $\beta\gamma$ dimer permits the latter to facilitate binding of receptor kinase to the plasma membrane (*arrow* from $\beta\gamma$ dimer to receptor kinase). Plasma membrane binding permits the receptor kinase to phosphorylate the agonist-bound GPCR (depicted here as occurring on the carboxyl-terminal tail of the GPCR, but sites on intracellular loops are also possible). GPCR phosphorylation in turn facilitates arrestin binding to GPCR, resulting in desensitization. Endocytic trafficking of arrestin-bound GPCR and recycling to the plasma membrane during resensitization are not depicted here.

extracellular amino terminus and an intracellular carboxyl terminus (see Fig. 5–8). This basic structure has now been verified by x-ray crystallography for rhodopsin.[112] Although there was already evidence that visual transduction in the retina and hormone activation of adenylyl cyclase shared common features, the discovery that the β-adrenergic receptor has the same topographic structure as rhodopsin came as a surprise.[111] Cloning of the complementary deoxyribonucleic acids (cDNAs) for a vast number of GPCRs followed elucidation of the primary sequence of the β-adrenergic receptor, and in every case the same core structure was predicted by hydropathy analysis.

In addition to the predicted core structure, certain other common features (with exceptions in some subsets of the GPCR superfamily) were noted[104]: (1) a disulfide bridge connecting the first and second extracellular loops; (2) one or more N-linked glycosylation sites, usually in the amino terminus but occasionally in extracellular loops; (3) palmitoylation of one or more cysteines in the carboxyl terminus, effectively creating a fourth intracellular loop; (4) potential phosphorylation sites in the carboxyl terminus and occasionally the third intracellular loop. Glycosylation appears to be important for proper folding and trafficking to the plasma membrane rather than for ligand binding. The disulfide bridge may help in proper arrangement of the transmembrane helices.

Superimposed on the basic structure of GPCRs are a number of variations relevant to differences in ligand binding, G protein coupling, and interaction with other proteins.[104] First, there are major differences in amino acid sequence among members of the GPCR superfamily. Sequence alignment, especially of the transmembrane helices, allows one to divide the superfamily into subfamilies (see Fig. 5–8). Of these, family 1 is the largest and itself can be subdivided. The largest subset includes opsins, odorant receptors, and monoamine, purinergic, and opiate receptors. These are characterized by a short amino terminus. The next subset includes chemokine, protease-activated, and certain peptide hormone receptors characterized by a slightly longer amino terminus. The last subset comprises receptors for the large glycoprotein hormones, TSH, luteinizing hormone, and follicle-stimulating hormone. These have an approximately 400-residue extracellular amino terminus.

Family 2 shows essentially no sequence homology to family 1 even within the transmembrane helices and is characterized by an approximately 100-residue amino terminus. Members include receptors for a number of peptide hormones such as parathyroid hormone (PTH), calcitonin, vasoactive intestinal peptide, and corticotropin-releasing hormone.

Family 3, in addition to a unique primary sequence, has other unique features such as an approximately 200-residue carboxyl terminus and an approximately 600-residue amino terminus. The latter consists of a putative "Venus flytrap–like" domain and a cysteine-rich domain. Members include the metabotropic glutamate receptors, an extracellular Ca^{2+}-sensing receptor, and putative taste and pheromone receptors.[113] The determination of the three-dimensional crystal structure of part of the extracellular amino terminus of one of the metabotropic glutamate receptors verifies the Venus flytrap structure.[113]

Ligand Binding

Given the diversity of ligands (>1000) that bind to GPCRs, it is not surprising that considerable diversity is evident in both the sequence and structure of presumptive GPCR ligand-binding domains. The opsins are unique among GPCRs in that the ligand, retinal, is covalently bound to a lysine in the seventh transmembrane helix.[112] Ligand binding for other members of family 1 with a short extracellular amino terminus, for example, adrenergic and other monoamine receptors, probably involves a pocket within the transmembrane helices as demonstrated for rhodopsin (see Fig. 5–8). For other family 1 GPCRs, the extracellular amino terminus, perhaps together with extracellular loops and portions of the transmembrane helices, is involved in ligand binding. In the case of the glycoprotein hormone receptors, the large extracellular amino terminus plays the principal role in hormone binding. Likewise, in family 2 receptors, the extracellular amino terminus is largely responsible for ligand binding. For family 3 GPCRs, the three-dimensional structure of the type 1 metabotropic glutamate receptor shows that agonist binding occurs within a cleft between the lobes of the Venus flytrap.[113]

G Protein Coupling

Because the number of potential G proteins to which GPCRs couple is much more limited than the number of ligands that bind GPCRs, more conservation of the domains involved in G protein coupling would be expected. Although GPCRs can be broadly divided into those that couple to Gs, those that couple to the Gq subfamily, and those that couple to the Gi-Go subfamily, the situation is probably more complicated. Specificity of coupling to the most recently identified G proteins, Gl2 and G13, is still uncertain. Also, some GPCRs evidently can couple to both Gs and Gq.

A vast number of studies have been performed to define the sites of ligand binding and G protein coupling of GPCRs.[114] Considerable evidence points to the third intracellular loop (particularly its membrane-proximal portions) and to the membrane-proximal portion of the carboxyl terminus as key determinants of G protein coupling specificity. For example, exchanging only the third intracellular loop between different GPCRs confers the G protein coupling specificity of the exchanged loop upon the recipient GPCR.[115] In contrast, the second intracellular loop, although important for G protein coupling, appears to play a role in the activation mechanism rather than in determining specificity of coupling.[115] A tripeptide motif (D/E, R, Y/W) at the start of the second intracellular loop that is highly conserved in family 1 GPCRs is critical for G protein activation.[114]

Mechanism of Activation

The precise mechanism of activation after agonist binding remains to be defined for most GPCRs, but studies of rhodopsin provide the clearest picture available. In the ground state, retinal covalently bound to the seventh transmembrane helix in rhodopsin holds the transmembrane helices in an inactive conformation. Isomerization of retinal upon absorption of light of the appropriate wavelength converts an antagonist ligand into an agonist. The rhodopsin crystal structure identifies the residues in the transmembrane helices that interact with retinal and suggests a mechanism for movement of the helices upon photoactivation of retinal.[112] Movement of the transmembrane helices in turn leads to changes in conformation of cytoplasmic loops that promote G protein activation.

For family 1 receptors related to rhodopsin, the determination of its three-dimensional structure validates the idea that a change in conformation of transmembrane helices is the direct result of agonist versus antagonist binding to residues within the helices. Further refinements in understanding the mechanism of activation for opsin-related GPCRs should come as additional three-dimensional structures are determined. Until then, molecular modeling by computer on the basis of the rhodopsin structure and then experimental testing offer a useful approach.[116] For other GPCRs whose presumptive site of agonist binding does not involve direct contact with transmembrane helices (families 2 and 3 and the glycoprotein hormone receptors in family 1), much remains to be learned about the mechanism of activation. Specifically, determining how agonist binding to the extracellular domain of such GPCRs leads to presumptive changes in conformation of transmembrane helices requires further studies of structure and function.

A general hypothesis of GPCR activation postulates that GPCRs are in equilibrium between an activated state and an inactive state. These states presumably differ in the disposition of the transmembrane helices and, in turn, the cytoplasmic domains that determine G protein coupling. Agonists, according to this model, are viewed as stabilizing the activated state. Antagonists may be neutral, that is, they simply compete with agonist for receptor binding but their binding does not influence this equilibrium. Alternatively, they may be "inverse" agonists; that is, their binding stabilizes the inactive state of the receptor. Naturally occurring, activating mutations of GPCRs lend support to this hypothesis.

Dimerization

Members of the tyrosine kinase receptor family have long been known to require dimerization as part of their activation mechanism. It is now apparent that many GPCRs likewise form homodimers and heterodimers.[104] Residues within transmembrane helix 6 may foster dimerization of small family 1 GPCRs,[117] and intermolecular disulfide bonds in the extracellular amino-terminal domain are involved in homodimerization of most family 3 GPCRs.[113, 118] A coiled-coil interaction in the carboxyl terminus of γ-aminobutyric acid B receptor subtypes is responsible for heterodimerization, and this is critical for proper receptor function.[119] Modifications of ligand binding, signaling, and receptor sequestration have been demonstrated upon heterodimerization of angiotensin with bradykinin receptors, of κ with δ opioid receptors, and of opioid with β-adrenergic receptors.[120, 121] Further studies are needed to elucidate the role of homodimerization and heterodimerization in GPCR function.

G Protein–Coupled Receptor Desensitization

Pharmacologists long ago appreciated that continued exposure to agonist leads to a diminished response, so-called desensitization. This phenomenon has been extensively studied in GPCRs. Two forms are defined: heterologous, in which binding of agonist to one GPCR leads to a diminished response of a different GPCR to its agonist, and homologous, in which desensitization occurs only for the GPCR to which agonist is bound. Both forms of desensitization involve GPCR phosphorylation but by different kinases and at different sites. Stimulation of cyclic adenosine monophosphate formation by agonist binding to a Gs-coupled GPCR leads to activation of protein kinase A, which in turn can phosphorylate and desensitize the GPCR. Such phosphorylation may also alter G protein coupling specificity.[104] Similarly, protein kinase C activation resulting from GPCR coupling to Gq family members may cause protein kinase C–catalyzed phosphorylation of GPCRs with desensitization.

In retinal photoreceptors, a specific rhodopsin kinase and a protein termed arrestin were implicated in attenuation of the light response. Just as parallels were identified between rhodopsin and GPCR structure, so were parallels identified in this desensitization mechanism. Rhodopsin kinase is but one member of a family of GPCR kinases and arrestin only one of a family of related proteins that function in desensitization of many members of the GPCR superfamily.[111] GPCR kinases preferentially phosphorylate the agonist-bound form of a GPCR, thus ensuring homologous desensitization. Upon GPCR phosphorylation by GPCR kinase, arrestins bind to the third intracellular loop and carboxyl-terminal tail of the GPCR, thereby blocking G protein binding (see Fig. 5–9). There is evidence that GPCR kinases and arrestins not only act to desensitize GPCRs but also mediate other functions including receptor internalization and interaction with other effectors (see next section).

G Protein–Coupled Receptor Interactions with Other Proteins

The initial paradigm of GPCR function postulated that G protein activation is the sole outcome of agonist binding to GPCRs. With the identification of GPCR interactions with GPCR kinases and arrestins, this concept was modified to include these proteins involved in GPCR desensitization. Later evidence, however, suggests that GPCR interaction with arrestins may also permit recruitment of other proteins to the GPCR. For example, the src tyrosine kinase may interact with the β-adrenergic receptor with β-arrestin serving as an adaptor.[122] Arrestins may also recruit proteins involved in endocytosis. GPCR kinases may also serve to recruit additional signaling proteins to the GPCR.[122]

Other classes of proteins may interact with specific GPCRs without recruitment by GPCR kinases and arrestins. These include SH2 domain–containing proteins, small GTP-binding proteins, and PDZ (for *p*ostsynaptic *d*ensity protein-95/*d*iscs large/*z*ona occluden-1) domain–containing proteins. Examples of the latter include binding of the Na^+/H^+ exchanger regulatory factor to the carboxyl terminus of the β-adrenergic receptor.[122] The long carboxyl terminus of family 3 GPCRs such as metabotropic glutamate receptors contains polyproline motifs involved in binding members of the Homer family. The latter can facilitate functional interactions with yet other proteins such as the inositol trisphosphate receptor.[123] Receptor activity–modifying proteins (RAMPs), a new family of single-transmembrane-domain proteins, appear to heterodimerize with certain GPCRs, assisting them in proper folding and membrane trafficking.[124] Interestingly, when the calcitonin receptor–like GPCR associates with RAMP1, it forms a calcitonin gene–related peptide receptor, whereas when it associates with RAMP2, it becomes an adrenomedullin receptor. Clearly, this rapidly evolving aspect of GPCR function holds many further interesting developments in store.

G Protein–Coupled Receptors in Disease Pathogenesis and Treatment

Because of their diverse and critical roles in normal physiology, their accessibility on the cell surface, and the ability to synthesize selective agonists and antagonists, GPCRs have long been a major target for drug development. One estimate is that about 65% of prescription drugs are targeted against GPCRs. With the cloning of GPCR cDNAs, much greater diversity of receptor subclasses became evident than had been anticipated on the basis of pharmacologic studies. For example, five muscarinic receptor subtypes and an even greater number of serotoninergic GPCRs were identified.[114] This has allowed the development of highly specific, subtype-selective drugs that have fewer side effects than those produced by previously available agents.

Another result of the cloning of GPCR cDNAs by homology screening and polymerase chain reaction–based approaches is the identification of "orphan" GPCRs, that is, receptors with the canonical, predicted seven-transmembrane-domain structure of GPCRs but without knowledge of their physiologic agonist. There have been substantial efforts to identify the relevant ligands for such orphan receptors. An example of the success of such efforts is the identification of an orphan GPCR as the neuromedin U receptor involved in regulation of feeding.[125] This will permit testing of candidate drugs targeting this receptor for obesity prevention and treatment.

Beyond drug development, defects in GPCRs are an important cause of a wide variety of human diseases.[126] GPCR mutations can cause loss of function by impairing any of several steps in the normal GPCR-GTPase cycle (see Fig. 5–9). These include failure to synthesize GPCR protein altogether, failure of synthesized GPCR to reach the plasma membrane, failure of GPCR to bind or be activated by agonist, and failure of GPCR to couple to or activate G protein. Because in most cases clinically significant impairment of signal transduction requires loss of both alleles of the GPCR gene, most such diseases are inherited in autosomal recessive fashion (Table 5–1).

Most of these diseases are manifested as resistance to the action of the normal agonist and thus mimic deficiency of the agonist. For example, TSH receptor loss-of-function mutations cause a form of hypothyroidism mimicking TSH deficiency, but serum TSH is actually elevated in such cases, reflecting resistance to the hormone's action caused by defective receptor function. Nephrogenic diabetes insipidus (renal vasopressin re-

Table 5–1. Diseases Caused by G Protein–Coupled Receptor Loss-of-Function Mutations

Receptor	Disease	Inheritance
V2 vasopressin	Nephrogenic diabetes insipidus	X-linked
ACTH	Familial ACTH resistance	Autosomal recessive
GHRH	Familial GH deficiency	Autosomal recessive
GnRH	Hypogonadotropic hypogonadism	Autosomal recessive
FSH	Hypergonadotropic ovarian dysgenesis	Autosomal recessive
LH	Male pseudohermaphroditism	Autosomal recessive
TSH	Familial hypothyroidism	Autosomal recessive
Ca^{2+} sensing	Familial hypocalciuric hypercalcemia, neonatal severe primary hyperparathyroidism	Autosomal dominant, autosomal recessive
Melanocortin 4	Obesity	Autosomal recessive
PTH/PTHrP	Blomstrand chondrodysplasia	Autosomal recessive

ACTH, adrenocorticotropic hormone; FSH, follicle-stimulating hormone; GH, growth hormone; GHRH, growth hormone–releasing hormone; GnRH, gonadotropin-releasing hormone; LH, luteinizing hormone; PTH, parathyroid hormone; PTHrP, parathyroid hormone–related protein; TSH, thyroid-stimulating hormone.

sistance) is caused by loss-of-function mutations in the V2 vasopressin receptor gene located on the X chromosome. Thus, males with a single copy of the gene experience the disease when they inherit a mutant gene, whereas most females do not show overt disease because random X inactivation leaves them with on average 50% of normal gene function. Most V2 vasopressin receptor mutations associated with nephrogenic diabetes insipidus cause loss of function by impairing normal synthesis or folding of the receptor, or both. A novel mechanism for receptor loss of function elucidated for a V2 vasopressin receptor missense mutation associated with nephrogenic diabetes insipidus involves constitutive arrestin-mediated desensitization.[127]

The extracellular Ca^{2+}-sensing receptor appears to be an interesting exception to the association between GPCR loss-of-function mutations and hormone resistance. Loss-of-function mutations of the Ca^{2+}-sensing receptor mimic a hormone hypersecretion state, primary hyperparathyroidism. In fact, Ca^{2+}-sensing receptor loss-of-function mutations do cause hormone resistance, but in this case extracellular Ca^{2+} is the hormonal agonist that acts through this receptor to inhibit PTH secretion. A loss-of-function mutation of one copy of the receptor gene typically causes mild resistance to extracellular Ca^{2+} manifested as familial hypocalciuric hypercalcemia. If two defective copies are inherited, extreme Ca^{2+} resistance causing neonatal severe primary hyperparathyroidism results (see Table 5–1). In some cases, a heterozygous receptor loss-of-function mutation may be associated with neonatal severe primary hyperparathyroidism, perhaps reflecting a dominant negative effect caused by dimerization of wild-type and mutant receptors.[128]

GPCR gain-of-function mutations (Table 5–2) are also an important cause of disease.[126] Given the dominant nature of activating mutations, most such diseases are inherited in an autosomal dominant manner. Activating TSH receptor mutations may be inherited in autosomal dominant fashion and cause diffuse thyroid enlargement in familial nonautoimmune hyperthyroidism, or they may occur as somatic mutations causing focal, sporadic hyperfunctional thyroid nodules.[129] Unlike

Table 5–2. Diseases Caused by G Protein–Coupled Receptor Gain-of-Function Mutations

Receptor	Disease	Inheritance
LH	Familial male precocious puberty	Autosomal dominant
TSH	Sporadic hyperfunctional thyroid nodules	Noninherited (somatic)
TSH	Familial nonautoimmune hyperthyroidism	Autosomal dominant
Ca^{2+} sensing	Familial hypocalcemic hypercalciuria	Autosomal dominant
PTH/PTHrP	Jansen's metaphyseal chondrodysplasia	Autosomal dominant

LH, luteinizing hormone; PTH, parathyroid hormone; PTHrP, parathyroid hormone–related protein; TSH, thyroid-stimulating hormone.

loss-of-function mutations, which may be missense as well as nonsense or frameshift mutations that truncate the normal receptor protein, GPCR gain-of-function mutations are almost always missense mutations. The location and nature of naturally occurring, disease-causing mutations offer important insights into GPCR structure and function. The basis for defective receptor function is clear with mutations that truncate receptor synthesis prematurely. More subtle missense mutations may impair function if they involve highly conserved residues in transmembrane helices critical for normal protein folding. Activating missense mutations often involve residues within or bordering transmembrane helices and are thought to disrupt normal inhibitory constraints that maintain the receptor in its inactive conformation.[130] Mutations disrupting these constraints mimic the effects of agonist binding and shift the equilibrium toward the activated state of the receptor.

Clinically, diseases caused by activating GPCR mutations therefore mimic states of agonist excess, but direct measurement shows that agonist concentrations are actually low, reflecting normal negative feedback mechanisms. Again, the Ca^{2+}-sensing receptor is an apparent exception, with activating mutations causing functional hypoparathyroidism. For most GPCRs, disease-associated gain-of-function mutations cause constitutive, agonist-independent, activation but with rare exceptions,[131] the Ca^{2+}-sensing receptor gain-of-function mutations cause increased sensitivity to extracellular Ca^{2+} rather than to Ca^{2+}-independent activation.

Naturally occurring animal models of human disease have revealed additional examples of etiologic GPCR mutations. For example, a loss-of-function mutation in the hypocretin (orexin) type 2 receptor gene was identified in canine narcolepsy.[132] Dozens of mouse GPCR gene knockout models have been created, many revealing interesting and in some cases unexpected phenotypes. Characterization of the phenotype resulting from disruption of a mouse GPCR gene may accurately predict the clinical picture resulting from the corresponding mutation in humans, such as with disruption of the melanocortin-4 receptor gene resulting in obesity in mouse[133] and human[134] and disruption of the PTH/PTH-related protein receptor gene impairing normal bone growth and development in mouse[135] and in the human disease Blomstrand chondrodysplasia.[136] Further knockout models and further detailed studies of these models can be expected to increase substantially our understanding of GPCR function and to address questions such as the unique roles of multiple subtypes of various GPCR subclasses, for example, the $\beta 3$-adrenergic receptor subtype.[137] Availability of mouse knockout models of human diseases such as nephrogenic diabetes insipidus[138] should also facilitate testing of novel therapies including gene transfer.

Screening of GPCR genes for mutations as the potential cause of additional human disorders may continue to turn up new examples, but it is also becoming clear that variations in GPCR gene sequence can have profound consequences beyond mutations causing diseases. One of the most striking examples is the discovery that homozygous loss-of-function mutations of the type 5 chemokine receptor (CCR5) confer resistance to human immunodeficiency virus (HIV) infection in individuals with this genotype.[139] The reason is that CCR5 serves as a coreceptor for HIV entry into cells. In the roundworm, two isoforms of a neuropeptide receptor are associated with profound differences in feeding behavior.[140]

As more polymorphisms are discovered in the human genome, many examples of variations in GPCR gene sequence will be found and the challenge will be to elucidate their possible functional significance. In vitro studies may reveal functional differences, such as differences in G protein coupling seen with a four-amino-acid polymorphism in the third intracellular loop of the α_{2C}-adrenergic receptor,[141] but further studies are required to determine whether such differences are important in individual variation in response to various drugs (pharmacogenomics) or in other subtle physiologic differences that could confer susceptibility to disease (complex disease genes). Given the high proportion of the human genome devoted to GPCR genes, it is clear that studies of this gene superfamily will play a prominent role in the postgenomic era.

References

1. Fradkin JE, Eastman RC, Lesniak MA, Roth J. Specificity spillover at the hormone receptor—exploring its role in human disease. N Engl J Med 1989; 320:640–645.
2. Hunter T. The Croonian Lecture 1997. The phosphorylation of proteins on tyrosine: its role in cell growth and disease. Philos Trans R Soc Lond B Biol Sci 1998; 353:583–605.
3. Ushiro H, Cohen S. Identification of phosphotyrosine as a product of epidermal growth factor–activated protein kinase in A-431 cell membranes. J Biol Chem 1980; 255:8363–8365.
4. Ullrich A, Coussens L, Hayflick JS, et al. Human epidermal growth factor receptor cDNA sequence and aberrant expression of the amplified gene in A431 epidermoid carcinoma cells. Nature 1984; 309:418–425.
5. Ullrich A, Gray A, Tam AW, et al. Insulin-like growth factor I receptor primary structure: comparison with insulin receptor suggests structural determinants that define functional specificity. EMBO J 1986; 5:2503–2512.
6. Weiss A, Schlessinger J. Switching signals on or off by receptor dimerization. Cell 1998; 94:277–280.
7. Westermark B, Claesson-Welsh L, Heldin CH. Structural and functional aspects of the receptors for platelet-derived growth factor. Prog Growth Factor Res 1989; 1:253–266.
8. Heldin CH, Ostman A, Ronnstrand L. Signal transduction via platelet-derived growth factor receptors. Biochim Biophys Acta 1998; 1378:F79–F113.
9. Wiesmann C, Fuh G, Christinger HW, et al. Crystal structure at 1.7 Å resolution of VEGF in complex with domain 2 of the Flt-1 receptor. Cell 1997; 91:695–704.
10. Cunningham BC, Ultsch M, De Vos AM, et al. Dimerization of the extracellular domain of the human growth hormone receptor by a single hormone molecule. Science 1991; 254:821–825.
11. de Vos AM, Ultsch M, Kossiakoff AA. Human growth hormone and extracellular domain of its receptor: crystal structure of the complex. Science 1992; 255:306–312.
12. Wells JA. Binding in the growth hormone receptor complex. Proc Natl Acad Sci USA 1996; 93:1–6.
13. Boni-Schnetzler M, Rubin JB, Pilch PF. Structural requirements for the transmembrane activation of the insulin receptor kinase. J Biol Chem 1986; 261:15281–15287.
14. Boni-Schnetzler M, Scott W, Waugh SM, et al. The insulin receptor: structural basis for high affinity ligand binding. J Biol Chem 1987; 262:8395–8401.
15. Taouis M, Levy-Toledano R, Roach P, et al. Structural basis by which a recessive mutation in the alpha-subunit of the insulin receptor affects insulin binding. J Biol Chem 1994; 269:14912–14918.
16. De Meyts P. The structural basis of insulin and insulin-like growth factor-I receptor binding and negative co-operativity, and its relevance to mitogenic versus metabolic signalling. Diabetologia 1994; 37:S135–S148.
17. Hubbard SR, Wei L, Ellis L, et al. Crystal structure of the tyrosine kinase domain of the human insulin receptor. Nature 1994; 372:746–754.
18. Hubbard SR. Crystal structure of the activated insulin receptor tyrosine kinase in complex with peptide substrate and ATP analog. EMBO J 1997; 16:5572–5581.
19. Hubbard SR, Mohammadi M, Schlessinger J. Autoregulatory mechanisms in protein-tyrosine kinases. J Biol Chem 1998; 273:11987–11990.
20. Herrera R, Rosen OM. Regulation of the protein kinase activity of the human insulin receptor. J Recept Res 1987; 7:405–415.
21. Tornqvist HE, Avruch J. Relationship of site-specific beta subunit tyrosine autophosphorylation to insulin activation of the insulin receptor (tyrosine) protein kinase activity. J Biol Chem 1988; 263:4593–4501.
22. Ullrich A, Schlessinger J. Signal transduction by receptors with tyrosine kinase activity. Cell 1990; 61:203–202.
23. Kavanaugh WM, Williams LT. An alternative to SH2 domains for binding tyrosine-phosphorylated proteins. Science 1994; 266:1862–1865.
24. Blaikie P, Immanuel D, Wu J, et al. A region in Shc distinct from the SH2 domain can bind tyrosine-phosphorylated growth factor receptors. J Biol Chem 1994; 269:32031–32034.
25. Gustafson TA, He W, Craparo A, et al. Phosphotyrosine-dependent interaction of SHC and insulin receptor substrate 1 with the NPEY motif of the insulin receptor via a novel non-SH2 domain. Mol Cell Biol 1995; 15:2500–2508.
26. Anderson D, Koch CA, Grey L, et al. Binding of SH2 domains of phospholipase Cg 1, GAP, and Src to activated growth factor receptors. Science 1990; 250:979–982.
27. Perrotti N, Accili D, Marcus-Samuels B, et al. Insulin stimulates phosphorylation of a 120-kDa glycoprotein substrate (pp120) for the receptor-associated protein kinase in intact H-35 hepatoma cells. Proc Natl Acad Sci USA 1987; 84:3137–3140.
28. Najjar SM, Philippe N, Suzuki Y, et al. Insulin-stimulated phosphorylation of recombinant pp120/HA4, an endogenous substrate of the insulin receptor tyrosine kinase. Biochemistry 1995; 34:9341–9349.
29. Kouhara H, Hadari YR, Spivak-Kroizman T, et al. A lipid-anchored Grb2-binding protein that links FGF-receptor activation to the Ras/MAPK signaling pathway. Cell 1997; 89:693–692.
30. White MF, Yenush L. The IRS-signaling system: a network of docking proteins that mediate insulin and cytokine action. Curr Top Microbiol Immunol 1998; 228:179–178.
31. Sun XJ, Rothenberg P, Kahn CR, et al. Structure of the insulin receptor substrate IRS-1 defines a unique signal transduction protein. Nature 1991; 352:73–77.
32. Sun XJ, Wang LM, Zhang Y, et al. Role of IRS-2 in insulin and cytokine signalling. Nature 1995; 377:173–177.
33. Lavan BE, Lane WS, Lienhard GE. The 60-kDa phosphotyrosine protein in insulin-treated adipocytes is a new member of the insulin receptor substrate family. J Biol Chem 1997; 272:11439–11443.
34. Sciacchitano S, Taylor SI. Cloning, tissue expression, and chromosomal localization of the mouse IRS-3 gene. Endocrinology 1997; 138:4931–4940.
35. Quon MJ, Chen H, Ing BL, et al. Roles of 1-phosphatidylinositol 3-kinase and ras in regulating translocation of GLUT4 in transfected rat adipose cells. Mol Cell Biol 1995; 15:5403–5411.
36. Kohn AD, Summers SA, Birnbaum MJ, et al. Expression of a constitutively active Akt Ser/Thr kinase in 3T3-L1 adipocytes stimulates glucose uptake and glucose transporter 4 translocation. J Biol Chem 1996; 271:31372–31378.
37. Cong LN, Chen H, Li Y, et al. Physiological role of Akt in insulin-stimulated translocation of GLUT4 in transfected rat adipose cells. Mol Endocrinol 1997; 11:1881–1890.
38. Standaert ML, Galloway L, Karnam P, et al. Protein kinase C-zeta as a downstream effector of phosphatidylinositol 3-kinase during insulin stimulation in rat adipocytes. Potential role in glucose transport. J Biol Chem 1997; 272:30075–30082.

39. Kitamura T, Ogawa W, Sakaue H, et al. Requirement for activation of the serine-threonine kinase Akt (protein kinase B) in insulin stimulation of protein synthesis but not of glucose transport. Mol Cell Biol 1998; 18:3708–3717.
40. Alessi DR, Deak M, Casamayor A, et al. 3-Phosphoinositide–dependent protein kinase-1 (PDK1): structural and functional homology with the *Drosophila* DSTPK61 kinase. Curr Biol 1997; 7: 776–779.
41. Alessi DR, Downes CP. The role of PI 3-kinase in insulin action. Biochim Biophys Acta 1998; 1436:151–154.
42. Cheatham B, Vlahos CJ, Cheatham L, et al. Phosphatidylinositol 3-kinase activation is required for insulin stimulation of pp70 S6 kinase, DNA synthesis, and glucose transporter translocation. Mol Cell Biol 1994; 14:4902–4911.
43. Watson R, Shigematsu S, Chiang S, et al. Lipid raft microdomain compartmentalization of TC10 is required for insulin signaling and GLUT4 translocation. J Cell Biol 2001; 154:829–840.
44. Baumann CA, Ribon V, Kanzaki M, et al. CAP defines a second signalling pathway required for insulin-stimulated glucose transport. Nature 2000; 407:202–207.
45. Chiang SH, Baumann CA, Kanzaki M, et al. Insulin-stimulated GLUT4 translocation requires the CAP-dependent activation of TC10. Nature 2001; 410:944–948.
46. Lowenstein EJ, Daly RJ, Batzer AG, et al. The SH2 and SH3 domain–containing protein GRB2 links receptor tyrosine kinases to ras signaling. Cell 1992; 70:431–432.
47. Pronk GJ, McGlade J, Pelicci G, et al. Insulin-induced phosphorylation of the 46- and 52-kDa Shc proteins. J Biol Chem 1993; 268:5748–5753.
48. Skolnik EY, Lee CH, Batzer A, et al. The SH2/SH3 domain–containing protein GRB2 interacts with tyrosine-phosphorylated IRS1 and Shc: implications for insulin control of ras signalling. EMBO J 1993; 12:1929–1936.
49. Li N, Batzer A, Daly R, et al. Guanine-nucleotide–releasing factor hSos1 binds to Grb2 and links receptor tyrosine kinases to Ras signalling. Nature 1993; 363:85–88.
50. Yarden Y, Escobedo JA, Kuang WJ, et al. Structure of the receptor for platelet-derived growth factor helps define a family of closely related growth factor receptors. Nature 1986; 323:226–232.
51. Clark SF, Martin S, Carozzi AJ, et al. Intracellular localization of phosphatidylinositide 3-kinase and insulin receptor substrate-1 in adipocytes: potential involvement of a membrane skeleton. J Cell Biol 1998; 140:1211–1225.
52. Carpentier JL. Insulin receptor internalization: molecular mechanisms and physiopathological implications. Diabetologia 1994; 37: S117–S124.
53. Carpentier JL, Hamer I, Gilbert A, et al. Molecular and cellular mechanisms governing the ligand-specific and non-specific steps of insulin receptor internalization. Z Gastroenterol 1996; 34:73–75.
54. Flier JS, Minaker KL, Landsberg L, et al. Impaired in vivo insulin clearance in patients with severe target-cell resistance to insulin. Diabetes 1982; 31:132–135.
55. Elchebly M, Payette P, Michaliszyn E, et al. Increased insulin sensitivity and obesity resistance in mice lacking the protein tyrosine phosphatase-1B gene. Science 1999; 283:1544–1548.
56. Klaman LD, Boss O, Peroni OD, et al. Increased energy expenditure, decreased adiposity, and tissue-specific insulin sensitivity in protein-tyrosine phosphatase 1B–deficient mice. Mol Cell Biol 2000; 20:5479–5489.
57. Hotamisligil GS, Peraldi P, Budavari A, et al. IRS-1–mediated inhibition of insulin receptor tyrosine kinase activity in TNF-alpha–and obesity-induced insulin resistance. Science 1996; 271: 665–668.
58. De Fea K, Roth RA. Modulation of insulin receptor substrate-1 tyrosine phosphorylation and function by mitogen-activated protein kinase. J Biol Chem 1997; 272:31400–31406.
59. Li J, DeFea K, Roth RA. Modulation of insulin receptor substrate-1 tyrosine phosphorylation by an Akt/phosphatidylinositol 3-kinase pathway. J Biol Chem 1999; 274:9351–9356.
60. Aguirre V, Uchida T, Yenush L, et al. The c-Jun NH_2 terminal kinase promotes insulin resistance during association with insulin receptor substrate-1 and phosphorylation of Ser(307). J Biol Chem 2000; 275:9047–9054.
61. Rui L, Aguirre V, Kim JK, et al. Insulin/IGF-1 and TNF-alpha stimulate phosphorylation of IRS-1 at inhibitory Ser307 via distinct pathways. J Clin Invest 2001; 107:181–189.
62. Taylor SI. Lilly lecture: molecular mechanisms of insulin resistance. Lessons from patients with mutations in the insulin-receptor gene. Diabetes 1992; 41:1473–1490.
63. Carlomagno F, Salvatore G, Cirafici AM, et al. The different RET-activating capability of mutations of cysteine 620 or cysteine 634 correlates with the multiple endocrine neoplasia type 2 disease phenotype. Cancer Res 1997; 57:391–395.
64. Drachman DB. Myasthenia gravis. N Engl J Med 1994; 330: 1797–1810.
65. Kahn CR, Flier JS, Bar RS, et al. The syndromes of insulin resistance and acanthosis nigricans: insulin-receptor disorders in man. N Engl J Med 1976; 294:739–745.
66. Flier JS, Kahn CR, Roth J, et al. Antibodies that impair insulin receptor binding in an unusual diabetic syndrome with severe insulin resistance. Science 1975; 190:63–65.
67. Taylor SI, Marcus-Samuels B. Anti-receptor antibodies mimic the effect of insulin to down-regulate insulin receptors in cultured human lymphoblastoid (IM-9) cells. J Clin Endocrinol Metab 1984; 58:182–186.
68. Weetman AP. Graves' disease. N Engl J Med 2000; 343:1236–1248.
69. Flier JS, Bar RS, Muggeo M, et al. The evolving clinical course of patients with insulin receptor autoantibodies: spontaneous remission or receptor proliferation with hypoglycemia. J Clin Endocrinol Metab 1978; 47:985–995.
70. Taylor SI, Grunberger G, Marcus-Samuels B, et al. Hypoglycemia associated with antibodies to the insulin receptor. N Engl J Med 1982; 307:1422–1426.
71. Taylor SI, Barbetti F, Accili D, et al. Syndromes of autoimmunity and hypoglycemia: autoantibodies directed against insulin and its receptor. Endocrinol Metab Clin North Am 1989; 18:123–143.
72. Amselem S, Duquesnoy P, Attree O, et al. Laron dwarfism and mutations of the growth hormone-receptor gene. N Engl J Med 1989; 321:989–995.
73. Clement K, Vaisse C, Lahlou N, et al. A mutation in the human leptin receptor gene causes obesity and pituitary dysfunction. Nature 1998; 392:398–401.
74. Smit LS, Meyer DJ, Argetsinger LS, et al. Molecular events in growth hormone–receptor interaction and signaling. In Handbook of Physiology (JS Kostyo and HM Goodman, eds). New York: Oxford University Press, 1999, pp 445–480.
75. Bravo J, Heath JK. Receptor recognition by gp130 cytokines. EMBO J 2000; 19:2399–2411.
76. Auernhammer CJ, Melmed S. Leukemia-inhibitory factor—neuroimmune modulator of endocrine function. Endocr Rev 2000; 21:313–345.
77. Lambert PD, Anderson KD, Sleeman MW, et al. Ciliary neurotrophic factor activates leptin-like pathways and reduces body fat, without cachexia or rebound weight gain, even in leptin-resistant obesity. Proc Natl Acad Sci USA 2001; 98:4652–4657.
78. Opal SM, DePalo VA. Anti-inflammatory cytokines. Chest 2000; 117:1162–1172.
79. Heim MH. The Jak-STAT pathway: cytokine signalling from the receptor to the nucleus. J Recept Signal Transduct Res 1999; 19: 75–120.
80. Campbell GS, Argetsinger LS, Ihle JN, et al. Activation of JAK2 tyrosine kinase by prolactin receptors in Nb2 cells and mouse mammary gland explants. Proc Natl Acad Sci USA 1994; 91: 5232–5236.
81. Argetsinger LS, Campbell GS, Yang X, et al. Identification of JAK2 as a growth hormone receptor–associated tyrosine kinase. Cell 1993; 74:237–244.
82. Livnah O, Stura EA, Middleton SA, et al. Crystallographic evidence for preformed dimers of erythropoietin receptor before ligand activation. Science 1999; 283:987–990.
83. Remy I, Wilson IA, Michnick SW. Erythropoietin receptor activation by a ligand-induced conformation change. Science 1999; 283:990–993.
84. Noguchi M, Yi H, Rosenblatt HM, et al. Interleukin-2 receptor gamma chain mutation results in X-linked severe combined immunodeficiency in humans. Cell 1993; 73:147–157.

85. Parganas E, Wang D, Stravopodis D, et al. Jak2 is essential for signaling through a variety of cytokine receptors. Cell 1998; 93: 385–395.
86. Ihle JN, Thierfelder W, Teglund S, et al. Signaling by the cytokine receptor superfamily. Ann NY Acad Sci 1998; 865:1–9.
87. Stahl N, Boulton TG, Farruggella T, et al. Association and activation of Jak-Tyk kinases by CNTF-LIF-OSM-IL-6 beta receptor components. Science 1994; 263:92–95.
88. Stocklin E, Wissler M, Gouilleux F, et al. Functional interactions between Stat5 and the glucocorticoid receptor. Nature 1996; 383: 726–728.
89. Danial NN, Rothman P. JAK-STAT signaling activated by Abl oncogenes. Oncogene 2000; 19:2523–2531.
90. Lin TS, Mahajan S, Frank DA. STAT signaling in the pathogenesis and treatment of leukemias. Oncogene 2000; 19:2496–2504.
91. Naka T, Narazaki M, Hirata M, et al. Structure and function of a new STAT-induced STAT inhibitor. Nature 1997; 387:924–929.
92. Yasukawa H, Misawa H, Sakamoto H, et al. The JAK-binding protein JAB inhibits Janus tyrosine kinase activity through binding in the activation loop. EMBO J 1999; 18:1309–1320.
93. Hansen JA, Lindberg K, Hilton DJ, et al. Mechanism of inhibition of growth hormone receptor signaling by suppressor of cytokine signaling proteins. Mol Endocrinol 1999; 13:1832–1843.
94. Ram PA, Waxman DJ. SOCS/CIS protein inhibition of growth hormone-stimulated STAT5 signaling by multiple mechanisms. J Biol Chem 1999; 274:35553–35561.
95. Mao Y, Ling PR, Fitzgibbons TP, et al. Endotoxin-induced inhibition of growth hormone receptor signaling in rat liver in vivo. Endocrinology 1999; 140:5505–5515.
96. Clevenger CV, Medaglia MV. The protein tyrosine kinase P59fyn is associated with prolactin (PRL) receptor and is activated by PRL stimulation of T-lymphocytes. Mol Endocrinol 1994; 8:674–681.
97. Rui L, Carter-Su C. Identification of SH2-Bb as a potent cytoplasmic activator of the tyrosine kinase Janus kinase 2. Proc Natl Acad Sci USA 1999; 96:7172–7177.
98. Shuai K. Modulation of STAT signaling by STAT-interacting proteins. Oncogene 2000; 19:2638–2644.
99. Hanks SK, Hunter T. Protein kinases 6. The eukaryotic protein kinase superfamily: kinase (catalytic) domain structure and classification. FASEB J 1995; 9:576–596.
100. Belham C, Wu S, Avruch J. Intracellular signalling: PDK1—a kinase at the hub of things. Curr Biol 1999; 9:R93–R96.
101. Avruch J, Khokhlatchev A, Kyriakis JM, et al. Ras activation of the Raf kinase: tyrosine kinase recruitment of the MAP kinase cascade. Recent Prog Horm Res 2001; 56:127–155.
102. Mulligan LM, Kwok JB, Healey CS, et al. Germ-line mutations of the *RET* proto-oncogene in multiple endocrine neoplasia type 2A. Nature 1993; 363:458–460.
103. Santoro M, Carlomagno F, Romano A, et al. Activation of *RET* as a dominant transforming gene by germline mutations of *MEN2A* and *MEN2B*. Science 1995; 267:381–383.
104. Bockaert J, Pin JP. Molecular tinkering of G protein–coupled receptors: an evolutionary success. EMBO J 1999; 18:1723–1729.
105. Neer EJ. Heterotrimeric G proteins: organizers of transmembrane signals. Cell 1995; 80:249–257.
106. Dessauer CW, Posner BA, Gilman AG. Visualizing signal transduction: receptors, G proteins and adenylate cyclases. Clin Sci 1996; 91:527.
107. Hamm H. The many faces of G protein signaling. J Biol Chem 1998; 273:669–672.
108. Bourne H. How receptors talk to trimeric G proteins. Curr Opin Cell Biol 1997; 9:134–142.
109. Rodbell M. The role of GTP-binding proteins in signal transduction: from the sublimely simple to the conceptually complex. Curr Top Cell Regul 1992; 32:1–47.
110. Ross EM, Wilkie TM. GTPase activating proteins for heterotrimeric G proteins: regulators of G protein signaling (RGS) and RGS-like proteins. Annu Rev Biochem 2000; 69:795–827.
111. Lefkowitz RJ. The superfamily of heptahelical receptors. Nat Cell Biol 2000; 2:E133-E136.
112. Palczewski K, Kumasaka T, Hori T, et al. Crystal structure of rhodopsin: a G protein–coupled receptor. Science 2000; 289: 739–745.
113. Kunishima N, Shimada Y, Tsuji Y, et al. Structural basis of glutamate recognition by a dimeric metabotropic glutamate receptor. Nature 2000; 407:971–977.
114. Wess J (ed). Structure-Function Analysis of G Protein–Coupled Receptors. New York, Wiley-Liss, 1999.
115. Yamashita T, Terakita A, Shichida Y. Distinct roles of the second and third cytoplasmic loops of bovine rhodopsin in G protein activation. J Biol Chem 2000; 275:34272–34279.
116. Gershengorn M, Osman R. Insights into G protein–coupled receptor function using molecular models. Endocrinology 2001; 142:2–10.
117. Herbert TE, Moffett S, Morello JP, et al. A peptide derived from a $\beta 2$-adrenergic receptor transmembrane domain inhibits both receptor dimerization and activation. J Biol Chem 1996; 271:16384–16392.
118. Ray K, Hauschild BC, Steinbach PJ, et al. Identification of the cysteine residues in the amino-terminal extracellular domain of the human Ca^{2+} receptor critical for dimerization. J Biol Chem 1999; 274:27642–27650.
119. Kaupmann K, Malitschek B, Schuler V, et al. GABA-B receptor subtypes assemble into functional heteromeric complexes. Nature 1998; 396:683–687.
120. Abdalla S, Lother H, Quitterer U. AT1-receptor heterodimers show enhanced G protein activation and altered receptor sequestration. Nature 2000; 407:94–98.
121. Jordan BA, Trapaidze N, Gomes I, et al. Oligomerization of opioid receptors with $\beta 2$-adrenergic receptors: a role in trafficking and mitogen-activated protein kinase activation. Proc Natl Acad Sci USA 2001; 98:343–348.
122. Hall RA, Premont RT, Lefkowitz RJ. Heptahelical receptor signaling: beyond the G protein paradigm. J Cell Biol 1999; 145: 927–932.
123. Tu JC, Xiao B, Yuan JP, et al. Homer binds a novel proline-rich motif and links group 1 metabotropic glutamate receptors with IP3 receptors. Neuron 1998; 21:717–726.
124. McLatchie L, Fraser N, Main M, et al. RAMPs regulate the transport and ligand specificity of the calcitonin-like receptor. Nature 1998; 393:333–339.
125. Howard AD, Wang R, Pong S-S, et al. Identification of receptors for neuromedin U and its role in feeding. Nature 2000; 406:70–74.
126. Spiegel AM (ed). G Proteins, Receptors, and Disease. Totawa, NJ, Humana Press, 1998.
127. Barak LS, Oakley RH, Laporte SA, et al. Constitutive arrestin-mediated desensitization of a human vasopressin receptor mutant associated with nephrogenic diabetes insipidus. Proc Natl Acad Sci USA 2001; 98:93–98.
128. Bai M, Trivedi S, Brown EM. Dimerization of the extracellular calcium-sensing receptor (CaR) on cell surface of CaR-transfected HEK293 cells. J Biol Chem 1998; 273:23605–23610.
129. Van Sande J, Parma J, Tonacchera M, et al. Somatic and germline mutations of the TSH receptor gene in thyroid diseases. J Clin Endocrinol Metab 1995; 80:2577–2585.
130. Javitch JA, Fu D, Liapakis G, Chen J. Constitutive activation of the $\beta 2$-adrenergic receptor alters the orientation of its sixth membrane-spanning segment. J Biol Chem 1997; 272:18546–18549.
131. Zhao XM, Hauache O, Goldsmith PK, et al. A missense mutation in the seventh transmembrane domain constitutively activates the human Ca^{2+} receptor. FEBS Lett 1999; 448:180–184.
132. Lin L, Faraco J, Li R, et al. The sleep disorder canine narcolepsy is caused by a mutation in the hypocretin (orexin) receptor 2 gene. Cell 1999; 98:365–376.
133. Huszar D, Lynch CA, Fairchild-Huntress V, et al. Targeted disruption of the melanocortin-4 receptor results in obesity in mice. Cell 1997; 88:131–141.
134. Vaisse C, Clement K, Durand E, et al. Melanocortin-4 receptor mutations are a frequent and heterogeneous cause of morbid obesity. J Clin Invest 2000; 106:253–262.
135. Lanske B, Karaplis AC, Lee K, et al. PTH/PTHrP receptor in early development and Indian hedgehog–regulated bone growth. Science 1996; 273:663–666.
136. Jobert AS, Zhang P, Couvineau A, et al. Absence of functional receptors for parathyroid hormone and parathyroid hormone–related peptide in Blomstrand chondrodysplasia. J Clin Invest 1998; 102:34–40.

137. Susulic VS, Frederich RC, Lawitts J, et al. Targeted disruption of the β3-adrenergic receptor gene. J Biol Chem 1995; 270:29483–29492.
138. Yun J, Schoneberg T, Liu J, et al. Generation and phenotype of mice harboring a nonsense mutation in the V2 vasopressin receptor gene. J Clin Invest 2000; 106:1361–1371.
139. Liu R, Paxton WA, Choe S, et al. Homozygous defect in HIV-1 coreceptor accounts for resistance of some multiply exposed individuals to HIV-1 infection. Cell 1996; 86:367–377.
140. de Bono M, Bargmann CI. Natural variation in a neuropeptide Y receptor homolog modifies social behavior and food response in *C. elegans*. Cell 1998; 94:679–689.
141. Small KM, Forbes SL, Rahman FF, et al. A four amino acid deletion polymorphism in the third intracellular loop of the human α2C-adrenergic receptor confers impaired coupling to multiple effectors. J Biol Chem 2000; 275:23059–23064.

6 Laboratory Techniques for Recognition of Endocrine Disorders

George Klee

Endocrinology is a practice of medicine that is highly dependent on accurate laboratory measurements because small changes in hormone levels often may be more specific and more sensitive for early disease than the classic physical signs and symptoms. Because most endocrinologists currently do not have facilities to develop and validate laboratory assays, they rely on commercial analytic assays or send a patient's specimen to specialized laboratories. Even most hospital and commercial laboratories have minimal expertise for developing analytic assays. This critical dependence on quality laboratory measurements, combined with minimal information about the performance of these tests, places endocrinologists in a potentially vulnerable position.

This chapter attempts to provide an overview of the strengths and weaknesses of the analytic techniques typically used for endocrine measurements in blood and urine. Concentrations of most hormones are much lower than those of general chemistry analytes, and specialized techniques are necessary to measure these low concentrations.

Three major types of assays for measuring hormones are described:

- Immunoassays (both competitive and sandwich)
- Chromatography
- Mass spectrometry

Nucleic acid measurements for evaluation of genetic alterations also are reviewed.

The minimal analytic performance validation required by the federal government for laboratories testing specimens of Medicare patients, along with explanations of these performance parameters, is outlined. This information should help endocrinologists better assess the performance of the analytic systems that they are using. Techniques to investigate discordant laboratory test values also are presented to help clinicians work with their laboratories to reconcile test values that do not match clinical presentations.

Hormone concentrations are reported in molar units, mass units, or standardized units, such as World Health Organization (WHO) International Units (IU). When these measurements are expressed in molar units, most hormones in blood and urine are present in concentrations of 10^{-6} to 10^{-12} M/L (Fig. 6–1). The terms used to describe these concentrations are micromolar (10^{-6} M/L), nanomolar (10^{-9} M/L), and picomolar (10^{-12} M/L). The range—from the lowest to highest concentrations—is more than a million-fold difference. Therefore, laboratory techniques must be targeted to the levels of each given hormone.

The major techniques for measuring picomolar concentrations are immunoassay and mass spectroscopy, whereas nanomolar and micromolar concentrations can be measured by these methods as well as chromatography and chemical detection systems. Some hormones, such as thyrotropin (TSH), have very low concentrations in the femtomolar (10^{-15} M/L) range in patients with diseases such as thyrotoxicosis. Exquisitely sensitive immunometric assays are usually needed to measure these very low concentrations.[1, 2]

TYPES OF ASSAYS

The four major techniques used for endocrine measurements are as follows:

- Antibody-based immunologic assays, of which there are two subcategories: competitive immunoassays and immunometric (sandwich) assays
- Chromatographic assays
- Mass spectroscopy
- Nucleic acid–based assays

Competitive Immunoassays

The term competitive radioimmunoassay refers to a measurement method in which an antigen (e.g., a hormone) in a specimen competes with radiolabeled reagent antigen for a limited number of binding sites on a reagent antibody. The three basic components of a competitive immunoassay are[3, 4]:

1. Antiserum specific for a unique epitope on a hormone or antigen.
2. Labeled antigen that binds to this antiserum.

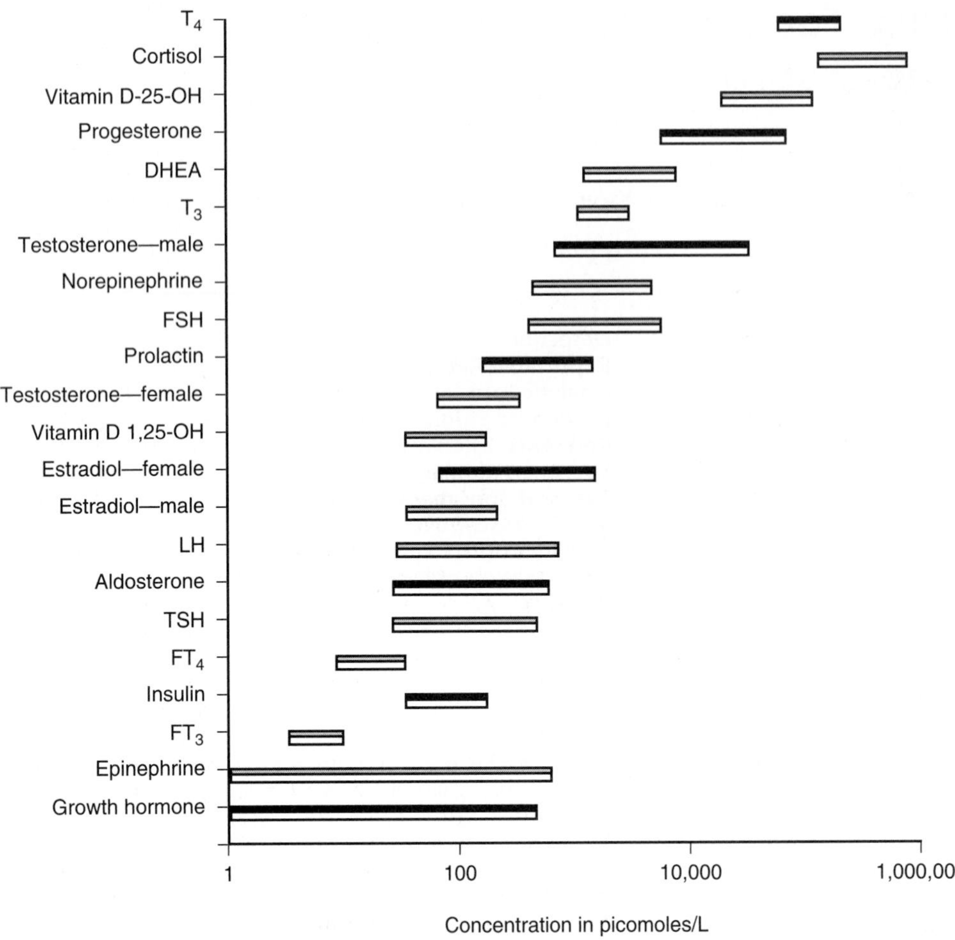

Figure 6–1. Seven-logarithm range of normal concentrations for the plasma concentrations of endocrine tests. DHEA, dehydroepiandrosterone; FSH, follicle-stimulating hormone; FT_4, free thyroxine; FT_3, free triiodothyronine; LH, luteinizing hormone; T_3, triiodothyronine; T_4, thyroxine; TSH, thyrotropin.

3. Unlabeled antigen in the specimen or standard that is to be measured.

The antiserum is diluted to a concentration in which the number of binding sites available on the antibodies is fewer than the number of antigen molecules (labeled and unlabeled) in the reaction mixture. The labeled and unlabeled antigens compete for these limited number of binding sites on the antiserum. The competition is not always equal because the labeled antigen *(tracer)* may react differently with the antibody compared with the native antigen. This disparity in reactivity may be caused by alteration of the antigen due to the chemical attachment of the label or by differences in the endogenous antigen versus the form of the antigen used in the reagents. As long as the reactions are reproducible, these differences in reactivity are not important because the reaction can be *calibrated* with standard reference materials having known concentrations.

Figure 6–2 illustrates the concepts of a competitive immunoassay. In the schematic diagram, 8 units of antibody react with 16 units of labeled antigen and 4 units of native antigen. At equilibrium (assuming equal reactivity), 6 units of label and 2 units of native antigen are bound to the limited supply of antibody. The antigen bound to the antibody is separated from the liquid antigen by any of several methods, and the amount of labeled antigen in the bound portion is quantitated. The assay is calibrated by measuring standards with known concentrations and cross-plotting the signal (i.e., counts of the gamma rays emitted from the radioactive label) versus the concentration of the standards to generate a dose-response curve. As the concentration increases, the signal decreases exponentially.

Typically, the antiserum used in a competitive assay is diluted to a titer that binds between 40% to 50% of the labeled antigen when no unlabeled antigen is present. Further dilution of the antiserum increases the analytic sensitivity but decreases the signal and range of the assay.

The precision of competitive immunoassays is related to the rate of change of the signal compared with the rate of change of concentration (i.e., the slope of the dose-response curve).[5] In Figure 6–2, the slope is much lower at higher concentrations, causing the assay precision to be less at higher concentrations. Most competitive immunoassays also have a relatively flat dose-response curve at very low concentrations, causing poor precision at the low end of the assay. Consequently, the precision profile for most immunoassays is U-shaped, having the best coefficients of variation in the center of the dose-response curve.

As shown in Figure 6–2, the higher the concentration of the unlabeled antigen, the lower the amount of radiolabeled antigen that binds to the limited amount of antiserum. The signal decreases exponentially from the approximately half-maximum at zero concentration to a minimum value at high concentrations. This minimal binding, or *nonspecific binding* (NSB), is a valuable control parameter. Elevations in NSB usually signify impurities in the label that bind to the sides of the tubes and are not competitively displaced. Most assays add surfactants and proteins to minimize the NSB. Monitoring of changes in the NSB provides an early warning of potential assay problems.

Statistical data-processing techniques are needed to translate the assay signals into concentrations. As illustrated, because these reactions are not linear, numerous curve-fitting algorithms have been developed. Before the introduction of micro-

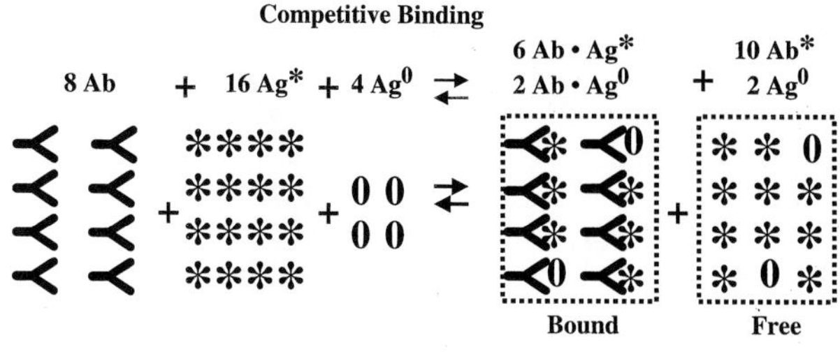

Calibration of Standards

Ab	+	Ag*	+	Ag0	Ab • Ag*	+ Ab • Ag0	+	Ag*	+ Ag0
8		16		0	8	0		8	0
8		16		4	6	2		10	2
8		16		12	4	4		12	8
8		16		36	2	6		14	30
Constant				Variable	Bound			Free	

A

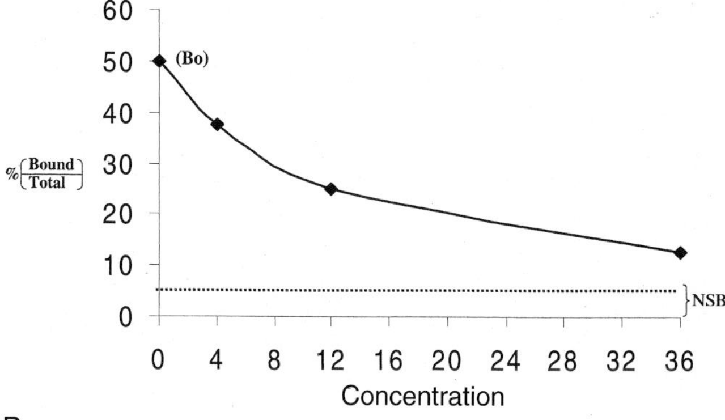

B

Figure 6–2. *A*, Principles of competitive binding assays. *B*, Typical dose-response curve.

processors, tedious error-prone, manual calculations were required to mathematically transform the data into linear models. A commonly used model was to cross-plot the logit of the normalized signal versus the logarithm of the concentration and to use linear regression lines to establish the dose-response curve.[5] Fortunately, today this procedure of curve fitting usually is accomplished electronically by using programs that automatically test the robustness of fit of multiparameter curves after statistically eliminating discordant data points.[6] However, users of these systems must understand the limitations and should pay attention to any warnings presented by the programs during processing of the data.

In radioimmunoassays, radioactive iodine (^{125}I) is usually used to label the antigen. The immune complexes are separated from the unbound molecules by precipitation with centrifugation after reaction with secondary antisera and precipitating reagents (e.g., polyethylene glycol).[7] These radioimmunoassays may require special handling and licensure to ensure safety of the radioisotopes and are labor-intensive. The statistical counting errors associated with the relatively low radioactive counts and the poor reproducibility associated with the multiple manual steps generally necessitate that most laboratories perform the measurements in duplicate.[8] Even when the averages of duplicate measurements are used, many manual radioimmunoassays have coefficients of variation between 10% and 15%.

It is important that key quality control parameters for radioimmunoassays be carefully monitored. In addition to NSB, another key quality control parameter is the percentage binding of the radiolabel when zero antigen (Bo) is present. As the label deteriorates, because of aging, the binding often decreases, resulting in a less reliable assay.

Another important quality control parameter is the slope of the dose-response curve. This parameter can be tracked by monitoring the concentration corresponding to half-maximum binding (50% of B/Bo). If this concentration increases significantly, the slope of the response curve decreases and the assay may not be capable of reliably measuring patient specimens at clinically important concentrations.

Many commercial kits and automated immunoassays today use nonisotopic signal systems to measure hormone concentrations. These assays often use colorimetric, fluorometric, or chemiluminescent signals rather than radioactivity to quantitate the response. The advantages of these alternate signals are biosafety, longer reagent self-life, and ease of automation. On the other hand, these signals are more subject to matrix interferences than radioactive iodine.

Radioactivity is not affected by changes in protein concentration, hemolysis, color, or drugs (except for other radioactive compounds), whereas many of the current signal systems may yield spurious results when such interferences are present. In addition, many of today's automated immunoassays are read kinetically before the reactions reach equilibrium. This step accentuates the effects of matrix differences between the reference standards and patient specimens. Later in this chapter potential trouble-shooting steps are outlined to help clinicians evaluate the integrity of test measurements when spurious results are suspected.

Solid-phase reactions often are used in current immunoassays to facilitate the separation of the bound antibody-antigen complexes from the free reactants.[9] Three frequently used solid-phase materials are (1) microtiter plates, (2) polystyrene beads, and (3) paramagnetic particles.[10] Typically, the antibody is attached to the solid phase, and the separation of the immune complexes from the unbound moieties is accomplished by plate washers, bead washers, or magnetic wash stations, eliminating the need for centrifugation. Other novel ways of accomplishing this separation is to attach high-affinity linkers to antiserum, which then can be coupled to a complementary linker on the solid phase.

An excellent pair of linkers are biotin and streptavidin. These compounds bind with affinity constants of approximately 10^{15} L/M.[11] Biotin is a relatively small molecule that can easily be covalently attached to antiserum and used with streptavidin (a 70-kD tetrameric nonglycosylated protein) conjugated to microtiter plates, beads, or paramagnetic particles to facilitate separation. This technique allows the antibody-antigen reaction to proceed faster with less stearic hindrance than when the antibody is directly coupled to the solid phase.

The antiserum used in these assays is a crucial component. Most earlier immunoassays used *polyclonal* antiserum produced in animals. The process of generating these antisera is a combination of art, science, and luck. Generally, a relatively pure form of the antigen is conjugated to a carrier protein (especially if the antigen is less than 10,000 d), mixed with adjuvant (e.g., Freud's complete adjuvant), and injected intradermally into the host animal. After several boosts with conjugated protein plus Freud's incomplete adjuvant, the host animal recognizes the material as foreign and develops immune responses. The antiserum then is harvested from the animal's blood. Under optimal conditions, moderate quantities of high-affinity antisera, which react only with the specific target antigen, are developed. The analytic sensitivity of a competitive immunoassay is approximately inversely related to the affinity of the antiserum, such that an antiserum with an affinity constant of

10^9 L/M can be used to measure analytes in the nanomolar concentration range.

The polyclonal antiserum developed by immunizing animals represents a composite of many immunologic clones, with each clone having a different affinity and different immunologic specificity. Most clones have affinities in the 10^7 to 10^8 L/M range, with only rare clones having affinities above 10^{12} L/M. Various techniques are used to develop a specific antiserum, including (1) altering the form of the antigen by blocking cross-reacting epitopes and (2) purifying the antiserum using affinity chromatography to select antibodies directed toward the epitope of interest. Affinity-column purification can also be used for immunoextraction of higher-affinity antisera by selectively eluting antiserum from the column by means of a series of buffers with increasing acidity.[12]

The major disadvantage of a polyclonal antiserum is the limited quantity. The large quantities needed by commercial suppliers of immunoassay reagents often require them to use multiple sources of antisera. These changes in antisera can cause significant changes in assay performance. In many instances, laboratories and clinicians are not informed about these changes, which may cause problems in medical decisions.

Monoclonal antisera are used in many current immunoassays. These antisera are made by immunizing animals (usually mice) using techniques similar to those used for polyclonal antisera; instead of harvesting the antisera from the blood, however, the animal is killed and the spleen is removed.[13] The lymphocytes in the spleen are fused with myeloma cells to make cells that will grow in culture and produce antisera.

These fused cells are separated into clones by means of serial plating techniques similar to those used in subculturing bacteria. The supernatant of these monoclonal cell lines (or ascites fluid if the cells are transplanted into carrier mice) contains monoclonal antisera. The selection processes used to separate the initial clones can be targeted to identify specific clones producing antisera with high affinities and low cross-reactivity to related compounds.

The high specificity of monoclonal antisera can cause problems for some endocrine assays. Many hormones circulate in the blood as heterogeneous mixtures of multiple forms. Some of these forms are caused by genetic differences in patients, whereas other forms are related to metabolic precursors and degradation products of the hormone. Genetic differences cause some patients to produce variant forms of a hormone such as luteinizing hormone (LH). These genetic differences can cause marked variations in measurements made using assays with specific monoclonal antisera compared with more uniform measurements made using assays with polyclonal antisera that cross-react with the multiple forms.[14] Well-characterized monoclonal antisera can be mixed together to make an "engineered polyclonal antiserum" with improved sensitivity and specificity.[15] Cross-reactivity with precursor forms of the analytes and with metabolic degradation products can cause major differences in assays. For example, cross-reactivity with precursor forms causes differences in insulin assays, and cross-reactivity with metabolic fragments causes major differences in carboxyl-terminal parathyroid hormone (PTH) assays.[16, 17]

Extraction of hormones from serum and urine specimens prior to measurement is a technique that can enhance both sensitivity and specificity of immunoassays. Numerous extraction systems have been developed, including (1) organic-aqueous partitioning to remove water-soluble interferences seen with steroids, (2) solid-phase extraction with absorption and selective elution from resins such as silica gels, and (3) immunoaffinity chromatography.[18, 19] Unfortunately, extraction and purification before immunoassay are seldom used in clinical assays. These techniques are difficult to automate and require skills and equipment not available in many clinical laboratories.

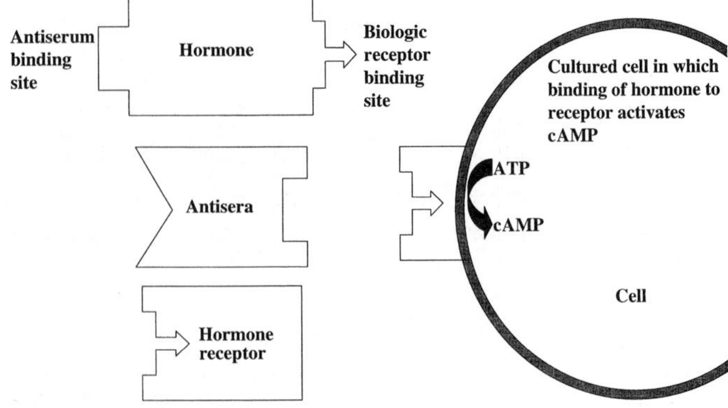

Figure 6–3. Comparison of an immunologic technique for measuring hormone concentration versus a receptor technique for measuring hormone activity. ATP, adenosine triphosphate; cAMP, cyclic adenosine monophosphate.

Although commercial assays generally use reagents having adequate sensitivity and specificity to measure *most* patient specimens, some patient specimens may give spurious results and some disease states may require more analytic sensitivity to ensure sound clinical decisions. In these cases, extraction of specimens prior to measurement may provide more reliable information.

Immunoassays measure concentrations rather than biologic activity. For most hormones, there is a strong correlation between the concentration of the protein or steroid being measured and the biologic activity, but this is not universally true. The reactive site for most antibodies is relatively small, about 5 to 10 amino acids for linear peptides. Some antiserum reactions are specific for the tertiary structure that corresponds to unique molecular configurations, but immunoassays seldom react with the exact antigenic structure that confers biologic activity.

Figure 6–3 presents a schematic illustration of the difference between immunologic binding site and biologic receptor binding site on a hormone. Indirect immunoassays have been developed using cultured cells that synthesize second messengers such as cyclic adenosine monophosphate (cAMP) at rates proportional to the concentration of hormone in the specimen. An example of this technique is the immunoassay measurement of cAMP produced by osteosarcoma cells to quantitate PTH bioactivity in serum.[20] Unfortunately, these assays are tedious and generally are not reproducible. More recent techniques using recombinant receptors as immunoassay binders may provide improved specificity with good reliability.[21–23]

Immunometric (Sandwich) Assays

A second immunologic technique used to measure hormones is the immunometric (sandwich) assay. The three basic components of a sandwich assay are:

1. An antigen large enough to allow two antibodies to bind concurrently on different binding sites.
2. A *capture* antiserum directed to one of the antigenic sites on the antigen. This antiserum is attached to a solid phase to permit immunologic extraction of the immune complexes.
3. A *signal* antiserum directed to a second antigenic site on the antigen. This antiserum is attached to an assay signal system.

In contrast to competitive immunoassays, these assays use a large excess of antiserum binding sites compared with the concentration of antigen. The capture antibody immunoextracts the antigen from the sample and the signal antibody binds to

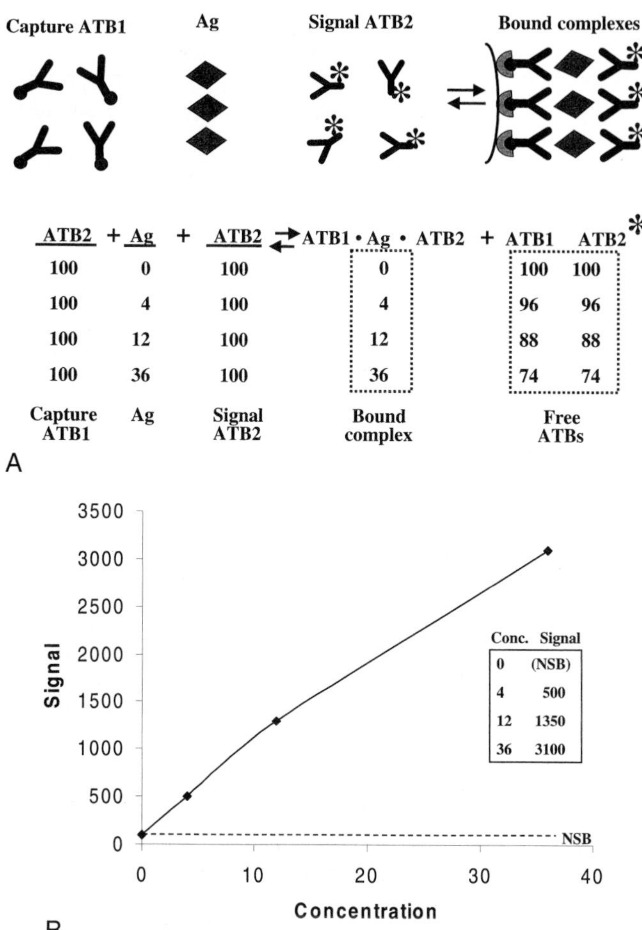

Figure 6–4. *A*, Principles of immunometric assays. Ag, antigen; ATB1, capture antiserum; ATB2, signal antiserum. *B*, Typical dose-response curve. NSB, nonspecific binding.

the capture antibody-antigen complex to form a tertiary complex. As the antigen concentration increases, the signal increases progressively.

Figure 6–4 schematically illustrates these concepts. The capture antiserum (ATB1) is attached to biotin (see solid circles). The signal antiserum (ATB2) is labeled with a detection system (see asterisks). The ATB1-antigen-ATB2 complexes are immunologically extracted using a streptavidin solid phase (see horizontal cups). After the complex is bound to the solid phase, most of the unbound signal antibody is washed away.

As shown in Figure 6–4, the signal increases progressively with the concentration. For lower concentrations, the signal generally increases proportional to the assay concentrations (after the offset caused by the NSB). At higher concentrations, the signal generally is less than proportional, so that nonlinear curve-fitting techniques are used to generate the dose-response curves. Again, the relative imprecision, expressed as a coefficient of variation, depends on the slope of the dose-response curve; consequently, the relative precision is less at higher concentrations.

In immunometric assays, the background level of signal is associated with very low concentrations. This background signal is caused by the NSB. The analytic sensitivity of immunometric assays is related to the ratio of the true signal to the NSB signal. Therefore, assays can be made more sensitive either by increasing the response signal or by decreasing NSB. Inadvertent increases in NSB caused by specimen interference or reagent deterioration can significantly alter the assay performance.

In immunometric assays, it is also important that a large excess of capture antibody be used. When the antigen concentration approaches the effective binding capacity of the capture antibody system, the signal no longer increases. If the antigen concentration exceeds the binding capacity of the capture antibody, the signal may actually decrease.

Figure 6–5 illustrates this *high-dose hook effect* for immunometric assays caused by insufficient amounts of capture or signal antiserum.[24] The signal increases progressively until the hormone concentration exceeds the binding capacity; the signal then decreases, apparently as a result of the removal of some of the weaker binding antigen-antibody complexes during the wash cycle on the assay.[25–27] This is a potentially dangerous phenomenon because very high concentrations can give the same "answer" as lower concentrations. If this artifact is suspected, the specimen can be diluted and reanalyzed. If the answer for the diluted specimen is higher than the original answer, a high-dose hook effect probably is present.

Most manufacturers are aware of this potential problem and configure assays with relatively large amounts of capture antibody; however, some patients produce high concentrations of hormones or antigens that may exceed assay limits. Laboratories are able to detect this phenomenon by analyzing specimens at two dilutions, but this practice generally is not cost-effective. Therefore, feedback to the laboratory about results that are inconsistent with clinical findings is essential.

Another potential problem for immunometric assays consists of endogenous heterophile antibodies that cross-react with reagent antiserum.[28] Normally, the signal antibody does not form a "sandwich" with the capture antibody unless the specific antigen is present; however, divalent heterophile antibodies may mimic the antigen by simultaneously binding to the signal and capture reagent antibodies.[29–31]

Figure 6–6 schematically illustrates this situation. The problem is most common with monoclonal antibodies but may also occur with polyclonal antibodies. Immunoglobulins contain both a *constant* (Fc) region and a *variable* (Fab) region. As implied in the name, the Fc region is constant, or similar, for all immunoglobulins from that species. Therefore, if a patient receives immunotherapy or imaging reagents containing mouse immunoglobulin, they are likely to develop human antimouse antibodies (HAMAs) directed to the Fc fragment.[32] Some patients may develop heterophile antibodies after exposure to foreign proteins from domestic pets or food contaminants. When these endogenous antibodies are present in a patient's specimen, they may bridge across the reagent antibodies used

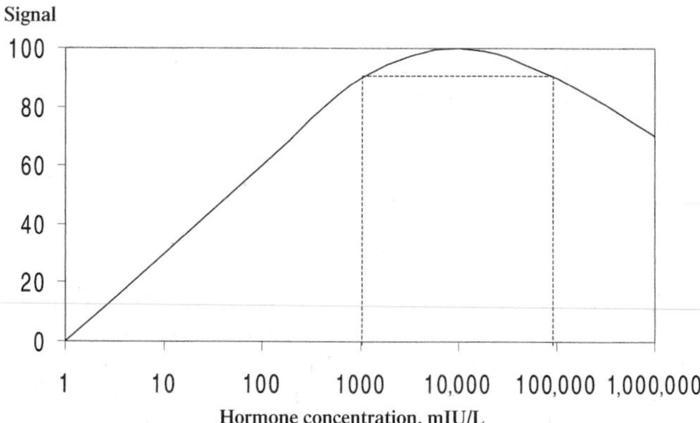

Figure 6–5. Immunometric "high-dose hook effect." The response signal reaches a maximum and then decreases when the antigen concentration exceeds the limit of the assay.

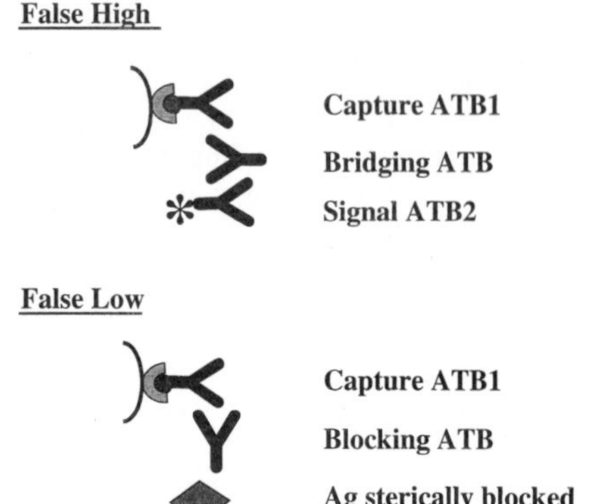

Figure 6–6. Assay interferences caused by heterophile antibodies, which result in either false high or false low results. Ag, antigen; ATB1, capture antiserum; ATB2, signal antiserum.

Table 6–1. Effect of Immunoassay Specificity on Calibration of Human Chorionic Gonadotropin (hCG) Assay

	Assay 1	Assay 2	Assay 3
Specificity for intact hCG standard	100%	100%	100%
Cross-reactivity with free β-hCG	0%	100%	200%
Value of specimen with no free β-hCG, IU/L	10.0	10.0	10.0
Value of specimen with 10% free β-hCG, IU/L	9.0	10.0	11.0
Value specimen with 50% free β-hCG, IU/L	5.0	10.0	15.0

in immunometric assays and may cause falsely high values. These antibodies also may bind to sites on the reagent antibodies, which sterically block the binding of the specific antigen and give falsely low test values. Most manufacturers include nonimmune immunoglobulin in the assays to help block these interferences; as with the high-dose hook effect, however, the amounts added are not always adequate and some patients with high titer antibodies thus may still show in vitro assay interference.

The combined specificity of the two antibodies used in an immunometric assay can produce exquisitely sensitive and specific immunoassays. In the past, a common problem with early competitive immunoassays was cross-reactivity among the structurally similar gonadotropins: LH, follicle-stimulating hormone (FSH), TSH, and human chorionic gonadotropin (hCG). The α subunits of each of these hormones are almost identical, and the β subunits have considerable structural homology. Many individual antisera (especially polyclonal antisera) used for measuring one of these hormones may have cross-reactivity for the other gonadotropins. The cross-reactivity of a pair of antibodies is less than the cross-reactivity of each of the individual antibodies because any cross-reacting substance must contain both of the binding epitopes in order to simultaneously bind to both antibodies.

For example, consider two antibodies for LH, each having 1% cross-reactivity with hCG. The cross-reactivity of the pair is less than the product of the two cross-reactivities or, in this case, less than 0.01%. Most current immunoassays for LH have cross-reactivity less than 0.01% because even this relatively low percentage of cross-reactivity would still cause significant assay interference in pregnant patients and patients with choriocarcinoma who have high hCG concentrations.

Multiple forms of most hormones circulate in the blood. Some hormones (e.g., prolactin, growth hormone) circulate with macro forms, which can cause difficulty in their analysis if specimens are not pretreated.[7] For hormones composed of subunits (e.g., the gonadotropins), both the intact and the free subunits circulate in blood. Immunometric assays can be made specific for intact molecules by pairing an antibody specific for the α-β bridge site of the subunits with a second antibody specific for the β subunit. Assays using these antibody pairs retain the two-antibody, low cross-reactivity needed for measuring gonadotropins and do not react with the free subunit forms of the hormones.

The heterogenous specificity characteristics of immunoassays make calibration and harmonization difficult. Two immunoassays calibrated with the same reference preparation can give widely varying measurements on patient specimens. Consider the example of hCG in Table 6–1. The three assays are calibrated with a pure preparation of intact hCG, such as the WHO Third International Reference Preparation.[33] The three assays differ in their cross-reactivity with free β-hCG (0, 100%, and 200%, respectively). These assays give identical measurements for a specimen containing only intact hCG but progressively disparate values as the percentage of free β-hCG in the specimen increases. In reality, the standardization issue is much more complex because multiple forms of hormones (i.e., intact, free subunits, nicked forms, glycosylated forms, degradation products) circulate in patients and each assay has different cross-reactivities for these forms.[33]

Free (Unbound) Hormone Assays

Many hormones are tightly bound to specific plasma-binding proteins and loosely bound to albumin. The unbound (free) forms as well as some of the loosely bound forms are biologically active.

Multiple methods are available to measure these free or biologically active forms of a hormone. Theoretically, the best procedure is direct measurement of the free hormone concentration after physical separation of free-form bound hormone by equilibrium dialysis, ultrafiltration, or gel filtration. Unfortunately, this method is difficult to perform and is thus not readily available and is subject to technical errors.

The two major clinical applications for free hormone measurements are for thyroid hormones (thyroxine [FT_4] and triiodothyronine [FT_3] and steroids (testosterone and estradiol). Four techniques are commonly used to estimate free thyroid hormone concentrations:

1. *Indirect index methods.* The *indirect indices* involve two measurements: one for total hormone concentration and another for the thyroxine-binding globulin (TBG), followed by calculation of the ratio or a normalized index (FT4I or FT3I). These methods correct for routine changes in TBG associated with estrogen levels, but they may produce inappropriately abnormal values in patients with extreme variations in TBG levels found in patients with congenital disorders of the TBG gene, familial dysalbuminemic hyperthyroxinemia, thyroid hormone autoantibodies, and nonthyroidal illnesses.

2. *Two-step labeled hormone methods.* These methods immunologically bind the free and loosely bound thyroid hormone to a solid phase. The other serum components are washed away, and the residual binding sites are back-titrated with labeled hormone. When calibrated with appropriate serum standards, these methods are thought to pose fewer problems with binding protein abnormalities.

3. *One-step labeled hormone analogue methods.* These methods use synthetic analogues of T_4 and T_3 that bind to the meas-

urement antibody but do not bind to normal TBG. These methods are seldom used because performance has been poor in patients with abnormal albumin concentrations, abnormal free fatty-acid concentrations, and all conditions that interfere with the indirect indices.[34]

4. *Labeled antibody methods.* These methods use kinetic reactions of antibodies with selected affinities that bind preferentially with the free form of the hormone. These methods work best for automated testing instruments and have become popular.

Each of these methods works well for correcting for minor changes in TBG levels, but each has problems with some patient sera, especially those containing interfering substances such as inhibitors and heterophilic antibodies. Unfortunately, most manufacturers have not fully validated their methods in patients with these abnormalities.[35]

Multiple methods are also available for measuring both the free and the biologically active forms of steroid hormones. The preferred method for measurement of free hormones consists of direct physical separation and high-sensitivity assays similar to those recommended for the thyroid hormones. One-step labeled hormone-analogue methods also have been developed, but these are associated with interference problems similar to the problems with free thyroid hormone assays.

Another complexity in regard to steroid hormones is that in addition to the free hormones, testosterone and estrogen bound to albumin also are biologically active. The concentration of the biologically active forms can be estimated using indirect indices calculated from measurements of the total hormones and sex hormone–binding globulin (SHBG) or by measurement of the residual free and albumin-bound steroids after separation of the SHBG-bound forms after differential precipitation with ammonium sulfate.[36]

Chromatographic Assays

Another major method of measuring hormone concentrations involves chromatographically separating the various biochemical forms and quantitating specific characteristics of the molecules. High-performance liquid chromatography (HPLC) systems utilize multiple forms of detection, including light absorption, fluorescence, electrochemical properties, and mass spectrometry.[37, 38]

There are two major advantages of these techniques: (1) they can be used to simultaneously measure multiple forms of an analyte, and (2) they are not dependent on unique immunologic reagents. Therefore, harmonization of measurements made with different assays is more feasible. The major disadvantages of these methods are their complexity and their limited availability.

Many chemical separation techniques are based on chromatography, but the two most commonly used for liquid chromatography are (1) *normal-phase* HPLC and (2) *reverse-phase* HPLC.[25] In both systems, a bonded solid-phase column is made that interacts with the analytes as they flow past in a liquid solvent. In normal-phase HPLC, the functional groups of the stationary phase are polar (e.g., amino or nitrile ions) relative to the nonpolar stationary phase (e.g., hexane); in reverse-phase HPLC, a nonpolar stationary phase (e.g., C-18 octadecylsilane molecules bonded to silica) is used.

More recently, polymeric packings made of mixed copolymers have been made with C4, C8, and C18 functional groups directly incorporated so that they are more stable over a wide pH range. The mobile and stationary phases are selected to optimize adherence of the analytes to the stationary phase. The adhered molecules can be eluted differentially from the solid phase after washing to separate specific forms of the analyte from interfering substances as follows:

1. When the composition of the mobile phase remains constant throughout the run, the process is called an *isocratic elution*.
2. If the mobile-phase composition is abruptly changed, a *step elution* occurs.
3. If the composition is gradually changed throughout the run, a *gradient elution* occurs.

The efficiency of separation in a chromatography system is a function of the flow rates of the different substances.[39] The resolution of the system is a measure of the separation of the two solute bands in terms of their relative retention volumes (V_r) and their bandwidths (W). Resolution (R_s) of solutes A and B is shown as

$$R_s = \frac{2[V_r(B) - V_r(A)]}{W(A) + W(B)}$$

Values of R_s less than 0.8 result in inadequate separation, and values greater than 1.25 correspond to baseline separation. The resolution of a chromatography column is a function of flow rates and thermodynamic factors.

The simultaneous measurement of the three catecholamines (epinephrine, norepinephrine, and dopamine) can be performed with reverse-phase HPLC with a C-18 column and electrochemical detection system[40] or fluorometric detection.[41] Prior extraction by absorption on activated alumina and acid elution helps to improve specificity. Dihydroxybenzylamine, a molecule similar to endogenous catecholamines, can be used as an internal standard.

Mass Spectrometry

The technique of mass spectrometry involves fragmentation of target molecules, followed by separation and measurement of the mass to charge ratio of the components.[39] When coupled with liquid chromatography, a mass spectrometer can function as a unique detector to provide structural information about the composition of individual solutes.[42] Inclusion of internal standards in the specimens, which are molecularly similar to the measured compounds, allows precise quantitation of the concentration of the eluting analytes. The measurement of specific mass fragments makes possible the quantitation of multiple specific analytes in complex mixtures.

A fundamental step in mass spectrometry is the fragmentation of the target compound into charged ions. Multiple techniques are used to generate these charged ions, including *chemical ionization* and *electron-impact ionization*.

Chemical ionization uses reagent gas molecules, such as methane, ammonia, water, and isobutane, to transfer protons. This process produces less fragmentation than other techniques because the process is not highly excited.

The electron impact bombards gas molecules from the sample, with electrons emitted from a heated filament. The process occurs in a vacuum to prevent the filament from burning out. *Electron-spray ionization* is a process in which a solution containing the analyte is introduced into a gas phase and is sprayed across an ionizing potential.[43] The charged droplets are desolvinated and analyzed in a mass spectrometer.

A *mass spectrum* is a bar graph in which the heights of the bars correspond to the relative abundance of a particular ion plotted as a function of the mass/charge ratio. Modern mass spectrometers can measure molecular masses so accurately and precisely that the elemental composition of a compound can be predicted by comparison with stored spectral libraries. When these systems are used to measure only a few select compounds having known spectrums, the mass spectrometer can be programmed to focus only on these selected ions.

Stable isotopes of the compounds of interest can be used as

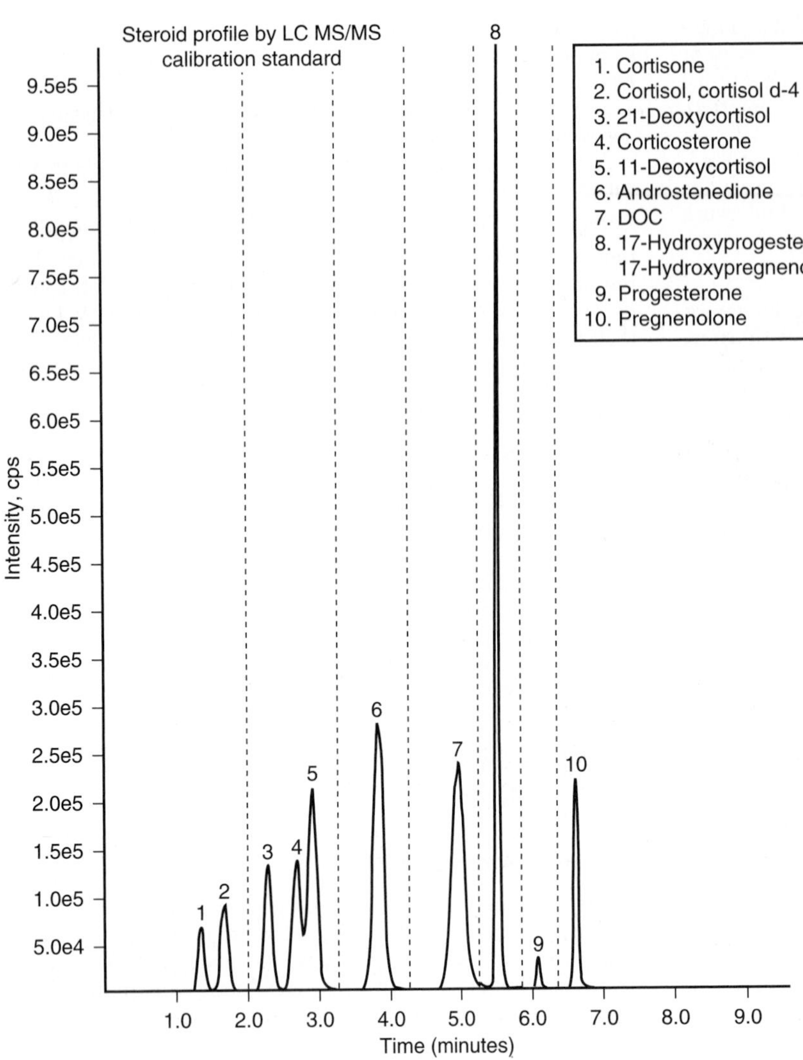

Figure 6–7. Mass spectrum illustrating the concurrent measurement of 10 cortisol-related compounds with one assay. cps, counts per second; LC, Supelcosil LC-18 column; MS/MS, tandem mass spectrometry. (Courtesy of Dr. R. Singh, Mayo Clinic.)

internal standards through a technique called *isotope dilution mass spectrometry*. Stable isotopes generally perform the same as the native compounds in terms of extraction, chromatography, and mass spectrometry and are thus ideal internal standards. However, they must have a sufficient number of isotopic atoms to ensure that their mass is different from naturally occurring substances that may be in the specimen.

Tandem mass spectrometry (MS/MS) is a powerful new tool consisting of two mass analyzers separated by an ion-activation device.[44, 45] The first analyzer is used to isolate and dissociate the ion of interest by activation, and the second mass analyzer is used to analyze its dissociation products. This technique can be used to provide rapid, definitive measurements of multiple endocrine analytes.[42] For example, liquid chromatography and tandem mass-spectrometry can be used to simultaneously quantitate multiple glucocorticoid-related compounds.[46, 47] In Figure 6–7, the chromatograph shows peaks for ten steroids that were first separated on reverse-phase liquid chromatography using a Supelcosil LC-18 column (Supelco, Bellefonte, Calif.) and a gradient elution of a 53% to 75% methanol/water mixture. The column eluate was fed directly into an electrospray ionization device in a triple-quadrapole mass spectrometer (API 3000, Perkin-Elmer Sciex, Foster City, Calif.). The stable isotopes were from Cambridge Isotope Laboratories (Andover, Mass.). A 10-minute analysis provides quantitation of the 10 compounds: cortisone, cortisol, 21-deoxycortisol, corticosterone, 11-deoxycortisol, androstenedione, deoxycorticosterone (DOC), 17-hydroxyprogesterone, progesterone, and pregnenolone. The sensitivity for cortisol using d_4 cortisol calibration is 0.1 μg/dL.

Nucleic Acid–Based Assays

The decoding of the human genome has set the stage for an enormous increase in nucleic acid–based gene assays. The basic principles of nucleic acid–based assays have been known for several decades, but the identification of specific genes and the mapping of gene defects to clinical disease states have now made these measurements clinically useful.[48, 49] Four concepts important for nucleic acid measurements are (1) hybridization, (2) amplification, (3) restriction fragment length polymorphisms (RFLPs), and (4) electrophoretic separation.[50]

Hybridization

Nucleic acid molecules have a unique ability to fuse with complementary base-pair sequences. When a fragment of a known sequence (probe) is mixed under specific conditions with a specimen containing a complementary sequence, hybridization occurs. This feature is analogous to the antibody-antigen binding used in immunoassays. Many of the formats used for immunoassay have been adopted to nucleic acid assays, including some of the same signal systems (e.g., radioactivity, fluorescence, chemiluminescence) and the same solid-phase capture systems (e.g., magnetic beads, biotin-streptavidin binding). In situ hybridization, which involves the binding of probes to intact tissue and cells, provides information about morphologic localization analogous to immunohistochemistry.

Amplification

Nucleic acid assays have an advantage that low concentrations can be amplified in vitro prior to quantitation. The best known amplification procedure is the polymerase chain reaction (PCR), first reported by Mullis and Faloona.[51] The three steps in the process (denaturation, annealing, and elongation) occur rapidly at different temperatures. Each "cycle" of amplification can occur in less than 90 seconds by cycling the temperature. The target double-stranded DNA is denatured at high temperature to make two single-stranded DNA fragments. Oligonucleotide primers, which are specific for target region, are annealed to the DNA when the temperature is lowered. Addition of DNA polymerase allows the primer DNA to extend across the amplification region, thus doubling the number of DNA copies.

At 85% to 90% efficiency, this process can amplify the DNA by about 250,000-fold in 20 cycles. This huge amplification is subject to major problems with contamination if special precautions are not taken. In one control technique, a psoralen derivative is used to prevent subsequent copying by polymerase during exposure to ultraviolet light.

Restriction Fragment Length Polymorphisms

Some diseases (e.g., sickle cell anemia) are associated with a specific gene mutation; generally, however, a series of deletions and additions of DNA are involved with the disease. A number of restriction enzymes that cleave DNA at specific locations have been identified. Changes in the sequence of DNA result in different fragment lengths. This technique, or RFLP, is particularly helpful in family studies for disorders that have a unique *genetic fingerprint*.

Electrophoretic Separation

E. M. Southern invented an electrophoretic separation technique known as *Southern blotting*.[52] Restriction enzymes are used to digest a sample of DNA into fragments, and the product is subjected to electrophoresis. The separated bands of DNA are then transferred to a solid support and hybridized. *Northern blotting* is a similar technique, in which RNA is used as the starting material. *Western blotting* refers to electrophoresis and transfer of proteins.

ANALYTIC VALIDATION

Clinicians generally assume that laboratory methods have been validated and that they function correctly. Although this assumption is generally true, it is helpful to understand the level of assay validation performed and the appropriateness of the validation criteria for each clinical application of a test.[53, 54]

In the United States, the federal government regulates all laboratories performing complex tests for patients receiving Medicare.[55] These regulations, published in the Federal Register, outline the validation requirements for both Food and Drug Administration (FDA)–approved instruments, kits, and test systems as well as methods developed in-house. Laboratories must document analytic accuracy, precision, reportable ranges, and reference ranges for all procedures. The regulations for in-house procedures and modifications of approved commercial procedures are more extensive and require laboratories to further document (1) analytic sensitivity; (2) analytic specificity, including interfering substances; and (3) other performance characteristics required for testing patient specimens.

Although the details of method validation may be unique to a specific procedure, the following analytic validation studies have proved valuable for most procedures: (1) method comparison, (2) precision, (3) linearity, (4) recovery, (5) detection limit, (6) reportable range, (7) analytic interference, (8) carryover, (9) reference interval, (10) specimen stability, and (11) specimen type. Laboratories should have documentation for each of these performance characteristics, either from the diagnostics manufacturer or from direct studies.

Method Comparison

Ideally, the system should be compared with an established reference method; however, many endocrine tests do not have reference methods and many laboratories do not have the facilities to perform reference methods when they exist. As a minimum, the assay should be compared with an analytic system that has been clinically validated with specimens from healthy subjects and specimens from patients with the diseases being investigated.[56] The system should be traceable to established reference standards, such as those from the WHO and the National Institute of Standards and Technology (NIST).[57–59] Between 100 and 200 different specimens distributed over the assay range are recommended for method comparisons.[60]

A cross-plot displaying the new method on the vertical axis versus the established method on the horizontal axis, along with the identity line, reference value lines, and regression statistics, is a useful way of displaying these comparisons. An alternative display method is the Bland-Altman difference plot, in which the difference between the test method and the reference method is plotted against the reference method values.

Although acceptable performance criteria for method comparisons are not well established, some important characteristics to examine are as follows:

1. Any grossly discordant test values.
2. The degree of scatter about the regression curve.
3. The size of the regression off-set on the vertical axis.
4. The number of points crossing between the low, normal, and high reference intervals for the two methods.

The European Union (EU) has enacted the In Vitro Diagnostics Directive, which requires manufacturers marketing in the EU after the year 2003 to establish that their products are "traceable to reference standards and reference procedures of a higher order" when these references exist.[61] This directive should serve to harmonize many test methods worldwide because most diagnostic companies market internationally.[62]

Precision

Precision is a measure of the replication of repeated measurements of the same specimen; it is a function of the time between repeats and the concentration of the analyte. Both short-term precision (within a run or within a day) and long-term precision (across calibrations and across batches of reagents) should be documented at clinically appropriate concentration levels.[63]

In general, normal range, abnormally low range, and abnormally high range targets are chosen for precision studies; however, targets focused on critical medical decision limits may be more appropriate for some analytes. Twenty measurements are recommended at each level for both short-term and long-term precision validations. Precision generally is expressed as the

Table 6–2. Recommended Analytic Performance Limits

Analyte	Biologic CVi (%)	Precision (%)	Accuracy (%)
Calcium	1.8*	0.9†	0.7*
Glucose	4.4*	2.2†	1.9*
Thyroxine	7.6*	3.4†	4.1*
Potassium	4.4*	2.4†	1.6*
Triiodothyronine	8.7†	4.0‡	5.5‡
Thyrotropin	20.2†	8.1‡	8.9‡
Cortisol	15.2†	(7.6)*	
Estradiol	21.7†	(10.9)	
Follicle-stimulating hormone	30.8†	(15.4)	
Luteinizing hormone	14.5†	(7.2)	
Prolactin	40.5†	(20.2)	
Testosterone	8.3†	(4.1)	
Insulin	15.2†	(7.6)	
Dehydroepiandrosterone	5.6†	(2.8)	
11-deoxycortisol	21.3†	(10.6)	

*Numbers in parentheses correspond to one-half of CVi (CVi = within individual coefficient of variation).

*Data from Stockl D, et al. Eur J Clin Chem Clin Biochem 1995; 33:157–169.[65]

†Data from Fraser CG. Arch Pathol Lab Med 1992; 116:916–923.[66]

‡Data from Fraser CG, et al. Eur J Clin Chem Clin Biochem 1992; 30:311–317.[67]

coefficient of variation, calculated as 100 times the standard deviation divided by the average of the replicate measurements.[64]

There is no universal agreement on the performance criteria for analytic precision, although numerous recommendations have been put forth. Two major approaches to defining these criteria have been (1) comparison with biologic variation and (2) expert opinion of clinicians based on their perceived impact of laboratory variation on clinical decisions.

The total variation clinically observed in test measurements is a combination of the analytic and biologic variations, for instance:

1. If the analytic standard deviation (SD) is less than one-fourth of the biologic SD, the analytic component increases the SD of the total error by less than 3%.
2. If the analytic precision is less than one-half of the biologic SD, the total error increases by only 12%.

These observations have led to recommendations for maintaining precision less than one quarter or one-half of the biologic variation. The expert opinion precision recommendations are based on estimates of the magnitude of change of a test value that would cause clinicians to alter their clinical decisions. Table 6–2 lists some precision recommendations for selected endocrine tests.[65–67]

Linearity

Patient specimens commonly contain several different forms of the hormones to be measured compared with the pure form contained in the reference standards and calibrators used to establish the assay dose-response curve.[68] When a patient specimen is diluted, the measured value for these dilutions should parallel the dose-response curve and give results proportional to the dilution. Linearity can be evaluated by measuring serial dilutions of patient specimens with high concentrations diluted in the appropriate assay diluent.[69, 70] The product of the measured value multiplied by the dilution factor should be approximately constant. There are no performance standards for linearity, but a reasonable expectation for most hormones is that dilutions are comparable within 10% of the undiluted value.

Recovery

Two methods of assessing the recovery of assays are (1) measuring the increase in test values after the reference analyte is added and (2) measuring the proportional changes caused by mixing high-concentration and low-concentration specimens. Some analytes circulate in the blood in multiple forms, and some of these forms may be bound to carrier proteins. The recovery rate of pure substances added to a specimen may be low if the assay does not measure some of the bound forms. Mixtures of patient specimens may not be measured correctly if one of the specimens contains cross-reacting substances such as autoantibodies. A thorough understanding of the chemical forms of the analyte and their cross-reactivities in the assay is important during assessment of recovery data.

Detection Limit

The minimal analytic detection limit is the smallest concentration that can be statistically differentiated from zero. This concentration is mathematically determined as the upper 95% limit of replicate measurements of the *zero standard*, calculated from the average signal plus 2.0 SD. This minimal detection limit is valid *only* for the average of multiple replicate measurements. When individual determinations are performed on a specimen having a true concentration exactly at the minimal detection limit, the probability that the measurement is above the noise level of the assay is only about 50%.

A second term for the lowest level of reliable measurement for an assay is the *functional detection limit*, or the *limit of quantitation*. For this parameter to be measured, multiple pools with low concentrations are made and analyzed in the replicate. A cross-plot of the coefficient of variation of the measurements versus the concentration allows one to generate a precision profile. The concentration corresponding to a coefficient of variation of 20% is the functional detection limit.[1] This term generally applies to across-assay variation, but it also can be calculated using within-assay variation if one uses the tests to evaluate results measured within one run (e.g., provocative and suppression tests).

Reportable Range

The reportable range of an assay generally spans from the functional detection limit to the concentration of the highest standard. Values above the highest standard may be reported if they are diluted and the measured value is multiplied by the dilution factor. The validity of the analytic range is documented by the linearity and recovery studies. Some laboratories erroneously report the exact values displayed by the test systems even if they are outside of the analytic range. Therefore, it is important for clinicians to understand the limitations of valid measurements and not inappropriately use meaningless numbers that may be reported.

Another potential source of error is failure of the technologist to multiply the measured value of diluted specimens by the dilution factor to correct for the dilution. In addition, care should be taken to define the number of significant figures used for reporting test values and to establish an appropriate algorithm for rounding test values to the significant number of digits.

Analytic Interference

The cross-reactivity and potential interference of other analytes that may react in a test system should be documented.[71]

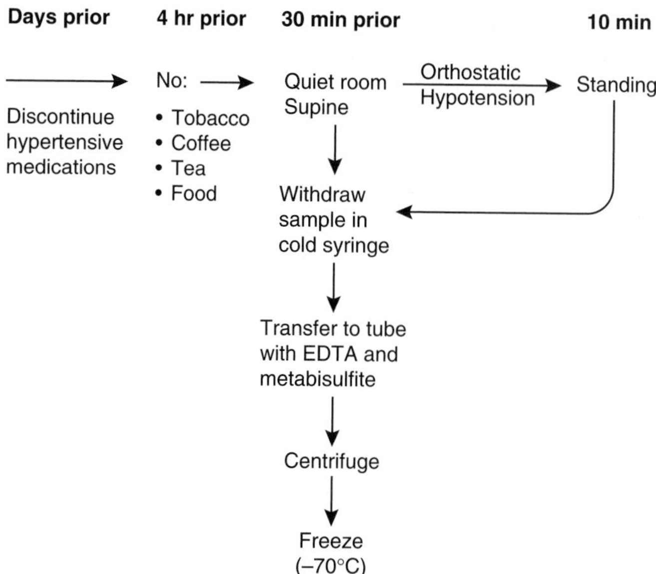

Figure 6–8. Flow diagram illustrating appropriate preanalytic conditions for measuring plasma catecholamines. EDTA, edetate.

The choice of potential interfering substances that must be evaluated requires an understanding of both the analytic system and the pathophysiology of the analyte being evaluated. In immunoassays, for example, compounds with similar structures as well as precursor forms and degradation products should be tested.[72–74] Drugs commonly prescribed for the diseases under evaluation should be assessed for interference both by addition of the drug to a specimen and by analysis of specimens from patients before and after receiving the drug.[75–77] Most assays also are evaluated for the effects of hemolysis, lipemia, and icterus.

Carry-over Studies

Many diagnostic systems use automated sample-handling devices. If a specimen to be tested is preceded by a specimen with a very high concentration, a trace amount of the first specimen may significantly increase the reported concentration of the second specimen. The choice of the concentration that should be tested for carry-over depends on the pathophysiology of the disease, but high values may need to be tested because some endocrine disorders may produce these high values. A prudent procedure would be to retest all specimens following a specimen with an extraordinarily high value. One also should document that carry-over from the sampling probe has not inadvertently contaminated subsequent specimen vials, thereby invalidating subsequently repeated measurements.

Reference Intervals

The development and validation of reference intervals for endocrine tests can be a very complex task.[78, 79] The normal reference interval for most laboratory tests is based on estimates of the central 95 percentile limits of measurements in healthy subjects.[80] A minimum of 120 subjects is needed to reliably define the 2.5 and 97.5 percentiles. The reference intervals for many endocrine tests depend on gender, age, developmental status, and other test values. Formal statistical consultation is recommended to determine the appropriate number of subjects to test and to develop statistical models for defining multivariate reference ranges.

Full evaluation of the adrenal, gonadal, and thyroid axes requires simultaneous measurement of the trophic and target hormones. Bivariate displays of these hormone concentrations along with their multivariate reference intervals facilitate the interpretation.[81] Preanalytic conditions should be well defined and controlled during evaluation of both healthy reference subjects and patients.

Figure 6–8 shows a recommended protocol to control preanalytic conditions for collection of plasma catecholamine specimens.

Specimen Stability

Analyte stability is a function of storage conditions and specimen type.[82] Although most hormones are relatively stable in serum or urine if they are rapidly frozen and stored in hermetically sealed vials at −70°C, multiple freeze/thaw cycles may damage analytes, and storage in frost-free freezers that repeatedly cycle through thawing temperatures can adversely affect stability. Blood specimens collected in edetate (EDTA) often are more stable than serum or heparinized specimens because edetate chelates calcium and magnesium ions, which function as coenzymes for some proteases. The addition of protease inhibitors (e.g., aprotinin) to blood specimens may also improve specimen stability.[83]

Types of Specimens

Most hormones are measured in blood or urine, but alternate testing sources, such as saliva and transdermal membrane monitors, are also used.

Urine Specimens

The 24-hour urine specimen is used for many endocrine tests. Urine specimens represent a time average that integrates over the multiple pulsatile spikes of hormone secretion occurring throughout the day. The 24-hour urine specimen also has the advantage of better analytic sensitivity for some hormones.[84, 85] Urine often contains not only the original hormone but also key metabolites that may or may not have biologic activity.

Drawbacks include the inconvenience of and delays in collecting the 24-hour specimen. Another limitation of urine specimens is the uncertainty of the completeness of the collection. Measurement of urinary creatinine concentrations helps in monitoring collection completeness, especially when it is compared with the patient's muscle mass. Many urinary hormones are conjugated to carrier proteins before excretion. Therefore, both hepatic function and, to a lesser degree, renal function may alter urinary hormone values.

Blood Specimens

Blood specimens have both the advantage and the limitation of time dependency. The ability to direct rapid changes to a provocative stimulus is a strong advantage, whereas the unsuspected changes due to pulsatile secretions may be a major limitation. Most hormones undergo significant biologic variations, including ultradian, diurnal, menstrual, and seasonal changes.[86–88] Many hormones have short half-lives and are thus rapidly cleared from the blood. The half-life is particularly important when one is attempting to measure the response to a provocative drug, such as the effect of gonadotropin-releasing hormone (GnRH).[89] The development of rapid intraoperative methods for measuring PTH and growth hormone has highlighted the importance of plasma specimens, which do not require extra waiting time for the blood to clot to make serum.[90, 91]

Saliva Specimens

Saliva has been used to measure some hormones. Methods of stimulation, collection, and storage of saliva should be standardized in order to ensure that the measurements are reproducible and meaningful.[92, 93] Saliva measurements correlate with blood measurements in some hormones like cortisol, progesterone, estradiol and testosterone but do not correlate well for others, (e.g., thyroid and pituitary hormones).[94–96] Unconjugated steroid hormones enter saliva by diffusion, and their concentrations are relatively independent of the rate of saliva production. The saliva concentration of conjugated steroids, thyroxine, chorionic gonadotropin, and many protein hormones generally do no correlate well with plasma concentrations.[97]

Blood Drops

Blood drops collected on filter paper from punctures of a finger or heel are a convenient system for collecting, transporting, and measuring hormones.[98, 99] If standardized collection conditions and extraction techniques are used, these measurements correlate well with serum measurements. Integration of immunochemistry with computer chip technology has also led to immunochips that can measure multiple analytes using a single drop of blood.[100]

Noninvasive Measurements

Noninvasive transcutaneous measurements also have been developed for some endocrine tests.[101] Transcutaneous glucose measurements using near-infrared spectroscopy correlate well with blood measurements.[102] The GlucoWatch device is also being marketed for noninvasive monitoring of glucose.[103]

QUALITY ASSURANCE

Quality Control Systems

Laboratory quality control programs are intended to ensure that the test procedures are being performed within defined limits. A critical component of control systems is the definition of acceptable performance criteria.[104, 105] Unfortunately, these criteria often are not well defined and many laboratories use floating criteria that change when assays change.[106] Control limits are often set at the mean *±2 or 3 SDs*, where the mean and SD are arbitrarily assigned based on measurements made in that laboratory. When reagents or equipment change, new limits are assigned. These types of control systems provide some assurance that the laboratory is functioning at a level of performance similar to that of the recent past, but they provide little assurance that measurements are adequate for clinical decisions.

Statistically, there are two major forms of analytic errors: random and systematic. *Random error* relates to reproducibility; *systematic error* relates to the offset or bias of the test values from the target or reference value. Performance criteria can be defined for each of these parameters, and quality control systems can be programmed to monitor compliance with these criteria. Control systems must have low false-positive rates as well as high statistical power to detect assay deviations. The multirule algorithms developed by Westgard and colleagues[107] use combinations of control rules, such as two consecutive controls outside of *warning limits*, one control outside of *action limits*, or moving average trend analyzers outside of limits to achieve good statistical error detection characteristics.[108]

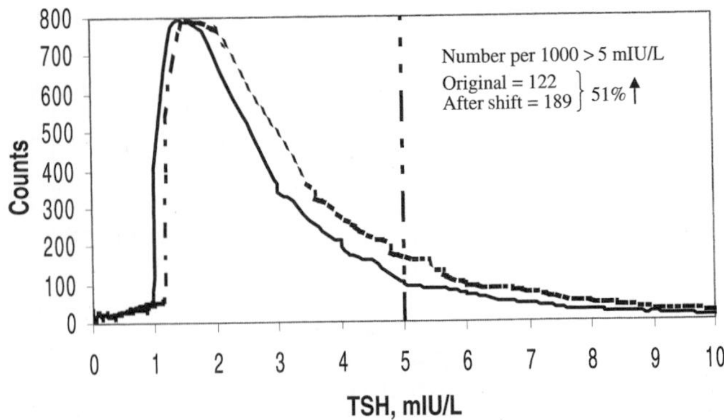

Figure 6–9. Effect of analytic bias, or shift, on the number of patients with elevated levels of thyrotropin (TSH).

Traditionally, quality control programs have focused primarily on precision; however, analytic bias also can cause major clinical problems. When fixed decision levels are used to trigger clinical actions, such as therapy and additional investigations, changes in the analytic set-point of an assay can cause major changes in the number of follow-up cases.[108] This concept is illustrated in Figure 6–9 for TSH measurements.

Under stable laboratory testing conditions, approximately 122 per 1000 patients tested have TSH values above 5.0 mIU/L. If the test shifts upward by 20%, the number of patients with TSH values above 5.0 mIU/L increases to 189, which equates to more than a 50% increase in the number of patients flagged as abnormal. These changes in test value distributions can often be sensed by clinicians who encounter multiple patients with unexpected elevated test values, causing them to call the laboratory and inquire whether the "test is running high today." Some modern quality control systems use moving averages of patient test values to help monitor changes in analytic bias.[109]

Some medical facilities are linking together into networks to provide more integrated patient care. This crossover of both physicians and patients is increasing the importance of *harmonized* testing systems. For endocrine tests, harmonization is best achieved when all the laboratories in the network use the same test systems. Differences in analytic specificity may cause across-method differences in patient test distributions even when the methods use the same reference standard. Full harmonization of testing requires not only standardization of equipment but also standardization of reagents (including using the same lot numbers) and standardization of laboratory protocols. Real-time quality control monitors with peer group comparisons across the laboratories in the health care network are necessary to ensure uniformity of testing.

Investigation of Discordant Test Values

The practice of modern endocrinology depends extensively on reliable and accurate test values; even in the best laboratories, however, erroneous results sometimes are reported. Careful correlation of pathophysiology with test values can help to identify values that are "discordant."[81] Some of these discordant test values may be analytically correct, but others may be erroneous. Clinicians can help investigate these suspicious test values by requesting laboratories to perform a few simple validation procedures.

Repeated testing of the same specimen is a valuable first step. If the specimen has been stored under stable conditions, the absolute value of the difference between the initial and the

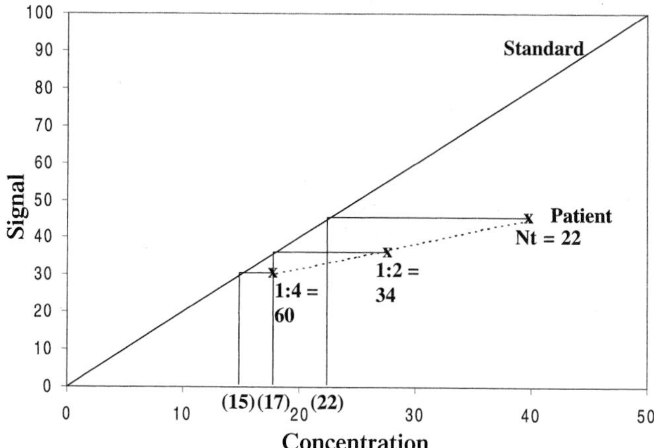

Figure 6-10. Nonproportional dilutions. Discordant values are produced when samples do not dilute linearly. (Nt = undiluted [neat].)

repeated measurements should be less than *3 analytic SDs* 95% of the time. Normally, the 95% confidence range is associated with the mean *±2 SDs*; with repeated laboratory tests, however, errors are associated with the first as well as the second measurement. The confidence interval for the uncertainty of the difference between two measurements can be calculated using the statistical rules for propagation of errors.

To better understand this propagation of error, consider that

$$D = X_1 - X_2$$

where X_1 is the first measurement, X_2 is the repeated measurement, and D is the difference.

The variance of D is the *sum* of the variance of X_1 and the variance of X_2. The SD of D is the square root of the variance of D, or the square root of twice the variance of X_1. The SD of D equates to 2 multiplied by the SDs of S. Therefore, 95% of the absolute values for D should be within $2\sqrt{2}$ SD(X), or approximately 3 SD(X). If a repeat measurement exceeds this 3 SD(X) limit, the initial (or reagent) measurement is probably in error.

Linearity and recovery are valuable techniques for evaluating test validity. If the initial test value is elevated, serially diluting the specimen in the assay diluent and reassaying should be considered. If the specimen dilutes nonproportionally (Fig. 6–10), no meaningful value can be reported with that assay.

In the example, the undiluted specimen reads 22, the twofold dilution multiplies back to 34 (2 × 17), and the fourfold dilution multiplies back to 60 (4 × 15). Therefore, the result depends on the dilution factor, so that no reliable answer can be reported.

If the initial value is low, one may consider adding known quantities of the analyte to part of the specimen. Analyzing these spiked or diluted specimens with the original specimen allows one to evaluate both reproducibility and recovery. It may be helpful to analyze the linearity or recovery of the assay standards at the same time to provide internal controls of the dilution or spiking procedures and the appropriateness of the diluent and spiking material.

If the replication, dilution, or recovery experiment appears successful, further analytic troubleshooting will vary according to the method used. Immunoassays may be affected by interference caused by heterophile antibodies. Addition of nonimmune mouse serum or heterophile antibody–blocking solutions may neutralize these effects.[110, 111] Chromatographic assays are usually more robust than immunoassays. Specimens with suspected interference on one type of assay can be reanalyzed by means of an alternative methodology.

Water-soluble interferences have been reported for some direct assays for steroid measurements.[18, 19, 112] Extraction of the hormones into organic solvents, followed by drying down and reconstitution in the assay zero standard, removes these interferences. Similarly, interferences with cross-reacting drugs and metabolic products can be minimized with selective extraction.

SUMMARY

The analytic methods of assessing endocrine problems in patients are continually expanding. The newer systems are often based on analytic techniques similar to those outlined in this chapter, but the configurations are generally more user-friendly. These advances make the systems more convenient, but they also become more of a "black box" that conceals most of the details of the system. The performance validation steps outlined in this chapter become important procedures for ensuring that these systems continue to provide the reliable measurements needed for quality medical care.

References

1. Spencer CA, LoPresti JS, Patel A, et al. Applications of a new chemiluminometric thyrotropin assay to subnormal measurement. J Clin Endocrinol Metab 1990; 70:453.
2. Klee GG, Hay ID. Biochemical testing of thyroid function. Endocrinol Metab Clin North Am 1997; 26:763–775.
3. Thorell JI, Larson SM. Radioimmunoassay and related techniques. St. Louis, CV Mosby, 1978.
4. Price CP, Newman DJ (eds). Principles and Practice of Immunoassay, 2nd ed. New York, Stockton Press, 1996.
5. Rodbard D. Data processing for radioimmunoassays: an overview. In Natelson S, Pesce AJ, Dietz AA (eds). Clinical Chemistry and Immunochemistry (AACC): Chemical and Cellular Bases and Applications in Disease. Washington, DC, AACC, 1978, pp 477–494.
6. Gosling JP. A decade of development in immunoassay methodology. Clin Chem 1990; 36:1408–1427.
7. Vieira JG, Tachibana TT, Obara LH, et al. Extensive experience and validation of polyethylene glycol precipitation as a screening method for macroprolactinemia. Clin Chem 1998; 44(8 Pt 1): 1758–1759.
8. Klee GG, Post G. Effect of counting errors on immunoassay precision. Clin Chem 1989; 35:1362–1366.
9. Butler JE (ed). Immunochemistry of Solid-Phase Immunoassay. Boston, CRC Press, 1991.
10. Hersh LS, Yaverbaum S. Magnetic solid-phase radioimmunoassay. Clin Chem Acta 1975; 63:69.
11. Suter M. Streptavidin: production, purification, and use in antibody immobilization. In Butler JE (ed). Immunochemistry of Solid-Phase Immunoassay. Boston, CRC Press, 1991, pp 269–276.
12. Hage DS. Survey of recent advances in analytical applications of immunoaffinity chromatography. J Chromatogr B Biomed Sci Appl 1998; 715:3–28.
13. Vetterlein D. Monoclonal antibodies: production, purification, and technology. Adv Clin Chem 1989; 27:303–354.
14. Pettersson KS, Soderholm JRM. Individual differences in lutropin immunoreactivity revealed by monoclonal antibodies. Clin Chem 1991; 37:333–340.
15. Ehrlich PH, Moyle WR. Cooperative immunoassays: ultrasensitive assays with mixed monoclonal antibodies. Science 1983; 221: 279–281.
16. Temple RC, Clark PMS, Nagi DK, et al. Radioimmunoassay may overestimate insulin in non–insulin-dependent diabetics. Clin Endocrinol 1990; 32:689–693.
17. Kao PC, van Heerden JA, Grant CS, et al. Clinical performance

of parathyroid hormone immunometric assays. Mayo Clin Proc 1992; 67:637–645.

18. Fitzgerald RL, Herold DA. Serum total testosterone: immunoassay compared with negative chemical ionization gas chromatography-mass spectrometry. Clin Chem 1996; 42:749–755.
19. Leung Y, Dees K, Cyr R, et al. Falsely increased serum estradiol results in direct estradiol assays. Clin Chem 1997; 43:1250–1251.
20. Klee GG, Preissner CM, Schloegel IW, et al. Bioassay of parathyrin: analytical characteristics and clinical performance in patients with hypercalcemia. Clin Chem 1988; 34:482–488.
21. Di Lorenzo D, Ruggeri G, Iacobello C, et al. Evaluation of a radioreceptor assay to assess exogenous estrogen activity in serum of patients with breast cancer. Int J Biol Markers 1991; 6:151–158.
22. Strasburger CJ, Wu Z, Pflaum CD, et al. Immunofunctional assay of human growth hormone (hGH) in serum: a possible consensus for quantitative hGH measurement. J Clin Endocrinol Metab 1996; 81:2613–2620.
23. Hoare SR, de Vries G, Usdin TB. Measurement of agonist and antagonist ligand-binding parameters at the human parathyroid hormone type 1 receptor: evaluation of receptor states and modulation by guanine nucleotide. J Pharm Exp Ther 1999; 289:1323–1333.
24. Zweig MH, Csako G. High-dose hook effect in a two-site IRMA for measuring thyrotropin. Ann Clin Biochem 1990; 27(Pt 5): 494–495.
25. Pesce MA. "High-dose hook effect" with the Centocor CA 125 assay. Clin Chem 1993; 39:1347.
26. Ooi DS, Escares EA. "High-dose hook effect" in IRMA-Count PSA assay of prostate-specific antigen. Clin Chem 1991; 37:771–772.
27. Wolf E, Brem G. 'High-dose hook effect' as a pitfall in quantifying transgene expression in metallothionein-human growth hormone (MT-hGH) transgenic mice. Clin Chem 1991; 37:763–765.
28. Kricka LJ. Human anti-animal antibody interferences in immunological assays. Clin Chem 1999; 45:942–956.
29. Klee GG. Human anti-mouse antibodies. Arch Pathol Lab Med 2000; 124:921–923.
30. Reinsberg J. Interference by human antibodies with tumor marker assays. Hybridoma 1995; 14:205–208.
31. Kricka LJ, Schmerfeid-Pruss D, Senior M, et al. Interference by human anti-mouse antibody in two-site immunoassays. Clin Chem 1990; 36:892–894.
32. Baum RP, Niesen A, Hertel A, et al. Activating anti-idiotypic human anti-mouse antibodies for immunotherapy of ovarian carcinoma. Cancer 1994; 73:1121–1125.
33. Cole LA. Immunoassay of human chorionic gonadotropin: its free subunits and metabolites. Clin Chem 1997; 43:2233–2243.
34. Ekins R. Analytic measurements of free thyroxine. Clin Lab Med 1993; 13:599–630.
35. Demers LM, Spencer CA (eds). In Laboratory Medicine Practice Guidelines. Laboratory Support for the Diagnosis and Monitoring of Thyroid Disease. National Academy of Clinical Biochemistry, Thyroid SOLP, 2000.
36. Klee GG, Heser DW. Techniques to measure testosterone in the elderly. Mayo Clin Proc 2000; 75(suppl):S19–S25.
37. Anderson DJ. High-performance liquid chromatography in clinical analysis. Anal Chem 1999; 71:742A–748A.
38. Volin P. High-performance liquid chromatographic analysis of corticosteroids. J Chromatogr B Biomed Appl 1995; 671(1–2): 319–340.
39. Ullman MD, Bowers LD, Burtis CA. Chromatography/mass spectrometry. In Burtis CA, Ashwood ER (eds). Tietz Textbook of Clinical Chemistry, 3rd ed. Philadelphia, WB Saunders, 1999, pp 164–204.
40. Clauson RC. High performance liquid chromatographic separation and determination of catecholamines. In Mark and Rodnight (eds). Research Methods in Neurochemistry, Vol 6. New York, Plenum, 1985.
41. Willemsem JJ, Ross HA, Jacobs MC, et al. Highly sensitive and specific HPLC with fluorometric detection for determination of plasma epinephrine and norepinephrine applied to kinetic studies in humans. Clin Chem 1995; 41:1455–1460.
42. Niessen WM. Advances in instrumentation in liquid chromatography-mass spectrometry and related liquid-introduction techniques. J Chromatogr A 1998; 794(1–2):407–435.
43. Strege MA. High-performance liquid chromatographic-electrospray ionization mass spectrometry analyses for the integration of natural products with modern high-throughput screening. J Chromatogr B 1999; 725:67–78.
44. Dongre AR, Eng JK, Yates JR 3rd. Emerging tandem mass spectrometry techniques for the rapid identification of proteins. Trends Biotechnol 1997; 15:418–425.
45. Magera MJ, Lacey JM, Casetta B, et al. Method for the determination of total homocysteine in plasma and urine by stable isotope dilution and electrospray tandem mass spectrometry. Clin Chem 1999; 45:1517–1522.
46. Park S, Magera MJ, Lacey JM, et al. Profiling of the conjugated forms of steroid hormones and their metabolites using HPLC-tandem mass spectrometry. Clin Chem 2000; 46(suppl 6):A127.
47. Machacek DA, Magera JM, Park S, et al. Diagnosis of adrenal dysfunction using liquid chromatography with tandem spectrometry. Clin Chem 2000; 46(suppl 6):A127.
48. Coleman WD, Tsongalis GJ. Molecular Diagnostics for the Clinical Laboratory. Totowa, NJ, Humana Press, 1997.
49. Stowasser M, Bachmann AW, Jonsson JR, et al. Clinical, biochemical and genetic approaches to the detection of familial hyperaldosteronism type 1. J Hypertens 1995; 13(12 Pt 2):1610–1613.
50. Unger ER, Piper MA. Nucleic acid biochemistry and diagnostic applications. In Burtis CA, Ashwood ER (eds). Tietz Textbook of Clinical Chemistry, 3rd ed. Philadelphia, WB Saunders, 1999, pp 421–443.
51. Mullis KB, Faloona FA. Specific synthesis of DNA in vitro via a polymerase-catalyzed chain reaction. Methods Enzymol 1987; 155:335–350.
52. Southern EM. Detection of specific sequences among DNA fragments separated by gel electrophoresis. J Mol Biol 1975; 98:503–517.
53. National Committee for Clinical Laboratory Standards (NCCLS). Preliminary Evaluation of Quantitative Clinical Laboratory Methods: Approved Guideline EP10-A. Wayne, Pa, NCCLS, 1998.
54. Carey RN, Garber CC. Evaluation of methods. In Kaplan LA, Pesce AJ (eds). Clinical Chemistry: Theory, Practice and Correlation, 2nd ed. St. Louis, CV Mosby, 1989, pp 290–310.
55. Department of Health and Human Services, Health Care Financing Administration. Clinical Laboratory Improvement Amendments of 1988: Final Rule. Federal Register, No. 7165[42CFR493.1217], February 28, 1992.
56. National Committee for Clinical Laboratory Standards (NCCLS). Method Comparison and Bias Estimation Using Patient Samples: Approved Guideline EP9-A. Wayne, Pa, NCCLS, 1995.
57. Taylor BN (U.S. ed). The International System of Units (SI). Special Publication 330. Gaithersburg, Md, National Institute of Standards and Technology (NIST), 1991, p 62.*
58. Hilleman MR. International biological standardization in historic and contemporary perspective. Dev Biol Stand 1999; 100:19–30.
59. Rose MP. Follicle-stimulating hormone international standards and reference preparations for the calibration of immunoassays and bioassays. Clin Chim Acta 1998; 273:103–117.
60. Linnet K. Necessary sample size for method comparison studies based on regression analysis. Clin Chem 1999; 45:882–894.
61. The European Parliament and the Council of the European Union Directive 98/79/EC of the European Parliament and of the Council of October 27, 1998, on in vitro diagnostic medical devices. OJ L 220, 30.8.1993:23.
62. Powers DM. Regulations and Standards: Traceability of assay calibrators: The EU's IVD Directive raises the bar. IVD Technol 2000; 26–33.
63. Fraser CG, Petersen PH. Analytical performance characteristics should be judged against objective quality specifications. Clin Chem 1999; 45:321–333.
64. National Committee for Clinical Laboratory Standards (NCCLS). Evaluation of Precision Performance of Clinical Chemistry Devices: Approved Guideline EP5-A. Wayne, Pa, NCCLS, 1999.

*Periodically revised; available from Superintendent of Documents, Code No. NSPUE2, U.S. Government Printing Office, Washington, DC 20402–9325.

65. Stockl D, Baadenhuijsen H, Fraser CG, et al. Desirable routine analytical goals for quantities assayed in serum. Eur J Clin Chem Clin Biochem 1995; 33:157–169.
66. Fraser CG: Biological variation in clinical chemistry: an update—collated data, 1988–1991. Arch Pathol Lab Med 1992; 116:916–923.
67. Fraser CG, Petersen PH, Ricos C, et al. Proposed quality specifications for the imprecision and inaccuracy of analytical systems for clinical chemistry. Eur J Clin Chem Clin Biochem 1992; 30: 311–317.
68. Kroll MH, Emancipator K. A theoretical evaluation of linearity. Clin Chem 1993; 39:405–413.
69. National Committee for Clinical Laboratory Standards (NCCLS). Evaluation of Matrix Effects: Proposed Guideline EP14-P. Wayne, Pa, NCCLS, 1998.
70. National Committee for Clinical Laboratory Standards (NCCLS). Evaluation of the Linearity of Quantitative Analytical Methods: Proposed Guideline EP6-P. Wayne, Pa, NCCLS, 1986.
71. National Committee for Clinical Laboratory Standards (NCCLS). Interference Testing in Clinical Chemistry: Proposed guideline EP7-P. Wayne, Pa, NCCLS, 1986.
72. Levine S, Noth R, Loo A, et al. Anomalous serum thyroxin measurements with the Abbott TDx procedure. Clin Chem 1990; 36:1838–1840.
73. Mbuyi-Kalala A, Ehrenstein G. Anomalous effects of hormone fragments on the measurement of parathyroid hormone by radioimmunoassay. Methods Find Exp Clin Pharmacol 1996; 18: 87–99.
74. Micallef JV, Hayes MM, Latif A, et al. Serum binding of steroid tracers and its possible effects on direct steroid immunoassay. Ann Clin Biochem 1995; 32:566–574.
75. Cook NJ, Read GF. Oestradiol measurement in women on oral hormone replacement therapy: the validity of commercial test kits. Br J Biomed Sci 1995; 52:97–101.
76. Cummings EA, Salisbyry SR, Givner ML, et al. Testolactone-associated high androgen levels: a pharmacologic effect or a laboratory artifact? J Clin Endocrinol Metab 1998; 83:784–787.
77. Thomas CM, van den Berg RJ, Segers MF, et al. Inaccurate measurement of 17 beta-estradiol in serum of female volunteers after oral administration of milligram amounts of micronized 17 beta-estradiol. Clin Chem 1993; 39(11 Pt 1):2341–2342.
78. O'Brien PC, Dyck PJ. Procedures for setting normal values. Neurology 1995; 45:17–23.
79. Solberg HE. Establishment and use of reference values. In Burtis CA, Ashwood ER (eds). Tietz Textbook of Clinical Chemistry, 2nd ed. Philadelphia, WB Saunders, 1994, pp 454–484.
80. National Committee for Clinical Laboratory Standards (NCCLS). How to Define and Determine Reference Intervals in the Clinical Laboratory: Approved Guideline C28-A2, 2nd ed. Wayne, Pa, NCCLS, 2000.
81. Klee GG. Maximizing efficacy of endocrine tests: Importance of decision-focused testing strategies and appropriate patient preparation. Clin Chem 1999; 45(8B):1323–1330.
82. Heins M, Heil W, Withold W. Storage of serum or whole blood samples? Effects of time and temperature on 22 serum analytes. Eur J Clin Chem Clin Biochem 1995; 33:231–238.
83. Tateishi K, Klee GG, Cunningham JM, Lennon VA. Stability of bombesin in serum, plasma, urine, and culture media. Clin Chem 1985; 31: 276–278.
84. Demir A, Alfthan H, Stenman UH, et al. A clinically useful method for detecting gonadotropins in children: assessment of luteinizing hormone and follicle-stimulating hormone from urine as an alternative to serum by ultrasensitive time-resolved immunofluorometric assays. Pediatr Res 1994; 36:221–226.
85. Hourd P, Edwards R. Current methods for the measurement of growth hormone in urine. Clin Endocrinol 1994; 40:155–170.
86. Maes M, Mommen K, Hendrickx D, et al. Components of biological variation, including seasonality, in blood concentrations of TSH, TT_3, FT_4, PRL, cortisol, and testosterone in healthy volunteers. Clin Endocrinol 1997; 46:587–598.
87. Sebastian-Gambaro MA, Liron-Hernandez FJ, Fuentes-Arderiu X. Intra- and interindividual biological variability bank. J Clin Chem Clin Biochem 1997; 35:845–852.
88. Leppaluoto J, Ruskoaho H. Atrial natriuretic peptide, renin activity, aldosterone, urine volume and electrolytes during a 24-hour sleep-wake cycle in man. Acta Physiol Scand 1990; 139:47–53.
89. Demers LM. Pituitary function. In Burtis CA, Ashwood ER (eds). Tietz Textbook of Clinical Chemistry, 3rd ed. Philadelphia, WB Saunders, 1999, pp 1470–1495.
90. Bergenfelz A, Isaksson A, Lindblom P, et al. Measurement of parathyroid hormone in patients with primary hyperparathyroidism undergoing first and reoperative surgery. Br J Surg 1998; 85: 1129–1132.
91. Abe T, Ludecke DK. Recent primary transnasal surgical outcomes associated with intraoperative growth hormone measurement in acromegaly. Clin Endocrinol 1999; 50:27–35.
92. Kruger C, Breunig U, Biskupek-Sigwart J, et al. Problems with salivary 17-hydroxyprogesterone determinations using the Salivette device. Eur J Clin Chem Clin Biochem 1996; 34:926–929.
93. Dabbs JM Jr. Salivary testosterone measurements: collecting, storing, and mailing saliva samples. Physiol Behav 1991; 49:815–817.
94. Vining RF, McGinley RA. The measurement of hormones in saliva: possibilities and pitfalls. Steroid Biochem 1987; 27:81–94.
95. Granger DA, Schwartz EB, Booth A, et al. Assessing dehydroepiandrosterone in saliva: a simple radioimmunoassay for use in studies of children, adolescents and adults. Psychoneuroendocrinology 1999; 24:567–579.
96. O'Rorke A, Kane MM, Gosling JP, et al. Development and validation of a monoclonal antibody enzyme immunoassay for measuring progesterone in saliva. Clin Chem 1994; 403:454–458.
97. Vining RF, McGinley RA, Symon RG. Hormones in saliva: mode of entry and consequent implication for clinical interpretation. Clin Chem 1983; 29:1752–1756.
98. Worthman CM, Stallings JF. Hormone measures in finger-prick blood spot samples: new field methods for reproductive endocrinology. Am J Phys Anthropol 1997; 104:1–21.
99. Howe CJ, Handelsman DJ. Use of filter paper for sample collection and transport in steroid pharmacology. Clin Chem 1997; 43: 1408–1415.
100. Kricka LJ. Miniaturization of analytical systems. Clin Chem 1998; 44:2008–2014.
101. Gabriely I, Kaplan J, Wozniak R. Transcutaneous glucose measurement using near-infrared spectroscopy during hypoglycemia. Diabetes Care 1999; 22:2026–2032.
102. Tamada JA, Garg S, Jovanovic L, et al. Noninvasive glucose monitoring: comprehensive clinical results. JAMA 1999; 282: 1839–1844.
103. Garg SK, Potts RO, Ackerman NR, et al. Correlation of fingerstick blood glucose measurements with GlucoWatch biographer glucose results in young subjects with type 1 diabetes. Diabetes Care 1999; 22:1708–1714.
104. Westgard JO, Klee GG. Quality management. In Burtis CA, Ashwood ER (eds). Tietz Textbook of Clinical Chemistry, 3rd ed. Philadelphia, WB Saunders, 1999, pp 384–420.
105. Browning MCK. Analytical goals for quantities used to assess thyrometabolic status. Ann Clin Biochem 1989; 26:1–2.
106. Tietz NW. Accuracy in clinical chemistry: does anybody care? Clin Chem 1994; 40:859–861.
107. Westgard JO, Barry PL, Hunt MR, et al. A multi-rule Shewhart chart for quality control on clinical chemistry. Clin Chem 1981; 27:493–501.
108. Klee GG, Schryver PG, Kisabeth RM. Analytic bias specifications based on the analysis of effects on performance of medical guidelines. Scand J Clin Lab Invest 1999; 59:509–512.
109. Smith FA, Kroft SH. Optimal procedures for detecting analytic bias using patient samples. Am J Clin Pathol 1997; 108:254–268.
110. Reinsberg J. Different efficacy of various blocking reagents to eliminate interferences by human antimouse antibodies with a two-site immunoassay. Clin Biochem 1996; 29:145–148.
111. Nicholson S, Fox M, Epenetos A, et al. Immunoglobulin inhibiting reagent: evaluation of a new method for eliminating spurious elevations in CA 125 caused by HAMA. Int J Biol Markers 1996; 11:46–49.
112. Wheeler MJ, D'Souza A, Matadeen J, et al. Ciba Corning ACS: 180 testosterone assay evaluated. Clin Chem 1996; 42:1445–1449.

HYPOTHALAMUS AND PITUITARY

7 Neuroendocrinology

Roger D. Cone, Malcolm J. Low, Joel K. Elmquist, and Judy L. Cameron

HISTORICAL PERSPECTIVE

The field of neuroendocrinology can be most broadly defined as the interaction between the central nervous system (CNS) and endocrine systems in the control of homeostasis. Much of this field, of course, has focused on the control of pituitary hormone secretion by the hypothalamus. At the beginning of the 21st century, we now appreciate the fundamental role of the hypothalamus in controlling anterior pituitary function. It is noteworthy that this concept is relatively recent, although the intimate interaction of the hypothalamus and the pituitary gland has been appreciated for some time.[1–3] For example, at the end of the 19th century, clinicians including Alfred Fröhlich described an obesity and infertility condition (often referred to as the adiposogenital dystrophic syndrome) in patients with pituitary tumors.[4] This condition subsequently became known as Fröhlich's syndrome and was most often associated with pituitary tumors and the accumulation of excessive subcutaneous fat and hypogonadism.[4, 5]

Whether this syndrome was due to injury to the pituitary gland itself or to the overlying hypothalamus was extremely controversial, however. Several leaders in the field of endocrinology, including Cushing and his colleagues, argued that the syndrome was due to disruption of the pituitary gland.[3, 6, 7] However, experimental evidence began to accumulate that the hypothalamus was somehow involved in the control of the pituitary gland. For example, Aschner[8] demonstrated in dogs that the precise removal of the pituitary gland without damage to the overlying hypothalamus did not result in obesity. Later, seminal studies by Hetherington and Ranson, using a stereotaxic apparatus, demonstrated that destruction of the medial basal hypothalamus with electrolytic lesions, without damage to the pituitary gland, resulted in morbid obesity and neuroendocrine derangements similar to those of the patients described by Fröhlich.[8, 9] This and subsequent studies clearly established that an intact hypothalamus is required for normal endocrine function. However, the mechanisms by which the hypothalamus was involved in endocrine regulation remained unsettled for years to come. We now know that the phenotypes of Fröhlich's syndrome and the ventromedial hypothalamic lesion syndrome are probably due to destruction of key hypothalamic neurons that respond to key metabolic signals including leptin[10] (see later).

The field of neuroendocrinology took a major step forward when it was recognized by several groups, especially Ernst and Berta Scharrer, that neurons in the hypothalamus were the source of the axons that constitute the neural lobe (see "Neurosecretion"). The hypothalamic control of the anterior pituitary gland remained unclear, however. For example, Popa and Fielding[11] are credited with the identification of the pituitary portal vessels linking the median eminence of the hypothalamus and the anterior pituitary gland. Although they appreciated the fact that this vasculature provided a link between hypothalamus and pituitary gland, they hypothesized at the time that blood flowed from the pituitary up to the brain. Anatomic studies by Wislocki and King[12] supported the concept that blood flow was from the hypothalamus to the pituitary. Later studies, including the seminal work of Geoffrey Harris,[13–15] established the flow of blood from the hypothalamus at the median eminence to the anterior pituitary gland. This supported the concept that the hypothalamus controlled anterior pituitary gland function indirectly and led to the now accepted hypophyseal-portal chemotransmitter hypothesis.[1, 16]

Later, several important studies, especially those from Schally and colleagues[17, 18] and the Guillemin group,[19–21] established that the anterior pituitary is tightly controlled by the hypothalamus. Both groups identified several putative peptide hormone releasing factors (see later sections). These fundamental studies resulted in the awarding of the Nobel Prize to Andrew Schally and Roger Guillemin. Of course, we now know that these releasing factors are the fundamental link between the CNS and the control of endocrine function. It is also established that these peptide hormones are highly conserved across species and are essential for reproduction, growth, and metabolism. The anatomy, physiology, and genetics of these factors constitute a major portion of this chapter.

Over the past two decades, work in the field of neuroendocrinology has continued to advance across several fronts. Cloning and characterization of the specific G protein–coupled rereceptors used by the hypothalamic releasing factors[22–25] have helped define signaling mechanisms utilized by the releasing factors. Furthermore, characterization of the distribution of these receptors has, in every case, demonstrated receptor expression in the brain and in peripheral tissues other than the pituitary, arguing for multifactorial roles for these factors. Finally, the last two decades have also seen tremendous advances in our understanding of both regulatory neuronal and humoral inputs to the hypophyseotropic neurons.

The adipostatic hormone leptin, discovered in 1994,[26] is an example of a humoral factor that has profound effects on multiple neuroendocrine circuits as the factor that suppresses the thyroid and reproductive axes during the starvation response. The subsequent discovery of ghrelin,[27, 28] a stomach peptide that regulates appetite and also acts on multiple neuroendocrine axes, demonstrates that much remains to be learned regarding the regulation of the hypothalamic releasing hormones. Traditionally, it has been extremely difficult to study the regulation of releasing factor gene expression or the specific regulation of the releasing factor neurons as a consequence of their small numbers and, in some cases, diffuse distribution. Transgenic experiments have resulted in the production of mice in which expression of fluorescent marker proteins has been specifically targeted to gonadotropin-releasing hormone (GnRH) neurons[29, 30] and arcuate pro-opiomelanocortin (POMC) neurons.[31] This technology will allow detailed study of important neuroendocrine neurons in the more native context of slice preparations or organotypic cultures. For example, investigators have already used this method to characterize directly the electrophysiologic properties of individual GnRH neurons.

As just described, much of the field of neuroendocrinology has focused on hypothalamic releasing factors and their control of reproduction, growth, development, fluid balance, and the stress response through their control of pituitary hormone production. More broadly, however, neuroendocrinology has become a rubric to define the study of interaction of the endocrine and nervous systems in the regulation of homeostasis. The rubric of neuroendocrinology has been further expanded, however, because many areas of basic research have often been fundamental to understanding the neuroendocrine system and thus championed by scientists in the field. These areas include studies of neuropeptide structure, function, and mechanism of action; neural secretion; hypothalamic neuroanatomy; G protein–coupled receptor structure, function, and signaling; transport of substances into the brain; and the action of hormones on the brain. Many homeostatic systems involve integrated endocrine, autonomic, and behavioral responses. Thus, many homeostatic systems exist in which the classical neuroendocrine axes are important but not autonomous pathways, such as energy homeostasis and immune function, and these subjects are also often studied in the context of neuroendocrinology.

This chapter first presents the concepts of neural secretion, the neuroanatomy of the hypothalamic-pituitary unit, and the CNS structures most relevant to the control of the neurohypophysis and hypophysis. The chapter then covers each classical hypothalamic-pituitary axis, followed by two homeostatic systems, energy homeostasis and immune function, which are heavily integrated with neuroendocrine function. Finally, the chapter reviews the pathophysiology of disorders of neural regulation of endocrine function.

NEURAL CONTROL OF GLANDULAR SECRETION

A fundamental principle of neuroendocrinology is the concept of regulated secretion of hormones, neurotransmitters, or neuromodulators by secretory cells.[16, 32] Endocrine cells and neurons are prototypical secretory cells, and both are characterized by the ability to be stimulated to cause the release of their products. In addition, secretory cells exist that can be broadly classified by their mechanisms of secretion. For example, endocrine cells secrete their contents directly into the blood stream, allowing these substances to act globally as hormones. In contrast, secretory cells in exocrine glands secrete substances into ductal systems. Cells classified as paracrine secrete their contents and affect the function of cells in the immediate vicinity. Similarly, autocrine secretory cells affect their own function by the local actions of their own secretions.

Neurosecretion

Neurons are specialized secretory cells that send their axons throughout the nervous system to release their neurotransmitters and neuromodulators into chemical synapses.[33] A specialized subset of neurons are the neurohumoral or neurosecretory cells. Two examples of neurosecretory cells are neurohypophyseal and hypophyseotropic cells.[34] The prototypical neurohypophyseal cells are the magnocellular neurons of the paraventricular and supraoptic nuclei in the hypothalamus. Hypophyseotropic cells are neurons that secrete their products into the pituitary portal vessels at the median eminence (Fig. 7–1) (see later).

In the most basic sense, neurosecretory cells are neurons that secrete substances directly into the blood stream to act as hormones. This concept of release is often referred to as neurosecretion (Fig. 7–2). The theory of neurosecretion evolved from the seminal work of Scharrer and Scharrer,[3, 32, 35, 36] who used morphologic techniques to identify stained secretory granules in the supraoptic and paraventricular hypothalamic neurons. They found that cutting the pituitary stalk led to an accumulation of these granules in the hypothalamus.[32, 35] These findings led them to hypothesize that the source of substances secreted by the neural lobe (posterior pituitary) was hypothalamic neurons. Of course, we now know that the axon terminals in the neural lobe arise from the supraoptic and paraventricular magnocellular neurons that contain oxytocin and arginine vasopressin (AVP).

The modern definition of neurosecretion has evolved to include the release of any neuronal secretory product from a neuron. Indeed, a basic principle of neuroscience is that all neurons in the CNS, including neurons that secrete AVP and oxytocin in the neural lobe, receive multiple synaptic inputs largely onto their dendrites and cell bodies. In addition, neu-

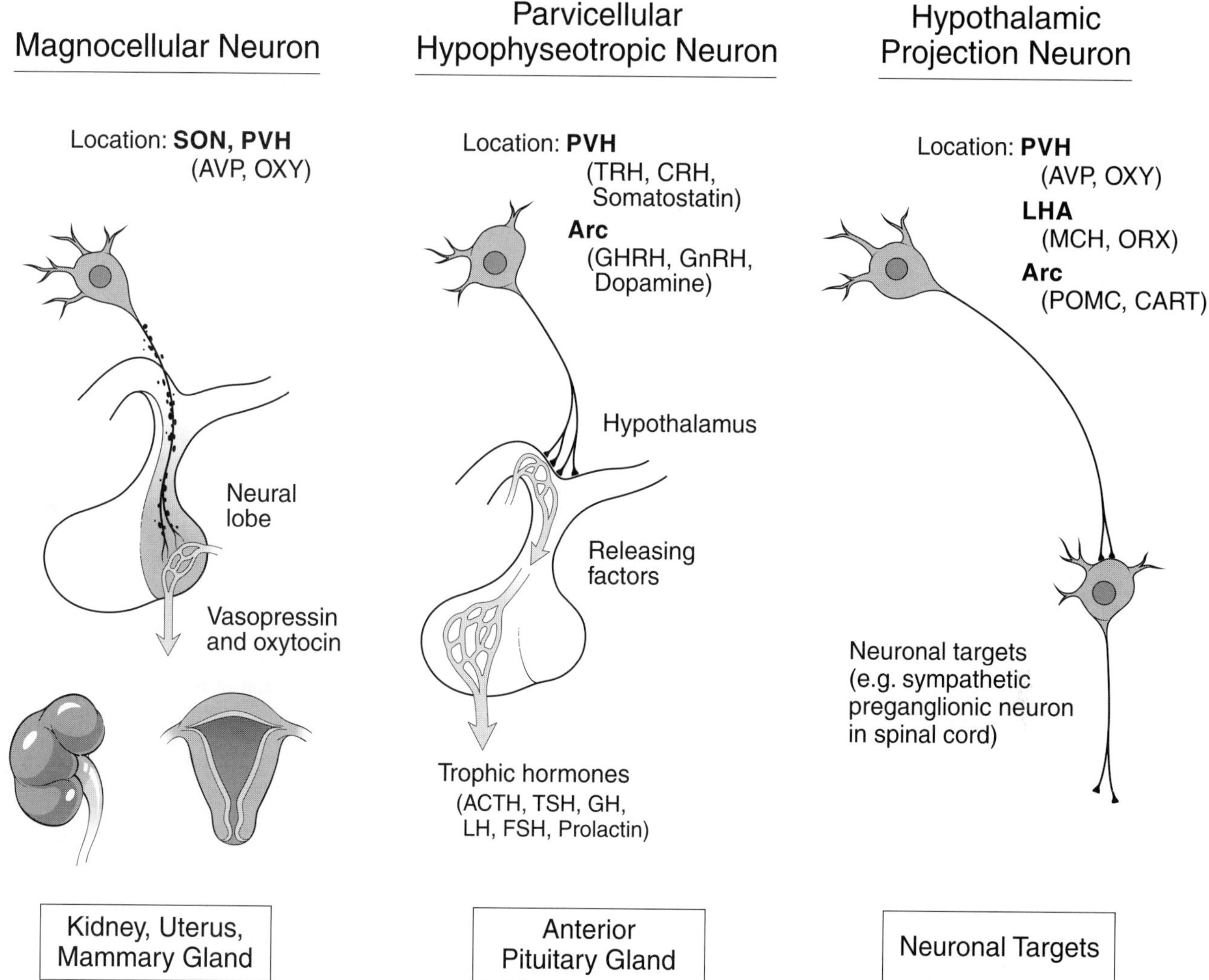

Figure 7–1. Three types of hypothalamic neurosecretory cells. *Left,* A magnocellular neuron that secretes arginine vasopressin or oxytocin (AVP, OXY). The cell body, which is located in the supraoptic or paraventricular hypothalamic nucleus (SON, PVH), projects its neuronal process into the neural lobe, and neurohormone is released from nerve endings. *Center,* Similar peptidergic neurons are located in the medial basal hypothalamus in nuclear groups including the PVH and arcuate nucleus of the hypothalamus (Arc). The neuropeptides in this case are released into the specialized blood supply to the pituitary to regulate its secretion. Similar in plan are neurosecretory neurons that terminate in relation to another neuron *(right).* These projection neurons are found in sites including the PVH, Arc, and lateral hypothalamic area (LHA) that project to autonomic preganglionic neurons in the brain stem and spinal cord. Such substances act as neurotransmitters or neuromodulators. ACTH, corticotropin; CART, cocaine and amphetamine–regulated transcript; CRH, corticotropin-releasing hormone; FSH, follicle-stimulating hormone; GH, growth hormone; GHRH, growth hormone–releasing hormone; GnRH, gonadotropin-releasing hormone; LH, luteinizing hormone; MCH, melanin-concentrating hormone; ORX, orexin-hypocretin; POMC, pro-opiomelanocortin; TRH, thyrotropin-releasing hormone; TSH, thyrotropin.

rons have the basic ability to respond and integrate input from multiple neurons through specific receptors.[33, 34] They in turn fire action potentials that result in the release of neurotransmitters and neuromodulators into synapses formed with postsynaptic neurons. The vast majority of communication between neurons is accomplished by "classical" neurotransmitters (e.g., glutamate, γ-aminobutyric acid [GABA], acetylcholine) and neuromodulators (e.g., neuropeptides) acting at chemical synapses (see Fig. 7–2).[33, 34, 37, 38] Thus, neurosecretion represents a fundamental concept in understanding the mechanisms used by the nervous system to control behavior and maintain homeostasis.

In the era of the elucidation of the human genome, the importance of these early observations is often not fully appreciated. However, accounts of these early studies are illuminating.[3] Moreover, it is not an overstatement that the confirmation of the neurosecretion hypothesis represented one of the major advances in the field of neuroscience and neuroendocrinology. Indeed, this and other early experiments, including the pioneering work of Geoffrey Harris,[13, 15, 39] led to the fundamental concept that the hypothalamus releases hormones directly into the blood stream (neurohypophyseal cells). These observations provided the principles on which the modern discipline of neuroendocrinology is built.

The Autonomic Nervous System Contribution to Endocrine Control

One of these fundamental principles of neuroendocrinology is that the nervous system controls or modifies, or both, the

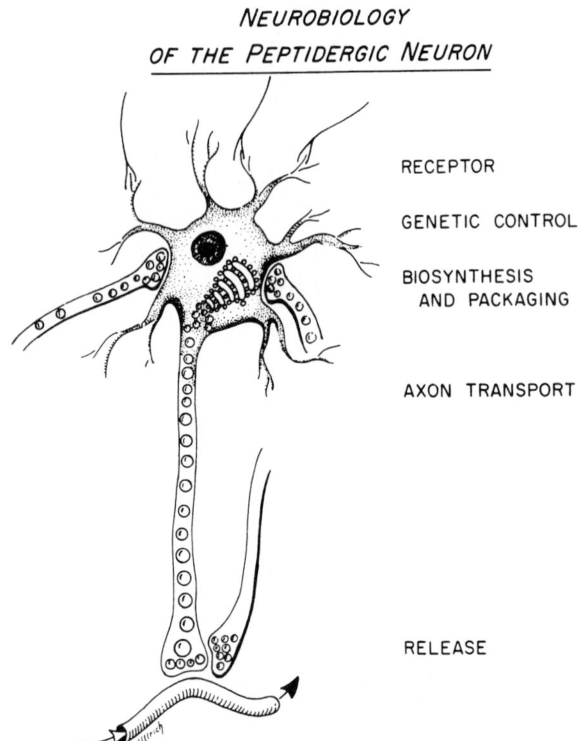

Figure 7–2. Neurobiologic features of the peptidergic neuron. Neurosecretory neurons can be regarded as having secretory functions that are in many ways analogous to those of glandular cells. A secretory product, which is formed on the endoplasmic reticulum under the direction of messenger ribonucleic acid, is packaged in granules and transported along the axon by axoplasmic flow to reach nerve terminals, where the granules are released. Virtually all neurons carry out similar functions. Some secrete neurotransmitters, such as acetylcholine or norepinephrine; others, such as motor nerves, secrete acetylcholine and myotropic factors. In all neurons there is a constant orthograde (forward) flow of cytoplasm and formed elements such as mitochondria. Retrograde flow also takes place to bring substances that enter nerve endings back to the body of the cell. In typical neurotransmitter neurons, the neurotransmitters are synthesized by enzymes and are packaged into secretory granules. These granules are transported in a manner similar to that of neuropeptide-containing granules. In many neurons cosecretion of one or two peptides may occur in association with secretion of a classic neurotransmitter. (From Reichlin S. Summarizing comments. In Gotto AM Jr, Peck EJ Jr, Boyd AE III, et al [eds]. Brain Peptides: A New Endocrinology. New York, Elsevier/North-Holland, 1979, pp 379–403.)

function of both endocrine and exocrine glands. The exquisite control of the anterior pituitary gland is accomplished by the release of releasing factor hormones (see later). Other endocrine and exocrine organs (e.g., pancreas, adrenal, pineal, salivary glands) are also regulated through direct innervation from the cholinergic and noradrenergic inputs from the autonomic nervous system.[40, 41] Although it is beyond the scope of this chapter, an appreciation of the functional anatomy and pharmacology of the parasympathetic and sympathetic nervous systems is fundamental in understanding the neural control of endocrine function.

The efferent arms of the autonomic nervous system comprise the sympathetic and parasympathetic systems. Both limbs are a classical two-neuron chain. Both are characterized by a preganglionic neuron that innervates a postganglionic neuron that targets an end organ. Preganglionic and postganglionic parasympathetic neurons are cholinergic. In contrast, preganglionic sympathetic neurons are cholinergic and postganglionic neurons are noradrenergic (except for those innervating sweat glands, which are cholinergic).[40, 41] Another basic concept is that autonomic neurons coexpress several neuropeptides. This coexpression is a common feature in neurons in both the central and peripheral nervous systems.[37, 38, 42] For example, postganglionic noradrenergic neurons coexpress somatostatin and neuropeptide Y (NPY). Postganglionic cholinergic neurons coexpress neuropeptides including vasoactive intestinal polypeptide and calcitonin gene-related peptide.

The majority of the sympathetic preganglionic neurons lie in the intermediolateral cell column in the thoracolumbar regions of the spinal cord.[40, 41] Most postganglionic neurons are located in sympathetic ganglia lying near the vertebral column (e.g., sympathetic chain and superior cervical ganglia). Postganglionic fibers, in turn, innervate target organs. Thus, as a rule, sympathetic preganglionic fibers are relatively short and the postganglionic fibers are long. In contrast, the parasympathetic preganglionic neurons lie in the midbrain (Edinger-Westphal nucleus of the third cranial nerve), the medulla oblongata (e.g., dorsal motor nucleus of the vagus and nucleus ambiguus), and the sacral spinal cord. Postganglionic neurons that innervate the eye and salivary glands arise from the ciliary, pterygopalatine, submandibular, and otic ganglia. Postganglionic neurons in thorax and abdomen typically lie in the target organs including the gut wall and pancreas.[40, 41] Thus, preganglionic neurons are relatively long and the postganglionic fibers are short.

The importance of coordinated neural control of endocrine organs is illustrated by the innervation of the pancreas. The endocrine pancreas receives both parasympathetic (cholinergic) innervation and sympathetic (noradrenergic) innervation.[40, 41, 43–45] The cholinergic innervation is provided by the vagus nerve (dorsal motor nucleus of the vagus). The activity in this innervation is an excellent example of neural modulation as it is clear that the secretory activity of insulin-producing beta cells is affected by the cholinergic tone of the beta cell.[43, 44] For example, vagal input is thought to modulate insulin secretion before (cephalic phase), during, and after ingestion of food.[46] In addition, noradrenergic stimulation of the endocrine pancreas can alter the secretion of glucagon and inhibits insulin release.[43, 44] It should be noted, of course, that a major regulator of insulin secretion by beta cells is glucose concentrations.[47] In fact, glucose can induce insulin secretion in the absence of neural input. However, the exquisite control by the nervous system is illustrated by the fact that populations of neurons in the brain stem and hypothalamus, like the beta cell, have the ability to sense glucose levels in the blood stream.[45, 48] This information is integrated by the hypothalamus and ultimately results in alterations in the activity of the autonomic nervous system innervating the pancreas. Thus, neural control of the endocrine pancreas probably contributes to the physiologic control of insulin secretion and may contribute to the pathophysiology of disorders such as diabetes mellitus. Certainly, an increased understanding of this complex interplay between the CNS and endocrine function is needed to diagnose and clinically manage endocrine disorders.

HYPOTHALAMIC-PITUITARY UNIT

The hypothalamus is one of the most evolutionarily conserved and essential regions of the mammalian brain. Indeed, the hypothalamus is the ultimate brain structure that allows mammals to maintain homeostasis, and destruction of the hypothalamus is not compatible with life.[2, 49, 50] Hypothalamic control of homeostasis stems from the ability of this collection of neurons to orchestrate coordinated endocrine, autonomic, and behavioral responses. A key principle is that the hypothalamus receives sensory inputs from the external environment (e.g., light, pain, temperature, odorants) and information regarding the internal environment (e.g., blood pressure, blood osmolality, blood glucose levels). In addition, of particular relevance to neuroendocrine control, hormones (e.g., glucocorticoids, estrogen, testosterone, thyroid hormone) exert negative feedback directly on the hypothalamus.[16, 49, 51, 52]

These sensory and hormonal cues are examples of a fundamental concept of neuroendocrinology: the hypothalamus *integrates* sensory and hormonal inputs and provides coordinated responses through motor outputs to key regulatory sites. These include the anterior pituitary gland, the posterior pituitary gland, the cerebral cortex, premotor and motor neurons in the brain stem and spinal cord, and autonomic (parasympathetic and sympathetic) preganglionic neurons. The patterned hypothalamic outputs to these effector sites ultimately result in coordinated endocrine, behavioral, and autonomic responses that maintain homeostasis. The focus of this section, the hypothalamic control of the pituitary gland, is an exquisitely controlled system and underlies the ability of mammals to coordinate endocrine functions that are necessary for survival.

Anatomy of the Hypothalamic-Pituitary Unit

The pituitary gland is regulated by three interacting elements: hypothalamic inputs (releasing factors or hypophyseotropic hormones), feedback effects of circulating hormones, and paracrine and autocrine secretions of the pituitary itself.[16, 51] In humans, the pituitary gland (hypophysis) can be divided into two major parts, the adenohypophysis and the neurohypophysis. The adenohypophysis in turn can be subdivided into three distinct lobes, the pars distalis (anterior lobe), pars intermedia (intermediate lobe), and pars tuberalis (Fig. 7–3).[53–55] Whereas a well-developed intermediate lobe is found in most mammals, only rudimentary vestiges of the intermediate lobe are detectable in adult humans with the bulk of intermediate lobe cells being dispersed in the anterior and posterior lobes.[55]

The neurohypophysis is composed of the pars nervosa (also known as the neural or posterior lobe), the infundibular stalk, and the median eminence. The infundibular stalk is surrounded by the pars tuberalis, and together they constitute the hypophyseal stalk. The pituitary gland lies in the sella turcica (the Turkish saddle) of the sphenoid bone and underlies the base of the hypothalamus.[1, 56] This anatomic location explains the hypothalamic damage described by Fröhlich.[4] In humans, the base of the hypothalamus forms a mound called the tuber cinereum, the central region of which gives rise to the median eminence (Fig. 7–4; see Fig. 7–3).

The anterior and intermediate lobes of the pituitary are derived from an outgrowth of the pharyngeal cavity called Rathke's pouch and migrate during development to surround the neural lobe. The intermediate lobe is in contact with the neural lobe and is the least prominent of the three lobes. With age, the intermediate lobe in humans decreases in size and is represented in the adult as a relatively small collection of POMC cells. In some species, these cells are responsible for secreting the POMC-derived product α-melanocyte-stimulating hormone (α-MSH).[55, 57]

In a strict sense, the neurohypophysis is made up of the neural lobe, the infundibular stalk, and the median eminence. The major component of the neural lobe is a collection of axon terminals arising from magnocellular secretory neurons from the paraventricular and supraoptic nuclei of the hypothalamus (Fig. 7–5; see Fig. 7–8*C*). These axon terminals are in close association with a capillary plexus, and they secrete substances including AVP and oxytocin into the hypophyseal veins and into the general circulation (Table 7–1).[58, 59] The blood supply to the neurohypophysis arises from the inferior hypophyseal artery (a branch of the internal carotid artery). Scattered among the nerve terminals are glial-like cells called pituicytes. As the source of AVP to the general circulation, the paraventricular and supraoptic nuclei and their axon terminals in the neural lobe are the effector arms of the central regulation of blood osmolality, fluid balance, and blood pressure[60–62] (see "Circumventricular Organs").

The secretion of oxytocin by magnocellular neurons is also well characterized and is critical at the time of parturition, resulting in uterine myometrial contraction. In addition, the secretion of oxytocin is regulated by the classical milk let-down reflex.[63, 64] The exact neuroanatomic substrate underlying the milk let-down response is still unclear. However, it is apparent that mechanosensory information from the nipple reaches the magnocellular neurons, directly or indirectly, from the dorsal horn of the spinal cord,[50, 65] resulting in release of oxytocin into the general circulation. Oxytocin acts on receptors on myoepithelial cells in the mammary gland acini, leading to release of milk into the ductal system and ultimately the release of milk from the mammary gland.

The Median Eminence and Hypophyseotropic Neuronal System

The median eminence lies in the center of the tuber cinereum; it is composed of an extensive array of blood vessels and nerve endings and is the functional link between the hypothalamus and the anterior pituitary gland (Figs. 7–6 to 7–9; see Fig. 7–5).[15, 36, 50, 65–74] The median eminence can be considered the functional link between the hypothalamus and pituitary and the site of the hypothalamus from which the pituitary portal vessels arise. The median eminence is characterized by an extremely rich blood supply that arises from the superior hypophyseal artery (from the internal carotid artery). The artery sends off many small branches that form capillary loops.[52] The small capillary loops extend into the internal and external zones (see later), form anastomoses, and drain into sinusoids that become the pituitary portal veins that enter the vascular pool of the pituitary gland.[68, 75, 76] The flow of blood in these short loops is thought to be predominantly (if not exclusively) in a hypothalamic-to-pituitary direction.[12, 15] This well-developed plexus results in a tremendous increase in the vascular surface area. In addition, the vessels are fenestrated, allowing diffusion of the peptide-releasing factors to their site of action in the anterior pituitary gland. This vascular complex in the base of the hypothalamus and its "arteriolized" venous drainage to the pituitary compose a circulatory system analogous to the portal vein system of the liver, hence the term *hypophyseal-portal circulation*.

Typically, three zones of the median eminence are discussed, the ependymal layer, the internal zone, and the external zone (see Fig. 7–8).[1] The innermost zone is made up of ependymal cells that form the floor of the third ventricle. These ependymal cells are unique in that they have microvilli rather than cilia. The ependymal layer also contains specialized cells called tanycytes that send processes into the other layers of the median eminence. There are tight junctions between the ependymal cells lining the floor of the third ventricle forming a barrier between the cerebrospinal fluid (CSF) and the blood in the median eminence. In addition, tight junctions exist between tanycytes at the lateral edges of the median eminence that are thought to prevent the diffusion of releasing factors back into the medial basal hypothalamus.[51]

The internal zone of the median eminence is composed of axons of passage of the supraoptic and paraventricular magnocellular neurons en route to the posterior pituitary (see Fig. 7–

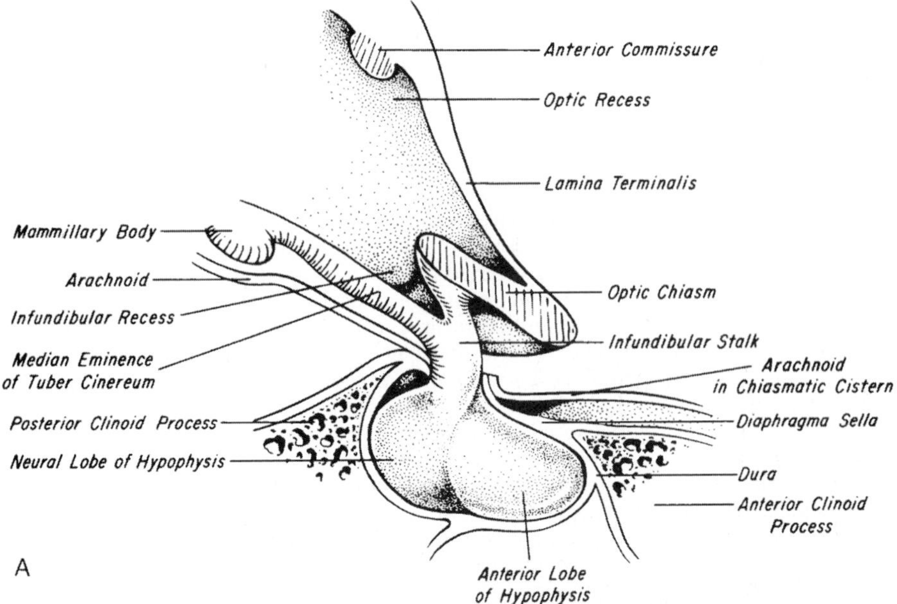

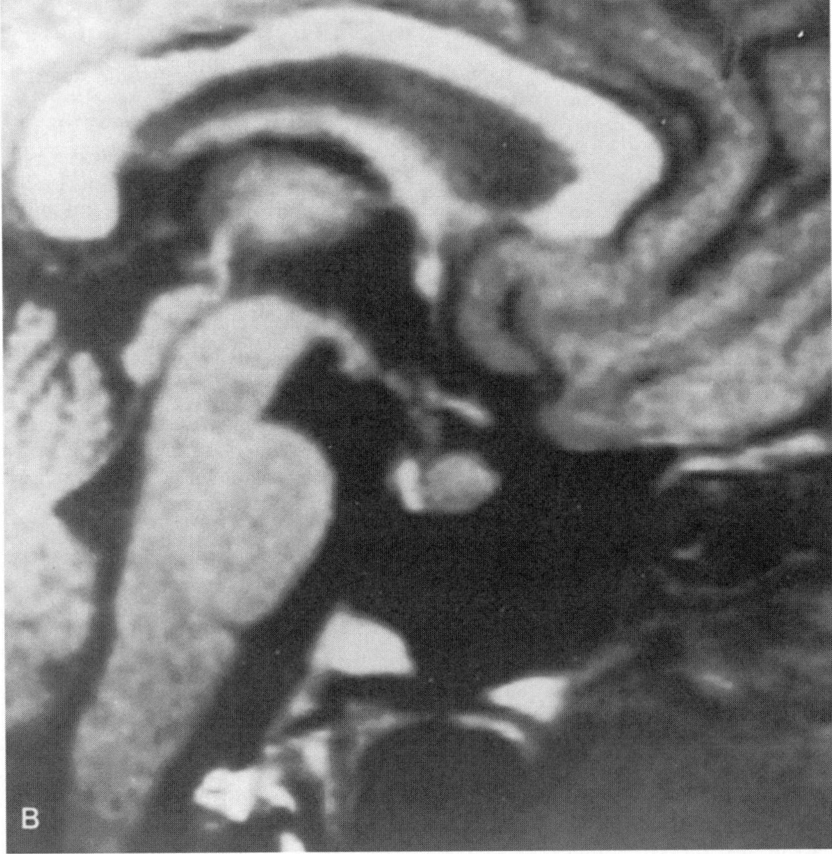

Figure 7–3. *A*, Human hypothalamic-pituitary unit showing the relationship to the sella turcica, brain membranes, and optic chiasm. *B*, Midsagittal nuclear magnetic resonance scan of the brain of a normal woman, which corresponds to the diagram in *A*. Note the location of the pituitary stalk, the intense signal from the posterior pituitary, and the anatomic relationship to the optic commissure and the optic nerve. (See also Fig. 7–4*A*.) (Courtesy of Dr. Samuel Wolpert.)

8*C*) and the axons of the hypophyseotropic neurons destined for the external layer of the median eminence (see Fig. 7–8*A* and *B*). In addition, supportive cells are found in this layer. Finally, the external zone represents the exchange point of the hypothalamic releasing factors and the pituitary portal vessels. The external zone contains terminals from two general types of releasing factors, peptides (discussed in detail later) and monoamines (dopamine and norepinephrine). This zone represents the site of convergence where the peptides come in contact with portal vessels.[75]

Two general types of tuberohypophyseal neurons project to the external zone of the median eminence: peptide-secreting (peptidergic) neurons (e.g., thyrotropin-releasing hormone [TRH], corticotropin-releasing hormone [CRH], and luteinizing hormone-releasing hormone [LHRH]; see Figs. 7–7 and 7–8) and neurons containing bioamines (e.g., dopamine and serotonin).[77] Although the secretion of these substances into the portal circulation is an important control mechanism, some peptides and neurotransmitters in nerve endings are not released into the hypophyseal-portal circulation[69] but instead

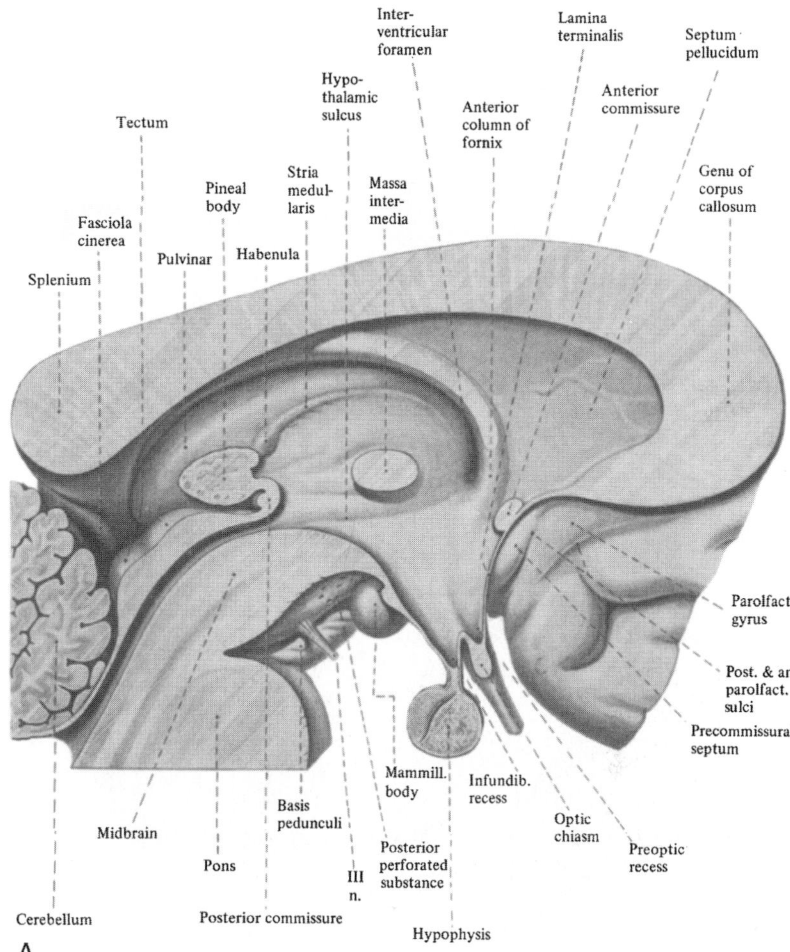

Figure 7–4. *A,* Midsagittal view of the human brain showing the hypothalamus and neighboring structures.

Figure continued on next page

function to regulate the secretion of other nerve terminals. The anatomic relationships of nerve endings, basement membranes, interstitial spaces, fenestrated (windowed) capillary endothelia, and glia in the median eminence are similar to those in the neural lobe. As in the case of the neurohypophysis, the release of neuropeptides is mediated by the depolarization of hypothalamic cells leading to secretion at the median eminence.[51, 52]

Non-neuronal supporting cells in the hypothalamus also play a dynamic role in hypophyseotropic regulation. For example, nerve terminals in the neurohypophysis are enveloped by glia (in the neural lobe they are called pituicytes); when the gland is inactive they surround the nerve endings, whereas the nerve ending is exposed when vasopressin secretion is enhanced as in states of dehydration. Within the median eminence, LHRH nerve endings are enveloped by the specialized ependymal cells called *tanycytes,* which also cover or uncover neurons with changes in functional status.[78] Thus, supporting elements, with their own sets of receptors, can change the neuroregulatory milieu within the hypothalamus, median eminence, and pituitary.

The site of production, the genetics, and the regulation of synthesis and release of peptide releasing factors are discussed in detail in the following. Briefly, the cell groups in the hypothalamus[79] that contain releasing factors that are secreted into the pituitary portal circulation are located in several cell groups of the medial hypothalamus (Table 7–2). These cell groups include the arcuate (infundibular) nucleus (see Fig. 7–9*D*), the paraventricular nucleus (see Fig. 7–9*A* and *C*), the periventricular nucleus, and a group of cells in the medial preoptic area near the organum vasculosum of the lamina terminalis (OVLT) (Fig. 7–10).[73, 80] As discussed, magnocellular neurons in the supraoptic and paraventricular nucleus send axon terminals that traverse the median eminence and make up the neural lobe of the pituitary. In addition, a projection from magnocellular neurons to the external zone of the median eminence has been described. However, its functional significance is not clear.

The third structure often grouped as a component of the median eminence is the pars tuberalis. The pars tuberalis is a subdivision of the adenohypophysis and is a thin glandular sheet of tissue that lies around the infundibulum and pituitary stalk. In some animals, the epithelial component may make up as much as 10% of the total glandular tissue of the anterior pituitary. The pars tuberalis contains cells making pituitary tropic hormones including luteinizing hormone (LH) and thyrotropin. A definitive physiologic function of the pars tuberalis is not established, but melatonin receptors are expressed in the pars tuberalis.

CIRCUMVENTRICULAR ORGANS

A fundamental principle of physiology and pharmacology is that the brain, including the hypothalamus, resides in an environment that is protected from humoral signals.[52, 60, 81–83] This exclusion of macromolecules is due to the structural vascular

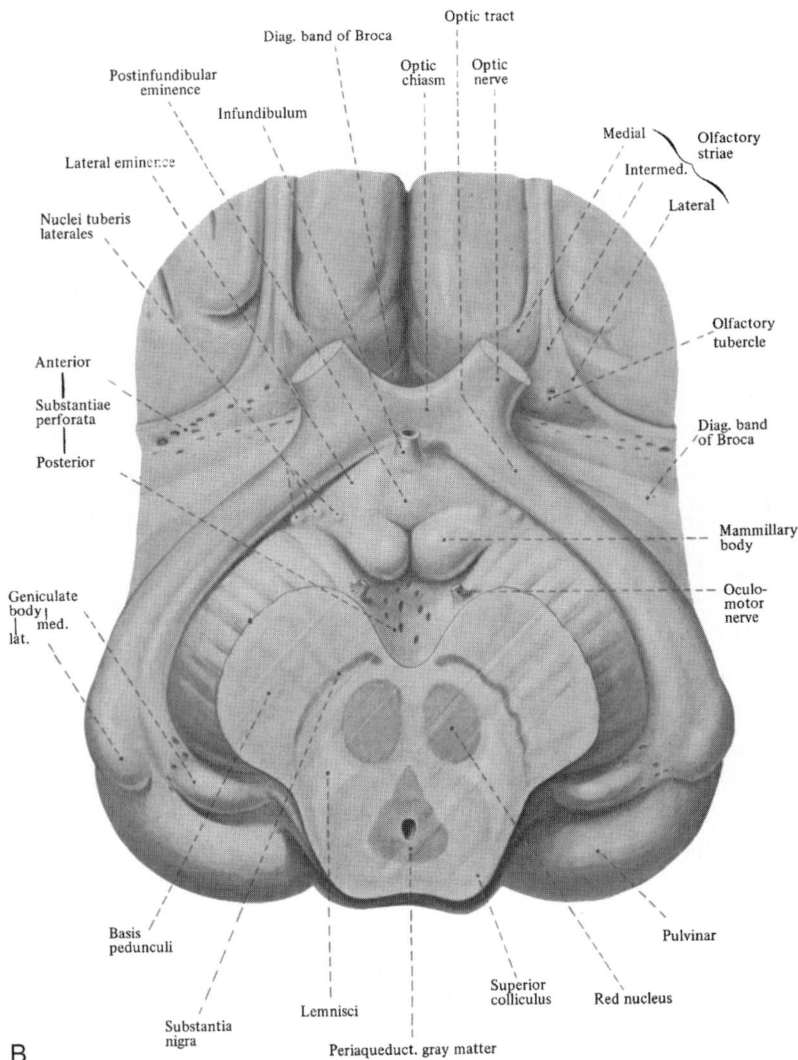

Figure 7–4 *Continued. B,* Base of the human brain, showing the hypothalamus and neighboring structures. On gross inspection, several landmarks outline the hypothalamus. It is bounded anteriorly by the optic chiasm, laterally by the sulci formed with the temporal lobes, and posteriorly by the mammillary bodies (in which the mammillary nuclei are located). Dorsally, the hypothalamus is delineated from the thalamus by the hypothalamic sulcus. The smooth, rounded base of the hypothalamus is the tuber cinereum; the pituitary stalk descends from its central region, which is termed the *median eminence.* The median eminence stands out from the rest of the tuber cinereum because of its dense vascularity, which is formed by the primary plexus of the hypophyseal-portal system. The long portal veins run along the ventral surface of the pituitary stalk. (From Nauta WJ, Haymaker W. Hypothalamic nuclei and fiber connections. In Haymaker W, Anderson E, Nauta WJ [eds]. The Hypothalamus. Springfield, Ill, Charles C Thomas, 1969, pp 136–209.)

specializations that make up the blood-brain barrier. These include tight junctions of brain vascular endothelial cells that preclude the free passage of polarized macromolecules including peptides and hormones. In addition, astrocytic foot processes and perivascular microglial cells contribute to the integrity of the blood-brain barrier.[52] However, to exert homeostatic control, the brain, especially the hypothalamus, must assess key sensory information from the blood stream including hormone levels, metabolites, and potential toxins.[84] For example, to monitor key signals the brain has "windows on the circulation" or circumventricular organs (CVOs) that serve as a conduit of peripheral cues into key neuronal cell groups that maintain homeostasis.[52, 60]

As the name implies, CVOs are specialized structures that lie on the midline of the brain along the third and fourth ventricles. These structures include the OVLT, subfornical organ (SFO), median eminence, neurohypophysis (posterior pituitary), subcommissural organ, and the area postrema (see Fig. 7–10). Unlike the vasculature in the rest of the brain, the blood vessels in CVOs have fenestrated capillaries that allow relatively free passage of molecules such as proteins and peptide hormones.[52, 60, 81–83] Thus, neurons and glial cells that reside within the CVOs have access to these macromolecules. In addition to the distinct nature of the vessels themselves, the CVOs have an unusually rich blood supply, allowing them to act as integrators at the interface of the blood-brain barrier. As discussed in more detail later, several of the CVOs have major projections to hypothalamic nuclear groups that regulate homeostasis.[50, 79] Thus, the CVOs serve as a critical link between peripheral metabolic cues, hormones, and potential toxins with cell groups within the brain that regulate coordinated endocrine, autonomic, and behavioral responses. Detailed discussion of the physiologic roles of individual CVOs is beyond the scope of this chapter, but several in-depth reviews have assessed the function of each.[50, 60, 61, 79, 81–83, 85–88]

Median Eminence

The median eminence and neurohypophysis contain the neurosecretory axons that control pituitary function. The role of the median eminence as a link between the hypothalamus and the pituitary gland is covered in greater detail in other sections of this chapter (see Figs. 7–8 and 7–9 and "Hypothalamic-Pituitary Unit"). However, it is important to understand that the anatomic location of the median eminence places it in a position to serve as an afferent sensory organ as well. Specifically, the median eminence is located adjacent to several neuroendocrine and autonomic regulatory nuclei at the tuberal level of the hypothalamus (see Fig. 7–9). These nuclear groups include the arcuate, ventromedial, dorsomedial, and paraventricular nuclei.[10, 89]

A role of cell groups surrounding the median eminence as afferent sensory centers is supported by several observations. For example, toxins such as monosodium glutamate and gold

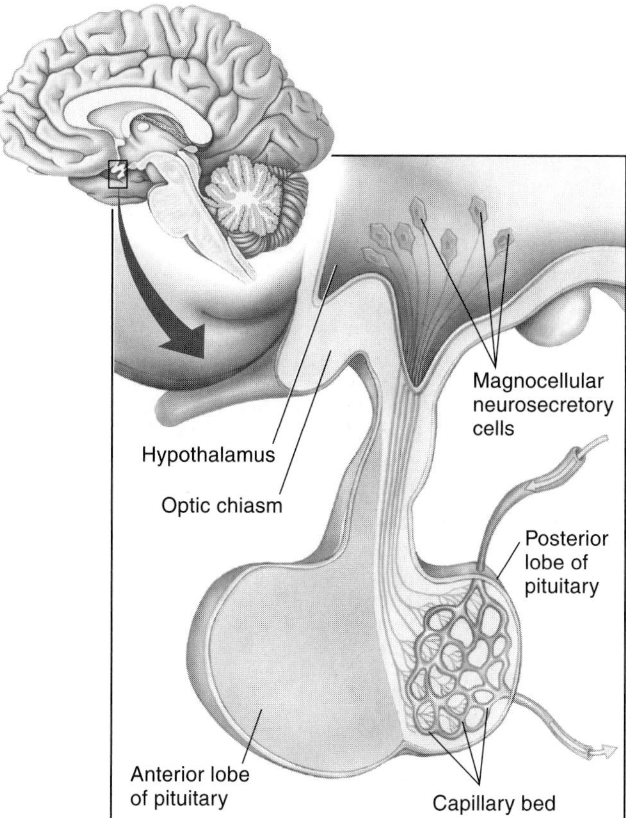

Figure 7–5. Hypothalamic magnocellular neurons and the posterior pituitary gland. This drawing of a midsagittal view of the hypothalamus and pituitary gland illustrates the concept that magnocellular neurons in the paraventricular and supraoptic nuclei secrete oxytocin and arginine vasopressin directly into capillaries in the posterior lobe of the pituitary gland. (From Bear MF, Connors BW, Paradiso MA. Neuroscience: Exploring the Brain. Baltimore, Williams & Wilkins, 1996, p 408.)

thioglucose damage neurons in cell groups overlying the median eminence, resulting in obesity and hyperphagia. Experimental evidence suggests that the median eminence is a portal of entry for hormones such as leptin. Indeed, administration of radiolabeled peptides or hormones, such as α-MSH or leptin, led to their accumulation around the median eminence.[90, 91] Moreover, leptin receptor messenger ribonucleic acid (mRNA) and leptin-induced gene expression are densely localized in the arcuate, ventromedial, dorsomedial, and ventral premammillary hypothalamic nuclei.[92–96] As discussed in detail in other sections of this chapter, leptin is an established mediator of body weight and neuroendocrine function that acts on several cells in the hypothalamus including POMC neurons that reside in the arcuate nucleus (see Fig. 8–67).[31, 97–100] Notably, POMC neurons are also found embedded within the median eminence. Thus, it is likely that the median eminence is involved in conveying information from humoral factors such as leptin to key hypothalamic regulatory neurons in the medial basal hypothalamus.

Organum Vasculosum of the Lamina Terminalis and the Subfornical Organ

The OVLT and the SFO are located at the front wall of the third ventricle, the lamina terminalis. The OVLT and SFO lie at the ventral and dorsal boundaries of the third ventricle, respectively (see Fig. 7–10).[60, 82] Because it lies at the rostral and ventral tip of the third ventricle, the OVLT is surrounded by cell groups of the preoptic region of the hypothalamus (see Fig. 8–66*A*). Like other CVOs, the OVLT is made up of neurons, glial cells, and tanycytes. It is also noteworthy that the OVLT is innervated by axons containing several neuropeptides and neurotransmitters including LHRH, somatostatin, angiotensin, dopamine, norepinephrine, serotonin, acetylcholine, oxytocin, vasopressin, and TRH.[79] In the rodent, neurons that contain GnRH (LHRH) surround the OVLT. In addition, the OVLT in the rat brain contains estrogen receptors and the application of estrogen or electric stimulation at this site is capable of stimulating ovulation through LHRH-containing neurons that project to the median eminence, suggesting that the region regulates sexual behavior in the rat.[78]

It is established that the region of the hypothalamus that immediately surrounds the OVLT regulates a diverse array of autonomic processes. However, as the OVLT is potentially involved in the maintenance of so many processes, definitive studies ascribing specific functions to the OVLT are inherently difficult. For example, lesions of the OVLT and surrounding preoptic area led to altered febrile responses after immunologic stimulation and disruptions in fluid and electrolyte balance, blood pressure, reproduction, and thermoregulation.[50] Indeed, large lesions of the OVLT attenuated lipopolysaccharide (LPS)-induced fever.[84, 101] Consistent with this finding, it has been demonstrated that receptors for prostaglandin E_2 (PGE_2) are located within and immediately surrounding the OVLT.[102] As PGE_2 is thought to be an obligate endogenous pyrogen (see "Neuroendocrine-Immune Interactions"), the OVLT may be a critical regulator of febrile responses.

The OVLT is also likely to be involved in sensing serum osmolality because lesions of the OVLT attenuate vasopressin and oxytocin secretion in response to osmotic stimuli.[81, 83] In addition, hypertonic saline administration to rats induced Fos (a marker of neuronal activation) in OVLT neurons.[103] The efferent projections of the OVLT are not well defined because of the inherent difficulty of injecting this small structure with specific neuroanatomic tracers without contaminating surrounding preoptic nuclei. However, the neurons in the OVLT apparently have a remarkably restricted range of projections that include the paraventricular and supraoptic nuclei, the dor-

Table 7–1. *Sequences of the Principal Peptides of the Neurohypophysis*

	1 2 3 4 5 6 7 8 9	1 2 3 4 5 6 7 8 9
Mammals (except pig)	Cys-Tyr-Ile-Gln-Asn-Cys-Pro-Leu-Gly-NH_2 Oxytocin	Cys-Tyr-Phe-Gln-Asn-Cys-Pro-Arg-Gly-NH_2 Arginine vasopressin
Pig	Cys-Tyr-Ile-Gln-Asn-Cys-Pro-Leu-Gly-NH_2 Oxytocin	Cys-Tyr-Phe-Gln-Asn-Cys-Pro-Lys-Gly-NH_2 Lysine vasopressin
Birds, reptiles, amphibians, lungfishes	Cys-Tyr-Ile-Gln-Asn-Cys-Pro-Ile-Gly-NH_2 Mesotocin	Cys-Tyr-Ile-Gln-Asn-Cys-Pro-Arg-Gly-NH_2 Vasotocin
Bony fishes (palcopteryglans and neopteryglans)	Cys-Tyr-Ile-Ser-Asn-Cys-Pro-Ile-Gly-NH_2 Isotocin	Cys-Tyr-Ile-Gln-Asn-Cys-Pro-Arg-Gly-NH_2 Vasotocin

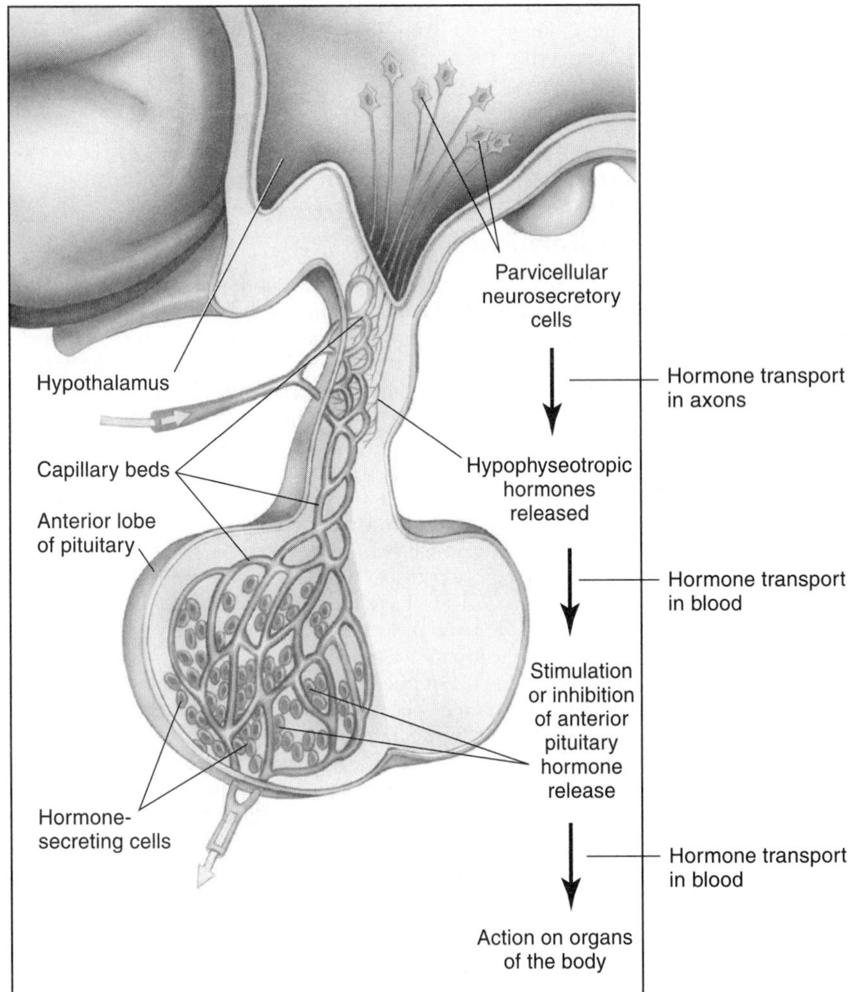

Figure 7–6. Hypothalamic parvicellular hypophyseotropic neurons and the anterior pituitary gland. This drawing of a midsagittal view of the hypothalamus and pituitary gland illustrates the concept that parvicellular neurosecretory cells secrete hypophyseotropic hormones (releasing factors) into capillaries of the pituitary portal system at the median eminence. These factors are transported to the anterior pituitary gland to regulate the secretion of pituitary hormones. (From Bear MF, Connors BW, Paradiso MA. Neuroscience: Exploring the Brain. Baltimore, Williams & Wilkins, 1996, p 9.)

somedial hypothalamic nucleus, and the lateral hypothalamic area (Elmquist JK, Sherin JE and Saper CB, unpublished observations).

The SFO is located in the roof of the third ventricle below the fornix. The SFO is known to be a critical regulator of fluid homeostasis, and it contributes to blood pressure regulation.[61, 81, 83] Consistent with this hypothesis, the SFO has receptors for angiotensin II and atrial natriuretic peptide.[85, 104, 105] In addition to expressing these key receptors, the SFO is thought to regulate fluid homeostasis because of its specific and massive projections to key hypothalamic regulatory sites. Notable among these are the inputs to oxytocin and vasopressin (AVP) magnocellular neurons in the supraoptic and paraventricular nuclei. Parvicellular neurons in the paraventricular nucleus concerned with neuroendocrine and autonomic control also receive innervation from the SFO. In addition, the SFO

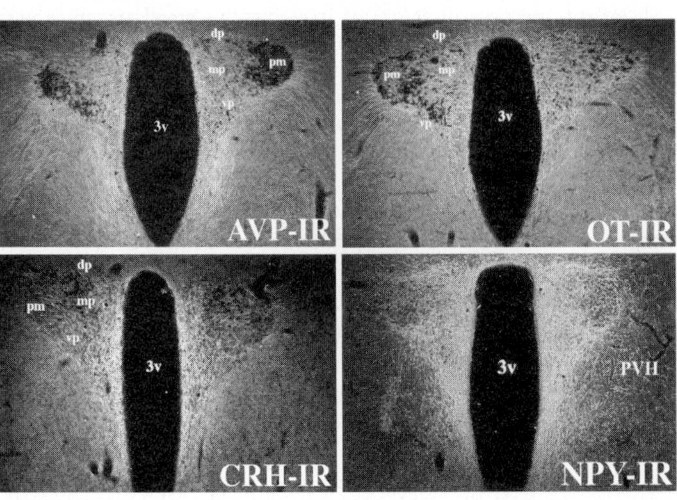

Figure 7–7. The paraventricular nucleus of the hypothalamus (PVH). A series of photomicrographs illustrate distinct subdivisions of the PVH and the presence of multiple neuropeptide mediators. Magnocellular neurons project to the posterior lobe of the pituitary gland to release arginine vasopressin or oxytocin (AVP, OT). Parvicellular hypophyseotropic neurons project to the median eminence and release releasing factors such as corticotropin-releasing hormone (CRH). In addition to neurons that make neuropeptides within the nucleus, the PVH receives a dense innervation from neurotransmitters and neuropeptide neurons, including neuropeptide Y (NPY). Note the subdivisions of the PVH including the dorsal (dp), ventral (vp), and medial (mp) parvicellular and posterior magnocellular (pm) divisions. IR, immunoreactivity; 3v, third ventricle.

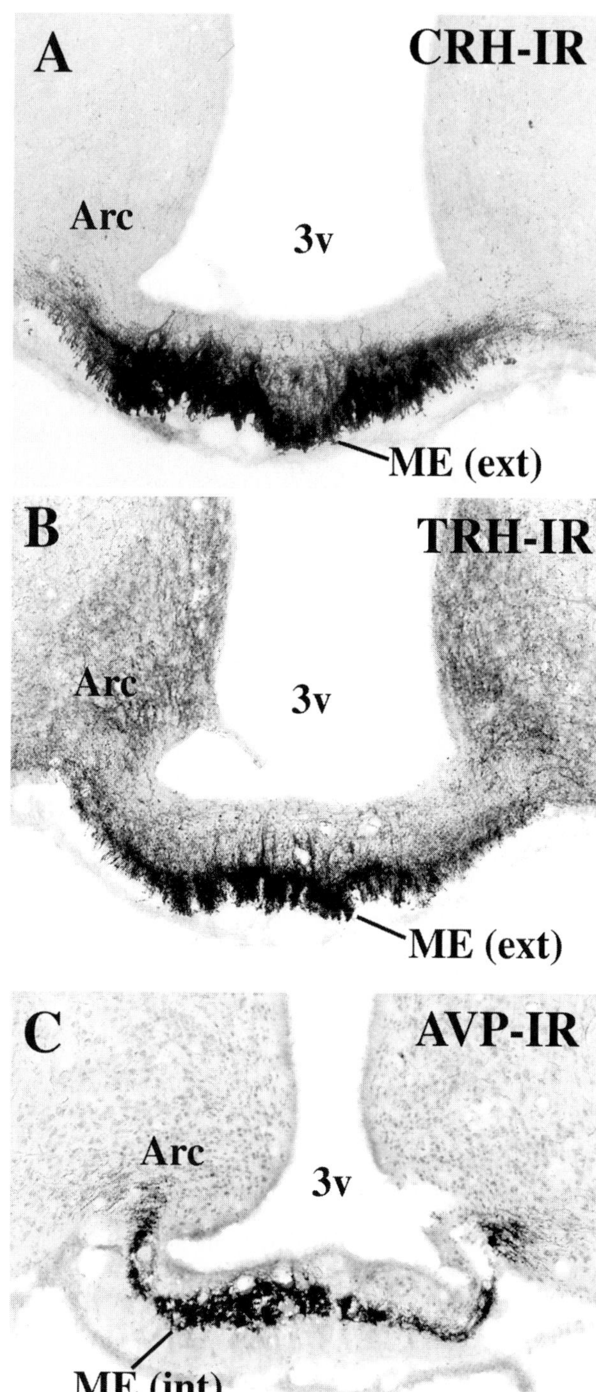

Figure 7–8. The median eminence is the functional connection of the hypothalamus and the pituitary gland. *A* and *B*, Distribution of corticotropin-releasing hormone and thyrotropin-releasing hormone (CRH-IR and TRH-IR) immunoreactivity in the external layer of the median eminence (ME ext) of the rat. CRH and TRH cell bodies reside in the medial division of the paraventricular hypothalamic nucleus. *C*, Arginine vasopressin (AVP) immunoreactivity in nerve endings in the internal layer of the median eminence (ME int). Arc, arcuate nucleus; 3v, third ventricle.

densely innervates the paramedian preoptic region of the hypothalamus (often known as the anteroventral third ventricular region) and other hypothalamic sites including the perifornical area of the lateral hypothalamus.[50] A major cell group within the anteroventral third ventricular region is the median preoptic nucleus, which receives dense innervation from the SFO.[105–107] Several neuroanatomic studies have demonstrated that the median preoptic nucleus is a major source of afferents to the magnocellular neuroendocrine neurons in the paraventricular and supraoptic hypothalamic nuclei.

In addition to the preceding neuroanatomic findings, physiologic evidence suggests that the SFO is critical in maintaining fluid balance. For example, Simpson and Routtenberg[108–110] demonstrated that substances such as angiotensin II induced drinking behavior only when the SFO was intact. Specifically, they found that low doses of angiotensin II when injected into the SFO elicited drinking. Later studies demonstrated that SFO neurons have electrophysiologic responses to angiotensin II.[83, 85] In addition, stimulation of the SFO elicited vasopressin secretion.[111] Like the OVLT, the SFO expressed Fos after hypertonic stimulation such as hypertonic saline administration.[103] Thus, the SFO provides dense direct and indirect innervation to the magnocellular neuroendocrine neurons in the paraventricular and supraoptic nuclei that are critical in the maintenance of fluid balance and blood pressure.

Area Postrema

The area postrema lies at the caudal end of the fourth ventricle adjacent to the nucleus of the solitary tract (see Figs. 7–10 and 8–66*D*). In experimental animals such as the rat and mouse, it is a midline structure lying above the nucleus of the solitary tract.[50, 52, 60, 112] However, in humans the area postrema is a bilateral structure. As the area postrema overlies the nucleus of the solitary tract, it also receives direct visceral afferent input from the glossopharyngeal nerve (including the carotid sinus nerve) and the vagus nerve. In addition, the area postrema receives direct input from several hypothalamic nuclei. The efferent projections of the area postrema include projections to the nucleus of the solitary tract, ventral lateral medulla, and the parabrachial nucleus. Consistent with a role as a sensory organ, the area postrema is enriched with receptors for several peptide hormones including glucagon-like peptide-1[113] and cholecystokinin.[114] It also contains chemosensory neurons that include osmoreceptors.[61, 82] Notably, the area postrema is thought to be critical in the detection of potential toxins and can induce vomiting in response to foreign substances. In fact, the area postrema is often referred to as the *chemoreceptor trigger zone*.[112]

The best-described physiologic role of the area postrema is probably the coordinated control of blood pressure.[52, 61, 82, 115, 116] For example, the area postrema contains binding sites for angiotensin II, AVP, and atrial natriuretic peptide. Moreover, lesions of the area postrema in rats blunt the rise in blood pressure induced by angiotensin II.[85, 115, 116] Finally, administration of angiotensin II induces the expression of Fos in neurons of the area postrema.[81, 117] The area postrema has also been hypothesized to play a role in responding to inflammatory cytokines during the acute febrile response (see Figs. 7–50 and 7–51 and "Neuroendocrine-Immune Interactions").

Subcommissural Organ

The subcommissural organ (SCO) is located below the posterior commissure near the junction of the third ventricle and cerebral aqueduct below the pineal gland (see Fig. 7–10).[82, 83] The SCO is composed of specialized ependymal cells that secrete a highly glycosylated protein of unknown function. The secretion of this protein leads to aggregation and formation of the so-called Reissner fibers.[87] The glycoproteins are extruded through the aqueduct, the fourth ventricle, and the spinal cord lumen to terminate in the caudal spinal canal. In humans, intracellular secretory granules are identifiable in the SCO but Reissner's fibers are absent. The SCO secretion in

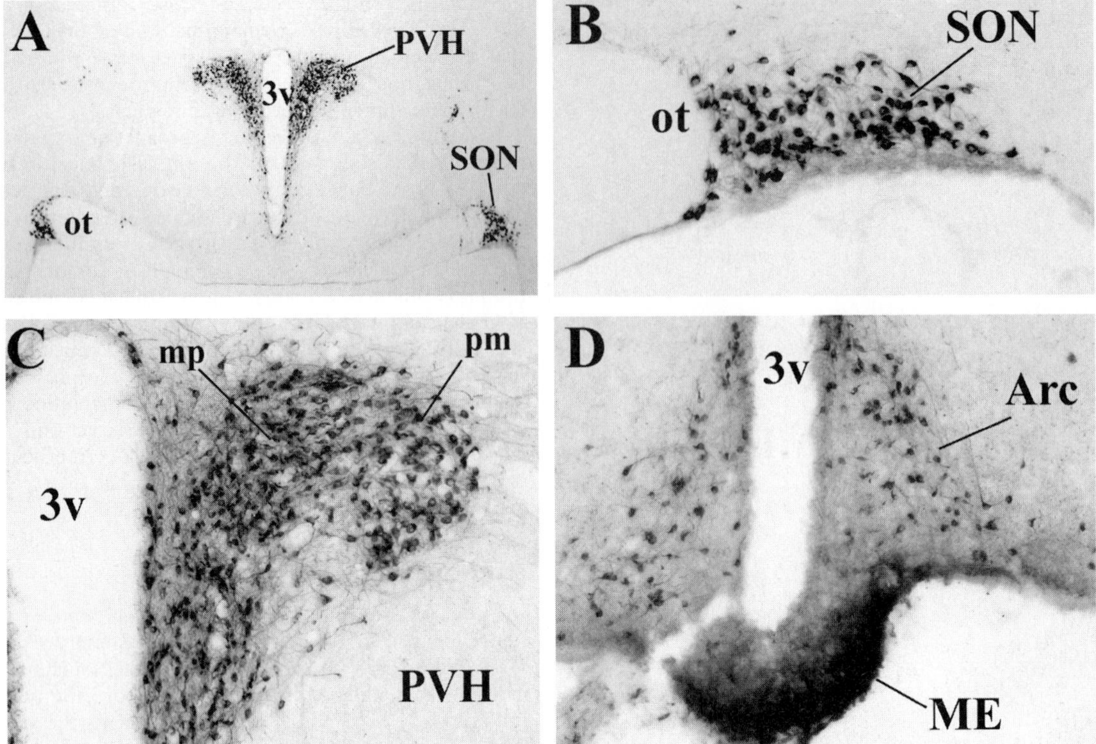

Figure 7–9. The tuberoinfundibular system is revealed by retrograde transport of cholera toxin subunit B (CtB). The location of hypothalamic cell bodies of neurons projecting to the median eminence (ME) and the posterior pituitary can be identified by microinjecting a small volume of retrograde tracer (CtB) into the median eminence of the rat (see Wiegand,[73] Lechan[80]). *A*, Retrogradely labeled cells can be seen in the paraventricular and supraoptic nuclei of the hypothalamus (PVH, SON). *B*, Magnocellular neurons are observed in the SON. *C*, Labeled neurons are found in the posterior magnocellular group (pm) as well as the medial parvicellular subdivision (mp). The labeled cells in the PVH include those that contain corticotrophin-releasing hormone and thyrotropin-releasing hormone. *D*, Retrogradely labeled cells are also found in the arcuate nucleus of the hypothalamus (Arc). These include neurons that release growth hormone–releasing hormone and dopamine. 3v, third ventricle; ot, optic tract.

humans is therefore presumed to be more soluble and to be absorbed directly from the CSF. Compared with other CVOs, relatively little is known about the physiologic role of the SCO. Hypothesized roles for the SCO include clearance of substances from the CSF.[86, 87]

PINEAL GLAND

Historically, the functional significance of the pineal gland has been difficult to discern. For example, Descartes called the pineal gland the "seat of the soul." The pineal gland is both an endocrine and a circumventricular organ; it is derived from cells from the roof of the third ventricle and lies above the posterior commissure near the level of the habenular complex and the sylvian aqueduct.[118–120] The pineal gland is composed of two cell types, pinealocytes and interstitial (glial-like) cells. Histologic studies suggest that the pineal gland cells are secretory in nature, and indeed the pineal is the source of melatonin in mammals.[121] As discussed subsequently, the pineal gland integrates information encoded by light into coordinated secretions that underlie biologic rhythmicity.[122, 123]

The pineal is an epithalamic structure and consists of primordial photoreceptive cells. The pineal retains its light sensitivity in lower vertebrates such as fish and amphibians but lacks photosensitivity in mammals and has evolved as a strictly secretory organ in higher vertebrates.[118, 120, 121] However, neuroanatomic studies have established that light-encoded information is relayed to the pineal in an indirect and multisynaptic fashion.[124] This series of synapses ultimately results in innervation of the gland by noradrenergic sympathetic nerve terminals that are critical regulators of melatonin production and release. Specifically, the retina provides direct innervation to the suprachiasmatic nucleus (SCN) of the hypothalamus through the retinohypothalamic tract.[125] The SCN in turn provides input to the paraventricular nucleus of the hypothalamus (PVH), a key cell group in neuroendocrine and autonomic control. This input is provided through direct and indirect pathways by intrahypothalamic projections.[126, 127] The PVH in turn provides direct innervation to sympathetic preganglionic neurons in the intermediolateral cell column of the thoracic regions of the spinal cord.[50, 128] Sympathetic preganglionic neurons innervate postganglionic neurons in the superior cervical ganglion,[129] which in turn provide the noradrenergic innervation to the pineal (see "Hypothalamic-Pituitary Unit"). This rather circuitous pathway is thought to represent the anatomic substrate for light to regulate the secretion of melatonin. It is important to note that in the absence of light input, the pineal gland rhythms persist but are not entrained to the external light-dark cycle.

The Pineal Is the Source of Melatonin

The predominant hormone secreted by the pineal gland is melatonin (Fig. 7–11). However, the pineal also contains biogenic amines, peptides, and GABA. Pineal-derived melatonin is synthesized from tryptophan, through serotonin, with the rate-

Table 7–2. Neuroactive Materials in the Paraventricular Nucleus and the Arcuate Nucleus

Paraventricular Nucleus
Magnicellular Division
Angiotensin II
Cholecystokinin
Glucagon
Oxytocin
Peptide 7B2
Proenkephalin B (dynorphin, rimorphin, α-neoendorphin)
Vasopressin
Nitric oxide (NO)
Parvicellular Division
γ-Aminobutyric acid (GABA)
Angiotensin II
Atrial natriuretic factor
Cholecystokinin
Corticotropin-releasing hormone
Dopamine
Follicle-stimulating hormone–releasing factor
Galanin
Glucagon
Neuropeptide Y
Neurotensin
Peptide 7B2
Proenkephalin A (met-enkephalin, leu-enkephalin, BAM 22P, metorphamide, met-enkephalin-Arg^6-Phe^7, met-enkephalin-Arg^6-Gly^7-Leu^8)
Somatostatin
Thyrotropin-releasing hormone (TRH)
Vasopressin
Interleukin-1 (IL-1)
Vasoactive intestinal peptide (VIP)–peptide-histidine-isoleucine (PHI)
Nitric oxide
Arcuate Nucleus
Acetylcholine (?)
γ-Aminobutyric acid
Dopamine
Galanin
Growth hormone–releasing hormone (GHRH)
Luteinizing hormone–releasing hormone (LHRH)
Neuropeptide Y
Neurotensin
Pancreatic polypeptide
Proenkephalin A
Prolactin
Melanocortins (corticotropin, α-melanocyte-stimulating hormone [α-MSH], γ-melanocyte-stimulating hormone [γ-MSH])
Endogenous opioids (β-endorphin, β-lipotropin [β-LPH])
Somatostatin
Substance P

Modified from Lechan RM. Neuroendocrinology of pituitary hormone regulation. Endocrinol Metab Clin North Am 1987; 16:475–502.

limiting step being catalyzed by the enzyme *N*-acetyltransferase (NAT)[130–132] (Fig. 7–12). The final step of melatonin synthesis is catalyzed by hydroxyindole-*O*-methyltransferase (HIOMT). These enzymes are expressed in a pineal specific manner; however, hydroxyindole-*O*-methyltransferase is also expressed in the retina and red blood cells. It is now established that melatonin plays a key role in regulating a myriad of circadian rhythms, and a fundamental principle of circadian biology is that the synthesis of melatonin is exquisitely controlled.[122, 133] This control is exerted at several levels. NAT mRNA levels, NAT activity, and melatonin synthesis and release are regulated in a circadian fashion and are entrained by the light-dark cycle, with darkness thought to be the most important signal.[130, 131, 134, 135] For example, melatonin and NAT levels are highest during the dark and decrease sharply with the onset of light. Melatonin is not thought to be stored to any degree and thus

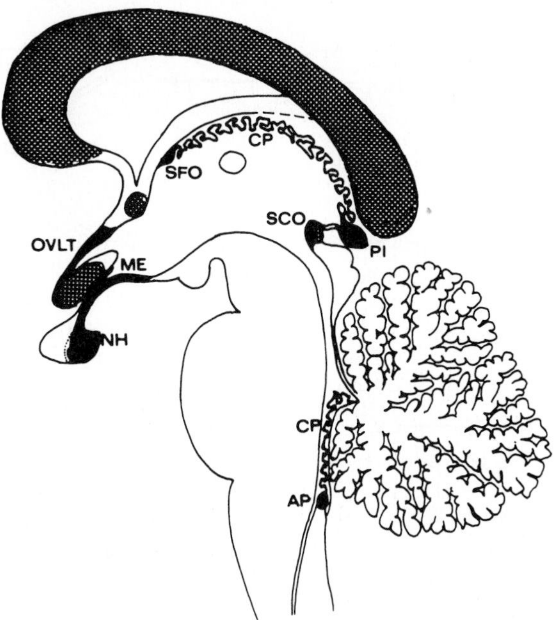

Figure 7–10. Median sagittal section through the human brain to show the circumventricular organs *(black)*. AP, area postrema; ME, median eminence; NH, neurohypophysis; OVLT, organum vasculosum of the lamina terminalis; PI, pineal body; SFO, subfornical organ; SCO, subcommissural organ; CP, choroid plexus. (From Weindl A. Neuroendocrine aspects of circumventricular organs. In Ganong WF, Martini L [eds]. Frontiers in Neuroendocrinology, vol 3. New York, Oxford University Press, 1973, pp 3–32.)

is released into blood or CSF directly.[136] Thus, this regulatory mechanism results in melatonin levels in the blood that are highest in the dark when NAT mRNA and activity are highest.

The CNS control of melatonin secretion during the dark is mediated by the neuroanatomic pathway already outlined. Lack of light ultimately results in the release of norepinephrine from postganglionic sympathetic nerve terminals that act on β-adrenergic receptors in pinealocytes, resulting in an increase in adenylate cyclase activity.[130, 137] The resultant increased levels of cyclic adenosine monophosphate (cAMP) activate signal transduction cascades, including increased protein kinase activity and phosphorylation of cAMP response element–binding protein. Notably, cAMP response elements have been identified in the promoter of NAT.[130, 138, 139] Thus, light (or lack of it) acting through the sympathetic nervous system induces an increase in cAMP, representing a fundamental regulator of NAT transcription and melatonin synthesis that ultimately results in a dramatic change of melatonin levels across the day.

Physiologic Roles of Melatonin

One of the best characterized roles of melatonin is the regulation of the reproductive axis, including gonadotropin secretion[140, 141] and the timing and onset of puberty (see "Gonadotropin-Releasing Hormone and Control of the Reproductive Axis"). The potent regulation of the reproductive axis by melatonin is established in rodents and domestic animals such as the sheep. It was observed experimentally with the demonstration that removal of the pineal leads to precocious puberty and ameliorates the effects of constant darkness to induce gonadal involution. In addition, male rats exposed to constant darkness or made blind experimentally display testicular atrophy and decreased levels of testosterone. These profound effects are normalized by removal of the pineal gland.[136, 142] The physiologic significance of melatonin is probably most important in species referred to as seasonal breeders. Indeed, the role of

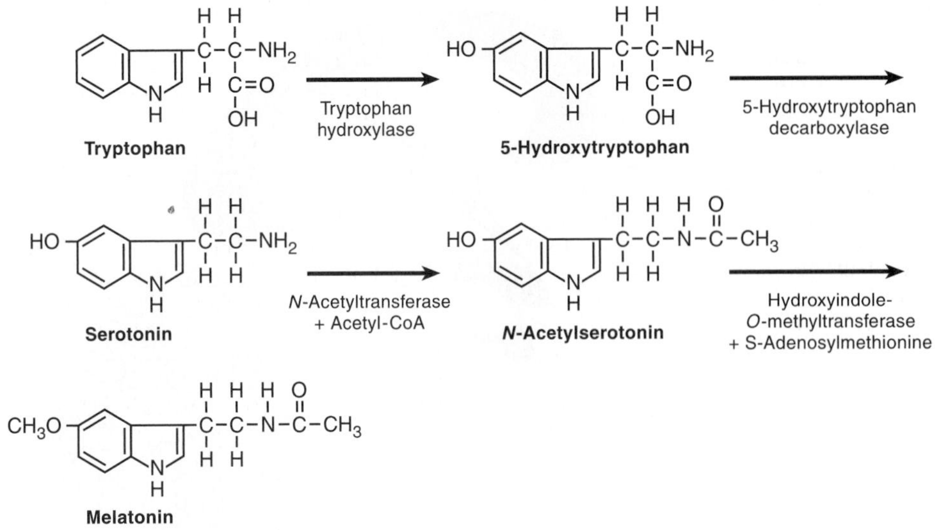

Tryptophan → Tryptophan hydroxylase → 5-Hydroxytryptophan → 5-Hydroxytryptophan decarboxylase →

Serotonin → N-Acetyltransferase + Acetyl-CoA → *N*-Acetylserotonin → Hydroxyindole-*O*-methyltransferase + S-Adenosylmethionine →

Melatonin

Figure 7–11. Biosynthesis of melatonin from tryptophan in the pineal gland. Step 1 is catalyzed by tryptophan hydroxylase, step 2 by aromatic-L-amino acid decarboxylase, step 3 by *N*-acetylating enzyme, and step 4 by hydroxyindole-*O*-methyltransferase. (From Wurtman RJ, Axelrod J, Kelly DE [eds]. Biochemistry of the pineal gland. In The Pineal. New York, Academic Press, 1968, pp 47–75.)

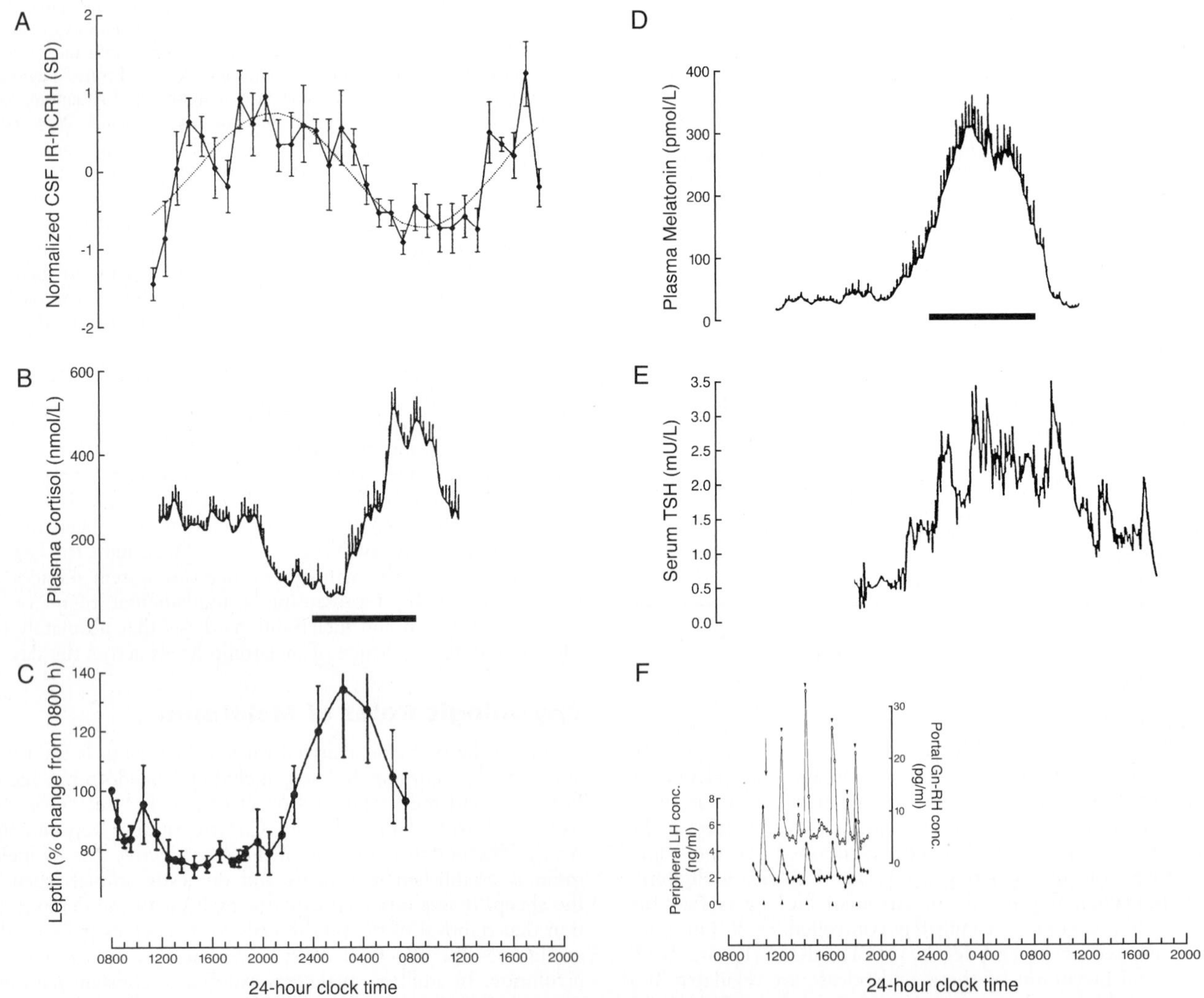

Figure 7–12. Diurnal rhythms of corticotropin-releasing hormone (CRH), cortisol, leptin, melatonin, thyrotropin (TSH), and luteinizing hormone (LH). CSF, cerebrospinal fluid; IR, immunoreactive. (From Kling et al. J Clin Endocrinol Metab 1994; 79:233, Fig 3; Van Coevorden et al. Am J Physiol 1991; 260:E651, Fig 1A; Sinha et al. J Clin Invest 1996; 97:1344, Fig 2; Van Coevorden et al. Am J Physiol 1991; 260:E651, Fig 1C; Brabant et al. J Clin Endocrinol Metab 1990; 70:403, Fig 2B; Clarke and Cummins. Endocrinology 1982; 111:1737, Fig 2A.)

melatonin in regulating reproductive capacity in species such as the sheep and the horse is now established.[143] This type of reproductive strategy probably evolved to synchronize the length of day with the gestational period of the species to ensure that the offspring are born at favorable times of the year and maximize the viability of the young.

Despite the potent effects of day length on reproduction in these species, exact mechanisms of melatonin regulation of GnRH release are unsettled. However, melatonin inhibits LH release from the rat pars tuberalis.[141] The role of the pineal in human reproduction is even more unsettled.[144] Earlier onset of menarche in blind women has been reported. In addition, a decline in melatonin at puberty has been described.[145] However, it was not found in other studies.[144, 146–148] Thus, the role of melatonin in human reproduction is not clear. Nonetheless, the therapeutic potential of melatonin in regulating and shifting biologic rhythms in humans has received great attention.[130, 133]

Melatonin Receptors

It is now established that melatonin mediates its effects by acting on a family of G protein–coupled receptors, which have been characterized by pharmacologic, neuroanatomic, and molecular approaches.[122, 149, 150] The first member of the family, Mel_{1a}, is a high-affinity receptor that was isolated originally from *Xenopus* melanophores. The second, Mel_{1b}, has approximately 60% homology with the Mel_{1a} receptor. A third receptor, the Mel_{1c} melatonin receptor, has been cloned from zebra fish, *Xenopus*, and chickens but not as yet from mammals.

The mechanisms for the effects of melatonin on regulating and entraining circadian rhythms are becoming increasingly understood. For example, melatonin inhibits the activity of neurons in the SCN of the hypothalamus, the master circadian pacemaker in the mammalian brain.[122, 150–153] Melatonin can entrain several mammalian circadian rhythms, probably by the inhibition of neurons in the SCN. Neuroanatomic evidence suggests that many of the effects of melatonin on circadian rhythms involve actions on Mel_{1a} receptors, as the distribution of Mel_{1a} mRNA overlaps with radiolabeled melatonin binding sites in the relevant brain regions. These sites include the SCN, the retina, and the pars tuberalis of the adenohypophysis. The Mel_{1b} melatonin receptor is also expressed in retina and brain; however, this is thought to be at much lower levels.[122, 150, 152]

Genetic studies in mice have also helped to illuminate the relative roles of each melatonin receptor in mediating the effects of this hormone. Targeted deletion (knockout) of the Mel_{1a} receptor abolished the ability of melatonin to inhibit the activity of SCN neurons.[152] Several studies have suggested that the inhibition of SCN neurons by melatonin is of great physiologic significance.[122, 152] For example, Reppert and colleagues have suggested that elevations of melatonin at night could decrease the responsiveness of the SCN to activity-related stimuli that could result in phase shifts. As noted, light potently inhibits melatonin synthesis and release. Thus, melatonin may underlie the mechanism by which light induces phase shifts. However, it should be noted that lack of the Mel_{1a} gene does not block the ability of melatonin to induce phase shifts. These unexpected and somewhat confusing results have resulted in the hypothesis that Mel_{1b} is involved in melatonin-induced phase shifts, as this receptor may be expressed in the human brain.[152]

Melatonin Therapy in Humans

The role of melatonin as a "wonder drug" has received great attention from the lay press.[133, 154] The proposed beneficial and therapeutic uses of melatonin include treatment of jet lag, slowing or reversing the progression of aging, and enhancing immune function. As noted earlier, the most studied and established role of melatonin is that of phase shifting and resetting circadian rhythms. In this context, melatonin has been used to treat jet lag and may be effective in treating circadian-based sleep disorders.[154] In addition, melatonin administration has been shown to regulate sleep in humans.[130, 133] Specifically, melatonin has a hypnotic effect at relatively low doses. Melatonin therapy has also been suggested as a way to treat seasonal affective disorders.

It is important to note that melatonin is now available over the counter and without a prescription throughout the United States. However, there is a striking paucity of controlled clinical studies of the relative efficacy and safety of melatonin administration. This should be viewed as problematic because melatonin is an endocrine hormone, and most hormones are not widely available without a prescription.[133, 152, 154] Clearly, controlled clinical studies are needed to assess fully the therapeutic potential and safety of melatonin in humans.

HYPOPHYSEOTROPIC HORMONES AND NEUROENDOCRINE AXES

With the demonstration by the first half of the 1900s that pituitary secretion was controlled by hypothalamic hormones released into the portal circulation, the search was on for the hypothalamic *releasing factors.* The search for hypothalamic neurohormones with anterior pituitary regulating properties focused on extracts of stalk, median eminence, neural lobe, and hypothalamus from sheep and pigs. To give some idea of the herculean nature of this effort, approximately 250,000 hypothalamic fragments were required to purify and characterize the first such factor, TRH.[20, 155] The identification and characterization of TRH in 1970 and of other releasing hormones ultimately led to the Nobel Prize in Medicine in 1977 for Andrew Schally and Roger Guillemin.[38, 156] Such hypophyseotropic substances were initially called releasing factors but are now more commonly called *releasing hormones.*

All of the hypothalamic-pituitary regulating hormones are peptides with the exception of dopamine, which is a biogenic amine that is the principal prolactin-inhibiting factor (PIF) (Table 7–3). All are now available for human investigation and treatment, and therapeutic analogues have been synthesized for dopamine, GnRH, and somatostatin.

In addition to regulating hormone release, some hypophyseotropic factors control pituitary cell differentiation and proliferation and hormone synthesis. Somatostatin and dopamine are inhibitory, and some act on more than one pituitary hormone. For example, TRH is a potent releaser of prolactin (PRL) and of thyrotropin and under some circumstances releases corticotropin and growth hormone (GH). GnRH releases both LH and follicle-stimulating hormone (FSH). Somatostatin inhibits the secretion of GH, thyrotropin, and a wide variety of nonpituitary hormones. The principal inhibitor of PRL secretion, dopamine, also inhibits secretion of thyrotropin, gonadotropin, and, under certain conditions, GH. Dual control is exerted by the interaction of inhibitory and stimulatory hypothalamic hormones. For example, somatostatin interacts with growth hormone–releasing hormone (GHRH) and TRH to control secretion of GH and thyrotropin, respectively, and dopamine interacts with prolactin-releasing factors (PRFs) to regulate PRL secretion. Some hypothalamic hormones act synergistically; for example, CRH and vasopressin act together to regulate the release of pituitary adrenocorticotropic hormone (ACTH).

Secretion of the releasing hormones in turn is regulated by

Table 7–3. Structural Formulas of Principal Human Hypothalamic Peptides Directly Related to Pituitary Secretion

Vasopressin
Cys-Tyr-Phe-Gln-Asn-Cys-Pro-Arg-Gly-NH_2 (MW = 1084.38)
Oxytocin
Cys-Tyr-Ile-Gln-Asn-Cys-Pro-Leu-Gly-NH_2 (MW = 1007.35)
Thyrotropin-releasing hormone
pGlu-His-Pro-NH_2 (MW = 362.42)
Gonadotropin-releasing hormone
pGlu-His-Trp-Ser-Tyr-Gly-Leu-Arg-Pro-Gly-NH_2 (MW = 1182.39)
Corticotropin-releasing hormone
Ser-Glu-Glu-Pro-Pro-Ile-Ser-Leu-Asp-Leu-Thr-Phe-His-Leu-Leu-Arg-Glu-Val-Leu-Glu-Met-Ala-Arg-Ala-Glu-Gln-Leu-Ala-Gln-Gln-Ala-His-Ser-Asn-Arg-Lys-Leu-Met-Glu-Ile-Ile-NH_2 (MW = 4758.14)
Growth hormone–releasing hormone (GHRH 1–40, 1–44-NH_2, Human)
Tyr-Ala-Asp-Ala-Ile-Phe-Thr-Asn-Ser-Tyr-Arg-Lys-Val-Leu-Gly-Gln-Leu-Ser-Ala-Arg-Lys-Leu-Leu-Gln-Asp-Ile-Met-Ser-Arg-Gln-Gln-Gly-Glu-Ser-Asn-Gln-Glu-Arg-Gly-Ala (MW = 4544.73), [-Arg-Ala-Arg-Leu-NH_2] (MW = 5040.4)
Somatostatin
Ala-Gly-Cys-Lys-Asn-Phe-Phe-Trp-Lys-Thr-Phe-Thr-Ser-Cys (MW = 1638.12)
Somatostatin-28
Ser-Ala-Asn-Ser-Asn-Pro-Ala-Met-Ala-Pro-Arg-Glu-Arg-Lys-Ala-Gly-Cys-Lys-Asn-Phe-Phe-Trp-Lys-Thr-Phe-Thr-Ser-Cys (MW = 3149.0)
Somatostatin-28 (1–12)
Ser-Ala-Asn-Ser-Asn-Pro-Ala-Met-Ala-Pro-Arg-Glu (MW = 1244.49)
Vasoactive intestinal peptide (human, pig, rat)
His-Ser-Asp-Ala-Val-Phe-Thr-Asp-Asn-Tyr-Thr-Arg-Leu-Arg-Lys-Gln-Met-Ala-Val-Lys-Lys-Tyr-Leu-Asn-Ser-Ile-Leu-Asn-NH_2 (MW = 3326.26)
Prolactin-releasing peptide (PrRP31, PrRP20)
Ser-Arg-Thr-His-Arg-His-Ser-Met-Glu-Ile-Arg-Thr-Pro-Asp-Ile-Asn-Pro-Ala-Trp-Tyr-Ala-Ser-Arg-Gly-Ile-Arg-Pro-Val-Gly-Arg-Phe-NH_2 (MW = 3665.16; 2273.58)
Ghrelin
Gly-Ser-Ser-Phe-Leu-Ser-Pro-Glu-His-Gln-Arg-Val-Gln-Gln-Arg-Lys-Glu-Ser-Lys-Lys-Pro-Pro-Ala-Lys-Leu-Gln-Pro-Arg (MW = 3314.9) [Ser 3 is *n*-octanoylated]

MW, molecular weight.

neurotransmitters and neuropeptides released by a complex array of neurons synapsing with hypophyseotropic neurons. Control of secretion is also exerted through feedback control by hormones such as glucocorticoids, gonadal steroids, thyroid hormone, anterior pituitary hormones (short-loop feedback control), and hypophyseotropic factors themselves (ultrashort-loop feedback control).

The distribution of the hypophyseotropic hormones is not limited to the hypothalamus. Most are also found in nonhypophyseotropic hypothalamic neurons, in extrahypothalamic regions of the brain, and in other organs where they may have functions (e.g., effects on behavior or homeostasis) unrelated to pituitary regulation. Most, although not all, of the peptides, hormones, and neurotransmitters involved in the regulation of hypothalamic-pituitary control belong to the G protein–coupled receptor family (Table 7–4).

Feedback Concepts in Neuroendocrinology

In order to understand the regulation of each hypothalamic-pituitary-target organ axis, it is important to understand some basic concepts of homeostatic systems. A simplified account of feedback control in relation to neuroendocrine regulation is presented in this section.[157–160] Hormonal systems form part of a feedback loop in which the *controlled variable* (generally the blood hormone level or some biochemical surrogate of the hormone) determines the rate of secretion of the hormone. In *negative feedback* systems the controlled variable inhibits hormone output, and in *positive feedback* control systems the controlled variable increases hormone secretion. Both negative and positive endocrine feedback control systems can be part of a *closed loop*, in which regulation is entirely restricted to the interacting regulatory glands, or an *open loop*, in which the nervous system influences the feedback loop. All pituitary feedback systems have nervous system inputs that either alter the *set-point* of the feedback control system or introduce open-loop elements that can influence or override the closed-loop control elements.

In *engineering* formulations of feedback, three controlled variables can be identified: a *sensing* element that detects the concentration of the controlled variable, a *reference input* that defines the proper control levels, and an *error signal* that determines the output of the system. The reference input is the set-point of the system.

Hormonal feedback control systems resemble engineering systems in that the concentration of the hormone in the blood (or some function of the hormone) regulates the output of the controlling gland. Hormonal feedback differs from engineering systems in that the sensor element and the reference input element are not readily distinguishable. The set-point of the controlled variable is determined by a complex cascade beginning with the kinetics of binding to a receptor and the activities of successive intermediate messengers. Sophisticated models incorporating control elements, compartmental analysis, and hormone production and clearance rates have been developed for many systems.

Endocrine Rhythms

Virtually all functions of living animals (regardless of their position on the evolutionary scale) are subject to periodic or cyclic changes, many of which are influenced mainly by the nervous system (see Table 7–5 for definitions).[161–164] Most periodic changes are *free-running*; that is, they are intrinsic to the organism independent of the environment and are driven by a biologic "clock."

Most free-running rhythms can be coordinated (*entrained*) by external signals (*cues*), such as light-dark changes, meal patterns, cycles of the lunar periods, or the ratio of the length of day to the length of night. External signals of this type (*zeitgeber* or time givers) do not bring about the rhythm but provide

Table 7–4. Receptors for Neurotransmitters and Neuropeptides Involved in Hypothalamic-Pituitary Control*

Group	Name	General Structure Transmembrane Sequences	Mode of Action
Classical Neurotransmitters			
Biogenic amines			
α_{1A}-Adrenoreceptors	α_{1A}	7	$G_{q/11}$
	α_{1B}	7	$G_{q/11}$
	α_{1D}	7	$G_{q/11}$
α_{2A}-Adrenoreceptors	α_{2A}	7	$G_{i/o}$
	α_{2B}	7	$G_{i/o}$
	α_{2C}	7	$G_{i/o}$
β-Adrenoreceptors	β_1	7	G_S
	β_2	7	G_S
	β_3	7	G_S
Serotonin (5-OH-tryptamine)	5-HT_{1A}	7	$G_{i/o}$
	5-HT_{1B}	7	$G_{i/o}$
	5-HT_{1D}	7	$G_{i/o}$
	5-HT_{1E}	7	$G_{i/o}$
	5-HT_{2A}	7	$G_{q/11}$
	5-HT_{2B}	7	$G_{q/11}$
	5-HT_{2C}	7	$G_{q/11}$
	5-HT_3	4	Cation channel
	5-HT_4	7	G_S
Dopamine	D_1	7	G_S
	D_2	7	$G_{i/o}$
	D_3	7	$G_{i/o}$
	D_4	7	$G_{i/o}$
	D_5	7	G_S
Histamine	H_1	7	$G_{q/11}$
	H_2	7	G_S
	H_3	7	$G_{i/o}$
Acetylcholine			
Muscarinic	M_1	7	$G_{q/11}$
	M_2	7	$G_{q/11}$
	M_3	7	$G_{q/11}$
	M_4	7	$G_{i/o}$
	M_5	7	$G_{q/11}$
Nicotinic	Muscle	4 Multiunit	Na/K/Ca
	Ganglionic	4 Multiunit	Na/K/Ca
	Central nervous system	4 Multiunit	Na/K/Ca
Excitatory amino acids (glutamate)			
Ionotropic	NMDA	Multiunit ?4TM	Na/K/Ca
	AMPA	Multiunit 3TM	Na/K/Ca
	Kainate	?	Na/K/Ca
Metabotropic	$mGlu_1$	7	$G_{q/11}$
	$mGlu_2$	7	$G_{i/o}$
	$mGlu_3$	7	$G_{i/o}$
	$mGlu_4$	7	$G_{i/o}$
	$mGlu_5$	7	$G_{q/11}$
	$mGlu_6$	7	$G_{i/o}$
	$mGlu_7$	7	$G_{i/o}$
Inhibitory amino acid (γ-Aminobutyric Acid [GABA])	$GABA_A$	Multiunit	Internal Cl
	$GABA_B$	7 Hetero-dimer gb1–gb2	$G_{i/o}$

Group	Name	General Structure Transmembrane Sequences	Mode of Action
Neuropeptides			
Neurohypophyseal hormones			
Vasopressin	V_{1A}	7	$G_{q/11}$
	V_{1B}	7	$G_{q/11}$
	V_2	7	G_S
Oxytocin	OT	7	$G_{q/11}$
Hypophyseotropic hormones			
TRH	TRH	7	$G_{q/11}$
GHRH	GHRH	7	G_S
LHRH	LHRH	7	$G_{q/11}$
CRH	CRH	7	G_S
Somatostatin	SST_1	7	$G_{i/o}$
	SST_{2A}	7	$G_{i/o}$
	SST_{2B}	7	$G_{i/o}$
	SST_3	7	$G_{i/o}$
	SST_4	7	$G_{i/o}$
	SST_5	7	$G_{i/o}$
Endogenous opioid peptides	μ	7	$G_{i/o}$
	δ	7	$G_{i/o}$
	κ	7	$G_{i/o}$
Melanocortins	MC1	7	G_S
	MC2 (corticotropin)	7	G_S
	MC3		
	MC4	7	G_S
	MC5	7	G_S
		7	G_S
Gut-brain peptides			
Tachykinins			
Substance P	NK_1	7	$G_{i/o}$
Substance K	NK_2	7	$G_{i/o}$
Neurokinin B	NK_3	7	$G_{i/o}$
Neurotensin	NT	7	$G_{q/11}$
VIP	VIP_1	7	G_S
	VIP_2	7	G_S
PACAP	PACAP	7	G_S
Galanin	G	7	$G_{i/o}$
Cholecystokinin	CCK_A	7	$G_{q/11}$
	CCK_B (gastrin receptor)	7	$G_{q/11}$
Neuropeptide Y	Y_1	7	$G_{i/o}$
	Y_2	7	$G_{i/o}$
Vasoactive peptides	Y_5	7	$G_{i/o}$
Angiotensin	AT_1	7	$G_{q/11}$
	AT_2	7	cGMP
Atrial natriuretic peptide	ANP_A	1	cGMP
	ANP_B	1	cGMP
Endothelin	ET_A	7	$G_{q/11}$
	ET_B	7	$G_{q/11}$

*Receptors cited are human or rat if human not available.

NMDA, *N*-methyl-D-aspartate; AMPA, α-amino-3-hydroxy-5-methyl-4-isoxazdeproprionic acid; TRH, thyrotropin-releasing hormone; GHRH, growth hormone-releasing hormone; LHRH, luteinizing hormone-releasing hormone; CRH, corticotropin-releasing hormone; NT, neurotensin; VIP, vasoactive peptide; PACAP, pituitary adenylate cyclase activating peptide; cGMP, cyclic guanosine monophosphate.

cGMP: Guanylate cyclase activity intrinsic to the receptor.

$G_{i/o}$: Receptor coupled to the $G_{i/o}$ family. Opens K^+ channel, closes Ca^{2+} channel, inhibits adenylate cyclase.

$G_{q/11}$: Receptor coupled to the $G_{q/11}$ family. Stimulates phosphoinositol cascade.

G_S: Receptor coupled to the G_S family. Stimulates adenylate cyclase and increases intracellular cAMP.

Some receptors have intrinsic tyrosine phosphorylase activity, others have intrinsic tyrosine hydroxylase activity. The former stimulate phosphorylation of tyrosine kinases; the latter stimulate breakdown of tyrosine kinase.

The designation of functional type is oversimplified. Many examples can be cited in which receptor activation can stimulate both adenylate cyclase and phosphoinositide turnover.

Adapted from Watson S, Girdlestone D. Receptor and channel nomenclature supplement. Trends Pharmacol Sci 1995; (Suppl 16):1–73.

Table 7–5. Terms Used to Describe Cyclic Endocrine Phenomena

Period:	length of the cycle
Circadian:	around a day
Diurnal:	exactly a day
Ultradian:	less than a day, i.e., minutes or hours
Infradian:	longer than a day, i.e., month or year
Mean:	arithmetic mean of all values within a cycle
Range:	difference between the highest and lowest values
Nadir:	minimal level (inferred from mathematical curve fitting calculations)
Acrophase:	time of maximal levels (inferred from curve fitting)
Zeitgeber:	"time-giver" (German), the external cue, usually the light-dark cycle that synchronizes endogenous rhythms
Entrainment:	the process by which an endogenous rhythm is regulated by a zeitgeber
Phase shift:	induced change in an endogenous rhythm
Intrinsic clock:	neural structures that possess intrinsic capacity for spontaneous rhythms; for circadian rhythms these are located in the suprachiasmatic nucleus

Adapted from Van Cauter E, Turek FW. Endocrine and other biological rhythms. In DeGroot LJ (ed). Endocrinology, 3rd ed. Philadelphia, WB Saunders, 1995, pp 2497–2548.

the synchronizing time cue. Many endogenous rhythms have a period of approximately 24 hours (*circadian* [around a day] or *diurnal* rhythms). Circadian changes follow an intrinsic program that is about 24 hours long, whereas diurnal rhythms can be either circadian or dependent on shifts in light and dark.[165] Rhythms that occur more frequently than once a day are *ultradian. Infradian* rhythms have a period longer than 1 day, as in the approximately 27-day human menstrual cycle and the yearly breeding patterns of some animals.

Most endocrine rhythms are circadian (see Fig. 7–12).[164] The secretion of GH and PRL is maximal shortly after an individual has gone to sleep, and that of cortisol is maximal between 2 and 4 AM. Thyrotropin secretion is lowest in the morning between 9 AM and 12 noon and maximal between 8 PM and midnight. Gonadotropin secretion in adolescents is increased at night.[162] Superimposed on the circadian cycle are ultradian bursts of hormone secretion. Gonadotropin secretion during adolescence is characterized by rapid, high-amplitude pulsations at night, whereas in sexually mature individuals secretory episodes are lower in amplitude and occur throughout the 24 hours.[162] GH, corticotropin,[164] and PRL[166] are also secreted in brief, fairly regular pulses. The short-term fluctuations in hormonal secretion have important functional significance. In the case of gonadotropins, the normal endogenous rhythm of pituitary secretion reflects the pulsatile release of LHRH. The period of approximately 90 minutes between the peak of pulses corresponds to the optimal timing to induce maximal pituitary stimulation. Episodic secretion of GH also enhances its biopotency, but for many rhythms the function is not clear. Most homeostatic activities are also rhythmic, including body temperature, water balance, blood volume, sleep, and activity.

Assessment of endocrine function must take into account the variability of hormone levels in the blood, and appropriately obtained samples at different times of day or night may provide useful dynamic indicators of hypothalamic-pituitary function. For example, the loss of diurnal rhythm of GH and corticotropin secretion may be an early sign of hypothalamic dysfunction. Furthermore, the optimal timing for the administration of glucocorticoids to suppress corticotropin secretion (as in therapy for congenital adrenal hyperplasia) must take into account the varying suppressibility of the pituitary at different times of day.

The best understood neural structures responsible for circadian rhythms are the suprachiasmatic nuclei, paired structures in the anterior hypothalamus above the optic chiasm.[157, 161] Individual cells of the suprachiasmatic nuclei have an intrinsic capacity to oscillate in a circadian pattern,[167] and the nucleus is organized to permit many reciprocal neuron-neuron interactions through direct synaptic contacts. It is especially rich in neuropeptides, including somatostatin, vasoactive intestinal polypeptide (VIP), NPY, and neurotensin, and microinjections of NPY into the SCN reset the timing cycle of some circadian rhythms in hamsters.[168] The SCN also responds to the pineal hormone melatonin through melatonin receptors.[149, 169]

The SCN receives neuronal input from many parts of the brain and from a direct projection from the retina that is distinct from the visual pathway, called the retinohypothalamic pathway, which is the route by which the nucleus is cued by light-dark changes.[161] Anatomic dissociation of pathways subserving subjective visual and nonvisual stimulation explains the finding that circadian hormonal rhythms in some blind individuals are entrained to the light-dark cycle.[170]

Circadian rhythms during fetal life are regulated by maternal circadian rhythms.[171] Circadian changes can be detected 2 to 3 days before birth, and suprachiasmatic nuclei from fetuses of this age display spontaneous rhythmicity in vitro. Maternal regulation of fetal circadian rhythms may be mediated by circulating melatonin or by cyclic changes in the food intake of the mother.

Metabolic changes in the SCN, such as increased uptake of 2-deoxyglucose and an increased level of VIP, accompany circadian rhythms. This nucleus projects to the pineal gland by way of the autonomic nervous system (see later in the section on the pineal gland) and regulates its activity.

In addition to determining patterns of pituitary secretion, the circadian pacemaker influences many homeostatic functions. In humans, the alteration of sleep brought about by jet lag and by working night shifts has profound effects on the sense of well-being and efficiency[172] and may be a factor in the pathogenesis of seasonal affective disorder, a condition characterized by depression in winter when days are short and levels of illumination are low.[173] Seasonal affective disorder has been treated by manipulating the light-dark cycle.[173]

The timing of the circadian pacemaker can be shifted in humans by the administration of triazolam, a short-acting benzodiazepine,[174] or melatonin, as described earlier, or by altered patterns of intense illumination.[172]

Thyrotropin-Releasing Hormone

Chemistry and Evolution

TRH, the smallest known peptide releasing hormone, is the tripeptide pyroGlu-His-Pro-NH_2. The TRH peptide sequence is repeated six times within the human TRH pre-prohormone gene (Fig. 7–13). The rat pro-TRH precursor contains five TRH peptide repeats flanked by dibasic residues (Lys-Arg or Arg-Arg), along with seven or more non-TRH peptides. Two prohormone convertases, PC1 and PC2, cleave the TRH tripeptides at the dibasic residues within the regulated secretory pathway. Carboxypeptidase E then removes the dibasic residues, leaving the sequence Gln-His-Pro-Gly. This peptide is then amidated at the C-terminus by peptidylglycine alpha-amidating monooxygenase, with Gly acting as the amide donor. The amino-terminal pyro-Glu residue results from cyclization of the Gln.

Although the TRH tripeptide is the only established hormone encoded within its large prohormone, the rat pro-TRH yields seven additional peptides that have unique tissue distributions.[175] Several biologic activities of these peptides have

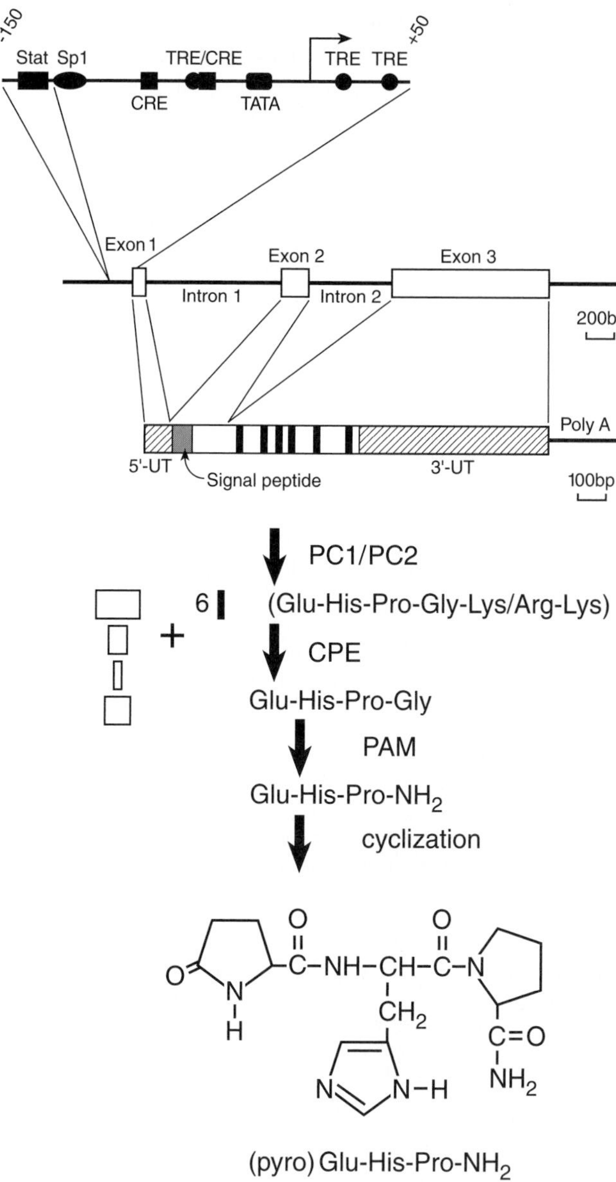

Figure 7–13. Structure of human thyrotropin-releasing hormone (TRH) gene and peptide, showing six repeating codons for the TRH sequence. CPE, carboxypeptidase E; PAM, peptidylglycine alpha-amidating monooxygenase; PC1, prohormone convertase 1. (From Yamada M, Radovick S, Wondisford FE, et al. Cloning and structure of human genomic DNA and hypothalamic cDNA encoding human preprothyrotropin-releasing hormone. Mol Endocrinol 1990; 4:551–556.)

been observed: pre-pro-TRH[160–169] may be a hypophyseotropic factor because it is released from hypothalamic slices[176] and potentiates the thyrotropin-releasing effects of TRH.[177] Pro-TRH[177–199] is also released from the median eminence[176] and appears to inhibit ACTH release.[178]

TRH is a phylogenetically ancient peptide, being found in primitive vertebrates, such as the lamprey, and even invertebrates such as the snail. TRH is widely expressed in both CNS and periphery in amphibians, reptiles, and fishes but does not stimulate thyrotropin release in these poikilothermic vertebrates.[179] Thus, TRH has multiple peripheral and central activities and was co-opted as a hypophyseotropic factor midway during the evolution of vertebrates, perhaps specifically as a factor needed for coordinate regulation of temperature homeostasis.

Effects on the Pituitary Gland and Mechanism of Action

After intravenous injection of TRH in humans, serum thyrotropin levels rise within a few minutes (Fig. 7–14),[180–182] followed by a rise in serum triiodothyronine (T_3) levels; there is an increase in thyroxine (T_4) release as well, but a change in blood levels of T_4 is usually not demonstrable because the pool of circulating T_4 (most of which is bound to carrier proteins) is so large. The clinical applications of TRH testing are covered later in this chapter and in Chapter 10. TRH action on the pituitary is blocked by previous treatment with thyroid hormone, which is a crucial element in feedback control of pituitary thyrotropin secretion.

TRH is also a potent PRF (Fig. 7–15).[180–182] The time course of response of blood PRL levels to TRH, the dose-response characteristics, and the suppression by thyroid hormone pretreatment (all of which parallel changes in thyrotropin secretion) suggest that TRH may be involved in the regulation of PRL secretion. Moreover, TRH is present in the hypophyseal-portal blood of lactating rats.[183] However, it is unlikely to be a physiologic regulator of PRL secretion[184, 185] because the PRL response to nursing in humans is unaccompanied by changes in plasma thyrotropin levels.[185] Nevertheless, TRH may occasionally cause hyperprolactinemia (with or without galactorrhea) in patients with hypothyroidism.

In normal individuals TRH has no influence on the secretion of pituitary hormones other than thyrotropin and PRL, but it enhances the release of human growth hormone (hGH) in acromegaly and of corticotropin in some patients with Cushing's disease. Furthermore, prolonged stimulation of the *normal* pituitary with GHRH can sensitize it to the hGH-releasing effects of TRH.[186, 187] TRH also causes the release of hGH in some patients with uremia, hepatic disease, anorexia

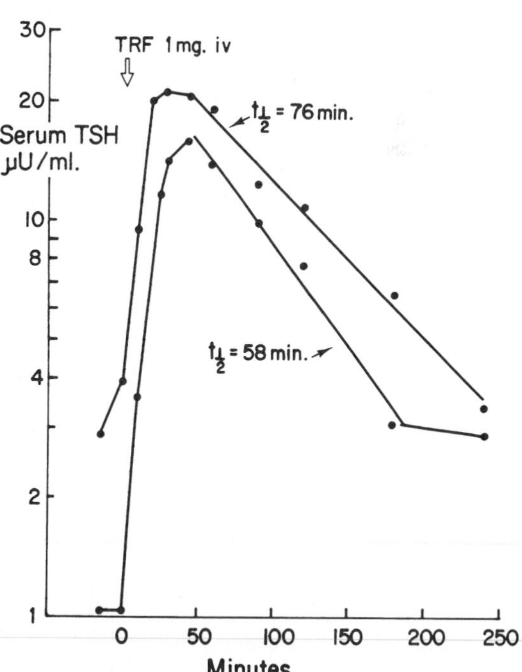

Figure 7–14. Effect of intravenous injection of thyrotropin-releasing hormone on serum thyrotropin levels in humans. TRF, thyrotropin-releasing hormone; TSH, thyrotropin. (From Hershman JM, Pittman JA Jr. Control of thyrotropin secretion in man. N Engl J Med 1971; 285:997–1006. Reprinted by permission of The New England Journal of Medicine.)

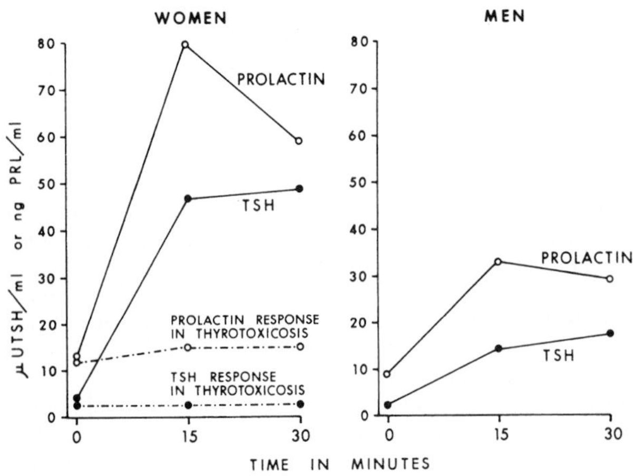

Figure 7–15. Prolactin (PRL) and thyrotropin (TSH) secretory responses to intravenous injection of 800 μg of thyrotropin-releasing hormone (TRH) in humans. This figure shows that TRH induces discharge of both PRL and thyrotropin, that the effect in females is greater than that in males (presumably owing to estrogen sensitization of the pituitary), and that thyrotoxicosis inhibits the response of both PRL and thyrotropin to TRH. An inhibitory effect on the TRH response is noted at the upper limit of the normal range of thyroid hormone levels and is a sensitive test of minor degrees of thyroid hormone excess. Although TRH is a potent prolactin-releasing factor (PRF), there is evidence that there is another PRF physiologically connected to PRL regulation. (Replotted from data of Bowers C, Friesen HG, Hwang P, et al. Prolactin and thyrotropin release in man by synthetic pyroglutamylhistidyl-prolinamide. Biochem Biophys Res Commun 1971; 45:1033–1041.)

nervosa, and psychotic depression[182] and in children with hypothyroidism. TRH inhibits sleep-induced hGH release through its actions in the CNS (see later in the section on extrapituitary actions of TRH).

Stimulatory effects of TRH are initiated by binding of the peptide to specific receptors on the plasma membrane of the thyrotroph.[24, 188] Neither thyroid hormone nor somatostatin, both of which antagonize the effects of TRH, interfere with its binding. TRH was originally thought to activate membrane adenylate cyclase to stimulate formation of cAMP,[182, 189] and cAMP in turn was thought to stimulate thyrotropin secretion. However, cAMP does not increase under all conditions of TRH-induced thyrotropin release,[190] and it is now clear that TRH action is mediated mainly through hydrolysis of phosphatidylinositol, with phosphorylation of key protein kinases and an increase in intracellular free Ca^{2+} as the crucial step in postreceptor activation (see Chapter 5).[190–192] TRH effects can be mimicked by exposure to a Ca^{2+} ionophore and are partially abolished by a Ca^{2+}-free medium. TRH stimulates the formation of mRNAs coding for thyrotropin[193] and PRL,[194] confirming that this peptide is trophic as well as a releasing factor.

TRH is degraded to acid TRH and to the dipeptide histidylprolineamide, which cyclizes nonenzymatically to histidylproline diketopiperazine (cyclic His-Pro).[195] Acid TRH has some behavioral effects in rats that are similar to those of TRH but no other proven actions. Cyclic His-Pro is reported to act as a PRF and to have other neural effects, including reversal of ethanol-induced sleep (TRH is also effective in this system), elevation of brain cyclic guanosine monophosphate levels, an increase in stereotypical behavior, modification of body temperature, and inhibition of eating behavior. Some of the effects of TRH may be mediated through cyclic His-Pro, but the fact that cyclic His-Pro is abundant in some areas and is not proportional to the amount of TRH suggests that the peptide may not be derived solely from TRH.[196, 197]

Extrapituitary Function

TRH is present in virtually all parts of the brain: cerebral cortex, circumventricular structures, neurohypophysis, pineal gland, and spinal cord.[182, 198–202] TRH is also found in pancreatic islet cells and in the gastrointestinal tract.[203] Although it exists in low concentration, the total amount in extrahypothalamic tissues exceeds the amount in the hypothalamus.

The extensive extrahypothalamic distribution of TRH, its localization in nerve endings, and the presence of TRH receptors in brain tissue suggest that TRH serves as a neurotransmitter or neuromodulator outside the hypothalamus. TRH is a general stimulant[182, 204–206] and induces hyperthermia on intracerebroventricular injection, suggesting a role in central thermoregulation.

Clinical Applications

The use of TRH for the diagnosis of hyperthyroidism is less common since the development of ultrasensitive assays for thyroid-stimulating hormone (TSH)[182] (see Chapter 10); its use to discriminate between hypothalamic and pituitary causes of thyrotropin deficiency has also declined because of the test's poor specificity,[182, 207] but the application of ultrasensitive assays in conjunction with the TRH test has not been fully evaluated.[208] TRH testing is also not of value in the differential diagnosis of causes of hyperprolactinemia[209] but is useful for the demonstration of residual abnormal somatotropin-secreting cells in acromegalic patients who release hGH in response to TRH before treatment.

Studies of the effect of TRH on depression have shown inconsistent results,[210] possibly because of poor blood-brain barrier penetration.[211] Intrathecal administration of TRH may improve responses in depressed patients,[211, 212] but its clinical utility is unknown. Although a role for TRH in depression is not established, many depressed patients have a blunted thyrotropin response to TRH and changes in TRH responsiveness correlate with the clinical course.[210] The mechanism by which blunting occurs is unknown.[213]

TRH has been proposed as a treatment for women with threatened premature labor to stimulate the production of lung surfactant in the preterm fetus. Despite encouraging results in early studies, several large-scale trials failed to show improvement in the survival of babies so treated.[214, 215]

TRH has been evaluated for the treatment of spinal muscle atrophy and amyotrophic lateral sclerosis; transient improvement in strength was reported in both disorders,[216–219] but the combined experience at many centers using a variety of treatment protocols including long-term intrathecal administration failed to confirm efficacy.[220–222] TRH administration also reduces the severity of experimentally induced spinal and ischemic shock[223–225]; preliminary studies in humans suggest that TRH treatment may improve recovery after spinal cord injury[226] and head trauma.[227] TRH has been used to treat children with neurologic disorders including West's syndrome, Lennox-Gastaut syndrome, early infantile epileptic encephalopathy, and intractable epilepsy.[228] TRH has been proposed to be an analeptic agent. Sleeping or drug-sedated animals were awakened by the administration of TRH,[229] TRH reportedly reversed sedative effects of ethanol in humans,[230] and TRH is said to have awakened a patient with a profound sleep disorder caused by a hypothalamic and midbrain eosinophilic granuloma.[231]

Regulation of Thyrotropin Release

The secretion of thyrotropin is regulated by two interacting elements: negative feedback by thyroid hormone and open-loop neural control by hypothalamic hypophyseotropic factors

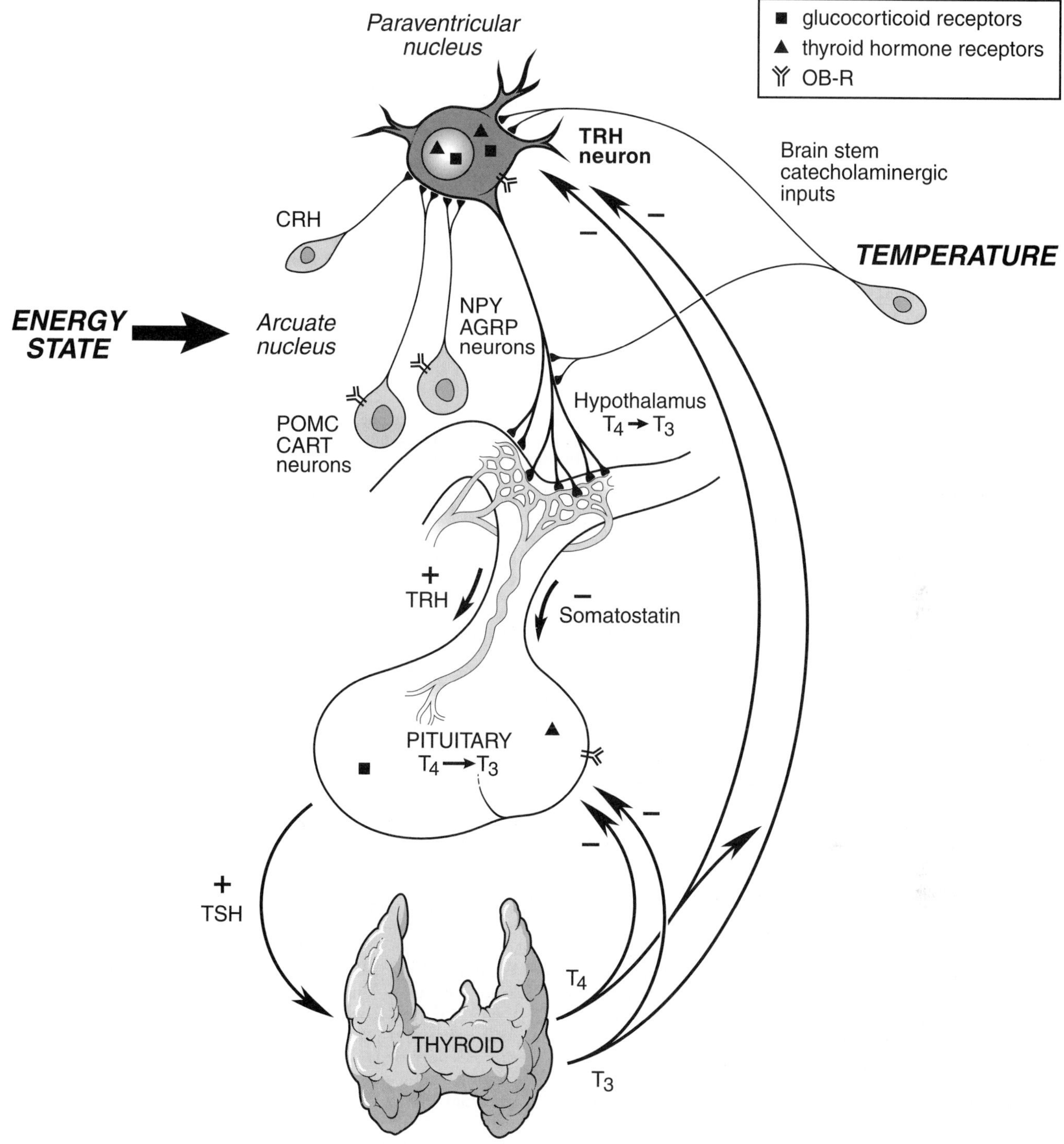

Figure 7–16. Regulation of the hypothalamic-pituitary-thyroid axis. AGRP, agouti-related protein; CART, cocaine and amphetamine–regulated transcript; CRH, corticotropin-releasing hormone; NPY, neuropeptide Y; POMC, pro-opiomelanocortin; T_3, triiodothyronine; T_4, thyroxine; TRH, thyrotropin-releasing hormone; TSH, thyrotropin; OB-R, leptin receptor.

(Fig. 7–16). Thyrotropin secretion is also modified by other hormones, including estrogens, glucocorticoids, and possibly GH, and is inhibited by cytokines in the pituitary and hypothalamus. Aspects of the pituitary-thyroid axis are also considered in Chapter 10.[182, 198, 232–236]

Feedback Control: Pituitary-Thyroid Axis

In the context of a *feedback system*, the level of thyroid hormone in blood or of its unbound fraction is the controlled variable and the set-point is the normal resting level of plasma thyroid hormone. Secretion of thyrotropin is inversely regulated by the level of thyroid hormone so that deviations from the set-point of control lead to appropriate changes in the rate of thyrotropin secretion (Fig. 7–17). Factors that determine the rate of thyrotropin secretion required to maintain a given level of thyroid hormone include the rate at which thyrotropin and thyroid hormone disappear from the blood (turnover rate) and the rate at which T_4 is converted to its more active form, T_3.

somatostatin in the regulation of thyrotropin secretion in humans is uncertain.

Dopamine has modest effects on thyrotropin secretion, and blockade of dopamine receptors (in the human) stimulates thyrotropin secretion slightly.[235] Changes in the metabolism of thyroid hormone also influence T_3 homeostasis within the brain. In states of thyroid hormone deficiency, brain T_3 levels are maintained by an increase in the deiodinase that converts T_4 to T_3.[254]

The pineal gland has been reported to inhibit thyroid function in some[255] but not all[256] studies. The pineal gland contains TRH, and in the frog its content changes with the season and with light and dark cycles independently of hypothalamic thyrotropin.[257]

Circadian Rhythm

Plasma thyrotropin in humans is characterized by a circadian periodicity, with a maximum between 9 PM and 5 AM and a minimum between 4 PM and 7 PM.[258] Smaller ultradian thyrotropin peaks occur every 90 to 180 minutes,[259] probably because of bursts of TRH release from the hypothalamus, and are physiologically important in controlling the synthesis and glycosylation of thyrotropin.[260] Glycosylation is a determinant of thyrotropin potency.

Temperature

External cold exposure activates and high ambient temperature inhibits the pituitary-thyroid axis in animals,[248] and analogous changes occur in humans under certain conditions. Exposure of infants to cold at the time of delivery causes an increase in blood thyrotropin levels, possibly because of alterations in the turnover and degradation of the thyroid hormones.[249] Blood thyroid hormone levels are higher in the winter than in the summer in individuals in cold climates[261] but not in other climates.[249] However, it is difficult to show that changes in environmental or body temperature in adults influence thyrotropin secretion. For example, exposure to cold ambient temperature or central hypothalamic cooling does not modify thyrotropin levels in young men.[262] Behavioral changes, activation of the sympathetic nervous system, and shivering appear to be more important in temperature regulation in adults than the thyroid response.[248]

The autonomic nervous system and the thyroid axis work together to maintain temperature homeostasis in mammals, and TRH plays a role in both pathways.[263] Hypothalamic TRH release is rapidly (30 to 45 minutes) increased in rats exposed to cold.[247] Rapid inhibition of somatostatin release in the median eminence has also been documented, and both changes appear to play important roles in the rise in plasma TSH induced by cold exposure. TRH mRNA is elevated within an hour of cold exposure (see Fig. 7–18*C* and *D*). The regulation of hypophyseotropic TRH release and expression by cold is largely mediated by catecholamines. Noradrenergic and adrenergic fibers, originating in the brain stem, are found in close proximity to TRH nerve endings in the median eminence, and a rapid rise in TRH release was seen after norepinephrine treatment of hypothalamic fragments containing mainly median eminence.[264] Brain stem adrenergic and noradrenergic fibers also make synaptic contacts with TRH neurons in the PVH (see Fig. 7–16),[265, 266] and thus catecholamines are likely to be involved in the regulation of TRH gene expression by cold. TRH neurons in the PVH are densely innervated by NPY terminals,[267] and a portion of the NPY terminals arising from the C1, C2, C3, and A1 cell groups of the brain stem and projecting to the PVH are known to be catecholaminergic.[268] Somatostatin, dopamine, and serotonin also play a variety of roles in the regulation of TRH.

Stress

Stress is another determinant of thyrotropin secretion.[232, 234] In humans physical stress inhibits thyrotropin release, as indicated by the finding that in the euthyroid sick syndrome low T_3 and T_4 do not cause compensatory increases in thyrotropin secretion as would occur in normal individuals.[269–271]

A number of observations demonstrate interactions between the thyroid and adrenal axes. Physiologically, the bulk of evidence suggests that glucocorticoids in humans[272] and rodents[273] act to blunt the thyroid axis through actions in the CNS. Some actions may be direct because the TRH gene (see Fig. 7–13) contains the glucocorticoid response element consensus sequence[196] and hypophyseotropic TRH neurons appear to contain glucocorticoid receptors.[274] The diurnal rhythm of cortisol is opposite that of TSH (see Fig. 7–12) and acute administration of glucocorticoids can block the nocturnal rise in TSH, but disruption of cortisol synthesis with metyrapone only modestly affects the TSH circadian rhythm.[275]

Several lines of evidence, however, identify conditions in which elevated glucocorticoids are associated with stimulation of the thyroid axis. Human depression is often associated with hypercortisolism and hyperthyroxinemia,[276] and TRH mRNA levels are elevated by glucocorticoids in a number of cell lines as well as in cultured fetal hypothalamic TRH neurons from the rat.[277] Thus, although glucocorticoids probably stimulate TRH production in TRH neurons, their overall inhibitory effect on the thyroid axis results from indirect glucocorticoid negative feedback on structures such as the hippocampus. Disruption of hippocampal suppression of the hypothalamic-pituitary-adrenal (HPA) axis is proposed to be involved in the hypercortisolemia commonly seen in affective illness,[278] and disruption of hippocampal inputs to the hypothalamus have been shown to produce a rise in hypophyseotropic TRH in the rat.[279]

Starvation

The thyroid axis is depressed during starvation, presumably to help conserve energy by depressing metabolism (see Fig. 7–18*E* to *G*). In humans, reduced T_3, T_4, and TSH are seen during starvation or fasting.[280] There are also changes in the thyroid axis in anorexia nervosa, such as low blood levels of T_3 and low normal levels of T_4 (see Chapter 33). Inappropriately low levels of TSH are found, suggesting defective activation of TRH production by low thyroid hormone levels. During starvation in rodents, reduced TRH release into hypophyseal portal blood[281] and reduced pro-TRH mRNA levels[282] are seen, despite lowered thyroid hormone levels. Reduced basal TSH levels are also usually present.

The hypothyroidism seen in fasting or in the leptin-deficient *Lep*^{ob}/*Lep*^{ob} mouse can be reversed by administration of leptin,[283] and the evidence suggests that the mechanism involves leptin's ability to up-regulate TRH gene expression in the PVH (see Fig. 7–18*E* to *G*).[284] Leptin appears to act both directly through leptin receptors on hypophyseotropic TRH neurons and indirectly through its actions on other hypothalamic cell groups, such as arcuate nucleus POMC and NPY–agouti-related peptide (AgRP) neurons.[285] TRH neurons in the PVH receive dense NPY–AgRP[267] and POMC projections[286] from the arcuate and express NPY and melanocortin-4 receptors,[287] and α-MSH administration partially prevents the fasting-induced drop in thyroid hormone levels.[286] Indeed, the TRH promoter contains a signal transducer and activator of transcription (STAT) response element and a cAMP response element that have been demonstrated to mediate induction of TRH gene expression by leptin and α-MSH, respectively, in a heterologous cell system (see Fig. 7–13).[287] The regulation of TRH by metabolic state is likely to be under redundant control, however, because, unlike rodents, leptin-deficient children are euthyroid,[288] and both melanocortin-4 receptor (MC4R)–deficient rodents[289] and humans are euthyroid.[290]

Central TRH outside the paraventricular nucleus also plays a role in thermoregulation through the autonomic nervous system.

Infection and Inflammation

The molecular basis of infection- or inflammation-induced thyrotropin suppression is now established. Sterile abscesses or the injection of interleukin-1β (IL-1β; endogenous pyrogen, a secretory peptide of activated lymphocytes)[291] or of tumor necrosis factor α (TNF-α) inhibits thyrotropin secretion,[292] and IL-1β stimulates the secretion of somatostatin.[293] TNF-α inhibits thyrotropin secretion directly and induces functional changes in the rat characteristic of the "sick euthyroid" state.[294] It is likely that the thyrotropin inhibition in animal models of the sick euthyroid syndrome is due to cytokine-induced changes in hypothalamic and pituitary function.[295] IL-6, IL-1, and TNF-α contribute to the suppression of TSH in the sick euthyroid syndrome.[296]

Corticotropin-Releasing Hormone

Chemistry and Evolution

The HPA axis is the humoral component of an integrated neural and endocrine system that functions to respond to internal and external challenges to homeostasis (stressors). The system comprises the neuronal pathways linked to release of catecholamines from the adrenal medulla (fight-or-flight response) and the hypothalamic-pituitary control of ACTH release in the control of glucocorticoid production by the adrenal cortex. Pituitary ACTH release is stimulated primarily by CRH and to a lesser extent by AVP (see Chapter 9). The hypophyseotropic CRH neurons are located in the parvicellular division of the PVH and project to the median eminence (see Figs. 7–6 to 7–9).

In a broader context, the CRH system in the CNS is also quite important in the behavioral response to stress. This complex system includes not only nonhypophyseotropic CRH neurons but also three CRH-like peptides (urocortin I, urocortin II or stresscopin-like peptide, and urocortin III or stresscopin), at least two cognate receptors (CRH-R1 and CRH-R2), and a high-affinity CRH-binding protein, each with distinct and complex distributions in the CNS.

The Schally and Guillemin laboratories demonstrated in 1955 that extracts from the hypothalamus stimulated ACTH release from the pituitary.[297, 298] The primary active principle, CRH, was purified and characterized from the sheep in 1981 by Vale and colleagues.[299] Human CRH is an amidated 41-amino-acid peptide that is cleaved from the carboxyl terminus of a 196-amino-acid pre-prohormone precursor by PC1 and PC2 and amidated (Fig. 7–19).[300] In general, the peptide is highly conserved; the human peptide is identical in sequence to the mouse and rat peptides but differs at seven residues from the ovine sequence. CRH and urocortin I, II, and III in mammals, fish urotensin, anuran sauvagine,[301] and the insect diuretic peptides[302] are members of an ancient family of peptides that evolved from an ancestral precursor early in the evolution of metazoans, approximately 500 million years ago. Comparison of peptide sequences in the vertebrate suggests grouping of the peptides into two families, CRH-urotensin-urocortin-sauvagine and urocortin II–urocortin III (Fig. 7–20).[303] Urocortin and sauvagine appear to represent tetrapod orthologues of fish urotensin. Sauvagine, isolated originally from *Phyllomedusa sauvagei*, is an osmoregulatory peptide produced in the skin of certain frogs; urotensin is an osmoregulatory peptide produced in the caudal neurosecretory system of the fish. Whereas isolation of CRH required 250,000 ovine hypothalami, the cloning of urocortin II and III[303–305] was accomplished by computer search of the human genome database.

The CRH peptides signal by binding to CRH-R1[306–308] and CRH-R2 receptors[309–312] that are members of the gut-brain family of G protein–coupled receptors and couple to Gs and activation of adenylyl cyclase. Two splice variants of the latter that differ in the extracellular amino-terminal domain, CRH-R2α and CRH-R2β, have been found in both rodents and humans,[313] and a third N-terminal splice variant, CRH-R2γ, has been reported in the human.[314]

CRH, urotensin, and sauvagine are all potent agonists of CRH-R1, urocortin is a potent agonist of both receptors, and urocortins II and III are specific agonists of CRH-R2. CRH-mediated activation of the HPA axis appears to be exclusively mediated through CRH-R1 expressed in the corticotroph. The PVH is the site of the majority of CRH neurons projecting to the median eminence, although some CRH neurons projecting to the median eminence are found in most hypothalamic nuclei (Fig. 7–21*A*). Some CRH fibers in the PVH also project to the brain stem, and CRH neurons are also found elsewhere, primarily in limbic structures involved in processing sensory information and in regulating the autonomic nervous system. Sites include the prefrontal, insular, and cingulate cortices; amygdala; substantia nigra; periaqueductal gray; locus coeruleus; nucleus of the solitary tract; and parabrachial nucleus. In the periphery, CRH is found in human placenta, where it is up-regulated 6-fold to 40-fold during the third trimester; lymphocytes; autonomic nerves; and gastrointestinal tract. Urocortin is found at highest levels in the Edinger-Westphal nucleus, lateral superior olive, and supraoptic nucleus of the rodent brain, with additional sites including the substantia nigra, ventral tegmental area, and dorsal raphe (Fig. 7–21*B*). In the human, urocortin is widely distributed with highest levels in the frontal cortex, temporal cortex, and hypothalamus[315] and has also been reported in the Edinger-Westphal and olivary nuclei.[316] In the periphery, urocortin is seen in placenta, mucosal inflammatory cells in the gastrointestinal tract, lymphocytes, and cardiomyocytes. The tissue distribution of urocortins II and III is not well characterized as of this writing.

In addition to its expression in pituitary corticotrophs, CRH-R1 is found in the neocortex and cerebellar cortex, subcortical limbic structures, and amygdala, with little to no expression in the hypothalamus (Fig. 7–21*C*). CRH-R1 is also found in a variety of peripheral sites in humans, including ovary, endometrium, and skin.[317] CRH-R2α is found mainly in the brain in rodents, with high levels of expression seen in the ventromedial hypothalamic nucleus and lateral septum (see Fig. 7–21*C*).[318] CRH-R2β is seen centrally in cerebral arterioles and peripherally in gastrointestinal tract, heart, and muscle.[309, 310, 312, 319] In contrast, in humans CRH-R2α is seen in brain and periphery, and the β and γ subtypes are primarily central.[313, 314] Little CRH-R2 message is seen in pituitary. Although CRH-R1 appears to be exclusively involved in regulation of pituitary ACTH synthesis and release, both receptors have been found to be expressed in the rodent adrenal cortex.[320] Data suggest that this intra-adrenal CRH-ACTH system may be involved in fine-tuning of adrenocortical corticosterone release.

The CRH system is also regulated in both brain and periphery by a 37-kd high-affinity CRH-binding protein.[321–323] This factor was initially postulated from the observation that CRH levels rise dramatically during the second and third trimesters of pregnancy without activating the pituitary-adrenal axis. Among hypophyseotropic factors, CRH is the only one for which a specific binding protein (in addition to the receptor) exists in tissue or blood. The placenta is the principal source of pregnancy-related CRH-binding protein. Human and rat

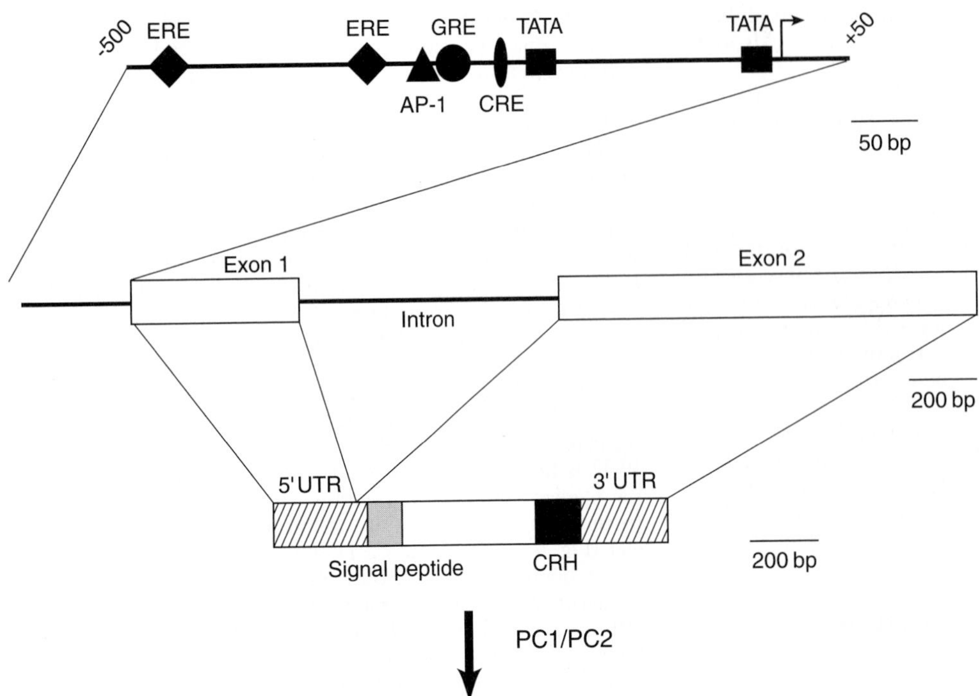

Ser - Glu - Glu - Pro - Pro - Ile - Ser - Leu - Asp - Leu - Thr - Phe - His - Leu - Leu -
Arg - Glu - Val - Leu - Glu - Met - Ala - Arg - Ala - Glu - Gln - Leu - Ala - Gln - Gln -
Ala - His - Ser - Asn - Arg - Lys - Leu - Met - Glu - Ile - Ile - Gly - Lys

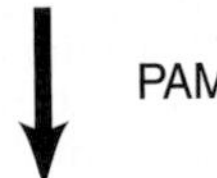

Ser - Glu - Glu - Pro - Pro - Ile - Ser - Leu - Asp - Leu - Thr - Phe - His - Leu - Leu -
Arg - Glu - Val - Leu - Glu - Met - Ala - Arg - Ala - Glu - Gln - Leu - Ala - Gln - Gln -
Ala - His - Ser - Asn - Arg - Lys - Leu - Met - Glu - Ile - Ile - NH_2

Figure 7–19. Structure of human corticotropin-releasing hormone (CRH) gene and protein. The sequence coding for CRH occurs at the terminus of the prohormone. Cleavage sites and the terminal Gly position are shown. PAM, peptidylglycine alpha-amidating monooxygenase; PC1/PC2, prohormone convertases 1 and 2; ERE, estrogen regulating element; GRE, glucocorticoid regulating element; CRE, cyclic AMP-responsive element; UTR, untranslated. (Redrawn from data of Shibahara S, Morimoto Y, Furutani Y, et al. Isolation and sequence analysis of the human corticotropin-releasing factor precursor gene. EMBO J 1983; 2:775–779.)

CRH-binding proteins are homologous (85% amino acid identity), but in the rat the protein is expressed only in brain.[324] The binding protein is species specific; bovine CRH, which is almost identical in sequence to rat-human CRH, has a lower affinity of binding to the human binding protein.

The functional significance of the CRH-binding protein is not fully understood.[325] CRH-binding protein does not bind to the CRH receptor but does inhibit CRH action. For this reason CRH-binding protein probably acts to modulate CRH actions at the cellular level. Corticotroph cells in the anterior pituitary have membrane CRH receptors and intracellular CRH-binding protein; conceivably, the binding protein acts to sequester or terminate the action of membrane-bound CRH. CRH-binding protein is present in many regions of the CNS, including cells that synthesize CRH and cells that receive innervation from CRH-containing neurons.[324] The anatomic distribution of the protein, the variability of its location in relation to the presence of CRH, and its relative sparseness in the CRH tuberohypophyseal neuronal system suggest a control system that is as yet poorly understood.

Structure-activity relationship studies have demonstrated that C-terminal amidation and an α-helical secondary structure[326] are both important for biologic activity of CRH. The first CRH antagonist described was termed α-helical CRH_{9-41}.[327] A second, more potent antagonist, termed astressin, had the structure cyclo(30–33)(D-Phe[12], Nle[12], Glu[12], Lys[12],)$hCRH_{12-41}$.[328] Both peptides are somewhat nonspecific, antagonizing both CRH-R1 and CRH-R2. Because of the anxiogenic activity of CRH and urocortin, a number of pharmaceutical companies have developed small molecule CRH antagonists; several of the

```
Frog  sauvagine        QGPPISIDLSLELLRKMIEIEKQEKEKQQAANNRLLLDTI
Carp  urotensin-I     NDDPPISIDLTFHLLRNMIEMARNENQREQAGLNRKYLDEV
Human urocortin        DNPSLSIDLTFHLLRTLLELARTQSQRERAEQNRIIFDSV
Human CRH             SEEPPISLDLTFHLLREVLEMARAEQLAQQAHSNRKLMEII
Human SRP           HPGSRIVLSLDVPIGLLQILLEQARARAAREQATTNARILARVGHC
Human SCP              TKFTLSLDVPTNIMNLLFNIAKAKNLRAQAAANAHLMAQIGRRK
```

Figure 7–20. Sequence comparison of members of the corticotropin-releasing hormone (CRH) peptide family. SPP, stresscopin related peptide; SCP, stresscopin.

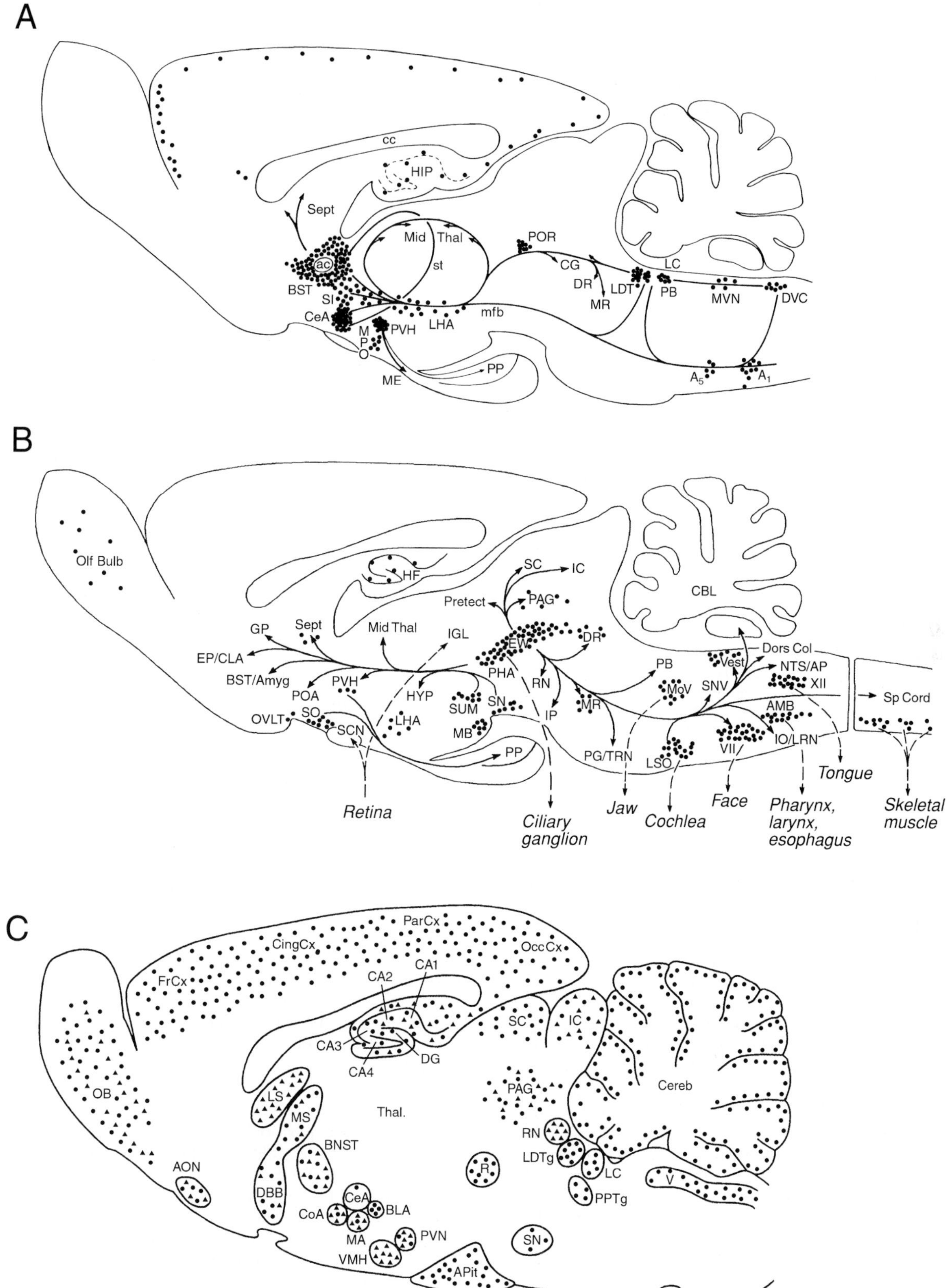

Figure 7–21. Distribution of corticotropin-releasing hormone (CRH), urocortin, and the CRH receptor 1 (CRH-R1) and CRH-R2 messenger ribonucleic acid sequences in the rat brain. A_1, noradrenergic cell group 1; A_5, noradrenergic cell group 5; ac, anterior commissure; BST, bed nucleus of the stria terminalis; cc, corpus callosum; CeA, central nucleus amygdala; CG, central gray; DR, dorsal raphe; DVC, dorsal vagal complex; HIP, hippocampus; LC, locus coeruleus; LDT, laterodorsal tegmental nucleus; LHA, lateral hypothalamic area; ME, median eminence; MID THAL, midline thalamic nuclei; mfb, medial forebrain bundle; MPO, medial preoptic area; MR, medial raphe; MVN, medial vestibular nucleus; PB, parabrachial nucleus; POR, perioculomotor nucleus; PP, posterior pituitary; PVH, periventricular nucleus; SEPT, septal region; SI, substantia innominata; st, stria. (From Swanson LW, Sawchenko PE, Rivier J, et al. Organization of ovine corticotropin-releasing factor immunoreactive cells and fibers in the rat brain: an immunohistochemical study. Neuroendocrinology 1983; 36:165–186; Bittencourt et al. J Comp Neurol 1999; 415:285, Fig. 17; Steckler and Holsboer. Biol Psychol 1999; 46:1480, Fig. 1.)

molecules are currently in clinical trials for anxiety and depression (discussed in more detail later). Thus far, this structurally diverse group of small molecule compounds, such as antalarmin, CP-154,526, and NBI27914, are potent antagonists of CRH-R1, with little activity at CRH-R2.[329] The efficacy of these compounds across the entire behavioral, neuroendocrine, and autonomic repertoire of response to stress has been demonstrated in a number of laboratory animal studies. For example, oral administration of antalarmin in a social stress model in the primate (introduction of strange males) reduced behavioral measures of anxiety such as lack of exploratory behavior, decreased plasma ACTH and cortisol, and reduced plasma epinephrine and norepinephrine.[330] A peptide antagonist with 100-fold selectivity for the CRH 2β receptor, (D-Phe,[11] His[12])sauvagine 11–40 or anti–sauvagine-30, has also been described.[331]

Effects on the Pituitary and Mechanism of Action

Administration of CRH to humans causes prompt release of corticotropin into the blood, followed by secretion of cortisol (Fig. 7–22) and other adrenal steroids including aldosterone.[332, 333] Most studies have used ovine CRH, which is more potent and longer acting than human CRH, but human and porcine CRHs appear to have equal diagnostic value.[332] The effect of CRH is specific to corticotropin release and is inhibited by glucocorticoids.

As mentioned before, CRH acts on the pituitary corticotroph primarily by binding to CRH-R1 and activating adenylyl cyclase. The concentration of cAMP in the tissue is increased in parallel with the biologic effects and is reduced by glucocorticoids. The rate of transcription of the mRNA that encodes the corticotropin prohormone POMC is also enhanced by CRH, indicating that CRH is a trophic factor as well as a releasing hormone.

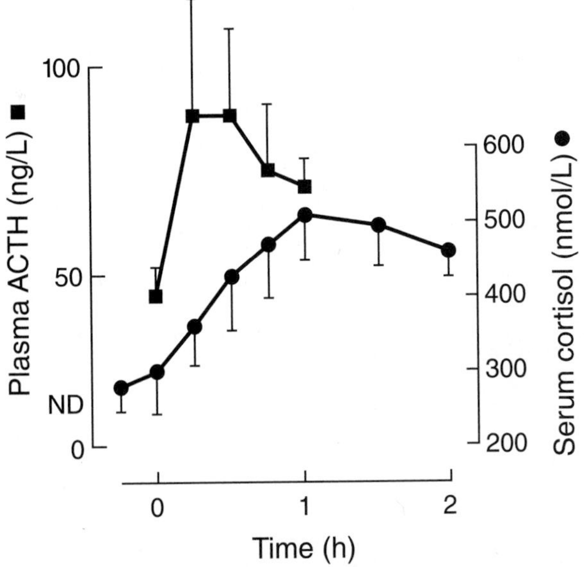

Figure 7–22. Changes in plasma levels of corticotropin and serum levels of cortisol after intravenous injection of corticotropin-releasing hormone in a group of six normal men. The initial prompt response in corticotropin is followed by a somewhat delayed secondary change in cortisol. To convert corticotropin values to picomoles per liter, multiply by 0.2202. To convert cortisol values to millimoles per liter, multiply by 27.59. ACTH, adrenocorticotropic hormone. (From Grossman A, Kruseman ACN, Perry L, et al. New hypothalamic hormone, corticotropin-releasing factor, specifically stimulates the release of adrenocorticotropic hormone and cortisol in man. Lancet 1982; 1:921–922.)

Extrapituitary Functions

CRH and the urocortin peptides have a wide range of biologic activities in addition to the hypophyseotropic role of CRH in regulating ACTH synthesis and release. Centrally, these peptides have behavioral activities in anxiety, mood, arousal, locomotion, reward, and feeding[334–336] and increase sympathetic activation. Many of the nonhypophyseotropic behavioral and autonomic functions of these peptides can be viewed as complementary to activation of the HPA axis in the maintenance of homeostasis under exposure to stress. In the periphery, activities have been reported in immunity, cardiac function, gastrointestinal function, and reproduction.

The CRH and urocortin peptides have a repertoire of behavioral and autonomic actions after central administration that suggests a role for these pathways in mediating the behavioral-autonomic components of the stress response. Hyperactivity of the HPA axis is a common neuroendocrine finding in affective disorders (Fig. 7–23) (for reviews see references [337] to [339]). Furthermore, normalization of HPA regulation is highly predictive of successful treatment. Defective dexamethasone suppression of CRH release, implying defective corticosteroid receptor signaling,[340] is seen not only in depressed patients but also in healthy subjects with a family history of depression.[341] Depressed patients also show elevated levels of CRH in the CSF.[342]

Central administration of CRH or urocortin activates neuronal cell groups involved in cardiovascular control and increases blood pressure, heart rate, and cardiac output.[343, 344] However, urocortin is expressed in cardiac myocytes,[345] and intravenous administration of CRH or urocortin decreases blood pressure and increases heart rate in most species, including humans.[346] This hypotensive effect is probably mediated peripherally because ganglion blockade did not disrupt the hypotensive effects of intravenous urocortin.[347] Furthermore, high levels of CRH-R2β have been seen in the cardiac atria and ventricles,[309, 310, 312, 319] and knockout of the CRH-R2 gene in the mouse removed the hypotensive effects of intravenous urocortin administration.[348, 349]

CRH and AVP also play an important role in the regulation of inflammatory responses. As described later ("Neuroendocrine-Immune Interaction"), cytokines have an important role in extinguishing inflammatory responses through activation of CRH and AVP neurons in the paraventricular nucleus and subsequent elevation of anti-inflammatory glucocorticoids. Interestingly, CRH is generally seen to be proinflammatory in the periphery, where it is found in sympathetic efferents, sensory afferent nerves, leukocytes, and in macrophages in some species.[350]

CRH is also made as a paracrine factor by the endometrium, where it may play a role in decidualization and implantation and act as a uterine vasodilator.[351]

The relative contributions of each of the CRH-urocortin peptides and receptors to the different biologic functions reported has been the topic of considerable analysis, given the receptor-specific antagonists already described as well as the CRH,[352] CRH-R1,[353, 354] and CRH-R2[348, 349, 355] knockout mice available for study.[356, 357] Examining three potent stressors—restraint, ether, and fasting—these studies demonstrated that other ACTH secretagogues, such as vasopressin, oxytocin, and catecholamines, could not replace CRH in its role in mounting the stress response. In contrast, augmentation of glucocorticoid secretion by a stressor after prolonged stress was not defective in the CRH knockout mouse, implicating CRH-independent mechanisms.[357]

Although CRH is a potent anxiogenic peptide,[358] the CRH knockout mouse exhibits normal anxiety behaviors in, for example, conditioned fear paradigms.[359] The nonpeptide CRH-R1 specific antagonist CP-154,526 was anxiolytic in a shock-

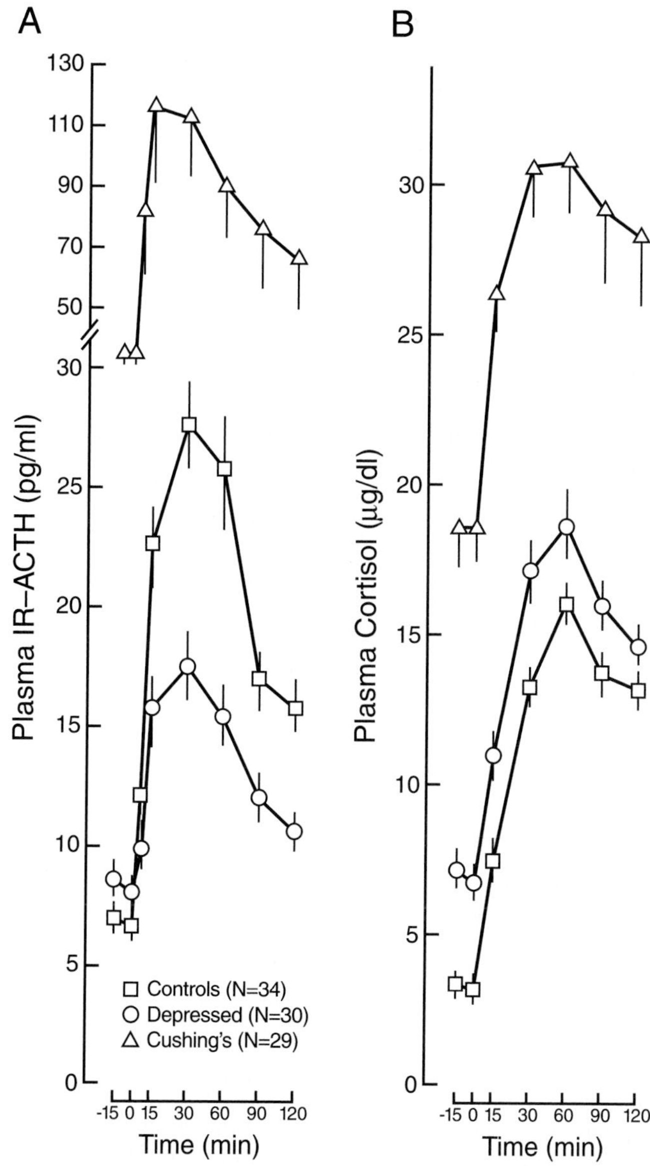

Figure 7–23. Comparison of plasma immunoreactive adrenocorticotropic hormone (IR-ACTH) *(A)* and cortisol *(B)* responses to ovine corticotropin-releasing hormone in control subjects, patients with depression, and patients with Cushing's disease. (From Gold PW, et al. N Engl J Med 1986; 314:1329.)

induced freezing paradigm in both wild-type and CRH knockout mice,[359] suggesting that the anxiogenic activity is a CRH-like peptide acting at the CRH-R1 receptor.

CRH and urocortin peptides also have potent anorexigenic activity, implicating the CRH system in stress-induced inhibition of feeding. Stress-induced inhibition of feeding remained intact, however, in the CRH knockout mouse.[360] Likewise, suppression of the proestrous LH surge by restraint was intact in the CRH knockout mouse.[361] Both CRH-R1 and CRH-R2 knockout strains had normal weight and feeding behavior but were distinctly different from wild-type mice in the anorexigenic response to centrally administered urocortin or CRH. The CRH-R1–deficient mice lacked the acute anorexigenic response (0 to 1.5 hours) to urocortin seen in wild-type mice.[362] Both wild-type and CRH-R1 −/− mice exhibited comparable reduction in feeding 3 to 11 hours after administration. In contrast, the late phase of urocortin responsiveness appeared to depend on the presence of CRH-R2.[348, 349, 355] Thus, signaling through CRH-R1 and CRH-R2 appears to play a complex role in the acute effects of stress on feeding behavior.

Clinical Applications

No useful therapeutic applications of CRH or CRH-like peptides have been reported, although the peptide has been demonstrated to have a number of activities in human and primate studies. For example, intravenous administration of CRH was found to stimulate energy expenditure and has been proposed for use in weight loss. The development of small molecule, orally available, CRH-R1 antagonists has, however, led to phase I clinical trials for anxiety and depression. An early study of 20 patients demonstrated significant reductions in scores of anxiety and depression, using ratings determined by either patient or clinician.[363]

Feedback Control

The administration of glucocorticoids inhibits corticotropin secretion; removal of the adrenals (or administration of drugs that impair secretion of glucocorticoids) leads to increased corticotropin release. The set-point of pituitary feedback is determined by the hypothalamus acting through hypothalamic releasing hormones CRH and vasopressin (see Chapters 8 and 9).[266, 333, 364–373] Glucocorticoids act on both the pituitary corticotrophs and the hypothalamic neurons that secrete CRH and vasopressin. These regulatory actions are analogous to the control of the pituitary-thyroid axis. However, whereas thyrotropin becomes completely unresponsive to TRH when thyroid hormone levels are sufficiently high, severe neurogenic stress and large amounts of CRH can break through the feedback inhibition by glucocorticoids. A still higher level of feedback control is exerted by glucocorticoid-responsive neurons in the hippocampus that project to the hypothalamus; these neurons affect the activity of CRH hypophyseotropic neurons and determine the set-point of pituitary responsiveness to glucocorticoids.[368]

Glucocorticoids are lipid soluble and enter the brain through the blood-brain barrier.[369] In brain and pituitary they can bind to two receptors, type I (the *mineralocorticoid* receptor, so named because it binds aldosterone and glucocorticoids with high affinity) and type II (*glucocorticoid* receptor, which has low affinity for mineralocorticoids).[266, 368–373] Glucocorticoid action involves binding of the steroid-receptor complex to regulator sequences in the genome.[370] Type I receptors are saturated by basal levels of glucocorticoids, whereas type II receptors are not saturated under basal conditions but approach saturation during peak phases of the circadian rhythm and during stress. These differences and differences in regional distribution within the brain suggest that type I receptors determine basal activity of the hypothalamic-pituitary axis and that type II receptors mediate stress responses.

In the pituitary, glucocorticoids inhibit secretion of corticotropin and the synthesis of POMC mRNA; in the hypothalamus, the secretion of CRH and vasopressin and the synthesis of their respective mRNAs are inhibited.[365, 366, 368–371] Neuron membrane excitability and ion transport properties are suppressed by changes in glucocorticoid-directed synthesis of intracellular protein. Glucocorticoids may also act directly on neuronal cell membranes to change corticotropin secretion rapidly.[374]

Glucocorticoids block stress-induced corticotropin release. The latency of the inhibitory effect is so short (less than 30 minutes)[367] that it is possible that gene regulation is not the sole basis of the response. Long-term suppression (more than 1 hour) clearly acts through genomic mechanisms.

Glucocorticoid receptors are also found outside the hypothalamus in the septum and amygdala,[368, 369, 373] structures that are involved in the emotional changes in hypercortisolism and hypocortisolism. Hippocampal neurons are damaged by prolonged elevation of glucocorticoids during prolonged stress.[368]

Neural Control

Significant physiologic or psychological stressors evoke an adaptive response that commonly includes activation of both the HPA axis and the sympathoadrenal axis. The end products of these pathways then help to mobilize resources to cope with the physiologic demands in emergency situations, acutely through the fight-or-flight response and over the long term through systemic effects of glucocorticoids on functions such as gluconeogenesis and energy mobilization (see Chapter 33). The HPA axis also has unique stress-specific homeostatic roles, the best example being the role of glucocorticoids in down-regulating immune responses after infection and other events that stimulate cytokine production by the immune system (see "Neuroendocrine-Immune Interactions").

The paraventricular nucleus is the primary hypothalamic nucleus responsible for providing the integrated whole-animal response to stress.[375–379] This nucleus contains three major types of effector neurons that are spatially distinct from one another within it: (1) magnocellular oxytocin and vasopressin neurons that project to the posterior pituitary and participate in the regulation of blood pressure, fluid homeostasis, lactation, and parturition; (2) neurons projecting to the brain stem and spinal cord that regulate a variety of autonomic responses including sympathoadrenal activation; and (3) parvocellular CRH neurons that project to the median eminence and regulate ACTH synthesis and release. Many CRH neurons coexpress AVP, which acts as an auxiliary ACTH secretagogue, synergistic with CRH. AVP is regulated quite differently in parvocellular versus magnocellular neurons but is also regulated somewhat differently from CRH by stressors in parvocellular cells expressing both peptides.[380] Different stressors result in different patterns of activation of the three major visceromotor cell groups within the paraventricular nucleus, as measured by the general neuronal activation marker c-fos (Fig. 7–24).[381] For example, salt loading down-regulates CRH mRNA in parvocellular CRH cells, up-regulates CRH in a small number of magnocellular CRH cells, but only activates magnocellular cells. Hemorrhage activates every division of the paraventricular nucleus, whereas cytokine administration primarily activates parvocellular CRH cells with some minor activation of magnocellular and autonomic divisions.

The synthesis and release of AVP, which regulates renal water absorption and vascular smooth muscle, are controlled mainly by the volume and tonicity of the blood. This information is relayed to the magnocellular AVP cell through the nucleus of the solitary tract and A1 noradrenergic cell group of the ventrolateral medulla and projections from a triad of CVOs lining the third ventricle, the SFO, MePO, and OVLT. Oxytocin is primarily involved in reproductive functions, such as parturition, lactation, and milk ejection, although it is cosecreted with AVP in response to osmotic and volume challenges, and oxytocin cells receive direct projections from the nucleus of the solitary tract as well as from the SFO, medial preoptic nucleus (MePO), and OVLT. In contrast to the neurosecretory neurons functionally defined by the three peptides, CRH, oxytocin, and AVP, PVH neurons projecting to brain stem and spinal cord include neurons expressing each of these peptides.

In the rodent, a wide variety of stressors have been determined to activate parvocellular CRH neurons, including cytokine injection, salt loading, hemorrhage, adrenalectomy, restraint, foot shock, hypoglycemia, fasting, and ether exposure. Thus, in contrast to the simplicity of inputs to magnocellular cells (Fig. 7–25*A*), it is not surprising that parvocellular CRH neurons receive a diverse and complex assortment of inputs (Fig. 7–26; see Fig. 7–25*B*). These may be divided into three major categories, brain stem, limbic forebrain, and hypothalamus. Because the PVH is not known to receive any direct projections from the cerebral cortex or thalamus, stressors involving emotional or cognitive processing must involve indirect relay to the PVH.

Visceral sensory input to the PVH involves primarily two pathways. The nucleus of the solitary tract, the primary recipient of sensory information from the thoracic and abdominal viscera, sends dense catecholaminergic projections to the PVH, both directly and through relays in the ventrolateral medulla.[382, 383] These brain stem projections account for about half of the NPY fibers present in the PVH,[268] described in more detail subsequently. A second major input responsible for transducing signals from blood-borne substances derives from three CVOs adjacent to the third ventricle, the SFO, OVLT, and MePO.[384, 385] These pathways account for activation of CRH neurons by what are referred to as *systemic* or *physiologic* stressors.[377]

By contrast, what are termed *neurogenic, emotional,* or *psychological* stressors involve, in addition, nociceptive or somatosensory pathways as well as cognitive and affective brain centers. Using elevation of c-fos as an indicator of neuronal activation, detailed studies have compared PVH-projecting neurons activated by IL-1 treatment (systemic stressor) versus foot shock (neurogenic stressor). Only catecholaminergic solitary tract nucleus and ventrolateral medulla neurons were activated by moderate doses of IL-1.[386] In contrast, foot shock activated neurons of the solitary tract nucleus and ventrolateral medulla but also cell groups in the limbic forebrain and hypothalamus.[387] Notably, pharmacologic or mechanical disruption of the ascending catecholaminergic fibers blocked IL-1–mediated activation but not foot shock–mediated activation of the HPA axis.[388] Data suggest that pathways activated by other neurogenic and systemic stressors may overlap significantly with those activated by foot shock and IL-1 treatment, respectively.[378]

Except for the catecholaminergic neurons of the nucleus of the solitary tract and ventrolateral medulla, parts of the bed nucleus of the stria terminalis, and the dorsomedial nucleus of the hypothalamus, many inputs to the paraventricular nucleus, such as those deriving from the prefrontal cortex and lateral septum, are thought to act indirectly through local hypothalamic glutamatergic[378] and GABAergic neurons[389] with direct synapses to the CRH neurons. The bed nucleus of the stria terminalis is the only limbic region with prominent direct projections to the PVH. With substantial projections from the amygdala, hippocampus, and septal nuclei, it may thus serve as a key integrative center for transmission of limbic information to the PVH.

Other Factors Influencing Secretion of Corticotropin

Circadian Rhythms

Levels of corticotropin and cortisol (in humans) peak in the early morning, fall during the day to reach a nadir at about midnight, and begin to rise between 1 AM and 4 AM (see Fig. 7–12).[164] Within the circadian cycle approximately 15 to 18 pulses of corticotropin can be discerned, their height varying with the time of day. The set-point of feedback control by glucocorticoids also varies in a circadian pattern. Pituitary-adrenal rhythms are entrained to the light-dark cycle and can be changed over several days by exposure to an altered light schedule. It has long been assumed that the rhythm of corticotropin secretion is driven by CRH rhythms, and CRH knockout mice were found to exhibit no circadian rhythm in corticosterone production.[390] Remarkably, however, a diurnal

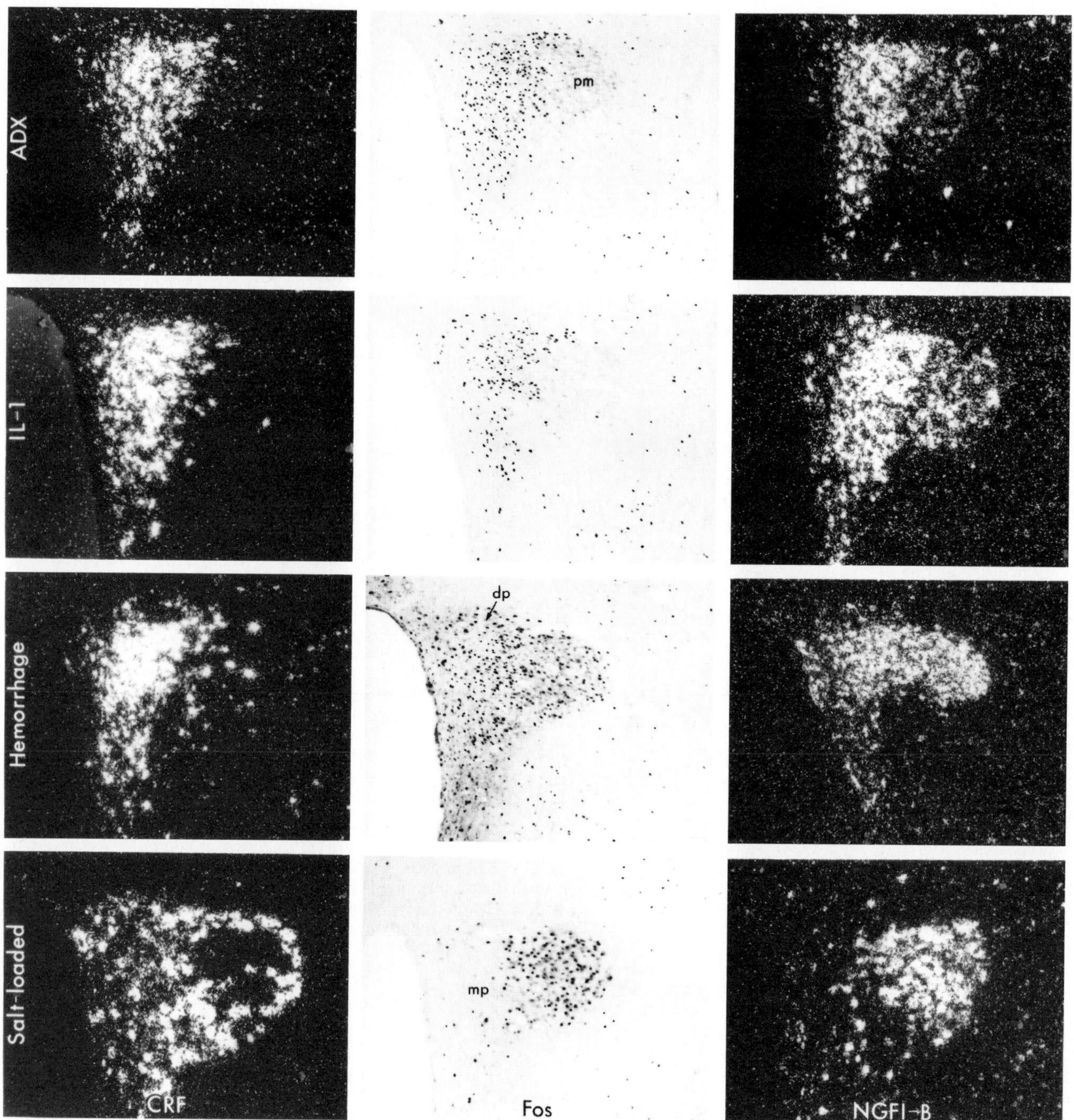

Figure 7–24. Regulation of neurons of the paraventricular nucleus (PVH) by diverse stressors. ADX, adrenalectomy; dp, dorsal PVH; IL-1, interleukin-1; mp, magnocellular PVH; NGFI-B, nerve growth factor I-B; pm, medial PVH. (Reprinted from Sawchentzo PE, et al. The paraventricular nucleus of the hypothalamus and the functional neuroanatomy of visceromotor responses to stress. Prog Brain Res 1996; 107:208. With permission from Elsevier Science.)

rhythm in corticosterone was restored by a constant infusion of CRH to the CRH knockout mouse,[390] suggesting that CRH is necessary to permit pituitary or adrenal responsiveness to another diurnal rhythm generator.

Corticotropin Release–Inhibiting Factor

Disconnection of the pituitary from the hypothalamus in several species leads to increased basal levels of corticotropin, and certain responses to physical stress (in contrast to psychological stress) are retained in such animals. These observations have led several investigators to postulate the existence of a *corticotropin inhibitory factor* analogous to dopamine in the control of PRL secretion and to somatostatin in the control of GH secretion.[391] Candidate hypothalamic peptides to inhibit corticotropin release at the level of the pituitary include atrial natriuretic peptide, activins and inhibins, and sequence 178 to 199 of the TRH prohormone.[178, 392] There is not yet a consensus on the existence of a physiologically relevant corticotropin release–inhibiting factor or on its identity.

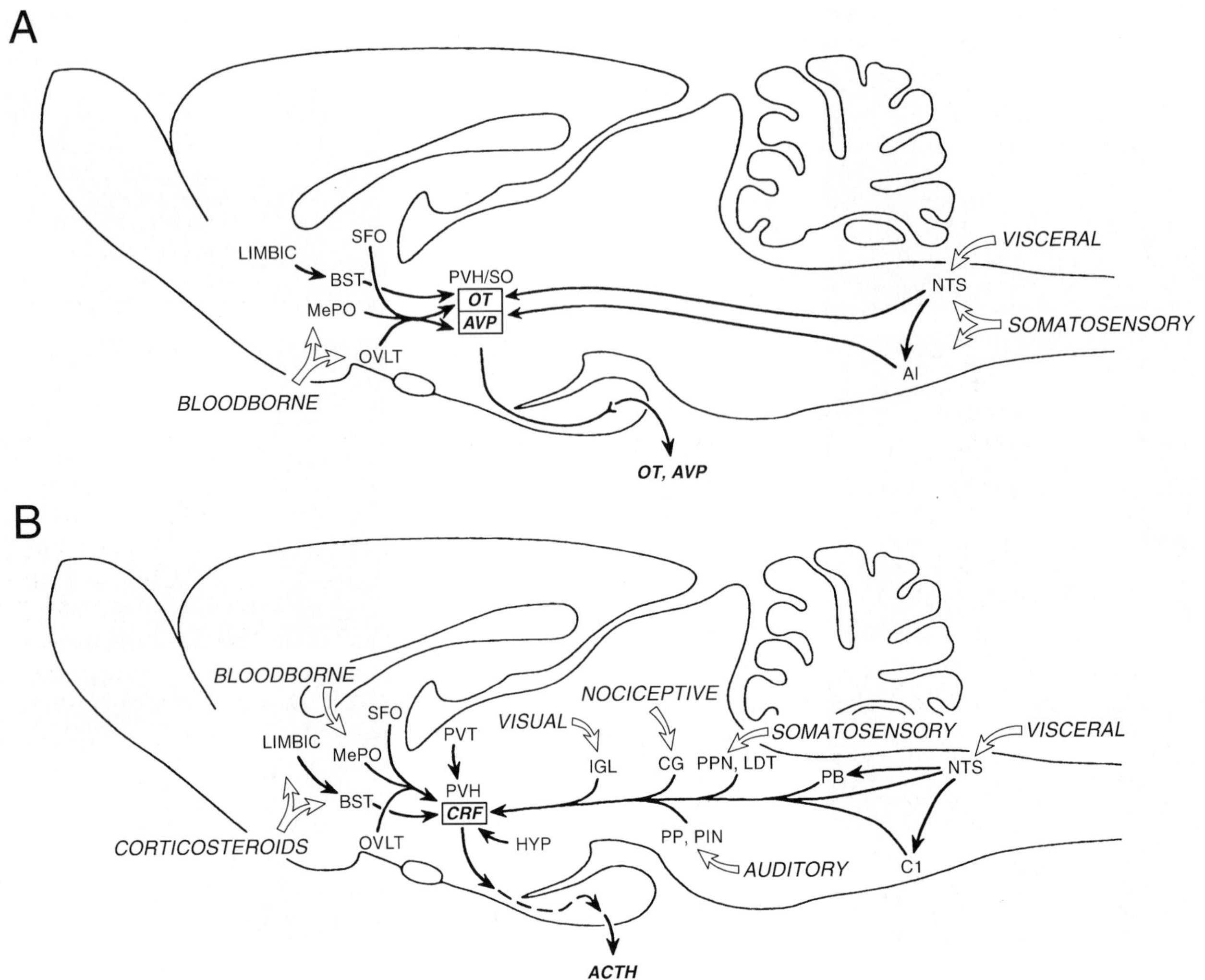

Figure 7–25. Neuronal inputs to neurons of the paraventricular nucleus. AVP, arginine vasopressin; BST, bed nucleus of the stria terminalis; CG, central gray; IGL, intergeniculate leaf; LDT, laterodorsal tegmental nucleus; MePO, medial preoptic nucleus; NTS, nucleus of the tractus solitarius; OT, oxytocin; OVLT, organum vasculosum of the lamina terminalis; PB, parabrachial nucleus; PIN, posterior intralaminar nucleus; PP, peripeduncular nucleus; PPN, pedunculopontine nucleus; SFO, subfornical organ. (Reprinted from Sawchentzo PE, et al. The paraventricular nucleus of the hypothalamus and the functional neuroanatomy of visceromotor responses to stress. Prog Brain Res 1996; 107:204. With permission from Elsevier Science.)

Growth Hormone–Releasing Hormone

Chemistry and Evolution

Evidence for neural control of GH secretion came from studies of its regulation in animals with lesions of the hypothalamus[393] and from the demonstration that hypothalamic extracts stimulate the release of GH from the pituitary. When it was shown that GH is released episodically, follows a circadian rhythm, responds rapidly to stress, and is blocked by pituitary stalk section, the concept of neural control of GH secretion became a certainty. However, it was only with the discovery of the paraneoplastic syndrome of ectopic GHRH secretion by pancreatic adenomas in humans that sufficient starting material became available for peptide sequencing and subsequent cloning of a complementary deoxyribonucleic acid (cDNA).[394–397]

Two principal molecular forms of GHRH occur in human hypothalamus: GHRH(1–44)-NH_2 and GHRH(1–40)-OH (Fig. 7–27).[398] As with other neuropeptides, the various forms of GHRH arise from post-translational modification of a larger prohormone.[397, 399] The NH_2-terminal tyrosine of GHRH (or histidine in rodent GHRHs) is essential for bioactivity, but a COOH-terminal NH_2 group is not. Fragments as short as (1–29)-NH_2 are active, but GHRH(1–27)-NH_2 is inactive. A circulating type IV dipeptidylpeptidase potently inactivates GHRH to its principal and more stable metabolite, GHRH(3–44)-NH_2,[400] which accounts for most of the immunoreactive peptide detected in plasma. As in the case of LHRH, there are species differences among GHRHs; the peptides from seven species range in sequence homology with the human peptide from 93% in the pig to 67% in the rat.[398] The COOH-terminal end of GHRH exhibits the most sequence diversity among species, consistent with the exon arrangement of the gene and dispensability of these residues for GHRH receptor binding.

Despite its importance for the elucidation of GHRH structure, ectopic secretion of the peptide is a rare cause of acromegaly. Fewer than 1% of acromegalic patients have elevated plasma levels of GHRH (see Chapter 8).[401] Approximately 20% of pancreatic adenomas and 5% of carcinoid tumors contain immunoreactive GHRH, but most are clinically silent.[402, 403]

In addition to expression in the hypothalamus, the GHRH

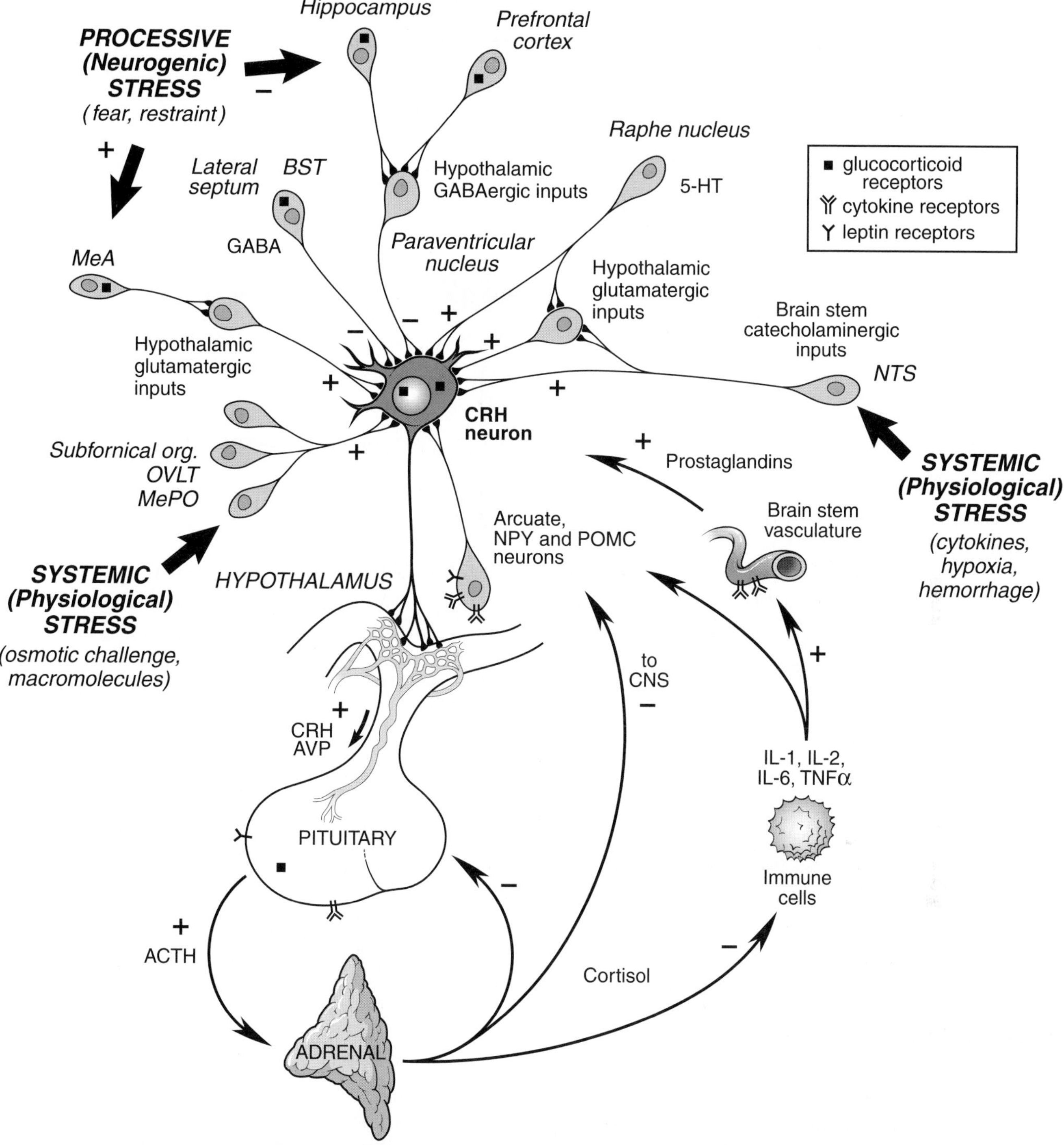

Figure 7–26. Regulation of the hypothalamic-pituitary-adrenal axis. ACTH, adrenocorticotropic hormone; AVP, arginine vasopressin; BST, bed nucleus of the stria terminalis; CNS, central nervous system; CRH, corticotropin-releasing hormone; CRIF, corticotropin release–inhibiting factor; GABA, γ-aminobutyric acid; 5-HT, 5-hydroxytryptamine; IL-1, interleukin-1; MeA, medial amygdala; MePO, medial preoptic; NPY, neuropeptide Y; NTS, nucleus of the tractus solitarius; OVLT, organum vasculosum of the lamina terminalis; POMC, pro-opiomelanocortin.

gene is expressed eutopically in human ovary, uterus, and placenta,[404] although its function in these tissues is not known. Studies in rat placenta indicate that an alternative transcriptional start site 10 kilobases upstream from the hypothalamic promoter is utilized together with an alternatively spliced exon 1a.[405]

Growth Hormone–Releasing Hormone Receptor

The GHRH receptor is a member of a subfamily of G protein–coupled receptors that includes receptors for VIP, pituitary adenylyl cyclase–activating peptide, secretin, glucagon, glucagon-like peptide 1, calcitonin, parathyroid hormone or

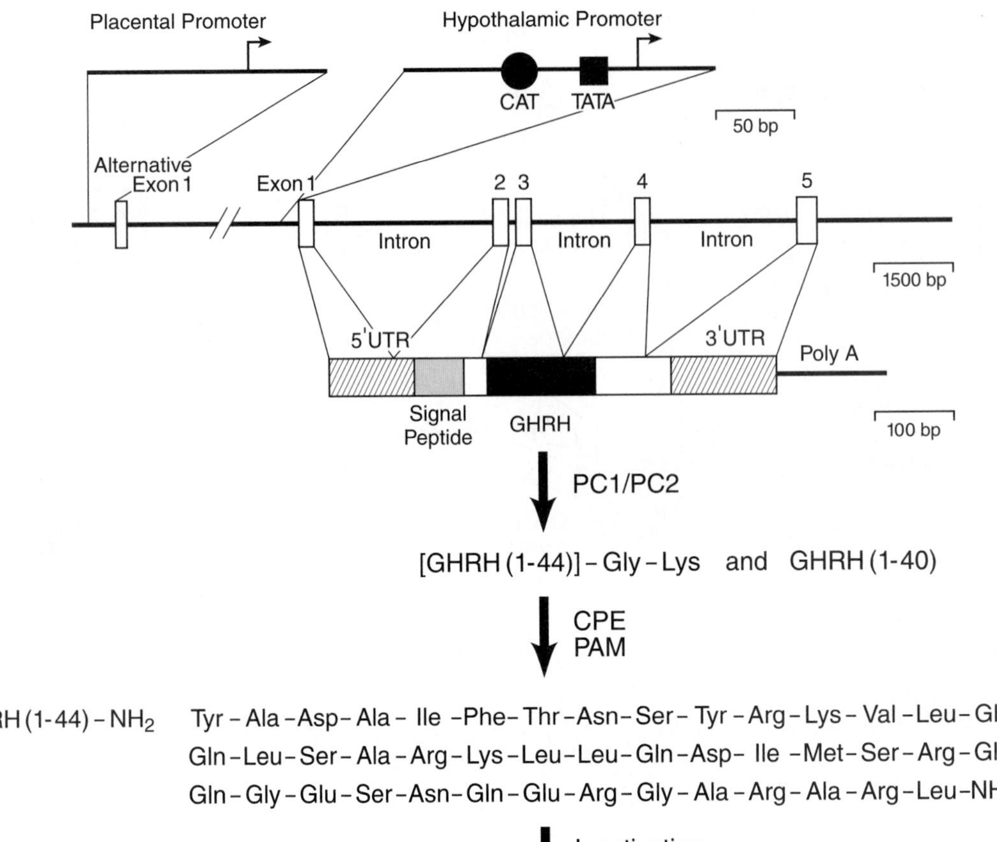

Figure 7–27. Diagram illustrating the genomic organization, messenger ribonucleic acid structure, and post-translational processing of the human growth hormone–releasing hormone (GHRH) prohormone. Few details are known about the transcriptional regulation of the GHRH gene except that distinct promoter sequences and alternative 5′ exons are utilized by hypothalamic neurons and extrahypothalamic tissues. All of the amino acid residues required for bioactive GHRH peptides are encoded by exon 3. An amino-terminal exopeptidase that cleaves the Tyr-Ala dipeptide is primarily responsible for the inactivation of GHRH peptides in extracellular compartments. CPE, carboxypeptidase E; PAM, peptidylglycine alpha-amidating monooxygenase; PC1/PC2, prohormone convertases 1 and 2; UTR, untranslated region. (Compiled from data of Mayo K, Cerelli GM, Lebo RV, et al. Gene encoding human growth hormone-releasing factor precursor: structure, sequence, and chromosomal assignment. Proc Natl Acad Sci USA 1985; 82:63–67; Frohman LA, Downs TR, Chomczynski P, Frohman MA. Growth hormone–releasing hormone: structure, gene expression and molecular heterogeneity. Acta Paediatr Scand [Suppl] 1990; 367:81–86; and González-Crespo S, Boronat A. Expression of the rat growth hormone–releasing hormone gene in placenta is directed by an alternative promoter. Proc Natl Acad Sci USA 1991; 88:8749–8753.)

parathyroid hormone–related peptide, and gastric inhibitory polypeptide.[406, 407] GHRH elevates intracellular cAMP by its receptor coupling to a stimulatory G protein (G_s), which activates adenylyl cyclase, increases intracellular free Ca^{2+}, releases preformed GH, and stimulates GH mRNA transcription and new GH synthesis (see Chapter 8).[408] GHRH also increases pituitary phosphatidylinositol turnover. Nonsense mutations in the human GHRH receptor gene are the cause of rare familial forms of GH deficiency[409, 410] and indicate that no other gene product can fully compensate for the specific receptor in pituitary.

Effects on the Pituitary and Mechanism of Action

Intravenous administration of GHRH to individuals with normal pituitaries caused a prompt, dose-related increase in serum GH that peaked between 15 and 45 minutes, followed by a return to basal levels by 90 to 120 minutes (Fig. 7–28).[411] A maximally stimulating dose of GHRH is approximately 1 μg/kg, but the response differs considerably between individuals and within the same individual tested on different occasions, presumably because of cosecretagogue and somatostatin tone that exists at the time of GHRH injection. Repeated bolus administration or sustained infusions of GHRH over several hours cause a modest decrease in the subsequent GH secretory response to acute GHRH administration. However, unlike the marked desensitization of the LHRH receptor and decline in circulating gonadotropins that occur in response to continuous LHRH exposure, pulsatile GH secretion and insulin-like growth factor I (IGF-I) production are maintained by constant GHRH in the human.[411] This response suggests the involvement of additional factors that mediate the intrinsic

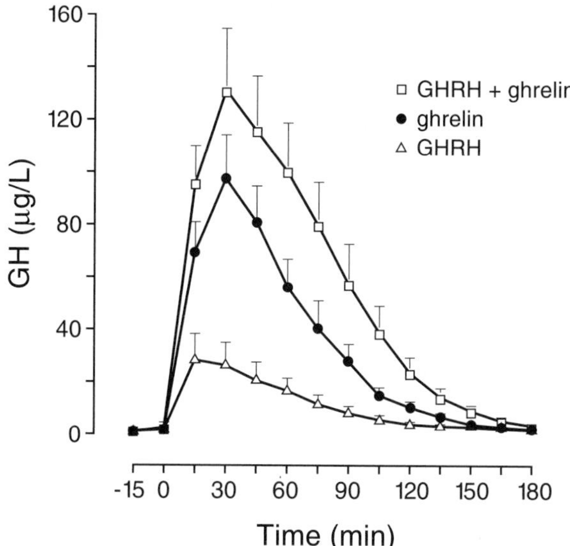

Figure 7–28. Response of normal men to growth hormone–releasing hormone (GHRH)(1–29) (1 μg/kg), ghrelin (1 μg/kg), or GHRH(1–29) and ghrelin administered by intravenous injection. Note the prompt release of GH, followed by a rather prolonged fall in hormone level in response to both secretagogues. Ghrelin alone was more efficacious than GHRH(1–29), and there was an additive effect from the two peptides administered simultaneously. (From Arvat E, Macario M, Di Vito L, et al. Endocrine activities of ghrelin, a natural growth hormone secretagogue (GHS), in humans: comparison and interactions with hexarelin, a nonnatural peptidyl GHS, and GH-releasing hormone. J Clin Endocrinol Metab 2001; 86:1169–1174.)

diurnal rhythm of GH, and these factors are addressed in the following sections.

The pituitary effects of a single injection of GHRH are almost completely specific for GH secretion, and there is minimal evidence for any interaction between GHRH and the other classical hypophyseotropic releasing hormones.[411] GHRH has no effect on gut peptide hormone secretion. The GH secretory response to GHRH is enhanced by estrogen administration, glucocorticoids, and starvation. Major factors known to blunt the response to GHRH in humans are somatostatin, obesity, and advancing age.

In addition to its role as a GH secretagogue, GHRH is a physiologically relevant growth factor for somatotrophs. Transgenic mice expressing a GHRH cDNA coupled to a suitable promoter developed diffuse somatotroph hyperplasia and eventually pituitary macroadenomas.[412, 413] The intracellular signal transduction pathways mediating the mitogenic action of GHRH are not known with certainty but probably involve an elevation of adenylyl cyclase activity. Several lines of evidence support this conclusion, including the association of activating mutations of the $G_s\alpha$ polypeptide in many human somatotroph adenomas.[414]

Extrapituitary Functions

GHRH has few known extrapituitary functions. The most important may be its activity as a sleep regulator. The administration of nocturnal GHRH boluses to normal men significantly increased the density of slow wave sleep, as also shown in other species.[415] Furthermore, there is a striking correlation between the age-related declines in slow wave sleep and daily integrated GH secretion in healthy men.[416] These and other data suggest that central GHRH secretion is under circadian entrainment and nocturnal elevations in GHRH pulse amplitude or frequency directly mediate sleep stage and sleep-induced increases in GH secretion.

GHRH has been reported to stimulate food intake in rats and sheep, and the effect is dependent on route of administration, time of administration, and macronutrient composition of the diet.[406] The neuropeptide's physiologic relevance to feeding in humans is unknown, although a study indicated that GHRH stimulated food intake in patients with anorexia nervosa but reduced it in patients with bulimia or in normal female control subjects.[417]

Growth Hormone–Releasing Peptides

In studies of the opioid control of GH secretion, several peptide analogues of met-enkephalin were found to be potent GH secretagogues. These include the GH-releasing peptide GHRP-6 (Fig. 7–29), hexarelin (His-D2MeTrp-Ala-Trp-DPhe-Lys-NH_2), and other more potent analogues including cyclic peptides and modified pentapeptides.[406, 418] Subsequently, a series of nonpeptidyl GHRP mimetics were synthesized with greater oral bioavailability, including the spiropiperidine MK-0677 and the shorter acting benzylpiperidine L-163,540 (see Fig. 7–29). Common to all these compounds, and the basis of their differentiation from GHRH analogues in pharmacologic activity screens, is their activation of phospholipase C and inositol 1,4,5-trisphosphate. This property was exploited in a cloning strategy that led to the identification of a G protein–coupled receptor GHS-R that is highly selective for the GH secretagogue class of ligands.[419] The GHS-R is unrelated to the GHRH receptor and is highly expressed in the anterior pituitary gland and multiple brain areas, including the medial basal hypothalamus, the hippocampus, and the mesencephalic nuclei that are centers of dopamine and serotonin production.

Peptidyl and nonpeptidyl GHSs are active when administered by intranasal and oral routes, are more potent on a weight basis than GHRH itself, are more effective in vivo than in vitro, synergize with coadministered GHRH and are almost ineffective in the absence of GHRH, and do not suppress somatostatin secretion.[406, 411] Prolonged infusions of GHRP amplify pulsatile GH secretion in normal men. GHRP administration, like that of GHRH, facilitates slow wave sleep. Patients with hypothalamic disease leading to GHRH deficiency have low or no response to hexarelin; similarly, pediatric patients with complete absence of the pituitary stalk have no GH secretory response to hexarelin.[420]

The potent biologic effects of GHRPs and the identification of the GHS-R suggested the existence of a natural ligand for the receptor that is involved in the physiologic regulation of GH secretion. A probable candidate for this ligand is the acylated peptide ghrelin, produced and secreted into the circulation from the stomach (see Fig. 7–29).[28] The effects of ghrelin on GH secretion in humans are identical to or more potent than those of the non-natural GHRPs (see Fig. 7–28).[421] In addition, ghrelin acutely increases circulating PRL, ACTH, cortisol, and aldosterone levels.[421] There is debate concerning the extent and localization of ghrelin expression in the brain that must be resolved before the implications of gastric-derived ghrelin in the regulation of pituitary hormone secretion are fully understood. A proposed role for ghrelin in appetite and regulation of food intake is discussed later in this chapter.

Clinical Applications

GHRH stimulates growth in children with intact pituitaries, but the optimal dosage, route, and frequency of administration, as well as possible usefulness by the nasal route, have not been determined. The availability of recombinant hGH (which re-

GHRP-6 His–$_D$Trp–Ala–Trp–$_D$Phe–Lys–NH_2

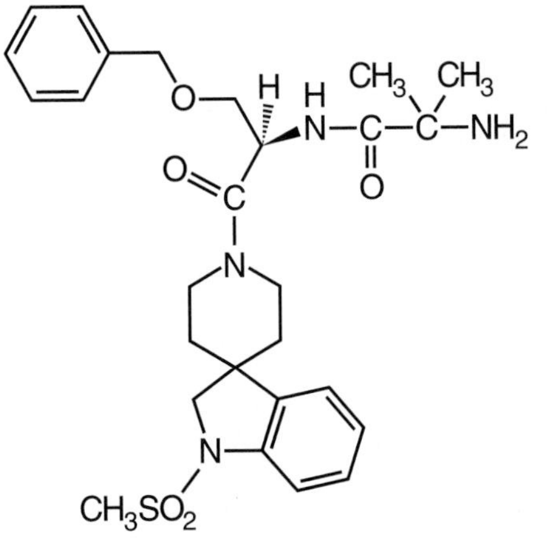

MK-0677

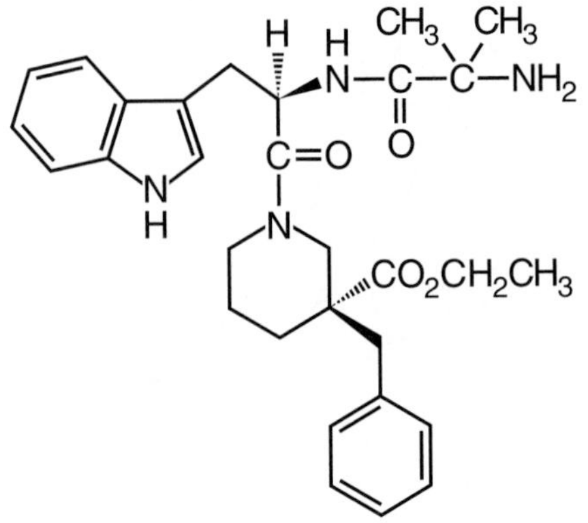

L-163,540

$O = C - (CH_2)_6 - CH_3$

ghrelin Gly – Ser – Ser – Phe – Leu – Ser – Pro – Glu – His – Gln – Arg – Val – Gln – Gln – Arg – Lys – Glu – Ser – Lys – Lys – Pro – Pro – Ala – Lys – Leu – Gln – Pro – Arg

Figure 7–29. Structure of a non-natural peptidyl (GHRP-6) and nonpeptidyl (MK-0677 and L-163,540) growth hormone secretagogues and a natural ligand (ghrelin) that all bind and activate the growth hormone secretagogue receptor. Ghrelin is an acylated 28-amino-acid peptide. The *O-n*-octanoylation at Ser3 is essential for biological activity and is a unique post-translational modification among the known neuropeptides. (Adapted from Smith RG, Feighner S, Prendergast K, et al. A new orphan receptor involved in pulsatile growth hormone release. Trends Endocrinol Metab 1999; 10:128–135; and Kojima M, Hosoda H, Date Y, et al. Ghrelin is a growth hormone–releasing acylated peptide from stomach. Nature 1999; 402:656–660.)

quires less frequent injections than GHRH) and the development of the more potent GHSs with improved oral bioavailability have reduced enthusiasm for the clinical use of GHRH or its analogues. GHRH is not useful for the differential diagnosis of hypothalamic and pituitary causes of GH deficiency in children. However, in adults a combined GHRH-GHRP challenge test may be ideal for the diagnosis of GH reserve. GH release in response to the combined secretagogues is not influenced by age, sex, or body mass index, and the test has a wider margin of safety than an insulin tolerance test.[422, 423]

The potential clinical applications of GHSs including MK-0677 are still being explored.[406, 418] An area of intense interest is the normal decline in GH secretion with age. GH administration in healthy older individuals has been associated with increased lean body mass, increased muscle strength, and decreased fat mass, although there is a high incidence of adverse side effects. The physiologic GH profile induced by MK-0677 may be better tolerated than GH injections. However, unlike treatment with GHRH, chronic administration of GHSs leads to significant desensitization of the GHS-R and attenuation of the GH response. The release of pituitary hormones other than GH may also limit the applicability of GHS therapy. Finally, apart from actions on GH secretion, both GHRH and GHSs are being investigated for the treatment of sleep disorders commonly associated with aging.

Neuroendocrine Regulation of Growth Hormone Secretion

GH secretion is regulated by hypothalamic GHRH and somatostatin interacting with circulating hormones and additional modulatory peptides at the level of both the pituitary and the hypothalamus (Fig. 7–30).[406, 411, 424] Additional background on somatostatin and its functions other than control of GH secretion are presented in a later section.

Feedback Control

Negative feedback control of GH release is mediated by GH itself and by IGF-I, which is synthesized in the liver under control of GH. Direct GH effects on the hypothalamus are produced by short-loop feedback, whereas those involving IGF-I and other circulating factors influenced by GH, including free fatty acids and glucose, are long-loop systems analo-

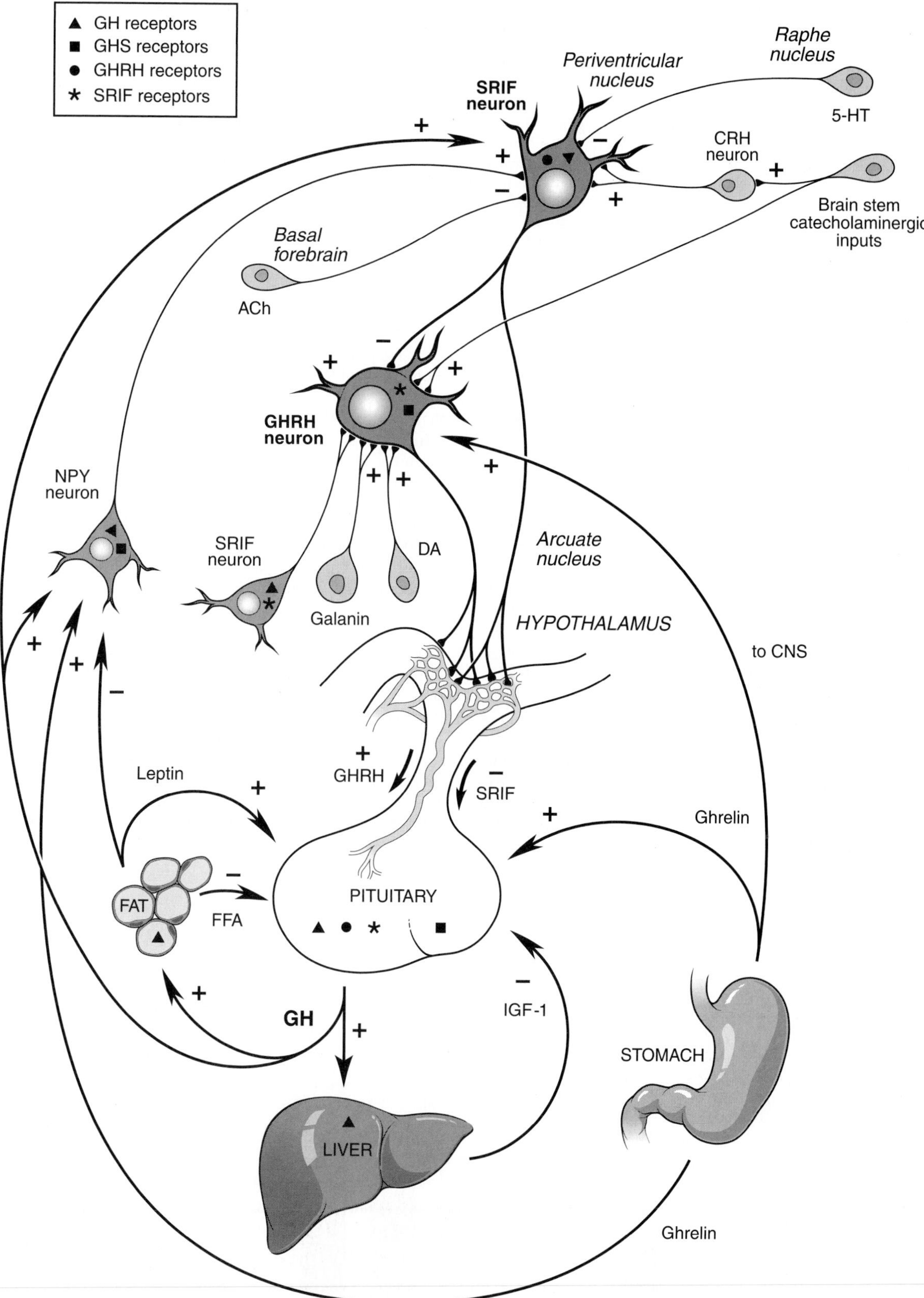

Figure 7–30. *See legend on following page*

Figure 7–30. *Continued.* Regulation of the hypothalamic-pituitary-growth hormone (GH) axis. GH secretion by the pituitary is stimulated by GH-releasing hormone (GHRH) and is inhibited by somatostatin (SRIF). Negative feedback control of GH secretion is exerted at the pituitary level by insulin-like growth factor I (IGF-I) and by free fatty acids (FFA). GH itself exerts a short-loop negative feedback by the activation of SRIF neurons in the hypothalamic periventricular nucleus. These SRIF neurons directly synapse on arcuate GHRH neurons and project to the median eminence. Neuropeptide Y (NPY) neurons in the arcuate nucleus also indirectly modulate GH secretion by integrating peripheral GH, leptin, and ghrelin signals and projecting to periventricular SRIF neurons. Ghrelin is secreted from the stomach and is a putative natural ligand for the GH secretagogue receptor that stimulates GH secretion at both the hypothalamic and pituitary levels. On the basis of indirect pharmacologic data, it appears that release of GHRH is stimulated by galanin, γ-aminobutyric acid (GABA), and α_2-adrenergic and dopaminergic stimuli and inhibited by somatostatin. Secretion of somatostatin is inhibited by acetylcholine (muscarinic receptors) and 5-HT (type 1D receptors), and increased by β_2-adrenergic stimuli and corticotropin-releasing hormone (CRH). ACh, acetylcholine; CNS, central nervous system; DA, dopamine.

gous to the pituitary-thyroid and pituitary-adrenal axes. Control of GH secretion thus includes two closed-loop systems (GH and IGF-I) and one open-loop regulatory system (neural).

Although most of the evidence for a direct role of GH in its own negative feedback has been derived from animals, an elegant study in normal men demonstrated that GH pretreatment blocks the subsequent GH secretory response to GHRH by a mechanism that is dependent on somatostatin.[425] The mechanism responsible for GH feedback through the hypothalamus has been largely elucidated in rodent models. GH receptors are selectively expressed on somatostatin neurons in the hypothalamic periventricular nucleus and on NPY neurons in the arcuate nucleus. C-fos gene expression is acutely elevated in both populations of GH receptor–positive neurons by GH administration, indicating an activation of hypothalamic circuitry that includes these neurons. Similarly, GHRH neurons in the arcuate nucleus are acutely activated by MK-0677 because of their selective expression of the GHS-R. Zheng and colleagues[426] showed in the latter group of neurons that c-fos induction after MK-0677 administration was blocked by pretreatment of mice with GH (Fig. 7–31). The effect must be indirect because there are no GH receptors on GHRH neurons. However, there are type 2 somatostatin receptors expressed on GHRH neurons, and the somatostatin analogue octreotide also significantly blocked c-fos activation in the arcuate nucleus by MK-0677. The inhibitory effects of either GH or octreotide pretreatment were abolished in knockout mice lacking the specific somatostatin receptor (see Fig. 7–31). Together with data from many other experiments, these results strongly support a model of GH negative feedback regulation that involves the primary activation of periventricular somatostatin neurons by GH. These tuberoinfundibular neurons then inhibit GH secretion directly by release of somatostatin in the median eminence, but they also indirectly inhibit GH secretion by way of collateral axonal projections to the arcuate nucleus that synapse on and inhibit GHRH neurons (see Fig. 7–30). It is probable from evidence in rodents that NPY and galanin also play a part in the short-loop feedback of GH secretion, but a definitive mechanism in humans is not yet established.

IGF-I has a major inhibitory action on GH secretion at the level of the pituitary gland.[406] IGF-I receptors are expressed on human somatotroph adenoma cells and inhibit both spontaneous and GHRH-stimulated GH release. In addition, gene expression of both GH and the pituitary-specific transcription factor Pit-1 is inhibited by IGF-I. Conflicting data among species suggest that circulating IGF-I may also regulate GH secretion by actions within the brain. The feedback effects of IGF-I account for the fact that in conditions in which circulating levels of IGF-I are low, such as anorexia nervosa, protein-

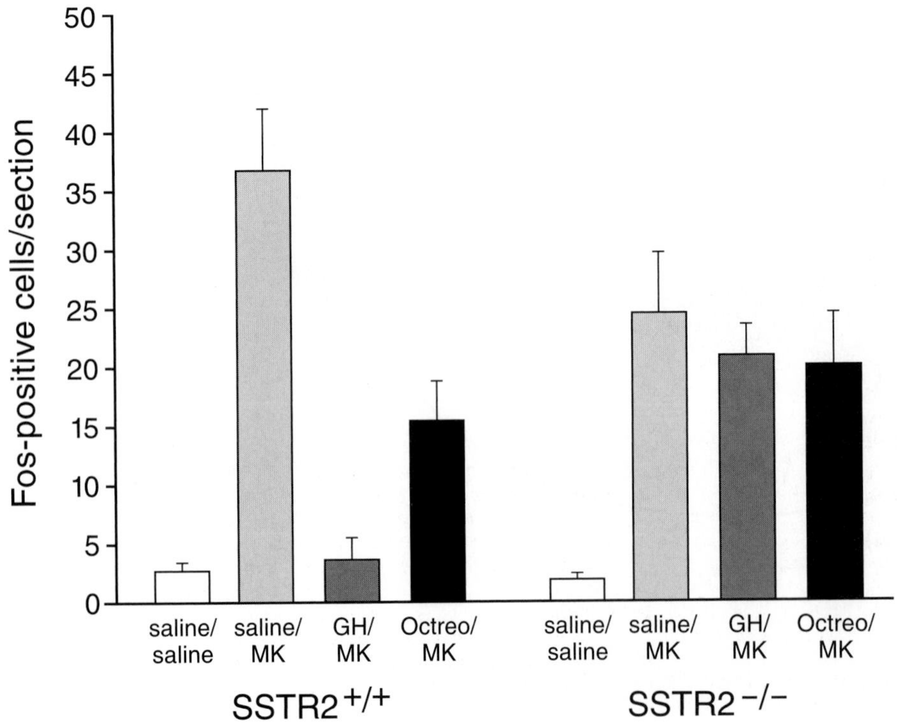

Figure 7–31. Somatostatin and the somatostatin receptor 2 subtype are involved in the short-loop inhibitory feedback of growth hormone (GH) on arcuate neurons. Activation of neurons in the arcuate nucleus was determined by the quantification of immunoreactive c-Fos–positive cells after administration of the growth hormone secretagogue MK-0677 (MK). Preliminary treatment of wild-type mice ($SSTR2^{+/+}$) with either GH or the somatostatin analogue octreotide (Octreo) significantly attenuated the neuronal activation by MK-0677. In contrast, GH and octreotide had no effect on MK-0677 neuronal activation in somatostatin receptor 2–deficient mice ($SSTR2^{-/-}$). (Adapted from Zheng H, Bailey A, Jian M-H, et al. Somatostatin receptor subtype 2 knockout mice are refractory to growth hormone-negative feedback on arcuate neurons. Mol Endocrinol 1997; 11: 1709–1717.)

calorie starvation,[427] and Laron dwarfism (the result of a defect in the GH receptor), serum GH levels are elevated.

Neural Control

The predominant hypothalamic influence on GH release is stimulatory, and section of the pituitary stalk or lesions of the basal hypothalamus cause reduction of basal and induced GH release. When the somatostatinergic component is inactivated (e.g., by antisomatostatin antibody injection in rats), basal GH levels and GH responses to the usual provocative stimuli are enhanced.

GHRH-containing nerve fibers that terminate adjacent to portal vessels in the external zone of the median eminence arise principally from within, above, and lateral to the infundibular nucleus in human hypothalamus, corresponding to rodent arcuate and ventromedial nuclei.[428] Perikarya of the tuberoinfundibular somatostatin neurons are located almost completely in the medial periventricular nucleus and parvocellular component of the anterior paraventricular nucleus. Neuroanatomic and functional evidence suggests a bidirectional synaptic interaction between the two peptidergic systems.[406]

Multiple extrahypothalamic brain regions provide efferent connections to the hypothalamus and regulate GHRH and somatostatin neuronal activity (Fig. 7–32; see Fig. 7–30). Somatosensory and affective information is integrated and filtered through the amygdaloid complex. The basolateral amygdala provides an excitatory input to the hypothalamus, and the central extended amygdala, which includes the central and medial nuclei of the amygdala together with the bed nucleus of the stria terminalis, provides a GABAergic inhibitory input. Many intrinsic neurons of the hypothalamus also release GABA, often with a peptide cotransmitter. Excitatory cholinergic fibers arise to a small extent from forebrain projection nuclei but mostly from hypothalamic cholinergic interneurons, which densely innervate the external zone of the median eminence. Similarly, the origin of dopaminergic and histaminergic neurons is local with their cell bodies located in the hypothalamic arcuate and tuberomammillary bodies, respectively. Two important ascending pathways to the medial basal hypothalamus regulate GH secretion and originate from serotoninergic neurons in the raphe nuclei and adrenergic neurons in the nucleus of the tractus solitarius and ventral lateral nucleus of the medulla.

Both GHRH and somatostatin neurons express presynaptic and postsynaptic receptors for multiple neurotransmitters and peptides (Table 7–6). The α_2-adrenoreceptor agonist clonidine reliably stimulates GH release, and for this reason a clonidine test was a standard diagnostic tool in pediatric endocrinology. The stimulatory effect is blocked by the specific α_2-antagonist yohimbine and appears to involve a dual mechanism of action, inhibition of somatostatin neurons and activation of GHRH neurons. In addition, partial attenuation of the effects of clonidine by mixed 5-hydroxytryptamine type 1 and type 2 antagonists suggests that some of the relevant α_2-receptors are located presynaptically on serotoninergic nerve terminals and increase serotonin release. Both norepinephrine and epinephrine play physiologic roles in the adrenergic stimulation of GH secretion. The α_1-agonists have no effect on GH secretion in humans, but β_2-agonists such as the bronchodilator salbutamol inhibit GH secretion by stimulating the release of somatostatin from nerve terminals in the median eminence. These effects are blocked by propranolol, a nonspecific β-antagonist. Dopamine generally has a net effect to stimulate GH secretion, but the mechanism is not clear because of multiple dopamine receptor subtypes and the apparent activation of both GHRH and somatostatin neurons.

Serotonin's effect on GH release in humans was difficult to decipher because of the large number of receptor subtypes. However, clinical studies with the receptor-selective agonist

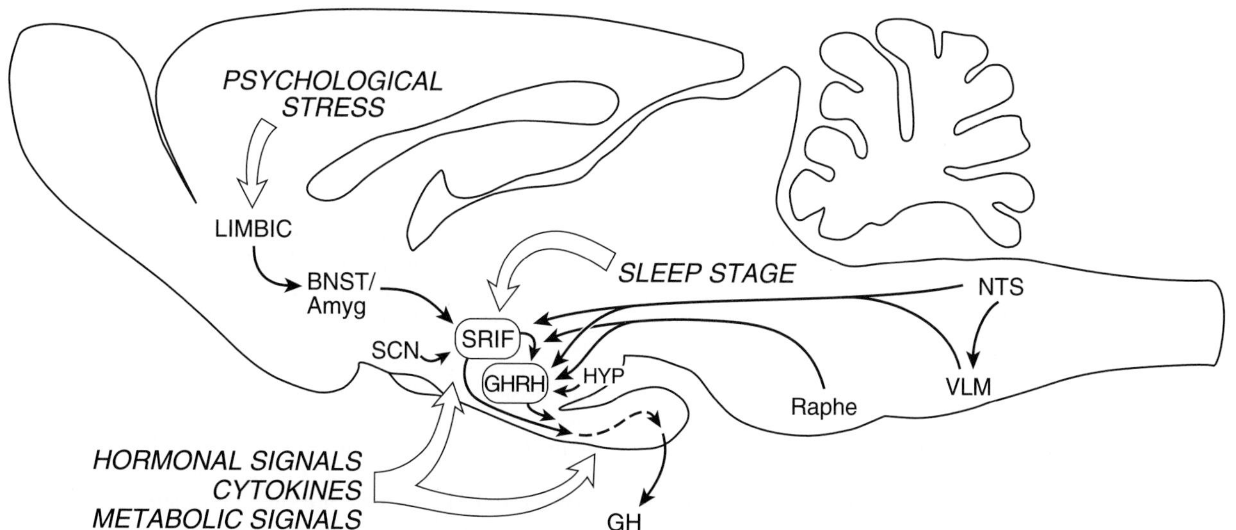

Figure 7–32. Neural pathways involved in growth hormone (GH) regulation. This diagram illustrates the varied pathways by which impulses from the limbic system and brain stem ultimately impinge on the hypothalamic periventricular and arcuate nuclei to stimulate GH release through the mediation of somatostatin (SRIF) and growth hormone–releasing hormone (GHRH). Psychological stress modulates hypothalamic function indirectly through the bed nucleus of the stria terminalis (BNST) and amygdalar complex (Amyg). Circadian rhythms are entrained in part by projections from the suprachiasmatic nucleus (SCN). Complex reciprocal interactions between sleep stage and GHRH release involve cortex and subcortical nuclei, but the detailed mechanisms are not known. Dopaminergic and histaminergic input are from neurons located in the arcuate and mammillary nuclei, respectively, of the hypothalamus (HYP). Ascending catecholaminergic projections arise in both the nucleus of the tractus solitarius (NTS) and ventral lateral medulla (VLM). Serotoninergic (5-HT) afferents are from the raphe nuclei. In addition to these neural pathways, a variety of peripheral hormonal and metabolic signals and cytokines influence GH secretion by actions within the medial basal hypothalamus and pituitary gland.

Table 7–6. Factors That Change Growth Hormone Secretion in Humans

Physiologic	Hormones and Neurotransmitters	Pathologic
	Stimulatory Factors	
Episodic, spontaneous release	Insulin hypoglycemia	Acromegaly
Exercise	2-Deoxyglucose	TRH
Stress	Amino acid infusions	LHRH
Physical	Arginine, lysine	Glucose
Psychological	Neuropeptides	Arginine
Slow wave sleep	GHRH	Interleukins 1, 2, 6
Postprandial glucose decline	Ghrelin	Protein depletion
Fasting	Galanin	Starvation
	Opioids (μ-receptors)	Anorexia nervosa
	Melatonin	Renal failure
	Classical neurotransmitters	Liver cirrhosis
	α_2-Adrenergic agonists	Type 1 diabetes mellitus
	β-Adrenergic antagonists	
	M1-cholinergic agonists	
	1D-serotonin agonists	
	H1-histamine agonists	
	GABA (basal levels)	
	Dopamine (? receptor)	
	Estrogen	
	Testosterone	
	Glucocorticoids (acute)	
	Inhibitory Factors*	
Postprandial hyperglycemia	Glucose infusion	Acromegaly
Elevated free fatty acids	Neuropeptides	L-Dopa
Elevated GH levels	Somatostatin	D2R DA agonists
Elevated IGF-I (pituitary)	Calcitonin	Phentolamine
Rapid eye movement (REM) sleep	Neuropeptide Y (NPY)†	Galanin
Senesence, aging	Corticotropin-releasing hormone (CRH)†	Obesity
	Classical neurotransmitters	Hypothyroidism
	$\alpha_{1/2}$-Adrenergic antagonists	Hyperthyroidism
	β_2-Adrenergic agonists	
	H1-histamine antagonists	
	Serotonin antagonist	
	Nicotinic cholinergic agonists	
	Glucocortioids (chronic)	

*In many instances, the inhibition can be demonstrated only as a suppression of GH release induced by a pharmacologic stimulus.

†The inhibitory actions of NPY and CRH on GH secretion are firmly established in the rodent and are secondary to increased somatostatin tone. Contradictory evidence exists in the human for both peptides and further studies are required.

TRH, thyrotropin-releasing hormone; LHRH, luteinizing hormone–releasing hormone; GHRH, growth hormone–releasing hormone; DA, dopamine; IGF-I, insulin-like growth factor I.

sumatriptan clearly implicated the 5-hydroxytryptamine 1D receptor subtype in the stimulation of basal GH levels.[429] The drug also potentiates the effect of a maximal dose of GHRH, suggesting the recurring theme of GH disinhibition by inhibition of hypothalamic somatostatin neurons in its mechanism of action. Histaminergic pathways acting through H1 receptors play only a minor, conditional stimulatory role in GH secretion in humans.

Acetylcholine appears to be an important physiologic regulator of GH secretion.[430] Blockade of acetylcholinergic muscarinic receptors reduces or abolishes GH secretory responses to GHRH, glucagon and arginine, morphine, and exercise. In contrast, drugs that potentiate cholinergic transmission increase basal GH levels and enhance the GH response to GHRH in normal individuals or in subjects with obesity or Cushing's disease. In vitro acetylcholine inhibits somatostatin release from hypothalamic fragments, and acetylcholine can act directly on the pituitary to inhibit GH release. There may even be a paracrine cholinergic control system within the pituitary. However, the sum of evidence suggests that the primary mechanism of action of M1 agonists is inhibition of somatostatin neuronal activity or the release of peptide from somatostatinergic terminals. Short-term cholinergic blockade with the M1 muscarinic receptor antagonist pirenzepine reduced the GH excess of patients with poorly controlled diabetes mellitus.[881] However, in the long term, cholinergic blockade did not prevent complications associated with the hypersomatotropic state.

Many neuropeptides in addition to GHRH and somatostatin are involved in the modulation of GH secretion in humans (see Table 7–6).[406, 411] Among these, the evidence is most compelling for a stimulatory role of galanin acting in the human hypothalamus by a GHRH-dependent mechanism.[431] Many GHRH neurons are immunopositive for galanin as well as neurotensin and tyrosine hydroxylase. Galanin's actions may be explained, in part, by presynaptic facilitation of catecholamine release from nerve terminals and subsequent direct adrenergic stimulation of GHRH release.[432] Opioid peptides also stimulate GH release, probably by activation of GHRH neurons, but under normal circumstances endogenous opioid tone in the hypothalamus is presumed to be low because opioid antagonists have little acute effect on GH secretion.

A larger number of neuropeptides are known or suspected to inhibit GH secretion in humans, at least under certain circumstances.[411] The list includes NPY, CRH, calcitonin, oxytocin, neurotensin, VIP, and TRH. Inhibitory actions of NPY are well established in the rat. The effect on GH secretion is secondary to stimulation of somatostatin neurons and is of particular interest because of the presumed role in GH auto-feedback (discussed earlier) and the integration of GH secretion with regulation of energy intake and expenditure (discussed in a later section). Finally, TRH has the well-established paradoxical effect of increasing GH secretion in patients with acromegaly, type 1 diabetes mellitus, hypothyroidism, or hepatic and renal failure.

Factors Influencing Secretion of Growth Hormone

Human Growth Hormone Rhythms

The unraveling of rhythmic GH secretion has relied on a combination of technical innovations in sampling and GH assay, and sophisticated mathematical modeling including deconvolution analysis and the calculation of approximate entropy as a measure of orderliness or regularity in minute-to-minute secretory patterns.[411] At least three distinct categories of GH rhythms, which differ markedly in their time scales, can be considered here. The daily GH secretion rate varies over two orders of magnitude from a maximum of nearly 2.0 mg/day in late puberty to a minimum of 20 μg/day in older or obese adults. The neonatal period is characterized by markedly amplified GH secretory bursts followed by a prepubertal decade of stable, moderate GH secretion of 200 to 600 μg/day. There is a marked increase in daily GH secretion during puberty that is accompanied by a commensurate rise in plasma IGF-I to levels that constitute a state of physiologic hypersomatotropism. This pubertal increase in GH secretion is due to increased GH mass per secretory burst and not to increased pulse frequency. Although the changes are clearly related to the increases in gonadal steroid hormones and can be mimicked by administration of estrogen or testosterone to hypogonadal children, the underlying neuroendocrine mechanisms are not fully understood. One hypothesis is that decreased sensitivity of the hypothalamic-pituitary axis to negative feedback of GH and IGF-I leads to increased GHRH release and action. Young adults have a return of daily GH secretion to prepubertal levels despite continued gonadal steroid elevation. The so-called somatopause is defined by an exponential decline in GH secretory rate with a half-life of 7 years starting in the third decade of life.

GH secretion in young adults exhibits a true circadian rhythm over a 24-hour period, characterized by a greater nocturnal secretory mass that is independent of sleep onset.[433] However, as discussed earlier, GH release is further facilitated when slow wave sleep coincides with the normal circadian peak. Under basal conditions GH levels are low most of the time, with an ultradian rhythm of about 10 (men) or 20 (women) secretory pulses per 24 hours as calculated by deconvolution analysis.[434] Both sexes have an increased pulse frequency during the nighttime hours, but the fraction of total daily GH secretion associated with the nocturnal pulses is much greater in men. Overall, women have more continuous GH secretion and more frequent GH pulses that are of more uniform size than men.[434] A complementary study using approximate entropy analysis concluded that the nonpulsatile regularity of GH secretion is also significantly different in men and women.[435] These sexually dimorphic patterns in the human are actually quite similar to those in the rat, although the sex differences are not as extreme in humans.[411, 435]

The neuroendocrine basis for sex differences in the ultradian rhythm of GH secretion is not fully understood. Gonadal sex steroids play both an organizational role during development of the hypothalamus and an activational role in the adult, regulating expression of the genes for many of the peptides and receptors central to GH regulation.[406, 411] In the human, unlike the rat, the hypothalamic actions of testosterone appear to be predominantly due to its aromatization to 17β-estradiol and interaction with estrogen receptors. Hypothalamic somatostatin appears to play a more prominent role in men than in women in the regulation of pulsatile GH secretion, and this difference is postulated to be a key factor in producing the sexual dimorphism.[434, 436, 437]

External and Metabolic Signals

The various peripheral signals that modulate GH secretion in humans are summarized in Table 7–6 (also see Figs. 7–30 and 7–32). Of particular importance are factors related to energy intake and metabolism because they provide a common signal between the peripheral tissues and hypothalamic centers regulating nonendocrine homeostatic pathways in addition to the classical hypophyseotropic neurons. It is also in this complex arena that species-specific regulatory responses are particularly prominent, making extrapolations between rodent experimental models and human GH regulation less reliable.[406, 411]

Important triggers of GH release include the normal decrease in blood glucose level after intake of a carbohydrate-rich meal, absolute hypoglycemia, exercise, physical and emotional stress, and high intake of protein (mediated by amino acids). Some of the pathologic causes of elevated GH represent extremes of these physiologic signals and include protein-calorie starvation, anorexia nervosa, liver failure, and type 1 diabetes mellitus. A critical concept is that many of these GH triggers work through the same final common mechanism of somatostatin withdrawal and consequent disinhibition of GH secretion. In contrast, postprandial hyperglycemia, glucose infusion, elevated plasma free fatty acids, type 2 diabetes mellitus (with obesity and insulin resistance), and obesity are all associated with inhibition of GH secretion. The role of leptin in mediating either increases or decreases in GH release is complicated by its multiple sites of action and coexistent secretory environment. Similarly, other members of the cytokine family including IL-1, IL-2, IL-6, and endotoxin have been inconsistently shown to stimulate GH in humans.

The actions of steroid hormones on GH secretion are complex because of their multiple loci of action within the proximal hypothalamic-pituitary components in addition to secondary effects on other neural and endocrine systems. Glucocorticoids in particular produce opposite responses that are dependent on the chronicity of administration. Moreover, glucocorticoid effects follow an inverted U-shaped dose-response curve. Both low and high glucocorticoid levels reduce GH secretion, the former because of decreased GH gene expression and somatotroph responsiveness to GHRH and the latter because of increased hypothalamic somatostatin tone and decreased GHRH. Similarly, physiologic levels of thyroid hormones are necessary to maintain GH secretion and promote GH gene expression. Excessive thyroid hormone is also inhibitory to the GH axis, and the mechanism is speculated to be a combination of increased hypothalamic somatostatin tone, GHRH deficiency, and suppressed pituitary GH production.

Somatostatin

Chemistry and Evolution

A factor that potently inhibited GH release from pituitary in vitro was unexpectedly identified during early efforts to isolate GHRH from hypothalamic extracts.[438] Somatostatin, the peptide responsible for this inhibition of GH secretion and the inhibition of insulin secretion by a pancreatic islet extract, was eventually isolated from hypothalamus and sequenced by Bra-

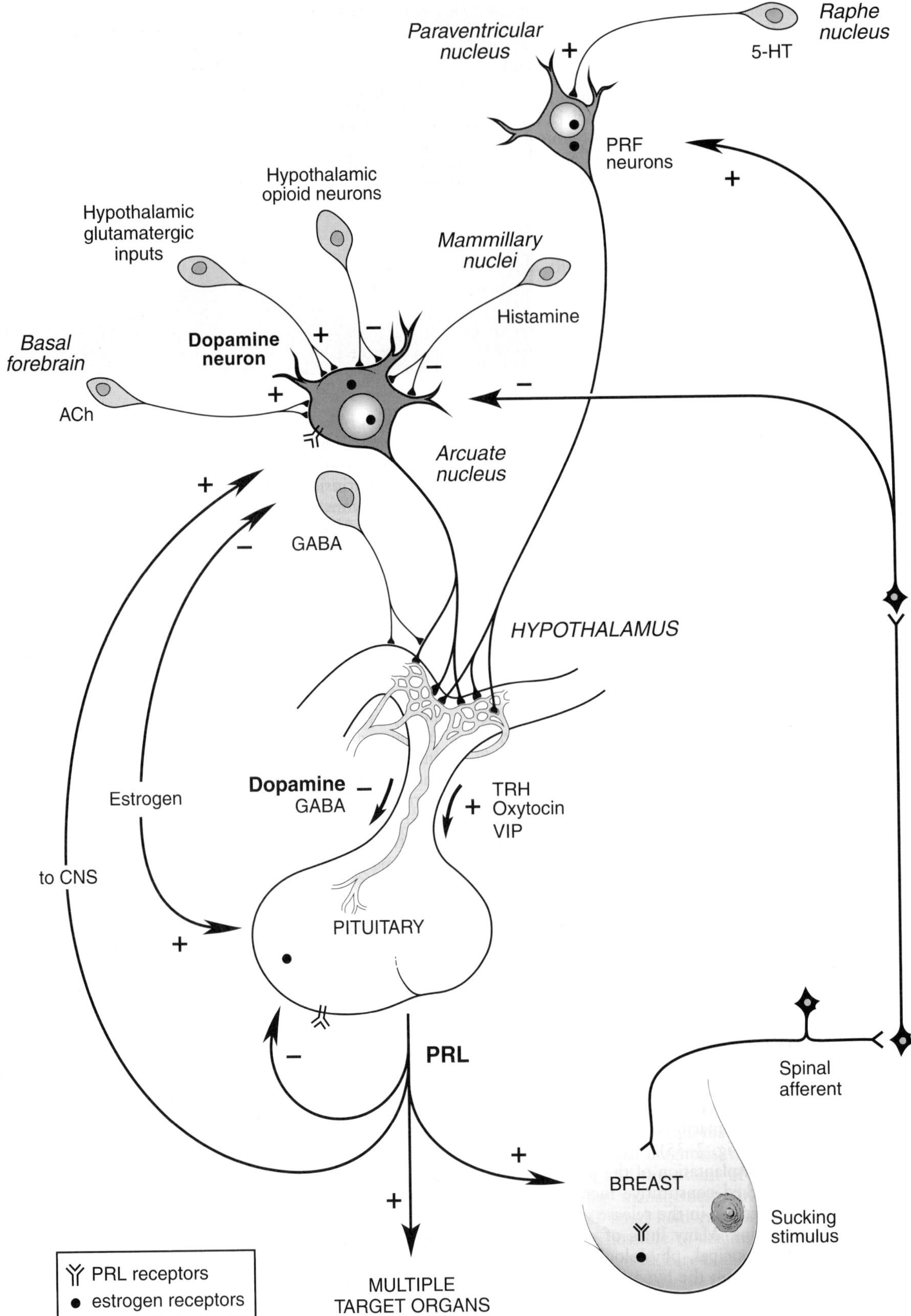

Figure 7–35. *See legend on opposite page*

Figure 7–35. *Continued.* Regulation of the hypothalamic-pituitary-prolactin (PRL) axis. The predominant effect of the hypothalamus is inhibitory, an effect mediated principally by dopamine secreted by the tuberohypophyseal dopaminergic neuron system. The dopamine neurons are stimulated by acetylcholine (ACh) and glutamate and inhibited by histamine and opioid peptides. One or more prolactin releasing factors (PRFs) probably mediate acute release of PRL as in suckling and stress. There are several candidate PRFs, including thyrotropin-releasing hormone (TRH), vasoactive intestinal polypeptide (VIP), and oxytocin. PRF neurons are activated by serotonin (5-HT). Estrogen sensitizes the pituitary to release PRL, which feeds back on the pituitary to regulate its own secretion (ultrashort-loop feedback) and also influences gonadotropin secretion by suppressing the release of luteinizing hormone–releasing hormone (LHRH). Short-loop feedback is also mediated indirectly by prolactin receptor regulation of hypothalamic dopamine synthesis, secretion, and turnover. CNS, central nervous system; DA, dopamine; GABA, γ-aminobutyric acid.

lation of Ets family transcription factors. Ets factors are important for the stimulatory responses of TRH, insulin, and epidermal growth factor on PRL expression[477–480] and they interact cooperatively with the pituitary-specific POU protein Pit1, which is essential for cAMP-mediated PRL gene expression.[481]

The second messenger pathways used by the D2 receptor to inhibit lactotroph cell division are also unsettled. A study using primary pituitary cultures from rats demonstrated that forskolin treatment, which activates protein kinase A and elevates intracellular cAMP, or insulin treatment, which activates a potent receptor tyrosine kinase, were both effective mitogenic stimuli for lactotrophs. Bromocriptine competitively antagonized the proliferative response caused by elevated cAMP. Furthermore, inhibition of MAPK signaling by PD98059 markedly suppressed the mitogenic action of both insulin and forskolin, suggesting an interaction of MAPK and protein kinase A signaling.[482]

Another study used immortalized mammosomatotroph tumor cells that were transfected with a D2 receptor expression vector and concluded that stimulation of a phosphotyrosine phosphatase activity was an important component of dopamine's antiproliferative action.[483] Therefore, it is clear that dopamine actions on lactotrophs involve multiple different intracellular signaling pathways linked to activation of the D2 receptor, but different combinations of these pathways are relevant for the inhibitory effects on PRL secretion, PRL gene transcription, and lactotroph proliferation.

The other major action of dopamine in the pituitary is the inhibition of hormone secretion from the POMC-expressing cells of the intermediate lobe, although, as noted earlier, the adult human differs from most other mammals in the rudimentary nature of this lobe.[57] THDA and PHDA axon terminals provide a dense plexus of synaptic-like contacts on melanotrophs. Dopamine release from these terminals is inversely correlated with serum MSH levels[484] and also regulates POMC gene expression and melanotroph proliferation.[485]

Other hypothalamic factors probably play a role secondary to that of dopamine as additional PIFs.[464] The primary reason to conjecture the existence of these PIFs is the frequent inconsistency between portal dopamine levels and circulating PRL in different rat models. GABA is the strongest candidate and most likely acts through $GABA_A$ inotropic receptors in the anterior pituitary. Melanotrophs, like lactotrophs, are inhibited by both dopamine and GABA but with the principal involvement of G protein–coupled, metabotropic $GABA_B$ receptors.[486] Because basal dopamine tone is high, the measurable inhibitory effects of GABA on PRL release are generally small under normal circumstances. Other putative PIFs include somatostatin and calcitonin.

Prolactin-Releasing Factors

Although tonic suppression of PRL release by dopamine is the dominant effect of the hypothalamus on PRL secretion, a number of stimuli promote PRL release, not merely by disinhibition of PIF effects but by causing release of one or more neurohormonal PRFs (see Fig. 7–35). The most important of the putative PRFs are TRH, oxytocin, and VIP, but vasopressin, angiotensin II, NPY, galanin, substance P, bombesin-like peptides, and neurotensin can also trigger PRL release under different physiologic circumstances.[464] TRH was discussed in a previous section of this chapter (see Fig. 7–15). In humans there is an imperfect correlation between pulsatile PRL and TSH release, suggesting that TRH cannot be the sole physiologic PRF under basal conditions.[487]

Like TRH, oxytocin, vasopressin, and VIP fulfill all the basic criteria for a PRF. They are produced in paraventricular hypothalamic neurons that project to the median eminence. Concentrations of the hormones in portal blood are much higher than in the peripheral circulation and are sufficient to stimulate PRL secretion in vitro.[488–490] Moreover, there are functional receptors for each of the neurohormones in the anterior pituitary gland and either pharmacologic antagonism or passive immunization against each hormone can decrease PRL secretion, at least under certain cirumstances.[491–495]

Vasopressin is released during stress and hypovolemic shock, as is PRL, suggesting a specific role for vasopressin as a PRF in these contexts. Similarly, another candidate PRF, peptide histidine isoleucine, may be specifically involved in the secretion of PRL in response to stress. Peptide histidine isoleucine and the human homologue PHM are structurally related to VIP and synthesized from the same prohormone precursor in their respective species.[496] Both peptides are coexpressed with CRH in parvocellular paraventricular neurons and presumably released by the same stimuli that cause release of CRH into the hypophyseal-portal vessels.[497]

There is evidence suggesting that dopamine itself may also act as a PRF, in contrast to its predominant function as a PIF.[464] At concentrations three orders of magnitude lower than that associated with maximal inhibition of PRL secretion, dopamine was shown to be capable of stimulating secretion from primary cultures of rat pituitary cells.[498] These studies were extended to an in vivo model by Arey and colleagues,[499] who demonstrated that low-dose dopamine infusion in cannulated rats caused a further increase in circulating PRL above the already elevated baseline produced by pharmacologic blockade of endogenous dopamine biosynthesis. The physiologic relevance of these findings to humans has yet to be established.

Finally, reports of "new" PRFs continue to be published. Much excitement was generated by the isolation of a peptide from bovine hypothalamus named prolactin-releasing peptide (PrRP).[500] PrRP binds with high affinity to an orphan G protein–coupled receptor (hGR3/GPR10) expressed specifically in human pituitary and selectively stimulates PRL release from rat pituitary cells with a potency similar to that of TRH. However, PrRP is expressed predominantly in a subpopulation of noradrenergic neurons in the medulla and a small population of non-neurosecretory neurons of the hypothalamus, raising the serious question of whether PrRP reaches the anterior pituitary and actually causes PRL secretion.[501] Subsequent studies found no direct evidence for release of PrRP in the arcuate nucleus–median eminence, further suggesting that the peptide is not a hypophyseotropic neurohormone.[502] However, PrRP probably does function as a neuromodulator within the

CNS at sites expressing its receptor and may be involved in the neural circuitry mediating satiety.[503]

Intrapituitary Regulation of Prolactin Secretion

Probably more than that of any other pituitary hormone, the secretion of PRL is regulated by autocrine-paracrine factors within the anterior lobe and by neurointermediate lobe factors that gain access to venous sinusoids of the anterior lobe by way of the short portal vessels. The wealth of local regulatory mechanisms within the anterior lobe has been reviewed extensively[464, 504, 505] and is also discussed in Chapter 8. Galanin, VIP, endothelin-like peptides, angiotensin II, epidermal growth factor, basic fibroblast growth factor, LHRH, and the cytokine IL-6 are among the most potent local stimulators of PRL secretion. Locally produced inhibitors include PRL itself, acetylcholine, transforming growth factor β, and calcitonin. Although none of these stimulatory or inhibitory factors plays a dominant role in the regulation of lactotroph function and much of the research in this area has not been directly confirmed in human pituitary, it seems apparent that the local milieu of autocrine and paracrine factors plays an essential modulatory role in determining the responsiveness of lactotrophs to hypothalamic factors in different physiologic states.

As noted earlier, a proportion of the inhibitory dopamine tone to the anterior lobe lactotrophs is derived from the neurointermediate lobe. It was therefore unanticipated that surgical removal of this structure in rats would block suckling-induced PRL release over the moderate basal increase attributed to partial dopamine disinhibition.[506] Further studies showed that exposure of the anterior pituitary to intermediate lobe extracts (devoid of VIP, vasopressin, and other known PRFs) stimulated PRL secretion. At least two kinds of PRF activity have been isolated from intermediate lobe tumors of the mouse, but the specific molecules involved have yet to be identified.[507] Other researchers have suggested a more passive role for the neurointermediate lobe in the regulation of PRL secretion. Melanotroph-derived *N*-acetylated MSH appears to act as a lactotroph responsiveness factor by recruiting nonsecretory cells to an active state and sensitizing secreting lactotrophs to the actions of other direct PRFs.[508] However, the relevance of the neurointermediate lobe for PRL regulation in primates (including humans) is not clear because of its attenuated structure in these species.

Neuroendocrine Regulation of Prolactin Secretion

Secretion of PRL, like that of other anterior pituitary hormones, is regulated by hormonal feedback and neural influences from the hypothalamus.[464, 465, 509] Feedback is exerted by PRL itself at the level of the hypothalamus. PRL secretion is regulated by many physiologic states including the estrous and menstrual cycles, pregnancy, and lactation. Furthermore, PRL is stimulated by several exteroceptive stimuli including light, ultrasonic vocalization of pups, olfactory cues, and various modalities of stress. Expression and secretion of PRL are also influenced strongly by estrogens at the level of both the lactotrophs and TIDA neurons[510] (see Fig. 7–35) and by paracrine regulators within the pituitary such as galanin and VIP.

Feedback Control

Negative feedback control of PRL secretion is mediated by a unique short-loop mechanism within the hypothalamus.[511] PRL activates PRL receptors, which are expressed on all three subpopulations of A12 and A14 dopamine neurons, leading to increased tyrosine hydroxylase expression and dopamine synthesis and release.[512, 513] Ames dwarf mice that secrete virtually no PRL, GH, or TSH have decreased numbers of arcuate dopamine neurons and this hypoplasia can be reversed by neonatal administration of PRL, suggesting a trophic action on the neurons.[514] However, another mouse model of isolated PRL deficiency generated by gene targeting appears to have normal numbers of hypofunctioning dopamine neurons secondary to the loss of PRL feedback.[515]

Neural Control

Lactotrophs have spontaneously high secretory activity, and therefore the predominant effect of the hypothalamus on PRL secretion is tonic suppression, which is mediated by regulatory hormones synthesized by tuberohypophyseal neurons. Secretory bursts of PRL are caused by the acute withdrawal of dopamine inhibition, stimulation by PRFs, or combinations of both events. At any given moment, locally produced autocrine and paracrine regulators further modulate the responsiveness of individual lactotrophs to neurohormonal PIFs and PRFs.

Multiple neurotransmitter systems impinge on the hypothalamic dopamine and PRF neurons to regulate their neurosecretion[464] (see Fig. 7–35). Nicotinic cholinergic and glutamatergic afferents activate TIDA neurons, whereas histamine, acting predominantly through H2 receptors, inhibits these neurons. An inhibitory peptidergic input to TIDA neurons of major physiologic significance is that associated with the endogenous opioid peptides enkephalin and dynorphin and their cognate μ- and κ-receptor subtypes.[516] Opioid inhibition of dopamine release has been associated with increased PRL secretion under virtually all physiologic conditions, including the basal state, different phases of the estrous cycle, lactation, and stress.

Ascending serotoninergic inputs from the dorsal raphe nucleus are the major activator of PRF neurons in the paraventricular nucleus.[517] There is still debate concerning the identity of the specific 5-hydroxytryptamine receptors involved in this activation.

The PRL regulatory system and its monoaminergic control have been scrutinized in detail because of the frequent occurrence of syndromes of PRL hypersecretion (see Chapter 8). Both the pituitary and the hypothalamus have dopamine receptors, and unfortunately the response to dopamine receptor stimulation and blockade does not distinguish between central and peripheral actions of the drug. Many commonly used neuroleptic drugs influence PRL secretion. Reserpine (a catecholamine depletor) and phenothiazines such as chlorpromazine and haloperidol enhance PRL release by disinhibition of dopamine action on the pituitary, and the PRL response is an excellent predictor of the antipsychotic effects of phenothiazines because of its correlation with D2 receptor binding and activation.[518] The major antipsychotic neuroleptic agents act on brain dopamine receptors in the mesolimbic system and in the pituitary-regulating tuberoinfundibular system. Consequently, treatment of such patients with dopamine agonists such as bromocriptine can reverse the psychiatric benefits of such drugs. A report of three patients with psychosis and concomitant prolactinomas recommended the combination of clozapine and quinagolide as the treatment of choice to manage both diseases simultaneously.[519]

Factors Influencing Secretion

Circadian Rhythm

PRL is detectable in plasma at all times during the day but is secreted in discrete pulses superimposed on basal secretion and exhibits a diurnal rhythm with peak values in the early morning hours.[520] There is a true circadian rhythm in humans because it is maintained in a constant environment independent of the sleep rhythm.[521] The combined body of data examining TIDA neuronal activity, dopamine concentrations in the median eminence, and manipulations of the SCN suggests that endogenous diurnal alterations in dopamine tone that are entrained by light constitute the major neuroendocrine mechanism underlying the circadian rhythm of PRL secretion.

External Stimuli

The suckling stimulus is the most important physiologic regulator of PRL secretion. Within 1 to 3 minutes of nipple stimulation, PRL levels rise and remain elevated for 10 to 20 minutes.[522] This reflex is distinct from the milk let-down, which involves oxytocin release from the neurohypophysis and contraction of mammary alveolar myoepithelial cells. These reflexes provide a mechanism by which the infant regulates both the production and the delivery of milk. The nocturnal rise in PRL secretion in nursing women and in non-nursing women may have evolved as a mechanism of milk maintenance during prolonged nonsuckling periods at night.[166]

Pathways involved in the suckling reflex arise in nerves innervating the nipple, enter the spinal cord by way of spinal afferent neurons, ascend the spinal cord through spinothalamic tracts to the midbrain, and enter the hypothalamus by way of the median forebrain bundle (see Fig. 7–35). In most of the pathway, neurons regulating the oxytocin-dependent milk let-down response accompany those involved in PRL regulation and then separate at the level of the paraventricular nuclei. The suckling reflex brings about an inhibition of PIF activity and a release of PRFs, although the identity of an undisputed suckling-induced PRF is unsettled.

Although the significance for PRL regulation in humans is not certain, environmental stimuli from seasonal changes in light duration and auditory and olfactory cues are clearly of great importance to many mammalian species.[464] Seasonal breeders, such as the sheep, exhibit a reduction in PRL secretion in response to shortened days. The specific ultrasound vocalization of rodent pups is among the most potent stimuli for PRL secretion in lactating and virgin female rats. Olfactory stimuli from pheromones also have potent actions in rodents. A prime example is the Bruce effect or spontaneous abortion induced by exposure of a pregnant female rat to an unfamiliar male. It is mediated by a well-studied neural circuitry involving the vomeronasal nerves, corticomedial amygdala, medial preoptic area of the hypothalamus, and finally activation of TIDA neurons and a reduction in circulating PRL that is essential for maintenance of luteal function in the first half of pregnancy.

Stress in many forms dramatically affects PRL secretion, although the teleologic significance is uncertain. It may be related to actions of PRL on cells of the immune system or some other aspect of homeostasis. Different stressors are associated with either a reduction or an increase in PRL secretion, depending on the local regulatory environment at the time of the stress. However, whereas well-documented changes in PRL are associated with relatively severe forms of stress in laboratory animal models, a study of academic stress in college students failed to show any significant correlation among the time periods before, during, or after final examinations and diurnal PRL levels.[523]

Gonadotropin-Releasing Hormone and Control of the Reproductive Axis

Chemistry and Evolution

The hypothalamic neuropeptide that controls the function of the reproductive axis is GnRH. GnRH is a 10-amino-acid

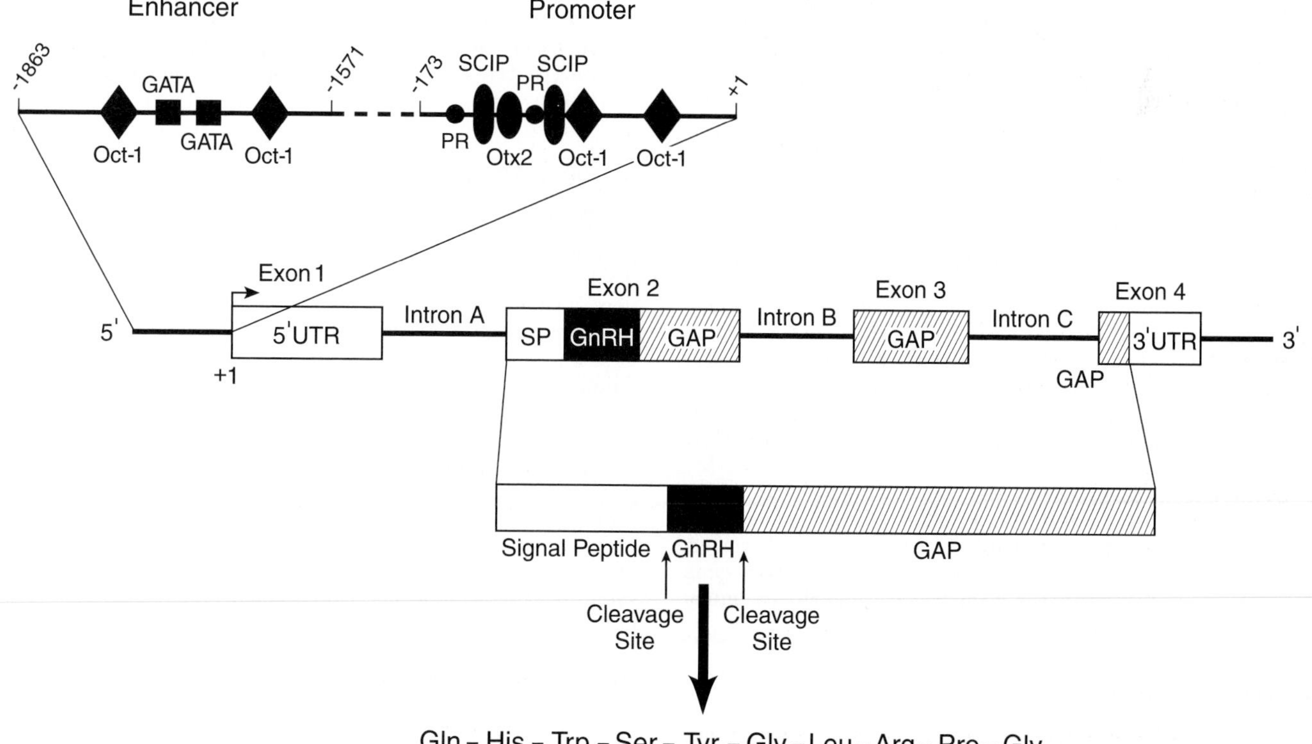

Figure 7–36. Schematic diagram of the gene for pre-pro-gonadotropin-releasing hormone (GnRH) and the GnRH peptide. Diagrams for the enhancer and promoter regions are specific to the rat gene.

peptide that is synthesized as part of a larger precursor molecule and is then enzymatically cleaved to remove a signal peptide from the N-terminus and GnRH-associated peptide (GAP) from the C-terminus (Fig. 7–36).[524–526] All forms of the decapeptide have a pyroGlu at the N-terminus and Gly-amide at the C-terminus, indicating the functional importance of the terminal regions throughout evolutionary biology.

Within mammals, two genes encoding GnRH have been identified.[527, 528] The first encodes a 92-amino-acid precursor protein. This form of GnRH is now referred to as GnRH-I and is the form found in hypothalamic neurons that serves as a releasing factor to regulate pituitary gonadotroph function.[529] The second GnRH gene, *GnRH-II*, encodes a decapeptide that differs from the first by three amino acids. This form of GnRH is found in the midbrain region and serves as a neurotransmitter rather than as a pituitary releasing factor. Both GnRH-I and GnRH-II are found in phylogenetically diverse species, from fish to mammals, suggesting that these multiple forms of GnRH diverged from one another early in vertebrate evolution.[529] A third form of GnRH, GnRH-III, has been identified in neurons of the telencephalon in teleost fish. This form of GnRH may have been lost in higher vertebrates or simply not yet discovered in other species.[529]

As discussed subsequently in more detail, GnRH-I and GnRH-III are found in cells that originate in the olfactory placode in early embryonic development. In contrast, GnRH-II–containing cells are derived from the midbrain ventricle. GnRH is also found in cells outside the brain. The roles of GnRH peptides produced outside the brain are not well understood but are an area of current investigation.[530]

All GnRH genes have the same basic structure, with the pre-prohormone mRNA encoded in four exons. Exon 1 contains the 5′ untranslated region of the gene; exon 2 contains the signal peptide, GnRH, and the N-terminus of GAP; exon 3 contains the central portion of GAP; and exon 4 contains the C-terminus of GAP and the 3′ untranslated region (see Fig. 7–36).[529, 531] Among species, the nucleotide sequences encoding the GnRH decapeptide are highly homologous.

Two transcriptional start sites have been identified in GnRH genes at +1 and −579, with the +1 promoter being active in hypothalamic neurons and the other promoter active in placenta. The first 173 base pairs of the promoter are highly conserved among species. In the rat, this promoter region has been shown to contain two Oct-1 binding sites; three regions that bind the POU domain family of transcription factors, SCIP, Oct-6, and Tst-1; and three regions that can bind the progesterone receptor.[532, 533] In addition, a variety of hormones and second messengers have been shown to regulate GnRH gene expression, and the majority of the *cis*-acting elements thus far characterized for hormonal control of GnRH transcription have been localized to the proximal promoter region.[533, 534] The 5′ untranslated region of the GnRH gene also contains a 300-base-pair enhancer region that is 1.8 kilobases upstream of the transcription start site.[535] It contains binding sites for POU homeodomain transcription factors and GATA factors.

In this chapter, we focus on the hypothalamic GnRH that is derived from GnRH-1 mRNA and plays an important role in the regulation of the hypothalamic-pituitary-gonadal axis. A mutant strain of mice with a deletion of the GnRH-1 gene have hypogonadism, and the homozygous animals are infertile.[536]

Anatomic Distribution

GnRH neurons are small, diffusely located cells that are not concentrated in a nucleus (Fig. 7–37*A*).[537, 538] They are generally bipolar and fusiform in shape, with long thin axons that can exhibit spines. The location of hypothalamic GnRH neurons is species-dependent. In the rat, hypothalamic GnRH neurons are concentrated in rostral areas including the medial preoptic area, the diagonal band of Broca, the septal areas, and the anterior hypothalamus. In primates, the majority of hypothalamic GnRH neurons are located more dorsally in the medial basal hypothalamus, the infundibulum, and periventricular to the third ventricle. Throughout the hypothalamus, neuroendocrine GnRH neurons, which extend their axon terminals to the median eminence, are interspersed with non-neuroendocrine GnRH neurons, which extend their axons to other regions of the brain including other hypothalamic regions and various regions of the cortex. GnRH secreted from non-neuroendocrine neurons has been implicated in the control of sexual behavior in rodents[539] but not in higher primates.[540]

Embryonic Development

GnRH neuroendocrine neurons are an unusual neuronal population in that they originate outside the CNS, from the epithelial tissue of the nasal placode.[541, 542] During embryonic development GnRH neurons migrate across the surface of the brain and into the hypothalamus, with the final hypothalamic location differing somewhat among species. Migration is dependent on a scaffolding of neurons and glial cells along which the GnRH neurons move, with neural cell adhesion molecules playing a critical role in guiding the migration process.[543]

Failure of GnRH neurons to migrate properly leads to a clinical condition, Kallmann's syndrome, in which GnRH neuroendocrine neurons do not reach their final destination and thus do not stimulate pituitary gonadotropin secretion.[544] Patients with Kallmann's syndrome do not enter puberty spontaneously. X-linked Kallmann's syndrome results from a deficiency of the *Kal-1* gene, which encodes a putative protein of 680 amino acids and contains four fibronectin type III repeats and a four-disulfide core motif.[545] However, this form of Kallmann's syndrome accounts for only a small percentage (about 8%) of cases, and the cause of other forms remains unknown. Administration of exogenous GnRH effectively treats this form of hypothalamic hypogonadism. Patients with Kallmann's syndrome often have other congenital midline defects, including anosmia, which results from hypoplasia of the olfactory bulb and tracts.

Action at the Pituitary

Receptors

GnRH binds to a membrane receptor on pituitary gonadotrophs and stimulates both LH and FSH synthesis and secretion. The GnRH receptor is a seven-transmembrane-domain G protein–coupled receptor, but it lacks a typical intracellular C-terminal cytoplasmic domain.[546–548] Under physiologic conditions, the GnRH receptor number varies and is usually directly correlated with the gonadotropin secretory capacity of pituitary gonadotrophs. For example, across the rat estrous cycle, a rise in GnRH receptors is seen just before the surge of gonadotropins that occurs on the afternoon of proestrus.[549, 550] GnRH receptor message levels are regulated by a variety of hormones and second messengers including steroid hormones (estradiol can both suppress and stimulate, and progesterone suppresses), gonadotropins (which suppress), and calcium and protein kinase C (which stimulate).

$G_{q/11\alpha}$ is the primary guanosine triphosphate–binding protein mediating GnRH responses; however, there is evidence that GnRH receptors can couple to other guanosine triphosphate–binding proteins including G_s and G_i.[548] With activation, the GnRH receptor couples to a phosphoinositide-specific phospholipase C, which leads to increases in calcium transport into gonadotrophs and calcium release from internal stores through a diacylglycerol–protein kinase C pathway. Increased calcium entry is a critical step in GnRH-stimulated release of gonadotropin secretion.[548, 551] However, the MAPK cascade is also stimulated by GnRH.[548]

When there is a decline in GnRH stimulation to the pituitary, as occurs in a variety of physiologic conditions including states of lactation, undernutrition, or seasonal periods of reproductive quiescence, the number of GnRH receptors on pituitary gonadotrophs declines dramatically.[549, 550] Subsequent exposure of the pituitary to pulses of GnRH restores receptor number by a Ca^{2+}-dependent mechanism that requires protein synthesis.[551, 552] The effect of GnRH to induce its own receptor is termed up-regulation or self-priming. Only certain physiologic frequencies of pulsatile GnRH can augment GnRH receptor production, and these frequencies appear to differ among species.[553] Up-regulation of GnRH receptors after a period of low GnRH stimulation to the pituitary can take hours to days of exposure to pulsatile GnRH, depending on the duration and extent of the prior decrease in GnRH. The self-priming effect of GnRH to up-regulate its own receptors also plays a crucial role in the production of the gonadotropin surge that occurs at midcycle in females of spontaneously ovulating species and triggers ovulation. Just before the gonadotropin surge, two factors, the increased frequency of pulsatile GnRH release[549, 550, 554–556] and a sensitization of the pituitary gonadotrophs by rising levels of estradiol,[557, 558] make the pituitary exquisitely sensitive to GnRH and allow an output of LH that is an order of magnitude greater than the release seen during the rest of the female reproductive cycle. This surge of LH triggers the ovulatory process at the ovary.

In contrast to up-regulation of GnRH receptors by pulsatile regimens of GnRH, continuous exposure to GnRH leads to down-regulation of GnRH receptors and an accompanying decrease in LH and FSH synthesis and secretion, termed *desensitization*.[559] Down-regulation does not require calcium mobilization or gonadotropin secretion.[559] It involves a rapid uncoupling of receptor from G proteins and sequestration of the receptors from the plasma membrane, followed by internalization and proteolytic degradation of the receptors.[548]

The concept of down-regulation has a number of clinical applications. For example, the most common current therapy for precocious puberty of hypothalamic origin (i.e., precocious GnRH secretion) is to treat the child with a long-acting GnRH agonist, which down-regulates pituitary GnRH receptors and effectively turns off the reproductive axis.[553, 560] Children with precocious puberty can be maintained with long-acting GnRH agonists for years to suppress the premature activation of the reproductive axis, and at the normal age of puberty agonist treatment can be withdrawn, allowing a reactivation of pituitary gonadotrophs and a downstream increase in gonadal steroid hormone production. Long-acting GnRH agonists are also used in the treatment of forms of breast cancer that are estrogen-dependent as well as other gonadal steroid–dependent cancers.[553, 561] Long-acting antagonists of GnRH have been developed that can also be used for these therapies.[562] Antagonists have the advantage of not having a flare effect, that is, an acute stimulation of gonadotropin secretion that is seen during the initial treatment of individuals with superagonists.

Pulsatile Gonadotropin-Releasing Hormone Stimulation

Because a single pulse of GnRH stimulates the release of both LH and FSH and chronic exposure of the pituitary to pulsatile GnRH supports the synthesis of both LH and FSH, many people believe that there is only one releasing factor regulating the synthesis and secretion of LH and FSH.[563] However, in a number of physiologic conditions there are divergent patterns of LH and FSH secretion, and thus a second FSH-releasing peptide has been proposed, but such a peptide has not been isolated to date.[564] Other mechanisms, discussed in more detail later, are likely to account for the differential regulation of LH and FSH release.

The ensemble of GnRH neurons in the hypothalamus that send axons to the portal blood system in the median eminence fire in a coordinated, repetitive, episodic manner, producing distinct pulses of GnRH in the portal blood stream.[565–567] The pulsatile nature of GnRH stimulation to the pituitary leads to the release of distinct pulses of LH into the peripheral blood stream.[568, 569] In experimental animals, in which it is possible to collect blood samples simultaneously from the portal and peripheral blood stream, GnRH and LH pulses have been found to correspond in about a one-to-one ratio at most physiologic rates of secretion (Fig. 7–38).[566, 567] Because the portal blood stream is generally inaccessible in humans, the collection of

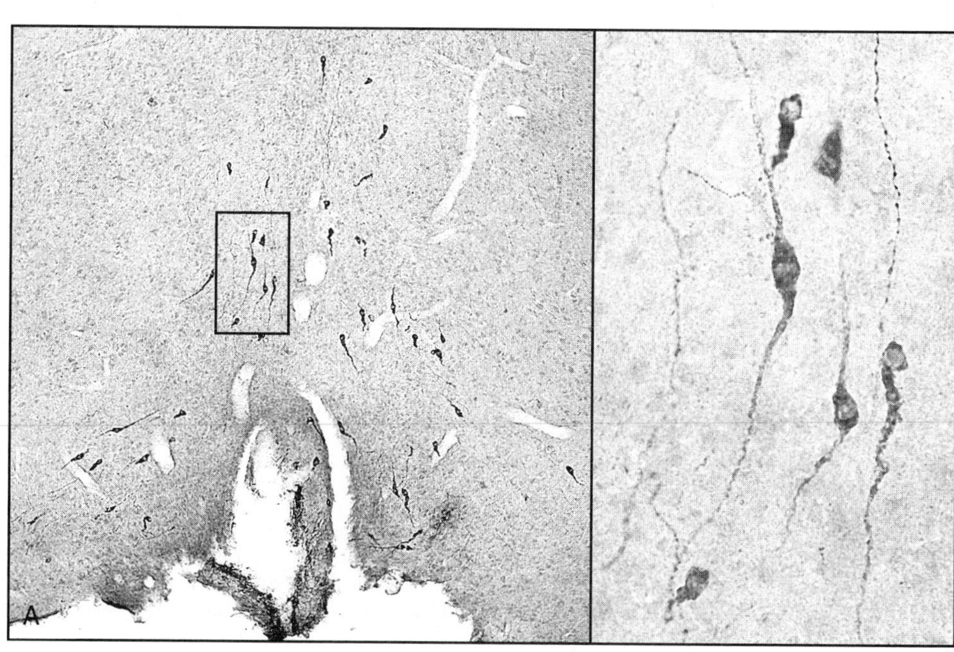

Figure 7–37. Regulation of the hypothalamic-pituitary-gonadal axis. *A*, Gonadotropin-releasing hormone (GnRH) neurons in a coronal section of the rat hypothalamus at 4× magnification. The inset is at 20× magnification. (Micrograph provided by Patricia Williamson and Kevin Grove, Oregon National Primate Center.)

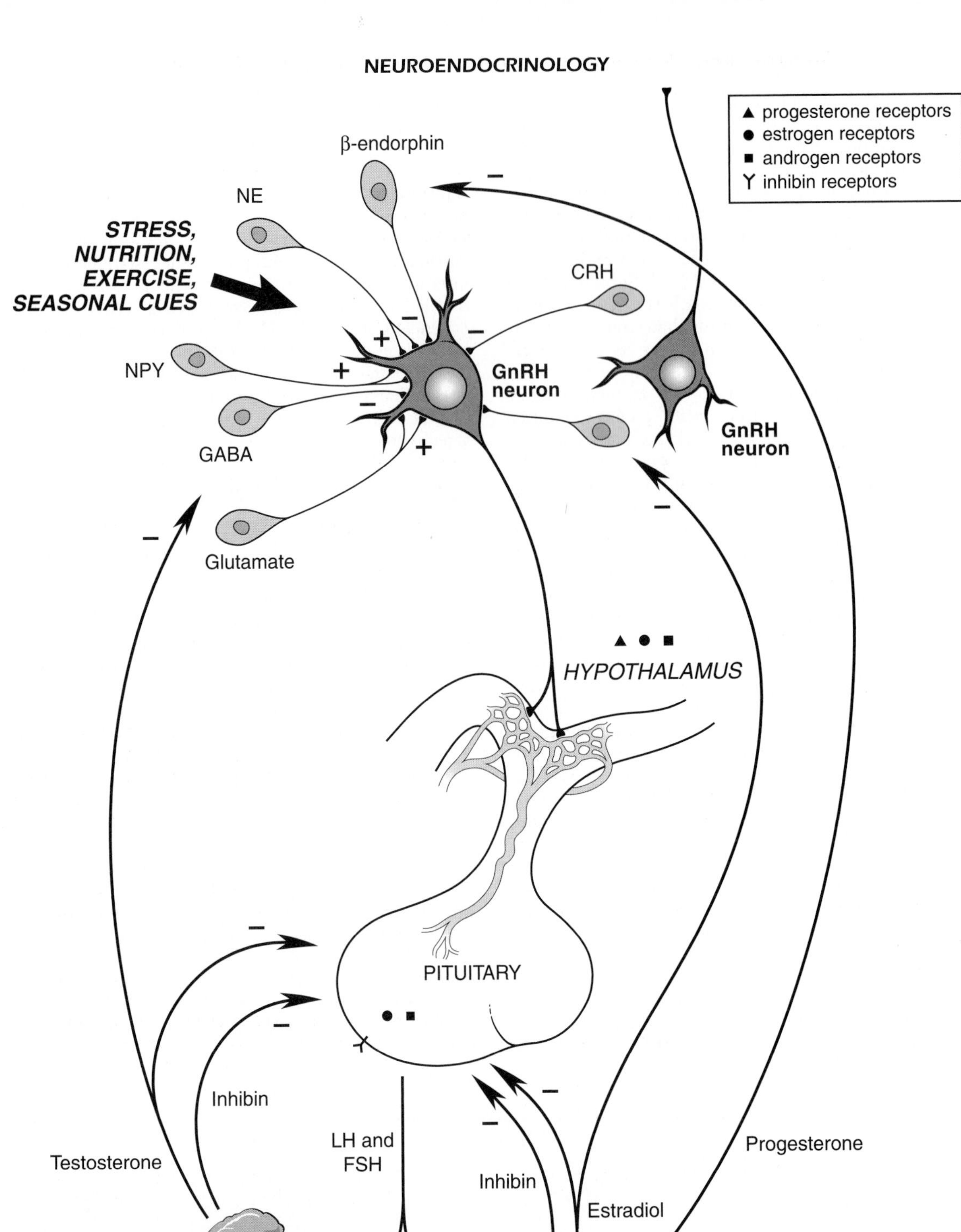

Figure 7–37 *Continued. B*, Schematic diagram of the hypothalamic-pituitary-gonadal axis showing neural systems that regulate GnRH secretion and feedback of gonadal steroid hormones at the level of the hypothalamus and pituitary. CRH, corticotropin-releasing hormone; FSH, follicle-stimulating hormone; GABA, γ-aminobutyric acid; LH, luteinizing hormone; NPY, neuropeptide Y.

frequent blood samples from the peripheral blood stream is used to define the pulsatile nature of LH secretion (i.e., frequency and amplitude of LH pulses), and pulsatile LH is used as an indirect measure of the activity of the GnRH secretory system. Indirect assessment of GnRH secretion by monitoring the rate of pulsatile LH secretion is also used in many animal studies examining the factors that govern the regulation of the pulsatile activity of the reproductive neuroendocrine axis. Un-

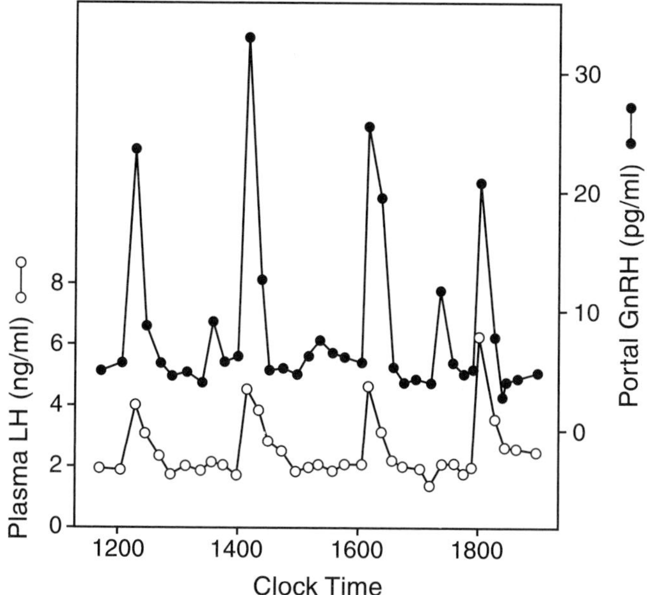

Figure 7–38. Simultaneous detection of pulses of gonadotropin-releasing hormone (GnRH) measured in blood collected from the hypothalamic-hypophyseal portal vessels and luteinizing hormone (LH) measured in blood collected from the peripheral vasculature of an oophorectomized ewe. (Redrawn from Clarke IJ, Cummins JT. Endocrinology 1982; 111:1737–1739).

like LH secretion, FSH secretion is not always pulsatile, and even when it is pulsatile, there is only partial concordance between LH and FSH pulses.[570]

It is possible to place multiple unit recording electrodes in the medial basal hypothalamus of monkeys and other species and find spikes of electrical activity that are concordant with the pulsatile discharge of LH secretion.[571–573] It is unknown, however, whether these bursts of electrical activity reflect the activity of GnRH neurons themselves or the activity of neurons that impinge on GnRH neurons and govern their firing. With the development of mice in which the gene for green fluorescent protein has been put under the regulation of the GnRH promoter, it has been possible to identify GnRH neurons in hypothalamic tissue slices using fluorescence microscopy and record from them intracellularly.[30] These studies have shown that many, but not all, GnRH neurons show a bursting pattern of electrical activity. A central, unsolved question in the field of reproductive neuroendocrinology is what causes GnRH neurons to pulse in a coordinated manner. Studies using a line of clonal GnRH neurons have shown that these neurons grown in culture can release GnRH in a pulsatile pattern, suggesting that the pulse-generating capacity of GnRH neurons may be intrinsic.[574] The term *GnRH pulse generator* is often used to acknowledge the fact that GnRH secretion occurs in pulses and to refer to the central mechanisms responsible for pulsatile GnRH release.[575]

A critical factor governing LH and FSH secretion and release is the rate of pulsatile GnRH stimulation of the gonadotrophs. Experimental studies in which the hypothalamus was lesioned and GnRH was replaced by pulsatile administration of exogenous GnRH showed that different frequencies of GnRH can lead to differential ratios of LH to FSH secretion from the pituitary.[576] Figure 7–39 shows that in a monkey with a hypothalamic lesion, replacement of one pulse of GnRH per hour led to a relatively low ratio of FSH to LH secretion. Subsequent institution of a slower pulse frequency of one pulse of GnRH every 3 hours led to a decrease in LH secretion but an increase in FSH secretion such that the ratio of FSH to LH secretion was greatly elevated. It is likely that this effect of pulse frequency on the ratio of FSH to LH secretion accounts, at least in part, for the clinical finding that at times when the GnRH pulse generator is just turning on, such as at the onset of puberty and during recovery from chronic undernutrition, the ratio of FSH to LH is higher than when it is measured in adults experiencing regular reproductive function.[577, 578] As discussed subsequently, steroid hormones act at both the hypothalamus and pituitary to influence strongly the rate of pulsatile GnRH release and amount of LH and FSH secreted from the pituitary.

GnRH pulse frequency not only influences the rate of pulsatile gonadotropin release and the ratio of FSH to LH secretion but also plays an important role in modulating the structural makeup of the gonadotropins. LH and FSH are structurally similar glycoprotein hormones.[579] Each of these hormones is made up of an α and a β subunit. LH, FSH, and TSH share a common α subunit, and each has a unique β subunit that conveys tissue specificity to the intact hormone. Before secretion of gonadotropins, terminal sugars are attached to each gonadotropin molecule.[579] The sugars include sialic acid, galactose, N-acetylglucosamine, and mannose, but the most important is sialic acid. The extent of glycosylation of

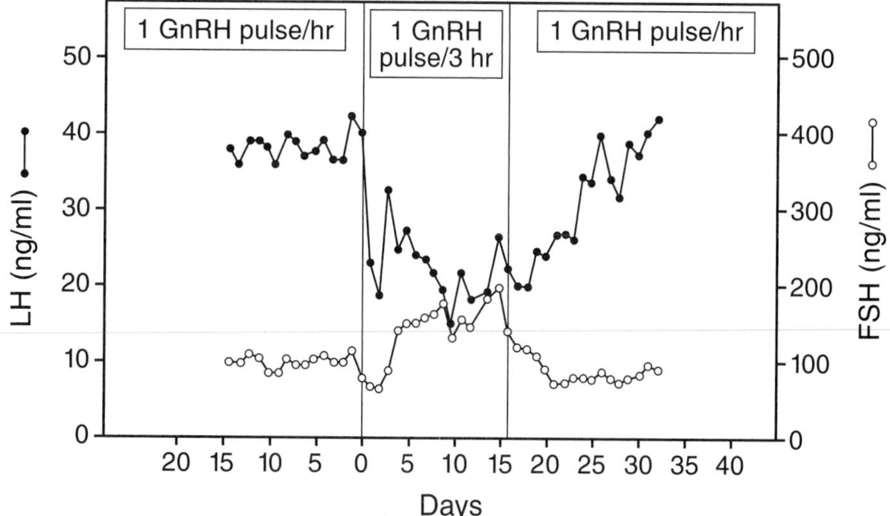

Figure 7–39. The influence of gonadotropin-releasing hormone (GnRH) pulse frequency on luteinizing hormone (LH) and follicle-stimulating hormone (FSH) secretion in a female rhesus monkey with an arcuate nucleus lesion ablating endogenous GnRH support of the pituitary. Decreasing GnRH pulse frequency from 1 pulse/hour to 1 pulse/3 hours leads to a decrease in plasma LH concentrations but an increase in plasma FSH concentrations. (Redrawn from Wildt L, Haulser A, Marshall G, et al. Endocrinology 1981; 109: 376–385.)

LH and FSH is important for the physiologic function of these hormones. Forms of gonadotropin with more sialic acid have a longer half-life because they are protected from degradation by the liver. Forms of gonadotropin with less sialic acid can have more potent effects at their biologic receptors. Both the rate of GnRH stimulation and ovarian hormone feedback at the level of the pituitary regulate the degree of LH and FSH glycosylation.[579, 580] For example, slow frequencies of GnRH, seen during follicular development, are associated with greater degrees of FSH glycosylation, which would provide sustained FSH support to growing follicles. In contrast, faster frequencies of GnRH, seen just before the midcycle gonadotropin surge, are associated with lesser degrees of FSH glycosylation, providing a more potent but shorter lasting form of FSH at the time of ovulation.[580]

Regulatory Systems

Many neurotransmitter systems from the brain stem, limbic system, and other areas of the hypothalamus convey information to GnRH neurons (see Fig. 7–37).[581] These afferent systems include neurons that contain norepinephrine, dopamine, serotonin, GABA, glutamate, endogenous opiate peptides, NPY, galanin, and a number of other peptide neurotransmitters. Glutamate and norepinephrine play important roles in providing stimulatory drive to the reproductive axis,[582, 583] whereas GABA and endogenous opioid peptides provide a substantial portion of the inhibitory drive to GnRH neurons.[584, 585] Influences of specific neurotransmitter systems are discussed where appropriate in later sections on the physiologic regulation of GnRH neurons.

GnRH neurons are surrounded by glial processes, and only a small percentage of their surface area is available to receive dendritic contacts from afferent neurons. Changes in the steroid hormone milieu influence the degree of glial sheathing and may play important roles in regulating afferent input to GnRH neurons by this mechanism.[586] Some glial cells also secrete substances that can modulate the activity of GnRH neurons. For example, at puberty there is an increase in the hypothalamic expression of transforming growth factor α, and transforming growth factor α can stimulate GnRH release by acting on astroglial cells to stimulate their release of PGE_2, which is stimulatory to GnRH neurons.[587]

Feedback Regulation

Steroid hormone receptors are abundant in the hypothalamus and in many neural systems that impinge on GnRH neurons, including noradrenergic, serotoninergic, β-endorphin–containing, and NPY neurons. Early studies identifying regions of the brain that bound labeled estrogens showed that in rodents the preoptic area and ventromedial hypothalamus had the highest concentrations of estrogen receptors in the brain.[588, 589] Further localization studies, identifying estrogen receptors by immunocytochemistry or in situ hybridization, confirmed the strong presence of estrogen receptors in the hypothalamus and in brain areas with strong connections to the hypothalamus, including the amygdala, septal nuclei, bed nucleus of the stria terminalis, medial part of the nucleus of the solitary tract, and lateral portion of the parabrachial nucleus.[590, 591] In 1986 a new member of the steroid hormone receptor superfamily with high sequence homology to the classical estrogen receptor (now referred to as estrogen receptor α) was isolated from rat prostate and named estrogen receptor β.[592, 593] This novel estrogen receptor was shown to bind estradiol and to activate transcription by binding to estrogen response elements.[593]

In situ hybridization studies examining the localization of estrogen receptor β mRNA have shown that these receptors are present throughout the rostral-caudal extent of the brain, with a high level of expression in the preoptic area, bed nucleus of the stria terminalis, paraventricular and supraoptic nuclei, amygdala, and laminae II to VI of the cerebral cortex.[594, 595] Specific receptors for progesterone are induced by estrogen in hypothalamic regions of the brain, including the preoptic area, the ventromedial and ventrolateral nuclei, and the infundibular-arcuate nucleus, although there is also evidence for constitutive expression of progesterone receptors in some regions.[596–599] Androgen receptor mapping studies have shown considerable overlap in the distribution of androgen and estrogen receptors throughout the brain. The highest density of androgen receptors was found in hypothalamic nuclei known to participate in the control of reproduction and sexual behaviors, including the arcuate nucleus, paraventricular nucleus, medial preoptic nucleus, ventromedial nucleus, and brain regions with strong connections to the hypothalamus including the amygdala, nuclei of the septal region, bed nucleus of the stria terminalis, nucleus of the solitary tract, and lateral division of the parabrachial nucleus.[591, 600, 601] The anterior pituitary also contains receptors for all of the gonadal steroid hormones.

Steroid hormones can dramatically alter the pattern of pulsatile release of GnRH and of the gonadotropins through actions at both the hypothalamus and the pituitary (Figs. 7–40 and 7–41). At the hypothalamus, estradiol, progesterone, and testosterone can all act to slow the frequency of GnRH release into the portal blood stream, an action referred to as negative feedback.[602–604] Because GnRH neurons have generally been shown to lack steroid hormone receptors, it is likely that the effects of steroid hormones on the firing rate of GnRH neurons are mediated by steroid hormone actions on other neural systems that provide afferent input to GnRH neurons. For example, progesterone-mediated negative feedback on GnRH secretion in primates appears to be regulated by β-endorphin–containing neurons in the hypothalamus, acting primarily through μ-opioid receptors.[603] If a μ-receptor antagonist, such as naloxone, is administered along with progesterone, the negative feedback action of progesterone on GnRH secretion can be blocked.[603]

Negative feedback of steroid hormones can also occur directly at the level of the pituitary.[602] For example, estradiol has been shown to be capable of binding to the pituitary, decreasing LH and FSH synthesis and release, and decreasing the sensitivity of pituitary gonadotrophs to the actions of GnRH such that less LH and FSH are released when a pulse of GnRH stimulates the pituitary. Evidence for such a direct pituitary action of estradiol came from studies with rhesus monkeys that had been rendered deficient in endogenous GnRH by a lesion in the arcuate nucleus and showed a decline in endogenous gonadotropin secretion. When these monkeys received a pulsatile regimen of GnRH gonadotropin secretion, subsequent estradiol infusions dramatically suppressed the responsiveness of the pituitary to GnRH and suppressed the gonadotropin secretion that was being driven by the pulsatile administration of GnRH.[606] Steroid hormones can have direct negative feedback actions at the pituitary; however, the extent of hypothalamic versus pituitary negative feedback actions is species-specific.[607] In primate species including humans, there is considerable feedback of estradiol at the pituitary, but most of the progesterone and testosterone negative feedback occurs at the level of the hypothalamus.[603, 607]

Most of the time, the hypothalamic-pituitary axis is under the negative feedback influence of gonadal steroid hormones. If the gonads are removed surgically or their normal secretion of steroid hormones is suppressed pharmacologically, there is a dramatic increase (10-fold to 20-fold) in circulating levels of LH and FSH secretion.[602, 607] This type of "castration response" occurs normally at the menopause in women, when

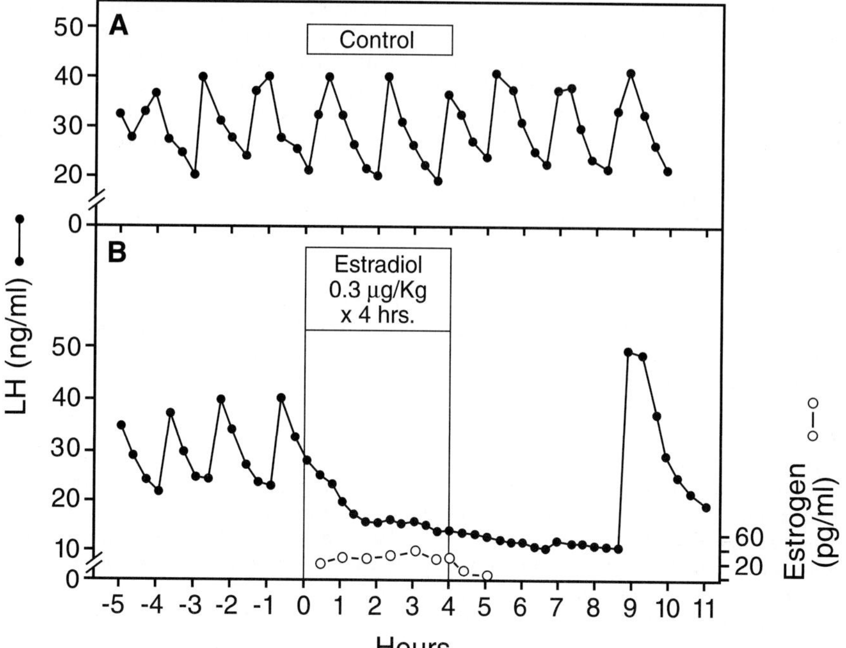

Figure 7–40. Pulsatile luteinizing hormone (LH) secretion in an ovariectomized rhesus monkey *(A)* and an ovariectomized rhesus monkey treated with estradiol *(B)*. Estradiol causes a rapid and sustained suppression of LH secretion. (Redrawn from Yamaji T, Dierschke DJ, Knobil E. Endocrinology 70: 771–777.)

ovarian follicular development and thus ovarian production of large quantities of estradiol and progesterone decrease and eventually cease.[608]

In addition to negative feedback, estradiol can have a positive feedback action at the level of the hypothalamus and pituitary to lead to a massive release of LH and FSH from the pituitary.[575, 602] This massive release of gonadotropins occurs once each menstrual cycle and is referred to as the LH-FSH surge. The positive feedback action of estradiol occurs as a response to the rising tide of estradiol that is produced during the process of dominant follicle development in the late follicular phase of the menstrual cycle. In women, elevated estradiol levels are generally maintained at about 500 pg/mL for about 36 hours prior to stimulation of the gonadotropin surge.

Experiments have shown that both a critical concentration of plasma estradiol and a critical duration of elevated estradiol are

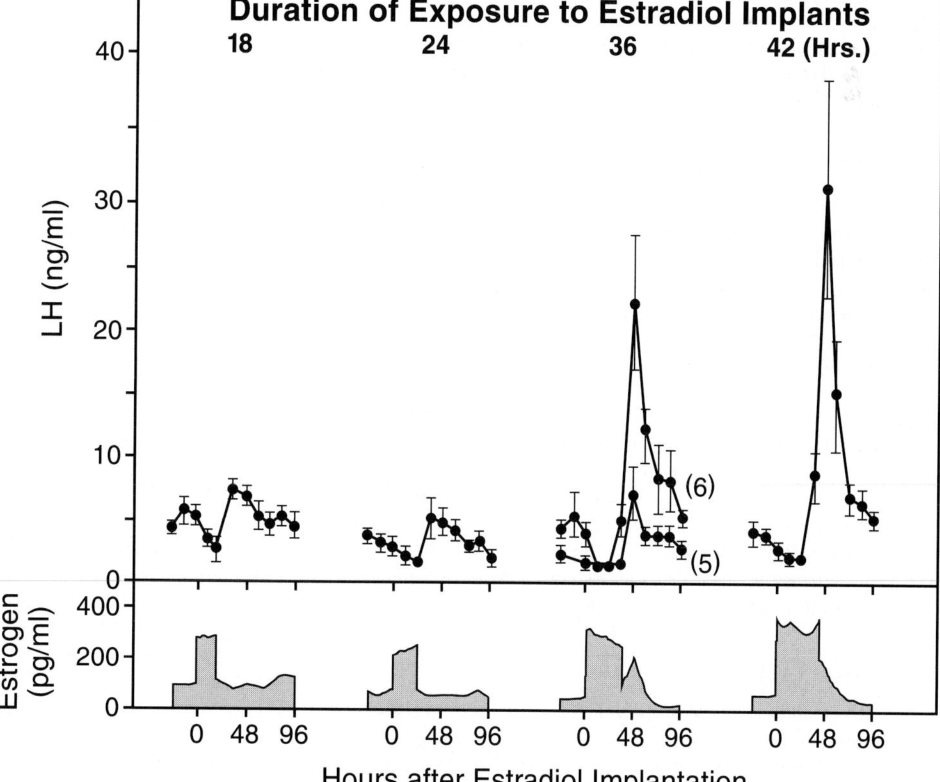

Figure 7–41. Dose and duration requirements for estradiol-induced negative and positive feedback on luteinizing hormone (LH) secretion. Varying amounts of estradiol were implanted into ovariectomized rhesus monkeys. Short-term exposure to estradiol led to negative feedback on LH secretion, 36 hours of exposure led to positive feedback in 6 of 11 monkeys, and 42 hours of exposure led to robust positive feedback resulting in a surge of LH secretion in all monkeys. (Redrawn from Karsch F, Weick RF, Butler WR, et al. Endocrinology 1973; 92:1740–1747.)

necessary to achieve positive feedback and a resulting gonadotropin surge (see Fig. 7–41). Moreover, the duration of estrogen elevation that is required to trigger a surge depends on the concentration of circulating estrogen.[609] If supraphysiologic doses of estradiol are administered, the surge can occur as early as 18 hours after their administration. Because the ovary is responsible for the production of estradiol and the time course and magnitude of estradiol release control the rate of positive feedback, the ovary has been referred to as the zeitgeber of the menstrual cycle.[575, 602] The dependence of the positive feedback system on the magnitude of estradiol production helps explain the fact that the portion of the menstrual cycle that varies most in length is the follicular phase. Production of higher levels of estradiol by a dominant follicle in one cycle would lead to a more rapid positive feedback action with earlier ovulation and thus a shorter follicular phase compared with a cycle in which the dominant follicle produced lower levels of estradiol.

As with negative feedback in response to estradiol, the positive feedback actions of estradiol occur both at the hypothalamus, to increase GnRH secretion, and at the pituitary, to enhance greatly pituitary responsiveness to GnRH. At the pituitary, estradiol increases pituitary sensitivity to GnRH by increasing the synthesis of new GnRH receptors and by enhancing the responsiveness to GnRH at a postreceptor site of action. At the level of the hypothalamus in rodent species, estradiol appears to act at a "surge center" to induce the ovulatory surge of GnRH. Lesions in areas adjacent to the medial preoptic area, near the anterior commissure and septal complex, block the ability of estradiol to induce a surge in these species without blocking negative feedback effects of estradiol.[610] In primate species, there does not appear to be a separate surge center mediating the positive feedback actions of estradiol.[575, 602] The cellular mechanisms that mediate the switch from negative to positive feedback of estrogen are not fully understood, but there is support for the concept that estrogen induction of various transcription factors and receptors (notably progesterone receptors) may play an important role in mediating this switch.[611, 612] Alternatively, estrogen has been shown to have biphasic actions on hypothalamic GABAergic neurons that impinge on GnRH neurons and are strong regulators of their activity, with the switch in action dependent on the duration of estradiol exposure.[613]

The molecular mechanisms by which estradiol influences GnRH gene expression are also not well understood, but it is likely that these influences occur through actions of neural systems afferent to GnRH because GnRH neurons do not appear to have estrogen receptors. Much more is known about the molecular mechanisms by which estradiol acts at the pituitary to regulate gonadotropin gene expression. Expression of LH β subunit is strongly regulated (10-fold to 14-fold) by estradiol, but expression of FSH β and α subunits is regulated to a lesser extent (4-fold to 8-fold and 2-fold to 3-fold, respectively).[614] Although in vivo studies indicate strong negative feedback actions of estradiol on LH gene transcription, such actions have not been replicated in in vitro studies with isolated pituitaries, leading to the conclusion that estradiol negative feedback on gonadotropin synthesis occurs predominantly by extrapituitary mechanisms.[614] In contrast, estradiol can stimulate LHβ mRNA transcription directly at the level of the pituitary, acting by binding to an estrogen response element in the 5′ promoter region of the LHβ gene.[614]

Regulation by Inhibins and Activins

Negative feedback of pituitary FSH secretion is also exerted by a family of peptide hormones produced by the gonads, the inhibins.[615] Inhibins are produced by follicular and luteal cells of the ovary and by Sertoli cells in the testes. Inhibins are members of the transforming growth factor β superfamily and comprise two subunits, an α and a β subunit. There are two forms of the β subunit, A and B. Inhibins selectively suppress FSH secretion without simultaneous suppression of LH secretion; thus, they provide one of the mechanisms whereby the pituitary can release differential amounts of LH and FSH, even though there appears to be only a single gonadotropin-releasing factor. Interestingly, the pituitary itself produces compounds related to inhibins that are dimers of the β B subunits. These are the activins.[615–618]

Activins received their name from their ability to facilitate FSH release. Activins have been shown to stimulate both basal and GnRH-induced FSH release from the anterior pituitary as well as increase FSHβ mRNA levels by enhancing transcription. An important role of endogenous activins in stimulating FSH secretion is supported by the finding that transgenic mice deficient in activin receptor IIA have reduced serum FSH levels.[619] Activins have other actions in pituitary gonadotrophs as well, including up-regulation of GnRH receptors and enhancement of GnRH-stimulated LH release.[618] Activins and inhibins also have local actions within the ovary influencing granulosa cell growth and differentiation, the responsiveness of the ovary to gonadotropins, steroid hormone production, follicular development, and oocyte maturation.[620]

Regulation of the Ovarian Cycle

Whereas in males spermatogenesis occurs continually throughout the adult years, females show a cyclic pattern of ovarian activity with intermittent maturation and release of ova from the ovaries. Cyclic activity in the ovary is controlled by an interplay between steroid hormones produced by the ovary and the hypothalamic-pituitary neuroendocrine components of the reproductive axis.[602, 621, 622] The duration of each phase of the ovarian cycle is species-dependent, but the general mechanisms controlling the cycle are similar in all species that have spontaneous ovarian cycles. In the human menstrual cycle, day 1 of the cycle is designated as the first day of menstrual bleeding. At this time, small and medium-sized follicles are present in the ovaries and only small amounts of estradiol are produced by the follicular cells. As a result, there is a low level of negative feedback to the hypothalamic-pituitary axis, LH pulse frequency is relatively fast (one pulse about every 60 minutes), and FSH concentrations are slightly elevated compared with much of the rest of the cycle (Fig. 7–42).[621, 622] FSH acts at the level of the ovarian follicles to stimulate development and causes an increase in follicular estradiol production, which in turn provides increased negative feedback to the hypothalamic-pituitary unit.

A result of the increased negative feedback is a slowing of pulsatile LH secretion over the course of the follicular phase to a rate of about one pulse every 90 minutes.[621, 622] However, as the growing follicle (or follicles, depending on the species) secretes more estradiol, a positive feedback action of estradiol is triggered that leads to an increase in GnRH release and a surge release of LH and FSH. The surge of gonadotropins acts at the fully developed follicle to stimulate the dissolution of the follicular wall and leads to ovulation of the matured ovum into the nearby fallopian tube, where fertilization takes place if sperm are present. Ovulation results in a reorganization of the cells of the follicular wall, which undergo hypertrophy and hyperplasia and start to secrete large amounts of progesterone and some estradiol. Progesterone and estradiol have a negative feedback effect at the level of the hypothalamus and pituitary, and thus LH pulse frequency becomes very slow during the luteal phase of the menstrual cycle.[621, 622] The corpus luteum has a fixed life span, and without additional stimulation in the form of chorionic gonadotropin from a developing embryo, the corpus luteum regresses spontaneously

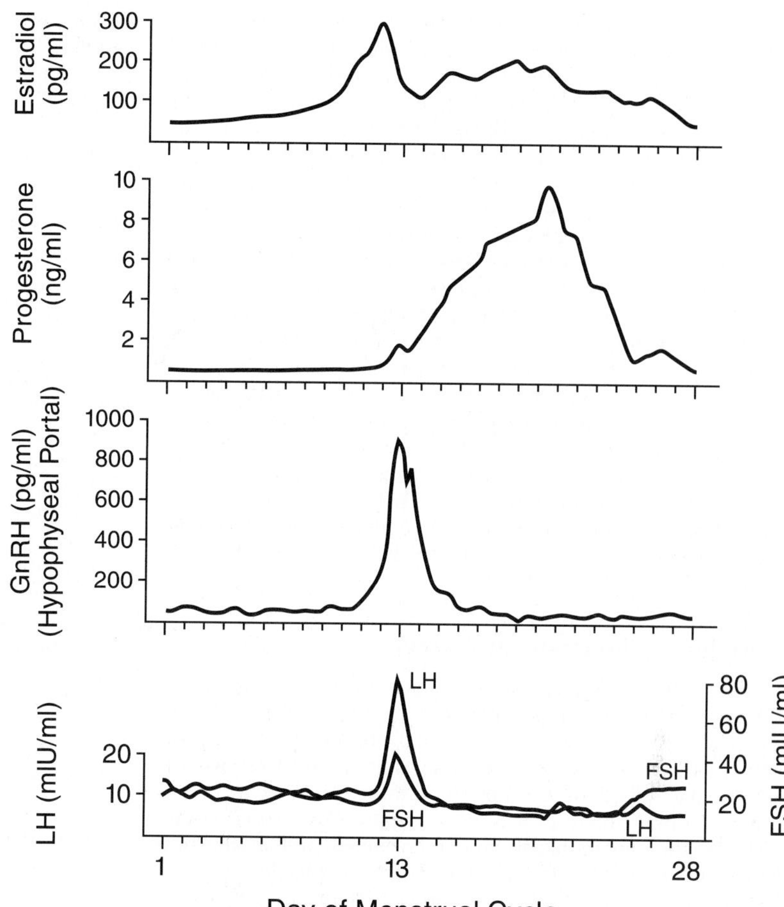

Figure 7-42. Diagrammatic representation of changes in plasma levels of estradiol, progesterone, luteinizing hormone (LH) and follicle-stimulating hormone (FSH) and portal levels of gonadotropin-releasing hormone (GnRH) over the human menstrual cycle.

after about 14 days and progesterone and estradiol secretion diminishes. This reduces the negative feedback signals to the hypothalamus and pituitary and allows an increase in FSH and LH secretion. The fall in progesterone is also a withdrawal of steroid hormone support to the endometrial lining of the uterus, and as a result the endometrium is shed as menses and a new cycle begins.

In other species, the interplay between the neuroendocrine and ovarian hormones is similar but the timing of events is different and other factors, such as circadian and seasonal regulatory factors, play a role in regulating the cycle. The rat has a 4- or 5-day ovarian cycle with no menses (the endometrial lining is absorbed rather than shed). The rat also shows strong circadian rhythmicity in the timing of the LH-FSH surge, with the surge always occurring in the afternoon of the day of proestrus.[623] Sheep are an example of a species that has a strongly seasonal pattern of ovarian cyclicity.[624] During the breeding season they have 15-day cycles, with a very short follicular phase and an extended luteal phase; during the nonbreeding season signals relaying information about day length through the visual system, pineal, and SCN cause a dramatic suppression of GnRH neuronal activity, and cyclic ovarian function is prevented by a decrease in trophic hormonal support from the pituitary.

Early Development and Puberty

Neuroendocrine stimulation of the reproductive axis is initiated during fetal development, and in primates in midgestation circulating levels of LH and FSH reach values similar to those in castrated adults.[625, 626] Later in gestational development, gonadotropin levels decline, restrained by rising levels of circulating gonadal steroids.[625–627] The steroids that have this effect are probably placental in origin in that after parturition there is a rise in circulating gonadotropin levels that is apparent for variable periods of the first year of life, depending on the species.[628, 629] The decline in reproductive hormone secretion in the postnatal period appears to be due to a decrease in GnRH stimulation of the reproductive axis because it occurs even in the castrate state and gonadotropin and gonadal steroid secretion can be supported by administration of pulses of GnRH.[629, 630]

Pubertal reawakening of the reproductive axis occurs in late childhood and is marked initially by nighttime elevations in gonadotropin and gonadal steroid hormone levels.[631, 632] The mechanisms controlling the pubertal reawakening of the GnRH pulse generator have been an area of intense investigation for the past two decades.[630, 633] Although the mechanisms are not fully understood, significant progress has been made in identifying central changes in the hypothalamus that appear to play a role in this process. There appear to be both a decrease in transsynaptic inhibition to the GnRH neuronal system at puberty and an increase in stimulatory input to GnRH neurons at this time. One of the major inhibitory inputs to the GnRH system is provided by GABAergic neurons. Studies in rhesus monkeys have shown that hypothalamic levels of GABA decrease during early puberty and that blocking GABAergic input before puberty, by intrahypothalamic administration of antisense oligodeoxynucleotides against the enzymes responsible for GABA synthesis, results in premature activation of the GnRH neuronal system.[584]

It has been suggested, on the basis of findings that a subset of glutamate receptors (i.e., kainate receptors) increase in the hypothalamus at puberty, that the pubertal decrease in GABA tone may be caused by an increase in glutamatergic transmission.[633] Further evidence for a role for glutamate comes from studies showing that administration of glutamate to prepubertal rhesus monkeys can drive the reawakening of the reproductive axis.[634] Increased stimulatory drive to the GnRH neuronal system also appears to come from increases in norepinephrine and NPY at the time of puberty.[583, 635] Furthermore, as discussed earlier, there is evidence that growth factors act through release of prostaglandin from glial cells at puberty to play a role in stimulating GnRH neurons.[633]

Despite an increased understanding of the neural changes occurring at puberty, the question of what signals trigger the pubertal awakening of the reproductive axis is unanswered at this time. Availability of food and nutritional status have been shown to affect the timing of puberty, but these signals appear to be only modulators of the pubertal process because puberty can be only moderately advanced by increasing food availability.[636] Determining whether there is a genetic timing mechanism that regulates the timing of puberty or whether other signals from the body or the brain are responsible for timing the reactivation of the reproductive axis awaits further research.

Reproductive Function and Stress

Many forms of physical stresses, such as energy restriction, exercise, temperature stress, infection, pain, and injury, as well as psychological stresses, such as being subordinate in a dominance hierarchy or being acutely psychologically stressed, can suppress the activity of the reproductive axis.[637–640] If the stress exposure is brief, there may be acute suppression of circulating gonadotropins and gonadal steroid hormones and in females disruption of normal menstrual cyclicity, but fertility is unlikely to be impaired.[639, 640] In contrast, prolonged periods of significant stress exposure can lead to complete impairment of reproductive function, also characterized by low circulating levels of gonadotropins and gonadal steroids.[637, 638] Stress appears to decrease the activity of the reproductive axis by decreasing GnRH drive to the pituitary because in all cases in which it has been examined, administration of exogenous GnRH can reverse the effects of the stress-induced decline in reproductive hormone secretion.[575] Although we do not know the neural circuits through which many forms of stress suppress GnRH neuronal activity, some forms of stress-induced suppression of reproductive function are better understood.

In the case of foot shock stress in rats[641] and immune stress (i.e., injection of IL-1α) in primates,[642] the suppression of gonadotropin secretion that occurs has been shown to be reversible by administration of a CRH antagonist, implying that endogenous CRH secretion mediates the effects of these stresses on GnRH neurons. In other studies, naloxone, a μ-opiate receptor antagonist, has been shown to be capable of reversing restraint stress–induced suppression of gonadotropin secretion in monkeys; however, naloxone is ineffective in reversing the suppression of gonadotropin secretion that occurs during insulin-induced hypoglycemia.[643, 644] In the case of metabolic stresses, multiple regulators appear to mediate changes in the neural drive to the reproductive axis.

Various metabolic fuels including glucose and fatty acids can regulate the function of the reproductive axis, and blocking cellular utilization of these fuels can lead to suppression of gonadotropin secretion and decreased gonadal activity.[645] Leptin, a hormone produced by fat cells, can also modulate the activity of the reproductive axis. Transgenic mice deficient in leptin or leptin receptors are infertile, and fertility can be restored by administration of leptin.[646] Moreover, leptin administration has been shown to reverse the suppressive effects of undernutrition on the reproductive axis in some situations.[647] Leptin receptors are found in several populations that are known to have a strong influence on the reproductive axis, notably NPY neurons.[648]

In summary, it appears that a number of neural circuits can mediate effects of stress on the GnRH neuronal system and that the neural systems involved are at least somewhat specific to the type of stress that is experienced.

Leptin and the Brain-Gut-Adipose Axis

Long-term energy, stored as fat in adipose tissue, is homeostatically maintained by a hypothalamic system termed the lipostat or adipostat.[649] Inputs to this system are many, including acute hormonal, nutritional, and vagal signals of hunger and satiety; the signal of long-term energy stores derived from the adipose hormone leptin; and powerful olfactory, visual, emotional, and cognitive inputs from higher brain centers. Outputs include those directed toward energy intake, primarily determined by feeding behavior, and energy expenditure, which can be broken down into basal metabolism, voluntary and involuntary activity, and diet-induced thermogenesis. As described throughout this chapter, energy homeostasis is maintained through the triad of behavioral, autonomic, and endocrine pathways. Thus, energy homeostasis is maintained by a complicated hypothalamic-brain stem-target organ axis that may be referred to as the brain-gut-adipose axis (Fig. 7–43).

The regulation of feeding behavior and metabolism is determined by both short-term and long-term control mechanisms. Short-term control involves the initiation and termination of meals. A major determinant of meal size is the perception of satiety that is produced by neural, endocrine, and nutritional inputs during ingestion of a meal. For example, gut distention and release of gastrointestinal peptides such as cholecystokinin lead to meal termination. Ghrelin, an orexigenic peptide, demonstrates a clear preprandial rise and postprandial fall in plasma levels supporting a possible physiologic role in meal initiation in humans.[650] Long-term signals that reflect the body's overall energy depots, such the adipocyte-derived hormone leptin, signal to the CNS to effect changes in feeding behavior and energy expenditure. Both these short-term and long-term factors are coordinated through the brain-gut-adipose axis to respond to changes in energy homeostasis (see Fig. 7–43).

Chemistry and Evolution of Leptin

A significant advance in understanding energy homeostasis in humans occurred with the identification of the basis for the monogenic obesity syndromes characterized in *ob/ob* and *db/db* mice.[26, 651] Parabiosis experiments in which mice were surgically fused to permit transfer of molecules from one to the other led to the hypothesis 30 years ago that *ob/ob* mice were deficient in a circulating signal of satiety whereas *db/db* mice were deficient in its cognate receptor. The *ob* gene was cloned in 1994 and encodes a unique member of the cytokine family now called leptin (from the Greek root *leptos*, meaning thin) (Fig. 7–44). Leptin protein has been highly conserved throughout evolution, as demonstrated by mouse and human leptin being 84% homologous.

Thus far, leptin has been found in birds but not in fish or amphibians. This 167-amino-acid protein has a mass of 16 kd and circulates in the blood at concentrations proportional to the amount of fat depots. Leptin circulates in the blood stream both as a free protein and bound to a soluble isoform of its receptor (Ob-Re). Its secretion is pulsatile and shows a rhythm with a nocturnal peak occurring between 1 and 2 AM and a nadir in the afternoon (Fig. 7–48).[652] Leptin is secreted primarily from the adipocyte; however, minor levels of regu-

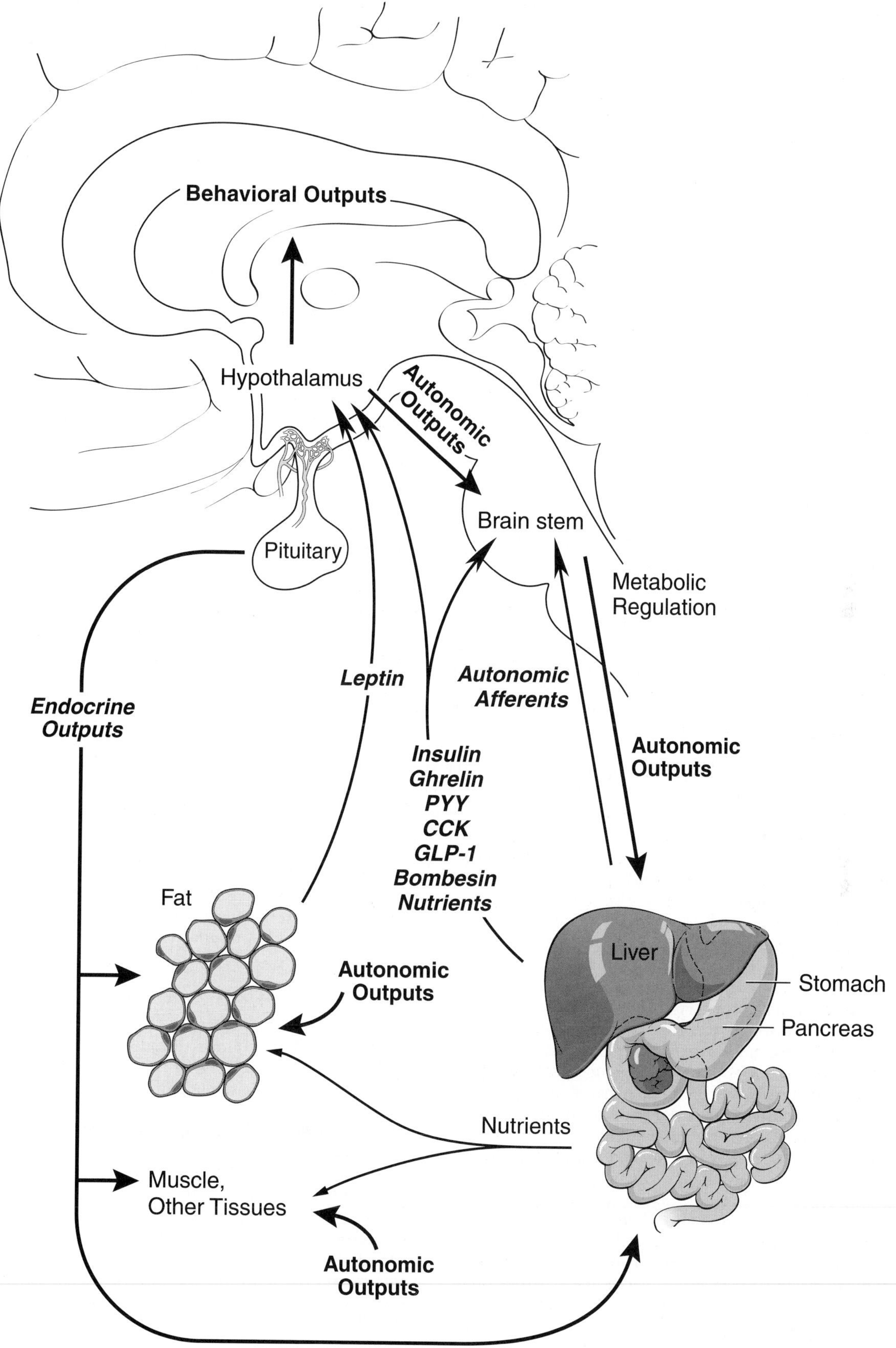

Figure 7–43. Regulation of energy homeostasis by the brain-gut-adipose axis. CCK, cholecystokinin; GLP-1, glucagon-like peptide 1; PYY, peptide YY.

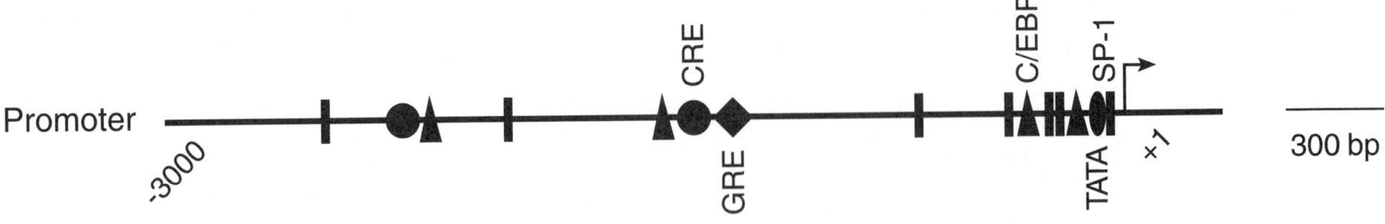

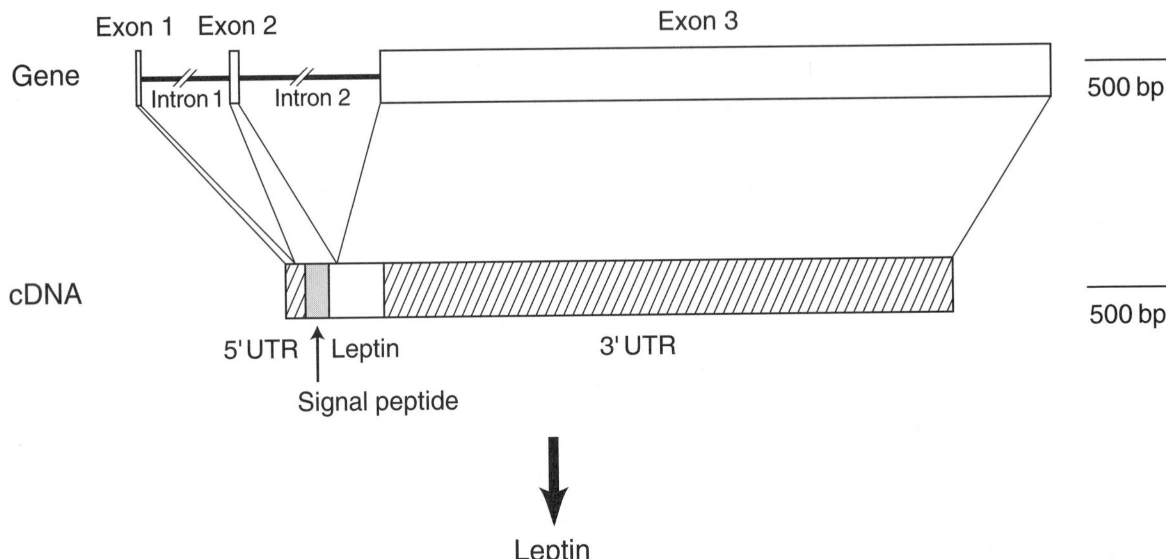

Figure 7–44. Structure of the human leptin gene. cDNA, complementary deoxyribonucleic acid; UTR, untranslated region; *rectangle*, SP-1 site; *triangle*, CCAAT/enhancer binding protein (C/EBP); *circle*, cyclic AMP-responsive element (CRE); *diamond*, glucorticoid response element (GRE).

lated leptin expression also occur in other sites such as skeletal muscle,[653] placenta, and stomach.

Effects of Leptin on the Hypothalamus and Neuroendocrine Axes

A reduction in leptin levels occurs because of loss of adipose mass such as in anorexia nervosa, weight loss induced by diet or exercise, or starvation and is crucial to metabolic adaptation to a state of negative energy balance. This metabolic adaptation includes a decrease in metabolic rate that allows extended survival periods; inhibition of the reproductive, GH, and thyroid axes[283]; and, at least in rodents, inhibition of the activity of the sympathetic nervous system[654, 655] and activation of the HPA axis.

In addition, leptin is a critical signal in the initiation of puberty. Leptin is a signal from the adipose tissue directed to the CNS that conveys readiness to proceed into puberty and is essential for fertility in the adult. Presumably, the leptin signal is a mechanism for the organism to determine whether adequate energy stores are present to maintain a pregnancy through term. For example, leptin administration restored fertility to *ob/ob* mice[646] and prevented the starvation-induced delay in ovulation in female mice and rats.[283, 656] In addition, leptin does not advance the onset of puberty beyond normal in animals fed a normal diet ad libitum, suggesting that leptin is not a trigger but rather a permissive signal in the complex process of initiation of puberty and reproductive competence. Furthermore, leptin exerted at least a permissive action on GnRH release from the hypothalamus and stimulated LH and FSH release from the pituitary in vitro.[657]

Mechanism of Action

After secretion, leptin circulates in plasma in both free and bound forms. It is assumed that the binding protein is a soluble form of the leptin receptor, but other alternatives are being evaluated.[658] In humans, the half-life of leptin is approximately 75 minutes.[659]

The precise mechanism of the transport of leptin into the CNS is unknown. Active uptake of leptin has been described in the capillary endothelium and microvasculature of brains from humans and mice, suggesting a role of short isoforms of the leptin receptor.[91] In addition, the transport of leptin into the choroid plexus is saturable.[91]

After its transport through the blood-brain barrier, leptin binds to specific receptors in the hypothalamus. Leptin receptor mRNA is densely concentrated in the arcuate nucleus, and lower levels are found in the ventromedial and dorsomedial hypothalamic nuclei.[96]

The leptin receptor is a member of the cytokine receptor superfamily. The leptin receptor binds Janus kinases (JAKs), tyrosine kinases involved in intracellular cytokine signaling. Activation of JAK leads to phosphorylation of members of the signal transducer and activator of transcription (STAT) family of proteins. In turn, these STAT proteins activate transcription of leptin target genes.

A great deal of effort has gone into characterizing the mechanism of leptin action in the hypothalamus. Leptin appears to inhibit feeding and stimulate metabolism by acting on a small number of nuclei in the hypothalamus and brain stem, including the ventromedial hypothalamus and the arcuate, dorsomedial, and paraventricular hypothalamic nuclei (Fig. 7–45).[660] In these neurons, leptin up-regulates the expression of an assortment of anorexigenic peptides, such as α-MSH, derived from the POMC pre-prohormone gene (Fig. 7–46), cocaine and amphetamine-regulated transcript (CART), and neuromedin U, and decreases the expression of orexigenic peptides, NPY, AgRP, and melanin-concentrating hormone. Furthermore, leptin has been shown to depolarize and activate the firing rate of the anorexigenic POMC neurons and hyperpolarize the adjacent orexigenic NPY-AgRP neurons.[31]

NPY, long known as a potent stimulator of feeding, was proved to have a role in leptin action when deletion of the NPY gene relieved a significant component of the obesity phenotype of the *ob/ob* mouse.[661] The role of the POMC neurons in energy homeostasis was originally discovered from studies on the agouti mouse,[289, 662, 663] one of the five naturally occurring monogenic obesity strains in the mouse.[664] Intracerebroventricular administration of α-MSH agonist and antagonist analogues inhibited and stimulated feeding behavior, respectively.[663] Furthermore, deletion of the melanocortin-4 receptor (MC4R), the primary neuronal receptor for the melanocortin peptides,[665] caused an obesity syndrome identical to that seen in the obese lethal yellow agouti animal.[289] The structure and distribution of the POMC and NPY-AgRP circuits are highly conserved in humans (Fig. 7–47). Furthermore, a null mutation in the POMC gene in humans caused an obesity syndrome similar to that seen in the lethal yellow mouse along with ACTH insufficiency and red hair[666] (see

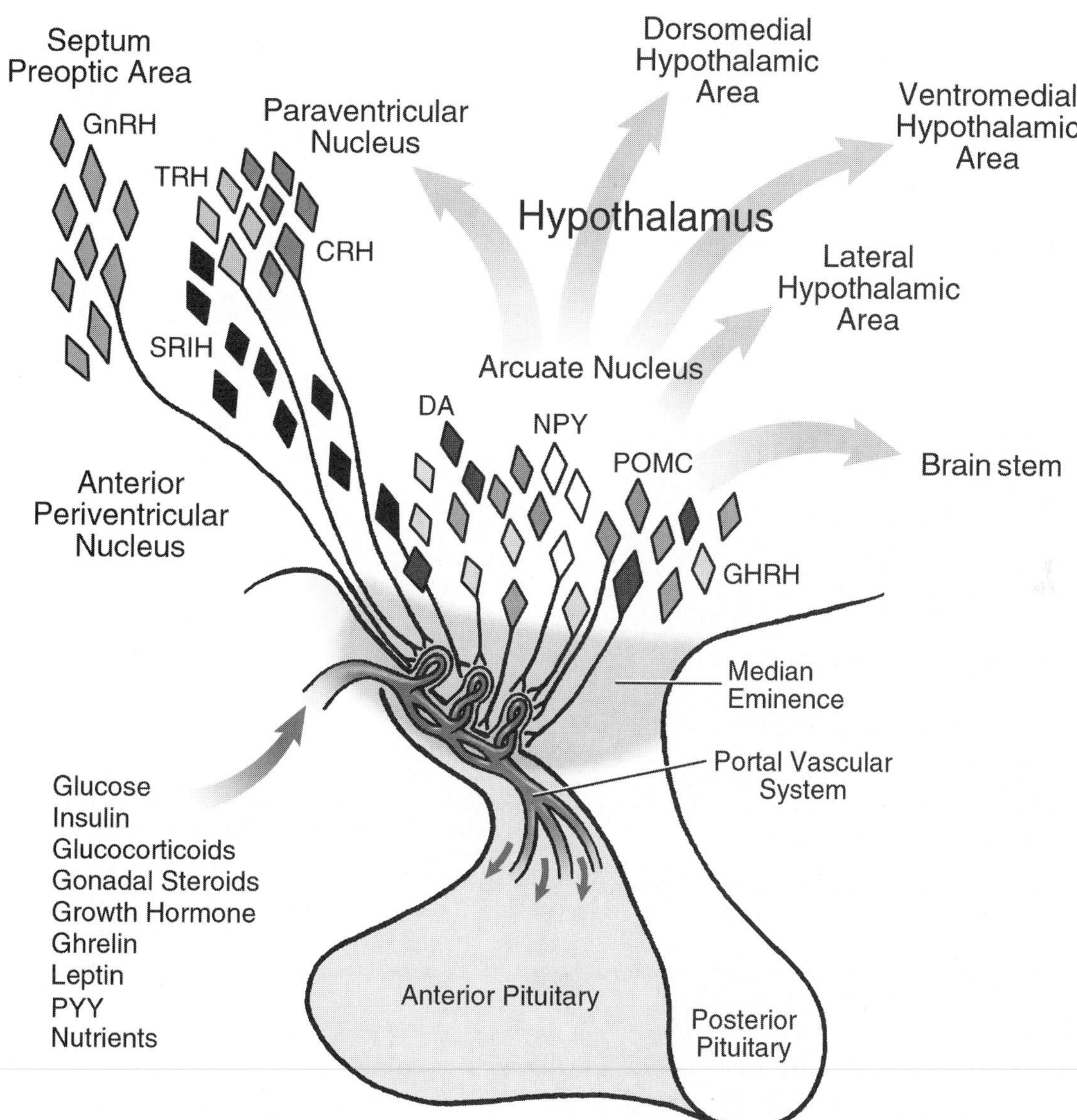

Figure 7–45. Role of the hypothalamus as a sensory organ in the regulation of energy homeostasis. CRH, corticotropin-releasing hormone; DA, dopamine; GHRH, growth hormone–releasing hormone; GnRH, gonadotropin-releasing hormone; NPY, neuropeptide Y; POMC, pro-opiomelanocortin; SRIH, somatotropin release–inhibiting hormone; TRH, thyrotropin-releasing hormone. (Modified with permission from Cone RD, Cowley MA, Buller AA, et al. The arcuate nucleus as a conduit for diverse signals relevant to energy homeostasis. Int J Obes 2001; 25:563–667.)

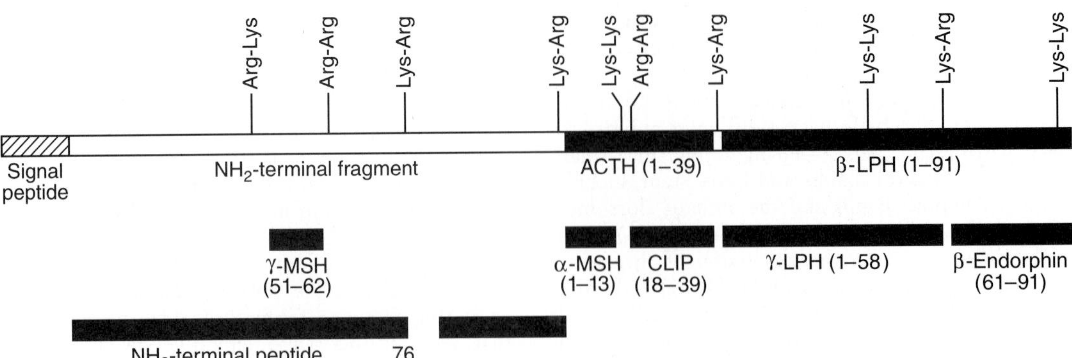

Figure 7–46. Organization of pro-opiomelanocortin (POMC), the precursor hormone of corticotropin (ACTH on figure), β-LPH, and related peptides. The precursor protein contains a leader sequence (signal peptide), followed by a long fragment that includes sequence 51–62 corresponding to α-MSH. This fragment is cleaved at Lys-Arg bonds to form corticotropin 1B39, which in turn includes the sequences for α-MSH (corticotropin 1B13) and corticotropin-like intermediate lobe peptide (CLIP) (corticotropin 17–39), and a sequence corresponding to β-LPH (1–91) that includes γ-LPH 1–58), and β-endorphin (61B91). The β-endorphin sequence also includes a sequence corresponding to met-enkephalin. The precursor molecule in the anterior lobe of the pituitary is processed predominantly to corticotropin and β-LPH. In the intermediate pituitary lobe (in the rat), corticotropin and β-LPH are further processed to α-MSH and a β-endorphin–like material. In all extrapituitary tissues, post-translational processing of the prohormone resembles that in the intermediate lobe. Hypothalamic processing is similar but not identical to that in the intermediate lobe. In the latter, β-endorphin and α-MSH are present predominantly in their acetylated forms. β-LPH, β-lipotropin; γ-MSH, γ-melanocyte-stimulating hormone; α-MSH, α-melanocyte-stimulating hormone; γ-LPH, γ-lipotropin.

"Neuroendocrine Disease"). Thus, it appears that the central melanocortin system subserves the same purposes in mouse and humans. Although obesity related to genetic defects in leptin or the leptin receptor is rare in humans, haploinsufficiency of the MC4R appears to be responsible for up to 3% to 5% of severe pediatric obesity.[290, 667, 668]

Thus, the arcuate nucleus, site of the POMC-CART and NPY-AgRP neurons described earlier, is an important site

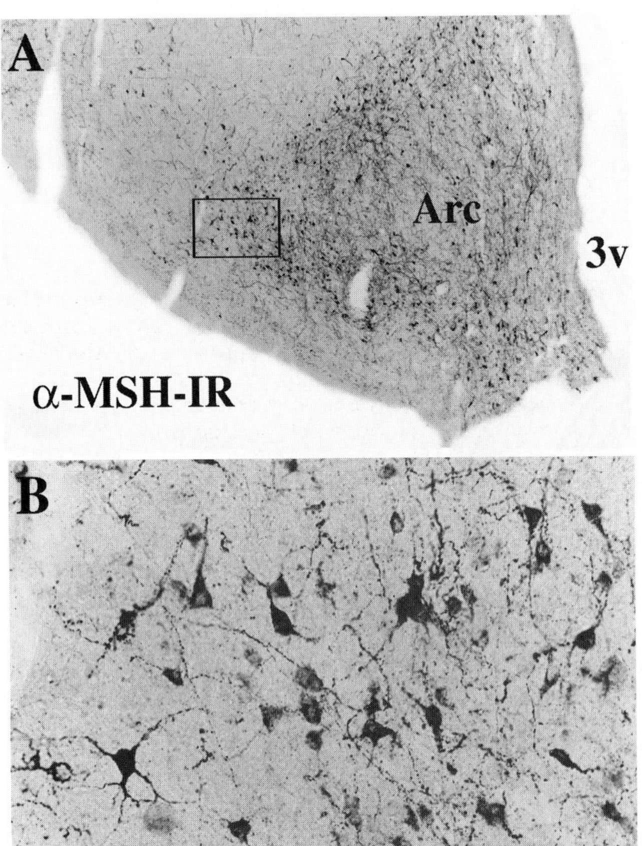

Figure 7–47. *A*, A series of photomicrographs demonstrate that α-melanocyte-stimulating hormone–immunoreactive (α-MSH-IR) neurons are present in the human hypothalamus. The neurons are found in the arcuate nucleus of the hypothalamus. Arc, infundibular nucleus; 3v, third ventricle.

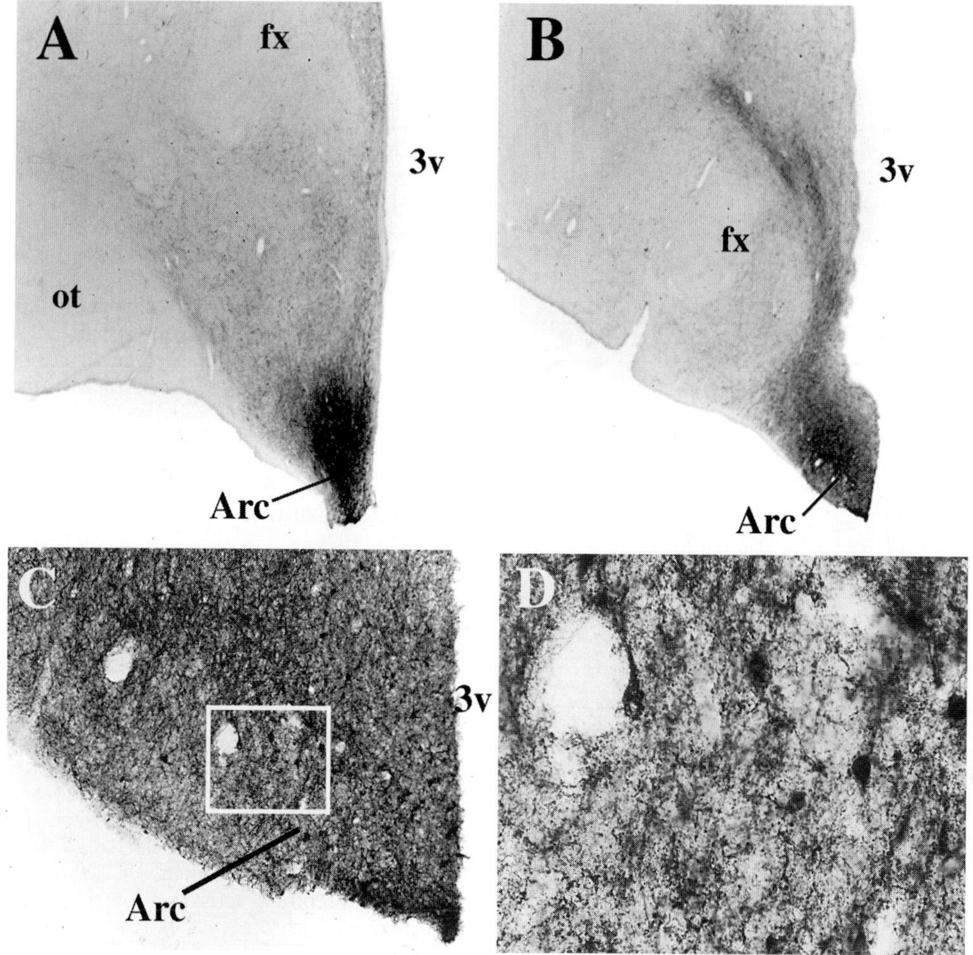

Figure 7–47 *Continued. B*, A series of photomicrographs demonstrate that agouti-related peptide–immunoreactive (AgRP-IR) neurons are present in the human hypothalamus. *A* and *B*, Two rostral to caudal low-power photomicrographs demonstrate that AgRP-IR neurons localize to the arcuate nucleus of the hypothalamus (Arc; infundibular nucleus). *B*, Immunoreactive fibers are also observed streaming dorsally out of the arcuate nucleus. *C* and *D*, AgRP-IR neurons are observed in the arcuate nucleus. *D* is a higher magnification of *C* (use box for orientation). 3v, third ventricle; fx, fornix; ot, optic tract. (Modified from Elias CF, Saper CB, Makatos-Flier E, et al. Chemically defined projections linking the mediobasal hypothalamus and the lateral hypothalamic area. J Comp Neurol 1998; 402:442–459.)

from which leptin exerts a subset of its actions on energy homeostasis. It is important to note that defective melanocortin signaling does not produce the severe neuroendocrine defects seen in leptin-deficient mice or people (e.g., infertility). Furthermore, as already described, the arcuate is adjacent to the median eminence, a CVO, and evidence suggests that acute signals of satiety and hunger may reach regulatory centers through the arcuate as well as vagal inputs to the brain stem.[669] The hormone ghrelin is proposed to be a hunger-initiating factor acting in part through receptor sites on arcuate NPY neurons.[670] The levels of serum ghrelin are potently decreased by food intake in humans (Fig. 7–48).

Clinical Applications

Leptin deficiency[288] and leptin receptor defects[671] in humans are rare. In fact, serum leptin levels in humans are generally proportional to adipose mass.[672] Thus, the vast majority of obese humans may be considered to manifest a leptin-resistant state rather than a deficient state.[673, 674] This concept of leptin resistance also remains poorly understood. However, it is thought that one mechanism of leptin resistance may be impaired leptin transport into the brain. Thus, suboptimal leptin transport through the blood-brain barrier may be one mechanism that underlies the development of leptin resistance in humans.[675] Furthermore, the concept of leptin resistance leads to some reservations concerning the ability of exogenously administered leptin to overcome this leptin resistance and cause effective weight reduction in obese humans.

Clinical studies have now demonstrated that leptin treatment is safe and well tolerated and clearly effective in individuals with congenital leptin deficiency.[676] In this study, low doses of methionyl leptin (met-leptin) were given to subjects with congenital deficiency that resulted in leptin levels 10% of that predicted on the basis of body fat. Leptin in this study was well tolerated and resulted in dramatic declines in appetite, body weight, and food intake.[676]

However, in individuals with common obesity, leptin had only modest effects on appetite and body weight. For example, studies evaluated the safety and efficacy of recombinant human met-leptin administration as well as pegylated human leptin. The first study was a double-blind, placebo-controlled, escalating-dose cohort trial in 54 lean and 73 obese subjects.[677] Higher doses of met-leptin (0.01 to 0.3 mg/kg daily) were also given for 4 to 24 weeks. Met-leptin treatment resulted in significant dose-dependent weight loss: −1.3 kg (placebo

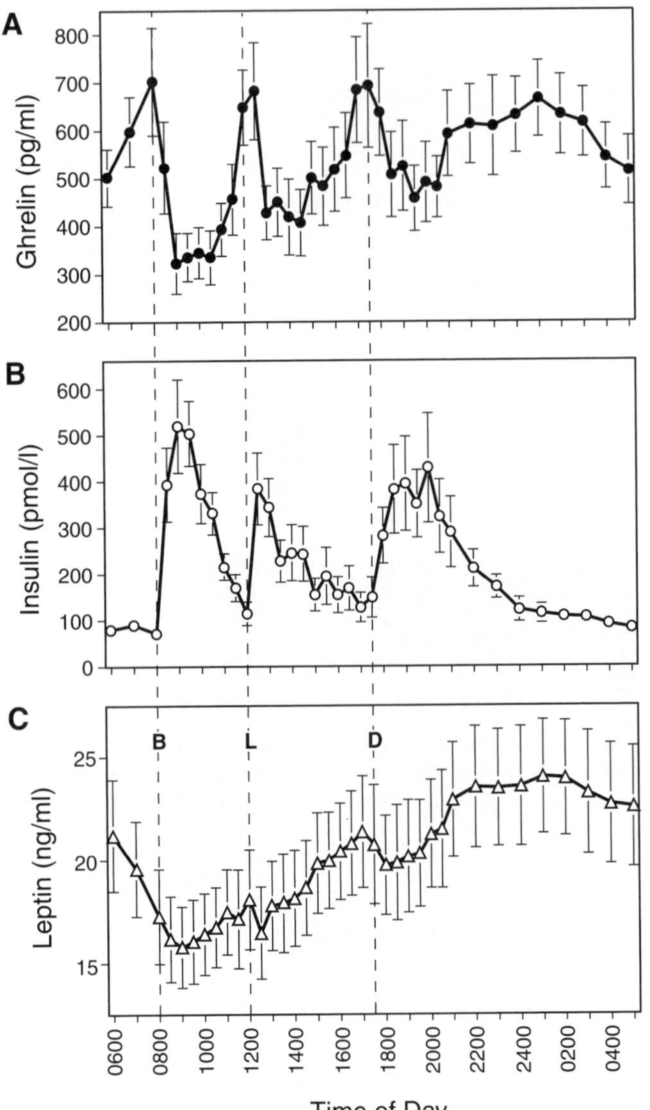

Figure 7–48. Average plasma ghrelin, insulin, and leptin concentrations during a 24-hour period in 10 human subjects consuming breakfast (B), lunch (L), and dinner (D) at the times indicated (0800, 1200, and 1730 hours, respectively) (Reprinted with permission from Cummings DE, et al. A preprandial rise in plasma ghrelin levels suggest a role in meal initiation in humans. Diabetes 2001; 50:1714–1719.).

group), −1.4 kg (0.03 mg/kg group), and −7.1 kg (0.30 mg/kg group) over a 24-week period.[677] Of note, 95% of the weight loss achieved in the two highest dose cohorts was due to loss of fat mass and not any significant changes in fat free mass. The findings have supported the idea that leptin resistance may be partially overcome by a high enough overall leptin concentration.

Another study evaluated the efficacy of another long-acting leptin compound (A-200) in 200 obese subjects in a 24-week randomized, placebo-controlled pilot study with mild dietary intervention (500 calories below daily requirement). Results indicated that A-200 was safe, well tolerated, and resulted in a statistically significant decline in body weight and fat mass.[678] Most of the weight loss again was determined to be secondary to decreases in fat mass. In a randomized, double-blind trial,[679, 680] 30 patients received either 20 mg of polyethylene glycol (PEG)-leptin or placebo weekly for 12 weeks. At the end of the study, patients receiving placebo had increased appetite and hunger levels in the fasting state, compared with reduced appetite and hunger in the treatment group. However, the treatment group did not experience reductions in daily food intake or body mass or changes in body composition compared with the control group. These findings led researchers to conclude that PEG-leptin has central rather than peripheral biologic activity in obese men.[680]

Studies in rodents have demonstrated that leptin is highly efficacious as an antidiabetic agent in lipodystrophy, in which leptin deficiency is directly responsible for a hyperinsulinemic diabetic syndrome.[681] The National Institute of Diabetes and Digestive and Kidney Diseases is currently studying the long-term efficacy of leptin replacement in patients with lipodystrophy (*www.clinicaltrials.gov*, National Institutes of Health protocols 02-DK-0146 and 02-DK-0022). Results from these studies are not yet available.

Feedback Control

Little is known about the cellular pathway involving leptin secretion. However, the rapid effects of β-adrenergic stimulation on leptin release from adipose tissue suggest that leptin secretion is regulated by cAMP. As well, leptin secretion is up-regulated by the hormones insulin and cortisol working synergistically and down-regulated by catecholamines, norepinephrine, and epinephrine. A report also suggests that cholecystokinin may regulate leptin secretion directly.[682] Finally, TNF may be an important paracrine regulator of leptin secretion.[683]

The interesting phenomenon of leptin resistance in obesity was initially suggested on the basis of the elevation of plasma leptin levels in obese humans. It turns out that, as with other cytokine receptors, activation of the leptin receptor induces expression of a protein called suppressor of cytokine signaling-3 (SOCS-3), which may inhibit further leptin signal transduction. The contribution of SOCS-3 to acquisition of leptin resistance and obesity remains an active area of investigation. As well, leptin receptors are expressed in the endothelial cells of the blood-brain barrier and it is plausible that dysfunction of this process may also lead to a state of obesity and leptin resistance.

Neuroendocrine-Immune Interactions

Stimulation of the immune system by foreign pathogens leads to a stereotyped set of responses orchestrated by the CNS. These responses are the result of the complex interaction of the immune system and the CNS and are often referred to as the cerebral component of the acute phase reaction.[84] This constellation of stereotyped responses is adaptive, is mediated in large part by the hypothalamus, and includes coordinated autonomic, endocrine, and behavioral components. These responses include fever, alterations in the activity of nearly every neuroendocrine axis, changes in the sleep-wake cycle, anorexia, and inactivity.

It is now clear that cytokines produced by white blood cells of the immune system mediate the CNS responses. Early evidence supporting this hypothesis was provided by the seminal observations that cytokines such as IL-1β can activate the HPA axis.[684–686] In fact, these and other observations provided the framework for a new area of research in neuroscience and neuroendocrinology. This discipline is often referred to as neuroimmunology. Thus, the term neuroimmunomodulation has been used to describe the study of the interactions of immune system cues and nervous system function.[687, 688]

Although it is established that cytokines modulate hypothalamic activity, it is also important to note that the immune system is modulated by the nervous system. This modulation occurs largely by two routes, endocrine mechanisms and direct innervation. The innervation includes lymphoid organs such as the thymus and spleen, which receive direct inputs from the autonomic nervous system.[689, 690] As noted earlier in the section on CRH, the hallmark of cytokine action on the hypothalamus is the activation of the HPA axis. The resultant glucocorticoid secretion acts as a classical negative feedback to the immune system to damp the immune response (Fig. 7–49). In general, glucocorticoids inhibit most limbs of the immune response, including lymphocyte proliferation, production of immunoglobulins, cytokines, and cytotoxicity. These inhibitory reactions form the basis of the anti-inflammatory actions of glucocorticoids.

Glucocorticoid feedback on immune responses is regulatory and beneficial because loss of this function makes animals with adrenal insufficiency vulnerable to inflammation. Moreover, this feedback response can have pathophysiologic consequences, as chronic activation of the HPA axis can certainly be detrimental.[687, 688] Indeed, it is now established that chronic stress can lead to immunosuppression. The fact that products of inflammation such as IL-1β can activate the HPA axis suggests the operation of a negative feedback control loop to regulate the intensity of inflammation. The role of the hypothalamus in regulating pituitary-adrenal function is an excellent example of neuroimmunomodulation.

This section addresses several of the hypothesized mechanisms by which cytokines engage neural pathways to mediate neuroendocrine and autonomic effects. In addition, some of the autonomic and endocrine pathways that are engaged by immune system cues are briefly discussed. It is important to note that many nonlymphocytic cells including endocrine and adipose cells and neurons also synthesize cytokines that exert effects independent of immunomodulation. Examples of cytokines secreted by adipocytes include leptin, adipsin, and TNF-α, which have profound effects on metabolism.[691]

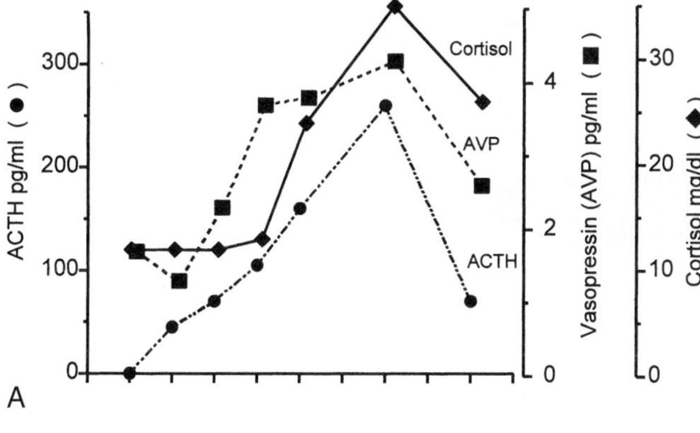

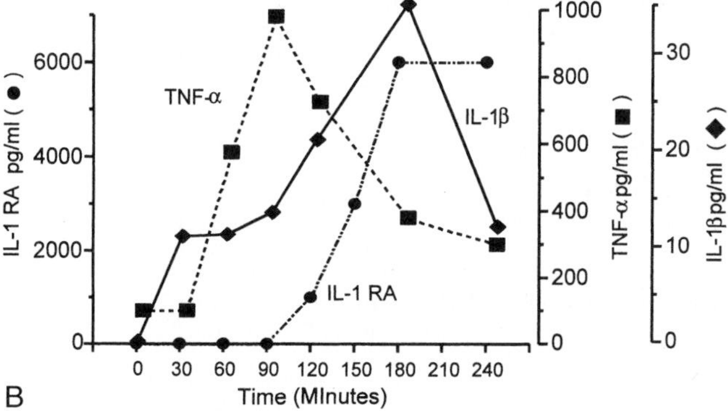

Figure 7–49. *A*, Effect of injection of *Escherichia coli* endotoxin (lipopolysaccharide [LPS]) on circulating levels of corticotropin, vasopressin, and cortisol. *B*, Effect of injection of LPS on circulating levels of IL-1β; IL-1RA; and TNF-α. AVP, vasopressin; ACTH, corticotropin; IL-1RA, interleukin-1 receptor antagonist; IL-1β, interleukin-1β; TNF-α, tumor necrosis factor α. (*A* redrawn from Michie HR, Majzoub JA, O'Dwyer ST, et al. Both cyclooxygenase-dependent and cyclooxygenase-independent pathways mediate the neuroendocrine response in humans. Surgery 1990; 108:254–259. *B* redrawn from Granowitz EV, Santos AA, Poutsiaka DD, et al. Production of interleukin-1-receptor antagonist during experimental endotoxaemia. Lancet 1991; 338:1423–1424, copyright by the Lancet Ltd. 1991; and Michie HR, Manoque KR, Spriggs DR, et al. Detection of circulating tumor necrosis factor after endotoxin injection. N Engl J Med 1988; 318:1481–1486. Copyright 1988. Massachusetts Medical Society. All rights reserved.)

Cytokines Signal the Central Nervous System

Cytokines made outside the CNS can alter the activity and function of populations of hypothalamic neurons. Although the interactions of cytokines with the nervous system have been studied extensively, the mechanisms by which immune signals influence the CNS remain unsettled. LPS (or endotoxin) is a cell wall component of all gram-negative bacteria that is a potent immune system stimulant. LPS administration is widely used as an experimental model and induces the secretion of several pyrogenic cytokines including IL-1β, TNF-α, and IL-6 that mimic the patterns of cytokine production seen in natural infections.[688, 692–694] Many other studies have used systemic injections of cytokines such as IL-1β and TNF-α to stimulate the CNS. Using methodologies such as these, at least four models have been proposed to explain how immune system signals might act upon the CNS (Fig. 7–50).

Interaction of Cytokines with the Circumventricular Organs

The CVOs, described in detail earlier, are specialized regions along the margins of the ventricular system that have fenestrated capillaries and therefore no blood-brain barrier.[695] Many circulating hormones such as angiotensin II act on neurons in the CVOs, converting blood-borne signals into CNS responses.[84] Several models of fever production have hypothesized that cytokines may enter the CNS through the CVOs, particularly at the OVLT (Fig. 7–51*A*; see Fig. 7–50).[101, 696–698] However, definitive evidence establishing this model as a predominant mechanism is still lacking.

Large lesions of the preoptic area of the hypothalamus including the OVLT block fever, but they inevitably damage nearby regions that are critical for thermoregulation.[101] Small lesions of the OVLT do not block fever or corticotropin responses.[699] However, an inherent limitation of this type of study is that the lesion itself breaches the blood-brain barrier, allowing entry of cytokines. Moreover, knife cuts just caudal to the OVLT, interrupting connections from the OVLT to the PVH, did not block activation of the HPA axis by IL-1.[386, 700] Other studies have focused on the area postrema, a CVO located in the medulla oblongata lying along the surface of the nucleus of the solitary tract at the caudal end of the fourth ventricle (see Figs. 7–50 and 7–51*D*). Lesions of the area postrema can block the IL-1–induced activation of the HPA axis and the induction of c-fos mRNA in the PVH.[701] How-

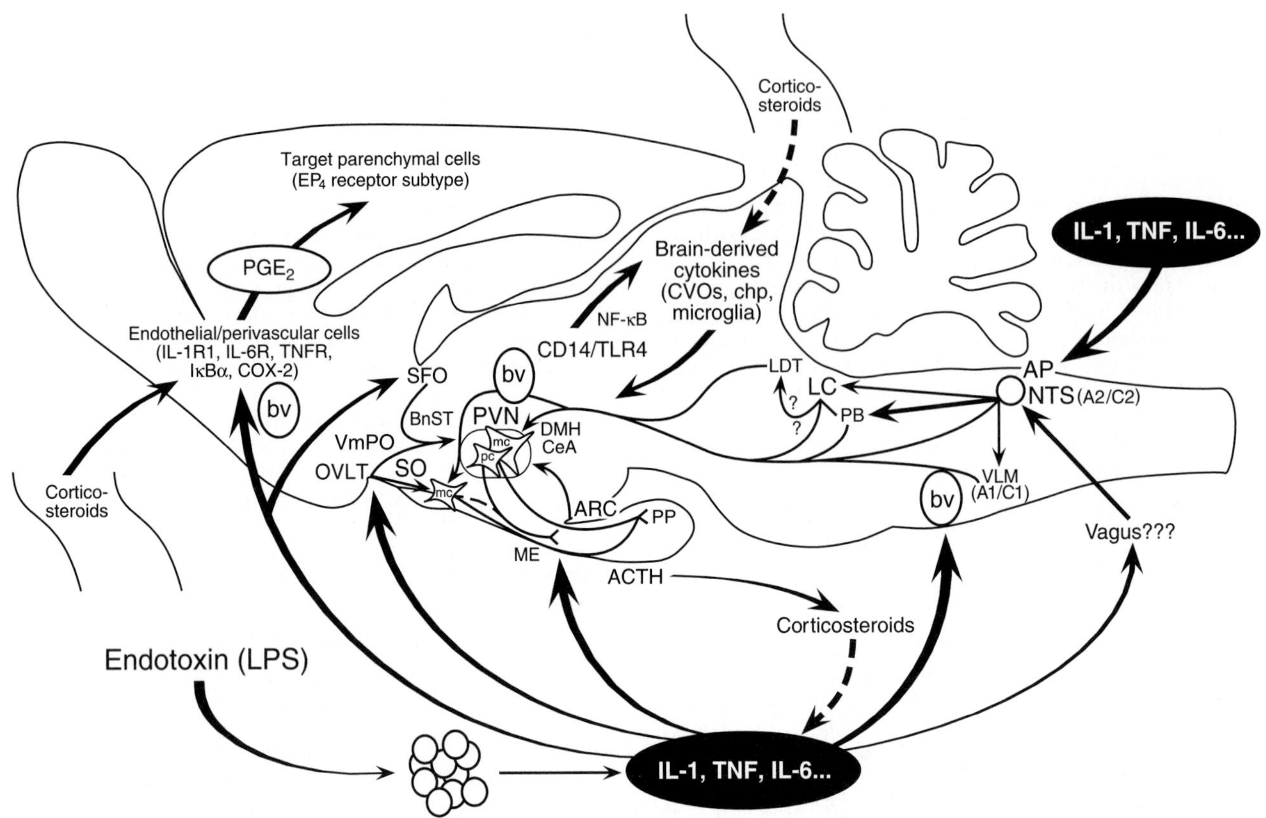

Figure 7–50. A model of the central nervous system circuitry mediating the activation of the paraventricular hypothalamic nucleus (PVN or PVH) and the hypothalamic-pituitary-adrenal (HPA) axis by immune system stimulation. The immune system probably uses several pathways and sites of entry to communicate with the brain. This model predicts that circumventricular organs (organs devoid of blood-brain barrier; CVOs) and the blood vessels (bv) are crucial target sites of cytokines of systemic origin produced during the acute-phase response, whereas activated regions of the brain stem and deep limbic system might play a determinate role in the integration of information received from the periphery. Among these integrative structures, the PVN is critical in coordinating autonomic and endocrine responses including the activity of the HPA axis. For example, corticotropin-releasing factor (CRF) neurons of the parvicellular PVN expressed c-*fos* messenger ribonucleic acid, and that transcription of the gene coding CRF is activated essentially in this hypothalamic nucleus indicates the importance and the specificity of this neuroendocrine nucleus in endotoxin-treated animals. The mechanisms and the circuitry controlling the CRF release and the activity of the HPA axis might also be different from those involved in the biosynthetic machinery of CRF during immune challenge. ACTH, adrenocorticotropic hormone; AP, area postrema; ARC, arcuate nucleus; BnST, bed nucleus of the stria terminalis; bv, blood vessels; chp, choroid plexus; CeA, central nucleus of the amygdala; COX-2, cyclooxygenase-2; DMH, dorsomedial nucleus of the hypothalamus; EP, prostaglandin E receptor; IL-1β, interleukin-1β; IL-1R1, IL-1 type 1 receptor; IL-6, interleukin-6; IκBα, NF-κB inhibitor; LC, locus coeruleus; LDT, laterodorsal tegmental nucleus; LPS, lipopolysaccharide; LRNm, lateral reticular nucleus medial; ME, median eminence; MPOA, medial preoptic area; NF-κB, nuclear factor κB; NTS, nucleus of the solitary tract; OVLT, organum vasculosum of the lamina terminalis; PGE$_2$, prostaglandin E$_2$; PB, parabrachial nucleus; PP, posterior pituitary; PVN, paraventricular nucleus of the hypothalamus (parvicellular [pc] and magnocellular [mc] divisions); SFO, subfornical organ; SON, supraoptic nucleus; TNF-α, tumor necrosis factor α; VLM, ventrolateral medulla. (Modified from Rivest S, Lacroix S, Vallieves L, et al. How the blood talks to the brain parenchyma and the paraventricular nucleus of the hypothalamus during systemic inflammatory and infectious stimuli. Proc Soc Exp Biol Med 2000; 223:22–38.)

ever, others have found that more circumscribed lesions, which do not injure the nucleus of the solitary tract, do not prevent CNS responses to intravenous IL-1[702]

Interactions of Cytokines at the Barriers of the Brain: The Requirement for Prostaglandins

One of the hallmarks of CNS responses to inflammation is that many of the components, including fever and activation of the HPA axis, can be prevented by blocking the production of prostaglandins. This is typically done by administration of nonsteroidal anti-inflammatory drugs such as aspirin and indomethacin.[703–705] Indeed, decades ago the work of Milton and Wendlandt[706, 707] demonstrated that central injections of prostaglandins increase body temperature. However, the site of action in the CNS of drugs such as aspirin that inhibit cyclooxygenase (COX), the enzyme that produces prostaglandins from arachidonic acid, has never been fully established. Two isoforms of COX exist. COX 1 is the constitutive form of the enzyme and is not thought to be regulated by inflammatory stimuli. COX 2 is an inducible isoform and is increased in several cell types in response to immunologic stimuli.[708, 709] In the normal brain, COX 2 mRNA and protein are found exclusively in neurons.[694, 710–712] In contrast, immune stimulation by LPS or cytokines induces COX 2 mRNA and protein throughout the brain in non-neuronal cells associated with blood vessels, the meninges, and the choroid plexus. In addition, systemic administration of IL-1β induces the expression of prostaglandin E synthase mRNA.[713] The cells probably include endothelial cells, perivascular microglial cells, and meningeal

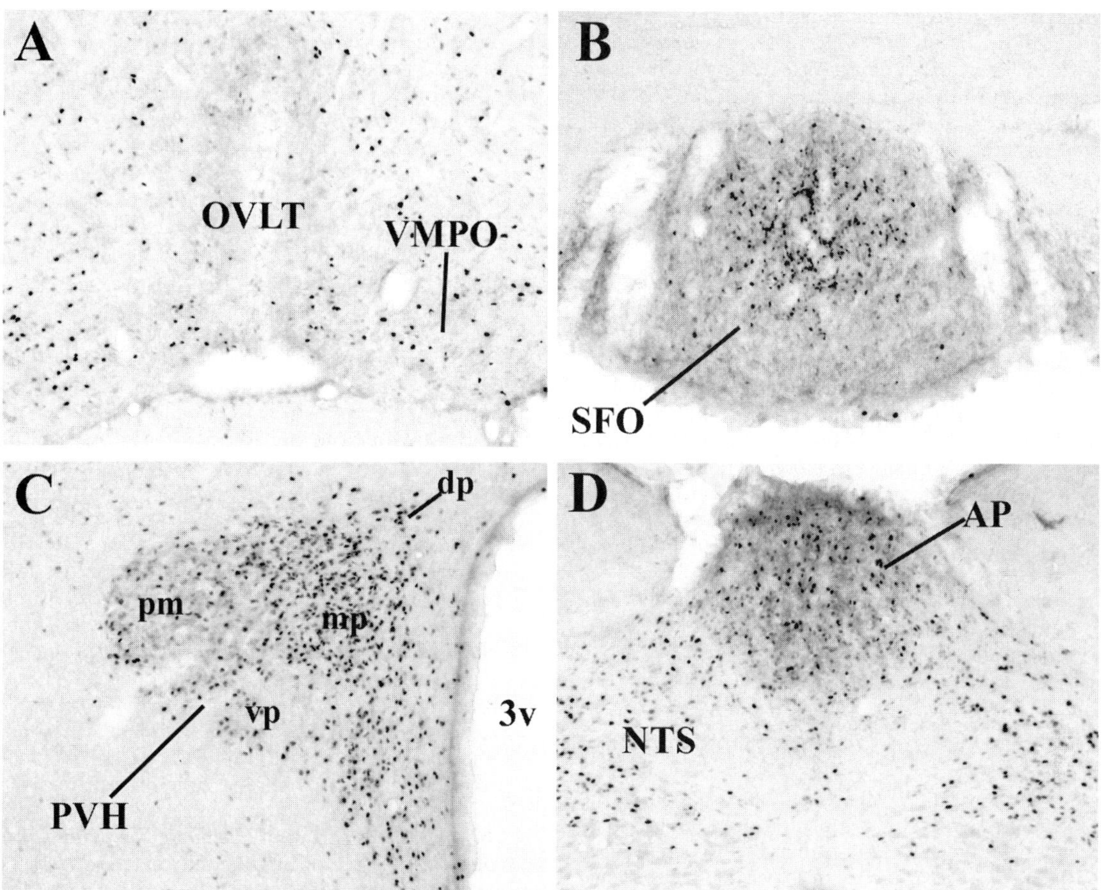

Figure 7–51. Immune stimulation activates key brain regions. A series of photomicrographs demonstrating the distribution of Fos-like immunoreactivity (Fos-IR) in the rat brain 2 hours after intravenous injections of lipopolysaccharide (LPS; 125 μg/kg). LPS administration is a commonly used model of immune stimulation, and Fos-IR is a widely used marker of neuronal activation. LPS activates (induces Fos-IR) in the ventral medial preoptic area and organum vasculosum of the lamina terminalis (VMPO and OVLT; *A*), in the subfornical organ (SFO; *B*), in the paraventricular nucleus of the hypothalamus (PVH; *C*), and in the area postrema and nucleus of the solitary tract in the brain stem (AP, NTS; *D*). Note that prominent Fos-IR is seen throughout the subdivisions of the PVH including the dorsal (dp), ventral (vp), and medial (mp) parvicellular and posterior magnocellular (pm) divisions. Also note that LPS activates neurons in the circumventricular organs (OVLT, SFO, AP). 3v, third ventricle.

macrophages (Fig. 7–62).[714–716] Regardless of the cell type, it seems clear that circulating LPS or cytokines induce COX 2 in cells in the perivascular space, which in turn may produce prostaglandins to stimulate nearby brain regions inside the blood-brain barrier.

PGE_2, the predominant endogenous isoform of PGE in the brain, is thought to be an essential mediator of cytokine modulation of hypothalamic function.[717] This claim is supported by the finding that microinjections of PGE receptor agonists into the brain of rats[698, 718, 719] and other species[720, 721] produce fever. The preoptic area of the hypothalamus surrounding the OVLT is thought to be critical in the response to PGE (see Fig. 7–51*A*). For example, microinjections of as little as 1 ng of PGE_2 into the anteroventral preoptic area of rats reliably produced fevers.[718] Conversely, the COX-2 inhibitor ketorolac attenuated LPS-induced fever with injections placed in the same region.[722] This PGE-sensitive zone is the same as the region containing the highest concentrations of PGE_2 binding sites.[723, 724] The cloning of the prostaglandin E (EP) receptors has allowed more definitive analysis of the receptors in the hypothalamus that mediate the effects of PGEs (see Fig. 7–50).

Four EP receptors have been identified, EP_1, EP_2, EP_3, and EP_4.[693, 725, 726] All four subtypes are expressed in the preoptic area of the hypothalamus.[102, 693, 727–730] Despite the established role of PGE_2 in producing fever and activating the HPA axis, the EP receptor subtypes that are crucial in the febrile response are not yet established.[102, 727, 731, 732] Pharmacologic evidence suggests that EP_1 and EP_3 receptor agonist administration has an effect mimicking PGE_2-induced fever.[731, 732] Moreover, an EP_1 receptor antagonist blocked PGE_2 fever.[732] In contrast, targeted deletion of the EP_3 gene resulted in mice that did not show an early phase of fever after intracerebroventricular injection of LPS or PGE_2.[726] Interestingly, there is up-regulation of EP_4 receptor expression in several areas of the brain, including the CRH neurons of the paraventricular nucleus, after immune challenge.[102, 729] In addition, paraventricular neurons that express Fos after intracerebroventricular PGE_2 also express EP_4 receptors.[729] Thus, production of PGE_2 is certainly an obligate step in the pathogenesis of the febrile response; the identity of the EP receptor subtypes required for distinct components of the response remains to be established.

Entry of Cytokines into the Brain

Circulating cytokines are proteins that cannot easily penetrate the blood-brain barrier. The kinetics of entry of cytokines into the brain have been examined, and evidence suggests that there is saturable transport of IL-1α, IL-1β , IL-6, and TNF-α into the brain.[733–735] However, it is not clear whether sufficient levels of cytokines are detectable in brain after acute intravenous administration to account for CNS responses to acute infection. Thus, the physiologic setting and significance of this mechanism remain to be established.

Moreover, it is noteworthy that levels of circulating IL-1β do not rise significantly during immune challenges.[736, 737] In contrast, large increases in circulating and brain IL-6 are found during fever. Although it is not completely understood, it appears that synthesis of IL-6 within the blood-brain barrier and not peripheral IL-6 crossing the barrier is critical in the production of fever.[738] Moreover, several studies have demonstrated that cells located at the blood-brain barrier and cells within the meninges respond to LPS stimulation with induction of IL-1β and TNF-α, the nuclear factor κB inhibitor IκBα, and the LPS receptor CD14 (Fig. 7–62).[693, 739–741] Cells with a similar morphology lining the blood vessels that penetrate the CNS and the meninges that cover it also have IL-1 receptors, suggesting that they may respond to cytokines as well.[742] Hence, endothelial and perivascular cells at the blood-brain interface may have the ability to elaborate cytokines after an LPS or cytokine signal. The physiologic role of centrally produced cytokines in the response to peripheral immune cues has been reviewed in detail.[693, 737]

Interactions of Cytokines with Peripheral Nerves

Another proposed model by which cytokines may alter the activity of CNS neurons involves stimulation of peripheral sensory nerves, the prototypical example being the vagus nerve (see Fig. 7–50).[743, 744] Several pieces of experimental evidence support the idea that the vagus may provide a conduit for cytokines to activate CNS pathways. For example, IL-1 receptor antagonist binds to vagal paraganglia.[743, 745] In addition, neurons in the nodose ganglia (vagal sensory neurons) expressed type 1 IL-1 receptor mRNA.[746] Peripheral administration of LPS induced Fos expression, a marker of neuronal activation, in the vagal sensory nodose ganglia, and this could be blocked by prior vagotomy.[745] Similarly, IL-1 administration induced the expression of Fos in neurons in the nodose ganglia and increased the firing rate of vagal afferent nerve fibers.[746] The IL-1–induced response was blocked by pretreatment with a COX inhibitor, demonstrating the need for prostaglandin production in this model as well.

Severing the vagus nerve below the diaphragm blocked fever, sickness behavior, and induction of IL-1β mRNA and Fos protein in the brain after intraperitoneal LPS or IL-1β.[743, 747–751] In contrast, the abdominal vagus nerve did not seem to be necessary for the CNS response to intravenous administration of LPS or IL-1β in rats.[747, 751] These observations suggest that, although vagal sensory mechanisms may contribute to CNS responses to immune stimuli, particularly with local infections in the abdominal or thoracic cavities, blood-borne immune challenge may activate the CNS by other routes. In the end, it is likely that redundant mechanisms exist by which the CNS is made aware of inflammatory signals in the periphery. The relative contribution of distinct mechanisms may depend upon the route of administration and dose of inflammatory mediators, and future studies should increase our understanding of these mechanisms.

Cell Groups Throughout the Brain Responsive to Cytokines

Many studies have used the expression of immediate early genes such as c-*fos* or its protein product, Fos,[752] as a marker of neuronal activity. In this way, investigators have assessed the involvement of extended neuronal systems during the complex physiologic responses after immune challenge. Mapping the patterns of activation in the CNS after either IL-1β or LPS administration has yielded new insights into the functional neuroanatomy underlying the coordinated autonomic, endocrine, and behavioral responses during the febrile response.[381, 386, 703, 747, 753–762] Immune activation using moderate to high doses of LPS and IL-1β activates central autonomic and endocrine structures at nearly every level of the neuraxis including several neuroendocrine regulator sites such as the central nucleus of the amygdala, paraventricular hypothalamic nucleus, arcuate nucleus of the hypothalamus, SFO, OVLT, and ventral medial preoptic area (see Fig. 7–51). Brain stem sites engaged include the parabrachial nucleus, nucleus of the solitary tract, area postrema, and the rostral and caudal levels of the ventrolateral medulla.[381, 386, 703, 747, 753–762] In the paraventricular nucleus, LPS and cytokines activate parvicellular CRH neurons.

Although it is established that the hypothalamus is responsible for inducing a febrile response, it is also important to note that there are hypothalamic systems that act to attenuate rises in body temperature. These include arcuate POMC neurons (see Figs. 7–45 and 7–47) and AVP neurons, both of which are thought to be endogenous antipyretic neuromodulators.[763–766] Thus, neuronal activation patterns elicited by LPS or cytokines probably include neurons engaged to limit rises in body temperature. Indeed, Tatro and colleagues[767] have found that exogenous α-MSH administration can block LPS-induced fever. Moreover, the central melanocortin system has been shown to contribute to anorexia during systemic illness.[768, 769] It is possible, therefore, that central melanocortin pathways may act in parallel to inhibit food intake and to reduce fever during immune challenge.

Experimental work has coupled neuroanatomic tract tracing with methods assessing immediate early gene expression to investigate the circuitry that is activated by peripheral immune signals. For example, intravenous administration of IL-1β induced Fos in C1 adrenergic neurons in the ventrolateral medulla that project to the PVH. The C1 adrenergic cell group targets the medial parvicellular subdivision of the PVH, the site of the CRH neurons (see Figs. 7–25 and 7–26).[386] Lesions interrupting the input from the C1 cells to the PVH prevent the HPA response to IL-1β. These studies suggest that the activation of C1 cells by locally produced prostaglandins[702] may play a critical role in activating the HPA axis in response to IL-1β.

Sympathetic preganglionic neurons in the intermediolateral cell column (IML), extending from the first thoracic through the upper lumbar segments of the spinal cord, also show Fos expression in response to LPS.[761] Preganglionic neurons in the upper thoracic (T1 to T4) levels mediate thermogenesis by brown adipose tissue,[770, 771] which is a key mechanism used by rats to control heat production and body temperature.[772] Sympathetic preganglionic neurons in the T2 to T5 levels are important for control of the heart,[773, 774] which is important because there are changes in cardiac output in the febrile state. Another important concept is that sympathetic preganglionic neurons receive direct, monosynaptic input from a series of well-defined nuclei in the brain stem and the hypothalamus (see Fig. 7–1). These cells provide another way in which the hypothalamus can contribute to the coordinated autonomic response to inflammatory signals. The major input to the sympathetic preganglionic column arises from neurons in the hypothalamus.[128] This innervation includes the paraventricular nucleus (dorsal, ventral, and lateral parvicellular subnuclei), the lateral hypothalamic area, and the arcuate nucleus and retrochiasmatic area.[50, 775] Direct projections to the intermediolateral cell column also arise in the brain stem from the A5 noradrenergic cell group in the ventral pons, the caudal part of the nucleus of the solitary tract, the ventromedial medulla including the medullary raphe nuclei, and the rostral ventrolateral medulla, including the C1 adrenergic cell group.[50, 774, 776]

Fos expression in hypothalamic and brain stem neurons projecting to the IML after LPS administration has been examined.[776] LPS-activated cells that innervate the IML are found in the rostral ventrolateral medulla (C1 adrenergic cell group) and the A5 noradrenergic cell group in the brain stem. Moreover, a prominent population of cells was found in the dorsal parvicellular division of the paraventricular nucleus in the hypothalamus. These results suggest that neurons in the parvicellular PVH specifically innervate sympathetic preganglionic neurons in the spinal cord that regulate LPS-induced fever. Furthermore, as noted earlier, activation of CRH neurons in the PVH is a signature of the CNS response to immune stimulation. Thus, the paraventricular hypothalamic nucleus is a key site for mediating both neuroendocrine and autonomic responses to immune stimulation.

NEUROENDOCRINE DISEASE

Disease of the hypothalamus can cause pituitary dysfunction, neuropsychiatric and behavioral disorders, and disturbances of autonomic and metabolic regulation (Fig. 7–52). In the diagnosis and treatment of suspected hypothalamic or pituitary disease, four issues must be kept in mind: the extent of the lesion, the physiologic impact, the specific cause, and the psychosocial setting. The etiology of hypothalamic neuroendocrine disorders categorized by age and syndrome is summarized in Tables 7–9 and 7–10.

Manifestations of pituitary insufficiency secondary to hypothalamic or pituitary stalk damage are not identical to those of primary pituitary insufficiency. Hypothalamic injury causes decreased secretion of most pituitary hormones but can cause hypersecretion of hormones normally under inhibitory control by the hypothalamus, as in hypersecretion of PRL after damage to the pituitary stalk and precocious puberty caused by loss of the normal restraint over gonadotropin maturation.[777] Impairment of inhibitory control of the neurohypophysis can lead to the syndrome of inappropriate vasopressin secretion (SIADH) (see Chapter 9). More subtle abnormalities in secretion can result from impairment of the control system. For example, loss of the normal circadian rhythm of corticotropin secretion may occur before loss of pituitary-adrenal secretory reserve,[778] and responses to physiologic stimuli may be paradoxical. Because hypophyseotropic hormone levels cannot be measured directly and pituitary hormone secretion is regulated by complex, multilayered controls, assay of pituitary hormones in blood does not necessarily give a meaningful picture of events at hypothalamic and higher levels. Rarely, tumors secrete excessive amounts of releasing peptides and cause hypersecretion of hormones from the pituitary.

Disorders of the hypothalamic-pituitary unit can result from lesions at several levels (Fig. 7–53). Defects can arise from destruction of the pituitary (as by tumor, infarct, inflammation, or autoimmune disease) or from a hereditary deficiency of a particular hormone as in rare cases of isolated FSH, GH, or POMC deficiency (Fig. 7–54). Selective loss of thyroid hormone receptors in the pituitary can give rise to increased thyrotropin secretion and thyrotoxicosis. Furthermore, disorders can arise through disruption of the stalk–median eminence contact zone, the stalk itself, or the nerve terminals of the tuberohypophyseal system; such disruption occurs after surgical stalk section, with tumors involving the stalk, and in some inflammatory diseases. At a higher level, tonic inhibitory and excitatory inputs can be lost as manifested by absence of circadian rhythms or the development of precocious puberty. Physical stress, cytokine products of inflammatory cells, toxins, and reflex inputs from peripheral homeostatic monitors also impinge on the tuberoinfundibular system. At the highest level of control, emotional stress and psychological disorders can activate the pituitary-adrenal stress response and suppress gonadotropin secretion (e.g., psychogenic amenorrhea) or inhibit GH secretion (e.g., psychosocial dwarfism) (see Chapter 23). Intrinsic disease of the anterior pituitary is reviewed in Chapter 8, and disturbances in neurohypophyseal function are discussed in Chapter 9. This chapter considers diseases of the hypothalamic-pituitary unit.

Pituitary Isolation Syndrome

Destructive lesions of the pituitary stalk, as occur with head injury, surgical transection, tumor, or granuloma, produce a characteristic pattern of pituitary dysfunction.[777, 779, 780] Central diabetes insipidus (DI) develops in a large percentage of patients, depending on the level at which the stalk has been sectioned. If the cut is close to the hypothalamus, DI is almost always produced, whereas if the section is low on the stalk, the incidence is lower. The extent to which nerve terminals in the upper stalk are preserved determines the clinical course. The

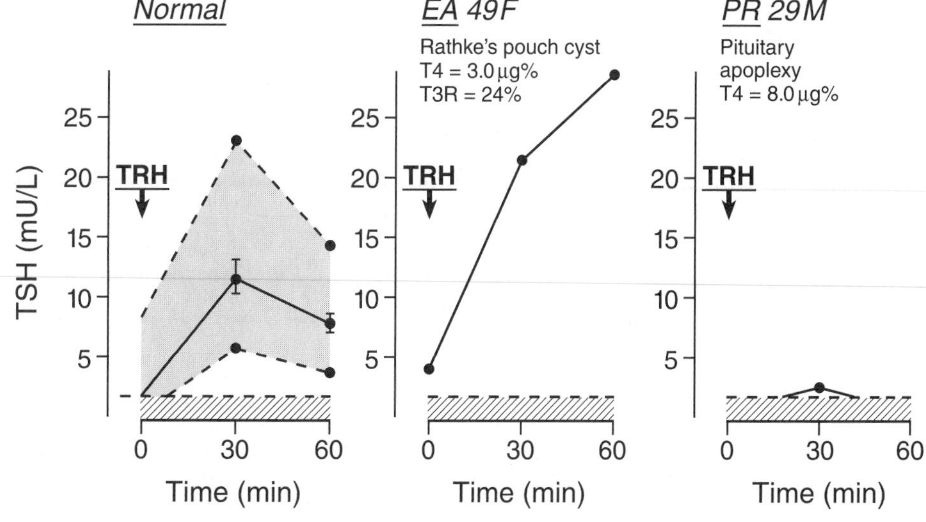

Figure 7–52. Typical pituitary response to thyrotropin-releasing hormone (TRH) administration in patients with hypothalamic-pituitary disease that has caused hypothyroidism. If there is intrinsic pituitary damage, the response is abnormally low. If there is hypothalamic damage, the response is normal or exaggerated. It must be emphasized that some patients with hypothalamic disease may not respond to TRH and that some patients with pituitary disease may respond to TRH. T_4, thyroxine; TSH, thyrotropin. (From Jackson IMD. Diagnostic tests for the evaluation of pituitary tumors. In Jackson IMD, Reichlin S [eds]. The Pituitary Adenoma. New York, Plenum, 1980, pp 219–238.)

Table 7–9. Etiology of Hypothalamic Disease by Age

Premature Infants and Neonates
- Intraventricular hemorrhage
- Meningitis: bacterial
- Tumors: glioma, hemangioma
- Trauma
- Hydrocephalus, kernicterus

1 mo–2 yr
- Tumors
  - Glioma, especially optic glioma
  - Histiocytosis X
  - Hemangioma
- Hydrocephalus
- Meningitis
- Familial disorders
  - Laurence-Moon-Biedl syndrome
  - Prader-Labhart-Willi syndrome

2–10 yr
- Neoplasms
  - Craniopharyngioma
  - Glioma, dysgerminoma, hamartoma
  - Histiocytosis X, leukemia
  - Ganglioneuroma, ependymoma
  - Medulloblastoma
- Meningitis
  - Bacterial
  - Tuberculous
- Encephalitis
  - Viral
  - Exanthematous demeyelinating
- Familial
  - Diabetes insipidus
- Radiation therapy
- Diabetic ketoacidosis
- Moyamoya disease, circle of Willis

10–25 yr
- Tumors
  - Craniopharyngioma
  - Glioma, hamartoma, dysgerminoma
  - Histiocytosis X, leukemia
- Dermoid, lipoma, neuroblastoma

10–25 yr (continued)
- Trauma
- Vascular
  - Subarachnoid hemorrhage
  - Aneurysm
  - Arteriovenous malformation
- Inflammatory disease
  - Meningitis
  - Encephalitis
  - Sarcoidosis
  - Tuberculosis
- Structural brain defect
  - Chronic hydrocephalus
  - Increased intracranial pressure

25–50 yr
- Nutritional: Wernicke's disease
- Tumors
  - Glioma, lymphoma, meningioma
  - Craniopharyngioma, pituitary tumors
  - Angioma, plasmacytoma, colloid cysts
  - Ependymoma, sarcoma, histiocytosis X
- Inflammatory disease
  - Sarcoidosis
  - Tuberculosis, viral encephalitis
- Vascular
  - Aneurysm, subarachnoid hemorrhage
  - Arteriovenous malformation
- Damage from pituitary radiation therapy

50 yr and Older
- Nutritional: Wernicke's disease
- Tumors: Pituitary tumors, sarcoma, glioblastoma, ependymoma, meningioma, colloid cysts, lymphoma
- Vascular disease
  - Infarct, subarachnoid hemorrhage
  - Pituitary apoplexy
- Inflammation: encephalitis, sarcoidosis, meningitis
- Damage from radiation therapy for ear-nose-throat carcinoma, pituitary tumors

Adapted from Plum F, Van Uitert R. Nonendocrine diseases and disorders of the hypothalamus. In Reichlin S, Baldessarini RJ, Martin JB (eds). The Hypothalamus, vol 56. New York, Raven Press, 1978, pp 415–473.

classical triphasic syndrome of initial polyuria followed by normal water control and then by vasopressin deficiency over a period of 1 week to 10 days is seen in less than half of the patients. The sequence is attributed to an initial loss of neurogenic control of the neural lobe, followed by autolysis of the neural lobe with release of vasopressin into the circulation and finally by complete loss of vasopressin. However, full expression of polyuria requires adequate cortisol levels; if cortisol is deficient, vasopressin deficiency may be present with only minimal polyuria. DI can also develop after stalk injury without an overt transitional phase. When DI occurs after head injury or operative trauma, varying degrees of recovery can be seen even after months or years. Sprouting of nerve terminals in the stump of the pituitary stalk may give rise to sufficient functioning tissue to maintain water balance. In contrast to the effects of stalk section, nondestructive injury to the neurohypophysis or stalk, as during surgical resection of optic chiasmatic astrocytomas, can sometimes give rise to transient SIADH.[781]

Although head injury, granulomas, and tumors are the most common causes of acquired DI, other cases develop in the absence of a clear-cut cause.[782] Some cases may be due to autoimmune disease of the hypothalamus as suggested by the finding of autoantibodies to neurohypophyseal cells in a third of cases of "idiopathic" DI in one series.[783] However, autoantibodies were also frequently found in association with histiocytosis-X. Later reports suggest the importance of continued vigilance in cases of idiopathic DI because a definite cause is frequently uncovered in time, including a high proportion of occult germinomas whose detection by magnetic resonance imaging may be preceded by elevated levels of human chorionic gonadotropin (hCG) in CSF.[784, 785]

Table 7–10. Etiology of Endocrine Syndromes of Hypothalamic Origin

Hypophyseotropic Hormone Deficiency
- Surgical pituitary stalk section
- Basilar meningitis and granuloma, sarcoidosis, tuberculosis, sphenoid osteomyelitis, eosinophilic granuloma
- Craniopharyngioma
- Hypothalamic tumor
  - Infundibuloma
  - Teratoma (ectopic pinealoma)
  - Neuroglial tumor, particularly astrocytoma
- Maternal deprivation syndrome, psychosocial dwarfism
- Isolated growth hormone–releasing hormone (GHRH) deficiency
- Hypothalamic hypothyroidism
- Panhypophyseotropic failure

Disorders of Regulation of Gonadotropin-Releasing Hormone Secretion
- Female
  - Precocious puberty
    - GnRH-secreting hamartoma
    - hCG-secreting germinoma
  - Delayed puberty
  - Neurogenic amenorrhea
  - Pseudocyesis
  - Anorexia nervosa
  - "Functional" amenorrhea
  - "Functional" oligomenorrhea
  - Drug-induced amenorrhea
- Male
  - Precocious puberty
  - Fröhlich's syndrome
  - Olfactory-genital dysplasia (Kallmann's syndrome)

Disorders of Regulation of Prolactin-Regulating Factors
- Tumor
- Sarcoidosis
- Drug-induced
- Reflex
- Herpes zoster of chest wall
- Post-thoracotomy
- Nipple manipulation
- Spinal cord tumor
- "Psychogenic"
- Hypothyroidism
- Carbon dioxide narcosis

Disorders of Regulation of Corticotropin-Releasing Hormone
- Paroxysmal corticotropin discharge (Wolff's syndrome)
- Loss of circadian variation
- Depression
- CRH-secreting gangliocytoma

CRH, corticotropin-releasing hormone; GnRH, gonadotropin-releasing hormone; hCG, human chorionic gonadotropin.

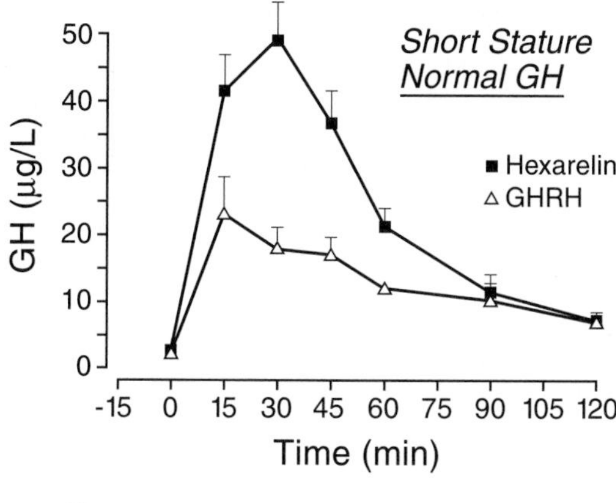

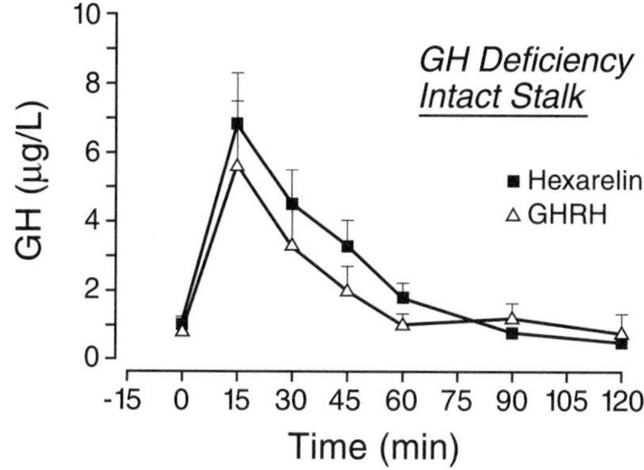

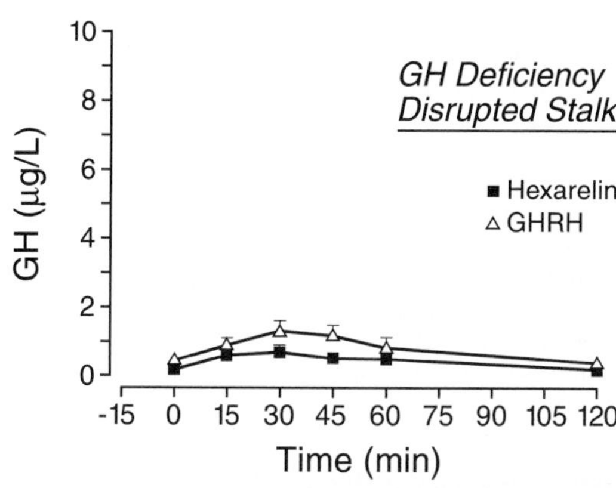

Figure 7–53. Effect of hypothalamic-pituitary disconnection on the growth hormone (GH) secretory responses to GH-releasing hormone (GHRH) (1 μg/kg) and hexarelin (2 μg/kg) administered intravenously to children with GH deficiency. *Top*, mean responses in a group of 24 prepubertal children with short stature secondary to familial short stature or constitutional growth delay. Children with GH deficiency and an intact vascular pituitary stalk as visualized by dynamic magnetic resonance imaging exhibited a clear, but blunted, GH response to both secretagogues *(middle)*. In contrast, children with pituitary stalk agenesis (both vascular and neural components) had no or a markedly attenuated response to both peptides *(bottom)*. (From Maghnie M, Spica-Russotto V, Cappa M, et al. The growth hormone response to hexarelin in patients with different hypothalamic-pituitary abnormalities. J Clin Endocrinol Metab 1998; 83:3886–3889.)

Congenital DI can be part of a hereditary disease. DI in the Brattleboro rat is due to an autosomal recessive genetic defect that impairs production of vasopressin but not of oxytocin.[786] Inherited forms of DI in humans have been attributed to mutations in the vasopressin V2 receptor gene or less frequently in the aquaporin or vasopressin genes.[787–790]

Menstrual cycles cease after stalk section although urinary gonadotropins may still be detectable, unlike the situation after hypophysectomy. Plasma glucocorticoid levels and urinary excretion of cortisol and 17-hydroxycorticoids decline after hypophysectomy and stalk section, but the change is slower after stalk section. A transient increase in cortisol secretion after stalk section is believed to be due to release of ACTH from preformed stores. The ACTH response to the lowering of blood cortisol is markedly reduced but ACTH release after stress may be normal, possibly because of CRH-independent mechanisms. Reduction in thyroid function after stalk section is similar to that seen with hypophysectomy. The fall in GH secretion is said to be the most sensitive indication of damage to the stalk; however, the insidious nature of this endocrinologic change in adults who have suffered traumatic brain injuries may cause it to be overlooked and therefore contribute to delayed rehabilitation.[791]

Humans with stalk sections or with tumors of the stalk region have widely varying levels of hyperprolactinemia and may have galactorrhea.[792] PRL responses to hypoglycemia and to TRH are blunted, in part because of loss of neural connections with the hypothalamus. PRL responses to dopamine agonists and antagonists in the pituitary isolation syndrome are similar to those in patients with prolactinomas. Interestingly, PRL secretion continues to show a diurnal variation in patients with either hypothalamopituitary disconnection or microprolactinoma.[520] Both forms of hyperprolactinemia are characterized by a similarly increased frequency of PRL pulses and a marked rise in nonpulsatile or basal PRL secretion, although the disruption is greater in the tumoral hyperprolactinemia.

An incomplete pituitary isolation syndrome may occur with the empty sella syndrome, intrasellar cysts, or pituitary adenomas.[793–795] Anterior pituitary failure after stalk section is in part due to loss of specific neural and vascular links to the hypothalamus and in part due to pituitary infarction.

Hypophyseotropic Hormone Deficiency

Selective pituitary failure can be due to a deficiency of specific pituitary cell types or a deficiency of one or more hypothalamic hormones. Isolated GnRH deficiency is the most common hypophyseotropic hormone deficiency. In Kallmann's syndrome (gonadotropin deficiency commonly associated with

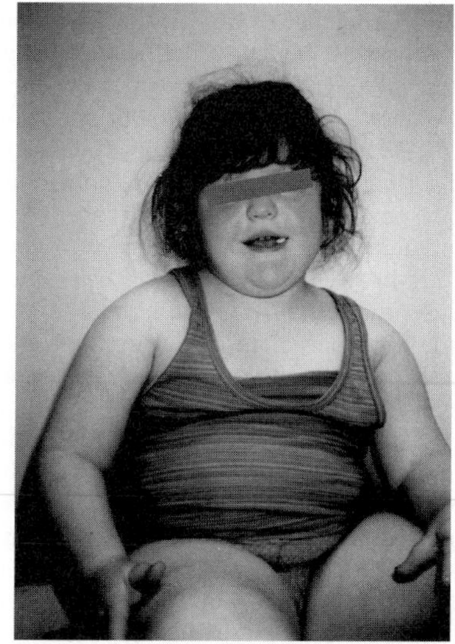

Figure 7–54. A neuroendocrine syndrome of adrenocorticotropic hormone insufficiency, obesity, and red hair resulting from a null mutation in the pro-opiomelanocortin gene. (Photo kindly provided by Dr. A. Gruters, Berlin.)

hyposmia),[796] hereditary agenesis of the olfactory lobe may be demonstrable by magnetic resonance imaging.[797] Abnormal development of the GnRH system is due to defective migration of the GnRH-containing neurons from the olfactory nasal epithelium in early embryologic life (see the earlier section on GnRH). Other malformations of the cranial midline structures, such as absence of the septum pellucidum in septo-optic dysplasia (De Morsier's syndrome), can cause hypogonadotropic hypogonadism (HH) or, less commonly, precocious puberty. A surprisingly large percentage of children with septo-optic dysplasia who otherwise have multiple hypothalamic-pituitary abnormalities actually retain normal gonadotropin function and enter puberty spontaneously.[798] The genetic basis of HH has now been established in approximately 10% of patients.[799, 800] Mutations in the *KAL* (Kallmann's syndrome) gene and the *AHC-DAX1* (adrenal hypoplasia congenita–HH) gene cause X-linked recessive disease. Autosomal recessive HH has been associated with mutations in the GnRH receptor, leptin, leptin receptor, FSH, LH, PROP-1 (combined pituitary deficiency), and *HESX* (septo-optic dysplasia) genes.

The GnRH response test is of little value in the differential diagnosis of hypothalamic hypogonadism. Most patients with GnRH deficiency show little or no response to an initial test dose, but normal responses are seen after repeated injection. This slow response has been attributed to down-regulation of GnRH receptors in response to prolonged GnRH deficiency. Furthermore, with intrinsic pituitary disease the response to GnRH may be absent or normal. Consequently, it is not possible to distinguish between hypothalamic and pituitary disease with a single injection of GnRH. Prolonged infusions or repeated administration of GnRH agonists after hormone replacement therapy priming may aid in the diagnosis or provide therapeutic options for women with Kallmann's syndrome wishing to become pregnant.[801, 802]

Deficiency of TRH secretion gives rise to hypothalamic hypothyroidism, also called tertiary hypothyroidism, which can occur in hypothalamic disease or more rarely as an isolated defect.[803] Molecular genetic analyses have revealed infrequent autosomal recessive mutations in the TRH and TRH receptor genes in the etiology of central hypothyroidism.[804] Hypothalamic and pituitary causes of TSH deficiency are most readily distinguished by imaging methods. Although theoretically reasonable, the TRH stimulation test for the differentiation of hypothalamic disease from pituitary disease is of limited value. The typical pituitary response to TRH administration in patients with TRH deficiency is an enhanced and somewhat delayed peak, whereas the response with pituitary failure is subnormal or absent. The hypothalamic type of response has been attributed to an associated GH deficiency that sensitizes the pituitary to TRH (possibly through suppression of somatostatin secretion), but GH also affects T_4 metabolism and may alter pituitary responses as well.[805] In practice, the responses to TRH in hypothalamic and pituitary disease overlap so much that they cannot be used reliably for a differential diagnosis. Persistent failure to demonstrate responses to TRH is good evidence for the presence of intrinsic pituitary disease, but the presence of a response does not mean that the pituitary is normal. Deficient TRH secretion leads to altered TSH biosynthesis by the pituitary, including impaired glycosylation. Poorly glycosylated TSH has low biologic activity, and dissociation of bioactive and immunoreactive TSH can lead to the paradox of normal or elevated levels of TSH in hypothalamic hypothyroidism.[803, 806]

GHRH deficiency appears to be the principal cause of hGH deficiency in children with idiopathic dwarfism.[807] This condition is frequently associated with abnormal electroencephalograms, a history of birth trauma, and breech delivery. Furthermore, magnetic resonance imaging scans show that a substantial proportion of children with idiopathic hGH deficiency have evidence of a torn pituitary stalk,[808, 809] which is presumed evidence for birth trauma as the cause. Human GH is the most vulnerable of the anterior pituitary hormones when the pituitary stalk is damaged. It can be difficult to differentiate between primary pituitary disease and GHRH deficiency by standard tests of GH reserve. However, a substantial GH secretory response to a single administration of hexarelin occurs only in the presence of at least a partially intact vascular stalk.[420]

In many children with dwarfism, the anatomic abnormalities of the intrasellar contents and pituitary stalk together with the frequent occurrence of other midline defects, such as those in septo-optic dysplasia, are consistent with the alternative hypothesis of a developmental defect occurring in embryogenesis.[808] There has been a remarkable advance in our understanding of the molecular ontogeny of the hypothalamic-pituitary unit, much of it based on mutant mouse models.[810, 811] Parallel genetic analyses have been conducted in children with isolated GH deficiency or combined pituitary hormone deficiencies. These studies have identified autosomal recessive mutations in both structural and regulatory genes including the GHRH receptor, *PIT1*, *PROP1*, and *HESX1* that are responsible for a sizable proportion of congenital hypothalamic-pituitary disorders once considered idiopathic.[409, 807, 812, 813]

Adrenal insufficiency is another manifestation of hypothalamic disease and can be due to CRH deficiency.[814, 815] Isolated ACTH deficiency is uncommon, but there is suggestive evidence in at least one family of genetic linkage to the CRH gene locus.[816] Later investigations have revealed mutations in the *TPIT* gene, a T box transcription factor expressed only in pituitary corticotrophs and melanotrophs, associated with cases of isolated ACTH deficiency.[817] The CRH stimulation test does not distinguish hypothalamic from pituitary failure as a cause of corticotropin deficiency.[818, 819]

Apart from intrinsic diseases of the hypothalamus such as tumors and granulomas, two environmental causes of central hypophyseotropic deficiencies are of increasing clinical importance. These are trauma to the brain,[777, 779, 791] particularly from motor vehicle accidents, and the sequelae of chemotherapy and radiation therapy for intracranial lesions in children and adults.[806, 820, 821] Improved short-term survival from head injuries associated with coma and CNS malignancies has greatly increased the prevalence of long-term neuroendocrine consequences.

Hypophyseotropic Hormone Hypersecretion

Pituitary hypersecretion is occasionally caused by tumors of the hypothalamus.[822] GnRH-secreting hamartomas can cause precocious puberty.[822] CRH-secreting gangliocytomas can cause Cushing's syndrome,[823] and GHRH-secreting gangliocytomas of the hypothalamus can cause acromegaly.[824] Although they do not arise from the hypothalamus, paraneoplastic syndromes can also cause pituitary hypersecretion, as with CRH-secreting tumors and GHRH-secreting tumors of the bronchi and pancreas. Bronchial carcinoids and pituitary islet cell tumors are the usual causes of this phenomenon.

Neuroendocrine Disorders of Gonadotropin Regulation

Precocious Puberty

The term *precocious puberty* is used when physiologically *normal* pituitary-gonadal function appears at an early age.[825, 826] By convention, the onset of androgen secretion and spermatogenesis must occur before the age of 9 or 10 in boys and the onset of estrogen secretion and cyclic ovarian activity before age 8 in girls.[827, 828] Central precocious puberty is due to disturbed CNS function, which may or may not have an identifiable structural basis. Pseudoprecocious puberty refers to premature sexual development resulting from excessive secretion of androgens, estrogens, or hCG caused by tumors (both gonadal and extragonadal), administration of exogenous gonadal steroids, or genetically determined activation of gonadotropin receptors (see Chapter 15). Central precocious puberty with neurogenic causes and pineal gland disease is discussed in this chapter.

Idiopathic Sexual Precocity

Familial occurrence is uncommon, but there is a hereditary form of idiopathic sexual precocity that is largely confined to males. Abnormal electroencephalograms and behavioral disturbances, suggesting the presence of brain damage, have been reported occasionally in girls with idiopathic precocious puberty. The pathogenesis may be related to the rate of hypothalamic development or other as yet undetermined nutritional, environmental, or psychosocial factors. Many cases previously thought to be idiopathic are due to small hypothalamic hamartomas discussed in more detail in the following. It has been argued that localized activation of discrete cellular subsets connected to GnRH neurons may be sufficient to initiate puberty.[829]

Neurogenic Precocious Puberty

Approximately two thirds of hypothalamic lesions that influence the timing of human puberty are located in the posterior hypothalamus, but in the subset of patients who come to autopsy, damage is extensive. Specific lesions known to cause precocity include craniopharyngioma (although delayed puberty is more common), astrocytoma, pineal tumors, subarachnoid cysts, encephalitis, miliary tuberculosis, tuberous sclerosis or neurofibromatosis type 1, the Sturge-Weber syndrome, porencephaly, craniostenosis, microcephaly, hydrocephalus, empty sella syndrome, and Tay-Sachs disease.[830, 831]

Hamartoma of the hypothalamus is an exception to the generalization that tumors of the brain cause precocious puberty by impairment of gonadotropin secretion (although hamartomas on occasion cause hypothalamic damage). A hamartoma is a tumor-like collection of normal-appearing nerve tissue lodged in an abnormal location. The *parahypothalamic* type consists of an encapsulated nodule of nerve tissue attached to the floor of the third ventricle or suspended from the floor by a peduncle and typically less than 1 cm in diameter. The *intrahypothalamic* or sessile type is enveloped by the posterior hypothalamus and can distort the third ventricle. These tend to be larger than the pedunculated variety, grow in the interpeduncular cistern, and are frequently accompanied by seizures, mental retardation, developmental delays, and roughly half the incidence of precocious puberty associated with the parahypothalamic lesions.[832, 833] Before the development of high-resolution scanning techniques, this tumor was considered rare, but small ones can now be visualized. Miniature hamartomas of the tuber cinereum are common at autopsy. Precocious puberty occurs when the hamartoma makes connections with the median eminence and thus serves as an accessory hypothalamus. Peptidergic nerve terminals containing GnRH have been found in the tumors.[834] Early pubertal development is presumably due to unrestrained GnRH secretion, although the hamartomas almost certainly have an intrinsic pulse generator of GnRH secretion because pulsatility is required for stimulation of gonadotropin secretion (see earlier section on GnRH).

Manifestations of premature puberty in patients with hamartomas are similar to those associated with other central causes of precocity. Hamartomas occur in both sexes and may be present as early as age 3 months. In the past most cases were thought to be fatal by age 20, but many hamartomas cause no brain damage and need not be excised.[833] The interpeduncular fossa of the brain is difficult to approach, and surgical experience is somewhat limited. Early in the course of illness, epilepsy manifested as "brief, repetitive, stereotyped attacks of laughter"[835] may provide a clue to the disease. Late in the course, hypothalamic damage can cause severe neurologic defects and intractable seizures.

Hypothyroidism

Hypothyroidism can cause precocious puberty in girls that is reversible with thyroid therapy. Hyperprolactinemia and galactorrhea may be present. One possibility is that elevated thyrotropin levels (in children with thyroid failure) cross-react with the FSH receptor.[836] Alternatively, low levels of thyroid hormone might simultaneously activate release of LH, FSH, and TSH. A third possibility is that hypothyroidism causes hypothalamic encephalopathy that impairs the normal tonic suppression of gonadotropin release by the hypothalamus. The high PRL levels that sometimes accompany this disorder may be due to a deficiency in PIF secretion, increased secretion of TRH, or increased sensitivity of the lactotrophs to TRH secretion.

Tumors of the Pineal Gland

Pineal gland tumors account for only a small percentage of intracranial neoplasms. They occur as a central midline mass with an enhancing lesion on magnetic resonance imaging frequently accompanied by hydrocephalus. Pinealomas cause a variety of neurologic abnormalities (Table 7–11). Parinaud's syndrome, which consists of paralysis of upward gaze, pupillary areflexia (to light), paralysis of convergence, and a wide-based gait, occurs with about half of pinealomas. Gait disturbances can also occur because of brain stem or cerebellar compression.

Several discrete cytopathologic entities account for mass lesions in the pineal region (Table 7–12).[836] The most common non-neoplastic conditions are degenerative pineal cysts, arachnoid cysts, and cavernous hemangioma. Pinealocytes give rise to primitive neuroectodermal tumors, the so-called small blue cell tumors that are immunopositive for the neuronal marker synaptophysin and negative for the lymphocyte marker CD45. True *pinealomas* can be relatively well-differentiated pineocytomas, intermediate mixed forms, or the less differentiated pineoblastomas,[837, 838] which are basically the same as medulloblastomas, neuroblastomas, and oat cell carcinomas of the lung.

The most common tumors of the pineal gland are actually germinomas (a form of teratoma), so designated because of their presumed origin in germ cells. Germinomas may also occur in the anterior hypothalamus or the floor of the third ventricle, where they are often associated with the clinical triad of DI, pituitary insufficiency, and visual abnormalities.[830] Identical tumors can be found in the testis and anterior mediastinum. Intracranial germinomas have a tendency to spread locally, infiltrate the hypothalamus, and metastasize to the spinal cord and CSF. Extracranial metastases (to the skin, lung, or liver) are rare. Teratomas derived from two or more germ cell layers also occur in the pineal region. Chorionic tissue in teratomas and germinomas may secrete hCG in sufficient amounts to cause gonadal maturation, and some of these tumors have histologic and functional characteristics of choriocarcinomas. Diagnosis is confirmed by the combination of a mass lesion, cytologic analysis of CSF, and radioimmunoassay detection of hCG in the CSF.

Precocious puberty is a relatively unusual manifestation of

Table 7–11. Classification of Tumors of the Pineal Region

A. Germ Cell Tumors
1. Germinoma
   a. Posterior third ventricle and pineal lesions
   b. Anterior third ventricle, suprasellar or intrasellar lesions
   c. Combined lesions in anterior and posterior third ventricle, apparently noncontiguous, with or without foci of cystic or solid teratoma
2. Teratoma
   a. Evidencing growth along two or three germ lines in varying degrees of differentiation
   b. Dermoid and epidermoid cysts with or without solid foci of teratoma
   c. Histologically malignant forms with or without differentiated foci of benign, solid, or cystic teratoma-teratocarcinoma, chorioepithelioma, embryonal carcinoma (endodermal-sinus tumor or yolk-sac carcinoma), combinations of these with or without foci of germinoma, chemodectoma

B. Pineal Parenchymal Tumors
1. Pinealocytes
   a. Pineocytoma
   b. Pineoblastoma
   c. Ganglioglioma and chemodectoma
   d. Mixed forms exhibiting transitions between these
2. Glia
   a. Astrocytoma
   b. Ependymoma
   c. Mixed forms and other less frequent gliomas (e.g., glioblastoma, oligodendroglioma)

C. Tumors of Supporting or Adjacent Structures
1. Meningioma
2. Hemangiopericytoma

D. Non-neoplastic Conditions of Neurosurgical Importance
1. "Degenerative" cysts of pineal lined by fibrillary astrocytes
2. Arachnoid cysts
3. Cavernous hemangioma

From DeGirolami U. Pathology of tumors of the pineal region. In Schmidek HH (ed). Pineal Tumors. New York, Masson, 1977, pp 1–19.

pineal gland disease. When it occurs, neuroanatomic studies suggest that the cause is secondary to pressure or destructive effects of the pineal tumor on the function of the adjacent hypothalamus or to the secretion of hCG. Most patients have other evidence of hypothalamic involvement such as DI, polyphagia, somnolence, obesity, or behavioral disturbance. Choriocarcinoma of the pineal gland is associated with high plasma levels of hCG. The hCG can stimulate testosterone secretion from the testis but not estrogen secretion by the ovary and hence causes premature puberty almost exclusively in boys. The prevalence of elevated hCG levels in children with premature puberty related to tumors in the pineal region is unknown, but the fact that this phenomenon occurs further challenges the theory that nonparenchymal tumors cause precocious puberty by damaging the normal pineal gland. Rarely, pinealomas cause *delayed* puberty, raising speculation about a role of melatonin in inhibiting gonadotropin secretion in these cases.

Table 7–12. Pinealomas: Frequency (%) of Presenting Symptoms and Signs

Increased intracranial pressure	85
Spasticity	35
Ataxia	30
Parinaud's syndrome	25
Cerebellar-type nystagmus	25
Syncope	20
Vertigo	20
Cranial nerve palsy (other than cranial nerves VI, VIII)	20
Intention tremor	15
Scotoma	10
Tinnitus	10
Other	10

From Brady WL. The role of radiation therapy. In Schmidek HH (ed). Pineal Tumors. New York, Masson, 1977, pp. 99–113.

Management of tumors in the pineal region is not straightforward.[837, 839] Operative mortality rates can be high, but the rationale for an aggressive approach to the pineal region is based on the need to make a histologic diagnosis, the variety of lesions found in this region, the possibility of cure of an encapsulated lesion, and the effectiveness of chemotherapeutic agents for germinomas and choriocarcinoma. Stereotaxic biopsy of the pineal region provided diagnosis in 33 of 34 cases in one series, suggesting that this is a useful alternative to open surgical exploration for diagnostic purposes.[840] Long-term palliation or cure of many pineal region tumors is possible by combinations of surgery, radiation, gamma knife, or chemotherapy, depending on the nature of the lesion.[841]

Approach to the Patient with Precocious Puberty

Several groups have reviewed the diagnostic approach to suspected central precocious puberty.[842–844] Although guidelines differ, the index of suspicion is clearly inversely proportional to the age of the patient. A GnRH stimulation test to assess gonadotropin release and thereby differentiate between primed and inactive gonadotrophs is probably the single most important endocrinologic measure. If LH and FSH levels are not stimulated and there is no evidence of gonadal germ cell maturation, the cause of precocious puberty lies outside the hypothalamic-pituitary axis and the diagnostic process should focus on the adrenal glands and gonads (see Chapters 13 and 15). Magnetic resonance imaging studies are central to the work-up for exclusion or characterization of organic lesions in the areas of the sella, optic chiasm, suprasellar hypothalamus, and interpeduncular cistern.[826]

Management of Sexual Precocity

Structural lesions of the hypothalamus are treated by surgery, radiation, chemotherapy, or combinations of these as indicated by the pathologic diagnosis and extent of disease. Endocrinologic manifestations of precocious puberty are best treated by GnRH agonists with the therapeutic goals of delaying sexual maturation to a more appropriate age and achieving optimal linear growth and bone mass, possibly with the combined use of GH treatment.[845–847] Other approaches include the use of cyproterone acetate, testolactone, or spironolactone to antagonize or inhibit gonadal steroid biosynthesis.[848, 849] Precocious puberty is stressful to both the child and the parents, and it is essential that psychological support be provided.

Psychogenic Amenorrhea

Menstrual cycles can cease in young nonpregnant women with no demonstrable abnormalities of the brain, pituitary, or ovary in several situations,[850, 851] including pseudocyesis (false pregnancy), anorexia nervosa, excessive exercise, psychogenic disorders, and hyperprolactinemic states (see Chapter 13). Psychogenic amenorrhea, the most common cause of secondary amenorrhea except for pregnancy, can occur with major psychopathology or minor psychic stress and is often temporary.

Psychogenic amenorrhea is probably mediated by excessive endogenous opioid activity because naloxone or naltrexone (opiate receptor blockers) can induce ovulation in some patients with this disorder.[850, 852]

Exercise-induced amenorrhea may be a variant of psychogenic amenorrhea or may result from loss of body fat.[851, 853] The syndrome is associated with intense and prolonged physical exertion such as running, swimming, or ballet dancing. Such women are always below ideal body weight and have low stores of fat. If the activity is begun before puberty, normal sexual maturation can be delayed for many years. The mass of fat may be a regulator of gonadotropin secretion with adipocyte-derived leptin as the principal mediator between peripheral energy stores and hypothalamic regulatory centers.[854] Studies in nonhuman primates showed a direct role of caloric intake in the pathogenesis of amenorrhea associated with long-distance running.[855] Exercise and psychogenic amenorrhea can have adverse effects because of the associated estrogen deficiency and accompanying osteopenia (also see Chapter 23).[856]

Neurogenic Hypogonadism in Males

A discussion of neurogenic hypogonadism in males should begin with an account of Fröhlich's syndrome (adiposogenital dystrophy), originally characterized as delayed puberty, hypogonadism, and obesity associated with a tumor that impinges on the hypothalamus. It was subsequently recognized that either hypothalamic or pituitary dysfunction can induce hypogonadism and the presence of obesity indicates that the appetite-regulating regions of the hypothalamus have been damaged. Several organic lesions of the hypothalamus can cause this syndrome, including tumors, encephalitis, microcephaly, Friedreich's ataxia, and demyelinating diseases. Other important causes of hypogonadotropic hypogonadism are Kallmann's syndrome, a disorder caused by failure of GnRH-containing neurons to migrate normally (see earlier in the section on GnRH and hypophyseotropic hormone deficiency), and a subset of the Prader-Willi syndrome.[857]

However, most males with delayed sexual development do not have serious neurologic conditions. Furthermore, most obese boys with delayed sexual development have no structural damage to the hypothalamus but have *constitutional delayed puberty*, which is commonly associated with obesity. It is not known whether there is a functional disorder of the hypothalamus in this condition. It is generally believed that psychosexual development of brain maturation depends on the presence of androgens and that hypogonadism in boys (regardless of cause) should be treated by the middle teen years (15 years at the latest).

In adult men, hypogonadism (including reduced spermatogenesis) can be induced by emotional stress or severe exercise,[858] but this abnormality is seldom diagnosed because the symptoms are more subtle than menstrual cycle changes in similarly stressed women. Prolonged physical stress and sleep and energy deficiency can also decrease testosterone and gonadotropin levels.[859] Chronic intrathecal administration of opiates for the control of intractable pain syndromes is strongly associated with hypogonadotropic hypogonadism, and to a lesser extent hypocorticism and GH deficiency, in both men and women.[860] Finally, critical illness with multiple causes is well known to be associated with hypogonadism and ineffectual altered pulsation of GnRH.[861]

Neurogenic Disorders of Prolactin Regulation

Neurogenic causes of hyperprolactinemia include irritative lesions of the chest wall (herpes zoster, thoracotomy), excessive tactile stimulation of the nipple, and lesions within the spinal cord such as ependymoma.[862, 863] Prolonged mechanical stimulation of the nipples by suckling or the use of a breast pump can initiate lactation in some women who are not pregnant, and neurologic lesions that interrupt the hypothalamic-pituitary connection can cause hyperprolactinemia, as discussed earlier. Hyperprolactinemia also occurs after certain forms of epileptic seizures. In one series, six of eight patients with temporal lobe seizures had a marked increase in PRL, whereas only one in eight frontal lobe seizures led to hyperprolactinemia.[864] Agents that block dopamine receptors (such as the phenothiazines) or prevent dopamine release (e.g., reserpine and methyldopa) must be excluded in all cases.

Because the nervous system exerts such profound effects on PRL secretion, patients with hyperprolactinemia (including those with adenomas) may have a deficit of PIF or an excess of PRF activity. In studies of PRL secretion in patients apparently cured of hyperprolactinemia by removal of a pituitary microadenoma, regulatory abnormalities persisted in some but not all patients. Persistence of regulatory abnormalities may be due to incomplete removal of tumor, abnormal function of the remaining part of the gland, or underlying hypothalamic abnormalities.[865]

Neurogenic Disorders of Growth Hormone Secretion

Hypothalamic Growth Failure

Loss of the normal nocturnal increase in GH secretion and loss of GH secretory responses to provocative stimuli occur early in the course of hypothalamic disease and may be the most sensitive endocrine indicator of hypothalamic dysfunction. As noted earlier, anatomic malformations of midline cerebral structures are associated with abnormal GH secretion, presumably related to failure of the development of normal GH regulatory mechanisms. Such disorders include optic nerve dysplasia and midline prosencephalic malformations (absence of the septum pellucidum, abnormal third ventricle, and abnormal lamina terminalis). Certain complex genetic disorders including Prader-Willi syndrome also commonly involve reduced GH secretory capacity.[866] Idiopathic hypopituitarism with GH deficiency was considered earlier in this chapter.

Maternal Deprivation Syndrome and Psychosocial Dwarfism

Infant neglect or abuse can impair growth and cause failure to thrive (the maternal deprivation syndrome). Malnutrition interacts with psychological factors to cause growth failure in children with the maternal deprivation syndrome, and each case should be carefully evaluated from this point of view. Older children with growth failure in a setting of abuse or severe emotional disturbance (termed psychosocial dwarfism) may also have abnormal circadian rhythms and deficient hGH release after insulin-induced hypoglycemia or arginine infusion (see Chapter 8).[867, 868] Deficient release of corticotropin and gonadotropins may also be present. A new variant termed hyperphagic short stature has been identified.[869] These disorders are reversible by placing the child in a supportive milieu where growth and neuroendocrine hGH responses rapidly return to normal.[870] The pathogenesis of altered GH secretion in children in response to deprivation is unknown. In the adult human, furthermore, physical or emotional stress usually causes an *increase* in hGH secretion, as noted earlier.

Neuroregulatory Growth Hormone Deficiency

The availability of biosynthetic hGH for treatment of short stature has brought into focus a group of patients who grow at low rates (below the third percentile) and have low levels of serum IGF-I but a normal hGH secretory reserve. Studies of 24-hour hGH secretion profiles indicate that many of these children do not have normal spontaneous hGH secretion (abnormal ultradian and circadian rhythms and decreased number or amplitude of secretory bursts, or both). These children with idiopathic short stature may have a functional regulatory disturbance of the hypothalamus and appear to grow normally when given exogenous hGH.[871]

There is considerable uncertainty about the criteria for the diagnosis of neuroregulatory hGH deficiency. Many normally growing children have profiles of hGH secretion that are indistinguishable from those in children with the postulated syndrome.[872] Patterns of hGH secretion do not predict which child will benefit from therapy, and there is a poor correlation between hGH secretion and growth. Furthermore, the results of repeated tests in children show considerable variability. It has been suggested that specific genetic defects may underlie the pathogenesis of a subset of children with this heterogeneous syndrome of growth failure.[873] The prevalence of an hGH neuroregulatory deficiency syndrome is thus unclear, and the decision to treat short children with hGH should be made cautiously.[874, 875]

Neurogenic Hypersecretion of Growth Hormone

Diencephalic Cachexia

Children and infants with tumors in and around the third ventricle frequently become cachectic, which is often associated with elevated hGH levels and paradoxical GH secretory responses to glucose and insulin.[876, 877] GH hypersecretion may be due to a hypothalamic abnormality[878] or to malnutrition. Deficits of pituitary-adrenal regulation are less common. A striking feature is an alert appearance and seeming euphoria despite the wasted state. A variety of associated neurologic abnormalities may be present (Table 7–13); the tumors that produce this syndrome are summarized in Table 7–14 and include a high proportion of chiasmatic-hypothalamic gliomas.[879]

Table 7–13. Clinical Features of Diencephalic Syndrome (Pooled Data of 67 Anatomically Defined Tumors)

Clinical Feature	%
Emaciation	100
Alert appearance	87
Increased vigor or hyperkinesis, or both	72
Vomiting	68
Euphoria	59
Pallor	55
Nystagmus	55
Irritability	32
Hydrocephalus*	33
Optic atrophy	24
Tremor	23
Sweating	15
Large hands, feet	5
Large genitalia	5
Polyuria	5
Papilledema	5
Positive pneumoencephalogram results	98
Endocrine anomalies†	90
Cerebrospinal fluid protein	64
Cerebrospinal fluid abnormal cells	23

*Hydrocephalus includes clinical plus radiologic findings.
†Positive in 9 of 10 cases with adequately recorded investigation. (Occasionally, patients had electrolyte and blood pressure anomalies and eosinophilia.)
Modified from Burr IM, Slonim AE, Danish RK, et al. Diencephalic syndrome revisited. J Pediatr 1976; 88:439–444.

Table 7–14. Tumors Producing Diencephalic Syndrome

Tumor	No. of Patients
Gliomas	56
Astrocytoma	37
Not subclassified	10
Spongioblastoma	5
Astroblastoma	1
Oligodendroglioma	1
Mixed astrocytoma-spongioblastoma	1
Mixed astrocytoma-oligodendroglioma	1
Ependymoma	2
Ganglioglioma	1
Dysgerminoma	1
No histology	10

From Burr IM, Slonim AE, Danish RK, et al. Diencephalic syndrome revisited. J Pediatr 1976; 88:439–444.

Syndrome of Inappropriate Growth Hormone Hypersecretion

Apparently inappropriate hGH hypersecretion (the *syndrome of inappropriate somatotropin secretion*) occurs with uncontrolled diabetes mellitus, hepatic failure, uremia, anorexia nervosa, and protein-calorie malnutrition. Nutritional factors are probably important in this response because in normal persons obesity inhibits and fasting stimulates episodic GH hypersecretion.[880] In diabetes mellitus cholinergic blockers reverse the abnormality,[881] possibly by inhibiting hypothalamic somatostatin secretion (see earlier in the section on neurotransmitter regulation of GH). Loss of inhibition of GH secretion by IGF-I may also play a role because most disorders in which this syndrome occurs are associated with low IGF-I levels.

Neurogenic Disorders of Corticotropin Regulation

Hypothalamic CRH hypersecretion is the likely cause of sustained pituitary-adrenal hyperfunction in at least two situations: Cushing's syndrome caused by the rare CRH-secreting gangliocytomas of the hypothalamus[882] and severe depression.

Severe depression is associated with pituitary-adrenal abnormalities, including inappropriately elevated corticotropin levels, abnormal cortisol circadian rhythms, and resistance to dexamethasone suppression.[883, 884] The dexamethasone suppression test has, in fact, been used as an aid to the diagnosis of depressive illness. Patients with depression also have diminished responses to CRH, suggesting that depressed individuals hypersecrete CRH (see earlier section on CRH). Another possible example of disordered neurogenic control of CRH associated with stress is the metabolic syndrome.[885–887] This syndrome is characterized by mild hypercortisolism, blunted dexamethasone suppression of the HPA axis, visceral obesity, and hypertension and may be strongly associated with greater risks for cardiovascular disease and stroke.

A unique syndrome of corticotropin hypersecretion termed *periodic hypothalamic discharge* (Wolff's syndrome) has been described in one young man. The patient had a recurring cyclic disorder characterized by high fever, paroxysms of glucocorticoid hypersecretion, and electroencephalographic abnormalities.[888]

Genetic Obesity Disorders Involving Hypothalamic Circuits

In the past 5 years there have been a number of important discoveries related to genetic mutations underlying certain human obesity disorders.[668, 889] These clinical advances have closely paralleled the advances of basic research in the neuroendocrine control of energy homeostasis discussed in an earlier section. Linkage studies and quantitative trait loci analyses have strongly implicated the *POMC* gene locus as an important determinant of weight homeostasis in humans of many, but not all, different ethnic populations, although specific alleles associated with obesity have not yet been demonstrated.[890–893] Because no mutations within the coding region of the *POMC* gene that alter peptide activity have been identified in these populations, a current hypothesis is that mutations in regulatory regions of the gene decrease the level of *POMC* expression in the brain.

However, a small number of children from consanguineous parents have been found to have null mutations in the *POMC* gene resulting in absence of detectable circulating ACTH.[666, 894] These children presented with a syndrome of red hair, adrenal insufficiency, and severe, early-onset obesity (see Fig. 7–54). In addition, both dominant and recessive mutations in the *MC4R* gene have been found in the human population, and MC4R mutations have been proposed to play a role in as many as 5% of pediatric obesity cases.[290, 667, 895–897] The genetic mirror image may also be true; an association between a polymorphism linked to the gene encoding the MC4R antagonist agouti-related protein and anorexia nervosa has been reported. Taking all these data into account, it is safe to say that obesity in a subpopulation of humans can be considered a genetic disorder of the hypothalamus.[668, 898]

Nonendocrine Manifestations of Hypothalamic Disease

The hypothalamus is involved in the regulation of diverse functions and behaviors (Table 7–15). Psychological abnormalities in hypothalamic disease include antisocial behavior; attacks of rage, laughing, and crying; disturbed sleep patterns; excessive sexuality; and hallucinations. Both somnolence (with posterior lesions) and pathologic wakefulness (with anterior lesions) occur, as do bulimia and profound anorexia. The abnormal eating patterns are analogous to the syndromes of hyperphagia produced in rats by destruction of the ventromedial nucleus or of connections to the paraventricular nucleus. Lateral hypothalamic damage causes profound anorexia.

Patients with hypothalamic damage may experience hyperthermia, hypothermia, unexplained fluctuations in body temperature, and poikilothermy. Disturbances of sweating, acrocyanosis, loss of sphincter control, and diencephalic epilepsy are occasional manifestations. Hypothalamic damage also causes loss of recent memory, believed to be due to damage of the mammillothalamic pathways. Severe memory loss, obesity, and personality changes (apathy, loss of ability to concentrate, aggressive antisocial behavior, severe food craving, inability to work or attend school) may occur with suprasellar extension of pituitary tumors, hypothalamic radiation, or damage incurred from surgical removal of parasellar tumors. Hypothalamic tumors grow slowly and may reach a large size while producing minimal disturbance of behavior or visceral homeostasis, whereas surgery of limited extent can produce striking functional abnormalities. Presumably, this is because slowly growing lesions permit compensatory responses to develop. These potential consequences should be weighed carefully with the neurosurgeon, patient, and patient's family in planning the therapeutic approach. Adverse effects of treatment have led to more conservative surgical guidelines for the treatment of craniopharyngioma.

Table 7–15. Neurologic Manifestations of Nonendocrine Hypothalamic Disease

Disorders of Temperature Regulation	**Hereditary Hypothalamic Disease**
Hyperthermia	Laurence-Moon-Biedl syndrome
Hypothermia	Prader-Willi syndrome
Poikilothermia	**Disorders of Psychic Function**
Disorders of Food Intake	Rage behavior
Hyperphagia (bulimia)	Hallucinations
Anorexia, aphagia	Hypersexuality
Disorders of Water Intake	**Disorders of Autonomic Nervous System**
Compulsive water drinking	Pulmonary edema
Adipsia	Cardiac arrhythmias
Essential hypernatremia	Sphincter disturbance
Disorders of Sleep and Consciousness	**Miscellaneous**
Narcolepsy	Diencephalic syndrome of infancy
Somnolence	Cerebral gigantism
Sleep rhythm reversal	
Akinetic mutism	
Coma	
Delirium	
Periodic Disease of Hypothalamic Origin	
Diencephalic epilepsy	
Kleine-Levin syndrome	
Periodic discharge syndrome of Wolff	

A convergence of functional genomics from two animal species, the dog and mouse, has refocused attention on neuropeptide circuits of the hypothalamus in the control of sleep. Positional cloning was used to identify mutations in the hypocretin-orexin receptor 2 as the cause of canine narcolepsy.[899] Knockout of the gene encoding the hypocretin-orexin peptide precursor produced an equivalent narcoleptic syndrome in mice,[900] further establishing this neuropeptide system as a major component of sleep-modulating neural circuits. Histaminergic neurons of the tuberomammillary nucleus express both forms of the orexin receptor and make reciprocal synaptic connections with orexin neurons in the lateral hypothalamus. Furthermore, orexin is an excitatory transmitter for the histamine neurons, suggesting that the two populations cooperate in the regulation of rapid eye movement sleep.[901] Targeted ablation of orexin neurons in the lateral hypothalamus of rats by means of a hypocretin receptor 2–saporin conjugate produced narcoleptic-like sleep behavior,[902] closely paralleling the clinical findings and selected loss of hypocretin-orexin neurons in the lateral hypothalamus of humans with narcolepsy.[903] These new discoveries add to the list of other neuropeptides including GHRH, somatostatin, and cortistatin with established function in modulation of the sleep cycle.

Acknowledgement

The authors are highly indebted to Dr. Seymour Reichlin, not only for text and figures he shared from the ninth edition of this text, but also for the inspiration and mentorship he provided to the current generation of neuroendocrinologists.

References

1. Riskind PN, Martin JB. Functional anatomy of the hypothalamic-anterior pituitary complex. In Degroot LJ, Besser M, Jameson JL. Endocrinology. Philadelphia, WB Saunders, 1984, pp 151–159.
2. Anderson E. Earlier ideas of hypothalamic function, including irrelevant concepts. In Haymaker W, Anderson E, Nauta WJH (eds). The Hypothalamus. Springfield, Ill, Charles C Thomas, 1968, pp 1–12.
3. Sawyer CH. Anterior pituitary neural control concepts. In McCann SM (ed). Endocrinology: People and Ideas. Bethesda, Md, American Physiological Society, 1988, pp 23–37.
4. Fröhlich A. Ein Fall von Tumor der Hypophysis cerebri ohne Akromegalie. Wien Klin Rundsch 1901; 15:883.
5. Bramwell B. Intracranial Tumours. Edinburgh, Pentland, 1888.
6. Longo LD. Classic pages in obstetrics and gynecology. Experimental hypophysectomy. Samuel James Crowe, Harvey Williams Cushing, and John Homans. Bulletin of the Johns Hopkins Hospital, vol. 21, pp. 128–169, 1910. Am J Obstet Gynecol 1978; 130:953–954.
7. Crowe SJ, Cushing H, Homans J. Experimental hypophysectomy. Bull Johns Hopkins Hosp 1910; 21:128–169.
8. Aschner B. Über die Funktion der Hypophyse. Pflugers Arch Physiol 1912; 146:1.
9. Hetherington AW, Ranson SW. Hypothalamic lesions and adiposity in the rat. Anat Rec 1940; 78:149–172.
10. Elmquist JK, Elias CF, Saper CB. From lesions to leptin: hypothalamic control of food intake and body weight. Neuron 1999; 22:221–232.
11. Popa G, Fielding U. A portal circulation from the pituitary to the hypothalamic region. J Anat 1930; 65:88.
12. Wislocki GB, King LS. Permeability of the hypophysis and hypothalamus to vital dyes, with study of hypophyseal blood supply. Am J Anat 1936; 58:421–472.
13. Harris GW. Neural control of the pituitary. Physiol Rev 1948; 28:139–179.
14. Harris GW. Neural Control of the Pituitary Gland. Monographs of the Physiological Society no 3. London, E Arnold, 1955, p 298.
15. Green JD, Harris GW. Neurovascular link between neurohypophysis and adenohypophysis. J Endocrinol 1947; 5:136–146.
16. Reichlin S. Neuroendocrinology of the pituitary gland. Toxicol Pathol 1989; 17:250–255.
17. Schally AV, Redding TW, Bowers CY, Barrett JF. Isolation and properties of porcine thyrotropin-releasing hormone. J Biol Chem 1969; 244:4077–4088.
18. Boler J, Enzmann F, Folkers K, et al. The identity of chemical and hormonal properties of the thyrotropin releasing hormone and pyroglutamyl-histidyl-proline amide. Biochem Biophys Res Commun 1969; 37:705–710.
19. Burgus R, Dunn TF, Desiderio D, Guillemin R. (Molecular structure of the hypothalamic hypophysiotropic TRF factor of ovine origin: mass spectrometry demonstration of the PCA-His-Pro-NH_2 sequence). C R Acad Sci Hebd Seances Acad Sci D 1969; 269:1870–1873.
20. Burgus R, Dunn TF, Desiderio D, et al. Characterization of ovine hypothalamic hypophysiotropic TSH-releasing factor. Nature 1970; 226:321–325.
21. Vale W, Grant G, Rivier J, et al. Synthetic polypeptide antagonists of the hypothalamic luteinizing hormone releasing factor. Science 1972; 176:933–934.
22. Mayo KE. Molecular cloning and expression of a pituitary-specific receptor for growth hormone-releasing hormone. Mol Endocrinol 1992; 10:1734–1744.
23. Chen R, Lewis KA, Perrin MH, Vale WW. Expression cloning of a human corticotropin-releasing-factor receptor. Proc Natl Acad Sci USA 1993; 90:8967–8971.
24. Straub R, Frech GC, Joho RH, Gershengom MC. Expression cloning of a cDNA encoding the mouse pituitary thyrotropin-releasing hormone receptor. Proc Natl Acad Sci USA 1990; 87: 9514–9518.
25. Tsutsumi M, Zhou W, Millar RP, et al. Cloning and functional expression of a mouse gonadotropin-releasing hormone receptor. Mol Endocrinol 1992; 6:1163–1169.
26. Zhang Y, Proenca R, Maffei M, et al. Positional cloning of the mouse obese gene and its human homologue. Nature 1994; 372: 425–432.
27. Kojima M, Hosoda H, Matsuo H, Kangawa K. Ghrelin: discovery of the natural endogenous ligand for the growth hormone secretagogue receptor. Trends Endocrinol Metab 2001; 12:118–122.
28. Kojima M, Hosoda H, Date Y, et al. Ghrelin is a growth-hormone-releasing acylated peptide from stomach. Nature 1999. 402:656–660.
29. Spergel DJ, Kruth U, Hanley DF, et al. GABA- and glutamate-activated channels in green fluorescent protein-tagged gonadotropin-releasing hormone neurons in transgenic mice. J Neurosci 1999; 19:2037–2050.
30. Suter K, Wuarin JP, Smith BN, et al. Whole-cell recordings from preoptic/hypothalamic slices reveal burst firing in gonadotropin-releasing hormone neurons identified with green fluorescent protein in transgenic mice. Endocrinology 2000; 141:3731–3736.
31. Cowley MA, Smart JL, Rubinstein M, et al. Leptin activates anorexigenic POMC neurons through a neural network in the arcuate nucleus. Nature 2001. 411:480–484.
32. Scharrer B. Neurosecretion: beginnings and new directions in neuropeptide research. Annu Rev Neurosci 1987; 10:1–17.
33. Kandel ER. Nerve cells and behavior. In Kandel ER, Schwartz JH, Jessell TM (eds). Principles of Neural Science. Norwalk, Conn, Appleton & Lange, 1991, pp 18–32.
34. Kupfermann I. Hypothalamus and limbic system: peptidergic neurons, homeostasis, and emotional behavior. In Kandel ER, Schwartz JH, Jessell TM (eds). Principles of Neural Science. Norwalk, Conn, Appleton & Lange, 1991, pp 735–749.
35. Scharrer E, Scharrer B. Secretory cells within the hypothalamus. In The Hypothalamus, vol xx. Publication of the ARNMD. New York, Hafner, 1940, pp 170–194.
36. Sawyer CH. History of the neurovascular concept of hypothalamo-hypophysial control. Biol Reprod 1978; 18:325–328.
37. Hokfelt T, Johansson O, Ljungdahl A, et al. Peptidergic neurons. Nature 1980; 284:515–521.
38. Guillemin R. Peptides in the brain: the new endocrinology of the neuron. Science 1978; 202:390–402.
39. Harris GW. Structure and function of the median eminence. Am J Anat 1970; 129:245–246.
40. Loewy AD. Anatomy of the autonomic nervous system: an overview. In Loewy AD, Spyer KM (eds). Central Regulation of Autonomic Functions. New York, Oxford University Press, 1990, pp 3–16.
41. Lefkowitz RJ, Hoffman BB, Taylor P. Neurotransmission. In Goodman LS, Gilman A, Hardman JG, Limbird LE (eds). Goodman & Gilman's The Pharmacological Basis of Therapeutics. New York, McGraw-Hill, 1996, pp 105–139.
42. Hokfelt T, Lundberg JM, Schultzberg M, et al. Coexistence of peptides and putative transmitters in neurons. Adv Biochem Psychopharmacol 1980; 22:1–23.
43. Edwards AV. Autonomic control of endocrine pancreatic and adrenal function. In Loewy AD, Spyer KM (eds). Central Regulation of Autonomic Functions. 1990, New York, Oxford University Press, 1990, pp 286–309.
44. Ahren B. Autonomic regulation of islet hormone secretion: implications for health and disease. Diabetologia 2000; 43:393–410.
45. Levin BE, Routh VH. Role of the brain in energy balance and obesity. Am J Physiol 1996; 271:R491–R500.
46. Berthoud HR, Fox EA, Powley TL. Localization of vagal preganglionics that stimulate insulin and glucagon secretion. Am J Physiol 1990; 258:R160–R168.
47. Saltiel AR. New perspectives into the molecular pathogenesis and treatment of type 2 diabetes. Cell 2001; 104:517–529.
48. Levin BE, Dunn-Meynell AA, Routh VH. Brain glucose sensing and body energy homeostasis: role in obesity and diabetes. Am J Physiol 1999; 276:R1223–R1231.
49. Reichlin S. Function of the hypothalamus. Am J Med 1967; 43: 477–485.
50. Saper CB. Central autonomic system. In Paxinos G (ed). The Rat Nervous System. 1995, San Diego, Academic Press, 1995, pp 107–135.
51. Lechan RM. Neuroendocrinology of pituitary hormone regulation. Endocrinol Metab Clin North Am 1987; 16:475–501.
52. Ganong WF. Circumventricular organs: definition and role in the regulation of endocrine and autonomic function. Clin Exp Pharmacol Physiol 2000; 27:422–427.

53. Page R. The anatomy of the hypothalamo-hypophysial complex. In Knobil E, Neill J (eds). The Physiology of Reproduction. New York, Raven Press, 1994, pp 1527–1619.
54. Halasz B. Hypothalamo-anterior pituitary system and pituitary portal vessels. In Imura H (ed). The Pituitary Gland. New York, Raven Press, 1994, pp 1–28.
55. Wingstrand KG. Microscopic anatomy, nerve supply, and blood supply of the pars intermedia. In Harris GW, Donovan BT (eds). The Pituitary Gland. London, Butterworth, 1966, pp 1–27.
56. Christ JF. Derivation and boundaries of the hypothalamus, with atlas of the hypothalamic grisea. In Haymaker W, Anderson E, Nauta WJH (eds). The Hypothalamus. Springfield, Ill, Charles C Thomas, 1968, pp 13–60.
57. Evans VR, Manning AB, Bernard LH, et al. Alpha-melanocyte-stimulating hormone and *N*-acetyl-beta-endorphin immunoreactivities are localized in the human pituitary but are not restricted to the zona intermedia. Endocrinology 1994; 134:97–106.
58. Lederis K. Neurosecretion and the functional structure of the neurohypophysis. In Greep R, Astwood EB, Knobil E, et al (eds). Handbook of Physiology. Sect 7: Endocrinology. Vol IV, The Pituitary Gland and Its Neuroendocrine Control, Part 1. Washington, DC, American Physiological Society, 1974, pp 81–102.
59. Zimmerman EA, et al. Anatomy of pituitary and extrapituitary vasopressin secretion system. In Reichlin S (ed). The Neurohypophysis. New York, Plenum, 1984, pp 5–27.
60. Johnson AK, Loewy AD. Circumventricular organs and their role in visceral functions. In Loewy AD, Spyer KM (eds). Central Regulation of Autonomic Functions. New York, Oxford University Press, 1990, pp 247–267.
61. Johnson AK, Zardetto-Smith AM, Edwards GL. Integrative mechanisms and the maintenance of cardiovascular and body fluid homeostasis: the central processing of sensory input derived from the circumventricular organs of the lamina terminalis. Prog Brain Res 1992;91:381–393.
62. Loewy AD. Forebrain nuclei involved in autonomic control. Prog Brain Res 1991; 87:253–268.
63. Lincoln DW, Paisley AC. Neuroendocrine control of milk ejection. J Reprod Fertil 1982; 65:571–586.
64. Wakerley JB, Lincoln DW. Proceedings: unit activity in the supra-optic nucleus during reflex milk ejection. J Endocrinol 1973; 59:xlvi–xlvii.
65. Burstein R, Cliffer KD, Giesler GJ Jr. Direct somatosensory projections from the spinal cord to the hypothalamus and telencephalon. J Neurosci 1987; 7:4159–4164.
66. Swanson LW, Sawchenko PE. Hypothalamic integration: organization of the paraventricular and supraoptic nuclei. Annu Rev Neurosci 1983; 6:269–324.
67. Swanson LW, Sawchenko PE, Rivier J, Vale WW. Organization of ovine corticotropin-releasing factor immunoreactive cells and fibers in the rat brain: an immunohistochemical study. Neuroendocrinology 1983; 36:165–186.
68. Flerko B. Fourth Geoffrey Harris Memorial Lecture: the hypophysial portal circulation today. Neuroendocrinology 1980; 30: 56–63.
69. Clarke I, Jessop D, Millar R, et al. Many peptides that are present in the external zone of the median eminence are not secreted into the hypophysial portal blood of sheep. Neuroendocrinology 1993; 57:765–775.
70. Page R. Directional pituitary blood flow: a microcinephotographic study. Endocrinology 1983; 112:157–165.
71. Page RB. The anatomy of the hypothalamo-hypophysial complex. In Knobil E, Neill JD (eds). The Physiology of Reproduction. New York, Raven Press, 1994, pp 1527–1619.
72. Lechan R, Lin HD, Ling N, et al. Distribution of immunoreactive growth hormone releasing factor (1–44)NH_2 in the tuberoinfundibular system of the rhesus monkey. Brain Res 1984; 309: 55–61.
73. Wiegand SJ, Price JL. Cells of origin of the afferent fibers to the median eminence in the rat. J Comp Neurol 1980; 192:1–19.
74. Fink G. The development of the releasing factor concept. Clin Endocrinol (Oxf) 1976; 5:245s–260s.
75. Knigge KM, Scott DE. Structure and function of the median eminence. Am J Anat 1970; 129:223–243.
76. Page RB. Pituitary blood flow. Am J Physiol 1982; 243:E427–E442.
77. Elde R, Hokfelt T. Localization of hypophysiotropic peptides and other biologically active peptides within the brain. Annu Rev Physiol 1979; 41:587–602.
78. King JC, Rubin BS. Dynamic alterations in luteinizing hormone-releasing hormone (LHRH) neuronal cell bodies and terminals of adult rats. Cell Mol Neurobiol 1995; 15:89–106.
79. Simerly RB. Anatomical substrates of hypothalamic integration. In Paxinos G (ed). The Rat Nervous System. San Diego, Academic Press, 1995, pp 353–376.
80. Lechan RM, Nestler JL, Jacobson S. The tuberoinfundibular system of the rat as demonstrated by immunohistochemical localization of retrogradely transported wheat germ agglutinin (WGA) from the median eminence. Brain Res 1982; 245:1–15.
81. McKinley MJ, Allen AM, Burns P, et al. Interaction of circulating hormones with the brain: the roles of the subfornical organ and the organum vasculosum of the lamina terminalis. Clin Exp Pharmacol Physiol Suppl 1998; 25:S61–S67.
82. Johnson AK, Gross PM. Sensory circumventricular organs and brain homeostatic pathways. FASEB J 1993; 7:678–686.
83. Ferguson AV, Bains JS. Electrophysiology of the circumventricular organs. Front Neuroendocrinol 1996; 17:440–475.
84. Saper C, Breder C. The neurologic basis of fever. N Engl J Med 1994; 330:1880–1886.
85. Ferguson AV, Bains JS. Actions of angiotensin in the subfornical organ and area postrema: implications for long term control of autonomic output. Clin Exp Pharmacol Physiol 1997; 24:96–101.
86. Rodriguez E, Oksche A, Hein S, Yulis CR. Cell biology of the subcommissural organ. Int Rev Cytol 1992; 135:39–121.
87. Rodriguez EM, Rodriguez S, Hein S. The subcommissural organ. Microsc Res Tech 1998; 41:98–123.
88. Gross PM. Circumventricular organ capillaries. Prog Brain Res 1992; 91:219–233.
89. Fei H, Okano HJ, Li C, et al. Anatomic localization of alternatively spliced leptin receptors (Ob-R) in mouse brain and other tissues. Proc Natl Acad Sci USA 1997; 94:7001–7005.
90. Tatro JB, Entwistle ML. Identification of a specific mammalian melanocortin receptor antagonist. Ann NY Acad Sci 1994; 739: 315–319.
91. Banks WA, Kastin AJ, Huang W, et al. Leptin enters the brain by a saturable system independent of insulin. Peptides 1996; 17: 305–311.
92. Hakansson ML, Hulting AL, Meister B. Expression of leptin receptor mRNA in the hypothalamic arcuate nucleus: relationship with NPY neurones. Neuroreport 1996; 7:3087–3092.
93. Cheung CC, Clifton DK, Steiner RA. Proopiomelanocortin neurons are direct targets for leptin in the hypothalamus. Endocrinology 1997; 138:4489–4492.
94. Mercer JG, Hoggard N, Williams LM, et al. Coexpression of leptin receptor and preproneuropeptide Y mRNA in arcuate nucleus of mouse hypothalamus. J Neuroendocrinol 1996; 8:733–735.
95. Mercer JG, Hoggard N, Williams LM, et al. Localization of leptin receptor mRNA and the long form splice variant (Ob-Rb) in mouse hypothalamus and adjacent brain regions by in situ hybridization. FEBS Lett 1996; 387:113–116.
96. Schwartz MW, Seeley RJ, Campfield LA, et al. Identification of targets of leptin action in rat hypothalamus. J Clin Invest 1996; 98:1101–1106.
97. Schwartz MW, Seeley RJ, Woods SC, et al. Leptin increases hypothalamic pro-opiomelanocortin mRNA expression in the rostral arcuate nucleus. Diabetes 1997; 46:2119–2123.
98. Mizuno TM, Makimura H, Silverstein J, et al. Fasting regulates hypothalamic neuropeptide Y, agouti-related peptide, and proopiomelanocortin in diabetic mice independent of changes in leptin or insulin. Endocrinology 1999; 140:4551–4557.
99. Thornton JE, Cheung CC, Clifton DK, Steiner RA. Regulation of hypothalamic proopiomelanocortin mRNA by leptin in *ob/ob* mice. Endocrinology 1997; 138:5063–5066.
100. Elias CF, Aschkenasi C, Lee C, et al. Leptin differentially regulates NPY and POMC neurons projecting to the lateral hypothalamic area. Neuron 1999; 23:775–786.
101. Blatteis CM. Role of the OVLT in the febrile response to circulating pyrogens. Prog Brain Res 1992; 91:409–412.
102. Oka T, Oka K, Scammell TE, et al. Relationship of EP(1–4) prostaglandin receptors with rat hypothalamic cell groups involved in lipopolysaccharide fever responses. J Comp Neurol 2000; 428:20–32.

103. Oldfield BJ, Bicknell RJ, McAllen RM, et al. Intravenous hypertonic saline induces Fos immunoreactivity in neurons throughout the lamina terminalis. Brain Res 1991; 561:151–156.
104. Standaert DG, Saper CB. Origin of the atriopeptin-like immunoreactive innervation of the paraventricular nucleus of the hypothalamus. J Neurosci 1988; 8:1940–1950.
105. Lind RW, Swanson LW, Ganten D. Angiotensin II immunoreactivity in the neural afferents and efferents of the subfornical organ of the rat. Brain Res 1984; 321:209–215.
106. Saper CB, Levisohn D. Afferent connections of the median preoptic nucleus in the rat: anatomical evidence for a cardiovascular integrative mechanism in the anteroventral third ventricular (AV3V) region. Brain Res 1983; 288:21–31.
107. Lind RW, Johnson AK. Subfornical organ-median preoptic connections and drinking and pressor responses to angiotensin II. J Neurosci 1982; 2:1043–1051.
108. Simpson JB, Routtenberg A. Subfornical organ lesions reduce intravenous angiotensin-induced drinking. Brain Res 1975; 88: 154–161.
109. Simpson JB, Routtenberg A. Subfornical organ: a dipsogenic site of action of angiotensin II. Science 1978; 201:379–381.
110. Simpson JB, Routtenberg A. Subfornical organ: site of drinking elicitation by angiotensin II. Science 1973; 181:1772–1775.
111. Mangiapane ML, Thrasher TN, Keil LC, et al. Role for the subfornical organ in vasopressin release. Brain Res Bull 1984; 13: 43–47.
112. Miller AD, Leslie RA. The area postrema and vomiting. Front Neuroendocrinol 1994; 15:301–320.
113. Merchenthaler I, Lane M, Shughrue P. Distribution of pre-pro-glucagon and glucagon-like peptide-1 receptor messenger RNAs in the rat central nervous system. J Comp Neurol 1999; 403: 261–280.
114. Moran TH, Robinson PH, Goldrich MS, McHugh PR. Two brain cholecystokinin receptors: implications for behavioral actions. Brain Res 1986; 362:175–179.
115. Osborn JW, Collister JP, Carlson SH. Angiotensin and osmoreceptor inputs to the area postrema: role in long-term control of fluid homeostasis and arterial pressure. Clin Exp Pharmacol Physiol 2000; 27:443–449.
116. Ferguson AV, Wall KM. Central actions of angiotensin in cardiovascular control: multiple roles for a single peptide. Can J Physiol Pharmacol 1992; 70:779–785.
117. Xu Z, Herbert J. Regional suppression by water intake of c-fos expression induced by intraventricular infusions of angiotensin II. Brain Res 1994; 659:157–168.
118. Wurtman R, Axelrod J, Kelly D. The Pineal. New York, Academic Press, 1968.
119. Rolleston HD. The Endocrine Organs in Health and Disease: With an Historical Review. London, Oxford University Press, 1936.
120. Pevet P. Anatomy of the pineal gland of mammals. In Relkin R (ed). The Pineal Gland. New York, Elsevier Biomedical, 1983, pp 1–76.
121. Kappers J, Smith A, De Vries R. The mammalian pineal gland and its control of hypothalamic activity. Prog Brain Res 1974; 41: 149–174.
122. Reppert SM. Melatonin receptors: molecular biology of a new family of G protein-coupled receptors. J Biol Rhythms 1997; 12: 528–531.
123. Czeisler CA. Commentary: evidence for melatonin as a circadian phase-shifting agent. J Biol Rhythms 1997; 12:618–623.
124. Moore RY. Circadian rhythms: basic neurobiology and clinical applications. Annu Rev Med 1997; 48:253–266.
125. Moore RY, Lenn NJ. A retinohypothalamic projection in the rat. J Comp Neurol 1972; 146:1–14.
126. Watts AG, Swanson LW. Efferent projections of the suprachiasmatic nucleus: II. Studies using retrograde transport of fluorescent dyes and simultaneous peptide immunohistochemistry in the rat. J Comp Neurol 1987; 258:230–252.
127. Watts AG, Swanson LW, Sanchez-Watts G. Efferent projections of the suprachiasmatic nucleus: I. Studies using anterograde transport of *Phaseolus vulgaris* leucoagglutinin in the rat. J Comp Neurol 1987; 258:204–229.
128. Saper CB, Loewy AD, Swanson LW, Cowan WM. Direct hypothalamo-autonomic connections. Brain Res 1976; 117:305–312.
129. Rando TA, Bowers CW, Zigmond RE. Localization of neurons in the rat spinal cord which project to the superior cervical ganglion. J Comp Neurol 1981; 196:73–83.
130. Borjigin J, Li X, Snyder SH. The pineal gland and melatonin: molecular and pharmacologic regulation. Annu Rev Pharmacol Toxicol 1999; 39:53–65.
131. Borjigin J, Wang MM, Snyder SH. Diurnal variation in mRNA encoding serotonin *N*-acetyltransferase in pineal gland. Nature 1995; 378:783–785.
132. Coon S, Roseboom PH, Baler R, et al. Pineal serotonin *N*-acetyltransferase: expression cloning and molecular analysis. Science 1995; 270:1681–1683.
133. Reppert S, Weaver D. Melatonin madness. Cell 1995; 83:1059–1062.
134. Klein DC, Weller JL. Rapid light-induced decrease in pineal serotonin *N*-acetyltransferase activity. Science 1972; 177:532–533.
135. Quay WB. Circadian rhythm in rat pineal substance effect on the rat ovary. Gen Comp Endocrinol 1963; 3:473–479.
136. Arendt J. The pineal gland: basic physiology and clinical implications In DeGroot LJ (ed). Endocrinology. Philadelphia, WB Saunders, 1995, pp 432–444.
137. Lewy A. Biochemistry and regulation of mammalian melatonin production. In Relkin R (ed). The Pineal Gland. New York, Elsevier Biomedical, 1983, pp 77–128.
138. Foulkes NS, Borjigin J, Snyder SH, Sassone-Corsi P. Transcriptional control of circadian hormone synthesis via the CREM feedback loop. Proc Natl Acad Sci USA 1996; 93:14140–14145.
139. Foulkes NS, Borjigin J, Snyder SH, Sassone-Corsi P. Rhythmic transcription: the molecular basis of circadian melatonin synthesis. Trends Neurosci 1997; 20:487–492.
140. Martin J, McKellar S, Klein D. Melatonin inhibition of the in vivo pituitary response to luteinizing hormone-releasing hormone in the neonatal rat. Neuroendocrinology 1980; 31:13–17.
141. Nakazawa K, Marubayashi U, McCann SM. Mediation of the short-loop negative feedback of luteinizing hormone (LH) on LH-releasing hormone release by melatonin-induced inhibition of LH release from the pars tuberalis. Proc Natl Acad Sci USA 1991; 88:7576–7579.
142. Reiter R. The pineal and its hormones in the control of reproduction in mammals. Endocr Rev 1980. 1:109–131.
143. Gerlach T, Aurich JE. Regulation of seasonal reproductive activity in the stallion, ram and hamster. Anim Reprod Sci 2000; 58: 197–213.
144. Reiter RJ. Melatonin and human reproduction. Ann Med 1998; 30:103–108.
145. Waldhauser F, Weiszenbacher G, Frisch H, et al. Fall in nocturnal serum melatonin during prepuberty and pubescence. Lancet 1984; 1:362–365.
146. Silman R, Leone RM, Hooper RJ, Preece MA. Melatonin, the pineal gland and human puberty. Nature 1979; 282:301–303.
147. Ehrenkranz JR, Tamerkin L, Comite F, et al. Daily rhythm of plasma melatonin in normal and precocious puberty. J Clin Endocrinol Metab 1982; 55:307–310.
148. Tetsuo M., Poth M, Markey S. Melatonin metabolite excretion during childhood and puberty. J Clin Endocrinol Metab 1982; 55:311–313.
149. Reppert S, Weaver D, Ebisawa T. Cloning and characterization of a mammalian melatonin receptor that mediates reproductive and circadian responses. Neuron 1994; 13:1177–1185.
150. Reppert SM, Godson C, Mahle CD, et al. Molecular characterization of a second melatonin receptor expressed in human retina and brain: the Mel1b melatonin receptor. Proc Natl Acad Sci USA 1995; 92:8734–8738.
151. McArthur AJ, Gillette MU, Prosser RA. Melatonin directly resets the rat suprachiasmatic circadian clock in vitro. Brain Res 1991; 565:158–161.
152. Liu C, Weaver DR, Jin X, et al. Molecular dissection of two distinct actions of melatonin on the suprachiasmatic circadian clock. Neuron 1997; 19:91–102.
153. Shibata S, Cassone VM, Moore RY. Effects of melatonin on neuronal activity in the rat suprachiasmatic nucleus in vitro. Neurosci Lett 1989; 97:140–144.
154. Arendt J. Melatonin, circadian rhythms, and sleep. N Engl J Med 2000; 343:1114–1116.
155. Bowers C, Schally AV, Enzmann F, et al. Porcine thyrotropin releasing hormone is (pyro)GluHisPro(NH_2). Endocrinology 1970; 86:1143–1153.

156. Schally AV. Aspects of hypothalamic regulation of the pituitary gland. Science 1978; 202:20–28.
157. Parkes D, Kasckoiw J, Vale W. Carbon monoxide modulates secretion of corticotropin-releasing factor from rat hypothalamic cell cultures. Brain Res 1994; 646:315–318.
158. DiStefano JI, Stubberud A, Williams I. Theory and Problems of Feedback and Control Systems. New York, Schaum Publishing, 1967.
159. Yates F. Modeling periodicities in reproductive, adrenocortical and metabolic systems. In Ferin M, Halberg F, Richart RM (eds). Biorhythms and Human Reproduction. New York, John Wiley & Sons, 1974, pp 133–142.
160. Houk J. Control strategies in physiological systems. FASEB J 1988; 2:97–107.
161. Moore R. The organization of the human circadian timing system. Prog Brain Res 1992; 93:101–115.
162. Boyar R. Sleep-related endocrine rhythms. In Reichlin S, Baldessarini R, Martin J (eds). The Hypothalamus. New York, Raven Press, 1978, pp 373–386.
163. Chadwick D, Ackrill K. Circadian clocks and their adjustment. Ciba Found Symp 1995.
164. Van Cauter E, Turek F. Endocrine and other biological rhythms. In DeGroot L (ed). Endocrinology. Philadelphia, WB Saunders, 1995, pp 2497–2548.
165. Star RA, Rajora N, Huang J, et al. Evidence of autocrine modulation of macrophage nitric oxide synthase by α-melanocyte-stimulating hormone. Proc Natl Acad Sci USA 1995; 92:8016–8020.
166. Stern J, Reichlin S. Prolactin circadian rhythm persists throughout lactation in women. Neuroendocrinology 1990; 51:31–37.
167. Welsh D, Logothetis DE, Meister M, Reppert SM. Individual neurons dissociated from rat suprachiasmatic nucleus express independently phased circadian firing rhythms. Neuron 1995; 14: 697–706.
168. Albers H, Ferris CF, Leeman SE, Goldman BP. Avian pancreatic polypeptide phase shifts hamster circadian rhythms when microinjected into the suprachiasmatic region. Science 1984; 223: 833–835.
169. Weaver D, Rivkees S, Reppert S. Localization and characterization of melatonin receptors in rodent brain by in vitro radioautography. J Neurosci 1989; 9:2581–2590.
170. Czeisler C, Shanahan T, Klerman E. Suppression of melatonin secretion in some blind patients by exposure to bright light. N Engl J Med 1995; 332:54–55.
171. Reppert S. Prenatal development of a hypothalamic biological clock. Prog Brain Res 1992; 93:119–132.
172. Czeisler C, Johnson MP, Duffy JF, et al. Exposure to bright light and darkness to treat physiologic maladaptation to night work. N Engl J Med 1990; 322:1253–1259.
173. Lewy A, Sack RL, Miller LS, Hoban TM. Antidepressant and circadian phase shifting effects of light. Science 1987; 235:352–354.
174. Turek F, Van Reeth O. Altering the mammalian circadian clock with the short-acting benzodiazepine, triazolam. Trends Neurosci 1988; 11:535–541.
175. Nillni EA, Sevarino KA. The biology of pro-thyrotropin-releasing hormone-derived peptides. Endocr Rev 1999; 20:599–648.
176. Valentijn K, Bunel DT, Liao N, et al. Release of pro-thyrotropin releasing hormone connecting peptides PS4 and PS5 from perfused rat hypothalamic slices. Neuroscience 1991; 44:223–233.
177. Bulant M, Roussel JP, Astier H, et al. Processing of thyrotropin releasing hormone prohormone (pro-TRH) generates a biologically active peptide, prepro-TRH(160–169) which regulates TRH-induced thyrotropin secretion. Proc Natl Acad Sci USA 1990; 87:4439–4443.
178. Redei E, Hilderbrand H, Aird F. Corticotropin release inhibiting factor is prepro-TRH 178–199. Endocrinology 1995; 136:3557–3563.
179. Barrington EJW. Hormones and Evolution. London, Academic Press, 1979, pp 1–989.
180. Bowers C, Friesen HG, Hwang P, et al. Prolactin and thyrotropin release in man by synthetic pyroglutamyl-histidyl-prolinamide. Biochem Biophys Res Commun 1971; 45:1033–1041.
181. Snyder J, Jacobs LS, Rabello MM, et al. Diagnostic value of thyrotropin-releasing hormone in pituitary and hypothalamic disease: assessment of thyrotropin and prolactin in 100 patients. Ann Intern Med 1974; 81:751–757.
182. Jackson I. Thyrotropin-releasing hormone. N Engl J Med 1982; 306:145–155.
183. Fink G, Koch Y, Ben Aroya N. Release of thyrotropin releasing hormone into hypophysial portal blood is high relative to other neuropeptides and may be related to prolactin secretion. Brain Res 1982; 243:186–189.
184. Reichlin S. Neuroendocrine regulation of prolactin secretion. Adv Biosci 1988; 69:277–292.
185. Gautvik K, Tashjian AH Jr, Kourides IA, et al. Thyrotropin-releasing hormone is not the sole physiologic mediator of prolactin release during suckling. N Engl J Med 1974; 290:1162–1165.
186. Thorner M, Perryman RL, Cronin MJ, et al. Somatotroph hyperplasia: successful treatment of acromegaly by removal of a pancreatic islet tumor secreting a growth hormone-releasing factor. J Clin Invest 1982; 70:965–977.
187. Borges J, Uskavitch DR, Kaiser DL, et al. Human pancreatic growth hormone-releasing factor-40 (hpGRF-40) allows stimulation of GH release by TRH. Endocrinology 1983; 113:1519–1521.
188. Halpern J, Hinkle P. Direct visualization of receptors for thyrotropin-releasing hormone with a fluorescein-labeled analog. Proc Natl Acad Sci USA 1981; 78:587–591.
189. Jun D, Ahn SK, Voon JH, et al. Involvement of a cAMP-responsive DNA element in mediating TRH responsiveness of the human thyrotropin alpha-subunit gene. Mol Endocrinol 1994; 8: 528–536.
190. Heinflink M, Nussenzveig DR, Friedman AM, Gershengom MC. Thyrotropin-releasing hormone receptor activation does not elevate intracellular cyclic adenosine 3′,5′-monophosphate in cells expressing high levels of receptors. J Clin Endocrinol Metab 1994; 79:650–652.
191. Tashjian AJ, Heslop J, Berridge M. Subsecond and second changes in inositol polyphosphates in GH4C1 cells induced by thyrotropin-releasing hormone. Biochem J 1987; 243:305–308.
192. Winiger B, Schlegel W. Rapid transient elevations of cytosolic calcium triggered by thyrotropin releasing hormone in individual cells of the pit line GH3B6. Biochem J 1988; 255:161–167.
193. Kim M, McClaskey JH, Bodemer DL, Weintraub BD. An AP1 like factor and the pituitary specific factor Pit1 are both necessary to mediate hormonal induction of human thyrotropin b gene expression. J Biol Chem 1993; 268:23366–23375.
194. Rosenfeld M, Amara SG, Birnberg NC, et al. Prolactin and growth hormone gene expression as model systems for the characterization of neuroendocrine regulation. Recent Prog Horm Res 1983; 39:305–352.
195. Peterkofsky A, Battaini F, Koch Y, et al. Histidyl-proline diketopiperazine: its biological role as a regulatory peptide. Mol Cell Biochem 1982; 42:45–63.
196. Lee S, Stewart K, Goodman R. Structure of the gene encoding rat thyrotropin releasing hormone. J Biol Chem 1988; 263: 16604–16609.
197. Myashita K, et al. Histidyl-proline diketopiperazine: novel formation that does not originate from thyrotropin-releasing hormone. J Biol Chem 1993; 268:20863–20865.
198. Toni R, Lechan RM. Neuroendocrine regulation of thyrotropin-releasing hormone (TRH) in the tuberoinfundibular system. J Endocrinol Invest 1993; 16:715–753.
199. Jackson I, Adelman LS, Munsat IL, et al. Amyotrophic lateral sclerosis: thyrotropin-releasing hormone and cerebrospinal fluid. Neurology 1986; 36:1218–1223.
200. Johansson O, Hokfelt T, Pernow B, et al. Immunohistochemical support for three putative transmitters in one neuron: coexistence of 5-hydroxytryptamine, substance P, and thyrotropin-releasing hormone-like immunoreactivity in medullary neurons projecting to the spinal cord. Neuroscience 1981; 6:1857–1881.
201. Lechan R, Snapper SB, Jacobson S, Jackson IM. The distribution of thyrotropin-releasing hormone (TRH) in the rhesus monkey spinal cord. Peptides 1984; 5(suppl 1):185–194.
202. Lechan R, et al. Organization of thyrotropin-releasing hormone (TRH) immunoreactivity in the human spinal cord. Soc Neurosci Abstr 1984; 431.
203. Engler D, Scanlon M, Jackson I. Thyrotropin releasing hormone in the systemic circulation of the neonatal rat is derived from the pancreas and other extraneural tissues. J Clin Invest 1981; 67: 800–808.
204. Jackson I, Metcalf G. TRH. Ann NY Acad Sci 1989; 553:1–631.

205. Griffiths E, Bennett G (eds). Thyrotropin-Releasing Hormone. New York, Raven Press, 1983.
206. Reichlin S. Neural functions of TRH. Acta Endocrinol (Copenh) 1986; 112:21–33.
207. Samuels H, Ridgway E. Central hypothyroidism. Endocrinol Metab Clin North Am 1992; 21:903–920.
208. Spencer C, Schwarzbein D, Guttler RB, et al. Thyrotropin (TSH)-releasing hormone stimulation test responses employing third and fourth generation TSH assays. J Clin Endocrinol Metab 1993; 76:494–498.
209. Molitch M. Pathogenesis of pituitary tumors. Endocrinol Metab Clin 1987; 16:503–527.
210. Loosen P, Prange AJ. The serum thyrotropin (TSH) response to thyrotropin-releasing hormone in psychiatric patients: a review. Am J Psychiatry 1982; 139:405–416.
211. Callahan AM, Frye MA, Marangell LB, et al. Comparative antidepressant effects of intravenous and intrathecal thyrotropin-releasing hormone: confounding effects of tolerance and implications for therapeutics. Biol Psychiatry 1997; 41:264–272.
212. Marangell LB, George MS, Callahan AM, et al. Effects of intrathecal thyrotropin-releasing hormone (protirelin) in refractory depressed patients. Arch Gen Psychiatry 1997; 54:214–222.
213. Rubinow D. Cerebrospinal fluid somatostatin and psychiatric illness. Biol Psychiatry 1986; 21:341–365.
214. Australian collaborative trial of antenatal thyrotropin-releasing hormone (ACTOBAT) for prevention of neonatal respiratory disease. Lancet 1995; 345:877–882.
215. Collaborative trial of prenatal thyrotropin-releasing hormone and corticosteroids for prevention of respiratory distress syndrome. Am J Obstet Gynecol 1998; 178:33–39.
216. Sobue I, Takayanagi T, Nakanishi T, et al. Controlled trial of thyrotropin-releasing hormone tartrate in ataxia of spinocerebellar degenerations. J Neurol Sci 1983; 61:235–248.
217. Engel W, Siddique T, Nicoloff J. Effect on weakness and spasticity in amyotrophic lateral sclerosis of thyrotropin-releasing hormone. Lancet 1983; 2:73–75.
218. Munsat T, Lechan R, Taft JM, et al. TRH and diseases of the motor system. Ann NY Acad Sci 1989; 553:388–398.
219. Tzeng AC, Cheng J, Fryczynski H, et al. A study of thyrotropin-releasing hormone for the treatment of spinal muscular atrophy: a preliminary report. Am J Phys Med Rehabil 2000; 79:435–440.
220. Brooks B. A summary of the current position of TRH in ALS therapy. Ann NY Acad Sci 1989; 553:431–461.
221. Askanas V, Engel WK, Eagleson K, Micaglio G. Influence of TRH and TRH analogues RGH2202 and DN1417 on cultured ventral spinal cord neurons. Ann NY Acad Sci 1989; 553:325–336.
222. Munsat T, Taft J, Jackson IM, et al. Intrathecal thyrotropin-releasing hormone does not alter the progressive course of ALS: experience with an intrathecal drug delivery system. Neurology 1992; 42:1049–1053.
223. Holaday J, Long JB, Martinez-Arizala A, et al., Effects of TRH in circulatory shock and central nervous system ischemia. Ann NY Acad Sci 1989; 445:370–379.
224. Faden A, Jacobs T, Holaday J. Thyrotropin-releasing hormone improves neurologic recovery after spinal trauma in cats. N Engl J Med 1981; 305:1063–1067.
225. Dumont RJ, Verma S, Okonkwo DO, et al. Acute spinal cord injury, part II: contemporary pharmacotherapy. Clin Neuropharmacol 2001; 24:265–279.
226. Pitts LH, Ross A, Chase GA, Faden AI. Treatment with thyrotropin-releasing hormone (TRH) in patients with traumatic spinal cord injuries. J Neurotrauma 1995; 12:235–243.
227. Maejima S, Katayama Y. Neurosurgical trauma in Japan. World J Surg 2001; 25:1205–1209.
228. Takeuchi Y, Takano T, Abe J, et al. Thyrotropin-releasing hormone: role in the treatment of West syndrome and related epileptic encephalopathies. Brain Dev 2001; 23:662–667.
229. Breese G, Cott JM, Cooper BR, et al. Effects of thyrotropin-releasing hormone (TRH) on the action of pentobarbital and other centrally acting drugs. J Pharmacol Exp Ther 1974; 193: 11–22.
230. Knutsen H, Dolva LO, Skrede S, et al. Thyrotropin-releasing hormone antagonism of ethanol inebriation. Alcohol Clin Exp Res 1989; 13:365–370.
231. Griffing G, Weiss CM, Bern M, et al. Thyrotropin (TRH) arousal and prolonged wakefulness in a hypersomnolent patient with histiocytosis-X (abstract). Clin Res 1989; 37:848A.
232. Reichlin S. Control of thyrotropic hormone secretion. In Martini L, Ganong W (eds). Neuroendocrinology. New York, Academic Press, 1966, pp 445–536.
233. Reichlin S, Martin J, Jackson I. Regulation of thyroid-stimulating hormone (TSH) secretion. In Jeffcoate S, Hutchinson J (eds). The Endocrine Hypothalamus. New York, Academic Press, 1978, pp 239–270.
234. Morley J. Neuroendocrine control of thyrotropin secretion. Endocr Rev 1981; 2:396–436.
235. Scanlon M, Hall R. Thyrotropin-releasing hormone: basic and clinical aspects. In DeGroot L (ed). Endocrinology. Philadelphia, WB Saunders, 1995, pp 208–217.
236. Wilber J. Control of thyroid function: the hypothalamic-pituitary-thyroid axis. In DeGroot L (ed). Endocrinology. Philadelphia, WB Saunders, 1995, pp 602–616.
237. Snyder P, Utiger R. Inhibition of thyrotropin response to thyrotropin releasing hormone by small quantities of thyroid hormones. J Clin Invest 1972; 51:2077–2084.
238. Vagenakis A, Rapoport B, Azizi F, et al. Hyper-response to thyrotropin releasing hormone accompanying small decreases in serum thyroid hormone concentration. J Clin Invest 1974; 54:913–918.
239. Segerson T, Kauer J, Wolfe HC, et al. Thyroid hormone regulates TRH biosynthesis in the paraventricular nucleus of the rat hypothalamus. Science 1987; 238:78–80.
240. Dyess E, Segerson TP, Liposits Z, et al. Triiodothyronine exerts direct cell-specific regulation of thyrotropin-releasing hormone gene expression in the hypothalamic paraventricular nucleus. Endocrinology 1988; 123:2291–2297.
241. Dahl G, Evans NP, Thrun LA, Karsch FJ. A central negative feedback action of thyroid hormones on thyrotropin-releasing hormone secretion. Endocrinology 1994; 135:2392–2397.
242. Schreiber G, Southwell B, Richardson S. Hormone delivery systems to the brain: transthyretin. Exp Clin Endocrinol 1995; 103: 75–80.
243. Lechan R, Qi Y, Jackson IM, Mahdavi V. Identification of thyroid hormone receptor isoforms in thyrotropin-releasing hormone neurons of the hypothalamic paraventricular nucleus. Endocrinology 1994; 135:92–100.
244. Lechan R, Kakucska I. Feedback regulation of thyrotropin-releasing hormone gene expression by thyroid hormone in the hypothalamic paraventricular nucleus. Ciba Found Symp 1992; 168: 144–158.
245. Kaplan M, Taft JA, Reichlin S, Munsat TL. Sustained rises in serum thyrotropin, thyroxine, and triiodothyronine during long term, continuous thyrotropin-releasing hormone treatment in patients with amyotrophic lateral sclerosis. J Clin Endocrinol Metab 1986; 63:808–814.
246. Kakucska I, Rand W, Lechan R. Thyrotropin-releasing hormone gene expression in the hypothalamic paraventricular nucleus is dependent on feedback regulation by both triiodothyronine and thyroxine. Endocrinology 1992; 130:2845–2850.
247. Arancibia S, Tapia-Arancibia L, Assenmacher I, Astier H. Direct evidence of short-term cold-induced TRH release in the median eminence. Neuroendocrinology 1983; 37:225–228.
248. Galton V. Environmental effects. In Ingbar S, Braverman L (eds). Werner's The Thyroid. Philadelphia, JB Lippincott, 1986, pp 407–413.
249. Sack J, Fisher D, Wang C. Serum thyrotropin, prolactin and growth hormone levels during the early neonatal period in the human infant. J Pediatr 1976; 89:298–300.
250. Arimura A, Schally A. Increases in basal and thyrotropin releasing hormone (TRH)–stimulated secretion of thyrotropin (TSH) by passive immunization with antiserum to somatostatin in rats. Endocrinology 1976; 98:1069–1072.
251. Ferland L, Labrie F, Jobin M, et al. Physiologic role of somatostatin in the control of growth hormone and thyrotropin secretion. Biochem Biophys Res Commun 1976; 68:149–151.
252. Berelowitz M, Maeda K, Harris S, Frohman LA. The effect of alterations in the pituitary-thyroid axis on hypothalamic content and in vitro release of somatostatin-like immunoreactivity. Endocrinology 1980; 107:24–29.
253. Rogers K, Vician L, Steiner RA, Clifton DK. The effect of hypophysectomy and growth hormone administration on pre-pro-

somatostatin messenger ribonucleic acid in the periventricular nucleus of the rat hypothalamus. Endocrinology 1988; 122:586–591.
254. Kaplan M. The role of thyroid hormone deiodination in the regulation of hypothalamo-pituitary function. Neuroendocrinology 1984; 38:254–260.
255. Relkin R. Pineal-hormonal interactions. In Relkin R (ed). The Pineal Gland. New York, Elsevier Biomedical, 1983, pp 225–246.
256. Brammer G, Morley JE, Geller E, et al. Hypothalamus-pituitary-thyroid axis interactions with pineal gland in the rat. Am J Physiol 1979; 236:E416–E420.
257. Jackson I, Sapirstein R, Reichlin S. Thyrotropin releasing hormone (TRH) in pineal and hypothalamus of the frog: effect of season and illumination. Endocrinology 1977; 100:97–100.
258. Brabant G, Prank K, Ranft U, et al. Physiological regulation of circadian and pulsatile thyrotropin secretion in normal man and woman. J Clin Endocrinol Metab 1990; 70:4403–4409.
259. Schallenberger E, Richardson D, Knobil E. Role of prolactin in the lactational amenorrhea of the rhesus monkey (*Macaca mulatta*). Biol Reprod 1981; 25:370–374.
260. Haisenleder D, Ortolano GA, Dalkin AC, et al. Differential actions of thyrotropin (TSH)-releasing hormone pulses in the expression of prolactin and TSH subunit messenger ribonucleic acid in rat pituitary cells in vitro. Endocrinology 1992; 130:2917–2923.
261. DuRuisseau J. Seasonal variation of PBI in healthy Montrealers. J Clin Endocrinol Metab 1965; 25:1513–1515.
262. Berg G, Utiger RD, Schalch DS, Reichlin S. Effect of central cooling in man on pituitary-thyroid function and growth hormone secretion. J Appl Physiol 1966; 21:1791–1794.
263. Arancibia S, Rage F, Astier H, et al., Neuroendocrine and autonomous mechanisms underlying thermoregulation in cold environment. Neuroendocrinology 1996; 64:257–267.
264. Tapia-Arancibia L, Arancibia S, Astier H. Evidence for α_1-adrenergic stimulatory control of in vitro release of immunoreactive thyrotropin-releasing hormone from rat median eminence: in vivo corroboration. Endocrinology 1985; 116:2314–2319.
265. Shioda S, Nakai Y, Sato A, et al. Electron-microscopic cytochemistry of the catecholaminergic innervation of TRH neurons in the rat hypothalamus. Cell Tissue Res 1986; 245:247–253.
266. Liposits Z, Uht RM, Harrison RW, et al. Ultrastructural localization of glucocorticoid receptor (GR) in hypothalamic paraventricular neurons synthesizing corticotropin releasing factor (CRF). Histochemistry 1987; 87:407–412.
267. Toni R, Jackson IM, Lechan RM. Neuropeptide-Y–immunoreactive innervation of thyrotropin-releasing hormone–synthesizing neurons in the rat hypothalamic paraventricular nucleus. Endocrinology 1990; 126:2444–2453.
268. Sawchenko PE, Swanson LW, Gizanna R, et al. Colocalization of neuropeptide Y immunoreactivity in brainstem catecholaminergic neurons that project to the paraventricular nucleus of the hypothalamus. J Comp Neurol 1985; 241:138–153.
269. Burger H, Patel Y. TSH and TRH: their physiological regulation and the clinical applications of TRH. In Martini L, Besser G (eds). Clinical Neuroendocrinology. New York, Academic Press, 1977, pp 67–131.
270. Wartofsky L, Burman K. Alterations in thyroid function in patients with systemic illness: the "euthyroid sick syndrome." Endocr Rev 1982; 3:164–217.
271. Peters J, Foord SM, Dieguez C, Scanlon MF. TSH neuroregulation and alterations in disease states. Clin Endocrinol Metab 1983; 12:669–695.
272. Nicoloff JT, Fischer D, Appleman MD. The role of glucocorticoids in the regulation of thyroid function in man. J Clin Invest 1970; 49:1922–1929.
273. Kakucska I, Qi Y, Lechan RM. Changes in adrenal status affect hypothalamic thyrotropin-releasing hormone gene expression in parallel with corticotropin releasing hormone. Endocrinology 1995; 136:2795–2802.
274. Cintra A, Fuxe K, Wikstrom AC, et al. Evidence for thyrotropin-releasing hormone and glucocorticoid receptor–immunoreactive neurons in various preoptic and hypothalamic nuclei of the male rat. Brain Res 1990; 506:139–144.
275. Salvador J, Dieguez C, Scanlon MF. The circadian rhythm of thyrotropin and prolactin secretion. Chronobiol Int 1988; 5:85–93.
276. Bauer MS, Whybrow PC. Thyroid hormones and the central nervous system in affective illness: interactions that may have clinical significance. Integr Psychiatry 1988; 6:75–100.
277. Jackson IMD, Luo L-G. Antidepressants inhibit the glucocorticoid stimulation of thyrotropin releasing hormone expression in cultured hypothalamic neurons. J Invest Med 1998; 46:470–475.
278. Axelson DA, Doraiswamy PM, McDonald WM, et al. Hypercortisolemia and hippocampal changes in depression. Psychiatry Res 1993; 47:163–173.
279. Shi Z-X, Levy A, Lightman SL. Hippocampal input to the hypothalamus inhibits thyrotrophin and thyrotrophin releasing hormone gene expression. Neuroendocrinology 1993; 57:576–580.
280. Spencer CA, Lum SM, Wilber JF, et al. Dynamics of serum thyrotropin and thyroid hormone changes in fasting. J Clin Endocrinol Metab 1983; 56:883–888.
281. Rondeel JMM, Heide R, de Greef WJ, et al. Effect of starvation and subsequent refeeding on thyroid function and release of hypothalamic thyrotropin-releasing hormone. Neuroendocrinology 1992; 56:348–353.
282. Blake NG, Eckland DJ, Foster OJ, Lightman SL. Inhibition of hypothalamic thyrotropin-releasing hormone messenger ribonucleic acid during food deprivation. Endocrinology 1991; 129: 2714–2718.
283. Ahima R, Prabakaran D, Mantzoros C, et al. Role of leptin in the neuroendocrine response to fasting. Nature 1996; 382:250–252.
284. Legradi G, Emerson CH, Ahima RS, et al. Leptin prevents fasting induced suppression of prothyrotropin-releasing hormone messenger ribonucleic acid in neurons of the hypothalamic paraventricular nucleus. Endocrinology 1997; 138:2569–2576.
285. Nillni EA, Vaslet C, Harris M, et al. Leptin regulates prothyrotropin-releasing hormone biosynthesis. J Biol Chem 2000; 275: 36124–36133.
286. Fekete C, Legradi G, Mihaly E, et al. α-Melanocyte-stimulating hormone is contained in nerve terminals innervating thyrotropin-releasing hormone–synthesizing neurons in the hypothalamic paraventricular nucleus and prevents fasting-induced suppression of prothyrotropin-releasing hormone gene expression. J Neurosci 2000; 20:1550–1558.
287. Harris M, Aschkenasi C, Elias CF, et al. Transcriptional regulation of the thyrotropin-releasing hormone gene by leptin and melanocortin signaling. J Clin Invest 2001; 107:111–120.
288. Montague CT, Farooqi IS, Whitehead JP, et al. Congenital leptin deficiency is associated with severe early-onset obesity in humans. Nature 1997; 387:903–908.
289. Huszar D, Lynch CA, Fairchild-Huntress V, et al. Targeted disruption of the melanocortin-4 receptor results in obesity in mice. Cell 1997; 88:131–141.
290. Farooqi IS, Yeo GS, Keogh JM, et al. Dominant and recessive inheritance of morbid obesity associated with melanocortin-4 receptor deficiency. J Clin Invest 2000; 106:271–279.
291. Dubois J, Dayer JM, Siegrist-Kaiser CA, et al. Human recombinant interleukin 1β decreases plasma thyroid hormone and thyroid stimulating hormone levels in rats. Endocrinology 1988; 123:2175–2181.
292. Cintra A, Fuxe K, Solfrini V, et al. Central peptidergic neurons as targets for glucocorticoid action: evidence for the presence of glycocorticoid receptor immunoreactivity in various types of classes of peptidergic neurons. J Steroid Biochem Mol Biol 1991; 40: 93–103.
293. Scarborough D, Lee SL, Dinarello CA, Reichlin S. Interleukin-1 beta stimulates somatostatin biosynthesis in primary cultures of fetal rat brain. Endocrinology 1989; 124:549–551.
294. Pang X, Hershman JM, Mirell CJ, Pekary AE. Impairment of hypothalamic-pituitary-thyroid function in rats treated with human recombinant tumor necrosis factor-alpha (cachectin). Endocrinology 1989; 125:76–84.
295. Koenig J, Snow K, Clark BD, et al. Intrinsic pituitary interleukin 1β is induced by bacterial lipopolysaccharide. Endocrinology 1990; 126:3053–3058.
296. Spath-Schwalbe E, Schrezenmeier H, Bornstein S, et al. Endocrine effects of recombinant interleukin 6 in man. Neuroendocrinology 1996; 63:237–243.
297. Saffran M, Schally A, Benfey B. Stimulation of the release of corticotropin from the adenohypophysis by a neurohypophysial factor. Endocrinology 1955; 57:439–444.

298. Guillemin R, Rosenberg B. Humoral hypothalamic control of anterior pituitary: study with combined tissue cultures. Endocrinology 1955; 57:599–607.
299. Spiess J, Rivier J, Rivier C, Vale W. Primary structure of corticotropin-releasing factor from ovine hypothalamus. Proc Natl Acad Sci USA 1981; 78:6517–6521.
300. Shibahara S, Morimoto Y, Furutani Y, et al. Isolation and sequence analysis of the human corticotropin-releasing factor precursor gene. EMBO J 1983; 2:775–779.
301. Lovejoy DA, Balment RJ. Evolution and physiology of the corticotropin-releasing factor family of neuropeptides in vertebrates. Gen Comp Endocrinol 1999; 115:1–22.
302. Coast GM. Insect diuretic peptides; structures, evolution, and actions. Am Zool 1998; 38:442–449.
303. Hsu SY, Hsueh AJW. Human stresscopin and stresscopin-related peptide are selective ligands for the type 2 corticotropin-releasing hormone receptor. Nat Med 2001; 7:605–611.
304. Reyes TM, Lewis K, Perrin MH, et al. Urocortin II: a member of the corticotropin-releasing factor (CRF) neuropeptide family that is selectively bound by type 2 CRF receptors. Proc Natl Acad Sci USA 2001; 98:2843–2848.
305. Lewis K, Li C, Perrin MH, et al. Identification of Urocortin III, an additional member of the corticotropin-releasing factor family with high affinity for the CRF2 receptor. Proc Natl Acad Sci USA 2001; 98:7570–7575.
306. Chen R, Lewis KA, Perrin MH, Vale WW. Expression cloning of a human corticotropin-releasing factor receptor. Proc Natl Acad Sci USA 1993; 90:8967–8971.
307. Vita N, Laurent P, Lefort S, et al. Primary structure and functional expression of mouse pituitary and human brain corticotrophin releasing factor receptors. Fed Eur Biochem Soc Meet Proc 1993; 335:1–5.
308. Chang C-P, Pearse RV 2nd, O'Connell S, Rosenfeld MG. Identification of a seven transmembrane helix receptor for corticotropin-releasing factor and sauvagine in mammalian brain. Neuron 1993; 11:1187–1195.
309. Stenzel P, Kesterson R, Yeung W, et al. Identification of a novel murine receptor for corticotropin-releasing hormone expressed in the heart. Mol Endocrinol 1995; 9:637–645.
310. Perrin M, Donaldson C, Chen R, et al. Identification of a second corticotropin-releasing factor receptor gene and characterization of a cDNA expressed in heart. Proc Natl Acad Sci USA 1995; 92:2969–2973.
311. Lovenberg TW, Liaw CW, Grigoriadis DE, et al. Cloning and characterization of a functionally distinct corticotropin-releasing factor receptor subtype from rat brain. Proc Natl Acad Sci USA 1995; 92:836–840.
312. Kishimoto T, Pearse RV 2nd, Lin CR, Rosenfeld MG. A sauvagine/corticotropin-releasing factor expressed in heart and skeletal muscle. Proc Natl Acad Sci USA 1995; 92:1108–1112.
313. Valdenaire O, Giller T, Breu V, et al. A new functional isoform of the human CRF2 receptor for corticotropin-releasing factor. Biochim Biophys Acta 1997; 1352:129–132.
314. Kostich WA, Chen A, Sperle K, Largent BL. Molecular identification and analysis of a novel human corticotropin-releasing factor (CRF) receptor: the CRF2gamma receptor. Mol Endocrinol 1998; 12:1077–1085.
315. Takahashi K, Totsune K, Sone M, et al. Regional distribution of urocortin-like immunoreactivity and expression of urocortin mRNA in the human brain. Peptides 1998; 19:643–647.
316. Iino K, Sasano H, Oki Y, et al. Urocortin expression in the human central nervous system. Clin Endocrinol (Oxf) 1999; 50: 107–114.
317. Perrin MH, Vale WW. Corticotropin releasing factor receptors and their ligand family. Ann NY Acad Sci 1999; 885:312–328.
318. Chalmers DT, Lovenberg TW, DeSouza EB. Localization of novel corticotropin-releasing receptor (CRF2) mRNA expression to specific subcortical nuclei in rat brain: comparison with CRF1 receptor mRNA expression. J Neurosci 1995; 15:6340–6350.
319. Lovenberg T, Chalmers DT, Liu C, DeSouza EB. CRF2a and CRF2b receptor mRNAs are differentially distributed between the rat central nervous system and peripheral tissues. Endocrinology 1995; 136:4139–4142.
320. Muller MB, Preil J, Renner U, et al. Expression of CRHR1 and CRHR2 in mouse pituitary and adrenal gland: implications for HPA system regulation. Endocrinology 2001; 142:4150–4153.
321. Orth DN, Mount CD. Specific high affinity binding protein for human corticotropin-releasing hormone in normal human plasma. Biochem Biophys Res Commun 1987; 143:411–417.
322. Behan DP, Linton EA, Lowry PJ. Isolation of the human plasma corticotropin-releasing factor–binding protein. J Endocrinol 1989; 122:23–31.
323. Linton E, Wolfe CD, Behan DP, Lowry PJ. Circulating corticotropin-releasing factor in pregnancy. Adv Exp Med Biol 1990; 274:147–164.
324. Potter E, Behan DP, Linton EA, et al. The central distribution of a corticotropin-releasing factor (CRF)–binding protein predicts multiple sites and modes of interaction with CRF. Proc Natl Acad Sci USA 1992; 89:4192–4196.
325. Seasholtz AF, Burrows HL, Karolyi IJ, Camper SA. Mouse models of altered CRH-binding protein expression. Peptides 2001; 22:743–751.
326. Pallai PV, Mabilia M, Goodman M, et al. Structural homology of corticotropin-releasing factor, sauvagine, and urotensin I: circular dichroism and prediction studies. Proc Natl Acad Sci USA 1983; 80:6770–6774.
327. Rivier J, Rivier C, Vale W. Synthetic competitive antagonists of corticotropin-releasing factor: effect on ACTH secretion in the rat. Science 1984; 224:889–891.
328. Maecker H, Desai A, Dash R, et al. Astressin, a novel and potent CRF antagonist, is neuroprotective in the hippocampus when administered after a seizure. Brain Res 1997; 744:166–170.
329. Gilligan PJ, Robertson DW, Zaczek R. Corticotropin releasing factor receptor modulators: progress and opportunities for new therapeutic agents. J Med Chem 2000; 43:1641–1660.
330. Habib KE, Weld KP, Rice KC, et al. Oral administration of a corticotropin releasing hormone receptor antagonist significantly attenuates behavioral, neuroendocrine, and autonomic responses to stress in primates. Proc Natl Acad Sci USA 2000; 97:6079–6084.
331. Ruhmann A, Bonk I, Lin CR, et al. Structural requirements for peptidic antagonists of the corticotropin-releasing factor receptor (CRFR): development of CRFR2beta-selective anti-sauvagine 30. Proc Natl Acad Sci USA 1998; 95:15264–15269.
332. Trainer P, Faria M, Newell-Price J, et al. A comparison of the effects of human and ovine corticotropin-releasing hormone on the pituitary-adrenal axis. J Clin Endocrinol Metab 1995; 80: 412–417.
333. Grossman A. Corticotropin-releasing hormone: basic physiology and clinical applications. In DeGroot LJ (ed). Endocrinology. Philadelphia, WB Saunders, 1995, pp 341–354.
334. Sutton RE, Koob GF, Le Moal M, et al. Corticotropin releasing factor produces behavioural activation in rats. Nature 1982; 297: 331–333.
335. Lenz H. Extrapituitary effects of corticotropin-releasing factor. Horm Metab Res 1987; 16(suppl):17–23.
336. Heilig M, Koob GF, Ekman R, Britton KT. Corticotropin-releasing factor and neuropeptide Y: role in emotional integration. Trends Neurosci 1994; 17:80–85.
337. Keck ME, Holsboer F. Hyperactivity of CRH neuronal circuits as a target for therapeutic interventions in affective disorders. Peptides 2001; 22:835–844.
338. Kasckow JW, Baker D, Geracioti TDJ. Corticotropin-releasing hormone in depression and post-traumatic stress disorder. Peptides 2001; 22:845–851.
339. Smagin GN, Heinrichs SC, Dunn AJ. The role of CRH in behavioral responses to stress. Peptides 2001; 22:713–724.
340. Modell S, Yassouridis A, Huber J, Holsboer F. Corticosteroid receptor function is decreased in depressed patients. Neuroendocrinology 1997; 65:216–222.
341. Modell S, et al. Hormonal response pattern in the combined DEX-CRH test is stable over time in subjects at high familial risks for affective disorders. Neuropsychopharmacology 1997; 18: 253–262.
342. Nemeroff CB, Widerlov E, Bissette G, et al. Elevated concentrations of CSF corticotropin-releasing factor–like immunoreactivity in depressed patients. Science 1984; 226:1342–1344.
343. Brown M, Fisher L. Central nervous system effects of corticotropin-releasing factor in the dog. Brain Res 1983; 280:75–79.
344. Fisher LA, Jessen G, Brown MR. Corticotropin-releasing factor (CRF): mechanism to elevate mean arterial pressure and heart rate. Regul Pept 1983; 5:153–161.

345. Okosi A, Brar BK, Chan M, et al. Expression and protective effects of urocortin in cardiac myocytes. Neuropeptides 1998; 32: 167–171.
346. Parkes DG, Weisinger RS, May CN. Cardiovascular actions of CRH and urocortin: an update. Peptides 2001; 22:821–827.
347. Parkes D, May C. Cardiac and vascular actions of urocortin. In Share L (ed). Hormones and the Heart in Health and Disease. 1999, Totowa, NJ, Humana Press, pp 39–52.
348. Bale L, Contarino A, Smith GW, et al. Mice deficient for corticotropin-releasing hormone receptor-2 display anxiety-like behavior and are hypersensitive to stress. Nat Genet 2000; 24:410–414.
349. Coste SC, Kesterson RA, Heldwein KA, et al. Abnormal adaptations to stress and impaired cardiovascular function in mice lacking corticotropin-releasing hormone receptor-2. Nat Genet 2000; 24:403–409.
350. Jessop DS, Harbuz MS, Lightman SL. CRH in chronic inflammatory stress. Peptides 2001; 22:803–807.
351. Gravanis A, Makrigiannakis A, Zoumakis E, Margioris AN. Endometrial and myometrial corticotropin-releasing hormone (CRH): its regulation and possible roles. Peptides 2001; 22:785–793.
352. Muglia L, Jacobson L, Dikkes P, Majzoub JA. Corticotropin-releasing hormone deficiency reveals major fetal but not adult glucocorticoid need. Nature 1995; 373:427–432.
353. Smith GW, Aubry JM, Dellu F, et al. Corticotropin releasing factor 1–deficient mice display decreased anxiety, impaired stress response, and aberrant neuroendocrine development. Neuron 1998; 20:1093–1102.
354. Timpl P, Spanagel R, Sillaber I, et al. Impaired stress response and reduced anxiety in mice lacking a functional corticotropin-releasing hormone receptor. Nat Genet 1998; 19:162–166.
355. Kishimoto T, Radulovic J, Radulovic M, et al. Deletion of Crhr2 reveals an anxiolytic role for corticotropin-releasing hormone receptor-2. Nat Genet 2000; 24:415–419.
356. Coste SC, Murray SE, Stenzel-Poore MP. Animal models of CRH excess and CRH receptor deficiency display altered adaptations to stress. Peptides 2001; 22:733–741.
357. Muglia LJ, Jacobson L, Weninger SC, et al. The physiology of corticotropin-releasing hormone deficiency in mice. Peptides 2001; 22:725–731.
358. Dunn AJ, Berridge CW. Physiological and behavioral responses to corticotropin-releasing factor administration: is CRF a mediator of anxiety or stress responses? Brain Res Rev 1990; 15:71–100.
359. Weninger SC, Dunn AJ, Muglia LJ, et al. Stress-induced behaviors require the corticotropin-releasing hormone (CRH) receptor, but not CRH. Proc Natl Acad Sci USA 1999; 96:8283–8288.
360. Weninger SC, Muglia LJ, Jacobson L, Majzoub JA. CRH-deficient mice have a normal anorectic-response to chronic stress. Regul Pept 1999; 84:69–74.
361. Jeong K-H, Jacobson L, Widmaier EP, Majzoub JA. Normal suppression of the reproductive axis following stress in corticotropin-releasing hormone-deficient mice. Endocrinology 1999; 140: 1702–1708.
362. Bradbury MJ, McBurnie MI, Denton DA, et al. Modulation of urocortin-induced hypophagia and weight loss by corticotropin-releasing factor receptor 1 deficiency in mice. Endocrinology 2000; in press.
363. Zobel AW, Nickel T, Kunzel HE, et al. Effects of the high-affinity corticotropin-releasing hormone receptor 1 antagonist R121919 in major depression: the first 20 patients treated. J Psychiatr Res 2000; 34:171–181.
364. Vale W, Rivier C, Brown MR, et al. Chemical and biological characterization of corticotropin releasing factor. Recent Prog Horm Res 1983; 39:245–270.
365. Antoni F. Hypothalamic control of adrenocorticotropin secretion: advances since the discovery of 41-residue corticotropin-releasing factor. Endocr Rev 1986; 7:351–378.
366. Imura H. Adrenocorticotropic hormone. In DeGroot L (ed). Endocrinology. Philadelphia, WB Saunders, 1995, pp 355–367.
367. Dallman M, Akana SF, Levin N, et al. Corticosteroids and the control of function in the hypothalamo-pituitary-adrenal (HPA) axis. Ann NY Acad Sci 1994; 746:22–31.
368. Sapolsky R, Krey L, McEwen B. The neuroendocrinology of stress and aging: the glucocorticoid cascade hypothesis. Endocr Rev 1986; 7:284–301.
369. deKloet E, Oitzl M, Joels M. Functional implications of brain corticosteroid receptor diversity. Cell Mol Neurobiol 1993; 13: 433–455.
370. Evans R. The steroid and thyroid hormone receptor superfamily. Science 1988; 240:889–895.
371. Joels M, deKloet E. Corticosteroid hormones: endocrine messengers in the brain. News Physiol Sci 1995; 10:71–76.
372. Arriza JL, Stoler MH, Angerer RC. The neuronal mineralocorticoid receptor as a mediator of glucocorticoid response. Neuron 1988; 1:887–900.
373. Fuxe K, Wikstrom AC, Okret S, et al. Mapping of glucocorticoid receptor immunoreactive neurons in the rat tel and diencephalon using a monoclonal antibody against rat liver glucocorticoid receptor. Endocrinology 1985; 117:1803–1812.
374. Hua S, Chen Y. Membrane receptor-mediated electrophysiological effects of glucocorticoid on mammalian neurons. Endocrinology 1989; 124:687–691.
375. Watts AG. The impact of physiological stimuli on the expression of corticotropin-releasing hormone (CRH) and other neuropeptide genes. Front Neuroendocrinol 1996; 17:281–326.
376. Sawchenko PE, Brown ER, Chan RK, et al. The paraventricular nucleus of the hypothalamus and the functional neuroanatomy of visceromotor responses to stress. Prog Brain Res 1996; 107:201–222.
377. Sawchenko PE, Li H-Y, Ericsson A. Circuits and mechanisms governing hypothalamic responses to stress: a tale of two paradigms. Prog Brain Res 2000; 122:61–78.
378. Herman JP. Neurocircuit control of the hypothalamo-pituitary adrenocortical axis during stress. Curr Opin Endocrinol Diabetes 1999; 6:3–9.
379. Herman JP, Cullinan WE. Neurocircuitry of stress: central control of the hypothalamo-pituitary-adrenocortical axis. Trends Neurosci 1997; 20:78–84.
380. Kovacs KJ. Functional neuroanatomy of the parvocellular vasopressinergic system: transcriptional responses to stress and glucocorticoid feedback. Prog Brain Res 1998; 119:31–43.
381. Chan RK, Brown ER, Ericsson A, et al. A comparison of two immediate-early genes, *c-fos* and *NGFI-B*, as markers for functional activation in stress-related neuroendocrine circuitry. J Neurosci 1993; 13:5126–5138.
382. Cunningham ET Jr, Bohn MC, Sawchenko PE. Organization of adrenergic inputs to the paraventricular and supraoptic nuclei of the hypothalamus in the rat. J Comp Neurol 1990; 292:651–667.
383. Cunningham ET Jr, Sawchenko PE. Anatomical specificity of noradrenergic inputs to the paraventricular and supraoptic nuclei of the rat hypothalamus. J Comp Neurol 1988; 274:60–76.
384. Sawchenko PE, Swanson LW. The organization of forebrain afferents to the paraventricular and supraoptic nuclei of the rat. J Comp Neurol 1983; 218:121–144.
385. Miselis RR, Shapiro RE, Hand PJ. Subfornical organ efferents to neural systems for control of body water. Science 1979; 205: 1022–1025.
386. Ericsson A, Kovacs KJ, Sawchenko PE. A functional anatomical analysis of central pathways subserving the effects of interleukin-1 on stress-related neuroendocrine neurons. J Neurosci 1994; 14: 897–913.
387. Li H-Y, Sawchenko PE. Hypothalamic effector neurons and extended circuitries activated in "neurogenic" stress: a comparison of footshock effects exerted acutely, chronically, and in animals with controlled glucocorticoid levels. J Comp Neurol 1998; 393: 244–266.
388. Li H-Y, Ericsson A, Sawchenko PE. Distinct mechanisms underlie activation of hypothalamic neurosecretory neurons and their medullary catecholaminergics afferents in categorically different stress paradigms. Proc Natl Acad Sci USA 1996; 93:2359–2364.
389. Roland BL, Sawchenko PE. Local origins of some GABAergic projections to the paraventricular and supraoptic nuclei of the hypothalamus in the rat. J Comp Neurol 1993; 332:123–143.
390. Muglia LJ, Jacobson L, Weninger SC, et al. Impaired diurnal adrenal rhythmicity restored by constant infusion of corticotropin-releasing hormone in corticotropin-releasing hormone deficient mice. J Clin Invest 1997; 99:2923–2929.
391. Engler D, Liu JP, Clarke IJ, et al. Corticotropin-release inhibitory factor: evidence for dual stimulatory and inhibitory hypothalamic regulation over adrenocorticotropin secretion and biosynthesis. Trends Endocrinol Metab 1994; 5:272–283.

392. Engler D, Redei E, Kola I. The corticotropin-release inhibitory factor hypothesis: a review of the evidence for the existence of inhibitory as well as stimulatory hypophysiotropic regulation of adrenocorticotropin secretion and biosynthesis. Endocr Rev 1999; 20:460–500.
393. Reichlin S. Growth and the hypothalamus. Endocrinology 1960; 67:760–773.
394. Frohman L, Szabo M, Berelowitz M, Stachura ME. Partial purification and characterization of a peptide with growth hormone–releasing activity from extrapituitary tumors in patients with acromegaly. J Clin Invest 1980; 65:43–54.
395. Guillemin R, Brazeau P, Bohlen P, et al. Growth hormone–releasing factor from a human pancreatic tumor that caused acromegaly. Science 1982; 218:585–587.
396. Rivier J, Spiess J, Thorner M, Vale W. Characterisation of a growth hormone-releasing factor from a human pancreatic islet tumour. Nature 1982; 300:276–278.
397. Mayo K, Vale W, Rivier J, et al. Expression-cloning and sequence of a cDNA encoding human growth hormone-releasing factor. Nature 1983; 306:86–88.
398. Frohman LA, Downs TR, Chomczynski P, Frohman MA. Growth hormone-releasing hormone: structure, gene expression and molecular heterogeneity. Acta Paediatr Scand Suppl 1990; 367:81–86.
399. Mayo KE, Cerilli GM, Lebo RV, et al. Gene encoding human growth hormone-releasing factor precursor: structure, sequence, and chromosomal assignment. Proc Natl Acad Sci USA 1985; 82: 63–67.
400. Frohman LA, Downs TR, Heimer EP, Felix AM. Dipeptidylpeptidase IV and trypsin-like enzymatic degradation of human growth hormone-releasing hormone in plasma. J Clin Invest 1989; 83:1533–1540.
401. Thorner M, Frohman LA, Leong DA, et al. Extrahypothalamic growth hormone-releasing factor (GRF) is a rare cause of acromegaly: plasma GRF levels in 177 acromegalic patients. J Clin Endocrinol Metab 1984; 59:846–849.
402. Asa S, Kovacs K, Thorner M, et al. Immunohistological localization of growth hormone-releasing hormone in human tumors. J Clin Endocrinol Metab 1985; 60:423–427.
403. Dayal Y, Lin HD, Tallberg K, et al. Immunocytochemical demonstration of growth hormone-releasing factor in gastrointestinal and pancreatic endocrine tumors. Am J Clin Pathol 1986; 85:13–20.
404. Khorram O, Garthwaite M, Grosen E, Golos T. Human uterine and ovarian expression of growth hormone-releasing hormone messenger RNA in benign and malignant gynecologic conditions. Fertil Steril 2001; 75:174–179.
405. Gonzalez-Crespo S, Boronat A. Expression of the rat growth hormone-releasing hormone gene in placenta is directed by an alternative promoter. Proc Natl Acad Sci USA 1991; 88:8749–8753.
406. Muller EE, Locatelli V, Cocchi D. Neuroendocrine control of growth hormone secretion. Physiol Rev 1999; 79:511–607.
407. Gaylinn BD, Harrison JK, Zysk JR, et al. Molecular cloning and expression of a human anterior pituitary receptor for growth hormone-releasing hormone. Mol Endocrinol 1993; 7:77–84.
408. Mayo KE, Godfrey PA, Suhr ST, et al. Growth hormone-releasing hormone: synthesis and signaling. Recent Prog Horm Res 1995; 50:35–73.
409. Wajnrajch MP, Gertner JM, Harbison MD, et al. Nonsense mutation in the human growth hormone-releasing hormone receptor causes growth failure analogous to the little (lit) mouse. Nat Genet 1996; 12:88–90.
410. Baumann G, Maheshwari H. The dwarfs of Sindh: severe growth hormone (GH) deficiency caused by a mutation in the GH-releasing hormone receptor gene. Acta Paediatr Suppl 1997; 423: 33–38.
411. Giustina A, Veldhuis JD. Pathophysiology of the neuroregulation of growth hormone secretion in experimental animals and the human. Endocr Rev 1998; 19:717–797.
412. Mayo KE, Hammer RE, Swanson LW, et al. Dramatic pituitary hyperplasia in transgenic mice expressing a human growth hormone-releasing factor gene. Mol Endocrinol 1988; 2:606–612.
413. Stefaneanu L, Kovacs K, Horvath E, et al. Adenohypophysial changes in mice transgenic for human growth hormone-releasing factor: a histological, immunocytochemical, and electron microscopic investigation. Endocrinology 1989; 125:2710–2718.
414. Vallar L, Spada A, Giannattasio G. Altered G_s and adenylate cyclase activity in human GH-secreting pituitary adenomas. Nature 1987; 330:566–568.
415. Steiger A, Guldner J, Hemmeter U, et al. Effects of growth hormone-releasing hormone and somatostatin on sleep EEG and nocturnal hormone secretion in male controls. Neuroendocrinology 1992; 56:566–573.
416. Van Cauter E, Leproult R, Plat L. Age-related changes in slow wave sleep and REM sleep and relationship with growth hormone and cortisol levels in healthy men. JAMA 2000; 284:861–868.
417. Vaccarino FJ, Kennedy SH, Ralevski E, Black R. The effects of growth hormone-releasing factor on food consumption in anorexia nervosa patients and normals. Biol Psychiatry 1994; 35:446–451.
418. Smith RG, Feighner S, Prendergast K, et al. A new orphan receptor involved in pulsatile growth hormone release. Trends Endocrinol Metab 1999; 10:128–135.
419. Howard AD, Feighner SD, Cully DF, et al. A receptor in pituitary and hypothalamus that functions in growth hormone release. Science 1996; 273:974–977.
420. Maghnie M, Spica-Russotto V, Cappa M, et al. The growth hormone response to hexarelin in patients with different hypothalamic-pituitary abnormalities. J Clin Endocrinol Metab 1998; 83: 3886–3889.
421. Arvat E, Maccario M, Di Vito L, et al. Endocrine activities of ghrelin, a natural growth hormone secretagogue (GHS), in humans: comparison and interactions with hexarelin, a nonnatural peptidyl GHS, and GH-releasing hormone. J Clin Endocrinol Metab 2001; 86:1169–1174.
422. Gasperi M, Aimaretti G, Scarcello G, et al. Low dose hexarelin and growth hormone (GH)-releasing hormone as a diagnostic tool for the diagnosis of GH deficiency in adults: comparison with insulin-induced hypoglycemia test. J Clin Endocrinol Metab 1999; 84:2633–2637.
423. Baldelli R, Otero X, Camino JP, et al. Growth hormone secretagogues as diagnostic tools in disease states. Endocrine 2001; 14: 95–99.
424. Veldhuis JD, Anderson SM, Shah N, et al. Neurophysiological regulation and target-tissue impact of the pulsatile mode of growth hormone secretion in the human. Growth Horm IGF Res 2001; 11(suppl A):S25–S37.
425. Ross RJ, Tsagarakis S, Grossman A, et al. GH feedback occurs through modulation of hypothalamic somatostatin under cholinergic control: studies with pyridostigmine and GHRH. Clin Endocrinol (Oxf) 1987; 27:727–733.
426. Zheng H, Bailey A, Jiang MH, et al. Somatostatin receptor subtype 2 knockout mice are refractory to growth hormone-negative feedback on arcuate neurons. Mol Endocrinol 1997; 11:1709–1717.
427. Soliman AT, ElZalabany MM, Salama M, Ansari BM. Serum leptin concentrations during severe protein-energy malnutrition: correlation with growth parameters and endocrine function. Metabolism 2000; 49:819–825.
428. Bloch B, Gaillard RC, Brazeau P, et al. Topographical and ontogenetic study of the neurons producing growth hormone-releasing factor in human hypothalamus. Regul Pept 1984; 8:21–31.
429. Mota A, Bento A, Penalva A, et al. Role of the serotonin receptor subtype 5-HT1D on basal and stimulated growth hormone secretion. J Clin Endocrinol Metab 1995; 80:1973–1977.
430. Muller EE. Cholinergic function and neural control of GH secretion: a critical reappraisal. Eur J Endocrinol 1997; 137:338–342.
431. Giustina A, Licini M, Schettino M, et al. Physiological role of galanin in the regulation of anterior pituitary function in humans. Am J Physiol 1994; 266:E57–E61.
432. Cella SG, Locatelli G, De Gennaro V, et al. Epinephrine mediates the growth hormone-releasing effect of galanin in infant rats. Endocrinology 1988; 122:855–859.
433. Van Cauter E, Kerkhofs M, Caufriez A, et al. A quantitative estimation of growth hormone secretion in normal man: reproducibility and relation to sleep and time of day. J Clin Endocrinol Metab 1992; 74:1441–1450.
434. Jaffe CA, Ocampo-Lim B, Guo W, et al. Regulatory mechanisms of growth hormone secretion are sexually dimorphic. J Clin Invest 1998; 102:153–164.

435. Pincus SM, Gevers EF, Robinson IC, et al. Females secrete growth hormone with more process irregularity than males in both humans and rats. Am J Physiol 1996; 270:E107–E115.
436. Wagner C, Caplan SR, Tannenbaum GS. Genesis of the ultradian rhythm of GH secretion: a new model unifying experimental observations in rats. Am J Physiol 1998; 275:E1046–E1054.
437. Low MJ, Otero-Corchon V, Parlow AF, et al. Somatostatin is required for masculinization of growth hormone-regulated hepatic gene expression but not of somatic growth. J Clin Invest 2001; 107:1571–1580.
438. Krulich L, Dhariwal A, McCann S. Stimulatory and inhibitory effects of purified hypothalamic extracts on growth hormone release from rat pituitary in vitro. Endocrinology 1968; 83:783–790.
439. Brazeau P, Vale W, Burgus R, et al. Hypothalamic polypeptide that inhibits the secretion of immunoreactive pituitary growth hormone. Science 1973; 179:77–79.
440. Galanopoulou AS, Kent G, Rabbani SN, et al. Heterologous processing of prosomatostatin in constitutive and regulated secretory pathways: putative role of the endoproteases furin, PC1, and PC2. J Biol Chem 1993; 268:6041–6049.
441. Shen LP, Rutter WJ. Sequence of the human somatostatin I gene. Science 1984; 224:168–171.
442. Conlon JM, Tostivint H, Vaudry H. Somatostatin- and urotensin II-related peptides: molecular diversity and evolutionary perspectives. Regul Pept 1997; 69:95–103.
443. de Lecea L, Criado JR, Prospero-Garcia O, et al. A cortical neuropeptide with neuronal depressant and sleep-modulating properties. Nature 1996; 381:242–245.
444. Spier AD, de Lecea L. Cortistatin: a member of the somatostatin neuropeptide family with distinct physiological functions. Brain Res Rev 2000; 33:228–241.
445. Fukusumi S, Kitada C, Takekawa S, et al. Identification and characterization of a novel human cortistatin-like peptide. Biochem Biophys Res Commun 1997; 232:157–163.
446. Schwartz PT, Vallejo M. Differential regulation of basal and cyclic adenosine 3′,5′- monophosphate-induced somatostatin gene transcription in neural cells by DNA control elements that bind homeodomain proteins. Mol Endocrinol 1998; 12:1280–1293.
447. Goudet G, Delhalle S, Biemar F, et al. Functional and cooperative interactions between the homeodomain PDX1, Pbx, and Prep1 factors on the somatostatin promoter. J Biol Chem 1999; 274:4067–4073.
448. Andersen FG, Jensen J, Heller RS, et al. Pax6 and Pdx1 form a functional complex on the rat somatostatin gene upstream enhancer. FEBS Lett 1999; 445:315–320.
449. Montminy M, Brindle P, Arias J, et al. Regulation of somatostatin gene transcription by cyclic adenosine monophosphate. Metabolism 1996; 45(8 suppl 1):4–7.
450. Capone G, Choi C, Vertifuille J. Regulation of the preprosomatostatin gene by cyclic-AMP in cerebrocortical neurons. Brain Res Mol Brain Res 1998; 60:247–258.
451. Schwartz PT, Perez-Villamil B, Rivera A, et al. Pancreatic homeodomain transcription factor IDX1/IPF1 expressed in developing brain regulates somatostatin gene transcription in embryonic neural cells. J Biol Chem 2000; 275:19106–19114.
452. Patel YC. Somatostatin and its receptor family. Front Neuroendocrinol 1999; 20:157–198.
453. Thoss VS, Perez J, Probst A, Hoyer D. Expression of five somatostatin receptor mRNAs in the human brain and pituitary. Naunyn Schmiedebergs Arch Pharmacol 1996; 354:411–419.
454. Strowski MZ, Parmer RM, Blake AD, Schaeffer JM. Somatostatin inhibits insulin and glucagon secretion via two receptors subtypes: an in vitro study of pancreatic islets from somatostatin receptor 2 knockout mice. Endocrinology 2000; 141:111–117.
455. Mathern GW, Babb TL, Pretorius JK, Leite JP. Reactive synaptogenesis and neuron densities for neuropeptide Y, somatostatin, and glutamate decarboxylase immunoreactivity in the epileptogenic human fascia dentata. J Neurosci 1995; 15:3990–4004.
456. Bissette G, Myers B. Somatostatin in Alzheimer's disease and depression. Life Sci 1992; 51:1389–1410.
457. Rohrer SP, Birzin ET, Mosley RT, et al. Rapid identification of subtype-selective agonists of the somatostatin receptor through combinatorial chemistry. Science 1998; 282:737–740.
458. Yang L, Berk SC, Rohrer SP, et al. Synthesis and biological activities of potent peptidomimetics selective for somatostatin receptor subtype 2. Proc Natl Acad Sci USA 1998; 95:10836–10841.
459. Lamberts SW, van der Lely AJ, de Herder WW, Hofland LJ. Octreotide. N Engl J Med 1996; 334:246–254.
460. Slooter GD, Mearadji A, Breeman WA, et al. Somatostatin receptor imaging, therapy and new strategies in patients with neuroendocrine tumours. Br J Surg 2001; 88:31–40.
461. Schirmer WJ, O'Dorisio TM, Schirmer TP, et al. Intraoperative localization of neuroendocrine tumors with ^{125}I-TYR(3)-octreotide and a hand-held gamma-detecting probe. Surgery 1993; 114: 745–751; discussion 751–752.
462. Henze M, Schuhmacher J, Hipp P, et al. PET imaging of somatostatin receptors using (^{68}Ga)DOTATOC. J Nucl Med 2001; 42:1053–1056.
463. Rochaix P, Delesque N, Esteve JP, et al. Gene therapy for pancreatic carcinoma: local and distant antitumor effects after somatostatin receptor sst2 gene transfer. Hum Gene Ther 1999; 10: 995–1008.
464. Freeman ME, Kanyicska B, Lerant A, Nagy G. Prolactin: structure, function, and regulation of secretion. Physiol Rev 2000; 80: 1523–1631.
465. Ben-Jonathan N, Hnasko R. Dopamine as a prolactin (PRL) inhibitor. Endocr Rev 2001; 22:724–763.
466. Ben-Jonathan N. Dopamine: a prolactin-inhibiting hormone. Endocr Rev 1985; 6:564–589.
467. Gibbs DM, Neill JD. Dopamine levels in hypophysial stalk blood in the rat are sufficient to inhibit prolactin secretion in vivo. Endocrinology 1978; 102:1895–1900.
468. MacLeod RM, Fontham EH, Lehmeyer JE. Prolactin and growth hormone production as influenced by catecholamines and agents that affect brain catecholamines. Neuroendocrinology 1970; 6:283–294.
469. Goldsmith PC, Cronin MJ, Weiner RI. Dopamine receptor sites in the anterior pituitary. J Histochem Cytochem 1979; 27:1205–1207.
470. Caron MG, Beaulieu M, Raymond V, et al. Dopaminergic receptors in the anterior pituitary gland: correlation of (^{3}H)dihydroergocryptine binding with the dopaminergic control of prolactin release. J Biol Chem 1978; 253:2244–2253.
471. Asa SL, Kelly MA, Grandy DK, Low MJ. Pituitary lactotroph adenomas develop after prolonged lactotroph hyperplasia in dopamine D2 receptor-deficient mice. Endocrinology 1999; 140: 5348–5355.
472. Kelly MA, Rubinstein M, Asa SL, et al. Pituitary lactotroph hyperplasia and chronic hyperprolactinemia in dopamine D2 receptor-deficient mice. Neuron 1997; 19:103–113.
473. Lerant A, Herman ME, Freeman ME. Dopaminergic neurons of periventricular and arcuate nuclei of pseudopregnant rats: semicircadian rhythm in Fos-related antigens immunoreactivities and in dopamine concentration. Endocrinology 1996; 137:3621–3628.
474. Peters LL, Hoefer MT, Ben-Jonathan N. The posterior pituitary: regulation of anterior pituitary prolactin secretion. Science 1981; 213:659–661.
475. Durham RA, Johnson JD, Eaton MJ, et al. Opposing roles for dopamine D1 and D2 receptors in the regulation of hypothalamic tuberoinfundibular dopamine neurons. Eur J Pharmacol 1998; 355:141–147.
476. Vallar L, Meldolesi J. Mechanisms of signal transduction at the dopamine D2 receptor. Trends Pharmacol Sci 1989; 10:74–77.
477. Chuang TT, Caccavelli L, Kordon C, Enjalbert A. Protein kinase C regulation of prolactin gene expression in lactotroph cells: involvement in dopamine inhibition. Endocrinology 1993; 132: 832–838.
478. Wang YH, Maurer RA. A role for the mitogen-activated protein kinase in mediating the ability of thyrotropin-releasing hormone to stimulate the prolactin promoter. Mol Endocrinol 1999; 13: 1094–1104.
479. Jacob KK, Wininger E, DiMinni K, Stanley FM. The EGF response element in the prolactin promoter. Mol Cell Endocrinol 1999; 152:137–145.
480. Yonehara T, Kanasaki H, Yamamoto H, et al. Involvement of mitogen-activated protein kinase in cyclic adenosine 3′,5′-monophosphate-induced hormone gene expression in rat pituitary GH(3) cells. Endocrinology 2001; 142:2811–2819.
481. Day RN, Liu J, Sundmark V, et al. Selective inhibition of prolactin gene transcription by the ETS-2 repressor factor. J Biol Chem 1998; 273:31909–31915.

482. Suzuki S, Yamamoto I, Arita J. Mitogen-activated protein kinase–dependent stimulation of proliferation of rat lactotrophs in culture by 3′,5′-cyclic adenosine monophosphate. Endocrinology 1999; 140:2850–2858.
483. Florio T, Pan MG, Newman B, et al. Dopaminergic inhibition of DNA synthesis in pituitary tumor cells is associated with phosphotyrosine phosphatase activity. J Biol Chem 1992; 267:24169–24172.
484. Lindley SE, Gunnet JW, Lookingland KJ, Moore KE. Effects of alterations in the activity of tuberohypophysial dopaminergic neurons on the secretion of alpha-melanocyte stimulating hormone. Proc Soc Exp Biol Med 1988; 188:282–286.
485. Chronwall BM, Millington WR, Griffin WS, et al. Histological evaluation of the dopaminergic regulation of proopiomelanocortin gene expression in the intermediate lobe of the rat pituitary, involving in situ hybridization and (^{3}H)thymidine uptake measurement. Endocrinology 1987; 120:1201–1211.
486. Chronwall BM, Davis TD, Severidt MW, et al. Constitutive expression of functional GABA(B) receptors in mIL-tsA58 cells requires both GABA(B(1)) and GABA(B(2)) genes. J Neurochem 2001; 77:1237–1247.
487. Samuels MH, Veldhuis J, Ridgway EC. Copulsatile release of thyrotropin and prolactin in normal and hypothyroid subjects. Thyroid 1995; 5:369–372.
488. Shimatsu A, Kato Y, Inoue T, et al. Peptide histidine isoleucine– and vasoactive intestinal polypeptide-like immunoreactivity coexist in rat hypophysial portal blood. Neurosci Lett 1983; 43:259–262.
489. Gibbs DM. High concentrations of oxytocin in hypophysial portal plasma. Endocrinology 1984; 114:1216–1218.
490. Holmes MC, Antoni FA, Aguilera G, Catt KJ. Magnocellular axons in passage through the median eminence release vasopressin. Nature 1986; 319:326–329.
491. Kjaer A. Vasopressin as a neuroendocrine regulator of anterior pituitary hormone secretion. Acta Endocrinol (Copenh) 1993; 129:489–496.
492. Shimatsu A, Kato Y, Ohta H, et al. Involvement of hypothalamic vasoactive intestinal polypeptide (VIP) in prolactin secretion induced by serotonin in rats. Proc Soc Exp Biol Med 1984; 175: 414–416.
493. Samson WK, Lumpkin MD, McCann SM. Evidence for a physiological role for oxytocin in the control of prolactin secretion. Endocrinology, 1986; 119:554–560.
494. Arey BJ, Freeman ME. Oxytocin, vasoactive-intestinal peptide, and serotonin regulate the mating-induced surges of prolactin secretion in the rat. Endocrinology 1990; 126:279–284.
495. Nagy GM, Gorcs TJ, Halasz B. Attenuation of the suckling-induced prolactin release and the high afternoon oscillations of plasma prolactin secretion of lactating rats by antiserum to vasopressin. Neuroendocrinology 1991; 54:566–570.
496. Itoh N, Obata K, Yanaihara N, Okamoto H. Human preprovasoactive intestinal polypeptide contains a novel PHI-27-like peptide, PHM-27. Nature 1983; 304:547–549.
497. Hokfelt T, Fahrenkrug J, Takemoto K, et al. The PHI (PHI-27)/corticotropin-releasing factor/enkephalin immunoreactive hypothalamic neuron: possible morphological basis for integrated control of prolactin, corticotropin, and growth hormone secretion. Proc Natl Acad Sci USA 1983; 80:895–898.
498. Denef C, Manet D, Dewals R. Dopaminergic stimulation of prolactin release. Nature 1980; 285:243–246.
499. Arey BJ, Burris TP, Basco P, Freeman ME. Infusion of dopamine at low concentrations stimulates the release of prolactin from alpha-methyl-*p*-tyrosine-treated rats. Proc Soc Exp Biol Med 1993; 203:60–63.
500. Hinuma S, Habata Y, Fujii R, et al. A prolactin-releasing peptide in the brain. Nature 1998; 393:272–276.
501. Morales T, Hinuma S, Sawchenko PE. Prolactin-releasing peptide is expressed in afferents to the endocrine hypothalamus, but not in neurosecretory neurones. J Neuroendocrinol 2000; 12: 131–140.
502. Watanobe H. In vivo release of prolactin-releasing peptide in rat hypothalamus in association with luteinizing hormone and prolactin surges. Neuroendocrinology 2001; 74:359–366.
503. Lawrence CB, Ellacott KL, Luckman SM. PRL-releasing peptide reduces food intake and may mediate satiety signaling. Endocrinology 2002; 143:360–367.
504. Schwartz J, Van de Pavert S, Clarke I, et al. Paracrine interactions within the pituitary gland. Ann NY Acad Sci 1998; 839: 239–243.
505. Lamberts SW, Macleod RM. Regulation of prolactin secretion at the level of the lactotroph. Physiol Rev 1990; 70:279–318.
506. Murai I, Ben-Jonathan N. Posterior pituitary lobectomy abolishes the suckling-induced rise in prolactin (PRL): evidence for a PRL-releasing factor in the posterior pituitary. Endocrinology 1987; 121:205–211.
507. Allen DL, Low MJ, Allen RG, Ben-Jonathan N. Identification of two classes of prolactin-releasing factors in intermediate lobe tumors from transgenic mice. Endocrinology 1995; 136:3093–3099.
508. Ellerkmann E, Nagy GM, Frawley LS. Alpha-melanocyte-stimulating hormone is a mammotrophic factor released by neurointermediate lobe cells after estrogen treatment. Endocrinology 1992; 130:133–138.
509. Voogt JL, Lee Y, Yang S, Arbogast L. Regulation of prolactin secretion during pregnancy and lactation. Prog Brain Res 2001; 133:173–185.
510. DeMaria JE, Livingstone JD, Freeman ME. Ovarian steroids influence the activity of neuroendocrine dopaminergic neurons. Brain Res 2000; 879:139–147.
511. Milenkovic L, Parlow AF, McCann SM. Physiological significance of the negative short-loop feedback of prolactin. Neuroendocrinology 1990; 52:389–392.
512. Arbogast LA, Voogt JL. Prolactin (PRL) receptors are colocalized in dopaminergic neurons in fetal hypothalamic cell cultures: effect of PRL on tyrosine hydroxylase activity. Endocrinology 1997; 138:3016–3023.
513. DeMaria JE, Lerant AA, Freeman ME. Prolactin activates all three populations of hypothalamic neuroendocrine dopaminergic neurons in ovariectomized rats. Brain Res 1999; 837:236–241.
514. Phelps CJ, Hurley DL. Pituitary hormones as neurotrophic signals: update on hypothalamic differentiation in genetic models of altered feedback. Proc Soc Exp Biol Med 1999; 222:39–58.
515. Phelps CJ, Horseman ND. Prolactin gene disruption does not compromise differentiation of tuberoinfundibular dopaminergic neurons. Neuroendocrinology 2000; 72:2–10.
516. Callahan P, Klosterman S, Prunty D, et al. Immunoneutralization of endogenous opioid peptides prevents the suckling-induced prolactin increase and the inhibition of tuberoinfundibular dopaminergic neurons. Neuroendocrinology 2000; 71:268–276.
517. Van de Kar LD, Bethea CL. Pharmacological evidence that serotonergic stimulation of prolactin secretion is mediated via the dorsal raphe nucleus. Neuroendocrinology 1982; 35:225–230.
518. Creese I, Burt D, Snyder S. Dopamine receptor binding predicts clinical and pharmacological potencies of antischizophrenic drugs. Science 1976; 192:481–483.
519. Melkersson K, Hulting AL. Prolactin-secreting pituitary adenoma in neuroleptic treated patients with psychotic disorder. Eur Arch Psychiatry Clin Neurosci 2000; 250:6–10.
520. Veldman RG, Frolich M, Pincus SM, et al. Basal, pulsatile, entropic, and 24-hour rhythmic features of secondary hyperprolactinemia due to functional pituitary stalk disconnection mimic tumoral (primary) hyperprolactinemia. J Clin Endocrinol Metab 2001; 86:1562–1567.
521. Waldstreicher J, Duffy JF, Brown EN, et al. Gender differences in the temporal organization of prolactin (PRL) secretion: evidence for a sleep-independent circadian rhythm of circulating PRL levels—a clinical research center study. J Clin Endocrinol Metab 1996; 81:1483–1487.
522. Diaz S, Seron-Ferre M, Cardenas H, et al. Circadian variation of basal plasma prolactin, prolactin response to suckling, and length of amenorrhea in nursing women. J Clin Endocrinol Metab 1989; 68:946–955.
523. Malarkey WB, Hall JC, Pearl DK, et al. The influence of academic stress and season on 24-hour concentrations of growth hormone and prolactin. J Clin Endocrinol Metab 1991; 73:1089–1092.
524. Matsuo H, Baba Y, Nair RM, et al. Structure of the porcine LH- and FSH-releasing hormone 1. The proposed amino acid sequence. Biochem Biophys Res Commun 1971; 43:1334–1339.
525. Seeburg P, Adelman J. Characterization of cDNA for precursor of human luteinizing hormone releasing hormone. Nature 1984; 311:666–668.
526. Amoss M, Burgus R, Blackwell R, et al. Purification, amino acid

composition and N-terminus of the hypothalamic luteinizing hormone releasing hormone factor (LRF) of ovine origin. Biochem Biophys Res Commun 1971; 44:205–210.
527. Sherwood N, Lovejoy D, Coe I. Origin of mammalian gonadotropin-releasing hormones. Endocr Rev, 1993; 14:241–254.
528. Urbanski H, White RB, Fernald RD, et al. Regional expression of mRNA encoding a second form of gonadotropin-releasing hormone in the macaque brain. Endocrinology 1999; 140:1945–1948.
529. Fernald R, White R. Gonadotropin-releasing hormone genes: phylogeny, structure, and functions. Front Neuroendocrinol 1999; 20:224–240.
530. Hsueh A, Jones B. Extrapituitary actions of gonadotropin-releasing hormone. Endocr Rev 1981; 2:437–461.
531. Lin Z-W, Otto C, Peter R. Evolution of neuroendocrine peptide systems: gonadotropin-releasing hormone and somatostatin. Comp Biochem Physiol 1998; 119:375–388.
532. Wierman M, Bruder J, Kepa J. Regulation of gonadotropin-releasing hormone (GnRH) gene expression in hypothalamic neuronal cells. Cell Mol Neurobiol 1995; 15:79–88.
533. Nelson S, Eraly S, Mellon P. The GnRH promoter: target of transcription factors, hormones, and signaling pathways. Mol Cell Endocrinol 1998; 140:151–155.
534. Gore AC, Roberts JL. Regulation of gonadotropin-releasing hormone gene expression in vivo and in vitro. Front Neuroendocrinol 1997; 18:209–245.
535. Clark M, Mellon P. The POU homeodomain transcription factor Oct-1 is essential for activity of the gonadotropin-releasing hormone neuron-specific enhancer. Mol Cell Biol 1995; 15:6169–6177.
536. Cattanach BM, Iddon CA, Charlton HM, et al. Gonadotropin-releasing hormone deficiency in a mutant mouse with hypogonadism. Nature 1977; 269:338–340.
537. Sternberger L, Hoffman G. Immunocytology of luteinizing hormone releasing hormone. Neuroendocrinology 1978; 25:111–128.
538. Silverman A, Krey L, Zimmerman E. A comparative study of the luteinizing hormone releasing hormone (LHRH) neuronal networks in mammals. Biol Reprod 1979; 20:98–110.
539. Moss R. Actions of hypothalamic-hypophysiotropic hormones on the brain. Annu Rev Physiol 1979; 41:617–631.
540. Phoenix C, Chambers K. Sexual performance of old and young male rhesus macaques following treatment with GnRH. Physiol Behav 1990; 47:513–517.
541. Wray S, Nieburgs A, Elkabes S. Spatiotemporal cell expression of luteinizing hormone-releasing hormone in the prenatal mouse: evidence for an embryonic origin in the olfactory placode. Dev Brain Res 1989; 46:309–318.
542. Schwanzel-Fukuda M, Pfaff D. Origin of luteinizing hormone-releasing hormone neurons. Nature 1989; 338:161–163.
543. Silverman A, Livne I, Witkin J. The gonadotropin-releasing hormone (GnRH) neuronal systems: immunocytochemistry and in situ hybridization. In Knobil E (ed). The Physiology of Reproduction. New York, Raven Press, 1994, pp 1683–1709.
544. Schwanzel-Fukuda M, Bick D, Pfaff D. Luteinizing hormone-releasing hormone (LHRH)-expressing cells do not migrate normally in an inherited hypogonadal (Kallmann) syndrome. Mol Brain Res 1989; 6:311–326.
545. Georgopoulos N, Pralong FP, Seidman CP, et al. Genetic heterogeneity evidenced by low incidence of KAL-1 gene mutations in sporadic cases of gonadotropin-releasing hormone deficiency. J Clin Endocrinol Metab 1997; 82:213–217.
546. Fan N, Jeung EB, Peng C, et al. The human gonadotropin-releasing hormone (GnRH) receptor gene: cloning, genomic organization and chromosomal assignment. Mol Cell Endocrinol 1994; 103:R1–R6.
547. Stojilkovic S, Reinhart J, Catt K. Gonadotropin-releasing hormone receptors: structure and signal transduction pathways. Endocr Rev 1994; 15:462–498.
548. Cheng K, Leung P. The expression, regulation and signal transduction pathways of the mammalian gonadotropin-releasing hormone receptor. Can J Physiol Pharmacol 2000; 78:1029–1052.
549. Clayton R, Solano AR, Garcia-Vela A, et al. Regulation of pituitary receptors for gonadotropin releasing hormone during the rat estrous cycle. Endocrinology 1980; 107:699–706.
550. Marian J, Cooper R, Conn P. Regulation of the rat pituitary GnRH-receptor. Mol Pharmacol 1981; 19:339–405.
551. Conn P. The molecular mechanism of gonadotropin-releasing hormone action in the pituitary. In Knobil E (ed). The Physiology of Reproduction. New York, Raven Press, 1994, pp 1815–1832.
552. Clayton R. Mechanism of GnRH action in gonadotrophs. Hum Reprod 1988; 3:479–483.
553. Conn P, Crowley WJ. Gonadotropin-releasing hormone and its analogs. Annu Rev Med 1994; 45:391–405.
554. Adams T, Spies H. Binding characteristics of gonadotropin-releasing hormone receptors throughout the estrous cycle of the hamster. Endocrinology 1981; 108:1592–1595.
555. Crowder M, Nett T. Pituitary content of gonadotropins and receptors for gonadotropin-releasing hormone (GnRH) and hypothalamic content of GnRH during the preovulatory period of the ewe. Endocrinology 1984; 114:234–239.
556. Nett T, Cermak D, Braden T, et al. Pituitary receptors for GnRH and estradiol, and pituitary content of gonadotropins in beef cows. I. Changes during the estrous cycle. Domest Anim Endocrinol 1987; 4:123–132.
557. Clarke I, Cummins JT, Crowder ME, Nett TM. Pituitary receptors for gonadotropin-releasing hormone in relation to changes in pituitary and plasma gonadotropins in ovariectomized hypothalamo/pituitary-disconnected ewes. II. A marked rise in receptor number during the acute feedback effects of estradiol. Biol Reprod 1988; 39:349–354.
558. Gregg D, Nett T. Direct effects of estradiol-17β on the number of gonadotropin-releasing hormone receptors in the ovine pituitary. Biol Reprod 1989; 40:288–293.
559. Conn P, Rogers D, Seay S. Biphasic regulation of the gonadotropin-releasing hormone receptor by receptor microaggregation and intracellular calcium levels. Mol Pharmacol 1984; 25:51–55.
560. Lahlou N, Carel JC, Chaussain JL, Roger M. Pharmacokinetics and pharmacodynamics of GnRH agonists: clinical implications in pediatrics. J Pediatr Endocrinol Metab 2000; 13(suppl 1):821–826.
561. Burger C, Prinssen H, Kenemans P. LHRH agonist treatment of breast cancer and gynecological malignancies: a review. Eur J Obstet Gynecol Reprod Biol 1996; 67:27–33.
562. Reissmann T, Schally AV, Bouchard P, et al. The LHRH antagonist cetrorelix: a review. Hum Reprod Update 2000; 6:322–331.
563. Wise P, Rance N, Barr G. Further evidence that luteinizing hormone-releasing hormone also is follicle-stimulating hormone-releasing hormone. Endocrinology 1979; 104:940–947.
564. McCann S, Mizunuma H, Samson W. Differential hypothalamic control of FSH secretion: a review. Psychoneuroendocrinology 1983; 8:299–308.
565. Carmel P, Araki S, Ferin M. Pituitary stalk portal blood collection in rhesus monkeys: evidence for pulsatile release of gonadotropin-releasing hormone (GnRH). Endocrinology 1976; 99:243–248.
566. Clarke I, Cummins J. The temporal relationship between gonadotropin-releasing hormone (GnRH) and luteinizing hormone (LH) in ovariectomized ewes. Endocrinology 1982; 111:1737–1739.
567. Caraty A, Locatelli A. Effect of time after castration on secretion of LHRH and LH in the ram. J Reprod Fertil 1988; 82:263–269.
568. Dierschke D, Bhattacharya AN, Atkinson LE, Knobil E. Circhoral oscillations of plasma LH in the ovariectomized rhesus monkey. Endocrinology 1970; 87:850–853.
569. Yen S, Tsai CC, Naftolin F, et al. Pulsatile patterns of gonadotropin release in subjects with and without ovarian function. J Clin Endocrinol Metab 1972; 34:671–675.
570. Fraser H, McNeilly A. Differential effects of LH-RH immunoneutralization on LH and FSH secretion in the ewe. J Reprod Fertil 1983; 69:569–577.
571. Wilson R, Kesner JS, Kaufman JM, et al. Central electrophysiologic correlates of pulsatile luteinizing hormone secretion in the rhesus monkey. Neuroendocrinology 1984; 39:256–260.
572. Kawakami M, Uemura T, Hayashi R. Electrophysiological correlates of pulsatile gonadotropin release in rats. Neuroendocrinology 1982; 35:63–67.
573. Mori Y, Nishihara M, Tanaka T, et al. Chronic recording of electrophysiological manifestation of the hypothalamic gonadotropin-releasing hormone pulse generator activity in the goat. Neuroendocrinology 1991; 53:392–395.

574. Martinez de la Escalera G, Choi A, Weiner R. Generation and synchronization of GnRH pulses: intrinsic properties of the Gt1-1 GnRH neuronal cell line. Proc Natl Acad Sci USA 1992; 89: 4149–4153.
575. Hotchkiss J, Knobil E. The menstrual cycle and its neuroendocrine control. In Knobil E (ed). The Physiology of Reproduction. New York, Raven Press, 1994, pp 711–749.
576. Belchetz P, Plant TM, Nakai Y, et al. Hypophysial responses to continuous and intermittent delivery of hypothalamic gonadotropin-releasing hormone. Science 1978; 202:631–633.
577. Burr I, Sizonenko PC, Kaplan SL, Grumbach MM. Hormonal changes in puberty. II. Correlation of serum luteinizing hormone and follicle stimulating hormone with stages of puberty, testicular size and bone age in normal boys. Pediatr Res 1970; 4:25–35.
578. Sizonenko P, Burr IM, Kaplan SL, Grumbach MM. Hormonal changes in puberty. II. Correlation of serum luteinizing hormone and follicle stimulating hormone with stages of puberty and bone age in normal girls. Pediatr Res 1970; 4:36–45.
579. Bousfield G, Perry W, Ward D. Gonadotropins: chemistry and biosynthesis. In Knobil E (ed). The Physiology of Reproduction. New York, Raven Press, 1994, pp 1749–1792.
580. Chappel S, Ulloa-Aguirre A, Coutifaris C. Biosynthesis and secretion of follicle-stimulating hormone. Endocr Rev 1983; 4:179–211.
581. Kordon C, et al. Role of classic and peptide neuromediators in the neuroendocrine regulation of luteinizing hormone and prolactin. In Knobil E (ed). The Physiology of Reproduction. New York, Raven Press, 1994, pp 1621–1681.
582. Wilson R, Knobil E. Acute effects of *N*-methyl-D,L-aspartate on the release of pituitary gonadotropins and prolactin in the adult female rhesus monkey. Brain Res 1982; 248:177–179.
583. Gore A, Terasawa E. A role for norepinephrine in the control of puberty in the female rhesus monkey, *Macaca mulatta*. Endocrinology 1991; 129:3009–3017.
584. Terasawa E. Mechanisms controlling the onset of puberty in primates: the role of GABAergic neurons. In Plant TM (ed). The Neurobiology of Puberty. Bristol, Journal of Endocrinology, 1995, p 139.
585. Ferin M, Van Vugt D, Chernick A. Central nervous system peptides and reproductive function in primates. In Norman RL (ed). Neuroendocrine Aspects of Reproduction. New York, Academic Press, 1983, pp 69–91.
586. Garcia-Segura L, Chowen JA, Duenas M, et al. Gonadal steroids and astroglial plasticity. Cell Mol Neurobiol 1996; 16:225–237.
587. Ojeda S. The neurobiology of mammalian puberty: has the contribution of glial cells been underestimated? J NIH Res 1994; 6: 51.
588. Pfaff D, Keiner M. Atlas of estradiol-concentrating cells in the central nervous system of the female rat. J Comp Neurol 1973; 151:128–158.
589. Stumpf W, Sar M, Keefer D. Atlas of estrogen target cells in the rat brain. In Stumpf W, Grant L (eds). Anatomical Neuroendocrinology. Basel, Karger, 1975, pp 104–119.
590. Fuxe K, Cintra A, Agnati LF, et al. Studies on the cellular localization and distribution of glucocorticoid receptor and estrogen receptor immunoreactivity in the central nervous system of the rat and their relationship to the monoaminergic and peptidergic neurons of the brain. J Steroid Biochem 1987; 27:159–170.
591. Simerly RB, Chang C, Muramatsu M, Swanson LW. Distribution of androgen and estrogen receptors mRNA-containing cells in the rat brain: an in situ hybridization study. J Comp Neurosci 1990; 294:76–95.
592. Kuiper G, Enmark E, Pelto-Huikko M, et al. Cloning of a novel estrogen receptor expressed in rat prostate. Proc Natl Acad Sci USA 1986; 493:5925–5930.
593. Kuiper G, Shughrue PJ, Merchenthaler I, et al. The estrogen receptor beta subtype: a novel mediator of estrogen action in neuroendocrine systems. Front Neuroendocrinol 1988; 19:254–286.
594. Shughrue P, Lane M, Merchenthaler I. The comparative distribution of estrogen receptor-α and β mRNA in rat central nervous system. J Comp Neurol 1997; 388:507–525.
595. Shughrue P, Merchenthaler I. Estrogen is more than just a "sex hormone": novel sites for estrogen action in the hippocampus and cerebral cortex. Front Neuroendocrinol 2000; 21:95–101.
596. Blaustein J, King JC, Toft DO, Turcotte J. Immunocytochemical localization of estrogen-induced progestin receptors in guinea pig brain. Brain Res 1988; 474:1–15.
597. DonCarlos L, Greene G, Morrell J. Estrogen plus progesterone increases progestin receptor immunoreactivity in the brain of ovariectomized guinea pigs. Neuroendocrinology 1989; 50:613–623.
598. Bethea C, Farrenbach WH, Sprangers SA, Freesh F. Immunocytochemical localization of progestin receptors in monkey hypothalamus: effect of estrogen and progestin. Endocrinology 1992; 130:895–905.
599. Bethea C, Brown N, Kohama S. Steroid regulation of estrogen and progestin receptor messenger ribonucleic acid in monkey hypothalamus and pituitary. Endocrinology 1996; 137:4372–4383.
600. Michael R, Clancy A, Zumpe D. Distribution of androgen receptor–like immunoreactivity in the brains of cynomolgus monkeys. J Neuroendocrinol 1995; 7:713–719.
601. Resko J, Roselli C. Prenatal hormones organize sex differences in the neuroendocrine reproductive system: observations on guinea pigs and nonhuman primates. Cell Mol Neurobiol 1997; 17:627–648.
602. Knobil E. On the control of gonadotropin secretion in the rhesus monkey. Recent Prog Horm Res 1974; 30:1–36.
603. Ferin M, Van Vugt D, Wardlaw S. The hypothalamic control of the menstrual cycle and the role of endogenous opioid peptides. Recent Prog Horm Res 1984; 40:441–480.
604. Steiner R, Bremner W, Clifton D. Regulation of luteinizing hormone pulse frequency and amplitude by testosterone in the male rat. Endocrinology 1982; 111:2055–2061.
605. Piva F, Limonta P, Dondi D, et al. Effects of steroids on the brain opioid system. J Steroid Biochem Mol Biol 1995; 53:343–348.
606. Nakai Y, Plant TM, Hess DL, et al. On the sites of the negative and positive feedback actions of estradiol in the control of gonadotropin secretion in the rhesus monkey. Endocrinology 1978; 102:1008–1014.
607. Plant T. Gonadal regulation of hypothalamic gonadotropin-releasing hormone release in primates. Endocr Rev 1986; 7:75–88.
608. Jaffe R. The menopause and perimenopausal period. In Yen SCC (ed). Reproductive Endocrinology. Philadelphia, WB Saunders, 1986, pp 406–440.
609. Karsch F, Dierschke DK, Weick RF, et al. Positive and negative feedback control by estrogen of luteinizing hormone secretion in the rhesus monkey. Endocrinology 1973; 92:799–804.
610. Bishop W, Kalra PS, Fawcett CP, et al. The effects of hypothalamic lesions on the release of gonadotropins and prolactin in response to estrogen and progesterone treatment in female rats. Endocrinology 1972; 91:1404–1410.
611. Chabbert-Buffet N, Skinne DC, Caraty A, et al. Neuroendocrine effects of progesterone. Steroids 2000; 65:613–620.
612. Levine J, Chappell PE, Schneider JS, et al. Progesterone receptors as neuroendocrine integrators. Front Neuroendocrinol 2001; 22:69–106.
613. Wagner E, Ronnekleiv OK, Bosch MA, Kelly MJ. Estrogen biophasically modifies hypothalamic GABAergic function concomitantly with negative and positive control of luteinizing hormone release. J Neurosci 2001; 21:2085–2093.
614. Shupnik M. Gonadotropin gene modulation by steroids and gonadotropin-releasing hormone. Biol Reprod 1996; 54:279–286.
615. Ying S. Inhibins and activins. In Martini L, Ganong W (eds). Frontiers in Neuroendocrinology. New York, Raven Press, 1988, pp 167–184.
616. DePaolo L. Inhibins, activins, and follistatins: the saga continues. Proc Soc Exp Biol Med 1997; 214:328–339.
617. Mather JP, Moore A, Li R-H. Activins, inhibins, and follistatins: further thoughts on a growing family of regulators. Proc Soc Exp Biol Med 1997; 215:209–222.
618. Peng C, Mukai S. Activins and their receptors in female reproduction. Biochem Cell Biol 2000; 78:261–279.
619. Matzuk M, Kumar TR, Shou W, et al. Transgenic models to study the roles of inhibins and activins in reproduction, oncogenesis, and development. Recent Prog Horm Res 1996; 51:123–154.
620. Knight P. Roles of inhibins, activins, and follistatin in the female reproductive axis. Annu Rev Physiol 1996; 57:219–244.

621. Zeleznik A, Fairchild Benyo D. Control of follicular development, corpus luteum function, and the recognition of pregnancy in higher primates. In Knobil E (ed). The Physiology of Reproduction. New York, Raven Press, 1994, pp 751–782.
622. Yen S, et al. Causal relationship between hormonal variables in the menstrual cycle. In Ferin M, Richart RM, Vande Wiele RL (eds). Biorhythms and Human Reproduction. New York, John Wiley & Sons, 1974, pp 219–238.
623. Freeman M. The neuroendocrine control of the ovarian cycle of the rat. In Knobil E (ed). The Physiology of Reproduction. New York, Raven Press, 1994, pp 613–658.
624. Goodman R. Neuroendocrine control of the ovine estrous cycle. In Knobil E (ed). The Physiology of Reproduction. New York, Raven Press, 1994, pp 659–709.
625. Kaplan S, Grumbach M, Aubert M. The ontogenesis of pituitary hormones and hypothalamic factors in the human fetus: maturation of central nervous system regulation of anterior pituitary function. Recent Prog Horm Res 1976; 32:161–234.
626. Ellinwood W, Resko J. Sex differences in biologically active and immunoreactive gonadotropins in the fetal circulation of rhesus monkeys. Endocrinology 1984; 107:902–907.
627. Resko J, Ellinwood W. Negative feedback regulation of gonadotropin secretion by androgens in fetal rhesus macaques. Biol Reprod 1985; 33:346–352.
628. Winter J, Faiman C, Hobson WC, et al. Pituitary-gonadal relations in infancy. I. Patterns of serum gonadotropin concentrations from birth to four years of age in man and chimpanzee. J Clin Endocrinol Metab 1975; 40:545–551.
629. Plant T. A striking sex difference in the gonadotropin response to gonadectomy during infantile development in the rhesus monkey (*Macaca mulatta*). Endocrinology 1986; 119:539–545.
630. Plant T. Neurobiological bases underlying the control of the onset of puberty in the rhesus monkey: a representative higher primate. Front Neuroendocrinol 2001; 22:107–139.
631. Boyar R, Rosenfeld RS, Kapen S, et al. Human puberty: simultaneous augmented secretion of luteinizing hormone and testosterone during sleep. J Clin Invest 1974; 54:609–618.
632. Boyar R, Wu RH, Roffwarg H, et al. Human puberty: 24-hour estradiol patterns in pubertal girls. J Clin Endocrinol Metab 1976; 43:1418–1421.
633. Ojeda S, Bilger M. Neuroendocrine regulation of puberty. In Conn FP (ed). Neuroendocrinology in Physiology and Medicine. Totowa, NJ, Humana Press, 2000, pp 197–224.
634. Gay V, Plant T. Sustained intermittent release of gonadotropin releasing hormone in the prepubertal male rhesus monkey induced by *N*-methyl-DL-aspartic acid. Neuroendocrinology 1988; 48:147–152.
635. El Majdoubi M, Sahu A, Ramaswamy S, Plant JM. Neuropeptide Y: a hypothalamic brake restraining the onset of puberty in primates. Proc Natl Acad Sci USA 2000; 97:6179–6184.
636. Frisch R, McArthur J. Menstrual cycles: fatness as a determinant of minimum weight for height necessary for their maintenance or onset. Science 1974; 185:949–951.
637. Laughlin G, Yenn S. Hypothalamic chronic anovulation. Am J Obstet Gynecol 1978; 130:825–831.
638. Pirke K, Wuttke W, Schweiger U. The Menstrual Cycle and Its Disorders. Berlin, Springer-Verlag, 1989.
639. Cameron J. Stress and behaviorally-induced reproductive dysfunction in primates. Semin Reprod Endocrinol 1997; 15:37–45.
640. Cameron J. Fasting and reproduction in non-human primates. In Hansel BG, Ryan DH (eds). Pennington Center Nutrition Series: Nutrition and Reproduction. Baton Rouge, University of Louisiana Press, 1998, pp 95–109.
641. Rivier C, Rivier J, Vale W. Stress induced inhibition of reproductive functions: role of endogenous corticotropin releasing factor. Science 1986; 231:607.
642. Feng Y, Shalts E, Xia LN, et al. An inhibitory effect of interleukin-1 on basal gonadotropin release in the ovariectomized rhesus monkey: reversal by a corticotropin-releasing factor antagonist. Endocrinology 1991; 128:2077–2082.
643. Norman R, Smith C. Restraint inhibits luteinizing hormone and testosterone secretion in intact male rhesus macaques: effects of concurrent naloxone administration. Neuroendocrinology 1992; 55:405–415.
644. Chen M, O'Byrne KT, Chiappini SE, et al. Hypoglycemic "stress" and gonadotropin releasing hormone pulse generator activity in the rhesus monkey: role of the ovary. Neuroendocrinology 1992; 56:666–673.
645. Wade G, Schneider J. Metabolic fuels and reproduction in female mammals. Neurosci Biobehav Rev 1992; 16:235–272.
646. Chehab FF, Lim ME, Lu R. Correction of the sterility defect in homozygous obese female mice by treatment with the human recombinant leptin. Nat Genet 1996; 12:318–320.
647. Schneider J, Zhou D, Blum R. Leptin and metabolic control of reproduction. Horm Behav 2000; 37:306–326.
648. Baskin DG, Schwartz MW, Seeley RJ, et al. Leptin receptor long-form splice-variant protein expression in neuron cell bodies of the brain and co-localization with neuropeptide Y mRNA in the arcuate nucleus. J Histochem Cytochem 1999; 47:353–362.
649. Kennedy GC. The role of depot fat in the hypothalamic control of food intake in the rat. Proc R Soc Lond B Biol Sci 1953; 140: 579–592.
650. Cummings DE, Purnell JO, Frayo RS, et al. A preprandial rise in plasma ghrelin levels suggest a role in meal initiation in humans. Diabetes 2001; 50:1714–1719.
651. Chen H, Charlat O, Tartaglia LA, et al. Evidence that the diabetes gene encodes the leptin receptor: identification of a mutation in the leptin receptor gene in *db/db* mice. Cell 1996; 84:491–495.
652. Licinio J, Mantzoros C, Negrao AB, et al. Human leptin levels are pulsatile and inversely related to pituitary-adrenal function. Nat Med 1997; 3:575–579.
653. Wang J, Liu R, Hawkins M, et al. A nutrient-sensing pathway regulates leptin gene expression in muscle and fat. Nature 1998; 393:684–688.
654. Haynes WG, Morgan DA, Djalali A, et al. Interactions between the melanocortin system and leptin in control of sympathetic nerve traffic. Hypertension 1999; 33:542–547.
655. Satoh N, Ogawa Y, Katsuura G, et al. Satiety effect and sympathetic activation of leptin are mediated by hypothalamic melanocortin system. Neurosci Lett 1998; 249:107–110.
656. Cheung CC, Thornton JE, Kuijper JL, et al. Leptin is a metabolic gate for the onset of puberty in the female rat. Endocrinology 1997; 138:855–858.
657. Yu WH, Kimura M, Walczewska A, et al. Role of leptin in hypothalamic-pituitary function. Proc Natl Acad Sci USA 1997; 94:1023–1028.
658. Sinha MK, Opentanova I, Ohannesian JP, et al. Evidence of free and bound leptin in human circulation. J Clin Invest 1996; 98: 1277–1282.
659. Hill RA, Margetic S, Pegg GG, Gazzola C. Leptin: Its pharmacokinetics and tissue distribution. Int J Obes Relat Metab Disord 1998; 22:765–770.
660. Elias CF, Kelly JF, Lee CE, et al. Chemical characterization of leptin-activated neurons in the rat brain. J Comp Neurol 2000; 423:261–281.
661. Erickson J, Hollopeter G, Palmiter JD. Attenuation of the obesity syndrome of *ob/ob* mice by the loss of neuropeptide Y. Science 1996; 274:1704–1707.
662. Lu D, Willard D, Patel IR, et al. Agouti protein is an antagonist of the melanocyte-stimulating hormone receptor. Nature 1994; 371:799–802.
663. Fan W, Boston BA, Kesterson RA, et al. Role of melanocortinergic neurons in feeding and the agouti obesity syndrome. Nature 1997; 385:165–168.
664. Robinson SW, Dinulescu DM, Cone RD. Genetic models of obesity and energy balance in the mouse. Annu Rev Genet 2000; 34:687–745.
665. Mountjoy KG, Mortrud MD, Low MJ, et al. Localization of the melanocortin-4 receptor (MC4-R) in neuroendocrine and autonomic control circuits in the brain. Mol Endocrinol 1994; 8: 1298–1308.
666. Krude H, Biebermann H, Luck W, et al. Severe early-onset obesity, adrenal insufficiency and red hair pigmentation caused by POMC mutations in humans. Nat Genet 1998; 19:155–157.
667. Vaisse C, Clement K, Durand E, et al. Melanocortin-4 receptor mutations are a frequent and heterogenous cause of morbid obesity. J Clin Invest 2000; 106:253–262.
668. Cone RD. Haploinsufficiency of the melanocortin-4 receptor: part of a thrifty genotype? J Clin Invest 2000; 106:185–187.
669. Butler AA, Marks DL, Fan W, et al. Melanocortin-4 receptor required for acute homeostatic responses to dietary fat. Nat Neurosci 2001; 4:605–611.

670. Inui A. Ghrelin: an orexigenic and somatotrophic signal from the stomach. Nat Rev Neurosci 2001; 2:1–10.
671. Clement K, Vaisse C, Lahlou N, et al. A mutation in the human leptin receptor gene causes obesity and pituitary dysfunction. Nature 1998; 392:398–401.
672. Considine RV, Inha MK, Heiman ML, et al. Serum immunoreactive-leptin concentrations in normal-weight and obese humans. N Engl J Med 1996; 334:292–295.
673. Friedman JM, Halaas JL. Leptin and the regulation of body weight in mammals. Nature 1998; 395:763–770.
674. Mantzoros CS. The role of leptin in human obesity and disease: a review of current evidence. Ann Intern Med 1999; 130:671–680.
675. Fujioka K, Patane J, Lubina J, Lau D. CSF leptin levels after exogenous administration of recombinant methionyl human leptin. JAMA 1999; 282:1517–1518.
676. Farooqi IS, Jebb SA, Langmack G, et al. Effects of recombinant leptin therapy in a child with congenital leptin deficiency. N Engl J Med 1999; 341:879–884.
677. Heymsfield SB, Greenberg AS, Fujioka K. Recombinant leptin for weight loss in obese and lean adults: a randomized, controlled, dose escalation trial. JAMA 1999; 282:1568–1575.
678. Fujioka K, et al. Significant body composition changes observed in obese subjects receiving chronic subcutaneous administration of a modified form of recombinant human leptin (abstract). North American Association for the Study of Obesity Annual Meeting, Long Beach, CA, October 29–November 2, 2000.
679. Hukshorn CJ, Saris WH, Westerterp-Plantenga MS, et al. Weekly subcutaneous pegylated recombinant native human leptin (PEG-OB) administration in obese men. J Clin Endocrinol Metab 2000; 85:4003–4009.
680. Westerterp-Plantenga MS, Saris WH, Hukshorn CJ, et al. Effects of weekly administration of pegylated recombinant human OB protein on appetite profile and energy metabolism in obese men. Am J Clin Nutr 2001; 74:426–434.
681. Shimomura I, Hammer RE, Ikemoto S, et al. Leptin reverses insulin resistance and diabetes mellitus in mice with congenital lipodystrophy. Nature 1999; 401:73–76.
682. Attoub S, Lavesseur S, Buyse M, et al. Physiological role of cholecystokinin B/gastrin receptor in leptin secretion. Endocrinology 1999; 140:4406–4410.
683. Kirchgessner TG, Uysal KT, Wiesbrock SM, et al. Tumor necrosis factor-alpha contributes to obesity-related hyperleptinemia by regulating leptin release from adipocytes. J Clin Invest 1997; 100:2777–2782.
684. Besedovsky H, del Rey A, Sorkin E, Dinarello CA. Immunoregulatory feedback between interleukin-1 and glucocorticoid hormones. Science 1986; 233:652–654.
685. Berkenbosch F, van Oers J, del Rey A, et al. Corticotropin-releasing factor–producing neurons in the rat activated by interleukin-1. Science 1987; 238:524–526.
686. Sapolsky R, Rivier C, Yamamoto G, et al. Interleukin-1 stimulates the secretion of hypothalamic corticotropin-releasing factor. Science 1987; 238:522–524.
687. Reichlin S. Neuroendocrine-immune interactions. N Engl J Med 1993; 329:1246–1253.
688. Reichlin S. Neuroendocrinology of infection and the innate immune system. Recent Prog Horm Res 1999; 54:133–181.
689. Ader R, Cohen N, Felten D. Psychoneuroimmunology: interactions between the nervous system and the immune system. Lancet 1995; 345:99–103.
690. Felten DL, Felten SY, Carlson SL, et al. Noradrenergic and peptidergic innervation of lymphoid tissue. J Immunol 1985; 135(2 suppl):755s–765s.
691. Spiegelman BM, Flier JS. Obesity and the regulation of energy balance. Cell 2001; 104:531–543.
692. Chen TY, Lei MG, Suzuki T, Morrison DC. Lipopolysaccharide receptors and signal transduction pathways in mononuclear phagocytes. Curr Top Microbiol Immunol 1992; 181:169–188.
693. Rivest S, Lacroix S, Vallieres L, et al. How the blood talks to the brain parenchyma and the paraventricular nucleus of the hypothalamus during systemic inflammatory and infectious stimuli. Proc Soc Exp Biol Med 2000; 223:22–38.
694. Elmquist JK, Scammell TE, Saper CB. Mechanisms of CNS response to systemic immune challenge: the febrile response. Trends Neurosci 1997; 20:565–570.
695. Broadwell RD, Brightman MW. Entry of peroxidase into neurons of the central and peripheral nervous systems from extracerebral and cerebral blood. J Comp Neurol 1976; 166:257–283.
696. Hellon R, Townsend Y. Mechanisms of fever. Pharmacol Ther 1982; 19:211–244.
697. Hunter WS, Sehic E, Blatteis CM. In Milton AS (ed). Temperature Regulation: Recent Physiological and Pharmacological Advances. Basel, Birkhauser, 1994, pp 75–85.
698. Stitt JT. Differential sensitivity in the sites of fever production by prostaglandin E1 within the hypothalamus of the rat. J Physiol (Lond) 1991; 432:99–110.
699. Katsuura G, Arimura A, Koves K, Gottschall PE. Involvement of organum vasculosum of lamina terminalis and preoptic area in interleukin 1 beta-induced ACTH release. Am J Physiol 1990; 258:E163–E171.
700. Kovacs KJ, Sawchenko PE. Mediation of osmoregulatory influences on neuroendocrine corticotropin-releasing factor expression by the ventral lamina terminalis. Proc Natl Acad Sci USA 1993; 90:7681–7685.#
701. Lee HY, Whiteside MB, Herkenham M. Area postrema removal abolishes stimulatory effects of intravenous interleukin-1beta on hypothalamic-pituitary-adrenal axis activity and c- fos mRNA in the hypothalamic paraventricular nucleus. Brain Res Bull 1998; 46:495–503.
702. Ericsson A, Arias C, Sawchenko PE. Evidence for an intramedullary prostaglandin-dependent mechanism in the activation of stress-related neuroendocrine circuitry by intravenous interleukin-1. J Neurosci 1997; 17:7166–7179.
703. Sagar SM, Price KJ, Kasting NW, Sharp FR. Anatomic patterns of Fos immunostaining in rat brain following systemic endotoxin administration. Brain Res Bull 1995; 36:381–392.
704. Vane JR. Inhibition of prostaglandin synthesis as a mechanism of action for aspirin-like drugs. Nat New Biol 1971; 231:232–235.
705. Johnson RW, von Borell E. Lipopolysaccharide-induced sickness behavior in pigs is inhibited by pretreatment with indomethacin [published erratum appears in J Anim Sci 1994; 72:801]. J Anim Sci 1994; 72:309–314.
706. Milton AS, Wendlandt S. A possible role for prostaglandin E1 as a modulator for temperature regulation in the central nervous system of the cat. J Physiol (Lond) 1970; 207:76P–77P.
707. Milton AS, Wendlandt E. Effects on body temperature of prostaglandins of the A, E and F series on injection into the third ventricle of unanaesthetized cats and rabbits. J Physiol (Lond) 1971; 218:325–336.
708. Goppelt-Struebe M. Regulation of prostaglandin endoperoxide synthase (cyclooxygenase) isozyme expression. Prostaglandins Leukot Essent Fatty Acids 1995; 52:213–222.
709. Robertson RP. Molecular regulation of prostaglandin synthesis: implications for endocrine systems. Trends Endocrinol Metab 1995; 6:293–297.
710. Breder CD, Dewitt D, Kraig RP. Characterization of inducible cyclooxygenase in rat brain. J Comp Neurol, 1995; 355:296–315.
711. Breder CD, Smith WL, Raz A, et al. Distribution and characterization of cyclooxygenase immunoreactivity in the ovine brain. J Comp Neurol 1992; 322:409–438.
712. Yamagata K, Andreasson KI, Kaufman WE, et al. Expression of a mitogen-inducible cyclooxygenase in brain neurons: regulation by synaptic activity and glucocorticoids. Neuron 1993; 11:371–386.
713. Ek M, Engblom D, Saha S, et al. Inflammatory response: pathway across the blood-brain barrier. Nature 2001; 410:430–431.
714. Elmquist JK, Breder CD, Sherin JE, et al. Intravenous lipopolysaccharide induces cyclooxygenase-II immunoreactivity in rat brain perivascular microglia. J Comp Neurol 1997; 381:119–129.
715. Elmquist JK, Ahima RS, Maratos-Flier E, et al. Leptin activates neurons in ventrobasal hypothalamus and brainstem. Endocrinology 1997; 138:839–842.
716. Rivest S. What is the cellular source of prostaglandins in the brain in response to systemic inflammation? Facts and controversies. Mol Psychiatry 1999; 4:500–507.
717. Blatteis CM, Sehic E. Cytokines and fever. Ann NY Acad Sci 1998; 840:608–618.
718. Scammell TE, Elmquist JK, Griffin JD, Saper CB. Ventromedial preoptic prostaglandin E_2 activates fever-producing autonomic pathways. J Neurosci 1996; 16:6246–6254.
719. Williams JW, Rudy TA, Yaksh TL, Viswanathan CT. An extensive exploration of the rat brain for sites mediating prostaglandin-induced hyperthermia. Brain Res 1977; 120:251–262.

720. Feldberg W, Saxena PN. Further studies on prostaglandin E1 fever in cats. J Physiol (Lond) 1971; 219:739–745.
721. Morimoto A, Nakamori T, Watanabe T, et al. Pattern differences in experimental fevers induced by endotoxin, endogenous pyrogen, and prostaglandins. Am J Physiol 1988; 254:R633–R640.
722. Scammell TE, Griffin JD, Elmquist JK, Saper CB. Microinjection of a cyclooxygenase inhibitor into the anteroventral preoptic region attenuates LPS fever. Am J Physiol 1998; 274:R783–789.
723. Watanabe Y, Watanabe Y, Hayaishi O. Quantitative autoradiographic localization of prostaglandin E_2 binding sites in monkey diencephalon. J Neurosci 1988; 8:2003–2010.
724. Matsumura K, Watanabe Y, Onoe H, et al. High density of prostaglandin E_2 binding sites in the anterior wall of the 3rd ventricle: a possible site of its hyperthermic action. Brain Res 1990; 533:147–151.
725. Coleman RA, Grix SP, Head SA, et al. A novel inhibitory prostanoid receptor in piglet saphenous vein. Prostaglandins 1994; 47: 151–168.
726. Ushikubi F, Segi E, Sugimoto Y, et al. Impaired febrile response in mice lacking the prostaglandin E receptor subtype EP3. Nature 1998; 395:281–284.
727. Ek M, Arias C, Sawchenko P, et al. Distribution of the EP3 prostaglandin E_2 receptor subtype in the rat brain: relationship to sites of interleukin-1-induced cellular responsiveness. J Comp Neurol 2000; 428:5–20.
728. Sugimoto Y, Shigemoto R, Namba T, et al. Distribution of the messenger RNA for the prostaglandin E receptor subtype EP3 in the mouse nervous system. Neuroscience 1994; 62:919–928.
729. Zhang J, Rivest S. A functional analysis of EP4 receptor-expressing neurons in mediating the action of prostaglandin E_2 within specific nuclei of the brain in response to circulating interleukin-1beta. J Neurochem 2000; 74:2134–2145.
730. Nakamura K, Kaneko T, Yamashita Y, et al. Immunocytochemical localization of prostaglandin EP3 receptor in the rat hypothalamus. Neurosci Lett 1999; 260:117–120.
731. Oka T, Hori T. EP1-receptor mediation of prostaglandin E_2-induced hyperthermia in rats. Am J Physiol 1994; 267:R289–R294.
732. Oka K, Oka T, Hori T. PGE_2 receptor subtype EP1 antagonist may inhibit central interleukin-1beta-induced fever in rats. Am J Physiol 1998; 275:R1762–R1765.
733. Banks WA, Kastin AJ, Durham DA. Bidirectional transport of interleukin-1 alpha across the blood-brain barrier. Brain Res Bull 1989; 23:433–437.
734. Banks WA, Ortiz L, Plotkin SR, Kastin AJ. Human interleukin (IL) 1 alpha, murine IL-1 alpha and murine IL-1 beta are transported from blood to brain in the mouse by a shared saturable mechanism. J Pharmacol Exp Ther 1991; 259:988–996.
735. Banks WA, Kastin AJ. Blood to brain transport of interleukin links the immune and central nervous systems. Life Sci 1991; 48: PL117–PL121.
736. Hopkins SJ, Rothwell NJ. Cytokines and the nervous system. I: Expression and recognition. Trends Neurosci 1995; 18:83–88.
737. Rothwell NJ, Hopkins SJ. Cytokines and the nervous system. II: Actions and mechanisms of action. Trends Neurosci 1995; 18: 130–136.
738. Klir JJ, McClellan JL, Kluger MJ. Interleukin-1 beta causes the increase in anterior hypothalamic interleukin-6 during LPS-induced fever in rats. Am J Physiol 1994; 266:R1845–R1848.
739. Breder CD, Hazuka C, Ghayur T, et al. Regional induction of tumor necrosis factor alpha expression in the mouse brain after systemic lipopolysaccharide administration. Proc Natl Acad Sci USA 1994; 91:11393–11397.
740. Quan N, Whiteside M, Kim L, Herkenham M. Induction of inhibitory factor kappaBalpha mRNA in the central nervous system after peripheral lipopolysaccharide administration: an in situ hybridization histochemistry study in the rat. Proc Natl Acad Sci USA 1997; 94:10985–10990.
741. Laflamme N, Lacroix S, Rivest S. An essential role of interleukin-1beta in mediating NF-kappaB activity and COX-2 transcription in cells of the blood-brain barrier in response to a systemic and localized inflammation but not during endotoxemia. J Neurosci 1999; 19:10923–10930.
742. Ericsson A, Liu C, Hart RP, Sawchenko PE. Type 1 interleukin-1 receptor in the rat brain: distribution, regulation, and relationship to sites of IL-1-induced cellular activation. J Comp Neurol 1995; 361:681–698.
743. Watkins LR, Goehler LE, Relton JK, et al. Blockade of interleukin-1 induced hyperthermia by subdiaphragmatic vagotomy: evidence for vagal mediation of immune-brain communication. Neurosci Lett 1995; 183:27–31.
744. Dantzer R. How do cytokines say hello to the brain? Neural versus humoral mediation. Eur Cytokine Netw 1994; 5:271–273.
745. Goehler LE, Busch CR, Tartaglia N, et al. Blockade of cytokine induced conditioned taste aversion by subdiaphragmatic vagotomy: further evidence for vagal mediation of immune-brain communication. Neurosci Lett 1995; 185:163–166.
746. Ek M, Kurosawa M, Lundeberg T, Ericsson A. Activation of vagal afferents after intravenous injection of interleukin-1beta: role of endogenous prostaglandins. J Neurosci 1998; 18:9471–9479.
747. Wan W, Wetmore L, Sorensen CM, et al. Neural and biochemical mediators of endotoxin and stress-induced c-fos expression in the rat brain. Brain Res Bull 1994; 34:7–14.
748. Bret-Dibat JL, Bluthe RM, Kent S, et al. Lipopolysaccharide and interleukin-1 depress food-motivated behavior in mice by a vagal-mediated mechanism. Brain Behav Immun 1995; 9:242–246.
749. Laye S, Bluthe RM, Kent S, et al. Subdiaphragmatic vagotomy blocks induction of IL-1 beta mRNA in mice brain in response to peripheral LPS. Am J Physiol 1995; 268:R1327–R1331.
750. Gaykema RP, Dijkstra I, Tilders FJ. Subdiaphragmatic vagotomy suppresses endotoxin-induced activation of hypothalamic corticotropin-releasing hormone neurons and ACTH secretion. Endocrinology 1995; 136:4717–4720.
751. Bluthe RM, Michaud B, Kelley KW, Dantzer R. Vagotomy blocks behavioural effects of interleukin-1 injected via the intraperitoneal route but not via other systemic routes. Neuroreport 1996; 7:2823–2827.
752. Sagar SM, Sharp FR, Curran T. Expression of c-fos protein in brain: metabolic mapping at the cellular level. Science 1988; 240: 1328–1331.
753. Elmquist JK, Ackermann MR, Register KB, et al. Induction of Fos-like immunoreactivity in the rat brain following Pasteurella multocida endotoxin administration. Endocrinology 1993; 133: 3054–3057.
754. Elmquist JK, Scammell TE, Jacobson CD, Saper CB. Distribution of Fos-like immunoreactivity in the rat brain following intravenous lipopolysaccharide administration. J Comp Neurol 1996; 371:85–103.
755. Elmquist JK, Saper CB. Activation of neurons projecting to the paraventricular hypothalamic nucleus by intravenous lipopolysaccharide. J Comp Neurol 1996; 374:315–331.
756. Wan W, Janz L, Vriend CY, et al. Differential induction of c-Fos immunoreactivity in hypothalamus and brain stem nuclei following central and peripheral administration of endotoxin. Brain Res Bull 1993; 32:581–587.
757. Brady LS, Lynn AB, Herkenham M, Gottesfeld Z. Systemic interleukin-1 induces early and late patterns of c-fos mRNA expression in brain. J Neurosci 1994; 14:4951–4964.
758. Hare AS, Clarke G, Tolchard S. Bacterial lipopolysaccharide-induced changes in FOS protein expression in the rat brain: correlation with thermoregulatory changes and plasma corticosterone. J Neuroendocrinol 1995; 7:791–799.
759. Rivest S, Rivier C. Stress and interleukin-1 beta-induced activation of c-fos, NGFI-B and CRF gene expression in the hypothalamic PVN: comparison between Sprague-Dawley, Fisher-344 and Lewis rats. J Neuroendocrinol 1994; 6:101–117.
760. Rivest S, Laflamme N. Neuronal activity and neuropeptide gene transcription in the brains of immune-challenged rats. J Neuroendocrinol 1995; 7:501–525.
761. Tkacs NC, Strack AM. Systemic endotoxin induces Fos-like immunoreactivity in rat spinal sympathetic regions. J Auton Nerv Syst 1995; 51:1–7.
762. Veening JG, van der Meer MJ, Joosten H, et al. Intravenous administration of interleukin-1 beta induces Fos-like immunoreactivity in corticotropin-releasing hormone neurons in the paraventricular hypothalamic nucleus of the rat. J Chem Neuroanat 1993; 6:391–397.
763. Huang QH, Entwistle ML, Alvaro JD, et al. Antipyretic role of endogenous melanocortins mediated by central melanocortin receptors during endotoxin-induced fever. J Neurosci 1997; 17: 3343–3351.

764. Kasting NW, Cooper KE, Veale WL. Antipyresis following perfusion of brain sites with vasopressin. Experientia 1979; 35:208–209.
765. Cooper KE, Kasting NW, Lederis K, Veale WL. Evidence supporting a role for endogenous vasopressin in natural suppression of fever in the sheep. J Physiol (Lond) 1979; 295:33–45.
766. Shih ST, Khorram O, Lipton JM, McCann SM. Central administration of alpha-MSH antiserum augments fever in the rabbit. Am J Physiol 1986; 250:R803–R806.
767. Huang QH, Hruby VJ, Tatro JB. Role of central melanocortins in endotoxin-induced anorexia. Am J Physiol 1999; 276:R864–R871.
768. Marks DL, Cone RD. Central melanocortins and the regulation of weight during acute and chronic disease. Recent Prog Horm Res 2001; 56:359–375.
769. Marks DL, Ling N, Cone RD. Role of the central melanocortin system in cachexia. Cancer Res 2001; 61:1432–1438.
770. Bamshad M, Aoki VT, Adkison MG, et al. Central nervous system origins of the sympathetic nervous system outflow to white adipose tissue. Am J Physiol 1998; 275:R291–R299.
771. Rothwell NJ, Stock MJ. Effects of denervating brown adipose tissue on the responses to cold, hyperphagia and noradrenaline treatment in the rat. J Physiol (Lond) 1984; 355:457–463.
772. Lowell BB, Flier JS. Brown adipose tissue, beta 3-adrenergic receptors, and obesity. Annu Rev Med 1997; 48:307–316.
773. Jansen AS, Wessendorf MW, Loewy AD. Transneuronal labeling of CNS neuropeptide and monoamine neurons after pseudorabies virus injections into the stellate ganglion. Brain Res 1995; 683:1–24.
774. Jansen AS, Nguyen XV, Karpitskiy V, et al. Central command neurons of the sympathetic nervous system: basis of the fight-or-flight response. Science 1995; 270:644–646.
775. Cechetto DF, Saper CB. Neurochemical organization of the hypothalamic projection to the spinal cord in the rat. J Comp Neurol 1988; 272:579–604.
776. Zhang YH, Lu J, Elmquist JK, Saper CB. Lipopolysaccharide activates specific populations of hypothalamic and brainstem neurons that project to the spinal cord. J Neurosci 2000; 20:6578–6586.
777. Benvenga S, Campenni A, Ruggeri RM, Trimarchi F. Clinical review 113: hypopituitarism secondary to head trauma. J Clin Endocrinol Metab 2000; 85:1353–1361.
778. Gudmundsson A, Carnes M. Pulsatile adrenocorticotropic hormone: an overview. Biol Psychiatry 1997; 41:342–365.
779. Yuan XQ, Wade CE. Neuroendocrine abnormalities in patients with traumatic brain injury. Front Neuroendocrinol 1991; 12: 209–230.
780. Honegger J, Buchfelder M, Fahlbusch R. Surgical treatment of craniopharyngiomas: endocrinological results. J Neurosurg 1999; 90:251–257.
781. Daaboul J, Steinbok P. Abnormalities of water metabolism after surgery for optic/chiasmatic astrocytomas in children. Pediatr Neurosurg 1998; 28:181–185.
782. Maghnie M, Cosi G, Genovese E, et al. Central diabetes insipidus in children and young adults. N Engl J Med 2000; 343:998–1007.
783. Scherbaum WA, Wass JA, Besser GM, et al. Autoimmune cranial diabetes insipidus: its association with other endocrine diseases and with histiocytosis X. Clin Endocrinol (Oxf) 1986; 25:411–420.
784. Mootha SL, Barkovich AJ, Grumbach MM, et al. Idiopathic hypothalamic diabetes insipidus, pituitary stalk thickening, and the occult intracranial germinoma in children and adolescents. J Clin Endocrinol Metab 1997; 82:1362–1367.
785. Al-Agha AE, Thomsett AJ, Ratcliffe JF, et al. Acquired central diabetes insipidus in children: a 12-year Brisbane experience. J Paediatr Child Health 2001; 37:172–175.
786. Bohus B, de Wied D. The vasopressin deficient Brattleboro rats: a natural knockout model used in the search for CNS effects of vasopressin. Prog Brain Res 1998; 119:555–573.
787. Nielsen S, Frpkiaer J, Marples D, et al. Aquaporins in the kidney: from molecules to medicine. Physiol Rev 2002; 82:205–244.
788. Birnbaumer M. The V2 vasopressin receptor mutations and fluid homeostasis. Cardiovasc Res 2001; 51:409–415.
789. Morello JP, Bichet DG. Nephrogenic diabetes insipidus. Annu Rev Physiol 2001; 63:607–630.
790. Nagasaki H, Ito M, Yuasa H, et al. Two novel mutations in the coding region for neurophysin-II associated with familial central diabetes insipidus. J Clin Endocrinol Metab 1995; 80:1352–1356.
791. Lieberman SA, Obero AL, Gilkison CR, et al. Prevalence of neuroendocrine dysfunction in patients recovering from traumatic brain injury. J Clin Endocrinol Metab 2001; 86:2752–2756.
792. Smith MV, Laws ER Jr. Magnetic resonance imaging measurements of pituitary stalk compression and deviation in patients with nonprolactin-secreting intrasellar and parasellar tumors: lack of correlation with serum prolactin levels. Neurosurgery 1994; 34:834–839; discussion 839.
793. Bjerre P. The empty sella: a reappraisal of etiology and pathogenesis. Acta Neurol Scand Suppl 1990; 130:1–25.
794. Voelker JL, Campbell RL, Muller J. Clinical, radiographic, and pathological features of symptomatic Rathke's cleft cysts. J Neurosurg 1991; 74:535–544.
795. Zucchini S, Ambrosetto P, Carla G, et al. Primary empty sella: differences and similarities between children and adults. Acta Paediatr 1995; 84:1382–1385.
796. Crowley WJ, Jameson J. Clinical counterpoint: gonadotropin-releasing hormone deficiency: perspectives from clinical investigation. Endocr Rev 1992; 13:635–640.
797. Klingmuller D, Dewes W, Krahe T, et al. Magnetic resonance imaging of the brain in patients with anosmia and hypothalamic hypogonadism (Kallmann's syndrome). J Clin Endocrinol Metab 1987; 65:581–584.
798. Nanduri VR, Stanhope R. Why is the retention of gonadotrophin secretion common in children with panhypopituitarism due to septo-optic dysplasia? Eur J Endocrinol 1999; 140:48–50.
799. Layman LC. Genetics of human hypogonadotropic hypogonadism. Am J Med Genet 1999; 89:240–248.
800. Layman LC, McDonough PG, Cohen DP, et al. Familial gonadotropin-releasing hormone resistance and hypogonadotropic hypogonadism in a family with multiple affected individuals. Fertil Steril 2001; 75:1148–1155.
801. Hayes FJ, Seminara SB, Crowley WF Jr. Hypogonadotropic hypogonadism. Endocrinol Metab Clin North Am 1998; 27:739–763, vii.
802. Chryssikopoulos A, Gregoriou O, Vitoratos N, et al. The predictive value of double Gn-RH provocation test in unprimed, Gn-RH-primed and steroid-primed female patients with Kallmann's syndrome. Int J Fertil Womens Med 1998; 43:291–299.
803. Samuels MH, Ridgway EC. Central hypothyroidism. Endocrinol Metab Clin North Am 1992; 21:903–919.
804. Winter WE, Signorino MR. Review: molecular thyroidology. Ann Clin Lab Sci 2001; 31:221–244.
805. Jorgensen JO, Pedersen SA, Laurberg P, et al. Effects of growth hormone therapy on thyroid function of growth hormone-deficient adults with and without concomitant thyroxine-substituted central hypothyroidism. J Clin Endocrinol Metab 1989; 69:1127–1132.
806. Rose SR. Cranial irradiation and central hypothyroidism. Trends Endocrinol Metab 2001; 12:97–104.
807. Argente J, Abusrewil SA, Bona G, et al. Isolated growth hormone deficiency in children and adolescents. J Pediatr Endocrinol Metab 2001; 14(suppl 2):1003–1008.
808. Triulzi F, Scotti G, di Natale B, et al. Evidence of a congenital midline brain anomaly in pituitary dwarfs: a magnetic resonance imaging study in 101 patients. Pediatrics 1994; 93:409–416.
809. Kikuchi K, Fujisawa I, Momoi T, et al. Hypothalamic-pituitary function in growth hormone-deficient patients with pituitary stalk transection. J Clin Endocrinol Metab 1988; 67:817–823.
810. Andersen B, Rosenfeld MG. POU domain factors in the neuroendocrine system: lessons from developmental biology provide insights into human disease. Endocr Rev 2001; 22:2–35.
811. Cushman LJ, Camper SA. Molecular basis of pituitary dysfunction in mouse and human. Mamm Genome 2001; 12:485–494.
812. Parks JS, Brown MR, Jurley DL, et al. Heritable disorders of pituitary development. J Clin Endocrinol Metab 1999; 84:4362–4370.
813. Pfaffle R, Blankenstein O, Wuller S, et al. Idiopathic growth hormone deficiency: a vanishing diagnosis? Horm Res 2000; 53(suppl 3):1–8.
814. Stacpoole P, Interlandi JW, Nicholson WE, Rabin D. Isolated ACTH deficiency: a heterogeneous disorder. Critical review and report of four new cases. Medicine (Baltimore) 1982; 61:13–24.

815. Nishihara E, Kimura H, Ishimaru T, et al. A case of adrenal insufficiency due to acquired hypothalamic CRH deficiency. Endocr J 1997; 44:121–126.
816. Kyllo JH, Collins MM, Vetter KL, et al. Linkage of congenital isolated adrenocorticotropic hormone deficiency to the corticotropin releasing hormone locus using simple sequence repeat polymorphisms. Am J Med Genet 1996; 62:262–267.
817. Lamolet B, Pulichino AM, Lamonerie T, et al. A pituitary cell-restricted T box factor, Tpit, activates POMC transcription in cooperation with Pitx homeoproteins. Cell 2001; 104:849–859.
818. Fukata J, Shimizu N, Imura H, et al. Human corticotropin-releasing hormone test in patients with hypothalamo-pituitary-adrenocortical disorders. Endocr J 1993; 40:597–606.
819. Fujiwara I, Igarashi Y, Ogawa E. A comparison of pituitary-adrenal responses to corticotropin-releasing hormone, hypoglycaemia and metyrapone in children with brain tumours and growth hormone deficiency. Eur J Pediatr 1995; 154:717–722.
820. Arlt W, Hove U, Muller B, et al. Frequent and frequently overlooked: treatment-induced endocrine dysfunction in adult long-term survivors of primary brain tumors. Neurology 1997; 49: 498–506.
821. Gleeson HK, Shalet SM. Endocrine complications of neoplastic diseases in children and adolescents. Curr Opin Pediatr 2001; 13: 346–351.
822. Asa SL, Ezzat S. The cytogenesis and pathogenesis of pituitary adenomas. Endocr Rev 1998; 19:798–827.
823. Asa S, Kovacs K, Tindall GT, et al. Cushing's disease associated with an intrasellar gangliocytoma producing corticotrophin-releasing factor. Ann Intern Med 1984; 101:789–793.
824. Asa S, Scheithauer BW, Bilbao JM, et al. A case for hypothalamic acromegaly: a clinicopathological study of six patients with hypothalamic gangliocytomas producing growth hormone-releasing factor. J Clin Endocrinol Metab 1984; 58:796–803.
825. Lee PA. Central precocious puberty. An overview of diagnosis, treatment, and outcome. Endocrinol Metab Clin North Am 1999; 28:901–918, xi.
826. Cassio A, Cacciari E, Zucchini S, et al. Central precocious puberty: clinical and imaging aspects. J Pediatr Endocrinol Metab 2000; 13(suppl 1):703–708.
827. Cisternino M, Arrigo T, Pasquino AM, et al. Etiology and age incidence of precocious puberty in girls: a multicentric study. J Pediatr Endocrinol Metab 2000; 13(suppl 1):695–701.
828. De Sanctis V, Corrias A, Rizzo V, et al. Etiology of central precocious puberty in males: the results of the Italian Study Group for Physiopathology of Puberty. J Pediatr Endocrinol Metab 2000; 13(suppl 1):687–693.
829. Ojeda SR, Heger S. New thoughts on female precocious puberty. J Pediatr Endocrinol Metab 2001; 14:245–256.
830. Rivarola, Belgorosky A, Mendilaharzu H, Vidal G. Precocious puberty in children with tumours of the suprasellar and pineal areas: organic central precocious puberty. Acta Paediatr 2001; 90: 751–756.
831. Virdis R, Sigorini M, Laiolo A, et al. Neurofibromatosis type 1 and precocious puberty. J Pediatr Endocrinol Metab 2000; 13(suppl 1):841–844.
832. Debeneix C, Bourgeois M, Trivin C, et al. Hypothalamic hamartoma: comparison of clinical presentation and magnetic resonance images. Horm Res 2001; 56:12–18.
833. Arita K, Ikawa F, Kurisu K, et al. The relationship between magnetic resonance imaging findings and clinical manifestations of hypothalamic hamartoma. J Neurosurg 1999; 91:212–220.
834. Hochman HI, Judge DM, Reichlin S. Precocious puberty and hypothalamic hamartoma. Pediatrics 1981; 67:236–244.
835. Berkovic SF, Andermann F, Melanson D, et al. Hypothalamic hamartomas and ictal laughter: evolution of a characteristic epileptic syndrome and diagnostic value of magnetic resonance imaging. Ann Neurol 1988; 23:429–439.
836. Anasti JN, Flack MR, Froelich J, et al. A potential novel mechanism for precocious puberty in juvenile hypothyroidism. J Clin Endocrinol Metab 1995; 80:276–279.
837. Fauchon F, Jouvet A, Paquis P, et al. Parenchymal pineal tumors: a clinicopathological study of 76 cases. Int J Radiat Oncol Biol Phys 2000; 46:959–968.
838. Jouvet A, Saint-Pierre G, Fauchon F, et al. Pineal parenchymal tumors: a correlation of histological features with prognosis in 66 cases. Brain Pathol 2000; 10:49–60.
839. Baumgartner JE, Edwards MS. Pineal tumors. Neurosurg Clin North Am 1992; 3:853–862.
840. Popovic EA, Kelly PJ. Stereotactic procedures for lesions of the pineal region. Mayo Clin Proc 1993; 68:965–970.
841. Dahlborg SA, Petrillo A, Crossen JR, et al. The potential for complete and durable response in nonglial primary brain tumors in children and young adults with enhanced chemotherapy delivery. Cancer J Sci Am 1998; 4:110–124.
842. Iughetti L, Predieri B, Ferrari M, et al. Diagnosis of central precocious puberty: endocrine assessment. J Pediatr Endocrinol Metab 2000; 13(suppl 1):709–715.
843. Chemaitilly W, Trivin C, Adan L, et al. Central precocious puberty: clinical and laboratory features. Clin Endocrinol (Oxf) 2001; 54:289–294.
844. Chalumeau M, Chemaitilly W, Trivin C, et al. Central precocious puberty in girls: an evidence-based diagnosis tree to predict central nervous system abnormalities. Pediatrics 2002; 109:61–67.
845. Shankar RR, Pescovitz OH. Precocious puberty. Adv Endocrinol Metab 1995; 6:55–89.
846. Tato L, Savage MO, Antoniazzi F, et al. Optimal therapy of pubertal disorders in precocious/early puberty. J Pediatr Endocrinol Metab 2001; 14(suppl 2):985–995.
847. Klein KO, Barnes KM, Jones JV, et al. Increased final height in precocious puberty after long-term treatment with LHRH agonists: the National Institutes of Health experience. J Clin Endocrinol Metab 2001; 86:4711–4716.
848. Feuillan P, Merke D, Leschek EW, Cutler EB Jr. Use of aromatase inhibitors in precocious puberty. Endocr Relat Cancer 1999; 6:303–306.
849. Laron Z, Kauli R. Experience with cyproterone acetate in the treatment of precocious puberty. J Pediatr Endocrinol Metab 2000; 13(suppl 1):805–810.
850. Yen SS. Female hypogonadotropic hypogonadism: hypothalamic amenorrhea syndrome. Endocrinol Metab Clin North Am 1993; 22:29–58.
851. Warren MP, Fried JL. Hypothalamic amenorrhea: the effects of environmental stresses on the reproductive system: a central effect of the central nervous system. Endocrinol Metab Clin North Am 2001; 30:611–629.
852. Khoury SA, Reame NE, Kelch RP, Marshall JC. Diurnal patterns of pulsatile luteinizing hormone secretion in hypothalamic amenorrhea: reproducibility and responses to opiate blockade and an alpha 2-adrenergic agonist. J Clin Endocrinol Metab 1987; 64: 755–762.
853. Cannavo S, Curto L, Trimarchi F. Exercise-related female reproductive dysfunction. J Endocrinol Invest 2001; 24:823–832.
854. Moschos S, Chan JL, Mantzoros CS. Leptin and reproduction: a review. Fertil Steril 2002; 77:433–444.
855. Williams NI, Helmreich DL, Parfitt DB, et al. Evidence for a causal role of low energy availability in the induction of menstrual cycle disturbances during strenuous exercise training. J Clin Endocrinol Metab 2001; 86:5184–5193.
856. Hobart JA, Smucker DR. The female athlete triad. Am Fam Physician 2000; 61:3357–3364, 3367.
857. Muller J. Hypogonadism and endocrine metabolic disorders in Prader-Willi syndrome. Acta Paediatr Suppl 1997; 423:58–59.
858. Hackney AC. Endurance exercise training and reproductive endocrine dysfunction in men: alterations in the hypothalamic-pituitary-testicular axis. Curr Pharm Des 2001; 7:261–273.
859. Opstad K. Circadian rhythm of hormones is extinguished during prolonged physical stress, sleep and energy deficiency in young men. Eur J Endocrinol 1994; 131:56–66.
860. Abs R, Verhelst J, Maeyaert J, et al. Endocrine consequences of long-term intrathecal administration of opioids. J Clin Endocrinol Metab 2000; 85:2215–2222.
861. Van den Berghe G. Novel insights into the neuroendocrinology of critical illness. Eur J Endocrinol 2000; 143:1–13.
862. Molitch ME. Pathologic hyperprolactinemia. Endocrinol Metab Clin North Am 1992; 21:877–901.
863. Biller BM, Luciano A, Crosignani PG, et al. Guidelines for the diagnosis and treatment of hyperprolactinemia. J Reprod Med 1999; 44(12 suppl):1075–1084.
864. Meierkord H, Shorvon S, Lightman S, Trimble M. Comparison of the effects of frontal and temporal lobe partial seizures on prolactin levels. Arch Neurol 1992; 49:225–230.
865. Molitch ME. Diagnosis and treatment of prolactinomas. Adv Intern Med 1999; 44:117–153.

866. Burman P, Ritzen EM, Lindgren AC. Endocrine dysfunction in Prader-Willi syndrome: a review with special reference to GH. Endocr Rev 2001; 22:787–799.
867. Blizzard RM, Bulatovic A. Psychosocial short stature: a syndrome with many variables. Baillieres Clin Endocrinol Metab 1992; 6: 687–712.
868. Gohlke BC, Khadilkar VV, Skuse D, Stanhope R. Recognition of children with psychosocial short stature: a spectrum of presentation. J Pediatr Endocrinol Metab 1998; 11:509–517.
869. Gilmour J, Skuse D. A case-comparison study of the characteristics of children with a short stature syndrome induced by stress (hyperphagic short stature) and a consecutive series of unaffected "stressed" children. J Child Psychol Psychiatry 1999; 40:969–978.
870. Albanese A, Hamill G, Jones J, et al. Reversibility of physiological growth hormone secretion in children with psychosocial dwarfism. Clin Endocrinol (Oxf) 1994; 40:687–692.
871. Bercu BB, Diamond FB Jr. Growth hormone neurosecretory dysfunction. Clin Endocrinol Metab 1986; 15:537–590.
872. Lin TH, Kirkland RT, Sherman BM, Kirkland JL. Growth hormone testing in short children and their response to growth hormone therapy. J Pediatr 1989; 115:57–63.
873. Attie KM. Genetic studies in idiopathic short stature. Curr Opin Pediatr 2000; 12:400–404.
874. Mehta A, Hindmarsh PC. The use of somatropin (recombinant growth hormone) in children of short stature. Paediatr Drugs 2002; 4:37–47.
875. Voss LD. Short normal stature and psychosocial disadvantage: a critical review of the evidence. J Pediatr Endocrinol Metab 2001; 14:701–711.
876. Burr IM, Slonim AE, Danish RK, et al. Diencephalic syndrome revisited. J Pediatr 1976; 88:439–444.
877. Poussaint TY, Barnes PD, Nichols K, et al. Diencephalic syndrome: clinical features and imaging findings. AJNR 1997; 18: 1499–1505.
878. Manski TJ, Haworth CS, Duval-Arnould BJ, Rushing EJ. Optic pathway glioma infiltrating into somatostatinergic pathways in a young boy with gigantism: case report. J Neurosurg 1994; 81: 595–600.
879. Gropman AL, Packer RJ, Nicholson HS, et al. Treatment of diencephalic syndrome with chemotherapy: growth, tumor response, and long term control. Cancer 1998; 83:166–172.
880. Ho KY, Veldhuis JD, Johnson ML, et al. Fasting enhances growth hormone secretion and amplifies the complex rhythms of growth hormone secretion in man. J Clin Invest 1988; 81:968–975.
881. Atiea J, Creagh F, Page M, et al. Early-morning hyperglycemia in IDDM: acute effects of cholinergic blockade. Diabetes Care 1989; 12:443–448.
882. Saeger W, Puchner MJ, Ludecke DK. Combined sellar gangliocytoma and pituitary adenoma in acromegaly or Cushing's disease: a report of 3 cases. Virchows Arch 1994; 425:93–99.
883. Gold PW, Goodwin FK, Chrousos GP. Clinical and biochemical manifestations of depression. Relation to the neurobiology of stress (2). N Engl J Med 1988; 319:413–420.
884. Posener JA, DeBattista C, Williams GH, et al. 24-Hour monitoring of cortisol and corticotropin secretion in psychotic and nonpsychotic major depression. Arch Gen Psychiatry 2000; 57:755–760.
885. Bjorntorp P, Rosmond R. The metabolic syndrome: a neuroendocrine disorder? Br J Nutr 2000; 83(suppl 1):S49–S57.
886. Rosmond R, Bjorntorp P. The hypothalamic-pituitary-adrenal axis activity as a predictor of cardiovascular disease, type 2 diabetes and stroke. J Intern Med 2000; 247:188–197.
887. Chrousos GP. The role of stress and the hypothalamic-pituitary-adrenal axis in the pathogenesis of the metabolic syndrome: neuro-endocrine and target tissue-related causes. Int J Obes Relat Metab Disord 2000; 24(suppl 2):S50–S55.
888. Wolff S. A syndrome of periodic hypothalamic discharge. Am J Med 1964; 36:956–967.
889. Wardlaw SL. Clinical review 127: obesity as a neuroendocrine disease: lessons to be learned from proopiomelanocortin and melanocortin receptor mutations in mice and men. J Clin Endocrinol Metab 2001; 86:1442–1446.
890. Comuzzie AG, Hixson JE, Almasy L, et al. A major quantitative trait locus determining serum leptin levels and fat mass is located on human chromosome 2. Nat Genet 1997; 15:273–276.
891. Hixson JE, Almasy L, Cole S, et al. Normal variation in leptin levels in associated with polymorphisms in the proopiomelanocortin gene, POMC. J Clin Endocrinol Metab 1999; 84:3187–3191.
892. Hager J, Dina C, Francke S, et al. A genome-wide scan for human obesity genes reveals a major susceptibility locus on chromosome 10. Nat Genet 1998; 20:304–308.
893. Rotimi CN, Comuzzie AG, Lowe WL, et al. The quantitative trait locus on chromosome 2 for serum leptin levels is confirmed in African-Americans. Diabetes 1999; 48:643–644.
894. Krude H, Gruters A. Implications of proopiomelanocortin (POMC) mutations in humans: the POMC deficiency syndrome. Trends Endocrinol Metab 2000; 11:1–5.
895. Vaisse C, Clement K, Guy-Grand B, Froguel P. A frameshift mutation in human MC4R is associated with a dominant form of obesity. Nat Genet 1998; 20:113–114.
896. Yeo GSH, Farooqi IS, Aminian S, et al. A frameshift mutation in MC4R associated with dominantly inherited human obesity. Nat Genet 1998; 20:111–112.
897. Farooqi IS, Yeo GS, Keogh AM, et al. Dominant and recessive inheritance of morbid obesity associated with melanocortin 4 receptor deficiency. J Clin Invest 2000; 106:271–279.
898. Vink T, Hinney A, van Elburg AA, et al. Association between an agouti-related protein gene polymorphism and anorexia nervosa. Mol Psychiatry 2001; 6:325–328.
899. Lin L, Faraco J, Li R, et al. The sleep disorder canine narcolepsy is caused by a mutation in the hypocretin (orexin) receptor 2 gene. Cell 1999; 98:365–376.
900. Chemelli RM, Willie JT, Sinton CM, et al. Narcolepsy in orexin knockout mice: molecular genetics of sleep regulation. Cell 1999; 98:437–451.
901. Eriksson KS, Sergeeva O, Brown RE, Haas HL. Orexin/hypocretin excites the histaminergic neurons of the tuberomammillary nucleus. J Neurosci 2001; 21:9273–9279.
902. Gerashchenko D, Kohls MD, Greco M, et al. Hypocretin-2-saporin lesions of the lateral hypothalamus produce narcoleptic-like sleep behavior in the rat. J Neurosci 2001; 21:7273–7283.
903. Thannickal TC, Moore RY, Nienhuis R, et al. Reduced number of hypocretin neurons in human narcolepsy. Neuron 2000; 27: 469–474.

8 Anterior Pituitary

Shlomo Melmed and David Kleinberg

DEVELOPMENT, ANATOMY, AND OVERVIEW OF CONTROL OF HORMONE SECRETION

The pituitary gland situated within the sella turcica derives its name from the Greek *ptuo* and Latin *pituita*, phlegm, reflecting its nasopharyngeal origin. Galen hypothesized that nasal phlegm originated from the brain and drained through the pituitary gland. It is now clear that together with the hypothalamus the pituitary orchestrates the structural integrity and function of endocrine glands, including the thyroid gland, adrenal gland, and gonads, in addition to target tissues including cartilage and breast. The pituitary stalk serves as an anatomic and functional connection to the hypothalamus. Preservation of the hypothalamic-pituitary unit is critical for integration of anterior pituitary control of sexual function and fertility, linear and organ growth, lactation, stress responses, energy, appetite, and temperature regulation and secondarily for carbohydrate and mineral metabolism.

Integration of vital body functions by the brain was first proposed by Descartes in the 17th century. In 1733, Morgagni recorded the absence of adrenal glands in an anencephalic neonate, providing early evidence for a developmental and functional connection between the brain and the adrenal glands. In 1849 Claude Bernard set the stage for the subsequent advances in neuroendocrinology by demonstrating that central lesions in the area of the fourth ventricle resulted in polyuria.[1] Subsequent studies led to the identification and chemical isolation of pituitary hormones, and astute clinical observations led to the realization that pituitary tumors were associated with functional hypersecretory syndromes, including acromegaly and Cushing's disease.[2–4] In 1948 Geoffrey Harris, the founder of modern neuroendocrinology, in reviewing anterior pituitary gland hormone control, proposed their hypothalamic regulation, predicting the subsequent discovery of specific hypothalamic regulating hormones.[5]

Anatomy

The pituitary gland comprises the predominant anterior lobe, the posterior lobe, and a vestigial intermediate lobe (Fig. 8–1). The gland is situated within the bony sella turcica and is overlain by the dural diaphragma sella, through which the stalk connects to the median eminence of the hypothalamus. The adult pituitary weighs approximately 600 mg (range, 400 to 900 mg) and measures about 13 mm in the longest transverse diameter, 6 to 9 mm in vertical height, and about 9 mm anteroposteriorly. Structural variation may occur in multiparous women, and gland volume also changes during the menstrual cycle. During pregnancy these measurements may be increased in either dimension, with pituitary weight increasing up to 1 g. Normal pituitary hypertrophy without evidence for the presence of an adenoma was described in seven eugonadal women with pituitary height greater than 9 mm and a convex upper gland boundary observed on magnetic resonance imaging (MRI).[6]

The sella turcica located at the base of the skull forms the thin bony roof of the sphenoid sinus. The lateral walls comprising either bone or dural tissue abut the cavernous sinuses, which are traversed by the third, fourth, and six cranial nerves and internal carotid arteries (Fig. 8–2). Thus, the cavernous sinus contents are vulnerable to increased intrasellar expansion. The dural roofing protects the gland from compression by fluctuant cerebrospinal fluid (CSF) pressure. The optic chiasm, located anterior to the pituitary stalk, is directly above the diaphragma sella. The optic tracts and central structures are therefore vulnerable to pressure effects by an expanding pituitary mass, which is likely to follow the path of least tissue resistance by lifting the diaphragma sella (Fig. 8–3). The intimate relationship of the pituitary and chiasm is borne out in optic chiasmal hypoplasia associated with developmental pituitary dysfunction seen in patients with septo-optic dysplasia. The posterior pituitary gland, in contrast to the anterior pituitary, is directly innervated by supraopticohypophyseal and tuberohypophyseal nerve tracts of the posterior stalk. Hypothalamic neuronal lesions, stalk disruption, or direct systemically derived metastases are therefore often associated with attenuated vasopressin (diabetes insipidus) or oxytocin secretion, or both.

The hypothalamus contains nerve cell bodies that synthesize hypophysiotropic releasing and inhibiting hormones as well as the neurohypophyseal hormones of the posterior pituitary (arginine vasopressin and oxytocin). Five distinct hormone-secret-

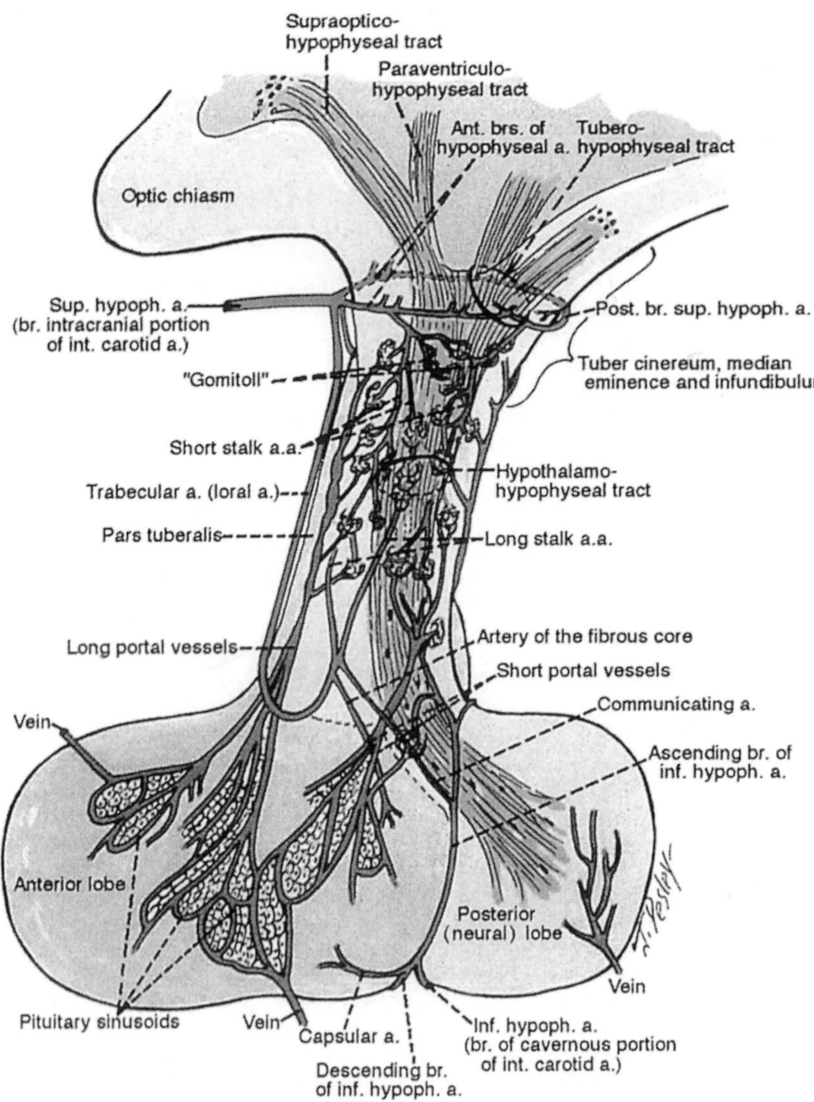

Figure 8–1. Schematic representation of the blood supply of the hypothalamus and pituitary. (From Scheithauer BW. The hypothalamus and neurohypophysis. In Kovacs K, Asa SL [eds]. Functional Endocrine Pathology. Boston, Blackwell Scientific, 1991, pp 170–244.)

ing cell types are present in the mature anterior pituitary gland. Corticotroph cells express pro-opiomelanocortin (POMC) peptides including adrenocorticotropic hormone (ACTH); somatotroph cells express growth hormone (GH); thyrotroph cells express the common glycoprotein α subunit and the specific thyrotropin (thyroid-stimulating hormone, TSH) β subunit; gonadotrophs express the α and β subunits for both follicle-stimulating hormone (FSH) and luteinizing hormone (LH); the lactotroph expresses prolactin (PRL). Each cell type is under highly specific signal controls that regulate their respective differentiated gene expression.

Pituitary Development

The pituitary gland arises from within the rostral neural plate. Rathke's pouch, a primitive ectodermal invagination an-

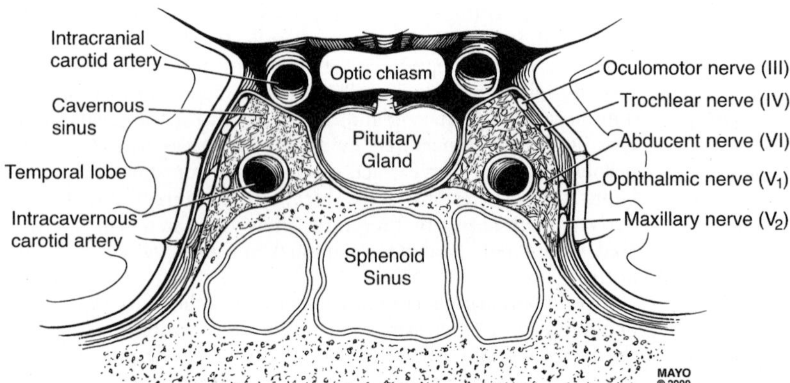

Figure 8–2. Coronal section of the sellar structures and cavernous sinus showing the relationship of the oculomotor (III), trochlear (IV), trigeminal ophthalmic and maxillary divisions (V_1 and V_2), and abducent (VI) cranial nerves to the pituitary gland. (From Stiver SI, Sharpe JA. Neuro-ophthalmologic evaluation of pituitary tumors. In Thapar K, Kovacs K, Schithauer BW, Lloyd RV [eds]. Diagnosis and Management of Pituitary Tumors. Totowa, NJ, Humana Press, 2001, pp 173–200.)

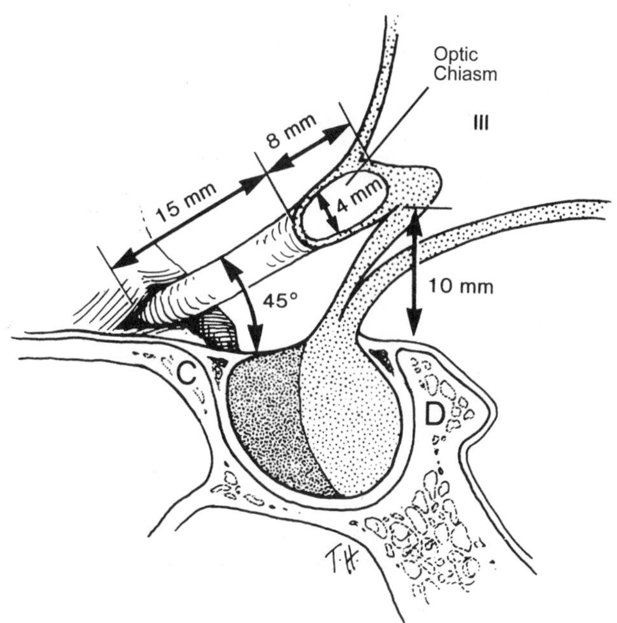

Figure 8–3. Relationship of the pituitary gland to the optic chiasm. *A*, The intracranial optic nerve/chiasmal complex lies up to 10 mm above the diaphragma sellae. C, Anterior clinoid process; D, dorsum of the sella turcica. *B*, Coronal section from magnetic resonance scan of patient with large pituitary adenoma tumor; suprasellar extension has elevated and distorted the chiasm. (From Miller NR, Newman NJ [eds]. Walsh and Hoyt's Clinical Neuro-Ophthalmology, vol 1, 4th ed. Baltimore, Williams & Wilkins, 1985, pp 60–69.)

terior to the roof of the oral cavity, is formed by the fourth to fifth week of gestation and gives rise to the anterior pituitary gland (Fig. 8–4).[7, 8] The pouch is directly connected to the stalk and hypothalamic infundibulum and ultimately becomes distinct from the oral cavity and nasopharynx. Rathke's pouch proliferates toward the third ventricle, where it fuses with the diverticulum and subsequently obliterates its lumen, which may persist as Rathke's cleft. The anterior lobe is formed from Rathke's pouch, and the diverticulum gives rise to the adjacent posterior lobe. Remnants of pituitary tissue may persist in the nasopharyngeal midline and rarely give rise to functional ectopic hormone-secreting tumors in the nasopharynx. The neurohypophysis arises from neural ectoderm associated with third-ventricle development.[9]

Functional development of the anterior pituitary cell types involves complex spatiotemporal regulation of cell lineage–specific transcription factors expressed in pluripotential pituitary stem cells as well as dynamic gradients of locally acting soluble factors.[10–12] Critical neuroectodermal signals for organizing the dorsal gradient of pituitary morphogenesis include infundibular bone morphogenetic protein 4 (BMP4) required for the initial pouch invagination,[8] fibroblast growth factor 8 (FGF-8), Wnt 5, and Wnt 4. Subsequent ventral developmental patterning and transcription factor expression are determined by spatial and graded expression of BMP2 and sonic hedgehog protein (shh), which appears critical for directing early patterns of cell proliferation.[13]

The human fetal Rathke pouch is evident at 3 weeks, and the pituitary grows rapidly in utero. By 7 weeks, the anterior pituitary vasculature begins to develop, and by 20 weeks the entire hypophyseal-portal system is already established. The anterior pituitary undergoes major cellular differentiation during the first 12 weeks, by which time all the major secretory cell compartments are structurally and functionally intact, except for lactotrophs. Totipotential pituitary stem cells give rise to acidophilic (mammosomatotroph, somatotroph, and lactotroph) and basophilic (corticotroph, thyrotroph, and gonadotroph) differentiated pituitary cell types, which appear at clearly demarcated developmental stages. Corticotroph cells are morphologically identifiable at 6 weeks, and immunoreactive ACTH is detectable by 7 weeks. At 8 weeks, somatotroph cells are evident with abundant immunoreactive cytoplasmic GH expression. Glycoprotein hormone–secreting cells express a common α subunit, and at 12 weeks differentiated thyrotrophs and gonadotrophs express immunoreactive β subunits for TSH, LH, and FSH. Interestingly, gonadotrophs expressing LH and FSH are equally distributed in females, whereas in the male fetus, LH-expressing gonadotrophs predominate.[14] Fully differentiated PRL-expressing lactotrophs are evident only late in gestation (after 24 weeks). Prior to that time, immunoreactive PRL is detectable only in mixed mammosomatotrophs, also expressing GH, reflecting the common genetic origin of these two hormones.[15]

Pituitary Transcription Factors

Determination of anterior pituitary cell type lineages results from a temporally regulated cascade of homeodomain transcription factors. Although most pituitary developmental information has been acquired from murine models,[16] histologic and pathogenetic observations in human subjects have largely corroborated these developmental mechanisms (see Fig. 8–4). Early cell differentiation requires intracellular Rpx and Ptx expression. Rathke's pouch expresses several transcription factors of the LIM homeodomain family, including Lhx3, Lhx4, and IsI-1,[17] which are early determinants of functional pituitary development. Pitx1 is expressed in the oral ectoderm and subsequently in all pituitary cell types, particularly those arising ventrally.[18] Rieger's syndrome, characterized by defective eye, tooth, umbilical cord, and pituitary development, is caused by defective related Pitx2.[19, 20]

Ptx behaves as a universal pituitary regulator and activates transcription of α-GSU (the α-subunit of gonadotroph hormones), POMC and LHβ (Ptx1), and GH (Ptx2). Lhx3 determines GH-PRL and TSH cell differentiation, and Prop-1 behaves as a prerequisite for Pit-1, which activates GH, PRL, TSH, and growth hormone-releasing hormone (GHRH) receptor transcription. TSH and gonadotropin-expressing cells share a common α subunit (αGSU) expression under developmental control of GATA-2.[11] These specific anterior pituitary transcription factors participate in a highly orchestrated cascade leading to the commitment of the five differentiated cell types (see Fig. 8–4). The major proximal determinant of pituitary cell lineage derived from a totipotential stem cell is thus Prop-1 expression, which determines subsequent development of Pit-1–dependent and gonadotroph cell lineages.[21]

POU1F1, the renamed Pit-1, is a POU-homeodomain transcription factor that determines development and appropriate temporal and spatial expression of cells committed to GH, PRL, TSH, and GHRH receptor expression. POU1F1 binds to specific deoxyribonucleic acid (DNA) motifs and activates and regulates somatotroph, lactotroph, and thyrotroph development and mature secretory function. Signal-dependent coactivating factors also cooperate with Pit-1 to determine specific hormone expression. Thus, in POU1F1-containing cells, high estrogen receptor levels induce a commitment to express PRL, whereas thyrotroph embryonic factor (TEF) favors TSH expression. Selective pituitary cell type specificity is also perpetuated by binding of POU1F1 to its own DNA regulatory elements as well as those contained within the GH, PRL, and TSH genes. Steroidogenic factor-1 (SF-1) and dosage-sensitive sex reversal, adrenal hypoplasia congenita, X-chromosome factor (DAX-1) determine subsequent gonadotroph development.[22, 23] Corticotroph cell commitment, although occurring earliest during fetal development, is independent of POU1F1-

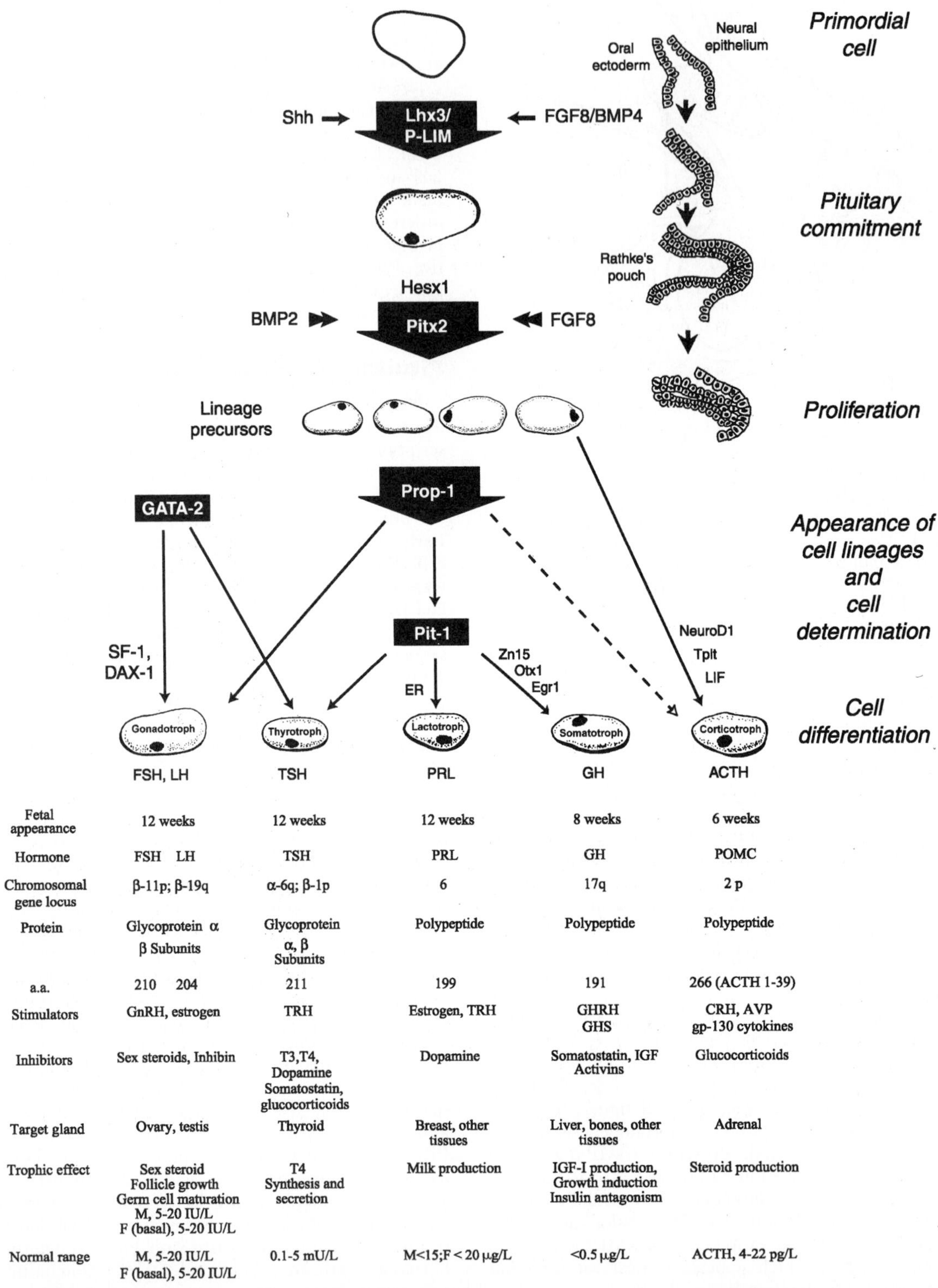

	FSH, LH	TSH	PRL	GH	ACTH
Fetal appearance	12 weeks	12 weeks	12 weeks	8 weeks	6 weeks
Hormone	FSH LH	TSH	PRL	GH	POMC
Chromosomal gene locus	β-11p; β-19q	α-6q; β-1p	6	17q	2 p
Protein	Glycoprotein α β Subunits	Glycoprotein α, β Subunits	Polypeptide	Polypeptide	Polypeptide
a.a.	210 204	211	199	191	266 (ACTH 1-39)
Stimulators	GnRH, estrogen	TRH	Estrogen, TRH	GHRH GHS	CRH, AVP gp-130 cytokines
Inhibitors	Sex steroids, Inhibin	T3,T4, Dopamine Somatostatin, glucocorticoids	Dopamine	Somatostatin, IGF Activins	Glucocorticoids
Target gland	Ovary, testis	Thyroid	Breast, other tissues	Liver, bones, other tissues	Adrenal
Trophic effect	Sex steroid Follicle growth Germ cell maturation M, 5-20 IU/L F (basal), 5-20 IU/L	T4 Synthesis and secretion	Milk production	IGF-I production, Growth induction Insulin antagonism	Steroid production
Normal range	M, 5-20 IU/L F (basal), 5-20 IU/L	0.1-5 mU/L	M<15;F < 20 μg/L	<0.5 μg/L	ACTH, 4-22 pg/L

Figure 8–4. Model for development of the human anterior pituitary gland and cell lineage determination by a cascade of transcription factors. Trophic cells are depicted with transcription factors known to determine cell-specific human or murine gene expression. (Adapted from Shimon I, Melmed S. In Conn P, Melmed S [eds]. Scientific Basis of Endocrinology. Totowa, NJ, Humana Press, 1996, pp 30–47; Amselem S. Perspectives on the molecular basis of developmental defects in the human pituitary region. In Rappaport R, Amselem S [eds]. Hypothalamic-Pituitary Development: Genetic and Clinical Aspects. Basel, Karger, 2001; and Dasen JS, Rosenfeld MG. Curr Opin Cell Biol 1999; 11:669–677.[849])

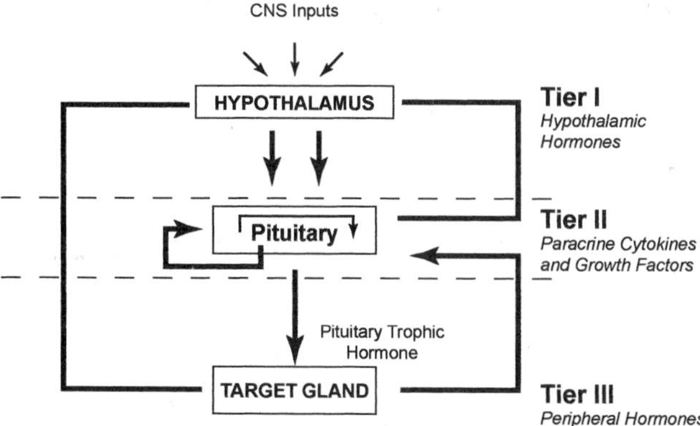

Figure 8–5. Model for regulation of anterior pituitary hormone secretion by three tiers of control. Hypothalamic hormones traverse the portal system and impinge directly upon their respective target cells. Intrapituitary cytokines and growth factors regulate tropic cell function by paracrine (and autocrine) control. Peripheral hormones exert negative feedback inhibition of respective pituitary trophic hormone synthesis and secretion. (From Ray D, Melmed S. Pituitary cytokine and growth factor expression and action. Endocr Rev 1997; 18:206–228.)

determined lineages, and Tpit protein appears to be a prerequisite for POMC expression.[24] Hereditary mutations arising within these transcription factors may result in isolated or combined pituitary hormone failure syndromes (see later).

Pituitary Blood Supply

The pituitary gland enjoys an abundant blood supply derived from several sources (see Fig. 8–1). The superior hypophyseal arteries branch from the internal carotid arteries to supply the hypothalamus, where they form a capillary network in the median eminence, external to the blood-brain barrier. Long and short hypophyseal portal vessels originate from infundibular plexuses and the stalk, respectively. These vessels form the hypothalamic-portal circulation, the predominant blood supply to the anterior pituitary gland. They deliver hypothalamic releasing and inhibiting hormones to the trophic hormone-producing cells of the adenohypophysis without significant systemic dilution, allowing the pituitary cells to be sensitively regulated by timed hypothalamic hormone secretion.

Vascular transport of hypothalamic hormones is also locally regulated by a contractile internal capillary plexus (gomitoli) derived from stalk branches of the superior hypophyseal arteries.[25] Retrograde blood flow toward the median eminence also occurs, facilitating bidirectional functional hypothalamic-pituitary interactions.[26] Systemic arterial blood supply is maintained by inferior hypophyseal arterial branches, which predominantly supply the posterior pituitary. Disruption of stalk integrity may lead to compromised pituitary portal blood flow, depriving the anterior pituitary cells of hypothalamic hormone access.

Pituitary Control

Three levels of control subserve the regulation of anterior pituitary hormone secretion (Fig. 8–5). Hypothalamic control is mediated by adenohypophysiotropic hormones secreted into the portal system and impinging directly upon anterior pituitary cell surface receptors. G protein–linked cell surface membrane binding sites are highly selective and specific for each of the hypothalamic hormones and elicit positive or negative signals mediating pituitary hormone gene transcription and secretion. Peripheral hormones also participate in mediating pituitary cell function, predominantly by negative feedback regulation of trophic hormones by their respective target hormones. Intrapituitary paracrine and autocrine soluble growth factors and cytokines act locally to regulate neighboring cell development and function.

The net result of these three tiers of complex intracellular signals is the controlled pulsatile secretion of the six pituitary trophic hormones, ACTH, GH, PRL, TSH, FSH, and LH, through the cavernous sinus, petrosal veins, and ultimately the systemic circulation through the superior vena cava (Fig. 8–6). The temporal and quantitative control of pituitary hormone secretion is critical for physiologic integration of peripheral hormonal systems such as the menstrual cycle, which relies on complex and precisely regulated pulse control.

PITUITARY MASSES

Pituitary Mass Effects

An expanding pituitary mass may inexorably alter the sellar size and shape by bone erosion and remodeling (Fig. 8–7). Although the exact time course of this process is unknown, it appears to be slowly progressive over years or decades. The tumor may invade soft tissue, and the dorsal sellar roof presents the least resistance to expansion from within the confines of the bony sella. Nevertheless, both suprasellar and parasellar compression and invasion may occur with an enlarging mass, with resultant clinical manifestations (Table 8–1). As tumors impinge upon the optic chiasm, they interfere with vision. Because of the anatomy of the chiasm, pressure from below affects temporal visual fields, starting superiorly and ultimately extending to the entire temporal field. Loss of nasal fields also occurs and may result in blindness. Long-standing optic chiasmal pressure results in optic disc pallor.

Lateral invasion of pituitary lesions may invade the dural

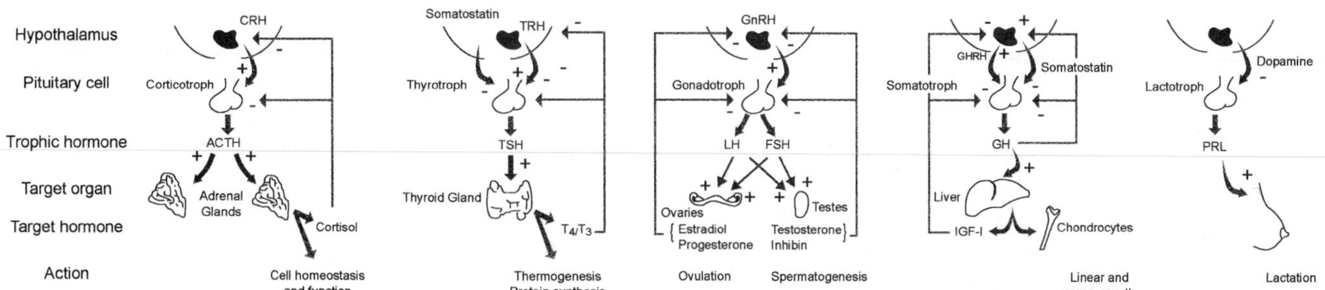

Figure 8–6. Control of hypothalamic-pituitary–target organ axes. (Reproduced from Melmed S. Disorders of anterior pituitary and hypothalamus. In Braunwald E, et al (eds). Harrison's Textbook of Medicine, 15th ed. New York, McGraw-Hill, 2001, p 2030.)

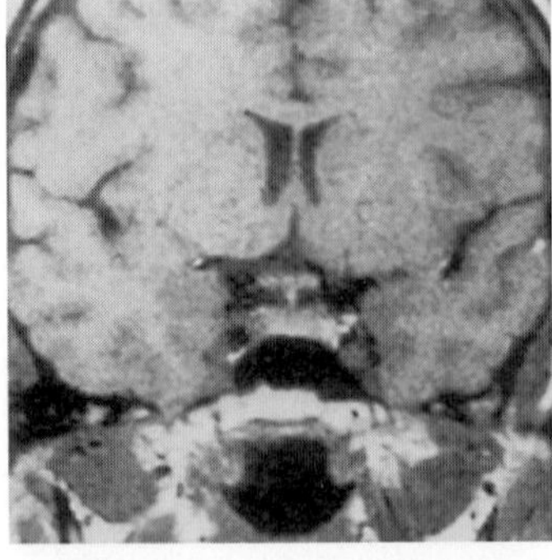

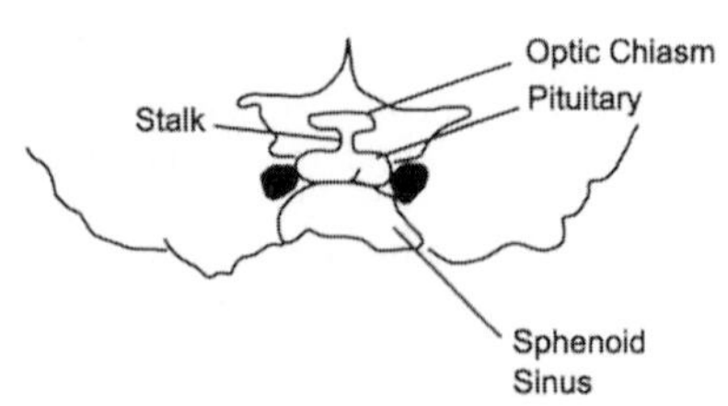

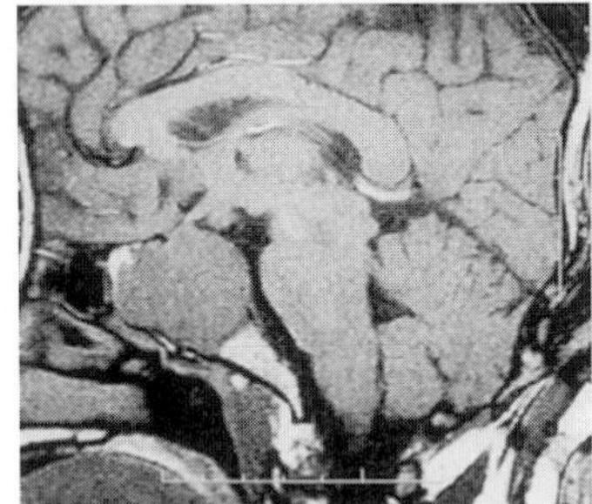

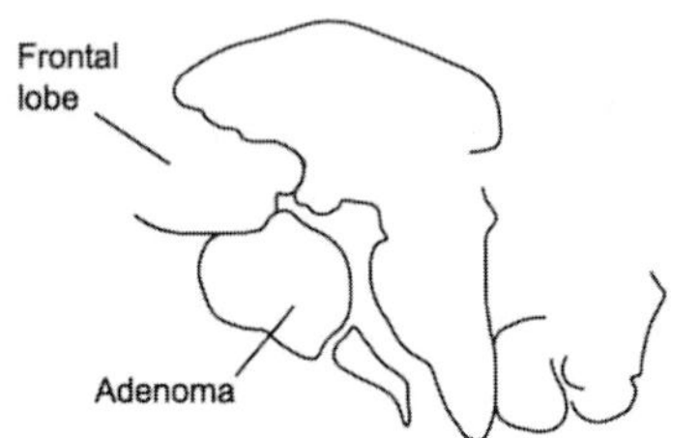

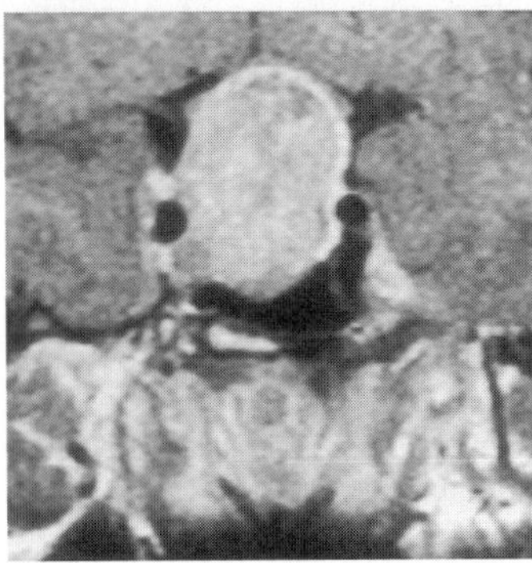

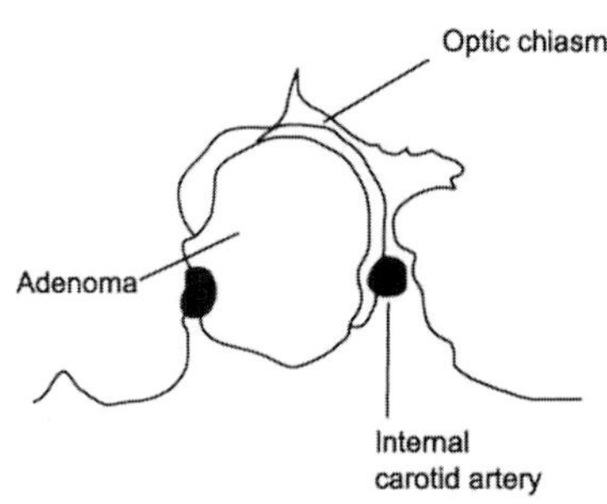

Figure 8–7. Magnetic resonance coronal section of a normal pituitary gland *(top)*. A large pituitary adenoma is seen lifting and distorting the optic chiasm *(arrow)* and is also invading the sphenoid sinus *(middle)*. A sagittal section of a large macroadenoma with bone invasion and impinging brain structures is shown *(bottom)*.

wall of the cavernous sinus affecting the third, fourth, and sixth cranial nerves as well as the ophthalmic and maxillary branches of the fifth cranial nerve and surround the internal carotid artery. Varying degrees of diplopia, ptosis, ophthalmoplegia, and decreased facial sensation may infrequently occur, depending on the extent of the neural involvement by the cavernous sinus mass. Downward extension into the sphenoid sinus indicates that the parasellar mass has eroded the bony sellar floor. Aggressive tumors may invade the roof of the palate and cause nasopharyngeal obstruction, infection, and CSF leakage. Infrequently, temporal or frontal lobes may be invaded, causing uncinate seizures, personality disorders, and anosmia. In addition to the anatomic lesions caused by the expanding mass, direct hypothalamic involvement of the encroaching mass may lead to important metabolic sequelae discussed in Chapter 7.

Patients with intrasellar tumors commonly present with headaches, even in the absence of demonstrable suprasellar extension. Small changes in intrasellar pressure caused by a microadenoma within the confined sella are sufficient to stretch the dural plate with resultant headache. Headache severity does not correlate with the size of the adenoma or the presence of suprasellar extension.[27] Relatively minor diaphragmatic distortions or dural impingement may be associated with persistent headache. Successful medical management of small functional pituitary tumors with dopamine agonists or somatostatin analogues is often accompanied by a remarkable improvement in or disappearance of headache.

Regardless of their etiology or size, pituitary masses, including adenomas, may be associated with compression of surrounding healthy tissue and resultant hypopituitarism. In 49 patients undergoing transsphenoidal resection of pituitary adenomas, mean intrasellar pressure was elevated twofold to threefold in patients with pituitary failure. Furthermore, prevalence of headache and elevated PRL levels correlated positively with intrasellar pressure levels,[28] suggesting interrupted portal delivery of hypothalamic hormones. Thus, surgical decompression of a sellar mass may lead to recovery of compromised anterior pituitary function. In the patients who do not recover pituitary function postoperatively, ischemic necrosis is likely to have occurred. Stalk compression may result in pituitary failure caused by encroachment of the portal vessels that normally provide pituitary access to the hypothalamic hormones. Stalk compression also usually leads to hyperprolactinemia and concomitant failure of other pituitary trophic hormones.

Pituitary Adenomas

Pathogenesis

Pituitary tumors account for about 15% of all intracranial neoplasms and are commonly encountered at autopsy. The Brain Tumor Registry of Japan reported that 15.8% of 28,424

Table 8–1. Local Effects of an Expanding Pituitary or Hypothalamic Mass

Affected Structure	Clinical Effect
Pituitary	Growth failure Adult hyposomatotrophism Hypogonadism Hypothyroidism Hypoadrenalism
Optic tract	Loss of red perception, bitemporal hemianopsia, superior or bitemporal field defect, scotoma, blindness
Hypothalamus	Temperature dysregulation, obesity, diabetes insipidus, thirst, sleep, appetite, behavioral and autonomic nervous system dysfunctions
Cavernous sinus	Ptosis, diplopia, ophthalmoplegia, facial numbness
Temporal lobe	Uncinate seizures
Frontal lobe	Personality disorder, anosmia
Central	Headache, hydrocephalus, psychosis, dementia, laughing seizures
Neuro-ophthalmologic tract	Field defects Bitemporal hemianopia (50%) Amaurosis with hemianopia (12%) Contralateral or monocular hemianopia (7%) Scotomas Junctional; monocular central, arcuate, altitudinal; hemianopic Homonymous hemianopia Acuity loss Snellen Contrast sensitivity Color vision Visual evoked potential Pupillary abnormality Impaired light reactivity Afferent defect Optic atrophy Papilledema Cranial nerve palsy—oculomotor, trachlear, abducens, sensory trigeminal Nystagmus Visual hallucinations Postfixation blindness

Adapted from Melmed S. In DeGroot LJ, Jameson JL (eds). Endocrinology. Philadelphia, WB Saunders, 2001; Arnold AC. Neuro-ophthalmologic evaluation of pituitary disorders. In Melmed S (ed) The Pituitary, 2nd ed. Malden, Mass, Blackwell Science, 2002, pp 687–708.

Table 8–2. Factors Involved in Pituitary Tumor Pathogenesis

Hereditary
- MEN-1
- Transcription factor defect (e.g., Prop-1 excess)
- Carney complex

Hypothalamic
- Excess GHRH or CRH production
- Receptor activation?
- Dopamine deprivation?

Pituitary
- Signal transduction mutations (e.g., gsp, CREB)
- Disrupted paracrine growth factor or cytokine action (e.g., FGF2, FGF4, LIF, EGF, NGF)
- Activated oncogene or cell cycle disruption (e.g., *PTTG*; *ras*; *p27*)
- Intrapituitary paracrine hypothalamic hormone action (e.g., GHRH, TRH)
- Loss of tumor suppressor gene function (11q13; 13)

Environmental
- Estrogens
- Irradiation

Peripheral
- Target failure (ovary, thyroid, adrenal)

CREB, cyclic adenosine monophosphate response element–binding protein; CRH, corticotropin-releasing hormone; EGF, epidermal growth factor; FGF, fibroblast growth factor; GHRH, growth hormone–releasing hormone; LIF, leukemia inhibitory factor; NGF, nerve growth factor; *PTTG*, primary tumor transforming gene; TRH, thyrotropin-releasing hormone.

Compiled from Heaney AP, Melmed S, PTTG: a novel factor in pituitary tumor formation. Baillieres Clin Endocrinol Metab 1999, 12:367.

cases were histologically confirmed pituitary adenomas.[29, 30] They are benign monoclonal adenomas that may express and secrete hormones autonomously, leading to hyperprolactinemia, acromegaly, and Cushing's disease, or may be functionally silent and initially diagnosed as a sellar mass. Although these adenomas are invariably benign, their neoplastic features represent a unique tumor biology that is reflected in their important local and systemic manifestations. These monoclonal neoplasms have a slow doubling time and, if small, may rarely resolve spontaneously. Nevertheless, they can be aggressive and locally invasive or compressive to vital central structures. They usually express a single gene product, but polyhormonal expression may reflect a primitive stem cell or mature bimorphous cellular origin.

Hypothalamic factors may have a specific role in the pathogenesis of pituitary tumors, in addition to regulating pituitary hormone gene expression and secretion (Table 8–2). Ectopic GHRH-secreting tumors (bronchial carcinoids, pancreatic islet cell tumors, or small cell lung carcinomas) result in GH hypersecretion, acromegaly, somatotroph hyperplasia, and occasionally somatotroph adenoma formation.[31, 32] In transgenic mice overexpressing a GHRH transgene, the pituitary size increased dramatically because of somatotroph hyperplasia, and older mice developed GH-secreting adenomas.[33] However, adenomatous hormonal secretion is usually independent of physiologic hypothalamic control, and the surgical resection of small well-defined adenomas usually results in definitive cure of hormonal hypersecretion. These observations imply that these tumors do not arise because of excessive polyclonal pituitary cell proliferation related to generalized hypothalamic stimulation.

Table 8–3. Candidate Genes in Pituitary Tumorigenesis

Gene	Protein	Tumor Type	Mechanism of Overexpression or Inactivaton	Function, Defect
Gsp	GNAS	40% GH-secreting tumors McCune-Albright syndrome Minority other types	Point mutation	Signal transduction, elevated cAMP
PTTG1	PTTG	All pituitary tumors	Unknown Estrogen?	Chromatid separation, regulates bFGF secretion, disrupted cell cycle, chromsomal instability, bFGF-mediated mitogenesis and angiogenesis
Hst	FGF4	Large prolactinomas	Unknown	Angiogenesis, overexpression Enhanced PRL transcription
CREB		GH-secreting	Increased Ser-phosphorylated CREB promoted by gsp overexpression	Dimerizes with cAMP response elements
H-ras	Ras	Metastatic pituitary carcinoma only	Point mutation, amplification	Signal transduction, stimulates tyrosine kinase pathway
Inactivating				
Men 1	Menin	Prolactinomas in familial MEN-1	11q13 loss of heterozygosity	Nuclear tumor suppressor, loss-of-function mutations
13q14	RB?	Highly invasive tumors	13q14 loss of heterozygosity	Inconsistent Rb protein loss, disrupted cell cycle regulation
CDKN2A	p16	All tumor types examined	Gene methylation leading to absent p16, allowing Rb phosphorylation and cell cycle progression	Cell cycle regulation, absent p16 protein leading to disrupted cell cycle regulation
CIP1/KIP1	p27	Transgenic mouse models	Gene methylation leading to absent p27	Regulate multiple CDK enzymes including CDK4/6-cyclin Ds, absent p27 protein

Adapted from Heaney AP, Melmed S. Molecular pathogenesis of pituitary tumors. In Wass J (ed). Oxford Textbook of Endocrinology: Endocrine-Related Career. New York, Oxford University Press, 2002.

However, hypothalamic factors may promote and maintain growth of already transformed pituitary adenomatous cells.

Normal and hyperplastic pituitary tissues are polyclonal, and pituitary adenomas arise as the result of monoclonal pituitary cell proliferation. Using X-chromosomal inactivation analysis, the monoclonal origin of adenomas secreting GH, PRL,[34] and ACTH[35, 36] and nonfunctioning pituitary tumors was confirmed in female patients heterozygous for variant alleles of the X-linked genes hypoxanthine phosphoribosyltransferase (*HPRT*) and phosphoglycerate kinase (*PGK*). Thus, an intrinsic somatic pituitary cell genetic alteration probably gives rise to clonal expansion of a single cell, resulting in adenoma formation (Table 8–3).

Activating *gsp* mutations are present in up to 40% of human GH-secreting adenomas.[37–39] These somatic heterozygous activating point mutations of the G protein α subunit (Gsα) gene involving either arginine 201 (replaced by cysteine or histidine) or glutamine 227 (replaced with arginine or leucine) constitutively activate the Gsα protein and convert it into an oncogene (*gsp*). This G protein activation increases cyclic adenosine monophosphate (cAMP) levels and activates protein kinase A, which in turn phosphorylates the cAMP response element–binding protein (CREB) and leads to sustained constitutive GH hypersecretion and cell proliferation. The *gsp*-bearing adenomas are smaller, have mildly lower GH levels and enhanced intratumoral cAMP, do not respond briskly to GHRH, and are extremely sensitive to the inhibitory effect of somatostatin.[39] These *gsp* activating mutations do not occur in PRL-secreting or in TSH-producing adenomas and are rarely present in nonfunctioning pituitary tumors or ACTH-secreting tumors (<10%).

Similar early postzygotic somatic mutations in codon 201 of Gsα were identified in tissues derived from patients with McCune-Albright syndrome, including GH-producing pituitary adenomas.[40] Transgenic mice overexpressing inactive pituitary CREB mutant exhibited a dwarf phenotype and somatotroph hypoplasia.[41] Thus, cAMP probably stimulates somatotroph proliferation by CREB phosphorylation. This was borne out by the observation that 15 human GH-secreting pituitary adenomas contained elevated levels of phosphorylated CREB.[42] However, only four of these tumors also contained the mutant *gsp* oncogene, and CREB phosphorylation was also demonstrated in adenomas overexpressing wild-type Gsα protein, suggesting a role of CREB independent of G protein actions.

Ras mutations are rare in pituitary adenomas. H-*ras* gene mutations were identified in an invasive prolactinoma[43] and in distant metastatic pituitary carcinomas but not in their respective primary pituitary tumors or in noninvasive adenomas.[44, 45] Thus, *ras* genetic alterations may be important in the rare progression to metastasis formation and growth. Pituitary tumor transforming gene (*PTTG*) was isolated from experimental pituitary tumors and shown to be highly abundant in all pituitary tumor types, especially prolactinomas.[46, 47] *PTTG*, a mammalian securin homologue, also induces FGF production and angiogenesis and is up-regulated by estrogen.[48] *PTTG* overexpression may lead to dysregulated separation and cell aneuploidy.[49, 50]

Multiple endocrine neoplasia type 1 (MEN-1) is an autosomal dominant hereditary disorder characterized by combined tumor formation or hyperfunction of pancreatic islets and anterior pituitary and, less commonly, carcinoid, thyroid, and adrenal tumors. The MEN-1 syndrome is fully described in Chapter 36. Unlike those in pituitary tumors constituting the MEN-1 syndrome, MEN-1 gene mutations were not identified in familial pituitary adenomas.[51, 52] Patients with sporadic pituitary adenomas do not demonstrate germ line or somatic pathogenic changes in the coding sequence of the MEN-1 gene, even in tumors with loss of heterozygosity of 11q13, and only two cases of sporadic pituitary adenomas (of 94 tumors stud-

Table 8–4. Genetic Syndromes Involving Pituitary Tumors

Syndrome	Clinical Features	Chromosomal Location	Gene	Protein	Proposed Function, Defect
Multiple endocrine neoplasia type 1 (MEN-1)	Parathyroid, endocrine pancreas, anterior pituitary (mostly prolactinomas) tumors	11q13	*Men1*	Menin	Nuclear, tumor suppressor protein interacts with junD
Familial acromegaly	GH-cell adenomas, acromegaly, gigantism	11q13 and other loci	Not *Men1*	—	—
McCune-Albright syndrome	Polyostotic fibrous dysplasia, pigmented skin patches; endocrine abnormalities: precocious puberty, GH-cell adenomas, acromegaly, gigantism, Cushing's syndrome	20q13.2 (mosaic)	*GNAS1* (*gsp*)	Gs α	Signal transduction, inactive GTPase results in constitutive cAMP elevation independent of GHRH
Carney, syndrome	Skin and cardiac myxomas, Cushing's syndrome, acromegaly	2p16	—	—	Protein kinase A signaling defect for activating GH

Adapted from Prezant TR, Melmed S. Pituitary oncogenes. In Webb S (ed). Pituitary Tumors: Epidemiology, Pathogenesis, and Management. Bristol, UK, Bioscientifica, 1998, pp 81–94.

ied) had specific MEN-1 mutations.[53, 54] Thus, MEN-1 gene mutations do not appear to play a role in pituitary tumorigenesis in most sporadic adenomas.

Loss of heterozygosity for chromosomes 11q13, 13, and 9 has been observed in about 15% of spontaneous pituitary adenomas, often correlating with tumor size and invasiveness. However, no distinct tumor suppressor gene has been identified for sporadic pituitary tumors. Loss of heterozygosity in proximity to the retinoblastoma (RB) locus on chromosome 13q14 was detected in malignant or highly invasive pituitary tumors and in their metastases, but immunohistochemical studies have shown the presence of RB protein in these malignant tumors with 13q14 allelic loss,[55] suggesting that the RB gene itself is not involved in pituitary adenoma development and that another suppressor gene located adjacent to the RB locus may play a role in invasive or malignant pituitary tumorigenesis. *p53* gene mutations were not detected in secreting and nonsecreting pituitary tumors or in pituitary carcinomas and their metastases.[45, 56]

Although no mutations in the GHRH, corticotropin-releasing hormone (CRH), thyrotropin-releasing hormone (TRH), or gonadotropin-releasing hormone (GnRH) receptor have been identified in pituitary adenomas,[57, 58] several GH-secreting adenomas express an alternatively spliced truncated GHRH receptor.[59] The insulin-like growth factor I (IGF-I) receptor β subunit in GH cell adenomas exhibited intact regions of the receptor critical for signal transduction.[60] The dopamine D2 receptor gene appears intact in PRL-producing and TSH-producing or nonfunctioning adenomas.[61] Therefore, there is no apparent role of pituitary cell surface receptor mutations of hypothalamic releasing and inhibitory factors in pituitary tumorigenesis.

FGF-2 (basic FGF) is expressed in pituitary tissues and induces basal and stimulated PRL secretion from normal and pituitary adenoma cells.[62, 63] Human pituitary adenomas express FGF-4, and transfected FGF-4 enhances PRL secretion[64–66] and tumor vascularity. FGF-4 is immunodetected in about a third of prolactinomas and is undetectable in normal pituitaries and other adenoma types.

Carney's complex is an autosomal dominant disorder comprising benign mesenchymal tumors including cardiac myxomas, schwannomas, and thyroid and pituitary adenomas associated with spotty skin pigmentation (Table 8–4).[67] The disorder has been mapped to chromosome 17q24 and results from a mutated RIα regulatory subunit of the cAMP-dependent protein kinase A (PRKARIA), an apparent tumor suppressor gene.[68]

In summary, multifactorial mechanisms subserve the multistep pathogenetic process of pituitary adenoma formation, including early initiating chromosomal mutations that result in mutated pituitary stem cells (see Table 8–2). The transformed pituitary cell is subjected to signals facilitating clonal expansion, and several permissive factors, including hypothalamic hormone receptor signals, intrapituitary growth factors, and disordered cell cycle regulation, may determine the ultimate biologic fate of the tumor. Autonomous anterior pituitary hormone production and secretion and cell proliferation, which are the hallmarks of pituitary adenomas, result. However, the subcellular events initiating the formation of most secreting and nonfunctional pituitary adenomas have not yet been elucidated.

Classification

Pituitary tumors arise from hormone-secreting adenohypophyseal cells, and their secretory products depend on the cell of origin (Table 8–5). Previously clinically inapparent pituitary adenomas are found in about 11% of autopsies (Table 8–6). They are often localized to unique areas of the gland, reflecting relative cell type abundance and intragland distribution (Fig. 8–8). Radiologic and surgical classifications are based on tumor localization, size, and degree of invasiveness (Fig. 8–9). Microadenomas are intrasellar and generally less than 10 mm in widest diameter. Macroadenomas are larger than 10 mm and usually impinge on adjacent sellar structures. Specific tumor types are considered subsequently for each respective cell type.

Immunocytochemistry detects pituitary cell gene products at both the light and electron microscopic level and allows classification of pituitary tumors on the basis of their function. Unlike the corticotroph, somatotroph, lactotroph, and thyrotroph cell tumors, which hypersecrete their respective hormones,[69] gonadotroph cell tumors are usually clinically silent and do not secrete their gene products efficiently.[70] Double immunostaining identifies mixed tumors expressing combinations of hormones, which are often macroadenomas secreting GH concomitantly with PRL, TSH, or ACTH. Generally, immunohistochemical identification of pituitary hormones correlates with tumor-specific messenger ribonucleic acid (mRNA) markers measured either in whole tissue extracts by Northern analysis or at the single-cell level by in situ hybridization techniques. With the exception of the glycoprotein α subunit, immunohistochemical positivity of more than 5% of cells making up the tumor is usually reflective of peripheral circulating hor-

Table 8–5. Clinical and Pathologic Characteristics of Pituitary Adenomas

Adenoma Type	Incidence (%) Pathologic	Incidence (%) Clinical	Incidence (new cases/ 10^6/yr)	Prevalence (total/ 10^6)	mRNA Expression	Immunohistochemistry	EM Secretory Granules (nm)	Clinical Syndrome
Lactotroph		29	6–10	60–100				
Sparsely granulated	28				PRL	PRL	150–500	Hypogonadism,
Densely granulated	1				PRL	PRL	400–1200	galactorrhea
Somatotroph		15	4–6	40–60				
Sparsely granulated	5				GH	GH	100–250	Acromegaly or
Densely granulated	5				GH	GH	300–700	gigantism
Combined		8						
GH/PRL cells	5				GH, PRL	GH, PRL	100–600	Hypogonadism
Mixed GH/PRL	1				GH, PRL	GH, PRL	350–2000	Acromegaly
Mammosomatotroph								
Acidophil stem cell	3				GH, PRL	GH, PRL	50–300	Galactorrhea
Corticotroph			2–3	20–30				
Cushing's	10	10			POMC	ACTH	250–700	Cushing's disease
Silent corticotroph	3	6			POMC	ACTH	Variable	None
Nelson's	2				POMC	ACTH	250–700	Local signs
Thyrotroph	1	0.9			TSH	TSH	50–250	Hyperthyroidism
Plurihormonal	10	4			GH, PRL	GH, PRL, glycoprotein	Mixed	Mixed
Nonfunctioning, null cell, gonadotroph		27	7–9	70–90				
Nononcocytic	14				FSH, LH αSU	Glycoprotein	<25% of cells 100–250	Silent or pituitary failure
Oncocytic	6				FSH, LH αSU	Glycoprotein	<25% of cells 100–250 many mitochondria	Pituitary failure
Gonadotroph	7–15				FSH, LH	FSH, LH	50–200	Silent or pituitary failure

Data are derived from studying a relatively stable 1 million catchment population surrounding Stoke-on-Trent, UK (Clayton RN, Clin Endo & Metab 13:451, 1999), and from Kovacs & Horvath 1986; Scheithauer 1994; Minderman & Wilson, Clin Endo 1994; Asa 1993. In Endocrine Tumours, Blackwell).

mone levels. Quantification of immunostaining intensity is subjective, and a scale of intensity should also include a description of the extent of staining, that is, whether occasional, scattered, or most tumor cells express the immunodetectable protein.

Electron microscopy is useful for assessing the ultrastructure of hormone secretory granules and their size and distribution. Other subcellular features important for diagnosis include large mitochondria in nonfunctioning oncocytomas and the secretory nature of Golgi and endoplasmic reticulum, especially for prolactinomas. Peroxidase or colloid gold particles of different diameters are also sensitive electron microscopic markers for identifying and localizing intracellular hormone signals. Because even invasive pituitary tumors grow slowly, use of mitotic markers including proliferating cell nuclear antigen (PCNA) and Ki-67 is of limited utility.[71]

Other Parasellar Masses

Clinical features of hypothalamic masses are fully described in Chapter 7, and parasellar masses (Table 8–7) are described here.[72]

Rathke's Cyst

The anterior and intermediate lobes of the pituitary gland arise embryologically from Rathke's pouch. Inadequate pouch obliteration results in the cysts or cystic remnants at the interface between the anterior and posterior pituitary lobes found in about 20% of pituitary glands at autopsy (Fig. 8–10).[73] Pituitary adenomas may also occasionally contain small cleft cysts.[74] They are lined by cuboidal or columnar ciliated epithelium surrounding mucoid cyst fluid, arise from midline rudiments of failed Rathke's cyst invagination, and account for about 3% of pituitary mass lesions.[75] In contrast, pituitary epidermoid cysts are lined by squamous epithelium, which rarely becomes malignant.

Rathke's cysts vary in size and may also extend to the suprasellar region. These lesions have heterogeneous MRI characteristics and may arise with panhypopituitarism with or without diabetes insipidus.[71] Most, however, are not symptomatic and should be observed expectantly. The extent of headache or visual disturbance is determined by the size and location of the cyst. Cyst formation is associated with sellar enlargement and hyperdense or hypodense masses seen on either T1-weighted or T2-weighted MR images, and computed tomography (CT) shows homogeneous hypodense areas that may be distinguished from pituitary adenomas.[71] These patients should all be evaluated for hypopituitarism. After surgical resection or drainage, MRI should be performed during long-term follow-up for signs of cyst recurrence.[73, 75]

Arachnoid, epidermoid, and dermoid cysts develop mainly in the cerebellopontine angle but may also arise in the suprasellar region. Dermoid cysts containing greasy sebaceous products or hair follicles are rarely encountered in the pituitary, and the cyst lining may be calcified. Acquired pituitary cysts may be secondary to intrapituitary hemorrhage, usually associated with an underlying adenoma, and these rarely cause pituitary fail-

Table 8–6. Frequency of Pituitary Adenomas Found at Autopsy

Study	No. of Pituitaries Examined	No. of Adenomas Found	Frequency (%)
Susman	260	23	9
Costello	1000	225	23
Sommers	400	26	7
McCormick	1600	140	9
Kovacs	152	20	13
Landolt	100	13	13
Mosca	100	24	24
Burrow	120	32	27
Parent	500	42	8
Muhr	205	3	2
Schwezinger	5100	485	9
Coulon	100	10	10
Chambers	100	14	14
Siqueira	450	39	9
El-Hamid	486	97	20
Scheithauer	251	41	16
Marin	210	35	16
Mosca	111	13	11
Sano	166	15	9
Teramoto	1000	51	5
Total	**12,411**	**1408**	**11**

Adapted from Molitch ME. Pituitary incidentalomas. In de Herder WW (ed). Functional and Morphological Imaging of the Endocrine System. Boston, Kluwer, 2000, pp 59–70.

ure.[76] Cyst compression causes internal hydrocephalus, visual disturbances, GH or ACTH deficiency, hyperprolactinemia, and diabetes insipidus. Rarely, squamous cell carcinoma may arise in the cyst.[77]

Granular Cell Tumors

Pituitary choristomas, or schwannomas, usually arise only after the age of 20. Their abundant cytoplasmic granules do not contain pituitary hormones, but these lesions may occur with diabetes insipidus. Pituitary adenomas are occasionally coincidentally associated with these tumors.[78]

Chordomas

These slow-growing cartilaginous tumors arise from midline notochord remnants, are locally invasive, and may metastasize.[79] Most arise from the vertebrae, and about one third involve the clivus region. Chordomas contain a mucin-rich matrix that allows diagnosis by fine-needle aspiration. Patients present with headaches, asymmetric visual disturbances, hormone deficiency, and occasional nasopharyngeal obstruction. The tumor mass is associated with osteolytic bone erosion and calcification, and MRI may allow the normal pituitary gland to be distinguished from the very heterogeneous and often flocculent tumor mass. At surgery, the tumors are rough, heterogeneous, and lobular. Markers for epithelial cells, including cytokeratin and vimentin, are present. Recurrences are common after surgical excision, and mean survival of patients is about 5 years. Rarely, chordomas undergo sarcomatous transformation with an aggressive natural history and require extensive surgical dissection.[80]

Craniopharyngiomas

This parasellar tumor constitutes about 3% of all intracranial tumors and up to 10% of childhood brain tumors. The tumor is commonly diagnosed during childhood and adolescence. Tumors arise from embryonic squamous remnants of Rathke's pouch extending dorsally toward the diencephalon; they may be large (>10 cm in diameter) and invade the third ventricle and associated brain structures. Over 60% arise from within the sella, with others arising from parasellar cell rests.[81–83] When intrasellar, they can often be distinguished from pituitary adenomas by a separate visible rim of normal pituitary tissue seen on MRI. The cystic mass is usually filled with cholesterol-rich viscous fluid, which may leak into the CSF and cause aseptic meningitis. The tumors may also contain calcifications and immunoreactive human chorionic gonadotropin (hCG).

Histologically, these tumors comprise two cell populations; cysts are lined with a squamous epithelium containing islands characterized by columnar cells, and a mixed inflammatory reaction may also occur with calcification. Although large craniopharyngiomas may obstruct CSF flow, they rarely undergo malignant transformation. Increased intracranial pressure results in headache, projectile vomiting, papilledema, and somnolence, especially in children. Only about one third of patients are older than 40 years, and they commonly present with asymmetric visual disturbances, including papilledema, optic atrophy, and field deficits. If cavernous sinus invasion is present, other cranial nerves may also be involved.

On CT imaging, most children and about half of all adults exhibit characteristic flocculent or convex calcifications. Rarely, however, pituitary adenomas, other parasellar tumors, and vascular lesions within the sella are also calcified. In contrast to pituitary adenomas, which rarely cause diabetes insipidus, craniopharyngiomas are often associated with this disorder as the earliest feature. These patients may also experience partial or complete pituitary deficiency. GH deficiency, with short stature and diabetes insipidus, and gonadal failure are common. Pituitary stalk compression or damage to hypothalamic dopaminergic neurons results in hyperprolactinemia. Thus, a craniopharyngioma may mimic a prolactinoma in terms of intrapituitary imaging, presence of hyperprolactinemia, and favorable biochemical response to dopamine agonists.

The treatment of these lesions may involve radical surgery, radiotherapy, or a combination of these modalities.[83] Stereotactic radiation has some success. A detailed discussion of the neurosurgical management of this disorder is beyond the scope of this text. Nevertheless, regardless of the form of therapy chosen, ablation of the mass invariably results in anterior or posterior pituitary hormone deficits. Postoperative recurrence may occur in about 20% of patients undergoing radical surgical excision, and there is no difference in outcome in those who undergo a subtotal surgical excision followed by radiotherapy. Pure papillary squamous cellular elements in the tumor may portend a higher surgical recurrence rate. Long-term effects of childhood radiation for these tumors are considered elsewhere (Chapter 23).

Meningiomas

Meningiomas arise from arachnoid and meningioendothelial cells, and those occurring in the sellar and parasellar region account for about one fifth of all meningiomas.[84] Sellar meningiomas are usually well circumscribed and do not attain the size of craniopharyngiomas. Suprasellar meningiomas may invade the pituitary ventrally, and intrasellar tumor origins are rare.[85] Coexisting functional pituitary adenomas have been described in patients with parasellar meningiomas. Secondary hyperprolactinemia occurs in up to half of patients, who usually present with local mass effects including headache and progressive visual disturbances accompanied by optic atrophy.

The differential distinction between a suprasellar menin-

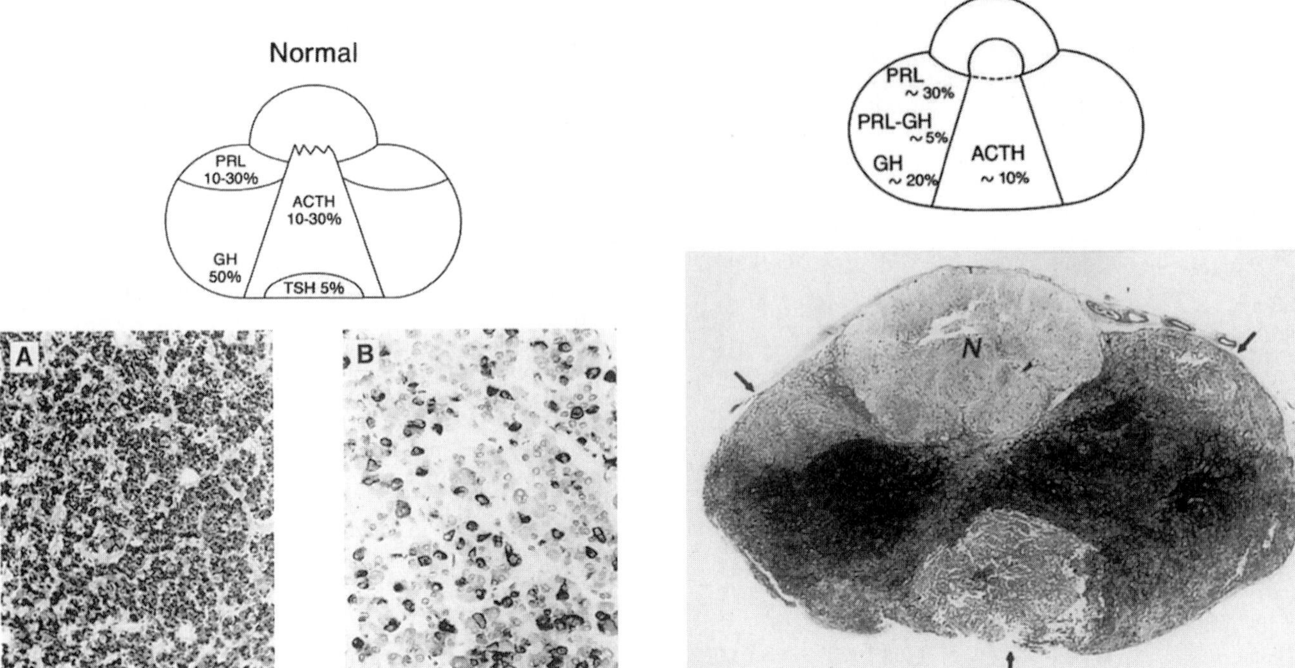

Figure 8–8. Schematic of the distribution of normal adenohypophyseal cells is reflected in that of pituitary adenomas. Nonfunctioning tumors, however, are typically macroadenomas that efface pituitary landmarks. The localization and frequency of functioning microadenomas reflect the maximal concentration of their corresponding normal pituitary cells. (From Scheithauer BW, Horvath E, Lloyd RV, Kovacs K. Pathology of pituitary adenomas and pituitary hyperplasia. In Thapar K, Kovacs K, Scheithauer BW, Lloyd RV [eds]. Diagnosis and Management of Pituitary Tumors. Totowa, NJ, Humana Press, 2001, pp 91–154.)

gioma with downward extension and an upwardly extending pituitary adenoma may be difficult. With MRI, meningiomas are isodense on both T1 and T2 imaging, in contrast to other parasellar lesions, which are usually hyperdense on T2 imaging. Dural calcification may be evident on CT scanning. Because of their rich vascularization, these tumors pose an intraoperative risk for hemorrhage and a resultant higher surgical mortality rate than usually encountered for pituitary adenoma resection.

Gliomas

Optic gliomas and low-grade astrocytomas arise from within the optic chiasm or optic tract and often infiltrate the optic nerve; less than one third are intraorbital. Von Recklinghausen's disease is the underlying cause in about one third of the patients. These tumors may occasionally be associated with growth retardation, delayed or precocious puberty, and mass effects including visual disturbances, diencephalic syndrome, diabetes insipidus, and hydrocephalus. Rarely, gliomas arise within the sella associated with hyperprolactinemia, and they should be considered in the uncommon differential diagnosis of a PRL-secreting pituitary adenoma.[86] Important distinguishing features include the young age of these patients (80% are younger than 10 years), relatively intact pituitary function, gross visual disturbances, and localization of the mass as visualized on MRI. Gliomas, unlike hamartomas, are usually enhanced after injection of contrast material.

Mucocele

Mucoceles are expanding accumulations of fluid within the sphenoid sinus and may compress parasellar structures. Headaches, visual disturbances (usually unilateral), and exophthalmos are characteristic features. On MRI, the homogeneous sphenoid mass may be quite prominent but may be distinguished from the pituitary gland dorsally.

Parasellar Aneurysms

Parasellar aneurysms may mimic pituitary adenomas and intraoperative rupture may be catastrophic, underlying the absolute need for preoperative diagnosis. Differentiating features of aneurysms from other pituitary masses may be subtle, including eye pain, intense headaches, and relatively sudden onset of cranial nerve palsies. Although imaging techniques usually distinguish blood and hemorrhage from solid tumor or tissue, a highly vascular meningioma may be confused with an aneurysm.

Pituitary Infections

Acute pituitary abscesses and perisellar arachnoiditis are encountered with sinus infections, especially after transsphenoidal surgery. Pituitary abscess may develop from hematogenous or direct local spread of infectious agents.[87] Abscesses may arise within a preexisting pituitary adenoma[88] and may be difficult to distinguish from an adenoma because these patients may not have fever or signs of meningitis.[89] On MRI imaging, an isointense central cavity with surrounding ring enhancement is characteristic of an abscess.[90]

Gram-positive streptococci or staphylococci may originate from nasopharyngeal passages.[89] Disseminated *Entamoeba histolytica* and *Pneumocystis carinii* may also seed to the pituitary.[91] Immunosuppressed patients may experience pituitary infections including cytomegalovirus infection, toxoplasmosis, aspergillosis, histoplasmosis, and coccidiosis. Syphilitic gumma may also

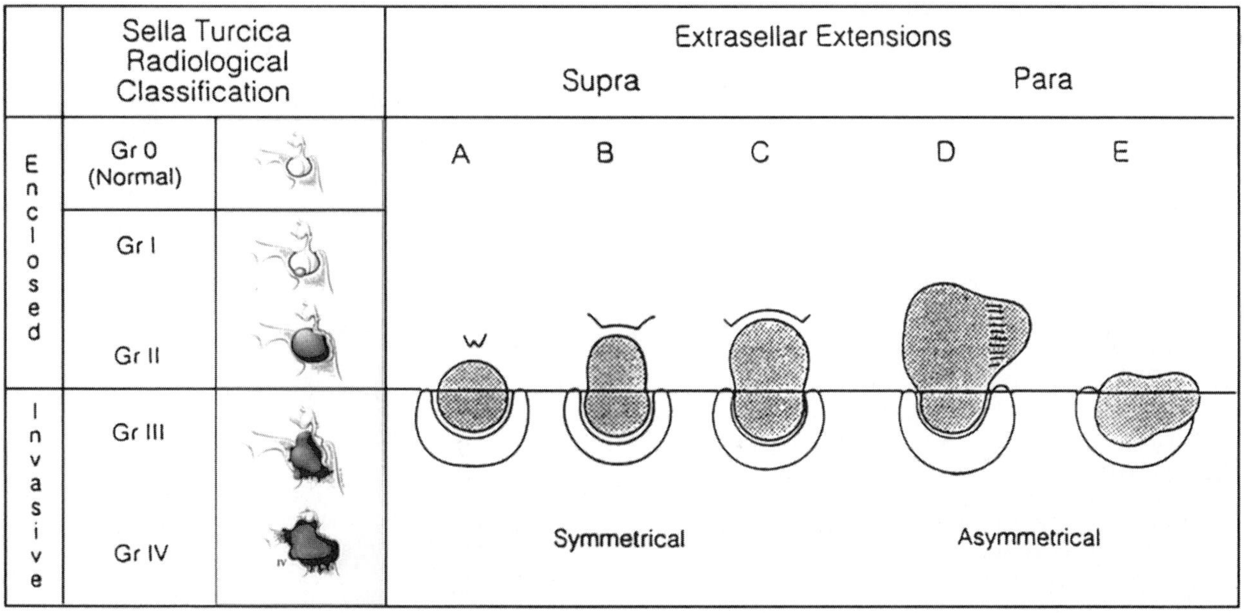

	Sella Turcica Radiological Classification		Extrasellar Extensions: Supra	Para
Enclosed	Gr 0 (Normal)		A B C	D E
	Gr I			
	Gr II			
Invasive	Gr III			
	Gr IV		Symmetrical	Asymmetrical

Hardy Classification of Pituitary Tumors

Radiologic	Anatomic	Surgical
Sella Turcica		
Grade 0	Intact, normal contour	Micro enclosed
Grade I	Intact, focal bulging	Micro enclosed
Grade II	Intact, enlarged	Macro enclosed
Grade III	Destroyed, partially	Macro invasive
Grade IV	Destroyed, totally	Macro invasive
Grade V	Distant spread via CSF or blood	Macro carcinoma

Extrasellar Extensions

Suprasellar *(Symmetrical)*	
A	Suprasellar cistern
B	Recesses of III ventricle
C	Whole anterior III ventricle
Parasellar *(Asymmetrical)*	
D	Intracranial intradural Anterior Midline Posterior
E	Extracranial extradural (lateral cavernous sinus)

Figure 8–9. Classification of pituitary tumors. (Adapted from Thapar K, Laws ER. Growth hormone–secreting pituitary tumors: operative management. In Krisht AF, Tindall GT [eds]. Pituitary Disorders. Philadelphia, Lippincott Williams & Wilkins, 1999; and Asa SL. In Tumors of the Pituitary Gland. Pituitary Adenomas. Atlas of Tumor Pathology. Washington, DC, Armed Forces Institute of Pathology, 1998, p 51.)

lead to pituitary damage and insufficiency. Common viral infections, including influenza, measles, mumps, and herpes, are rarely associated with pituitary damage and insufficiency. Although tuberculosis is rarely confined to the pituitary gland, most of the fewer than 20 reported patients exhibited suprasellar extension of the pituitary mass, compromised pituitary function, and visual defects.[92–94] Although evidence for systemic tuberculosis is usually present, isolated *sellar tuberculomas* have been described.

Hematologic Malignancies

Primary central nervous system lymphomas are usually B-cell non-Hodgkin's types, and nine such patients with pituitary lymphoma have been described.[95, 96] The pituitary mass may be an isolated presentation of the underlying disease. The disorder is usually diagnosed by histologic examination of tissue obtained by excision biopsy. Six of nine patients had headache, and five had cranial nerve abnormalities with varying degrees of hypopituitarism. MRI reveals cavernous sinus invasion and isointense T1-weighted and T2-weighted images that are enhanced by gadolinium. Patients with solitary pituitary plasmacytomas have been reported who did not have classical multiple myeloma. Acute lymphoblastic leukemia may be associated with periglandular pituitary infiltrates with minimal pituitary dysfunction.

Pituitary Granulomas

Sarcoidosis

Infiltrative sarcoidosis of the hypothalamic-pituitary region occurs in most patients with central nervous system sarcoid involvement. These patients may present with varying degrees of anterior pituitary failure with or without diabetes insipidus.[97] Hypothalamic granulomatous involvement is commonly encountered in patients with central nervous system sarcoidosis and may be the sole manifestation of the disease.[98] The hypothalamus, pituitary stalk, and posterior pituitary are diffusely invaded by noncaseating granulomas, consisting of giant cells, macrophages, and lymphocytes.[99] Sarcoidosis may be progressive and eventually result in pituitary damage and even an empty sella. Onset of diabetes insipidus with no obvious features of a pituitary disorder should alert the physician to exclude hypothalamic sarcoid deposits, especially in the presence of a thickened stalk on MRI.[100]

Hand-Schüller-Christian Disease

Hand-Schüller-Christian disease (histiocytosis X) may comprise sleep disorders, adipsia, and morbid obesity. Other features of granulomatous involvement, including axillary skin rash, history of recurrent pneumothorax, and classical bone lesions, should be sought, especially in young patients with

Table 8–7. Parasellar Masses

Genetic
Transcription factor mutations (e.g., PROP-1)
Cysts
Rathke's
Arachnoid
Epidermoid
Dermoid
Tumors
Hormone-secreting or nonfunctional pituitary adenoma
Granular cell tumor
Craniopharyngioma
Chordoma
Meningioma
Sarcomas
Glioma
Schwannoma
Germ cell tumor
Vascular tumor
Solid or hematologic metastases
Malformation and Hamartomas
Ectopic pituitary, neurohypophyseal, or salivary tissue
Hypothalamic hamartoma
Gangliocytoma
Miscellaneous Lesions
Aneurysms
Hypophysitis
Infections
Sarcoidosis
Giant cell granuloma
Histiocytosis X

new-onset diabetes insipidus.[101] The disorder may be associated with granulomatous damage to the hypothalamus or posterior pituitary, or both, with characteristic diabetes insipidus.[102] The pituitary lesions consist of dendritic Langerhans cells, and pituitary MRI may reveal stalk thickening or a diminished posterior pituitary bright spot.[103] Adults with the disorder should be carefully evaluated for anterior pituitary hormone deficits, which should be appropriately replaced.

Metastases to the Pituitary Region

Pituitary metastases are found in up to 3.5% of patients with cancer.[104, 105] As the vascular supply to the posterior pituitary is derived directly from the systemic circulation through the internal carotid arteries, the posterior pituitary is the preferred site for blood-borne metastatic spread. Carcinomas that metastasize to the pituitary include breast, lung, and gastrointestinal tract cancers. Up to one quarter of patients with metastatic breast cancer have pituitary metastases. Symptomatic pituitary metastases (usually diabetes insipidus) may be the presenting sign of occult malignancy and of malignancy of unknown origin. Rarely, isolated metastatic stalk deposits may also occur with pituitary failure.

If extensive bone erosion is present and disease onset is rapid, the diagnosis is more readily apparent. However, pituitary imaging may not clearly distinguish metastatic deposits from a pituitary adenoma, these lesions may masquerade as an adenoma, and the diagnosis is made only by histologic study of the resected specimen.[106] When the diagnosis is clear-cut in the presence of a primary cancer, relatively low-dose pituitary radiation may be sufficient to shrink the metastasis and decrease morbidity.

Iron storage diseases, including hemochromatosis and hemosiderosis, result in predominantly gonadotroph cell damage.

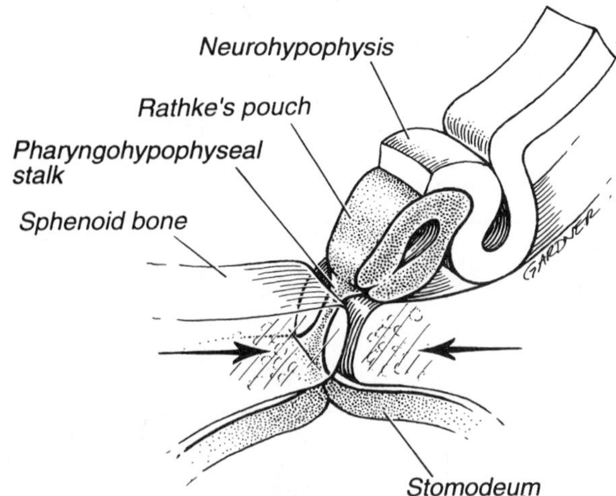

Figure 8–10. Pathogenesis of Rathke's cysts. Schematic of the embryologic progenitors of sellar and parasellar structures. Rathke's pouch arises from an outpocketing of stomodeum (ectoderm) and gives rise to the adenohypophysis. The pharyngohypophyseal stalk, which connects the stomodeum and Rathke's pouch, is divided by the sphenoid bone as it grows together *(arrows)*, isolating Rathke's pouch and the neurohypophysis within the sella. (From Harrison MJ, Morgello S, Post KD. Epithelial cystic lesions of the sellular and parasellular region: a continuum of ectodermal derivates? J Neurosurg 1994; 80: 1018-1025.)

Idiopathic retroperitoneal fibrosis may also be associated with a suprasellar mass and hypothalamic panhypopituitarism.[107]

Primary Hypophysitis

Pituitary mass lesions composed of inflammatory cells may arise as primary disorders exclusively confined to the hypophysis. At least three distinct clinicopathologic forms have been described.

Lymphocytic Hypophysitis

This apparently autoimmune inflammatory disorder occurs predominantly during pregnancy or in postpartum women[108] but has also been reported after menopause,[109] and about 15% of reported cases occurred in men.[110, 111] Of the disorders that develop in association with pregnancy, about 50% occur during the first 6 postpartum months.[112] The disorder is characterized by a lymphocytic and plasma cell pituitary infiltrate, which may be isolated or associated with other recognized endocrinopathies. Circulating antipituitary antibodies have occasionally been reported, and the presence of isolated pituitary hormone deficiency may imply an autoimmune process selectively targeted to pituitary cell types.

Although the natural history is often brief, the few comprehensive pathologic evaluations suggest that secondary adenohypophyseal cell atrophy, with a resultant empty sella, is a frequent outcome. Pathologic criteria for diagnosis include islands of anterior pituitary cells surrounded by diffuse lymphocytic (T-cell and B-cell) infiltrates. Over 125 cases have been reported, and the diagnosis has been definitively confirmed by histology in only about 10%.[113] Some patients have been reported with lymphocytic, plasma cell, and macrophage infiltrates ultimately resulting in cell destruction, fibrosis, and an irreversible chronic hypophysitis.[112]

Clinical Features. More than half the patients present with headache and visual field impairment, and pituitary deficiency accounts for the remaining cases (Table 8–8). MRI reveals a

Table 8-8. Features of Lymphocytic Hypophysitis

Feature	Frequency (%)
Pituitary enlargement	80–95
Headache, visual disturbances	55–70
Hypopituitarism	63–68
Hyperprolactinemia	20–38
Associated autoimmune disease	30
Diabetes insipidus	14–19

pituitary mass, often indistinguishable from an adenoma. An associated partially empty sella and contrast enhancement of the pituitary mass may be helpful in distinguishing MRI features.[114] The inflammatory process often resolves with time, and pituitary function may be restored or remain chronically compromised. Limited numbers of patients have been reported with histologically proven lymphocytic hypophysitis and documented spontaneous regression of pituitary mass on follow-up imaging. In two patients with histologically proven hypophysitis, spontaneous resolution of the pituitary mass was followed by subsequent successful pregnancies.[115, 116] Diabetes insipidus, encountered in 20% of patients, may be attributed to posterior pituitary or stalk infiltration.[117] In one third of patients, other autoimmune conditions, including thyroiditis, hypoadrenalism, parathyroid failure, atrophic gastritis, systemic lupus erythematosus, and Sjögren's syndrome, are also present.[118] The differential diagnosis includes prolactinoma and other sellar masses, and a careful history and demonstrated loss of the posterior pituitary bright spot on MRI are useful for supporting the diagnosis.

Laboratory Results. The erythrocyte sedimentation rate is often elevated; antibodies to a 49-kd cytosolic protein were detected in 70% of patients with histologically confirmed lymphocytic hypophysitis and in 10% of control subjects.[119] Although the specificity of this antibody and two additional antibodies to 68- and 43-kd human pituitary membrane antigens is high, all three were detected in only 5 of 13 patients with lymphocytic hypophysitis and 1 of 12 patients with infundibuloneurohypophysitis.[120] PRL levels are usually elevated in both female and male patients, hyperprolactinemia is expected during pregnancy and during the early postpartum period, and the mass effect of the infiltrate may also contribute to stalk compression and secondary hyperprolactinemia. GH and ACTH responses to hypothalamic hormone challenges may be blunted. Rarely, isolated ACTH or TSH deficiencies have been reported.[121, 122]

Treatment. If the diagnosis is convincingly supported and compressive visual field disturbances are absent, surgical therapy should be withheld, pituitary hormone deficits appropriately replaced, and spontaneous resolution of the inflammatory mass observed expectantly. Treatment with adrenal steroids is advocated; it often resolves the sellar mass and improves endocrine dysfunction. Steroids are also indicated if adrenal reserve is compromised. Transsphenoidal surgery may be required to confirm a tissue diagnosis and may also relieve compression symptoms,[123] but the degree of surgical resection should be constrained by the need to conserve viable pituitary tissue, particularly in view of frequent spontaneous resolution.

Granulomatous Hypophysitis

Granulomatous hypophysitis is not usually associated with pregnancy and has an equal female-male incidence. Rarely, the condition may coexist with lymphocytic hypophysitis in the same gland.[123] Pituitary histology shows histiocytes, multinucleated giant cells, and other features of chronic inflammation and granuloma.[124] Patients present with headache and may have aseptic meningitis. MRI can reveal a thickened pituitary stalk or a characteristic tongue-shaped extension of the lesion under the hypothalamus. Granulomatous hypophysitis may reflect an underlying systemic disorder such as sarcoidosis[125] or Takayasu's disease.[126]

Xanthomatous Hypophysitis

This least common primary pituitary inflammatory process also occurs with the same frequency in both sexes and consists of lipid-laden macrophages, which resemble postinfectious cell debris. MRI often reveals a highly cystic lesion, leading to the suggestion that this entity reflects an inflammatory response to a damaged or ruptured pituitary cyst.[127]

Hemorrhage and Infarction

Intrapituitary hemorrhage and infarction are usually caused by ischemic damage to the hypophyseal-portal system and may be catastrophic. These acute events cause significant damage to the pituitary gland, and small clinically silent microinfarcts are found in up to 5% of unselected autopsies. Pituitary cells are relatively resilient to vascular insult, and pituitary insufficiency is clinically apparent only when about 75% of the gland is chemically damaged. Ten percent residual functional pituitary cell mass appears sufficient to mask complete pituitary failure. Ischemic damage is limited to the anterior lobe and posterior pituitary function usually remains intact, reflecting the predominant neural control of oxytocin and arginine vasopressin secretion. Acute intrapituitary hemorrhage can cause significant life-threatening damage to the pituitary and its surrounding vital structures.[128]

Postpartum Pituitary Infarction. During pregnancy, the pituitary gland normally enlarges in response to estrogen stimulation. The hypervascular gland is thus particularly vulnerable to arterial pressure changes and prone to hemorrhage. Sheehan's syndrome, classically described after severe postpartum hemorrhage, is less commonly encountered with modern obstetric care.[129] Development of hypovolemic shock in these women results in adenohypophyseal vessel vasospasm and pituitary necrosis.[130]

Pituitary Apoplexy

Pituitary apoplexy may result from spontaneous hemorrhage into a pituitary adenoma or occur after head trauma, skull base fracture, or in association with hypertension and diabetes mellitus, sickle cell anemia, or acute hypovolemic shock.[131, 132]

Clinical Features. Pituitary apoplexy is an endocrine emergency. The condition may evolve over 1 to 2 days with severe headache, neck stiffness, and progressive cranial nerve damage, cardiovascular collapse, and change in consciousness. Signs include severe hypotension, bilateral visual disturbances, hypoglycemia, fever, central nervous system hemorrhage, and coma. Acute adrenal insufficiency may also be superimposed because of disordered intravascular clotting disorders, heparin administration, or acute effects of central nervous system hemorrhage. Pituitary imaging without contrast usually reveals signs of intrapituitary or intra-adenoma hemorrhage, stalk deviation, compression of normal pituitary tissue, and, in severe cases, signs of parasellar hemorrhage.[133]

Management. Most patients recover spontaneously but may experience long-term pituitary insufficiency. Patients who are fully alert and conscious with no visual symptoms may be observed. The decision to initiate therapy with high-dose glucocorticoids depends on the clinical status.[128] Ophthalmoplegia, which is common, may resolve spontaneously over time. Failure of optic tract pressure to resolve or signs of progressive pituitary compression are indications for urgent transsphenoidal surgical decompression.[128] Postoperative recovery of visual function correlates inversely with the time elapsed since the acute hemorrhage.[134] Cranial nerve palsies, however, often improve whether or not surgery is undertaken. Pituitary function does not commonly recover after resolution of the acute hemorrhage, and patients require adrenal, thyroid, or gonadal steroid hormone replacement.[135] The subsequent atrophy of infarcted pituitary tissue often results in the development of a complete or partially empty sella evident on MRI.

Evaluation of Pituitary Masses

Approach to the Patient Harboring a Pituitary Mass

Ninety-one percent of 1120 patients undergoing transsphenoidal surgery for sellar masses were diagnosed with pituitary adenomas.[90] Thus, the differential diagnosis of a pituitary mass should be aimed at excluding the diagnosis of a pituitary adenoma before considering other rare sellar lesions. The management of and prognosis for anterior pituitary adenomas differ markedly from those for other nonpituitary masses, and an important diagnostic challenge is to distinguish a pituitary adenoma from other parasellar masses.

Several physiologic states are associated with pituitary enlargement. Lactotroph hyperplasia is seen during pregnancy, and thyrotroph or gonadotroph hyperplasia occurs in the presence of long-standing primary thyroid or gonadal failure, respectively. Pituitary enlargement may also occur as a result of ectopic GHRH or CRH secretion with resultant hyperplasia of somatotroph or corticotroph cells. Autopsy series show that up to 20% of subjects harbor an incidental clinically silent pituitary adenoma. Incidental pituitary cysts, hemorrhages, and infarctions are also discovered at autopsy.

With the widespread use of sensitive imaging techniques for nonpituitary indications including head trauma, chronic sinusitis, or headaches, previously inapparent pituitary lesions are being identified with increasing frequency. Pituitary abnormalities compatible with the diagnosis of microadenoma are detectable in about 10% of the normal adult population undergoing MRI. Recognizing that approximately 90% of observed pituitary lesions represent pituitary adenomas, initial assessment should determine whether the mass is hormonally functional and whether local mass effects are apparent at the time of diagnosis or likely to develop in the future.

As clinical features associated with disordered hormone secretion have an insidious onset and may be unnoticed for years or decades, endocrine function should always be tested (Table 8–9). Clinical evaluation for changes compatible with hypersecretion or hyposecretion of GH, gonadotropins, PRL, or ACTH may reveal unique long-term sequelae requiring distinct therapies. In the absence of clinical features of a humoral hypersecretory syndrome, cost-effective laboratory screening should be performed. Serum PRL levels higher than 200 μg/L strongly suggest the presence of a prolactinoma, whereas lower PRL levels would indicate secondary stalk interruption by a pituitary mass. Elevated age-matched and gender-matched IGF-I levels indicate the presence of a GH-secreting adenoma, and a high 24-hour urinary free cortisol level is an effective screen for most patients with Cushing's disease. Nevertheless, the incidence of functional hormone-secreting tumors in asymptomatic subjects with incidentally discovered pituitary masses is low.

Table 8–9. Screening Tests for Functional Pituitary Adenomas

Condition	Test	Comments
Acromegaly	IGF-I	Interpret IGF-I relative to age- and gender-matched controls
	OGTT with GH obtained at 0, 30 and 60 min	Normal subjects should suppress growth hormone to <1 μg/L
Prolactinoma	Serum PRL level Exclude medications	MRI of the sella should be ordered if PRL levels elevated
Cushing's disease	24-hr urinary free cortisol	Ensure urine collection is total and accurate
	Dexamethasone (1 mg) at 11 PM and fasting plasma cortisol measured at 8 AM	Normal subjects suppress to <5 μg/dL
	ACTH assay	Distinguishes adrenal adenoma from ectopic ACTH or Cushing's disease.

ACTH, adrenocorticotropic hormone; IGF-I, insulin-like growth factor I; MRI, magnetic resonance imaging; OGTT, oral glucose tolerance test; PRL, prolactin.

The presence of, or the potential for, local compressive effects must also be considered. Because the risk of microadenoma enlargement toward a compressive macroadenoma is low, no direct intervention may be warranted. For parasellar masses of uncertain origin, histologic tissue examination may be the best approach to obtain an accurate diagnosis. Although MRI or CT imaging features may be helpful in diagnosing a nonpituitary sellar mass, the final diagnosis may remain elusive until pathologic confirmation is obtained.

Parasellar masses include neoplastic and nonneoplastic lesions and are manifest clinically by local compression of surrounding vital structures or metabolic or hormonal derangements (see Table 8–9). Rarely, sellar masses may be the presenting feature of a previously undiagnosed systemic disorder such as lymphoma or tuberculosis.[136] Fever with or without associated sterile or septic meningitis may rarely be caused by fluid leakage into the subarachnoid space from Rathke's cleft, dermoid and epidermoid cysts, and craniopharyngioma and apoplexy.[128, 135, 137, 138] Patients with pituitary masses may present with hemorrhage and infarction, especially during pregnancy when the normal pituitary is adenomatous and swollen; diabetes mellitus; and hypertension or hypotension, which may be found in elderly people with unsuspected pituitary tumors. Rarely, these adenomas occur with CSF leakage, which may predispose to meningitis. Pituitary masses may also undergo silent infarction leading to development of a partially or totally empty pituitary sella with normal pituitary reserve, implying that the surrounding rim of pituitary tissue is fully functional. Large sellar cysts may be mistaken for an empty sella.

Rarely, functional pituitary adenomas may arise within the remnant pituitary tissue, and these tumors may not be visible by sensitive MRI (i.e., <2 mm in diameter) despite their endocrine hyperactivity. Acute or chronic infection with abscess formation rarely occurs within the mass. Compromised pituitary hormone hyposecretion may be due to direct pressure effects of the expanding mass on hormone-secreting cells or to parasellar pressure effects that attenuate synthesis or secretion of hypothalamic hormones, with resultant pituitary failure. Hypothalamic masses (gangliocytomas) may overproduce a specific releasing hormone with resultant stimulation of secretion of a specific pituitary hormone.

Imaging

Tumors of the pituitary gland are best diagnosed with MRI because it has better resolution than other radiologic modalities for identifying soft tissue changes (see Fig. 8–7). When a pituitary tumor or other parasellar mass is suspected, MRI specifically focused on the pituitary should be requested because brain MRI is often inadequate for optimal visualization of pituitary tumors and may miss the tumor completely.[139, 140] This technique permits high-contrast, detailed visualization of tumor mass effects on neighboring soft tissue structures, including the cavernous sinus[141] or optic chiasm. Pituitary MRI includes images of the optic chiasm, hypothalamus, pituitary stalk, and cavernous and sphenoid sinuses.[142, 143] High-resolution T1-weighted sections in the coronal and sagittal planes both before and after administration of gadolinium pentetic acid for contrast distinguish most pituitary masses.[144] Slice thickness should be less than 3 mm to obtain a pixel of 1 mm. Contiguous sections are therefore required to diagnose lesions of 1 to 3 mm.[145] If necessary, especially for diagnosing high-signal hemorrhage, T2-weighted images provide additional diagnostic information.

MRI thus clearly delineates the pituitary gland, stalk, optic tracts, and surrounding soft tissues. The gland may be concave, convex, or flat. The posterior pituitary lobe exhibits a discrete bright spot of high signal intensity on T1-weighted images, which declines with age and is absent in diabetes insipidus and most posterior pituitary lesions. This T1 shortening may reflect the presence of arginine vasopressin localized within neurosecretory vesicles.[146] The pituitary gland may enlarge transiently during adolescence, during pregnancy, and after childbirth, and teenage girls exhibit increasing gland convexity during the menstrual cycle.[147, 148] During pregnancy, the gland should normally not exceed 10 to 12 mm and the stalk should not exceed 4 mm in diameter. A thickened stalk may indicate the presence of hypophysitis, granuloma, or atypical chordomas.

After gadolinium administration, microadenomas are usually hypodense compared with the normal gland, especially when multiple thin-section echo sequences are examined in the first few minutes after injection of the contrast agent. It has been suggested that this hypointensity may reflect compromised microadenoma vasculature.[149] Microadenomas may also cause gland asymmetry or stalk deviation. In contrast, macroadenomas, which are significantly more vascular than microadenomas, have a higher affinity for gadolinium. They often enlarge the sella turcica by remodeling the bony fossa, suggesting a gradual long-term process. These tumors can grow upward toward the optic apparatus and cause draping of the nerves over the tumor, often accompanied by visual field abnormalities. Tumors can also extend into the sphenoid sinus and not infrequently invade connective tissue separating the pituitary from the cavernous sinus.

Radiologically, visible tumor tissue surrounding the carotid artery confirms cavernous sinus invasion. Infrequently, these patients experience palsies of third, fourth, or sixth cranial nerves. MRI may readily distinguish pituitary adenomas from other masses, including hyperplasias, craniopharyngiomas, meningiomas, chordomas, cysts, and hypophysitis. Secondary distinguishing features such as visualization of distinct noninvolved pituitary tissue, mass consistency, calcification, hemorrhage, and suprasellar involvement usually allow an imaging diagnosis of these masses, but these can often be confirmed only by direct tissue histology. Preoperative localization of carotid artery aneurysms can also be confirmed by MRI or magnetic resonance angiography.

Pituitary CT allows visualization of bony structures, including the sellar floor and clinoid bones, and their invasion. CT also recognizes calcifications that characterize craniopharyngiomas, meningiomas, and rarely aneurysms. Calcifications are not evident on MRI. Occasionally, pituitary adenomas may calcify. Pituitary CT scanning is indicated for discovery of hemorrhagic lesions, metastatic deposits, and chordomas and evidence of calcification.

Receptor Imaging

Because prolactinomas express D2 receptors, they can be imaged with a radiolabeled D2 receptor antagonist by using iodine 123-labeled iodobenzamine single photon emission scanning. Failure to visualize nonfunctioning tumors by this technique has led some to advocate its use to distinguish the two tumor types.[150] Radiolabeled indium pentetreotide has been used for in vivo tumor imaging. Most pituitary adenomas express somatostatin receptor subtypes to a varying degree, thus limiting the specificity of the procedure. Single photon emission CT (SPECT) has a sensitivity of about 1 cm and can detect normal pituitary tissue receptor expression. Because most adenomas and normal tissue are identified by this technique, its utility is limited for tumor detection, but it may be helpful for imaging ectopic ACTH-secreting tumors.

Neuro-ophthalmologic Assessment of Pituitary Masses

The optic tracts are particularly vulnerable to compression by expanding pituitary masses, and expanding pituitary tumors affect mostly the chiasm. Accurate neuro-ophthalmologic evaluation is helpful for tumor diagnosis, for determining pretreatment baseline visual status, and for post-treatment monitoring or detection of mass recurrence.[151] The relationships of the optic chiasm and the intracranial components of the optic nerves with the pituitary gland and surrounding vessels are depicted in Figure 8–2. A 10-mm posteriorly angled gap separates the optic chiasm and diaphragma sellae (see Fig. 8–3). Therefore, extensive suprasellar mass extension is required before visual function is compromised. Decussation of neural fibers originating from the nasal half of each retina occurs at the chiasm, and those originating from the temporal retinal halves are situated ipsilaterally.[152] Fibers from the superior and inferior retinal aspect are segregated in the corresponding chiasmal regions. Local vascular compromise or chiasmal stretching contributes to the pathogenesis of selective visual compromise. Reversibility of visual effects may correlate inversely with acuteness of the compressive insult.

Visual Symptoms. An abnormal visual examination may unmask the presence of a pituitary mass in an asymptomatic patient. Before the availability of sophisticated assay and imaging techniques, patients with virtually all pituitary masses presented with visual loss.[153] Currently, less than 10% of patients present with visual loss,[154] and most of these harbor clinically nonfunctioning pituitary adenomas often detected by incidental imaging. Unilateral or bilateral temporal or central visual loss is usually asymmetric and may be quite insidious, remitting, or recurring. Rarely, sudden visual loss occurs in a previously asymptomatic patient. Other symptoms include diplopia, impaired depth perception, and rarely visual hallucinations (Fig. 8–11).[155]

Clinical Signs. Impingement of the inferior crossing chiasmal fibers leads to bitemporal visual loss, especially in the superior field portions, accounting for about half of all pituitary-related visual defects. Pituitary-related defects preferentially marginate at the vertical field midline,[151] whereas bitemporal defects of other causes tend to occur away from the midline (Fig. 8–12). Despite prominent field defects, many of which can be directly correlated with defined tumor location by MRI, visual acuity

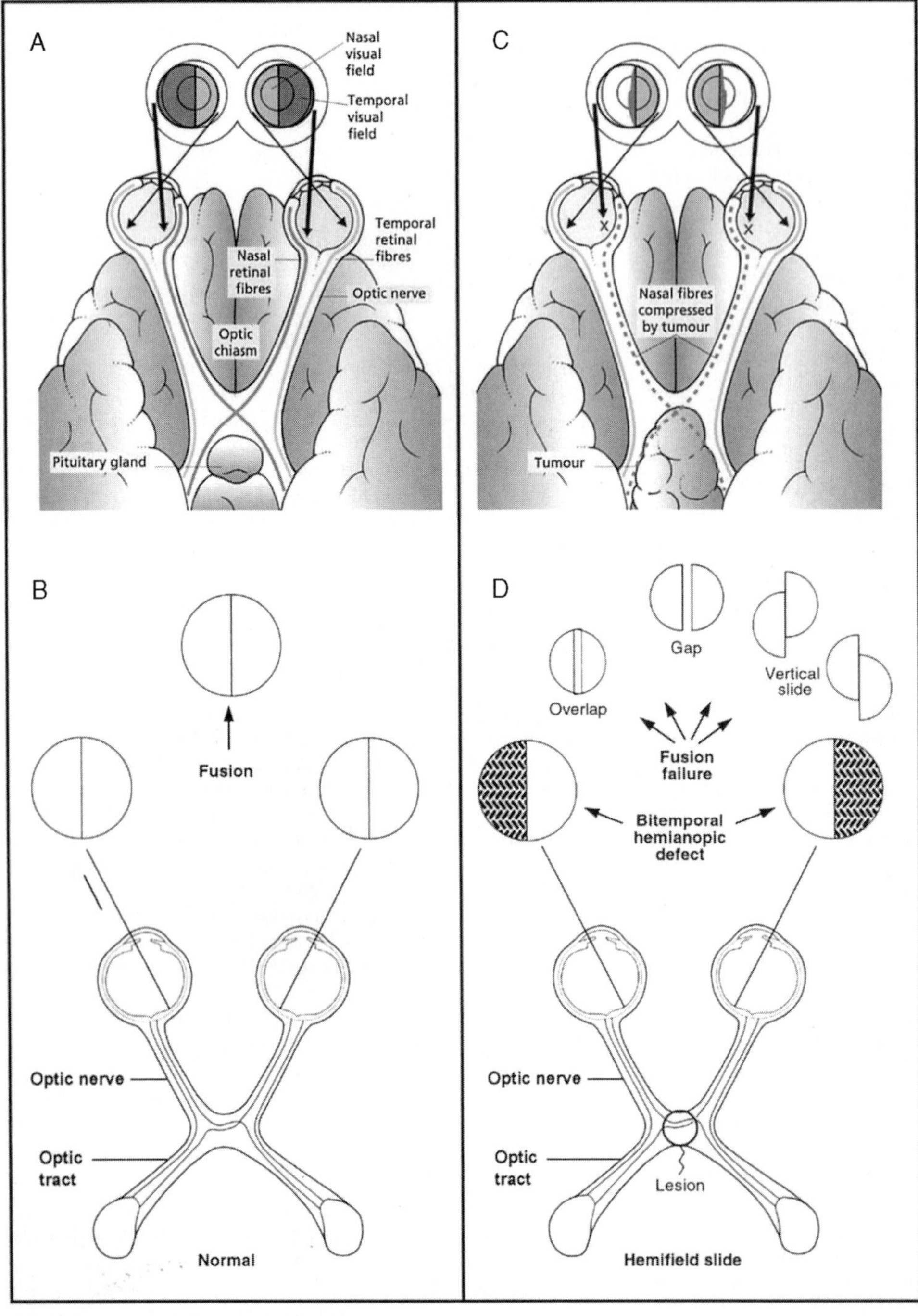

Figure 8–11. Local effects of an expanding pituitary tumor causing visual field defects: normal vision *(A)*; bitemporal hemianopsia *(C)*. Hemifield slide phenomena arising in the setting of bitemporal hemianopia *(B)* and *(D)* from fusion instability. The nasal and temporal fields lose their linkage, resulting in overlap of the preserved visual fields. (*A* and *C*, From Newell-Price J. Endocrine Assessment. In Sheaves R, Jenkins PJ, Wass JAH [eds]. Clinical Endocrine Oncology. Cambridge, Mass, Blackwell Science, 1997, pp 152–157; *B* and *D*, from Stiver SI, Sharpe JA. Neuro-ophthalmologic evaluation of pituitary tumors. In Thapar K, Kovacs K, Scheithauer BW, Lloyd RV [eds]. Diagnosis and Management of Pituitary Tumors. Totowa, NJ, Humana Press, 2001, pp 173–200.)

in the remaining fields is invariably normal in over 95% of patients.[156] Anterior tumor extension may damage central visual acuity, and this is detected by using the Snellen chart or by loss of color discrimination, especially in the red-green spectrum. Rarely, pupillary abnormalities, optic atrophy, papilledema, cranial nerve palsies, and nystagmus may be encountered. Visual fields are assessed by bedside confrontational testing, Goldmann perimetry, the Amsler grid, and automated quantitative perimetry.

Management of Pituitary Masses

The goals of therapy for masses are to alleviate local compressive mass effects, to suppress hormone hypersecretion, and to relieve hormone hyposecretion while maintaining intact pituitary trophic function. The three modes of therapy available are surgical, radiotherapeutic, and medical approaches. In general, the benefits of each therapy should be weighed against the respective risks, and comprehensive awareness on the part of the physician and the patient is required to individualize treatment approaches.

Surgical Management of Pituitary Tumors and Sellar Masses

Pituitary surgery is indicated for excision of mass lesions causing central pressure effects, primary correction of hormonal hypersecretion (other than prolactinomas), or functional

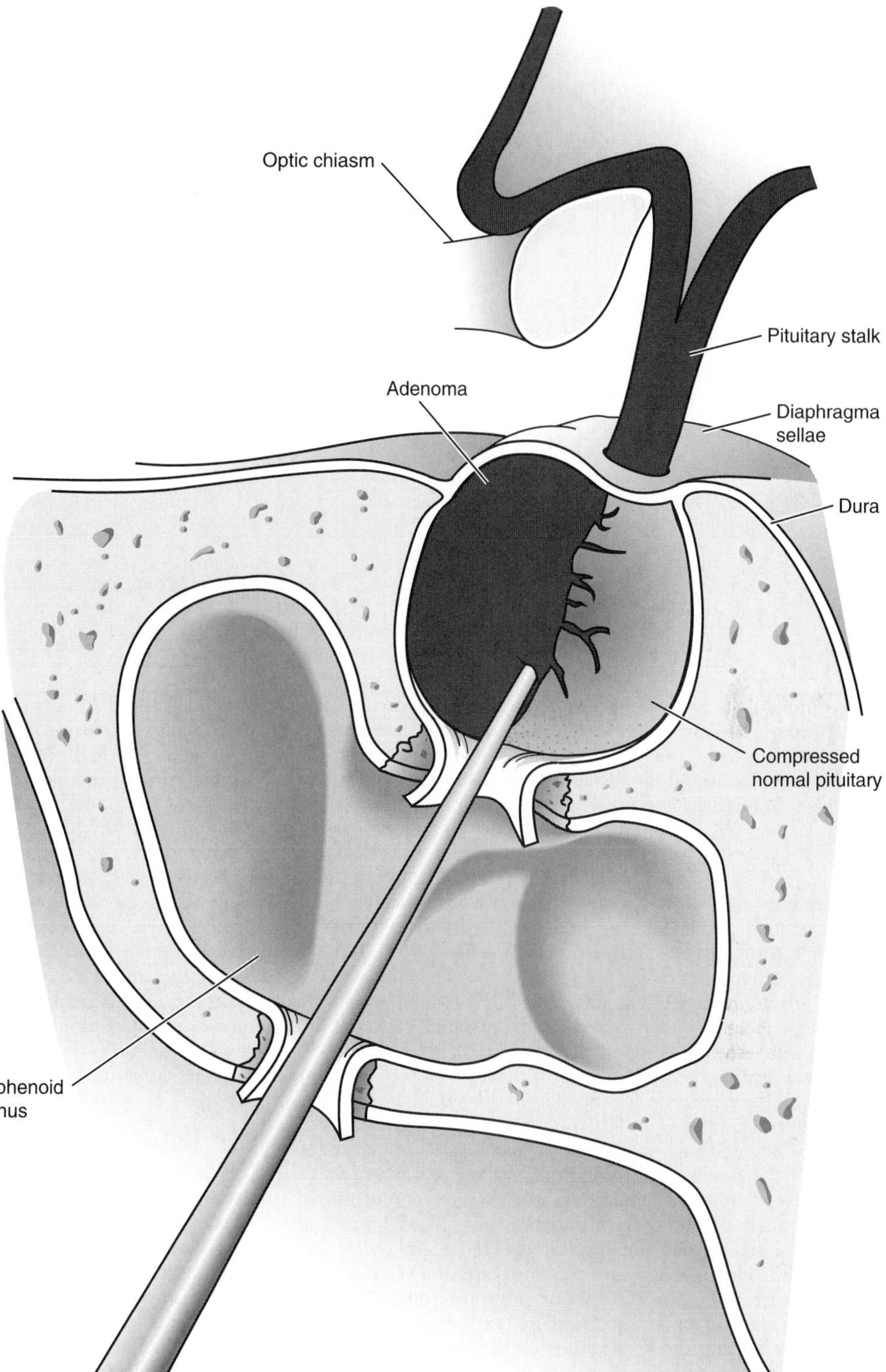

Figure 8–14. Transsphenoidal resection of pituitary adenoma. (Modified from BMI Quarterly 6:5, 1990.)

enable intraoperative surgical neuronavigation by three-dimensional imaging. Intraoperative ultrasonography and MRI technologies allow real-time assessment of the dimensions and extent of the pituitary mass and the progress of surgery. Intraoperative MRI is performed while the surgical field is still open, allowing the surgeon to assess directly the need for further dissection, and also provides an excellent baseline for postoperative follow-up.[159] In contrast, postoperative image stabilization may not be evident for months after surgery.

Endonasal transsphenoidal endoscopy avoids use of a retractor or speculum, does not require nasal packing, and sometimes leads to a shorter operating time, resulting in decreased postoperative morbidity and a shorter hospital stay (Fig. 8–15). The advantages of the technique include a clear panoramic

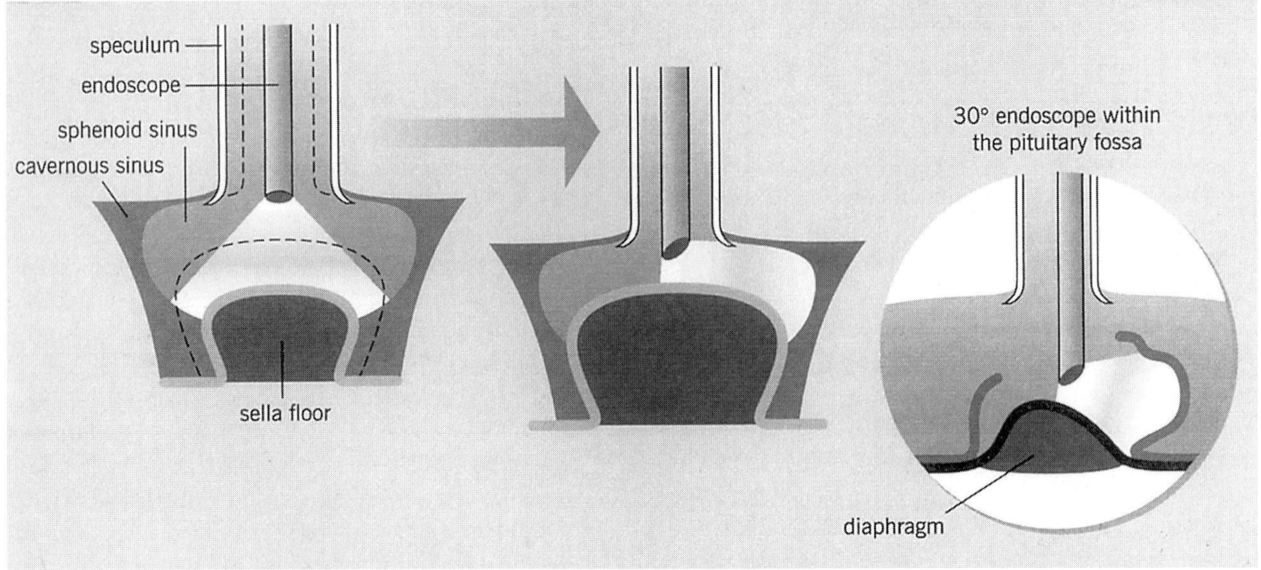

Figure 8–15. Endoscope-assisted microsurgery provides a panoramic view of the sphenoid sinus. Using a 30-degree endoscope, a view "around the corner" is possible. Parasellar structures can be visualized and residual tumor detected and resected. (From Fahlbusch R, Buchfelder M, Kreutzer J, Nomikos P. Surgical management of acromegaly. In Wass JAH [ed]. Handbook of Acromegaly. Bristol, UK, BioScientifica, 2001, p. 46.)

view of bone landmarks and access to suprasellar and parasellar tumor extensions into the cavernous sinuses. Disadvantages of this relatively new approach include the need for management of perioperative intrasellar bleeding and CSF leaks as well as the added requirement for a preoperative CT scan.[160]

Indications for Transsphenoidal Surgery

A pituitary mass that may or may not be compressing local vital structures should be evaluated for surgical resection (Table 8–10). Although surgical resection offers a rapid resolution of hormone hypersecretion and many of the resultant clinical features of functioning adenomas, indications for the procedure differ depending on the tumor type (see later). In general, patients who are intolerant of or resistant to medical therapy require surgery. Surgery is indicated primarily for well-circumscribed GH-secreting adenomas and all ACTH-secreting, TSH-secreting, and nonfunctioning macroadenomas. Surgery may also be indicated when tissue histology is required to determine the nature of an enigmatic sellar mass. Progressive compressive features, including visual field loss, compromised pituitary function, or other central nervous system functional change, are indications for surgical debulking and sellar decompression. Hemorrhage into the encased bony sella turcica, usually occurring within a known or previously unknown adenoma, may require immediate surgical decompression. Urgent surgical decompression is required for acute pituitary hemorrhage that may result in apoplexy related to partial or complete infarction, especially in patients with signs of progressive compressive signs.

When pituitary function after surgery was assessed in 234 patients, 52 patients had new trophic hormone dysfunction and 45 of 93 patients with preoperative evidence for hypopituitarism had recovered between one and three previously suppressed axes. Significant factors determining restoration of postoperative pituitary function were no visible tumor remnants as assessed by MRI (P = .001) and no tumor invasion as determined by the neurosurgeon as well as by pathologic examination of surrounding tissue (P <.049).[161] Therefore, because about half of all patients with preoperative pituitary failure recover function, depending on the clinical circumstance, patients should be considered for retesting before initiating postoperative substitution therapy except for adrenal steroid replacement, which requires greater caution. Indications for second surgery in the same patient include tumor recurrence, persistent hormonal hypersecretion by tumor remnants, or repair of a CSF leak.

After surgery, patients should be kept in bed rest at an angle of 30 to 45 degrees and urine and serum osmolality and serum electrolytes should be measured every 6 hours. Indications for postoperative vasopressin replacement include urine output greater than 300 mL/hour for 3 consecutive hours with serum osmolality above 285 mOsm/L, elevated serum sodium concentrations, and inappropriately low urine osmolality. Postoperative polyuria alone is not an indication for vasopressin replacement unless it is a reflection of compromised posterior pituitary function.

Side Effects

The success of surgery is largely determined by the skill and experience of the neurosurgeon. Tumor size, degree of invasiveness, preoperative hormone levels, and previous pituitary surgery are all determinants of surgical outcome. CSF leakage, transient diabetes insipidus, and inappropriate arginine vasopressin secretion are the most commonly encountered transient side effects, occurring in up to 20% of patients (see Table 8–10). Local damage may also result in arachnoiditis, vascular bleeding, hematoma formation, and epistaxis. Rarely, pulmonary embolism, narcolepsy, and local abscess have been reported. Iatrogenic hypopituitarism, diabetes insipidus, and syndrome of inappropriate antidiuretic hormone (SIADH) have been reported in up to 10% of patients. Rarely, the central nervous system may be permanently damaged with hemiparesis, cranial nerve palsies, or encephalopathy.

A triphasic postoperative diabetes insipidus has been described in which the transient disorder is followed by an interphase on days 6 to 11 with no polydipsia or polyuria. During this later phase, hyponatremia with features of inappropriate antidiuretic hormone secretion has also been reported.[162, 163] Cognitive dysfunction, including deficits in anterograde memory and executive function, has been reported in several retro-

Table 8–10. Transsphenoidal Pituitary Surgery

Primary Indications
General
Visual tract or central nervous compression arising from within sella
Relief of compressive hypopituitarism by presenting, residual, or recurrent tumor tissue
Tumor recurrence after surgery or radiation
Pituitary hemorrhage
Cerebrospinal fluid leak
Resistance to medical therapy
Intolerance of medical therapy
Personal choice
Desire for immediate pregnancy with macroadenoma
Requirement for diagnostic tissue histology
Specific
Acromegaly
Cushing's disease
Clinically nonfunctioning macroadenoma
Prolactinoma (rarely indicated)
Nelson's syndrome
TSH-secreting adenoma
Side Effects
Transient
Diabetes insipidus
Cerebrospinal fluid leak and rhinorrhea
Inappropriate ADH secretion
Arachnoiditis
Meningitis
Postoperative psychosis
Local hematoma
Arterial wall damage
Epistaxis
Local abscess
Pulmonary embolism
Narcolepsy
Permanent (up to 10%)
Diabetes insipidus
Total or partial hypopituitarism
Visual loss
Inappropriate ADH secretion
Vascular occlusion
CNS damage
  Oculomotor palsy
  Hemiparesis
  Encephalopathy
Nasal septum perforation
Surgery-Related Mortality (up to 1%)
Brain, hypothalamic injury
Vascular damage
Postoperative meningitis
Cerebrospinal leak
Pneumocephalus
Acute cardiopulmonary disease
Anesthetic
Seizure

ADH, antidiuretic hormone; CNS, central nervous system; TSH, thyroid-stimulating hormone.

spective studies after transsphenoidal surgery.[164, 165] Mortality has been reported in less than 1% of patients undergoing pituitary surgery and may be related to direct hypothalamic or cerebrovascular damage, meningitis, pneumocephalus formation, or anesthetic complications. Surgical failure may result from a non–pituitary-related event, including anesthesia-related complication or bleeding disorder. Incomplete tumor removal may also be due to inaccurate preoperative MRI localization or identification. Rarely, a previously undiagnosed functioning pituitary tumor or ectopic source of ACTH may be unmasked after initially unsuccessful pituitary surgery.

Pituitary Radiation

Principles

High-energy ionizing radiation can be delivered to deep tissues by megavoltage techniques. The challenge of this approach is to provide maximal localized necrotizing radiation to the pituitary lesion while minimally exposing surrounding normal structures to radiation damage. Several advances have improved both efficacy and safety, including highly precise tumor localization, a high-voltage (6 to 15 MEv) linear accelerator, and accurate simulation models with isocentric rotational arcing that allow repeated head positioning at exactly the same points in the patient's subsequent visits. Up to a maximum of 4500 rads is administered as 180-rad daily fractions for about 5 to 6 weeks. High-precision techniques such as stereotactic conformal radiotherapy[166] and the gamma knife[167] allow delivery of high energy to the pituitary lesion while minimizing the mass of normal brain exposed to radiation (Fig. 8–16).

Indications

The use of radiation for treating pituitary tumors is highly individualized and depends on the expertise of the treating center, conviction of the treating physician in weighing the potential benefits and risks of the procedure, and the patient's preference based on informed choice (Table 8–11). In general, radiation techniques are indicated for persistent hormone hypersecretion or residual mass effects after surgery or when surgery for a compressive mass is contraindicated. As GH-secreting and PRL-secreting tumors are generally amenable to medical therapy, indications for radiation are rare. Most indications for radiation are adjuvant to either surgical or medical treatment. Radiation may be indicated after resection of a potentially recurring or inadequately resected pituitary mass, such as a nonfunctioning pituitary adenoma, craniopharyngioma, or chordoma. In acromegaly, use of radiation as primary treatment is generally not recommended,[168] but for resistant, aggressively growing prolactinomas the procedure may prevent further local invasion. Recurrent pituitary-dependent Cushing's disease appears to be particularly amenable to radiation, especially in younger patients.

Side Effects

Hypopituitarism. Pituitary failure occurs commonly in patients who have received pituitary radiation. Within 10 years after radiation, up to 80% of patients may have gonadotroph, somatotroph, thyrotroph, or corticotroph deficits.[168–171] The mechanism for hypopituitarism appears to involve damage to hypothalamic releasing hormone cells as well as direct pituitary damage. These patients require lifelong endocrine follow-up for pituitary reserve testing and hormone replacement when appropriate.

Second Brain Tumors. Thirty-two cases of glioma occurring after conventional pituitary radiation for adenomas and craniopharyngioma have been reported with a mean latency period of 11.5 years from initial diagnosis.[172] In a meta-analysis of results of irradiation for pituitary tumors, the standardized incidence ratio for second brain tumors was approximately 6 (confidence interval 3.16 to 10.69). This analysis was based on 12 diagnosed second tumors with a latency of 6 to 24 years in three separate cohorts.[173–175] Because patients harboring pituitary tumors are more likely to undergo routine brain imaging during follow-up, it is not clear whether observed meningiomas are coincidental findings. As this complication, which occurs in less than 5% of patients, also appears dose-related, fractionated doses not exceeding 4500 rads should be given. Use of conformal radiation techniques to irradiate a smaller

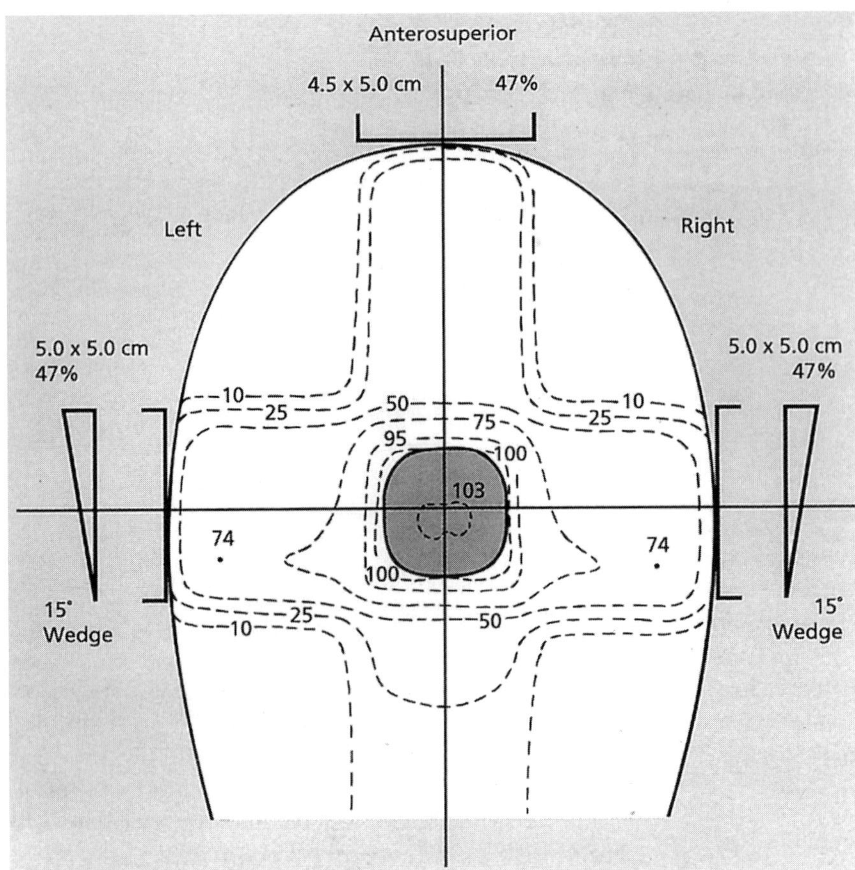

Figure 8–16. Pituitary radiotherapy: 8-mV x-ray isodosimetric plan. The three fields restrict high dose volume to the target. (From Plowman PN. Pituitary radiotherapy: techniques and potential complications. In Sheaves R, Jenkins PJ, Wass JAH [eds]. Clinical Endocrine Oncology. Cambridge, Mass, Blackwell Science, 1997, p 186.)

tissue volume, including radiosurgery, fractionated stereotactic radiotherapy, and proton beam radiation, may minimize this adverse effect. Nevertheless, prospectively controlled surveillance studies are required to evaluate this critical question rigorously.

Visual Damage. Approximately 2% of patients experience impaired vision related to optic nerve damage.[176] The risk of visual damage is minimized by fractionating dosages to less than 200 rads per treatment session. Consequent blindness, however, has been reported in two patients who received 4500 rads in 180-rad fractions.[177]

Brain Necrosis. Dose-related radiation-induced brain necrosis was documented by MRI in 14 of 45 patients, with temporal lobe atrophy and cystic and diffuse cerebral atrophy.[178] Cognitive dysfunction, especially memory loss, has also been reported.[179]

Radiosurgery

The proton beam, the gamma knife using focused cobalt 60 emissions, and the linear accelerator deliver high-dose radiation while sparing surrounding tissue. Delivery of high energy by gamma knife directly targeted at the pituitary tumor minimizes the radiation exposure of surrounding tissues. Early reports indicated more rapid reduction of hormone hypersecretion, although long-term efficacy and safety outcomes are not yet apparent.[167] It appears that this procedure is best suited for intrasellar and cavernous lesions distant from the optic nerves.

Medical

Pituitary tumors often express receptors mediating hypothalamic control of hormone secretion, and appropriate ligands for the dopamine D2 receptor and the somatotropin release-inhibiting factor (SRIF) receptor subtype 2 are employed to suppress PRL or GH hypersecretion, to block tumor growth, and often to shrink tumor size. A novel approach has employed a peripheral receptor antagonist to block GH action without targeting the pituitary tumor source. Medical ablation of target glands, including thyroid and adrenal, may also be useful in mitigating the deleterious impact of pituitary tumor hypersecretion. Each of these medical approaches is fully considered in the following.

PHYSIOLOGY AND DISORDERS OF PITUITARY HORMONE AXES

Prolactin

Lactotroph Cells

Lactotroph cells constitute about 15% to 25% of functioning anterior pituitary cells (Fig. 8–17). Although their absolute number does not change with age, lactotroph hyperplasia does occur during pregnancy and lactation[180] and resolves within several months of delivery (Fig. 8–18). Most PRL-expressing cells appear to arise from GH-producing cells. Ablation of somatotrophs by expression of GH–diphtheria toxin and GH–thymidine kinase fusion genes inserted into the germ line of transgenic mice eliminated most lactotrophs, suggesting that the majority of PRL-producing cells arose from postmitotic somatotrophs.[181]

Two cell forms expressing the PRL gene are large polyhedral cells found throughout the gland and smaller angulated or

Table 8–11. Pituitary Radiation

Indications

Pituitary adenoma
- Acromegaly
- Cushing's disease
- Nonfunctioning adenoma
- Prolactinoma

Craniopharyngioma
Nelson's syndrome
Nonadenomatous invasive sellar mass
Tumor recurrence
Hormone hypersecretion recurrence

Side Effects

Hypopituitarism
- Deficient GH, gonadotropin, TSH, and ACTH reserve

Eye
- Visual loss
- Optic neuritis

Brain
- Brain necrosis
- Temporal lobe deficits
- Cognitive dysfunction

Relative Risk of Second Brain Tumor Post-radiation

Second Tumor	Incidence		SIR	95% Confidence Intervals	Reference
	Observed	Expected			
Astrocytoma (2) Meningioma (1) Meningeal sarcoma (1)	5	0.53	9.4	3.05–21.98	(Brada, 1992)
Gliomas	4	0.25	16	4.4–41	(Tsang, 1993)
Astrocytoma (2) Meningioma (1)	3	1.13	2.7	0.55–7.76	(Erfurth, 2001)*
Meta-analysis	12	1.96	6.1	3.16–10.69	

*Excludes patients with acromegaly.

ACTH, adrenocorticotropic hormone; GH, growth hormone; SIR, standardized incidence ratio for person-years at risk; TSH, thyroid-stimulating hormone.

Adapted from Erfurth EM, Bulow B, Mikoczy Z, Hagman L. Is there an increase in second brain tumors after surgery and irradiation for a pituitary tumor. Clin Endocrinol 2001, 55:613–616.

elongated cells clustered mainly in the lateral wings and median wedge. Large PRL secretory granules (250 to 800 nm) are present in the evenly distributed cells, and the laterally localized cells are sparsely populated by smaller (200 to 350 nm) granules (Fig. 8–19). Occasional mammosomatotroph cells may also cosecrete both PRL and GH, often stored within the same granule (Fig. 8–20). In animal models, lactotroph cell function is heterogeneous. Thus, dopamine or TRH responsiveness and shifting proportions of PRL-secreting and GH-secreting cells may depend on cell localization within the pituitary as well as the surrounding hormonal milieu, especially that of estrogen.[182]

Prolactin History

Shortly after its discovery and partial characterization,[183–185] PRL was prominently featured in *The New York Times* on December 3, 1937, indicating that it held the "key to peace in the world." The article, based on a lecture delivered by Prof. C. R. Stockard, proposed that "higher forms of life" were "governed by a 'glandocracy,' with the glands of internal secretion as the supreme rulers [in this instance PRL], exerting absolute control not only over the functioning of the individual from conception to death but also over the relationship of men and other vertebrate animals to each other."

The identification of PRL in humans was elusive until 1970 because human GH is highly lactogenic and active in bioassays used to isolate and measure PRL.[186] Furthermore, GH is present in human pituitary glands in much higher concentrations (5 to 10 mg) than PRL (~100 μg).[187, 188] To distinguish human PRL from GH, lactogenic activity was neutralized with GH antiserum; sera from postpartum women and patients with galactorrhea had high lactogenic activity in the presence of GH antibodies.[189, 190] Human PRL, bioassayed by stimulating pregnant mouse mammary milk production,[191] was elevated in patients with nonpuerperal galactorrhea resulting from pituitary tumors, exposure to phenothiazines, and withdrawal from oral contraceptives. The purification and isolation of PRL by Friesen and colleagues and the development of a specific radioimmunoassay underscored the new place of PRL in understanding human disease.[192, 193]

Prolactin Structure

The human PRL gene, located on chromosome 6,[194] apparently arose from a single common ancestral gene giving rise to the relatively homologous PRL, GH, and placental lactogen–related proteins (Fig. 8–21).[195] Several factors influence PRL gene expression, including estrogen, dopamine, TRH, and thyroid hormones.[196] PRL is a 199-amino-acid polypeptide containing three intramolecular disulfide bonds. It circulates in blood in various sizes: monomeric PRL ("little" PRL; 23 kd), dimeric PRL ("big" PRL; 48 to 56 kd), and polymeric forms (also known as "big, big" PRL; >100 kd).[197–199] The monomeric form is the most bioactive PRL. In response to TRH, the proportion of the more active monomeric form increases.

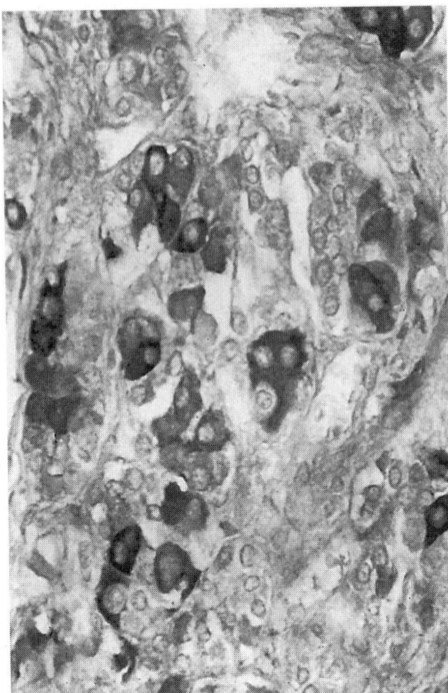

Figure 8–17. Lactotroph cell. Normal prolactin-secreting cells express strong positivity for prolactin within the cytoplasm of polyhedral cells, which have elongated cell processes. Some processes surround adjacent immunonegative cells that correspond to gonadotrophs. (From Asa SL. In Tumors of the Pituitary Gland. Atlas of Tumor Pathology. Washington, DC, Armed Forces Institute of Pathology, 1997, p 15.)

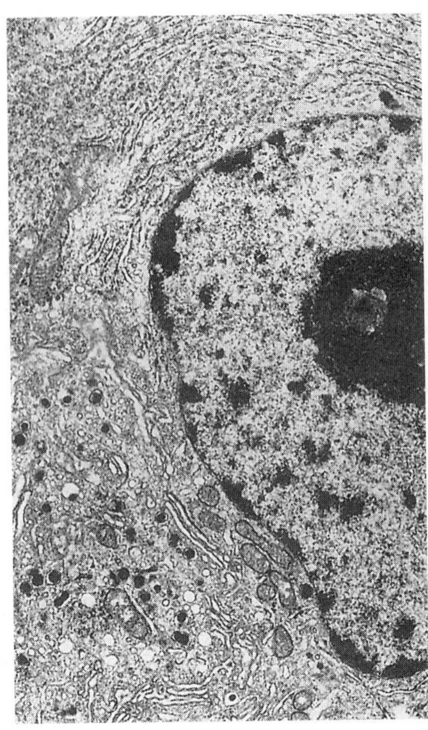

Figure 8–19. Electron micrograph of a normal lactotroph shows a well-developed rough endoplasmic reticulum that forms concentric whorls. A prominent Golgi complex is seen in a juxtanuclear location and harbors forming pleomorphic secretory granules. The cytoplasm is otherwise sparsely granulated. (From Asa SL. In Tumors of the Pituitary Gland. Atlas of Tumor Pathology. Washington, DC, Armed Forces Institute of Pathology, 1997, p 16.)

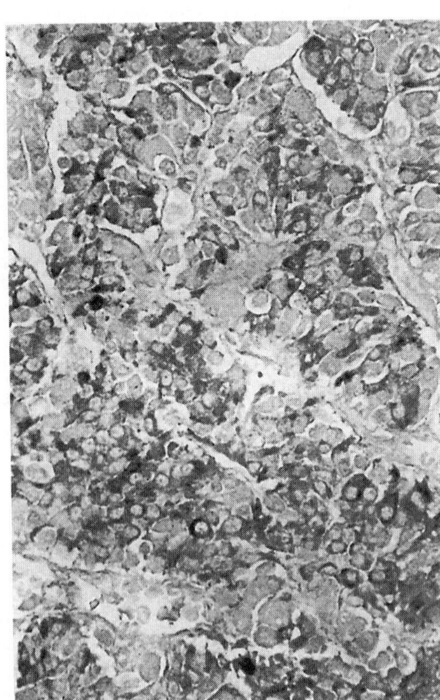

Figure 8–18. Prolactin cell hyperplasia. In the third trimester of pregnancy, prolactin cell hyperplasia occurs; cells containing immunoreactive prolactin make up almost 50% of the cell population of the gland. (From Asa SL. In Tumors of the Pituitary Gland. Atlas of Tumor Pathology. Washington, DC, Armed Forces Institute of Pathology, 1997, p 15.)

A glycosylated form of PRL identified in pituitary extracts is less biologically active than little PRL.[200] Monomeric PRL is cleaved into 8- and 16-kd forms,[201] and the 16-kd variant is antiangiogenic.[202, 203] A circulating PRL-binding protein corresponds to the extracellular domain of the PRL receptor.[204]

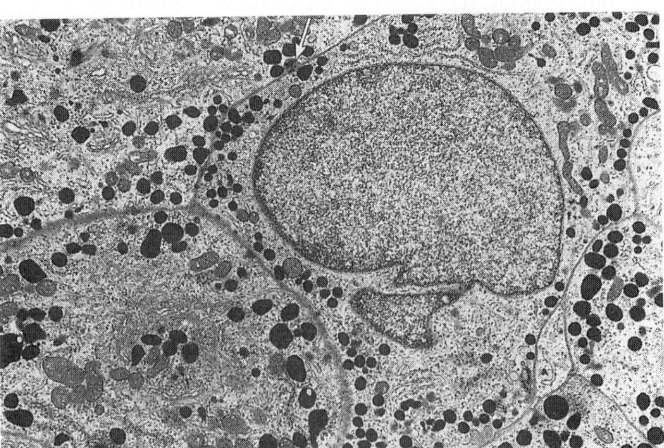

Figure 8–20. Normal mammosomatotroph. Occasional cells resembling densely granulated somatotrophs exhibit atypical features consistent with prolactin secretion; the secretory granules are highly pleomorphic and there is misplaced exocytosis, that is, extrusion of secretory material along the lateral cell border *(arrow)*. (From Asa SL. In Tumors of the Pituitary Gland. Atlas of Tumor Pathology. Washington, DC, Armed Forces Institute of Pathology, 1997, p 17.)

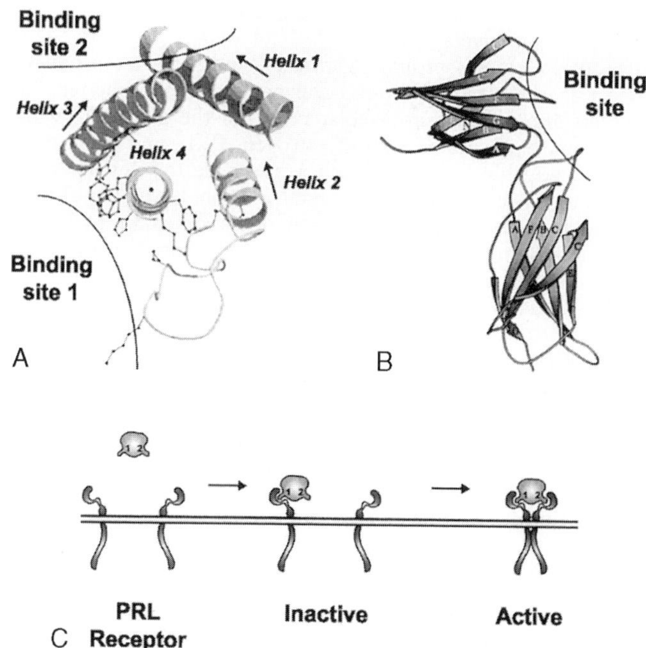

Figure 8–21. Molecular structure of prolactin and its interaction with the dimerized receptor. (From Bole-Feysot C, Goffin V, Edery M, et al. Prolactin (PRL) and its receptors: actions, signal transduction pathways and phenotypes observed in PRL receptor knockout mice. Endocr Rev 1998; 19:225–268.)

Regulation of Prolactin Secretion

PRL secretion is under the inhibitory control of dopamine, which is largely produced by the tuberoinfundibular (TIDA) cells, and the hypothalamic tuberohypophyseal dopaminergic system.[205, 206] DA reaches the lactotrophs through the hypothalamic pituitary portal system and inhibits PRL secretion by binding to the D2 receptors on pituitary lactotrophs.[207] PRL, in turn, participates in negative feedback to control its release by increasing tyrosine hydroxylase activity in the TIDA neurons.[206] In PRL-deficient animals, DA was decreased in the median eminence.[208] Mice lacking the D2 receptor experienced hyperprolactinemia and lactotroph proliferation.[207]

Factors other than DA inhibit PRL secretion, including endothelin-1 and transforming growth factor β1, which act as paracrine PRL inhibitors.[209, 210] and calcitonin, which may be derived from the hypothalamus.[211] Several substances act as PRL-releasing factors. Basic FGF and epidermal growth factor induce PRL synthesis and secretion. Vasoactive intestinal polypeptide (VIP) stimulates PRL synthesis through cAMP.[212] A hypothalamic PRL-releasing peptide produced in the hypothalamus acts through a specific receptor[213] in normal pituitary glands and in a subset of PRL-secreting tumors.[214] Oxytocin and pituitary adenylate cyclase activating protein also release PRL.[206] TRH stimulates PRL[215] but probably does not play an important role in PRL secretion. Estrogen stimulates PRL gene transcription and secretion,[216] explaining why women have higher PRL levels and why cycling women have a higher PRL pulse frequency than postmenopausal women and men.[217] Galanin is synthesized in both the pituitary and hypothalamus and may act as a PRL releasing factor.[218] The physiologic role of γ-aminobutyric acid, neurotensin, substance P, bombesin, and cholecystokinin in regulating human PRL secretion is unresolved.[206]

Serotonin may be additive with VIP in releasing PRL, and infusion of 5-hydroxytryptophan, a serotonin precursor, elicits PRL release. Nocturnal PRL secretion is attenuated by cyproheptadine. Thus, serotonin may mediate nocturnal PRL secretion and also participate with VIP in the suckling reflex. Opiates acutely induce PRL release, although naloxone does not consistently suppress PRL levels. GHRH, when administered in high doses, moderately induces PRL secretion, and patients harboring ectopic GHRH-producing tumors have mild to moderate hyperprolactinemia. GnRH also stimulates PRL in women, especially during the periovulatory menstrual phase. Although posterior pituitary hormones have been shown to regulate rat PRL secretion,[219] the role of vasopressin or oxytocin or other neurohypophyseal molecules in regulating human PRL remains unresolved. Histamine may act on the hypothalamus to regulate PRL, and H_2 blockers induce PRL secretion. A short-loop feedback of PRL has been proposed, and transgenic mice with deleted PRL were found to have a decreased hypothalamic dopamine content.[220] In humans, the existence of this regulatory loop has been difficult to prove.

Prolactin Receptor

The PRL receptor gene is a member of the cytokine receptor superfamily,[221] localizes to chromosome 5p13, and has 10 exons. The receptor gene has two 5′ promoters that direct transcription of a 598-amino-acid peptide[222] comprising an extracellular domain, a hydrophobic transmembrane domain, and an intracytoplasmic region homologous to the GH receptor.[223] Similarly, PRL receptor dimerization occurs with ligand binding and subsequent phosphorylation of intracellular Janus kinase/signal transducer and activator of transcription (JAK/STAT) molecules. Two binding sites encompassing helices 1 and 4 and helices 1 and 3 on the PRL molecule are critical for formation of the trimeric ligand-receptor complex and subsequent signaling (see Fig. 8–21).[224, 225]

The PRL receptor induces protein tyrosine phosphorylation and activation of JAK2 kinase and STATS 1 to 5.[226, 227] STAT5 phosphorylation mediates transcriptional activation of the β-casein gene.[228] PRL receptors are expressed in breast, pituitary, liver, adrenal cortex, kidneys, prostate, ovary, testes, intestine, epidermis, pancreatic islets, lung, myocardium, brain, and lymphocytes. Estrogen also induces liver PRL receptor expression.[224] Regulation of milk production occurs through a cascade of intracellular events. Homozygous mice in whom the PRL receptor was inactivated were infertile[224]; heterozygous animals were fertile but unable to nurse their first litters, presumably because of inadequate PRL receptor expression after the first but not subsequent pregnancies.

Functions of Prolactin

PRL is essential for human survival because of its role in milk production during pregnancy and lactation. Additional biologic functions ascribed to PRL include reproductive and metabolic effects, mammary development, pigeon crop sac activity, fresh water survival, melanin synthesis, water-seeking behavior of newts, molting, and parental behavior.[184] Although PRL and its receptor are clearly crucial in lower animals,[229] the impact of PRL on maternal behavior in humans has not been fully delineated.

Mammary Gland Development and Lactation

Puberty. PRL is not essential for pubertal mammary development, which appears to require GH, whose action is mediated by IGF-I.[230–234] Studies of mammary development have, for the most part, been carried out in rodents.[235] At birth, the mammary gland consists of a fat pad with small areas of ductal anlagen, which differentiate into pubertal mammary glandular

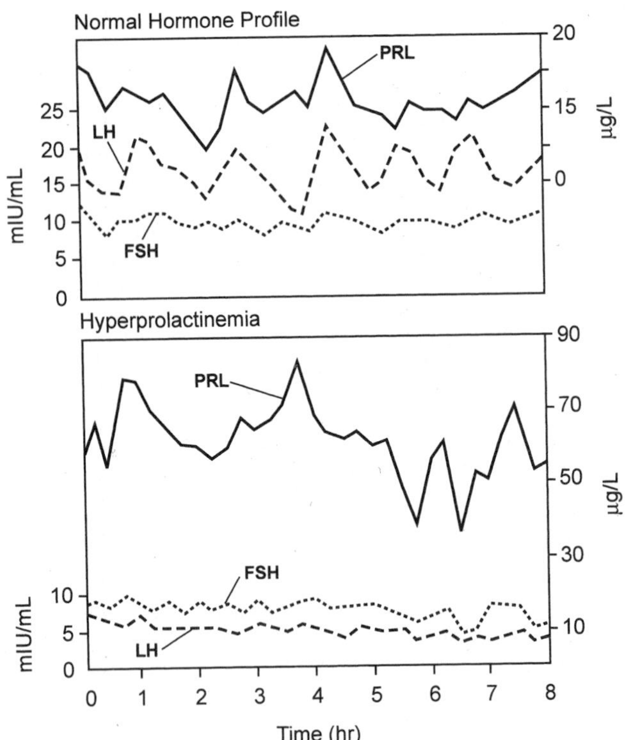

Figure 8–22. Effect of hyperprolactinemia on suppressing follicle-stimulating hormone (FSH) and luteinizing hormone (LH) secretory patterns leading to hypogonadotropism in a female patient. (Adapted from Tolis G. Prolactin: physiology and pathology. Hosp Pract 1980; 15: 85–95.)

elements under the influence of estrogen, GH, and IGF-I. At puberty, a surge of estrogen begins the process. Terminal end buds form and lead the process of mammary development by branching and extending into the substance of the mammary fat pad, leaving a network of ducts that virtually fill the mouse mammary fat pad.[235, 236] Interestingly, estrogen does not affect this process in the absence of GH and IGF-I.[237, 238]

These hormones are also responsible for most of ductal morphogenesis. Thus, GH acts on the mammary stromal compartment to produce IGF-I, which, in turn, stimulates formation of terminal end buds and ducts in synergy with estrogen.[232, 239] Parathyroid hormone–related protein is essential for fetal mammary development[240] and epidermal growth factor is essential for pubertal mammary development,[241] but their relationships to other hormones are as yet unclear. Once fully developed, the pubertal mammary gland remains quiescent until pregnancy, although cyclic changes occur during the menstrual cycle. Progesterone, possibly in association with GH and PRL, causes the formation of lobular "decorations" along ducts, which are precursors to true glands, and progestins have similar effects.[242] Pubertal mammary development begins in girls between the ages of 8 and 13 (see Tanner's developmental scale, Chapter 24).

Pregnancy. During pregnancy, the size of the normal pituitary gland may double or more than double,[180] the result of a marked increase in the number of PRL-producing cells and a relative decrease in other hormone-secreting cells. Serum PRL concentrations rise to a mean of 207 μg/L during pregnancy,[243] and amniotic fluid PRL concentrations are 100 times those of maternal or fetal blood.[243] In pregnancy, mammary alveolar elements proliferate and begin to produce milk proteins and colostrum. At 3 to 4 weeks of gestation, terminal ductal sprouting occurs, followed by lobular-alveolar formation. Epithelial buds invade and replace the surrounding fat pad, and true alveoli form at the end of the first trimester. Glandular elements proliferate further, and secretory products appear in the alveolar lumina. During the third trimester, fat droplets are seen within alveolar cells and the glands fill with colostrum.[244] A combination of estrogen, PRL, and progesterone and possibly IGF-I is largely responsible for this phase of mammary development.[245] Placental protein hormones (PRL, GH-V, human placental lactogen)[246] may contribute to mammary development and milk formation. In the absence of PRL, formation of alveolar structures is impaired, as demonstrated in mice with targeted disruption of the PRL gene.[207] Likewise, women with isolated PRL deficiency are unable to lactate.[247]

Alveolar formation and milk production also require progesterone, and lobular-alveolar formation does not occur in mice lacking the progesterone receptor.[248] Interestingly, only a minority of women have expressible milk during pregnancy, most likely because of inhibitory effects of estradiol[249] and progesterone[250] on PRL-induced milk production. Hormone perturbations during pregnancy also act on fetal mammary gland, causing prominent neonatal nipples and secretion of "witch's milk."

Lactation. Mechanisms of milk production are similar in all mammals, but milk composition differs.[251] Active lactation is due in part to a falloff in estrogen and progesterone and elevation of PRL levels after delivery. Suckling also increases milk production after parturition and is essential for continued lactation because of its distal effect on pituitary hormone production and because it empties the mammary gland of milk.[252] Milk accumulation further inhibits milk synthesis, explaining why a certain level of nursing activity is necessary for successful breast-feeding. In the absence of suckling, PRL concentrations, which rise throughout gestation, return to normal by 7 postpartum days.[243] Suckling increases serum PRL levels approximately 8.5-fold in actively nursing mothers,[253, 254] and the milk let-down phenomenon is not associated with increased PRL. As nursing continues, PRL concentrations fall, but each suckling episode causes a subsequent episodic rise in serum PRL. Mean serum concentrations were 162 μg/L at 2 to 4 postpartum weeks, 130 μg/L at 5 to 14 weeks, and 77 μg/L at 15 to 24 weeks.[255]

It is unclear why active milk production continues despite progressively lower PRL levels after parturition. Although PRL is essential for milk production, the milk yield does not closely correlate with serum PRL levels.[256] In addition to its effects on PRL, suckling stimulates posterior pituitary oxytocin release. Unlike those of PRL, oxytocin responses to suckling do not decline as nursing continues for up to 6 months. Mothers who breast-fed exclusively had mean stimulated oxytocin levels significantly higher during late than during early lactation.[255] Oxytocin induces myoepithelial cell contraction, thereby causing milk ejection.[257] Oxytocin also has important effects on alveolar proliferation.[258] Mice deficient in oxytocin are unable to nurse their young, and oxytocin replacement permits dams to nurse.

Lactational Amenorrhea

Lactational amenorrhea is a form of contraception that depends on the frequency and duration of breast-feeding. The Kung hunter-gatherer women were suckled approximately four times an hour and at will during the night and bore a mean of 4.7 children during their reproductive years.[259] In contrast, the Hutterites of North America bore a mean of 10.6 children during their lifetimes, presumably because they nursed according to a rigid schedule, used supplemental feedings, and weaned at 1 year. In Edinburgh, resumption of menses, albeit anovulatory, occurred in 28 weeks and the first ovulation occurred at a mean of 34 postpartum weeks because of persistently abnormal LH pulsatile secretion.[260]

Immune Function

Several lines of evidence indicate that PRL is a lymphocyte growth factor and stimulates immune responsiveness.[261] PRL levels change in concert with immune disease, as seen in patients with lupus erythematosus. In immunosuppressed mice, PRL stimulated immune cell functions.[262] Although PRL has been suggested as an immunomodulatory hormone,[263] there is evidence that PRL may not be important for immune function[264] because innate immunity was not altered in mice that lacked either the PRL receptor ($PRLR^{(-/-)}$) or the PRL gene ($PRL^{(-/-)}$).[207, 264, 265]

Prolactin Effects on Reproductive Function

In mice with disrupted PRL receptor expression, both ovulation and the number of primary follicles are reduced.[208, 266] These findings underscore the luteotrophic function of PRL but do not explain the suppressed gonadal function observed in patients with hyperprolactinemia.[267] These include a short luteal phase, reduced central FSH and LH levels, decreased granulosa cells, decreased estradiol levels, and ultimately amenorrhea (Fig. 8–22). Clearly, attenuated gonadotropin secretion is also a major determinant of ovarian dysfunction in these patients. Male mice with disrupted PRL receptors are fertile with low gonadotropin and normal testosterone levels. In male subjects with hyperprolactinemia, LH and FSH pulsatility is attenuated, testosterone levels are suppressed, and sperm counts and motility are low.

Prolactin Assays

The PRL radioimmunoassay (RIA) is highly specific and clearly distinguishes PRL from GH. PRL measurements are standardized using reference preparations provided by the National Institute for Biological Standards and Control in London and the National Hormone and Pituitary Program. Improvements in assay efficiency and turnaround time, reproducibility, and sensitivity have been achieved by immunoradiometric assay (IRMA) and chemiluminescent PRL assays. Because these samples are usually assayed at a single dilution, extremely high PRL concentrations may saturate their ability to detect very high PRL levels, resulting in a falsely low value being reported.[268] This "hook" effect may result in PRL-secreting macroadenomas diagnosed as clinically nonfunctioning adenomas, with "normal" PRL levels reported in about 5% of patients. In patients harboring macroadenomas with clear-cut clinical features of hyperprolactinemia, serum samples should be subjected to at least a 1:100 dilution before assay.

Prolactin Secretion

The calculated production rate of PRL ranges from 200 to 536 μg/day/m^2, and the metabolic clearance rate ranges from 40 to 71 mL/min/m^2.[269] PRL is cleared rapidly with a calculated disappearance half-life ranging from 26 to 47 minutes. PRL secretion occurs episodically in 4 to 14 secretory pulses, each lasting 67 to 76 minutes, over 24 hours.[270–272] PRL is secreted episodically during the day, with the highest levels achieved during sleep and the lowest occurring between 10 AM and noon.[273] The nocturnal elevation is sleep entrained and a temporal relationship exists between rapid eye movement (REM) and non-REM sleep cycles,[274] and PRL may cause periods of REM. VIP stimulates both REM sleep and PRL, and when VIP was given to rats together with a PRL antiserum, REM sleep was inhibited. PRL levels fall with age in both men and women. In older men, less PRL is produced with each secretory burst than in younger men.[275] Likewise, postmenopausal women have lower mean serum PRL levels and a lower PRL pulse frequency than premenopausal women or men, suggesting a stimulatory effect of estrogen on both of these parameters.[217]

Hyperprolactinemia

In the absence of a prolactinoma, hyperprolactinemia may be caused by other pituitary or sellar tumors that inhibit dopamine because of pressure on the pituitary stalk or interruption of the vascular connections between the pituitary and hypothalamus (Table 8–12).

Idiopathic Hyperprolactinemia

An elevated circulating PRL level in patients in whom no cause is identified is considered idiopathic, and these patients are relatively resistant to dopamine.[276] The mean serum PRL level in 41 patients with idiopathic hyperprolactinemia was 57 μg/L, with only 3 patients having PRL concentrations over 100 μg/L.[277] Patients were observed for up to 11 years, and 33 had both galactorrhea and amenorrhea or galactorrhea and oligomenorrhea. Hyperprolactinemia ultimately resolved spontaneously in 14 patients.

Macroprolactinemia

PRL is a 23-kd single-chain polypeptide but may also be produced in higher molecular mass forms (50 and 150 kd). Macroprolactinemia reflects a predominant larger circulating PRL molecule (particularly the 150-kd variety) with markedly reduced bioactivity, and few of the expected clinical abnormalities usually associated with hyperprolactinemia (sexual dysfunction, galactorrhea, osteoporosis) occur.[278] The high-molecular-weight PRL variant may represent 85% or more of the total PRL, whereas under usual circumstances the 22-kd variety predominates. Screening for macroprolactinemia can be accomplished by polyethylene glycol precipitation of serum samples.[279]

Other Causes of Hyperprolactinemia

Mild hyperprolactinemia occurs in up to 30% of women with *polycystic ovarian syndrome.*[280] No definite cause-and-effect relationship between the two disorders is apparent.[281] Dopamine agonists reduced PRL and LH levels in patients with polycystic ovarian syndrome in the presence or absence of hyperprolactinemia, and indeed a subset of patients with amenorrhea experienced a return of menses after treatment with these drugs.[282] *Breast stimulation* has only a minimal effect on serum PRL levels. In 18 normal women serum PRL rose from a mean of 10 to 15 μg/L during breast pump stimulation,[253] and no increase was observed in men. Up to 20% of patients with *hypothyroidism* have elevated PRL levels.[283] Although the cause of this elevation is not known, studies of hypothyroid animals suggest increased pituitary TRH.[284] Treatment of hypothyroidism with thyroid hormone normalizes serum PRL if the hyperprolactinemia is due to thyroid hormone deprivation.[285] PRL is moderately elevated (mean 28 μg/L) in patients with *chronic renal failure* and those receiving dialysis.[286] The increase is largely a result of an increase in little PRL related in part to a decreased glomerular filtration rate. A specific pituitary defect is also suggested by the observation that TRH failed to evoke PRL in these patients.[287] Sexual dysfunction is common, and reducing PRL with dopamine agonists improved sexual function in men receiving dialysis[288] but did not normal-

Table 8–12. Etiology of Hyperprolactinemia

Physiologic
Pregnancy
Lactation
Stress
Sleep
Coitus
Exercise

Pathologic
Hypothalamic-Pituitary Stalk Damage
Tumors
- Craniopharyngioma
- Suprasellar pituitary mass extension
- Meningioma
- Dysgerminoma
- Hypothalamic metastases

Granulomas
Infiltrations
Rathke's cyst
Irradiation
Trauma
- Pituitary stalk section
- Suprasellar surgery

Pituitary
Prolactinoma
Acromegaly
Macroadenoma (compressive)
Idiopathic
Plurihormonal adenoma
Lymphocytic hypophysitis or parasellar mass
Macroprolactinemia
Surgery
Trauma

Systemic Disorders
Chronic renal failure
Polycystic ovarian disease
Cirrhosis
Pseudocyesis
Epileptic seizures
Cranial radiation
Chest—neurogenic chest wall trauma, surgery, herpes zoster

Pharmacologic
Neuropeptides
Thyrotropin-releasing hormone
PRL-releasing peptide

Drug-Induced Hypersecretion
Dopamine receptor blockers
- Phenothiazines: chlorpromazine, perphenazine
- Butyrophenones: haloperidol
- Thioxanthenes
- Metoclopramide

Dopamine synthesis inhibitors
- α-Methyldopa

Catecholamine depletors
- Reserpine

Cholinergic Agonists
Physostigmine

Antihypertensives
Labetolol
Reserpine
Verapamil

H_2 Antihistamines
Cimetidine
Ranitidine

Estrogens

Oral Contraceptives

Oral Contraceptive Withdrawal

Anticonvulsants
Phenytoin

Anesthetics

Neuroleptics
Chlorpromazine
Promazine
Promethazine
Trifluoperazine
Fluphenazine
Butaperazine
Perphenazine
Thiethylperazine
Thioridazine
Haloperidol
Pimozide
Thiothixene
Molindone

Opiates and Opiate Antagonists
Heroin
Methadone
Apomorphine
Morphine

Antidepressants
Tricyclic antidepressants
- Chlorimipramine
- Amitriptyline

Selective serotononin re-uptake inhibitors
- Fluoxetine

ize menses.[289] Side effects of dopamine agonists in patients with renal failure may be exacerbated because of fluid shifts and interactions of multiple medications.

PRL levels rise in response to stress, correlate with the degree of stress, and generally return to normal as stress abates. The mean peak serum PRL in 19 women undergoing general anesthesia was 39 μg/L immediately before surgery, was 173 μg/L at surgery, and was still elevated 24 hours after surgery at 47 μg/L.[290] Severe *head trauma* also results in hyperprolactinemia, often accompanied by diabetes insipidus or SIADH and other anterior pituitary hormone deficiencies. Fifty percent of patients experienced moderate hyperprolactinemia after *cranial and hypothalamic radiation*.[291] A variety of *medications* cause minimal or moderate PRL elevations and may cause galactorrhea, amenorrhea, or reduced male sexual function. Neuroleptic drugs elevate PRL because of their dopamine antagonist properties. Chlorpromazine stimulated PRL acutely after an intramuscular injection[191] and chronically during oral administration.[292] Neuroleptics, which act by antagonizing both serotonin and dopamine receptors, including clozapine and olanzapine, weakly induce PRL, whereas others such as risperidone are potent stimulators of PRL.[293]

Treatment of Drug-Induced Hyperprolactinemia

Unless patients exhibit sexual dysfunction, related osteoporosis, or troublesome galactorrhea, no treatment may be advised.

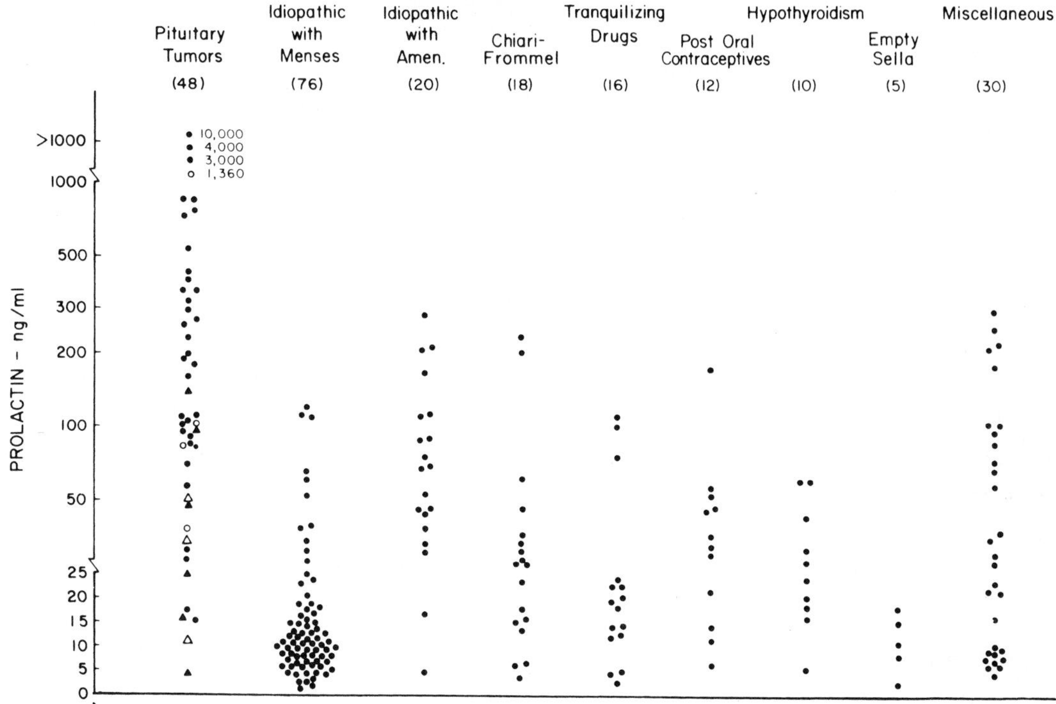

Figure 8–23. Prolactin levels in 235 patients with galactorrhea of various causes. Triangles denote patients with acromegaly; open circles or triangles denote patients studied after radiotherapy or surgery. (From Kleinberg DL, et al. Galactorrhea: a study of 235 cases including 48 with pituitary tumors. N Engl J Med 1977, 296:589–600.)

It should not always be assumed that hyperprolactinemia in patients receiving drugs known to elevate PRL is due to those medications. Prolactinoma, other pituitary or hypothalamic lesions, hypothyroidism, or renal failure should be considered. In patients taking neuroleptic medications, if the clinical situation permits, temporary drug withdrawal might be considered to determine whether PRL levels become normal. If not, pituitary MRI should be performed. When neuroleptics elevate PRL, olanzapine may be tried because it does not elevate PRL.[294] In determining to discontinue a drug or use an alternative medication, the benefits should be weighed against the risks of drug replacement or cessation. Although combined use of dopamine antagonists and dopamine agonists is not usually advised because of the increased risk of side effects, such as postural hypotension and worsening of psychosis, some advocate the use of both simultaneously.[293, 295]

Galactorrhea

The Talmud describes a man who nursed his baby after his wife's untimely death, probably representing the first recorded case of male galactorrhea. Galactorrhea and amenorrhea were reported in the 19th century by Chiari,[296] and only in the 1950s did Argonz[297] and Forbes[298] and their colleagues associate galactorrhea and amenorrhea with pituitary tumors and PRL. Galactorrhea, inappropriate secretion of milk-like substances from the nipples of either men or women,[234] may persist after childbirth or discontinuation of nursing for as long as 6 months. Thereafter, continued milk production is considered abnormal and other etiologies for galactorrhea should be investigated.

Galactorrhea can occur either unilaterally or bilaterally, be profuse or sparse, and vary in color and thickness. If blood is present in the galactorrhea fluid, it could be the harbinger of an underlying pathologic process, such as a ductal papilloma or carcinoma, and mammography or sonography is indicated. Blood may also appear in galactorrhea fluid with no underlying tumor, such as during pregnancy. Conversely, the absence of blood does not rule out an underlying tumor, particularly when galactorrhea is unilateral and the fluid emanates from a single duct.

The most common cause of galactorrhea is hyperprolactinemia[283] (Fig. 8–23). It is likely that most patients with so-called idiopathic galactorrhea with amenorrhea harbor microprolactinomas. Fifty percent of patients with acromegaly also have hyperprolactinemia. Even in the absence of hyperprolactinemia, human GH is a potent lactogen and can cause galactorrhea when elevated.[299] Twenty-nine of 48 patients with pituitary tumors and galactorrhea had PRL concentrations less than 200 μg/L, suggesting that they had pituitary tumors other than prolactinomas on the basis of stalk compression.

Idiopathic Galactorrhea with Regular Menses

This diagnosis represents the largest single cause of galactorrhea. In two thirds of patients, galactorrhea begins after parturition persists, despite the resumption of menses, and probably does not represent a pathologic entity. Normal PRL levels may still permit milk production because treatment of such patients with dopamine agonists alleviates galactorrhea.

Chiari-Frommel Syndrome

The syndrome, first described by Chiari and later in the 19th century by Frommel,[296] consists of postpartum galactorrhea, amenorrhea, and "utero-ovarian atrophy" in patients not nursing. Eighteen such patients had galactorrhea and amenorrhea for up to 11 years after parturition.[283] The mean PRL level was 45 μg/L. This disorder is usually self-limiting, and patients eventually become spontaneously fertile, sometimes without having had an intervening menstrual period. Individual patients with postpartum amenorrhea, hyperprolactinemia, and

Table 8–13. Signs and Symptoms of Prolactinomas

Signs and Symptoms Associated with Tumor Mass	Signs and Symptoms Associated with Hyperprolactinemia
Visual field abnormalities	Amenorrhea, oligomenorrhea, primary amenorrhea, infertility
Blurred vision or decreased visual acuity	Decreased libido, impotence, premature ejaculation, erectile dysfunction, oligospermia
Symptoms of hypopituitarism	
Headaches	Galactorrhea
Cranial nerve palsies	
Pituitary apoplexy	Osteoporosis
Seizures (temporal lobe)	
Hydrocephalus (rare)	
Unilateral exophthalmos (rare)	

galactorrhea have also been found subsequently to harbor prolactinomas.

Management of Galactorrhea

Treating the underlying cause of galactorrhea is usually effective. Treating prolactinomas with dopamine agonists reduces tumor size and PRL, normalizes abnormal sexual function, and alleviates galactorrhea. If a pituitary tumor is not PRL-secreting, high PRL levels are normalized and galactorrhea reduced by dopamine agonists but the underlying disorder is not addressed. For medication-induced galactorrhea, an alternative medication might be tried. Galactorrhea related to hypothyroidism should be treated with thyroid hormone replacement. If the galactorrhea is entirely due to inadequate thyroid hormone, thyroxine (T_4) therapy should normalize both TSH and PRL secretion and suppress nonpuerperal galactorrhea. If hyperprolactinemia persists after T_4 therapy, the existence of two coexisting disorders is likely. It may not be necessary to treat all patients with galactorrhea unless it is profuse or troublesome to the patient or is associated with sexual dysfunction.[300]

Prolactin-Secreting Adenomas

With the development of a human PRL assay in 1970,[190, 192] it became apparent that prolactinomas were the most frequently encountered secretory pituitary tumors, occurring with an annual incidence of approximately 6 in 100,000 (Table 8–13). The incidence would be much higher if the estimate included microadenomas discovered in 23% to 27% of pituitaries at autopsy, 42% of which immunostain positively for PRL.[301] The female/male ratio for microprolactinomas is 20:1, whereas for macroadenomas the gender ratio is roughly 1.[302] Both PRL levels and tumor size generally remain stable when followed prospectively.[303, 304] Although in some patients PRL levels fall over time and microadenomas may disappear on MRI, 7% to 14% of microadenomas continue to grow.[305, 306]

Macroprolactinomas have a greater propensity to grow and are typically larger in men than in women. Tumor size correlates positively with serum PRL levels, and a PRL level higher than 200 ng/mL is strongly indicative of a PRL-secreting pituitary tumor. In 45 men and 51 women with prolactinomas, the mean serum PRL levels were 2789 ± 572 and 292 ± 74 ng/mL, respectively. Tumor size was also larger in men than women (26 ± 2 mm versus 10 ± 1 mm). Tumors in men are more invasive and show histologic evidence of more rapid growth.[307] However, PRL levels above 200 ng/mL are not always indicative of a prolactinoma and may reflect use of a drug such as risperidol. In contrast, a PRL concentration less than 200 ng/mL in a patient harboring a macroadenoma indicates that the tumor is probably not producing PRL. In that case, it is likely that PRL elevation occurs as a result of mass pressure on the pituitary stalk or portal circulation, presumably interrupting inhibitory control by dopamine.[308]

Pathology and Pathogenesis

Although more than 99% of prolactinomas are benign and often sharply demarcated without evidence of invasion, about half invade local structures[309] as evidenced by pathologic examination.[310] Invasive tumors may have higher mitotic activity and are more cellular and pleomorphic. Invasion into adjacent dura, bone, or venous structures may represent an intermediate form of prolactinoma between the sharply demarcated benign variety and the exceedingly rare malignant tumor. Invasive tumors that do not metastasize are considered benign.[311] Immunostaining for PRL confirms the diagnosis of prolactinoma, which is usually distinct from the adjacent normal pituitary but is not truly encapsulated. These tumors have a "pseudocapsule" composed of compressed adenohypophyseal cells and a reticulin fiber network.[311] To consider a prolactinoma malignant, a distant extracranial metastasis must be demonstrated.[312, 313]

For the most part, prolactinomas grow slowly, arise sporadically, usually occur singly, and are monoclonal.[34] Infrequently, more than one prolactinoma arises within the gland.[314] Prolactinomas are the most common pituitary tumors associated with MEN-1, occurring in approximately 20% of a large kindred,[315] although the occurrence of prolactinomas is not evenly distributed. Familial prolactinomas have been described with no other features of MEN-1.[316]

Clinical Features

Prolactinomas usually come to attention because of symptoms or signs associated with either hyperprolactinemia or tumor size or invasiveness (see Table 8–13).

Hyperprolactinemia

Patients with both large and small PRL-secreting tumors can present with signs and symptoms of hyperprolactinemia. Menstrual irregularities, sexual dysfunction, galactorrhea,[283] and osteopenia[300] are attributable to elevated PRL levels. Elevated PRL causes sexual dysfunction through a short-loop feedback effect on gonadotropin pulsatilty,[317] presumably inhibiting GnRH[318] (see Fig. 8–22). In oophorectomized rats, high PRL decreased LH pulse frequency and amplitude.[319] High PRL also directly inhibits ovarian and testicular function. Increased opioid LH inhibition has also been implicated as a cause of amenorrhea in hyperprolactinemic patients.[320] Women with prolactinomas may present with primary or secondary amenorrhea, oligomenorrhea, menorrhagia, delayed menarche, or regular menses with a short luteal phase that may cause infertility. Patients may also report changes in libido and vaginal dryness. Sexual dysfunction in men is usually manifest as loss of or decrease in libido, impotence, premature ejaculation, or loss of erection. If men have oligospermia or azoospermia as a result of hyperprolactinemia, it usually occurs only after many years.

Up to 50% of women and 35% of men with prolactinomas have galactorrhea.[188] This gender difference may occur because male mammary tissue is less susceptible to the lactogenic effects of hyperprolactinemia.[234] Galactorrhea can be overlooked unless actively elicited. Bone density may decrease in both men and women as a result of hyperprolactinemia-induced sex steroid deficiency.[321]

Tumor Mass Effects

Prolactinomas may be found as a result of tumor size or invasiveness, or both. Microadenomas range from entirely asymptomatic tumors as small as 2 to 3 mm in diameter found at autopsy to larger ones that are still less than 10 mm in diameter. These tumors can be invasive despite their small size. The incidence of headaches in patients with a microadenoma is twice that of normal control subjects.[322] In contrast, macroadenomas range in size from noninvasive or diffuse tumors approximately 1 cm in diameter to huge tumors that may impinge on parasellar structures. Signs and symptoms caused by large or invasive tumors are often related to compressive effects on visual structures.

The most frequent ophthalmic complaint in a series of 1000 patients with tumors was loss of vision.[323] The most frequent objective findings were bitemporal hemianopsia, superior bitemporal defects, and decreased visual acuity. Headaches are common, but seizures (a result of extension into the temporal lobe) and hydrocephalus[324] are rare, as is unilateral exophthalmos.[325] Interestingly, many tumors invade the cavernous sinuses and yet cranial nerve palsies are rarely encountered. A sudden insult, such as pituitary apoplexy, is the more common cause of such palsies and may be a presenting symptom. Prolactinomas can also be found inadvertently by MRI or CT performed for another purpose.

Evaluation

All patients with pituitary tumors should have serum PRL levels measured. Conversely, patients with elevated serum PRL levels, not fully explicable by an obvious cause (such as pregnancy or exposure to neuroleptic medications), should be evaluated for the presence of a pituitary tumor. Prolactinomas may also coexist with another cause of hyperprolactinemia, such as neuroleptic drug administration. It is important to investigate even minimal to moderate PRL elevations because they may indicate the presence of a large pituitary tumor that does not secrete PRL. PRL levels correlate strongly with tumor size and are usually higher in male patients (Fig. 8–24). Occasionally, a patient with a very high serum PRL level may be found to have a normal result if dilutions of the patient's serum are not assayed, a phenomenon called the *high-dose hook effect*.[268]

A careful history often unmasks symptoms or signs of a space-related mass such as visual field abnormalities, impaired visual acuity, blurred or double vision, CSF rhinorrhea, headaches, diabetes insipidus, rare hydrocephalus,[324] and hypopituitarism. Patients should also be questioned carefully about sexual history, including onset of menarche, regularity of menses, fertility, libido, potency, and ability to maintain an erection. A history of galactorrhea should also be ascertained. The coexistence of galactorrhea and amenorrhea should lead the physician to make a diagnosis of pituitary adenoma until otherwise proved. A change in posture or history of bone fracture should be elucidated.

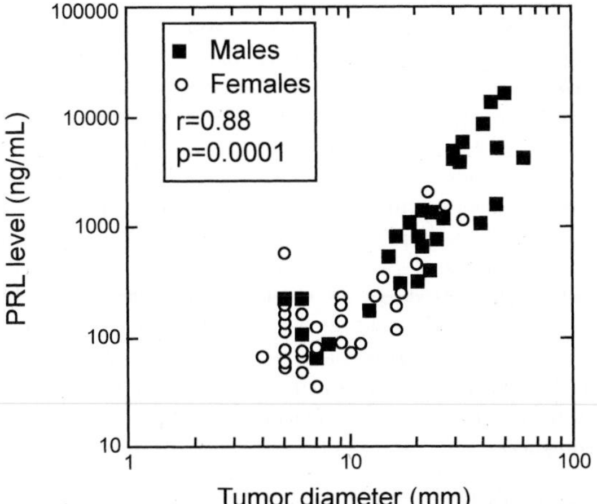

Figure 8–24. Prolactin-secreting tumors are more often macroadenomas in men ($n = 31$) than in women ($n = 45$). Serum prolactin levels highly correlate with tumor size. (Adapted from Danila DC, Klibanski, A. Prolactin secreting pituitary tumors in men. Endocrinologist 2001; 11:105–111.)

PRL is elevated in up to 50% of patients with acromegaly.[283] Patients in the early stages of acromegaly or with mild disease or those harboring acidophil stem cell adenomas may have few obvious signs of GH excess. Because human GH is as lactogenic as PRL by weight,[326] signs and symptoms of a prolactinoma may be mimicked by a purely GH-secreting tumor. Therefore, serum IGF-I should be measured. Elevated PRL levels are occasionally encountered in patients with TSH-secreting tumors. Other pituitary hormone functions should be ascertained to determine the presence of hypopituitarism. MRI is required to make a definitive diagnosis of a prolactinoma.

Treatment

Optimal outcomes of treatment for a prolactinoma include normalization of PRL levels (and associated signs and symptoms) and complete tumor removal or shrinkage with a reversal of tumor mass effects (Table 8–14). Specifically, previously abnormal sexual function and fertility should be restored, galactorrhea stopped, impaired bone density improved, tumor eliminated or reduced in size without impairing pituitary or hypothalamic function, and vision normalized, if impaired.

Medical Management

Medical management of prolactinomas with dopamine agonist drugs has been widely recommended as the treatment of choice.

Bromocriptine. Bromocriptine, a semisynthetic ergot alkaloid dopamine agonist, lowers elevated PRL levels, restores abnormal menstrual function in 80% to 90% of patients,[327, 328] shrinks prolactinomas, restores impaired sexual function, and improves galactorrhea.[306, 329, 330] Improvement in visual field abnormalities occurs in approximately 90% of affected patients.[331, 332] Drug withdrawal can result in rapid tumor expansion.[333] In contrast, occasional tumors that have shrunk during bromocriptine therapy do not become larger after drug withdrawal.[334] In a subset of patients, hyperprolactinemia disappeared spontaneously after long-term observation.[335] Occasionally, bromocriptine lowers PRL despite continued tumor expansion,[336] although when tumors grow during dopamine agonist therapy there is usually a simultaneous PRL elevation.

Despite high doses of bromocriptine, some patients are entirely or partially resistant to its effects. In bromocriptine-resistant patients, there is reduced bromocriptine binding to dopamine receptors on cell membranes.[337] Not infrequently, it is difficult to normalize PRL levels completely in patients with initially very high levels, although these patients have impressive tumor shrinkage and sometimes improved sexual function. Although higher doses or a change in the form of dopamine agonist has been reported to normalize PRL further in some cases,[249, 338] many such patients continue to have elevated PRL levels regardless of the treatment employed.

Bromocriptine shrinks prolactinomas by reducing tumor cell size, including cytoplasmic, nuclear, and nucleolar areas.[339–341] Histologic sections appear quite dense as a result of the small cell size and clumping of nuclei (Fig. 8–25). PRL mRNA and synthesis is inhibited, exocytoses are reduced, PRL secretory

Table 8–14. Treatment of Macroadenomas with Cabergoline

Study	Number of Patients	Time	Effect on PRL	Effect on Tumor Size	Method of Measurement
Cannavo S, 1999[1]	11	24 months	Normalized in 11/11 Mean 408 μg/L (range: 122–978) to 11.1 μg/L (range: 6.4–30)	Mean decrease from 16 to 6.9 (43%)	Maximum diameter (mm)
Biller B, 1996[2]	15	48 weeks	Normalized in 11/15 Mean PRL fell from 727 ng/mL (range: 160–3087) to 94 ng/mL (range: <1–926)	Decreased by a mean of 31% in 11/15 (range: 5–95)	Maximal gland craniocaudal height in the coronal plane and width (cm)—percent change from baseline
Colao 2000[3]	26 Naïve patients, 37 "resistant" patients	At least 52 weeks	Mean PRL fell from 1013 ng/mL (range: 186–5611) to the normal range in 21/26 naïve, and from 602 ng/mL (range: 148–3511) to normal in 19/37 "resistant" patients	Tumor volume reduced by a mean of 92% in naïve patients and by 58% in "resistant" ones	DiChiro and Nelson formula: volume = height × length × width × π/6 (mm^3)
Di Sarno A, 2001[4]	56	24 months	46/56 normalized from mean of 2069 ng/mL (ranges: N/A) to 5.7 ng/ml (N/A) in "responders" and from 2069 ng/mL to 69 ng/mL (ranges: N/A) in "non-responders"	Mean decrease from 19.9–7.4 mm in "responders" and from 23.6 to 11.9 mm in "non-responders"	Maximal tumor diameter (mm)
Overall	Total = 145		108/145 patients had normalization of PRL	Tumor shrinkage occurred in 115/132 patients*	

*Information regarding number of patients in whom tumors shrank was not available for the Cannavo study, and all ranges were not available for the Colao and Di Sarno studies.

[1]Cannavo S, Curto L, Squadrito S, et al. Cabergoline: a first-choice treatment in patients with previously untreated prolactin-secreting pituitary adenoma. J Endocrinol Invest 1999; 22(5):354–359.

[2]Biller BMK, Molitch ME, Vance ML, et al. Treatment of prolactin-secreting macroadenomas with the once-weekly dopamine agonist cabergoline. J Clin Endocrinol Metab 1996; 81:2338–2343.

[3]Colao A, Di Sarno A, Landi ML, et al. Macroprolactinoma shrinkage during cabergoline treatment is greater in naive patients than in patients pretreated with other dopamine agonists: a prospective study in 110 patients. J Clin Endocrinol Metab 2000; 85(6):2247–2252.

[4]Di Sarno A, Landi ML, Cappabianca P, et al. Resistance to cabergoline as compared with bromocriptine in hyperprolactinemia: prevalence, clinical definition, and therapeutic strategy. J Clin Endocrinol Metab 2001; 86(11):5256–5261.

granules decrease, and rough endoplasmic reticulum and Golgi apparatus involute. The net effect is reduced cell volume.[306] Tumor necrosis may also occur.[342]

Perivascular fibrosis was noted in prolactinomas derived from patients treated with bromocriptine[343] and it was proposed that this led to difficulty in tumor removal. However, others found no effect of prior treatment with bromocriptine on surgical success rates.[344, 345] In contrast, bromocriptine was a helpful adjunct to transsphenoidal microsurgery for macroprolactinomas.[346] Even the largest tumors or those with the highest PRL levels respond well to treatment with 2.5 mg of bromocriptine three times daily. Higher doses are often not more effective.[188] When positive effects on tumor size and amenorrhea and galactorrhea are established, some patients can be satisfactorily maintained with smaller doses[347] but rarely without medication.

Cabergoline. Cabergoline has a longer duration of action than other available dopamine agonists and is usually administered once or twice weekly. Since its introduction, it has surpassed bromocriptine as the first-line therapeutic choice for most patients. The long half-life of cabergoline is a result of its high affinity for D2 receptors on lactotrophs[306] and a greater propensity of the drug to remain in pituitary tissue.[306, 348]

In pharmacokinetic studies, cabergoline lowered PRL in a dose-related manner.[349, 350] PRL levels were normalized in 83% of 459 women with hyperprolactinemia treated with cabergoline (0.5 to 1 mg twice weekly) and in 52% of women receiving bromocriptine (2.5 to 5 mg twice daily). Cabergoline was also more effective than bromocriptine in restoring ovulatory cycles and fertility (72% versus 52%; $P < .001$), was better tolerated than bromocriptine, and caused fewer but similar side effects (Fig. 8–26) (see Table 8–14). Tumor size decreased in 11 of 15 patients with macroadenomas, and menses resumed in three of four premenopausal women.[351] In our experience, bromocriptine or pergolide is as effective or almost as effective as cabergoline. In 85 patients with macroprolactinomas treated with cabergoline (0.25 to 10.5 mg/week), PRL concentrations were normalized in 61% of patients, decreased by at least 75% in an additional 24 patients, and tumor size decreased in 66% of patients. Nine patients were resistant to cabergoline despite doses of up to 7 mg/week.[352, 353] Despite the continued experience that a subset of hyperprolactinemic patients are resistant to most or all dopamine agonists, a report indicated that cabergoline normalized PRL in 15 of 19 patients with macroprolactinomas previously resistant to other dopamine agonists.[338]

Pergolide Mesylate. Pergolide, a long-acting ergot derivative with dopamine agonist properties, has an estimated potency 100 times that of bromocriptine.[354] Pergolide is administered at an initial dose of 25 μg/day, and then at 50 μg/day with gradual dose escalation depending on the extent of serum PRL normalization. Menses resumed in 76% of women and serum

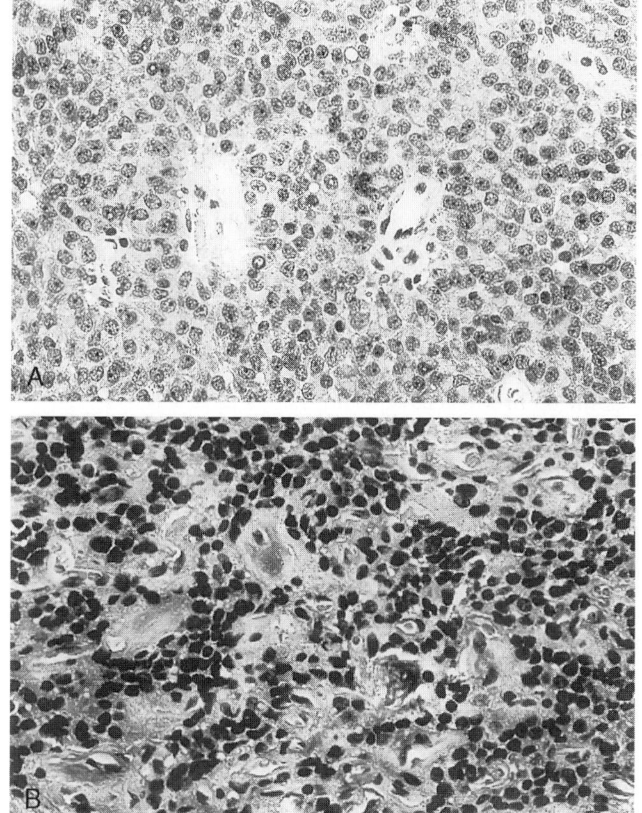

Figure 8-25. *Top,* A prolactin-secreting adenoma removed at surgery with no preoperative dopamine agonist therapy. *Bottom,* Prolactin-producing pituitary adenoma removed by surgery from a patient treated with dopamine agonist in the preoperative period. The adenoma cells are small with dark nuclei and a narrow rim of cytoplasm. Accumulation of interstitial connective tissue is apparent. (Hematoxylin-eosin stain; original magnification ×400.) (Courtesy of Kalman Kovacs.)

testosterone increased in 10 of 14 men not receiving testosterone, and tumor size decreased in 10 of 13 patients with macroadenomas.[249] In 22 patients with macroadenomas, pergolide lowered PRL from a mean of 2938 to 59 ng/mL. PRL became normal in 15 of 22 patients, and tumor shrinkage was observed in 95%.[355] The efficacies and side effect profiles of pergolide and bromocriptine were similar in a study of 96 patients with prolactinomas.[356]

Quinagolide. This nonergot dopamine agonist (CV 205-502), administered once daily (mean daily dose of 0.09 mg), normalized PRL in 5 of 10 patients previously intolerant of or resistant to bromocriptine.[357] Side effects, principally nausea, occurred in 6 of 10 women. In 26 patients similarly evaluated,[358] quinagolide normalized PRL levels in 13 but the post-treatment mean remained above normal (30 ng/mL). Thirteen had a return of menses, and galactorrhea was reduced in 12 of 15 women. The effect of this medication on tumor shrinkage is similar to that of other dopamine antagonists, but it is not available in the United States.

Administration. Attention to administration of dopamine agonists helps avoid or minimize potential adverse effects. Usual starting doses are 1.25 mg of bromocriptine (daily), 0.025 mg of pergolide (daily), and 0.25 mg of cabergoline (weekly). Doses of medication are either increased gradually as tolerated or decreased depending on tolerability, and treatment should be initiated with a small dose with food before bedtime. Patients should initially avoid activities that cause peripheral vasodilatation (e.g., hot showers or baths), thereby decreasing the risk of postural hypotension. If side effects are troublesome, the next dose should be halved and doses subsequently increased gradually to reach effective levels. Switching from one medication to another may be beneficial,[299] as evidenced by the success of pergolide in patients intolerant of bromocriptine. Intravaginal bromocriptine administration has been used with some success to reduce adverse events.[359]

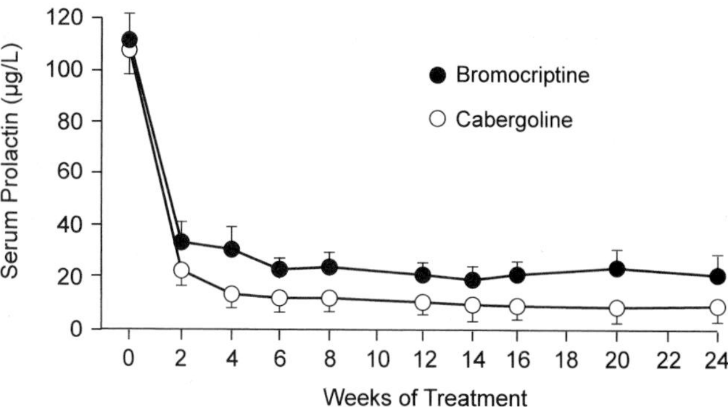

Figure 8-26. Comparison of bromocriptine and cabergoline in suppressing prolactin levels in women with hyperprolactinemia. (From Webster J, et al. A comparison of cabergoline and bromocriptine in the treatment of hyperprolactinemic amenorrhea. N Engl J Med 1994; 331:904–909.)

Adverse Events of Dopamine Agonists. Side effects of dopamine agonists are common. Nausea occurs in 31% to 50% of patients; nasal stuffiness, depression, and digital vasospasm also occur, the latter more frequently with higher doses, as in patients with Parkinson's disease. The most serious side effect, postural hypotension, which can cause loss of consciousness, occurs infrequently and can often be avoided by careful dosing. Signs and symptoms of psychosis or exacerbation of preexisting psychosis can be encountered in up to 1.3% of patients taking bromocriptine.[360] Psychosis also occurs with other dopamine agonists, including cabergoline (personal experience).

A history of present or past psychotic symptoms should raise concerns about using these medications. If psychosis occurs in a patient in whom dopamine agonists are clearly the treatment of choice, a judicious combination of the agent and antipsychotic medication can be effective. A neuroleptic that is not a potent PRL stimulator, such as olanzapine, is preferred. The combined use of dopamine agonists and antagonists may increase the occurrence of side effects, particularly postural hypotension. Other rarely reported serious side effects include CSF rhinorrhea,[361] hepatic dysfunction,[249] and cardiac arrythmias.[299] Retroperitoneal fibrosis, pleural effusions, and thickening have been reported in patients taking high doses of bromocriptine.[306, 362]

Radiation Therapy

Linear accelerator radiotherapy is effective in controlling or reducing the size of prolactinomas.[363, 364] However, this therapy takes years to achieve its maximal effect. The usual recommended radiation dose is 4500 to 4600 cGy, and higher doses are associated with a greater complication rate.[365] Normalization of PRL was achieved in 7 of 12 patients during 3 to 8 years after radiotherapy[363] and in 18 of 36 patients at a mean of 7.3 years after treatment in another study.[366]

Hypopituitarism is a side effect of radiation. Of 165 patients after radiotherapy (3750 to 4250 cGy),[367] all patients were GH-deficient, 91% were gonadotropin-deficient, 77% were

ACTH-deficient, and 42% were TSH-deficient by 5 years. Of 36 patients with prolactinomas, 83% of whom had normal GH responses to insulin-induced hypoglycemia before therapy, 34 were GH-deficient 9 to 12 years after radiotherapy.[366] The incidence of other forms of hypopituitarism was lower.

Thus, although radiotherapy is useful in the control of tumor growth, it is not nearly as effective as dopamine agonists on endocrine function. Stereotactic conformal radiotherapy with a linear accelerator can provide greater tumor focus and a smaller radiation field.[166] There are as yet no reports on large-scale studies of treatment of prolactinomas with gamma knife radiotherapy.

Surgery

Surgical removal of prolactinomas by the transsphenoidal route was repopularized in the early 1970s.[368] As with other functioning pituitary tumors, the success rate of surgery correlates inversely with tumor size and serum PRL concentrations.[344, 369] In a compilation of results in 31 published surgical series, serum PRL was normalized in 71% of 1224 patients with microprolactinomas.[306] Although surgical cure rates for microprolactinomas are high, the rate of hyperprolactinemia recurrence is also relatively high,[370] now estimated to be 17% in patients initially considered cured.[371] In contrast, complete removal of macroprolactinomas, especially large invasive ones, is difficult to achieve; postoperative serum PRL was normalized in only 32% of patients with macroadenomas, with a recurrence rate of 19%. The experience of the surgeon is of major importance, as the cure rate is not nearly as favorable for neurosurgeons who perform a limited number of procedures.[372]

Although results of medical therapy are better than those of surgery, there remains a role for surgery in these patients. Patients with prolactinomas who are resistant to dopamine agonist therapy are particularly well suited for surgery. If tumor removal is only partial, adjunctive radiation therapy should be considered. Prophylactic transsphenoidal surgery should also be considered in women whose prolactinomas are large enough to be a potential threat to vision during pregnancy. A subset of patients cannot tolerate available dopamine agonists, and others prefer surgery and refuse medication (Fig. 8–27).

Pregnancy

The normal pituitary gland enlarges during pregnancy and by the end of pregnancy may increase in size by 136%.[373] Prolactinomas may also increase in size during pregnancy.[374] Pregnancy-associated tumor enlargement, as determined by the development of abnormal visual fields, has been estimated to occur in 1.4% of women with microadenomas and 16% of women with macroadenomas.[375] In other reports, the risk of macroadenoma enlargement has been estimated to be as high as 36%. In a prospective analysis in which 57 patients with microprolactinomas were observed by formal visual field examinations during pregnancy, none experienced visual disturbances. In contrast, six of eight primiparous women with macroadenomas had visual loss.[376] The results for patients with macroadenomas are probably skewed because these patients were recommended for surgery before pregnancy.

Although dopamine agonists have been used during pregnancy to prevent tumor growth (Fig. 8–28),[377, 378] it seems prudent to reduce fetal exposure to medication if possible. It is recommended that menstrual periods be allowed to occur naturally for a period of time (3 to 4 months) long enough to predict that a missed period might be a result of pregnancy (Table 8–15). Barrier contraception is recommended during this period. Within several days to a week of obtaining a positive hCG test, medication should be discontinued. In 6239 pregnancies of patients managed in this manner, bromocriptine therapy was not associated with increased abortions or terminations, prematurity, multiple births, or infant malformations above those expected in the control population.[306] There is no evidence that other dopamine agonists are less safe, but exposure to the other agonist forms in pregnancy is less comprehensively documented. Treatment options for patients harboring prolactinomas whose vision becomes impaired during pregnancy include bromocriptine, high-dose steroids, and surgery.[375, 379] One study reported that for 53 pregnant women receiving bromocriptine, mean offspring birth weight was normal, congenital abnormalities occurred in four babies, and the physical and intellectual development of the children was normal for up to 9 years.[378]

To avoid neurologic complications of tumor enlargement during pregnancy, it is recommended that women with prolactinomas be tested for sensitivity to dopamine agonists before proceeding with a pregnancy. If tumors are insensitive to dopamine agonist–related tumor shrinkage, prophylactic surgery would be appropriate. If the tumor is a macroadenoma approximating the optic chiasm, the likelihood of visual difficulties is greater and therefore surgery would be prudent before pregnancy.[380]

Gonadotropins

Gonadotroph cells secreting FSH and LH constitute about 10% to 15% of the functional anterior pituitary cells. Two classes of electrodense secretory granules are evident; large 350- to 450-nm and smaller 150- to 250-nm granules are packaged in vesicles (Figs. 8–29 and 8–30). They contain large, round cell bodies with prominent rough endoplasmic reticulum and Golgi apparatus. LH secretory granules often accumulate peripherally, and their Golgi may be less prominent. SF-1 and DAX-1 orphan nuclear receptors determine gonadotroph-specific gene expression.

Biosynthesis

In concert with peripheral hormones and paracrine soluble factors, FSH and LH function to regulate gonadal steroid hormone biosynthesis and initiate and maintain germ cell development. The four glycoprotein hormones LH, FSH, TSH, and hCG share structural homology, having evolved from a common ancestral gene. Although the homologous LH and FSH molecules are cosecreted by the single gonadotroph cell, their regulatory mechanisms are not uniformly concordant. The α and β subunits are encoded by different genes located on chromosomes 6, 11, and 19 (Fig. 8–4). The heterodimeric structure of the common α and unique β subunit is essential for their biologic activity. Disulfide linkages maintain noncovalent subunit linkages, which also determine the ultrastructure of the mature folded molecule (Fig. 8–31).[381] After processing of hormonal protein precursors, glycosylation occurs by transferring oligosaccharide complexes to asparaginyl residues.[382] Post-translational processing of carbohydrate side chains is critical for hormone signaling and may be species specific and not uniformly similar for both human LH and FSH.

The complex human LH-β gene cluster comprises seven CG-like genes, one of which encodes LH-β? whose promoter and transcriptional start site differ from those of hCG.[383, 384] The three exons and two introns encode a 24-amino-acid leader peptide and a 121-amino-acid mature protein. Unlike β-LH, hCG is present only in primate and equine species, and the hCG peptide product contains a 24-amino-acid carboxyl-

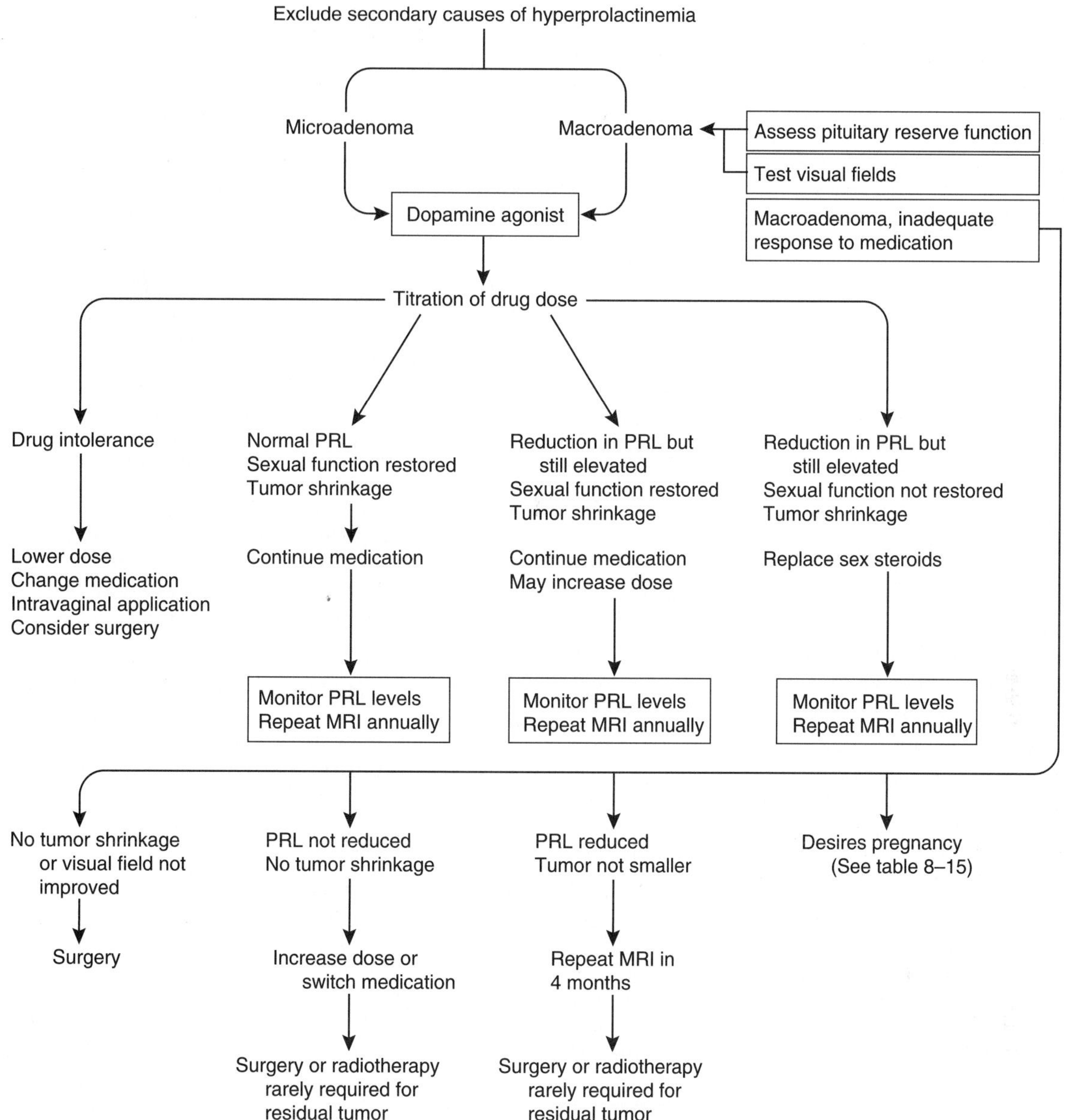

Figure 8–27. Prolactinoma management. After secondary causes of hyperprolactinemia have been excluded, subsequent management decisions are based on clinical imaging and biochemical criteria. MRI, magnetic resonance imaging; PRL, prolactin.

terminal extension.[385] Cell-specific LH gene expression and GnRH responsiveness of LH are subserved by different transcriptional mechanisms.[386, 387] GnRH induces LH-β transcription, as does SF-1.[388] The rat LH-β promoter contains an estrogen-responsive motif and a nuclear factor Y binding site, which appears to be important for basal but not GnRH-mediated trancription.[386] The FSH-β gene comprises three exons and two introns located on chromosome 11.[389] The gene promoter is dissimilar to that of LH-β, and structure-function mechanisms for transcriptional regulation of the human gene by GnRH and sex steroids are not well clarified.[390]

Gonadotropin Assays

Because of the high homology of the glycoprotein hormones, development of highly specific assays, especially to distinguish free α subunit from intact hormones, has been challenging. Heterogeneity of circulating LH and FSH molecules, insufficient assay sensitivity especially for measurements in normal healthy individuals, and lack of rigorously pure reference preparations have hampered assay development. Immunofluorometric assays detect LH with a sensitivity of 0.1 mIU/mL.[391] Differences in carbohydrate moieties result in isoelectric charge heterogeneity for LH, accounting for some of the disparities in biologic and immunoreactive LH ratios observed with GnRH agonist treatment, acute critical illness, or aging.

LH bioassays include assessing testosterone generation by cell cultures,[392] and FSH bioassays include measuring granulosa cell or Sertoli cell aromatase generation.[393] Because only intact molecules, but not free α or β subunits, are biologically active, these cumbersome assays are nevertheless useful for measuring bioactive hormone without potential cross-reaction with free subunits.

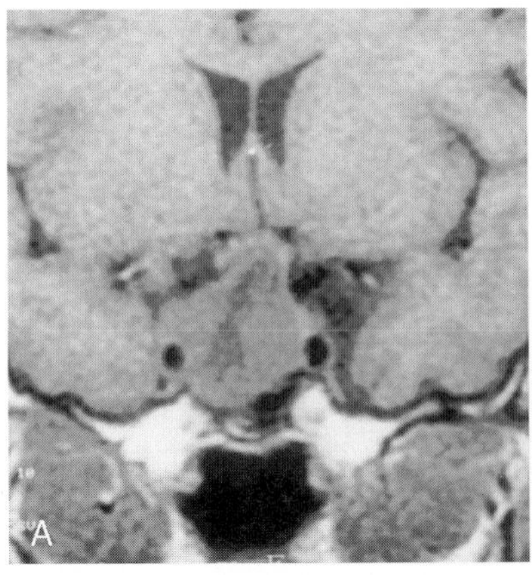

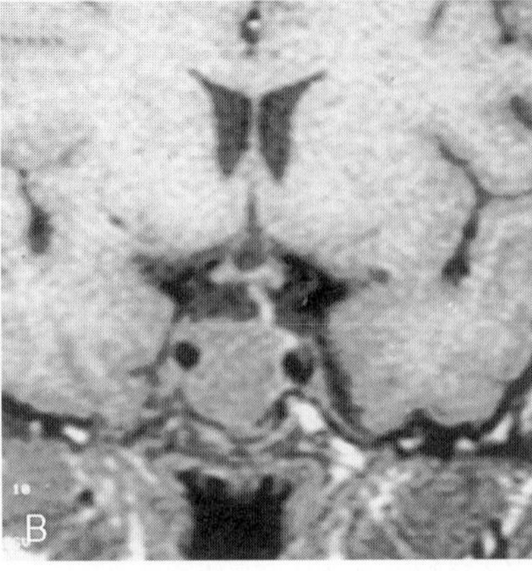

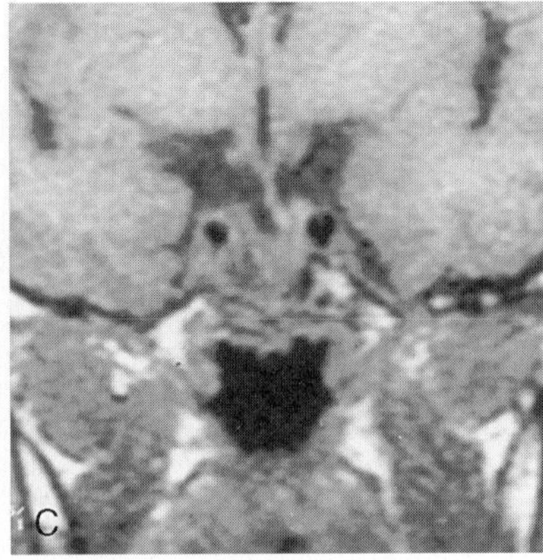

Figure 8–28. Shrinkage of macroadenoma by cabergoline in a woman harboring a macroadenoma *(A)* at 22 weeks of gestation when prolactin (PRL) was 488 μg/L *(B)* and further reduction at 3 postpartum weeks *(C)*. (From Liu C, Tyrrell JB. Successful treatment of a large macroprolactinoma with cabergoline during pregnancy. Pituitary 2002; 4:3.)

α Subunit Secretion

Both GnRH and TRH increase circulating levels of free α subunit derived from either gonadotrophs or thyrotrophs, especially in patients with hypothyroidism, after castration, and during the menopause. GnRH agonist treatment, TSH-secreting tumors, or nonfunctioning pituitary adenomas may result in discordant ratios of free α subunit from intact LH dimer secretion.

Regulation of FSH and LH Secretion

FSH and LH secretion patterns reflect the integration of sensitive complex hypothalamic, pituitary, and peripheral signals. Both GnRH pulse amplitude and frequency determine the physiologic patterns of LH and FSH secretion (Fig. 8–32).[394] In patients with hypothalamic GnRH deficiency, intravenous GnRH injections (25 ng/kg) that achieve GnRH levels similar to those present in primate hypophyseal-portal blood replicate the physiologic pattern of LH secretion.[395] The magnitude of the LH response exceeds that of FSH. Decreasing GnRH pulse frequency enhances LH pulse amplitudes, whereas increasing GnRH pulse frequency to more than every 2 hours down-regulates the subsequent LH response. The interpulse LH secretory interval is 55 minutes, and the pulse amplitude is approximately 40% of basal tonic secretion. Changes in gonadotropin secretion during infancy, childhood, puberty, and aging are described in Chapters 21 and 25 (Fig. 8–33). A log-linear relationship is evident between GnRH dose and the amounts of LH, FSH, and free α subunit pituitary secretion.

Both pituitary and hypothalamic targets for testosterone signals mediate FSH and LH regulation, and testosterone attenuates gonadotropin secretion in males. Thus, after castration, elevated gonadotropin levels can be partially overcome by testosterone replacement. The mechanisms involved are complex, as testosterone also exerts a stimulatory effect on FSH-β mRNA levels. Although estrogen administration decreases LH pulse amplitude in normal and GnRH-deficient male subjects,[396, 397] depending on the clinical situation, estrogen may either stimulate or inhibit pituitary gonadotropin synthesis and secretion and also inhibit GnRH synthesis and or action. This

Table 8–15. Management of Prolactinomas in Patients Planning Pregnancies*

Microadenoma	Macroadenoma
Discontinue dopamine agonist when pregnancy test positive	Consider surgery prior to pregnancy
↓	
Periodic visual field examinations during pregnancy	Ensure bromocriptine sensitivity prior to pregnancy
↓	↓
Postpartum MRI after 6 weeks	Follow visual fields expectantly and frequently
	↓
	Administer bromocriptine if vision becomes compromised
	↓
	Or, continue bromocriptine throughout pregnancy if tumor previously affected vision
	↓
	Consider high-dose steroids or surgery during pregnancy if vision threatened or adenoma hemorrhage
	Postpartum MRI after 6 weeks

*Pituitary MRI may be required during pregnancy if deemed necessary.
MRI, magnetic resonance imaging.

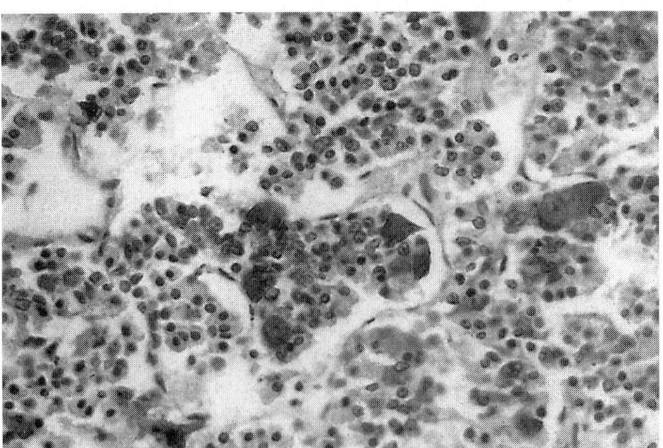

Figure 8–29. Normal gonadotroph cells contain immunoreactive β-follicle-stimulating hormone scattered throughout acini of the nontumorous pituitary. These round cells have evenly dispersed cytoplasmic immunoreactivity for α and β gonadotrophic subunits. (From Asa SL. In Tumors of the Pituitary Gland. Atlas of Tumor Pathology. Washington, DC, Armed Forces Institute of Pathology, 1997, p. 26.)

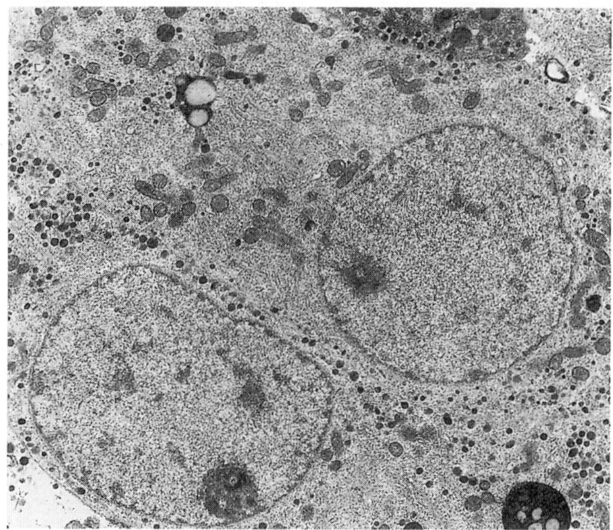

Figure 8–30. Electron micrograph of gonadotroph cell showing large round to elongated cells with ovoid nuclei with occasional nucleoli. Short profiles of rough endoplasmic reticulum are scattered throughout the cytoplasm and are dilated and frequently contain electron-lucent material. The Golgi complex is usually well developed and in a juxtanuclear location. Secretory granules are highly variable in size, shape, and electron density and lysosomes are prominent. (From Asa SL. In Tumors of the Pituitary Gland. Atlas of Tumor Pathology. Washington, DC, Armed Forces Institute of Pathology, 1997, p 26.)

pattern is manifest in the cyclic control of gonadotropin secretion during the menstrual cycle and during puberty.

LH, FSH, free α subunit, and testosterone pulses are usually concordant in male subjects (Bhasin 2002). Deconvolution pulse analysis allows estimation of "real-time" hormone secretion rates, with an assumed disappearance rate constant. The characteristic secretory episodes characterized for LH and FSH indicate daily production rates of 1000 and 200 IU, respectively, and a disappearance half-life of 90 and 500 minutes for the respective β subunits.[269, 398]

Gonadal Peptides

Pituitary gonadotropin secretion is regulated by gonadal peptides including inhibin A, an α:βA heterodimer, and inhibin B, an α:βB heterodimer, and follistatin peptides. The activin A (βA) and activin AB (βB) homodimers stimulate in vitro FSH secretion.[399] These proteins, related to transforming growth factor β and müllerian-inhibiting factor, are fully described in Chapter 16.

Follicle-Stimulating Hormone and Luteinizing Hormone Action

Female

Luteal cell LH receptors signal to enhance cAMP levels and induce cholesterol availability for ovarian steroidogenesis (Fig. 8–34). The steroidogenic acute regular (StAR) protein[400] is induced by LH and mediates cholesterol delivery to the inner membrane. LH enhances cytochrome P450–linked enzyme activity to synthesize pregnenolone and induces 3β-hydroxysteroid dehydrogenase, 17α-hydroxylase, and 17,20-ylase synthesis. The FSH receptor, a G protein–linked molecule with seven transmembrane domains shares 50% extracellular domain and 80% transmembrane homology with the LH receptor.[401] FSH regulates ovarian estrogen synthesis by inducing 17β-hydroxysteroid dehydrogenase and aromatase and also induces follicular growth. Estrogens are also permissive for FSH action and enhance FSH-induced cAMP levels.[402]

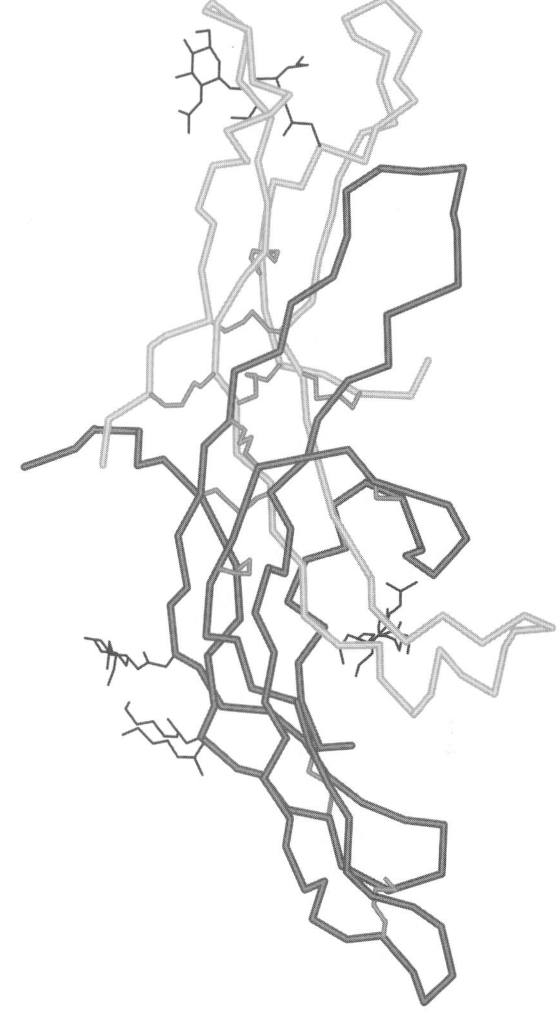

Figure 8–31. Schematic depiction of the subunit structure and glycosylation sites of the four glycoprotein hormone heterodimers (α subunit, *light gray;* β subunit, *dark gray*). (From *http://www.chem.gla.ac.uk/protein/glyco/GPH.html.)*

Male

Leydig cell LH receptor signaling induces intratesticular testosterone synthesis mediated by enhanced cAMP production. FSH function in male subjects is not readily apparent but probably mediates spermatozoa development from spermatids in concert with testosterone, especially as failed spermatogenesis leads to elevated FSH levels.

Gonadotropin-Releasing Hormone Stimulation Test

A single bolus of GnRH (25 to 100 μg) dose dependently evokes serum LH and FSH levels within 20 to 30 minutes. LH rises more abundantly than FSH, and peak values range from 8 to 34 mIU/mL; patients with low testosterone levels exhibit more exuberant responses.[403] In contrast, patients with hypogonadotropic hypogonadism and no demonstrable hypothalamic-pituitary lesion have blunted LH responses and reversal of the LH/FSH ratio. The test, however, cannot adequately distinguish hypothalamic from pituitary lesions, and similar

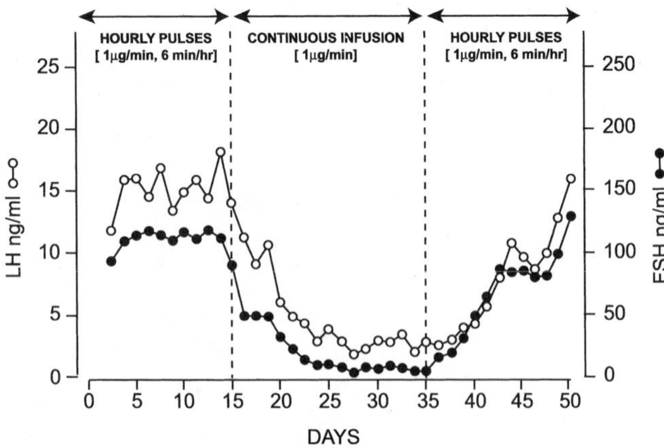

Figure 8–32. Effects of pulsatile or continuous administration of gonadotropin-releasing hormone (GnRH) to ovariectomized monkeys rendered GnRH-deficient by placement of a lesion in the hypothalamus. Gonadotropin secretion was restored by hourly GnRH pulses, reduced during a continuous GnRH infusion, and again increased after reinstitution of pulsatile GnRH administration. FSH, follicle-stimulating hormone. (From Belchetz PE, Plant TM, Nakai Y, et al. Hypophyseal responses to continuous and intermittent delivery of hypothalamic gonadotropin-releasing hormone. Science 1978; 202:631–633. Copyright 1978 by the American Association for the Advancement of Science.)

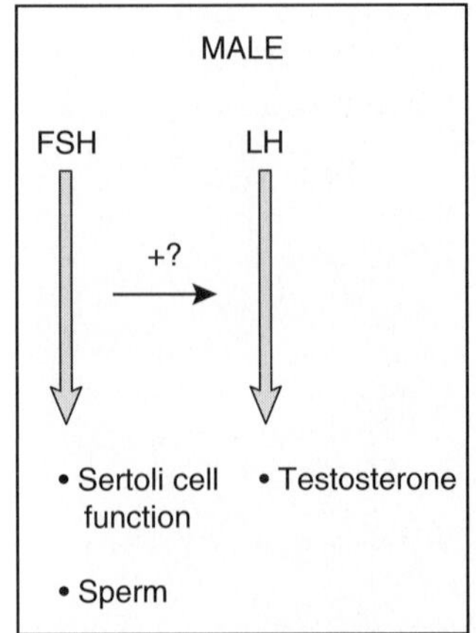

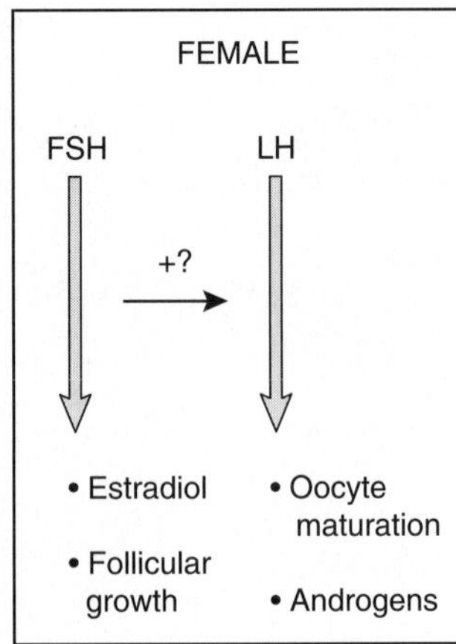

Figure 8–34. Functions of follicle-stimulating hormone (FSH) in the male and female. *Plus signs* and *horizontal arrows* indicate potentially unrecognized new functions of FSH since the discovery of FSHβ gene mutations. LH, luteinizing hormone. (Modified from Layman LC. Genetics of human hypogonadotropic hypogonadism. Am J Med Genet [Semin Med Genet] 1999; 89:240–248; Bhasin. Follicle-stimulating hormone and luteinizing hormone. In Melmed S (ed). The Pituitary, 2nd ed. Malden, Mass, Blackwell Scientific, 2002, pp 216–278.)

patterns are observed in patients with anorexia nervosa. Repetitive GnRH pulses may, in fact, normalize responses, as would be expected from an intact hypothalamic-pituitary unit. GnRH responses may vary during the stages of puberty, reflecting altered pituitary sensitivity.

Clomiphene (100 mg) administered daily for up to 4 weeks usually doubles LH levels, and FSH increases about 50% over baseline levels. Because an abnormal or absent response does not distinguish hypothalamic from pituitary lesions, the utility of this test is limited.

Gonadotropin Deficiency

Gonadotropin deficiency causes hypogonadism with decreased sex steroid production of varying degree, depending on the severity of the insult (Table 8–16). This disorder may occur at any stage of life. In its complete form (e.g., panhypopituitarism, Kallmann's syndrome), primary amenorrhea or total failure of male sexual development may occur. Later in life a varying spectrum of sexual dysfunction develops, ranging from luteal abnormalities or oligomenorrhea to amenorrhea in women and absence of libido, potency, and fertility in men. Women exhibit secondary amenorrhea, vaginal dryness, hot flushes, decreased bone density, decreased breast tissue, and infertility. Men have impotence, testicular hypoplasia or atrophy, decreased libido, low energy, infertility, loss of secondary sexual characteristics, decreased muscle strength and mass, decreased bone mass, decreased body hair growth, and fine facial wrinkling.

In both men and women, serum gonadotropin levels are inappropriately low in the presence of decreased sex steroids and sexual dysfunction. In women with amenorrhea or oligomenorrhea, serum LH, FSH, and estradiol levels should be measured. A vaginal cytologic study is helpful in determining the adequacy of gonadotropin function. Endogenous estrogen

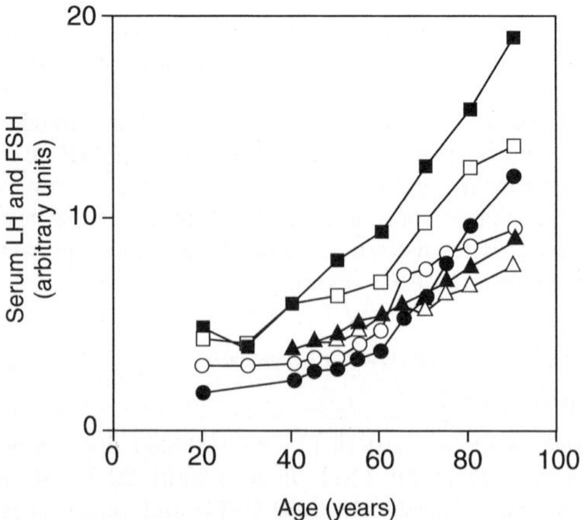

Figure 8–33. Serum luteinizing hormone (LH) levels *(open symbols)* and follicle-stimulating hormone (FSH) levels *(solid symbols)* in men as a function of age from three studies. (From Tenover JL. Male hormone replacement therapy including "andropause." Endocrinol Metab Clin North Am 1998; 27:969–987; Bhasin. In Melmed S (ed). The Pituitary, 2nd ed. Malden, Mass, Blackwell Scientific, 2002.)

Table 8–16. Clinical Features of Hypogonadotrophism

Prepubertal Onset
High-pitched voice
Terminal facial hair
Decreased or absent body hair
Eunuchoidal body proportions
Female escutcheon
Testicular volume <6 cm^3, hypoplastic
Testicular length <2.5 cm
Penile length <5 cm
Smooth scrotum with no rugae
Small prostate
Postpubertal Onset
Decreased libido
Slow beard growth
Decreased body hair
Testes atrophic if long-standing
Normal voice pitch
Decreased muscle and bone mass
Normal: skeletal proportions, penis length, scrotal rugae, prostate size

Table 8–17. Mutations Affecting Genes of the Hypothalamic-Pituitary-Gonadal Axis

Hypothalamus		Anterior Pituitary		Ovary		Testes	
Gene	**Phenotype**	**Gene**	**Phenotype**	**Gene**	**Phenotype**	**Gene**	**Phenotype**
Kal-1	HH Anosmia	*GnRH-R*	Partial or complete HH	*FSH-R*	Primary or secondary amenorrhea Delayed puberty	*FSH-R*	Defective spermatogenesis
Dax-1	HH AHC	*Dax-1*	HH AHC	*LH-R*	Normal puberty	*LH-R*	Pseudohermaphroditism
PC-1	HH Amenorrhea Obesity	*FSH-β*	Primary amenorrhea Defective spermatogenesis			*DAX-1*	Genital ambiguity Defective spermatogenesis
Lep	HH	*LH-β*	Delayed puberty			*AR*	Androgen insensitivity
Lep-R	HH Obesity Short stature					*DAZ*	OTA
						RBM	OTA

AR=Androgen receptor; DAZ=deleted in azoospermia; RBM=RNA binding motif protein; OTA=oligoteratoazoospermia; HH=hypogonadotropic hypogonadism.
Adapted from Pralong FP. Genetic basis of hypothalamic-pituitary hypogonadism. In Rappaport R, Amselem S (eds). Hypothalamic-Pituitary Development. Basel, Karger, p 125.

sufficiency can also be assessed by the response to a progesterone challenge (100 mg intramuscularly or 10 mg medroxyprogesterone [Provera] orally daily for 5 days). Men should have serum gonadotropin and testosterone levels measured.

Hypogonadotropic hypogonadism may result from hypothalamic or pituitary defects. Hypothalamic damage including Kallmann's syndrome, radiation, anorexia nervosa, and excessive stress result in deficient GnRH secretion and action. Pituitary damage from tumors, infarction, or hyperprolactinemia may directly or indirectly attenuate FSH and LH secretion patterns. These acquired causes of central hypogonadism are considered fully in Chapters 16 and 18, and genetic causes are listed in Table 8–17.

Because FSH is required for quantitatively normal spermatogenesis, isolated FSH deficiency is associated with oligospermia or azoospermia in normally androgenized men in the presence of normal testosterone and LH levels.[404] Isolated LH deficiency may be manifest by eunuchoidal body proportions and low testosterone levels. Low LH levels in these patients lead to low intratesticular testosterone concentrations with resultant decreased spermatogenesis.[405] Serum testosterone levels are restored in this "fertile eunuch" syndrome by hCG administration. Isolated hypogonadotropic hypogonadism[406] occurring after apparently normal puberty is manifest with relatively mature secondary sex characteristics or even secondary infertility. These patients have abundant gonadotropin responses to pulsatile GnRH therapy, which restores reproductive function and fertility.

Evaluation

In evaluating hypogonadal patients in the absence of an obvious pituitary or gonadal disorder, the primary diagnostic challenge is to distinguish constitutional pubertal delay from other causes of hypogonadotropism.[407] When puberty is delayed beyond 14 years of age, a primary developmental disorder, hypogonadotropic hypogonadism, or acquired disorders of reproductive function should be considered. The presence of midline defects, a pituitary mass lesion, anosmia, a history of radiation or pituitary damage, drug ingestion, or other systemic illness should be excluded. Patients with chronic liver disease or sickle cell disease may present with impaired pituitary reserve as well as primary testicular dysfunction.

No single test clearly distinguishes constitutional delayed puberty and true hypogonadotropism, and expectant follow-up is often helpful as many patients enter puberty spontaneously. To provide androgenization, testosterone replacement should be intermittently provided until age 18 with periodic interruptions to unmask physiologic pubertal advance. In adults presenting with features of hypogonadotropic hypogonadism, hyperprolactinemia, hemochromatosis, and sarcoidosis should also be excluded before the diagnosis of the idiopathic variety. Pituitary MRI, GH, TSH, and ACTH reserve testing should be performed selectively.

Management

Sex steroid replacement therapy is required to induce and maintain primary and secondary sexual functions, minimize cardiovascular risk factors, and maintain normal body composition and integrity of bone mineral density and muscle mass. For patients not desirous of fertility, sex steroid therapy is warranted to correct central hypogonadism. However, monitoring of LH and FSH responses does not accurately reflect adequate steroid hormonal replacement because basal gonadotropin levels are already low or undetectable.

For women, estrogens are administered as a tablet, patch, gel, or implant. For premenopausal women with pituitary deficiency, a combined oral contraceptive (20 to 35 μg ethynyl estradiol) may be used. Conjugated equine estrogens (0.625 mg) and estradiol valerate (2 mg) provide relatively physiologic steroid replenishment. Estrogen patches or transcutaneous gels usually enable daily absorption of 50 to 100 μg of estradiol. Concomitant cyclic progesterone therapy is indicated for women with an intact uterus to prevent unopposed endometrial proliferation and bleeding.

Although early replacement lowers the risk of developing osteoporosis, effects of estrogen replacement on cardiovascular function are unresolved. In patients with hypopituitarism, estrogen replacement should be maintained at least until the age of 50, after which continuation should be determined on an individual basis by assessing risks and benefits especially in terms of bone mineral integrity, cardiovascular function, and cancer risk. In women with ovarian deficiency, combined estrogen and testosterone replacement may improve libido and sexual function. Estrogen treatment may be associated with thromboembolic disease, breast tenderness, and possibly an enhanced risk of breast cancer.

For males not desiring fertility, intramuscular injection of testosterone 17α-hydroxyl esters (testosterone enanthate and testosterone cypionate) at 200 mg intramuscularly every 2 or 3 weeks is effective but may be associated with fluctuations in sexual potency, energy level, and mood reflecting dynamic changes in circulating testosterone concentrations.[408] Administration of lower doses more frequently (e.g., 100 mg weekly or 150 mg every 14 days) may stabilize hormone fluctuations. Elderly men require lower doses, as do boys with delayed puberty. Scrotal and nonscrotal transdermal testosterone patch systems deliver 4 to 6 mg and sustain testosterone profiles. These preparations require adequate shaved scrotal skin for application. Nonscrotal patch sites may develop skin irritation, blisters, and vesicles in about 25% of patients.[409] Some patients require combined patches or low-dose injection to maintain adequate potency and energy levels.[410, 411] There is no apparent cost-benefit advantage of patch delivery over intramuscular injection. Oral androgen replacement therapy with 17α-hydroxyl ester testosterone undecanoate requires frequent dosing (two to four times daily) and, because absorption is not uniform, testosterone levels may not be adequately maintained. Oral 17α-methyltestosterone is associated with hepatotoxicity and not recommended. Testosterone may cause acne, gynecomastia, rarely urine retention related to prostatic obstruction, and polycythemia. Although there is no compelling evidence that testosterone replacement causes prostate cancer, benign prostatic hypertrophy may be exacerbated, especially in elderly patients. Testosterone replacement should not be administered to men with diagnosed prostate cancer.

In patients with hypogonadotropic hypogonadism, fertility may be achieved with gonadotropin or GnRH therapy. In males, coexistence of primary testicular dysfunction precludes the success of direct gonadotropin replacement or GnRH, although the relatively low sperm counts induced may be adequate for impregnation when fertility is induced by gonadotropin or GnRH. Because testosterone therapy may suppress spermatogenesis, the steroid should be discontinued prior to initiating treatment. To induce spermatogenesis, hCG is administered subcutaneously or intramuscularly (500 to 2000 IU two to three times weekly). Lower doses may also be effective.[412] If necessary, after 6 months, human menopausal gonadotropin or purified FSH (75 IU three times weekly) should be added to improve sperm quantity, and doses may be doubled after a further 6 months. If testosterone levels are increased, subsequent conversion to estradiol may be enhanced, resulting in gynecomastia. Gonadotropin therapy may also cause androgenized oily skin and acne. Therefore, both testosterone and estradiol levels should be monitored.

Pulsatile GnRH therapy is indicated for patients with normal pituitary function, that is, those with idiopathic hypogonadotropic hypogonadism or Kallmann's syndrome. GnRH is infused subcutaneously by continuous minipump (5 mg every 2 hours) with the dose titrated to maintain normal gonadotropin and testosterone levels and may be marginally more effective and cause less gynecomastia. These approaches require strong commitment of the patient because adequate spermatogenesis may not be attained for 2 years or longer despite normalized testosterone levels. Aliquots of successfully generated sperm samples should be frozen for future impregnation.

In women with central hypogonadism, fertility may be effectively achieved by GnRH or gonadotropin therapy (fully discussed in Chapter 17). Although ovulation is often induced and pregnancy achieved with gonadotropin treatment, a high rate of multiple follicle development remains a concern. A pregnancy rate of 83% was achieved in 77 patients with hypogonadotropic hypogonadism treated by gonadotropins or pulsatile GnRH.[413] If the residual pituitary gonadotroph reserve is sufficiently robust, GnRH therapy is more likely to result in ovulation of a single rather than multiple follicles, thereby reducing the chances of multiple gestation.[414] The beneficial role of adding GH to these treatments remains unresolved,[415] except for women with known hypopituitarism and GH deficiency (GHD).

Gonadotropin-Producing Pituitary Tumors (Clinically Nonfunctioning Pituitary Tumors)

Approximately 25% to 35% of pituitary tumors are nonfunctioning.[416] Most arise from gonadotroph cells and are monoclonal[34, 36] and usually chromophobic. Although they most frequently occur as clinically nonfunctioning masses and are not associated with elevated serum gonadotropins, they produce sufficient gonadotropin subunits to be detectable by immunohistochemistry. Thirteen of 14 nonfunctioning gonadotroph tumors produced gonadotropic hormone subunits detected by immunohistochemistry.[417]

In another series of nonfunctioning adenomas, 42% of tumors immunostained for TSHβ, 83% for LHβ, 75% for FSHβ, and 92% for α subunit[272] some also express chromogranin A.[418] Although LH, FSH, or α subunit is released from these nonfunctioning tumors when maintained in culture, production is usually not sufficient to elevate blood levels.[70] In the past, when immunochemistry was unavailable, these tumors were often classified as null cell adenomas, which do not express glycoprotein subunits.[419] A small subset of tumors secrete sufficient hormone to elevate serum gonadotropin or α subunit levels, which occasionally cause clinical syndromes.

Presentation

Clinically Nonfunctioning Gonadotroph Tumors. Clinically nonfunctioning tumors generally come to attention because of their large size or are detected incidentally (Table 8–18).[420] A gradual visual deficit arising from optic chiasmal compression is common, and patients are often unaware of the disturbance. Recognition of visual field deficits is often delayed because formal visual fields are not routinely evaluated unless a defect is suspected clinically. In the absence of associated space-occupying or hormonal disorders, these large tumors may go unrecognized for many years and be inadvertently detected on scans or radiographs obtained for other purposes (incidentaloma). Sinusitis evaluation, pituitary apoplexy, or performance of a brain MRI for an unrelated indication (e.g., head trauma) may bring these tumors to clinical attention. Although these tumors are not often the initial presenting complaint, the patients are commonly deficient in one or more pituitary hormones,[161, 421] as noted in two thirds of 56 patients with nonfunctioning macroadenomas.[161] The most common endocrine symptoms are related to gonadotropin deficiency.

Functioning Gonadotroph Tumors. The small subset of gonadotroph adenomas producing elevated serum FSH, LH, or α subunit concentrations are considered functioning adenomas

Table 8–18. Presentation of Gonadotroph Adenomas

Common	Uncommon
Clinically nonfunctioning macroadenomas	Intact gonadotropin overproduction
Immunostain for gonadotropin subunits (usually more than one)	Immunostain for subunits or intact hormone being hypersecreted
Usually discovered because of space-occupying effects or inadvertently	Usually discovered because of space-occupying effects or inadvertently
Pituitary deficiency	May cause clinical syndrome related to hormone overproduction
	Other pituitary hormones may be deficient

but are not often associated with specific endocrine syndromes. High serum FSH, usually with low LH levels, is usually the only sign that a pituitary tumor secretes FSH. Paradoxically, these patients may present with hypogonadism related to gonadal down-regulation. Female patients with such tumors may present with pelvic pain caused by ovarian hyperstimulation.[422] High gonadotropin levels associated with menopause or testicular failure may complicate interpretation of gonadotropin levels, but both LH and FSH are high in primary gonadal failure. LH-producing tumors are exceedingly rare and in males cause elevations of serum testosterone with acne and skin oiliness.

Evaluation

MRI, visual field examination, and pituitary hormone evaluation should be performed, the last not only to detect hypopituitarism but also to exclude hormone overproduction that may not be clinically apparent. LH, FSH, α subunit, PRL, T_4, triiodothyronine (T_3), TSH, cortisol, and IGF-I levels should be measured. A 24-hour urinary free cortisol measurement by RIA is useful to exclude inapparent ACTH hypersecretion. The extent of hormonal evaluation requires clinical judgment. When LH or FSH is elevated, the values must be interpreted in light of the patient's physiologic state. Elevated serum FSH in a woman with regular menstrual cycles would be interpreted differently than that detected in a menopausal patient; gonadotropin elevations in patients with primary gonadal failure are not generally limited to one hormone, and elevation of circulating α subunit is consistent with a pituitary tumor but not gonadal failure. TRH stimulation may differentiate elevated gonadotropin levels ascribed to end-organ failure from those related to independent tumor production. In patients harboring gonadotroph adenomas, increases in FSH, LH, LHβ subunit, or α subunit are evoked in response to TRH.[423] Calculating the molar ratio of LH or FSH to α subunit may assist in the diagnosis.

Treatment

Clinical judgment should be used in determining appropriate therapy including surgery, surgery followed by radiotherapy, radiotherapy alone, or expectant observation. Unfortunately, no reliable tumor marker is predictive of mass growth or recurrence (Fig. 8–35).

Surgery and Radiotherapy. If tumors threaten vision or are macroadenomas whose size threatens vital structures, transsphenoidal surgery is recommended. Vision improved in approximately 75% of patients whose vision was impaired.[420, 424] Of 100 patients undergoing transsphenoidal surgery, 72 had visual disturbances, 61 hypopituitarism, and 36 headache. Vision improved in 53 of 72 patients after surgery, and headache improved in all. Of 50 patients who underwent surgery followed by radiotherapy, 9 had tumor recurrences at a mean of 73 months after radiotherapy and there were 5 recurrences in 42 patients who did not receive radiotherapy.[425] An expectant follow-up of 65 patients after pituitary surgery for nonfunctioning adenomas showed that 32% of tumors grew during a mean follow-up period of 76 months.[426] In a retrospective comparison of 126 patients undergoing surgery alone or surgery with radiation, early postoperative radiotherapy (within 12 months) significantly reduced the risk of tumor regrowth by about 15% at 10 years.[427] Despite the relatively high incidence of postoperative tumor regrowth, even after apparently complete resection, most neurosurgeons avoid routine postoperative radiation therapy. Radiation can be offered if the tumor mass reexpands.[424] This approach requires advising careful follow-up with periodic annual MRI studies and visual evaluations. Because patients experience tumor regrowth even after

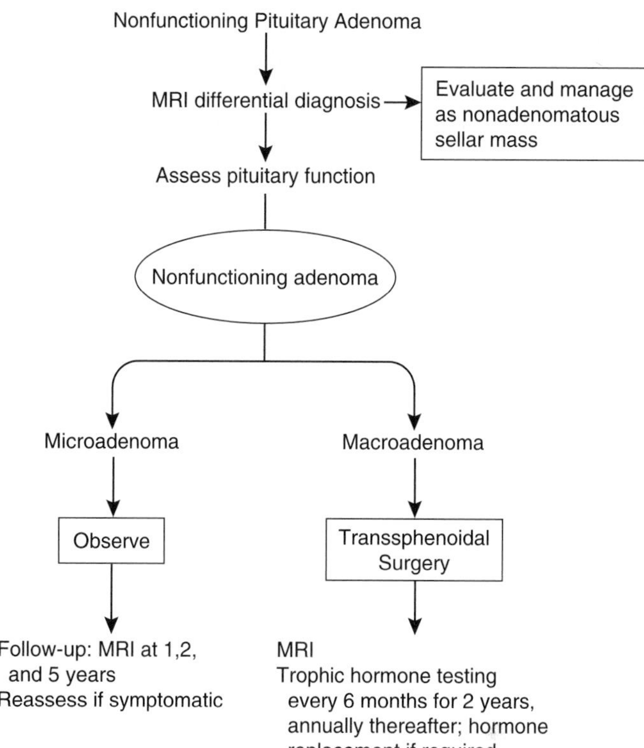

Figure 8–35. Management of nonfunctioning pituitary adenomas. Skilled MRI interpretation is crucial to diagnose non-adenomatous mass (e.g., meningioma, aneurysm, or other sellar lesion). MRI, magnetic resonance imaging.

radiation therapy, all should undergo periodic post-treatment MRI, although less frequently.

Expectant Observation. For nonfunctioning microadenomas or small macroadenomas (incidentalomas), patients may be observed expectantly.[428] Some tumors do not grow over years or even decades. However, regular follow-up with MRI is necessary because these tumors may grow insidiously and are usually asymptomatic until they are large enough to affect vision. Periodic but less frequent endocrine evaluation is also suggested according to the clinical situation. Microadenomas rarely impair vision during pregnancy, whereas macroadenomas do so with greater frequency.[376] Because macroadenomas do not respond to medical therapy, the risks of visual impairment arising during a pregnancy must be weighed carefully and resection prior to pregnancy may be indicated.

Medications. Medications are not effective in reducing tumor size and visual compromise. Although dopamine agonists,[429] GnRH antagonists,[430] and somatostatin analogues[431] modestly reduce tumor size in a few patients, they are not sufficiently effective to be recommended as therapy.

Growth Hormone

Somatotroph Cells

Mammosomatotroph cells expressing both PRL and GH arise from the acidophilic stem cell and immunostain mainly for PRL. Somatotrophs are located predominantly in the lateral wings of the anterior pituitary gland and constitute 35% to 45% of pituitary cells (Fig. 8–36). These ovoid cells contain prominent secretory granules up to 700 μm in diameter. Juxtanuclear Golgi is particularly prominent with secretory granules

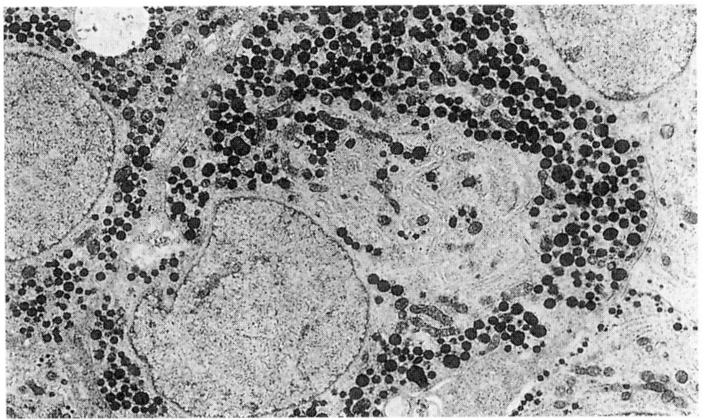

Figure 8–36. Normal somatotroph. A somatotroph in the nontumorous pituitary is large, round to ovoid, and contains numerous electron-dense secretory granules whose diameter ranges from 250 to 700 μm. Short profiles of rough endoplasmic reticulum are scattered throughout the cytoplasm. The prominent juxtanuclear Golgi complex harbors forming secretory granules. (From Asa SL. In Tumors of the Pituitary Gland. Atlas of Tumor Pathology. Washington, DC, Armed Forces Institute of Pathology, 1997, p 14.)

in formation. The gland contains a total of 5 to 15 mg of GH.[432]

Growth Hormone Biosynthesis

The human GH (hGH) genome locus spans approximately 66 kb and contains a cluster of five highly conserved genes located on the long arm of human chromosome 17q22-24.[433] These are *hGH-N*, *hCS-L*, *hCS-A*, *hGH-V*, and *hCS-B*,[434] all of which consist of five exons separated by four introns. The *hGH-N* gene is selectively transcribed in pituitary somatotrophs and encodes a 22-kd (191-amino-acid) protein. The *hCS-A* and *hCS-B* genes are expressed in placental trophoblasts.[435] Approximately 10% of pituitary GH is a 20-kd variant lacking amino acid residues 32 to 46. *hGH-V*, expressed in placental syncytiotrophoblasts, encodes a 22-kd protein detected in the maternal circulation from midpregnancy and a minor form, hGH-V2. Elevated maternal hGH-V serum concentrations are accompanied by a decline in hGH-N, suggesting feedback regulation of the maternal hypothalamic-pituitary axis. After childbirth, circulating GH-V levels drop rapidly and are undetectable after 1 hour.[436]

The hGH promoter region contains *cis* elements that mediate both pituitary-specific and hormone-specific signaling. The POUIFI transcription factor confers tissue-specific GH expression, and a second, ubiquitous factor binds to a distal Pit-1 site containing a consensus sequence for the Sp1 transcription factor. Pit-1 and Sp1 both contribute to GH promoter activation because mutation of the Sp1 binding site attenuates promoter activity.[437] Deoxyribonuclease hypersensitive sites of a locus control region of the hGH gene determine somatotroph and lactotroph GH expression, which involves regulation of a chromatin domain in these pituitary cells.[438] GH synthesis and release are under control of a variety of hormonal agents, including GHRH, somatostatin, ghrelin, IGF-I, thyroid hormone, and glucocorticoids. GHRH stimulates GH synthesis and release mediated by cAMP. CREB binding protein is phosphorylated by protein kinase A and is a cofactor for Pit-1–dependent human GH activation. IGF-I attenuates basal and stimulated GH gene expression.

The GH molecule, a single-chain polypeptide hormone consisting of 191 amino acids, is synthesized, stored, and secreted by somatotroph cells. The crystal structure of human GH reveals four alpha helices.[439] Circulating GH molecules comprise several heterogeneous forms: 22- and 20-kd monomers, acetylated 22K, and two des-amino GH molecules. The 22-kd peptide is the major physiologic GH component, accounting for 75% of pituitary GH secretion. Amino acids 32 to 46 are deleted by alternative splicing of the GH gene to yield 20-kd GH, accounting for about 10% of pituitary GH. The 20-kd GH has slower metabolic clearance,[440] accounting for the 20-kd/22-kd ratio being higher in plasma than in the pituitary gland. The 22-kd peptide retains growth-promoting activity but lacks diabetogenic effects, which are more pronounced with the 20-kd form.

GHRH and SRIF Interaction in Regulating Growth Hormone Secretion

The somatotroph cell expresses specific receptors for GHRH,[441] GH secretagogues, and SRIF receptor subtypes 2 and 5 that mediate GH secretion.[442, 443] Hypothalamic SRIF and GHRH are secreted in independent waves and interact together with additional GH secretagogues to generate pulsatile GH release. GHRH selectively induces GH gene transcription and hormone release and does not induce other anterior pituitary or gut hormones.[444, 445] SRIF suppresses both basal and GHRH-stimulated GH pulse amplitude and frequency but does not affect GH biosynthesis. GHRH administered to normal adults elicits a prompt rise in serum GH levels, with higher levels occurring in female subjects.[446] Although mature GHRH comprises 44 amino acids, GH-releasing activity resides in shorter proteolyzed forms involving amino acids 1 to 37 and 1 to 40 and the N-terminus. GHRH is also a determinant of somatotroph mitotic activity.

The rat hypothalamus releases GHRH and SRIF 180 degrees out of phase every 3 to 4 hours, resulting in pulsatile GH levels. SRIF antibody administration elevates GH levels, with intact intervening GH pulses,[447] implying that hypothalamic SRIF secretion generates GH troughs. Similarly, GHRH antibodies eliminate spontaneous GH surges. In humans, GH pulsatility persists when GHRH is tonically elevated as with ectopic tumor GHRH production or during GHRH infusion,[358] suggesting that hypothalamic SRIF is largely responsible for GH pulsatility. Preexposure to SRIF enhances somatotroph sensitivity to GHRH stimulation. Hence, during a normal GH trough period, the high SRIF level probably primes the somatotroph to respond maximally to a subsequent GHRH pulse, thus optimizing GH release. SRIF also inhibits central GHRH release through direct synaptic connections with hypothalamic SRIF-containing neurons.

Chronic GHRH stimulation, by either continuous infusion or repeated bolus administration, eventually desensitizes GH release in vitro and in vivo, possibly through depletion of a GHRH-sensitive pool of GH. GHRH pretreatment also decreases somatotroph GHRH binding sites.[448] GH stimulates hypothalamic SRIF, GHRH and SRIF autoregulate their own secretion, and GHRH also stimulates SRIF release.[449–451] GH secretion is further regulated by its target growth factor, IGF-I, which participates in a hypothalamic-pituitary peripheral regulatory feedback system.[452] GH stimulates IGF-I, which exerts a negative feedback effect on the hypothalamus and pituitary. IGF-I stimulates hypothalamic SRIF release and inhibits pituitary GH gene transcription and secretion.

Growth Hormone Secretagogues and Ghrelin

The isolation of ghrelin indicates a control system in addition to GHRH and SRIF in regulation of GH secretion (see Chapter 23). Ghrelin is a 28-amino-acid peptide that binds the GH secretagogue (GHS) receptor[453] to induce hypothalamic GHRH and pituitary GH.[454] A unique *n*-octanoylated serine 3 residue confers GH-releasing activity to the molecule. Ghrelin

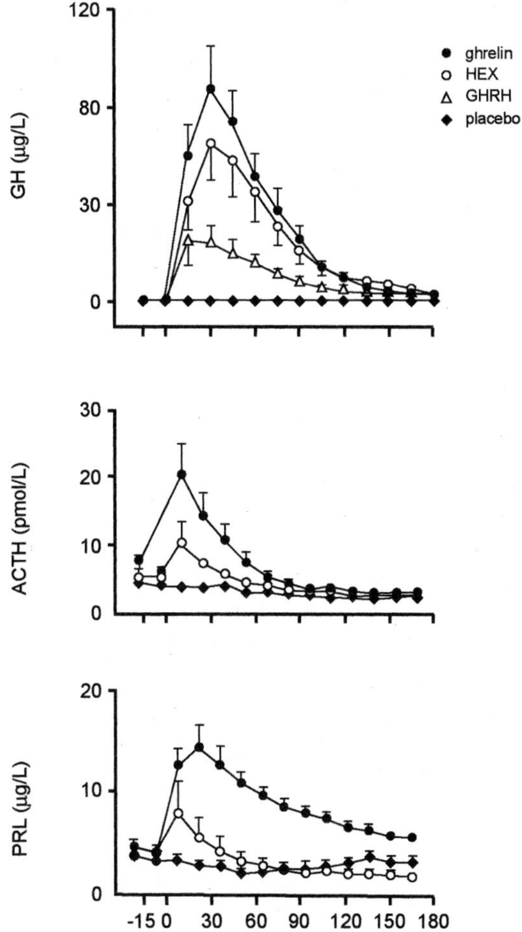

Figure 8–37. Effect of growth hormone (GH) secretagogues on GH, adrenocorticotropic hormone (ACTH) and prolactin (PRL) secretion in healthy subjects. Mean (+ SEM) curve responses after administration of ghrelin (1.0 μg/kg), hexarelin (HEX) (1.0 μg/kg), growth hormone–releasing hormone (GHRH) (1.0 μg/kg), or placebo. (Adapted from Arvat E, Maccario M, Di Vito L, et al. Endocrine activities of ghrelin, a natural growth hormone secretagogue (GHS), in humans: comparison and interactions with hexarelin, a nonnatural peptidyl GHS, and GH-releasing hormone. J Clin Endocrinol Metab 2001; 86: 1169–1174.)

is synthesized primarily in peripheral tissues, especially gastric mucosal neuroendocrine cells. Ghrelin administration dose dependently evokes GH release and also induces food intake and obesity development (Fig. 8–37). It is thought that ghrelin controls GH secretion and peripheral sources may have additional nutritional effects requiring further elucidation.[454a] Current evidence suggests that the dual control of GH secretion postulated for GHRH and SRIF should be expanded to incorporate ghrelin.[455]

Synthetic hexapeptides (artificial GHSs) recognize the GHS receptor, induce potent and reproducible GH release, and are useful for the diagnosis of GHD.[456] GHSs stimulate GH secretion, and GHRH and GHSs act though distinct receptors and different intracellular signaling pathways on somatotroph subpopulations.[457] GHSs require the presence of a functional hypothalamus to evoke GH, as evidenced in patients with an intact pituitary but disordered hypothalamic function, in whom GHS does not induce GH.[458] GHSs potentiate GH release in response to a maximal stimulating dose of exogenous GHRH,[459] and after a saturating dose of GHRH, when subsequent GHRH administration is ineffective, GHSs remain fully effective.[460]

Functional GHS receptors are expressed in the human fetal pituitary by the fifth week of gestation.[353] GHS-mediated GH release is demonstratable at birth, continues through infancy, increases at puberty, and decreases thereafter. Estrogen and testosterone increase GHS-mediated GH release in childhood.[461] Because GHS-evoked GH secretion is minimally altered by age, sex, or adiposity and is devoid of potential side effects (unlike insulin-induced hypoglycemia), GHSs may become a useful diagnostic tool in the diagnosis of adult GHD. Slight PRL and ACTH or cortisol increases have been reported with some GHSs, leading to the development of novel GHSs with more selective somatotroph actions.[462]

Regulation of Growth Hormone Secretion

Multiple factors regulate the integrated secretion of GH (Fig. 8–38). Major GH secretory pulses accounting for up to 70% of daily GH secretion occur with the first episode of slow wave sleep.[463] The decline in slow wave sleep from early adulthood to midlife is paralleled by a major decline in GH secretion, suggesting that age-related alterations in the GH axis may partially reflect decreased sleep quality.[464] "Jet lag" transiently increases GH peak amplitude, resulting in a transient increase of 24-hour GH secretion. Exercise and physical stress, including trauma with hypovolemic shock and sepsis, increase GH levels.[465] Emotional deprivation is associated with sup-

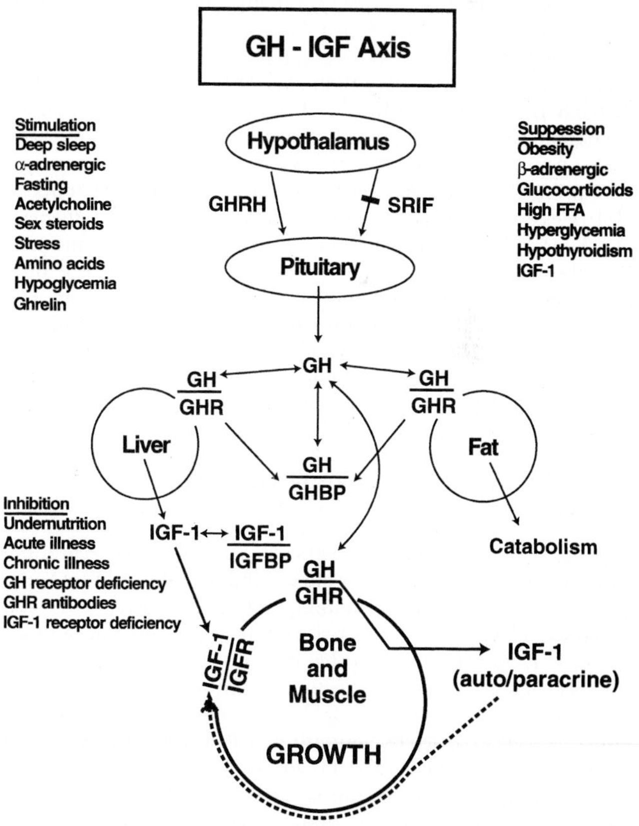

Figure 8–38. Growth hormone (GH) axis. Simplified diagram of GH–IGF-I axis involving hypophysiotropic hormones controlling pituitary GH release, circulating GH-binding protein and its GH receptor source, IGF-I and its largely GH-dependent binding proteins, and cellular responsiveness to GH and IGF-I interacting with their specific receptors. FFA, free fatty acids; IGFR, insulin-like growth factor I (IGF-I) receptor. Ghrelin, probably of predominantly gastric origin, also stimulates pituitary GH secretion. (From Rosenbloom A. Growth hormone insensitivity: physiologic and genetic basis, phenotype and treatment. J Pediatr 1999; 135:280–289.)

pressed GH secretion, and attenuated GH responses to provocative stimuli occur in endogenous depression.[466] Chronic malnutrition and prolonged fasting are associated with elevated GH pulse frequency and amplitude (Fig. 8–39).[467]

Obesity decreases basal and stimulated GH secretion, insulin-induced hypoglycemia stimulates GH, and hyperglycemia inhibits GH secretion. Chronic hyperglycemia is, however, not associated with low GH levels, and poorly controlled diabetes is associated with increased basal and exercise-induced GH levels.[468] Central glucoreceptors appear to sense glucose fluctuations rather than absolute levels. High-protein meals, and intravenous single amino acids (including arginine and leucine) stimulate GH secretion. Increased serum free fatty acids blunt the effects of arginine infusion, sleep, L-dopa, and exercise on GHRH-stimulated GH release.[469] Leptin plays a key role in regulation of body fat mass,[470] regulating food intake and energy expenditure, and may act as a metabolic signal to regulate GH secretion. Leptin- and neuropeptide Y–producing hypothalamic neurons synapse with somatostatin neurons, and antisera to neuropeptide Y and somatostatin reverse starvation-induced GH release.[471] In GH-deficient hypopituitary adults, leptin concentrations are higher than would be expected from their body fat mass.[472]

Neuropeptides, neurotransmitters, and opiates impinge on the hypothalamus and modulate GHRH and somatostatin (SRIF) release. Integrated effects of these complex neurogenic influences determine the final secretory pattern of GH. Apomorphine, a central dopamine receptor agonist, stimulates GH secretion,[473] as does levodopa treatment. Oral levodopa administration evokes a brisk serum GH response within an hour in healthy young subjects. Norepinephrine increases GH secretion through α-adrenergic pathways and inhibits GH release through β-adrenergic pathways. Insulin-induced hypoglycemia, clonidine, arginine administration, exercise, levodopa, and arginine vasopressin facilitate GH secretion through α-adrenergic effects.[474] β-Adrenergic blockade increases GHRH-induced GH release, possibly by a direct pituitary action or by decreasing hypothalamic somatostatin release. Endorphins and enkephalins stimulate GH and may account for GH release during severe physical stress and extreme exercise.[474] Galanin, a 29-amino-acid neuropeptide, induces GH release and responses to GHRH. Cholinergic and serotoninergic neurons and several neuropeptides stimulate GH, including neurotensin, VIP, motilin, cholecystokinin, and glucagon.

Other Hormones Facilitating Growth Hormone Secretion

Acute glucocorticoid administration stimulates GH secretion, whereas chronic steroid treatment inhibits GH. Three hours after acute glucocorticoid administration, GH levels rose and remained elevated for 2 hours.[475] However, supraphysiologic glucocorticoid exposure retarded growth, and Cushing's disease was also associated with growth retardation, decreased serum GH, and decreased pituitary GH content surrounding the adenoma.[476] Glucocorticoids administered to normal subjects dose dependently inhibited GHRH-simulated GH secretion in a manner similar to that seen in Cushing's syndrome.[475] Furthermore, cortisol antagonizes peripheral GH action.

GH levels are decreased in hyperthyroid patients but become normal when patients are rendered euthyroid, suggesting that thyroid hormone suppresses GH secretion. Elevated circulating gonadal steroids observed during puberty may also account for higher pubertal GH levels. Estrogen stimulates GH secretory rates, and testosterone increases GH secretory mass per pulse with resultant IGF-I induction.[474] TRH does not stimulate GH secretion in normal subjects but does induce GH secretion in about 70% of patients with acromegaly.[477]

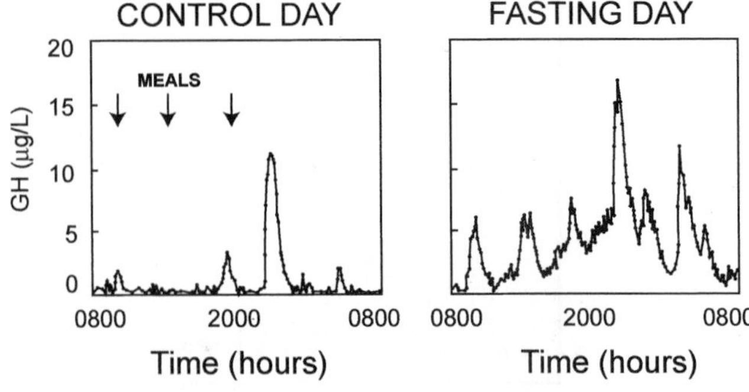

Figure 8–39. Effect of fasting on growth hormone (GH) secretion patterns in a healthy male subject. (From Hartman ML, Veldhuis JD, Johnson ML, et al. Augmented growth hormone (GH) secretory burst frequency and amplitude mediate enhanced GH secretion during a two-day fast in normal men. J Clin Endocrinol Metab 1992; 74:757–765.)

Discordant GH responses to TRH are evoked in patients with liver disease, renal disease, ectopic GHRH-releasing carcinoid tumors,[31] anorexia nervosa, and depression. Intravenous CRH modestly increases GH in some patients with acromegaly or chronic depression. GnRH stimulates GH secretion in about one third of patients with acromegaly.

Growth Hormone Binding Proteins

Circulating GH binding proteins (GHBPs) include a 20-kd low-affinity BP and a 60-kd high-affinity BP, which corresponds to the extracellular domain of the hepatic GH receptor and binds half of the circulating 22-kd GH form.[478, 479] The 20-kd GH binds preferentially to the low-affinity BP, which is unrelated to the GH receptor. The GHBPs function to damp acute oscillations in serum GH levels associated with pulsatile pituitary GH secretion, and the plasma half-life of GH is prolonged by decreased renal clearance of bound GH. The high-affinity BP also prevents GH binding to surface GH receptors by competing for the GH ligand. Patients with hypopituitarism or acromegaly have normal BP concentrations. GH resistance, as demonstrated in malnutrition, chronic liver disease, short stature, Laron dwarfism, and some African pygmies, is characterized by decreased BP levels in plasma. High BP levels are encountered in obese or pregnant subjects or those receiving estrogens or undergoing refeeding.[480]

Peripheral Growth Hormone Action

GH acts to mediate growth and metabolic functions (Fig. 8–40). GH elicits intracellular signaling though a peripheral receptor and initiates a phosphorylation cascade involving the JAK/STAT pathway.[481] The liver contains abundant GH receptors, and several peripheral tissues also express modest amounts of receptor, including muscle and fat (Fig. 8–41).[482] The GH receptor is a 620-amino-acid, 70-kd protein of the class I cytokine-hematopoietin receptor superfamily consisting of an extracellular ligand-binding domain, a single membrane-spanning domain, and a cytoplasmic signaling component.[483] The GH receptor superfamily is homologous with receptors for PRL, interleukins 2 to 7, erythropoietin, interferon, and colony-stimulating factor.

GH complexes with two GH receptor components leading to receptor dimerization critical for subsequent GH signaling. Dimerization is followed by rapid JAK2 tyrosine kinase activation leading to phosphorylation of intracellular signaling molecules, including the signal-transducing activators of transcription proteins (STATs 1, 3, and 5), critical signaling com-

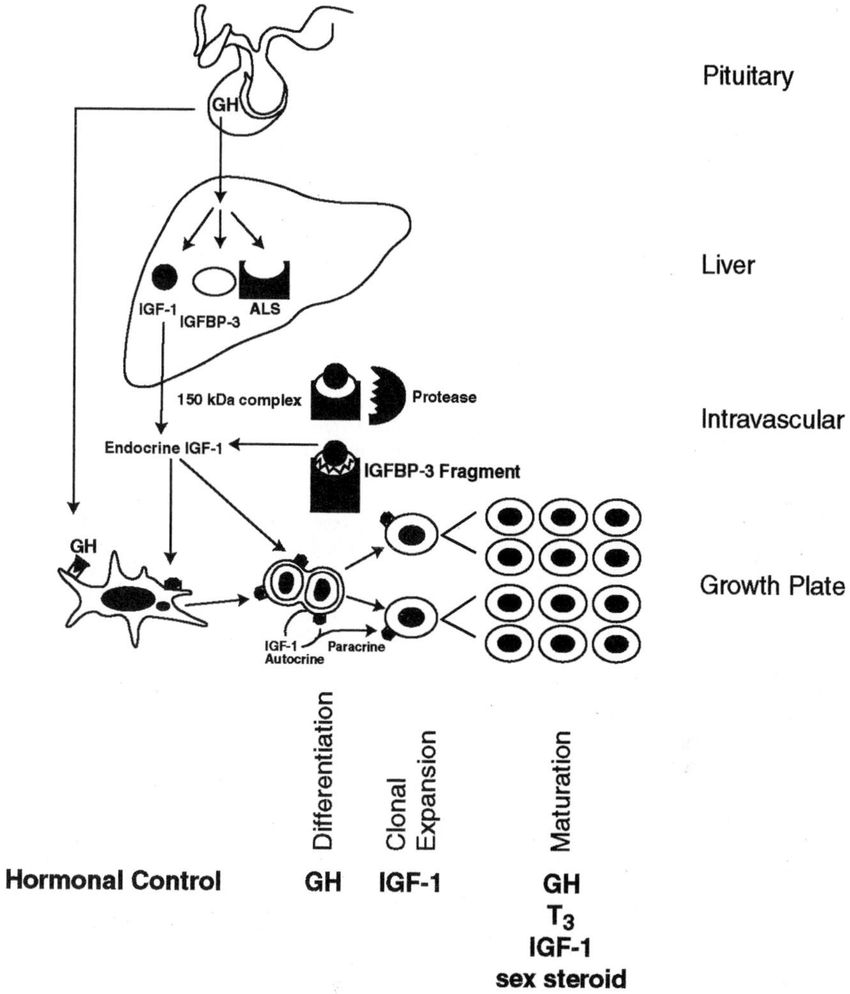

Figure 8–40. Integrated model of the growth hormone-insulin-like growth factor binding protein-IGF (GH–IGF-BP-IGF) axis in the growth process. Three mechanisms are proposed: (1) GH stimulates IGF-I production, and circulating IGF-I (endocrine IGF-I) acts at the growth plate; (2) GH regulates hepatic production of IGF-BP3 and acid-liable subunit (ALS): IGF-I binds to IGFBP-3 and thereafter with ALS, forming the 150-kd ternary complex; proteases cleave into fragments that release IGF-BP3 into fragments that release IGF-I in the intravascular space and at the growth plate; and (3) GH induces differentiation local IGF-I production, and IGF-I acts through an autocrine and paracrine mechanism to stimulate cell division. (From Spagnoli A, Rosenfeld RG. The mechanism by which growth hormone brings about growth: The relative contributions of growth hormone and insulin-like growth factors. Endocrinol Metab Clin North Am 1996; 25: 615–631.)

ponents for GH action.[484] Phosphorylated STAT proteins are directly translocated to the cell nucleus, where they elicit GH-specific target gene expression by binding to nuclear DNA. STAT1 and STAT5 may also interact directly with the GH receptor molecule.[484] GH also induces c-fos, insulin receptor substrate 1 (IRS-1) phosphorylation, and insulin synthesis. Additional intracellular signaling pathways induced by GH include mitogen-activated protein kinase, protein kinase C, SH2-Bβ, SHP-2, SIRPα, Shc, FAK, CrK, C-Src, paxillin, and tensin. How these seemingly overlapping pathways converge to integrate the net cellular effects of GH is at present unclear.[481]

IGF-I, a critical growth factor induced by GH, is probably responsible for most growth-promoting activities of GH[452] and also directly regulates GH receptor function.[483] Paracrine IGF-I produced in extrahepatic tissues appears critical for growth because growth persists even when hepatic IGF-I is deleted in mice.[485] GH receptor mutations are associated with partial or complete GH insensitivity and growth failure. These syndromes are associated with normal or high circulating GH levels, decreased circulating GHBP levels, and low levels of circulating IGF-I. Multiple homozygous or heterozygous exonic and intronic GHR mutations have been described. These occur mostly in the extracellular ligand-binding receptor domain (see Chapter 23).

Tissue responses to GH signaling are determined by the pattern of GH secretion in addition to the absolute amount of circulating hormone. Gender-specific patterns of GH secretion profiles determine sex-specific expression of cytochrome P450 enzymes. In turn, circulating steroids regulate neuroendocrine release of GH. SRIF, by suppressing interpulse GH levels, serves to masculinize the ultradian GH rhythm. In mice harboring a disrupted SRIF gene, plasma GH secretory patterns were elevated and liver enzyme induction lost its gender-specific dimorphism but the animals retained sexually dimorphic growth patterns.[486]

Linear growth patterns and liver enzyme induction are phenotypically gender-specific because of higher GH pulse frequency rates and also show gender-specific STAT5b activity.[487] Sexually dimorphic patterns of GH secretion and tissue targeting appear to be determined by STAT5b, which is sensitive to repeated pulses of injected GH,[488] whereas other GH-induced responses are desensitized by repeated GH administration. Disruption of STAT5b in transgenic mice caused impaired male-pattern body growth[489] associated with female-pattern IGF-I and testosterone levels. Appropriate GH pulsatility is also required to determine body growth mediated by STAT5b[490, 491] but not for metabolic effects of GH on carbohydrate metabolism.

Intracellular GH signaling is abrogated by suppressor of cytokine signaling (SOCS) proteins, which disrupt the JAK/STAT pathway and thus disrupt GH action.[492] In transgenic mice with deletion of SOCS-2, gigantism develops, presumably because of unrestrained GH action. Because SOCS proteins are also induced by proinflammatory cytokines, critically ill patients or those with renal failure may experience GH resistance related to cytokine-induced SOCS proteins.[493] Unraveling STAT-SOCS regulation in syndromes associated with disordered GH signaling should yield mechanistic insights into

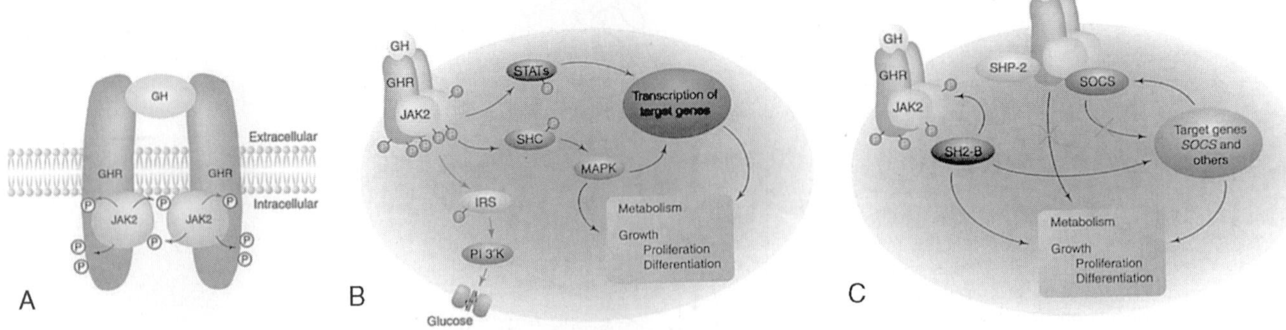

Figure 8-41. Growth hormone (GH) receptors. (See also Color Plate.)

A, Model of GH activation of JAK2 tyrosine kinase. GH binding to two GH receptors increases the affinity to each receptor for JAK2. The two receptor-associated JAK2 molecules are in close proximity, so that each JAK2 can phosphorylate the activating tyrosine of the other JAK2 molecule *(blue arrows)*, thereby activating it. Activated JAK2 then phosphorylates itself *(red arrow)* and the cytoplasmic domain of the GH receptor *(purple arrows)* on tyrosines. These phosphotyrosines within the GH receptor and JAK2 form binding sites for signaling proteins. GH, growth hormone; GHR, growth hormone receptor; JAK2, Janus kinase 2; P, phosphate.

B, Regulation of GH receptor-JAK2 signaling. SH2 enhances GH receptor signaling by increasing the activity of JAK2. GH-induced expression of SOCS proteins inhibits further GHR signaling by decreasing the activity of JAK2. Tyrosine phosphatases, such as SHP-2, might also contribute to inhibiting GH receptor signaling by dephosphorylating tyrosines in the GH receptor and/or JAK2. GH, growth hormone; GHR, growth hormone receptor; JAK2, Janus kinase 2; P, phosphatase; SHP-2, src homology 2 domain-containing protein tyrosine phosphatase 2; SOCS, suppressor of cytokine signaling.

C, GH receptors signaling pathways. Some of the signaling pathways initiated by GH activation of JAK2 are shown. JAK2 phosphorylates SHC, leading to activation of MAPK *(blue arrows)*. JAK2 also phosphorylates STAT transcription factors. MAPK and STATs are important for GH regulation of gene transcription *(purple arrows)*. JAK2 phosphorylates IRS proteins, which are thought to lead to activation of PI 3′-kinase (PI3 K: *red arrows*). GH activation of PI 3′ kinase via IRS protein might be important for GH stimulation of glucose transport.

GH, growth hormone, GHR, growth hormone receptor; IRS, insulin receptor substrates; JAK2, Janus kinase 2; MAPK, mitogen-activated protein kinase; P, phosphate; PI 3′K, phosphatidylinositol 3-kinase, STAT, signal transducers and activators of transcription.

(*A–C*, From Herrington J, Carter-Su C. Signaling pathway activated by the growth hormone receptor. Trends Endocrinol Metab 2001; 12:252-257.)

dysregulated GH action. The impact of GH on growth is fully reviewed in Chapter 23. Extrapituitary GH and GH secretagogues may complement the classical endocrine action between the GH-releasing factors, GH, and target tissues. Although GH immunoreactivity and mRNA expression have been documented in placenta, mammary gland, muscle, spleen, and lymphocytes,[494] their physiologic role is not yet apparent.

Metabolic Actions of Growth Hormone

GH continues to be secreted in adulthood after growth cessation, implying important metabolic functions of GH in adult life. Although acute, transient, insulin-like effects of GH have been demonstrated, chronic GH exposure has potent anti-insulin effects at both hepatic and peripheral sites resulting in decreased glucose utilization, increased lipolysis, and tissue refractoriness of the acute insulin-like effects of GH. Endogenous GH concentrations antagonize insulin action. GH secretion increases 3 to 5 hours after glucose ingestion, resulting in decreased disposal of a subsequent oral glucose challenge associated with hyperinsulinemia occurring 2 hours after the GH peak. GH-deficient children have decreased fasting glucose levels, decreased insulin secretion, and increased insulin sensitivity with increased glucose utilization and blunted hepatic glucose release. GH replacement increases fasting glucose and insulin levels and restores hepatic glucose production. GH-deficient adults have elevated fasting insulin levels, and enhanced visceral fat mass, suggesting insulin resistance, which has been confirmed by hyperinsulinemic euglycemic clamp studies.[495]

GH is anabolic and causes urinary nitrogen retention, decreased plasma urea levels, and increased muscle mass. GH increases fat mobilization, decreases fat deposition, and activates hormone-sensitive lipase, resulting in increased triglyceride hydrolysis to free fatty acids and glycerol (lipolysis) and also decreased fatty acid reesterification. Replacement of GH in GH-deficient adults leads to decreased body fat and decreased adipocyte size and lipid content. As GH is degraded in the kidney, GH levels are elevated in patients with chronic renal failure and GH rises paradoxically in response to a glucose load in these patients.

Growth Hormone Secretion Patterns

Frequent serum sampling for measurements of GH concentrations has revealed a pattern of pulsatile secretion separated by troughs, during which GH is undetectable (<0.4 μg/L) (Table 8–19). Using currently available assays, random GH levels are undetectable in 50% of samples obtained from healthy subjects. GH secretion is high in the fetal circulation, peaking at about 150 μg/L during midgestation. Neonatal levels are lower ($\sim$30 μg/L), possibly reflecting negative feedback control by rising levels of circulating IGF. GH levels during childhood (up to 7 μg/L) are characterized by enhanced pubertal GH pulse amplitude and mass with unchanged GH pulse frequency. GH pulse amplitudes decline inexorably with age, and GH levels in middle age are about 15% of pubertal levels. Healthy adult males produce GH at about 0.25 to 0.52 mg/m^2 per 24 hours.[451] Obesity is associated with decreased GH pulse frequency and blunted evoked GH responses to

Table 8-19. Adult Growth Hormone Secretion*

Observation	Young Adult (μg/24 hr)	Fasting	Obesity	Middle-Age
24-hr secretion	540±44	2171±333	77±20	196±65
Secretory bursts	12±1	32±2	3±0.5	10±1
Growth hormone burst	45±4	64±9	24±5	10±6

*Deconvolution analysis of growth hormone (GH) secretion in adult males.
From Thorner MO, Varee ML, Horvath E, Kovcs K. The anterior pituitary. In Wilson JD, Foster DW (eds). Williams Textbook of Endocrinology. Philadelphia, WB Saunders, 1992, pp 221–310.

secretagogues. In contrast, fasting is associated with enhanced GH pulse frequency and amplitude, possibly reflecting altered feedback regulation by nutritionally mediated changes in IGF binding protein concentrations and free IGF-I availability.

Measurement of Spontaneous Growth Hormone Secretion

Because pituitary GH secretion occurs episodically, accurate quantification of integrated GH secretion requires continuous measurement of secretion over 24 hours. This procedure requires insertion of a continuous withdrawal pump or patent indwelling catheter with unrestricted food intake and physical activity. Increasing sampling frequencies from every 20 minutes to 5-minute or 30-second sampling intervals enhances the threshold for detecting more pulses per hour. Although cumbersome and expensive, this method eliminates the error of isolated peak or trough measurements that might otherwise be obtained by single or multiple random GH samplings.

The discriminating power of continuous 24-hour GH measurement in the diagnosis of GHD in children has been disputed.[496] With no clear diagnostic advantage over GH stimulation tests, integrated GH levels in young healthy subjects may overlap those of patients with organic hypopituitary disorders, which limits the utility of the measurement in the diagnosis of acquired adult GHD. However, fasted subjects may exhibit a clear distinction of deficient integrated GH levels measured over 8 hours.[497]

Urinary Growth Hormone Measurement

Immunoassay methods for urinary GH measurement do not reliably reflect pharmacologic GH testing or adequately discriminate between normal and abnormal GH secretion. Clinical utility of urinary GH measurements requires rigorous age-matched and gender-matched control subjects and standardized expression of GH concentrations relative to body weight or creatinine excretion.[498]

Variability of Growth Hormone Assays

Plasma GH is measured by RIA (polyclonal or monoclonal) or by IRMA (dual monoclonal), but comparative GH measurements obtained using 11 commercial immunoassays varied by a factor of 3.[499] Measured GH concentrations are antibody-dependent, and different antibodies bind to a heterogeneous spectrum of GH isoforms.[500] Furthermore, GH isoform patterns vary between individuals and not all circulating GH forms are routinely detectable in GH assays adding further variation to comparison of results from different GH immunoassays. Monomeric 22-kd GH, the most abundant circulating form, is the only GH standard of sufficient purity and quantity and is used as the basis for GH measurement; however, it accounts for only about 25% of circulating immunoreactivity.[501] Other GH forms are recognized to varying and largely unknown degrees. Polyclonal antibodies used in earlier RIAs recognized several molecular forms of GH as compared with newer immunometric assays employing highly specific monoclonal antibodies.[502]

GH standards also affect comparison of GH values. In 1994, the first World Health Organization international standard for somatotropin, IRP 88/624,[503] used recombinant technology, whereas previous standards were prepared from pituitary extracts. GHBPs may also interfere because approximately 50% of GH is complexed to GHBP and noncompetitive immunometric assays may lead to low estimates of GH. In competitive assays employing antibodies directed against GH molecular epitopes that bind GHBP, spuriously high GH values may be reported.[504] The heterogeneity of GH immunoassay results poses a challenge in the definition of accepted standards for diagnosis of GHD. However, the RIA is now infrequently used and clinicians should be aware of the nature of the GH assay employed and how values compare with those previously obtained by polyclonal RIA. New GH assays based on measuring GH bioactivity have been developed, including the eluted stain assay (ESTA) and the immunofunctional assay (IFA). The 22-kd exclusion assay (GHEA) also measures circulating GH isoforms.[502]

Growth Hormone Deficiency

GHD in adults is recognized as a distinct adult syndrome (Table 8–20).[505] GH is the most frequently deficient of the pituitary hormones in patients with pituitary disease, and GHD has negative effects on body composition, cardiovascular risk factors, and quality of life.[506, 507] Life expectancy is reduced in hypopituitary patients with GHD[508–510] largely as a consequence of cardiovascular and cerebrovascular events, especially in female subjects.[511] Although neither estrogen nor thyroid deficiency accounts for these risk factors and reduced survival, it has not yet been rigorously confirmed that the observed increased mortality and morbidity are solely a result of GHD.

Pathophysiology

Adult GHD is most frequently encountered in patients with pituitary or hypothalamic disease.[512] Although pituitary tumors and craniopharyngiomas are associated with GHD, these patients may also experience GHD as a result of head or neck radiotherapy. GHD in children is typically isolated GHD or results from rare genetic causes (see Chapter 23) or other central structural abnormalities. Isolated GHD may be complete or partial, and up to 67% of children initially diagnosed with "idiopathic" GHD had normal GH responses when retested for GHD after cessation of GH treatment as adults.[513] Children with GHD should be retested before GH treatment is continued into adulthood unless they have clearly documented panhypopituitarism or a defined genetic or developmental abnormality that causes complete and irreversible GHD. Mutations in the GH[514] and GHRH receptor genes[515] and GH insensitivity as a result of primary GH receptor dysfunction[516] result in GHD. Other genetic abnormalities such as Prop1 or POU1F1 mutations cause GHD with concomitant deficiencies of other pituitary hormones.[517]

Evaluation

As GH is secreted in a pulsatile manner,[474] the diagnosis of GHD requires tests of evoked GH sufficiency in response to

Table 8–20. Adult Somatotropin Deficiency

Observation	Effects of Growth Hormone Replacement
Clinical	
Impaired quality of life	
Decreased energy and drive	Mood and energy uplift
Poor concentration	Enhanced vitality
Low self-esteem	Improved physical mobility
Social isolation	Social isolation improved
Body composition changes	
Increased body fat mass with altered distribution	Increased lean body mass Decreased fat mass
Increased waist-hip ratio	Increased bone mass
Decreased lean body mass	
Reduced exercise capacity	
Reduced maximum O_2 uptake	Increased maximum O_2 uptake
Impaired cardiac function	Increased maximum power
Reduced muscle mass	
Cardiovascular risk factors	
Cardiovascular structure and function impaired	Increased stroke volume
Abnormal lipid profile	Increased diastolic volume
Decreased fibrinolytic activity	Increased left ventricular wall mass
Atherosclerosis	Atherosclerosis impact
Omental obesity	
Insulin resistance	
Sialic acid increased	
Lower exercise frequency and duration	
Imaging	
Pituitary: mass or structural damage	Decreased adipocyte size Increased lipolysis
Bone: reduced density	Decreased lipogenesis
Abdomen: excess omental adiposity	
Laboratory	
Evoked GH response (see Table 8–21)	Increased IGF-I levels Increased BMR
IGF-I and IGF-BP3 low or normal	Decreased LDL with probable increased HDL
Lipid disorders	Transient hyperglycemia
Concomitant gonadotrophin, TSH, and/or ACTH reserve deficits	Increased T_3 levels Salt and water retention

ACTH, adrenocorticotropic hormone; BMR, basal metabolic rate; GH, growth hormone; HDL, high-density lipoprotein: IGF-I, insulin-like growth factor I; IGF-BP3; IGF-binding protein 3; LDL low-density lipoprotein; T_3, triiodothyronine; T_4, thyroxine.

specific GH secretagogues. The insulin tolerance test (ITT) has remained the "gold standard" test for GHD. Although some GH secretagogues reliably differentiate normal GH reserve from GHD, others are not as effective in clearly distinguishing between normal and deficient because of overlapping GH values (Table 8–21).

Differences in published responses can also be accounted for by gender, weight, or possibly age. For example, the mean peak GH response to arginine plus GHRH in control subjects was 70 μg/L. In contrast, the peak response in older and more obese men was 18 μg/L. In normal control subjects, much higher GH responses were noted when arginine plus GHRH, GHRH plus hexarelin, or GHRH plus GH-releasing peptide 6 was administered than when insulin-induced hypoglycemia was employed.[518] Although a GH response of less than 3 μg/L has been considered consistent with GHD according to a current consensus,[519, 520] the recommended cutoff points below which adult patients should be considered to have GHD vary according to the test employed (Fig. 8–42).[456] Not unexpectedly, patients with pituitary disease with no or one pituitary hormone deficiency have a lower incidence of GHD than patients with multiple hormone deficiencies. When 3 or more pituitary hormones are deficient, or if patients had pituitary disease associated with low IGF-I levels, a GH stimulation test may not be required to diagnose adult GHD.[837a]

Use of ghrelin, an endogenous ligand for the GH-releasing peptide receptor,[454] may also be proposed as a test for GHD because ghrelin is a potent GH secretagogue.[521] The requirement to test patients with proven panhypopituitarism has been questioned because virtually all patients with more than two trophic hormone deficiencies are also GH-deficient.[522] Although mean serum IGF-I levels are low in adults with GHD and very low IGF-I levels may indicate GHD, IGF-I is not useful in a screening test in adults because about 60% of GH-deficient adults have normal IGF-I levels for their age and gender.[523] Forty percent of patients older than 60 years with GHD had IGF-I concentrations that were normal for their age.[524] Measurement of IGF-BP3 is also not a reliable screening procedure for adult GHD.[525]

Presentation

Symptoms of GHD are nonspecific and may include fatigue, lack of energy, social isolation, poor concentration, and memory loss.[526] Signs include increased fat mass (especially abdominal and visceral),[527] decreased lean body mass, decreased body water,[505] and decreased bone density, particularly in patients with more severe GHD[528] and long-standing childhood-onset GHD.[529] Other features include hyperlipidemia,[530, 531] reduced exercise capacity,[506] and an increase in cardiovascular risk factors[511] including abdominal adiposity, insulin resistance,[532] and increased carotid intimal thickness.[533, 534] GHD may also be associated with heart abnormalities including reduced left ventricular mass.[526, 535–537] Cardiovascular parameters of GHD are often more pronounced in adults who had childhood-onset GHD than in those who acquired the deficiency during adulthood, who have more pronounced disorders involving quality of life, lipids, and body composition.[497, 526, 538, 539]

Many symptoms of GHD are nonspecific, and clinical judgment should be exercised in selecting patients for testing. Patients with pituitary or hypothalamic disease should be considered for diagnosis of GHD and replacement with GH even in the absence of other pituitary hormone deficiencies. Deficiencies in sex hormones also lead to body composition changes similar to those observed in GHD. For example, testosterone deficiency causes decreased lean body and bone mass and increased fat mass, each of which can be partially improved when testosterone is administered.[540] That GH has additional positive effects on body composition is suggested by observations that many patients with GHD whose body composition parameters improved after GH replacement were already receiving sex steroids. A study of healthy volunteers also demonstrated inhibition of catabolic effects when hGH was given along with prednisone.[541]

Growth Hormone Replacement Therapy

See Table 8–20. Treatment of GH-deficient adults with recombinant hGH for 4 to 6 months increased lean body mass and decreased fat mass (Figs. 8–43 and 8–44).[505] In a composite review of nine placebo-controlled trials, hGH (in doses ranging from 2.6 to 26 μg/kg/day) increased lean body mass by a mean of 3.4 kg and reduced fat mass by 4.4%.[526] GH also increased bone density[542] and parameters of both bone formation and bone resorption.[543] The GH-induced reduction in abdominal and visceral fat suggests an associated improvement in cardiovascular risk factors.

Table 8–21. Responses to Growth Hormone Stimulation Tests*

Test (Reference)	Controls, Growth Hormone Deficiency	Sex	Mean Age	Mean Body Mass Index (kg/m²)	Dose	Serum Sampling	Controls, Peak Mean (Range) (μg/L)	Growth Hormone Deficiency Peak Mean (RANGE) μg/L	Reference
ITT	33	M:12 F:21	34.1	NA	Insulin	q15 min	22.1	0.6	836
	19	M:10 F:9	39.99	24.5	0.1–0.15 U/kg IV	– 15 to 90	(3–84)	(0.1–1.8)	
Arginine-GHRH	77	M:40 F:37	28.1	NA	0.5 g/kg IV 30	q15 min	69.5	3.6	
	19	M:10 F:9	39.9	24.5	1 μg/kg IV	– 15 to 90	(13.8–171)	(0.1–16.5)	836
ITT	34	M:20 F:14	47.2	30.3	Insulin (R)	20–30 min	17.8	0.95	
	39	M:26 F:13	48.9	30.5	0.1–0.15 U/kg IV	for 2.5 hr	(0.025–52)	(0.025–7.9)	837
Arginine-GHRH	34	M:20 F:14	47.2	30.3	30 g over	q30 min for	18.4	1.44	
	39	M:26 F:13	48.9	30.5	30 min IV, 1 μg/kg IV	2.5 hr	(1.2–127)	(0.025–7.7)	837
Hexarelin-GHRH	25	M:18 F:7	28.5	NA	0.25 μg/kg IV	q15 min	83.6	2.6	
	19	M:10 F:9	39.9	24.5	1 μg/kg IV	– 15 to 90	(49–124)	(0.1–11.1)	836
GHRH-GHRP-6	125	M:65 F:60	39.9	23.5	1 μg/kg IV	q15–30 min	59.2	4.1	
	125	M:73 F:52	39.6	26.9	1 μg/kg IV	– 30 to 120	(15–139)	(0.01–15)	456

Recommended test sensitivity by 95% confidence limits* or recommended by investigator to diagnose adult GH deficiency**

Test	Value <μg/L	References
ITT	5.1*	Biller, 2002
Arginine + GHRH	4.1*	Biller, 2002
Arginine + GHRH	9.0**	Gasperi, 1999
Arginine + L-Dopa	1.7*	Biller, 2002
Hexarelin + GHRH	9.0**	Gasperi, 1999
GHRH + GHRP-6	10.0**	Popovic, 2000

*Results from two studies on the effects of insulin-induced hypoglycemia and the combination of arginine and GHRH illustrate the effect of body weight on GH responses.

The effect of hGH replacement on lipid abnormalities is variable.[544] The hGH had a significant effect on raising high-density lipoprotein cholesterol[531] and overall the most consistent change was an improvement in the ratio of cholesterol to high-density lipoprotein cholesterol. Some have reported increases in cardiac output,[545, 546] reduction in intima media thickness,[533] and improved energy, mood, and quality of life,[547] but not all investigators concur.[548] Improved quality of life, including a significant reduction in sick days, hospitalization length, and physician visits, has been reported in some studies.[548a] There may be a latency period up to 3 months before patients recognize the benefits of hGH replacement, which are most obvious in those with the most profound symptoms and signs of GHD.[522] Beneficial effects of GH replacement persist for at least 10 years.[549]

GH Administration. GH is administered by nightly subcutaneous injection, the recommended dose for adults is much lower than for children,[550] and children experience fewer side effects of GH than adults. Men, particularly older ones, are more sensitive to GH and require lower GH doses than women. The maintenance dose of hGH in 665 adult patients with GHD was 0.43 mg/day for men and 0.53 mg/day for women.[512] Women with GHD require higher doses of hGH with oral than with transdermal estrogen (Fig. 8–45).[551, 552] It is recommended that replacement be initiated with relatively low doses.[538] Most adults tolerate a starting dose of 300 μg/day or lower, which is then titrated according to serum IGF-I concentrations and side effects of the medication.[553] If side effects occur, the dose should be reduced. If no side effects are reported, the therapeutic goal is to maintain IGF-I levels in the normal range for age and gender while avoiding levels in the upper quintile.

Precautions and Caveats of Treating with Human Growth Hormone

The most common side effects of hGH are edema, arthralgias, and myalgias which occurred in up to one third of patients when the drug was administered at a weight-based dosage (Table 8–22). Using total daily doses titrated for IGF-I levels, the incidence of side effects is much lower.[531] Patients with active malignancies should not be treated with GH, nor should patients with active carpal tunnel syndrome or other fluid retention disorders. The possibility that hGH might initi-

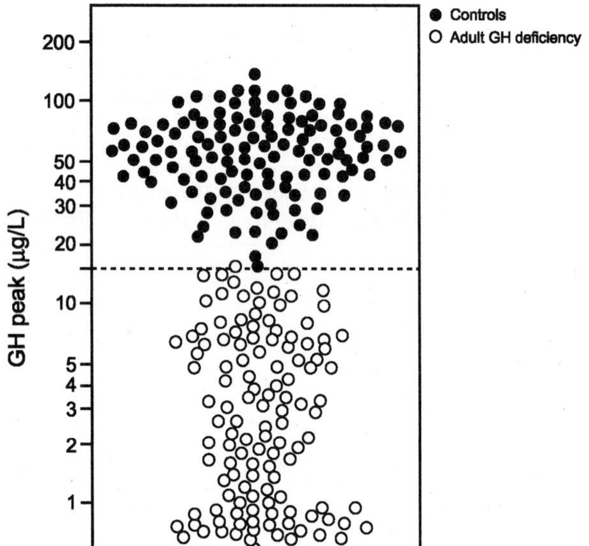

Figure 8–42. Individual growth hormone–releasing hormone (GHRH) plus GHRP-6–mediated GH peaks in control subjects *(black dots)* and GH-deficient adults *(white dots)*. GH secretion was a continuum between excessive secretion and abnormally low secretion, although a transition concentration between normality and abnormality may be seen at about the 15 μg/L concentration. Logarithmic representation (From Popovic V, Leal A, Micic D, et al. GH-releasing hormone and GH-releasing peptide-6 for diagnostic testing in GH-deficient adults. Lancet 2000; 356:1137–1142.)

ate new cancers or stimulate growth of preexisting benign tumors is an important theoretical issue. An epidemiologic association between higher, albeit normal, IGF-I levels and later risk of development of prostate cancer,[554] breast cancer in premenopausal women,[555] and colon and lung cancer[556] has been reported. In contrast, patients with acromegaly, who have very high serum levels of IGF-I, do not have an increased incidence of either breast or prostate cancer or cancer in general. In fact, the overall risk for cancer in acromegaly is lower than expected. However, these patients have significantly increased mortality from colon cancer.[557–559]

The possibility that hGH treatment might cause new or recurrent malignancies has been best examined in children in whom GHD developed as a result of treatment for their malignancies.[560] When the relative risk of brain tumor recurrence in 180 children treated with hGH versus 891 who did not receive hGH was analyzed, the risk of recurrence after a mean of 6.4 years was lower in the treated group than those not receiving hGH.[561] Nevertheless, long-term surveillance with adequate control groups and avoidance of high IGF-I levels in adults being treated for GHD are required to ensure that GH replacement in adults does not increase the incidence of new

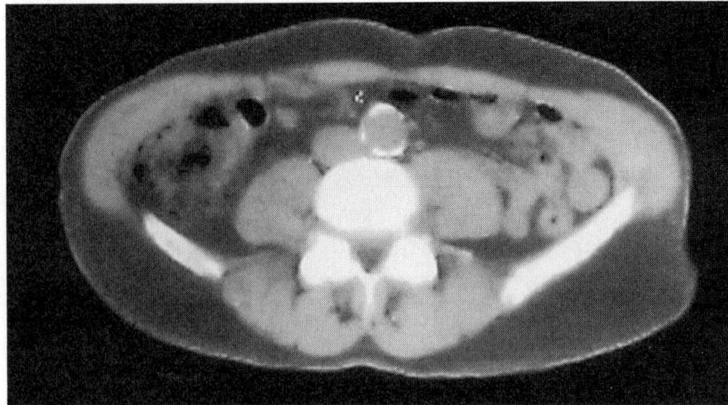

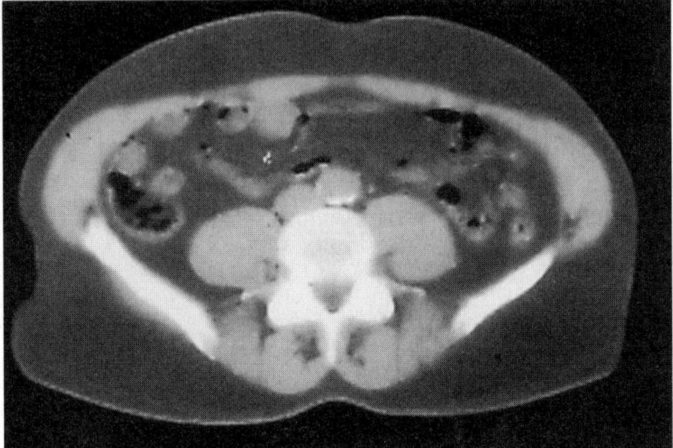

Figure 8–44. Abdominal subcutaneous and visceral adipose tissue determined with computed tomography at the level of L4–5 in one man before *(top)* and after *(bottom)* 9 months of rhGH treatment. The scan shows the reduction in both visceral and subcutaneous adipose tissue. (Figures and caption kindly provided by B.A. Bengtsson.)

cancers or growth of existing benign tumors. Blood glucose levels should also be monitored carefully, especially in patients also being treated for diabetes (Fig. 8–46).

Growth Hormone Treatment of Catabolic States

The well-recognized anabolic actions of GH have prompted use of GH in catabolic states including those associated with surgery, trauma, burns, parenteral nutrition, and organ failure. These potential indications for GH are not approved in the United States. The negative nitrogen balance in critically ill patients is partly attributable to GH resistance as well as to decreased IGF-I production and action.[562] GH administered to postsurgical patients as well as to normal subjects receiving

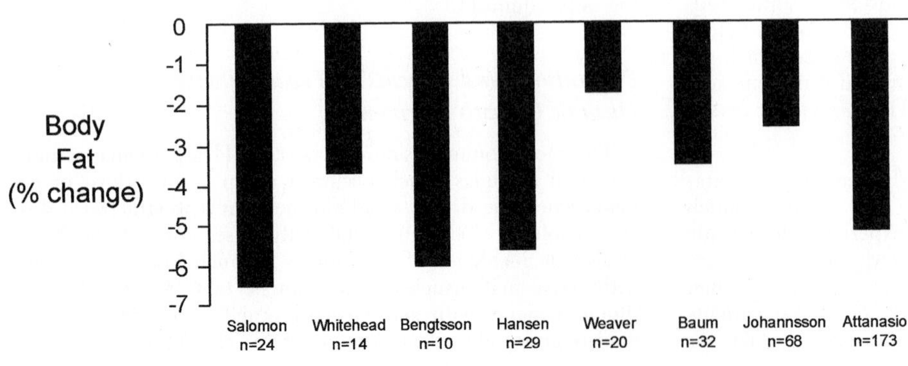

Figure 8–43. Effect of treatment with human growth hormone (hGH) on body fat in eight studies. (Adapted from Newman CB, Kleinberg DL. Adult growth hormone deficiency. Endocrinologist 1998; 8:178–186.)

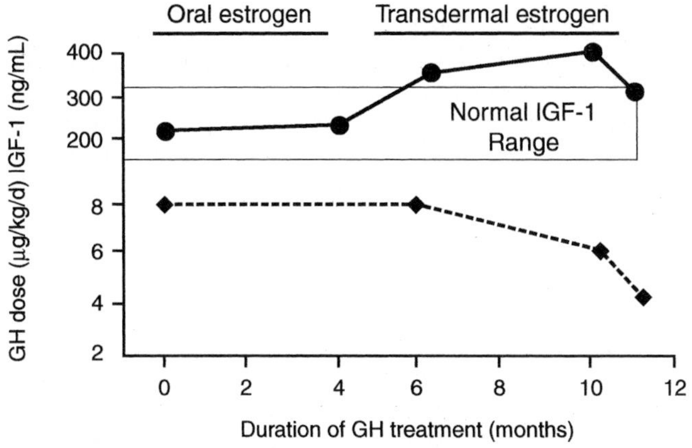

Figure 8-45. Time course of growth hormone (GH) dose and serum insulin-like growth factor I (IGF-I) concentration in a representative patient (38-year-old female) who was switched from oral to transdermal estrogen therapy during the course of GH replacement. (From Cook DM, Ludlam WH, Cook MB. Route of estrogen administration helps to determine growth hormone [GH] replacement dose in GH-deficient adults. J Clin Endocrinol Metab 1999; 84:3956–3960.)

Table 8-22. Side Effects of Growth Hormone Treatment

Edema
Arthralgias
Myalgias
Muscle stiffness
Paresthesias
Carpal tunnel syndrome
Hypertension
Atrial fibrillation
Headache
Tinnitus
Benign intracranial hypertension
Increase in melanocytic nevi

hypocaloric intravenous alimentation results in reversion to positive nitrogen balance.

Beneficial effects of GH have been reported in patients with extensive burns, chronic high-dose glucocorticoid treatment, chronic obstructive pulmonary disease, cancer, and cardiac failure. Nevertheless, published end points for these studies have not been definitive. When GH was administered to elderly malnourished patients, it was found to be an effective adjuvant for dietary augmentation.[563] A study in which critically ill patients received very high doses of GH (up to 7 mg/day) was prematurely terminated because of unexplained increased mortality.[564] It was suggested that GH may have had an adverse effect on acute phase protein synthesis in these patients.[565]

Growth Hormone Treatment for Osteoporosis

As declining GH secretion has been implicated in the pathogenesis of osteoporosis, GH was administered to otherwise healthy subjects with idiopathic osteoporosis in an attempt to decrease bone loss.[566] GH increased indices of bone formation and resorption, but a modest increase in spine bone mineral density was observed only in male subjects. A longer study in osteoporotic female subjects showed that GH together with calcitonin increased spine and total hip bone mineral density[567] after 2 years of treatment, although the response was less marked than that observed with estrogen or bisphosphonate therapy. Limited proven efficacy, unclear side effects, and lack

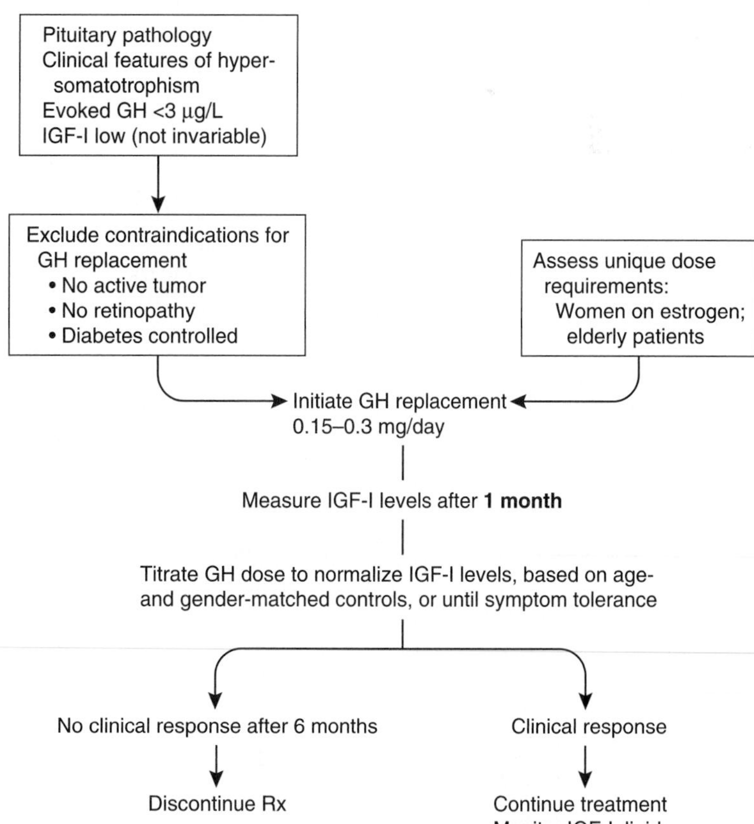

Figure 8-46. Management of adult somatotropin deficiency. Patients older than 60 years require lower maintenance doses. Women receiving transdermal estrogen require lower doses than those receiving oral estrogen preparations. GH, growth hormone; IGF-I, insulin-like growth factor I; Rx, treatment.

of comparative studies with other beneficial therapies for osteoporosis indicate a need for further study of the potential use of GH in treating osteoporosis.

Growth Hormone Treatment in Human Immunodeficiency Virus Infection

GH is approved by the Food and Drug Administration for administration to adult patients with human immunodeficiency virus (HIV)–associated cachexia. The GH treatment resulted in positive nitrogen balance, increased lean body mass, decreased body fat, and improved work output.[568] Ten HIV-infected subjects with fat redistribution syndrome associated with protease inhibitor therapy received GH at 6 mg/day subcutaneously for 12 weeks and showed decreased weight/hip ratios and enhanced midthigh circumference.[569, 570] However, long-term beneficial effects of GH on survival and quality of life in HIV infection have not yet been reported.

Growth Hormone Use in Competitive Sports

The public policy issues of GH abuse in competitive sports have received much attention. GH has been used by athletes to enhance muscle mass.[571] Whether persistent GH use is accompanied by increased muscle strength is unclear. Continued use of pharmacologic GH doses by athletes could result in adverse effects of acromegaly, which would decrease performance.

Decreased Insulin-like Growth Factor I Levels

Short-term fasted normal healthy subjects have moderately elevated basal GH levels, and protein-calorie malnutrition, starvation, and anorexia nervosa are associated with low IGF-I and markedly elevated GH levels.[540] This observation may reflect uncoupling of IGF-I feedback regulation of GH secretion. Low IGF-I levels in normal fasting subjects are normalized by caloric refeeding to a greater degree than by protein intake alone.[572]

Acromegaly

In 1886 Pierre Marie[2] published the first clinical description of disordered somatic growth and proportion and proposed the name *acromegaly*. He also recognized cases previously described by others. When the relation of this syndrome to a pituitary tumor was later recognized, Benda[573] showed in 1900 that these tumors comprise mainly adenohypophyseal eosinophilic cells, which he proposed to be hyperfunctioning. Cushing, Davidoff, and Bailey documented the clinicopathologic features of acromegaly and demonstrated clinical remission of soft tissue signs after adenoma resection.[3] Evans and Long[574] induced gigantism in rats injected with anterior pituitary extracts, confirming the association of a pituitary factor with somatic growth. Establishment of the unequivocal pathophysiologic link between hyperfunctioning adenoma and acromegaly represented the earliest example of a pituitary disorder being clinically and pathologically recognized and appropriately managed by surgical excision of a hypersecreting source.

Incidence

The prevalence of acromegaly is estimated to range from 38 to 69 cases per million, and the annual incidence of new patients is 3 to 4 cases per million.[575–577] On the basis of these largely Western European studies, it is estimated that over 1000 new cases of acromegaly are diagnosed annually in the United States.

Pathogenesis

GH and IGF-I act both independently and dependently in inducing features of hypersomatotropism. Acromegaly is caused by pituitary tumors secreting GH or rarely by extrapituitary disorders (Fig. 8–47).[578] Regardless of the etiology, the disease is characterized by elevated levels of GH and IGF-I with resultant signs and symptoms of hypersomatotropism.

Pituitary Acromegaly

More than 95% of patients with acromegaly harbor a GH-secreting pituitary adenoma (Table 8–23). *Pure GH cell adenomas* contain either densely or sparsely staining cytoplasmic GH granules, and these two variants grow slowly (densely granulated) or rapidly (sparsely granulated).[579, 580] The former arise insidiously and occur during or after middle age, whereas the latter arise in younger subjects with more florid disease. Mixed GH cell and PRL cell adenomas are composed of distinct somatotrophs expressing GH and lactotrophs expressing PRL. Monomorphous acidophil stem cell adenomas arise from the common GH and PRL stem cell and also often contain giant mitochondria and misplaced GH granule exocytosis. They grow rapidly, are invasive, and arise with predominant features of hyperprolactinemia.[581] Monomorphous mammosomatotroph cell adenomas express both GH and PRL from a single cell, and plurihormonal tumors may express GH with any combination of PRL, TSH, ACTH, or α subunit.[582] These patients present with clinical features of acromegaly as well as hyperprolactinemia, Cushing's disease, or rarely hyperthyroxinemia.

Somatotroph hyperplasia is difficult to distinguish from a GH cell adenoma, and silver staining displays a well-preserved reticulin network without a surrounding pseudocapsule. The rigorous morphologic diagnosis of GH cell hyperplasia is usually associated with stimulation by ectopic GHRH derived from an extrapituitary tumor causing acromegaly. *Silent somatotroph adenomas* immunostain positively for GH and are apparently clinically nonfunctional, although GH or PRL levels, or both, may be modestly elevated in over 50% of these patients.

Pathogenesis of Somatotroph Cell Adenomas

Both pituitary and hypothalamic factors influence pituitary tumor pathogenesis.[583, 584] Even when exhibiting marked nuclear pleomorphism, mitotic activity, and invasiveness, these tumors are usually benign.

Disordered GHRH Secretion or Action. Adenomas express receptors for GHRH, ghrelin,[453] and SRIF,[585] but activating mutations of the GHRH or SRIF receptor have not been reported. GHRH directly stimulates GH gene expression and also induces somatotroph mitotic activity. Transgenic GHRH expression causes somatotroph hyperplasia and ultimately adenoma. Clinically, GHRH production by hypothalamic, abdominal or chest neuroendocrine tumors causes somatotroph hyperplasia and occasionally adenoma with resultant unrestrained GH secretion and acromegaly.[32] However, histologic examination of most pituitary GH cell adenoma tissue specimens does not show hyperplastic somatotroph tissue surrounding the adenoma, implying no generalized hypothalamic overstimulation. Failure to down-regulate GH secretion during prolonged GHRH stimulation also points to a role for GHRH in maintaining persistent GH hypersecretion. Expression of intra-adenomatous GHRH correlates with tumor size and activity, implying a paracrine role for GHRH in mediating adenoma pathogenesis.[586] GHRH modestly stimulates PRL secretion, and up to 40% of patients with acromegaly also have hyperprolactinemia.

Complete surgical resection of well-defined GH-secreting

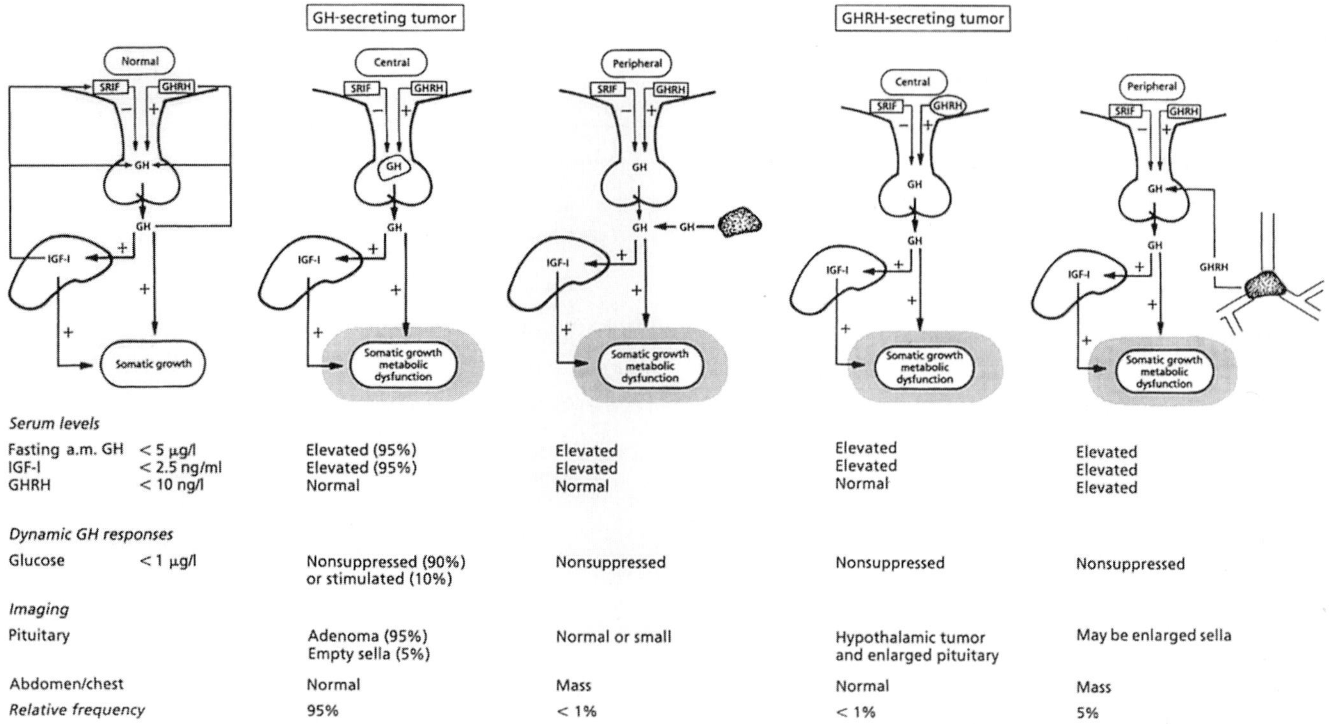

	Normal	GH-secreting tumor: Central	GH-secreting tumor: Peripheral	GHRH-secreting tumor: Central	GHRH-secreting tumor: Peripheral
Serum levels					
Fasting a.m. GH	< 5 μg/l	Elevated (95%)	Elevated	Elevated	Elevated
IGF-I	< 2.5 ng/ml	Elevated (95%)	Elevated	Elevated	Elevated
GHRH	< 10 ng/l	Normal	Normal	Normal	Elevated
Dynamic GH responses					
Glucose	< 1 μg/l	Nonsuppressed (90%) or stimulated (10%)	Nonsuppressed	Nonsuppressed	Nonsuppressed
Imaging					
Pituitary		Adenoma (95%) Empty sella (5%)	Normal or small	Hypothalamic tumor and enlarged pituitary	May be enlarged sella
Abdomen/chest		Normal	Mass	Normal	Mass
Relative frequency		95%	< 1%	< 1%	5%

Figure 8–47. Pathogenesis and diagnosis of acromegaly. GH, growth hormone; GHRH, growth hormone–releasing hormone; IGF, insulin-like growth factor type I; SRIF, somatostatin. (From Melmed S. Acromegaly. N Engl J Med 1990; 322:966–977.)

microadenomas usually results in a definitive cure of excess hormone secretion with low postoperative tumor recurrence rates, strongly suggestive of intact hypothalamic function in these patients. Although basal GH levels are usually high in acromegaly, the episodic pulsatile pattern of GH release is intact and the nocturnal GH surge usually preserved.[587] Patients treated with SRIF analogues also retain GH pulsatility, and GH pulse amplitude and sensitivity to GHRH appear intact.

Disordered Somatotroph Cell Function. A somatotroph mutation may be a prerequisite for the abnormal growth response to disordered GHRH secretion or action. The monoclonal origin of somatotroph adenomas was determined by X-chromosome inactivation analysis of somatotroph tumor DNA.[588] An altered Gsα protein identified in a subset of GH-secreting pituitary adenomas led to high levels of intracellular cAMP and GH hypersecretion.[589, 590] Point mutations in two critical sites, Arg201, the site for adenosine diphosphate ribosylation, and Gly227, the guanosine triphosphate binding domain of Gsα proteins, prevent guanosine triphosphatase activity and result in constitutive adenyl cyclase activation. This dominant *gsp* mutant mimics GHRH effects, results in elevated cAMP levels, and is present in about 30% of GH-secreting tumors. Loss of heterozygosity has been observed for chromosomes 11, 13, and 9,[45, 55, 585] especially in larger, more invasive macroadenomas. However, no defined tumor suppressor gene has been isolated for these sporadic nonfamilial tumors. An activating pituitary tumor transforming gene (*PTTG*) isolated from pituitary tumors is overexpressed in GH-secreting tumors, and its abundance correlates with tumor size and invasiveness.[46–48] PTTG participates as a securin protein, regulating sister chromatid separation during the cell cycle, and its overexpression may lead to cell aneuploidy.[49]

The sequence of events leading to somatotroph clonal expansion appears multifactorial. An activated oncogene may be required for initiating tumorigenesis, and promotion of tumor growth may require GHRH and other growth factor stimulation. The cellular mutation may not by itself be sufficient to provide a growth advantage for a GH-secreting adenoma without additional disordered hypothalamic or paracrine growth factor signaling.

Extrapituitary Acromegaly

Excess GH secretion in acromegaly may not necessarily be pituitary in origin.[591] Because management of ectopic acromegaly differs from that of pituitary GH hypersecretion, rigorous clinical and biochemical criteria should be fulfilled to confirm the diagnosis of ectopic acromegaly.[592] These criteria include demonstration of elevated circulating GHRH or GH levels in the absence of a primary pituitary lesion, a significant arteriovenous hormone gradient across the ectopic tumor source, biochemical and clinical cure of acromegaly after resection of the ectopic hormone-producing tumor, and normalization of the GHRH–GH–IGF-I axis. Finally, GHRH or GH gene product expression should be shown. Patients with inconclusive imaging, biochemical, or clinical features of pituitary acromegaly may inadvertently be diagnosed as harboring a nonpituitary source of excess GH secretion and be inappropriately treated.

GHRH Hypersecretion. Hypothalamic tumors, including hamartomas, choristomas, gliomas, and gangliocytomas, may produce GHRH with subsequent somatotroph hyperplasia or even a pituitary GH cell adenoma and resultant acromegaly.[32] Primary mammosomatotroph hyperplasia with no evidence for pituitary adenoma or an extrapituitary tumor source of GHRH has been described in gigantism.[593] The structure of hypothalamic GHRH was, in fact, elucidated from material extracted from pancreatic GHRH-secreting tumors in patients with acromegaly.[31]

Table 8–23. Causes of Acromegaly

Cause	Prevalence (%)	Hormonal Product/s	Clinical Features	Pathologic Characteristics
Excess Growth Hormone Secretion				
Pituitary	98	GH	Slow growing	Resemble normal somatotrophs, numerous, large secretory granules
Densely granulated GH cell adenoma	30		Clinically insidious	
Sparsely granulated adenoma	30	GH	Rapidly growing Often invasive	Cellular pleomorphism Characteristic ultrastructure
Mixed GH cell and PRL cell adenoma	25	GH and PRL	Variable	Densely granulated somatotrophs sparsely granulated lactotrophs
Mammosomatotroph cell adenoma	10	GH and PRL	Common in children. Gigantism, mild hyperprolactinemia	Both GH and PRL in same cell, often same secretory granule
Acidophil stem cell adenoma		PRL and GH	Rapidly growing invasive, hyperprolactinemia dominant	Distinctive ultrastructure Giant mitochondria
Plurihormonal adenoma		GH (PRL w/αGSU, FSH/LH, TSH, or ACTH	Often secondary hormonal products are clinically silent	Variable—either monomorphous or plurimorphous
GH cell carcinoma or metastases		GH	Usually aggressive	Documented metastasis
Multiple endocrine neoplasia-type 1 (adenoma)				
McCune-Albright syndrome (rarely adenoma)		GH, PRL	Classic triad	
Ectopic sphenoid or parapharyngeal sinus pituitary adenoma		GH	Ectopic mass	Adenoma
Familial acromegaly (adenoma)		GH		
Carney's syndrome (adenoma)		GH		
Extrapituitary tumor				
Pancreatic islet cell tumor	<1			
Excess Growth Hormone Releasing–Hormone Secretion				
Central	<1		Hypothalamic mass	Somatotroph hyperplasia
Hypothalamic hamartoma, choristoma, ganglioneuroma				
Peripheral	1	GH, PRL	Systemic features	Somatotroph hyperplasia Rarely adenoma
Bronchial carcinoid, pancreatic islet cell tumor, small cell lung cancer, adrenal adenoma, medullary thyroid carcinoma, pheochromocytoma				

Adapted from Melmed S. N Engl J Med 1990; 322:966–977[578]; Melmed S. Pathophysiology of acromegaly. Endocr Rev 1983; 4:271–290.

GHRH immunoreactivity is detectable in about 25% of carcinoid tumor samples. Acromegaly in these patients is uncommon, however. In a retrospective survey of 177 patients with acromegaly, only a single patient was identified with elevated plasma GHRH levels.[445] Bronchial carcinoids make up most tumors associated with ectopic GHRH secretion. Pancreatic cell tumors, small cell lung cancers, adrenal adenoma, pheochromocytoma, and medullary thyroid, endometrial, and breast cancers have rarely been described to express GHRH and cause acromegaly.[594, 595] Surgical resection of the tumor secreting ectopic GHRH should reverse the GH hypersecretion, and pituitary surgery is not required in these patients. Carcinoid syndrome with ectopic GHRH secretion can also be managed with somatostatin analogues, which lower GH and IGF-I levels and suppress ectopic tumor elaboration of GHRH.[596, 597]

Ectopic Pituitary Adenomas. GH-secreting adenomas may arise from ectopic pituitary remnants in the sphenoid sinus, petrous temporal bone, or nasopharyngeal cavity.[598, 599] Rarely, pituitary carcinoma may spread to the meninges, CSF, or cervical lymph nodes, resulting in functional GH-secreting metastases that may be diagnosed by radiolabeled octreotide imaging (indium In 111 pentetreotide [OctreoScan]).[428]

Peripheral GH-Secreting Tumors. Lung adenocarcinoma, breast cancer, and ovarian tissues contain immunoreactive GH without clinical evidence of acromegaly. Rarely, a GH-secreting intramesenteric pancreatic islet cell tumor causes acromegaly; these patients present with an intra-abdominal mass, a normal-sized or small pituitary gland on MRI, no GH response to TRH injection, and normal levels of circulating plasma GHRH.[592]

Acromegaloidism. Rarely, conditions exhibiting soft tissue and skin changes usually associated with acromegaly and normal baseline and dynamic GH and IGF-I with no demonstrable pituitary or extrapituitary tumor have been termed *acromegaloid.* Pachydermoperiostosis should be considered in the differential diagnosis. Insulin resistance and defective IGF-I binding have been demonstrated in cells derived from some patients with acanthosis nigricans, and treatment is symptomatic.

McCune-Albright Syndrome. This rare hypersecretory syndrome consists of polyostotic fibrous dysplasia, cutaneous pigmentation, sexual precocity, hyperthyroidism, hypercortisolism, hyperprolactinemia, and acromegaly. Although few patients have definitive evidence of a pituitary adenoma, Gsα mutations have been detected in both endocrine and nonendocrine tissues.[600] GH hypersecretion can be controlled by somatostatin analogues or pituitary irradiation.

Multiple Endocrine Neoplasia. GH cell pituitary adenoma is a well-documented component of the autosomal dominant MEN-1 syndrome, which also includes parathyroid and pancreatic tumors (see Chapter 36). MEN-1, associated with germ cell inactivation of the *MENIN* tumor suppressor gene located on chromosome 11q13,[601] appears intact in sporadic GH cell adenomas.[54, 602] Rarely, functional pancreatic tumors in patients with MEN-1 also express GHRH.

Familial Acromegaly. Familial acromegaly may occur in association with the Carney complex, which maps to chromosome 2p.[603] Several families with isolated familial acromegaly comprise related cases of acromegaly and gigantism and harbor loss of heterozygosity in chromosome 11q13, distinct from *MENIN* (see Table 8–4).[604]

Clinical Features

Manifestations of acromegaly are caused by either central pressure effects of the pituitary mass or peripheral actions of excess GH and IGF-I. Central features of the expanding pituitary mass are common to all pituitary masses[302] and have already been described. In acromegaly, headache is often severe and debilitating. Local signs are especially important presenting features because a preponderance of macroadenomas (>65%) is encountered in acromegaly, compared with mostly microadenomas for PRL-secreting tumors.[605]

Gigantism

Tall stature may be caused by a GH-secreting pituitary tumor or hyperplasia. About 20% of patients have the McCune-Albright syndrome with somatotroph hyperplasia or rarely pituitary adenomas. Somatotroph hyperplasia and acidophilic stem cell adenomas may cause gigantism in infancy or early childhood, suggesting early hypersecretion of GHRH or disordered pituicyte cell differentiation.[593, 606] Pituitary gigantism should be considered in children who are more than 3 standard deviations (SD) above normal mean height for age or more than 2 SD above their adjusted mean parental height.

The biochemical diagnosis is similar to that for acromegaly; that is, GH levels are in excess of 1 μg/L after a glucose load and serum IGF-I concentrations are elevated. In children undergoing pubertal growth spurts, GH responses to glucose may be paradoxical and serum IGF-I concentrations are often physiologically elevated. Thus, the diagnosis requires clear-cut MRI evidence for a pituitary lesion. The differential diagnosis includes familial tall stature, redundancy of Y chromosomes, Marfan's syndrome, and homocystinuria.

Table 8–24. Presentation of Acromegaly*

Presenting Chief Complaint	Frequency (%)
Menstrual disturbance	13
Change in appearance, acral growth	11
Headaches	8
Paresthesias, carpal tunnel syndrome	6
Diabetes mellitus, impaired glucose tolerance	5
Heart disease	3
Visual impairment	3
Decreased libido, impotence	3
Arthopathy	3
Thyroid disorder	2
Hypertension	1
Gigantism	1
Fatigue	0.3
Hyperhidrosis	0.3
Somnolence	0.3
Other	5
Chance (detected by unrelated physical or dental examination or radiograph)	40
Total	100
Causes of Death	
Cardiovascular	60
Respiratory	25
Malignancy	15

*From Molitch ME. Clinical manifestations of acromegaly. Endocrinol Metab Clin North Am 1992; 21:597–614, based on 310 patients.

Data integrated from Holdaway, 1998; Wright, 1969; Alexander, 1980; Nabarro, 1987; Bengtsson, 1988; Bates, 1993; Extabe, 1993; Rajasoorya, 1994.

Clinical Features of Acromegaly

Effects of hypersomatotropism on acral and soft tissue growth and metabolic function occur insidiously over several years (Table 8–24; Figs. 8–48 and 8–49).[607] The slow onset and elusive symptoms often result in a delay in diagnosis ranging from 6.6 to 10.2 years, with a mean delay of almost 9 years.[608] Patients may seek care for dental, orthopedic, rheumatologic, or cardiac disorders. Only 13% of 256 patients diagnosed during a 20-year period presented with primary symptoms of altered facial appearance or enlarged extremities.[609] In a review of several hundred patients presenting with acromegaly worldwide, 98% had acral enlargement and hyperhidrosis was prominent in 70%.[607]

When patients present early, facial and peripheral features are usually not obvious and a serial review of old photographs often reveals the progress of subtle physical changes. Characteristic features include large fleshy lips and nose, spade-like hands, frontal skull bossing, and cranial ridges. Enlarged tongue, bones, salivary glands, thyroid, heart, liver, and spleen are the effects of generalized visceromegaly. Clinically apparent hepatosplenomegaly, however, is rare. Increases in shoe, ring, or hat size are commonly reported. Progressive acral changes may lead to facial and skeletal disfigurement, especially if excess GH secretion begins prior to epiphyseal closure.[610] These include mandibular overgrowth with prognathism, maxillary widening, teeth separation, jaw malocclusion and overbite, and nasal bone hypertrophy.[611] Sonorous voice deepening occurs in association with laryngeal hypertrophy and enlarged paranasal sinuses.

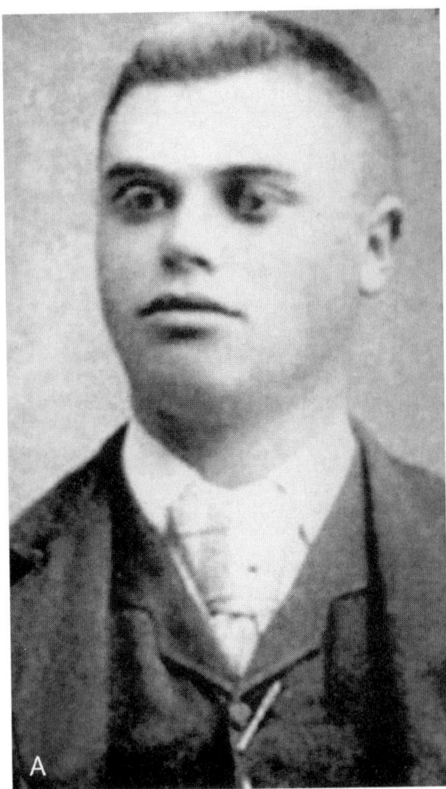

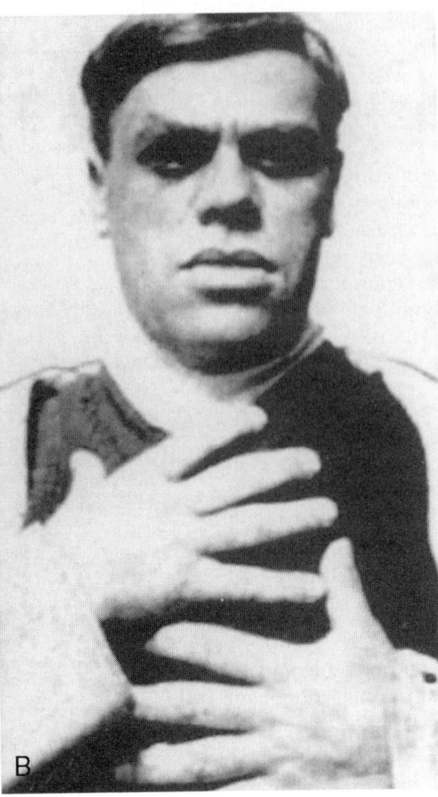

Figure 8–48. Harvey Cushing's first acromegaly patient. *(A)* Some years before presentation and *(B)* at admission. (From Jane JA, Laws ER. History of Acromegaly. In Wass JAH (ed). Handbook of acromegaly. Bristol, UK, BioScientifica, 2001, pp 3–15.)

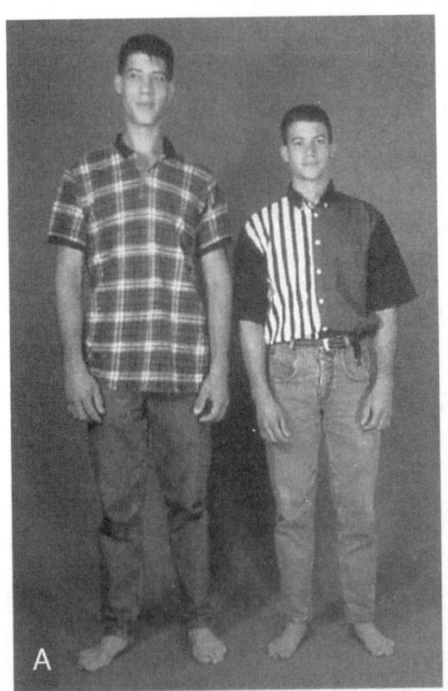

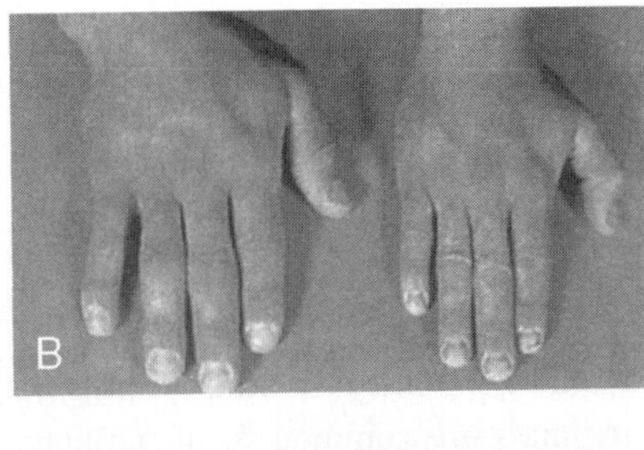

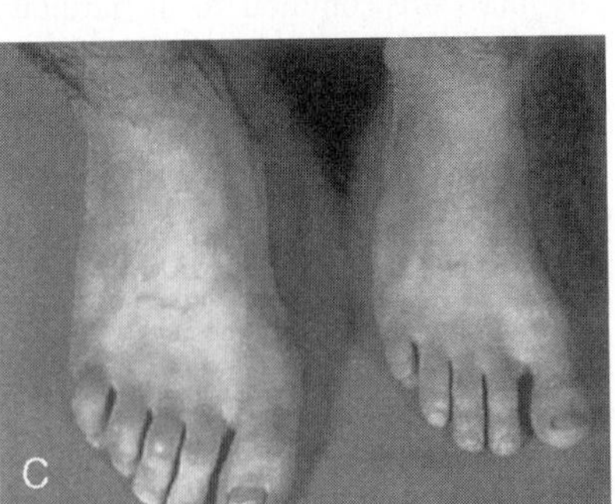

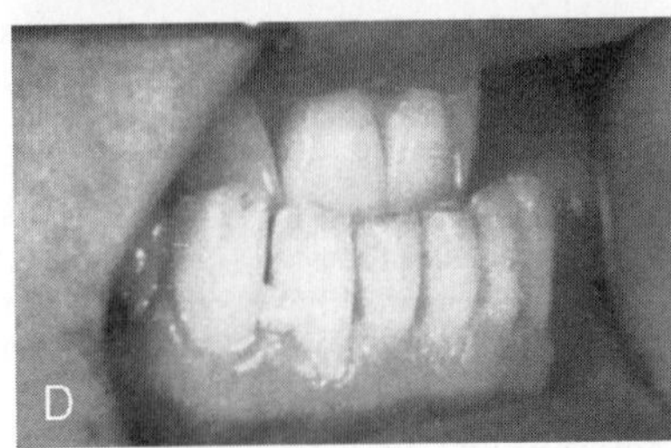

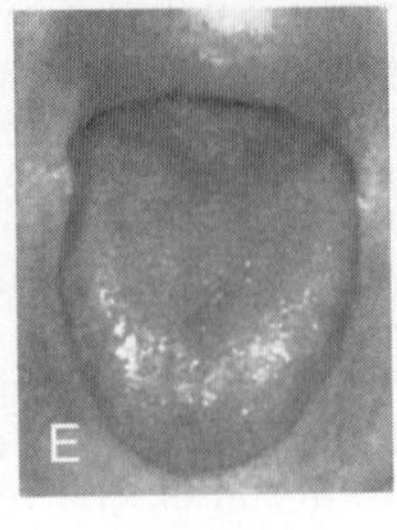

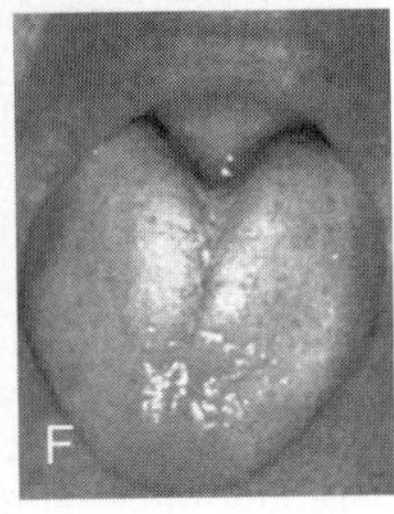

Figure 8–49. Clinical features of acromegaly. *A* to *C*, Features of acromegaly or gigantism in two identical twins. A 22-year-old man with gigantism related to excess growth hormone is shown to the left of his identical twin. The increased height and prognathism *(A)* and enlarged hand *(B)* and foot *(C)* of the affected twin are apparent. Their clinical features began to diverge at the age of approximately 13 years. *D* to *F*, Increased incisor spacing and prognathism *(D)*, macroglossia *(E)*, and a normal tongue *(F)*. (*A–C*, From Gagel R, McCutcheon IE. Images in clinical medicine: pituitary gigantism. N Engl J Med 1999; 324:524; *D–F*, from Turner. Clinical features, investigation and complications of acromegaly. In Wass J [ed]. Handbook of Acromegaly. Bristol, UK, BioScientifica, 2001.)

Up to half of the patients may experience joint symptoms severe enough to limit daily activities. Arthropathy occurs in about 70% of patients, most of whom exhibit joint swelling, hypermobility, and cartilaginous thickening.[612] Local periarticular fibrous tissue thickening may cause joint stiffening or deformities and nerve entrapment. Knees, hips, shoulders, lumbosacral joints, elbows, and ankles are affected with monoarticular or polyarticular arthritides, but joint effusions rarely develop.[613] Spinal involvement includes osteophytosis, disc space widening, and increased anteroposterior vertebral length, which may result in dorsal kyphosis.

Neural enlargement and wrist tissue swelling may lead to carpal tunnel syndrome in up to half of all patients. Chondrocyte proliferation with an increased joint space occurs early, and ulcerations and fissures of weight-bearing cartilage areas are often accompanied by new bone formation. Debilitating osteoarthritis may result in bone remodeling, osteophyte formation, subchondral cysts, narrowed joint spaces, and lax periarticular ligaments. Osteophytes commonly occur at the phalangeal tufts and over the anterior aspects of spinal vertebrae. Ligaments may ossify, and periarticular calcium pyrophosphate deposition occurs. Although the duration of hypersomatotropism correlates with clinical severity of the joint changes, it is unclear whether higher GH levels correlate with increased articular disease activity. Therapeutic responses usually depend on the degree of irreversible bone changes already in place.

Hyperhidrosis and malodorous oily skin are common early signs, occurring in up to 70% of patients. Facial wrinkles, nasolabial folds, and heel pads thicken and body hair may become coarse,[614] attributed to glycosaminoglycan deposition and increased connective tissue collagen production.[615] Skin tags are common and may be markers for the adenomatous colonic polyps.[616] Raynaud's phenomenon is reported in up to one third of patients.

Symptomatic cardiac disease is present in about 20% of patients and is a major cause of morbidity and mortality.[617, 618] Hypertension is present in about 50% of patients with active acromegaly, and half of these have evidence of left ventricular dysfunction.[619] Left ventricular hypertrophy is also observed in about half of normotensive patients with acromegaly. Asymmetric septal hypertrophy is common, and cardiac failure may occur with early or mild cardiomegaly. Subclinical left ventricular diastolic dysfunction is due to myocardial hypertrophy, interstitial fibrosis, and lymphocytic myocardial infiltrates. Resting electrocardiograms are abnormal in about 50% of patients, with S-T segment depression, T-wave abnormalities, conduction defects, and arrhythmias. Plasma renin levels are suppressed, and endogenous plasma digitalis-like activity with chronic volume expansion has been identified in acromegaly.[620] Cardiovascular disease accounts for approximately 60% of deaths in patients with acromegaly,[621] and the presence of cardiovascular disease at the time of diagnosis portends high mortality rates despite improved cardiac function after effective GH and IGF-I control.[352]

Prognathism, thick lips, macroglossia, and hypertrophied nasal structures may obstruct aiways.[622, 623] Irregular laryngeal mucosa, cartilage hypertrophy, tracheal calcification, and cricoarytenoid joint arthropathy lead to unilateral or bilateral vocal cord fixation or laryngeal stenosis with voice changes and upper airway obstruction or stridor. Tracheal intubation may be particularly difficult in patients undergoing anesthesia, and tracheostomy may be required. Both central respiratory depression and airway obstruction lead to paroxysmal daytime sleep (narcolepsy), sleep apnea, and habitual excessive snoring. Obstructive sleep apnea, characterized by excessive daytime sleepiness with at least five episodes of apnea per hour of sleep, causes daytime somnolence, especially in men with acromegaly, who may also have a ventilation-perfusion defect with hypoxemia. Sleep apnea may also be central in origin and associated with higher GH and IGF-I levels.[623]

Synovial edema leads to hyperplastic wrist ligaments and tendons that contribute to painful median nerve compression. Peripheral acroparesthesias and symmetric peripheral neuropathy should be distinguished from diabetic neuropathy, which may be secondary to acromegaly.[624] Proximal myopathy may also be accompanied by myalgias, cramps, and nonspecific myopathic changes on electromyography. Exophthalmos may be present but may be masked by frontal bossing. Hypertrophied tissue surrounding the canal of Schlemm may impede aqueous filtration, leading to open-angle glaucoma. Progressive facial and bodily disfigurement often leads to lowered self-esteem. Depression, mood swings, and apathy may be secondary to physical deformity.[625]

Growth Hormone and Tumor Formation

The early practice of hypophysectomy for managing metastatic carcinoma was based on evidence implicating GH as a factor in tumor development. GH or IGF-I, or both, may have direct or indirect mitogenic effects on mammalian cells and act as permissive growth stimulators of cells previously exposed to other growth factors.[626] IGF-BP3, also induced by GH (see Chapter 23), inhibits cell proliferation and promotes apoptosis.[627, 628] Thus, the ultimate impact of elevated GH levels on cell proliferation reflects a balance of apoptotic versus growth-promoting signals.[558]

A compelling cause-effect relationship of acromegaly with cancer has not been established.[557, 629–631] Benign colon polyps have been reported in 45% of 678 patients in 12 prospective studies (Table 8–25). A controlled study of 161 patients revealed no increase in polyp incidence in acromegaly.[559] More than three skin tags in patients older than 50 years may be peripheral markers for the presence of adenomatous colon polyps, unrelated to GH or IGF-I serum levels.[632] Hypertrophic mucosal folds and colonic hypertrophy are commonly present; colonoscopy is warranted every 3 to 5 years after diagnosis, depending on the presence of other risk factors. Mortality from colon cancer is largely related to GH levels rather than the enhanced incidence of the disease in acromegaly (Table 8–26).

Analysis of nine retrospective reports (1956 to 1998) encompassing 21,470 person-years of risk yielded no significant increase in cancer incidence.[558] Cancer incidence was, in fact, lower than expected in 1362 patients with acromegaly in the United Kingdom, and the enhanced colon cancer mortality observed in this study correlated with GH levels.[557] Thus, although disordered cell proliferation and increased risk for promotion of coexisting neoplasms could be anticipated, there is little evidence for an increased cancer incidence in acromegaly (Table 8–27). Although elevated IGF-I levels may correlate with colon polyp prevalence when patients are retested,[629] a controlled prospective study showed no increased colon polyp incidence in acromegaly.[558, 559] Patients are now living longer with improved biochemical control, and long-term prospective controlled studies are required to resolve this question in an aging population.

Endocrine Complications

About 30% of patients exhibit elevated serum PRL levels (up to 100 μg/L or more) with or without galactorrhea.[633] Functional pituitary stalk compression by a pituitary mass prevents lactotroph access of hypothalamic dopamine, releasing the cell from tonic hypothalamic inhibition. GH-secreting adenoma subtypes may also concomitantly secrete PRL. Because GH behaves as an agonist for breast PRL binding sites, the

Table 8–25. Colon Polyps in Acromegaly*

n	M/F	Mean Age	Polyps: Adenoma	Polyps: Hyperplastic	Polyps: Total	Carcinoma	Reference
17	10/7	49	5	3	8	2	838
12	11/11	56	2	1	3	2	839
29	n.a.	n.a.	4	0	4	2	840
23	12/11	47	8	1	9	0	632
54	26/28	47	5	11	19	0	631
50	25/25	25–70	11	12	23	1	688
49	30/19	54	11	5	16	0	841
31	11/20	52	11	8	16	0	842
103	49/54	51	23	25	48	0	630
129	68/60	57	33	42	75	6	843
115	63/69	54.8‡	27	18	45	3	559
66†	NA	32.7	25	18	43	1	629
678			165 (24%)	144 (21%)	309 (45%)	17 (2.5%)	

*Incidence of colonic lesions in 678 patients prospectively evaluated in 12 studies. Of note, up to 45% of asymptomatic males age older than 50 years harbor colon adenomas. (Lieberman. Use of colonoscopy to screen asymptomatic adults for colon cancer. N Eng J Med 2000; 343:162–168.)

†Repeated colonoscopy.

‡Median age.

Derived from Melmed S. Acromegaly and cancer: not a problem. J Clin Endocrinol Metab 2001; 86:2924–2934.

tumor may cause galactorrhea in the presence of normal PRL levels. Tumor mass compressing surrounding normal pituitary tissue may also cause hypopituitarism. Over half of all patients have amenorrhea or impotence,[605, 634, 635] and secondary thyroid or adrenal failure is present in about 20% of patients. Gonadal dysfunction may result in reduced bone.[636]

The direct anti-insulin effects of GH cause carbohydrate intolerance, and insulin-requiring diabetes mellitus may also develop. Carbohydrate intolerance and insulin requirements improve rapidly with lowering of GH after surgery or somatostatin analogue therapy. Hypertriglyceridemia (type IV), hypercalciuria, and hypercalcemia also occur. Thyroid dysfunction in acromegaly may be caused by diffuse or nodular toxic or nontoxic goiter or Graves' disease, especially as IGF-I is a major determinant of thyroid cell growth.[637] Associated MEN-1 features may be present in affected individuals, including hypercalcemia with hyperparathyroidism or pancreatic tumors. Benign prostatic hypertrophy has been documented in acromegaly with no apparent increase in prostate cancer rates.[638, 639]

Morbidity and Mortality

Cardiovascular disease, respiratory disorders, diabetes, and malignancy account for the threefold enhanced mortality in acromegaly.[557, 575, 576, 621, 640–644] In a retrospective study reported in 1966, cardiovascular disease was the leading cause of death and 50% of patients died before the age of 50. Life expectancy was reduced in 194 patients with acromegaly, with cardiovascular disorders accounting for 24% of deaths followed by respiratory (18%) and cerebrovascular (14%) disease. Diabetes mellitus, occurring in 20% of patients, was associated with 2.5 times the predicted mortality, and hypertension was present in about 50% of all patients.[621] The most significant mortality determinants are GH levels and the presence of coexisting cardiac disease. Moreover, control of GH levels to less than 2.5 μg/L after surgery or medical treatments significantly reduces both morbidity and mortality (Fig. 8–50).

Diagnosis

Measurement of Growth Hormone Levels

The diagnosis of acromegaly requires measurement of a random GH higher than 0.4 μg/L or a GH nadir greater than 1 μg/L during an oral glucose tolerance test.[645] In healthy subjects, serum GH levels initially fall after oral glucose and subsequently increase as plasma glucose declines. However, in patients with acromegaly, oral glucose fails to suppress GH; GH levels may increase, remain unchanged, or fall modestly in approximately one third of patients. Basal morning (AM) and random GH levels are usually elevated in acromegaly. Because of the episodic nature of GH secretion, however, serum concentrations may normally fluctuate from undetectable up to 30 μg/L. In contrast to the largely undetectable nadir GH levels

Table 8–26. Post-treatment Growth Hormone Levels and Mortality in Acromegaly*

Mortality Ratio	Post-treatment Growth Hormone (ng/mL): <2.5 (n = 541)	2.5–9.9 (n = 493)	>10 (n = 207)	P
Overall	1.10 (0.89–1.15)	1.41 (1.16–1.69)	2.12 (1.70–2.62)	<.0001
Cancer-related	0.96 (0.63–1.41)	0.81 (0.50–1.24)	1.81 (1.13–2.74)	<.05

*Post-treatment GH levels correlate with mortality in acromegaly. Standardized mortality ratios are depicted for overall mortality and for cancer-related mortality.

Adapted from Orme S, McNally RJQ, Cartwright RA, Belchetz PE. Mortality and cancer incidence in acromegaly: a retrospective cohort study. J Clin Endocrinol Metab 1998; 83:2730–2734.

Table 8–27. Acromegaly and Cancer Incidence: Multicenter Analyses*

A.	n	Person-Years at Risk	Cancers Observed	Cancers O/E	p
Females	95	1351	8	1.33	NS
Males	128	1630	5	1.30	NS
Total	223	2981	13	1.3	
B.	4822	21,740	178	0.76–3.4	NA

*A. Multicenter analysis of cancer incidence in patients with acromegaly ranging in age from 1–79 years. Adapted from Mustacchi, Cancer 10:100, 1957. B. Analysis of retrospective published reports (1956–1998) of cancer incidence in patients with acromegaly. Included are data from 844, 575, 576, 609, 845–847 (Mustacchi 1957)[848, 557] O/E, observed/expected ratio. From Melmed S. J Clin Endocrinol Metab 2001; 86:2929–2934.

in normal subjects, detectable levels of GH (>2 μg/L) were found in those with acromegaly sampled over 24 hours.[646]

Evoked GH responses to GHRH administration are not of diagnostic utility. A higher episodic GH pulse frequency occurs, which often persists after surgical adenoma resection. Random GH levels measured with sensitive assays in acromegaly may be as low as 0.37 μg/L with persistently elevated postoperative IGF-I levels.[644] Serum IGF-I levels are high[647] and correlate with the logarithm of serum GH determinations. IGF-I elevations for age and gender may persist for several months after GH levels are biochemically controlled after treatment.[648] Elevated IGF-I levels are also encountered during pregnancy and late puberty. A high IGF-I level is thus highly specific for acromegaly and correlates with clinical indices of disease activity. IGF-BP3 levels are also elevated but provide little added diagnostic information. GH-secreting adenomas exhibit discordant GH responses to TRH and GnRH administration in up to 50% of patients, but these adjunctive tests are rarely required to confirm the diagnosis.

Differential Diagnosis of Acromegaly

The overwhelming majority of patients with acromegaly harbor a GH cell pituitary adenoma; rarely, extrapituitary acromegaly should be considered. Nevertheless, distinguishing between pituitary and extrapituitary acromegaly is important for planning effective management. Regardless of the cause of unrestrained GH secretion, IGF-I levels are invariably elevated and GH levels are not suppressed (<1 μg/L) after an oral glucose load.[649] When clinical features of acromegaly are associated with normal GH and IGF-I levels, "burned out" acromegaly associated with an infarcted pituitary adenoma, often with a secondary empty sella, should be considered. About 5% of consecutive patients with proven GH cell adenomas have normal GH and elevated IGF-I levels. It is likely that improved GH assay sensitivity will unmask abnormal GH secretion in these patients.

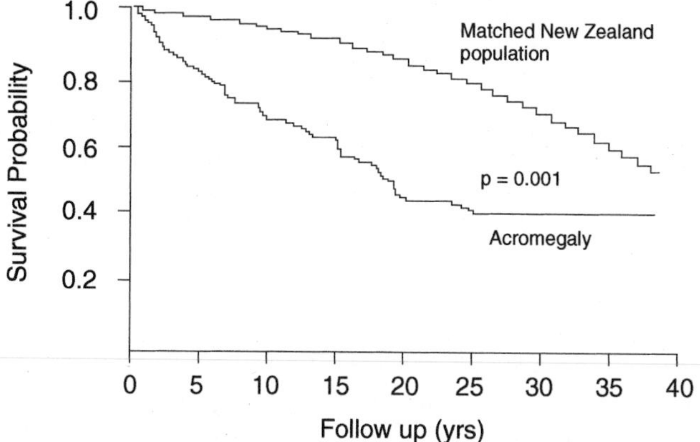

Figure 8–50. Mortality in acromegaly. Documented determinants of mortality outcome in retrospective studies of acromegaly include GH level, cardiovascular disease, diabetes, and duration of disease. (From Holdaway IM, et al. Natural history of treated functional pituitary adenomas. In Webb S [ed]. Pituitary Tumors. Bristol, UK, BioScientifica, 1998, pp 31–43.)

Dynamic pituitary testing (with TRH, dopamine) does not differentiate patients with pituitary adenomas from those harboring extrapituitary tumors.[650] Plasma GHRH levels are invariably elevated in patients with peripheral GHRH-secreting tumors but are normal or low in patients with pituitary adenomas.[651] GHRH plasma level measurement is precise and cost-effective for diagnosis of ectopic acromegaly. Peripheral GHRH levels are not elevated in patients with hypothalamic GHRH-secreting tumors, presumably because eutopic hypothalamic GHRH secreted into the hypophyseal portal system does not appreciably enter the systemic circulation.

Unique or unexpected clinical features, including respiratory wheezing or dyspnea, facial flushing, peptic ulcers, or renal stones, sometimes indicate the diagnosis of a nonpituitary endocrine tumor. Hypoglycemia, hyperinsulinemia, hypergastrinemia, and rarely hypercortisolism, all not usually encountered in pituitary acromegaly, should justify an evaluation for an extrapituitary source of GH excess. MRI and CT scanning are employed to localize a pituitary or extrapituitary tumor. Routine abdominal or chest imaging of all patients yields a low incidence of true positive cases of ectopic tumor, and such screening is not recommended as cost-effective.

A normal-sized or small pituitary gland or clinical and biochemical features of other tumors known to be associated with extrapituitary acromegaly and elevated circulating GHRH levels are indications for extrapituitary imaging. An enlarged pituitary is, however, often present in patients with peripheral GHRH-secreting tumors, and the radiologic diagnosis of a pituitary adenoma may be difficult to exclude. The McCune-Albright syndrome should be considered after definitive exclusion of pituitary and extrapituitary tumors.

Treatment

Aims

A comprehensive strategy for treating patients with acromegaly should aim to manage the pituitary mass, suppress GH and IGF-I hypersecretion, and prevent long-term clinical sequelae of hypersomatotropism while maintaining normal anterior pituitary function.[645, 652] As elevated GH levels per se are associated with threefold increased morbidity and account for the single most important determinant of mortality,[621, 640–643, 653] it is important to reverse the mortality rate to that of age-matched healthy subjects by aiming for tight GH control.[652]

Table 8–28. Transsphenoidal Surgery for Growth Hormone–Secreting Pituitary Adenomas

Series	Number of Cases	Total Cure Rate (%)	Microadenomas (%)	Macroadenomas (%)	Definition of "Cure"
Ross and Wilson, 1988	153	56	NA	NA	GH <5 μg/L(<10 mU/l)
Losa et al., 1989	29	55	NA	NA	GH <1 μg/L (<2 mU/l) and normal IGF-I levels
Fahlbusch et al., 1992	222	57	72	49	GH <2 μg/L (<4 mU/l) after OGTT
		71	81	65	GH <5 μg/L (<10 mU/l)
Tindall et al., 1993	91	82	NA	NA	GH <5 μg/L (<10 mU/l) and/or normal IGF-I levels
Davis et al., 1993	174	52	NA	NA	GH ≤2 μg/L (<4 mU/l; basal or OGTT)
Sheaves et al., 1996	100	42	61	23	GH ≤2.5 μg/L (<5 mU/l)
Abosch et al., 1998	254	76	75	71	GH <5 μg/L (<10 mU/l)
Freda et al., 1998	115	61	88	53	GH <2 μg/L (<4 mU/l) OGTT or normal IGF-I levels
Swearingen, 1998	162	57	91	48	Normal IGF-I levels
Lissett, 1998	73	18	39	12	GH <5 μg/L OGTT
Ahmed et al., 1999	97	—	90	56	Basal GH ≤2.5 μg/L(<5 mU/l), OGTT GH <1 μg/L (<2 mU/l), normal IGF-I levels
Laws et al., 2000	117	67	87	51	Basal GH <2.5 μg/L (<5 mU/l), OGTT GH <1 μg/L (<2 mU/l), normal IGF-I levels
Fahlbusch, 2001	490	56	78	50	Basal GH ≤5 μg/L (<10 mU/l), OGTT GH <2 μg/L (≤4 mU/l), normal IGF-I levels

Compiled from Fahlbusch. Surgical management of acromegaly. In Wass J (ed). Handbook of Acromegaly. Bristol, UK, BioScientifica, 2001, p 44; Lissett, 1998; Swearingen, 1998.

Serum GH levels should be suppressed to less than 1 μg/L after an oral glucose load and serum IGF-I levels normalized for age and gender. A patient whose condition is controlled should also have a normal 24-hour integrated secretion of GH (<2.5 μg/L). GH may not be measurable for most of the day, but the tumor may still be hypersecreting as reflected by elevated IGF-I levels. Current therapeutic modes for acromegaly management, including surgery, irradiation, and medical treatment, do not comprehensively fulfill these goals.

Surgical Management

Well-circumscribed somatotroph cell adenomas should preferably be resected by transsphenoidal surgery.[427, 654–660] Successful resection alleviates preoperative compression effects and compromised trophic hormone secretion, and the skilled surgeon balances the extent of maximal tumor tissue removal with preserving anterior pituitary function. Within 2 hours of successful resection, metabolic dysfunction and soft tissue swelling start to improve, and GH levels are often controlled within an hour. Surgical outcome correlates well with adenoma size and preoperative serum GH levels and particularly with the experience of the surgeon.

Smaller tumors (less than 5 mm), those totally confined within the sella, and preoperative serum GH levels lower than 40 μg/L portend a favorable surgical outcome. Up to 90% of patients with microadenomas achieved postoperative GH levels less than 2.5 μg/L, and less than 50% of those with all-sized macroadenomas had postoperative GH levels below 2 μg/L after glucose administration[658] (Table 8–16). Less than one third of all patients achieve control after resection of adenomas larger than 10 mm, and about 75% of patients with preoperative GH less than 5 μg/L have normalized IGF-I. Overall, in 17 studies of 1284 patients published between 1995 and 1999, 82% of patients harboring microadenomas had normalized IGF-I levels compared with less than 50% of those with macroadenomas (Table 8–28).

A review of 2665 patients from a single center showed that 72% of patients with microadenomas and 50% harboring macroadenomas had GH levels below 1.0 μg/L during glucose loading and normal serum IGF-I levels.[661] Eight percent of these patients had recurrences after 10 years. Endoscopic transnasal surgery offers promise as a less invasive procedure for resection of pituitary tumors[160] and access to cavernous sinus tumor mass, although long-term comparative results are not yet available. Difficulties in endotracheal intubation related to macroglossia or severe kyphosis, or both, may necessitate tracheostomy for anesthesia.

Side Effects. Although often transient, surgical complications may require lifelong pituitary hormone replacement. New hypopituitarism develops in up to 20% of patients, reflecting operative damage to the surrounding normal pituitary tissue.[662] Permanent diabetes insipidus, CSF leaks, hemorrhage, and meningitis occur in up to 10% of patients (Table 8–10). The extent and prevalence of local complications depend on tumor size and invasiveness. Experienced pituitary surgeons report more favorable postoperative complication rates. Biochemical or anatomic recurrence (~7% over 10 years) or postoperative tumor persistence may indicate incomplete resection of adenomatous tissue, surgically inaccessible cavernous sinus tissue, or nesting of functional tumor tissue within the dura.

Radiation

Primary or adjuvant radiation of GH-secreting tumors may be achieved by conventional external deep x-ray therapy as well as heavy-particle (proton beam) therapy.[168, 171, 663–665] Maximal tumor radiation should ideally be attained with minimal soft tissue damage. Precise MRI localization, accurate simulation and isocentral rotational techniques, and high-voltage (6 to 15 MEv) delivery have improved radiation efficacy. Radiation is a highly individual choice, depending on the expertise and experience of the treating radiotherapist as well as the

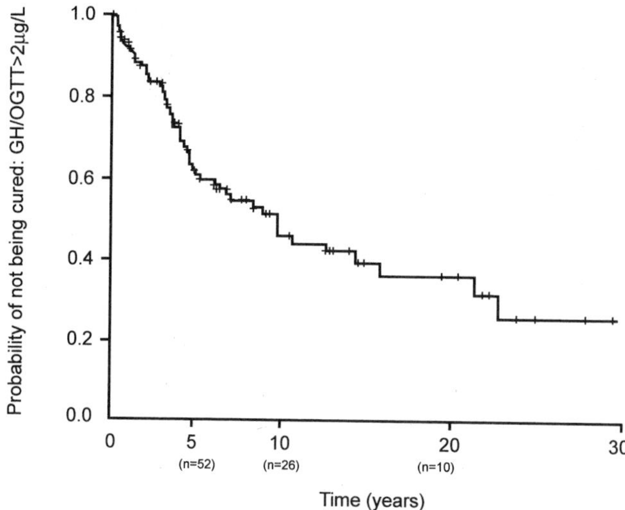

Figure 8–51. Radiation treatment of acromegaly. Long-term effects of radiation therapy on growth hormone (GH) secretion using a GH nadir after an oral glucose load below 2 μg/L as the cure criterion and the probability of not being cured with time after radiotherapy. The numbers of patients not cured at 5, 10, and 20 years after pituitary irradiation are indicated in *parentheses*. Each step represents one cure; each cross *(+)* denotes a patient not cured at the latest follow-up. (From Barrande G, Pittino-Lungo M, Coste J, et al. Hormonal and metabolic effects of radiotherapy in acromegaly: long term results in 128 patients followed in a single center. J Clin Endocrinol Metab 2000; 85:3779–3785.)

physician's and patient's choice of the benefits of therapy weighed against potential risks.

For radiation treatment, up to 5000 rads are administered in split doses of 180-cGy fractions divided over 6 weeks. Radiation arrests tumor growth, and most pituitary adenomas ultimately shrink.[171] GH levels fall gradually during the first year after treatment, and levels are less than 10 μg/L in 70% of patients after 10 years. The National Institutes of Health experience is that over 90% of patients have GH levels less than 5 μg/L after 20 years (Fig. 8–51).[663] When pretreatment GH levels were greater than 100 μg/L, only 60% of patients had GH less than 5 μg/L after 18 years. During the first 7 years after irradiation less than 5% of patients had normal IGF-I levels[664] but about 70% of patients exhibited normal IGF-I levels when tested during longer follow-up.[665]

Radiotherapy does not normalize GH secretory patterns, probably accounting for persistently elevated IGF-I levels in the presence of apparently controlled GH levels.[666] Thus, during the initial years after irradiation, most patients are still exposed to unacceptably high levels of circulating GH and IGF-I. Promising stereotactic pituitary tumor ablation by the gamma knife has been reported. Long-term outcomes and potential long-term side effects are not yet available.[667]

Side Effects

After 10 years about half of all patients receiving radiotherapy have signs of pituitary trophic hormone disruption, and the prevalence increases annually thereafter,[668] requiring gonadal steroids, thyroid hormone, or cortisone replacement. Side effects of conventional radiation, including hair loss, cranial nerve palsies, tumor necrosis with hemorrhage, and rarely loss of vision or pituitary apoplexy, have been documented in up to 2% of patients.[176, 668, 669] Lethargy, impaired memory, and personality changes may also occur.[670, 671] The incidence and extent of local complications have been markedly diminished by use of highly reproducible simulators, precise rotational isocentric arc capability, and doses less than 5000 cGy. Proton beam therapy (Bragg peak) is contraindicated in patients with suprasellar tumor extension because of unacceptable optic tract exposure to the radiation field. The rare development of second brain tumors in these patients has been reported at a cumulative risk frequency of 1.9% over 20 years.[174, 175]

Radiation therapy effectively shrinks over 95% of GH cell adenomas and lowers GH levels over 20 years in more than 90% of patients. In fact, GHD may result from radiation.[672] Because of the side effects, radiation therapy should be employed as an adjuvant for patients not controlled by surgery or medical management or for those who refuse these therapies.

Dopamine Agonists

Because dopamine attenuates GH secretion in about one third of patients with acromegaly, D2 receptor agonists, including bromocriptine and cabergoline, have been used as either primary or adjuvant therapy for acromegaly.[332, 338] Bromocriptine may lower GH at a dose of 20 mg/day or more, which is higher than required to suppress PRL in patients harboring prolactinomas. Approximately 15% of patients worldwide have been reported to have suppressed GH levels below 5 μg/L when taking the medication (7.5 to 80 mg/day),[673] and IGF-I became normal in 10% of patients. The drug causes minimal tumor shrinkage, but most patients experience subjective clinical improvement and report reduced perspiration, decreased soft tissue swelling, and improved fatigue and headache despite persistently elevated serum GH or IGF-I levels, or both. Side effects of bromocriptine are more marked, especially as high doses are required. These include gastrointestinal upset, transient nausea and vomiting, headache, transient postural hypotension with dizziness, nasal stuffiness, and rarely cold-induced peripheral vasospasm (see earlier).

Cabergoline, a long-acting dopamine agonist, is highly effective in suppressing PRL hypersecretion and shrinking prolactinomas. The drug has been reported to suppress GH to less than 2 μg/L and to normalize IGF-I in up to a third of patients with acromegaly.[674] Side effects include gastrointestinal symptoms, dizziness, headache, and mood disorders. Patients with hyperprolactinemia and minimal GH elevation may benefit most from dopamine agonist treatment.

Somatotropin Release-Inhibiting Factor Receptor Ligands

Of the five SRIF receptor subtypes, SSTR2 and SSTR5 are preferentially expressed on somatotroph and thyrotroph cell surfaces and mediate suppression of GH and TSH secretion.[585] Several SRIF ligands have been employed as approved or investigational drugs for acromegaly (Fig. 8–52). For over 15 years, these analogues have proved safe and effective for controlling acromegaly.

Octreotide (D-Phe-Cys-Phe-D-Trp-Lys-Thr-Cys-Thr-OH), an octapeptide SRIF analogue, binds predominantly to SSTR2 and SSTR5 and inhibits GH secretion with a potency 45 times greater than that of native SRIF, whereas its potency for inhibiting insulin release is only 1.3-fold that of SRIF.[675] The in vivo half-life of the analogue is prolonged (up to 2 hours) because of its relative resistance to enzymatic degradation. The rebound GH hypersecretion seen after SRIF infusion does not occur after octreotide injection. These properties are highly advantageous for long-term use in acromegaly.[676] A single subcutaneous dose (50 or 100 μg) suppresses GH secretion for up to 5 hours. In patients harboring microadenomas, integrated GH and IGF-I levels almost invariably became normal,[677] but the response in larger tumors was less pronounced. In a double-blind, placebo-controlled trial, octreotide (8-hourly injec-

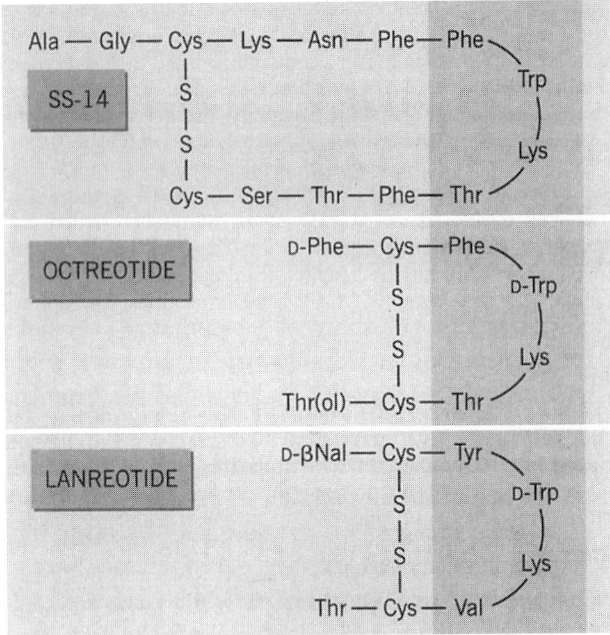

Figure 8–52. Amino acid sequences of somatotropin release-inhibiting factor (SRIF) receptor ligands. Amino acid sequences of the three available somatostatin analogues compared with endogenous somatostatin-14. (From van der Lely AJ, Lamberts S. Medical therapy for acromegaly. In Wass J [ed]. Handbook of Acromegaly. BioScientifica, 2001, pp 51–64.)

tions) significantly attenuated GH and IGF-I levels overall in over 90% of patients.[677]

A combination of octreotide and bromocriptine or cabergoline may provide added efficacy. In vivo OctreoScan imaging visualizing SRIF receptors demonstrated that GH responsiveness directly correlates with the abundance of pituitary receptors and patients resistant to octreotide do not have visible in vivo receptor binding sites.[678] Efficacy of octreotide action is determined by the frequency of drug administration, total daily dose, tumor size, and pretreatment GH levels. Smaller tumors secreting less GH may, in fact, harbor more abundant SRIF receptors. Increasing the frequency of administration more effectively suppresses GH levels,[679] and continuous subcutaneous infusion (up to 600 μg/day) provides sustained GH control.[679] Total daily octreotide doses of 300 to 1500 μg are optimal, and further dose increases are usually not beneficial for resistant patients. Elderly male patients are particularly sensitive to the GH-lowering effects of octreotide, and in the long term desensitization does not occur.[680]

Long-acting somatostatin analogue formulations are convenient, enhance compliance and allow sustained biochemical control (Fig. 8–53). Serum levels of octreotide (Sandostatin LAR; 20 to 30 mg intramuscularly), a sustained-release octreotide depot preparation,[681] peaked at 28 days and integrated GH levels were effectively suppressed for up to 49 days. Monthly injections for 18 months in patients known to be octreotide-responsive reduced integrated serum GH levels to less than 2 μg/L in 9 of 14 patients.[682] In an open-label study of 151 patients responsive to octreotide, the analogue suppressed serum GH levels to less than 2.5 μg/L in about 70% of all patients.[683, 684] Overall, IGF-I levels became normal in 60% to 70% of patients.[685] Lanreotide is a slow-release, long-acting depot preparation administered as fixed 30-mg injectable dose every 7, 10, or 14 days. GH levels less than 2.5 μg/L were achieved in 60% of 56 patients treated for 48 weeks and in about one third of 22 patients treated for up to 3 years, and IGF-I levels were normalized in almost two thirds of patients.[686] Lanreotide is not yet approved for use in the United States.

Effects of SRIF Receptor Ligands on Pituitary Adenoma

Invariably, tumor growth does not occur while patients receive depot preparations of SRIF analogues, and adenomas shrink by 20% to 80% in about one third of patients receiving these analogues.[687] Interestingly, tumor shrinkage was observed after up to 2 years in 12 of 15 patients receiving octreotide LAR as primary treatment, whereas no shrinkage was observed in 4 of 9 patients after surgery.[685] Fifty-nine patients undergoing pituitary surgery were randomly assigned to treatment with or without octreotide, and 22 who received preoperative octreotide for 3 to 6 months demonstrated improved postoperative biochemical control and reduced hospital length of stay.[688, 689]

Effects on Clinical Features

Over 70% of patients experience improved general well-being, and soft tissue swelling dissipates within several days of treatment.[677] Headache, a common symptom in acromegaly, usually resolves within minutes of injection,[690] reflecting a specific central analgesic effect. Asymptomatic patients experience a significant decrease of blood pressure, heart rate, and left ventricular wall thickness.[691] In patients with cardiac failure, octreotide reversibly reduces systemic arterial resistance, oxygen consumption, and fluid volume and restores functional activity. In 30 patients, an improved left ventricular ejection fraction with unchanged diastolic filling was associated with octreotide-induced GH suppression to less than 2.5 μg/L. Persistently elevated GH levels after a year were associated with increased systolic blood pressure.[692] Control of IGF-I and GH levels is associated with improved left ventricular ejection function; in patients in whom the levels were not controlled, cardiac performance worsened.[693] Joint function and crepitus improve, ultrasonography shows evidence of bone or cartilage repair, and after several months sleep apnea improves.[611]

Side Effects

SRIF receptor ligands are generally safe and well tolerated. Gastrointestinal side effects predominate and include transient loose stools, nausea, mild malabsorption, and flatulence, reported in about one third of patients. Hypoglycemia and hyperglycemia are not commonly encountered, and insulin requirements in diabetic patients with acromegaly are dramatically reduced within hours of receiving octreotide, concomitant with GH lowering. The drug attenuates gallbladder contractility, delays emptying, and leads to reversible sludge formation evidenced by ultrasonography in up to 25% of patients.[694] Frank cholecystitis is rarely reported in these patients. The incidence of gallbladder sludge or stones is geographically variable, with higher rates reported in China, Australia, and the United Kingdom. In the United States, up to 30% of patients have demonstrable evidence of echogenic gallbladder deposits within the first 18 months of treatment. Thereafter, further sludge formation is not usually encountered.[681] Octreotide may interact with several drugs including cyclosporine, enhancing transplant rejection risk. SRIF receptor ligand dose adjustments should be carefully titrated in patients requiring insulin or oral hypoglycemic agents, calcium channel blockers, and β-blockers. Asymptomatic sinus bradycardia has also been recognized.

Growth Hormone Receptor Antagonist

GH action through the surface membrane GH receptor is mediated by ligand-induced GH receptor dimerization and

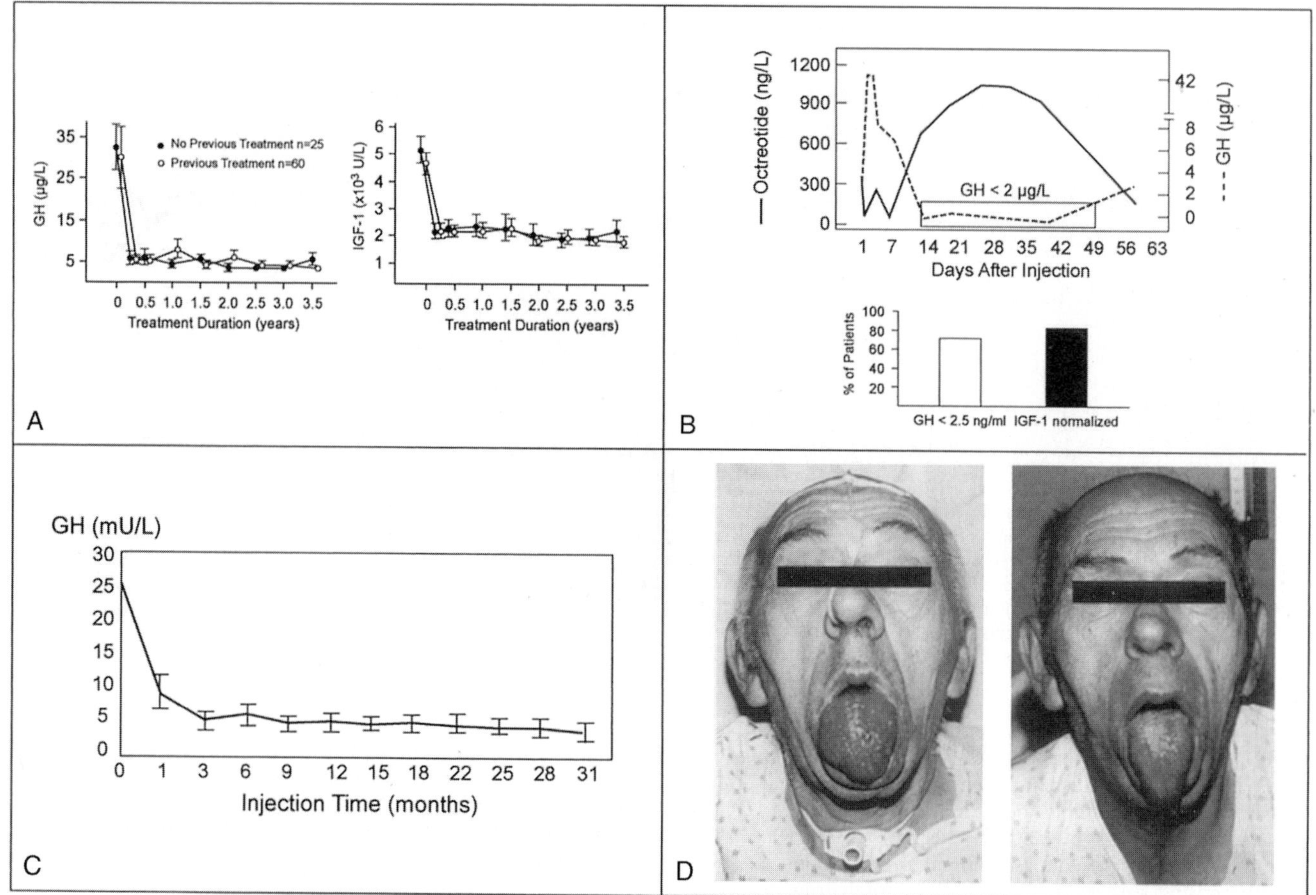

Figure 8–53. Medical management of acromegaly. *A*, Growth hormone (GH) and insulin-like growth factor I (IGF-I) concentrations with long-term octreotide treatment. Comparison of primary octreotide treatment in 25 previously untreated patients and in 80 patients who had previously undergone surgical resection or irradiation, or both. (From Newman C, Melmed S, George A, et al. Octreotide as primary therapy for acromegaly. J Clin Endocrinol Metab 1998; 83:3034–3040.) *B*, Pharmacodynamics of octreotide LAR twelve-hour mean serum octreotide and GH concentrations in a representative patient treated with a single 30-mg injection of Sandostatin LAR and observed for 60 days. After injection, drug levels peak at 28 days, and nadir GH levels are sustained for 4 weeks. (Adapted from Lancranjan I, Bruns C, Grass P, et al. Sandostatin LAR: a promising therapeutic tool in the management of acromegalic patients. Metabolism 1996; 45:67–71.)

C, Mean growth hormone (GH) concentration with octreotide (long-acting release) long-term treatment. Serum GH levels in acromegaly following monthly LAR octreotide injections in 12 patients for 1 year, and 8 patients for 31 months. (From Davies PH, Stewart SE, Lancranjan I, et al. Long-term therapy with long-acting octreotide [Sandostatin-LAR] for the management of acromegaly. Clin Endocrinol (Oxf) 1998; 48:311–316.)

D, Clinical impact of octreotide in reducing soft tissue swelling. Acromegaly in a patient suffering from obstructive sleep apnea before octreotide. Note the macroglossia, tracheotomy for airway obstruction, and intranasal feeding tube. After 6 months of treatment with octreotide, tongue size was reduced by half. Tracheotomy and nasal tube have been removed and sleep apnea has resolved. (Courtesy of S. Reichlin.)

subsequent receptor signaling.[695] The postreceptor GH signal is not elicited if the receptor fails to dimerize (Fig. 8–54). Pegvisomant, a GH receptor antagonist, blocks receptor dimerization and subsequent IGF-I generation.[695] The pegylated molecule also binds to the GH receptor dimer and interacts with GHBP.[696] Daily injections (20 mg) of this pegylated GH mutant molecule normalized IGF-I levels in over 90% of patients and dose dependently improved fatigue, decreased soft tissue swelling as assessed by ring size, and diminished perspiration.[695] The drug, not yet approved in the United States, may be particularly useful in patients resistant to somatostatin receptor ligand therapy as it effectively normalizes IGF-I levels in these patients.[697] Long-term side effects are not yet known, but the action of the medication increases levels of GH, which are bioinactive because of receptor blockade. Long-term surveillance should also include monitoring of liver function and pituitary adenoma size.[698]

Choice of Therapy

Tight control of GH secretion should be achieved because adverse mortality rates correlate strongly with GH levels. Each treatment modality has respective advantages and disadvantages that should be weighed in order to individualize patients' care (Table 8–29). Selective surgical excision of a well-defined pituitary microadenoma is recommended for most patients. Remission rates are unacceptably low for patients with macroadenomas and locally invasive tumors. Attempted medical debulking of the sellar mass prior to surgery would be desirable, although controlled prospective studies are required to confirm the validity of this approach to improve surgical morbidity and possibly enhance subsequent postoperative outcomes, especially for patients with surgically inaccessible tumor tissue and cavernous sinus invasion (Fig. 8–55).

Postoperatively, patients who do not achieve control can be

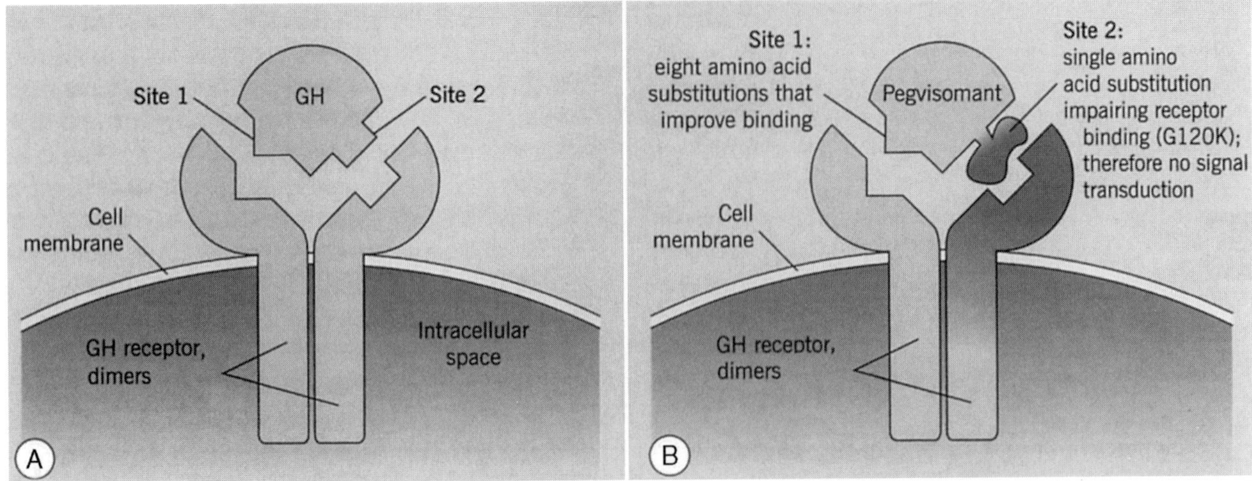

Figure 8–54. Action of growth hormone (GH) receptor antagonist. *A*, Normally, a single molecule of GH binds two GH receptors through sites 1 and 2, and the GH signal transduction pathway is activated. *B*, Pegvisomant increases binding of GH receptor to site 1 and blocks binding at site 2 to prevent functional GH-receptor dimerization, initiation of GH action, and induction of insulin-like growth factor I (IGF-I) synthesis and secretion. The peripheral effects of excess GH are antagonized at the cellular level, independent of the presence of somatostatin or dopamine receptors on the pituitary tumor. (Adapted from van der Lely AJ, Lamberts S. Medical therapy for acromegaly. In Wass J [ed]. Handbook of Acromegaly. Bristol, UK, BioScientifica, 2001, pp 51–54.)

treated with bromocriptine; although the efficacy of this drug is low, it is relatively inexpensive and free of major side effects. An SRIF analogue should be administered, GH and IGF-I measured after 2 hours, and Sandostatin LAR (10, 20, or 30 mg) initiated if patients are shown to be responsive. More frequent dosing rather than increases in total drug dose may be more efficacious and beneficial, and some may benefit by addition of bromocriptine or cabergoline with octreotide. Gallbladder ultrasonography should be performed only in symptomatic patients, and those with demonstrable sludge or gallstones may require prophylactic anticholelithogenic agents or laparoscopic cholecystectomy if symptoms develop.

Primary therapy with SRIF receptor ligands may be offered to patients who refuse surgery or in whom the risks of surgery or anesthesia are unacceptable. Invasive macroadenomas invariably hypersecrete GH postoperatively and require somatostatin

Table 8–29. Treatment Options for Acromegaly

Surgery	Somatostatin Analogue	Radiotherapy	Dopamine Agonists (High Dose)	Growth Hormone-Receptor Antagonist
Efficacy				
80% of microadenomas: GH controlled	GH controlled in ~65% of patients	GH <5 μg/L in 90% of patients in 18 yr	GH <5μg/L in 15%	Elevated bioinactive GH
<50% of macroadenomas: GH controlled	Normal IGF-I in ~70%	Normal IGF-I in <7 yr 24%, >10 yr 54%	Normal IGF-I in ~10%	Normal IGF-I in >90%
IGF-I normalized in ~50%				
Advantages				
Rapid onset	No hypopituitarism	Permanent	Oral administration	Rapid onset
One-time cost	Rapid onset	One-time cost	Low cost	No hypopituitarism
Maybe permanent control	Sustained long-term efficacy	Good compliance by patients	No hypopituitarism	Sustained efficacy
Disadvantages				
New hypopituitarism (10%)	Cost of drug and monitoring	Ineffective and slow onset	Relatively ineffective	Long-term safety unknown
Diabetes insipidus (2–3%)	Asymptomatic gallstones (25%)	Hypopituitarism (70%)	Adverse events (~30%)	
Local complications (~6%)	Injections required	Visual and CNS dysfunction (~2%)	High dose required	Not yet approved (2002)
Cranial nerve or CNS damage (~1%)		Cost of interim medical therapy		
Tumor persistence				

CNS, central nervous system; GH, growth hormone; IGF-I, insulin-like growth factor I.
Adapted from Melmed S, Jackson I, Kleinberg D, Klibanski A. Current treatment guidelines for acromegaly. J Clin Endocrinol Metab 1998; 83:2646–2652.

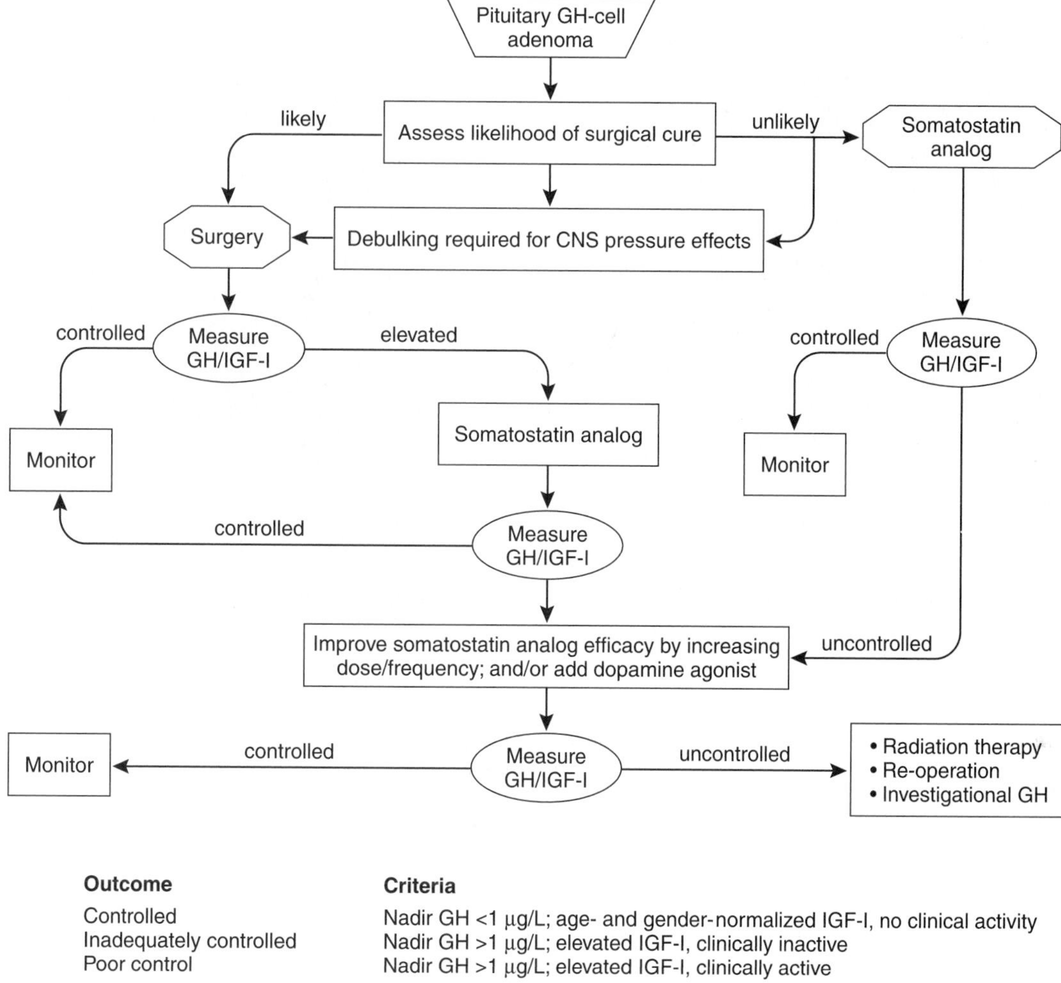

Figure 8–55. Treatment of acromegaly. CNS, central nervous system; GH, growth hormone; IGF-I, insulin-like growth factor I. (Adapted from Giustina A, Barkan A, Casanueva FF, et al. Criteria for cure of acromegaly: a consensus statement. J Clin Endocrinol Metab 2000; 85:526–529; from Ben-Shlomo A, Melmed S. Acromegaly. Endocrinology and Metabolism Clinics 2001; 30:565–583; and from Melmed S. Acromegaly. In Melmed S (ed). The Pituitary. Blackwell Scientific, 2002, pp 419–454.)

analogue treatment. In patients whose pituitary lesion does not compress vital structures, primary medical management may therefore be an appropriate therapeutic option.[699] Radiation should be administered to patients who are resistant to or cannot tolerate the medication, prefer not to receive long-term injections, or cannot afford the medication. After radiation, medications are required for several years until GH levels are effectively controlled.

Tumors that recur despite medical therapy or radiation may rarely require reoperation. Although tight GH control is critical, these patients also require counseling for anxiety engendered by disfigurements and interpretation of laboratory test results. Patients should be observed quarterly until biochemical control is achieved. Thereafter, hormone evaluation is performed semiannually, and for patients who are biochemically in remission and in whom no residual tumor tissue is present, MRI should be repeated every 1 to 2 years.[353] Follow-up evaluation includes documenting and treating new skin tag and lipoma growth; nerve entrapments; jaw overbites; rheumatologic, dental, and cardiac evaluations; and metabolic assessment. Visual field perimetry and pituitary reserve testing should be repeated semiannually and pituitary MRI annually, especially in patients with residual tumor or those requiring hormone replacement or medical treatment. Mammography and colonoscopy should be performed as clinically indicated for patients older than 50 or those harboring polyps. Maximal and sustained long-term GH and IGF-I control should ameliorate the deleterious effects of these hormones by judicious use of available treatment modalities.

Adrenocorticotropic Hormone

Corticotroph Cells

Corticotroph cells constitute about 20% of functional anterior pituitary cells and are the earliest detectable human fetal pituitary cell type, appearing by the eighth week of gestation. Corticotrophs are clustered mainly in the central median pituitary wedge and are readily identified by immunostaining with ACTH or β-lipotropin antibodies. They are large, irregular cells with ultrastructural features including prominent neurosecretory granules (150 to 400 nm), endoplasmic reticulum, and Golgi bodies (Figs. 8–56 and 8–57).[700] These cells produce the *POMC* gene products including ACTH 1 to 39, β-lipotropin, and endorphins. Because of the rich carbohydrate moiety of these molecules, the cells are strongly positive for periodic

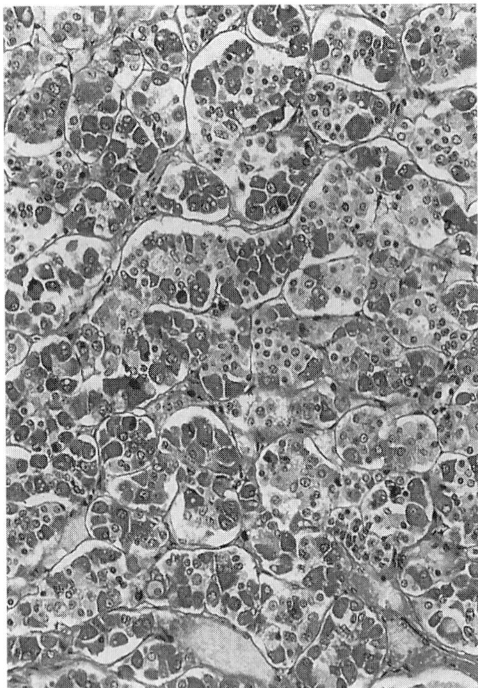

Figure 8-56. Corticotroph cell. The periodic acid–Schiff stain documents the presence of corticotrophs in the normal pituitary, reflecting glycosylation of the adrenocorticotropic hormone peptide. Some cells have clear cytoplasmic vacuoles corresponding to the "enigmatic body." (From Asa SL. In Tumors of the Pituitary Gland. Atlas of Tumor Pathology. Washington, DC, Armed Forces Institute of Pathology, 1997, p 21.)

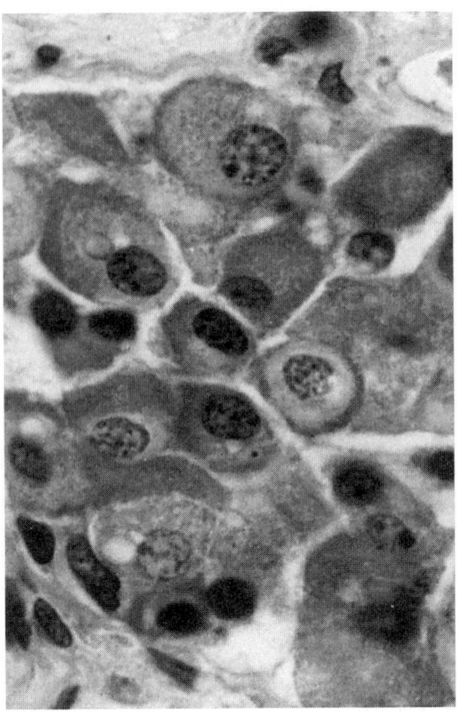

Figure 8-58. Crooke's hyalinization. Pituitary corticotrophs exposed to glucocorticoid excess develop cytoplasmic hyalinization that displaces adrenocorticotropic hormone (ACTH)–positive secretory material to the cell periphery. Clear vacuoles correspond to complex lysosomes (enigmatic bodies). (From Asa SL. In Tumors of the Pituitary Gland. Atlas of Tumor Pathology. Washington, DC, Armed Forces Institute of Pathology, 1997, p 23.)

acid–Schiff stain. In the presence of excess glucocorticoid, characteristic hyaline deposits are evident (Fig. 8–58).

Adrenocorticotropic Hormone Biosynthesis

The 8-kb human *POMC* gene, located on chromosome 2p23,[701] consists of three exons with two intervening introns (Fig. 8–59). The first exon encodes a leader sequence, the second encodes the signal initiation sequence and the N-terminal portion of the POMC peptide, and the third exon encodes most of the mature peptide sequences including ACTH and β-lipotropin.[702] A pituitary-selective promoter region for *POMC* generates an approximately 1200-nucleotide *POMC* mRNA transcript; an upstream promoter generates a longer, about 1350-nucleotide transcript. A downstream promoter generates a shorter, 800-nucleotide transcript arising from the 5′ end of exon 3, predominantly in extrapituitary tissues including the gonads, placenta, gastrointestinal tissues, liver, kidney, adrenal medulla, lung, and lymphocytes. Elements of the promoter regions mediate POMC regulation by glucocorticoids, cAMP, activator protein 1 (AP-1), and STAT signaling molecules.[493] A corticotroph-specific factor, Tpit, has been described.[24]

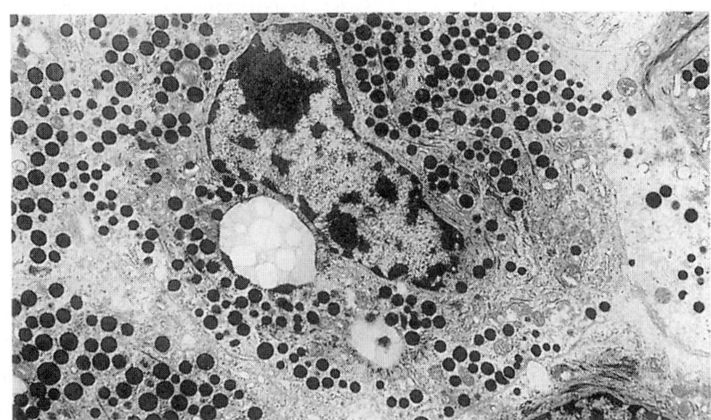

Figure 8-57. Electron micrograph of normal corticotroph that contains dispersed profiles of rough endoplasmic reticulum; numerous secretory granules of variable size, shape, and electron density; and conspicuous juxtanuclear complex lysosomes. Small bundles of intermediate filaments representing keratin are perinuclear. (From Asa SL. In Tumors of the Pituitary Gland. Atlas of Tumor Pathology. Washington, DC, Armed Forces Institute of Pathology, 1997, p 22.)

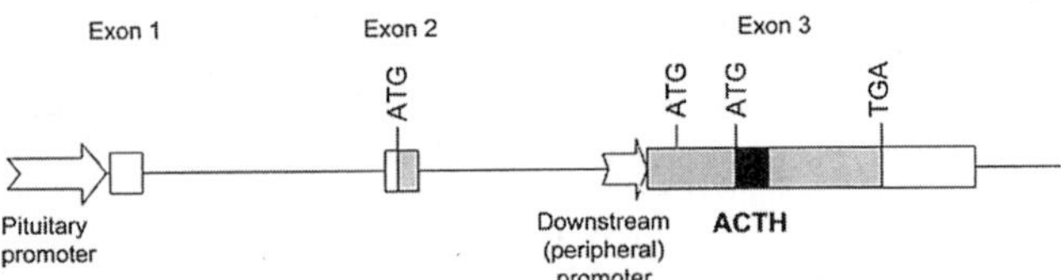

Figure 8-59. Structure of pro-opiomelanocortin (POMC) gene. Exon 1 encodes the RNA leader sequence, exon 2 encodes the initiator methionine (ATG), the signal peptide and several N-terminal residues of the precursor peptide, the remainder of which is encoded by exon 3. Corticotroph expression is determined by the upstream "pituitary" promoter *(longer white arrowhead)*, whereas peripheral expression of the short POMC mRNA is determined by the "downstream" promoter *(shorter white arrowhead)*. Translation of these shorter transcripts initiates from the initiator methionines (ATG) indicated in exon 3. The precursor peptide coding region is shaded light gray and the ACTH coding region is black. (From Clark AJL, Swords FM. Molecular pathology of corticotroph function. In Rappaport R, Amselem S [eds]. Hypothalamic-Pituitary Development: Genetic and Clinical Aspects. Basel, Karger, 2001, pp 140–161.)

POMC is the precursor of ACTH, which acts on the adrenal glands to induce synthesis and secretion of adrenal steroids. The primary translation product of POMC is a 266-amino-acid POMC pre-prohormone molecule encoding corticotrophic, opioid, and melanotropic peptides. The peptide contains a leader sequence and multiple dibasic proteolytic cleavage sites for glycosylation, acetylation, and amidation. Products of this processing include ACTH 1 to 39 and β-lipotropin, which in turn give rise to α-lipotropin and β-endorphin, also containing met-enkephalin. ACTH itself may also be cleaved to α-melanocyte-stimulating hormone (1 to 13) and corticotropin-like intermediate lobe peptide (CLIP; 18 to 39). The neurointermediate pituitary lobe is not developed in humans and is not normally a source of circulating POMC-derived peptides.

Multiple signals act in synergy to activate *POMC* gene expression. These include CRH, cytokines, arginine vasopressin, catecholamines, and VIP. Glucocorticoids inhibit *POMC* gene expression. The CRH type 1 receptor is predominantly expressed on the corticotroph,[703, 704] and receptor activation increases cAMP, protein kinase A, and CREB induction of CRHBP binding to the promoter leading to *POMC* transcription.[705] CRH also activates an AP-1 site within the first exon by a mitogen-activated protein kinase–mediated pathway. In addition to mediating ACTH secretion, this receptor appears critical for fear and anxiety responses, possibly through a related ligand, urocortin.[706] The type 2 CRH receptor is predominantly important for cardiovascular function.[707]

Leukemia inhibitory factor (LIF), a proinflammatory cytokine also expressed in the pituitary and hypothalamus, signals through the JAK/STAT pathway, acts in synergy with CRH, and induces direct STAT3 binding to POMC.[708] Glucocorticoid receptor activation leads to transcriptional suppression through two cooperative binding sites. The intracellular glucocorticoid receptor binds directly to 5′-regulatory elements to suppress *POMC* transcription.[709] CRH action is also potentiated by vasopressin (acting through phospholipase C) and β-adrenergic catecholamines by enhancing *POMC* mRNA levels, increasing ACTH secretion, or both. The net effects of these intracellular signals are to regulate *POMC* gene transcription, peptide synthesis, and ACTH secretion for mediating appropriate neuroendocrine responses.[710]

Pro-opiomelanocortin Processing

Several post-translational POMC modification steps are required for ultimate polypeptide hormone secretion (Fig. 8–60).

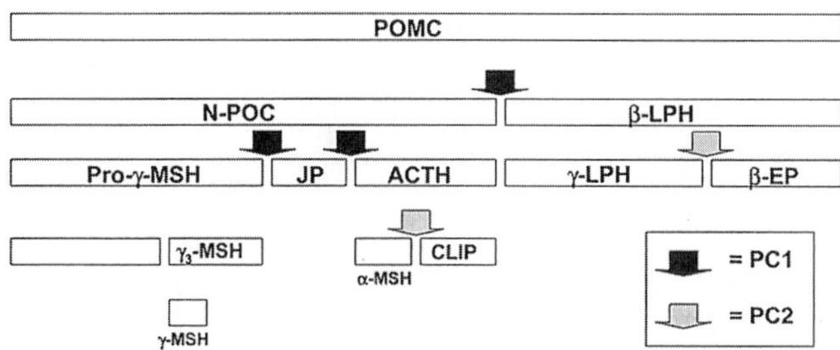

Figure 8–60. Processing and cleavage of pro-opiomelanocortin (POMC). The mature POMC precursor peptide is sequentially cleaved by PC-1 in the anterior pituitary corticotroph. In the neurointermediate lobe and other cell types, cleavage by PC2 allows release of β-MSH and/or β-endorphin. Carboxypeptidase H (not shown) removes residual basic amino acids at cleavage sites. β-LPH, β-lipotropin; JP, joining peptide; γ-LPH, γ-lipotropin, CLIP, corticotropin-like intermediate lobe peptide. (From Clark AJL, Swords FM. Molecular pathology of corticotroph function. In Rappaport R, Amselem S [eds]. Hypothalamic-Pituitary Development: Genetic and Clinical Aspects. Basel, Karger, 2001, pp 140–161.)

First, the N-terminal signal sequence is removed followed by glycosylation through an O linkage to Thr45 and N linkage to Asn65.[711] Serine phosphorylation then occurs within the Golgi apparatus. After being transported to secretory vesicles, the constituent peptides are cleaved at dibasic amino acid residues and ACTH-related peptides stored in dense secretory granules for ultimate regulated release. Some POMC products also undergo C-terminal amidation mediated by peptidylglycine-amidating monooxygenase and peptidylhydroxyglycine-amidating lyase[712] and N-terminal acetylation. POMC proteolytic processing occurs at Lys-Arg or Arg-Arg residues. Prohormone convertase 1 (PC1) or prohormone convertase 2 (PC2), related to the subtilisin-kexin proteinases, exert tissue-specific cleavage activities at dibasic sites. PC1 is most abundant in the pituitary and hypothalamus, and PC2 is present in the central nervous system and pancreatic islets but absent in the pituitary. Heterozygous mutations of the PC1 gene have been associated with childhood obesity, adrenal insufficiency, hyperproinsulinemia, and postprandial hypoglycemia[713] with elevated levels of plasma ACTH precursors.

Extrapituitary Tumor Adrenocorticotropic Hormone Synthesis

Tissue POMC is also expressed in the gonads, lung, gastrointestinal and adrenal medullary neuroendocrine cells, and white blood cells. Nevertheless, most circulating ACTH is derived from the anterior pituitary or from neuroendocrine tumor ectopic production. Extrapituitary neuroendocrine tumors associated with ectopic ACTH secretion do not process the prohormone efficiently. As ACTH is synthesized in nontumorous neuroendocrine cells, "ectopic" tumor hormone production may in fact reflect inappropriate ACTH processing. These patients also exhibit a higher ratio of circulating ACTH precursors as well as smaller peptides, including CLIP.

Adrenocorticotropic Hormone Secretion

The complex control of ACTH secretion patterns is critical for maintenance of adrenal cortex function and reflects the neuroendocrine control of stress homeostasis. Essential metabolic and endocrine functions require a sensitively controlled nonstress pattern of hypothalamic-pituitary-adrenal (HPA) axis function. This baseline pattern allows the axis to mount an appropriate stress response, with a well-buffered reserve capacity to counteract life-threatening insults.

The 4.5-kd ACTH polypeptide consists of 39 amino acids. The highly conserved 12 N-terminal amino acid residues are critical for adrenal gland steroid synthesis. Several variables characterize the central and peripheral control of ACTH secretion. The ACTH circadian rhythm is generated in the suprachiasmatic nucleus, which signals CRH release. The hormone is secreted with both circadian periodicity and ultradian pulsatility, and this centrally controlled pattern is influenced by peripheral corticosteroids. ACTH pulse amplitudes may vary by 40% over 24 hours. The circadian pattern of ACTH secretion typically begins at about 4 AM and peaks before 7 AM, with both ACTH and adrenal steroid levels reaching their nadir between 11 PM and 3 AM. Within this overall diurnal cycle, periodic ACTH secretory bursts occur at a frequency of 40 pulses per 24 hours, with changing pulse amplitudes throughout the day.[714] Each pulse contains an average ACTH level of 24 ng/L.

Pulse amplitude changes, rather than frequency, appear to determine ACTH circadian rhythm.[715] ACTH circadian rhythm is entrained by visual cues and the light-dark cycle and is centrally controlled by CRH and other factors.[716] Although continuous CRH administration desensitizes the ACTH response, prolonged pulsatile CRH administration restores cortisol secretion without depleting the pituitary ACTH pool.[717] The 24-hour ACTH but not cortisol secretion is higher in males, who also exhibit higher pulse frequency and peak amplitudes,[718] possibly reflecting gender-specific set-points for cortisol feedback or a relative male adrenal insensitivity to ACTH. Endogenous and exogenous stresses, including hypoglycemia, act centrally to increase ACTH pulse amplitude, and corticosteroids directly suppress basal or stimulated corticotroph ACTH pulse amplitude.[719]

Adrenocorticotropic Hormone Action

The primary action of ACTH is to maintain adrenal gland size, structure, and function; ACTH induces adrenal steroidogenesis by activating ACTH receptors situated on the adrenal cortex cell surface. ACTH signals through adenyl cyclase to regulate P450 enzyme transcription, cortisol aldosterone (10%), 17-hydroxyprogesterone, and to a lesser extent adrenal androgen synthesis and secretion.[720] ACTH stimulates mitochondrial cholesterol transport and regulates the rate-limiting side-chain cleavage of cholesterol to pregnenolone.[721] Secretory cortisol pulses follow ACTH pulses within 5 to 10 minutes, with a linear dose dependence, especially evident after physiologic CRH stimulation.[722] However, circulating cortisol levels reach a plateau when pharmacologic levels of ACTH are attained by cosyntropin (Cortrosyn; Synacthen) injection.

The adrenal cortisol response to ACTH is sensitive to the background ambient ACTH milieu. In states of chronic ACTH deficiency, adrenal reserve is compromised, whereas during ongoing ACTH hypersecretion the gland is primed so that a given ACTH bolus elicits a higher cortisol response. Both basal ACTH secretion and stimulated (e.g., by CRH) ACTH secretion are blunted by glucocorticoids. Conversely, low or absent circulating glucocorticoids (e.g., after adrenalectomy) result in exaggerated ACTH secretion[723, 724] and corticotroph cell hyperplasia.[725] The HPA axis is inhibited by a long feedback inhibition whereby cortisol rapidly inhibits hypothalamic CRH and pituitary ACTH. These effects may also be delayed by 30 to 60 minutes by inhibition of ACTH release rather than synthesis,[726] especially after a single glucocorticoid bolus. After chronic glucocorticoid exposure (>24 hours), HPA suppression may persist for days or longer. In a short feedback loop, pituitary ACTH inhibits hypothalamic CRH, and in an ultrashort loop it may also suppress the corticotroph itself.

Physiologic Adrenocorticotropic Hormone Regulation

Exercise enhances ACTH and β-endorphin levels, especially if it is exhausting and of short duration. Exercising up to 90% of maximum oxygen capacity causes a significant elevation of ACTH, similar to levels observed during surgery or hypoglycemia.[727] Levels may remain elevated for up to 6 minutes after exercise cessation, and lower intensity exercise does not evoke ACTH.[728] Well-trained athletes exhibit hypercortisolism, possibly a result of decreased adrenal ACTH sensitivity. Other causes of elevated ACTH include acute hemorrhage, surgery, and emotional stress. Acute illness is associated with increased ACTH and cortisol levels with loss of diurnal secretory patterns.

Stress Response

Both exogenous and endogenous stress stimuli activate the HPA axis to produce sufficient glucocorticoid in an attempt to counteract the insult. The HPA stress response occurs in the context of a wide variety of peripheral and central adaptors to stress, including vasovagal and catecholamine activation and cytokine secretion and action. A tightly controlled immunoneuroendocrine interface regulates the ACTH response to peripheral stressors, which include pain, infection, inflammation, hypovolemia, trauma, psychologic stress, and hypoglycemia. These signals vary in their ability to generate ACTH secretion and to sensitize the ACTH response to glucocorticoids. In addition to CRH, peripheral and centrally released proinflammatory cytokines potently induce *POMC* transcription and ACTH secretion.[493] Sensitive intracellular signals within the corticotroph also serve to override the ACTH response to stress, thus preventing persistent and chronic hypercortisolemia.

Cytokines such as interleukin-6 and LIF activate the HPA axis and enhance glucocorticoid production, thus protecting the organism against lethality by constraining the inflammatory response.[493] Thus, mice with inactivated CRH or LIF genes mount an inadequate neuroendocrine response to stress, inflammation, or endotoxins.[493] During stress, glucocorticoid inhibition of ACTH is also prevented by nuclear factor κB activation, which interferes with pituitary glucocorticoid receptor function, thus further exaggerating enhanced ACTH secretion.[729]

Integrated Regulation of Adrenocorticotropic Hormone Secretion

As with other anterior pituitary hormones, ACTH regulation is subserved by at least three tiers of control. First, the brain and hypothalamus release regulatory molecules (including CRH, vasopressin, and other peptides) that traverse the portal system and directly signal for corticotroph secretory and mitotic activity. Second, intrapituitary cytokines and growth factors act locally to regulate ACTH either in concert with hypothalamic factors or independently. These paracrine controls often overlap and are redundant, and they have been shown to induce sensitive intracellular molecules that limit the ACTH response and prevent chronic ACTH hypersecretion. Third, peripheral hormones, especially glucocorticoids, maintain potent feedback inhibition control of corticotroph secretion and replication.

Measurement of Adrenocorticotropic Hormone

Both RIA and IRMA employ antisera specifically directed against intact ACTH (1 to 39) or other POMC fragments. Generally, the IRMA is more sensitive, reproducible, and rapid.[730] Most IRMAs have a sensitivity of less than 0.5 ng/L with precise variations of less than 10%. Intact ACTH or POMC precursor peptides are detectable, depending on the sequence specificity of the assay employed. Awareness of the peptide specificity may be especially critical when evaluating ectopic POMC products secreted by lung tumors. ACTH precursors are assessed by a specific IRMA employing unique monoclonal antibodies to ACTH, N-POMC, β-lipotropin (β-LPH), or β-endorphin.[731]

Ideally, nonstressed resting subjects should have venous blood withdrawn between 6 and 9 AM. Because ACTH is relatively unstable at room temperature and has a propensity to adhere to glass, plasma samples should be separated immediately in iced siliconized glass tubes containing ethylenediaminetetraacetic acid (EDTA) and stored below −20°C for transport. The plasma ACTH levels at 8 AM range from 8 to 25 ng/L as measured by IRMA. Episodic secretion and short plasma half-life result in wide and rapid fluctuation of plasma measurements. Cortisol values at 4 PM are about half of morning levels, and at 11 PM levels are usually less than 5 μg/dL.

Altered corticosteroid-binding globulin (CBG) levels and stress may influence measured cortisol values.

Random ACTH values do not provide an accurate assessment of HPA function unless concurrent cortisol levels are obtained. Thus, an integrated assessment of both hormone levels is required for interpreting the significance of an appropriately obtained ACTH value. Often, measurement of cortisol levels alone may provide a useful surrogate end-point for ACTH action and HPA axis integrity. Plasma ACTH levels fluctuate broadly within the same individual and are highly sensitive to stress, time of collection, and gender. Men exhibit greater ACTH pulse frequency and amplitude[718] and pregnant women have higher ambient ACTH levels, possibly related to placental CRH secretion.[732]

Dynamic Testing for Adrenocorticotropic Hormone Reserve

Hypothalamic

Insulin hypoglycemia is a potent endogenous stressor that evokes ACTH secretion.[733] Thus insulin (0.1 to 0.15 U/kg) is injected intravenously after an overnight fast to achieve symptomatic hypoglycemia and a blood glucose level less than 40 mg/dL. This test correlates well with other indices of ACTH reserve. A normal HPA response to this stressor evokes cortisol levels above 20 μg/dL. As hypoglycemia acts centrally, a normal response implies integrity of all three tiers of HPA axis control. Up to 20% of patients may require insulin up to 0.3 U/kg or more to achieve symptoms of glucopenia including sweating, hunger, palpitations, and tremors.[734] Venous samples are collected at −15, 0, 15, 30, 45, 60, 90, and 120 minutes for measurement of glucose, ACTH, and cortisol levels. GH can also be measured. After the test, oral glucose should be administered. Intraindividual variations in blood glucose levels attained at a given dose of insulin, fluctuations in central sensitivity to glucose, and activation of catecholamines may lead to difficulties in reproducibility. The test is contraindicated in subjects with a history of seizures, those with active coronary or cerebral ischemia, and in pregnancy. If pronounced adrenal insufficiency is likely, insulin injection may provoke an adrenal crisis because of inadequate adrenal reserve, and hydrocortisone (100 mg) should be available for urgent intravenous use if required.

Metyrapone blocks cortisol synthesis by inhibiting adrenal 11β-hydroxylase. Thus, the drug releases the HPA axis from negative feedback by cortisol, normally resulting in an ACTH surge and elevated levels of 11-deoxycortisol (compound S). A single oral dose (2 to 3 g) is given at midnight, and serum levels of ACTH, 11-deoxycortisol, and cortisol are measured at 8 AM the next morning. The test is valid only in the presence of documented suppressed cortisol levels less than 10 μg/dL. In normal subjects, peak ACTH values higher than 200 ng/L are achieved. Side effects include nausea, gastrointestinal upset, and insomnia.[735] False-positive results may be obtained when phenytoin is being administered because the drug prevents adequate enzymatic blockade. This test should be performed under observation in hospital because acute adrenal insufficiency may ensue.

Pituitary Stimulation

Pituitary ACTH secretion may be evoked by injecting either CRH or arginine vasopressin. Ovine or human CRH (100 μg or 1 μg/kg) is administered intravenously, and cortisol and ACTH are measured at −5, −1, 0, 15, 30, 60, 90, and 120 minutes. Normally, maximal ACTH responses (twofold to fourfold above baseline) are evoked at 30 minutes[736] and cortisol levels peak (over 20 μg/dL) at 60 minutes or increase more than 10 μg/dL above baseline. Although CRH readily induces ACTH secretion and demonstrates ACTH deficiency or ACTH excess, the wide variation of responses observed has limited its utility.

A useful application of the CRH test is in making the diagnosis of Cushing's disease with or without dexamethasone pretreatment and in the context of petrosal venous sampling for diagnosing ACTH-secreting pituitary adenoma. CRH injection allows a sensitive and specific ACTH gradient to be established, which effectively distinguishes peripheral from pituitary sources of excessive ACTH secretion.[737] Because of the suppressive impact of circulating glucocorticoids on pituitary CRH responsiveness, it may be difficult to distinguish a corticotroph adenoma from pseudo-Cushing's disease, as hypercortisolism is associated with both conditions. In these circumstances, combining this test with dexamethasone suppression may be useful.

In the combined dexamethasone-CRH test, dexamethasone is administered at 0.5 mg every 6 hours for 48 hours starting at noon and ending at 6 AM and then CRH is administered intravenously at 8 AM.[738] In normal subjects or those with pseudo-Cushing's disorder, cortisol levels do not rise and are less than 1.4 μg/dL. If cortisol levels elicited at 15 minutes exceed 4 μg/dL, an ACTH-secreting pituitary tumor is invariably present with 100% sensitivity and specificity.[738] CRH responsiveness (at least a 35% cortisol rise) is usually retained in ACTH-secreting adenomas but is not apparent in more than 90% of ectopic ACTH-producing tumors, with which ACTH increases of less than 35% above baseline are usually encountered. Although this approach has 100% specificity, only 90% sensitivity is achieved, and the test does not distinguish ACTH-secreting adenomas from pseudo-Cushing's disorder.[739]

Adrenal Stimulation

The acute response of the adrenal gland to a bolus ACTH injection reflects ambient ACTH concentrations to which the gland has been exposed. Thus, the cortisol response to an acute ACTH injection is blunted if the subject has had chronic pituitary ACTH hyposecretion with resultant adrenal atrophy and diminished cortisol reserve. Conversely, persistently elevated ACTH levels lead to adrenal hypertrophy and augmented cortisol responses.[736] The utility of this test in diagnosing a diminished pituitary ACTH reserve has been challenged because the commonly employed dose of Cortrosyn (ACTH 1 to 24, 250 μg) or Synacthen is high and may evoke a "normal" cortisol response in hypopituitary subjects. An unacceptably high false-negative rate (about 65%) has been determined in a large series,[740] although peak cortisol levels at 30 minutes do, in fact, correlate well with peak responses to an ITT.[741]

A normal cortisol response is greater than 20 μg/dL or a doubling of baseline values. Basal cortisol levels correlate inversely with the incremental response to ACTH.[742] Low-dose stimulation with 1 μg of Synacthen evoked maximal serum cortisol levels at 30 minutes, and these correlated well with values observed after insulin or high-dose ACTH administration.[741] A cutoff of greater than 500 nmol/L provides almost 100% sensitivity and a specificity of 80% to 100%.[743] Failure to respond to low-dose ACTH should be corroborated by a standard dose insulin or ACTH test stimulation.

Test. A 250-μg dose of Cortrosyn (ACTH 1 to 24) is injected intramuscularly or intravenously, and cortisol levels are measured before and 30 and 60 minutes after injection. Cortisol values higher than 20 μg/dL reflect a normal adrenal reserve response.

Interpretation. Fluctuation of CBG levels may confound interpretation of cortisol values. Thus, cirrhosis and hyperthyroidism lower CBG and cortisol levels, whereas estrogens elevate CBG concentrations.

Secondary Adrenal Insufficiency

ACTH deficiency is usually reflective of already profound pituitary insufficiency with disordered GH, gonadotropin, and TSH reserve. Rarely, isolated ACTH deficiency is manifest later in life, is more common in males, but may occur after childbirth associated with autoimmune thyroiditis and diabetes mellitus. Two families with recessive mutations in the corticotroph-specific *TPIT* gene have been described with congenital adrenal insufficiency and ACTH deficiency.[24] Insufficient ACTH secretion leads to attenuated adrenal corticosteroid production, with relative mineralocorticoid preservation.

Patients present with slowly progressive weight and appetite loss, anorexia, and generalized fatigue. Because adrenal mineralocorticoid is largely unimpaired, salt wasting, volume contraction, and hyperkalemia, commonly encountered features in Addison's disease, are not present. Furthermore, the hyperpigmentation usually associated with exuberant ACTH-related peptide secretion in the presence of adrenal damage does not occur. Morning serum cortisol levels less than 3 μg/dL suggest ACTH deficiency, and basal morning cortisol levels greater than 18 μg/dL usually indicate a normal ACTH reserve. Patients with ACTH deficiency have low to normal serum cortisol levels and low to normal plasma ACTH levels. Blunted responses to provocative tests such as insulin-induced hypoglycemia or metyrapone are required to document a partial deficiency.

Treatment. Hydrocortisone is used to replace deficient glucocorticoid hormone directly. The normal secretory rate of cortisol is about 20 mg/day, which is the recommended total daily dose for correcting hypoadrenalism and maintaining blood pressure. The plasma circulating half-life of cortisol is less than 2 hours, and twice-daily dosing regimens may result in very low cortisol levels in the late afternoon with impaired quality of life. Hydrocortisone dosing three times daily for a total daily requirement of 20 mg (10 mg in the morning, 5 mg at noon, and 5 mg in the evening) is most effective for starting replacement.[522] Although excessive dosing leads to iatrogenic Cushing's syndrome, doses should be increased during stress or prior to operative procedures. Cortisone acetate is metabolized to cortisol and has a slower onset of action and longer biologic activity than hydrocortisone. Other synthetic glucocorticoids, including prednisolone and dexamethasone, are less useful because they are difficult to monitor biochemically. Even modest cortisol overreplacement may result in bone mineral loss.[744]

Mineralocorticoid replacement is rarely required. Central diabetes insipidus may rarely be unmasked after initial glucocorticoid replacement.

Adrenocorticotropic Hormone–Secreting Tumors

The evaluation and management of Cushing's disease are described fully in Chapter 14. Briefly, the diagnosis of an ACTH-secreting pituitary tumor is suggested by features of hypercortisolism, elevated 24-hour urinary free cortisol levels, and failure to suppress morning cortisol levels to less than 3 μg/dL after 1 mg of dexamethasone administered at 11 PM. In healthy subjects, glucocorticoid feedback suppresses CRH and ACTH, attenuating cortisol secretion.

Surgical resection of an ACTH-secreting adenoma is the treatment of choice. Because these tumors are usually small, sometimes less than 2 mm in diameter, they may be localized incorrectly, or not at all, by venous sampling for ACTH (see earlier) and sensitive MRI. Therefore, these tumors pose a significant challenge even for the experienced surgeon. Furthermore, the disorder is also characterized by venous hypertension leading to turgid venous sinuses[745] requiring control by the anesthetist.

Bilateral petrosal venous sampling for ACTH levels and cavernous sinus venography should ideally be performed before surgery. However, if sellar venous sinus drainage is predominantly unilateral, left-right ACTH gradients may not reliably lateralize the lesion. Cavernous sinus venography may also outline a filling defect representing the tumor.[746] If an ACTH gradient is indeed detected with normal venous drainage patterns, hemihypophysectomy may be curative in 80% of such patients with clearly defined biochemical features of ACTH-dependent Cushing's disease. Meticulous surgical exploration of both anterior and posterior lobes is required for these tiny tumors, which are often off-white and speckled by petechiae and may be inadvertently suctioned. Unfortunately, even carefully performed preoperative lateralization is not infallible and the so-called normal side should also be carefully explored.

Assessment of Surgical Outcome

Transsphenoidal adenoma resection is the preferred treatment for these adenomas. After selective adenomectomy of a clearly identifiable adenoma, remission was achieved in 75% of 295 patients. However, partial hypophysectomy performed in 31 patients in whom an adenoma could not be identified resulted in biochemical remission in only 10 patients.[158] On the third postoperative day, 1 mg of dexamethasone can be given at 10 PM and cortisol levels measured the following morning, prior to initiating hydrocortisone therapy. If the immediate postoperative cortisol level is less than 3 μg/dL, a 95% 5-year remission rate can be expected. In 21 of 27 patients tested prior to glucocorticoid administration, postoperative cortisol levels below 10 mg/dL or less than those obtained with preoperative midnight sampling were predictive of remission.[747]

Silent Corticotroph Adenoma

These basophilic tumors are generally nonfunctional and yet exhibit POMC, β-lipotropin, and β-endorphin immunoreactivity. ACTH secretion is apparently unaltered, with no associated clinical or biochemical features of hypercortisolism, although these tumors are morphologically indistinguishable from adenomas associated with Cushing's disease. They may represent up to 7% of all surgically removed adenomas[700] and are usually hemorrhagic and invariably macroadenomas. Unlike Cushing's disease, they have a 2:1 male preponderance, often occur with mass effects, and about one third have preoperative evidence of pituitary insufficiency. About half exhibit cavernous sinus or bone invasion, hemorrhage, necrosis, and cyst formation. These tumors often recur, and postoperative radiation and reoperation are required to eradicate tumor regrowth or residual mass.[748] Unless appropriate immunostaining is performed, many of these tumors remain undiagnosed and are classified as recurrent nonfunctioning macroadenomas.

Thyroid-Stimulating Hormone

Thyrotroph cells constitute about 5% of the functional anterior pituitary cells and are situated predominantly in the anteromedial areas of the gland. They are smaller than the other cell types and are irregularly shaped with flattened nuclei and relatively small secretory granules ranging from 120 to 150 μm (Figs. 8–61 and 8–62).

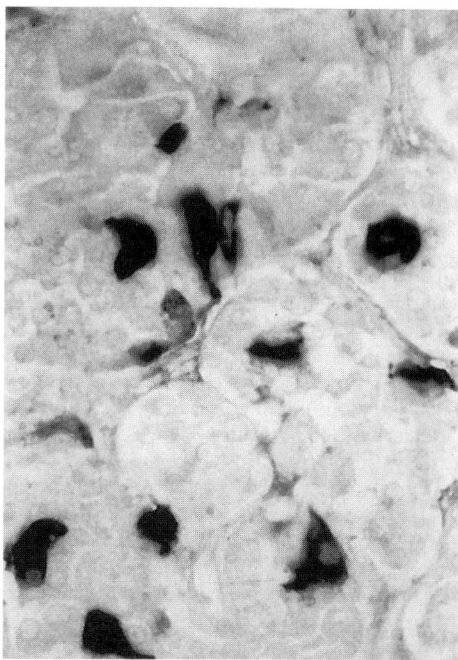

Figure 8–61. Normal thyrotrophs have angular cell bodies with elongated processes. (From Asa SL. In Tumors of the Pituitary Gland. Atlas of Tumor Pathology. Washington, DC, Armed Forces Institute of Pathology, 1997, p 19.) (See also Color Plate.)

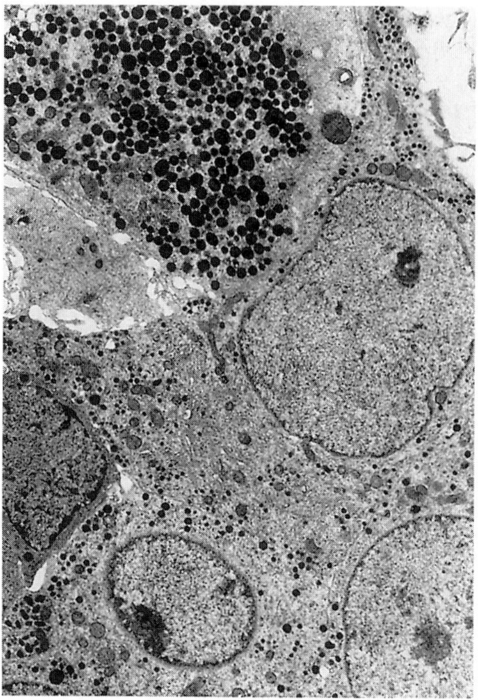

Figure 8–62. Electron micrograph of normal thyrotrophs showing angular cell bodies with elongated processes. (From Asa SL. In Tumors of the Pituitary Gland. Atlas of Tumor Pathology. Washington, DC, Armed Forces Institute of Pathology, 1997, p 19.)

Thyroid-Stimulating Hormone Biosynthesis

TSH is a glycoprotein hormone that is a heterodimer of two noncovalently linked α and β subunits.[749] The α subunit is common to TSH, LH, FSH, and hCG, but the β subunit is unique and confers specificity of action.[750] The α subunit is the earliest hormone gene expressed embryonically; activation of the β subunit gene occurs later under the influence of GATA-2 and Pit-1.[11] The 13.5-kb α subunit gene is located on chromosome 6 and comprises four exons and three introns.[751] Although the α subunit gene is expressed in thyrotroph, gonadotroph, and placental cells, its regulation is uniquely cell-specific. The downstream promoter region (−200 and below) is required for placental expression, intermediate sequences are required for gonadotroph expression, and upstream promoter elements are required for thyrotroph-specific expression.[752] The α subunit transcription is inhibited by T_3 at regions close to the transcriptional initiation site, in concert with other nuclear corepressors.[753] The 4.9-kb TSH β subunit gene located on chromosome 1 comprises three exons and two introns.[754] Pit-1 binds directly to the gene promoter to confer tissue-specific expression.[755] TSH-β gene transcription is suppressed by the thyroid hormone receptor acting directly on exon 1.[756]

This potent suppression is evident within 30 minutes of T_3 exposure and is a critical determinant of TSH synthesis and ultimate secretion. Transcription of both α and β TSH subunit genes is induced by TRH, and depletion of cAMP by dopamine leads to suppressed gene transcription.[757] Intrapituitary TSH is stored in secretory granules, and the mature hormone (28 kd) is released into the venous circulation primarily in response to hypothalamic TRH. The predicted structural model of the TSH molecule is that of a cystine knot growth factor. The tertiary TSH structure comprises three hairpin loops separated by central disulfide bonds, with the longer loop straddling one side.[758, 759]

Production of the mature heterodimeric TSH molecule requires complex cotranslational glycosylation and folding of nascent α and β subunits.[750] After subunit translation and signal peptide cleavage, glycosylation occurs at asparagine 23 on the β subunit and at two asparagine residues, 52 and 78, on the α subunit.[760] Appropriate glycosylation is required for accurate molecular folding and subsequent combination of α and β subunits within the rough endoplasmic reticulum and Golgi apparatus. Both TRH and T_3 regulate TSH glycosylation, albeit in opposite directions. TRH administration or T_3 deprivation, such as occurs in hypothyroidism or T_3 resistance, enhances oligosaccharide addition to the TSH molecule.[761]

Thyroid-Stimulating Hormone Secretion

The TSH production rate is normally 100 to 400 mU/day,[762] with a calculated circulating half-life of about 50 minutes. Secretion rates are enhanced up to 15-fold in hypothyroid subjects and are suppressed in states of hyperthyroidism. The degree of TSH glycosylation determines the metabolic clearance rate as well as bioactivity, and in hypothyroidism the molecule appears highly sialylated.[760] Immunoreactive fetal pituitary TSH is detectable by 12 weeks. Immediately after full-term birth, there is a brisk rise in TSH, which remains elevated for up to 5 days before stabilizing at adult levels.[763]

Although TSH secretion is pulsatile, the low pulse amplitudes and long TSH half-life result in modest circulating variances. Secretory pulses every 2 to 3 hours are interspersed with periods of tonic, nonpulsatile TSH secretion.[272] Circadian TSH secretion peaks between 11 PM and 5 AM, mainly because of increased pulse amplitude, which does not appear to be sleep-entrained.[764] Pulsatile and circadian TSH secretory patterns are largely determined by ambient thyroid hormone levels, TRH release, dopamine, and cortisol. Primary hypothyroidism is associated with enhanced TSH pulse amplitudes occurring throughout the day, and nocturnal TSH surges are abrogated in patients with critical illness.[765]

Thyrotropin-Releasing Hormone and Thyroid Hormone Regulation

Because feedback control of TSH secretion by peripheral thyroid hormones is so sensitive, most thyrotroph disorders can be diagnosed by measuring basal TSH and thyroid hormone levels. However, evoked dynamic TSH measurements may be required to assess fully the integrity of the hypothalamic-pituitary-thyroid axis.[766] TRH (200 to 500 μg) is administered intravenously, and TSH levels are measured at -15, 0, 15, 30, 60, and 120 minutes.

In euthyroid subjects, peak TSH levels (up to 22-fold higher than basal) are observed after 30 minutes.[767] Because feedback suppression of TSH by elevated thyroid hormone levels overrides positive hypothalamic signals, hyperthyroid subjects have undetectable basal TSH levels that do not respond to TRH. In subjects with primary thyroid failure, the TSH response is exuberant, but in those with secondary thyroid failure related to pituitary disease TSH levels do not change in response to TRH.

Sustained TRH infusions for up to 4 hours result in biphasic TSH increases, reflecting early release of preformed TSH, followed later by newly synthesized hormone. Further prolonged TRH infusions elevate thyroid hormone levels, which subsequently suppress pituitary TSH synthesis and release.[768] Within hours of T_3 administration, basal TSH levels are suppressed and TRH-evoked TSH levels are attenuated. Thyroid hormones suppress tonic TSH secretion and pulse amplitude but do not appear to regulate TSH pulse frequency. T_3 also suppresses hypothalamic TRH synthesis and decreases pituitary TRH receptor number, thus further limiting TSH biosynthesis.

Other Factors

SRIF inhibits TSH pulse amplitude, blocks the nocturnal TSH surge[769] directly at the pituitary level, and may also suppress TRH release and possibly TRH receptor abundance.[770] Although SRIF analogues are used to treat TSH-secreting pituitary adenomas (see later), long-term SRIF treatment for acromegaly does not lead to hypothyroidism in adult subjects although T_4 levels may be lowered within the normal range.[680] Dopamine inhibits TSH β subunit gene expression, and dopamine infusions suppress TSH pulse amplitude by 70% and abrogate the nocturnal TSH surge.[771] Prolonged use of dopamine agonists, however, does not result in hypothyroidism.

Glucocorticoids suppress TSH secretion, and in patients with adrenal failure without autoimmune thyroid damage, TSH levels may be elevated. Sex steroids and cytokines alter TSH secretion in animal models, but their contribution to human TSH physiology is unclear. Nonsteroidal anti-inflammatory agents, especially meclofenamate and fenclofenac, decrease serum TSH levels, albeit still within the normal range. The mechanism may involve displacement of thyroid hormone ligands from their binding proteins or direct inhibition of pituitary TSH.[772]

Thyroid-Stimulating Hormone Action

TSH acts on the thyroid gland to induce thyroid hormone synthesis and release and to maintain trophic thyroid cell integrity.[773] The TSH G protein-coupled (GPC) receptor is located on the thyrocyte plasma membrane and is encoded by a gene on chromosome 11q31. Its regulation is comprehensively described in Chapter 10.

Thyroid-Stimulating Hormone Assays

The challenge for a clinically compelling robust TSH assay is to differentiate circulating TSH levels in euthyroid subjects from those in both hyperthyroid and hypothyroid patients. The development of immunoradiometric TSH assays has provided high specificity with little or no cross-reactivity with other glycoprotein hormones. These assays detect quantifiable TSH levels in euthyroid control subjects with no overlap with the low values associated with hyperthyroidism.[767, 774] The most sensitive commercially available third-generation assays have a functional sensitivity of 0.01 to 0.02 mU/L, and newer fourth-generation assays should have greatly enhanced sensitivity (0.001 to 0.002 mU/L). Levels of free α subunit (normal range 0.1 to 1.6 μg/L) are elevated in patients harboring TSH-secreting or nonfunctional pituitary adenomas, choriocarcinomas, and several malignancies.

TSH deficiency results in childhood mental or growth retardation, or both, and hypothyroidism in adults is associated with a broad spectrum of clinical features including hypothermia, fluid retention, voice and skin changes, and ultimately frank myxedema and death. Pituitary damage may result in functional TSH deficiency, often without a clearly demonstrable reduction in serum TSH levels. Although impractical to measure, nocturnal TSH pulse amplitudes may be attenuated in patients with pituitary dysfunction.[775] TSH deficiency should be diagnosed by measuring free T_4 levels because TSH measurements are not helpful in diagnosing central hypothyroidism. In fact, only about one third of patients with secondary hypothyroidism have abnormally low basal TSH levels.[776] TSH deficiency is thus associated with low T_4 levels concomitant with low, normal, or even minimally elevated TSH levels. This biochemical profile may also be encountered in critically ill patients with low TSH and T_4 levels without evidence of pituitary disease.

Treatment

L-Thyroxine is used for replacement therapy, and dosing variables are similar to those required for treating primary hypothyroidism. Hypothyroid features are effectively ameliorated by T_4 (0.05 to 0.25 mg/day). The molecule is converted peripherally into the active T_3 and has a 7-day half-life with stable blood levels. The dose of levothyroxine in hypopituitary patients is titrated to achieve midnormal clinically euthyroid serum free T_4 levels because serum TSH levels are low or undetectable in patients with damaged pituitary function.

Measurement of TSH levels is not useful in determining thyroid hormone replacement because the damaged thyrotroph is unlikely to reflect appropriate feedback suppression. Many women with pituitary failure also receive estrogen replacement, and measuring free T_4 levels is required because of increased TBG levels. T_4 overdosing may also lead to osteopenia and cardiac arrhythmias. Some patients may have associated ACTH deficiency, and thyroid hormone replacement should not be initiated until adrenal reserve has been evaluated and, if necessary, treated. Thyroid hormone replacement may also accelerate cortisol metabolism or requirements, or both, and may therefore exacerbate primary hypoadrenalism or precipitate adrenal crisis in patients with perturbed adrenal function.

Thyrotropin-Secreting Tumors

TSH-producing pituitary tumors are rare. Most older series indicate that they represent less than 1% of pituitary tumors.[540, 777, 778] From 1979 to 1992, Mindermann and Wilson analyzed tumor type by immunohistochemistry and found that the overall prevalence of TSH-secreting tumors was 19 in

2225 (0.85%). Between 1989 and 1991, they found a prevalence of 2.8%.[777] It is not clear whether the incidence of this tumor type is increasing or whether tumors are now more readily recognized. Enhanced recognition may be a result of the development of high-sensitivity TSH assays that distinguish between normal TSH levels that are, in fact, inappropriately elevated for thyroid hormone levels in some patients with TSH-producing tumors and frankly low ones. TSH-secreting tumors can also cosecrete other hormones including GH, PRL, and rarely ACTH.[779]

Pathology

These tumors are invasive, but for the most part benign, and distant metastases are extremely rare. The secretory pattern is determined by a panel of antibodies to TSH β, α subunit, GH, PRL, and ACTH. TSH-secreting tumors exhibit positive immunostaining for α subunit and TSHβ in 20% to 75% of cells and for Pit-1.[780, 781]

Presentation

Patients with TSH-secreting tumors present with symptoms related to tumor size (e.g., visual field abnormalities, cranial nerve palsies or headache) or to hormone overproduction. Signs and symptoms of hyperthyroidism, including palpitations, arrhythmias, weight loss, tremor, and nervousness, or a goiter are common. A case of periodic paralysis has been reported.[782] Serum TSH is often but not invariably elevated, and the combination of abnormally high thyroid hormone and TSH within the normal range points to a TSH-producing pituitary tumor. A relatively long period of hyperthyroidism, initially thought to represent Graves' disease and treated accordingly, often predates the realization that the hyperthyroidism is a result of a TSH-secreting pituitary tumor. Alternatively, thyroid hormone insensitivity can exist with similar laboratory profiles.[783, 784]

TSH-secreting tumors are usually large. A review of six reports indicates that 88% of TSH-secreting tumors are macroadenomas and 12% microadenomas. Over 60% are also locally invasive.[785] From an analysis of 10 reports on a total of 153 patients, we estimate that TSH is frankly elevated in 58% of patients, with the remainder having normal although inappropriately elevated levels. Patients previously treated with radioactive iodine for presumed Graves' disease present with significantly higher TSH levels than patients not previously radioablated (mean of 56 and 9 mU/L, respectively).[776] An ectopic TSH-producing tumor has also been reported.[786] Serum T_4 is high in the majority of patients, as is the glycoprotein hormone α subunit. Approximately two thirds[776] of patients with TSH-producing pituitary tumors have a goiter with elevated radioactive iodine uptakes. Signs or symptoms of acromegaly or hyperprolactinemia may also be presenting complaints.

Evaluation

The T_4, T_3, TSH (by high-sensitivity assay), and α subunit should be measured. The combination of high T_4, T_3, and α subunit; high or inappropriately normal TSH; and a pituitary tumor strongly confirms the diagnosis of a TSH-producing pituitary adenoma. TRH stimulation distinguishes between TSH overproduction by a TSH-secreting tumor and thyroid hormone insensitivity. With TSH-secreting tumors, the TSH response to TRH is blunted. In contrast, TSH usually rises in response to TRH in thyroid hormone insensitivity and in normal subjects. Concomitant measurement of α subunit at each point during the TRH test is helpful because the molar ratio of α subunit to TRH is high (>1) in almost 85% of patients with TSH-secreting tumors. Ratios greater than 1 can also be seen in normal subjects.[787]

A T_3 suppression test is helpful in that complete inhibition of TSH does not occur in patients with TSH-secreting tumors. This test can also differentiate subclinical hypothyroidism in a patient treated with radioactive iodine for hyperthyroidism in the past but found to have an incidental pituitary tumor. TSH elevation may also result from inadequate thyroid hormone replacement. Pituitary MRI should be performed and IGF-I and PRL levels determined to exclude acromegaly or hyperprolactinemia. The presence of other pituitary hormones in immunostained histologic sections does not necessarily imply that their serum levels are elevated.

The degree of hyperthyroidism should be assessed to determine whether control of these signs and symptoms should be undertaken prior to further evaluation or treatment of the pituitary tumor. One report characterized the hyperthyroidism in this condition as being severe in 14 of 25 patients and having been present in most patients for years before the diagnosis was made.[785] Perioperative deaths in patients with TSH-secreting tumors have been reported, which might be attributed to poorly controlled hyperthyroidism.

Management

Surgery

Surgery is recommended as the first-line treatment,[188] but surgical cures occur in no more than 40% of patients (Table 8–30).[788, 789] However, the rarity of this tumor type has precluded large controlled studies. Fourteen of 22 patients had cavernous or sphenoid sinus invasion and tumors were fibrous and unusually hard. Eight patients were considered cured after surgery.[779] In another study, surgery resulted in normalization of T_4 in 15 and of parameters of cure in 7 of 17 patients. Over half of the patients, when assessed by MRI 6 months after surgery, exhibited evidence of residual tumor.[790]

Radiation Therapy

There are no large series reporting treatment of TSH-secreting tumors with radiotherapy alone. Radiation has mostly been employed as adjunctive therapy to surgery, especially when the latter was not curative.

Somatostatin Analogues

Octreotide, used as either primary or adjunctive treatment, normalized T_4 and T_3 and reduced TSH levels by half.[791] In 25 patients treated with octreotide (100 to 500 μg/day) for up to 61 months, 84% had controlled thyroid function. However, tachyphylaxis developed in five patients, and three escaped the effect of the drug. Overall, tumor shrinkage occurs in about a third of patients. In 18 patients with TSH-secreting adenomas, lanreotide (30 mg every 10 or 14 days), significantly decreased TSH levels from 2.72 to 1.89 mU/L, decreased T_4 levels, but did not shrink tumors. Responsiveness to octreotide LAR (up to 30 mg monthly) appeared similar to that observed for the subcutaneous preparation in seven patients.[792]

Unless vision is threatened, patients should be evaluated to determine whether the clinical signs of hyperthyroidism warrant immediate treatment (Fig. 8–63). Propranolol, radioactive iodine thyroid ablation, thyroidectomy, antithyroid medications including methimazole (Tapazole) and propylthiouracil, and somatostatin analogues are employed.[793] Both radioactive iodine and antithyroid medications are targeted to the thyroid gland rather than the pituitary seat of the disorder. Both also

Table 8–30. Results of Treatment of Thyrotropin-Secreting Tumors

Source	Number of Patients	Micro-adenomas	Macro-adenomas	Extrasellar Extension	Visual Field Deficit	Cured by Surgery	Immunostain	Radia-tion	Cured by Radia-tion
Grisoli, 1987 (776b)	6	0/6	6/6	4/6	3/6	2/5	4/4 TSH 2/4 TSH, PRL	3/6	1/3
Gesundheit, 1989 (776a)	9	2/9	7/9			3/5*	5/7 TSH 3/7 α subunit	3/8	0/3
McCutcheon, 1990 (779)	8	1/8	7/8	6/7	4/8	4/8	6/7 TSH 2/7 PRL	3/8	0/3
Beckers, 1991 (788)	7	1/7	6/7			3/4	2/7 pure TSH 1/7 TSH, PRL 1/7 TSH, PRL, GH		
Chanson, 1992 (789a)	37	2/37	35/37					8/37	0/8
Chanson, 1993 (789)	52							9/52	0/9
Mindermann, 1993 (777)	19	0/19	19/19	12/19	6/19	NA	6/14 pure TSH 4/14 TSH, GH, PRL, ACTH 1/14 TSH, GH, PRL 1/14 TSH, PRL 1/14 TSH, GH 1/14 TSH, ACTH	9/19 E	NA
Losa, 1996 (740)	17	3/17	14/17	10/14	3/17	7/17	14 TSH 2 GH 3 PRL 1LH 13/14 α subunit		
Brucker-Davis, 1999 (785)	25	2/25	23/25	20/25	7/18	8/22	5/25 GH 4/25 PRL 3/25 FSH	11	
Kuhn, 2000 (785a)	16	5/16	11/16	8/11					
Total (%)	164	15/136 11%	121/136 89%	60/82 73%	23/66 35%	24/56 43%			

ACTH, adrenocorticotropic hormone; GH, growth hormone; PRL, prolactin; TSH, thyrotropin.

inhibit the remaining negative feedback of T_3 on TSH and lead to increased tumor TSH production.[791]

Surgery and somatostatin analogues simultaneously treat hyperthyroidism and tumor TSH hypersecretion. Propranolol is important for inhibiting peripheral hyperthyroid manifestations.[784, 794] Somatostatin analogues lower TSH, α subunit, and T_4 and are recommended as first-line drugs in the initial control of hyperthyroidism related to TSH-secreting tumors because they act more rapidly than other therapeutic approaches and tumor shrinkage occurs in up to 40% of patients. If these drugs are ineffective or only partially effective, other therapeutic modalities should be used. Thus, no single treatment is expected to cure patients with TSH-secreting adenomas. Surgery is curative in only a minority of patients, and although tumor bulk removal may normalize thyroid function when invasive tumor tissue persists, patients continue to have abnormal TSH responses to TRH and require somatostatin analogue therapy.

PITUITARY FAILURE

Impaired synthesis of one or more anterior pituitary hormones may result from heritable genetic factors, acquired anatomic insults, inflammation, or vascular damage (Tables 8–31 and 8–32). Because of its close anatomic contiguity, impaired hypothalamic hormone synthesis or secretion may also occur as a component of the pituitary gland insult, especially after external radiation. Furthermore, distinct hypothalamic lesions may result in diminished pituitary hormone secretion by abrogating hypothalamic hypophysiotropic signals.

Developmental and Genetic Causes of Pituitary Failure

Developmental Pituitary Dysfunction

Congenital pituitary gland absence (aplasia), partial hypoplasia, or ectopic tissue rudiments are rarely encountered. Pituitary development follows midline cell migration from Rathke's pouch, and impaired midline anomalies including failed forebrain cleavage and anterior commissure and corpus callosum defects lead to structural pituitary anomalies. Craniofacial developmental anomalies including anencephaly result in cleft lip and palate, basal encephalocele, hypertelorism, and optic nerve hypoplasia with varying degrees of pituitary dysplasia and aplasia. If these infants survive, appropriate lifelong pituitary hormone replacement is required. Children with mild forms of midline anomalies are also more susceptible to GH deficiencies.

With sensitive MRI techniques for pituitary visualization, several anatomic features characteristic of hypopituitarism are now apparent. Evidence for acquired pituitary gland damage or destruction is often clearly visible on MRI, and patients presenting with hypopituitarism of undetermined etiology may exhibit decreased gland volume, partial or complete empty sella, disturbed sella turcica architecture, absent or transected pituitary stalk, and an absent or ectopic posterior pituitary bright intensity signal.[795] An absent infundibulum noted on MRI is associated with pituitary hormone deficits, and about

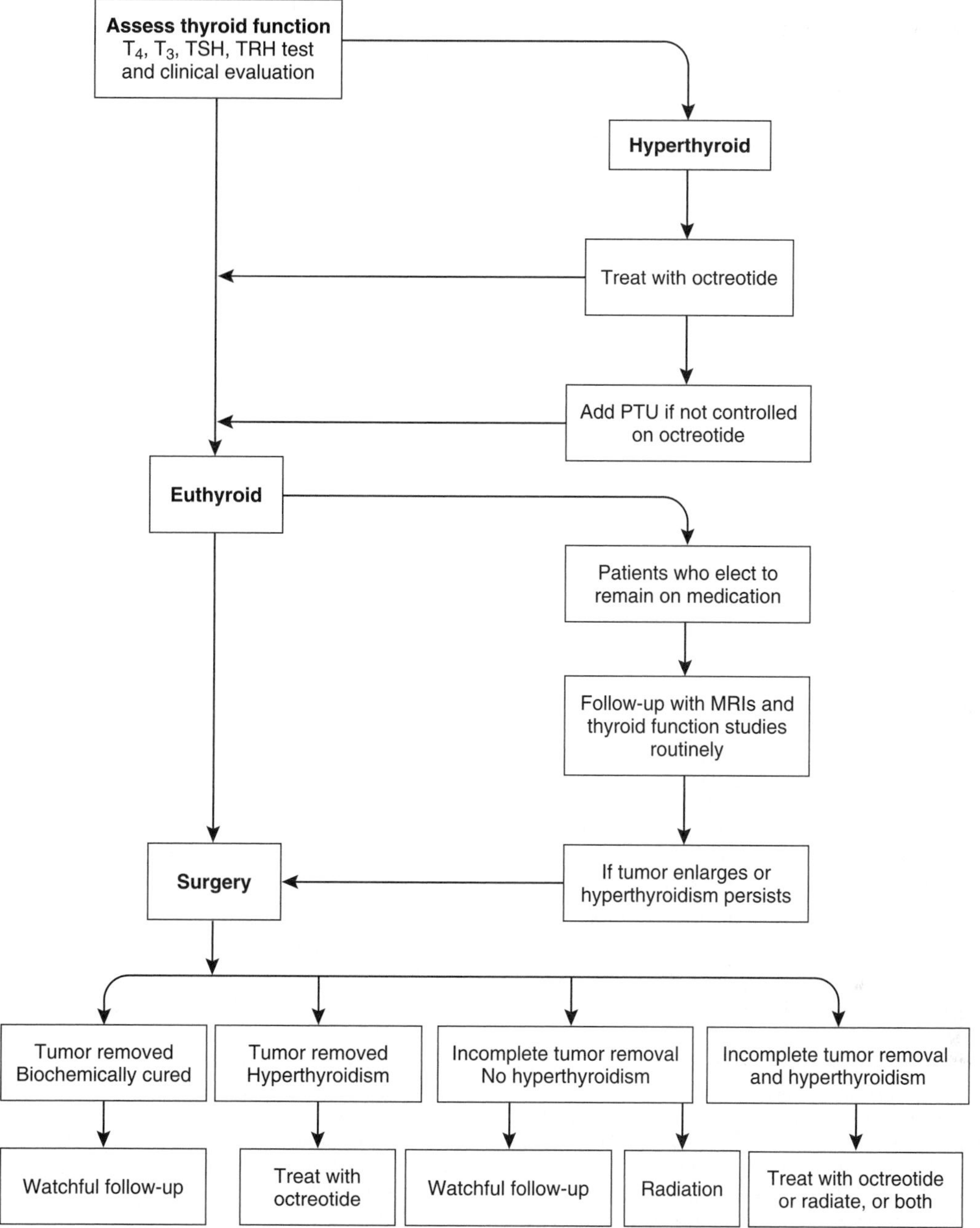

Figure 8–63. Management of thyroid-stimulating hormone (TSH)-secreting pituitary tumors. PTU, propylthiouracil; T_3, triiodothyronine; T_4, thyroxine; TRH, thyrotropin-releasing hormone.

40% of patients with GHD of unclear cause show imaging evidence of mild stalk defects, reflecting a midline developmental anomaly. Congenital basal encephalocele may result in the pituitary herniating through the sphenoid sinus roof, resulting in pituitary failure and diabetes insipidus.

Heritable Disorders of Pituitary Failure

Mutations of transcription factors that determine anterior pituitary development may lead to pituitary deficiency syndromes (Table 8–33). Patients heretofore diagnosed with idiopathic isolated or polyhormonal pituitary failure may, in fact, harbor such a mutation. As the genetic control of pituitary development has been clarified, increasing numbers of mutant genes have become apparent (Chapter 23).

PROP1

PROP1 (Online Mendelian Inheritance in Man [OMIM] 601538) gene expression is required for subsequent Pit-1 activation. The gene, located on chromosome 5q, encodes a 223-amino-acid protein expressed in cells secreting GH, PRL, and TSH.[796] The Ames dwarf mouse harbors a missense *PROP1* mutation (Ser83Pro) and exhibits a hypoplastic pituitary gland with combined GH, PRL, and TSH deficiency. This mutation abrogates Pit-1 activation and results in failed development of Pit-1–dependent cell lineages.[797] At least eight human mutations have been associated with GH, PRL, TSH, and gonadotrophin deficiencies. The most commonly encountered mutation is a 2-bp deletion at position 296 (301-302delAG), resulting in early translation termination and a nonfunctional

Table 8–31. Etiology of Inherited Pituitary Deficiency

Developmental Factor	Hormone Deficit
Genetic	
KAL mutation	FSH, LH
Prader-Willi syndrome	FSH, LH
Lawrence-Moon-Biedl syndrome	FSH, LH
Receptor	
Melanocortin receptor	
GHRH receptor	GH
CRH receptor	ACTH
GnRH receptor	FSH, LH
Leptin and leptin receptor defect	LH, FSH
Structural	
Pituitary aplasia	Any
Pituitary hypoplasia	Any
CNS masses; encephalocele	Any
Transcription factor defect	
PITX2	
Prop1	GH, PRL, TSH, LH, FSH, ACTH
Pit-1 (POU1F1)	PRL, GH, TSH
HESX1	GH, PRL, TSH, LH, FSH, ACTH
LHX3	GH, PRL, TSH, LH, FSH
DAX1	Adrenal, LH, FSH
Hormone mutation	
GH-1	GH
Bioinactive GH	GH
FSHβ	FSH
LHβ	LH
POMC	ACTH
POMC processing defect	ACTH
TSHβ	TSH

ACTH, adrenocorticotropic hormone; FSH, follicle-stimulating hormone; GH, growth hormone. Functional defects include missense or frameshifts leading to truncated or deleted protein, DNA binding abnormality, inactivated protein, or impaired coactivation. *POU1F1* mutations result in varying phenotype of early growth failure with or without hypothyroidism. *PROP1* mutations may be fully manifest only in adulthood. *HESX1* is critical for corpus development and associated with structural brain defects.

protein product. The clinical spectrum of combined pituitary hormone deficiency associated with *PROP1* mutations varies with both the type of mutation and the age of the patient.[798]

Human *PROP1* mutations are associated with deficiencies in Pit-1–dependent lineages (GH, PRL, and TSH) as well as impaired FSH, LH, and ACTH reserve function.[517] Because the development and mature function of the latter cell types are not Pit-1–dependent, it appears that additional critical developmental factors are disrupted in these patients, leading to the clinical phenotype. Over 50 patients with *PROP1* mutations leading to combined pituitary hormone deficiency have been described since the original report in 1996,[799] and this disorder appears to be the most common heritable cause of combined pituitary hormone deficiency.

Molecular Analysis

Modes of inheritance of *PROP1* mutations usually reflect autosomal recessive patterns. Thus, patients are usually homozygous for either deletion or missense frameshift mutations leading to truncated PROP1 protein products devoid of functional activity.[517, 800] A "hot spot" in *PROP1* has been identified at a GA repeat in exon 2. Combination of a GA or AG deletion in this repeat results in a coding frameshift and premature termination at codon 109. Nonafflicted siblings are heterozygous or bear a normal *PROP1* sequence on both alleles.

Table 8–32. Etiology of Acquired Pituitary Insufficency

Traumatic
- Surgical resection
- Radiation damage
- Head trauma

Infiltrative or inflammatory
- Primary hypophysitis
  - Lymphocytic
  - Granulomatous
  - Xanthomatous
- Secondary hypophysitis
  - Sarcoidosis
  - Histiocytosis X
  - Infections
  - Wegener's granulomatosis
  - Takayasu's disease
- Hemochromatosis

Infections
- Tuberculosis
- *Pneumocystis carinii*
- Fungal (histoplasmosis, aspergillosis)
- Parasites (toxoplasmosis)
- Viral (cytomegalovirus)

Vascular
- Pregnancy-related
- Aneurysm
- Apoplexy
- Diabetes
- Hypotension
- Arteritis
- Sickle cell disease

Neoplastic
- Pituitary adenoma
- Parasellar mass
  - Rathke's cyst
  - Dermoid cyst
  - Meningioma
  - Germinoma
  - Ependymoma
  - Glioma
- Craniopharyngioma
- Hypothalamic harmatoma, gangliocytoma
- Pituitary metastatic deposits
- Hematologic malignancy
  - Leukemia
  - Lymphoma

Functional
- Nutritional
  - Caloric restriction
  - Malnutrition
- Excessive exercise
- Critical illness
  - Acute illness
  - Chronic renal failure
  - Chronic liver failure
- Hormonal
  - Hyperprolactinemia
  - Hypothyroidism
  - After treatment of Cushing's disease

Drugs
- Anabolic steroids
- Glucocorticoid excess
- Gonadotropin-releasing hormone agonists
- Estrogen
- Dopamine
- Somatostatin analogue
- Thyroid hormone excess

Causes of acquired growth hormone deficiency in 1034 hypopituitary adult patients*

Cause	%
Pituitary tumor	53.9
Craniopharyngioma	12.3
Idiopathic	10.2
Central nervous system tumor	4.4
Empty sella syndrome	4.2
Sheehan's syndrome	3.1
Head trauma	2.4
Hypophysitis	1.6
Surgery other than for pituitary treatment	1.5
Granulomatous diseases	1.3
Irradiation other than for pituitary treatment	1.1
Central nervous system malformation	1.0
Perinatal trauma or infection	0.5
Other	2.5

*From Abs R, Bengtsson BA, Hernberg-Stahl E, et al. GH replacement in 1034 growth hormone deficient adults: demographic and clinical characteristics, dosing and safety. Clin Endocrinol (OXF) 1999; 50:703–713.

Clinical Features

The frequency of *PROP1* gene mutations in patients with combined pituitary hormone deficiency is high, the mutations occurring in approximately 50% of affected subjects. However, in families with multiple affected subjects, *PROP1* mutations account for virtually all affected individuals. Patients harboring *PROP1* mutations exhibit a predominantly hypogonadal phenotype. Puberty is often delayed or absent, with markedly attenuated LH and FSH responses to GnRH stimulation.[437] Some patients enter puberty spontaneously and develop subsequent

Table 8–33. Imaging and Clinical Evaluation of Hereditary Pituitary Deficiency

Gene*	Pituitary Deficiency	Magnetic Resonance Imaging	Associated Malformations	Inheritance Mode
POU1F1	GH, PRL, ± TSH	Normal or hypoplastic anterior pituitary		Recessive Dominant
PROP1	GH, PRL, TSH, LH, FSH, ± ACTH	Normal, hypoplastic, hyperplastic, or cystic anterior pituitary		Recessive
HESX1	GH, PRL, TSH, LH, FSH, ACTH Posterior defects	Hypoplastic or hyperplastic anterior pituitary; normal or ectopic posterior pituitary	Septo-optic dysplasia	Recessive
LHX3	GH, PRL, TSH, LH, FSH	Hypoplastic or hyperplastic anterior pituitary	Stubby neck with rigid cervical spine	

ACTH, adrenocorticotropic hormone; FSH, follicle-stimulating hormone; GH, growth hormone; LH, luteinizing hormone; PRL, prolactin; TSH, thyrotropin.
Adapted from Netchine I. Magnetic resonance imaging of the hypothalamic-pituitary region in nontumoral hypopituitarism. In Rappaport R, Amselem S (eds). Hypothalamic Pituitary Development. Basel, Karger, 2001, pp 94–108.

features of central hypogonadism, akin to an acquired presentation.[800]

A broad spectrum of variable time of onset and degree of pituitary loss is characteristic of the syndrome. Some older patients also exhibit blunted cortisol responses to Cortrosyn administration, and others present with panhypopituitarism.[801] Although the pituitary gland is small or normal in size, patients have been described with grossly hyperplastic pituitary glands with cystic changes and development of a secondary empty sella. Slowing of linear growth usually becomes apparent after the age of 3 years, and these patients usually do not enter puberty. Height SDs may be severely impaired and may range to −10 with eunuchoidal proportions and reduced upper body/lower body ratios. Affected adults are short and have infantile external genitalia. The onset of clinically evident pituitary failure is usually characterized by GHD (~80%) and thyroid failure (TSH deficiency, ~20%), followed by hypogonadism and later subclinical or overt adrenal insufficiency.[802]

Features of PROP1 excess have been described in a mouse model.[803] These animals have hypothyroidism, hypogonadism, and persistent Rathke's cleft cysts and, after 1 year, develop pituitary adenomas.

Evaluation

Combined hypothalamic hormone stimulation (GnRH, TRH, CRH, and GHRH) or insulin-evoked hypoglycemia reveals blunted responses consistent with varying degrees of pituitary hormone deficiencies. Serum IGF-I and IGF-BP3 levels are usually low, and peripheral thyroid hormone levels are low or at the lower limits of normal ranges. In the presence of low or absent TSH responses, these findings are consistent with secondary hypothyroidism. Most older patients also exhibit blunted cortisol responses to CRH or ACTH or insulin stimulation.[804]

Pituitary Size

Heterogeneous changes in pituitary size may reflect a combination of apoptotic signals for the Pit-1 lineage, compensatory cystic expansion of nonaffected pituitary cell types with subsequent autoinfarction, and the absence of other unknown factors required for mature pituitary function.[805]

POU1F1

The *POU1F1* gene (Pit-1) is located on chromosome 3p11 (OMIM 173110) and encodes a 290-amino-acid protein. The N-terminal POU-specific domain activates gene transcription, and two DNA-binding domains recognize a TATNCAT consensus sequence present in the GH, PRL, and TSH hormones and the GHRH receptor gene.[806] The Pit-1 nuclear protein activates transcription of the GH, PRL, and TSH genes and the GHRH receptor gene and also interacts with coactivators including thyroid hormone, estrogen, and retinoic acid receptors as well as other transcription factors including CREB, P-Lim, Ptx-1, HESX-1, and Zn-15. Pit-1 autoregulates its own expression and is therefore critical for maintaining appropriate Pit-1 expression. Because of the absolute requirement of Pit-1 for GH, PRL, and TSH cell development and specific gene expression, inactivating mutations of the gene result in a spectrum of pituitary hormone deficiencies.[12] Two dwarf mouse strains harbor *POU1F1* gene mutations. The Snell dwarf mouse harbors a tryptophan cysteine missense mutation (Trp261Cys).[807] The Jackson mouse, also a dwarf, harbors a truncated POU1F1 protein with defective DNA binding.

Several *POU1F1* mutations have been described, each of which is associated with a characteristic clinical phenotype.[808] Arg172Tyr mutants are associated with neonatal hypothyroidism and GH and PRL deficiency. Both sporadic patients and multiplex families with multiple pituitary hormone defects have been described, and at least 10 recessive and 3 dominant Pit-1 mutations have been identified so far. Recessive mutations result in a varied spectrum of loss of DNA binding or transcriptional activation of TSH, GH, or PRL. Impaired retinoic acid activation of the Pit-1 distal enhancer has been described for a Pit-1 Lys261Glu mutation. This mutant protein also behaves as a dominant negative inhibitor of Pit-1 activation. A sporadic mutation (Arg271Try) results in a protein that binds to DNA but dominantly inhibits pituitary gene transcription. Compound heterozygosity for a 1-bp deletion (747delA) and a missense mutation (Trp193Arg) causes defective DNA binding and transcriptional activation with severe combined GH, PRL, and TSH deficiencies.[809]

Hesx1

Hesx1 (Rpx) is an early transcriptional marker of the primitive pituitary, with expression restricted to Rathke's pouch.[810] Coincidentally with the appearance of specific pituitary cell types, Hesx1 expression declines and is extinguished in the mature anterior pituitary.[811] The gene is located on chromosome 3p212, encodes a 185-amino-acid protein, and competes with PROP1 protein for DNA binding. The heterogeneous syndrome of septo-optic dysplasia (hypoplastic optic nerves, absent corpus callosum and septum pellucidum, and panhypopituitarism) is associated with a homozygous Arg53Cys homeodomain mutation. Although the mutant molecule exhibits reduced DNA binding, no specific hormonal target gene is yet apparent, and panhypopituitarism may be secondary to the profound anatomic defects in midline development. The reason for GHD in these patients is not apparent.

LHX3

Missense and deletion mutations of *LHX3* are associated with panhypopituitarism except for intact ACTH reserve. These patients also exhibit defective neck rotation because of a rigid cervical spine.[812] PtX2 Rieger's syndrome (anterior eye, teeth, and umbilical maldevelopment) may be associated with GHD and haploinsufficiency of the *RIEG* (PtX2) homeobox gene.

The frequency of heritable combined pituitary hormone deficiencies is rare. Nevertheless, within this cohort of patients, *PROP1* mutations appear to be the most prevalent, accounting for well over 50% of retrospective reports and over 90% of patients with more than one affected sibling. Pit-1 mutations are less commonly encountered. Patients with a family history of pituitary dysfunction and those who exhibit blunted hormonal responses to TRH, GHRH, or GnRH stimulation should be subjected to molecular screening for PROP1 or Pit-1 defects. The pronounced clinical phenotype of Hesx-1 mutations determines the need for further molecular analysis.

Lawrence-Moon-Biedl Syndrome

This autosomal recessive disorder is characterized by hypogonadotropic hypogonadism, mental retardation, obesity, retinitis pigmentosa, hexadactyly, brachydactyly, or syndactyly. By age 30, most patients are blind.[813] Although most patients have evidence of GnRH deficiency, about 25% of afflicted males may have primary testicular failure.

Prader-Willi Syndrome

These patients have marked hyperphagia and obesity with retarded mental development, muscle hypotonia, and diabetes mellitus. Related conditions include micrognathia, absent auricular cartilage, and acromicria.[814] The condition has been ascribed to deletion or translocation of chromosome 15. In hypogonadal patients, bilateral cryptorchidism and absent scrotal folds are accompanied by evidence for attenuated GnRH secretion.[815] LH and FSH levels have been restored in some patients with chronic GnRH treatment. Defective oxytocin and vasopressin synthesis has also been reported.

Kallmann's Syndrome

Kallmann's syndrome consists of defective GnRH synthesis with olfactory nerve agenesis or hypoplasia and variable anosmia. Associated developmental disorders include optic atrophy, color blindness, eighth-nerve deafness, cleft palate, renal agenesis, cryptorchidism, and movement disorders.[816] This X-linked recessive disorder has been ascribed to a defective *KAL* gene located on chromosome Xp22.3.[817] The KAL protein mediates hypothalamic migration of GnRH cells from the primitive olfactory placode, and its absence leads to defective GnRH synthesis and anosmia.[818, 819] Both autosomal recessive and dominant forms of the disorder have been described, indicating the involvement of additional genetic factors in the pathogenesis of the disorder.

Clinical Features

These patients are exposed to low or absent sex steroids from birth. Consequently, females are tall and present with primary amenorrhea and absent secondary sexual development and males have delayed puberty and micropenis.[820]

Laboratory

Absent GnRH secretory pulses result in characteristically low LH and FSH levels in the presence of very low concentrations of estradiol or testosterone. Because the nonprimed normal pituitary may not respond initially to GnRH stimulation (25 to 100 μg intravenously), this test is of little value in distinguishing the hypothalamic defect. In some patients, repetitive GnRH priming may elicit normal pituitary LH and FSH responses, indicating a hypothalamic defect in GnRH secretion.

The differential diagnosis of congenital hypogonadotropic hypogonadism includes Kallmann's syndrome (*KAL* gene mutation), congenital adrenal hypoplasia (*DAX1* mutation),[821] GnRH receptor mutations, leptin and leptin receptor mutations, *PROP1* gene mutations, and mutations of the LH or FSH molecules themselves. These conditions are characterized by absent or low GnRH-mediated LH secretory patterns in the presence of a structurally normal pituitary gland. The cause of hypogonadotropic hypogonadism still remains elusive in over 80% of patients (see earlier). In the absence of a structural pituitary defect, genetic evaluation of these patients should be undertaken.

Acquired Pituitary Failure

Causes

In the absence of demonstrable hypothalamic-pituitary anatomic damage and after excluding genetic and syndromic causes of pituitary insufficiencies, acquired, often transient, causes of pituitary failure should be considered (Table 8–32). Causes of pituitary insufficiency including pituitary tumors, parasellar masses, hypophysitis, aneurysms, and pituitary apoplexy have already been discussed. Hypothalamic damage reflected by the presence of a large parasellar mass leading to decreased GnRH production is associated with hyperphagia, obesity, and central hypogonadism with low levels of FSH and LH (Fröhlich's syndrome). Marked caloric restriction, anorexia,[822, 823] weight loss of other etiologies, and strenuous exercise may attenuate GnRH secretion or action, or both. Hypogonadotropic hypogonadism may occur in both men and women (see Chapters 16 and 18). Exogenous anabolic steroid and glucocorticoid therapies suppress the reproductive and adrenal axes, respectively.

Patients with severe critical illnesses or chronic debilitating disease (including cirrhosis) may have impaired GH–IGF-I, adrenal, and gonadal axes. Hyperprolactinemia causes sexual dysfunction by inhibiting GnRH pulsatility through a short feedback loop. Hypothyroidism, hypoadrenalism, or hypogonadism causes hyperplasia of specific trophic cells related to lack of negative feedback and sometimes actual pituitary tumor formation.[824] The acquired immunodeficiency syndrome (AIDS) is associated with suppressed pituitary function independent of other associated infections. Drugs such as estrogens, which suppress FSH and LH, and GnRH analogues used for treating prostate cancer inhibit gonadotropin action. In addition to pituitary apoplexy, other vascular accidents such as aneurysms, strokes, cavernous sinus thrombosis, and arteritis can cause pituitary hormone insufficiency. Isolated pituitary hormone deficiencies may also occur as a manifestation of vascular abnormalities including arteritis.

Head Trauma

The pituitary gland may be partially or totally damaged by birth trauma, cranial hemorrhage, fetal asphyxia, or breech delivery. Head trauma may lead to direct pituitary damage by a sella turcica fracture, pituitary stalk section, trauma-induced

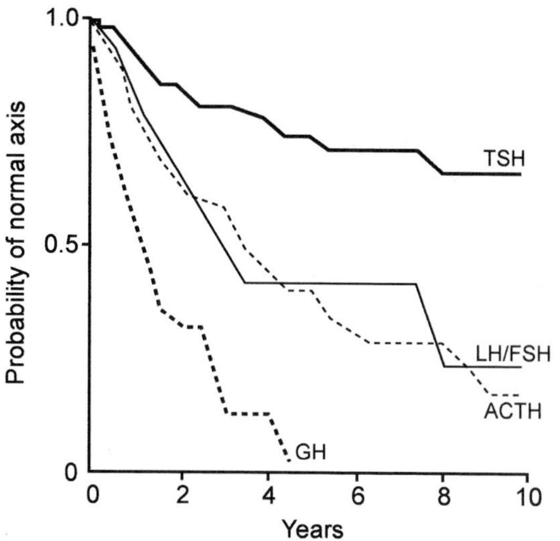

Figure 8–64. Life-table analysis indicating probabilities of initially normal hypothalamic–pituitary–target gland axes remaining normal after radiotherapy (3750 to 4250 cGy). Growth hormone (GH) secretion is the most sensitive of the anterior pituitary hormones to the effects of external radiotherapy, and TSH secretion is the most resistant. In two thirds of patients, gonadotropin deficiency develops before adrenocorticotropic hormone (ACTH) deficiency. The reverse occurs in the remaining third. (From Littley MD, Shalet SM, Beardwell CG, et al. Hypopituitarism following external radiotherapy for pituitary tumors in adults. Q J Med 1989; 70:145–160.)

vasospasm, or ischemic infarction after blunt trauma.[825] The most common traumatic cause of compromised pituitary function in the adult is iatrogenic neurosurgical trauma. Advertent or inadvertent pituitary manipulation or damage during surgery leads to transient or permanent diabetes insipidus and varying degrees of anterior pituitary dysfunction.

Although hypopituitarism after head trauma is usually manifest within a year after the insult, some patients may have overtly manifest signs of pituitary failure only after several decades. Seventy-five percent of patients with post-traumatic pituitary failure are men younger than 40 years who were involved in a motor vehicle accident within a year of diagnosis. Virtually all patients with subsequent pituitary failure have a history of loss of consciousness after trauma, and half of all such patients have documented skull fracture.[825] One third of these patients have demonstrable signs of hypothalamic or posterior pituitary hemorrhage or anterior lobe infarction on MRI. Diabetes insipidus is the most common endocrine disorder, encountered in about 30% of these patients. Gonadotropin failure, amenorrhea, and hyperprolactinemia may occur in the months following trauma or even years later.[826] Pituitary testing performed within the first 48 hours of hospital admission shows that about 75% of patients have evidence of hypopituitarism,[827] and the degree of pituitary failure correlates with the severity of head trauma.

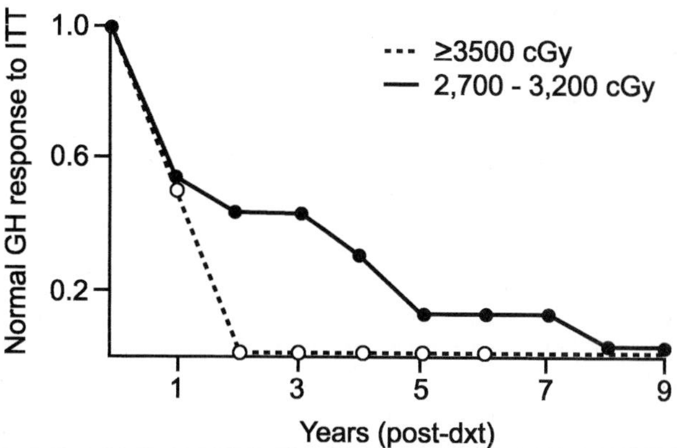

Figure 8–65. Incidence of growth hormone (GH) deficiency in children receiving 27 to 32 Gy or 35 Gy of cranial irradiation for a brain tumor in relation to time from irradiation (dxt). This illustrates that the speed at which individual pituitary hormone deficits develop is dose-dependent; the higher the radiation dose, the earlier GH deficiency occurs (Courtesy of the Department of Medical Illustrations, Wilkington Hospital, Manchester, England. From Shalet S. Pituitary failure. In DeGroot LJ, Jameson JL [eds]. Endocrinology, 4th ed. Philadelphia, WB Saunders, 2001.)

Radiation

Pituitary radiation, usually indicated as therapy for pituitary adenoma, directly causes atrophy of the gland in addition to the damaging impact of radiation on hypothalamic synthesis of hypophysiotropic hormones. Pituitary function in children and adolescents is particularly sensitive to head and neck therapeutic radiation.[291] Radiation dose exposure, time interval after completion of radiotherapy, and distance of the pituitary or hypothalamus from the central energy field correlate with the development of pituitary hormone deficits (Figs. 8–64 and 8–65).

After a median dose of 5000 rads directed at the skull base, nasopharynx, or cranium, up to 75% of patients experience pituitary insufficiency within 10 years.[828] Later manifestations of pituitary failure usually reflect hypothalamic damage rather than atrophy of irradiated pituitary cells. Although the degree of hormone loss after radiation is variable, the pattern of loss usually occurs sequentially with GH before FSH and LH followed by ACTH and TSH.[829] Thus, evidence for secondary thyroid or adrenal failure usually implies that the GH and gonadotropin axes are also compromised. Previously irradiated patients should therefore undergo lifelong periodic anterior pituitary hormone testing. Ideally, rigorous long-term screening should unmask incipient pituitary failure before the onset of morbidity.[830]

Empty Sella Syndrome

Damage to the sellar diaphragm may lead to arachnoid herniation into the sellar space. An empty sella may develop as a consequence of a primary congenital weakness of the diaphragm in patients in whom no secondary cause is evident. Up to 50% of patients with primary empty sella have associated benign intracranial hypertension.[831] A secondary empty sella may develop after infarction of a pituitary adenoma or surgical or radiation-induced damage to the sellar diaphragm. MRI usually exhibits demonstrable pituitary tissue compressed against the sellar floor with lateral stalk deviation. Although an empty sella is usually an incidental finding, if more than 90% of pituitary tissue is compressed or atrophied, pituitary failure occurs. About 10% of patients may have small adenomas secreting GH or PRL within the rim of compressed pituitary tissue.

Clinical Features of Hypopituitarism

The spectrum of clinical features of pituitary insufficiency depends on several factors. In acquired pituitary insufficiency, the clinical spectrum depends on the degree of hormone deficiency, the number of hormones impaired, and the rapidity of onset. In congenital forms, the earlier the age of onset, the greater the severity of thyroid, gonadal, adrenal, growth, or water disturbances. Heritable genetic disorders invariably exhibit the most severe phenotypic changes, although later changes may also occur in these disorders, as seen with *PROP1* mutations.

The resilience of the individual pituitary cell lineages in the presence of compressive, inflammatory, vascular, radiation, and invasive insults also differs. The lactotroph cell is often hyperfunctional as a result of decreased tonic inhibitory signals. PRL deficiency is thus exceedingly rare except for complete pituitary destruction or genetic syndromes. The order of diminished trophic hormone reserve function with pituitary compression usually is GH prior to the other trophic hormones. The corticotroph and thyrotroph cells appear particularly resistant to hypothalamic or pituitary destruction and are usually the last to lose function. The qualitative phenotypic manifestations of pituitary failure are determined by which specific trophic hormones are lost (see the preceding descriptions of individual hormone deficiencies) (Table 8–34).

Adrenocorticotropic Hormone

Clinical symptoms and signs of ACTH deficiency are most profound and life-threatening. With acute pituitary failure, such as may occur with pituitary apoplexy, patients with ACTH deficiency may present with hypotension, shock, hypoglycemia, nausea and vomiting, extreme fatigue and asthenia, and dilutional hyponatremia. Serum potassium is normal because these patients are deficient in glucocorticoids but usually not mineralocorticoids.

When acute ACTH deficiency is suspected clinically, treatment with steroids should not be withheld. Serum cortisol and ACTH should be determined before glucocorticoid administration and would be expected to be low. In an acute setting, such as sudden apoplexy, responses to Synacthen stimulation may be normal and misleading because the blunted response of cortisol usually seen in secondary adrenal insufficiency is due to loss of glucocorticoid-producing cells, which requires at least several weeks after the onset of ACTH deficiency. When ACTH deficiency occurs gradually, features are more insidious and include weight loss, asthenia, weakness, fatigue, nausea, and dilutional hyponatremia. This may be due to corticotroph dysfunction arising as a result of an enlarging pituitary tumor, delayed effects of radiation, damage related to pituitary tumor surgery, or removal of parasellar masses. In these cases, tests for ACTH reserve are likely to be blunted. If unsuspected or untreated, this form of adrenal insufficiency may also lead to death. Caution must be exercised in performing an ITT or metyrapone test because the latter can cause worsening of adrenal insufficiency and the former seizures and nausea. These tests should be done only in a hospital setting under supervision with available intravenous cortisone and glucose.

Steroid replacement doses should be appropriate to the clinical situation. Under conditions of major stress, such as pituitary apoplexy or pituitary surgery, maximal cortisone requirements range from 200 to 300 mg daily. Because the adrenal glands are incapable of increasing cortisol production during stress in the presence of deficient ACTH, an initial intravenous dose of 100 mg of hydrocortisone (Solu-Cortef) in acute adrenal insufficiency or an intravenous infusion of the same dose during pituitary surgery is followed by 50 mg intravenously every 6 hours for the first day. Similar doses are employed for other forms of major stress in patients with established secondary adrenal insufficiency.

Clinical judgment must be used in determining how long patients should be exposed to supraphysiologic doses of steroids. In our view, doses should be lowered to maintenance as soon as clinically feasible without endangering the patient. We employ replacement doses of 10 to 20 mg of hydrocortisone daily, usually 10 mg in the morning and 5 mg in the evening. An additional 5 mg is administered in the afternoon if needed clinically. Because surgical decompression may lead to recovery from hormone deficiencies,[161, 308] a clinical decision should be made postoperatively about whether to wean patients from hormonal replacement therapy and retest them hormone by hormone. Great care must be taken when secondary adrenal insufficiency has been previously documented.

Thyroid-Stimulating Hormone

Because the half-life of serum T_4 is 6.8 days, hypothyroidism may not become apparent for several weeks in patients with acute pituitary insufficiency; therefore, thyroid function should be tested expectantly. TSH is not elevated in secondary hypothyroidism and it cannot be used to assess the adequacy of thyroid hormone replacement, nor is a TRH test helpful. Severity of symptoms of hypothyroidism depends on the degree of hypothyroidism and length of time it has been present. Even in the absence of symptoms, T_4 should be administered if thyroid function studies are consistent with hypothyroidism. Glucocorticoids should be replaced before thyroid hormone because thyroid hormone in hypothyroid individuals increases the requirement for glucocorticoids in stressful situations.

Gonadotropins

Sexual dysfunction related to gonadotropin deficiency is far more common than hypothyroidism or hypoadrenalism in patients with pituitary disease. Its presence is established by the constellation of abnormal menses or amenorrhea with no elevated LH and FSH levels in women and sexual dysfunction in men with low testosterone and normal or low gonadotropin levels. Because even mild hyperprolactinemia may cause sexual dysfunction, it should be determined whether PRL is causing hypogonadism. Treatment with dopamine agonists may result in normal sexual function without the need to replace sex steroids. A GnRH stimulation test rarely differentiates causes of gonadotropin deficiency and is usually not indicated.

Sex steroid replacement in deficient patients has important effects on body composition in addition to normalizing sexual function. Testosterone replacement may not be as effective in normalizing sexual function in men with long-standing secondary hypogonadism and loss of libido as it is in men whose sexual dysfunction is recent. Osteoporosis is common in women deficient in estrogen and men deficient in testosterone,[832] and replacement improves bone density. Testosterone reduces abdominal and visceral fat and improves muscle mass in testosterone-deficient men.[833] Therefore, sex hormone replacement is important even though sexual function may not be normalized or is not desired.

Growth Hormone

GHD is discussed comprehensively earlier and is invariably present when two or more other trophic hormones are deficient.[837a]

Prolactin

PRL deficiency is extremely rare because it occurs only when the anterior pituitary is completely destroyed, as in patients after apoplexy, or in patients with congenital causes of PRL deficiency. When present, PRL deficiency prevents lactation.[234] In fact, PRL is often elevated in most forms of pituitary insufficiency. For example, many patients with preopera-

Table 8–34. Assessment of Anterior Pituitary Hyperfunction and Hypofunction

Name of Test	Method	Response
	TSH-Secreting Tumors	
TSH		Frankly elevated in 58% Measurable in normal range in others
Serum T_4		Elevated in most patients
Free T_4		Elevated in most patients
T_3		Elevated in most patients
α subunit		May be elevated
T_3 suppression test	RAI uptake before and after T_3 25 μg tid for 8 days	Incomplete suppression
TRH stimulation	200–500 μg IV over 1 min TSH and α subunit at 0, 30, 60, and 90 min	TSH response is blunted Molar ratio of α subunit/TSH >1
Pituitary MRI		Mostly macroadenomas, some microadenomas
Thyroid ultrasound		Goiter present in majority
IGF-I		Can be elevated if GH co-secreted
GH		Can be co-secreted
PRL		Can be co-secreted
ACTH		Can be co-secreted
	Acromegaly	
Serum GH		**Random measurement is not helpful because fluctuations are too wide.**
Serum IGF-I		Elevated for age and sex-matched controls
IGFBP-3		Elevated in most acromegaly patients; not as reliable as IGF-I
OGTT	75 g glucose solution hGH at 0, 30, 60, and 120 min	<1 ng/mL is probably within normal limits >1 ng/mL in most but not all acromegaly patients
TRH test	200–500 μg IV over 1 min hGH at 0, 30, 60 min	A minority of acromegaly patients have inappropriate GH elevation
Thyroid ultrasound		Often reveals goiter
Sleep studies		Consistent with obstructive sleep apnea
MRI of pituitary		Most have macroadenomas, a minority have microadenomas
EMG of wrists		Sometimes consistent with carpal tunnel syndrome
	ACTH Overproduction	
24-hour urinary free cortisol	HPLC RIA	Elevated Sometimes intermittent elevation
8 AM and 4 PM serum cortisol		Abnormal diurnal variation
Overnight 1 mg dexamethasone suppression test	1 mg dexamethasone at 11 PM the night before blood test	Should be <5 μg/dL Above 10 μg/dL c/w Cushing's syndrome
2 mg and 8 mg dexamethasone suppression test	Nothing on days, 1 and 2 0.5 mg q6h for 2 days 2.0 mg q6h for 2 days	2 mg: no suppression or partial suppression 8 mg: >90% suppression
CRH stimulation	100 μg IV draw ACTH and cortisol at 0, 15, and 30 min	ACTH: ≥34% increase c/w Cushing's syndrome Cortisol: 20% increase
CRH stimulation after 2 days of dexamethasone	100 μg IV or IM after 0.5 mg q6h	In Cushing's disease, cortisol >4 μg/dL
Bilateral inferior petrosal sinus sampling	CRH—measure ACTH from left and right petrosal sinuses and peripheral blood before and 3, 5, and 10 min after ovine CRH 1 μg/kg IV	Gradient post-CRH above 2.4–3.2 indicative of central Cushing's disease
	Gonadotropin-Secreting Tumors	
FSH	RIA	Usually normal, sometimes elevated—in which case LH is normal
LH	RIA	Usually normal, rarely elevated—with normal FSH
α-subunit		May be elevated
TRH	200–500 μg TRH IV over 1 min	LH, FSH, or α-subunit may be increased
	ACTH Deficiency	
ITT	0.1–0.15 U/kg IV	Peak cortisol response >20 μg/dL or increase by 10 μg/dL
Metyrapone test	Oral administration of 30 mg/kg at 11 PM	Peak 11-DOC ≥7 μg/dL

Table continued on following page

Table 8–34. Assessment of Anterior Pituitary Hyperfunction and Hypofunction *Continued*

Name of Test	Method	Response
CRH stimulation (limited utility)	100 μg IV	Peak ACTH ≥2–4-fold increase
Cortrosyn stimulation	250 μg IV or IM	Peak cortisol ≥20 μg/dL
Cortrosyn stimulation (low dose)	1 μg IV cortisol at 0, 30, and 60 min	>20 μg is normal
8 AM cortisol		>18 μg/dL goes firmly against ACTH deficiency
Urinary free cortisol 24-hour	RIA (only)	Normal range: 10 or 20 to 80 or 90 μg/24 hr depending on laboratory normal range; may be low in 2° secondary adrenal insufficiency
	TSH Deficiency	
Serum T_4		Low
Free T_4		Low
Serum T_3		Low
Serum TSH		Normal or low (not a good screening test for secondary or tertiary hypothyroidism)
RAI uptake		Not indicated
TRH test	200–500 μg IV over 1 min, TSH at 0, 30, and 60 min	Blunted in secondary hypothyroidism; partially blunted in tertiary with delayed response
	Growth Hormone Deficiency	**Mean Peak in GHD Patients**
ITT	See Table 8–21	0.6–0.95 ng/mL, depending on series
Arginine-GHRH	See Table 8–21	1.44 or 3.6 ng/mL, depending on series
Arginine-GHRH		3.6 ng/mL, depending on series
Hexarelin GHRH	See Table 8–21	2.6 ng/mL
L-Dopa	500 mg L-Dopa PO	1.4 ng/mL (median response) Not recommended for diagnosis
Arginine	IV over 30 min	2.6 ng/mL (median response) Not recommended as single test
IGF-I		IGF-I of <84 ng/mL strongly predicts GHD
Lipid panel		GHD patients frequently have hyperlipidemia
	Gonadotropin Deficiency	
LH and FSH		Normal or low in secondary hypogonadism High in primary hypogonadism
Testosterone		Below normal in presence of normal or low gonadotropins
GnRH test	100 μg IV	LH ≥2–3-fold FSH ≥1.5–2-fold
Clomiphene	50–100 mg PO bid for 5 days	LH ≥2–fold (F) (day 10–14) FSH ≥1.5–2-fold (F) (day 10–14) LH ≥ 50–250% (M) FSH ≥30–200% (M)

ACTH, adrenocorticotropic hormone; CRH, corticotropin-releasing hormone; FSH, follicle-stimulating hormone; GH, growth hormone; GHD, growth hormone deficiency; GHRH, GH-releasing hormone; GnRH, gonadotropin-releasing hormone; PRL, prolactin; T_3, triiodothyronine; T_4, thyroxine; TRH, thyrotropin-releasing hormone; TSH, thyrotropin. PRL hypersecretion is diagnosed by single serum measurement.

*Not a good screening test for secondary or tertiary hypothyroidism.

tive hyperprolactinemia related to tumor pressure on stalk structures continue to have hyperprolactinemia even after tumors are surgically debulked. Likewise, hyperprolactinemia occurs in 50% of patients treated with whole-brain radiation, the most common endocrine disturbance.[291]

Posterior Pituitary

Diabetes insipidus occurs frequently after pituitary surgery. Hyponatremia may also develop as the second of three phases of postoperative diabetes insipidus or may develop without evidence of diabetes insipidus after surgery. This subject is comprehensively covered in Chapter 9.

Screening for Pituitary Failure

The onset of hypopituitarism may be extremely slow, and subclinical pituitary failure is often not apparent to the patient or physician. Screening for pituitary dysfunction should be undertaken in patients with hypothalamic or pituitary mass lesions, developmental craniofacial abnormalities, inflammatory disorders, brain granulomatous disease, prior head or neck radiation, head trauma, prior skull base surgery, and newly discovered empty sella and in those who previously experienced pregnancy-associated hemorrhage or blood pressure changes.

Because hypopituitarism may develop insidiously and is often not readily clinically apparent, screening of appropriate patients is important to prevent long-term morbidity. Therefore, all patients harboring hypothalamic or pituitary masses should be screened for hypopituitarism. PRL should be measured because many patients with hypopituitarism also present with secondary hyperprolactinemia. Up to two thirds of patients harboring pituitary macroadenomas, craniopharyngiomas, and other parasellar lesions have compromised pituitary reserve function. Less commonly, patients with intrasellar aneurysms, pituitary metastases, parasellar meningiomas, optic gliomas, and hypothalamic astrocytomas also have pituitary failure. Although about a third of patients with hypopituitarism undergoing pituitary surgery recover function after decompression, about 25% of patients experience further loss of pituitary function after surgery and therefore should be screened annually. Treatment of pituitary failure was described fully earlier.

References

1. Bernard C. Physiologie; chiens rendus diabétiques. C R Soc Biol 1849; 1:60.
2. Marie P. On two cases of acromegaly: marked hypertrophy of the upper and lower limbs and the head. Rev Med 1886; 6:297–333.
3. Cushing H. Partial hypophysectomy for acromegaly: with remarks on the function of the hypophysis. Ann Surg 1909; 50: 1002–1017.
4. Cushing H. Surgical experiences with pituitary disorders. J Am Med Assoc 1914; 63:1515–1525.
5. Harris GW. Neural control of pituitary gland. Physiol Rev 1948; 28:139–179.
6. Chanson P, Daujat F, Young J, et al. Normal pituitary hypertrophy as a frequent cause of pituitary incidentaloma: a follow-up study. J Clin Endocrinol Metab 2001; 86:3009–3015.
7. Etchevers HC, Vincent C, Le Douarin NM, Couly GF. The cephalic neural crest provides pericytes and smooth muscle cells to all blood vessels of the face and forebrain. Development 2001; 128:1059–1068.
8. Takuma N, Sheng HZ, Furuta Y, et al. Formation of Rathke's pouch requires dual induction from the diencephalon. Development 1998; 125:4835–4840.
9. Gleiberman AS, Fedtsova NG, Rosenfeld MG. Tissue interactions in the induction of anterior pituitary: role of the ventral diencephalon, mesenchyme, and notochord. Dev Biol 1999; 213: 340–353.
10. Sheng HZ, Westphal H. Early steps in pituitary organogenesis. Trends Genet 1999; 15:236–240.
11. Dasen JS, O'Connell SM, Flynn SE, et al. Reciprocal interactions of Pit1 and GATA2 mediate signaling gradient- induced determination of pituitary cell types. Cell 1999; 97:587–598.
12. Andersen B, Rosenfeld MG. POU domain factors in the neuroendocrine system: lessons from developmental biology provide insights into human disease. Endocr Rev 2001; 22:2–35.
13. Treier M, Gleiberman AS, O'Connell SM, et al. Multistep signaling requirements for pituitary organogenesis in vivo. Genes Dev 1998; 12:1691–1704.
14. Asa SL, Kovacs K, Laszlo FA, et al. Human fetal adenohypophysis: histologic and immunocytochemical analysis. Neuroendocrinology 1986; 43:308–316.
15. Dubois PM, Hemming FJ. Fetal development and regulation of pituitary cell types. J Electron Microsc Tech 1991; 19:2–20.
16. Sheng HZ, Moriyama K, Yamashita T, et al. Multistep control of pituitary organogenesis. Science 1997; 278:1809–1812.
17. Sheng HZ, Zhadanov AB, Mosinger B Jr, et al. Specification of pituitary cell lineages by the LIM homeobox gene *Lhx3*. Science 1996; 272:1004–1007.
18. Lanctot C, Gauthier Y, Drouin J. Pituitary homeobox 1 (Ptx1) is differentially expressed during pituitary development. Endocrinology 1999; 140:1416–1422.
19. Semina EV, Datson NA, Leysens NJ, et al. Exclusion of epidermal growth factor and high-resolution physical mapping across the Rieger syndrome locus. Am J Hum Genet 1996; 59:1288–1296.
20. Lu MF, Pressman C, Dyer R, et al. Function of Rieger syndrome gene in left-right asymmetry and craniofacial development. Nature 1999; 401:276–278.
21. Martin D, Camper S. Genetic regulation of forebrain and pituitary development. In Rappaport R, Anselem S (eds). Hypothalamic-Pituitary Development: Genetic and Clinical Aspects, vol 4. Basel, Karger, 2001, p 1.
22. Muscatelli F, Strom TM, Walker AP, et al. Mutations in the *DAX-1* gene give rise to both X-linked adrenal hypoplasia congenita and hypogonadotropic hypogonadism. Nature 1994; 372: 672–676.
23. Tabarin A, Achermann JC, Recan D, et al. A novel mutation in *DAX1* causes delayed-onset adrenal insufficiency and incomplete hypogonadotropic hypogonadism. J Clin Invest 2000; 105:321–328.
24. Lamolet B, Pulichino AM, Lamonerie T, et al. A pituitary cell–restricted T box factor, Tpit, activates POMC transcription in cooperation with Pitx homeoproteins. Cell 2001; 104:849–859.
25. Stanfield JP. The blood supply of the human pituitary gland. J Anat 1960; 94:257–273.
26. Bergland RM, Page RB. Pituitary-brain vascular relations: a new paradigm. Science 1979; 204:18–24.
27. Musolino NR, Marino R Jr, Bronstein MD. Headache in acromegaly: dramatic improvement with the somatostatin analogue SMS 201–995. Clin J Pain 1990; 6:243–245.
28. Arafah BM, Prunty D, Ybarra J, et al. The dominant role of increased intrasellar pressure in the pathogenesis of hypopituitarism, hyperprolactinemia, and headaches in patients with pituitary adenomas. J Clin Endocrinol Metab 2000; 85:1789–1793.
29. Sano K. Incidence of primary tumors (1969–1983) In Brain Tumor Registry of Japan. Neurol Med Chir 1992; 37(Special Issue): 391–441.
30. Randall RV, Scheithauer BW, Kovacs K. Pituitary adenomas. In Thapar K, Kovacs K, Scheithauer BW, Lloyd RV (eds). Diagnosis and Management of Pituitary Tumors. Totowa, NJ, Humana Press, 2001, pp 1–12.
31. Thorner MO, Perryman RL, Cronin MJ, et al. Somatotroph hyperplasia: successful treatment of acromegaly by removal of a pancreatic islet tumor secreting a growth hormone–releasing factor. J Clin Invest 1982; 70:965–977.
32. Sano T, Asa SL, Kovacs K. Growth hormone–releasing hormone–producing tumors: clinical, biochemical, and morphological manifestations. Endocr Rev 1988; 9:357–373.
33. Mayo KE, Hammer RE, Swanson LW, et al. Dramatic pituitary hyperplasia in transgenic mice expressing a human growth hormone-releasing factor gene. Mol Endocrinol 1988; 2:606–612.
34. Herman V, Fagin J, Gonsky R, et al. Clonal origin of pituitary adenomas. J Clin Endocrinol Metab 1990; 71:1427–1433.
35. Schulte HM, Oldfield EH, Allolio B, et al. Clonal composition of pituitary adenomas in patients with Cushing's disease: determination by X-chromosome inactivation analysis. J Clin Endocrinol Metab 1991; 73:1302–1308.
36. Alexander JM, Biller BM, Bikkal H, et al. Clinically nonfunctioning pituitary tumors are monoclonal in origin. J Clin Invest 1990; 86:336–340.
37. Boggild MD, Jenkinson S, Pistorello M, et al. Molecular genetic studies of sporadic pituitary tumors. J Clin Endocrinol Metab 1994; 78:387–392.
38. Spada A, Vallar L. G-protein oncogenes in acromegaly. Horm Res 1992; 38:90–93.
39. Faglia G, Arosio M, Spada A. GS protein mutations and pituitary tumors: functional correlates and possible therapeutic implications. Metabolism 1996; 45:117–119.
40. Dotsch J, Kiess W, Hanze J, et al. Gs alpha mutation at codon 201 in pituitary adenoma causing gigantism in a 6-year-old boy with McCune-Albright syndrome. J Clin Endocrinol Metab 1996; 81:3839–3842.
41. Struthers RS, Vale WW, Arias C, et al. Somatotroph hypoplasia and dwarfism in transgenic mice expressing a non-phosphorylatable CREB mutant. Nature 1991; 350:622–624.
42. Bertherat J, Chanson P, Montminy M. The cyclic adenosine 3′,5′-monophosphate–responsive factor CREB is constitutively

activated in human somatotroph adenomas. Mol Endocrinol 1995; 9:777–783.
43. Karga HJ, Alexander JM, Hedley-Whyte ET, et al. *Ras* mutations in human pituitary tumors. J Clin Endocrinol Metab 1992; 74: 914–919.
44. Pei L, Melmed S, Scheithauer B, et al. H-*ras* mutations in human pituitary carcinoma metastases. J Clin Endocrinol Metab 1994; 78:842–846.
45. Herman V, Drazin NZ, Gonsky R, Melmed S. Molecular screening of pituitary adenomas for gene mutations and rearrangements. J Clin Endocrinol Metab 1993; 77:50–55.
46. Pei L, Melmed S. Isolation and characterization of a pituitary tumor-transforming gene (*PTTG*). Mol Endocrinol 1997; 11:433–441.
47. Zhang X, Horwitz GA, Heaney AP, et al. Pituitary tumor transforming gene (*PTTG*) expression in pituitary adenomas. J Clin Endocrinol Metab 1999; 84:761–767.
48. Heaney AP, Horwitz GA, Wang Z, et al. Early involvement of estrogen-induced pituitary tumor transforming gene and fibroblast growth factor expression in prolactinoma pathogenesis. Nat Med 1999; 5:1317–1321.
49. Zou H, McGarry TJ, Bernal T, Kirschner MW. Identification of a vertebrate sister-chromatid separation inhibitor involved in transformation and tumorigenesis. Science 1999; 285:418–422.
50. Yu R, Heaney AP, Lu W, et al. Pituitary tumor transforming gene causes aneuploidy and p53-dependent and p53-independent apoptosis. J Biol Chem 2000; 275:36502–36505.
51. Tanaka C, Kimura T, Yang P, et al. Analysis of loss of heterozygosity on chromosome 11 and infrequent inactivation of the *MEN1* gene in sporadic pituitary adenomas. J Clin Endocrinol Metab 1998; 83:2631–2634.
52. Tanaka C, Yoshimoto K, Yamada S, et al. Absence of germ-line mutations of the multiple endocrine neoplasia type 1 (*MEN1*) gene in familial pituitary adenoma in contrast to *MEN1* in Japanese. J Clin Endocrinol Metab 1998; 83:960–965.
53. Clayton RN, Boggild M, Bates AS, et al. Tumour suppressor genes in the pathogenesis of human pituitary tumours. Horm Res 1997; 47:185–193.
54. Prezant TR, Levine J, Melmed S. Molecular characterization of the men1 tumor suppressor gene in sporadic pituitary tumors. J Clin Endocrinol Metab 1998; 83:1388–1391.
55. Pei L, Melmed S, Scheithauer B, et al. Frequent loss of heterozygosity at the retinoblastoma susceptibility gene (RB) locus in aggressive pituitary tumors: evidence for a chromosome 13 tumor suppressor gene other than RB. Cancer Res 1995; 55:1613–1616.
56. Levy A, Hall L, Yeudall WA, Lightman SL. p53 gene mutations in pituitary adenomas: rare events. Clin Endocrinol (Oxf) 1994; 41:809–814.
57. Faccenda E, Melmed S, Bevan JS, Eidne KA. Structure of the thyrotrophin-releasing hormone receptor in human pituitary adenomas. Clin Endocrinol (Oxf) 1996; 44:341–347.
58. Kaye PV, Hapgood J, Millar RP. Absence of mutations in exon 3 of the GnRH receptor in human gonadotroph adenomas. Clin Endocrinol (Oxf) 1997; 47:549–554.
59. Hashimoto K, Koga M, Motomura T, et al. Identification of alternatively spliced messenger ribonucleic acid encoding truncated growth hormone–releasing hormone receptor in human pituitary adenomas. J Clin Endocrinol Metab 1995; 80:2933–2939.
60. Greenman Y, Prager D, Melmed S. The IGF-I receptor submembrane domain is intact in GH-secreting pituitary tumours. Clin Endocrinol (Oxf) 1995; 42:169–172.
61. Friedman E, Adams EF, Hoog A, et al. Normal structural dopamine type 2 receptor gene in prolactin-secreting and other pituitary tumors. J Clin Endocrinol Metab 1994; 78:568–574.
62. Atkin SL, Landolt AM, Jeffreys RV, et al. Basic fibroblastic growth factor stimulates prolactin secretion from human anterior pituitary adenomas without affecting adenoma cell proliferation. J Clin Endocrinol Metab 1993; 77:831–837.
63. Li Y, Koga M, Kasayama S, et al. Identification and characterization of high molecular weight forms of basic fibroblast growth factor in human pituitary adenomas. J Clin Endocrinol Metab 1992; 75:1436–1441.
64. Shimon I, Huttner A, Said J, et al. Heparin-binding secretory transforming gene (*hst*) facilitates rat lactotrope cell tumorigenesis and induces prolactin gene transcription. J Clin Invest 1996; 97: 187–195.
65. Gonsky R, Herman V, Melmed S, Fagin J. Transforming DNA sequences present in human prolactin-secreting pituitary tumors. Mol Endocrinol 1991; 5:1687–1695.
66. Shimon I, Hinton DR, Weiss MH, Melmed S. Prolactinomas express human heparin-binding secretory transforming gene (*hst*) protein product: marker of tumour invasiveness. Clin Endocrinol (Oxf) 1998; 48:23–29.
67. Casey M, Vaughan CJ, He J, et al. Mutations in the protein kinase A R1alpha regulatory subunit cause familial cardiac myxomas and Carney complex. J Clin Invest 2000; 106:R31-R38.
68. Kirschner LS, Carney JA, Pack SD, et al. Mutations of the gene encoding the protein kinase A type I-alpha regulatory subunit in patients with the Carney complex. Nat Genet 2000; 26:89–92.
69. Kovacs K, Horvath E, Stefaneanu L, et al. Pituitary adenoma producing growth hormone and adrenocorticotropin: a histological, immunocytochemical, electron microscopic, and in situ hybridization study. Case report. J Neurosurg 1998; 88:1111–1115.
70. Saccomanno K, Bassetti M, Lania A, et al. Immunodetection of glycoprotein hormone subunits in nonfunctioning and glycoprotein hormone–secreting pituitary adenomas. J Endocrinol Invest 1997; 20:59–64.
71. Mukherjee JJ, Islam N, Kaltsas G, et al. Clinical, radiological and pathological features of patients with Rathke's cleft cysts: tumors that may recur. J Clin Endocrinol Metab 1997; 82:2357–2362.
72. Saeki N, Tamaki K, Murai H, et al. Long-term outcome of endocrine function in patients with neurohypophyseal germinomas. Endocr J 2000; 47:83–89.
73. el-Mahdy W, Powell M. Transsphenoidal management of 28 symptomatic Rathke's cleft cysts, with special reference to visual and hormonal recovery. Neurosurgery 1998; 42:7–16; discussion 16–17.
74. Inoue T, Fukui M, Nishio S, et al. Hyperosmotic blood-brain barrier disruption in brains of rats with an intracerebrally transplanted RG-C6 tumor. J Neurosurg 1987; 66:256–263.
75. Freda PU, Wardlaw SL, Post KD. Unusual causes of sellar/parasellar masses in a large transsphenoidal surgical series. J Clin Endocrinol Metab 1996; 81:3455-3459.
76. Cohen JE, Abdallah JA, Garrote M. Massive rupture of suprasellar dermoid cyst into ventricles: case illustration. J Neurosurg 1997; 87:963.
77. Lewis AJ, Cooper PW, Kassel EE, Schwartz ML. Squamous cell carcinoma arising in a suprasellar epidermoid cyst: case report. J Neurosurg 1983; 59:538–541.
78. Schaller B, Kirsch E, Tolnay M, Mindermann T. Symptomatic granular cell tumor of the pituitary gland: case report and review of the literature. Neurosurgery 1998; 42:166–170; discussion 170–171.
79. Volpe R, Mazabraud A. A clinicopathologic review of 25 cases of chordoma (a pleomorphic and metastasizing neoplasm). Am J Surg Pathol 1983; 7:161–170.
80. Rosenberg AE, Nielsen GP, Keel SB, et al. Chondrosarcoma of the base of the skull: a clinicopathologic study of 200 cases with emphasis on its distinction from chordoma. Am J Surg Pathol 1999; 23:1370–1378.
81. Weiner HL, Wisoff JH, Rosenberg ME, et al. Craniopharyngiomas: a clinicopathological analysis of factors predictive of recurrence and functional outcome. Neurosurgery 1994; 35:1001–1010; discussion 1010–1011.
82. Fahlbusch R, Honegger J, Paulus W, et al. Surgical treatment of craniopharyngiomas: experience with 168 patients. J Neurosurg 1999; 90:237–250.
83. Honegger J, Buchfelder M, Fahlbusch R. Surgical treatment of craniopharyngiomas: endocrinological results. J Neurosurg 1999; 90:251–257.
84. Nozaki K, Nagata I, Yoshida K, Kikuchi H. Intrasellar meningioma: case report and review of the literature. Surg Neurol 1997; 47:447–452; discussion 452–454.
85. Beems T, Grotenhuis JA, Wesseling P. Meningioma of the pituitary stalk without dural attachment: case report and review of the literature. Neurosurgery 1999; 45:1474–1477.
86. Collet-Solberg PF, Sernyak H, Satin-Smith M, et al. Endocrine outcome in long-term survivors of low-grade hypothalamic/chiasmatic glioma. Clin Endocrinol (Oxf) 1997; 47:79–85.
87. Gokalp HZ, Deda H, Baskaya MK, et al. Pituitary abscesses: report of three cases. Neurosurg Rev 1994; 17:199–203.
88. Wolansky LJ, Gallagher JD, Heary RF, et al. MRI of pituitary

abscess: two cases and review of the literature. Neuroradiology 1997; 39:499–503.
89. Jain KC, Varma A, Mahapatra AK. Pituitary abscess: a series of six cases. Br J Neurosurg 1997; 11:139–143.
90. Freda PU, Post KD. Differential diagnosis of sellar masses. Endocrinol Metab Clin North Am 1999; 28:81–117, vi.
91. Telzak EE, Cote RJ, Gold JW, et al. Extrapulmonary *Pneumocystis carinii* infections. Rev Infect Dis 1990; 12:380–386.
92. Ashkan K, Papadopoulos MC, Casey AT, et al. Sellar tuberculoma: report of two cases. Acta Neurochir 1997; 139:523–525.
93. Berger SA, Edberg SC, David G. Infectious disease in the sella turcica. Rev Infect Dis 1986; 8:747–755.
94. Gazioglu N, Ak H, Oz B, et al. Silent pituitary tuberculoma associated with pituitary adenoma. Acta Neurochir 1999; 141: 785–786.
95. Landman RE, Wardlaw SL, McConnell RJ, et al. Pituitary lymphoma presenting as fever of unknown origin. J Clin Endocrinol Metab 2001; 86:1470–1476.
96. Au WY, Kwong YL, Shek TW, et al. Diffuse large-cell B-cell lymphoma in a pituitary adenoma: an unusual cause of pituitary apoplexy. Am J Hematol 2000; 63:231–232.
97. Newman LS, Rose CS, Maier LA. Sarcoidosis. N Engl J Med 1997; 336:1224–1234.
98. Bell NH. Endocrine complications of sarcoidosis. Endocrinol Metab Clin North Am 1991; 20:645–654.
99. Sharma OP. Neurosarcoidosis: a personal perspective based on the study of 37 patients. Chest 1997; 112:220–228.
100. Pitale SU, Camacho PM, Gordon DL. Central nervous system involvement in sarcoidosis presenting as a recurrent pituitary mass. Endocrinologist 2000; 10:429–431.
101. Kaltsas GA, Powles TB, Evanson J, et al. Hypothalamo-pituitary abnormalities in adult patients with Langerhans cell histiocytosis: clinical, endocrinological, and radiological features and response to treatment. J Clin Endocrinol Metab 2000; 85:1370–1376.
102. Braunstein GD, Kohler PO. Pituitary function in Hand-Schüller-Christian disease: evidence for deficient growth-hormone release in patients with short stature. N Engl J Med 1972; 286:1225–1229.
103. Vadakekalam J, Stamos T, Shenker Y. Sometimes the hooves do belong to zebras! An unusual case of hypopituitarism. J Clin Endocrinol Metab 1995; 80:17–20.
104. Max MB, Deck MD, Rottenberg DA. Pituitary metastasis: incidence in cancer patients and clinical differentiation from pituitary adenoma. Neurology 1981; 31:998–1002.
105. Losa M, Grasso M, Giugni E, et al. Metastatic prostatic adenocarcinoma presenting as a pituitary mass: shrinkage of the lesion and clinical improvement with medical treatment. Prostate 1997; 32:241–245.
106. Schubiger O, Haller D. Metastases to the pituitary-hypothalamic axis: an MR study of 7 symptomatic patients. Neuroradiology 1992; 34:131–134.
107. Braun J, Schuldes H, Berkefeld J, et al. Panhypopituitarism associated with severe retroperitoneal fibrosis. Clin Endocrinol (Oxf) 2001; 54:273–276.
108. Asa SL, Bilbao JM, Kovacs K, et al. Lymphocytic hypophysitis of pregnancy resulting in hypopituitarism: a distinct clinicopathologic entity. Ann Intern Med 1981; 95:166–171.
109. Cosman F, Post KD, Holub DA, Wardlaw SL. Lymphocytic hypophysitis: report of 3 new cases and review of the literature. Medicine (Baltimore) 1989; 68:240–256.
110. Lee JH, Laws ER Jr, Guthrie BL, et al. Lymphocytic hypophysitis: occurrence in two men. Neurosurgery 1994; 34:159–162; discussion 162–163.
111. Ezzat S. Acromegaly. Endocrinol Metab Clin North Am 1997; 26:703–723.
112. Thodou E, Asa SL, Kontogeorgos G, et al. Clinical case seminar: lymphocytic hypophysitis: clinicopathological findings. J Clin Endocrinol Metab 1995; 80:2302–2311.
113. Gillam M. Lymphocytic hypophysitis. In Bronstein MD (ed). Pituitary Tumor in Pregnancy, vol 131. Boston, Kluwer, 2001, pp 131–148.
114. Unluhizarci K, Bayram F, Colak R, et al. Distinct radiological and clinical appearance of lymphocytic hypophysitis. J Clin Endocrinol Metab 2001; 86:1861–1864.
115. Gagneja H, Arafah B, Taylor HC. Histologically proven lymphocytic hypophysitis: spontaneous resolution and subsequent pregnancy. Mayo Clin Proc 1999; 74:150–154.
116. Ishihara T, Hino M, Kurahachi H, et al. Long-term clinical course of two cases of lymphocytic adenohypophysitis. Endocr J 1996; 43:433–440.
117. Lee YJ, Lin JC, Shen EY, et al. Loss of visibility of the neurohypophysis as a sign of central diabetes insipidus. Eur J Radiol 1996; 21:233–235.
118. Muir A, Maclaren NK. Autoimmune diseases of the adrenal glands, parathyroid glands, gonads, and hypothalamic-pituitary axis. Endocrinol Metab Clin North Am 1991; 20:619–644.
119. Crock PA. Cytosolic autoantigens in lymphocytic hypophysitis. J Clin Endocrinol Metab 1998; 83:609–618.
120. Nishiki M, Murakami Y, Ozawa Y, Kato Y. Serum antibodies to human pituitary membrane antigens in patients with autoimmune lymphocytic hypophysitis and infundibuloneurohypophysitis. Clin Endocrinol (Oxf) 2001; 54:327–333.
121. Jensen MD, Handwerger BS, Scheithauer BW, et al. Lymphocytic hypophysitis with isolated corticotropin deficiency. Ann Intern Med 1986; 105:200–203.
122. Burke CW, Moore RA, Rees LH, et al. Isolated ACTH deficiency and TSH deficiency in the adult. J R Soc Med 1979; 72: 328–335.
123. Honegger J, Fahlbusch R, Bornemann A, et al. Lymphocytic and granulomatous hypophysitis: experience with nine cases. Neurosurgery 1997; 40:713–722; discussion 722–723.
124. Shimizu C, Kubo M, Kijima H, et al. Giant cell granulomatous hypophysitis with remarkable uptake on gallium- 67 scintigraphy. Clin Endocrinol (Oxf) 1998; 49:131–134.
125. Hayashi H, Yamada K, Kuroki T, et al. Lymphocytic hypophysitis and pulmonary sarcoidosis: report of a case. Am J Clin Pathol 1991; 95:506–511.
126. Toth M, Szabo P, Racz K, et al. Granulomatous hypophysitis associated with Takayasu's disease. Clin Endocrinol (Oxf) 1996; 45:499–503.
127. Daily PO, Jones B, Folkerth TL, et al. Comparison of myocardial temperatures with multidose cardioplegia versus single-dose cardioplegia and myocardial surface cooling during coronary artery bypass grafting. J Thorac Cardiovasc Surg 1989; 97:715–724.
128. Maccagnan P, Macedo CL, Kayath MJ, et al. Conservative management of pituitary apoplexy: a prospective study. J Clin Endocrinol Metab 1995; 80:2190–2197.
129. Abucham J, Castro V, Maccagnan P, Vieira JG. Increased thyrotrophin levels and loss of the nocturnal thyrotrophin surge in Sheehan's syndrome. Clin Endocrinol (Oxf) 1997; 47:515–522.
130. Yen SSC. Chronic anovulation due to CNS-hypothalamic dysfunction. In Yen SSC, Jaffe RB (eds). Reproductive Endocrinology: Physiology, Pathophysiology and Clinical Management, 3rd ed. Philadelphia, WB Saunders, 1991, pp 631–688.
131. Arafah BM, Harrington JF, Madhoun ZT, Selman WR. Improvement of pituitary function after surgical decompression for pituitary tumor apoplexy. J Clin Endocrinol Metab 1990; 71:323–328.
132. Wakai S, Fukushima T, Teramoto A, Sano K. Pituitary apoplexy: its incidence and clinical significance. J Neurosurg 1981; 55:187–193.
133. Cardoso ER, Peterson EW. Pituitary apoplexy: a review. Neurosurgery 1984; 14:363–373.
134. Ebersold MJ, Laws ER Jr, Scheithauer BW, Randall RV. Pituitary apoplexy treated by transsphenoidal surgery: a clinicopathological and immunocytochemical study. J Neurosurg 1983; 58: 315–320.
135. Bills DC, Meyer FB, Laws ER Jr, et al. A retrospective analysis of pituitary apoplexy. Neurosurgery 1993; 33:602–608; discussion 608–609.
136. Lam KS, Sham MM, Tam SC, et al. Hypopituitarism after tuberculous meningitis in childhood. Ann Intern Med 1993; 118: 701–706.
137. Case records of the Massachusetts General Hospital. Weekly clinicopathological exercises. Case 17-1980. N Engl J Med 1980; 302:1015–1023.
138. Van Hilten BJ, Roos RA, De Bakker HM, De Beer FC. Periodic fever: an unusual manifestation of a recurrent Rathke's cleft. J Neurol Neurosurg Psychiatry 1990; 53:533.
139. Macpherson P, Hadley DM, Teasdale E, Teasdale G. Pituitary microadenomas: does gadolinium enhance their demonstration? Neuroradiology 1989; 31:293–298.

140. Witte RJ, Mark LP, Daniels DL, Haughton VM. Radiographic evaluation of the pituitary and anterior hypothalamus. In DeGroot LJ, Jameson JL (eds). Endocrinology. Philadelphia, WB Saunders, 2001, pp 257–268.
141. Kucharczyk W, Peck WW, Kelly WM, et al. Rathke cleft cysts: CT, MR imaging, and pathologic features. Radiology 1987; 165: 491–495.
142. Elster AD, Chen MY, Williams DW III, Key LL. Pituitary gland: MR imaging of physiologic hypertrophy in adolescence. Radiology 1990; 174:681–685.
143. Wolpert SM, Molitch ME, Goldman JA, Wood JB. Size, shape, and appearance of the normal female pituitary gland. AJR 1984; 143:377–381.
144. FitzPatrick M, Tartaglino LM, Hollander MD, et al. Imaging of sellar and parasellar pathology. Radiol Clin North Am 1999; 37: 101–121, x.
145. Pressman BD. Pituitary imaging. In Melmed S (ed). The Pituitary, 2nd ed. Malden, Mass, Blackwell Scientific, 2002, pp 663–686.
146. Kucharczyk W, Lenkinski RE, Kucharczyk J, Henkelman RM. The effect of phospholipid vesicles on the NMR relaxation of water: an explanation for the MR appearance of the neurohypophysis? AJNR 1990; 11:693–700.
147. Elster AD, DiPersio DA. Cranial postoperative site: assessment with contrast-enhanced MR imaging. Radiology 1990; 174:93–98.
148. Elster AD, Sanders TG, Vines FS, Chen MY. Size and shape of the pituitary gland during pregnancy and post partum: measurement with MR imaging. Radiology 1991; 181:531–535.
149. Turner HE, Nagy Z, Gatter KC, et al. Angiogenesis in pituitary adenomas and the normal pituitary gland. J Clin Endocrinol Metab 2000; 85:1159–1162.
150. de Herder WW, Reijs AE, Kwekkeboom DJ, et al. In vivo imaging of pituitary tumours using a radiolabelled dopamine D2 receptor radioligand. Clin Endocrinol (Oxf) 1996; 45:755–767.
151. Arnold A. Neuroophthalmologic evaluation of pituitary disorders. In Melmed S (ed). The Pituitary, 2nd ed. Malden, Mass, Blackwell Scientific, 2002, pp 687–708.
152. Hoyt WF. Correlative functional anatomy of the optic chiasm—1969. Clin Neurosurg 1970; 17:189–208.
153. Henderson WR. The pituitary adenomata: a follow-up study of the surgical results in 338 cases. Br J Surg 1939; 26:811–921.
154. Anderson D, Faber P, Marcovitz S, et al. Pituitary tumors and the ophthalmologist. Ophthalmology 1983; 90:1265–1270.
155. Poon A, McNeill P, Harper A, O'Day J. Patterns of visual loss associated with pituitary macroadenomas. Aust NZ J Ophthalmol 1995; 23:107–115.
156. Ikeda H, Yoshimoto T. Visual disturbances in patients with pituitary adenoma. Acta Neurol Scand 1995; 92:157–160.
157. Schloffer H. Erfolgreiche operation eines hypohysentumors auf nasalem wege. Wien Klin Wochenschr 1907; 20:621.
158. Fahlbusch R, Thapar K. New developments in pituitary surgical techniques. Baillieres Best Pract Res Clin Endocrinol Metab 1999; 13:471–484.
159. Steinmeier R, Fahlbusch R, Ganslandt O, et al. Intraoperative magnetic resonance imaging with the magnetom open scanner: concepts, neurosurgical indications, and procedures: a preliminary report. Neurosurgery 1998; 43:739–747; discussion 747–748.
160. Jho HD, Carrau RL, Ko Y, Daly MA. Endoscopic pituitary surgery: an early experience. Surg Neurol 1997; 47:213–222; discussion 222–223.
161. Webb SM, Rigla M, Wagner A, et al. Recovery of hypopituitarism after neurosurgical treatment of pituitary adenomas. J Clin Endocrinol Metab 1999; 84:3696–3700.
162. Cusick JF, Hagen TC, Findling JW. Inappropriate secretion of antidiuretic hormone after transsphenoidal surgery for pituitary tumors. N Engl J Med 1984; 311:36–38.
163. Olson BR, Rubino D, Gumowski J, Oldfield EH. Isolated hyponatremia after transsphenoidal pituitary surgery. J Clin Endocrinol Metab 1995; 80:85–91.
164. Guinan EM, Lowy C, Stanhope N, et al. Cognitive effects of pituitary tumours and their treatments: two case studies and an investigation of 90 patients. J Neurol Neurosurg Psychiatry 1998; 65:870–876.
165. Peace KA, Orme SM, Padayatty SJ, et al. Cognitive dysfunction in patients with pituitary tumour who have been treated with transfrontal or transsphenoidal surgery or medication. Clin Endocrinol (Oxf) 1998; 49:391–396.
166. Jalali R, Brada M, Perks JR, et al. Stereotactic conformal radiotherapy for pituitary adenomas: technique and preliminary experience. Clin Endocrinol (Oxf) 2000; 52:695–702.
167. Landolt AM, Haller D, Lomax N, et al. Stereotactic radiosurgery for recurrent surgically treated acromegaly: comparison with fractionated radiotherapy. J Neurosurg 1998; 88:1002–1008.
168. Barrande G, Pittino-Lungo M, Coste J, et al. Hormonal and metabolic effects of radiotherapy in acromegaly: long-term results in 128 patients followed in a single center. J Clin Endocrinol Metab 2000; 85:3779–3785.
169. McCord MW, Buatti JM, Fennell EM, et al. Radiotherapy for pituitary adenoma: long-term outcome and sequelae. Int J Radiat Oncol Biol Phys 1997; 39:437–444.
170. Brada M, Rajan B, Traish D, et al. The long-term efficacy of conservative surgery and radiotherapy in the control of pituitary adenomas. Clin Endocrinol (Oxf) 1993; 38:571–578.
171. Biermasz NR, van Dulken H, Roelfsema F. Long-term follow-up results of postoperative radiotherapy in 36 patients with acromegaly. J Clin Endocrinol Metab 2000; 85:2476–2482.
172. Simmons NE, Laws ER Jr. Glioma occurrence after sellar irradiation: case report and review. Neurosurgery 1998; 42:172–178.
173. Erfurth EM, Bulow B, Mikoczy Z, Hagmar L. Incidence of a second tumor in hypopituitary patients operated for pituitary tumors. J Clin Endocrinol Metab 2001; 86:659–662.
174. Brada M, Ford D, Ashley S, et al. Risk of second brain tumour after conservative surgery and radiotherapy for pituitary adenoma. BMJ 1992; 304:1343–1346.
175. Tsang RW, Laperriere NJ, Simpson WJ, et al. Glioma arising after radiation therapy for pituitary adenoma: a report of four patients and estimation of risk. Cancer 1993; 72:2227–2233.
176. Millar JL, Spry NA, Lamb DS, Delahunt J. Blindness in patients after external beam irradiation for pituitary adenomas: two cases occurring after small daily fractional doses. Clin Oncol (R Coll Radiol) 1991; 3:291–294.
177. Jones JI, D'Ercole AJ, Camacho-Hubner C, Clemmons DR. Phosphorylation of insulin-like growth factor (IGF)-binding protein 1 in cell culture and in vivo: effects on affinity for IGF-I. Proc Natl Acad Sci USA 1991; 88:7481–7485.
178. al-Mefty O, Kersh JE, Routh A, Smith RR. The long-term side effects of radiation therapy for benign brain tumors in adults. J Neurosurg 1990; 73:502–512.
179. Peace KA, Orme SM, Sebastian JP, et al. The effect of treatment variables on mood and social adjustment in adult patients with pituitary disease. Clin Endocrinol (Oxf) 1997; 46:445–450.
180. Scheithauer BW, Sano T, Kovacs KT, et al. The pituitary gland in pregnancy: a clinicopathologic and immunohistochemical study of 69 cases. Mayo Clin Proc 1990; 65:461–474.
181. Burrows HL, Birkmeier TS, Seasholtz AF, Camper SA. Targeted ablation of cells in the pituitary primordia of transgenic mice. Mol Endocrinol 1996; 10:1467–1477.
182. Boockfor FR, Hoeffler JP, Frawley LS. Estradiol induces a shift in cultured cells that release prolactin or growth hormone. Am J Physiol 1986; 250:E103-E105.
183. Stricker S, Grueter F. Action du lobe antérieur de l'hypophyse sur la montée laiteuse. C R Soc Biol 1928; 99:1978–1980.
184. Riddle O. Prolactin in vertebrate function and organization. J Natl Cancer Inst 1963; 31:1039–1110.
185. Riddle O, Bates RW, Dykshorn SW. The preparation, identification and assay of prolactin: a hormone of the anterior pituitary. Am J Physiol 1933; 105:191–216.
186. Wilhelmi AE. Fractionation of human pituitary glands. Can J Biochem 1961; 39:1659–1668.
187. Suganuma N, Seo H, Yamamoto N, et al. Ontogenesis of pituitary prolactin in the human fetus. J Clin Endocrinol Metab 1986; 63:156–161.
188. Thorner MO, Vance ML, Laws ER Jr, et al. The anterior pituitary. In Wilson JD, Foster DW (eds). Williams Textbook of Endocrinology. Philadelphia, WB Saunders, 1998, pp 249–340.
189. Kleinberg DL, Frantz AG. A sensitive in vitro assay for prolactin. Program of the 51st Meeting of the Endocrine Society, 1969, pp 32–32.
190. Frantz AG, Kleinberg DL. Prolactin: evidence that it is separate from growth hormone in human blood. Science 1970; 170:745–747.

191. Kleinberg DL, Frantz AG. Human prolactin: measurement in plasma by in vitro bioassay. J Clin Invest 1971; 50:1557–1568.
192. Hwang P, Guyda H, Friesen H. A radioimmunoassay for human prolactin. Proc Natl Acad Science USA 1971; 68:1902–1906.
193. Friesen HG. The discovery of human prolactin: a very personal account. Clin Invest Med 1995; 18:66–72.
194. Owerbach D, Rutter WJ, Cooke NE, et al. The prolactin gene is located on chromosome 6 in humans. Science 1981; 212:815–816.
195. Cooke NE, Coit D, Weiner RI, et al. Structure of cloned DNA complementary to rat prolactin messenger RNA. J Biol Chem 1980; 255:6502–6510.
196. Lamberts SW, Macleod RM. Regulation of prolactin secretion at the level of the lactotroph. Physiol Rev 1990; 70:279–318.
197. Farkouh NH, Packer MG, Frantz AG. Large molecular size prolactin with reduced receptor activity in human serum: high proportion in basal state and reduction after thyrotropin-releasing hormone. J Clin Endocrinol Metab 1979; 48:1026–1032.
198. Sinha YN. Structural variants of prolactin: occurrence and physiological significance. Endocr Rev 1995; 16:354–369.
199. Suh HK, Frantz AG. Size heterogeneity of human prolactin in plasma and pituitary extracts. J Clin Endocrinol Metab 1974; 39:928–935.
200. Lewis UJ, Singh RN, Sinha YN, VanderLaan WP. Glycosylated human prolactin. Endocrinology 1985; 116:359–363.
201. Mittra I. A novel "cleaved prolactin" in the rat pituitary: part I. Biosynthesis, characterization and regulatory control. Biochem Biophys Res Commun 1980; 95:1750–1759.
202. Lee H, Struman I, Clapp C, et al. Inhibition of urokinase activity by the antiangiogenic factor 16K prolactin: activation of plasminogen activator inhibitor 1 expression. Endocrinol 1998; 139:3696–3703.
203. Ferrara N, Clapp C, Weiner R. The 16K fragment of prolactin specifically inhibits basal or fibroblast growth factor stimulated growth of capillary endothelial cells. Endocrinology 1991; 129:896–900.
204. Kline JB, Clevenger CV. Identification and characterization of the prolactin-binding protein in human serum and milk. J Biol Chem 2001; 276:24760–24766.
205. Liu JW, Ben Jonathan N. Prolactin-releasing activity of neurohypophysial hormones: structure-function relationship. Endocrinology 1994; 134:114–118.
206. Horseman ND. Prolactin. In DeGroot LJ, Jameson JL (eds). Endocrinology. Philadelphia, WB Saunders, 2001 pp 209–220.
207. Horseman ND, Zhao W, Montecino-Rodriguez E, et al. Defective mammopoiesis, but normal hematopoiesis, in mice with targeted disruption of the prolactin gene. EMBO J 1997; 16:6926–6935.
208. Steger RW, Chandrashekar V, Zhao W, et al. Neuroendocrine and reproductive functions in male mice with targeted disruption of the prolactin gene. Endocrinology 1998; 139:3691–3695.
209. Kanyicska B, Lerant A, Freeman ME. Endothelin is an autocrine regulator of prolactin secretion. Endocrinology 1998; 139:5164–5173.
210. Sarkar DK, Kim KH, Minami S. Transforming growth factor-beta 1 messenger RNA and protein expression in the pituitary gland: its action on prolactin secretion and lactotropic growth. Mol Endocrinol 1992; 6:1825–1833.
211. Shah GV, Pedchenko V, Stanley S, et al. Calcitonin is a physiological inhibitor of prolactin secretion in ovariectomized female rats. Endocrinology 1996; 137:1814–1822.
212. Ben Jonathan N. Regulation of prolactin secretion. In Imura H (ed). The Pituitary Gland. New York, Raven Press, 1994, pp 261–283.
213. Hinuma S, Habata Y, Fujii R, et al. A prolactin-releasing peptide in the brain [published erratum appears in Nature 1998; 394:302]. Nature 1998; 393:272–276.
214. Rubinek T, Hadani M, Barkai G, et al. Prolactin (PRL)-releasing peptide stimulates PRL secretion from human fetal pituitary cultures and growth hormone release from cultured pituitary adenomas. J Clin Endocrinol Metab 2001; 86:2826–2830.
215. Reichlin S. TRH: historical aspects. Ann NY Acad Sci 1989; 553:1–6.
216. Cooke NE. Prolactin: normal synthesis, regulation, and actions. In DeGroot LJ, Besser GM, Cahill GFJ (eds). Endocrinology. Philadelphia, WB Saunders, 1989, pp 384–407.
217. Katznelson L, Riskind PN, Saxe VC, Klibanski A. Prolactin pulsatile characteristics in postmenopausal women. J Clin Endocrinol Metab 1998; 83:761–764.
218. Bredow S, Kacsoh B, Obal F Jr, et al. Increase of prolactin mRNA in the rat hypothalamus after intracerebroventricular injection of VIP or PACAP. Brain Res 1994; 660:301–308.
219. Peters LL, Hoefer MT, Ben-Jonathan N. The posterior pituitary: regulation of anterior pituitary prolactin secretion. Science 1981; 213:659–661.
220. Asa SL, Kelly MA, Grandy DK, Low MJ. Pituitary lactotroph adenomas develop after prolonged lactotroph hyperplasia in dopamine D2 receptor–deficient mice. Endocrinology 1999; 140:5348–5355.
221. Bazan JF. Structural design and molecular evolution of a cytokine receptor superfamily. Proc Natl Acad Sci USA 1990; 87:6934–6938.
222. Arden KC, Boutin JM, Djiane J, et al. The receptors for prolactin and growth hormone are localized in the same region of human chromosome 5. Cytogenet Cell Genet 1990; 53:161–165.
223. Hu ZZ, Zhuang L, Meng J, et al. The human prolactin receptor gene structure and alternative promoter utilization: the generic promoter hPIII and a novel human promoter hP(N). J Clin Endocrinol Metab 1999; 84:1153–1156.
224. Bole-Feysot C, Goffin V, Edery M, et al. Prolactin (PRL) and its receptor: actions, signal transduction pathways and phenotypes observed in PRL receptor knockout mice. Endocr Rev 1998; 19:225–268.
225. de Vos AM, Ultsch M, Kossiakoff AA. Human growth hormone and extracellular domain of its receptor: crystal structure of the complex. Science 1992; 255:306–312.
226. Gao J, Hughes JP, Auperin B, et al. Interactions among Janus kinases and the prolactin (PRL) receptor in the regulation of a PRL response element. Mol Endocrinol 1996; 10:847–856.
227. Hynes NE, Cella N, Wartmann M. Prolactin mediated intracellular signaling in mammary epithelial cells. J Mammary Gland Biol Neoplasia 1997; 2:19–27.
228. Goffin V, Kelly PA. The prolactin/growth hormone receptor family: structure/function relationships. J Mammary Gland Biol Neoplasia 1997; 2:7–17.
229. Lucas BK, Ormandy CJ, Binart N, et al. Null mutation of the prolactin receptor gene produces a defect in maternal behavior. Endocrinology 1998; 139:4102–4107.
230. Kleinberg DL, Ruan W, Catanese V, et al. Non-lactogenic effects of growth hormone on growth and insulin-like growth factor-I messenger ribonucleic acid of rat mammary gland [published erratum appears in Endocrinology 1990; 127:1977]. Endocrinology 1990; 126:3274–3276.
231. Feldman M, Ruan WF, Cunningham BC, et al. Evidence that the growth hormone receptor mediates differentiation and development of the mammary gland. Endocrinology 1993; 133:1602–1608.
232. Ruan W, Catanese V, Wieczorek R, et al. Estradiol enhances the stimulatory effect of insulin-like growth factor-I (IGF-I) on mammary development and growth hormone–induced IGF-I messenger ribonucleic acid. Endocrinology 1995; 136:1296–1302.
233. Ruan W, Newman CB, Kleinberg DL. Intact and amino-terminally shortened forms of insulin-like growth factor I induce mammary gland differentiation and development. Proc Natl Acad Sci USA 1992; 89:10872–10876.
234. Kleinberg DL. Endocrinology of mammary development, lactation and galactorrhea. In DeGroot LJ, Jameson JL (eds). Endocrinology. Philadelphia, WB Saunders, 2000, pp 2464–2475.
235. Cunha GR. Role of mesenchymal-epithelial interactions in normal and abnormal development of the mammary gland and prostate. Cancer 1994; 74:1030–1044.
236. Daniel CW, Silberstein GB. Postnatal development of the rodent mammary gland. In Neville MC, Daniel CW (eds). The Mammary Gland. New York, Plenum Press, 1987, pp 3–36.
237. Kleinberg DL, Ruan W. The crucial roles of insulin-like growth factor I and growth hormone in mammary gland development. In LeRoith D (ed). Advances in Molecular and Cellular Endocrinology. Stamford, Conn, JAI Press, 1999, pp 225–238.
238. Ruan W, Kleinberg DL. Insulin-like growth factor I is essential for terminal end bud formation and ductal morphogenesis during mammary development. Endocrinology 1999; 140:5075–5081.
239. Walden PD, Ruan W, Feldman M, Kleinberg DL. Evidence that

growth hormone acts on stromal tissue to stimulate pubertal mammary gland development. Program 79th Annual Meeting of the Endocrine Society, 1997, abstract.
240. Wysolmerski JJ, Stewart AF. The physiology of parathyroid hormone–related protein: an emerging role as a developmental factor. Annu Rev Physiol 1998; 60:431–460.
241. Wiesen JF, Young P, Werb Z, Cunha GR. Signaling through the stromal epidermal growth factor receptor is necessary for mammary ductal development. Development 1999; 126:335–344.
242. Anderson TJ, Battersby S, King RJB, et al. Oral contraceptive use influences resting breast proliferation. Hum Pathol 1989; 20: 1139–1144.
243. Tyson JE, Hwang P, Guyda H. Studies of prolactin secretion in human pregnancy. Am J Obstet Gynecol 1972; 113:14–20.
244. Vorherr H. Hormonal and biochemical changes of pituitary and breast during pregnancy. Semin Perinatol 1979; 3:193–198.
245. Richert MM, Wood TL. The Insulin-like growth factors (IGF) and the IGF type I receptor during postnatal growth of the murine mammary gland: sites of messenger ribonucleic acid expression and potential functions. Endocrinology 1999; 140:454–461.
246. Pepe GJ, Albrecht ED. Actions of placental and fetal adrenal steroid hormones in primate pregnancy. Endocr Rev 1995; 16: 608–648.
247. Falk RJ. Isolated prolactin deficiency: a case report. Fertil Steril 1992; 58:1060–1062.
248. Humphreys RC, Lydon J, O'Malley BW, Rosen JM. Mammary gland development is mediated by both stromal and epithelial progesterone receptors. Mol Endocrinol 1997; 11:801–811.
249. Kleinberg DL, Boyd AE II, Wardlaw S, et al. Pergolide for the treatment of pituitary tumors secreting prolactin or growth hormone. N Engl J Med 1983; 309:704–709.
250. Graham JD, Clarke CL. Physiological action of progesterone in target tissues. Endocr Rev 1997; 18:502–519.
251. Neville MC. Mammary gland biology and lactation: a short course. International Society for Research in Human Milk and Lactation, 1997.
252. Vorherr H. Galactopoiesis, galactosecretion, and onset of lactation. In Vorherr H (ed). The Breast. New York, Academic Press, 1974, pp 71–127.
253. Noel GL, Suh HK, Frantz AG. Prolactin release during nursing and breast stimulation in postpartum and nonpostpartum subjects. J Clin Endocrinol Metab 1974; 38:413–423.
254. Diaz S, Seron-Ferre M, Cardenas H, et al. Circadian variation of basal plasma prolactin, prolactin response to suckling, and length of amenorrhea in nursing women. J Clin Endocrinol Metab 1989; 68:946–955.
255. Johnston JM, Amico JA. A prospective longitudinal study of the release of oxytocin and prolactin in response to infant suckling in long term lactation. J Clin Endocrinol Metab 1986; 62:653–657.
256. Howie PW, McNeilly AS, McArdle T, et al. The relationship between suckling-induced prolactin response and lactogenesis. J Clin Endocrinol Metab 1980; 50:670–673.
257. Leite V, Cowden EA, Friesen HG. Endocrinology of lactation and nursing: disorders of lactation. In DeGroot LJ (ed). Endocrinology. Philadelphia, WB Saunders, 1995, pp 2224–2233.
258. Wagner KU, Young WS, Liu X, et al. Oxytocin and milk removal are required for post partum mammary-gland development. Genes Funct 1997; 1:233–244.
259. Short RV. Breast feeding. Sci Am 1984; 250(4):35–41.
260. Glasier A, McNeilly AS. Physiology of lactation. Baillieres Clin Endocrinol Metab 1990; 4:379–395.
261. Walker SE, Allen SH, McMurray RW. Prolactin and autoimmune disease. Trends Endocrinol Metab 1993; 4:147–151.
262. Zellweger R, Zhu XH, Wichmann MW, et al. Prolactin administration following hemorrhagic shock improves macrophage cytokine release capacity and decreases mortality from subsequent sepsis. J Immunol 1996; 157:5748–5754.
263. Richards SM, Murphy WJ. Use of human prolactin as a therapeutic protein to potentiate immunohematopoietic function. J Neuroimmunol 2000; 109:56–62.
264. Dorshkind K, Horseman ND. The roles of prolactin, growth hormone, insulin-like growth factor-I, and thyroid hormones in lymphocyte development and function: insights from genetic models of hormone and hormone receptor deficiency. Endocr Rev 2000; 21:292–312.
265. Ormandy CJ, Camus A, Barra J, et al. Null mutation of the prolactin receptor gene produces multiple reproductive defects in the mouse. Genes Dev 1997; 11:167–178.
266. Clement-Lacroix P, Ormandy C, Lepescheux L, et al. Osteoblasts are a new target for prolactin: analysis of bone formation in prolactin receptor knockout mice. Endocrinology 1999; 140: 96–105.
267. Demura R, Ono M, Demura H, et al. Prolactin directly inhibits basal as well as gonadotropin-stimulated secretion of progesterone and 17 beta-estradiol in the human ovary. J Clin Endocrinol Metab 1982; 54:1246–1250.
268. Barkan AL, Chandler WF. Giant pituitary prolactinoma with falsely low serum prolactin: the pitfall of the 'high-dose hook effect': case report. Neurosurgery 1998; 42:913–915.
269. Cooper DS, Ridgway EC, Kliman B, et al. Metabolic clearance and production rates of prolactin in man. J Clin Invest 1979; 64: 1669–1680.
270. Veldhuis JD, Johnson ML. Operating characteristics of the hypothalamo-pituitary-gonadal axis in men: circadian, ultradian, and pulsatile release of prolactin and its temporal coupling with luteinizing hormone. J Clin Endocrinol Metab 1988; 67:116–123.
271. Greenspan SL, Klibanski A, Rowe JW, Elahi D. Age alters pulsatile prolactin release: influence of dopaminergic inhibition. Am J Physiol 1990; 258:E799–E804.
272. Samuels MH, Henry P, Kleinschmidt-DeMasters BK, et al. Pulsatile glycoprotein hormone secretion in glycoprotein-producing pituitary tumors. J Clin Endocrinol Metab 1991; 73:1281–1288.
273. Sassin JF, Frantz AG, Weitzman ED, Kapen S. Human prolactin: 24-hour pattern with increased release during sleep. Science 1972; 177:1205–1207.
274. Parker DC, Rossman LG, Vanderlaan EF. Relation of sleep-entrained human prolactin release to REM-nonREM cycles. J Clin Endocrinol Metab 1974; 38:646–651.
275. Iranmanesh A, Mulligan T, Veldhuis JD. Mechanisms subserving the physiological nocturnal relative hypoprolactinemia of healthy older men: dual decline in prolactin secretory burst mass and basal release with preservation of pulse duration, frequency, and interpulse interval—a General Clinical Research Center study. J Clin Endocrinol Metab 1999; 84:1083–1090.
276. Webb CB, Thominet JL, Barowsky H, et al. Evidence for lactotroph dopamine resistance in idiopathic hyperprolactinemia. J Clin Endocrinol Metab 1983; 56:1089–1093.
277. Martin TL, Kim M, Malarkey WB. The natural history of idiopathic hyperprolactinemia. J Clin Endocrinol Metab 1985; 60: 855–858.
278. Kleinberg DL. Pharmacologic therapies and surgical options in the treatment of hyperprolactinemia. Endocrinologist 1997; 7(Suppl):379–384.
279. Fahie-Wilson MN. Polyethylene glycol precipitation as a screening method for macroprolactinemia. Clin Chem 1999; 45:436–437.
280. Franks S. Polycystic ovary syndrome [published erratum appears in N Engl J Med 1995; 333:1435]. N Engl J Med 1995; 333: 853–861.
281. Bracero N, Zacur HA. Polycystic ovary syndrome and hyperprolactinemia. Obstet Gynecol Clin North Am 2001; 28:77–84.
282. Falaschi P, Rocco A, del Pozo E. Inhibitory effect of bromocriptine treatment on luteinizing hormone secretion in polycystic ovary syndrome. J Clin Endocrinol Metab 1986; 62:348–351.
283. Kleinberg DL, Noel GL, Frantz AG. Galactorrhea: a study of 235 cases, including 48 with pituitary tumors. N Engl J Med 1977; 296:589–600.
284. Lam KS, Lechan RM, Minamitani N, et al. Vasoactive intestinal peptide in the anterior pituitary is increased in hypothyroidism. Endocrinology 1989; 124:1077–1084.
285. Biller BM, Sesmilo G, Baum HB, et al. Withdrawal of long-term physiological growth hormone (GH) administration: differential effects on bone density and body composition in men with adult-onset GH deficiency. J Clin Endocrinol Metab 2000; 85:970–976.
286. Travaglini P, Moriondo P, Togni E, et al. Effect of oral zinc administration on prolactin and thymulin circulating levels in patients with chronic renal failure. J Clin Endocrinol Metab 1989; 68:186–190.
287. LeRoith D, Danovitz G, Trestan S, Spitz IM. Dissociation of prolactin response to thyrotropin-releasing hormone and meto-

clopramide in chronic renal failure. J Clin Endocrinol Metab 1979; 49:815–817.
288. Ramirez G, Butcher DE, Newton JL, et al. Bromocriptine and the hypothalamic hypophyseal function in patients with chronic renal failure on chronic hemodialysis. Am J Kidney Dis 1985; 6: 111–118.
289. Lim VS, Henriquez C, Sievertsen G, Frohman LA. Ovarian function in chronic renal failure: evidence suggesting hypothalamic anovulation. Ann Intern Med 1980; 93:21–27.
290. Noel GL, Suh HK, Stone JG, Frantz AG. Human prolactin and growth hormone release during surgery and other conditions of stress. J Clin Endocrinol Metab 1972; 35:840–851.
291. Constine LS, Woolf PD, Cann D, et al. Hypothalamic-pituitary dysfunction after radiation for brain tumors. N Engl J Med 1993; 328:87–94.
292. Kleinberg DL, Noel GL, Frantz AG. Chlorpromazine stimulation and L-dopa suppression of prolactin. J Clin Endocrinol Metab 1971; 33:873–876.
293. Tollin SR. Use of the dopamine agonists bromocriptine and cabergoline in the management of risperidone-induced hyperprolactinemia in patients with psychotic disorders. J Endocrinol Invest 2000; 23:765–770.
294. Crawford AM, Beasley CMJ, Tollefson GD. The acute long-term effect of olanzapine compared with placebo and haloperidol on serum prolactin concentrations. Schizophr Res 1997; 26:41–54.
295. Perovich RM, Lieberman JA, Fleischhacker WW, Alvir J. The behavioral toxicity of bromocriptine in patients with psychiatric illness. J Clin Psychopharmacol 1989; 9:417–422.
296. Sharp EA. Historical review of a syndrome embracing utero-ovarian atrophy with persistent lactation (Frommel's disease). Am J Obstet Gynecol 1935; 30:411–414.
297. Argonz J, del Castillo EB. A syndrome characterized by estrogenic insufficiency, galactorrhea and decreased urinary gonadotropin. J Clin Endocrinol Metab 1953; 13:79–87.
298. Forbes AP, Henneman PH, Griswold GC, Albright F. Syndrome characterized by galactorrhea, amenorrhea and low urinary FSH: comparison with acromegaly and normal lactation. J Clin Endocrinol Metab 1954; 14:265–271.
298a. Kleinberg DL, Noel GL, Franz AG. Galactorrhea: a study of 235 cases, including 48 with pituitary tumors. N Engl J Med 1977; 296:589–600.
299. Kleinberg DL, Lieberman A, Todd J, et al. Pergolide mesylate: a potent day-long inhibitor of prolactin in rhesus monkeys and patients with Parkinson's disease. J Clin Endocrinol Metab 1980; 51:152–154.
300. Klibanski A, Neer RM, Beitins IZ, et al. Decreased bone density in hyperprolactinemic women. N Engl J Med 1980; 303:1511–1514.
301. McComb DJ, Ryan N, Horvath E, Kovacs K. Subclinical adenomas of the human pituitary: new light on old problems. Arch Pathol Lab Med 1983; 107:488–491.
302. Melmed S, Braunstein GD, Chang RJ, Becker DP. Pituitary tumors secreting growth hormone and prolactin. Ann Intern Med 1986; 105:238–253.
303. Koppelman MCS, Jaffe MJ, Rieth KG, et al. Hyperprolactinemia, amenorrhea, and galactorrhea. Ann Intern Med 1984; 100:115–121.
304. Sisam DA, Sheehan JP, Sheeler LR. The natural history of untreated microprolactinomas. Fertil Steril 1987; 48:67–71.
305. Schlechte J, Dolan K, Sherman B, et al. The natural history of untreated hyperprolactinemia: a prospective analysis. J Clin Endocrinol Metab 1989; 68:412–418.
306. Molitch ME. Medical treatment of prolactinomas. Endocrinol Metab Clin North Am 1999; 28:143–69, vii.
307. Delgrange E, Trouillas J, Maiter D, et al. Sex-related difference in the growth of prolactinomas: a clinical and proliferation marker study. J Clin Endocrinol Metab 1997; 82:2102–2107.
308. Arafah BM, Nekl KE, Gold RS, Selman WR. Dynamics of prolactin secretion in patients with hypopituitarism and pituitary macroadenomas. J Clin Endocrinol Metab 1995; 80:3507–3512.
309. Kovacs K, Horvath E. Pathology of pituitary tumors. Endocrinol Metab Clin North Am 1987; 16:529–551.
310. Kovacs K, Horvath E, Asa SL. Classification and pathology of pituitary tumors. In Wilkins RH, Rengachary SS (eds). Neurosurgery. New York, McGraw-Hill, 1985, pp 834–842.
311. Scheithauer BW, Kovacs KT, Laws ER Jr, Randall RV. Pathology of invasive pituitary tumors with special reference to functional classification. J Neurosurg 1986; 65:733–744.
312. Pernicone PJ, Scheithauer BW, Sebo TJ, et al. Pituitary carcinoma: a clinicopathologic study of 15 cases. Cancer 1997; 79: 804–812.
313. Hurel SJ, Harris PE, McNicol AM, et al. Metastatic prolactinoma: effect of octreotide, cabergoline, carboplatin and etoposide; immunocytochemical analysis of proto-oncogene expression. J Clin Endocrinol Metab 1997; 82:2962–2965.
314. Kontogeorgos G, Kovacs K, Horvath E, Scheithauer BW. Multiple adenomas of the human pituitary: a retrospective autopsy study with clinical implications. J Neurosurg 1991; 74:243–247.
315. Burgess JR, Shepherd JJ, Parameswaran V, et al. Spectrum of pituitary disease in multiple endocrine neoplasia type 1 (MEN 1): clinical, biochemical, and radiological features of pituitary disease in a large MEN 1 kindred. J Clin Endocrinol Metab 1996; 81: 2642–2646.
316. Berezin M, Karasik A. Familial prolactinoma. Clin Endocrinol (Oxf) 1995; 42:483–486.
317. Sauder SE, Frager M, Case GA, et al. Abnormal patterns of pulsatile luteinizing hormone secretion in women with hyperprolactinemia and amenorrhea: responses to bromocriptine. J Clin Endocrinol Metab 1984; 59:941–948.
318. Milenkovic L, D'Angelo G, Kelly PA, Weiner RI. Inhibition of gonadotropin hormone–releasing hormone release by prolactin from GT1 neuronal cell lines through prolactin receptors. Proc Natl Acad Sci USA 1994; 91:1244–1247.
319. Cohen-Becker IR, Selmanoff M, Wise PM. Hyperprolactinemia alters the frequency and amplitude of pulsatile luteinizing hormone secretion in the ovariectomized rat. Neuroendocrinology 1986; 42:328–333.
320. Matera C, Freda PU, Ferin M, Wardlaw SL. Effect of chronic opioid antagonism on the hypothalamic-pituitary-ovarian axis in hyperprolactinemic women. J Clin Endocrinol Metab 1995; 80: 540–545.
321. Klibanski A, Biller BMK, Rosenthal DI, Saxe V. Effects of prolactin and estrogen deficiency in amenorrheic bone loss. J Clin Endocrinol Metab 1988; 67:124–130.
322. Kemmann E, Jones JR. Hyperprolactinemia and headaches. Am J Obstet Gynecol 1983; 145:668–671.
323. Hollenhorst RW, Younge BR. Ocular manifestations produced by adenomas of the pituitary gland: analysis of 1000 cases. In Kohler PO, Ross GT (eds). Diagnosis and Treatment of Pituitary Tumors. New York, American Elsevier, 1973, pp 53–64.
324. Zikel OM, Atkinson JL, Hurley DL. Prolactinoma manifesting with symptomatic hydrocephalus. Mayo Clin Proc 1999; 74:475–477.
325. Krassas GE, Pontikides N, Kaltsas T. Giant prolactinoma presented as unilateral exophthalmos in a prepubertal boy: response to cabergoline. Horm Res 1999; 52:45–48.
326. Kleinberg DL, Todd J. Evidence that human growth hormone is a potent lactogen in primates. J Clin Endocrinol Metab 1980; 51: 1009–1015.
327. Thorner MO, Martin WH, Rogol AD, et al. Rapid regression of pituitary prolactinomas during bromocriptine treatment. J Clin Endocrinol Metab 1980; 51:438–445.
328. Besser GM, Thorner MO. Bromocriptine in the treatment of the hyperprolactinaemia-hypogonadism syndromes. Postgrad Med J 1976; 52(Suppl 1):64–70.
329. Shimon I, Yan X, Melmed S. Human fetal pituitary expresses functional growth hormone–releasing peptide receptors. J Clin Endocrinol Metab 1998; 83:174–178.
330. Bevan JS, Webster J, Burke CW, Scanlon MF. Dopamine agonists and pituitary tumor shrinkage. Endocr Rev 1992; 13:220–240.
331. Weiss MH. Treatment options in the management of prolactin-secreting pituitary tumors. Clin Neurosurg 1986; 33:547–552.
332. Vance ML, Evans WS, Thorner MO. Drugs five years later: bromocriptine. Ann Intern Med 1984; 100:78–91.
333. Thorner MO, Perryman RL, Rogol AD, et al. Rapid changes of prolactinoma volume after withdrawal and reinstitution of bromocriptine. J Clin Endocrinol Metab 1981; 53:480–483.
334. Kovacs K, Stefaneanu L, Horvath E, et al. Effect of dopamine agonist medication on prolactin producing pituitary adenomas: a morphological study including immunocytochemistry, electron

microscopy and in situ hybridization. Virchows Arch A Pathol Anat Histopathol 1991; 418:439–446.
335. Jeffcoate WJ, Pound N, Sturrock ND, Lambourne J. Long-term follow-up of patients with hyperprolactinaemia. Clin Endocrinol (Oxf) 1996; 45:299–303.
336. Kupersmith MJ, Kleinberg DL, Warren A, et al. Growth of prolactinoma despite lowering of serum prolactin by bromocriptine. Neurosurgery 1989; 24:417–423.
337. Pellegrini I, Rasolonjanahary R, Gunz G, et al. Resistance to bromocriptine in prolactinomas. J Clin Endocrinol Metab 1989; 69:500–509.
338. Colao A, Di Sarno A, Sarnacchiaro F, et al. Prolactinomas resistant to standard dopamine agonists respond to chronic cabergoline treatment. J Clin Endocrinol Metab 1997; 82:876–883.
339. Tindall GT, Kovacs K, Horvath E, Thorner MO. Human prolactin-producing adenomas and bromocriptine: a histological, immunocytochemical, ultrastructural, and morphometric study. J Clin Endocrinol Metab 1982; 55:1178–1183.
340. Bassetti M, Spada A, Pezzo G, Giannattasio G. Bromocriptine treatment reduces the cell size in human macroprolactinomas: a morphometric study. J Clin Endocrinol Metab 1984; 58:268–273.
341. Saitoh Y, Mori S, Arita N, et al. Cytosuppressive effect of bromocriptine on human prolactinomas: stereological analysis of ultrastructural alterations with special reference to secretory granules. Cancer Res 1986; 46:1507–1512.
342. Hallenga B, Saeger W, Ludecke DK. Necroses of prolactin-secreting pituitary adenomas under treatment with dopamine agonists: light microscopical and morphometric studies. Exp Clin Endocrinol 1988; 92:59–68.
343. Landolt AM, Osterwalder V. Perivascular fibrosis in prolactinomas: is it increased by bromocriptine? J Clin Endocrinol Metab 1984; 58:1179–1183.
344. Tyrrell JB, Lamborn KR, Hannegan LT, et al. Transsphenoidal microsurgical therapy of prolactinomas: initial outcomes and long-term results. Neurosurgery 1999; 44:254–261.
345. Hubbard JL, Scheithauer BW, Abboud CF, Laws ER Jr. Prolactin-secreting adenomas: the preoperative response to bromocriptine treatment and surgical outcome. J Neurosurg 1987; 67:816–821.
346. Fahlbusch R, Buchfelder M, Schrell U. Short-term preoperative treatment of macroprolactinomas by dopamine agonists. J Neurosurg 1987; 67:807–815.
347. Liuzzi A, Dallabonzana D, Oppizzi G, et al. Low doses of dopamine agonists in the long-term treatment of macroprolactinomas. N Engl J Med 1985; 313:656–659.
348. DiSalle E, Ornati G, Giudici D. A comparison of the in vivo and in vitro duration of prolactin lowering effect in rats of FCE 21336, pergolide and bromocriptine. J Endocrinol Invest 1984; 7: 32–32.
349. Andreotti AC, Pianezzola E, Persiani S, et al. Pharmacokinetics, pharmacodynamics, and tolerability of cabergoline, a prolactin-lowering drug, after administration of increasing oral doses (0.5, 1.0, and 1.5 milligrams) in healthy male volunteers. J Clin Endocrinol Metab 1995; 80:841–845.
350. Webster J, Piscitelli G, Polli A, et al. A comparison of cabergoline and bromocriptine in the treatment of hyperprolactinemic amenorrhea. N Engl J Med 1994; 331:904–909.
351. Biller BM, Molitch ME, Vance ML, et al. Treatment of prolactin-secreting macroadenomas with the once-weekly dopamine agonist cabergoline. J Clin Endocrinol Metab 1996; 81:2338–2343.
352. Colao A, Di Sarno A, Landi ML, et al. Long-term and low-dose treatment with cabergoline induces macroprolactinoma shrinkage. J Clin Endocrinol Metab 1997; 82:3574–3579.
353. Shimon I, Melmed S. Management of pituitary tumors. Ann Intern Med 1998; 129:472–483.
354. Goldstein M, Lieberman A, Lew JY, et al. Interaction of pergolide with central dopaminergic receptors. Proc Natl Acad Sci USA 1980; 77:3725–3728.
355. Freda PU, Andreadis CI, Khandji AG, et al. Long-term treatment of prolactin-secreting macroadenomas with pergolide. J Clin Endocrinol Metab 2000; 85:8–13.
356. Lamberts SWJ, Quik RFP. A comparison of the efficacy and safety of pergolide and bromocriptine in the treatment of hyperprolactinemia. J Clin Endocrinol Metab 1991; 72:635–641.
357. Newman CB, Hurley AM, Kleinberg DL. Effect of CV 205-502 in hyperprolactinemic patients intolerant of bromocriptine. Clin Endocrinol (Oxf) 1989; 31:391–400.
358. Vance ML, Cragun JR, Reimnitz C, et al. CV205-502 treatment of hyperprolactinemia. J Clin Endocrinol Metab 1989; 68:336–339.
359. Kletzky OA, Vermesh M. Effectiveness of vaginal bromocriptine in treating women with hyperprolactinemia. Fertil Steril 1989; 51:269–272.
360. Turner TH, Cookson JC, Wass JA, et al. Psychotic reactions during treatment of pituitary tumours with dopamine agonists. Br Med J (Clin Res Ed) 1984; 289:1101–1103.
361. Leong KS, Foy PM, Swift AC, et al. CSF rhinorrhoea following treatment with dopamine agonists for massive invasive prolactinomas. Clin Endocrinol (Oxf) 2000; 52:43–49.
362. Melmed S, Braunstein GD. Bromocriptine and pleuropulmonary disease. Arch Intern Med 1989; 149:258–259.
363. Rush SC, Newall J. Pituitary adenoma: the efficacy of radiotherapy as the sole treatment. Int J Radiat Oncol Biol Phys 1989; 17: 165–169.
364. Halberg FE, Sheline GE. Radiotherapy of pituitary tumors. Endocrinol Metab Clin 1987; 16:667–684.
365. Littley MD, Shalet SM, Beardwell CG, et al. Radiation-induced hypopituitarism is dose-dependent. Clin Endocrinol 1989; 31: 363–373.
366. Tsagarakis S, Grossman A, Plowman PN, et al. Megavoltage pituitary irradiation in the management of prolactinomas: long-term follow-up. Clin Endocrinol (Oxf) 1991; 34:399–406.
367. Littley MD, Shalet SM, Beardwell CG, et al. Hypopituitarism following external radiotherapy for pituitary tumours in adults. Q J Med 1989; 70:145–160.
368. Hardy J. Transsphenoidal hypophysectomy. J Neurosurg 1971; 34:582–591.
369. Randall RV, Laws ER Jr, Abboud CF, et al. Transsphenoidal microsurgical treatment of prolactin-producing pituitary adenomas: results in 100 patients. Mayo Clin Proc 1983; 58:108–121.
370. Serri O, Rasio E, Beauregard H, et al. Recurrence of hyperprolactinemia after selective transsphenoidal adenomectomy in women with prolactinoma. N Engl J Med 1983; 309:280–283.
371. Molitch ME. Management of prolactinomas. Annu Rev Med 1989; 40:225–232.
372. Clayton RN, Stewart PM, Shalet SM, Wass JA. Pituitary surgery for acromegaly: should be done by specialists. BMJ 1999; 319: 588–589.
373. Gonzalez JG, Elizondo G, Saldivar D, et al. Pituitary gland growth during normal pregnancy: an in vivo study using magnetic resonance imaging. Am J Med 1988; 85:217–220.
374. Molitch ME, Thorner MO, Wilson C. Management of prolactinomas. J Clin Endocrinol Metab 1997; 82:996–1000.
375. Molitch ME, Elton RL, Blackwell RE, et al. Bromocriptine as primary therapy for prolactin-secreting macroadenomas: results of a prospective multicenter study. J Clin Endocrinol Metab 1985; 60:698–705.
376. Kupersmith MJ, Rosenberg C, Kleinberg D. Visual loss in pregnant women with pituitary adenomas. Ann Intern Med 1994; 121:473–477.
377. Liu C, Tyrrell JB. Successful treatment of a large macroprolactinoma with cabergoline during pregnancy. Pituitary 2002; 4:3–6.
378. Krupp P, Turkalj I. Surveillance of Parlodel (bromocriptine) in pregnancy. In Jacobs HS, Harrison RF, Bonnar J (eds). Prolactinomas and Pregnancy. Lancaster; Boston, MTP Press, 1983, pp 45–50.
379. Maeda T, Ushiroyama T, Okuda K, et al. Effective bromocriptine treatment of a pituitary macroadenoma during pregnancy. Obstet Gynecol 1983; 61:117–121.
380. Laws ER Jr, Fode NC, Randall RV, et al. Pregnancy following transsphenoidal resection of prolactin-secreting pituitary tumors. J Neurosurg 1983; 58:685–688.
381. Gharib SD, Wierman ME, Shupnik MA, Chin WW. Molecular biology of the pituitary gonadotropins. Endocr Rev 1990; 11: 177–199.
382. Sairam MR, Bhargavi GN. A role for glycosylation of the alpha subunit in transduction of biological signal in glycoprotein hormones. Science 1985; 229:65–67.
383. Albanese C, Colin IM, Crowley WF, et al. The gonadotropin genes: evolution of distinct mechanisms for hormonal control. Recent Prog Horm Res 1996; 51:23–58.
384. Shupnik MA. Gonadotropin gene modulation by steroids and gonadotropin-releasing hormone. Biol Reprod 1996; 54:279–286.

385. Ezashi T, Hirai T, Kato T, et al. The gene for the beta subunit of porcine LH: clusters of GC boxes and CACCC elements. J Mol Endocrinol 1990; 5:137–146.
386. Keri RA, Bachmann DJ, Behrooz A, et al. An NF-Y binding site is important for basal, but not gonadotropin-releasing hormone–stimulated, expression of the luteinizing hormone beta subunit gene. J Biol Chem 2000; 275:13082–13088.
387. Duan WR, Shin JL, Jameson JL. Estradiol suppresses phosphorylation of cyclic adenosine 3′,5′- monophosphate response element binding protein (CREB) in the pituitary: evidence for indirect action via gonadotropin-releasing hormone. Mol Endocrinol 1999; 13:1338–1352.
388. Halvorson LM, Ito M, Jameson JL, Chin WW. Steroidogenic factor-1 and early growth response protein 1 act through two composite DNA binding sites to regulate luteinizing hormone beta-subunit gene expression. J Biol Chem 1998; 273:14712–14720.
389. Glaser T, Lewis WH, Bruns GA, et al. The beta-subunit of follicle-stimulating hormone is deleted in patients with aniridia and Wilms' tumour, allowing a further definition of the WAGR locus. Nature 1986; 321:882–887.
390. Brown P, McNeilly AS. Transcriptional regulation of pituitary gonadotrophin subunit genes. Rev Reprod 1999; 4:117–124.
391. Jaakkola T, Ding YQ, Kellokumpu-lehtinen P, et al. The ratios of serum bioactive/immunoreactive luteinizing hormone and follicle-stimulating hormone in various clinical conditions with increased and decreased gonadotropin secretion: reevaluation by a highly sensitive immunometric assay. J Clin Endocrinol Metab 1990; 70:1496–1505.
392. Lucky AW, Rich BH, Rosenfield RL, et al. LH bioactivity increases more than immunoreactivity during puberty. J Pediatr 1980; 97:205–213.
393. Jia XC, Hsueh AJ. Granulosa cell aromatase bioassay for follicle-stimulating hormone: validation and application of the method. Endocrinology 1986; 119:1570–1577.
394. Knobil E. The neuroendocrine control of the menstrual cycle. Recent Prog Horm Res 1980; 36:53–88.
395. Crowley WF Jr, Whitcomb RW, Jameson JL, et al. Neuroendocrine control of human reproduction in the male. Recent Prog Horm Res 1991; 47:27–62.
396. Finkelstein JS, O'Dea LS, Whitcomb RW, Crowley WF Jr. Sex steroid control of gonadotropin secretion in the human male. II. Effects of estradiol administration in normal and gonadotropin-releasing hormone–deficient men. J Clin Endocrinol Metab 1991; 73:621–628.
397. Finkelstein JS, Whitcomb RW, O'Dea LS, et al. Sex steroid control of gonadotropin secretion in the human male. I. Effects of testosterone administration in normal and gonadotropin-releasing hormone–deficient men. J Clin Endocrinol Metab 1991; 73:609–620.
398. Veldhuis JD, Pincus SM, Garcia-Rudaz MC, et al. Disruption of the synchronous secretion of leptin, LH, and ovarian androgens in nonobese adolescents with the polycystic ovarian syndrome. J Clin Endocrinol Metab 2001; 86:3772–3778.
399. Vale W, Rivier C, Hsueh A, et al. Chemical and biological characterization of the inhibin family of protein hormones. Recent Prog Horm Res 1988; 44:1–34.
400. Stocco DM. Tracking the role of a star in the sky of the new millennium. Mol Endocrinol 2001; 15:1245–1254.
401. Sprengel R, Braun T, Nikolics K, et al. The testicular receptor for follicle stimulating hormone: structure and functional expression of cloned cDNA. Mol Endocrinol 1990; 4:525–530.
402. Hsueh AJ, Adashi EY, Jones PB, Welsh TH Jr. Hormonal regulation of the differentiation of cultured ovarian granulosa cells. Endocr Rev 1984; 5:76–127.
403. Mortimer CH, Besser GM, McNeilly AS, et al. Luteinizing hormone and follicle stimulating hormone–releasing hormone test in patients with hypothalamic-pituitary-gonadal dysfunction. Br Med J 1973; 4:73–77.
404. Zirkin BR, Awoniyi C, Griswold MD, et al. Is FSH required for adult spermatogenesis? J Androl 1994; 15:273–276.
405. McCullagh DR. Dual endocrine activity of the testes. Science 1932; 76:19–23.
406. Nachtigall LB, Boepple PA, Pralong FP, Crowley WF Jr. Adult-onset idiopathic hypogonadotropic hypogonadism: a treatable form of male infertility. N Engl J Med 1997; 336:410–415.
407. Anawalt BD, Bremner WJ. Diagnosis and treatment of male gonadotropin insufficiency. In Lamberts SW (ed). The Diagnosis and Treatment of Pituitary Insufficiency. Bristol, UK, BioScientifica, 1997, pp 163–207.
408. Snyder PJ, Lawrence DA. Treatment of male hypogonadism with testosterone enanthate. J Clin Endocrinol Metab 1980; 51:1335–1339.
409. Handelsman DJ, Conway AJ, Boylan LM. Pharmacokinetics and pharmacodynamics of testosterone pellets in man. J Clin Endocrinol Metab 1990; 71:216–222.
410. Whitsel EA, Boyko EJ, Matsumoto AM, et al. Intramuscular testosterone esters and plasma lipids in hypogonadal men: a meta-analysis. Am J Med 2001; 111:261–269.
411. Anawalt BD, Bebb RA, Bremner WJ, Matsumoto AM. A lower dosage levonorgestrel and testosterone combination effectively suppresses spermatogenesis and circulating gonadotropin levels with fewer metabolic effects than higher dosage combinations. J Androl 1999; 20:407–414.
412. Bhasin S, Salehian B. Gonadotropin therapy of men with hypogonadotropic hypogonadism. Curr Ther Endocrinol Metab 1997; 6:349–352.
413. Balen AH, Braat DD, West C, et al. Cumulative conception and live birth rates after the treatment of anovulatory infertility: safety and efficacy of ovulation induction in 200 patients. Hum Reprod 1994; 9:1563–1570.
414. Martin KA, Hall JE, Adams JM, Crowley WF Jr. Comparison of exogenous gonadotropins and pulsatile gonadotropin-releasing hormone for induction of ovulation in hypogonadotropic amenorrhea. J Clin Endocrinol Metab 1993; 77:125–129.
415. Suikkari A, MacLachlan V, Koistinen R, et al. Double-blind placebo controlled study: human biosynthetic growth hormone for assisted reproductive technology. Fertil Steril 1996; 65:800–805.
416. Horvath E, Kovacs K. Ultrastructural diagnosis of human pituitary adenomas. Microsc Res Tech 1992; 20:107–135.
417. Jameson JL, Klibanski A, Black PM, et al. Glycoprotein hormone genes are expressed in clinically nonfunctioning pituitary adenomas. J Clin Invest 1987; 80:1472–1478.
418. Nobels FR, Kwekkeboom DJ, Coopmans W, et al. A comparison between the diagnostic value of gonadotropins, alpha-subunit, and chromogranin-A and their response to thyrotropin-releasing hormone in clinically nonfunctioning, alpha-subunit-secreting, and gonadotroph pituitary adenomas. J Clin Endocrinol Metab 1993; 77:784–789.
419. Kovacs K, Horvath E, Ryan N, Ezrin C. Null cell adenoma of the human pituitary. Virchows Arch A Pathol Anat Histol 1980; 387:165–174.
420. Snyder PJ. Clinically nonfunctioning pituitary adenomas. Endocrinol Metab Clin North Am 1993; 22:163–175.
421. Greenman Y, Woolf P, Coniglio J, et al. Remission of acromegaly caused by pituitary carcinoma after surgical excision of growth hormone–secreting metastasis detected by 111-indium pentetreotide scan. J Clin Endocrinol Metab 1996; 81:1628–1633.
422. Valimaki MJ, Tiitinen A, Alfthan H, et al. Ovarian hyperstimulation caused by gonadotroph adenoma secreting follicle-stimulating hormone in 28-year-old woman. J Clin Endocrinol Metab 1999; 84:4204–4208.
423. Daneshdoost L, Gennarelli TA, Bashey HM, et al. Recognition of gonadotroph adenomas in women. N Engl J Med 1991; 324: 589–594.
424. Boelaert K, Gittoes NJ. Radiotherapy for non-functioning pituitary adenomas. Eur J Endocrinol 2001; 144:569–575.
425. Ebersold MJ, Quast LM, Laws ER Jr, et al. Long-term results in transsphenoidal removal of nonfunctioning pituitary adenomas. J Neurosurg 1986; 64:713–719.
426. Turner HE, Stratton IM, Byrne JV, et al. Audit of selected patients with nonfunctioning pituitary adenomas treated without irradiation: a follow-up study. Clin Endocrinol (Oxf) 1999; 51: 281–284.
427. Gittoes NJ, Bates AS, Tse W, et al. Radiotherapy for non-function pituitary tumours. Clin Endocrinol (Oxf) 1998; 48:331–337.
428. Greenman Y, Melmed S. Diagnosis and management of nonfunctioning pituitary tumors. Annu Rev Med 1996; 47:95–106.
429. Kwekkeboom DJ, Lamberts SW. Long-term treatment with the dopamine agonist CV 205-502 of patients with a clinically non-

functioning, gonadotroph, or alpha-subunit secreting pituitary adenoma. Clin Endocrinol (Oxf) 1992; 36:171–176.
430. McGrath GA, Goncalves RJ, Udupa JK, et al. New technique for quantitation of pituitary adenoma size: use in evaluating treatment of gonadotroph adenomas with a gonadotropin-releasing hormone antagonist. J Clin Endocrinol Metab 1993; 76:1363–1368.
431. Plockinger U, Reichel M, Fett U, et al. Preoperative octreotide treatment of growth hormone–secreting and clinically nonfunctioning pituitary macroadenomas: effect on tumor volume and lack of correlation with immunohistochemistry and somatostatin receptor scintigraphy. J Clin Endocrinol Metab 1994; 79:1416–1423.
432. Frohman LA, Burek L, Stachura MA. Characterization of growth hormone of different molecular weights in rat, dog and human pituitaries. Endocrinology 1972; 91:262–269.
433. Cooke NE, Ray J, Watson MA, et al. Human growth hormone gene and the highly homologous growth hormone variant gene display different splicing patterns. J Clin Invest 1988; 82:270–275.
434. Miller WL, Eberhardt NL. Structure and evolution of the growth hormone gene family. Endocr Rev 1983; 4:97–130.
435. Lewis UJ, Dunn JT, Bonewald LF, et al. A naturally occurring structural variant of human growth hormone. J Biol Chem 1978; 253:2679–2687.
436. Frankenne F, Closset J, Gomez F, et al. The physiology of growth hormones (GHs) in pregnant women and partial characterization of the placental GH variant. J Clin Endocrinol Metab 1988; 66:1171–1180.
437. Parks JS, Brown MR, Hurley DL, et al. Heritable disorders of pituitary development. J Clin Endocrinol Metab 1999; 84:4362–4370.
438. Bennani-Baiti IM, Asa SL, Song D, et al. DNase I–hypersensitive sites I and II of the human growth hormone locus control region are a major developmental activator of somatotrope gene expression. Proc Natl Acad Sci USA 1998; 95:10655–10660.
439. Cunningham BC, Ultsch M, De Vos AM, et al. Dimerization of the extracellular domain of the human growth hormone receptor by a single hormone molecule. Science 1991; 254:821–825.
440. Baumann G, MacCart JG, Amburn K. The molecular nature of circulating growth hormone in normal and acromegalic man: evidence for a principal and minor monomeric forms. J Clin Endocrinol Metab 1983; 56:946–952.
441. Mayo KE, Miller T, DeAlmeida V, et al. Regulation of the pituitary somatotroph cell by GHRH and its receptor. Recent Prog Horm Res 2000; 55:237–266.
442. Shimon I, Taylor JE, Dong JZ, et al. Somatostatin receptor subtype specificity in human fetal pituitary cultures: differential role of SSTR2 and SSTR5 for growth hormone, thyroid-stimulating hormone, and prolactin regulation. J Clin Invest 1997; 99: 789–798.
443. Shimon I, Yan X, Taylor JE, et al. Somatostatin receptor (SSTR) subtype–selective analogues differentially suppress in vitro growth hormone and prolactin in human pituitary adenomas: novel potential therapy for functional pituitary tumors. J Clin Invest 1997; 100:2386–2392.
444. Barinaga M, Yamonoto G, Rivier C, et al. Transcriptional regulation of growth hormone gene expression by growth hormone–releasing factor. Nature 1983; 306:84–85.
445. Thorner MO, Frohman LA, Leong DA, et al. Extrahypothalamic growth-hormone–releasing factor (GRF) secretion is a rare cause of acromegaly: plasma GRF levels in 177 acromegalic patients. J Clin Endocrinol Metab 1984; 59:846–849.
446. Gelato MC, Pescovitz O, Cassorla F, et al. Effects of a growth hormone releasing factor in man. J Clin Endocrinol Metab 1983; 57:674–676.
447. Tannenbaum GS, Ling N. The interrelationship of growth hormone (GH)–releasing factor and somatostatin in generation of the ultradian rhythm of GH secretion. Endocrinology 1984; 115: 1952–1957.
448. Bilezikjian LM, Seifert H, Vale W. Desensitization to growth hormone–releasing factor (GRF) is associated with down-regulation of GRF-binding sites. Endocrinology 1986; 118:2045–2052.
449. Kineman RD, Teixeira LT, Amargo GV, et al. The effect of GHRH on somatotrope hyperplasia and tumor formation in the presence and absence of GH signaling. Endocrinology 2001; 142: 3764–3773.
450. Gaykema RP, Compaan JC, Nyakas C, et al. Long-term effects of cholinergic basal forebrain lesions on neuropeptide Y and somatostatin immunoreactivity in rat neocortex. Brain Res 1989; 489:392–396.
451. Pombo M, Pombo CM, Garcia A, et al. Hormonal control of growth hormone secretion. Horm Res 2001; 55:11–16.
452. Melmed S, Yamashita S, Yamasaki H, et al. IGF-I receptor signalling: lessons from the somatotroph. Recent Prog Horm Res 1996; 51:189–215.
453. Howard AD, Feighner SD, Cully DF, et al. A receptor in pituitary and hypothalamus that functions in growth hormone release. Science 1996; 273:974–977.
454. Kojima M, Hosoda H, Date Y, et al. Ghrelin is a growth-hormone–releasing acylated peptide from stomach. Nature 1999; 402:656–660.
454a. Pinkney J, Williams G. Ghrelin gets hungry. Lancet 2002; 359: 1360–1361.
455. Casanueva FF, Dieguez C. Growth hormone secretagogues: physiological role and clinical utility. Trends Endocrinol Metab 1999; 10:30–38.
456. Popovic V, Leal A, Micic D, et al. GH-releasing hormone and GH-releasing peptide-6 for diagnostic testing in GH-deficient adults. Lancet 2000; 356:1137–1142.
457. Chang CH, Rickes EL, McGuire L, et al. Growth hormone (GH) and insulin-like growth factor I responses after treatments with an orally active GH secretagogue L-163,255 in swine. Endocrinology 1996; 137:4851–4856.
458. Popovic V, Damjanovic S, Micic D, et al. Blocked growth hormone–releasing peptide (GHRP-6)–induced GH secretion and absence of the synergic action of GHRP-6 plus GH-releasing hormone in patients with hypothalamopituitary disconnection: evidence that GHRP-6 main action is exerted at the hypothalamic level. J Clin Endocrinol Metab 1995; 80:942–947.
459. Penalva A, Pombo M, Carballo A, et al. Influence of sex, age and adrenergic pathways on the growth hormone response to GHRP-6. Clin Endocrinol (Oxf) 1993; 38:87–91.
460. Jaffe CA, Friberg RD, Barkan AL. Suppression of growth hormone (GH) secretion by a selective GH-releasing hormone (GHRH) antagonist: direct evidence for involvement of endogenous GHRH in the generation of GH pulses. J Clin Invest 1993; 92:695–701.
461. Loche S, Colao A, Cappa M, et al. The growth hormone response to hexarelin in children: reproducibility and effect of sex steroids. J Clin Endocrinol Metab 1997; 82:861–864.
462. Raun K, Hansen BS, Johansen NL, et al. Ipamorelin, the first selective growth hormone secretagogue. Eur J Endocrinol 1998; 139:552–561.
463. Van Cauter E, Plat L, Copinschi G. Interrelations between sleep and the somatotropic axis. Sleep 1998; 21:553–566.
464. Van Cauter E. Slow wave sleep and release of growth hormone. JAMA 2000; 284:2717–2718.
465. Vigas M, Malatinsky J, Nemeth S, Jurcovicova J. Alpha-adrenergic control of growth hormone release during surgical stress in man. Metabolism 1977; 26:399–402.
466. Sachar EJ, Mushrush G, Perlow M, et al. Growth hormone responses to L-dopa in depressed patients. Science 1972; 178: 1304–1305.
467. Ho KY, Veldhuis JD, Johnson ML, et al. Fasting enhances growth hormone secretion and amplifies the complex rhythms of growth hormone secretion in man. J Clin Invest 1988; 81:968–975.
468. Vigneri R, Squatrito S, Pezzino V, et al. Growth hormone levels in diabetes: correlation with the clinical control of the disease. Diabetes 1976; 25:167–172.
469. Casanueva FF, Dieguez C. Neuroendocrine regulation and actions of leptin. Front Neuroendocrinol 1999; 20:317–363.
470. Carro E, Senaris R, Considine RV, et al. Regulation of in vivo growth hormone secretion by leptin. Endocrinology 1997; 138: 2203–2206.
471. Okada K, Sugihara H, Minami S, Wakabayashi I. Effect of parenteral administration of selected nutrients and central injection of gamma-globulin from antiserum to neuropeptide Y on growth hormone secretory pattern in food-deprived rats. Neuroendocrinology 1993; 57:678–686.
472. al-Shoumer KA, Anyaoku V, Richmond W, Johnston DG. Elevated leptin concentrations in growth hormone–deficient hypopituitary adults. Clin Endocrinol (Oxf) 1997; 47:153–159.

473. Lal S, Martin JB, De la Vega CE, Friesen HG. Comparison of the effect of apomorphine and L-DOPA on serum growth hormone levels in normal men. Clin Endocrinol (Oxf) 1975; 4:277–285.
474. Giustina A, Veldhuis JD. Pathophysiology of the neuroregulation of growth hormone secretion in experimental animals and the human. Endocr Rev 1998; 19:717–797.
475. Casanueva FF, Burguera B, Muruais C, Dieguez C. Acute administration of corticoids: a new and peculiar stimulus of growth hormone secretion in man. J Clin Endocrinol Metab 1990; 70: 234–237.
476. Suda T, Demura H, Demura R, et al. Anterior pituitary hormones in plasma and pituitaries from patients with Cushing's disease. J Clin Endocrinol Metab 1980; 51:1048–1053.
477. Irie M, Tsushima T. Increase of serum growth hormone concentration following thyrotropin-releasing hormone injection in patients with acromegaly or gigantism. J Clin Endocrinol Metab 1972; 35:97–100.
478. Herington AC, Ymer S, Stevenson J. Identification and characterization of specific binding proteins for growth hormone in normal human sera. J Clin Invest 1986; 77:1817–1823.
479. Leung DW, Spencer SA, Cachianes G, et al. Growth hormone receptor and serum binding protein: purification, cloning and expression. Nature 1987; 330:537–543.
480. Baumann G, Shaw MA, Amburn K. Regulation of plasma growth hormone–binding proteins in health and disease. Metabolism 1989; 38:683–689.
481. Carter-Su C, Schwartz J, Smit LS. Molecular mechanism of growth hormone action. Annu Rev Physiol 1996; 58:187–207.
482. Barnard R, Waters MJ. The serum growth hormone binding protein: pregnant with possibilities. J Endocrinol 1997; 153:1–14.
483. Leung KC, Waters MJ, Markus I, et al. Insulin and insulin-like growth factor-I acutely inhibit surface translocation of growth hormone receptors in osteoblasts: a novel mechanism of growth hormone receptor regulation. Proc Natl Acad Sci USA 1997; 94: 11381–11386.
484. Xu BC, Wang X, Darus CJ, Kopchick JJ. Growth hormone promotes the association of transcription factor STAT5 with the growth hormone receptor. J Biol Chem 1996; 271:19768–19773.
485. Yakar S, Liu JL, Stannard B, et al. Normal growth and development in the absence of hepatic insulin-like growth factor I. Proc Natl Acad Sci USA 1999; 96:7324–7329.
486. Low MJ, Otero-Corchon V, Parlow AF, et al. Somatostatin is required for masculinization of growth hormone–regulated hepatic gene expression but not of somatic growth. J Clin Invest 2001; 107:1571–1580.
487. Udy GB, Towers RP, Snell RG, et al. Requirement of STAT5b for sexual dimorphism of body growth rates and liver gene expression. Proc Natl Acad Sci USA 1997; 94:7239–7244.
488. Ram PA, Park SH, Choi HK, Waxman DJ. Growth hormone activation of Stat 1, Stat 3, and Stat 5 in rat liver: differential kinetics of hormone desensitization and growth hormone stimulation of both tyrosine phosphorylation and serine/threonine phosphorylation. J Biol Chem 1996; 271:5929–5940.
489. Teglund S, McKay C, Schuetz E, et al. Stat5a and Stat5b proteins have essential and nonessential, or redundant, roles in cytokine responses. Cell 1998; 93:841–850.
490. Davey HW, Park SH, Grattan DR, et al. STAT5b-deficient mice are growth hormone pulse-resistant: role of STAT5b in sex-specific liver p450 expression. J Biol Chem 1999; 274:35331–35336.
491. Park SH, Liu X, Hennighausen L, et al. Distinctive roles of STAT5a and STAT5b in sexual dimorphism of hepatic P450 gene expression: impact of STAT5a gene disruption. J Biol Chem 1999; 274:7421–7430.
492. Starr R, Hilton DJ. SOCS: suppressors of cytokine signalling. Int J Biochem Cell Biol 1998; 30:1081–1085.
493. Auernhammer CJ, Melmed S. Leukemia-inhibitory factor: neuroimmune modulator of endocrine function. Endocr Rev 2000; 21:313–345.
494. Harvey S, Hull KL. Growth hormone: a paracrine growth factor? Endocrine 1997; 7:267–279.
495. Johansson JO, Fowelin J, Landin K, et al. Growth hormone–deficient adults are insulin-resistant. Metabolism 1995; 44:1126–1129.
496. Rose SR, Ross JL, Uriarte M, et al. The advantage of measuring stimulated as compared with spontaneous growth hormone levels in the diagnosis of growth hormone deficiency. N Engl J Med 1988; 319:201–207.
497. Aimaretti G, Colao A, Corneli G, et al. The study of spontaneous GH secretion after 36-h fasting distinguishes between GH-deficient and normal adults. Clin Endocrinol (Oxf) 1999; 51:771–777.
498. Rosenfeld RG, Albertsson-Wikland K, Cassorla F, et al. Diagnostic controversy: the diagnosis of childhood growth hormone deficiency revisited. J Clin Endocrinol Metab 1995; 80:1532–1540.
499. Granada ML, Sanmarti A, Lucas A, et al. Assay-dependent results of immunoassayable spontaneous 24-hour growth hormone secretion in short children. Acta Paediatr Scand Suppl 1990; 370:63–70.
500. Reiter EO, Morris AH, MacGillivray MH, Weber D. Variable estimates of serum growth hormone concentrations by different radioassay systems. J Clin Endocrinol Metab 1988; 66:68–71.
501. Baumann G, Shaw M, Amburn K, et al. Heterogeneity of circulating growth hormone. Nucl Med Biol 1994; 21:369–379.
502. Strasburger CJ, Dattani MT. New growth hormone assays: potential benefits. Acta Paediatr Suppl 1997; 423:5–11.
503. Bristow AF, Gaines-Das R, Jeffcoate SL, Schulster D. The first international standard for somatropin: report of an international collaborative study. Growth Regul 1995; 5:133–141.
504. Fisker S, Orskov H. Factors modifying growth hormone estimates in immunoassays. Horm Res 1996; 46:183–187.
505. Salomon F, Cuneo RC, Hesp R, Sonksen PH. The effects of treatment with recombinant human growth hormone on body composition and metabolism in adults with growth hormone deficiency. N Engl J Med 1989; 321:1797–1803.
506. de Boer H, Blok GJ, van der Veen EA. Clinical aspects of growth hormone deficiency in adults. Endocr Rev 1995; 16:63–86.
507. Stavrou S, Kleinberg DL. Diagnosis and management of growth hormone deficiency in adults. Endocrinol Metab Clin North Am 2001; 30:545-563.
508. Rosen T, Bengtsson BA. Premature mortality due to cardiovascular disease in hypopituitarism. Lancet 1990; 336:285–288.
509. Bates AS, Van't Hoff W, Jones PJ, Clayton RN. The effect of hypopituitarism on life expectancy. J Clin Endocrinol Metab 1996; 81:1169–1172.
510. Tomlinson JW, Holden N, Hills RK, et al. Association between premature mortality and hypopituitarism. West Midlands Prospective Hypopituitary Study Group. Lancet 2001; 357:425–431.
511. Bulow B, Hagmar L, Eskilsson J, Erfurth EM. Hypopituitary females have a high incidence of cardiovascular morbidity and increased prevalence of cardiovascular risk factors. J Clin Endo Metab 2000; 85:574–584.
512. Bengtsson BA, Abs R, Bennmarke H, et al. The effect of treatment and the individual's responsiveness to GH replacement. KIMS Study Group international board. J Clin Endocrinol Metab 1999; 84:3929–3935.
513. Tauber M, Moulin P, Pienkowski C, et al. Growth hormone retesting and auxological data in 131 GH-deficient patients after completion of treatment. J Clin Endocrinol Metab 1997; 82:352–356.
514. Cogan JD, Phillips JA, Schenkman SS, et al. Familial growth hormone deficiency: a model of dominant and recessive mutations affecting a monomeric protein. J Clin Endocrinol Metab 1994; 79:1261–1265.
515. Baumann G. Mutations in the growth hormone releasing hormone receptor: a new form of dwarfism in humans. Growth Horm IGF Res 1999; 9(Suppl B):24–29; discussion 29–30.
516. Rosenfeld RG, Rosenbloom AL, Guevara-Aguirre J. Growth hormone (GH) insensitivity due to primary GH receptor deficiency. Endocr Rev 1994; 15:369–390.
517. Wu W, Cogan JD, Pfaffle RW, et al. Mutations in *PROP1* cause familial combined pituitary hormone deficiency. Nat Genet 1998; 18:147–149.
518. Sesmilo G, Biller BM, Llevadot J, et al. Effects of growth hormone (GH) administration on homocyst(e)ine levels in men with GH deficiency: a randomized controlled trial. J Clin Endocrinol Metab 2001; 86:1518–1524.
519. Consensus guidelines for the diagnosis and treatment of adults with growth hormone deficiency: summary statement of the Growth Hormone Research Society Workshop on Adult Growth

Hormone Deficiency. J Clin Endocrinol Metab 1998; 83:379–381.

520. Carroll PV, Christ ER, Bengtsson BA, et al. Growth hormone deficiency in adulthood and the effects of growth hormone replacement: a review. Growth Hormone Research Society Scientific Committee. J Clin Endocrinol Metab 1998; 83:382–395.
521. Arvat E, Di Vito L, Broglio F, et al. Preliminary evidence that ghrelin, the natural GH secretagogue (GHS)-receptor ligand, strongly stimulates GH secretion in humans. J Endocrinol Invest 2000; 23:493–495.
522. Drake WM, Howell SJ, Monson JP, Shalet SM. Optimizing GH therapy in adults and children. Endocr Rev 2001; 22:425–450.
523. Marzullo P, Di Somma C, Pratt KL, et al. Usefulness of different biochemical markers of the insulin-like growth factor (IGF) family in diagnosing growth hormone excess and deficiency in adults. J Clin Endocrinol Metab 2001; 86:3001–3008.
524. Hilding A, Hall K, Wivall-Helleryd IL, et al. Serum levels of insulin-like growth factor I in 152 patients with growth hormone deficiency, aged 19–82 years, in relation to those in healthy subjects. J Clin Endocrinol Metab 1999; 84:2013–2019.
525. Gill MS, Toogood AA, O'Neill PA, et al. Urinary growth hormone (GH), insulin-like growth factor I (IGF-I), and IGF-binding protein-3 measurements in the diagnosis of adult GH deficiency. J Clin Endocrinol Metab 1998; 83:2562–2565.
526. Newman CB, Kleinberg DL. Adult growth hormone deficiency. Endocrinologist 1998; 8:178–186.
527. Rosen T, Bosaeus I, Tolli J, et al. Increased body fat mass and decreased extracellular fluid volume in adults with growth hormone deficiency. Clin Endocrinol (Oxf) 1993; 38:63–71.
528. Colao A, Di Somma C, Pivonello R, et al. Bone loss is correlated to the severity of growth hormone deficiency in adult patients with hypopituitarism. J Clin Endocrinol Metab 1999; 84:1919–1924.
529. Kaufman JM, Taelman P, Vermeulen A, Vanderweghe M. Bone mineral status in growth hormone deficient males with isolated and multiple pituitary deficiencies of childhood onset. J Clin Endocrinol Metab 1992; 74:118–123.
530. Sesmilo G, Biller BM, Llevadot J, et al. Effects of growth hormone administration on inflammatory and other cardiovascular risk markers in men with growth hormone deficiency: a randomized, controlled clinical trial. Ann Intern Med 2000; 133:111–122.
531. Attanasio AF, Lamberts SWJ, Matranga AMC, et al. Adult growth hormone (GH)–deficient patients demonstrate heterogeneity between childhood onset and adult onset before and during human GH treatment. J Clin Endocrinol Metab 1997; 82:82–88.
532. Christopher M, Hew FL, Oakley M, et al. Defects of insulin action and skeletal muscle glucose metabolism in growth hormone–deficient adults persist after 24 months of recombinant human growth hormone therapy. J Clin Endocrinol Metab 1998; 83:1668–1681.
533. Pfeifer M, Verhovec R, Zizek B, et al. Growth hormone (GH) treatment reverses early atherosclerotic changes in GH-deficient adults. J Clin Endocrinol Metab 1999; 84:453–457.
534. Borson-Chazot F, Serusclat A, Kalfallah Y, et al. Decrease in carotid intima-media thickness after one year growth hormone (GH) treatment in adults with GH deficiency. J Clin Endocrinol Metab 1999; 84:1329–1333.
535. Merola B, Cittadini A, Colao A, et al. Cardiac structural and functional abnormalities in adult patients with growth hormone deficiency. J Clin Endocrinol Metab 1993; 77:1658–1661.
536. Amato G, Carella C, Fazio S, et al. Body composition, bone metabolism, and heart structure and function in growth hormone (GH)–deficient adults before and after GH replacement therapy at low doses. J Clin Endocrinol Metab 1993; 77:1671–1676.
537. Valcavi R, Gaddi O, Zini M, et al. Cardiac performance and mass in adults with hypopituitarism: effects of one year of growth hormone treatment. J Clin Endocrinol Metab 1995; 80:659–666.
538. Murray RD, Skillicorn CJ, Howell SJ, et al. Dose titration and patient selection increases the efficacy of GH replacement in severely GH deficient adults. Clin Endocrinol (Oxf) 1999; 50:749–757.
539. Murray RD, Skillicorn CJ, Howell SJ, et al. Influences on quality of life in GH deficient adults and their effect on response to treatment. Clin Endocrinol (Oxf) 1999; 51:565–573.
540. Wang TC, Koh TJ, Varro A, et al. Processing and proliferative effects of human progastrin in transgenic mice. J Clin Invest 1996; 98:1918–1929.
541. Horber FF, Haymond MW. Human growth hormone prevents the protein catabolic side effects of prednisone in humans. J Clin Invest 1990; 86:265–272.
542. Baum HB, Biller BM, Finkelstein JS, et al. Effects of physiologic growth hormone therapy on bone density and body composition in patients with adult-onset growth hormone deficiency: a randomized, placebo-controlled trial. Ann Intern Med 1996; 125:883–890.
543. Kotzmann H, Riedl M, Bernecker P, et al. Effect of long-term growth-hormone substitution therapy on bone mineral density and parameters of bone metabolism in adult patients with growth hormone deficiency. Calcif Tissue Int 1998; 62:40–46.
544. Cuneo RC, Judd S, Wallace JD, et al. The Australian Multicenter Trial of Growth Hormone (GH) Treatment in GH-Deficient Adults. J Clin Endocrinol Metab 1998; 83:107–116.
545. Boger RH, Skamira C, Bode-Boger SM, et al. Nitric oxide may mediate the hemodynamic effects of recombinant growth hormone in patients with acquired growth hormone deficiency: a double-blind, placebo-controlled study. J Clin Invest 1996; 98:2706–2713.
546. Colao A, Marzullo P, Di Somma C, Lombardi G. Growth hormone and the heart. Clin Endocrinol (Oxf) 2001; 54:137–154.
547. Burman P, Broman JE, Hetta J, et al. Quality of life in adults with growth hormone (GH) deficiency: response to treatment with recombinant human GH in a placebo-controlled 21-month trial. J Clin Endocrinol Metab 1995; 80:3585–3590.
548. Baum HB, Katznelson L, Sherman JC, et al. Effects of physiological growth hormone (GH) therapy on cognition and quality of life in patients with adult-onset GH deficiency. J Clin Endocrinol Metab 1998; 83:3184–3189.
548a. Stavrou S, Kleinberg D. Diagnosis and management of GH deficiency in adults. Endocrin Metab Clin 2001; 30:545–563.
549. Gibney J, Wallace JD, Spinks T, et al. The effects of 10 years of recombinant human growth hormone (GH) in adult GH-deficient patients. J Clin Endocrinol Metab 1999; 84:2596–2602.
550. Blethen S. Dosing, monitoring, and safety of growth hormone–replacement therapy in adults with growth hormone deficiency. Endocrinologist 1998; 8:36S–40S.
551. Cook DM, Ludlam WH, Cook MB. Route of estrogen administration helps to determine growth hormone (GH) replacement dose in GH-deficient adults. J Clin Endocrinol Metab 1999; 84:3956–3960.
552. Hoffman DM, Pallasser R, Duncan M, et al. How is whole body protein turnover perturbed in growth hormone–deficient adults? J Clin Endocrinol Metab 1998; 83:4344–4349.
553. de Boer H, Blok GJ, Popp-Snijders C, et al. Monitoring of growth hormone replacement therapy in adults, based on measurement of serum markers. J Clin Endocrinol Metab 1996; 81:1371–1377.
554. Chan JM, Stampfer MJ, Giovannucci E, et al. Plasma insulin-like growth factor-I and prostate cancer risk: a prospective study. Science 1998; 279:563–566.
555. Hankinson SE, Willett WC, Colditz GA, et al. Circulating concentrations of insulin-like growth factor-I and risk of breast cancer. Lancet 1998; 351:1393–1396.
556. Yu H, Rohan T. Role of the insulin-like growth factor family in cancer development and progression. J Natl Cancer Inst 2000; 92:1472–1489.
557. Orme S, McNally RJQ, Cartwright RA, Belchetz PE. Mortality and cancer incidence in acromegaly: a retrospective cohort study. J Clin Endocrinol Metab 1998; 83:2730–2734.
558. Melmed S. Acromegaly and cancer: not a problem? J Clin Endocrinol Metab 2001; 86:2929–2934.
559. Renehan AG, Bhaskar P, Painter JE, et al. The prevalence and characteristics of colorectal neoplasia in acromegaly. J Clin Endocrinol Metab 2000; 85:3417–3424.
560. Sklar C. Paying the price for cure: treating cancer survivors with growth hormone. J Clin Endocrinol Metab 2000; 85:4441–4443.
561. Swerdlow AJ, Reddingius RE, Higgins CD, et al. Growth hormone treatment of children with brain tumors and risk of tumor recurrence. J Clin Endocrinol Metab 2000; 85:4444–4449.
562. Jenkins RC, Ross RJ. Growth hormone therapy for protein catabolism. QJM 1996; 89:813–819.
563. Chu LW, Lam KS, Tam SC, et al. A randomized controlled trial

of low-dose recombinant human growth hormone in the treatment of malnourished elderly medical patients. J Clin Endocrinol Metab 2001; 86:1913–1920.
564. Takala J, Ruokonen E, Webster NR, et al. Increased mortality associated with growth hormone treatment in critically ill adults. N Engl J Med 1999; 341:785–792.
565. Hoiden-Guthenberg I, Flores-Morales A, Norstedt G, Fryklund L. Anabolic actions of growth hormone in catabolic states: analysis of differential gene expression in rats treated with GH and LPS using cDNA microarrays. The Endocrine Society's 83rd Annual Meeting, Denver, 2001.
566. Johansson AG, Lindh E, Blum WF, et al. Effects of growth hormone and insulin-like growth factor I in men with idiopathic osteoporosis. J Clin Endocrinol Metab 1996; 81:44–48.
567. Holloway L, Kohlmeier L, Kent K, Marcus R. Skeletal effects of cyclic recombinant human growth hormone and salmon calcitonin in osteopenic postmenopausal women. J Clin Endocrinol Metab 1997; 82:1111–1117.
568. Schambelan M, Mulligan K, Grunfeld C, et al. Recombinant human growth hormone in patients with HIV-associated wasting: a randomized, placebo-controlled trial. Serostim Study Group. Ann Intern Med 1996; 125:873–882.
569. Wanke C, Gerrior J, Kantaros J, et al. Recombinant human growth hormone improves the fat redistribution syndrome (lipodystrophy) in patients with HIV. AIDS 1999; 13:2099–3103.
570. Lo JC, Mulligan K, Noor MA, et al. The effects of recombinant human growth hormone on body composition and glucose metabolism in HIV-infected patients with fat accumulation. J Clin Endocrinol Metab 2001; 86:3480–3487.
571. Sonksen PH. Insulin, growth hormone and sport. J Endocrinol 2001; 170:13–25.
572. Isley WL, Underwood LE, Clemmons DR. Dietary components that regulate serum somatomedin-C concentrations in humans. J Clin Invest 1983; 71:175–182.
573. Benda C. Beitrage zur normalen und pathologischen histologic der menschhchen hypophysis cerebri. Klin Wochenschr 1900; 36: 1205.
574. Evans HM, Long JA. The effect of the anterior lobe of the pituitary administered intra-peritoneally upon growth, maturity and oestrus cycle of the rat. Anat Rev 1921; 21:62.
575. Alexander L, Appleton D, Hall R, et al. Epidemiology of acromegaly in the Newcastle region. Clin Endocrinol (Oxf) 1980; 12: 71–79.
576. Bengtsson BA, Eden S, Ernest I, et al. Epidemiology and long-term survival in acromegaly: a study of 166 cases diagnosed between 1955 and 1984. Acta Med Scand 1988; 223:327–335.
577. Ritchie CM, Atkinson AB, Kennedy AL, et al. Ascertainment and natural history of treated acromegaly in Northern Ireland. Ulster Med J 1990; 59:55–62.
578. Melmed S. Acromegaly. N Engl J Med 1990; 322:966–977.
579. Asa SL, Kovacs K. Pituitary pathology in acromegaly. Endocrinol Metab Clin North Am 1992; 21:553–574.
580. Lloyd RV, Cano M, Chandler WF, et al. Human growth hormone and prolactin secreting pituitary adenomas analyzed by in situ hybridization. Am J Pathol 1989; 134:605–613.
581. Maheshwari HG, Prezant TR, Herman-Bonert V, et al. Long-acting peptidomimergic control of gigantism caused by pituitary acidophilic stem cell adenoma. J Clin Endocrinol Metab 2000; 85:3409–3416.
582. Kovacs K, Horvath E, Asa SL, et al. Pituitary cells producing more than one hormone. Trends Endocrinol Metab 1989; 1:104–108.
583. Melmed S. Pituitary function and neoplasia. In Jameson JL (ed). Principles of Molecular Medicine. Totowa, NJ, Humana Press, 1998, pp 443–449.
584. Heaney AP, Melmed S. Molecular pathogenesis of pituitary tumors. In Wass J (ed). Oxford Textbook of Endocrinology: Endocrine-Related Cancer. New York, Oxford University Press, 2002.
585. Shimon I, Melmed S. Genetic basis of endocrine disease: pituitary tumor pathogenesis. J Clin Endocrinol Metab 1997; 82: 1675–1681.
586. Thapar K, Kovacs K, Stefaneanu L, et al. Overexpression of the growth-hormone–releasing hormone gene in acromegaly-associated pituitary tumors: an event associated with neoplastic progression and aggressive behavior. Am J Pathol 1997; 151:769–784.
587. Thorner MO, Vance ML. Growth hormone, 1988. J Clin Invest 1988; 82:745–747.
588. Herman I, Gonsky R, Fagin J. Clonal origin of secretory and non-secretory pituitary tumors. Clin Res 1990; 38:296A–296A.
589. Vallar L, Spada A, Giannattasio G. Altered Gs and adenylate cyclase activity in human GH-secreting pituitary adenomas. Nature 1987; 330:566–568.
590. Landis CA, Harsh G, Lyons J, et al. Clinical characteristics of acromegalic patients whose pituitary tumors contain mutant Gs protein. J Clin Endocrinol Metab 1990; 71:1416–1420.
591. Frohman LA, Jansson JO. Growth hormone–releasing hormone. Endocr Rev 1986; 7:223–253.
592. Melmed S, Ezrin C, Kovacs K, et al. Acromegaly due to secretion of growth hormone by an ectopic pancreatic islet-cell tumor. N Engl J Med 1985; 312:9–17.
593. Moran A, Asa SL, Kovacs K, et al. Gigantism due to pituitary mammosomatotroph hyperplasia. N Engl J Med 1990; 323:322–327.
594. Faglia G, Arosio M, Bazzoni N. Ectopic acromegaly. Endocrinol Metab Clin North Am 1992; 21:575–595.
595. Frohman LA, Szabo M, Berelowitz M, Stachura ME. Partial purification and characterization of a peptide with growth hormone–releasing activity from extrapituitary tumors in patients with acromegaly. J Clin Invest 1980; 65:43–54.
596. Drange MR, Melmed S. Long-acting lanreotide induces clinical and biochemical remission of acromegaly caused by disseminated growth hormone–releasing hormone–secreting carcinoid. J Clin Endocrinol Metab 1998; 83:3104–3109.
597. Barkan AL, Shenker Y, Grekin RJ, Vale WW. Acromegaly from ectopic growth hormone–releasing hormone secretion by a malignant carcinoid tumor: successful treatment with long-acting somatostatin analogue SMS 201-995. Cancer 1988; 61:221–226.
598. Lloyd RV, Chandler WF., Kovacs K, et al. Ectopic pituitary adenomas with normal anterior pituitary glands. Am J Surg Pathol 1986; 10:546–552.
599. Madonna D, Kendler A, Soliman AM. Ectopic growth hormone–secreting pituitary adenoma in the sphenoid sinus. Ann Otol Rhinol Laryngol 2001; 110:99–101.
600. Weinstein LS, Shenker A, Gejman PV, et al. Activating mutations of the stimulatory G protein in the McCune- Albright syndrome. N Engl J Med 1991; 325:1688–1695.
601. Chandrasekharappa SC, Guru SC, Manickam P, et al. Positional cloning of the gene for multiple endocrine neoplasia-type 1. Science 1997; 276:404–407.
602. Teh BT, Kytola S, Farnebo F, et al. Mutation analysis of the MEN1 gene in multiple endocrine neoplasia type 1, familial acromegaly and familial isolated hyperparathyroidism. J Clin Endocrinol Metab 1998; 83:2621–2626.
603. Stratakis CA, Carney JA, Lin JP, et al. Carney complex, a familial multiple neoplasia and lentiginosis syndrome: analysis of 11 kindreds and linkage to the short arm of chromosome 2. J Clin Invest 1996; 97:699–705.
604. Gadelha MR, Prezant TR, Une KN, et al. Loss of heterozygosity on chromosome 11q13 in two families with acromegaly/gigantism is independent of mutations of the multiple endocrine neoplasia type I gene. J Clin Endocrinol Metab 1999; 84:249–256.
605. Drange MR, Fram NR, Herman-Bonert V, Melmed S. Pituitary tumor registry: a novel clinical resource. J Clin Endocrinol Metab 2000; 85:168–174.
606. Daughaday WH. Pituitary gigantism. Endocrinol Metab Clin North Am 1992; 21:633–647.
607. Molitch ME. Clinical manifestations of acromegaly. Endocrinol Metab Clin North Am 1992; 21:597–614.
608. Jadresic A, Banks LM, Child DF, et al. The acromegaly syndrome: relation between clinical features, growth hormone values and radiological characteristics of the pituitary tumours. Q J Med 1982; 51:189–204.
609. Nabarro JD. Acromegaly. Clin Endocrinol (Oxf) 1987; 26:481–512.
610. Colao A, Marzullo P, Vallone G, et al. Reversibility of joint thickening in acromegalic patients: an ultrasonography study. J Clin Endocrinol Metab 1998; 83:2121–2125.
611. Scillitani A, Chiodini I, Carnevale V, et al. Skeletal involvement in female acromegalic subjects: the effects of growth hormone excess in amenorrheal and menstruating patients. J Bone Miner Res 1997; 12:1729–1736.

612. Lieberman SA, Bjorkengren AG, Hoffman AR. Rheumatologic and skeletal changes in acromegaly. Endocrinol Metab Clin North Am 1992; 21:615–631.
613. Dons RF, Rosselet P, Pastakia B, et al. Arthropathy in acromegalic patients before and after treatment: a long-term follow-up study. Clin Endocrinol (Oxf) 1988; 28:515–524.
614. Matsuoka LY, Wortsman J, Kupchella CE, et al. Histochemical characterization of the cutaneous involvement of acromegaly. Arch Intern Med 1982; 142:1820–1823.
615. Verde GG, Santi I, Chiodini P, et al. Serum type III procollagen propeptide levels in acromegalic patients. J Clin Endocrinol Metab 1986; 63:1406–1410.
616. Leavitt J, Klein I, Kendricks F, et al. Skin tags: a cutaneous marker for colonic polyps. Ann Intern Med 1983; 98:928–930.
617. Lombardi G, Colao A, Marzullo P, et al. Is growth hormone bad for your heart? Cardiovascular impact of GH deficiency and of acromegaly. J Endocrinol 1997; 155(Suppl 1):S33-S37; discussion S39.
618. Colao A, Cuocolo A, Marzullo P, et al. Impact of patient's age and disease duration on cardiac performance in acromegaly: a radionuclide angiography study. J Clin Endocrinol Metab 1999; 84:1518–1523.
619. Lopez-Velasco R, Escobar-Morreale HF, Vega B, et al. Cardiac involvement in acromegaly: specific myocardiopathy or consequence of systemic hypertension? J Clin Endocrinol Metab 1997; 82:1047–1053.
620. Deray G, Rieu M, Devynck MA, et al. Evidence of an endogenous digitalis-like factor in the plasma of patients with acromegaly. N Engl J Med 1987; 316:575–580.
621. Rajasoorya C, Holdaway IM, Wrightson P, et al. Determinants of clinical outcome and survival in acromegaly. Clin Endocrinol (Oxf) 1994; 41:95–102.
622. Rosenow F, Reuter S, Deuss U, et al. Sleep apnoea in treated acromegaly: relative frequency and predisposing factors. Clin Endocrinol (Oxf) 1996; 45:563–569.
623. Grunstein RR, Ho KK, Sullivan CE. Effect of octreotide, a somatostatin analog, on sleep apnea in patients with acromegaly. Ann Intern Med 1994; 121:478–483.
624. Jenkins PJ, Sohaib SA, Akker S, et al. The pathology of median neuropathy in acromegaly. Ann Intern Med 2000; 133:197–201.
625. Furman K, Ezzat S. Psychological features of acromegaly. Psychother Psychosom 1998; 67:147–153.
626. Stewart CE, Rotwein P. Growth, differentiation, and survival: multiple physiological functions for insulin-like growth factors. Physiol Rev 1996; 76:1005–1026.
627. Grinspoon S, Clemmons D, Swearingen B, Klibanski A. Serum insulin-like growth factor–binding protein-3 levels in the diagnosis of acromegaly. J Clin Endocrinol Metab 1995; 80:927–932.
628. Cohen P, Peehl DM, Graves HC, Rosenfeld RG. Biological effects of prostate specific antigen as an insulin-like growth factor binding protein-3 protease. J Endocrinol 1994; 142:407–415.
629. Jenkins PJ, Frajese V, Jones AM, et al. Insulin-like growth factor I and the development of colorectal neoplasia in acromegaly. J Clin Endocrinol Metab 2000; 85:3218–3221.
630. Delhougne B, Deneux C, Abs R, et al. The prevalence of colonic polyps in acromegaly: a colonoscopic and pathological study in 103 patients. J Clin Endocrinol Metab 1995; 80:3223–3226.
631. Ladas SD, Thalassinos NC, Ioannides G, Raptis SA. Does acromegaly really predispose to an increased prevalence of gastrointestinal tumours? Clin Endocrinol (Oxf) 1994; 41:597–601.
632. Ezzat S, Strom C, Melmed S. Colon polyps in acromegaly. Ann Intern Med 1991; 114:754–755.
633. Barkan AL, Stred SE, Reno K, et al. Increased growth hormone pulse frequency in acromegaly. J Clin Endocrinol Metab 1989; 69:1225–1233.
634. Katznelson L, Kleinberg D, Vance ML, et al. Hypogonadism in patients with acromegaly: data from the multi-centre acromegaly registry pilot study. Clin Endocrinol (Oxf) 2001; 54:183–188.
635. Kaltsas GA, Mukherjee JJ, Jenkins PJ, et al. Menstrual irregularity in women with acromegaly. J Clin Endocrinol Metab 1999; 84:2731–2735.
636. Lesse GP, Fraser WD, Farquharson R, et al. Gonadal status is an important determinant of bone density in acromegaly. Clin Endocrinol (Oxf) 1998; 48:59–65.
637. Kasagi K, Shimatsu A, Miyamoto S, et al. Goiter associated with acromegaly: sonographic and scintigraphic findings of the thyroid gland. Thyroid 1999; 9:791–796.
638. Colao A, Marzullo P, Ferone D, et al. Prostatic hyperplasia: an unknown feature of acromegaly. J Clin Endocrinol Metab 1998; 83:775–779.
639. Colao A, Marzullo P, Spiezia S, et al. Effect of growth hormone (GH) and insulin-like growth factor I on prostate diseases: an ultrasonographic and endocrine study in acromegaly, GH deficiency, and healthy subjects. J Clin Endocrinol Metab 1999; 84: 1986–1991.
640. Jenkins D, O'Brien I, Johnson A, et al. The Birmingham pituitary database: auditing the outcome of the treatment of acromegaly. Clin Endocrinol (Oxf) 1995; 43:517–522.
641. Bates AS, Van't Hoff W, Jones JM, Clayton RN. An audit of outcome of treatment in acromegaly. Q J Med 1993; 86:293–299.
642. Swearingen B, Barker FG, Katznelson L, et al. Long-term mortality after transsphenoidal surgery and adjunctive therapy for acromegaly. J Clin Endocrinol Metab 1998; 83:3419–3426.
643. Abosch A, Tyrrell JB, Lamborn KR, et al. Transsphenoidal microsurgery for growth hormone-secreting pituitary adenomas: initial outcome and long-term results. J Clin Endocrinol Metab 1998; 83:3411–3418.
644. Freda PU, Post KD, Powell JS, Wardlaw SL. Evaluation of disease status with sensitive measures of growth hormone secretion in 60 postoperative patients with acromegaly. J Clin Endocrinol Metab 1998; 83:3808–3816.
645. Giustina A, Barkan A, Casanueva FF, et al. Criteria for cure of acromegaly: a consensus statement. J Clin Endocrinol Metab 2000; 85:526–529.
646. Duncan E, Wass JA. Investigation protocol: acromegaly and its investigation. Clin Endocrinol (Oxf) 1999; 50:285–293.
647. Clemmons DR, Van Wyk JJ, Ridgway EC, et al. Evaluation of acromegaly by radioimmunoassay of somatomedin-C. N Engl J Med 1979; 301:1138–1142.
648. Drange MR. IGFs in the evaluation of acromegaly. In Rosenfeld RG, Roberts CT (eds). Contemporary Endocrinology. The IGF System: Molecular Biology, Physiology, and Clinical Applications. Totowa, NJ, Humana Press, 1999, pp 699–720.
649. Melmed S, Ho K, Klibanski A, et al. Clinical review 75: recent advances in pathogenesis, diagnosis, and management of acromegaly. J Clin Endocrinol Metab 1995; 80:3395–3402.
650. Melmed S. Extrapituitary acromegaly. Endocrinol Metab Clin North Am 1991; 20:1–9.
651. Frohman LA. Ectopic hormone production by tumors. Clin Neuroendocrinol Perspect 1984; 3:201–224.
652. Melmed S, Jackson I, Kleinberg D, Klibanski A. Current treatment guidelines for acromegaly. J Clin Endocrinol Metab 1998; 83:2646–2652.
653. Freda PU, Wardlaw SL, Post KD. Long-term endocrinological follow-up evaluation in 115 patients who underwent transsphenoidal surgery for acromegaly. J Neurosurg 1998; 89:353–358.
654. Lissett CA, Peacey SR, Laing I, et al. The outcome of surgery for acromegaly: the need for a specialist pituitary surgeon for all types of growth hormone (GH) secreting adenoma. Clin Endocrinol (Oxf) 1998; 49:653–657.
655. Ahmed S, Elsheikh M, Stratton IM, et al. Outcome of transsphenoidal surgery for acromegaly and its relationship to surgical experience. Clin Endocrinol (Oxf) 1999; 50:561–567.
656. Sheaves R, Jenkins P, Blackburn P, et al. Outcome of transsphenoidal surgery for acromegaly using strict criteria for surgical cure. Clin Endocrinol (Oxf) 1996; 45:407–413.
657. Ross DA, Wilson CB. Results of transsphenoidal microsurgery for growth hormone–secreting pituitary adenoma in a series of 214 patients. J Neurosurg 1988; 68:854–867.
658. Fahlbusch R, Honegger J, Buchfelder M. Surgical management of acromegaly. Endocrinol Metab Clin North Am 1992; 21:669–692.
659. Stewart PM. Current therapy for acromegaly. Trends Endocrinol Metab 2000; 11:128–132.
660. Laws ER, Thapar K. Pituitary surgery. Endocrinol Metab Clin North Am 1999; 28:119–131.
661. Thapar K, Laws ER. Pituitary surgery. In Thapar K, Kovacs K, Scheithauer BW, Lloyd RV (eds). Diagnosis and Management of Pituitary Tumors. Totowa, NJ, Humana Press, 2001, pp 225–246.
662. Tindall GT, Oyesiku NM, Watts NB, et al. Transsphenoidal adenomectomy for growth hormone-secreting pituitary adenomas

in acromegaly: outcome analysis and determinants of failure. J Neurosurg 1993; 78:205–215.
663. Eastman RC, Gorden P, Glatstein E, Roth J. Radiation therapy of acromegaly. Endocrinol Metab Clin North Am 1992; 21:693–712.
664. Barkan AL, Halasz I, Dornfeld KJ, et al. Pituitary irradiation is ineffective in normalizing plasma insulin-like growth factor I in patients with acromegaly. J Clin Endocrinol Metab 1997; 82: 3187–3191.
665. Powell JS, Wardlaw SL, Post KD, Freda PU. Outcome of radiotherapy for acromegaly using normalization of insulin-like growth factor I to define cure. J Clin Endocrinol Metab 2000; 85:2068–2071.
666. Peacey SR, Toogood AA, Veldhuis JD, et al. The relationship between 24-hour growth hormone secretion and insulin-like growth factor I in patients with successfully treated acromegaly: impact of surgery or radiotherapy. J Clin Endocrinol Metab 2001; 86:259–266.
667. Laws ER, Vance ML. Radiosurgery for pituitary tumors and craniopharyngiomas. Neurosurg Clin North Am 1999; 10:327–336.
668. van der Lely AJ, de Herder WW, Lamberts SW. The role of radiotherapy in acromegaly. J Clin Endocrinol Metab 1997; 82: 3185–3186.
669. Pan L, Zhang N, Wang E, et al. Pituitary adenomas: the effect of gamma knife radiosurgery on tumor growth and endocrinopathies. Stereotact Funct Neurosurg 1998; 70(Suppl 1):119–26.
670. Alexander MJ, DeSalles AA, Tomiyasu U. Multiple radiation-induced intracranial lesions after treatment for pituitary adenoma: case report. J Neurosurg 1998; 88:111–115.
671. Crossen JR, Garwood D, Glatstein E, Neuwelt EA. Neurobehavioral sequelae of cranial irradiation in adults: a review of radiation-induced encephalopathy. J Clin Oncol 1994; 12:627–642.
672. Murray RM, Grill V, Crinis N, et al. Hypocalcemic and normocalcemic hyperparathyroidism in patients with advanced prostatic cancer. J Clin Endocrinol Metab 2001; 86:4133–4138.
673. Jaffe CA, Barkan AL. Treatment of acromegaly with dopamine agonists. Endocrinol Metab Clin North Am 1992; 21:713–735.
674. Abs R, Verhelst J, Maiter D, et al. Cabergoline in the treatment of acromegaly: a study in 64 patients. J Clin Endocrinol Metab 1998; 83:374–378.
675. Lamberts SW, van der Lely AJ, de Herder WW, Hofland LJ. Octreotide. N Engl J Med 1996; 334:246–254.
676. Lamberts SW, Uitterlinden P, Verschoor L, et al. Long-term treatment of acromegaly with the somatostatin analogue SMS 201-995. N Engl J Med 1985; 313:1576–1580.
677. Ezzat S, Snyder PJ, Young WF, et al. Octreotide treatment of acromegaly: a randomized, multicenter study. Ann Intern Med 1992; 117:711–718.
678. Ur E, Mather SJ, Bomanji J, et al. Pituitary imaging using a labelled somatostatin analogue in acromegaly. Clin Endocrinol (Oxf) 1992; 36:147–150.
679. Wang C, Lam KS, Arceo E, Chan FL. Comparison of the effectiveness of 2-hourly versus 8-hourly subcutaneous injections of a somatostatin analog (SMS 201-995) in the treatment of acromegaly. J Clin Endocrinol Metab 1989; 69:670–677.
680. Newman CB, Melmed S, Snyder PJ, et al. Safety and efficacy of long-term octreotide therapy of acromegaly: results of a multicenter trial in 103 patients—a clinical research center study. J Clin Endocrinol Metab 1995; 80:2768–2775.
681. Gillis JC, Noble S, Goa KL. Octreotide long-acting release (LAR): a review of its pharmacological properties and therapeutic use in the management of acromegaly. Drugs 1997; 53:681–699.
682. Flogstad AK, Halse J, Bakke S, et al. Sandostatin LAR in acromegalic patients: long-term treatment. J Clin Endocrinol Metab 1997; 82:23–28.
683. Lancranjan I, Atkinson AB. Results of a European multicentre study with Sandostatin LAR in acromegalic patients. Sandostatin LAR Group. Pituitary 1999; 1:105–114.
684. Baldelli R, Colao A, Razzore P, et al. Two-year follow-up of acromegalic patients treated with slow release lanreotide (30 mg). J Clin Endocrinol Metab 2000; 85:4099–4103.
685. Colao A, Ferone D, Marzullo P, et al. Long-term effects of depot long-acting somatostatin analog octreotide on hormone levels and tumor mass in acromegaly. J Clin Endocrinol Metab 2001; 86:2779–2786.
686. Caron P, Morange-Ramos I, Cogne M, Jaquet P. Three year follow-up of acromegalic patients treated with intramuscular slow-release lanreotide. J Clin Endocrinol Metab 1997; 82:18–22.
687. Flogstad AK, Halse J, Haldorsen T, et al. Sandostatin LAR in acromegalic patients: a dose-range study. J Clin Endocrinol Metab 1995; 80:3601–3607.
688. Colao A, Ferone D, Cappabianca P, et al. Effect of octreotide pretreatment on surgical outcome in acromegaly. J Clin Endocrinol Metab 1997; 82:3308–3314.
689. Biermasz NR, van Dulken H, Roelfsema F. Direct postoperative and follow-up results of transsphenoidal surgery in 19 acromegalic patients pretreated with octreotide compared to those in untreated matched controls. J Clin Endocrinol Metab 1999; 84: 3551–3555.
690. Pascual J, Freijanes J, Berciano J, Pesquera C. Analgesic effect of octreotide in headache associated with acromegaly is not mediated by opioid mechanisms: case report. Pain 1991; 47:341–344.
691. Colao A, Marzullo P, Ferone D, et al. Cardiovascular effects of depot long-acting somatostatin analog Sandostatin LAR in acromegaly. J Clin Endocrinol Metab 2000; 85:3132–3140.
692. Colao A, Cuocolo A, Marzullo P, et al. Effects of 1-year treatment with octreotide on cardiac performance in patients with acromegaly. J Clin Endocrinol Metab 1999; 84:17–23.
693. Colao A, Cuocolo A, Marzullo P, et al. Is the acromegalic cardiomyopathy reversible? Effect of 5-year normalization of growth hormone and insulin-like growth factor I levels on cardiac performance. J Clin Endocrinol Metab 2001; 86:1551–1557.
694. Melmed S, Dowling RH, Frohman L, et al. Consensus statement: benefits vs. risks of medical therapy for acromegaly. Am J Med 1994; 97:468.
695. Trainer PJ, Drake WM, Katznelson L, et al. Treatment of acromegaly with the growth hormone-receptor antagonist pegvisomant. N Engl J Med 2000; 342:1171–1177.
696. Ross RJ, Leung KC, Maamra M, et al. Binding and functional studies with the growth hormone receptor antagonist, B2036-PEG (pegvisomant), reveal effects of pegylation and evidence that it binds to a receptor dimer. J Clin Endocrinol Metab 2001; 86: 1716–1723.
697. Herman-Bonert VS, Zib K, Scarlett JA, Melmed S. Growth hormone receptor antagonist therapy in acromegalic patients resistant to somatostatin analogs. J Clin Endocrinol Metab 2000; 85: 2958–2961.
698. van der Lely AJ, Muller A, Janssen JA, et al. Control of tumor size and disease activity during cotreatment with octreotide and the growth hormone receptor antagonist pegvisomant in an acromegalic patient. J Clin Endocrinol Metab 2001; 86:478–481.
699. Newman CB, Melmed S, George A, et al. Octreotide as primary therapy for acromegaly. J Clin Endocrinol Metab 1998; 83:3034–3040.
700. Scheithauer BW, Horvath E, Lloyd RV, Kovacs K. Pathology of pituitary adenomas and pituitary hyperplasia. In Thapar K, Kovacs K, Scheithauer BW, Lloyd RV (eds). Diagnosis and Management of Pituitary Tumors. Totowa, NJ, Humana Press, 2001, pp 91–154.
701. Zabel BU, Naylor SL, Sakaguchi AY, et al. High-resolution chromosomal localization of human genes for amylase, proopiomelanocortin, somatostatin, and a DNA fragment (D3S1) by in situ hybridization. Proc Natl Acad Sci USA 1983; 80:6932–6936.
702. Cochet M, Chang AC, Cohen SN. Characterization of the structural gene and putative 5′-regulatory sequences for human proopiomelanocortin. Nature 1982; 297:335–339.
703. Chen WY, Wight DC, Wagner TE, Kopchick JJ. Expression of a mutated bovine growth hormone gene suppresses growth of transgenic mice. Proc Natl Acad Sci USA 1990; 87:5061–5065.
704. Arai M, Assil IQ, Abou-Samra AB. Characterization of three corticotropin-releasing factor receptors in catfish: a novel third receptor is predominantly expressed in pituitary and urophysis. Endocrinology 2001; 142:446–454.
705. Jin WD, Boutillier AL, Glucksman MJ, et al. Characterization of a corticotropin-releasing hormone–responsive element in the rat proopiomelanocortin gene promoter and molecular cloning of its binding protein. Mol Endocrinol 1994; 8:1377–1388.
706. Weninger SC, Dunn AJ, Muglia LJ, et al. Stress-induced behaviors require the corticotropin-releasing hormone (CRH) receptor, but not CRH. Proc Natl Acad Sci USA 1999; 96:8283–8288.

707. Coste SC, Kesterson RA, Heldwein KA, et al. Abnormal adaptations to stress and impaired cardiovascular function in mice lacking corticotropin-releasing hormone receptor-2. Nat Genet 2000; 24:403–409.
708. Bousquet C, Zatelli MC, Melmed S. Direct regulation of pituitary proopiomelanocortin by STAT3 provides a novel mechanism for immuno-neuroendocrine interfacing. J Clin Invest 2000; 106: 1417–1425.
709. Eberwine JH, Roberts JL. Glucocorticoid regulation of pro-opiomelanocortin gene transcription in the rat pituitary. J Biol Chem 1984; 259:2166–2170.
710. Loeffler JP, Kley N, Pittius CW, Hollt V. Calcium ion and cyclic adenosine 3′,5′-monophosphate regulate proopiomelanocortin messenger ribonucleic acid levels in rat intermediate and anterior pituitary lobes. Endocrinology 1986; 119:2840–2847.
711. Seidah NG, Chretien M. Complete amino acid sequence of a human pituitary glycopeptide: an important maturation product of pro-opiomelanocortin. Proc Natl Acad Sci USA 1981; 78: 4236–4240.
712. Fenger M, Johnsen AH. Alpha-amidated peptides derived from pro-opiomelanocortin in normal human pituitary. Biochem J 1988; 250:781–788.
713. Jackson RS, Creemers JW, Ohagi S, et al. Obesity and impaired prohormone processing associated with mutations in the human prohormone convertase 1 gene. Nat Genet 1997; 16:303–306.
714. Veldhuis JD, Iranmanesh A, Johnson ML, Lizarralde G. Twenty-four-hour rhythms in plasma concentrations of adenohypophyseal hormones are generated by distinct amplitude and/or frequency modulation of underlying pituitary secretory bursts. J Clin Endocrinol Metab 1990; 71:1616–1623.
715. Veldhuis JD, Iranmanesh A, Johnson ML, Lizarralde G. Amplitude, but not frequency, modulation of adrenocorticotropin secretory bursts gives rise to the nyctohemeral rhythm of the corticotropic axis in man. J Clin Endocrinol Metab 1990; 71:452–463.
716. Gomez MT, Magiakou MA, Mastorakos G, Chrousos GP. The pituitary corticotroph is not the rate limiting step in the postoperative recovery of the hypothalamic-pituitary-adrenal axis in patients with Cushing syndrome. J Clin Endocrinol Metab 1993; 77:173–177.
717. Desir D, Van Cauter E, Beyloos M, et al. Prolonged pulsatile administration of ovine corticotropin-releasing hormone in normal man. J Clin Endocrinol Metab 1986; 63:1292–1299.
718. Horrocks PM, Jones AF, Ratcliffe WA, et al. Patterns of ACTH and cortisol pulsatility over twenty-four hours in normal males and females. Clin Endocrinol (Oxf) 1990; 32:127–134.
719. Dorin RI, Ferries LM, Roberts B, et al. Assessment of stimulated and spontaneous adrenocorticotropin secretory dynamics identifies distinct components of cortisol feedback inhibition in healthy humans. J Clin Endocrinol Metab 1996; 81:3883–3891.
720. Keeney DS, Waterman MR. Regulation of steroid hydroxylase gene expression: importance to physiology and disease. Pharmacol Ther 1993; 58:301–317.
721. Ilvesmaki V, Voutilainen R. Interaction of phorbol ester and adrenocorticotropin in the regulation of steroidogenic P450 genes in human fetal and adult adrenal cell cultures. Endocrinology 1991; 128:1450–1458.
722. Orth DN. Corticotropin-releasing hormone in humans. Endocr Rev 1992; 13:164–191.
723. Debold CR, Jackson RV, Kamilaris TC, et al. Effects of ovine corticotropin-releasing hormone on adrenocorticotropin secretion in the absence of glucocorticoid feedback inhibition in man. J Clin Endocrinol Metab 1989; 68:431–437.
724. Sonino N, Zielezny M, Fava GA, et al. Risk factors and long-term outcome in pituitary-dependent Cushing's disease. J Clin Endocrinol Metab 1996; 81:2647–2652.
725. Kubota T, Hayashi M, Kabuto M, et al. Corticotroph cell hyperplasia in a patient with Addison disease: case report. Surg Neurol 1992; 37:441–447.
726. Keller-Wood ME, Dallman MF. Corticosteroid inhibition of ACTH secretion. Endocr Rev 1984; 5:1–24.
727. Kanaley JA, Weltman JY, Pieper KS, et al. Cortisol and growth hormone responses to exercise at different times of day. J Clin Endocrinol Metab 2001; 86:2881–2889.
728. Luger A, Deuster PA, Kyle SB, et al. Acute hypothalamic-pituitary-adrenal responses to the stress of treadmill exercise: physiologic adaptations to physical training. N Engl J Med 1987; 316: 1309–1315.
729. Urban RJ, Kaiser DL, van Cauter E, et al. Comparative assessment of objective pulse detection algorithms. II. Studies in men. Am J Physiol 1988; 254:E113–E119.
730. White A, Smith H, Hoadley M, et al. Clinical evaluation of a two-site immunoradiometric assay for adrenocorticotrophin in unextracted human plasma using monoclonal antibodies. Clin Endocrinol (Oxf) 1987; 26:41–51.
731. Crosby SR, Stewart MF, Ratcliffe JG, White A. Direct measurement of the precursors of adrenocorticotropin in human plasma by two-site immunoradiometric assay. J Clin Endocrinol Metab 1988; 67:1272–1277.
732. Allolio B, Gunther RW, Benker G, et al. A multihormonal response to corticotropin-releasing hormone in inferior petrosal sinus blood of patients with Cushing's disease. J Clin Endocrinol Metab 1990; 71:1195–1201.
733. Erturk E, Jaffe CA, Barkan AL. Evaluation of the integrity of the hypothalamic-pituitary-adrenal axis by insulin hypoglycemia test. J Clin Endocrinol Metab 1998; 83:2350–2354.
734. Abdu TA, Elhadd TA, Neary R, Clayton RN. Comparison of the low dose short synacthen test (1 microg), the conventional dose short synacthen test (250 microg), and the insulin tolerance test for assessment of the hypothalamo-pituitary-adrenal axis in patients with pituitary disease. J Clin Endocrinol Metab 1999; 84: 838–843.
735. Hartzband PI, Van Herle AJ, Sorger L, Cope D. Assessment of hypothalamic-pituitary-adrenal (HPA) axis dysfunction: comparison of ACTH stimulation, insulin-hypoglycemia and metyrapone. J Endocrinol Invest 1988; 11:769–776.
736. l'Allemand D, Penhoat A, Lebrethon MC, et al. Insulin-like growth factors enhance steroidogenic enzyme and corticotropin receptor messenger ribonucleic acid levels and corticotropin steroidogenic responsiveness in cultured human adrenocortical cells. J Clin Endocrinol Metab 1996; 81:3892–3897.
737. Oldfield EH, Doppman JL, Nieman LK, et al. Petrosal sinus sampling with and without corticotropin-releasing hormone for the differential diagnosis of Cushing's syndrome. N Engl J Med 1991; 325:897–905.
738. Yanovski JA, Cutler GB Jr, Chrousos GP, Nieman LK. Corticotropin-releasing hormone stimulation following low-dose dexamethasone administration: a new test to distinguish Cushing's syndrome from pseudo-Cushing's states. JAMA 1993; 269:2232–2238.
739. Nieman LK, Oldfield EH, Wesley R, et al. A simplified morning ovine corticotropin-releasing hormone stimulation test for the differential diagnosis of adrenocorticotropin-dependent Cushing's syndrome. J Clin Endocrinol Metab 1993; 77:1308–1312.
740. Hurel SJ, Thompson CJ, Watson MJ, et al. The short Synacthen and insulin stress tests in the assessment of the hypothalamic-pituitary-adrenal axis. Clin Endocrinol (Oxf) 1996; 44:141–146.
741. Rasmuson S, Olsson T, Hagg E. A low dose ACTH test to assess the function of the hypothalamic-pituitary-adrenal axis. Clin Endocrinol (Oxf) 1996; 44:151–156.
742. Kukreja SC, Williams GA. Corticotrophin stimulation test: inverse correlation between basal serum cortisol and its response to corticotrophin. Acta Endocrinol (Copenh) 1981; 97:522–524.
743. Shankar RR, Jakacki RI, Haider A, et al. Testing the hypothalamic-pituitary-adrenal axis in survivors of childhood brain and skull-based tumors. J Clin Endocrinol Metab 1997; 82:1995–1998.
744. Peacey SR, Guo CY, Robinson AM, et al. Glucocorticoid replacement therapy: are patients over treated and does it matter? Clin Endocrinol (Oxf) 1997; 46:255–261.
745. Wilson CB. Surgical management of pituitary tumors. J Clin Endocrinol Metab 1997; 82:2381–2385.
746. Wilson CB, Mindermann T, Tyrrell JB. Extrasellar, intracavernous sinus adrenocorticotropin-releasing adenoma causing Cushing's disease. J Clin Endocrinol Metab 1995; 80:1774–1777.
747. Simmons NE, Alden TD, Thorner MO, Laws ER Jr. Serum cortisol response to transsphenoidal surgery for Cushing disease. J Neurosurg 2001; 95:1–8.
748. Scheithauer BW, Jaap AJ, Horvath E, et al. Clinically silent corticotroph tumors of the pituitary gland. Neurosurgery 2000; 47:723–729; discussion 729–730.
749. Pierce JG, Parsons TF. Glycoprotein hormones: structure and function. Annu Rev Biochem 1981; 50:465–495.
750. Grossmann M, Weintraub BD, Szkudlinski MW. Novel insights

into the molecular mechanisms of human thyrotropin action: structural, physiological, and therapeutic implications for the glycoprotein hormone family. Endocr Rev 1997; 18:476–501.

751. Fiddes JC, Goodman HM. The gene encoding the common alpha subunit of the four human glycoprotein hormones. J Mol Appl Genet 1981; 1:3–18.
752. Sarapura VD, Strouth HL, Wood WM, et al. Activation of the glycoprotein hormone alpha-subunit gene promoter in thyrotropes. Mol Cell Endocrinol 1998; 146:77–86.
753. Tagami T, Madison LD, Nagaya T, Jameson JL. Nuclear receptor corepressors activate rather than suppress basal transcription of genes that are negatively regulated by thyroid hormone. Mol Cell Biol 1997; 17:2642–2648.
754. Wondisford FE, Radovick S, Moates JM, et al. Isolation and characterization of the human thyrotropin beta-subunit gene: differences in gene structure and promoter function from murine species. J Biol Chem 1988; 263:12538–12542.
755. Steinfelder HJ, Hauser P, Nakayama Y, et al. Thyrotropin-releasing hormone regulation of human TSHB expression: role of a pituitary-specific transcription factor (Pit-1/GHF-1) and potential interaction with a thyroid hormone-inhibitory element. Proc Natl Acad Sci USA 1991; 88:3130–3134.
756. Bodenner DL, Mroczynski MA, Weintraub BD, et al. A detailed functional and structural analysis of a major thyroid hormone inhibitory element in the human thyrotropin beta-subunit gene. J Biol Chem 1991; 266:21666–21673.
757. Ross DS, Downing MF, Chin WW, et al. Changes in tissue concentrations of thyrotropin, free thyrotropin beta, and alpha-subunits after thyroxine administration: comparison of mouse hypothyroid pituitary and thyrotropic tumors. Endocrinology 1983; 112:2050–2053.
758. Abel ED, Kaulbach HC, Campos-Barros A, et al. Novel insight from transgenic mice into thyroid hormone resistance and the regulation of thyrotropin. J Clin Invest 1999; 103:271–279.
759. Beck-Peccoz P, Persani L. Variable biological activity of thyroid-stimulating hormone. Eur J Endocrinol 1994; 131:331–340.
760. Lania A, Persani L, Ballare E, et al. Constitutively active Gs alpha is associated with an increased phosphodiesterase activity in human growth hormone-secreting adenomas. J Clin Endocrinol Metab 1998; 83:1624–1628.
761. Papandreou MJ, Persani L, Asteria C, et al. Variable carbohydrate structures of circulating thyrotropin as studied by lectin affinity chromatography in different clinical conditions. J Clin Endocrinol Metab 1993; 77:393–398.
762. Ridgway EC, Weintraub BD, Maloof F. Metabolic clearance and production rates of human thyrotropin. J Clin Invest 1974; 53: 895–903.
763. Vanhole C, Aerssens P, Naulaers G, et al. L-Thyroxine treatment of preterm newborns: clinical and endocrine effects. Pediatr Res 1997; 42:87–92.
764. Goichot B, Weibel L, Chapotot F, et al. Effect of the shift of the sleep-wake cycle on three robust endocrine markers of the circadian clock. Am J Physiol 1998; 275:E243-E248.
765. Van den Berghe G, de Zegher F, Veldhuis JD, et al. Thyrotrophin and prolactin release in prolonged critical illness: dynamics of spontaneous secretion and effects of growth hormone-secretagogues. Clin Endocrinol (Oxf) 1997; 47:599–612.
766. Faglia G. The clinical impact of the thyrotropin-releasing hormone test. Thyroid 1998; 8:903–908.
767. Spencer CA, Schwarzbein D, Guttler RB, et al. Thyrotropin (TSH)-releasing hormone stimulation test responses employing third and fourth generation TSH assays. J Clin Endocrinol Metab 1993; 76:494–498.
768. Samuels MH, Henry P, Luther M, Ridgway EC. Pulsatile TSH secretion during 48-hour continuous TRH infusions. Thyroid 1993; 3:201–206.
769. Samuels MH, Henry P, Ridgway EC. Effects of dopamine and somatostatin on pulsatile pituitary glycoprotein secretion. J Clin Endocrinol Metab 1992; 74:217–222.
770. Siler TM, Yen SC, Vale W, Guillemin R. Inhibition by somatostatin on the release of TSH induced in man by thyrotropin-releasing factor. J Clin Endocrinol Metab 1974; 38:742–745.
771. Cooper DS, Klibanski A, Ridgway EC. Dopaminergic modulation of TSH and its subunits: in vivo and in vitro studies. Clin Endocrinol (Oxf) 1983; 18:265–275.
772. Wang R, Nelson JC, Wilcox RB. Salsalate administration: a potential pharmacological model of the sick euthyroid syndrome. J Clin Endocrinol Metab 1998; 83:3095–3099.
773. Rapoport B, Chazenbalk GD, Jaume JC, McLachlan SM. The thyrotropin (TSH) receptor: interaction with TSH and autoantibodies. Endocr Rev 1998; 19:673–716.
774. Nicoloff JT, Spencer CA. Clinical review 12: the use and misuse of the sensitive thyrotropin assays. J Clin Endocrinol Metab 1990; 71:553–558.
775. Adriaanse R, Romijn JA, Brabant G, et al. Pulsatile thyrotropin secretion in nonthyroidal illness. J Clin Endocrinol Metab 1993; 77:1313–1317.
776. Beck-Peccoz P, Persani L. TSH-producing adenomas. In DeGroot LJ, Jameson JL (eds). Endocrinology. Philadelphia, WB Saunders, 2001, pp 321–328.
776a. Gesundheit N, Patrick PA, Nissim M, et al. Thyrotropin-Secreting pituitary adenomas. Ann Int Med 1989; 111:827–835.
776b. Grisoli F, LeClercq P, Winteler JP. Thyroid stimulating hormone pituitary adenomas. Surg Neurol 25:361–368, 1986.
777. Mindermann T, Wilson CB. Thyrotropin-producing pituitary adenomas. J Neurosurg 1993; 79:521–527.
778. Saeger W, Ludecke DK. Pituitary adenomas with hyperfunction of TSH: frequency, histological classification, immunocytochemistry and ultrastructure. Virchows Arch A Pathol Anat Histol 1982; 394:255–267.
779. McCutcheon IE, Weintraub BD, Oldfield EH. Surgical treatment of thyrotropin-secreting pituitary adenomas. J Neurosurg 1990; 73:674–683.
780. Sanno N, Teramoto A, Matsuno A, et al. GH and PRL gene expression by nonradioisotopic in situ hybridization in TSH-secreting pituitary adenomas. J Clin Endocrinol Metab 1995; 80: 2518–2522.
781. Sanno N, Teramoto A, Matsuno A, et al. Clinical and immunohistochemical studies on TSH-secreting pituitary adenoma: its multihormonality and expression of Pit-1. Mod Pathol 1994; 7: 893–899.
782. Alings AM, Fliers E, de Herder WW, et al. A thyrotropin-secreting pituitary adenoma as a cause of thyrotoxic periodic paralysis. J Endocrinol Invest 1998; 21:703–706.
783. Weintraub BD, Gershengorn MC, Kourides IA. Inappropriate secretion of thyroid-stimulating hormone. Ann Intern Med 1981; 95:339–351.
784. Beck-Peccoz P, Brucker-Davis F, Persani L, et al. Thyrotropin-secreting pituitary tumors. Endocr Rev 1996; 17:610–638.
785. Brucker-Davis F, Oldfield EH, Skarulis MC, et al. Thyrotropin-secreting pituitary tumors: diagnostic criteria, thyroid hormone sensitivity, and treatment outcome in 25 patients followed at the National Institutes of Health. J Clin Endocrinol Metab 1999; 84: 476–486.
785a. Kuhn JM, Arlot S, Lefebvre H, et al. Evaluation of treatment of TSH-secreting adenomas with slow release formulation of somatostatin analog lanreotide. J Clin Endocrinol Metab 2000; 85: 1487–1491.
786. Cooper DS, Wenig BM. Hyperthyroidism caused by an ectopic TSH-secreting pituitary tumor. Thyroid 1996; 6:337–343.
787. Kourides IA, Ridgway EC, Weintraub BD, et al. Thyrotropin-induced hyperthyroidism: use of alpha and beta subunit levels to identify patients with pituitary tumors. J Clin Endocrinol Metab 1977; 45:534–543.
788. Beckers A, Abs R, Mahler C, et al. Thyrotropin-secreting pituitary adenomas: report of seven cases. J Clin Endocrinol Metab 1991; 72:477–483.
789. Chanson P, Weintraub BD, Harris AG. Octreotide therapy for thyroid-stimulating hormone–secreting pituitary adenomas: a follow-up of 52 patients. Ann Intern Med 1993; 119:236–240.
789a. Chanson P, Warnet A. Treatment of TSH-secreting adenomas with octreotide. Metabolism 1992; 41:62–65.
790. Losa M, Giovanelli M, Persani L, et al. Criteria of cure and follow-up of central hyperthyroidism due to thyrotropin-secreting pituitary adenomas. J Clin Endocrinol Metab 1996; 81:3084–3090.
791. Beck-Peccoz P, Mariotti S, Guillausseau PJ, et al. Treatment of hyperthyroidism due to inappropriate secretion of thyrotropin with the somatostatin analog SMS 201-995. J Clin Endocrinol Metab 1989; 68:208–214.
792. Caron P, Arlot S, Bauters C, et al. Efficacy of the long-acting octreotide formulation (octreotide-LAR) in patients with thyro-

tropin-secreting pituitary adenomas. J Clin Endocrinol Metab 2001; 86:2849–2853.
793. Samuels MH, Wood WM, Gordon DF, et al. Clinical and molecular studies of a thyrotropin-secreting pituitary adenoma. J Clin Endocrinol Metab 1989; 68:1211–1215.
794. Warnet A, Timsit J, Chanson P, et al. The effect of somatostatin analogue on chiasmal dysfunction from pituitary macroadenomas. J Neurosurg 1989; 71:687–690.
795. Root AW. Neonatal screening for 21-hydroxylase deficient congenital adrenal hyperplasia: the role of CYP21 analysis. J Clin Endocrinol Metab 1999; 84:1503–1504.
796. Duquesnoy P, Roy A, Dastot F, et al. Human Prop-1: cloning, mapping, genomic structure. Mutations in familial combined pituitary hormone deficiency. FEBS Lett 1998; 437:216–220.
797. Sornson MW, Wu W, Dasen JS, et al. Pituitary lineage determination by the Prophet of Pit-1 homeodomain factor defective in Ames dwarfism. Nature 1996; 384:327–333.
798. Fofanova O, Takamura N, Kinoshita E, et al. Compound heterozygous deletion of the *PROP-1* gene in children with combined pituitary hormone deficiency. J Clin Endocrinol Metab 1998; 83: 2601–2604.
799. Cohen LE, Wondisford FE, Radovick S. Role of Pit-1 in the gene expression of growth hormone, prolactin, and thyrotropin. Endocrinol Metab Clin North Am 1996; 25:523–540.
800. Deladoey J, Fluck C, Bex M, et al. Aromatase deficiency caused by a novel P450arom gene mutation: impact of absent estrogen production on serum gonadotropin concentration in a boy. J Clin Endocrinol Metab 1999; 84:4050–4054.
801. Agarwal G, Bhatia V, Cook S, Thomas PQ. Adrenocorticotropin deficiency in combined pituitary hormone deficiency patients homozygous for a novel PROP1 deletion. J Clin Endocrinol Metab 2000; 85:4556–4561.
802. Rosenbloom AL, Almonte AS, Brown MR, et al. Clinical and biochemical phenotype of familial anterior hypopituitarism from mutation of the *PROP1* gene. J Clin Endocrinol Metab 1999; 84: 50–57.
803. Cushman LJ, Watkins-Chow DE, Brinkmeier ML, et al. Persistent Prop1 expression delays gonadotrope differentiation and enhances pituitary tumor susceptibility. Hum Mol Genet 2001; 10: 1141–1153.
804. Fluck C, Deladoey J, Rutishauser K, et al. Phenotypic variability in familial combined pituitary hormone deficiency caused by a *PROP1* gene mutation resulting in the substitution of ArgCys at codon 120 (R120C). J Clin Endocrinol Metab 1998; 83:3727–3734.
805. Pernasetti F, Toledo SP, Vasilyev VV, et al. Impaired adrenocorticotropin-adrenal axis in combined pituitary hormone deficiency caused by a two-base pair deletion (301-302delAG) in the prophet of Pit-1 gene. J Clin Endocrinol Metab 2000; 85:390–397.
806. Voss JW, Rosenfeld MG. Anterior pituitary development: short tales from dwarf mice. Cell 1992; 70:527–530.
807. Li S, Crenshaw EB 3rd, Rawson EJ, et al. Dwarf locus mutants lacking three pituitary cell types result from mutations in the POU-domain gene *pit-1*. Nature 1990; 347:528–533.
808. Cohen LE, Wondisford FE, Salvatoni A, et al. A “hot spot” in the Pit-1 gene responsible for combined pituitary hormone deficiency: clinical and molecular correlates. J Clin Endocrinol Metab 1995; 80:679–684.
809. Hendriks-Stegeman BI, Augustijn KD, Bakker B, et al. Combined pituitary hormone deficiency caused by compound heterozygosity for two novel mutations in the POU domain of the Pit1/POU1F1 gene. J Clin Endocrinol Metab 2001; 86:1545–1550.
810. Dattani MT, Martinez-Barbera JP, Thomas PQ, et al. Mutations in the homeobox gene *HESX1/Hesx1* associated with septo-optic dysplasia in human and mouse. Nat Genet 1998; 19:125–133.
811. Thomas PQ, Dattani MT, Brickman JM, et al. Heterozygous *HESX1* mutations associated with isolated congenital pituitary hypoplasia and septo-optic dysplasia. Hum Mol Genet 2001; 10: 39–45.
812. Netchine I, Sobrier ML, Krude H, et al. Mutations in *LHX3* result in a new syndrome revealed by combined pituitary hormone deficiency. Nat Genet 2000; 25:182–186.
813. Green JS, Parfrey PS, Harnett JD, et al. The cardinal manifestations of Bardet-Biedl syndrome, a form of Laurence-Moon-Biedl syndrome. N Engl J Med 1989; 321:1002–1009.
814. Bray GA, Dahms WT, Swerdloff RS, et al. The Prader-Willi syndrome: a study of 40 patients and a review of the literature. Medicine (Baltimore) 1983; 62:59–80.
815. Ledbetter DH, Mascarello JT, Riccardi VM, et al. Chromosome 15 abnormalities and the Prader-Willi syndrome: a follow-up report of 40 cases. Am J Hum Genet 1982; 34:278–285.
816. Kallmann F, Schonfeld WA, Barrera WS. Genetic aspects of primary eunuchoidism. Am J Ment Defic 1944; 48:203.
817. Rugarli EI, Ballabio A. Kallmann syndrome: from genetics to neurobiology. JAMA 1993; 270:2713–2716.
818. Hardelin JP, Levilliers J, Young J, et al. Xp22.3 deletions in isolated familial Kallmann's syndrome. J Clin Endocrinol Metab 1993; 76:827–831.
819. Prager D, Braunstein GD. X-chromosome-linked Kallmann's syndrome: pathology at the molecular level. J Clin Endocrinol Metab 1993; 76:824–826.
820. Lieblich JM, Rogol AD, White BJ, Rosen SW. Syndrome of anosmia with hypogonadotropic hypogonadism (Kallmann syndrome): clinical and laboratory studies in 23 cases. Am J Med 1982; 73:506–519.
821. Zhang YH, Guo W, Wagner RL, et al. *DAX1* mutations map to putative structural domains in a deduced three- dimensional model. Am J Hum Genet 1998; 62:855–864.
822. Stoving RK, Veldhuis JD, Flyvbjerg A, et al. Jointly amplified basal and pulsatile growth hormone (GH) secretion and increased process irregularity in women with anorexia nervosa: indirect evidence for disruption of feedback regulation within the GH-insulin-like growth factor I axis. J Clin Endocrinol Metab 1999; 84: 2056–2063.
823. Stoving RK, Hangaard J, Hansen-Nord M, Hagen C. A review of endocrine changes in anorexia nervosa. J Psychiatr Res 1999; 33:139–152.
824. Kleinberg DL. Pituitary tumors and failure of endocrine target organs. Arch Intern Med 1979; 139:969–970.
825. Benvenga S, Campenni A, Ruggeri RM, Trimarchi F. Clinical review 113: hypopituitarism secondary to head trauma. J Clin Endocrinol Metab 2000; 85:1353–1361.
826. Benvenga S, Lo Giudice F, Campenni A, et al. Post-traumatic selective hypogonadotropic hypogonadism. J Endocrinol Invest 1997; 20:675–680.
827. King LR, Knowles HC Jr, McLaurin RL, et al. Pituitary hormone response to head injury. Neurosurgery 1981; 9:229–235.
828. Clayton PE, Shalet SM. Dose dependency of time of onset of radiation-induced growth hormone deficiency. J Pediatr 1991; 118:226–228.
829. Rose SR, Lustig RH, Pitukcheewanont P, et al. Diagnosis of hidden central hypothyroidism in survivors of childhood cancer. J Clin Endocrinol Metab 1999; 84:4472–4479.
830. Lissett CA, Shalet SM. Hypopituitarism. In DeGroot LJ, Jameson JL (eds). Endocrinology, vol 1, 4th ed. Philadelphia, WB Saunders, 2001, pp 289–299.
831. Vance ML. Hypopituitarism. N Engl J Med 1994; 330:1651–1662.
832. Finkelstein JS, Klibanski A, Neer RM, et al. Increases in bone density during treatment of men with idiopathic hypogonadotropic hypogonadism. J of Clin Endocrinol Metab 1989; 69:776–783.
833. Wang C, Eyre DR, Clark R, et al. Sublingual testosterone replacement improves muscle mass and strength, decreases bone resorption, and increases bone formation markers in hypogonadal men: a clinical research center study. J Clin Endocrinol Metab 1996; 81:3654–3662.
834. Webster J, Piscitelli G, Polli A, et al. A comparison of cabergoline and bromocriptine in the treatment of hyperprolactinemic amenorrhea. Cabergoline Comparative Study Group. N Engl J Med 1994; 331:904–909.
835. Thorner MO, Vance ML, Horvath E, Kovacs K. The anterior pituitary. In Wilson JD, Foster DW (eds). Williams Textbook of Endocrinology. Philadelphia, WB Saunders, 1992, pp 221–310.
836. Gasperi M, Aimaretti G, Scarcello G, et al. Low dose hexarelin and growth hormone (GH)–releasing hormone as a diagnostic tool for the diagnosis of GH deficiency in adults: comparison with insulin-induced hypoglycemia test. J Clin Endocrinol Metab 1999; 84:2633–2637.
837. Biller BM, Vance ML, Kleinberg DL, et al. Clinical and reimbursement issues in growth hormone use in adults. Am J Manag Care 2000; 6:S817-S827.

837a. Hartman MC, Crowe BJ, Biller BM, et al. Which patients do not require a GH stimulation test for the diagnosis of adult GH deficiency. J Clin Endocrinol Metab 2002; 87:477–485.
838. Klein I, Parveen G, Gavaler JS, Vanthiel DH. Colonic polyps in patients with acromegaly. Ann Intern Med 1982; 97:27–30.
839. Ituarte EA, Petrini J, Hershman JM. Acromegaly and colon cancer. Ann Intern Med 1984; 101:627–628.
840. Brunner JE, Johnson CC, Zafar S, et al. Colon cancer and polyps in acromegaly: increased risk associated with family history of colon cancer. Clin Endocrinol (Oxf) 1990; 32:65–71.
841. Vasen HF, van Erpecum KJ, Roelfsema F, et al. Increased prevalence of colonic adenomas in patients with acromegaly. Eur J Endocrinol 1994; 131:235–237.
842. Terzolo M, Tappero G, Borretta G, et al. High prevalence of colonic polyps in patients with acromegaly: influence of sex and age. Arch Intern Med 1994; 154:1272–1276.
843. Jenkins PJ, Fairclough PD, Richards T, et al. Acromegaly, colonic polyps and carcinoma. Clin Endocrinol (Oxf) 1997; 47:17–22.
844. Wright AD, Hill DM, Lowy C, Fraser TR. Mortality in acromegaly. Q J Med 1970; 39:1–16.
845. Cheung NW, Boyages SC. Increased incidence of neoplasia in females with acromegaly. Clin Endocrinol (Oxf) 1997; 47:323–327.
846. Popovic V, Damjanovic S, Micic D, et al. Increased incidence of neoplasia in patients with pituitary adenomas. The Pituitary Study Group. Clin Endocrinol (Oxf) 1998; 49:441–445.
847. Barzilay J, Heatley GJ, Cushing GW. Benign and malignant tumors in patients with acromegaly. Arch Intern Med 1991; 151: 1629–1632.
848. Ron E, Gridley G, Hrubec Z, et al. Acromegaly and gastrointestinal cancer. Cancer 1991; 68:1673–1677.
849. Dasen JS, Rosenfeld MG. Signaling mechanisms in pituitary morphogenesis and cell fate determination. Curr Opin Cell Biol 1999; 11:669–677.
850. Hartman ML, Veldhuis JD, Johnson ML, et al. Augmented growth hormone (GH) secretory burst frequency and amplitude mediate enhanced GH secretion during a two-day fast in normal men. J Clin Endocrinol Metab 1992; 74:757–765.

9 Posterior Pituitary Gland

Alan G. Robinson and Joseph G. Verbalis

ANATOMY

Normal Anatomy

The posterior pituitary gland is neural tissue and consists only of the distal axons of the hypothalamic magnicellular neurons that make up the neurohypophysis. The perikarya (cell bodies) of these axons are located in the paired supraoptic nuclei and the paired paraventricular nuclei of the hypothalamus.

During embryogenesis,[1] neuroepithelial cells of the lining of the third ventricle mature into magnicellular neurons while migrating laterally to and above the optic chiasm to form the *supraoptic nuclei* (SON) and to the walls of the third ventricle to form the *paraventricular nuclei* (PVN). The axon tracts in the hypothalamus are shown in Figure 9–1. In the posterior pituitary gland, the axon terminals of the magnicellular neurons contain neurosecretory granules, membrane-bound packets of hormones stored for subsequent release. The blood supply for the anterior pituitary is through the hypothalamic-pituitary portal system but the posterior pituitary blood supply is directly from the inferior hypophyseal arteries, which are branches of the posterior communicating and internal carotid arteries. The drainage is into the cavernous sinus and internal jugular vein.

The hormones of the posterior pituitary gland—*oxytocin* and *vasopressin*—are synthesized in individual hormone-specific magnicellular neurons. In addition, the magnicellular neurons that synthesize vasopressin and oxytocin, respectively, are clustered into subdivisions of the supraoptic and paraventricular nuclei.[2–4] The synthesis of oxytocin and vasopressin in separate neurons and the organization of the magnocellular neurons into clusters of oxytocinergic and vasopressinergic cells are compatible with the idea that the secretion and function of each hormone are distinct and individually controlled. Virtually all of the oxytocinergic neurons and vasopressinergic neurons in the supraoptic nucleus project their axons to the posterior pituitary.[1, 5–7] The organization of the paraventricular nuclei, however, is much more complex and varies among species. In addition to at least three distinct magnicellular divisions consisting of oxytocinergic neurons and vasopressinergic neurons, parvicellular (smaller cells) divisions synthesize other peptides (e.g., corticotropin-releasing hormone, thyrotropin-releasing hormone, somatostatin)[8] and opioids.[6] The parvicellular neurons project to the median eminence, brain stem, and spinal cord,[9] where they play a role in a variety of neuroendocrine autonomic functions. The supraoptic nucleus is a more discrete nucleus, but there are concentrations of oxytocin-containing cells in its dorsal portion and vasopressin-containing cells in its ventral portion.[10]

Dorsally and laterally, the supraoptic nucleus is surrounded by a cell-poor, fiber-rich area (the perinuclear zone). This zone contains GABAergic (γ-aminobutyric acid)-secreting neurons that project outside the general area and to the supraoptic nucleus, where they are reported to have an inhibitory function.[11] Another nucleus that contains many vasopressin but not oxytocin neurons is the suprachiasmatic nucleus located in the midline at the base of and anterior to the third ventricle.[5] The suprachiasmatic nucleus controls circadian as well as seasonal rhythms.[12–14]

Ectopic Posterior Pituitary

With the development of magnetic resonance imaging (MRI) scans of the brain, it was discovered that T1-weighted MR images showed a bright signal in the posterior pituitary.[15] This new diagnostic imaging technology (see later) allowed the identification of a group of patients in whom there was abnormal anatomy of the posterior pituitary, and the *bright spot* was recognized in the base of the hypothalamus. These cases are referred to as *ectopic posterior pituitary*. Most of these cases are recognized in children with growth retardation and anterior pituitary deficiency rather than posterior pituitary deficiency. Although most of these patients do not have clinically apparent diabetes insipidus,[16–19] when specifically and systematically

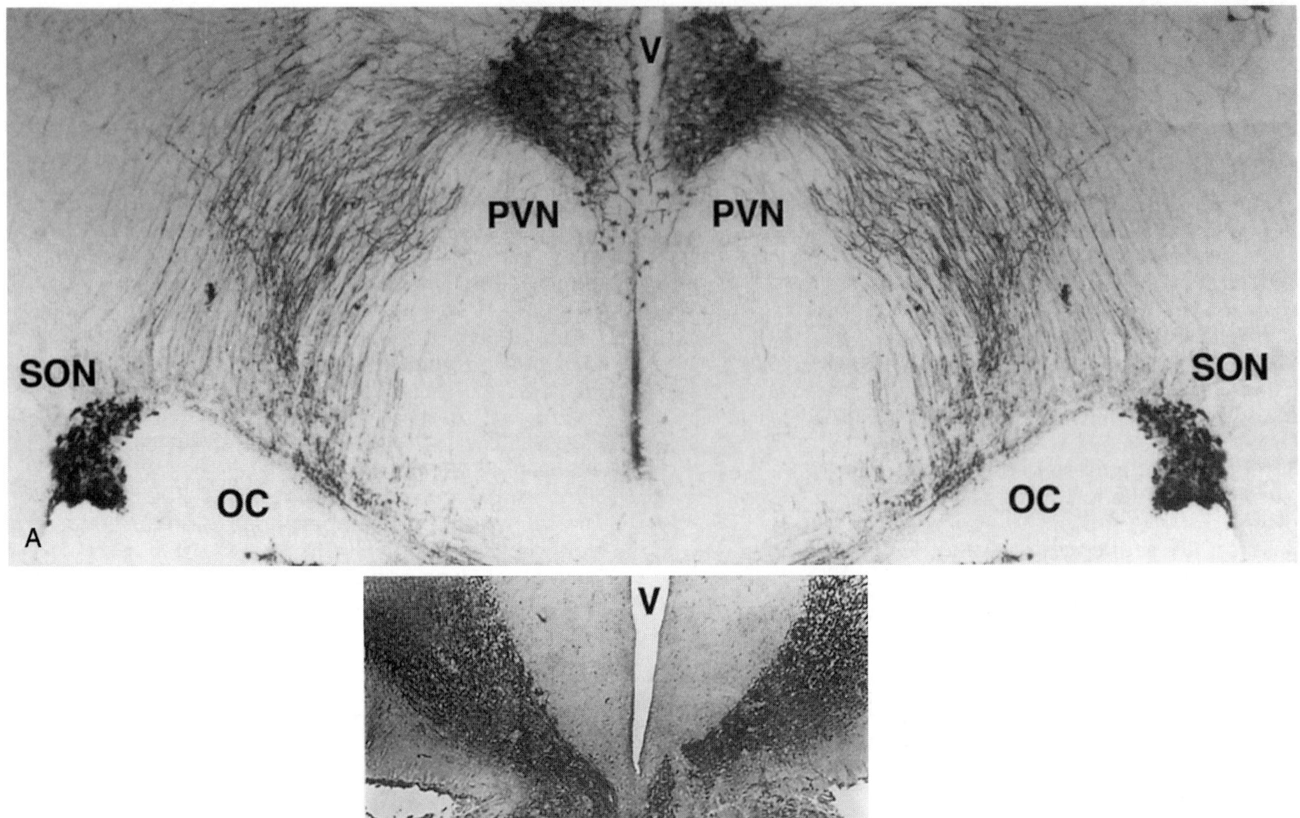

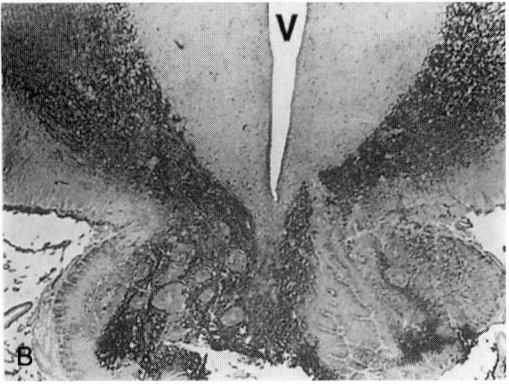

Figure 9–1. Magnicellular neurons and axon tracts in the hypothalamus.

A, Coronal section of the hypothalamus in which neurophysin antibodies are used in an immunoperoxidase technique to demonstrate the magnicellular neurons and axons. The paired paraventricular nuclei (PVN) are at the top in the walls of the third ventricle (V). The axons course laterally and ventrally to the supraoptic nucleus (SON) at the lateral extremes of the optic chiasm (OC) and then inferiorly to the median eminence. (Adapted from Zimmerman EA. Anatomy of vasopressin in producing cells. In Czernichow P, Robinson AG [eds]. Diabetes Insipidus in Man. Basel, Karger, 1985, pp 1–21. Modified to add right SON by A. G. Robinson, University of California, Los Angeles.)

B, In the median eminence, the axons from the two sides coalesce to form the supraopticohypophyseal tract that descends through the stalk to the axon terminals in the posterior pituitary. (Adapted from Robinson AG, Zimmerman EA. Cerebrospinal fluid and ependymal neurophysin. J Clin Invest 1973; 52:1260–1267. Modified to remove tissue tear by A. G. Robinson, University of California, Los Angeles.)

tested for quantitative abnormalities of thirst or vasopressin secretion, subnormal responses have been noted.[20]

The degree of anterior pituitary deficit depends on the persistence of a pituitary stalk and a retained portal vasculature from the hypothalamus to the anterior pituitary.[18, 19, 21, 22] Most authors believe that this condition is not a traumatic but a congenital abnormality with an undescended[19, 22] posterior pituitary that may be at any level along the pituitary stalk.[22]

SYNTHESIS AND RELEASE OF NEUROHYPOPHYSEAL HORMONES

Vasopressin and oxytocin are nonapeptides consisting of a six-amino-acid ring with a cysteine-to-cysteine bridge and a three-amino-acid tail (Fig. 9–2). All mammals have arginine vasopressin and oxytocin (see Fig. 9–2) with the exception of the pig. In the pig, a lysine is substituted for arginine in position 8 of vasopressin, producing lysine vasopressin. Both genes are found on chromosome 20,[23] although they are situated in a tail-to-tail position and transcribed in opposite directions. The cellular anatomy and biochemistry of synthesis are illustrated in Figure 9–3.[23, 24] For oxytocin, the peptide products are the nonapeptide and a neurophysin but no glycopeptide. The neurophysin is distinct for each hormone but with high homology.[25]

When a stimulus for secretion of vasopressin or oxytocin acts on the appropriate magnicellular cell body, an action potential is generated and propagates down the long axon to the posterior pituitary. The action potential causes an influx of calcium, which induces a movement of neurosecretory granules to fuse with the cell membrane and extrude the entire contents of the neurosecretory granule into the perivascular space and subsequently into the capillary system of the posterior pituitary. At the physiologic pH of plasma, there is no binding of

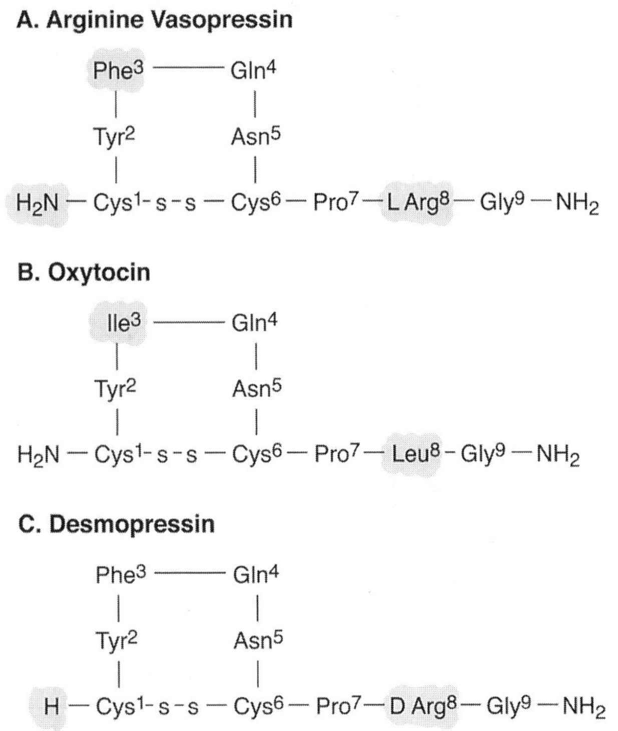

A. Arginine Vasopressin

Phe3 — Gln4
Tyr2 Asn5
H2N — Cys1- s - s — Cys6 — Pro7 — L Arg8 — Gly9 — NH2

B. Oxytocin

Ile3 — Gln4
Tyr2 Asn5
H2N — Cys1- s - s — Cys6 — Pro7 — Leu8 - Gly9 — NH2

C. Desmopressin

Phe3 — Gln4
Tyr2 Asn5
H — Cys1- s - s — Cys6 — Pro7 — D Arg8 — Gly9 — NH2

Figure 9–2. Comparison of the chemical structures of arginine vasopressin, oxytocin, and desmopressin. The differences are illustrated by the *shaded areas*. Oxytocin differs from vasopressin in position 3 (Ile for Phe) and position 8 (Leu for Arg). Desmopressin differs from arginine vasopressin in that the terminal cystine is deaminated and the arginine in position 8 is a D rather than an L isomer. (© 2003, UCLA, AG Robinson.)

hormones (vasopressin and oxytocin) to their respective neurophysins and each peptide circulates independently in the blood stream.[26, 27]

The control of hormone synthesis resides at the level of transcription. Stimuli for secretion of vasopressin or oxytocin also stimulate transcription and increase the messenger ribonucleic acid (mRNA) content in the magnocellular neurons. This has been studied in most detail in rats, in which dehydration[28] accelerates transcription and increases the levels of vasopressin (and oxytocin) mRNA[29–32] and hypo-osmolality produces a decrease in the content of vasopressin mRNA.[33]

The transport of neurosecretory vesicles from the site of synthesis to the posterior pituitary along microtubule tracks[34, 35] is also regulated. When synthesis is turned off, transport stops, and when synthesis is increased transport is up-regulated.[35] Thus, there is coordination of stimulated release of hormone, transport of hormone, and synthesis of new hormone. There is, however, asynchrony in the timing of these events. The asynchrony is demonstrated by changes in the content of vasopressin stored in the posterior pituitary. The absolute content varies considerably among species but is quite a remarkable store, generally equivalent to the amount of hormone required to sustain basal release for 30 to 50 days or maximum release for 5 to 10 days.[36]

In animals, prolonged and intense stimulation of vasopressin release, such as dehydration or salt loading,[32, 37–42] produces a depletion of stored hormone in the posterior pituitary. There is then a gradual recovery of pituitary content back to baseline (or above) 7 to 14 days after animals are returned to normal water intake. This phenomenon has been modeled by Fitzsimmons and colleagues,[43] who provided experimental evidence that a long half-life of the vasopressin message, approximately 2 days, is (from a minimalist point of view) a plausible explanation for the events. When a strong or sustained stimulus releases vasopressin, there is an immediate stimulus to the synthesis of new mRNA. However, because it requires several days for the peak level of mRNA to be reached, synthesis increases slowly. When the stimulus is removed, the elevated mRNA synthesizes hormone to replete the store in the posterior pituitary. The mRNA slowly declines to the previous baseline, and synthesis of vasopressin returns to a basal rate.

The magnicellular neurons specific for oxytocin and vasopressin have intrinsic individual characteristic electrical firing patterns. These patterns are modulated by the paracrine and autocrine action of hormone released by the dendrites into the extracellular space surrounding the magnicellular neurons in the supraoptic nucleus and paraventricular nuclei.[44, 45] Oxytocin neurons develop a pattern of high-amplitude bursting activity (hormone release) followed by long pauses,[46] a pattern that may facilitate the pumping action of muscular contraction of myoepithelial cells in the breast.[47, 48] For vasopressin, weakly active neurons and highly active neurons are brought to a medium level of alternate phasic firing and resting that facilitates optimal secretion of vasopressin.[49, 50]

Structural plasticity also enhances secretion. When stimulated to secrete, the neurons retract dendrites to become more compact, which may allow more efficient propagation of inputs and decrease nonspecific synaptic inputs.[51, 52] Retraction of glia around the magnicellular perikarya increases juxtaposition of like neurons to enhance recruitment of neighboring neurons and to synchronize firing.[53–55] At the level of the posterior pituitary, retraction of pituicytes surrounding axon terminals removes an immediate barrier between the axons and the perivascular space and facilitates diffusion of peptides into capillaries.[54]

PHYSIOLOGY OF SECRETION OF VASOPRESSIN AND THIRST

The physiologic regulation of vasopressin synthesis and secretion involves two systems: osmotic and pressure-volume (Fig. 9–4). The functions of these two systems are so distinct that historically it was thought there were two hormones—an antidiuretic hormone and a vasopressor hormone. Hence, the two names that are used interchangeably for (8-arginine) vasopressin.

There are separate systems at the level of the receptors on the end organs of response. V1 receptors on blood vessels are distinct from V2 receptors on renal collecting duct epithelia. A third receptor, V3, is responsible for the nontraditional biologic action of vasopressin to stimulate adrenocorticotropic hormone (ACTH) secretion from the anterior pituitary, and V2 receptors regulate the nontraditional action of vasopressin to stimulate factor VIII production.

Vasopressin is the main hormone involved in regulation of water in humans, and all mammals control water to regulate osmolality. On the other hand, the main hormones involved in pressure-volume in humans are renin, angiotensin, and aldosterone; and controlling serum sodium concentration ([Na^+]) largely regulates pressure-volume. Therefore, the pathology of disorders of the neurohypophysis is expressed primarily as abnormalities of osmolality produced by abnormal excretion or retention of water. In the case of osmoreceptors, the magnicellular neurons are chronically under some mild input to stimulate release of vasopressin, and the regulation of vasopressin in response to osmolality is relatively uncomplicated, with small decreases in osmolality causing a parallel decrease in

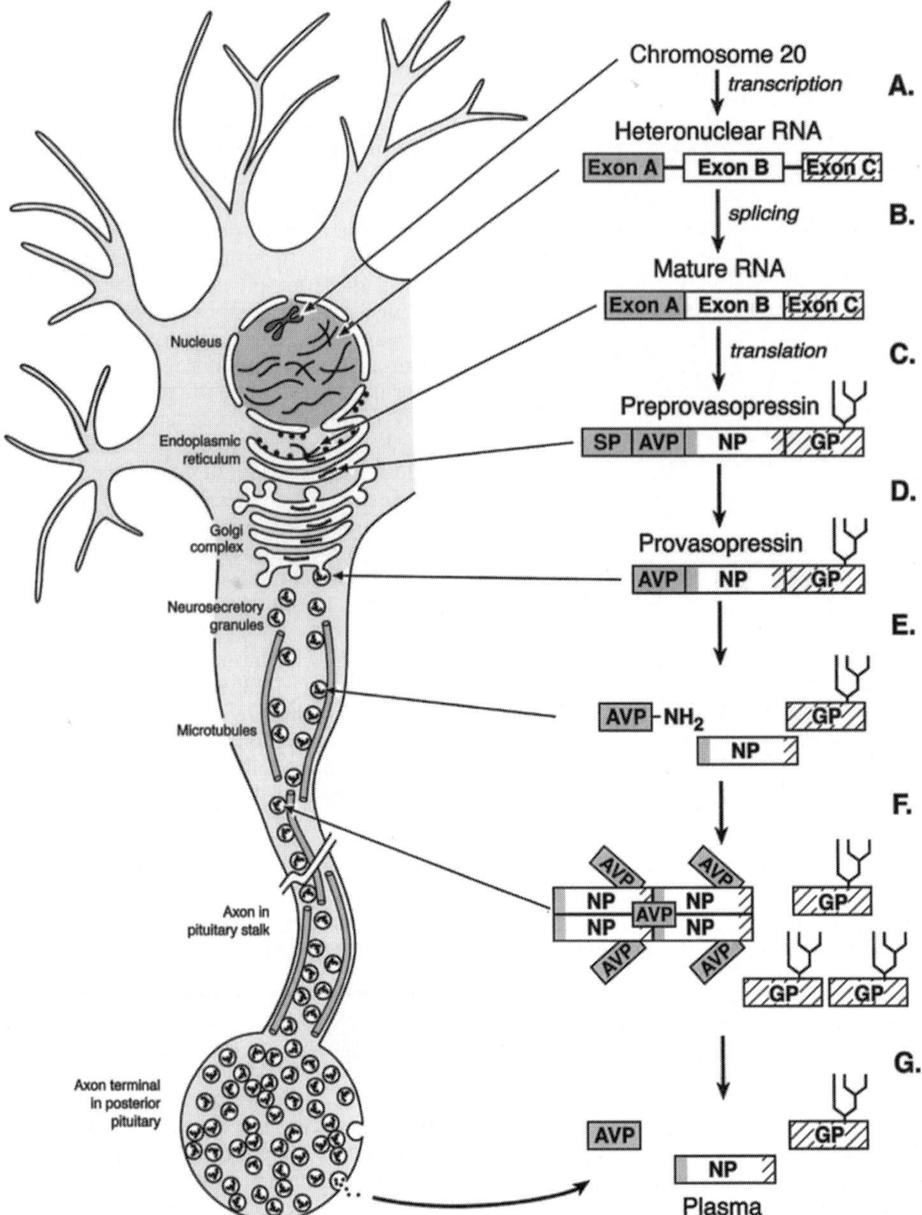

Figure 9–3. Vasopressin synthesis in a magnicellular neuron.

A, The vasopressin gene is located on the short arm of chromosome 20. In the nucleus, the gene is transcribed to heteronuclear ribonucleic acid (RNA).

B, The introns are then excised, and the three exons are spliced to form mature RNA, which consists of exon A, exon B, and exon C. The mature RNA exits the nucleus to the cytoplasm. It is targeted to the endoplasmic reticulum, where it is attached to ribosomes.

C and *D*, There is translation of the three exons into pre-provasopressin. Exon A is translated to the 19-amino-acid signal peptide (SP), the nonapeptide arginine vasopressin (AVP), and the amino-terminal portion of the 93- to 95-amino-acid neurophysin (NP). Exon B encodes the highly conserved middle region of neurophysin. Exon C encodes the variable carboxyl terminus of neurophysin and a 39-amino-acid glycopeptide (GP). The pre-provasopressin is transferred across the endoplasmic reticulum, the glycopeptide is glycosylated, and the signal peptide is cleaved *(D)*.

E, Provasopressin enters the Golgi apparatus, where the entire provasopressin complex is packaged into neurosecretory granules. The neurosecretory granules attach to microtubules and are transported along the microtubules to the posterior pituitary, where the neurosecretory granules are stored.

F, During transport, enzymes in the acidic granules cleave the prohormone to vasopressin (which is amidated), to neurophysin, and to the glycopeptide. Neurophysins form dimers and, subsequently, tetramers with one vasopressin attached to each neurophysin. There is an auxiliary fifth binding site for vasopressin, which spans the four neurophysin molecules of the tetramer.

G, When there is an action potential signaling release, a neurosecretory granule fuses with the axon membrane and the vasopressin, neurophysin, and glycopeptide are secreted into the extracellular space and, hence, into plasma, where they circulate independently of each other. (© 2003, UCLA, AG Robinson.)

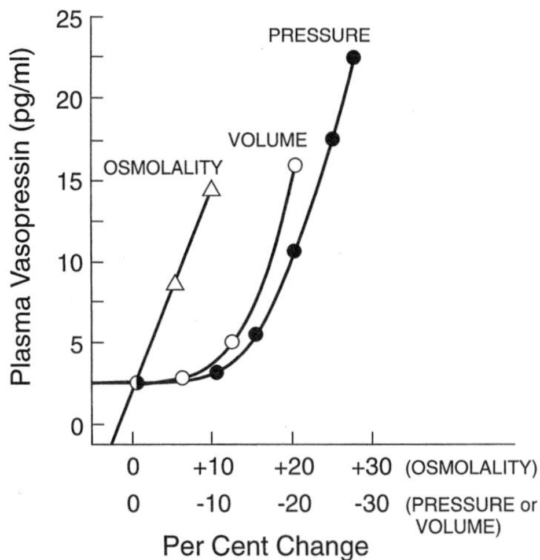

Figure 9–4. Comparison in humans of the release of vasopressin in response to percentage changes of osmolality (increase) and pressure or volume (decrease). *Note:* To increase plasma vasopressin, the change in osmolality is much more sensitive, responding to as little as a 1% increase in osmolality, whereas volume and pressure require greater than a 10% to 15% change to stimulate release of vasopressin. (Redrawn from Robertson GL, Berl T. Water metabolism. In Brenner BM, Rector FC Jr [eds]. The Kidney, vol 1, 3rd ed. Philadelphia, WB Saunders, 1986, p 385.)

vasopressin and small increases in osmolality a parallel increase in vasopressin.

The regulation of volume and blood pressure is complicated (see Thrasher[56]), and experimental models of vasopressin and baroreceptor regulation in animals often involve inhibiting or measuring other concurrent sympathetic inputs to the system in order to determine any direct effect of a stimulus on secretion of vasopressin (see Fig. 9–4). Other influences on secretion of vasopressin, such as the inhibiting influence of glucocorticoids and the potent stimulus of nausea and vomiting, are less important as physiologic regulators of vasopressin but may be important in the differential diagnosis of the syndrome of inappropriate secretion of antidiuretic hormone (SIADH), discussed later.

Volume and Pressure Regulation

High-pressure arterial baroreceptors are located in the carotid sinus and aortic arch and low-pressure volume receptors in the atria and pulmonary venous system.[56, 57] The afferent signals from these receptors are carried from the chest to the brain stem through cranial nerves IX and X. Interruption of the vagal input by vagotomy or vagal cold block[58–60] in dogs and destruction of the A1 area of the medulla, which receives input from IX and X,[61–63] in rabbits leads to an increase in vasopressin secretion.

These and other data led to the concept that baroreceptors and volume receptors normally inhibit the magnicellular neurons and that decreases in this tonic inhibition result in release of vasopressin. Arterial and venous constriction induced by vasopressin action on V1 receptors causes the vessels around the existing plasma volume to contract and effectively increase plasma volume and reestablish the inhibition of secretion of vasopressin. Although the action of vasopressin at the kidney to retain water helps to replace volume, the major hormonal regulation to control volume actually involves the renin-angiotensin system, which stimulates sodium reabsorption in the kidney (see Chapter 15).

The concept of tonic inhibition of vasopressin by baroreceptors has been questioned,[56, 64] but most agree that the volume receptor and baroreceptor responses leading to an increase in vasopressin in humans are much less sensitive than are the osmoreceptor responses (see Fig. 9–4). It has been interpreted that the lesser response occurs because changes in volume and central venous pressure have little effect to increase vasopressin in humans as long as arterial pressure is maintained by sympathetic reflexes.[56, 65] When hypovolemia is sufficient to cause a decrease in blood pressure, there is a sudden and exponential increase in the level of vasopressin in plasma (see Fig. 9–4).[56, 66]

It is also agreed that changes in volume or pressure that are insufficient to cause increases in vasopressin nonetheless modify the response of the vasopressin system to osmoregulation.[66, 67] Increases in pressure and central volume decrease the secretion of vasopressin,[68] but, again, the response of the renin-angiotensin system to cause sodium excretion is much more sensitive to increases of pressure and volume than the response to decrease secretion of vasopressin.[56, 69] Thus, both excitatory and inhibitory influences exist from the brain stem to the magnocellular neurons, with the dominant influence depending on the physiologic circumstances.

Osmotic Regulation

The primary receptors for sensing changes in osmolality are located in the brain. Most of the brain is within the blood-brain barrier, which is impermeable to polar solutes. Because the osmostat is insensitive to urea and glucose, which readily cross cellular membranes (but not the blood-brain barrier), the osmoreceptors must be outside the blood-brain barrier.

Studies of experimental brain lesions in animals strongly suggest that cells in the organum vasculosum of the lamina terminalis (OVLT) and in areas of the adjacent anterior hypothalamus near the anterior wall of the third cerebral ventricle are osmoreceptors. These organs are perfused by fenestrated capillaries and are thus outside the blood-brain barrier. Surgical destruction of the OVLT abolishes vasopressin secretion and thirst responses to hyperosmolality but not responses to other stimuli such as hypovolemia.[70]

Essentially the same conclusion was drawn from clinical observations of human subjects with brain damage that destroyed the region around the OVLT, who are often unable to maintain normal plasma osmolalities even under basal conditions.[71] In contrast, destruction of the magnicellular neurons of the supraoptic nucleus and paraventricular nuclei eliminates dehydration-induced secretion of vasopressin but does not alter thirst, clearly indicating that osmotically stimulated thirst must be generated proximal to the magnocellular cells.

Extracellular fluid (ECF) osmolality (determined predominantly by sodium concentration) in normal subjects varies from 280 to 295 mOsm/kg but in any individual is maintained in a narrow range. The ability to maintain this narrow range depends on (1) the sensitive response of plasma vasopressin to changes in plasma osmolality, (2) the sensitive response of urine osmolality to changes in plasma vasopressin, and (3) the gain in the system by the response of urine volume to change in plasma vasopressin (Fig. 9–5). Basal plasma vasopressin is in the range of 0.5 to 2 pg/μL. As little as a 1% increase or decrease in plasma osmolality causes[66] a rapid increase in plasma vasopressin by release of vasopressin from the store of hormone in the posterior pituitary. For levels of vasopressin in plasma to decrease rapidly requires rapid metabolism of vasopressin, and this is also characteristic of the hormone, which circulates freely in plasma and has a half-life of approximately 15 minutes. Thus, small increases in osmolality produce a concentrated urine and small decreases in osmolality produce a water diuresis.

Figure 9–5 illustrates the linear relationship between plasma osmolality and plasma vasopressin that has been described in

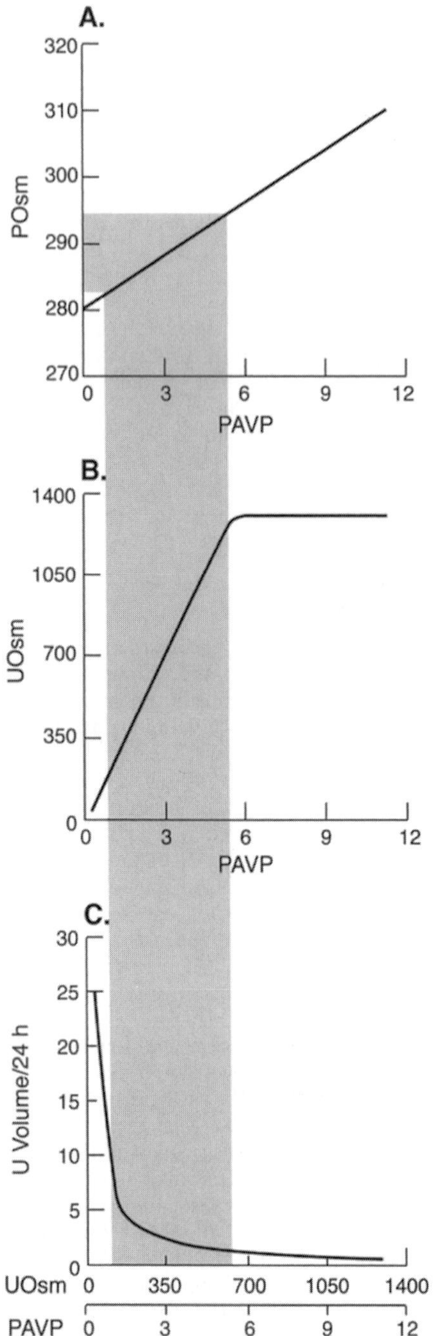

Figure 9–5. Relationship of plasma osmolality (mOsm/kg of H_2O) to plasma vasopressin (pg/mL) to urine osmolality (mOsm/kg of H_2O) to urine volume (L/day). AVP, arginine vasopressin; P, plasma; U, urine.

A, Small changes in osmolality induce changes in vasopressin from less than 0.5 to 5 to 6 pg/mL.

B, These small changes in plasma vasopressin induce changes in urine osmolality through the full range from maximally dilute to maximally concentrated urine. Plasma vasopressin can rise to higher levels than 6 pg/mL, as illustrated in *A*, but this does not translate into increased urine osmolality, which has a maximum determined by the osmolality of an inner medulla of the kidney.

C, The relationship of volume to urine osmolality is logarithmic, assuming a constant osmolar load and the urine volume that would excrete that osmolar load at the urine osmolality indicated.

The interrelationship between the three graphs is illustrated by the *shaded area* that represents the normal range. Urine volume changes relatively little with small changes in the other parameters until there is nearly complete absence of vasopressin, and the urine volume then increases dramatically.

(Calculated from formulas in Robertson GL, Shelton RL, Athar S. The osmoregulation of vasopressin. Kidney Int 1976; 10:25–37.)

humans.[66] The linear relationship exists for osmolalities well above the normal excursion of osmolalities, as demonstrated when the increase is induced by infusion of hypertonic saline or is observed during dehydration of patients with nephrogenic diabetes insipidus.[72] Similarly, Figure 9–5 shows the presence of a sensitive and linear relationship between the level of vasopressin in plasma and the induced osmolality of the urine. In this case, however, although plasma vasopressin may increase out of the normal physiologic range, the urine osmolality levels off at approximately 1000 to 1200 mOsm/kg. This occurs because the maximum concentration reached by the fluid in the collecting duct is determined by the osmolality of the inner medulla.

Figure 9–5 also shows the relationship of plasma vasopressin to urine volume. This relationship is calculated on the basis of the urine volume necessary to excrete a fixed quantity of osmolytes (800 mOsm) at the urine osmolality produced by the change in plasma vasopressin. These graphs demonstrate the gain in the system when the changes in urine volume relative to plasma vasopressin are considered. With a decrease of plasma vasopressin, for example, from 5 to 1 pg/mL, urine volume is maintained at less than 4 L/day; however, urine volume increases dramatically to 18 to 20 L/day when plasma vasopressin is decreased further.

In the kidney, water is conserved by the combined functions of the loop of Henle and the collecting duct. The loop of Henle generates a high osmolality in the renal medulla through the countercurrent multiplier system. Vasopressin acts in the collecting duct to increase water permeability, thereby allowing osmotic equilibration between the urine and the hypertonic medullary interstitium. The net effect of this process is to extract water from the urine into the medullary interstitial blood vessels (vasa recta), resulting in increased urine concentration and decreased urine volume (antidiuresis). Vasopressin produces antidiuresis by its effects on the epithelial principal cells of the collecting tubule, which have vasopressin receptors of the V2 type.

The intracellular organelles responsible for water reabsorption across the collecting duct cells are called *aquaporins*, a widely expressed family of water channels that mediate rapid water transport across some cell membranes.[73] *Aquaporin-2* is regulated by vasopressin and mediates water transport across the apical plasma membrane of the principal cells of the collecting ducts. In contrast, *aquaporin-3* and *aquaporin-4* are expressed at high levels in the basolateral plasma membranes of principal cells and are responsible for the constitutively high water permeability of the basolateral plasma membrane.[74]

Vasopressin binding to the V2 receptor increases intracellular cyclic adenosine monophosphate (cAMP) levels by activating adenylate cyclase. The cAMP induces a fusion of aquaporin-2–containing intracytoplasmic vesicles with the apical plasma membranes of the principal cells, a process that increases apical water permeability by markedly increasing the number of water-conducting pores in the apical plasma membrane.[75] Dissociation of vasopressin from the V2 receptor allows intracellular cAMP levels to decrease, and the water channels are reinternalized into the intracytoplasmic vesicles, thereby terminating the increased water permeability.

The aquaporin-containing vesicles remain just below the apical membrane and can be quickly "shuttled" into and out of the membrane in response to changes in intracellular cAMP levels. This mechanism therefore allows minute-to-minute regulation of renal water excretion through changes in ambient levels of vasopressin in plasma. There is also long-term regulation of collecting duct water permeability in response to prolonged high levels of circulating vasopressin. This response requires at least 24 hours to elicit and is not as rapidly reversible. The long-term effect is due to the ability of vasopressin to induce large increases in the abundance of aquaporin-2 and aquaporin-3 water channels in the collecting duct principal cells.[76, 77] Greater total expression of the number of aquaporin-2 and aquaporin-3 water channels, when combined with the short-term effect of vasopressin to shift aquaporin-2 into the apical plasma membrane, allows the collecting ducts to achieve extremely high water permeabilities during conditions of prolonged dehydration, thereby further enhancing the ability to conserve water in response to equivalent levels of circulating vasopressin.

Thirst

Urine volume can be reduced to a minimum but not eliminated, and insensible water loss is a continuous process. To maintain water balance, one must consume water to replace the obligate urinary and insensible fluid losses, and this consumption is regulated by thirst. Thirst represents the body's defense mechanism to increase water consumption in response to perceived deficits of body fluids.

Like vasopressin, thirst can be stimulated by increases in osmolality of the ECF or by decreases in intravascular volume. Furthermore, there is evidence that the receptors are similar, that is, osmoreceptors in the anterior hypothalamus and low-pressure or high-pressure, or both, baroreceptors (with a likely contribution from circulating angiotensin II during more severe degrees of intravascular hypovolemia and hypotension).[78] Studies in animals have consistently reported thresholds for osmotically induced drinking ranging from 1% to 4% increases in plasma osmolality above basal levels, and analogous studies in humans using quantitative estimates of subjective symptoms of thirst have confirmed that increases in plasma osmolality of 2% to 3% are necessary to produce an unequivocal sensation described as thirst.[71, 79]

As with vasopressin, the threshold for producing thirst by hypovolemia is significantly higher. Studies in multiple species have shown that sustained decreases in plasma volume or blood pressure of at least 4% to 8%, and in some species 10% to 15%, are necessary to stimulate drinking consistently. In humans, it is difficult to demonstrate an effect of mild to moderate hypovolemia to stimulate thirst independently of osmotic changes occurring with dehydration. This blunted sensitivity to changes in ECF volume or blood pressure in humans probably represents an adaptation that occurred as a result of the erect posture of primates, which predisposes them to wider fluctuations in blood and atrial filling pressures as a result of orthostatic pooling of blood in the lower body. Stimulation of thirst (and secretion of vasopressin) by transient postural changes in blood pressure may lead to overdrinking and inappropriate antidiuresis in situations in which the ECF volume was actually normal but transiently maldistributed.

Although osmotic changes clearly are effective stimulants of thirst, it is not likely that changes in plasma osmolality are responsible for the major part of day-to-day fluid intakes. Most humans consume the bulk of their ingested water as a result of the relatively unregulated components of fluid intake, such as the consumption of beverages in association with food intake, for reasons of palatability or desired secondary effects (e.g., caffeine), or for social or habitual reasons (e.g., sodas or alcoholic beverages). As a result, both animals and humans generally ingest volumes in excess of what can be considered to be an actual need for fluid.

Consistent with this observation is the fact that, under most conditions, plasma osmolalities in humans remain within 1% to 2% of basal levels, and these relatively small changes in plasma osmolality are generally below the threshold levels that have been found to stimulate thirst. This suggests that despite the obvious vital importance of thirst during pathologic situations of hyperosmolality and hypovolemia, under normal physiologic conditions water balance in humans is accomplished more by free water excretion regulated by vasopressin than by water intake regulated by thirst. This also demonstrates why water intake must be consciously restricted in cases of persistent unregulated secretion of vasopressin.

Clinical Consequences of Osmotic and Volume Regulation

In most physiologic situations, there is concurrence and synergy between the effects of increased osmolality and decreased volume to stimulate release of vasopressin. For example, with dehydration, osmolality increases and volume decreases and each stimulates the release of vasopressin. Furthermore, there is good evidence that a decrease in volume shifts the plasma vasopressin–plasma osmolality response curve to the left, resulting in a greater release of vasopressin at a given osmolality.[56, 80] Similarly, excess of fluid produces a decrease in osmolality and an increase in volume, and both cause a decrease in vasopressin secretion.

The physiology underlying the relationships between plasma osmolality, plasma vasopressin, and especially urine volume determines some of the pathophysiology of decreased or increased secretion of vasopressin. In Figure 9–5, we see that a regular loss of vasopressin neurons, which may decrease the secretory capacity of the neurohypophysis from that able to produce a blood vasopressin level of 10 to 20 pg/mL down to a secretory capacity sufficient only to maintain a blood level of 5 pg/mL, may produce no change in the ability to attain a maximum urine osmolality. Below 5 pg/mL, there is a linear decrease in the ability to concentrate the urine maximally. However, from the volume curve we see that this results in only a modest increase in urine volume because of the logarithmic relationship of urine volume to urine osmolality and plasma vasopressin. Then, when the last few vasopressinergic neurons are lost and the maximum vasopressin level drops from 1 to 0.5 pg/mL, there might be a great increase in urine volume.

These responses might be viewed as protective, allowing water conservation, even with minimal ability to secrete vasopressin. This may be why even in idiopathic hypothalamic diabetes insipidus there is often a sudden onset of symptoms. The same physiologic considerations may explain why patients with diabetes insipidus that has persisted for a relatively long period of time (e.g., after surgery or head injury) may eventually be able to discontinue vasopressin treatment. The number of vasopressinergic neurons that need to recover to maintain an asymptomatic urine volume is small. The same pathophysiology is important in regard to SIADH. In this situation, however, one might consider the consequences of an inability to suppress vasopressin to less than 1 pg/mL. Note that the maximum urine volume with a standard osmolar load at 1 pg/mL can be as little as 2 L/day. If a patient's fluid intake is greater than that which can be excreted with the fixed level of vasopressin of 1 pg/mL, the extra fluid is retained and the sequence of events that causes hyponatremia in SIADH is initiated.

A synthesis of what is known about the regulation of thirst and secretion of vasopressin in humans contributes to our understanding of this simple but elegant system to maintain water balance. Under normal physiologic conditions, the sensitivity of the osmoregulatory system for secretion of vasopressin accounts for maintenance of plasma osmolality within narrow limits by adjusting renal water excretion to small changes in osmolality. Stimulated thirst does not represent a major regulatory mechanism under these conditions, and unregulated fluid ingestion and water from metabolized food supply water in excess of true need. Excess water is then excreted using osmoregulated secretion of vasopressin. However, when unregulated water intake does not supply body needs, even with plasma levels of vasopressin sufficient to produce maximal antidiuresis, plasma osmolality rises to levels that stimulate thirst and produce water intake proportional to the elevation of osmolality. Thirst thus represents a backup mechanism that is called into play when pituitary and renal mechanisms are insufficient to maintain plasma osmolality within a few percentage points of basal levels.

This arrangement has the advantage of freeing animals and humans from frequent episodes of thirst that would require a diversion of activities toward behavior oriented to seeking water when the water deficiency is sufficiently mild to be compensated for by renal water conservation, but it does stimulate water ingestion when water deficiency reaches a potentially harmful level. This system of differential effective thresholds for thirst and secretion of vasopressin therefore nicely complements the excess unregulated, or need-free, drinking in both humans and animals demonstrated in many studies.

Reset Osmostat during Pregnancy

During pregnancy, major shifts of fluid produce a decreased plasma osmolality of about 10 mmol/kg and an increase in plasma volume.[81, 82] This decrease in osmolality is a normal consequence of pregnancy and is probably the best example of a true resetting of the osmostat. A true resetting of the osmostat must regulate both increases and decreases of secretion of vasopressin at a lower than normal plasma osmolality. These criteria are met in pregnant women, and there is a resetting of the osmostat for thirst in parallel with the resetting of the osmostat for release of vasopressin.[83]

Figure 9–6 shows the relationship of plasma vasopressin to plasma osmolality in normal and pregnant women. In pregnant women, as in nonpregnant women, the plasma vasopressin level is increased with as little as a 1% increase in plasma osmolality, but the entire curve with a normal slope is shifted to the left.[81] The shift in osmotic threshold appears at about 5 to 8 weeks of gestation and persists throughout pregnancy, returning to normal by 2 weeks after delivery.[81] Although the osmotic threshold is constant throughout pregnancy, there is a change in sensitivity at about 28 to 33 weeks of gestation. At this time, the threshold to release vasopressin occurs at the same plasma osmolality; however, the slope changes, so that for increases in osmolality, there is less vasopressin (see Fig. 9–6, slope C).

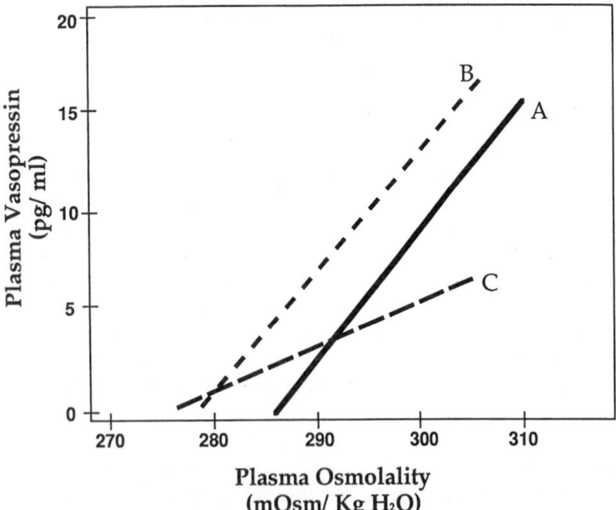

Figure 9–6. Comparison of the normal response of plasma vasopressin to plasma osmolality (A) with that in midgestation (B) and late gestation (C). During midgestation (B), there is a reset of the osmostat to a lower level, shifting the curve to the left. In late gestation, the osmotic threshold remains the same but there is a change in the slope and less vasopressin is secreted. (Adapted from Davison JM, Shiells EA, Phillips PR, Lindheimer MD. Serial evaluation of vasopressin release and thirst in human pregnancy: role of human chorionic gonadotrophin in the osmoregulatory changes of gestation. J Clin Invest 1988; 81:798–806.)

The physiology of the reset osmostat has been considered in relation to the expanded plasma volume. Total body water in pregnant women is also increased by 7 to 8 L as a result of profound vasodilatation.[84] This volume is sensed as normal, and vasopressin responds normally to decreases and increases of volume.[81, 85, 86] Both the changes in volume and the changes in regulation of osmolality have been reproduced by infusion of relaxin (a normal hormone of pregnancy that is a member of the insulin-like growth factor family) into virgin female and normal rats[87, 88] and reversed in pregnant rats by immunoneutralization of relaxin[89]; therefore, relaxin is a proposed mediator of the effect.

In women, the placenta produces an enzyme, cysteine aminopeptidase, that is released into the plasma and is known as oxytocinase.[81, 82] This enzyme is as potent in degrading vasopressin as in degrading oxytocin and in making vasopressin biologically inactive. The activity of vasopressinase increases markedly around 20 weeks of gestation and increases further to 40 weeks, returning slowly to normal over a few weeks after delivery.[90] The data are consistent with the supposition that the change in the sensitivity of the plasma vasopressin–plasma osmolality response in late pregnancy (see Fig. 9–6, line C) may be due to accelerated degradation of vasopressin.

Aging

Many physiologic processes are compromised in aging humans, and numerous studies have reported that elderly people are at risk for both hypernatremia and hyponatremia.[91–93] In many older subjects, there is a decrease in glomerular filtration rate (GFR),[93] and the collecting duct in the aged kidney may be less sensitive to vasopressin,[93] limiting the ability to excrete free water. Many other abnormalities of fluid and electrolyte balance in elderly people are due to co-morbid conditions or to the numerous pharmacologic agents to which these patients are often exposed. Studies of responses to dehydration, osmolar stimulation, or volume stimulation in older people are complicated by the fact that by age 75 to 80 years the total body water level declines to 50% of the level in normal young adults.[94]

Although some have reported altered morphology of the neurohypophyseal system in aged humans,[95, 96] there appears to be no change in the number of magnocellular neurons in normal elderly people[97] or in patients with Alzheimer's disease.[98] There is a greater range of normal levels of vasopressin and a less direct correlation of plasma vasopressin with plasma osmolality,[99, 100] but changes in levels of vasopressin in response to acute increases in serum sodium are either normal[101] or increased.[93, 102, 103] An increased response of vasopressin to changes in plasma osmolality has been ascribed to a decreased ability of vasopressin to stimulate levels of aquaporin-2 in the kidney.[74, 93] The decrease in renal sensitivity has also been interpreted as causing a chronic increase in secretion of vasopressin and a depletion of hormone stores in the posterior pituitary. This may be why elderly patients demonstrate a decreased incidence of visualization of the bright spot on T1-weighted MRI scans; in more than 70% of elderly subjects, the spot was not observed.[104]

A number of studies have indicated that elderly people have decreased thirst with dehydration and less fluid intake to return their volume to normal during recovery from dehydration.[101, 105–107] At the other end of the spectrum, elderly patients have been found to excrete a water load less well than younger subjects and at least part of this is due to decreased suppression of vasopressin.[108] Elderly people are also reported to have a decreased ability to shut off vasopressin in response to drinking and stimulation of oral-pharyngeal receptors.[105, 109]

In summary, there are age-related changes in body volumes and renal function that probably predispose elderly people to abnormalities in water and electrolyte balance. Diseases that are more common in elderly persons exacerbate this and, in addition to therapy for these diseases, affect water balance. Healthy older humans probably have at least a normal ability to secrete vasopressin but a decreased appreciation for thirst and a decreased ability to achieve either a maximum concentration of urine to retain water or a maximum dilution of urine to excrete water. Thus, it is necessary to pay attention to fluid balance problems in older people as undetected hypernatremia or hyponatremia can lead to increased morbidity and mortality.[110, 111]

DIABETES INSIPIDUS

Diabetes insipidus is a disorder in which there is a large volume of urine (diabetes) that is hypotonic, dilute, and tasteless (insipid). This is in contrast to the hypertonic and sweet urine of diabetes mellitus (honey). Four pathophysiologic mechanisms related to vasopressin produce large volumes of dilute urine and polydipsia, resulting from the following conditions:

1. *Hypothalamic* (central or neurohypophyseal) diabetes insipidus, with inability to secrete and usually to synthesize vasopressin in the neurohypophyseal system.
2. *Nephrogenic* diabetes insipidus, in which there is an inappropriate renal response to vasopressin.
3. *Transient* diabetes insipidus of pregnancy, produced by the accelerated metabolism of vasopressin.
4. *Primary polydipsia*, in which the initial pathophysiology involves the ingestion of fluid rather than the excretion of fluid.

Differential Diagnosis

To determine whether there is a large volume of urine, one can measure a 24-hour urine collection or the patient can keep a diary for 24 hours, recording the volume and the time of each voided urine. Simultaneously, it must be determined whether polyuria is due to an osmotic agent, such as glucose, or to intrinsic renal disease. Usually, routine laboratory studies and the clinical setting distinguish these diseases or disorders from consideration of diabetes insipidus. If the thirst mechanism is intact, most patients are ambulatory with normal serum sodium levels and no evidence of dehydration. All agree that the diagnosis of diabetes insipidus is confirmed by the presence of some dehydration to stimulate the normal release of vasopressin and then by the absence of the ability to concentrate the urine.

The test most commonly used clinically is a *dehydration test* in a controlled environment, followed by a response to administered vasopressin or to the analogue desmopressin. If the patient has mild polyuria, the test may begin in the evening with the majority of dehydration taking place overnight. If the patient gives a history of large volumes of urine during the night, it is best to perform the test during the day when the patient can be observed.

The patient is weighed at the beginning of test in attire that can be worn throughout the study and on a clinical quality scale that can be used for all repeated weighings. The patient voids, and the starting weight is recorded. A serum sodium level is obtained, and nothing is allowed by mouth (certainly no fluid) during the test. Each voided urine is then recorded and urine osmolality measured. The patient is weighed after each liter of urine is excreted.

When two consecutive measures of urine osmolality differ by no more than 10% and the patient has lost 2% of the body weight, plasma is drawn for Na^+, osmolality, and vasopressin determinations. The patient is given 2 μg of desmopressin intravenously or intramuscularly (or 5 units of aqueous vasopressin subcutaneously), and urine output and osmolality are recorded hourly for an additional 2 hours.[112, 113] The test is discontinued if the patient loses more than 3% of the body weight or at any time that serum Na^+ is elevated above the normal range. The duration of the test varies; patients with complete diabetes insipidus reach a maximum but very low urine osmolality within a few hours; patients with other disorders reach a maximum in up to 18 hours.

There is no difficulty in determining the diagnosis of severe hypothalamic or severe nephrogenic diabetes insipidus. In the former, urine has minimal concentration despite dehydration and there is a marked increase in urine osmolality in response to administered desmopressin, at least a 50% but often a 200% to 400% increase. At the end of the test, these patients have undetectable vasopressin in plasma. In patients with nephrogenic diabetes insipidus, there is also little concentration of the urine despite achieving dehydration, but the urine osmolality also shows little or no response to the administered desmopressin. These patients are unequivocally distinguished from those with hypothalamic diabetes insipidus by high levels of vasopressin in plasma, often greater than 5 pg/μL, at the end of the dehydration phase.

The difficulty is in differentiating partial hypothalamic diabetes insipidus from primary polydipsia. In both disorders, the urine shows some concentration (often above plasma osmolality) with dehydration but the urine osmolality does not approach the 800 to 1000 mOsm/kg characteristic of normal subjects. In response to the administered desmopressin, patients with partial hypothalamic diabetes insipidus usually show a further concentration of the urine of at least 10%, whereas patients with primary polydipsia show no further increase. The reliability of the response to desmopressin is debated. Some patients with primary polydipsia may achieve a plateau level in urine osmolality before reaching their maximum attainable urine osmolality and hence respond to desmopressin. Alternatively, some patients with partial hypothalamic diabetes insipidus may, with severe dehydration, secrete sufficient vasopressin to achieve the maximum attainable urine osmolality and do not respond with a further increase to administered desmopressin.

Investigators who have a highly sensitive radioimmunoassay for vasopressin are able to distinguish between partial hypothalamic diabetes insipidus and primary polydipsia by the measurement of vasopressin at the end of the dehydration phase[114, 115] and further report that one of these disorders may be inappropriately diagnosed using the standard dehydration test.[114, 115] However, a longitudinal clinical study of patients with autoimmune hypothalamic diabetes insipidus reported good correlation between results of the dehydration test and measured vasopressin to diagnose partial diabetes insipidus occurring over time.[116]

There is concern about making the diagnosis of partial diabetes insipidus in patients with primary polydipsia because patients given desmopressin may experience symptomatic hyponatremia as they continue to drink fluid despite desmopressin-induced water conservation. Therefore, when the diagnosis is in doubt, patients should have adequate follow-up to ensure that a good therapeutic response is obtained and that hyponatremia does not develop. This clinical follow-up and response have been considered a continuation of the diagnosis with the trial of desmopressin as a test agent. If a standard dose of desmopressin produces a decrease in polyuria, a decrease in thirst, and no reduction of sodium, the patient almost certainly has partial hypothalamic diabetes insipidus. If polydipsia does not improve and hyponatremia develops, the patient has some abnormality of thirst, and the diagnosis may be primary polydipsia.[114, 117]

The clinical presentation is often helpful in the differential diagnosis. In a patient with no previous history of polyuria or polydipsia who is found to have these symptoms immediately after surgery in the hypothalamic-pituitary area or after head trauma (especially with skull fracture and loss of consciousness), the diagnosis of hypothalamic diabetes insipidus is highly probable. Sometimes diuresis after surgery is the result of water retention during the procedure. Vasopressin is released during surgical procedures, and administered fluid may be retained. As the stress of surgery abates, the vasopressin level falls and administered fluid is excreted. If an attempt is made to match the urine output with further fluid infusion, persistent polyuria occurs and may be mistaken for diabetes insipidus.

Because these patients may be unconscious and may be unable to sense thirst, it is crucial that the diagnosis be established and that patients be treated appropriately to prevent severe dehydration. Because these patients do not sense thirst, it is easy to withhold fluids until there is a modest increase in sodium and then to measure urine osmolality and determine the response to administered desmopressin. If urine output decreases and the serum sodium level remains normal, the response was excretion of physiologically retained fluid. If the serum sodium begins to rise, a response to desmopressin should be determined and the diagnosis of diabetes insipidus established.[118]

Patients with hypothalamic diabetes insipidus often experience a sudden onset of symptoms and persistent thirst throughout the day and night, whereas patients with renal disease experience a more gradual onset of disease and patients with primary polydipsia may have decreased thirst and urination during the night. Hypothalamic diabetes insipidus is associated more with a desire for cold liquids,[119] probably because of dehydration. Patients with diabetes insipidus often have serum sodium levels in the high range of normal, whereas patients with primary polydipsia have serum sodium levels in the low range of normal. Blood urea nitrogen (BUN) concentration is often low in both hypothalamic diabetes insipidus and primary polydipsia because of the high renal clearance, but there is a difference in serum uric acid concentrations.

Serum uric acid is elevated in hypothalamic diabetes insipidus because of modest volume contraction and because vasopressin acts on V1 receptors in the kidney to increase urate clearance. Therefore, in patients with no vasopressin, the uric acid level is high; a value greater than 5 μg/dL has been reported to separate hypothalamic diabetes insipidus from primary polydipsia. Presumably, in patients with primary polydipsia, there is modest volume expansion and intermittent secretion of vasopressin to act on V1 receptors to clear serum urate.[120] Urine volume greater than 18 L suggests primary polydipsia because the volume exceeds the amount of urine delivered to the collecting duct. In fact, most patients with hypothalamic diabetes insipidus have modest dehydration, have a decreased GFR, and excrete urine volumes in the range of 6 to 12 L/day.

Imaging of the Neurohypophysis

When MRI began to be used to evaluate the pituitary gland and hypothalamus, a bright spot in the sella was reported on T1-weighted images.[15] The bright spot is due to stored hormone in neurosecretory granules in the posterior pituitary.[41, 42, 121] The interest in the posterior pituitary bright spot as a diagnostic tool was heightened by reports that the bright spot was absent in patients with diabetes insipidus.[122–124]

Many studies using small numbers of normal subjects have demonstrated this bright spot in all normal subjects; when larger numbers were evaluated, however, the bright spot was not seen in some normal subjects. In one study of 500 normal subjects, it was calculated that the bright spot would be present in 84% of normal youth.[125] Although it had been suggested that the intensity of this bright spot might vary with the physiologic state of water balance in humans,[125, 126] this would occur only with a prolonged stimulus.

Absence of the bright spot is characteristic of diabetes insipidus,[122, 127, 128] but some studies have reported the presence of a bright spot in patients with clinical evidence of diabetes insipidus.[129] This may be of most interest in patients with familial hypothalamic diabetes insipidus (see later). In these cases, the posterior pituitary bright spot may be seen early in the disease (especially when the diabetes insipidus is partial) but usually disappears over time with increasing severity of the diabetes insipidus.[130]

The role of stored oxytocin as a source of the pituitary bright spot has been largely ignored. Oxytocin is synthesized in the same nuclear groups and is transported and stored in the posterior pituitary in a manner similar to that with vasopressin. In humans, secretion of oxytocin is less responsive to changes in hydration. Therefore, it is possible that a persistent bright spot in patients with diabetes insipidus might be due to the pituitary content of oxytocin. Furthermore, oxytocinergic neurons are more resistant to destruction by trauma compared with vasopressinergic neurons in rats[131] and humans.[132]

The presence of a positive posterior pituitary bright spot has been variably reported in other polyuric disorders considered in the differential diagnosis of diabetes insipidus. The bright spot is usually seen in patients with primary polydipsia.[123, 133] This observation is consistent with studies in animals, in which even prolonged lack of secretion of vasopressin caused by hyponatremia did not produce a decreased content of hormone in the posterior pituitary.[33] In nephrogenic diabetes insipidus, the bright spot has been reported to be absent in some patients[123] but present in others.[123, 128, 133] Because these patients have high levels of vasopressin in plasma and are chronically dehydrated, the posterior pituitary might be depleted of vasopressin and the bright spot might be absent.

Imaging of the hypothalamus is also an important diagnostic tool for diseases of the neurohypophysis. As noted earlier, the hormones of the neurohypophysis are synthesized in the paired paraventricular nuclei, located bilaterally in the walls of the third ventricle, and in the supraoptic nuclei, located at the extremes of the optic chiasm. When this anatomic information is coupled with the knowledge that 90% of the vasopressinergic neurons must be destroyed to produce symptomatic diabetes insipidus,[134, 135] it is apparent that for a mass lesion or a destructive lesion to produce diabetes insipidus, it either must destroy a large area of the hypothalamus or must be specifically located where the tracks converge in the base of the hypothalamus at the origin of the pituitary stalk (see Fig. 9–1). Furthermore, the hormones are synthesized in cell bodies quite distant from the site of release in the posterior lobe, and with section or damage of the axons at the level of the posterior lobe there is a reaccumulation of neurosecretory material and regeneration of a posterior lobe above the site of injury. Thus, tumors confined to the sella do not cause diabetes insipidus,[135] and the area of interest is the discrete area immediately above the diaphragm sella at the base of the hypothalamus.

The pituitary stalk can also be readily identified by MRI and has been an additional tool in the differential diagnosis of diseases of the neurohypophysis. Enlargement of the stalk beyond 2 to 3 mm has been reported as pathologic.[122, 136] The most common tumor to enlarge the stalk is suprasellar germinoma.[124, 136] Metastatic tumors may be seen as enlargements of the pituitary stalk, probably related to seating of metastases in the long portal capillary system. Infiltrative diseases of the neurohypophysis, such Langerhans cell histiocytosis,[82, 133, 137, 138] Wegener's granulomatosis,[139] and lymphocytic infundibulohypophysitis, may enlarge the stalk.[140] Sarcoidosis and tuberculosis are infiltrative lesions that can cause widening of the stalk.[136] Even cases that remain idiopathic may involve enlargement of the stalk.[82]

When the etiologic diagnosis of diabetes insipidus is in doubt and MRI reveals thickening of the stalk, especially with absence of the posterior pituitary bright spot, a search for systemic diseases is indicated. This search may result in a diagnosis of Langerhans cell histiocytosis, sarcoidosis, or tuberculosis. Further evaluation of cerebrospinal fluid (CSF) and plasma for secretion of human chorionic gonadotropin (hCG) and α-fetoprotein may indicate suprasellar germinoma.[137, 141, 142]

When a diagnosis is still in doubt, MRI should be repeated every 3 to 6 months, especially in children, in whom enlargement may indicate a germinoma.[137, 142] Decrease in size of the stalk with follow-up is more likely indicative of lymphocytic infundibulohypophysitis or idiopathic diabetes insipidus (but many of these cases may be infundibulitis), although it may also occur with specific treatment of infiltrative diseases.

Finally, MRI may show formation of a new "posterior pituitary" after stalk transection. It has been known for many years that section of the neurohypophyseal stalk at a low level may produce transient diabetes insipidus with eventual return of function. Reaccumulation of neurosecretory material above the transection has been noted histiologically.[82, 143, 144] Indeed, the accumulation of neurosecretory products above the site of section was early evidence proving that neurosecretory material was transported along axons. Postoperative patients with diabetes insipidus or patients in whom the posterior pituitary was destroyed by compression of an adjacent anterior pituitary adenoma may "lose" the bright spot on MRI but may demonstrate reappearance of a bright spot at the level of the remaining stalk.[122, 145]

Clinical Syndromes of Hypothalamic Diabetes Insipidus

Hereditary Hypothalamic Diabetes Insipidus

Hereditary hypothalamic (central or neurohypophyseal) diabetes insipidus is characterized by the onset of classic diabetes insipidus, thirst, polydipsia, and polyuria in childhood,[82, 146–148] but during infancy those who carry the genetic defect may be asymptomatic.[148, 149] In contrast, in cases of familial nephrogenic diabetes insipidus, the defect is expressed as a polyuric disease at birth (see later). The relatively late onset of hereditary hypothalamic diabetes insipidus is also supported by MRI findings, which, although variable, have shown a positive bright spot suggesting vasopressin stores early in the disease but a loss of the bright spot (or a greatly diminished one) late in the disease.[127, 130, 137, 150, 151]

More than 30 different families with autosomal dominant hypothalamic (neurohypophyseal) diabetes insipidus have been studied and the genetic defect identified.[148–168] Only one defect has been described in the vasopressin gene itself[169]; this was reported as autosomal recessive with heterozygotic parents and late onset of the disease related to a biologically less active mutated vasopressin hormone. A number of families have been described with a genetic abnormality in the signal peptide of the pre-prohormone, most commonly at the extreme carboxyl terminus at the site of cleavage of the signal peptide from vasopressin (see Fig. 9–3). Disruption of the cleavage is thought to cause the disease. Except for the rare mutants involving the vasopressin hormone, all of the other defects have been in the neurophysin molecule. None have been reported for the glycopeptide.

Most authors have suggested that abnormalities of the folding of neurophysin might by some mechanism be toxic to the magnicellular neurons and that over time (consistent with the late onset of an autosomal dominant disease) may cause neuronal cell death. Of the few postmortem studies, some findings have been consistent with degeneration of magnicellular neurons[170, 171] but others have shown normal neurons with decreased expression of vasopressin[172] or no hypothalamic abnormality.[173] The mutant deoxyribonucleic acid (DNA) of the vasopressin neurophysin precursor has been expressed in neurogenic cell lines[146, 174, 175]; all showed abnormal trafficking and accumulation of mutant prohormone in the endoplasmic reticulum with low or absent expression in the Golgi apparatus, suggesting difficulty with packaging into neurosecretory granules (see Fig. 9–3). The mechanism whereby this may lead to cell death has not been defined, but cell death may not be necessary to decrease available vasopressin.[176]

Normally, proteins retained in the endoplasmic reticulum are selectively degraded, but if excess mutant is produced and the selective normal degradative process is overwhelmed, an alternative nonselective degradative system (autophagy) is activated. As more and more mutant precursor builds up in the endoplasmic reticulum, the normal wild type is trapped with the mutant protein and degraded by the activated nonspecific degradative system. By this mechanism, the amount of vasopressin that matures and is packaged is markedly reduced. This explanation is consistent with the cases in which little pathology is found in the magnicellular neurons and also with cases of diabetes insipidus in which some small amount of vasopressin can be detected.[149]

Diabetes Insipidus Produced by Solid Tumors or Hematologic Malignancies

Some tumors such as craniopharyngioma and suprasellar germinoma or pinealoma characteristically occur in a suprasellar basal hypothalamic area and are regularly associated with diabetes insipidus.[177–179] The latter are often diagnosed by accompanying precocious puberty or serum markers such as hCG or α-fetoprotein in spinal fluid or plasma.[141, 180] It is not uncommon with pinealomas and suprasellar germinomas for diabetes insipidus to be the presenting complaint, although other evidence of hypopituitarism may be present. MRI may not demonstrate a mass in the suprasellar area for a few months,[181–183] but the tumor is usually apparent within the first few years of follow-up.[184] Rarely, it is not apparent for several years.[137, 183]

Metastatic disease involving the pituitary is usually found in association with widespread metastatic disease and is reported at autopsy but is often not symptomatic during life. Metastases are twice as likely to involve the posterior pituitary as the anterior pituitary,[185, 186] which is thought to be due to a more direct arterial blood supply to the posterior pituitary. It is also possible that any potential metastases to the anterior pituitary lodge in the portal system and occur as hypothalamic tumors. In either case, with metastatic tumors, diabetes insipidus is more common than is deficiency of anterior pituitary hormones.

The diagnosis is usually made in a patient who is known to have primary cancer with metastases elsewhere. MRI of the brain usually demonstrates the pituitary metastasis, often with other metastases in the brain or skull.[187–189] Occasionally, only micrometastases are found at autopsy and enlargement of the stalk may be the presenting finding.[190] Most primary tumors in the hypothalamic-pituitary area that cause diabetes insipidus grow relatively slowly, and any tumor in this area that shows rapid growth in a short period of time should be considered a possible metastatic tumor. Carcinoma of the breast is the most common primary cancer in women,[189] and carcinoma of the lung is the most common primary tumor in men.[191, 192] Other tumors that have been reported in the area include adenocarcinoma of the stomach, pancreas, uterus, thyroid, and bladder.[191, 193]

Diabetes insipidus has been reported with lymphomas in the hypothalamic-pituitary area. Usually, lymphoma is recognized elsewhere,[194–196] but rarely it is a primary central nervous system (CNS) lymphoma.[197] There may be an increased incidence of lymphoma with diabetes insipidus because of the increased incidence of lymphoproliferative disease with human immunodeficiency virus (HIV) and hepatitis C infection.[196] Occasionally, MRI findings are normal and a vasculitis may be the cause of diabetes insipidus,[198] but it has been emphasized that infiltrative lesions may leave the anatomy of the hypothalamic area intact and be missed on MRI examination if a contrast agent such as gadolinium is not used.[197]

Diabetes insipidus is also associated with leukemia. The mechanism is thought to be infiltration of the hypothalamus, thrombosis, or infection.[199, 200] Although acute lymphocytic leukemia is as common as nonlymphocytic leukemia and is well known to involve the CNS, diabetes insipidus is distinctly more common with nonlymphocytic leukemia.[201–206] As many as 75% of the cases of diabetes insipidus with leukemia involve nonlymphocytic leukemia. There is also a suggested association with monosomy 7,[205, 207] although a mechanism has not been defined.[207] MRI results in leukemia may show infiltration or an infundibular mass[202] but are often normal even when leukemic cells are found in CSF.[201] In other cases, the CSF has no leukocytes and thrombosis of small vessels in the hypothalamus might be a more likely cause of the diabetes insipidus.[204] Posterior pituitary deficiency may be associated with panhypopituitarism,[201, 206] and the diabetes insipidus may not be apparent because of coexisting adrenal insufficiency and hypothyroidism. Indeed, in some patients symptomatic diabetes insipidus occurs only when prednisone therapy is initiated as treatment for the leukemia.[206]

Response of the Neurohypophyseal System to Surgery or Trauma

Although diabetes insipidus is well known to occur after hypothalamic-pituitary surgery, this diagnosis should be made with caution.[118, 208] Vasopressin is normally secreted in the stress of surgical procedures,[132] and fluid may be retained and then normally excreted after surgery (see "Differential Diagnosis"). The stress of surgery may also induce insulin resistance and may exacerbate diabetes mellitus, producing an osmotic diuresis resulting from glucose. The patterns of diabetes insipidus after surgery have been described in detail.[135] As many as 50% to 60% of patients have some transient diabetes insipidus within 24 hours of pituitary surgery that usually resolves, especially with transsphenoidal surgery in which the resection of a tumor is confined to the sella.

If there is complete section of the stalk, patients may exhibit a pattern known as *triphasic diabetes insipidus* (Fig. 9–7):

The first phase, diabetes insipidus, occurs within the first 24 hours of surgery and is thought to be due to axon shock and inability to propagate action potentials from the cell body to the axon terminals in the posterior pituitary.

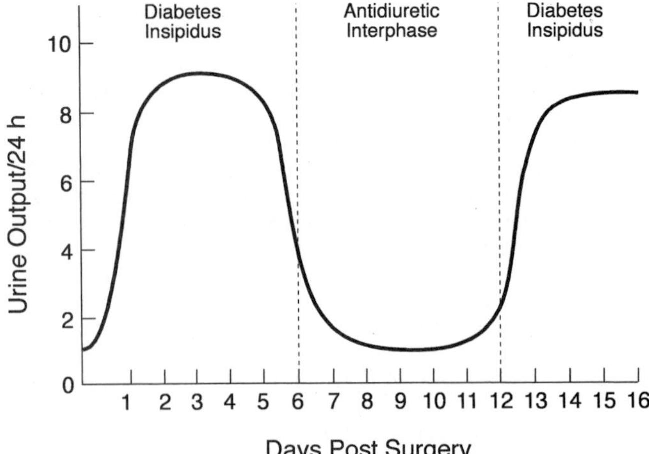

Figure 9–7. Typical triphasic response of urine volume after section of the pituitary stalk induced by surgery or head trauma. The first phase of diabetes insipidus occurs immediately after operation and continues to day 6. The second phase of antidiuresis occurs from day 7 and continues to day 12. The third stage is the recurrence of diabetes insipidus on day 13. (Durations vary; see text for discussion.)

The second (antidiuretic) phase, although originally described as a normal interphase, is not normal and is thought to be due to unregulated release of vasopressin from the store of hormone in the axons of the posterior pituitary as these axons degenerate. Because the release of vasopressin in this phase is unregulated, excess administration of fluids produces hyponatremia as in other forms of SIADH.

The third phase, the return of diabetes insipidus, occurs when all of the hormone has been released from the posterior pituitary. The course of diabetes insipidus may be permanent or may subsequently resolve to partial or clinically inapparent disease.

Magnicellular neurons are unique in that, after the axons are sectioned, the neurons survive and there is outgrowth of dendrites and regeneration of new axons.[131, 209–211] A factor contributing to the ability of magnicellular neurons to regenerate is the close association of these neurons with specialized glial cells. The glial cells in the area of magnicellular neurons and the median eminence synthesize and release growth factors that may stimulate nerve growth. The newly formed axons grow along fixed glial cells *(tanycytes)* that span the median eminence from the third ventricle to the external zone of the median eminence.[212] Thus, the regenerating axons and sprouting axons create neurosecretory processes in the CSF of the third ventricle as well as in the perivascular region of the external zone of the median eminence.[209–211, 213]

The transected neurosecretory axons may promote capillary sprouting, but its importance in the return of function is uncertain. These newly formed capillaries may have tight interendothelial junctions similar to those elsewhere in the brain,[211] whereas the capillaries that are already present in the external zone of the median eminence are fenestrated capillaries capable of receiving secreted peptides.[211] Several studies have shown that oxytocin neurons survive better than vasopressin neurons after transection of the pituitary stalk.[131, 209, 210, 212] In studies in the rat, the activity of the magnicellular vasopressin neurons had a dramatic effect on recovery. After stalk compression in the rat, if synthesis of vasopressin was inhibited, fewer vasopressin neurons survived,[131] and if vasopressin synthesis was stimulated, more vasopressin neurons survived. However, because the magnitude and duration of both the hypernatremia and the hyponatremia in the rat studies exceeded those seen in patients, the application of the findings to clinical medicine is uncertain.

An important observation is that the second phase of the triphasic response—uncontrolled release of vasopressin related to axon trauma—may occur without preceding or subsequent diabetes insipidus.[214, 215] This has been observed clinically and has been produced experimentally in the rat by unilateral lesion of the supraopticohypophyseal tract.[215] The interpretation is that if the trauma is only to some of the axons coursing to the posterior pituitary, the remaining intact axons have sufficient vasopressin function to avoid clinically apparent diabetes insipidus characteristic of the first and third phases of the triphasic response. However, the store of hormone in the posterior pituitary is sufficiently large that degeneration and necrosis of even a fraction of these vasopressin neurons cause enough uncontrolled release of vasopressin to produce hyponatremia if excess fluid is administered. The hyponatremia becomes apparent because it is often symptomatic with new-onset headache, nausea, and emesis.[216] When all the vasopressin from the damaged neurons has been secreted, the stimulus for water retention resolves and the retained water is excreted, resulting in recovery from the hyponatremia.

Thus, the clinical picture is one of hyponatremia occurring about 7 days after pituitary surgery, persisting for a few days, and then returning to normal. This syndrome of transient hyponatremia has been referred to as an *isolated second phase*[215] to emphasize the pathophysiologic etiology. In one series, isolated hyponatremia occurred in as many as 25% of patients after pituitary surgery.[217] The hyponatremia was associated with lack of suppression of vasopressin, inability to excrete a water load, and inappropriate natriuresis[217] and was observed in spite of normal levels of cortisol or glucocorticoid replacement.[216] In larger series, including various sizes and etiologic mechanisms of tumors, isolated hyponatremia was reported in about 10%, with only 2% symptomatic.[218]

The same patterns of diabetes insipidus that occur after surgery can be seen in patients after closed-head trauma.[135, 219] Seventy-five percent of these cases are due to motor vehicle accidents[135, 219] and there is a great preponderance of male patients, usually young men with a mean age in the 20s. More than 90% of patients experience coma and a high percentage have associated skull fracture.[135, 219–221] Computed tomography (CT) or MRI in a large group of patients with post-traumatic hypopituitarism including diabetes insipidus showed hemorrhage in the hypothalamus or posterior pituitary in 55% and stalk resection or infarction of the posterior pituitary in approximately 5%.[219]

Several important clinical points should be emphasized concerning diabetes insipidus induced by head trauma:

1. These patients are virtually always unconscious and do not have the normal ability to sense thirst.
2. In this situation, large volumes of fluid may be given because of blood loss or other volume deficits; this fluid loss or stress may induce diabetes mellitus and an osmotic diuresis (see "Differential Diagnosis").
3. There may be a greater risk if the second phase is unrecognized because hyponatremia may produce cerebral edema and worsen any edema related to trauma. Therefore, in administering desmopressin, the effect of one dose should be allowed to wane before another dose is administered in order to ensure that the patient has not entered the second phase.
4. There is a high incidence of anterior pituitary deficiency in association with diabetes insipidus induced by head trauma.[219]

The possibility of cortisol deficiency should be considered immediately, as it may be life-threatening in these patients. It is also well known that anterior pituitary deficiency and, especially, decreased ACTH and adrenal function interfere with the ability to dilute the urine maximally.[222, 223] Cortisol deficiency should also be considered subsequently if diabetes insipidus appears to improve because of a decrease of water excretion in the absence of an administered antidiuretic agent.[135]

Finally, in the long-term follow-up of these patients, the possibility of late development of anterior pituitary deficiency should be kept in mind[219] as well as the possible return of sufficient vasopressin function that the patient no longer has symptomatic diabetes insipidus.[135, 224]

Granulomatous Diseases

Langerhans Cell Histiocytosis

The term Langerhans cell histiocytosis is now applied to a spectrum of diseases from the severe fulminant visceral Letterer-Siwe disease to the multifocal Hand-Schüller-Christian disease to benign eosinophilic granuloma. The etiology is unknown, but the condition is characterized by proliferation of monoclonal Langerhans cells. It may have an acute fulminant course or be marked by spontaneous remission and recurring disease.[225–227]

In patients with Langerhans cell histiocytosis, diabetes insipidus occurs as a manifestation of CNS involvement and usually in association with other involvements of the head, including cranial bones, oral mucosa, or other areas of the brain.[228–230] Diabetes insipidus is also more common when there is systemic disease, especially involving the lung,[228, 231] but occasionally diabetes insipidus may be the only systemic manifestation other than diffuse involvement of the skin[232, 233] and may even precede the diagnosis of Langerhans cell histiocytosis.[228, 234] A variety of disorders of water balance may be produced, including complete hypothalamic diabetes insipidus (the most common), partial diabetes insipidus, abnormalities of thirst, and the disorder of essential hypernatremia.

The reported frequency of diabetes insipidus with Langerhans cell histiocytosis depends on whether it is routinely sought by endocrine tests and MRI of the brain or noted only on the basis of the diagnosis in retrospective series. Higher incidences were reported in earlier reviews, possibly because the new definition of Langerhans cell histiocytosis includes more mild disease. Later reviews reported an incidence of 5% to 25%.[227–231] MRI of the hypothalamus usually shows absence of a posterior pituitary bright spot on T1-weighted images and widening of the stalk with contrast.[138, 226, 229, 235–237] Irradiation of the hypothalamus has been used to treat diabetes insipidus associated with Langerhans cell histiocytosis, but the value has been questioned.[227, 231] Success is difficult to determine from published reviews because a decreased requirement for desmopressin has been considered a positive response; as noted later, however, this decrease in requirement for medication may not be a manifestation of lessened disease.[238] In addition, patients with Langerhans cell histiocytosis may experience spontaneous remissions, which confounds the interpretation of response to therapy.[231]

Most patients with complete diabetes insipidus and Langerhans cell histiocytosis have permanent disease, and recommendations for therapy suggest that radiation therapy (if considered to treat the diabetes insipidus) be reserved for patients with partial diabetes insipidus.[227, 239] Yet other studies have stressed the benefit of aggressive chemotherapy[229] and suggest that it may prevent the progression to diabetes insipidus that often occurs within the first 2 years after diagnosis.[231] Anterior pituitary deficiency, especially growth hormone deficiency, may coexist with diabetes insipidus,[138, 225, 230] and there is concern that irradiation of the hypothalamic-pituitary area might worsen anterior pituitary deficiency.[227] Treatment of the water balance problems associated with Langerhans cell histiocytosis does not differ from treatment of abnormalities of diabetes insipidus and thirst produced by other causes.

Wegener's Granulomatosis

Wegener's granulomatosis is a necrotizing granulomatous vasculitis that typically affects the lung and kidneys, although it may affect other organs; in 15% to 30% of cases, there is neurologic involvement[240, 241] with the predominant manifestations of peripheral neuropathy. The involvement of the kidney may make it difficult to diagnose the cause of polyuria and polydipsia in Wegener's granulomatosis, but several reports have demonstrated hypothalamic diabetes insipidus and radiologic evidence of inflammation of the hypothalamus and pituitary.[139, 242–245] When hypothalamic diabetes insipidus is found, MRI usually demonstrates absence of the pituitary bright spot and widening of the stalk. As with other disorders, the degree of involvement is better demonstrated with the administration of contrast agents[242, 243] but occasionally the MRI is completely normal and the pathology is thought to be a vasculitis that is not apparent on imaging studies.[245]

A number of cases have shown complete resolution of diabetes insipidus with appropriate therapy and response of Wegener's granulomatosis; others have demonstrated persistent diabetes insipidus in spite of response of peripheral manifestations of the disease and even decreased granulomatous lesions in the hypothalamus. Other less specifically defined granulomatous diseases of the periphery have also rarely been reported with hypothalamic diabetes insipidus[246, 247]; however, when diabetes insipidus and abnormalities of the pituitary stalk and posterior pituitary are the only findings, these nonspecific inflammatory disorders may be indistinguishable from infundibulohypophysitis.[248]

Sarcoidosis

Although only about 5% of patients with sarcoidosis have symptoms of neurosarcoidosis,[249] neurologic symptoms are the presenting complaint in about 50% of those patients,[250, 251] and about 25% of the patients with neurosarcoidosis have hypothalamic diabetes insipidus.[251] MRI findings may mimic those with other causes of hypothalamic diabetes insipidus and consist of a widened stalk with contrast and absence of a posterior pituitary bright spot.[252, 253] Thus, in cases considered as idiopathic diabetes insipidus or infundibuloneurohypophysitis, sarcoidosis should be considered and possible systemic manifestations of the disease should be sought. The study would include at a minimum chest radiography, erythrocyte sedimentation rate (EFR), and serum and CSF levels of angiotensin-converting enzyme and serum calcium. Tuberculosis should also be considered and a PPD test done.[252–254]

Because early treatment of neurosarcoidosis is recommended, it is desirable to make the diagnosis.[255] Although hypothalamic diabetes insipidus is the most common water balance problem in sarcoidosis, disordered regulation of thirst and nephrogenic diabetes insipidus related to the disease or hypercalcemia have also been noted.[256] Whereas neurosarcoidosis may be treated with a variety of mechanisms leading to remission of the disease, diabetes insipidus, once established, is usually permanent.[252]

Lymphocytic Infundibulohypophysitis

When obvious causes of diabetes insipidus are not present, most cases of diabetes insipidus are idiopathic. As in other endocrine systems in which loss of function is not associated with a specific etiology, the possibility of an autoimmune process has been considered.[177, 257] Vasopressin antibodies have been reported in serum in up to one third of patients with idiopathic diabetes insipidus and in two thirds of those with Langerhans cell histiocytosis but were absent in patients with tumors.[258] Furthermore, a relatively high incidence of other autoimmune diseases has been reported.[259] In one study, 878 patients with autoimmune endocrine diseases, but without hypothalamic diabetes insipidus, were screened for vasopressin antibodies and 9 patients were found to have them. With careful testing, four of these patients were found to have partial diabetes insipidus and five were normal. After a 4-year follow-up, though, three of the normal subjects had experienced partial diabetes insipidus and one, complete diabetes insipidus. Interestingly, two of the patients who had partial diabetes insipidus at entry were treated with desmopressin and after 1 year no longer had vasopressin antibodies and had normal posterior pituitary function.[116]

A rare but now well-recognized cause of autoimmune diabetes insipidus is lymphocytic infundibulohypophysitis. Lymphocytic infiltration of the anterior pituitary, lymphocytic hypophysitis, has been recognized as a cause of anterior pituitary deficiency for a number of years, but it was not until an autopsy called attention to a similar finding in the posterior pituitary of a patient with diabetes insipidus that this pathology was recognized for the neurohypophysis.[260] Since that report, a number of cases have been described, including cases in the postpartum period, which is characteristic of lymphocytic hypophysitis.[261, 262] Since the advent of MRI, lymphocytic infundibulohypophysitis has been diagnosed on the basis of the appearance of a thickened stalk or enlargement of the posterior pituitary mimicking a pituitary tumor, or both. In these cases, the characteristic bright spot on T1-weighted MRI images is lost.

Enlargement of the stalk so resembled pituitary tumor that before lymphocytic infundibulohypophysitis was known to produce stalk enlargement, some of these patients underwent operations because of a suspicion of a pituitary tumor.[263, 264] Recently, a number of patients with suspected infundibulohypophysitis and no other obvious cause of diabetes insipidus have been monitored and have shown regression of the thickened pituitary stalk and tumor-like appearance.[257, 263, 265] Treatment of these patients with prednisone may be associated with a decrease in size of the stalk, but a decrease may also occur spontaneously.[265]

Some cases show coexistence of infundibulohypophysitis and adenohypophysitis.[266, 267] Autoimmune diseases may affect more than one endocrine organ without any specific link to explain the association, such as diabetes insipidus in association with systemic lupus erythematosus[268–270] or Behçet's disease.[271, 272]

Diabetes Insipidus in Pregnancy

In rare cases, women with normal regulation of vasopressin have symptoms of diabetes insipidus during pregnancy because of extremely elevated activity of cysteine aminopeptidase (vasopressinase). This syndrome has been referred to as *vasopressin-resistant diabetes insipidus of pregnancy*.[273] Levels of vasopressinase are markedly elevated above levels in normal pregnancy in such patients,[274, 275] and the concurrence of preeclampsia, acute fatty liver, and coagulopathies has been noted.[84, 276–278] That the excess vasopressinase is due to the condition of the pregnancy (i.e., *preeclampsia*) is further shown by the report that subsequent pregnancies of these women are uncomplicated by either diabetes insipidus or acute fatty liver.[278] It has been suggested that the products of vasopressin degradation produced by vasopressinase might be biologically active in increasing blood pressure, but during testing they were not thought to be causative in the preeclampsia.[275]

Because of the accelerated metabolic clearance of vasopressin in pregnancy, symptomatic diabetes insipidus may also develop in patients with borderline vasopressin function resulting from a specific disease. Therefore, in patients presenting with diabetes insipidus during pregnancy, one should not assume that the diabetes insipidus is due solely to oxytocinase. Instead, these patients must be evaluated to establish an etiologic diagnosis.[82, 279] In a few cases, the diabetes insipidus is specifically related to the pregnancy (e.g., as when it occurs with Sheehan's syndrome and infarction of the neurohypophysis).[280, 281] One might anticipate an increased incidence of lymphocytic infundibuloneurohypophysitis in pregnancy because other autoimmune diseases occur during or just after pregnancy. Although such cases have been reported,[282, 283] there does not appear to be a significant association of infundibulohypophysitis with pregnancy.

Desmopressin is clearly the treatment of choice for diabetes insipidus in pregnant women (see "Treatment of Diabetes Insipidus"). In general, labor and parturition proceed normally, and patients have no trouble with lactation.[284] There is a possibility of chronic and severe dehydration when diabetes insipidus is unrecognized, and this may pose a threat in pregnant women. In one case of severe oligohydramnios found to be due to unrecognized diabetes insipidus, the patient responded promptly to therapy with desmopressin.[285]

Essential Hypernatremia

One variant of diabetes insipidus is the *syndrome of absent osmostat with intact baroreceptors*. Because of the dysfunction of the osmostat, patients do not sense thirst and do not drink water. Unlike the situation with normal subjects, however, as the serum sodium level rises, there is no (or there is a markedly subnormal) release of vasopressin and a hypotonic polyuria continues. Even when patients are made euvolemic with the infusion of normal saline and the serum sodium concentration is allowed to rise to high levels, appropriate secretion of vasopressin is not present. Vasopressin is synthesized and stored, however, because maneuvers to stimulate baroreceptors cause secretion of vasopressin and concentration of the urine.[286, 287]

The proposed pathophysiologic mechanism is that the inadequate water intake and excess water excretion produce a degree of dehydration with hypernatremia. When dehydration is sufficient to stimulate the baroreceptors, vasopressin is released, urine is concentrated, and patients remain in a steady state of hypernatremia with modest dehydration. The increased concentration of sodium per se also causes sodium excretion to help maintain the new steady state.[288]

Infectious Diseases

Infectious granulomatous diseases (tuberculosis, syphilis) are rare causes of diabetes insipidus in the United States. Occasional cases of tuberculosis are still reported,[289] however, and it is important to consider the diagnosis, because a tuberculoma in the suprasellar area may mimic an endocrine tumor[290, 291] or sarcoidosis. It is desirable to make the diagnosis on the basis of peripheral manifestations or CSF findings rather than at surgery.

Diabetes Insipidus and Brain Death

Endocrine failure has been a topic of several clinical reports of brain death.[292–294] Diabetes insipidus is virtually universal in animal models of brain death.[295] It is extremely common in clinical series, with the incidence ranging from 30% to 80%,[292, 293, 296, 297] higher in series involving only adults than in series including children, and obviously dependent on the rigor with which the diagnosis is sought in patients with diuresis. Important clinical considerations are whether coexistent anterior pituitary deficiency exists, especially whether steroids should be administered, and whether the diabetes insipidus should be treated.

The subject of treatment is controversial. Although there is no firm evidence that treating the diabetes insipidus affects the quality of donor organs,[292, 293, 298] there is also no evidence that treating diabetes insipidus results in any complications.[299] It is important to bear in mind that not all brain death is accompanied by diabetes insipidus and that diabetes insipidus in a comatose patient does not necessarily connote brain death and even severely injured comatose patients may survive[300] (see earlier discussion of diabetes insipidus after head injury). The treatment of diabetes insipidus with brain death is similar to that of acute head injury.

Primary Polydipsia

Primary polydipsia and subsequent polyuria must be differentiated from diabetes insipidus and may also contribute to SIADH. Primary polydipsia may be induced by an organic structural lesion in the hypothalamus identical to that in any of the disorders described as causes of diabetes insipidus and may be especially associated with sarcoidosis of the hypothalamus.[256, 301] It may also be produced by drugs that cause a dry mouth or by any peripheral disorder causing an elevation of renin or angiotensin, or both.[177] If the pathologic etiology is not identifiable, the disorder may be habitual throughout a lifetime or, more commonly, may be associated with psychiatric syndromes.

Series involving patients with polydipsia in psychiatric hospitals have shown an incidence as high as 42% of patients with some form of polydipsia, and for more than 50% of these, the cause of the polydipsia remained unexplained.[302, 303] In some cases, the unexplained presence of polydipsia represented a resetting of the osmotic threshold for thirst independent of the osmotic threshold for vasopressin and these patients responded to administered desmopressin producing SIADH and hyponatremia.[304] Usually, the patient's condition was refractory to attempts to restrict fluid.[177] Propranolol has been used with some success, presumably because of its ability to inhibit the renin-angiotensin system.[305]

Clinical Syndromes of Nephrogenic Diabetes Insipidus

Congenital Nephrogenic Diabetes Insipidus

Babies with nephrogenic diabetes insipidus present with vomiting, constipation, failure to thrive, fever, and polyuria. Symptoms usually occur during the first week of life,[306–308] and on testing the patients are found to have hypernatremia and a low urine osmolality. Historically, the patients were reported to have mental retardation, complications of urinary tract dilatation,[306, 307] and intracranial calcification. An association between intracranial calcification and mental retardation has not been established, and the calcification may be a consequence of hypernatremia rather than of congenital disease.[309, 310]

The diagnosis is established by high levels of vasopressin in the plasma in the presence of hypotonic polyuria and, subsequently, by the absence of a response to administered desmopressin. There are two causes: (1) mutation in the V2 receptor and (2) mutations in the aquaporin-2 water channels; however, the presentation of diabetes insipidus is independent of the genotype.[306–308] In patients with the aquaporin defect, one can detect other V2 responses (e.g., stimulation of factor VIII secretion).[307] As genetic testing becomes more widely available, it may be unnecessary to perform extensive clinical testing to establish the diagnosis; instead, treatment may be initiated when the syndrome is suspected and direct genetic testing of the child and of the parents performed.[311]

Nephrogenic Diabetes Insipidus Caused by Mutation of the V2 Receptor

More than 90% of cases of congenital nephrogenic diabetes insipidus are X-linked disorders occurring in males and are caused[308, 312, 313] by one of more than 132 different V2 receptor mutations.[313] Most mutations occur in the part of the receptor that is highly conserved among species or that is conserved among similar receptors (e.g., homology with V1 vasopressin receptors or oxytocin receptors). Mutations at other locations on the gene may cause mild abnormalities of urinary concentration, but mild defects in concentrating ability may not cause polyuria and may escape clinical detection.[314]

Most reported receptor abnormalities produce disruption of protein folding of the V2 receptor, and the receptor is trapped in the endoplasmic reticulum, destroyed in the cell, or improperly inserted into the cell membrane.[307, 314–318] In a few cases, the receptors reached the cell membrane and were inserted; the defect was due to inhibition of binding of vasopressin to the receptor or to improper signaling of G proteins and subsequent generation of cAMP.[313, 315, 319] When the V2 receptor is inserted in the cell membrane, cloning and expressing the mutant gene in cell culture may show that the receptor responds to high concentrations of vasopressin or desmopressin,[314] yet only a few of these are sufficiently responsive to physiologic levels of vasopressin to express congenital nephrogenic diabetes insipidus as a partial disorder.[315, 320, 321]

In clinical series, approximately 10% of the V2 receptor defects causing congenital nephrogenic diabetes insipidus are thought to be de novo. This high incidence of de novo cases, coupled with the large number of mutations that have been identified, hinders the clinical use of genetic identification because it is necessary to sequence the entire open reading frame of the receptor gene rather than short sequences of DNA. This degree of sophistication exceeds the level of expertise that is found in most clinical laboratories.[313]

Although most female carriers of the X-linked V2 receptor defect have no clinical disease, some females were reported to have symptomatic nephrogenic diabetes insipidus. Carriers may have a decreased maximum urine osmolality in response to the plasma level of vasopressin that they obtain but are asymptomatic because of normal urine volume.[322] Female carriers respond to desmopressin with an increase in factor VIII, although the response may be only a fraction of the normal response.[323, 324] Some girls have as severe a defect as boys, and this is thought to be due to inactivation of the normal X chromosome.[308, 311, 325] In some cases, there may be some heterogeneity of X inactivation in various tissues, so that there is symptomatic nephrogenic diabetes insipidus but a normal response to stimulate factor VIII.[323]

Nephrogenic Diabetes Insipidus Caused by Mutation of Aquaporin-2

When the proband is a girl, it is likely that the defect is a mutation of the aquaporin-2 water channel gene on chromosome 12,q12-13 producing an autosomal recessive disease.[326] This should be especially considered when consanguinity is known in the family and the family history shows disease expressed in men and women. The phenotype of nephrogenic diabetes insipidus is identical to the receptor defect when the abnormality is in the aquaporin-2 protein.[327] More than 20 different mutations of the aquaporin-2 protein have been described.[328] The patients may be heterozygous for two different recessive mutations[329] or homozygous for the same abnormality from both parents.[330]

The biologic mechanism responsible for the defect in the aquaporin proteins may be related to the site of the mutation. In some mutations, aquaporins are not properly processed in the endoplasmic reticulum or released into the cytoplasm.[328] In other mutations, aquaporins are processed but are not appropriately inserted in the cell membrane. Mutations in the C-terminal portion of the aquaporin-2 protein produce an autosomal dominant nephrogenic diabetes insipidus. A mutant aquaporin-2 protein produces oligomers with the wild-type protein in the Golgi apparatus, and no functional aquaporin-2 proteins are produced. This form is similar to the autosomal dominant form of congenital hypothalamic diabetes insipidus described earlier.[326, 331–333]

Acquired Nephrogenic Diabetes Insipidus

The ability to produce a concentrated urine depends on maintaining hyperosmolality of the inner medulla of the kidney. The following conditions are necessary to produce and maintain hyperosmolality of the inner medulla:

1. An intact kidney architecture, with an intact tubular structure of the descending limb and ascending limb of the loop of Henle (essential to the development of the countercurrent multiplier) and a normal anatomy of the collecting duct to pass back through the inner medulla.
2. Active sodium transport in the thick ascending limb and functional aquaporins, to allow water transport across membranes.
3. An anatomically intact vascular structure so that the hyperosmolality of the inner medulla is not washed away by normal blood flow.

Acquired nephrogenic diabetes insipidus without the capacity to produce a concentrated urine may be caused by numerous chronic renal diseases that distort the architecture of the kidney (e.g., polycystic kidney disease; renal infarcts with neovascularization, such as produced by sickle cell anemia; and infiltrative disease of the kidney). Washout of the medullary gradient may be produced by excessive water intake of primary polydipsia or by forced sodium and water loss related to administration of a diuretic.[334] A low-protein diet may be associated with reduced medullary urea concentration, causing inability to produce maximum concentration of the urine.[335–337] Aquaporin is decreased in chronic renal failure, and other more specific disorders of acquired nephrogenic diabetes insipidus are related to abnormalities of aquaporins.[338]

Studies have shown that the polyuria associated with potassium deficiency develops in parallel with decreased expression of renal aquaporin-2.[339, 340] Repletion of potassium reestablished the normal urinary concentrating mechanism and normalized the expression of aquaporin-2.[340] Hypercalcemia was also associated with down-regulation of aquaporin-2.[336, 341] A low-protein diet diminished the ability to concentrate the urine primarily by decreased delivery of urea to the inner medulla, thus decreasing the hypertonicity of the medulla, but rats on a low-protein diet also down-regulated aquaporin-2, which may be an additional component of the decreased ability to concentrate the urine.[335] Bilateral urinary tract obstruction caused inability to produce a maximum concentration of the urine,[336, 337] and rat models demonstrated a down-regulation of aquaporin-2 that persisted for several days after release of the obstruction. In addition, the washout of accumulated waste products contributed to postobstructive polyuria.[337, 342, 343]

Drug-Induced Nephrogenic Diabetes Insipidus

Administration of lithium to treat psychiatric disorders is the most common cause of drug-induced nephrogenic diabetes insipidus and illustrates the mechanisms.[344, 345] As many as 10% to 20% of patients receiving chronic lithium therapy may have nephrogenic diabetes insipidus.[345, 346] Lithium is known to interfere with the production of cAMP,[345, 347] and it has been demonstrated in studies of animals that lithium produces a dramatic reduction in aquaporin-2 levels.[340] The defect is both of aquaporin-2 on the luminal surface of the collecting duct and of aquaporin-3 on the basal lateral membrane, producing a severe defect in aquaporin production that parallels the lithium-induced polyuria.[340] There is as much as a 95% decrease in aquaporin-2 content, and even the 5% of aquaporin-2 that persists is not normally transported to the collecting duct membrane.[345] Sodium transporters either show no change or are up-regulated in an effort to compensate for the water loss.[348]

The defect of aquaporins is slow to correct in both experimental animals and humans, may be permanent,[346] and may be associated with glomerular or tubulointerstitial nephropathy.[349] Lithium may also cause nephrogenic diabetes insipidus by inducing hypercalcemia. Other drugs that are known to induce renal concentrating defects or disorders such as nephrotic syndrome may be associated with abnormalities of aquaporin synthesis.[336, 350–352] Demeclocycline is another drug known to cause nephrogenic diabetes insipidus and is used clinically to treat SIADH (discussed later). See Bendz and Aurell[353] for a list of drugs also known to induce diabetes insipidus.

Deficient Vasopressin

There may be an element of nephrogenic diabetes insipidus associated with severe central diabetes insipidus related to decreased aquaporin-2. Indeed, even physiologic suppression of vasopressin by chronic administration of water may produce down-regulation of aquaporin-2 in the renal collecting duct.[354] As discussed earlier in this chapter, when a dehydration test is followed by administration of desmopressin to differentiate various causes of diabetes insipidus, the ability to concentrate the urine maximally is impaired both for central diabetes insipidus and for primary polydipsia. Although this has long been attributed to washout of the medullary concentration gradient, part of the decreased response to vasopressin is due to the down-regulation of aquaporin-2. In addition, it takes some time to restore normal expression of aquaporin-2, and this may contribute to the long time it takes patients with primary polydipsia and central diabetes insipidus to achieve maximum concentration of urine after water restriction (or treatment) is initiated.[339, 355]

Treatment

Patients with diabetes insipidus and inadequate thirst can rapidly become dehydrated and may experience severe hypernatremia with devastating effects on the CNS. Hypertonic encephalopathy with obtundation, coma, and seizures may be produced by brain shrinkage. A decreased volume of brain in the skull may lead to subarachnoid hemorrhage, intracerebral bleeding, or petechial hemorrhage.[356–358] Fortunately, these problems associated with severe hypernatremia are not observed in patients with diabetes insipidus who are ambulatory and have an intact thirst mechanism. Furthermore, they are not a part of the syndromes of hypodipsia (e.g., essential hypernatremia) in ambulatory patients, probably because of the chronic and slower onset of hypernatremia in these cases.

Thus, although hypernatremia is a commonly observed clinical event in hospitalized patients,[359] in most cases the dehydration is due to increased insensible water loss or gastrointestinal loss in elderly or young patients at admission (e.g., with fever)[359–361] rather than diabetes insipidus. Hypernatremic encephalopathy is a risk in patients with diabetes insipidus only when patients cannot respond to thirst because of either age or level of consciousness. Patients with diabetes insipidus should carry a medical card and wear a medical alert tag indicating that they have this disorder; because diabetes insipidus is rare, the name of a physician who is familiar with the disorder and whom one can notify in an emergency should be included.

Most patients with diabetes insipidus have intact thirst and drink sufficient fluid to maintain relatively normal fluid balance. The absence of vasopressin per se does not produce pathology, and a major goal of therapy is to decrease the thirst and polyuria to an acceptable level to allow the patient to maintain a normal lifestyle. The therapeutic regimen should be easy for the patient to accommodate, and the timing and quantity of dosage should be individually prescribed. The safety of the prescribed agent and a regimen that avoids any detrimental effects of overtreatment are primary considerations because of the relatively benign course of diabetes insipidus and the adverse consequences of hyponatremia.

The therapeutic agents used to treat diabetes insipidus are shown in Table 9–1. Water is considered a therapeutic agent for this disease; when water is taken in sufficient quantity, there is no metabolic abnormality. As noted, therapy is designed to reduce the necessary water intake (and polyuria) to an acceptable level, but occasional lapses in pharmacologic therapy are not detrimental, may avoid overtreatment producing hyponatremia, and may allow recognition of any spontaneous recovery.

Table 9–1. Therapeutic Agents for Treatment of Diabetes Insipidus

Water
Water-Retaining Agents
Arginine vasopressin
1-(3-Mercaptopropanoic acid)-8-D-arginine vasopressin
Chlorpropamide
Carbamazepine*
Clofibrate*
Indomethacin
Natriuretic Agents
Thiazide diuretics
Amiloride
Indapamide

*Not recommended.

Chronic Severe Hypothalamic Diabetes Insipidus

In severe diabetes insipidus, there is virtually no vasopressin in the circulation and no ability to concentrate the urine with dehydration. An antidiuretic hormone is required, and the drug of choice is desmopressin.[114, 362] In this synthetic analogue, the substitution of D-arginine markedly reduced pressor activity, and removing the terminal amine increased the half-life (see Fig. 9–2). The two changes produced an agent nearly 2000 times more specific for antidiuresis than naturally occurring L-arginine vasopressin.[363] Most patients prefer the desmopressin tablets (0.1 and 0.2 mg), although many patients continue to be treated successfully with the desmopressin intranasal spray.

Because of the variability among patients, it is desirable to determine the duration of action of individual doses in each patient.[364, 365] First the patient is allowed to be cleared from the effects of any previous medication, and for each voided urine the time can be recorded and the volume and (if possible) osmolality measured. The patient is allowed to drink fluid ad libitum. A dose is administered; a decrease in urine volume is noted in 1 to 2 hours; and the total duration of action usually ranges from 6 to 18 hours. A satisfactory schedule can usually be determined with a modest dose, and the maximum dose needed is rarely above 0.2 mg orally or 20 μg (two sprays) given two or three times a day (usually two).[364–367]

Tablets allow considerable flexibility in dosage because they can be used either whole or split. For intranasally administered desmopressin, there is less flexibility with the metered spray, which is fixed at 10 μg in 100 μL. If more flexibility is necessary, the patient should be taught to use the rhinal catheter (see Robinson and Verbalis[362] for specific directions). When a dose is sufficient to elicit a stable therapeutic response, further increasing the dose (e.g., doubling it) produces only a moderate increase in duration of few hours,[364–366] consistent with the half-life of desmopressin in plasma.[366, 367]

The medication is expensive, and in many patients a smaller dose given more often is more cost-effective than a larger dose given less often. Rarely is it necessary to resort to parenterally administered desmopressin (2-mL vials, 1-mL ampules, or 10-mL vials of 4 μg/mL) for ambulatory patients. If an intercurrent illness or allergy makes this desirable, a dose of 0.5 to 2.0 μg can be administered subcutaneously using an insulin (low dose if necessary) syringe and needle.[364]

Parenterally administered desmopressin gives virtually the same therapeutic response when given as an intravenous bolus or intramuscularly or subcutaneously,[364] and the parenterally administered dose is 5 to 20 times as potent as an intranasally administrated dose.[362, 364] *Note:* When other therapeutic agents are administered to patients with diabetes insipidus for specific indications (see Table 9–1), the effect of administered desmopressin may be augmented, exposing the patients to the possibility of excess water retention and hyponatremia.

Hyponatremia is a rare complication of desmopressin therapy and occurs only if the patient is continually antidiuretic while maintaining a fluid intake sufficient to become volume-expanded and natriuretic. Thirst may be protective, and most patients with diabetes insipidus receiving standard therapy may not be continuously maximally antidiuretic. Hyponatremia has been reported in patients with normal thirst and normal vasopressin function after taking desmopressin for treatment of von Willebrand's disease[368–371] and in children treated for primary enuresis.[372–379] Hyponatremia is often indicated first by the onset of convulsions and coma. Hyponatremia in patients with diabetes insipidus who are receiving desmopressin[380, 381] may be avoided by ensuring, either with routine therapy or by occasionally delaying a dose of desmopressin, that polyuria recurs once or twice a week, so that any excess fluid can be excreted.

Chronic Partial Hypothalamic Diabetes Insipidus

Patients with *partial* diabetes insipidus have some ability to secrete vasopressin and to concentrate the urine, but the function is inadequate to maintain normal water intake and urine output. These patients are more likely to respond to therapeutic agents such as chlorpropamide or thiazide diuretics because only a modest decrease in urine volume may make them asymptomatic. The major action of chlorpropamide is on the renal tubule to increase the hydro-osmotic action of vasopressin.[382, 383] The agent can also produce significant antidiuresis even in patients with severe hypothalamic diabetes insipidus.[114]

The usual dose is 250 to 500 mg/day, with a response noted in 1 to 2 days and a maximum antidiuresis in 4 days.[114, 362] This is an off-label use of the drug. This agent should not be used in pregnancy and is not recommended for children, especially those with concurrent hypopituitarism, because of the possibility of severe hypoglycemia. These patients also respond to desmopressin; guidelines for initiating and maintaining therapy are essentially the same as those described earlier for patients with severe diabetes insipidus.

Chronic Diabetes Insipidus with Inadequate Thirst

The presence of diabetes insipidus in a patient with inadequate thirst is a difficult management problem because patients with lack of thirst can experience severe hypernatremia and, if given an antidiuretic agent and encouraged to drink, can become hyponatremic. Thus, these patients are subject not only to wide swings in osmolality but also, most characteristically, to persistent hypernatremia. The spectrum of disorders includes that described as *essential hypernatremia.*

The first therapeutic agent to try is chlorpropamide; it has been found useful for treating diabetes insipidus and for increasing the thirst response.[384, 385] If chlorpropamide does not produce adequate control, the appropriate therapy is a fixed dose of desmopressin and a prescribed quantity of water. These patients usually require encouragement to drink. A constant antidiuresis is maintained by a rigid regimen of desmopressin and water intake prescribed for every 6 to 8 hours during a 24-hour period. Regular follow-up with measurement of serum sodium concentrations is essential to prevent development of water intoxication with hyponatremia or recurrent dehydration with hypernatremia.

Diabetes Insipidus in Pregnancy

Desmopressin is the only therapeutic agent recommended for treatment of diabetes insipidus during pregnancy. Desmopressin has 2% to 25% of the oxytocic activity of lysine vasopressin or arginine vasopressin[363] and can be used with minimal stimulation of the oxytocin receptors in the uterus.[284, 386] The physician must note the volume expansion and the reset osmostat that occur naturally in pregnancy (see earlier) and must give sufficient therapy to satisfy thirst and to maintain serum sodium at the low level that is normal during pregnancy. Desmopressin is not destroyed by the cysteine aminopeptidase (oxytocinase) in the plasma of pregnant women[284, 387, 388] and is reported to be safe for both mother and child.[389, 390]

During delivery, these patients should maintain adequate oral intake and continued administration of desmopressin. Physicians should be cautious about overadministration of fluid parenterally during delivery because these patients are not able to excrete the fluid and may experience water intoxication and hyponatremia.

After delivery, oxytocinase decreases in plasma and, depending on the cause of the diabetes insipidus, the disorder may disappear or the patient may become asymptomatic with regard to fluid intake and urine volume.

Diabetes Insipidus after Hypothalamic or Pituitary Surgery and after Head Injury

Pituitary Surgery

The surgeon often knows how severely the posterior pituitary or stalk has been injured. The difficulty in making the diagnosis in this clinical setting has been discussed under "Differential Diagnosis." Sometimes the duration of diabetes insipidus is transient, and the surgeon may prefer to treat only with fluid replacement parenterally or orally (if the patient is awake and able to respond to thirst).

To treat diabetes insipidus, desmopressin may be given at 0.5 to 2 μg subcutaneously, intramuscularly, or intravenously. The intravenous route may be preferable because (1) there is no question about absorption and (2) with the lack of pressor activity, desmopressin is safe. Urine output is reduced in 1 to 2 hours, and the duration of effect is 6 to 24 hours. If the patient is alert, thirst is a good guide to fluid replacement. Because diabetes insipidus may be transient and some patients may experience the triphasic pattern described previously, it is desirable to allow polyuria to return before administering subsequent doses of desmopressin.

Head Injury

The treatment of acute diabetes insipidus after blunt trauma to the head, usually from a motor vehicle accident, is similar to that in the postoperative situation, except that the patient with head injury is more likely to be comatose and unable to respond to thirst. Therefore, hypotonic polyuria is more likely to be associated with hypernatremia. Because a comatose patient must be given fluids parenterally, some clinicians prefer to use a continuous infusion of low-dose vasopressin. The vasopressin can either be added directly to the crystalloid solution that is being administered[391] or infused separately to maintain a constant antidiuresis while fluid intake is adjusted appropriately to any persistent polyuria and to cover insensible water loss. Doses of 0.25 to 2.7 mU/kg per hour have been described.[392–394]

With this method, there is a potential to produce hyponatremia,[391, 394] and serum sodium levels must be checked regularly. Furthermore, with continuous replacement, one does not know whether normal function has returned or whether a patient is entering the second phase of a triphasic pattern.

Nephrogenic Diabetes Insipidus

Adequate water intake should always be maintained; indeed, appropriate water intake may be lifesaving in congenital nephrogenic diabetes insipidus. By definition, these forms of diabetes insipidus do not respond to vasopressin or desmopressin, although there may be rare partial defects with some response to high doses of desmopressin.[315]

Therapy is aimed at reducing symptomatic polyuria by reducing the volume of urine output. The volume is reduced primarily by causing an element of volume contraction. For congenital nephrogenic diabetes insipidus, volume contraction has been produced by a low-sodium diet and a thiazide diuretic. Thiazide diuretics act at the distal convoluted tubule to inhibit sodium chloride absorption, producing sodium (and water) diuresis. The antidiuretic effect has been attributed to ECF volume contraction, decreased GFR, proximal sodium and water reabsorption, and decreased delivery of fluid to the collecting duct resulting in a decreased volume of urine.[395] However, studies have demonstrated that thiazide diuretics also induce water reabsorption in the collecting duct of rats independent of vasopressin.[396, 397] All of the thiazide diuretics appear to have similar effects.

Potassium replacement or coadministration of a potassium-sparing antidiuretic, or both, may be desirable. An added effect is obtained by coadministration of indomethacin[398] or the potassium-sparing diuretic amiloride.[306, 399, 400] Addition of amiloride therapy is now recommended because of the absence of duodenal ulcer and gastrointestinal hemorrhage that may be produced by nonsteroidal anti-inflammatory agents. If the condition is recognized early and treated vigorously, complications such as intracerebral calcification, mental retardation, growth failure, and hydronephrosis are largely preventable.[306, 400]

Drug-induced nephrogenic diabetes insipidus should be treated by stopping the offending agent if possible. Persistence of nephrogenic diabetes insipidus can be similarly treated by hydrochlorothiazide and amiloride. With the induced volume contraction, the patient should be closely monitored for the development of renal or other toxicity of the drug causing the diabetes insipidus.[401] For example, volume contraction produced by thiazide diuretics, when used to treat lithium-induced nephrogenic diabetes insipidus, may decrease lithium excretion and predispose to lithium toxicity.[353, 402] Amiloride has the advantage of decreasing lithium entrance into cells in the distal tubule and may have a specific and preferable action for the treatment of lithium-induced nephrogenic diabetes insipidus.[353, 402–405] Indapamide is an antihypertensive diuretic agent with a structure similar to that of hydrochlorothiazides and chlorpropamide. It has been reported to reduce urine volume in patients with hypothalamic diabetes insipidus.[406]

Diabetes Insipidus in Association with Other Therapeutic Decisions

Routine Surgical Procedures

In most routine surgical procedures, the patient is not unconscious long enough to require anything more than administration of the usual dose of desmopressin and careful monitoring of fluids during the surgery to avoid overhydration. If the patient has been taking desmopressin orally and is to be given nothing by mouth, a nasal or a parenteral dose can be administered before the procedure.

Panhypopituitarism

Because hypothyroidism and adrenal insufficiency act directly on the kidney to inhibit the ability to excrete water, any patient who has anterior pituitary deficiency in association with diabetes insipidus is at risk for hyponatremia if treatment for diabetes insipidus is continued but treatment with thyroid hormone and (more dramatically) hydrocortisone is stopped. For such patients, it is important to maintain treatment of all anterior and posterior pituitary deficiencies continuously as the balance of these replacements is essential.

Promoting a Saline Diuresis

In some clinical situations, such as chemotherapy or use of some contrast agents, diuresis is desirable to minimize renal toxicity. Continuing desmopressin while giving a large volume of normal saline induces a prompt natriuresis and hyponatremia. Withholding desmopressin and replacing with 5% dextrose in water may lead to hyperglycemia, and replacing with normal saline may lead to hypernatremia. It has been reported that continuous intravenous administration of low-dose vasopressin in a manner similar to that described earlier for comatose patients can be used. In this case, the dose of vasopressin is even lower (e.g., 0.08 to 0.1 mU/kg per hour) to allow a moderate and controlled diuresis.[407] As with any situation in which vasopressin is given continuously, serum sodium levels must be checked regularly and the amount of fluids infused monitored carefully.

Hypertonic Encephalopathy

Conditions other than diabetes insipidus are the more common causes of hypernatremia with coma and hypernatremic encephalopathy. These conditions often affect older patients with concurrent renal problems or who are receiving treatment with diuretics, in whom total body sodium may be decreased despite hypernatremia,[359] or children with insensible loss or diarrhea and who are taking sodium-containing fluids.[358, 360, 408, 409] In patients with severe hypernatremia and hypernatremic encephalopathy, overaggressive treatment of the hypernatremia may cause cerebral edema and may worsen the neurologic condition.[358, 361, 410, 411] Sodium is mainly an extracellular cation, and hypernatremia invariably leads to movement of water out of cells and to cellular dehydration.

In the brain, *idiogenic* osmoles are generated intracellularly, and the degree of cell shrinkage is less than would be expected on the basis of the degree of hypernatremia. The idiogenic osmoles are in three organic classes: (1) polyols, (2) trimethylamines, and (3) amino acids and their derivatives. The increase in these organic osmoles has occurred within 1 to 2 hours in experimental animals[410, 412] but may be somewhat slower in humans.[358] The important clinical observation is that when fluid is replaced, these organic osmoles decrease much more slowly intracellularly than the decrease in osmolality of the ECF. This asynchrony increases the potential for cerebral edema and worsening of the neurologic condition with overzealous treatment of hypernatremia.[358, 408, 412]

In most cases of diabetes insipidus that are seen immediately after surgery or that are identified promptly after head injury, the diagnosis is made within a few hours and therapy is instituted promptly. When the duration of the hypernatremia is not known, the degree of correction of hypernatremia should not exceed 0.5 mEq/L per hour to prevent cerebral edema and convulsions.[358, 408]

Organ Donors

As noted earlier, diabetes insipidus is commonly associated with brain death. Because the patient may be a candidate for organ donation, regulating fluid homeostasis is thought to be desirable for maintaining the health of the organs. Although this is controversial, some degree of treatment of diabetes insipidus is not unreasonable. This may be a situation in which continuous administration of vasopressin in a low dose is easier than maintaining antidiuresis with intermittent doses of desmopressin.

THE SYNDROME OF INAPPROPRIATE ANTIDIURETIC HORMONE SECRETION

SIADH is produced when plasma levels of arginine vasopressin are elevated at times during which the physiologic secretion of vasopressin from the posterior pituitary would normally be suppressed. Because the clinical abnormality is a decrease in the osmotic pressure of body fluids, the hallmark of SIADH is hypo-osmolality. In 1957, this finding led to the identification of the first well-described cases of this disorder[413] and the subsequent clinical investigations that resulted in delineation of the essential characteristics of the syndrome.[414] It is thus necessary to summarize general issues concerning hypo-osmolality and hyponatremia before we present details specific to SIADH.

Hypo-osmolality and Hyponatremia

Incidence

Hypo-osmolality is one of the most common disorders of fluid and electrolyte balance in hospitalized patients. The incidence and prevalence of hypo-osmolar disorders depend on the nature of the population of patients studied as well as the laboratory methods and criteria used to diagnose hyponatremia. Most investigators have used serum Na^+ to determine the clinical incidence of hypo-osmolality. When hyponatremia was defined as a serum Na^+ less than 135 mEq/L, incidences as high as 15% to 30% were observed in studies of both acutely and chronically hospitalized patients. However, incidences decreased to the range of 1% to 4% when only patients with serum Na^+ under 130 to 131 mEq/L were included, which represents a more appropriate level at which to define the occurrence of clinically significant cases of this disorder. Even when these more stringent criteria have been used, incidences from 7% to 53% have been reported in institutionalized geriatric patients.[415]

All studies to date have noted a high proportion of iatrogenic or hospital-acquired hyponatremia, which has accounted for as many as 40% to 75% of all patients studied.[416] Therefore, although hyponatremia and hypo-osmolality are quite common, most cases are relatively mild and most are acquired during the course of hospitalization. Nonetheless, hyponatremia is important clinically because:

1. Severe hypo-osmolality (serum $Na^+ < 120$ mEq/L) is associated with substantial morbidity and mortality.[417]
2. Even relatively mild hypo-osmolality can quickly progress to more dangerous levels during the therapeutic management of other disorders.
3. Overly rapid correction of hyponatremia can itself cause severe neurologic morbidity and mortality.[418]
4. Mortality rates are much higher (threefold to 60-fold higher) in patients with even asymptomatic degrees of hypo-osmolality compared with normonatremic patients.[419]

In many but not all cases, hypo-osmolality is more an indicator of the severity of underlying illnesses than an independent factor contributing to mortality.

Osmolality, Tonicity, and Serum Sodium

As discussed previously, the osmolality of body fluid is normally maintained within narrow limits by osmotically regulated vasopressin secretion and thirst. Although basal plasma osmolality can vary appreciably among individuals, the range in the general population under conditions of normal hydration is between 280 and 295 mOsm/kg H_2O. Plasma osmolality can be determined directly by measuring the freezing-point depression or the vapor pressure of plasma. Alternatively, it can be calculated indirectly from the concentrations of the three major solutes in plasma:

$$\text{plasma osmolality (mOsm/kg } H_2O) = 2 \times [Na^+] \text{ (mEq/L)} + \text{glucose (mg/dL)}/18 + \text{BUN (mg/dL)}/2.8$$

Both methods produce comparable results under most conditions.

Although either method produces valid measures of *total* osmolality, this is not always equivalent to the *effective* osmolality, commonly referred to as the *tonicity* of the plasma. Only cell solutes such as Na^+ and Cl^- that cannot permeate the cell membrane and remain relatively compartmentalized within the ECF space are effective solutes because they create osmotic gradients across cell membranes and regulate the osmotic movement of water between the *intracellular fluid* (ICF) compartment and the ECF compartment. Solutes that readily permeate cell membranes (e.g., urea, ethanol, methanol) are not effective solutes. Therefore, only the concentrations of effective solutes in plasma should be used to ascertain whether clinically significant hyperosmolality or hypo-osmolality is present.[420]

Because sodium and its accompanying anions are the major effective plasma solutes, hyponatremia and hypo-osmolality are usually synonymous. However, there are two situations in which hyponatremia does not reflect true hypo-osmolality:

1. *Pseudohyponatremia*, produced by marked elevations of either lipids or proteins in plasma. When Na^+ is measured by flame photometry, the concentration of Na^+ per liter of plasma is artifactually decreased because of the larger relative proportion of plasma volume that is occupied by the excess lipids or proteins.[421] However, because the increased protein or lipid does not appreciably change the total number of solute particles in solution, the directly measured plasma osmolality is not significantly affected. Measurement of serum [Na^+] by ion-specific electrodes, now commonly performed by most clinical laboratories, is less influenced by high concentrations of lipids or proteins than is measurement of serum [Na^+] by flame photometry.
2. *Presence of high concentrations of effective solutes other than Na^+ in plasma*. The initial hyperosmolality produced by the additional solute causes an osmotic shift of water from ICF to ECF, which in turn produces a dilutional decrease in serum [Na^+]. When equilibrium between both fluid compartments is achieved, the total effective osmolality remains relatively unchanged. This situation most commonly occurs with hyperglycemia and is a frequent cause of hyponatremia in hospitalized patients, accounting for up to 10% to 20% of all cases.[419]

Misdiagnosis of true hypo-osmolality in such cases can be avoided by measuring plasma osmolality directly or by correcting the measured serum [Na^+] for the glucose elevation; traditionally, the correction factor has been 1.6 mEq/L for each 100 mg/dL increase in serum glucose concentration above normal levels,[422] but later studies showed a more complex relation between hyperglycemia and serum [Na^+] and suggested that a more accurate correction factor is closer to 2.4 mEq/L.[423] When the plasma contains significant amounts of unmeasured solutes, such as osmotic diuretics, radiographic contrast agents, and some toxins (ethanol, methanol, and ethylene glycol), plasma osmolality cannot be calculated accurately. In these situations, osmolality must be ascertained by direct measurement, although even this method does not yield an accurate measure of the true effective osmolality if the unmeasured solutes are noneffective solutes that freely permeate cell membranes (e.g., ethanol).

Because of these potential confounders, determining whether true hypo-osmolality is present can sometimes be difficult. A straightforward and relatively simple approach is as follows:

1. The effective plasma osmolality should be calculated from the measured serum [Na^+] and glucose concentration ($2 \times [Na^+] + \text{glucose}/18$); alternatively, the measured serum [Na^+] can simply be corrected by 1.6 to 2.4 mEq/L for each 100 mg/dL increase in serum glucose concentration above normal levels (100 mg/dL).
2. If the calculated effective plasma osmolality is less than 275 mOsm/kg H_2O or if the corrected serum [Na^+] is less than 135 mEq/L, significant hypo-osmolality exists, provided that large concentrations of unmeasured solutes or pseudohyponatremia secondary to hyperlipidemia or hyperproteinemia is not present.
3. To eliminate the latter possibilities, plasma osmolality should also be measured directly when the hyponatremia cannot be accounted for by elevated serum glucose levels. The absence of a discrepancy between the calculated and measured total plasma osmolalities (<10 mOsm/kg H_2O) confirms the absence of significant amounts of unmeasured solutes; if a significant discrepancy between these measures is found (an osmolal gap), appropriate tests must be conducted to rule out pseudohyponatremia or to identify possible unmeasured plasma solutes.

Pathogenesis of Hypo-osmolality

Because water moves freely between ICF and ECF, osmolality is always equivalent in both of these fluid compartments. Because the bulk of body solute consists of electrolytes, namely the exchangeable Na^+ (Na^+_E) in ECF and the exchangeable K^+ (K^+_E) in ICF along with their associated anions, total body osmolality is largely a function of these parameters[424]:

$$OSM_{ECF} = OSM_{ICF} = \text{total body osmolality} = \\ (\text{ECF solute} + \text{ICF solute})/\text{body water} = \\ (2 \times Na^+_E + 2 \times K^+_E + \text{nonelectrolyte solute})/\text{body water}$$

According to this definition, the presence of plasma hypo-osmolality indicates a relative excess of water to solute in the ECF. The excess can be produced either by an excess of body water, resulting in dilution of remaining body solute, or by a depletion of body solute, either Na^+ or K^+, relative to body water. This classification is an oversimplification because most hypo-osmolar states involve significant components of both solute depletion and water retention. Nonetheless, it is conceptually useful for understanding the mechanisms underlying the pathogenesis of hypo-osmolality and as a framework for therapy of hypo-osmolar disorders.

Solute Depletion

Depletion of body solute can result from any significant losses of ECF. Body fluid losses by themselves rarely cause hypo-osmolality because excreted or secreted body fluids are usually isotonic or hypotonic relative to plasma and therefore tend to increase plasma osmolality. When hypo-osmolality accompanies ECF losses, it is the result of replacement of body fluid losses by more hypotonic solutions either by drinking or by infusion, thereby diluting the remaining body solutes. If the solute losses are marked, these patients show signs of volume depletion (e.g., addisonian crisis). However, such patients often have a more deceptive clinical presentation because the volume deficits were partially replaced. Moreover, they may not manifest signs or symptoms of cellular dehydration because osmotic gradients draw water into the relatively hypertonic ICF.

Therefore, clinical evidence of hypovolemia strongly supports solute depletion as the cause of plasma hypo-osmolality, but absence of clinically evident hypovolemia never completely eliminates this as a possibility. Although ECF solute losses are responsible for most cases of depletion-induced hypo-osmolality, ICF solute loss can also cause hypo-osmolality as a result of osmotic water shifts from the ICF into the ECF. This mechanism probably contributes to some cases of diuretic-induced hypo-osmolality, in which depletion of total body K^+ often occurs.[425]

Water Retention

Despite the importance of solute depletion in some patients, most cases of clinically significant hypo-osmolality are caused by increases in total body water rather than by primary losses of extracellular solute. Such increases can occur because of either impaired renal free water excretion or excessive free water intake. However, the former accounts for most hypo-osmolar disorders because normal kidneys have sufficient diluting capacity to allow excretion of free water up to approximately 18 L/day. Intakes of this magnitude are occasionally seen in some psychiatric patients but not in most patients with

SIADH, in whom fluid intakes average only 2 to 3 L/day.[426] Consequently, dilutional hypo-osmolality is usually the result of an abnormality of renal free water excretion. The renal mechanisms responsible for impairments in free water excretion can be subgrouped according to whether the *major* impairment in free water excretion occurs in proximal or distal parts of the nephron, or both.

Any disorder that leads to a decrease in GFR causes increased reabsorption of both Na^+ and water in the proximal tubule. As a result, the ability to excrete free water is limited because of decreased delivery of tubular fluid to the distal nephron. Disorders causing solute depletion through nonrenal mechanisms (e.g., gastrointestinal fluid losses) also produce this effect. Disorders that cause a decreased GFR in the absence of significant ECF fluid losses are, for the most part, edema-forming states associated with decreased effective arterial blood volume (EABV) and secondary hyperaldosteronism.[427]

Even though these conditions are characterized by increased proximal reabsorption of both Na^+ and fluid, water retention also results from increased distal reabsorption caused by non-osmotic baroreceptor-mediated stimulated increases in plasma vasopressin levels. Distal nephron impairments in free water excretion are characterized by inability to dilute tubular fluid maximally. These disorders are usually associated with abnormalities in the secretion of vasopressin from the posterior pituitary. However, just as depletion-induced hypo-osmolar disorders usually include an important component of secondary impairments of free water excretion, most dilution-induced hypo-osmolar disorders involve significant degrees of secondary solute depletion. This is described later with SIADH.

Some dilutional disorders do not fit well into either category, specifically the hyponatremia that sometimes occurs in patients who ingest large volumes of beer with little food intake for prolonged periods, called *beer potomania*.[428] Even though the volume of fluid ingested may not seem sufficiently excessive to overwhelm renal diluting mechanisms, free water excretion is limited by low urinary solute excretion, thereby causing water retention and dilutional hyponatremia. A case in which hyponatremia occurred in an ovolactovegetarian with a very low protein intake but no beer ingestion is consistent with this pathophysiology.[429]

Adaptation to Hyponatremia: Intracellular Fluid and Extracellular Fluid Volume Regulation

Many past studies have indicated that the combined effects of water retention and urinary solute excretion cannot adequately explain the degree of plasma hypo-osmolality observed in patients.[414, 430] This observation led to the *theory of cellular inactivation of solute*.[414] The theory suggested that as ECF osmolality falls, water moves into cells along osmotic gradients, causing the cells to swell. At some point during this volume expansion, the cells osmotically inactivate some of their intracellular solutes as a defense mechanism to prevent continued cellular swelling and detrimental effects on cell function and survival. This inactivation decreases the intracellular osmolality and water shifts back out of the ICF into the ECF, further worsening the dilution-induced hypo-osmolality. Despite the appeal of this theory, its validity has never been demonstrated conclusively in either human or animal studies.

An appealing alternative theory is that cell volume is maintained under hypo-osmolar conditions by extrusion of potassium.[431] Whole-brain volume regulation through electrolyte losses was first described by Yannet[432] and has long been recognized as the mechanism by which the brain is able to adapt to hyponatremia and limit brain edema to sublethal levels.[433] After the recognition that low-molecular-weight organic compounds (called *organic osmolytes*) are a significant osmotic component of a wide variety of cell types, studies demonstrated accumulation of these compounds in response to hyperosmolality in both kidney[434] and brain[435] tissue (see hypernatremic encephalopathy earlier). Conversely, the brain loses organic osmolytes in addition to electrolytes during volume regulation to hypo-osmolar conditions in experimental animals[436, 437] and human patients.[438] These losses occur relatively quickly (within 24 to 48 hours in rats) and can account for as much as one third of the brain solute losses during hyponatremia.[439] Such coordinate losses of both electrolytes (K^+) and organic osmolytes from brain tissue allow effective regulation of brain volume during chronic hyponatremia. Consequently, it is now clear that cellular volume regulation in brain tissue occurs predominantly through depletion of a variety of intracellular solutes rather than intracellular osmotic inactivation.

Although contemporary studies of volume regulation during hyponatremia have focused on the brain, all cells regulate volume by cellular losses of both electrolytes and organic solutes to varying degrees.[440] However, volume regulatory processes are not limited to cells. In most cases of hyponatremia induced by stimulated antidiuresis and water retention, natriuresis also regulates the volumes of the ECF and intravascular spaces.

Many experimental and clinical observations are consistent with ECF volume regulation through secondary solute losses, as described next.

First, the concentrations of most blood constituents other than Na^+ and Cl^- are not decreased in patients with SIADH[441]; this suggests that plasma volume is not nearly as expanded as would be predicted simply by the measured decreases in serum [Na^+].

Second, an increased incidence of hypertension has never been observed in patients with SIADH; again, this is evidence against significant expansion of the arterial blood volume.

Third, results of animal studies in both dogs[442] and rats[443] have indicated that a significant component of chronic hyponatremia is attributable to secondary Na^+ losses rather than water retention. The relative contributions of water retention and sodium loss vary with the duration and severity of the hyponatremia; water retention was found to be the major cause of decreased serum [Na^+] in the first 24 hours of induced hyponatremia in rats, but Na^+ depletion became the predominant etiologic factor after longer periods (7 to 14 days) of sustained hyponatremia, particularly at low ($<$115 mEq/L) serum Na^+ levels.[443]

Finally, multiple studies of body fluid compartment volumes in hyponatremic patients have not shown either plasma or ECF expansion. For example, a report of body fluid space measurements using isotope dilution techniques in hyponatremic and normonatremic patients with small cell lung carcinoma showed no differences between the two groups with regard to exchangeable sodium space, ECF volume determined by $^{35}SO_4$ distribution, or total body water.[444]

Such results have generally been explained by the relative insensitivity of isotope dilution techniques for measurement of body fluid compartment spaces, but an equally plausible possibility is that body fluid compartments have regulated back toward normal through a combination of extracellular (predominantly electrolyte) and intracellular (electrolyte and organic osmolyte) solute losses.[445] Figure 9–8 schematically illustrates some of the volume regulatory processes that probably occur in response to water retention induced by inappropriate antidiuresis. The degree to which solute losses versus water retention contribute to the resulting hyponatremia depends on many different factors, including:

1. The cause of the hyponatremia.

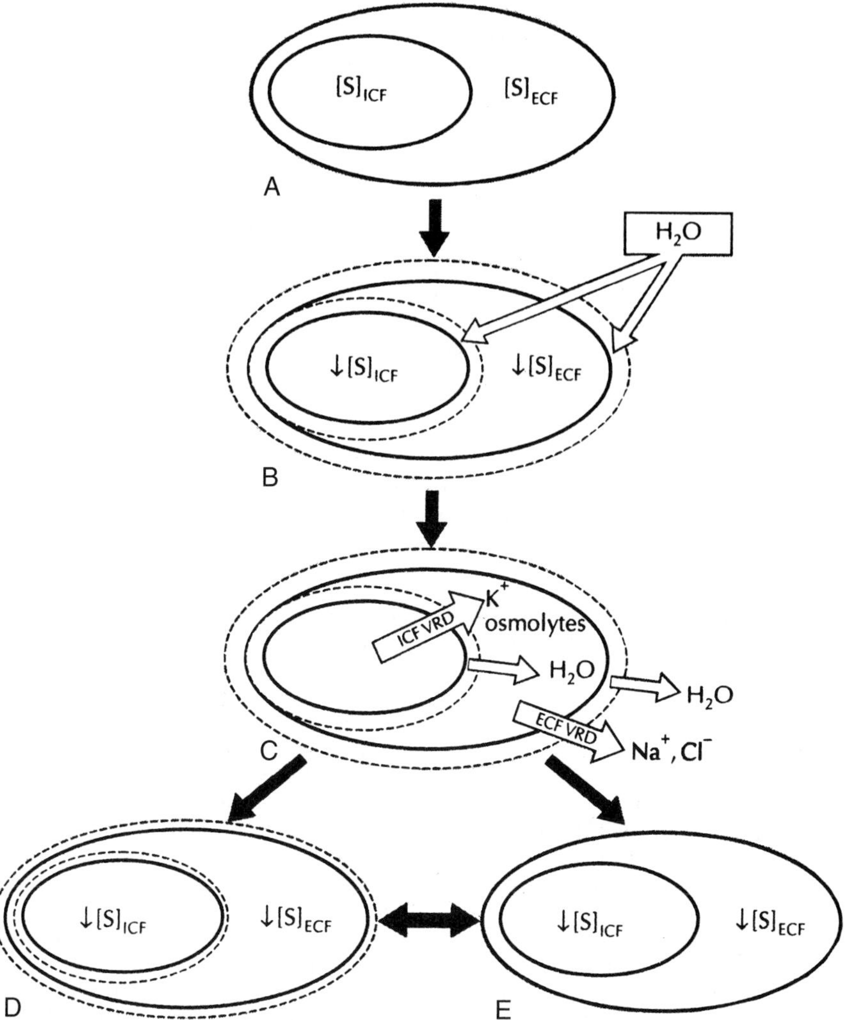

Figure 9–8. Schematic illustration of potential changes in whole-body fluid compartment volumes at various times during adaptation to hyponatremia.

A, Under basal conditions the concentrations of effective solutes in the extracellular fluid ($[S]_{ECF}$) and the intracellular fluid ($[S]_{ICF}$) are in osmotic balance.

B, During the first phase of water retention resulting from inappropriate antidiuresis, the excess water distributes across total body water, causing expansion of both ECF and ICF volumes *(dashed lines)* with equivalent dilutional decreases in $[S]_{ICF}$ and $[S]_{ECF}$.

C, In response to the volume expansion, compensatory volume regulatory decreases (VRD) occur to reduce the effective solute content of both the ECF (through pressure diuresis and natriuretic factors) and ICF (through increased electrolyte and osmolyte extrusion mediated by stretch-activated channels and down-regulation of synthesis of osmolytes and osmolyte uptake transporters).

D and *E*, If both processes go to completion, such as under conditions of fluid restriction, a final steady state can be reached in which ICF and ECF volumes have returned to normal levels but $[S]_{ICF}$ and $[S]_{ECF}$ remain low *(E)*. In most cases, this final steady state is not reached and moderate degrees of ECF and ICF expansion persist but are significantly less than would be predicted from the decrease in body osmolality *(D)*. Consequently, the degree to which hyponatremia is due to dilution from water retention versus solute depletion from volume regulatory processes can vary markedly depending on which phase of adaptation the patient is in and also on the relative rates at which the different compensatory processes occur (e.g., delayed ICF VRD can worsen hyponatremia related to shifts of intracellular water into the ECF as intracellular organic osmolytes are extruded and subsequently metabolized, probably accounting for some component of the hyponatremia unexplained by the combination of water retention and sodium excretion in previous clinical studies).

(From Verbalis JG. Hyponatremia: epidemiology, pathophysiology, and therapy. Curr Opin Nephrol Hypertens 1993; 2:626–652.)

2. The rapidity of hyponatremia development.
3. The chronicity of the hyponatremia.
4. The volume of daily water loading and subsequent volume expansion.
5. Undoubtedly, some degree of individual variability as well.

Differential Diagnosis of Hyponatremia and Hypo-osmolality

Because of the multiplicity of disorders causing hypo-osmolality and the fact that many involve more than one pathologic mechanism, a definitive diagnosis is not always possible at the

Table 9–2. Differential Diagnosis of Hyponatremia

Extracellular Fluid Volume	Urinary $[Na^+]$*	Presumptive Diagnosis
↓	Low	*Depletion (nonrenal)*: GI, cutaneous, or blood ECF loss
	High	*Depletion (renal)*: diuretics, mineralocorticoid insufficiency (Addison's disease), salt-losing nephropathy
→	Low	*Depletion (nonrenal)*: any cause + hypotonic fluid replacement *Dilution (proximal)*: hypothyroidism, early decreased effective arterial blood volume *Dilution (distal)*: SIADH + fluid restriction
	High	*Dilution (distal)*: SIADH, glucocorticoid insufficiency *Depletion (renal)*: any cause + hypotonic fluid replacement (especially diuretic treatment)
↑	Low	*Dilution (proximal)*: decreased effective arterial blood volume (CHF, cirrhosis, nephrosis)
	High	*Dilution (proximal)*: any cause + diuretics or improvement in underlying disease, renal failure

*Urinary $[Na^+]$ values <30 mEq/L are generally considered to be low and values ≥ 30 mEq/L to be high, based on studies of responses of hyponatremic patients to infusions of isotonic saline.

CHF, congestive heart failure; ECF, extracellular fluid; GI, gastrointestinal; SIADH, syndrome of inappropriate antidiuretic hormone secretion.

(Data from Chung HM, Kluge R, Schrier RW, et al. Clinical assessment of extracellular fluid volume in hyponatremia. Am J Med 1987; 83:905–908.

time of initial presentation. Nonetheless, an approach based on clinical parameters of ECF volume status and urinary sodium concentration generally allows sufficient categorization for appropriate decisions regarding initial therapy and further evaluation (Table 9–2).

Decreased Extracellular Fluid Volume

Clinically detectable hypovolemia always signifies total body solute depletion. A low urinary $[Na^+]$ indicates a nonrenal cause and an appropriate renal response. A high urinary $[Na^+]$ indicates that renal causes of solute depletion are more likely. Therapy with thiazide diuretics is the most common cause of renal solute losses,[425] particularly in elderly people,[446] but mineralocorticoid deficiency as a result of adrenal insufficiency[447] or mineralocorticoid resistance[448] must be considered as well as (less commonly) renal solute losses related to salt-wasting nephropathy (e.g., polycystic kidney disease), interstitial nephritis, or chemotherapy.

Increased Extracellular Fluid Volume

Clinically detectable hypervolemia always signifies total body Na^+ excess. In these patients, hypo-osmolality results from an even greater expansion of total body water caused by a marked reduction in the rate of water excretion (and sometimes an increased rate of water ingestion). The impairment in water excretion is secondary to a decreased effective arterial blood volume,[427] which increases the reabsorption of glomerular filtrate not only in the proximal nephron but also in the distal and collecting tubules by stimulated secretion of vasopressin. These patients generally have a low urinary $[Na^+]$ because of secondary hyperaldosteronism. Under certain conditions, however, urinary $[Na^+]$ may be elevated if there is concurrent diuretic therapy or a solute diuresis (e.g., glucosuria in diabetic patients) or after successful treatment of the underlying disease (e.g., inotropic therapy in patients with congestive heart failure).

An additional disorder that can produce hypo-osmolality and hypervolemia is acute or chronic renal failure with fluid overload (although in early stages of renal failure polyuria resulting from vasopressin resistance is more likely).[449] Urinary $[Na^+]$ in these cases is usually elevated, but it can be variable, depending on the stage of renal failure. It is important to remember that primary polydipsia is not accompanied by signs of hypervolemia because water ingestion alone, in the absence of Na^+ retention, does not produce clinically apparent degrees of ECF volume expansion.

Normal Extracellular Fluid Volume

Many different hypo-osmolar disorders occur with euvolemia, and measurement of urinary $[Na^+]$ is an especially important first step.[450] A high urinary $[Na^+]$ usually implies a distally mediated, dilution-induced hypo-osmolality such as that in SIADH. However, glucocorticoid deficiency can mimic SIADH so closely that these two disorders are often indistinguishable in terms of water balance. Hyponatremia resulting from diuretic use can also occur without clinically evident hypovolemia, and urinary $[Na^+]$ is usually elevated.[425] A low urinary $[Na^+]$ suggests a depletion-induced hypo-osmolality resulting from ECF losses with subsequent volume replacement by water or other hypotonic fluids. The solute loss is often nonrenal, but an important exception is recent cessation of diuretic therapy because urinary $[Na^+]$ can decrease to low values within 12 to 24 hours after discontinuation of the drug.

The presence of low serum $[K^+]$ is an important clue to diuretic use. Low urinary $[Na^+]$ can also be seen in some cases of hypothyroidism, in the early stages of decreased effective arterial blood volume before the development of clinically apparent salt retention and fluid overload, or during the recovery phase of SIADH. Hence, a low urinary $[Na^+]$ is less meaningful diagnostically than a high value.

Clinical Syndrome of Inappropriate Antidiuretic Hormone Secretion

SIADH is the most common cause of euvolemic hypo-osmolality; it is also the single most common cause of hypo-osmolality of all etiologic mechanisms encountered in clinical practice, with prevalence rates from 20% to 40% among all hypo-osmolar patients.[419, 426] The clinical criteria necessary to diagnose SIADH remain basically as set forth by Bartter and Schwartz in 1967[414]:

1. *Decreased effective osmolality of the ECF (plasma osmolality $<$ 275 mOsm/kg H_2O).* Pseudohyponatremia or hyperglycemia alone must be excluded.
2. *Inappropriate urinary concentration (urine osmolality $>$ 100 mOsm/kg H_2O with normal renal function) at some level of hypo-osmolality.* This does not mean that urine osmolality is greater than plasma osmolality; rather, the urine is less than maximally

dilute (i.e., urine osmolality > 100 mOsm/kg H_2O). Also, urine osmolality need not be elevated inappropriately at all levels of plasma osmolality because in the reset osmostat variant form of SIADH, vasopressin secretion can be suppressed with resultant maximal urinary dilution if plasma osmolality is decreased to sufficiently low levels.[451]

3. *Clinical euvolemia as defined by the absence of signs of hypovolemia (orthostasis, tachycardia, decreased skin turgor, dry mucous membranes) or hypervolemia (subcutaneous edema, ascites).* Hypovolemia or hypervolemia strongly suggests different causes of hypo-osmolality. Patients with SIADH can become hypovolemic or hypervolemic for other reasons, but in such cases it is impossible to diagnose the underlying inappropriate antidiuresis until the patient is rendered euvolemic and is found to have persistent hypo-osmolality.

4. *Elevated urinary sodium excretion with a normal salt and water intake.* This criterion is included because of its utility in differentiating between hypo-osmolality caused by a decreased effective arterial blood volume, in which case renal Na^+ conservation occurs, and distal dilution-induced disorders, in which urinary Na^+ excretion is normal or increased secondary to ECF volume expansion. Patients with SIADH can have low urinary Na^+ excretion if they subsequently become hypovolemic or solute-depleted, conditions that sometimes follow severe salt and water restriction. Consequently, high urinary Na^+ excretion is the rule in most patients with SIADH, its presence does not guarantee this diagnosis, and its absence does not rule out the diagnosis.

5. *Absence of other potential causes of euvolemic hypo-osmolality:* hypothyroidism, hypercorticalism (Addison's disease or pituitary ACTH insufficiency), and diuretic use.

Several other criteria support, but are not essential for, a diagnosis of SIADH. Because volume expansion and vasopressin acting on V1 receptors in the kidney increase the clearance of uric acid, hypouricemia is found with SIADH. In hyponatremic patients, values of uric acid have been less than 4 mg/dL (<0.24 mmol/L).[452, 453] A water-loading test is of value when there is uncertainty about the etiology of modest degrees of hypo-osmolality in euvolemic patients, but it does not add useful information if the plasma osmolality is already less than 275 mOsm/kg H_2O.

Inability to excrete a standard water load normally (with normal excretion defined as a cumulative urine output of at least 90% of the administered water load within 4 hours to suppress urine osmolality to <100 mOsm/kg H_2O) confirms the presence of an underlying defect in free water excretion. However, water excretion is abnormal in almost all disorders that cause hypo-osmolality, whether dilutional or depletion-induced with secondary impairments in free water excretion. Two exceptions are primary polydipsia, in which hypo-osmolality can rarely be secondary to excessive water intake alone, and the reset osmostat variant of SIADH, in which normal excretion of a water load can occur when plasma osmolality falls below the new set-point for vasopressin secretion.

The water load test may also be used to assess water excretion after treatment of an underlying disorder thought to be causing SIADH. For example, after discontinuation of a drug associated with SIADH, a normal water load test can confirm the absence of persistent inappropriate antidiuresis. Despite its limitations as a diagnostic clinical test, water loading remains an extremely useful tool in clinical research for quantitating changes in free water excretion in response to physiologic or pharmacologic manipulations.

A second supportive criterion is an inappropriately elevated plasma vasopressin level in relation to plasma osmolality. With the development of sensitive vasopressin radioimmunoassays capable of detecting the small physiologic concentrations of this peptide that circulate in plasma,[454] it had been hoped that measurement of plasma vasopressin levels might become the definitive test for diagnosis of SIADH. This has not occurred for several reasons:

First, although plasma vasopressin levels are elevated in most patients with this syndrome, the elevations generally remain within the normal physiologic range and are abnormal only in relation to plasma osmolality (see Fig. 9–2).

Second, 10% to 20% of patients with SIADH do not have measurably elevated plasma vasopressin levels (see Fig. 9–2), and the levels are at the limits of detection by radioimmunoassay.[455]

Third, most disorders causing solute and volume depletion or decreased effective arterial blood volume are associated with elevations of plasma vasopressin levels secondary to nonosmotic hemodynamic stimuli.

Finally, the response to fluid restriction or volume expansion can be helpful in distinguishing between causes of hyponatremia. Infusion of isotonic sodium chloride (NaCl) in patients with SIADH provokes a natriuresis with little correction of osmolality, whereas fluid restriction allows gradual achievement of solute and water balance through insensible free water losses. By contrast, isotonic saline is the treatment of choice in disorders of solute depletion; when volume deficits are corrected, the stimulus to continued secretion of vasopressin and free water retention is eliminated. The diagnostic value of this therapeutic response is limited somewhat by the fact that patients with proximal types of dilution-induced disorders may show a response similar to that found in patients with SIADH.

Etiology

Although the list of disorders associated with SIADH is long (Table 9–3), they can be divided into four major etiologic groups: tumors, CNS disorders, drugs, and pulmonary disorders.

Tumors

The most common association of SIADH is with tumors. Although many different types of tumors have been associated with SIADH, bronchogenic carcinoma of the lung has been uniquely associated with SIADH since the first description of this disorder in 1957.[413] In virtually all cases, the bronchogenic carcinomas causing this syndrome have been of the small cell (or oat cell) variety. Incidences of hyponatremia as high as 11% of all patients with small cell carcinoma[456] or 33% of those with more extensive disease[457] have been reported.

The unusually high incidence of small cell carcinoma of the lung, together with the relatively favorable therapeutic response of this type of tumor, makes it imperative that all adult patients presenting with an otherwise unexplained SIADH be investigated thoroughly and aggressively for a possible lung tumor. The evaluation should include a chest CT scan or MRI study and bronchoscopy with cytologic analysis of bronchial washings even if the results of routine chest radiography are normal, because several studies have reported hypo-osmolality that predated radiographic abnormality by 3 to 12 months.[458] Head and neck cancers are another group of malignancies associated with relatively higher incidences of SIADH,[459] and some of these tumors have been shown to synthesize vasopressin.[460] A report from a large cancer hospital showed an incidence of hyponatremia for all malignancies combined of 3.7%, with approximately one third of these related to SIADH.[461]

Central Nervous System Disorders

A large number of CNS disorders are associated with SIADH; no common denominator links them. This is not surprising when one considers the neuroanatomy described earlier. Mag-

Table 9–3. Common Causes of Syndrome of Inappropriate Antidiuretic Hormone Secretion

Tumors
1. Pulmonary-mediastinal (bronchogenic carcinoma; mesothelioma; thymoma)
2. Nonchest (duodenal carcinoma; pancreatic carcinoma; ureteral/prostate carcinoma; uterine carcinoma; nasopharyngeal carcinoma; leukemia)

Central Nervous System Disorders
1. Mass lesions (tumors; brain abscesses; subdural hematoma)
2. Inflammatory diseases (encephalitis; meningitis; systemic lupus; acute intermittent porphyria; multiple sclerosis)
3. Degenerative-demyelinative diseases (Guillain-Barré; spinal cord lesions)
4. Miscellaneous (subarachnoid hemorrhage; head trauma; acute psychosis; delirium tremens; pituitary stalk section; transsphenoidal adenomectomy; hydrocephalus)

Drug Induced
1. Stimulated AVP release (nicotine; phenothiazines; tricyclics)
2. Direct renal effects and/or potentiation of AVP antidiuretic effects (dDAVP; oxytocin; prostaglandin synthesis inhibitors)
3. Mixed or uncertain actions (angiotensin-converting enzyme inhibitors; carbamazepine and oxcarbazepine; chlorpropamide; clofibrate; clozapine; cyclophosphamide; 3,4-methylenedioxymethamphetamine [Ecstasy]; omeprazole; serotonin reuptake, inhibitors; vincristine)

Pulmonary Diseases
1. Infections (tuberculosis; acute bacterial and viral pneumonia; aspergillosis; empyema)
2. Mechanical-ventilatory (acute respiratory failure; COPD; positive-pressure ventilation)

Other
1. Acquired immunodeficiency syndrome (AIDS) and AIDS-related complex
2. Prolonged strenuous exercise (marathon; triathlon; ultramarathon; hot-weather hiking)
3. Senile atrophy
4. Idiopathic

AVP, arginine vasopressin; COPD, chronic obstructive pulmonary disease; dDAVP, 1-deamino(8-D-arginine) vasopressin.

nicellular vasopressin neurons receive excitatory inputs from osmoreceptive cells in the anterior hypothalamus but also a major innervation from brain stem cardiovascular regulatory and emetic centers. Although various components of these pathways have yet to be elucidated fully, many of them appear to have inhibitory as well as excitatory components.[462] Consequently, any diffuse CNS disorder can potentially cause vasopressin hypersecretion either by nonspecifically exciting these pathways through irritative foci or by disrupting them and thereby decreasing the level of inhibition. The wide variety of CNS processes that can potentially cause SIADH stands in contrast to CNS causes of diabetes insipidus, which are limited to lesions of the suprasellar hypothalamus.

Drugs

Drug-induced hyponatremia is a common cause of hypo-osmolality.[463] Table 9–3 lists some of the agents that have been associated with SIADH, but new drugs are added continually. Pharmacologic agents may stimulate secretion of vasopressin, activate V2 renal receptors, or potentiate the antidiuretic effect of vasopressin. Not all of the drug effects are fully understood, however, and many appear to work through a combination of mechanisms.

A particularly interesting and clinically important class of agents is the *selective serotonin reuptake inhibitors* (SSRIs). In studies in rats, serotoninergic agents increased secretion of vasopressin[464] but more directly oxytocin.[465] In humans, SSRIs have generally not had significant effects on secretion of vasopressin.[466] However, hyponatremia after SSRI administration has been reported almost exclusively in elderly persons, with rates as high as 22% to 28%, although in larger series the incidence was closer to 1 in 200.[467] Elderly patients are uniquely hypersensitive to serotonin stimulation of vasopressin secretion. A similar effect is probably also responsible for the severe fatal hyponatremia caused by use of the recreational drug 3,4-methylenedioxymethamphetamine, Ecstasy,[468] which has substantial serotoninergic activity[469] and activated hypothalamic magnocellular neurons in rats.[470]

Pulmonary Disorders

Various pulmonary disorders have been associated with SIADH; other than tuberculosis, acute pneumonia, and advanced chronic obstructive lung disease, however, the occurrence of hypo-osmolality has been noted only sporadically. One reported case of pulmonary tuberculosis suggested that tuberculous lung tissue might synthesize vasopressin,[471] but reports of the reset osmostat with advanced pulmonary tuberculosis[472, 473] and others indicated nonosmotic stimulation of secretion of vasopressin. Hypoxia stimulated secretion of vasopressin in animals,[474] but in humans[475] hypercarbia was more associated with abnormal water retention.[476] Elevated vasopressin levels may be limited to the initial days of hospitalization, when respiratory failure is most marked.[477] Therefore, with SIADH in nontumor pulmonary disease, pulmonary disease is obvious with severe dyspnea or extensive radiographically evident infiltrates and the inappropriate antidiuresis is usually limited to the period of respiratory failure. Mechanical ventilation can cause inappropriate secretion of vasopressin and can worsen SIADH caused by other factors. The mechanism is thought to be decreased venous return.

Other Causes

In patients with acquired immunodeficiency syndrome (AIDS) or AIDS-related complex and human immunodeficiency virus (HIV) infection, the incidence of hyponatremia has been reported to be as high as 30% to 38% in adults[478] and children.[479] Although there are many potential etiologic mechanisms, including dehydration, adrenal insufficiency, and pneumonitis, 12% to 68% of AIDS patients with hyponatremia appear to meet criteria for a diagnosis of SIADH.[478, 480] Not unexpectedly, some of the medications used to treat these conditions may cause the hyponatremia through direct renal tubular toxicity or induced SIADH.[481, 482]

Elderly patients sometimes experience SIADH without any apparent underlying etiologic factor,[483] and the incidence of hyponatremia in geriatric patients[415, 484] suggests that the normal aging process may be accompanied by abnormalities of regulation of secretion of vasopressin. Such an effect may potentially account for the fact that drug-induced hyponatremia occurs much more frequently in older patients. In a series of 50 consecutive elderly patients meeting criteria for SIADH, 60% remained idiopathic despite rigorous evaluation, leading the authors to conclude that extensive diagnostic procedures were not warranted in such elderly patients if routine history, physical examination, and laboratory evaluation failed to suggest an underlying cause.[485]

Some well-known stimuli for vasopressin secretion are notable primarily because of their exclusion from Table 9–3. Despite unequivocal stimulation of vasopressin secretion by nicotine,[486] cigarette smoking has been associated with SIADH rarely and primarily in psychiatric patients who have several other potential causes of inappropriate vasopressin secretion.[487]

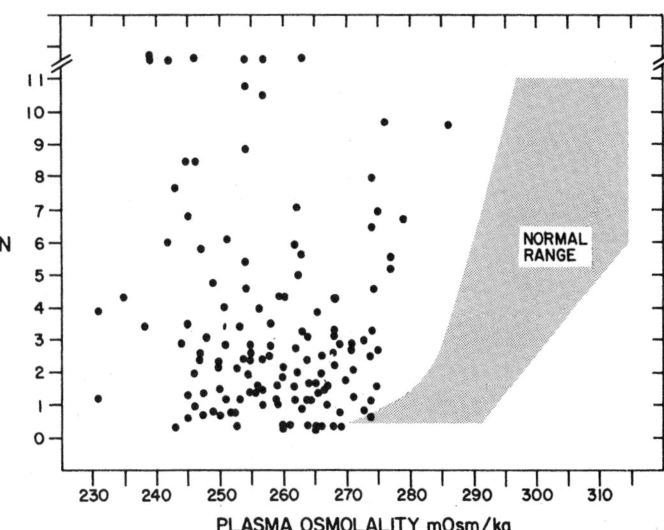

Figure 9–9. Plasma arginine vasopressin (AVP) levels in patients with syndrome of inappropriate antidiuretic hormone secretion as a function of plasma osmolality. Each point depicts one patient at a single point in time. The *shaded area* represents AVP levels in normal subjects over physiologic ranges of plasma osmolality. The lowest measurable plasma AVP level using this radioimmunoassay was 0.5 pg/mL. (From Robertson GL, Aycinena P, Zerbe RL. Neurogenic disorders of osmoregulation. Am J Med 1982; 72:339–353.)

The reasons for this include chronic adaptation to the effects of nicotine and the short half-life of vasopressin in plasma (~15 minutes in humans), which limits the duration of antidiuresis produced by smoking. Similarly, although nausea remains the most potent stimulus of vasopressin secretion known in humans,[488] chronic nausea is rarely associated with hypo-osmolality unless it is accompanied by vomiting and ingestion of hypotonic fluids. Nausea may be a factor contributing to the hyponatremia that often occurs in cancer patients receiving chemotherapy and intravenous fluids.

Pathophysiology

Sources of Vasopressin Secretion

Elevated plasma levels of vasopressin can be broadly divided into those associated with *paraneoplastic (ectopic) secretion* of vasopressin and those associated with *pituitary hypersecretion* of vasopressin. There is substantial cumulative evidence that tumor tissue can synthesize vasopressin,[489, 490] but it is not certain whether all tumors associated with SIADH do so, because only about half of small cell carcinomas have been found to contain vasopressin immunoreactivity and many of the tumors listed in Table 9–3 have not been so studied.

Pituitary Vasopressin Secretion: Inappropriate versus Appropriate

In most cases of SIADH, vasopressin secretion originates from the posterior pituitary. This is also true of more than 90% of all cases of hyponatremia, including hypovolemic and hypervolemic hyponatremia.[419] This raises the question: What is *inappropriate* secretion of vasopressin?

Secretion of vasopressin in response to a hypovolemic stimulus is clearly physiologically appropriate, but when it leads to symptomatic hyponatremia it can be considered inappropriate for the osmolality. Despite these semantic difficulties, the diagnosis of SIADH should rest on the original criteria and should specifically exclude other clinical conditions known to cause impairments in free water excretion *even when* these are mediated by secondary stimulation of vasopressin. Without maintaining these distinctions, arguable as some may be, the definition of SIADH becomes too broad to retain any practical clinical utility.

In most cases of SIADH, plasma levels of vasopressin are within normal physiologic ranges and abnormal only relative to the osmolality (Fig. 9–9). This is important for two main reasons:

1. Because the well-known vasoconstrictive effects of vasopressin do not come into play until much higher plasma levels are achieved (see "Physiology of Secretion of Vasopressin and Thirst"), hyponatremia can be ascribed to vasopressor effects of vasopressin.
2. Normal or low but nonsuppressible levels of vasopressin can cause sufficient impairment of free water excretion to produce hypo-osmolality, depending on exogenous fluid intake, as in psychiatric patients with polydipsia.[491]

Patterns of Vasopressin Secretion

Studies of plasma vasopressin levels in patients with SIADH during graded increases in plasma osmolality produced by hypertonic saline administration have defined four patterns of secretion (Fig. 9–10)[455, 492]:

1. Random hypersecretion of vasopressin.
2. Inappropriate nonsuppressible basal vasopressin release but normal secretion in response to osmolar changes above basal plasma osmolality.
3. A reset osmostat system whereby vasopressin is secreted at an abnormally low threshold of plasma osmolality but otherwise displays a normal response to relative changes in osmolality.
4. Low or even undetectable plasma vasopressin levels despite classic clinical characteristics of SIADH.

The first pattern, unregulated vasopressin secretion, is often observed in patients with paraneoplastic vasopressin production. Resetting of the osmotic threshold for vasopressin secretion has been well described with volume depletion[493] and edema-forming states with effective arterial blood volume,[427, 494] but most patients with a reset osmostat are clinically euvolemic[451] and may have SIADH. It has been suggested that chronic hypo-osmolality itself may over time reset the intracellular threshold for osmoreceptor firing, but in animals chronic hyponatremia did not significantly alter the osmotic threshold for vasopressin secretion.[495]

The best physiologic example of a reset osmostat is pregnancy, as discussed earlier. Perhaps the most perplexing aspect of the reset osmostat pattern is its occurrence in patients with tumors, which suggests that in some of these cases a tumor-

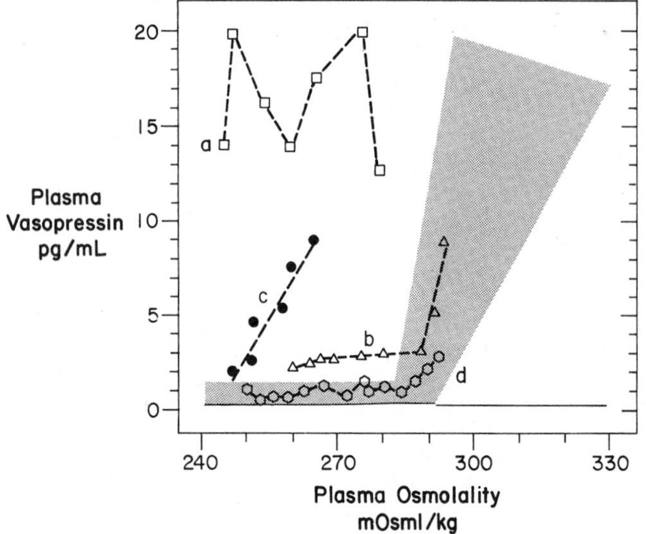

Figure 9–10. Schematic summary of different patterns of arginine vasopressin (AVP) secretion in patients with syndrome of inappropriate antidiuretic hormone secretion. Each line (a to d) represents the relation between plasma AVP and plasma osmolality of individual patients in whom osmolality was increased by infusion of hypertonic NaCl. The *shaded area* represents plasma AVP levels in normal subjects over physiologic ranges of plasma osmolality. (From Robertson GL. Thirst and vasopressin function in normal and disordered states of water balance. J Lab Clin Med 1983; 101:351–371.)

related mechanism may affect pituitary vasopressin secretion.[455, 492] The pattern of SIADH that occurs without measurable vasopressin secretion is not yet well understood, but the positive response of one such patient to a vasopressin V2 receptor antagonist suggests that it may represent increased renal sensitivity to low circulating levels of vasopressin.[496]

It is surprising that no correlation has been found between any of these patterns of secretion of vasopressin and the various causes of SIADH.[455] It seems likely that in many cases a heterogeneous group of CNS processes are involved, including osmotic and nonosmotic and stimulatory and inhibitory pathways, rather than a single dominant cause.

Contribution of Natriuresis to the Hyponatremia of SIADH

Since the original cases studied by Bartter and Schwartz,[414] increased renal Na^+ excretion has been one of the cardinal manifestations of SIADH and later became embedded in the requirements for its diagnosis. That the natriuresis accompanying administration of antidiuretic hormone is due not to vasopressin itself but, rather, to the volume expansion produced as a result of water retention was unequivocally shown by Leaf and co-workers[497] even before the description of the disorder. Although a negative sodium balance occurs during the development of hyponatremia in patients with SIADH, eventually urinary sodium excretion simply reflects daily sodium intake.[413] Thus, renal sodium wasting is excretion of sodium despite hyponatremia, but in reality there is a new steady state in which there is a neutral sodium balance.

Studies of long-term antidiuretic-induced hyponatremia in dogs and rats indicated that a large proportion of the hyponatremia was attributable to secondary Na^+ losses rather than to water retention.[442, 443] However, the natriuresis did not actually worsen the hyponatremia; rather, it allowed volume regulation of ECF. Because of the secondary natriuresis in patients with SIADH, expanded plasma or ECF volumes are not found with tracer dilution techniques.[444] Intrinsic renal mechanisms produced both diuresis and natriuresis in response to increases in renal perfusion pressures (so-called pressure diuresis) when vasopressin-infused animals were continually fluid loaded.[498] However, it has not yet been proved that this mechanism is sensitive enough to detect the relatively mild degrees of volume expansion that accompany dilutional hyponatremias.

Another possibility is that natriuresis is mediated through increases in circulating natriuretic peptides such as atrial natriuretic peptide (ANP), which are elevated in SIADH into ranges capable of promoting renal sodium excretion.[499] These possibilities are not mutually exclusive.

The degree to which hyponatremia may occur primarily as a result of natriuresis is controversial. Cerebral salt-wasting syndrome was first proposed by Peters and colleagues in 1950[500] as an explanation for the natriuresis and hyponatremia that sometimes accompany intracranial disease, particularly subarachnoid hemorrhage (SAH), in which up to one third of patients experience hyponatremia. After the description of SIADH in 1957, such patients were generally assumed to have hyponatremia secondary to vasopressin hypersecretion with a secondary natriuresis.[501] However, clinical and experimental data have suggested that some patients with SAH and other intracranial diseases indeed have a primary natriuresis leading to volume contraction rather than SIADH[502–504] and the elevated plasma vasopressin levels may be physiologically appropriate for the degree of volume contraction. Some studies indicate that there is insufficient evidence of hypovolemia despite ongoing natriuresis,[505] whereas others argue that the combined measures used to estimate ECF volume do support hypovolemia.[506]

With regard to the potential mechanisms of natriuresis, both plasma and CSF ANP levels are elevated in many patients with SAH[504] and have been found to correlate variably with hyponatremia in patients with intracranial diseases.[504, 507] However, because SIADH is also frequently associated with elevated plasma ANP levels, this finding does not prove causality. In other disorders of hyponatremia related to Na^+ wasting (e.g., Addison's disease) and diuretic-induced hyponatremia, infusion of saline restores normal ECF volume and plasma tonicity by shutting off the secondary vasopressin secretion. In SAH, however, large volumes of isotonic saline sufficient to maintain plasma volume did not change the incidence of hyponatremia.[508] In contrast, mineralocorticoid therapy to inhibit natriuresis reduced the incidence of hyponatremia in patients with SAH,[509] but elderly patients with SIADH responded similarly to mineralocorticoid therapy.[510] It seems most likely that SAH and other intracranial diseases represent a mixed disorder in which some patients have *both* exaggerated natriuresis and inappropriate vasopressin secretion; which effect predominates in the clinical presentation depends on their relative intensities as well as the effects of concomitant therapy.

The possibility that ANP-induced natriuresis may exacerbate hyponatremia is not confined to intracranial diseases, and it has been suggested that ectopic ANP production may contribute to or even cause the hyponatremia accompanying some small cell lung cancers.[511] In several studies, small cell lung carcinoma was reported to produce ANP in addition to, or (in some cases) instead of, vasopressin.[512] However, hyponatremia appeared to correlate more with plasma vasopressin levels than plasma ANP levels.[513] Consequently, such cases may represent a mixture of inappropriate secretion of both hormones, and the ANP may further exacerbate the secondary natriuresis produced primarily by vasopressin-induced water retention.

Renal Adaptation

In addition to excretion of osmoles to bring volumes back toward normal, some adaptations allow excretion of more water. As stated earlier, vasopressin stimulates water retention by increasing the activity and content of aquaporin-2 water channels in the renal collecting duct epithelium. Chronic action of vasopressin in SIADH produces dramatic increases above normal of aquaporin-2 content and insertion into the epithelial cell membranes. This increases the efficiency of water retention and worsens the pathology. However, when vasopressin induces volume expansion and hypotonicity, the volume expansion and hypotonicity per se, by ill-defined mechanisms, act on the tubular cells of the collecting duct to decrease the content and action of aquaporin-2, thus decreasing the amount of water resorbed in spite of high vasopressin. This *renal escape* is another adaptation (besides natriuresis) that allows a patient with persistent SIADH to achieve a new steady state of Na^+ and water balance with a low serum sodium level.[514, 515]

Clinical Manifestations of Hypo-osmolar Disorders

Regardless of the etiology of hypo-osmolality, most clinical manifestations are similar. Non-neurologic symptoms are relatively uncommon, but a number of cases of rhabdomyolysis have been reported, presumably secondary to osmotically induced swelling of muscle fibers. Hypo-osmolality is primarily associated with a broad spectrum of neurologic manifestations, ranging from mild nonspecific symptoms (e.g., headache, nausea) to more significant disorders (e.g., disorientation, confusion, obtundation, focal neurologic deficits, seizures).[416] This neurologic symptom complex has been termed *hyponatremic encephalopathy*[516] and primarily reflects brain edema resulting from osmotic water shifts into the brain because of decreased effective plasma osmolality.

Significant neurologic symptoms generally do not occur until serum [Na^+] falls below 125 mEq/L, and the severity of symptoms is roughly correlated with the degree of hypo-osmolality.[416, 517] Individual variability is marked, however, and for any single patient the level of serum [Na^+] at which symptoms appear cannot be predicted. When the brain has volume-adapted through solute losses, thereby reducing brain edema, neurologic symptoms may even be virtually absent.[517, 518] From animal studies, the rate of serum [Na^+] decline is often more strongly correlated with morbidity and mortality than is the actual magnitude of the decrease.[416] The reason is that the volume-adaptation process takes a finite period of time to complete, and the more rapid the decline in serum [Na^+], the more brain edema is accumulated before the brain can volume-regulate.

Thus, there is a much higher incidence of neurologic symptoms as well as a higher mortality rate in patients with acute hyponatremia than in patients with chronic hyponatremia.[416, 519] For example, the most dramatic cases of death related to hyponatremic encephalopathy have generally been reported in postoperative patients in whom hyponatremia developed rapidly as a result of intravenous infusion of hypotonic fluids.[417, 520] In such cases, nausea and vomiting are frequently overlooked as potential early signs of increased intracranial pressure; however, because hypo-osmolality does not have any direct effects on the gastrointestinal tract, unexplained nausea or vomiting in a hypo-osmolar patient should be assumed to have a CNS origin. Similarly, critically ill patients with unexplained seizures should be immediately evaluated for possible hyponatremia, because as many as one third of such patients have [Na^+] below 125 mEq/L as the cause of the seizure activity.[521] Underlying neurologic disease and non-neurologic metabolic disorders (e.g., hypoxia,[522] acidosis, hypercalcemia) can raise the level of plasma osmolality at which CNS symptoms occur.

In the most severe cases of hyponatremic encephalopathy, death results from respiratory failure after tentorial cerebral herniation and brain stem compression. One quarter of patients with severe postoperative hyponatremic encephalopathy manifested hypercapnic respiratory failure, the expected result of brain stem compression, but three quarters had pulmonary edema as the apparent cause of the hypoxia.[523]

Studies of acute hyponatremia after marathon races have shown hypoxia and pulmonary edema in association with brain edema.[524] These results therefore suggest that hypoxia resulting from noncardiogenic pulmonary edema may be an early sign of developing cerebral edema even before the brain stem compression and tentorial herniation.

Clinical studies also suggest that menstruating women[520] and young children[525] may be particularly susceptible to the development of neurologic morbidity and mortality during hyponatremia, especially in the acute postoperative setting.[516] However, other studies have failed to corroborate these findings.[526, 527] Consequently, the true clinical incidence and the mechanisms responsible for these sometimes catastrophic cases are not certain.

Therapy of Hypo-osmolar Disorders

Despite some areas of continuing controversy regarding correction of osmolality in hypo-osmolar patients, a relative consensus has evolved concerning the most appropriate treatment of this disorder. The following recommendations are summarized in the diagnostic and therapeutic flow diagram shown in Figure 9–11.

Initial Evaluation

ECF volume status determines treatment of hyponatremia. If volume is expanded, the treatment of the underlying disease should take precedence over correction of plasma osmolality. This treatment often involves diuretic therapy, which should simultaneously improve plasma tonicity by stimulating excretion of hypotonic urine. If hypovolemia is present, the patient must be considered to have depletion-induced hypo-osmolality, in which case volume repletion with isotonic saline (0.9% NaCl) at a rate appropriate for the estimated fluid deficit should be initiated.

If diuretic use is known or suspected, the isotonic saline should be supplemented with potassium (30 to 40 mEq/L) even if serum [K^+] is not low because of the propensity for total body potassium depletion to occur in such patients. Although generally the hypo-osmolar patient is clinically euvolemic, if a possibility of depletion-induced, rather than dilution-induced, hypo-osmolality exists, it is then appropriate to treat the patient initially with isotonic saline whether or not signs of hypovolemia are present. Improvement in and eventual correction of the hyponatremia verify solute and volume depletion. If the SIADH rather than solute depletion is present, administration of a limited volume (e.g., 1 to 2 L) of isotonic saline produces Na^+ and water excretion without significantly changing plasma osmolality.[413]

A patient who meets the essential criteria for SIADH but has a low urine osmolality should be observed with a trial of modest fluid restriction. If the hypo-osmolality is attributable to transient SIADH or severe polydipsia, the urine remains dilute and the plasma osmolality is fully corrected as free water is excreted. If the patient has the reset osmostat form of the disorder, however, the urine becomes concentrated at some point before the plasma osmolality and serum [Na^+] return to normal ranges.

If either primary or secondary adrenal insufficiency is suspected, glucocorticoid replacement should be initiated immediately after the completion of a rapid ACTH stimulation test. A prompt water diuresis after initiation of glucocorticoid treatment supports a diagnosis of glucocorticoid deficiency, but

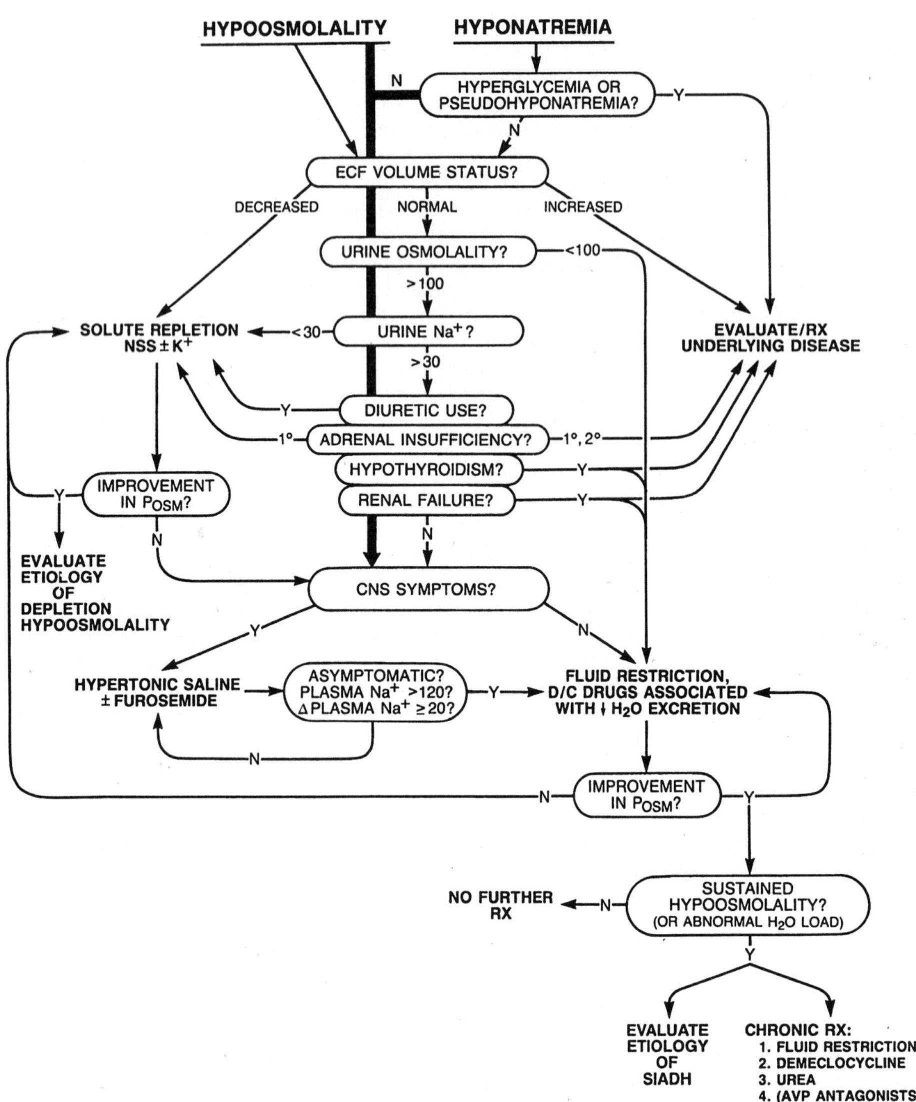

Figure 9–11. Schematic summary of the evaluation and therapy of hypo-osmolar patients. The *dark arrow* in the center emphasizes that the presence of central nervous system dysfunction related to hyponatremia should always be assessed immediately so that appropriate therapy can be started as soon as possible in symptomatic patients while the outlined diagnostic evaluation is proceeding. (From Verbalis JG. Inappropriate antidiuresis and other hypoosmolar states. In Becker KL [ed]. Principles and Practice of Endocrinology and Metabolism. Philadelphia, JB Lippincott, 1995, pp 265–276.)

absence of a quick response does not necessarily negate this diagnosis because several days of glucocorticoid replacement are sometimes required for normalization of plasma osmolality.[528] If hypothyroidism is suspected, thyroid function tests should be performed. Replacement therapy is usually withheld pending these results unless the patient is obviously myxedematous.

If renal failure is present in a patient with hypo-osmolality, a more extensive evaluation of renal function is necessary before a course of treatment is selected.

Acute Treatment

For any significantly hyponatremic patient, one must decide how quickly the plasma osmolality should be increased and to what level. This decision depends on the risks of uncorrected hyponatremia and the risks of the correction. It has become clear that correcting severe hyponatremia too rapidly is dangerous because it is sometimes associated with pontine and extrapontine myelinolysis, a brain demyelinating disease that causes severe neurologic morbidity and mortality.[418] Consequently, appreciation of the appropriate therapy of this disorder requires understanding this disease as well as the pathophysiology underlying hyponatremic encephalopathy.

Pontine and Extrapontine Myelinolysis

It has become apparent that the demyelinating disease of central pontine myelinolysis (CPM) occurs with a significantly higher incidence in patients with hyponatremia,[529] and in both animal[530] and human[418] studies brain demyelination has been associated with the correction of existing hyponatremia. In animal models of chronic hyponatremia, this pathologic disorder is probably precipitated by the brain dehydration that has been demonstrated to occur after correction of serum [Na^+] toward normal ranges.[531–533] MRI in animals has shown that chronic hypo-osmolality predisposes to opening of the blood-brain barrier in rats after rapid correction of hyponatremia[534] and that the disruption of the blood-brain barrier is highly correlated with subsequent demyelination.[535] Opening the blood-brain barrier can lead to subsequent myelinolysis through an influx of complement, which is toxic to the oligodendrocytes that manufacture and maintain myelin sheaths of neurons.[536]

Although there has been considerable debate in the literature, studies in both patients[537] and experimental animals[530, 538] support the concept that both the rate of correction of hyponatremia and the total magnitude of the correction over the first few days determine the risk of demyelination. In rats, an initial rate of correction of hyponatremia less than 20 mEq/L in 24 hours[539] involved less risk, and clinical data indicate that the initial magnitude of correction represents the major risk factor related to subsequent neurologic morbidity and mortality. Initial reports implicated increases in serum [Na+] greater than 25 mEq/L over the first 24 to 48 hours of treatment,[540] but later studies suggested the occurrence of CPM with increases in serum [Na+] of more than 12 mEq/L in 24 hours or 18 mEq/hour in 48 hours.[541] Although overcorrection of hyponatremia to supranormal levels is also clearly a risk factor for neurologic deterioration, both clinical and experimental studies have found that demyelination occurred after corrections to serum [Na+] levels still below normal ranges. Both experimental studies[530] and clinical reports[418, 542, 543] have demonstrated that demyelination occurs regardless of the method used to correct the hyponatremia.

The susceptibility to demyelination after correction of hyponatremia is strongly influenced by the severity and duration of the preexisting hyponatremia. The more severe and prolonged the hyponatremia, the more solute loss that occurs during the process of brain volume regulation, and the loss of larger amounts of solute impairs the ability of the brain to buffer volume in response to subsequent increases in plasma osmolality. Clinical studies show that CPM rarely occurs in patients with a starting serum [Na+] above 120 mmol/L, does not appear to occur in patients with psychogenic polydipsia in whom hyponatremia develops acutely as a result of massive water ingestion, and is corrected rapidly by diuresis of the excess fluid.[544]

Other independent risk factors for the occurrence of CPM are chronic alcoholism and malnutrition.[545] It seems likely that the threshold for increases in serum [Na+] that increase the risk for CPM is lower in alcoholic and malnourished patients, and a case report of myelinolysis in a patient with beer potomania in whom the rate of correction stayed within the recommended guidelines supports this likelihood.[546] Interestingly, uremia appears to protect hyponatremic patients from myelinolysis after rapid correction of hyponatremia, purportedly because urea acts as an intracellular osmolyte to stabilize intracellular volume and thereby reduces the degree of brain dehydration produced after rapid correction of hyponatremia.[547]

The term *central pontine myelinolysis* is historically correct but anatomically too limited.[529] Demyelination after correction of hyponatremia frequently occurs in white matter areas of the brain other than the pons. This occurrence led to the term *osmotic demyelination syndrome*,[418] but the term *pontine and extrapontine myelinolysis* (PEM) would be more accurate. Apropos of the widespread nature of the neuropathologic lesions, a much broader range of neurologic disorders is now being reported in patients after correction of hyponatremia, including cognitive, behavioral, and neuropsychiatric disorders, presumably as a result of demyelination in subcortical, corpus callosal, and hippocampal white matter, and movement disorders, as a result of demyelination in the basal ganglia.

The presence of positive MRI findings strongly supports a diagnosis of PEM, but scans often fail to demonstrate the characteristic demyelinative lesions because scans are usually negative until sufficient time has passed (generally 3 to 4 weeks) after correction of hyponatremia and onset of neurologic symptoms.[548, 549] Although most cases of osmotically induced PEM have been associated with rapid correction of hyponatremia, the disorder has also been reported with severe hypernatremia in both animal models[550] and patients.[551] It is clear that one cannot predict with any degree of certainty which patients will develop demyelination. Many patients undergo rapid and large changes of serum [Na+] without subsequent neurologic complications,[552] which is true of experimental animals as well.[530, 539] Consequently, overly rapid correction of hyponatremia should be viewed as a factor that puts patients *at risk* for PEM but does not inevitably precipitate this disorder.

Individualization of Therapy

From the previous discussions of hyponatremic encephalopathy and PEM, it follows that optimal treatment of hyponatremia must entail balancing the risks of hyponatremia against the risks of correction for each patient individually.[553, 554] Three factors should be considered when one is making a treatment decision for a hypo-osmolar patient: (1) the severity of the hyponatremia, (2) the duration of the hyponatremia, and (3) the patient's neurologic symptoms.

Acute Hyponatremia

Cases of acute hyponatremia, arbitrarily defined as 48 hours in duration, are usually symptomatic if the hyponatremia is severe (i.e., $<$ 120 mEq/L). These patients are at greatest risk for neurologic complications from the hyponatremia but rarely have demyelination,[544] presumably because sufficient brain volume regulation has not yet occurred. Consequently, serum [Na+] in such patients should be corrected relatively quickly.

Figure 9–11 (see dark black arrow) emphasizes that hypo-osmolar patients should always be evaluated quickly for the presence of neurologic symptoms so that appropriate therapy can be initiated, if indicated, even while other results of the diagnostic evaluation are pending. Postoperative patients,[555] and particularly young women and children in some studies,[520, 525] appear to be at somewhat greater risk for rapidly progressing hyponatremic encephalopathy. They should be treated especially promptly, and administration of hypotonic fluids should be avoided in such patients postoperatively.[516]

Chronic Asymptomatic Hyponatremia

Conversely, patients with chronic hyponatremia (arbitrarily defined as more than 48 hours in duration) who have minimal neurologic symptoms are at little risk from complications of hyponatremia itself, but demyelination can develop after rapid correction because of greater degrees of brain volume regulation through electrolyte and osmolyte losses.[439] There is no indication to correct the hyponatremia rapidly, regardless of the initial serum [Na+], and these patients should be treated by slower-acting therapies, such as fluid restriction.

Chronic Symptomatic Hyponatremia

Although the first two extremes have clear treatment indications, most hypo-osmolar patients have hyponatremia of indeterminate duration and varying degrees of neurologic symptoms. Such patients should be treated promptly, because of their symptoms, but with methods that allow a *controlled and limited increase* of hypo-osmolality.[554] Some studies have suggested that correction parameters should consist of a maximal rate of correction of serum [Na+] in the range of 1 to 2 mEq/L per hour as long as the total magnitude of correction does not exceed 25 mEq/L over the first 48 hours.[540] Others recommend even more conservative parameters, with maximal correction rates of 0.5 mEq/L per hour or less and magnitudes of correction that do not exceed 12 mEq/L in the first 24 hours and 18 mEq/L in the first 48 hours.[541]

A reasonable approach for treatment of individual patients would therefore entail choosing correction parameters within these limits, depending on the symptoms. In patients who are only minimally symptomatic, one should proceed at the lower recommended limits of 0.5 mEq/L per hour or less. In patients with more severe neurologic symptoms, initial correction at a rate of 1 to 2 mEq/L per hour (or even 3 to 5 mEq/L per hour in comatose or seizing patients who are at risk for imminent tentorial herniation and respiratory arrest) would be more appropriate.

Regardless of the initial rate of correction chosen, acute treatment should be interrupted when any of three end-points is reached:

1. The patient's symptoms are abolished.
2. A safe serum [Na+] (>120 mEq/L) is achieved.
3. A total magnitude of correction of 20 mEq/L is achieved.

At such a point, the active correction should be stopped and the patient treated with slower-acting therapies (e.g., oral rehydration, fluid restriction), depending on the cause of the hypo-osmolality. From these recommendations, it follows that serum [Na+] levels must be carefully monitored at frequent intervals (at least every 4 hours) during the active phases of treatment to adjust therapy to keep the correction within these guidelines.

Interventional (Active) Therapies for Acute Corrections

Controlled limited corrections can be accomplished with either isotonic or hypertonic saline infusions, depending on the etiology of the hypo-osmolality. Patients with volume-depletion hypo-osmolality (e.g., clinical hypovolemia, diuretic use, or urine [Na+] < 30 mEq/L) usually respond well to isotonic (0.9%) NaCl.[450] However, patients with diuretic-induced hyponatremia are especially susceptible to rapid corrections for several reasons:

1. Such patients are usually only minimally volume-depleted.
2. They are often small, elderly women with correspondingly small plasma volumes.
3. With cessation of diuretic therapy, these patients often have a free water diuresis as their urinary diluting defect dissipates.[556]
4. The hypokalemia that frequently accompanies the hyponatremia in such patients appears to be an additional risk factor for demyelination after correction.[557]

Consequently, in the absence of marked neurologic symptoms, such patients should simply be prescribed a regular sodium diet (4 to 8 g/day) and should discontinue diuretics. If isotonic saline is infused, it should be done so judiciously (e.g., 50 to 75 mL/hour) with potassium replacement. Patients with euvolemic hypo-osmolality (including those with SIADH) generally do not respond to isotonic NaCl[413, 450] and are best treated with hypertonic (3%) NaCl solution given by continuous infusion. An initial infusion rate can be estimated by multiplying the patient's body weight in kilograms by the desired rate of increase in serum [Na+] in milliequivalents per liter per hour. For example, in a 70-kg patient, an infusion of 3% NaCl at 70 mL/hour increases serum [Na+] by approximately 1 mEq/L per hour and an infusion of 35 mL/hour increases serum [Na+] by about 0.5 mEq/L per hour.

In patients with known cardiovascular disease, furosemide can be used to treat volume overload.[558] It cannot be emphasized too strongly that it is necessary only to correct plasma osmolality acutely to a *safe* range rather than completely to normonatremia.

Spontaneous (Passive) Correction

In rare circumstances, hyponatremia may be corrected spontaneously by means of a water diuresis. If the hyponatremia is acute, such as that caused by water intoxication in psychogenic polydipsia, spontaneous correction appears to involve little risk for subsequent demyelination.[544]

When hyponatremia has been chronic, patients are at risk for demyelination[542, 559] and one might consider intervention (e.g., administration of desmopressin or intravenous infusion of hypotonic fluid) to limit the rate and magnitude of correction of serum [Na+]. A report of such a case demonstrates the utility of interrupting a spontaneous free water diuresis with desmopressin.[560] In some cases, an overcorrection occurs spontaneously before it is noticed. Animal models in this situation have shown that delayed lowering of the serum [Na+] can prevent subsequent brain damage,[561] which would be consistent with the occurrence of a delayed immunologic demyelination as a result of complement influx into the brain after sustained blood-brain barrier disruption.[536] A clinical case in which delayed lowering of serum [Na+] was associated with a reversal of symptoms suggestive of early myelinolysis supports this as a potential therapy in similar cases.[562]

Chronic Treatment

Fluid Restriction

The treatment of chronic SIADH entails a choice among several suboptimal therapeutic regimens. Any drugs known to be associated with SIADH should be discontinued or changed. Continued fluid restriction represents the least toxic treatment choice and is the preferred treatment for most cases of mild to moderate SIADH. Several points should be remembered when this approach is used:

1. All fluids, not only water, must be included in the restriction.
2. The degree of restriction required depends on urine output plus insensible fluid loss (generally, discretionary, nonfood fluids should be limited to 500 mL a day below the average daily urine volume).
3. Several days of restriction are usually necessary before a significant increase in plasma osmolality occurs.
4. Only fluid, not salt, should be restricted.

Because of the ongoing natriuresis, patients with chronic SIADH often have a negative total body [Na+] balance and therefore should be maintained with relatively high NaCl intakes unless otherwise contraindicated. Failure to improve after several days of confirmed negative fluid balance prompts reconsideration of other possible causes, including solute depletion and clinically inapparent hypovolemia.

Although it has not been confirmed in humans, in animals the expanded volume and hypotonicity of SIADH decrease the vasopressin-induced increase of aquaporin-2 water channels in the collecting duct and this escape allows more water excretion.[514, 515] Unfortunately, from a therapeutic standpoint, correction of expanded volume and hyponatremia by restriction of fluid would reduce the escape phenomenon. Aquaporin content and action increase again in response to the persistent level of vasopressin, and the efficiency of extracting free water increases. This is a plausible explanation for the clinical observation that a patient with stable hyponatremia with modest fluid intake may require severe water restriction to correct the hyponatremia permanently.

Treatment of Polydipsia

When hyponatremia is caused primarily by polydipsia, ideally therapy should be directed at reducing fluid intake to normal ranges. Unfortunately, fluid restriction has proved difficult to accomplish in many cases. Patients with a reset thirst threshold are resistant to fluid restriction because of the thirst resulting from stimulation of brain thirst centers at higher plasma osmolalities.[563] In some cases, the use of alternative methods to ameliorate the sensation of thirst (e.g., wetting the mouth with ice chips or using sour candies to increase salivary flow) can help to reduce fluid intake.

Fluid intake in patients with psychogenic causes of polydipsia is driven by psychiatric factors that have responded variably to behavioral modification and pharmacologic therapy. Several reports have suggested potential efficacy of the antipsychotic drug clozapine as an agent to reduce polydipsia and to prevent recurrent hyponatremia in at least a subset of these patients.[564]

Pharmacologic Therapy

Pharmacologic intervention is reserved for refractory cases in which the degree of fluid restriction required to avoid hypo-osmolality is so severe that the patient is unable or unwilling to maintain it. Pharmacologic intervention should also be avoided initially in patients with SIADH that is secondary to tumors because successful treatment of the underlying malignant lesion often eliminates or reduces the inappropriate vasopressin secretion.

When pharmacologic management is necessary, the preferred drug is the tetracycline derivative demeclocycline.[565] This agent causes nephrogenic diabetes insipidus,[566] thereby decreasing urine concentration even in the presence of high plasma vasopressin levels. Appropriate doses of demeclocycline range from 600 to 1200 mg/day administered in divided doses. Treatment must be continued for several days to achieve maximal diuretic effects; consequently, one should wait 3 to 4 days before deciding to increase the dose. Demeclocycline can cause reversible azotemia and sometimes nephrotoxicity, especially in patients with cirrhosis.[567] Renal function should therefore be monitored on a regular basis in patients receiving demeclocycline, and the medication discontinued if increasing azotemia is noted.

Other agents, such as lithium, have similar renal effects but are less desirable because of inconsistent results and significant side effects.[568] Urea has also been described as an alternative mode of treatment for SIADH as well as other hyponatremic disorders.[569]

Several drugs appear to decrease vasopressin hypersecretion in some cases (e.g., diphenylhydantoin, opiates, ethanol), but responses have been erratic and unpredictable. Potential exceptions are agonists selective for kappa opioid receptors, which appeared to be more specific for inhibition of vasopressin hypersecretion in animal studies[570] and in clinical trials successfully produced an aquaresis in patients with cirrhosis.[571]

Vasopressin Antagonists

An antagonist of the kidney vasopressin V2 receptors would be the ideal agent for treatment of dilutional hyponatremia.[572] Previous attempts at using peptide vasopressin receptor antagonists in humans were frustrated by species variability with regard to partial agonistic effects of such compounds.[573] Several nonpeptide V2 receptor antagonists have been described that appear to overcome these problems.[574–576] As of this writing, several of these compounds were already in clinical trials with promising results.[577] It thus appears that we are poised to begin a new era in both the evaluation and treatment of patients with SIADH.

When selective V2 receptor antagonists are eventually approved for clinical use, clinical trials should enable investigators to answer some long-standing questions about the role of vasopressin receptor activation in producing antidiuresis as well as other potential effects in various disease states (e.g., hyponatremic patients without measurable vasopressin levels) and should provide better therapy for patients with chronic hyponatremia. Patients whose hyponatremia is corrected too rapidly with vasopressin receptor antagonists will still be at risk for PEM, which has already been documented in animals,[578] but appropriate dosing and monitoring should allow successful adherence to the same guidelines for limited controlled correction that apply to other methods of treatment.

OXYTOCIN

Synthesis of oxytocin and electrophysiology of oxytocinergic neurons have been described earlier in the chapter. The normal physiologic regulation of oxytocin secretion and action is complicated by the fact that secretion and function of oxytocin vary markedly among different experimental mammals. There are sites of synthesis in the ovary and in various tissues of the uterus that differ among species. Because it is difficult to study pregnant women and human tissue, physiologic regulation of oxytocin secretion and function is less well known in humans than other species. The classic roles of oxytocin are uterine myometrial contraction at parturition and smooth muscle activation promoting milk let-down with nursing.[579–582]

Parturition

The isolation of oxytocin was followed quickly by the description of its ability to stimulate uterine contractions, and this was soon followed by clinical use of oxytocin as a uterotonic agent.[583] Indeed, oxytocin is the most potent known stimulator of myometrial contraction.[584] The uterine myometrial cells have intrinsic contractile activity, and it is necessary during pregnancy to maintain the uterus in a quiet state. In most species, this is accomplished by action of progesterone and by relaxin (produced by the corpus luteum and decidual tissue), which decrease uterine contraction.[581, 585, 586] Late in pregnancy, parturition is initiated by synchronizing the myometrial activity so that contractures become contractions, with softening and dilatation of the cervix and rupture of the fetal membranes.[585, 587] Parturition is then completed by separation of the placenta and involution of the uterus.[585]

Estrogen activates many of the events required to initiate and progress through parturition, whereas progesterone tends to inhibit these events. In several species, progesterone withdrawal may be an initiating factor of parturition. The mechanism of the increase of the estrogen/progesterone ratio, however, may vary considerably among species. In sheep, an increase in corticotropin-releasing hormone and vasopressin in the fetus near term produces a remarkable increase in ACTH and cortisol. The increased cortisol leads to decreased progesterone in the ewe, and this triggers parturition.[587, 588] In mice, the corpus luteum makes progesterone and estradiol throughout pregnancy. There is also a decrease in progesterone at delivery, but the progesterone decrease is not dependent on glucocorticoids.[589]

In some species, such as mice and sheep, the corpus luteum is maintained throughout pregnancy and secretes progesterone. Luteolysis at the time of parturition causes an abrupt fall in progesterone. In humans and nonhuman primates, the corpus luteum is present only during the first trimester[589] and estrogen and progesterone rise throughout pregnancy, although the rate of increase of estrogen is greater than that of progesterone as parturition approaches.[590] A decreasing effect of progesterone and increasing effect of estrogen in humans may be more important at a paracrine level in fetal membranes, where progesterone is inactivated and estrogen synthesis increased.[582, 591] It has also been reported that estrogen receptor increases in human fetal membranes at parturition whereas progesterone receptor remains stable.[585, 592] Thus, the cycle of events that are observed in plasma in some species may be reproduced distally as a paracrine action in primates.[591, 593, 594]

Levels of oxytocin in plasma may not be indicative of the role of oxytocin in parturition. In humans, there is a dramatic increase in the responsiveness of the uterus to oxytocin as parturition approaches.[582] This increased responsiveness, which may be as much as 200-fold, is accompanied by a similar increase in oxytocin receptor density.[586, 595] Another major influence on uterine contractility late in pregnancy is the formation of gap junctions between myometrial cells. Gap junctions are a prerequisite for synchronous contraction of the uterus and, like other events, gap junction formation is inhibited by progesterone and stimulated by estrogens.[595]

In various species, several other hormones play a role in initiation of or completion of parturition, or both, including prostaglandins, endothelins, adrenergic agonists, glucocorticoids, and cytokines.[582, 585, 586, 595] The role of oxytocin in the complex interplay of these various agents is not well understood in humans.

The importance of *prostaglandins* is increasingly recognized in numerous species. The predominant prostaglandin, prostaglandin $F_{2\alpha}$ ($PGF_{2\alpha}$), is responsible for luteolysis of the corpus luteum in sheep and rodents, causing the decrease in progesterone described earlier.[582, 589, 595, 596] In fetal membranes, cyclooxygenase enzymes that stimulate synthesis of prostaglandins from arachidonic acid are increased at parturition[582, 595] and release prostaglandins from the uterus to act on the ovary to cause luteolysis.[589, 596] Prostaglandins may also help promote a controlled inflammatory response in the cervix to assist in thinning and dilatation.[589, 597–599]

In nonhuman primates, as parturition approaches, synchronized nocturnal contractions begin but revert to asynchronous contractures during the day. These synchronized nocturnal contractions correlate with plasma oxytocin levels[600] and are blocked by administration of an oxytocin antagonist. Similarly, the response of the uterus to administered oxytocin in the monkey is greater at night than during the day,[601] and fetal dehydroepiandrosterone sulfate (DHEAS) levels are also highest at night.[602] DHEAS secretion by the fetus may be an important source of estrogen because the DHEAS is converted to estradiol by the placenta. Estradiol stimulates oxytocin synthesis in decidua and also stimulates synthesis of $PGF_{2\alpha}$ in decidua.

As mentioned earlier, at this time there is an increase in estrogen receptors, which would favor the action of DHEAS to increase the estrogen response. Furthermore, there is a feed-forward mechanism whereby increased $PGF_{2\alpha}$ stimulates oxytocin, which in turn stimulates increased production of $PGF_{2\alpha}$. Teleologically, it makes sense that the developing fetus, upon reaching maturation, would be a controlling factor in the initiation of labor. It was previously noted that in the sheep there is an absolute requirement for the fetal hypothalamic-pituitary-adrenal axis to initiate labor, and the interaction of fetal DHEAS, estrogen, oxytocin, and progesterone provides a potential similar mechanism in primates (and humans?).

Although the role of oxytocin in the initiation of parturition is still debated, it is agreed that oxytocin is released explosively in a pulsatile fashion after the initiation of parturition and as parturition continues. This release of oxytocin is brought about by vaginal and cervical dilatation and is known as the *Fergusson reflex*. In animals with multiple births, the reflex release of oxytocin after one fetus passes the cervicovaginal canal may assist in the delivery of subsequent pups,[603] but in humans this second phase of delivery is usually only to deliver the placenta[582, 585, 586] and may be more important in stimulating a clamping down of the uterine muscle to decrease blood loss.

Interestingly, studies with mice to "knock out" synthesis of oxytocin have found that in oxytocin-deficient mice parturition is initiated on time and proceeds normally,[584, 604, 605] whereas mice deficient in cyclooxygenase and in prostaglandins have markedly prolonged labor. Administration of $PGF_{2\alpha}$ to the deficient animals resulted in delivery of viable pups at the appropriate time.[606, 607]

From this brief review, it is clear that parturition is a complicated cascade of events that interact with each other at parturition and feed forward with cross-stimulation. It is not surprising that physiologic events as important to the species as pregnancy and parturition would have many redundant systems to ensure survival of the species. In addition, the complicated interaction of these various redundant systems and the feedforward nature of the responses make it unlikely that interrupting any single hormonal response after parturition is initiated would be sufficient to inhibit completion of delivery.[588]

In all of these discussions, there has been an obvious lack of understanding of the role of cysteine aminopeptidase (oxytocinase) in the physiology of pregnancy in humans. If this enzyme developed as a protective mechanism, one would assume that oxytocin secretion by the neurohypophysis was increased throughout pregnancy, but the presence of this enzyme and the inability to do studies of the hypothalamus in vivo make this possibility uncertain. However, the presence of the oxytocin-associated neurophysin throughout pregnancy supports this point of view.[608] Furthermore, the presence of circulating cysteine aminopeptidase provides a teleologic explanation for the development of oxytocin synthesis and secretion in fetal membranes in a manner that serves a paracrine function possibly protected from the degradative activity of the cysteine aminopeptidase in plasma.

Lactation

The hypothalamic-pituitary hormones critical to lactation are prolactin and oxytocin. Prolactin storage and secretion from the anterior pituitary and its action to promote milk production are described in Chapter 8. Oxytocin is critical for milk secretion through the characteristic milk let-down response. Each of these hormones is influenced and regulated by gonadal steroid hormones. The milk-producing unit of the breast is the *alveolar system*, with multiple clusters of milk-producing cells surrounded by specialized myoepithelial cells. The alveoli are directly connected to ductules, and the ducts converge and lead to the nipple.

Milk is synthesized in the glandular cells of the alveoli.[609] Oxytocin receptors are localized on glandular cells and oxytocin in the systemic circulation acts on these receptors to cause myoepithelial contraction. Oxytocin also acts on myoepithelial cells along the duct to shorten and widen the ducts, enhancing milk flow through the ducts to the nipple.[610] Interestingly, in humans there are also oxytocin receptors on the epithelium of the gland and ducts, and oxytocin may have other indirect effects that enhance milk transport.[611]

When an infant begins sucking at the breast, an afferent signal is transmitted from the mechanoreceptors or tactile receptors in the breast to the spinal cord and from the spinal cord to the lateral cervical nucleus. These ascending fibers cross in the medulla and eventually ascend to the oxytocinergic magnocellular neurons in the supraoptic nucleus and the paraventricular nucleus.[580, 610, 612] Numerous neurotransmitters and neuropeptides are activated by different inputs to stimulate or inhibit the magnocellular neurons.[610] Oxytocin itself is a regulator of oxytocin neurons. Oxytocin released by the dendrites acts on the same magnocellular neuron in an autocrine fashion, and an oxytocin antagonist infused into the hypothalamus decreases milk yield.[613]

Although the exact role of each of these neurotransmitters or neuropeptides and their cooperative and competitive interactions has not been clarified in any animal (especially in humans), it is agreed that the final result is synchronous pulsatile depolarization of oxytocin neurons.[613–615] The pulsatile release of oxytocin by the posterior pituitary can produce a pumping action on the alveoli, promoting maximal emptying of milk from the alveoli.[609, 616] Complete emptying of the breast is important to increase milk yield,[617, 618] and if milk is not released from the breast there is involution of synthetic and secretory capacity.

The importance of oxytocin in maintaining milk secretion has been demonstrated by transgenic mice with a neurophysin construct that inhibited oxytocin synthesis. These animals delivered their young normally and had normal milk production, but there was no milk release despite normal suckling. The pups died of dehydration with no milk in the stomach.[619, 620] Administration of oxytocin to these oxytocin-deficient mice restored the ability to secrete milk and allowed the pups to survive. Similarly, oxytocin may promote successful lactation in women who have difficulty with lactation and milk production.[621]

Whereas in most species suckling must occur for the sequence of events leading to milk let-down and, indeed, let-down may require several minutes of suckling,[622] in humans suckling is not essential because oxytocin secretion and milk let-down are elicited by psychological stimuli such as preparing for nursing or hearing a baby cry.[579, 623, 624] Suckling is, however, important in women because only suckling causes release of prolactin[579] and suckling causes pulsatile release of oxytocin, whereas artificial massage of the breast produces continuous secretion of oxytocin.[624] In women, if oxytocin is not secreted, only 20% to 30% of stored milk is released during nursing and secretion of oxytocin can be markedly inhibited by stress.[625]

The role of steroids in oxytocin secretion is complex. Estrogen stimulates oxytocin release by dendrites,[626] and progesterone withdrawal in an estrogen-primed animal stimulates oxytocin synthesis.[627, 628] Changes in these steroid hormones at the time of parturition probably modulate the lactation response both by modulating oxytocin synthesis and secretion and by modulating oxytocin receptors. Vaginal delivery and the pulses of oxytocin that are produced during the second phase of labor may enhance the pulses of oxytocin that later occur with suckling and lactation.[629]

As breast-feeding continues in humans, the basal levels of oxytocin decrease but pulses of oxytocin in response to suckling continue and may increase.[630] Women with diabetes insipidus have been able to breast-feed infants, and this has caused some to question the importance of oxytocin in humans.[631] As noted earlier, however, oxytocin secretion may be preserved in the absence of vasopressin in patients with diabetes insipidus, even in those with traumatic section of the stalk.

The literature supports an interaction of oxytocin and prolactin. Receptors for prolactin have been described in the supraoptic nucleus,[632] and prolactin enhances oxytocin release at the level of the pituitary and enhances synthesis of oxytocin when applied to magnocellular neurons.[632] The importance of these findings has been questioned because prolactin probably does not cross the blood-brain barrier. Systemic administration of prolactin has been reported to stimulate release of oxytocin and immunoneutralization of prolactin to eliminate suckling-induced oxytocin release.[622] Oxytocin was also reported to act as a prolactin-releasing factor. There may be a reinforcing interaction of oxytocin to stimulate release of prolactin and prolactin to enhance the release of oxytocin, producing a feed-forward interaction.[610, 622]

Behavior

In addition to the actions in the periphery to stimulate milk let-down and uterine contraction during parturition, oxytocin is reported to have numerous actions on the CNS. The separate functions, peripheral and central, are mirrored anatomically by two sets of neurons: the magnocellular neurons and the smaller parvocellular neurons, respectively.[633] Because the role of oxytocin secreted peripherally is to regulate physiologic events of reproduction, most of the emphasis regarding CNS effects has been on various aspects of maternal behavior. Maternal behavior is coincident with parturition and lactation in most mammalian species and is not seen with other physiologic events that produce changes only in gonadal steroid secretion. Therefore, it is likely that something in addition to or in place of gonadal steroids is active in inducing maternal behavior.[634]

The most studied species regarding maternal behavior are sheep[635] and rats.[633, 634, 636–638] Studies have found that oxytocin is increased in various areas of the brain that are thought to be sites of regulation of maternal behavior, such as the olfactory lobes of rats.[634] In some species, injection of oxytocin into the cerebral ventricles can initiate maternal behavior and injection of oxytocin antagonists can inhibit such behavior. However, the findings regarding oxytocin and reproductive behavior vary markedly among species and among strains within a given species.

Oxytocin has also been reported to play a role in males, but this is much less certain. In rodents, oxytocin administered in the CNS induced arousal and penile erection; in some species, oxytocin has been reported to increase sperm transport.[639–641]

Other Actions of Oxytocin

In a number of reproductive tissues in a variety of species, oxytocin stimulates prostaglandin production.[642] In several species, oxytocin is produced in peripheral organs rather than in the hypothalamus. There is some evidence for action of oxytocin in the menstrual cycle of humans, although this evidence is not as clear as that for the involvement of oxytocin in the estrous cycle of ruminants. Nonetheless, it is suggested that oxytocin may participate in a paracrine or autocrine fashion between cells in the human corpus luteum to stimulate the synthesis of progesterone.[643, 644]

In addition to accepted and postulated roles of oxytocin in reproductive behavior, numerous other central functions may be affected by central secretion of oxytocin, including the following:

1. Feeding behavior and satiety.[645–647]
2. Gastric acid secretion.
3. Regulation of autonomic functions such as blood pressure, temperature, and heart rate.
4. Stimulation of glucagon to increase glucose.
5. Gonadotropin secretion.[648]
6. Response to stress.[649]
7. Decreasing stress.[633, 636, 639, 640]
8. Stimulation of contractions of tubules and sperm transfer in the testes.[650, 651]

Some generalizations concerning these various central actions of oxytocin are that many of the purported actions are modulated by gonadal steroids, opioids appear to have a generally suppressive effect on oxytocin action,[638] and there is great variability in the pattern of oxytocin receptors among species and considerable plasticity of the oxytocin receptors that may accompany physiologic changes.[641] Oxytocin may have direct actions on receptors in the brain and may serve as a neurotransmitter or may modulate the response of classic neurotransmitters.

References

1. Makarenko IG, Ugrumov MV, Derer P, et al. Projections from the hypothalamus to the posterior lobe in rats during ontogene-

sis: 1,1′-dioctadecyl-3,3,3′,3′-tetramethylindocarbocyanine perchlorate tracing study. J Comp Neurol 2000; 422:327–337.
2. Sofroniew MV, Weindl A, Schinko I, et al. The distribution of vasopressin-, oxytocin-, and neurophysin-producing neurons in the guinea pig brain. I. The classical hypothalamo-neurohypophyseal system. Cell Tissue Res 1979; 196: 367–384.
3. Dierickx K, Vandesande F. Immunocytochemical demonstration of separate vasopressin-neurophysin and oxytocin-neurophysin neurons in the human hypothalamus. Cell Tissue Res 1979; 196: 203–212.
4. Zimmerman EA, Defendini R, Sokol HW, et al. The distribution of neurophysin-secreting pathways in the mammalian brain: light microscopic studies using the immunoperoxidase technique. Ann NY Acad Sci 1975; 248:92–111.
5. Sofroniew MV. Morphology of vasopressin and oxytocin neurones and their central and vascular projections. Prog Brain Res 1983; 60:101–114.
6. Sawchenko PE, Swanson LW. The organization and biochemical specificity of afferent projections to the paraventricular and supraoptic nuclei. Prog Brain Res 1983; 60:19–29.
7. Swanson LW, Sawchenko PE. Hypothalamic integration: organization of the paraventricular and supraoptic nuclei. Annu Rev Neurosci 1983; 6:269–324.
8. Treier M, Rosenfeld MG. The hypothalamic-pituitary axis: codevelopment of two organs. Curr Opin Cell Biol 1996; 8:833–843.
9. Swanson LW, Sawchenko PE. Paraventricular nucleus: a site for the integration of neuroendocrine and autonomic mechanisms. Neuroendocrinology 1980; 31:410–417.
10. Defendini R, Zimmerman EA. The magnocellular neurosecretory system of the mammalian hypothalamus. Res Publ Assoc Res Nerv Ment Dis 1978; 56:137–154.
11. Armstrong WE, Stern JE. Electrophysiological distinctions between oxytocin and vasopressin neurons in the supraoptic nucleus. Adv Exp Med Biol 1998; 449:67–77.
12. Swaab DF. Development of the human hypothalamus. Neurochem Res 1995; 20:509–519.
13. Hofman MA, Swaab DF. Seasonal changes in the suprachiasmatic nucleus of man. Neurosci Lett 1992; 139:257–260.
14. Hofman MA, Swaab DF. Alterations in circadian rhythmicity of the vasopressin-producing neurons of the human suprachiasmatic nucleus (SCN) with aging. Brain Res 1994; 651:134–142.
15. Mark L, Pech P, Daniels D, et al. The pituitary fossa: a correlative anatomic and MR study. Radiology 1984; 153:453–457.
16. Root AW, Martinez CR, Muroff LR. Subhypothalamic high-intensity signals identified by magnetic resonance imaging in children with idiopathic anterior hypopituitarism: evidence suggestive of an 'ectopic' posterior pituitary gland. Am J Dis Child 1989; 143:366–367.
17. Kikuchi K, Fujisawa I, Momoi T, et al. Hypothalamic-pituitary function in growth hormone–deficient patients with pituitary stalk transection. J Clin Endocrinol Metab 1988; 67:817–823.
18. Ultmann MC, Siegel SF, Hirsch WL, et al. Pituitary stalk and ectopic hyperintense T1 signal on magnetic resonance imaging: implications for anterior pituitary dysfunction. Am J Dis Child 1993; 147:647–652.
19. Maghnie M, Triulzi F, Larizza D, et al. Hypothalamic-pituitary dysfunction in growth hormone–deficient patients with pituitary abnormalities. J Clin Endocrinol Metab 1991; 73:79–83.
20. Lukezic M, Righini V, Di Natale B, et al. Vasopressin and thirst in patients with posterior pituitary ectopia and hypopituitarism. Clin Endocrinol (Oxf) 2000; 53:77–83.
21. Maghnie M, Genovese E, Villa A, et al. Dynamic MRI in the congenital agenesis of the neural pituitary stalk syndrome: the role of the vascular pituitary stalk in predicting residual anterior pituitary function. Clin Endocrinol (Oxf) 1996; 45:281–290.
22. Chen S, Leger J, Garel C, et al. Growth hormone deficiency with ectopic neurohypophysis: anatomical variations and relationship between the visibility of the pituitary stalk asserted by magnetic resonance imaging and anterior pituitary function. J Clin Endocrinol Metab 1999; 84:2408–2413.
23. Gainer H, Wray S. Cellular and molecular biology of oxytocin and vasopressin. In Knobil E, Neill JD (eds). The Physiology of Reproduction, 2nd ed. New York, Raven Press, 1994, pp 1099–1129.
24. Chen LQ, Rose JP, Breslow E, et al. Crystal structure of a bovine neurophysin II dipeptide complex at 2.8 Å determined from the single-wavelength anomalous scattering signal of an incorporated iodine atom. Proc Natl Acad Sci USA 1991; 88:4240–4244.
25. Acher R. Evolution of neurohypophysial control of water homeostasis: integrative biology of molecular, cellular and organismal aspects. In Saito T, Kurokawa K, Yoshida S (eds). Neurohypophysis: Recent Progress of Vasopressin and Oxytocin Research. Amsterdam, Elsevier, 1995, pp 39–54.
26. Nowycky MC, Seward EP, Chernevskaya NI. Excitation-secretion coupling in mammalian neurohypophysial nerve terminals. Cell Mol Neurobiol 1998; 18:65–80.
27. Giovannucci DR, Stuenkel EL. Regulation of secretory granule recruitment and exocytosis at rat neurohypophysial nerve endings. J Physiol (Lond) 1997; 498:735–751.
28. Herman JP, Schafer MK, Watson SJ, et al. In situ hybridization analysis of arginine vasopressin gene transcription using intron-specific probes. Mol Endocrinol 1991; 5:1447–1456.
29. Majzoub JA, Rich A, van Boom J, et al. Vasopressin and oxytocin mRNA regulation in the rat assessed by hybridization with synthetic oligonucleotides. J Biol Chem 1983; 258:14061–14064.
30. Majzoub JA. Vasopressin biosynthesis. In Schrier RW (ed). Vasopressin. New York, Raven Press, 1985, pp 465–474.
31. Sherman TG, Akil H, Watson SJ. Vasopressin mRNA expression: a northern and in situ hybridization analysis. In Schrier RW (ed). Vasopressin. New York, Raven Press, 1985, pp 475–483.
32. Zingg HH, Lefebvre D, Almazan G. Regulation of vasopressin gene expression in rat hypothalamic neurons: response to osmotic stimulation. J Biol Chem 1986; 261:12956–12959.
33. Robinson AG, Roberts MM, Evron WA, et al. Hyponatremia in rats induces downregulation of vasopressin synthesis. J Clin Invest 1990; 86:1023–1029.
34. Porter KR. Cytoplasmic microtubules and their functions. In Wolstenholme GEW, O'Conner M (eds). Principles of Biomolecular Organization. Boston, Little, Brown, 1966, pp 308–356.
35. Roberts MM, Robinson AG, Hoffman GE, et al. Vasopressin transport regulation is coupled to the synthesis rate. Neuroendocrinology 1991; 53:416–422.
36. Lederis K, Jayasena K. Storage of neurohypophysial hormones and the mechanism for their release. In Heller H, Pickering BT (eds). Pharmacology of the Endocrine System and Related Drugs. London, Pergamon, 1970, pp 111–154.
37. Jones CW, Pickering BT. Comparison of the effects of water deprivation and sodium chloride imbibition on the hormone content of the neurohypophysis of the rat. J Physiol (Lond) 1969; 203:449–458.
38. Robinson AG, Fitsimmons MD, Roberts MM, et al. Steadily increasing posterior pituitary vasopressin content in the rat is related to aging not to weight. Endocrinol Soc Abstr 1991; 43: 139.
39. Zingg HH, Lefebvre DL, Almazan G. Regulation of poly(A) tail size of vasopressin mRNA. J Biol Chem 1988; 263:11041–11043.
40. Sato N, Tanaka S, Tateno M, et al. Origin of posterior pituitary high intensity on T1-weighted magnetic resonance imaging: immunohistochemical, electron microscopic, and magnetic resonance studies of posterior pituitary lobe of dehydrated rabbits. Invest Radiol 1995; 30:567–571.
41. Kurokawa H, Fujisawa I, Nakano Y, et al. Posterior lobe of the pituitary gland: correlation between signal intensity on T1-weighted MR images and vasopressin concentration. Radiology 1998; 207:79–83.
42. Fujisawa I, Asato R, Kawata M, et al. Hyperintense signal of the posterior pituitary on T1-weighted MR images: an experimental study. J Comput Assist Tomogr 1989; 13:371–377.
43. Fitzsimmons MD, Roberts MM, Sherman TG, et al. Models of neurohypophyseal homeostasis. Am J Physiol 1992; 262:R1121–R1130.
44. Pow DV, Morris JF. Dendrites of hypothalamic magnocellular neurons release neurohypophysial peptides by exocytosis. Neuroscience 1989; 32:435–439.
45. Ludwig M, Callahan MF, Neumann I, et al. Systemic osmotic stimulation increases vasopressin and oxytocin release within the supraoptic nucleus. J Neuroendocrinol 1994; 6:369–373.
46. Richard P, Moos F, Dayanithi G, et al. Rhythmic activities of hypothalamic magnocellular neurons: autocontrol mechanisms. Biol Cell 1997; 89:555–560.

47. Moos F, Gouzenes L, Brown D, et al. New aspects of firing pattern autocontrol in oxytocin and vasopressin neurones. Adv Exp Med Biol 1998; 449:153–162.
48. Meyer C, Freund-Mercier MJ, Guerne Y, et al. Relationship between oxytocin release and amplitude of oxytocin cell neurosecretory bursts during suckling in the rat. J Endocrinol 1987; 114: 263–270.
49. Shaw FD, Bicknell RJ, Dyball RE. Facilitation of vasopressin release from the neurohypophysis by application of electrical stimuli in bursts: relevant stimulation parameters. Neuroendocrinology 1984; 39:371–376.
50. Gouzenes L, Desarmenien MG, Hussy N, et al. Vasopressin regularizes the phasic firing pattern of rat hypothalamic magnocellular vasopressin neurons. J Neurosci 1998; 18:1879–1885.
51. Stern JE, Armstrong WE. Reorganization of the dendritic trees of oxytocin and vasopressin neurons of the rat supraoptic nucleus during lactation. J Neurosci 1998; 18:841–853.
52. Deleuze C, Duvoid A, Hussy N. Properties and glial origin of osmotic-dependent release of taurine from the rat supraoptic nucleus. J Physiol (Lond) 1998; 507:463–471.
53. Theodosis DT, el Majdoubi M, Pierre K, et al. Factors governing activity-dependent structural plasticity of the hypothalamo-neurohypophysial system. Cell Mol Neurobiol 1998; 18:285–298.
54. Theodosis DT, Poulain DA. Contribution of astrocytes to activity-dependent structural plasticity in the adult brain. Adv Exp Med Biol 1999; 468:175–182.
55. Hatton GI. Function-related plasticity in hypothalamus. Annu Rev Neurosci 1997; 20:375–397.
56. Thrasher TN. Baroreceptor regulation of vasopressin and renin secretion: low-pressure versus high-pressure receptors. Front Neuroendocrinol 1994; 15:157–196.
57. Hainsworth R. Reflexes from the heart. Physiol Rev 1991; 71: 617–658.
58. Share L, Levy MN. Cardiovascular receptors and blood titer of antidiuretic hormone. Am J Physiol 1962; 203:425–428.
59. Thames MD, Schmid PG. Cardiopulmonary receptors with vagal afferents tonically inhibit ADH release in the dog. Am J Physiol 1979; 237:H299–H304.
60. Bishop VS, Thames MD, Schmid PG. Effects of bilateral vagal cold block on vasopressin in conscious dogs. Am J Physiol 1984; 246:R566–R569.
61. Blessing WW, Sved AF, Reis DJ. Destruction of noradrenergic neurons in rabbit brainstem elevates plasma vasopressin, causing hypertension. Science 1982; 217:661–663.
62. Sved AF, Blessing WW, Reis DJ. Caudal ventrolateral medulla can alter vasopressin and arterial pressure. Brain Res Bull 1985; 14:227–232.
63. Blessing WW, Sved AF, Reis DJ. Arterial pressure and plasma vasopressin: regulation by neurons in the caudal ventrolateral medulla of the rabbit. Clin Exp Hypertens A 1984; 6:149–156.
64. Schreihofer AM, Stricker EM, Sved AF. Chronic nucleus tractus solitarius lesions do not prevent hypovolemia-induced vasopressin secretion in rats. Am J Physiol 1994; 267:R965–R973.
65. Bie P, Secher NH, Astrup A, et al. Cardiovascular and endocrine responses to head-up tilt and vasopressin infusion in humans. Am J Physiol 1986; 251:R735–R741.
66. Robertson GL. Thirst and vasopressin function in health and disease. Recent Prog Horm Res 1977; 33:333–385.
67. Callahan MF, Ludwig M, Tsai KP, et al. Baroreceptor input regulates osmotic control of central vasopressin secretion. Neuroendocrinology 1997; 65:238–245.
68. Pump B, Gabrielsen A, Christensen NJ, et al. Mechanisms of inhibition of vasopressin release during moderate antiorthostatic posture change in humans. Am J Physiol 1999; 277:R229–R235.
69. Schrier RW, Martin PY. Recent advances in the understanding of water metabolism in heart failure. In Zingg HH, Bourque CW, Bichet DG (eds). Vasopressin and Oxytocin: Molecular, Cellular, and Clinical Advances. New York, Plenum Press, 1998, pp 415–426.
70. Johnson AK, Thunhorst RL. The neuroendocrinology of thirst and salt appetite: visceral sensory signals and mechanisms of central integration. Front Neuroendocrinol 1997; 18:292–353.
71. Baylis PH, Thompson CJ. Osmoregulation of vasopressin secretion and thirst in health and disease. Clin Endocrinol (Oxf) 1988; 29:549–576.
72. Baylis PH. Investigation of suspected hypothalamic diabetes insipidus. Clin Endocrinol (Oxf) 1995; 43:507–510.
73. Borgnia M, Nielsen S, Engel A, et al. Cellular and molecular biology of the aquaporin water channels. Annu Rev Biochem 1999; 68:425–458.
74. Nielsen S, Kwon TH, Christensen BM, et al. Physiology and pathophysiology of renal aquaporins. J Am Soc Nephrol 1999; 10:647–663.
75. Nielsen S, Chou CL, Marples D, et al. Vasopressin increases water permeability of kidney collecting duct by inducing translocation of aquaporin-CD water channels to plasma membrane. Proc Natl Acad Sci USA 1995; 92:1013–1017.
76. DiGiovanni SR, Nielsen S, Christensen EI, et al. Regulation of collecting duct water channel expression by vasopressin in Brattleboro rat. Proc Natl Acad Sci USA 1994; 91:8984–8988.
77. Ecelbarger CA, Terris J, Frindt G, et al. Aquaporin-3 water channel localization and regulation in rat kidney. Am J Physiol 1995; 269:F663–F672.
78. Stocker SD, Sved AF, Stricker EM. Role of renin-angiotensin system in hypotension-evoked thirst: studies with hydralazine. Am J Physiol 2000; 279:R576–R585.
79. Robertson GL. Thirst and vasopressin function in normal and disordered states of water balance. J Lab Clin Med 1983; 101: 351–371.
80. Robertson GL, Berl T. Water metabolism. In Brenner BM, Rector FC Jr (eds). The Kidney, 3rd ed. Philadelphia, WB Saunders, 1986, pp 385–432.
81. Lindheimer MD, Davison JM. Osmoregulation, the secretion of arginine vasopressin and its metabolism during pregnancy. Eur J Endocrinol 1995; 132:133–143.
82. Robinson AG, Fitzsimmons MD. Diabetes insipidus. In Mazzaferri EL, Bar RS, Kreisberg RA (eds). Advances in Endocrinology and Metabolism. St. Louis, Mosby, 1994, pp 261–296.
83. Davison JM, Gilmore EA, Durr J, et al. Altered osmotic thresholds for vasopressin secretion and thirst in human pregnancy. Am J Physiol 1984; 246:F105–F109.
84. Lindheimer MD, Barron WM. Water metabolism and vasopressin secretion during pregnancy. Baillieres Clin Obstet Gynaecol 1994; 8:311–331.
85. Barron WM, Stamoutsos BA, Lindheimer MD. Role of volume in the regulation of vasopressin secretion during pregnancy in the rat. J Clin Invest 1984; 73:923–932.
86. Davison JM, Shiells EA, Philips PR, et al. Influence of humoral and volume factors on altered osmoregulation of normal human pregnancy. Am J Physiol 1990; 258:F900–F907.
87. Danielson LA, Sherwood OD, Conrad KP. Relaxin is a potent renal vasodilator in conscious rats. J Clin Invest 1999; 103:525–533.
88. Danielson LA, Kercher LJ, Conrad KP. Impact of gender and endothelin on renal vasodilation and hyperfiltration induced by relaxin in conscious rats. Am J Physiol 2000; 279:R1298–R1304.
89. Novak J, Danielson LA, Kerchner LJ, et al. Relaxin is essential for renal vasodilation during pregnancy in conscious rats. J Clin Invest 2001; 107:1469–1475.
90. Davison JM, Sheills EA, Barron WM, et al. Changes in the metabolic clearance of vasopressin and in plasma vasopressinase throughout human pregnancy. J Clin Invest 1989; 83:1313–1318.
91. Stout NR, Kenny RA, Baylis PH. A review of water balance in ageing in health and disease. Gerontology 1999; 45:61–66.
92. Davies I. Ageing in the hypothalamo-neurohypophysial-renal system. Compr Gerontol [C] 1987; 1:12–23.
93. Davis PJ, Davis FB. Water excretion in the elderly. Endocrinol Metab Clin North Am 1987; 16:867–875.
94. Fulop T Jr, Worum I, Csongor J, et al. Body composition in elderly people. II. Comparison of measured and predicted body composition in healthy elderly subjects. Gerontology 1985; 31: 150–157.
95. Schultz C, Koppers D, Braak H, et al. Cytoskeletal alterations in the aged human neurohypophysis. Neurosci Lett 1997; 237:93–96.
96. Hofman MA, Goudsmit E, Purba JS, et al. Morphometric analysis of the supraoptic nucleus in the human brain. J Anat 1990; 172:259–270.
97. Hofman MA. Lifespan changes in the human hypothalamus. Exp Gerontol 1997; 32:559–575.
98. Goudsmit E, Neijmeijer-Leloux A, Swaab DF. The human hypothalamo-neurohypophyseal system in relation to development, aging and Alzheimer's disease. Prog Brain Res 1992; 93:237–247.

99. Johnson AG, Crawford GA, Kelly D, et al. Arginine vasopressin and osmolality in the elderly. J Am Geriatr Soc 1994; 42:399–404.
100. Faull CM, Holmes C, Baylis PH. Water balance in elderly people: is there a deficiency of vasopressin? Age Ageing 1993; 22(2): 114–120.
101. Phillips PA, Bretherton M, Johnston CI, et al. Reduced osmotic thirst in healthy elderly men. Am J Physiol 1991; 261:R166–R171.
102. Davies I, O'Neill PA, McLean KA, et al. Age-associated alterations in thirst and arginine vasopressin in response to a water or sodium load. Age Ageing 1995; 24(2):151–159.
103. Ayus JC, Arieff AI. Abnormalities of water metabolism in the elderly. Semin Nephrol 1996; 16:277–288.
104. Terano T, Seya A, Tamura Y, et al. Characteristics of the pituitary gland in elderly subjects from magnetic resonance images: relationship to pituitary hormone secretion. Clin Endocrinol (Oxf) 1996; 45:273–279.
105. Phillips PA, Johnston CI, Gray L. Disturbed fluid and electrolyte homoeostasis following dehydration in elderly people. Age Ageing 1993; 22:S26–S33.
106. Takamata A, Ito T, Yaegashi K, et al. Effect of an exercise-heat acclimation program on body fluid regulatory responses to dehydration in older men. Am J Physiol 1999; 277:R1041–R1050.
107. Kugler JP, Hustead T. Hyponatremia and hypernatremia in the elderly. Am Fam Physician 2000; 61:3623–3630.
108. Crowe MJ, Forsling ML, Rolls BJ, et al. Altered water excretion in healthy elderly men. Age Ageing 1987; 16:285–293.
109. Phillips PA, Bretherton M, Risvanis J, et al. Effects of drinking on thirst and vasopressin in dehydrated elderly men. Am J Physiol 1993; 264:R877–R881.
110. Roberts MM, Robinson AG. Hyponatremia in the elderly. Geriatr Nephrol Urol 1993; 3:43–50.
111. Hoffman NB. Dehydration in the elderly: insidious and manageable. Geriatrics 1991; 46(6):35–38.
112. Miller M, Dalakos T, Moses AM, et al. Recognition of partial defects in antidiuretic hormone secretion. Ann Intern Med 1970; 73:721–729.
113. Baylis PH, Cheetham T. Diabetes insipidus. Arch Dis Child 1998; 79:84–89.
114. Robertson GL. Diabetes insipidus. Endocrinol Metab Clin North Am 1995; 24:549–572.
115. Zerbe RL, Robertson GL. A comparison of plasma vasopressin measurements with a standard indirect test in the differential diagnosis of polyuria. N Engl J Med 1981; 305:1539–1546.
116. De Bellis A, Colao A, Di Salle F, et al. A longitudinal study of vasopressin cell antibodies, posterior pituitary function, and magnetic resonance imaging evaluations in subclinical autoimmune central diabetes insipidus. J Clin Endocrinol Metab 1999; 84: 3047–3051.
117. Baylis PH. Diabetes insipidus. J R Coll Physicians Lond 1998; 32:108–111.
118. Bononi PL, Robinson AG. Central diabetes insipidus: management in the postoperative period. Endocrinologist 1991; 1(3): 180–185.
119. Salata RA, Verbalis JG, Robinson AG. Cold water stimulation of oropharyngeal receptors in man inhibits release of vasopressin. J Clin Endocrinol Metab 1987; 65:561–567.
120. Decaux G, Prospert F, Namias B, et al. Hyperuricemia as a clue for central diabetes insipidus (lack of V1 effect) in the differential diagnosis of polydipsia. Am J Med 1997; 103:376–382.
121. Arslan A, Karaarslan E, Dincer A. High intensity signal of the posterior pituitary: a study with horizontal direction of frequency-encoding and fat suppression MR techniques. Acta Radiol 1999; 40(2):142–145.
122. Tien R, Kucharczyk J, Kucharczyk W. MR imaging of the brain in patients with diabetes insipidus. AJNR 1991; 12:533–542.
123. Moses AM, Clayton B, Hochhauser L. Use of T1-weighted MR imaging to differentiate between primary polydipsia and central diabetes insipidus. AJNR 1992; 13:1273–1277.
124. Gudinchet F, Brunelle F, Barth MO, et al. MR imaging of the posterior hypophysis in children. Am J Nucl Radiol 1989; 10: 511–514.
125. Brooks BS, el Gammal T, Allison JD, et al. Frequency and variation of the posterior pituitary bright signal on MR images. AJNR 1989; 10:943–948.
126. Fujisawa I, Murakami N, Furuto-Kato S, et al. Plasma and neurohypophyseal content of vasopressin in diabetes mellitus. J Clin Endocrinol Metab 1996; 81:2805–2809.
127. Ozata M, Tayfun C, Kurtaran K, et al. Magnetic resonance imaging of posterior pituitary for evaluation of the neurohypophyseal function in idiopathic and autosomal dominant neurohypophyseal diabetes insipidus. Eur Radiol 1997; 7:1098–1102.
128. Sato N, Ishizaka H, Yagi H, et al. Posterior lobe of the pituitary in diabetes insipidus: dynamic MR imaging. Radiology 1993; 186: 357–360.
129. Maghnie M, Genovese E, Bernasconi S, et al. Persistent high MR signal of the posterior pituitary gland in central diabetes insipidus. AJNR 1997; 18:1749–1752.
130. Miyamoto S, Sasaki N, Tanabe Y. Magnetic resonance imaging in familial central diabetes insipidus. Neuroradiology 1991; 33: 272–273.
131. Dohanics J, Hoffman GE, Verbalis JG. Chronic hyponatremia reduces survival of magnocellular vasopressin and oxytocin neurons after axonal injury. J Neurosci 1996; 16:2373–2380.
132. Robinson AG, Haluszczak C, Wilkins JA, et al. Physiologic control of two neurophysins in humans. J Clin Endocrinol Metab 1977; 44:330–339.
133. Maghnie M, Villa A, Arico M, et al. Correlation between magnetic resonance imaging of posterior pituitary and neurohypophyseal function in children with diabetes insipidus. J Clin Endocrinol Metab 1992; 74:795–800.
134. Heinbecker P, White HL. Hypothalamico-hypophysial system and its relation to water balance in the dog. Am J Physiol 1944; 133:582–593.
135. Verbalis JG, Robinson AG, Moses AM. Postoperative and posttraumatic diabetes insipidus. In Czernichow P, Robinson AG (eds). Diabetes Insipidus in Man. Basel, Karger, 1985, pp 247–265.
136. Bonneville JF, Cattin F, Dietemann JL. The pituitary stalk. In Bonneville JF (ed). Computed Tomography of the Pituitary Gland. New York, Springer-Verlag, 1986, pp 106–114.
137. Leger J, Velasquez A, Garel C, et al. Thickened pituitary stalk on magnetic resonance imaging in children with central diabetes insipidus. J Clin Endocrinol Metab 1999; 84:1954–1960.
138. Maghnie M, Bossi G, Klersy C, et al. Dynamic endocrine testing and magnetic resonance imaging in the long-term follow-up of childhood Langerhans cell histiocytosis. J Clin Endocrinol Metab 1998; 83:3089–3094.
139. Rosete A, Cabral AR, Kraus A, et al. Diabetes insipidus secondary to Wegener's granulomatosis: report and review of the literature. J Rheumatol 1991; 18:761–765.
140. Ahmed SR, Aiello DP, Page R, et al. Necrotizing infundibulohypophysitis: a unique syndrome of diabetes insipidus and hypopituitarism. J Clin Endocrinol Metab 1993; 76:1499–1504.
141. Pomarede R, Chernichow P, Brauner R, et al. Intracranial germinoma in children and diabetes insipidus: clinical description and search for tumor markers. In Czernichow P, Robinson AG (eds). Diabetes Insipidus in Man. Basel, Karger, 1985, pp 240–246.
142. Czernichow P, Garel C, Leger J. Thickened pituitary stalk on magnetic resonance imaging in children with central diabetes insipidus. Horm Res 2000; 53(Suppl 3):61–64.
143. Daniel PM, Prichard MM. Regeneration of hypothalamic nerve fibres after hypophysectomy in the goat. Acta Endocrinol (Copenh) 1970; 64:696–704.
144. Lipsett MB, MacLean IP, West CD, et al. An analysis of the polyurea induced by hypophysectomy in the goat. J Clin Endocrinol Metab 1956; 16:183–195.
145. el Gammal T, Brooks BS, Hoffman WH. MR imaging of the ectopic bright signal of posterior pituitary regeneration. AJNR 1989; 10:323–328.
146. Siggaard C, Rittig S, Corydon TJ, et al. Clinical and molecular evidence of abnormal processing and trafficking of the vasopressin preprohormone in a large kindred with familial neurohypophyseal diabetes insipidus due to a signal peptide mutation. J Clin Endocrinol Metab 1999; 84:2933–2941.
147. Baylis PH, Robertson GL. Vasopressin function in familial cranial diabetes insipidus. Postgrad Med J 1981; 57:36–40.
148. Grant FD, Ahmadi A, Hosley CM, et al. Two novel mutations of the vasopressin gene associated with familial diabetes insipidus and identification of an asymptomatic carrier infant. J Clin Endocrinol Metab 1998; 83:3958–3964.

149. McLeod JF, Kovacs L, Gaskill MB, et al. Familial neurohypophyseal diabetes insipidus associated with a signal peptide mutation. J Clin Endocrinol Metab 1993; 77:599A–599G.
150. Gagliardi PC, Bernasconi S, Repaske DR. Autosomal dominant neurohypophyseal diabetes insipidus associated with a missense mutation encoding Gly23Val in neurophysin II. J Clin Endocrinol Metab 1997; 82:3643–3646.
151. Rutishauser J, Boni-Schnetzler M, Boni J, et al. A novel point mutation in the translation initiation codon of the pre-pro-vasopressin–neurophysin II gene: cosegregation with morphological abnormalities and clinical symptoms in autosomal dominant neurohypophyseal diabetes insipidus. J Clin Endocrinol Metab 1996; 81:192–198.
152. Fujii H, Iida S, Moriwaki K. Familial neurohypophyseal diabetes insipidus associated with a novel mutation in the vasopressin–neurophysin II gene. Int J Mol Med 2000; 5:229–234.
153. Calvo B, Bilbao JR, Rodriguez A, et al. Molecular analysis in familial neurohypophyseal diabetes insipidus: early diagnosis of an asymptomatic carrier. J Clin Endocrinol Metab 1999; 84:3351–3354.
154. Calvo B, Bilbao JR, Urrutia I, et al. Identification of a novel nonsense mutation and a missense substitution in the vasopressin–neurophysin II gene in two Spanish kindreds with familial neurohypophyseal diabetes insipidus. J Clin Endocrinol Metab 1998; 83:995–997.
155. Rittig S, Robertson GL, Siggaard C, et al. Identification of 13 new mutations in the vasopressin–neurophysin II gene in 17 kindreds with familial autosomal dominant neurohypophyseal diabetes insipidus. Am J Hum Genet 1996; 58:107–117.
156. Rutishauser J, Kopp P, Gaskill MB, et al. A novel mutation (R97C) in the neurophysin moiety of prepro-vasopressin–neurophysin II associated with autosomal-dominant neurohypophyseal diabetes insipidus. Mol Genet Metab 1999; 67:89–92.
157. Repaske DR, Medlej R, Gultekin EK, et al. Heterogeneity in clinical manifestation of autosomal dominant neurohypophyseal diabetes insipidus caused by a mutation encoding Ala-1Val in the signal peptide of the arginine vasopressin/neurophysin II/copeptin precursor. J Clin Endocrinol Metab 1997; 82:51–56.
158. Repaske DR, Summar ML, Krishnamani MR, et al. Recurrent mutations in the vasopressin–neurophysin II gene cause autosomal dominant neurohypophyseal diabetes insipidus. J Clin Endocrinol Metab 1996; 81:2328–2334.
159. Repaske DR, Browning JE. A de novo mutation in the coding sequence for neurophysin-II (Pro24Leu) is associated with onset and transmission of autosomal dominant neurohypophyseal diabetes insipidus. J Clin Endocrinol Metab 1994; 79:421–427.
160. Bahnsen U, Oosting P, Swaab DF, et al. A missense mutation in the vasopressin-neurophysin precursor gene cosegregates with human autosomal dominant neurohypophyseal diabetes insipidus. EMBO J 1992; 11:19–23.
161. Heppner C, Kotzka J, Bullmann C, et al. Identification of mutations of the arginine vasopressin–neurophysin II gene in two kindreds with familial central diabetes insipidus. J Clin Endocrinol Metab 1998; 83:693–696.
162. Ueta Y, Taniguchi S, Yoshida A, et al. A new type of familial central diabetes insipidus caused by a single base substitution in the neurophysin II coding region of the vasopressin gene. J Clin Endocrinol Metab 1996; 81:1787–1790.
163. Nagasaki H, Ito M, Yuasa H, et al. Two novel mutations in the coding region for neurophysin-II associated with familial central diabetes insipidus. J Clin Endocrinol Metab 1995; 80:1352–1356.
164. Yuasa H, Ito M, Nagasaki H, et al. Glu-47, which forms a salt bridge between neurophysin-II and arginine vasopressin, is deleted in patients with familial central diabetes insipidus. J Clin Endocrinol Metab 1993; 77:600–604.
165. Ito M, Oiso Y, Murase T, et al. Possible involvement of inefficient cleavage of preprovasopressin by signal peptidase as a cause for familial central diabetes insipidus. J Clin Invest 1993; 91: 2565–2571.
166. Ito M, Mori Y, Oiso Y, et al. A single base substitution in the coding region for neurophysin II associated with familial central diabetes insipidus. J Clin Invest 1991; 87:725–728.
167. Abbes AP, Bruggeman B, van Den Akker EL, et al. Identification of two distinct mutations at the same nucleotide position, concomitantly with a novel polymorphism in the vasopressin–neurophysin II gene (AVP-NP II) in two Dutch families with familial neurohypophyseal diabetes insipidus. Clin Chem 2000; 46:1699–1702.
168. Krishnamani MR, Phillips JA III, Copeland KC. Detection of a novel arginine vasopressin defect by dideoxy fingerprinting. J Clin Endocrinol Metab 1993; 77:596–598.
169. Willcutts MD, Felner E, White PC. Autosomal recessive familial neurohypophyseal diabetes insipidus with continued secretion of mutant weakly active vasopressin. Hum Mol Genet 1999; 8: 1303–1307.
170. Braverman LE, Mancini JP, McGoldrick DM. Hereditary idiopathic diabetes insipidus: a case report with autopsy findings. Ann Intern Med 1965; 63:503–508.
171. Bergeron C, Kovacs K, Ezrin C, et al. Hereditary diabetes insipidus: an immunohistochemical study of the hypothalamus and pituitary gland. Acta Neuropathol (Berl) 1991; 81:345–348.
172. Nagai I, Li CH, Hsieh SM, et al. Two cases of hereditary diabetes insipidus, with an autopsy finding in one. Acta Endocrinol (Copenh) 1984; 105:318–323.
173. Forssman H. On hereditary diabetes insipidus with special regard to a sex-linked form. Acta Med Scand Suppl 1945; 159:1–196.
174. Olias G, Richter D, Schmale H. Heterologous expression of human vasopressin-neurophysin precursors in a pituitary cell line: defective transport of a mutant protein from patients with familial diabetes insipidus. DNA Cell Biol 1996; 15:929–935.
175. Ito M, Jameson JL, Ito M. Molecular basis of autosomal dominant neurohypophyseal diabetes insipidus: cellular toxicity caused by the accumulation of mutant vasopressin precursors within the endoplasmic reticulum. J Clin Invest 1997; 99:1897–1905.
176. Si-Hoe S, De Bree FM, Nijenhuis M, et al. Endoplasmic reticulum derangement in hypothalamic neurons of rats expressing a familial neurohypophyseal diabetes insipidus mutant vasopressin transgene. FASEB J 2000; 14:1680–1684.
177. Moses AM. Clinical and laboratory observations in the adult with diabetes insipidus and related syndromes. In Czernichow P, Robinson AG (eds). Diabetes Insipidus in Man. Basel, Karger, 1985, pp 156–175.
178. Sklar CA, Grumbach MM, Kaplan SL, et al. Hormonal and metabolic abnormalities associated with central nervous system germinoma in children and adolescents and the effect of therapy: report of 10 patients. J Clin Endocrinol Metab 1981; 52:9–16.
179. Pomarede R, Czernichow P, Finidori J, et al. Endocrine aspects and tumoral markers in intracranial germinoma: an attempt to delineate the diagnostic procedure in 14 patients. J Pediatr 1982; 101:374–378.
180. Carella C, Rotondi M, Del Buono A, et al. Diabetes insipidus and increased serum levels of leptin and lactate- dehydrogenase (LDH) in an adolescent boy with a primary intracranial germinoma: case report and an endocrinological revaluation of literature. J Endocrinol Invest 1999; 22:558–561.
181. Saeki N, Uchida D, Tatsuno I, et al. MRI detection of suprasellar germinoma causing central diabetes insipidus. Endocr J 1999; 46:263–267.
182. Cho DY, Wang YC, Ho WL. Primary intrasellar mixed germ-cell tumor with precocious puberty and diabetes insipidus. Childs Nerv Syst 1997; 13:42–46.
183. Tarng DC, Huang TP. Diabetes insipidus as an early sign of pineal tumor. Am J Nephrol 1995; 15:161–164.
184. Czernichow P, Pomarede R, Brauner R, et al. Neurogenic diabetes insipidus in children. In Czernichow P, Robinson AG (eds). Diabetes Insipidus in Man. Basel, Karger, 1985, pp 190–209.
185. Max MB, Deck MD, Rottenberg DA. Pituitary metastasis: incidence in cancer patients and clinical differentiation from pituitary adenoma. Neurology 1981; 31:998–1002.
186. Kovacs K. Metastatic cancer of the pituitary gland. Oncology 1983; 27:533–542.
187. Marinella MA. Metastatic adenocarcinoma presenting with central diabetes insipidus. Tumori 1998; 84:85–86.
188. Koshimoto Y, Maeda M, Naiki H, et al. MR of pituitary metastasis in a patient with diabetes insipidus. AJNR 1995; 16(4 Suppl):971–974.
189. Van de Velde A, Wassenaar H, Strubbe A, et al. Metastatic breast cancer presenting with diabetes insipidus. JBR -BTR 2000; 83(2):68–70.
190. Matsuda R, Chiba E, Kawana I, et al. Central diabetes insipidus caused by pituitary metastasis of lung cancer. Intern Med 1995; 34:913–918.

191. Nelson PB, Robinson AG, Martinez AJ. Metastatic tumor of the pituitary gland. Neurosurgery 1987; 21:941–944.
192. Huinink DT, Veltman GA, Huizinga TW, et al. Diabetes insipidus in metastatic cancer: two case reports with review of the literature. Ann Oncol 2000; 11:891–895.
193. Salpietro FM, Romano A, Alafaci C, et al. Pituitary metastasis from uterine cervical carcinoma: a case presenting as diabetes insipidus. Br J Neurosurg 2000; 14:156–159.
194. Breidert M, Schimmelpfennig C, Kittner T, et al. Diabetes insipidus in a patient with a highly malignant B-cell lymphoma and stomatitis. Exp Clin Endocrinol Diabetes 2000; 108:54–58.
195. Merlo EM, Maiolo A, Brocchieri A, et al. Hypophyseal non-Hodgkin's lymphoma presenting with diabetes insipidus: a case report. J Neurooncol 1999; 42:69–72.
196. Agarwal S, Gockerman JP, Aldous MD, et al. Primary central nervous system lymphoma, presenting as diabetes insipidus, as a sequela of hepatitis C (letter). Am J Med 1999; 107:303–304.
197. Balmaceda CM, Fetell MR, Selman JE, et al. Diabetes insipidus as first manifestation of primary central nervous system lymphoma. Neurology 1994; 44:358–359.
198. Ramsahoye BH, Griffiths DF, Whittaker JA. Angiocentric T-cell lymphoma associated with diabetes insipidus (letter). Eur J Haematol 1996; 56:100–103.
199. Castagnola C, Morra E, Bernasconi P, et al. Acute myeloid leukemia and diabetes insipidus: results in 5 patients. Acta Haematol 1995; 93:1–4.
200. Foresti V, Casati O, Villa A, et al. Central diabetes insipidus due to acute monocytic leukemia: case report and review of the literature. J Endocrinol Invest 1992; 15:127–130.
201. Ra'anani P, Shpilberg O, Berezin M, et al. Acute leukemia relapse presenting as central diabetes insipidus. Cancer 1994; 73: 2312–2316.
202. Dilek I, Uysal A, Demirer T, et al. Acute myeloblastic leukemia associated with hyperleukocytosis and diabetes insipidus. Leuk Lymphoma 1998; 30:657–660.
203. Nieboer P, Vellenga E, Adriaanse R, et al. Central diabetes insipidus preceding acute myeloid leukemia with t(3;12)(q26;p12). Neth J Med 2000; 56(2):45–47.
204. Yen CC, Tzeng CH, Liu JH, et al. Acute myelomonocytic leukemia preceded by secondary amenorrhea and presenting with central diabetes insipidus: a case report. Chung Hua I Hsueh Tsa Chih 1997; 60:213–218.
205. Kanabar DJ, Betts DR, Gibbons B, et al. Monosomy 7, diabetes insipidus and acute myeloid leukemia in childhood. Pediatr Hematol Oncol 1994; 11:111–114.
206. Endo T, Tamai Y, Takami H, et al. Acute myeloid leukaemia with trilineage myelodysplasia complicated by masked diabetes insipidus. Clin Lab Haematol 2000; 22:233–235.
207. Mozersky RP, Bahl VK, Meisner D, et al. Diabetes insipidus, acute myelogenous leukemia, and monosomy 7. J Am Osteopath Assoc 1996; 96(2):116–118.
208. Buonocore CM, Robinson AG. The diagnosis and management of diabetes insipidus during medical emergencies. Endocrinol Metab Clin North Am 1993; 22:411–423.
209. Huang YS, Dellmann HD. Chronic intermittent salt loading enhances functional recovery from polydipsia and survival of vasopressinergic cells in the hypothalamic supraoptic nucleus following transection of the hypophysial stalk. Brain Res 1996; 732:95–105.
210. Alonso G, Bribes E, Chauvet N. Survival and regeneration of neurons of the supraoptic nucleus following surgical transection of neurohypophysial axons depend on the existence of collateral projections of these neurons to the dorsolateral hypothalamus. Brain Res 1996; 711:34–43.
211. Dellmann HD, Carithers J. Development of neural lobe–like neurovascular contact regions after intrahypothalamic transection of the hypothalamo-neurohypophysial tract. Brain Res 1992; 585: 19–27.
212. Scott DE, Wu W, Slusser J, et al. Neural regeneration and neuronal migration following injury. I. The endocrine hypothalamus and neurohypophyseal system. Exp Neurol 1995; 131:23–38.
213. Chauvet N, Parmentier ML, Alonso G. Transected axons of adult hypothalamo-neurohypophysial neurons regenerate along tanycytic processes. J Neurosci Res 1995; 41:129–144.
214. Cusick JF, Hagen TC, Findling JW. Inappropriate secretion of antidiuretic hormone after transsphenoidal surgery for pituitary tumors. N Engl J Med 1984; 311:36–38.
215. Ultmann MC, Hoffman GE, Nelson PB, et al. Transient hyponatremia after damage to the neurohypophyseal tracts. Neuroendocrinology 1992; 56:803–811.
216. Olson BR, Rubino D, Gumowski J, et al. Isolated hyponatremia after transsphenoidal pituitary surgery. J Clin Endocrinol Metab 1995; 80:85–91.
217. Olson BR, Gumowski J, Rubino D, et al. Pathophysiology of hyponatremia after transsphenoidal pituitary surgery. J Neurosurg 1997; 87:499–507.
218. Hensen J, Henig A, Fahlbusch R, et al. Prevalence, predictors and patterns of postoperative polyuria and hyponatraemia in the immediate course after transsphenoidal surgery for pituitary adenomas. Clin Endocrinol (Oxf) 1999; 50:431–439.
219. Benvenga S, Campenni A, Ruggeri RM, et al. Clinical review 113: hypopituitarism secondary to head trauma. J Clin Endocrinol Metab 2000; 85:1353–1361.
220. Goldman KP, Jacobs A. Anterior and posterior pituitary failure after head injury. Br Med J 1960; 5217:1924–1926.
221. Daniel PM, Treip C. The pathology of the pituitary gland in head injury. In Gardiner-Hill H (ed). Modern Trends in Endocrinology. New York, Hoeber, 1961, pp 55–69.
222. Mandell IN, DeFronzo RA, Robertson GL, et al. Role of plasma arginine vasopressin in the impaired water diuresis of isolated glucocorticoid deficiency in the rat. Kidney Int 1980; 17:186–195.
223. Linas SL, Berl T, Robertson GL, et al. Role of vasopressin in the impaired water excretion of glucocorticoid deficiency. Kidney Int 1980; 18:58–67.
224. Moses AM. Long-standing posttraumatic diabetes insipidus. Medical Grand Rounds. New York, Plenum Publishing, 1983, pp 117–128.
225. Rami B, Schneider U, Wandl-Vergesslich K, et al. Primary hypothyroidism, central diabetes insipidus and growth hormone deficiency in multisystem Langerhans cell histiocytosis: a case report. Acta Paediatr 1998; 87:112–114.
226. Proietto G, Amatetti M, Amerio P, et al. Langerhans cell histiocytosis associated with diabetes insipidus: magnetic resonance imaging. Int J Dermatol 1996; 35:730–732.
227. Broadbent V, Pritchard J. Diabetes insipidus associated with Langerhans cell histiocytosis: is it reversible?. Med Pediatr Oncol 1997; 28:289–293.
228. Minehan KJ, Chen MG, Zimmerman D, et al. Radiation therapy for diabetes insipidus caused by Langerhans cell histiocytosis. Int J Radiat Oncol Biol Phys 1992; 23:519–524.
229. Grois N, Flucher-Wolfram B, Heitger A, et al. Diabetes insipidus in Langerhans cell histiocytosis: results from the DAL-HX 83 study. Med Pediatr Oncol 1995; 24:248–256.
230. Lin KD, Lin JD, Hsu HH, et al. Endocrinological aspects of Langerhans cell histiocytosis complicated with diabetes insipidus. J Endocrinol Invest 1998; 21:428–433.
231. Dunger DB, Broadbent V, Yeoman E, et al. The frequency and natural history of diabetes insipidus in children with Langerhans-cell histiocytosis. N Engl J Med 1989; 321:1157–1162.
232. Hoeger PH, Janka-Schaub G, Mensing H. Late manifestation of diabetes insipidus in "pure" cutaneous Langerhans cell histiocytosis. Eur J Pediatr 1997; 156:524–527.
233. Weston WL, Travers SH, Mierau GW, et al. Benign cephalic histiocytosis with diabetes insipidus. Pediatr Dermatol 2000; 17: 296–298.
234. Catalina PF, Rodr'iguez GM, de la Torre C, et al. Diabetes insipidus for five years preceding the diagnosis of hypothalamic Langerhans cell histiocytosis. J Endocrinol Invest 1995; 18:663–666.
235. Tien RD. Intraventricular mass lesions of the brain: CT and MR findings. AJR 1991; 157:1283–1290.
236. Rosenfield NS, Abrahams J, Komp D. Brain MR in patients with Langerhans cell histiocytosis: findings and enhancement with Gd-DTPA. Pediatr Radiol 1990; 20:433–436.
237. Maghnie M, Genovese E, Arico M, et al. Evolving pituitary hormone deficiency is associated with pituitary vasculopathy: dynamic MR study in children with hypopituitarism, diabetes insipidus, and Langerhans cell histiocytosis. Radiology 1994; 193:493–499.
238. Ercan O, Hatemi S, Kutlu E, et al. 'Diabetes insipidus associated with Langerhans cell histiocytosis: is it reversible? (Broadbent and Pritchard, Med Pediatr Oncol 28:289–293)' (letter; comment). Med Pediatr Oncol 1998; 30:197–198.

239. Rosenzweig KE, Arceci RJ, Tarbell NJ. Diabetes insipidus secondary to Langerhans' cell histiocytosis: is radiation therapy indicated? Med Pediatr Oncol 1997; 29:36–40.
240. Nishino H, Rubino FA, DeRemee RA, et al.: Neurological involvement in Wegener's granulomatosis: an analysis of 324 consecutive patients at the Mayo Clinic. Ann Neurol 1993; 33:4–9.
241. Hoffman GS, Kerr GS, Leavitt RY, et al. Wegener granulomatosis: an analysis of 158 patients. Ann Intern Med 1992; 116:488–498.
242. Miesen WM, Janssens EN, van Bommel EF. Diabetes insipidus as the presenting symptom of Wegener's granulomatosis. Nephrol Dial Transplant 1999; 14:426–429.
243. Hama S, Arita K, Kurisu K, et al. Parasellar chronic inflammatory disease presenting Tolosa-Hunt syndrome, hypopituitarism and diabetes insipidus: a case report. Endocr J 1996; 43:503–510.
244. Czarnecki EJ, Spickler EM. MR demonstration of Wegener granulomatosis of the infundibulum, a cause of diabetes insipidus. AJNR 1995; 16(4 Suppl):968–970.
245. Hajj-Ali RA, Uthman IW, Salti IA, et al. Wegener's granulomatosis and diabetes insipidus (letter). Rheumatology (Oxf) 1999; 38:684–685.
246. Rossi GP, Pavan E, Chiesura-Corona M, et al. Bronchocentric granulomatosis and central diabetes insipidus successfully treated with corticosteroids. Eur Respir J 1994; 7:1893–1898.
247. van der Lee I, Slee PH, Elbers JR. A patient with diabetes insipidus and periorbital swellings; Erdheim-Chester disease. Neth J Med 1999; 55:76–79.
248. Hoshimaru M, Hashimoto N, Kikuchi H. Central diabetes insipidus resulting from a nonneoplastic tiny mass lesion localized in the neurohypophyseal system. Surg Neurol 1992; 38:1–6.
249. Scott TF. Neurosarcoidosis: progress and clinical aspects. Neurology 1993; 43:8–12.
250. Stern BJ, Krumholz A, Johns C, et al. Sarcoidosis and its neurological manifestations. Arch Neurol 1985; 42:909–917.
251. Oksanen V. Neurosarcoidosis: clinical presentations and course in 50 patients. Acta Neurol Scand 1986; 73:283–290.
252. Bullmann C, Faust M, Hoffmann A, et al. Five cases with central diabetes insipidus and hypogonadism as first presentation of neurosarcoidosis. Eur J Endocrinol 2000; 142:365–372.
253. Loh KC, Green A, Dillon WP Jr, et al. Diabetes insipidus from sarcoidosis confined to the posterior pituitary. Eur J Endocrinol 1997; 137:514–519.
254. Oksanen V, Gronhagen-Riska C, Fyhrquist F, et al. Systemic manifestations and enzyme studies in sarcoidosis with neurologic involvement. Acta Med Scand 1985; 218:123–127.
255. Chapelon C, Ziza JM, Piette JC, et al. Neurosarcoidosis: signs, course and treatment in 35 confirmed cases. Medicine (Baltimore) 1990; 69:261–276.
256. Bell NH. Endocrine complications of sarcoidosis. Endocrinol Metab Clin North Am 1991; 20:645–654.
257. Maghnie M, Cosi G, Genovese E, et al. Central diabetes insipidus in children and young adults. N Engl J Med 2000; 343:998–1007.
258. Scherbaum WA, Bottazzo GF, Czernichow P, et al. Role of autoimmunity in central diabetes insipidus. In Czernichow P, Robinson AG (eds). Diabetes Insipidus in Man. Basel, Karger, 1985, pp 232–239.
259. Scherbaum WA, Wass JA, Besser GM, et al. Autoimmune cranial diabetes insipidus: its association with other endocrine diseases and with histiocytosis X. Clin Endocrinol (Oxf) 1986; 25:411–420.
260. Kojima H, Nojima T, Nagashima K, et al. Diabetes insipidus caused by lymphocytic infundibuloneurohypophysitis. Arch Pathol Lab Med 1989; 113:1399–1401.
261. Van Havenbergh T, Robberecht W, Wilms G, et al. Lymphocytic infundibulohypophysitis presenting in the postpartum period: case report. Surg Neurol 1996; 46:280–284.
262. Nishioka H, Ito H, Sano T, et al. Two cases of lymphocytic hypophysitis presenting with diabetes insipidus: a variant of lymphocytic infundibulo-neurohypophysitis. Surg Neurol 1996; 46: 285–290.
263. Imura H, Nakao K, Shimatsu A, et al. Lymphocytic infundibuloneurohypophysitis as a cause of central diabetes insipidus. N Engl J Med 1993; 329:683–689.
264. Tsujii S, Takeuchi J, Koh M, et al. A candidate case for lymphocytic infundibulo-neurohypophysitis mimicking a neurohypophysial tumor. Intern Med 1997; 36:293–297.
265. Takahashi M, Otsuka F, Miyoshi T, et al. An elderly patient with transient diabetes insipidus associated with lymphocytic infundibulo-neurohypophysitis. Endocr J 1999; 46:741–746.
266. Hashimoto K, Takao T, Makino S. Lymphocytic adenohypophysitis and lymphocytic infundibuloneurohypophysitis. Endocr J 1997; 44:1–10.
267. Thodou E, Asa SL, Kontogeorgos G, et al. Clinical case seminar: lymphocytic hypophysitis: clinicopathological findings. J Clin Endocrinol Metab 1995; 80:2302–2311.
268. Sanchez-Roman J, Castillo-Palma MJ, Ocana MC, et al. Neurogenic diabetes insipidus in patients with systemic lupus erythematosus (letter). Ann Rheum Dis 1998; 57:261–262.
269. Harada M, Yoshida H, Mimura Y, et al. Systemic sclerosis associated with diabetes insipidus. Intern Med 1997; 36:73–76.
270. Tekin N, Kural N, Kocak AK, et al. Diabetes insipidus in a pediatric patient with systemic lupus erythematosus: a case report. Turk J Pediatr 1997; 39:281–284.
271. Jin-No M, Fujii T, Jin-no Y, et al. Central diabetes insipidus with Behçet's disease. Intern Med 1999; 38:995–999.
272. Otsuka F, Amano T, Ogura T, et al. Diabetes insipidus with Behçet's disease (letter). Lancet 1995; 346:1494–1495.
273. Barron WM, Cohen LH, Ulland LA, et al. Transient vasopressin-resistant diabetes insipidus of pregnancy. N Engl J Med 1984; 310:442–444.
274. Durr JA, Hoggard JG, Hunt JM, et al. Diabetes insipidus in pregnancy associated with abnormally high circulating vasopressinase activity. N Engl J Med 1987; 316:1070–1074.
275. Gordge MP, Williams DJ, Huggett NJ, et al. Loss of biological activity of arginine vasopressin during its degradation by vasopressinase from pregnancy serum. Clin Endocrinol (Oxf) 1995; 42:51–58.
276. Durr JA. Diabetes insipidus syndromes of pregnancy. In Cowley AJ, Liard JF, Ausiello DA (eds). Vasopressin: Cellular and Integrative Functions. New York, Raven Press, 1988, pp 257–263.
277. Krege J, Katz VL, Bowes WA Jr. Transient diabetes insipidus of pregnancy. Obstet Gynecol Surv 1989; 44:789–795.
278. Kennedy S, Hall PM, Seymour AE, et al. Transient diabetes insipidus and acute fatty liver of pregnancy. Br J Obstet Gynaecol 1994; 101:387–391.
279. Hashimoto M, Ogura T, Otsuka F, et al. Manifestation of subclinical diabetes insipidus due to pituitary tumor during pregnancy. Endocr J 1996; 43:577–583.
280. Kan AK, Calligerous D. A case report of Sheehan syndrome presenting with diabetes insipidus. Aust NZ J Obstet Gynaecol 1998; 38:224–226.
281. Briet JW. Diabetes insipidus, Sheehan's syndrome and pregnancy. Eur J Obstet Gynecol Reprod Biol 1998; 77:201–203.
282. Leggett DA, Hill PT, Anderson RJ. 'Stalkitis' in a pregnant 32-year-old woman: a rare cause of diabetes insipidus. Australas Radiol 1999; 43:104–107.
283. Enomoto J, Murakami Y, Koshimura K, et al. Unique female case of hypothalamic hypopituitarism associated with MRI abnormalities in the pituitary stalk. Endocr J 1996; 43(Suppl):S141–S143.
284. Amico JA. Diabetes insipidus and pregnancy. In Czernichow P, Robinson AG (eds). Diabetes Insipidus in Man. Basel, Karger, 1985, pp 266–277.
285. Hanson RS, Powrie RO, Larson L. Diabetes insipidus in pregnancy: a treatable cause of oligohydramnios. Obstet Gynecol 1997; 89:816–817.
286. DeRubertis FR, Michelis MF, Beck N, et al. 'Essential' hypernatremia due to ineffective osmotic and intact volume regulation of vasopressin secretion. J Clin Invest 1971; 50:97–111.
287. Halter JB, Goldberg AP, Robertson GL, et al. Selective osmoreceptor dysfunction in the syndrome of chronic hypernatremia. J Clin Endocrinol Metab 1977; 44:609–616.
288. Oh MS, Carroll HJ. Essential hypernatremia: is there such a thing? Nephron 1994; 67:144–145.
289. Lam KS, Sham MM, Tam SC, et al. Hypopituitarism after tuberculous meningitis in childhood. Ann Intern Med 1993; 118: 701–706.
290. Altunbasak S, Baytok V, Alhan E, et al. Suprasellar tuberculoma causing endocrinologic disorders and imitating craniopharyngioma. Pediatr Neurosurg 1995; 23:328–331.
291. Iraci G, Giordano R, Gerosa M, et al. Tuberculoma of the anterior optic pathways: case report. J Neurosurg 1980; 52:129–133.

292. Gramm HJ, Meinhold H, Bickel U, et al. Acute endocrine failure after brain death? Transplantation 1992; 54:851–857.
293. Howlett TA, Keogh AM, Perry L, et al. Anterior and posterior pituitary function in brain-stem-dead donors: a possible role for hormonal replacement therapy. Transplantation 1989; 47:828–834.
294. Wijnen RM, van der Linden CJ. Donor treatment after pronouncement of brain death: a neglected intensive care problem. Transpl Int 1991; 4:186–190.
295. Bittner HB, Kendall SW, Chen EP, et al. Endocrine changes and metabolic responses in a validated canine brain death model. J Crit Care 1995; 10:56–63.
296. Fiser DH, Jimenez JF, Wrape V, et al. Diabetes insipidus in children with brain death. Crit Care Med 1987; 15:551–553.
297. Staworn D, Lewison L, Marks J, et al. Brain death in pediatric intensive care unit patients: incidence, primary diagnosis, and the clinical occurrence of Turner's triad. Crit Care Med 1994; 22:1301–1305.
298. Guesde R, Barrou B, Leblanc I, et al. Administration of desmopressin in brain-dead donors and renal function in kidney recipients. Lancet 1998; 352:1178–1181.
299. Wong MF, Chin NM, Lew TW. Diabetes insipidus in neurosurgical patients. Ann Acad Med Singapore 1998; 27:340–343.
300. Barzilay Z, Somekh E. Diabetes insipidus in severely brain damaged children. J Med 1988; 19:47–64.
301. Stuart CA, Neelon FA, Lebovitz HE. Disordered control of thirst in hypothalamic-pituitary sarcoidosis. N Engl J Med 1980; 303:1078–1082.
302. De Leon J, Dadvand M, Canuso C, et al. Polydipsia and water intoxication in a long-term psychiatric hospital. Biol Psychiatry 1996; 40:28–34.
303. Siegel AJ, Baldessarini RJ, Klepser MB, et al. Primary and drug-induced disorders of water homeostasis in psychiatric patients: principles of diagnosis and management. Harv Rev Psychiatry 1998; 6(4):190–200.
304. Mellinger RC, Zafar MS. Primary polydipsia: syndrome of inappropriate thirst. Arch Intern Med 1983; 143:1249–1251.
305. Kishi Y, Kurosawa H, Endo S: Is propranolol effective in primary polydipsia? Int J Psychiatry Med 1998; 28:315–325.
306. van Lieburg AF, Knoers NV, Monnens LA. Clinical presentation and follow-up of 30 patients with congenital nephrogenic diabetes insipidus. J Am Soc Nephrol 1999; 10:1958–1964.
307. Bichet DG. Nephrogenic diabetes insipidus. Am J Med 1998; 105:431–442.
308. Knoers NV, Monnens LL. Nephrogenic diabetes insipidus. Semin Nephrol 1999; 19:344–352.
309. Di Rocco M, Picco P, Gandullia P, et al. Intracranial calcifications and nephrogenic diabetes insipidus. Eur J Pediatr 1991; 150:599–600.
310. Tohyama J, Inagaki M, Koeda T, et al. Intracranial calcification in siblings with nephrogenic diabetes insipidus: CT and MRI. Neuroradiology 1993; 35:553–555.
311. Wildin RS, Cogdell DE. Clinical utility of direct mutation testing for congenital nephrogenic diabetes insipidus in families. Pediatrics 1999; 103:632–639.
312. Arthus MF, Lonergan M, Crumley MJ, et al. Report of 33 novel *AVPR2* mutations and analysis of 117 families with X-linked nephrogenic diabetes insipidus. J Am Soc Nephrol 2000; 11:1044–1054.
313. Birnbaumer M. Vasopressin receptors. Trends Endocrinol Metab 2000; 11:406–410.
314. Wildin RS, Cogdell DE, Valadez V. *AVPR2* variants and V2 vasopressin receptor function in nephrogenic diabetes insipidus. Kidney Int 1998; 54:1909–1922.
315. Postina R, Ufer E, Pfeiffer R, et al. Misfolded vasopressin V2 receptors caused by extracellular point mutations entail congenital nephrogenic diabetes insipidus. Mol Cell Endocrinol 2000; 164:31–39.
316. Bichet DG, Turner M, Morin D. Vasopressin receptor mutations causing nephrogenic diabetes insipidus. Proc Assoc Am Physicians 1998; 110:387–394.
317. Schulein R, Zuhlke K, Oksche A, et al. The role of conserved extracellular cysteine residues in vasopressin V2 receptor function and properties of two naturally occurring mutant receptors with additional extracellular cysteine residues. FEBS Lett 2000; 466:101–106.
318. Pasel K, Schulz A, Timmermann K, et al. Functional characterization of the molecular defects causing nephrogenic diabetes insipidus in eight families. J Clin Endocrinol Metab 2000; 85:1703–1710.
319. Albertazzi E, Zanchetta D, Barbier P, et al. Nephrogenic diabetes insipidus: functional analysis of new *AVPR2* mutations identified in Italian families. J Am Soc Nephrol 2000; 11:1033–1043.
320. Kamperis K, Siggaard C, Herlin T, et al. A novel splicing mutation in the V2 vasopressin receptor. Pediatr Nephrol 2000; 15:43–49.
321. Sadeghi H, Robertson GL, Bichet DG, et al. Biochemical basis of partial nephrogenic diabetes insipidus phenotypes. Mol Endocrinol 1997; 11:1806–1813.
322. Schoneberg T, Schulz A, Biebermann H, et al. V2 vasopressin receptor dysfunction in nephrogenic diabetes insipidus caused by different molecular mechanisms. Hum Mutat 1998; 12:196–205.
323. Moses AM, Sangani G, Miller JL. Proposed cause of marked vasopressin resistance in a female with an X-linked recessive V2 receptor abnormality. J Clin Endocrinol Metab 1995; 80:1184–1186.
324. Bichet DG, Razi M, Arthus MF, et al. Epinephrine and dDAVP administration in patients with congenital nephrogenic diabetes insipidus: evidence for a pre-cyclic AMP V2 receptor defective mechanism. Kidney Int 1989; 36:859–866.
325. Chan Seem CP, Dossetor JF, Penney MD. Nephrogenic diabetes insipidus due to a new mutation of the arginine vasopressin V2 receptor gene in a girl presenting with non-accidental injury. Ann Clin Biochem 1999; 36:779–782.
326. Deen PM, Knoers NV. Vasopressin type-2 receptor and aquaporin-2 water channel mutants in nephrogenic diabetes insipidus. Am J Med Sci 1998; 316:300–309.
327. Rocha JL, Friedman E, Boson W, et al. Molecular analyses of the vasopressin type 2 receptor and aquaporin-2 genes in Brazilian kindreds with nephrogenic diabetes insipidus. Hum Mutat 1999; 14:233–239.
328. Tamarappoo BK, Yang B, Verkman AS. Misfolding of mutant aquaporin-2 water channels in nephrogenic diabetes insipidus. J Biol Chem 1999; 274:34825–34831.
329. Canfield MC, Tamarappoo BK, Moses AM, et al. Identification and characterization of aquaporin-2 water channel mutations causing nephrogenic diabetes insipidus with partial vasopressin response. Hum Mol Genet 1997; 6:1865–1871.
330. van Os CH, Deen PM. Aquaporin-2 water channel mutations causing nephrogenic diabetes insipidus. Proc Assoc Am Physicians 1998; 110:395–400.
331. Deen PM, Croes H, van Aubel RA, et al. Water channels encoded by mutant aquaporin-2 genes in nephrogenic diabetes insipidus are impaired in their cellular routing. J Clin Invest 1995; 95:2291–2296.
332. Rutishauser J, Kopp P. Aquaporin-2 water channel mutations and nephrogenic diabetes insipidus: new variations on a theme. Eur J Endocrinol 1999; 140:137–139.
333. Mulders SM, Bichet DG, Rijss JP, et al. An aquaporin-2 water channel mutant which causes autosomal dominant nephrogenic diabetes insipidus is retained in the Golgi complex. J Clin Invest 1998; 102:57–66.
334. Saito T, Ishikawa SE, Sasaki S, et al. Urinary excretion of aquaporin-2 in the diagnosis of central diabetes insipidus. J Clin Endocrinol Metab 1997; 82:1823–1827.
335. Sands JM, Naruse M, Jacobs JD, et al. Changes in aquaporin-2 protein contribute to the urine concentrating defect in rats fed a low-protein diet. J Clin Invest 1996; 97:2807–2814.
336. Martin PY, Schrier RW. Role of aquaporin-2 water channels in urinary concentration and dilution defects. Kidney Int Suppl 1998; 65:S57–S62.
337. Frokiaer J, Marples D, Knepper MA, et al. Pathophysiology of aquaporin-2 in water balance disorders. Am J Med Sci 1998; 316:291–299.
338. Kwon TH, Laursen UH, Marples D, et al. Altered expression of renal AQPs and Na^+ transporters in rats with lithium-induced NDI. Am J Physiol 2000; 279:F552–F564.
339. Knepper MA, Verbalis JG, Nielsen S. Role of aquaporins in water balance disorders. Curr Opin Nephrol Hypertens 1997; 6:367–371.
340. Marples D, Christensen S, Christensen EI, et al. Lithium-induced downregulation of aquaporin-2 water channel expression in rat kidney medulla. J Clin Invest 1995; 95:1838–1845.

341. Earm JH, Christensen BM, Frokiaer J, et al. Decreased aquaporin-2 expression and apical plasma membrane delivery in kidney collecting ducts of polyuric hypercalcemic rats. J Am Soc Nephrol 1998; 9:2181–2193.
342. Frokiaer J, Marples D, Knepper MA, et al. Bilateral ureteral obstruction downregulates expression of vasopressin-sensitive AQP-2 water channel in rat kidney. Am J Physiol 1996; 270: F657–F668.
343. Frokiaer J, Christensen BM, Marples D, et al. Downregulation of aquaporin-2 parallels changes in renal water excretion in unilateral ureteral obstruction. Am J Physiol 1997; 273:F213–F223.
344. Peet M, Pratt JP. Lithium: current status in psychiatric disorders. Drugs 1993; 46:7–17.
345. Marples D, Frokiaer J, Knepper MA, et al. Disordered water channel expression and distribution in acquired nephrogenic diabetes insipidus. Proc Assoc Am Physicians 1998; 110:401–406.
346. Bendz H, Sjodin I, Aurell M. Renal function on and off lithium in patients treated with lithium for 15 years or more: a controlled, prospective lithium-withdrawal study. Nephrol Dial Transplant 1996; 11:457–460.
347. Christensen S, Kusano E, Yusufi AN, et al. Pathogenesis of nephrogenic diabetes insipidus due to chronic administration of lithium in rats. J Clin Invest 1985; 75:1869–1879.
348. Kwon SC, Ozaki H, Karaki H. NO donor sodium nitroprusside inhibits excitation-contraction coupling in guinea pig taenia coli. Am J Physiol 2000; 279:G1235–G1241.
349. Markowitz GS, Radhakrishnan J, Kambham N, et al. Lithium nephrotoxicity: a progressive combined glomerular and tubulointerstitial nephropathy. J Am Soc Nephrol 2000; 11:1439–1448.
350. Apostol E, Ecelbarger CA, Terris J, et al. Reduced renal medullary water channel expression in puromycin aminonucleoside-induced nephrotic syndrome. J Am Soc Nephrol 1997; 8:15–24.
351. Navarro JF, Quereda C, Quereda C, et al. Nephrogenic diabetes insipidus and renal tubular acidosis secondary to foscarnet therapy. Am J Kidney Dis 1996; 27:431–434.
352. Fernandez-Llama P, Andrews P, Ecelbarger CA, et al. Concentrating defect in experimental nephrotic syndrome: altered expression of aquaporins and thick ascending limb Na^+ transporters. Kidney Int 1998; 54:170–179.
353. Bendz H, Aurell M. Drug-induced diabetes insipidus: incidence, prevention and management. Drug Saf 1999; 21:449–456.
354. Terris J, Ecelbarger CA, Nielsen S, et al. Long-term regulation of four renal aquaporins in rats. Am J Physiol 1996; 271:F414–F422.
355. Kishore BK, Terris JM, Knepper MA. Quantitation of aquaporin-2 abundance in microdissected collecting ducts: axial distribution and control by AVP. Am J Physiol 1996; 271:F62–F70.
356. Riggs JE. Neurologic manifestations of fluid and electrolyte disturbances. Neurol Clin 1989; 7:509–523.
357. Ross EJ, Christie SB: Hypernatremia. Medicine (Baltimore) 1969; 48:441–473.
358. Adrogue HJ, Madias NE. Hypernatremia. N Engl J Med 2000; 342:1493–1499.
359. Palevsky PM, Bhagrath R, Greenberg A. Hypernatremia in hospitalized patients. Ann Intern Med 1996; 124:197–203.
360. Ng PC, Chan HB, Fok TF, et al. Early onset of hypernatraemic dehydration and fever in exclusively breast-fed infants. J Paediatr Child Health 1999; 35:585–587.
361. Brown WD, Caruso JM. Extrapontine myelinolysis with involvement of the hippocampus in three children with severe hypernatremia. J Child Neurol 1999; 14:428–433.
362. Robinson AG, Verbalis JG. Diabetes insipidus. Curr Ther Endocrinol Metab 1997; 6:1–7.
363. Robinson AG. DDAVP in the treatment of central diabetes insipidus. N Engl J Med 1976; 294:507–511.
364. Richardson DW, Robinson AG: Desmopressin. Ann Intern Med 1985; 103:228–239.
365. Fjellestad A, Czernichow P. Central diabetes insipidus in children. V. Oral treatment with a vasopressin hormone analogue (DDAVP). Acta Paediatr Scand 1986; 75:605–610.
366. Lam KS, Wat MS, Choi KL, et al. Pharmacokinetics, pharmacodynamics, long-term efficacy and safety of oral 1-deamino-8-D-arginine vasopressin in adult patients with central diabetes insipidus. Br J Clin Pharmacol 1996; 42:379–385.
367. Fjellestad-Paulsen A, Hoglund P, Lundin S, et al. Pharmacokinetics of 1-deamino-8-D-arginine vasopressin after various routes of administration in healthy volunteers. Clin Endocrinol (Oxf) 1993; 38:177–182.
368. Francis JD, Leary T, Niblett DJ. Convulsions and respiratory arrest in association with desmopressin administration for the treatment of a bleeding tonsil in a child with borderline haemophilia. Acta Anaesthesiol Scand 1999; 43:870–873.
369. Humphries JE, Siragy H. Significant hyponatremia following DDAVP administration in a healthy adult. Am J Hematol 1993; 44:12–15.
370. Dunn AL, Powers JR, Ribeiro MJ, et al. Adverse events during use of intranasal desmopressin acetate for haemophilia A and von Willebrand disease: a case report and review of 40 patients. Haemophilia 2000; 6:11–14.
371. Bertholini DM, Butler CS. Severe hyponatraemia secondary to desmopressin therapy in von Willebrand's disease. Anaesth Intensive Care 2000; 28:199–201.
372. Apakama DC, Bleetman A. Hyponatraemic convulsion secondary to desmopressin treatment for primary enuresis. J Accid Emerg Med 1999; 16:229–230.
373. Yaouyanc G, Jonville AP, Yaouyanc-Lapalle H, et al. Seizure with hyponatremia in a child prescribed desmopressin for nocturnal enuresis. J Toxicol Clin Toxicol 1992; 30:637–641.
374. Beach PS, Beach RE, Smith LR. Hyponatremic seizures in a child treated with desmopressin to control enuresis: a rational approach to fluid intake. Clin Pediatr (Phila) 1992; 31:566–569.
375. Kallio J, Rautava P, Huupponen R, et al. Severe hyponatremia caused by intranasal desmopressin for nocturnal enuresis. Acta Paediatr 1993; 82:881–882.
376. Schwab M, Wenzel D, Ruder H. Hyponatraemia and cerebral convulsion due to short term DDAVP therapy for control of enuresis nocturna. Eur J Pediatr 1996; 155:46–48.
377. Robson WL, Norgaard JP, Leung AK. Hyponatremia in patients with nocturnal enuresis treated with DDAVP. Eur J Pediatr 1996; 155:959–962.
378. Neuhaus TJ, der Heiden-Ranz M. Hyponatraemia and cerebral convulsion after a single dose of intranasal DDAVP (letter). Pediatr Nephrol 1997; 11:527.
379. Donoghue MB, Latimer ME, Pillsbury HL, et al. Hyponatremic seizure in a child using desmopressin for nocturnal enuresis. Arch Pediatr Adolesc Med 1998; 152:290–292.
380. Williford SL, Bernstein SA. Intranasal desmopressin-induced hyponatremia. Pharmacotherapy 1996; 16:66–74.
381. Bernstein SA, Williford SL. Intranasal desmopressin-associated hyponatremia: a case report and literature review. J Fam Pract 1997; 44:203–208.
382. Pokracki FJ, Robinson AG, Seif SM. Chlorpropamide effect: measurement of neurophysin and vasopressin in humans and rats. Metabolism 1981; 30:72–78.
383. Moses AM, Numann P, Miller M. Mechanism of chlorpropamide-induced antidiuresis in man: evidence for release of ADH and enhancement of peripheral action. Metabolism 1973; 22:59–66.
384. Nandi M, Harrington AR. Successful treatment of hypernatremic thirst deficiency with chlorpropamide. Clin Nephrol 1978; 10:90–95.
385. Bode HH, Harley BM, Crawford JD. Restoration of normal drinking behavior by chlorpropamide in patients with hypodipsia and diabetes insipidus. Am J Med 1971; 51:304–313.
386. Edwards CR, Kitau MJ, Chard T, et al. Vasopressin analogue DDAVP in diabetes insipidus: clinical and laboratory studies. Br Med J 1973; 3:375–378.
387. Davison JM, Sheills EA, Philips PR, et al. Metabolic clearance of vasopressin and an analogue resistant to vasopressinase in human pregnancy. Am J Physiol 1993; 264:F348–F353.
388. Burrow GN, Wassenaar W, Robertson GL, et al. DDAVP treatment of diabetes insipidus during pregnancy and the post-partum period. Acta Endocrinol (Copenh) 1981; 97:23–25.
389. Ray JG. DDAVP use during pregnancy: an analysis of its safety for mother and child. Obstet Gynecol Surv 1998; 53:450–455.
390. Kallen BA, Carlsson SS, Bengtsson BK. Diabetes insipidus and use of desmopressin (Minirin) during pregnancy. Eur J Endocrinol 1995; 132:144–146.
391. Ralston C, Butt W. Continuous vasopressin replacement in diabetes insipidus. Arch Dis Child 1990; 65:896–897.
392. Lugo N, Silver P, Nimkoff L, et al. Diagnosis and management algorithm of acute onset of central diabetes insipidus in critically ill children. J Pediatr Endocrinol Metab 1997; 10:633–639.

393. Lee YJ, Yang D, Shyur SD, et al. Neurogenic diabetes insipidus in a child with fatal Coxsackie virus B1 encephalitis. J Pediatr Endocrinol Metab 1995; 8:301–304.
394. Chanson P, Jedynak CP, Dabrowski G, et al. Ultralow doses of vasopressin in the management of diabetes insipidus. Crit Care Med 1987; 15:44–46.
395. Magaldi AJ. New insights into the paradoxical effect of thiazides in diabetes insipidus therapy. Nephrol Dial Transplant 2000; 15: 1903–1905.
396. Gronbeck L, Marples D, Nielsen S, et al. Mechanism of antidiuresis caused by bendroflumethiazide in conscious rats with diabetes insipidus. Br J Pharmacol 1998; 123:737–745.
397. Cesar KR, Magaldi AJ. Thiazide induces water absorption in the inner medullary collecting duct of normal and Brattleboro rats. Am J Physiol 1999; 277:F756–F760.
398. Hochberg Z, Even L, Danon A. Amelioration of polyuria in nephrogenic diabetes insipidus due to aquaporin-2 deficiency. Clin Endocrinol (Oxf) 1998; 49:39–44.
399. Uyeki TM, Barry FL, Rosenthal SM, et al. Successful treatment with hydrochlorothiazide and amiloride in an infant with congenital nephrogenic diabetes insipidus. Pediatr Nephrol 1993; 7:554–556.
400. Kirchlechner V, Koller DY, Seidl R, et al. Treatment of nephrogenic diabetes insipidus with hydrochlorothiazide and amiloride. Arch Dis Child 1999; 80:548–552.
401. Bendz H, Aurell M, Balldin J, et al. Kidney damage in long-term lithium patients: a cross-sectional study of patients with 15 years or more on lithium. Nephrol Dial Transplant 1994; 9:1250–1254.
402. Singer I, Oster JR, Fishman LM. The management of diabetes insipidus in adults. Arch Intern Med 1997; 157:1293–1301.
403. Batlle DC, von Riotte AB, Gaviria M, et al. Amelioration of polyuria by amiloride in patients receiving long-term lithium therapy. N Engl J Med 1985; 312:408–414.
404. Sonnenberg H, Honrath U, Wilson DR. Effects of amiloride in the medullary collecting duct of rat kidney. Kidney Int 1987; 31: 1121–1125.
405. Knoers N, Monnens LA. Nephrogenic diabetes insipidus: clinical symptoms, pathogenesis, genetics and treatment. Pediatr Nephrol 1992; 6:476–482.
406. Tetiker T, Sert M, Kocak M. Efficacy of indapamide in central diabetes insipidus. Arch Intern Med 1999; 159:2085–2087.
407. Bryant WP, O'Marcaigh AS, Ledger GA, et al. Aqueous vasopressin infusion during chemotherapy in patients with diabetes insipidus. Cancer 1994; 74:2589–2592.
408. Kahn A, Brachet E, Blum D. Controlled fall in natremia and risk of seizures in hypertonic dehydration. Intensive Care Med 1979; 5:27–31.
409. Ross O. The management of extreme hypernatraemia secondary to salt poisoning in an infant (letter; comment). Paediatr Anaesth 2000; 10:110–111.
410. Lien YH, Shapiro JI, Chan L. Effects of hypernatremia on organic brain osmoles. J Clin Invest 1990; 85:1427–1435.
411. Fall PJ. Hyponatremia and hypernatremia: a systematic approach to causes and their correction. Postgrad Med 2000; 107:75–82.
412. Ayus JC, Armstrong DL, Arieff AI. Effects of hypernatraemia in the central nervous system and its therapy in rats and rabbits. J Physiol (Lond) 1996; 492:243–255.
413. Schwartz WB, Bennett S, Curelop S, et al. A syndrome of renal sodium loss and hyponatremia probably resulting from inappropriate secretion of antidiuretic hormone. Am J Med 1957; 23: 529–542.
414. Bartter FC, Schwartz WB. The syndrome of inappropriate secretion of antidiuretic hormone. Am J Med 1967; 42:790–806.
415. Miller M, Morley JE, Rubenstein LZ. Hyponatremia in a nursing home population. J Am Geriatr Soc 1995; 43:1410–1413.
416. Arieff AI, Llach F, Massry SG. Neurological manifestations and morbidity of hyponatremia: correlation with brain water and electrolytes. Medicine (Baltimore) 1976; 55:121–129.
417. Arieff AI. Hyponatremia, convulsions, respiratory arrest, and permanent brain damage after elective surgery in healthy women. N Engl J Med 1986; 314:1529–1535.
418. Sterns RH, Riggs JE, Schochet SS Jr. Osmotic demyelination syndrome following correction of hyponatremia. N Engl J Med 1986; 314:1535–1542.
419. Anderson RJ, Chung HM, Kluge R, et al. Hyponatremia: a prospective analysis of its epidemiology and the pathogenetic role of vasopressin. Ann Intern Med 1985; 102:164–168.
420. Oster JR, Singer I. Hyponatremia, hyposmolality, and hypotonicity: tables and fables. Arch Intern Med 1999; 159:333–336.
421. Weisberg LS. Pseudohyponatremia: a reappraisal. Am J Med 1989; 86:315–318.
422. Katz MA. Hyperglycemia-induced hyponatremia: calculation of expected serum sodium depression. N Engl J Med 1973; 289: 843–844.
423. Hillier TA, Abbott RD, Barrett EJ. Hyponatremia: evaluating the correction factor for hyperglycemia. Am J Med 1999; 106:399–403.
424. Rose BD. New approach to disturbances in the plasma sodium concentration. Am J Med 1986; 81:1033–1040.
425. Spital A. Diuretic-induced hyponatremia. Am J Nephrol 1999; 19:447–452.
426. Gross PA, Pehrisch H, Rascher W, et al. Pathogenesis of clinical hyponatremia: observations of vasopressin and fluid intake in 100 hyponatremic medical patients. Eur J Clin Invest 1987; 17:123–129.
427. Schrier RW. Body fluid volume regulation in health and disease: a unifying hypothesis. Ann Intern Med 1990; 113:155–159.
428. Demanet JC, Bonnyns M, Bleiberg H, et al. Coma due to water intoxication in beer drinkers. Lancet 1971; 2:1115–1117.
429. Thaler SM, Teitelbaum I, Berl T. "Beer potomania" in non-beer drinkers: effect of low dietary solute intake. Am J Kidney Dis 1998; 31:1028–1031.
430. Cooke CR, Turin MD, Walker WG. The syndrome of inappropriate antidiuretic hormone secretion (SIADH): pathophysiologic mechanisms in solute and volume regulation. Medicine (Baltimore) 1979; 58:240–251.
431. Grantham J, Linshaw M. The effect of hyponatremia on the regulation of intracellular volume and solute composition. Circ Res 1984; 54:483–491.
432. Yannet H. Changes in the brain resulting from depletion of extracellular electrolytes. Am J Physiol 1940; 128:683–689.
433. Holliday MA, Kalayci MN, Harrah J. Factors that limit brain volume changes in response to acute and sustained hyper- and hyponatremia. J Clin Invest 1968; 47:1916–1928.
434. Garcia-Perez A, Burg MB. Renal medullary organic osmolytes. Physiol Rev 1991; 71:1081–1115.
435. Heilig CW, Stromski ME, Blumenfeld JD, et al. Characterization of the major brain osmolytes that accumulate in salt-loaded rats. Am J Physiol 1989; 257:F1108–F1116.
436. Lien YH, Shapiro JI, Chan L. Study of brain electrolytes and organic osmolytes during correction of chronic hyponatremia: implications for the pathogenesis of central pontine myelinolysis. J Clin Invest 1991; 88:303–309.
437. Verbalis JG, Gullans SR. Hyponatremia causes large sustained reductions in brain content of multiple organic osmolytes in rats. Brain Res 1991; 567:274–282.
438. Videen JS, Michaelis T, Pinto P, et al. Human cerebral osmolytes during chronic hyponatremia: a proton magnetic resonance spectroscopy study. J Clin Invest 1995; 95:788–793.
439. Gullans SR, Verbalis JG. Control of brain volume during hyperosmolar and hypoosmolar conditions. Annu Rev Med 1993; 44: 289–301.
440. Grantham JJ. Pathophysiology of hyposmolar conditions: a cellular perspective. In Andreoli TE, Grantham JJ, Rector FC (eds). Disturbances in Body Fluid Osmolality. Bethesda, Md, American Physiological Society, 1977, pp 217–225.
441. Graber M, Corish D. The electrolytes in hyponatremia. Am J Kidney Dis 1991; 18:527–545.
442. Smith MJ Jr, Cowley MJ Jr, Guyton AC, et al. Acute and chronic effects of vasopressin on blood pressure, electrolytes, and fluid volumes. Am J Physiol 1979; 237:F232–F240.
443. Verbalis JG. Pathogenesis of hyponatremia in an experimental model of the syndrome of inappropriate antidiuresis. Am J Physiol 1994; 267:R1617–R1625.
444. Southgate HJ, Burke BJ, Walters G. Body space measurements in the hyponatraemia of carcinoma of the bronchus: evidence for the chronic 'sick cell' syndrome? Ann Clin Biochem 1992; 29:90–95.
445. Verbalis JG. Hyponatremia: epidemiology, pathophysiology, and therapy. Curr Opin Nephrol Hypertens 1993; 2:636–652.

446. Clark BA, Shannon RP, Rosa RM, et al. Increased susceptibility to thiazide-induced hyponatremia in the elderly. J Am Soc Nephrol 1994; 5:1106–1111.
447. Werbel SS, Ober KP. Acute adrenal insufficiency. Endocrinol Metab Clin North Am 1993; 22:303–328.
448. Zennaro MC. Mineralocorticoid resistance. Steroids 1996; 61: 189–192.
449. Teitelbaum I, McGuinness S. Vasopressin resistance in chronic renal failure: evidence for the role of decreased V2 receptor mRNA. J Clin Invest 1995; 96:378–385.
450. Chung HM, Kluge R, Schrier RW, et al. Clinical assessment of extracellular fluid volume in hyponatremia. Am J Med 1987; 83: 905–908.
451. Michelis MF, Fusco RD, Bragdon RW, et al. Reset of osmoreceptors in association with normovolemic hyponatremia. Am J Med Sci 1974; 267:267–273.
452. Beck LH. Hypouricemia in the syndrome of inappropriate secretion of antidiuretic hormone. N Engl J Med 1979; 301:528–530.
453. Decaux G, Prospert F, Cauchie P, et al. Dissociation between uric acid and urea clearances in the syndrome of inappropriate secretion of antidiuretic hormone related to salt excretion. Clin Sci (Colch) 1990; 78:451–455.
454. Robertson GL, Mahr EA, Athar S, et al. Development and clinical application of a new method for the radioimmunoassay of arginine vasopressin in human plasma. J Clin Invest 1973; 52: 2340–2352.
455. Zerbe R, Stropes L, Robertson G. Vasopressin function in the syndrome of inappropriate antidiuresis. Annu Rev Med 1980; 31: 315–327.
456. List AF, Hainsworth JD, Davis BW, et al. The syndrome of inappropriate secretion of antidiuretic hormone (SIADH) in small-cell lung cancer. J Clin Oncol 1986; 4:1191–1198.
457. Maurer LH, O'Donnell JF, Kennedy S, et al. Human neurophysins in carcinoma of the lung: relation to histology, disease stage, response rate, survival, and syndrome of inappropriate antidiuretic hormone secretion. Cancer Treat Rep 1983; 67:971–976.
458. Gschwantler M, Weiss W. [Hyponatremic coma as the first symptom of a small cell bronchial carcinoma]. Dtsch Med Wochenschr 1994; 119:261–264.
459. Ferlito A, Rinaldo A, Devaney KO. Syndrome of inappropriate antidiuretic hormone secretion associated with head neck cancers: review of the literature. Ann Otol Rhinol Laryngol 1997; 106: 878–883.
460. Kavanagh BD, Halperin EC, Rosenbaum LC, et al. Syndrome of inappropriate secretion of antidiuretic hormone in a patient with carcinoma of the nasopharynx. Cancer 1992; 69:1315–1319.
461. Berghmans T, Paesmans M, Body JJ. A prospective study on hyponatraemia in medical cancer patients: epidemiology, aetiology and differential diagnosis. Support Care Cancer 2000; 8(3): 192–197.
462. Renaud LP. Hypothalamic magnocellular neurosecretory neurons: intrinsic membrane properties and synaptic connections. Prog Brain Res 1994; 100:133–137.
463. Moses AM, Miller M. Drug-induced dilutional hyponatremia. N Engl J Med 1974; 291:1234–1239.
464. Gibbs DM, Vale W. Effect of the serotonin reuptake inhibitor fluoxetine on corticotropin-releasing factor and vasopressin secretion into hypophysial portal blood. Brain Res 1983; 280:176–179.
465. Mikkelsen JD, Jensen JB, Engelbrecht T, et al. D-fenfluramine activates rat oxytocinergic and vasopressinergic neurons through different mechanisms. Brain Res 1999; 851:247–251.
466. Faull CM, Rooke P, Baylis PH. The effect of a highly specific serotonin agonist on osmoregulated vasopressin secretion in healthy man. Clin Endocrinol (Oxf) 1991; 35:423–430.
467. Wilkinson TJ, Begg EJ, Winter AC, et al. Incidence and risk factors for hyponatraemia following treatment with fluoxetine or paroxetine in elderly people. Br J Clin Pharmacol 1999; 47:211–217.
468. O'Connor A, Cluroe A, Couch R, et al. Death from hyponatraemia-induced cerebral oedema associated with MDMA ('Ecstasy') use. NZ Med J 1999; 112:255–256.
469. Burgess C, O'Donohoe A, Gill M: Agony and ecstasy: a review of MDMA effects and toxicity. Eur Psychiatry 2000; 15:287–294.
470. Stephenson CP, Hunt GE, Topple AN, et al. The distribution of 3,4-methylenedioxymethamphetamine Ecstasy-induced c-fos expression in rat brain. Neuroscience 1999; 92:1011–1023.
471. Vorherr H, Massry SG, Fallet R, et al. Antidiuretic principle in tuberculous lung tissue of a patient with pulmonary tuberculosis and hyponatremia. Ann Intern Med 1970; 72:383–387.
472. DeFronzo RA, Goldberg M, Agus ZS. Normal diluting capacity in hyponatremic patients: reset osmostat or a variant of the syndrome of inappropriate antidiuretic hormone secretion. Ann Intern Med 1976; 84:538–542.
473. Hill AR, Uribarri J, Mann J, et al. Altered water metabolism in tuberculosis: role of vasopressin. Am J Med 1990; 88:357–364.
474. Kelestimur H, Leach RM, Ward JP, et al. Vasopressin and oxytocin release during prolonged environmental hypoxia in the rat. Thorax 1997; 52:84–88.
475. Baylis PH, Stockley RA, Heath DA. Effect of acute hypoxaemia on plasma arginine vasopressin in conscious man. Clin Sci Mol Med 1977; 53:401–404.
476. Reihman DH, Farber MO, Weinberger MH, et al. Effect of hypoxemia on sodium and water excretion in chronic obstructive lung disease. Am J Med 1985; 78:87–94.
477. Dhawan A, Narang A, Singhi S. Hyponatraemia and the inappropriate ADH syndrome in pneumonia. Ann Trop Paediatr 1992; 12:455–462.
478. Tang WW, Kaptein EM, Feinstein EI, et al. Hyponatremia in hospitalized patients with the acquired immunodeficiency syndrome (AIDS) and the AIDS-related complex. Am J Med 1993; 94:169–174.
479. Tolaymat A, Al Mousily F, Sleasman J, et al. Hyponatremia in pediatric patients with HIV-1 infection. South Med J 1995; 88: 1039–1042.
480. Cusano AJ, Thies HL, Siegal FP, et al. Hyponatremia in patients with acquired immune deficiency syndrome. J Acquir Immune Defic Syndr 1990; 3:949–953.
481. Noto H, Kaneko Y, Takano T, et al. Severe hyponatremia and hyperkalemia induced by trimethoprim-sulfamethoxazole in patients with *Pneumocystis carinii* pneumonia. Intern Med 1995; 34(2):96–99.
482. Yeung KT, Chan M, Chan CK. The safety of i.v. pentamidine administered in an ambulatory setting. Chest 1996; 110:136–140.
483. Miller M. Hyponatremia: age-related risk factors and therapy decisions. Geriatrics 1998; 53(7):32–38, 41.
484. Miller M, Hecker MS, Friedlander DA, et al. Apparent idiopathic hyponatremia in an ambulatory geriatric population. J Am Geriatr Soc 1996; 44:404–408.
485. Hirshberg B, Ben Yehuda A. The syndrome of inappropriate antidiuretic hormone secretion in the elderly. Am J Med 1997; 103:270–273.
486. Rowe JW, Kilgore A, Robertson GL. Evidence in man that cigarette smoking induces vasopressin release via an airway-specific mechanism. J Clin Endocrinol Metab 1980; 51:170–172.
487. Vieweg WV, Karp BI. Severe hyponatremia in the polydipsia-hyponatremia syndrome. J Clin Psychiatry 1994; 55:355–361.
488. Rowe JW, Shelton RL, Helderman JH, et al. Influence of the emetic reflex on vasopressin release in man. Kidney Int 1979; 16: 729–735.
489. Ishikawa S, Kuratomi Y, Saito T. A case of oat cell carcinoma of the lung associated with ectopic production of ADH, neurophysin and ACTH. Endocrinol Jpn 1980; 27:257–263.
490. Rosenbaum LC, Neuwelt EA, van Tol HH, et al. Expression of neurophysin-related precursor in cell membranes of a small-cell lung carcinoma. Proc Natl Acad Sci USA 1990; 87:9928–9932.
491. Goldman MB, Luchins DJ, Robertson GL. Mechanisms of altered water metabolism in psychotic patients with polydipsia and hyponatremia. N Engl J Med 1988; 318:397–403.
492. Robertson GL, Aycinena P, Zerbe RL. Neurogenic disorders of osmoregulation. Am J Med 1982; 72:339–353.
493. Robertson GL, Athar S. The interaction of blood osmolality and blood volume in regulating plasma vasopressin in man. J Clin Endocrinol Metab 1976; 42:613–620.
494. Bichet D, Szatalowicz V, Chaimovitz C, et al. Role of vasopressin in abnormal water excretion in cirrhotic patients. Ann Intern Med 1982; 96:413–417.
495. Verbalis JG, Dohanics J. Vasopressin and oxytocin secretion in chronically hyposmolar rats. Am J Physiol 1991; 261:R1028–R1038.
496. Kamoi K. Syndrome of inappropriate antidiuresis without involving inappropriate secretion of vasopressin in an elderly woman:

effect of intravenous administration of the nonpeptide vasopressin V2 receptor antagonist OPC-31260. Nephron 1997; 76:111–115.
497. Leaf A, Bartter FC, Santos RF, et al. Syndrome in man that urinary electrolyte loss induced by pitressin is a function of water retention. J Clin Invest 1953; 32:868–878.
498. Hall JE, Montani JP, Woods LL, et al. Renal escape from vasopressin: role of pressure diuresis. Am J Physiol 1986; 250:F907–F916.
499. Kamoi K, Ebe T, Kobayashi O, et al. Atrial natriuretic peptide in patients with the syndrome of inappropriate antidiuretic hormone secretion and with diabetes insipidus. J Clin Endocrinol Metab 1990; 70:1385–1390.
500. Peters JP, Welt KG, Sims EAH, et al. A salt-wasting syndrome associated with cerebral disease. Trans Assoc Am Physicians 1950; 63:57–64.
501. Doczi T, Tarjanyi J, Huszka E, et al. Syndrome of inappropriate secretion of antidiuretic hormone (SIADH) after head injury. Neurosurgery 1982; 10:685–688.
502. Nelson PB, Seif S, Gutai J, et al. Hyponatremia and natriuresis following subarachnoid hemorrhage in a monkey model. J Neurosurg 1984; 60:233–237.
503. Wijdicks EF, Ropper AH, Hunnicutt EJ, et al. Atrial natriuretic factor and salt wasting after aneurysmal subarachnoid hemorrhage. Stroke 1991; 22:1519–1524.
504. Diringer MN, Lim JS, Kirsch JR, et al. Suprasellar and intraventricular blood predict elevated plasma atrial natriuretic factor in subarachnoid hemorrhage. Stroke 1991; 22:577–581.
505. Oh MS, Carroll HJ. Cerebral salt-wasting syndrome: we need better proof of its existence. Nephron 1999; 82:110–114.
506. Maesaka JK, Gupta S, Fishbane S. Cerebral salt-wasting syndrome: does it exist? Nephron 1999; 82:100–109.
507. Weinand ME, O'Boynick PL, Goetz KL. A study of serum antidiuretic hormone and atrial natriuretic peptide levels in a series of patients with intracranial disease and hyponatremia. Neurosurgery 1989; 25:781–785.
508. Diringer MN, Wu KC, Verbalis JG, et al. Hypervolemic therapy prevents volume contraction but not hyponatremia following subarachnoid hemorrhage. Ann Neurol 1992; 31:543–550.
509. Mori T, Katayama Y, Kawamata T, et al. Improved efficiency of hypervolemic therapy with inhibition of natriuresis by fludrocortisone in patients with aneurysmal subarachnoid hemorrhage. J Neurosurg 1999; 91:947–952.
510. Ishikawa S, Fujita N, Fujisawa G, et al. Involvement of arginine vasopressin and renal sodium handling in pathogenesis of hyponatremia in elderly patients. Endocr J 1996; 43:101–108.
511. Kamoi K, Ebe T, Hasegawa A, et al. Hyponatremia in small cell lung cancer: mechanisms not involving inappropriate ADH secretion. Cancer 1987; 60:1089–1093.
512. Gross AJ, Steinberg SM, Reilly JG, et al. Atrial natriuretic factor and arginine vasopressin production in tumor cell lines from patients with lung cancer and their relationship to serum sodium. Cancer Res 1993; 53:67–74.
513. Johnson BE, Chute JP, Rushin J, et al. A prospective study of patients with lung cancer and hyponatremia of malignancy. Am J Respir Crit Care Med 1997; 156:1669–1678.
514. Verbalis JG, Murase T, Ecelbarger CA, et al. Studies of renal aquaporin-2 expression during renal escape from vasopressin-induced antidiuresis. Adv Exp Med Biol 1998; 449:395–406.
515. Murase T, Ecelbarger CA, Baker EA, et al. Kidney aquaporin-2 expression during escape from antidiuresis is not related to plasma or tissue osmolality. J Am Soc Nephrol 1999; 10:2067–2075.
516. Fraser CL, Arieff AI. Epidemiology, pathophysiology, and management of hyponatremic encephalopathy. Am J Med 1997; 102: 67–77.
517. Daggett P, Deanfield J, Moss F. Neurological aspects of hyponatraemia. Postgrad Med J 1982; 58:737–740.
518. Sterns RH. Severe symptomatic hyponatremia: treatment and outcome. A study of 64 cases. Ann Intern Med 1987; 107: 656–664.
519. Kleeman CR. The kidney in health and disease: X. CNS manifestations of disordered salt and water balance. Hosp Pract 1979; 14(5):59–68, 73.
520. Ayus JC, Wheeler JM, Arieff AI. Postoperative hyponatremic encephalopathy in menstruant women. Ann Intern Med 1992; 117:891–897.
521. Wijdicks EF, Sharbrough FW. New-onset seizures in critically ill patients. Neurology 1993; 43:1042–1044.
522. Vexler ZS, Ayus JC, Roberts TP, et al. Hypoxic and ischemic hypoxia exacerbate brain injury associated with metabolic encephalopathy in laboratory animals. J Clin Invest 1994; 93:256–264.
523. Ayus JC, Arieff AI. Pulmonary complications of hyponatremic encephalopathy: noncardiogenic pulmonary edema and hypercapnic respiratory failure. Chest 1995; 107:517–521.
524. Ayus JC, Varon J, Arieff AI. Hyponatremia, cerebral edema, and noncardiogenic pulmonary edema in marathon runners. Ann Intern Med 2000; 132:711–714.
525. Arieff AI, Ayus JC, Fraser CL. Hyponatraemia and death or permanent brain damage in healthy children. BMJ 1992; 304: 1218–1222.
526. Wattad A, Chiang ML, Hill LL. Hyponatremia in hospitalized children. Clin Pediatr (Phila) 1992; 31:153–157.
527. Wijdicks EF, Larson TS. Absence of postoperative hyponatremia syndrome in young, healthy females. Ann Neurol 1994; 35:626–628.
528. Carroll PB, McHenry L, Verbalis JG. Isolated adrenocorticotrophic hormone deficiency presenting as chronic hyponatremia. NY State J Med 1990; 90:210–213.
529. Wright DG, Laureno R, Victor M. Pontine and extrapontine myelinolysis. Brain 1979; 102:361–385.
530. Verbalis JG, Martinez AJ. Neurological and neuropathological sequelae of correction of chronic hyponatremia. Kidney Int 1991; 39:1274–1282.
531. Verbalis JG, Baldwin EF, Robinson AG. Osmotic regulation of plasma vasopressin and oxytocin after sustained hyponatremia. Am J Physiol 1986; 250:R444–R451.
532. Sterns RH, Thomas DJ, Herndon RM. Brain dehydration and neurologic deterioration after rapid correction of hyponatremia. Kidney Int 1989; 35:69–75.
533. Cserr HF, DePasquale M, Patlak CS. Regulation of brain water and electrolytes during acute hyperosmolality in rats. Am J Physiol 1987; 253:F522–F529.
534. Adler S, Verbalis JG, Williams D. Effect of rapid correction of hyponatremia on the blood-brain barrier of rats. Brain Res 1995; 679:135–143.
535. Adler S, Martinez J, Williams DS, et al. Positive association between blood brain barrier disruption and osmotically-induced demyelination. Mult Scler 2000; 6:24–31.
536. Baker EA, Tian Y, Adler S, et al. Blood-brain barrier disruption and complement activation in the brain following rapid correction of chronic hyponatremia. Exp Neurol 2000; 165:221–230.
537. Sterns RH. The management of symptomatic hyponatremia. Semin Nephrol 1990; 10:503–514.
538. Ayus JC, Krothapalli RK, Armstrong DL, et al. Symptomatic hyponatremia in rats: effect of treatment on mortality and brain lesions. Am J Physiol 1989; 257:F18–F22.
539. Soupart A, Penninckx R, Stenuit A, et al. Treatment of chronic hyponatremia in rats by intravenous saline: comparison of rate versus magnitude of correction. Kidney Int 1992; 41:1662–1667.
540. Ayus JC, Krothapalli RK, Arieff AI. Treatment of symptomatic hyponatremia and its relation to brain damage: a prospective study. N Engl J Med 1987; 317:1190–1195.
541. Sterns RH, Cappuccio JD, Silver SM, et al. Neurologic sequelae after treatment of severe hyponatremia: a multicenter perspective. J Am Soc Nephrol 1994; 4:1522–1530.
542. Verbalis JG. Hyponatremia: endocrinologic causes and consequences of therapy. Trends Endocrinol Metab 1992; 3:1–7.
543. Ellis SJ. Extrapontine myelinolysis after correction of chronic hyponatraemia with isotonic saline. Br J Clin Pract 1995; 49:49–50.
544. Cheng JC, Zikos D, Skopicki HA, et al. Long-term neurologic outcome in psychogenic water drinkers with severe symptomatic hyponatremia: the effect of rapid correction. Am J Med 1990; 88: 561–566.
545. Adams RD, Victor M, Mancall EL. Central pontine myelinolysis: a hitherto undescribed disease occurring in alcoholic and malnourished patients. Arch Neurol Psych 1959; 81:154–172.
546. Kelly J, Wassif W, Mitchard J, et al. Severe hyponatraemia secondary to beer potomania complicated by central pontine myelinolysis. Int J Clin Pract 1998; 52:585–587.
547. Soupart A, Penninckx R, Stenuit A, et al. Azotemia (48 h) de-

creases the risk of brain damage in rats after correction of chronic hyponatremia. Brain Res 2000; 852:167–172.
548. Brunner JE, Redmond JM, Haggar AM, et al. Central pontine myelinolysis and pontine lesions after rapid correction of hyponatremia: a prospective magnetic resonance imaging study. Ann Neurol 1990; 27:61–66.
549. Kumar SR, Mone AP, Gray LC, et al. Central pontine myelinolysis: delayed changes on neuroimaging. J Neuroimaging 2000; 10:169–172.
550. Soupart A, Penninckx R, Namias B, et al. Brain myelinolysis following hypernatremia in rats. J Neuropathol Exp Neurol 1997; 55:106–113.
551. McComb RD, Pfeiffer RF, Casey JH, et al. Lateral pontine and extrapontine myelinolysis associated with hypernatremia and hyperglycemia. Clin Neuropathol 1989; 8:284–288.
552. Ayus JC, Olivero JJ, Frommer JP. Rapid correction of severe hyponatremia with intravenous hypertonic saline solution. Am J Med 1982; 72:43–48.
553. Berl T. Treating hyponatremia: damned if we do and damned if we don't. Kidney Int 1990; 37:1006–1018.
554. Verbalis JG. Adaptation to acute and chronic hyponatremia: implications for symptomatology, diagnosis, and therapy. Semin Nephrol 1998; 18:3–19.
555. Ayus JC, Arieff AI. Brain damage and postoperative hyponatremia: the role of gender. Neurology 1996; 46:323–328.
556. Sterns RH, Ocdol H, Schrier RW, et al. Hyponatremia: pathophysiology, diagnosis, and therapy. In Narins RG (ed). Disorders of Fluid and Electrolytes. New York, McGraw-Hill, 1994, pp 583–615.
557. Lohr JW. Osmotic demyelination syndrome following correction of hyponatremia: association with hypokalemia. Am J Med 1994; 96:408–413.
558. Hantman D, Rossier B, Zohlman R, et al. Rapid correction of hyponatremia in the syndrome of inappropriate secretion of antidiuretic hormone: an alternative treatment to hypertonic saline. Ann Intern Med 1973; 78:870–875.
559. Tanneau RS, Henry A, Rouhart F, et al. High incidence of neurologic complications following rapid correction of severe hyponatremia in polydipsic patients. J Clin Psychiatry 1994; 55: 349–354.
560. Goldszmidt MA, Iliescu EA. DDAVP to prevent rapid correction in hyponatremia. Clin Nephrol 2000; 53:226–229.
561. Soupart A, Penninckx R, Stenuit A, et al. Reinduction of hyponatremia improves survival in rats with myelinolysis-related neurologic symptoms. J Neuropathol Exp Neurol 1996; 55:594–601.
562. Soupart A, Ngassa M, Decaux G. Therapeutic relowering of the serum sodium in a patient after excessive correction of hyponatremia. Clin Nephrol 1999; 51:383–386.
563. Robertson GL. Abnormalities of thirst regulation. Kidney Int 1984; 25:460–469.
564. Canuso CM, Goldman MB. Clozapine restores water balance in schizophrenic patients with polydipsia-hyponatremia syndrome. J Neuropsychiatry Clin Neurosci 1999; 11:86–90.
565. De Troyer A. Demeclocycline: treatment for syndrome of inappropriate antidiuretic hormone secretion. JAMA 1977; 237:2723–2726.
566. Dousa TP, Wilson DM. Effects of demethylchlortetracycline on cellular action of antidiuretic hormone in vitro. Kidney Int 1974; 5:279–284.
567. Miller PD, Linas SL, Schrier RW. Plasma demeclocycline levels and nephrotoxicity: correlation in hyponatremic cirrhotic patients. JAMA 1980; 243:2513–2515.
568. Forrest JN Jr, Cox M, Hong C, et al. Superiority of demeclocycline over lithium in the treatment of chronic syndrome of inappropriate secretion of antidiuretic hormone. N Engl J Med 1978; 298:173–177.
569. Decaux G, Mols P, Cauchi P, et al. Use of urea for treatment of water retention in hyponatraemic cirrhosis with ascites resistant to diuretics. Br Med J [Clin Res] 1985; 290:1782–1783.
570. Brooks DP, Valente M, Petrone G, et al. Comparison of the water diuretic activity of kappa receptor agonists and a vasopressin receptor antagonist in dogs. J Pharmacol Exp Ther 1997; 280:1176–1183.
571. Gadano A, Moreau R, Pessione F, et al. Aquaretic effects of niravoline, a kappa-opioid agonist, in patients with cirrhosis. J Hepatol 2000; 32:38–42.
572. Schrier RW. New treatments for hyponatremia. N Engl J Med 1978; 298:214–215.
573. Kinter LB, Ileson BE, Caltabinol S, et al. Antidiuretic hormone antagonism in humans: are there predictors? In Jard S, Jamison R (eds). Vasopressin. Paris, John Libbey Eurotext, 1991, pp 321–329.
574. Yamamura Y, Ogawa H, Yamashita H, et al. Characterization of a novel aquaretic agent, OPC-31260, as an orally effective, nonpeptide vasopressin V2 receptor antagonist. Br J Pharmacol 1992; 105:787–791.
575. Serradeil-Le Gal C, Lacour C, Valette G, et al. Characterization of SR 121463A, a highly potent and selective, orally active vasopressin V2 receptor antagonist. J Clin Invest 1996; 98:2729–2738.
576. Tahara A, Tomura Y, Wada KI, et al. Pharmacological profile of YM087, a novel potent nonpeptide vasopressin V1A and V2 receptor antagonist, in vitro and in vivo. J Pharmacol Exp Ther 1997; 282:301–308.
577. Saito T, Ishikawa S, Abe K, et al. Acute aquaresis by the nonpeptide arginine vasopressin (AVP) antagonist OPC-31260 improves hyponatremia in patients with syndrome of inappropriate secretion of antidiuretic hormone (SIADH). J Clin Endocrinol Metab 1997; 82:1054–1057.
578. Verbalis JG, Martinez AJ. Determinants of brain myelinolysis following correction of chronic hyponatremia in rats. In Jard S, Jamison RL (eds). Vasopressin. Paris, John Libbey Eurotext, 1991, pp 539–547.
579. Jenkins JS, Nussey SS. The role of oxytocin: present concepts. Clin Endocrinol (Oxf) 1991; 34:515–525.
580. Giraldi A, Enevoldsen AS, Wagner G. Oxytocin and the initiation of parturition: a review. Dan Med Bull 1990; 37:377–383.
581. Evans JJ. Oxytocin in the human: regulation of derivations and destinations. Eur J Endocrinol 1997; 137:559–571.
582. Russell JA, Leng G. Sex, parturition and motherhood without oxytocin? J Endocrinol 1998; 157:343–359.
583. Robinson AG, Amico JA. Remarks on the history of oxytocin. In Amico JA, Robinson AG (eds). Oxytocin: Clinical and Laboratory Studies: Proceedings of the Second International Conference on Oxytocin, Lac Beauport, Quebec, Canada, June 29 to July 1, 1984. Amsterdam, Excerpta Medica, 1985, pp xvii–xxiv.
584. Nishimori K, Young LJ, Guo Q, et al. Oxytocin is required for nursing but is not essential for parturition or reproductive behavior. Proc Natl Acad Sci USA 1996; 93:11699–11704.
585. Olson DM, Mijovic JE, Sadowsky DW. Control of human parturition. Semin Perinatol 1995; 19:52–63.
586. Steer PJ. The endocrinology of parturition in the human. Baillieres Clin Endocrinol Metab 1990; 4:333–349.
587. Nathanielsz PW. Comparative studies on the initiation of labor. Eur J Obstet Gynecol Reprod Biol 1998; 78:127–132.
588. Nathanielsz PW. A time to be born: implications of animal studies in maternal-fetal medicine. Birth 1994; 21:163–169.
589. Muglia LJ. Genetic analysis of fetal development and parturition control in the mouse. Pediatr Res 2000; 47:437–443.
590. Moran DJ, McGarrigle HH, Lachelin GC. Lack of normal increase in saliva estriol/progesterone ratio in women with labor induced at 42 weeks' gestation. Am J Obstet Gynecol 1992; 167: 1563–1564.
591. Mitchell BF, Chibbar R. Synthesis and metabolism of oxytocin in late gestation in human decidua. Adv Exp Med Biol 1995; 395: 365–380.
592. Mitchell BF, Chibbar R, Miller FD, et al. Estrogen regulates oxytocin gene expression in term human fetal membranes and decidua. Presented at the meeting of the Society for Gynecologic Investigation, Toronto, 1992.
593. Chibbar R, Miller FD, Mitchell BF. Synthesis of oxytocin in amnion, chorion, and decidua may influence the timing of human parturition. J Clin Invest 1993; 91:185–192.
594. Mitchell BF, Fang X, Wong S. Oxytocin: a paracrine hormone in the regulation of parturition? Rev Reprod 1998; 3:113–122.
595. Keelan JA, Coleman M, Mitchell MD. The molecular mechanisms of term and preterm labor: recent progress and clinical implications. Clin Obstet Gynecol 1997; 40:460–478.
596. Jenkin G. Oxytocin and prostaglandin interactions in pregnancy and at parturition. J Reprod Fertil Suppl 1992; 45:97–111.
597. Kelly RW. Pregnancy maintenance and parturition: the role of

prostaglandin in manipulating the immune and inflammatory response. Endocr Rev 1994; 15:684–706.
598. Uozumi N, Kume K, Nagase T, et al. Role of cytosolic phospholipase A2 in allergic response and parturition. Nature 1997; 390: 618–622.
599. Grazzini E, Guillon G, Mouillac B, et al. Inhibition of oxytocin receptor function by direct binding of progesterone. Nature 1998; 392:509–512.
600. Hirst JJ, Haluska GJ, Cook MJ, et al. Comparison of plasma oxytocin and catecholamine concentrations with uterine activity in pregnant rhesus monkeys. J Clin Endocrinol Metab 1991; 73: 804–810.
601. Honnebier MB, Myers T, Figueroa JP, et al. Variation in myometrial response to intravenous oxytocin administration at different times of the day in the pregnant rhesus monkey. Endocrinology 1989; 125:1498–1503.
602. Walsh SW, Stanczyk FZ, Novy MJ. Daily hormonal changes in the maternal, fetal, and amniotic fluid compartments before parturition in a primate species. J Clin Endocrinol Metab 1984; 58: 629–639.
603. Gilbert CL, Goode JA, McGrath TJ. Pulsatile secretion of oxytocin during parturition in the pig: temporal relationship with fetal expulsion. J Physiol (Lond) 1994; 475:129–137.
604. Young WS III, Shepard E, Amico J, et al. Deficiency in mouse oxytocin prevents milk ejection, but not fertility or parturition. J Neuroendocrinol 1996; 8:847–853.
605. Gross G, Imamura T, Muglia LJ. Gene knockout mice in the study of parturition. J Soc Gynecol Invest 2000; 7:88–95.
606. Gross GA, Imamura T, Luedke C, et al. Opposing actions of prostaglandins and oxytocin determine the onset of murine labor. Proc Natl Acad Sci USA 1998; 95:11875–11879.
607. Sugimoto Y, Yamasaki A, Segi E, et al. Failure of parturition in mice lacking the prostaglandin F receptor. Science 1997; 277: 681–683.
608. Robinson AG, Archer DF, Tolstoi LF. Neurophysin in women during oxytocin-related events. J Clin Endocrinol Metab 1973; 37:645–652.
609. Glasier A, McNeilly AS. Physiology of lactation. Baillieres Clin Endocrinol Metab 1990; 4:379–395.
610. Crowley WR, Armstrong WE. Neurochemical regulation of oxytocin secretion in lactation. Endocr Rev 1992; 13:33–65.
611. Kimura T, Ito Y, Einspanier A, et al. Expression and immunolocalization of the oxytocin receptor in human lactating and nonlactating mammary glands. Hum Reprod 1998; 13:2645–2653.
612. Uvnas-Moberg K, Eriksson M. Breastfeeding: physiological, endocrine and behavioural adaptations caused by oxytocin and local neurogenic activity in the nipple and mammary gland. Acta Paediatr 1996; 85:525–530.
613. Neumann I, Koehler E, Landgraf R, et al. An oxytocin receptor antagonist infused into the supraoptic nucleus attenuates intranuclear and peripheral release of oxytocin during suckling in conscious rats. Endocrinology 1994; 134:141–148.
614. Brown D, Moos F. Onset of bursting in oxytocin cells in suckled rats. J Physiol (Lond) 1997; 503:625–634.
615. McKenzie DN, Leng G, Dyball RE. Electrophysiological evidence for mutual excitation of oxytocin cells in the supraoptic nucleus of the rat hypothalamus. J Physiol (Lond) 1995; 485: 485–492.
616. McNeilly AS, Robinson IC, Houston MJ, et al. Release of oxytocin and prolactin in response to suckling. Br Med J [Clin Res] 1983; 286:257–259.
617. Uvnas-Moberg K, Widstrom AM, Werner S, et al. Oxytocin and prolactin levels in breast-feeding women: correlation with milk yield and duration of breast-feeding. Acta Obstet Gynecol Scand 1990; 69:301–306.
618. Chatterton RT Jr, Hill PD, Aldag JC, et al. Relation of plasma oxytocin and prolactin concentrations to milk production in mothers of preterm infants: influence of stress. J Clin Endocrinol Metab 2000; 85:3661–3668.
619. Young WS III, Shepard E, DeVries AC, et al. Targeted reduction of oxytocin expression provides insights into its physiological roles. Adv Exp Med Biol 1998; 449:231–240.
620. Wagner KU, Young WS III, Liu X, et al. Oxytocin and milk removal are required for post-partum mammary-gland development. Genes Funct 1997; 1:233–244.
621. Renfrew MJ, Lang S, Woolridge M. Oxytocin for promoting successful lactation. Cochrane Database Syst Rev 2000; (2): CD000156.
622. Crowley WR, Parker SL, Armstrong WE, et al. Neurotransmitter and neurohormonal regulation of oxytocin secretion in lactation. Ann NY Acad Sci 1992; 652:286–302.
623. Lindow SW, Hendricks MS, Nugent FA, et al. Morphine suppresses the oxytocin response in breast-feeding women. Gynecol Obstet Invest 1999; 48:33–37.
624. Yokoyama Y, Ueda T, Irahara M, et al. Releases of oxytocin and prolactin during breast massage and suckling in puerperal women. Eur J Obstet Gynecol Reprod Biol 1994; 53:17–20.
625. McNeilly AS, Tay CC, Glasier A. Physiological mechanisms underlying lactational amenorrhea. Ann NY Acad Sci 1994; 709: 145–155.
626. Wang H, Ward AR, Morris JF. Oestradiol acutely stimulates exocytosis of oxytocin and vasopressin from dendrites and somata of hypothalamic magnocellular neurons. Neuroscience 1995; 68: 1179–1188.
627. Thomas A, Crowley RS, Amico JA. Effect of progesterone on hypothalamic oxytocin messenger ribonucleic acid levels in the lactating rat. Endocrinology 1995; 136:4188–4194.
628. Leng G. Steroidal influences on oxytocin neurones (comment). J Physiol (Lond) 2000; 524:315.
629. Nissen E, Uvnas-Moberg K, Svensson K, et al. Different patterns of oxytocin, prolactin but not cortisol release during breastfeeding in women delivered by caesarean section or by the vaginal route. Early Hum Dev 1996; 45:103–118.
630. Johnston JM, Amico JA. A prospective longitudinal study of the release of oxytocin and prolactin in response to infant suckling in long term lactation. J Clin Endocrinol Metab 1986; 62:653–657.
631. De Coopman J. Breastfeeding after pituitary resection: support for a theory of autocrine control of milk supply? J Hum Lact 1993; 9:35–40.
632. Ghosh R, Sladek CD. Prolactin modulates oxytocin mRNA during lactation by its action on the hypothalamo-neurohypophyseal axis. Brain Res 1995; 672:24–28.
633. De Wied D, Diamant M, Fodor M. Central nervous system effects of the neurohypophyseal hormones and related peptides. Front Neuroendocrinol 1993; 14:251–302.
634. Pedersen CA. Oxytocin control of maternal behavior: regulation by sex steroids and offspring stimuli. Ann NY Acad Sci 1997; 807:126–145.
635. Kendrick KM, Keverne EB. Control of synthesis and release of oxytocin in the sheep brain. Ann NY Acad Sci 1992; 652:102–121.
636. Giovenardi M, Padoin MJ, Cadore LP, et al. Hypothalamic paraventricular nucleus, oxytocin, and maternal aggression in rats. Ann NY Acad Sci 1997; 807:606–609.
637. Giovenardi M, Padoin MJ, Cadore LP, et al. Hypothalamic paraventricular nucleus modulates maternal aggression in rats: effects of ibotenic acid lesion and oxytocin antisense. Physiol Behav 1998; 63:351–359.
638. Landgraf R, Neumann I, Russell JA, et al. Push-pull perfusion and microdialysis studies of central oxytocin and vasopressin release in freely moving rats during pregnancy, parturition, and lactation. Ann NY Acad Sci 1992; 652:326–339.
639. Argiolas A, Gessa GL. Central functions of oxytocin. Neurosci Biobehav Rev 1991; 15:217–231.
640. Uvnas-Moberg K. Oxytocin may mediate the benefits of positive social interaction and emotions. Psychoneuroendocrinology 1998; 23:819–835.
641. Insel TR, Young L, Wang Z. Central oxytocin and reproductive behaviours. Rev Reprod 1997; 2:28–37.
642. Soloff MS, Jeng YJ, Copland JA, et al. Signal pathways mediating oxytocin stimulation of prostaglandin synthesis in select target cells. Exp Physiol 2000; 85(Spec No):51S–58S.
643. Khan-Dawood FS. Oxytocin in intercellular communication in the corpus luteum. Semin Reprod Endocrinol 1997; 15:395–407.
644. Khan-Dawood FS, Yang J, Dawood MY. Potential role of oxytocin in cell to cell communication in the corpus luteum. Adv Exp Med Biol 1995; 395:507–516.
645. Verbalis JG, McHale CM, Gardiner TW, et al. Oxytocin and vasopressin secretion in response to stimuli producing learned taste aversions in rats. Behav Neurosci 1986; 100:466–475.

646. Verbalis JG, McCann MJ, McHale CM, et al. Oxytocin secretion in response to cholecystokinin and food: differentiation of nausea from satiety. Science 1986; 232:1417–1419.
647. Nelson EE, Alberts JR, Tian Y, et al. Oxytocin is elevated in plasma of 10-day-old rats following gastric distension. Brain Res Dev Brain Res 1998; 111:301–303.
648. O'Conner JL, Wade MF. Evidence that the posterior pituitary plays a role in neuropeptide Y and luteinizing hormone–releasing hormone–stimulated gonadotropin secretion in vitro. Proc Soc Exp Biol Med 1996; 213:59–64.
649. Onaka T, Palmer JR, Yagi K. A selective role of brainstem noradrenergic neurons in oxytocin release from the neurohypophysis following noxious stimuli in the rat. Neurosci Res 1996; 25:67–75.
650. Assinder SJ, Carey M, Parkinson T, et al. Oxytocin and vasopressin expression in the ovine testis and epididymis: changes with the onset of spermatogenesis. Biol Reprod 2000; 63:448–456.
651. Einspanier A, Ivell R. Oxytocin and oxytocin receptor expression in reproductive tissues of the male marmoset monkey. Biol Reprod 1997; 56:416–422.

10 Thyroid Physiology and Diagnostic Evaluation of Patients with Thyroid Disorders

P. Reed Larsen, Terry F. Davies,
Martin-Jean Schlumberger, and Ian D. Hay

Dysfunction and anatomic abnormalities of the thyroid are among the most common diseases of the endocrine glands. This chapter provides an up-to-date physiologic and biochemical background and describes the various tests for evaluating patients with suspected disease of the thyroid gland.

PHYLOGENY, EMBRYOLOGY, AND ONTOGENY

Phylogeny

The phylogeny, embryogenesis, and certain aspects of thyroid function are closely interlinked with the gastrointestinal (GI) tract. The capacity of the thyroid gland to metabolize iodine and incorporate it into a variety of organic compounds occurs widely throughout the animal and plant kingdoms.

Monoiodotyrosine (3′-monoiodo-L-tyrosine [MIT]) and diiodotyrosine (3,5′-diiodo-L-tyrosine [DIT]) are present in a variety of invertebrate species, including mollusks, crustaceans, coelenterates, annelids, insects, and certain marine algae (Fig. 10–1). In these lower forms, however, no recognizable thyroid tissue is present. Thyroid tissue is confined to and is present in all vertebrates. A close link to the thyroid of higher vertebrates is evident in the ammocoete, the larval form of the lamprey. Here the endostyle is capable of carrying out iodinations, but prior to metamorphosis a protease is expressed in the endostyle that can hydrolyze the iodoprotein formed. Presumably, this permits the endostyle to lose its connection with the pharynx during metamorphosis and to assume its adult function as an endocrine organ that secretes iodothyronines, including 3,5,3′,5′-tetraiodo-L-thyronine (thyroxine, T_4, and 3,5,3′-triiodo-L-thyronine [T_3]) (Fig. 10–1).

The phylogenetic association of the thyroid gland and the GI tract is evident in several functions. The salivary and gastric glands, like the thyroid, are able to concentrate iodide in their secretions, although iodide transport in these sites is not responsive to stimulation by thyrotropin (also called thyroid-stimulating hormone [TSH]). The salivary gland contains enzymes that are capable of iodinating tyrosine in the presence

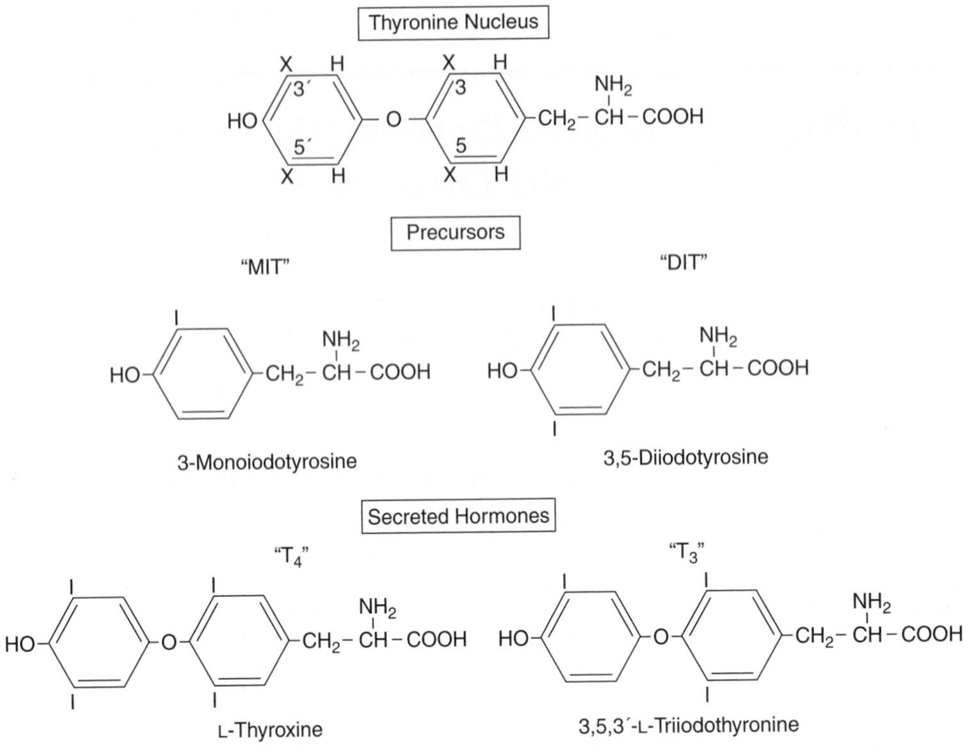

Thyronine Nucleus

Precursors

"MIT" 3-Monoiodotyrosine

"DIT" 3,5-Diiodotyrosine

Secreted Hormones

"T_4" L-Thyroxine

"T_3" 3,5,3′-L-Triiodothyronine

Figure 10–1. Structure of thyroid hormone and related compounds. The thyronine nucleus, the precursor iodinated amino acids, and the secreted hormones, thyroxine (T_4) and triiodothyronine (T_3). Iodinated thyronines are formed by the oxidative coupling of the precursor iodotyrosines monoiodotyrosine (MIT) and diiodotyrosine (DIT) in the thyroglobulin molecule.

of hydrogen peroxide (H_2O_2), although it forms insignificant quantities of iodoproteins under normal circumstances.

Structural Embryology

The human thyroid anlage is first recognizable about 1 month after conception, when the embryo is approximately 3.5 to 4.0 mm in length. The primordium begins as a thickening of epithelium in the pharyngeal floor, which later forms a diverticulum. With continuing development, the median diverticulum is displaced caudad and the primitive stalk connecting the primordium with the pharyngeal floor elongates (thyroglossal duct). During its caudal displacement, the primordium assumes a bilobate shape, coming into contact and fusing with the ventral aspect of the fourth pharyngeal pouch.

Normally, the thyroglossal duct undergoes dissolution and fragmentation by about the second month after conception, leaving at its point of origin a small dimple at the junction of

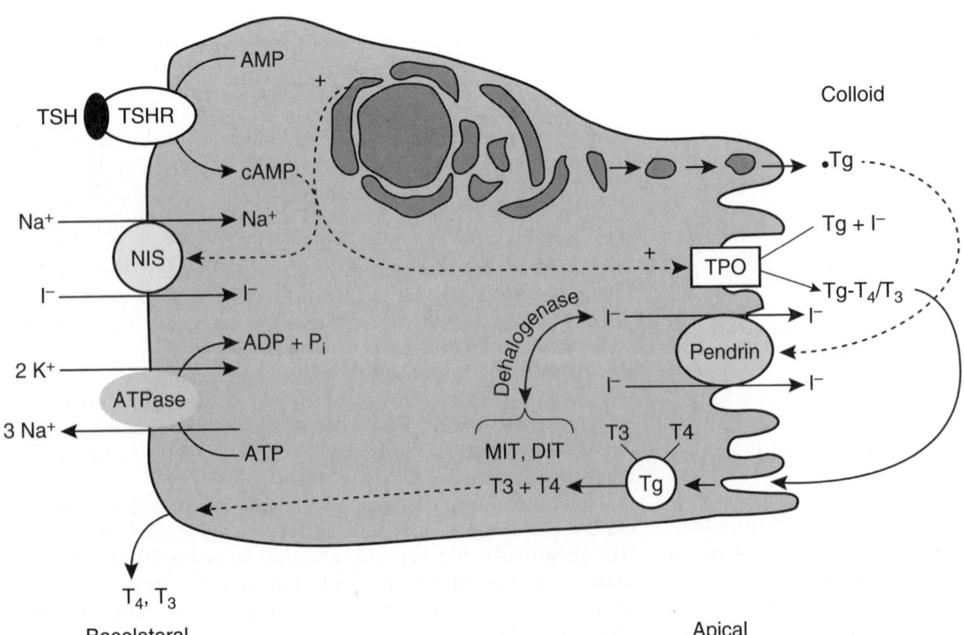

Figure 10–2. Schematic illustration of a thyroid follicular cell showing the key aspects of thyroid iodine transport and thyroid hormone synthesis. AMP, adenosine monophosphate; cAMP, cyclic AMP; DIT, diiotyrosine; MIT, monoiodotyrosine; NIS, sodium iodide symporter; T_3, triiodothyronine; T_4, thyroxine; Tg, thyroglobulin; TPO, thyroid peroxidase; TSH, thyrotropin; TSHR, thyrotropin receptor. (Modified from Spitzweg C, Heufelder AE, Morris JC. Thyroid iodine transport. Thyroid 2000; 10:321–330.)

the middle and posterior thirds of the tongue, the *foramen caecum*. Cells of the lower portion of the duct differentiate into thyroid tissue, forming the pyramidal lobe of the gland. Concomitantly, histologic alterations occur throughout the gland. Complex interconnecting cord-like arrangements of cells interspersed with vascular connective tissue replace the solid epithelial mass and become tubule-like structures at about the third month of fetal life; shortly thereafter, follicular arrangements devoid of colloid appear and eventually the follicles fill with colloid.

Functional Ontogeny

The ontogeny of thyroid function and its regulation in the human fetus are fairly well defined.[1] Future follicular cells acquire the capacity to form thyroglobulin (Tg) as early as the 29th day of gestation, whereas the capacities to concentrate iodide and synthesize T_4 are delayed until about the 11th week. Radioactive iodine inadvertently given to the mother would be accumulated by the fetal thyroid soon thereafter.

Because the capacity of the pituitary to synthesize and secrete TSH is not apparent until the 10th to 12th weeks, early growth and development of the thyroid do not seem to be TSH-dependent. Subsequently, rapid changes in pituitary and thyroid function take place. Probably as a consequence of hypothalamic maturation and increasing secretion of thyrotropin-releasing hormone (TRH), the serum TSH concentration increases between 18 and 26 weeks of gestation, after which levels remain higher than those in the mother.[1, 2] The higher levels may reflect a higher set-point of the negative feedback control of TSH secretion during fetal life than at maturity.

Thyroxine-binding globulin (TBG), the major thyroid hormone–binding protein in plasma, is detectable in serum by the 10th gestational week and increases in concentration progressively to term. This increase accounts, in part, for the progressive increase in the serum T_4 concentration during the second and third trimesters, but increased secretion of T_4 must also play a role because the concentration of unbound, or free, T_4 also rises. The peripheral metabolism of T_4 in the human fetus differs markedly from that in the adult both quantitatively and qualitatively. Overall, rates of production and degradation of T_4 in unit per body mass exceed those in the adult by 10-fold. In addition, the enzymatic pathways by which T_4 is metabolized differ from those in the adult, favoring the formation of the inactive 3,3′,5′-triiodo-L-thyronine (reverse T_3 [rT_3]) at the expense of T_3.

From the clinical standpoint, several aspects of thyroid development are notable.[3] In rare circumstances, thyroid tissue may develop from remnants of the thyroglossal duct near the base of the tongue. Such lingual thyroid tissue may be the sole functioning thyroid tissue present, and thus its surgical removal would lead to hypothyroidism. More commonly, elements of the thyroglossal duct may persist and later give rise to thyroglossal duct cysts, or thyroid tissue progenitors may migrate to occupy a place within the mediastinum.

ANATOMY AND HISTOLOGY

The thyroid gland is one of the largest of the endocrine organs, weighing approximately 15 to 20 g in North American adults. Moreover, the potential of the thyroid for growth is tremendous. The enlarged thyroid, commonly termed a *goiter*, can weigh many hundreds of grams.

The normal thyroid gland is made up of two lobes joined by a thin band of tissue, the isthmus. The latter is approximately 0.5 cm thick, 2 cm wide, and 2 cm high. The individual lobes normally have a pointed superior pole and a poorly defined, blunt inferior pole that merges medially with the isthmus. Each lobe is approximately 2.0 to 2.5 cm in thickness and width at its largest diameter and is approximately 4.0 cm in length. Occasionally, especially when the remainder of the gland is goitrous, a pyramidal lobe is discernible as a finger-like projection directed upward from the isthmus, generally just lateral to the midline, usually on the left. The right lobe is normally more vascular than the left, is often the larger of the two, and tends to enlarge more in disorders associated with a diffuse increase in size.

Two pairs of vessels constitute the major arterial blood supply: (1) the superior thyroid artery, arising from the external carotid artery, and (2) the inferior thyroid artery, arising from the subclavian artery. Estimates of thyroid blood flow range from 4 to 6 mL/minute per g, well in excess of the blood flow to the kidney (3 mL/minute per g). In diffuse toxic goiter due to Graves' disease, blood flow may exceed 1 L/minute and may be associated with an audible bruit or even a palpable thrill.

The gland is composed of closely packed spherical units *(follicles)*, which are invested with a rich capillary network. The interior of the follicle is filled with the clear, proteinaceous colloid that normally is the major constituent of the total thyroid mass (Fig. 10–2). On cross-section, thyroid tissue appears as closely packed, ring-shaped structures consisting of a single layer of thyroid cells surrounding a lumen. The diameter of the follicles varies considerably, even within a single gland, but averages about 200 μm. The follicular cells vary in height with the degree of glandular stimulation, becoming columnar when active and cuboidal when inactive. The epithelium rests on a basement membrane that is rich with glycoproteins separating the follicular cells from the surrounding capillaries. From 20 to 40 follicles are demarcated by connective tissue septa to form a lobule supplied by a single artery. The function of a given lobule may vary from that of its neighbors.

Under electron microscopy, the thyroid follicular epithelium has many features in common with other secretory cells and some peculiar to the thyroid. From the apex of the follicular cell, numerous microvilli extend into the colloid. It is at or near this surface of the cell that iodination, exocytosis, and the initial phase of hormone secretion, namely colloid resorption, occur (see Fig. 10–2).[4] The nucleus has no distinctive features, and the cytoplasm contains an extensive endoplasmic reticulum laden with microsomes. The endoplasmic reticulum is composed of a network of wide, irregular tubules that contain the precursor of Tg. The carbohydrate component of Tg is added to this precursor in the Golgi apparatus, which is located apically. Lysosomes and mitochondria are scattered throughout the cytoplasm. Stimulation by TSH results in enlargement of the Golgi apparatus, formation of pseudopodia at the apical surface, and the appearance in the apical portion of the cell of many droplets that contain colloid taken up from the follicular lumen (see Fig. 10–2).

The thyroid also contains parafollicular cells *(C cells)* that are the source of the calcium-lowering hormone, calcitonin. These cells arise during embryonic development from the last pair of pharyngeal pouches but ultimately come to rest either among the cells of the follicular epithelium or in the thyroid interstitium. They differ from the cells of the follicular epithelium in never bordering on the follicular lumen and in being rich in mitochondria. The C cells undergo hyperplasia early in the syndrome of familial medullary carcinoma of the thyroid and give rise to this tumor in both its familial and its sporadic forms (see Chapter 36).

IODINE AND THE SYNTHESIS AND SECRETION OF THYROID HORMONES

Overview

The function of the thyroid gland is to generate the quantity of thyroid hormone necessary to meet the demands of the peripheral tissues. This requires the daily thyroidal uptake of sufficient iodide and its oxidation by thyroid peroxidase (TPO) to allow the synthesis of approximately 110 nmoles (85 μg) of T_4, which is 65% iodine by weight. This requires the synthesis of a 660-kd glycoprotein homodimer, Tg. Tg contains specific tyrosine residues that are then iodinated at the apical portion of the thyroid cell to form mono- and diiodotyrosine (MIT and DIT) (see Fig. 10–2).

TPO-catalyzed coupling of two molecules of DIT, or one of DIT and one of MIT, leads to formation of T_4 and T_3, respectively, which are then stored as colloid, still as part of the Tg molecule. Pinocytosis of stored colloid leads to the formation of phagolysosomes, the colloid droplets in which Tg is digested, releasing T_4, T_3, DIT, and MIT as the droplet is translocated toward the basal portion of the cell. Thyroxine and T_3 exit the cell into the capillaries, and DIT and MIT are deiodinated by an iodotyrosine deiodinase to allow recycling of the iodide to iodinate newly synthesized Tg.

The synthesis of thyroid hormones requires the expression of a number of thyroid cell–specific proteins. In addition to Tg and TPO, the TSH receptor is also required to transduce the effects of extracellular TSH for efficient hormone synthesis. Several thyroid cell–specific proteins—thyroid transcription factors 1 and 2 (TTF-1 and TTF-2) and PAX-8—stimulate transcription of the Tg and TPO genes. One or more of these proteins may also influence expression of the TSH receptor.[5–7]

Although the biochemical details of these processes are beyond the scope of this discussion, those aspects with clinical relevance are detailed in the following sections. Excellent detailed reviews of these topics may be found elsewhere.[8–11]

Dietary Iodine

Formation of normal quantities of thyroid hormone requires the availability of adequate quantities of exogenous iodine to allow thyroidal uptake of about 60 μg daily, taking into account the fecal losses of about 10 to 20 μg iodine of iodothyronines as glucuronides and about 100 to 150 μg as urinary iodine in iodine-sufficient populations. Plasma iodide (I^-), the form of the element in biologic solutions, is completely filterable with about 60% to 70% of the filtered load reabsorbed passively. At least 100 μg of iodine per day is required to eliminate all signs of iodine deficiency (Table 10–1).

In North America, the daily dietary iodine intake is in the range of 150 to 300 μg daily, largely owing to the iodination of salt; in Japan, where large quantities of foods rich in iodine are consumed, intakes may be as high as several milligrams per day. Notably, iodine intake in the United States is decreasing as a result of a reduction in salt intake, with median urinary iodine of 15 μg/dL but a low urinary iodine (<5 μg/dL) in 12% of the population.[12–14]

The daily dietary intake of iodine varies widely throughout the world, depending on the iodine content of soil and water and on dietary practice (see Table 10–1). Even in a single area, iodine intake varies among different individuals and in the same individual from day to day. Iodine may also enter the body via medications, diagnostic agents, dietary supplements, and food additives.

Table 10–1. Recommended and Typical Values for Dietary Iodine Intake

	μg I/day
Recommended Daily Intake	
Adults	150
During pregnancy	200
Children	90–120
Typical iodine intakes	
North America (1992)	75–300
Chile (1981)	<50–150
Belgium (1993)	50–60
Germany (1993)	20–70
Switzerland (1993)	130–160

As detailed later under the heading "Regulation of Thyroid Function," iodine deficiency is common, especially in mountainous and in formerly glaciated regions of the earth. An estimated 1 billion people live in iodine-deficient areas of the world, and individuals living in such areas often develop TSH-induced compensatory enlargement of the thyroid *(endemic goiter)*. If iodine deficiency is severe during pregnancy, fetal thyroid hormone production falls with irreparable damage to the developing central nervous system (CNS). This is manifested by varying degrees of mental retardation and is termed *endemic cretinism*. Thus, *iodine-deficiency disorders* (IDDs), including endemic goiter and cretinism, are the most common thyroid-related human illnesses—indeed, the most common endocrine disorders worldwide.

Plasma iodide is partly replenished by that lost from the thyroid gland into the blood and by iodide liberated through deiodination of iodothyronines in peripheral tissues. Ultimately, however, the diet is its most important source. Iodine is ingested in both inorganic and organically bound forms. Iodide is rapidly and efficiently absorbed from the GI tract (within 30 minutes), and little is lost in the stool. In the body, iodide is confined largely to the extracellular fluid; however, it is also found in red blood cells and is concentrated in the intraluminal fluids of the GI tract, notably the saliva and gastric juice, from which it is reabsorbed, thus reentering the extracellular fluid. Iodide is also concentrated in milk.

Until it is oxidized and bound to tyrosyl residues in Tg, iodide entering the thyroid by active transport is in rapid equilibrium with the main iodide pool. The concentration of iodide in the extracellular fluid is normally 10 to 15 μg/L ($\sim 10^{-7}$ M), and the content of the peripheral pool is approximately 250 μg. The thyroid gland contains the largest pool of body iodine (normally ~8000 μg), most of which is in the form of DIT and MIT. Generally, this pool of iodine turns over slowly (~1%/day).

Iodide Metabolism by the Thyroid Cell

Because the concentration of iodide in plasma is extremely low, a mechanism is required for the thyroid cell to concentrate the required amounts of this element. This process, called *iodide trapping*, is accomplished by a membrane protein, the *sodium-iodide symporter* (NIS).[15, 16] Human NIS is a 643 amino acid protein with 13 membrane-spanning domains.

The transport of iodide is an active process, depending on the presence of sodium gradient across the basal membrane of the thyroid cell such that downhill transport of 2 Na^+ ions results in the entry of one iodide atom against an electrochemical gradient (see Fig. 10–2). In addition to being expressed in the basolateral membrane of the thyroid cell, NIS has also been identified in other iodide concentrating cells, including salivary and mammary glands, choroid plexus, gastric mucosa, and in the cytotrophoblast and syncytiotrophoblast.[15–17] The iodide transport system generates an iodide gradient of 20 to 40 over the cell membrane and NIS also transports TcO_4^-, ClO_4^-, and SCN^-, accounting for the utility of radioactive TcO_4^- as a thyroid scanning tool and the capacity of potassium perchlorate ($KClO_4^-$) to block iodide uptake.[18] In fact, these anions have a higher affinity for NIS than does iodide itself. On the other hand, the affinity of NIS for iodide is much higher than it is for the other inorganic anions, such as bromide and chloride, accounting for the selectivity of the thyroid transport mechanism.

It has been known for decades that the iodide-concentrating mechanism is required for normal thyroid function, as its absence is associated with congenital hypothyroidism and goiter unless large quantities of inorganic iodide are provided.[19] A number of families have now been identified in which various mutations in the NIS gene are associated with congenital hypothyroidism and an iodide transport defect.[20–22] Transcription of the NIS gene is increased by TSH. The mechanism for this has not been completely elucidated, but studies of the rat NIS promoter suggest that there is an NIS *upstream enhancer*, which confers a cyclic adenosine monophosphate (cAMP) response but also contains binding sites for the thyroid specific transcription factors PAX-8 and TTF-1, as well as a degenerate cAMP response element sequence.[15] Importantly, several studies have documented decreases in NIS expression in human thyroid adenomas and carcinomas that contribute to the loss of iodine uptake in neoplastic thyroid cells, which thus present as "cold" nodules on radioisotopic imaging.[22, 23]

A second thyroid cell protein involved in iodide metabolism, *pendrin*, the product of the *PDS gene*, has now been identified by positional cloning using genomic DNA from families with the autosomal recessive disorder, *Pendred's syndrome*. This is a long-recognized inherited condition in which sensorineural hearing loss is combined with varying degrees of impaired thyroid hormone synthesis, leading to goiter. Pendrin is a transmembrane protein, a member of the sulfate transport protein family. Initially thought to be a sulfate transporter, it is now recognized to transport chloride, iodide, and bicarbonate (HCO_3^-).[24, 25] Pendrin is expressed in the apical border of the thyroid cell, the inner ear, and the kidney (see Fig. 10–2). Mutations in pendrin cause an inner ear malformation, although not all patients have goiter.[25] It is postulated that pendrin is required for iodide transport across the apical membrane of the thyrocyte into the follicular lumen, where it is then oxidized and coupled to tyrosine in Tg (see Fig. 10–2).

The presence of thyroid dysfunction in Pendred's syndrome can be ascertained by the *perchlorate discharge test*, which illustrates the physiologic role of pendrin in thyroidal iodine metabolism. In normal individuals, more than 90% of thyroidal radioiodine is present as iodotyrosine and iodothyronine within minutes of its entry into the thyroid. It is then no longer in the intracellular iodide pool. In patients with Pendred's syndrome, or with other disorders inhibiting the iodination of tyrosine (see later topics, such as Hashimoto's thyroiditis), this process is delayed, as shown by the exit (discharge) of more than 10% of the thyroidal radioiodine within 2 hours of administration of 500 mg of $KClO_4$.[18] Perchlorate inhibits NIS function by an as yet unidentified mechanism eliminating the iodide gradient, which is required for maintaining the radioiodide in the gland. This illustrates that both iodide transport by NIS at the basal pole of the thyrocyte and its efflux across the apical membrane by pendrin are required for thyroid hormone synthesis. Deafness in patients with Pendred's syndrome is due to formation of a common cavity in the upper coils of the cochlea with dilatation of the vestibular aqueducts, not to the hypothyroidism per se.[25]

In addition to being brought into the thyroid gland by active transport from the extracellular fluid, thyroidal iodide is generated by the deiodination of iodotyrosines liberated during the hydrolysis of Tg. A portion of this iodide is oxidized and used to iodinate tyrosine, and the remainder is lost from the gland as the *iodide leak* (see Fig. 10–2). This conservation process is interrupted when antithyroid drugs—which inhibit iodide oxidation, such as methimazole (MMI), carbimazole (CB) or propylthiouracil (PTU)—are given, thus further enhancing the effectiveness of these thyroid peroxidase inhibitors in blocking thyroid hormone synthesis.

Iodide Oxidation and Organification of Iodide

Within the thyroid gland, iodide participates in a series of reactions that lead to the synthesis of the active thyroid hormones. The first of these involves oxidation of iodide and incorporation of the resulting intermediate into the hormonally inactive iodotyrosines MIT and DIT, a process termed *organification*. Iodide is normally oxidized rapidly, immediately appearing in organic combination in Tg. The iodinations that lead to formation of iodotyrosines occur within Tg rather than on the free amino acids.

Oxidation of thyroidal iodide is mediated by the heme-containing protein TPO. The complementary DNA (cDNA) for human TPO encodes 933 amino acids with a molecular size of 103 kd, 10% of which is due to carbohydrate. The protein contains a membrane spanning region near the COOH terminus, and it is oriented in the apical membrane of the thyroid cell with residues 1 to 844 in the follicular lumen (see Fig. 10–2).[26] TPO is the major *thyroid microsomal antigen*, and recombinant human TPO is now used for the detection of *anti-thyroid microsomal antibodies*, commonly present in the serum of patients with Hashimoto's thyroiditis.

Because TPO is a heme protein, organic iodinations require molecular oxygen and are inhibited by cyanide and azide. In vitro, TPO, in the presence of H_2O_2, iodinates Tg as well as other proteins. The reaction catalyzed by peroxidase in vitro has many properties of the iodination reaction in vivo, including inhibition by PTU and MMI and by high concentrations of iodide (the Wolff-Chaikoff effect).[27] The evanescent product of the peroxidation of iodide (i.e., the active iodinating form) may be free hypoiodous acid, iodine, or iodinium (I^+).[9] The H_2O_2 that serves as the oxidant of iodide is generated through the auto-oxidation of flavin enzymes acting as NADH—and particularly NADPH—oxidases. In this way, generation of H_2O_2 is linked to electron transfers due to substrate oxidations within the thyroid. Radioautographic and histochemical evidence suggests that the iodination reactions occur at the cell colloid interface (see Fig. 10–2).[28] Thus mitochondrial systems provide a source of H_2O_2, cell membranes contain TPO, and the cytoplasmic fraction the regulatory inhibitors of organic iodinations.

The rate of organic iodinations depends on the degree of thyroid stimulation by TSH (see later). Iodinations are susceptible to inhibition by a number of pharmacologic agents, including the thiourea derivatives, PTU, MMI, and CB, which are inhibitors of peroxidase and have intrinsic reducing activity.[9] Defects in the organic binding mechanism cause goitrous congenital hypothyroidism or, if less severe, goiter without hypothyroidism. In some families, thyroidal TPO is absent.[29] In others, the defect may reside in inadequate production of H_2O_2 or in abnormalities in Tg that render it less readily iodinated (see Chapter 12).[30, 31]

Iodothyronine Synthesis

The MIT and DIT formed via oxidation and organic binding of iodide are precursors of the hormonally active iodothyronines T_4 and T_3. Because noniodinated thyronine cannot be demonstrated in Tg, T_4 and T_3 must arise from iodinated tyrosine precursors. Synthesis of T_4 from DIT requires the fusion of two DIT molecules to yield a structure with two diiodinated rings linked by an ether bridge and is catalyzed by TPO. Concomitantly, a residual dehydroalanine is formed at the site of the DIT residue contributing the phenolic hydroxyl group (beta or outer ring).[32] This process is termed the *coupling reaction*.

Efficient synthesis of T_4 and T_3 in the thyroid requires Tg. The large (>260 kb) Tg gene is on chromosome 8. The Tg messenger RNA is 8 to 8.5 kb in length and encodes a 330-kd 12S subunit that is 10% carbohydrate by weight. There are 134 tyrosyl residues in the 660-kd homodimer. Only 25 to 30 of these are iodinated, but only residues 5, 1290, and 2553 form T_4 and residue 2746, T_3.[8, 33] The T_4-forming, readily iodinated, and iodothyronine-forming acceptor residues of Tg from different species are in a Glu/Asp-Tyr or a Thr/Ser-TyrSer sequence, suggesting an important role of primary sequence in these reactions.

There are three to four T_4 molecules in each molecule of human Tg under conditions of normal iodination (~25 atoms per Tg molecule, ~0.5% iodine by weight), but only about one in five molecules of human Tg contains a T_3 residue.[28] In Tg from patients with untreated Graves' disease, the content of T_4 residues remains approximately the same, but the number of T_3 residues doubles to an average of 0.4 per molecule. This difference is independent of the iodination state of the Tg and is a consequence of thyroidal stimulation. Because the coupling reaction is catalyzed by TPO, virtually all agents that inhibit organic binding also inhibit coupling.

Storage and Release of Thyroid Hormone

The thyroid gland is unique among the endocrine glands by virtue of the large store of hormone it contains and the low rate at which the hormone turns over (1%/day). This aspect of thyroid hormone economy has homeostatic value, in that the reservoir provides prolonged protection against depletion of circulating hormone should synthesis cease. In normal humans, administration of antithyroid agents for as long as 2 weeks has little effect on the serum T_4 concentration. There are approximately 250 μg T_4/g wet weight in normal human thyroid or 5000 μg of T_4 in a 20-g gland.[34] This is sufficient to maintain a euthyroid state for at least 50 days. When T_4 is released rapidly in an uncontrolled fashion during subacute or painless thyroiditis, this can cause significant transient thyrotoxicosis. Tg is present in the plasma of normal individuals at concentrations up to 50 ng/mL, leaving the thyroid gland through the lymphatics. However, peripheral hydrolysis of Tg does not contribute significantly to the T_4 and T_3 in the circulation, even during thyroiditis, when large quantities of this protein are released.[35]

The first step in thyroid hormone release is the endocytosis of colloid from the follicular lumen by two processes: *macropinocytosis* by pseudopods formed at the apical membrane, and *micropinocytosis* by small coated vesicles that form at the apical surface (see Fig. 10–2). Both processes are stimulated by TSH, but the relative importance of the two pathways varies among species. Micropinocytosis is thought to predominate in humans.

Following endocytosis, endocytotic vesicles fuse with lysosomes, and proteolysis is catalyzed by cathepsin L- and D-like thiol proteases, all of which are active at the acidic pH of the lysosome. The iodotyrosines released from Tg are rapidly deiodinated by an NADPH-dependent iodotyrosine deiodinase, and the released iodine is recycled. The T_4 is released from Tg, but it is not clear how its transfer into the plasma is regulated. Release is acutely stimulated by TSH, as may be the 5′-monodeiodination of small amounts of T_4 to T_3 by the types 1 and 2 iodothyronine deiodinases (D1 and D2), which are both expressed in human thyroid.[36–38]

Although basal and TSH-stimulated conversion of T_4 to T_3 is easily demonstrated in the perfused canine thyroid gland, the contribution of thyroidal T_4 deiodination to T_3 secretion in humans under physiologic conditions is not known. The 15/1 ratio of T_4 to T_3 in human Tg, as compared with the 10/1 ratio of the secreted hormones, suggests minor T_4 monodeiodination. However, stimulation of D2-catalyzed T_4 5′-deiodination in Graves' thyroid may enhance that pathway and contribute to the relative increase in the ratio of T_3 to T_4 production in that condition.[39]

Tg proteolysis and T_4 release are inhibited by several agents, the most important of which is iodide. Inhibition of hormone release is responsible for the rapid improvement that iodide induces in hyperthyroid patients. The mechanism by which this effect is mediated is uncertain, but iodide inhibits the stimulation of thyroid adenylate cyclase by TSH and by the stimulatory immunoglobulins of Graves' disease. Increasing iodination of Tg also increases its resistance to hydrolysis by acid proteases in the lysosomes. Lithium inhibits thyroid hormone release, although its mechanism of action is poorly understood and may differ from that of iodide.[40–42]

Role and Mechanism of Thyrotropin Effects

All steps in the formation and release of thyroid hormones are stimulated by TSH secreted by the pituitary thyrotrophs (see Chapter 8). Thyroid cells express the TSH receptor (TSHR), a member of the glycoprotein G protein–coupled-receptor family. The deduced amino acid sequence of this protein predicts a large extracellular NH_2-terminal domain, seven membrane-spanning domains, and an intracellular domain that transduces the signal to the Gs (adenylyl cyclase) and G qIII (phospholipase C [PL-C]) pathways (Table 10–2).[10] The TSHR also binds thyroid-stimulating antibody (TSAb) and thyroid-blocking antibodies (TBAb) (see Chapter 11).[43] In addition, the closely related luteinizing hormone (LH) and chorionic gonadotropin (CG) also bind to and activate TSHR signaling. CG accounts for the physiologic hyperthyroidism of early pregnancy.[1, 10, 43, 44]

Besides the thyrocyte, TSHR is also expressed in adipocytes in human neonates as well as in orbital adipocytes in adults.[45, 46] Interestingly, certain "activating mutations," either germline or somatic, have been identified in the membrane spanning or intracellular portions of the TSHR molecule that cause generalized or nodular hyperfunction.[47, 48] Even more subtle changes may occur. In one family, a replacement of lysine 183 with arginine in the extracellular domain increased the activation of TSHR by human chorionic gonadotropin (hCG), causing recurrent *gestational hyperthyroidism*.[49] Curiously, the TSHR may be cleaved into A and B subunits to varying extents, but the physiologic significance of cleaved and uncleaved receptors is unclear.[50]

Studies of the rate-limiting intracellular reactions stimulated by TSH are complicated by the fact that the intrathyroidal events are stimulated by protein kinase A (PKA)–related mechanisms in one species or cell model and by PL-C–directed pathways in another (see Table 10–2).[50] The effects on

Table 10–2. Thyroid Cell Functions Stimulated by Thyrotropin

Function Affected	General Mechanism
Iodide Metabolism	
Increase I^- in follicular lumen	PL-C
Delayed increase in NIS expression	cAMP
Increase thyroid blood flow	↑ Nitric oxide synthesis (↓ cellular iodide)
Increase in I^- efflux from thyroid cell	?
Thyroid Hormone Synthesis	
↑ Hydrogen peroxide	PL-C
↑ Thyroglobulin and TPO synthesis	cAMP
↑ NADPH via pentose-phosphate pathway	?
Thyroid Hormone Secretion	
↑ Pinocytosis of thyroglobulin	cAMP
↑ Release of thyroglobulin into plasma via basolateral membrane	cAMP (?)
Mitogenesis	cAMP, PL-C, and IGF-I– and FGF-mediated kinase activation

cAMP, cyclic adenosine monophosphate; FGF, follicular growth factor; IGF-I, insulin-like growth factor I; NIS, sodium-iodide symporter; PL-C, phospholipase C; TPO, thyroid peroxidase.

iodide kinetics include both an early stimulation of iodide efflux into the follicular lumen and a later increase in the V_{max} for iodide transport. The latter is likely due to enhanced expression of NIS.[15, 16, 22]

Peroxidase generation in human thyrocytes is activated by Ca^{2+} and diacylglycerol, although 10-fold higher concentrations of TSH are required for activation of this limb of the TSHR pathways than for activation of adenylate cyclase. TSH increases the levels of both TPO messenger RNA (mRNA) and protein, even though no cAMP response element-binding protein (CREB) sequences have been identified in the promoter of this gene.[11] The effect on TPO may be secondary to cAMP stimulation of thyroid cell–specific proteins, such as TTF-1, TTF-2, or PAX-8 (see earlier), but this remains to be shown. Similarly, transcription of the Tg gene is also stimulated by cAMP through indirect pathways, perhaps involving the same mechanism.[11]

Interestingly, TSH can increase TSHR mRNA in human thyroid cells, although at high TSH concentrations there may be a modest decrease in receptor expression. Nonetheless, the persistence of a functional TSHR that is not down-regulated by autophosphorylation can explain the hyperthyroidism of Graves' disease and that associated with TSH-producing thyrotroph tumors.[43, 51] TSH, via cAMP, also stimulates the ingestion and hydrolysis of colloid and the release of T_4 (and Tg) from the thyroid cell.

Thyroid cell proliferation is stimulated by cAMP, phorbol esters, and epidermal growth factor (EGF) through tyrosine kinases.[11] However, cAMP causes proliferation while maintaining differentiated function, whereas EGF and phorbol esters lead to dedifferentiation. Similarly, insulin-like growth factor I (IGF-I) and fibroblast growth factor (FGF) stimulate cell division and dedifferentiation, although species differences exist in the effects of these agents.[10, 11, 52] In human thyrocytes, the events stimulated by the adenylate cyclase pathway are probably the most crucial for thyroid growth and explain the goitrous changes associated with prolonged TSH stimulation, such as those occurring during iodine deficiency.

THYROID HORMONES IN PERIPHERAL TISSUES

Plasma Transport

The metabolic transformations of thyroid hormones in peripheral tissues determine their biologic potency and regulate their biologic effects. Consequently, an understanding of thyroid physiopathology requires a knowledge of the pathways of thyroid hormone metabolism.

A wide variety of iodothyronines and their metabolic derivatives exist in plasma. Of these, T_4 is highest in concentration and the only one that arises solely from direct secretion by the thyroid gland. In normal people, T_3 is also released from the thyroid but about 80% is derived from the peripheral tissues by the enzymatic removal of a single 5′-iodine atom (outer ring or 5′-monodeiodination) from T_4.[53] The remaining iodothyronines and their derivatives are generated in the peripheral tissues from T_4 and T_3. Principal among them are 3,3′,5′-triiodothyronine (rT_3) and 3,3′-diiodo-L-thyronine (3,3′-T_2) (Fig. 10–3). Trace concentrations of other diiodothyronines, monoiodothyronines, and conjugates thereof with glucuronic or sulfuric acid are also present.[54, 55] Deaminated derivatives of T_4 and T_3 that bear an acetic acid rather than an alanine side chain (tetrac and triac) are also present in low concentrations (Fig. 10–4).

The major iodothyronines are poorly soluble in water and thus bind reversibly to plasma proteins. The plasma proteins with which T_4 is mainly associated are TBG and transthyretin (TTR), formerly termed T_4-binding prealbumin (TBPA), and albumin (Table 10–3). About 75% to 80% of T_3 is bound by TBG, with the remainder bound by TTR and albumin.

Thyroxine-Binding Globulin

TBG is a glycoprotein with a molecular mass of about 54 kDa, about 20% of which is carbohydrate. The gene that encodes the protein is on the X chromosome.[56] The protein sequence of TBG resembles that of the SERPIN family of serine antiproteases.[57, 58] Because there is one iodothyronine binding site per TBG molecule, the T_4 or T_3 binding capacity of TBG in normal human serum is equivalent to its concentration, approximately 270 nmol/L (21 μg T_4/dL). The half-life of the protein in plasma is about 5 days, and the *metabolic clearance rate* (MCR) is approximately 800 mL/day.

Congenital deficiencies of TBG are common, occurring in 1/5000 newborns, and are associated with the complete absence of the protein in males.[59, 60] Other abnormalities of TBG can alter the susceptibility to heat denaturation or the capacity to bind thyroid hormone. One such variant has been described in Australian aborigines, and a TBG protein with increased heat lability occurs in Africans. All of these abnormalities are inherited in an X-linked fashion. L-Asparaginase blocks the synthesis of TBG, which explains the low serum T_4 and TBG concentrations in patients receiving this agent.[61, 62]

The glycosylation of TBG influences its clearance from the plasma and its behavior during isoelectric focusing.[63, 64] Four to six bands are present; after exposure to neuraminidase, however, these differences are lost, indicating that they are due to variations in the numbers of sialic acid residues. In estrogen-treated patients, the prevalence of the more acidic bands of TBG is increased. The more highly sialylated TBG, compared with the more positively charged TBG, is cleared more slowly from plasma because increased sialylation inhibits the hepatic uptake of glycoproteins. The sera of pregnant patients, women receiving oral contraceptives, and patients with acute hepatitis have increased fractions of acidic TBG. Patients with inherited

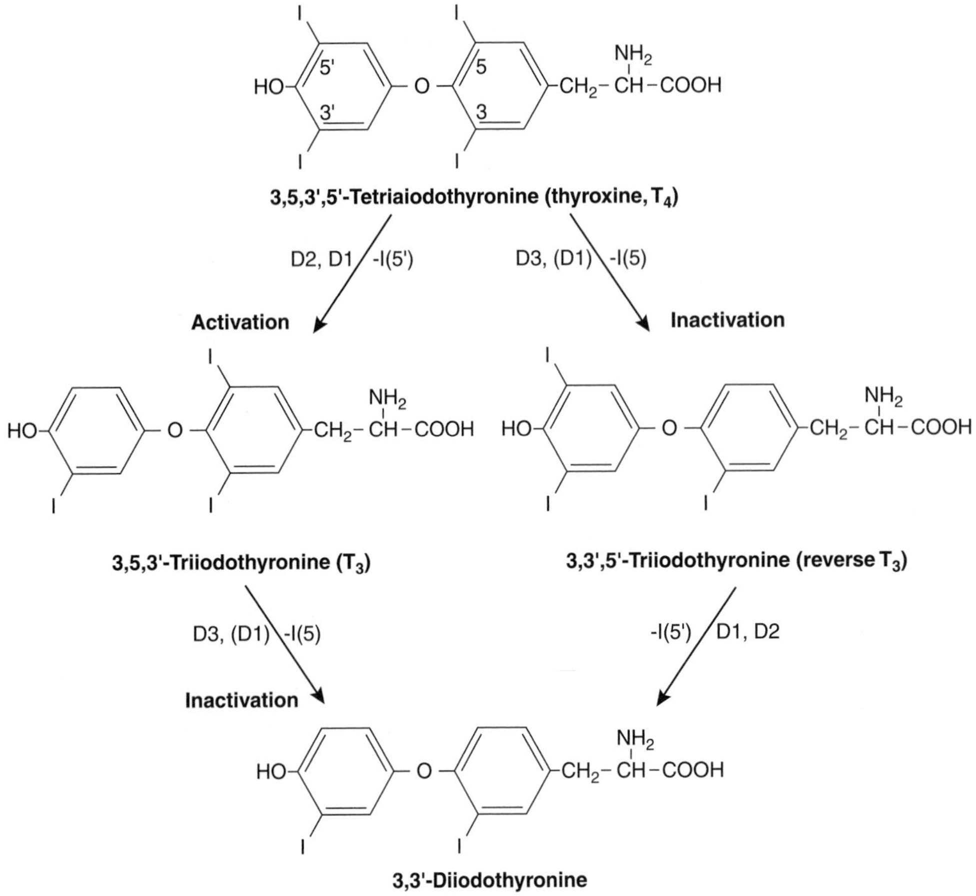

Figure 10–3. Pathways for thyroid hormone activation and inactivation catalyzed by human iodothyronine selenodeiodinases. Numbers refer to the iodine positions in the iodothyronine nucleus. The iodothyronine deiodinases are abbreviated D1, D2, and D3 for types 1, 2, and 3 deiodinases, respectively. *Arrows* refer to monodeiodination of the outer or inner ring of the iodothyronine nucleus, termed 5′ or 5 by convention. The parentheses around D1 emphasize that D3, not D1, is probably the major enzyme catalyzing inner ring deiodination of T_4 and T_3.

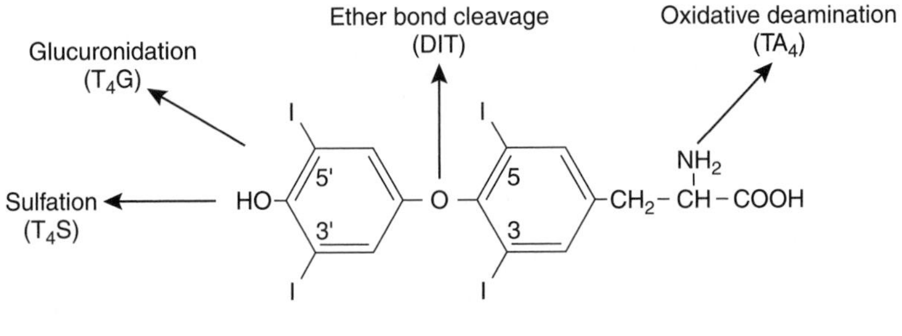

Figure 10–4. Important nondeiodinative pathways of thyroid hormone metabolism. DIT, diiodotyrosine; S, sulfate; TA_4, tetraiodothyroacetic acid; T_4, thyroxine; T_3, triiodothyronine. (Modified from Visser TJ. Pathways of thyroid hormone metabolism. Acta Med Austriaca 1996; 23:10–16.)

Table 10–3. Comparison of the Major Human Thyroid Hormone-Binding Proteins

	Thyroxine-Binding Globulin	Transthyretin	Albumin
Mol wt of holoprotein (kDa)	54,000	54,000 (4 subunits)	66,000
Plasma concentrations (μmol/L)	0.27	4.6	640
T_4 binding capacity as μg T_4/dL	21	350	50,000
Association constants of the major binding site (L/M)			
T_4	1×10^{10}	7×10^7	7×10^5
T_3	5×10^8	1.4×10^7	1×10^5
Fraction of sites occupied by T_4 in euthyroid plasma	0.31	0.02	<0.001
Distribution volume (L)	7	5.7	7.8
Turnover rate (%/d)	13	59	5
Distribution of iodothyronines (%/protein)			
T_4	68	11	20
T_3	80	9	11

TBG excess have normal amounts of highly sialylated TBG, as do men and nonpregnant women. Because TBG is the principal T_4- and T_3-binding protein, changes in TBG or in its binding are paralleled by changes in total plasma T_4 and T_3 even though T_4 and T_3 production is little changed.

Another post-translational modification affecting TBG occurs in patients with sepsis or in patients after cardiopulmonary bypass surgery.[65–67] TBG is subjected to cleavage by a serine protease released from polymorphonuclear leukocytes resulting in the release of a 5-kD COOH terminal loop with a consequent decrease in affinity for T_4. An analogous reaction has been described for CBG that releases cortisol at the site of inflammation.[68] It has been postulated that the released T_4 might play a critical role in the response to injury, perhaps by providing a supply of iodine for antibacterial purposes.[65, 69] The cleaved TBG (~49 kd) circulates, and because it binds T_4 with lower avidity, this may explain the increased ratio of free T_4 to bound T_4 in acute illness, even when TBG saturation studies or immunoassays indicate a normal TBG concentration (see "Thyroid Function during Fasting or Illness").[56]

Transthyretin

TTR exists in part as a complex with retinol (vitamin A)-binding protein, hence its name. It consists of four identical polypeptide chains, with a total molecular mass of approximately 55 kDa, and is not glycosylated. Its concentration in plasma is approximately 4 mmol/L (250 μg/mL). Each mole of TTR binds 1 mole of T_4 with high affinity, and a second T_4 molecule is bound with lower affinity at high concentrations of T_4.[59] Binding of T_4 by TTR is independent of the association with retinol-binding protein. Its half-life in plasma is normally about 2 days, but this decreases during illness.[70]

TTR is expressed in the choroid plexus and is the major thyroid hormone–binding protein in the cerebrospinal fluid (CSF).[71] Targeted TTR gene disruption in mice shows that—aside from the predictable 50% decrease in total plasma T_4 concentration and reciprocal increase in the free T_4 fraction (since TTR is a major T_4-binding protein in mice)—the absence of the gene causes no developmental abnormality. There is also no evidence of impaired uptake of T_4 into the brain, leaving the role of TTR in CSF undefined in regard to thyroid physiology.[72, 73]

Variant forms of TTR are associated with familial amyloidotic polyneuropathy.[59, 60] In affected families, the TTR monomer has one of several different point mutations and TTR accumulates in amyloid tissue deposits. Neither thyroid dysfunction nor altered vitamin A metabolism has been reported, although there is altered affinity of some of the mutant proteins for T_4. Families with both high-affinity TTR and a few with increased TTR levels have been reported.[74]

Comparison of Thyroxine and Triiodothyronine Binding by Thyroxine-Binding Globulin and Transthyretin

The TBG-binding site has an affinity for T_3 that is about 20-fold less than that for T_4 (see Table 10–3). TBG binds both the dextroisomer of T_4 and the naturally occurring levoisomer. Deamination of the iodothyronine molecule reduces binding to TBG and increases the affinity for TTR; the acetic and propionic acid analogues of T_4 and T_3 bind poorly, if at all, to this protein. Binding of T_4 by TBG is inhibited by phenytoin,[75] salicylate,[76] salsalate,[77, 78] furosemide,[79] fenclofenac,[80] and mitotane. The affinity of these compounds for TBG is much weaker than is that of T_4 or T_3, but their concentration in plasma may be sufficient to interfere with T_4 and T_3 binding and reduce total hormone levels. Inhibitors of the T_4 TTR interaction include salicylate, salsalate and some of its congeners, penicillin, and plant flavonoids.[81]

Albumin

The affinity of albumin for T_4 and T_3 binding is much lower than that of either TBG or TTR, but the high concentration of this protein results in the binding of 10% of the plasma thyroid hormones (see Table 10–3). Changes in albumin concentration per se have little influence on the total hormone levels unless they are accompanied by alterations in TBG and TTR, all three of which are synthesized in the liver. Hepatic failure or nephrotic syndrome leads to a decreased plasma concentration of all three, and the albumin concentration serves as a surrogate for estimating TBG concentrations.

The role of albumin in thyroid physiology becomes chemically important in patients with *familial dysalbuminemic hyperthyroxinemia* (FDH).[82, 83] In this autosomal dominant disorder, the plasma contains high amounts of a usually minor albumin variant that binds T_4 (but not T_3) with increased avidity. This increases total T_4 levels, but free T_4 and total and free T_3 levels remain normal in an otherwise euthyroid patient. In one family, the albumin variant was reported to bind T_3, but not T_4, with 40-fold higher affinity, resulting in dysalbuminemic hypertriiodothyroxinemia.[84]

Other Plasma Thyroid Hormone–Binding Proteins

Between 3% and 6% of plasma T_4 and T_3 are bound to lipoproteins.[85] The T_4-binding lipoprotein is 27-kDa homodimer with an affinity for T_4 that is lower than that of TBG. This binding is of uncertain physiologic significance but may play a role in targeting T_4 delivery to specific tissues.

Free Thyroid Hormones

Because most of the circulating T_4 and T_3 is bound to TBG, its concentration and degree of saturation are the major determinants of the free fraction of T_4. Binding of the thyroid hormones to the plasma proteins alters their metabolism. The negligible urinary excretion of T_3 and T_4 is due to the limited filterability of the hormone-binding protein complexes at the glomerulus. The volume of distribution and rate of turnover of the hormones are also affected by their protein associations.

In vitro, the interaction between the thyroid hormones and their binding proteins conforms to a reversible binding equilibrium that can be expressed by conventional equilibrium equations. For the formulations that follow, T_4 is used as the prototype, with the understanding that similar interactions apply in the case of T_3. The interaction between T_4 and TBG can be expressed as follows:

$$T_4 + TBG \overset{K}{\rightleftharpoons} T_4 \cdot TBG$$

where TBG is the *unoccupied* binding protein, K is the equilibrium association constant for the interaction, and T_4 is the concentration of *free* T_4.

$T_4 \cdot TBG$ is T_4 bound to TBG (almost equal to 68% of total T_4). This interaction can also be expressed by the mass action relationship, wherein

$$\frac{T_4 \cdot TBG}{(T_4)\,(TBG)} = K$$

Rearranging

$$\frac{T_4}{T_4 \cdot TBG} = \frac{1}{(TBG)K}$$

Thus, the free fraction of T_4 is inversely proportional to the concentration of unoccupied TBG-binding sites. Estimates of the free T_4 concentration in serum can be generated by direct or indirect assay. For example, with the aid of radiolabeled T_4, the proportion that is unbound by protein is determined by dialysis, and the concentration of free T_4 can then be calculated as the product of the total hormone concentration and the fraction that is free. In normal serum, the free T_4 is approximately 0.02% of the total (~20 pmol/L, 1.5 ng/dL). The approximately 20-fold lower affinity of TBG for T_3 results in a higher proportion of T_3 free (0.30%).

It is the free hormone that is available to the tissues for intracellular transport and feedback regulation, that induces its metabolic effects, and that undergoes degradation. The bound hormone acts merely as a reservoir. It follows that the concentration of the free hormone is the determinant of the metabolic state, and it is this concentration that is defended by homeostatic mechanisms. If an increase in the overall net binding affinity for T_4 occurs, the free T_4 concentration can be maintained at normal levels only if the bound T_4 increases. This is true whether or not the causative factor is an increase in the concentration of TBG or the presence of abnormal T_4-binding proteins.

The plasma concentration of T_4 is determined by its rate of entry into, and exit from, the plasma. The MCR relates the quantity of T_4 removed from the plasma per unit time to the quantity available for removal (i.e., its plasma concentration). Thus,

$$MCR = D/[P]$$

where MCR is the metabolic clearance rate (volume/time), D is the absolute disposal or removal rate (amount/time), and [P] is the plasma concentration (amount/volume). Transposing,

$$[P] = D/MCR$$

However, under steady-state conditions, the production rate (PR) of T_4 and the disposal rate (D) are equal. Hence,

$$[P] = PR/MCR$$

Thus, for any level of T_4 production, be it increased, normal, or decreased, the total plasma T_4 level varies inversely with its MCR. However, if only the free T_4 leaves the plasma and enters the cells while the bound T_4 is confined largely to the intravascular space, changing the fraction of total T_4 that is free, by changing the fraction that is available to the tissues, changes the MCR in a parallel manner. This explains, in part, why a primary increase in thyroid hormone binding, such as occurs when TBG concentrations are increased during pregnancy or by administration of excess estrogen, transiently reduces the free T_4 level and its clearance, causing an increase in the plasma total T_4 concentration.

The transient decrease in free thyroid hormones also reduces the negative feedback on the hypothalamic-pituitary-thyroid axis. This results in an increase in TSH secretion with a consequent increase in thyroid hormone production as an additional compensation.[86, 87] This can explain a portion of the increased levothyroxine (L-thyroxine) requirement in the first trimester of pregnancy and the adaptation of the normal thyroid gland that occurs during estrogen administration.[88, 89]

This formulation is called the *free thyroid hormone hypothesis*.[90, 91] If it is free hormone that is available for cellular entry, what is the role, if any, of the hormone-binding proteins? These proteins permit distribution of the hydrophobic thyroid hormones throughout the vascular system. For example, if a protein-free solution containing tracer T_3 is perfused through rat liver via the portal vein, there is a steep concentration gradient with a decreasing quantity of T_3 in cells as the distance from the center of the portal lobule increases.[92] In fact, virtually all of the T_3 is taken up by the first cells to be contacted by the bolus. In contrast, if serum albumin is added to the perfusate, the distribution of tracer is uniform throughout the lobule, with only 46% of the tracer removed from the bolus. Both influx and efflux of thyroid hormone from tissues are rapid. Thus, intracellular free T_3 and T_4 are in equilibrium with the free hormone pool in plasma. In the steady state, the rate of T_3 and T_4 metabolism (not the dissociation rate from plasma proteins) determines the rate of removal of these hormones from the plasma.

Cellular Uptake and Intracellular Binding

Carrier-mediated, energy-dependent transport of thyroid hormones has now been demonstrated in many cell lines.[93] The carrier transport system for T_3 and T_4 is saturable, stereospecific, and requires adenosine triphosphate (ATP), but the two iodothyronines typically do not compete for uptake.

The proteins mediating this transport are the Na^+/taurocholate cotransporting polypeptide (NTCP), members of the Na^+ independent organic anion transporter (OATP) family[94–96] and the L type amino acid transporters.[97–100] Information is still available only in preliminary form, but it is likely that there will be a variety of overlapping mechanisms for thyroid hormone transport and that different transporters will be present in different cell types.[93]

In patients receiving a low-calorie diet for 1 week, T_3 and T_4 uptake into both rapidly equilibrating (liver and kidney) and slowly equilibrating pools (muscle) is decreased.[101] Thus, inhibition of T_4 (and rT_3) transport into these organs may well explain the low production of T_3 and the elevation of rT_3 concentrations in the serum of sick or fasting individuals (see later). The processes regulating efflux of thyroid hormones from cells are less well understood but appear to involve a verapamil-sensitive mechanism.[102, 103] Our knowledge of the mechanisms regulating both T_4 and T_3 influx and efflux is expected to increase rapidly over the next few years now that these transporters have been cloned.

Cellular-Binding Proteins

Proteins that bind T_4 and T_3 are present in the cytosol, and some studies suggest that the cytosol-binding proteins for T_4 and T_3 are distinct from one another. The intracellular free T_3 concentration can be estimated by evaluating the binding affinity of intracellular and nuclear binding proteins and by measuring the T_3 concentration in cytosol.[104] Such analyses suggest that there is a free hormone gradient of twofold to threefold across the plasma membrane. This concentration gradient, however, is not nearly as high as that calculated for the nuclear/cytosolic ratios in liver, kidney, heart, and brain, which are 50:1 to 250:1.

The mechanisms for maintaining these gradients have not been defined and have not been verified by direct methods. It is surprising that, despite such high ratios for free T_3 between the nucleus and cytoplasm, only 10% of the intracellular T_3 is present in the nucleus except in pituitary cells, where T_3 is equally divided between the nuclear and cytoplasmic compartments.[105]

Thyroid Hormone Activation and Inactivation by the Selenodeiodinases

The most important pathway for T_4 metabolism is its *outer ring* (5′) monodeiodination to the active thyroid hormone, T_3.

Table 10–4. Human Iodothyronine Selenodeiodinases

Parameter	Type 1 (Outer and Inner Ring)	Type 2 (Outer Ring)	Type 3 (Inner Rings)
Physiologic Role	rT_3 and T_3S degradation, source of plasma T_3 especially in hyperthyroid patients	Provide intracellular T_3 in specific tissues, source of plasma T_3	Inactivate T_3 and T_4
Tissue location	Liver, kidney, thyroid, pituitary (?) (not CNS)	CNS, pituitary, brown adipose tissue, placenta, thyroid, skeletal muscle, heart	Placenta, CNS, hemangiomas, fetal liver
Subcellular location	Plasma membrane	Endoplasmic reticulum	?
Preferred substrates (position)	rT_3 (5′), T_3S (5)	T_4, rT_3 (5′)	T_3, T_4 (5)
K_m	10^{-7} (rT_3), 10^{-6} (T_4)	10^{-9} (T_4 and rT_3)	10^{-9} (T_3 and T_4)
Susceptibility to PTU inhibition	High	Absent	Absent
Response to increased T_4	↑	↓	↑

CNS, central nervous system; PTU, propylthiouracil; rT_3, reverse T_3.

This reaction is catalyzed by type 1 and type 2 deiodinases *(D1* and *D2)* (see Fig. 10–3). *Inner ring* deiodination, catalyzed primarily by type 3 deiodinase *(D3)*, inactivates T_4 and T_3 (see Fig. 10–3).[53, 106] These reactions can be considered physiologically activating and inactivating pathways that control T_3 concentrations in peripheral tissues.

The structures of the three human deiodinases are similar to one another and are conserved from tadpoles to humans.[53] All three contain selenocysteine in the active catalytic center and hence are termed *selenodeiodinases* (Table 10–4). Selenocysteine has nucleophilic properties that make it ideal for catalysis of oxidoreductive reactions such as iodothyronine deiodination and the reduction of H_2O_2 by another family of selenoenzymes, the glutathione peroxidases.[107, 108] Selenium acts as the iodine acceptor during deiodination reactions (Fig. 10–5).

Mutagenesis of selenocysteine in D1 to cysteine (e.g., replacing Se with S) reduces the reaction velocity by 100-fold.[109] Synthesis of selenoproteins is a complex process because the normal STOP translation function of the UGA codon which encodes selenocysteine must be overridden by the cell. This is accomplished by a combination of a specific structural feature, the SECIS element, in the 3′-untranslated region of the mRNAs encoding these proteins together with a specific group of selenocysteine-incorporating gene products.[53, 110–112]

Comparative Enzymology and Regulation of the Selenodeiodinases

Types 1 and 2

Type 1 deiodinase has several characteristics that distinguish it from D2 and D3 (see Table 10–4). It can catalyze both 5′- and 5-deiodination of T_4 to form T_3 and rT_3, respectively, but the K_m for these reactions is about three orders of magnitude greater than that of D2 and D3 for this substrate. In fact, the preferred substrates of D1 are rT_3 (5′-deiodination) and T_3-SO_4 (5-deiodination).[113]

Unlike the deiodinations catalyzed by D2 and D3, D1-catalyzed reactions are susceptible to inhibition by PTU (see Fig. 10–5). D1 also differs from D2 in being markedly increased by excess thyroid hormone through increased gene transcription, whereas D2 mRNA and protein are reduced during thyrotoxicosis and increased during hypothyroidism.[114–116]

The half-life of D2 is 20 to 30 minutes, whereas the half-life of D1 is more than 12 hours. The short half-life of D2 is due to the rapid ubiquitination of D2, a process that is accelerated by interaction with its preferred substrates, T_4 or rT_3.[117] D1 is not ubiquitinated though prolonged exposure to high substrate concentrations or iodinated inhibitors of deiodinases such as iopanoic acid cause inactivation but not loss of enzyme protein.[118]

D1 and D2 are also expressed in different tissues; D1 is highly expressed in human liver and kidney, but human D2 is widely distributed in skeletal and cardiac muscle, the CNS, skin, and the pituitary gland.[119, 120] Furthermore, in some cell types, the subcellular location of D1 is the plasma membrane whereas that of D2 is the endoplasmic reticulum.[121]

It is likely based on its subcellular location that the T_3 produced by D1 is formed close to the cell surface, whereas that generated by D2 is near the nucleus. This may explain why the T_3 produced by D1-catalyzed reactions readily enters the plasma whereas that generated by D2 enters the nucleus.[122]

Type 3

Type 3 deiodinase is most highly expressed in placenta and in the gravid uterus in rats; it is also found in the CNS.[123, 124] The highest expression identified to date in humans is in infantile hemangiomas. In infants with extensive visceral lesions, thyroid hormone inactivation by D3 may overwhelm the secretory capacity of the infant's thyroid, causing hypothyroidism.[125] D3 expression is increased by thyroid hormone at a transcriptional level thus providing a feedback loop to maintain T_3 homeostasis.

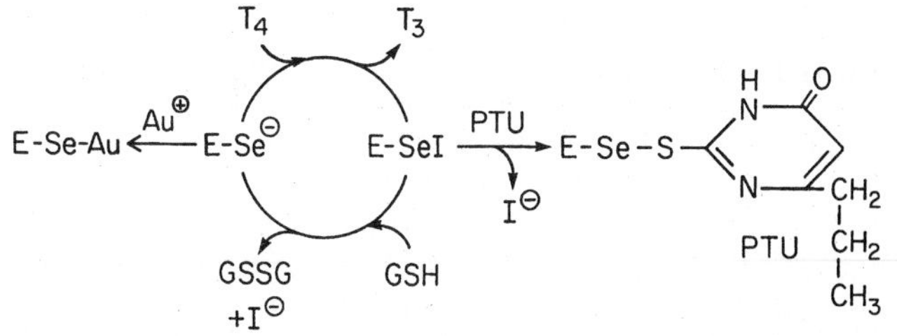

Figure 10–5. Schematic diagram of thyroxine (T_4) 5′-deiodination reaction as catalyzed by the type 1 iodothyronine deiodinase (D1). The reaction assumes the formation of a selenolyl-iodide intermediate, which requires a cystolic cofactor that is likely to be an -SH compound, such as reduced glutathione (GSH). Heavy metals with a single positive charge, such as gold (Au^+), inhibit deiodination by interaction with the negatively charged selenium atom. Propylthiouracil (PTU) is thought to form a relatively stable Se-S complex, thereby blocking regeneration of the active enzyme. (Modified from Leonard JL, Visser TJ. Biochemistry of deiodination. In Hennemann G [ed]. Thyroid Hormone Metabolism. New York, Marcel Dekker, 1986, pp 189–229.)

Quantitative Aspects of Thyroid Hormone Metabolism

Thyroid Hormone Turnover

In normal adults, T_4 has a distribution volume of approximately 10 L (Table 10–5). Because the concentration of total T_4 in plasma is approximately 100 nmol/L (8 μg/dL), the extrathyroidal T_4 pool is approximately 1 μmol (about 800 μg). In the adult, the fractional rate of turnover of T_4 in the periphery is about 10%/day (half-life, 6.7 days). Thus, about 1.1 L of the peripheral T_4 distribution space is cleared of hormone daily, a volume containing approximately 110 nmol (85 μg) of T_4.

The kinetics of T_3 metabolism differ from those of T_4, partly because of the 10-fold to 15-fold lower affinity of T_3 for TBG. The volume of distribution of T_3 in the normal adult is about 40 L, about four times that of T_4, and its fractional turnover rate is about 60%/day. Hence, the MCR of T_3 is about 24 L/day. At a mean normal serum T_3 concentration of 1.8 nmol/L (120 ng/dL), 50-fold lower than T_4, the daily production of T_3 is approximately 50 nmol (33 μg), or about 46% that of T_4 (see Table 10–4). The rapid MCR of reverse T_3 and a low concentration in plasma (0.25 nmol/L, 15 ng/dL) combine to yield daily production rates for rT_3 of about 45 nmol. The turnover of 3,3′-T_2 (see Fig. 10–3) is even more rapid than that of rT_3.

About 40% of secreted T_4 is monodeiodinated in the 5′-position to yield T_3, and a similar fraction is deiodinated in the 5-position to yield rT_3, the latter largely by D3 (see Fig. 10–3). With a normal T_4 production rate of approximately 110 nmol (85 μg)/day, about 44 nmol (28 μg) of T_3 and rT_3 is produced by peripheral deiodination. Thus, 80% to 85% of T_3 and all of rT_3 production in humans can be accounted for by peripheral deiodination of T_4, findings consonant with the high ratio of T_4 to T_3 (15:1) and rT_3 (>100:1) in human Tg.

Of the T_3 generated via T_4 5′-deiodination in euthyroid humans, only 20% to 25% is inhibited by PTU.[126, 127] This suggests that in the euthyroid state, thyroidal T_3 secretion and D1-catalyzed T_3 production may only account for about 40% of T_3 produced. Alternatively, the inhibition by PTU may be incomplete and D1-generated T_3 thereby underestimated. Whatever the contribution, the remainder of T_3 production is derived from D2-catalyzed T_4 deiodination, perhaps catalyzed by the large pool of D2 in skeletal muscle. This is consistent with the increase in fractional T_4 to T_3 conversion in hypothyroid or hypothyroxinemic subjects characteristic of D2-mediated deiodination.[128, 129] In contrast, PTU inhibits about 50% of peripheral T_3 production in the hyperthyroid patient consistent with an up-regulation of D1 and down-regulation of D2, which would be anticipated under these circumstances.[39, 53]

Table 10–5. Comparison of Triiodothyroxine (T_3) and Thyroxine (T_4) in Humans

	T_3	T_4
Production rate (nmol/day)	50	110
Fraction from thyroid	0.2	1.0
Relative metabolic potency	1.0	0.3
Serum concentration		
Total (nmol/L)	1.8	100
Free (pmol/L)	5	20
Fraction of total hormone in free form (× 10^{-2})	0.3	0.02
Distribution volume (L)	40	10
Fraction intracellular	0.64	0.15
Half-life (days)	0.75	6.7

To convert T_4 from nmol/L to μg/dL (total) or pmol/L to ng/dL (free), divide by 12.87. To convert T_3 from nmol/L to ng/dL (total) or pmol/L to pg/dL (free), multiply by 65.1.

Although much of the T_3 and rT_3 produced from T_4 in peripheral tissues exits those tissues and enters the blood, an uncertain fraction of both are degraded intracellularly prior to their exit. As discussed later, in some D2-containing tissues a significant fraction of T_3 in the cell nucleus is derived from intracellular local T_3 generation rather than from the plasma.

Other pathways are also involved in T_4 and T_3 metabolism. T_4 and T_3 undergo glucuronidation of the phenolic hydroxyl by the UDP-glucuronyltransferases (UDPGT) (see Fig. 10–4). This pathway is clinically significant because certain pharmacotherapeutic agents such as phenytoin, rifampin and phenobarbital may enhance glucuronide conjugation, leading to biliary excretion into the intestine.[54, 55]

Because T_4-G and T_3-G are not easily reabsorbed from intestinal contents, the significance of this pathway is that therapy with such agents generally increases L-thyroxine requirements.[130, 131] In patients with an intact thyroid, this is not apparent, because internal adjustments increase the thyroid hormone production rate to compensate for the accelerated biliary excretion. In patients with hypothyroidism, however, an increase in L-thyroxine dosage is required. Deamination and decarboxylation reactions that produce tetrac and triac and sulfation of T_4 and T_3 at the phenolic hydroxyl account for an as-yet-unidentified fraction of T_4 and T_3 metabolism in humans (see Fig. 10–4).

T_3 is metabolized mainly by 5-monodeiodination, either by D3 or—after sulfation in the liver—by D1. rT_3 is metabolized by 5′-monodeiodination, primarily by D1 (see Table 10–4). Both pathways yield 3,3′-T_2 (see Fig. 10–3), which is then rapidly degraded to monoiodothyronines and thyronine.[132] Thyronine and the iodide which escapes uptake by the thyroid gland are excreted in the urine.

Sources of Intracellular Triiodothyronine

In view of the differential tissue distribution of the various deiodinases, their various K_m values, and their differential regulation, it is not surprising that tissues may derive intracellular T_3 via several deiodinative pathways. Because T_3 regulates gene expression, it is especially relevant to analyze the quantity and source of nuclear T_3 in various tissues (Fig. 10–6).

In rat kidney and liver, D1-expressing tissues, most nuclear T_3 is derived from plasma T_3. In the rat cerebral cortex, pituitary gland, and brown fat, all of which express D2, half or more of intracellular T_3 is generated locally from T_4 within the tissue. This may be due in part to the differences in the subcellular localization between D2 and D1 that were mentioned earlier. In the rat, tissues depending on D2 for nuclear T_3 are those in which a constant supply of thyroid hormone is crucial for either normal development (cerebral cortex), thyroid function (pituitary), or survival during cold stress (brown adipose tissue). These tissues are also characterized by a high degree of saturation of the nuclear T_3 receptors in comparison with other tissues (liver, kidney) in which nuclear T_3 receptor sites are only about 50% occupied at normal serum T_3 concentrations (see Fig. 10–6). This arrangement allows multiple levels of regulation of thyroid hormone action.

Intracellular D2-catalyzed T_3 production has important implications for thyroid hormone physiology. First, because the T_3 produced from T_4 occupies a significant fraction of the receptors in those tissues, changes in either serum T_4 or T_3 can change receptor occupancy. However, because a fall in T_4 also increases D2 protein half-life by decreasing the rate of ubiquitination and its proteasomal degradation, a rise in D2 activity mitigates the impact of a reduction of serum T_4 in D2-

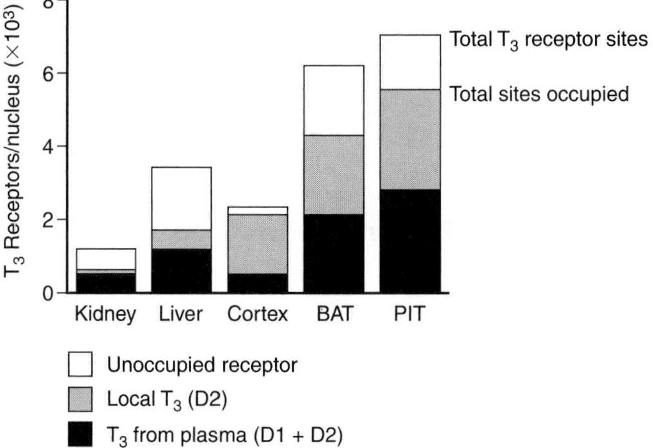

Figure 10–6. Schematic diagram of the origin of the specifically bound nuclear triiodothyronine (T_3) in various rat tissues. Data are derived from studies in which double-isotope labeling techniques were used to esimate the sources of specifically bound nuclear T_3. In tissues having a receptor saturation significantly greater than 50%, the additional T_3 is provided by D2-catalyzed T_4 to T_3 conversion. T3 in rat plasma is derived from thyroid secretion (~40%) with the remainder from D1- and D2-catalyzed T_4 to T_3 conversion. BAT, brown adipose tissue; PIT, pituitary gland.

expressing tissues, helping to maintain T_3 homeostasis.[53] Second, the requirement for both T_3 and T_4 for normal saturation of pituitary gland and CNS T_3 receptors permits a response of the hypothalamic-pituitary axis to a reduction in plasma T_4, which is the earliest manifestation of iodine deficiency or primary hypothyroidism (see "Regulation of Thyroid Function").

Because the D2 gene is positively regulated by cAMP, D2 activity and T_3 production increase rapidly in brown adipose tissue under stimulation by the sympathetic nervous system during exposure to cold.[133] This response is critical to adaptive thermogenesis during cold exposure in the human neonate and lifelong in the rodent.[134, 135]

Physiologic, Pathologic, and Pharmacologic Influences on Thyroid Hormone Deiodination

There are a number of circumstances in which thyroid hormone activation is either inhibited or the degradation of thyroid hormone is accelerated via deiodination pathways. There are several categories: (1) physiologic, (2) pathologic, and (3) pharmacologic (Table 10–6).

Physiologic Influences

Physiologic activation of T_4 to T_3, particularly by D1, is impaired during fetal life. In experimental animals, however, D3 activity is increased in the fetus, particularly in the skin and in other tissues as well, contributing to a reduced serum T_3 level in the fetal state. In contrast, D2 action is sufficient to provide intracellular T_3 in those tissues, such as the brain, where thyroid hormone is absolutely required for normal development.

Careful chronologic activation of D2 or D3 has been demonstrated in several animal models. These include a short-lived burst of D2 activity in the cochlea of the newborn mouse and the increased D3 activity in the retina during metamorphosis in the tadpole.[136, 137] Similar, although not yet documented, events may occur in humans.

Pathologic Influences

Alterations in iodothyronine deiodination occur during fasting and illness.[138] This group of conditions is associated with a marked decrease in T_3, elevated serum rT_3 levels, and a decrease in T_4 clearance.[53] These changes in thyroid hormone metabolism probably reflect both decreased T_4 transport and D1 and D2 actions. Tumor necrosis factor-α (TNF-α) and interleukin-1 decrease D1 expression in isolated hepatocytes, and TNF-α decreases D2 expression in human skeletal muscle cells.[139, 140] TNF and IL might be playing a role in the fasting or illness-induced reductions in T_4 activation. These events are part of the global response that reduces plasma T_3 during illness (see "Thyroid Function during Fasting or Illness").

Selenium deficiency may be due to endemic deficiency (e.g., as in western China) or to the effects of protein-restricted diets. Because of the differential retention of selenium in various organs, selenium deficiency predominantly affects the liver and kidney, organs expressing D1. Under these circumstances, the serum T_4 level and the serum T_4/T_3 ratio are increased, a compensatory response to decreased T_3 production via the D1 pathway during this condition.

In Zaire, where both iodine and selenium are deficient, repletion of selenium prior to repletion of iodine led to a deterioration in overall thyroid function, presumably because of the acceleration of T_4 degradation by D1, and perhaps by D3, in the selenium-deficient subject.[141, 142] Hepatic dysfunction may reduce T_4 activation as a consequence of the decrease in D1-containing cells or because of the effects of the accompanying illness on deiodinase activity. Changes in deiodinase function with altered thyroid states have been reviewed in Table 10–4.

Pharmacologic Influences

A number of commonly used drugs have significant effects on thyroid hormone deiodination. PTU causes a dose-related inhibition of T_3 production, which is most readily seen in the thyrotoxic patient in whom T_4 to T_3 conversion via the D1 pathway is markedly increased.[39, 143] This inhibitory capacity is not shared by methimazole or carbimazole.

Table 10–6. Factors Altering the Peripheral Activation or Inactivation of Thyroid Hormones

Factor or Condition	Tissue Uptake	Effect on Deiodination		
		D1	D2	D3
Physiologic				
Fetus	?	↓	N*	↑
Pathologic				
Fasting	↓	↓	↓	?
Illness	↓	↓	↓	?
Selenium deficiency	N	↓	N	N
Hepatic dysfunction	↓	↓	?	N
Thyrotoxicosis	N	↑	↓	↑
Hypothyroidism	?	↓	↑	↓
Hemangioma	?	↓	↑	↑↑
Pharmacologic				
Propylthiouracil	N	↓	N	N
Amiodarone	↓	↓	↓	?
Iopanoic or iopodipic acid	↓	↓	↓	↓
Growth hormone	?	↑ (?)	↑ (?)	↓
Gold thioglucose	?	↓	N	N
Thyroid hormone	?	↑	↓	↑

*Normal.

The antiarrhythmic drug amiodarone shares sufficient structural similarity with T_4 that it can inhibit deiodination of T_4 and rT_3 (Fig. 10–7). Patients receiving this agent develop a compensatory increase in plasma T_4 to maintain serum T_3 in the normal range. There is also a corresponding increase in TSH within the first weeks of therapy that gradually returns to normal as the thyroid axis reequilibrates.[144, 145] The T_4 and rT_3 MCRs are reduced by 20% to 25%, with a reduction in the fractional T_4 to T_3 conversion rate of about 50%.[146–148] There is direct evidence of inhibition of D1 activity in rats given this agent, but no studies have examined its effects on D2. The mechanism is probably due to competitive inhibition either by the drug or by one of its metabolites, but inactivation of D1 and accelerated D2 degradation may also occur.[149] Amiodarone also inhibits the active transport of T_4 and T_3 into hepatocytes,[150] and the drug or one of its products may interfere with T_3 binding to thyroid hormone receptors.[151]

The effects of amiodarone resemble those observed with the iodoaniline derivatives formerly used for visualization of the gallbladder (see Fig. 10–7).[152, 153] Iopanoic or iopodipic acid inhibits the deiodinases by competing with the iodothyronine substrates.[53] This makes these agents useful in the acute treatment of patients with severe hyperthyroidism, in whom they cause a rapid decrease in T_3.[154]

High dosages of glucocorticoids (10 times replacement) acutely reduce the T_3/T_4 ratio in plasma, suggesting that T_4 to T_3 conversion is blocked. The rT_3/T_4 ratio increases, suggesting that D3 action is also increased.[155] These effects resolve during chronic therapy such that thyroid function is little affected, and thyroid hormone requirements are not increased by chronic glucocorticoid therapy.

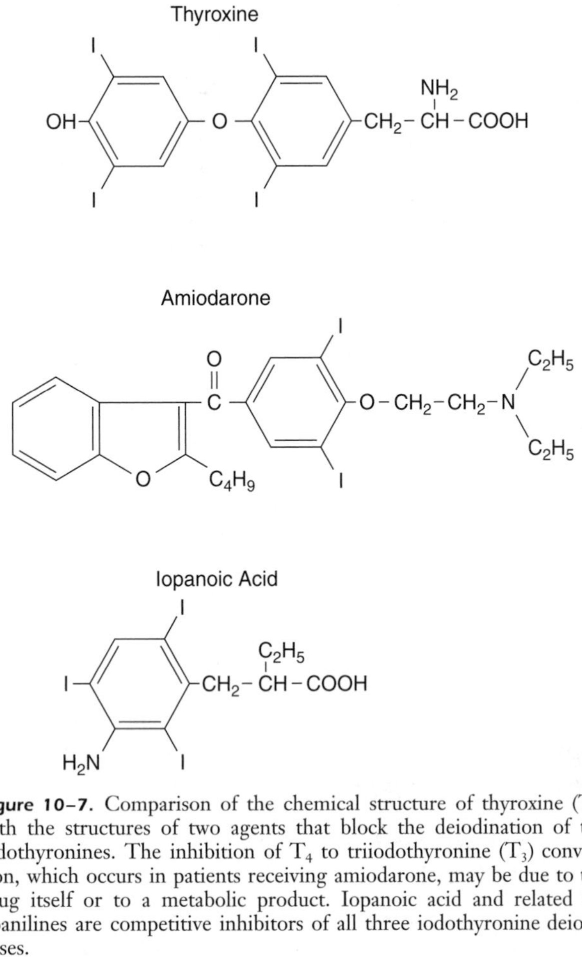

Thyroxine

Amiodarone

Iopanoic Acid

Figure 10–7. Comparison of the chemical structure of thyroxine (T_4) with the structures of two agents that block the deiodination of the iodothyronines. The inhibition of T_4 to triiodothyronine (T_3) conversion, which occurs in patients receiving amiodarone, may be due to the drug itself or to a metabolic product. Iopanoic acid and related iodoanilines are competitive inhibitors of all three iodothyronine deiodinases.

Recombinant growth hormone increases circulating T_3 and T_4 levels and reduces rT_3/T_4 ratios.[156] This result is also seen in patients with hypothyroidism who are receiving L-thyroxine, indicating it is a peripheral effect. In the chick, growth hormone reduces D3 activity, suggesting that a similar effect on this enzyme may be the explanation for its effect in humans; however, direct evidence is lacking.[157]

Mechanism of Thyroid Hormone Action

Thyroid hormone acts by binding to a specific nuclear DNA-bound *thyroid hormone receptor* (TR), usually as a heterodimer with *retinoid X receptor* (RXR) at specific sequences (*thyroid hormone response elements* [TREs]) dictated by the DNA binding-site preferences of the RXR-TR complex (Fig. 10–8). The general mechanism by which nuclear receptor-activating ligands, such as T_3, produce their effects is discussed in Chapter 4.

T_3 has a 15-fold higher binding affinity for TRs than does T_4, which explains its function as the active thyroid hormone. In humans, two TR genes (α and β) are found on different chromosomes (TRα on chromosome 17, TRβ on chromosome 3). Several alternatively spliced gene products from each of these genes form both active and inactive gene products. The active proteins are TRα-1 and TRs β1, β2, and β3.[158] The structure of the TRs conforms to a protein with three major functional domains, one binding DNA, one binding ligand, and two major transcriptional activation domains (Fig. 10–9). These activation domains of the TRα and β are similar to, but not identical with, the major differences in the amino-terminal portion of the molecule.

There are tissue-specific preferences in expression of the various TRs, suggesting that they subserve different functions in various tissues.[159] In general, TRβ, particularly TRβ-2, is thought to be important in the hypothalamus and pituitary gland, where regulation of thyroid function occurs.[160] In addition to differences in the amino-terminus between TRβ-1 and β2, the two proteins are under the regulation of different promoters that can function in tissue-specific patterns.

TRβ-2 is down-regulated by T_3, whereas TRβ-1 mRNA expression is not affected.[161] TRβ-2 is also expressed in the cochlea. TRβ-1 is expressed in all tissues, although its mRNA is especially highly expressed in the kidney, liver, brain, and heart. TRα-1 mRNA is also expressed in the brain and at lower levels in skeletal muscle, lungs, and heart. TRβ-3 mRNA is expressed at very low levels but is more abundant in the liver or kidneys and lungs in comparison with other tissues.

It is instructive to examine the effects of gene targeting of TRα and TRβ in order to understand their different physiologic roles.[161, 162] A disruption of the TRβ gene (both TRβ-1 and β2) causes deafness, a marked reduction in feedback sensitivity of hypothalamic-pituitary-thyroid axis, and a decrease in hepatic D1.[159, 163, 164] Thus, in these mice, both TSH and thyroid hormone levels are elevated. However, TSH levels are further increased if thyroid hormone levels are reduced, indicating a feedback suppression of TSH release is present, albeit attenuated by this genetic manipulation. Phenotypically, thyroid function in these mice resembles that in families with *resistance to thyroid hormone* (RTH) in which TRβ mutations markedly reduce its binding affinity for T_3.[165] Curiously, the clinical manifestations in these individuals may resemble thyrotoxicosis for reasons discussed in Chapter 12.

Despite evidence of impaired feedback regulation, there is relatively little abnormality in the brain and heart of the TRβ-deficient mice. The effect of a TRα-1 disruption in the mouse is quite different. The predominant phenotypic effects are modest bradycardia and hypothermia.[166, 167] These animals have

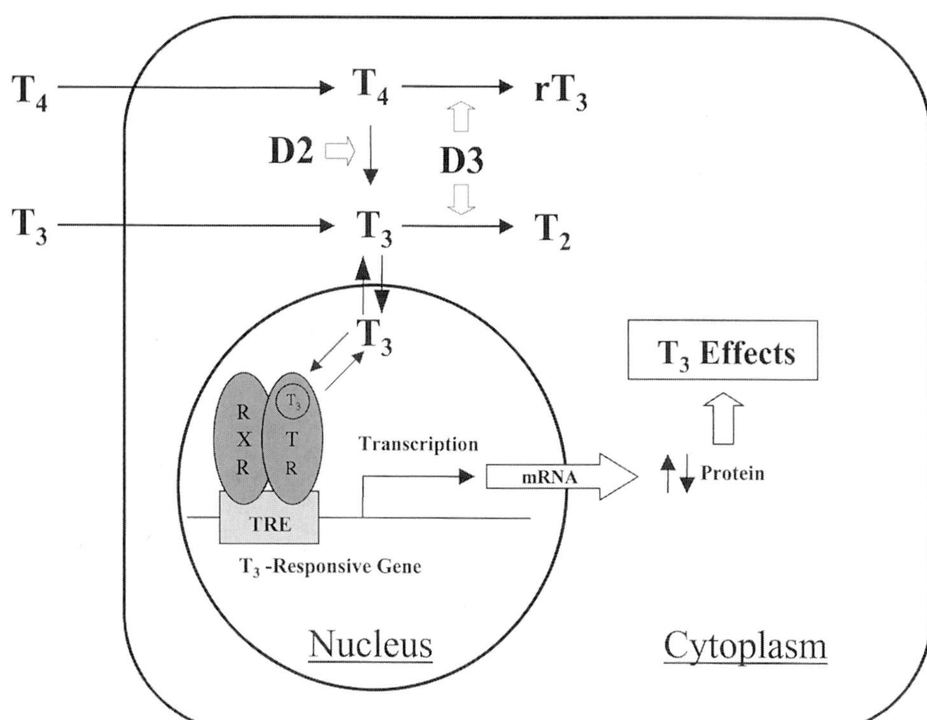

Figure 10–8. Schematic diagram of thyroid hormone activation and inactivation in a cell expressing D2 and D3, such as an astroglial cell or a neuron. The triiodothyronine (T_3) that enters the cell can either be deiodinated to 3,3′ T_2 (diodothyronine) or can enter the nucleus and bind to the thyroid hormone receptor. An additional source of T_3 is that generated by outer ring deiodination of thyroxine (T_4) within the cell. The interaction of T_3 with the thyroid hormone receptor (TR) bound as a heterodimer with a retinoid X receptor (RXR) to the thyroid hormone response element (TRE), causes either an increase or a decrease in the transcription of that gene. This leads to parallel changes in the concentrations of critical proteins, thus producing the thyroid hormone response of a given cell. mRNA, messenger RNA; rT_3, reverse T_3. (See Chapter 4 for specific details.)

subtle but significant abnormalities in myocardial function and electrical activity and, despite the basal hypothermia, have normal responses to cold exposure.[166]

These studies have led to the generalization that feedback regulation of thyroid hormone effects, along with cochlear development, are functions of TRβ, whereas cardiac functions and energy metabolism are probably regulated by TRα. However, this is a generalization, and further experimental studies of these animals, as well as animals with specific mutations in the TRβ gene analogous to those in families with thyroid hormone resistance, are currently in progress. It is also likely that small differences in the ligand-binding domains of TRα and TRβ will allow design of thyroid hormone analogues selective for one or the other of these receptors.[168, 169] The result may be agents (such as GC-1) that can suppress TSH in patients with thyroid cancer without inducing tachycardia.[170, 171]

The binding of T_3 to the TR-TRE complex of a gene positively regulated by T_3 initiates a conformational change in the TR such that one or more repressors of transcription are dissociated from the receptor and replaced by coactivator proteins (see Figs. 4–5 and 4–6 in Chapter 4).[172] Some of these coactivating proteins induce DNA acetylation, or *histone acetyltransferase* activity, making the neighboring thyroid hormone–regulated genes dissociate from nucleosomes and available for binding of the transcriptional initiation complex.[173, 174] The action of T_3 is terminated by its dissociation from the receptor or by ubiquitination and proteasomal degradation of the T_3-TR complex.[175, 176]

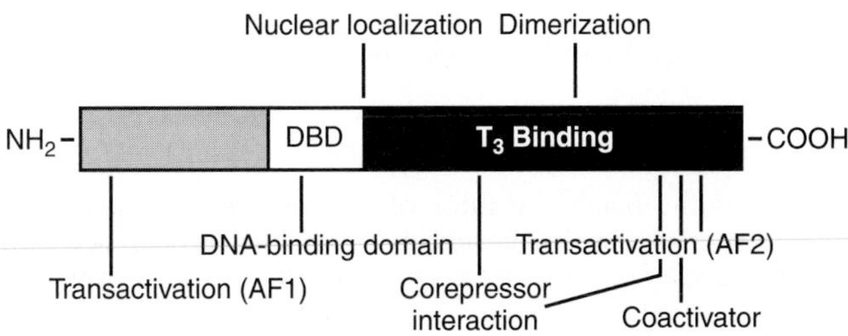

Figure 10–9. The functional domains in the thyroid hormone receptor are similar in both α_1 and β isoforms of the thyroid hormone receptors. These isoforms differ primarily in their NH_2-terminal domains. AF, activating factor; DBD, DNA-binding domain; T_3, triiodothyronine.

Another group of genes, as exemplified by those encoding the TSH β subunit, the α-glycoprotein subunit, and TRH, are negatively regulated by T_3. Negative regulation by thyroid hormone is still poorly understood but may involve specific negative TREs located in the promoter or even the coding regions of target genes. In one scenario, the complexing of T_3 with DNA-bound TRs recruits corepressors and *histone deacetylases* to these binding sites. An example of this mechanism is that regulating the β subunit of TSH.[177] In the absence of T_3, a gene containing a TR bound to a negative TRE is activated by association of coactivator and histone acetylating activator proteins, which then dissociate as a result of T_3. Other mechanisms of negative regulation by T_3 have also been suggested, including TR trapping and sequestration of coactivators to prohibit positive regulation of these genes.[178]

Other potential mechanisms of thyroid hormone action by interaction with the membrane are under investigation.[179–181] The pivotal role of T_3 in the activation of thyroid hormone–dependent genes indicates that T_4 serves primarily as a prohormone. Because T_4 down-regulates D2 and inactivates D1, however, it might be considered an active hormone in the sense that it negatively regulates its own activation.[53]

REGULATION OF THYROID FUNCTION

Hypothalamic-Pituitary-Thyroid Axis

The thyroid gland participates with the hypothalamus and pituitary gland in a classic feedback control loop (Fig. 10–10).

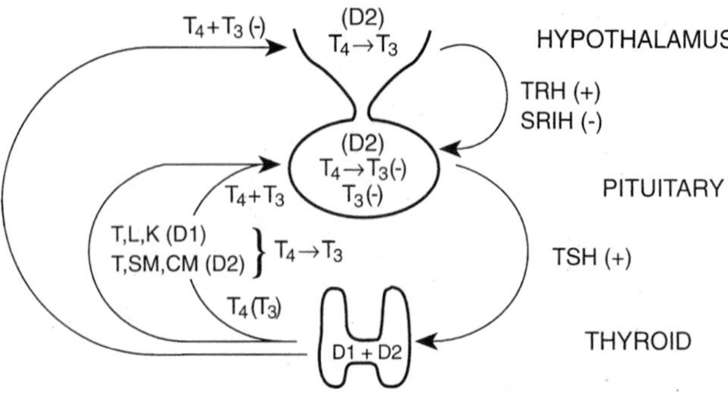

Figure 10–10. Role of thyroxine and triiodothyronine (T_4 and T_3) in the feedback regulation of thyrotropin-releasing hormone (TRH) and thyrotropin (TSH) secretion. Secreted T_4 must be converted to T_3 to produce its effects. This conversion may take place in tissues such as the liver (L) and kidney (K) and thyroid (T) catalyzed by D1 or D2 in the human thyroid gland (T), skeletal muscle (SM), and, possibly, cardiac muscle (CM). SRIH, somatostatin.

In addition, there is an inverse relationship between the glandular organic iodine level and the rate of hormone formation. Such autoregulatory mechanisms serve to stabilize the rate of hormone synthesis despite fluctuations in the availability of iodine. Stability in hormone production is achieved, in part, because the large intraglandular store of hormone buffers the effect of acute increases or decreases in hormone synthesis. Autoregulatory mechanisms within the gland, in turn, tend to maintain the constancy of the thyroid hormone pool.

Finally, the hypothalamic-pituitary feedback mechanism senses variations in the availability of free thyroid hormones, however small, and acts to correct them. There is a close relationship between the hypothalamus, the anterior pituitary gland, the thyroid gland, and still higher centers in the brain, with the function of the entire complex being modified in a typical negative-feedback manner by the availability of the thyroid hormones. Additional hormones and neuropeptides also influence this axis (see Chapters 7 and 8).

Thyrotropin-Releasing Hormone Synthesis and Secretion

TRH, a modified tripeptide (pyroglutamyl-histidyl-proline-amide), is derived from a large pre-pro-TRH molecule that contains five progenitor sequences. The TRH peptides are released from the pre-pro molecule by a peptidase that acts at flanking lysine/arginine residues. TRH is expressed in the hypothalamus, the brain, the C cells of the thyroid gland, the beta cells of the pancreas, the myocardium, the reproductive organs (including prostate and testis), and the spinal cord. The parvocellular region of the paraventricular nuclei of the hypothalamus is the source of the TRH that regulates TSH secretion. The 5′-flanking region of the gene encoding TRH has sequences for mediating responses to glucocorticoids and cAMP. In addition, at least two elements in this region of the gene can confer negative regulation of thyroid hormone receptor complexes.[182]

TRH travels in the axons of the peptidergic neurons through the median eminence and is released close to the hypothalamic-pituitary portal plexus. The neuron bodies that produce TRH are innervated by catecholamine, neuropeptide Y, and somatostatin-containing axons, all of which potentially influence the rate of synthesis of the pre-pro-TRH molecule.

A complex series of interactions with neuropeptides involving leptin, agouti-related peptide (AgRP), and melanocyte-stimulating hormone (α-MSH) regulates pre-pro-TRH synthesis in the rat. The acute decrease in TRH synthesis that occurs in the starved rodent and leads to central hypothyroidism can be reversed by leptin infusion.[183, 184] Leptin directly increases pro-TRH biosynthesis in rat hypothalamic neurons, as does α-MSH, whereas neuropeptide Y and melanocortin-4 receptor (MC4R) suppress TRH synthesis as well.[185, 186] Thus, a fall in leptin, directly and indirectly, can reduce TRH synthesis.

Although leptin and α-MSH can also activate the human TRH promoter through MC4R and the leptin receptor (ObRb), there is no acute reduction of TSH in fasted humans despite a decline in leptin levels.[187] In humans, fasting causes a slight decrease in the amplitude of the pulsatile TSH release, which may be due to a decrease in TRH synthesis owing to reduced leptin.[188] In addition, whereas a human leptin gene–inactivating mutation causes morbid obesity and hypogonadism, it does not cause central hypothyroidism.[189] Thus, current results suggest that the major role of leptin in regulating thyroid function in rodents in response to fasting is not shared by humans.[190, 191]

T_3 suppresses the levels of pre-pro-TRH mRNA by T_3 in the hypothalamus,[192, 193] but normal feedback regulation of pre-pro-TRH mRNA synthesis by thyroid hormone requires a combination of T_3 and T_4 in the circulation, with the latter giving rise to T_3 via T_4 5′-deiodination in the CNS.[194] In rats, there is a dense expression of D2 in the specialized ependymal cells *(tanycytes)* in the inferior portion of the third ventricle.[195–197] These cells have processes extending into the median eminence and arcuate nucleus, where active conversion of T_4 to T_3 releases T_3 in the region of the hypothalamic-pituitary portal system. Thus, part of the negative feedback induced by T_4 may be generated both indirectly at the level of the paraventricular nucleus by suppressing TRH and at the median eminence and arcuate nucleus at a point where neuropeptides and T_3 enter the pituitary portal system.

TRH binds to a receptor in the thyrotroph membrane, and calcium and cyclic guanosine monophosphate (cGMP) are the second messengers for induction of the thyrotroph response.[198] The calcium is derived from endoplasmic reticulum, owing to increases in inositol triphosphate (IP_3) secondary to G protein activation of PL-C. Both phorbol ester and calcium ionophores can stimulate TSH gene transcription.[199] In addition to inhibiting the synthesis of pre-pro-TRH mRNA, thyroid hormone also blocks the capacity of TRH to stimulate TSH release from the thyrotroph. The mechanism for this effect is unknown, but the stimulating effects of both phorbol esters and calcium ionophores are blocked by prior incubation with thyroid hormone.[200, 201]

Exogenous TRH elicits the secretion of prolactin at threshold doses that are the same as those for stimulation of TSH secretion. As with TSH, the prolactin response to TRH is modified by the prevailing levels of thyroid hormones, although not to as marked an extent. The role of TRH as a physiologic modulator of prolactin secretion is uncertain, however. For example, nursing increases the serum prolactin concentration, but the serum TSH concentration is unchanged.

Thyrotropin Synthesis and Secretion

TSH is the major regulator of the morphologic and functional states of the thyroid gland. It is a glycoprotein secreted by thyrotrophs in the anteromedial portion of the adenohypophysis (see Chapter 8) composed of an α subunit of 14 kd (92 amino acids) that is common to LH, follicle-stimulating hormone (FSH), and hCG as well as a specific β subunit, a 112–amino acid protein synthesized in thyrotrophs. The peptide sequence cysteine-alanine-glycine-tyrosine-cysteine (CAGYC) is highly conserved in the β subunits of TSH, FSH, LH, and hCG and is required for heterodimerization with the α subunit.[202] An autosomal recessive form of hypothyroidism is associated with a glycine to arginine mutation in this sequence of the TSH β subunit, which blocks its capacity to heterodimerize and renders it nonfunctional.[203]

In normal thyrotrophs and in thyrotroph tumors, synthesis of the α subunit is in excess, indicating that the quantity of the β subunit is rate-limiting for TSH secretion. TRH increases and thyroid hormone suppresses the transcription of both subunits; these are the most important influences on TSH synthesis.

The physiologic glycosylation of TSH involves addition of preformed asparagine-linked oligosaccharides in the rough endoplasmic reticulum, modifications in proximal and distal Golgi apparatus, and the appearance of the intact, folded hormone in the secretory granules.[204] The glycosylation of the subunits protects them from intracellular degradation and permits normal folding of the protein chains so that internal disulfide linkages are correctly formed. Glycosylation is also required for full biologic activity, and sialylation protects circulating TSH from interaction with hepatic galactose receptors, thus increasing its half-life.[205, 206] The biologic activity of TSH in the serum of patients with pituitary tumors or hypothalamic disorders is inappropriately low compared with immunologic activity, suggesting the formation of an abnormal product.[51, 207] Long-term administration of TRH can enhance the biologic activity of TSH in patients with hypothalamic hypothyroidism and may lead to increased thyroid hormone levels, suggesting that this is due to TRH deficiency.[205] Thus, in humans, TRH regulates not only α and β TSH subunit synthesis but also post-translational processing.

Levels of α subunit in serum range from 0.5 to 5 μg/L but are elevated in postmenopausal women. In normal serum, TSH is present at concentrations between 0.5 and 5 mU/L. The level is increased in hypothyroidism and reduced in hyperthyroidism (see later). The plasma TSH half-life is about 30 minutes, and production rates in humans are 40 to 150 mU/day.

Circulating TSH displays two types of variations. *Pulsatile* variations are characterized by fluctuations at 1- to 2-hour intervals. The magnitude of TSH pulsations is decreased during fasting, illness, or after surgery.[188, 208, 209] *Circadian* variations are characterized by a nocturnal surge that precedes the onset of sleep and appears to be independent of the cortisol rhythm and fluctuations in serum and in T_4 and T_3 concentrations. When the onset of sleep is delayed, the nocturnal TSH surge is enhanced and prolonged, and the early onset of sleep results in a surge of lesser magnitude and shorter duration.

The degree of thyroid hypofunction after destruction of the hypothalamus is less severe than that following hypophysectomy, and residual thyroid function in the former circumstance can be altered by raising or lowering the concentration of thyroid hormones in the blood. Thus, thyroid hormones mediate the feedback regulation of TSH secretion, and TRH determines its set-point. The relationship between circulating T_4 and T_3 and pituitary TSH release is illustrated in Fig. 10–10. The acute inhibition of TSH release by in vivo administration of physiologic quantities of T_4 is mediated by the T_3 produced by D2 in the pituitary gland (and perhaps the hypothalamus), since it is blocked by a general deiodinase inhibitor, but not by PTU, the specific D1 inhibitor.[210, 211] A decrease in either plasma T_3 or T_4 causes an increase in TSH secretion because both T_3 directly, and T_4 via intrapituitary and intracerebral T_4 to T_3 conversion, contribute to T_3 in the hypothalamus and pituitary gland (see Fig. 10–10).[122] It follows that exogenous T_4 is an effective suppressor of TSH secretion because (1) it is converted to plasma T_3 and (2) it serves as the prohormone for T_3 in the CNS and the pituitary gland. There is a linear relationship between the serum T_4 concentration and the log of the TSH (Fig. 10–11). Thus, the serum TSH concentration is an exquisitely sensitive indicator of the thyroid state of most patients.

Somatostatin (SRIH, or somatotropin release-inhibiting hormone), acting through inhibitory G protein (G_i), decreases TSH secretion in vitro and in vivo, but prolonged treatment with a somatostatin analogue does not cause hypothyroidism.[212, 213] Similar acute effects occur during dopamine infusion and administration of bromocriptine, a dopamine agonist. Both of these agents inhibit adenylate cyclase. Conversely, blockade of the dopamine receptor by metoclopramide increases the basal serum TSH concentration in both euthyroid and hypothyroid patients. These findings suggest that dopamine is a regulator of TSH secretion, but chronic administration of dopamine agonists (e.g., for the treatment of prolactinoma) does not cause central hypothyroidism, indicating that compensatory mechanisms negate these acute effects.[214] The neuroendocrine regulation of TSH secretion is detailed in Chapter 7.

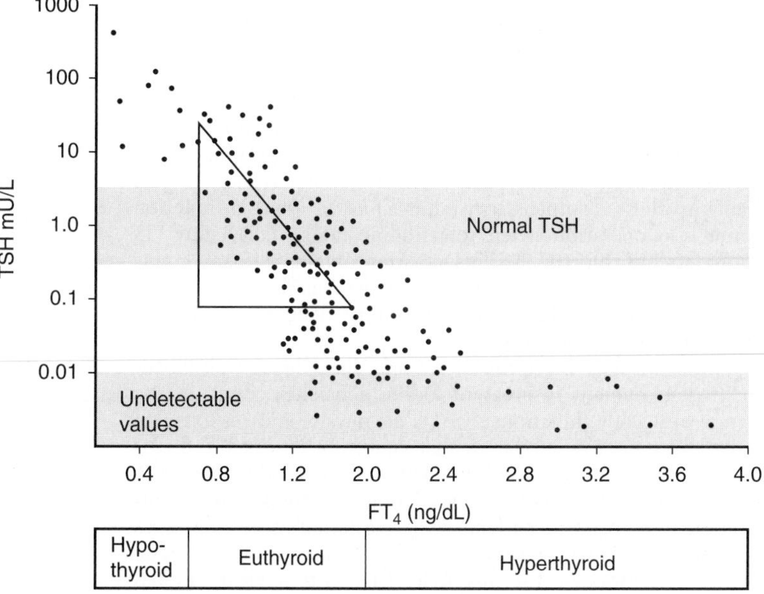

Figure 10–11. The log/linear relationship between thyrotropin (TSH) (vertical axis) and free thyroxine (FT_4) concentrations. Typical free T_4 concentrations in hypothyroid, euthyroid, and hyperthyroid patients are shown. (Modified from Spencer CA, LoPresti JS, Patel A, et al. Applications of a new chemiluminometric thyrotropin assay to subnormal measurement. J Clin Endocrinol Metab 1990; 70:453–460.)

Table 10–7. Endogenous and Exogenous Agents That May Suppress Thyrotropin Secretion

Thyroid hormones and analogues
Dopamine and dopamine agonists
Somatostatin and somatostatin analogues
Dobutamine
Glucocorticoids (acute, high-dose)
Interleukin-1β, interleukin-6
Tumor necrosis factor-α
Bexarotene (retinoid X receptor agonist)
Phenytoin

A number of drugs or hormones can suppress TSH secretion (Table 10–7). Glucocorticoids given in high doses acutely suppress TSH secretion transiently, although prolonged therapy is not associated with central hypothyroidism.[215] Patients with Cushing's disease have subnormal TSH production but with minimal effects on T_4 production.[215, 216] Bexarotene, an RXR agonist used for treatment of T cell lymphoma, suppresses TSH sufficiently to cause central hypothyroidism, presumably by reducing TSH β gene transcription.[217]

Iodine Deficiency

The response of vertebrates to a deficiency of iodine is designed to conserve this limited resource and to improve the efficiency of its utilization. These adjustments occur at the hypothalamic, pituitary, thyroid, and peripheral tissue levels. Removal of iodine from the diet causes a rapid decrease in serum T_4 concentrations and a simultaneous increase in serum TSH (Fig 10–12).[218] Interestingly, no detectable decrease in T_3 occurs, suggesting that the signal to increase TSH must derive from a decrease in the T_3 generated intracellularly from T_4 in the pituitary gland, the hypothalamus, or both. TSH increases NIS, Tg, and TPO synthesis and iodine organification and Tg turnover (see Fig. 10–2). Because of the decrease in iodide supply and in the DIT/MIT ratio, the T_4/T_3 ratio in Tg decreases and the rate of thyroidal T_3 secretion is probably increased despite a decline in T_4 secretion.

TSH also stimulates cell division, leading to goiter. In the rat model, the fall in plasma T_4 increases D2 from fivefold to 20-fold in the CNS, hypothalamus, and pituitary gland, increasing the efficiency of T_4 conversion to T_3. With moderately severe iodine deficiency, D3 in the CNS is also reduced, prolonging the mean residence time of T_3 in that organ.[219, 220] This permits serum T_3 to remain normal and the CNS T_3 to be only moderately reduced even with up to a 10-fold decrease in circulating T_4.[221]

Despite the TSH elevation and nearly undetectable serum T_4, growth, oxygen (O_2) consumption and thermal homeostasis can be maintained.[222, 223] If iodine deficiency is prolonged and severe, however, frank hypothyroidism will supervene.[224, 225] In humans, these compensatory alterations in thyroid function come into operation when total iodine intake falls below 75 μg/day (see Table 10–1). This situation obtains in many countries in Europe and South America as well as for several hundred million individuals in areas of iodine deficiency in China, India, Indonesia, and Africa.[226, 227]

These changes in serum hormones have been well documented in humans in areas of iodine deficiency[228] and in patients with NIS mutations.[19, 229] The physiologic response to iodine deficiency is similar to that occurring during the development of primary hypothyroidism in humans.[230] It is also reproduced when the efficiency of iodide trapping and organification is reduced in patients with Hashimoto's disease or in patients with Graves' disease receiving thiourea drugs.[28, 34] The physiologic rationale for this series of events is clear. T_3 has approximately three times the potency of the prohormone T_4 and contains only three iodine atoms. In terms of metabolic potency, this results in a fourfold more efficient use of iodine. Maintenance of normal circulating T_3 levels provides hormone for tissues in which nuclear T_3 is completely derived from the plasma (see Fig. 10–6).

Iodine Excess

Besides being protected against iodine deficiency, the thyroid gland is protected against an excess of iodine that might otherwise lead to hyperthyroidism. As with the response to iodine deficiency, there are multiple levels of defense against this eventuality. The usual source of excess iodine is pharmaceutical, with angiographic dyes, amiodarone, and povidone-iodine the most common sources (Table 10–8).

Effects of Increased Iodine Intake on Thyroid Hormone Synthesis

The quantity of iodine undergoing organification displays a biphasic response to increasing doses of iodide, at first increasing and then decreasing as a result of a relative blockade of organic binding. This decreasing yield of organic iodine from increasing doses of iodide (the *Wolff-Chaikoff effect*) results from a high concentration of inorganic iodide within the thyroid cell.[27, 231, 232] The susceptibility to the Wolff-Chaikoff effect can be increased by (1) stimulation of the iodide-trapping mechanism (as in patients with Graves' disease) or during per-

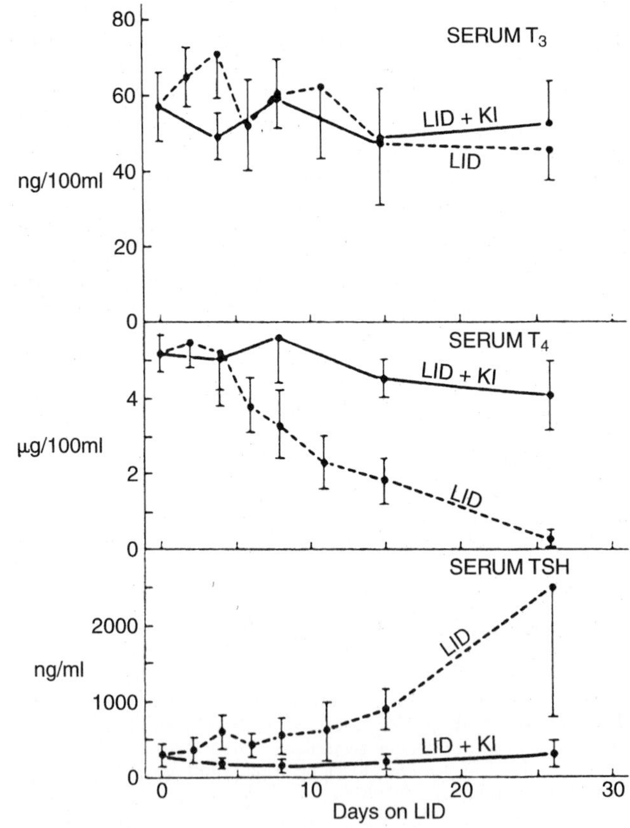

Figure 10–12. Effects of acute depletion of dietary iodine on serum triiodothyronine (T_3), thyroxine (T_4), and thyrotropin (TSH) in rats. Animals received a low-iodine diet (LID) without or with supplementation of potassium iodide (KI) in drinking water. (From Riesco G, Taurog A, Larsen PR, Krulich L. Acute and chronic responses to iodine deficiency in rats. Endocrinology 1977; 100:303–313. © The Endocrine Society.)

Table 10–8. Iodine Content of Various Iodinated Pharmaceuticals*

Saturated solution of potassium iodide	38-mg/drop
Lugol's solution	6-mg/drop
Iodized salt (1 part KI/10,000 NaCl)	760 μg/10 g
Amiodarone	75 mg/200-mg tablet
Iopanoate, ipodate	350-mg/tablet
Angiographic and CT dyes	400–4000 mg/dose
Povidone-iodine	10 mg/mL
Kelp tablets	150-μg/tablet
Prenatal vitamins	150-μg/tablet
Iodinated glycerol	25 mg/mL
Quantity of iodine required to suppress radioactive iodine to < 2%	> 30 mg/day

CT, computed tomography; KI, potassium iodide; NaCl, sodium chloride.
*Typical iodide intake in the United States is 100 to 400 μg/day.

sistent TSH stimulation or (2) in patients with impairment of iodine organification, as may occur during thiourea drug treatment, in Hashimoto's disease, or in thyroid glands previously irradiated by either ^{131}I or external beam therapy (e.g., for Hodgkin's disease).

In such situations, goiter and hypothyroidism can develop if excess iodide is given for long periods. The mechanism for inhibition of organification may involve the effects of high iodide concentrations on TPO-catalyzed organifications as well as a consequence of the formation of one or more inhibitory iodolipids in the thyroid cells.[233, 234]

In patients with normal thyroid glands given moderate or large doses of iodide, the relative inhibition of organic binding and inhibition of iodothyronine formation are partially relieved. This *escape* or *adaptation phenomenon* occurs because iodide transport activity decreases, probably through a reduction in NIS expression.[235] Consequently, thyroidal iodide falls to levels insufficient to maintain the full Wolff-Chaikoff effect.[236, 237] This adaptation prevents the development of hypothyroidism, iodide goiter, or myxedema. Of note, it does *not* occur in the third trimester fetus; thus, chronic high iodine intake during pregnancy must be avoided because it causes fetal hypothyroidism and compensatory, obstructive goiter (Fig. 10–13).

Effects on Thyroid Hormone Release

An important practical effect of pharmacologic doses of iodine is the prompt inhibition of thyroid hormone release. Iodine decreases not only the fractional turnover of thyroidal iodine but also the T_4 secretion rate. This effect is the mechanism by which iodine rapidly lowers the serum T_4 concentration in patients with diffuse toxic goiter or toxic nodules (see Chapter 11). The mechanism by which iodide inhibits secretion of thyroid hormones is unknown, but the effect is mediated at the thyroid cell level rather than through an action on TSH. Iodine also diminishes the hypervascularity and hyperplasia that characterize the diffuse toxic goiter of Graves' disease. This effect facilitates surgical therapy for the disorder.[238, 239]

Thyroid Function in Pregnancy and in the Fetus and Newborn

Pregnancy affects virtually all aspects of thyroid hormone economy (Table 10–9).[1, 240, 241] Total serum T_4 and T_3 concentrations rise to levels twice those of nonpregnant women owing to the increase in TBG concentration in the first trimester (Fig. 10–14).[63, 64] Free T_4 and T_3 levels also increase slightly during the first trimester but return to normal by

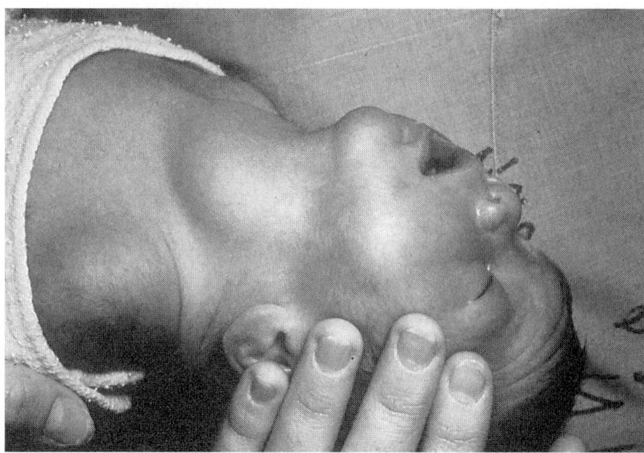

Figure 10–13. Newborn infant with iodide-induced goiter due to Lugol's solution treatment of the mother during the third trimester. This illustration shows the danger of chronic excess iodide administration during gestation.

about 20 weeks of gestation and remain so until delivery. This increase is due to hCG, which is a weak agonist for the TSH receptor.[242] The slight decrease in serum TSH during the first trimester indicates that the free T_4 and T_3 changes are not dependent on the hypothalamic-pituitary axis. This decrease in serum TSH is all the more surprising, since it coincides with a number of events that act to increase maternal requirements for thyroid hormone.

In addition to an increase in serum TBG, there is also an increased plasma volume as well as accelerated inactivation of T_3 and T_4 by D3 expression in placenta and, perhaps, in the uterus as well.[123] On the basis of changes in requirements for L-thyroxine during gestation in women with primary hypothyroidism, the estimated increase in T_4 production required during this period is approximately 50%.[88, 243]

During pregnancy, the requirement for increased T_4 production increases iodine requirements. This need is compounded by the fact that the increased glomerular filtration rate during pregnancy enhances renal iodide clearance, leading to higher fractional urinary excretion of circulating iodide. In addition, maternal iodine intake must be increased to supply the iodide requirements of the fetal thyroid gland during the second and third trimesters (see Table 10–9). If these in-

Table 10–9. Effects of Pregnancy on Thyroid Physiology

Physiologic Change	Thyroid-Related Consequences
↑ Serum thyroxine-binding globulin	↑ Total T_4 and T_3; ↑ T_4 production
↑ Plasma volume	↑ T_4 and T_3 pool size; ↑ T_4 production; ↑ cardiac output
D3 expression in placenta and (?) uterus	↑ T_4 production
First trimester ↑ in hCG	↑ Free T_4; ↓ basal thyrotropin; ↑ T_4 production
↑ Renal I^- clearance	↑ Iodine requirements
↑ T_4 production; fetal T_4 synthesis during second and third trimesters	
↑ Oxygen consumption by fetoplacental unit, gravid uterus, and mother	↑ Basal metabolic rate; ↑ cardiac output

hCG, human chorionic gonadotropin.

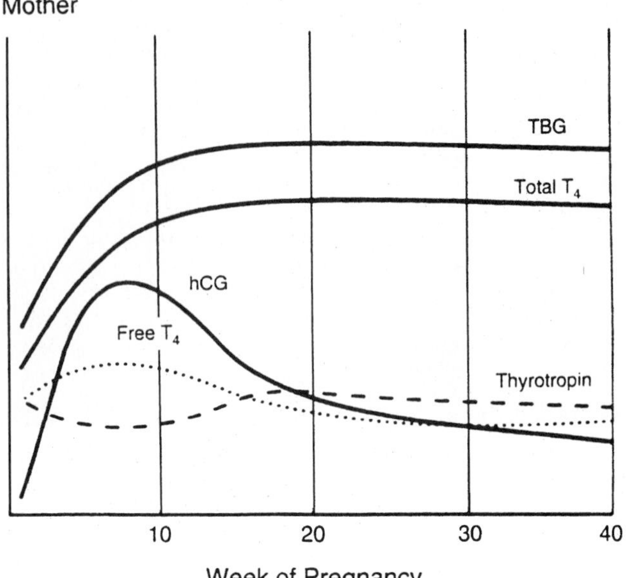

Figure 10–14. Changes in various critical components of the thyroid-pituitary axis during pregnancy. Note the early increase in free thyroxine (T_4), probably due to thyroidal stimulation by human chorionic gonadotropin (hCG), which causes a reciprocal modest suppression of serum thyrotropin (TSH) during the late first trimester. TBG, thyroxine-binding globulin. (From Burrow GN, Fisher DA, Larsen PR. Mechanisms of disease: maternal and fetal thyroid function. N Engl J Med 1994; 331:1072–1078. © 1994, Massachusetts Medical Society.)

creased requirements for iodide are not met, serum T_4 levels fall, TSH levels rise, and goiter ensues. This series of events is well documented in areas of endemic iodine deficiency or a borderline iodine supply, such as in Brussels.[240] In that city, 70% of pregnant women carefully monitored throughout their pregnancy had a 20% or greater increase in thyroid volume during gestation.[244] This contrasts with the lack of goiter during pregnancy in studies in North America.[245] After delivery, the changes in thyroid function gradually return to normal, with serum TBG values reaching their normal levels 6 to 8 weeks post partum.

Pregnancy exerts a number of effects on the immune system. These changes may have striking effects on the natural history of patients with autoimmune thyroid disease, including both Graves' disease and Hashimoto's thyroiditis.[246] In general, thyroid stimulation in women with Graves' disease is exacerbated during the first trimester but then is reduced gradually during the second and third, only to exacerbate again in the first several months post partum. Other than the increase in L-thyroxine requirements in hypothyroid pregnant women, there is no evidence of a clinically significant change in patients with Hashimoto's disease during pregnancy, except that thyroid antibody levels fall. On the other hand, the marked rebound in the immune system occurring in the postpartum period leads to a phase of acute thyroid cell destruction, *postpartum thyroid disease* (PPTD), in about 30% of these patients (see Chapters 11 and 12).[247]

The basal metabolic rate (BMR) increases during the second trimester owing to the increase in the total mass of body tissue consequent to the pregnancy. The changes of pregnancy, together with the decreased peripheral vascular resistance, vasodilatation, and modest tachycardia, may suggest thyrotoxicosis (see Table 10–9). It is important that physicians remember that such changes are normal in pregnancy, especially when treating the hyperthyroid pregnant patient.

Fetal Thyroid Function

Fetal thyroid function begins at about the end of the first trimester. Thereafter, there are steady increases in fetal TBG and in total T_4 and T_3.[248, 249]

Throughout gestation, serum TSH values are greater than are present in maternal circulation and higher than would be expected in adults with normal thyroid function. This indicates that there is increasing hypothalamic-pituitary resistance to T_4 during fetal development; it is speculated that this may be a consequence of increased TRH secretion.[249, 250]

Circulating T_3 levels remain relatively low, in contrast to the fetal free T_4 concentrations that approximate those in the maternal circulation from gestational age 28 weeks onward. This is explained primarily by the high D3 in fetal tissues, especially the liver.[251]

Maternal-Fetal Interactions

The fetal pituitary-thyroid axis functions as a unit that is essentially independent of the mother.[1, 2, 250, 252] Transplacental passage of TSH from mother to fetus is negligible, but the same is not true of maternal T_4. In infants with congenital hypothyroidism caused by either TPO deficiency or athyreosis, serum concentrations of T_4 in umbilical cord blood are usually one third to one half of normal.[29]

Thus, at least when the maternal-fetal concentration gradient is high, significant transfer of T_4 to the fetal circulation occurs. This transfer may be significant, given the capacity of the fetal brain to increase the efficiency of T_4 to T_3 conversion.[253] Furthermore, T_4 can be found in coelomic and amniotic fluids prior to the onset of thyroid function.[254]

The major factor limiting T_4 and T_3 transport from mother to fetus is the D3 expressed in the placenta.[255] Blocking D3 activity in a perfused human placental lobule markedly increases the quantity of T_4 crossing into the equivalent of the fetal circulation.[255] Placental D3 activity is present throughout gestation, although its activity, expressed per milligram of placental protein, decreases.[256] Nonetheless, the increase in placental size results in progressive increases in total D3 content throughout gestation. This can account, at least in part, for the sudden decrease in maternal L-thyroxine requirements that occurs immediately upon delivery.[88]

Thyroid Function in the Newborn

Mean total T_4 levels in cord sera are 150 nmol/L (12 μg/dL). Serum TBG concentrations are elevated, but not as high as in the maternal serum. At term, free T_4 concentrations are slightly lower than those in the mother. Cord serum T_3 concentrations are low ($\sim 0.8 \times 10^{-9}$M, 50 ng/dL), and rT_3 and T_3 S are elevated.[1, 250, 257] After delivery, the neonate's serum TSH level increases rapidly to a peak at 30 minutes of extrauterine life, returning to its initial value within 48 hours.[258] This neonatal TSH surge is thought to occur in response to marked reduction in environmental temperature after delivery. Serum T_4, T_3, and Tg concentrations increase rapidly during the first few hours after delivery and are in the hyperthyroid range by 24 hours of life.[259] The TSH surge doubtless contributes to the increase in serum T_3 concentration, but enhancement of extrathyroidal conversion of T_4 to T_3 by D1 or D2 is thought to be a major factor as well.[53] The adrenergic stimulation of D2 in brown adipose tissue may also contribute to the increase in serum T_3.[133, 135]

Serum rT_3 concentrations increase during the first 24 hours of postnatal life as a result of the increased T_4 but decrease to normal values by the fifth postnatal day. By the 10th day or so, the serum T_4 and T_3 concentrations are lower but still exceed normal adult values. Serum T_3 levels are slightly higher in the first year of life but gradually fall to the normal adult range.[250, 260]

Premature infants have an immature hypothalamic-pituitary-thyroid axis with low levels of T_4, T_3, and TSH.[261] Serum T_4 TBG, and free T_4 all tend to correlate with gestational age. Preterm infants do have a TSH surge after delivery, but this is attenuated relative to that of full-term infants. In addition, when prematurity is accompanied by complications, such as respiratory distress syndrome or nutritional problems, serum T_4, and especially T_3, may fall to low levels because of a combination of reduced TBG production, immaturity of the thyroid gland, and suppression of the hypothalamic-pituitary axis owing to illness.[262] These changes are, in many respects, similar to those in adults who are severely ill. The physician must take all of these issues into account when evaluating the thyroid status of the preterm infant, particularly given the increased prevalence of congenital hypothyroidism in this age group.[263, 264]

Thyroid hormone production rates are higher per unit of body weight in neonatal infants and children than in adults. The daily L-thyroxine requirement is about 10 μg/kg in the newborn, decreasing to about 1.6 μg/kg in the adult.[249]

Aging and the Thyroid Gland

Reproducible thyroid function abnormalities are observed in aging patients. In the healthy patient, there is a normal free T_4 but a relatively lower serum TSH than in younger individuals. In addition, although some disagree, it appears that serum T_3 levels decline, especially in individuals older than age 100 years.[265] The serum T_3/T_4 ratio also tends to be reduced in individuals in their eighth and ninth decades; in addition, the daily secretion rate of TSH is reduced.[266]

Although these changes resemble those occurring in patients who are ill, serum rT_3 concentrations are not nearly as elevated as they are in hospitalized individuals, and whether the reductions in serum T_3 are pathologic or physiologic is still unclear.[265, 267, 268] A decreased requirement of about 20% for thyroid hormone replacement in the hypothyroid elderly becomes apparent in the eighth decade.[269]

Thyroid Function during Fasting or Illness

A number of changes may take place in thyroid function during nutritional deprivation or illness. The changes that are induced in these two conditions are similar and, therefore, are best discussed in concert. Many of the changes involve alterations in thyroid hormone metabolism and are alluded to in that discussion.

Effects of Nutritional Deprivation

Both short-term and long-term alterations in nutritional state affect various aspects of thyroid hormone economy, especially peripheral hormone metabolism, as previously discussed. When euthyroid lean or obese subjects are starved, the serum total and free T_3 levels decrease to subnormal levels.[132] In general, the serum total and free T_4 concentration remains essentially unchanged, or total T_4 may decrease slightly because of a modest decrease in iodothyronine-binding proteins. As serum T_3 concentrations decrease, concentrations of rT_3 increase reciprocally, usually to values about twice normal, not because of a major increase in the production of rT_3 but because of a decrease in its clearance.[53] The abnormal T_3 and rT_3 concentrations in serum are quickly restored to normal by administration of small quantities (200 kcal) of carbohydrate. Similar quantities of protein have no effect on the serum T_3 level but may lower the serum rT_3 level. Calories given as fat are ineffective.[270]

Despite the decrease in free T_3 concentration with starvation, the basal serum TSH and the free T_4 concentration and its response to TRH infusion are essentially unchanged. This occurs despite a decrease in leptin, suggesting that this hormone is less crucial in maintaining TRH production in humans than in rats despite its positive stimulation of the human TRH promoter.[183, 185, 187, 191]

Basal oxygen consumption and heart rate decline, nitrogen balance returns toward normal, and peripheral steroid metabolism shifts toward the pattern seen in hypothyroidism. In some, but not all studies, these changes are partially reversed by administration of exogenous T_3 while fasting continues.[271] The decrease in T_3 during fasting is viewed by many as a beneficial energy-sparing and nitrogen-sparing adaptation.[272]

Chronic malnutrition, as in protein-calorie malnutrition and anorexia nervosa, is also associated with a decreased serum T_3 concentration. Serum T_4 levels also tend to be slightly decreased, but serum TSH concentrations and their response to exogenous TRH are usually normal. In contrast, overfeeding, particularly with carbohydrate, increases T_3 production rate, increases the serum T_3 level, lowers the serum rT_3 concentration, and increases basal thermogenesis.[273]

Effects of Illness

The changes in circulating thyroid hormones in illness resemble those during fasting, except that they may be much more severe. In addition, in the severely ill patient, there is often a suppression of the pituitary hormone release, which is either endogenous, because of loss of hypothalamic input, or worsened by some agents, such as dopamine and glucocorticoids, often given to very ill patients.[274, 275] This condition has come to be called the *euthyroid sick syndrome*, *nonthyroid illness*, or *the low T_3 syndrome*. These terms refer to the global pattern of changes in thyroid physiology that occur during illness.

The changes in thyroid function are a continuum, with the abnormalities becoming progressively more severe in accordance with the patient's clinical condition. The disruption in thyroid function in sick patients can be arbitrarily divided into three stages (Table 10–10):

Table 10–10. Modifications of Thyroid-Related Hormones during Fasting or Illness

Severity of Illness	Thyroid-Related Hormone			
	Free T_4	Free T_3	Total Reverse T_3	Thyrotropin
Stage 1 (mild)	Normal	Reduced up to 50%	Increased up to twofold	Normal
Stage 2 (moderate)	Increased	Reduced up to 90%	Increased up to severalfold	Normal
Stage 3 (severe)	Reduced	Almost undetectable	Variable	Reduced

Stage 1. In patients with mild illness, generally there is a reduction of up to 50% in circulating T_3, a modest increase in serum rT_3, but no change in serum free T_4, total T_4, or TSH.[21, 276]

Stage 2. The clearance of T_4 is significantly reduced, but pulsatile TSH secretion persists, leading to a modest increase in free T_4. This is generally accompanied by further decreases in serum T_3 and increases in rT_3.

Stage 3. These changes occur in addition to loss of pulsatile secretion of TSH and a fall in T_4 and T_3 levels.[274] Depending on how rapidly the patient enters this phase, levels of serum free T_4 may be normal but eventually are reduced. Serum rT_3 levels may be elevated earlier and then return to normal later if T_4 levels fall, but total serum T_3 may be almost undetectable. Patients are quite ill, and the changes may be seen as a preagonal phase of severe illness, since mortality in such patients is high.[277, 278]

In addition to the central changes in TSH regulation and the abnormalities in peripheral hormone metabolism, patients may also have abnormalities in thyroid function that may be attributed to changes in the circulating binding proteins and, especially in the case of sepsis, those caused by the marked reduction the TBG affinity due to the serpin cleavage of the carboxy-terminal fragment of TBG.[65, 69] In addition to these endogenous changes, the TSH-suppressive effects of therapeutic agents (e.g., dopamine, dobutamine, glucocorticoids) on the central thyroid axis may complicate and exacerbate the abnormality. Illness and surgery decrease the nocturnal pulsatile TSH surge, presumably by reducing TRH release.[274, 279]

After the initial recognition of this syndrome, a large number of studies were performed using the starved rat as a model. As we have come to recognize, thyroid physiology in the rat, especially during fasting, differs from that in humans.[53] Therefore, many of the studies pointing to an effect of illness or starvation to impair D1 activity, either through reductions in D1 or a D1 cofactor, may have limited applicability in humans. In addition, the role of leptin appears to be much more important in maintaining TRH synthesis in rodents than in humans.[191] Patients with severe illness have high leptin levels despite suppression of the central hypothalamic-pituitary-thyroid axis.[190] In humans, rT_3 production remains normal as long as T_4 secretion is maintained.[276] Therefore, the elevation in rT_3 indicates an impairment of its clearance and rT_3 uptake into D1-expressing tissues is impaired during illness or fasting.[280] This decreased transport is due either to ATP depletion or, perhaps, to substances that compete with rT_3 for cellular entry.[93, 281]

Because the serum T_3 can fall to undetectable levels during illness, it seems likely that all three pathways for T_3 production, T_3 secretion and T_4 outer ring deiodination by D1 and D2, may be reduced.[53] Again, it is not certain whether the changes, particularly in D2, are a result of (1) decreased enzyme levels (e.g., as in skeletal muscle induced by TNF-α),[282] (2) decreased uptake into the slowly equilibrating D2-containing tissue pool,[101] or (3) a reduction in D2 due to accelerated proteolysis of this enzyme via the ubiquitin-proteasome pathway.[117] T_4 uptake into rapidly equilibrating pools, such as those in the liver and kidney, is also reduced during fasting or in illness.[101]

Although serum TSH concentrations in severely ill patients are reduced, an increase in TSH above the normal range may appear during recovery, with the elevation in TSH concentration persisting until circulating free T_4 and T_3 levels return to normal.[283–285] This pattern can be confusing if the elevated TSH concentration is associated with the still-reduced concentrations of free T_4. Such patients meet all laboratory criteria for primary hypothyroidism with the exception of the clinical context. Follow-up generally reveals a normalization of TSH and T_4 within 1 to 2 months.

Despite the severity of the abnormalities, particularly in serum T_3, it is still debatable whether therapeutic intervention should be initiated even in the most severely ill patients.[281, 286, 287] This is because most controlled studies have not shown beneficial effects of T_4 or T_3 supplementation in such individuals.[288, 289] The one exception is the possible beneficial effect of T_3 therapy in patients after coronary artery bypass grafting; one study showed a positive effect but a second showed no beneficial effect.[290–292]

A promising alternative strategy has been initiated in a series of studies of patients with prolonged critical illness.[274, 275, 293–295] In an attempt to correct the inappropriate catabolism and failure of fat mobilization of prolonged critical illness, infusions of GH-releasing peptide-2 (GHRP-2) and TRH have been given for 5-day periods in a randomized fashion.[295] Increases in TSH, T_3, and T_4 (as well as in IGF-I) insulin and IGF-binding proteins 1, 3, and 5 and leptin occurred and were associated with positive effects on osteocalcin, and decreases in the urinary/urea creatinine ratio.

These results suggested that restoration of somatotroph and thyrotroph function simultaneously by replacement of deficient neuroendocrine peptides had significant beneficial effects on the disordered metabolism of severe chronic illness that cannot be achieved by isolated and supraphysiologic replacement of either thyroid hormone or growth hormone alone.[296] Whether these encouraging results will be associated with an improved outcome remains to be demonstrated, but the results suggest that in prolonged critical illness the central hypothyroidism is not beneficial.

The Thyroid Axis and Neuropsychiatric Illness

Patients with neuropsychiatric disease can present with any of a number of abnormalities in thyroid function. Patients with bipolar disorders may show slight elevations in serum TSH and reductions in free T_4, whereas patients with severe depression have slightly elevated serum T_4 and reduced serum TSH levels.[297] Other acutely psychotic patients may have either high or low serum TSH concentrations and tend to have elevated free T_4 levels.[298, 299]

The etiologic mechanism of these minor abnormalities is not clear, but the thyroid function test results of such patients may resemble the results of those with primary thyroid disease and must be differentiated from these.

Hormonal Effects on Thyroid Function

Glucocorticoids

The acute administration of pharmacologic doses of glucocorticoid eliminates pulsatile release of serum TSH concentrations in normal patients, presumably by reducing TRH release.[300] With continued administration, there is an escape from this suppression (Table 10–11). Pharmacologic doses of glucocorticoid decrease serum T_3 concentration in normal and hyperthyroid patients as well as in hypothyroid patients maintained on L-thyroxine. The latter finding and the accompanying increase in rT_3 production suggest that glucocorticoids increase D3 activity.[155] The decreases in TBG and TTR have only modest effects on total T_4 concentrations.

Primary adrenal insufficiency may be associated with reduced serum T_4 and elevated serum TSH concentrations, suggesting the coexistence of primary hypothyroidism. However, treatment of the adrenal insufficiency can lead to complete

Table 10–11. Effects of Hormones on Thyroid Function

Glucocorticoids
Excess
Decrease TSH, TBG, TTR (high-dose)
Decrease serum T_3/T_4 and increase rT_3/T_4 ratios
Increase rT_3 production (? ↑ D3)
Decrease T_4 and T_3 secretion in Graves' disease
Deficiency
Increase TSH
Estrogen
Increase TBG sialylation and half-life in serum
Increase TSH in postmenopausal women
Increase T_4 requirement in hypothyroid patients
Androgen
Decrease TBG
Decrease T_4 turnover in women and reduce T_4 requirements in hypothyroid patients
Growth Hormone
Decrease D3 activity

D3, type 3 deoidinase; T_3, T_4, reverse T_3 and T_4; TBG, thyroxine-binding globulin; TSH, thyrotropin; TTR, transthyretin.

resolution of the abnormalities in thyroid function, suggesting that in some patients they are a consequence of glucocorticoid deficiency rather than primary thyroid disease.[301] Nevertheless, the prevalence of primary hypothyroidism is increased in patients with autoimmune hypoadrenalism, so the two causes must be differentiated (see Chapter 37). Similarly, thyroid autoimmunity can develop in patients successfully treated for Cushing's disease.[302]

Gonadal Steroids

Estrogen increases TBG by mechanisms already mentioned.[63] Estrogen administration to postmenopausal women causes an increase of 15% to 20% in TSH.[86] Presumably, this increases T_4 secretion, since total T_4 increases and free T_4 is unchanged. It is not certain whether this is a transient or persisting phenomenon. Estrogen also increases the L-thyroxine requirement in patients with primary hypothyroidism.[89]

In contrast, administration of androgens to women decreases TBG and decreases T_4 turnover and levothyroxine requirements in patients with primary hypothyroidism.[303] Again, the cause of this change is unclear.

Growth Hormone

Growth hormone increases the serum free T_3 and decreases free T_4 in both L-thyroxine-treated and normal individuals, suggesting either suppression of D3 activity or increased T_4 to T_3 conversion.[156] This change would reduce requirements for L-thyroxine in patients receiving exogenous hormone.

LABORATORY ASSESSMENT OF THYROID STATUS

In considering the laboratory assessment of the patient with known or suspected thyroid disease, the physician should seek to arrive at both functional and anatomic diagnoses. Laboratory determinations will confirm whether there is an excess, normal, or an insufficient supply of thyroid hormone to verify the inferences from the clinical history and physical examination. The second is to ascertain the presence or absence of anatomic abnormalities in the thyroid gland itself.

Laboratory evaluation can be divided into five major categories:

1. Tests that assess the state of the hypothalamic-pituitary-thyroid axis.
2. Estimates of the free T_4 or T_3 concentrations in the serum.
3. Tests that reflect the impact of thyroid hormone on tissues.
4. Tests for evidence of the presence of autoimmune thyroid disease.
5. Tests that provide information about thyroidal iodine metabolism.

Techniques for evaluation of anatomic abnormalities of the thyroid gland (thyroid ultrasound) and thyroid isotopic scanning are covered in Chapter 13.

Tests of the Hypothalamic-Pituitary-Thyroid Axis

Thyrotropin

While they are an inherently indirect reflection of thyroid hormone supply, tests that assess the state of the hypothalamic-pituitary-thyroid axis play a critical role in the diagnosis of thyroid disease. This is because the rate of TSH secretion is exquisitely sensitive to plasma concentrations of free thyroid hormones, thus providing a precise and specific barometer of the patient's thyroid status (see Fig. 10–11). Exceptions to this rule do occur (see later) but are rare. For example, the feedback of TSH secretion in premature infants and children is less sensitive to free T_4 than is that of the adult, probably due to higher TRH secretion rates.[250]

Immunometric assay technology now makes it possible to define the normal range for serum TSH and, hence, to ascertain (1) when thyroid function is inadequate and (2) when the hormone supply is excessive.[304–306] This assay uses the TSH molecule as a link between a TSH antibody bound to an inert surface (e.g., particles, the side of a test tube) and a second antibody directed against a different TSH epitope that is labeled with a detectable marker (^{125}I, an enzyme, or a chemiluminescent reagent) (see Chapter 6). Thus, the signal generated is proportional to the concentration of TSH in the serum. This technique is more specific, sensitive, and rapid than radioimmunoassay.

The normal range of serum TSH concentration varies slightly in different laboratories but is most commonly 0.5 to 5 mU/L or 0.3 to 4.0 mU/L, depending on the TSH reference preparation and assay used. Not all immunometric TSH assays are equally sensitive and specific.[307] A useful functional categorization is in terms of the minimal detectable TSH that can be quantified with a less than 20% coefficient of variation.

The term *generation* has been employed to categorize each assay with respect to its sensitivity. Each successive generation offers about a 10-fold improvement in sensitivity (Fig. 10–15). The *first* generation (TSH radioimmunoassay) has lower limits of detectability of approximately 1 mU/L, whereas the *third* generation assay has minimal detectable limits of about 0.004 mU/L. A minimally suitable TSH assay should be able to quantitate concentrations of TSH of 0.1 mU/L with a coefficient of variation of less than 20%, thus falling into the second-generation or third-generation category.

An artifactually elevated result may be obtained using the immunometric technique with serum containing heterophilic antimouse immunoglobulin G antibodies (HAMA).[308] Such antibodies may substitute for TSH and cause falsely high values

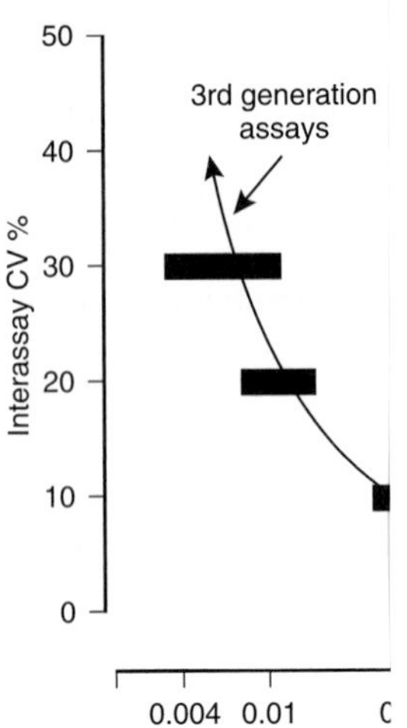

Figure 10–15. With the d
assays with greater sensitiv
normal thyrotropin concent
thyroidism. Each generatio
ment in functional sensitiv
variation (CV) value. *Black*
measurement at different t
JT, Spencer CA. Clinical r
tive thyrotropin assays. J Cl

(see Chapter 6). Most m
ulin G (IgG) to the assa
the quantity added may
with high HAMA titers
are elevated out of pro
free hormone concentrat
factual.
The free α subunit c
is generally detectable in
$\mu g/L^{309}$, but the TSH β
production are increase
or when TSH product
hypothyroidism), the fre
α subunit level may als
protein-producing tumo
ter 8). Its measurement
hyperthyroidism and a
differentiate tumorous f
cess.[51, 309]

Thyrotropin in Patie
Dysfunction

In patients with *hyper*
cretion) and/or *thyrotoxi*
cause), the TSH level is
fall into two general cat
normal and 0.1 mU/L a
in the former category a
clinical hyperthyroidism),
almost invariably have s
icant elevation in free T
Patients with hypothal
cally have normal, not
sometimes the TSH is e
the circulating TSH g
because of abnormal gly
pothalamic-pituitary rel

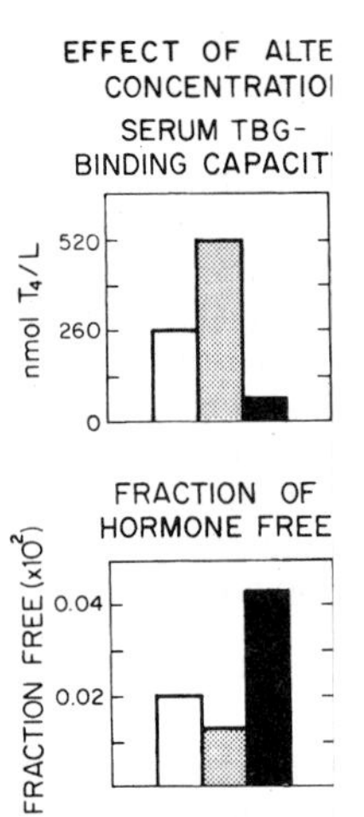

Figure 10–16. Patter
centrations and thyro
patients with alterati
binding globulin (TB
or pmol/L (free), divi

the reduced THBR
creased total T_4, t
reflection of the fr
rum T_4 concentrat
concentration of u
even greater extent.
free T_4 (and T_3) fr
and the FT_4I remai
The THBR is lir
hormones except a
maximum informat
both the calculated
total hormone and
of binding proteins
measurements from
of the THBR (see
stance, one should
rather than an alt
responsible for the
level. However, wh
T_4 secretion or exo
cupied TBG-bindin
and the THBR are
FT_4I are increased
would be suggeste
level.
The changes in h
but of lower mag
TBG-binding sites
T_4 level decreases
nmol/L, and the
THBR are not larg
ism is due predomi
a decrease in its fre
17 show the parall
and THBR when t
Simultaneous ab
mone production n
suspected during p
high and the TH
concentration in th
pregnant woman,
the THBR, indicat

ties in the hypothalamic-pituitary-thyroid axis, although these findings are rarely associated with clinical symptoms. Typically, TSH is suppressed but in some patients it may be spontaneously elevated.[299] A small fraction of the elderly population may have suppressed TSH, either without hyperthyroidism or associated with mild thyrotoxicosis due to Graves' disease, multinodular goiter, autonomous thyroid nodules, or excessive thyroid hormone replacement.[266, 325] Although acute treatment with glucocorticoids may transiently suppress TSH, chronic treatment does not. Rarely, patients with genetic deficiency of the PIT1 protein or with a mutation in the TSH-α subunit have severe hypothyroidism and no detectable TSH (see Chapter 12).[203, 326, 327]

Elevated Thyrotropin Levels

Elevations in TSH nearly always suggest a reduced supply of T_4 or T_3, which may be permanent or transient. Acutely ill patients may have elevated serum TSH levels, as in renal insufficiency,[328] or may experience an asynchronous return of the hypothalamic-pituitary and thyroid axes to normal as they recover from acute illness; the latter case, patients have a transient form of primary hypothyroidism.[284] Iodine deficiency is the most common cause of elevated TSH worldwide, but this does not occur in North America.

Patients with resistance to thyroid hormone may be clinically hyperthyroid, euthyroid, or hypothyroid. The most common laboratory pattern is a serum TSH that is *normal* in absolute terms but inappropriately high for the elevated FT_4I. Individuals with a more marked *pituitary* than *general* resistance to thyroid hormone (sometimes called pituitary RTH or PRTH) have symptoms suggesting hyperthyroidism, an elevated FT_4I, and a normal or even elevated serum TSH.[329–331] These patients must be differentiated from the equally rare patients with a thyrotroph tumor in whom the persistent secretion of TSH causes hyperthyroidism (see Chapter 8).[51]

Patients with hypothalamic-pituitary dysfunction may have clinical and chemical hypothyroidism but low-normal or even elevated serum TSH concentrations. The explanation for this paradox is that the biologic effectiveness of the circulating TSH is impaired because of abnormal glycosylation secondary to reduced TRH stimulation of the thyrotrophs. Nonetheless, the abnormal TSH is a suitable antigen in the immunometric assay.

Some patients with psychiatric illness may have elevated TSH levels for reasons that are not understood.[299] In adrenal insufficiency, TSH levels may be modestly elevated but return to normal with glucocorticoid replacement.[301] In patients with antimouse IgG antibodies, TSH is usually artifactually elevated, often greatly so (see Chapter 6).[332]

Despite the utility and general efficacy of the serum TSH measurement alone as a screening tool for identifying patients with thyroid dysfunction, a patient should *not* receive treatment for this dysfunction solely on the basis of an abnormal TSH level. The TSH assay is an *indirect reflection* of thyroid hormone supply and does not, by itself, permit a conclusive diagnosis of a specific disorder of thyroid hormone production.

Concordant and Divergent Abnormalities of Serum Thyroxine and Triiodothyronine Concentrations

One suspects that millions of dollars might be saved each year by the judicious selection of thyroid tests. In the authors' experience, far too many serum T_3 measurements are performed. Serum T_3 is rarely required for the accurate evaluation of the patient with an abnormal TSH level and is almost always an indirect reflection of the serum T_4 supply. Serum T_3 results are virtually useless in the hospitalized patient. Nonetheless, the endocrinologist is often asked to interpret abnormal or discordant serum T_4 and T_3 values (Table 10–14).

Table 10–14. Causes of Concordant and Divergent Changes in Serum Thyroxine (T_4) and Triiodothyronine (T_3) Levels

T_4 and T_3 Increased
Increased TBG (see Table 10–12)
Thyrotoxicosis
Thyroid hormone resistance (RTH)
T_4 Increased, T_3 Normal or Low
Familial dysalbuminemic hyperthyroxinemia (FDH)
Increased TTR or TTR binding
Amiodarone, high-dose propranolol, or oral cholecystographic agents
Illness, especially psychiatric
Amphetamine abuse
T_4 thyrotoxicosis, thyrotoxicosis with decreased T_4-to-T_3 conversion (see Table 10–6)
T_4 Normal, T_3 Increased
T_3 thyrotoxicosis
T_4 Normal, T_3 Decreased
Most patients with significant illness or during fasting (see Table 10–10)
T_4 Decreased, T_3 Increased
Thyrotoxicosis due to ingestion of liothyronine (T_3)
Euthyroid patients taking desiccated thyroid or liotrix (see text on hypothyroidism)
T_4 Decreased, T_3 Normal
Mild or moderate thyroid failure
Iodine deficiency
Phenytoin, carbamazepine
T_4 and T_3 Decreased
Severe hypothyroidism
Severe systemic illness (euthyroid patient)
Decreased TBG
Salicylates in high doses (>2.0 g/day)

TBG, thyroxine-binding globulin; TTR, transthyretin.

Increased Thyroxine, Increased Triiodothyronine

An increase in serum TBG concentration secondary to increased estrogen is the most common cause of simultaneous elevations of serum total T_4 and T_3. Other causes of TBG elevation are listed in Table 10–12. Thyrotoxicosis due to hyperthyroidism is usually associated with an increased T_3/T_4 ratio, whereas that due to thyroiditis or exogenous L-thyroxine is associated with a decreased T_3/T_4 ratio. In patients with RTH, serum total and free T_4 and T_3 concentrations are elevated, although typical clinical features of thyrotoxicosis are often lacking, and both basal serum TSH concentrations and the response to TRH are normal or increased.[329, 331]

Increased Thyroxine, Normal or Low Triiodothyronine

Almost all severe illnesses and fasting reduce the T_3/T_4 ratio in the circulation, producing the *low T_3 syndrome* (see earlier). Serum T_4 levels are also increased relative to T_3 in the rare patient with FDH, glucagon-secreting tumors of the pancreatic islet cells, and in the patient with an increase in the binding affinity of TTR.[59, 60] In all these conditions, serum T_3 concentrations are normal.

Certain pharmacotherapeutic agents may elevate the serum T_4 concentration by inhibiting the conversion of T_4 to T_3 by

D1 and D2 or by interfering with the cellular uptake of T_4. Agents that inhibit peripheral T_3 production include amiodarone and oral cholecystographic agents, such as iopanoic acid, sodium ipodate, tyropanoate, and iobenzamic acid (see Fig. 10–7).[144, 151, 152] Propranolol in high doses, but not other β-adrenergic agents, can inhibit D1 and, at doses greater than 160 ng/day, can lower serum T_3.[333, 334] The T_4 increase is a compensatory response to the blockade of T_3 production attributed to these agents, and the T_3 and TSH eventually normalizes with a T_4 level that is elevated as long as thyroid function is normal.

Decreased Thyroxine, Increased Triiodothyronine

Patients receiving replacement therapy with either liothyronine (T_3) or with agents with a higher T_3/T_4 ratio than in human thyroid secretion (~11/1 by weight), including liotrix and desiccated thyroid, usually have a low-normal FT_4I when doses are titered to return serum concentrations of TSH to normal. T_3 levels are transiently elevated if serum is drawn between 1 and 4 hours after the patient ingests the medication.[335–337]

Increased Thyroxine, Normal Triiodothyronine

The reasons for the decreased T_4 and normal T_3 in early hypothyroidism or during iodine deficiency have been discussed earlier (see "Iodine Deficiency"). Many drugs lower the serum T_4 concentration by interfering with the binding of T_4 to plasma proteins or by accelerating T_4 metabolism or both.[81] Therapeutic doses of phenytoin lower the serum FT_4I concentration, sometimes into the hypothyroid range. Although high concentrations of the drug can inhibit the binding of T_4 and T_3 to TBG in vitro, a drug-induced acceleration of T_4 disposal and, perhaps, central TSH suppression appear to be responsible for the reduced T_4.[81]

Enhancement of hepatic disposal of T_4 by induction of cytochrome CYP3A4 in patients receiving carbamazepine, rifampin, phenobarbital, and phenytoin causes increased gluconuride conjugation of T_4 and T_3. This does not pose a problem in euthyroid patients. In hypothyroid patients, however, the levothyroxine dose must be increased.[54, 338–340] Serum T_3 concentrations usually remain at low-normal levels.

Decreased Thyroxine, Decreased Triiodothyronine

Hypothyroidism of any origin and TBG deficiency are the most common causes of parallel reductions in serum T_4 and T_3 (see Table 10–12). In addition, salicylates, especially salsalate, inhibit the binding of T_4 and T_3 by serum proteins in vitro and have comparable effects in vivo when given in high doses.[76–78] Initially, serum free T_4 and T_3 concentrations increase, but the consequent increased MCRs of the hormones, combined with the suppression of the hypothalamic-pituitary axis, lead to a new equilibrium in which serum total T_4 and T_3 values are decreased and free T_4, free T_3, and TSH values return to normal.

Marked lowering of the serum T_4 concentration and moderate decreases in the serum T_3 level may also occur in patients receiving the nonsteroidal anti-inflammatory drug (NSAID) fenclofenac.[341] Patients are clinically euthyroid, and serum TSH levels are normal. Administration of L-asparaginase has the same rapid effect owing to inhibition of TBG synthesis.[61] Stage 3 (severe) illness reduces both serum T_4 and T_3 (see Table 10–10).

Tests That Assess the Metabolic Impact of Thyroid Hormones

Abnormalities in the supply of thyroid hormone to the peripheral tissues are associated with alterations in a number of metabolic processes that can be quantitated. Some of these may be useful in the rare patient in whom serum TSH is not an accurate barometer of thyroid status, such as the patient with RTH. Such tests may be the sole means of evaluating the metabolic response of the peripheral tissues to thyroid hormones in such patients.

Basal Metabolic Rate

Thyroid hormones increase energy expenditure and heat production, as manifested by weight loss, increased caloric requirement, and heat intolerance. Because it is impractical to measure heat production directly, the basal metabolic rate measures oxygen consumption under specified conditions of fasting, rest, and tranquil surroundings. Under these conditions, the energy equivalent of 1 L of oxygen is equivalent to 4.83 kcal.

Under basal conditions, approximately 25% of oxygen consumption is due to energy expenditure in visceral organs, including the liver, kidneys, and heart; 10% in the brain; 10% in respiratory activity; and the remainder in skeletal muscle. Because energy expenditure is related to functioning tissue mass, oxygen consumption is related to some index thereof, most often body surface area. Calculated in this way, basal oxygen consumption (resting energy expenditure) is higher in men than in women and declines rapidly from infancy to the third decade and more slowly thereafter.

Values in patients, calculated as a percentage of established normal means for gender and age, normally range from −15% to +5%. In severely hypothyroid patients, values may be as low as −40%. In thyrotoxic patients, these values may reach +25% to 50%. Abnormal, usually elevated values, are seen in patients with burns and with systemic disorders (e.g., febrile illnesses, pheochromocytoma, myeloproliferative disorders, anxiety, and disorders associated with involuntary muscular activity). Interestingly, the changes in resting energy expenditure correlate well with the FT_4I and TSH in hypothyroid patients who are taking varying doses of levothyroxine.[342]

Biochemical Markers of Thyroid Status

Occasionally, a diagnosis of thyroid dysfunction is first suspected as a result of an abnormality in a laboratory test performed in the course of an evaluation for an unrelated medical problem. Classical examples are a markedly elevated creatine kinase MM isoenzyme or LDL cholesterol level leading to the recognition of hypothyroidism.[343, 344] Other similar markers are listed in Table 10–15. These tests are not useful in the diagnosis of thyroid disease, but some, such as sex hormone–binding globulin (SHBG), ferritin, or LDL cholesterol, have been used as end points in clinical studies of the responsivity of the liver to thyroid hormone in patients with RTH.[345, 346]

Serum Thyroglobulin

The sensitivity of modern Tg assays is 1 ng/mL or even less.[347] The results can be artifactually altered by serum anti-Tg antibodies, and serum should be screened for Tg antibodies with a sensitive Tg-antibody immunoassay. In immunoradiometric assays, interferences lead to underestimations or false-negative values. Tg is normally present in serum, with the concentration ranging up to 90 pmol/L (50 ng/mL); mean normal values vary with the assay used but are on the order of 30 pmol/L (20 ng/mL).[348]

Table 10–15. Biochemical Markers of Thyroid Status

Thyrotoxicosis
Increased
Osteocalcin
Urine pyridinium collagen cross-links
Alkaline phosphatase (bone or liver)
Atrial natriuretic hormone
Sex hormone–binding globulin
Ferritin
von Willebrand's factor
Decreased
Low-density-lipoprotein cholesterol
Lp(a)
Hypothyroidism
Increased
Creatine kinase (MM isoform)
Low-density-lipoprotein cholesterol
Lp(a)
Plasma norepinephrine
Decreased
Vasopressin

Lp(a), lipoprotein a.

Concentrations are somewhat higher in women than in men and are elevated several-fold in pregnant women and in newborns. Levels are elevated in three types of thyroid disorders:

- Goiter and thyroid gland hyperfunction
- Inflammatory or physical injury to the thyroid gland
- Differentiated follicular cell–derived thyroid tumors

Values are elevated in both endemic and sporadic nontoxic goiter, and the degree of elevation correlates with the thyroid size. Transient elevations occur in patients with subacute thyroiditis and as a result of trauma to the gland during thyroid surgery or after ^{131}I therapy.[35, 349] Subnormal or undetectable concentrations are found in patients with thyrotoxicosis factitia and aid in differentiating this disorder from other causes of thyrotoxicosis with a low radioactive iodine uptake (RAIU).[350] Antithyroglobulin antibodies interfere with measurements of the Tg concentration, thus precluding its use in patients with Hashimoto's disease.[351]

A major clinical value of measuring the level of serum Tg is in the management,[349, 352] but not in the diagnosis, of differentiated thyroid carcinoma.[347] Serum Tg concentrations are increased in patients with both benign and differentiated malignant follicular cell–derived tumors of the thyroid and do not serve to distinguish between the two. After total thyroid ablation for papillary or follicular thyroid carcinoma, Tg should not be detectable and its subsequent appearance signifies the presence of persistent or recurrent disease.[353] Secretion of Tg is TSH-dependent. Therefore, the serum Tg level may rise when suppressive therapy is withdrawn or after injections of rhTSH,[354, 355] and this increases the sensitivity of the marker for the detection of persistent or recurrent thyroid carcinoma, even when ^{131}I scans are negative (see Chapter 13).[354]

Tests for Thyroid Autoantibodies

Graves' disease and Hashimoto's disease are well characterized and interrelated *autoimmune thyroid disorders* (AITDs). Thus, circulating antibodies and T cells against one or another thyroid antigen are often present.

Three varieties of thyroid autoantibodies are useful and widely available for clinical diagnostic use receptor (Table 10–16). In this section, antibodies to Tg and thyroid peroxidase (TPO) are discussed. Antibodies directed against the TSH receptor, the cause of hyperthyroidism in patients with Graves' disease, are covered in greater detail in Chapter 11.

Table 10–16. Common Thyroid Autoantibodies (Ab)

Antigen	Molecular Size	Abbreviation	Notes
TSH receptor	100 kd	TSHRAb	Antibody that causes Graves' disease
		TSHR-blocking Ab	Present in some thyroiditis patients
Thyroglobulin	330 kd	TgAb	Often undetectable using older techniques
Thyroid peroxidase	107 kd	TPOAb	Useful diagnostic marker

TSH, thyrotropin.

Autoantibodies to Thyroid Peroxidase and Thyroglobulin

Table 10–17 summarizes some advantages and disadvantages of available techniques for measuring thyroid autoantibodies. The original technique of hemagglutination has many disadvantages, including lack of IgG specificity, low sensitivity, and operator dependency. Modern assay techniques have good precision because they depend on the direct measurement of the interaction between autoantibody and autoantigen (i.e., the interaction between labeled thyroid antigen and the patient's serum). In general, the more sensitive an assay, the more it tends to be specific and precise. However, because many normal individuals exhibit low levels of autoantibodies, the clinical specificity of the more sensitive tests is reduced and the absolute concentration becomes more important; the higher the concentration of autoantibody, the greater the clinical specificity.

The prevalence of detectable thyroid autoantibodies in various disorders is shown in Table 10–18; however, data on concentration tend to vary from assay to assay even with the use of standardization.[351]

Standardization

To compare levels of thyroid antibodies from one office visit to the next and to compare results between patients and

Table 10–17. Advantages and Disadvantages of Different Methods for Measurement of Autoantibodies to Thyroid Peroxidase and Thyroglobulin

Technique	Precision	Sensitivity	Specificity	Cost
Immunofluorescence	Low	Low	High	High
Hemagglutination	Low	Low	Variable	High
ELISA	Variable	High	High	Low
Radioassay	High	High	High	Low

ELISA, enzyme-linked immunosorbent assay.

Table 10–18. Prevalence of Thyroid Autoantibodies (Ab)

Group	TSHRAb (%)	hTgAb (%)	hTPOAb (%)
General population	0	5–20	8–27
Graves' disease	80–95	50–70	50–80
Autoimmune thyroiditis	10–20	80–90	90–100
Relatives of patients	0	40–50	40–50
Patients with IDDM	0	40	40
Pregnant women	0	14	14

IDDM, insulin-dependent diabetes mellitus; Tg, thyrogobulin; TPO, thyroid peroxidase.

among laboratories, assays for thyroid autoantibodies should be standardized (i.e., results should be expressed in relation to a widely available standard preparation, as with hormone immunoassays). Although there are no formal "international standards" for human thyroid autoantibodies, TgAb and TPOAb standard sera are available from the National Institute for Biological Standards in the United Kingdom and are an essential component of many thyroid autoantibody assays. Such results can then be expressed in units per milliliter.

The actual standard serum preparation, however, cannot be included in every assay. Instead, a serum pool is usually compared and normalized to the original standard. Yet autoantibodies differ considerably in their affinity and epitope recognition of antigen. Hence, despite this attempt at standardization, assay results from different commercial assays may still vary considerably. When following antibody titers (e.g., after the treatment of thyroid cancer), it is important to use the same autoantibody assay.

Pathogenic Role of Thyroglobulin and Thyroid Peroxidase Antibodies

Tg and TPO autoantibodies are a secondary response to thyroid injury and do not cause disease themselves. Both types of antibodies are polyclonal, and although they are of the IgG class, are not restricted to one particular IgG subclass. Polyclonality mitigates against a primary role in disease, but these antibodies may be important in determining the end-organ effects and may also be determinants of chronicity.

Whereas both TPOAb and TgAb levels correlate with lymphocytic infiltration of the thyroid gland, they do not transfer disease from mother to fetus or between animals. Thus, thyroid antibodies to Tg and TPO do not initiate disease. Both antibodies, however, may have complement-fixing cytotoxic activity, and TPOAb autoantibodies, in particular, correlate with thyroidal damage and lymphocytic infiltration. Patients with AITDs have autoantibody "fingerprints," a characteristic spectrum of Tg and TPO autoantibodies belonging to IgG1, IgG2, IgG3, and IgG4 subclasses. This pattern may be inherited as an autosomal dominant trait within families.[356, 357]

Because IgG1 antibodies fix complement, whereas IgG4 antibodies do not, for example, this pattern of distribution may affect the disease phenotype.

Thyroid Autoantibodies in Hashimoto's Disease

The disease most associated with TgAb and TPOAb is *autoimmune thyroiditis*, a term that embraces both goitrous Hashimoto's disease and atrophic thyroid failure. The titers of these antibodies correlate with the degree of thyroidal lymphocytic infiltration. Immunoassays show that both TgAb and TPOAb are found in almost 100% of such patients, but TPO antibodies are of higher affinity and in higher concentrations. This may be because TgAb is bound by circulating Tg, causing its concentration to be underestimated. In an unclear clinical situation, positive TgAb and TPOAb levels are diagnostic of primary autoimmune thyroid disease.

Antibody measurements may also be useful prognostically in mildly (subclinically) hypothyroid patients (i.e., with elevated TSH and normal T_4 levels), since the rate of overt hypothyroidism is about 3% to 5% per year in patients with a mildly increased TSH level and positive thyroid autoantibodies.[358] Falling titers of TgAb indicate a good prognosis in treated thyroid cancer patients who show this autoantibody (~20% of patients)[351] and TPOAb has been shown to be an important predictor of postpartum thyroiditis, a transient form of autoimmune thyroiditis found in 8% to 10% of all women and in 33% or more of TPOAb-positive mothers.[356]

Thyroid Autoantibodies in Graves' Disease

Antibodies to Tg and TPO are also detectable in 50% to 90% of patients with Graves' disease, indicative of the associated thyroiditis that is evident histologically. Hence, Graves' disease may occur on a background of autoimmune thyroiditis. Although the presence of such autoantibodies favors a diagnosis of an autoimmune cause for the hyperthyroidism over other causes, the tests are neither sensitive nor specific in this setting and are interpretable only as part of the clinical scenario.

TSH receptor antibodies remain the test of choice in such patients (see Chapter 11). Limited data suggest that higher titers of TgAb and TPOAb in patients with hyperthyroid Graves' disease are predictive of future hypothyroidism after treatment with antithyroid drugs.[359]

Thyroid Autoantibodies in Non-autoimmune Thyroid Disorders

Antibodies to Tg and TPO are more common in patients with sporadic goiter, multinodular goiter, and isolated thyroid nodules and cancer than in the general population. This finding usually represents an associated thyroiditis on histologic examination. Low levels of thyroid autoantibodies may occur transiently in patients with subacute (de Quervain's) thyroiditis but correlate poorly with disease course and are probably a nonspecific response to thyroid injury. There is also a higher prevalence of thyroid autoantibodies in other autoimmune diseases, such as insulin-dependent diabetes mellitus (IDDM), indicative of a common genetic susceptibility and etiology.

The "Normal" Population

Although the prevalence of thyroid autoantibodies depends on the technique used for detection, autoantibodies to Tg and TPO are common in the general population (see Table 10–18) and, at all ages, are almost five times more common in women than in men. The tendency to secrete thyroid autoantibodies is inherited in a mendelian-dominant manner and has been linked to polymorphisms in the CTLA-4 gene.[357, 360] Selected groups at risk include younger women and relatives of patients with an AITD, in whom the incidence is higher.

Low levels of autoantibodies to TPO and Tg are of uncertain significance in the presence of normal thyroid function; however, within a family with an AITD, they remain a significant risk factor.

Clinical Utility: Establishment of Disease Etiology

Thyroid failure has a variety of causes, and autoimmune thyroid disease can be inferred by the presence of a family history of Graves' disease or Hashimoto's disease. However, the only simple way of confirming the autoimmune diathesis, other than biopsy, is the presence of significant levels of thyroid autoantibodies. The measurement of thyroid autoantibodies also allows the generation of data regarding the prevalence of AITDs within the patient's family.

Prediction of Disease Onset

Patients with increased TSH and normal T_4 levels progress to overt thyroid failure at a rate of about 5% per year if thyroid autoantibody levels are elevated.[358] Hence, patients with mild (subclinical) hypothyroidism (increased TSH levels but apparently normal free T_4 values) and thyroid autoantibodies are at twice the risk for development of thyroid failure as patients without thyroid antibodies.

Thyroid Cancer

Approximately 20% to 40% of patients with thyroid cancer have thyroid autoantibodies, and their presence (indicating underlying immunoreactivity against thyroid cell antigens) may suggest a better prognosis for these patients.[351, 361] After total thyroidectomy and radioiodine ablation, a sensitive assay should show a serum Tg level below 1 ng/mL. The presence of TgAb significantly interferes with this assessment, and attempts to correct for the presence of TgAb using Tg recovery from the serum are not always helpful.[352] A falling titer or total loss of TgAb in such patients, however, is an important and reliable prognostic sign indicating the absence of thyroid cell antigens.[351]

Risk Analysis for Postpartum Thyroid Disease

The prevalence of PPTD is 8% to 10% in the first 4 to 12 months after delivery. More than 33% of women who are TPOAb-positive early in pregnancy, particularly patients with high thyroid autoantibody levels, develop some form of PPTD.[362] Hence, the measurement of TPOAb is important in pregnancy screening (see Chapter 12).

Risk Analysis for Early Pregnancy Loss

Thyroid autoantibodies are markers of an at-risk pregnancy[363, 364] but do not imply that thyroid dysfunction causes the increased risk. Many studies have shown double the rate of pregnancy loss in women with these antibodies. However, the presence of thyroid autoantibodies appears to be a signal of immune uncertainty. The role of placental megalin receptors, which may be activated by TgAb, is also of interest.[365]

Thyroid Disease Screening in Associated Autoimmune Conditions

AITDs occur commonly with other forms of autoimmune disease. For example, patients with IDDM are at particular risk, and the presence of thyroid autoantibodies is helpful in selecting patients for monitoring of thyroid function.

Radioiodine Uptake

The only direct test of thyroid function employs a radioactive isotope of iodine as a tag for the body's stable form of iodine, ^{127}I. Most often the test involves the measurement of the fractional uptake by the thyroid of a tracer (i.e., a chemically inconsequential) dose of radioiodine. However, several factors have caused this test to be less frequently used and less valuable for diagnosis of thyroid disorders than in the past; specifically, (1) the improvement in indirect methods for assessing thyroid status and (2) the decrease in normal values for thyroid RAIU consequent to the widespread increase in daily dietary iodine intake.[366]

Both ^{131}I (half-life, 8.1 days) and ^{123}I (half-life, 0.55 days) emit gamma radiation, which permits their external detection and quantitation at sites of accumulation, such as the thyroid gland. These isotopes (I*) are physiologically indistinguishable, not only from one another but also from the naturally occurring ^{127}I, which permits their use as valid tracers. The shorter half-life of ^{123}I is preferable because the radiation delivered to the thyroid per amount of administered ^{123}I is only about 1% of that delivered by ^{131}I.

Physiologic Basis

When tracer quantities of inorganic radioiodine are administered either orally or intravenously, the isotope quickly mixes with the endogenous stable iodide in the extracellular fluid and begins to be removed by the two major sites of clearance, the thyroid gland and the kidneys. As this process continues, the plasma level of I* decreases exponentially. Normally, low values are reached by 24 hours, and inorganic I* is virtually undetectable in the plasma 72 hours after its administration. The thyroid content of I* increases rapidly during the early hours, then at a decreasing rate until a plateau is approached. The proportion of administered I* that is ultimately accumulated by the thyroid gland is a function of the clearance of iodide by the thyroid and kidneys. The relation is simply expressed as follows:

$$\text{RAIU at plateau} = \frac{C_T}{C_T + C_K}$$

where C_T is the thyroid iodide clearance rate and C_K is the renal iodide clearance rate.

The normal thyroid iodide clearance rate is approximately 0.4 L/hour, and the renal iodide clearance rate is 2.0 L/hour. Thus, the uptake of I* normally approximates 0.17 of the administered dose.

Measurements of the RAIU are generally made at 24 hours, both as a matter of convenience and because the value at 24 hours is usually near the plateau. The RAIU usually indicates the rate of thyroid hormone synthesis and, by inference, the rate of thyroid hormone release into the blood.

Radioactive Iodine Uptake

Little difference is noted if the uptake is measured at any time during the day following that on which the isotope was administered. For calculating therapeutic radioiodine doses in treating thyrotoxic Graves' disease, an uptake at 3 to 6 hours may produce results comparable to those found at 20 to 28 hours.[367] With the use of this modified early RAIU measurement, diagnosis and treatment of thyrotoxic Graves' disease can be accomplished on the same day.

In general, the range of normal values for the 24 hr radioiodine uptake in North America is approximately 5% to 25%. Higher values may indicate iodine deficiency or thyroid hyperfunction. As with other procedures, however, values in patients with mild hyperthyroidism may be at or just above the upper limit of the normal range (Table 10–19).

Table 10-19. Factors That Influence 24-Hour Thyroid Iodide Uptake

Factors That Increase Uptake
Increased hormone synthesis
Hyperthyroidism
Response to glandular hormone depletion
Recovery from thyroid suppression
Recovery from subacute thyroiditis
Antithyroid agents
Excessive hormone losses
Nephrotic syndrome
Chronic diarrheal states
Soybean ingestion
Normal hormone synthesis
Iodine deficiency
Dietary insufficiency
Excessive loss (dehalogenase defect, pregnancy)
Hormone biosynthetic defects
Factors That Decrease Uptake
Decreased hormone synthesis
Primary hypofunction
Primary hypothyroidism
Antithyroid agents
Hormone biosynthetic defects
Hashimoto's disease
Subacute thyroiditis
Secondary hypofunction
Exogenous thyroid hormones
Not reflecting decreased hormone synthesis
Increased availability of iodine
Diet or drugs
Cardiac or renal insufficiency
Increased hormone release
Very severe hyperthyroidism (rare)

States Associated with Increased Radioactive Iodine Uptake

Hyperthyroidism

Hyperthyroidism causes an increased RAIU unless body iodide stores are increased. Such increases in uptake are always evident except in patients with severe thyrotoxicosis, in whom release of hormone can be so rapid that the thyroid content of I* has decreased to the normal range by the time the measurement is made. This condition is rare and is usually associated with obvious thyrotoxicosis.

Aberrant Hormone Synthesis

The RAIU can be increased in the absence of hyperthyroidism in disorders in which iodine accumulation is normal but the secretion of hormone is impaired, such as in patients with abnormal thyroglobulin synthesis.[368] The magnitude of the increase in uptake and the time at which the plateau is achieved vary with the nature and severity of the disorder. Differentiation of these states from hyperthyroidism is generally not difficult; in the former, clinical findings and laboratory evidence of hyperthyroidism are lacking, and indeed hypothyroidism may be present.

Iodine Deficiency

The RAIU is increased in acute or chronic iodine deficiency, as demonstrated by measurement of urinary iodine excretion, with urinary iodine values lower than 100 μg/day indicating deficiency. Chronic iodine deficiency is usually the result of an inadequate content of iodine in the food and water (endemic iodine deficiency). Patients with cardiac, renal, or hepatic disease may develop iodine deficiency if given diets severely restricted in salt, especially if diuretic agents are administered.

Response to Thyroid Hormone Depletion

Rebound increases in the RAIU are seen after withdrawal of antithyroid therapy, after subsidence of transient or subacute thyroiditis, and after recovery from prolonged suppression of thyroid function by exogenous hormone. A striking increase in RAIU occurs in patients with iodide-induced myxedema after cessation of iodide administration. The duration of the rebound depends on the time required to replenish thyroid hormone stores.

Excessive Hormone Losses

In patients with nephrotic syndrome, excessive losses of hormone in the urine occurring in association with urinary loss of binding protein cause a compensatory increase in hormone synthesis and in the RAIU. A similar sequence may occur when losses of hormone via the gastrointestinal tract are abnormal, as in chronic diarrheal states or during ingestion of agents (e.g., soybean protein, cholestyramine) that bind T_4 in the gut.

States Associated with Decreased Radioactive Iodine Uptake

A general increase in iodine intake has made RAIU values in hypothyroidism indistinguishable from those at the lower end of the normal range. Therefore, the major indication for measuring the RAIU is to establish the causes of thyrotoxicosis associated with decreased values of the RAIU.

Hypothyroidism

The problems involved in using the RAIU as an aid to the diagnosis of hypothyroidism have been discussed.

Exogenous Thyroid Hormone: Thyrotoxicosis Factitia

Except in disorders in which homeostatic control is disrupted or overridden (e.g., with Graves' disease or autonomously functioning thyroid nodules), administration of exogenous thyroid hormone suppresses TSH secretion and reduces the RAIU, usually to values below 5%.

Low values of the RAIU in a patient who is clinically thyrotoxic may indicate the presence of *thyrotoxicosis factitia*, the syndrome produced by the ingestion of excess thyroid hormone. The unmeasurably low level of Tg in serum differentiates thyrotoxicosis factitia from other causes of thyrotoxicosis with a decreased RAIU.[350]

Disorders of Hormone Storage

The RAIU is usually low in the early phase of subacute thyroiditis and in chronic thyroiditis with transient hyperthyroidism. In these instances, inflammatory follicular disruption leads to loss of the normal storage function of the gland and leakage of hormone into the blood. In the early stage of subacute thyroiditis, leakage of hormone is usually sufficient to suppress TSH secretion and the RAIU. Transient hypothyroidism often occurs late in both diseases, when stores of preformed hormone are depleted; the RAIU may return to normal or increased values at that time.

Exposure to Excessive Iodine

Exposure to excessive iodine is the most common cause of a subnormal RAIU. Such decreases are spurious in the clinical sense because they do not indicate decreased absolute iodine uptake or decreased hormone production but can be produced by the introduction of excessive iodine in any form—inorganic, organic, or elemental. Special offenders are organic iodinated dyes used as x-ray contrast media and amiodarone (see Table 10–8). The duration of suppression of the uptake varies among individuals and with the compound administered. In general, dyes used for pyelography or computed tomography are cleared within weeks, whereas amiodarone may influence the uptake for up to 12 months because of its storage in fat.

A single large dose of inorganic iodide can decrease the uptake for several days, and chronic ingestion of iodide may depress the uptake for many weeks. Lugol's solution or saturated solution of potassium iodide (SSKI) in the usual dosage (2 to 5 drops three times/day) can deliver up to about 500 mg of iodine daily, as opposed to the customary intake of about 200 μg/day in the United States. Excessive quantities of iodine may also be present in vitamin and mineral preparations, vaginal or rectal suppositories, and iodinated antiseptics such as povidone (see Table 10–8). In patients with thyrotoxicosis, the RAIU may help to differentiate excessive hormone synthesis with an increased RAIU from destructive thyrotoxicosis with a subnormal RAIU. Inhibition of uptake by excess stable iodine is of shorter duration in hyperthyroid than in normal individuals.

The measurement of urinary iodine excretion is an invaluable means of establishing or excluding the existence of excessive body iodide stores; a random urine sample can be obtained, and the 24-hour iodine excretion can be extrapolated from the iodine/creatinine ratio. Values in excess of several milligrams per day can explain a low RAIU value, whereas values less than 1 mg/day suggest that a low RAIU value is due to one of the other disorders discussed in this section.

CLINICAL EVALUATION AND INITIAL LABORATORY TESTING

Manifestations of thyroid disease are usually due to (1) excessive or insufficient production of thyroid hormone, (2) local symptoms in the neck (principally goiter but occasionally pain or compression of adjacent structures), or, (3) in the case of Graves' disease, ophthalmopathy or dermopathy. Although attention is directed initially at the major features, it is crucial to define the metabolic state and to ascertain the nature of the underlying disorder. A functional diagnosis of thyroid disease is based on a carefully taken history, a thorough search for the physical signs of hypothyroidism or thyrotoxicosis, and an appraisal of the results of laboratory tests. Although conditioned by the functional diagnosis, the anatomic diagnosis depends largely on the examination of the thyroid gland itself (Fig. 10–18).

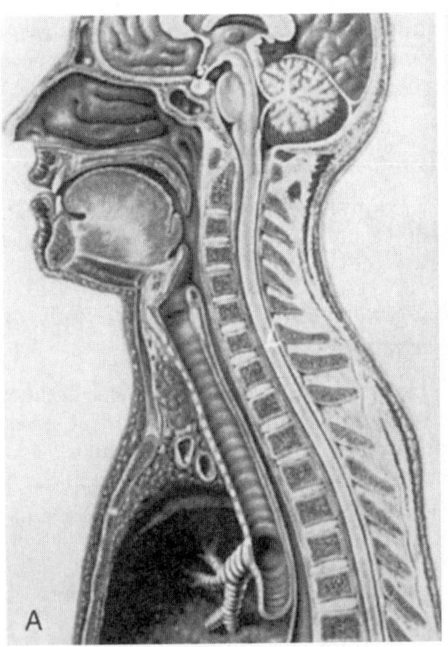

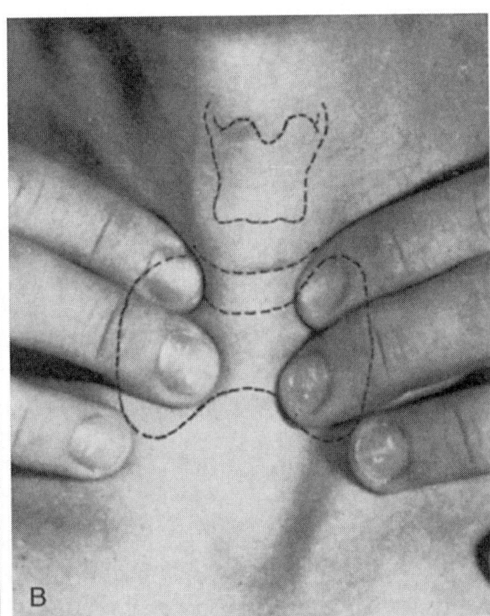

Figure 10–18. Examination of the thyroid gland.

A, Sagittal section demonstrates relations of the isthmus of the normal thyroid gland. The superior border is inferior to the cricoid cartilage. The inferior thyroid border is essentially at the level of the superior surface of the manubrium. The inferior portions of the lateral lobes (not shown) extend more inferiorly than the isthmus.

B, The cricoid cartilage is regarded as an important landmark. Especially when the thyroid gland is thought to be essentially normal or subnormal in size, the cricoid should be located. This is easily accomplished. The index fingers are then inserted so that their superior portion rests against the inferior portion of the cricoid while the inferior portion of these fingers is over the superior portion of the thyroid. The second and third fingers are rotated over other portions of the gland to evaluate its size, contour, consistency, possible adherence to surrounding structures, and other features. Because there is marked variation among different subjects in the length and thickness of the neck and in the length of the trachea superior to the level of the manubrium, the relative position of the thyroid may vary. In some cases, essentially all of the thyroid gland rests posterior to the sternum. In most instances, however, by having the patient moderately extend the neck (short of tightening the anterior neck muscles) and swallow repeatedly, it is possible to palpate most or all of the gland. Despite marked variations in neck-chest relations, thyroid tissue, when present, is found within 1 cm of the cricoid. By concentrating the palpation meticulously in the area where the thyroid is normally found, with rare exceptions the examiner can outline small as well as enlarged glands.

Physical Examination

Local examination of the neck is best accomplished with the patient seated in a good light and with the neck moderately extended. The patient must be provided with a cup of water to facilitate swallowing.

The physician first inspects the neck from the front and on the sides, especially while the patient swallows, with the neck slightly extended. The presence of old surgical scars, distended veins, and redness or fixation of the overlying skin should be noted. If a mass is present, attention should be directed to its location and to whether it moves when the patient swallows.

The position of the trachea is noted. Movement on swallowing is a characteristic of the thyroid gland because it is ensheathed in the pretracheal fascia; this feature distinguishes a goiter from most other neck masses. If a goiter is so large, however, that it occupies all the available space in the neck or if the thyroid gland is the seat of an invasive carcinoma or Riedel's thyroiditis that has caused fixation to adjacent structures, movement on swallowing may be lost. The physician should also inspect the dorsum of the tongue, which is the origin of the thyroglossal duct and rarely the seat of lingual thyroid tissue.

Standing behind the seated patient, the physician may examine the thyroid gland by palpating with the fingertips of both hands. The position of the cricoid cartilage is determined first because the superior border of the isthmus lies just below it (see Fig. 10–18). The isthmus is a band of tissue crossing the front of the trachea joining the two lobes. The examiner then attempts to outline the thyroid gland and to determine the limits of the lower borders of the lateral lobes while the patient swallows sips of water at appropriate intervals. With practice, a normal thyroid gland can usually be palpated, particularly in women.

An alternative approach to the thyroid gland examination is for the physician to face the seated patient and use gentle pressure with the thumb to locate the thyroid isthmus. The right thumb is then moved laterally, without release of pressure, to compress the right lobe of the thyroid against the trachea as the patient again swallows sips of water. This strategy allows the palpating thumb to slide under and laterally displace the medial border of the sternocleidomastoid muscle. A similar strategy with the left thumb is employed for the left lobe. This technique is especially useful as an aid in detecting small nodules that may not be easily appreciated with the posterior approach.

The examiner notes the shape of the gland, its size in relation to normal, and its consistency, which is usually slightly more firm than adipose tissue. The normal thyroid lobe is approximately the same in size in frontal projection as the terminal phalanx of the patient's thumb. Whereas the diffuse colloid goiter and the hyperplastic gland in Graves' disease tend to be softer than normal, the gland in Hashimoto's disease is usually firm. In rare circumstances, the gland that is the seat of carcinoma or Riedel's thyroiditis may be "stony" hard. Irregularities of the surface, variations in consistency, and tender areas should be noted. If nodules are palpated, their shape, size, position, translucency, and consistency in relation to the surrounding tissue should be determined.

A search should be made for the pyramidal lobe, a thin band of tissue extending upward from the isthmus to the thyroid cartilage to the right or left of the midline. The pyramidal lobe may be mistaken for a pretracheal lymph node that sometimes accompanies thyroid carcinoma or thyroiditis. It is usually palpable in patients with generalized thyroid disease, such as Hashimoto's or Graves' disease. Thyroglossal cysts are midline masses that remain attached to the base of the tongue by the fibrotic thyroglossal duct and that move upward when the tongue is protruded.

During palpation, a vascular thrill may be felt that, in the absence of cardiac disease, is suggestive of hyperthyroidism. Finally, palpation should always include examination of the regional lymph nodes.

Auscultation of the neck can indicate the vascularity of an enlarged gland. A systolic or continuous bruit is sometimes heard over a hyperplastic gland. The physician should take care to distinguish a thyroid bruit from a murmur transmitted from the base of the heart or from a venous hum that can be obliterated by gentle compression of the external jugular vein or by turning the patient's head. A venous hum is generally found in younger patients with high cardiac output, such as in Graves' disease or severe anemia.

An arm-raising test is useful when a retrosternal goiter is suspected. The basis for this maneuver is that if the size of the thoracic inlet is already reduced by a retrosternal goiter, raising both arms until they touch the sides of the head further narrows the thoracic inlet and causes congestion and venous engorgement of the face and, sometimes, respiratory distress (Pemberton's sign) or even (rarely) syncope.

In addition to examination of the thyroid gland and the regional lymph nodes, the physician should seek evidence of compression or displacement of adjacent structures. Hoarseness may indicate compression of the recurrent laryngeal nerve, usually by a malignant thyroid neoplasm, and this possibility should be confirmed by laryngoscopy. Displacement of the trachea may be evident, and inspiratory stridor may indicate compression of the trachea.

Laboratory Evaluation

Initial laboratory tests for any patient with suspected thyroid disease should include an immunometric TSH assay. If the physician is reasonably confident that a functional disorder of the thyroid is present, an FT_4I or FT_4 should be included as an initial test to confirm the presence and assess the degree of the abnormality inferred from the TSH result. There is rarely reason to measure total T_3 in the initial evaluation unless the patient is receiving liothyronine or liotrix. More extensive guidelines for laboratory procedures relevant to specific thyroid conditions are discussed in Chapters 11 to 13.

References

1. Burrow GN, Fisher DA, Larsen PR. Mechanisms of disease: maternal and fetal thyroid function. N Engl J Med 1994; 331:1072–1078.
2. Thorpe-Beeston JG, Nicolaides KH, Felton CV, et al. Maturation of the secretion of thyroid hormone and thyroid-stimulating hormone in the fetus. N Engl J Med 1991; 324:532–536.
3. Mansberger AR, Wei JP. Surgical embryology and anatomy of the thyroid and parathyroid glands. Surg Clin North Am 1993; 73:727–746.
4. Ericson LE. Exocytosis and endocytosis in the thyroid follicle cell. Mol Cell Endocrinol 1981; 22:1–24.
5. Missero C, Cobellis G, De Felice M, et al. Molecular events involved in differentiation of thyroid follicular cells. Mol Cell Endocrinol 1998; 140:37–43.
6. Damante G, Tell G, Di Lauro R. A unique combination of transcription factors controls differentiation of thyroid cells. Prog Nucleic Acid Res Mol Biol 2000; 66:307–356.
7. Pasca Di Magliano M, Di Lauro R, Zannini M. Pax8 has a key role in thyroid cell differentiation. Proc Natl Acad Sci USA 2000; 97:13144–13149.
8. Gentile F, Ferranti P, Mamone G, et al. Identification of hormonogenic tyrosines in fragment 1218–1591 of bovine thyroglobulin by mass spectrometry: hormonogenic acceptor TYR-12donor TYR-1375. J Biol Chem 1997; 272:639–646.
9. Taurog A, Dorris ML, Doerge DR. Mechanism of simultaneous iodination and coupling catalyzed by thyroid peroxidase. Arch Biochem Biophys 1996; 330:24–32.

10. Vassart G, Dumont JE. The thyrotropin receptor and the regulation of thyrocyte function and growth. Endocr Rev 1992; 13: 596–611.
11. Dumont JE, Lamy F, Roger P, et al. Physiological and pathological regulation of thyroid cell proliferation and differentiation by thyrotropin and other factors. Physiological Review 1992; 72: 667–697.
12. Hollowell JG, Staehling NW, Hannon WH, et al. Iodine nutrition in the United States: Trends and public health implications—iodine excretion data from National Health and Nutrition Examination Surveys I and III (1971–1974 and 1988–1994) J Clin Endocrinol Metab 1998; 83:3401–3408.
13. Glinoer D. Maternal and fetal impact of chronic iodine deficiency. Clin Obstet Gynecol 1997; 40:102–116.
14. Glinoer D, Delange F. The potential repercussions of maternal, fetal, and neonatal hypothyroxinemia on the progeny. Thyroid 2000; 10: 871–887.
15. De La Vieja A, Dohan O, Levy O, et al. Molecular analysis of the sodium/iodide symporter: impact on thyroid and extrathyroid pathophysiology. Physiol Rev 2000; 80:1083–1105.
16. Kosugi S, Inoue S, Matsuda A, et al. Novel, missense and loss-of-function mutations in the sodium/iodide symporter gene causing iodide transport defect in three Japanese patients. J Clin Endocrinol Metab 1998; 83:3373–3376.
17. Bidart JM, Lacroix L, Evain-Brion D, et al. Expression of Na+/I- symporter and Pendred syndrome genes in trophoblast cells. J Clin Endocrinol Metab 2000; 85:4367–4372.
18. Wolff J. Perchlorate and the thyroid gland. Pharmacol Rev 1998; 50:89–105.
19. Wolff J. Congenital goiter with defective iodide transport. Endocrinology Rev 1983; 4:240.
20. Pohlenz J, Rosenthal IM, Weiss RE, et al. Congenital hypothyroidism due to mutations in the sodium/iodide symporter: identification of a nonsense mutation producing a downstream cryptic 3′ splice site. J Clin Invest 1998; 101:1028–1035.
21. Kosugi S, Sato Y, Matsuda A, et al. High prevalence of T354P sodium/iodide symporter gene mutation in Japanese patients with iodide transport defect who have heterogeneous clinical pictures. J Clin Endocrinol Metab 1998; 83:4123–4129.
22. Spitzweg C, Heufelder AE, Morris JC. Thyroid iodine transport. Thyroid 2000; 10:321–330.
23. Filetti S, Bidart JM, Arturi F, et al. Sodium/iodide symporter: a key transport system in thyroid cancer cell metabolism. Eur J Endocrinol 1999; 141:443–457.
24. Scott DA, Wang R, Kreman TM, et al. The Pendred syndrome gene encodes a chloride-iodide transport protein. Nat Genet 1999; 21: 440–443.
25. Scott DA, Wang R, Kreman TM, et al. Functional differences of the PDS gene product are associated with phenotypic variation in patients with Pendred syndrome and non-syndromic hearing loss (DFNB4). Hum Mol Genet 2000; 9:1709–1715.
26. Yokoyama N, Taurog A. Porcine thyroid peroxidase: relationship between the native enzyme and an active, highly purified tryptic fragment. Mol Endocrinol 1988; 2:838–844.
27. Wolff J, Chaikoff IL. Plasma inorganic iodide as a homeostatic regulator of thyroid function. J Biol Chem 1948; 174:555.
28. Izumi M, Larsen PR. Triiodothyronine, thyroxine, and iodine in purified thyroglobulin from patients with Graves' disease. J Clin Invest 1977; 59:1105–1112.
29. Vulsma T, Gons MH, DeVijlder JMM. Maternal fetal transfer of thyroxine in congenital hypothyroidism due to a total organification defect of thyroid dysgenesis. N Engl J Med 1989; 321:13–16.
30. LaFranchi S. Congenital hypothyroidism: etiologies, diagnosis, and management. Thyroid 1999; 9:735–740.
31. Bakker B, Bikker H, Vulsma T, et al. Two decades of screening for congenital hypothyroidism in The Netherlands: TPO gene mutations in total iodide organification defects (an update). J Clin Endocrinol Metab 2000; 85:3708–3712.
32. Ohmiya Y, Hayashi H, Kondo T, et al. Location of dehydroalanine residues in the amino acid sequence of bovine thyroglobulin: identification of "donor" tyrosine sites for hormonogenesis in thyroglobulin. J Biol Chem 1990; 265:9066–9071.
33. Dunn AD, Corsi CM, Myers HE, et al. Tyrosine 130 is an important outer ring donor for thyroxine formation in thyroglobulin. J Biol Chem 1998; 273:25223–25229.
34. Larsen PR. Thyroidal triiodothyronine and thyroxine in Graves' disease: correlation with presurgical treatment, thyroid status, and iodine content. J Clin Endocrinol Metab 1975; 41:1098–1104.
35. Izumi M, Larsen PR. Correlation of sequential changes in serum thyroglobulin, triiodothyronine, and thyroxine in patients with Graves' disease and subacute thyroiditis. Metabolism 1978; 27: 449–460.
36. Salvatore D, Tu H, Harney JW, et al. Type 2 iodothyronine deiodinase is highly expressed in human thyroid. J Clin Invest 1996; 98:962–968.
37. Gereben B, Salvatore D, Harney JW, et al. The human, but not rat, dio2 gene is stimulated by thyroid transcription factor-1 (TTF-1). Mol Endocrinol 2001; 15:112–124.
38. Laurberg P. Mechanisms governing the relative proportions of thyroxine and 3,5,3′-triiodothyronine in thyroid secretion. Metabolism 1984; 33:379–392.
39. Abuid J, Larsen PR. Triiodothyronine and thyroxine in hyperthyroidism: comparison of the acute changes during therapy with antithyroid agents. J Clin Invest 1974; 54:201–208.
40. Berens SC, Bernstein RS, Robbins J, et al. Antithyroid effects of lithium. J Clin Invest 1970; 49:1357–1367.
41. Lazarus JH. The effects of lithium therapy on thyroid and thyrotropin-releasing hormone. Thyroid 1998; 8:909–913.
42. Temple R, Berman M, Robbins J, et al. The use of lithium in the treatment of thyrotoxicosis. J Clin Invest 1972; 51:2746–2756.
43. Rapoport B, Chazenbalk GD, Jaume JC, et al. The thyrotropin (TSH) receptor: interaction with TSH and autoantibodies. Endocr Rev 1998; 19:673–716.
44. Glinoer D. What happens to the normal thyroid during pregnancy? Thyroid 1999; 9:631–635.
45. Valyasevi RW, Erickson DZ, Harteneck DA, et al. Differentiation of human orbital preadipocyte fibroblasts induces expression of functional thyrotropin receptor. J Clin Endocrinol Metab 1999; 84:2557–2562.
46. Lu R, Wang P, Wartofsky L, et al. Oxygen free radicals in interleukin-1β–induced glycosaminoglycan production by retro-ocular fibroblasts from normal subjects and Graves' ophthalmopathy patients. Thyroid 1999; 9:297–303.
47. Van Sande J, Parma J, Tonacchera M, et al. Somatic and germline mutations of the TSH receptor gene in thyroid diseases. J Clin Endocrinol Metab 1995; 80:2577–2585.
48. Duprez L, Parma J, Van Sande J, et al. Germline mutations in the thyrotropin receptor gene cause non-autoimmune autosomal dominant hyperthyroidism. Nat Genet 1994; 7:396–401.
49. Rodien P, Bremont C, Sanson ML, et al. Familial gestational hyperthyroidism caused by a mutant thyrotropin receptor hypersensitive to human chorionic gonadotropin. N Engl J Med 1998; 339:1823–1826.
50. Allgeier A, Offermanns S, Van Sande J, et al. The human thyrotropin receptor activates G-proteins Gs and Gq/11. J Biol Chem 1994; 269:13733–13735.
51. Brucker-Davis F, Oldfield EH, Skarulis MC, et al. Thyrotropin-secreting pituitary tumors: diagnostic criteria, thyroid hormone sensitivity, and treatment outcome in 25 patients followed at the National Institutes of Health. J Clin Endocrinol Metab 1999; 84: 476–486.
52. Deleu S, Pirson I, Coulonval K, et al. IGF-1 or insulin, and the TSH cyclic AMP cascade separately control dog and human thyroid cell growth and DNA synthesis, and complement each other in inducing mitogenesis. Mol Cell Endocrinol 1999; 149:41–51.
53. Bianco AC, Slavatore D, Gereben B, et al. Biochemistry, cellular and molecular biology and physiological roles of the iodothyronine selenodeiodinases. Endocr Rev 2002; 23:38–89.
54. Curran PG, DeGroot LJ. The effect of hepatic enzyme-inducing drugs on thyroid hormones and the thyroid gland. Endocr Rev 1991; 12: 135–150.
55. Findlay KA, Kaptein E, Visser TJ, et al. Characterization of the uridine diphosphate-glucuronosyltransferase–catalyzing thyroid hormone glucuronidation in man. J Clin Endocrinol Metab 2000; 85:2879–2883.
56. Schussler GC. The thyroxine-binding proteins. Thyroid 2000; 10:141–149.
57. Grasberger H, Buettner C, Janssen OE. Modularity of serpins: a bifunctional chimera possessing alpha$_1$-proteinase inhibitor and thyroxine-binding globulin properties. J Biol Chem 1999; 274: 15046–15051.

58. Buettner C, Grasberger H, Hermansdorfer K, et al. Characterization of the thyroxine-binding site of thyroxine-binding globulin by site-directed mutagenesis. Mol Endocrinol 1999; 13:1864–1872.
59. Bartalena L. Recent achievements in studies on thyroid hormone-binding proteins. Endocr Rev 1990; 11:47–64.
60. Bartalena L. Thyroid hormone-binding proteins: update 1994. Endocr Rev 1994; 3:140–142.
61. Garnick MB, Larsen PR. Acute deficiency of thyroxine-binding globulin during L-asparaginase therapy. N Engl J Med 1979; 301: 252–253.
62. Bartalena L, Martino E, Antonelli A, et al. Effect of the antileukemic agent L-asparaginase on thyroxine-binding globulin and albumin synthesis in cultured human hepatoma (HEP G2) cells. Endocrinology 1985; 119:1185–1188.
63. Ain KB, Mori Y, Refetoff S. Reduced clearance rate of thyroxine-binding globulin (TBG) with increased sialylation: a mechanism for estrogen-induced elevation of serum TBG concentration. J Clin Endocrinol Metab 1987; 65:689–696.
64. Ain KB, Refetoff S. Relationship of oligosaccharide modification to the cause of serum thyroxine-binding globulin excess. J Clin Endocrinol Metab 1988; 66:1037–1043.
65. Jirasakuldech B, Schussler GC, Yap MG, et al. A characteristic serpin cleavage product of thyroxine-binding globulin appears in sepsis sera. J Clin Endocrinol Metab 2000; 85:3996–3999.
66. Afandi B, Schussler GC, Arafeh AH, et al. Selective consumption of thyroxine-binding globulin during cardiac bypass surgery. Metabolism 2000; 49:270–274.
67. Afandi B, Vera R, Schussler GC, et al. Concordant decreases of thyroxine and thyroxine binding protein concentrations during sepsis. Metabolism 2000; 49:753-1754.
68. Pemberton PA, Stein PE, Pepys MB, et al. Hormone binding globulins undergo serpin conformational change in inflammation. Nature 1988; 336:257–258.
69. Robbins J. New ideas in thyroxine-binding globulin biology (editorial). J Clin Endocrinol Metab 2000; 85:3994–3995.
70. Surks MI, Oppenheimer JH. Postoperative changes in the concentration of thyroxine-binding prealbumin and serum free thyroxine. J Clin Endocrinol 1964; 24:794–801.
71. Dickson PW, Aldred AR, Marley PD, et al. Rat choroid plexus specializes in the synthesis and secretion of transthyretin (prealbumin). J Biol Chem 1985; 261:3475.
72. Palha JA, Episkopou V, Maeda S, et al. Thyroid hormone metabolism in a transthyretin-null mouse strain. J Biol Chem 1994; 269:33135–33139.
73. Palha JA, Fernandes R, de Escobar GM, et al. Transthyretin regulates thyroid hormone levels in the choroid plexus, but not in the brain parenchyma: study in a transthyretin-null mouse model. Endocrinology 2000; 141:3267–3272.
74. Rosen HN, Moses AC, Murrell JR, et al. Thyroxine interactions with transthyretin: a comparison of 10 different naturally occurring human transthyretin variants. J Clin Endocrinol Metab 1993; 77:370–374.
75. Chin W, Schussler GC. Decreased serum free thyroxine concentration in patients treated with diphenylhydantoin. J Clin Endocrinol 1968; 28:181–186.
76. Larsen PR. Salicylate-induced increases in free triiodothyronine in human serum: evidence of inhibition of triiodothyronine binding to thyroxine-binding globulin and thyroxine-binding prealbumin. J Clin Invest 1972; 51:1125–1134.
77. Wang R, Nelson JC, Wilcox RB. Salsalate and salicylate binding to and their displacement of thyroxine from thyroxine-binding globulin, transthyretin, and albumin. Thyroid 1999; 9:359–364.
78. McConnell RJ. Changes in thyroid function tests during short-term salsalate use. Metabolism 1999; 48:501–503.
79. Stockigt JR, Lim CF, Barlow JW, et al. Interaction of furosemide with serum thyroxine binding sites: in vivo and in vitro studies and comparison with other inhibitors. J Clin Endocrinol Metab 1985; 60:1025–1031.
80. Kurtz AB, Capper SJ, Clifford J, et al. The effect of fenclofenac on thyroid function. Clin Endocrinol 1981; 15:117–124.
81. Surks MI, Sievert R. Drugs and thyroid function. N Engl J Med 1995; 333:1688–1694.
82. Docter R, Bos G, Krenning EP, et al. Inherited thyroxine excess: a serum abnormality due to an increased affinity for modified albumin. Clin Endocrinol 1981; 15:363–371.
83. Mendel CM, Cavalieri RR. Thyroxine distribution and metabolism in familial dysalbuminemic hyperthyroxinemia. J Clin Endocrinol Metab 1984; 59:499–504.
84. Sunthornthepvarakul T, Likitmaskul S, Ngowngarmratana S, et al. Familial dysalbuminemic hypertriiodothyroninemia: a new, dominantly inherited albumin defect. J Clin Endocrinol Metab 1998; 83:1448–1454.
85. Benvenga S. A thyroid hormone binding motif is evolutionarily conserved in apolipoproteins. Thyroid 1997; 7:605–611.
86. Marqusee E, Braverman LE, Lawrence JE, et al. The effect of droloxifene and estrogen on thyroid function in postmenopausal women. J Clin Endocrinol Metab 2000; 85:4407–4410.
87. Muller AF, Verhoeff A, Mantel MJ, et al. Decrease of free thyroxine levels after controlled ovarian hyperstimulation. J Clin Endocrinol Metab 2000; 85:545–548.
88. Mandel SJ, Larsen PR, Seely EW, et al. Increased need for thyroxine during pregnancy in women with primary hypothyroidism N Engl J Med 1990; 323:91–96.
89. Arafah BM. Increased need for thyroxine in women with hypothyroidism during estrogen therapy. N Engl J Med 2001; 344: 1743–1749.
90. Robbins J, Rall JE. The interaction of thyroid hormones and protein in biological fluids. Rec Prog Horm Res 1957; 13:161.
91. Mendel CM. The free hormone hypothesis: a physiologically based matematical model. Endocr Rev 1989; 103:232–274.
92. Mendel CM, Weisiger RA, Jones AL, et al. Thyroid hormone–binding proteins in plasma facilitate uniform distribution of thyroxine within tissues: a perfused rat liver study. Endocrinology 1987; 120:1742–1749.
93. Hennemann G, Docter R, Friesema ECH, et al. Plasma membrane transport of thyroid hormones and its role in thyroid hormone metabolism and bioavailibility. Endocr Rev 2001; 22:451–476.
94. Friesema EC, Docter R, Moerings EP, et al. Identification of thyroid hormone transporters. Biochem Biophys Res Commun 1999; 254:497–501.
95. Hagenbuch B. Molecular properties of hepatic uptake systems for bile acids and organic anions. J Membr Biol 1997; 160: 1–8.
96. Kullak-Ublick GA. Regulation of organic anion and drug transporters of the sinusoidal membrane. J Hepatol 1999; 31:563–573.
97. Abe T, Kakyo M, Sakagami H, et al. Molecular characterization and tissue distribution of a new organic anion transporter subtype (oatp3) that transports thyroid hormones and taurocholate and comparison with oatp2. J Biol Chem 1998; 273:22395–22401.
98. Cattori V, Hagenbuch B, Hagenbuch N, et al. Identification of organic anion transporting polypeptide 4 (Oatp4) as a major full-length isoform of the liver-specific transporter-1 (rlst-1) in rat liver. FEBS Lett 2000; 474:242–245.
99. Abe T, Kakyo M, Tokui T, et al. Identification of a novel gene family encoding human liver-specific organic anion transporter LST-1. J Biol Chem 1999; 274:17159–17163.
100. Hsiang B, Zhu Y, Wang Z, et al. A novel human hepatic organic anion transporting polypeptide (OATP2): identification of a liver-specific human organic anion transporting polypeptide and identification of rat and human hydroxymethylglutaryl-CoA reductase inhibitor transporters. J Biol Chem 1999; 274:37161–37168.
101. van der Heyden JTM, Docter R, van Toor H, et al. Effects of caloric deprivation on thyroid hormone tissue uptake and generation of low-T_3 syndrome. Am J Physiol 1986; 251:E156–E163.
102. Ribeiro RCJ, Cavalieri RR, Lomri N, et al. Thyroid hormone export regulates cellular hormone content and response. J Biol Chem 1996; 271:17147–17151.
103. Cavalieri RR, Simeoni LA, Park SW, et al. Thyroid hormone export in rat FRTL-5 thyroid cells and mouse NIH-3T3 cells is carrier-mediated, verapamil-sensitive, and stereospecific. Endocrinology 1999; 140:4948–4954.
104. Oppenheimer JH, Schwartz HL. Stereospecific transport to triiodothyronine from plasma to cytosol and from cytosol to nucleus in rat liver, kidney, brain, and heart. J Clin Invest 1985; 75:147–154.
105. Oppenheimer JH, Schwartz HL, Surks MI. Tissue differences in the concentration of triiodothyronine nuclear binding sites in the rat: liver, kidney, pituitary, heart, brain, spleen, and testis. Endocrinology 1974; 95:897–903.
106. St. Germain DL, Galton VA. The deiodinase family of selenoproteins. Thyroid 1997; 7:655–668.

107. Berry MJ, Banu L, Larsen PR. Type I iodothyronine deiodinase is a selenocysteine-containing enzyme. Nature 1991; 349:438–440.
108. Berry MJ, Larsen PR. The role of selenium in thyroid hormone action. Endocr Rev 1992; 13:207–219.
109. Berry MJ, Kieffer JD, Harney JW, et al. Selenocysteine confers the biochemical properties characteristic of the type I iodothyronine deiodinase. J Biol Chem 1991; 266:14155–14158.
110. Berry MJ, Banu L, Chen YY, et al. Recognition of UGA as a selenocysteine codon in type I deiodinase requires sequences in the 3′-untranslated region. Nature 1991; 353:273–276.
111. Tujebajeva RM, Copeland PR, Xu XM, et al. Decoding apparatus for eukaryotic selenocysteine incorporation. EMBO R 2000; 2:158–163.
112. Low SC, Berry MJ. Knowing when not to stop: selenocysteine incorporation in eukaryotes. Trends Biochem Sci 1996; 21:203–208.
113. Toyoda N, Kaptein E, Berry MJ, et al. Structure-activity relationships for thyroid hormone deiodination by mammalian type I iodothyronine deiodinases. Endocrinology 1997; 138:213–219.
114. Nishikawa M, Toyoda N, Yonemoto T, et al. Quantitative measurements for type 1 deiodinase messenger ribonucleic acid in human peripheral blood mononuclear cells: mechanism of the preferential increase of T_3 in hyperthyroid Graves' disease. Biochem Biophys Res Commun 1998; 250:642–646.
115. Toyoda N, Zavacki AM, Maia AL, et al. A novel retinoid X receptor–independent thyroid hormone response element is present in the human type 1 deiodinase gene. Mol Cell Biol 1995; 15:5100–5112.
116. Kim SW, Harney JW, Larsen PR. Studies of the hormonal regulation of type 2,5′-iodothyronine deiodinase messenger ribonucleic acid in pituitary tumor cells using semiquantitative reverse transcription–polymerase chain reaction. Endocrinology 1998; 139:4895–4905.
117. Gereben B, Goncalves C, Harney JW, et al. Selective proteolysis of human type 2 deiodinase: a novel ubiquitin-proteasomal mediated mechanism for regulation of hormone activation. Mol Endocrinol 2000; 14:1697–1708.
118. St. Germain DL. Dual mechanisms of regulation of type I iodothyronine 5′-deiodinase in the rat kidney, liver, and thyroid gland: implications for the treatment of hyperthyroidism with radiographic contrast agents. J Clin Invest 1988; 81:1476–1484.
119. Croteau W, Davey JC, Galton VA, et al. Cloning of the mammalian type II iodothyronine deiodinase: a selenoprotein differentially expressed and regulated in human and rat brain and other tissues. J Clin Invest 1996; 98:405–417.
120. Salvatore D, Bartha T, Harney JW, et al. Molecular biological and biochemical characterization of the human type 2 selenodeiodinase. Endocrinology 1996; 137:3308–3315.
121. Baqui MM, Gereben B, Harney JW, et al. Distinct subcellular localization of transiently expressed types 1 and 2 iodothyronine deiodinases as determined by immunofluorescence confocal microscopy. Endocrinology 2000; 141:4309–4312.
122. Larsen PR, Silva JE, Kaplan MM. Relationships between circulating and intracellular thyroid hormones: physiological and clinical implications. Endocr Rev 1981; 2:87–102.
123. Galton VA, Martinez E, Hernandez A, et al. Pregnant rat uterus expresses high levels of the type 3 iodothyronine deiodinase. J Clin Invest 1999; 103:979–987.
124. Campos-Barros A, Hoell T, Musa A, et al. Phenolic and tyrosyl ring iodothyronine deiodination and thyroid hormone concentrations in the human central nervous system. J Clin Endocrinol Metab 1996; 81:2179–2185.
125. Huang SA, Tu HM, Harney JW, et al. Severe hypothyroidism caused by type 3 iodothyronine deiodinase in infantile hemangiomas. N Engl J Med 2000; 343:185–189.
126. Saberi M, Sterling FH, Utiger RD. Reduction in extrathyroidal triiodothyronine production by propylthiouracil in man. J Clin Invest 1975; 55:218–223.
127. Geffner DL, Azukizawa M, Hershman JM. Propylthiouracil blocks extrathyroidal conversion of thyroxine to triiodothyronine and augments thyrotropin secretion in man. J Clin Invest 1975; 55:224–229.
128. Inada M, Kasagi K, Kurata S, et al. Estimation of thyroxine and triiodothyronine distribution and of the conversion rate of thyroxine to triiodothyronine in man. J Clin Invest 1975; 55:1337–1348.
129. Lum SM, Nicoloff JT, Spencer CA, et al. Peripheral tissue mechanism for maintenance of serum triiodothyronine values in a thyroxine-deficient state in man. J Clin Invest 1984; 73:570–575.
130. Cavalieri RR, Pitt-Rivers R. The effects of drugs on the distribution and metabolism of thyroid hormones. Pharmacol Rev 1981; 33:55–80.
131. Eiris-Punal J, Del Rio-Garma M, Del Rio-Garma MC, et al. Long-term treatment of children with epilepsy with valproate or carbamazepine may cause subclinical hypothyroidism. Epilepsia 1999; 40:1761–1766.
132. Engler D, Burger AG. The deiodination of the iodothyronines and of their derivatives in man. Endocr Rev 1984; 5:151–184.
133. Silva JE, Larsen PR. Adrenergic activation of triiodothyronine production in brown adipose tissue. Nature 1983; 305:712–713.
134. Hull D. Brown adipose tissue and the newborn infant's response to cold. In Philipp EE, Barnes J, Newton M (eds). Scientific Foundation of Obstetrics and Gynaecology. London, William Heinemann, 1977, pp 545–550.
135. Houstek J, Vizek K, Pavelka S, et al. Type II iodothyronine 5′-deiodinase and uncoupling protein in brown adipose tissue of human newborns. J Clin Endocrinol Metab 1993; 77:382–387.
136. Campos-Barros A, Amma LL, Faris JS, et al. Type 2 iodothyronine deiodinase expression in the cochlea before the onset of hearing. Proc Natl Acad Sci USA 2000; 97:1287–1292.
137. Marsh-Armstrong N, Huang H, Remo BF, et al. Asymmetric growth and development of the *Xenopus laevis* retina during metamorphosis is controlled by type III deiodinase. Neuron 1999; 24: 871–878.
138. Vignati L, Finley RJ, Hagg S, et al. Protein conservation during prolonged fast: a function of triiodothyronine levels. Trans Assoc Am Physicians 1978; 91:169–179.
139. Nagaya T, Fujieda M, Otsuka G, et al. A potential role of activated NF-kappa B in the pathogenesis of euthyroid sick syndrome. J Clin Invest 2000; 106:393–402.
140. Yu J, Koenig RJ. Regulation of hepatocyte thyroxine 5′-deiodinase by T_3 and nuclear receptor coactivators as a model of the sick euthyroid syndrome. J Biol Chem 2000; 275:38296–38301.
141. Contempre B, Dumont JE, Ngo B, et al. Effect of selenium supplementation in hypothyroid subjects of an iodine and selenium deficient area: the possible danger of indiscriminate supplementation of iodine-deficient subjects with selenium. J Clin Endocrinol Metab 1991; 73:213–215.
142. Contempre B, Duale NL, Dumont JE, et al. Effect of selenium supplementation on thyroid hormone metabolism in an iodine and selenium deficient population. Clin Endocrinol (Oxf) 1992; 36:579–583.
143. Toyoda N, Zavacki AM, Maia AL, et al. A novel retinoid X receptor–independent thyroid hormone response element is present in the human type 1 deiodinase gene. Mol Cell Biol 1995; 15:5100–5112.
144. Trip MD, Wiersinga W, Plomp TA. Incidence, predictability, and pathogenesis of amiodarone-induced thyrotoxicosis and hypothyroidism. Am J Med 1991; 91:507–511.
145. Harjai KJ, Licata AA. Effects of amiodarone on thyroid function. Ann Intern Med 1997; 126:63–73.
146. Lambert MJ, Burger AG, Galeazzi RL, et al. Are selective increases in serum thyroxine (T_4) due to iodinated inhibitors of T_4 monodeiodination indicative of hyperthyroidism? J Clin Endocrinol Metab 1982; 55:1058–1065.
147. Borowski GD, Garofano CD, Rose LI, et al. Effect of long-term amiodarone therapy on thyroid hormone levels and thyroid function. Am J Med 1985; 78:443–450.
148. Hershman JM, Nademanee K, Sugawara M, et al. Thyroxine and triiodothyronine kinetics in cardiac patients taking amiodarone. Acta Endocrinol (Copenh) 1986; 111:193–199.
149. Ha HR, Stieger B, Grassi G, et al. Structure-effect relationships of amiodarone analogues on the inhibition of thyroxine deiodination. Eur J Clin Pharmacol 2000; 55:807–814.
150. Krenning EP, Docter R, Bernard HF, et al. Decreased transport of thyroxine (T_4), 3,3′,5-triiodothyronine (T_3) and 3,3′,5′-triiodothyronine (rT3) into rat hepatocytes in primary culture due to a decrease of cellular ATP contnent and various drugs. FEBS Lett 1982; 140:229–233.
151. Wiersinga WM, Trip MD. Amiodarone and thyroid hormone metabolism. Postgrad Med J 1986; 62:909–914.
152. Burgi H, Wimpfheimer C, Burger A, et al. Changes of circulat-

ing thyroxine, triiodothyronine, and reverse triiodothyronine after radiographic contrast agents. J Clin Endocrinol Metab 1976; 43: 1203–1210.

153. Suzuki H, Kadena N, Takeuchi K, et al. Effects of three-day oral cholecystography on serum iodothyronines and TSH concentrations: comparison of the effects among some cholecystographic agents and the effects of iopanoic acid on the pituitary-thyroid axis. Acta Endocrinol (Copenh) 1979; 92:477–488.
154. Wu SY, Chopra IJ, Solomon DH, et al. The effect of repeated administration of ipodate (Oragrafin) in hyperthyroidism. J Clin Endocrinol Metab 1978; 47:1358–1362.
155. LoPresti JS, Eigen A, Kaptein E, et al. Alterations in 3,3′5′-triiodothyronine metabolism in response to propylthiouracil, dexamethasone, and thyroxine administration in man. J Clin Invest 1989; 84:1650–1656.
156. Jorgensen JOL, Pedersen SA, Laurberg P, et al. Effects of growth hormone therapy on thyroid function of growth hormone–deficient adults with and without concomitant thyroxine-substituted central hypothyroidism. J Clin Endocrinol Metab 1989; 69:1127–1132.
157. Van der Geyten S, Buys N, Sanders JP, et al. Acute pretranslational regulation of type III iodothyronine deiodinase by growth hormone and dexamethasone in chicken embryos. Mol Cell Endocrinol 1999; 147:49–56.
158. Williams GR. Cloning and characterization of two novel thyroid hormone receptor beta isoforms. Mol Cell Biol 2000; 20:8329–8342.
159. Amma LL, Campos-Barros A, Wang Z, et al. Distinct tissue-specific roles for thyroid hormone receptors beta and alpha$_1$ in regulation of type 1 deiodinase expression. Mol Endocrinol 2001; 15:467–475.
160. Abel ED, Kaulbach HC, Campos-Barros A, et al. Novel insight from transgenic mice into thyroid hormone resistance and the regulation of thyrotropin. J Clin Invest 1999; 103:271–279.
161. Forrest D, Golarai G, Connor J, et al. Genetic analysis of thyroid hormone receptors in development and disease. Recent Prog Horm Res 1996; 51:1–22.
162. Forrest D, Vennstrom B. Functions of thyroid hormone receptors in mice. Thyroid 2000; 10:41–52.
163. Forrest D, Hanebuth E, Smeyne RJ, et al. Recessive resistance to thyroid hormone in mice lacking thyroid hormone receptor beta: evidence for tissue-specific modulation of receptor function. EMBO J 1996; 15:3006–3015.
164. Rusch A, Erway LC, Oliver D, et al. Thyroid hormone receptor beta–dependent expression of a potassium conductance in inner hair cells at the onset of hearing. Proc Natl Acad Sci USA 1998; 95:15758–15762.
165. Beck-Peccoz P, Chatterjee VKK. The variable clinical phenotype in thyroid hormone resistance syndrome. Thyroid 1994; 4:225–231.
166. Wikstrom L, Johansson C, Salto C, et al. Abnormal heart rate and body temperature in mice lacking thyroid hormone receptor alpha 1. EMBO J 1998; 17:455–461.
167. Passonneau JV, Lowry OH. Enzymatic Analysis: A Practical Guide. Tatowa, NJ, Humana Press, 1993.
168. Wagner RL, Huber BR, Shiau AK, et al. Hormone selectivity in thyroid hormone receptors. Mol Endocrinol 2001; 15:398–410.
169. Wagner RL, Apriletti JW, McGrath ME, et al. A structural role for hormone in the thyroid hormone receptor. Nature 1995; 378: 690–697.
170. Chiellini G, Apriletti JW, al Yoshihara H, et al. A high-affinity subtype-selective agonist ligand for the thyroid hormone receptor. Chem Biol 1998; 5:299–306.
171. Trost SU, Swanson E, Gloss B, et al. The thyroid hormone receptor-beta–selective agonist GC-1 differentially affects plasma lipids and cardiac activity Endocrinology 2000; 141:3057–3064.
172. Glass CK, Rosenfeld MG. The coregulator exchange in transcriptional functions of nuclear receptors. Genes Dev 2000; 14: 121–141.
173. Wolffe AP, Collingwood TN, Li Q, et al. Thyroid hormone receptor, v-ErbA, and chromatin. Vitam Horm 2000; 58:449–492.
174. Urnov FD, Wolffe AP. An array of positioned nucleosomes potentiates thyroid hormone receptor action in vivo. J Biol Chem 2001; 23:23.
175. Kim SW, Ahn IM, Larsen PR. In vivo genomic footprinting of thyroid hormone–responsive genes in pituitary tumor cell lines. Mol Cell Biol 1996; 16:4465–4477.
176. Dace A, Zhao L, Park KS, et al. Hormone binding induces rapid proteasome-mediated degradation of thyroid hormone receptors. Proc Natl Acad Sci USA 2000; 97:8985–8990.
177. Sasaki S, Lesoon-Wood LA, Dey A, et al. Ligand-induced recruitment of a histone deacetylase in the negative-feedback regulation of the thyrotropin beta gene. EMBO J 1999; 18:5389–5398.
178. Tagami T, Park Y, Jameson JL. Mechanisms that mediate negative regulation of the thyroid-stimulating hormone alpha gene by the thyroid hormone receptor. J Biol Chem 1999; 274:22345–22353.
179. Davis PJ, Davis FB. Nongenomic actions of thyroid hormone. Thyroid 1996; 6:497–504.
180. Davis PJ, Shih A, Lin HY, et al. Thyroxine promotes association of mitogen-activated protein kinase and nuclear thyroid hormone receptor (TR) and causes serine phosphorylation of TR. J Biol Chem 2000; 275:38032–38039.
181. Lin HY, Davis FB, Gordinier JK, et al. Thyroid hormone induces activation of mitogen-activated protein kinase in cultured cells. Am J Physiol 1999; 276:C1014–C1024.
182. Hollenberg AN, Monden T, Flynn TR, et al. The human thyrotropin-releasing hormone gene is regulated by thyroid hormone through two distinct classes of negative thyroid hormone response elements. Mol Endocrinol 1995; 9:540–550.
183. Legradi G, Emerson CH, Ahima RS, et al. Leptin prevents fasting-induced suppression of prothyrotropin-releasing hormone messenger ribonucleic acid in neurons of the hypothalamic paraventricular nucleus. Endocrinology 1997; 138:2569–2576.
184. Ahima RS, Prabakaran D, Mantzoros C, et al. Role of leptin in the neuroendocrine response to fasting. Nature 1996; 382:250–252.
185. Nillni EA, Vaslet C, Harris M, et al. Leptin regulates prothyrotropin-releasing hormone biosynthesis. Evidence for direct and indirect pathways. J Biol Chem 2000; 275:36124–36133.
186. Kim MS, Small CJ, Stanley SA, et al. The central melanocortin system affects the hypothalamo-pituitary thyroid axis and may mediate the effect of leptin. J Clin Invest 2000; 105:1005–1011.
187. Harris M, Aschkenasi C, Elias CF, et al. Transcriptional regulation of the thyrotropin-releasing hormone gene by leptin and melanocortin signaling. J Clin Invest 2001; 107:111–120.
188. Romijn JA, Adriaanse R, Brabant G, et al. Pulsatile secretion of thyrotropin during fasting: a decrease of thyrotropin pulse amplitude. J Clin Endocrinol Metab 1990; 70:1631–1636.
189. Ozata M, Ozdemir IC, Licinio J. Human leptin deficiency caused by a missense mutation: multiple endocrine defects, decreased sympathetic tone, and immune system dysfunction indicate new targets for leptin action, greater central than peripheral resistance to the effects of leptin, and spontaneous correction of leptin-mediated defects. J Clin Endocrinol Metab 1999; 84:3686–3695.
190. Bornstein SR, Torpy DJ, Chrousos GP, et al. Leptin levels are elevated despite low thyroid hormone levels in the 'euthyroid sick' syndrome. J Clin Endocrinol Metab 1997; 82:4278–4279.
191. Himms-Hagen J. Physiological roles of the leptin endocrine system: differences between mice and humans. Crit Rev Clin Lab Sci 1999; 36:575–655.
192. Segerson TP, Kauer J, Wolfe H, et al. Thyroid hormone regulates TRH biosynthesis in the paraventricular nucleus of the rat hypothalamus. Science 1987; 238:78–80.
193. Dyess EM, Segerson TP, Liposits Z, et al. Triiodothyronine exerts direct cell-specific regulation of thyrotropin-releasing hormone gene expression in the hypothalamic paraventricular nucleus. Endocrinology 1988; 123:2291–2297.
194. Kakucska I, Rand W, Lechan RM. Thyrotropin-releasing hormone (TRH) gene expression in the hypothalamic paraventricular nucleus is dependent upon feedback regulation by both triiodothyronine and thyroxine. Endocrinology 1992; 130:2845–2850.
195. Riskind PN, Kolodny JM, Larsen PR. The regional hypothalamic distribution of type II 5′-monodeiodinase in euthyroid and hypothyroid rats. Brain Res 1987; 420:194–198.
196. Tu HM, Kim SW, Salvatore D, et al. Regional distribution of type 2 thyroxine deiodinase messenger ribonucleic acid in rat hypothalamus and pituitary and its regulation by thyroid hormone. Endocrinology 1997; 138:3359–3368.
197. Guadano-Ferraz A, Obregon MJ, St. Germain DL, et al. The

297. Kirkegaard C, Faber J. The role of thyroid hormones in depression. Eur J Endocrinol 1998; 138:1–9.
298. Jackson IM. The thyroid axis and depression. Thyroid 1998; 8: 951–956.
299. Nader S, Warner MD, Doyle S, et al. Euthyroid sick syndrome in psychiatric inpatients. Biol Psychiatry 1996; 40:1288–1293.
300. Brabant G, Brabant A, Ranft U. Circadian and pulsatile thyrotropin secretion in euthyroid man under the influence of thyroid hormone and glucocorticoid administration. J Clin Endocrinol Metab 1987; 65:83.
301. Topliss DJ, White EL, Stockigt JR. Significance of thyrotropin excess in untreated primary adrenal insufficiency. J Clin Endocrinol Metab 1980; 50:52–56.
302. Colao A, Pivonello R, Faggiano A, et al. Increased prevalence of thyroid autoimmunity in patients successfully treated for Cushing's disease. Clin Endocrinol (Oxf) 2000; 53:13–19.
303. Arafah BM. Decreased levothyroxine requirement in women with hypothyroidism during androgen therapy for breast cancer. Ann Intern Med 1994; 121:247–251.
304. Spencer CA, LoPresti JS, Patel A, et al. Applications of a new chemiluminometric thyrotropin assay to subnormal measurement. J Clin Endocrinol Metab 1990; 70:453–460.
305. Spencer CA, Schwarzbein D, Guttler RB, et al. Thyrotropin (TSH)-releasing hormone stimulation test responses employing third and fourth generation TSH assays. J Clin Endocrinol Metab 1993; 76:494–498.
306. Spencer CA, Takeuchi M, Kazarosyan M, et al. Interlaboratory/intermethod differences in functional sensitivity of immunometric assays of thyrotropin (TSH) and impact on reliability of measurement of subnormal concentrations of TSH. Clin Chem 1995; 41: 367–374.
307. Laurberg P. Persistent problems with the specificity of immunometric TSH assays. Thyroid 1993; 3:279–283.
308. Kahn BB, Weintraub BD, Csako G, et al. Factitious elevation of thyrotropin in a new ultrasensitive assay: implications for the use of monoclonal antibodies in 'sandwich' immunoassay. J Clin Endocrinol Metab 1988; 66:526–533.
309. Kuzuya N, Kinji I, Ishibashi M. Endocrine and immunohistochemical studies on thyrotropin (TSH)-secreting pituitary adenomas: responses of TSH, α-subunit, and growth hormone to hypothalamic releasing hormones and their distribution in adenoma cells. J Clin Endocrinol Metab 1990; 71:1103–1111.
310. Nystrom E, Caidahl K, Fager G, et al. A double-blind cross-over 12-month study of L-thyroxine treatment of women with 'subclinical' hypothyroidism. Clin Endocrinol 1988; 29:63–76.
311. Bell GM, Todd WTA, Forfar JC, et al. End-organ responses to thyroxine therapy in subclinical hypothyroidism. Clin Endocrinol 1985; 22:83–89.
312. Snyder PJ, Utiger RD. Repetitive administration of thyrotropin-releasing hormone results in small elevations of serum thyroid hormones and in marked inhibition of thyrotropin response. J Clin Invest 1973; 52:2305.
313. Saberi M, Utiger RD. Augmentation of thyrotropin responses to thyrotropin-releasing hormone following small decreases in serum thyroid hormone concentrations. J Clin Endocrinol Metab 1975; 40:435.
314. Wu SY, Jordan M, Nguyen JH. Compound W: a potential marker in maternal serum for assessing fetal thyroid function. Compr Ther 1995; 21:594–596.
315. Cortelazzi D, Morpurgo PS, Zamperini P, et al. Maternal compound W serial measurements for the management of fetal hypothyroidism. Eur J Endocrinol 1999; 141:570–578.
316. Nelson JC, Weiss RM, Wilcox RB. Underestimates of serum free thyroxine (T_4) concentrations by free T_4 immunoassays. J Clin Endocrinol Metab 1994; 79:76–79.
317. Nelson JC, Wilcox RB, Pandian MR. Dependence of free thyroxine estimates obtained with equilibrium tracer dialysis on the concentration of thyroxine-binding globulin. Clin Chem 1992; 38:1294–1300.
318. Wang R, Nelson JC, Weiss RM, et al. Accuracy of free thyroxine measurements across natural ranges of thyroxine binding to serum proteins. Thyroid 2000; 10:31–39.
319. Hay ID, Bayer MF, Kaplan MM, et al. American Thyroid Association assessment of current free thyroid hormone and thyrotropin measurements and guidelines for future clinical assays: The Committee on Nomenclature of the American Thyroid Association. Clin Chem 1991; 37:2002–2008.
320. Steele BW, Witte DL, Whitley RJ, et al. The effects of modifying proficiency testing materials on thyroid function test results: A College of American Pathologists Ligand Assay Survey Study. Arch Pathol Lab Med 1997; 121:1241–1246.
321. Faix JD, Rosen HN, Velazquez FR. Indirect estimation of thyroid hormone–binding proteins to calculate free thyroxine index: comparison of nonisotopic methods that use labeled thyroxine ('T-uptake'). Clin Chem 1995; 41:41–47.
322. Nelson JC, Weiss RM. The effect of serum dilution on free thyroxine (T_4) concentrations in the low T_4 syndrome of nonthyroidal illness. J Clin Endocrinol Metab 1985; 61:239–246.
323. Toft AD, Irvine WJ, Hunter WM, et al. Anomalous plasma TSH levels in patients developing hypothyroidism in the early months after ^{131}I therapy for thyrotoxicosis. J Clin Endocrinol Metab 1974; 39:607.
324. Davies P, Franklyn JA, Daykin J, et al. The significance of TSH values measured in a sensitive assay in the follow-up of hyperthyroid patients treated with radioiodine. J Clin Endocrinol Metab 1992; 74:1189–1194.
325. Sawin CT, Geller A, Wolf PA, et al. Low serum thyrotropin concentrations as a risk factor for atrial fibrillation in older persons. N Engl J Med 1994; 331:1249–1252.
326. Cohen LE, Wondisford FE, Radovick S. Role of Pit-1 in the gene expression of growth hormone, prolactin, and thyrotropin. Endocrinol Metab Clin North Am 1996; 25:523–540.
327. Radovick S, Cohen LE, Wondisford FE. The molecular basis of hypopituitarism. Horm Res 1998; 49:30–36.
328. Kaptein EM. Thyroid hormone metabolism and thyroid diseases in chronic renal failure. Endocr Rev 1996; 17:45–63.
329. Nagaya T, Seo H. Molecular basis of resistance to thyroid hormone (RTH). Endocr J 1998; 45:709–718.
330. Weiss RE, Refetoff S. Treatment of resistance to thyroid hormone: primum non nocere. J Clin Endocrinol Metab 1999; 84: 401–404.
331. Refetoff S, Weiss RE, Usala SJ. The syndromes of resistance to thyroid hormone. Endocr Rev 1993; 14:348–399.
332. Kricka LJ. Human anti-animal antibody interferences in immunological assays. Clin Chem 1999; 45:942–956.
333. Cooper DS, Daniels GH, Ladenson PW, et al. Hyperthyroxinemia in patients treated with high-dose propranolol. Am J Med 1982; 73:867–871.
334. Perrild H, Molhom Hansen J, Skovsted L, et al. Different effects of propranolol, alprenolol, sotalol, atenolol, and metoprolol on serum T_3 and serum rT_3 in hyperthyroidism. Clin Endocrinol 1983; 18:139–142.
335. LeBoff MS, Kaplan MM, Silva JE, et al. Bioavailability of thyroid hormones from oral replacement preparations. Metabolism 1982; 31:900–905.
336. Rees-Jones RW, Larsen PR. Triiodothyronine and thyroxine content of desiccated thyroid tablets. Metabolism 1977; 26:1213–1218.
337. Rees-Jones RW, Rolla AR, Larsen PR. Hormonal content of thyroid replacement preparations. JAMA 1980; 243:549–550.
338. Smith PJ, Surks MI. Multiple effects of 5,5′-diphenylhydantoin on the thyroid hormone system. Endocr Rev 1984; 5:514–524.
339. Liewendahl K, Tikanoja S, Helenius T, et al. Free thyroxine and free triiodothyronine as measured by equilibrium dialysis and analog radioimmunoassay in serum of patients taking phenytoin and carbamazepine. Clin Chem 1985; 31:1993–1996.
340. Christensen HR, Simonsen K, Hegedus L, et al. Influence of rifampicin on thyroid gland volume, thyroid hormones, and antipyrine metabolism. Acta Endocrinol (Copenh) 1989; 121:406–410.
341. Capper SJ, Humphrey MJ, Kurtz AB. Inhibition of thyroxine binding to serum proteins by fenclofenac and related compounds. Clin Chim Acta 1981; 112:77–83.
342. al-Adsani H, Hoffer LJ, Silva JE. Resting energy expenditure is sensitive to small dose changes in patients on chronic thyroid hormone replacement. J Clin Endocrinol Metab 1997; 82:1118–1125.
343. Klein I, Mantell P, Parker M, et al. Resolution of abnormal muscle enzyme studies in hypothyroidism. Am J Med Sci 1980; 279:159.
344. Becker C. Hypothyroidism and atherosclerotic heart disease: pathogenesis, medical management, and the role of coronary artery bypass surgery. Endocr Rev 1985; 6:432–440.

345. Brenta G, Schnitman M, Gurfinkiel M, et al. Variations of sex hormone–binding globulin in thyroid dysfunction. Thyroid 1999; 9:273–277.
346. Smallridge RC, Parker RA, Wiggs EA, et al. Thyroid hormone resistance in a large kindred: physiologic, biochemical, pharmacologic, and neuropsychologic studies. Am J Med 1989; 86:289–296.
347. Schlumberger M, Baudin E. Serum thyroglobulin determination in the follow-up of patients with differentiated thyroid carcinoma. Eur J Endocrinol 1998; 138:249–252.
348. Spencer CA, Wang CC. Thyroglobulin measurement: techniques, clinical benefits, and pitfalls. Endocrinol Metab Clin North Am 1995; 24:841–863.
349. Spencer CA. Serum thyroglobulin measurements: clinical utility and technical limitations in the management of patients with differentiated thyroid carcinomas. Endocr Pract 2000; 6:481–484.
350. Mariotti S, Martino E, Cupini C, et al. Low serum thyroblobulin as a clue to the diagnosis of thyrotoxicosis factitia. N Engl J Med 1982; 307:410–412.
351. Spencer CA, Takeuchi M, Kazarosyan M, et al. Serum thyroglobulin autoantibodies: prevalence, influence on serum thyroglobulin measurement, and prognostic significance in patients with differentiated thyroid carcinoma. J Clin Endocrinol Metab 1998; 83:1121–1127.
352. Spencer CA, LoPresti JS, Fatemi S, et al. Detection of residual and recurrent differentiated thyroid carcinoma by serum thyroglobulin measurement. Thyroid 1999; 9:435–441.
353. Tenenbaum F, Corone C, Schlumberger M, et al. Thyroglobulin measurement and postablative iodine-131 total body scan after total thyroidectomy for differentiated thyroid carcinoma in patients with no evidence of disease. Eur J Cancer 1996; 32A:1262.
354. Schneider AB, Ikekubo K. Sequential serum thyroglobulin determinations, ^{131}I scans, and ^{131}I uptakes after triiodothyronine withdrawal in patients with thyroid cancer. J Clin Endocrinol Metab 1981; 53:1199–1206.
355. Haugen BR, Pacini F, Reiners C, et al. A comparison of recombinant human thyrotropin and thyroid hormone withdrawal for the detection of thyroid remnant or cancer. J Clin Endocrinol Metab 1999; 84:3877–3885.
356. Stagnaro-Green A. Recognizing, understanding, and treating postpartum thyroiditis. Endocrinol Metab Clin North Am 2000; 29:417–430, ix.
357. Phillips D, Prentice L, Upadhyaya M, et al. Autosomal dominant inheritance of autoantibodies to thyroid peroxidase and thyroglobulin: studies in families not selected for autoimmune thyroid disease. J Clin Endocrinol Metab 1991; 72:973–975.
358. Vanderpump MPJ, Tunbridge WMG, French JM, et al. The incidence of thyroid disorders in the community: a twenty-year follow-up of the Whickham survey. Clin Endocrinol 1995; 43: 55–68.
359. Wood LC, Ingbar SH. Hypothyroidism as a late sequela in patients with Graves' disease treated with antithyroid agents. J Clin Invest 1979; 64:1429–1436.
360. Tomer Y, Greenberg DA, Barbesino G, et al. CTLA-4 and not CD28 is a susceptibility gene for thyroid autoantibody production. J Clin Endocrinol Metab 2001; 86:1687–1693.
361. Baker J, Fosso CK. Immunological aspects of cancers arising from thyroid follicular cells. Endocr Rev 1993; 14:729–746.
362. Stagnaro-Green A, Roman SH, Cobin RH, et al. A prospective study of lymphocyte-initiated immunosuppression in normal pregnancy: evidence of a T-cell etiology for postpartum thyroid dysfunction. J Clin Endocrinol Metab 1992; 74:645–653.
363. Stagnaro-Green A, Roman SH, Cobin RH, et al. Detection of at-risk pregnancy by means of highly sensitive assays for thyroid autoantibodies. JAMA 1990; 264:1422–1426.
364. Lejeune B, Grun JP, de Nayer P, et al. Antithyroid antibodies underlying thyroid abnormalities and miscarriage or pregnancy induced hypertension. Br J Obstet Gynaecol 1993; 100:669–672.
365. Marino M, Pinchera A, McCluskey RT, et al. Megalin in thyroid physiology and pathology. Thyroid 2001; 11:47–56.
366. Pittman JA Jr, Dailey GE III, Beschi RJ. Changing normal values for thyroidal radioiodine uptake. N Engl J Med 1969; 280:1431–1441.
367. Hayes AA, Akre CM, Gorman CA. Iodine-131 treatment of Graves' disease using modified early iodine-131 uptake measurements in therapy dose calculations. J Nucl Med 1990; 31:519–522.
368. Medeiros-Neto G, Kim PS, Vono J, et al. Congenital hypothyroid goiter with deficient thyroglobulin. J Clin Invest 1996; 98: 2838–2844.

11 Thyrotoxicosis

Terry F. Davies and P. Reed Larsen

OVERVIEW

The term *thyrotoxicosis* refers to the biochemical and physiologic manifestations of excessive quantities of the thyroid hormones. We prefer the term *thyrotoxicosis* rather than *hyperthyroidism* to describe this disorder, because it need not originate in the thyroid gland. The term *hyperthyroidism* is reserved for disorders that result from overproduction of hormone by the thyroid gland itself, of which Graves' disease is the most common (Table 11–1). The manifestations depend on the severity of the disease, the age of the patient, the presence or absence of extrathyroidal manifestations, and the specific disorder producing the thyrotoxicosis.

Peripheral Clinical Manifestations

(Table 11–2)

Skin and Hair

The most characteristic change in thyrotoxicosis is the warm, moist feel of the skin that results from cutaneous vasodilatation and excessive sweating. Although the hands are usually warm and moist, the texture of the hands may be altered by occupational or environmental factors; hence, texture is best assessed on the inner aspect of the arm or over the chest. The elbows are smooth and pink, the complexion is rosy, and the patient blushes readily. Palmar erythema may resemble "liver palms," and telangiectasia may be present. Increased diffuse pigmentation resembles that in adrenal insufficiency, but buccal pigmentation does not occur. The hair is fine and friable, and hair loss may be excessive. A history of early graying in the patient or in relatives is said to be common in Graves' disease. The nails are often soft and friable. A characteristic finding is *Plummer's nails*, a term applied to separation of the distal margin of the nail from the nail bed, with irregular recession of the junction (onycholysis).

Eyes

Retraction of the upper eyelid, evident as the presence of a rim of sclera between the lid and the limbus, is common in all forms of thyrotoxicosis, regardless of the underlying cause, and is responsible for the bright-eyed "stare" or "fish eyes" of the patient with thyrotoxicosis. *Lid lag* is the phenomenon in which the upper lid lags behind the globe when the patient is asked to gaze slowly downward, and *globe lag* occurs when the globe lags behind the upper lid when the patient gazes slowly upward. The movements of the lids may be jerky and spasmodic, and a fine tremor of the lightly closed lids can often be observed in severe cases. These ocular manifestations appear to be the result of increased adrenergic activity. It is important to differentiate these ocular manifestations, which occur in all forms of thyrotoxicosis, from those of infiltrative orbitopathy, which are characteristic of hyperthyroid Graves' disease (see later).

Cardiovascular System

Alterations in cardiovascular function are due to increased circulatory demands that result from the hypermetabolism and the need to dissipate the excess heat produced.[1] At rest, peripheral vascular resistance is decreased and cardiac output is increased as a result of an increase in stroke volume and heart rate. Thyroid hormones in excess have a direct inotropic effect mediated by alterations of contractile proteins. Tachycardia is almost always present, and tachycardia during sleep (pulse rate >90 beats/minute) serves to distinguish tachycardia of thyrotoxic origin from that of psychogenic causes. Widening of the pulse pressure is due to an increase in systolic pressure and a decrease in diastolic pressure.

Table 11–1. Varieties of Thyrotoxicosis

*Sustained Hormone Overproduction (Hyperthyroidism)**
Graves' disease
Toxic multinodular goiter
Toxic adenoma
Iodine-induced (Jod-Basedow)
Trophoblastic tumor
Increased TSH secretion

No Associated Hyperthyroidism†
Thyrotoxicosis factitia
Subacute thyroiditis
Thyroiditis with transient thyrotoxicosis (painless thyroiditis, silent thyroiditis, postpartum thyroiditis)
Ectopic thyroid tissue (struma ovarii, functioning metastatic thyroid cancer)

*Except for iodine-induced hyperthyroidism, associated with increased values of RAIU.
†Associated with decreased values of RAIU.
RAIU, radioactive iodine uptake; TSH, thyrotropin.

The increased force of cardiac contraction is often felt by the patient as palpitations and may be evident on inspection or palpation of the precordium. Because of the diffuse and forceful nature of the apex beat, the heart may seem enlarged but echocardiographic findings are usually normal. Heart sounds are loud and ringing, and a systolic or even a late diastolic or presystolic murmur (Means-Lerman scratch) may be present at the apex. A scratchy systolic sound along the left sternal border, resembling a pleuropericardial friction rub, may also be heard. These manifestations usually abate when a normal metabolic state is restored. Mitral valve prolapse occurs more frequently than in the normal population and may persist indefinitely.[2]

Cardiac arrhythmias are almost invariably supraventricular. Approximately 10% of patients with thyrotoxicosis have atrial fibrillation, and a similar percentage of patients with otherwise unexplained atrial fibrillation are thyrotoxic. In a study of more than 2000 individuals 60 years of age or older, atrial fibrillation developed in 28% of those with a suppressed thyrotropin (TSH, or thyroid-stimulating hormone) level.[3] Paroxysmal supraventricular tachycardia may be demonstrable or may be suggested by the history. Systolic time intervals are altered in thyrotoxicosis, the pulse-wave propagation is accelerated, the pre-ejection period is shortened, and the ratio of pre-ejection period to left ventricular ejection time is decreased.

The adequacy of the circulation is an important issue. The increased cardiovascular cost of a standard workload or metabolic challenge is adequately met if the patient is not or has not previously been in heart failure. Thus, *in most patients without underlying heart disease, cardiac competence is maintained.* Mild edema may occur in the absence of heart failure. Thyrotoxicosis may lead to congestive heart failure, but even so, the circulation time may remain short. Heart failure usually occurs in patients with preexisting heart disease, but it may not be possible to determine whether underlying heart disease is present until after thyrotoxicosis is relieved.

Atrial fibrillation decreases the efficiency of the cardiac response to any increased circulatory demand and may play a role in causing cardiac failure. Attempts to convert atrial fibrillation to sinus rhythm are usually of no avail while thyrotoxicosis is present. Regardless of the type of rhythm, the response to digitalis is decreased, possibly because of accelerated metabolism of the drug, and large quantities may be required to produce a clinical effect. Resistance to digitalis and failure of cardiac decompensation to respond to a usually adequate regimen should suggest the possibility of thyrotoxicosis. It is obviously important to deal definitively with thyrotoxicosis in a patient with concomitant heart disease.

Table 11–2. Manifestations of Thyrotoxicosis

Symptom	Percent	Sign	Percentage
Nervousness	99	Tachycardia*	100
Increased sweating	91	Goiter†	100
Hypersensitivity to heat	89	Skin changes	97
Palpitation	89	Tremor	97
Fatigue	88	Bruit over thyroid	77
Weight loss	85	Eye signs‡	71
Tachycardia	82	Atrial fibrillation	10
Dyspnea	75	Splenomegaly‡	10
Weakness	70	Gynecomastia	10
Increased appetite	65	Liver palms	8
Eye complaints‡	54		
Swelling of legs	35		
Hyperdefecation (without diarrhea)	33		
Diarrhea	23		
Anorexia	9		
Constipation	4		
Weight gain	2		

*In other studies, thyrotoxic patients with normal pulse rate have been observed.
†In our experience, enlargement of the thyroid may be lacking in fewer than 5% of patients with thyrotoxicosis.
‡These manifestations are much more common or, in the case of splenomegaly, exclusively present, in patients with Graves' disease.
Data from Williams RH. Thiouracil treatment of thyrotoxicosis. J Clin Endocrinol 1946; 6:1–22.

Sympathetic Nervous System

Many of the manifestations of thyrotoxicosis and sympathetic nervous system activation are similar. As judged from the plasma concentrations of epinephrine and norepinephrine, as well as their urinary excretion and that of their metabolites, the activity of the sympathetic nervous system is not increased in patients or animals with thyrotoxicosis, and thyroid hormones may exert effects separate from, but similar and additive to, those of the catecholamines. Consideration of the relationship between catecholamines and thyroid hormone excess and deficiency reveals the futility of attempting a generalization in this area.[4]

The reduction in heart rate and in some clinical manifestations of hyperthyroidism induced by β-blockade in patients with this condition has led to the concept of an increased sympathetic tone or increased cardiac sensitivity to the sympathetic nervous system. Careful studies have shown that this is clearly not the case in terms of the heart.[5, 6] Adequate β-adrenergic blockade reduces the basal level of cardiac output, but the slope of the epinephrine dose-response curve is not altered in hyperthyroidism. In other tissues, the situation may be even more complex and species differences may exist.

In hyperthyroid patients, there are no alterations in β-adrenergic receptor number on lymphocytes and no changes in lymphocyte β-adrenergic responsiveness, suggesting that clinical effects are direct on the target cell. However, the α_1-adrenergic receptor is down-regulated by thyroid hormone.[7]

In normal subjects given thyroid hormone for 10 days, the β-adrenergic receptor number in fat and skeletal muscle increased 60% and 30%, respectively, but metabolic and hemodynamic sensitivity to infused epinephrine in vivo were not altered.[8, 9] There was no evidence of increased glycemic, lipolytic, glycogenolytic, or ketogenic sensitivity to catecholamines, possibly because of a concomitant increase in endogenous insulin secretion that compensated for these changes.

Respiratory System

Dyspnea is common in severe thyrotoxicosis, and several factors may contribute to this condition. Vital capacity is commonly reduced; this reduction appears to result mainly from weakness of the respiratory muscles, but decreased pulmonary compliance may also play a role. During exercise, ventilation is increased out of proportion to the increase in oxygen uptake, although the diffusing capacity of the lung is normal. Pulmonary function returns to normal when a normal metabolic state is restored.

Alimentary System

An increase in appetite is common but is usually not seen in patients with mild disease. In severe disease, the increased intake of food is usually inadequate to meet the increased caloric requirements, and weight is lost at a variable rate. In the occasional, usually younger, patient with mild disease, however, weight gain may occur when caloric intake exceeds the metabolic demand. Anorexia, rather than hyperphagia, occurs in about one third of elderly thyrotoxic patients and contributes to the picture of *apathetic* thyrotoxicosis.

Stools are frequently soft and the frequency of bowel movements is increased, but diarrhea is rare. When constipation has preceded the development of thyrotoxicosis, bowel function may become normal. Anorexia, nausea, and vomiting are uncommon but may occur with severe disease. These symptoms, as well as abdominal pain, may be forerunners of accelerated thyrotoxicosis. The increased gastric emptying and intestinal motility in thyrotoxicosis appear to be responsible for slight malabsorption of fat, and these functions return to normal when a normal metabolic state has been restored. Celiac disease and Graves' disease may coexist, and a high proportion of patients have gastric achlorhydria. In most cases, acid secretion returns after relief of the thyrotoxicosis. Autoantibodies against gastric parietal cells are detectable in some patients with Graves' disease, and approximately 3% have pernicious anemia. In the oral glucose tolerance test, the glycemic peak is frequently delayed.

Hepatic dysfunction occurs, particularly when thyrotoxicosis is severe; hypoproteinemia and increases in serum alanine aminotransferase and alkaline phosphatase levels may be present. Hepatomegaly and jaundice occasionally develop. Splanchnic oxygen consumption is increased, whereas splanchnic blood flow is essentially unchanged. As a result, the arteriovenous oxygen difference across the splanchnic bed is increased; hence, hypoxia may contribute to hepatic dysfunction.[10] Hypoxia and the relative caloric deprivation may partly account for the depletion of hepatic glycogen that is evident both in the response to glycogenolytic agents and on direct analysis. In the absence of severe thyrotoxicosis or congestive heart failure, the liver usually appears normal on light microscopic examination. Ultramicroscopic examination of the liver reveals enlarged mitochondria and hypertrophic smooth endoplasmic reticulum. Graves' disease and autoimmune hepatitis may also coexist.

Nervous System

Alterations in nervous system function in patients with thyrotoxicosis are manifested by nervousness, emotional lability, and hyperkinesia. The nervousness is not typical of the patient who is chronically anxious but, rather, is characterized by restlessness, shortness of attention span, and a compulsion to be moving around, sometimes referred to as almost "levitating." Unlike the patient with neurocirculatory asthenia, the thyrotoxic patient wishes to be active but is hampered by fatigue and is tired from the neck down rather than from the top of the head down. Fatigue may be due both to muscle weakness and to the insomnia that is commonly present. In some patients, severe wasting and fatigue impair overall activity. Emotional lability causes patients to lose their temper easily and to have episodes of crying with only slight provocation. In rare cases, mental disturbance may be severe; manic-depressive, schizoid, or paranoid reactions may emerge.

The hyperkinesia of the thyrotoxic patient is characteristic. During the interview, the patient cannot sit still, may drum on the table, may tap a foot, or may shift positions frequently. Movements are quick, jerky, exaggerated, and often purposeless. In children, in whom such manifestations tend to be more severe, Sydenham's chorea may be suggested. Examination also reveals a fine, rhythmic tremor of the hands, tongue, or lightly closed eyelids. With the aid of a magnifying glass, a tremor of the eyeballs may be seen. The tremor may sometimes mimic that of parkinsonism, and a preexisting parkinsonian tremor can be accentuated. The electroencephalogram reveals an increase in fast-wave activity, and in patients with convulsive disorders, the frequency of seizures is increased.

The physiologic basis of these nervous system findings is not well understood; they may reflect increased adrenergic activity because some improvement occurs during treatment with adrenergic antagonists. The widespread distribution of thyroid hormone receptors in the brain makes it likely that alterations in cerebral metabolism are induced by thyroid hormone excess. Nevertheless, oxygen consumption by the brain is not altered.

Muscle

Weakness and fatigability are usually not accompanied by objective evidence of muscle disease except for the generalized wasting associated with loss of weight. Often the weakness is most prominent in the proximal muscles of the limbs, causing difficulty in climbing stairs or in maintaining the leg in an extended position. The latter maneuver can be employed to assess the degree of muscle weakness.

Occasionally, in severe untreated cases, muscle wasting that again tends to be proximal develops out of proportion to the overall loss of weight *(thyrotoxic myopathy)*. In the extreme form, the patient may be unable to rise from a sitting or lying position and may be virtually unable to walk. This disorder may resemble progressive muscular atrophy or polymyositis; however, fasciculation is absent, and little if any inflammatory change is evident on biopsy. Instead, the muscle is atrophic and infiltrated with fat cells and lymphocytes. Electron microscopy reveals abnormal mitochondria and dilatations of the myotubular system. Electromyograms reveal a decreased duration of action potentials and an increased number of polyphasic potentials. The biochemical basis of the muscle weakness is uncertain but may be related to the impaired ability to phosphorylate creatine.

Myopathy affects men with thyrotoxicosis more commonly than women and may overshadow the other manifestations of the syndrome. In the most severe forms, the myopathy may involve the more distal muscles of the extremities and the muscles of the trunk and face. Although myopathy of ocular muscles is unusual, the disorder may mimic myasthenia gravis or the ophthalmic form of myasthenia. Muscular strength returns to normal when a normal metabolic state is restored, but muscle mass takes longer to recover.

Graves' disease occurs in about 3% to 5% of patients with myasthenia gravis, and myasthenia gravis develops in about 1% of patients with Graves' disease. Antibodies and T cells specific for receptors—the TSH receptor (TSHR) and the acetylcholine receptor—are involved in the pathogenesis of the two diseases. Unlike thyrotoxic myopathy, the association of myasthenia gravis with Graves' disease has a distinct female preponderance. Although the effect of both thyrotoxicosis and its alleviation on the course of myasthenia gravis is variable, in most instances myasthenia is accentuated during the thyrotoxic state and improves when a normal metabolic state is restored.

Periodic paralysis of the hypokalemic type may occur together with thyrotoxicosis, and its severity is accentuated by the latter disorder. The coincidence of the two disorders is particularly common in Asian and Latino men.[11–14]

Skeletal System: Calcium and Phosphorus Metabolism

Thyrotoxicosis is generally associated with the following[15–17]:

1. Increased excretion of calcium and phosphorus in urine and stool.
2. Demineralization of bone, as demonstrated by routine bone densitometry.
3. Occasionally, pathologic fractures, especially in older women.

In these instances, the pathologic changes are variable and may include osteitis fibrosa, osteomalacia, and osteoporosis.

Urinary excretion of collagen breakdown products is increased, indicating increased turnover of collagen. Kinetic studies indicate an increase in the exchangeable calcium pool and acceleration of both bone resorption and accretion, particularly the former. The changes lead to decreased bone density and a propensity to hip fractures in later years. As thyrotoxicosis is treated, bone density may improve.[16, 18, 19] Postmenopausal women, however, may have a permanent reduction in bone density that may require treatment with agents that increase bone density (see Chapter 26).

Much controversy has existed over the induction of decreased bone density by thyroid hormone replacement therapy in hypothyroidism and thyroid hormone suppression therapy in patients with thyroid cancer. Suffice it to say that postmenopausal women who receive excessive thyroid hormone are at certain risk of bone damage, but careful replacement therapy does no harm to anyone.

Hypercalcemia can occur in patients with thyrotoxicosis. The total serum calcium concentration is increased in as many as 27% of patients, and the ionized serum calcium level is elevated in 47%.[20] The concentrations of heat-labile serum alkaline phosphatase and osteocalcin may also be elevated.[21] These findings resemble those of primary hyperparathyroidism, but the concentration of immunoreactive parathyroid hormone in serum is decreased in most thyrotoxic patients with hypercalcemia.[20] True primary hyperparathyroidism and thyrotoxicosis may sometimes coexist. Hypercalcemia may be severe enough to induce anorexia, nausea, vomiting, polyuria, and occasionally impairment of renal function. The alterations in calcium metabolism in thyrotoxicosis may be due to a direct effect of thyroid hormones in stimulating bone resorption and are reversed when the eumetabolic state is restored. Plasma 25-hydroxyvitamin D_3 (25-hydroxycholecalciferol) levels are decreased in thyrotoxic patients, and this alteration may contribute to the decreased intestinal absorption of calcium and osteomalacia noted in some patients.

Renal Function: Water and Electrolyte Metabolism

Thyrotoxicosis produces no symptoms referable to the urinary tract other than mild polyuria. Nevertheless, renal blood flow, glomerular filtration, and tubular reabsorptive rates are increased. Total amounts of body water and exchangeable potassium are decreased, possibly because of a decrease in lean body mass, but the amount of exchangeable sodium tends to be increased. Serum sodium, potassium, and chloride concentrations are normal. In patients with thyrotoxicosis, the level of exchangeable magnesium is normal, the serum magnesium concentration is often decreased, and urinary magnesium excretion is increased.

Hematopoietic System

Red blood cells are usually normal, as judged by the usual indices, but red blood cell mass is increased. The increase in erythropoiesis appears to be due both to the direct effect of thyroid hormones on the erythroid marrow and to increased production of erythropoietin. A parallel increase in plasma volume also occurs, resulting in a normal hematocrit value. Other abnormalities in thyrotoxicosis include a reduced content of zinc and carbonic anhydrase and an increased content of sodium in red blood cells, probably because the activity of Na^+,K^+-ATPase is impaired (in contrast with the increased Na^+,K^+-ATPase activity sometimes seen in other tissues).

Approximately 3% of patients with Graves' disease have pernicious anemia, and an additional 3% have antibodies to intrinsic factor but normal absorption of vitamin B_{12}. Autoantibodies against gastric parietal cells may also be present in patients with Graves' disease, and the requirements for vitamin B_{12} and folic acid appear to be increased. Rarely, thyrotoxicosis is associated with a mild hypochromic anemia characterized by adequate stores of iron in marrow and responsive to large doses of pyridoxine (vitamin B_6).

The total white blood cell count is often low because of a decrease in the number of neutrophils. The absolute lymphocyte count is normal or increased, leading to a relative lymphocytosis. The numbers of monocytes and eosinophils may also be increased. Splenic enlargement occurs in about 10% of the patients, and thymic and lymph node enlargement is common.[22] These abnormalities are thought to be a reflection of the autoimmune aspects of Graves' disease because they do not occur in thyrotoxicosis stemming from other causes.

Platelet levels and the intrinsic clotting mechanism are normal, but factor VIII concentrations are often elevated and return to normal when the thyrotoxicosis is treated.[23] Despite this elevation, there is an enhanced sensitivity to anticoagulants of the coumarin series because of accelerated clearance of the vitamin K–dependent clotting factors. Somewhat paradoxically, the dosage of such anticoagulants may have to be reduced in thyrotoxic patients and is increased in hypothyroid patients.[24] Coincidental autoimmune thrombocytopenia may also occur.

Pituitary and Adrenocortical Function

The thyrotoxic state imposes several challenges on pituitary and adrenocortical function. The inactivation of cortisol is accelerated, including reduction of the A ring, which is rapidly followed by conjugation, and oxidation of the 11-hydroxy group to a keto group as a result of an increase in 11-β-hydroxysteroid dehydrogenase (HSD) activity. As a result of these changes the disposal of cortisol is accelerated, but its rate of secretion is also increased, so the plasma cortisol concentration remains normal. The concentration of corticosteroid-binding globulin in plasma is normal. Urinary excretion of free cortisol and 17-hydroxycorticosteroids is normal or slightly increased, whereas urinary excretion of 17-ketosteroids may be reduced.[25, 26]

Basal pituitary-adrenal function is adequate, as indicated by normal plasma cortisol concentrations, and the response to an acute challenge, such as that imposed by insulin-induced hypoglycemia, is adequate. The rate of turnover of aldosterone is increased, but the plasma level is normal. Plasma renin activity is increased, and sensitivity to angiotensin II is reduced.

The response of plasma growth hormone concentration to insulin-induced hypoglycemia is subnormal, particularly in those with severe disease. This observation may not indicate deficient growth hormone production but, rather, may reflect depletion of pituitary stores from caloric inadequacy or accelerated removal of growth hormone from plasma. Incomplete suppression of plasma growth hormone concentration by induced hyperglycemia may also reflect prolonged caloric deprivation.

Reproductive Function

Thyrotoxicosis in early life may cause delayed sexual maturation, although physical development is normal and skeletal growth may be accelerated. Thyrotoxicosis after puberty influences reproductive function, especially in women. An increase in libido sometimes occurs in both men and women. The intermenstrual interval may be prolonged or shortened, and menstrual flow is initially diminished and ultimately ceases. Fertility may be reduced, and if conception takes place, the risk of miscarriage is increased. The association of thyroid autoantibodies and increased pregnancy loss is not related to changes in thyroid function[27]; the thyroid autoantibodies are thought to represent a marker of immune instability predisposing to pregnancy interruption, as seen in an animal model.[28]

In some patients, menstrual cycles are predominantly anovulatory with oligomenorrhea; in most patients, however, ovulation occurs, as indicated by a secretory endometrium. In the former situation, a subnormal midcycle surge of luteinizing hormone (LH) may be responsible. In premenopausal women with thyrotoxicosis, basal plasma concentrations of LH and follicle-stimulating hormone (FSH) are reportedly normal but may display enhanced responsiveness to gonadotropin-releasing hormone (GnRH).

Thyrotoxicosis, whether spontaneous or induced by triiodothyronine (T_3), is accompanied by an increase in the concentration of sex hormone–binding globulin in plasma. As a result, the plasma concentrations of total testosterone, dihydrotestosterone (DHT), and estradiol are increased, but their unbound fractions are normal or transiently decreased. The increased binding in plasma is responsible for the decreased metabolic clearance rate of testosterone and DHT. In the case of estradiol, however, the metabolic clearance rate is normal, suggesting that tissue metabolism of the hormone is increased.

Conversion rates of androstenedione to testosterone, estrone, and estradiol and of testosterone to DHT are increased. The increased rate of conversion of androgens to estrogens may be the mechanism of gynecomastia and erectile dysfunction in about 10% of thyrotoxic men and may be one mechanism of menstrual irregularities in women. Another more likely mechanism of menstrual changes is the disruption in amplitude and frequency of LH/FSH pulses due to thyroid hormone influences on GnRH signaling.

Catecholamines and Serotonin

Many effects induced by thyroid hormones are reminiscent of those induced by epinephrine, including tachycardia, increased cardiac output, and enhanced glycogenolysis, lipolysis, and calorigenesis (see earlier). Moreover, the fact that some of the manifestations of thyrotoxicosis—among them eyelid retraction, tremor, excessive sweating, and tachycardia—are at least partly alleviated by adrenergic antagonists has been interpreted as indicating that a state of increased adrenergic activity exists in the thyrotoxic organism. As discussed earlier, however, this apparent adrenergic hyperactivity appears to be a consequence of a direct effect of thyroid hormones on these tissues or due to decreased vagal tone.[4–8, 29–32] Plasma levels of epinephrine and norepinephrine are normal but 24-hour catecholamine secretion may be increased.[30, 33, 34]

Some manifestations of thyrotoxicosis, such as flushing, sweating, tachycardia, and gastrointestinal hypermotility, are also reminiscent of those of carcinoid syndrome. However, plasma serotonin levels, urinary 5-hydroxyindoleacetic acid excretion, and platelet monoamine oxidase activity are normal.

Energy (Protein, Carbohydrate, and Lipid) Metabolism

The stimulation of energy metabolism and heat production is reflected in the increased basal metabolic rate, increased appetite, and heat intolerance and in a sometimes slightly elevated basal body temperature.[35] Despite an increased food intake, a state of chronic caloric and nutritional inadequacy often ensues, depending on the degree of increased metabolism. Both synthesis and degradation of protein are increased (the latter to a greater extent than the former), with the result that there is a net decrease in tissue protein, as indicated by negative nitrogen balance, loss of weight, muscle wasting, weakness, and mild hypoalbuminemia. The oral glucose tolerance curve is often abnormal and varies from one in which the peak glycemia is increased and somewhat delayed to one that is frankly diabetic. Plasma insulin concentrations, however, are increased, suggesting insulin resistance. The pathogenesis of these alterations remains to be defined. Preexisting diabetes mellitus is exacerbated by thyrotoxicosis, one cause being increased degradation of insulin.

Both synthesis and degradation of triglycerides and of cholesterol are increased, but the net effect is one of lipid degradation, as reflected by an increase in the plasma concentration of free fatty acids and glycerol and a decrease in the serum cholesterol level; serum triglyceride levels are usually slightly decreased. Postheparin lipolytic activity is reported to be decreased in some studies and increased in others. The enhanced mobilization and oxidation of free fatty acids in response to fasting, catecholamines, and growth hormone are probably due to activation of adenylate cyclase and result in a tendency to ketosis and to fatty infiltration of the liver, depending on the degree of caloric deprivation.

Composite Clinical Picture and Laboratory Tests in Thyrotoxic States

The effects of thyrotoxicosis on the major organ systems are the same, regardless of the underlying cause. Their frequency and intensity and other findings with which they are associated are influenced by the nature of the underlying disorder. To a large extent, the same is true of laboratory test results. Consequently the clinical picture, laboratory features, and differential diagnosis are considered in relation to the specific etiologic mechanisms (see Table 11–1).

ROBERT GRAVES' DISEASE

Background

Robert Graves' disease, although first described by Parry in 1825,[36] is best known as *Graves' disease* in the English-speaking world and as *von Basedow's disease* on the continent of Europe because of the prominence of the disease reports by these eminent physicians. It is the most enigmatic and, in areas of iodine abundance, one of the most common of thyroid diseases.

Presentation

Graves' disease is characterized by diffuse goiter, thyrotoxicosis, infiltrative orbitopathy and ophthalmopathy, and occasionally infiltrative dermopathy. In the individual patient, thyroid disease and the infiltrative phenomena may occur singly or together but run courses that are largely independent. The thyroid component is closely related to autoimmune thyroiditis *(Hashimoto's disease)* in its pathogenesis and clinical course. In Graves' disease, hyperthyroidism occurs in the presence of some degree of chronic thyroiditis and may ultimately be replaced, in the long term, by thyroid hypofunction. Conversely, hyperthyroidism may occasionally supervene in patients with preexisting Hashimoto's thyroiditis.[37, 38] Both of these diseases may occur within the same family.

Autoimmune Characteristics

Autoimmune thyroid disease is characterized by the occurrence in the serum of antibodies against thyroid peroxidase (TPO) (the "microsomal" antigen), thyroglobulin (Tg), and the TSHR.[39] T-cell–mediated autoimmunity can also be demonstrated against the three primary thyroid antigens, as judged by a variety of criteria, including the ability of the T cells to elaborate various lymphokines and to exhibit a mitogenic response when exposed to thyroid antigens or to peptide sequences from the antigens. Autoimmune thyroid disease is also characterized by lymphocytic infiltration of the thyroid gland or remnant thyroid bed. In patients and their relatives, there is an increased frequency of other disorders of autoimmune origin, such as insulin-dependent diabetes mellitus, pernicious anemia, myasthenia gravis, adrenal atrophy, Sjögren's syndrome, lupus erythematosus, rheumatoid arthritis, and idiopathic thrombocytopenic purpura (see Chapter 37).

Circulating autoantibodies specific to hyperthyroid Graves' disease are directed against the TSHR (TSHRAbs) and behave as thyroid-stimulating antibodies.[40] These antibodies can compete for the binding of TSH to its specific receptor site in the cell membrane (Fig. 11–1) and can activate adenylate cyclase as TSH agonists (Fig. 11–2). Similar but distinct autoantibodies in the sera of some patients with autoimmune thyroiditis do not stimulate the thyroid cell and may block the ligand-binding site and act as TSH antagonists[41] (Fig. 11–3).

The thyroid gland itself is a site of thyroid autoantibody secretion in autoimmune thyroid disease via the B cells that form part of the intrathyroidal infiltrate. Transplantation of Graves' thyroid tissue into T cell–deficient and B cell–deficient mice with severe combined immunodeficiency (scid mice) results in the appearance of human thyroid autoantibodies, including TSHRAb, in the serum.[42] Additional evidence for a role of the thyroid itself in antibody production comes from animal models of thyroiditis and from the decline in thyroid autoantibody levels after antithyroid drug treatment,[43, 44] thyroidectomy, or radioiodine ablation.[45] After thyroidectomy and radioiodine treatment, however, some patients show no decline in autoantibody secretion, which suggests extrathyroidal sources of continued production.

Pathology

In patients with Graves' disease, the thyroid gland is characterized by a nonhomogeneous lymphocytic infiltration with an absence of follicular destruction (Fig. 11–4).[46] Antithyroid drug treatment may reduce the degree of infiltration.[47] Although the intrathyroidal lymphocyte population is mixed, most are T lymphocytes; B-cell germinal centers are less common than in

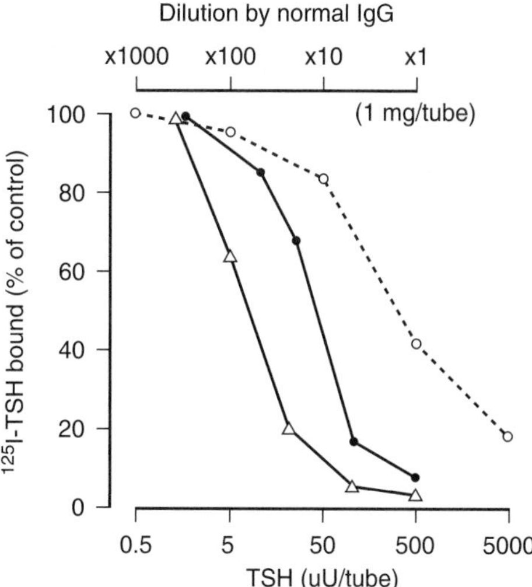

Figure 11–1. Inhibition of the binding of ^{125}I-labeled thyrotropin (TSH) to human thyroid TSH receptors by increasing concentrations of bovine TSH (○—○) and by increasing concentrations of immunoglobulin G (IgG)-containing TSH receptor antibodies referred to here as TSH-binding inhibitory immunoglobulin (TBII) activity (△—△ and ●—●. (From Endo K, Kashagi K, Konishi J, et al. Detection and properties of TSH-binding inhibitor immunoglobulins in patients with Graves' disease and Hashimoto's thyroiditis. J Clin Endocrinol Metab 1978; 46:734–739. © 1978, The Endocrine Society.)

autoimmune thyroiditis.[48] However, both intraepithelial T cells and plasma cells can be seen in peripolesis within the thyroid follicles.[48–50] Follicular epithelial cell size correlates with the intensity of the local infiltrate, suggesting local thyroid cell stimulation by TSHRAb.[51] Memory T cells may predominate within the T-cell population, but this finding can vary from patient to patient. Activated B-cell and T-cell markers are more frequent in intrathyroidal lymphocyte cultures than in peripheral blood cultures.

Prevalence

In the United States, the prevalence of Graves' disease is uncertain but is assumed to be similar to that of the one well-designed epidemiologic survey published. This survey came from Whickham, a small town in the northeast of England (~2800 in population), an area thought to be representative of the United Kingdom. The results indicated a prevalence of 2.7%, past and present, in women and a prevalence about one tenth as frequent in men. Overall, the incidence was estimated, in women, to be 1 case per 1000 per year over a 20-year follow-up.[52] Graves' disease is the most common cause of spontaneous hyperthyroidism in patients younger than 40 years of age, and the hazard rate does not change with age. The overall prevalence of autoimmune thyroid disease, comprising Graves' disease and autoimmune thyroiditis, approaches or exceeds that of diabetes mellitus (Table 11–3).

Pathogenesis

The Major Antigen of Graves' Disease—the Thyrotropin Receptor

The TSH receptor (TSHR) is G protein–linked with seven transmembrane domains and employs cyclic adenosine monophosphate (cAMP) and the phosphoinositol pathways for signal transduction.[40] The human TSHR (hTSHR) is the primary autoantigen of Graves' disease, as shown by the development of hyperthyroidism in mice and hamsters after immunization

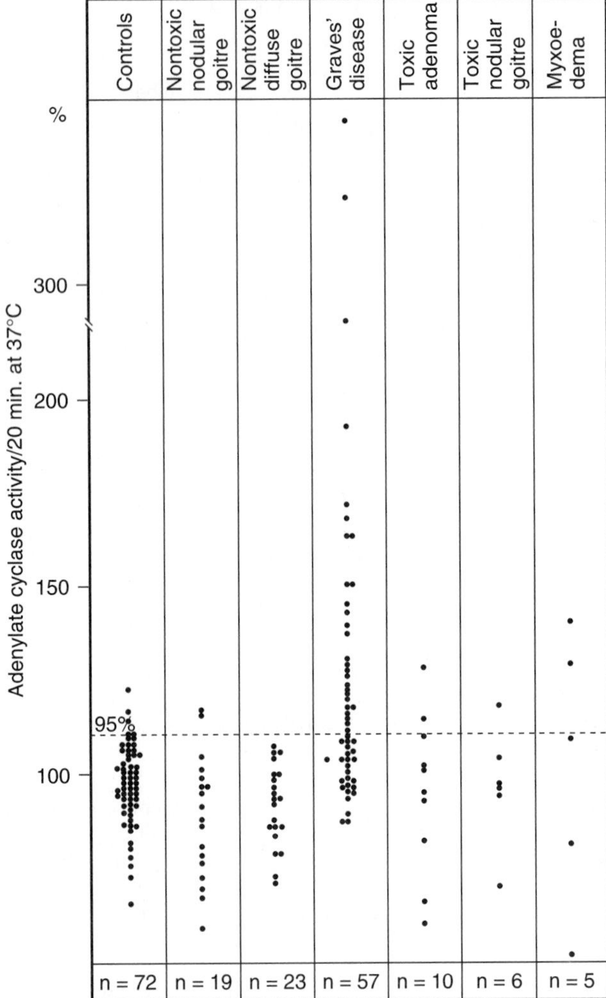

Figure 11–2. Stimulation of adenylate cyclase activity in human thyroid membranes by serum immunoglobulin G in normal control subjects and patients with thyroid disease. (From Bech K, Nistrup Madsen SN. Thyroid adenylate cyclase–stimulating immunoglobulins in thyroid disease. Clin Endocrinol 1979; 11:47–58.)

with hTSHR antigen (Fig. 11–5) (see also Color Plate).[53, 54] Putative extrathyroidal TSHR messenger RNA (mRNA) and receptor protein have been reported in many other tissues, including retro-orbital adipocytes, muscle cells, lymphocytes, and fibroblasts, but the physiologic and pathologic role of TSH receptors in these sites is still under investigation.[55, 56]

Molecular Biology of the Human Thyrotropin Receptor

Cloning of TSHR complementary DNA (cDNA) of animals and humans[57–59] made it possible to define the structure of the hTSHR gene and its chromosomal location (14q31).[60, 61] The hTSHR gene spans more than 60 kb and is split into 10 exons (Fig. 11–6). Seven hydrophobic transmembrane spanning regions in the hTSHR indicate that it is a member of the G protein–coupled receptor gene superfamily, and those receptors with large extracellular domains have been designated *subgroup B*. The hTSHR-specific mRNA of human thyroid consists of a major 4.3-kb transcript and additional smaller species, indicating that mRNA undergoes alternate splicing.[62]

Protein Structure of the Human Thyrotropin Receptor

The hTSHR holoreceptor consists of a 100-kd, glycosylated, 744–amino acid sequence and a 20–amino acid signal peptide. ProTSHR is cleaved into two subunits, α (or A) and β (or B), which are linked by disulfide bonds to form the physiologic receptor (Fig. 11–7)[63, 64] The 50-kd α subunit is water-soluble and may contain the TSH-binding site, previously referred to as long-acting thyroid stimulator (LATS)-absorbing activity (LAA).[65] The 30-kd β subunit is water-insoluble, contains the membrane spanning domain[40] with its three extracellular loops and three cytoplasmic loops, and is 70% to 75% homologous with the LH/human chorionic gonadotropin (hCG) receptor. Shedding of the α subunit has been suggested in vitro. The TSHR forms dimers and multimeric complexes on the thyroid cell surface, and these are of unclear physiologic significance.[66]

Autoantibodies to the Thyrotropin Receptor

In Graves' disease, TSHRAbs bind to the TSH receptor, activate adenylate cyclase, induce thyroid growth, increase vascularity, and cause an increased rate of thyroid hormone production and secretion (see Fig. 11–3).[40] TSHRAbs in patients with Graves' disease are referred to as *stimulating* or *agonist types of TSHRAbs*, as first described by Adams and Purves.[67, 68] Other varieties of TSHRAbs may also be present, namely a receptor antibody that acts as a TSH antagonist and referred to as *blocking TSHRAbs* or a *neutral* form of antibody with no functional effect on the receptor. Blocking TSHRAbs may be coincident with the stimulating type and may also predominate in certain patients after treatment with radioiodine, antithyroid drugs, or surgery. Blocking TSHRAbs can also be found in 15% of patients with autoimmune thyroiditis, particularly in patients without a goiter (the atrophic variety).[41] TSHRAbs are not detectable in the normal population with the use of currently available methods.

Bioactivity of Thyrotropin Receptor Autoantibody

The self-infusion of sera from patients with Graves' disease caused thyroid stimulation and was the first demonstration of the role of TSHRAbs in the induction of human hyperthyroidism.[69] Another example of the in vivo effects of TSHRAbs came from studies in neonates demonstrating the transplacen-

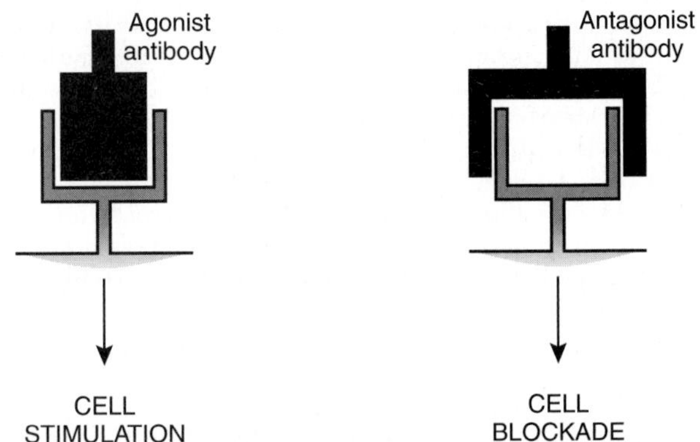

Figure 11–3. Schematic diagram of thyroid cell stimulation and blockade by antibodies to the thyrotropin-stimulating hormone receptor. Such autoantibodies may act as agonists or antagonists, depending on how they interact within the extracellular domain.

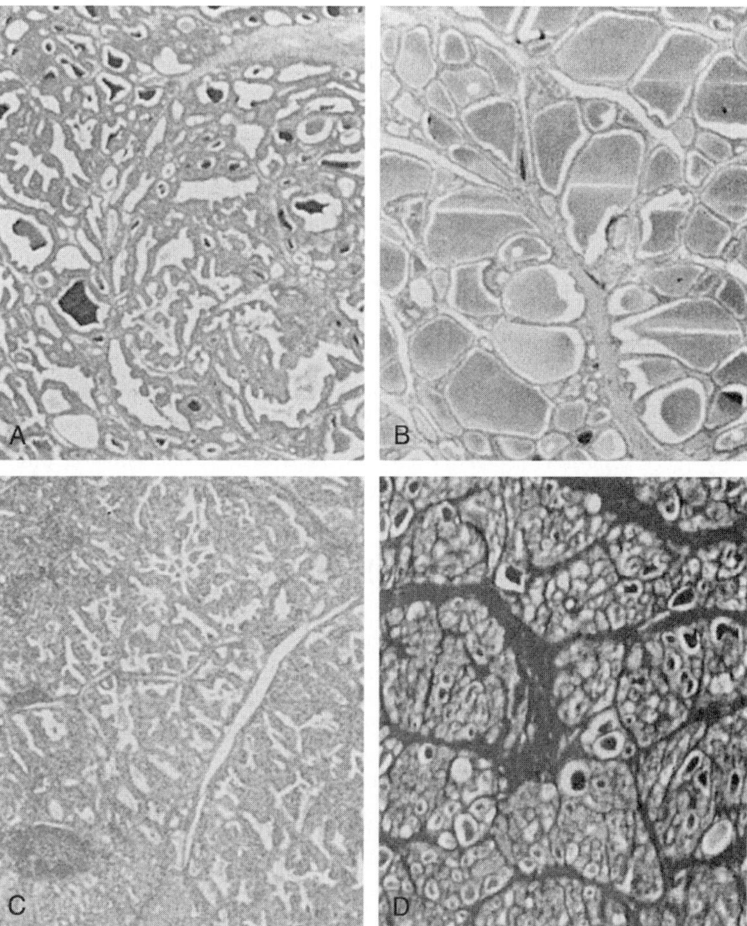

Figure 11–4. Section of thyroid gland of four patients with Graves' disease. *A*, Untreated. *B*, After therapy with potassium iodide for 3 weeks. *C*, After treatment with thiouracil for 5 weeks. *D*, Three months after three treatments with radioiodine. Note the marked hypertrophy and hyperplasia of the acinar cells and scant amount of colloid in sections *A*, *C*, and *D*. A lymph follicle is present in *C*. Note the broad bands of scar tissue in *D*. Section *B* is almost normal in appearance. Each patient, except the first one, was euthyroid at the time of thyroidectomy.

tal stimulation of the fetal thyroid in mothers with high titers of TSHRAbs.[70] TSHRAbs show light chain restriction in many patients with Graves' disease, and TSHRAbs that exhibit TSH agonist bioactivity are in the immunoglobulin G1 (IgG1) subclass; both observations suggest oligoclonality.[70, 71]

As discussed earlier, autoantibodies that bind to the TSHR may or may not activate adenylate cyclase and may thus be either TSHR-stimulating or TSHR-blocking (see Fig. 11–3).[41] Further complicating this issue is the fact that many patients have both TSHR-stimulating and TSHR-blocking antibodies; the degree of thyroid stimulation depends on the relative concentration and bioactivity of the different autoantibodies.[72]

Prevalence of Thyrotropin Receptor Autoantibodies in Graves' Disease

The fact that TSHRAbs are detectable only in patients with autoimmune thyroid disease indicates that the autoantibodies are disease-specific, in contrast with the high prevalence of Tg antibodies and TPO antibodies in the normal population. Furthermore, TSHRAbs are unique human autoantibodies and do not occur in natural animal disease. A total of 80% to 100% of untreated hyperthyroid patients with Graves' disease have detectable TSHRAbs with thyroid-stimulating activity. The levels of TSHRAbs are decreased by treatment of the disease[44] and, when they persist, are predictive of failure of response to antithyroid drug treatment.[73–75] With time, TSHR-blocking autoantibodies may become the prevalent type after treatment of Graves' disease.

Table 11–3. Incidence of Thyroid Dysfunction*

Status	Females	Males
Hypothyroidism	4.1	0.6
Hyperthyroidism	0.8	<0.1

*Per 1000 population per year over a 20-year period.
From Vanderpump MP, Tunbridge WM, French JM, et al. The incidence of thyroid disorders in the community: a 20-year follow-up of the Whickham Survey. Clin Endocrinol 1995; 43:55–68.

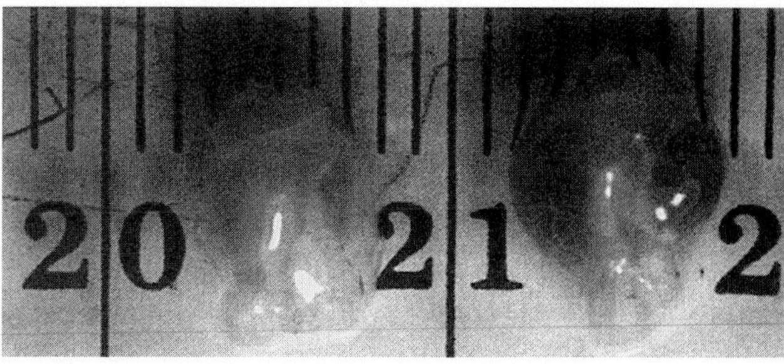

Figure 11–5. Thyroid glands from hyperthyroid mice immunized with fibroblasts expressing the human thyrotropin-stimulating hormone receptor. *Left*, A thyroid gland from a control mouse. *Right*, An enlarged thyroid from a hyperthyroid mouse. Ruler is in centimeters. (From Kita ML, Ahmad RC, Marians H, et al. Regulation and transfer of a murine model of thyrotropin receptor antibody–mediated Graves' disease. Endocrinology 1999; 140:1392–1398.) (See also Color Plate.)

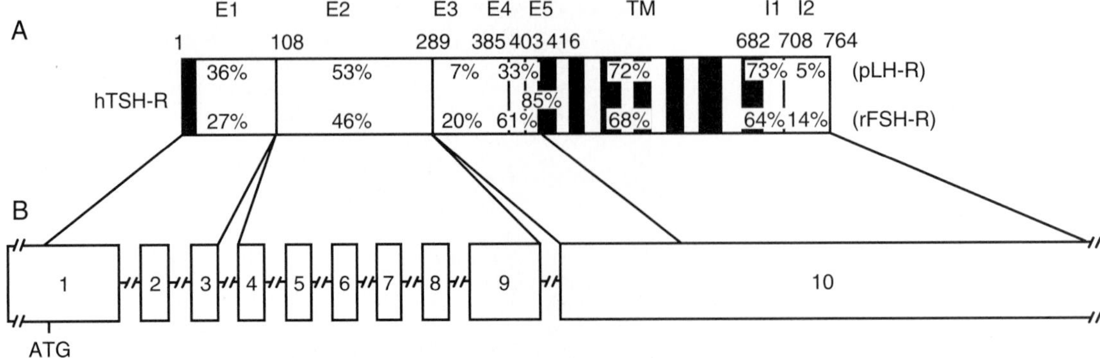

Figure 11–6. Human thyrotropin receptor (hTSH-R) exon structure. Outline structure of the TSHR *(A)* in comparison with the porcine luteinizing hormone receptor (pLH-R) and rat follicle-stimulating hormone receptor (rFSH-R) genes and *(B)* the exon/intron organization of the TSHR gene. *A* shows the similarity (%) between the hTSHR and the pLH and rFSH receptors, respectively. (From Gross B, Misrahi M, Sar S, et al. Composite structure of the human TSH receptor gene. Biochem Biophys Res Comm 1991; 177:679–687.)

Thyrotropin Receptor Autoantibody Epitopes

The extracellular domain of the TSHR is the major site of TSHRAb binding (see Fig. 11–7). The difference in functional activity of different TSHRAbs also depends on receptor conformation and affinity. The use of recombinant chimeric TSH/LH receptors has suggested at least two major regions of TSHRAb binding that may convey thyroid-stimulating activity (the N-terminal end) and thyroid-blocking activity (the C-terminal end)[76, 77]; however, the situation is probably more complex than this. Prokaryotic TSHR–extracellular domain has also been used to identify immunogenic regions using antibodies from immunized mice and from patients with Graves' disease.[78] These data suggested that some TSHRAbs may also recognize linear epitopes, but these may be neutral rather than pathologic antibodies.

Control of Thyrotropin Receptor Function in Graves' Disease

Like TSH, TSHRAbs cause cAMP-mediated generation of thyroid hormone and Tg, uptake and release of iodine, stimulation of protein synthesis, and cell growth. Desensitization of the thyroidal cAMP response by prolonged exposure to TSHRAbs can be observed in vitro but cannot be complete in vivo, or else patients would not remain hyperthyroid.[79, 80] At lower levels of stimulation, the TSHR is positively regulated by TSH both in vivo and in vitro,[81, 82] and such resistance to desensitization by low levels of TSH may allow the hyperthyroid state to persist.

Principles of Antigenic Recognition

Antibodies interact with either *linear* (conformationally independent) or *nonlinear* (conformationally dependent) areas of a target molecule called the *epitope*. The strength of the binding of antibodies to target antigen (affinity of the antibody) depends largely on the number of binding sites the antibody has with the antigen. These sites contribute to the binding energy, which is therefore likely to be greater for large nonlinear epitopes than for small linear peptides.[83] High-affinity antibodies are thus most likely to interact with nonlinear epitopes and to depend on the natural conformation of the target molecule.

The T-cell receptor is also a member of the Ig receptor superfamily[84] but interacts only with a complex of antigen and HLA molecule. The $CD8^+$ T cells recognize target antigen complexed with HLA class I molecules (A, B, and C), and $CD4^+$ T cells recognize antigen complexed with HLA class II molecules (D, P, and Q). The antigen that interacts with T cells when complexed with autologous HLA molecules is a ~15–amino acid linear peptide derived from the whole antigen molecule.[85] Thyroid antigens are endocytosed by antigen-presenting cells (APCs), such as macrophages and dendritic cells; peptide breakdown products are then bound to HLA molecules, and the entire complex is transported to the cell surface where the peptide lies within a clearly defined binding groove within the HLA molecule.[86]

In addition to the recognition of antigen (the first immune cell signal), immune cells (both T and B) also depend on secondary signals to enter an active proliferative and secretory state.[87] Cytokines originating from T cells serve as secondary B-cell signals. Important second signals for the T cells include the CD80 (B7) family of cell surface molecules found on APCs (e.g., macrophages and dendritic cells) that combine with CD28 on the T-cell surface and the CD40/CD40 ligand interaction, where CD40 is found more often on nonprofessional APCs (e.g., fibroblasts and thyroid cells).[88] B cells and T cells

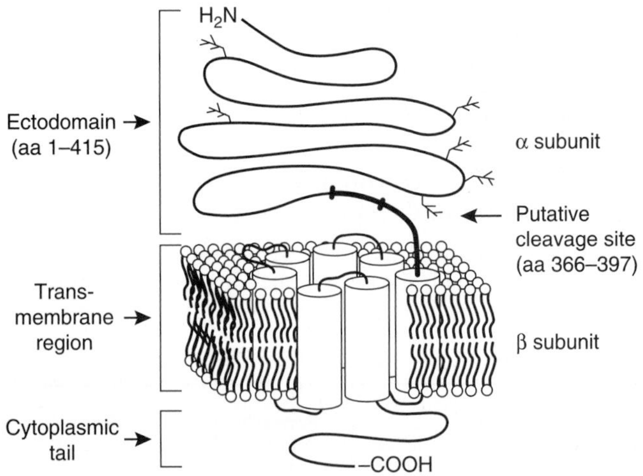

Figure 11–7. A current model of the human thyrotropin-stimulating hormone receptor structure. The TSHR has seven transmembrane domains, a large extracellular domain, and a small intracellular domain. The receptor is cleaved, probably after activation, into A (or α) and B (or β) subunits. The α subunit is thought to be shed from the cell surface.

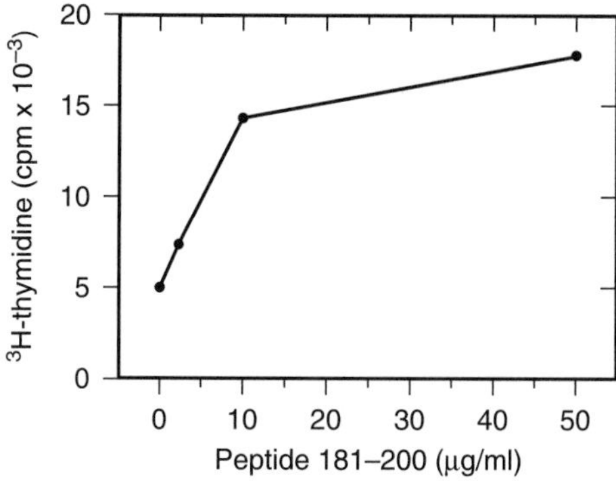

Figure 11–8. T cells from a patient with Graves' disease demonstrate a dose-related proliferative response to a thyrotropin-stimulating hormone receptor peptide (aa 181–200). Data shown as ^{3}H-thymidine uptake at 18 hours.

that interact with specific antigen in the absence of a second signal may be *deleted* by apoptosis or may survive in a state of *anergy* (i.e., desensitized). Hence, deletion and anergy combine to help define the repertoire of immune responses in an individual.

The Autoimmune Response

It is helpful to know whether autoimmune reactions are *multireactive* (representative of a secondary polyclonal immune response) or more *focused*, involving a restricted number of B cells and T cells.[89] In autoimmune disease, a restricted immune response has been observed at the onset of the disease. The following discussion presents some of the evidence for this in Graves' disease.

Intrathyroidal T Cells

As described earlier, T cells in patients with autoimmune thyroid disease are reactive to thyroid antigens and to peptides derived from these antigens (Fig. 11–8).90[89–94] About 10% of activated T cells infiltrating the thyroid gland in patients with autoimmune thyroid disease proliferate in response to thyroid cell antigens.[95] Intrathyroidal T cells from patients with Graves' disease exhibit characteristics of helper T-cell subset 1 (Th1) (which secrete interleukin-2 [IL-2] and interferon α) and Th2 (which secrete IL-4).[96] Such T-cell populations enhance thyroid autoantibody secretion. Memory T cells enhance thyroid autoantibody secretion and may have both helper and cytotoxic (apoptosis-inducing) T-cell activity. The thyroid gland in patients with Graves' disease exhibits a small degree of apoptosis.[97–99]

T-Cell Receptor V Gene Repertoire

T-cell receptors (TCRs) consist of two noncovalently linked chains (α and β, or, less commonly, γ and δ), each with variable (V), diversity (D, mainly β), and junctional (J) regions (Fig. 11–9). The V, D, and J genes code for the antigen recognition sites on the TCR that determine antigen specificity. In addition to the many V (>100) and J (>50) genes, random nucleotide (N) additions and deletions to the D region (the CDR3 region or NDN region) provide additional complexity to the TCR repertoire.[84, 100] Studies of the V_α and V_β families expressed by intrathyroidal T cells from patients with Graves' disease[101, 102] have demonstrated that human TCR V gene expression by T cells from within the thyroid gland differed from hTCR V gene expression found in peripheral blood from the same individuals. Additional evidence has been obtained in the thyroid gland for the presence of clonally expanded T cells based on the presence of multiple identical sequences within the generated fragments.[103–106] Such information further documents that Graves' disease is an antigen-driven disorder that causes oligoclonal T-cell expansion. Similar data have been obtained in rheumatoid arthritis, multiple sclerosis, and other autoimmune diseases.[107, 108]

Regulatory T Cells

The presence of reduced levels of circulating CD8+ (suppressor/cytotoxic) T cells in patients with Graves' disease suggested that a lack of suppressor/cytotoxic T cells might be responsible for the breakdown of tolerance in Graves' disease.[109] However, thyroid hormone excess itself may give rise to changes in T-cell numbers.[110] The immune system does exert some of its overall control via "regulatory" cells, including the secretion of T-cell cytokines and the suppressive influence of "anergized" T cells. In addition to these regulatory cells, other important mechanisms include both positive and negative selection of T cells and B cells in the thymus, and deletion of immature immune cells via antigen-initiated apoptosis, which takes place in the peripheral immune system.[111, 112] Deletion probably occurs when T cells and B cells see antigen in the absence of second signals (see earlier). When a mature immune cell sees antigen in the absence of second signal, it may become desensitized rather than deleted, a phenomenon known as *anergy*. Together, deletion, anergy, and apoptosis account for immunosuppression. However, certain HLA-DR haplotypes are associated with reduced suppressor T-cell function. For example, normal individuals with HLA-DR3 have reduced suppressor activity compared with non-DR3 individuals.[113, 114]

The Insult

Initiation is thought to occur with an insult that leads to an immune response (Fig. 11–10). This may take the form of a direct insult to the thyroid gland by a viral infection or another external influence, including trauma leading to activation of T cells[115, 115a] or may be initiated elsewhere in the body. In

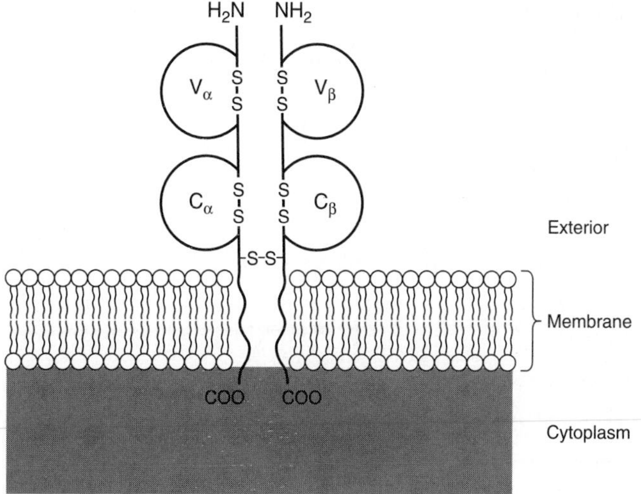

Figure 11–9. Schematic diagram of a T-cell receptor dimer showing the alpha and beta chains retained by transmembrane regions. V, variable region; C, constant region. (From Davis MM, Chien YH, Gascoigne NR, et al. A murine T cell receptor gene complex. Immunol Rev 1984; 81:235–258.)

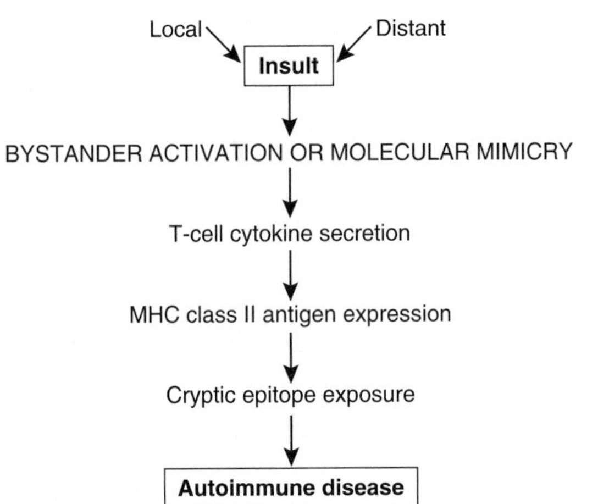

Figure 11–10. Possible mechanisms involved in the cause and precipitation of Graves' disease. MHC, major histocompatibility complex.

the latter case, it would be the arrival of activated T cells in the thyroid gland that would start the process. Such an arrival may be nonspecific because the same T cells may arrive in many glands but the patient has a particular susceptibility to autoimmune thyroid disease (see "Risk Factors" later).

Bystander Activation

Evidence has mounted from a model of insulitis that bystander activation of local resident antigen-specific T cells may initiate autoimmunity.[116] The presence of activated T cells within the thyroid gland following an insult may induce, via cytokine secretion, the activation of local thyroid-specific T cells. This series of events can occur only in a susceptible individual with the right immune repertoire. Bystander activation would arise from any activated T cells within the thyroid gland, which may be activated by many different infections and antigens unrelated to the thyroid gland itself. The attractiveness of this model is that many different types of infections would lead to the same clinical disease phenotype. There is much evidence for residual thyroid-resident T cells in the glands of patients with Graves' disease.[104]

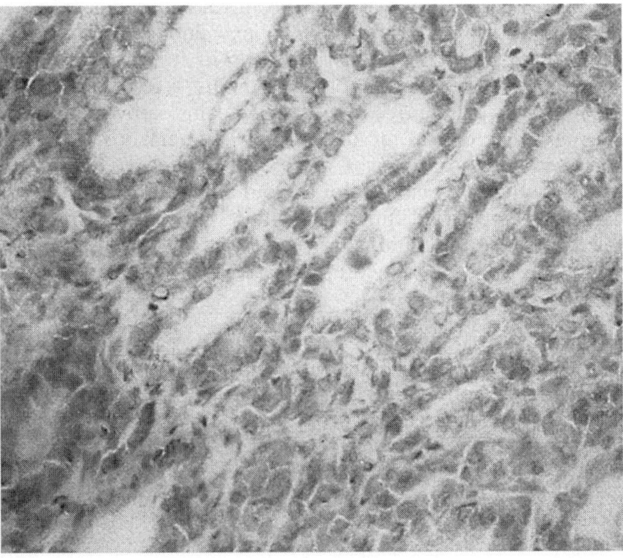

Figure 11–11. Photomicrograph of Graves' thyroid tissue stained for HLA class II (DR) antigen expression using the immunoperoxidase technique. Note the brown thyroid epithelial cells indicating the presence of DR antigen. Note also the relative lack of lymphocytic infiltration in this region. (See also Color Plate.)

Molecular Mimicry (Specificity Crossover)

In addition to the effects of the direct release of cytokines from T cells activated elsewhere via the bystander effect, intrathyroidal T cells may become activated in another nonspecific way. Structural similarity between different antigens can lead to specificity crossover (or *molecular mimicry*). Antigenic similarity between bacteria and viruses and human proteins is common, and in one study 4% of monoclonal antibodies raised against a variety of viruses cross-reacted with antigens in tissues.[117] Furthermore, mice infected with reovirus type 1 developed an autoimmune polyendocrinopathy with autoantibodies directed against normal pancreas, pituitary, thyroid, and gastric mucosa, suggesting molecular mimicry between a reoviral antigen and a common tissue antigen.[118] Molecular mimicry has also been reported between *Yersinia enterocolitica* and the TSHR based on the observed cross-reaction between sera from patients with *Yersinia* infection and sera from patients with Graves' disease and between retroviral sequences and the TSH receptor.[119]

Thyroid Cell Involvement by Aberrant Expression of Class II HLA Antigens

Normal thyroid epithelial cells do not express HLA class II antigens, but they are expressed in thyroid glands from patients with autoimmune thyroid disease (Fig. 11–11) (see also Color Plate).[120] As proposed by Hanafusa and colleagues,[121] a local insult, such as a viral infection of the thyroid gland, can cause production of interferon γ or other cytokines in the thyroid gland, which in turn would induce HLA class II expression. This first-time expression would lead to enhanced presentation of thyroid autoantigens to the immune system and activation of local autoreactive thyroid-specific T cells in a susceptible individual. Support for this concept comes from the in vivo induction of MHC class II molecules on mouse thyrocytes by interferon γ that also induced autoimmune thyroiditis[122] and the demonstration of the necessity for MHC class II antigen expression on TSH receptor expressing fibroblasts used in the induction of Graves' disease in mice.[123] A number of viruses may also induce MHC class II expression independent of immune cell cytokine secretion,[124] including reovirus types 1 and 3[125] and cytomegalovirus.[126]

Cryptic Antigenic Epitopes

T-cell tolerance depends on the visualization of self-antigens in sufficient amounts to initiate continuous T-cell deletion and anergy induction. However, many molecules are not seen in sufficient concentrations to cause the removal of T cells that may react to them. These antigens contain what are sometimes called *cryptic epitopes*. Hence, T cells specific for these cryptic epitopes may be present in normal immune repertoires. They may then induce autoaggressive T cells if such an epitope is uncovered or increased in concentration by a local insult. HLA class II antigen expression in a situation where it normally does not occur, such as the thyroid epithelial cell, would then allow the presentation of these normally cryptic thyroid antigens to local autoreactive T cells if they are present.

Risk Factors for Graves' Disease

Genetic Susceptibility

The development and the subsequent course of Graves' disease are greatly influenced by heredity. The role of hereditary factors is evidenced by the increased incidence in members of patients' families of other autoimmune disorders, such as Hashimoto's disease, insulin-dependent diabetes (type 1) or pernicious anemia, and of autoantibodies against endocrine tissues, gastric parietal cells, and intrinsic factor. Indeed, the propensity for development of thyroid autoantibodies appears to be an autosomal dominant trait linked to the *CTLA4* gene that codes for a modulator of the second signal to T cells, as discussed earlier.[79, 127] In addition, monozygotic twins have a higher concordance rate of Graves' disease than do dizygotic twins,[128] and this is true despite the rearrangement of B-cell and T-cell V genes that cause the immune repertoires of identical twins to differ (see also Chapter 37).

Hence, Graves' disease appears to be an oligogenic disorder with a number of genetic loci that may contribute to disease susceptibility. However, no thyroid-specific genes have been found to be involved, and only chromosomal loci, not actual genes, have been linked to the disease.[129, 130] There is an increased frequency of the HLA DR3 and DQA10501 haplotypes in whites with Graves' disease, although the HLA region provides less than 5% of the genetic susceptibility because it is associated but not linked.[131–134]

Infection

It is not known whether a specific infection initiates Graves' disease. If infection were the cause of Graves' disease, an identifiable agent should be present in most patients, and transfer of the agent to susceptible recipients should transfer the disease. It has been suggested that Graves' disease is "associated" with infectious agents (e.g., *Y. enterocolitica*),[135, 136] but no studies meet the necessary criteria to prove this. Infections of the thyroid gland itself (e.g., subacute thyroiditis, congenital rubella) are associated with thyroid autoimmune phenomena.[115] Nevertheless, a causative role of infectious agents has not been definitively demonstrated in Graves' disease, although thyroid disease can be induced in experimental animals by certain viral infections.[115, 137] Reports of retroviral sequences in the thyroid glands of patients with Graves' disease[138–140] have not been confirmed.[138, 141, 142]

Stress

Graves' disease commonly appears to become evident either after severe emotional stress, such as the actual or threatened separation from a loved one, or after an acute fright, such as an automobile accident. There are, in fact, many clinical experiences and reports associating major stress with the onset of Graves' disease, including data on the high incidence of thyrotoxicosis among refugees from Nazi prison camps.[143] Some data suggest that stress induces an overall state of immune suppression by nonantigen-specific mechanisms,[144] perhaps secondary to the effects of cortisol and corticotropin-releasing hormone action at the level of the immune cell. Furthermore, more patients with Graves' disease are said to give a history of major stress in the 12 months before disease onset compared with control groups.[145–147]

Following the acute immune suppression by stress, there is presumably an overcompensation by the immune system when the suppression is released. This would then precipitate autoimmune thyroid disease, as in the postpartum period during which Graves' disease may occur 3 to 9 months after delivery.[80, 148] The rebound phenomenon would result in greater immune activity than normal and would initiate disease if the individual were genetically susceptible.

Gender and Gonadal Steroids

Graves' disease is more common in women than in men (7 to 10:1) and tends to become more prevalent after puberty (see Table 11–3). The female preponderance and the fact that the disorder is uncommon before puberty have suggested that gonadal steroids may be responsible for this difference. Indeed, androgens may suppress experimental autoimmune thyroiditis.[149] Estrogen has been shown to influence the immune system, particularly the B-cell repertoire, and may be a reason for this susceptibility.[150, 151] However, Graves' disease continues to occur after the menopause and is still seen in men. In fact, when the disease develops in men, it tends to occur at a later age, to be more severe, and to be accompanied more often by ophthalmopathy. Such observations have suggested that perhaps it is the X chromosome rather than sex steroids that is the responsible element in female susceptibility. Women have two X chromosomes and, therefore, would receive twice the gene dose. A locus on the X chromosome has indeed been linked to Graves' disease, but the gene responsible has not yet been located. The phenomenon of X-gene inactivation has also been invoked in autoimmune disease.[152] Female cells may inactivate different X chromosomes, leading to potentially differing gene expression between somatic cells and immune cells.

Pregnancy

Graves' disease is uncommon during pregnancy because hyperthyroidism is associated with reduced fertility and increased pregnancy loss. In addition, pregnancy is a time of immunosuppression, so that the disease tends to improve as pregnancy progresses.[153, 154] Both T-cell and B-cell functions are diminished, and the rebound from this immunosuppression may contribute to the development of postpartum thyroid disease.[80] As many as 30% of young women give a history of pregnancy in the 12 months before the onset of Graves' disease,[155] indicating that postpartum Graves' disease is a surprisingly common presentation and that pregnancy is a major risk factor in susceptible women.

Iodine and Drugs

Iodine and iodine-containing drugs, such as amiodarone, may precipitate Graves' disease or its recurrence in a susceptible individual. Iodine is most likely to precipitate thyrotoxicosis in an iodine-deficient population simply by allowing TSHRAbs to be effective in stimulating more thyroid hormone to be formed. Whether there is any other precipitating event is unclear. Iodine may also damage thyroid cells directly and release thyroid antigens to the immune system.[156, 157]

Irradiation

There is no evidence that radiation exposure itself is a risk factor for Graves' disease. However, there is evidence that thyroid autoantibodies are more prevalent in the radiation-exposed population and thus this fact should be considered.[158, 159] In addition, radioactive iodine (RAI) treatment may cause the onset or worsening of clinical ophthalmopathy, but often this is transient (see later).[160]

Pathogenesis of Graves' Orbitopathy and Dermopathy

The pathogenesis of the orbitopathy and dermopathy is now better understood than ever before. The extraocular muscle and adipose tissue are swollen by the accumulation in the extracellular matrix of glycosaminoglycans that are secreted by fibroblasts under the influence of cytokines such as interferon γ from local lymphocytes (Figs. 11–12 and 11–13) (see also Color Plate).[160–162] This accumulation disrupts and impairs the function of muscle. As the disease runs its course and inflam-

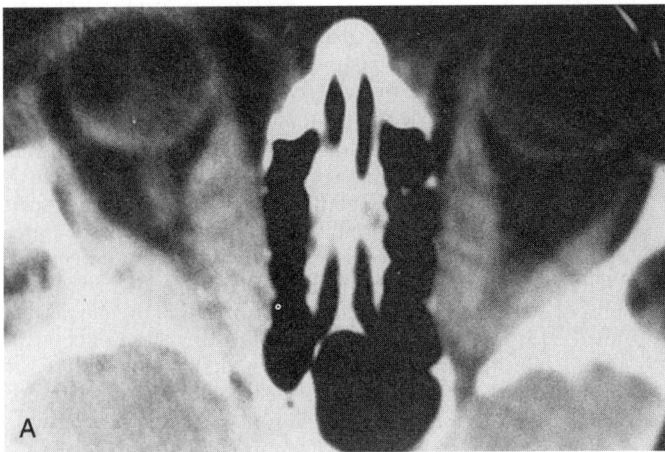

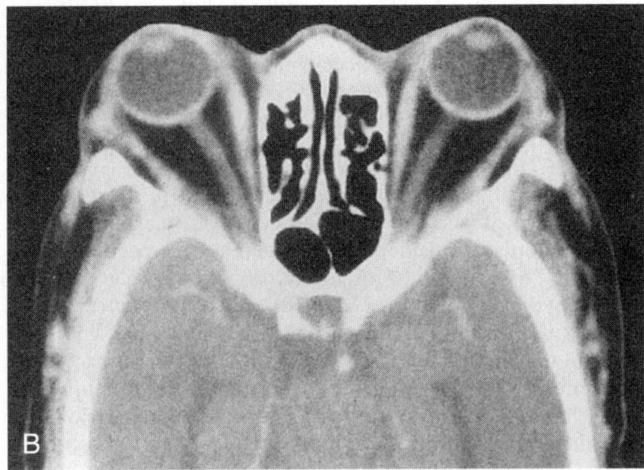

Figure 11–12. CT scans of orbits in two patients with Graves' orbitopathy. *A*, Note the obviously grossly swollen medial rectus extraocular muscles in both orbits and the resulting proptosis. *B*, The patient shows considerable proptosis with only minimal muscle enlargement, suggesting the presence of a large amount of retro-orbital fat. (Courtesy of Dr. Peter Som, New York, NY.)

mation decreases, the damaged muscles become fibrosed. Hence, histologic examination shows a patchy muscle infiltrate predominantly of T cells, and some muscle cells exhibit HLA class II antigen as seen within the thyroid gland. Such T cells react in vitro with retro-orbital tissue.[163] The antigen to which they react may be the TSH receptor itself.

The TSHR mRNA and protein are expressed in fibroblasts and adipocytes and in many other cells.[56] However, retro-orbital tissues seem to express more TSHR than other sites, and/or the TSHR-specific T cells have a propensity for the retro-orbital tissues. Whatever the mechanism, the current working hypothesis is that the immune system recognizes an antigen common to the thyroid gland and retro-orbital tissues (and skin) and is likely to be the TSHR itself, the main antigen of Graves' disease. Furthermore, patients with the most severe orbitopathy have the highest titers of TSHRAbs, and the level of TSHRAbs correlates with the severity of the eye disease. There is currently no convincing evidence that specific antibodies against orbital tissue contents play a primary pathogenic role. More likely, antigen-specific T cells have the major role in initiating the disorder. However, such antibodies may serve as markers of extraocular muscle inflammation.[164]

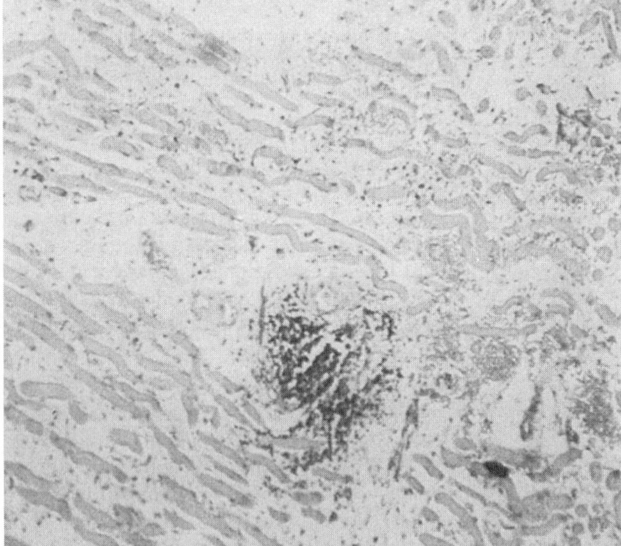

Figure 11–13. Section of extraocular muscle from a biopsy taken from a patient with severe Graves' orbitopathy. Note that within the muscle fibers is a patch of lymphocytic infiltration. (Courtesy of Dr. D. Kendler, University of British Columbia, Vancouver, Canada.) (See also Color Plate.)

Risk Factors in Ophthalmic Graves' Disease

There is no evidence that a separate and distinct genetic risk can be ascribed to severe ophthalmic Graves' disease, suggesting that it is mainly environmental factors that lead to the enhanced retro-orbital inflammation in some patients.[164a] All of the same risk factors (e.g., infection, stress, gender and gonadal steroids, pregnancy, and drugs) apply to the onset of both thyroid and eye involvement in Graves' disease.

For example, it is well known that eye disease in men may be worse than expected.[165] However, there are two distinct risk factors that deserve attention. The first is smoking, which may increase the risk for ophthalmic involvement in many studies, perhaps by causing anoxia or simply direct inflammation.[166–168] The second is radioiodine, which in controlled clinical trials accentuates ophthalmic Graves' disease.[169, 170] However, this worsening is typically mild and transient and can be ameliorated with corticosteroid treatment for the subsequent 3 to 4 months. For this reason, some physicians are reluctant to prescribe radioiodine to patients with severe eye disease unless the patients are receiving corticosteroids.

Natural History and Course of Graves' Disease

The course of the thyrotoxic component of Graves' disease is variable and often erratic. In some patients, thyrotoxicosis persists, although it may vary in severity. In others, the course may be cyclic, exhibiting remissions of varying frequency, intensity, and duration. This cyclic feature has an important bearing on treatment. With the passage of months or years, thyrotoxicosis tends to give way to euthyroidism. Approximately one third of patients become hypothyroid within 20 years of treatment with antithyroid agents.[171]

The orbitopathy may or may not commence together with the thyrotoxic component. Thus, thyrotoxic patients may initially be free from eye disease but are affected by it months or years later or not at all. Conversely, Graves' disease may begin

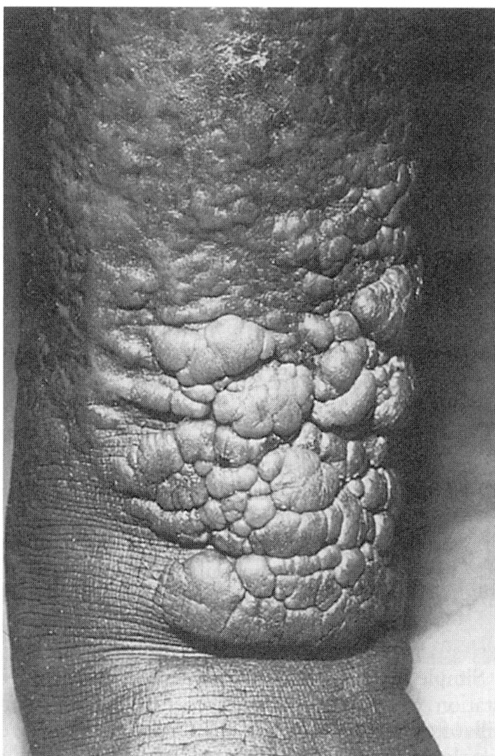

Figure 11–14. Chronic pretibial myxedema in a patient with Graves' disease and orbitopathy. The lesions are firm and nonpitting, with a clear edge to feel. (Courtesy of Dr. Andrew Werner, New York, N.Y.) (See also Color Plate.)

with orbitopathy and only later, if at all, be associated with thyrotoxicosis. In euthyroid patients with orbitopathy, so-called euthyroid Graves' disease, evidence of a thyroid abnormality, as judged from thyroid function tests and tests for TSHRAbs and other thyroid autoantibodies is common. Some such patients become hypothyroid within a few years, some become hyperthyroid, and a few remain euthyroid. Many euthyroid patients do have evidence of chronic thyroiditis.[172] The course of thyroid function in many of these patients is therefore unpredictable.

Histopathology

Thyroid Gland

The older designation for Graves' disease, *diffuse toxic goiter*, denoted that the gland was both enlarged and uniformly affected. The gland might vary in consistency from softer than normal to firm and rubbery. The outer surface is usually smooth but may be somewhat lobular; rarely, the gland is grossly nodular prior to treatment. The cut surface is red and glistening. Microscopically, the follicles are small and lined with hyperplastic columnar epithelium and contain scant colloid that displays much marginal scalloping and vacuolization (see Fig. 11–4). Nuclei are vesicular and basally located and exhibit occasional mitoses. Papillary projections of the hyperplastic epithelium extend into the lumina of the follicles. Vascularity is increased, and there is a varying infiltration by lymphocytes and plasma cells that collect in aggregates and may form germinal centers. In such regions, thyroid epithelial cells express HLA class II antigens not seen in normal thyroid glands and are large, perhaps due to local stimulation by TSHRAbs (see Fig. 11–11).

When the patient is given iodine or antithyroid drugs, the thyroid gland may undergo *involution* if TSHRAbs decrease. Then hyperplasia and vascularity regress, papillary projections recede, and follicles enlarge and become filled with colloid once again.

Eyes

In patients with infiltrative orbitopathy, the volume of orbital contents is increased because of an increase both in retrobulbar connective tissue and in extraocular muscle mass (see Fig. 11–11). Some of the increase in connective tissue is due to edema resulting from accumulation in the ground substance of hyaluronic acid and chondroitin sulfates, which are hydrophilic.[173] The extraocular muscles are swollen, and some fibers exhibit loss of striation, fragmentation, and lymphocytic infiltration. The lacrimal glands may also be involved. Ultimately, the tissues fibrose.

Skin

Dermopathy (Fig. 11–14) (see also Color Plate) is usually a late manifestation, and 99% of patients with infiltrative dermopathy have Graves' orbitopathy.[174] The content of hyaluronic acid and chondroitin sulfates in the dermis is increased, presumably by lymphokine activation of fibroblasts, causing compression of the dermal lymphatics and nonpitting edema[175]; the collagen fibers are separated and fragmented, and early lesions contain lymphocytic infiltrate. TSH receptor expression can be demonstrated in fibroblasts and adipocytes,[176] and TSHRAbs are high. Nodule and plaque formation may occur in chronic lesions. The cause of the characteristic location of the dermopathy is unclear but, presumably, depends on trauma to the exposed areas.

Pathophysiology

In patients with Graves' disease, all aspects of thyroid hormone economy are abnormal, including disruption of the regulatory control of thyroid function; alterations in thyroid function itself; changes in the concentration, binding, and metabolism of thyroid hormones; and manifestations of thyroid hormone excess in the peripheral tissues. Abnormalities in these parameters also occur in other forms of thyrotoxicosis but may differ in kind or amount.

An abnormality or override of normal regulatory control is inherent in all forms of thyrotoxicosis, as illustrated by the reemergence of TSH secretion when thyrotoxicosis is relieved. In Graves' disease, regulatory mechanisms are overridden by the action of TSHR autoantibodies of the stimulating variety. The resulting hyperfunction of the thyroid gland leads to suppression of TSH secretion that is reflected in a suppressed or an undetectable serum TSH level. The basal TSH level may also be suppressed in patients with euthyroid Graves' disease (indicating the presence of mild excess of thyroid hormone) and in patients in apparent remission, indicating that thyroid hormone excess is not necessarily associated with clinical thyrotoxicosis.

In this context, the term *functional autonomy* is often misused when the intent is to imply that thyroid function is independent of TSH stimulation. True functional autonomy occurs when the thyroid gland is capable of functioning at a normal or an increased pace in the absence of both TSH and any other circulating thyroid stimulator. Defined in this way, functional autonomy occurs with toxic multinodular goiter and toxic adenoma but *not* in Graves' disease. In Graves' disease, the thyroid gland is controlled by an abnormal stimulator, the TSHRAbs (as in molar pregnancy, in which hCG is responsible). When that stimulator is withdrawn (i.e., when the disease enters remission), hyperfunction subsides, and the nonauton-

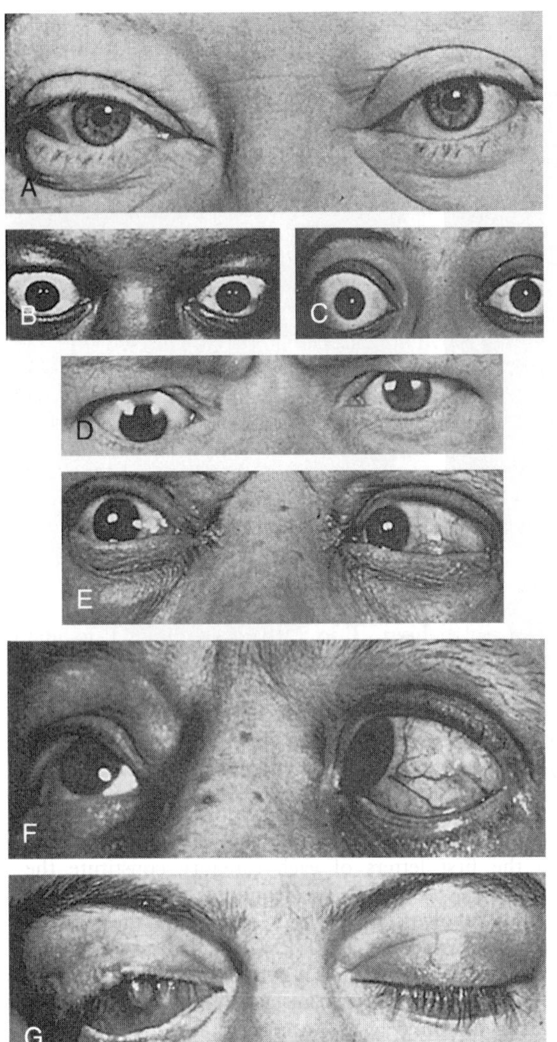

Figure 11–16. Graves' orbitopathy. *A*, Palpebral edema. This patient's eyes protruded anteriorly 1 cm more than normal, but there is no "popeye" appearance, owing to edema of the surrounding structures. *B*, Marked widening of palpebral fissures and slight palpebral swelling. *C*, Unequal degrees of ophthalmopathy. *D*, Unilateral lid retraction. *E*, Palpebral swelling, presumably because of fat pads and edema, and paralysis of the right external rectus muscle. *F*, Marked conjunctival injection and chemosis, together with ophthalmoplegia. *G*, Failure to close lid on the right because of marked exophthalmos, corneal scarring, and panophthalmitis; the eye had to be enucleated.

develop on the face, elbows, or dorsa of the hands. Clubbing of the digits is occasionally associated with long-standing thyrotoxicosis (thyroid acropachy) (Fig. 11–18) (see also Color Plate).

Laboratory Tests

In moderate or severe Graves' disease, laboratory findings are consonant with the pathophysiology. The serum TSH level, when measured by a sensitive immunoassay, is almost totally suppressed, and serum T_4 and T_3 levels are elevated (see Table 10–13). The free T_4 and free T_3 indices are increased more than are the T_4 and T_3 levels. The serum T_3 concentration is proportionally more elevated than the serum T_4 level. The increase in thyroid iodide uptake and clearance rate is reflected in the increased radioactive iodine uptake (RAIU). In patients with severe accompanying illness, conversion of T_4 to T_3 may be impaired, permitting the return to normal of the serum T_3 concentration but usually not the free T_4 (T_4 toxicosis); a similar effect on the relation between serum T_4 and T_3 levels can be seen in patients with Graves' disease who have been exposed to iodine. Occasionally, the discrepancy between T_4 and T_3 levels is exaggerated, the serum T_4 concentration being normal and the serum T_3 concentration alone being elevated (T_3 toxicosis).

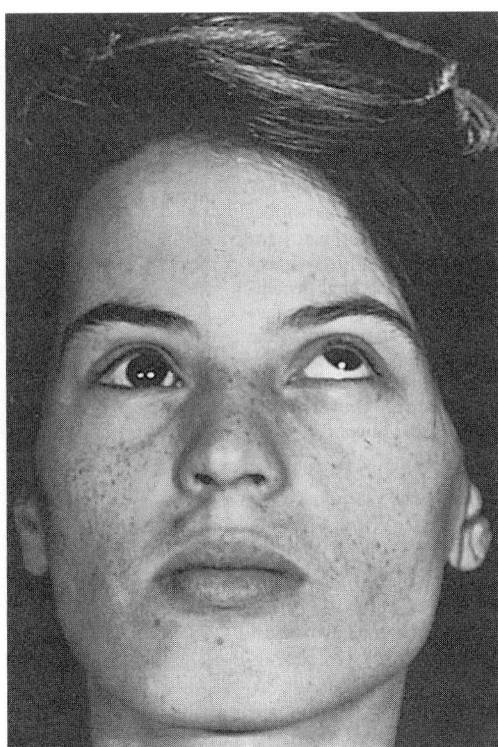

Figure 11–17. Ophthalmoplegia in Graves' disease. Other than slight conjunctival injection, the only ocular abnormality was paralysis of upward gaze on the right in this woman with severe Graves' disease.

The physiologic basis of these tests and the manner in which they are affected by factors other than thyroid disease have been discussed earlier (Chapter 10, Laboratory Assessment of Thyroid Status). Some practical aspects of the use of the tests in the diagnosis of Graves' disease deserve emphasis. It is neither desirable nor feasible that all the major laboratory tests be used to make the diagnosis. Documentation that the serum TSH concentration is suppressed by an appropriate assay establishes the diagnosis of hyperthyroidism in most cases and excludes the possibility of TSH-induced hyperthyroidism (see later). Because there are other causes of suppressed serum TSH, such as depression and hypothalamic-pituitary disease

Table 11–4. American Thyroid Association Classification of Eye Changes in Graves' Disease

Class	Definition
0	*N*o physical signs or symptoms
1	*O*nly signs, no symptoms (signs limited to upper lid retraction, stare, lid lag, and proptosis to 22 mm)
2	*S*oft tissue involvement (symptoms and signs)
3	*P*roptosis > 22 mm
4	*E*xtraocular muscle involvement
5	*C*orneal involvement
6	*S*ight loss (optic nerve involvement)

Table 11–5. Assessment of Severity of Eye Disease by Orbitopathy Activity Score

Characteristic	Score
Soft tissue inflammation	
Slight	1
Moderate	2
Severe	3
Exophthalmos (mm)	
16	0.2
17	0.4
18	0.6
19	0.8
20	1
21	2
22	3
≥ 23	4
Palpebral aperture (mm)	
8	0.15
9	0.45
10	0.75
11	1.05
12	1.35
13	1.65
14	1.95
15	2.25
16	2.55
17	2.85
18	3.00
Differential IOP (mm Hg)	
1	0.1
2	0.2
3	0.3
4	0.4
5	0.5
6	0.6
7	0.7
8	0.8
9	0.9
10	1.0
Diplopia	
Intermittent	1
Inconstant	2
Constant	3
Cornea	
Initial lesions	1
Ulcers	2
Clouding/perforation	3
Optic neuropathy	
Abnormal VEP	3
VA = 0.5–0.9	5
VA = 0.1–0.4	7
VA < 0.1	9

IOP, intraocular pressure; VA, visual acuity; VEP, visual evoked potential.
From Perros P, Crombie AL, Matthews JNS, et al. Age and gender influence the severity of thyroid-associated ophthalmopathy: a study of 101 patients attending a combined thyroid-eye clinic. Clin Endocrinol 1993; 38:367–372.

(see Table 10–13), and to exclude the possibility that an increase in serum T_4 concentration is the result of an increase in hormone binding in the blood, either the free T_4 concentration or the free T_4 index should also be measured. When values for serum total or free T_4 concentrations are not increased, the serum T_3 or T_3 free index should be measured to exclude T_3 thyrotoxicosis.

The diagnostic accuracy of the RAIU in hyperthyroidism does not approach that of the serum TSH plus free T_4 index measurement. Therefore, determining the RAIU is not useful in straightforward Graves' disease but is useful for excluding thyrotoxicosis not caused by hyperthyroidism. Very low values of the RAIU in association with thyrotoxicosis signal the presence of *thyrotoxicosis factitia*, ectopic thyroid tissue, subacute thyroiditis, or the thyrotoxic phase of autoimmune (silent) thyroiditis. A low value may also alert one to unsuspected iodine-induced hyperthyroidism, in which, of course, production of hormone by the thyroid gland is indeed increased.

Mild (Subclinical) Graves' Disease

In subtle or mild cases of thyrotoxicosis, laboratory tests are most important, particularly when values are only slightly abnormal. With the improved sensitivity of TSH assays, there is now no indication for the thyrotropin-releasing hormone (TRH) stimulation test. In the office setting, a TSH concentration below 0.2 mU/L (normal range, 0.5 to 5.0 mU/L) is virtually pathognomonic of an excessive thyroid hormone supply. A value between 0.2 and 0.4 mU/L suggests a supranormal exposure to thyroid hormones but not a condition likely to be associated with significant clinical manifestations. Even when no clinical signs of thyrotoxicosis are present, there are often good reasons to treat subclinical Graves' disease once the correct diagnosis is made (see later).

Measuring Thyrotropin Receptor Autoantibodies

Two types of tests are usually employed for the detection of TSHRAbs. The first test assesses the capacity of patient serum or IgG to inhibit the binding of ^{125}I-labeled TSH to TSH receptors from thyroid membrane preparations (available commercially) or to Chinese hamster ovary (CHO) cells expressing recombinant human TSHR. This protein-binding inhibition assay is of low cost and good precision, and the frequency of positive results in patients with active and untreated disease is on the order of 80% to 90%. Enhanced assays of this type have recently been evaluated but not yet independently.[184, 185]

The second test assesses the capacity of patient's serum or IgG to stimulate adenylate cyclase or to enhance thyroid hormone or Tg secretion or iodine uptake in isolated thyroid epithelial cells or CHO-TSHR cells.[107] Tests of this type are more expensive, have relatively poor precision, and are positive in 80% to 90% of the patients with active untreated Graves' disease. Because of the proliferation of acronyms describing these antibodies, the authors encourage the designation of the specific assay used.[186]

Both types of tests are now available commercially. New techniques are now available for measuring TSHRAbs using recombinant antigens and chemiluminescent tags, but whether they are more sensitive remains to be determined.[14]

Standardization

As with all autoantibody tests, it is important to use an internationally accepted standard to allow comparison of results from different laboratories. A TSHRAb standard from the Medical Research Council (MRC) in Britain is sometimes employed. Results may be reported in MRC units. Alternatively, results have often been reported in terms of equivalent TSH units. However, the hTSHRAbs from different patients may not give parallel results with the MRC standards or TSH standards when measured in different dilutions. This means that the conversion of hTSHRAb data into MRC units or TSH units can be erroneous.

Indications for Measuring Thyrotropin Receptor Autoantibodies

Quantitations of TSHRAbs may be a useful indicator of the degree of disease activity in an individual patient and confirm the clinical diagnosis of Graves' disease. However, a bioassay is

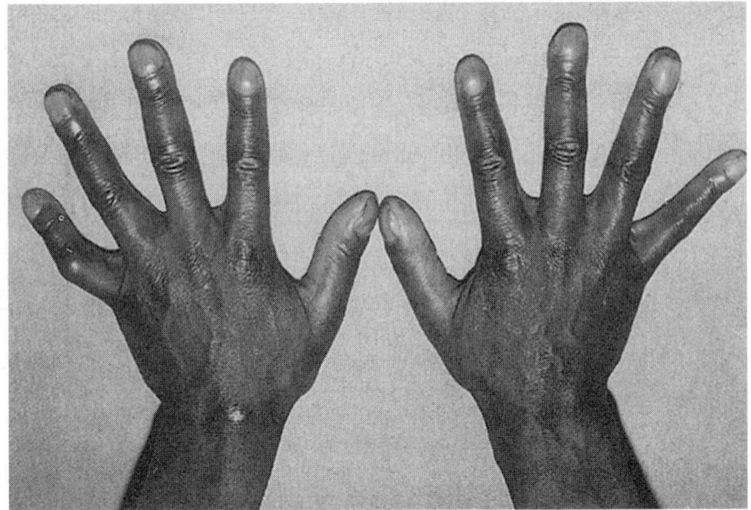

Figure 11-18. Rare thyroid acropachy in a patient with Graves' disease. The hypermetabolic state leads to axial bone destruction, presumably secondary to enhanced osteoclast activity. Acropachy is not to be confused with clubbing, which is usually painless. (Courtesy of Dr. Andrew Werner, New York, NY.) (See also color section.)

not needed in a hyperthyroid patient because the patient is already demonstrating antibody bioactivity. Demonstration of TSHRAbs may also be of diagnostic value in the euthyroid patient with exophthalmos, especially when it is unilateral. High TSHRAbs in a pregnant woman with Graves' disease increase the likelihood that neonatal thyrotoxicosis will be present in her offspring, and in this situation a bioassay is preferred to a radioassay.

Another use of TSHRAb testing is in the prognosis of patients with Graves' disease who are treated with antithyroid agents. A persisting high level of TSHRAbs is a useful predictor of relapse on cessation of the drug. Unfortunately, in patients with low or negative titers, the test is much less helpful.[75] Furthermore, the presence of iodine deficiency may also interrupt the development of hyperthyroidism despite the presence of TSHRAbs, and this has raised unjustified criticism of the usefulness of this test.

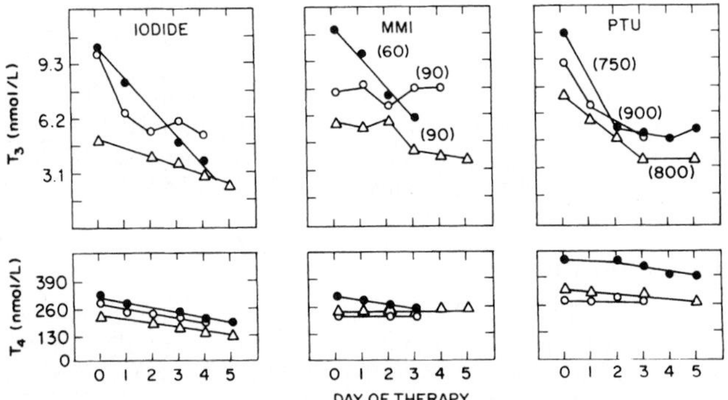

Figure 11-19. Effects of antithyroid agents on the serum levels of triiodothyronine (T_3) and thyroxine (T_4) in patients with Graves' disease. The *left panels* show the effects of potassium iodide (SSKI, 5 drops every 8 hours). A rapid reduction in T_3 concentration occurs in all patients over the first 5 days of therapy. Methimazole (MMI) at the indicated doses has a variable effect on serum T_3 concentrations. In one patient the serum T_3 level falls rapidly over the first 3 days, whereas in the other two individuals, despite an even larger dosage, there is no change. Serum T_4 concentration does not change significantly over this time interval. The *right panels* show that the administration of high-dose propylthiouracil (PTU) causes a marked decrease in serum T_3 concentrations to one third to one half of initial levels. This decrease is due to the PTU-induced inhibition of type 1 iodothyronine 5′-deiodinase. (Data from Abuid J, Larsen PR. Triiodothyronine and thyroxine in thyrotoxicosis: acute response to therapy with antithyroid agents. J Clin Invest 1974; 39:263–268.)

Differential Diagnosis

The patient with major manifestations of Graves' disease (namely thyrotoxicosis, goiter, and infiltrative orbitopathy) does not pose a diagnostic problem. In some patients, however, one of the major manifestations either dominates the clinical picture or is present alone, and the disorder may mimic another disease. All of these issues can be resolved by appropriate laboratory testing (see Table 10–13).

The diffuse goiter of Graves' disease may rarely be confused with that of other thyroid diseases if thyrotoxicosis is present. In subacute thyroiditis, particularly the painless variant, asymmetry of the gland, tenderness, and systemic evidence of inflammation assist in the diagnosis. The very low RAIU distinguishes this disease from Graves' disease. When Graves' disease is in a latent or inactive phase and thyrotoxicosis is absent, the goiter may require differentiation from Hashimoto's thyroiditis or simple nontoxic goiter as possible diagnoses. The goiter of Hashimoto's disease is somewhat lobulated and firmer and rubbery compared with that of Graves' disease. Serum levels of thyroid antibodies are generally higher in Hashimoto's disease but may not be helpful in distinguishing individual patients. In the absence of thyrotoxicosis, the diffuse goiter of Graves' disease cannot be distinguished from nontoxic, or simple, goiter. An abnormal serum TSH concentration and the presence of TSHRAbs indicate underlying Graves' disease, but their absence does not exclude quiescent disease.

Eye Disease

The orbitopathy of Graves' disease, if bilateral and associated with thyrotoxicosis past or present, does not require differentiation from exophthalmos of any other origin. However, unilateral exophthalmos, even when associated with thyrotoxicosis, should alert the physician to the possibility of a local cause. Other diseases that may produce either unilateral or bilateral exophthalmos include orbital neoplasms, carotid-cavernous sinus fistulae, cavernous sinus thrombosis, infiltrative disorders affecting the orbit, and pseudotumor of the orbit. Mild bilateral exophthalmos, generally without infiltrative signs, is occasionally present on a familial basis and also sometimes occurs in patients with Cushing's syndrome, cirrhosis,

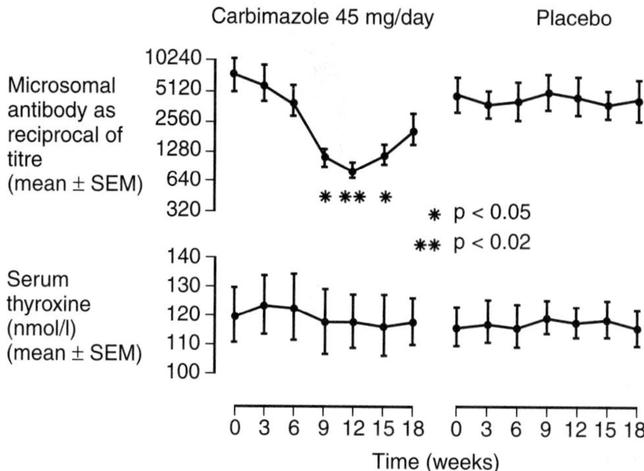

Figure 11–20. Influence of carbimazole and placebo treatment on thyroid peroxidase antibody levels (measured as antimicrosomal antibodies) in patients with Hashimoto's thyroiditis. These data illustrate the immunosuppressive effect of carbimazole in patients who remained euthyroid throughout observation. SEM, standard error of the mean. (From McGregor AM, Ibbertson HK, Smith BR, Hall R. Carbimazole and autoantibody synthesis in Hashimoto's thyroiditis. Br Med J 1980; 281:968–970.)

uremia, chronic obstructive pulmonary disease, and superior vena cava syndrome.

Ophthalmoplegia as the sole manifestation of the orbitopathy of Graves' disease requires exclusion of diabetes mellitus and other disorders affecting the brain stem and its connections. The demonstration of swelling of the extraocular muscles by orbital ultrasonography, CT, or MRI is diagnostic of Graves' orbitopathy,[180, 181] as is the detection of TSHRAbs in serum or the demonstration of a suppressed TSH level.

Treatment of Hyperthyroidism

It is not yet possible to treat the basic pathogenetic factors in Graves' disease. Existing therapies for both the thyrotoxic and the ophthalmic manifestations are only palliative.

The lack of general agreement as to which therapy is the best is due to the fact that none is ideal, as reflected in the treatment guidelines of the American Thyroid Association.[188] Because the therapeutic problems posed by thyrotoxicosis and orbitopathy differ, and because they run independent courses, their treatments are discussed separately. Treatment of thyrotoxicosis is designed to impose restraint on hormone secretion either by means of chemical agents that inhibit hormone synthesis or release or by reducing the quantity of thyroid tissue.

Antithyroid Agents

The mechanisms of action of the various antithyroid drugs are discussed in the section on the formation and secretion of thyroid hormones in Chapter 10.

Iodide Transport Inhibitors

Both thiocyanate and perchlorate inhibit thyroid iodide transport. As discussed earlier, however, theoretical and practical disadvantages attend their use except in special circumstances.

Thionamides

The major agents for treating thyrotoxicosis are drugs of the thionamide class, most commonly propylthiouracil, methimazole, and carbimazole.[189] These agents inhibit the oxidation and organic binding of thyroid iodide and, therefore, produce intrathyroidal iodine deficiency that further increases the ratio of T_3 to T_4 in the thyroid secretion, as reflected in the high T_3/T_4 ratio in the serum. In addition large doses of propylthiouracil, but not methimazole, impair the conversion of T_4 to T_3 by deiodinase type 1 in the peripheral tissues. Because of this additional action, large doses of propylthiouracil may provide rapid alleviation of severe thyrotoxicosis (Fig. 11–19).[189–192]

The half-life in plasma of methimazole is about 6 hours, whereas that of propylthiouracil is about 1.5 hours, and both drugs are accumulated by the thyroid gland. A single dose of methimazole may exert an antithyroid effect for longer than 24 hours. This provides a rational basis for the single-daily-dose regimen of methimazole for mild or moderate thyrotoxicosis.[193] The propylthiouracil concentration in serum correlates with the extent of blockade of organic binding of iodine within the thyroid gland.[189] These drugs cross the placenta and can inhibit thyroid function in the fetus. Some evidence suggests that methimazole may cross the placenta more readily than propylthiouracil, but both drugs have been used highly effectively in pregnancy (see discussion hyperthyroidism and thyrotoxicosis in pregnancy later).

Immunosuppressive Action of Thionamides

Thionamide drugs may also directly influence the immune response in patients with autoimmune thyroid disease.[44] This action occurs within the thyroid gland, where the drugs are concentrated. The action on the thyroid cells themselves decreases thyroid antigen expression and decreases prostaglandin and cytokine release from thyroid cells.[47, 194, 195] Thionamides also inhibit the generation of oxygen radicals in T cells, B cells, and particularly the APCs and hence may cause a further decline in antigen presentation.[196] More recently, it has been shown that methimazole induces the expression of Fas ligand on the thyroid epithelial cell,[197] thus inducing apoptosis of infiltrating lymphocytes such as T cells that express Fas[198] and decreasing the lymphocytic infiltration (see Fig. 12–7 in Chapter 12).

The clinical importance of immunosuppression and induction of apoptosis compared with inhibition of thyroid hormone formation is unclear. However, the decrease in the immune infiltration of patients on such drugs and the fall in autoantibody levels after their introduction to a patient is powerful evidence of their effect (Fig. 11–20).

Use of Thionamides

An initial dose of methimazole commonly employed is 10 to 15 mg twice a day. An equivalent dose of propylthiouracil is 150 mg every 8 hours. Carbimazole, which is converted to methimazole in vivo and is equivalent in potency, is widely used in Europe but not in the United States. These doses are effective in most patients, but in some no therapeutic response is seen, and in some patients doses of up to 60 mg of methimazole or an equivalent amount of propylthiouracil daily may be required.

It is unlikely that a true state of complete resistance to these agents ever occurs. The higher doses are required in patients with severe thyrotoxicosis and large thyroid glands, or possibly because of more rapid degradation of the drug within the gland or extrathyroidally. When large amounts are required, doses of propylthiouracil should be administered at 4- to 6-hour intervals.

The therapeutic response to effective antithyroid therapy invariably occurs after a latent period because the agents inhibit the synthesis but not the release of hormone; hence reduction in the supply of hormone to the tissues does not occur until glandular hormone stores are depleted (see Figs. 11–4 and 11–19). Although propylthiouracil differs from methimazole in having the additional effect of inhibiting the peripheral conversion of T_4 to T_3, there appears to be little difference in the duration of the latent period when either of these agents is employed alone in the usual dosage because the extrathyroidal effect of propylthiouracil on conversion of T_4 to T_3 is more apparent at dosages greater than 600 mg/day. This effect may be an advantage in the acute treatment of severe hyperthyroidism.[190]

Factors that influence the duration of the latent period include the quantity of hormone initially stored in the thyroid gland, its inherent rate of release, and the effectiveness of blockade of new hormone synthesis achieved. In an iodine-rich thyroid gland, as when the patient has received medications containing iodine, the clinical response to antithyroid agents may be delayed for months. As would be expected, the latent period is shortened by administration of large doses (more than 600 mg daily of propylthiouracil), and such doses should be given when a more rapid therapeutic response is required. Generally, improvement within the first 2 weeks includes decreased nervousness and palpitations, increased strength, and weight gain. Usually, the metabolic state becomes normal within about 6 weeks. At this time, the dosage can often be reduced substantially to maintain a normal metabolic state.

During treatment, the size of the thyroid gland decreases in one third to one half of the patients. In the remainder, it may remain unchanged or even enlarge. In the latter situation, the change signals either an intensification of the disease process, which often requires that the dosage of drug be increased, or the production of hypothyroidism and increased TSH secretion as a result of excessive dosage.

It is important to differentiate between these causes. Clinical criteria are the main guidelines by which the adequacy of treatment is judged, but confirmation may be sought in the serum T_4 and T_3 levels. Mild thyrotoxicosis may persist despite a serum T_4 concentration in the normal range because the serum T_3 concentration may still be elevated. The latter phenomenon may also account for maintenance of a normal metabolic state in the setting of a subnormal serum T_4 level. The serum TSH concentration may remain subnormal for many months, presumably secondary to accelerated conversion of T_4 to T_3. An enlarging thyroid gland in a treated patient with Graves' disease may indicate the presence of a neoplasm and should be investigated appropriately.

Antithyroid agents can cause hypothyroidism if given in excessive amounts over long periods. When this occurs, the patient often complains of gain in weight, sluggishness, and fatigue, and signs of mild hypothyroidism may be present, especially a delay in the relaxation phase of the deep tendon reflexes. One major sign of incipient hypothyroidism is enlargement of the thyroid gland secondary to increased TSH. The hypothyroidism can be reversed by reducing the dosage of the antithyroid drug or by administering supplemental thyroid hormone. To forestall this development, which may also have adverse effects on preexisting orbitopathy, some physicians employ supplemental thyroid hormone routinely, the "block-and-replace" approach.

Block-and-Replace Regimens

The logic behind prescribing a full dose of a thionamide drug and adding T_4 supplements to prevent the patient from becoming hypothyroid is twofold. First, a few patients are difficult to keep euthyroid with thionamide therapy alone, and a block-and-replace regimen can be helpful and requires fewer office visits. Second, the immunosuppressive action of the thionamides may be helpful in attenuating the natural history of the autoimmune thyroid diseases directly.

Although some investigators found the relapse rate after the block-and-replace approach to be much reduced,[199] others have found no difference.[200, 201] One group has reported that continuing levothyroxine replacement after withdrawal of antithyroid drugs also increased the remission rate,[202] possibly because suppression of pituitary TSH inhibited expression of thyroid antigens and reduced immune stimulation (an effect influenced by the level of TSHRAbs). Such studies have not been reproduced,[200, 203] and this approach is not recommended.

Predicting the Response to Drug Withdrawal

A central question in the treatment of Graves' disease to which there is no simple answer is the appropriate duration of antithyroid drug treatment. As discussed earlier, antithyroid therapy may alter the course of the underlying autoimmune process, but remission after withdrawal of treatment will persist only if the disorder has entered a latent or inactive phase. This latter transition and the natural decline in the levels of TSHRAbs are more likely to occur the longer the course of treatment. This reasoning is the basis for the traditional practice of continuing antithyroid treatment for 6 to 12 months or longer. However, persistence of high levels of circulating TSHRAbs during treatment of Graves' disease portends recurrence after withdrawal of antithyroid drugs in iodine-replete areas.[75]

Factors preventing a recurrence include (1) a change from stimulating antibody to blocking antibody, which occurs rarely, and (2) the progression of concomitant thyroiditis. Furthermore, iodine deficiency itself may prevent the recurrence of Graves' disease. These factors may explain why some authors have been unable to confirm the predictive value of TSHRAb measurement.[204] The use of poorly validated assays for TSHRAbs may compound this problem. However, most patients do not have persisting high levels of TSHRAb, and predicting their outcome is more difficult; additional factors need to be taken into account.[73]

Other features associated with the likelihood of long-term remission after withdrawal of therapy (Table 11–6) include (1) the initial presence of T_3 toxicosis, (2) a small thyroid gland (less than twice normal), (3) a decrease in the size of the thyroid gland, and (4) in particular, return of the TSH concentration to normal during treatment. HLA typing is not helpful in such predictions.[205]

Hence, treatment should generally be continued for about 6 to 12 months and then withdrawn if the TSHRAbs disappear. Alternatively, if the patient's condition can be easily controlled with low doses of antithyroid drugs and the serum TSH has returned to the normal range, antithyroid drugs may be withdrawn and the serum TSH concentration measured at monthly intervals. About 75% of relapses occur in the first 3 months after withdrawal of therapy, and most of the remainder occur during the subsequent 6 months. Suppression of the TSH

Table 11–6. Factors Favoring Long-Term Remission after Antithyroid Therapy for Graves' Disease

T_3 toxicosis
Small goiter
Decrease in goiter size during therapy
Normal thyroid function tests and normal serum TSH
Negative tests for TSH receptor autoantibody

TSH, thyrotropin.

concentration is the first signal of relapse even in the presence of a normal serum T_4 level.

Long-Term Remission

The frequency with which long-term remission occurs after withdrawal of antithyroid therapy has decreased over the past 30 years,[206, 207] in part because of the increase in dietary iodine intake, but this decrease has also occurred in geographic regions where iodine intake has remained constant and low. Nevertheless, about one third of patients experience a lasting remission. This fact alone indicates that antithyroid agents have a significant role as a sole therapy in the initial treatment of thyrotoxicosis.

Adverse Reactions

Adverse reactions occur in a small number of patients taking thionamide drugs (Table 11–7). Agranulocytosis occurs in fewer than 1% of the patients, generally within the first few weeks or months of treatment. It is accompanied by fever and sore throat. When therapy is begun, the patient should be instructed to discontinue the drug and to notify the physician immediately should these symptoms develop. This precaution is more important than the frequent measurement of leukocyte counts because agranulocytosis may develop within a day or two. Because of the frequency of lymphopenia in hyperthyroidism, a complete blood count with differential is recommended before antithyroid drug therapy is started. If the absolute neutrophil count falls below 1500 cells/μL, the drug should be withdrawn. If agranulocytosis occurs, the drug should be discontinued immediately and the patient treated with antibiotics as appropriate. Granulocyte colony-stimulating factor has been used to speed the recovery that invariably takes place.[208] Lymphocytes of patients who have developed agranulocytosis while taking propylthiouracil undergo blast transformation when exposed in vitro to propylthiouracil or methimazole[209]; consequently, they should not be given a thionamide drug again. Granulocytopenia occurs during antithyroid therapy and is sometimes a forerunner of agranulocytosis, but, as already mentioned, it can also be a manifestation of thyrotoxicosis itself. For this reason, and as noted previously, a total white blood cell count with differential should be obtained before initiation of treatment with thionamide drugs. Granulocytopenia that develops during the first few weeks of therapy may be difficult to interpret. In this circumstance, serial measurements of the leukocyte count should be made. If they display a downward trend, the antithyroid drugs should be discontinued. When serial measurements of the white blood cell count remain constant or return to normal, treatment need not be interrupted.

A rash that can take many forms, including hives, occurs in as many as 10% of patients. Less frequent reactions include arthralgia, myalgia, neuritis, hepatitis (with propylthiouracil) or cholestasis (with methimazole) and rare liver necrosis necessitating transplantation, thrombocytopenia, loss of or abnormal pigmentation of the hair, loss of taste sensation, enlargement of lymph nodes or salivary glands, edema, a lupus-like syndrome, and toxic psychoses. The mechanisms underlying these reactions are not known, although some reactions disappear with continuance of treatment. It is obviously helpful to have a baseline complete blood count and liver function studies before initiation of antithyroid drugs to help interpret the presence of some of these side effects. We believe that the suspicion of any serious manifestation should be an indication for abandonment of antithyroid therapy and a recourse to surgery or ^{131}I.

Table 11–7. Incidence of Toxic Reactions with Antithyroid Drugs

Drug	All Reactions (%)	Agranulocytosis (%)
Methimazole	7.1	0.1
Carbimazole	1.9	0.8
Propylthiouracil	3.3	0.4

Iodine and Iodine-Containing Agents

Iodine is now rarely used as a sole therapy. The mechanism of action of iodine in relieving thyrotoxicosis differs from that of the thionamides. Although quantities of iodine in excess of several milligrams can acutely inhibit organic binding (acute Wolff-Chaikoff effect), this transient phenomenon probably does not contribute to the therapeutic effect. Instead, the major action of iodine is to inhibit hormone release (see Chapter 10). Administration of iodine increases glandular stores of organic iodine, but the beneficial effect of iodine is evident more quickly than the effects of even large doses of agents that inhibit hormone synthesis (Fig. 11–19). In patients with Graves' disease, iodine acutely retards the rate of secretion of T_4, an effect that is rapidly lost when iodine is withdrawn. These features of iodine action provide both disadvantages and advantages. The enrichment of glandular organic iodine stores that occurs when this agent is given alone may retard the clinical response to subsequently administered thionamide, and the decrease in RAIU produced by iodine prevents the use of radioiodine as treatment for several weeks. Furthermore, if iodine is withdrawn, resumption of accelerated release of hormone from an enriched glandular hormone pool may exacerbate the disorder.

Another reason for not using iodine alone is that the therapeutic response on occasion is either incomplete or absent, and even if initially effective iodine may lose its effect with time. (This phenomenon, which has been termed *iodine escape*, should not be confused with the escape from the acute Wolff-Chaikoff effect [see Chapter 10].) Nevertheless, the rapid slowing of hormone release by iodine makes it more effective than the thionamide drugs when prompt relief of thyrotoxicosis is mandatory (see Fig. 11–19). Therefore, aside from its use in preparation for subtotal thyroidectomy, iodine is useful mainly in patients with actual or impending thyrotoxic crisis, severe thyrocardiac disease, or acute surgical emergencies.

If iodine is used in these circumstances, it should be administered with large doses of a thionamide, as the severity of the thyrotoxicosis itself indicates. The dose of iodine required for control of thyrotoxicosis is approximately 6 mg daily, a quantity much less than that usually given. Six milligrams of iodine is present in one eighth of a drop of saturated solution of potassium iodide (SSKI) or an 0.8 drop of Lugol's solution; many physicians, however, prescribe 5 to 10 drops of one of these agents three times daily. Although it is advisable to administer amounts larger than the suggested minimal effective dose, huge quantities of iodine are more likely to produce adverse reactions, including iodide myxedema. We recommend the use of a maximum of 3 drops of SSKI three times daily.

In patients who are so ill that medications cannot be taken by mouth, antithyroid agents can be triturated and administered by stomach tube; iodine can be given by the same route or can be absorbed through the mucosa. When use of a stomach tube is contraindicated, thionamide drugs cannot be administered because no parenteral preparations are available. Here, the disadvantages attendant on administration of iodine may be accepted if the clinical situation is sufficiently serious. Iodine appears to be particularly effective after administration of a therapeutic dose of ^{131}I for the rapid alleviation of thyrotoxicosis.

Reactions to Iodine

Adverse reactions to iodine are unusual and are generally not serious[210, 211] but may include rash, which may be acneiform; drug fever; sialadenitis; conjunctivitis and rhinitis; vasculitis; and a leukemoid eosinophilic granulocytosis. Sialadenitis may respond to reduction of dosage; in the case of the other reactions, iodine should be stopped.

Ipodate

In doses of 1 g daily, the iodine-containing cholecystographic contrast agent sodium ipodate (or iopanoate) causes a prompt decrease in serum T_4 and serum T_3 concentrations in patients with hyperthyroidism.[212] These effects are the result of both the release of iodine and the ability of the agent to inhibit peripheral T_3 production from T_4, a combination that can be useful in the seriously ill patient. As with iodine itself, however, withdrawal of the drug carries the risk of an exacerbation. Hence, if the patient is sufficiently ill to warrant treatment with ipodate, large doses of antithyroid agents should be administered concomitantly.

Other Antithyroid Agents

Lithium

Lithium carbonate also inhibits thyroid hormone secretion, but, unlike iodine, it does not interfere with the accumulation of radioiodine. Lithium, 300 to 450 mg every 8 hours, is employed only to provide temporary control of thyrotoxicosis in patients who are allergic to both thionamide and iodide.[212] This is because the blocking effect is often lost with time. The goal is to maintain a serum concentration of 1 mEq/L.

Dexamethasone

Dexamethasone, 2 mg every 6 hours, inhibits the glandular secretion of hormone, inhibits the peripheral conversion of T_4 to T_3, and has immunosuppressive effects.[213] The inhibitory effect of dexamethasone on the conversion of T_4 to T_3 is additive to that of propylthiouracil, suggesting a different mechanism of action. Concurrent administration of propylthiouracil, SSKI, and dexamethasone to the patient with severe thyrotoxicosis effects a rapid reduction in serum T_3 concentration, often to within the normal range in 24 to 48 hours.[214]

Beta-Blocking Agents

Agents that block the response to catecholamines at the receptor site (e.g., propranolol) ameliorate some of the manifestations of thyrotoxicosis and are often used as adjuncts in management. Tremulousness, palpitations, excessive sweating, eyelid retraction, and heart rate decrease; effects are rapidly manifested and appear to be mediated largely through the adrenergic nervous system, although propranolol may also impair the conversion of T_4 to T_3.

Adrenergic antagonists are most useful in the interval when a response to thionamide or radioiodine therapy is being awaited. They are of limited usefulness in patients with mild to moderate disease but are useful in patients with severe thyrotoxicosis, such as those with impending or actual thyrotoxic crisis (see special aspects of thyrotoxicosis later). Adrenergic antagonists are especially useful when tachycardia is contributing to cardiac insufficiency. However, the fact that β-adrenergic blockers can reduce cardiac output without altering oxygen consumption can have adverse effects in some organs, such as the liver, where the arteriovenous oxygen difference is already elevated in the hyperthyroid state.[10] Moreover, because thyroid hormone has a direct effect on the myocardium independent of the adrenergic nervous system, adrenergic antagonists reduce the heart rate by an independent mechanism (see earlier discussion of catecholamine-thyroid interrelationships).[4–7, 29–32]

Propranolol is the most widely used agent because it is relatively free from adverse effects and can be given orally in a dose of 20 to 80 mg every 6 or 8 hours. For intravenous use, a shorter-acting agent may be preferable (see treatment of "Thyrotoxic Crisis [Thyroid Storm]"). Propranolol is contraindicated in patients with asthma or chronic obstructive pulmonary disease because it aggravates bronchospasm. Because of its myocardial depressant action, it is also contraindicated in patients with heart block and in patients with congestive failure, unless severe tachycardia is a contributory factor. Whether propranolol should be given chronically to pregnant women with hyperthyroidism has been questioned, and we avoid it where possible. Some studies indicate that its use causes no significant complications,[72, 215, 216] whereas others report an association with small size of the fetus, low Apgar scores, and postnatal bradycardia and hypoglycemia.

Another β-blocking agent is metoprolol, a longer-acting drug that allows a once-a-day regimen when treatment is likely to be prolonged. Calcium channel–blocking agents such as diltiazem may also be used when β-blocking agents are contraindicated.[217]

Surgery

Both types of ablative therapy—surgery and radioiodine—ameliorate thyrotoxicosis by permanent removal or destruction of thyroid tissue, impairing the capacity of the gland to synthesize hormone. Antithyroid therapy, aimed at preserving the thyroid gland, and ablative therapy are different, and their opposite properties may be advantageous or disadvantageous, depending on one's point of view. The impermanence of antithyroid therapy leads to a relatively frequent recurrence, whereas recurrence is uncommon with ablative therapy. However, antithyroid therapy probably does not cause permanent hypothyroidism, whereas the frequency of permanent hypothyroidism is very high with ablative therapy.

The surgical procedure of choice for the treatment of Graves' disease is a bilateral subtotal thyroidectomy that avoids the dangers of hypoparathyroidism and laryngeal nerve injury. Surgery is effective in relieving hyperthyroidism, the frequency of recurrent hyperthyroidism after subtotal thyroidectomy in adults being less than 5% when the procedure is performed by experienced surgeons. Nevertheless the high prevalence of postoperative hypothyroidism makes surgery an imperfect treatment.

Table 11–8 is taken from summaries of results of surgery that have not changed significantly in recent years except for the large decline in mortality to near zero in most reports.[218, 219] The incidence of permanent hypothyroidism

Table 11–8. Effects of Surgery for Hyperthyroidism

Result	Percent
Recurrent hyperthyroidism	0.6–9.8
Vocal cord paralysis	0.0–3.4
Permanent hypoparathyroidism	0.0–3.6
Permanent hypothyroidism	5.8–75.0

ranged in frequency from 4% to approximately 30% and was highest in clinics in which internists did the follow-up examinations. In a study conducted by internists, a mean frequency of postoperative hypothyroidism of 28% was found in patients followed for 1 to 16 years, and the frequency in patients followed for 10 years was 43%.

Although it was previously assumed that hypothyroidism usually develops within 1 year after operation, long-term studies indicated a progressive increase in the cumulative incidence with time, similar to that produced by radioiodine but of lesser magnitude. It is likely that the frequency of partial impairment of thyroid function (as revealed by small increases in serum TSH) is even higher than that of hypothyroidism because the aim of subtotal thyroidectomy is to decrease thyroid reserve. The increasing frequency with time of hypothyroidism may result from progressive restriction of blood supply or from autoimmune destruction of the thyroid remnant.[171] If eventual thyroid failure is a frequent consequence of the Graves' disease process itself, the increase in the cumulative frequency with time of hypothyroidism after either surgery or radioiodine therapy is to be expected and is unavoidable. Treatment that destroys thyroid tissue would accelerate the emergence of hypothyroidism resulting from the disease process itself.

There is an inverse relationship between the frequency of recurrence and that of hypothyroidism, and both partly depend on the amount of thyroid tissue left in place. When one considers that thyroid glands vary in size and degree of hyperfunction and that the techniques of surgeons vary to a considerable extent, it is remarkable that a normal metabolic state is restored for long periods in most patients. The reason for this favorable outcome may be that the amount of tissue remaining after operation is insufficient to sustain a normal metabolic state and hence becomes stimulated by endogenous TSH. In this way, the patient's homeostatic mechanism provides the adjustment in thyroid function that surgery alone could not. This hypothesis is supported by the return of serum TSH levels to normal in patients restored to a normal metabolic state by surgery. However, this explanation would suffice only in the absence of TSHRAbs, which rapidly decrease and disappear in many patients after surgery. How the autoimmune disease is suppressed following surgery is unclear, but clearly the release of thyroid antigen during the procedure must induce apoptosis of many of the clones of TSHR-specific T cells and B cells.

Complications of Surgery

Because the hazards of subtotal thyroidectomy are inversely related to the experience and skill of the surgical team, it is impossible to generalize about the frequency of complications. Furthermore, data from the era in which surgery was common are probably no longer applicable (see Table 11–8). Unless circumstances are otherwise compelling, thyroidectomy should not be performed by surgeons who do the operation only occasionally. Bleeding into the operative site, the most serious postoperative complication, can rapidly produce death by asphyxia and requires immediate evacuation of the blood and ligation of the bleeding vessel. Even with subtotal surgery, the recurrent laryngeal nerve can be damaged. If such damage is unilateral, it causes dysphonia that usually improves in a few weeks but that may leave the patient slightly hoarse. If laryngeal nerve damage is bilateral, obstruction of the airway can cause stridor within hours; tracheostomy is then required, at which time the nature of the damage to the nerves should be explored.

Hypoparathyroidism can be either transient or permanent. Transient hypoparathyroidism results from inadvertent removal of some parathyroids and impairment of blood supply to those that remain. Depending on the severity of these insults, symptoms and signs of hypocalcemia appear, usually within 1 to 7 days after surgery. The earliest evidence of hypoparathyroidism may be anxiety and mental depression, followed by paresthesias and heightened neuromuscular excitability, such as Chvostek's and Trousseau's signs and carpopedal spasm. The serum calcium level is subnormal, and the serum inorganic phosphate level is increased.

Severe hypoparathyroidism should be treated with intravenous calcium gluconate. Milder cases can be treated with oral calcium carbonate in a dose of 1 g three times daily. It is impossible at the onset to predict whether hypoparathyroidism will be permanent or will regress within a few weeks, as usually occurs. Some surgeons insist on prophylactic calcium and vitamin D after every thyroidectomy. Of course, this approach may hide any developing deficiency. With the increasing use of ambulatory thyroid surgery, it is likely that this approach will grow.

However, the hypocalcemia that occurs immediately after surgery for thyrotoxicosis may not be due to transient hypoparathyroidism, because it occurs more frequently here than after surgery for other thyroid disorders. Instead, it may be due to retention of calcium by bone[220] because of the demineralization of bone that occurs in hyperthyroidism,[221–223] which begins to be reversed after cure of the hyperthyroid state and may contribute to the modest elevation in alkaline phosphatase during recovery. The frequency of permanent hypoparathyroidism correlates with the proportion of the thyroid gland removed and with the frequency of postoperative hypothyroidism. The incidence of mild hypoparathyroidism (or diminished parathyroid reserve) detectable years after surgery is probably greater than is generally supposed. The treatment of hypoparathyroidism is discussed in Chapter 26.

Preparation for Surgery

Preoperative use of antithyroid agents has greatly decreased the morbidity and mortality rates of surgery for Graves' disease because these drugs deplete glandular hormone stores and restore the metabolic state to normal surgery. However, these agents do not improve the hyperplasia and hypervascularity of the gland unless TSHRAb levels fall. Iodine, however, is reported to cause a decrease in height of the follicular cells, enlargement of follicles with retention of colloid, and reduction of hypervascularity. Hence, the aim of preoperative management is to restore the metabolic state to normal with antithyroid agents and then to induce involution of the gland with iodine.

Patients who are to undergo subtotal thyroidectomy are first given antithyroid therapy in the manner described earlier. Often, relatively large doses are given in order to hasten the clinical response and because surgical candidates are often patients with severe disease or large goiters. After the metabolic state is restored to normal, SSKI is added (3 drops three times daily) for a further 7 to 10 days. During this period, a preexisting bruit or thrill may decrease in intensity or disappear entirely and the gland usually becomes firm.

Several cautions should be observed:

1. No date for surgery should be set until a normal metabolic state has been restored. Much too often, the operation is planned well in advance and the patient is given a standardized regimen independent of the clinical progress.
2. Therapy with iodine should not be started until a normal metabolic state has been restored; iodine should not be relied on to complete an as yet incomplete response to antithyroid therapy because iodine will enrich glandular hormone stores if the antithyroid drug is not entirely effective.

3. Antithyroid agents should not be withdrawn when iodine therapy is begun.

Thyroid Surgery in the Hyperthyroid Patient

Propranolol may be a useful adjunct in controlling signs and symptoms (see earlier) while the patient is being prepared for surgery. Propranolol has been used alone in preoperative preparation of the patient in whom surgery is to be undertaken,[224] and although this mode of therapy is probably safe and effective in many patients with mild disease, thyroid crises can occur in patients receiving propranolol alone. Therefore, we believe that unless there is some compelling indication for the use of propranolol alone, restoration of the patient to a eumetabolic state, as outlined earlier, is appropriate before subjecting the patient to the stress of surgery.

Radioiodine

Radioiodine produces thyroid ablation without the complications of surgery. The principal disadvantages of radioiodine are the influence of radiation on Graves' ophthalmopathy and the high frequency of late hypothyroidism. Previously, there was concern that this form of therapy might also produce thyroid carcinoma, leukemia, or an increase in mutation rates. However, during the half-century in which radioiodine has been in use, no increased prevalence of thyroid or other carcinoma in treated patients has been noted.[225, 226] This phenomenon is to be contrasted with the increased prevalence of thyroid carcinoma in patients treated with low amounts of radiation in childhood or adolescence as exemplified by the results of the Chernobyl radiation leak.[158] The prevalence of leukemia is also no greater in adults treated with radioiodine, and the frequency of genetic damage in the offspring of patients treated earlier with radioiodine does not appear to be increased. Indeed, the conventional dose of radioiodine employed in the treatment of thyrotoxicosis delivers to the gonads a radiation dose about equivalent to that delivered by a barium enema examination or intravenous urogram.

In view of the lack of evidence of serious toxicity from radioiodine in doses generally employed for treating hyperthyroidism, the age limit for the use of radioiodine has been lowered progressively from the initial limit of 40 years, and in some clinics it is now employed in children and adolescents. Experience from the Chernobyl nuclear accident, which caused a large increase in the number of childhood thyroid cancers, may alter this trend, particularly for adolescents,[227–230] and many physicians think that the use of any radioactivity in children should be avoided if possible. Hence, there is regional and international variation in the use of radioiodine therapy.

Attempts have been made to standardize the radiation delivered to the thyroid gland by varying the dose of radioiodine according to the size of the gland, the uptake of ^{131}I, and its subsequent rate of release (dosimetry). However, such calculations do not provide uniform results, probably because of variations in individual sensitivity. Hence, many physicians have settled on an arbitrary dose calculated to result in the delivery of 300 MBq (~8 mCi) of ^{131}I to the thyroid gland 24 hours after administration. Others aim to deliver 50 to 100 Gy (5000 to 10,000 rad) to the gland.[231]

Hypothyroidism after Radioiodine

Many reports have documented that the incidence of hypothyroidism is significant during the first year or two after treatment with RAI and continues to increase at a rate of approximately 5% per year thereafter. The incidence of postradioiodine hypothyroidism at 5 years is approximately 30% and at 10 years is approximately 40%, although values as high as 70% have been reported (Fig. 11–21). Such values, of course, also depend on the dose delivered in the different centers.

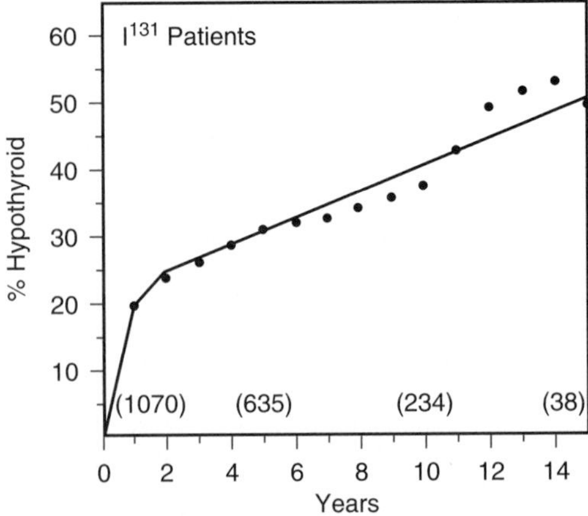

Figure 11–21. Incidence of postradioiodine hypothyroidism in relation to the duration of follow-up. The total number of patients followed for each of the indicated time periods is shown in parentheses. (From Dunn JT, Chapman EM. Rising incidence of hypothyroidism after radioactive iodine therapy in thyrotoxicosis. Reprinted by permission of The New England Journal of Medicine, 1964; 271:1037–1042.)

The beneficial effect of radioiodine and the early induction of hypothyroidism are both consequences of radiation-induced destruction of thyroid parenchyma. Radiation thyroiditis may develop within the first few weeks of treatment, as evidenced by epithelial swelling and necrosis, disruption of follicular architecture, edema, and infiltration with mononuclear cells. Resolution of the acute phase is followed by fibrosis, vascular narrowing, and further lymphocytic infiltration. These changes account for the early response to radioiodine, be it favorable or excessive, but do not appear sufficient to account for the continuing development of hypothyroidism with time.

In some studies, the likelihood of hypothyroidism is increased by the presence of high levels of thyroid antibodies and, presumably, of thyroid specific T cells, at the time of treatment and with increasing age of the patient. The two predisposing factors may be related to one another. If this is true, it is unlikely that the early ablative effects can be obtained free from subsequent late effects, and doses of radioiodine sufficient to exert an early therapeutic action will inevitably be associated with a high frequency of delayed hypothyroidism.

This therapeutic dilemma with respect to radioiodine therapy is handled differently in different practices. Some continue to administer the conventional dose because of its effectiveness and because hypothyroidism, when it eventually occurs, can be easily treated. A disadvantage of such an approach is that the onset and progression of hypothyroidism may still be insidious, that prolonged follow-up of patients may not be possible, and that patients may not associate symptoms arising long after therapy with a complication. The advantage of this approach is that it minimizes the dangers of persistent or recurrent thyrotoxicosis, which may be hazardous, especially in the elderly.

One way to minimize the frequency of hypothyroidism is to administer a dose per gram of estimated weight that is larger the greater the gland size. In this way, many patients with large thyroid glands are given large doses, and the converse is true for thyroid glands that are small. However, regimens of this type do not appear to improve the treatment of hyperthyroidism in the short run, and it is not known whether the rate of later hypothyroidism is changed.

In a controlled, prospective study, the effects of a single conventional dose of approximately 5.2 MBq/g (140 μCi/g) of estimated glandular weight were compared with the effects of half the dose.[232] Although the therapeutic effect of radioiodine developed more slowly in patients receiving the half-dose, and although a greater proportion required antithyroid drug therapy until this effect became apparent, the frequency of remission after 2 years was the same as that in patients receiving the conventional dose, and recurrence of thyrotoxicosis was no more common. In the full-dose group, the incidence of hypothyroidism was 8% at 1 year and 29% at 5 years, whereas in the half-dose group the corresponding values were 4% and 7%. However, thereafter the cumulative frequency with time with the low dose was similar to that observed with conventional doses. For these reasons, some physicians advocate an ablative approach to treatment.[231, 233]

The use of antithyroid drugs before RAI treatment is widely used to theoretically decrease a post-RAI increase in thyroid hormone release. This is considered especially dangerous in older age groups with ischemic heart disease in which cardiac deaths have been reported. Antithyroid drugs may also prevent the post-RAI increase in thyroid autoantibodies that may affect ophthalmopathy.[234, 235] Clearly, it is important to monitor free T4 and free T3 levels in at-risk patients and to consider β-adrenergic blockade whether or not antithyroid drugs are used before RAI treatment.

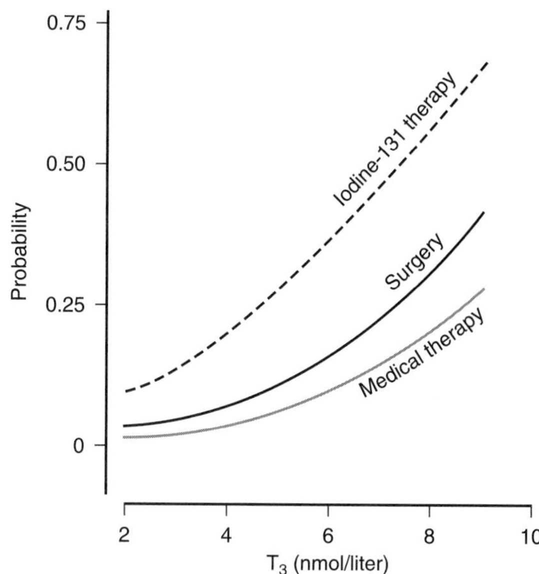

Figure 11–22. Probability of the development of worsening of orbitopathy in patients with Graves' disease. The serum triiodothyronine (T_3) levels are shown before treatment, and the type of therapy is shown as a variable. (From Tallestedt L, Lundell G, Torring O, et al. Occurrence of ophthalmopathy after treatment for Graves' disease. N Engl J Med 1992; 326:1733–1738. Copyright © 1992, Massachusetts Medical Society. All rights reserved.)

Orbitopathy and Radioiodine

As discussed earlier, Graves' orbitopathy is probably the result of a crossover specificity between retro-orbital and thyroid antigens, perhaps the TSH receptor itself. Any worsening of the autoimmune thyroid response might therefore worsen the orbital immune response. Following radioiodine therapy, the levels of circulating TSHRAbs are elevated strikingly,[45] perhaps secondary to impairment of immune restraint caused by the intrathyroidal irradiation where regulatory cells may be more sensitive. This change is in keeping with exacerbation of pretibial myxedema after radioiodine administration.[236] Similarly, carefully conducted studies indicate that eye disease worsens in about 10% of patients with Graves' orbitopathy who are treated with radioiodine (Fig. 11–22),[169, 170] although others disagree.[237, 238] Such changes, if any, are usually mild and temporary but on occasion can involve dramatic deterioration.

Some physicians advocate the use of glucocorticoids at the time of radioiodine treatment to prevent such effects.[239] One regimen involves prednisone, 0.4 to 0.5 mg/kg 1 month before ^{131}I treatment, with a gradual tapering over 3 to 4 months. Others suggest that radioiodine may not be the treatment of choice in patients with significant orbitopathy. However, maneuvers such as careful control of thyroid function before and after therapy and cessation of smoking by the patient may minimize ocular changes.

Other Side Effects of Radioiodine

Additional hazards may attend the use of radioiodine, particularly large doses. The parathyroid glands are exposed to radiation in patients treated with radioiodine. Although parathyroid reserve may be diminished in some patients, development of overt hypoparathyroidism is rare. The effect of radioiodine on other tissues that concentrate iodide (e.g., the salivary glands, the gastric glands, and the breasts) has received little attention.

Radiation thyroiditis itself may lead to an exacerbation of thyrotoxicosis 10 to 14 days after radioiodine is administered, with occasionally serious consequences, including precipitation of thyrotoxic crisis and aggravation of patients with severe thyrotoxicosis or cardiac insufficiency. In thyrocardiac disease, therefore, antithyroid drugs should be given for several weeks before radioiodine is given to deplete glandular hormone stores. This prevents an outpouring of hormone if severe radiation thyroiditis occurs. The antithyroid agent is withdrawn about 3 to 5 days before administration of the radioiodine; if the clinical condition warrants, the agent can be begun again 7 days later.

Because ^{131}I administration is contraindicated during pregnancy, a pregnancy test should be carried out in women of childbearing age before ^{131}I therapy is initiated if there is any possibility of pregnancy.

General Measures

Several general measures may contribute to the well-being of the patient with severe thyrotoxicity. Help with family responsibilities and avoidance of physical exertion are also important. In addition, a diet rich in protein, calories, and vitamins may repair the nutritional deficiencies that are common in thyrotoxic patients.

Choice of Therapy

The choice of therapy for thyrotoxicosis is influenced by emotional attitudes, economic considerations, and family and personal issues. Our choice of therapy takes into account the natural history of the disease, the advantages and disadvantages of the available therapies, and the features of the population group in which the patient falls. Apart from patients directly requesting surgery, this procedure is recommended only when the shortcomings of other modes of therapy are of particular importance (e.g., patients with antithyroid drug allergy, a cold nodule, patients with very large goiters, and patients with the need for a rapid return to normal). Occasionally, in young adults, it is necessary to remove a diffuse toxic goiter because of obstructive symptoms or cosmetic disfigurement. Nevertheless, only a small percentage of patients with Graves' disease are recommended for surgery. The choice, therefore, is among antithyroid drugs, RAI, or a mixture of both.

In one common approach to therapy in adults, the physician initiates treatment with antithyroid drugs in all patients to produce a euthyroid state before reaching a final decision regarding a definitive therapeutic strategy. This allows the patient to return to a euthyroid status as rapidly as possible and provides an estimate of the antithyroid drug dose requirement. The magnitude of the drug requirement and the size of the thyroid gland are two of a number of factors considered in the evaluation of the patient with regard to the likelihood of a remission. The options for treatment are explained to the patient during these first months of contact, and individual recommendations are then formulated. This approach allows the establishment of a workable physician-patient relationship, which is especially important in addressing anxieties about the use of radioiodine. Such concerns lead many patients, especially those younger than 50 years of age, to elect a trial of antithyroid drugs before definitive therapy with ^{131}I.

Patients with a large thyroid gland, a maintenance thionamide dose requirement of more than 400 mg/day of propylthiouracil, and high titers of TSHRAbs require prolonged antithyroid treatment and are advised that the chance of spontaneous remission is less than 30%. A therapeutic trial is generally pursued for 6 to 12 months if long-term thionamide therapy is selected. One can, in theory, treat forever unless side effects become a problem. When a decision in favor of radioiodine is made, ^{131}I may be prescribed at a dose designed to result in the retention of about 300 MBq (8 mCi) ^{131}I in the thyroid gland at 24 hours. This estimate is based on a ^{123}I uptake test performed immediately before treatment and at least 5 days after stopping thionamides. Patients with a larger goiter (more than four times normal) or those who have received large doses of propylthiouracil may require more radioiodine.[231, 240, 241] Because ^{131}I is given when the patient is euthyroid and this is a relatively large dose, no additional therapy is required immediately after treatment except for patients in whom a recurrence of hyperthyroidism poses a medical risk (e.g., patients with coronary artery disease or congestive heart failure).

Patients are seen at 4-week intervals after ^{131}I administration, and hypothyroidism is treated when it appears with an elevated TSH level, generally within 3 months. Women planning to become pregnant are advised to wait for an arbitrary period of 6 months after ^{131}I therapy to allow for resolution of any transient effects of gonadal radiation. If, after a period of 6 months, hyperthyroidism is still present and the patient is symptomatic, the treatment is repeated, generally with about 1.5 times the initial dose of ^{131}I.

Although the foregoing reflects our approach to therapy, the opinions of thyroidologists differ widely.[242] In view of the several approaches to treatment available, each with its advantages and disadvantages, it is incumbent on the physician to explain these factors thoroughly to patients, to indicate a preference and the reasons for it, and to allow the final choice to rest with the patient when appropriate.

Hypothyroidism in the Recently Hyperthyroid Patient

The early onset of hypothyroidism may cause distinct symptoms in the previously thyrotoxic patient after ^{131}I or surgical treatment or even with high doses of thionamide drugs. Such patients may develop severe muscle cramps, often in large muscle groups such as the trapezius or latissimus dorsi or the proximal muscles of the extremities. Such symptoms can develop even when the serum hormone levels are only low-normal or slightly decreased and before the TSH concentration has risen. It is possible to mistake a symptom such as back pain for an unrelated illness unless the patient is warned in advance. It is also not unusual for patients to complain of hypothyroid symptoms when thyroid function test results return to within the normal range. Such patients appear to have trouble adjusting to the normal thyroid hormone levels after being exposed to excessive amounts for long periods.

Treatment of Infiltrative Orbitopathy or Infiltrative Dermopathy

Infiltrative orbitopathy varies in severity from the common mild form to a severe form that threatens vision. The latter type is rare but remains difficult to treat. Indeed, the most effective therapies are merely palliative. The natural course of the disorder, which is variable and characterized by exacerbations and remissions, makes conclusions about the efficacy of any treatment difficult. A further source of confusion is the variable terminology for describing the manifestations of orbitopathy and the lack of rigid criteria for defining their severity. Use of the American Thyroid Association classification and its expanded indices, described earlier, is strongly recommended (see Tables 11–4 and 11–5).

Effect of Treatment of the Thyroid Gland on Orbitopathy

The first question that arises is whether different treatments for thyrotoxicosis affect the course of the eye disease differently. Subtotal thyroidectomy and thionamide drug therapy do not influence ophthalmopathy unless they lead to the development of hypothyroidism.[243] Hypothyroidism has an adverse effect on the disorder and should be treated fully when it occurs. However, exogenous thyroid hormone in the absence of hypothyroidism does not improve the ophthalmopathy.

As discussed earlier, controlled studies suggest that radioiodine treatment may lead to a slight but significant worsening of orbitopathy (see earlier discussion),[239] and it may be best to avoid radioiodine in patients with severe eye disease. Alternatively, as mentioned earlier, coincidental glucocorticoid therapy may prevent deterioration of orbitopathy after radioiodine but may itself cause significant side effects.[169] Controlled, prospective studies of the influence of antithyroid drug treatment prior to radioiodine on ocular changes are needed.

Symptomatic Treatment

Treatment modalities can be those that are largely symptomatic (useful mainly in the mild form) and those that attempt to arrest or reverse the progression of the disorder. With milder forms, little treatment is required.[244] The patient who experiences photophobia and sensitivity to wind or cold air can benefit by wearing dark glasses, which also afford protection from foreign bodies. Elevation of the head of the bed at night and instillation of lubricants, such as 1% methylcellulose, may help when the eyelids do not appose completely during sleep. Artificial tears can be used during the day. Because the ophthalmic manifestations tend to be self-limited and the progression to a more severe form is uncommon, such measures usually suffice to tide the patient over until the disorder regresses spontaneously.

Glucocorticoids

The appearance of increasing proptosis with inability to appose the eyelids or of severe infiltrative manifestations such as chemosis warrants the use of more vigorous therapeutic measures. Such changes, even when severe, may respond favorably and rapidly to glucocorticoids. Some physicians use massive doses of prednisone (120 to 140 mg/day). If improvement occurs, the dose is decreased to the lowest level at which improvement is maintained. The latter dose is still likely to be large, but it is hoped that a halt to the progression or actual regression of the disease will occur before untoward effects make withdrawal of the drug necessary. Other physicians find that much smaller doses of prednisone (20 to 30 mg/day) can be highly effective with rapid reduction to a longer-term maintenance dose (10 to 15 mg/day). Intravenous hydrocortisone pulse therapy is said to have the advantage of fewer side effects than high doses of prednisone.[245, 246]

To circumvent the inevitable side effects of large doses of glucocorticoids, periodic injection of depot preparations of glucocorticoids subconjunctivally or into the retro-orbital space has been tried but is not recommended. Such treatment may have a dramatic effect on irritative symptoms as well as on diplopia, but the efficacy varies, and systemic effects of the glucocorticoids are sometimes seen. Moreover, this treatment entails the risk of puncture of the globe or a retro-orbital hematoma. It is important to protect the patient's bones during corticosteroid treatment, especially with a postmenopausal woman, and preferably with a bisphosphonate drug such as alendronate, given at 70 mg once a week (see Chapter 27).

External Radiation

The value of external radiation to the orbits has been established by some, but not all, controlled trials.[160, 246] In fact, this treatment is steroid-sparing rather than steroid-replacing therapy and is said by some to work best in combination.[165] Whether it is more effective than prednisone therapy is unclear; as a result, the combined therapy has long been advocated.[247] The safe administration of highly collimated supervoltage radiation to the retro-orbital space requires experienced personnel. Exophthalmos and ophthalmoparesis are usually affected minimally.[248] There is a clear need for a reliable disease marker to monitor the effects of such treatment. A recent trial in mild eye disease failed to show any advantage to this approach.[248a]

Orbital Decompression

If glucocorticoid therapy and external radiation do not halt progression of the disease and if loss of vision is threatened either by ulceration or infection of the cornea or by changes in the retina or optic nerve, orbital decompression can be performed by a variety of techniques.[249] In some patients, a desire for a nearly complete cosmetic correction may be such that decompression surgery is the only therapy. This procedure usually involves removal of either the lateral wall or the roof of the orbit or resection of the lateral wall of the ethmoid sinus and the roof of the maxillary sinus.[250] This operation may cause diplopia, and even in the best of hands corrective muscle surgery may be necessary later.

An Approach to the Treatment of Orbitopathy

There are no controlled trials to support the suggestion that infiltrative orbitopathy is benefited or that its progression is retarded by total ablation of the thyroid gland, whether surgery, radioiodine, or a combination of the two is used. Hence, we recommend a trial of oral glucocorticoid therapy for patients with severe or progressive orbitopathy. If effective doses cannot be tolerated, a course of external radiation may be attempted if edema predominates.

Along with these major forms of treatment local measures should be employed. Ulceration and infection of the cornea should be treated with antibiotics, lubricants, and protective shields. An attempt to appose the eyelids by means of sutures (tarsorrhaphy) should be performed only by an experienced ophthalmologist because sutures may be torn out and cause scarring.

The management of severe orbitopathy should never be undertaken by the endocrinologist or by the ophthalmologist acting alone. Close, coordinated observation of the effects of medical therapy and the progress of the disease is necessary to determine whether and when surgery is appropriate. Surgery almost invariably halts the progress of the disease and preserves vision if it is performed in time. This decision is influenced by the ability of the available surgical team because the degree of success of such procedures is proportional to experience.

Treatment of Infiltrative Dermopathy

Treatment of infiltrative dermopathy is necessary as soon as the condition is recognized. The application of a topical, high-potency glucocorticoid preparation with an occlusive dressing may cause regression or disappearance of the lesion. Long-standing untreated dermopathy is more resistant to treatment.

Hyperthyroidism and Thyrotoxicosis in Pregnancy

As discussed earlier, postpartum thyroiditis with transient thyrotoxicosis may occur with some frequency (~5% to 10%) during the postpartum period. An overactive thyroid gland, however, is much less common in pregnancy itself. When thyrotoxicosis is present during pregnancy, it is usually more severe and is usually due to Graves' disease. Difficulty in conception and fetal wastage are increased in women with Graves' disease, but occasional patients become pregnant despite antecedent untreated hyperthyroidism. More commonly, a woman under treatment for hyperthyroidism becomes pregnant, or hyperthyroidism develops after pregnancy is under way. Whatever the sequence, pregnancy complicates the diagnosis and treatment of hyperthyroidism in Graves' disease and influences its severity and course.[251]

Diagnosis

Pregnancy and hyperthyroidism are both accompanied by thyroid enlargement, a hyperdynamic circulation, and hypermetabolism. Amenorrhea may occur in thyrotoxicosis not associated with pregnancy. In pregnancy, serum TBG levels are increased by changes in glycosylation, and thus in both conditions, the total serum T_4 and T_3 levels are elevated. The most useful laboratory tests in their differentiation are measurement of the serum TSH and free T_4 levels. Serum TSH is suppressed in hyperthyroidism during pregnancy, just as it is in nonpregnant individuals. However, there is sometimes a modest suppression of TSH (between 0.1 and 0.4 mU/L) during the 8th to 14th weeks of normal pregnancy because of stimulation of the thyroid gland by hCG during this interval.[252–255] A serum TSH below 0.1 mU/L and an elevated free T_4 or free T_3 level strongly suggests coexistent hyperthyroidism.

Treatment During Pregnancy

The management of hyperthyroidism during pregnancy can be an even greater problem than the diagnosis; however, pregnancy has an attenuating influence on the hyperthyroid state because of the immunosuppression associated with pregnancy, manifested here by a decrease in the level of thyroid autoantibodies (including levels of TSHRAbs).[256–259] Pregnancy is also one of the few clinical situations in which the biologic activity of the TSHRAbs is helpful in predicting its effect on the newborn.

Surgery

Surgery during the last trimester, and probably during the first trimester as well, is not desirable because of the possible induction of premature labor. Although surgery may be successful during the middle trimester, it is best to avoid major surgery during pregnancy if possible.

Antithyroid Drugs

Because antithyroid drug treatment poses no greater risk to the mother or fetus than does surgery and possibly involves less risk, medical therapy is the method of choice. Yet because of the usual improvement in the disease, the dosage of antithyroid drug required to control the disease in the latter phases of pregnancy is generally much less than that required in the same patient when she is not pregnant.

Certain aspects of placental physiology are relevant to the use of antithyroid drugs. Propylthiouracil and methimazole readily cross the placenta,[260] are concentrated in the fetal thyroid, and in excess quantity can cause goitrous hypothyroidism in the fetus. The administration of as little as 100 to 300 mg/day of propylthiouracil to the mother causes a slight decrease in serum T_4 concentration and an elevated TSH level in neonates.[261, 262] The long-term complication of this mild hypothyroidism is unknown but should be kept in mind in view of the observations of reduced childhood intelligence when mothers have increased TSH levels.[263] Although maternal T_4 crosses the placenta (as obviously evidenced by infants born normal with congenital hypothyroidism), placental transfer is not efficient and varies from patient to patient.[9] For these reasons, the flux of antithyroid agent to the fetus should be limited by giving the mother the smallest dosage of antithyroid agent that induces a physiologic state consistent with normal pregnancy. The serum free T_4 level should be maintained in the upper normal range. However, the concentration of hormone is not as critical as the clinical status of the patient. A modest tachycardia is a physiologic response to the increased metabolic demands of pregnancy; and pulse rates of 90 to 100 beats/minute are well tolerated without evidence of myocardial decompensation during delivery.

In most cases, the daily maintenance dose of propylthiouracil should be 200 mg or less, although maintenance doses up to 600 mg may occasionally be required. Propylthiouracil has been generally preferred to methimazole because of the greater transplacental passage of the latter drug,[260] but both drugs have proven equally safe in millions of pregnancies throughout the world and accumulate equally in breast.[264–267] In a compliant patient, a dose requirement in excess of 400 mg/day of propylthiouracil is a reasonable threshold for considering subtotal thyroidectomy, preferably in the second trimester.

All pregnant patients with significant Graves' disease should be managed in close cooperation with obstetricians experienced with modern techniques for monitoring the fetus for intrauterine thyroid dysfunction. These techniques normally include fetal heart rate monitoring and ultrasonographic assessment of fetal growth rate. With advanced ultrasonography it is usually possible to examine the fetus for the presence of goiter. Convincing evidence of fetal hyperthyroidism may be an indication to switch the mother to methimazole to attempt more effective in utero treatment of the fetus.[257] The concern regarding a rare congenital defect, *aplasia cutis*, in infants of mothers receiving methimazole or carbimazole has been allayed to some extent but cannot be dismissed.[268–271]

Iodine and Beta-Blockers

Obviously, radioiodine is contraindicated in pregnancy, although no harm has been shown by diagnostic doses.[272] Iodine itself should also not be used as therapy for any length of time in the pregnant woman because it readily crosses the placenta and can induce in the fetus an extremely large goiter that may cause airway obstruction and even death. Whether propranolol should be used in the pregnant woman with hyperthyroidism is a matter of debate. In the experience of some, it can cause intrauterine growth retardation and neonatal hypoglycemia or depression, but other studies suggest that it can be employed with safety.[215, 216]

Thyrotropin Receptor Antibodies in Pregnancy

Assays for TSHRAbs in the serum of pregnant women with Graves' disease may be of value in selected cases.[257, 273, 274] Because maternal antibodies cross the placenta, there is a correlation between the maternal level of stimulatory TSHRAbs, as measured by bioassay, and the development of fetal thyrotoxicosis. Although thyrotoxicosis occurs in only 1% of infants of mothers with Graves' disease, it is helpful to know the level of maternal TSHRAbs by radioassay, and in those women in whom the level remains high in the third trimester a formal bioassay should be obtained to estimate the stimulatory capacity of the TSHRAbs. Pregnant women at risk include those with more severe hyperthyroidism and those with significant Graves' orbitopathy or infiltrative dermopathy. In addition, the prior ablative treatment of the mother with either surgery or radioiodine may not always be accompanied by a reduction in TSHRAbs. Thus, the fetus of a treated patient with Graves' disease is still at risk for development of neonatal thyrotoxicosis and might require in utero antithyroid drug treatment, as described earlier.

Graves' Disease in the Postpartum Period

Changes in the Immune Response

Pregnancy induces a variety of immune changes that are responses to the paternal foreign antigens that must not be rejected.[153] These include a T-cell shift from Th1 to Th2 autoimmune responses and an overall decrease in all autoimmune responses as evidenced by marked decreases in thyroid autoantibodies.[275] Following delivery, these immune changes are slowly lost and a return to normal is observed but only after a period of exacerbated autoimmune reactivity in which large increases in T-cell and autoantibody activity occur.[154] It is at this time—3 to 9 months' post partum—that autoimmune thyroid disease recurrence or new onset is seen. The mechanisms behind these changes are not fully understood, but maternal microchimerism has been invoked, among other theories, and appears to be associated with Graves' disease–susceptible HLA haplotypes.[276, 276a]

Presentation

A high percentage of women in the 20- to 35-year age group give a history of pregnancy in the 12 months before the onset of Graves' disease.[155] Pregnancy and the postpartum state also apparently influence the course of hyperthyroidism in Graves' disease. Patients in clinical remission during pregnancy are prone to postpartum relapse.[258, 277] In 41 pregnancies in 35 patients in remission, 78% were followed by development of thyrotoxicosis during the postpartum period. The patients with

Graves' disease and postpartum thyrotoxicosis were classified into three categories:

1. Some patients had persistent recurrent hyperthyroidism with an elevated RAIU (*classic* Graves' disease).
2. Some had a transient disorder associated with a normal or an elevated RAIU (*transient* Graves' disease).
3. Some patients, especially those with the highest titers of TPOAb, experienced a *transient* thyrotoxicosis with a decreased RAIU that is the *thyrotoxic phase* of postpartum thyroiditis. This phase, in turn, may be followed by a hypothyroid phase (see later).

The Desire for Pregnancy

A special problem related to hyperthyroidism and pregnancy is presented by the patient who is in early remission after a course of antithyroid drug treatment or is being treated with antithyroid agents and wants to become pregnant in the near future. Management with antithyroid agents can be continued through pregnancy or reinstituted should hyperthyroidism recur, but in such instances definitive therapy (radioiodine or surgery) should be considered to forestall the complexities of managing hyperthyroidism during pregnancy. As with the therapy of Graves' disease in general, such decisions must involve education of the patient so that the risks and benefits of the various alternatives are clearly appreciated.

Nursing and Antithyroid Drugs

Older studies suggested that relatively more methimazole than propylthiouracil appeared in breast milk of women receiving these drugs,[278] but more recent evidence shows little difference between them (see earlier). However, it is generally recommended that women who take antithyroid drugs should be advised not to nurse their infants because of the difficulty in monitoring young babies. No serious drug side effects have been reported in neonates whose mothers were taking antithyroid drugs, although periodic thyroid function tests would seem appropriate if the mother continues to breast-feed.[267]

Treatment of Graves' Disease in Children and Adolescents

Thyrotoxicosis in childhood and adolescence is almost always the result of Graves' disease. Thyrotoxicosis in this age group is worthy of special consideration because treatment is less satisfactory than in adults. Hence, there is more uncertainty concerning its management, probably because the disease tends to be more severe in children.[279, 279a]

Radioiodine

For several reasons, we do not often use radioiodine in the treatment of childhood thyrotoxicosis. At least three factors weigh against such use:

1. The enhanced carcinogenic potential of radiation in the thyroid gland of the infant or child is evidenced by the correlation between childhood thyroid carcinoma and a history of radiation therapy to the head, neck, or chest in childhood[280] and the increased incidence of thyroid cancer in children exposed to radiation from the Chernobyl nuclear accident.[158]
2. Among patients with thyrotoxicosis, those treated in childhood or adolescence are thought to be at greatest risk for transmitting genetic damage, although available data suggest that this may not be likely.[281]
3. Postradioiodine hypothyroidism is a particularly undesirable complication in young children because inadequate or interrupted therapy can impair growth, development, and scholastic performance.

Antithyroid Drugs

The choice between destructive and antithyroid drug therapy may be a difficult one. The data indicate that children have a lower incidence of long-term remission after antithyroid therapy than adults,[282] although some believe that thyrotoxicosis often undergoes remission after adolescence. A course of 1 to 2 years of antithyroid therapy seems reasonable, and a second course of antithyroid therapy is regularly employed if recrudescence or relapse occurs after the first course. Measuring TSHRAbs may be helpful in assessing the child's progress. If sustained remission does not follow a second course of therapy and particularly if the patient has passed through adolescence during this period, radioiodine therapy or surgery may be considered.

Surgery

Most surgical series reveal a relatively high frequency of postoperative hypothyroidism in children. Recurrences are also more frequent, presumably as a result of attempts to avoid hypothyroidism. Complications such as hypoparathyroidism and recurrent laryngeal nerve damage must be borne over a long life span. All this leads to surgery's being less appropriate than antithyroid drugs for most children.

OTHER CAUSES OF THYROTOXICOSIS

Toxic Multinodular Goiter

Toxic multinodular goiter is a disorder in which hyperthyroidism arises in a multinodular goiter, usually of long standing, and is the result of one of several pathogenetic factors. It is important to avoid the term *toxic nodular goiter* because this confuses toxic multinodular goiter, as here described, with a toxic adenoma of the thyroid gland (see later).

Pathogenesis

The pathogenesis of toxic multinodular goiter cannot be considered apart from that of its invariable forerunner, nontoxic multinodular goiter, from which it emerges slowly and surreptitiously. Two hallmarks of the disorder—structural and functional heterogeneity and functional autonomy—evolve over time; the increase in the extent of autonomous function causes the disease to move from the nontoxic to the toxic phase, but the mechanisms of this change in all cases are uncertain. The somatic mutations in the *TSHR* gene demonstrated in toxic adenomas have been demonstrated in some cases of toxic multinodular goiter and appeared to differ from nodule to nodule.[283] However, only about 60% of toxic nodules have *TSHR* mutations, and only a few have G protein mutations. Hence, there are many nodules with undetermined causes of their autonomy.

Studies show that radioiodine becomes localized in one or more discrete nodules, whereas iodine accumulation in the remainder of the gland is usually suppressed.[284] No further suppression is produced by exogenous thyroid hormone, but TSH stimulates iodine uptake in the previously inactive areas, indicating that the suppression is due to the lack of TSH.

Histopathologically, the functioning areas resemble adenomas in being reasonably well demarcated from surrounding tissue. They generally consist of large follicles, sometimes with hyperplastic epithelium. The remaining tissue appears inactive, and zones of degeneration are present in both functioning and nonfunctioning areas. Hence, from the pathophysiologic standpoint, these thyroids harbor multiple solitary hyperfunctioning and hypofunctioning adenomas interspersed by suppressed normal thyroid tissue. The hyperfunctioning areas probably represent adenomas, with somatic mutations in the *TSHR* gene or G protein genes.

Presentation

The overproduction of thyroid hormone in toxic multinodular goiter is usually less than that in Graves' disease. First, the clinical manifestations of thyrotoxicosis are rarely flagrant. Second, the serum T_4 and T_3 concentrations may be only marginally increased, and a suppressed serum TSH level may be the only abnormality.[285] Finally, the total RAIU is only slightly increased or within the normal range.

The mildness of the hyperthyroidism is consistent with either of its presumed pathogenetic origins. The effectiveness of any stimulus to hyperfunction may be blunted in a thyroid gland that is the seat of a preexisting nontoxic multinodular goiter because of the associated impairment in the efficiency of hormone synthesis. Toxic multinodular goiter is a common complication of nontoxic multinodular goiter, but its precise incidence is unknown. It usually occurs after the age of 50 years in patients who have had nontoxic multinodular goiter for many years. Like its forerunner, toxic multinodular goiter is many times more common in women than in men. Sometimes hyperthyroidism develops abruptly, usually after exposure to increased quantities of iodine, which permits autonomous foci to increase hormone secretion to excessive levels and which may simply exacerbate already established mild hyperthyroidism (iodine-induced hyperthyroidism, von Basedow's disease). In addition, Graves' disease may either present or develop in a multinodular gland, as confirmed by the presence of TSHRAbs of the stimulating variety.[286]

Toxic multinodular goiter is almost never accompanied by infiltrative ophthalmopathy, and when the two coexist, it represents the emergence of Graves' disease. Graves' disease in the presence of multinodular goiter is a well-defined variant.[286] The clinical manifestations of toxic multinodlular goiter also differ from those in Graves' disease. Cardiovascular manifestations tend to predominate, possibly because of the age of the patients, and include atrial fibrillation or tachycardia, with or without heart failure. Surveys have indicated that TSH was suppressed in 26% of elderly patients with atrial fibrillation (Table 11–9; see also Table 11–2).[3]

A decreased response to digitalis may alert the physician to the presence of thyrotoxicosis. Weakness and wasting of muscles are common. The nervous manifestations are less prominent than in younger patients with thyrotoxicosis, but emotional lability may be pronounced. Because of the physical characteristics of the thyroid gland and its frequent retrosternal extension, obstructive symptoms are more common than in Graves' disease. On palpation, the characteristics of the goiter are the same as those of the more common nontoxic multinodular goiter (see later). In as many as 20% of elderly patients with thyrotoxicosis, the thyroid gland is firm and irregular but not distinctly enlarged. Ultrasonographic examination confirms the diagnosis as toxic multinodular goiter rather than a single toxic adenoma or Graves' disease.

Table 11–9. Atrial Fibrillation and Thyrotoxicosis

Total no. of patients examined	443
Euthyroid patients	303
Hypothyroid patients	23
Hyperthyroid patients	117 (26.4%)

From Donatelli M, Abbadi V, Bucalo ML, et al. [Atrial fibrillation and hyperthyroidism: the results of a retrospective study.] Minerva Cardioangiol 1998; 48: 157–162.

Laboratory Tests and Differential Diagnosis

The challenge to determine whether the patient with a multinodular goiter is thyrotoxic can be resolved only with laboratory tests. If the free T_4 index or free T_3 index is elevated and the TSH level is suppressed, the diagnosis of hyperthyroidism is established. TSH levels intermediate between 0.1 and the 0.5 mU/L lower limit of normal are not usually associated with significant symptoms. Such patients have thyroid autonomy but are not thyrotoxic. The pituitary-hypothalamic axis provides the most sensitive indicator of the level of thyroid hormone that is specifically relevant to the individual patient. Monitoring the concentration of serum TSH takes advantage of this sensitivity and is one of the most useful ways of establishing the existence of autonomous thyroid function. The RAIU is of little help because thyrotoxicosis may exist in association with values that are normal or only slightly increased.

Treatment

Radioiodine

Radioiodine is the treatment of choice for most patients with toxic multinodular goiter despite disagreement about the size and number of doses required to achieve a therapeutic response.[287, 288] Along the eastern seaboard of the United States, the responsiveness of toxic multinodular goiter to radioiodine may differ little from that of the diffuse toxic goiter of Graves' disease. However, in areas where goiter was formerly endemic, such as the Great Lakes area of the United States, toxic multinodular goiter is said to be more resistant to radioiodine. The more resistant variety of toxic multinodular goiter may be a reflection of low radioiodine uptake for a variety of reasons ranging from increased iodine consumption to low sodium-iodide symporter (NIS) activity.

Because of the age of the patient and variations in sensitivity to radioiodine, increased doses of RAI are often administered. These doses are likely to be larger than those used in Graves' disease because the uptake of ^{131}I tends to be lower and the gland larger. Many patients with this disorder have underlying heart disease. Therefore, the administration of radioiodine should be preceded by a course of antithyroid therapy until a eumetabolic state is achieved. Medication is then discontinued for at least 3 days before radioiodine is administered. Seven days thereafter, the antithyroid drug is reinstituted so that the thyrotoxicosis is controlled until radioiodine takes effect. After 6 to 8 weeks, the antithyroid drug is gradually withdrawn; if thyrotoxicosis recurs, a second course of therapy is given. This entire treatment sequence should be accompanied by adequate β-blockade if the cardiac status permits.

Surgery

Surgical therapy is often recommended after adequate preoperative preparation in patients with obstructive manifestations or when it is feared that such manifestations may result from the temporary thyroid enlargement that radioiodine sometimes produces, particularly in patients with retrosternal extensions of the goiter. In these patients, MRI is recommended to define the extent of the goiter and the adequacy of the tracheal walls. Respiratory function studies may also be helpful in assessing the need for surgery. When surgery is contraindicated, even significant obstructive symptoms can be relieved by adequate radioiodine therapy.[289]

Toxic Adenoma (Plummer's Disease)

A third, less common form of hyperthyroidism is caused by one or more autonomous adenomas of the thyroid gland. As herein employed, the term *toxic adenoma* refers to a tumor in a thyroid that is otherwise intrinsically normal. The disorder is usually caused by a single adenoma that is palpable as a solitary nodule and therefore is sometimes referred to as *hyperfunctioning solitary nodule* or *toxic nodule.* Occasionally, two or three adenomas of similar character are present.

Pathogenesis

Toxic adenomas are true follicular adenomas (for histopathologic characteristics, see Chapter 13). The basic pathogenesis of a large fraction of them is one of several somatic point mutations in the *TSHR* gene, commonly in the third transmembrane loop. These single nucleotide substitutions cause amino acid changes that lead to constitutive activation of the TSH receptor in the absence of TSH (Fig. 11–23).[285, 290] It appears therefore that the TSHR is "tripped" from an *off state* to an *on state.* Similarly, loss of function rather than gain of function mutations may also occur in the *TSHR* gene and may cause hypothyroidism (see later). A small number of autonomous adenomas have mutations in the G protein genes that lead to a similar state of constitutive activation.[291]

The course is one of progressive growth and increasing function over many years. At first, the adenoma may be present as a small nodule or may be impalpable; in either case, it can be detected in a radioiodine thyroid scan as a localized area of increased radioiodine accumulation (Fig. 11–24) and much of the remainder of the gland may be suppressed. With further growth, a progressively increasing share of glandular function is assumed by the adenoma, with the result that the remaining tissue is increasingly suppressed. Ultimately the remainder of the gland is completely suppressed and atrophic,

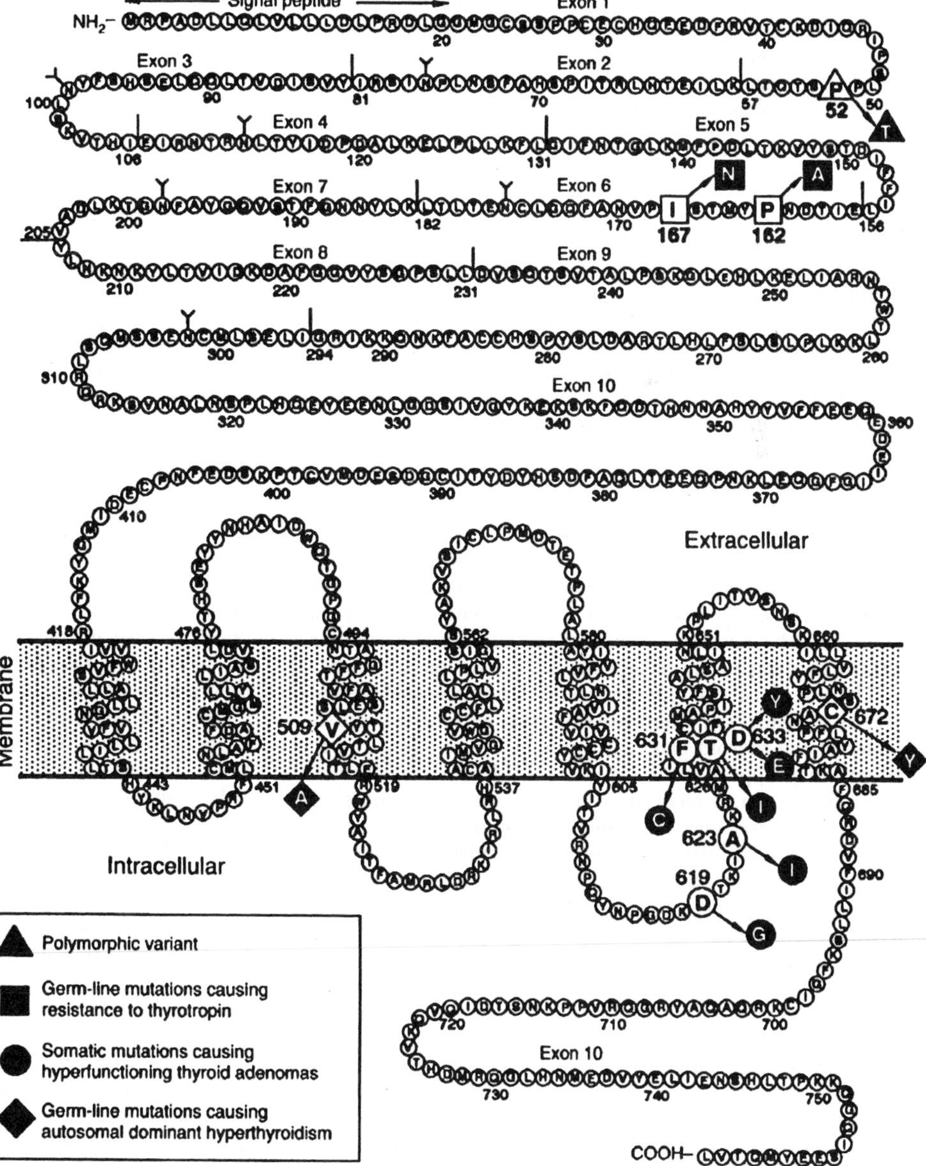

Figure 11–23. This diagram shows the thyrotropin (TSH) receptor and its ectodomain, transmembrane loops, and intracellular segment and illustrates activating and inactivating mutations of the TSH receptor. The amino acids are indicated by the single-letter code and numbered consecutively, starting with the transcription initiation codon. The *vertical lines* indicate exon boundaries. (From Sunthornthepvarakul T, Gottschalk ME, Hayashi Y, et al. Resistance to thyrotropin caused by mutations in the thyrotropin-receptor gene. N Engl J Med 1995; 332: 155–161.)

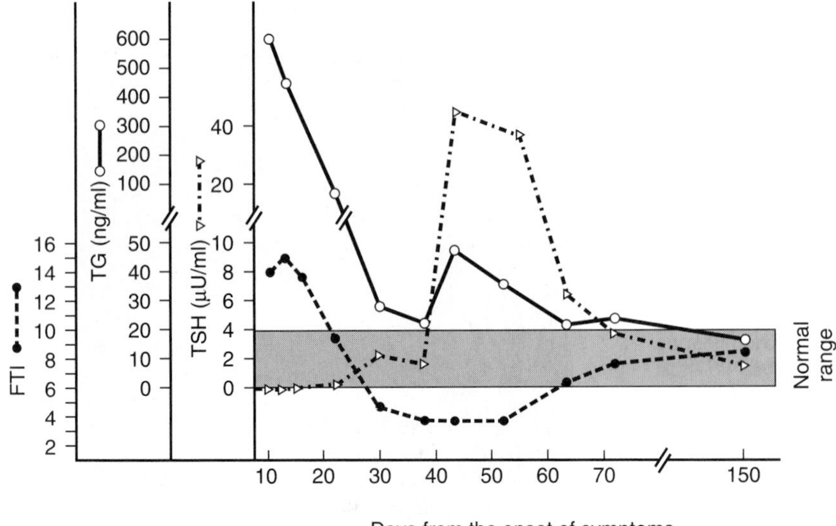

Figure 11–26. Thyroid function in a patient in the course of de Quervain's (subacute) thyroiditis. During the thyrotoxic phase (days 10 to 20) the serum thyroglobulin (TG) concentration was elevated, the free thyroxine index (FTI) was high, and thyrotropin (TSH) was suppressed. The erythrocyte sedimentation rate was 86 mm/hour, and the thyroidal radioactive iodine uptake was 2%. The Tg level and FTI declined in parallel. During the phase of hypothyroidism (days 30 to 63), when the FTI was below normal, the serum Tg level transiently increased in parallel with the increase in serum TSH. All parameters of thyroid function were normal by day 150, 5 months after the onset of symptoms. (From DeGroot LJ, Larsen PR, Hennemann G [eds]. Acute and subacute thyroiditis. In The Thyroid and Its Diseases, 6th ed. New York, Churchill Livingstone, 1996, p 705.)

moderately enlarged, firm, even nodular, and usually exquisitely tender, one lobe frequently being more severely affected than the other. Indeed, the symptoms may be truly unilateral. The overlying skin may be warm and red. Occasionally the locus of maximal involvement migrates over the course of a few weeks to other parts of the gland.

The disease usually subsides within a few months, leaving no residual deficiency of thyroid function, but often passes through a transient phase of hypothyroidism, resembling the syndrome of transient silent autoimmune thyroiditis preceded by transient thyrotoxicosis (see Fig. 11–26). In rare cases, the disease may smolder, with repeated exacerbations over many months and with hypothyroidism sometimes being the final result.

Laboratory Tests

The laboratory findings vary with the phase of the disease. During the active phase, the erythrocyte sedimentation rate (ESR) can be increased to a remarkable extent. Indeed, a diagnosis of active subacute thyroiditis is hardly tenable when the ESR is normal. The leukocyte count is normal or, at most, moderately increased. The serum Tg level is characteristically high, in keeping with the degree of thyroid destruction.

Subacute thyroiditis is one of several causes of *low-uptake thyrotoxicosis*; the others are so-called silent thyroiditis (the early phase of Hashimoto's disease [described earlier]), thyrotoxicosis factitia, and iodine-induced hyperthyroidism. For reasons described earlier, the RAIU is subnormal, despite the presence of normal, or often elevated, values of serum T_4 and T_3 concentrations. At this point in the course, basal serum TSH levels are suppressed. In the typical patient, TPO and Tg autoantibodies either are not detectable or are present in low levels. In milder cases, some uptake of radioiodine may persist in unaffected portions of the gland, as revealed by a radioiodine scan; however, this is unusual, and a diagnosis of active, subacute thyroiditis should be viewed with suspicion if the RAIU is normal.

In the hypothyroid phase, serum T_4 and T_3 concentrations are low and the serum TSH concentration is appropriately

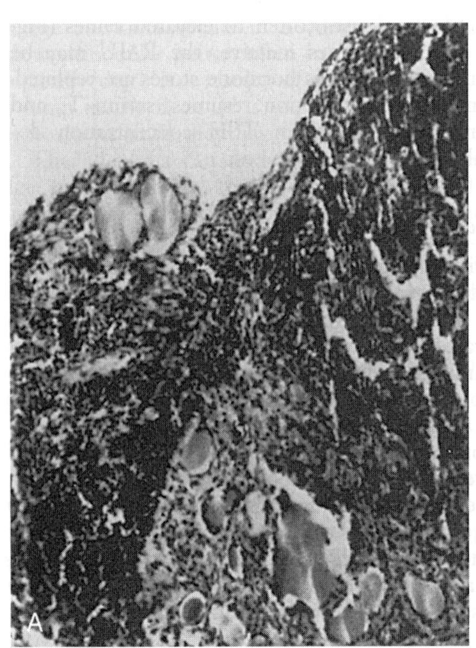

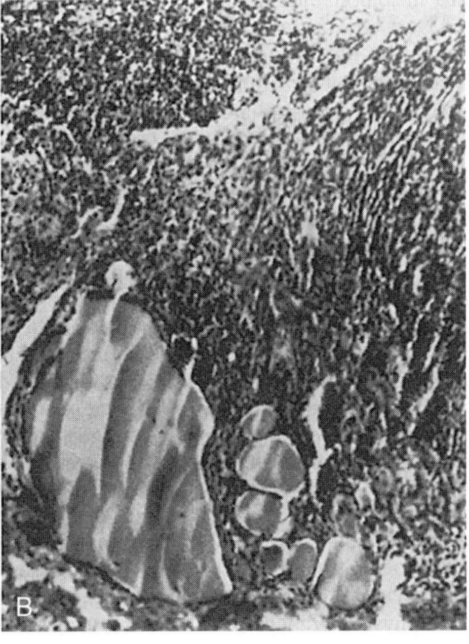

Figure 11–27. Low-power *(A)* and high-power *(B)* magnification of a thyroid gland biopsy during the hypothyroid phase of "silent thyroiditis." Note the extensive lymphocytic infiltration and patchy distribution of poorly preserved follicles. (From Woolf PD. Transient painless thyroiditis with hyperthyroidism: a variant of lymphocytic thyroiditis? Endocr Rev 1980; 1:411–420. © 1980, The Endocrine Society.)

elevated (see Fig. 11–26). With recovery, the RAIU returns to normal or high levels, and values for serum T_4 and T_3 concentrations are restored to normal.

Differential Diagnosis

Subacute thyroiditis must be differentiated from (1) acute hemorrhagic degeneration in a preexisting thyroid nodule, (2) Hashimoto's disease of acute onset, and (3) acute pyogenic thyroiditis.

Differentiation from *hemorrhage into a nodule* presents no difficulty when this occurs in a multinodular goiter, because other nontender nodules can be felt. Detection is more difficult when there is hemorrhage into a solitary nodule, but this should be easily seen on ultrasonography. In both varieties of hemorrhage, function in the remainder of the gland persists, and the ESR is rarely elevated.

Hashimoto's disease of acute onset may be accompanied by pain and tenderness in the thyroid gland, but the gland usually is diffusely affected and may present as a truly painless thyroiditis with thyrotoxicosis and a decreased RAIU but with a histologic picture of autoimmune thyroiditis and no giant cells, often termed *hashitoxicosis*. This may be difficult to distinguish from painless, subacute thyroiditis. Lack of elevation of the ESR and high titers of thyroid autoantibodies strongly suggest the former.

Acute pyogenic thyroiditis is distinguished by the presence of a septic focus elsewhere, by a greater inflammatory reaction in the tissues adjacent to the thyroid gland, and by much greater leukocytic and febrile responses. The RAIU is usually preserved in acute pyogenic thyroiditis. Rarely, widespread infiltrating thyroid cancer can present with a clinical and laboratory picture almost indistinguishable from that of subacute thyroiditis.[302]

Treatment

In mild cases, aspirin, nonsteroidal anti-inflammatory drugs, or cyclooxygenase-2 inhibitors generally control the symptoms. In more severe cases, glucocorticoids (e.g., prednisone up to 40 mg/day) alleviate the manifestations but do not influence the underlying disease process. Hence, the symptoms may be exacerbated if treatment is withdrawn too early but do again respond if treatment is reinstituted. The chance of relapse may be minimized if glucocorticoid therapy is continued at a dose that maintains the patient in an asymptomatic state until the RAIU has returned to normal.[303] Thyroid hormone replacement therapy may decrease the size of the gland by suppressing TSH and by relieving the pressure on the thyroid capsule. Because TSH is needed for thyroid cell regeneration, however, such therapy should be decreased as the symptoms subside.

Thyrotoxicosis in Silent Thyroiditis

Thyrotoxicosis is associated with the early phase of subacute thyroiditis in both painful and painless variants. In addition, thyrotoxicosis can also occur without pain in early autoimmune thyroiditis (Hashimoto's disease), in which biopsy of the thyroid gland reveals the histopathologic changes of Hashimoto's disease rather than those of subacute thyroiditis (Fig. 11–27).[304] This syndrome has variously been alluded to as silent thyroiditis with thyrotoxicosis, *hyperthyroiditis*, or *hashitoxicosis*, and cannot be distinguished from the early phase of postpartum thyroiditis (see later).

The cardinal features are thyrotoxicosis associated with depressed values of the RAIU in the absence of excess body iodide stores, lack of pain or tenderness in the thyroid area, and spontaneous resolution of the thyrotoxic phase of the disease. There is a tendency to pass through a transient euthyroid phase and then a hypothyroid phase before a long-term return to euthyroidism and a tendency for the syndrome to recur (Fig. 11–28). The thyroid gland is enlarged in only about 50% of cases, and enlargement is usually mild and unaccompanied by nodularity. Thyrotoxicosis is usually mild, and this is reflected in the extent of elevation of serum T_4 and T_3 levels. High levels of TPO autoantibodies can be detected in most patients by sensitive assays. Systemic manifestations of inflammation are lacking, and the ESR is normal or nearly normal.

Several aspects of the pathophysiology of this disorder are instructive. As in subacute thyroiditis, because of widespread apoptosis and TSH suppression the rate of ongoing synthesis of thyroid hormones is negligible, justifying the classification of this disorder among those that lead to "thyrotoxicosis without hyperthyroidism." Decreased values of the RAIU are due partly to suppression of TSH secretion by the excess of circulating hormones because the serum TSH level is suppressed; function of the thyroid follicular cell is also impaired, however, because the RAIU does not increase after administration of TSH, presumably secondary to T cell–mediated and antibody-mediated thyroid cell death.

The tendency of the disorder to pass through a hypothyroid phase is not surprising, in view of the extensive depletion of glandular hormone stores that occur while hormone is leaking from the gland and new hormone synthesis is impaired.

The duration of the thyrotoxic phase averages about 1 to 2 months. About 50% of patients return to a euthyroid phase and remain well, at least for some time. In the remaining 50%, a hypothyroid phase may follow and may last from 2 to 9 months. In most instances, euthyroidism is eventually restored, but permanent hypothyroidism may develop in some patients years later.[305] About one third of patients retain a goiter, usually with persistence of thyroid autoantibodies in the serum. The opposite sequela—recurrence of thyrotoxicosis—may also occur months or years after restoration of a euthyroid state, and some patients experience multiple recurrences.

Treatment of the thyrotoxic phase consists of alleviation of the peripheral manifestations through the use of β-blockers or sedatives. Reportedly, prednisone (30 to 50 mg/day) decreases the duration of the thyrotoxic phase without the risk of relapse on its withdrawal but is not needed.[306] If the hypothyroid phase is mild and brief, patients may not require treatment. When treatment with levothyroxine is needed, it should be undertaken with the understanding that it will be withdrawn approximately 6 months later, because the hypothyroidism is unlikely to be permanent.

The underlying nature of the disorder is an autoimmune

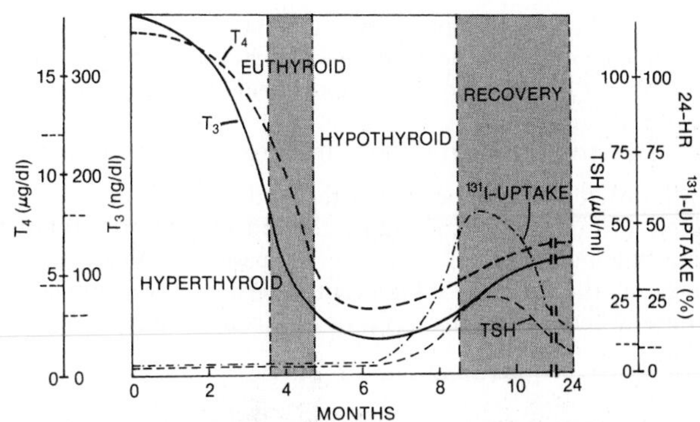

Figure 11–28. Schematic of the typical course in chronic thyroiditis with transient thyrotoxicosis. The duration of each phase may vary, and some patients do not experience a discernible hyperthyroid or hypothyroid phase. (From Woolf PD. Transient painless thyroiditis with hyperthyroidism: a variant of lymphocytic thyroiditis? Endocr Rev 1980; 1:411–420. © 1980, The Endocrine Society.)

dysregulation. Extensive lymphocytic infiltration and the presence of plasma cells within the thyroid are similar to those seen in more classic Hashimoto's thyroiditis, as are the circulating thyroid autoantibodies. The latter, however, may merely reflect a response to the inflammatory release of antigens. The occurrence of the syndrome in patients known to also have Graves' disease, which we and others have observed, and the later emergence of hypothyroidism (Hashimoto's disease) are also consonant with an autoimmune etiology. On the other hand, the absence of high levels of circulating antithyroid antibodies in many patients and the permanent resolution indicate that the immune system regains its equilibrium in these patients. This provides a great opportunity to further our understanding of these control mechanisms.

Thyrotoxicosis in Postpartum Thyroiditis

The postpartum thyroiditis syndrome is similar in presentation, course, and pathophysiology to silent thyroiditis (Fig. 11–29).[307] Transient thyrotoxicosis with low RAIU may develop within 3 to 6 months after delivery and is often followed by a period of hypothyroidism of several months' duration and an eventual return to a euthyroid state. In some patients, only a hypothyroid phase is evident. The incidence of postpartum thyroiditis varies geographically but may occur in as many as 10% of women and in more than 30% of those with positive TPO autoantibodies.[308, 309] This argues for prenatal assessment for the presence of TPO antibodies. In women found to be positive for TPO antibodies, postpartum assessment of thyroid function is recommended at 2, 4, 6, and 12 months.

As in the similar syndrome of silent thyroiditis, not temporally related to pregnancy, recurrences are common after subsequent pregnancies. Most patients have a small goiter and positive tests for TPO antibodies, although levels may be low. The syndrome has also been observed post partum in patients known to have prepartum Graves' disease. There is a strong association with the HLADR3 and HLADR5 haplotypes,[309] which are also associated with autoimmune thyroid disease. The occurrence of the disorder after delivery is probably due to a rebound of immune activity after its suppression during pregnancy.[154, 256] However, the role of fetal microchimerism has also been implicated in the initiation of disease.[276a]

Hyperthyroidism Caused by Thyrotropin or Thyrotropin Receptor Agonists

Rarely hyperthyroidism results from hypersecretion of TSH or TSH-like activity because of three causative factors:

1. A TSH-secreting pituitary adenoma.
2. Inappropriate hypersecretion of TSH secondary to localized pituitary resistance to thyroid hormones or increased secretion of TRH.
3. Excessive secretion of hCG from trophoblastic tumors.

All varieties are associated with a diffuse, hyperfunctioning goiter. Features of autoimmune thyroid disease are absent in these patients and in the families of patients. When TSH is the cause, the serum TSH concentrations are not suppressed at a time when serum free T_4 or T_3 concentrations are elevated.[310]

Thyrotropin-Secreting Pituitary Tumors

In the adenomatous variety, a mass lesion is present in the pituitary gland (see Chapter 8). The concentration of free α subunits of TSH in serum is elevated, and serum TSH concentrations may fail to increase after TRH administration. In patients with nonadenomatous TSH hypersecretion, in contrast, α subunits are not present in the blood in high concentrations and the response to TRH is usually normal.[310–312] In addition, patients with thyroid hormone resistance may respond to oral T_3 rather than T_4.

Patients with excess TSH in the absence of resistance present a difficult therapeutic problem. In some cases, TSH secretion can be suppressed if somewhat large doses of thyroid hormone are administered, but this results in worsening of the thyrotoxicosis. Hyperthyroidism can be controlled, of course, by thyroid ablation, but serum TSH levels then increase still further, raising the question as to whether a TSH-producing adenoma may ultimately develop. Bromocriptine, a dopamine agonist, may suppress TSH secretion and alleviate the hyperthyroidism in this disorder.[313] Somatostatin analogues have also been used. However, TSH-producing tumors usually require surgical resection.[314, 315] Treatment with 3,5,3′–triiodothyroacetic acid has also been successful.[316]

The occurrence of TSH-induced hyperthyroidism further supports the argument that a serum TSH concentration should be measured as part of the initial work-up of every patient who is hyperthyroid and has a diffuse goiter. The remote possibility that a patient with Graves' disease might have an artifactual elevation of TSH concentration because of a heterophilic antibody cross-reacting with mouse immunoglobulin (see Chapter 6) must be kept in mind.[317] For some sera, the use of a different assay kit may confirm the elevated level. Alternatively, mouse serum may be added to the assay tube to absorb the heterophile antibody.

A Note on Pituitary Resistance to Thyroid Hormone

In some patients with inherited thyroid hormone resistance due to mutations in the β thyroid hormone receptor, the hypothalamic pituitary feedback mechanism may be more resistant to the effects of thyroid hormone compared with peripheral tissues, such as the heart.[318–321] These patients may have a hyperthyroid appearance with tachycardia, nervousness, and goiter associated with an elevated free T_4 index. Because the thyroid hormone hyperproduction is TSH-driven, however, serum TSH concentrations are detectable (>0.1 mU/L) or even elevated inappropriately for the circulating thyroid hormone levels (see Chapter 12).

In general, the manifestations are due not to excessive but to inadequate thyroid hormone action, and these individuals may require treatment with thyroid hormone or thyroid hormone analogues and β-adrenergic receptor–blocking agents rather than antithyroid drugs.[319, 320, 322] This argues again for the appropriateness of at least one serum TSH measurement in every hyperthyroid patient because this is the only way that an accurate diagnosis can be achieved (see discussion of thyroid hormone resistance in topic of hypothyroidism). Rarely, families with just pituitary resistance to thyroid hormone (PRTH) may respond to treatment with liothyronine.[323]

Hyperthyroidism in Trophoblastic Disease

Thyroid hyperfunction often accompanies hydatidiform mole, choriocarcinoma, or metastatic embryonal carcinoma of the testis. Such neoplasms, particularly hydatidiform mole, elaborate differentially glycosylated hCG molecules that exhibit crossover specificity for binding to the TSH receptor and can induce thyroid overactivity.[253, 324–326] Some patients have clinically overt thyrotoxicosis; however, clinical manifestations are usually not prominent, and goiter is absent or minimal despite laboratory evidence of a hyperthyroid state. Free T_4 or free T_3

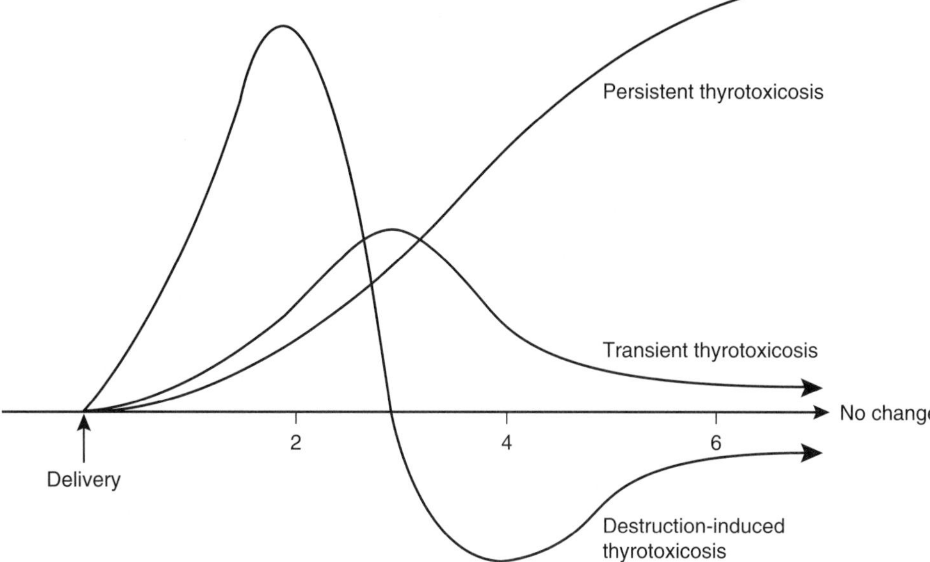

Figure 11–29. Changes in free thyroxine in various types of postpartum thyroid disease. Numbers indicate the number of months post partum. (Adapted from Davies TF [ed]. Autoimmune Endocrine Disease. New York, John Wiley & Sons, 1983, p 255.)

levels are increased, and TSH values are suppressed. The reason for this discordance between the clinical and the laboratory indices is not known but the discordance may be due to the relatively short duration of thyroid hormone excess. The possibility of a molar pregnancy should always be considered in a young woman with thyrotoxicosis, because appropriate therapy is evacuation of the uterus.

Iodine-Induced Hyperthyroidism

Administration of supplemental iodine to subjects with endemic iodine deficiency goiter can result in iodine-induced hyperthyroidism and even Graves' disease. This response, termed *iodine-induced hyperthyroidism* or the *Jod-Basedow effect,* occurs in only a small fraction of individuals at risk. The best-studied experience has been in Tasmania, where a temporary increase in thyrotoxicosis occurred shortly after the addition of small quantities of iodine to bread as a means of correcting iodine deficiency.

Studies revealed two major patterns of underlying thyroid disorder. In the first, especially common in older individuals, nodular goiter with areas of autonomous function were present and TSHRAbs of the type found in Graves' disease were not detectable in the blood. In the second pattern, which occurred in younger individuals with diffuse goiter, stimulating TSHRAbs were often present. These findings suggest that the Jod-Basedow effect occurs only in thyroid glands in which function is independent of TSH stimulation. The occurrence of the Jod-Basedow effect should not be construed as a reason for failing to treat endemic iodine deficiency. Apart from the many other benefits that accrue from iodine treatment and prophylaxis, over the long run the frequency of spontaneous hyperthyroidism associated with the development of autonomous nodules is diminished.

Iodine-induced hyperthyroidism is an important disorder in areas of the world where dietary iodine intake is high.[211] In regions where iodine intake is marginal but overt iodine deficiency is absent, moderate increments in iodine intake may induce hyperthyroidism in patients with autonomous thyroid nodules, and large pharmacologic doses of iodine, can do so in geographic areas where the iodine intake is more than adequate. Consequently, the physician must be alert to the possibility of inducing hyperthyroidism when administering large quantities of iodine in expectorants, radiographic contrast media, medications containing iodine (e.g., amiodarone), or any other form to patients with nodular goiter. Because nodular goiter is generally a disease of older people, induction of the Jod-Basedow phenomenon can have serious consequences, because enrichment of the thyroid gland with iodine forestalls administration of ^{131}I and delays the response to antithyroid agents. In these patients, serum T_3 concentration is sometimes normal, although total and free T_4 concentrations are increased and TSH is suppressed. Confirmation that the patient has been exposed to large quantities of iodine can be obtained by demonstrating that the RAIU is low and urinary iodine excretion increased (more than several milligrams per day).

The treatment of these individuals may be difficult. Even after discontinuation of exogenous iodide, uptake of ^{131}I by the thyroid gland may remain low, not adequate for conventional doses of radioiodine. The elevated thyroid hormone content also makes thionamide drugs less effective. In some cases, it may be necessary to treat such individuals for prolonged periods (6 to 9 months) before administering radioiodine therapy; if uptake is detectable, however, larger doses of radioiodine may be given to destroy thyroid tissue.

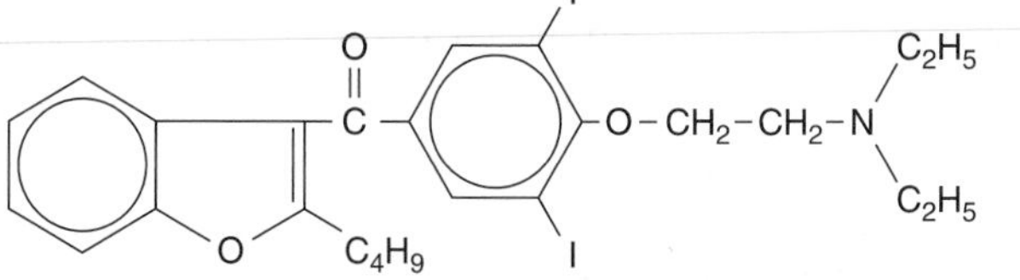

I O C O–CH$_2$–CH$_2$–N C$_2$H$_5$ C$_2$H$_5$ O C$_4$H$_9$ I

Figure 11–30. The structure of amiodarone illustrating the characteristics of thyroid hormone. The molecule is 37% iodine by weight.

Amiodarone

Amiodarone is an iodine-rich drug that has become increasingly popular because of its effectiveness in combating severe cardiac arrhythmias. The drug has complex effects on the thyroid gland, although most patients(~80%) remain euthyroid.[327–329] Structurally, the drug resembles T_4 (Fig. 11–30) and contains 37% iodine. It has been estimated that a huge amount (~200 mg/day) of iodide is made available in a daily dose of 600 mg. It has a half-life of 50 to 60 days and therefore remains available for a long period even after drug withdrawal.

Amiodarone inhibits types 1 and 2 5′-deiodinases and increases T_4 levels at the same time as it increases TSH. The drug may also compete for the T_3 receptor. Amiodarone also has a direct cytotoxic effect on thyroid cells via induction of apoptosis. In addition, an iodine load may precipitate thyroid autoimmune disease, as discussed earlier, in susceptible individuals and induces most commonly autoimmune hypothyroidism, but Graves' disease may also be precipitated. Most commonly, however, it is the influence of the iodine load that causes the clinical effects, particularly in areas of iodine deficiency where thyrotoxicosis is most commonly seen and in areas of iodine sufficiency where hypothyroidism is most commonly seen.

Amiodarone-induced hyperthyroidism may develop either rapidly in a patient or even after a few years of treatment. The different presentations have been divided as follows[330]:

Type I occurs in abnormal thyroid glands secondary to iodine excess.

Type II is secondary to drug-induced destructive thyroiditis, sometimes resulting in high serum IL-6 levels that can be checked in the serum.

Both types may occur together, and treatment is often a major challenge. Antithyroid drugs and radioiodine may be ineffective because of the large intrathyroidal iodine load. Thyroidectomy is therefore the treatment of choice if the patient's clinical condition permits. This allows the continuation of the drug. The use of combined potassium perchlorate (1 g daily) and methimazole (40 mg daily) may be tried if surgery is not possible.[331] A complete blood count must be checked regularly with such treatment, which is fraught with side effects. If Type II predominates, steroids may control the destructive thyroiditis (2 to 6 mg of dexamethasone daily). In contrast, when hypothyroidism is the presentation, due to thyroid destruction at the onset of Hashimoto's disease or the failure to escape from iodine blockade, levothyroxine replacement is effective. TSH should be monitored appropriately. If the drug is discontinued, there may be spontaneous remission. Potassium perchlorate may provide increased speed of recovery by discharging intrathyroidal iodide.

Hamburger Thyrotoxicosis

An unusual form of exogenous thyrotoxicosis occurred in the midwestern portion of the United States in 1984 and 1985. The source was the inclusion of large quantities of bovine thyroid in ground beef preparations.[332] When the slaughtering practices were changed, this condition, called hamburger thyrotoxicosis, disappeared. Such a possibility, however remote, should be considered, especially if one is confronted with epidemic exogenous thyrotoxicosis. Here the cause was probably the direct ingestion of large amounts of thyroid hormone, but the additional iodine load and its consequences should also be considered.

Thyrotoxicosis Caused by Nonthyroid Sources of Thyroid Hormone

Thyrotoxicosis Factitia

Thyrotoxicosis that arises from the (usually chronic) ingestion of excessive quantities of thyroid hormone usually occurs in individuals with a background of underlying psychiatric disease, especially in paramedical personnel who have access to thyroid hormone or in patients for whom thyroid hormone medication has been prescribed in the past.[333] Generally, the patient is aware of taking thyroid hormone but may adamantly deny it. In other instances, large doses of thyroid hormone or other thyroactive material, such as iodocasein, may be given without the knowledge of the patient, usually as part of a regimen for weight reduction. Symptoms are typical of thyrotoxicosis and may be severe.

In the absence of preexisting thyroid disease, the diagnosis is made from the combination of typical thyrotoxic manifestations, together with thyroid atrophy and hypofunction. Infiltrative ophthalmopathy never occurs, but lid lag, stare, and other "thyrotoxic" eye signs may be present. Hypofunction of the thyroid gland is evidenced by suppressed serum Tg levels and subnormal values of RAIU, which can be increased by administration of TSH. Serum T_4 concentrations are increased unless the patient is taking T_3, in which case they will be subnormal. Serum T_3 concentrations are increased in either case. TSH levels are suppressed. The presence of low, rather than elevated, values of serum Tg concentration is a clear indication that the thyrotoxicosis results from exogenous hormone rather than thyroid hyperfunction.[334] This disorder may be confused with other varieties of thyrotoxicosis associated with a subnormal RAIU and absence of goiter, including the syndrome of Hashimoto's disease preceded by transient thyrotoxicosis (silent thyroiditis), ectopic thyroid tissue, and hyperfunctioning metastatic follicular carcinoma. Evidence for the latter two disorders can be obtained by demonstration of the ectopic focus or foci by external radioiodine scanning and the fact that serum thyroglobulin is increased in both conditions.

Differentiation from silent and painless thyroiditis may be difficult. The presence of circulating TPO and Tg antibodies points to painless chronic autoimmune thyroiditis, whereas a firm thyroid gland and a brief history suggest the painless variant of subacute thyroiditis.

Treatment consists of withdrawing the offending medication. Psychiatric help may be necessary.

Ectopic Thyroid Tissue

Thyroid tissue may be present in teratomas, especially in the ovary (struma ovarii), and such foci may produce thyrotoxicosis.[335] Rarely, hyperfunctioning metastases of follicular carcinoma can produce thyrotoxicosis. The distinguishing features of such lesions have been discussed earlier.

Special Aspects of Thyrotoxicosis

T_3 Toxicosis

Concurrent measurements of T_4 and T_3 production rates have revealed a disproportionate increase in T_3 production in most patients with hyperthyroidism.[336] Whether this phenomenon results solely from the preferential increase in thyroid synthesis of T_3, preferential intrathyroidal T_4 to T_3 conversion or from a disproportionate increase in peripheral conversion of T_4 to T_3 is uncertain, but the preferential synthesis is probably responsible in most instances.[178] In the extreme case, the production rate of T_3 alone is increased, resulting in the thyrotoxic state designated T_3 toxicosis. In some patients, T_3 toxicosis may be the forerunner of the usual form of thyrotoxicosis in which production of both T_3 and T_4 is increased, and in other patients it persists as such. T_3 toxicosis may occur with Graves' disease, toxic multinodular goiter, or toxic adenoma. (See Table 10–14.)

The prevalence is not known, but T_3 toxicosis appears to be more common than the conventional types of hyperthyroidism in areas of iodine deficiency. In our experience, it tends to be more frequent in older people.

The diagnosis should be suspected in a patient with clinical manifestations of thyrotoxicosis in whom the serum T_4 level and free T_4 concentration or index are normal or decreased while the serum TSH concentration is suppressed. Documentation of an elevated free T_3 level confirms the diagnosis. The presence of a palpable goiter and a normal or increased RAIU excludes the diagnosis of thyrotoxicosis factitia induced by ingestion of T_3. Experience suggests that patients with T_3 toxicosis are more likely to have a long-term remission after withdrawal of antithyroid drug therapy than patients with the usual form of thyrotoxicosis.

T_4 Toxicosis

T_4 toxicosis refers to thyrotoxicosis with an increased serum T_4 concentration and free T_4 concentration or index but a normal or decreased serum T_3 concentration. This phenomenon occurs in two circumstances. One is iodine-induced thyrotoxicosis,[211] in which about one third of the patients have a normal serum T_3 concentration and the remainder display proportionate elevations of serum T_3 and T_4 concentrations.[337] The second is thyrotoxicosis accompanied by severe intercurrent illness.[338, 339] (See Table 10–14.) Here, that component of the serum T_3 usually contributed by peripheral T_4 5′−monodeiodination is decreased or lacking, so the serum T_3 concentration, sustained mainly or entirely by direct thyroid secretion, is normal or low, although the serum T_4 concentration is high.

Concomitantly, the serum rT_3 concentration is increased, often markedly, owing to inhibition of its 5′−monodeiodination. With recovery from the intercurrent illness, serum rT_3 concentration declines and serum T_3 concentration increases into the thyrotoxic range.[340] T_4 toxicosis of this type is to be differentiated from the low serum T_3 level and elevated serum T_4 concentration that are occasionally found in the euthyroid sick syndrome.[341] A reduced serum TSH level may not distinguish patients who are mildly hyperthyroid from those who are not. Some of these changes are thought to be cytokine-mediated.

Thyrotoxic Crisis (Thyroid Storm)

Thyrotoxic crisis, also called *accelerated hyperthyroidism* or *thyroid storm*, is an extreme accentuation of thyrotoxicosis. The crisis, however, may be exaggerated by an inexperienced physician. It is an uncommon but serious complication, usually occurring in association with Graves' disease but sometimes with toxic multinodular goiter. Before the availability of adequate means for achieving full preoperative control, crisis frequently followed subtotal thyroidectomy *(surgical crisis)*.

Thyrotoxic crisis is usually of abrupt onset and occurs in patients in whom preexisting thyrotoxicosis has been treated incompletely or has not been treated at all. Crisis is usually precipitated by infection, trauma, surgical emergencies, or operations and, less commonly, by radiation thyroiditis, diabetic ketoacidosis, toxemia of pregnancy, or parturition. The mechanism by which such factors worsen thyrotoxicosis may be related to cytokine release and acute immunologic disturbance caused by the precipitating condition. The serum thyroid hormone levels in crisis are not appreciably greater than those in uncomplicated thyrotoxicosis.

The clinical picture is one of severe hypermetabolism. Fever is almost invariable and may be severe; sweating is profuse. Marked tachycardia of sinus or ectopic origin and arrhythmias may be accompanied by pulmonary edema or congestive heart failure. Tremulousness and restlessness are present; delirium or frank psychosis may supervene. Nausea, vomiting, and abdominal pain may occur early in the course. As the disorder progresses, apathy, stupor, and coma may supervene, and hypotension can develop. If unrecognized, the condition may be fatal. This clinical picture in a patient with a history of preexisting thyrotoxicosis or with goiter or exophthalmos or both is sufficient to establish the diagnosis, and emergency treatment should not await laboratory confirmation.

There are no foolproof criteria by which severe thyrotoxicosis complicated by some other serious disease can be distinguished from thyrotoxic crisis induced by that disease. In any event, the differentiation between these alternatives is of no great significance because treatment of the two is the same.

Treatment aims to correct both the severe thyrotoxicosis and the precipitating illness and to provide general support. The patient thought to have thyroid crisis should be monitored in a medical intensive care unit during the initial phases of therapy. The therapy itself is designed to inhibit hormone synthesis and release and to antagonize the adrenergically mediated aspects of peripheral thyroid hormone action.

Large doses of an antithyroid agent (300 to 400 mg of propylthiouracil every 4 hours) are given by mouth, by stomach tube, or, if necessary, per rectum. Propylthiouracil may be preferable to methimazole because it has the additional action of inhibiting the peripheral generation of T_3 from T_4 by Type 1 iodothyronine deiodinase.[190–192] Administration of propylthiouracil initiates therapy for the postcrisis period and prevents enrichment of glandular hormone stores by the iodine, whose administration is of more immediate importance. The latter agent, administered either as SSKI (5 drops every 6 hours), ipodate (0.5 g twice daily) or, if available, sodium iodide intravenously (0.250 g every 6 hours), acutely retards the release of hormone from the thyroid gland.

Propylthiouracil should be administered before iodine to inhibit the synthesis of additional thyroid hormones from the administered iodine. Nonetheless, because iodine blocks release of preformed thyroid hormones from the thyroid gland, its administration *should not be delayed or omitted* in the severely toxic patient if propylthiouracil (or methimazole) is not immediately available. The latter agents may be given by intragastric infusion if necessary.

Large doses of dexamethasone (2 mg orally every 6 hours) are given to inhibit both the release of hormone from the gland and the peripheral generation of T_3 from T_4, synergizing with iodide and propylthiouracil, respectively, in these actions. Indeed, the combined use of propylthiouracil, iodide, and dexamethasone restores the serum T_3 concentration to within the normal range in 24 to 48 hours,[342] and the substitution of sodium ipodate or iopanoate for iodide may be even more effective.[212] In the absence of cardiac insufficiency a β-adrenergic blocking agent should be given to ameliorate the manifestations. Most experience has been with propranolol given at a dose of 40 to 80 mg orally every 6 hours, but a short-acting β-adrenergic blocker such as labetalol may be safer than propranolol in this situation. High-output congestive heart failure can develop in patients with severe thyrotoxicosis, and a β-adrenergic antagonist may further reduce cardiac output.

Supportive measures include correction of dehydration and hypernatremia, if present, and administration of glucose. Hyperpyrexia should be treated vigorously. In mild cases, acetaminophen may suffice, but wet packs, fans, or ice packs may be required. Salicylates should be avoided because they compete with T_3 and T_4 for binding to TBG and transthyretin (TTR) and therefore increase the free hormone levels.[343] In addition, in large doses, salicylates increase the metabolic rate. If heart failure or pulmonary congestion is present, appropriate diuretics are indicated. In patients with atrial fibrillation, the rapid ventricular response requires appropriate blockade of atrioventricular node conduction.

When treatment is successful, improvement is usually manifested within 1 or 2 days and recovery occurs within a week. At this time, iodide and dexamethasone are gradually withdrawn and plans for long-term management are made.

Subclinical Hyperthyroidism

With the advent of thyroid function screening and the presence of highly sensitive TSH assays, many patients with mild thyroid disease now consult physicians for advice.[344] The presence of a chronically suppressed serum level TSH with peripheral free thyroid hormone levels within the normal range has been defined as mild or "subclinical" hyperthyroidism. In a study of more than 25,000 people attending a health fair, 0.9% were found to have this condition.[345]

Subclinical hyperthyroidism may occur with clinical symptoms and signs that include weight loss, anxiety, atrial fibrillation, and osteoporosis or with no symptoms at all.[3] All of the causes of thyrotoxicosis may be associated with such a mild presentation, most often Graves' disease and toxic multinodular goiter. Indeed, it is these patients who are the ones with precipitated severe thyrotoxicosis after an increase in their iodine intake.

Making the correct diagnosis is helpful in deciding treatment and excluding transient thyroiditis. When there are symptoms or obvious risks, treatment is required. If there are no signs or symptoms and the diagnosis has been made biochemically, watchful observation may be appropriate. In patients with mild Graves' disease, a short course of low-dose antithyroid drugs may cure the condition. In the presence of toxic nodules, radioiodine may be more appropriate, particularly in elderly populations, whose risk of cardiac arrhythmias is increased.

References

1. Woeber KA. Thyrotoxicosis and the heart. N Engl J Med 1992; 327:94–98.
2. Channick BJ, Adlin EV, Marks AD. Hyperthyroidism and mitral valve prolapse. N Engl J Med 1981; 305:497–500.
3. Sawin CT, Geller A, Wolf PA, et al. Low serum thyrotropin concentrations as a risk factor for atrial fibrillation in older persons. N Engl J Med 1994; 331:1249–1252.
4. Bilezekian J, Loeb J. The influence of hyperthyroidism and hypothyroidism on the alpha and beta adrenergic receptor system and adrenergic responsiveness. Endocr Rev 1983; 4:378–388.
5. Aoki VS, Wilson WR, Theilen EO. The effects of triiodothyrinine on hemodynamic responses to epinephrine and norepinephrine in man. J Pharmacol Exp Ther 1967; 157:62–68.
6. Landsberg L. Catecholamines and hyperthyroidism. Clin Endocrinol Metab 1977; 6:697–718.
7. Metz LD, Seidler FJ, McCook EC, Slotkin TA. Cardiac alpha-adrenergic receptor expression is regulated by thyroid hormone during a critical developmental period. J Mol Cell Cardiol 1996; 28:1033–1044.
8. Liggett SB, Cryer PE. Increased fat and skeletal muscle beta adrenergic receptors but unaltered metabolic and hemodynamic sensitivity to epinephrine in vivo in experimental human thyrotoxicosis. J Clin Invest 1989; 83:803–809.
9. Penela P, Barradas M, Alvarez-Dolado M, et al. Effect of hypothyroidism on G protein–coupled receptor kinase 2 expression levels in rat liver, lung, and heart. Endocrinology 2001; 142:987–991.
10. Myers JD, Brannon ES, Holland BC. A correlative study of the cardiac output and the hepatic circulation in hyperthyroidism. J Clin Invest 1950; 29:1069–1077.
11. Ober KP. Thyrotoxic periodic paralysis in the United States: report of seven cases and review of the literature. Medicine (Baltimore) 1992; 71:109–120.
12. Tamai H, Tanaka K, Komaki G, et al. HLA and thyrotoxic periodic paralysis in Japanese patients. J Clin Endocrinol Metab 1987; 64:1075–1078.
13. Kodali VR, Jeffcote B, Clague RB. Thyrotoxic periodic paralysis: a case report and review of the literature. J Emerg Med 1999; 17: 43–45.
14. Costagliola S, Morgenthaler NG, Hoermann R, et al. Second-generation assay for thyrotropin receptor antibodies has superior diagnostic sensitivity for Graves' disease. J Clin Endocrinol Metab 1999; 84:90–97.
15. Wakasugi M, Wakao R, Tawata M, et al. Bone mineral density in patients with hyperthyroidism measured by dual energy X-ray absorptiometry. Clin Endocrinol (Oxf) 1993; 38:283–286.
16. Wakasugi M, Wakao R, Tawata M, et al. Change in bone mineral density in patients with hyperthyroidism after attainment of euthyroidism by dual energy X-ray absorptiometry. Thyroid 1994; 4:179–182.
17. Kumeda Y, Inaba M, Tahara H, et al. Persistent increase in bone turnover in Graves' patients with subclinical hyperthyroidism. J Clin Endocrinol Metab 2000; 85:4157–4161.
18. Wejda B, Hintze G, Katschinski B, et al. Hip fractures and the thyroid: a case-control study. J Intern Med 1995; 237:241–247.
19. Diamond T, Vine J, Smart R, Butler P. Thyrotoxic bone disease in women: a potentially reversible disorder. Ann Intern Med 1994; 120:8–11.
20. Burman RD, Monchik JM, Earll JM, et al. Ionized and total serum calcium and parathyroid hormone in hyperthyroidism. Ann Intern Med 1976; 84:668–671.
21. Rhone DP, Berlinger FG, White FM. Tissue sources of elevated serum alkaline phosphatase activity in hyperthyroid patients. Am J Clin Pathol 1980; 74:381–386.
22. Bergman TA, Mariash CN, Oppenheimer JH. Anterior mediastinal mass in a patient with Graves' disease. J Clin Endocrinol Metab 1982; 55:587–588.
23. Rogers JS, Shane SR, Jencks FS. Factor VIII activity and thyroid function. Ann Intern Med 1982; 97:713.
24. Self TH, Straughn AB, Weisburst MR. Effect of hyperthyroidism on hypoprothrombinemic response to warfarin. Am J Hosp Pharm 1976; 33:387–389.
25. Gordon GG, Southren AL. Thyroid hormone effects on steroid hormone metabolism. Bull NY Acad Med 1977; 53:241–259.
26. Taniyama M, Honma K, Ban Y. Urinary cortisol metabolites in the assessment of peripheral thyroid hormone action: application for diagnosis of resistance to thyroid hormone. Thyroid 1993; 3: 229–233.
27. Stagnaro-Green A. Recognizing, understanding, and treating postpartum thyroiditis. Endocrinol Metab Clin North Am 2000; 29:417–30, ix.
28. Imaizumi M, Pritsker A, Kita M, et al. Pregnancy and murine thyroiditis: thyroglobulin immunization leads to fetal loss in specific allogeneic pregnancies. Endocrinology 2001; 142:823–829.
29. Ojamaa K, Klein I, Sabet A, Steinberg SF. Changes in adenylyl cyclase isoforms as a mechanism for thyroid hormone modulation of cardiac beta-adrenergic receptor responsiveness. Metabolism 2000; 49(2):275–279.
30. Burggraaf J, Tulen JH, Lalezari S, et al. Sympathovagal imbalance in hyperthyroidism. Am J Physiol Endocrinol Metab 2001; 281(1):E190–195.
31. Faber J, Wiinberg N, Schifter S, Mehlsen J. Haemodynamic changes following treatment of subclinical and overt hyperthyroidism. Eur J Endocrinol 2001; 145(4):391–396.
32. Napoli R, Riondi B, Guardasole V, et al. Impact of hyperthyroidism and its correction on vascular reactivity in humans. Circulation 2001; 104(25):3076–3080.
33. Coulombe P, Dussault JH, Walker P. Plasma catecholamine concentrations in hyperthyroidism and hypothyroidism. Metabolism 1976; 25:973–979.
34. Moghetti P, Castello R, Tosi F, et al. Glucose counterregulatory response to acute hypoglycemia in hyperthyroid human subjects. J Clin Endocrinol Metab 1994; 78(1):169–173.
35. Silva JE. Thyroid hormone control of thermogenesis and energy balance. Thyroid 1995; 5:481–492.
36. Parry CH. Disease of the heart. In Collections from the Unpublished Writings, Vol 2. London, Underwoods, 1825, pp 111–125.
37. Tamai H, Kasagi K, Mizuno O, et al. Thyroid-stimulating antibody and thyrotropin-binding inhibitory immunoglobulin activity in hypothyroid patients who subsequently developed thyrotoxicosis. Acta Endocrinol (Copenh) 1990; 122:499–504.
38. Kohut WD, Gharib H, Anderson MW. Triiodothyronine thyro-

toxicosis complicating primary hypothyroidism in a patient with autoimmune thyroiditis. Am J Med 1982; 72:843–846.
39. Salvi M, Fukazawa H, Bernard N, et al. Role of autoantibodies in the pathogenesis and association of endocrine autoimmune disorders. Endocr Rev 1988; 9:450–466.
40. Rees Smith B, McLachlan SM, Furmaniak J. Autoantibodies to the thyrotropin receptor. Endocr Rev 1988; 9:106–121.
41. Kraiem Z, Lahat N, Glaser B, et al. Thyrotropin receptor-blocking antibodies: incidence, characterization and in vitro synthesis. Clin Endocrinol 1987; 27:409–421.
42. Martin A, Valentine M, Unger P, et al. Engraftment of human lymphocytes and thyroid tissue into Scid and Rag2-deficient mice: absent progression of lymphocytic infiltration. J Clin Endocrinol Metab 1994; 79:716–723.
43. McGregor AM, Petersen MM, McLachlan SM, et al. Carbimazole and the autoimmune response in Graves' disease. N Engl J Med 1980; 303:302–304.
44. Weetman AP. The immunomodulatory effects of antithyroid drugs. Thyroid 1994; 4:145–146.
45. McGregor AM, Petersen MM, Capiferri R, et al. Effects of radioiodine on thyrotrophin binding inhibiting immunoglobulins in Graves' disease. Clin Endocrinol 1979; 11:437–444.
46. Livolsi VA. Surgical Pathology of the Thyroid, 2nd ed. Philadelphia WB Saunders, 2001.
47. Weetman AP, McGregor AM, Hall R. Evidence for an effect of antithyroid drugs on the natural history of Graves' disease. Clin Endocrinol 1984; 21:163–172.
48. Martin A, Goldsmith NK, Friedman EW, et al. Intrathyroidal accumulation of T cell phenotypes in autoimmune thyroid disease. Autoimmunity 1990; 6:269–281.
49. Paschke R, Bruckner N, Schmeidl R, et al. Predominant intraepithelial localization of primed T cells and immunoglobulin-producing lymphocytes in Graves' disease. Acta Endocrinol 1991; 124:630–636.
50. Roman SH, Goldsmith NK, Leiderman IZ, Davies TF. Induction of microsomal antigen and comparison with histologic localization of HLA-DR in Graves' thyroid tissue. Autoimmunity 1989; 2:253–263.
51. Paschke R, Bruckner N, Eck T, et al. Regional stimulation of thyroid epithelial cells in Graves' disease by lymphocytic aggregates and plasma cells. Acta Endocrinol 1991; 125:459–465.
52. Tunbridge WMG, Evered DC, Hall R, et al. The spectrum of thyroid disease in a community. Clin Endocrinol 1977; 7:483–493.
53. Shimojo N, Kohno Y, Yamaguchi K, et al. Induction of Graves-like disease in mice by immunization with fibroblasts transfected with the thyrotropin receptor and a class II molecule. Proc Natl Acad Sci USA 1996; 93:11074–11079.
54. Kita M, Ahmad L, Marians RC, et al. Regulation and transfer of a murine model of thyrotropin receptor antibody mediated Graves' disease. Endocrinology 1999; 140:1392–1398.
55. Janson A, Karlsson FA, Micha-Johansson G, et al. Effects of stimulatory and inhibitory thyrotropin receptor antibodies on lipolysis in infant adipocytes. J Clin Endocrinol Metab 1995; 80: 1712–1716.
56. Davies TF. The TSH receptors spread themselves around. J Clin Endocrinol Metab 1995; 79:1232–1233.
57. Parmentier M, Libert F, Maenhaut C, et al. Molecular cloning of the TSH receptor. Science 1989; 246:1620–1622.
58. Misrahi M, Loosfelt H, Atger M, et al. Cloning, sequencing, and expression of human TSH receptor. Biochem Biophys Res Comm 1990; 166:394–403.
59. Libert F, Lefort A, Gerard C, et al. Cloning, sequencing and expression of the human TSH receptor: evidence for binding of autoantibodies. Biochem Biophys Res Comm 1989; 165:1250–1255.
60. Kaufman SC, Gross TP, Kennedy DL. Thyroid hormone use: trends in the United States from 1960 through 1988. Thyroid 1991; 1:285–291.
61. Libert F, Passage E, Lefort A, et al. Localization of human thyrotropin receptor gene to chromosome 14q31 by in situ hybridization. Cytogen Cell Genet 1991; 54:82–83.
62. Graves PN, Tomer Y, Davies TF. Cloning and sequencing of a 1.3 kb variant of human thyrotropin receptor mRNA lacking the transmembrane domain. Biochem Biophys Res Commun 1992; 187:1135–1143.
63. Loosfelt H, Pichon C, Jolivet A, et al. Two-subunit structure of the human thyrotropin receptor. Proc Natl Acad Sci USA 1992; 89:3765–3769.
64. Graves P, Pritsker A, Davies TF. Post-translational processing of the natural human thyrotropin receptor: demonstration of more than two cleavage sites. J Clin Endocrinol Metab 1999; 84:2177–2181.
65. Rees Smith B. Characterisation of long-acting thyroid stimulator gamma globulin binding protein. Biochem Biophys Acta 1971; 229:649–662.
66. Graves P, Pritsker A, Davies TF. Post-translational processing of the natural human TSH receptor: demonstration of more than two cleavage sites. Endocrinology 1999; 84:2177–2181.
67. Adams DD. The presence of an abnormal thyroid-stimulating hormone in the serum of some thyrotoxic patients. J Clin Endocrinol Metab 1958; 18:699–712.
68. Adams DD, Purves HD. Abnormal responses in the assay of thyrotropin. Proc Univ Otago Med School 1956; 34:11–12.
69. Adams DD, Fastier FN, Howie JB, et al. Stimulation of the human thyroid by infusions of plasma containing LATS protector. J Clin Endocrinol Metab 1974; 39:826–832.
70. Zakarija MJ. Immunochemical characterization of the thyroid-stimulating antibody (TSab) of Graves' disease: evidence for restricted heterogeneity. J Clin Lab Immunol 1983; 10:77–85.
71. Weetman AP, Yateman ME, Ealey PA, et al. Thyroid-stimulating antibody activity between different immunoglobulin G subclasses. J Clin Invest 1990; 86:723–727.
72. Zakarija M, McKenzie JM, Eidson MS. Transient neonatal hypothyroidism: characterization of maternal antibodies to the thyrotropin receptor. J Clin Endocrinol Metab 1990; 70:1239–1246.
73. Davies TF, Yeo PP, Evered DC, et al. Value of thyroid-stimulating antibody determinations in predicting short-term thyrotoxic relapse in Graves' disease. Lancet 1977; 1:1181–1182.
74. Wilson R, McKillop JH, Henderson N, et al. The ability of the serum TSH receptor antibody index and HLA status to predict long-term remission of thyrotoxicosis following medical therapy for Graves' disease. Clin Endocrinol 1986; 25:151–156.
75. Davies TF. Thyroid-stimulating antibodies predict hyperthyroidism. J Clin Endocrinol Metab 1998; 83:3777–3781.
76. Nagayama Y, Wadsworth HL, Russo D, et al. Binding domains of stimulatory and inhibitory TSH receptor autoantibodies determined with chimeric TSH-LH/CG receptors. J Clin Invest 1991; 88:336–340.
77. Kosugi S, Ban T, Akamizu T, Kohn LD. Site-directed mutagenesis of a portion of the extracellular domain of the rat thyrotropin receptor important in autoimmune thyroid disease and nonhomologous with gonadotropin receptors: relationship of functional and immunogenic domains. J Biol Chem 1991; 266:19413–19418.
78. Vlase H, Graves PN, Magnusson R, Davies TF. Human autoantibodies to the TSH receptor: recognition of linear, folded and glycosylated recombinant extracellular domain. J Clin Endocrinol Metab 1995; 80:46–53.
79. Phillips D, Prentice L, Upadhyaya M, et al. Autosomal dominant inheritance of autoantibodies to thyroid peroxidase and thyroglobulin: studies in families not selected for autoimmune thyroid disease. J Clin Endocrinol Metab 1991; 72:973–975.
80. Stagnaro-Green A, Roman SH, Cobin RH, et al. A prospective study of lymphocyte-initiated immunosuppression in normal pregnancy: evidence of a T-cell etiology for postpartum thyroid dysfunction. J Clin Endocrinol Metab 1992; 74:645–653.
81. Davies TF. Positive regulation of the guinea pig thyrotropin receptor. Endocrinology 1985; 117:201–207.
82. Huber G, Concepcion LE, Graves P, Davies TF. Positive regulation of the human TSH receptor mRNA by recombinant human TSH is at the nuclear level. Endocrinology 1992; 130:2858–2864.
83. Tainer JA, Deal CD, Geysen HM, et al. Defining antibody-antigen recognition: towards engineered antibodies and epitopes. Int Rev Immunol 1991; 7:165–188.
84. Weiss A. Structure and function of the T cell antigen receptor. J Clin Invest 1990; 86:1015–1022.
85. Brown JH, Jardetzky S, Gorga JC, et al. Three-dimensional structure of the human class II histocompatibility antigen HLA-DR1. Nature 1993; 364:33–39.
86. Bjorkman PJ, Saper MA, Samraoui B, et al. Structure of the

human class I histocompatibility antigen, HLA-A2. Nature 1987; 329:506–512.
87. Schwartz RH. T-cell anergy. Sci Am 1993; 269:66–71.
88. Smith TJ, Sciaky D, Phipps RP, Jennings TA. CD40 expression in human thyroid tissue: evidence for involvement of multiple cell types in autoimmune and neoplastic diseases. Thyroid 1999; 9: 749–755.
89. Martin A, Davies TF. T cells and human autoimmune thyroid disease: emerging data show lack of need to invoke suppressor T-cell problems. Thyroid 1992; 2:247–261.
90. Male DK, Champion BR, Pryce G, et al. Antigenic determinants of human thyroglobulin differentiated using antigen fragments. Immunology 1985; 54:419–427.
91. Dayan CM, Londei M, Corcoran AE, et al. Autoantigen recognition by thyroid-infiltrating T cells in Graves' disease. Proc Natl Acad Sci USA 1991; 88:7415–7419.
92. Acuto O, Reinhertz EL. The human T cell receptor: structure and function. N Engl J Med 1985; 312:1100–1111.
93. Benacerraf B. Role of MHC gene products in immune regulation. Science 1981; 212:1229–1238.
94. Tandon N, Freeman MA, Weetman AP. T-cell response to synthetic TSH receptor peptides in Graves' disease. Clin Exp Immunol 1992; 89:468–473.
95. Mackenzie WA, Schwartz AE, Friedman EW, Davies TF. Intrathyroidal T cell clones from patients with autoimmune thyroid disease. J Clin Endocrinol Metab 1987; 64:818–824.
96. Grubeck Loebenstein B, Turner M, Pirich K, et al. CD4+ T-cell clones from autoimmune thyroid tissue cannot be classified according to their lymphokine production. Scand J Immunol 1990; 32:433–440.
97. Stassi G, Di Liberto D, Todaro M, et al. Control of target cell survival in thyroid autoimmunity by T helper cytokines via regulation of apoptotic proteins. Nat Immunol 2000; 1:483–488.
98. Del Prete GF, Tiri A, Mariotti S, et al. Enhanced production of gamma-interferon by thyroid-derived T cell clones from patients with Hashimoto's thyroiditis. Clin Exp Immunol 1987; 69:323–331.
99. Watson PF, Pickerill AP, Davies R, Weetman AP. Analysis of cytokine gene expression in Graves' disease and multinodular goiter. J Clin Endocinol Metab 1994; 79:355–360.
100. Davis MM, Bjorkman PJ. T-cell antigen receptor genes and T-cell recognition. Nature 1988; 334:395–402.
101. Davies TF, Martin A, Concepcion ES, et al. Evidence of limited variability of antigen receptors on intrathyoidal T cells in autoimmune thyroid disease. N Engl J Med 1991; 325:238–244.
102. Davies T, Concepcion E, Ben Nun A, et al. T-cell receptor V gene usage in autoimmune thyroid disease: direct assessment by thyroid aspiration. J Clin Endocrinol Metab 1993; 76:660–666.
103. Matsuoka N, Martin A, Concepcion ES, et al. Preservation of functioning human thyroid organoids in the Scid mouse: II. Biased use of intrathyroidal T cell receptor V genes. J Clin Endocrinol Metab 1993; 77:311–315.
104. De Riu A, Martin A, Valentine M, et al. Graves' disease thyroid transplants in Scid mice: persistent selectivity in hTcR V alpha gene family use. Autoimunity 1994; 19:271–277.
105. Nakashima M, Martin A, Davies TF. Intrathyroidal T cell accumulation in Graves' disease: delineation of mechanisms based on in situ T cell receptor analysis. J Clin Endocrinol Metab 1996; 81:3346–3351.
106. Heufelder AE, Wenzel BE, Scriba PC. Antigen receptor variable region repertoires expressed by T cells infiltrating thyroid, retroorbital, and pretibial tissue in Graves' disease. J Clin Endocrinol Metab 1996; 81:3733–3739.
107. Oksenberg JR, Stuart S, Begovich AB, et al. Limited heterogeneity of rearranged T cell receptor V alpha transcripts in brains of multiple sclerosis patients. Nature 1990; 345:344–346.
108. Ben-Nun A, Liblau RS, Cohen L, et al. Restricted T cell receptor V beta usage by myelin basic protein-specific T cell clones in multiple sclerosis: predominant genes vary in individuals. Proc Natl Acad Sci USA 1991; 88:2466–2470.
109. Sridama V, Pacini V, DeGroot LJ. Decreased suppressor T lymphocytes in autoimmune thyroid diseases detected by monoclonal antibodies. J Clin Endocrinol Metab 1982; 54:316–329.
110. Ludgate ME, McGregor AM, Weetman AP, et al. Analysis of T cell subsets in Graves' disease: alterations associated with carbimazole. BMJ 1984; 288:526–530.
111. Jenkins M. The role of cell division in the induction of clonal anergy. Immunol Today 1992; 13:69–73.
112. Morahan G, Hoffmann M, Miller J. A nondeletional mechanism of peripheral tolerance in T-cell receptor transgenic mice. Proc Natl Acad Sci USA 1992; 88:11421–11425.
113. Ambinder JM, Chiorazzi N, Gibofsky A, et al. Special characteristics of cellular immune function in normal individuals of the HLA-DR3 type. Clin Immunol Immunopathol 1982; 23:269–274.
114. Kallenberg CGM, Klaassen RJL, Beelen JM, et al. HLA-B8/DR3 phenotype and the primary immune response. Clin Immunol Immunopathol 1985; 34:135–140.
115. Tomer Y, Davies TF. Infection, thyroid disease, and autoimmunity. Endocr Rev 1993; 14:107–120.
115a. Davies TF. Trauma and pressure explain the clinical presentation of the Graves' disease triad. Thyroid 2000; 10:629–630.
116. Horwitz MS, Bradley LM, Harbertson J, et al. Diabetes induced by Coxsackie virus: initiation by bystander damage and not molecular mimicry. Nat Med 1998; 4:781–785.
117. Srinivasappa J, Saegusa J, Prabhakar BS, et al. Molecular mimicry: frequency of reactivity of monoclonal antiviral antibodies with normal tissues. J Virol 1986; 57:397–401.
118. Haspel MV, Onodera T, Prabhakar BS, et al. Virus-induced autoimmunity: monoclonal antibodies that react with endocrine tissues. Science 1983; 220:304–306.
119. Burch HB, Nagy EV, Lukes YG, et al. Nucleotide and amino acid homology between the human thyrotropin receptor and HIV-1 nef protein: identification and functional analysis. Biochem Biophys Res Comm 1991; 181:498–505.
120. Bottazzo GF, Pujol Borrell R, Hanafusa T, Feldmann M. Role of aberrant HLA-DR expression and antigen presentation in induction of endocrine autoimmunity. Lancet 1983; 2:1115–1119.
121. Hanafusa T, Pujol Borrell R, Chiovato L, et al. Aberrant expression of HLA-DR antigen on thyrocytes in Graves' disease: relevance for autoimmunity. Lancet 1983; 2:1111–1115.
122. Kawakami Y, Kuzuya N, Watanebe T, et al. Induction of experimental thyroiditis in mice by recombinant interferon gamma administration. Acta Endocrinol 1990; 122:41–48.
123. Shimojo N, Kohno Y, Yamaguchi KI, et al. Induction of Graves'-like disease in mice by immunization with fibroblasts transfected with the thyrotropin receptor and a class II molecule. Proc Natl Acad Sci USA 1996; 93:11074–11079.
124. Massa PT, Dorries R, Meulen V. Viral particles induce Ia antigen expression on astrocytes. Nature 1986; 320:543–546.
125. Neufeld DS, Platzer M, Davies TF. Reovirus induction of MHC class II antigen in rat thyroid cells. Endocrinology 1988; 124: 543–545.
126. Khoury E, Pereira L, Greenspan F. Induction of HLA-DR expression on thyroid follicular cells by cytomegalovirus infection in vitro. Am J Pathol 1991; 138:1209–1223.
127. Tomer Y, Greenberg DA, Barbesino G, et al. Ctla-4 and not cd28 is a susceptibility gene for thyroid autoantibody production. J Clin Endocrinol Metab 2001; 86:1687–1693.
128. Brix TH, Christensen K, Holm NV, et al. A population-based study of Graves' disease in Danish twins. Clin Endocrinol 1998; 48:397–400.
129. Tomer Y, Barbesino G, Greenberg DA, et al. Mapping the major susceptibility loci for familial Graves' and Hashimoto's diseases: evidence for genetic heterogeneity and gene interactions. J Clin Endocrinol Metab 1999; 84:4656–4664.
130. Wass J, Shalet S (eds). Oxford Textbook of Endocrinology. Oxford, UK, Oxford University Press, 2000.
131. Dahlberg PA, Holmlund G, Karlsson FA, Safwenberg J. HLA-A, -B, -C and -DR antigens in patients with Graves' disease and their correlation with signs and clinical course. Acta Endocrinol (Copenh) 1981; 97:42–47.
132. Roman SH, Greenberg D, Rubinstein P, et al. Genetics of autoimmune thyroid disease: lack of evidence for linkage to HLA within families. J Clin Endocrinol Metab 1992; 74:496–503.
133. O'Connor G, Neufeld DS, Greenberg DA, et al. Lack of disease associated HLA-DQ restriction fragment length polymorphisms in families with autoimmune thyroid disease. Autoimmunity 1993; 14:237–241.
134. Barbesino G, Tomer Y, Concepcion ES, et al. Linkage analysis of candidate genes in autoimmune thyroid disease: I. Selected immunoregulatory genes. J Clin Endocrinol Metab 1998; 83: 1580–1584.

135. Lidman K, Eriksson U, Norberg R, Fagraeus A. Indirect immunofluorescence staining of human thyroid by antibodies occurring in *Yersinia enterocolitica* infections. Clin Exp Immunol 1976; 23: 429–435.
136. Wenzel BE, Heeseman J, Wenzel KW, Scriba PC. Antibodies to plasmid-encoded proteins of enteropathogenic *Yersinia* in patients with autoimmune thyroid disease. Lancet 1988; 1:56–59.
137. Carter JK, Smith RE. Rapid induction of hypothyroidism by an avian leukosis virus. Infect Immun 1983; 40:795–805.
138. Ciampolillo A, Mirakian R, Schulz T, et al. Retrovirus-like sequences in Graves' disease: implications for human autoimmunity. Lancet 1989; 1:1096–1099.
139. Wick G, Trieb K, Aguzzi A, et al. Possible role of human foamy virus in Graves' disease. Intervirology 1993; 35:101–107.
140. Lagaye S, Vexiau P, Morozov V, et al. Human spumaretrovirus-related sequences in the DNA of leukocytes from patients with Graves' disease. Proc Natl Acad Sci USA 1992; 89:10070–10074.
141. Humphrey M, Baker JR Jr, Carr FE, et al. Absence of retroviral sequences in Graves' disease. Lancet 1991; 337:17–18.
142. Neumann-Haefelin D, Fleps U, Renne R, Schweizer M. Foamy viruses. Intervirology 1993; 35:196–207.
143. Weisman SA. Incidence of thyrotoxicosis among refugees from Nazi prison camps. J Clin Endocrinol Metab 1958; 48:747–752.
144. Locke S, Ader R, Besedovsky H, et al. Foundations of Psychoneuroimmunology. New York, Aldine, 1985.
145. Leclere J, Weryha S. Stress and autoimmune diseases. Horm Metab Res 1989; 31:90–93.
146. Winsa B, Adami HO, Bergstrom R, et al. Stressful life events and Graves' disease. Lancet 1991; 338:1475–1479.
147. Sonino N, Girelli M, Boscaro M, et al. Life events in the pathogenesis of Graves' disease: a controlled study. Acta Endocrinol 1993; 128:293–296.
148. Amino N, Miyai K. Postpartum autoimmune endocrine syndromes. In Davies TF (ed). Autoimmune Endocrine Disease. New York, John Wiley & Sons, 1983, pp 247–272.
149. Ansar AS, Young PR, Penhale WJ. Beneficial effect of testosterone in the treatment of chronic autoimmune thyroiditis in rats. J Immunol 1986; 136:143–147.
150. Paavonen T. Hormonal regulation of immune responses. Ann Med 1994; 26:255–258.
151. Da Silva JAP. Sex hormones, glucocorticoids, and autoimmunity: facts and hypotheses. Ann Rheum Dis 1995; 54:6–16.
152. Stewart JJ. The female X-inactivation mosaic in systemic lupus erythematosus. Immunol Today 1998; 19:352–357.
153. Weetman AP. The immunology of pregnancy. Thyroid 1999; 9: 643–646.
154. Davies TF. The thyroid immunology of the postpartum period. Thyroid 1999; 9:675–684.
155. Jansson R, Dahlberg PA, Winsa B, et al. The postpartum period constitutes an important risk for the development of clinical Graves' disease in young women. Acta Endocrinol 1987; 116: 321–325.
156. Di Matola T, D'Ascoli F, Fenzi G, et al. Amiodarone induces cytochrome c release and apoptosis through an iodine-independent mechanism. J Clin Endocrinol Metab 2000; 85:4323–4330.
157. Burikhanov RB, Matsuzaki S. Excess iodine induces apoptosis in the thyroid of goitrogen-pretreated rats in vivo. Thyroid 2000; 10:123–129.
158. Pacini F, Vorontsova T, Molinaro E, et al. Thyroid consequences of the Chernobyl nuclear accident. Acta Paediatr Suppl 1999; 88: 23–27.
159. Vermiglio F, Castagna MG, Volnova E, et al. Post-Chernobyl increased prevalence of humoral thyroid autoimmunity in children and adolescents from a moderately iodine-deficient area in Russia. Thyroid 1999; 9:781–786.
160. Bartalena L, Pinchera A, Marcocci C. Management of Graves' ophthalmopathy: reality and perspectives. Endocr Rev 2000; 21: 168–199.
161. Bahn RS. Understanding the immunology of Graves' ophthalmopathy: is it an autoimmune disease? Endocrinol Metab Clin North Am 2000; 29:287–96, vi.
162. Rapoport B, McLachlan S M. Keeping our eyes open. Thyroid 2001; 11:165–166.
163. Grubeck-Loebenstein B, Trieb K, Holter W, et al. Retrobulbar T cells from patients with Graves' ophthalmopathy are CD8+ and specifically autologous fibroblasts. J Clin Invest 1993; 93: 2738–2743.
164. Hosal BM, Swanson JK, Thompson CR, Kubota S, et al. Significance of serum antibodies reactive with flavoprotein subunit of succinate dehydrogenase in thyroid-associated orbitopathy. Br J Ophthalmol 1999; 83:605–608.
164a. Villaneuva R, Inzerillo AM, Tomer Y. Limited genetic susceptibility to severe Graves' ophthalmopathy: no role for CTLA-4 but evidence for an environmental etiology. Thyroid 2000; 10:791–798.
165. Bartalena L, Pinchera A, Marcocci C. Management of Graves' ophthalmopathy: reality and perspectives. Endocr Rev 2000; 21: 168–199.
166. Yoshiuchi K, Kumano H, Nomura S, et al. Stressful life events and smoking were associated with Graves' disease in women, but not in men. Psychosom Med 1998; 60:182–185.
167. Shine B, Fells P, Edwards OM, Weetman AP. Association between Graves' ophthalmopathy and smoking. Lancet 1990; 335: 1261–1263.
168. Bartalena L, Martino E, Marcocci C, et al. More on smoking habits and Graves' ophthalmopathy. J Endocrinol Invest 1989; 12:733–737.
169. Bartalena L, Marcocci C, Bogazzi F, et al. Use of corticosteroids to prevent progression of Graves' ophthalmopathy after radioiodine therapy for hyperthyroidism. N Engl J Med 1989; 321: 1349–1352.
170. Tallestedt L, Lundell G, Torring O, et al. Occurrence of ophthalmopathy after treatment for Graves' disease. N Engl J Med 1992; 326:1733–1738.
171. Wood LC, Ingbar SH. Hypothyroidism as a late sequela in patients with Graves' disease treated with antithyroid agents. J Clin Invest 1979; 64:1429–1436.
172. Solomon DH, Chopra IJ, Chopra U, et al. Identification of subgroups of euthyroid Graves' ophthalmopathy. N Engl J Med 1977; 296:181–186.
173. Bahn RS, Heufelder AE. Pathogenesis of Graves' ophthalmopathy. N Engl J Med 1993; 329:1468–1475.
174. Fatourechi V, Fransway AF. Dermopathy of Graves' disease (pretibial myxedema). Medicine 1994; 73:1–7.
175. Bull RH, Coburn PR, Mortimer PS. Pretibial myxedema: a manifestation of lymphoedema? Lancet 1993; 341:403–404.
176. Rapoport B, Alsabeh R, Aftergood D, McLachlan SM. Elephantiasic pretibial myxedema: insight into and a hypothesis regarding the pathogenesis of the extrathyroidal manifestations of Graves' disease. Thyroid 2000; 10:685–692.
177. Sato K, Yamazaki K, Shizume K, et al. Stimulation by TSH and Graves' immunoglobulin G of vascular endothelial growth factor mRNA expression in human thyroid follicles in vitro and fit mRNA expression in the rat thyroid in vivo. J Clin Invest 1995; 96:1295–1302.
178. Izumi M, Larsen PR. Triiodothyronine, thyroxine, and iodine in purified thyroglobulin from patients with Graves' disease. J Clin Invest 1977; 59:1105–1112.
179. Marks AD, Bertram BJ, Channick J, et al. Chronic thyroiditis and mitral valve prolapse. Ann Intern Med 1995; 102:479–483.
180. Forrester JV, Sutherland GR, McDougall IR. Dysthyroid ophthalmopathy: orbital evaluation with B-scan ultrasonography. J Clin Endocrinol Metab 1977; 45:221–224.
181. Dallow RH, Momose KJ, Weber AL, et al. Comparison of ultrasonography, computerized tomography (EMI scan) and radiographic techniques in evaluation of exophthalmos. Trans Am Acad Ophthalmol Otolaryngol 1976; 81:305–322.
182. Wartofsky L. Classification of eye changes of Graves' disease. Thyroid 1992; 3:235–236.
183. Perros P, Crombie AL, Matthews JNS, Kendall-Taylor P. Age and gender influence the severity of thyroid-associated ophthalmopathy: a study of 101 patients attending a combined thyroid-eye clinic. Clin Endocrinol 1993; 38:367–372.
184. Massart C, Orgiazzi J, Maugendre D. Clinical validity of a new commercial method for detection of TSH-receptor binding antibodies in sera from patients with Graves' disease treated with antithyroid drugs. Clin Chim Acta 2001; 304:39–47.
185. Bolton J, Sanders J, Oda Y, et al. Measurement of thyroid-stimulating hormone receptor autoantibodies by ELISA. Clin Chem 1999; 45:2285–2287.
186. Larsen PR, Alexander NM, Chopra IJ, et al. Revised nomenclature for tests of thyroid hormones and thyroid-related proteins in serum. J Clin Endocrinol Metab 1987; 64:1089–1094.

187. Tomer Y, Greenberg DA, Davies TF. Genetic susceptibility to type 1 diabetes mellitus and the autoimmune thyroid diseases. In Volpe R (ed). Autoimmune Endocrinopathies. Ottawa, Humana Press, 1999, pp 57–90.
188. Singer PA, Cooper DS, Levy E, et al. Treatment guidelines for patients with hyperthyroidism and hypothyroidism. JAMA 1995; 273:808–812.
189. Cooper DS. Antithyroid drugs for the treatment of hyperthyroidism caused by Graves' disease. (Review) Endocrinol Metab Clin North Am 1998; 27(1):225–247.
190. Abuid J, Larsen PR. Triiodothyronine and thyroxine in hyperthyroidism: comparison of the acute changes during therapy with antithyroid agents. J Clin Invest 1974; 54:201–208.
191. Bianco AC, Salvatore D, Gereben B, et al. Biochemistry, cellular and molecular biology, and physiological roles of the iodothyronine selenodeiodinases. Endocr Rev 2002; 23:38–89.
192. Laurberg P, Weeke J. Dynamics of inhibition of iodothyronine deiodination during propylthiouracil treatment of thyrotoxicosis. Hormone Metab Res 1981; 13:289–292.
193. Jansson R, Dahlberg PA, Johansson H, Lindstrom B. Intrathyroidal concentrations of methimazole in patients with Graves' disease. J Clin Endocrinol Metab 1983; 57:129–132.
194. Weetman AP, McGregor AP, Hall R. Methimazole inhibits thyroid autoantibody production by an action on accessory cells. Clin Immunol Immunopathol 1983; 28:39–45.
195. Volpe R. Evidence that the immunosuppressive effects of antithyroid drugs are mediated through actions on the thyroid cell, modulating thyrocyte-immunocyte signaling: a review. Thyroid 1994; 4:217–223.
196. McGregor AM, Ibbertson HK, Rees Smith B, Hall R. Carbimazole and autoantibody synthesis in Hashimoto's thyroiditis. BMJ 1995; 281:968–969.
197. Mitsiades N, Poulaki V, Tseleni-Balafouta S, et al. Fas ligand expression in thyroid follicular cells from patients with thionamide-treated Graves' disease. Thyroid 2000; 10:527–532.
198. Stassi G, Todaro M, Bucchieri F, et al. Fas/Fas ligand-driven T cell apoptosis as a consequence of ineffective thyroid immunoprivilege in Hashimoto's thyroiditis. J Immunol 1999; 162:263–267.
199. Romaldini JH, Bromberg N, Werner RS, et al. Comparison of effects of high- and low-dosage regimens of antithyroid drugs in the management of Graves' hyperthyroidism. J Clin Endocrinol Metab 1983; 57:563–570.
200. Tamai H, Hayaki I, Kawai K, et al. Lack of effect of thyroxine administration on elevated thyroid-stimulating hormone receptor antibody levels in treated Graves' disease. J Clin Endocrinol Metab 1995; 80:1481–1484.
201. McIver B, Rae P, Beckett G, et al. Lack of effect of thyroxine in patients with Graves' hyperthyroidism who are treated with an antithyroid drug. N Engl J Med 1996; 334:220–224.
202. Hashizume K, Ichikawa K, Sakurai A, et al. Administration of thyroxine in treated Graves' disease: effects on the level of antibodies to thyroid stimulating hormone receptors and on the risk of recurrence of hyperthyroidism. N Engl J Med 1991; 324:947–953.
203. Rittmaster RS, Abbott EC, Douglas R, et al. Effect of methimazole, with or without L -thyroxine, on remission rates in Graves' disease. J Clin Endocrinol Metab 1998; 83:814–818.
204. Feldt-Rasmussen U, Schleusner H, Carayon P. Meta-analysis evaluation of the impact of thyrotropin receptor antibodies on long-term remission after medical therapy of Graves' disease. J Clin Endocrinol Metab 1994; 78:98–102.
205. Weetman AP, Ratanachaiyavong S, Middleton GW, et al. Prediction of outcome in Graves' disease after carbimazole treatment. Q J Med 1986; 59:409–419.
206. Greer MA, Kammer H, Bouma DJ. Short-term antithyroid drug therapy for the thyrotoxicosis of Graves' disease. N Engl J Med 1977; 297:173–176.
207. Solomon BL, Evaul JE, Burman KD, et al. Remission rates with antithyroid drug therapy: continuing influence of iodine intake? Ann Intern Med 1987; 107:510–512.
208. Bartalena L, Bogazzi F, Martino E. Adverse effects of thyroid hormone preparations and antithyroid drugs. Drug Saf 1996; 15: 53–63.
209. Wall JR, Fang SL, Kuroki T, et al. In vitro immunoreactivity to propylthiouracil, methimazole, and carbimazole in patients with Graves' disease: a possible cause of antithyroid drug-induced agranulocytosis. Clin Endocrinol Metab 1984; 58:868–872.
210. Becker DV, Braverman LE, Dunn JT, et al. The use of iodine as a thyroidal blocking agent in the event of a reactor accident. JAMA 1984; 252:659–661.
211. Fradkin JE, Wolff J. Iodide-induced thyrotoxicosis. Medicine 1983; 62:1–20.
212. Wu SY, Shyh TP, Chopra I, et al. Comparison of sodium ipodate (Orografin) and propylthiouracil in early treatment of hyperthyroidism. J Clin Endocrinol Metab 1982; 54:630–634.
213. Williams DF, Chopra IJ, Orgiazzi J, Solomon DH. Acute effects of corticosteroids on thyroid activity in Graves' disease. J Clin Endocrinol Metab 1975; 41:354–358.
214. Pfaffle RW, DiMattia GE, Parks JS, et al. Mutation of the POU-specific domain of Pit-1 and hypopituitarism without pituitary hypoplasia. Science 1992; 257:1118–1121.
215. Rubin PC. Beta-blockers in pregnancy. N Engl J Med 1981; 305: 1323–1326.
216. Gladstone R, Hordf A, Gersony WM. Propranolol administration during pregnancy: effects on the fetus. J Pediatr 1975; 86:962–964.
217. Milner MR, Gelman KM, Phillips RA, et al. Double-blind crossover trial of diltiazem versus propranolol in the management of thyrotoxic symptoms. Pharmacotherapy 1990; 10:100–106.
218. Alsanea O, Clark OH. Treatment of Graves' disease: The advantages of surgery. Endocrinol Metab Clin North Am 2000; 29(2): 321–337.
219. Weetman AP. The role of surgery in primary hyperthyroidism. J R Soc Med 1998; 91(Suppl 33):7–11.
220. Michie W, Stowers JM, Duncan T, et al. Mechanism of hypocalcemia after thyroidectomy for thyrotoxicosis. Lancet 1971; 1: 508–514.
221. Garrel DR, Delmas PD, Malaval L, et al. Serum bone Gla protein: a marker of bone turnover in hyperthyroidism. J Clin Endocrinol Metab 1986; 62:1052–1055.
222. Eriksen EF, Mosekilde L, Melsen F. Trabecular bone remodeling and bone balance in hyperthyroidism. Bone 1985; 6:421–428.
223. Rhone DP, Berlinger FG, White FM. Tissue sources of elevated serum alkaline phosphatase activity in hyperthyroid patients. Am J Clin Pathol 1980; 74:381–386.
224. Toft AD, Irvine WJ, McIntosh D, et al. Propranolol in the treatment of thyrotoxicosis by subtotal thyroidectomy. J Clin Endocrinol Metab 1976; 43:1312–1316.
225. Franklyn JA, Maisonneuve P, Sheppard M, et al. Cancer incidence and mortality after radioiodine treatment for hyperthyroidism: a population-based cohort study. Lancet 1999; 353:2111–2115.
226. Franklyn JA, Maisonneuve P, Sheppard MC, et al. Mortality after the treatment of hyperthyroidism with radioactive iodine. N Engl J Med 1998; 338:712–718.
227. Kazakov VS, Demidchik EP, Astakhova LN. Thyroid cancer after Chernobyl (letter). Nature 1992; 359:21–22.
228. Nikiforov Y, Gnepp DR. Pediatric thyroid cancer after the Chernobyl disaster: pathomorphologic study of 84 cases (1991–1992) from the Republic of Belarus. Cancer 1994; 74:748–766.
229. Baverstock KF. Thyroid cancer in children in Belarus after Chernobyl. World Health Stat Q 1993; 46:204–208.
230. Williams ED. Fallout from Chernobyl: thyroid cancer in children increased dramatically in Belarus [letter]. BMJ 1994; 309:1298–1299.
231. Alexander EK, Larsen PR. High dose of (131)I therapy for the treatment of hyperthyroidism caused by Graves' disease. J Clin Endocrinol Metab 2002; 87:1073–1077.
232. Smith RN, Wilson GM. Clinical trial of different doses of ^{131}I in the treatment of thyrotoxicosis. BMJ 1967; 1:129–132.
233. Wise PH, Ahmad A, Burnet RB, et al. Intentional radioiodine ablation for Graves' disease. Lancet 1975; 2:1231–1233.
234. Nakazato N, Yoshida K, Mori K, et al. Antithyroid drugs inhibit radioiodine-induced increases in thyroid autoantibodies in hyperthyroid Graves' disease. Thyroid 1999; 9:775–779.
235. Andrade VA, Gross JL, Maia AL. Effect of methimazole pretreatment on serum thyroid hormone levels after radioactive treatment in Graves' hyperthyroidism. J Clin Endocrinol Metab 1999; 84:4012–4016.
236. Harvey RD, Metclafe RA, Morteo C, et al. Acute pre-tibial myxedema following radioiodine therapy for thyrotoxic Graves' disease. Clin Endocrinol 1995; 42:657–660.
237. Bartley GB, Fatourechi V, Kadrmas EF, et al. Chronology of

Graves' ophthalmopathy in an incidence cohort. Am J Ophthalmol 1996; 121:426–434.
238. Gorman CA. Therapeutic controversies: radioiodine therapy does not aggravate Graves' ophthalmopathy. J Clin Endocrinol Metab 1995; 80:340–342.
239. Wartofsky L. Therapeutic controversies: summation, commentary, and overview: concerns over aggravation of Graves' ophthalmopathy by radioactive iodine treatment and the use of retrobulbar radiation therapy. J Clin Endocrinol Metab 1995; 80:347–349.
240. Imseis RE, Vanmiddlesworth L, Massie JD, et al. Pretreatment with propylthiouracil but not methimazole reduces the therapeutic efficacy of iodine-131 in hyperthyroidism. J Clin Endocrinol Metab 1998; 83:685–687.
241. Tuttle RM, Patience T, Budd S. Treatment with propylthiouracil before radioactive iodine therapy is associated with a higher treatment failure rate than therapy with radioactive iodine alone in Graves' disease. Thyroid 1995; 5:243–247.
242. Dunn JT. Choice of therapy in young adults with hyperthyroidism of Graves' disease. Ann Intern Med 1984; 100:891–893.
243. Sridama V, DeGroot LJ. Treatment of Graves' disease and the course of ophthalmopathy. Am J Med 1989; 87:70–73.
244. Jacobson DH, Gorman CA. Endocrine ophthalmopathy: current ideas concerning etiology, pathogenesis, and treatment. Endocr Rev 1984; 5:200–220.
245. Burch HB, Wartofsky L. Graves' ophthalmopathy: current concepts regarding pathogenesis and management. Endocr Rev 1993; 14:747–793.
246. Prummel MF, Wiersinga WM. Medical management of Graves' ophthalmopathy. Thyroid 1995; 5:231–234.
247. Bartalena L, Marcocci C, Chiovato L, et al. Orbital cobalt irradiation combined with systemic corticosteroids for Graves' ophthalmopathy: comparison with systemic corticosteroids alone. J Clin Endocrinol Metab 1983; 56:1139–1144.
248. Teng CS, Crombie AL, Hall R, et al. An evaluation of supervoltage orbital irradiation for Graves' disease. Clin Endocrinol 1980; 13:545–551.
248a. Gorman CA, Garrity JA, Fatourechi V, et al. A prospective, randomized, double-blind, placebo-controlled study of orbital radiotherapy for Graves' ophthalmopathy. Ophthalmology 2001; 108:1523–1534.
249. Lyons CJ, Rootman J. Orbital decompression for disfiguring exophthalmos in thyroid orbitopathy. Ophthalmopathy 1994; 101: 223–230.
250. Ogura J, Wessler S, Avioli LV, et al. Surgical approach to the ophthalmopathy of Graves' disease. JAMA 1971; 216:1627–1631.
251. Davis LE, Lucas MJ, Hankins GDV, et al. Thyrotoxicosis complicating pregnancy. Am J Obstet Gynecol 1989; 160:63–70.
252. Guillaume J, Schussler GC, Goldman J. Components of the total serum thyroid hormone concentrations during pregnancy: high free thyroxine and blunted thyrotropin (TSH) response to TSH-releasing hormone in the first trimester. J Clin Endocrinol Metab 1985; 60:678–684.
253. Pekonen F, Alfthan H, Stenman UH, Ylikorkala O. Human chorionic gonadotropin (hCG) and thyroid function in early human pregnancy: circadian variation and evidence for intrinsic thyrotropic activity of hCG. J Clin Endocrinol Metab 1988; 66:853–856.
254. Hershman JM, Lee HY, Sugawara M, et al. Human chorionic gonadotropin stimulates iodide uptake, adenylate cyclase, and deoxyribonucleic acid synthesis in cultured rat thyroid cells. J Clin Endocrinol Metab 1988; 67:74–79.
255. Yoshikawa N, Nishikawa M, Horimoto M, et al. Thyroid-stimulating activity in sera of normal pregnant women. J Clin Endocrinol Metab 1989; 69:891–895.
256. Amino N, Kuro R, Tanizawa O, et al. Changes of serum antithyroid antibodies during and after pregnancy in autoimmune thryoid diseases. Clin Exp Immunol 1978; 31:30–37.
257. Zakarija M, McKenzie JM, Hoffman WH. Prediction and therapy of intrauterine and late-onset neonatal hyperthyroidism. J Clin Endocrinol Metab 1986; 62:368–371.
258. Yabu Y, Amino N, Mori H, et al. Postpartum recurrence of hyperthyroidism and changes of thyroid-stimulating immunoglobulins in Graves' disease. J Clin Endocrinol Metab 1980; 51:1454–1458.
259. Amino N, Tanizawa O, Mori H, et al. Aggravation of thyrotoxicosis in early pregnancy and after delivery in Graves' disease. J Clin Endocrinol Metab 1982; 55:108–111.
260. Marchant B, Brownlie BEW, Hart DM, et al. The placental transfer of propylthiouracil, methimazole, and carbamizole. J Clin Endocrinol Metab 1977; 45:1187–1193.
261. Cheron RG, Kaplan M, Larsen PR, et al. Neonatal thyroid function after propylthiouracil therapy for maternal Graves' disease. N Engl J Med 1981; 304:525–528.
262. Momotani N, Noh J, Oyanagi H, et al. Antithyroid drug therapy for Graves' disease during pregnancy: optimal regimen for fetal thyroid status. N Engl J Med 1986; 315:24–28.
263. Haddow JE, Palomaki GE, Allan WC, et al. Maternal thyroid deficiency during pregnancy and subsequent neuropsychological development of the child. N Engl J Med 1999; 341:549–555.
264. Cooper DS. Antithyroid drugs: to breast-feed or not to breast-feed. Am J Obstet Gynecol 1987; 157:234–235.
265. Myres AW. Thyroid and antithyroid drugs and breast-feeding. Can Med Assoc J 1987; 136:921.
266. Azizi F, Khoshniat M, Bahrainian M, Hedayati M. Thyroid function and intellectual development of infants nursed by mothers taking methimazole. J Clin Endocrinol Metab 2000; 85:3233–3238.
267. Mandel SJ, Cooper DS. The use of antithyroid drugs in pregnancy and lactation. J Clin Endocrinol Metab 2001; 86:2354–2359.
268. van Dijke CP, Heydendael RJ, de Kleine MJ. Methimazole, carbimazole, and congenital skin defects. Ann Intern Med 1987; 106:60–61.
269. Signore A, Pozzilli P, Mario UD, et al. Inhibition of the receptor for interleukin-2 induced by carbimazole: relevance for the therapy of autoimmune thyroid disease. Isr J Med Sci 1985; 60:111–116.
270. Kalb RE, Grossman ME. The association of aplasia cutis congenita with therapy of maternal thyroid disease. Pediatr Dermatol 1986; 3:327–330.
271. Mandel SJ, Brent GA, Larsen PR. Review of antithyroid drug use during pregnancy and report of a case of aplasia cutis. Thyroid 1994; 4:129–133.
272. Gorman CA. Radioiodine and pregnancy. Thyroid 1999; 9:721–726.
273. Nygaard B, Laurberg P, Glinoer D, et al. [Guidelines for measurement of TSH receptor antibodies in pregnant women. Results from an evidence based symposium organized by the European Thyroid Society]. Ugeskr Laeger 1999; 161:6037–6038.
274. Glinoer D. Thyroid hyperfunction during pregnancy. Thyroid 1998; 8:859–864.
275. Stagnaro-Green A, Roman SH, Cobin RH, et al. A prospective study of lymphocyte-initiated immunosuppression in normal pregnancy: evidence of a T-cell etiology for postpartum thyroid dysfunction. J Clin Endocrinol Metab 1992; 74:645–653.
276. Lambert NC, Evans PC, Hashizumi TL, et al. Cutting edge: persistent fetal microchimerism in T lymphocytes is associated with HLA-DQA1*0501: implications in autoimmunity. J Immunol 2000; 164:5545–5548.
276a. Imaizumi M, Pritsker A, Unger P, Davies TF. Intrathyroidal fetal microchimerism in pregnancy and postpartum. Endocrinology 2002; 143:247–253.
277. Amino N, Tanizawa O, Mori H, et al. Aggravation of thyrotoxicosis in early pregnancy and after delivery in Graves' disease. J Clin Endocrinol Metab 1982; 55:108–112.
278. Low LCK, Lang J, Alexander WD. Excretion of carbimazole and propylthiouracil in breast milk. Lancet 1979; 2:1011.
279. Gruters A. Treatment of Graves' disease in children and adolescents. Horm Res 1998; 49(6):255–257.
279a. Hanna CE, LaFranchi SH. Adolescent thyroid disorders. Adolesc Med 2002; 13(1):13–36.
280. Favus MJ, Schneider AB, Stachura ME, et al. Thyroid cancer occurring as a late consequence of head-and-neck irradiation. N Engl J Med 1976; 294:1019–1025.
281. Safa AM, Schneider AB, Stachura ME, et al. Long-term follow-up results in children and adolescents treated with radioactive iodine (^{131}I) for hyperthyroidism. N Engl J Med 1975; 292:167–171.
282. Kraiem Z, Newfield RS. Graves' disease in childhood. J Pediatr Endocrinol Metab 2001; 14:229–243.
283. Tonacchera M, Agretti P, Chiovato L, et al. Activating thyrotro-

pin receptor mutations are present in nonadenomatous hyperfunctioning nodules of toxic or autonomous multinodular goiter. J Clin Endocrinol Metab 2000; 85:2270–2274.
284. Krohn K, Wohlgemuth S, Gerber H, Paschke R. Hot microscopic areas of iodine-deficient euthyroid goitres contain constitutively activating TSH receptor mutations. J Pathol 2000; 192: 37–42.
285. Van Sande J, Parma J, Tonacchera M, et al. Somatic and germline mutations of the TSH receptor gene in thyroid diseases. J Clin Endocrinol Metab 1995; 80:2577–2585.
286. Kraiem Z, Glaser B, Yigla M, et al. Toxic multinodular goiter: a variant of autoimmune hyperthyroidism. J Clin Endocrinol Metab 1987; 65:659–664.
287. Nygaard B, Hegedus L, Gervil M, et al. Radioiodine treatment of multinodular non-toxic goitre. BMJ 1993; 307:828–832.
288. Bonnema SJ, Bennedbaek FN, Wiersinga WM, Hegedus L. Management of the nontoxic multinodular goitre: a European questionnaire study. Clin Endocrinol (Oxf) 2000; 53:5–12.
289. Huysmans DA, Hermus RMM, Corstens FHM, et al. Large, compressive, goiters treated with radioiodine. Ann Intern Med 1994; 121:757–762.
290. Tonacchera M, Agretti P, Chiovato L, et al. Activating thyrotropin receptor mutations are present in nonadenomatous hyperfunctioning nodules of toxic or autonomous multinodular goiter. J Clin Endocrinol Metab 2000; 85(6):2270–2274.
291. Clapham DE. Mutations in G protein–linked receptors: novel insights on disease. Cell 1993; 75:1237–1239.
292. Ross DS, Ridgway EC, Daniels GH. Successful treatment of solitary toxic thyroid nodules with relatively low-dose iodine-131, with low prevalence of hypothyroidism. Ann Intern Med 1984; 101:488–490.
293. Goldstein R, Hart IA. Follow-up of solitary autonomous thyroid nodules treated with ^{131}I. N Engl J Med 1983; 309:1473–1476.
294. Gorman CA, Robertson JS. Radiation dose in the selection of ^{131}I or surgical treatment for toxic thyroid adenoma. Ann Intern Med 1978; 89:85–90.
295. Duprez L, Parma J, Van Sande J, et al. Germline mutations in the thyrotropin receptor gene cause non-autoimmune autosomal dominant hyperthyroidism. Nature Genetics 1994; 7:396–401.
296. Biebermann H, Schoneberg T, Krude H, et al. Constitutively activating TSH-receptor mutations as a molecular cause of non-autoimmune hyperthyroidism in childhood. Langenbecks Arch Surg 2000; 385:390–392.
297. Parma J, Van Sande J, Swillens S, et al. Somatic mutations causing constitutive activity of the thyrotropin receptor are the major cause of hyperfunctioning thyroid adenomas: identification of additional mutations activating both the cyclic adenosine 3′5′-monophosphate and inositol phosphate: Ca^{2+} cascades. Mol Endocrinol 1995; 9:725–733.
298. Stancek D, Stancekova-Gressnerova M, Janotka M, et al. Isolation and some serological and epidemiological data on the viruses recovered from patients with subacute thyroiditis de Quervain. Med Microbiol Immunol 1975; 161:133–144.
299. Wall JR, Fang SL, Ingbar SH, Braverman LE. Lymphocyte transformation in response to human thyroid extract in patients with subacute thyroiditis. J Clin Endocrinol Metab 1976; 43:587–590.
300. Weetman AP, Smallridge RC, Nutman TB, Burman KD. Persistent thyroid autoimmunity after subacute thyroiditis. J Clin Lab Immunol 1987; 23:1–6.
301. Papapetrou PD, Jackson IMD. Thyrotoxicosis due to "silent" thyroiditis. Lancet 1975; 361:363.
302. Rosen IB, Strawbridge HG, Walfish PG, et al. Malignant pseudothyroiditis: a new clinical entity. Am J Surg 1978; 136:445–449.
303. Vagenakis AG, Abreau CM, Braverman LE. Prevention of recurrence in acute thyroiditis following corticosteroid withdrawal. J Clin Endocrinol Metab 1970; 31:705–708.
304. Woolf PD. Transient painless thyroiditis with hyperthyroidism: a variant of lymphocytic thyroiditis? Endocr Rev 1980; 1:411–420.
305. Nikolai TF, Coombs GJ, McKenzie AK. Lymphocytic thyroiditis with spontaneously resolving hyperthyroidism and subacute thyroiditis. Arch Intern Med 1981; 141:1455–1458.
306. Nikolai TF, Brosseau J, Kettrick MA, et al. Lymphocytic thyroiditis with spontaneously resolving hyperthyroidism (silent thyroiditis). Arch Intern Med 1980; 140:478–482.
307. Jansson R, Bernander S, Karlsson A, et al. Autoimmune thyroid dysfunction in the postpartum period. J Clin Endocrinol Metab 1984; 58:681–687.
308. Freeman R, Rosen H, Thysen B. Incidence of thyroid dysfunction in an unselected postpartum population. Arch Intern Med 1986; 146:1361–1364.
309. Tachi J, Amino N, Tamaki H, et al. Long-term follow-up and HLA association in patients with postpartum hypothyroidism. J Clin Endocrinol Metab 1986; 66:480–484.
310. Smallridge RC. Thyrotropin-secreting pituitary tumors. Endocrinol Metab Clin North Am 1987; 16:765–792.
311. Kourides IA, Ridgway EC, Weintraub BD, et al. Thyrotropin-induced hyperthyroidism: use of alpha and beta subunit levels to identify patients with pituitary tumors. J Clin Endocrinol Metab 1977; 45:534.
312. Faglia G, Beck-Peccoz P, Piscitelli G, Medri G. Inappropriate secretion of thyrotropin by the pituitary. Hormone Res 1987; 26: 79–99.
313. Kourides IA. A patient with thyroid-stimulating hormone (TSH) hypersecretion. Med Grand Rounds 1983; 2:222–228.
314. Wemeau JL, Dewailly D, Leroy R, et al. Long-term treatment with the somatostatin analog SMS 201-995 in a patient with a thyrotropin- and growth hormone-secreting pituitary adenoma. J Clin Endocrinol Metab 1988; 66:636–639.
315. Oppenheim DS, Klibanski A. Medical therapy of glycoprotein hormone-secreting pituitary tumors. Endocrinol Metab Clin North Am 1989; 18:339–358.
316. Beck-Peccoz P, Piscitelli G. Successful treatment of hyperthyroidism due to neoplastic pituitary TSH secretion with 3,5,3′triiodothyroacetic acid (TRIAC). Endocrinol Invest 1983; 6: 217–223.
317. Kahn BB, Weintraub BD, Csako G, et al. Factitious elevation of thyrotropin in a new ultrasensitive assay: implications for the use of monoclonal antibodies in "sandwich" immunoassay. J Clin Endocrinol Metab 1988; 66:526–533.
318. Refetoff S, Weiss RE, Usala SJ. The syndromes of resistance to thyroid hormone. Endocr Rev 1993; 14:348–399.
319. Refetoff S, Weiss RE, Usala SJ, Hayashi Y. The syndromes of resistance to thyroid hormone: update 1994. Endocr Rev 1994; 3: 336–342.
320. Beck-Peccoz P, Chatterjee VKK. The variable clinical phenotype in thyroid hormone resistance syndrome. Thyroid 1994; 4:225–231.
321. O'Shanick GD, Ellinwood EH Jr. Persistent elevation of thyroid-stimulating hormone in women with bipolar affective disorder. Am J Psychiatry 1982; 139:513–514.
322. Refetoff S. Resistance to thyroid hormone: an historical overview. Thyroid 1994; 4:345–349.
323. Rosler A, Litvin Y, Hage C, et al. Familial hyperthyroidism due to inappropriate thyrotropin secretion successfully treated with triiodothyronine. J Clin Endocrinol Metab 1982; 54:76–82.
324. Davies TF, Platzer M. hCG-induced TSH receptor activation and growth acceleration in FRTL-5 thyroid cells. Endocrinology 1986; 118:2149–2151.
325. Tomer Y, Huber GK, Davies TF. Human chorionic gonadotropin (hCG) interacts directly with recombinant human TSH receptors. J Clin Endocrinol Metab 1992; 74:1477–1479.
326. Hershman JM. Human chorionic gonadotropin and the thyroid: hyperemesis gravidarum and trophoblastic tumors. Thyroid 1999; 9:653–657.
327. Martino E, Bartalena L, Bogazzi F, Braverman LE. The effects of amiodarone on the thyroid. Endocr Rev 2001; 22:240–254.
328. Newman CM, Price A, Davies DW, et al. Amiodarone and the thyroid: a practical guide to the management of thyroid dysfunction induced by amiodarone therapy. Heart 1998; 79:121–127.
329. Loh KC. Amiodarone-induced thyroid disorders: a clinical review. Postgrad Med J 2000; 76:133–140.
330. Bartalena L, Brogioni S, Grasso L, et al. Interleukin-6: a marker of thyroid-destructive processes? J Clin Endocrinol Metab 1994; 79:1424–1427.
331. Bartalena L, Brogioni S, Grasso L, et al. Treatment of amiodarone-induced thyrotoxicosis, a difficult challenge: results of a prospective study. J Clin Endocrinol Metab 1996; 81:2930–2933.
332. Hedberg CW, Fishbein DB, Janssen RS, et al. An outbreak of thyrotoxicosis caused by the consumption of bovine thyroid gland in ground beef. N Engl J Med 1987; 316:993–998.

333. Cohen JH, Ingbar SH, Braverman LE. Thyrotoxicosis due to ingestion of excess thyroid hormone. Endocr Rev 1989; 10:113–124.
334. Mariotti S, Martino E, Cupini C, et al. Low serum thyroglobulin as a clue to the diagnosis of thyrotoxicosis factitia. N Engl J Med 1982; 307:410–412.
335. Brown WW, Shetty KR, Rosenfeld PS. Hyperthyroidism due to struma ovarii: demonstration by radioiodine scan. Acta Endocrinol (Copenh) 1973; 73:266–272.
336. Wiersinga WM, Trip MD. Amiodarone and thyroid hormone metabolism. Postgrad Med J 1986; 62:909–914.
337. Sobrinho LG, Limbert ES, Santos MA. Thyroxine toxicosis in patients with iodine-induced thyrotoxicosis. J Clin Endocrinol Metab 1977; 45:25–29.
338. Gavin LA, Rosenthal M, Cavalieri RR. The diagnostic dilemma of isolated hyperthyroxinemia in acute illness. JAMA 1979; 242: 251–253.
339. Birkhauser M, Burer T, Busset R, et al. Diagnosis of hyperthyroidism when serum thyroxine alone is raised. Lancet 1977; 2: 53–56.
340. Engler D, Donaldson EB, Stockight JR, et al. Hyperthyroidism without triiodothyronine excess: an effect of severe non-thyroidal illness. J Clin Endocrinol Metab 1978; 46:77–82.
341. Burman KD, Borst GC, Eil C. Euthyroid hyperthyroxinemia. Ann Intern Med 1983; 98:366–378.
342. Croxson MS, Hall TD, Nicoloff JT. Combination drug therapy for treatment of hyperthyroid Graves' disease. J Clin Endocrinol Metab 1977; 45:623–630.
343. Larsen PR. Salicylate-induced increases in free triiodothyronine in human serum: evidence of inhibition of triiodothyronine binding to thyroxine-binding globulin and thyroxine-binding prealbumin. J Clin Invest 1972; 51:1125–1134.
344. Danese MD, Powe NR, Sawin CT, Ladenson PW. Screening for mild thyroid failure at the periodic health examination: a decision and cost-effectiveness analysis. JAMA 1996; 276:285–92.
345. Canaris GJ, Manowitz NR, Mayor G, Ridgway EC. The Colorado thyroid disease prevalence study. Arch Intern Med 2000; 160:526–534.
346. Toft AD. Clinical practice. Subclinical hyperthyroidism. N Engl J Med 2001; 345(7):512–516.
347. Shrier DK, Burman KD. Subclinical hyperthyroidism: Controversies in management. Am Fam Physician 2002; 65(3):431–438.

12 Hypothyroidism and Thyroiditis

P. Reed Larsen and Terry F. Davies

HYPOTHYROIDISM

Many structural or functional abnormalities can impair the production of thyroid hormones and cause the clinical state termed *hypothyroidism*. The causes can be divided into six main categories:

1. Hypothyroidism with compensatory thyroid enlargement due to transient or progressive impairment of hormone biosynthesis (goitrous hypothyroidism).
2. Permanent loss or atrophy of thyroid tissue (atrophic hypothyroidism).
3. Transient hypothyroidism.
4. Consumptive hypothyroidism.
5. Central hypothyroidism, that is, hypothyroidism due to insufficient stimulation of a normal gland as a result of hypothalamic or pituitary disease or defects in the thyroid-stimulating hormone (TSH) molecule itself.
6. Resistance to thyroid hormone (RTH).

Primary hypothyroidism accounts for approximately 99% of cases, with fewer than 1% being due to TSH deficiency. Central hypothyroidism is discussed in Chapters 7 and 8.

Clinically apparent acquired impairment of thyroid function affects about 2% of adult women and about 0.1 to 0.2% of adult men.[1, 2] Subclinical hypothyroidism, an elevated TSH level in an asymptomatic patient, was recently found in 9.5% of a self-selected U.S. population of approximately 26,000.[3] Neonatal screening programs for congenital hypothyroidism discover hypothyroidism in almost 1 in 3500 newborns.[4]

Clinical Presentation

Hypothyroidism can affect all organ systems, and these manifestations are largely independent of the underlying disorder but are a function of the degree of hormone deficiency. The following sections discuss the pathophysiology of each organ system at various levels of thyroid hormone deficiency, from mild to severe. The term *myxedema*, formerly used as a synonym for hypothyroidism, refers to the appearance of the skin and subcutaneous tissues in the patient in a severely hypothyroid state (Fig. 12–1). Hypothyroidism of this severity is rarely seen today, and the term should be reserved to describe the physical signs.

Skin and Appendages

Hypothyroidism causes an accumulation of hyaluronic acid that alters the composition of the ground substance in the dermis and other tissues.[5] This material is hygroscopic, producing the mucinous edema that is responsible for the thickened features and puffy appearance (myxedema) with full-blown hypothyroidism. Myxedematous tissue is characteristically boggy and nonpitting and is apparent around the eyes, on the dorsa of the hands and feet, and in the supraclavicular fossae (see Fig. 12–1). It causes enlargement of the tongue and thickening of the pharyngeal and laryngeal mucous membranes.

A histologically similar deposit may occur in patients with Graves' disease, usually over the pretibial area (infiltrative dermopathy or pretibial myxedema). In addition to having a puffy appearance, the skin is pale and cool as a result of cutaneous vasoconstriction. Anemia may contribute to the pallor; hypercarotenemia gives the skin a yellow tint but does not cause scleral icterus (see Fig. 12–1). The secretions of the sweat glands and sebaceous glands are reduced, leading to dryness and coarseness of the skin, which in extreme cases may resemble ichthyosis.

Wounds of the skin tend to heal slowly. Easy bruising is due to an increase in capillary fragility. Head and body hair is dry and brittle, lacks luster, and tends to fall out. Hair may be lost from the temporal aspects of the eyebrows, although this is not specific for hypothyroidism (see Fig. 12–1*B*). Growth of hair is retarded so that haircuts and shaves are required less often. The nails are brittle and grow slowly.

In secondary hypothyroidism, the degree of hypothyroidism is less severe and the changes in the skin and its appendages may be less striking than in primary hypothyroidism. The skin is pale and cool and tends to be thinner and finely wrinkled, and infiltration of the tissues is less prominent. Depigmentation of areas that are normally pigmented, such as the areolae, occurs in central but not primary hypothyroidism.

Histopathologic examination of the skin reveals hyperkeratosis with plugging of hair follicles and sweat glands. The dermis is edematous, and the connective tissue fibers are separated by an increased amount of metachromatically staining, periodic acid–Schiff positive mucinous material. This material consists of protein complexed with two mucopolysaccharides: hyaluronic acid and chondroitin sulfate B. The glycosaminoglycans

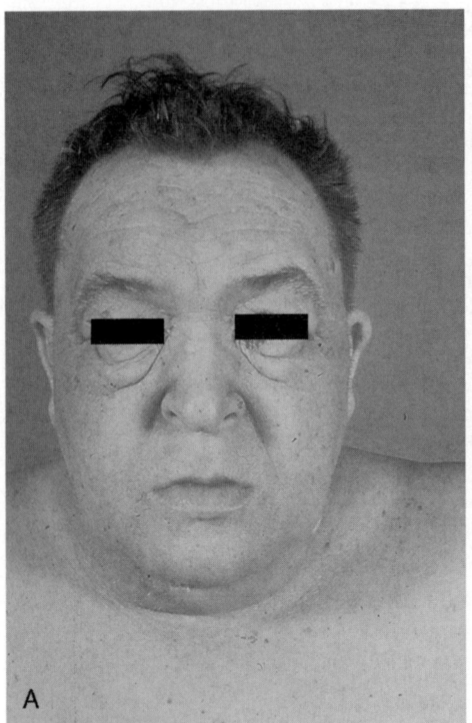

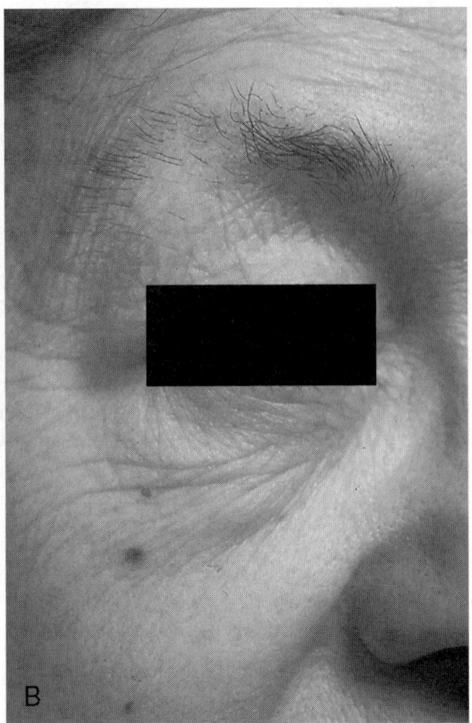

Figure 12–1. *A* and *B*, Typical appearance of patients with moderately severe primary hypothyroidism or myxedema. Note dry skin, sallow complexion, with the absence of scleral pigmentation differentiating the carotenemia from jaundice. Both individuals demonstrate periorbital myxedema. The patient in *B* illustrates the loss of the lateral aspect of the eyebrow, sometimes termed *Queen Anne's sign*. That finding is not unusual in the age group that is commonly affected by severe hypothyroidism and should not be considered to be a specific sign of the condition. (See also Color Plate.)

are mobilized early during treatment with thyroid hormone, leading to an increase in urinary excretion of nitrogen and hexosamine.[6]

Cardiovascular System

The cardiac output at rest is decreased because of reduction in both stroke volume and heart rate, reflecting loss of the inotropic and chronotropic effects of thyroid hormones. Peripheral vascular resistance at rest is increased, and blood volume is reduced. These hemodynamic alterations cause narrowing of pulse pressure, prolongation of circulation time, and decrease in blood flow to the tissues.[7, 8] The decrease in cutaneous circulation is responsible for the coolness and pallor of the skin and the sensitivity to cold. In most tissues, the decrease in blood flow is proportional to the decrease in oxygen consumption, so the arteriovenous oxygen difference remains normal. The hemodynamic alterations at rest resemble those of congestive heart failure. However, in hypothyroidism, cardiac output increases and peripheral vascular resistance decreases normally in response to exercise unless the hypothyroid state is severe and of long standing.

In severe primary hypothyroidism the cardiac silhouette is enlarged (Fig. 12–2), and the heart sounds are diminished in intensity. These findings are the result largely of effusion into the pericardial sac of fluid rich in protein and glycosaminogly-

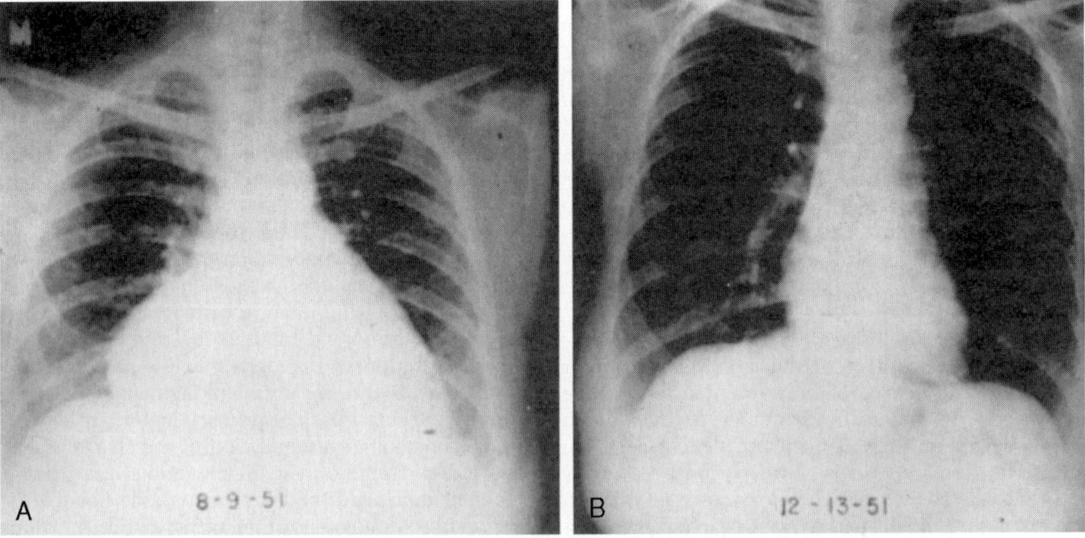

Figure 12–2. *A* and *B*, Chest roentgenograms in a patient with myxedema heart disease. The patient had signs of severe congestive heart failure and was given thyroid hormone alone. Within 4 months, the heart had returned to normal size and there was no evidence of underlying heart disease.

cans, but the "flabby" myocardium may also be dilated.[7, 9] Pericardial effusion is rarely of sufficient magnitude to cause tamponade. In central hypothyroidism, the heart is typically small.

Angina pectoris is uncommon, but it may appear or worsen during treatment of the hypothyroid state with thyroid hormone.[7, 10, 11] There is considerable controversy over whether hypothyroidism is a risk factor for atherosclerosis. The Whickham Study[1] showed no increase in cardiovascular mortality in patients with subclinical hypothyroidism over 20 years, whereas the Rotterdam Study[12] suggested that there was a twofold increase in risk. Systemic vascular resistance is increased, and hypertension is more common.[13]

Electrocardiographic changes include sinus bradycardia, prolongation of the PR interval, low amplitude of the P wave and QRS complex, alterations of the ST segment, and flattened or inverted T waves. Pericardial effusion is probably responsible for the low amplitude in severe hypothyroidism. Rarely, complete heart block may be present, but this disappears when hypothyroidism is treated.[7] Systolic time intervals are altered; the pre-ejection period is prolonged, and the ratio of pre-ejection period to left ventricular ejection time is increased. Echocardiographic studies have revealed a high frequency of asymmetrical septal hypertrophy and apparent obstruction of the left ventricular outflow tract, suggesting idiopathic hypertrophic subaortic stenosis. These findings disappear when the hypothyroidism is treated, and their hemodynamic significance is uncertain.

Serum levels of homocysteine, creatine kinase, aspartate aminotransferase, and lactate dehydrogenase may be increased.[14–16] Typically, the isoenzyme patterns suggest that the source of the increased creatine kinase and lactate dehydrogenase is skeletal, not cardiac, muscle. All levels return to normal with therapy.

The combination of large heart, hemodynamic and electrocardiographic alterations, and the serum enzyme changes has been termed *myxedema heart.* Myxedema heart rarely causes heart failure by itself because the usual hemodynamic response to exercise in hypothyroidism is typically normal, although exceptions have been reported.[7, 8, 17] In the patient with hypothyroidism, as in the normal individual, the Valsalva maneuver leads to a decrease in pulse pressure, whereas in the patient with heart failure the pulse pressure does not decrease but displays the so-called square-wave response. In the absence of coexisting organic heart disease, treatment with thyroid hormone corrects the hemodynamic, electrocardiographic, and serum enzyme alterations of myxedema heart and restores heart size to normal (see Fig. 12–2).

Respiratory System

Pleural effusions usually are evident only on radiologic examination but in rare instances may cause dyspnea. Lung volumes are usually normal, but maximal breathing capacity and diffusing capacity are reduced. In severe hypothyroidism, myxedematous involvement of respiratory muscles and depression of both the hypoxic and the hypercapnic ventilatory drives may cause alveolar hypoventilation and carbon dioxide retention, which in turn can contribute to the development of myxedema coma.[18] Obstructive sleep apnea is common but is reversible with restoration of a euthyroid state.[19]

Alimentary System

Although most patients experience a modest gain in weight, appetite is usually reduced. The weight gain that occurs is caused partly by retention of fluid by the hydrophilic glycoprotein deposits in the tissues. Peristaltic activity is decreased and, together with the decreased food intake, is responsible for the frequent complaint of constipation. The latter may lead to fecal impaction (myxedema megacolon). Gaseous distention of the abdomen (myxedema ileus), if accompanied by colicky pain and vomiting, may mimic mechanical ileus.

Elevations in the serum levels of carcinoembryonic antigen, which may occur on the basis of hypothyroidism alone,[20] add to the impression that an organic obstruction is present. Ascites in the absence of another cause is unusual in hypothyroidism, but it can occur, usually in association with pleural and pericardial effusions. Like pericardial and pleural effusions, the ascitic fluid is rich in protein and glycosaminoglycans.

Achlorhydria after maximal histamine stimulation may be present in patients with primary hypothyroidism. Circulating antibodies against gastric parietal cells have been found in about one third of patients with primary hypothyroidism and may be secondary to atrophy of the gastric mucosa. Overt pernicious anemia is reported in about 12% of patients with primary hypothyroidism. The coexistence of pernicious anemia and other autoimmune diseases, such as gluten enteropathy, with primary hypothyroidism reflects the fact that autoimmunity plays the central role in the pathogenesis of these diseases (see Chapter 37).

Hypothyroidism has complex effects on intestinal absorption. Although the rates of absorption for many substances are decreased, the total amount absorbed may be normal or even increased because the decreased bowel motility may allow more time for absorption. Malabsorption is occasionally overt.

Liver function test results are usually normal, but levels of aminotransaminases may be elevated, probably because of impaired clearance. The gallbladder contracts sluggishly and may be distended, but whether these changes predispose to the development of gallstones is unknown.

Atrophy of the gastric and intestinal mucosa and myxedematous infiltration of the bowel wall may be demonstrated on histologic examination. The colon may be greatly distended, and the volume of fluid in the peritoneal cavity is usually increased. The liver and pancreas are normal.

Central and Peripheral Nervous System

Thyroid hormone is essential for the development of the central nervous system. Deficiency in fetal life or at birth causes retention of the infantile characteristics of the brain, hypoplasia of cortical neurons with poor development of cellular processes, retarded myelination, and reduced vascularity.[21, 22] If the deficiency is not corrected in early postnatal life, the damage is irreversible. Deficiency of thyroid hormone beginning in adult life causes less severe manifestations that usually respond to treatment with the hormone. Cerebral blood flow is reduced, but cerebral oxygen consumption is usually normal; this finding is in accord with the conclusion that the oxygen consumption of isolated brain tissue in vitro, unlike that of most other tissues, is not stimulated by administration of thyroid hormones. In severe cases, decreased cerebral blood flow may lead to cerebral hypoxia.

All intellectual functions, including speech, are slowed. Loss of initiative is present, slow-wittedness and memory defects are common, lethargy and somnolence are prominent, and dementia in elderly patients may be mistaken for senile dementia. Psychiatric disorders are common and are usually of the paranoid or depressive type and may induce agitation (myxedema madness).[23, 24] Headaches are frequent. Cerebral hypoxia due to circulatory alterations may predispose to confusional attacks and syncope, which may be prolonged and lead to stupor or coma. Other factors predisposing to coma in hypothyroidism include exposure to severe cold, infection, trauma, hypoventilation with carbon dioxide retention, and depressant drugs.

Epileptic seizures have been reported and tend to occur in myxedema coma. Night blindness is due to deficient synthesis of the pigment required for dark adaptation. Hearing loss of the perceptive type is frequent due to myxedema of the eighth cranial nerve and serous otitis media. Perceptive deafness may also occur in association with a defect in the organic binding of thyroidal iodide (Pendred's syndrome) (see discussion of iodine metabolism), but in these instances it is not due to hypothyroidism per se.

Thick, slurred speech and hoarseness are due to myxedematous infiltration of the tongue and larynx, respectively. Body movements are slow and clumsy, and cerebellar ataxia may occur. Numbness and tingling of the extremities are frequent; in the fingers these symptoms may be due to compression by glycosaminoglycan deposits in and around the median nerve in the carpal tunnel (carpal tunnel syndrome).[25, 26] The tendon reflexes are slow, especially during the relaxation phase, producing the characteristic "hung-up reflexes"; this phenomenon is due to a decrease in the rate of muscle contraction and relaxation rather than a delay in nerve conduction.[27, 28]

The presence of extensor plantar responses or diminished vibration sense should alert the physician to the possibility of coexisting pernicious anemia with combined system disease. Electroencephalographic changes include slow alpha wave activity and general loss of amplitude. The concentration of protein in the cerebrospinal fluid is often increased, but cerebrospinal pressure is normal.

Histopathologic examination of the brain in patients with untreated hypothyroidism reveals that the nervous system is edematous with mucinous deposits in and around nerve fibers. In patients with cerebellar ataxia, neural myxedematous infiltrates of glycogen and mucinous material are present in the cerebellum. There may be foci of degeneration and an increase in glial tissue. The cerebral vessels show atherosclerosis, but this is much more common if the patient has had coexistent hypertension.

Muscular System

Stiffness and aching of muscles are common and are worsened by cold temperatures. Delayed muscle contraction and relaxation cause the slowness of movement and delayed tendon jerks. Muscle mass may be reduced or enlarged due to interstitial myxedem.[29] Muscle mass may be slightly increased, and the muscles tend to be firm. Rarely, a profound increase in muscle mass with slowness of muscular activity may be the predominant manifestation (the Kocher-Debré-Sémélaigne, or Hoffmann, syndrome). Myoclonus may be present. The electromyogram may be normal or may exhibit disordered discharge, hyperirritability, and polyphasic action potentials.

On histopathologic examination, the muscles appear pale and swollen. The muscle fibers may show swelling, loss of normal striations, and separation by mucinous deposits. Type I muscle fibers tend to predominate.[28]

Skeletal System: Calcium and Phosphorus Metabolism

Thyroid hormone is essential for normal growth and maturation of the skeleton, and growth failure is due both to impaired general protein synthesis and to a reduction in growth hormone, but especially of insulin-like growth factor I (Fig. 12–3).[30–34] Before puberty, thyroid hormone plays a major role in the maturation of bone. Deficiency of thyroid hormone in early life leads to both a delay in the development of, and an abnormal, stippled appearance of the epiphyseal centers of ossification (epiphyseal dysgenesis) (Fig. 12–4). Impairment of linear growth leads to dwarfism in which the limbs are disproportionately short in relation to the trunk but cartilage growth is unaffected (see Fig. 12–3).[30, 31]

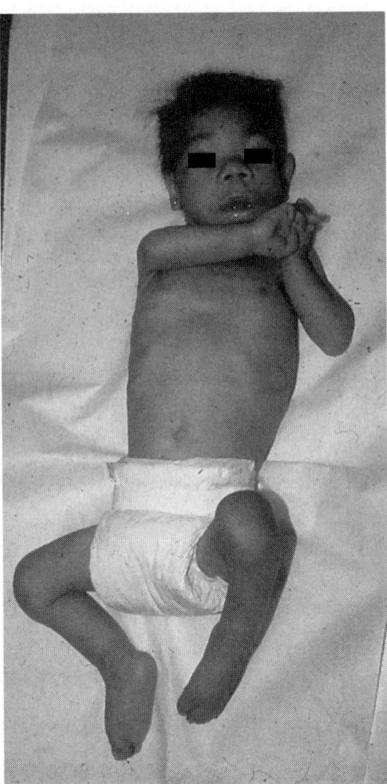

Figure 12–3. The consequences of untreated congenital hypothyroidism are demonstrated in this 17-year-old girl. Her condition had been diagnosed at birth but, through a series of misunderstandings, was not treated with thyroid hormone. Note her size, the poorly developed nasal bridge, the wide-set eyes, and the ears, which are larger than are appropriate for head size. Her tongue is enlarged, and her extremities are inappropriately short in relation to her trunk. (Courtesy of Dr. Ronald B. Stein.)

Urinary excretion of calcium is decreased, as is the glomerular filtration rate, whereas fecal excretion of calcium and both urinary and fecal excretion of phosphorus are variable. Calcium balance is also variable, and any changes are slight. The exchangeable pool of calcium and its rate of turnover are reduced, changes that reflect decreased bone formation and resorption.[35, 36] Because levels of parathyroid hormone are often slightly increased, some degree of resistance to its action may be present; levels of $1,25(OH)_2D$ are also increased.

Levels of calcium and phosphorus in serum are usually normal, but calcium may be slightly elevated. The alkaline phosphatase level is usually below normal in infantile and juvenile hypothyroidism. Bone density may be increased. The radiologic appearance of the skeleton in cretinism and juvenile hypothyroidism are discussed subsequently.

Renal Function: Water and Electrolyte Metabolism

Renal blood flow, glomerular filtration rate, and tubular reabsorptive and secretory maxima are reduced. Blood urea nitrogen and serum creatinine levels are normal, but uric acid levels may be increased. Urine flow is reduced, and delay in the excretion of a water load may result in reversal of the normal diurnal pattern of urine excretion. The delay in water excretion appears to be due to decreased volume delivery to the distal diluting segment of the nephron as a result of the diminished renal perfusion; evidence supporting inappropriate secretion of vasopressin (syndrome of inappropriate antidiuretic

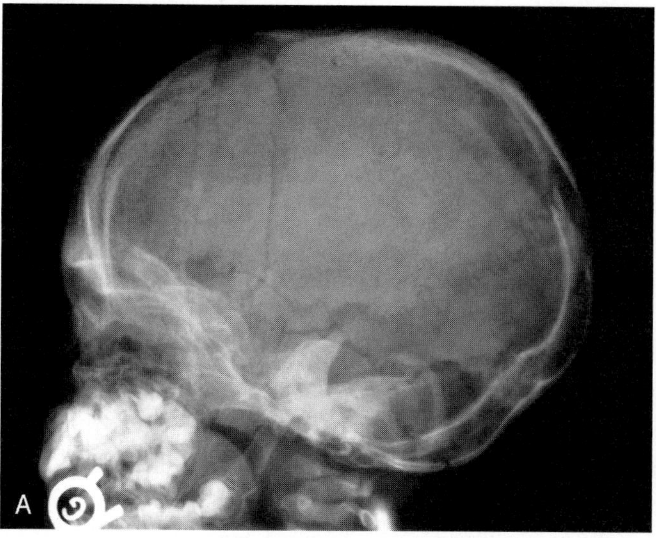

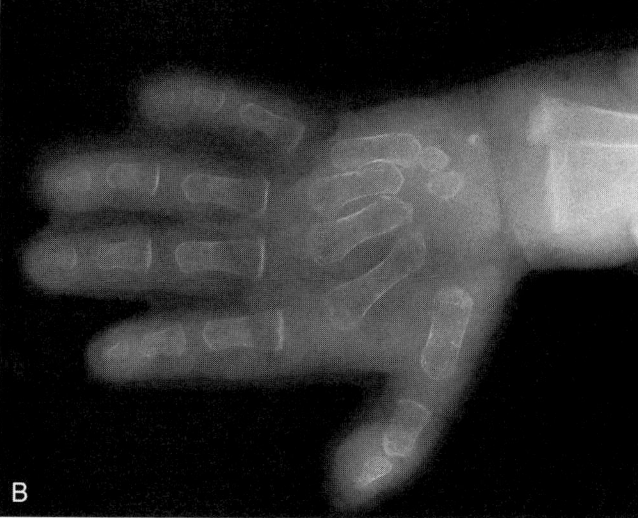

Figure 12–4. X-ray films of the skull and hand of the 17-year-old patient illustrated in Figure 12–3. *A*, Skull film showing that the posterior and anterior fontanelles are open and that the sutures are not fused. The deciduous and permanent teeth are present. *B*, Radiograph of the wrist and hand showing the delayed appearance of the epiphyseal centers of the bones of the hand and the absence of the distal radial epiphysis. The estimated bone age is 9 months. (Courtesy of Dr. Ronald B. Stein.)

hormone) is less compelling.[37] These changes are reversed by treatment with thyroid hormone. The ability to concentrate urine may be slightly impaired. Mild proteinuria may occur.

The impaired renal excretion of water and the retention of water by the hydrophilic deposits in the tissues result in an increase in total body water, even though plasma volume is reduced. This increase accounts for the hyponatremia occasionally noted because the level of exchangeable sodium is increased. The amount of exchangeable potassium is usually normal in relation to lean body mass. Serum magnesium concentration may be increased, but exchangeable magnesium levels and urinary magnesium excretion are decreased.

Hematopoietic System

In response to the diminished oxygen requirements and decreased production of erythropoietin, the red blood cell mass is decreased; this is evident in the mild normocytic, normochromic anemia that often occurs. Less commonly, the anemia is macrocytic, sometimes from deficiency of vitamin B_{12}. Reference has already been made to the high incidence of pernicious anemia (and of achlorhydria and vitamin B_{12} deficiency without overt anemia) in primary hypothyroidism (see Chapter 37). Conversely, overt and subclinical hypothyroidism is present in 12% and 15% of patients, respectively, with pernicious anemia. Folate deficiency from malabsorption or dietary inadequacy may also cause macrocytic anemia. The frequent menorrhagia and the defective absorption of iron resulting from achlorhydria may contribute to a microcytic, hypochromic anemia.

The total and differential white blood cell counts are usually normal, and platelets are adequate, although platelet adhesiveness may be impaired. If pernicious anemia or significant folate deficiency is present, the characteristic changes in peripheral blood and bone marrow will be found. The intrinsic clotting mechanism may be defective because of decreased concentrations in plasma of factors VIII and IX, and this, together with an increase in capillary fragility and the decrease in platelet adhesiveness, may account for the bleeding tendency that sometimes occurs.[38–41]

Pituitary and Adrenocortical Function

In long-standing hypothyroidism of thyroid origin, hyperplasia of the thyrotropes may cause the pituitary gland to be enlarged. This feature can be detected radiologically as an increase in the volume of the pituitary fossa.[42] Rarely, the pituitary enlargement compromises the function of other pituitary cells and causes pituitary insufficiency or visual field defects. Patients with severe hypothyroidism may have increased serum prolactin levels that correlate with the level of serum TSH, and galactorrhea may develop in some patients.[43] Treatment with thyroid hormone corrects serum prolactin and TSH levels and causes disappearance of galactorrhea, if present. The cause of hyperprolactinemia in hypothyroidism is uncertain but may result from enhanced sensitivity of the lactotropes to thyrotropin-releasing hormone (TRH). In severe primary hypothyroidism, the response of growth hormone to provocative stimuli, such as insulin-induced hypoglycemia or growth hormone–releasing hormone may be subnormal.[30, 44]

As a result of the decreased rate of turnover of cortisol due to decreased hepatic 11β-hydroxysteroid dehydrogenase, type 1 (11β-HSD-1), the 24-hour urinary excretion of cortisol and 17-hydroxycorticosteroids is decreased but the plasma cortisol level is usually normal (see Chapter 14). The responses of urinary 17-OH-corticosteroid to exogenous adrenocorticotropic hormone and metyrapone are usually normal but may be decreased. The response of plasma cortisol to insulin-induced hypoglycemia may be impaired.[44]

In severe, long-standing primary hypothyroidism, pituitary and adrenal function may be secondarily decreased and adrenal insufficiency may be precipitated by stress or by rapid replacement therapy with thyroid hormone.[45] The rate of turnover of aldosterone is decreased, but the plasma level is normal. Plasma renin activity is decreased, and sensitivity to angiotensin II is increased (see Chapter 15).

Reproductive Function

In both sexes, thyroid hormones influence sexual development and reproductive function. Infantile hypothyroidism, if untreated, leads to sexual immaturity, and juvenile hypothyroidism causes a delay in the onset of puberty followed by anovulatory cycles. Paradoxically, primary hypothyroidism may also cause precocious sexual development and galactorrhea.

In adult women, severe hypothyroidism may be associated with diminished libido and failure of ovulation. Secretion of progesterone is inadequate, and endometrial proliferation persists, resulting in excessive and irregular breakthrough menstrual bleeding.[46] These changes may be due to deficient secretion of luteinizing hormone. Rarely, in primary hypothyroidism, secondary depression of pituitary function may lead to ovarian atrophy and amenorrhea. Fertility is reduced, and spontaneous abortion may result, although many pregnancies are successful.[47, 48] Hypothyroidism in men may cause diminished libido, impotence, and oligospermia.

Values for plasma gonadotropins are usually in the normal range in primary hypothyroidism; in postmenopausal women, levels are usually somewhat lower than in euthyroid women of the same age but are nevertheless within the menopausal range. This provides a valuable means of differentiating primary from secondary hypothyroidism.

The metabolism of both androgens and estrogens is altered in hypothyroidism. Secretion of androgens is decreased, and the metabolism of testosterone is shifted toward etiocholanolone rather than androsterone. With respect to estradiol and estrone, hypothyroidism favors metabolism of these steroids via 16α-hydroxylation over that via 2-oxygenation, with the result that formation of estriol is increased and that of 2-hydroxyestrone and its derivative, 2-methoxyestrone, is decreased. The sex hormone–binding globulin in plasma is decreased, with the result that the plasma concentrations of both testosterone and estradiol are decreased, but the unbound fractions are increased. The alterations in steroid metabolism are corrected by restoration of the euthyroid state.[49]

Catecholamines

The plasma cyclic adenosine monophosphate (cAMP) response to epinephrine is decreased, suggesting a state of decreased adrenergic activity. The fact that the responses of plasma cAMP to glucagon and parathyroid hormone are also decreased suggests that thyroid hormones have a general modulating influence on cAMP generation. The mechanism underlying the decreased adrenergic responsiveness is uncertain but probably results from impaired cAMP responses to norepinephrine.[50, 51] The secretion rate and plasma concentration of epinephrine are normal, but the corresponding norepinephrine functions are increased.[52–54]

Energy Metabolism: Protein, Carbohydrate, and Lipid Metabolism

The decrease in energy metabolism and heat production is reflected in the low basal metabolic rate, decreased appetite, cold intolerance, and slightly low basal body temperature. Both the synthesis and the degradation of protein are decreased, the latter especially so, with the result that nitrogen balance is usually slightly positive. The decrease in protein synthesis is reflected in retardation of both skeletal and soft tissue growth. In addition, thyroid hormone deficiency impairs both the secretion and effectiveness of growth hormone, the latter perhaps related to impaired formation of insulin-like growth factor I.[30–33]

Permeability of capillaries to protein is increased, accounting for the high levels of protein in effusions and in cerebrospinal fluid. In addition, the albumin pool is increased because of the greater decrease in albumin degradation than in albumin synthesis. A greater than normal fraction of exchangeable albumin is in the extravascular space. The total concentration of serum proteins may be increased.

The oral glucose tolerance curve is characteristically flat, and the insulin response to glucose is delayed. These alterations may be due to a decreased rate of absorption of glucose from the gut. The disappearance from plasma of an intravenous (IV) load of glucose is delayed because of the slow rate of glucose uptake by tissues. Insulin sensitivity of skeletal muscle is normal.[55] Degradation of insulin is slow, so the sensitivity to exogenous insulin may be increased. Increased insulin sensitivity and the decrease in appetite presumably account for the decrease in insulin requirement when hypothyroidism develops in a patient with preexisting diabetes mellitus.[56] Hepatic glycolysis is unaffected by hypothyroidism.[55]

Both the synthesis and the degradation of lipid are depressed, the latter especially so, the net effect being one of lipid accumulation, especially of low-density lipoprotein (LDL) and triglycerides.[57–59] The decrease in the lipid degradation rate may reflect the decrease in post-heparin lipolytic activity, as well as reduced LDL receptors.[60] High-density lipoprotein (HDL) concentrations are reduced. The increase in serum cholesterol in primary (but not central) hypothyroidism is accompanied by increased levels of serum phospholipids, serum triglycerides, and LDL. Plasma free fatty acid levels are decreased, and the mobilization of free fatty acids in response to fasting, catecholamines, and growth hormone is impaired. All of these abnormalities are relieved by treatment.[61, 62]

In a random group of 1149 Dutch women, 11% were found to have subclinical hypothyroidism (TSH > 4.0 μU/L with normal free thyroxine. There was an increased prevalence of aortic atherosclerosis (odds ratio, 1.7; confidence interval, 1.1 to 2.6) and myocardial infarction (odds ratio, 2.3; confidence interval, 1.3 to 4.0).[12] Also, hyperhomocysteinemia, a risk factor for vascular disease, is present in patients with primary hypothyroidism and responds rapidly to levothyroxine replacement.[15, 63]

Current Clinical Picture

In the adult, the onset of hypothyroidism is usually so insidious that the typical manifestations may take months or years to appear and go unnoticed by family and friends. The gradual development of the hypothyroid state is due to slow progression both of thyroid hypofunction and of the clinical manifestations after thyroid failure is complete. This course is in contrast with the more rapid development of the hypothyroid state when replacement therapy is discontinued in a patient with treated primary hypothyroidism or when the thyroid gland of a normal subject is surgically removed. In such patients, manifestations of frank hypothyroidism are present by 6 weeks; by 3 months myxedema appears.

The clinical picture of hypothyroidism in the third millennium is, in general, much milder than that described 50 years ago in the first edition of this textbook. New scales for assessment of clinical symptoms suggesting hypothyroidism have been developed (Fig. 12–5).[64] In general, many of the symptoms are similar but much less prevalent than they were and do not significantly discriminate the hypothyroid from the euthyroid patient (e.g., cold intolerance or pulse rate). The reason for this is largely the ready availability of sensitive and specific laboratory tests for hypothyroidism that allow recognition of the primary form of the disease long before severe symptoms have developed. Nonetheless, early symptoms are variable and nonspecific. There should be a low threshold for screening patients for primary hypothyroidism with a TSH determination because in every series there are a number of patients with significant biochemical abnormalities who do not score high on symptom and sign testing.[64]

With respect to physical signs of hypothyroidism, the pres-

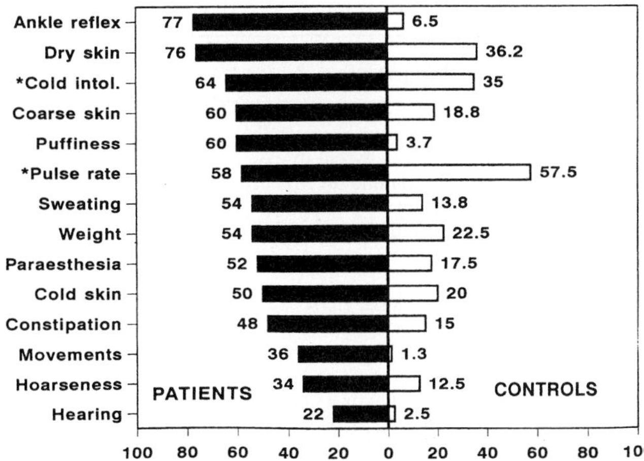

Figure 12–5. Frequency of hypothyroid symptoms and signs (percentage) in 50 patients with overt hypothyroidism and in 80 euthyroid controls. Two symptoms (pulse rate and cold intolerance, marked by asterisks) showed positive and negative predictive values of less than 70% and were thus excluded from the new score. (From Zulewski H, Müller B, Exer P, et al. Estimation of tissue hypothyroidism by a new clinical score: evaluation of patients with various grades of hypothyroidism and controls. J Clin Endocrinol Metab 1997; 82:771–776.)

ence of coarse skin, periorbital puffiness that obscures the curve of the malar bone (see Fig. 12–1), cold skin, and delayed ankle reflex relaxation phase all are signs that should lead to appropriate diagnostic tests.

The unusual syndrome of acute hypothyroidism in the previously hyperthyroid patient that is characterized by painful cramping of large muscle groups is discussed under the topic "Treatment of Graves' Disease" (see Chapter 11).

Severe hypothyroidism is seldom apparent at birth, hence the requirement for systematic screening.[4, 65] The age at which symptoms appear depends on the degree of impairment of thyroid function (see Figs. 12–3 and 12–4). Severe hypothyroidism in infancy is termed *cretinism*. As the age at onset increases, the clinical picture of cretinism merges imperceptibly with that of juvenile hypothyroidism. Retardation of mental development and growth, the hallmark of cretinism, becomes manifest only in later infancy and is largely irreversible. Consequently, early recognition is crucial and can be achieved by population screening by measuring serum T_4 or TSH concentrations routinely in neonates. During the first few months of life, symptoms of hypothyroidism include feeding problems, failure to thrive, constipation, a hoarse cry, and somnolence. In succeeding months, especially in severe cases, protuberance of the abdomen, dry skin, poor growth of hair and nails, and delayed eruption of the deciduous teeth become evident. Retardation of mental and physical development is manifested by delay in reaching the normal milestones of development, such as holding up the head, sitting, walking, and talking.[4]

Impairment of linear growth results in dwarfism, with the limbs disproportionately short in relation to the trunk (see Fig. 12–3). Delayed closure of the fontanelles causes the head to be large in relation to the body. The naso-orbital configuration remains infantile. Maldevelopment of the femoral epiphyses results in a waddling gait. The teeth are malformed and susceptible to caries. The characteristic appearance includes a broad, flat nose; widely set eyes; periorbital puffiness; large protruding tongue; sparse hair; rough skin; short neck; and protuberant abdomen with an umbilical hernia. Mental deficiency is usually severe.

Radiologic examination of the skeleton is diagnostic. The skull shows a poorly developed base; delayed closure of the fontanelles; widely set orbits; and a short, flat nasal bone. The pituitary fossa may be enlarged. Shedding of deciduous teeth and eruption of permanent teeth are delayed (see Fig. 12–4).

The radiologic picture of epiphyseal dysgenesis is virtually pathognomonic of hypothyroidism in infancy and childhood and may involve any center of endochondral ossification, depending on the age at onset of the hypothyroid state; it is usually best seen in the femoral and humeral heads and the navicular bone of the foot. The centers of ossification appear late, so bone age is retarded in relation to chronologic age, and when they eventually appear, instead of a single center, multiple small centers are scattered through a misshapen epiphysis (see Fig. 12–4). These small centers of ossification eventually coalesce and form a single center with an irregular outline and a stippled appearance (stippled epiphysis). Epiphyseal dysgenesis is evident only in centers that normally ossify at a time after the onset of the hypothyroidism. After a normal metabolic state is restored by treatment, centers destined to ossify at a later age develop normally.

Hypothyroidism that begins in childhood is termed *juvenile hypothyroidism*. The clinical manifestations are intermediate, between those of infantile and those of adult hypothyroidism, in that the developmental retardation is not as severe as that of cretinism and the manifestations of full-blown adult myxedema are rarely seen. Growth and sexual development are affected predominantly. Linear growth is severely retarded, and the rate of linear growth is usually less than that of weight gain. Sexual maturation and the onset of puberty are delayed. The result is a child who appears much younger than the chronologic age. Rarely, precocious puberty and galactorrhea occur. Intellectual performance is poor, but the mental deficiency is not as severe as that in cretinism.

The manifestations of adult hypothyroidism are present to a varying, but usually milder, degree. On radiologic examination, epiphyseal dysgenesis may be present and epiphyseal union is always delayed, resulting in a bone age that is retarded in relation to chronologic age.

Laboratory Evaluation

Primary and Central Hypothyroidism

A decrease in secretion of the thyroid hormones is common to all varieties of hypothyroidism, except for *consumptive hypothyroidism* and *resistance to thyroid hormone* (see later). In patients with primary thyroid disease, the cause of hypothyroidism in more than 99% of the patients, there is a significant increase in basal serum TSH concentration. A strategy for evaluating the patient suspected of hypothyroidism involves an initial TSH determination (Table 12–1). If the suspicion of hypothyroidism is strong, a goiter is present or central hypothyroidism is part of the differential diagnosis, a free T_4 or free T_4 index (FT_4I) should be included (see Chapter 10). If hypothyroidism is thought to be unlikely but must be excluded, only a TSH determination is required because primary hypothyroidism is almost always the cause. If TSH is elevated, an FT_4I can be added to the same determination (Fig. 12–6). As hypothyroidism becomes more severe, the serum TSH increases and serum FT_4I, and later serum triiodothyronine (T_3), concentrations become subnormal, the former more rapidly than the latter (see Table 12–1). The persistence of a normal serum T_3 is, in part, due to preferential synthesis and secretion of T_3 by residual functioning thyroid tissue under the influence of the increased plasma TSH. In addition, the efficiency of conversion of T_4 to T_3 by D2 is increased as the serum T_4 level falls.[66, 67] Consequently, the serum T_3 concentration may remain within the normal range and is not a useful index of thyroid function in the hypothyroid patient.

The differentiation of hypothyroidism due to intrinsic thyroid failure from hypothyroidism due to diminished TSH se-

Table 12–1. Laboratory Evaluation of Patients with Suspected Hypothyroidism

TSH, Free T_4 Index	TPO Antibodies	Diagnosis
TSH > 10 mU/L		
Low	+	Primary hypothyroidism due to autoimmune thyroid disease
Low-normal	+	Primary "subclinical" hypothyroidism (autoimmune)
Low or low-normal	−	Recovery from systemic illness
		External irradiation, drug-induced, congenital hypothyroidism
		Iodine deficiency
		Seronegative autoimmune thyroid disease
		Rare thyroid disorders (amyloidosis, sarcoidosis, etc.)
		Recovery from subacute granulomatous thyroiditis
Normal	+, −	Consider TSH or T_4 assay artifacts
Elevated	−	Thyroid hormone resistance
		Blockade of T_4-to-T_3 conversion (amiodarone) or a congenital 5′-deiodinase deficiency
		Consider assay artifacts
TSH 5–10 mU/L		
Low, low-normal	+	Early primary autoimmune hypothyroidism
Low, low-normal	−	Milder forms of nonautoimmune hypothyroidism (see above)
		Central hypothyroidism with impaired TSH bioactivity
Elevated	−(+)	Consider thyroid hormone resistance
		T_4-to-T_3 conversion blockade (e.g., amiodarone)
TSH 0.5–5 mU/L		
Low, low-normal	−(+)	Central hypothyroidism
		Salicylate or phenytoin therapy
		Desiccated thyroid or T_3 replacement
TSH <0.5 mU/L		
Low, low-normal	−(+)	"Posthyperthyroid" hypothyroidism (^{131}I or surgery), central hypothyroidism
		T_3 or desiccated thyroid excess
		Post–excess levothyroxine withdrawal

Initial tests: Serum TSH, serum free T_4 index, antibodies to TPO. A parenthesis indicates that the result is less common but may occur.
TSH, thyroid-stimulating hormone; T_3, triiodothyronine; T_4, thyroxine; TPO, thyroid peroxidase.
Results are grouped with respect to the serum TSH concentration. The different diagnoses possible for low, normal, or elevated free T_4 index and TPO antibody results are indicated.

cretion from hypothalamic or pituitary disease (central or secondary hypothyroidism) is the most critical decision point in this pathway (see Fig. 12–6). A low thyroid hormone level with a normal or low TSH level should lead to an evaluation for the possibility of failure of other endocrine systems that require trophic pituitary hormones for normal function (Table 12–2) (see Chapters 7and 8). The only exception to this is *posthyperthyroid* hypothyroidism, in which TSH levels may remain suppressed for several months even though hypothyroidism has been induced by ^{131}I, surgery, or antithyroid drugs (see Table 12–1). In some patients with central hypothyroidism, the basal serum TSH concentration (and the response to TRH) may even be somewhat elevated, but the TSH has reduced biologic potency even though it is immunologically reactive.[68]

In patients with an elevated TSH level and a reduced FT_4I, the presence or absence of thyroid peroxidase (TPO) antibodies should be ascertained (see Fig. 12–6). The presence of TPO antibodies generally points to autoimmune thyroid disease (Hashimoto's disease) as the cause of the hypothyroidism. On the other hand, the absence of TPO antibodies requires a search for less common causes of hypothyroidism such as transient hypothyroidism, infiltrative thyroid disorders, and external irradiation, as discussed later (see Table 12–1).

Tests that employ radioiodine to assess the function of the thyroid gland display a variable pattern, depending on the underlying thyroid disorder. When the amount of thyroid tissue is reduced, the radioactive iodine uptake (RAIU) is subnormal. However, the diagnostic value of this finding in North America is minimized by the low normal range resulting from the high dietary iodine intake. Yet when hypothyroidism results primarily from a biochemical defect in thyroid hormone synthesis rather than thyroid cell destruction (thus leading to compensatory goitrogenesis), RAIU may be normal or increased. Specific functional patterns in relation to the causes of hypothyroidism are discussed later. Nonetheless, measurement of RAIU is almost never required in the diagnostic evaluation of the hypothyroid patient.

Differential Diagnosis

The clinical picture of fully developed hypothyroidism is characteristic enough to leave the diagnosis in little doubt. Despite the availability of inexpensive and specific tests, it is still surprising how often what is retrospectively obvious, severe, primary hypothyroidism is overlooked by experienced clinicians. If the diagnosis is not considered during the first meeting with the patient, it may take another 6 months before it is recognized that multiple, seemingly disparate complaints are due to hypothyroidism. A high index of suspicion is required to avoid this oversight.

For the milder forms of hypothyroidism, it may be necessary to differentiate them from several other states. The fact that these disorders often occur in older patients is partly responsible for the diagnostic uncertainty. In some cases, slowing of mental and physical activity, dry skin, and loss of hair may mimic similar findings in hypothyroidism. Furthermore, older people often become hypothermic with cold exposure. In patients with chronic renal insufficiency, anorexia, torpor, periorbital puffiness, sallow complexion, and anemia (e.g., see Fig. 12–1) may suggest hypothyroidism and may call for specific testing. Distinguishing nephrotic states from hypothyroidism by clinical examination alone may be even more difficult. In this disorder, waxy pallor, edema, hypercholesterolemia, and

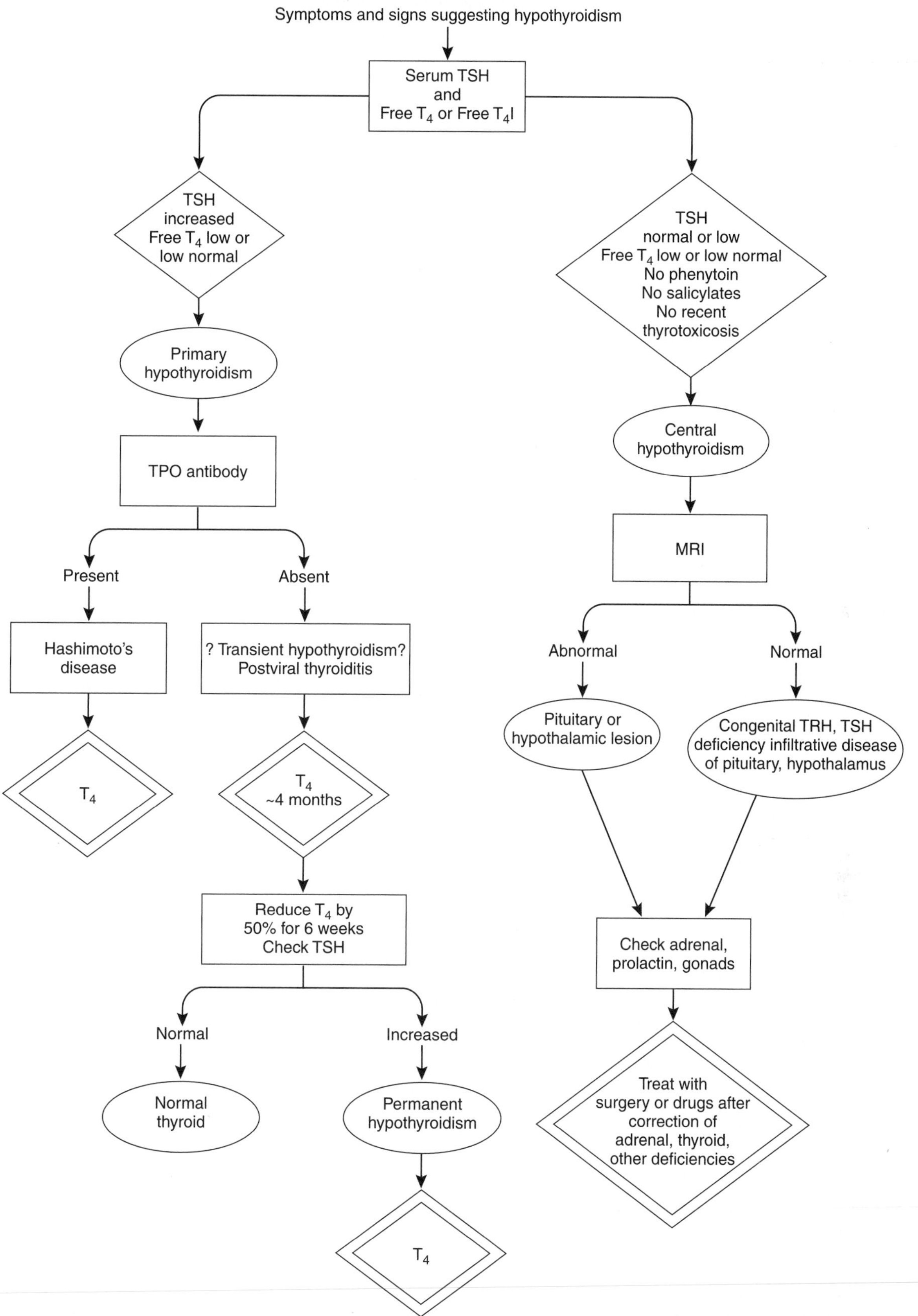

Figure 12–6. Strategy for the laboratory evaluation of patients with suspected hypothyroidism. The principal differential diagnosis is between primary and central hypothyroidism (see Chapter 8). The serum thyrotropin (TSH) concentration is the critical laboratory determination that, in general, allows recognition of the cause of the disease. An exception is the individual with a recent history of thyrotoxicosis (and suppressed TSH) in whom a low free thyroxine (T_4) level may be associated with a reduced TSH level for several months after relief of the thyrotoxicosis. In patients with primary hypothyroidism, the absence of thyroid peroxidase (TPO) antibodies raises a possible diagnosis of transient hypothyroidism following an undiagnosed episode of subacute or postviral thyroiditis. In such patients, a trial of a reduced levothyroxine dosage after 4 months may reveal recovery of thyroid function thus avoiding permanent levothyroxine replacement. MRI, magnetic resonance imaging.

Table 12–2. Causes of Hypothyroidism

Primary Hypothyroidism with Goiter
Acquired
- Hashimoto's thyroiditis (autoimmune thyroiditis type 2A)
- Iodine deficiency (endemic goiter)
- Drugs blocking synthesis or release of T_4 (e.g., lithium, ethionamide, sulfonamides, iodide)
- Goitrogens in foodstuffs or as endemic substances or pollutants
- Cytokines (interferon α, interleukin-2)
- Thyroid infiltration (amyloidosis, hemochromatosis, sarcoidosis, Riedel's struma, cystinosis, scleroderma)

Congenital
- Iodide transport or utilization defect (NIS or pendrin mutations)
- Iodotyrosine dehalogenase deficiency
- Organification disorders (TPO deficiency or dysfunction)
- Defects in thyroglobulin synthesis or processing

Atrophic Hypothyroidism
Acquired
- Hashimoto's disease (autoimmune thyroiditis type 2B)
- Postablative due to ^{131}I, surgery, or therapeutic irradiation for nonthyroidal malignancy

Congenital
- Thyroid agenesis or dysplasia
- TSH receptor defects
- Thyroidal Gs protein abnormalities (pseudohypoparathyroidism type 1a)
- Idiopathic TSH unresponsiveness

Transient (Post-thyroiditis) Hypothyroidism
Following subacute, painless, or postpartum thyroiditis

Consumptive Hypothyroidism
Rapid destruction of thyroid hormone due to D3 expression in large hemangiomas or hemangioendotheliomas

Central Hypothyroidism
Acquired
- Pituitary origin (secondary)
- Hypothalamic disorders (tertiary)
- Bexarotene (*RXR* receptor agonist)
- Dopamine and/or severe illness

Congenital
- TSH deficiency or structural abnormality
- TSH receptor defect

Resistance to Thyroid Hormone
Generalized
"Pituitary" dominant

TPO, thyroid peroxidase; TSH, thyroid-stimulating hormone.

hypometabolism may suggest hypothyroidism. In addition, the total serum T_4 concentration may be decreased if significant thyroglobulin is lost in the urine but the FT_4I and TSH would be normal.

In patients with pernicious anemia, psychiatric abnormalities, pallor, and numbness and tingling of the extremities may mimic similar findings in hypothyroidism. Although there is a clinical and immunologic overlap between primary hypothyroidism and pernicious anemia, this association is not invariable (see Chapter 37). The presence of hypothyroidism is often suspected in patients who are severely ill, especially in the elderly.[69] In such patients, the total T_4 concentration may be decreased, often markedly so, but the FT_4I is generally normal unless the patient is severely ill (see Chapter 10). These features, together with the absence of an elevation of serum TSH, usually serve to differentiate the ill euthyroid patient from one with primary hypothyroidism.

Hypothyroidism may develop either because of some extrinsic factor or acquired condition or because of a congenital defect impairing thyroid hormone biosynthesis (see Table 12–2). Inadequate synthesis of hormone leads to hypersecretion of TSH, which in turn produces both goiter and stimulation of all steps in hormone biosynthesis capable of response. If the compensatory response is inadequate, goitrous hypothyroidism results. In some instances, however, the compensatory response overcomes the impairment in hormone biosynthesis, and the patient is euthyroid with a compensatory goiter. The latter condition is discussed in Chapter 13 under the topic "Simple or Nontoxic Goiter." Less commonly, hypothyroidism is associated with an atrophic gland or, in the case of a congenital abnormality, one that never developed properly. From a clinical standpoint, it is useful to classify patients with hypothyroidism into those with and those without goiter (see Table 12–2).

Classification

Goitrous Hypothyroidism

Acquired Causes

Hashimoto's Thyroiditis

Hashimoto's disease, or autoimmune thyroiditis type 2A, is the most common cause of goitrous hypothyroidism in areas of the world in which dietary iodine is sufficient. Before discussing this entity, it is important to redefine the term *autoimmune thyroid disease* (Table 12–3). Many use the term *autoimmune*

Table 12–3. Classification of Autoimmune Thyroiditis

Type 1 Autoimmune Thyroiditis (Hashimoto's Disease Type 1)
- 1A Goitrous
- 1B Nongoitrous

Status
Euthyroid with normal TSH level. Autoantibodies to Tg and TPO usually present

Type 2 Autoimmune Thyroiditis (Hashimoto's Disease Type 2)
- 2A Goitrous (classic Hashimoto's disease)
- 2B Nongoitrous (primary myxedema, atrophic thyroiditis)

Status
Persistent hypothyroidism with increased TSH levels. Autoantibodies to Tg and TPO usually present. Some type 2B is associated with blocking-type TSH receptor autoantibodies

- 2C Transient aggravation of thyroiditis

Status
May start as transient thyrotoxicosis (increased serum thyroid hormones with low thyroidal radioactive iodine uptake). Often followed by transient hypothyroidism. However, patients may show transient hypothyroidism without the preceding thyrotoxicosis. Autoantibodies to Tg and TPO present. Example: postpartum thyroiditis

Type 3 Autoimmune Thyroiditis (Graves' Disease)
- 3A Hyperthyroid Graves' disease
- 3B Euthyroid Graves' disease

Status
Hyperthyroid or euthyroid with suppressed TSH. Stimulatory autoantibodies to the TSH receptor are present. Autoantibodies to Tg and TPO are also usually present

- 3C Hypothyroid Graves' disease

Status
Orbitopathy with hypothyroidism. Diagnostic levels of autoantibodies to the TSH receptor of the blocking or stimulating variety may be detected. Autoantibodies to Tg and TPO are usually present

TSH, thyroid-stimulating hormone; Tg, thyroglobulin; TPO, thyroid peroxidase.

From Davies TF, Amino N. A new classification for human autoimmune thyroid disease. Thyroid 1993; 3:332.

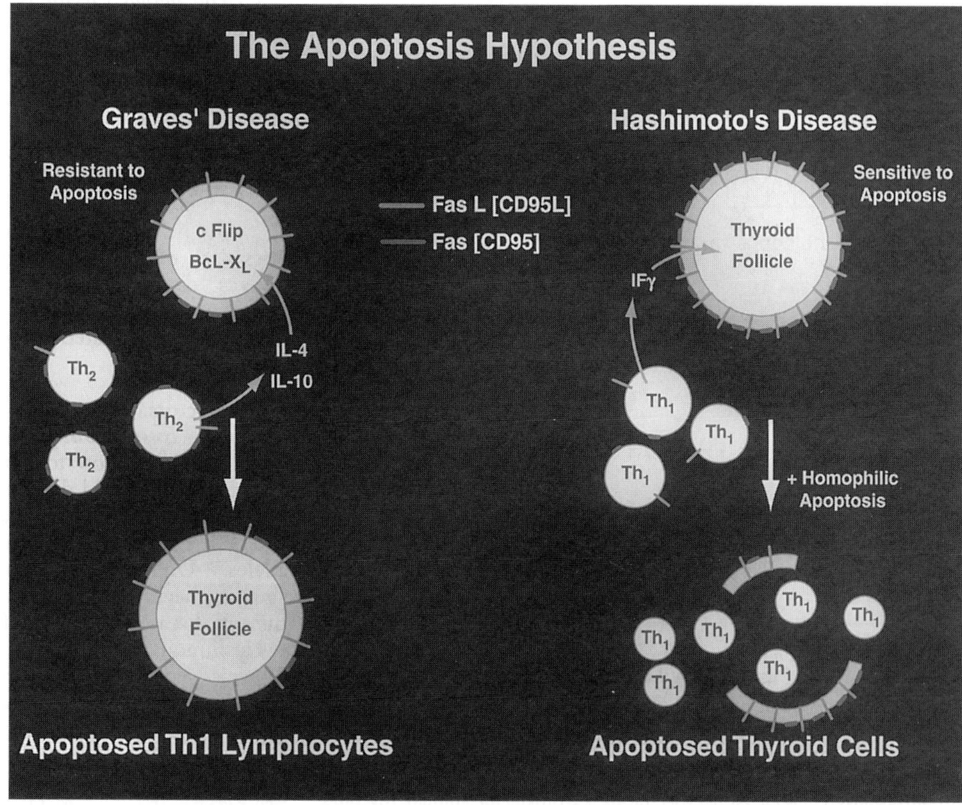

Figure 12–7. Possible involvement of Fas-Fasl in the apoptosis of Hashimoto's thyroiditis. In Graves' disease, the thyroid follicles thrive because the thyroid cells do not express many functional Fas molecules (shown in red) and, therefore, the thyroid cells are resistant to the Fasl (Fas ligand) on both the thyroid cells themselves and on the Th2 T cells (shown in blue). Further apoptotic resistance may be driven by Th2 cytokines, such as interleukin-4 (IL-4) and IL-10. However, the Th2 cells express Fas and may themselves be deleted by the Fasl constitutively expressed on the thyroid cells. The result is thyroid cell survival with T-cell destruction. In contrast, in Hashimoto's disease, the thyroid cell expresses many functional Fas molecules, perhaps induced by gamma interferon from the Th1 type T cells associated with this disease. The expression of thyroid cell Fas may lead to self (homophilic) apoptosis via thyroid cell Fasl, or apoptosis may result from attack by the Fasl armed Th1 cells. The result is thyroid follicle destruction and T-cell proliferation. (See also Color Plate.)

thyroiditis to cover both primary myxedema (nongoitrous) and classic Hashimoto's disease (goitrous).[70] These are differing clinical manifestations of the same disorder that is also closely related to autoimmune hyperthyroidism—Graves' disease.

Autoantibodies to the TSH receptor that act as TSH antagonists may be the cause of some cases of the thyroid atrophy seen in primary myxedema and are seen less often in goitrous Hashimoto's disease.[71, 72] However, both Graves' and Hashimoto's diseases may occur within the same families and may share human leukocyte antigen (HLA) and other genetic susceptibility haplotypes.[73–75] Furthermore, thyroid failure occurs in some patients with Graves' disease,[76] and hyperthyroidism and even orbitopathy develop in some patients with Hashimoto's disease.[77, 78] Both types of patients may have autoantibodies to thyroglobulin, TPO, and the TSH receptor. Hence, the diseases must be closely related, and autoimmune thyroid disease can be viewed as a spectrum from hyperthyroidism to hypothyroidism.

To bring some clarity to this situation, we should also redefine the term *chronic thyroiditis.* [79] In pathologic terms, thyroiditis implies the presence of both a mononuclear cell infiltrate and destruction of thyroid follicles. However, these are arbitrary criteria. The term *chronic thyroiditis* is more appropriately defined simply as evidence of "intrathyroidal lymphocytic infiltration" without the necessity of follicular damage. Because by this definition patients with both Graves' disease and Hashimoto's disease have thyroiditis, replacement of the term *autoimmune thyroid disease* with the more correct term *autoimmune thyroiditis* allows a simple classification for autoimmune thyroid disease (see Table 12–3).

Until the demonstration of circulating thyroid antigen–specific T cells and thyroid autoantibodies, the diagnosis of Hashimoto's disease could be confirmed only by biopsy of the thyroid. The ease with which we can now demonstrate high levels of circulating antibodies and thyroid antigen–specific T cells in most patients with Hashimoto's disease led to the use of the term *autoimmune thyroiditis,* which, as explained earlier, we prefer to use for any mononuclear infiltrate.

Hashimoto's disease is common and may be increasing in frequency. The mean incidence in women is in the order of 3.5 cases per 1000 people per year and in men is 0.8 cases per 1000 people per year.[1] No age group is exempt, although the prevalence increases with age. Hashimoto's disease is the most common cause of goitrous hypothyroidism in areas of iodine sufficiency.

Pathophysiology. Impairment of hormone synthesis is due to apoptotic destruction of the thyroid cells. The sick cells exhibit a defect in organic binding of thyroid iodide, as evidenced by a positive perchlorate discharge test (see Chapter 10 for a discussion of pendrin). In addition, release of iodoproteins, mostly thyroglobulin, is enhanced by cell lysis. Approximately 90% of the thyroid gland must be destroyed before hypothyroidism develops. The presence of lymphocytic infiltration of the thyroid (hence the older term *lymphocytic thyroiditis*), circulating thyroid autoantibodies, and clinical or immunologic overlap with other diseases with autoimmune components indicate that Hashimoto's disease is an autoimmune thyroid disorder.

The current understanding of autoimmune mechanisms has been discussed earlier in Chapter 11. However, autoimmune thyroiditis is characterized by thyroid cell apoptosis leading to follicular destruction rather than thyroid stimulation and thyroid cell hyperplasia. Although both autoantibodies to thyroid peroxidase (TPOAb) and thyroglobulin (TgAb) may be complement-fixing and cytotoxic, the thyroid gland is infiltrated by both B cells and by T cells; the latter are armed with Fas ligand and capable of destroying thyroid cells expressing Fas via apoptosis (Fig. 12–7) (see also Color Plate).[80, 81] In addition, other cell death pathways may be involved.[82] Fas expression on thyroid cells may be secondary to elaboration of a variety of cytokines from T cells that undergo blast transformation when exposed to thyroid antigens (thyrotropin recep-

thyroid gland enlarges rapidly and, when accompanied by pain and tenderness, may mimic de Quervain's or subacute thyroiditis. Some patients, particularly those with the fibrous variant, are hypothyroid when first seen. The goiter is generally moderate in size and firm in consistency and moves freely on swallowing. The surface is either smooth or scalloped, but well-defined nodules are unusual. Both lobes are enlarged, but the gland may be asymmetrical. The pyramidal lobe may be enlarged, and adjacent structures, such as the trachea, esophagus, and recurrent laryngeal nerves, may be compressed. Enlargement of regional lymph nodes is unusual.

Although nongoitrous Hashimoto's disease (atrophic hypothyroidism) (see later) is thought to be the end result of autoimmune destruction of the thyroid, the progression of goitrous Hashimoto's disease to the atrophied state is not commonly seen in the individual patient. Indeed, the histopathologic picture tends to remain rather static except for an increase in fibrous tissue.

Clinically, the untreated goiter remains unchanged or enlarges gradually over many years. The manifestations of hypothyroidism may develop over several years in patients who are initially euthyroid. Some, but not all, studies also suggest an increased prevalence of thyroid carcinoma in Hashimoto's disease.[111] As mentioned earlier, the presence of coexistent Hashimoto's disease may be a favorable prognostic factor in patients with papillary carcinoma.[112]

Occasionally, hyperthyroidism develops in patients with Hashimoto's disease. In other patients with early autoimmune thyroiditis, transitory thyrotoxicosis (painless or silent thyroiditis with thyrotoxicosis) occurs as the result of thyroid cell destruction. In such cases, evidence of ongoing thyroid hyperfunction is lacking because the thyroid RAIU is depressed. As described earlier, a phase of transient hypothyroidism begins 3 to 6 months post partum in 30% of women with autoimmune thyroiditis, as evidenced by the presence of TPOAb.[113–117] The history may suggest earlier mild thyrotoxicosis (see syndromes associated with transient hyperthyroidism in Chapter 11).

Laboratory Tests. The results of the common tests of thyroid function depend on stage of disease (see Table 12–1). Rarely, the tests may suggest thyroid hyperfunction with a suppressed TSH but without overproduction of hormone. The RAIU may be increased, but serum T_4 and T_3 levels may remain normal. At this stage, the patient may be eumetabolic. As the TSH level rises, the glandular response at first compensates for the impairment of hormone biosynthesis. With time, the ability of the thyroid to respond to TSH diminishes, and the RAIU and serum T_4 level decline to subnormal values. The serum T_3 concentration, however, may be slightly increased, probably reflecting maximal stimulation of the failing thyroid by the increased serum TSH level. The foregoing sequence, with still normal T_4 and T_3 and increased TSH levels, reflects the development of mild (subclinical) hypothyroidism (see Table 12–1).

The diagnosis of Hashimoto's disease is confirmed by the presence of thyroid autoantibodies in the serum, usually in high levels. TPO autoantibodies are more common and in higher concentrations than thyroglobulin autoantibodies. Sometimes part of a gland with autoimmune thyroiditis may look and feel like a firm thyroid nodule, and ultrasonography should be performed to resolve the issue.

Differential Diagnosis. Differentiation of Hashimoto's disease from other uncomplicated disorders of the thyroid is facilitated by the demonstration that high levels of thyroid autoantibodies occur more commonly in Hashimoto's disease than in other thyroid disorders. The frequent coexistence of hypothyroidism and Hashimoto's disease serves to distinguish this disease from nontoxic goiter and thyroid neoplasms.

Differentiation of euthyroid Hashimoto's disease from a diffuse nontoxic goiter is often difficult, although diffuse nontoxic goiter tends to be softer than that of Hashimoto's disease and ultrasound examination may reveal the heterogeneity of Hashimoto's disease. In adolescents, differentiation of Hashimoto's disease from diffuse nontoxic goiter is even more difficult because in this age group Hashimoto's disease may not be accompanied by such high levels of thyroid autoantibodies. The presence of well-defined nodules usually distinguishes nontoxic multinodular goiter from Hashimoto's disease.

Differentiation between Hashimoto's disease and thyroid carcinoma can sometimes be made on clinical grounds. Thyroid carcinoma is usually nodular and firm or hard and may be fixed to adjacent structures. Compression of the recurrent laryngeal nerve with hoarseness is virtually pathognomonic of thyroid carcinoma but occurs late in the disease progression. A history of a recent enlargement of the goiter is more common in thyroid carcinoma than in Hashimoto's disease. Enlargement of regional lymph nodes also suggests thyroid carcinoma. In thyroid carcinoma, ultrasound examination or radioiodine scanning of the thyroid may reveal only the isolated lesion. In Hashimoto's disease, activity is usually heterogeneous.

Treatment. In many patients, no treatment is required because the goiter is small and the disease is asymptomatic, with the TSH level remaining in the normal range (autoimmune thyroiditis type 1). In other patients, treatment with thyroid hormone is directed at alleviating goiter, hypothyroidism, or both (autoimmune thyroiditis type 2A).

Levothyroxine treatment is indicated in patients when the goiter presses on adjacent structures or is unsightly, and it is most effective in goiters of recent onset. In long-standing goiter, treatment with thyroid hormone is usually ineffective, possibly because of fibrosis.

Glucocorticoids may cause regression of the goiter and decrease autoantibody levels, but these agents are not recommended in the usual case because of untoward side effects and the return of activity after treatment is withdrawn.

Full-replacement doses of thyroid hormone should be given when hypothyroidism or subclinical hypothyroidism supervenes. Surgery is justified if pressure symptoms or unsightly enlargement persists after a trial of suppressive therapy. Administration of levothyroxine should be continued after surgery because hypothyroidism is inevitable. The importance of maintaining the serum TSH level within the normal range is covered later, under Treatment.

Iodine Deficiency (Endemic Goiter)

The term endemic goiter denotes any goiter occurring in a region where goiter is prevalent.[118–120] As mentioned, endemic goiter almost always occurs in areas of environmental iodine deficiency. Although this condition is estimated to affect more than 200 million people throughout the world and is of major public health significance, it is most common in mountainous areas, such as the Alps, Himalayas, and Andes, or in the Great Lakes and Mississippi Valley regions of the United States, owing to the depletion of iodine consequent to the persistent glacial run-off in these regions.

The causative role of iodine deficiency in the genesis of endemic goiter is supported by the inverse correlation between the iodine content of soil and water and the incidence of goiter, the kinetics of iodine metabolism in patients with the disorder, and a decrease in incidence after iodine prophylaxis. The latter accounts for its absence in the population residing in the Great Plains region of the United States.

The occurrence of endemic goiter can be spotty, even within an area of known iodine deficiency; the role of dietary minerals or naturally occurring goitrogens and of pollution of water supplies has been suggested in instances of this type. For example, in the Cauca Valley of Colombia, waterborne goitrogens have been implicated, and in many areas of endemic iodine deficiency, consumption of cassava meal, which gives rise to thiocyanate, aggravates the iodine-deficient state by inhibiting thyroid iodide transport.[121]

Most abnormalities in iodine metabolism in patients with endemic goiter are consistent with the expected effects of iodine deficiency (see Chapter 10, "Iodine Metabolism"). Thyroid iodide clearance rates and RAIU are increased in proportion to the decrease in the urinary excretion of stable iodine. The absolute iodine uptake is normal or low. In areas of moderate iodine deficiency, the serum T_4 concentration is usually in the lower range of normal; in areas of severe deficiency, however, values are decreased. Nevertheless, most patients in these areas do not appear to be in a hypothyroid state because of an increase in the synthesis of the calorigenically more efficient T_3 at the expense of T_4 and because of an increase in the activity of thyroidal D1 and D2 (see Fig. 10–12).

The incidence and severity of endemic goiter and the metabolic state of the goitrous patient depend mainly on the degree of iodine deficiency. In the absence of hypothyroidism, the effects of the goiter are mainly cosmetic. When the goiter becomes nodular, however, hemorrhage into a nodule may cause acute pain and swelling, mimicking subacute thyroiditis or neoplasia. The goiter may also compress adjacent structures, such as the trachea, esophagus, and recurrent laryngeal nerves. The borderline nature of the iodine supply in many countries of western Europe is exemplified by the development in Belgium of compensatory goiter during pregnancy due to the increased requirement for thyroid hormone during gestation.[122, 123]

The incidence of endemic goiter has been greatly reduced in many areas by the introduction of iodized salt. In the United States, table salt is enriched with potassium iodide to a concentration of 0.01%, which, if the intake of salt is average, would provide an iodine intake of approximately 500 μg/day, the desired amount in an adult (see Table 10–1). As mentioned, iodine intake in the United States has been decreasing in recent decades because of reduced salt consumption.[124] It is now possible that some pregnant patients may have inadequate iodine supplies. An annual injection of iodized oil is another effective means of administering iodine, and endemic goiter can be treated by the addition of iodine to communal drinking water.

Administration of iodine has little, if any, effect on a long-standing endemic goiter, but it causes the early endemic hyperplastic goiter of iodine deficiency to regress.[125] Similarly, thyroid hormone usually has no effect on long-standing goiter or on established mental or skeletal changes, but it should be given in full-replacement doses if there is evidence of hypothyroidism. This is of paramount importance in pregnant women. Surgical treatment is indicated if the adjacent structures are compressed or if the goiter is either very large or is enlarging rapidly.

Endemic Cretinism

Endemic cretinism is a developmental disorder that occurs in regions of severe endemic goiter.[22, 119, 126] Both parents of an endemic cretin are usually goitrous, and in addition to the features of sporadic cretinism described earlier, endemic cretins often have deaf-mutism, spasticity, motor dysfunction, and abnormalities in the basal ganglia demonstrable by magnetic resonance imaging.[127, 128]

Three types of cretins can be discerned: (1) hypothyroid cretins, (2) neurologic cretins, and (3) cretins with combined features of the two. The pathogenesis of neurologic cretinism is obscure but may be due to severe thyroid hormone deficiency during a critical early phase of central nervous system development in utero.[22] Some cretins are goitrous, but the thyroid may also be atrophic, possibly as a consequence of exhaustion atrophy from continuous overstimulation or the lack of iodine.

Iodide Excess

Goiter and hypothyroidism, either alone or in combination, are sometimes induced by chronic administration of large doses of iodine in either organic or inorganic form (see Table 10–8).[129–131] Iodide-induced goiter was formerly seen in patients with chronic respiratory disease, who were given potassium iodide as an expectorant. The development of iodide goiter has also been reported after a single administration of radiographic contrast medium from which iodide is released slowly over a long period and may also occur during amiodarone administration.[132, 133] Iodide goiter without hypothyroidism may occur endemically, such as on the island of Hokkaido, Japan, where seaweed products are consumed in large quantities.

From an analysis of reported cases and from the fact that only a small percentage of patients who receive iodides chronically develop goiter, it appears that the disorder evolves on a background of underlying thyroid dysfunction. Categories of susceptible individuals include the following:

1. Patients with Hashimoto's disease.
2. Patients with Graves' disease, especially after its treatment with radioiodine.
3. Patients with cystic fibrosis.

Among these groups, many, but not all, individuals display a positive iodide-perchlorate discharge test, indicating a defect in the thyroid organic binding mechanism (see Chapter 10, "Iodine Metabolism"). However, intrinsic thyroid disease need not be present because a propensity to develop iodide goiter and hypothyroidism has also been demonstrated in patients who have undergone hemithyroidectomy for a solitary thyroid nodule in whom the remaining lobe was histologically normal. In these patients, as in those with Hashimoto's disease or Graves' disease studied prospectively, individuals with the highest basal serum TSH concentrations, even within the normal range, were those who developed iodide goiter. Iodinated contrast material, amiodarone and povidone iodine are common sources.[134]

Goiter and hypothyroidism commonly occur in newborn infants born to women given large quantities of iodine during pregnancy, and death from neonatal asphyxia has been reported (see Fig. 10–13). In such cases, the mother is usually free from goiter. Pregnant women should not receive large doses of iodine (>1 mg/ day) over prolonged periods (>10 days), especially near term. Maternal amiodarone therapy causes thyroidal dysfunction in up to 20% of newborns.[135] It is not known whether iodide goiter in newborns results from an inherent hypersensitivity of the fetal thyroid or from the fact that the placenta concentrates iodide several-fold or both.[129, 136]

As discussed earlier (see Chapter 10, "Regulation of Thyroid Function"), large doses of iodine cause an acute inhibition of organic binding that abates in the normal individual, despite continued iodine administration (acute Wolff-Chaikoff effect and escape).[137] Iodide goiter appears to result from a more pronounced inhibition of organic binding and the failure of the escape phenomenon. As a consequence of decreased hormone synthesis and the consequent increase in TSH, iodide transport is enhanced. Because inhibition of organic binding is a function of the intrathyroidal concentration of iodide, a vicious circle, augmented by this increase in serum TSH, is set in motion.

The disorder usually appears as a goiter with or without

hypothyroidism, although in rare instances iodine may produce hypothyroidism unaccompanied by goiter. Usually the thyroid gland is firm and diffusely enlarged, often greatly so. Histopathologic examination reveals intense hyperplasia. The FT_4I concentration is low, TSH concentration is increased, and the 24-hour urinary iodine excretion and the serum inorganic iodide concentration are increased. The disorder regresses after iodine is withdrawn. Thyroid hormone may also be given to relieve severe symptoms.

Drugs Blocking Thyroid Hormone Synthesis or Release

Ingestion of compounds that block thyroid hormone synthesis or release may cause goiter with or without hypothyroidism. Apart from the agents used in the treatment of hyperthyroidism, antithyroid agents may be encountered either as drugs for the treatment of disorders unrelated to the thyroid gland or as natural agents in foodstuffs.[132]

Goiter with or without hypothyroidism can occur in patients given lithium, usually for bipolar manic-depressive psychosis.[138] Like iodide, lithium inhibits thyroid hormone release, and in high concentrations can inhibit organic binding reactions. At least acutely, iodide and lithium act synergistically in the latter respect. The mechanisms underlying the several effects of lithium are uncertain; what differentiates patients who develop goiter during lithium therapy from those who do not is also unclear. Underlying autoimmune thyroiditis may be at least one factor because many patients with this combination have autoimmune thyroid disease.

Other drugs that occasionally produce goitrous hypothyroidism include para-aminosalicylic acid, phenylbutazone, aminoglutethimide, and ethionamide.[139, 140] Like the thionamides, these drugs interfere with both the organic binding of iodine and the later steps in hormone biosynthesis. Although soybean flour is not an antithyroid agent, soybean products in feeding formulas formerly resulted in goiter in infants by enhancing fecal loss of hormone, which, together with the low iodine content of soybean products, produced a state of iodine deficiency. Feeding formulas containing soybean products are now enriched with iodine.

Cigarette smoking increases the risk of hypothyroidism in patients with underlying autoimmune thyroid disease. Although the mechanism is unclear, certain components of cigarette smoke, including thiocyanate, hydroxyperidine, and benzopyrene derivatives, may be responsible.[141, 142]

Both the goiter and the hypothyroidism usually subside after the antithyroid agent is withdrawn. If continued administration of pharmacologic goitrogens is required, however, replacement therapy with thyroid hormone causes the goiter to regress.

Goitrogens in Foodstuffs or as Endemic Substances or Pollutants

Antithyroid agents also occur naturally in foods. These are widely distributed in the family Cruciferae or Brassicaceae, particularly in the genus *Brassica*, including cabbages, turnips, kale, kohlrabi, rutabaga, mustard, and various plants that are not eaten by humans but that serve as animal fodder. It is likely that some thiocyanate is present in such plants (particularly cabbage).[143] Cassava meal, a dietary staple in many regions of the world, contains linamarin, a cyanogenic glycoside, the metabolism of which leads to the formation of thiocyanate. Ingestion of cassava can accentuate goiter formation in areas of endemic iodine deficiency. Except for thiocyanate, dietary goitrogens influence thyroid iodine metabolism in the same manner as do the thionamides, which they resemble chemically; their role in the induction of disease in humans is uncertain. Waterborne, sulfur-containing goitrogens of mineral origin are believed to contribute to the development of endemic goiter in certain areas of Colombia.[121]

A number of synthetic chemical pollutants have been implicated in causing goitrous hypothyroidism, including polychlorinated biphenyls and resorcinol derivatives. Perchlorate has also been noted in high concentrations in geographic regions in which explosives were made. It is not clear whether the concentrations are significant enough to produce hypothyroidism.[144–146]

Cytokines

Patients with chronic hepatitis C or various malignancies may be given interferon α or interleukin-2. Such patients may experience hypothyroidism, which is usually transient but may persist. These agents activate the immune system and can induce a clinical picture suggesting an exacerbation of underlying autoimmune disease such as occurs during postpartum thyroiditis (see Chapters 11 and 37).[100, 101, 147] Graves' disease with hyperthyroidism may also develop, and ablative therapy may be required to treat this condition. Patients with preexisting evidence of autoimmune thyroid disease who have positive TPO antibodies are probably at higher risk for this complication and should be monitored carefully during and after a course of treatment with either of these cytokines. Autoimmune hypothyroidism may also develop after successful treatment of Cushing's disease, presumably as a result of the release of the glucocorticoid-induced immunosuppression.[148]

Congenital Causes

Inherited defects in hormone biosynthesis are rare causes of goitrous hypothyroidism and account for only about 10% to 15% of the 1 in 3500 newborns with congenital hypothyroidism.[4] In most instances, the defect appears to be transmitted as an autosomal recessive trait. Individuals with goitrous hypothyroidism are believed to be homozygous for the abnormal gene, whereas euthyroid relatives with slightly enlarged thyroids are presumably heterozygous. In the latter group, appropriate functional testing may disclose a mild abnormality of the same biosynthetic step that is defective in the homozygous individual. In contrast with nontoxic goiter, which is more common in females than in males, these defects, as a group, affect females only slightly more commonly than males.

Although goiter may be present at birth, it usually does not appear until several years later. Therefore, the absence of goiter in a child with functioning thyroid tissue does not exclude the presence of hypothyroidism. The goiter is initially diffusely hyperplastic, often intensely so, suggesting papillary carcinoma, but eventually becomes nodular. In general, the more severe the biosynthetic defect, the earlier the goiter appears, the larger it is, and the greater the likelihood of early development of hypothyroidism or even cretinism. Five specific defects in the pathways of hormone synthesis have been identified.

Iodide Transport Defect

Iodide transport defect is rare, a result of impaired iodide transport by the sodium-iodide symporter (NIS) protein mechanism and is reflected by defective iodide transport in the thyroid, salivary gland, and gastric mucosa.[149–151] Administration of iodide, by raising the plasma concentration, increases the intrathyroidal concentration of iodide sufficiently to permit the synthesis of normal quantities of hormone, demonstrating that this is the cause of the deficiency.[152]

Defects in Expression or Function of Thyroid Peroxidase

TPO is a protein that is required for normal synthesis of iodothyronines. Quantitative or qualitative abnormalities of TPO have been identified in 1 in 66,000 infants in the Netherlands.[153] The most common of the 16 mutations identified in 35 families was a GGCC insertion in exon 8, leading to premature termination of TPO synthesis.

Pendred's Syndrome

The most common presentation in patients with Pendred's syndrome is a defect in iodine organification accompanied by sensory nerve deafness. The abnormality is in the *PDS* gene encoding pendrin, which is involved in the apical secretion of iodide into the follicular lumen (see Fig. 10–2 and Chapter 10, "Iodine Metabolism").[154–156] Thyroid function is only mildly impaired in this disorder.[157]

Defects in Thyroglobulin Synthesis

Defects in the synthesis of thyroglobulin due to genetic causes are rare, having been identified only in a small number of families with congenital hypothyroidism.[158–161] Some defects lead to premature termination of translation, whereas another defect causes deficiency in endoplasmic reticulum processing of the thyroglobulin molecule.[160] The complex regulation and huge size of this gene makes screening for mutations a difficult task, and considerable work is still required to unravel the extent of the defects in this gene.

Iodotyrosine Dehalogenase Defect

The pathogenesis of goiter and hypothyroidism in the iodotyrosine dehalogenase defect is complex. The major abnormality is an impairment of both intrathyroidal and peripheral deiodination of iodotyrosines, presumably because of a lack (or dysfunction) of the iodotyrosine dehalogenase. The gene encoding this enzyme has yet to be identified.

As a consequence of intense thyroid stimulation and lack of intrathyroidal recycling of iodide derived from dehalogenation, iodide is rapidly accumulated by the thyroid gland and is rapidly released; monoiodotyrosine (MIT) and diiodotyrosine (DIT) are elevated in plasma and, together with their deaminated derivatives, in the urine. Hypothyroidism is presumed to result from the loss of large quantities of MIT and DIT in the urine and to secondary iodine deficiency. The goiter and hypothyroidism are relieved by administration of large doses of iodine.

Thyroid Infiltration

A number of infiltrative or fibrosing conditions may cause hypothyroidism. Some are often associated with goiter, such as Riedel's struma (see later).[162–164] Others, such as amyloidosis,[165, 166] hemochromatosis,[167, 168] or scleroderma[169] may not be. Although the other manifestations of these conditions are usually obvious and hypothyroidism is only a complication, the presence of significant hypothyroidism without evidence of autoimmune thyroiditis should lead to a consideration of these rare causes of this condition.

Atrophic Hypothyroidism

In some patients, manifestations of hypothyroidism are apparent but there is no obvious thyroid enlargement (atrophic hypothyroidism). This may be due to either acquired or congenital abnormalities, prominent among the former being Autoimmune Thyroiditis Type 2B (Table 12–3). The pathophysiology and thyroid function tests are similar to those found when goiter is present.

Acquired Causes

Nongoitrous Hypothyroidism

Hypothyroidism in the absence of a classic Hashimoto's goiter has often been termed *primary hypothyroidism* (or *myxedema*); this condition is more common in women than in men and occurs most often between the ages of 40 and 60 years. Many years ago, the presence of circulating thyroid autoantibodies in almost all patients and the clinical and immunologic overlap with autoimmune diseases indicated that this represented the end stage of an autoimmune thyroiditis in which goiter either did not develop or went unnoticed (Autoimmune Thyroiditis 2B). Although most cases are due to autoimmune-induced apoptosis of the thyroid epithelial cells (see Figs. 12–7 and 12–8), some cases of nongoitrous hypothyroidism are also associated with TSH receptor antibodies that block the response of thyroid cells to endogenous TSH (see Chapter 11).[170–172] In primary thyroid failure, the thyroid gland is not usually palpable but may be normal in size or even somewhat enlarged on sonography and of firm consistency. Circulating TPOAbs or TgAbs are detectable in most patients but may be absent in long-standing disease.

Postablative Hypothyroidism

Postablative hypothyroidism is a common cause of thyroid failure in adults. One type follows total thyroidectomy usually performed for thyroid carcinoma. Although functioning remnants may be present, as indicated by foci of radioiodine accumulation, hypothyroidism invariably develops. Another etiologic mechanism is subtotal resection of the diffuse goiter of Graves' disease or multinodular goiter. Its frequency depends on the amount of tissue remaining, but continued autoimmune destruction of the thyroid remnant in patients with Graves' disease may be a factor because some studies suggest a correlation between the presence of circulating thyroid autoantibodies in thyrotoxicosis and the development of hypothyroidism after surgery. Hypothyroidism can be manifested during the first year after surgery, but, as with postradioiodine hypothyroidism, the incidence increases with time to approach 100%. In some patients, mild hypothyroidism appears during the early postoperative period and then may occasionally remit, as also occurs after radioiodine treatment.[173]

Hypothyroidism after destruction of thyroid tissue with radioiodine is common and is the one established disadvantage of this form of treatment for hyperthyroidism in adults. Its frequency is determined, in large part, by the dose of radioiodine but is also influenced by variations in individual susceptibility, including autoimmune factors.[76] The incidence of postradioiodine hypothyroidism increases with time, approaching 100%. Although the FT_4I is low in patients with postablative hypothyroidism, serum TSH levels may be anomalously low for several months after either surgical or ^{131}I-induced hypothyroidism if TSH synthesis has been suppressed for a long period prior to treatment.[173–175]

Primary atrophic thyroid failure may also develop in patients with Hodgkin's disease after treatment with mantle irradiation[176] or after high-dose neck irradiation for other forms of lymphoma or carcinoma.[176–178] Surgical, radioiodine, or external beam therapy may also lead to a state of subclinical hypothyroidism, which usually represents an interim phase in the evolution of thyroid failure. During this phase, the patient is eumetabolic but has a modest increase in the serum TSH level

(5 to 15 mU/L), low-to-normal FT_4I, and a normal serum T_3 concentration (see Table 12–1).

Congenital Causes

Thyroid Agenesis or Dysplasia

Developmental defects of the thyroid are often responsible for the hypothyroidism that occurs in 1 in 3500 newborns.[4] These defects may take the form of complete absence of thyroid tissue or failure of the thyroid to descend properly during embryologic development. Thyroid tissue may then be found anywhere along its normal route of descent from the foramen caecum at the junction of the anterior two thirds and posterior third of the tongue (lingual thyroid) to the normal site or below. Absence of thyroid tissue or its ectopic location can be ascertained by scintiscanning.

As indicated, a number of proteins are known to be crucial for normal thyroid gland development. These include the thyroid-specific transcription factor *PAX8* as well as thyroid transcription factors 1 and 2 (TTF1 and 2). It might be anticipated that defects in one or more of these proteins may explain abnormalities in thyroidal development. These have been identified in several patients with *PAX8* mutations,[179] and a mutation in the human *TTF2* gene was associated with thyroid agenesis, cleft palate, and choanal atresia.[180] Despite a specific search, no mutations have been found in the *TTF1* gene in infants with congenital hypothyroidism.[181, 182]

Thyroid Aplasia Due to Thyrotropin Receptor Unresponsiveness

Several families exist in which thyroid hypoplasia, high TSH concentrations, and a low free T_4 level are associated with loss-of-function mutations in the TSH receptor.[183–185] The thyroid glands were in the normal location but did not trap pertechnetate (TCO_4^-). Somewhat surprisingly, thyroglobulin levels were still detectable. The molecular details of these patients are still under study.

A second type of abnormality that may cause TSH unresponsiveness is a mutation in the Gs protein that occurs in pseudohypoparathyroidism type 1A. These patients have inactivating mutations in the α-subunit of the Gs protein and, consequently, mild hypothyroidism.[186] Other as yet unexplained patients with elevated TSH levels and hypothyroidism in which the molecular nature of the defect has not been defined have been reported.[187]

Transient Hypothyroidism

Transient hypothyroidism is defined as a period of reduced FT_4I with suppressed, normal, or elevated TSH levels that are eventually followed by a euthyroid state. This unusual form of hypothyroidism usually occurs in the clinical context of a patient with subacute (postviral), lymphocytic (painless), autoimmune, or postpartum thyroiditis. These conditions are reviewed in detail in Chapter 11.

The patient reports mild to moderate symptoms of hypothyroidism of short duration, and serum TSH concentrations are typically elevated, although not greatly so. The patient often has a preceding episode of symptoms consistent with mild or moderate thyrotoxicosis. If these symptoms cannot be elucidated from the history, it may be difficult to distinguish such patients from those with a permanent form of hypothyroidism. In the early phases of post-thyroiditis hypothyroidism, TSH concentrations may still be suppressed even though the FT_4I is low because of the delayed recovery of pituitary TSH synthesis, such as in patients with Graves' disease or with toxic nodules who have undergone surgery and who have experienced rapid relief of hypothyroidism (see Table 12–1). In that situation, the TSH response to hypothyroidism may be suppressed for many months; in post-thyroiditis hypothyroidism, this period is rarely longer than a few weeks.

A significant fraction (~33%) of women with autoimmune thyroiditis but normal thyroid function have episodes of hypothyroidism during the postpartum period.[93, 117, 188] In some, the preceding hyperthyroidism is relatively asymptomatic, which can make an accurate clinical diagnosis difficult. Patients who have had an episode of typical subacute postviral thyroiditis with pain, tenderness, and hyperthyroidism are not difficult to recognize.

Diagnostic evaluation should include a determination of TSH, FT_4I, and TPOAbs. Negative or low antibodies argue strongly for a nonautoimmune cause. This is significant, in that it may be possible for the patient not to be treated only temporarily for hypothyroidism. In such patients, a trial of a lower levothyroxine dosage after 3 to 6 months may reveal that thyroid function has recovered (see Fig. 12–6). This may also occur in patients with hypothyroidism that follows acute autoimmune thyroiditis (e.g., in the postpartum period), but it is somewhat less likely to occur because of the underlying progressive nature of the autoimmune thyroiditis.

In patients with hypothyroidism due to postviral thyroiditis, the thyroid gland is usually relatively small and atrophic. In patients with hypothyroidism that follows an episode of acute lymphocytic thyroiditis, the gland is usually slightly enlarged and somewhat firm, reflecting the underlying scarring and infiltration associated with that condition.

Consumptive Hypothyroidism

Consumptive hypothyroidism is the term given to an unusual cause of hypothyroidism that has been identified in infants with visceral hemangiomas or related tumors.[67, 189] The first patient reported with this syndrome presented with abdominal distention caused by a large hepatic hemangioma with respiratory compromise secondary to upward displacement of the diaphragm. However, clinical signs suggested hypothyroidism, which was confirmed by finding a markedly elevated TSH level and undetectable T_4 and T_3 levels. The infant's response to an initial IV infusion of liothyronine was transient, leading to the decision to use parenteral thyroid hormone replacement to relieve the clinical hypothyroidism. The accelerated degradation of thyroid hormone was apparent from the fact that it required 96 μg of liothyronine plus 50 μg of levothyroxine to normalize the TSH level. The equivalent dosage as levothyroxine alone is roughly nine times that ordinarily required for treatment of infants with congenital hypothyroidism. The infant succumbed to complications of the hemangioma, and a postmortem tumor biopsy showed type 3 iodothyronine deiodinase (D3) activity in the tumor at levels eightfold higher than those normally present in term placenta. The serum reverse T_3 was extremely elevated (400 ng/dL), and the serum thyroglobulin was higher than 1000 ng/mL.

Retrospective search revealed two other patients with similar pathophysiology in whom the cause of the hypothyroidism had not been recognized. Significant D3 expression has subsequently been noted in all proliferating cutaneous hemangiomas studied to date. The cutaneous hemangiomas of infancy, although they express D3, are not associated with hypothyroidism owing to their small size. Because a significant fraction of hemangiomas remit with glucocorticoid and interferon α therapy, it is important to treat such patients with adequate doses of thyroid hormone to prevent the permanent neurologic complications associated with untreated hypothyroidism during the critical phase of neurologic development. A recent report described a similar syndrome in a 21-year-old with epithelioid hemangioendothelioma.[189a]

Central Hypothyroidism

Central hypothyroidism is due to TSH deficiency caused by either acquired or congenital hypothalamic or pituitary gland disorders (see Chapters 7 and 8). The causes of TSH deficiency may be classified as those of pituitary (*secondary* hypothyroidism) and hypothalamic (*tertiary* hypothyroidism) origins, but this distinction is not necessary in the initial separation of primary from central hypothyroidism.

In many cases, hyposecretion of TSH is accompanied by decreased secretion of other pituitary hormones, with the result that evidence of somatotroph, gonadotroph, and corticotroph failure is also present. Hyposecretion of TSH as the sole demonstrable abnormality (monotropic deficiency) is less common but does occur in both acquired and congenital forms. Hypothyroidism due to pituitary insufficiency varies in severity from instances in which it is mild and overshadowed by features of gonadal and adrenocortical failure to those in which the features of the hypothyroid state are predominant. Because a small but significant fraction of thyroid gland function is independent of TSH (~10% to 15%), hypothyroidism due to central causes is less severe than primary hypothyroidism.

The causes of central hypothyroidism are both acquired and congenital. The general subject has been discussed in Chapters 7 and 8, and those causes with relatively specific thyroid-related deficiencies are mentioned here for completeness. In addition to pituitary tumors, hypothalamic disorders, and the like, an unusual cause of secondary hypothyroidism occurs in individuals given bexarotene (a retinoid X [RXR] receptor agonist) for T-cell lymphoma.[190] This drug suppresses the activity of the human TSH β-subunit promoter in vitro. Serum T_4 concentrations are reduced about 50%, and patients experience clinical benefit from thyroid hormone replacement. Dopamine, dobutamine, high-dose glucocorticoids, or severe illness may suppress TSH release transiently, leading to a pattern of thyroid hormone abnormalities suggesting central hypothyroidism. As discussed earlier (see Chapter 10, "Changes in Thyroid Function During Severe Illness"), this severe state of hypothalamic-pituitary-thyroid suppression is a manifestation of stage 3 illness (see Table 10–10). Although these agents might be expected to have similar effects when given chronically, they do not; nor does somatostatin have a similar effect when given for acromegaly, although it does block the response of TSH to TRH and it has been administered to patients with thyrotropin-secreting pituitary adenomas.[191, 192]

Congenital defects in either the stimulation or the synthesis of TSH or in its structure have been identified as rare causes of congenital hypothyroidism. These include the consequences of defects in several of the homeobox genes, including *POU1F1* (formerly termed *Pit-1*), *PROP1*, and *HESX1*. The latter factor is necessary for the development of the hypothalamus, pituitary, and olfactory portions of the brain, and its targeted deficiency in the mouse produces a condition resembling septo-optic dysplasia in humans.[193] Defects in *POU1F1* and *PROP1* cause hereditary hypothyroidism, usually accompanied by deficiencies in growth hormone and prolactin.[194–198] One patient has been identified with a familial defect in the TRH receptor gene.[199] All of these conditions are associated with the typical pattern of reduced FT_4I and TSH.

Structural defects in TSH have also been described. These include those with a mutation in the CAGYC peptide sequence of the β-subunit, thought to be necessary for its association with the α-subunit[200] or defects that produce premature termination of the TSH β-subunit gene.[201, 202] As mentioned, some of these abnormalities may be associated with elevations in TSH, suggesting the diagnosis of primary hypothyroidism, but the TSH molecule is immunologically, but not biologically, intact.

Resistance to Thyroid Hormone

Patients with resistance to thyroid hormone (RTH) may have features of hypothyroidism if the resistance is severe and affects all tissues. Alternatively, patients with RTH may have hyperthyroidism if the resistance is more severe in the hypothalamic-pituitary axis than in the remainder of the tissues. In clinical terms, patients in the former group are said to have *generalized resistance to thyroid hormone*, whereas patients in the latter group are said to have *pituitary resistance to thyroid hormone*.[203–206] Patients with both forms almost always have mutations in one allele of the *TR-beta (TRβ)* gene that interfere with the capacity of that receptor to respond normally to T_3, usually by reducing its binding affinity (see Fig. 10–9).

The mutations in the *TRβ* gene causing RTH cluster in three areas of the thyroid hormone receptor, which have been recognized to have important contacts with the hydrophobic ligand-binding domain cavity of *TRβ* as recognized from its crystal structure.[207–209] The mutations do not interfere with the function of the DNA-binding domain, its co-repressor binding domain, or its region of heterodimerization with RXR. Some mutations affect the activation domain in the carboxy-terminus of the *TRβ* receptor.

RTH is probably produced by the heterodimerization of the mutant TRβ with RXR or homodimerization with a normal TRβ or TRα. These mutant TRβ-containing dimers compete with wild-type TR-containing dimers for binding to the thyroid hormone response elements (TREs) of thyroid hormone–dependent genes (see Fig. 10–8). Because these complexes bind co-repressor molecules that cannot be released in the absence of T_3 binding, genes containing these TREs are more repressed than they would be normally at the prevailing concentrations of circulating thyroid hormones. Receptors that contain mutations in the activation domain may have a combination of both decreased affinity for T_3 as well as impaired activating potential.

Thus, the mutant TRβ complex can interfere with the function of the three normal TR-expressing genes, producing a pattern termed *dominant negative inhibition* with an autosomal dominant pattern of inheritance. At least 400 families have been identified with this condition, and there are probably many more unreported cases. The gene frequency estimate is about 1 : 50,000, and the study of the function of the mutant receptors in this disorder has provided valuable insights into the mechanism of thyroid hormone action.[205, 208–212]

Patients with RTH usually are recognized because of thyroid enlargement, which is present in about two thirds of these individuals. Despite one's expectations, patients usually report a peculiar mixture of symptoms of hyperthyroidism and hypothyroidism. With respect to the heart, palpitations and tachycardia are more common than a reduced heart rate; however, patients may also demonstrate growth retardation and retarded skeletal maturation. This has been attributed to the fact that thyroid hormone effects in the heart appear to be primarily dependent on TRα rather than TRβ, whereas the hypothalamic-pituitary axis is primarily regulated through TRβ, particularly TRβ2.[205]

Abnormalities in neuropsychological development exist, with an increased prevalence of attention deficient hyperactivity disorder, which is found in approximately 10% of such individuals. Other neuropsychological abnormalities have also been described.[213–216] Deafness in patients with RTH reflects the important role of TRβ and thyroid hormone in the normal development of auditory function.[214] The mixture of symptoms, some suggesting hypothyroidism and others suggesting hyperthyroidism, may even differ in individuals within the same family, despite the identical mutation, thus confusing the clinical picture.

Because patients may present with symptoms suggesting hyperthyroidism, it is important to keep this diagnosis in mind in a patient with tachycardia, goiter, and elevated thyroid hormones. RTH is discussed here because a reduced response to thyroid hormone is the biochemical basis for the condition. However, the laboratory results may be the first clear evidence that a patient otherwise thought to have hyperthyroidism has RTH. These tests show the unusual combination of an increased FT_4I accompanied by normal or slightly increased TSH levels. Thus, the principal differential diagnosis is between a TSH-secreting pituitary tumor and RTH.[214, 217]

Factors that may assist in the differential diagnosis are as follows:

1. Absence of a family history in patients with TSH-producing tumors.
2. Normal thyroid hormone levels in family members of individuals with TSH-induced hyperthyroidism due to pituitary tumor.
3. Presence of an elevated glycoprotein α-subunit in patients with pituitary tumor but not in those with thyroid hormone resistance.

A definitive diagnosis requires sequencing of the *TRβ* gene demonstrating the abnormality. Although virtually all patients with RTH have such abnormalities, in a few individuals this is not the case, suggesting that there may be mutations in coactivator proteins or one of the RXR receptors, which can also present in a similar fashion.[218]

Treatment is difficult because thyroid hormone analogues designed to suppress TSH, thereby relieving the hyperthyroxinemia, may lead to worsening of the cardiovascular manifestations of the condition.[203, 219] Therapy with 3,5,3′-triiodothyroacetic acid (TRIAC) has been used in several patients.[220–222] The development of analogues of thyroid hormone with TRβ, as opposed to mixed or TRα preferential effects, may eventually prove useful in treatment.[223]

Treatment

Hypothyroidism, either primary or central, is gratifying to treat because of the ease and completeness with which it responds to thyroid hormone. Treatment is nearly always with levothyroxine, and the proper use of this medication has been reviewed extensively.[122, 224, 225] A primary advantage of levothyroxine therapy is that the peripheral deiodination mechanisms can continue to produce the amount of T_3 required under physiologic control. If one accepts the principle that replicating the natural state is the goal of hormone replacement, it is logical to provide the "prohormone" and allow the peripheral tissues to activate it by physiologically regulated mechanisms.

Pharmacologic and Physiologic Considerations

Levothyroxine has a 7-day half-life; about 80% of the hormone is absorbed relatively slowly and equilibrates rapidly in its distribution volume, therefore avoiding large postabsorptive perturbations in FT_4I levels.[226] With its long half-life, omission of a single day's tablet has no significant effect and the patient may safely take an omitted tablet the following day. In fact, the levothyroxine dosage can be calculated almost as satisfactorily on a weekly, as on a daily, basis.

According to the U.S. Pharmacopeia, the levothyroxine content of replacement tablets must be between 90% and 110% of the stated amount, although narrower restrictions are being introduced in the United States. The availability in many countries of a multiplicity of tablet strengths with content ranging from 25 to 300 μg allows precise titration of the daily levothyroxine dosage for most patients with a single tablet, improving compliance significantly.

The typical dose of levothyroxine, approximately 1.6 to 1.8 μg/kg ideal body weight per day (0.7 to 0.8 μg/pound), generally results in the prescription of between 75 and 112 μg/day for women and 125 to 200 μg/day for men. Replacement doses need not be adjusted upward in obese patients. This dosage is about 20% greater than the T_4 production rate owing to incomplete absorption of the levothyroxine. In patients with primary hypothyroidism, these amounts usually result in serum TSH concentrations that are within the normal range. Because of the 7-day half-life, approximately 6 weeks is required before there is complete equilibration of the FT_4I and the biologic effects of levothyroxine. Accordingly, assessments of the adequacy of a given dose or the effects of a change in dosage should not be made until this interval has passed.

By and large, levothyroxine products are clinically equivalent, although problems do occur.[227, 228] However, the variation permitted by the U.S. Food and Drug Administration in tablet content can result in slight variations in serum TSH in patients with primary hypothyroidism even when the same brand is used. Although the serum TSH level is an *indirect reflection* of the levothyroxine effect in patients with primary hypothyroidism, it is superior to any other readily available method of assessing the adequacy of therapy. Return of the serum TSH level to normal is therefore the goal of levothyroxine therapy in the patient with primary hypothyroidism. Some patients may require slightly higher or lower doses than generally used, owing to individual variations in absorption, and a number of conditions or associated medications may change levothyroxine requirements in patients with established hypothyroidism (see later).

In decades past, desiccated thyroid was successfully employed for the treatment of hypothyroidism and still accounts for a small fraction of the prescriptions written for thyroid replacement in the United States. Although this approach was successful, desiccated thyroid preparations contain thyroid hormone derived from animal thyroid glands that have significantly higher ratios of T_3 to T_4 than the 1:11 value in normal human thyroid gland.[229, 230] Accordingly, such preparations may lead to supraphysiologic levels of T_3 in the immediate postabsorptive period (2 to 4 hours) owing to the rapid release of T_3 from thyroglobulin, its immediate and nearly complete absorption, and the 1-day period required for T_3 to equilibrate with its 40-L volume of distribution (see Table 10–5).[231]

Mixtures of liothyronine and levothyroxine (*liotrix*) contain in a 1-grain (64-mg) equivalent tablet (Thyrolar in the United States), the amounts of T_3 (~12.5 μg) and T_4 (~50 μg) present in the most popular desiccated thyroid tablet.[232] The levothyroxine equivalency of a 1-grain desiccated thyroid tablet or its liotrix equivalent can be estimated as follows. The 12.5 μg of liothyronine (T_3) is completely absorbed from desiccated thyroid or from liotrix tablets.[231] Levothyroxine is approximately 80% absorbed,[233, 234] and about 36% of the 40 μg of levothyroxine absorbed is converted to T_3, with the molecular weight of T_3 (651) being 84% that of T_4 (777). Accordingly, a 1-grain tablet should provide about 25 μg of T_3 (12.5 + 12.1), which would be approximately equivalent to that obtained from 100 μg of levothyroxine. This equivalency ratio can be used as an initial guide in switching patients from desiccated thyroid or liotrix to levothyroxine.

As indicated earlier, the use of levothyroxine as thyroid hormone replacement is a compromise with the normal pathway of T_3 production, in which about 80% of T_3 is derived from T_4 5′-monodeiodination and approximately 20% (~6 μg) is secreted directly from the thyroid gland.[235] Studies in thyroidectomized rats, for example, show that it is not possible to normalize T_3 simultaneously in all tissues by an IV infusion of T_4.[236] However, it should be recalled from the earlier discussion of T_4 deiodination that the ratio of T_3/T_4 in the human thyroid gland is about 0.09 but is 0.17 in the rat thyroid gland.[237] Thus, about 40% of the rat's daily T_3 production is derived from the thyroid versus about 20% in humans.[67] Accordingly, the demonstration that T_4 alone cannot provide normal levels of T_3 in all tissues in the rat is of interest but is not strictly applicable to thyroid hormone replacement in humans.[236, 238] Nonetheless, the ratio of T_3/T_4 in the serum of a patient receiving levothyroxine as the only source of T_3 must be about 20% lower than is that in a normal individual.

Similarly, the quantity of levothyroxine required to normalize TSH in an athyreotic patient results in a slightly higher serum T_4 concentration than is present in normal individuals.[226] Although this may, to some extent, compensate for the lack of T_3 secretion, the fact that T_4 has an independent mechanism for TSH suppression owing to the intracellular generation of T_3 in the hypothalamic-pituitary-thyroid axis results in a portion of the feedback regulation being independent of the plasma T_3 concentration.

Does this slightly lower T_3 concentration in patients receiving levothyroxine make any difference physiologically? Probably not, although the question is difficult to answer definitively because the most readily measurable end point, TSH, cannot be used. In one study, patients who received 12.5 μg of T_3 as a substitution for 50 μg of their levothyroxine preparation scored, on average, somewhat higher on tests of mood than when they were taking levothyroxine alone.[239] The dosage of thyroid hormone used in these studies was excessive, as judged by the fact that 20% of the group had serum TSH values below normal on either regimen and the test period was only a few months, making it difficult to extrapolate to the chronic replacement setting.

On the other hand, another study showed that the FT_4I correlated as closely with the resting energy expenditure, as did TSH levels in a group of patients in whom small supplements or decrements in their ideal replacement levothyroxine dosage were made.[240] The correlation with serum T_3 was not statistically significant, suggesting that in humans, perhaps as a result of differences in the peripheral metabolism of T_4 from that in rodents, the FT_4I may be as accurate as the TSH value as an index of satisfactory thyroid hormone replacement. The practical difficulty with the design of tablets providing combinations of T_3 and T_4 is that the approximate dose of 6 μg of T_3 provided would need to be released in a sustained fashion over 24 hours, which is quite different from the rapid absorption of T_3 with a peak at 2 to 4 hours when given in its conventional form.[231] Thus, for the present, it appears that the current approach to thyroid replacement using levothyroxine, although not a perfect replication of the normal physiology, is satisfactory for most patients.

Institution of Replacement Therapy

The initial dose of levothyroxine prescribed depends on the degree of hypothyroidism and the age and general health of the patient. Patients who are young or middle-aged and otherwise healthy with no associated cardiovascular or other abnormalities and mild to moderate hypothyroidism (TSH concentrations 5 to 50 mU/L) can be given a complete replacement dose of about 1.7 μg/kg of ideal body weight. The resulting increase in serum T_4 concentration to normal requires 5 to 6 weeks, and the biologic effects of T_3 are sufficiently delayed that these patients do not experience adverse effects. At the other extreme, the older patient with heart disease, particularly angina pectoris, without reversible coronary lesions, should be given small initial doses of levothyroxine (25 or even 12.5 μg/day), and the dosage should be increased in 12.5 μg increments at 2- to 3-month intervals with careful clinical and laboratory evaluation.[241]

The goal in the patient with primary hypothyroidism is to return serum TSH concentrations to normal, reflecting normalization of that patient's thyroid hormone supply. This usually results in a mid to high-normal serum FT_4I. The serum TSH should be evaluated 6 weeks after a theoretically complete replacement dose has been instituted to allow minor adjustments to optimize the individual dose. In patients with central hypothyroidism, serum TSH is not a reliable index of adequate replacement and the serum FT_4I should be restored to a concentration in the upper half of the normal range. Such patients should also be evaluated and treated for glucocorticoid deficiency before institution of thyroid replacement (see Chapter 8).

Although the adverse effects of the rapid institution of therapy are unusual, pseudotumor cerebri has been reported in profoundly hypothyroid juveniles between ages 8 and 12 years who were given even modest initial levothyroxine replacement.[242] This complication appears 1 to 10 months after initiation of treatment and responds to acetazolamide and dexamethasone.

The interval between the initiation of treatment and the first evidence of improvement depends on the strength of dose given and the degree of the deficit. An early clinical response in moderate to severe hypothyroidism is a diuresis of 2 to 4 kg. The serum sodium (Na^+) level increases even sooner if hyponatremia was present initially. Thereafter, pulse rate and pulse pressure increase, appetite improves, and constipation may disappear. Later, psychomotor activity increases and the delay in the deep tendon reflex disappears. Hoarseness abates slowly, and changes in skin and hair do not disappear for several months. In individuals started on a complete replacement dose, the serum FT_4I level should return to normal after 6 weeks; a somewhat longer period may be necessary for serum TSH levels to return to normal, perhaps up to 3 months.

In addition to myxedema coma (see later), it is sometimes clinically appropriate to alleviate hypothyroidism rapidly. For example, patients with severe hypothyroidism withstand acute infections or other serious illnesses poorly and myxedema coma may develop as a complication. In such circumstances, rapid repletion of the peripheral hormone pool in the average adult can be accomplished by a single IV dose of 500 μg of levothyroxine. Alternatively, by virtue of its rapid onset of action, liothyronine (25 μg orally every 12 hours) can be administered if the patient can take medication by mouth. With both approaches, an initial effect is achieved within 24 hours. Parenteral therapy with levothyroxine is then continued with a dose that is 80% of the appropriate oral dose but not in excess of 1.4 μg/kg of ideal body weight. Because of the possibility that rapid increases in metabolic rate will overtax the existing pituitary-adrenocortical reserve, supplemental glucocorticoid (IV hydrocortisone 5 mg/hour) should also be given to patients with severe hypothyroidism receiving high initial doses of thyroid hormones. Finally, in view of the tendency of hypothyroid patients to retain free water, IV fluids containing only dextrose should not be given.

When replacement therapy is withdrawn for short periods (4 to 6 weeks) for purposes of evaluating therapy for thyroid cancer, rapid reinstitution of levothyroxine using a loading dose of three times the daily replacement dose for 3 days can usually be given unless there are other complicating medical illnesses.

When hypothyroidism results from administration of iodine-containing or antithyroid drugs, withdrawal of the offending agent usually relieves both the hypothyroidism and the accompanying goiter, although it is appropriate to provide interim tial diagnosis lie between that and pyogenic thyroiditis. In that context, subacute thyroiditis is also mentioned later.

Acute Infectious Thyroiditis

Although the thyroid gland is remarkably resistant to infection, congenital abnormalities of the piriform sinus, underlying autoimmune disease, or immunocompromise of the host may lead to the development of an infectious disease of the thyroid gland.[307, 308] The etiology may be any bacterium, including *Staphylococcus*, *Pneumococcus*, *Salmonella*, or *Mycobacterium tuberculosis*.[309–311] In addition, infections with certain fungi, including *Coccidioides immitis*, *Candida*, or *Aspergillus* and *Histoplasma* have been reported.[312]

The most common cause of repeated childhood pyogenic thyroiditis, particularly in the left lobe, is a consequence of an internal fistula extending from the piriform sinus to the thyroid.[313, 314] This sinus is the residual connection following the path of migration of the ultimobranchial body from the fifth pharyngeal pouch to the thyroid gland. The predominance of thyroiditis of the left lobe is explained by the fact that the right ultimobranchial body is often atrophic, whereas this is not the case for the left side. Nonetheless, a patient with a completely normal thyroid gland may develop bacterial thyroiditis. This is an extremely rare disease even as a complication of direct puncture of the thyroid gland, such as in fine-needle aspiration. In individuals with midline infections, persistence of the thyroglossal duct should be considered.

Incidence

Infectious thyroiditis is extremely rare, with no more than a few cases being seen in large tertiary care centers.

Clinical Manifestations

The clinical manifestations of infectious thyroiditis are dominated by local pain and tenderness in the affected lobe or entire gland. This is accompanied by painful swallowing and difficulty on swallowing. Because of the tendency for referral of pain to the pharynx or ear, the patient may not recognize the tenderness in the anterior neck. Depending on the virulence of the organism and the presence of septicemia, symptoms such as fever and chills may also accompany the condition.

The major differential diagnosis lies between an infectious form of thyroiditis and subacute, nonsuppurative thyroiditis. It is instructive to compare the principal features of these two diseases to arrive at an accurate diagnosis (Table 12–6). By and large, patients with acute thyroiditis caused by a bacterium are much sicker than patients with subacute thyroiditis; they have more severe and localized tenderness and are less likely to have laboratory evidence of hyperthyroidism, which is present in approximately 60% of patients with subacute thyroiditis. Ultrasonographic examination often reveals the abscess in the thyroid gland or evidence of swelling, and needle aspiration may help pinpoint the responsible organism.[310, 315] A gallium scan will be positive as a result of the diffuseness of the inflammation and, particularly in children with thyroiditis of the left lobe, a barium swallow showing a fistula connecting the piriform sinus and left lobe of the thyroid is diagnostic.[316, 317]

Occasionally, pertechnetate scanning is useful in showing normal function of one lobe of the thyroid gland, which is much less common in subacute thyroiditis (which more often affects the entire gland). Needle aspiration should be used to drain the affected lobe, although occasionally surgical drainage may be required. If a piriform sinus fistula can be demonstrated, it must be removed to prevent recurrence of the problem.

Table 12–6. Features Useful in Differentiating Acute Suppurative Thyroiditis and Subacute Thyroiditis

	Characteristic	Acute Thyroiditis	Subacute Thyroiditis
History	Preceding upper respiratory infection	88%	17%
	Fever	100%	54%
	Symptoms of thyrotoxicosis	Uncommon	47%
	Sore throat	90%	36%
Physical examination of the thyroid	Painful thyroid swelling	100%	77%
	Left side affected	85%	Not specific
	Migrating thyroid tenderness	Possible	27%
	Erythema of overlying skin	83%	Not usually
Laboratory	Elevated white blood cell count	57%	25–50%
	Elevated erythrocyte sedimentation rate (>30 mm/hr)	100 %	85%
	Abnormal thyroid hormone levels (elevated or depressed)	5–10%	60%
	Alkaline phosphatase, transaminases increased	Rare	Common
Needle aspiration	Purulent, bacteria or fungi present	~100%	0
	Lymphocytes, macrophages, some polyps, giant cells	0	~100%
	^{123}I uptake low	Uncommon	~100%
Radiologic	Abnormal thyroid scan	92%	—
	Thyroid scan or ultrasound helpful in diagnosis	75%	—
	Gallium scan positive	~100%	~100%
	Barium swallow showing fistula	Common	0
	CT scan useful	Rarely	Not indicated
Clinical course	Clinical response to glucocorticoid treatment	Transient	100%
	Incision and drainage required	85%	No
	Recurrence following operative drainage	16%	No
	Piriform sinus fistula discovered	96%	No

From DeGroot LJ, Larsen PR, Hennemann G. Acute and subacute thyroiditis. In The Thyroid and Its Diseases, 6th ed. New York, Churchill Livingstone, 1996, p 700.

Antibiotics should be administered appropriate to the offending organism. Fungal infections should be treated appropriately, especially because many of these individuals are immunocompromised. Endemic organisms should be kept in mind as a cause, since both *Echinococcus* and *Trypanosomiasis* infections of the thyroid gland have been reported.

The prognosis is excellent with preservation of thyroid function in general, although post-thyroiditis thyroid function tests should be monitored to ascertain that thyroid failure has not occurred.

Riedel's Thyroiditis

Riedel's chronic sclerosing thyroiditis is rare and dramatic and occurs chiefly in middle-aged women.[318, 319] The etiologic mechanism is uncertain, although some cases are considered to be an advanced state of Hashimoto's disease.[320, 321] This condition is characterized by fibrosis of the thyroid gland and adjacent structures and may be associated with fibrosis elsewhere, especially in the retroperitoneal area.[318] The presence of eosinophils has been demonstrated histologically, suggesting a unique autoimmune response to fibrous tissue.[322]

Symptoms develop insidiously and are related chiefly to compression of adjacent structures, including the trachea, esophagus, and recurrent laryngeal nerves. Constitutional evidence of inflammation is uncommon. The thyroid gland is moderately enlarged, stony hard, and usually asymmetrical. The consistency of the gland and the invasion of adjacent structures suggest carcinoma, but there is no enlargement of regional lymph nodes. Temperature, pulse, and leukocyte count are normal. Severe hypothyroidism is unusual but does occur, as does loss of parathyroid function. The RAIU may be normal or low. Circulating thyroid autoantibodies are less common and are found in lower titers than in Hashimoto's disease.

Surgery may be required to preserve tracheal and esophageal function. If extensive involvement of perithyroid tissues is present, resection of the isthmus may relieve some symptoms. Treatment with thyroid hormone relieves the hypothyroidism but has no effect on the primary process, which may progress inexorably. Immunosuppressive treatment and even chemotherapy has been tried in individual cases.

Miscellaneous Causes

Only a few causes of generalized inflammation of the thyroid gland have been reported. These include inflammation arising after ^{131}I treatment of individuals for Graves' disease, a residual thyroid lobe in a patient with thyroid cancer of the contralateral lobe, and thyroiditis arising from external-beam therapy for conditions such as Hodgkin's or non-Hodgkin's lymphoma, breast carcinoma, or other lesions of the oropharynx. In general, only radioiodine-induced thyroiditis is associated with pain and glucocorticoid treatment may be useful in symptomatic therapy.

References

1. Vanderpump MPJ, Tunbridge WMG, French JM, et al. The incidence of thyroid disorders in the community: a twenty-year follow-up of the Whickham survey. Clin Endocrinol (Oxf) 1995; 43:55–68.
2. Danese MD, Powe NR, Sawin CT, et al. Screening for mild thyroid failure at the periodic health examination: a decision and cost-effectiveness analysis. JAMA 1996; 276:285–292.
3. Canaris GJ, Manowitz NR, Mayor G, et al. The Colorado thyroid disease prevalence study. Arch Intern Med 2000; 160:526–534.
4. LaFranchi S. Congenital hypothyroidism: etiologies, diagnosis, and management. Thyroid 1999; 9:735–740.
5. Smith TJ, Bahn RS, Gorman CA. Connective tissue, glycosaminoglycans, and diseases of the thyroid. Endocr Rev 1989; 10:366–391.
6. Smith TJ, Horwitz AL, Refetoff S. The effect of thyroid hormone on glycosaminoglycan accumulation in human skin fibroblasts. Endocrinology 1981; 108:2397–2399.
7. Klein I, Ojamaa K. Thyroid hormone and the cardiovascular system. N Engl J Med 2001; 344:501–509.
8. Ladenson PW, Sherman SI, Baughman KL, et al. Reversible alterations in myocardial gene expression in a young man with dilated cardiomyopathy and hypothyroidism. Proc Natl Acad Sci USA 1992; 89:5251–5255.
9. Hardisty CA, Naik DR, Munro DS. Pericardial effusion in hypothyroidism. Clin Endocrinol (Oxf) 1980; 13:349–354.
10. Keating FR, Parkin TW, Selby JB, et al. Treatment of heart disease associated with myxedema. Prog Cardiovasc Dis 1961; 3:364–381.
11. Levine HD. Compromise therapy in the patient with angina pectoris and hypothyroidism: a clinical assessment. Am J Med 1980; 69:411–418.
12. Hak AE, Pols HA, Visser TJ, et al. Subclinical hypothyroidism is an independent risk factor for atherosclerosis and myocardial infarction in elderly women: the Rotterdam Study. Ann Intern Med 2000; 132:270–278.
13. Polikar R, Burger AG, Scherrer U, et al. The thyroid and the heart. Circulation 1993; 87:1435–1441.
14. Sap J, de Magistris L, Stunnenberg H, et al. A major thyroid hormone response element in the third intron of the rat growth hormone gene. EMBO J 1990; 9:887–896.
15. Hussein WI, Green R, Jacobsen DW, et al. Normalization of hyperhomocysteinemia with L-thyroxine in hypothyroidism. Ann Intern Med 1999; 131:348–51.
16. Hickman PE, Silvester W, McLellan GH, et al. Cardiac enzyme changes in myxedema coma. Clin Chem 1987; 33:622.
17. Crowley WF Jr, Ridgeway EC, Bough EW, et al. Noninvasive evaluation of cardiac function in hypothyroidism. N Engl J Med 1977; 296:1–6.
18. Zwillich CW, Pierson DJ, Hofeldt FD, et al. Ventilatory control in myxedema and hypothyroidism. N Engl J Med 1975; 292:662–665.
19. Orr WC, Males JL, Imes NK. Myxedema and obstructive sleep apnea. Am J Med 1981; 70:1061–1066.
20. Amino N, Kuro R, Yabu Y, et al. Elevated levels of circulating carcinoembryonic antigen in hypothyroidism. J Clin Endocrinol Metab 1981; 52:457–462.
21. Rosman NP. Neurological and muscular aspects of thyroid dysfunction in childhood. Pediatr Clin North Am 1976; 23:575–594.
22. Porterfield SP, Hendrich CE. The role of thyroid hormones in prenatal and neonatal neurological development: current perspectives. Endocr Rev 1993; 14:94–106.
23. Hall RCW. Psychiatric effects of thyroid hormone disturbance. Psychosomatics 1983; 24:7.
24. Esposito S, Prange AJ Jr, Golden RN. The thyroid axis and mood disorders: overview and future prospects. Psychopharmacol Bull 1997; 33:205–217.
25. Bland JH, Frymoyer JW. Rheumatic syndromes of myxedema. N Engl J Med 1970; 282:1171–1174.
26. Frymoyer JW, Bland JH. Carpal tunnel syndrome in patients with myxedematous arthropathy. J Bone Joint Surg Am 1973; 55A:78–82.
27. Sanders V. Neurologic manifestations of myxedema. N Engl J Med 1962; 266:547–552, 599–603.
28. Khaleeli AA, Griffith DG, Edwards RHT. The clinical presentation of hypothyroid myopathy. Clin Endocrinol (Oxf) 1983; 19:365–376.
29. Duyff RF, Van den Bosch J, Laman DM, et al. Neuromuscular findings in thyroid dysfunction: a prospective clinical and electrodiagnostic study. J Neurol Neurosurg Psychiatry 2000; 68:750–755.
30. Balkman C, Ojamaa K, Klein I. Time course of the in vivo effects of thyroid hormone on cardiac gene expression. Endocrinology 1992; 130:2001–2006.
31. Chernausek SD, Turner R. Attenuation of spontaneous nocturnal growth hormone secretion in children with hypothyroidism and its correlation with plasma insulin-like growth factor I concentrations. J Pediatr 1989; 114:968–972.

32. Valcavi R, Jordon V, Kieguez C, et al. Growth hormone responses to GRF 1–29 in patients with primary hypothyroidism before and during replacement therapy with thyroxine. Clin Endocrinol (Oxf) 1986; 24:693–696.
33. Cavaliere H, Knobel M, Medeiros-Neto G. Effect of thyroid hormone therapy on plasma insulin-like growth factor I levels in normal subjects, hypothyroid patients, and endemic cretins. Hormone Res 1987; 25:132–139.
34. Greenspan SL, Greenspan FS. The effect of thyroid hormone on skeletal integrity. Ann Intern Med 1999; 130:750–758.
35. Eriksen EF, Mosekilde L, Melsen F. Trabecular bone remodeling and bone balance in hyperthyroidism. Bone 1985; 6:421–428.
36. Eriksen EF. Normal and pathological remodeling of human trabecular bone: three-dimensional reconstruction of the remodeling sequence in normals and in metabolic bone disease. Endocr Rev 1986; 7:379–408.
37. Iwasaki Y, Oiso Y, Yamauchi K, et al. Osmoregulation of plasma vasopressin in myxedema. J Clin Endocrinol Metab 1990; 70: 534–539.
38. Rogers JS, Shane SR, Jencks FS. Factor VIII activity and thyroid function. Ann Intern Med 1982; 97:713.
39. Dalton RG, Dewar MS, Savidge GF, et al. Hypothyroidism as a cause of acquired von Willebrand's disease. Lancet 1987; 1:1007–1009.
40. Tachman ML, Guthrie GP Jr. Hypothyroidism: diversity of presentation. Endocr Rev 1984; 5:456–465.
41. Edson JR, Fecher DR, Doe RP. Low platelet adhesiveness and other hemostatic abnormalities in hypothyroidism. Ann Intern Med 1975; 82:342.
42. Lecky BRF, Williams TDM, Lightman SL, et al. Myxoedema presenting with chiasmal compression: resolution after thyroxine replacement. Lancet 1987; 1:1347–1350.
43. Onishi T, Miyai K, Aono T, et al. Primary hypothyroidism and galactorrhea. Am J Med 1977; 63:373–378.
44. Bigos ST, Ridgway EC, Kourides IA, et al. Spectrum of pituitary alterations with mild and severe thyroid impairment. J Clin Endocrinol Metab 1978; 46:317.
45. Kamilaris TC, DeBold CR, Pavlou SN, et al. Effect of altered thyroid hormone levels on hypothalamic-pituitary-adrenal function. J Clin Endocrinol Metab 1987; 65:994–999.
46. Koutras DA. Disturbances of menstruation in thyroid disease. Ann N Y Acad Sci 1997; 816:280–284.
47. Allan WC, Haddow JE, Palomaki GE, et al. Maternal thyroid deficiency and pregnancy complications: implications for population screening. J Med Screen 2000; 7:127–130.
48. Leung AS, Millar LK, Koonings PP, et al. Perinatal outcome in hypothyroid pregnancies. Obstet Gynecol 1993; 81:349–353.
49. Brenta G, Schnitman M, Gurfinkiel M, et al. Variations of sex hormone-binding globulin in thyroid dysfunction. Thyroid 1999; 9:273–277.
50. Levine MA, Feldman AM, Robishaw JD, et al. Influence of thyroid hormone status on expression of genes encoding G protein subunits in the rat heart. J Biol Chem 1990; 265:3553–3560.
51. Michel-Reher MB, Gross G, Jasper JR, et al. Tissue- and subunit-specific regulation of G-protein expression by hypo- and hyperthyroidism. Biochem Pharmacol 1993; 45:1417–1423.
52. Coulombe P, Dussault JH, Walker P. Catecholamine metabolism in thyroid disease: II. Norepinephrine secretion rate in hyperthyroidism and hypothyroidism. J Clin Endocrinol Metab 1977; 44: 1185–1189.
53. Bramnert M, Hallengren B, Lecerof H, et al. Decreased blood pressure response to infused noradrenaline in normotensive as compared to hypertensive patients with primary hypothyroidism. Clin Endocrinol (Oxf) 1994; 40:317–321.
54. Manhem P, Bramnert M, Hallengren B, et al. Increased arterial and venous plasma noradrenaline levels in patients with primary hypothyroidism during hypothyroid as compared to euthyroid state. J Endocrinol Invest 1992; 15:763–765.
55. Harris PE, Walker M, Clark F, et al. Forearm muscle metabolism in primary hypothyroidism. Eur J Clin Invest 1993; 23:585–588.
56. Clausen N, Lins PE, Adamson U, et al. Counterregulation of insulin-induced hypoglycaemia in primary hypothyroidism. Acta Endocrinol (Copenh) 1986; 111:516–521.
57. Dullaart RPF, Hoogenberg K, Groener JEM, et al. The activity of cholesteryl ester transfer protein is decreased in hypothyroidism: a possible contribution to alterations in high-density lipoproteins. Eur J Clin Invest 1990; 20:581–587.
58. Danese MD, Ladenson PW, Meinert CL, et al. Clinical review 115: effect of thyroxine therapy on serum lipoproteins in patients with mild thyroid failure—a quantitative review of the literature. J Clin Endocrinol Metab 2000; 85:2993–3001.
59. Pearson G, Robinson F, Beers Gibson T, et al. Mitogen-activated protein (map) kinase pathways: regulation and physiological functions. Endocr Rev 2001; 22:153–183.
60. Scarabottolo L, Trezzi E, Roma P, et al. Experimental hypothyroidism modulates the expression of the low-density lipoprotein receptor by the liver. Atherosclerosis 1986; 59:329–333.
61. Franklyn JA, Daykin J, Betteridge J, et al. Thyroxine replacement therapy and circulating lipid concentrations. Clin Endocrinol (Oxf) 1993; 38:453–459.
62. O'Brien T, Katz K, Hodge D, et al. The effect of the treatment of hypothyroidism and hyperthyroidism on plasma lipids and apolipoproteins AI, AII, and E. Clin Endocrinol (Oxf) 1997; 46:17–20.
63. Eikelboom JW, Lonn E, Genest J, et al. Homocyst(e)ine and cardiovascular disease: a critical review of the epidemiologic evidence. Ann Intern Med 1999; 131:363–375.
64. Zulewski H, Müller B, Exer P, et al. Estimation of tissue hypothyroidism by a new clinical score: evaluation of patients with various grades of hypothyroidism and controls. J Clin Endocrinol Metab 1997; 82:771–776.
65. LaFranchi SH, Murphey WH, Foley TP Jr, et al. Neonatal hypothyroidism detected by the Northwest Regional Screening Program. Pediatrics 1979; 63:180–191.
66. Lum SM, Nicoloff JT, Spencer CA, et al. Peripheral tissue mechanism for maintenance of serum triiodothyronine values in a thyroxine-deficient state in man. J Clin Invest 1984; 73:570–575.
67. Bianco AC, Slavatore D, Gereben B, et al. Biochemistry, cellular and molecular biology, and physiological roles of the iodothyronine selenodeiodinases. Endocr Rev 2001; 23:38–39.
68. Gesundheit N, Petrick PA, Nissim M, et al. Thyrotropin-secreting pituitary adenomas: clinical and biochemical heterogeneity. Ann Intern Med 1989; 11:827–835.
69. Mariotti S, Franceschi C, Cossarizza A, et al. The aging thyroid. Endocr Rev 1995; 16:686–715.
70. Doniach D. Hashimoto's thyroiditis and primary myxedema viewed as separate entities. Eur J Clin Invest 1981; 11:245–246.
71. Konishi J, Iida Y, Kasagi K, et al. Primary myxedema with thyrotrophin-binding inhibitor immunoglobulins. Ann Intern Med 1985; 103:26–31.
72. Arikawa K, Ichikawa Y, Yoshida T, et al. Blocking type antithyrotropin receptor antibody in patients with nongoitrous hypothyroidism: its incidence and characteristics of action. J Clin Endocrinol Metab 1985; 60:953–959.
73. Roman SH, Greenberg D, Rubinstein P, et al. Genetics of autoimmune thyroid disease: lack of evidence for linkage to HLA within families. J Clin Endocrinol Metab 1992; 74:496–503.
74. Tamai H, Uno H, Hirota Y, et al. Immunogenetics of Hashimoto's and Graves' diseases. J Clin Endocrinol Metab 1985; 60: 62–66.
75. Sellers EA, You SS. Role of the thyroid in metabolic responses to a cold environment. Am J Physiol 1950; 163:81–91.
76. Wood LC, Ingbar SH. Hypothyroidism as a late sequela in patients with Graves' disease treated with antithyroid agents. J Clin Invest 1979; 64:1429–1436.
77. Bell PM, Sinnamon DG, Smyth PPA, et al. Hyperthyroidism following primary hypothyroidism in association with polyendocrine autoimmunity. Acta Endocrinol (Copenh) 1996; 108:491–497.
78. Weetman AP. Thyroid-associated ophthalmopathy. Autoimmunity 1992; 12:215–222.
79. DeGroot LJ, Reed Larsen P, Refetoff S, et al (eds). The Thyroid and Its Diseases. New York, John Wiley, 1984, pp 1–907.
80. Giordano C, Stassi G, De Maria R, et al. Potential involvement of Fas and its ligand in the pathogenesis of Hashimoto's thyroiditis. Science 1997; 275:960–963.
81. Stassi G, Di Liberto D, Todaro M, et al. Control of target cell survival in thyroid autoimmunity by T-helper cytokines via regulation of apoptotic proteins. Nat Immunol 2000; 1:483–488.
82. Phelps E, Wu P, Bretz J, Baker JR Jr. Thyroid cell apoptosis: a new understanding of thyroid autoimmunity. Endocrinol Metab Clin North Am 2000; 29:375–388.

83. Doniach D, Botttazo GF, Russell RCG. Goitrous autoimmune thyroiditis. Clin Endocrinol (Oxf) 1979; 8:63–80.
84. Martin A, Davies TF. T cells and human autoimmune thyroid disease: emerging data show lack of need to invoke suppressor T-cell problems. Thyroid 1992; 2:247–261.
85. Atkins MB, Mier JW, Parkinson DR, et al. Hypothyroidism after treatment with interleukin-2 and lymphokine-activated killer cells. N Engl J Med 1988; 318:1558–1563.
86. Klingenspor M, Ivemeyer M, Wiesinger H, et al. Biogenesis of thermogenic mitochondria in brown adipose tissue of Djungarian hamsters during cold adaptation. Biochem J 1996; 316:607–613.
87. Stenszky V, Kozma L, Balazs C, et al. The genetics of Graves' disease: HLA and disease susceptibility. J Clin Endocrinol Metab 1985; 61:735–740.
88. Shi Y, Zou M, Robb D, et al. Typing for major histocompatability complex class II antigens in thyroid tissue blocks: association of Hashimoto's thyroiditis with HLA-DQA0301 and DQB0201 alleles. J Clin Endocrinol Metab 1992; 75:943–946.
89. Nicholson LB, Wong FS, Ewins DL, et al. Susceptibility to autoimmune thyroiditis in Down's syndrome is associated with the major histocompatibility class II DQA 0301 allele. Clin Endocrinol (Oxf) 1994; 41:381–383.
90. Bottazzo GF, Pujol Borrell R, Hanafusa T, et al. Role of aberrant HLA-DR expression and antigen presentation in induction of endocrine autoimmunity. Lancet 1983; 2:1115–1119.
91. Tomer Y, Greenberg DA, Barbesino G, et al. CTLA-4 and not CD28 is a susceptibility gene for thyroid autoantibody production. J Clin Endocrinol Metab 2001; 86:1687–1693.
92. Nistico L, Buzzetti R, Pritchard LE, et al. The CTLA-4 gene region of chromosome 2q33 is linked to, and associated with, type 1 diabetes. Belgian Diabetes Registry. Hum Mol Genet 1996; 5:1075–1080.
93. Amino N, Tada H, Hidaka Y, et al. Therapeutic controversy: screening for postpartum thyroiditis. J Clin Endocrinol Metab 1999; 84:1813–1821.
94. Lambert NC, Evans PC, Hashizumi TL, et al. Cutting edge: persistent fetal microchimerism in T lymphocytes is associated with HLA-DQA1*0501: implications in autoimmunity. J Immunol 2000; 164:5545–5548.
95. Stagnaro-Green A. Recognizing, understanding, and treating postpartum thyroiditis. Endocrinol Metab Clin North Am 2000; 29:417–430, ix.
96. Hall R, Lazarus JH. Changing iodine intake and the effect on thyroid disease. Br Med J 1987; 294:721–722.
97. Sundick RS, Herdegen DM, Brown TR, et al. The incorporation of dietary iodine into thyroglobulin increases its immunogenicity. Endocrinology 1987; 120:2078–2084.
98. Allen EM, Appel MC, Braverman LE. Iodine-induced thyroiditis and hypothyroidism in the hemithyroidectomized BB/W rat. Endocrinology 1987; 121:481–485.
99. Champion BR, Page KR, Parish N, et al. Identification of a thyroxine-containing self-epitope of thyroglobulin which triggers thyroid autoreactive T cells. J Exp Med 1991; 174:363–370.
100. Vialettes B, Guillerand MA, Viens P, et al. Incidence rate and risk factors for thyroid dysfunction during recombinant interleukin-2 therapy in advanced malignancies. Acta Endocrinol (Copenh) 1993; 129:31–38.
101. Preziati D, La Rosa L, Covini G, et al. Autoimmunity and thyroid function in patients with chronic active hepatitis treated with recombinant interferon alpha-2a. Eur J Endocrinol 1995; 132: 587–593.
102. Marazuela M, Garcia-Buey L, Gonzalez-Fernandez B, et al. Thyroid autoimmune disorders in patients with chronic hepatitis C before and during interferon-alpha therapy. Clin Endocrinol (Oxf) 1996; 44:635–642.
103. Custro N, Montalto G, Scafidi V, et al. Prospective study on thyroid autoimmunity and dysfunction related to chronic hepatitis C and interferon therapy. J Endocrinol Invest 1997; 20:374–380.
104. Pacini F, Vorontsova T, Molinaro E, et al. Thyroid consequences of the Chernobyl nuclear accident. Acta Paediatr Suppl 1999; 88: 23–27.
105. Vermiglio F, Castagna MG, Volnova E, et al. Post-Chernobyl increased prevalence of humoral thyroid autoimmunity in children and adolescents from a moderately iodine-deficient area in Russia. Thyroid 1999; 9:781–786.
106. Bonar BD, McColgan B, Smith DF, et al. Hypothyroidism and aging: the Rosses' survey. Thyroid 2000; 10:821–827.
107. Czarnocka B, Szabolcs I, Pastuszko D, et al. In old age the majority of thyroid peroxidase autoantibodies are directed to a single TPO domain irrespective of thyroid function and iodine intake. Clin Endocrinol (Oxf) 1998; 48:803–808.
108. Potocka-Plazak K, Pituch-Noworolska A, Kocemba J. Prevalence of autoantibodies in the very elderly: association with symptoms of ischemic heart disease. Aging (Milano) 1995; 7:218–220.
109. Tomer Y, Davies TF. Infection, thyroid disease, and autoimmunity. Endocr Rev 1993; 14:107–120.
110. Weetman AP, Smallridge RC, Nutman TB, et al. Persistent thyroid autoimmunity after subacute thyroiditis. J Clin Lab Immunol 1987; 23:1–6.
111. Crile JG. Struma lymphomatosa and carcinoma of the thyroid. Surg Gynecol Obstet 1978; 147:350–352.
112. Baker J, Fosso CK. Immunological aspects of cancers arising from thyroid follicular cells. Endocr Rev 1993; 14:729–746.
113. Amino N, Kuro R, Tanizawa O, et al. Changes of serum antithyroid antibodies during and after pregnancy in autoimmune thyroid diseases. Clin Exp Immunol 1978; 31:30–37.
114. Jansson R, Bernander S, Karlsson A, et al. Autoimmune thyroid dysfunction in the postpartum period. J Clin Endocrinol Metab 1984; 58:681–687.
115. Freeman R, Rosen H, Thysen B. Incidence of thyroid dysfunction in an unselected postpartum population. Arch Intern Med 1986; 146:1361–1364.
116. Tachi J, Amino N, Tamaki H, et al. Long-term follow-up and HLA association in patients with postpartum hypothyroidism. J Clin Endocrinol Metab 1986; 66:480–484.
117. Amino N, Mori H, Iwatani Y, et al. High prevalence of transient post-partum thyrotoxicosis and hypothyroidism. N Engl J Med 1982; 306:849–852.
118. Boyages SC. Clinical review 49: iodine deficiency disorders. J Clin Endocrinol Metab 1993; 77:587–591.
119. Boyages SC, Halpern JP. Endemic cretinism: toward a unifying hypothesis. Thyroid 1993; 3:59–69.
120. Porter BA, Refetoff S, Rosenfeld RL, et al. Abnormal thyroxine metabolism in hyposomatotrophic dwarfism and inhibition of responsiveness to TRH during GH therapy. Pediatrics 1975; 51: 668.
121. Meyer JD, Gaitan E, Merino H, et al. Geologic implications in the distribution of endemic goiter in Colombia, South America. Int J Epidemiol 1978; 7:25–30.
122. Mandel SJ, Brent GA, Larsen PR. Levothyroxine therapy in patients with thyroid disease. Ann Intern Med 1993; 119:492–502.
123. Glinoer D. Maternal and fetal impact of chronic iodine deficiency. Clin Obstet Gynecol 1997; 40:102–116.
124. Hollowell JG, Staehling NW, Hannon WH, et al. Iodine nutrition in the United States—trends and public health implications: iodine excretion data from National Health and Nutrition Examination Surveys I and III (1971–1974 and 1988–1994). J Clin Endocrinol Metab 1998; 83:3401–3408.
125. Wolff J. Physiology and pharmacology of iodized oil in goiter prophylaxis. Medicine (Baltimore) 2001; 80:20–36.
126. Delange F. The disorders induced by iodine deficiency. Thyroid 1994; 4:107–128.
127. Halpern JP, Boyages SC, Maberly GF. The neurology of endemic cretinism. A study of two endemias. Brain 1991; 114:825–841.
128. Ma T, Lian ZC, Qi SP, et al. Magnetic resonance imaging of brain and the neuromotor disorder in endemic cretinism. Ann Neurol 1993; 34:91–94.
129. Wolff J. Iodide goiter and the pharmacologic effects of excess iodide. Am J Med 1969; 47:101–124.
130. Silva JE. Effects of iodine and iodine-containing compounds on thyroid function. Med Clin North Am 1985; 69:881–898.
131. Namba H, Yamashita S, Kimura H, et al. Evidence of thyroid volume increase in normal subjects receiving excess iodide. J Clin Endocrinol Metab 1993; 76:605–608.
132. Surks MI, Sievert R. Drugs and thyroid function. N Engl J Med 1995; 333:1688–1694.
133. Martino E, Safran M, Aghini-Lombardi F, et al. Environmental iodine intake and thyroid dysfunction during chronic amiodarone therapy. Ann Intern Med 1984; 101:28–34.
134. Martino E, Bartalena L, Bogazzi F, et al. The effects of amiodarone on the thyroid. Endocr Rev 2001; 22:240–254.
135. Bartalena L, Bogazzi F, Braverman LE, et al. Effects of amioda-

content of desiccated thyroid tablets. Metabolism 1977; 26:1213–1218.
230. Rees-Jones RW, Rolla AR, Larsen PR. Hormonal content of thyroid replacement preparations. JAMA 1980; 243:549–550.
231. LeBoff MS, Kaplan MM, Silva JE, et al. Bioavailability of thyroid hormones from oral replacement preparations. Metabolism 1982; 31:900–905.
232. Blumberg KR, Mayer WJ, Parikh DK, et al. Liothyronine and levothyroxine in Armour thyroid. J Pharm Sci 1993; 76:346–347.
233. Hays MT. Localization of human thyroxine absorption. Thyroid 1991; 3:241–248.
234. Hays MT. Thyroid hormone and the gut. Endocrine Res 1988; 14:203–224.
235. Pilo A, Iervasi G, Vitek F, et al. Thyroidal and peripheral production of 3,5,3′-triiodothyronine in humans by multicompartmental analysis. Am J Physiol 1990; 258:E715–E726.
236. Escobar-Morreale HF, Óbregon MJ, Escobar del Ray F, et al. Replacement therapy for hypothyroidism with thyroxine alone does not ensure euthyroidism in all tissues, as studied in thyroidectomized rats. J Clin Invest 1995; 96:2828–2838.
237. Riesco G, Taurog A, Larsen R, et al. Acute and chronic responses to iodine deficiency in rats. Endocrinology 1977; 100: 303–313.
238. Escobar-Morreale HF, Rey F, Obregon MJ, et al. Only the combined treatment with thyroxine and triiodothyronine ensures euthyroidism in all tissues of the thyroidectomized rat. Endocrinology 1996; 137:2490–2502.
239. Bunevicius R, Kazanavicius G, Zalinkevicius R, et al. Effects of thyroxine as compared with thyroxine plus triiodothyronine in patients with hypothyroidism. N Engl J Med 1999; 340:424–429.
240. Toru-Delbauffe D, Baghdassarian-Chalaye D, Gavaret JM, et al. Effects of transforming growth factor $beta_1$ on astroglial cells in culture. J Neurochem 1990; 54:1056–1061.
241. Carr K, Mcleod DT, Parry G, et al. Fine adjustment of thyroxine replacement dosage: comparison of the thyrotrophin releasing hormone tests using a sensitive thyrotrophin assay with measurement of free thyroid hormones and clinical assessment. Clin Endocrinol (Oxf) 1988; 28:325–333.
242. Van Dop C, Conte FA, Koch TK, et al. Pseudotumor cerebri associated with initiation of levothyroxine therapy for juvenile hypothyroidism. N Engl J Med 1983; 308:1076–1080.
243. Burrow GN, Fisher DA, Larsen PR. Mechanisms of disease: maternal and fetal thyroid function. N Engl J Med 1994; 331: 1072–1078.
244. Sato T, Suzuki Y, Taketani T, et al. Age-related change in pituitary threshold for TSH release during thyroxine replacement therapy for cretinism. J Clin Endocrinol Metab 1977; 44:553–559.
245. Fisher DA, Schoen EJ, La Franchi S, et al. The hypothalamic-pituitary-thyroid negative feedback control axis in children with treated congenital hypothyroidism. J Clin Endocrinol Metab 2000; 85:2722–2727.
246. Rosenbaum RL, Barzel US. Levothyroxine replacement dose for primary hypothyroidism decreases with age. Ann Intern Med 1982; 96:53–55.
247. Arafah BM. Decreased levothyroxine requirement in women with hypothyroidism during androgen therapy for breast cancer. Ann Intern Med 1994; 121:247–251.
248. Mandel SJ, Larsen PR, Seely EW, et al. Increased need for thyroxine during pregnancy in women with primary hypothyroidism N Engl J Med 1990; 323:91–96.
249. Kaplan MM. Monitoring thyroxine treatment during pregnancy. Thyroid 1992; 2:147–152.
250. Marqusee E, Braverman LE, Lawrence JE, et al. The effect of droloxifene and estrogen on thyroid function in postmenopausal women. J Clin Endocrinol Metab 2000; 85:4407–4410.
251. Koopdonk-Kool JM, deVijlder JJM, Veenboer GJM, et al. Type II and type III deiodinase activity in human placenta as a function of gestational age. J Clin Endocrinol Metab 1996; 81:2154–2158.
252. Galton VA, Martinez E, Hernandez A, et al. Pregnant rat uterus expresses high levels of the type 3 iodothyronine deiodinase. J Clin Invest 1999; 103:979–987.
253. Vulsma T, Gons MH, DeVijlder JMM. Maternal fetal transfer of thyroxine in congenital hypothyroidism due to a total organification defect of thyroid dysgenesis. N Engl J Med 1989; 321:13–16.
254. Haddow JE, Palomaki GE, Allan WC, et al. Maternal thyroid deficiency during pregnancy and subsequent neuropsychological development of the child. N Engl J Med 1999; 341:549–555.
255. Havrankova J, Lahaie R. Levothyroxine binding by sucralfate. Ann Intern Med 1992; 117:445–446.
256. Schneyer CR. Calcium carbonate and reduction of levothyroxine efficacy. JAMA 1998; 279:750.
257. Campbell NRC, Hasinoff BB, Stalts H, et al. Ferrous sulfate reduces thyroxine efficacy in patients with hypothyroidism. Ann Intern Med 1992; 117:1010–1013.
258. Demke DM. Drug interaction between thyroxine and lovastatin. N Engl J Med 1989; 321:1341–1342.
259. Harmon SM, Seifert CF. Levothyroxine-cholestyramine interaction reemphasized. Ann Intern Med 1991; 115:658–659.
260. McLean M, Kirkwood I, Epstein M, et al. Cation-exchange resin and inhibition of intestinal absorption of thyroxine. Lancet 1993; 341:1286.
261. Isley WL. Effect of rifampin therapy on thyroid function tests in a hypothyroid patient on replacement L-thyroxine. Ann Intern Med 1987; 107:517–518.
262. DeLuca F, Arrigo T, Pandullo E, et al. Changes in thyroid function tests induced by 2-month carbamazepine treatment in L-thyroxine–substituted hypothyroid children. Eur J Pediatr 1986; 145:77–79.
263. Faber J, Lumholtz IB, Kirkegaard C, et al. The effects of phenytoin on the extrathyroidal turnover of thyroxine, 3,5,3′-triiodothyronine, 3,3′,5′-triiodothyronine, and 3′,5′-diiodothyronine in man. J Clin Endocrinol Metab 1985; 61:1093–1099.
264. McCowen KC, Garber JR, Spark R. Elevated serum thyrotropin in thyroxine-treated patients with hypothyroidism given sertraline. N Engl J Med 1997; 337:1010–1011.
265. Arafah BM. Increased need for thyroxine in women with hypothyroidism during estrogen therapy. N Engl J Med 2001; 344: 1743–1749.
266. Figge J, Dluhy RG. Amiodarone-induced elevation of thyroid stimulating hormone in patients receiving levothyroxine for primary hypothyroidism. Ann Intern Med 1990; 113:553–555.
267. Jochum F, Terwolbeck K, Meinhold H, et al. Effects of a low selenium state in patients with phenylketonuria. Acta Paediatr 1997; 86:775–777.
268. Lombeck I, Jochum F, Terwolbeck K. Selenium status in infants and children with phenylketonuria and in maternal phenylketonuria. Eur J Pediatr 1996; 155:S140–S144.
269. Kauf E, Dawczynski H, Jahreis G, et al. Sodium selenite therapy and thyroid-hormone status in cystic fibrosis and congenital hypothyroidism. Biol Trace Elem Res 1994; 40:247–253.
270. Ross DS. Hyperthyroidism, thyroid hormone therapy, and bone. Thyroid 1994; 4:319–326.
271. Marcocci C, Golia F, Bruno-Bosoro G, et al. Carefully monitored levothyroxine suppressive therapy is not associated with bone loss in premenopausal women. J Clin Endocrinol Metab 1994; 78:818–823.
272. Biondi B, Fazio S, Carella C, et al. Control of adrenergic overactivity by β-blockade improves the quality of life in patients receiving long-term suppressive therapy with levothyroxine. J Clin Endocrinol Metab 1994; 78:1028–1033.
273. Biondi B, Palmieri E, Fazio S, et al. Endogenous subclinical hyperthyroidism affects quality of life and cardiac morphology and function in young and middle-aged patients. J Clin Endocrinol Metab 2000; 85:4701–4705.
274. Kaplan MM, Swartz SL, Larsen PR. Partial peripheral resistance to thyroid hormone. Am J Med 1981; 70:1115–1121.
275. Weetman AP. Hypothyroidism: screening and subclinical disease. BMJ 1997; 314:1175–1178.
276. Cooper DS, Halpern R, Wood LC, et al. L-Thyroxine therapy in subclinical hypothyroidism: a double-blind, placebo-controlled trial. Ann Intern Med 1984; 101:18–24.
277. Nystrom E, Caidahl K, Fager G, et al. A double-blind cross-over 12-month study of L-thyroxine treatment of women with "subclinical" hypothyroidism. Clin Endocrinol (Oxf) 1988; 29:63–76.
278. Forfar JC, Wathen CG, Todd WTA, et al. Left ventricular performance in subclinical hypothyroidism. Q J Med 1985; 224:857–865.
279. Biondi B, Fazio S, Palmieri EA, et al. Left ventricular diastolic dysfunction in patients with subclinical hypothyroidism. J Clin Endocrinol Metab 1999; 84:2064–2067.

280. Ayala AR, Danese MD, Ladenson PW. When to treat mild hypothyroidism. Endocrinol Metab Clin North Am 2000; 29:399–415.
281. Sherman SI, Ladenson PW. Complications of surgery in hypothyroid patients. Am J Med 1991; 90:367–370.
282. Weinberg AD, Brennan MD, Gorman CA, et al. Outcome of anesthesia and surgery in hypothyroid patients. Arch Intern Med 1983; 143:893–897.
283. Ladenson PW, Levin AA, Ridgway EC, et al. Complications of surgery in hypothyroid patients. Am J Med 1984; 77:261–266.
284. Hay ID, Duick DX, Vlietstra RE, et al. Thyroxine therapy in hypothyroid patients undergoing coronary revascularization: a retrospective analysis. Ann Intern Med 1981; 95:456–457.
285. Sherman SI, Ladenson PW. Percutaneous transluminal coronary angioplasty in hypothyroidism. Am J Med 1991; 90:367–370.
286. Klemperer JD, Klein I, Gomez M, et al. Thyroid hormone treatment after coronary artery bypass surgery. N Engl J Med 1995; 333:1522–1527.
287. Rossant J, Moens CB, Nagy A. Genome manipulation in embryonic stem cells. Philos Trans R Soc Lond Biol 1993; 339:207–215.
288. Hamilton MA, Stevenson LW, Fonarow GC, et al. Safety and hemodynamic effects of intravenous triiodothyronine in advanced congestive heart failure. Am J Cardiol 1998; 81:443–447.
289. Moruzzi P, Doria E, Agostoni PG. Medium-term effectiveness of L-thyroxine treatment in idiopathic dilated cardiomyopathy. Am J Med 1996; 101:461–467.
290. Klemperer JD, Klein IL, Ojamaa K, et al. Triiodothyronine therapy lowers the incidence of atrial fibrillation after cardiac operations. Ann Thorac Surg 1996; 61:1323–1327; discussion 1328–1329.
291. Mullis-Jansson SL, Argenziano M, Corwin S, et al. A randomized double-blind study of the effect of triiodothyronine on cardiac function and morbidity after coronary bypass surgery. J Thorac Cardiovasc Surg 1999; 117:1128–1134.
292. Chowdhury D, Parnell VA, Ojamaa K, et al. Usefulness of triiodothyronine (T3) treatment after surgery for complex congenital heart disease in infants and children. Am J Cardiol 1999; 84: 1107–1109, A10.
293. Hamilton MA, Stevenson LW, Luu M, et al. Altered thyroid hormone metabolism in advanced heart failure. J Am Coll Cardiol 1990; 16:91–95.
294. Bennett-Guerrero E, Jimenez JL, White WD, et al. Cardiovascular effects of intravenous triiodothyronine in patients undergoing coronary artery bypass graft surgery. A randomized, double-blind, placebo-controlled trial. Duke T3 Study Group. JAMA 1996; 275:687–692.
295. Danese D, Sciacchitano S, Farsetti A, et al. Diagnostic accuracy of conventional versus sonography-guided fine-needle aspiration biopsy of thyroid nodules. Thyroid 1998; 8:15–21.
296. Helfand M, Redfern CC. Clinical guideline: II. Screening for thyroid disease: an update. American College of Physicians. Ann Intern Med 1998; 129:144–158.
297. Bona M, Santini F, Rivolta G, et al. Cost effectiveness of screening for subclinical hypothyroidism in the elderly: a decision-analytical model. Pharmacoeconomics 1998; 14:209–216.
298. Klein RZ, Haddow JE, Faix JD, et al. Prevalence of thyroid deficiency in pregnant women. Clin Endocrinol (Oxf) 1991; 35: 41–46.
299. Pop VJ, Kuijpens JL, van Baar AL, et al. Low maternal free thyroxine concentrations during early pregnancy are associated with impaired psychomotor development in infancy. Clin Endocrinol (Oxf) 1999; 50:149–155.
300. Jordan RM. Myxedema coma: the prognosis is improving. Endocrinologist 1993; 3:149–153.
301. Reinhardt W, Mann K. Incidence, clinical picture, and treatment of hypothyroid coma: results of a survey. Med Klin 1997; 92: 521–524.
302. Nicoloff JT, LoPresti JS. Myxedema coma: a form of decompensated hypothyroidism. Endocrinol Metab Clin North Am 1993; 22:279–290.
303. Blackburn CM, McConahey WM, Keating RF, et al. Calorigenic effects of single intravenous doses of L-triiodothyronine and L-thyroxine in myxedematous persons. J Clin Invest 1954; 33:819–824.
304. MacKerrow SD, Osborn LA, Levy H, et al. Myxedema-associated cardiogenic shock treated with intravenous triiodothyronine. Ann Intern Med 1992; 117:1014–1015.
305. Hylander B, Rosenquist U. Treatment of myxedema coma: factors associated with fatal outcome. Acta Endocrinol (Copenh) 1985; 108:65–71.
306. Szabo SM, Allen DB. Thyroiditis—differentiation of acute suppurative and subacute: case report and review of the literature. Clin Pediatr 1989; 28:171–174.
307. Singer PA. Thyroiditis: acute, subacute, and chronic. Med Clin North Am 1991; 75:61–77.
308. Fernandez JF, Anaissie EJ, Vassilopoulou-Sellin R, et al. Acute fungal thyroiditis in a patient with acute myelogenous leukemia. J Intern Med 1991; 230:539–541.
309. Nieuwland Y, Tan KY, Elte JW. Miliary tuberculosis presenting with thyrotoxicosis. Postgrad Med J 1992; 68:677–679.
310. Das DK, Pant CS, Chachra KL, et al. Fine-needle aspiration cytology diagnosis of tuberculous thyroiditis: a report of eight cases. Acta Cytol 1992; 36:517–522.
311. Chiovato L, Canale G, Maccherini D, et al. *Salmonella brandenburg*: a novel cause of acute suppurative thyroiditis. Acta Endocrinol (Copenh) 1993; 128:439–442.
312. Goldani LZ, Klock C, Diehl A, et al. Histoplasmosis of the thyroid. J Clin Microbiol 2000; 38:3890–3891.
313. Miyauchi A, Matsuzuka F, Kuma K, et al. Piriform sinus fistula: an underlying abnormality common in patients with acute suppurative thyroiditis. World J Surg 1990; 14:400–405.
314. Lucaya J, Berdon WE, Enriquez G, et al. Congenital pyriform sinus fistula: a cause of acute left-sided suppurative thyroiditis and neck abscess in children. Pediatr Radiol 1990; 21:27–29.
315. Gandhi RT, Tollin SR, Seely EW. Diagnosis of *Candida* thyroiditis by fine-needle aspiration. J Infect 1994; 28:77–81.
316. Bernard PJ, Som PM, Urken ML, et al. The CT findings of acute thyroiditis and acute suppurative thyroiditis. Otolaryngol Head Neck Surg 1988; 99:489–493.
317. Hatabu H, Kasagi K, Yamamoto K, et al. Acute suppurative thyroiditis associated with piriform sinus fistula: sonographic findings. Am J Med 1990; 155:845–847.
318. Bartholomew LG, Cain JC, Woolner LB, et al. Sclerosing cholangitis: its possible association with Riedel's struma and fibrous retroperitonitis—report of two cases. N Engl J Med 1963; 269: 8–13.
319. Chopra D, Wool MS, Grossen A, et al. Riedel's struma associated with subacute thyroiditis, hypothyroidism, and hypoparathyroidism. J Clin Endocrinol Metab 1978; 46:869–871.
320. Zelmanovitz F, Zelmanovitz T, Beck M, et al. Riedel's thyroiditis associated with high titers of antimicrosomal and antithyroglobulin antibodies and hypothyroidism. J Endocrinol Invest 1994; 17: 733–737.
321. Julie C, Vieillefond A, Desligneres S, et al. Hashimoto's thyroiditis associated with Riedel's thyroiditis and retroperitoneal fibrosis. Pathol Res Pract 1997; 193:573–577.
322. Heufelder AE, Goellner JR, Bahn RS, et al. Tissue eosinophilia and eosinophil degranulation in Riedel's invasive fibrous thyroiditis. J Clin Endocrinol Metab 1996; 81:977–984.

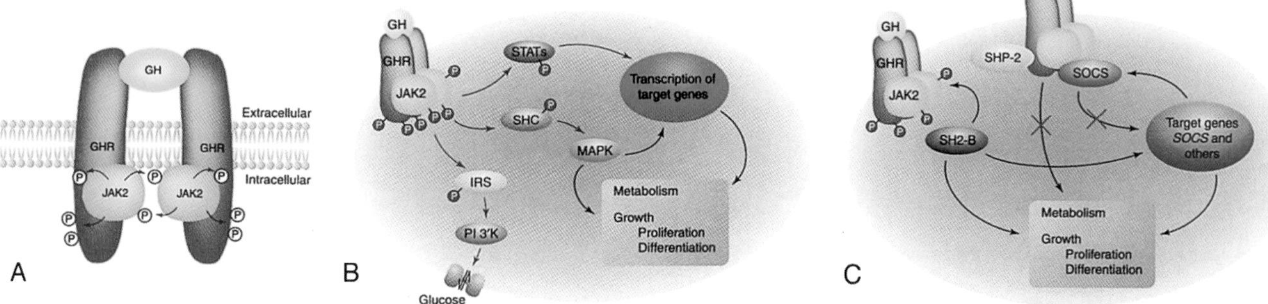

Figure 8–41. Growth hormone (GH) receptors.

A, Model of GH activation of JAK2 tyrosine kinase. GH binding to two GH receptors increases the affinity to each receptor for JAK2. The two receptor-associated JAK2 molecules are in close proximity, so that each JAK2 can phosphorylate the activating tyrosine of the other JAK2 molecule *(blue arrows)*, thereby activating it. Activated JAK2 then phosphorylates itself *(red arrow)* and the cytoplasmic domain of the GH receptor *(purple arrows)* on tyrosines. These phosphotyrosines within the GH receptor and JAK2 form binding sites for signaling proteins. GH, growth hormone; GHR, growth hormone receptor; JAK2, Janus kinase 2; P, phosphate.

B, Regulation of GH receptor-JAK2 signaling. SH2 enhances GH receptor signaling by increasing the activity of JAK2. GH-induced expression of SOCS proteins inhibits further GHR signaling by decreasing the activity of JAK2. Tyrosine phosphatases, such as SHP-2, might also contribute to inhibiting GH receptor signaling by dephosphorylating tyrosines in the GH receptor and/or JAK2. GH, growth hormone; GHR, growth hormone receptor; JAK2, Janus kinase 2; P, phosphatase; SHP-2, src homology 2 domain-containing protein tyrosine phosphatase 2; SOCS, suppressor of cytokine signaling.

C, GH receptors signaling pathways. Some of the signaling pathways initiated by GH activation of JAK2 are shown. JAK2 phosphorylates SHC, leading to activation of MAPK *(blue arrows)*. JAK2 also phosphorylates STAT transcription factors. MAPK and STATs are important for GH regulation of gene transcription *(purple arrows)*. JAK2 phosphorylates IRS proteins, which are thought to lead to activation of PI 3′-kinase (PI3 K: *red arrows*). GH activation of PI 3′-kinase via IRS protein might be important for GH stimulation of glucose transport.

GH, growth hormone, GHR, growth hormone receptor; IRS, insulin receptor substrates; JAK2, Janus kinase 2; MAPK, mitogen-activated protein kinase; P, phosphate; PI 3′K, phosphatidylinositol 3-kinase, STAT, signal transducers and activators of transcription.

(*A–C,* From Herrington J, Carter-Su C. Signaling pathway activated by the growth hormone receptor. Trends Endocrinol Metab 2001; 12:252-257.)

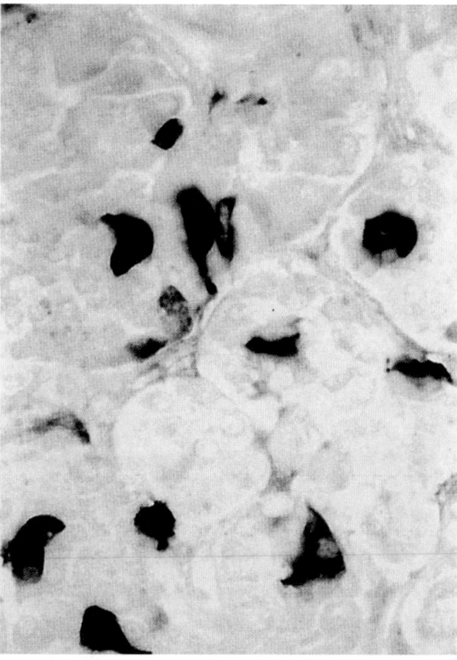

Figure 8–61. Normal thyrotrophs have angular cell bodies with elongated processes. (From Asa SL. In Tumors of the Pituitary Gland. Atlas of Tumor Pathology. Washington, DC, Armed Forces Institute of Pathology, 1997, p 19.)

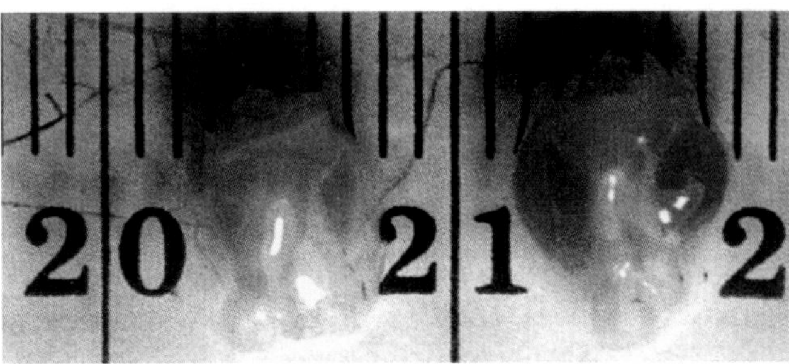

Figure 11–5. Thyroid glands from hyperthyroid mice immunized with fibroblasts expressing the human thyrotropin-stimulating hormone receptor. *Left*, A thyroid gland from a control mouse. *Right*, An enlarged thyroid from a hyperthyroid mouse. Ruler is in centimeters. (From Kita ML, Ahmad RC, Marians H, et al. Regulation and transfer of a murine model of thyrotropin receptor antibody–mediated Graves' disease. Endocrinology 1999; 140:1392–1398.)

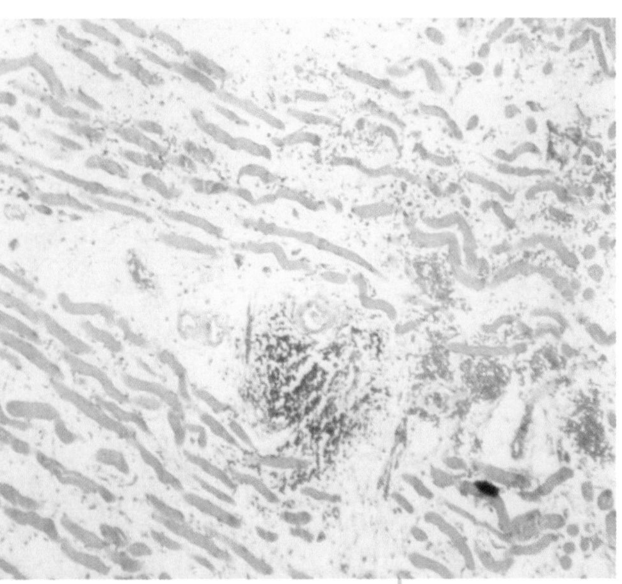

Figure 11–13. Section of extraocular muscle from a biopsy taken from a patient with severe Graves' orbitopathy. Note that within the muscle fibers is a patch of lymphocytic infiltration. (Courtesy of Dr. D. Kendler, University of British Columbia, Vancouver, Canada.)

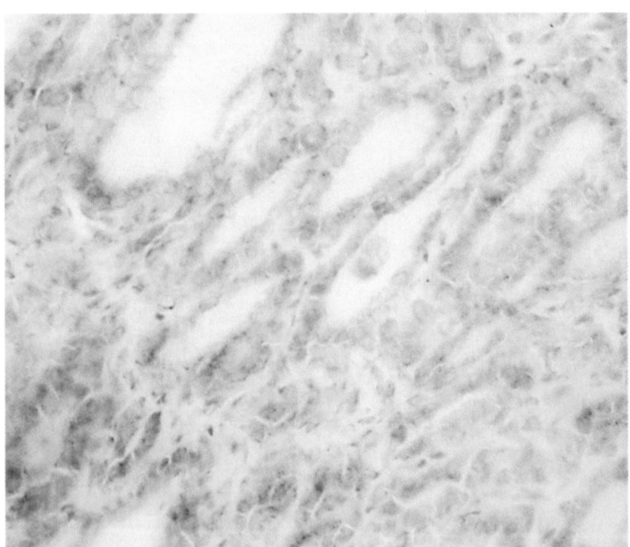

Figure 11–11. Photomicrograph of Graves' thyroid tissue stained for HLA class II (DR) antigen expression using the immunoperoxidase technique. Note the brown thyroid epithelial cells indicating the presence of DR antigen. Note also the relative lack of lymphocytic infiltration in this region.

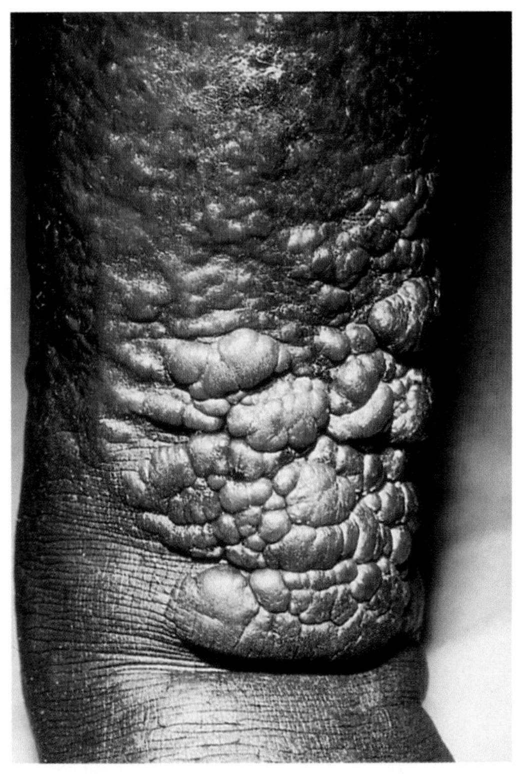

Figure 11–14. Chronic pretibial myxedema in a patient with Graves' disease and orbitopathy. The lesions are firm and nonpitting, with a clear edge to feel. (Courtesy of Dr. Andrew Werner, New York, N.Y.)

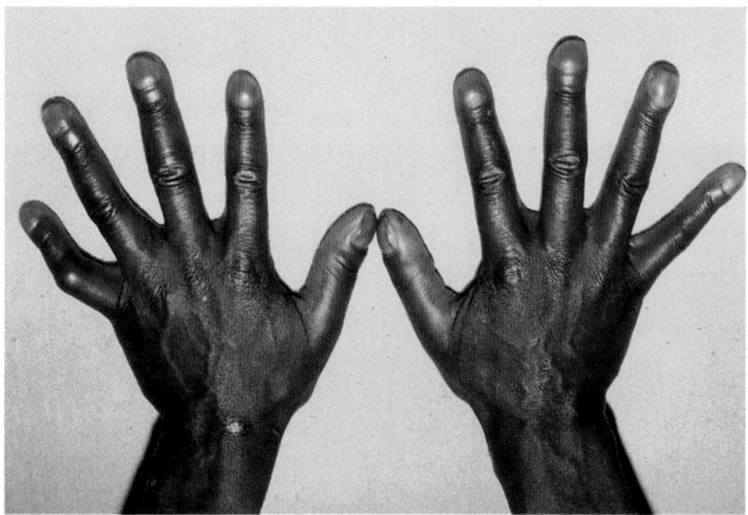

Figure 11–18. Rare thyroid acropachy in a patient with Graves' disease. The hypermetabolic state leads to axial bone destruction, presumably secondary to enhanced osteoclast activity. Acropachy is not to be confused with clubbing, which is usually painless. (Courtesy of Dr. Andrew Werner, New York, N.Y.)

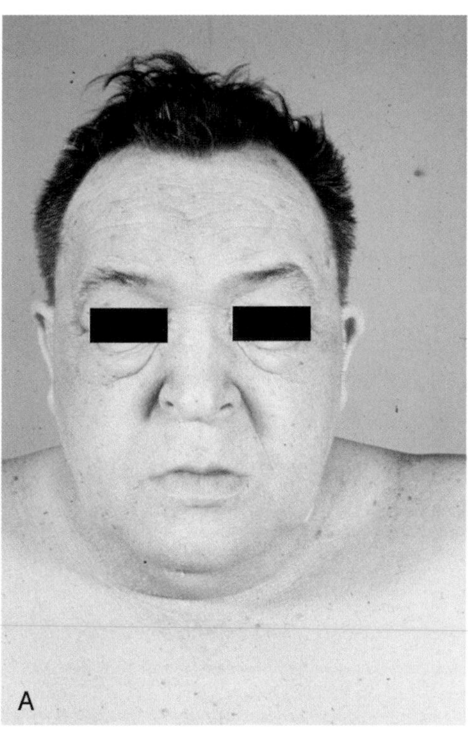

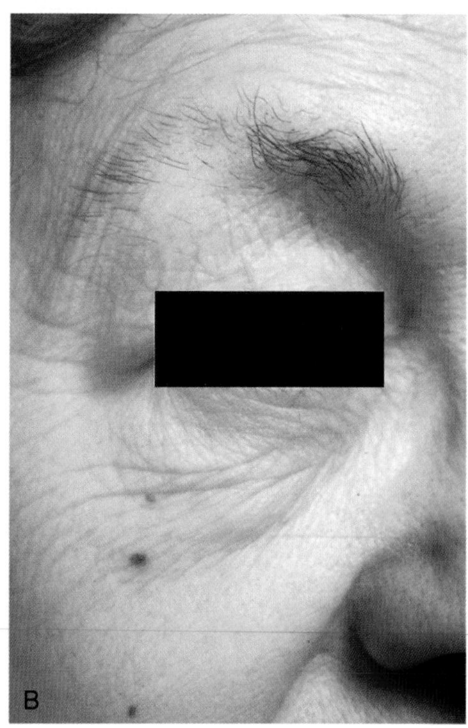

Figure 12–1. *A* and *B*, Typical appearance of patients with moderately severe primary hypothyroidism or myxedema. Note dry skin, sallow complexion, with the absence of scleral pigmentation differentiating the carotenemia from jaundice. Both individuals demonstrate periorbital myxedema. The patient in *B* illustrates the loss of the lateral aspect of the eyebrow, sometimes termed *Queen Anne's sign*. That finding is not unusual in the age group that is commonly affected by severe hypothyroidism and should not be considered to be a specific sign of the condition.

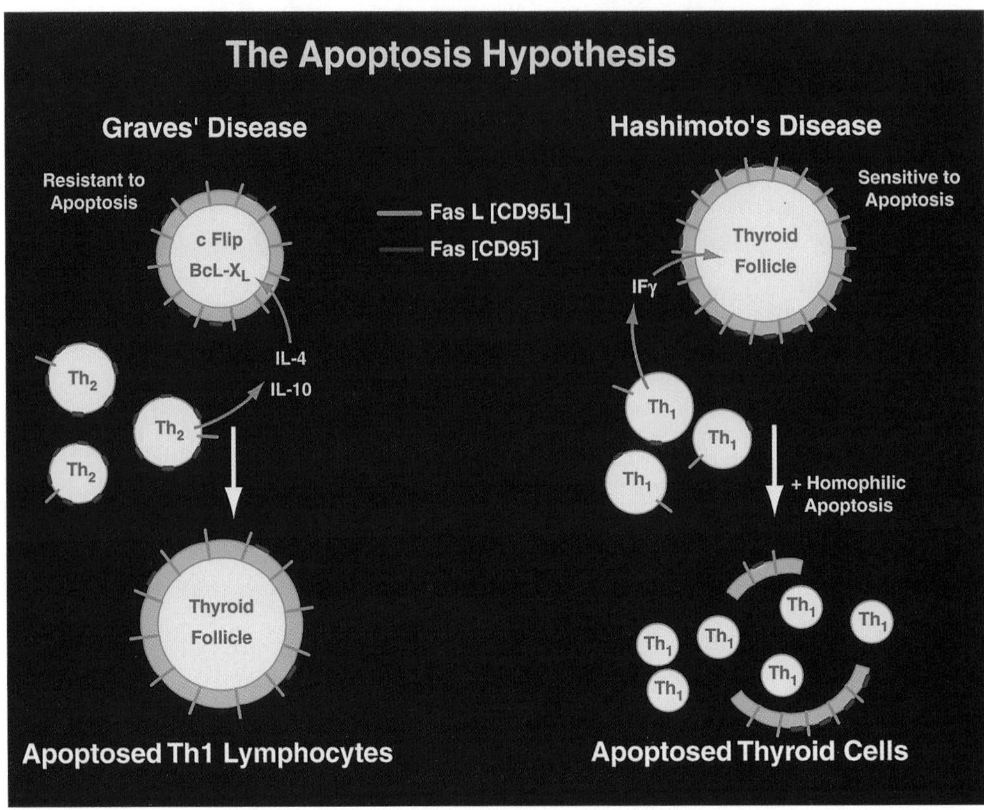

Figure 12–7. Possible involvement of Fas-Fasl in the apoptosis of Hashimoto's thyroiditis. In Graves' disease, the thyroid follicles thrive because the thyroid cells do not express many functional Fas molecules (shown in red) and, therefore, the thyroid cells are resistant to the Fasl (Fas ligand) on both the thyroid cells themselves and on the Th2 T cells (shown in blue). Further apoptotic resistance may be driven by Th2 cytokines, such as interleukin-4 (IL-4) and IL-10. However, the Th2 cells express Fas and may themselves be deleted by the Fasl constitutively expressed on the thyroid cells. The result is thyroid cell survival with T-cell destruction. In contrast, in Hashimoto's disease, the thyroid cell expresses many functional Fas molecules, perhaps induced by gamma interferon from the Th1 type T cells associated with this disease. The expression of thyroid cell Fas may lead to self (homophilic) apoptosis via thyroid cell Fasl, or apoptosis may result from attack by the Fasl armed Th1 cells. The result is thyroid follicle destruction and T-cell proliferation.

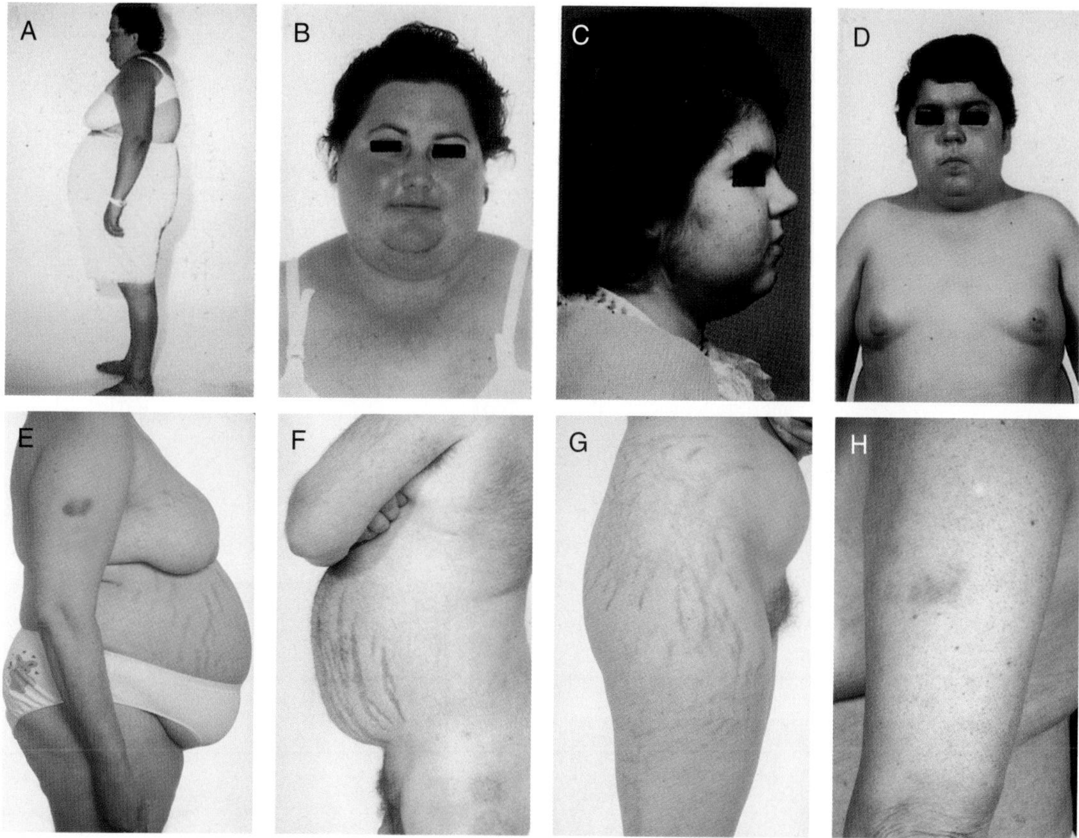

Figure 14–16. Clinical features of Cushing's syndrome. *A*, Centripetal and some generalized obesity and dorsal kyphosis in a 30-year-old woman with Cushing's disease. *B*, Same woman as in *A*, showing moon facies, plethora, hirsutism, and enlarged supraclavicular fat pads. *C*, Facial rounding, hirsutism, and acne in a 14-year-old girl with Cushing's disease. *D*, Central and generalized obesity and moon facies in a 14-year-old boy with Cushing's disease. *E* and *F*, Typical centripetal obesity with livid abdominal striae seen in a 41-year-old woman *(E)* and a 40-year-old man *(F)* with Cushing's syndrome. *G*, Striae in a 24-year-old patient with congenital adrenal hyperplasia treated with excessive doses of dexamethasone as "replacement" therapy. *H*, Typical bruising and thin skin of Cushing's syndrome. In this case, the bruising has occurred without obvious injury.

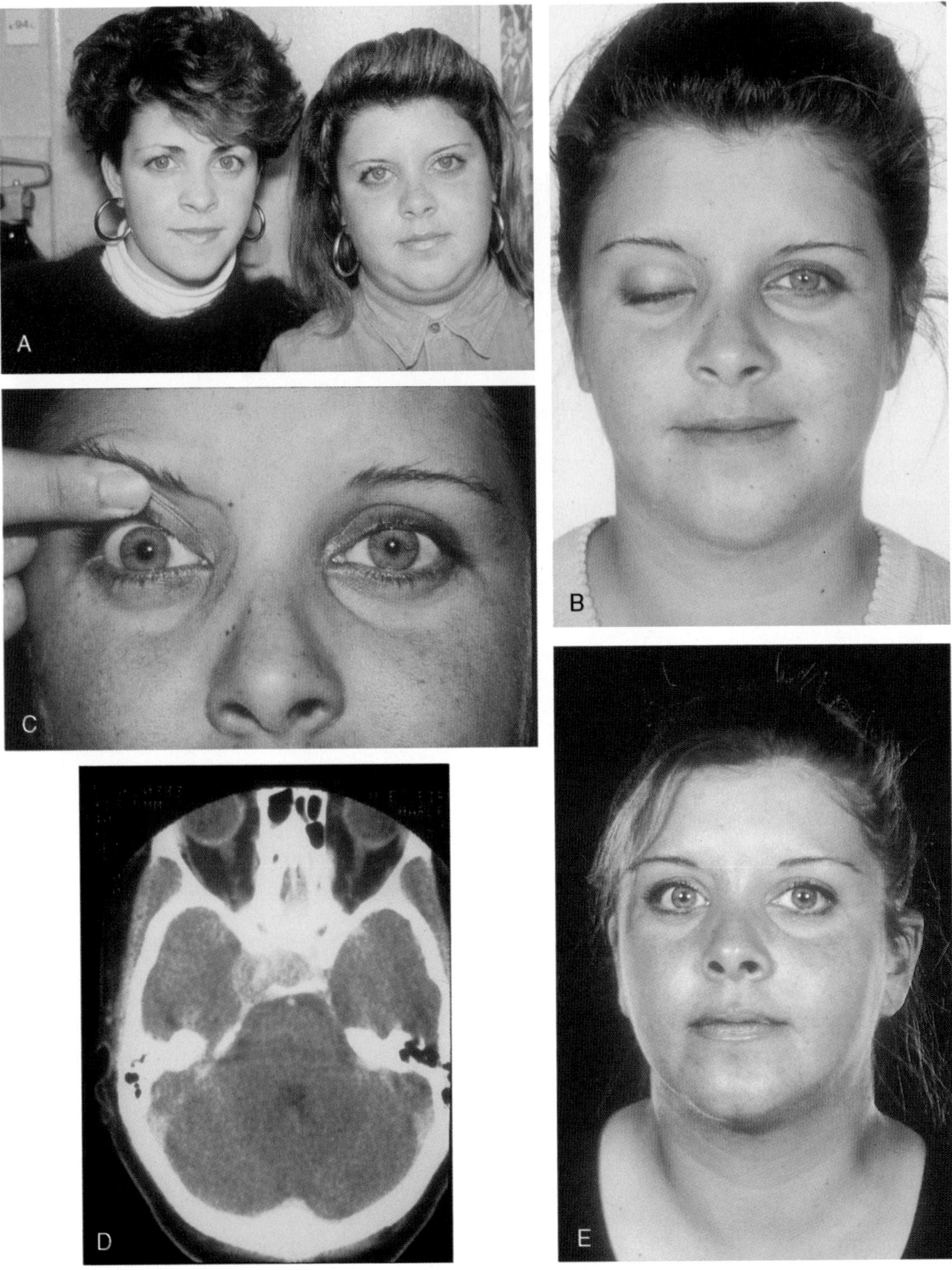

Figure 14–27. A young woman with Cushing's disease, photographed initially beside her identical twin sister *(A)*. In this case, treatment with bilateral adrenalectomy was undertaken. Several years later, the patient presented with Nelson's syndrome and a right third cranial nerve palsy (*B* and *C*) related to cavernous sinus infiltration from a locally invasive corticotropinoma *(D)*. Hypophysectomy and radiotherapy were performed with reversal of the third nerve palsy *(E)*. Note the advancing skin pigmentation of Nelson's syndrome.

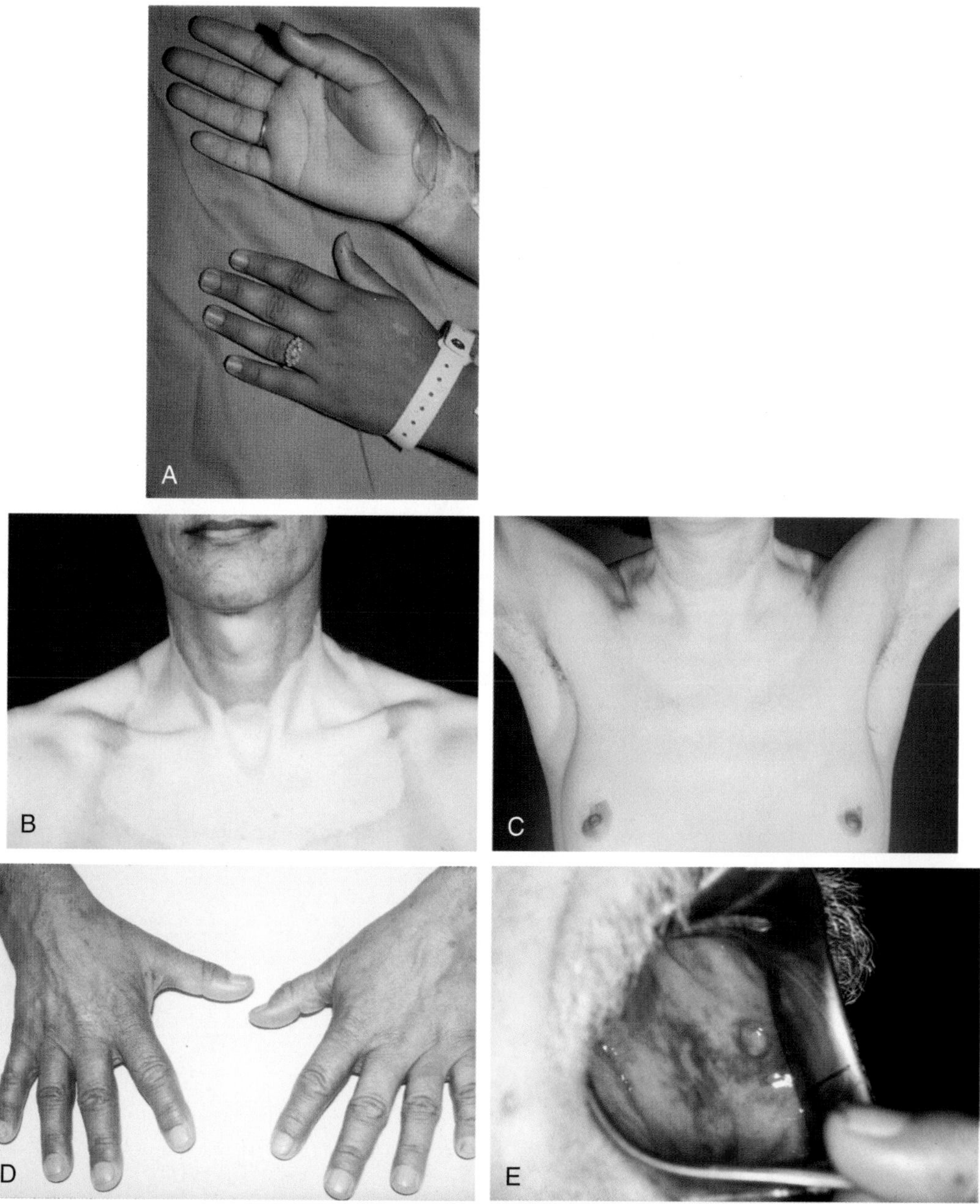

Figure 14–30. Pigmentation in Addison's disease. *A*, Hands of an 18-year-old woman with autoimmune polyendocrine syndrome and Addison's disease. Pigmentation in a patient with Addison's disease before (*B*) and after (*C*) treatment with hydrocortisone and fludrocortisone. Note the additional presence of vitiligo. *D*, Similar changes also seen in a 60-year-old man with tuberculous Addison's disease before and after corticosteroid therapy. *E*, Buccal pigmentation in the same patient. (*B* and *C*, courtesy of Professor C.R.W. Edwards.)

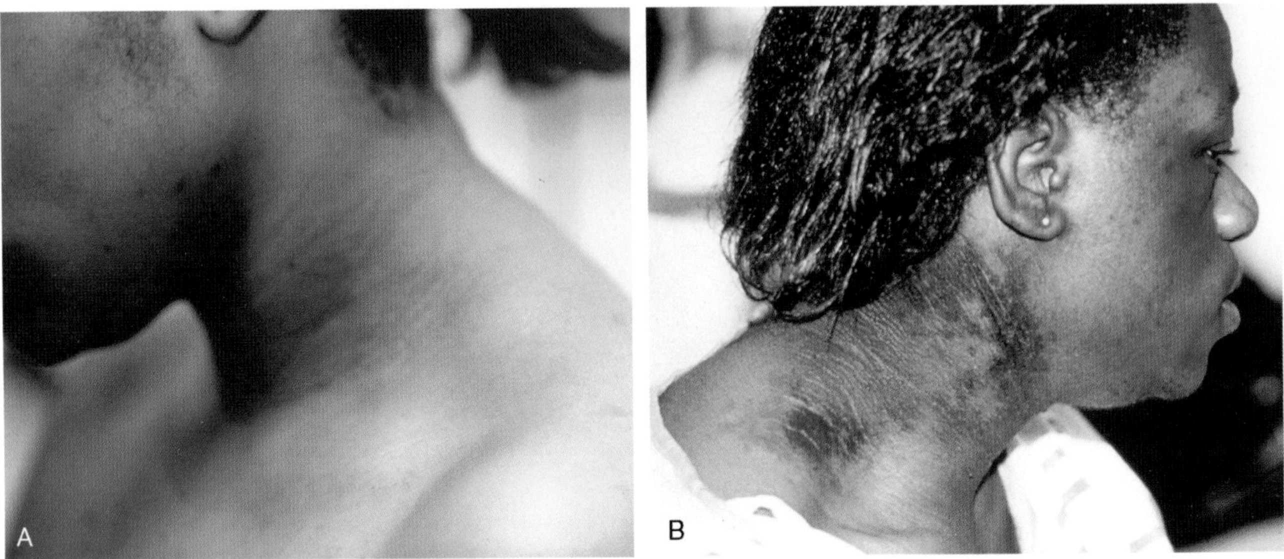

Figure 16–34. Acanthosis nigricans. *A*, Moderate acanthosis nigricans (darkening and thickening of skin) at the lateral lower fold of the neck. Note facial hirsutism (sideburns) in the same patient. *B*, Severe acanthosis nigricans in another patient with severe insulin resistance. (*B*, courtesy of Dr. R. Ann Word.)

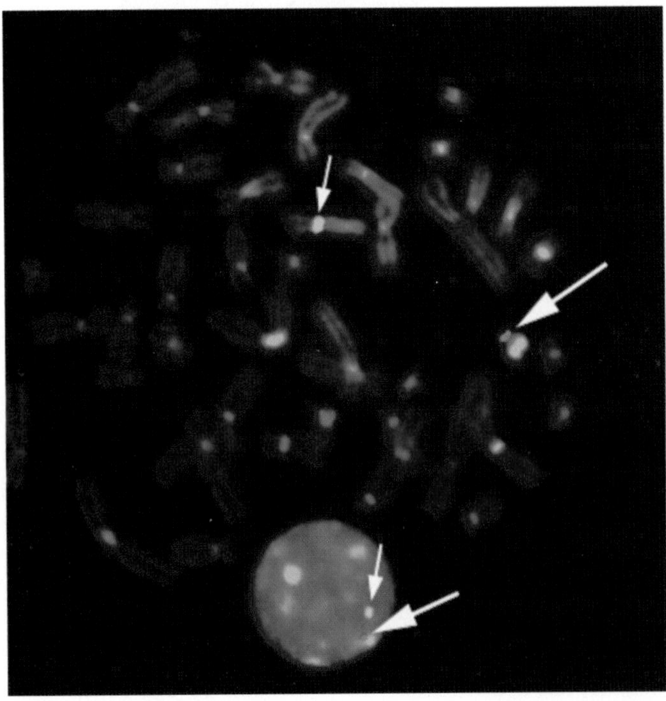

Figure 22–3. FISH for *SRY* analysis in metaphase and interphase 46,XY cells. FISH images illustrating localization of the Vysis SRY probe on the distal short arm of the Y chromosome (Yp11.3) shown in SpectrumOrange and Vysis CEPX, a probe for the X centromere shown in SpectrumGreen. Note the localization of the X (green) and Y (orange) in an interphase nucleus (*right*). (Courtesy of Philip Cotter and Helen Jenks.)

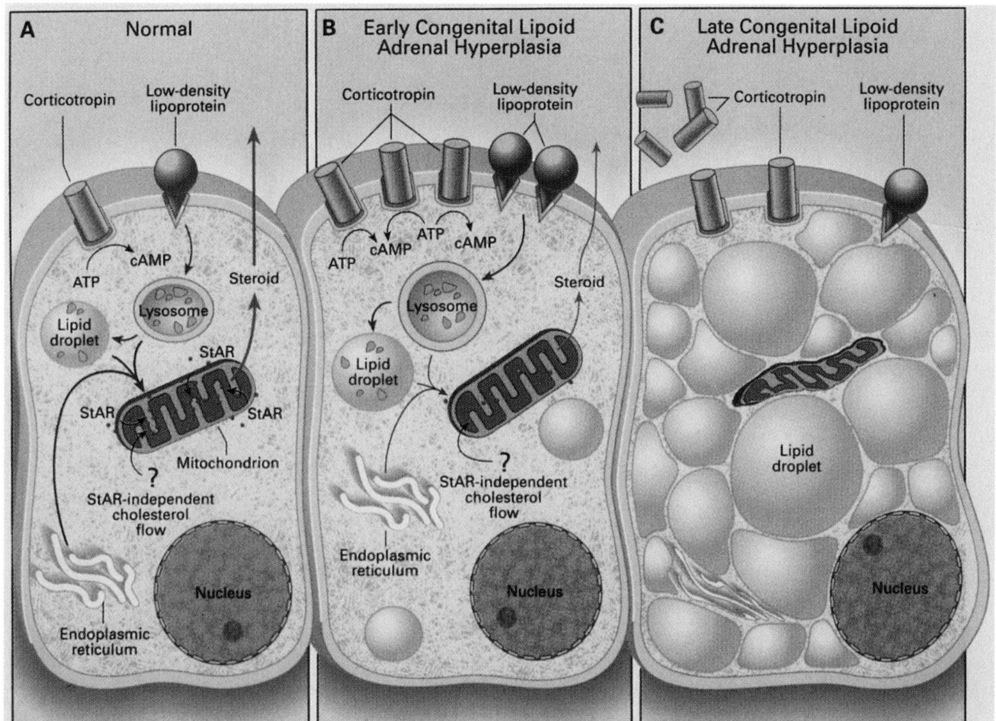

Figure 22–64. Model of the steroid-synthesizing cell (adrenal/gonadal) showing conversion of cholesterol to steroids. *A*, Cholesterol from low-density lipoprotein, from cholesterol esters stored in lipid droplets, and from endogenous synthesis in the endoplasmic reticulum is transported from the outer mitochondrial membrane to the inner membrane. This transport, which is a rate-limiting step in steroid synthesis, is facilitated by StAR (steroidogenic acute regulatory protein) as well as by other, StAR-independent mechanisms. In the mitochondria, steroid synthesis then ensues as a result of the conversion of cholesterol to Δ^5-pregnenolone by the enzyme CYP11A1 ($P450_{scc}$). *B*, In patients with congenital lipoid adrenal hyperplasia, a mutation in the gene encoding StAR results in little or no activity of the mutant StAR, causing greatly diminished cholesterol transport into the mitochondria. Low levels of steroidogenesis via mechanisms independent of StAR can occur; however, increased ACTH (LH/FSH) secretion results in cholesterol accumulation in the cells as lipid droplets. *C*, Continued stimulation and resultant accumulation of cholesterol causes engorgement of these cells, with both mechanical and chemical perturbation of the cell function. Females with congenital lipoid adrenal hyperplasia feminize at puberty and menstruate but have progressive hypergonadotropic hypogonadism. It has been hypothesized by Bose and co-workers that this occurs because the follicular cells are relatively quiescent in utero and before puberty; hence, they are undamaged. At the beginning of each cycle, they are recruited, and a small amount of estradiol can be produced as a result of StAR-independent mechanisms. This can occur until the follicular cells are engorged and rendered nonfunctional. (From Bose HS, Sujiwara T, Strauss JF III, Miller WL. The pathophysiology and genetics of congenital lipoid adrenal hyperplasia. N Engl J Med 1996; 335:1870–1878. Copyright 1996, Massachusetts Medical Society. All rights reserved.) (See text.)

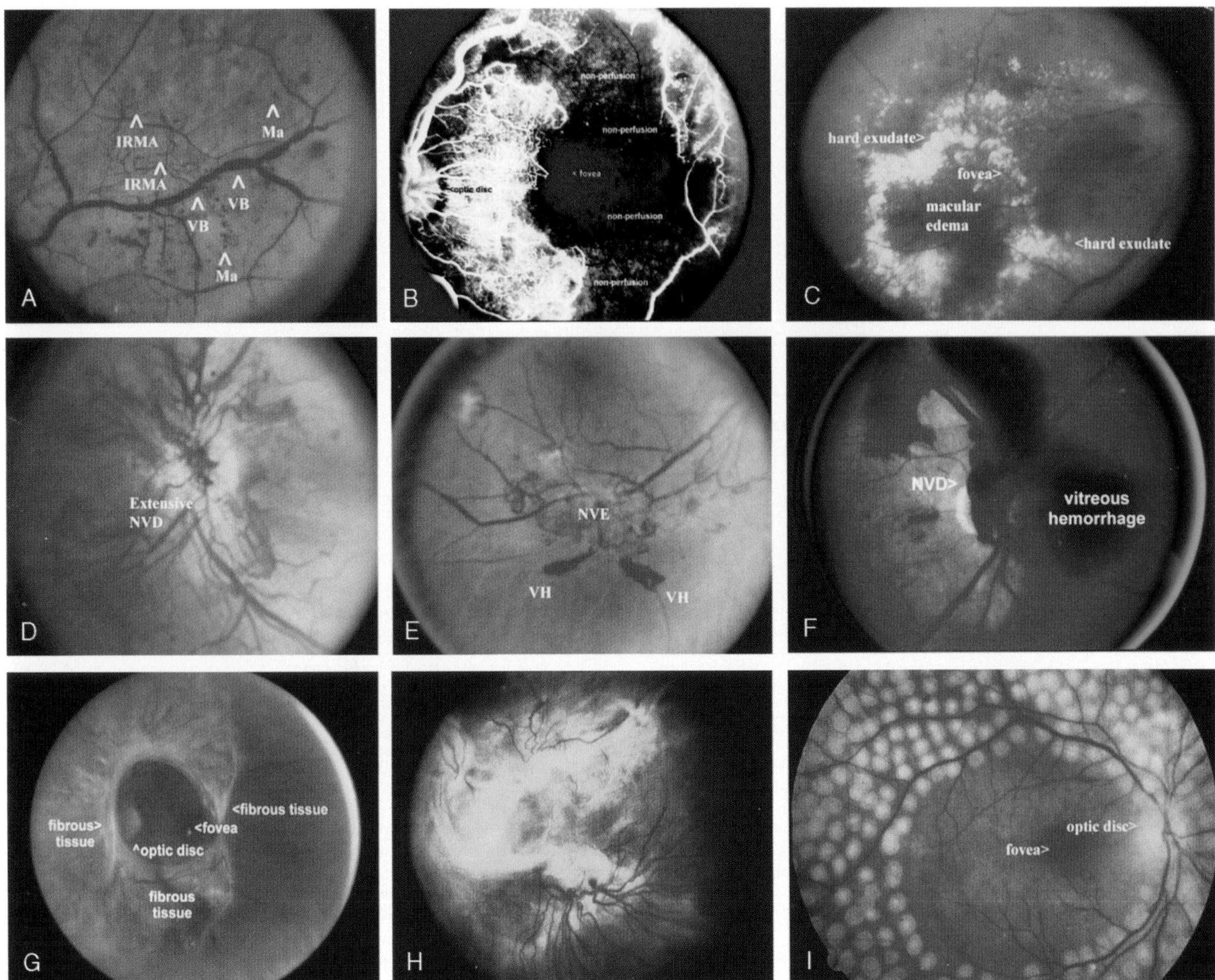

Figure 31–19. Clinical features of diabetic retinopathy: some typical findings in human diabetic retinopathy. *A*, Findings in severe nonproliferative diabetic retinopathy, including microaneurysms (Ma), venous beading (VB), and intraretinal microvascular abnormalities (IRMA). *B*, Fluorescein angiogram showing marked capillary nonperfusion. *C*, Clinically significant macular edema with retinal thickening and hard exudates involving the fovea. *D*, Extensive neovascularization of the optic disc (NVD). This is high-risk proliferative diabetic retinopathy. *E*, Neovascularization elsewhere (NVE) and two small vitreous hemorrhages (VH). *F*, Extensive vitreous hemorrhage arising from severe neovascularization of the disc (NVD). *G*, Severe fibrovascular proliferation surrounding the fovea. *H*, Traction retinal detachment from extensive fibrovascular proliferation. *I*, Panretinal (scatter) laser photocoagulation. The macula and fovea and optic disc are not treated to preserve central vision. Laser burns are evident as white retinal lesions. (*A* to *I*, Adapted from Aiello LP. Eye complications of diabetes. In Korenman SG, Kahn CR [eds]. Atlas of Clinical Endocrinology. Vol 2: Diabetes. Philadelphia, Blackwell Scientific, 1999.)

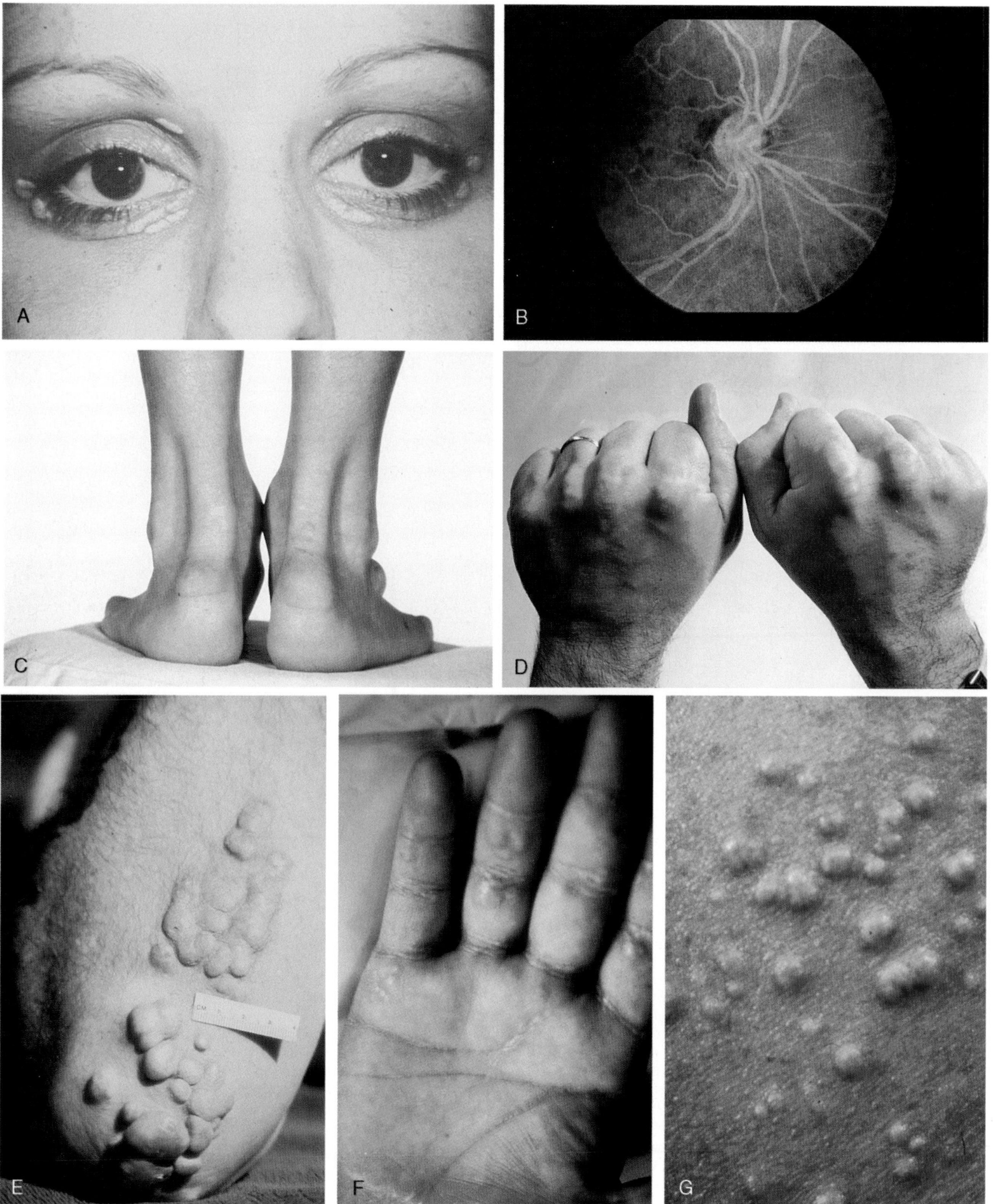

Figure 34–26. Physical examination findings associated with hyperlipidemia. *A*, Xanthelasma. *B*, Lipemia retinalis. *C*, Achilles tendon xanthomas. Note the marked thickening of the tendons. *D*, Tendon xanthomas. *E*, Tuberous xanthomas. *F*, Palmar xanthomas. *G*, Eruptive xanthomas. (*A* and *B*, Courtesy of Dr. Mark Dresner and Hospital Practice [May 1990, p 15]. *C*, *D*, *E*, and *F*, Courtesy of Dr. Tom Bersot. *G*, Courtesy of Dr. Alan Chait.)

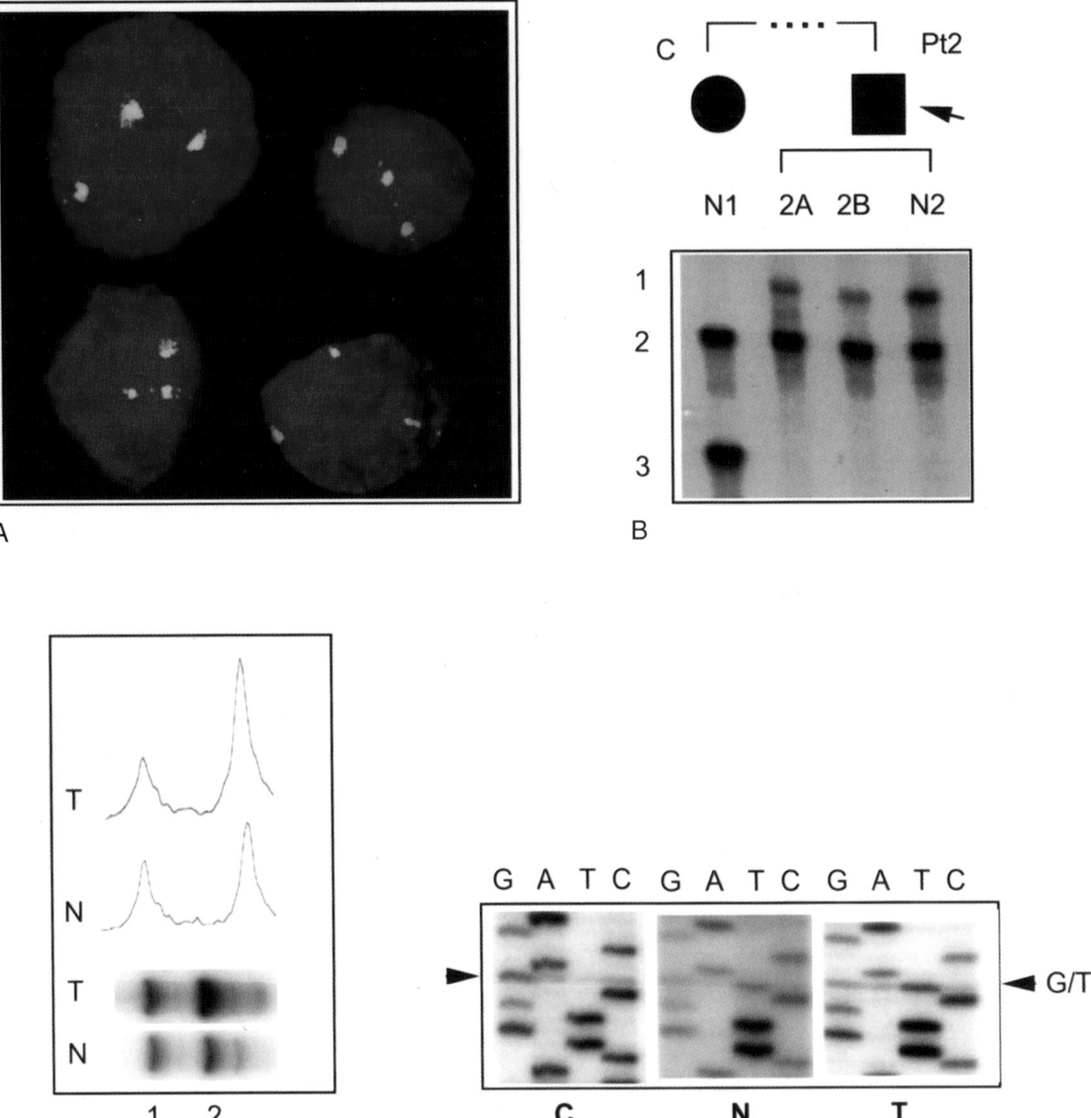

Figure 36–17. Trisomy 10 with nonrandom duplication of the mutant *RET* allele in pheochromocytoma associated with multiple endocrine neoplasia type 2 (MEN2). *A*, Representative interphase fluorescence in situ hybridization analysis of tumor touch preparation from patient 2 (tumor 2A). Three copies of chromosome 10 are shown using a centromeric satellite probe (fluorescein isothiocyanate, green signal) specific for chromosome 10. *B*, Combined pedigree and tumor allelic analysis of patient 2 (Pt2). *Arrow*, patient 2. *Filled symbols*, individuals with MEN2. Genotypes are shown for the chromosome 10 microsatellite marker *D10S1239* linked to the *RET* locus. Allele 2 of *D10S1239* is coinherited with the disease in this patient's family. In patient 2, allele 2 shows greater intensity in lanes 2A and 2B (tumors) than allele 1, representing the wild-type allele, as compared with lane N2 (blood DNA). Lane N1 (blood DNA) shows equal intensities of mutant and wild-type allele in the patient's affected cousin (C). *C*, Representative results of microsatellite and phosphorimage analyses. After polymerase chain reaction amplification using marker *D10S1239*, quantitative measurement of allelic intensity was performed using phosphorimage analysis. In tumor tissue (T), allele 2 is more intense than allele 1. Phosphorimage densitometry shows a 2:1 imbalance between the two alleles in the tumor (T) compared with the normal tissue (N). *D*, Representative results of sequencing analysis of *RET* in tumor 3A. Blood DNA from an unaffected healthy individual (C, *left*) shows the wild-type *RET* sequence (codon 631 GAC). Blood DNA from patient 3 (N, *middle*) shows the germ line mutation (G/T). Tumor DNA (T, *right*) shows a higher intensity of the mutant nucleotide (T) compared with the wild type. (From Huang SC, Koch CA, Vortmeyer AO, et al. Duplication of the mutant *RET* allele in trisomy 10 or loss of the wild-type allele in multiple endocrine neoplasia type 2–associated pheochromocytomas. Cancer Res 2000; 60:6223–6226.)

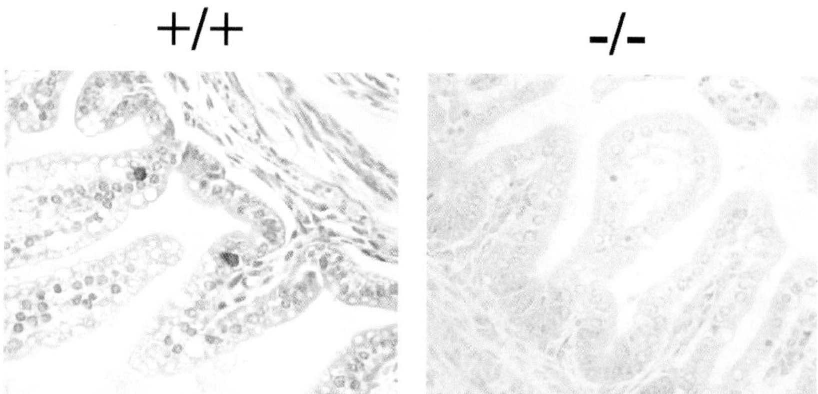

Figure 38–1. Essential requirement for *Pax6* for glucagon-positive enteroendocrine cell formation in the murine intestine. *Pax6* SEY^{NEU} mutant mice (−/−) exhibit markedly reduced numbers of glucagon-immunopositive cells in the small and large intestine.

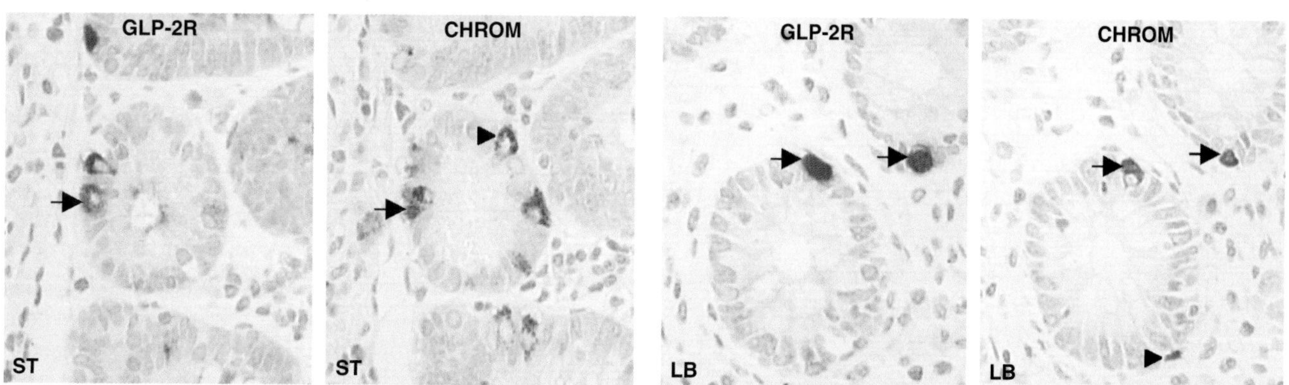

Figure 38–2. Glucagon-like peptide II receptor (GLP-2R) expression in subsets of endocrine cells in the human stomach (ST) and large bowel (LB). Most cells exhibiting positivity with antisera against the human GLP-2R also exhibited immunopositivity for an endocrine marker such as chromogranin (CHROM). In contrast, most endocrine cells in the stomach and both small and large intestine did not express the GLP-2R. *Arrows* denote cells positive for both the GLP-2R and chromogranin, and *arrowheads* denote cells positive for the GLP-2R or chromogranin. (From Yusta B, Huang L, Munroe D, et al. Endocrine localization of GLP-2 expression in humans and rodents. Gastroenterology 2000; 119:744–755.)

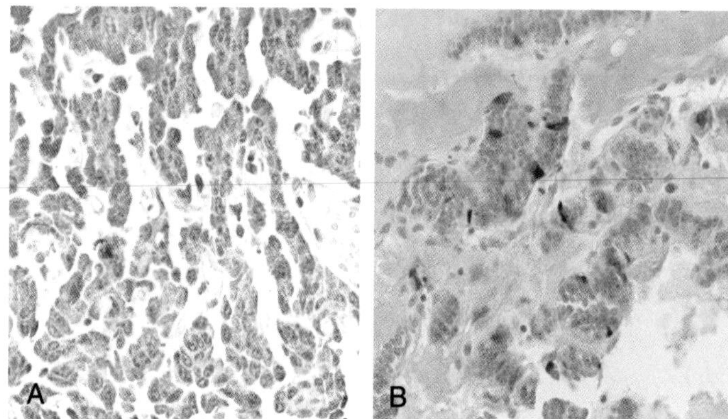

Figure 38–3. Clinically "nonfunctioning" tumors are often found to express one or more peptide hormones after immunocytochemical analyses. The photomicrographs represent histologic sections from the identical nonfunctioning human pancreatic endocrine tumor that exhibit immunopositivity for glucagon (*A*) and pancreatic polypeptide (*B*). (Courtesy of Dr. G. Rindi, Brescia, Italy.)

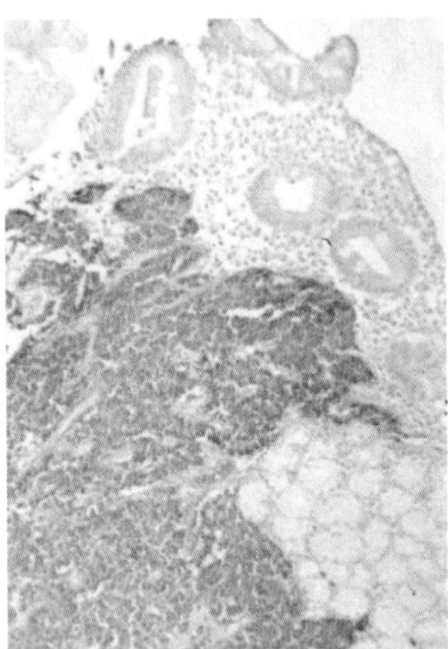

Figure 38–5. Somatostatin immunoreactivity in a human duodenal D cell tumor. The low-power micrograph illustrates the diffuse somatostatin immunoreactivity. Brunner's glands and the partly eroded mucosa are seen in the lower and upper right areas, respectively, in relation to the immunopositive endocrine tumor.

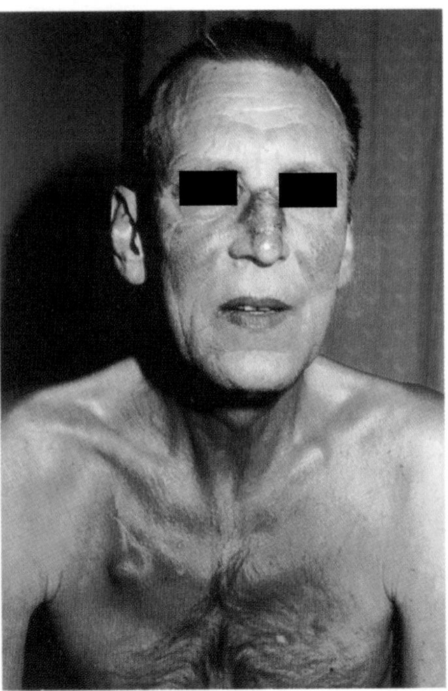

Figure 41–9. Long-lasting chronic flushing in a patient with long-standing carcinoid disease. Note the telangiectases.

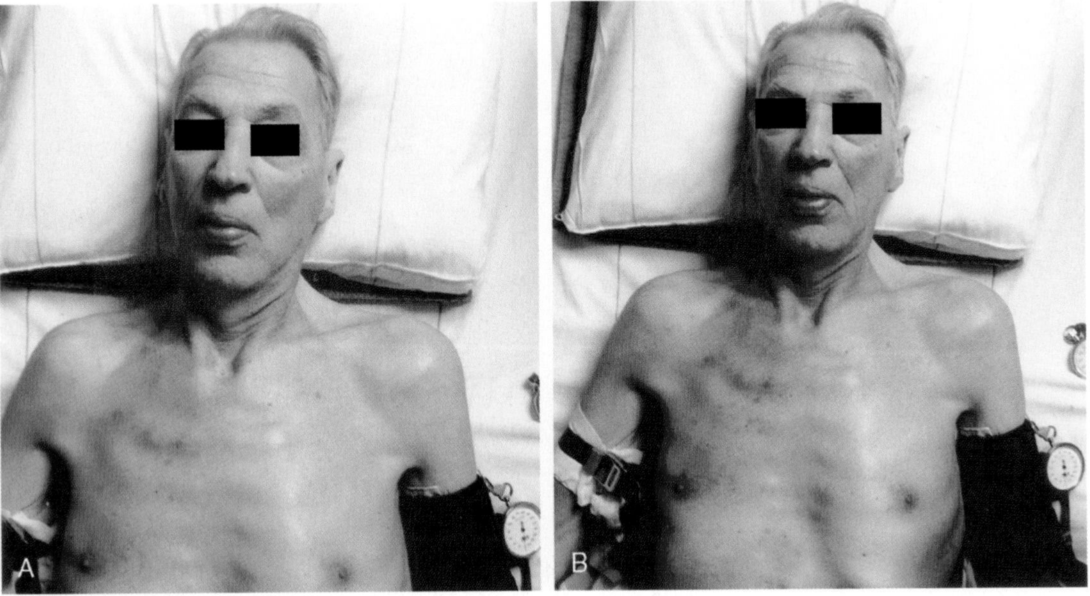

Figure 41–8. Carcinoid syndrome before and after provocation. *A*, Before flush provocation. *B*, Same patient after pentagastrin-stimulated flush.

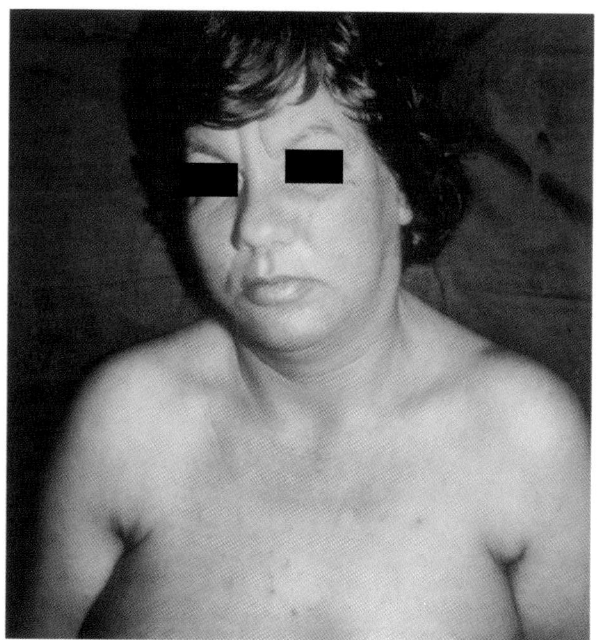

Figure 41–10. The patient has lung carcinoid and carcinoid syndrome with severe, long-standing flushing, lacrimation, and a swollen face.

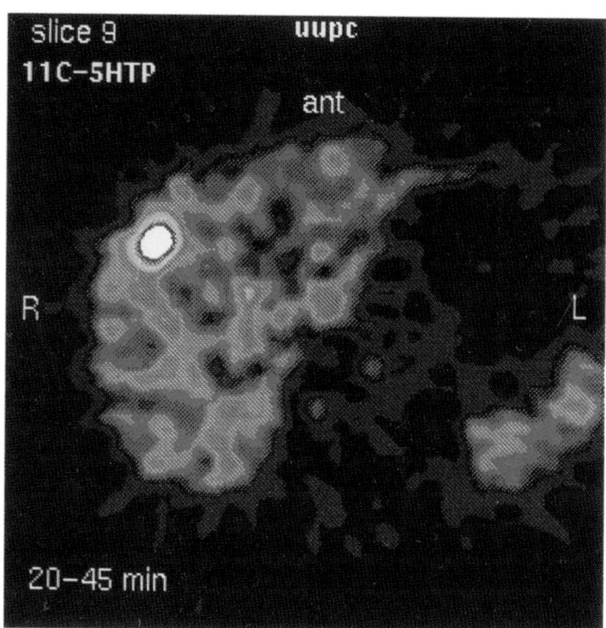

Figure 41–14. Positron emission tomography (PET) with ^{11}C-5-hydroxytryptophan. Note the metastasis in the liver.

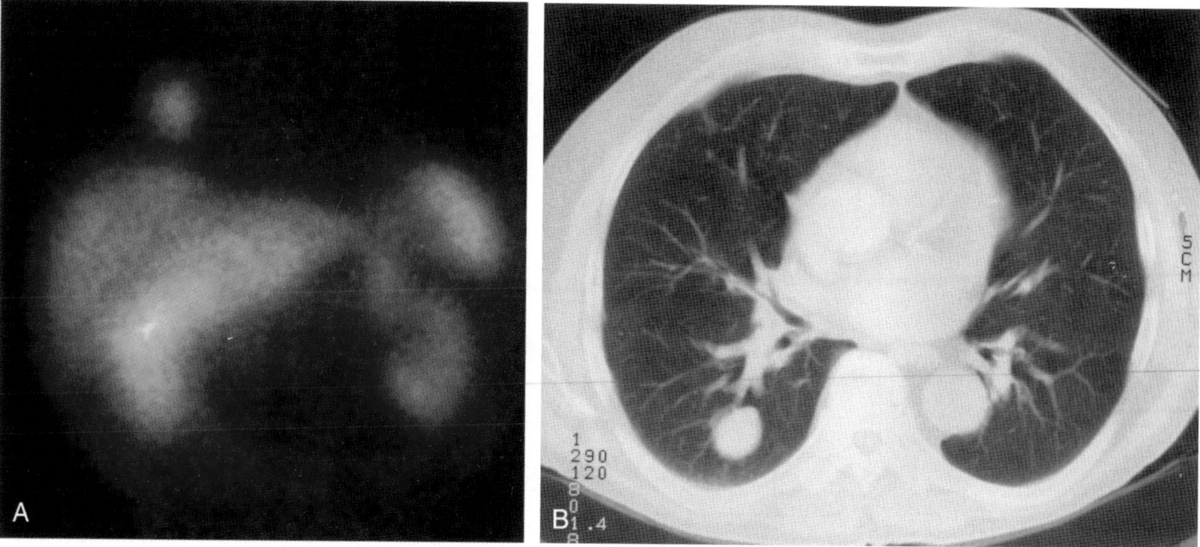

Figure 41–13. Bronchial carcinoid. *A,* Somatostatin-receptor scintigraphy in a patient with a bronchial carcinoid. *B,* CT scan in the same patient.

13 Nontoxic Goiter and Thyroid Neoplasia

Martin-Jean Schlumberger, Sebastiano Filetti, and Ian D. Hay

After thyroid dysfunction and neck pain, the discovery of an apparent structural abnormality of the thyroid gland is the most common reason for a patient to seek the expertise of a clinical thyroidologist. In this chapter, we review the imaging techniques available for evaluating thyroid structural abnormalities; the units of measurement used in evaluation of the radiation dose and radioactivity are defined in Table 13–1.

Goiter resulting in thyrotoxicosis and other thyroid conditions arising from autoimmune thyroid disease are considered in Chapters 11 and 12.

This chapter describes simple or nontoxic goiter in addition to the increasingly recognized problem of nodular thyroid disease. Moreover, thyroid neoplasia, both benign and malignant, is discussed authoritatively. We consider an appropriate histologic classification and staging of thyroid cancer and present a management program for the most common thyroid cancer types.

EVALUATION OF STRUCTURAL ABNORMALITIES BY IMAGING TECHNIQUES

External Scintiscanning

Localization of functioning or nonfunctioning thyroid tissue in the area of the thyroid gland or elsewhere is made possible by techniques of external scintiscanning. The underlying principle is that isotopes that are selectively accumulated by thyroid tissue can be detected and quantified in situ and the data transformed into a visual display. Two types of apparatus are available.

The *rectilinear scanner* is a device that moves a highly collimated (focused) scintillation detector back and forth across the area of study in a series of parallel tracks. A printing device records a mark whenever a predetermined number of counts has been received to provide a visual representation of the localization of radioactivity.

The *stationary scintillation camera* has now replaced the rectilinear scanner in most centers. It is equipped with a pinhole collimator that views the entire field of interest and translates the counting rates from specific areas of the field into images. Radioactivity in specific areas can be quantified. These cameras provide better resolution than rectilinear scanners, but anatomic localization may be more difficult.[1]

Several radioisotopes are employed in thyroid imaging. Technetium 99m (^{99m}Tc) pertechnetate is a monovalent anion that is actively concentrated by the thyroid gland but undergoes negligible organic binding and diffuses out of the thyroid gland as its concentration in the blood decreases. The short physical half-life of ^{99m}Tc (6 hours), its low fractional uptake, and its transient stay within the thyroid make the radiation delivered to the thyroid gland by a standard dose very low. Consequently, the intravenous administration of large doses (>37 MBq [1 mCi]) permits, about 30 minutes later, adequate imaging of the thyroid.

Two radioactive isotopes of iodine have been used in thyroid imaging. Iodine 131 (^{131}I) was commonly used in the past and is still useful when functioning metastases of thyroid carcinoma are being sought; however, ^{131}I is a beta emitter, its physical half-life is 8.1 days, and the energy of its main gamma ray is high and thus poorly adapted for its detection. ^{123}I is, in many respects, ideal but is expensive. The energy of its main gamma ray is adapted for its detection by gamma cameras. Its short half-life (0.55 day) and the absence of beta radiation result in a radiation dose to the thyroid that is about 1% of that delivered by a comparable activity of ^{131}I.[2, 3] It is the isotope of choice for thyroid scintigraphy in pediatric practice.

Table 13–1. Radiation Nomenclature: Traditional and International System (SI) Units

Radiation dose	*Abbreviation*
1 Gy = 100 rad = absorption of 1 joule/kg	Gy = gray
1 rad = 0.01 Gy = 1 cGy	rad = radiation absorbed dose
1 Sv = 100 rem	rem = roentgen-equivalent-man
Radioactivity	
1 Bq = 1 disintegration per second	mCi = millicurie
	Bq = becquerel
1 mCi = 37 MBq	kBq = kilobecquerel
1 GBq = 10^3 MBq = 10^6 kBq = 10^9 Bq	MBq = megabecquerel
	GBq = gigabecquerel

The most important use of scintigraphic imaging of thyroid tissue is to define areas of increased or decreased function ("hot" or "cold" areas, respectively) relative to function of the remainder of the gland, provided that they are 1 cm in diameter or larger. Almost all malignant nodules are hypofunctioning, but more than 80% of benign nodules are also nonfunctioning. Conversely, functioning nodules (hot nodules), particularly if they are either more active than surrounding tissue or the sole functioning tissue, are rarely malignant.

In the past, several nuclear medical tests were used to evaluate thyroid disorders. In patients with a single area of thyroid uptake, scintiscans after administration of exogenous thyrotropin (TSH) may demonstrate the presence of hemiagenesis of the thyroid or document the functional capability of suppressed thyroid tissue. Conversely, scans performed after a period of exogenous thyroid hormone administration (suppression scans) can reveal areas of autonomous function that may not be detectable in baseline studies. These tests should no longer be used because the use of sensitive TSH assays and of scanning with a gamma camera permits the diagnosis of most of these hot nodules. Scintiscanning with radioactive iodine can also be used to demonstrate that intrathoracic masses represent thyroid tissue, to detect ectopic thyroid tissue in the neck, and to detect functioning metastases of thyroid carcinoma.

The choice of the scanning agent depends on many factors. ^{99m}Tc pertechnetate delivers a small dose of radiation to the thyroid gland, is readily available, and is inexpensive. Because imaging is performed soon after administration of the scanning agent, the entire procedure requires only a single visit to the laboratory. However, 5% to 10% of thyroid tumors appear to be functioning when examined with ^{99m}Tc pertechnetate but not with radioiodine. Because ^{99m}Tc pertechnetate imaging is done early, the intravascular activity and the activity in salivary tissue may obscure or confuse the findings. For the same reason, ^{99m}Tc pertechnetate is inappropriate for scanning substernal or intrathoracic goiter or for detecting ectopic tissue in the neck. In these cases, radioactive iodine should be used.

Total-body scanning is performed with ^{131}I in the follow-up of patients with papillary and follicular thyroid carcinoma. As detailed subsequently, radioiodine uptake by neoplastic tissue may be found only after TSH stimulation and is always lower than in normal thyroid tissue. For this reason, sufficiently high doses of ^{131}I should be given, and scanning should be performed 2 to 3 days after the dose (or even later), when background blood activity is low and when the contrast is optimal. Scanning conditions should be optimized, preferably by use of a gamma camera with two opposed heads equipped with thick crystals and high-energy collimators.

Scanning at low speed with spot images on regions of interest is performed. There are two aims: (1) to verify the completeness of ablation and to detect and localize foci of uptake, and (2) to quantify any uptake. This quantification permits a dosimetric evaluation that indicates the usefulness of ^{131}I treatment.

Fluorescent Scan

Fluorescent scanning provides information concerning the content of stable iodine within the gland.[4] In this technique, discrete zones of the thyroid gland are subjected to radiation from radioactive americium (^{241}Am) or from an x-ray tube. When incident radiation encounters ^{127}I, a fluorescent x-ray, registered by a suitable detector, is emitted. Nonfunctioning nodules generally have a low iodine content and are therefore cold on fluorescent scan; thyroid iodine is depleted during subacute thyroiditis[5] and increased during chronic iodine overload, such as with amiodarone treatment. The technique has limited clinical utility.

Ultrasonography

Sonography is noninvasive, is less expensive than computed tomography (CT) or magnetic resonance imaging (MRI), and produces no known tissue damage. No special preparation of the patient is necessary, and the technique requires only portable equipment, allowing it to be performed in the physician's examining room. A major limitation of ultrasonography is a high degree of observer dependence.

High-frequency sound waves are emitted by a transducer and reflected as they pass through the body, whereupon the returning echoes are received by the transducer, which also acts as a receiver. The amplitude of the reflections of the sound waves is influenced by differences in the acoustic impedance of the tissues encountered by the sound; for example, *fluid-filled* structures reflect few echoes and therefore have no or few internal echoes and well-defined margins; *solid* structures reflect varying amounts of sound and thus have varying degrees of internal echoes and less well-defined margins; and *calcified* structures reflect virtually all incoming sound and yield pronounced echoes with an acoustic "shadow" posteriorly.

High-frequency sound waves, such as those used in current thyroid sonography, are attenuated rapidly in the body tissues. Therefore, they cannot be used to image structures deeper than about 5 cm from the skin. Fortunately, the thyroid gland is usually well within this limit and can be completely imaged.[6]

High-frequency (7 to 13 MHz), small-parts instruments have become widely available since the middle 1980s and provide good spatial resolution and image quality.[7] The theoretical axial resolution of these systems is about 1 mm; no other thyroid imaging method can achieve this degree of resolution.[6] Intrathyroidal nodules as small as 3 mm in diameter and cystic nodules as small as 2 mm can be readily detected.[8] Color flow Doppler ultrasonography allows visualization of very small vessels, so that vascularity of thyroid nodules can be assessed, but its diagnostic performance for malignancy is lower, as compared with fine-needle aspiration biopsy (FNAB).

Thyroid sonography is typically performed with the patient supine. The patient's neck is hyperextended by a pad centered under the scapulae to provide optimal exposure. The examiner usually sits at the head of the examining table and can steady the transducer by resting an elbow or a forearm on the table next to the patient's head. The thyroid gland must be examined thoroughly in transverse and longitudinal planes. Imaging of the lower poles can be enhanced by swallowing, which momentarily raises the thyroid gland in the neck. The examination should cover the entire gland, including the isthmus. Imaging should also include the region of the carotid artery and jugular vein to identify enlarged cervical lymph nodes.[6]

The normal thyroid parenchyma has a characteristic homogeneous medium-level echogenicity, with little identifiable in-

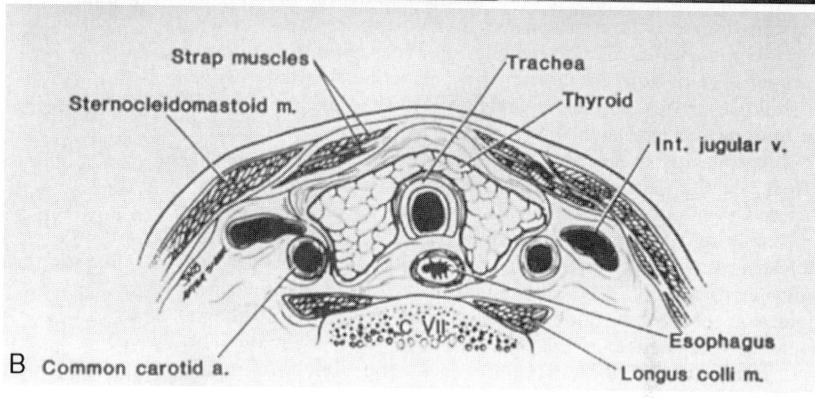

Figure 13–1. Transverse composite sonogram (*A*) and corresponding anatomic map (*B*) of the normal thyroid gland. C, common carotid artery; CVII, seventh cervical vertebra; LC, longus colli muscle; SM, strap muscles; SCM, sternocleidomastoid muscle; T, thyroid; TR, trachea. (From Rifkin MD, Charboneau JW, Laing FC. Special course: ultrasound 1991. In Reading CC [ed]. Syllabus: Thyroid, Parathyroid, and Cervical Lymph Nodes. Oak Brook, Ill, Radiological Society of North America, 1991, pp 363–377.)

ternal architecture (Fig. 13–1). The surrounding muscles have the appearance of hypoechoic structures. The air-filled trachea in the midline gives a characteristic curvilinear reflecting surface with an associated reverberation artifact. The esophagus is usually hidden from sonographic visualization by the tracheal air shadow. A portion of the esophagus, however, may swing laterally, usually toward the left, where it may lie adjacent to the posteromedial surface of the thyroid.

Neck ultrasonography may confirm the presence of a thyroid nodule when the findings on physical examination are equivocal. A diagrammatic representation of the neck showing the location or locations of any abnormal finding is a useful supplement to the routine film images recorded during an ultrasound examination.[6] Such a cervical map (Fig. 13–2) can help communicate the anatomic relationships of the pathology more clearly to the referring clinician and serves as a reference for the sonographer on follow-up examinations.

In patients with known thyroid cancer, sonography can be useful in evaluating the extent of disease, both preoperatively and postoperatively. In most instances, sonography is not performed routinely before thyroidectomy but can be useful in patients with large cervical masses for evaluation of nearby structures (e.g., the carotid artery and internal jugular vein) to exclude the possibility of direct invasion or encasement by the tumor.

Alternatively, in patients who present with cervical lymphadenopathy caused by papillary thyroid carcinoma (PTC) but in whom the gland is palpably normal, sonography may be used preoperatively to detect an occult, primary intrathyroid focus. Some surgeons do regularly obtain a preoperative sonogram in patients with PTC or medullary thyroid carcinoma (MTC) in order to identify prior to surgery the anatomic locations of any sonographically suspicious regional lymph nodes and thereby to permit planning of the extent of nodal dissection. Occasionally, a hand-held ultrasound probe can be used intraoperatively to identify impalpable residual cancer that has been identified by preoperative ultrasonography and proved to be cytologically positive by ultrasound-guided FNAB.

After surgery for thyroid cancer, sonography is the preferred method for detecting residual, recurrent, or metastatic disease in the neck.[9] In patients who have undergone less than a near-total thyroidectomy, the sonographic appearance of the remaining thyroid tissue may be an important factor in the decision whether to recommend completion thyroidectomy. Also, it is more sensitive than neck palpation in detecting recurrent disease within the thyroid bed and metastatic disease in cervical lymph nodes.[10, 11] The location at the lower part of the neck and the sonographic appearance (hypoechoic, without a central echogenic line), the size (>1 cm in diameter), the

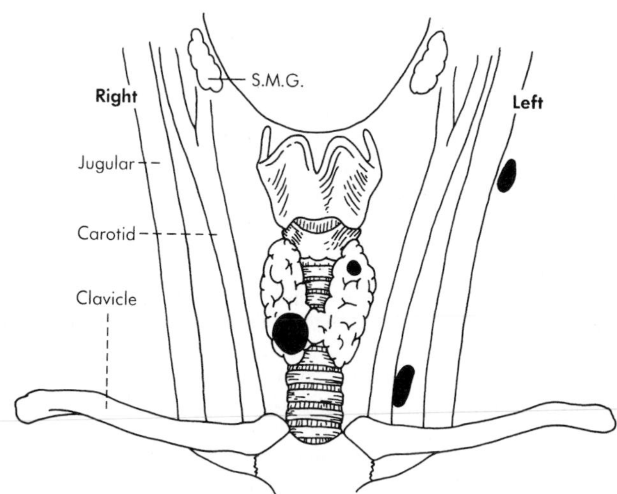

Figure 13–2. Cervical map, derived from sonographic images, helps to communicate anatomic relationships of pathology to clinicians and serves as a reference for follow-up examinations. SMG, submandibular gland. (From James EM, Charboneau JW, Hay ID. The thyroid. In Rumack CM, Wilson SR, Charboneau JW [eds]. Diagnostic Ultrasound, vol 1. St. Louis, Mosby–Year Book, 1991, pp 507–528.)

shape (round), the presence of fine microcalcifications or a cystic component, and the use of color Doppler ultrasonography (hypervascularization) may aid in recognition of lymph node metastases. Sonography may also be useful to guide fine-needle biopsy of thyroid bed masses and lymph nodes, especially when these abnormalities are not palpable.[10–12]

Computed Tomography

The CT appearance of the anatomic structures depends on the attenuation of the tissue examined. The thyroid gland, because of its high concentration of iodine, has higher attenuation than do the surrounding soft tissues.[13]

The diagnostic utility of CT in the evaluation of nodular thyroid disease is limited because thyroid masses, whether benign or malignant, may be hypodense, hyperdense, or isodense compared with adjacent normal thyroid tissue.[14] In aggressive pathologic processes, such as anaplastic thyroid carcinoma, CT can define the extension of the tumor to the mediastinum and its relationships to surrounding structures, such as the carotid artery, jugular vein, and trachea, before attempted surgical excision. In patients with known thyroid cancer, CT is less useful in evaluating recurrence in the neck because of the difficulty in detecting small masses in the indistinct tissue planes in the postoperative neck.[15] CT imaging can, however, improve the detection of lymph node metastases in the neck, although there is considerable overlap in the appearance of malignant and inflammatory nodes and CT lacks the ability to guide fine-needle biopsy of minimally enlarged nodes.[7] In patients with thyroid cancer, CT is used most frequently to search for lymph node metastases in the mediastinum and for distant metastases in the chest and abdomen.

CT scanning can provide useful information regarding the presence and extent of intrathoracic (substernal) goiters. The CT findings of an intrathoracic mass in continuity with the thyroid gland, with high attenuation on non–contrast-enhanced images and marked enhancement after intravenous contrast material injection, all suggest intrathoracic goiter.[16] Radionuclide scanning can also be performed in this clinical setting, but false-negative results can occur when little or no functional tissue is present in the intrathoracic goiter. Because of the necessity of infusing iodine-containing contrast agents, CT should be performed at least 4 weeks before any radioiodine therapy.[15]

Magnetic Resonance Imaging

Because the hydrogen atoms of different tissues have different relaxation times (termed T1 and T2), a computer-assisted analysis of T1-weighted and T2-weighted signals is used to differentiate the thyroid gland from skeletal muscles, blood vessels, or regional lymph nodes. Normal thyroid tissue tends to be slightly more intense than muscle on a T1-weighted image, and tumors often appear more intense than normal thyroid tissue.

MRI is rapidly evolving, with improvements in spatial resolution, reduction of artifacts, and development of new contrast agents. Currently obtained MR images have superior tissue contrast resolution but poorer spatial resolution than comparable CT images. Like CT, MRI does not distinguish benign from malignant nodules and does not assess functional status[17]; however, it can define the anatomic extent of large goiters with great clarity.[18] Coronal and sagittal images provide a simultaneous view of the cervical and thoracic components of substernal goiters. The relation of the goiter to surrounding vessels in the mediastinum is also well visualized.[19]

Recurrent neoplasms in the thyroid bed or regional lymph nodes can be detected with MRI; MRI is more accurate than palpation and comparable in accuracy to CT.[20] Recurrence is characterized by a mass with low to medium intensity on T1-weighted images and medium to high signal intensity on T2-weighted images. Conversely, scar tissue or fibrous tissue has low signal intensity on both T1-weighted and T2-weighted images. Tumor invasion of adjacent skeletal muscle has high signal intensity on T2-weighted images.[21] Edema or inflammation in the muscle can cause a similar appearance and can be difficult to differentiate from recurrent tumor.[17]

Positron Emission Tomography

Positron emission tomography (PET) is a special nuclear medical imaging technique that is both quantitative and tomographic. The radionuclide used emits a positron that is converted into a pair of photons after a short path of a few millimeters in the tissue. The coincidence detection of the two photons, which travel on a line in opposite directions, permits the localization of the site of the radionuclide decay.

The agent most widely used with PET is [^{18}F]fluorodeoxyglucose (^{18}FDG). This agent is transported and phosphorylated as a glucose substitute but remains metabolically trapped inside tumor cells because of its inability to undergo glycolysis.

PET scanners with a large field of view permit in vivo images related to regional glucose metabolism, with high sensitivity and a spatial resolution less than 5 mm. Superimposition of CT and PET images greatly improves both the sensitivity and specificity of the technique and the anatomic localization of any focus of abnormal uptake. Elevated glucose metabolism is present in most malignant tumor tissues, and PET scanning has been shown to be particularly useful for the detection of lymph node metastases in the neck or mediastinum in patients with papillary and follicular thyroid carcinoma who have no tumoral radioiodine uptake.[22–24] High uptake has also been observed in several thyroid diseases, such as thyroiditis, but PET cannot be used to differentiate benign from malignant thyroid nodules.

SIMPLE (NONTOXIC) GOITER: DIFFUSE AND MULTINODULAR

Simple, or nontoxic, goiter may be defined as any thyroid enlargement that is not associated with hyperthyroidism or hypothyroidism and that does not result from inflammation or neoplasia. The term is usually restricted to the form that occurs sporadically or in regions that are not the locus of endemic goiter (i.e., where more than 10% of the children in the population have a thyroid enlargement) as a result of iodine deficiency. Although the term *simple goiter* is useful in indicating the presence of the characteristics just noted, the condition can be a result of different underlying abnormalities.[25]

Pathogenesis and Pathophysiology

Goiter has been traditionally regarded as the adaptive response of the thyroid follicular cell to any factor that impairs thyroid hormone synthesis. This classic concept no longer appears to encompass the many aspects of goiters. Indeed, goiter is characterized by a variety of clinical, functional, and morphologic presentations, and whether this heterogeneity represents different entities remains to be clarified. Also, iodine deficiency as the sole factor responsible for goiter appears to be an oversimplification. Thus, not all inhabitants in an iodine-deficient region develop goiter; moreover, endemic goiter has been observed in countries with no iodine deficiency, and even with iodine excess, and has not been observed in some regions with severe iodine deficiency. These findings suggest that other factors, both genetic and environmental, may play a role in the genesis of simple and nodular goiter, and some of these factors may act synergistically.

The role of genetic factors is suggested by several lines of evidence,[26, 27] such as

1. The clustering of goiters within families.
2. The higher concordance rate for goiters in monozygotic than in dizygotic twins.
3. The female/male ratio (1 : 1 in endemic versus 7 : 1 to 9 : 1 in sporadic goiters).
4. The persistence of goiters in areas where a widespread iodine prophylaxis program has been properly implemented.

By studying families affected by goiter, researchers have been able to detect several gene abnormalities involving proteins related to thyroid hormone synthesis, such as mutations in thyroglobulin (*Tg*),[28] sodium/iodide symporter (*NIS*),[29] thyroid peroxidase (*TPO*),[30] pendrin syndrome (*PDS*),[31] and TSH receptor (*TSHR*)[32] genes. In addition, two loci for this disorder have been identified. The first locus, identified on chromosome 14q, was designated *MNG1* (Online Mendelian Inheritance in Man [OMIM] 138800) for multinodular goiter 1[33]; the other, *MNG2* (OMIM 300273), maps to chromosome Xp22.[34] Although an autosomal dominant inheritance has been demonstrated in several families, multiple genes may be involved in other families. This may explain why predisposing gene alterations remain unidentified in most patients with simple goiter. Such genetic predispositions are believed to cause abnormalities in thyroid hormone synthesis. Thus, in some cases, defects can be detected by abnormalities of perchlorate discharge (see Chapter 10); more often, however, no abnormality can be demonstrated.[35]

Goiter should thus be regarded as a complex trait in which both genetic susceptibility and environmental factors probably contribute to the development of disease. Whereas iodine deficiency represents the main environmental factor in the genesis of endemic goiter, other factors, such as cigarette smoking, infections, drugs, and goitrogens, may play a role in the genesis of goitrous disease together with a genetic background of susceptibility. Interestingly, in a population-based twin study, a critical role of the genetic background in the etiology of goiter was demonstrated in females.[27]

TSH has long been considered the major agent determining thyroid growth in response to any factor that impairs thyroid hormone synthesis. When such factors are operative, hypersecretion of TSH stimulates thyroid growth and increases the aspects of hormone biosynthesis that are capable of response. As a consequence of the increase in thyroid mass and functional activity, a normal rate of hormone secretion is restored and the patient is goitrous but eumetabolic. Indeed, in the rare clinical setting of functioning TSH-secreting pituitary tumor, the increased blood TSH levels typically cause an enlargement of the thyroid gland.[36]

It is interesting that goiter is also a typical part of the clinical picture of Graves' disease, in which a stimulatory growth effect on thyroid tissue is induced by thyroid-stimulating antibody through TSHR activation.[37] Moreover, thyroid enlargement may appear during the course of Graves' disease when increased TSH levels result from overtreatment with antithyroid drugs. In addition, toxic thyroid hyperplasia is usually present in non-autoimmune autosomal dominant hyperthyroidism, a disorder related to germ line–activating mutations of the *TSHR* gene.[32] This clinical condition further emphasizes the role of TSH-TSHR system activation in the genesis of thyroid hyperplasia in diffuse nontoxic or toxic goiter.

This concept of the pathogenesis of nontoxic goiter is inconsistent with the fact that the serum TSH concentration is normal in most patients with nontoxic goiter.[38, 39] Nonetheless, a participatory role of TSH in the maintenance of goiter is indicated by the regression of goiter that sometimes follows administration of suppressive doses of thyroid hormone.

Several possible mechanisms may accommodate these apparently divergent findings. The mechanism with experimental support in rats is that iodine depletion enhances the promotion of thyroid growth by TSH.[39] Hence, any factor that impairs intrathyroidal iodine levels may lead to gradual development of goiter in response to normal concentrations of TSH.

A second possibility is that the increase in serum TSH concentration is significant but too small to be detected by immunoassay methods.

Finally, a goitrogenic stimulus may have been present in the past but may no longer be detectable at the time of study. Thus, the residual normal TSH concentration can maintain—but not initiate—the goiter. However, this primary, if not exclusive, role for TSH in determining thyroid growth and hyperplasia has been challenged.[40–42] Indeed, a complex network of both TSH-dependent and TSH-independent pathways directs thyroid follicular cell growth and function and plays a role in the goitrogenic process. In particular, a variety of growth factors, derived either from the blood stream or through autocrine or paracrine secretion, may serve to regulate thyroid cell proliferation and differentiation processes.[43] Among these factors, epidermal growth factor (EGF) and insulin-like growth factor (IGF) have been recognized as thyroid growth–promoting substances in different species.

IGF-I stimulates cell proliferation and differentiation (i.e., thyroglobulin expression) in thyroid tissue both in vitro and in vivo. Indeed, enhanced IGF-I expression may play a role in the goitrogenic process. In this regard, it is worth emphasizing that acromegalic patients with elevated levels of serum growth hormone and IGF-I and normal TSH levels have an increased prevalence of goiter.[44] Similarly, fibroblast growth factor (FGF) stimulates thyroid function, and its expression has been associated with thyroid hyperplasia. Interestingly, the proliferation effect of these growth factors also occurs through stimulation of their respective receptors in thyrocytes. Other factors, including IGF-binding proteins (IGF-BPs), transforming growth factor α and β, cytokines, prostaglandins, norepinephrine, acetylcholine, and vasoactive intestinal peptide, may also participate in the regulation of thyroid cell proliferation. However, the relative contribution of these factors to the goitrogenic process has not yet been clarified.

In the propylthiouracil-induced goiter in the rat, Wollman and colleagues[45] recognized the importance of the development of new blood vessels in goiter formation and demonstrated that growth of perifollicular blood vessels was induced by angiogenic factors produced by follicular cells. Indeed, many molecules involved in promoting or inhibiting thyroid angiogenesis, including vascular endothelial growth factor, angiopoietins 1 and 2, hepatocyte growth factor, endothelin, angiogenin or thrombospondin, angiostatin, and endostatin, have now been identified.[46]

Goitrogenesis, therefore, appears to be a complex process in which TSH, growth factors, and angiogenic substances either play a distinct and separate role or act synergistically through complex interaction mechanisms.

Another pathogenetic concept is based on autoradiographic and clinical studies of normal thyroid tissue and nontoxic and toxic multinodular goiters.[47] Early in the course of goiter formation, areas of microheterogeneity of structure and function are intermixed and include areas of functional autonomy and small areas of focal hemorrhage. Indeed, as judged from the presence of scattered foci of persistent radioiodine uptake in the thyroid glands of patients given suppressive doses of thy-

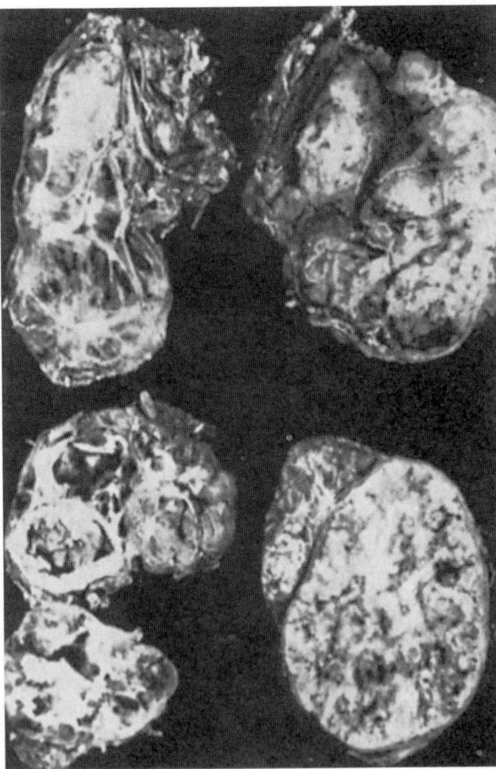

Figure 13–3. Outer and cut surfaces of a nontoxic nodular goiter of 15 years' duration. Note variations in size and structure of the nodules; there are thick areas of fibrous tissue, flecks of calcium, scattered areas of thyroid tissue, cysts, and small hemorrhages.

roid hormone before surgery, some cells with functional autonomy are present in the normal thyroid gland; this is in accordance with the heterogeneous staining for NIS observed in normal thyroid and goitrous tissues.[48] Thus, in addition to the variability in thyroid microcirculation, heterogeneity may result from clonal differences among cells that give rise to thyroid follicles, some being more and some less responsive to external stimulation factors, including TSH, and others being autonomous from the outset. This concept implies that the anatomic and functional heterogeneity observed within the thyroid at the outset of the disease is exaggerated by prolonged stimulation.

Further insights into the pathogenesis of sporadic multinodular goiter have been gained by assessment of the clonality of individual thyroid nodules. *Polyclonality* implies a multicellular origin related to the proliferation of a group of cells, whereas a *monoclonal* tumor is thought to be formed by expansion of a single cell.[49] Studies involving X-chromosome inactivation analysis have produced variable results in multinodular goiters. Some dominant nodules are monoclonal, especially if they showed evidence of recent rapid growth.[50] Other researchers have found a monoclonal pattern in only a minority of large nodules.[51]

Two groups reported that in multinodular glands more than one nodule can be monoclonal, and both monoclonal and polyclonal nodules can coexist within the same gland.[52, 53] Analysis of hyperplastic nodules by rigid criteria[54] also indicated that morphologically indistinguishable hyperplastic thyroid nodules may be either monoclonal or polyclonal. Monoclonal adenomas within hyperplastic thyroid glands may reflect a stage in progression along the hyperplasia-neoplasia spectrum; accumulation of multiple somatic mutations may subsequently confer a selective growth advantage to this single-cell clone.[54]

Cytogenetic[55] and in situ hybridization[56] studies also support the idea of a biologic continuum and karyotypic evolution between hyperplastic nodules and true follicular adenomas.[57]

Eventually, the amount of functionally autonomous tissue in a multinodular goiter may be sufficient to suppress TSH secretion.[38, 58] Ultimately, autonomous hyperfunction may be sufficient to produce subclinical or overt thyrotoxicosis, or thyrotoxicosis may supervene when the patient is exposed to an iodine load. For this reason, patients with nontoxic multinodular goiter should not be given medications that contain iodine and should be observed after radiologic procedures that involve administration of iodinated contrast media. Some investigators administer antithyroid agents to patients with nodular goiter who are to receive agents containing iodine. This is a reasonable suggestion, especially in areas of iodine deficiency where jodbasedow is likely to occur.

Nontoxic goiter has a female preponderance (7:1 to 9:1) and seems to be common during adolescence or pregnancy. There appears to be no physiologic increase in thyroid volume during normal adolescence, and development of a goiter during adolescence is a pathologic rather than a physiologic process.[59] However, as evidenced by sonographic measurement of thyroid volume in women living in an area of moderate iodine intake, normal pregnancy is goitrogenic, especially in women with preexisting thyroid disorders.[60] The increased thyroid volume during pregnancy is associated with biochemical features of thyroid stimulation (i.e., an increased triiodothyronine/thyroxine [T_3/T_4] ratio) owing to slightly elevated serum TSH levels at delivery or a high human chorionic gonadotropin (hCG) concentration during the first trimester.[60–62] Repeated pregnancies may play a role in the development of later thyroid disorders, a relation that might explain the high prevalence of thyroid disorders in women.[63]

Pathology

Simple goiter is a noninflammatory, non-neoplastic, diffuse or nodular enlargement of the thyroid gland without hyperthyroidism.[64] The gland is usually large and may have a distorted shape (Fig. 13–3). The cut surface shows areas of nodularity, fibrosis, hemorrhage, and calcification. The nodules vary in size, number, and appearance, the last according to their colloid or cellular content. Single or multiple cystic areas may contain colloid or brown fluid, representing previous hemorrhage.

Histologically, nodules contain irregularly enlarged, involuted follicles distended with colloid or clusters of smaller follicles lined by taller epithelium and containing small colloid droplets. These microfollicles may be surrounded by an edematous or a fibrous stroma. Large nodules tend to compress the surrounding parenchyma and may have a partially developed fibrous capsule. Markedly distended follicles may coalesce to form colloid cysts several millimeters in diameter.

The nodules tend to be incompletely encapsulated and are poorly demarcated from and merge with the internodular tissue, which also has an altered architecture. However, the nodules in some glands appear to be localized, with areas of apparently normal architecture elsewhere. Here, the distinction from a follicular adenoma may be difficult, and some pathologists apply terms such as *colloid* or *adenomatous* nodules to such lesions. Studies of clonality may be helpful in distinguishing between focal or nodular hyperplasia and true adenomas.[65, 66] Whereas nodular goiters are polyclonal in origin, solitary thyroid nodules are monoclonal and therefore true benign neoplasms.[51]

Clinical Picture

Diffuse or nodular goiters are usually not associated with abnormal thyroid hormone secretion. Therefore, affected patients do not exhibit clinical symptoms or signs of thyroid dysfunction. The only clinical features of nontoxic goiter are those of thyroid enlargement. Nearly 70% of patients with sporadic nontoxic goiter complain of neck discomfort; the remainder have cosmetic concerns or a fear of possible malignancy.[67]

Large goiter, which may displace or compress the trachea, esophagus, and neck vessels, can be associated with symptoms and signs including inspiratory stridor, dysphagia, and a choking sensation. These obstructive symptoms may be accentuated by the so-called Pemberton maneuver. This maneuver, which consists of "elevating both arms until they touch the sides of the head," is considered positive if, after a minute or so, congestion of the face, some cyanosis, and lastly distress become apparent.[68] Compression of the recurrent laryngeal nerve, with hoarseness, suggests carcinoma rather than nontoxic goiter, but vocal cord paralysis can occasionally result from benign nodular goiters.[69] Hemorrhage into a nodule or cyst produces acute, painful enlargement locally and may enhance or induce obstructive symptoms.

Endogenous subclinical thyrotoxicosis caused by autonomously functioning nodules should be carefully investigated. It is particularly relevant in elderly patients, whose cardiac morphology and function may be affected, thereby increasing their risk of developing cardiac arrhythmias.[70]

Laboratory Tests

Serum TSH, measured in a highly sensitive immunometric assay, combined with a single measurement of free thyroid hormone concentrations may be used as a first-line screening test. Serum free thyroid hormones and TSH are, by definition, within the normal range. However, the T_3/T_4 ratio may be increased, perhaps reflecting defective iodination of Tg. Patients with sporadic nontoxic goiter tend to have high-normal free T_4 and T_3 concentrations and low TSH levels.[67] The prevalence of so-called subclinical hyperthyroidism is higher when patients with nodular goiter have clear-cut autonomous areas on scintigraphy.[71]

An undetectable serum TSH, even associated with normal free thyroid hormone levels, should suggest the possibility of toxic, autonomously functioning nodular areas in the goiter. Such a finding should prompt further cardiac investigation, especially in elderly patients, whose risk of atrial fibrillation may be increased as much as threefold when serum TSH levels are less than 0.1 mU/L.[72] Moreover, it has been demonstrated that this condition, by affecting cardiac morphology and function, has a relevant clinical impact even in young patients and that many patients are, in fact, symptomatic. Therefore, this disorder should be considered a mild form of tissue thyrotoxicosis that may necessitate treatment.[73]

In a cross-sectional study of 102 patients with sporadic nontoxic goiter, the serum TSH level correlated negatively with the thyroid volume, which in turn correlated positively with both the age of the patient and the duration of the goiter.[67] In a prospective study of 242 patients with nodular goiter, no correlation was found between thyroid volume and any thyroid biochemical parameters, but there were significant negative correlations between the number of nodules identified by ultrasonography and the levels of basal TSH and the TSH response to thyrotropin-releasing hormone (TRH) stimulation.[71]

Imaging in Goiter Evaluation

A diagnosis of goiter usually does not warrant the use of imaging procedures. When a nodular goiter is present, however, both scintigraphy and sonography provide useful information for disease management and treatment. Indeed, the former should be used to detect hot or warm nodules in the thyroid tissue. This finding affects the therapeutic approach. Sonography should be used to assess both morphology and size of the goiter.[74] Thus, sonography in patients with a nodular goiter may allow a determination of the number and the individual features of the nodules and serve as guidance for FNAB.[75] Sonography also permits an accurate, objective measure of goiter growth over time or after treatment.

Conventional radiography of the neck and the upper mediastinum should be used to determine the presence of tracheal compression. CT and MRI are indicated in the presence of intrathoracic goiter to define the relationships with surrounding structures.

Differential Diagnosis

The differential diagnosis of nontoxic goiter can be considered in functional and anatomic terms. As indicated, the same factors that lead to goitrous hypothyroidism can, if they are less severe, cause nontoxic goiter. Consequently, some patients with putative nontoxic goiter are slightly hypothyroid. On the other hand, foci of autonomous function may develop in multinodular goiters in which the spectrum of function can range from clinical euthyroidism with intact regulatory control to euthyroidism with some degree of functional autonomy to thyrotoxicosis.[76]

Anatomically, the diffuse stage of nontoxic goiter can resemble the thyroid of either Graves' or Hashimoto's disease. If Graves' disease is not in an actively thyrotoxic phase, and if the ocular manifestations are lacking, there is no way to distinguish between the two except to demonstrate the presence of TSHR antibody in the serum. In one study of 108 patients with diffuse nontoxic goiter observed for more than 5 years, 33% had a family history of autoimmune thyroid disease and five patients developed Graves' disease during follow-up.[77] Diffuse nontoxic goiter is sometimes also difficult to differentiate from Hashimoto's disease, although the thyroid of Hashimoto's disease is usually firmer and more irregular. Demonstration of high titers of antithyroid antibodies should indicate autoimmune disease.

In its multinodular stage, nontoxic goiter may suggest thyroid carcinoma. The approach to distinguishing between the two is discussed in the following section on thyroid neoplasms.

Treatment

Patients with small, asymptomatic goiters can be monitored by clinical examination and evaluated periodically with ultrasound measurements. In fact, goiter growth can be variable, and some patients have stable goiters for many years.

For more than a century, thyroid "feeding" has been employed to reduce the size of nontoxic goiters.[78] The 1953 report of Greer and Astwood, in which two thirds of patients' goiters regressed with thyroid therapy, led to widespread acceptance of suppressive therapy[79] despite some doubts about the value of such therapy.[80, 81] An overview of studies performed from 1960 to 1992 suggested that 60% or more of sporadic nontoxic goiters respond to suppressive therapy.[80] In a prospective placebo-controlled, double-blind randomized clinical trial, 58% of the thyroxine-treated group had a significant response at 9 months, as measured by ultrasonography, in contrast with 5% after placebo.[82] However, ultrasonographic measurement of goiter size demonstrated a return to pretherapy values within 3 months of treatment discontinuation.[83]

Therefore, maintenance of the size reduction may require continuous long-term treatment. Nodular goiters appear to be less responsive than diffuse goiters, and the therapeutic efficacy of thyroxine treatment is increased in younger patients and in those with small or recently diagnosed goiters.[80]

It has been proposed that a basal serum TSH greater than

1 mU/L in a patient with sporadic nontoxic goiter is an indication to administer levothyroxine to lower the serum TSH level to the low-normal range (0.5 to 1.0 mU/L). Others[84] have suggested that TSH levels on treatment should be subnormal but not profoundly suppressed (0.1 to 0.3 mU/L). The validity of this approach remains to be ascertained. If the goiter size decreases or remains stable, treatment should be continued indefinitely, with periodic monitoring of serum TSH levels to detect possible development of functional autonomy.[85]

A major concern in relation to long-term thyroxine suppression therapy is the possibility of detrimental effects on the skeleton and heart.[86] It has been reported that TSH suppression therapy is associated with variable degrees of bone loss, particularly in postmenopausal women.[87, 88] However, other studies did not demonstrate significant change in bone mass after long-term thyroxine therapy.[89, 90] Furthermore, although marginal cardiac changes may occur with levothyroxine therapy, there is no evidence that levothyroxine per se is detrimental to the heart.[86] It is now generally accepted that TSH should be suppressed with the lowest effective dose of levothyroxine,[80, 85, 86, 89] usually between 1.5 and 2.0 μg/kg body weight per day; the risk of deleterious effects may be minimized by monitoring serum TSH and free T_3 concentrations.[86]

Surgery for simple nontoxic goiter is physiologically unsound because it further restricts the ability of the thyroid to meet hormone requirements. Nevertheless, surgery may become necessary because of persistence of obstructive manifestations despite a trial of levothyroxine. Surgery, which should consist of a near-total or total thyroidectomy, rapidly and effectively removes the goiter, but recurrence is seen in about 10% to 20% within 10 years.[91] Surgical complications have been reported in 7% to 10% of cases and are more common with large goiters and with reoperation.[92] Prophylactic treatment with levothyroxine after goiter resection probably does not prevent recurrence of goiter.[93, 94]

Traditionally, the role of ^{131}I therapy for nontoxic goiter was to reduce the size of a massive goiter in elderly patients who were poor candidates for surgery[95, 96] or to treat goiter that recurs after resection.[97] However, several studies have demonstrated that primary treatment of multinodular goiter with ^{131}I is followed by a reduction in thyroid volume (Fig. 13–4).[98, 99] In one study, thyroid volume (assessed by ultrasonography) was reduced by 40% after 1 year and 55% after 2 years with no further reduction thereafter,[98] and 60% of the total reduction occurred within the first 3 months.

A randomized trial comparing levothyroxine at suppressive doses with radioactive iodine treatment (120 μCi/g corrected for 24-hour thyroid uptake) showed impressive differences in outcome. After ^{131}I therapy, 97% of patients responded, with a mean decrease in goiter size of 39% at 1 year and 46% at 2 years; the initial side effects were neck tenderness and slight thyrotoxic symptoms in 12% of patients, and at 2 years 35% of patients were hypothyroid and 10% had subclinical thyrotoxicosis. In contrast, with levothyroxine therapy 43% of patients responded with a mean decrease of 23% at 1 year and 22% at 2 years; the initial side effect was a mild thyrotoxicosis in 30% of patients and at 2 years a significant decrement in spine bone density.[88]

It was formerly argued that treatment of large goiters or goiters with substernal extension with ^{131}I should be avoided because of the risks of acute swelling of the gland and consequent tracheal compression.[100] Ultrasonographic studies of thyroid volume after ^{131}I have failed to demonstrate significant early volume increase.[101] Moreover, decreased tracheal deviation and increased tracheal lumen size were demonstrable by MRI in patients who had compression by nontoxic goiters with substernal extension.[96]

Therefore, it appears that ^{131}I treatment of nontoxic multinodular goiter is effective and safe,[81] but hypothyroidism may occur in 22% to 40% within 5 years after ^{131}I therapy.[98, 99] Regular follow-up, preferably by a systematic annual recall scheme, is necessary.[102] Although reassuring data are available on the long-term thyroid and nonthyroidal cancer risk after ^{131}I treatment in hyperthyroidism,[103, 104] the follow-up of patients with ^{131}I-treated nontoxic goiters is short-term and involves small numbers of patients. Children and adolescents should not be treated with ^{131}I. Stimulation with low doses of recombinant human TSH (rhTSH) (0.01 to 0.03 mg) increases the thyroid ^{131}I uptake and therefore may allow the administration of a lower dosage of ^{131}I.[105] Long-term randomized studies comparing the effects, side effects, and costs and benefits of surgery and ^{131}I treatment need to be performed.[81]

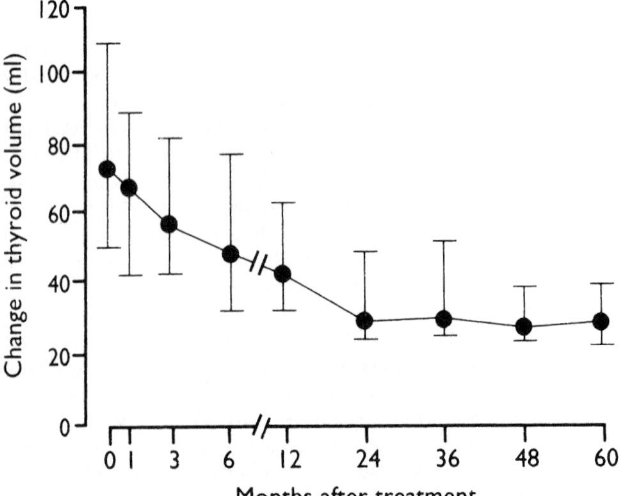

Figure 13–4. Median changes in thyroid volume alterations after iodine 131 treatment in 39 patients with nontoxic multinodular goiter who remained euthyroid after a single dose. *Bars* represent quartiles. (From Nygaard B, Hegedus L, Gervil M, et al. Radioiodine treatment of multinodular nontoxic goiter. BMJ 1993; 307:828–832.)

THYROID NEOPLASIA

In an era when patients are advised on self-examination to detect cancer at an early stage, the finding of a palpable mass in such a superficial location as the thyroid gland can be disconcerting. The affected patient is likely to seek medical evaluation. At the end of an appropriate investigation, the clinician can usually reassure the patient that the nodule is benign. Alternatively, if the evaluation does suggest malignancy, the patient can be advised that the management of typical thyroid cancer is effective and usually consists of surgical resection,[106] followed by medical therapy[107] and regular surveillance.[108] The major challenge in this circumstance is to determine whether the discovered thyroid nodule is malignant.

Some degree of consensus has been achieved with regard to both the initial evaluation of nodular thyroid disease[109–111] and the management of differentiated thyroid cancer,[112–114] but important clinical and biologic questions remain unanswered.[115–117] In the following discussion, we describe a clinical approach to nodular thyroid disease and present a widely used scheme for classifying and staging tumors of the thyroid gland. We also review the features of the principal types of benign and malignant thyroid neoplasms and the controversies in the management of differentiated thyroid carcinoma.

Initial Investigation

Thyroid tumors are the most common endocrine neoplasms. They usually arise as anterior neck nodules that usually can be localized to the thyroid gland by palpation. Most of these nodules are benign hyperplastic (or colloid) nodules or benign follicular adenomas, but about 5% to 10% of nodules coming to medical attention are carcinomas. Differentiating true neoplasms from hyperplastic nodules and distinguishing between benign and malignant tumors are major challenges.

Moreover, with the widespread practice of medical checkups in healthy individuals and the increasing use of imaging technology, this problem is likely to become more common. High-resolution ultrasound studies suggest that the prevalence of nodular thyroid disease in healthy adults is above 60%.[118] However, during 2001 in the United States, only about 19,500 new cases of thyroid cancer were likely to be diagnosed.[119] Therefore, most of these so-called thyroid incidentalomas are obviously benign and do not progress to clinical tumors.[120]

In identifying the nodules that are likely to be malignant, a thorough history and a careful physical examination should be supplemented with laboratory testing, imaging procedures, and, most important, FNAB of the nodule in question. With the use of this approach, it is possible to assess the likelihood of malignancy and to advise appropriate treatment in the majority of patients.

History and Physical Examination

Historical features that favor benign disease include the following:

1. A family history of Hashimoto's thyroiditis, benign thyroid nodule, or goiter.
2. Symptoms of hypothyroidism or hyperthyroidism.
3. A sudden increase in size of the nodule with pain or tenderness, suggesting a cyst or localized subacute thyroiditis.

Historical features that suggest malignancy include the following:

1. Young (<20 years old) or old (>70 years old) age;
2. Male sex;
3. A history of external neck radiation during childhood or adolescence;
4. Recent changes in speaking, breathing, or swallowing;
5. A family history of thyroid cancer or multiple endocrine neoplasia (MEN) type 2.

On physical examination, manifestations of thyroid malignancy should be sought, including firm consistency of the nodule, irregular shape, fixation to underlying or overlying tissues, and suspicious regional lymphadenopathy.

In both prospective[121] and retrospective[122, 123] studies, the sensitivity and specificity rates for detecting thyroid malignancy by history and physical examination were about 60% and 80%, respectively. In these historical series, only about 20% of patients with later confirmed malignancy had, when initially seen, neither suspicious historical features nor evidence of potential malignancy on neck examination. Further testing may include assessment of thyroid function, measurement of tumor markers, genetic screening, thyroid imaging, and the only decisive parameter, FNAB.

Laboratory Evaluation

The serum TSH level is measured to exclude thyroid dysfunction. Patients with thyroid cancer rarely have abnormalities in serum TSH levels. A low (suppressed) serum TSH level may indicate a toxic nodule and should lead to thyroid scintigraphy. Measurement of serum anti-TPO antibody and anti-Tg antibody levels may be helpful in diagnosis of chronic autoimmune thyroiditis, especially if the serum TSH level is elevated. In chronic autoimmune thyroiditis, the thyroid gland's size and consistency may simulate either a solitary nodule or bilateral nodules. Evidence of autoimmune thyroiditis, however, does not preclude the presence of cancer in the gland.

Follicular cell–derived thyroid cancers (FCTCs) may release increased amounts of Tg into the blood stream. Unfortunately, there is overlap of serum Tg levels in FCTCs and in a number of benign conditions, and measurement of serum Tg levels is not useful in the initial work-up of nodular thyroid disease.[111] Similarly, some investigators[124] routinely measure calcitonin (Ct) levels in all patients with nodular thyroid disease to identify cases of MTC. In fact, the calcitonin level is increased in virtually all patients with clinical MTC. However, because of the rarity of unsuspected MTC, the high frequency of false-positive results that may prompt a thyroidectomy despite a reassuring cytologic result, and the unknown clinical relevance of medullary microcarcinomas, it is neither cost-effective nor necessary to measure calcitonin levels in patients with nodular thyroid disease in the absence of clinical suspicion of MTC or abnormal cytologic findings.

The molecular abnormality in more than 95% of familial MTC cases is a germline mutation of the *RET* proto-oncogene that is located on the long arm of chromosome 10.[125] Many investigators advocate *RET* mutation testing in all patients with MTC, including apparently sporadic cases, because 4% to 6% of such patients have germline mutations of the gene (see Chapter 36).[126] Such tests are highly accurate, reproducible, and reliable. If a mutation is found, family members at risk are then tested to identify affected individuals. A negative result obviates the need for any further testing, and individuals who harbor such mutations should undergo prophylactic total thyroidectomy to prevent later development of the multicentric MTC that occurs in this disorder.[127]

Thyroid Imaging

The traditional imaging procedure is thyroid scintigraphy using ^{131}I, ^{123}I, or ^{99m}Tc. Most thyroid carcinomas are inefficient in trapping and organifying iodine and appear on scans as areas of diminished isotope uptake, so-called cool or cold nodules. Unfortunately, most benign nodules also do not concentrate iodine and therefore are cold nodules. Furthermore, not all nodules with normal or slightly increased ^{99m}Tc uptake are benign and may appear cold on a thyroid scan with radioactive iodine.

The only situation in which an iodine scan can exclude malignancy with reasonable certainty is in the case of a toxic adenoma, which is characterized by significantly increased uptake within the nodule and markedly suppressed or absent uptake in the remainder of the gland. These lesions account for fewer than 10% of thyroid nodules and are almost invariably benign.[128] When isotopic thyroid scanning is compared with history and physical examination, most authors have found scanning to be of negligible or no value for the diagnosis of malignancy.[129, 130]

In an attempt to improve the performance of isotopic scanning, a number of radioisotopes other than iodine-related compounds have been tried, such as thallium 201 (^{201}Tl)[131, 132] and ^{99m}Tc-labeled methoxyisobutyl isonitrile (MIBI). In the hands of dedicated experts, these techniques may be valuable, but they are expensive and their widespread use must await more extensive evaluation.

Ultrasonography is capable of detecting even minute thyroid nodules and increases the sensitivity of carcinoma detection but does little to enhance specificity. In fact, of 1000 normal control subjects, 65% had detectable nodularity on high-resolution scanning.[118] Attempts have been made to develop crite-

Table 13-2. Probability of Malignancy at Histology Based on Fine-Needle Aspiration Biopsy Cytology (Summary of the Literature)

Cytology	Percent of Results (%), Mean (Range)	Probability of Malignancy (%), Range
Inadequate or nondiagnostic	16 (15–20)	10–20
Benign	70 (53–90)	1–2
Suspicious*	10 (5–23)	10–20
Malignant	4 (1–10)	>95

*The suspicious category includes follicular neoplasms (hyperplastic nodules, follicular adenomas, and follicular carcinomas) and some Hürthle cell tumors.

ria for distinguishing benign and malignant nodules. Echo-free (cystic) and homogeneously hyperechoic lesions are reputed to carry a low risk of malignancy.[133, 134] Positive predictive criteria of malignancy include solid hypoechoic nodules, presence of calcifications, irregular shape, absence of halo, and absence of cystic elements; however, in one study only 64% of malignant nodules displayed patterns typical of malignancy.[135] In addition, nodules that can be clearly identified as benign by sonography are uncommon, limiting the usefulness of ultrasound scanning.

Ultrasonography is useful in identifying hypoechoic nodules that should be submitted to FNAB and also in examining the rest of the thyroid gland and lymph node areas.[75] It may also be used in case of nonpalpable nodules to guide FNAB, especially when the diameter of the nodule is 1 cm or more.[12] Cystic lesions may be treated by aspiration of the fluid and ethanol injection to avoid recurrence; this is optimally performed under ultrasonographic guidance.[136]

CT scanning and MRI in the initial diagnosis of thyroid malignancy do not provide higher-quality images of the thyroid and cervical nodes than those of ultrasonography. CT examination of the lower central neck is preferable when tracheal or mediastinal invasion is suspected.

Fine-Needle Aspiration Biopsy

FNAB of thyroid nodules has eclipsed all other techniques for diagnosing thyroid cancer, with reported overall rates of sensitivity and specificity exceeding 90% in iodine-sufficient areas.[137, 138] The technique is easy to perform and safe, with only a handful of complications having been reported in the literature,[139, 140] and causes little discomfort. However, care must be taken to obtain an adequate specimen; most authors recommend between three and six aspirations.[137, 138] A satisfactory specimen contains at least five or six groups of 10 to 15 well-preserved cells. The cells are categorized by their cytologic appearances into *benign*, *indeterminate* or *suspicious*, and *malignant* (Table 13–2).

The diagnosis of PTC by FNAB on the basis of characteristic nuclear changes is particularly reliable and accurate, with sensitivity and specificity both approaching 100%. For follicular neoplasms, however, the performance of FNAB is inferior. If strict criteria for malignancy are used, sensitivity may be as low as 8%.[123] If any follicular neoplasm that is not clearly benign on cytologic examination is classified as cancerous, sensitivity rises to about 90% or more. Unfortunately, this increase is associated with a considerable drop in specificity to less than 50% (i.e., a large number of false-positive results). This seriously limits the usefulness of FNAB in iodine-deficient regions, where the incidence of follicular thyroid carcinoma (FTC) approaches that of PTC and where both follicular adenomas and hyperplastic adenomatous nodules are prevalent.

TPO immunochemistry with a monoclonal antibody (MoAb 47) shows promise in improving the accuracy of FNAB for follicular lesions.[141] For 100% sensitivity, a specificity of almost 70% has been achieved with this technique. Pending independent confirmation of these results, TPO immunocytochemistry may be a valuable adjunct to the standard cytologic techniques. The use of large-needle biopsy in addition to standard FNAB has improved diagnostic accuracy in difficult FNA cases,[142, 143] but the technique is more exacting than FNAB alone and is associated with increased morbidity and, possibly, increased complication rates.

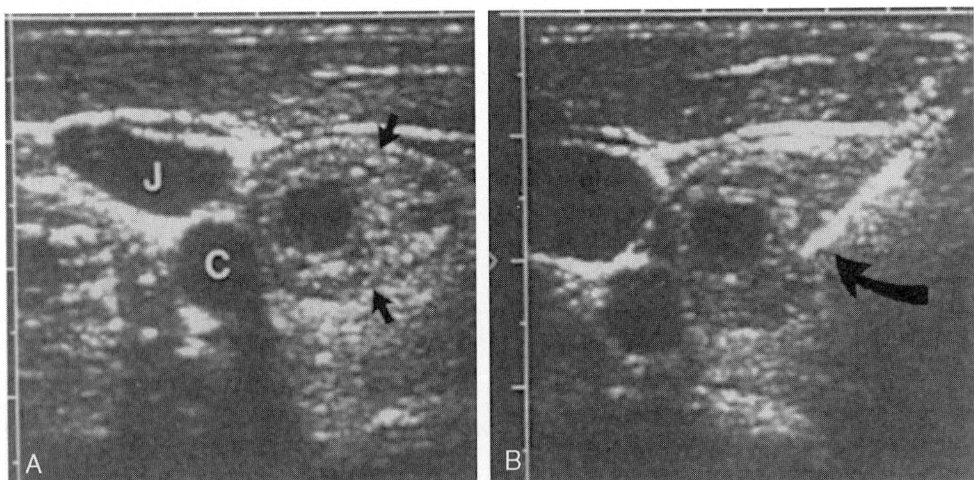

Figure 13-5. Sonographically guided thyroid nodule fine-needle aspiration. Transverse sonogram of the right thyroid lobe (*A*, left panel) shows a 1.5-cm solid thyroid nodule *(arrows)* containing a central cystic component. *C*, common carotid artery; J, jugular vein. Palpation-guided aspiration biopsy obtained nondiagnostic fluid only. *B*, right panel, shows sonographically guided needle aspiration biopsy *(curved arrow)* of the solid portion of the nodule, which proved that this was a benign adenomatous nodule. (From Rifkin MD, Charboneau JW, Laing FC. Special course: ultrasound 1991. In Reading CC [ed]. Syllabus: Thyroid, Parathyroid, and Cervical Lymph Nodes. Oak Brook, Ill, Radiological Society of North America, 1991, pp 363–377.)

Particularly for cystic thyroid nodules, sampling from the margin of the nodule, rather than from the cystic fluid and debris in the center, increases accuracy.[137] Ultrasonographically guided FNA can be used for this purpose (Fig. 13–5). Although such guided biopsies are sometimes helpful, routine use of ultrasound-guided biopsy for clinically palpable nodules is not any better than "freehand" aspiration.[12, 144] However, some centers are evaluating this approach to allow recognition and FNA of nonpalpable nodules 1 cm or smaller in size and to reduce the number of passes to three.[75]

In some European centers, both preoperative FNAB and intraoperative frozen section are combined in endemic goitrous regions with high rates of follicular tumors.[145] In the hands of experienced surgeon-pathologist teams, this approach results in less than 5% misdiagnoses, as evidenced by subsequent review of paraffin-embedded specimens. The approach avoids unnecessarily extensive surgery in patients with benign tumors, achieves resection of nearly all malignant tumors, and rarely necessitates a second operation for completion thyroidectomy.[145] Such an approach is employed at the Mayo Clinic and at the Institut Gustave Roussy, where intraoperative frozen section is routine.

Apart from its limited utility in the evaluation of follicular neoplasms, the only other limitation of FNAB is nondiagnostic specimens, which may be obtained in up to 20% of cases.[138] Although repeated aspiration increases both the accuracy and the rate of diagnostic aspirations, even repeated attempts may sometimes fail. Many persistently nondiagnostic FNAB specimens may be neoplastic, possibly 50%.[146] Hence, either close observation or surgical removal of the nodule is probably the best option. Some authorities recommend a trial of TSH suppression, which can sometimes shrink benign nodules.[137] However, a significant proportion of benign nodules do not shrink, and some carcinomas do shrink; consequently, the diagnostic value of TSH suppression is doubtful. Whether ultrasound-guided FNAB can help overcome this problem is unclear, but confirmation is required.[12, 75, 144] Figure 13–6 is an algorithm for the management of nodular thyroid disease in which FNAB is the first diagnostic test and subsequent management is based on cytologic results.

The most expeditious way to diagnose thyroid malignancy is to obtain a thorough history and physical examination, followed by FNAB and evaluation of the sample by an experienced cytologist. In some cases, FNAB should be performed under ultrasound guidance. Imaging procedures, in addition to ultrasonography, and other tests may occasionally be helpful, but diagnostic thyroid scintiscanning, as traditionally practiced, is of little or no value and should be abandoned.

In iodine-sufficient areas with a high relative prevalence of PTC, the combination of history and physical examination and FNAB is usually sufficient to confirm malignancy. Conversely, if history and physical examination, FNAB, and ultrasonography do not suggest malignancy, the chances of missing PTC are probably less than 1%.[123] In areas where the prevalence of follicular tumors is higher, more patients may require neck exploration because FNAB may not be conclusive; in experienced hands, however, intraoperative frozen sections can limit the number of unnecessarily extensive, bilateral procedures.

Surgery should also be considered for large tumors (>4 cm), especially in young subjects, in order to avoid repeated evaluations; in addition, because these tumors may be composed of various cell populations, results of FNAB may be less reliable. Finally, micronodules less than 1 cm in diameter, found incidentally during imaging, do not need to be tested any further, unless there are sonographic features suggestive of PTC or MTC. The usual advice is to repeat ultrasonography of such lesions after an interval of 6 to 12 months.[120]

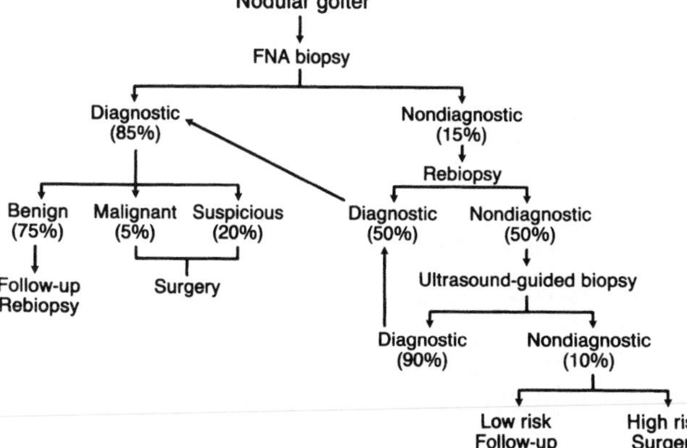

Figure 13–6. Management of nodular goiter based on fine-needle aspiration (FNA) biopsy as the first diagnostic test. Subsequent management is based on cytologic results. Percentages in parentheses indicate satisfactory or unsatisfactory biopsy results. (From Gharib H. Fine-needle aspiration biopsy of thyroid nodules: advantages, limitations, and effect. Mayo Clin Proc 1994; 69:44–49.)

Classification of Thyroid Tumors

Histologic Classification

Two monographs have had a major impact on the histologic classification of thyroid tumors. One is from the World Health Organization (WHO),[147] the other, from the Armed Forces Institute of Pathology (AFIP).[148] The classification described in Table 13–3 is modified from the guidelines described by these organizations.[147, 148]

Lesions of follicular cell origin constitute more than 95% of the cases, and the remainder are largely made up of tumors exhibiting C cell differentiation.[149] Mixed medullary and follicular carcinomas, made up of cells with both C-cell and follicular differentiation, are rare and of uncertain histogenesis.[147] Nonepithelial thyroid tumors mainly include malignant lymphomas, which may involve the thyroid gland as the only manifestation of the disease or as part of a systemic disease. True sarcomas and malignant hemangioendotheliomas are exceptional. Blood-borne metastases to the thyroid are not uncommon at autopsy in patients with widespread malignancy but rarely cause clinically detectable thyroid enlargement.

Staging of Thyroid Carcinoma

In addition to the histologic classification of thyroid tumors developed by WHO and AFIP groups, the International Union Against Cancer (UICC) and the American Joint Commit-

Table 13–3. Classification of Thyroid Neoplasms

Primary Epithelial Tumors	*Tumors of C Cells*
Tumors of Follicular Cells	Medullary carcinoma
Benign: follicular adenoma	*Tumors of Follicular and C Cells*
Malignant: carcinoma	Mixed medullary-follicular carcinoma
Differentiated	
Papillary	
Follicular	***Primary Nonepithelial Tumors***
Poorly differentiated	*Malignant Lymphomas*
Insular	*Sarcomas*
Others	*Others*
Undifferentiated (anaplastic)	***Secondary Tumors***

Table 13–4. American Joint Committee on Cancer Stage Groupings for Thyroid Carcinoma*

Stage	Papillary or Follicular (Age <45 yr)	Papillary or Follicular (Age ≥45 yr)	Medullary (Any Age)	Anaplastic (Any Age)
I	M0	T1	T1	—
II	M1	T2–T3	T2–T4	—
III	—	T4 or N1	N1	—
IV	—	M1	M1	Any

*T, size of primary thyroid tumor (T1, ≤1 cm; T2, >1≤4 cm; T3, >4 cm; T4, extrathyroid invasion); N, regional nodal metastases (0, absent; 1, present); M, distant metastases (0, absent; 1, present).

tee on Cancer (AJCC) have agreed on a staging system in thyroid cancer.[150] As stated by the AJCC,

> "the principal purpose served by international agreement on the classification of cancer cases by extent of disease was to provide a method of conveying clinical experience to others without ambiguity."[150]

The AJCC based its system of classification on the TNM system, which relies on assessing three components: (1) extent of the primary tumor (T), (2) absence or presence of regional lymph node metastases (N), and (3) absence or presence of distant metastases (M).

The TNM system allows a reasonably precise description and recording of the anatomic extent of disease. The classification may be either *clinical* (cTNM), based on evidence (including biopsy) acquired before treatment, or *pathologic* (pTNM), by which intraoperative and surgical pathology data are available. Obviously, pTNM classification is preferable because a precise size can be assigned to the primary tumor, the histotype is identified, and extrathyroid invasion is demonstrated unequivocally.

Typically, the primary thyroid tumor (T) status is defined according to the size of the primary lesion:

- T1, greatest diameter 1 cm or smaller
- T2, larger than 1 cm but not larger than 4 cm
- T3, larger than 4 cm
- T4, direct (extrathyroidal) extension or invasion through the thyroid capsule

A thyroid tumor with four degrees of T, two degrees of N, and two degrees of M can have 16 different TNM categories.

For purposes of tabulation and analysis, these categories have been condensed into a convenient number of TNM stage-groupings (Table 13–4). Whereas head and neck cancer is usually staged entirely on the basis of anatomic extent, in thyroid cancer staging both the histologic diagnosis and the age of the patient for PTC and FTC are included because of their importance in predicting the behavior and prognosis of thyroid cancer.

According to this staging scheme, all patients younger than age 45 years with PTC or FTC are in stage I, unless they have distant metastases (DM), in which case they would be in stage II. In young patients and especially in children, the risk of recurrence is high[151] and may be underestimated by the TNM staging system. Older patients (aged 45 years or more) with node-negative papillary or follicular microcarcinoma (T1 N0 M0) are in stage I. Tumors between 1.1 and 4.0 cm are classified as stage II, and those with either nodal spread (N1) or extrathyroidal invasion (T4), stage III.

For MTC, the scheme is similar, in that microcarcinoma is stage I and a node-positive tumor is stage III. There is no age distinction for MTC, although age is a significant independent prognostic indicator in most multivariate analyses,[152–155] and local (extrathyroidal) invasion is grouped within stage II. For patients with MTC and older patients with PTC or FTC, stage IV denotes the presence of DMs. Independent of age or tumor extent, all patients with undifferentiated (anaplastic) cancer are considered to be in stage IV.

Follicular Adenoma

Follicular adenoma is a benign, encapsulated tumor with evidence of follicular cell differentiation.[147, 148] It is the most common thyroid neoplasm and may be found in 4% to 20% of glands examined at autopsy.[156, 157] The tumor has a well-defined fibrous capsule that is grossly and microscopically complete. There is a sharp demarcation and distinct structural difference from the surrounding parenchyma. These adenomas vary in size, but most have a diameter of 1 to 3 cm at the time of excision. Degenerative changes, including necrosis, hemorrhage, edema, fibrosis, or calcification, are common features, particularly in larger tumors.

Follicular adenomas can be classified into subtypes (Table 13–5) according to the size or presence of follicles and degree of cellularity. Each adenoma tends to have a consistent architectural pattern. *Microfollicular*, *normofollicular*, and *macrofollicular* adenomas owe their names to the size of their follicles compared with follicles in the neighboring, non-neoplastic areas of the gland. *Trabecular adenomas* are cellular and consist of columns of cells arranged in compact cords. They show little follicle formation and rarely contain colloid. A variant, the *hyalinizing trabecular adenoma*, has unusually elongated cells and prominent hyaline changes in the extracellular space.[158]

The histologic differences between these subtypes are striking but of no clinical importance. The only practical value of the classification is that the more cellular a follicular nodule is, the more one should search for evidence of malignancy in the form of invasion of blood vessels and capsule, either singly or in combination.[148] Atypical adenomas are hypercellular or heterogeneous, or both, with gross and histologic appearances

Table 13–5. Subtypes of Follicular Adenoma

Conventional
- Trabecular/solid (embryonal) adenoma
- Microfollicular (fetal) adenoma
- Normofollicular (simple) adenoma
- Macrofollicular (colloid) adenoma

Variants
- Hyalinizing trabecular adenoma
- Oncocytic (oxyphilic or Hürthle cell) tumor
- Adenomas with papillary hyperplasia
- Hyperfunctioning ("toxic") adenoma
- Atypical (hypercellular) adenoma

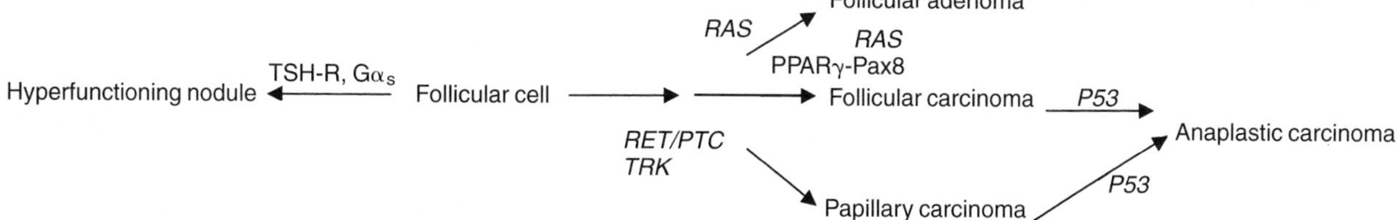

Figure 13–7. Genetic events in thyroid tumorigenesis. Activating point mutations of the *RAS* genes are found with a similar frequency in follicular adenomas and follicular carcinomas and are considered an early event in follicular tumorigenesis. The PPARγ-PAX8 rearrangement was found only in follicular carcinomas. Rearrangements of transmembrane receptors with tyrosine kinase activity (*RET, TRK* genes) are found only in papillary thyroid carcinomas. Inactivating point mutations of the *P53* gene are found only in poorly differentiated and anaplastic thyroid carcinomas. Activation of the cyclic adenosine monophosphate pathway, by point mutation of the thyrotropin receptor (TSH-R) or the α subunit of the G protein genes, leads to the appearance of hyperfunctioning thyroid nodules. Gα_s stimulatory guanyl nucleotide protein.

that suggest the possibility of malignancy but not invasion. They account for fewer than 3% of all follicular adenomas. Follow-up indicates that this lesion behaves in a benign fashion. The fact that the tumor does not recur or produce metastases after removal does not prove that it is actually benign; removal may have interrupted a natural history that would have culminated in invasion and metastases.[64]

The most important cytologic variant is the *oxyphilic* or *oncocytic (Hürthle cell) adenoma*, which is composed predominantly (at least 75%) or entirely of large cells with granular, eosinophilic cytoplasm.[159] Ultrastructurally, the cells are rich in mitochondria and may exhibit nuclear pleomorphism with distinct nucleoli. Although all such neoplasms are thought by some to be potentially malignant,[160] the biologic behavior and clinical course of oncocytic tumors correlate closely with the histology and the size of the initial lesion. The absence of invasion predicts a benign outcome,[161, 162] but larger tumors may rarely be associated with later recurrence or metastases, even in the absence of obvious microscopic evidence of invasion; fortunately, such an occurrence is extremely rare, and generally a diagnosis of benign Hürthle cell adenoma can be reliable.[163, 164] Some normofollicular adenomas may contain pseudopapillary structures that can be confused with the papillae of papillary carcinoma. These structures are probably an expression of localized hyperactivity and are most common in adenomas that show autonomous function.

In the majority of hyperfunctioning follicular adenomas, activating point mutations have been identified in the TSHR[32, 165] or in the α subunit of the stimulatory guanyl nucleotide protein (Gα_s) (Fig. 13–7). Such mutations may impair guanosine triphosphatase (GTP) activity, trapping the G protein in a state of constitutive activation, resulting in enhanced cyclic adenosine monophosphate (cAMP) production and constitutive hyperstimulation of the cells.[166, 167]

Papillary Thyroid Carcinoma

PTC has been defined as "a malignant epithelial tumor showing evidence of follicular cell differentiation, and characterized by the formation of papillae and/or a set of distinctive nuclear changes."[168] The most common thyroid malignancy, PTC constitutes 50% to 90% of differentiated FCTCs worldwide.[169]

Papillary thyroid microcarcinoma (PTM) is defined by the WHO as a PTC 1.0 cm in diameter or smaller.[147, 170, 171] The incidence rates for clinically diagnosed PTC in the United States are approximately 5 per 100,000 for tumors larger than 1 cm in diameter and 1 per 100,000 for PTM. By contrast, the incidence of PTM in autopsy material from various continents ranges from 4% to 36%.[168]

Typically, PTC shows a predominance of papillary structures, consisting of a fibrovascular core lined by a single layer of epithelial cells, but the papillae are usually admixed with neoplastic follicles having characteristic nuclear features.

The nuclei of PTC cells have a distinctive appearance that has a diagnostic significance comparable to that of the papillae. Indeed, the preoperative diagnosis of PTC can often be made on the basis of the characteristic nuclear changes seen in FNA material: Nuclei are larger than in normal follicular cells and overlap, they may be fissured like coffee beans, chromatin is hypodense (ground glass nuclei), limits are irregular, and they frequently contain an inclusion corresponding to a cytoplasmic invagination.

Several subtypes exist:

1. The tumor is designated a *follicular variant* of PTC when the lining cells of the neoplastic follicles have the same nuclear features as seen in typical PTC and the follicular predominance over the papillae is complete.[147–149]
2. The *diffuse sclerosing variant* is characterized by diffuse involvement of one or both thyroid lobes, widespread lymphatic permeation, prominent fibrosis, and lymphoid infiltration.
3. The *tall cell variant* is characterized by well-formed papillae that are covered by cells twice as tall as they are wide.
4. The *columnar cell variant* differs from other forms of PTC because of the presence of prominent nuclear stratification.

The tall cell and columnar cell variants are more aggressive,[168] but controversy exists regarding outcome for the diffuse sclerosing variant.[172]

Molecular Pathogenesis

The thyroid follicular cell may give rise to both benign and malignant tumors, and the malignancy can be of either papillary or follicular histotype. There is no evidence that benign tumors ever undergo malignant transformation into classic PTC. Structural abnormalities of the chromosomes may occur in about 50% of PTCs, frequently involving the long arm of chromosome 10.[173] The *RET* proto-oncogene is located on chromosome 10q11-2. It encodes a transmembrane receptor with a tyrosine kinase domain. Its ligands are the glial cell line–derived neutrophilic factor (GDNF) and the neurturin, both of which induce protein dimerization. *RET* activation was first demonstrated in transfection experiments and has been found only in PTC tumors.[174–179] It was therefore called *RET/PTC.*

All activated forms of the *RET* proto-oncogene are the consequence of oncogenic rearrangements fusing the tyrosine kinase domain of the *RET* gene with the 5′ domain of different genes. The foreign gene is constitutively expressed, and its 5′ domain acts as a promoter, resulting in permanent expression of the *RET* gene. Furthermore, these genes have domains that induce *RET* activation by permanent dimerization; because of this fusion, the chimeric protein is localized in the cytoplasm and not in the plasma cell membrane.

Three major classes of *RET/PTC* have been identified:

1. *RET/PTC*$_1$ is formed by an intrachromosomal rearrangement fusing the *RET* tyrosine kinase domain to a gene designated *H4* (D10S170), whose function is still unknown.
2. *RET/PTC*$_2$ is formed by an interchromosomal rearrangement fusing the *RET* tyrosine kinase domain to a gene located on chromosome 17 encoding the RIα regulatory subunit of protein kinase A.
3. *RET/PTC*$_3$ is formed by an intrachromosomal rearrangement fusing the *RET* tyrosine kinase domain to a gene designated *ELE1*, whose function is still unknown.

Several variants of *RET/PTC* have been observed in post-Chernobyl thyroid tumors, including rearrangements formed by fusing the tyrosine kinase domain of the RET gene at other breakpoint sites or with other partners.

The frequency of *RET/PTC* rearrangements occurring in PTC patients without prior childhood neck irradiation varies between 2.5% and 35%. In these tumors, the frequencies of *RET/PTC*$_1$ and *RET/PTC*$_3$ were similar and that of *RET/PTC*$_2$ was lower. The *RET/PTC* rearrangements were more frequently found (in 60% to 80% of cases) in PTC cases occurring either after external irradiation in childhood or in children after the Chernobyl accident.[174–176] *RET/PTC*$_3$ was more frequently found in aggressive tumors that occurred early after the accident and *RET/PTC*$_1$ in less aggressive tumors that occurred later. The finding of *RET/PTC* rearrangement in micropapillary thyroid carcinomas suggests that it constitutes an early event in thyroid carcinogenesis.[177] On the other hand, *RET/PTC*-positive tumors lack evidence of progression to poorly or undifferentiated tumor phenotypes.[176]

Several additional oncogenes may occasionally be involved in PTC, including *NTRK1* (also named *TRKA*), which codes for a neural growth factor receptor with a tyrosine kinase domain and which is activated by rearrangement in about 10% of PTCs.[174] The receptor for hepatocyte growth factor is a transmembrane tyrosine kinase encoded by the *MET* oncogene; it is overexpressed in some patients with PTC, and low expression has been associated with the occurrence of DM.[180, 181]

A high incidence of PTC has been reported in patients with adenomatous polyposis coli and Cowden's disease (the multiple hamartoma syndrome), suggesting that the predisposing genes may play a role in the occurrence of papillary carcinoma. About 3% of cases of PTC are familial; their behavior is similar to or slightly more aggressive than that of nonfamilial cases.[182] The gene predisposing to familial thyroid tumors with cellular oxyphilia has been mapped to chromosome 19q13.2, and in a family with PTC and renal carcinoma a separate gene was mapped to chromosome 1q21.[183, 184]

The expression of thyroid-specific genes has been studied at the messenger ribonucleic acid (mRNA) and protein levels in a large series of human thyroid tumors. Expression of *NIS* was profoundly decreased in both benign and malignant thyroid hypofunctioning nodules; moreover, in malignant nodules, low expression of TPO, PDS, and Tg was also found.[185] These abnormalities clearly explain many of the metabolic defects typically observed in thyroid cancer tissues: a low iodine concentration, a low rate of iodine organification, low hormonal synthesis, and a short intrathyroidal half-life of iodine.[186] However, Tg is expressed in all FCTCs and can be shown by immunohistochemistry, which can prove useful in cases with atypical histology.

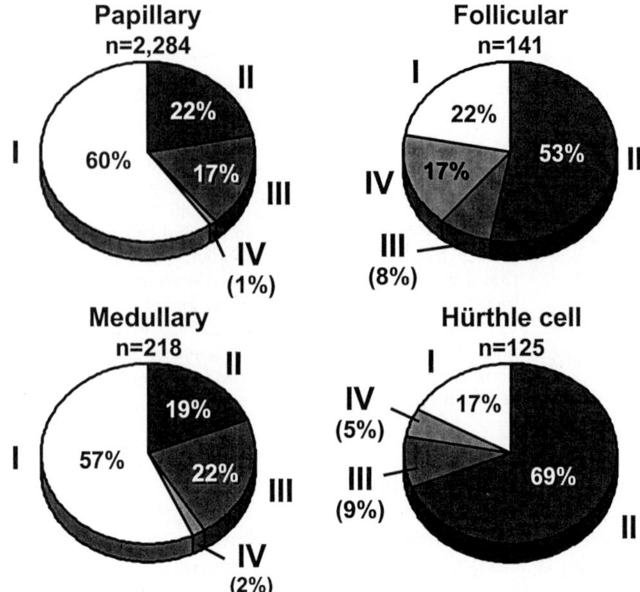

Figure 13–8. Distribution of pathologic-Tumor-Node-Metastases (pTNM) stages in 2284 patients with papillary thyroid carcinoma (*upper left*), 218 patients with medullary thyroid cancer (*lower left*), 141 patients with follicular thyroid cancer (*upper right*), and 125 patients with Hürthle cell cancer (*lower right*) undergoing primary surgical treatment at the Mayo Clinic from 1940 to 1997.

Presenting Features

Although PTCs can occur at any age, most occur in patients between 30 and 50 years of age (mean age, 45 years). Women are affected more frequently (female predominance, 60% to 80%). Most primary tumors are 1 to 4 cm in size; they average about 2 to 3 cm in greatest diameter.[169, 187] Extrathyroidal invasion of adjacent soft tissues is present in about 15% (range 5% to 34%) at primary surgery, and about one third of PTC patients have clinically evident lymphadenopathy at presentation.[187] About 35% to 50% of excised neck nodes have histologic evidence of involvement, and in patients 17 years of age or younger nodal involvement may be present in up to 90%.[151, 188] Only 1% to 7% of PTC patients have DM at diagnosis.[169, 187] Spread to superior mediastinal nodes is usually associated with extensive neck nodal involvement.

The TNM classification is a widely used system for tumor staging.[189] Most PTC patients present with either stage I (60%) or stage II (22%). Patients aged 45 years or older with either nodal metastases or extrathyroidal extension (stage III) account for fewer than 20% of cases.[169] As already noted, few (1% to 7%) of PTC patients present with DM and have stage IV disease (age 45 years or older with any T, any N, M1). Figure 13–8 (upper left) illustrates the distribution of TNM stages in 2284 PTC cases seen at the Mayo Clinic, and Figure 13–9 demonstrates survival by TNM stage in this cohort of PTC patients treated from 1940 to 1997.

Recurrence and Mortality

Three types of tumor recurrence may occur with PTC:

- Postoperative *nodal metastases* (NM)
- *Local recurrence* (LR)
- Postoperative *distant metastases* (DM)

LR may be defined as "histologically confirmed tumor occurring in the resected thyroid bed, thyroid remnant, or other adjacent tissues of the neck (excluding lymph nodes)" after

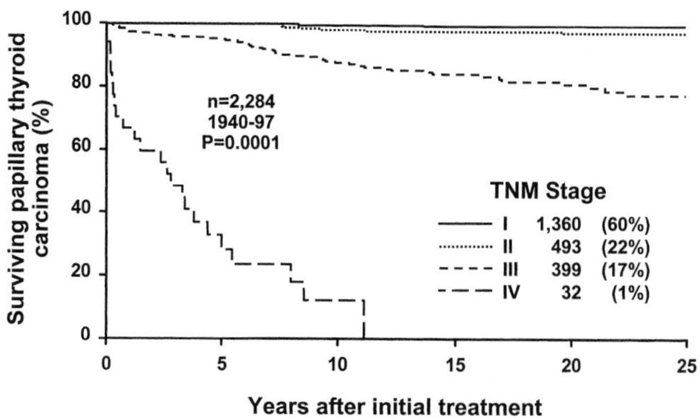

Figure 13–9. Cause-specific survival according to pathologic-Tumor-Node-Metastases (pTNM) stage in a cohort of 2284 patients with papillary thyroid carcinoma treated at the Mayo Clinic from 1940 to 1997. The numbers in parentheses represent the percentages of patients in each pTNM stage grouping.

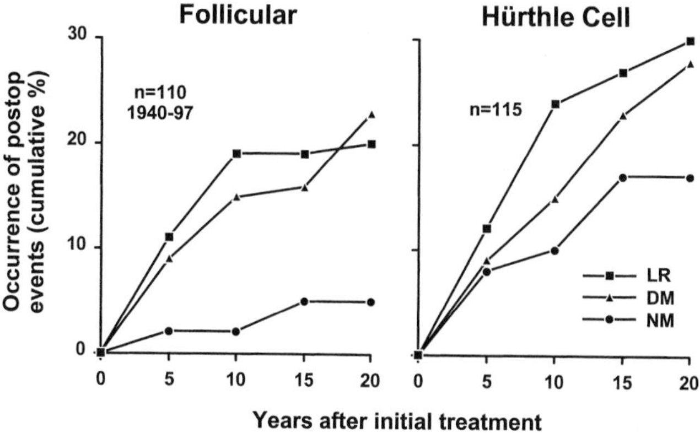

Figure 13–11. Development of neck nodal metastases (NM), local recurrences (LR), and distant metastases (DM) in the first 20 years after definitive surgery for follicular thyroid cancer (FTC) or Hürthle cell cancer (HCC) performed at the Mayo Clinic from 1940 to 1997. Based on 110 consecutive FTC patients (*left*) and 115 HCC patients (*right*) who had complete surgical resection and were without distant metastases on initial examination.

complete surgical removal of the primary tumor.[190] Nodal or distant spread may be considered postoperative if the metastases are discovered within 180 or 30 days, respectively.[169] Ideally, tumor recurrence should be considered only as it occurs in patients without initial DM who had complete surgical resection of the primary tumors.

Figure 13–10 illustrates rates of PTC recurrence at local, nodal, and distant sites in 2150 patients with PTC treated at one institution from 1940 to 1997. After 20 years of follow-up, postoperative NM had been discovered in 9%, and LR and DM occurred in 5% and 4%, respectively. Both LR and DM are less common in PTC than in FTC (Fig. 13–11). However, postoperative cases of NM were more frequent in PTC than in FTC.

Cause-specific mortality (CSM) rates for differentiated thyroid cancer are shown in Figure 13–12. CSM rates for PTC were 2% at 5 years, 4% at 10 years, and 5% at 20 years. Among those with lethal PTC, 20% of deaths occurred in the first year after diagnosis, and 80% of the deaths occurred within 10 years. The 25-year cause-specific survival rate of 95% for PTC was significantly higher than the 79%, 71%, and 66% rates seen with MTC, Hürthle cell cancer (HCC), and FTC, respectively.

Outcome Prediction

Only a fraction (~15%) of patients with PTC are likely to experience relapse of disease, and even fewer (~5%) have a lethal outcome. Exceptional patients, who have an aggressive course, tend to experience relapse early (Fig. 13–13), and the rare fatalities usually occur within 5 to 10 years of diagnosis.[169, 170, 187, 188] Multivariate analyses have been used to identify variables predictive of CSM.[191–194] Increasing age of the patient and the presence of extrathyroidal invasion are independent prognostic factors in all studies.[191–194]

The presence of initial DM and large size of the primary tumor are also significant variables in most studies,[191, 193, 194] and some groups[169, 191, 192, 195] have reported that histopathologic grade (degree of differentiation) is an independent variable. The completeness of initial tumor resection (postoperative status) is also a predictor of mortality.[169, 193, 196] The presence of initial neck NM, although relevant to future nodal recurrence, does not influence CSM (Fig. 13–14).[169, 187, 196]

Several scoring systems based on these significant prognostic indicators have been devised. Each system allows one to assign the majority of PTC patients (80% or more) to a low-risk

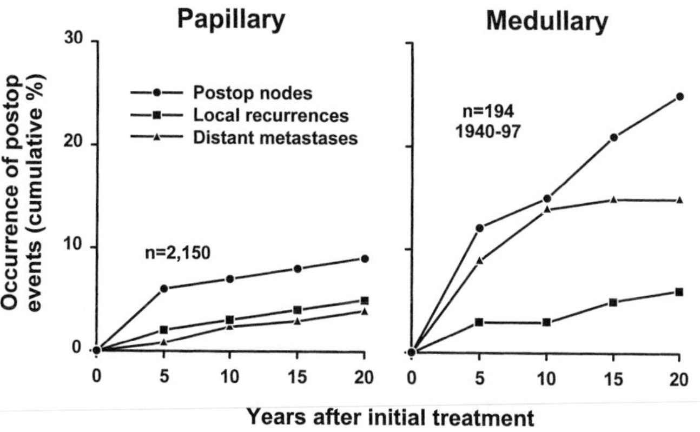

Figure 13–10. Development of neck nodal metastases, local recurrences, and distant metastases in the first 20 years after definitive surgery for papillary thyroid cancer (PTC) or medullary thyroid cancer (MTC) performed at the Mayo Clinic from 1940 to 1997. Based on 2150 consecutive PTC (*left*) and 194 MTC (*right*) patients who had complete surgical resection (i.e., had no gross residual disease) and were without distant metastases on initial examination. Postop, postoperative.

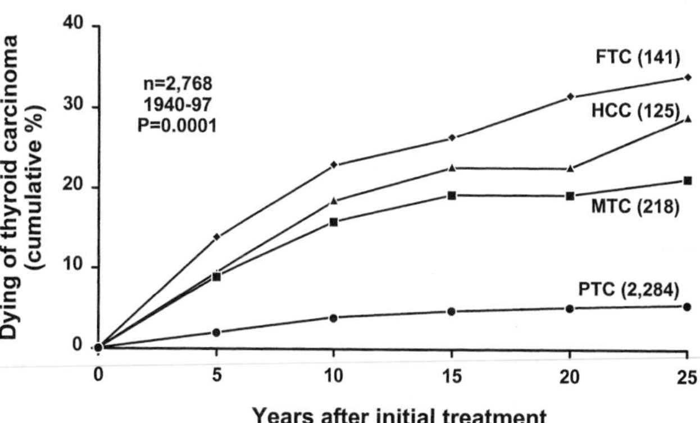

Figure 13–12. Cumulative cause-specific mortality rates for patients with differentiated thyroid carcinoma in the first 25 years after treatment with initial surgery performed at the Mayo Clinic from 1940 to 1997. Based on 2768 consecutively treated patients (2284 with papillary thyroid carcinoma [PTC], 141 with follicular thyroid cancer [FTC], 125 with Hürthle cell cancer [HCC], and 218 with medullary thyroid cancer [MTC]).

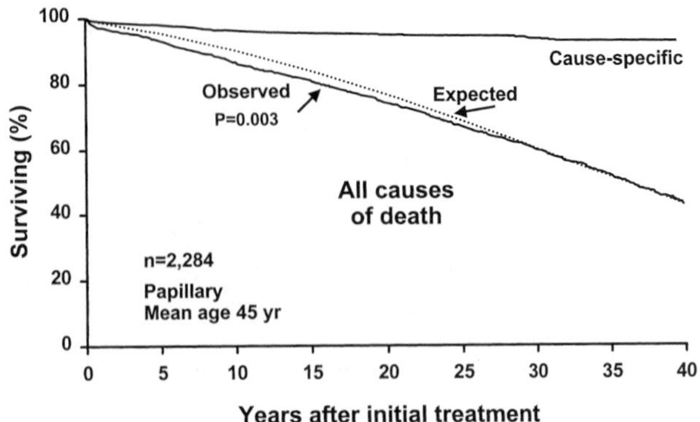

Figure 13–13. Survival to death from all causes and to death from thyroid cancer (cause-specific mortality) in 2284 consecutive patients with papillary thyroid carcinoma undergoing initial management at the Mayo Clinic from 1940 to 1997. Also plotted is the expected survival (all causes) of persons of the same age and sex and with the same date of treatment but living under mortality conditions of the northwest central United States.

group, in which the CSM at 25 years is less than 2%, and the others (a small minority) to a high-risk group, in which almost all cancer-related deaths are observed. In general, these systems provide prediction of postoperative events comparable to that of the internationally accepted TNM staging system.[197]

A scoring index devised to assign PTC patients to prognostic risk groups[191] was named the AGES scheme after the four independent variables: patient's *a*ge, tumor grade, tumor *e*xtent (local invasion, DM), and tumor *s*ize. With the use of such a scoring system, 86% of patients were in the minimal risk group (AGES score < 4) and they experienced a 20-year CSM rate of only 1%.[169] By contrast, patients with AGES scores of 4+ (high-risk; 14% of the total) had a 20-year CSM of 36%.

Figure 13–15 compares the AGES scores with TNM stage and with two other subsequently introduced schemes designed to stratify PTC patients into groups at either minimal risk or high risk of cancer-related death. Such a prognostic scoring system makes it possible to counsel patients and to aid in the planning of individualized postoperative management programs in PTC.[191, 196]

Although the AGES scheme had the potential for universal application, some academic centers could not include the differentiation (G) variable because their surgical pathologists did not recognize higher-grade PTC tumors.[198] Accordingly, a

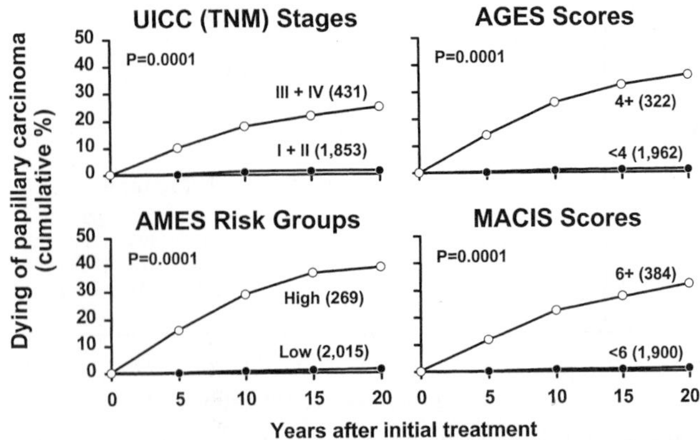

Figure 13–15. Cumulative mortality from papillary thyroid carcinoma in patients at either minimal risk or higher risk of cancer-related death as defined by International Union Against Cancer (UICC) pathologic-Tumor-Node-Metastases (pTNM) stages (*upper left*), AGES scores (*upper right*), AMES risk groups (*lower left*), and MACIS scores (*lower right*). The minimal risk group constitutes 81% of the 2284 patients when defined by pTNM stages I and II, 86% as defined by AGES scores less than 4, 88% as defined by AMES low-risk, and 83% when defined by a MACIS score less than 6. The cause-specific mortality (CSM) rates at 20 years were 25% for stages III and IV, 36% for AGES scores of 4+, 39% for AMES high-risk, and 32% for patients with MACIS scores of 6+. The CSM ratios between the high-risk and low-risk groups at 20 years were 19 for pTNM, 36 for AGES, 35 for AMES, and 40 for MACIS.

prognostic scoring system for predicting PTC mortality rates was devised with the use of candidate variables that included completeness of primary tumor resection but excluded histologic grade.[196] Cox model analysis and stepwise variable selection led to a final prognostic model that included five variables: *m*etastasis, *a*ge, *c*ompleteness of resection, *i*nvasion, and *s*ize (MACIS). The final score was defined as

3.1 (age 39 years or younger) or
0.08 × age (age 40 years or older)
+0.3 × tumor size (in centimeters)
+1 (if tumor not completely resected)
+1 (if locally invasive)
+3 (if DM present)

As illustrated by Figure 13–16, the MACIS scoring system

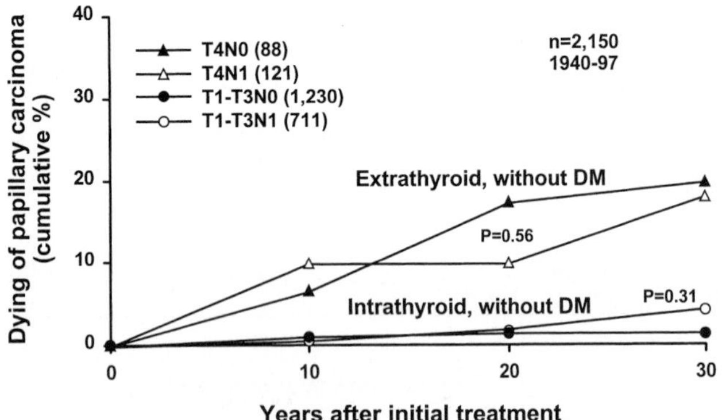

Figure 13–14. Lack of influence of nodal metastases at initial operation on cumulative mortality from papillary thyroid carcinoma in 1941 patients with pT1-3 intrathyroidal tumors (completely confined to the thyroid gland) and 209 pT4 patients with extrathyroidal (locally invasive) tumors. All patients had initial surgical treatment at the Mayo Clinic from 1940 to 1997. DM, distant metastases.

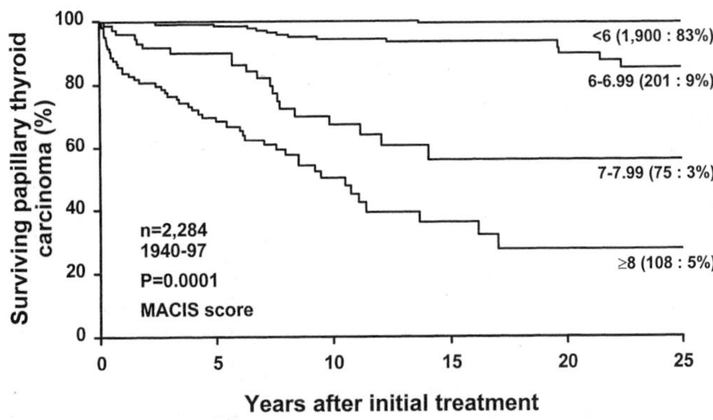

Figure 13–16. Cause-specific survival according to MACIS (*m*etastases, *a*ge, *c*ompleteness of resection, *i*nvasion, and *s*ize) scores of less than 6, 6 to 6.99, 7 to 7.99, and 8+ in a cohort of 2284 consecutive patients with papillary thyroid carcinoma (PTC) undergoing initial treatment at the Mayo Clinic from 1940 to 1997. The numbers in parentheses represent the numbers and percentages of PTC patients in each of the four risk groups.

permits identification of groups of patients with a broad range of risk of death from PTC. Twenty-year cause-specific survival rates for patients with MACIS scores of less than 6, 6 to 6.99, 7 to 7.99, and 8+ were 99%, 89%, 56%, and 27%, respectively ($P < .0001$). When cumulative mortality from all causes of death was considered, approximately 85% of PTC patients with AGES scores below 4 or MACIS scores below 6 had no excess mortality over rates predicted for control subjects.[191, 196]

It should be emphasized that the five variables in MACIS scoring are easy to define after primary operation; consequently, the system can be applied in any clinical setting. The MACIS system can be used for counseling individual PTC patients and can help guide decision making concerning the intensity of the postoperative tumor surveillance and the appropriateness of adjunctive radioiodine therapy. Because the CIS (*c*ompleteness of *r*esection, *i*nvasion, and *s*ize) variables require information obtained at surgery, the system probably should not be used to decide the extent of primary surgery.[198]

Follicular Thyroid Carcinoma

FTC is "a malignant epithelial tumor showing evidence of follicular cell differentiation but lacking the diagnostic features of papillary carcinoma."[147] Such a definition excludes the follicular variant of PTC, and it is also customary to exclude both the poorly differentiated insular carcinoma[199] and the rare mixed medullary and follicular carcinoma.[200] The correct classification of tumors with predominant oncocytic features (Hürthle cell carcinomas) is controversial.[159] The WHO committee has taken the stance that this tumor is an oxyphilic variant of FTC.[147] The AFIP monograph, by contrast, states that "the tumors made up of this cell type have gross, microscopic, behavioral, cytogenetic (and conceivably etiopathogenic) features that set them apart from all others and justify discussing them in a separate section."[148]

Thus categorized, FTC is a relatively rare neoplasm whose identification requires invasion of the capsule, blood vessel, or adjacent thyroid. In epidemiologic surveys, FTC constituted from 5% to 50% of differentiated thyroid cancers and tended to be more common in areas with iodine deficiency.[201] Owing to a combination of changing diagnostic criteria and an increase in the incidence of PTC associated with dietary iodine supplementation, the diagnosis of FTC has decreased in frequency; in one North American experience, minimally invasive nonoxyphilic FTC made up fewer than 2% of thyroid malignancies.[202]

The microscopic appearance of FTC varies from well-formed follicles to a predominantly solid growth pattern.[147–149] Poorly formed follicles and atypical patterns (e.g., cribriform) may occur, and multiple architectural types may coexist. Mitotic activity is not a useful indicator of malignancy.

FTC is best divided into two categories on the basis of degree of invasiveness:

- Minimally invasive or encapsulated
- Widely invasive

There is little overlap between these two types.

Minimally invasive FTC is an encapsulated tumor whose growth pattern resembles that of a trabecular or solid, microfollicular, or atypical adenoma. The diagnosis of malignancy depends on the demonstration of blood vessel or capsular invasion, or both. The criteria for invasion must therefore be strict.[149] Blood vessel invasion is almost never seen grossly.

Microscopically, the vessels "should be of venous caliber, be located in or immediately outside of the capsule and contain one or more clusters of tumor cells attached to the wall and protruding into the lumen."[149] Interruption of the capsule must involve the full thickness to qualify as capsular invasion. Penetration of only the inner half or the presence of tumor cells embedded in the capsule does not qualify for the diagnosis of FTC. Foci of capsular invasion must be distinguished from the capsular rupture that can result from FNA. The acronym WHAFFT (worrisome histologic alterations following FNA of the thyroid) is applied to such changes.[203]

In contrast, the rare, *widely invasive* form of FTC can be distinguished easily from benign lesions. Although the tumor may be partially encapsulated, the margins are infiltrative even on gross examination and vascular invasion is often extensive. The structural features are variable, with solid and trabecular areas, but a follicular element is always present. When follicular differentiation is poor or absent, the tumor may be classified as a poorly differentiated (insular) carcinoma.[64, 149]

Focal or extensive clear-cell changes can occur. A rare clear cell variant of FTC has been described in which glycogen accumulation or dilatation of the granular endoplasmic reticulum is responsible for the clear cells.[204] When more than 75% of cells in an FTC exhibit Hürthle cell (or oncocytic) features, the tumor is classified as a Hürthle cell or an oncocytic carcinoma[148, 205] or an oxyphilic variant FTC.[64, 147]

Molecular Pathogenesis

There is still no accepted paradigm for the pathogenesis of follicular thyroid cancer. A multistep adenoma-to-carcinoma pathogenesis, similar to that for colon cancer and other adenocarcinomas,[176, 206] is not universally accepted because pathologists do not recognize follicular carcinoma in situ and documentation of the evolution of adenoma to carcinoma is rare. Nevertheless, several facts about the pathogenesis of FTC are firmly established.

First, most follicular adenomas and all FTCs are probably of monoclonal origin.[51, 65, 66] Second, oncogene activation, particularly by point mutation of the *RAS* oncogene, is common both in follicular adenomas and in FTCs (~40%), supporting a role in early tumorigenesis.[167, 206] Such *RAS* mutations are not specific for follicular tumors and also occur in PTC. The *RET* oncogene does not appear to be significantly involved in follicular tumors.[207] Third, cytogenetic abnormalities and evidence of genetic loss are more common in FTC than in PTC and also occur in follicular adenomas.[208–211] Losses in FTC are particularly associated with chromosomes 3, 10, 11, and 17.[209, 212]

Of the cytogenetic abnormalities described in FTC,[213] the most common are deletions, partial deletions, and deletion-rearrangements involving the p arm of chromosome 3.[211, 214] Loss of heterozygosity (LOH) on chromosome 3p appears to be limited to FTC because no evidence for 3p LOH has been found in follicular adenomas or PTC.[209, 210] A translocation, t(2;3)(q13;p25), resulting in the fusion of the deoxyribonucleic acid (DNA) binding domains of the thyroid transcription factor PAX-8 to domains of the peroxisome proliferator–activated receptor (PPAR) $\gamma 1$, was detected in five of eight FTCs but not in follicular adenomas, PTCs, or multinodular hyperplasia. The chimeric protein may retard growth inhibition and follicular differentiation normally induced by PPAR $\gamma 1$.[215]

Presenting Features

FTC tends to occur in older people, with the mean age in most studies being more than 50 years, about 10 years older than that for typical PTC.[201, 216] The average median age of patients with oxyphilic FTC (HCC) is about 60 years.[201, 205] As in most thyroid malignancies, women outnumber men by more than 2 to 1. Most patients with FTC present with a painless thyroid nodule, with or without background thyroid nodularity, and they rarely (4% to 6%) have clinically evident lymphadenopathy at presentation.[201] Lymph node metastases to the neck in FTC are so exceptional that "wherever they are observed, the alternative possibilities of follicular variant papil-

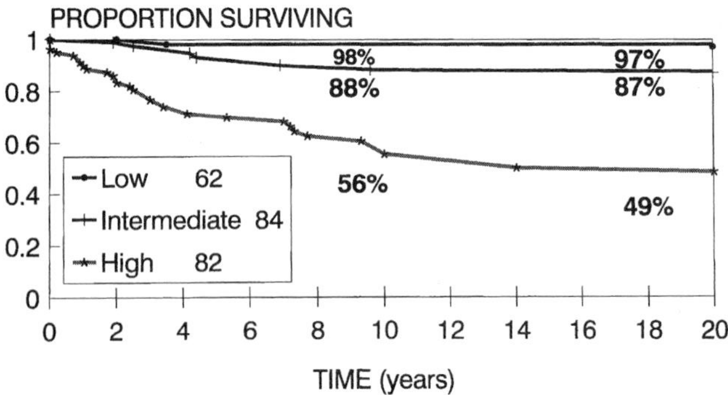

Figure 13–22. Survival differences in low-risk, intermediate-risk, and high-risk groups for 228 consecutive patients with follicular thyroid carcinoma who were seen and treated at the Memorial Sloan-Kettering Cancer Center during a period of 55 years from 1930 to 1985. (From Shaha AR, Loree TR, Shah JP. Prognostic factors and risk group analyses in follicular carcinoma of the thyroid. Surgery 1995; 118: 1131–1138.)

56% of patients died from their tumor within 8 years of initial therapy.[199] The tumor is viewed by the WHO committee[147] as a morphologic variant of FTC, but others view it as a poorly differentiated variant of either PTC or FTC.[64, 149] Some tumors formerly classified as the compact form of undifferentiated small cell carcinoma probably belonged to this category.[64] The AFIP group also considers that a large proportion of "low-risk" young patients with aggressive PTC or FTC belong to this category of high-grade poorly differentiated FTC.[148]

Undifferentiated (Anaplastic) Carcinoma

Anaplastic carcinoma constitutes about 5% of all thyroid carcinomas, usually occurs after the age of 60 years, and is slightly more common in women (1.3 : 1 to 1.5 : 1).[226] This carcinoma is highly malignant, nonencapsulated, and extends widely. Evidence of invasion of adjacent structures, such as the skin, muscles, nerves, blood vessels, larynx, and esophagus, is common. DM occur early in the course of the disease in lungs, liver, bones, and brain.

On histopathologic examination, the lesion is composed of atypical cells that exhibit numerous mitoses and form a variety of patterns. Spindle-shaped cells, multinucleate giant cells, and squamoid cells usually predominate. Areas of necrosis and polymorphonuclear infiltration are common, and the presence of PTC or FTC suggests that they may be the precursors of anaplastic carcinoma. Mutations of the *p53* gene are present in many undifferentiated carcinomas but may not be found in the residual well-differentiated component,[227, 228] suggesting that these mutations occurred after the development of the original tumor and may have played a key role in tumor progression.

The usual clinical complaint is of a rapid, often painful enlargement of a mass that may have been present in the thyroid gland for many years. The tumor invades adjacent structures, causing hoarseness, inspiratory stridor, and difficulty in swallowing. On examination, the overlying skin is often warm and discolored. The mass is tender and is often fixed to adjacent structures. It is stony hard in consistency, but some areas may be soft or fluctuant. The regional lymph nodes are enlarged, and there may be evidence of DM. Anaplastic carcinomas do not accumulate iodine and do not typically produce thyroglobulin.

Treatment should be initiated rapidly to avoid death from locally infiltrative disease and possible suffocation. It consists of surgical resection of the tumor tissue present in the neck, when this is feasible, followed by a combination of external irradiation and chemotherapy. When the extent of disease is limited and when these protocols can be applied, local control may be obtained in about two thirds of the patients and long-term survival in about 20%.[229]

Medullary Thyroid Carcinoma

MTC accounts for less than 10% of thyroid malignancies (see Chapter 36). It arises from the parafollicular or C cells of the thyroid gland, and the tumor cells typically produce an early biochemical signal (hypersecretion of calcitonin).[230] MTC readily invades the intraglandular lymphatics and spreads to other parts of the gland, in addition to the pericapsular and regional lymph nodes. It also regularly spreads through the blood stream to the lungs, bone, and liver.[152–155]

MTC tumors are firm and usually unencapsulated. On histopathologic examination, the tumor is composed of cells that vary in morphologic features and arrangement. Round, polyhedral, and spindle-shaped cells form a variety of patterns, which may vary from solid, trabecular to endocrine or glandular-like structures. An amyloid stroma is commonly present.[231] Gross or microscopic foci of carcinoma may be present in other parts of the gland, and blood vessels may be invaded. The histopathologic appearance of the metastases resembles that of the primary lesion. In all cases, the diagnosis can be confirmed by positive immunostaining of tumor tissue for calcitonin and carcinoembryonic antigen (CEA).

MTC first appears either as a hard nodule or mass in the thyroid gland or as an enlargement of the regional lymph nodes. Occasionally, a metastatic lesion in a distant site is found first. The neck masses are frequently painful; they are sometimes bilateral and are often localized to the upper two thirds of each lobe of the gland, which reflects the anatomic location of the parafollicular cells.

The tumor occurs in both sporadic and hereditary forms, the latter making up about 20% of the total. The hereditary variety can be transmitted as a single entity, familial MTC, or it can arise as part of MEN syndrome type 2A or 2B. The hereditary form is typically bilateral[232] and is usually preceded by a premalignant C cell hyperplasia. Total thyroidectomy at this premalignant stage can cure the disease in more than 90% of cases.[126, 127, 233, 234] *RET* proto-oncogene testing should be performed in all MTC patients. The finding of a germline mutation in this gene indicates a hereditary disease; the mutation should then be sought in all first-degree family members.

Early series of MTC mainly described sporadic cases, in which 80% of patients presented with TNM stage II or III.[231] As more patients with familial MTC[235] or MEN 2A have been diagnosed, more patients have curable (stage I) disease, and the survival rate has improved, a trend that should continue with widespread application of *RET* proto-oncogene testing.[236] Patients with MTC now have outcomes similar to or better than those of patients with nonpapillary FCTC (see Fig. 13–10). The cause-specific survival curves for 218 consecutive MTC cases treated from 1940 to 1997 at the Mayo Clinic, according to TNM stage, are presented in Figure 13–23.

Prognostic factors relevant to outcome in MTC include (1) age at diagnosis, (2) male gender, (3) initial extent of the disease, such as NM and DM, (4) tumor size, (5) extrathyroidal invasion, (6) vascular invasion, (7) calcitonin immunoreactivity and amyloid staining in tumor tissue, (8) postoperative gross residual disease, and (9) postoperative plasma calcitonin levels.[231]

In multivariate analysis, only the age of the patient at initial treatment and the stage of the disease remain significantly independent indicators of survival. This suggests that, in rou-

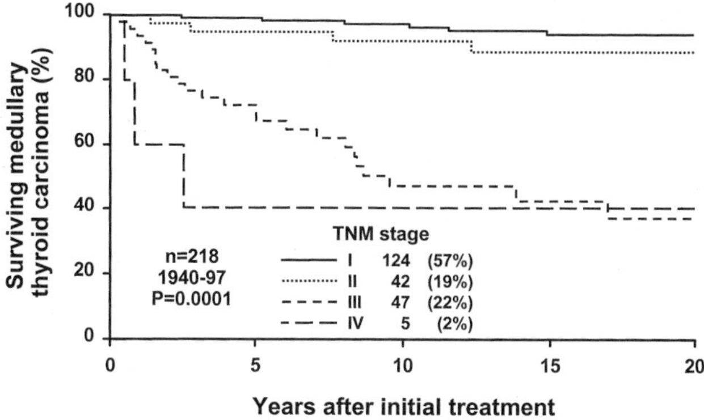

Figure 13–23. Cause-specific survival according to pathologic-Tumor-Node-Metastases (pTNM) stage in a cohort of 218 patients with medullary thyroid carcinoma treated at the Mayo Clinic from 1940 to 1997. Numbers in parentheses represent the percentages of patients in each pTNM stage grouping.

tine practice, clinicians attempting to predict outcome in MTC should take into account not only the presenting disease stage, as assessed by the pTNM system (see Fig. 13–23), but also the age of the patient at diagnosis.[153–155]

In patients with MTC, Cushing's syndrome may occur because of secretion of corticotropin by the tumor. Prostaglandins, serotonin, kinins, and vasoactive intestinal peptide may also be secreted and are variously responsible for flushing and for the attacks of watery diarrhea that about one third of patients experience, usually at an advanced stage of the disease.[154] In MEN-2A, hyperparathyroidism occurs late and is usually due to parathyroid hyperplasia rather than adenoma. Pheochromocytomas invariably occur later than MTC; they are often bilateral and may be clinically silent, and patients at risk should be screened with measurements of urinary metanephrine excretion. In MEN-2B, MTC and pheochromocytomas are associated with multiple mucosal neuromas *(bumpy lip syndrome)*, a marfanoid habitus, and typical facies, but such patients do not regularly have hyperparathyroidism.[234]

Differentiation of sporadic MTC from other types of thyroid nodule on clinical grounds alone may be difficult. In patients with a family history of thyroid cancer associated with hypertension or hyperparathyroidism, the MEN-2A syndrome should be suspected. FNAB has made it possible to diagnose MTC before surgery. In some patients, however, cytologic findings may be misleading because the type of carcinoma is difficult to determine and HCC may occasionally be confused with MTC.

Positive immunocytochemical staining for calcitonin allows confirmation of the diagnosis. Basal plasma calcitonin levels are elevated in virtually all patients with clinical MTC. Infusions of pentagastrin or calcium elicit secretion of calcitonin, and the response may be exaggerated in patients with either MTC or the antecedent C-cell hyperplasia; its use should be restricted to patients with an undetectable or borderline plasma calcitonin level (see Chapter 36).

When the diagnosis of MTC is made from calcitonin measurements or FNAB, patients should be evaluated for hyperparathyroidism and for pheochromocytoma. If these diagnoses are satisfactorily excluded, a total thyroidectomy with removal of regional nodes can safely be performed.[230] In patients with MEN, surgery should be performed for pheochromocytomas before surgery for MTC is performed. First-degree relatives of patients with MEN or familial MTC should undergo DNA testing for the presence of the mutant *RET* gene (see Chapter 36). Gene carriers should undergo a prophylactic total thyroidectomy between 5 and 7 years of age.[232, 233]

Primary Malignant Lymphoma

Primary lymphomas of the thyroid are uncommon tumors, constituting fewer than 2% of all thyroid malignancies. The peak incidence is in the seventh decade, and the male/female ratio is 1:3.[237–240] Thyroid lymphomas are almost invariably seen as a rapidly enlarging, painless neck mass, fixed to surrounding tissues; they cause compressive symptoms and should be differentiated from anaplastic carcinoma. Unilateral or bilateral lymph node enlargement is present in about 50% of affected patients. Clinically evident distant disease is uncommon. The palpated mass is solid and, if studied by imaging, would be hypoechoic on ultrasonography and nonfunctioning on thyroid scintiscan. Most primary thyroid lymphomas arise in patients who have chronic autoimmune thyroiditis. Nonetheless, the disease is a rare complication of Hashimoto's thyroiditis.[241]

Primary thyroid lymphomas should be distinguished from generalized lymphomas with thyroid involvement. FNAB can be useful in distinguishing lymphoid proliferation from epithelial tumors. However, differentiating lymphoma from chronic autoimmune thyroiditis by thyroid cytology may be difficult.[242] Therefore, surgical specimens are needed for diagnosis. Immunohistochemical studies identify lymphoid proliferation if findings are positive for leukocyte common antigen.

Because chronic autoimmune thyroiditis reproduces the exact features of a mucosa-associated lymphoid tissue (MALT), most cases of thyroid lymphoma are considered MALT lymphomas.[243] Those small cell lymphomas are characterized by a low grade of malignancy, slow growth, and a tendency for recurrence in other MALT sites, such as the gastrointestinal or respiratory tract, the thymus, or the salivary glands.

A large proportion of clinical cases are large cell lymphomas and have an aggressive course. With immunohistochemistry, nearly all of them show B-cell markers. Monoclonality for light chain immunoglobulin is considered a strong indication of malignant lymphoma. Usually, immunohistochemistry is positive for BCL2 in small cell and negative in large cell lymphomas.

Although accurate staging is very important for planning treatment, patients are often elderly, in poor condition, or may require urgent therapy to relieve symptoms, thus making a full staging investigation before treatment impractical. Staging includes physical examination; complete blood count; serum lactate dehydrogenase and β_2-microglobulin measurements; liver function tests; bone marrow biopsy; CT scanning of the neck, thorax, abdomen, and pelvis; and appropriate biopsies at sites where tumor is suspected. Involvement of Waldeyer's ring and of the gastrointestinal tract has been associated with thyroid lymphomas, and for this reason upper gastrointestinal radiography or endoscopy should be performed.

Disseminated disease necessitates chemotherapy. In patients with disease apparently confined to the neck, therapy is guided by the histologic features of the lymphoma. Chemotherapy with an anthracycline-based regimen and involved-field radiotherapy should be given to all patients with large cell thyroid lymphoma and in some series has provided long-term survival rates of nearly 100%. For small cell MALT lymphomas, radiation alone may be adequate if the disease is determined to be localized after accurate staging.[238–240]

SURGICAL TREATMENT OF THYROID CARCINOMA

The extent of surgery appropriate for thyroid malignancy is a matter of controversy.[190, 191] Factors that influence this decision include the histologic diagnosis, the size of the original lesion, the presence of DM, the patient's age, and the risk group category.[221, 223] Obviously, the surgeon must be appropriately skilled in thyroid surgery, and the goal of surgery should be to remove all the malignant neoplastic tissue present in the neck. Therefore, the thyroid gland and affected neck lymph nodes should all be carefully identified and adequately resected.

In the case of PTC and FTC, although some debate still exists regarding the extent of thyroid surgery, many favor a near-total (leaving no more than 2 to 3 g of thyroid tissue) thyroidectomy for all patients.[169, 187] Near-total thyroidectomy reduces the recurrence rate, compared with more limited surgery, because many PTCs are both multifocal and bilateral. Removal of most, if not all, of the thyroid gland facilitates postoperative remnant ablation with ^{131}I.

For extremely low-risk patients (i.e., those with unifocal intrathyroidal PTM and possibly small [$<$2 cm] FTC with only capsular invasion), a lobectomy may be an appropriate primary surgical procedure.[171, 219] In patients who have undergone a previous unilateral lobectomy for a supposedly benign tumor that proves to be an angioinvasive FTC, a completion thyroidectomy is advisable because it facilitates future follow-up.

Surgery of lymph nodes is routinely performed in patients with PTC. It should include dissection of the central compartment (paratracheal and tracheoesophageal areas) and may also include dissection of the supraclavicular area and the lower third of the jugulocarotid chain. A modified neck dissection is performed if palpable lymph node metastases are present in the jugulocarotid chain. Dissection is preferable to lymph node picking. Although this type of lymph node dissection has not been shown to improve the recurrence and survival rates,[218, 244] several arguments support its routine use in patients with papillary carcinomas. These include the fact that histologic evidence of lymph node metastases is present in about two thirds of PTC patients, of whom more than 80% have involvement of the central compartment, and metastases are difficult to detect by palpation in lymph nodes located behind the vessels or in the paratracheal groove. The knowledge of initial lymph node status, acquired by such a routine, helps in the interpretation of any cervical abnormality identified during the subsequent postoperative follow-up. In the case of FTC, lymph node metastases are less frequent, but a lymph node dissection should be performed if FTC has already been diagnosed and palpable lymph nodes are present.

MTC is usually treated by total thyroidectomy, with a dissection of the central compartment of the neck and the lower two thirds of the jugulocarotid chains. A modified neck dissection may be required for MTC affecting the lateral neck nodes.[230, 245]

Ideally, patients with anaplastic carcinoma should be treated with near-total thyroidectomy and lymph node dissection,[229] but lesions are usually too extensive for any procedure but palliative surgery.[226] In these cases, surgery may be performed later in the case of tumor regression after a combination of chemotherapy and external radiotherapy.

In recommending surgery, the endocrinologist should discuss potential operative complications with the patient. Unilateral lobectomy virtually never causes permanent hypocalcemia but can cause vocal cord paralysis in as many as 3% of patients. Near-total thyroidectomy causes temporary hypocalcemia in 7% to 10% of patients and permanent hypocalcemia in 0.5% to 1%; temporary vocal cord paralysis occurs in about 1% to 2%. A total extracapsular thyroidectomy may lead to hypoparathyroidism in as many as 30% of individuals, an unacceptable complication rate for patients with indolent malignancy. In addition, vocal cord paralysis is more common after such a procedure. The experience of the surgeon is important in terms of the finer technical points of thyroidectomy, including preservation of the external branch of the recurrent laryngeal nerve, which is important in the fine regulation of voice pitch.

A history of radiation in childhood increases the risk of both benign and malignant thyroid nodules in later life.[246] The risk increases with a younger age at exposure and larger radiation dose.[247, 248] Several issues are relevant for the thyroidologist. First, given that surgical exploration may be required for patients with a history of thyroid radiation and suspicious thyroid nodules, what should the extent of initial surgery be and how should such patients be treated subsequently?

With respect to the extent of surgery, the protocol described previously should be applied to patients with a thyroid carcinoma. In cases with benign lesions, individuals with bilateral nodular disease should have a near-total thyroidectomy; when the opposite lobe is macroscopically normal, one must weigh the relative risk of complications associated with a more extensive surgical procedure against the possibility of recurrence of thyroid nodules in the residual thyroid tissue.

In one irradiated population, both benign and malignant nodules recurred after previous subtotal thyroidectomy.[249] The overall risk of recurrence in this study was approximately 20% and was lower in those who had more thyroid tissue removed than in those who had less extensive procedures. In those patients, suppression of TSH by thyroid hormone led to a reduction in recurrence from 35% to approximately 8%, but TSH suppression had no influence on the occurrence of malignant nodules.

Thus, the recommendations for such patients must take into account the estimated risk of developing a thyroid nodule and the experience of the operating surgeon. All irradiated patients who have had thyroid nodules removed should receive TSH-suppressive doses of levothyroxine regardless of the extent of surgery. The appearance of new thyroid nodules is, however, fairly common, and such patients should be monitored indefinitely for this possibility.

It is not clear whether this experience should be extrapolated to prescribe routine TSH suppression therapy for all irradiated patients, even if nodularity is not present, because its beneficial effects have not been quantified and the risks of long-term TSH suppression in women, especially vis-à-vis osteoporosis, have not been clearly defined and may be significant.[88–90] At present, this approach cannot be recommended for all irradiated patients but can be recommended for patients at high risk of developing a thyroid nodule.[246]

POSTOPERATIVE MANAGEMENT

In view of the foregoing uncertainties and the different needs of individual patients, postoperative treatment of thyroid carcinoma cannot always accord with a rigid algorithm.[250] One must consider the extent of disease at surgery, the histotype and differentiation of the tumor, the age of the patient, and the risk group category.[108, 126, 223]

Iodine 131 Therapy

^{131}I is an effective agent for delivering high radiation doses to the thyroid tissue with low spillover to other portions of the body. The radiation dose to the thyroid tissue is related to the tissue concentration, the ratio between the total tissue uptake and the volume of functional tissue, and the effective half-life of ^{131}I in the tissue. Thyroid tissue is able to concentrate iodine only after TSH stimulation, but even after optimal TSH stimulation, iodine uptake in neoplastic tissue is always lower than in normal thyroid tissue and may not be detectable in about one third of cases.

^{131}I therapy is given postoperatively for three reasons. First, it destroys normal thyroid remnants, thereby increasing the sensitivity of subsequent ^{131}I total-body scanning and the specificity of measurements of serum Tg for the detection of persistent or recurrent disease. Second, it may destroy occult microscopic carcinoma, thereby potentially decreasing the long-term recurrence rate. Finally, it makes it possible to perform a postablative ^{131}I total-body scan, a sensitive tool for detecting persistent carcinoma.

It cannot be emphasized too strongly that postoperative ^{131}I therapy should be used *selectively* and that not all patients with a diagnosis of FCTC benefit from routine postoperative radioiodine ablative therapy.[117] For low-risk patients, the long-term prognosis after surgery alone is so favorable that ^{131}I ablation is not usually recommended. However, patients who are at high risk of recurrence (Table 13–6) are routinely treated with ^{131}I because such therapy can potentially decrease both recurrence and death rates. Young children are also usually candidates for postoperative radioiodine therapy because they may have extensive neck lymph node involvement and frequently harbor pulmonary metastases that may not be detectable with standard radiographs or even with CT imaging of the chest.[251, 252]

Postoperatively, no levothyroxine treatment is given for 4 to 6 weeks but liothyronine can be substituted for at least 3 to 4 weeks and then discontinued for 2 weeks before radioiodine studies. At that time, the serum TSH level should be greater than 25 to 30 mU/L. Neck uptake may be measured with a tracer dose of ^{131}I; high uptake (>10%) should lead to completion surgery. ^{131}I therapy can be administered to the other patients, usually with 24-hour uptakes considerably less than 10%. A total body scan is performed 4 to 7 days after the treatment dose, and levothyroxine suppressive therapy is initiated. Total ablation (defined as no visible uptake) may be verified by an ^{131}I total-body scan 6 to 12 months later, typically with 2 to 5 mCi (74 to 185 MBq).[253]

Total ablation is achieved after administration of either 100 mCi (3700 MBq) or 30 mCi (1100 MBq) in more than 80% of patients who had at least a near-total thyroidectomy. After less extensive surgery, ablation is achieved in only two thirds of patients with 30 mCi (1100 MBq). Therefore, a near-total thyroidectomy should be performed in all patients who are to be treated with ^{131}I. Total ablation requires that a dose of at least 300 Gy (30,000 rad) is delivered to thyroid remnants, and a dosimetric study can allow a more precise estimate of the ^{131}I dose to be administered.[253] Obviously, the only patients eligible for such a protocol would be those selected high-risk patients with either PTC or FTC. ^{131}I ablation therapy does not play a regular role in the management of patients with anaplastic thyroid cancer, MTC, or thyroid lymphoma.

Table 13–6. Indications for ^{131}I Treatment in Patients with Papillary, Follicular, or Hürthle Cell Thyroid Carcinoma after Initial Definitive Near-Total Thyroidectomy

No indication
- Patients at low risk of cause-specific mortality or of relapse (e.g., PTC patients with MACIS scores < 6 and pTNM stage I FTC or HCC patients)

Indications
- **Definite**
  - Distant metastasis at diagnosis
  - Incomplete tumor resection
  - Patients at high risk for mortality or recurrence (e.g., PTC with MACIS 6+ and pTNM stage II/III FTC or HCC)
- **Probable**
  - PTC or FTC in children younger than 16 years
  - Tall cell or columnar cell variant of PTC
- **Possible**
  - Diffuse sclerosing variant PTC
  - Bulky bilateral nodal metastases
  - Elevated Tg at 3+ months postoperatively

FTC, follicular thyroid carcinoma; HCC, Hürthle cell carcinoma; MACIS, metastasis, age, completeness of resection, invasion, and size; PTC, papillary thyroid carcinoma; pTNM, pathologic-Tumor-Node-Metastasis; Tg, thyroglobulin.

External Radiotherapy

External radiotherapy to the neck and mediastinum is indicated only for older patients with extensive PTC in whom complete surgical excision is impossible and in whom the tumor tissue does not take up ^{131}I. Retrospective studies have shown that in these selected patients, external radiotherapy decreases the risk of neck recurrence.[254–256] The target volume encompasses the thyroid bed, bilateral neck lymph node areas, and the upper part of the mediastinum. Typically, 50 Gy (5000 rad) would be delivered in 25 fractions over 5 weeks.

In patients with MTC, this protocol may be applied after incomplete resection of the tumor and also after apparently complete surgery, when plasma calcitonin remains detectable in the absence of DM. In these patients, it may decrease the risk of neck recurrence by a factor of 2 to 4.[153, 254]

In patients with anaplastic thyroid carcinoma, when the extent of disease is limited and surgery is feasible, accelerated external radiotherapy in combination with chemotherapy permits local control of the disease in two thirds of the patients and long-term survival in about 20%.[229]

Levothyroxine Treatment

The growth of thyroid tumor cells is controlled by TSH, and inhibition of TSH secretion with levothyroxine is thought to improve the recurrence and survival rates. Therefore, levothyroxine should be given to all patients with FCTC, whatever the extent of thyroid surgery and other treatment. The initial effective dose is about 2.5 μg/kg body weight in adults; children require a higher dose. The adequacy of therapy is monitored by measuring serum TSH 3 months after it is begun, the initial goal being a serum TSH concentration of 0.1 mU/L or less. In some centers, the serum free T_3 concentration is also documented to be within the normal range.[257] When these guidelines are followed, levothyroxine therapy does not have deleterious effects on the heart or bone.[89]

In patients with anaplastic thyroid carcinoma, MTC, or thyroid lymphoma, a replacement dose of levothyroxine is given with the aim of obtaining a serum TSH level in the normal range.

FOLLOW-UP

In patients with PTC or FTC, the goals of follow-up after initial therapy are to maintain adequate levothyroxine suppressive therapy and to detect persistent or recurrent thyroid carcinoma. Most recurrences occur during the first years of follow-up, but some occur late. Therefore, follow-up is necessary throughout the patient's life.

Early Detection of Recurrent Disease

Clinical and Ultrasonographic Examinations

Palpation of the thyroid bed and lymph node areas should be routinely performed at all follow-up visits in patients with thyroid cancer. Ultrasonography should be performed in patients at high risk of recurrence and in any patient with clinically suspicious findings. Palpable lymph nodes that are small, thin, or oval; in the posterior neck chains; and especially if they decrease in size after an interval of 3 months are considered benign. By contrast, round shape, hypoechogenicity and absence of a central echogenic line, microcalcifications, a cystic component, and hypervascularization on color Doppler ultrasonography are suspicious findings.

Serum Tg is undetectable in 20% of patients receiving levothyroxine treatment who have isolated lymph node metastases, and undetectable values do not exclude metastatic lymph node disease. If in doubt, ultrasound-guided node biopsy for cytology and Tg measurement in the fluid aspirate may be performed.[258] Sensitive reverse transcriptase–polymerase chain reaction (RT-PCR) to amplify Tg mRNA appears to be even more sensitive but is not yet being used by commercial laboratories.[259]

Radiographs

Bone and chest radiographs are no longer routinely obtained for patients with undetectable serum Tg concentrations. The reason is that virtually all patients with abnormal radiographs have readily detectable serum Tg concentrations.

Serum Thyroglobulin Determinations

Tg is a glycoprotein that is produced only by normal or neoplastic thyroid follicular cells. Methods used for serum Tg determination and serum interferences are detailed in Chapter 10. It should not be detectable in patients who have had total thyroid ablation, and its detection in that setting probably signifies the presence of persistent or recurrent disease (Table 13–7). In patients who are in complete remission after total thyroid ablation, serum Tg antibodies decline gradually to low or undetectable levels. Their persistence or their reappearance during follow-up should be considered suspicious for persistent or recurrent disease.[260]

Table 13–7. Percentages of Patients with Detectable (>1 ng/mL) Serum Thyroglobulin Concentrations during Thyroxine Treatment and after Discontinuation of Thyroxine According to the Presence or Absence of Normal Thyroid Tissue*

Thyroid Tumor Status	Total Ablation		Total Thyroidectomy	
Thyroxine treatment	On	Off	On	Off
Complete remission†	<2	10	7	20
Lymph node metastases	80	~90	—	—
Distant metastases with normal radiographs	95	~100	—	—
Large distant metastases‡	~100	~100	—	—

*Detectable serum thyroglobulin concentrations are above 1 ng/mL. Serum thyroglobulin values are highly dependent on the assay. In this study, an immunoradiometric method with a sensitivity of 1 ng/mL was used.

†Most detectable serum thyroglobulin concentrations were below 5 ng/mL.

‡Most serum thyroglobulin concentrations were above 10 ng/mL.

From Schlumberger MJ. Papillary and follicular thyroid carcinoma. N Engl J Med 1998; 338:297–306.

The production of Tg by both normal and neoplastic thyroid tissue is in part TSH dependent. When serum Tg is detectable during levothyroxine treatment, it increases after TSH stimulation obtained either after the treatment is discontinued or with injections of rhTSH. After rhTSH stimulation, the peak of serum Tg is usually obtained 3 days after the second injection.[261–263]

The serum Tg concentration is an excellent prognostic indicator. Most patients with undetectable serum Tg concentrations who were not receiving levothyroxine therapy remained free of relapse after more than 15 years of follow-up, and only 2% had a neck lymph node recurrence. Conversely, 60% to 80% of patients with serum Tg concentrations above 10 ng/mL after levothyroxine withdrawal and with no other evidence of disease had detectable foci of ^{131}I uptake in the neck or at distant sites after administration of a large dose (3700 MBq, 100 mCi) of ^{131}I.[264]

Several researchers have developed sensitive RT-PCR assays to amplify circulating Tg mRNA. The technique appeared sensitive in that the test was positive in most patients with thyroid tissue, but results were not related to the extent of the disease.[265, 266] This technique may be useful in patients with Tg antibodies.

Iodine 131 Total-Body Scan

The results of a ^{131}I total-body scan depend on the ability of neoplastic thyroid tissue to take up ^{131}I in the presence of high serum TSH concentrations, which are achieved by withdrawing levothyroxine for 4 to 6 weeks. However, the resulting hypothyroidism is poorly tolerated by some patients. This effect can be attenuated by substituting the more rapidly metabolized liothyronine for levothyroxine for 3 to 4 weeks and withdrawing it for 2 weeks or simply by reducing the dose of levothyroxine by 50%.[267]

The serum TSH concentration should be above some arbitrary value (>25 to 30 mU/L) in patients treated in this way; if it is not, ^{131}I administration should be delayed until it is. Intramuscular injections of rhTSH (0.9 mg for 2 consecutive days) are an alternative because levothyroxine treatment need not be discontinued and side effects are minimal. When combining serum Tg measurement and ^{131}I total-body scanning, its efficiency is comparable to that of levothyroxine withdrawal in most patients.[261–263]

Table 13–8. Nonthyroidal Conditions Associated with ^{131}I Accumulation

Contamination
- Skin, hair, clothes

Physiologic accumulations
- Salivary glands (mouth, nose)
- Stomach, esophagus, colon
- Bladder
- Breast
- Diffuse hepatic uptake (^{131}I-labeled iodoproteins)

Inflammatory processes
- Lung or bronchial, cutaneous, dental, sinusoidal

Various conditions
- Nonthyroidal neoplasms: salivary glands, stomach, lung, meningioma, struma ovarii
- Cysts: renal, pleuropericardial, hepatic, salivary, mammary, testicular hydrocele
- Thymus: normal or hyperplastic
- Ectasia of the common carotid artery with stasis
- Esophagus: dilatation, hiatal hernia
- Pericardial effusion, cardiac insufficiency

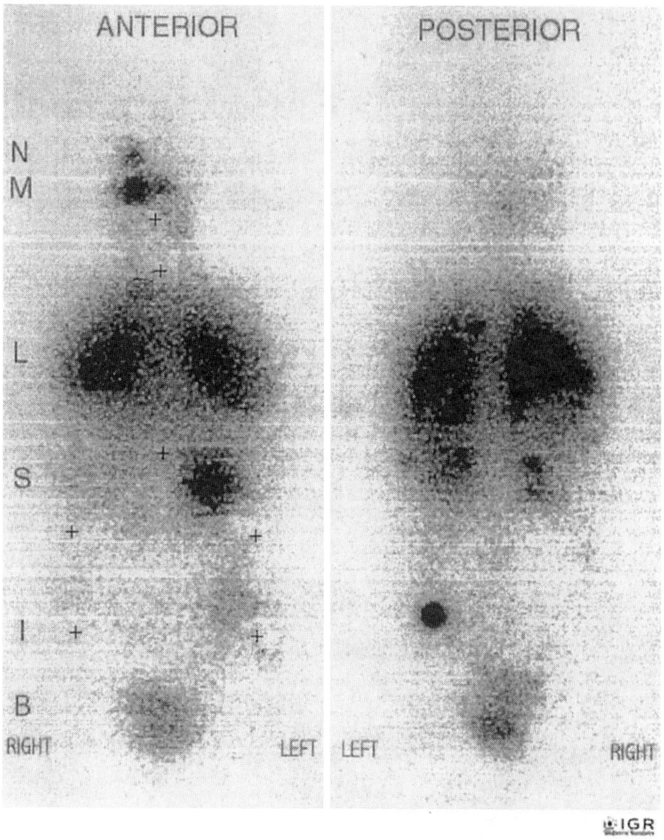

Figure 13–24. Total-body scan performed 5 days after administration of 100 mCi (3700 MBq) of radioactive iodine (^{131}I). The chest radiograph of this asymptomatic 34-year-old patient, who was being monitored for a papillary thyroid carcinoma, was normal; the only abnormality was an elevated serum thyroglobulin level, at 45 ng/mL, during levothyroxine suppressive treatment. Note the presence of diffuse uptake in the lungs (L) and in the left iliac bone (I). After four treatments with 100 mCi of ^{131}I, metastatic uptake disappeared and the thyroglobulin level became undetectable during levothyroxine therapy. B, bladder; M, mouth; N, nose; S, stomach.

When ^{131}I scanning is planned, patients should be instructed to avoid iodine-containing medications and iodine-rich foods, and urinary iodine should be measured in doubtful cases. Pregnancy must be excluded in women of childbearing age. For routine diagnostic scans, from 2 to 5 mCi (74 to 185 MBq) of ^{131}I is given; higher doses may reduce the uptake of a subsequent therapeutic dose of ^{131}I.[268] The scan is done and uptake, if any, is measured 48 to 72 hours after the dose, preferably using a double-head gamma camera equipped with thick crystals and high-energy collimators. False-positive results are rare and are usually easily recognized (Table 13–8).

Post–Iodine 131 Therapy Total-Body Scans

Assuming equivalent fractional uptake after administration of either a diagnostic or a therapeutic dose of ^{131}I, uptake too low to be detected with 2 to 5 mCi (74 to 185 MBq) may be detectable after the administration of 100 mCi (3700 MBq). Thus, a total-body scan should be routinely performed 4 to 7 days after a high dose (Fig. 13–24). This is also the rationale for administering a large dose of ^{131}I in patients with elevated Tg levels (>10 ng/mL in the absence of levothyroxine treatment), even if the diagnostic scan is negative.[264]

Other Tests

These should be performed only in selected cases and may include spiral CT or MR imaging of the neck and chest, bone scintigraphy, PET scanning using ^{18}FDG, and scintigraphy using a less specific tracer (e.g., thallium, MIBI, tetrofosmin). The FDG PET scan is more frequently positive in patients with no detectable ^{131}I uptake in the metastases and is particularly sensitive for the discovery of neck lymph nodes (Fig. 13–25); a spiral CT scan is more sensitive than a FDG PET scan for the discovery of small lung metastases.[22–24]

Follow-up Strategy

If the total-body scan performed after administration of ^{131}I to destroy the thyroid remnants does not show any uptake outside the thyroid bed, physical examination is performed and serum TSH and Tg are measured during levothyroxine treatment 3 months later (Fig. 13–26). In most centers, the serum Tg level is measured and a diagnostic ^{131}I total-body scan is done after thyroid hormone withdrawal or rhTSH stimulation 6 to 12 months later. Visible uptake in the thyroid bed that is too low to be quantified should not be considered evidence of disease in the absence of any other abnormality.

If any significant uptake is detected outside the thyroid bed, a therapeutic dose of 100 mCi (3700 MBq) of ^{131}I is given. Serum Tg determination after TSH stimulation, obtained after either thyroid hormone withdrawal or injections of rhTSH, may help to select for scanning with a large amount of ^{131}I those patients with negative diagnostic ^{131}I total-body scans who have detectable serum Tg levels.[269]

In low-risk patients considered cured, the dose of levothyroxine is decreased to maintain a low but detectable serum TSH concentration (0.1 to 0.5 mU/L). In high-risk patients, higher doses of levothyroxine are given, the goal being a serum TSH concentration less than 0.1 mU/L.[270] Clinical and biochemical evaluations are performed annually; neck ultrasonography is frequently performed in case of doubt or in high-risk patients, but any other testing is unnecessary as long as the patient's serum Tg concentration is undetectable and the patient does not produce an interfering anti-Tg autoantibody.

In patients receiving levothyroxine in whom serum Tg becomes detectable, neck ultrasonography is performed and serum Tg may be measured again after levothyroxine is discontinued or after rhTSH stimulation. If residual neck disease is found on sonography, the diagnosis should be confirmed by guided biopsy and consideration given to surgical reexploration

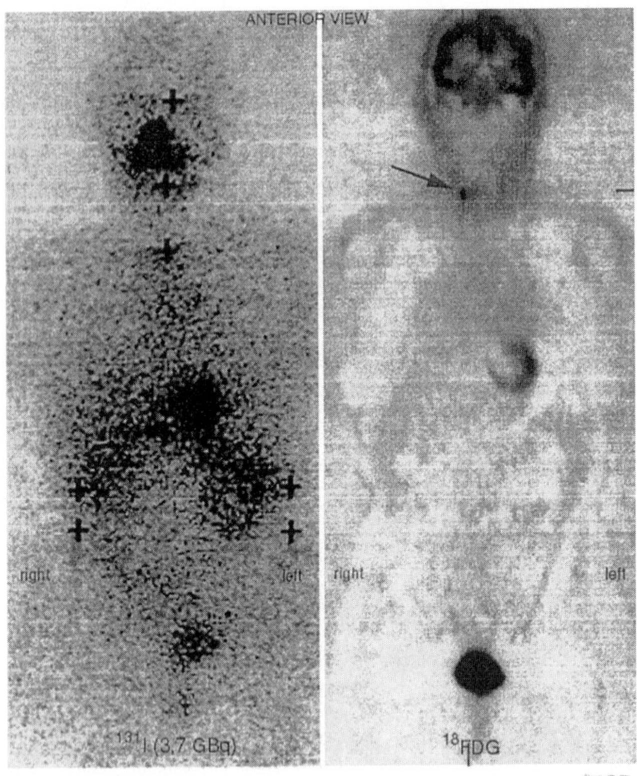

Figure 13–25. The patient was being monitored for a papillary thyroid carcinoma. The serum thyroglobulin level was 22 ng/mL during levothyroxine suppressive treatment, and local imaging modalities were not interpretable because of three previous extensive neck operations. *Left*, Total-body scan performed 4 days after administration of 100 mCi (3.7 GBq); there is no visible uptake in the neck. *Right*, Positron emission tomography scan using [^{18}F]fluorodeoxyglucose (^{18}FDG) demonstrating significant uptake in a paratracheal lymph node *(arrow)* that measured 12 mm in diameter at surgery.

of the neck. If there is no demonstrable neck disease but the stimulated serum Tg concentration increases above 10 ng/mL, even if no uptake is seen on a diagnostic ^{131}I total-body scan performed with 2 to 5 mCi, consideration should be given to the administration of a therapeutic dose of 100 mCi of ^{131}I. In the absence of ^{131}I uptake, spiral CT of the neck and lungs, bone scintigraphy, and FDG PET scanning can be useful in localizing hitherto unrecognized sites of recurrent disease. In patients whose serum Tg levels are initially undetectable during levothyroxine treatment but later become detectable (levels <10 ng/mL) after TSH stimulation, another Tg determination should be obtained after TSH stimulation every 2 to 5 years, depending on Tg levels and on prognostic factors.

In low-risk PTC patients who have had a near-total thyroidectomy but who were not given ^{131}I postoperatively, the intensity of the follow-up strategy depends largely on the serum Tg level. If the Tg is not detectable and a neck ultrasound is negative, ^{131}I total-body scanning may be avoided. However, if despite adequate TSH suppression, the Tg is readily detectable, a ^{131}I total-body scan may be performed 6 to 12 months after surgery. An ablative ^{131}I treatment may rarely be necessary in some of those patients who have either an elevated serum Tg level or abnormal findings on ^{131}I total-body scanning. The follow-up protocol previously described is then applied on the basis of serum Tg determinations.

In low-risk PTC patients who have initially undergone only a unilateral lobectomy for small (<15 mm) tumors, yearly follow-up should consist of a careful neck examination and serum Tg determination during levothyroxine treatment. With time, ultrasonography is likely to show focal nodular abnormalities in the remaining lobe in most patients with detectable Tg concentrations. Usually, biopsies of these lesions can be performed under sonographic guidance, and most prove to be cytologically benign. However, if recurrent PTC is found on biopsy, a completion thyroidectomy should be performed.

For MTC patients, the tumor marker for follow-up is the plasma calcitonin level. In more than 90% of young patients whose disease is treated at a preclinical stage on the basis of a *RET* oncogene mutation, the postoperative calcitonin level returns to normal and peak levels after stimulation with either pentagastrin or calcium are absent.[233] Patients with a negative pentagastrin stimulation test after two follow-up evaluations are likely to be cured, despite the fact that about 5% of them have subsequent biologic recurrence of the disease.

In adults with sporadic MTC, who most often present with TNM stage III (node-positive) disease, postoperative calcitonin levels are rarely normal, and normal responsiveness to pentagastrin stimulation is unusual.[271] In general, basal and stimulated calcitonin levels correlate with MTC tumor mass,[230, 233] but many MTC patients who have surgery with a curative intent still have postoperative elevations in calcitonin levels without clinical or imaging evidence of persistent disease.[230, 271] In these patients, the localization of neoplastic foci may be difficult and may require a venous sampling catheterization with calcitonin measurements. Reinterventions based on the

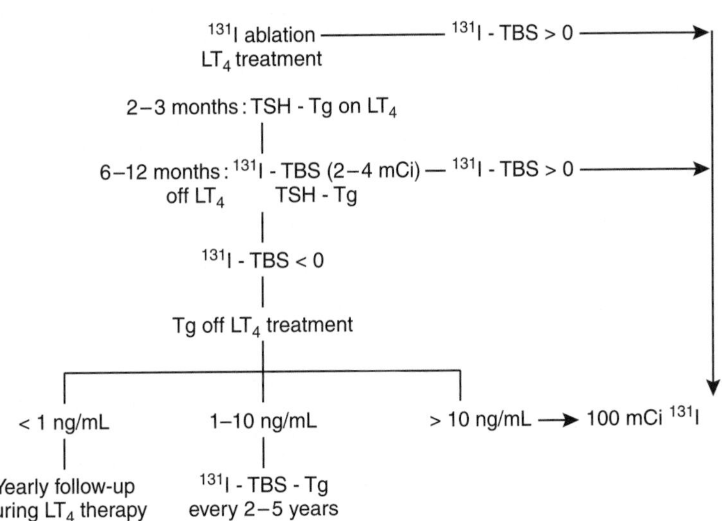

Figure 13–26. Follow-up of high-risk patients with papillary or follicular thyroid carcinoma after near-total thyroidectomy based on serum thyroglobulin (Tg) measurements and ^{131}I ablation, total-body scanning. LT_4, levothyroxine; TBS, total-body scan; TSH, thyrotropin. Thyroglobulin values are method specific, and the normal range should be determined in each assay. For the total-body scan, above 0 is positive, with ^{131}I uptake indicative of neoplastic foci; below 0 is negative.

results of selective venous sampling catheterization allow the removal of neoplastic foci in most patients, but they are not likely to improve the cure rate by more than 5% to 30%.[272, 273] Such a situation may exist for several postoperative years, and slowly rising calcitonin levels may not necessarily imply a prognosis worse than that indicated by the presenting stage of disease.[271]

A second major tumor marker for MTC is CEA. In general, serum CEA levels are higher in more malignant MTC, whereas the plasma calcitonin level is higher in those with better differentiated tumors, leading some authorities to suggest that a rising CEA level postoperatively correlates better with the emergence of a potentially aggressive tumor recurrence.[274, 275]

Papillary and Follicular Thyroid Carcinoma

Locoregional Recurrences

Locoregional recurrences occur in 5% to 20% of patients with PTC and FTC. A recurrence that is palpable or easily visualized with ultrasonography or CT scanning should be excised.[276–278] Total excision may be facilitated by total-body scanning 4 days after administration of 100 mCi (3700 MBq) of ^{131}I because additional tissue that should be excised may be identified. In some selected centers, surgery is performed 1 day later, typically using an intraoperative probe. The completeness of resection is verified 1 to 2 days after surgery by another total-body scan, and in one series this was achieved in 92% of cases.[278] External radiotherapy is indicated only in FCTC patients with soft tissue recurrences that cannot be completely excised and that do not take up ^{131}I.[254]

Recently, it has been reported that patients with PTC who were not eligible for further surgery or ^{131}I therapy have been treated for regional nodal recurrence with ultrasound-guided radiofrequency ablation[279] or percutaneous ethanol injections (PEI).[280] Both techniques appear promising in selected PTC patients with recurrent nodal disease that is not amenable to conventional retreatment with surgery, ^{131}I, or external irradiation.

Distant Metastases

In a large group of patients with differentiated carcinoma (PTC, FTC, and HCC), only 9% developed DM.[281] Mortality rates at 5 and 10 years after the diagnosis of metastasis were 65% and 75% for all patients with DM, and nearly 80% of the deaths were due to thyroid cancer. Thus, the development of DM in FCTC portends an ominous prognosis. Lung metastases are more frequent in young patients with PTC, and the lung is almost the only site of distant spread in children.[151, 252] Bone metastases are more common in older patients and in those with FTC. Other less common sites are the brain, liver, and skin.

Clinical symptoms of lung involvement are uncommon. By contrast, pain, swelling, or fracture occurs in more than 80% of patients with bone metastases. The pattern of lung involvement may vary from macronodular to diffuse infiltrates. The latter, when not detected by chest radiography, are usually diagnosed with ^{131}I total-body scan and may be confirmed by spiral CT; enlarged mediastinal lymph nodes are often present in patients with PTC, especially children. Bone metastases are osteolytic and are often difficult to visualize on radiographs; bone scintigraphy may show decreased or moderately increased uptake, and bone involvement is better visualized by CT or MRI. Nearly all patients with DM have high serum Tg concentrations unless the lung metastases are not visible on radiographs, and two thirds of such patients have ^{131}I uptake in their sites of metastasis.

Palliative surgery is required for bone metastases when there are neurologic or orthopedic complications or a high risk of such complications. Surgery may also be performed with a curative intent in patients with a single or a few bone metastases.[282–284]

Patients with DM that take up ^{131}I should be treated with 100 to 150 mCi (3700 to 5550 MBq) every 4 to 6 months. Between ^{131}I treatments, suppressive doses of levothyroxine are given. The radiation dose to the tumor tissue and outcome of ^{131}I therapy are correlated.[285] A radiation dose higher than 80 Gy (8000 rads) should be delivered to obtain cure; with radiation doses less than 35 Gy (3500 rads), there is little chance for success. For treatment to be effective in this clinical setting, appropriate levels of TSH stimulation and absence of iodine contamination are essential. For this reason, higher doses (200 mCi [7400 MBq] or more) have been advocated in patients with bone metastases, but their effectiveness remains to be demonstrated. Lower doses (1 mCi [37 MBq]/kg body weight) are given to children.

There is no limit to the cumulative dose of ^{131}I that can be given to patients with DM, although the risk of leukemia rises slightly above a cumulative dose of 500 mCi (18,500 MBq); furthermore, above this dose, further ^{131}I therapy may rarely provide benefit. External radiotherapy is given to bone metastases visible on radiographs, even in the presence of iodine uptake.[254] Alternatively, embolization or cement injection may be considered.[286] Chemotherapy is poorly effective and should be given only to patients with progressing and nonfunctioning metastases.[287, 288] Retinoic acid analogues increased iodine uptake by neoplastic tissue and decreased its growth rate in several in vitro models.[289] Further clinical trials are still warranted to assess the role of such therapies.

Complete responses have been obtained overall in about 45% of patients with DM showing avidity for ^{131}I, and responses are even more frequent in younger patients and in those with small pulmonary metastases.[290, 291] It was shown by PET scanning that large DM with high FDG uptake almost never respond to ^{131}I therapy.[23] When response was judged to have been complete after ^{131}I therapy, subsequent relapse rarely occurred even though serum Tg levels were persistently detectable in some patients.

Overall survival after the discovery of DM is more favorable in young patients with well-differentiated tumors that take up ^{131}I and have metastases that are small when discovered. When the tumor mass is considered, the location of the DM, be it in the lungs or bone, has no independent prognostic influence. The poor prognosis of patients with bone metastases is linked to the large size of their lesions.[283, 290, 291] The prognostic importance of the small size of the metastases at their discovery has led to the administration of 100-mCi (3700-MBq) doses of ^{131}I to patients with elevated serum Tg concentrations and no other evidence of disease. Some believe that there is no conclusive evidence that ^{131}I treatment of these asymptomatic patients meaningfully prolongs life.[292] Others recently have reported a 33% complete remission rate in treated patients who had a positive post-^{131}I therapy total-body scan.[293]

Complications of Treatment with Iodine 131

Acute side effects (nausea, sialadenitis) after treatment with ^{131}I are common but are typically mild and resolve rapidly. Radiation thyroiditis is usually trivial, but if the thyroid remnant is large, the patient may have enough pain to warrant corticosteroid therapy for a few days. Tumor in certain locations, such as the brain, spinal cord, and paratrachea, may swell in response to TSH stimulation or after ^{131}I therapy, causing compressive symptoms. Radiation fibrosis may develop in patients with diffuse lung metastases and can eventually prove fatal if high doses (>150 mCi [5550 MBq]) are administered at short intervals (<3 months).

Particular attention must be paid to avoid administration of ^{131}I to pregnant women. After ^{131}I treatment, spermatogenesis may be transiently depressed, and women may have transient ovarian failure. Genetic damage induced by exposure to ^{131}I before conception has been a major subject of concern. However, the only anomaly reported to date is an increased frequency of miscarriages in women treated with ^{131}I during the year preceding the conception. Therefore, it is recommended that conception be postponed for 1 year after treatment with ^{131}I. There is no evidence that pregnancy affects tumor growth in women receiving adequate levothyroxine therapy.[294] During pregnancy, the serum TSH level should be measured every 2 months, and this frequently leads to an increase in the daily dose of levothyroxine.

Mild pancytopenia may occur after repeated ^{131}I therapy, especially in patients with bone metastases also treated with external radiotherapy. The overall relative risk of leukemia was found to be increased only in patients treated with a high cumulative dose of ^{131}I (>500 mCi [18,500 MBq]) or in association with external radiotherapy.[295, 296] In contrast, there is no significant increased risk of solid carcinoma in these patients.[293]

Medullary Thyroid Carcinoma

For patients with locoregional recurrence of MTC, a complete diagnostic work-up should be obtained, principally to exclude DM. Surgery is performed when feasible and is typically followed by external radiotherapy.

DM are usually multifocal in each involved organ and frequently involve multiple organs, including liver, lungs, and bones. They may progress slowly and may be compatible with decades of survival. Systemic chemotherapy is poorly efficient and may be indicated only in cases of rapid tumor progression.[297]

References

1. Nishiyama H, Sodd VJ, Berke RA, et al. Evaluation of clinical value of ^{123}I and ^{131}I in thyroid disease. J Nucl Med 1974; 15: 261–265.
2. Paltiel HJ, Summerville DA, Treves ST. Iodine-123 scintigraphy in the evaluation of pediatric thyroid disorders: a ten-year experience. Pediatr Radiol 1992; 22:251–256.
3. Price DC. Radioisotopic evaluation of the thyroid and the parathyroids. Radiol Clin North Am 1993; 31:991–1015.
4. Hoffer PB, Goltschalk A, Refetoff S. Thyroid scanning technics: the old and the new. Curr Probl Radiol 1972; 2:1–26.
5. Rapoport B, Block MB, Hofer PB, et al. Depletion of thyroid iodine during subacute thyroiditis. J Clin Endocrinol Metab 1973; 36:610–611.
6. James EM, Charboneau JW, Hay ID. The thyroid. In Rumack CM, Wilson SR, Charboneau JW (eds). Diagnostic Ultrasound. St. Louis, Mosby Year Book, 1991, pp 507–523.
7. Reading CC, Gorman CA. Thyroid imaging techniques. Clin Lab Med 1993; 13:711–724.
8. James EM, Charboneau JW. High-frequency (10 MHz) thyroid ultrasonography. Semin Ultrasound CT MR 1985; 6:294–309.
9. Simeone JF, Daniels GH, Hall DA, et al. Sonography in the follow-up of 100 patients with thyroid carcinoma. AJR 1987; 148: 45–49.
10. Sutton RT, Reading CC, Charboneau JW, et al. US-guided biopsy of neck masses in postoperative management of patients with thyroid cancer. Radiology 1988; 168:769–772.
11. Boland GW, Lee MJ, Mueller PR, et al. Efficacy of sonographically-guided biopsy of thyroid masses and cervical lymph nodes. AJR 1993; 161:1053–1056.
12. Leenhardt L, Hejblum G, Franc B, et al. Indications and limits of ultrasound-guided cytology in the management of nonpalpable thyroid nodules. J Clin Endocrinol Metab 1999; 84:24–28.
13. Reede DL, Berceron RT. The CT evaluation of the normal diseased neck. Semin Ultrasound CT MR 1986; 22:239–250.
14. Silverman PM, Newman GE, Korobkin M. Computed tomography in the evaluation of thyroid disease. AJR 1984; 141:897–902.
15. Blum M, Reede DL, Seltzer TF, et al. Computerized tomography in the diagnosis of thyroid and parathyroid disorders. Am J Med Sci 1984; 287:34–39.
16. Bashist B, Ellis K, Gold RP. Computed tomography of intrathoracic goiters. AJR 1983; 140:455–460.
17. Higgins CB, Aufferman W. MR imaging of thyroid and parathyroid glands: a review of current status. AJR 1988; 151:1095–1106.
18. Mountz JM, Glazer GM, Dmuchowski C, et al. MR imaging of the thyroid: comparison with scintigraphy in the normal and diseased gland. J Comput Tomogr 1987; 11:612–621.
19. Brown LR, Aughenbaugh GL. Masses of the anterior mediastinum: CT and MR imaging. AJR 1991; 157:1171–1180.
20. van den Brekel MW, Castelijns JA, Stel HV, et al. Modern imaging techniques and ultrasound-guided aspiration cytology for the assessment of neck node metastases: a prospective comparative study. Eur Arch Otorhinolaryngol 1993; 250:11–17.
21. Toubert ME, Cyna-Gorse F, Zagdanski AM, et al. Cervicomediastinal magnetic resonance imaging in persistent or recurrent papillary thyroid carcinoma: clinical use and limits. Thyroid 1999; 9:591–597.
22. Wang W, Macapinlac H, Larson SM, et al. ^{18}F-2-fluoro-2-deoxy-D-glucose positron emission tomography localizes residual thyroid cancer in patients with negative diagnostic ^{131}I whole body scans and elevated serum thyroglobulin levels. J Clin Endocrinol Metab 1999; 84:2291–2302.
23. Wang W, Larson SM, Fazzari M, et al. Prognostic value of [^{18}F]fluorodeoxyglucose positron emission tomographic scanning in patients with thyroid cancer. J Clin Endocrinol Metab 2000; 85:1107–1113.
24. Dietlen M, Scheidhauer K, Voth E, et al. Fluorine-18-fluorodeoxyglucose positron emission tomography and iodine-131 whole-body scintigraphy in the follow-up of differentiated thyroid cancer. Eur J Nucl Med 1997; 24:1342–1348.
25. Thomas GA, Williams ED. Aetiology of simple goiter. Baillieres Clin Endocrinol Metab 1988; 2:703–718.
26. Greig WR, Boyle JA, Duncan A, et al. Genetic and non-genetic factors in simple goiter formation: evidence from a twin study. Q J Med 1967; 36:175–185.
27. Brix TH, Kyvik KO, Hegedus L. Major role of genes in the etiology of simple goiter in females: a population-based twin study. J Clin Endocrinol Metab 1999; 84:3071–3075.
28. Medeiros-Neto G, Kim PS, Vono J, et al. Congenital hypothyroid goiter with deficient thyroglobulin. J Clin Invest 1996; 98: 2838–2844.
29. Pohlenz J, Rosenthal IM, Weiss RE, et al. Congenital hypothyroidism due to mutations in the sodium/iodide symporter: identification of a nonsense mutation producing a downstream cryptic 3′ splice site. J Clin Invest 1998; 101:1028–1035.
30. Bikker H, Baas F, De Vijlder JJ. Molecular analysis of mutated thyroid peroxidase detected in patients with total iodide organification defects. J Clin Endocrinol Metab 1997; 82:649–653.
31. Sheffield VC, Kraiem Z, Beck JC, et al. Pendred syndrome maps to chromosome 7q21-34 and is caused by an intrinsic defect in thyroid iodine organification. Nat Genet 1996; 12:424–426.
32. Van Sande J, Parma J, Tonacchera M, et al. Somatic and germline mutations of the TSH receptor gene in thyroid diseases. J Clin Endocrinol Metab 1995; 80:2577–2585.
33. Bignell GR, Canzian F, Shayeghi M, et al. Familial nontoxic multinodular thyroid goiter locus maps to chromosome 14q but does not account for familial nonmedullary thyroid cancer. Am J Hum Genet 1997; 61:1123–1130.
34. Capon F, Tacconelli A, Giardina E, et al. Mapping a dominant form of multinodular goiter to chromosome Xp22. Am J Hum Genet 2000; 67:1004–1007.
35. Billerbeck AAC, Cavaliere H, Goldberg AC, et al. Clinical and molecular genetics studies in Pendred's syndrome. Thyroid 1994; 4:279–284.
36. Abs R, Stevenaert A, Beckers A. Autonomously functioning thyroid nodules in a patient with a thyrotropin-secreting pituitary

adenoma: possible cause-effect relationship. Eur J Endocrinol 1994; 131:355–358.
37. Salvi M, Fukazawa H, Bernard N, et al. Role of autoantibodies in the pathogenesis and association of endocrine autoimmune disorders. Endocr Rev 1988; 9:450–466.
38. Dige-Petersen H, Hummer L. Serum thyrotropin concentrations under basal conditions and after stimulation with thyrotropin-releasing hormone in idiopathic non-toxic goiter. J Clin Endocrinol Metab 1977; 44:1115–1120.
39. Bray GA. Increased sensitivity of the thyroid in iodine-depleted rats to the goitrogenic effects of thyrotropin. J Clin Invest 1968; 47:1640–1647.
40. Vassart G, Dumont JE. The thyrotropin receptor and the regulation of thyrocyte function and growth. Endocr Rev 1992; 13: 596–611.
41. Dumont JE, Lamy F, Roger P, et al. Physiological and pathological regulation of thyroid cell proliferation and differentiation by thyrotropin and other factors. Physiol Rev 1992; 72:667–697.
42. Derwahl M, Broecker M, Kraiem Z. Clinical review 101: thyrotropin may not be the dominant growth factor in benign and malignant thyroid tumors. J Clin Endocrinol Metab 1999; 84: 829–834.
43. Tansey WP, Schaufele F, Heslewood M, et al. Distance-dependent interactions between basal, cyclic AMP, and thyroid hormone response elements in the rat growth hormone promoter. J Biol Chem 1993; 268:14906–14911.
44. Wuster C, Steger G, Schmelzle A, et al. Increased incidence of euthyroid and hyperthyroid goiters independently of thyrotropin in patients with acromegaly. Horm Metab Res 1991; 23:131–134.
45. Wollman SH, Herveg JP, Zeligs JD, et al. Blood capillary enlargement during the development of thyroid hyperplasia in the rat. Endocrinology 1978; 103:2306–2314.
46. Ramsden JD. Angiogenesis in the thyroid gland. J Endocrinol 2000; 166:475–480.
47. Studer H, Ramelli F. Simple goiter and its variants: euthyroid and hyperthyroid multinodular goiters. Endocr Rev 1982; 3:40–61.
48. Caillou B, Troalen F, Baudin E, et al. Na^+/I^- symporter distribution in human thyroid tissues: an immunohistochemical study. J Clin Endocrinol Metab 1998; 83:4102–4106.
49. Wainscoat JS, Fey MF. Assessment of clonality in human tumors: a review. Cancer Res 1990; 50:1355–1360.
50. Aeschimann S, Kopp PA, Kimura ET, et al. Morphological and functional polymorphism within clonal thyroid nodules. J Clin Endocrinol Metab 1993; 77:846–851.
51. Thomas GA, Williams D, Williams ED. The clonal origin of thyroid nodules and adenomas. Am J Pathol 1989; 134:141–147.
52. Bamberger AM, Bamberger CM, Barth J, et al. Clonal composition of thyroid nodules from patients with multinodular goiters, determination of X-chromosome inactivation analysis with M27 beta. Exp Clin Endocrinol 1992; Suppl 1:73–70.
53. Kopp P, Kimura ET, Aeschimann S, et al. Polyclonal and monoclonal thyroid nodules coexist within human multinodular goiter. J Clin Endocrinol Metab 1994; 79:134–139.
54. Apel RL, Ezzat S, Bapat BV, et al. Clonality of thyroid nodules in sporadic goiter. Diagn Mol Pathol 1995; 4:113–121.
55. Roque L, Gomes P, Correia C, et al. Thyroid nodular hyperplasia: chromosomal studies in 14 cases. Cancer Genet Cytogenet 1993; 69:31–34.
56. Criado B, Barros A, Suijkerbuijk RF, et al. Detection of numerical alterations for chromosomes 7 and 12 in benign thyroid lesions by in situ hybridization. Am J Pathol 1995; 147:136–144.
57. Studer H, Derwahl M. Mechanisms of nonneoplastic endocrine hyperplasia—a changing concept: a review focused on the thyroid gland. Endocr Rev 1995; 16:411–426.
58. Bartalena L, Martino E, Vellozzi F, et al. The lack of nocturnal serum TSH surge in patients with nontoxic nodular goiter may predict the subsequent occurrence of hyperthyroidism. J Clin Endocrinol Metab 1991; 72:604–609.
59. Foley TP. Goiter in adolescents. Endocrinol Metab Clin North Am 1993; 22:593–606.
60. Glinoer D, Leome M. Goiter and pregnancy: a new insight into an old problem. Thyroid 1992; 2:65–69.
61. Glinoer D, De Nayer P, Bourdoux P, et al. Regulation of maternal thyroid during pregnancy. J Clin Endocrinol Metab 1990; 71: 276–287.
62. Glinoer D, Delange F, Laboureur I, et al. Maternal and neonatal thyroid function at birth in an area of marginally low iodine intake. J Clin Endocrinol Metab 1992; 75:800–805.
63. Hennemann G. Goiter and pregnancy: a new insight into an old problem: comment. Thyroid 1992; 2:71–72.
64. Murray D. The thyroid gland. In Kovacs K, Asa S (eds). Functional Endocrine Pathology. Boston, Blackwell Scientific Publications, 1991, pp 293–374.
65. Hicks DG, Livolsi VA, Neidich JA, et al. Clonal analysis of solitary follicular nodules in the thyroid. Am J Pathol 1990; 137: 553–562.
66. Namba H, Matsuo K, Fagin JA. Clonal composition of benign and malignant human thyroid tumors. J Clin Invest 1990; 86: 120–125.
67. Berghout A, Wiersinga WM, Smits NJ, et al. Interrelationships between age, thyroid volume, thyroid nodularity, and thyroid function in patients with sporadic nontoxic goiter. Am J Med 1990; 89:602–608.
68. Wallace C, Siminoski K. The Pemberton sign. Ann Intern Med 1996; 125:568–569.
69. Collazo-Clavell ML, Gharib H, Maragos NE. Relationship between vocal cord paralysis and benign thyroid disease. Head Neck 1995; 17:24–30.
70. Biondi B, Fazio S, Palmieri EA, et al. Effects of chronic subclinical hyperthyroidism from levothyroxine on cardiac morphology and function. Cardiologia 1999; 44:443–449.
71. Rieu M, Bekka S, Sambor B, et al. Prevalence of subclinical hyperthyroidism and relationship between thyroid hormonal states and thyroid ultrasonographic parameters in patients with nontoxic nodular goiter. Clin Endocrinol (Oxf) 1993; 39:67–71.
72. Sawin CT, Geller A, Wolf PA, et al. Low serum thyrotropin concentrations as a risk factor for atrial fibrillation in older persons. N Engl J Med 1994; 331:1249–1252.
73. Biondi B, Palmieri E, Fazio S, et al. Endogenous subclinical hyperthyroidism affects quality of life and cardiac morphology and function in young and middle-aged patients. J Clin Endocrinol Metab 2000; 85:4701–4705.
74. Peterson S, Sanga A, Eklof H, et al. Classification of thyroid size by palpation and ultrasonography in field surveys. Lancet 2000; 355:106–110.
75. Marqusee E, Benson CB, Frates MC, et al. Usefulness of ultrasonography in the management of nodular thyroid disease. Ann Intern Med 2000; 133:696–700.
76. Kristensen HL, Vadstrup S, Knudsen N, et al. Development of hyperthyroidism in nodular goiter and thyroid malignancies in an area of relatively low iodine intake. J Endocrinol Invest 1995; 18: 41–43.
77. Hara T, Tamai H, Mukata T, et al. A long-term follow-up study of patients with nontoxic diffuse goitre in Japan. Clin Endocrinol (Oxf) 1993; 39:541–546.
78. Bruns P. Ueber die Kropfbehandlung mit Schilddrusenfutterung. Beitr Klin Chir 1894; 12:847–853.
79. Greer MA, Astwood EB. Treatment of simple goiter with thyroid. J Clin Endocrinol 1953; 13:1312–1331.
80. Ross DS. Thyroid hormone suppressive therapy of sporadic nontoxic goiter. Thyroid 1992; 2:263–269.
81. Nygaard B, Faber J, Hegedus L, et al. ^{131}I treatment of nodular nontoxic goitre. Eur J Endocrinol 1996; 134:15–20.
82. Berghout A, Wiersinga WM, Drexhage HA, et al. Comparison of placebo with L-thyroxine alone or with carbimazole for treatment of sporadic nontoxic goitre. Lancet 1990; 336:193–197.
83. Perrild H, Hansen JM, Hegedus L. Triiodothyronine and thyroxine treatment of diffuse nontoxic goitre evaluated by ultrasound scanning. Acta Endocrinol (Copenh) 1982; 100:382–387.
84. Baran DT, Braverman LE. Thyroid hormone and bone mass. J Clin Endocrinol Metab 1991; 72:1182–1184.
85. Mandel SJ, Brent GA, Larsen PR. Levothyroxine therapy in patients with thyroid disease. Ann Intern Med 1993; 119:492–502.
86. Bartalena L, Pinchera A. Levothyroxine suppressive therapy: harmful and useless or harmless and useful? J Endocrinol Invest 1994; 17:675–677.
87. Faber J, Galloe AM. Changes in bone mass during prolonged subclinical hyperthyroidism due to L-thyroxine treatment: a meta-analysis. Eur J Endocrinol 1994; 130:350–356.
88. Wesche MFT, Tiel-V Buul MCC, Lips P, et al. A randomized trial comparing levothyroxine with radioactive iodine in the treat-

ment of sporadic nontoxic goiter. J Clin Endocrinol Metab 2001; 86:998–1005.
89. Marcocci C, Golia F, Bruno-Bosoro G, et al. Carefully monitored levothyroxine suppressive therapy is not associated with bone loss in premenopausal women. J Clin Endocrinol Metab 1994; 78:818–823.
90. Muller CG, Baylel TA, Harrison JE, et al. Possible limited bone loss with suppressive thyroxine therapy is unlikely to have clinical relevance. Thyroid 1995; 5:81–87.
91. Berghout A, Wiersinga WM, Drexhage HA, et al. The long-term outcome of thyroidectomy for sporadic nontoxic goitre. Clin Endocrinol (Oxf) 1989; 31:193–199.
92. Agerback H, Pilegaard HK, Watt-Boolsen S, et al. Complications of 2,028 operations for benign thyroid disease. Ugeskr Laeger 1988; 150:533–536.
93. Berglund J, Bondesson L, Christensen SB, et al. Indications for thyroxine therapy after surgery for nontoxic benign goitre. Acta Chir Scand 1990; 156:433–438.
94. Bistrup C, Nielsen JD, Gregersen G, et al. Preventive effect of levothyroxine in patients operated for nontoxic goitre: a randomized trial of one hundred patients with nine years follow-up. Clin Endocrinol (Oxf) 1994; 40:323–327.
95. Verelst J, Bonnyns M, Glinoer D. Radioiodine therapy in voluminous multinodular nontoxic goiter. Acta Endocrinol (Copenh) 1990; 122:417–421.
96. Huysmans DAKC, Hermus RMM, Corstens FHM, et al. Large, compressive, goiters treated with radioiodine. Ann Intern Med 1994; 121:757–762.
97. Kay TW, d'Emden MC, Andrews JT, et al. Treatment of nontoxic multinodular goiter with radioactive iodine. Am J Med 1988; 84:19–22.
98. Nygaard B, Hegedus L, Gervil M, et al. Radioiodine treatment of multinodular nontoxic goiter. Br Med J 1993; 307:828–832.
99. Wesche MF, Tiel-V Buul MM, Smits NJ, et al. Reduction in goiter size by ^{131}I therapy in patients with nontoxic multinodular goiter. Eur J Endocrinol 1995; 132:86–87.
100. DeGroot LJ, Larsen PR, Hennemann G. The Thyroid and Its Diseases. New York, Churchill Livingstone, 1996.
101. Nygaard B, Faber J, Hegedus L. Acute changes in thyroid volume and function following ^{131}I therapy of multinodular goiter. Clin Endocrinol (Oxf) 1994; 41:715–718.
102. Glinoer D. Radioiodine therapy of nontoxic multinodular goiter. Clin Endocrinol (Oxf) 1994; 41:713–714.
103. Holm LE, Hall P, Wiklund K, et al. Cancer risk after iodine-131 therapy for hyperthyroidism. J Natl Cancer Inst 1991; 83:1072–1077.
104. Hall P, Berg G, Bjelkengren G, et al. Cancer mortality after iodine-131 therapy for hyperthyroidism. Int J Cancer 1992; 50: 886–890.
105. Huysmans DA, Nieuwlaat WA, Erdtsieck RJ, et al. Administration of a single low dose of recombinant human thyrotropin significantly enhances thyroid radioiodide uptake in nontoxic nodular goiter. J Clin Endocrinol Metab 2000; 85:3592–3596.
106. Tezelman S, Clark OH. Current management of thyroid cancer. Adv Surg 1995; 28:191–221.
107. Dulgeroff AJ, Hershman JM. Medical therapy for differentiated thyroid carcinoma. Endocr Rev 1994; 15:500–515.
108. Schlumberger MJ. Papillary and follicular thyroid carcinoma. N Engl J Med 1998; 338:297–306.
109. Mazzaferri EL. Management of a solitary thyroid nodule. N Engl J Med 1993; 328:553–559.
110. Woeber KA. Cost-effective evaluation of the patient with a thyroid nodule. Surg Clin North Am 1995; 75:357–363.
111. Feld S, Garcia M, Baskin HJ, et al. AACE clinical practice guidelines for the diagnosis and management of thyroid nodules. Endocrinol Pract 1996; 2:78–84.
112. Van De Velde CJH, Hamming JF, Goslings BM, et al. Report of the consensus development conference on the management of differentiated thyroid cancer in the Netherlands. Eur J Cancer Clin Oncol 1988; 24:287–292.
113. Baldet L, Manderscheid JC, Glinoer D, et al. The management of differentiated thyroid cancer in Europe in 1988: results of an international survey. Acta Endocrinol (Copenh) 1989; 120:547–558.
114. Pasieka JL, Rotstein LE. Consensus conference on well-differentiated thyroid cancer: a summary. Can J Surg 1993; 36:298–301.
115. DeGroot LJ. Long-term impact of initial and surgical therapy on papillary and follicular thyroid cancer. Am J Med 1994; 97:499–500.
116. Solomon BL, Wartofsky L, Burman KD. Current trends in the management of well differentiated papillary thyroid carcinoma. J Clin Endocrinol Metab 1996; 81:333–339.
117. Wartofsky L, Sherman SI, Gopal J, et al. The use of radioactive iodine in patients with papillary and follicular thyroid cancer. J Clin Endocrinol Metab 1998; 83:4195–4203.
118. Bruneton JN, Balu-Maestro C, Marcy PY, et al. Very high frequency (13 MHz) ultrasonographic examination of the normal neck: detection of normal lymph nodes and thyroid nodules. J Ultrasound Med 1994; 13:87–90.
119. Greenlee RT, Hill-Harmon MB, Murray T, et al. Cancer statistics, 2001. CA Cancer J Clin 2001; 51:15–36.
120. Tan GH, Gharib H. Thyroid incidentalomas: management approaches to nonpalpable nodules discovered incidentally on thyroid imaging. Ann Intern Med 1997; 126:226–231.
121. Blum M, Rothschild M. Improved nonoperative diagnosis of the solitary 'cold' thyroid nodule: surgical selection based on risk factors and three months of suppression. JAMA 1980; 243:242–245.
122. Piromalli D, Martelli G, DelPrato I, et al. The role of fine needle aspiration in the diagnosis of thyroid nodules: analysis of 795 consecutive cases. J Surg Oncol 1992; 50:247–250.
123. Okamato T, Yamashita T, Harasawa A, et al. Test performances of three diagnostic procedures in evaluating thyroid nodules: physical examination, ultrasonography and fine needle aspiration cytology. Endocr J 1994; 41:243–247.
124. Pacini F, Fontanelli M, Fugazzola L, et al. Routine measurement of serum calcitonin in nodular thyroid diseases allows the preoperative diagnosis of unsuspected sporadic medullary thyroid carcinoma. J Clin Endocrinol Metab 1994; 78:826–829.
125. Ledger GA, Khosla S, Lindor NM, et al. Genetic testing in the diagnosis and management of multiple endocrine neoplasia type II. Ann Intern Med 1995; 122:118–124.
126. Gagel RF, Goepfert H, Callender DL. Changing concepts in the pathogenesis and management of thyroid carcinoma. CA Cancer J Clin 1996; 46:261–283.
127. Wells SA, Chi DD, Toshima K, et al. Predictive DNA testing and prophylactic thyroidectomy in patients at risk for multiple endocrine neoplasia type 2A. Ann Surg 1994; 220:237–250.
128. Christensen SB, Bondeson L, Ericsson UB, et al. Prediction of malignancy in the solitary thyroid nodule by physical examination, thyroid scan, fine-needle biopsy and serum thyroglobulin: a prospective study of 100 surgically treated patients. Acta Chir Scand 1984; 150:433–439.
129. Nelson RL, Wahner HW, Gorman CA. Rectilinear thyroid scanning as a predictor of malignancy. Ann Intern Med 1978; 88:41–44.
130. Hughes FC, Baudet M, Laccourreye H. Le nodule thyroidien. Une étude rétrospective de 200 observations. Ann Otolaryngol Chir Cervicofac 1989; 106:77–81.
131. Hermans J, Schmitz A, Merlo P, et al. Le thallium 201 permet-il de différencier le nodule thyroidien bénin du nodule malin? Ann Endocrinol (Paris) 1993; 54:248–254.
132. Kumar A, Ahuja MM, Chattopadhyay TK, et al. Fine needle aspiration cytology, sonography and radionuclide scanning in solitary thyroid nodule. J Assoc Physicians India 1992; 40:302–306.
133. Leisner B. Ultrasound evaluation of thyroid diseases. Horm Res 1987; 26:33–41.
134. Solbiati L, Volterrani L, Rizzatto G, et al. The thyroid gland with low uptake lesions: evaluation by ultrasound. Radiology 1985; 155:187–191.
135. Seya A, Oeda T, Terano T, et al. Comparative studies on fine-needle aspiration cytology with ultrasound scanning in the assessment of thyroid nodule. Jpn J Med 1990; 29:478–480.
136. Zingrillo M, Torlontano M, Chiarella R, et al. Percutaneous ethanol injection may be a definitive treatment for symptomatic thyroid cystic nodules not treatable by surgery: five-year follow-up study. Thyroid 1999; 9:763–767.
137. Hamburger JI. Diagnosis of thyroid nodules by fine needle biopsy: use and abuse. J Clin Endocrinol Metab 1994; 79:335–339.
138. Gharib H. Changing concepts in the diagnosis and management of thyroid nodules. Endocrinol Metab Clin North Am 1997; 26: 777–800.

139. Hales MS, Hsu FS. Needle tract implantation of papillary carcinoma of the thyroid following aspiration biopsy. Acta Cytol 1990; 34:801–804.
140. Keyhani-Rofagha S, Kooner DS, Keyhani M, et al. Necrosis of Hürthle cell tumor of the thyroid following fine needle aspiration: case report and literature review. Acta Cytol 1990; 34:805–808.
141. DeMicco C, Vasko V, Garcia S, et al. Fine needle aspiration of thyroid follicular neoplasm: diagnostic use of thyroid peroxidase immunochemistry with monoclonal antibody 47. Surgery 1994; 116:1031–1034.
142. Carpi A, Ferrari E, DeGaudio C, et al. The value of aspiration needle biopsy in evaluating thyroid nodules. Thyroidology 1994; 6:5–9.
143. Liu Q, Castelli M, Gattuso P, et al. Simultaneous fine-needle aspiration and core-needle biopsy of thyroid nodules. Am Surg 1995; 61:628–632.
144. Takashima S, Fukuda H, Kobayashi T. Thyroid nodules: clinical effect of ultrasound-guided fine-needle aspiration biopsy. J Clin Ultrasound 1994; 22:535–542.
145. Schmid KW, Ladurner D, Zechmann W, et al. Clinicopathologic management of tumors of the thyroid gland in an endemic goiter area: combined use of preoperative fine needle aspiration biopsy and intraoperative frozen section. Acta Cytol 1989; 33:27–30.
146. McHenry CR, Walfish PG, Rosen IB. Non-diagnostic fine needle aspiration biopsy: a dilemma in management of nodular thyroid disease. Am Surg 1993; 59:415–419.
147. Hedinger C, Williams ED, Sobin LH. Histological typing of thyroid tumours, 2nd ed, no 11. In International Histological Classification of Tumours, World Health Organization. New York, Springer-Verlag, 1988, pp 1–20.
148. Rosai J, Carganio ML, Delellis RA. Tumors of the Thyroid Gland. Washington, DC, Armed Force Institute of Pathology, 1992.
149. Rosai J. Thyroid gland. In Rosai J (ed). Ackerman's Surgical Pathology, 8th ed. St Louis, Mosby, 1996, pp 493–567.
150. Beahrs OH, Henson DE, Hutter RVP, et al. Manual for Staging of Cancer. Philadelphia, JB Lippincott, 1992.
151. Schlumberger M, de Vathaire F, Travagli JP, et al. Differentiated thyroid carcinoma in childhood: long term follow-up of 72 patients. J Clin Endocrinol Metab 1987; 65:1088–1094.
152. Gharib H, McConahey WM, Tiegs RD, et al. Medullary thyroid carcinoma: clinicopathologic features and long-term follow-up of 65 patients treated during 1946 through 1970. Mayo Clin Proc 1992; 67:934–940.
153. Brierley J, Tsang R, Simpson WJ, et al. Medullary thyroid cancer: analyses of survival and prognostic factors and the role of radiation therapy in local control. Thyroid 1996; 6:305–310.
154. Kebebew E, Ituarte PH, Siperstein AE, et al. Medullary thyroid carcinoma: clinical characteristics, treatment, prognostic factors, and a comparison of staging systems. Cancer 2000; 88:1139–1148.
155. Modigliani E, Cohen R, Campos JM, et al. Prognostic factors for survival and for biochemical cure in medullary thyroid carcinoma: results in 899 patients. The GETC Study Group. Groupe d'étude des tumeurs à calcitonine. Clin Endocrinol (Oxf) 1998; 48:265–273.
156. Doniach I. The thyroid gland. In Symmers W St C (ed). Systemic Pathology, Vol 14, 2nd ed. Edinburgh, Churchill Livingstone, 1978, 198: 1976–2037.
157. Bisi H, Fernandes VS, Asato de Camargo RY, et al. The prevalence of unsuspected thyroid pathology in 300 sequential autopsies, with special reference to the incidental carcinoma. Cancer 1989; 64:1888–1893.
158. Carney JA, Ryan J, Goellner JR. Hyalinizing trabecular adenoma of the thyroid gland. Am J Surg Pathol 1987; 11:583–592.
159. Tallini G, Carcangiu ML, Rosai J. Oncocytic neoplasms of the thyroid gland. Acta Pathol Jpn 1992; 42:305–315.
160. Gundry SR, Burney RE, Thompson NW, et al. Total thyroidectomy for Hürthle cell neoplasm of the thyroid. Arch Surg 1983; 118:529–532.
161. Ryan JJ, Hay ID, Grant CS, et al. Flow cytometric DNA measurements in benign and malignant Hürthle cell tumors of the thyroid. World J Surg 1988; 12:482–487.
162. Carcangiu ML, Bianchi S, Savino D, et al. Follicular Hürthle cell neoplasms of the thyroid gland: a study of 153 cases. Cancer 1991; 68:1944–1953.
163. Grant CS, Barr D, Goellner JR, et al. Benign Hürthle cell tumors of the thyroid: a diagnosis to be trusted? World J Surg 1988; 12:488–494.
164. Chen H, Nicol TL, Zeiger MA, et al. Hürthle cell neoplasms of the thyroid: are there factors predictive of malignancy? J Nucl Med 1998; 34:1626–1631.
165. Parma J, Duprez L, Van Sande J, et al. Somatic mutations of the thyrotropin receptor gene cause hyperfunctioning thyroid adenomas. Nature 1993; 365:649–651.
166. Duh Q-Y, Grossman RF. Thyroid growth factors, signal transduction pathways, and oncogenes. Surg Clin North Am 1995; 75: 421–437.
167. Suarez HG. Genetic alterations in human epithelial thyroid tumours. Clin Endocrinol (Oxf) 1998; 48:531–546.
168. Rosai J. Papillary carcinoma. Monogr Pathol 1993; 35:138–165.
169. Hay ID. Papillary thyroid carcinoma. Endocrinol Metab Clin North Am 1990; 19:545–576.
170. Hay ID, Grant CS, vanHeerden JA, et al. Papillary thyroid microcarcinoma: a study of 535 cases observed in a 50-year period. Surgery 1992; 112:1139–1147.
171. Baudin E, Travagli J, Ropers J, et al. Microcarcinoma of the thyroid gland: the Gustave Roussy Institute experience. Cancer 1998; 83:553–559.
172. Mazzaferri EL, Kloos RT. Clinical review 128: current approaches to primary therapy for papillary and follicular thyroid cancer. J Clin Endocrinol Metab 2001; 86:1447–1463.
173. Teyssier JR, Liautaud-Roger F, Ferre D, et al. Chromosomal changes in thyroid tumors: relation with DNA content, karyotypic features, and clinical data. Cancer Genet Cytogenet 1990; 50:249–263.
174. Bounacer A, Wicker R, Caillou B, et al. High prevalence of activating *ret* proto-oncogene rearrangements, in thyroid tumors from patients who had received external radiation. Oncogene 1997; 15:1263–1273.
175. Rabes HM, Demidchik EP, Sidorow JD, et al. Pattern of radiation-induced *RET* and *NTRK1* rearrangements in 191 post-Chernobyl papillary thyroid carcinomas: biological, phenotypic, and clinical implications. Clin Cancer Res 2000; 6:1093–1103.
176. Santoro M, Grieco M, Melillo R, et al. Molecular defects in thyroid carcinomas: role of the *RET* oncogene in thyroid neoplastic transformation. Eur J Endocrinol 1995; 133:513–522.
177. Viglietto G, Chiappetta G, Martineztello FJ, et al. *RET*/PTC oncogene activation is an early event in thyroid carcinogenesis. Oncogene 1995; 11:1207–1210.
178. Tallini G, Santoro M, Helie M, et al. *RET*/PTC oncogene activation defines a subset of papillary thyroid carcinomas lacking evidence of progression to poorly differentiated or undifferentiated tumor phenotypes. Clin Cancer Res 1998; 4:287–294.
179. Bongarzone I, Pierotti MA, Monzini N, et al. High frequency of activation of tyrosine kinase oncogenes in human papillary thyroid carcinoma. Oncogene 1989; 4:1457–1462.
180. Di Renzo MF, Olivero M, Ferro S, et al. Overexpression of the c-Met/HGF receptor gene in human thyroid carcinomas. Oncogene 1992; 7:2549–2553.
181. Belfiore A, Gangemi P, Costantino A, et al. Negative/low expression of the Met/hepatocyte growth factor receptor identifies papillary thyroid carcinomas with high risk of distant metastases. J Clin Endocrinol Metab 1997; 82:2322–2328.
182. Alsanea O, Wada N, Ain K, et al. Is familial non-medullary thyroid carcinoma more aggressive than sporadic thyroid cancer? A multicenter series. Surgery 2000; 128:1043–1050.
183. Canzian F, Amati P, Harach HR, et al. A gene predisposing to familial thyroid tumors with cell oxyphilia maps to chromosome 19p13.2. Am J Hum Genet 1998; 63:1743–1748.
184. Malchoff CD, Sarfarazi M, Tendler B, et al. Papillary thyroid carcinoma associated with papillary renal neoplasia: genetic linkage analysis of a distinct heritable tumor syndrome. J Clin Endocrinol Metab 2000; 85:1758–1764.
185. Lazar V, Bidart JM, Caillou B, et al. Expression of the Na^+/I^- symporter gene in human thyroid tumors: a comparison study with other thyroid-specific genes. J Clin Endocrinol Metab 1999; 84:3228–3234.
186. Filetti S, Bidart JM, Arturi F, et al. Sodium/iodide symporter: a key transport system in thyroid cancer cell metabolism. Eur J Endocrinol 1999; 141:443–457.
187. McConahey WM, Hay ID, Woolner LB, et al. Papillary thyroid

cancer treated at the Mayo Clinic, 1946 through 1970: initial manifestations, pathologic findings, therapy and outcome. Mayo Clin Proc 1986; 61:978–996.
188. Zimmerman D, Hay ID, Gough IR, et al. Papillary thyroid carcinoma in children and adults: long-term follow-up of 1,039 patients conservatively treated at one institution during three decades. Surgery 1988; 104:1157–1166.
189. Kukkonen ST, Haapiainen RK, Fransila KO, et al. Papillary thyroid carcinoma: the new, age-related TNM classification system in a retrospective analysis of 199 patients. World J Surg 1990; 14:837–842.
190. Grant CS, Hay ID, Gough IR, et al. Local recurrence in papillary thyroid carcinoma: is extent of surgical resection important? Surgery 1988; 104:954–962.
191. Hay ID, Grant CS, Taylor WF, et al. Ipsilateral lobectomy versus bilateral lobar resection in papillary thyroid carcinoma: a retrospective analysis of surgical outcome using a novel prognostic scoring system. Surgery 1987; 102:1088–1095.
192. Simpson WJ, McKinney SE, Carruthers JS, et al. Papillary and follicular thyroid cancer: prognostic factors in 1,578 patients. Am J Med 1987; 83:479–488.
193. DeGroot LJ, Kaplan EL, McCormick M, et al. Natural history, treatment and course of papillary thyroid carcinoma. J Clin Endocrinol Metab 1990; 71:414–424.
194. Shah JP, Loree TR, Dharker D, et al. Prognostic factors in differentiated carcinoma of the thyroid gland. Am J Surg 1992; 164:658–661.
195. Akslen LA, Livolsi VA. Prognostic significance of histologic grading compared with subclassification of papillary thyroid carcinoma. Cancer 2000; 88:1902–1908.
196. Hay ID, Bergstralh EJ, Goellner JR, et al. Predicting outcome in papillary thyroid carcinoma: development of a reliable prognostic scoring system in a cohort of 1,779 patients surgically treated at one institution during 1940 through 1989. Surgery 1993; 114: 1050–1058.
197. Brierley JD, Panzarella T, Tsang RW, et al. A comparison of different staging systems predictability of patient outcome: thyroid carcinoma as an example. Cancer 1997; 79:2414–2423.
198. DeGroot LJ, Kaplan EL, Straus FH, et al. Does the method of management of papillary thyroid carcinoma make a difference in outcome? World J Surg 1994; 18:123–130.
199. Carcangiu MC, Zempi G, Rosai J. Poorly differentiated ("insular") thyroid carcinoma: a reinterpretation of Langhans "wuchernde Struma." Am J Surg Pathol 1984; 8:655–668.
200. Sobrinho-Simoes M. Mixed medullary and follicular carcinoma of the thyroid. Histopathology 1993; 23:187–189.
201. Grebe SKG, Hay ID. Follicular thyroid cancer. Endocrinol Metab Clin North Am 1996; 24:761–801.
202. Livolsi VA, Asa SL. The demise of follicular carcinoma of the thyroid gland. Thyroid 1994; 4:233–236.
203. Livolsi VA, Merino MJ. Worrisome histologic alterations following fine-needle aspiration of the thyroid. Pathol Annu 1994; 29: 99–120.
204. Ishimaru Y, Fukuda S, Kurano R, et al. Follicular thyroid carcinoma with clear cell change showing unusual ultrastructural features. Am J Surg Pathol 1988; 12:240–246.
205. Watson RG, Brennan MD, Goellner JR, et al. Invasive Hürthle cell carcinoma of the thyroid: natural history and management. Mayo Clin Proc 1984; 59:851–855.
206. Farid NR, Zou M, Shi Y. Genetics of follicular thyroid cancer. Endocrinol Metab Clin North Am 1995; 24:865–883.
207. Santoro M, Carlomagno F, Hay ID, et al. *Ret* oncogene activation in human thyroid neoplasms is restricted to the papillary cancer subtype. J Clin Invest 1992; 89:1517–1522.
208. Hay ID. Cytometric DNA ploidy analysis in thyroid cancer. Diagn Oncol 1991; 1:181–185.
209. Herrmann MA, Hay ID, Bartlet DH, et al. Cytogenetic and molecular genetic studies of follicular and papillary thyroid cancers. J Clin Invest 1991; 88:1596–1603.
210. Matsuo K, Tang SH, Fagin JA. Allelotype of human thyroid tumors: loss of chromosome 11q13 sequences in follicular neoplasms. Mol Endocrinol 1991; 5:1873–1879.
211. Roque L, Cestedo S, Clode A, et al. Deletion of 3p25→pter in a primary thyroid follicular thyroid carcinoma and its metastasis. Genes Chromosomes Cancer 1993; 8:199–203.
212. Zedenius J, Wallin G, Svensson A, et al. Deletions of the long arm of chromosome 10 in progression of follicular thyroid tumors. Hum Genet 1996; 97:299–303.
213. Soares P, Sobrinhoe-Simoes M. Recent advances in cytometry, cytogenetics and molecular genetics of thyroid tumors and tumor-like lesions. Pathol Res Pract 1995; 191:304–317.
214. Jenkins RB, Hay ID, Herath JF, et al. Frequent occurrence of cytogenetic abnormalities in sporadic nonmedullary thyroid carcinoma. Cancer 1990; 66:1213–1220.
215. Kroll TG, Sarraf P, Pecciarini L, et al. PAX8-PPARgamma1 fusion oncogene in human thyroid carcinoma. Science 2000; 289: 1357–1360.
216. Brennan MD, Bergstralh EJ, van Heerden JA, et al. Follicular thyroid cancer treated at the Mayo Clinic, 1946 through 1970: initial manifestations, pathologic findings, therapy and outcome. Mayo Clin Proc 1991; 66:11–19.
217. Paul SJ, Sisson JC. Thyrotoxicosis caused by thyroid cancer. Endocrinol Metab Clin North Am 1990; 19:593–612.
218. Grebe SKG, Hay ID. Thyroid cancer nodal metastases: biologic significance and therapeutic considerations. Surg Oncol Clin North Am 1996; 5:43–63.
219. van Heerden JA, Hay ID, Goellner JR, et al. Follicular thyroid carcinoma with capsular invasion alone: a non-threatening malignancy. Surgery 1992; 112:1130–1136.
220. Mueller-Gaertner HW, Brzac HT, Rehpenning W. Prognostic indices for tumor relapse and tumor mortality in follicular thyroid carcinoma. Cancer 1991; 67:1903–1908.
221. Cady R, Rossi R. An expanded view of risk-group definition in differentiated thyroid carcinoma. Surgery 1985; 98:1171–1176.
222. Shaha AR, Loree TR, Shah JP. Prognostic factors and risk group analysis in follicular carcinoma of the thyroid. Surgery 1995; 118: 1131–1138.
223. Loree TR. Therapeutic implications of prognostic factors in differentiated carcinoma of the thyroid gland. Semin Surg Oncol 1995; 11:246–255.
224. Emerick GT, Duh QY, Siperstein AE, et al. Diagnosis, treatment, and outcome of follicular thyroid carcinoma. Cancer 1993; 72:3287–3294.
225. Davis NL, Bugis SD, McGregor GI, et al. An evaluation of prognostic scoring systems in patients with follicular thyroid cancer. Am J Surg 1995; 170:476–480.
226. McIver B, Hay ID, Giuffrida DF, et al. Anaplastic thyroid carcinoma: a 50-year experience at a single institution. Surgery 2001; 130:1028–1034.
227. Fagin JA, Matsuo K, Karmakar A, et al. High prevalence of mutation of the *p53* gene in poorly differentiated human thyroid carcinomas. J Clin Invest 1993; 91:179–184.
228. Ito T, Segama T, Mizuno T, et al. Unique associations of *p53* mutations with undifferentiated but not with differentiated carcinoma of the thyroid gland. Cancer Res 1992; 52:1369–1371.
229. Schlumberger M, Caillou B. Miscellaneous tumors of the thyroid. In Braverman LE, Utiger RD (eds). The Thyroid: A Fundamental and Clinical Text. Philadelphia, Lippincott Williams & Wilkins, 2000, pp 945–948.
230. Moley JF. Medullary thyroid cancer. Surg Clin North Am 1995; 75:405–420.
231. Pyke CM, Hay ID, Goellner JR, et al. Prognostic significance of calcitonin immunoreactivity, amyloid staining, and flow cytometric DNA measurements in medullary thyroid carcinoma. Surgery 1991; 110:964–970; discussion 970–971.
232. Wohllk N, Cote GJ, Evans DB, et al. Applications of genetic screening information to the management of medullary thyroid carcinoma and multiple endocrine neoplasia type 2. Endocrinol Metab Clin North Am 1996; 25:1–25.
233. Lips CJM, Landsvater RM, Hoppener JWM, et al. Clinical screening as compared with DNA analysis in families with multiple endocrine neoplasia type 2A. N Engl J Med 1994; 331:828–835.
234. Chong GC, Beahrs OH, Sizemore GW. Medullary carcinoma of the thyroid gland. Cancer 1975; 35:695–704.
235. Farndon JR, Leight GS, Dilley WG, et al. Familial medullary thyroid carcinoma without associated endocrinopathies: a distinct clinical entity. Br J Surg 1986; 73:278–281.
236. Wohllk N, Cote GJ, Bugalho MMJ, et al. Relevance of *RET* proto-oncogene mutations in sporadic medullary thyroid carcinoma. J Clin Endocrinol Metab 1996; 81:3740–3745.
237. Matsuzuka F, Migauchi A, Katayama S, et al. Clinical aspects of

primary thyroid lymphoma: diagnosis and treatment based on our experience of 119 cases. Thyroid 1993; 3:93–98.
238. Doria R, Jekel JF, Cooper DL. Thyroid lymphoma: the case for combined modality therapy. Cancer 1994; 73:200–206.
239. Laing RW, Hoskin P, Hudson BV, et al. The significance of MALT histology in thyroid lymphoma: a review of patients from the BNLI and Royal Marsden Hospital. Clin Oncol (R Coll Radiol) 1994; 6:300–304.
240. Tsang RW, Gospodarowicz MK, Sutcliffe SB, et al. Non-Hodgkin's lymphoma of the thyroid gland: prognostic factors and treatment outcome. The Princess Margaret Hospital Lymphoma Group. Int J Radiat Oncol Biol Phys 1993; 27:599–604.
241. Holm LE, Blomgren H, Lowhagen T. Cancer risks in patients with chronic lymphocytic thyroiditis. N Engl J Med 1985; 312: 601–604.
242. Pyke CM, Grant CS, Habermann TM, et al. Non-Hodgkin's lymphoma of the thyroid: is more than biopsy necessary? World J Surg 1992; 16:604–609.
243. Harris NL, Jaffe ES, Stein H, et al. A revised European-American classification of lymphoid neoplasms: a proposal from the International Lymphoma Study Group. Blood 1994; 84:1361–1392.
244. Hay ID, Bergstralh EJ, Grant CS, et al. Impact of primary surgery on outcome in 300 patients with pathologic tumor-node-metastasis stage III papillary thyroid carcinoma treated at one institution from 1940 through 1989. Surgery 1999; 126:1173–1181.
245. Buhr HJ, Kallinowski F, Raue F, et al. Microsurgical neck dissection for metastasizing medullary thyroid carcinoma. Eur J Surg Oncol 1995; 21:195–197.
246. Sarne D, Schneider A. External radiation and thyroid neoplasia. Endocrinol Metab Clin North Am 1996; 25:181–195.
247. Ron E, Lubin JH, Shore RE, et al. Thyroid cancer after exposure to external radiation: a pooled analysis of seven studies. Radiat Res 1995; 141:259–277.
248. de Vathaire F, Hardiman C, Shamsaldin A, et al. Thyroid carcinomas after irradiation for a first cancer during childhood. Arch Intern Med 1999; 159:2713–2719.
249. Fogelfeld L, Wiviott MBT, Shore-Freedman P, et al. Recurrence of thyroid nodules after surgical removal in patients irradiated in childhood for benign conditions. N Engl J Med 1989; 320:835–840.
250. Singer PA, Cooper DS, Daniels GH, et al. Treatment guidelines for patients with thyroid nodules and well-differentiated thyroid cancer. Arch Intern Med 1996; 156:2165–2172.
251. Schlumberger M, Arcangioli O, Piekarski JD, et al. Detection and treatment of lung metastases of differentiated thyroid carcinoma in patients with normal chest x-rays. J Nucl Med 1988; 29: 1790–1794.
252. Vassilopoulou-Sellin R, Klein MJ, Smith TH, et al. Pulmonary metastases in children and young adults with differentiated thyroid cancer. Cancer 1993; 71:1348–1352.
253. Maxon HR, Englaro EE, Thomas SR, et al. Radioiodine-131 therapy for well-differentiated thyroid cancer—a quantitative radiation dosimetric approach: outcome and validation in 85 patients. J Nucl Med 1992; 33:1132–1140.
254. Tubiana M, Haddad E, Schlumberger M, et al. External radiotherapy in thyroid cancers. Cancer 1985; 55:2062–2071.
255. Farahati J, Reiners C, Stuschke M, et al. Differentiated thyroid cancer: impact of adjuvant external radiotherapy in patients with perithyroidal tumor infiltration (stage pT4). Cancer 1996; 77: 172–180.
256. Tsang RW, Brierley JD, Simpson WJ, et al. The effects of surgery, radioiodine, and external radiation therapy on the clinical outcome of patients with differentiated thyroid carcinoma. Cancer 1998; 82:375–388.
257. Bartalena L, Martino E, Pacchiarotti A, et al. Factors affecting suppression of endogenous thyrotropin secretion by thyroxine treatment: retrospective analysis in athyreotic and goitrous patients. J Clin Endocrinol Metab 1987; 64:849–855.
258. Pacini F, Fugazzola L, Lippi F, et al. Detection of thyroglobulin in fine needle aspirates of nonthyroidal neck masses: a clue to the diagnosis of metastatic differentiated thyroid cancer. J Clin Endocrinol Metab 1992; 74:1401–1404.
259. Arturi F, Russo D, Giuffrida D, et al. Early diagnosis by genetic analysis of differentiated thyroid cancer metastases in small lymph nodes. J Clin Endocrinol Metab 1997; 82:1638–1641.
260. Spencer CA, Takeuchi M, Kazarosyan M, et al. Serum thyroglobulin autoantibodies: prevalence, influence on serum thyroglobulin measurement, and prognostic significance in patients with differentiated thyroid carcinoma. J Clin Endocrinol Metab 1998; 83:1121–1127.
261. Ladenson PW, Braverman LE, Mazzaferri EL, et al. Comparison of administration of recombinant human thyrotropin with withdrawal of thyroid hormone for radioactive iodine scanning in patients with thyroid carcinoma. N Engl J Med 1997; 337:888–896.
262. Schlumberger M, Ricard M, Pacini F. Clinical use of recombinant human TSH in thyroid cancer patients. Eur J Endocrinol 2000; 143:557–563.
263. Haugen BR, Pacini F, Reiners C, et al. A comparison of recombinant human thyrotropin and thyroid hormone withdrawal for the detection of thyroid remnant or cancer. J Clin Endocrinol Metab 1999; 84:3877–3885.
264. Schlumberger M, Mancusi F, Baudin E, et al. ^{131}I therapy for elevated thyroglobulin levels. Thyroid 1997; 7:273–276.
265. Ringel MD, Balducci-Silano PL, Anderson JS, et al. Quantitative reverse transcription–polymerase chain reaction of circulating thyroglobulin messenger ribonucleic acid for monitoring patients with thyroid carcinoma. J Clin Endocrinol Metab 1999; 84:4037–4042.
266. Paula R, Biscolla M, Cerutti JM, et al. Detection of recurrent thyroid cancer by sensitive nested reverse transcription–polymerase chain reaction of thyroglobulin and sodium/iodide symporter messenger ribonucleic acid transcripts in peripheral blood. J Clin Endocrinol Metab 2000; 85:3623–3627.
267. Guimares V, De Groot LJ. Moderate hypothyroidism as preparation for whole body ^{131}I scintiscans and thyroglobulin testing. Thyroid 1996; 6:69–73.
268. Park HM, Perkins O, Edmondson J, et al. Influence of diagnostic radioiodines on the uptake of ablative dose of iodine-131. Thyroid 1994; 4:49–54.
269. Cailleux AF, Baudin E, Travagli JP, et al. Is diagnostic iodine-131 scanning useful after total thyroid ablation for differentiated thyroid cancer? J Clin Endocrinol Metab 2000; 85:175–178.
270. Cooper DS, Specker B, Ho M, et al. Thyrotropin suppression and disease progression in patients with differentiated thyroid cancer: results from the National Thyroid Cancer Treatment Cooperative Registry. Thyroid 1998; 8:737–744.
271. van Heerden JA, Grant CS, Gharib H, et al. Long-term course of patients with persistent hypercalcitoninemia after apparent curative primary surgery for medullary thyroid carcinoma. Ann Surg 1990; 212:395–400.
272. Abdelmoumene N, Schlumberger M, Gardet P, et al. Selective venous sampling catheterisation for localisation of persisting medullary thyroid carcinoma. Br J Cancer 1994; 69:1141–1144.
273. Kebebew E, Kikuchi S, Duh QY, et al. Long-term results of reoperation and localizing studies in patients with persistent or recurrent medullary thyroid cancer. Arch Surg 2000; 135:895–901.
274. Saad MF, Fritsche HA, Samaan NA. Diagnostic and prognostic values of carcinoembryonic antigen in medullary carcinoma of the thyroid. J Clin Endocrinol Metab 1984; 58:889–894.
275. Mendelsohn G, Wells SA, Baylin SB. Relationship of tissue carcinoembryonic antigen and calcitonin to tumor virulence in medullary thyroid carcinoma. Cancer 1984; 54:657–664.
276. Pacini F, Cetani F, Miccoli P, et al. Outcome of 309 patients with metastatic differentiated thyroid carcinoma treated with radioiodine. World J Surg 1994; 18:600–604.
277. Coburn M, Teates D, Wanebo HJ. Recurrent thyroid cancer: role of surgery versus radioactive iodine (I-131). Ann Surg 1994; 219:587–593.
278. Travagli JP, Cailleux AF, Ricard M, et al. Combination of radioiodine (^{131}I) and probe-guided surgery for persistent or recurrent thyroid carcinoma. J Clin Endocrinol Metab 1998; 83:2675–2680.
279. Dupuy DE, Monchik JM, Decrea C, Pisharodi L. Radiofrequency ablation of regional recurrence from well-differentiated thyroid malignancy. Surgery 2001; 130:971–977.
280. Lewis BD, Hay ID, Charboneau JW, et al. Percutaneous ethanol injection for treatment of cervical lymph node metastases in patients with papillary thyroid carcinoma. Am J Radiol 2002; 178: 301–306.

281. Ruegemer JJ, Hay ID, Bergstralh EJ, et al. Distant metastases in differentiated thyroid carcinoma: a multivariate analysis of prognostic variables. J Clin Endocrinol Metab 1988; 63:960–967.
282. Roher HD, Goretzki PE. Surgical treatment of distant metastases from differentiated thyroid cancer. Prog Surg 1988; 19:113–132.
283. Bernier MO, Leenhardt L, Hoang C, et al. Survival and therapeutic modalities in patients with bone metastases of differentiated thyroid carcinomas. J Clin Endocrinol Metab 2001; 86: 1568–1573.
284. Marcocci C, Pacini F, Elisei R, et al. Clinical and biologic behavior of bone metastases from differentiated thyroid carcinoma. Surgery 1989; 106:960–966.
285. Maxon HR, Thomas SR, Hertzberg VS, et al. Relation between effective radiation dose and outcome of radioiodine therapy for thyroid cancer. N Engl J Med 1983; 309:937–941.
286. Smit JWA, Vielvoye GJ, Goslings BM. Embolization for vertebral metastases of follicular thyroid carcinoma. J Clin Endocrinol Metab 2000; 85:989–994.
287. Shimaoka K, Schoenfeld DA, DeWys WD, et al. A randomized trial of doxorubicin versus doxorubicin plus cisplatin in patients with advanced thyroid carcinoma. Cancer 1985; 56:2155–2160.
288. Williams SD, Birch R, Einhorn LH. Phase II evaluation of doxorubicin plus cisplatin in advanced thyroid cancer: a Southeastern Cancer Study Group Trial. Cancer Treat Rep 1986; 70:405–407.
289. Schmutzler C, Koehrle J. Innovative strategies for the treatment of thyroid cancer. Eur J Endocrinol 2000; 143:15–24.
290. Schlumberger M, Challeton C, de Vathaire F, et al. Radioactive iodine treatment and external radiotherapy for lung and bone metastases from thyroid carcinoma. J Nucl Med 1996; 37:598–605.
291. Casara D, Rubello D, Saladini G, et al. Different features of pulmonary metastases in differentiated thyroid cancer: natural history and multivariate statistical analysis of prognostic variables. J Nucl Med 1993; 34:1626–1631.
292. McDougall IR. ^{131}I treatment of ^{131}I negative whole body scan and positive thyroglobulin in differentiated thyroid carcinoma: what is being treated? Thyroid 1997; 7:669–672.
293. Pacini F, Agate L, Elisel R, et al. Outcome of differentiated thyroid cancer with detectable serum Tg and negative diagnostic ^{131}I whole-body scan: comparison of patients treated with high ^{131}I activities versus untreated patients. J Clin Endocrinol Metab 2001; 86:4092–4097.
294. Schlumberger M, de Vathaire F, Ceccarelli C, et al. Exposure to radioactive iodine-131 for scintigraphy or therapy does not preclude pregnancy in thyroid cancer patients. J Nucl Med 1996; 37: 606–612.
295. Hall P, Holm LE, Lundell G, et al. Cancer risks in thyroid cancer patients. Br J Cancer 1991; 64:159–163.
296. de Vathaire F, Schlumberger M, Delisle MJ, et al. Leukaemias and cancers following iodine-131 administration for thyroid cancer. Br J Cancer 1997; 75:734–739.
297. Nocera M, Baudin E, Pellegriti G, et al. Treatment of advanced medullary thyroid cancer with an alternating combination of doxorubicin-streptozocin and 5 FU-dacarbazine. Groupe d'Étude des Tumeurs a Calcitonine (GETC). Br J Cancer 2000; 83:715–718.

SECTION FOUR

ADRENAL CORTEX AND ENDOCRINE HYPERTENSION

14 The Adrenal Cortex

Paul M. Stewart

HISTORICAL MILESTONES

The anatomy of the adrenal glands was described almost 450 years ago by Bartholomeo Eustacius,[1] and the zonation of the gland and its distinction from the medulla were elucidated shortly thereafter. However, a functional role for the adrenal glands was not accurately defined until the pioneering work of Thomas Addison, who described the clinical and autopsy findings in 11 cases of "Addison's disease" in his classical monograph in 1855.[2] Just a year later, Brown-Séquard demonstrated that the adrenal glands were "organs essential for life" by performing adrenalectomies in dogs, cats, and guinea pigs.[3] In 1896, William Osler first administered adrenal extract to a patient with Addison's disease,[4] a feat that was repeated by others in both animal and human studies over the next 40 years. As a consequence, between 1937 and 1955 the adrenocorticosteroid hormones were isolated, their structures defined, and the hormones synthesized,[5] notable breakthroughs being the discovery of cortisone and the clinical evaluation of its anti-inflammatory effect in patients with rheumatoid arthritis (Reichstein, Hench, Kendall, and Slocumb)[6] and the isolation of aldosterone (Simpson and Tait).[7]

The control of adrenocortical function by a pituitary factor was demonstrated in the 1920s, and this led to the isolation of sheep adrenocorticotropic hormone (ACTH) in 1943.[8] Such a concept was supported through clinical studies, notably in 1932 by Harvey Cushing, who associated his original clinical observations of 1912 (a "polyglandular syndrome" caused by pituitary basophilism) with adrenal hyperactivity.[9] The neural control of pituitary ACTH secretion by corticotropin-releasing hormone (CRH) was defined by Harris and other workers in the 1940s,[10] but CRH was not characterized and synthesized until 1981 in the laboratory of Wylie Vale.[11] Jerome Conn described primary aldosteronism in 1956,[12] and the control of adrenal aldosterone secretion by angiotensin II was confirmed shortly afterward. Advances in radioimmunoassays and particularly molecular biology have facilitated an exponential increase in our understanding of adrenal physiology and pathophysiology (Table 14–1).

ANATOMY

The adrenal cortex derives from mesenchymal cells attached to the coelomic cavity lining adjacent to the urogenital ridge. The fetal adrenal is evident from 6 to 8 weeks of gestation and rapidly increases in size so that by midgestation it is larger than its adjacent kidney. In fetal life and up to 12 months post partum two distinct zones are evident, an inner prominent fetal zone and an outer definitive zone that differentiates into the adult adrenal gland. Post partum the fetal zone regresses and the definitive zone containing an inner zona fasciculata and outer glomerulosa proliferates.[13, 14] The innermost zone, the zona reticularis, is evident after 1 year of life. The differentiation of the adrenal cortex into distinct zones has important functional consequences (discussed later) and is thought to be dependent upon the temporal expression of transcription factors including Pref-1/ZOG, inner zone antigen, and steroidogenic factor-1.[15, 16]

The adult gland is a pyramidal structure approximately 4 g in weight, 2 cm wide, 5 cm long, and 1 cm thick lying immediately above the kidney on its posteromedial surface. Beneath the capsule, the zona glomerulosa constitutes approximately 15% of the cortex (depending upon sodium intake) (Fig. 14–1). Cells are clustered in spherical nests and are small with smaller nuclei in comparison with other zones. The zona fasciculata makes up 75% of the cortex; cells are large and lipid-laden and form radial cords between the fibrovascular radial network. The innermost zona reticularis is sharply demarcated from both the zona fasciculata and adrenal medulla. Cells here are irregular with little lipid content. The maintenance of normal adrenal size appears to involve a progenitor cell population lying between the zona glomerulosa and zona fasciculata[17]; cell migration and differentiation occur within the fasciculata and senescence within the reticularis, but the factors regulating this important aspect of adrenal regeneration are unknown. ACTH administration results in glomerulosa cells adopting a fasciculata phenotype; in turn, the innermost fasciculata cells adopt a reticularis phenotype, which is reversible upon withdrawal of ACTH.

Table 14–1. History of the Adrenal Cortex: Important Milestones

1563	Eustachius describes the adrenals (published by Lancisi in 1714).
1849	Thomas Addison, while searching for the cause of pernicious anemia, "stumbles" on a bronzed appearance associated with the adrenal glands—"melasma suprarenale."
1855	Thomas Addison describes the clinical features and autopsy findings of 11 cases of diseases of the suprarenal capsules, at least 6 of which were tuberculous in origin.
1856	In adrenalectomy experiments, Brown-Séquard demonstrates that the adrenal glands are essential for life.
1896	William Osler gives an oral glycerine extract derived from pig adrenals and demonstrates clinical benefit in patients with Addison's disease.
1905	Bulloch and Sequeria describe patients with congenital adrenal hyperplasia.
1929	Liquid extracts of cortical tissue are used to keep adrenalectomized cats alive indefinitely (Swingle and Pfiffner). Subsequently, this extract was used successfully to treat a patient with Addison's disease (Rowntree and Greene).
1932	Harvey Cushing associates the "polyglandular syndrome" of pituitary basophilism first described by him in 1912 with hyperactivity of the pituitary-adrenal glands.
1936	Concept of stress and its effect upon pituitary-adrenal function described by Seyle.
1937–1952	Isolation and structural characterisation of adrenocortical hormones (Kendall, Reichstein).
1943	Li and colleagues isolate pure adrenocorticotropic hormone from sheep pituitary.
1950	Hench, Kendall, and Reichstein share Nobel Prize in medicine for describing the anti-inflammatory effects of cortisone in patients with rheumatoid arthritis.
1953	Isolation and analysis of the structure of aldosterone (Simpson and Tait).
1956	Conn describes primary aldosteronism.
1981	Characterization and synthesis of corticotropin-releasing hormone (Vale)
1980–present	The "molecular era." Cloning and functional characterization of steroid receptors, steroidogenic enzymes, and adrenal transcription factors. Definition of the molecular basis for human adrenal diseases.

The vasculature of the adrenal cortex is complex. Arterial supply is conveyed by up to 12 small arteries from the aorta, inferior phrenic, renal, and intercostal arteries. These branch to form a subcapsular arteriolar plexus from which radial capillaries penetrate deeper into the cortex. In the zona reticularis, a dense sinusoidal plexus is created that empties into a central vein. The right adrenal vein is short, draining directly into the inferior vena cava; the longer left adrenal vein usually drains into the left renal vein.[18]

ADRENAL STEROIDS AND STEROIDOGENESIS

Three main types of hormones are produced by the adrenal cortex: glucocorticoids (cortisol, corticosterone), mineralocorticoids (aldosterone, deoxycorticosterone [DOC]), and sex steroids (mainly androgens). All steroid hormones are derived from the cyclopentanoperhydrophenanthrene structure, that is, three cyclohexane rings and a single cyclopentane ring (Fig. 14–2).

Steroid nomenclature is defined in two ways: either by trivial names (e.g., cortisol, aldosterone) or by the chemical structure as defined by the International Union of Pure and Applied Chemistry (IUPAC).[19] The IUPAC classification is inappropriate for clinical use but does provide invaluable insight into steroid structure. The basic structure and trivial and IUPAC names of some common steroids are given in Figure 14–2 and Table 14–2. Estrogens have 18 carbon atoms (C_{18} steroids), androgens have 19 carbon atoms (C_{19}), and glucocorticoids and progestagens are C_{21} steroid derivatives.

Cholesterol is the precursor for all adrenal steroidogenesis. Most of this cholesterol is provided from the circulation in the form of low-density lipoprotein (LDL) cholesterol.[20] Uptake is by specific cell surface LDL receptors present on adrenal tissue[21]; LDL is then internalized by receptor-mediated endocytosis,[22] the resulting vesicles fuse with lysozymes, and free cholesterol is produced after hydrolysis. However, it is clear that this cannot be the sole source of adrenal cholesterol; patients with abetalipoproteinemia who have undetectable circulating LDL[23] and patients with defective LDL receptors in the setting of familial hypercholesterolemia[24] still have normal basal adrenal steroidogenesis. Cholesterol can be generated de novo within the adrenal cortex from acetyl coenzyme A.[25] In addition, there is evidence that the adrenal can utilize HDL cholesterol after uptake through the putative HDL receptor, the class B, type I scavenger receptor (SR-BI).[26, 27]

The biochemical pathways involved in adrenal steroidogenesis are shown in Figure 14–3. The initial hormone-dependent rate-limiting step is the transport of intracellular cholesterol from the outer to the inner mitochondrial membrane for conversion to pregnenolone by cytochrome $P450_{scc}$. Human experiments of nature have confirmed the importance of a 30-kd protein, steroidogenic acute regulatory protein (StAR), in mediating this effect (see later). StAR is induced by an increase in intracellular cyclic adenosine monophosphate after binding of ACTH to its cognate receptor, providing the first important rate-limiting step in adrenal steroidogenesis.[28, 29] Other transporters, including the peripheral benzodiazepine-like receptor, may be involved.[30]

Steroidogenesis involves the concerted action of several enzymes, including a series of cytochrome P450 enzymes, all of which have been cloned and characterized (Table 14–3). Cholesterol side-chain cleavage enzyme and the CYP11B enzymes are localized to the mitochondria and require an electron shuttle system, provided through adrenodoxin–adrenodoxin reductase, to oxidize and hydroxylate steroids.[30–32] 17α-Hydroxylase and 21-hydroxylase are localized to the microsomal–endoplasmic reticulum fraction and are dependent upon a distinct electron shuttle system involving a flavoprotein, cytochrome b_5[33, 34] (Fig. 14–4). Mutations in the genes encoding these enzymes result in human disease, so some understanding of the underlying pathways and steroid precursors is required.[35]

After uptake of cholesterol to the mitochondrion, cholesterol is cleaved by the P450 cholesterol side-chain cleavage enzyme to form pregnenolone.[36, 37] In the cytoplasm, pregnenolone is converted to progesterone by the type II isozyme of 3β-hydroxysteroid dehydrogenase (3β-HSD) by a reaction involving dehydrogenation of the 3-hydroxyl group and isomerization of the double bond at C5.[38, 39] Progesterone is hydroxylated to 17-OHP through the activity of CYP 17α-hydroxylase. 17-Hydroxylation is a prerequisite for glucocorticoid synthesis, and the zona glomerulosa does not express 17-hydroxylase. CYP17 also possesses 17,20-lyase activity, which results in the

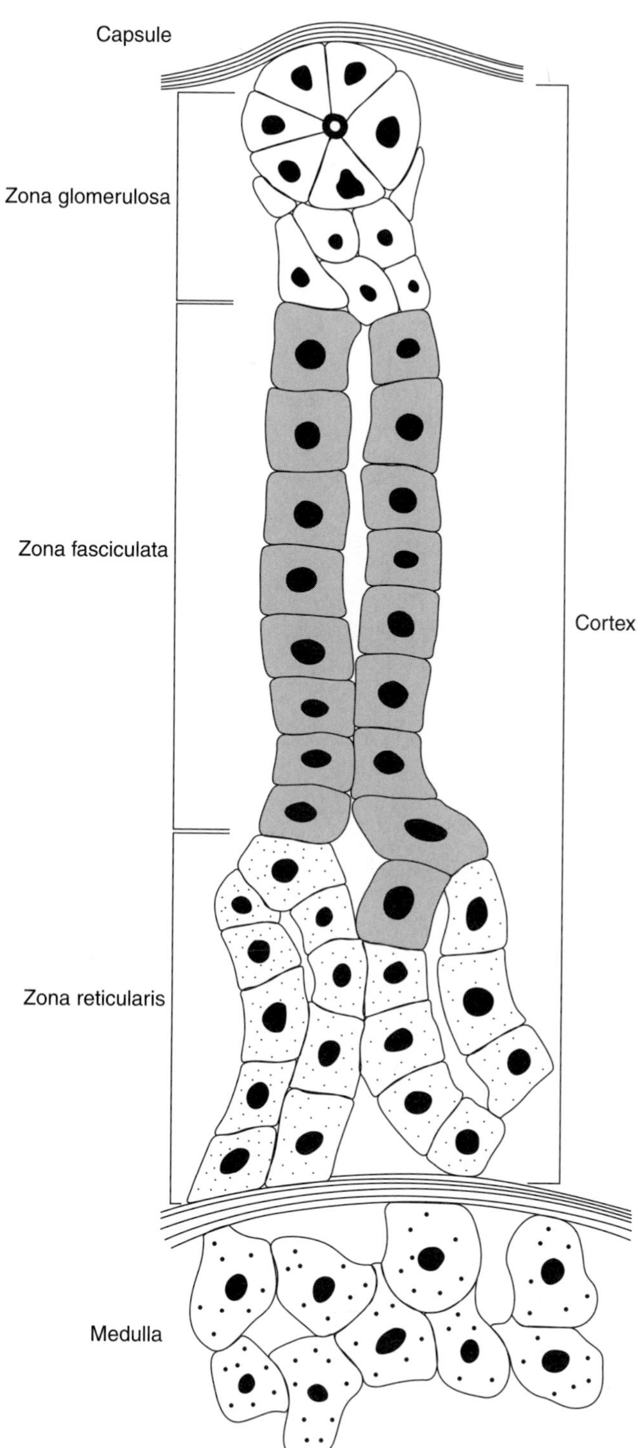

Figure 14–1. Schematic diagram of the structure of the human adrenal cortex, depicting the outer zona glomerulosa and inner zona fasciculata and zona reticularis.

production of the C_{19} adrenal androgens, dehydroepiandrosterone (DHEA) and androstenedione.[40, 41] In humans, however, 17-OHP is not an efficient substrate for CYP17, and there is negligible conversion of 17-OHP to androstenedione. Adrenal androstenedione secretion is dependent on the conversion of DHEA to androstenedione by 3β-HSD; this enzyme also converts 17-hydroxypregnenolone to 17-OHP, but the preferred substrate is pregnenolone.

21-Hydroxylation of either progesterone (zona glomerulosa) or 17-OHP (zona fasciculata) is carried out by the product of the *CYP21A2* gene, 21-hydroxylase, to yield DOC or 11-deoxycortisol, respectively.[42–44] The final step in cortisol biosynthesis takes place in the mitochondria and involves the conversion of 11-deoxycortisol to cortisol by the enzyme CYP11B1, 11β-hydroxylase.[45, 46] In the zona glomerulosa, 11β-hydroxylase may also convert DOC to corticosterone. However, the enzyme CYP11B2 or aldosterone synthase may also carry out this reaction and, in addition, is required for the conversion of corticosterone to aldosterone through the intermediate 18-OH corticosterone.[47–49] Thus, CYP11B2 can carry out 11β-hydroxylation, 18-hydroxylation, and 18-methyl oxidation to yield the characteristic C11-18 hemiacetal structure of aldosterone.

Regulation of Adrenal Steroidogenesis

"Functional Zonation" of the Adrenal Cortex

Glucocorticoids are secreted in relatively high amounts (cortisol 10 to 20 mg/day) from the zona fasciculata under the control of ACTH, and mineralocorticoids are secreted in low amounts (aldosterone 100 to 150 μg/day) from the zona glomerulosa under the principal control of angiotensin II. As a class, adrenal androgens (DHEA, dehydroepiandrosterone sulfate [DHEAS], androstenedione) are the most abundant steroids secreted from the adult adrenal gland (>20 mg/day). In each case, this is facilitated through the expression of steroidogenic enzymes in a specific zonal manner. The zona glomerulosa cannot synthesize cortisol because it does not express 17α-hydroxylase. In contrast, aldosterone secretion is confined to the outer zona glomerulosa through the restricted expression of CYP11B2. Although CYP11B1 and CYP11B2 share 95% homology, the 5′ promoter sequences differ and permit regulation of the final steps in glucocorticoid and mineralocorticoid biosynthesis by ACTH and angiotensin II, respectively. DHEA is sulfated only in the zona reticularis to form DHEAS.

In the fetal adrenal, steroidogenesis occurs primarily within the inner fetal zone.[50] Because of a relative lack of 3β-HSD and high sulfotransferase activity, the principal steroidogenic products are DHEA and DHEAS,[51] which are then aromatized by placental trophoblast to estrogens. Thus, the majority of maternal estrogen across pregnancy is, indirectly, fetally derived.[52] The control and ontogeny of human fetal steroidogenesis are discussed further in Chapter 21.

Classical endocrine feedback loops are in place to control the secretion of both hormones; cortisol inhibits the secretion of both CRF and ACTH from the hypothalamus and pituitary, respectively, and the aldosterone-induced sodium retention inhibits renal renin secretion.

Glucocorticoid Secretion: The Hypothalamo-Pituitary-Adrenal Axis

Pro-opiomelanocortin and Adrenocorticotropic Hormone

ACTH is the principal hormone stimulating adrenal glucocorticoid biosynthesis and secretion. ACTH has 39 amino acids but is synthesized within the anterior pituitary as part of a much larger 241-amino-acid precursor, pro-opiomelanocortin (POMC). POMC is cleaved in a tissue-specific fashion to yield smaller peptide hormones. In the anterior pituitary this results in the secretion of β-lipoprotein and pro-ACTH, the latter being further cleaved to an N-terminal peptide, joining peptide, and ACTH itself[53–55] (Fig. 14–5). The functions of the N-terminal peptide and β-lipoprotein are unknown, although

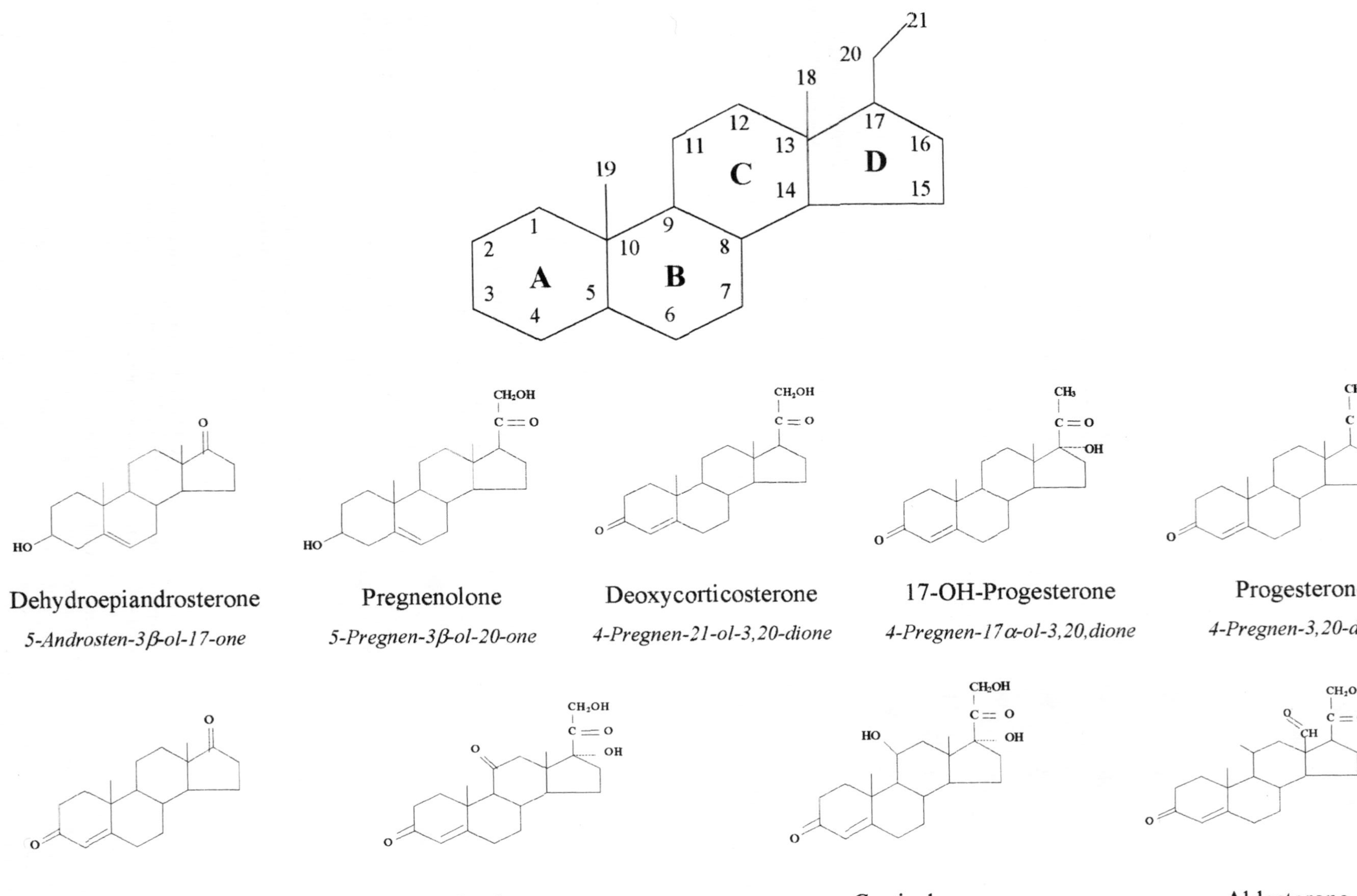

Figure 14–2. The cyclopentanoperhydrophenanthrene structure of corticosteroid hormones highlighting the structure of some endogenous steroid hormones together with their nomenclature.

Table 14–2. IUPAC and Trivial Names of Several Natural and Synthetic Steroids

Trivial Name	IUPAC Name
Aldosterone	4-Pregnen-11β,21-diol-3,18,20-trione
Androstenedione	4-Androsten-3,17-dione
Cortisol	4-Pregnen-11β,17α,21-triol-3,20-dione
Cortisone	4-Pregnen-17α,21-diol-3,11,20-trione
Dehydroepiandrosterone	5-Androsten-3β-ol-17-one
Deoxycorticosterone	4-Pregnen-21-ol-3,20-dione
Dexamethasone	1,4-Pregnadien-9α-fluoro-16α-methyl-11β,17α,21-triol-3,20-dione
Dihydrotestosterone	5α-Androstan-17β-ol-3-one
Estradiol	1,3,5(10)-Estratrien-3,17β-diol
Fludrocortisone	4-Pregnen-9α-fluoro-11β,17α,21-triol-3,20-dione
17-Hydroxyprogesterone	4-Pregnen-17α-ol-3,20-dione
Methylprednisolone	1,4-Pregnadien-6α-methyl-11β,17α,21-triol-3,20-dione
Prednisolone	1,4-Pregnadien-11β,17α,21-triol-3,20-dione
Prednisone	1,4-Pregnadien-17α,21-diol-3,11,20-trione
Pregnenolone	5-Pregnen-3β-ol-20-one
Progesterone	4-Pregnen-3,20-dione
Testosterone	4-Androsten-17β-ol-3-one
Triamcinolone	1,4-Pregnadien-9α-fluoro-11β,16α,17α,21-tetrol-3,20-dione

IUPAC, International Union of Pure and Applied Chemistry.

Table 14–3. Nomenclature for Adrenal Steroidogenic Enzymes and Their Genes and Chromosomal Localization

Enzyme Name	Gene	Chromosome
Cholesterol side-chain cleavage (SCC) (desmolase)	*CYP11A1*	15q23–q24
3β-Hydroxysteroid dehydrogenase (3β-HSD) (type II isozyme)	*HSD3B2*	1p13.1
17α-Hydroxylase/17,20 lyase	*CYP17*	10q24.3
21-Hydroxylase	*CYP21A2*	6p21.3
11β-Hydroxylase	*CYP11B1*	8q24.3
Aldosterone synthase	*CYP11B2*	8q24.3

they have weak steroidogenic activity of their own and may augment the effect of ACTH, particularly on stimulating adrenal growth. Indeed, recent studies have cloned a serine protease expressed in the outer adrenal cortex that leaves pro-gamma MSH, releasing shorter fragments that promote adrenal growth.[56] The first 24 amino acids of ACTH are common to all species, and synthetic ACTH 1 to 24 (Synacthen) is available commercially for clinical testing of the hypothalamo-pituitary-adrenal (HPA) axis and assessment of adrenal glucocorticoid reserve. Melanocyte-stimulating hormones (MSHs, α, β, and γ) are also cleaved products from POMC, but the increased pigmentation characteristic of Addison's disease is thought to arise directly from increased ACTH concentrations binding to the melanocortin-2 receptor rather than the result of α-MSH secretion.[57]

POMC is also transcribed in many extrapituitary tissues, notably brain, liver, kidney, gonad, and placenta.[54, 58, 59] In these normal tissues, POMC messenger ribonucleic acid (mRNA) is usually shorter than the pituitary 1200-bp species

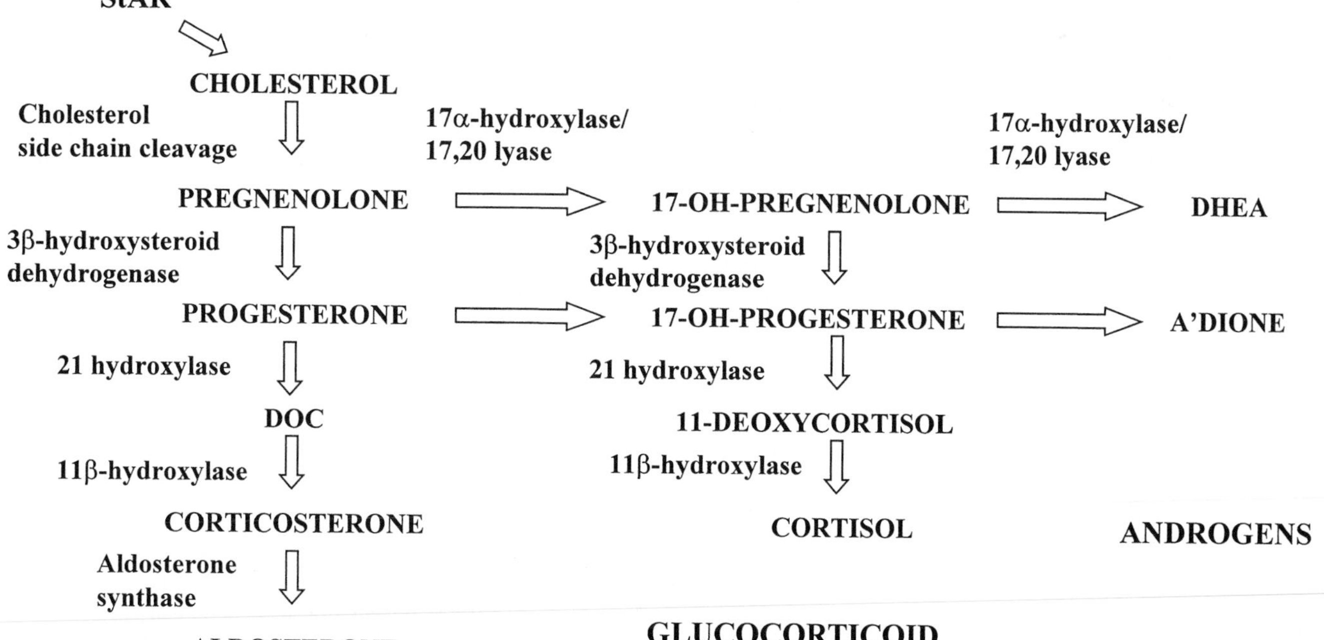

Figure 14–3. Adrenal steroidogenesis. After the steroidogenic acute regulatory (StAR) protein–mediated uptake of cholesterol into mitochondria within adrenocortical cells, aldosterone, cortisol, and adrenal androgens are synthesized through the coordinated action of a series of steroidogenic enzymes in a zone-specific fashion. A'dione, androstenedione; DHEA, dehydroepiandrosterone; DOC, deoxycorticosterone.

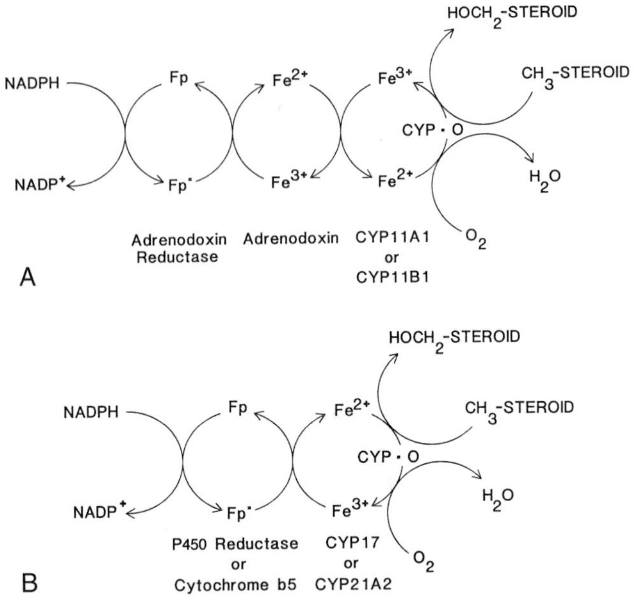

Figure 14–4. *A*, Electron shuttle system for the mitochondrial enzymes, CYP11A1 and CYP11B1. Adrenodoxin reductase receives electrons from reduced nicotinamide adenine dinucleotide phosphate (NADPH) and reduces adrenodoxin, which transfers reducing equivalents to the CYP enzyme. The enzyme then transfers electrons, by way of oxygen, to the steroid. Fp, flavoprotein; Fp$^{\bullet}$, reduced form of flavoprotein. *B*, Electron shuttle system for the microsomal enzymes, CYP17 and CYP21A2. P450 reductase, a flavoprotein, accepts electrons from NADPH and transfers them to the NADPH-P450 enzyme. The enzyme then transfers electrons, by way of oxygen, to the steroid. A second reducing equivalent may be supplied to CYP17 by NADPH-P450 reductase or cytochrome b_5.

because of lack of exons 1 and 2 and the 5′ region of exon 3.[60] As a result, it is probable that this POMC-like peptide is neither secreted nor active. However, in ectopic ACTH syndrome, additional POMC mRNA species are described that are longer than normal pituitary 1200-bp POMC species (typically 1450 bp) because of the use of alternative promoters in the 5′ region of the gene.[61, 62] This may in part explain the resistance of POMC secretion to glucocorticoid feedback in these tumors. Others factors, including interaction with tissue-specific transcription factors[63] and POMC methylation, may explain the ectopic expression of ACTH in some malignant tissues. The cleavage of POMC is also tissue-specific[64] and, at least in some cases of ectopic ACTH syndrome, it is possible that circulating ACTH precursors, notably pro-ACTH, may cross-react in current ACTH radioimmunoassays.[65, 66] The biologic activity of POMC itself upon adrenal function is thought to be negligible.

POMC expression within the hypothalamus and its cleavage to MSHs appear to be of crucial importance in regulating hair pigmentation and appetite control (see later).

Corticotropin-Releasing Hormone and Arginine Vasopressin

POMC secretion is tightly controlled by numerous factors, notably corticotropin-releasing hormone (CRH) and arginine vasopressin (AVP)[67, 68] (Fig. 14–6). Additional control is provided through an endogenous circadian rhythm, stress, and feedback inhibition by cortisol itself. CRH is a 41-amino-acid peptide that is synthesized in neurons within the paraventricular nucleus of the hypothalamus.[11, 69–71] Human[72] and rat[73] CRHs are identical, but ovine[74] CRH differs by seven amino acids; in humans it is slightly more potent than human CRH in stimulating ACTH secretion but has a longer half-life and is therefore used diagnostically. CRH is secreted into the hypophyseal portal blood, where it binds to specific type I CRH receptors on anterior pituitary corticotrophs[75] to stimulate POMC gene transcription through a process that includes the activation of adenylate cyclase.[76] It is unclear whether hypothalamic CRH contributes in any way to circulating levels. CRH is also synthesized in other tissues, and it is likely that circulating CRH reflects synthesis from testis, gastrointestinal tract, adrenal medulla,[77, 78] and particularly the placenta,[79] where the increased secretion during pregnancy results in a threefold increase in circulating CRH levels.[80]

In the circulation, CRH is bound to CRH-binding protein; levels of CRH-binding protein also increase during pregnancy so that cortisol secretion is not markedly elevated.[81] CRH is the principal stimulus for ACTH secretion[82, 83] but AVP is able to potentiate CRH-mediated secretion.[84, 85] In this case, AVP acts through the V1B receptor to activate protein kinase C.[86] The peak response of ACTH to CRH does not differ throughout the day, but it is affected by endogenous function of the HPA axis in that responsiveness is reduced in subjects treated with corticosteroids but increased in subjects with Cushing's disease. Other reported ACTH secretagogues, including angiotensin II, cholecystokinin, atrial natriuretic factor, and vasoactive peptides, probably act to modulate the CRH control of ACTH secretion.[87, 88]

The Stress Response and Immune-Endocrine Axis

The proinflammatory cytokines, notably interleukin-1, interleukin-6, and tumor necrosis factor α, also increase ACTH secretion either directly or by augmenting the effect of CRF.[89, 90] Leukemia inhibitory factor, a cytokine of the interleukin-6 family, is a further activator of the HPA axis.[91] This explains the response of the HPA axis to an inflammatory stimulus and is an important immune-endocrine interaction (Chapter 3). Physical stresses increase ACTH and cortisol secretion, again through central actions mediated by CRH and AVP. Thus, cortisol secretion rises in response to fever, surgery,[92] burn injury,[93] hypoglycemia,[94] hypotension, and exercise.[95] In all of these cases, this can be viewed as a normal counterregulatory response to the insult. Acute psychological stress raises cortisol levels, but secretion rates appear to be normal in patients with chronic anxiety states and underlying psychotic illness. However, depression is associated with high circulating cortisol concentrations, and this an important consideration in the differential diagnosis of Cushing's syndrome (see later).[96–98]

Circadian Rhythm

ACTH is secreted in a pulsatile fashion with a circadian rhythm so that levels are highest on waking and decline throughout the day, reaching nadir values in the evening[99] (Fig. 14–7). ACTH pulse frequency is higher in normal adult men than in women (on average 18 pulses versus 10 pulses per 24 hours), and the circadian ACTH rhythm appears to be mediated principally by an increased ACTH pulse amplitude between 5 and 9 AM but also by a reduction in ACTH pulse frequency between 6 and 12 PM.[100–102] Food ingestion is a further stimulus to ACTH secretion.[103] Circadian rhythm is dependent upon both day-night[104] and sleep-wake[105] patterns and is disrupted by alternating day-night shift working patterns and by long-distance travel across time zones.[106] It may take up to 2 weeks for circadian rhythm to reset to an altered day-night cycle.

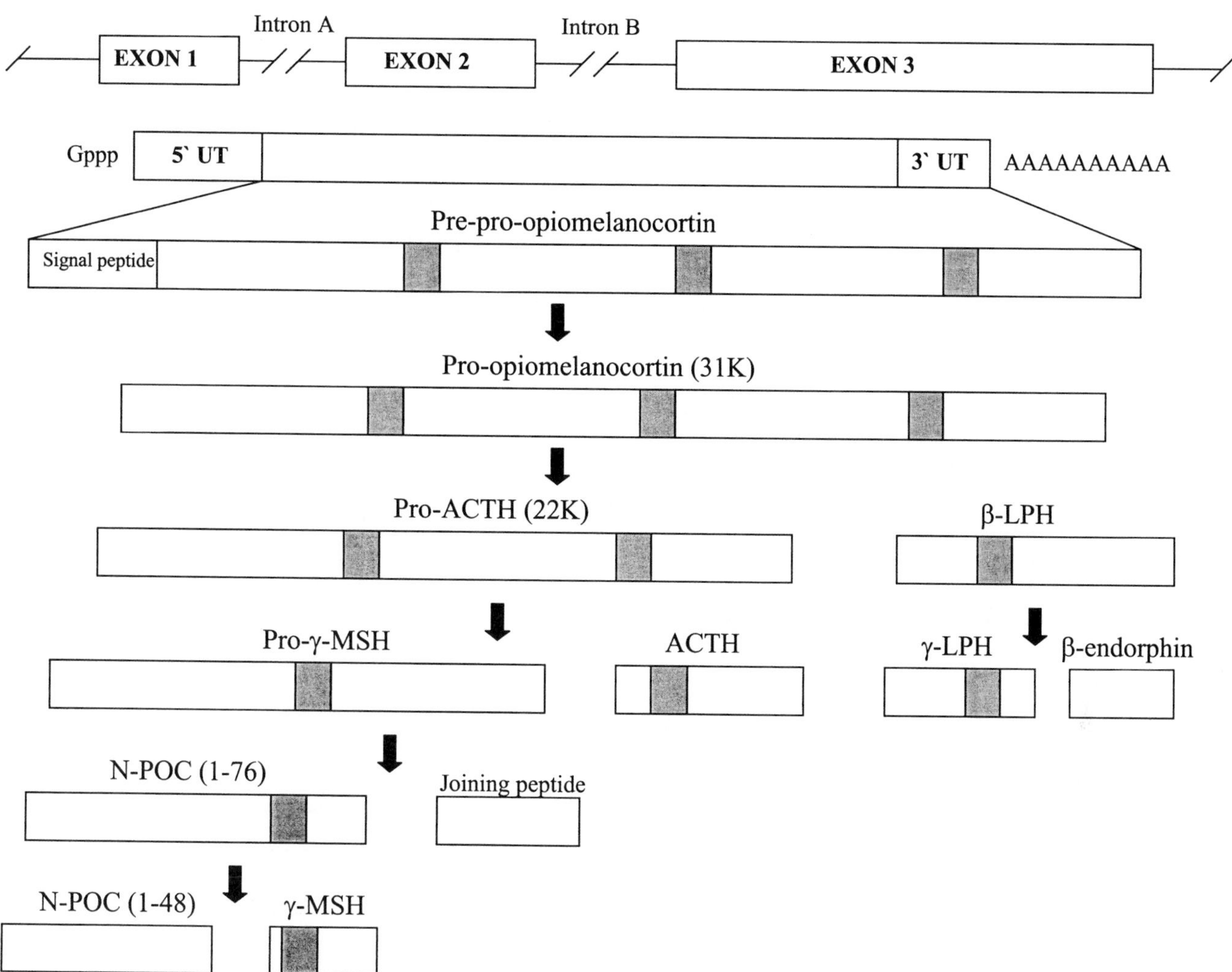

Figure 14–5. Synthesis and cleavage of pro-opiomelanocortin (POMC) within the human anterior pituitary gland. Prohormone convertase enzymes sequentially cleave POMC to adrenocorticotropic hormone (ACTH). *Shaded areas* represent melanocyte-stimulating hormone (MSH) structural units. β-LPH, β-lipoprotein; γ-LPH, γ-lipoprotein; N-POC, amino-terminal pro-opiomelanocortin.

Negative Feedback

An important aspect of CRH and ACTH secretion is the negative feedback control exerted by glucocorticoids themselves. Glucocorticoids inhibit POMC gene transcription in the anterior pituitary[67] and CRH and AVP mRNA synthesis and secretion in the hypothalamus.[107–109] This negative feedback effect is dependent upon the dose, potency, half-life, and duration of administration of the glucocorticoid and has important physiologic and diagnostic consequences. Suppression of the HPA axis by pharmacologic corticosteroids may persist for many months after cessation of therapy, and adrenocortical insufficiency should be anticipated. Diagnostically, the feedback mechanism in Addison's disease explains ACTH hypersecretion and undetectable ACTH levels in patients with a cortisol-secreting adrenal adenoma. Feedback inhibition is principally mediated by the glucocorticoid receptor (GR); patients with glucocorticoid resistance caused by mutations in the GR[110] and mice lacking the GR gene[111] have ACTH and cortisol hypersecretion related to perceived lack of negative feedback.

The Adrenocorticotropic Hormone Receptor and ACTH Effects on the Adrenal

ACTH binds to a G protein–coupled, melanocortin-2 receptor,[112, 113] of which there are approximately 3500 on each adrenocortical cell. Signal transduction is mediated principally through the stimulation of adenylate cyclase and intracellular cyclic adenosine monophosphate,[114, 115] although both extracellular and intracellular Ca^{2+} play a role.[116] Other factors synergize with or inhibit the effects of ACTH on the adrenal cortex, including angiotensin II, activin, inhibin, and cytokines (tumor necrosis factor α and leptin).[117] Cell-to-cell communication through gap junctions is also important in mediating the effects of ACTH.[118]

The effects of ACTH on the adrenal include both immediate and chronic effects; the end result is the stimulation of adrenal steroidogenesis and growth. Acutely, steroidogenesis is stimulated through a StAR-mediated increase in cholesterol delivery to the CYP11A1 enzyme in the inner mitochondrial membrane.[28] Chronically (within 24 to 26 hours of exposure), ACTH acts to increase the synthesis of all steroidogenic CYP

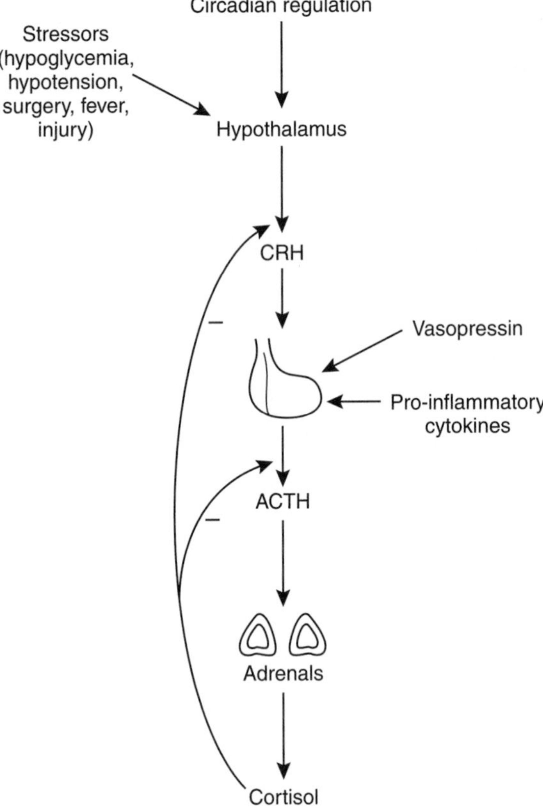

Figure 14–6. Normal regulation of adrenal glucocorticoid secretion. Adrenocorticotropic hormone (ACTH) is secreted from the anterior pituitary under the influence of two principal secretagogues, corticotropin-releasing hormone (CRH) and arginine vasopressin; other factors including cytokines also play a role. CRH secretion is regulated by an inbuilt circadian rhythm and additional stressors operating through the hypothalamus. Secretion of both CRH and ACTH is inhibited by cortisol, highlighting the importance of negative feedback control.

enzymes (CYP11A1, CYP17, CYP21A2, CYP11B1) in addition to adrenodoxin,[31, 119, 120] effects that are mediated at the transcriptional level. ACTH also increases synthesis of the LDL and HDL receptors and possibly also 3-hydroxy-3-methylglutaryl coenzyme A reductase, the rate-limiting step in cholesterol biosynthesis. ACTH increases adrenal weight by inducing both hyperplasia and hypertrophy. Adrenal atrophy is a feature of ACTH deficiency.

Mineralocorticoid Secretion: The Renin-Angiotensin-Aldosterone Axis

Aldosterone is secreted from the zona glomerulosa under the control of three principal secretagogues, angiotensin II, potassium, and to a lesser extent ACTH. Other factors, notably somatostatin, heparin, atrial natriuretic factor, and dopamine, can directly inhibit aldosterone synthesis. The secretion of aldosterone and its intermediary 18-hydroxylated metabolites is restricted to the zona glomerulosa because of the zonal-specific expression of CYP11B2 (aldosterone synthase).[121] Corticosterone and DOC, although synthesized in both the zona fasciculata and zona glomerulosa, can act as mineralocorticoids; this becomes significant in some clinical diseases, notably some forms of congenital adrenal hyperplasia (CAH) and adrenal tumors. Similarly, it is now established that cortisol can act as a mineralocorticoid in the setting of impaired metabolism to cortisone carried out by the enzyme 11β-HSD; this is impor-

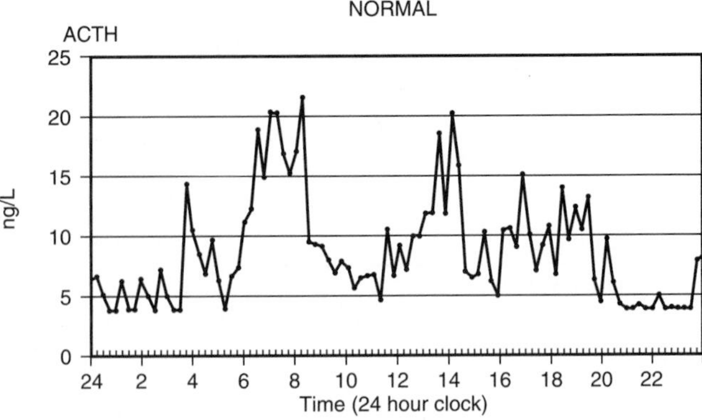

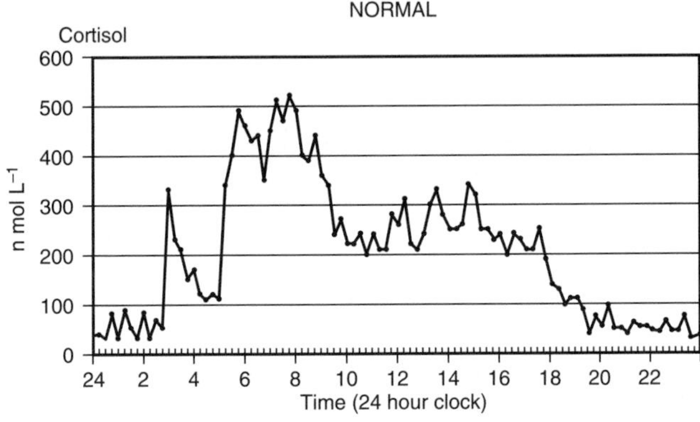

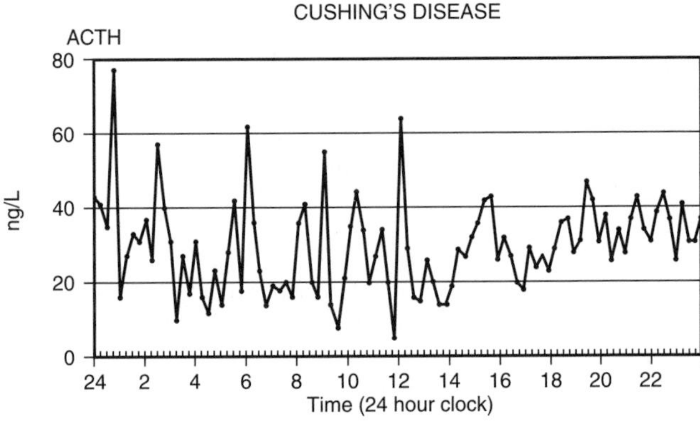

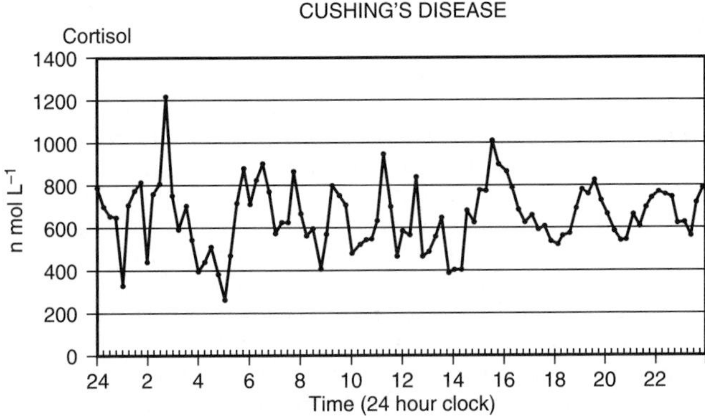

Figure 14–7. Circadian and pulsatile secretion of adrenocorticotropic hormone (ACTH) and cortisol in a normal subject *(top two panels)* and in a patient with Cushing's disease. In a normal subject, secretion of ACTH and cortisol is highest in early morning and falls to a nadir at midnight. ACTH pulse frequency and pulse amplitude are increased in Cushing's disease, and circadian rhythm secretion is lost.

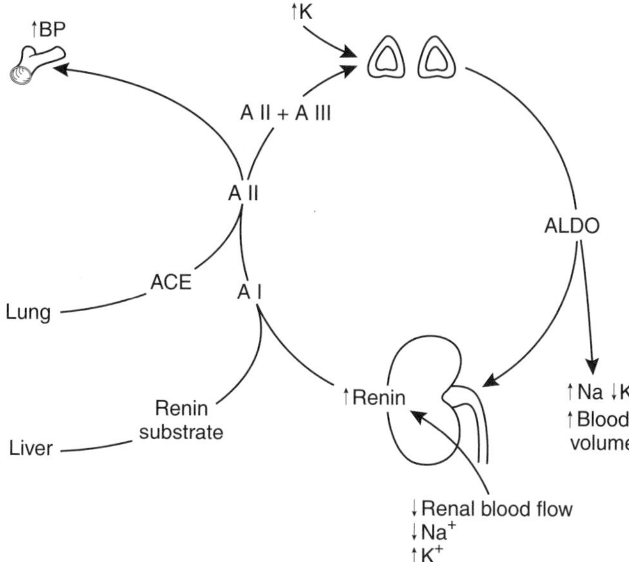

Figure 14–8. The normal renin-angiotensin-aldosterone regulatory system. Renin, secreted by the kidney, cleaves angiotensin I (A I) from renin substrate (angiotensinogen), an α_2-globulin produced by the liver. Angiotensin I is converted into biologically active angiotensin II by angiotensin-converting enzyme (ACE), mainly in the lung. Angiotensin II increases peripheral vascular resistance, and, together with angiotensin III, stimulates aldosterone (ALDO) secretion, which results in sodium retention and increased plasma volume.

tant in patients with hypertension, ectopic ACTH syndrome, and renal disease (see Chapter 15).

Angiotensin II is generated through the renin-angiotensin system (Fig. 14–8). Angiotensinogen is an α_2-globulin synthesized within the liver and is cleaved by renin to form angiotensin I. Angiotensin I is converted to angiotensin II by angiotensin-converting enzyme in lung and many other peripheral tissues; further cleavage to angiotensin III may also occur. Angiotensin I has no apparent biologic activity, but both angiotensin II and angiotensin III are potent in stimulating aldosterone secretion. In addition, angiotensin II is a potent vasoconstrictor.

The rate-limiting step in the renin-angiotensin system is the secretion of renin, which is also controlled through a negative feedback loop.[122, 123] Renin is secreted from juxtaglomerular epithelial cells within the macula densa of the renal tubule in response to underlying renal arteriolar pressure, oncotic pressure, and sympathetic drive. Thus, low perfusion pressure or low tubular fluid sodium content, as seen in hemorrhage, renal artery stenosis, dehydration, or salt loss, increases renin secretion. Conversely, secretion is suppressed by a high-salt diet and by factors that increase blood pressure. Autoregulation is therefore maintained because the increase in renin secretion stimulates angiotensin II and aldosterone production; the concomitant increase in blood pressure and renal sodium retention results in feedback inhibition of renin secretion.

Hypokalemia increases and hyperkalemia decreases renin secretion; in addition, potassium exerts a direct effect on the adrenal cortex to increase aldosterone secretion. The sensitivity of the renin-angiotensin system to changes in circulating potassium is high, with changes in potassium concentrations of only 0.1 to 0.5 mmol/L producing marked changes in aldosterone concentrations. Potassium concentrations also determine the sensitivity of the aldosterone response to a given infusion of angiotensin II, with high potassium intake increasing responsiveness.[124]

Norepinephrine increases renin secretion, and β-blockers inhibit renin release. In the clinical assessment of the renin-angiotensin-aldosterone axis, α-blockers have a minimal effect on endogenous renin levels and can be given concomitantly if required to control hypertension so that renin and aldosterone concentrations can be measured. Prostaglandins also play a role in modulating renin secretion, and indomethacin inhibits renin release.

Angiotensin II and potassium stimulate aldosterone secretion principally by increasing the transcription of CYP11B2 through common intracellular signaling pathways. Cyclic adenosine monophosphate response elements in the 5′ region of the *CYP11B2* gene are activated after an increase in intracellular Ca^{2+} and activation of calmodulin kinases. The potassium effect is mediated through membrane depolarization and opening of calcium channels and the angiotensin II effect following binding of angiotensin II to the surface angiotensin I receptor and activation of phospholipase C.[121]

The effect of ACTH on aldosterone secretion is modest and differs in the acute and chronic situations. An acute bolus of ACTH increases aldosterone secretion, principally by stimulating the early pathways of adrenal steroidogenesis (see earlier), but circulating levels increase by no more than 10% to 20% above baseline values.[125] ACTH has no effect on *CYP11B2* gene transcription or enzyme activity. Chronic continual ACTH stimulation has either no effect or an inhibitory effect on aldosterone production, possibly because of receptor down-regulation or suppression of angiotensin II–stimulated secretion because of a mineralocorticoid effect of cortisol, DOC, or corticosterone.[126] Dopamine[127] and atrial natriuretic peptide[128] inhibit aldosterone secretion, as does heparin.

The separate control of glucocorticoid biosynthesis through the HPA axis and mineralocorticoid synthesis through the renin-angiotensin system has important clinical consequences. Patients with primary adrenal failure invariably have both cortisol and aldosterone deficiency, whereas patients with ACTH deficiency related to pituitary disease have glucocorticoid deficiency but normal aldosterone concentrations because the renin-angiotensin system is intact.

Adrenal Androgen Secretion

Adrenal androgens represent an important component (>50%) of circulating androgens in premenopausal females.[129] In males this contribution is much smaller because of the testicular production of androgens, but adrenal androgen excess even in males may be of clinical significance, notably in patients with CAH. The adult adrenal secretes DHEA at approximately 4 mg/day, DHEAS at 7 to 15 mg/day, androstenedione at 1.5 mg/day, and testosterone at 0.05 mg/day. DHEA is a weak sex steroid but can be converted to androgens and estrogens through the activities of 3β-HSD, a superfamily of 17β-HSD isozymes, and aromatase, expressed in peripheral target tissues, and this is of clinical importance in many diseases.[130]

ACTH stimulates androgen secretion; DHEA (but not DHEAS because of its increased plasma half-life) and androstenedione demonstrate a similar circadian rhythm to cortisol.[131] However, there are many discrepancies between adrenal androgen and glucocorticoid secretion, which has led to the suggestion of an additional androgen-stimulating hormone (Table 14–4). Many putative androgen-stimulating hormones have been proposed including POMC derivatives such as joining peptide, prolactin, and insulin-like growth factor-I (IGF-I), but conclusive proof is lacking. Adrenal androgen steroidogenesis is dependent upon the relative activities of 3β-HSD and 17α-hydroxylase and in particular upon the 17,20-lyase activity of 17α-hydroxylase. Factors that determine whether 17-hydroxylated substrates, 17-hydroxypregnenolone and 17-OHP, undergo 21-hydroxylation to form glucocorticoid or side-chain

Table 14–4. Dissociation of Adrenal Androgen and Glucocorticoid Secretion: Evidence for an Adrenal-Stimulating Hormone

Dexamethasone studies: Complete cortisol suppression with chronic high-dose dexamethasone. DHEA falls by only 20%. Greater sensitivity of DHEA to acute low-dose dexamethasone administration.
Adrenarche: Rise in circulating DHEA at 6–8 years of age. Cortisol production unaltered.
Aging: Reduction in DHEA production, no change in cortisol.
Anorexia nervosa and illness: Fall in DHEA, no change (or increase) in cortisol.

DHEA, dehydroepiandrosterone.

cleavage by 17α-hydroxylase to form DHEA and androstenedione are unresolved and seem likely to be important in defining the activity of any putative androgen-stimulating hormone.[131]

CORTICOSTEROID HORMONE ACTION

Receptors and Gene Transcription

Both cortisol and aldosterone exert their effects after uptake of free hormone from the circulation and binding to intracellular receptors, termed the glucocorticoid and mineralocorticoid receptors (GR and MR).[132–134] These are both members of the thyroid/steroid hormone receptor superfamily of transcription factors comprising a C-terminal ligand-binding domain, a central deoxyribonucleic acid (DNA) binding domain interacting with specific DNA sequences on target genes, and an N-terminal hypervariable region. In both cases, although there is only a single gene encoding the GR and MR, splice variants have been described resulting in α and β variants[135, 136] (Fig. 14–9).

Glucocorticoid hormone action has been studied in more depth than mineralocorticoid action. The binding of steroid to the GRα in the cytosol results in activation of the steroid-receptor complex through a process that involves the dissociation of heat shock proteins (HSP 90 and HSP 70).[137] After translocation to the nucleus, gene transcription is stimulated or repressed following binding of dimerized GR-ligand complexes to specific DNA sequences in the promoter regions of target genes.[138, 139] This glucocorticoid response element is invariably a palindromic CGTACAnnnTGTACT sequence that binds with high affinity to two loops of DNA within the DNA binding domain of the GR (zinc fingers). This stabilizes the RNA polymerase II complex, facilitating gene transcription. The GRβ variant may act as a dominant negative regulator of GRα transactivation.[140]

Naturally occurring mutations in the GR (as seen in patients with glucocorticoid resistance, discussed later) and GR mutants generated in vitro have highlighted critical regions of the receptor responsible for binding and transactivation,[141–143] but numerous others factors are also required (coactivators, corepressors[144]) that may confer tissue specificity of response. This is a rapidly evolving field and is reviewed in Chapter 4. However, the interactions between GR and two particular transcription factors are important in mediating the anti-inflammatory effects of glucocorticoids and explain the effect of glucocorticoids on genes that do not contain obvious glucocorticoid response elements in their promoter regions. Activator protein-1 (AP-1) comprises Fos and Jun subunits and is a proinflammatory transcription factor induced by a series of cytokines and phorbol ester. The GR-ligand complex can bind to c-jun and prevent interaction with the AP-1 site to repress AP-1 and GR *trans*-activation functions.[145, 146] Similarly, functional antagonism exists between the GR and nuclear factor κB (NF-κB). NF-κB is a ubiquitously expressed transcription factor that activates a series of genes involved in lymphocyte development, inflammatory response, host defense, and apoptosis[146] (Fig. 14–10). In keeping with the diverse array of actions of cortisol, many hundred glucocorticoid-responsive genes have been identified. Some glucocorticoid-induced genes and repressed genes are given in Table 14–5.

In contrast to the diverse actions of glucocorticoids, mineralocorticoids have a more restricted role, principally to stimulate

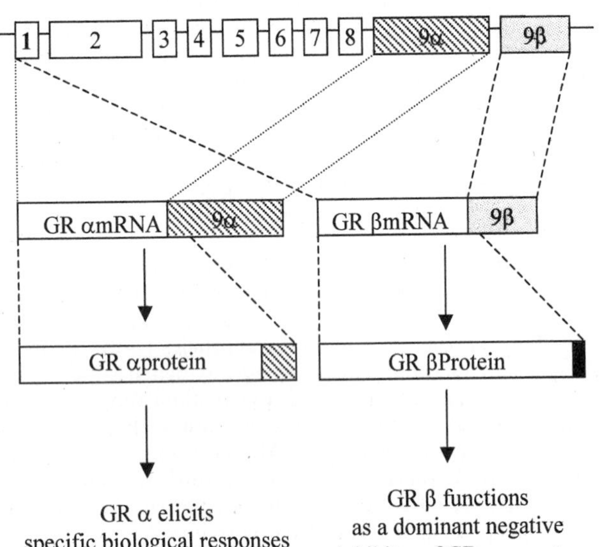

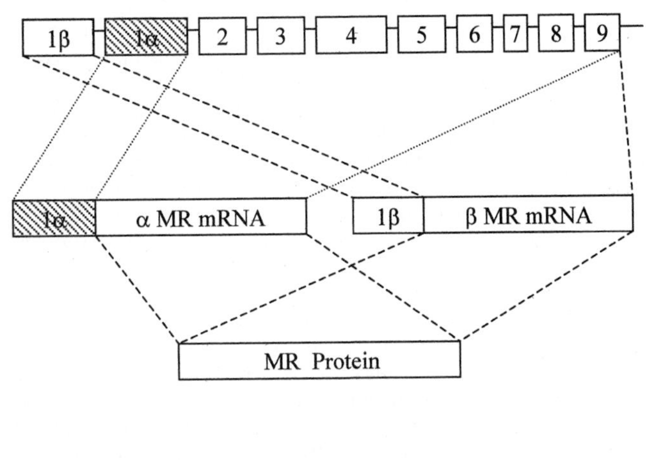

Figure 14–9. Schematic structure of the human genes encoding the glucocorticoid receptor (GR) and mineralocorticoid receptor (MR). In both cases splice variants have been described; in the case of the GR, there is evidence that the GRβ isoform can act as a dominant negative inhibitor of GRα action. mRNA, messenger ribonucleic acid.

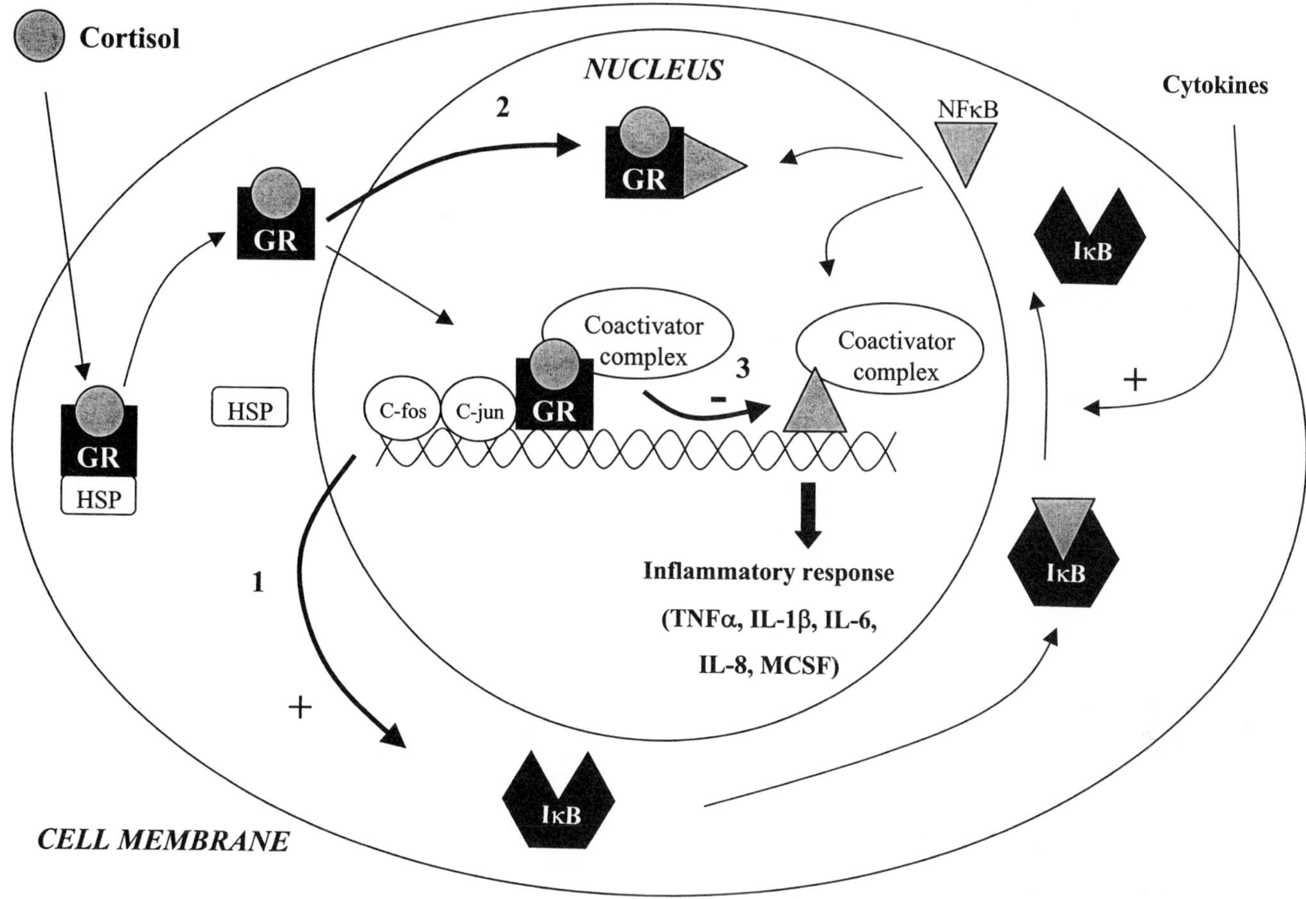

Figure 14–10. The anti-inflammatory action of glucocorticoids. Cortisol binds to the cytoplasmic glucocorticoid receptor (GR). Conformational changes in the receptor-ligand complex result in dissociation from heat shock proteins (HSPs) 70 and 90 and migration to the nucleus. Binding occurs to specific DNA motifs—glucocorticoid response elements in association with the activator protein-1 (AP-1) comprising c-fos and c-jun. Glucocorticoids mediate their anti-inflammatory effects through several mechanisms: (1) The inhibitory protein IκB, which binds and inactivates nuclear factor κB (NFκB), is induced. (2) The GR-cortisol complex is able to bind NFκB and thus prevent initiation of an inflammatory process. (3) Both GR and NFκB compete for the limited availability of coactivators that include cyclic adenosine monophosphate response element binding protein (CREB) binding protein and steroid receptor coactivator-1.

epithelial sodium transport in the distal nephron, distal colon, and salivary glands.[147] This stimulation is mediated through the induction of the apical sodium channel (comprising three subunits, α, β and γ)[148] and the α_1 and β_1 subunits of the basolateral Na^+,K^+-adenosine triphosphatase[149] through transcriptional regulation of an aldosterone-induced gene, serum and glucocorticoid-induced kinase (*SGK*).[150] Aldosterone binds to the MR, principally in the cytosol (although there is evidence for expression of the unliganded MR in the nucleus), followed by translocation of the hormone-receptor complex to the nucleus (Fig. 14–11).

The MR and GR share considerable homology: 57% in the steroid binding domain and 94% in the DNA binding domain. It is perhaps not surprising, therefore, that there is promiscuity of ligand binding with aldosterone (and the synthetic mineralocorticoid fludrocortisone) binding to the GR and cortisol binding to the MR. For the MR this is particularly impressive—in vitro the MR has the same inherent affinity for aldosterone, corticosterone, and cortisol.[133, 151] Specificity upon the MR is conferred through the "prereceptor" metabolism of cortisol through the enzyme 11β-HSD, which inactivates cortisol and corticosterone to inactive 11-keto metabolites, enabling aldosterone to bind to the MR.[152, 153]

For both glucocorticoids and mineralocorticoids there is accumulating evidence for so-called nongenomic effects involving hormone responses obviating the genomic GR or MR. A series of responses have been reported within seconds or minutes of exposure to corticosteroids and are thought to be mediated by as yet uncharacterized membrane-coupled receptors.[154, 155]

Cortisol-Binding Globulin and Corticosteroid Hormone Metabolism

Over 90% of circulating cortisol is bound, predominantly to the α_2-globulin cortisol-binding globulin (CBG).[156] This 383-amino-acid protein is synthesized in the liver and binds cortisol with high affinity. Affinity for synthetic corticosteroids (except prednisolone, which has an affinity for CBG about 50% of that of cortisol) is negligible. Circulating CBG concentrations are approximately 26 mg/dL (700 nmol/L); levels are increased by estrogens and in some patients with chronic active hepatitis but reduced by glucocorticoids and in patients with cirrhosis, nephrosis, and hyperthyroidism.[157] The estrogen effect can be marked, with levels increasing twofold to threefold during pregnancy, and this should also be taken into account when measuring plasma "total" cortisol in pregnancy and in women taking estrogens.

Table 14–5. Some of the Genes Regulated by Glucocorticoids or Glucocorticoid Receptors

Site of Action	Induced Genes	Repressed Genes
Immune system	IκB (NFκB inhibitor) Haptoglobin TCR ζ p21, p27, and p57 Lipocortin	Interleukins TNF-α IFN-γ E-selectin ICAM-1 Cyclooxygenase 2 iNOS
Metabolic	PPAR-γ Tyrosine aminotransferase Glutamine synthase Glycogen synthase Glucose-6-phosphatase PEPCK Leptin γ-Fibrinogen Cholesterol 7α-hydroxylase C/EBP/β	Tryptophan hydroxylase Metalloprotease
Bone	Androgen receptor Calcitonin receptor Alkaline phosphatase IGF-BP-6	Osteocalcin Collagenase
Channels and transporters	Epithelial sodium channel (ENaC) α, β, γ Serum and glucocorticoid–induced kinase (SGK) Aquaporin 1	
Endocrine	bFGF VIP Endothelin RXR GHRH receptor Natriuretic peptide receptors	GR PRL POMC/CRH PTHrP Vasopressin
Growth and development	Surfactant protein A, B, C	Fibronectin α-Fetoprotein NGF Erythropoietin G1 cyclins Cyclin-dependent kinases

Modified from McKay LI, Cidlowski JA. Molecular control of immune/inflammatory responses: interactions between nuclear factor–κB and steroid receptor–signalling pathways. Endocr Rev 1999; 20:435–459.

bFGF, basic fibroblast growth factor; CRH, corticotropin-releasing hormone; C/EBP/β, CAAT-enhancer binding protein-beta; GR, glucocorticoid receptor; GHRH, growth hormone–releasing hormone; ICAM, intercellular adhesion molecule; IFN, interferon; IGF-BP, insulin-like growth factor–binding protein; IκB, inhibitory kappa B; iNOS, inducible nitric oxide synthase; NFκB, nuclear factor κB; NGF, nerve growth factor; PEPCK, phosphoenolpyruvate carboxykinase; POMC, pro-opiomelanocortin; PPAR, peroxisome proliferator–activated receptor; PTHrP, parathyroid hormone–related protein; RXR, retinoid X receptor; SGK, serum and glucocorticoid-induced kinase; TCR, T-cell receptor; TNF-α, tumor necrosis factor-alpha; VIP, vasoactive intestinal peptide.

Inherited abnormalities in CBG synthesis are much rarer than those described for thyroxine-binding globulin but include elevated CBG, partial and complete deficiency of CBG, or CBG variants with reduced affinity for cortisol.[158, 159] In each case, alterations in CBG concentrations change total circulating cortisol concentrations accordingly but free cortisol concentrations are normal. Only this free circulating fraction is available for transport into tissues for biologic activity.[160] The free cortisol excreted through the kidneys is termed urinary free cortisol and represents only 1% of the total cortisol secretion rate.

The circulating half-life of cortisol varies between 70 and 120 minutes.[161] The major steps for cortisol metabolism are depicted in Figure 14–12.[162, 163] These comprise:

1. The interconversion of the 11-hydroxyl (cortisol, Kendall's compound F) to the 11-oxo group (cortisone, compound E) through the activity of 11β-HSD (EC 1.1.1.146).[164, 165] The metabolism of cortisol and cortisone then follow similar pathways.

2. Reduction of the C4-C5 double bond to form dihydrocortisol or dihydrocortisone followed by hydroxylation of the 3-oxo group to form tetrahydrocortisol (THF) and tetrahydrocortisone (THE). The reduction of the C4-C5 double bond can be carried out by either 5β-reductase[166] or 5α-reductase[167] to yield, respectively, 5β-THF (THF) or 5α-THF (allo-THF). In normal subjects the 5β metabolites predominate (5β:5α-THF 2:1). THF, allo-THF, and THE are rapidly conjugated with glucuronic acid and excreted in the urine.[168]

3. Further reduction of the 20-oxo group by either 20α–HSD or 20β-HSD to yield α- and β-cortols and cortolones from cortisol and cortisone, respectively. Reduction of the C20 position may also occur without A ring reduction, giving rise to 20α-hydroxycortisol and 20β-hydroxycortisol.[163]

4. Hydroxylation at C6 to form 6β-hydroxycortisol.[169]

5. Cleavage of THF and THE to the C_{19} steroids 11-hydroxy and 11-oxo androsterone or etiocholanolone.

6. Oxidation of the C21 position of cortols and cortolones to form the extremely polar metabolites cortolic and cortolonic acids.[170]

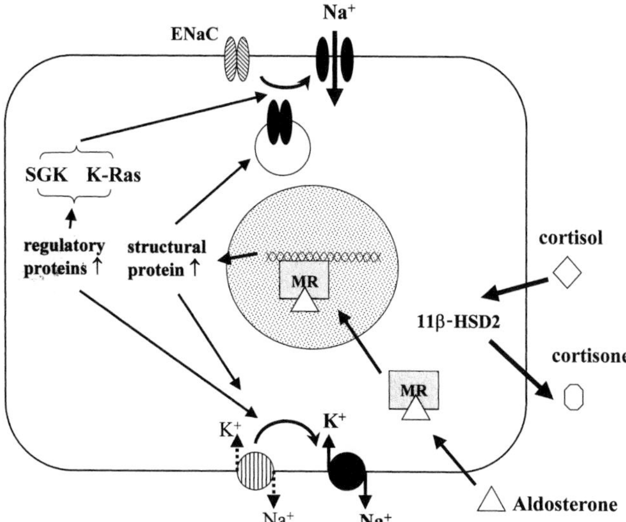

Figure 14–11. Mineralocorticoid hormone action. An epithelial cell is depicted in the distal nephron or distal colon, or both. The much higher concentrations of cortisol are inactivated by the type 2 isozyme of 11β-hydroxysteroid dehydrogenase (11β-HSD2) to cortisone, permitting the endogenous ligand, aldosterone, to bind to the mineralocorticoid receptor (MR). Relatively few mineralocorticoid target genes have been identified, but these include serum and glucocorticoid-induced kinase (SGK), subunits of the epithelial sodium channel (ENaC), and basolateral Na^+,K^+-adenosine triphosphatase.

Approximately 50% of secreted cortisol appears in the urine as THF, allo-THF, and THE; 25% as cortols and cortolones; 10% as C_{19} steroids; and 10% as cortolic and cortolonic acids. The remaining metabolites are free, unconjugated steroids (cortisol, cortisone, 6β- and 20α/20β-metabolites of THF and THE).[162, 163]

The principal site of cortisol metabolism has been considered to be the liver, but many of the preceding enzymes have been described in the mammalian kidney, notably in the inactivation of cortisol to cortisone by 11β-HSD. Quantitatively, the interconversion of cortisol to cortisone by 11β-HSD is also the most important pathway. Furthermore, the bioactivity of glucocorticoids is in part related to the hydroxyl group at C11; cortisone with a C11 oxo group is an inactive steroid so that 11β-HSD expressed in peripheral tissues plays a crucial role in regulating corticosteroid hormone action. Two distinct 11β-HSD isozymes have been reported: a type 1 oxoreductase dependent on reduced nicotinamide adenine dinucleotide phosphate and expressed principally in the liver, which confers bioactivity upon orally administered cortisone by converting it to cortisol, and a type 2, nicotinamide adenine dinucleotide–dependent dehydrogenase. It is 11β-HSD2, coexpressed with the MR in the kidney, colon, and salivary gland, that inactivates cortisol to cortisone and permits aldosterone to bind to the MR in vivo. If this enzyme-protective mechanism is impaired, cortisol is able to act as a mineralocorticoid; this explains some forms of endocrine hypertension (apparent mineralocorticoid excess, licorice ingestion; see Chapter 15) and the mineralocorticoid excess state that characterizes the ectopic ACTH syndrome (see later).[164, 165]

Hyperthyroidism results in increased cortisol metabolism and clearance and hypothyroidism the converse, principally because of an effect of thyroid hormone on hepatic 11β-HSD and 5α/5β-reductases.[164, 171, 172] IGF-I increases cortisol clearance by inhibiting hepatic 11β-HSD (conversion of cortisone to cortisol).[173, 174] 6β-Hydroxylation is normally a minor pathway, but cortisol itself induces 6β-hydroxylase so that 6β-hydroxycortisol excretion is markedly increased in patients with Cushing's syndrome.[169] Furthermore, some drugs, notably rifampicin[175] and phenytoin,[176] increase cortisol clearance through this pathway. Patients with renal disease have impaired cortisol clearance because of reduced renal conversion of cortisol to cortisone.[177] These observations have clinical implications for patients with thyroid disease, acromegaly, and renal disease and for patients taking cortisol replacement therapy. Adrenal crisis has been reported in steroid-replaced addisonian patients given rifampicin,[178] and hydrocortisone replacement therapy may need to be increased in treated patients in whom hyperthyroidism develops.

Aldosterone is also metabolized in the liver and kidneys. In the liver it undergoes tetrahydro reduction and is excreted in the urine as a 3-glucuronide tetrahydroaldosterone derivative; however, glucuronide conjugation at the 18 position occurs directly in the kidney, as does 3α and 5α/5β metabolism of the free steroid.[179] Because of the aldehyde group at the C18 position, aldosterone is not metabolized by 11β-HSD. Hepatic aldosterone clearance is reduced in patients with cirrhosis, ascites, and severe congestive heart failure

Effects of Glucocorticoids (Fig. 14–13)

Carbohydrate, Protein, and Lipid Metabolism

Glucocorticoids increase blood glucose concentrations through their action on glycogen, protein, and lipid metabolism. In the liver, cortisol stimulates glycogen deposition by increasing glycogen synthase and inhibiting the glycogen-mobilizing enzyme glycogen phosphorylase.[180] Hepatic glucose output increases through the activation of key enzymes involved in gluconeogenesis, principally glucose-6-phosphatase and phosphoenolpyruvate carboxykinase.[181, 182] In peripheral tissues (muscle, fat), cortisol inhibits glucose uptake and utilization.[183] In adipose tissue lipolysis is activated, resulting in the release of free fatty acids into the circulation.[184] An increase in total circulating cholesterol and triglycerides is observed, but HDL cholesterol levels fall. Glucocorticoids also have a permissive effect on other hormones including catecholamines and glucagon. The resultant effect is to cause insulin resistance and an increase in blood glucose concentrations at the expense of protein and lipid catabolism.

Glucocorticoids stimulate adipocyte differentiation, promoting adipogenesis through the transcriptional activation of key differentiation genes including lipoprotein lipase, glycerol-3-phosphate dehydrogenase, and leptin.[185] Chronically, the effects of glucocorticoid excess on adipose tissue are more complex, at least in humans, in whom the deposition of visceral or central adipose tissue is stimulated,[186] providing a useful discriminatory sign for the diagnosis of Cushing's syndrome. The explanation for the predilection for visceral obesity may be related to the increased expression of both the GR[187] and type 1 isozyme of 11β-HSD (generating cortisol from cortisone) in omental compared with subcutaneous adipose tissue.[188]

Skin, Muscle, and Connective Tissue

In addition to inducing insulin resistance in muscle tissue, glucocorticoids cause catabolic changes in muscle, skin, and connective tissue. In the skin and connective tissue, glucocorticoids inhibit epidermal cell division and DNA synthesis and reduce collagen synthesis and production.[189] In muscle, glucocorticoids cause atrophy (but not necrosis), and this seems to be specific for type II or "phasic" muscle fibers. Muscle protein synthesis is reduced.

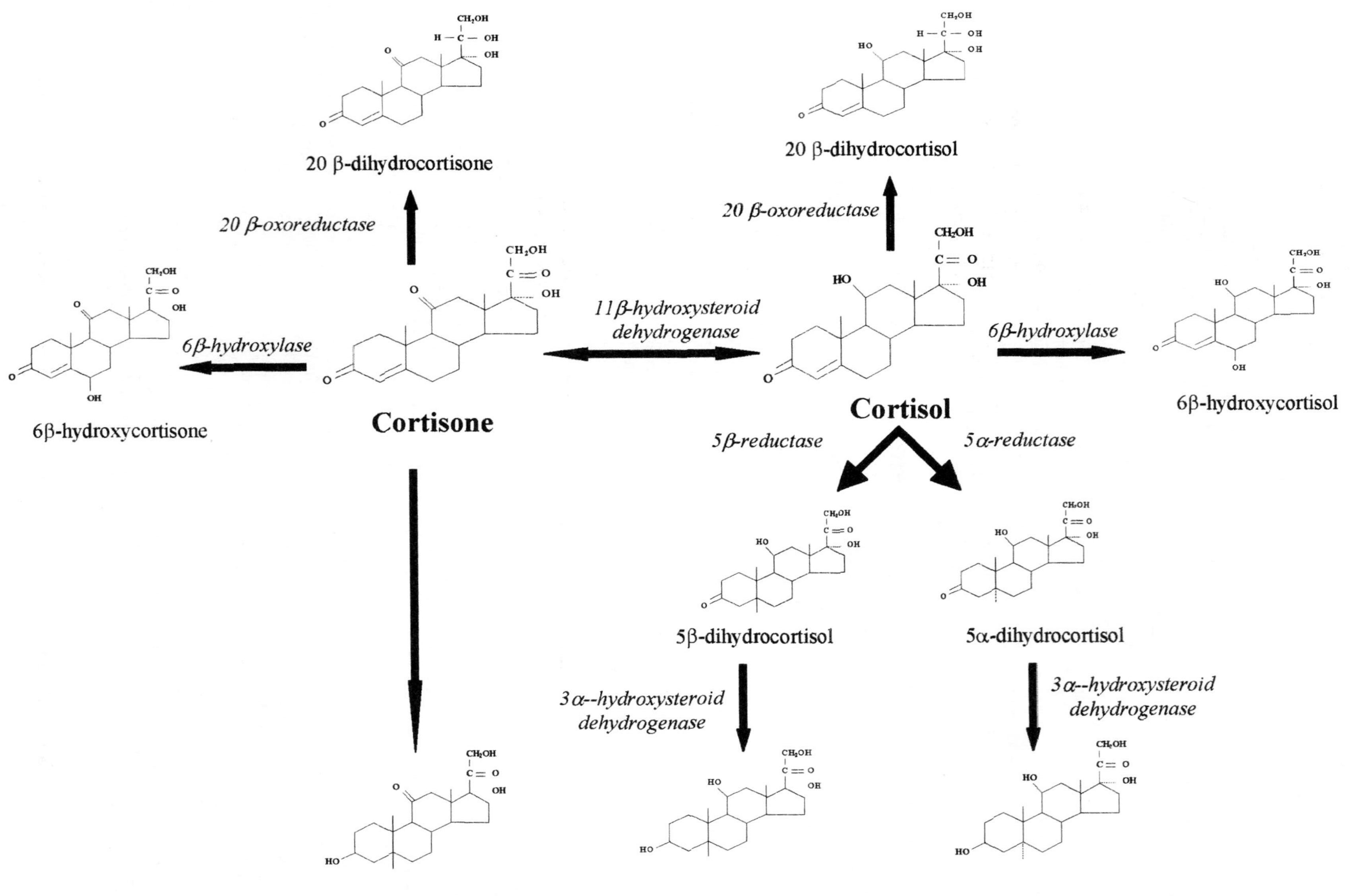

Figure 14–12. The principal pathways of cortisol metabolism. Interconversion of hormonally active cortisol to inactive cortisone is catalyzed by two isozymes of 11β-hydroxysteroid dehydrogenase (11β-HSD), 11β-HSD1 principally converting cortisone to cortisol and 11β-HSD2 the reverse. Cortisol can be hydroxylated at the C6 and C20 positions. A ring reduction is undertaken by 5α-reductase or 5β-reductase and 3α-hydroxysteroid dehydrogenase.

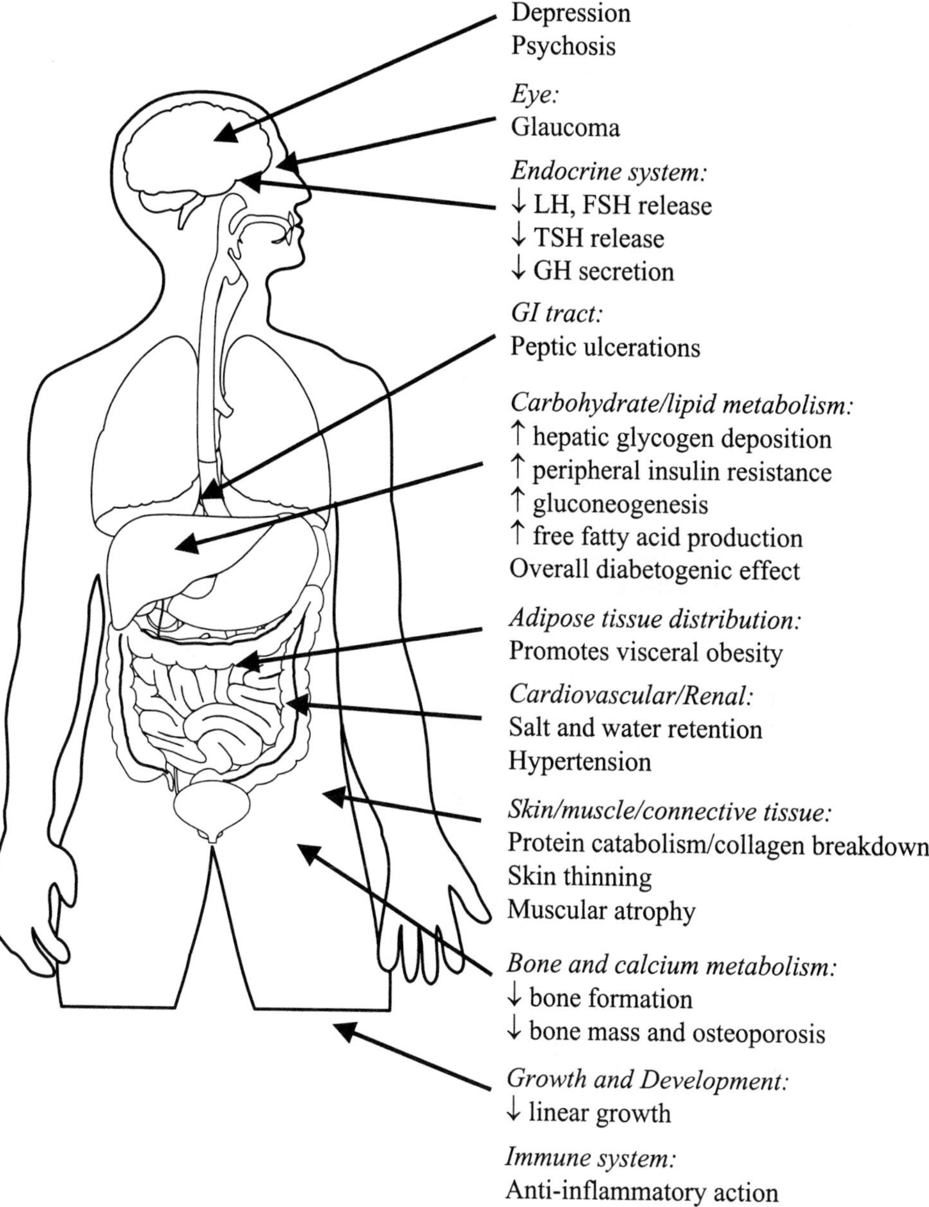

Figure 14–13. The principal sites of action of glucocorticoids in humans highlighting some of the consequences of glucocorticoid excess. CNS, central nervous system; GI, gastrointestinal; FSH, follicle-stimulating hormone; GH, growth hormone; LH, luteinizing hormone; TSH, thyroid-stimulating hormone.

Bone and Calcium Metabolism

The effects of glucocorticoids on osteoclast function are debated, but osteoblast function is inhibited by glucocorticoids, and this is thought to explain the osteopenia and osteoporosis that characterize glucocorticoid excess.[190, 191] With 0.25% to 0.5% of Western populations receiving chronic glucocorticoid therapy,[192] glucocorticoid-induced osteoporosis is becoming a prevalent health concern.[193] Glucocorticoids also induce a negative calcium balance by inhibiting intestinal calcium absorption[194] and increasing renal calcium excretion.[195] As a consequence, parathyroid hormone secretion is usually increased.

Salt and Water Homeostasis and Blood Pressure Control

Glucocorticoids increase blood pressure by a variety of mechanisms involving actions on the kidney and vasculature.[196] In vascular smooth muscle they increase sensitivity to pressor agents such as catecholamines and angiotensin II while reducing nitric oxide–mediated endothelial dilatation.[197, 198] Angiotensinogen synthesis is increased by glucocorticoids.[198, 199] In the kidney, depending on the activity of the type 2 isozyme of 11β-HSD, cortisol can act on the distal nephron to cause sodium retention and potassium loss (mediated by the MR).[164] Elsewhere across the nephron, glucocorticoids increase glomerular filtration rate, proximal tubular epithelial sodium transport, and free water clearance.[200] The last effect involves antagonism of the action of vasopressin and explains the dilutional hyponatremia seen in patients with glucocorticoid deficiency.[201, 202]

Anti-Inflammatory Actions and the Immune System

Glucocorticoids suppress immunologic responses, and this has been the stimulus to develop a series of highly potent pharmacologic glucocorticoids to treat a variety of autoimmune and inflammatory conditions. The inhibitory effects are mediated at many levels. In the peripheral blood, glucocorticoids reduce lymphocyte counts acutely (T lymphocytes > B lymphocytes) by redistributing lymphocytes from the intravascular compartment to spleen, lymph nodes, and bone marrow.[203] Conversely, neutrophil counts increase after glucocorticoid administration. Eosinophil counts fall rapidly, an effect that was used historically as a bioassay for glucocorticoids.

The immunologic actions of glucocorticoids involve direct actions on both T and B lymphocytes that include inhibition of immunoglobulin synthesis and stimulation of lymphocyte apoptosis.[204] Inhibition of cytokine production from lymphocytes is mediated through inhibition of the action of NF-κB. NF-κB plays a crucial and generalized role in inducing cytokine gene transcription; glucocorticoids can bind directly to NF-κB to prevent nuclear translocation and can induce NF-κB inhibitor, which sequesters NF-κB in the cytoplasm, thereby inactivating its effect.[146, 205–207]

Additional anti-inflammatory effects involve inhibition of monocyte differentiation into macrophages and macrophage phagocytosis and cytotoxic activity. Glucocorticoids reduce the local inflammatory response by preventing the action of histamine and plasminogen activators. Prostaglandin synthesis is impaired through the induction of lipocortins, which inhibit phospholipase A_2 activity.[208, 209]

Central Nervous System and Mood

Clinical observations of patients with glucocorticoid excess and deficiency reveal that the brain is an important target tissue for glucocorticoids, with depression, euphoria, psychosis, apathy, and lethargy being important manifestations (see the following). Both glucocorticoid and mineralocorticoid receptors are expressed in discrete regions of the rodent brain including hippocampus, hypothalamus, cerebellum, and cortex.[210] Glucocorticoids cause neuronal death notably in the hippocampus,[211] and this may underlie the interest in glucocorticoids and cognitive function, memory, and neurodegenerative diseases such as Alzheimer's. In the eye, glucocorticoids act to raise intraocular pressure through an increase in aqueous humor production and deposition of matrix within the trabecular meshwork, which inhibits aqueous drainage. Steroid-induced glaucoma appears to have a genetic predisposition, but the underlying mechanisms are unknown.[212, 213]

Gut

Chronic but not acute administration of glucocorticoids increases the risk of developing peptic ulcer disease.[214] Pancreatitis with fat necrosis is reported in patients with glucocorticoid excess. The GR is expressed throughout the gastrointestinal tract and the MR in the distal colon, and these mediate the corticosteroid control of epithelial ion transport.[215]

Growth and Development

Although glucocorticoids stimulate growth hormone (GH) gene transcription in vitro,[216] glucocorticoids in excess inhibit linear skeletal growth,[217, 218] probably as a result of catabolic effects on connective tissue, muscle, and bone and inhibition of the effects of IGF-I. Experiments on mice lacking the GR gene[111] emphasize the role of glucocorticoids in normal fetal development. In particular, glucocorticoids stimulate lung maturation through the synthesis of surfactant proteins (SP-A, SP-B, SP-C),[219, 220] and mice lacking the GR die shortly after birth as a result of hypoxia from lung atelectasis. Glucocorticoids also stimulate the enzyme phenylethanolamine *N*-methyltransferase,[221] which converts norepinephrine to epinephrine in adrenal medulla and chromaffin tissue. Mice lacking the GR do not develop an adrenal medulla.

Endocrine Effects

Glucocorticoids suppress the thyroid axis, probably through a direct action on thyroid-stimulating hormone (TSH) secretion. In addition, they inhibit 5′ deiodinase activity, mediating the conversion of thyroxine to active triiodothyronine. Glucocorticoids also act centrally to inhibit gonadotropin-releasing hormone pulsatility and release of luteinizing hormone (LH) and follicle-stimulating hormone (FSH) (see later).

THERAPEUTIC CORTICOSTEROIDS

Since the dramatic anti-inflammatory effect of cortisone was first demonstrated in the 1950s, a series of synthetic corticosteroids have been developed for therapeutic purposes. These are used to treat a diverse variety of human diseases and rely principally on their anti-inflammatory and immunologic actions (Table 14–6). The main corticosteroids used in clinical practice, together with their relative glucocorticoid and mineralocorticoid potencies, are listed in Table 14–7.

The structures of common synthetic steroids are depicted in Figure 14–14. Biologic activity of a corticosteroid is dependent upon a Δ4-3-keto, 11β-hydroxy, 17α,21-trihydroxyl configuration.[222] Conversion of the C11 hydroxyl group to a C11 keto group (cortisol to cortisone) inactivates the steroid. The addition of a 1,2 unsaturated bond to cortisol results in prednisolone, which is four times more potent than cortisol in classical glucocorticoid bioassays such as hepatic glycogen deposition, suppression of eosinophils, and anti-inflammatory actions. Prednisone is the "cortisone equivalent" of prednisolone and relies upon conversion by 11β-HSD type 1 in the liver for bioactivity.[223] Potency is further increased by the addition of a 6α-methyl group to prednisolone (methylprednisolone). Fludrocortisone is a synthetic mineralocorticoid that has 125-fold greater potency than cortisol in stimulating sodium reabsorption.[224] This is achieved through the addition of a 9α-fluoro group to cortisol. Interestingly, fludrocortisone also has glucocorticoid potency (12-fold greater than cortisol), and the addition of a 16α-methyl group and 1,2 saturated bond to fludrocortisone results in dexamethasone, a highly potent glucocorticoid (25-fold greater than cortisol) but with negligible mineralocorticoid activity.[225] Betamethasone has the same structure but with a 16β-methyl group and is widely used in respiratory and nasal aerosol sprays.

Table 14–6. Therapeutic Use of Corticosteroids

Endocrine: Replacement therapy (Addison's disease, pituitary disease, congenital adrenal hyperplasia), Graves' ophthalmopathy
Skin: Dermatitis, pemphigus
Hematology: Leukemia, lymphoma, hemolytic anemia, idiopathic thrombocytopenic purpura
Gastrointestinal: Inflammatory bowel disease (Ulcerative colitis, Crohn's disease)
Liver: Chronic active hepatitis, transplantation, organ rejection
Renal: Nephrotic syndrome, vasculitides, transplantation, rejection
Central nervous system: Cerebral edema, raised intracranial pressure
Respiratory: Angioedema, anaphylaxis, asthma, sarcoidosis, tuberculosis, obstructive airway disease
Rheumatology: Systemic lupus erythematosus, polyarteritis, temporal arteritis, rheumatoid arthritis
Muscle: polymyalgia rheumatica, myasthenia gravis

Table 14–7. Relative Biologic Potencies of Synthetic Steroids in Bioassay Systems

Steroid	Anti-inflammatory Action	Hypothalamic-Pituitary-Adrenal Suppression	Salt Retention
Cortisol	1	1	1
Prednisolone	3	4	0.75
Methylprednisolone	6.2	4	0.5
Fludrocortisone	12	12	125
Δ^1 Fludrocortisone	14		225
Triamcinolone	5	4	0
Dexamethasone	26	17	0

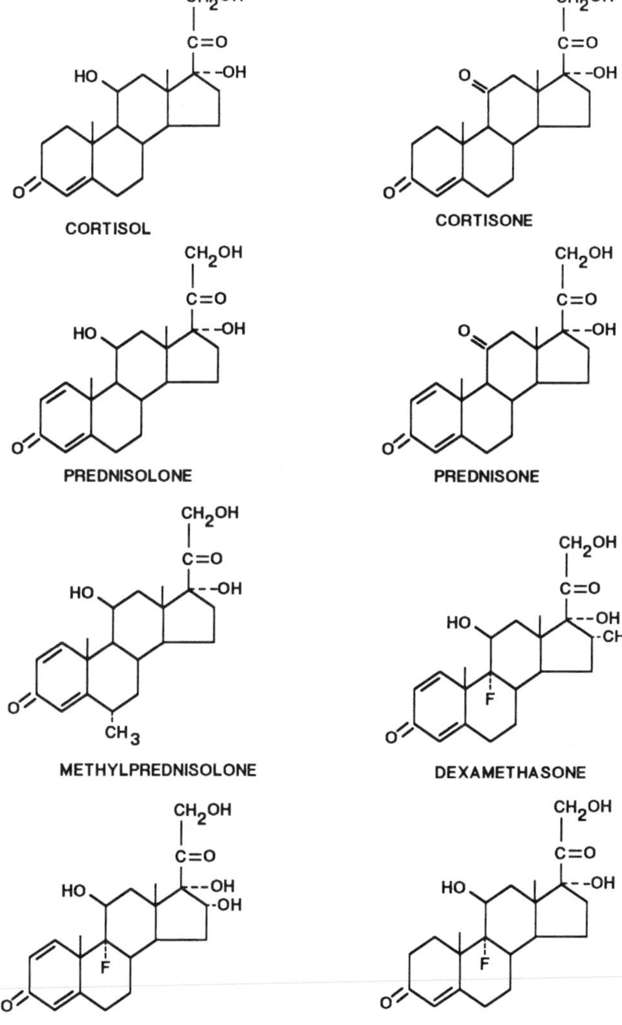

Figure 14–14. Structures of the natural glucocorticoid cortisol, some of the more commonly prescribed synthetic glucocorticoids, and the mineralocorticoid fludrocortisone. Note that triamcinolone is identical to dexamethasone except that a 16α-hydroxyl group is substituted for the 16α-methyl group. Betamethasone, another widely used glucocorticoid, has a 16β-methyl group.

Corticosteroids are given orally, parenterally, and by numerous topical routes (e.g., eyes, skin, nose, inhalation, rectal suppositories).[226] Unlike hydrocortisone, which has a high affinity for CBG, most synthetic steroids have low affinity for this binding protein and circulate as free steroid (~30%) or bound to albumin (~70%). Circulating half-lives vary depending upon individual variability and underlying disease, particularly renal and hepatic impairment. Cortisone acetate should not be used parenterally as it requires metabolism by the liver to active cortisol.

It is beyond the consideration of this chapter to describe which steroid should be given and by which route for the nonendocrine conditions listed in Table 14–6. The acute and chronic administration of corticosteroid therapy in patients with hypoadrenalism and CAH is discussed in these sections. In addition to the undoubted benefit that corticosteroids provide, there is increasingly a misuse of corticosteroid therapy, particularly in patients with respiratory or rheumatologic disease, to such an extent that up to 0.5% of the population is now prescribed chronic corticosteroid therapy. Because of their established euphoric effect, corticosteroids often make patients feel better but without any objective measures of improvements in underlying disease parameters. In view of the long-term sequelae of chronic glucocorticoid excess, decisions regarding treatment should be evidence-based and subject to constant review for efficacy and side effects. The endocrinologic consequences, notably suppression of the HPA axis, are an important aspect of modern clinical practice. Endocrinologists need to be aware of the effects of chronic therapy and advise on steroid withdrawal.

Chronic Corticosteroid Therapy, Hypothalamo-Pituitary-Adrenal Axis Suppression, and Steroid Withdrawal

The negative feedback control of the HPA axis by endogenous cortisol has already been detailed. Synthetic corticosteroids similarly suppress the function of the HPA axis through a process that is dependent on both dose and duration of treatment. As a result, sudden cessation of corticosteroid therapy may result in adrenal failure.[226] This may also occur after treatment with high doses of the synthetic progestagen medroxyprogesterone acetate, which possesses glucocorticoid agonist activity.[227] In patients taking any steroid dose for less than 3 weeks, clinically significant suppression of the HPA axis is rarely a problem and patients can withdraw from steroids suddenly with no ill effect.[228] The possible exception to this is the patient who receives frequent short courses of corticosteroid therapy, for example, patients with recurrent episodes of severe asthma. Conversely, suppression of the HPA axis is invariable in patients taking the equivalent of 15 mg or more of prednis-

Table 14–8. Duration of Glucocorticoid Treatment

Dose (mg pred/day)	≤3 wk*	>3 wk		
≥7.5 mg	Can stop	Reduce rapidly e.g., 2.5 mg every 3–4 days THEN		
5–7.5 mg	Can stop	Reduce by 1 mg every 2–4 wk THEN	OR	Convert 5 mg pred to HC 20 mg and ↓ by 2.5 mg/wk to 10 mg for 2–3 mo ↓ SST/ITT ↙ ↘ Pass: Withdraw Fail: Continue
<5 mg	Can stop	Reduce by 1 mg every 2–4 wk		

*Beware frequent steroid courses, e.g., in asthma.
Pred, prednisolone; SST, short Synacthen test; ITT, insulin tolerance test.

olone per day chronically.[229] In patients taking lower doses of corticosteroid chronically (prednisolone 5 to 15 mg/day or equivalent), suppression of the HPA axis is variable. Defects in response of the HPA axis to insulin-induced hypoglycemia or exogenous ACTH have been reported in patients taking prednisolone doses as low as 5 mg/day,[230] but clinically significant suppression at these doses is debatable.[228] Alternate-day therapy is associated with less suppression of the HPA axis.[231]

All patients treated chronically with corticosteroids should be treated in a similar fashion to patients with chronic ACTH deficiency; they should carry steroid cards and be offered Steroid Alert bracelets or necklaces. In the event of an intercurrent stress (infection, surgery), supplemental steroid cover should be given, equivalent to hydrocortisone at 100 to 150 mg/day. If the patient is unable to take drugs orally, parenteral therapy is required.

Recovery from suppression may take 6 to 9 months. CRH secretion returns to normal, and within a few weeks ACTH levels begin to increase and indeed rise above normal values until adrenal steroidogenesis recovers.[232] In the interim, and without replacement therapy, patients may experience symptoms of glucocorticoid deficiency including anorexia, nausea, weight loss, arthralgia, lethargy, skin desquamation and postural dizziness[233] (see Glucocorticoid Insufficiency). To avoid symptoms of glucocorticoid deficiency, steroids should be withdrawn cautiously over a period of months.[234] Assuming the underlying disease permits steroid reduction, doses should be reduced from pharmacologic levels to physiologic levels (equivalent to prednisolone at 7.5 mg/day) over a few weeks. Thereafter doses should be reduced by 1 mg/day prednisolone every 2 to 4 weeks depending on the patient's well-being. An alternative approach is to change to hydrocortisone at 20 mg/day and reduce the daily dose by 2.5 mg/day every week to 10 mg/day. Doses at nighttime should be avoided as they result in greater suppression of early morning ACTH secretion.

After 2 to 3 months of these reduced doses of corticosteroids, endogenous function of the HPA axis can be assessed through a corticotropin (ACTH, Synacthen) stimulation test or an insulin-induced hypoglycemia test (see later). A pass response to these tests indicates adequacy of function of the HPA axis, and corticosteroid therapy can be safely withdrawn. In patients taking physiologic doses of prednisolone (less than 5 to 7.5 mg/day) or equivalent, a corticotropin stimulation test 12 to 24 hours after having omitted steroid therapy will provide an immediate answer on whether sudden or gradual withdrawal of steroid therapy is indicated (Table 14–8).

Iatrogenically induced Cushing's syndrome occurs in patients taking suppressive doses of corticosteroids for more than 3 weeks.[226, 235] The rapidity of onset of clinical features is dependent upon the administered dose but can occur within 1 month of therapy.

Table 14–9. Adrenocortical Diseases

Glucocorticoid Excess
Cushing's syndrome
Pseudo-Cushing's syndromes

Glucocorticoid Resistance

Glucocorticoid Deficiency
Primary hypoadrenalism
Secondary hypoadrenalism
Post-chronic corticosteroid replacement therapy

Congenital Adrenal Hyperplasia
21-Hydroxylase, 3β-hydroxysteroid dehydrogenase, 17α-hydroxylase, 11β-hydroxylase, and StAR deficiencies

Mineralocorticoid Excess

Mineralocorticoid Deficiency
Defects in aldosterone synthesis
Defects in aldosterone action
Hyporeninemic hypoaldosteronism

Adrenal Incidentalomas, Adenomas, and Carcinomas

StAR, steroidogenic acute regulatory (protein).

ADRENOCORTICAL DISEASES

Adrenocortical diseases are relatively rare, but their importance lies in their morbidity and mortality if untreated coupled with the relative ease of diagnosis and the availability of effective therapy. The diseases are most readily classified on the basis of whether there is hormone excess or deficiency (Table 14–9).

Glucocorticoid Excess

In 1912 Harvey Cushing first described a 23-year-old woman with obesity, hirsutism, and amenorrhea and 20 years later postulated that this "polyglandular syndrome" was due to a primary pituitary abnormality causing adrenal hyperplasia.[9] Adrenal tumors were shown to cause the syndrome in some cases,[236] but ectopic ACTH production was not characterized until much later in 1962.[237] The term *Cushing's syndrome* is used to describe all causes, and *Cushing's disease* is reserved for cases of pituitary-dependent Cushing's syndrome.

Cushing's syndrome comprises the symptoms and signs associated with prolonged exposure to inappropriately elevated levels of free plasma glucocorticoids (Fig. 14–15). The use of the term glucocorticoid in the definition covers both endogenous (cortisol) and exogenous (e.g., prednisolone, dexamethasone) excess (Table 14–10). Iatrogenic Cushing's syndrome is common,[226, 235] occurring to some degree in the majority of patients taking chronic corticosteroid therapy. Endogenous causes of Cushing's syndrome result in loss of the normal feedback mechanism of the HPA axis and the normal circadian rhythm of cortisol secretion and are rare.

The incidence of pituitary-dependent Cushing's syndrome is estimated to be 5 to 10 cases per million population per year. The incidence of ectopic ACTH syndrome parallels that of bronchogenic carcinoma, and although 0.5% of lung cancer patients have ectopic ACTH syndrome,[238] the rapid progression of the underlying disease often precludes an early diagnosis. Cushing's disease and adrenal adenomas are four times commoner in women, and ectopic ACTH syndrome is commoner in men.

Table 14–10. Classification of Causes of Cushing's Syndrome

ACTH-Dependent
Cushing's disease (pituitary-dependent)
Ectopic ACTH syndrome
Ectopic CRH syndrome
Macronodular adrenal hyperplasia
Iatrogenic (treatment with ACTH 1–24)
ACTH-Independent
Adrenal adenoma and carcinoma
Primary pigmented nodular adrenal hyperplasia and Carney's syndrome.
McCune-Albright syndrome
Aberrant receptor expression (gastric inhibitory polypeptide, interleukin-1β).
Iatrogenic (e.g., pharmacologic doses of prednisolone, dexamethasone)
Pseudo-Cushing's Syndromes
Alcoholism
Depression
Obesity

ACTH, adrenocorticotrophic hormone; CRH, corticotropin-releasing hormone.

Clinical Features of Cushing's Syndrome

The classical features of Cushing's syndrome with centripetal obesity, moon face, hirsutism, and plethora are well known following Cushing's initial descriptions in 1912 and 1932 (Figs. 14–15 and 14–16). However, this gross clinical picture is not always present and a high index of suspicion is required in many cases. When the normal physiologic effects of glucocorticoids are appreciated (see Fig. 14–13), the clinical features of glucocorticoid excess are easier to define. These are summarized in Table 14–11 together with the most discriminatory features that assist in distinguishing Cushing's syndrome from simple obesity.[239]

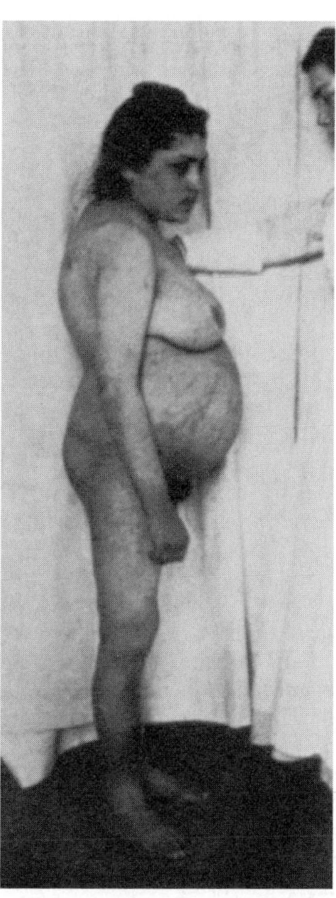

Figure 14–15. Minnie G., Cushing's index patient, at age 23 years. (From Cushing H. The basophil adenomas of the pituitary body and their clinical manifestations [pituitary basophilism]. Bull Johns Hopkins Hosp 1932; 50:137–195.)

Obesity

Weight gain and obesity are the commonest sign, and at least in adults this is invariably centripetal in nature.[186, 240] Indeed, generalized obesity is commoner in the general population than in patients with Cushing's syndrome. One exception to this is childhood, in which glucocorticoid excess may result in generalized obesity. In addition to centripetal obesity, patients develop fat depots over the thoracocervical spine ("buffalo hump"), in the supraclavicular region, and over the cheeks and temporal regions, giving rise to the rounded "moon-like" facies. The epidural space is another site of abnormal fat deposition, and this may lead to neurologic deficits.

Reproductive Dysfunction

Gonadal dysfunction is common, with menstrual irregularity in females and loss of libido in both sexes.[241–243] Hirsutism is frequently found in female patients, as is acne. The commonest form of hirsutism is vellous hypertrichosis on the face and should be distinguished from darker terminal differentiated hirsutism, which may occur but usually signifies concomitant androgen excess (as may occur secondary to ACTH-mediated adrenal androgen secretion). Hypogonadism occurs because of a direct inhibitory effect of cortisol upon gonadotropin-releasing hormone pulsatility and LH or FSH secretion and is reversible upon correction of the hypercortisolism.

Psychiatric Abnormalities

Psychiatric abnormalities occur in approximately 50% of patients with Cushing's syndrome regardless of cause.[244–246] Agitated depression and lethargy are among the commonest problems,[247] but paranoia and overt psychosis are also well

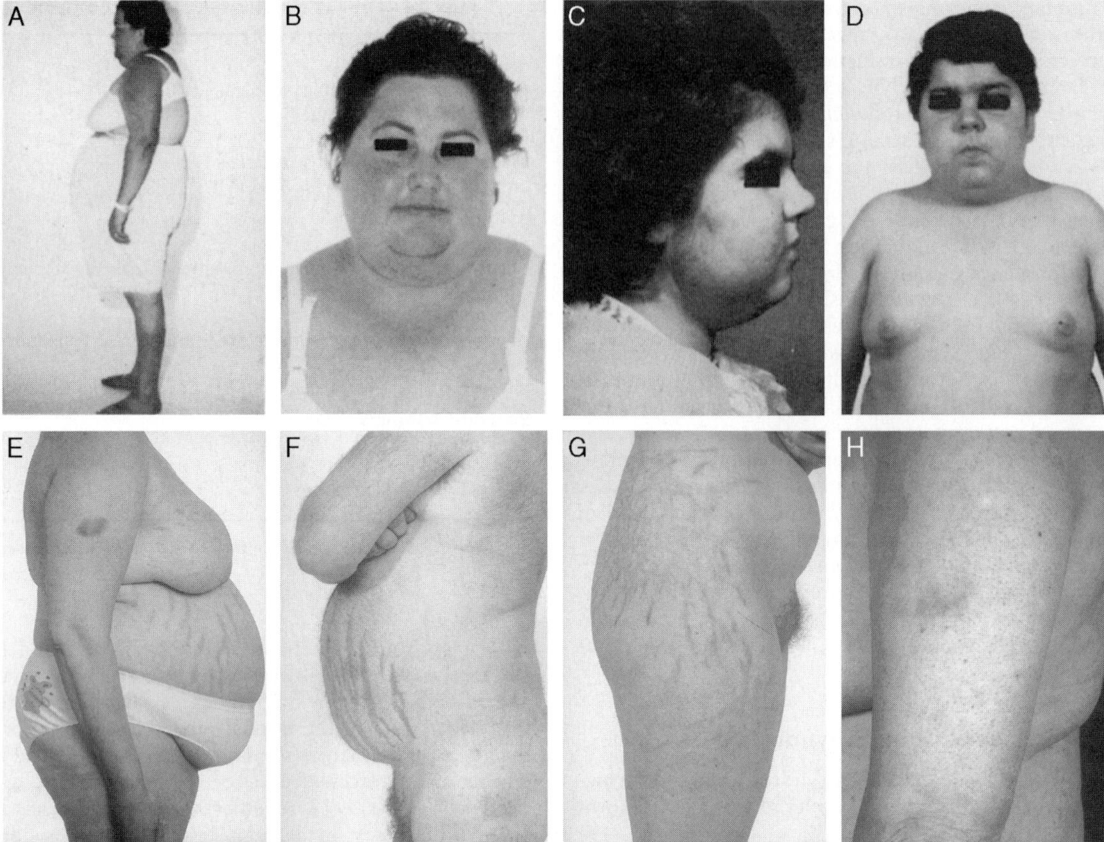

Figure 14–16. Clinical features of Cushing's syndrome (see also Color Plate). *A*, Centripetal and some generalized obesity and dorsal kyphosis in a 30-year-old woman with Cushing's disease. *B*, Same woman as in *A*, showing moon facies, plethora, hirsutism, and enlarged supraclavicular fat pads. *C*, Facial rounding, hirsutism, and acne in a 14-year-old girl with Cushing's disease. *D*, Central and generalized obesity and moon facies in a 14-year-old boy with Cushing's disease. *E* and *F*, Typical centripetal obesity with livid abdominal striae seen in a 41-year-old woman *(E)* and a 40-year-old man *(F)* with Cushing's syndrome. *G*, Striae in a 24-year-old patient with congenital adrenal hyperplasia treated with excessive doses of dexamethasone as "replacement" therapy. *H*, Typical bruising and thin skin of Cushing's syndrome. In this case, the bruising has occurred without obvious injury.

recognized. Memory and cognitive function may also be affected, and increased irritability may be an early feature. Insomnia is common, and both rapid eye movement and delta wave sleep patterns are reduced.[248, 249] Lowering of plasma cortisol by medical or surgical therapy usually results in a rapid improvement in the psychiatric state.[245, 246]

Bone

In childhood the commonest presentation is with poor linear growth and weight gain; as discussed earlier, glucocorticoids have profound effects on growth and development.[218] Many patients with long-standing Cushing's syndrome have lost height because of osteoporotic vertebral collapse. This can be assessed by measuring the patient's height and comparing it with the patient's span; in normal subjects these measurements should be equal. Pathologic fractures, either spontaneous or after minor trauma, are not uncommon. Rib fractures, in contrast to those of the vertebrae, are often painless. The radiographic appearances are typical, with exuberant callus formation at the site of the healing fracture. In addition, aseptic necrosis of the femoral and humeral heads, a recognized feature of high-dose exogenous corticosteroid therapy, can occur in endogenous Cushing's syndrome (Fig. 14–17). Hypercalciuria may lead to renal calculi, but hypercalcemia is not a feature.

Skin

Hypercortisolism results in skin thinning, separation, and exposure of the subcutaneous vascular tissue. On examination, wrinkling of the skin on the dorsum of the hand may be seen resulting in a "cigarette paper" appearance (Liddle's sign). Minimal trauma may result in bruising, which frequently resembles the appearance of "senile purpura." The plethoric appearance of the patient with Cushing's syndrome is secondary to the thinning of the skin[250] combined with loss of facial subcutaneous fat and is not due to true polycythemia. Acne and papular lesions may occur over the face, chest, and back.

The typical, almost pathognomonic red-purple livid striae greater than 1 cm in diameter are most frequently found on the abdomen but may also be present on the upper thighs, breasts, and arms. They are common in younger patients and less so in those older than 50 years.[251] They must be differentiated from the paler, less pigmented striae that occur post partum (striae gravidarum) or in association with rapid weight loss.

Increased skin pigmentation is rare in Cushing's disease but common in the ectopic ACTH syndrome and arises because of overstimulation of melanocyte receptors by ACTH.

Muscle

Myopathy and bruising are two of the most discriminatory features of the syndrome.[239] The myopathy of Cushing's syn-

Table 14–11. Prevalence of Symptoms and Signs in Cushing's Syndrome and Discriminant Index Compared with Prevalence of Features in Patients with Simple Obesity

Findings	%	Discriminant Index
Symptoms		
Weight gain	91	
Menstrual irregularity	84	1.6
Hirsutism	81	2.8
Psychiatric dysfunction	62	
Backache	43	
Muscle weakness	29	8.0
Fractures	19	
Loss of scalp hair	13	
Signs		
Obesity	97	
Truncal	46	1.6
Generalized	55	0.8
Plethora	94	3.0
Moon face	88	
Hypertension	74	4.4
Bruising	62	10.3
Red-purple striae	56	2.5
Muscle weakness	56	
Ankle edema	50	
Pigmentation	4	
Other findings		
Hypertension	74	
Diabetes	50	
Overt	13	
Impaired glucose tolerance test	37	
Osteoporosis	50	
Renal calculi	15	

Data from Ross EJ, Linch DC. Cushing's syndrome–killing disease: discriminatory value of signs and symptoms aiding early diagnosis. Lancet 1982; 2:646–649.

drome involves the proximal muscles of the lower limb and the shoulder girdle.[240, 252] Complaints of weakness such as inability to climb stairs or get up from a deep chair are relatively uncommon, but testing for proximal myopathy by asking the patient to rise from a crouching position often reveals the problem.

Cardiovascular

Hypertension is another prominent feature, occurring in up to 75% of cases; even though epidemiologic data show a strong association between blood pressure and obesity, hypertension is much more common in patients with Cushing's syndrome than in those with simple obesity.[198] This, together with the established metabolic consequences of the disease (diabetes, hyperlipidemia; see the following), is thought to explain the increased cardiovascular mortality in untreated cases. In addition, thromboembolic events may be commoner in Cushing's patients.

Infections

Infections are more common in patients with Cushing's syndrome.[253, 254] In many instances these are asymptomatic and occur because the normal inflammatory response is suppressed. Reactivation of tuberculosis has been reported[255] and has even been the presenting feature in some cases. Fungal infections of the skin (notably tinea versicolor) and nails may occur, as may opportunistic fungal infections. Bowel perforation is commoner in patients with extreme hypercortisolism, and the hypercortisolism may mask the usual symptoms and signs of the condition. Wound infections are commoner and contribute to poor wound healing.

Metabolic and Endocrine

Glucose intolerance occurs, and overt diabetes mellitus is present in up to one third of patients in some series. Hepatic lipoprotein synthesis is stimulated, and increases in circulating cholesterol and triglycerides may be found.[256] Hypokalemic alkalosis is found in 10% to 15% of patients with Cushing's disease but over 95% of patients with ectopic ACTH syndrome.[257] Severe factors may contribute to this mineralocorticoid excess state, including corticosterone and DOC excess, but the principal culprit is thought to be cortisol itself. Depending on the prevailing cortisol production rate, cortisol swamps the normal metabolizing enzyme, 11β-HSD type 2 in the kidney, to act as a mineralocorticoid. Hypokalemic alkalosis is commoner in ectopic ACTH syndrome because cortisol production rates are higher than in patients with Cushing's disease.[258, 259] This can be diagnosed by documenting an increase in the ratio of urinary cortisol to cortisone metabolites. In addition, hepatic 5α-reductase activity is inhibited, resulting in greater excretion of 5β-cortisol metabolites.[259]

The function of both the pituitary-thyroid axis and the pituitary-gonadal axis is suppressed in patients with Cushing's syndrome because of a direct effect of cortisol on TSH and gonadotrophin secretion.[260, 261] Cortisol causes a reversible form of hypogonadotropic hypogonadism but also directly inhibits Leydig cell function. GH secretion is reduced, possibly mediated through an increase in somatostatinergic tone.

Eye

Ocular effects include raised intraocular pressure[262] and exophthalmos[263] (in up to one third of patients in Cushing's original series), the latter occurring because of increased retro-orbital fat deposition. Cataracts, a well-recognized complication of corticosteroid therapy, seem to be uncommon[264] except as a complication of diabetes. In the author's experience chemosis is a sensitive and underreported feature of Cushing's syndrome.

Classification and Pathophysiology of Cushing's Syndrome

The condition is most readily classified into ACTH-dependent and ACTH-independent causes (see Table 14–10).

Adrenocorticotropic Hormone–Dependent Causes

Cushing's Disease

When iatrogenic causes are excluded, the commonest cause of Cushing's syndrome is Cushing's disease, accounting for approximately 70% of cases. The adrenal glands in these patients show bilateral adrenocortical hyperplasia with widening of the zona fasciculata and zona reticularis.

Etiology. Cushing himself raised the question of whether this disease was a primary pituitary condition or secondary to an abnormality in the hypothalamus, and there has been an ongoing debate on this issue ever since.[265] The hypothalamic theory states that ACTH-secreting adenomas arise because of dysfunctional regulation of corticotrophs through chronic stimulation by CRH (or AVP), but other studies provide data to support a primary pituitary defect as the cause of the condition (Table 14–12).[266–275]

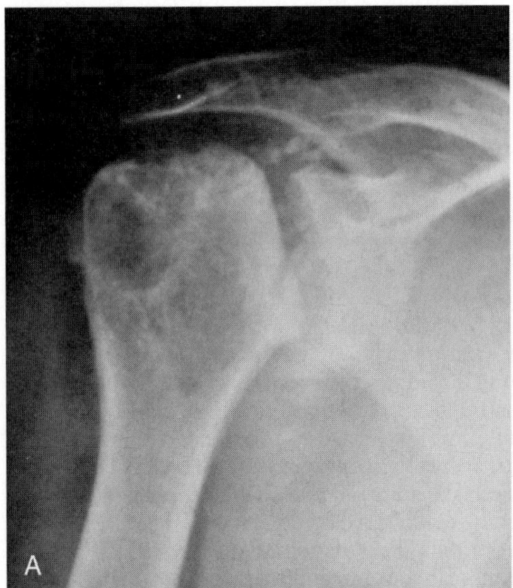

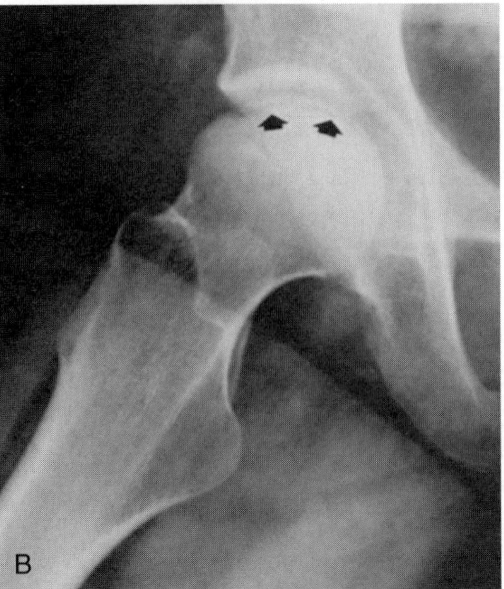

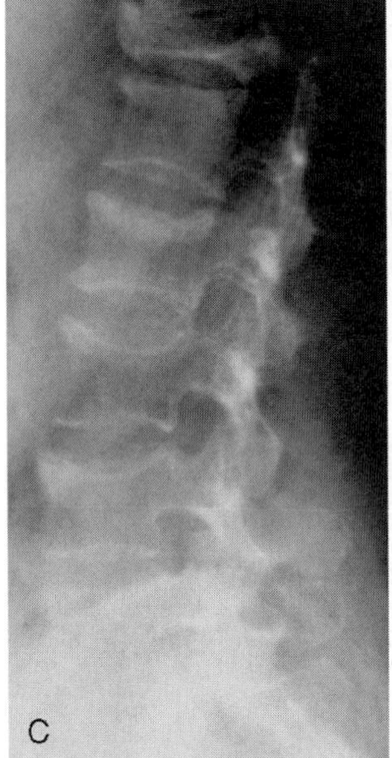

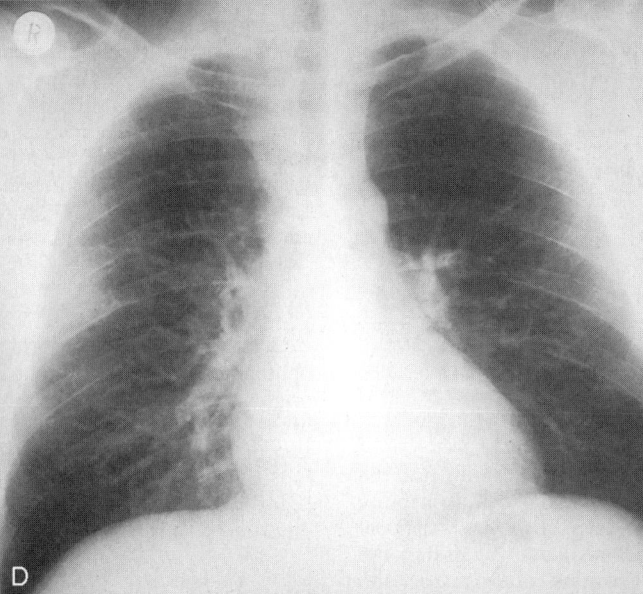

Figure 14–17. Bone abnormalities in Cushing's disease. *A*, Aseptic necrosis of the right humeral head of a 43-year-old woman with Cushing's disease of about 8 months' duration. *B*, Aseptic necrosis of the right femoral head in a 24-year-old woman with Cushing's disease of about 4½ years' duration. The *arrows* indicate the crescent subchondral radiolucency, best seen in this lateral view. *C*, Diffuse osteoporosis, vertebral collapse, and subchondral sclerosis in the patient whose shoulder is shown in *A*. *D*, Rib fracture in a 38-year man with Cushing's disease. (*A–C* from Phillips KA, Nance EP Jr, Rodriguez RM, et al. Avascular necrosis of bone: a manifestation of Cushing's disease. Reprinted by permission from the Southern Medical Journal 1986; 79:825–829.)

Table 14–12. Hypothalamic versus Pituitary Theory Underpinning the Etiology of Cushing's Disease

Hypothalamic Theory	Pituitary Theory
Neuroendocrine abnormalities[266,267] Loss of circadian rhythm, sleep disturbance, other "hypothalamic defects" (TSH, LH-FSH secretion)	Lack of "cure" after pituitary stalk section Circulating and CSF CRH levels are suppressed[268] Reversal of "hypothalamic defects" upon correction of hypercortisolism
Efficacy of centrally acting drugs[269,270] Bromocriptine, cyprohepatadine, sodium valproate	
Recurrences after pituitary surgery	High surgical cure rate (recurrences resulting from regrowth of initial inadequately resected tumor rather than "real" recurrence)[271,272] Secondary hypoadrenalism after successful pituitary surgery (may be prolonged and associated with reduced ACTH expression in surrounding adjacent normal corticotrophs)[273]
Ectopic CRH-secreting tumors cause Cushing's disease,[265] but pathology shows basophil hyperplasia, not adenomas	Pituitary ACTH-secreting adenoma in almost 90% of cases are monoclonal in origin[274,275]

ACTH, adrenocorticotropic hormone; CRH, corticotropin-releasing hormone; CSF, cerebrospinal fluid; FSH, follicle-stimulating hormone; LH, luteinizing hormone; TSH, thyroid-stimulating hormone.

The hypothalamus may have an initiating role, but the overwhelming evidence is that, at presentation, the condition is pituitary-dependent. In 85% to 90% of cases the disease is due to a pituitary adenoma of monoclonal origin[274, 275]; basophil hyperplasia alone is found in 9% to 33% of pathologic series.[265] The majority of tumors are small microadenomas, but larger macroadenomas occur in up to 10% of cases and usually signify a more invasive tumor.[276] Selective surgical removal of a microadenoma results in cure with a low recurrence rate. However, it is possible, particularly in cases with no identifiable pituitary adenoma, that Cushing's disease may be heterogeneous with different subtypes.[277, 278]

A key biochemical hallmark of the disease is a relative resistance of ACTH secretion to normal glucocorticoid feedback inhibition.[279] ACTH-secreting pituitary adenomas function at a higher than normal set-point for cortisol feedback. In Cushing's disease the predominant finding is an increase in ACTH pulse amplitude with loss of normal circadian rhythm, but ACTH pulse frequency is also increased in some cases (see Fig. 14–7).[280, 281]

Ectopic Adrenocorticotropic Hormone Syndrome

In 15% of cases, Cushing's syndrome may be associated with nonpituitary tumors secreting ACTH—the ectopic ACTH syndrome.[238, 282–285] On clinical grounds, this condition can be divided into two entities, cases occurring in the setting of highly malignant tumors such as small cell carcinoma of bronchus (Table 14–13) and more indolent cases occurring in patients with underlying neuroendocrine tumors such as bronchial carcinoids. In the former case, the clinical presentation more commonly resembles Addison's disease than Cushing's syndrome. Circulating ACTH concentrations and cortisol secretion rates can be extremely high. As a result, the duration of symptoms from onset to presentation is short (<3 months); patients are commonly pigmented, and the metabolic manifestations of glucocorticoid excess are often rapid and progressive. Weight loss, myopathy, and glucose intolerance are prominent symptoms and signs. The association of these features with hypokalemic alkalosis and peripheral edema should alert the clinician to the diagnosis.

Depending on local referral practice, approximately 20% of cases of ectopic ACTH syndrome are explained by indolent tumors, such as benign bronchial carcinoids that produce ACTH.[286, 287] In these cases, symptoms and signs are commonly present for 18 months from onset to clinical presentation. Such patients present with the typical features of Cushing's syndrome and may be biochemically similar to patients with Cushing's disease. Thus, once a diagnosis of Cushing's syndrome is established, the principal diagnostic dilemma is in the distinction of pituitary-dependent Cushing's from these indolent causes of ectopic ACTH syndrome.[283]

Table 14–13. Tumors Associated with the Ectopic Adrenocorticotropic Hormone Syndrome

Tumor Type	Approximate Incidence (%)
Small cell lung carcinoma	50
Non–small cell lung carcinoma	5
Pancreatic tumors (including carcinoids)	10
Thymic tumors (including carcinoids)	5
Lung carcinoids	10
Other carcinoids	2
Medullary carcinoma of thyroid	5
Pheochromocytoma and related tumors	3
Rare carcinomata of prostate, breast, ovary, gallbladder, colon	10

Etiology. POMC is expressed in some normal extrapituitary tissues and many tumors (lung, testis) irrespective of the presence of Cushing's syndrome, raising the appropriateness of the term "ectopic" ACTH syndrome.[288] Tumors most commonly associated with ectopic ACTH syndrome arise from neuroendocrine tissues, the cells of which have the ability to take up and decarboxylate amine precursors (APUD cells). However, in the case of small cell lung cancer, only 0.5% to 1% of tumors are associated with ectopic ACTH syndrome and the explanation for the development of ectopic ACTH secretion remains unclear.[289, 290] POMC mRNA transcripts are usually shorter in tumors not associated with ectopic ACTH syndrome, whereas those with the syndrome express larger POMC mRNA species in addition to the "pituitary" size transcript. In addition to aberrant transcriptional regulation of the POMC gene, interaction with tissue-specific transcription factors or methylation status of the POMC gene may be involved (see earlier). Once secreted, POMC is cleaved in the pituitary by specific serine endoproteases to produce ACTH precursors; in ectopic ACTH syndrome, aberrant peripheral processing of POMC may lead to increased circulating ACTH precursor concentrations (pro-ACTH, amino-terminal POMC [N-POMC]). In contrast to ACTH-secreting pituitary adenomas, ectopic POMC or ACTH production is not responsive to normal glucocorticoid feedback[291] because of a defective GR or GR signaling mechanism.[292–294] However, this sensitivity to glucocorticoid feedback is far from clear-cut, which is one reason why the differential diagnosis of ACTH-dependent Cushing's syndrome can be challenging.[283]

Ectopic Corticotropin-Releasing Hormone Production

This is a rare cause of pituitary-dependent Cushing's syndrome. A number of cases have now been described in which a tumor (usually bronchial carcinoid, medullary thyroid, or prostate carcinoma) has been shown to contain CRH but not ACTH.[295–303] Where available, pituitary histology reveals corticotroph hyperplasia but not adenoma formation. Biochemically, these patients usually are similar to patients with ectopic ACTH syndrome with loss of the normal negative glucocorticoid feedback mechanism; 50% are resistant to high-dose dexamethasone therapy. It has been suggested that ectopic CRH production may explain the suppression of cortisol secretion after high-dose dexamethasone found in some patients with the ectopic ACTH syndrome.

Macronodular Adrenal Hyperplasia

In 10% to 40% of patients with Cushing's disease, there is bilateral adrenocortical hyperplasia associated with one or more nodules that may be up to several centimeters in diameter.[304, 305] Patients tend to be older and have had symptoms for a longer time but otherwise present with the classical clinical features of Cushing's syndrome. Pathologically, the nodules are lobulated and can be markedly enlarged, but internodular hyperplasia is invariably found. Macronodular adrenal hyperplasia is thought to result from long-standing adrenal ACTH stimulation that leads to autonomous adrenal adenoma formation. Thus, as the adrenals in a patient with Cushing's disease become more hyperplastic, they secrete more cortisol for a given ACTH level and this may ultimately lead to autosuppression. Individual clinical cases support this hypothesis, and macronodular adrenal hyperplasia should be regarded as an ACTH-dependent form of Cushing's syndrome, even though ACTH levels may be relatively low and dexamethasone suppressibility less marked than in other cases of Cushing's disease.[306–308] The adenomas can be a trap for the unwary as they may be mistaken for primary adrenal tumors.

Adrenocorticotropic Hormone–Independent Causes

Cortisol-Secreting Adrenal Adenoma and Carcinoma

With the exclusion of iatrogenic Cushing's syndrome, adrenal adenomas are responsible for about 10% to 15% of cases and carcinomas for less than 5%. By contrast, in children 65% of cases of Cushing's syndrome have an adrenal etiology (15% adenomas, 50% carcinoma).[309–312] Onset of clinical features is gradual in patients with adenomas but often rapid in adrenal carcinoma. In addition to the features of hypercortisolism, patients may complain of loin or abdominal pain and a tumor may be palpable. The tumor may secrete other steroids, such as androgens or mineralocorticoids. Thus, in females, there may be features of virilization, with hirsutism, clitorimegaly, breast atrophy, deepening of the voice, temporal recession, and severe acne. With "pure" cortisol-secreting adenomas, hirsutism is uncommon. Subclinical Cushing's syndrome has been reported in patients with adrenal "incidentalomas" (see later).

Primary Pigmented Nodular Adrenal Hyperplasia and Carney Complex

About 100 cases of ACTH-independent Cushing's syndrome have been reported in association with bilateral, small pigmented adrenal nodules. Pathologically, these nodules are usually 2 to 4 mm in diameter (but can be larger) and black or brown on cut section. Adjacent adrenal tissue is atrophic, distinguishing this condition from macronodular adrenal hyperplasia. Presentation is with typical features of Cushing's syndrome but is always before 30 years of age and before 15 years of age in 50% of cases.[313–315] Cases of primary pigmented nodular adrenocortical disease (PPNAD) have been reported without Cushing's syndrome. Bilateral adrenalectomy is curative.

In 20% of cases, there is a family history, and it is known that PPNAD forms part of the familial autosomal dominant condition called Carney complex (Table 14–14). This comprises mesenchymal tumors (especially atrial myxomas), spotty skin pigmentation, peripheral nerve tumors, and various tumors including breast lesions and testicular and GH-secreting pituitary tumors.[316, 317] Genetic linkage studies in affected kindreds have mapped the disease to two separate loci on chromosomes 2p16 (some distance from the POMC gene) and 17q24.[318, 319] Recent reports have identified mutations in a gene encoding the R1-alpha regulatory subunit of cAMP-dependent protein kinase A (PRKAR1-alpha) in affected cases.[320, 321]

Table 14–14. Clinical Features of the Carney Complex

Feature	Prevalence (%)
Skin lesions	80
Pigmented lesions	
Blue nevi	
Cutaneous myxomas	
Cardiac myxomas	72
Pigmented nodular adrenal hyperplasia	45
Breast lesions	
Bilateral fibroadenomas	45 (females only)
Testicular tumors	56 (males only)
Pituitary lesions, usually growth hormone–secreting	10
Neural lesions (gastric schwannomas)	<5
Miscellaneous	
Thyroid cancer	Rare
Acoustic neuromas	Rare
Hepatoma	Rare

McCune-Albright Syndrome

In this condition, fibrous dysplasia and cutaneous pigmentation may be associated with pituitary, thyroid, adrenal, and gonadal hyperfunction. The commonest manifestation is with sexual precocity and GH excess, but Cushing's syndrome has been reported.[322] The underlying abnormality is a somatic mutation in the α subunit of the stimulatory G protein that is linked to adenyl cyclase.[323] The mutation results in the G protein being constitutively activated, mimicking constant ACTH stimulation at the level of the adrenal. ACTH levels are suppressed, and adrenal adenomas may occur.

Macronodular Hyperplasia and Aberrant Receptor Expression

Although macronodular hyperplasia commonly occurs in patients with ACTH-dependent Cushing's syndrome (see earlier), truly ACTH-independent macronodular disease is also recognized as a distinct entity.[324, 325] The nodules are nonpigmented and over 5 mm in diameter; occasionally the adrenals may be massively enlarged. The pathogenesis is unknown in many cases, but in one kindred activating mutations of the ACTH–G protein–coupled receptor may have caused the phenotype.[326] It is likely that many cases may be explained on the basis of aberrant receptor expression within the adrenal cortex. Patients have been described with macronodular hyperplasia, ACTH-independent Cushing's syndrome, and enhanced adrenal responsiveness to gastric inhibitory polypeptide (GIP).[327, 328] Biochemically, plasma cortisol levels are subnormal in the morning and rise after food because of the normal increase in GIP after eating. The adrenocortical tissue of these patients responded in vitro to low doses of GIP, whereas there was no such effect in normal adrenal cortex, suggesting that adrenal GIP receptors are linked to steroidogenesis in these patients.[329] It remains to be seen whether abnormalities of adrenal sensitivity to GIP play a subtle role in other types of Cushing's syndrome. Similarly, Cushing's syndrome related to a cortisol-secreting adrenal adenoma has been attributed to aberrant expression of receptors for interleukin-1.[330]

Iatrogenic Cushing's Syndrome

The basis for this condition is discussed under "Therapeutic Corticosteroids." Development of the features of Cushing's syndrome depends on the dose, duration, and potency of corticosteroid used in clinical practice. ACTH is rarely prescribed but chronically also results in cushingoid features. Some features such as increased intraocular pressure, cataracts, benign intracranial hypertension, aseptic necrosis of the femoral head, osteoporosis, and pancreatitis are commoner in iatrogenic compared with endogenous Cushing's syndrome, whereas other features, notably hypertension, hirsutism, and oligomenorrhea or amenorrhea, are rarer.

Special Features of Cushing's Syndrome

Cyclic Cushing's Syndrome

Of particular clinical interest has been a group of patients with cyclic Cushing's syndrome, characterized by periods of excess cortisol production interspersed with intervals of normal cortisol production (Fig. 14–18). Some of these patients demonstrate a paradoxical rise in plasma ACTH and cortisol when treated with dexamethasone, and occasional patients show benefit with dopamine agonist (bromocriptine) or serotonin antagonist (cyproheptadine) therapy. The majority of cases have been thought to have pituitary-dependent disease, and in many of these patients basophil adenomas have been removed, some with long-term cure.[331, 332] However, cortisol secretion may show some evidence of cyclicity in patients with an ectopic source of ACTH syndrome.[333, 334]

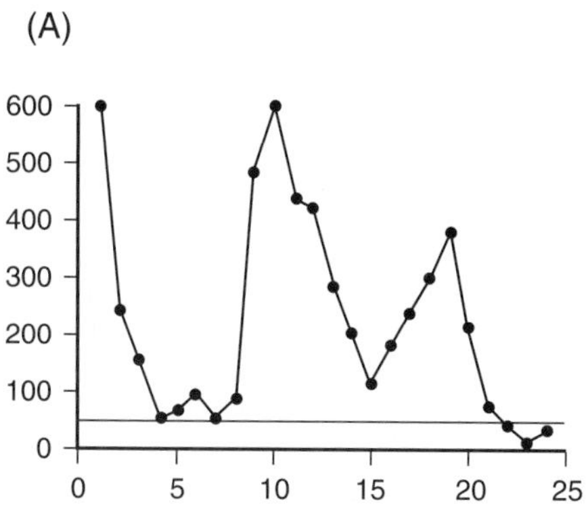

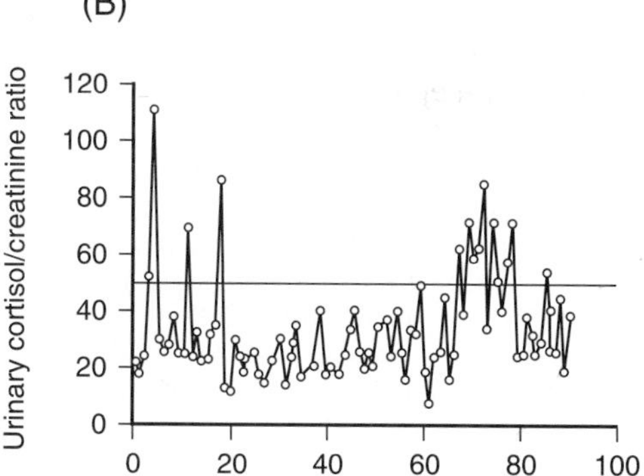

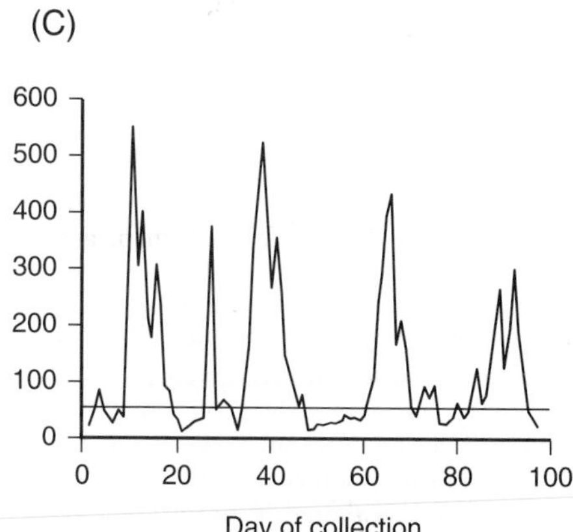

Figure 14–18. Patterns of cortisol secretion in three patients with cyclical Cushing's syndrome. In each case, ratios of early morning urinary cortisol (nmol/L) to creatinine (mmol/L) are plotted against time. Variable periodicity in cortisol hypersecretion is shown. (From Atkinson AB, McCance DR, Kennedy L, et al. Cyclical Cushing's syndrome first diagnosed after pituitary surgery: a trap for the unwary. Clin Endocrinol 1992; 36:297–299.)

Children

In children, in addition to the preceding features, growth arrest is almost invariable.[335] The dissociation between height and weight on the growth chart is obvious. If the patient is growing along the same centile line, the diagnosis of Cushing's syndrome is highly unlikely. In addition to glucocorticoid-induced growth arrest, androgen excess may result in precocious puberty. Adrenal causes account for 65% of all cases.

Pregnancy

Pregnancy is rare in women with Cushing's syndrome because of associated amenorrhea related to androgen excess or hypercortisolism. However, approximately 100 such cases have been reported, 50% of which were due to adrenal adenomas.[336] A few cases of true pregnancy-induced Cushing's syndrome have been described with regression post partum.[337, 338] In these cases, the etiology is unknown. Establishing a diagnosis and cause can be difficult; clinically, striae, hypertension, and gestational diabetes are common features in pregnancy, yet hypertension and diabetes are the commonest signs of Cushing's syndrome in pregnant women (70% and 30% of all cases, respectively). Furthermore, biochemically, normal pregnancy is associated with a threefold increase in plasma cortisol because of increased cortisol production rates and increases in CBG. Urinary free cortisol also rises, and dexamethasone does not suppress plasma cortisol to the same degree as in the nonpregnant state. Untreated, the condition results in high maternal and fetal morbidity and mortality. Adrenal or pituitary adenomas should be excised. Metyrapone, which is not teratogenic, has been effective in many cases in controlling the hypercortisolism.[338]

Pseudo-Cushing's Syndromes

A pseudo-Cushing's state can be defined as some or all of the clinical features of Cushing's syndrome together with some evidence for hypercortisolism. Resolution of the underlying cause results in disappearance of the cushingoid state. Several causes have been described.

Alcohol

In the original description of this syndrome, urinary and plasma cortisol levels were elevated and not suppressed by dexamethasone. Plasma ACTH has been found to be normal or suppressed. The condition is rare but should be suspected in a patient with an ongoing history of heavy alcohol intake and biochemical or clinical evidence of chronic liver disease.[339–341] The pathogenesis of this condition remains unknown, but a "two-hit" hypothesis has been put forward to explain its etiology. Chronic liver disease of any cause is associated with impaired cortisol metabolism, but in alcoholics this is associated with an increase in cortisol secretion rate rather than concomitant suppression in the presence of impaired metabolism.[342] In some studies, alcohol has directly stimulated cortisol secretion; alternatively, vasopressin levels are elevated in patients with decompensated liver disease and may stimulate the HPA axis. With abstinence from alcohol the biochemical abnormalities rapidly revert to normal.

Depression

Although the cause is unknown, it is recognized that patients with depression may exhibit the hormonal abnormalities of patients with Cushing's syndrome.[343] These abnormalities are reversible on correction of the psychiatric condition. Conversely, patients with Cushing's syndrome are frequently depressed, and a careful clinical and endocrinologic assessment is required.

Obesity

Although one of the commonest referrals to a clinical endocrinologist is to exclude an underlying endocrine cause in a patient with obesity, the diagnosis of Cushing's syndrome in such patients should not cause difficulties. Patients with obesity have mildly increased cortisol secretion rates, and the data suggest that this is due to activation of the hypothalamo-pituitary axis.[344–346] However, circulating cortisol concentrations are invariably normal and urinary free cortisol concentrations are either normal or only slightly elevated. The stimulus for the increased secretion rate appears to be increased peripheral metabolism and hence clearance of cortisol (principally reduced hepatic conversion of cortisone to cortisol by 11β-HSD type 1 and increased conversion of cortisol to 5α-reduced derivatives).[347, 348]

Investigation of Suspected Cushing's Syndrome

There are two stages in the investigation of suspected Cushing's syndrome. (1) Does the patient have Cushing's syndrome? (2) If the answer is yes, then what is the cause? Unfortunately, many investigators fail to make this distinction and ill-advisedly use tests that are relevant to question 2 to try to answer question 1. In particular, it is essential that radiologic investigations not be undertaken until Cushing's syndrome has been confirmed biochemically. The major tests are listed in Table 14-15[349, 350] and their application in Figure 14–19.

Does the Patient Have Cushing's Syndrome?

Circadian Rhythm of Plasma Cortisol

In normal subjects, plasma cortisol levels are at their highest first thing in the morning and reach a nadir at about midnight (<50 nmol/L (2 μg/dL) in a nonstressed subject).[351] This circadian rhythm is lost in patients with Cushing's syndrome so that in the majority of patients the 9 AM plasma cortisol is normal but nocturnal levels are raised. Random morning plasma cortisol levels are therefore of little value in making the diagnosis, and a midnight cortisol level greater than 200 nmol/L (7 μg/dL) indicates Cushing's syndrome. However, various factors such as stress of venipuncture, intercurrent illness, and admission to the hospital may result in false-positive results. Ideally, patients should be hospitalized for 24 to 48 hours before measuring cortisol at midnight, but some centers have reported discriminant results from measurements of midnight values on an outpatient basis. Salivary cortisol concentrations may offer a sensible alternative in patients who are unable to go to the hospital.[352, 353]

Few laboratories have developed methods for the measurement of free levels of plasma cortisol. Because more than 90% of plasma cortisol is protein bound, the results of the conventional assay are affected by drugs or conditions that alter CBG levels. Thus, estrogen therapy or pregnancy may elevate CBG and total plasma cortisol. Loss of circadian rhythm is a sensitive diagnostic test but for the preceding reasons is not a widely used screening test.

Table 14–15. Tests Used in the Diagnosis and Differential Diagnosis of Cushing's Syndrome

Diagnosis
Does the patient have Cushing's syndrome?
- Circadian rhythm of plasma cortisol
- Urinary free cortisol excretion*
- Low-dose dexamethasone suppression test*

Differential Diagnosis
What is the cause of the Cushing's syndrome?
- Plasma ACTH
- Plasma potassium, bicarbonate
- High-dose dexamethasone suppression test
- Metyrapone test
- Corticotropin-releasing hormone
- Inferior petrosal sinus sampling
- CT, MRI scanning of pituitary, adrenals
- Scintigraphy
- Tumor markers

*Valuable outpatient screening tests (see text).
ACTH, adrenocorticotropic hormone; CT, computed tomography; MRI, magnetic resonance imaging.

Urinary Free Cortisol Excretion

For many years the diagnosis of Cushing's syndrome was based on the measurement of urinary metabolites of cortisol (24-hour urinary 17-hydroxycorticosteroid or 17-oxogenic steroid excretion, depending on the method used). However, the sensitivity and specificity of these methods are poor and most centers have replaced these assays with the more sensitive measurement of urinary free cortisol excretion. Urinary free cortisol is an integrated measure of plasma free cortisol; as cortisol secretion increases, the binding capacity of CBG is exceeded, resulting in a disproportionate rise in urinary free cortisol. Normal values are less than 220 to 330 nmol (80 to 120 μg) per 24 hours depending on the assay used.

Patients should make two or three complete consecutive collections to account for error in collecting samples and episodic cortisol secretion, notably from adrenal adenomas. Simultaneous creatinine excretion (which differs by no more than 10% on a day-to-day basis) may be used to ensure adequacy of collection. Urinary free cortisol is a useful screening test, but it is accepted that urinary free cortisol may be normal in up to 8% to 15% of patients with Cushing's syndrome.[354, 355] Conversely, moderately elevated results should always be endorsed by further testing before making a diagnosis of Cushing's syndrome.

Measurement of the cortisol/creatinine ratio in the first urine specimen passed on waking obviates the need for a timed collection and has been used as a screening test, particularly if cyclic Cushing's syndrome is suspected. Urine aliquots can be sent by post to the local endocrinology laboratory, which should provide normal reference ranges.

Low-Dose and Overnight Dexamethasone Suppression Tests

In normal subjects, the administration of a supraphysiologic dose of glucocorticoid results in suppression of ACTH and cortisol secretion. In Cushing's syndrome of any cause there is failure of this suppression when low doses of the synthetic glucocorticoid dexamethasone are given.[279]

The overnight test is a useful outpatient screening test.[356] Various doses of dexamethasone have been used, but 1 mg of dexamethasone is usually given at midnight. A normal response is a plasma cortisol less than 140 nmol/L (5 μg/dL) between 8 and 9 AM the following morning. A dose of 1.5 or 2 mg gives a 30% false-positive rate, whereas after 1 mg this is reduced to 12.5% with a false-negative rate less than 2%. In addition, sensitivity can be improved by reducing the plasma cortisol cutoff value; a postdexamethasone cortisol value of less than 50 nmol/L (2 μg/dL) effectively excludes Cushing's syndrome.[350] Thus, the outpatient overnight test has high sensitivity (95%)

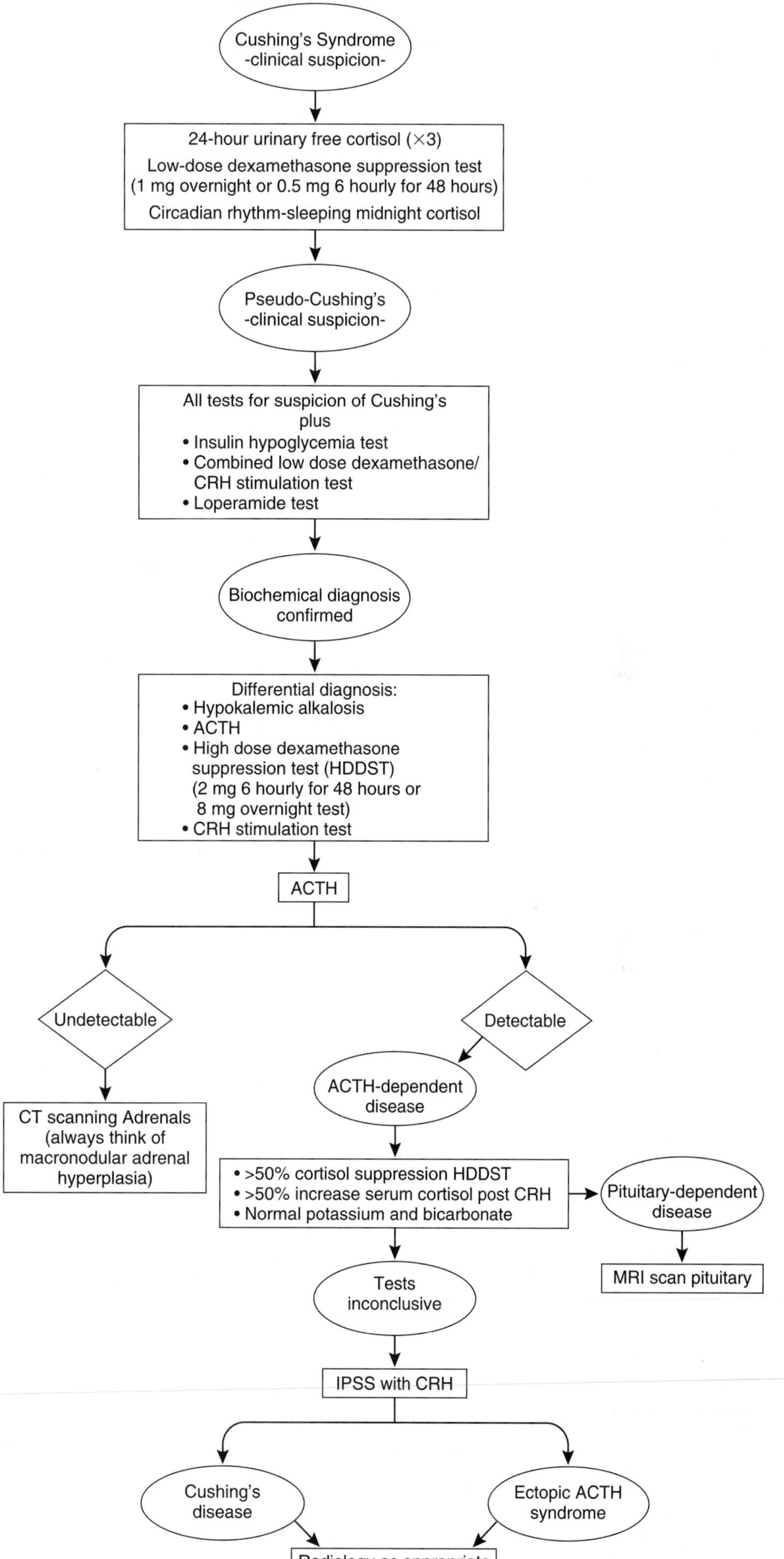

Figure 14–19. Investigation of a patient with suspected Cushing's syndrome. The laboratory diagnosis of Cushing's syndrome and the differential diagnosis of its cause are debatable and differ in any given center depending on many factors, including familiarity, turn-around time of hormone assays, and local expertise in techniques such as inferior petrosal sinus sampling (IPSS). Depicted here is an algorithm in use within many endocrine units based upon the reported sensitivity and specificity of each endocrine test.

but low specificity, and further investigation is often required.[357–359]

In the 48-hour low-dose dexamethasone test, plasma cortisol is measured at 9 AM on day 0 and 48 hours later following dexamethasone given at a dose of 0.5 mg every 6 hours for 48 hours. Using a postdexamethasone plasma cortisol concentration of less than 50 nmol/L (2 μg/dL), this test is reported as having a 97% to 100% true-positive rate and a false-positive rate less than 1%.[350, 359] Sensitivity is higher if plasma rather than urinary cortisol is measured.

Certain drugs (phenytoin, rifampicin) may increase the metabolic clearance rate of dexamethasone and lead to false-positive results. Simultaneous measurement of plasma dexamethasone may be useful here and also detects patients who failed to take the drug.[360]

Pseudo-Cushing's or True Cushing's Syndrome?

In patients with depression, urinary free cortisol concentrations may be elevated and overlap those seen in patients with true Cushing's syndrome. Compared with patients with Cushing's disease, depressed patients have greater suppressibility after dexamethasone and a reduced response to CRH, but neither of these tests is diagnostic.[350, 361] However, by performing a CRH test after the standard 2-day low-dose dexamethasone suppression test, separation of true versus pseudo-Cushing's syndrome has been possible. In normal subjects and in patients with endogenous depression, insulin-induced hypoglycemia results in a rise in ACTH and cortisol levels, a response that is usually not seen in Cushing's syndrome. Finally, loperamide lowers cortisol values in patients with pseudo-Cushing's but not in true Cushing's syndrome.[350]

Having Confirmed Cushing's Syndrome Clinically and Biochemically, What Is the Cause?

When the biochemical diagnosis has been made, a series of investigations are required to determine the cause of the Cushing's syndrome.

9 AM Plasma ACTH

Ideally, ACTH should be measured using a modern two-site immunoradiometric assay, which differentiates ACTH-dependent from ACTH-independent causes. In Cushing's disease, 50% of patients have a 9 AM ACTH within the normal reference range (2 to 12 pmol/L [9 to 54 pg/mL]); in the remainder it is modestly elevated. ACTH levels in the ectopic ACTH syndrome are high (usually > 20 pmol/L [90 pg/mL]) but nevertheless overlap values seen in Cushing's disease in 30% of cases[362] and cannot therefore be used to differentiate these two conditions (Fig. 14–20). The most discriminatory time of day to measure ACTH is actually between 11 PM and 1 AM, when ACTH-cortisol secretion is at a nadir, and in our practice ACTH is usually measured with cortisol in the circadian rhythm studies. A midnight ACTH result greater than 5 pmol/L (23 pg/mL) in a patient with biochemical hypercortisolism confirms that the underlying disease is ACTH-dependent. The measurement of ACTH precursors (pro-ACTH, POMC) is not routinely available but may be more useful in detecting an ectopic source of ACTH; more data are required on patients with occult tumors causing the syndrome.

In patients with adrenal tumors, plasma ACTH is invariably undetectable (<1 pmol/L [4.5 pg/mL]). This can also occur with degradation of ACTH; as a result, nonhemolyzed blood samples should be taken on ice and immediately separated.

Problem patients are those in whom plasma ACTH levels are low normal or intermittently detectable. This may occur in macronodular hyperplasia. The danger is that in some patients the asymmetry of the nodular hyperplasia may lead to a diagnosis of adrenal adenoma, the plasma ACTH is ignored, and an inappropriate adrenalectomy is performed. Conversely, in some patients with this syndrome an autonomous adrenal tumor develops and, despite detectable ACTH, unilateral adrenalectomy is required.

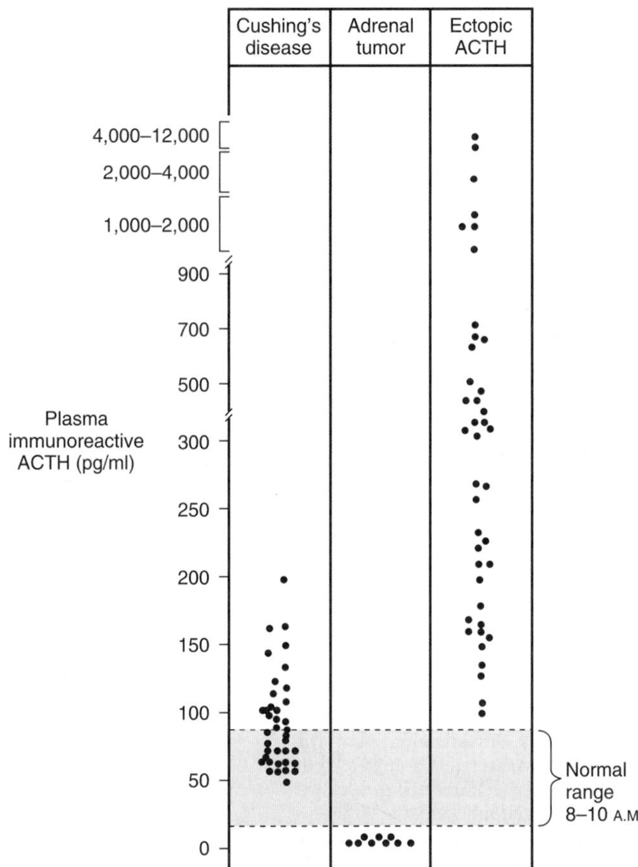

Figure 14–20. Plasma adrenocorticotropic hormone (ACTH) concentrations in patients with Cushing's disease and Cushing's syndrome associated with adrenocortical tumors and ectopic ACTH syndrome. To convert values to pmol/L, multiply by 0.2202. (From Besser GM, Edwards CRW. Cushing's syndrome. Clin Endocrinol Metab 1972; 1: 451–490.)

Plasma Potassium

Hypokalemic alkalosis is present in more than 95% of patients with the ectopic ACTH syndrome but is present in fewer than 10% of patients with Cushing's disease.[283] As discussed earlier ("Metabolic and Endocrine"), the etiology of this mineralocorticoid excess state is now established. Patients with the ectopic syndrome usually have higher cortisol secretion rates that saturate the renal protective 11β-HSD type 2 enzyme, resulting in cortisol-induced, mineralocorticoid hypertension (see Chapter 15). In addition, these patients have higher levels of the ACTH-dependent mineralocorticoid DOC.[257–259]

High-Dose Dexamethasone Suppression Test

The rationale for this test is that in Cushing's disease there is a resetting of the negative feedback control of ACTH to a higher level than normal. Thus, cortisol levels are not suppressed with low-dose but are suppressed with high-dose dexamethasone. The original test introduced by Liddle[279] was based on giving dexamethasone at 2 mg every 6 hours for 48 hours and demonstrating a greater than 50% fall in urinary 17-hydroxycorticosteroids after dexamethasone. In the modern test, plasma or urinary free cortisol, or both, are measured at 0 and +48 hours and a greater than 50% suppression of plasma cortisol in comparison with the basal sample defines a positive response. In all cases, response is graded and dependent upon the original cortisol secretion rate; greater suppression is often observed in patients with lower basal cortisol values.[363]

In Cushing's disease about 90% of patients have a positive 48-hour test in comparison with 10% with the ectopic ACTH syndrome. The robustness of the test can be improved by altering the cortisol cutoff value; thus, the test has 100% specificity for diagnosing pituitary disease if more than 90% suppression in urinary free cortisol is used. Less commonly, 8 mg of dexamethasone is given orally at 11 PM and plasma cortisol taken at 8 AM on the same day (basal sample) and 8 AM on the following morning.[364] A further variation on this test is the timed (5- to 7-hour) infusion of dexamethasone (1 mg/hour).[365]

Up to 50% of patients with ectopic ACTH syndrome related to indolent bronchial carcinoid tumors exhibit some suppression after high-dose dexamethasone. Conversely, some patients with Cushing's disease, usually those with large invasive ACTH-secreting pituitary macroadenomas, may show no suppression after high-dose dexamethasone.[366]

Metyrapone Test

Metyrapone blocks the conversion of 11-deoxycortisol to cortisol and DOC to corticosterone by inhibiting 11β-hydroxylase (see Fig. 14–3). This effect lowers plasma cortisol and, through negative feedback control, increases plasma ACTH. This, in turn, stimulates an increase in the secretion of adrenal steroids proximal to the block. When metyrapone is given in doses of 750 mg every 4 hours for 24 hours, patients with Cushing's disease exhibit an exaggerated rise in plasma ACTH with 11-deoxycortisol levels at 24 hours exceeding 1000 nmol/L (35 μg/dL). In most patients with the ectopic ACTH syndrome there is little or no response, but occasional patients (possibly those producing both ACTH and CRH) have an 11-deoxycortisol response that may be similar to that observed in Cushing's disease.[367]

The metyrapone test was originally used to distinguish patients with Cushing's disease from those with a primary adrenal cause. However, these can be more reliably distinguished by measuring plasma ACTH and subsequent computed tomographic (CT) scanning of the adrenals. As indicated, the test does not reliably distinguish between Cushing's disease and the ectopic ACTH syndrome, and the value of this test in modern endocrine practice has been questioned. It should be reserved for patients when the results of other tests are equivocal.

Corticotropin-Releasing Hormone (CRH) Test

CRH is a 41-amino-acid peptide identified by Vale in 1981 from ovine hypothalami. The ovine sequence differs by seven amino acid residues from that of the human but, despite this, is slightly more effective in stimulating the release of ACTH in humans.[368] The test involves the intravenous injection of either ovine or human CRH in a dose of 1 μg/kg body weight or a single dose of 100 μg (Fig. 14–21). In some centers CRH is combined with AVP, which results in an augmented ACTH response. The test can be performed in the morning or afternoon, and, after basal sampling, blood samples for ACTH and cortisol are taken every 15 minutes for 1 to 2 hours following the administration of CRH.[355, 369–373]

In normal subjects, CRH produces a rise in ACTH and cortisol (approximately 15% to 20%), but this response is exaggerated in Cushing's disease, where typically an ACTH rise greater than 50% and a cortisol rise greater than 20% over baseline values are seen. No response is seen in the ectopic ACTH syndrome, but false-positive results have been reported. In distinguishing pituitary-dependent Cushing's from the ectopic ACTH syndrome, the response of ACTH and cortisol to CRH has a specificity and sensitivity of approximately 90%. However, using an ACTH increase of 100% or a cortisol rise of 50% over baseline values, a positive response effectively eliminates a diagnosis of ectopic ACTH syndrome, and this is the real benefit of this test. Up to 10% of patients with Cushing's disease do not respond to CRH.

Inferior Petrosal Sinus Sampling and Selective Venous Catheterization

The most robust test to distinguish Cushing's disease from the ectopic ACTH syndrome is inferior petrosal sinus sampling (IPSS). As blood from each half of the pituitary drains into the ipsilateral inferior petrosal sinus, catheterization and venous sampling of both sinuses simultaneously can distinguish a pituitary from an ectopic source[366] (Fig. 14–22). In virtually all patients with the ectopic ACTH syndrome, the ratio of ACTH concentrations between the inferior petrosal sinus and simultaneously drawn peripheral venous level is less than 1.4:1. In contrast, in Cushing's disease this ratio is elevated at greater than 2.0.[366] However, because of the problem of intermittent ACTH secretion, it is useful to make measurements before and at intervals (for example, 2, 5, and 15 minutes) after intravenous injection of 100 μg of synthetic ovine CRH.[374–376] Using this approach, an ACTH petrosal sinus/peripheral ratio greater than 3.0 after CRH has a sensitivity of 97% and specificity of 100% in diagnosing Cushing's disease.[376]

IPSS may also be of value in lateralizing a pituitary tumor in a patient in whom imaging techniques have failed to demonstrate a microadenoma, although other centers have found that this is of little value in predicting tumor location. Coadministration of desmopressin with CRH may help in localizing the tumor. However, it should be remembered that many tumors are central and may drain into both sinuses; current evidence suggests that it would unwise to base the surgical procedure on the results of IPSS studies alone.

IPSS is a useful technique for establishing the differential diagnosis of ACTH-dependent Cushing's syndrome. However, it is technically demanding, has been associated with complications (referred aural pain, thrombosis), and is expensive. In our practice, it is reserved for cases in which the differential diagnosis is still in doubt after conducting the preceding tests (see Fig. 14–19).

Rarely, selective catheterization of vascular beds may be required to identify the source of ectopic ACTH secretion, for example, from a small pulmonary carcinoid or thymic tumor.

Tumor Markers

Many tumors responsible for the ectopic ACTH syndrome also produce peptide hormones other than ACTH or its precursors.

Imaging

Computed Tomographic and Magnetic Resonance Imaging Scanning of Pituitary and Adrenals. High-resolution, thin-section contrast-enhanced imaging using either CT or magnetic resonance imaging (MRI) has revolutionized the investigation of Cushing's syndrome.[377, 378] However, the results of any imaging technique must always be interpreted alongside the biochemical results if mistakes are to be avoided. In imaging the

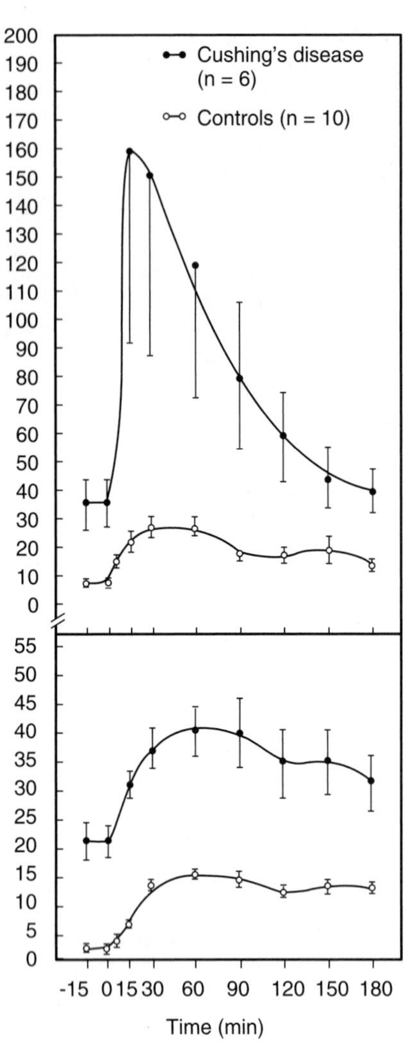

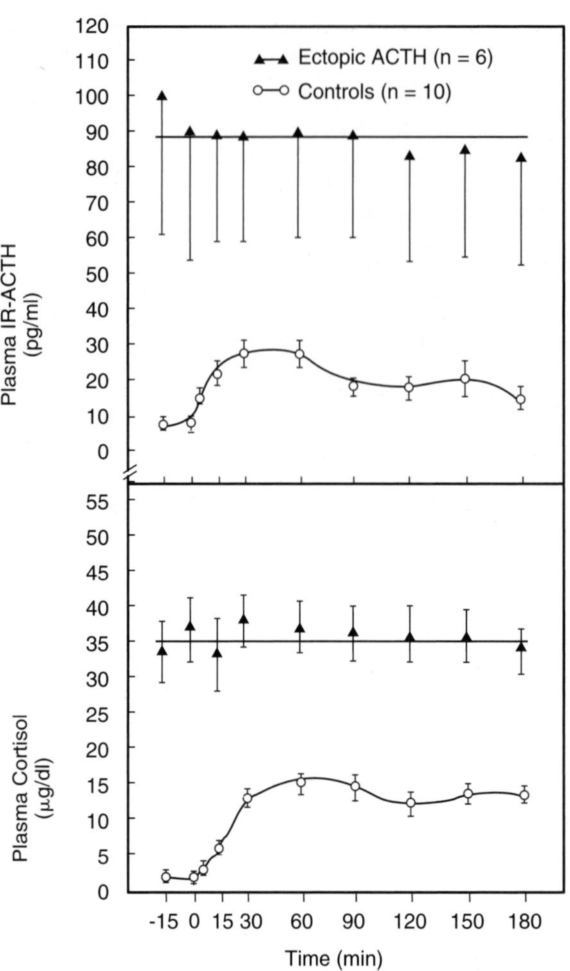

Figure 14–21. Comparison of the cortisol and adrenocorticotropic hormone (ACTH) responses to an intravenous injection of ovine corticotropin-releasing hormone (1 μg/kg) in normal subjects, patients with Cushing's disease, and patients with ectopic ACTH. (From Chrousos GP, Schulte HM, Oldfield EH, et al. The corticotropin-releasing factor stimulation test: an aid in the evaluation of patients with Cushing's syndrome. N Engl J Med 1984; 310:622–626.)

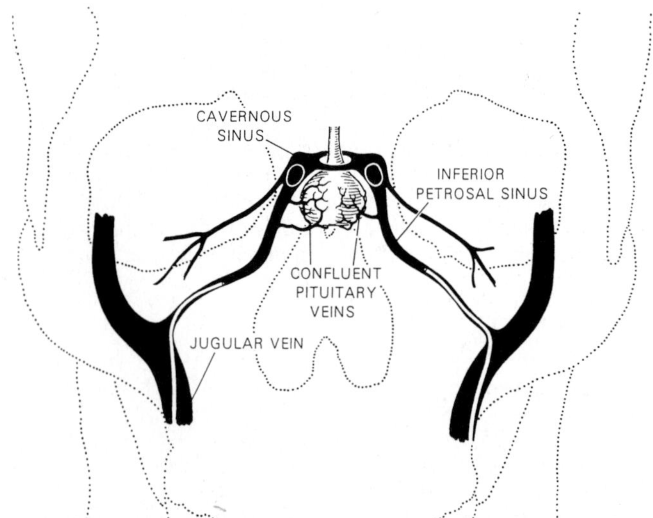

Figure 14–22. Anatomy of the venous drainage of the pituitary gland through the inferior petrosal venous sinuses. (From Oldfield EH, Chrousos GP, Schulte HM, et al. Preoperative lateralization of ACTH-secreting pituitary microadenomas by bilateral and simultaneous inferior petrosal sinus sampling. Reprinted by permission of The New England Journal of Medicine 1985; 312:100–103.)

adrenals, asymmetric nodular hyperplasia may lead to a false diagnosis of adrenal adenoma. Because of the presence of pituitary incidentalomas,[379] pituitary CT or MRI scanning may produce false-positive results, particularly for lesions less than 5 mm in diameter.

Pituitary MRI is the investigation of choice when the biochemical tests suggest Cushing's disease, with a sensitivity of 70% and specificity of 87% (Fig. 14–23). About 90% of ACTH-secreting pituitary tumors are microadenomas (i.e., less than 10 mm in diameter). The classical features of a pituitary microadenoma are a hypodense lesion after contrast, associated with deviation of the pituitary stalk and a convex upper surface of the pituitary gland (see Fig. 14–23). With such small tumors it is not surprising that the sensitivity of CT scanning is relatively low (20% to 60%) with a similar specificity.

By contrast, for adrenal imaging, CT rather than MRI is the investigation of choice, offering better spatial resolution (Fig. 14–24),[380] but MRI scanning may provide diagnostic information in patients with suspected adrenal carcinoma. Once again, it is stressed that adrenal incidentalomas are present in up to 5% of normal subjects (see later), and thus adrenal imaging should not be performed unless biochemical investigation suggests a primary adrenal cause (undetectable ACTH concentrations). Adrenal carcinomas are large and often associated with metastatic spread at presentation (Fig. 14–25).

In patients with occult ectopic ACTH syndrome, high-definition CT or MRI scanning of thorax, abdomen, and pelvis

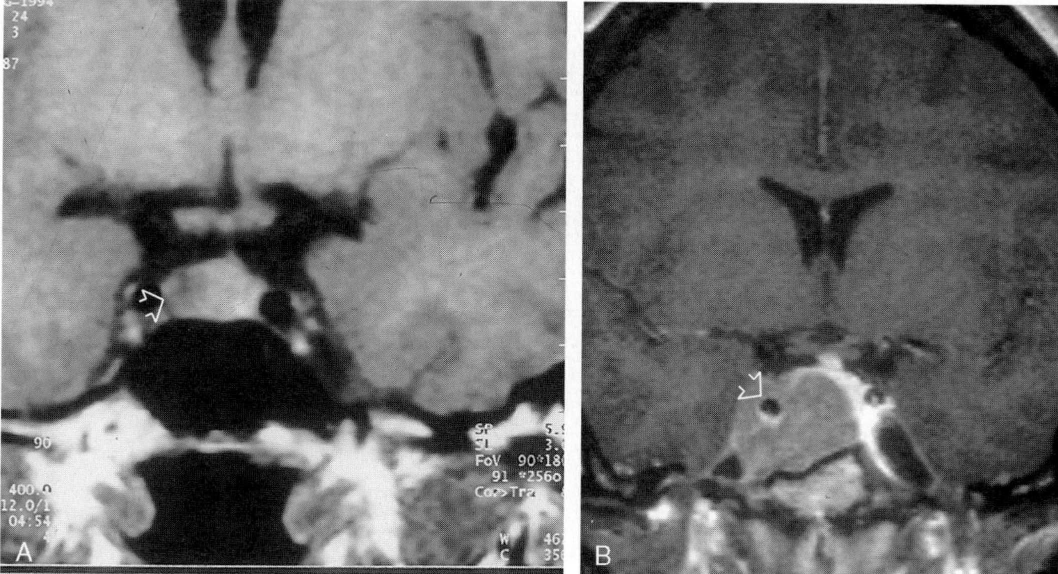

Figure 14–23. *A*, Magnetic resonance imaging (MRI) scan of pituitary demonstrating the typical appearance of a pituitary microadenoma. A hypodense lesion is seen in the right side of the gland with deviation of the pituitary stalk away from the lesion. After a biochemical diagnosis of Cushing's disease, this patient was cured following transsphenoidal hypophysectomy. *B*, MRI scan of the pituitary gland demonstrating a large macroadenoma in a patient with Cushing's disease. In contrast to smaller tumors, these tumors are invariably invasive and recur after surgery.

with images every 0.5 cm may be required to detect small ACTH-secreting carcinoid tumors (Fig. 14–26).

Scintigraphy Studies. Scintigraphy is of value in certain patients with primary adrenal pathology. The most commonly used agent is ^{131}I-labeled 6β-iodomethyl-19-norcholesterol.[381] This is a marker of adrenocortical cholesterol uptake. In patients with adrenal adenomas, the isotope is taken up by the adenoma but not by the contralateral suppressed adrenal. Adrenal scintigraphy is useful for suspected adrenocortical macronodular hyperplasia, in which CT scanning may be misleading by suggesting unilateral pathology, whereas with isotope scanning the bilateral adrenal involvement is identified.

Many neuroendocrine tumors giving rise to the ectopic ACTH syndrome express somatostatin receptors and can be imaged by administering radiolabeled analogues of somato-

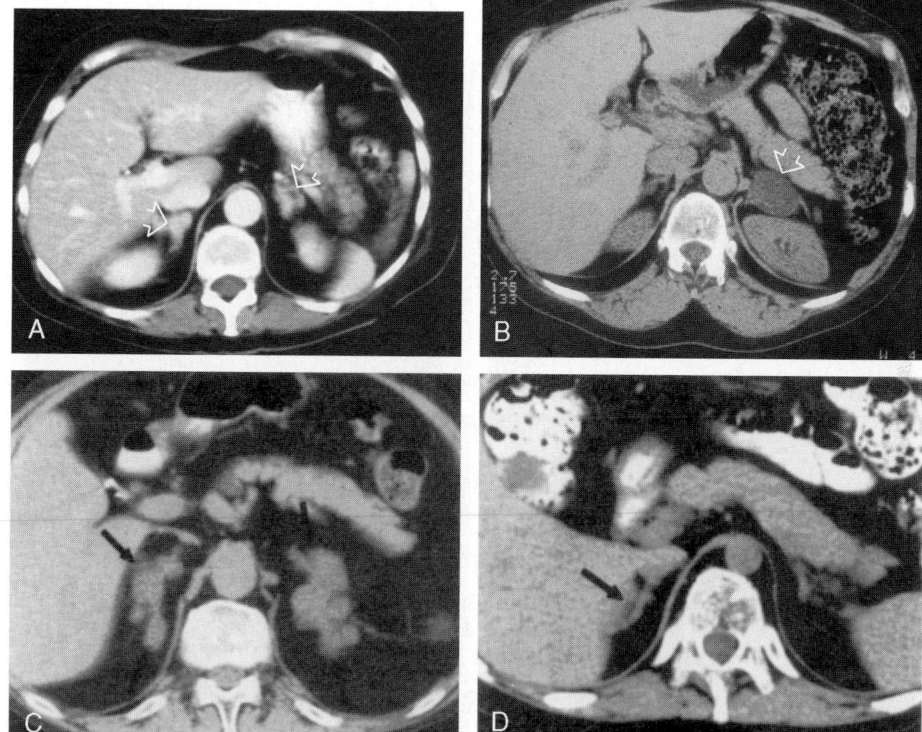

Figure 14–24. *A*, Adrenal computed tomographic (CT) scan demonstrating bilateral adrenal hyperplasia in a patient with Cushing's disease. *B*, CT scan of a typical solitary left adrenal adenoma causing Cushing's syndrome. *C*, Cushing's syndrome caused by massive macronodular hyperplasia. Adrenal glands are replaced by multiple nodules *(arrows)*. Combined weight of adrenal glands was over 100 g. *D*, Cushing's syndrome caused by surgically proven primary pigmented nodular adrenal disease in a 21-year-old patient. Notice the multiple small nodules with the relatively atrophic internodular adrenocortical tissue involving the medial limb of the right adrenal gland *(arrow)*. (*C* and *D* from Findling JW, Doppman JL. Biochemical and radiologic diagnosis of Cushing's syndrome. Endocrinol Metab Clin North Am 1994; 23:511–537.)

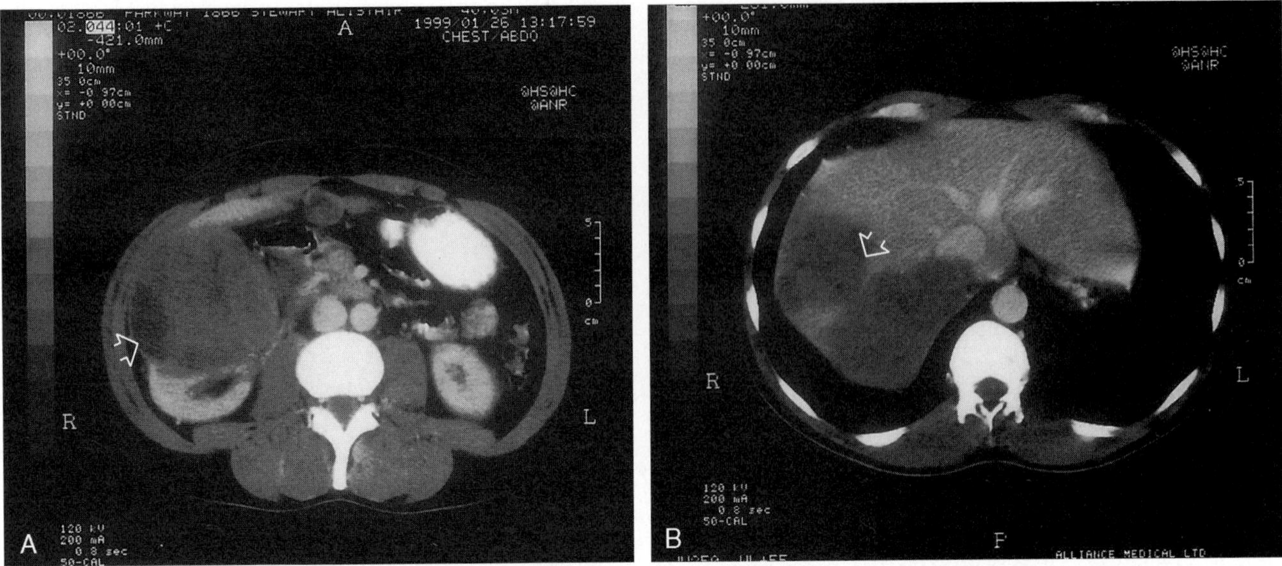

Figure 14–25. Computed tomographic scan of a patient with rapidly progressing Cushing's syndrome caused by an adrenal carcinoma. An irregular right adrenal mass is shown *(A)* with a large liver metastasis *(B)*.

statin (most commonly ^{111}In-labeled octreotide). This technique can detect tumors only a few millimeters in diameter and should be considered for patients with ACTH-dependent Cushing's syndrome in whom pituitary disease has been excluded.[382, 383]

Treatment of Cushing's Syndrome

Adrenal Causes

Adrenal adenomas should be removed by unilateral adrenalectomy, which has a 100% cure rate.[311, 384] With the increasing experience of laparoscopic adrenalectomy in most tertiary centers, this has now become the surgical treatment of choice for unilateral tumors, reducing surgical morbidity and postoperative hospital stay compared with traditional open approaches.[385, 386] After operation it may take many months or even years for the contralateral suppressed adrenal to recover. It is wise, therefore, to give slightly suboptimal replacement therapy with dexamethasone at 0.5 mg in the morning, with intermittent measurement of morning plasma cortisol before taking dexamethasone. When the morning plasma cortisol is above 180 nmol/L (6 μg/dL), dexamethasone can be stopped. A subsequent insulin tolerance test may then demonstrate whether the response to stress is normal. In the interim, all patients should carry a Steroid Alert card and increase their dose of replacement therapy in the event of an intercurrent illness (see earlier).

Adrenal carcinomas have a poor prognosis, and most patients are dead within 2 years of diagnosis.[312] It is usual prac-

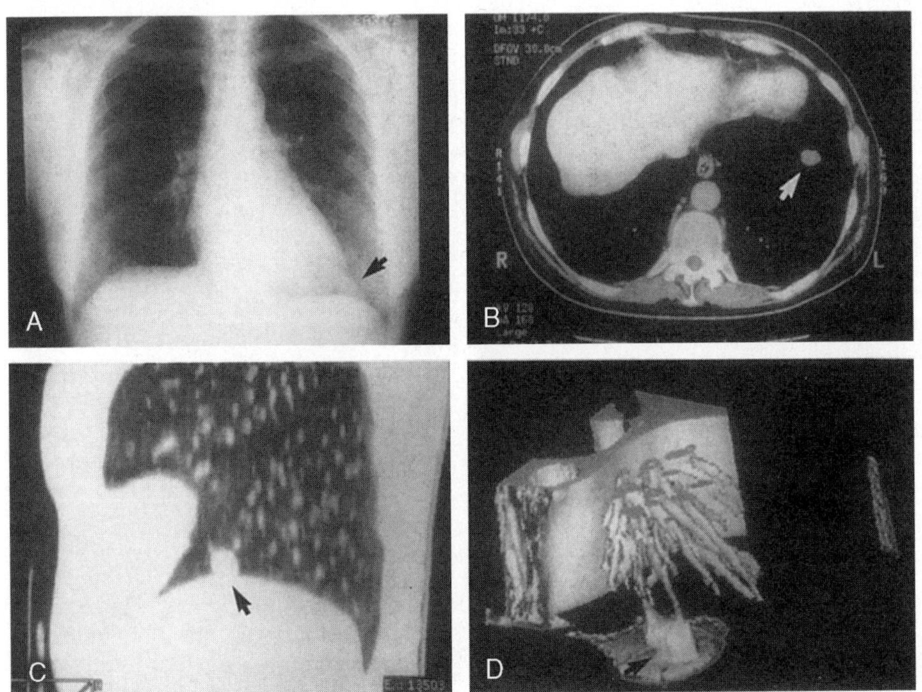

Figure 14–26. Imaging of the thorax in the ectopic adrenocorticotropic hormone (ACTH) syndrome. *A*, Plain chest radiograph demonstrating suspicious lesion behind the left heart border *(arrow)*. *B* and *C*, Axial and sagittal computed tomographic images demonstrating a bronchial carcinoid tumor *(arrow)* abutting the diaphragm. *D*, Three-dimensional reconstruction illustrating adherence of the tumor to the diaphragm *(arrow)*, which was confirmed at surgery. (From Newell-Prince J, Trainer P, Besser M, et al. The diagnosis and differential diagnosis of Cushing's syndrome and pseudo-Cushing's states. Endocr Rev 1998; 19:647–672.)

tice to try to remove the primary tumor even though metastases may be present so as to enhance the response to the adrenolytic agent *o,p'*-dichlorodiphenyldichloroethane (*o,p'*-DDD, mitotane; see later). Radiotherapy to the tumor bed and to some metastases, such as those in the spine, may be of limited value.

Pituitary-Dependent Cushing's Syndrome

The treatment of Cushing's disease has been significantly enhanced through transsphenoidal surgery conducted by an experienced surgeon. Before the selective removal of a pituitary microadenoma, the treatment of choice was bilateral adrenalectomy. This had an appreciable mortality even in the best centers (up to 4%) and significant morbidity. The major risk was the subsequent development of Nelson's syndrome (postadrenalectomy hyperpigmentation with a locally aggressive pituitary tumor) (Fig. 14–27), which was attributed to loss of any negative feedback after adrenalectomy.[387] In an attempt to avoid this, pituitary radiation was often carried out at the time of bilateral adrenalectomy.[388] In addition, these patients required lifelong replacement therapy with hydrocortisone and fludrocortisone. Today, bilateral adrenalectomy is rarely indicated for patients with Cushing's disease but may be performed when pituitary surgery has failed or when the condition has recurred.

The surgical outcome for transsphenoidal hypophysectomy is center-dependent and related to surgical expertise. Because of the hazards of untreated Cushing's disease and potential complications of surgery, the endocrinologist should refer cases only to a recognized surgical specialist where outcome data have been established. In optimal centers, cure rates are 80% to 90% for microadenomas and 50% for macroadenomas.[271, 272, 389] Rates for hypopituitarism and permanent diabetes insipidus postoperatively depend on how aggressive the surgeon has been in removing pituitary tissue. The ideal outcome is a cured patient with intact pituitary function, but this may not be possible in a patient with Cushing's disease in whom a pituitary adenoma was not identified preoperatively or during the operation itself.

At the time of surgery, patients should be treated with corticosteroids as for any other potential or confirmed deficit of the HPA axis (see later). Postoperatively, hydrocortisone can be withdrawn to maintenance replacement doses, usually within 3 to 7 days. On day 5 postoperatively, plasma cortisol should be measured at 9 AM with the patient having omitted hydrocortisone for 24 hours. After selective removal of a microadenoma, the surrounding corticotrophs are normally suppressed (Fig. 14–28). In these cases plasma cortisol levels are less than 30 nmol/L (1 μg/dL) postoperatively and glucocorticoid replacement therapy is required. Using the dexamethasone regimen described earlier after removal of an adrenal adenoma, there is usually (but not invariably) gradual recovery of the HPA axis (Fig. 14–29). A nonsuppressed plasma cortisol postoperatively suggests that the patient is not cured even though cortisol secretion may have fallen to normal or subnormal values.[390, 391] The recurrence rate in patients with an established cure after pituitary surgery is 2%, but this value is higher in children (up to 40%).[392] A detailed assessment of residual pituitary function is required in each case, and close follow-up of such individuals is warranted.

In the past, pituitary radiation was often used in the treatment of Cushing's disease. However, the improvements in pituitary surgery have resulted in far fewer patients being so treated. In children, pituitary radiation appears to be more effective.[393] Radiotherapy is not recommended as a primary treatment but is reserved for patients who do not respond to pituitary microsurgery, those in whom bilateral adrenalectomy has been performed, or patients with established Nelson's syndrome.

Ectopic Adrenocorticotropic Hormone Syndrome

Treatment of the ectopic ACTH syndrome depends on the cause. If the tumor can be found and has not spread, then its removal can lead to cure (e.g., bronchial carcinoid or thymoma). However, the prognosis for small cell lung cancer associated with the ectopic ACTH syndrome is poor. The cortisol excess and associated hypokalemic alkalosis and diabetes mellitus can be ameliorated by medical therapy. The treatment of the small cell tumor itself also, at least initially, produces improvement. Sometimes, if the ectopic source of ACTH cannot be found, it may be necessary to perform bilateral adrenalectomy and then observe the patient carefully (sometimes for several years) before the primary tumor becomes apparent.

Medical Treatment of Cushing's Syndrome

Several drugs have been used in the treatment of Cushing's syndrome. Metyrapone inhibits 11β-hydroxylase and has been most commonly given, often to lower cortisol concentrations prior to definitive therapy or while awaiting benefit from pituitary radiation. The daily dose has to be determined by measuring either plasma or urinary free cortisol. The aim should be to achieve a mean plasma cortisol of about 300 nmol/L (11 μg/dL) during the day or a normal urinary free cortisol. The drug is usually given in doses ranging from 250 mg twice daily to 1.5 g every 6 hours. Nausea is a side effect that can be helped (if it is not due to adrenal insufficiency) by giving the drug with milk.[394]

Aminoglutethimide is a more toxic drug that, in high doses, blocks earlier enzymes in the steroidogenic pathway and thus affects the secretion of steroids other than cortisol. In doses of 1.5 to 3 g daily (start with 250 mg every 8 hours) it commonly produces nausea, marked lethargy, and a high incidence of skin rash.[395] It is commonly prescribed as combination therapy with metyrapone.

Trilostane, a 3β-HSD inhibitor, is ineffective in Cushing's disease, as the block in steroidogenesis is overcome by the rise in ACTH. However, it can be effective in patients with adrenal adenomas.[396]

Ketoconazole is an imidazole that has been widely used as an antifungal agent but causes abnormal liver function tests in about 15% of patients. Ketoconazole blocks a variety of steroidogenic cytochrome P450–dependent enzymes and thus lowers plasma cortisol levels. For effective control of Cushing's syndrome, 400 to 800 mg daily has been required.[397]

Mitotane is an adrenolytic drug that is taken up by both normal and malignant adrenal tissue, causing adrenal atrophy and necrosis.[312] Because of its toxicity, it has been used mainly in the management of adrenal carcinoma. Doses of up to 10 to 20 g/day are required to control glucocorticoid excess, although evidence that it causes tumor shrinkage or improves long-term survival is lacking. The drug also produces mineralocorticoid deficiency, and concomitant glucocorticoid and mineralocorticoid replacement therapy may be required. Side effects are common and include fatigue, skin rashes, and gastrointestinal disturbance.

Prognosis of Cushing's Syndrome

Studies carried out before the introduction of effective therapy indicated that 50% of patients with untreated Cushing's syndrome died within 5 years, principally from vascular disease.[398, 399] Even with modern management, an increased prev-

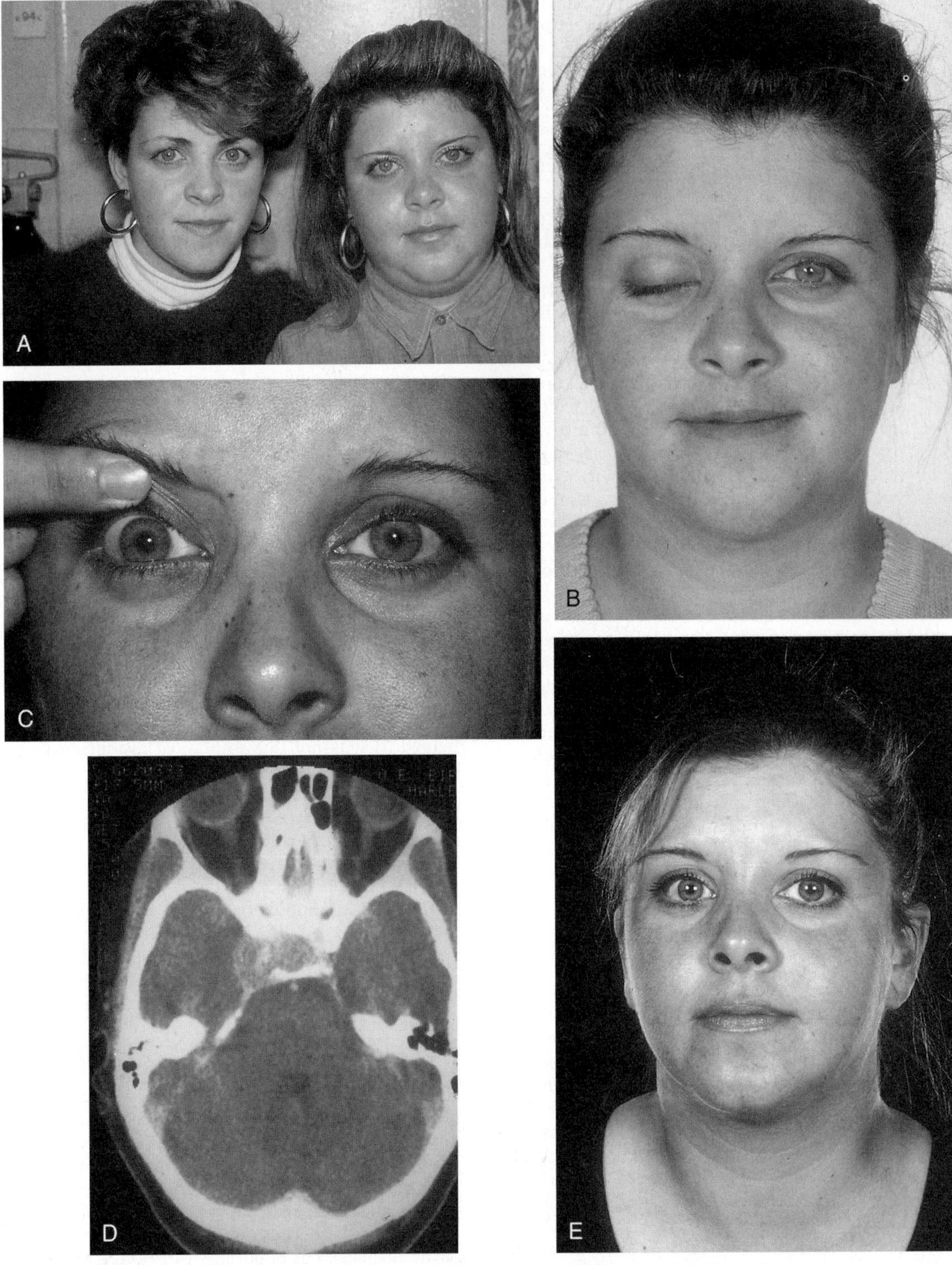

Figure 14–27. A young woman with Cushing's disease, photographed initially beside her identical twin sister *(A)*. In this case, treatment with bilateral adrenalectomy was undertaken. Several years later, the patient presented with Nelson's syndrome and a right third cranial nerve palsy (*B* and *C*) related to cavernous sinus infiltration from a locally invasive corticotropinoma *(D)*. Hypophysectomy and radiotherapy were performed with reversal of the third nerve palsy *(E)*. Note the advancing skin pigmentation of Nelson's syndrome. (See also Color Plate.)

alence of cardiovascular risk factors persists for many years after an apparent cure.[400] Paradoxically, upon correction of the hypercortisolism, patients can often feel worse. Skin desquamation, steroid withdrawal arthropathy, profound lethargy, and mood changes may occur and take several weeks or months to resolve.[243] In the author's experience, these features, together with postural hypotension, are particularly severe in cured patients who may also be rendered vasopressin-deficient. They can usually be ameliorated by a transient increase in glucocorticoid replacement therapy. Patients are invariably GH-deficient, and GH replacement therapy may produce clinical benefit.

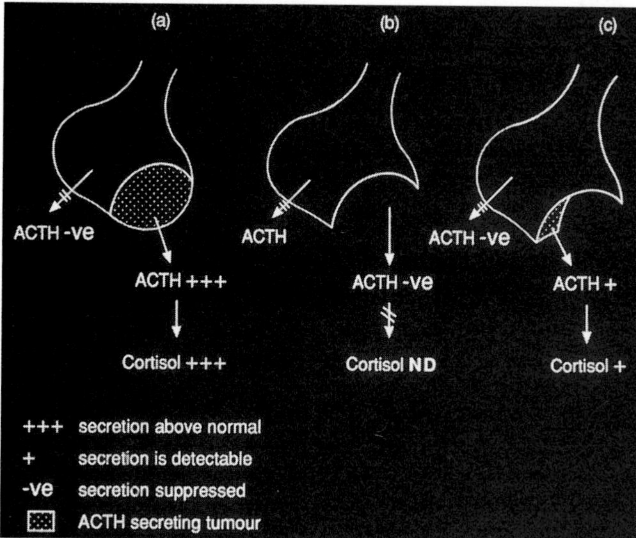

Figure 14–28. Selective removal of a microadenoma and its effect on the hypothalamic-pituitary-adrenal axis. Because the surrounding normal pituitary corticotrophs are suppressed in a patient with an adrenocorticotropic hormone (ACTH)–secreting pituitary adenoma, successful removal of the tumor results in ACTH and hence adrenocortical deficiency with an undetectable (<50 nmol/L [2 μg/dL]) plasma cortisol level. A plasma cortisol level higher than 50 nmol/L (2 μg/dL) postoperatively implies that the patient is not cured. (Courtesy of Dr. Peter Trainer.)

Features of Cushing's syndrome disappear over a period of 2 to 12 months. Hypertension and diabetes mellitus improve but, as with other secondary causes, may not resolve completely. The osteopenia of Cushing's syndrome improves rapidly in the first 2 years after treatment but resolves more slowly thereafter.[401] Vertebral fractures and aseptic necrosis are irreversible, and permanent deformity results. Visceral obesity and myopathy are both reversible features. Reproductive and sexual functions return to normal within 6 months provided anterior pituitary function was not compromised.

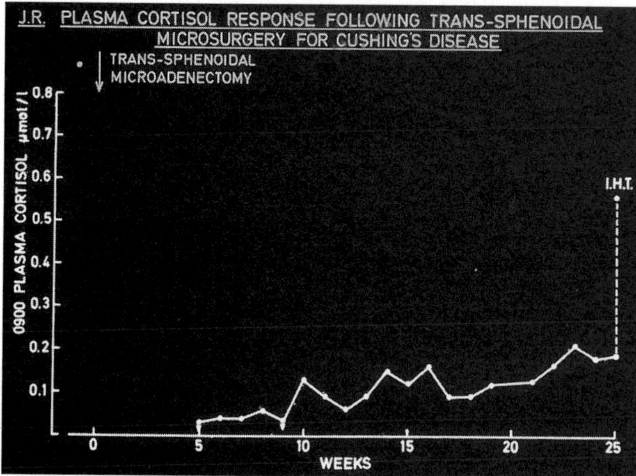

Figure 14–29. Gradual recovery of function of the hypothalamic-pituitary-adrenal axis after removal of a pituitary adrenocorticotropic hormone–secreting microadenoma. The insulin hypoglycemia test (I.H.T.) eventually demonstrated the return of a normal stress response.

Glucocorticoid Resistance

A small number of patients have been described who have increased cortisol secretion but without the stigmata of Cushing's syndrome.[110, 402, 403] These patients are resistant to suppression of cortisol with low-dose dexamethasone but respond to high doses. ACTH levels are elevated and lead to increased adrenal production of androgens and DOC. Thus, patients may present with the features of androgen or mineralocorticoid excess, or both. Treatment with a dose of dexamethasone adequate to suppress ACTH (usually 3 mg/day) results in a fall in adrenal androgens and often return of plasma potassium and blood pressure to normal levels. Many of these patients have been found to have point mutations in the steroid-binding domain of the GR, with consequent reduction of glucocorticoid-binding affinity,[110, 403] but this is not invariable.[404] A useful clinical discriminatory test to differentiate this condition from Cushing's syndrome is to measure bone mineral density; this is preserved in patients with glucocorticoid resistance or even increased in female patients because of the androgen excess. In addition, circadian rhythm for ACTH and cortisol is preserved in patients with glucocorticoid resistance.

Glucocorticoid Deficiency

Primary and Secondary Hypoadrenalism

Primary hypoadrenalism refers to glucocorticoid deficiency occurring in the setting of adrenal disease; secondary hypoadrenalism arises because of deficiency of ACTH (Table 14–16). A major distinction between these two is that mineralocorticoid deficiency invariably accompanies primary hypoadrenalism but does not occur in secondary hypoadrenalism because only ACTH is deficient; the renin-angiotensin-aldosterone axis is intact. A further important cause of adrenal insufficiency where there may be dissociation of glucocorticoid and mineralocorticoid secretion is congenital adrenal hyperplasia (CAH) (see later).

Primary Hypoadrenalism

Addison's Disease

Thomas Addison described this condition in his classical monograph published in 1855.[2]

Etiology. This is a rare condition with an estimated incidence in the developed world of 0.8 cases per 100,000 and prevalence of 4 to 11 cases per 100,000 population. It is associated with significant morbidity and mortality, but when the diagnosis is made it can be easily treated.[405, 406] The causes of Addison's disease are listed in Table 14–16.

Autoimmune Adrenalitis. In the Western world, autoimmune adrenalitis accounts for over 70% of all cases.[407] Pathologically, the adrenal glands are atrophic, with loss of most of the cortical cells, but the medulla is usually intact. In 75% of cases adrenal autoantibodies can be detected. Fifty percent of patients with this form of Addison's disease have an associated autoimmune disease (Table 14–17), thyroid disease being the commonest.[408] Conversely, only 1% to 2% of patients with commoner autoimmune diseases such as insulin-dependent diabetes mellitus or thyrotoxicosis have antiadrenal autoantibodies and adrenal disease. This figure is higher in patients with autoimmune hypoparathyroidism (16%).

These autoimmune polyendocrine syndromes (APS) I and II have been classified into two distinct variants.[409, 410] APS type I is inherited as an autosomal recessive condition and comprises Addison's disease, chronic mucocutaneous candidiasis, and hypoparathyroidism. Also called autoimmune polyendocrinopa-

Table 14–16. Etiology of Adrenocortical Insufficiency (Excluding CAH)

Primary: Addison's Disease
Autoimmune
  Sporadic
  Autoimmune polyendocrine syndrome type I (Addison's disease, chronic mucocutaneous candidiasis, hypoparathyroidism, dental enamel hypoplasia, alopecia, primary gonadal failure, see Chapter 37)
  Autoimmune polyendocrine syndrome type II (Schmidt's syndrome) (Addison's disease, primary hypothyroidism, primary hypogonadism, insulin-dependent diabetes, pernicious anaemia, vitiligo, Chapter 37)
Infections
  Tuberculosis
  Fungal infections
  Cytomegalovirus
  HIV
Metastatic tumor
Infiltrations
  Amyloid
  Hemochromatosis
Intra-adrenal haemorrhage (Waterhouse-Friderichsen syndrome) after meningococcal septicemia
Adrenoleukodystrophies
Congenital adrenal hypoplasia
  DAX-1 mutations
  SF-1 mutations
ACTH resistance syndromes
  Mutations in *MC2-R*
  Triple A syndrome
Bilateral adrenalectomy

Secondary
Exogenous glucocorticoid therapy
Hypopituitarism
Selective removal of ACTH-secreting pituitary adenoma
Pituitary tumors and pituitary surgery, craniopharyngiomas
Pituitary apoplexy
Granulomatous disease (tuberculosis, sarcoid, eosinophilic granuloma)
Secondary tumor deposits (breast, bronchus)
Postpartum pituitary infarction (Sheehan's syndrome)
Pituitary irradiation (effect usually delayed for several years)
Isolated ACTH deficiency
Idiopathic
Lymphocytic hypophysitis
POMC processing defect
POMC gene mutations

ACTH, adrenocorticotropic hormone; HIV, human immunodeficiency virus; POMC, pro-opiomelanocortin.

thy–candidiasis–ectodermal dysplasia (APECED) (Table 14–18), the condition is rare and is usually seen in childhood with either candidiasis or hypoparathyroidism.[409, 411] Other autoimmune conditions such as pernicious anemia, thyroid disease, chronic active hepatitis, and gonadal failure may occur but are rare (see also Chapter 37). The adrenal autoantibodies characterizing PGA type I are to the steroidogenic enzymes side-chain cleavage and 17-hydroxylase but not to 21-hydroxylase.[412, 413] The disease has been mapped to chromosome 21q22.3, and mutations in a transcription regulation gene designated *AIRE* (autoimmune regulator) have been defined.[414, 415]

APS II is commoner and comprises Addison's disease, autoimmune thyroid disease, diabetes mellitus, and hypogonadism[406, 407] (see Table 14–18). The condition has an inherited basis with linkage to the human leukocyte antigen (HLA) major histocompatibility complex, notably HLA DR3 and HLA DR4.[416] Autoantibodies to 21-hydroxylase are usually present and are predictive of the development of adrenal destruction.[412, 416–418]

Other features may accompany APS I and APS II (see Table 14–18). Patients with APS are more likely to be female (70%); conversely, patients presenting with isolated autoimmune adrenalitis are usually male.

Table 14–17. Incidence of Other Endocrine and Autoimmune Diseases in Patients with Autoimmune Adrenal Insufficiency (N = 448)

Disease	Incidence (%)
Thyroid disease	
Hypothyroidism	8
Nontoxic goiter	7
Thyrotoxicosis	7
Gonadal failure	
Ovarian	20
Testicular	2
Insulin-dependent diabetes mellitus	11
Hypoparathyroidism	10
Pernicious anemia	5
None	53

Infections. Worldwide, infectious diseases are the commonest cause of primary adrenal insufficiency and comprise tuberculosis, fungal infections (histoplasmosis, cryptococcosis), and cytomegalovirus infection. Adrenal failure may also occur in the acquired immunodeficiency syndrome.

Tuberculous Addison's disease results from hematogenous spread of the infection from elsewhere in the body, and extra-adrenal disease is usually evident.[419] The adrenals are initially enlarged with extensive epithelioid granulomas and caseation, and both the cortex and the medulla are affected. Fibrosis ensues, and the adrenals become normal or smaller in size with calcification evident in 50% of cases.

The adrenals are frequently involved in patients with ac-

Table 14–18. Clinical Manifestations of Autoimmune Polyendocrine Syndromes (APS) Associated with Adrenal Insufficiency

Disorder	Prevalence (%)
APS, Type I	
Endocrine	
Hypoparathyroidism	89
Chronic mucocutaneous candidiasis	75
Adrenal insufficiency	60
Gonadal failure	45
Hypothyroidism	12
Insulin-dependent diabetes mellitus	1
Hypopituitarism	<1
Diabetes insipidus	<1
Nonendocrine	
Malabsorption syndromes	25
Alopecia totalis or areata	20
Pernicious anemia	16
Chronic active hepatitis	9
Vitiligo	4
APS, Type II	
Endocrine	
Adrenal insufficiency	100
Autoimmune thyroid disease	70
Insulin-dependent diabetes mellitus	50
Gonadal failure	5–50
Diabetes insipidus	<1
Nonendocrine	
Vitiligo	4
Alopecia, pernicious anemia, myasthenia gravis, immune thrombocytopenia purpura, Sjögren's syndrome, rheumatoid arthritis	<1

quired immunodeficiency syndrome (AIDS)[420]; adrenalitis may occur after infection with cytomegalovirus or atypical mycobacterium, and Kaposi's sarcoma may result in adrenal replacement. The onset is often insidious,[421] but if tested, over 10% of patients with AIDS demonstrate a subnormal cortisol response following a short Synacthen test. Adrenal insufficiency may be precipitated through the concomitant administration of appropriate anti-infectives such as ketoconazole (inhibits cortisol synthesis) or rifampicin (increases cortisol metabolism). Rarely, patients with AIDS and features of adrenal insufficiency are found to have elevated circulating ACTH and cortisol concentrations that are not suppressed normally by low-dose dexamethasone administration. This is thought to reflect an acquired form of glucocorticoid resistance related to reduced GR affinity, but the underlying cause remains unknown.[422]

Miscellaneous. With the exception of tuberculosis and autoimmune adrenal failure, other causes of Addison's disease are rare (see Table 14–16). Adrenal metastases (commonest primary being lung and breast) are often found at postmortem examination, but adrenal insufficiency resulting from these is uncommon,[423] perhaps because over 90% of the adrenal cortex needs to be compromised before symptoms and signs become apparent. Necrosis of the adrenals related to intra-adrenal hemorrhage should be considered in any severely sick patient, particularly those with underlying infection, trauma, or coagulopathy.[424] Intra-adrenal bleeding may be found with any cause of severe septicemia, particularly in children, in whom a common cause is infection with *Pseudomonas aeruginosa*. When Addison's disease is caused by meningococcus, the association with adrenal insufficiency is known as the Waterhouse-Friderichsen syndrome.[425] Adrenal replacement may also occur with amyloidosis and hemochromatosis.

Adrenal hypoplasia congenita is an X-linked disorder comprising congenital adrenal insufficiency and hypogonadotropic hypogonadism. The condition is caused by mutations in the dosage-sensitive sex reversal, adrenal hypoplasia congenita, X-chromosome factor (*DAX-1*) gene, a member of the nuclear receptor family of unknown function that is expressed in the adrenal cortex, gonads, and hypothalamus.[426–428] Mutations in another transcription factor, steroidogenic factor-1, also results in adrenal insufficiency related to lack of development of a functional adrenal cortex.[429] The transcriptional regulation of many P450 steroidogenic enzymes is dependent upon steroidogenic factor-1.[16] Congenital adrenal hypoplasia may also occur in association with glycerol kinase deficiency and muscular dystrophy.[430]

Adrenoleukodystrophy has a prevalence of 1 in 20,000 and is a cause of adrenal insufficiency in association with demyelination within the nervous system related to a failure of beta oxidation of fatty acids within peroxisomes because of reduced activity of very-long-chain acyl-CoA synthetase (VLCS).[431, 432] Increased accumulation of very-long-chain fatty acids occurs in many tissues, and serum assays can be used diagnostically. Only males have the fully expressed condition, and carrier females are usually normal. Several forms are recognized: a childhood cerebral form (30% to 40% of cases), adult adrenomyeloneuropathy (40% of cases), and Addison's disease only (7% of cases).

The childhood-onset form occurs at 5 to 10 years of age with eventual progression to a blind, mute, and severely spastic tetraplegic state. Adrenal insufficiency is usually present but does not appear to correlate with the neurologic deficit. Nevertheless, this is the commonest form of adrenal insufficiency in a child younger than 7 years.[431] Adrenomyeloneuropathy, by contrast, arises later in life with the gradual development of spastic paresis and peripheral neuropathy. Both the childhood and adult conditions result from mutations in a gene on chromosome Xq28 that encodes a peroxisomal membrane protein with homology to the adenosine triphosphate–binding transmembrane transporter proteins. At present, there are no genotype-phenotype correlations and it is uncertain how these mutations affect the activity of VLCS.[433, 434] Treatment is unsuccessful. Monounsaturated fatty acids that block the synthesis of the saturated very-long-chain fatty acids have been used. A combination of erucic acid and oleic acid (Lorenzo's oil) has led to normal levels of very-long-chain fatty acids, but this has not altered the rate of neurologic deterioration. However, more promising results have been obtained after bone marrow transplantation.[435]

Familial glucocorticoid deficiency is a rare, autosomal recessive cause of hypoadrenalism that is usually seen in childhood. The renin-angiotensin-aldosterone axis is intact, and children usually present either with neonatal hypoglycemia or later with increasing pigmentation, often with enhanced growth velocity. Patients have glucocorticoid deficiency with very high plasma ACTH levels; this occurs because of mutations in the melanocortin-2 or ACTH receptor (MC2R) on chromosome 18p11.2 in some but not all cases.[436] A variant is called triple A or Allgrove's syndrome[437] and refers to the triad of adrenal insufficiency related to ACTH resistance, achalasia, and alacrima. It is not caused by mutations in the MC2R; studies have mapped this disease to chromosome 12q13, and mutations in a novel gene have been reported.[438]

Secondary Hypoadrenalism (Adrenocorticotropic Hormone Deficiency)

This is a common clinical problem and is most often due to sudden cessation of exogenous glucocorticoid therapy. Such therapy suppresses the hypothalamic-pituitary-adrenal axis with consequent adrenal atrophy, and this may last for months after stopping glucocorticoid treatment. Adrenal atrophy and subsequent deficiency should be anticipated in any subject who has taken more than the equivalent of 30 mg of hydrocortisone per day orally (~7.5 mg/day prednisolone or 0.75 mg/day dexamethasone) for more than 3 weeks. In addition to the magnitude of the dose of glucocorticoid, the timing of administration of the dose may affect the degree of adrenal suppression. Thus, prednisolone in a dose of 5 mg given last thing at night and 2.5 mg in the morning produces more marked suppression of the hypothalamic-pituitary-adrenal axis than 2.5 mg at night and 5 mg in the morning because the larger evening dose blocks the early morning surge of ACTH. Secondary hypoadrenalism may also occur after failure to give adequate glucocorticoid replacement therapy for intercurrent stress in a patient who has received long-term glucocorticoid therapy.

Other causes of secondary adrenal insufficiency (see Table 14–16) reflect inadequate ACTH production from the anterior pituitary gland. In many of these, other pituitary hormones are deficient in addition to ACTH and the patient presents with partial or complete hypopituitarism. The clinical features of hypopituitarism make this a relatively easy diagnosis (see also Chapter 8). Isolated ACTH deficiency is rare but a difficult diagnosis to make.[439] It may occur in patients with lymphocytic hypophysitis. A rare but fascinating cause is related to a defect in the normal post-translational processing of POMC to ACTH by the prohormone convertase enzymes (PC1 and PC2).[440] Such patients may have more generalized defects in peptide processing (e.g., cleavage of proinsulin to insulin) giving rise to diabetes mellitus.[441]

Patients have also been described with mutations in the POMC gene that interrupt the synthesis of ACTH and causes ACTH deficiency. The elucidation of the phenotype of these cases, however, has uncovered a novel role for POMC peptides in regulating appetite and hair color. A central role for α-MSH in regulating food intake through the hypothalamic melanocortin-4 receptor has been established. Thus, in addition to adrenal insufficiency, mutations in the POMC gene result in severe obesity and red hair pigmentation.[442] In recombinant mice lacking the POMC gene, the obese phenotype can be reversed by giving an α-MSH agonist peripherally.[443]

Secondary hypoadrenalism is also observed in patients with Cushing's disease after successful and selective removal of the ACTH-secreting pituitary adenoma. The function of adjacent "normal" pituitary corticotrophs is suppressed and may remain so for many months after surgery.[390, 391]

Clinical Features of Adrenal Insufficiency

Patients with primary adrenal failure usually have both glucocorticoid and mineralocorticoid deficiency. In contrast, those with secondary adrenal insufficiency have an intact renin-angiotensin-aldosterone system. This accounts for differences in salt and water balance in the two groups of patients, which in turn result in different clinical presentations. The most obvious feature that differentiates primary from secondary hypoadrenalism is skin pigmentation (Table 14–19 and Fig. 14–30), which is nearly always present in primary adrenal insufficiency (unless of short duration) and absent in secondary insufficiency. The pigmentation is seen in sun-exposed areas, recent rather than old scars, axillae, nipples, palmar creases, pressure points, and in mucous membranes (buccal, vaginal, vulval, anal). The cause of the pigmentation has long been debated, but it is thought to reflect increased stimulation of the melanocortin-2 receptor by ACTH itself. In autoimmune Addison's disease there may be associated vitiligo (see Fig. 14–30).

The clinical features are related to the rate of onset and severity of adrenal deficiency.[445] In many cases, the disease has an insidious onset and a diagnosis is made only when the patient presents with an acute crisis during an intercurrent illness. Acute adrenal insufficiency or an adrenal or addisonian crisis is a medical emergency manifesting as hypotension and acute circulatory failure (Table 14–20). Anorexia may be an early feature, which progresses to nausea, vomiting, diarrhea, and sometimes abdominal pain. Fever may be present, and hypoglycemia may occur. Patients presenting acutely with adrenal hemorrhage have hypotension; abdominal, flank, or lower chest pain; anorexia; and vomiting. The condition is difficult to diagnose, but evidence of occult hemorrhage (rapidly falling hemoglobin), progressive hyperkalemia, and shock should alert the clinician to the diagnosis.

Alternatively, the patient may present with vague features of chronic adrenal insufficiency—weakness, tiredness, weight loss, nausea, intermittent vomiting, abdominal pain, diarrhea or constipation, general malaise, muscle cramps, arthralgia, and symptoms suggestive of postural hypotension (see Table 14–19). Salt craving may be a feature, and there may be a low-grade fever. Supine blood pressure is usually normal, but almost invariably there is a fall in blood pressure on standing. Although adrenal androgen secretion is lost, this is clinically more apparent in women, who may complain of loss of axillary and pubic hair. Psychiatric symptoms may occur in long-standing cases and include memory impairment, depression, and psychosis.[445] Patients may be inappropriately diagnosed as suffering from chronic fatigue syndrome or anorexia nervosa. These features regress upon treatment with replacement corticosteroids.

In secondary adrenal insufficiency associated with hypopituitarism, the presentation may be related to deficiency of hormones other than ACTH, notably LH or FSH (infertility, oligomenorrhea or amenorrhea, poor libido) and TSH (weight gain, cold intolerance). Fasting hypoglycemia occurs because of loss of the gluconeogenic effects of cortisol. It is rare in adults unless there is concomitant alcohol abuse or additional GH deficiency. However, hypoglycemia is a common presenting feature of ACTH or adrenal insufficiency in childhood.[446] In addition, patients with ACTH deficiency present with malaise, weight loss, and other features of chronic adrenal insufficiency. Rarely, the presentation may be more acute in patients with pituitary apoplexy.

Table 14–19. Clinical Features of Primary Adrenal Insufficiency

Symptom, Sign, or Laboratory Finding	Frequency (%)
Symptom	
Weakness, tiredness, fatigue	100
Anorexia	100
Gastrointestinal symptoms	92
Nausea	86
Vomiting	75
Constipation	33
Abdominal pain	31
Diarrhea	16
Salt craving	16
Postural dizziness	12
Muscle or joint pains	6–13
Sign	
Weight loss	100
Hyperpigmentation	94
Hypotension (<110 mm Hg systolic)	88–94
Vitiligo	10–20
Auricular calcification	5
Laboratory Finding	
Electrolyte disturbances	92
Hyponatremia	88
Hyperkalemia	64
Hypercalcemia	6
Azotemia	55
Anemia	40
Eosinophilia	17

Investigation of Hypoadrenalism

Routine Biochemical Profile

In established primary adrenal insufficiency, hyponatremia is present in about 90% of cases and hyperkalemia in 65%. The blood urea concentration is usually elevated. Hyperkalemia occurs because of aldosterone deficiency and is therefore usually absent in patients with secondary adrenal failure. Hyponatremia may be depletional in an addisonian crisis, but in addition vasopressin levels are elevated, resulting in increased free water retention.[447] Thus, in secondary adrenal insufficiency there may be a dilutional hyponatremia with normal or low blood urea. Reversible abnormalities in liver transaminases frequently occur. Hypercalcemia occurs in 6% of all cases[448] and may be particularly marked in patients with coexisting thyrotoxicosis. However, free thyroxine concentrations are usually low or normal but TSH values are frequently moderately elevated.[449] This is a direct effect of glucocorticoid deficiency and reverses with replacement therapy. Persistent elevation of TSH in association with positive thyroid autoantibodies suggests concomitant autoimmune thyroid disease.

Mineralocorticoid Status

In primary hypoadrenalism, mineralocorticoid deficiency usually occurs with elevated plasma renin activity and either low or low normal plasma aldosterone. The investigation of zona glomerulosa activity is frequently neglected in Addison's

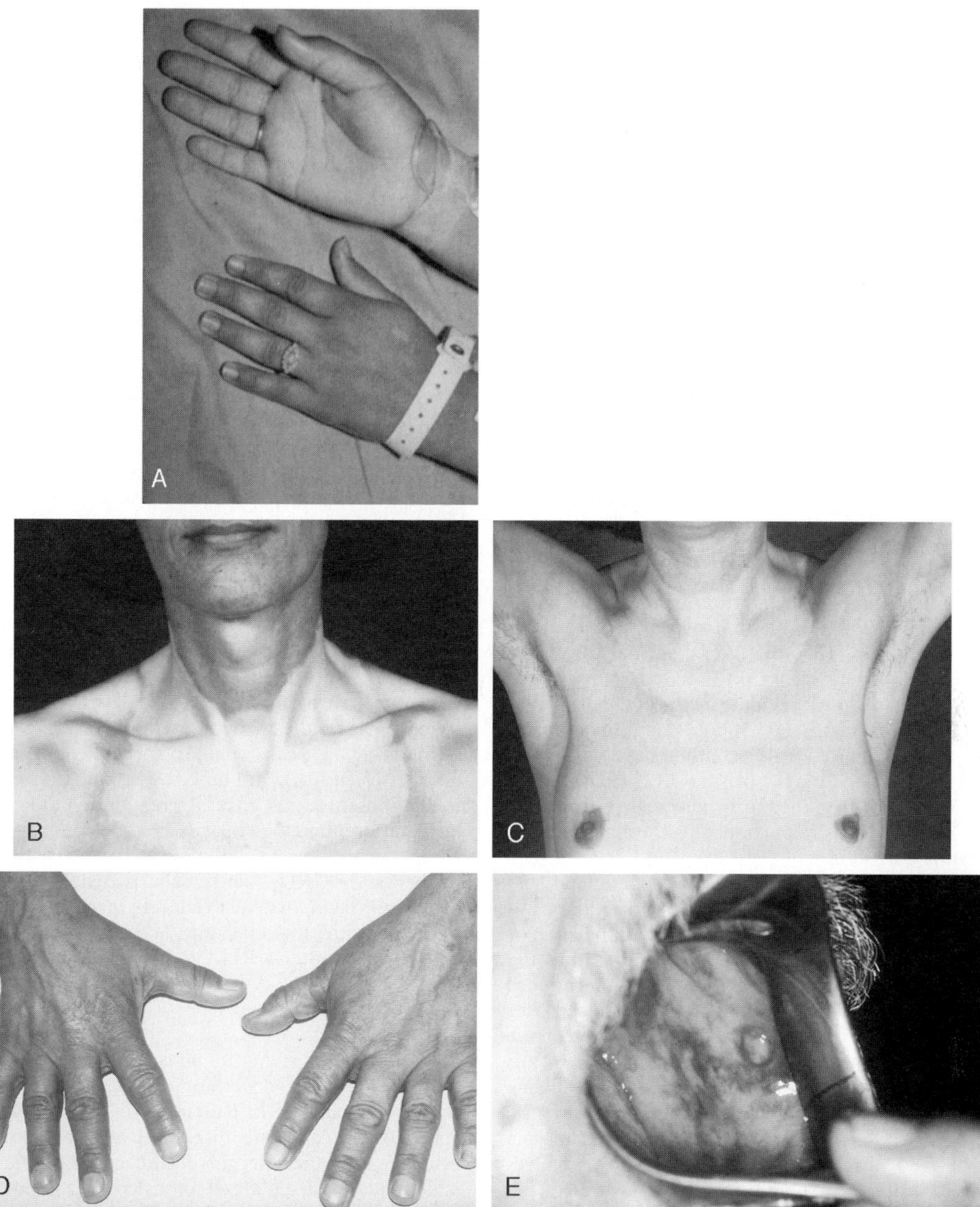

Figure 14–30. Pigmentation in Addison's disease. *A*, Hands of an 18-year-old woman with autoimmune polyendocrine syndrome and Addison's disease. Pigmentation in a patient with Addison's disease before (*B*) and after (*C*) treatment with hydrocortisone and fludrocortisone. Note the additional presence of vitiligo. *D*, Similar changes also seen in a 60-year-old man with tuberculous Addison's disease before and after corticosteroid therapy. *E*, Buccal pigmentation in the same patient. (*B* and *C*, courtesy of Professor C.R.W. Edwards.) (See also Color Plate.)

Table 14–20. Clinical and Laboratory Features of an Adrenal Crisis

Dehydration, hypotension, or shock out of proportion to severity of current illness
Nausea and vomiting with a history of weight loss and anorexia
Abdominal pain, so-called acute abdomen
Unexplained hypoglycemia
Unexplained fever
Hyponatremia, hyperkalemia, azotemia, hypercalcemia, or eosinophilia
Hyperpigmentation or vitiligo
Other autoimmune endocrine deficiencies, such as hypothyroidism or gonadal failure

disease as compared with assessment of zona fasciculata function. In secondary adrenal insufficiency, the renin-angiotensin-aldosterone system is intact.

Assessing Adequacy of Function of the Hypothalamo-Pituitary-Adrenal Axis

Clinical suspicion of the diagnosis should be confirmed with definitive diagnostic tests. Basal plasma cortisol and urinary free cortisol levels are often in the low normal range and cannot be used to exclude the diagnosis. However, a basal cortisol value greater than 400 nmol/L (15 μg/dL) invariably indicates an intact HPA axis.[450] In practice, rather than waiting for results of insensitive basal tests, all patients suspected of having adrenal insufficiency should have an ACTH stimulation test, although in patients with an addisonian crisis treatment should be instigated immediately and stimulation tests conducted at a later stage.

The ACTH stimulation test involves intramuscular or intravenous administration of 250 μg of tetracosactrin (Synacthen), comprising the first 24 amino acids of normally secreted ACTH 1 to 39.[451] Plasma cortisol levels are measured at 0 and 30 minutes after ACTH, and a normal response is defined by a peak plasma cortisol level greater than 525 nmol/L (19 μg/dL).[452] This value equates to the fifth percentile response in normal subjects but is assay-dependent, with different cortisol radioimmunoassays giving different results. Incremental responses (i.e., the difference between peak and basal values) are of no value in defining a pass response and should not be used. Response is unaffected by the time of day of the test, and the test can be performed in patients who have commenced corticosteroid replacement therapy provided this is of short duration and does not include hydrocortisone (which would cross-react in the cortisol assay).

A prolonged ACTH stimulation test, involving the administration of depot or intravenous infusions of tetracosactrin for 24 to 48 hours, differentiates primary from secondary hypoadrenalism. In normal subjects the plasma cortisol at 4 hours is greater than 1000 nmol/L (36 μg/dL), and beyond this time there is no further increase. Patients with secondary hypoadrenalism show a delayed response with usually a much higher value at 24 and 48 hours than at 4 hours, but in primary hypoadrenalism there is no response at either time. However, the test is now rarely required if plasma ACTH has been appropriately measured at baseline. In primary adrenal insufficiency the ACTH level is disproportionately elevated in comparison with plasma cortisol.[453]

Although there is agreement about the investigation of suspected primary adrenal failure, the diagnosis of secondary hypoadrenalism, notably in patients with existing hypothalamic or pituitary disease, is contentious. Based on correlations with the response of circulating cortisol to surgery, the insulin-induced hypoglycemia test or insulin tolerance test was introduced over 30 years ago as a laboratory test to assess the integrity of the HPA axis and should be considered the "gold standard" in this regard.[454] It should not be performed in patients with ischemic heart disease (always check an electrocardiogram before the test), epilepsy, or severe hypopituitarism (that is, 9 AM plasma cortisol less than 180 nmol/L [6 μg/dL]). The test involves intravenous administration of soluble insulin in a dose of 0.1 to 0.15 U/kg body weight with measurement of plasma cortisol at 0, 30, 45, 60, 90, and 120 minutes. Adequate hypoglycemia (blood glucose less than 39 μg/dL (2.2 mmol/L) with signs of neuroglycopenia—sweating and tachycardia) is essential. In normal subjects the peak plasma cortisol exceeds 500 nmol/L (18 μg/dL).

However, the cortisol response to hypoglycemia can be reliably predicted by the response to acute ACTH stimulation (see earlier), a safer, cheaper, and quicker test.[451, 455] This test relies on the principle that the cortisol response to an exogenous bolus of ACTH is determined by the endogenous ACTH trophic drive to the adrenal cortex, impaired ACTH secretion from the anterior pituitary resulting in an impaired cortisol response after Synacthen. However, the ACTH test should not be used to diagnose secondary hypoadrenalism in patients with a recent pituitary insult (surgery, apoplexy). Total hypophysectomy would result in a failed cortisol response to an insulin tolerance test immediately thereafter, but it takes 2 to 3 weeks for the adrenal cortex to readjust to the reduced level of ACTH secretion; in the interim, a false-positive cortisol response would be seen.

The short Synacthen test should also be avoided in patients with a primary diagnosis of Cushing's disease, in whom an exaggerated cortisol response to ACTH may persist. In clinical practice, if the ACTH test is normal, insulin hypoglycemia testing is not necessary in the vast majority of cases unless there is also a need to document endogenous GH reserve in a patient with pituitary disease. In our practice, an insulin tolerance test is performed if, in a patient with suspected hypopituitarism, there is a subnormal response to ACTH. Some patients have an inadequate response to ACTH but then respond normally to hypoglycemia.[455] They do not require corticosteroid replacement therapy. This approach is open to debate, and even taking into account the preceding caveats, false-positive results have been reported for the short Synacthen test[456, 457]; although these are rare (<2% of cases) this should be noted, particularly in patients with ongoing symptoms and signs indicative of hypoadrenalism.

A low-dose ACTH stimulation test giving only 1 μg of ACTH has been proposed as a screen for adequacy of function of the HPA axis with the suggestion that it may be more sensitive than the conventional 250-μg test.[458–460] Further validation of this test is required to support such a concept.

Two other tests have been advocated to assess adequacy of function of the HPA axis, but their use in modern clinical practice should be restricted to difficult diagnostic cases. In the overnight metyrapone test, metyrapone is given at 30 mg/kg (maximum 3 g) at midnight and plasma cortisol and 11-deoxycortisol are measured at 8 AM the following morning. In patients with an intact axis, ACTH levels rise after the blockade of cortisol synthesis by metyrapone and a normal result is signified by a peak 11-deoxycortisol value greater than 200 nmol/L (7 μg/dL).[461] The CRH stimulation test has been used to diagnose adrenal insufficiency and, unlike the metyrapone test, differentiates primary from secondary causes. Patients with primary adrenal failure have high ACTH levels that rise further after CRH. Conversely, patients with secondary adrenal failure have low ACTH levels that fail to respond to CRH. Patients with hypothalamic disease show a steady rise in ACTH levels after CRH.

Other Tests

Radioimmunoassays to detect autoantibodies such as those against the 21-hydroxylase antigen are now available and should be analyzed in patients with primary adrenal failure. In autoimmune Addison's disease, it is also important to look for evidence of other organ-specific autoimmune disease. A CT scan may reveal enlarged or calcified adrenals, suggesting an infective, hemorrhagic, or malignant diagnosis (Fig. 14–31). Chest radiograph, tuberculin testing, and early morning urine samples cultured for *Mycobacterium tuberculosis* should be obtained if tuberculosis is suspected. CT-guided adrenal biopsy may reveal an underlying diagnosis in patients with suspected malignant deposits in the adrenal. Adrenoleukodystrophy can be diagnosed by measuring circulating levels of very-long-chain fatty acids. Finally, appropriate investigations, including pituitary MRI scans and an assessment of anterior function, are required for patients suspected of having secondary hypoadrenalism who are not receiving corticosteroid therapy.

Treatment of Acute Adrenal Insufficiency

Acute adrenal insufficiency is a life-threatening emergency, and treatment should not be delayed while waiting for definitive proof of diagnosis (Table 14–21). However, in addition to measurement of plasma electrolytes and blood glucose, appropriate samples for ACTH and cortisol should be taken before giving corticosteroid therapy. If the patient is not critically ill, an acute ACTH stimulation test can be performed.

Intravenous hydrocortisone should be given in a dose of 100

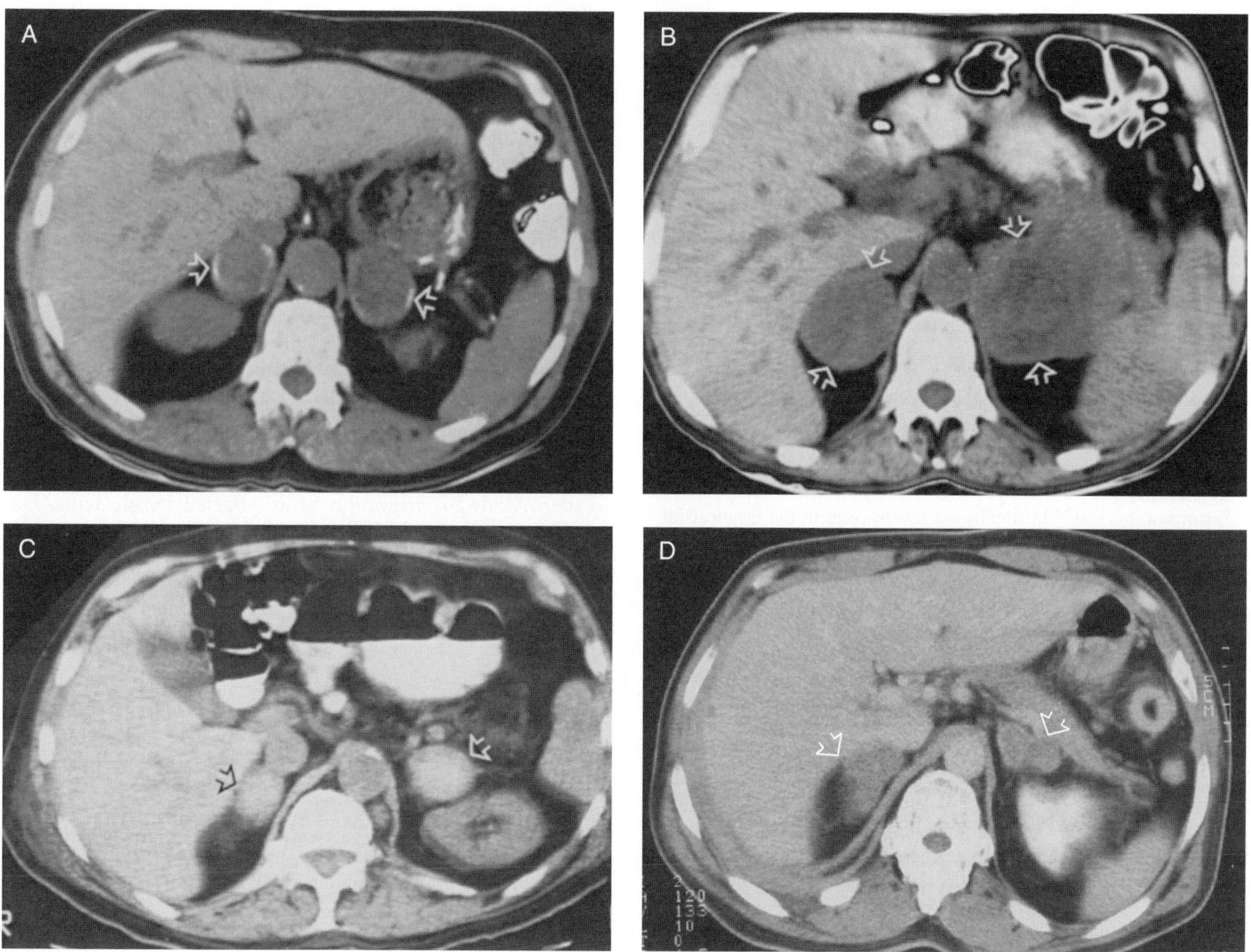

Figure 14–31. Computed tomographic (CT) scans of patients with primary adrenal insufficiency. The affected adrenal glands are indicated by *arrows*. *A*, CT scan of a 59-year-old man with histoplasmosis. Note the subcapsular calcium in both glands. *B*, CT scan of a 59-year-old man with metastatic melanoma. *C*, CT scan of an 80-year-old man with bilateral adrenal hemorrhage resulting from anticoagulation for pulmonary emboli. *D*, Bilateral adrenal tuberculomas in a 79-year-old man with tuberculosis affecting the urogenital tract. (*A* and *B* courtesy of Dr. William D. Salmon, Jr.; *C* courtesy of Dr. Craig R. Sussman.)

mg every 6 hours. If this is not possible, the intramuscular route should be used. In the shocked patient, 1 L of normal saline should be given intravenously over the first hour. Because of possible hypoglycemia, it is usual to give 5% dextrose saline. Subsequent saline and dextrose therapy depends on biochemical monitoring and the patient's condition. Clinical improvement, especially in the blood pressure, should be seen within 4 to 6 hours if the diagnosis is correct. It is important to recognize and treat any associated condition, such as an infection, which may have precipitated the acute adrenal crisis.

After the first 24 hours the dose of hydrocortisone can be reduced, usually to 50 mg intramuscularly every 6 hours, and then, if the patient can take it by mouth, to oral hydrocortisone, 40 mg in the morning and 20 mg at 6 PM. This can then be rapidly reduced to a more standard replacement dose of 20 mg on wakening and 10 mg at 6 PM.

Chronic Replacement Therapy

The aim is to give replacement doses of hydrocortisone to mimic the normal cortisol secretion rate (Table 14–22). Initially this was thought to be approximately 25 to 30 mg/day, but stable isotope studies indicate lower normal cortisol production rates of 22 to 41 μmol/day (8 to 15 mg/day).[463] Increasingly, most patients can cope with less than 84 μmol/day (30 mg/day) (usually 15 to 25 mg/day in divided doses). Doses are usually given on wakening, with a smaller dose in the late afternoon, but some patients may feel better with dosing three times daily. In primary adrenal failure, cortisol day curves with simultaneous ACTH measurements may provide some insight into the adequacy of replacement therapy,[464] but unfortunately there are no good objective tests in secondary adrenal failure. Decisions about doses of replacement therapy are largely based on crude but nevertheless important end points such as weight, well-being, and blood pressure. Bone mineral density may be reduced with conventional hydrocortisone doses of 30 mg/day, highlighting the need to strive for minimally effective but safe doses.[465, 466]

In primary adrenal failure, mineralocorticoid replacement is usually also required in the form of fludrocortisone (or 9α-fluorinated hydrocortisone) at 0.05 to 0.2 mg/day. The mineralocorticoid activity of this is about 125 times that of hydrocortisone. After the acute phase has passed, the adequacy of mineralocorticoid replacement should be assessed by measuring electrolytes and supine and erect blood pressure and plasma renin activity[467]; too little fludrocortisone may cause postural

Table 14–21. Treatment of Acute Adrenal Insufficiency (Adrenal Crisis)

Emergency Measures
1. Establish intravenous access with a large-gauge needle.
2. Draw blood for stat serum electrolytes and glucose and routine measurement of plasma cortisol and ACTH. Do not wait for laboratory results.
3. Infuse 2 to 3 L of 154 mmol/L NaCl (0.9% saline) solution or 50 g/L (5%) dextrose in 154 mmol/L NaCl (0.9% saline) solution as quickly as possible. Monitor for signs of fluid overload by measuring central or peripheral venous pressure and listening for pulmonary rales. Reduce infusion rate if indicated.
4. Inject intravenous hydrocortisone (100 mg immediately and every 6 hr)
5. Use supportive measures as needed.

Subacute Measures After Stabilization of the Patient
1. Continue intravenous 154 mmol/L NaCl (0.9% saline) solution at a slower rate for next 24 to 48 hr.
2. Search for and treat possible infectious precipitating causes of the adrenal crisis.
3. Perform a short ACTH stimulation test to confirm the diagnosis of adrenal insufficiency, if patient does not have known adrenal insufficiency.
4. Determine the type of adrenal insufficiency and its cause if not already known.
5. Taper glucocorticoids to maintenance dosage over 1 to 3 days, if precipitating or complicating illness permits.
6. Begin mineralocorticoid replacement with fludrocortisone (0.1 mg by mouth daily) when saline infusion is stopped.

ACTH, adrenocorticotropic hormone.

hypotension with elevated plasma renin activity and too much may cause the converse. Mineralocorticoid replacement therapy is all too frequently neglected in patients with adrenal failure.[468]

Patients receiving glucocorticoid replacement therapy should be advised to double the daily dose in the event of intercurrent febrile illness, accident, or mental stress such as an important examination. If the patient is vomiting and cannot take medication by mouth, parenteral hydrocortisone must be given urgently, as indicated earlier. For minor surgery, 50 to 100 mg of hydrocortisone hemisuccinate is given with the premedication. For major operations, this is then followed by the same regimen as for acute adrenal insufficiency (see Table 14–22). Pregnancy proceeds normally in patients taking replacement therapy, but daily doses of hydrocortisone are usually increased modestly (5 to 10 mg/day) in the last trimester. During labor, patients should be well hydrated with a saline drip and receive hydrocortisone at 50 mg intramuscularly every 6 hours until delivery. Thereafter, doses can be rapidly tapered off to usual maintenance regimens.

Every patient receiving glucocorticoid therapy should be advised to register for a Medic Alert bracelet or necklace and must carry a Steroid Alert card.

For patients with both primary and secondary adrenal failure, beneficial effects of adrenal androgen replacement therapy with DHEA at 25 to 50 mg/day have been reported. To date, the reported benefit is principally confined to female patients and includes improvement in sexual function and well-being.[469, 470]

Congenital Adrenal Hyperplasia

These inherited syndromes are caused by deficient adrenal corticosteroid biosynthesis. In each case, there is reduced negative feedback inhibition of cortisol and, depending on the steroidogenic pathway involved, alteration in adrenal mineralocorticoid and androgen secretion (Table 14–23).

21-Hydroxylase Deficiency

Ninety percent of cases of CAH are due to 21-hydroxylase deficiency.[471] In Western societies the incidence varies from 1 in 5000 to 1 in 15,000 live births, but in isolated communities the incidence may be much higher (1 in 300 in Alaskan Eskimos, for example). The condition arises because of defective conversion of 17α-hydroxyprogesterone to 11-deoxycortisol. Reduced cortisol biosynthesis results in reduced negative feedback drive and increased ACTH secretion; as a consequence, adrenal androgens are produced in excess (Fig. 14–32). Seventy-five percent of cases have mineralocorticoid deficiency because of failure to convert progesterone to DOC in the zona glomerulosa. Clinically, several distinct variants of 21-hydroxylase deficiency have been recognized (Table 14–24).

Simple Virilizing Form

The enhanced ACTH drive to adrenal androgen secretion in utero leads to virilization of an affected female fetus. Depending on the severity, clitoral enlargement, labial fusion, and development of a urogenital sinus may occur, leading to sexual ambiguity at birth and even inappropriate sex assignment. Rarely, the diagnosis is not made in the neonatal period, especially in boys, who may be phenotypically normal at birth.

Table 14–22. Treatment of Chronic Primary Adrenal Insufficiency

Maintenance Therapy

Glucocorticoid Replacement
- Hydrocortisone 15–20 mg on awakening and 5–10 mg in early afternoon.
- Monitor clinical symptoms and morning plasma ACTH.

Mineralocorticoid Replacement
- Fludrocortisone 0.1 (0.05–0.2) mg orally.
- Liberal salt intake.
- Monitor lying and standing blood pressure and pulse, edema, serum potassium, and plasma renin activity.
- Educate patient about the disease, how to manage minor illnesses and major stresses, and how to inject steroid intramuscularly.
- Obtain Medic Alert bracelet/necklace, Emergency Medical Information Card.

Treatment of Minor Febrile Illness or Stress
- Increase glucocorticoid dose twofold to threefold for the few days of illness; do not change mineralocorticoid dose.
- Contact physician if illness worsens or persists for more than 3 days or if vomiting develops.
- No extra supplementation is needed for most uncomplicated, outpatient dental procedures under local anesthesia. General anesthesia or intravenous sedation should not be used in the office.

Emergency Treatment of Severe Stress or Trauma
- Inject contents of prefilled dexamethasone (4-mg) syringe intramuscularly.
- Get to physician as quickly as possible.

Steroid Coverage for illness or Surgery in Hospital
- For moderate illness give hydrocortisone 50 mg twice a day orally or intravenously. Taper rapidly to maintenance dose as patient recovers.
- For severe illness give hydrocortisone 100 mg intravenously every 8 hr. Taper dose to maintenance level by decreasing by half every day. Adjust dose according to course of illness.
- For minor procedures under local anesthesia and most radiologic studies, no extra supplementation is needed.
- For moderately stressful procedures, such as barium enema, endoscopy, or arteriography, give a single 100 mg intravenous dose of hydrocortisone just before the procedure.
- For major surgery, give hydrocortisone 100 mg intravenously just before induction of anesthesia and continue every 8 hr for first 24 hr. Taper dose rapidly, decreasing by half per day, to maintenance level.

Table 14–23. Congenital Adrenal Hyperplasia: Features for Each Enzyme Defect

Feature	21-Hydroxylase Deficiency	11β-Hydroxylase Deficiency	17α-Hydroxylase Deficiency	3β-Hydroxysteroid Defeciency	Lipoid Hyperplasia	Aldosterone Synthase Deficiency
Defective gene	*CYP21*	*CYP11B1*	*CYP17*	*HSD3B2*	*StAR*	*CYP11B2*
Chromosomal localization	6p21.3	8q24.3	10q24.3	1p13.1	8p11.2	8q24.3
Ambiguous genitalia	+(female)	+(female)	+(male) Absent puberty (female)	+(male) Mild in female	+(male) Absent puberty (female)	No
Acute adrenal insufficiency	+	Rare	No	+	++	Salt wasting only
Incidence	1:15,000	1:100,000	Rare	Rare	Rare	Rare
Hormones						
Glucocorticoids	Reduced	Reduced	Reduced	Corticosterone normal	Reduced	Normal
Mineralocorticoids	Reduced	Increased	Reduced	Increased	Reduced	Reduced
Androgens	Increased	Increased	Reduced	Reduced (male) Increased (female)	Reduced	Normal
Elevated metabolite	17-Hydroxy-progesterone	DOC, 11-deoxycortisol	B, DOC	DHEA, $17\Delta^5$-pregnenolone	None	B, 18-OHB
Blood pressure, sodium balance	Decreased	Increased	Decreased	Increased	Decreased	Decreased
Potassium	Increased	Decreased	Increased	Decreased	Increased	Increased

B, corticosterone; DHEA, dehydroepiandrosterone; DOC, deoxycorticosterone; 18-OHB, 18-hydroxycorticosterone.

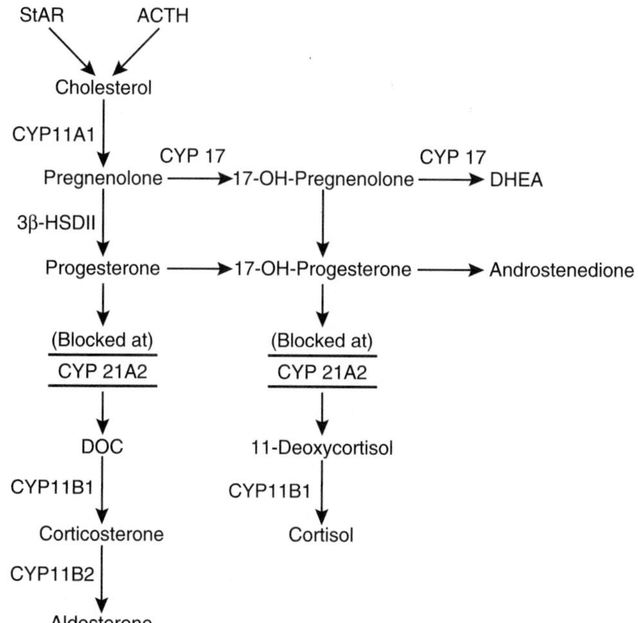

Figure 14–32. Congenital adrenal hyperplasia related to 21-hydroxylase deficiency. The normal synthesis of cortisol is impaired, and adrenocorticotropic hormone (ACTH) levels increase because of loss of normal negative feedback inhibition resulting in an increase in adrenal steroid precursors proximal to the block. The results are cortisol deficiency, variable mineralocorticoid deficiency, and excessive secretion of adrenal androgens. DHEA, dehydroepiandrosterone; DOC, deoxycorticosterone; HSD, hydroxysteroid dehydrogenase; StAR, steroidogenic acute regulatory protein.

Such patients may present in early childhood with sexual precocity and pubic hair development. Initially, linear growth is accelerated because of premature androgen excess, but if left untreated this stimulates epiphyseal closure and final adult height is invariably diminished.[472, 473]

Salt-Wasting Form

Seventy-five percent of cases in both sexes also have concomitant aldosterone deficiency. In addition to the preceding features, neonates may present within the first week of life with a salt-wasting crisis and hypotension. Indeed, this may alert the clinician to the diagnosis in a male, but unfortunately the diagnosis is still delayed in many cases and the condition carries a significant neonatal mortality rate.

Cryptic or "Late-Onset" 21-Hydroxylase Deficiency

Patients present in childhood or early adulthood with premature pubarche or with a phenotype that may masquerade as polycystic ovary syndrome (PCOS).[471, 474] Indeed, late-onset CAH is a recognized secondary cause of PCOS and appears to be commoner than the classical variety.[475] In some series from tertiary referral centers, late-onset 21-hydroxylase deficiency may account for up to 12% of all patients with PCOS, but more realistic prevalence rates are probably 1% to 3%. Females present with hirsutism, primary or secondary amenorrhea or anovulatory infertility.[476] Androgenic alopecia and acne may be other presenting features. Males may develop enlargement of the testes related to adrenal rests, that is, ectopic adrenal tissue within the testes that regresses after glucocorticoid suppression of ACTH secretion.[477]

Heterozygote Deficiency

Salt-wasting, simple virilizing, and late-onset 21-hydroxylase deficiencies are all caused by homozygous or compound het-

Table 14–24. Different Forms of 21-Hydroxylase Deficiency

Phenotype	Classical Salt Wasting	Simple Virilizing	Nonclassical
Age at diagnosis	Newborn–6 mo	Newborn–2 yr (female) 2–4 yr (male)	Child–adult
Genitalia	Males normal; females ambiguous	Males normal; females ambiguous	Males normal, females virilized
Incidence	1:20,000	1:60,000	1:1000
Hormones			
Aldosterone	Reduced	Normal	Normal
Renin	Increased	Normal or increased	Normal
Cortisol	Reduced	Reduced	Normal
17-Hydroxyprogestrone	>5000 nmol/L	2500–5000 nmol/L	500–2500 nmol/L (ACTH stimulation)
Testosterone	Increased	Increased	Variable, increased
Growth	−2–3 SD	−1–2 SD	Probably normal
21-Hydroxylase activity (% of wild type)	0%	1%	20%–50%
Typical *CYP21A2* mutations	Deletions, conversions, nt656g G110Δ8nt, R356W I236N, V237E, M239K, Q318X	I172N nt656g	V281L P30L

ACTH, adrenocorticotropic hormone; SD, standard deviation.

erozygous mutations in the human *CYP21A2* gene, whereas in the carrier, heterozygote state, only one allele is mutated. The clinical significance of the heterozygote state is uncertain; it does not appear to affect reproductive capability but may cause signs of hyperandrogenism in women.[471]

Two *CYP21A2* genes are located within 50 kb of the short arm of chromosome 6 within the major histocompatibility locus, a 3′ *CYP21A2B* gene encoding the functional enzyme and a pseudogene, *CYP21A2A* (Fig. 14–33). These two genes are closely homologous, and at least 25% of cases of 21-hydroxylase deficiency arise because of unequal crossover and genetic recombination of these two genes at meiosis. Although mutations have been identified within the *CYP21A2B* gene in affected kindreds (point mutations, gene conversions, and deletions[471, 478]), the relationship between genotype and phenotype is complex.[479] Severe mutations within the gene do not correlate with a severe phenotype either within families or in individual cases. Phenotypic variability (e.g., salt wasting, age of onset) seems likely to depend on other interacting genes rather than *CYP21A2B* itself. The condition is inherited as an autosomal recessive trait, and the higher incidence of the condition in some ethnic communities is almost certainly related to consanguinity.

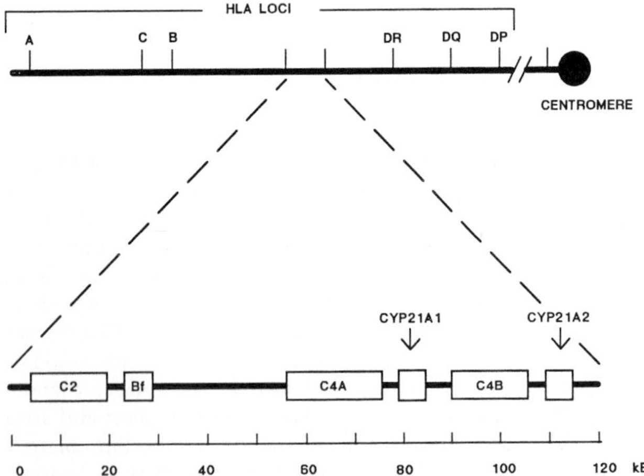

Figure 14–33. Map of the short arm of human chromosome 6 *(upper bar)*, showing the relative positions of the genes encoding the major histocompatibility proteins A, C, B, DR, DQ, and DP. The detail *(lower bar)* shows the approximately 120-kilobase region containing the genes for complement component C2, properdin factor B (Bf), and the duplicated complement C4 gene (C4A and C4B). The pseudogene *CYP21A1* and the functional gene *CYP21A2* are in tandem array with the two C4 genes. HLA, human leukocyte antigen.

A *diagnosis of 21-hydroxylase deficiency* should be considered in any newborn infant with genital ambiguity, salt wasting, or hypotension. Hyponatremia and hyperkalemia with raised plasma renin activity are found in salt wasters. In later life, adrenal androgen excess (DHEAS, androstenedione) is found in patients presenting with sexual precocity or a PCOS-like phenotype. 17-Hydroxyprogesterone (17-OHP) is invariably elevated, and clinically useful nomograms have been developed comparing circulating concentrations of 17-OHP before and 60 minutes after exogenous ACTH.[480] This separates patients with classical and nonclassical 21-hydroxylase deficiency from heterozygote carriers and normal subjects, but there is some overlap between values seen in heterozygotes and normal people. 17-OHP is measured basally and then 60 minutes after 250 μg of Synacthen. Stimulated values are invariably grossly elevated in patients with classical and nonclassical varieties (in excess of 35 nmol/L [11 μg/dL]). Heterozygote patients usually have stimulated values between 10 and 30 nmol/L (3 to 9 μg/dL) (Fig. 14–34). Stimulation tests are not always required to make a diagnosis; for example, a basal 17α-OHP concentration less than 5 nmol/L in the follicular phase of the menstrual cycle effectively excludes late-onset 21-hydroxylase deficiency.[476] Increasingly, genotyping programs will form a useful adjunct to hormonal measurements. Androgen excess in 21-hydroxylase deficiency is readily suppressed after glucocorticoid administration.

Prenatal diagnosis of 21-hydroxylase deficiency has been advocated because treatment of an affected female may prevent masculinization in utero.[481] 17-OHP can be assayed in amniotic fluid, but the most robust approach is the rapid genotyping of fetal cells obtained by chorionic villus sampling in early gestation. Unlike hydrocortisone, which is inactivated by placental 11β-HSD, maternally administered dexamethasone can cross the placenta to suppress the fetal HPA axis. One approach is to advocate dexamethasone therapy as soon as pregnancy is confirmed in high-risk cases and to continue this until the diagnosis is excluded in the fetus. If the fetus is affected, only those of female sex require dexamethasone therapy during

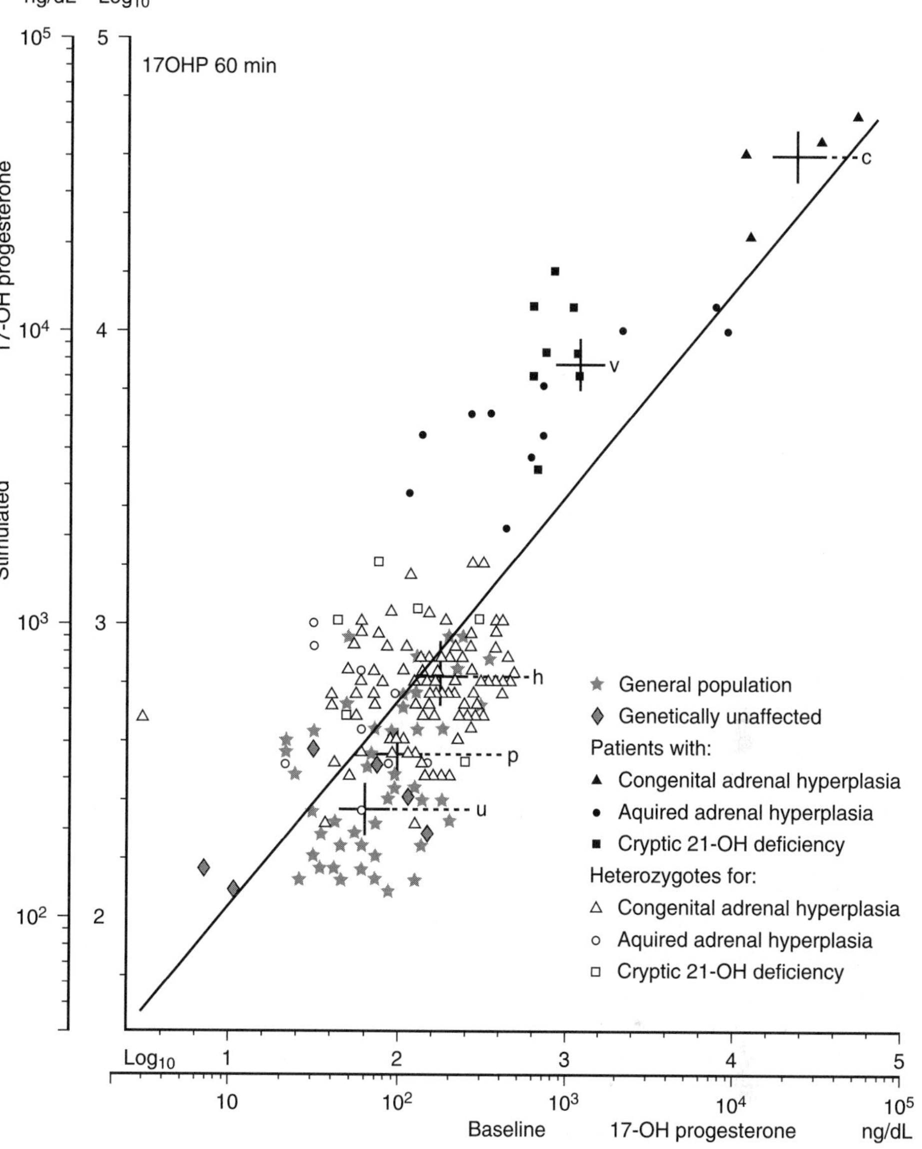

Figure 14–34. Basal and stimulated plasma 17α-hydroxyprogesterone (17OHP) concentrations in patients with CYP21A2 (21-hydroxylase) deficiency. To convert values to nmol/L, multiply by 0.0303. The mean for each group is indicated by a large cross and the adjacent letter: c, patients with classical CYP21A2 deficiency; v, patients with nonclassical (acquired and cryptic) CYP21A2 deficiency; h, heterozygotes for all forms of CYP21A2 deficiency; p, general population; u, known unaffected persons (e.g., siblings of patients with CYP21A2 deficiency who carry neither affected parental haplotype as determined by human leukocyte antigen typing). (From White PC, New MI, Dupont B. Congenital adrenal hyperplasia: part 1. Reprinted by permission of The New England Journal of Medicine 1987; 316:1519–1524.)

gestation. Therapy must be initiated before 8 to 10 weeks of gestation to be effective. However, because only one in eight cases treated in this way have an affected female fetus, the use of steroid therapy in this setting has been questioned.[482] Dexamethasone can lead to maternal cushingoid effects in pregnancy[483] and may in turn have long-term, deleterious effects on the fetus.

In patients with known cases requesting fertility (be they male or female), determination of 17-OHP levels through a Synacthen test in the partner before conception uncovers late-onset or heterozygote cases and provides the endocrinologist or geneticist with some assignment of risk before pregnancy.

Treatment

The objectives in treating 21-hydroxylase deficiency differ with age, but at all ages treatment and overall management can be fraught with difficulties. In childhood the overall goal is to replace glucocorticoid and mineralocorticoid, thereby preventing further salt-wasting crises, but also to suppress adrenal androgen secretion so that normal growth and skeletal maturation can proceed.[473] Accurate replacement is essential; glucocorticoids in excess suppress growth, and inadequate replacement results initially in accelerated linear growth but ultimately in short stature because of premature epiphyseal closure.[471] Response is best monitored through growth velocity and bone age, with biochemical markers (17-OHP, DHEAS, testosterone) being useful adjuncts. In difficult cases, a day curve study as described for patients with primary adrenal failure, but measuring the ACTH and 17-OHP response before and after corticosteroid replacement, may confirm overreplacement or underreplacement. Corrective surgery is frequently required (clitoral reduction, vaginoplasty) during childhood.

In late childhood and adolescence, appropriate replacement therapy is equally important. Overtreatment may result in obesity and delayed menarche or puberty with sexual infantilism, whereas underreplacement results in sexual precocity. Compliance with regular medication is often an issue through adolescence.

Although much has been written about adequate control in childhood, adults with CAH often provide an ongoing dilemma for the endocrinologist. The follow-up of such patients should involve multidisciplinary clinics, initially with transition adolescence clinics to facilitate transfer from pediatric to adult care. Problems in adulthood are related to fertility concerns, hirsutism and menstrual irregularity in women, obesity and impact of short stature, sexual dysfunction, and psychological problems[471, 484, 485]; counseling is often required in addition to endocrine support.

In the absence of any evidence-based data, there are no prescriptive steroid regimens to treat patients with CAH at any age, and as a result many individualized regimens are used in clinical practice. Usual starting doses of hydrocortisone in childhood are 10 to 25 mg/m^2 per day in divided doses. Reverse-phase therapy may be appropriate, giving the largest dose of hydrocortisone at night to suppress early morning ACTH secretion. Long-acting steroids such as dexamethasone are more effective in this regard, but care should be taken to avoid oversuppression and reduction in linear growth. Fludrocortisone is required for patients with salt wasting (although this may improve spontaneously with age); doses of 0.1 to 0.2 mg/day should be given and blood pressure, electrolytes, and supine-erect plasma renin activity monitored to assess response. Fludrocortisone may improve linear growth in patients with simple virilizing CAH even if they are not salt wasters.[486]

In women with hyperandrogenism and untreated late-onset CAH, there is no evidence that final height is affected. In this setting, glucocorticoid suppression in isolation rarely controls hirsutism and additional antiandrogen therapy is often required (cyproterone acetate, spironolactone, flutamide together with an oral estrogen contraceptive pill). However, ovulation induction rates with gonadotropin therapy are improved after suppression of nocturnal ACTH levels with 0.25 to 0.5 mg of dexamethasone. Once final height is achieved in adult males, strict control is required only for patients with adrenal rests within the testes or to ensure fertility; inadequate replacement therapy may result in adrenal androgen excess suppressing pituitary FSH secretion and lowering sperm counts.[487]

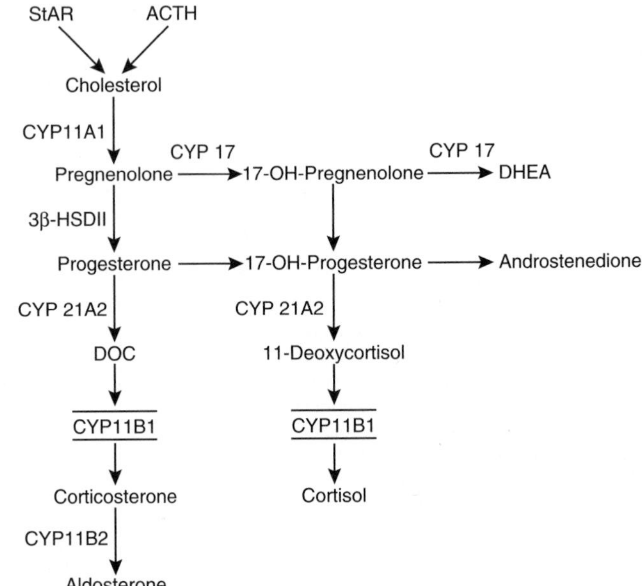

Figure 14–35. Congenital adrenal hyperplasia related to 11β-hydroxylase deficiency. The normal synthesis of cortisol is impaired, and adrenocorticotropic hormone (ACTH) levels increase because of loss of normal negative feedback inhibition resulting in an increase in adrenal steroid precursors proximal to the block. The results are cortisol deficiency, mineralocorticoid excess related to excessive deoxycorticosterone (DOC) secretion, and excessive secretion of adrenal androgens. DHEA, dehydroepiandrosterone; StAR, steroidogenic acute regulatory protein.

11β-Hydroxylase Deficiency

11β-Hydroxylase deficiency accounts for 7% of all cases of CAH with an incidence of 1 per 100,000 live births.[488] The incidence is higher in Israel (1 per 30,000). The condition arises because of mutations in the *CYP11B1* gene that result in loss of enzyme activity and a block in the conversion of 11-deoxycortisol to cortisol. As reported for 21-hydroxylase deficiency, there remains a poor correlation between genotype and phenotype. There is loss of negative cortisol feedback and enhanced ACTH-mediated adrenal androgen excess (Fig. 14–35). Clinical features are therefore similar to those reported in the simple virilizing form of CAH (virilized female fetus, sexual ambiguity), and again milder cases can present later in childhood or even young adulthood. The principal difference compared with 21-hydroxylase deficiency is hypertension, and this is thought to be secondary to the mineralocorticoid effect of DOC excess (see Table 14–23). However, there is a poor correlation between DOC secretion and the presence of hypertension; furthermore, unexplained salt wasting has been reported in a few cases.[489, 490]

On this clinical background, the diagnosis can be made by demonstrating a plasma ACTH-stimulated 11-deoxycortisol value that is more than three times the 95th percentile for an age-matched normal group. Although established heterozygotes do not demonstrate a rise in 11-deoxycortisol above normal after Synacthen[491] (unlike the 17-OHP response observed in heterozygote 21-hydroxylase patients), exaggerated ACTH-stimulated responses have been observed in patients with hirsutism[492] and in patients with essential hypertension,[493] suggesting partial defects in 11β-hydroxylase activity. As reported for 21-hydroxylase deficiency, treatment is with replacement glucocorticoid therapy; with suppression of DOC secretion, plasma renin activity (suppressed at baseline) increases into the normal range.

17α-Hydroxylase Deficiency

Fewer than 150 cases of 17α-hydroxylase deficiency have been reported.[494, 495] Mutations within the CYP17 gene result in the failure to synthesize cortisol (17α-hydroxylase activity), adrenal androgens (17,20-lyase activity), and gonadal steroids[496] (Fig. 14–36). Thus, in contrast to 21-hydroxylase and 11-hydroxylase deficiencies, 17α-hydroxylase deficiency results in adrenal and gonadal insufficiency. A single enzyme is expressed in adrenal and gonad and possesses both 17-hydroxylation and 17,20-lyase activities,[41] but patients with isolated deficiency in the hydroxylation of 17-OHP or 17,20-lyase deficiency have rarely been reported.[497] Loss of negative feedback results in increased secretion of steroids proximal to the block, and mineralocorticoid synthesis is enhanced. However, aldosterone levels are variable and the mineralocorticoid excess state that characterizes this condition is thought to be induced by DOC excess in over 80% of cases.[498]

The genetic basis for the disease has been established in many cases, involving point mutations, gene deletions, and conversions in the *CYP17* gene.[499, 500] Relative hydroxylase and lyase activities of mutant *CYP17* complementary DNAs vary in in vitro transfection assays, but correlations with clinical phenotype are lacking. Thus, patients with clinically pure 17,20-lyase deficiency may have mutant *CYP17* complementary DNAs that exhibit compromised 17-hydroxylase activity.[494]

The diagnosis is usually made at the time of puberty when patients present with hypertension, hypokalemia, and hypogonadism, the latter occurring because of lack of *CYP17* expression within the gonad and impaired gonadal steroidogene-

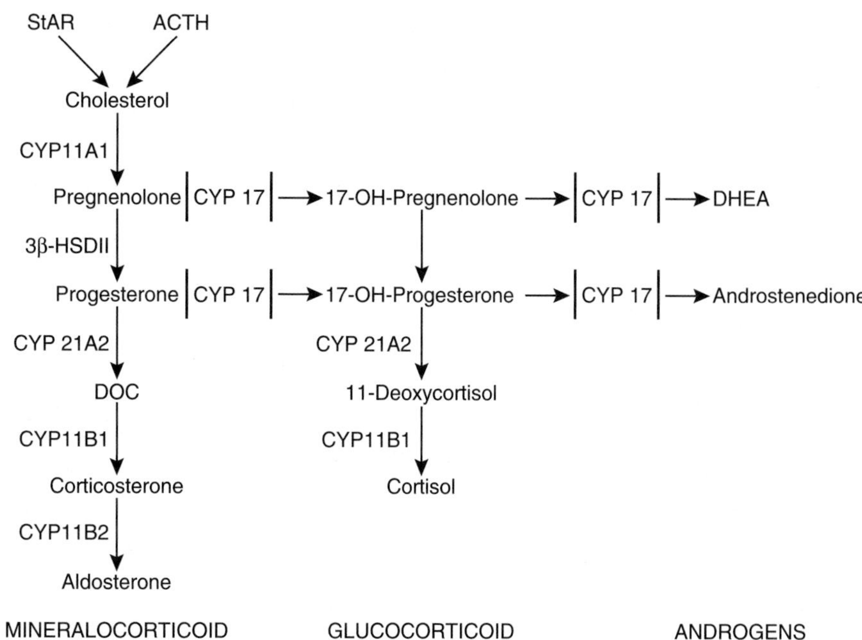

Figure 14–36. Congenital adrenal hyperplasia related to 17-hydroxylase deficiency. The normal synthesis of cortisol is impaired, and adrenocorticotropic hormone (ACTH) levels increase because of loss of normal negative feedback inhibition resulting in an increase in adrenal steroid precursors proximal to the block. The result is cortisol deficiency and mineralocorticoid excess usually related to deoxycorticosterone (DOC) excess. Because gonadal 17-hydroxylase activity is also absent, sex steroid secretion in addition to adrenal androgen secretion is severely impaired, resulting in hypogonadism. DHEA, dehydroepiandrosterone; StAR, steroidogenic acute regulatory protein.

sis. As a result, LH and FSH levels are elevated. Female patients (XX) have primary amenorrhea with absent sexual characteristics, and males (46,XY) have complete pseudohermaphroditism with female external genitalia but absent uterus and fallopian tubes. The intra-abdominal testes should be removed, and such patients are usually reared as female.

Glucocorticoid replacement reverses the DOC-induced suppression of the renin-angiotensin system and lowers blood pressure. Additional sex steroid replacement is required from puberty onward.

3β-Hydroxysteroid Dehydrogenase Deficiency

In this rare form of CAH, the secretion of all classes of adrenal and ovarian steroids is impaired because of mutations within the *HSD3B2* gene encoding 3β-HSDII.[501, 502] Patients usually present in early infancy with adrenal insufficiency. Loss of mineralocorticoid secretion results in salt wasting, although this is absent in 30% to 40% of cases (Fig. 14–37). As with 21-hydroxylase deficiency, absence of salt wasting may delay the presentation into childhood or puberty.[503] The correlation between genotype and phenotype is once again poor; identical mutations have been found in the *HSD3B2* gene in both salt wasters and non–salt wasters.[501] The spectrum of genital development is variable in both sexes. In males, because the 3β-HSDII enzyme is also expressed within the gonad, male pseudohermaphroditism may occur with female external genitalia. In milder cases, hypospadias may be found or even normal male genitalia. In females, genital development can be normal but there is usually evidence of mild virilization, presumably because of enhanced adrenal secretion of DHEA, which is converted peripherally to testosterone. A late-onset form has been described in patients with premature pubarche[504] and a PCOS-like phenotype (hirsutism, oligomenorrhea, amenorrhea).[505]

Because activity of the 3β-HSDI enzyme present in skin and other peripheral tissues is intact, circulating Δ4 steroid levels (progesterone, 17α-hydroxyprogesterone, androstenedione) may be normal (or even increased). However, a diagnosis is established by demonstrating an increased ratio of Δ5 steroids (pregnenolone, 17α-hydroxypregnenolone, DHEA) to Δ4 steroids in plasma or urine. ACTH stimulation may be required to detect a late-onset presentation. Treatment is with replacement glucocorticoids, fludrocortisone (if indicated), and sex steroids from puberty onward.

Steroidogenic Acute Regulatory Protein Deficiency

Mutations in the gene encoding StAR result in a failure of transport of cholesterol from the outer to the inner mitochon-

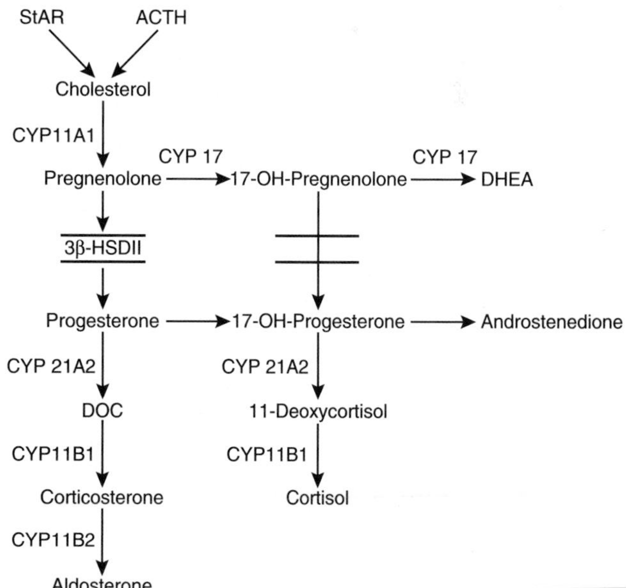

Figure 14–37. Congenital adrenal hyperplasia related to 3β-hydroxysteroid dehydrogenase (3β-HSD) deficiency resulting in cortisol deficiency and variable mineralocorticoid deficiency. Gonadal 3β-HSD activity is also absent, resulting in male pseudohermaphroditism and hypogonadism or primary amenorrhea in females. ACTH, adrenocorticotropic hormone; DOC, deoxycorticosterone; DHEA, dehydroepiandrosterone; StAR, steroidogenic acute regulatory protein.

drial membrane in steroidogenic tissues; as a result, there is deficiency of all adrenal and gonadal steroid hormones.[28, 506] Presentation is with acute adrenal insufficiency in the neonatal period, and males exhibit pseudohermaphroditism because of absent gonadal steroids. The condition is fatal in infancy in two thirds of all cases. The adrenal glands are often massively enlarged and full of lipid; prior to the characterization of StAR, the condition was termed congenital "lipoid" hyperplasia and the candidate gene was thought to be cholesterol side-chain cleavage (*CYP11A1*).[506] In fact, to date, no mutations have been reported in the *CYP11A1* gene; such mutations are thought to be lethal in utero. This clinical phenotype is endorsed by recombinant mouse models lacking the StAR gene.[507]

Apparent Cortisone Reductase Deficiency

In this condition, adrenal glands become hyperplastic because of ACTH stimulation resulting from a defect in cortisol metabolism rather than an inherent defect within the gland itself. Patients with apparent cortisone reductase deficiency have a defect in the conversion of cortisone to cortisol, suggesting inhibition of 11-oxoreductase activity and, by implication, inhibition of the type 1 isozyme of 11β-hydroxysteroid dehydrogenase (11β-HSD1) (see Fig. 14–12). Eight cases have been described; with one exception, all are female (Table 14–25). Cortisol clearance is increased, and ACTH secretion is elevated to maintain normal circulating cortisol concentrations but at the expense of adrenal androgen excess. As a consequence, patients described are usually women who present with hirsutism, menstrual irregularity, or androgenic alopecia.

Dexamethasone treatment to suppress ACTH has been used with some success to control the hyperandrogenism in these cases. Urinary tetrahydro metabolites of cortisol and cortisone show almost exclusively THE with little or no detectable THF or allo-THF (ratio of THF + allo-THF to THE less than 0.05, reference range 0.8 to 1.3). Further studies have also shown impaired plasma cortisol concentrations after an oral dose of cortisone acetate. Despite this biochemical evidence implicating a defect in 11β-HSD1, investigations have revealed no mutations to date in the *HSD11B1* gene in affected cases.[508–514]

Patients with PCOS share many of the same clinical characteristics as those with apparent cortisone reductase deficiency. Although there is evidence to support increased cortisol secretion rates in PCOS, perhaps indicative of a defect in conversion of cortisone to cortisol, there remains to be a consensus with respect to THF + allo-THF/THE ratios. Both normal and reduced ratios have been reported in the literature.

Table 14–25. Clinical and Biochemical Characteristics of Reported Cases of Apparent Cortisone Reductase Deficiency

Age	Sex	Clinical Features	Serum Androgens	THF + allo THF: THE ratio	Comments	Reference
28	F	Hirsuitism	↑ Testosterone ↑ DHEAS ↑ Androstenedione	—	Marked fall in serum androgens on treatment with dexamethasone	510
17	F	Oligomenorrhea, hirsuitism, acne, obesity	↑ Testosterone ↑ DHEAS	0.039	Fall in androgens with dexamethasone treatment although developed cushingoid side effects.	511
18	F	Oligomenorrhea, hirsuitism, acne		0.045	Sibling of preceding patient. Fall in androgens with treatment.	511
30	F	Oligomenorrhea, hirsuitism, infertility	↑ Testosterone	—	Fall in testosterone with treatment.	512
	M	Excess body hair (sibling of preceding patient)		—	Sibling of preceding patient. No mutations on genetic sequence analysis of *HSD11B1*	508
37	F	Obesity, oligomenorrhea, hirsuitism	↑ Testosterone ↑ DHEAS ↑ Androstenedione	0.03 (0.5–1.15)	No mutations on genetic sequence analysis of *HSD11B1*	514
	F	Congenital adrenal hyperplasia diagnosed shortly after birth (21-hydroxylase deficiency). 17-Hydroxyprogesterone levels unresponsive to cortisone acetate		↓	17-OHP levels suppressed completely with prednisolone, indicative of an inability to activate cortisone acetate. No mutations on genetic sequence analysis of *HSD11B1*	513
55	F	Androgenetic alopecia, mild hirsutism	↑ Testosterone	0.04 (0.5–0.8)	No mutations on genetic sequence analysis of *HSD11B1*	509

DHEAS, dehydroepiandrosterone sulfate; allo-THF, 5α-tetrahydrocortisol; THE, tetrahydrocortisone; THF, 5β-tetrahydrocortisol.

Mineralocorticoid Deficiency

These syndromes are listed in Table 14–26. They can be divided into those that are congenital and others that are acquired. Mineralocorticoid deficiency may occur in some forms of CAH and with other causes of adrenal insufficiency (e.g., Addison's disease and congenital adrenal hypoplasia) (see preceding).

Primary Defects in Aldosterone Biosynthesis: Aldosterone Synthase Deficiency

Failure of conversion of corticosterone to 18-hydroxycorticosterone or of 18-hydroxycorticosterone to aldosterone usually results in a salt-wasting crisis in neonatal life. Hyperkalemia, metabolic acidosis, dehydration, and hyponatremia are found. The condition has been called corticosterone methyl oxidase (CMO) deficiency, but this was before the final enzyme or enzymes involved in the conversion of DOC to aldosterone were characterized and cloned.[515, 516] In fact, a single enzyme, aldosterone synthase, carries a multistep reaction involving 11-hydroxylation of DOC to corticosterone and 18-hydroxylation of corticosterone to 18-hydroxycorticosterone followed by 18-dehydrogenation to aldosterone (see Fig. 14–3).

Two variants of CMO deficiency are described; CMO I is characterized by low 18-hydroxycorticosterone and aldosterone levels, whereas patients with CMO II deficiency have hypoaldosteronism but high 18-hydroxycorticosterone levels. In both cases, mutations in the gene encoding aldosterone synthase have been described and the discrepant 18-hydroxycorticosterone levels seem likely to be explained on the basis of variable 18-hydroxylase activity of the related CYP45011β-hydroxylase enzyme.[488, 517, 518] CMO II is much more common in Iranian Jews than the white population.

Defects in Aldosterone Action: Pseudohypoaldosteronism

Pseudohypoaldosteronism type I may occur in neonatal life with respiratory difficulties but is usually found in infancy with severe salt wasting and failure to thrive, with very high plasma aldosterone and plasma renin activity levels and inappropriate urinary sodium loss.[519, 520] The MR appears to be defective, as judged by studies evaluating the binding of aldosterone to monocytes, but molecular studies have failed to show any abnormality in the MR itself.[521] Rather, inactivating mutations in the α, β, and γ subunits of the epithelial sodium channel have been shown to explain the condition.[522] Acquired forms of pseudohypoaldosteronism can occur in patients after renal transplantation, following obstructive uropathy, and in premature infants.

Pseudohypoaldosteronism type II or Gordon's syndrome is an autosomal dominant disorder characterized by hyperkalemia but not salt wasting, in contrast to the type I condition. Patients have resistance to the mineralocorticoid effects of aldosterone on tubular potassium transport but not to those of sodium and chloride transport. As a result, affected individuals have hyperchloremia, hypertension, and suppression of plasma renin activity.[523] Recently, deletions in the WNK4 gene (a member of the WNK family of serine-threonine kinases) have been described in affected cases.[524]

Table 14–26. Causes of Mineralocorticoid Deficiency

Addison's disease
Adrenal hypoplasia
Congenital adrenal hyperplasia (21-hydroxylase and 3β-hydroxysteroid dehydrogenase deficiencies)
Pseudohypoaldosteronism types I and II
Hyporeninmic hypoaldosteronism
Aldosterone biosynthetic defects
Drug induced

Hyporeninemic Hypoaldosteronism

Angiotensin II is a key stimulus to aldosterone secretion, and damage or blockade of the renin-angiotensin system may result in mineralocorticoid deficiency. Various renal conditions have been associated with damage to the juxtaglomerular apparatus and hence renin deficiency. These include systemic lupus erythematosus, myeloma, amyloid, AIDS, and use of nonsteroidal anti-inflammatory drugs, but the most common (greater than 75% cases) is diabetic nephropathy.[525–527]

The usual picture is of an elderly patient with hyperkalemia, acidosis, and mild to moderate impairment of renal function. Plasma renin activity and aldosterone are low and fail to respond to sodium depletion, the erect posture, or furosemide administration. In contrast to those with adrenal insufficiency, patients have normal or elevated blood pressure and no postural hypotension. Muscle weakness and cardiac arrhythmias may also occur. Other factors may contribute to the hyperkalemia, including the use of potassium-sparing diuretics, potassium supplementation, insulin deficiency, and β-adrenoceptor blocking drugs and prostaglandin synthetase inhibitors, which inhibit renin release.

Treatment of primary renin deficiency is with fludrocortisone in the first instance together with dietary potassium restriction. However, these patients are not salt depleted and may become hypertensive with fludrocortisone. In such a scenario, the addition of a loop-acting diuretic such as furosemide is appropriate. This increases acid excretion and improves the metabolic acidosis.

Adrenal Adenomas, Incidentalomas, and Carcinomas

Etiology of Adrenal Tumors

The underlying basis for adrenal tumorigenesis is unknown. Clonal analysis suggests progression from a normal to adenomatous to carcinomatous lesion, but the molecular pathways involved remain obscure. Several factors have been associated with malignant transformation including genes encoding p53, p57 cyclin-dependent kinase, menin, IGF-II, MC2R, and inhibin-α.[528] Mice lacking the inhibin-α gene develop adrenal tumors through a process that is also gonadotropin-dependent.[529]

Adenomas

Cortisol-secreting adrenal adenomas have been discussed in detail ("Cortisol-Secreting Adrenal Adenoma and Carcinoma"), and aldosterone-secreting adenomas (Conn's syndrome) are discussed in Chapter 15.

Pure virilizing benign adrenal adenomas are rare, with approximately 50 cases reported in the literature. The majority of cases occur in women; male cases are restricted to childhood, when presentation is with sexual precocity and accelerated bone age. In females, the majority of cases arise before the menopause with marked hirsutism, deepening of the voice, and amenorrhea. Clitorimegaly is found in 80% of cases. Testosterone is usually strikingly elevated, but gonadotropin levels may not be suppressed. By definition, urinary free cortisol is

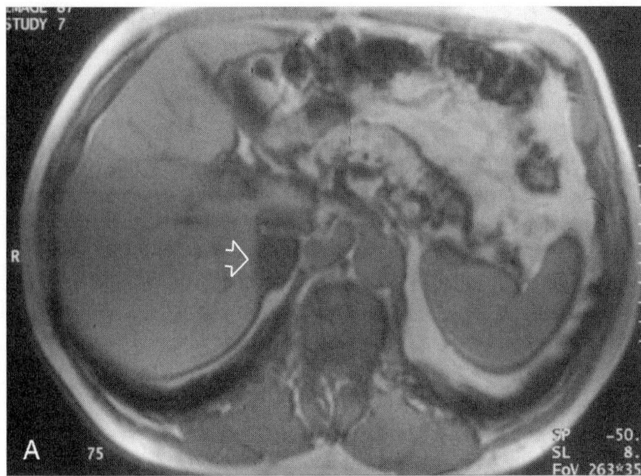

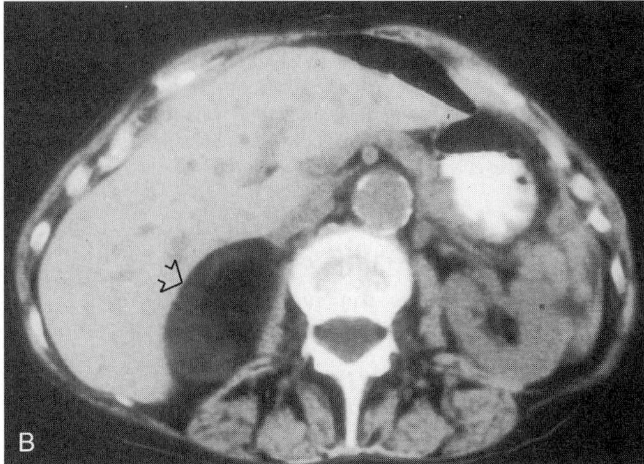

Figure 14–38. *A*, Adrenal incidentaloma discovered in a woman undergoing investigation for abdominal pain. *B*, Incidentally discovered right adrenal myelolipoma.

normal. Tumors vary in size and should be treated surgically. Postoperatively, clinical features invariably improve and normal menses return.[530]

Incidentalomas

Autopsy series had defined the prevalence of adrenal adenomas more than 1 cm in diameter to be between 1.5% and 7%. It is perhaps not surprising, therefore, that with the advent of high-resolution imaging procedures (CT, MRI), incidentally discovered adrenal masses have become a common clinical problem. An adrenal mass is uncovered in up to 4% of patients imaged for nonadrenal pathology.[531] Incidentalomas are uncommon in patients younger than 30 years but increase in frequency with age; they occur equally in males and females. In more than 85% of cases these lesions are nonfunctioning, benign adenomas. Occasionally they may represent myelolipomas, hamartomas, or granulomatous infiltrations of the adrenal and result in a characteristic CT or MRI appearance (Fig. 14–38). Functioning tumors (pheochromocytomas or those secreting cortisol, aldosterone, or sex steroids) and carcinomas make up the remainder.

In addition, it is established that some incidentalomas may cause abnormal hormone secretion without obvious clinical manifestations of a hormone excess state; the best example of this is "preclinical" Cushing's syndrome, which may occur in up to 20% of all cases.[532] This may explain why incidentalomas appear to be commoner in patients with obesity and diabetes mellitus. As a result, all patients with incidentally discovered adrenal masses should undergo appropriate endocrine screening tests. These should comprise 24-hour urinary catecholamine collection, 24-hour urinary free cortisol, and overnight dexamethasone suppression tests. Because of the reported poor sensitivity of serum potassium measurements in detecting primary aldosteronism, our practice has been to measure supine circulating plasma renin activity and aldosterone levels. DHEAS should be measured as a marker of adrenal androgen secretion. Low levels may occur in patients with suppressed ACTH concentrations related to autonomous cortisol secretion from the adenoma,[533] and it is important that DHEAS not be measured during the overnight dexamethasone study. Some studies have also documented high levels of 17-OHP after ACTH stimulation tests, suggesting partial defects in 21-hydroxylase in some tumors.[534]

The possibility of malignancy should be considered in each case. In patients with a known extra-adrenal primary, the incidence of malignancy is obviously much higher (up to 20% of patients with lung cancer, for example, have adrenal metastases on CT scanning). In those with no evidence of malignancy, adrenal carcinoma is rare; in one study, only 26 of 630 incidentalomas were found to be adrenal carcinomas.[531] In true incidentalomas, size appears to be predictive of malignancy; a lesion less than 5 cm in diameter is most unlikely to be malignant. The majority of nonfunctioning lesions less than 5 cm can therefore be treated conservatively and patients followed up with annual imaging. Even incidentalomas larger than 5 cm are more likely to be benign than malignant, but because of an increased risk of malignancy many centers recommend removal of tumors more than 5 cm in diameter, preferably by laparoscopic adrenalectomy. Additional characteristic MRI appearances or scintigraphy studies may aid in differentiating malignant from nonmalignant lesions. CT-guided biopsy is useful in differentiating adrenal from nonadrenal tissue in the case of a suspected metastasis but is poor in differentiating benign adenomas from malignant adrenal lesions.

Carcinomas

Primary adrenal carcinoma is rare, with an incidence of 1 per million population per year. Women are more commonly affected than men (2.5:1); mean age of onset is 40 to 50 years, although men tend to be older at presentation. Eighty percent of tumors are functional, most commonly secreting glucocorticoids alone (45%), glucocorticoids and androgens (45%), or androgens alone (10%). Less than 1% of all cases secrete aldosterone. Patients present with features of the hormone excess state (glucocorticoid or androgen excess, or both), but abdominal pain, weight loss, anorexia, and fever occur in 25% of cases. An abdominal mass may be palpable.[310–312]

Current treatments for what is often an aggressive tumor are poor. Surgery offers the only chance of cure for patients with local disease, but metastatic spread is evident in 75% of cases at presentation. Radiotherapy is ineffective, as are most chemotherapeutic regimens. Mitotane in high doses offers transient benefit in reducing tumor growth in 25% to 30% of cases and controlling hormonal hypersecretion in 75% of cases.[311] Overall, the prognosis is poor, with 5-year survival rates of less than 20%.[535]

References

1. Eustachius B. Tabulae Anatomicae. Lancisius B, ed. Amsterdam, 1774.

2. Addison T. On the Constitutional and Local Effects of Disease of the Supra-Renal Capsules. London, Highley, 1855.
3. Brown-Séquard CE. Recherches expérimentales sur la physiologie et la pathologie des capsules surrénales. Arch Gen Med 1856; ser 5, no 8:385–401.
4. Osler W. On six cases of Addison's disease with the report of a case greatly benefited by the use of suprarenal extract. Int Med Mag 1896.
5. Medvei VC. A History of Clinical Endocrinology. Pearl River, NY, Parthenon, 1993.
6. Hench PS, Kendall EC, Slocumb CH, et al. The effect of a hormone of the adrenal cortex (17-hydroxy-11-dehydrocorticosterone: compound E) and of pituitary adrenocorticotropic hormone on rheumatoid arthritis. Mayo Clin Proc 1949; 24:181–197.
7. Simpson SA, Tait JF. Recent progress in methods of isolation, chemistry, and physiology of aldosterone. Recent Prog Horm Res 1955; 11:183–210.
8. Li CH, Simpson ME, Evans HM. Adrenocorticotrophic hormone. J Biol Chem 1943; 149:413–424.
9. Cushing H. The basophil adenomas of the pituitary body and their clinical manifestations (pituitary basophilism). Bull Johns Hopkins Hosp 1932; 50:137–195.
10. Harris GW. Neural control of the pituitary gland. Physiol Rev 1948; 28:139–179.
11. Vale W, Spiess J, Rivier C, et al. Characterization of a 41-residue ovine hypothalamic peptide that stimulates secretion of corticotropin and β-endorphin. Science 1981; 213:1394–1397.
12. Conn JW. Primary aldosteronism, a new clinical entity. J Lab Clin Med 1955; 45:3–17.
13. Mesiano S, Jaffe RB. Developmental and functional biology of the primate fetal adrenal cortex. Endocr Rev 1997; 18:378–404.
14. Jaffe RB, Mesiano S, Smith R, et al. The regulation and role of fetal adrenal development in human pregnancy. Endocr Res 1998; 24:919–926.
15. Okamoto M, Takemori H. Differentiation and zonation of the adrenal cortex. Curr Opin Endocrinol Diabetes 2000; 7:122–127.
16. Luo X, Ikeda Y, Parker KL. A cell-specific nuclear factor is essential for adrenal and gonadal development and sexual differentiation. Cell 1994; 77:481–490.
17. Neville AM, O'Hare MJ. Histopathology of the human adrenal cortex. Clin Endocrinol Metab 1985; 14:791–820.
18. Dobbie JW, Symington T. The human adrenal gland with special reference to the vasculature. J Endocrinol 1966; 34:479–489.
19. International Union of Pure and Applied Chemistry. Definitive rules for the nomenclature of steroids. Pure Appl Chem 1972; 31:285–322.
20. Gwynne JT, Strauss JF III. The role of lipoprotein in steroidogenesis and cholesterol metabolism in steroidogenic glands. Endocr Rev 1982; 3:299–329.
21. Faust JR, Goldstein JL, Brown MS. Receptor-mediated uptake of low density lipoprotein and utilization of its cholesterol for steroid synthesis in cultured mouse adrenal cells. J Biol Chem 1977; 252:4861–4871.
22. Goldstein JL, Anderson RGW, Brown MS. Coated pits, coated vesicles, and receptor-mediated endocytosis. Nature 1979; 279: 679–685.
23. Illingworth DR, Kenny TA, Orwoll ES. Adrenal function in heterozygous and homozygous hypobetalipoproteinemia. J Clin Endocrinol Metab 1982; 54:27–33.
24. Illingworth DR, Lees AM, Lees RS. Adrenal cortical function in homozygous familial hypercholesterolemia. Metabolism 1983; 32: 1045–1052.
25. Borkowski AJ, Levin S, Delcroix C, et al. Blood cholesterol and hydrocortisone production in man: quantitative aspects of the utilization of circulating cholesterol by the adrenals at rest and under adrenocorticotropin stimulation. J Clin Invest 1967; 46: 797–811.
26. Acton S, Rigotti A, Landschulz KT, et al. Identification of scavenger receptor SR-BI as a high density lipoprotein receptor. Science 1996; 27:518–520.
27. Landschulz KT, Pathak RK, Rigotti A, et al. Regulation of scavenger receptor, class B, type I, a high density lipoprotein receptor, in liver and steroidogenic tissues of the rat. J Clin Invest 1996; 98:984–995.
28. Lin D, Sugawara T, Strauss JF, et al. Role of steroidogenic acute regulatory protein in adrenal and gonadal steroidogenesis. Science 1995; 267:1828–1831.
29. Stocco DM, Clark BJ. Regulation of the acute production of steroids in steroidogenic cells. Endocr Rev 1996; 17:221–244.
30. Amri H, Li H, Culty M, et al . The peripheral-type benzodiazepine receptor and adrenal steroidogenesis. Curr Opin Endocrinol Diabetes 1999; 6:179–184.
31. Chu JW, Kimura T. Molecular and catalytic properties of adrenodoxin reductase (a flavoprotein). J Biol Chem 1973; 248:2089–2094.
32. Bernhardt R. The role of adrenodoxin in adrenal steroidogenesis. Curr Opin Endocrinol Diabetes 2000; 7:109–115.
33. Onoda M, Hall PF. Cytochrome b_5 stimulates purified testicular microsomal cytochrome P450 (C_{21} side-chain cleavage). Biochem Biophys Res Commun 1982; 108:454–460.
34. Yanigabashi K, Hall PF. Role of electron transport in the regulation of lyase activity of C_{21} side-chain cleavage P450 from porcine adrenal and testicular microsome. J Biol Chem 1986; 261: 8429–8433.
35. Miller WL. Molecular biology of steroid hormone synthesis. Endocr Rev 1988; 9:295–318.
36. John ME, John MC, Ashley P, et al. Identification and characterization of cDNA clones specific for cholesterol side-chain cleavage cytochrome P-450. Proc Natl Acad Sci USA 1984; 81:5628–5632.
37. Chung B, Matteson KJ, Voutilainen R, et al. Human cholesterol side-chain cleavage enzyme, P450scD: cDNA cloning, assignment of the gene to chromosome 15, and expression in the placenta. Proc Natl Acad Sci USA 1986; 83:8962–8966.
38. Lorence MC, Murray BA, Trant JM, Mason JI. Human 3β-hydroxysteroid dehydrogenase/Δ^5-Δ^4 isomerase from placenta: expression in nonsteroidogenic cells of a protein that catalyses the dehydrogenation/isomerization of C21 and C19 steroids. Endocrinology 1990;126:2493–2498.
39. Rheaume E, Lachance Y, Zhao HF, et al. Structure and expression of a new complementary DNA encoding the almost exclusive 3β-hydroxysteroid dehydrogenase/Δ^5-Δ^4 in human adrenals and gonads. Mol Endocrinol 1991; 5:1147–1157.
40. Bradshaw KD, Waterman MR, Couch RT, et al. Characterization of complementary deoxyribonucleic acid for human adrenocortical 17α-hydroxylase: a probe for analysis of 17α-hydroxylase deficiency. Mol Endocrinol 1987; 1:348–354.
41. Chung B-C, Picado-Leonard J, Haniu M, et al. Cytochrome P450C17 (steroid 17α-hydroxylase/17,20-lyase): cloning of human adrenal and testis cDNAs indicates the same enzyme is expressed in both tissues. Proc Natl Acad Sci USA 1987; 84:407–411.
42. White PC, New MI, Dupont B. Cloning and expression of cDNA encoding a bovine adrenal cytochrome P450 specific for steroid 21-hydroxylation. Proc Natl Acad Sci USA 1984; 81: 1986–1990.
43. White PC, Chaplin DD, Weis JH, et al. Two steroid 21-hydroxylase genes are located in the murine S region. Nature 1984; 312: 465–467.
44. Yoshioka H, Morohashi K, Sogawa K, et al. Structural analysis of cloned cDNA for mRNA of microsomal cytochrome P450 (C_{21}) which catalyzes steroid 21-hydroxylation in bovine adrenal cortex. J Biol Chem 1986; 261:4106–4109.
45. Chua SC, Szabo P, Vitek A, et al. Cloning of cDNA encoding steroid 11β-hydroxylase (P450c11). Proc Natl Acad Sci USA 1987; 84:7193–7197.
46. John ME, John MC, Simpson ER, et al. Regulation of cytochrome P-450-11β gene expression by adrenocorticotropin. J Biol Chem 1985; 260:5760–5767.
47. Mornet E, Dupont J, Vitek A, et al. Characterization of two genes encoding human steroid 11β-hydroxylase (P-450(11)β). J Biol Chem 1989; 264:20961–20967.
48. Curnow KM, Tusie-Luna MT, Pascoe L, et al. The product of the CYP11B2 gene is required for aldosterone biosynthesis in the human adrenal cortex. Mol Endocrinol 1991; 5:1513–1522.
49. Ogishima T, Shibata H, Shimada H, et al. Aldosterone synthase cytochrome P-450 expressed in the adrenals of patients with primary aldosteronism. J Biol Chem 1991; 266:10731–10734.
50. Branchaud CL, Goodyer CG, Shore P, et al. Functional zonation of the midgestation human fetal adrenal cortex: fetal versus definitive zone use of progesterone for cortisol synthesis. Am J Obstet Gynecol 1985; 151:271–277.

51. Goldman AS, Yackovas WC, Bongiovanni AM. Development of activity of 3β-hydroxysteroid dehydrogenase in human fetal tissues and in two anencephalic newborns. J Clin Endocrinol Metab 1966; 26:14–22.
52. Siiteri PK, MacDonald PC. The utilization of dehydroisoandrosterone sulphate for estrogen synthesis during human pregnancy. Steroids 1963; 2:713–730.
53. Seidah NG, Chretien M. Complete amino acid sequence of a human pituitary glycopeptide: an important maturation product of pro-opiomelanocortin. Proc Natl Acad Sci USA 1981; 78: 4236–4340.
54. Smith AI, Funder JW. Proopiomelanocortin processing in the pituitary, central nervous system, and peripheral tissues. Endocr Rev 1988; 9:159–179.
55. Donald RA. ACTH and related peptides. Clin Endocrinol (Oxf) 1980; 12:491–524.
56. Bicknell AB, Lomthaisong K, Woods RJ, et al. Characterization of a serine protease that cleaves pro-gamma-melanotropin at the adrenal to stimulate growth. Cell 2001; 105:903–912.
57. Suzuki I, Cone RD, Im S, et al. Binding of melanotropic hormones to the melanocortin receptor MC1R on human melanocytes stimulates proliferation and melanogenesis. Endocrinology 1996; 137:1627–1633.
58. DeBold CR, Nicholson WE, Orth DN. Immunoreactive proopiomelanocortin (POMC) peptides and POMC-like messenger ribonucleic acid are present in many rat nonpituitary tissues. Endocrinology 1988; 122:2648–2657.
59. de Keyzer Y, Lenne F, Massias JF, et al. Pituitary-like proopiomelanocortin transcripts in human Leydig cell tumours. J Clin Invest 1990; 86:871–877.
60. Clark AJ, Lavender PM, Coates P, et al. In vitro and in vivo analysis of the processing and fate of the peptide products of the short proopiomelanocortin mRNA. Mol Endocrinol 1990; 4: 1737–1743.
61. de Keyzer Y, Bertagna X, Luton JP, Kahn A. Variable modes of proopiomelanocortin gene transcription in human tumors. Mol Endocrinol 1989; 3:215–223.
62. Clark AJL, Lavender PM, Besser GM, Rees LH. Pro-opiomelanocortin mRNA size heterogeneity in ACTH-dependent Cushing's syndrome. J Mol Endocrinol 1989; 2:3–9.
63. Picon A, Bertagna X, de Keyzer Y. Analysis of the human proopiomelanocortin gene promoter in a small cell lung carcinoma cell line reveals an unusual role for E2F transcription factors. Oncogene 1999; 18:2627–2633.
64. Mains RE, Eipper BA. The tissue specific processing of pro-ACTH/endorphin. Trends Endocrinol Metab 1990; 2:388–394.
65. Hale AC, Besser GM, Rees LH. Characterisation of pro-opiomelanocortin–derived peptides in pituitary and ectopic adrenocorticotropin-secreting tumours. J Endocrinol 1985; 108:49–56.
66. Stewart PM, Gibson S, Crosby SR, et al. ACTH precursors characterize the ectopic ACTH syndrome. Clin Endocrinol (Oxf) 1994; 40:199–204.
67. Lundblad JR, Roberts JL. Regulation of proopiomelanocortin gene expression in pituitary. Endocr Rev 1988; 9:135–158.
68. Orth DN. Corticotropin-releasing hormone in humans. Endocr Rev 1992; 13:164–191.
69. Rivier J, Spiess J, Vale W. Characterization of rat hypothalamic corticotropin-releasing factor. Proc Natl Acad Sci USA 1983; 80: 4851–4855.
70. Taylor AL, Fishman LM. Corticotropin-releasing hormone. N Engl J Med 1988; 319:213–222.
71. Antoni FA. Hypothalamic control of adrenocorticotropin secretion: advances since the discovery of 41-residue corticotropin-releasing factor. Endocr Rev 1986; 7:351–378.
72. Shibahara S, Morimoto Y, Furutani Y, et al. Isolation and sequence analysis of the human corticotropin-releasing factor precursor gene. EMBO J 1983; 2:775–779.
73. Jingami H, Mizuno N, Takahashi H, et al. Cloning and sequence analysis of cDNA for rat corticotropin-releasing factor precursor. FEBS Lett 1985; 191:63–66.
74. Furutani Y, Morimoto Y, Shibahara S, et al. Cloning and sequence analysis of cDNA for ovine corticotropin releasing factor precursor. Nature 1983; 301:537–540.
75. Chen R, Lewis KA, Perrin MH, et al. Expression cloning of a human corticotropin-releasing-factor receptor. Proc Natl Acad Sci USA 1993; 90:8967–8971.
76. Giguere V, Labrie F, Cote J, et al. Stimulation of cyclic AMP accumulation and corticotropin release by synthetic ovine corticotropin-releasing factor in rat anterior pituitary cells: site of glucocorticoid action. Proc Natl Acad Sci USA 1982; 79:3466–3469.
77. Suda T, Tomori N, Tozawa F, et al. Distribution and characterization of immunoreactive corticotropin-releasing factor in human tissues. J Clin Endocrinol Metab 1984; 59:861–866.
78. Sasaki A, Sato S, Murakami O, et al. Immunoreactive corticotropin-releasing hormone present in human plasma may be derived from both hypothalamic and extrahypothalamic sources. J Clin Endocrinol Metab 1987; 65:176–182.
79. Grino M, Chrousos GP, Margioris AN. The corticotropin releasing hormone gene is expressed in human placenta. Biochem Biophys Res Commun 1987; 148:1208–1214.
80. Campbell EA, Linton EA, Wolfe CD, et al. Plasma corticotropin-releasing hormone concentrations during pregnancy and parturition. J Clin Endocrinol Metab 1987; 64:1054–1059.
81. Linton EA, Wolfe CD, Behan DP, et al. A specific carrier substance for human corticotrophin releasing factor in late gestational maternal plasma which could mask the ACTH-releasing activity. Clin Endocrinol (Oxf) 1988; 28:315–324.
82. Rivier C, Rivier J, Vale W. Inhibition of adrenocorticotropic hormone secretion in the rat by immunoneutralization of corticotropin-releasing factor. Science 1982; 218:377–379.
83. Bruhn TO, Sutton RE, Rivier CL, et al. Corticotropin-releasing factor regulates proopiomelanocortin messenger ribonucleic acid levels in vivo. Neuroendocrinology 1984; 39:170–175.
84. DeBold CR, Sheldon WR, DeCherney GS, et al. Arginine vasopressin potentiates adrenocorticotropin release induced by ovine corticotropin-releasing factor. J Clin Invest 1984; 73:533–538.
85. Hauger RL, Aguilera G. Regulation of pituitary corticotropin releasing hormone (CRH) receptors by CRH: interaction with vasopressin. Endocrinology 1993; 133:1708–1714.
86. Sugimoto T, Saito M, Mochizuki S, et al. Molecular cloning and functional expression of a cDNA encoding the human V1b vasopressin receptor. J Biol Chem 1994; 269:27088–27092.
87. Rivier C, Vale W. Effect of angiotensin II on ACTH release in vivo: role of corticotropin-releasing factor. Regul Pept 1983; 7: 253–258.
88. Watanabe T, Oki Y, Orth DN. Kinetic actions and interactions of arginine vasopressin, angiotensin-II, and oxytocin on adrenocorticotropin secretion by rat anterior pituitary cells in the microperfusion system. Endocrinology 1989; 125:1921–1931.
89. Bateman A, Singh A, Kral T, et al. The immune-hypothalamic-pituitary-adrenal axis. Endocr Rev 1989; 10:92–112.
90. Chrousos GP. The hypothalamo-pituitary-adrenal axis and immune-mediated inflammation. N Engl J Med 1998 332:1351–1362.
91. Ray DW, Ren SG, Melmed S. Leukemia inhibitory factor (LIF) stimulates proopiomelanocortin (POMC) gene expression in a corticotroph cell line: role of STAT pathway. J Clin Invest 1996; 97:1852–1859.
92. Udelsman R, Norton JA, Jelenich SE, et al. Responses of the hypothalamic-pituitary-adrenal and renin-angiotensin axes and the sympathetic system during controlled surgical and anesthetic stress. J Clin Endocrinol Metab 1987; 64:986–994.
93. Vaughan GM, Becker RA, Allen JP, et al. Cortisol and corticotropin in burned patients. J Trauma 1982; 22:263–272.
94. Fish HR, Chernow B, O'Brian JT. Endocrine and neurophysiologic responses of the pituitary to insulin-induced hypoglycemia: a review. Metabolism 1986; 35:763–780.
95. Luger A, Deuster PA, Kyle SB, et al. Acute hypothalamic-pituitary-adrenal responses to the stress of treadmill exercise: physiologic adaptations to physical training. N Engl J Med 1987; 316: 1309–1315.
96. Aguilera G. Regulation of pituitary ACTH secretion during chronic stress. Front Neuroendocrinol 1994; 15:321–350.
97. Streeten DHP, Anderson GH Jr, Dalakos TG, et al. Normal and abnormal function of the hypothalamic-pituitary-adrenocortical system in man. Endocr Rev 1984; 5:371–394.
98. Linkowski P, Mendlewicz J, Kerkhofs M, et al. 24-hour profiles of adrenocorticotropin, cortisol, and growth hormone in major depressive illness: effect of antidepressant treatment. J Clin Endocrinol Metab 1987; 65:141–152.
99. Krieger DT, Allen W, Rizzo F, et al. Characterization of the normal temporal pattern of plasma corticosteroid levels. J Clin Endocrinol Metab 1971; 32:266–284.

100. Weitzman ED, Fukushima DK, Nogeire C, et al. Twenty-four hour pattern of the episodic secretion of cortisol in normal subjects. J Clin Endocrinol Metab 1971; 33:14–22.
101. Veldhuis JD, Iranmanesh A, Johnson ML, et al. Amplitude, but not frequency, modulation of adrenocorticotropin secretory bursts gives rise to the nyctohemeral rhythm of the corticotropic axis in man. J Clin Endocrinol Metab 1990; 71:452–463.
102. Horrocks PM, Jones AF, Ratcliffe WA, et al. Patterns of ACTH and cortisol pulsatility over twenty four hours in normal males and females. Clin Endocrinol (Oxf) 1990; 32:127–134.
103. Slag MF, Ahmed M, Gannon MC, et al. Meal stimulation of cortisol secretion: a protein induced effect. Metabolism 1981; 30: 1104–1108.
104. Boivin DB, Duffy JF, Kronauer RE, et al. Dose-response relationships for resetting of human circadian clock by light. Nature 1996; 379:540–542.
105. Czeisler CA, Dumont M, Duffy JF, et al. Association of sleep-wake habits in older people with changes in output of circadian pacemaker. Lancet 1992; 340:933–936.
106. Desir D, Van Cauter E, Fang VS, et al. Effects of "jet lag" on hormonal patterns: I. Procedures, variations in total plasma proteins, and disruption of adrenocorticotropin-cortisol periodicity. J Clin Endocrinol Metab 1981; 52:628–641.
107. Davis LG, Arentzen R, Reid JM, et al. Glucocorticoid sensitivity of vasopressin mRNA levels in the paraventricular nucleus of the rat. Proc Natl Acad Sci USA 1986; 83:1145–1149.
108. Eberwine JH, Jonassen JA, Evinger MJ, et al. Complex transcriptional regulation by glucocorticoids and corticotropin-releasing hormone of proopiomelanocortin gene expression in rat pituitary cultures. DNA Cell Biol 1987; 6:483–492.
109. Keller-Wood ME, Dallman MF. Corticosteroid inhibition of ACTH secretion. Endocr Rev 1984; 5:1–24.
110. Lamberts SWJ, Koper JW, Biemond P, et al. Cortisol receptor resistance: the variability of its clinical presentation and response to treatment. J Clin Endocrinol Metab 1992;74:313–321.
111. Cole TJ, Blendy JA, Monaghan AP, et al. Targeted disruption of the glucocorticoid receptor gene blocks adrenergic chromaffin cell development and severely retards lung maturation. Genes Dev 1995; 9:1608–1621.
112. Catalano RD, Stuve L, Ramachandran J. Characterization of corticotropin receptors in human adrenocortical cells. J Clin Endocrinol Metab 1986; 62:300–304.
113. Mountjoy KG, Robbins LS, Mortrud MT, et al. The cloning of a family of genes that encode the melanocortin receptors. Science 1992; 257:1248–1251.
114. Rae PA, Gutmann NS, Tsao J, et al. Mutations in cyclic AMP–dependent protein kinase and corticotropin (ACTH)-sensitive adenylate cyclase affect adrenal steroidogenesis. Proc Natl Acad Sci USA 1979; 76:1896–1900.
115. Cooke BA. Signal transduction involving cyclic AMP–dependent and cyclic AMP–independent mechanisms in the control of steroidogenesis. Mol Cell Endocrinol 1999; 151:25–35.
116. Enyeart JJ, Mlinar B, Enyeart JA. T-type Ca^{2+} channels are required for adrenocorticotropin-stimulated cortisol production by bovine adrenal zona fasciculata cells. Mol Endocrinol 1993; 7: 1031–1040.
117. Ehrhart-Bornstein M, Hinson JP, Bornstein SR, et al. Intra-adrenal interactions in the regulation of adrenocortical steroidogenesis. Endocr Rev 1998; 19:101–143.
118. Munari-Silem Y, Lebrethon MC, Morand I, et al. Gap junction–mediated cell-to-cell communication in bovine and human adrenal cells: a process whereby cells increase their responsiveness to physiological corticotropin concentrations. J Clin Invest 1995; 95: 1429–1439.
119. Simpson ER, Waterman MR. Regulation of the synthesis of steroidogenic enzymes in adrenal cortical cells by ACTH. Annu Rev Physiol 1988; 50:427–440.
120. Waterman MR, Biscoff LJ. Cytochromes P450 12: diversity of ACTH (cAMP)-dependent transcription of bovine steroid hydroxylase genes. FASEB J 1997; 11:419–427.
121. Rainey WE, White PC. Functional adrenal zonation and regulation of aldosterone biosynthesis. Curr Opin Endocrinol Diabetes 1998; 5:175–182.
122. Gibbons GH, Dzau VJ, Farhl ER, et al. Interaction of signals influencing renin release. Annu Rev Physiol 1984; 46:291–308.
123. Quinn SJ, Williams GH. Regulation of aldosterone secretion. Annu Rev Physiol 1988; 50:409–426.
124. Dluhy RG, Axelrod L, Underwood RH, et al. Studies of the control of plasma aldosterone concentration in normal man: effect of dietary potassium and acute potassium infusion. J Clin Invest 1972; 51:1950–1957.
125. Rayfield EJ, Rose LI, Dluhy RG, et al. Aldosterone secretory and glucocorticoid excretory responses to alpha 1–24 ACTH (Cortrosyn) in sodium-depleted normal man. J Clin Endocrinol Metab 1973; 36:30–35.
126. Abayasekara DRE, Vazir H, Whitehouse BJ, et al. Studies on the mechanisms of ACTH-induced inhibition of aldosterone biosynthesis in the rat adrenal cortex. J Endocrinol 1989; 122:625–632.
127. Carey RM. Acute dopaminergic inhibition of aldosterone secretion is independent of angiotensin II and adrenocorticotropin. J Clin Endocrinol Metab 1982; 54:463–469.
128. Chartier L, Schiffrin EL. Role of calcium in effects of atrial natriuretic peptide on aldosterone production in adrenal glomerulosa cells. Am J Physiol 1987; 252:E485–E491.
129. Longcope C. Adrenal and gonadal secretion in normal females. Clin Endocrinol Metab 1986; 15:213–228.
130. Labrie F, Belanger A, Simard J, et al. DHEA and peripheral androgen and estrogen formation: intracrinology. Ann NY Acad Sci 1995; 774:16–28.
131. McKenna TJ, Fearon U, Clarke D, Cunningham SK. A critical review of the origin and control of adrenal androgens. Baillieres Clin Obstet Gynaecol 1997; 11: 229–248.
132. Weinberger C, Hollenberg SM, Rosenfeld MG, et al. Domain structure of the human glucocorticoid receptor and its relationship to the v-*erb-A* oncogene product. Nature 1985; 318:670–672.
133. Arriza JL, Weinberger C, Cerelli G, et al. Cloning of human mineralocorticoid receptor complementary DNA: structural and functional kinship with the glucocorticoid receptor. Science 1987; 237:268–275.
134. Gustafsson J-AD, Carlstedt-Duke J, Poellinger L, et al. Biochemistry, molecular biology, and physiology of the glucocorticoid receptor. Endocr Rev 1987; 8:185–234.
135. Encio IJ, Detera-Wadleigh SD. The genomic structure of the human glucocorticoid receptor. J Biol Chem 1991; 266:7182–7188.
136. Zennaro M-C, Farman N, Bonvalet JP, Lombes M. Tissue-specific expression of α and β mRNA isoforms of the human mineralocorticoid receptor in normal and pathological states. J Clin Endocrinol Metab 1997; 82:1345–1352.
137. Pratt WB. The role of heat shock protein in regulating the function, folding and trafficking of the glucocorticoid receptor. J Biol Chem 1993; 268:21455–21458.
138. Luisi BF, Xu WX, Otwinowski Z, et al. Crystallographic analysis of the interaction of the glucocorticoid receptor with DNA. Nature 1991; 352:497–505.
139. Beato M, Sanchez-Pacheco A. Interaction of steroid hormone receptors with the transcription initiation complex. Endocr Rev 1996; 17:587–609.
140. Oakley RH, Sar M, Cidlowski JA. The human glucocorticoid receptor β isoform: expression, biochemical properties, and putative function. J Biol Chem 1996; 271:9550–9559.
141. Hollenberg SM, Giguere V, Segui P, et al. Colocalization of DNA-binding and transcriptional activation functions in the human glucocorticoid receptor. Cell 1987; 49:39–46.
142. Rusconi S, Yamamoto KR. Functional dissection of the hormone and DNA binding activities of the glucocorticoid receptor. EMBO J 1987; 6:1309–1315.
143. Bamberger CM, Schulte HM, Chrousos GP. Molecular determinants of glucocorticoid receptor function and tissue sensitivity to glucocorticoids. Endocr Rev 1996; 17:245–261.
144. McKenna NJ, Lanz RB, O'Malley BW. Nuclear receptor coregulators: cellular and molecular biology. Endocr Rev 1999; 20:321–344.
145. Schule R, Rangarajan P, Kliewer S, et al. Functional antagonism between oncoprotein c-Jun and the glucocorticoid receptor. Cell 1990; 62:1217–1226.
146. McKay LI, Cidlowski JA. Molecular control of immune/inflammatory responses: interactions between nuclear factor-κB and steroid receptor–signalling pathways. Endocr Rev 1999; 20:435–459.
147. Funder JW. Aldosterone action. Annu Rev Physiol 1993; 55:115–130.

148. Rossier BC, Alpern RJ. Cell and molecular biology of epithelial transport. Curr Opin Nephrol Hypertens 1999; 8:579–580.
149. Verrey F, Kraehenbuhl JP, Rossier BC. Aldosterone induces a rapid increase in the rate of Na,K-ATPase gene transcription in cultured kidney cells. Mol Endocrinol 1989; 3:1369–1376.
150. Chen SY, Bhargava A, Mastroberardino L, et al. Epithelial sodium channel regulated by aldosterone-induced protein sgk. Proc Natl Acad Sci USA 1999; 93:6025–6030.
151. Krozowski ZS, Funder JW. Renal mineralocorticoid receptors and hippocampal corticosterone-binding species have identical intrinsic steroid specificity. Proc Natl Acad Sci USA 1983; 80: 6056–6060.
152. Edwards CRW, Stewart PM, Burt D, et al. Localisation of 11β-hydroxysteroid dehydrogenase: tissue specific protector of the mineralocorticoid receptor. Lancet 1988; 2:836–841.
153. Funder JW, Pearce PT, Smith R, Smith AI. Mineralocorticoid action: target tissue specificity is enzyme, not receptor, mediated. Science 1988; 242:583–585.
154. Iwasaki Y, Aoki Y, Katahira M, et al. Non-genomic mechanisms of glucocorticoid inhibition of adrenocorticotropin secretion: possible involvement of GTP-binding protein. Biochem Biophys Res Commun 1997; 235:295–299.
155. Christ M, Haseroth K, Falkenstein E, Wehling M. Nongenomic steroid actions: fact or fancy? Vitam Horm 1999; 57:325–373.
156. Hammond GL. Molecular properties of corticosteroid binding globulin and the sex-steroid binding proteins. Endocr Rev 1990; 11:65-79.
157. Brien TG. Human corticosteroid binding globulin. Clin Endocrinol (Oxf) 1981; 14:193-212.
158. Roitman A, Bruchis S, Bauman B, et al. Total deficiency of corticosteroid binding globulin. Clin Endocrinol (Oxf) 1984; 21: 541–548.
159. Smith CL, Power SG, Hammond GL. A Leu-His substitution at residue 93 in human corticosteroid binding globulin results in reduced affinity for cortisol. J Steroid Biochem Mol Biol 1992; 42:671–676.
160. Mendel CM. The free hormone hypothesis: a physiologically based mathematical model. Endocr Rev 1989; 10:232–274.
161. Peterson RE, Wyngaarden JB, Guerra SL, et al. The physiological disposition and metabolic fate of hydrocortisone in man. J Clin Invest 1955; 34:1779–1794.
162. Fukushima DK, Bradlow HL, Hellman L, et al. Metabolic transformation of hydrocortisone ^{14}C in man. J Biol Chem 1960; 235: 2246–2252.
163. Shackleton CHL. Mass spectrometry in the diagnosis of steroid-related disorders and hypertension research. J Steroid Biochem Mol Biol 1993; 45:127–140.
164. Stewart PM, Krozowski ZS. 11β-Hydroxysteroid dehydrogenase. Vitam Horm 1999; 57:249–324.
165. White PC, Mune T, Agarwal AK. 11β-Hydroxysteroid dehydrogenase and the syndrome of apparent mineralocorticoid excess. Endocr Rev 1997; 18:135–136.
166. Okuda A, Okuda K. Purification and characterization of Δ^4-3-ketosteroid 5β-reductase. J Biol Chem 1984; 259:7519–7524.
167. Russell DW, Wilson JD. Steroid 5α-reductase: two genes/two enzymes. Annu Rev Biochem 1994; 63:25–61.
168. Cope CL. Metabolic breakdown. In Cope CL (ed). Adrenal Steroids and Disease. 2nd ed. London, Pitman Medical 1972, pp 80–104.
169. Voccia E, Saenger P, Peterson RE, et al. 6β-Hydroxycortisol excretion in hypercortisolemic states. J Clin Endocrinol Metab 1979; 48:467–471.
170. Monder C, Bradlow LH. Cortoic acids: explorations at the frontier of corticosteroid metabolism. Recent Prog Horm Res 1980; 36:345–400.
171. Zumoff B, Bradlow HL, Levin J, et al. Influence of thyroid function on the in vivo cortisol-cortisone equilibrium in man. J Steroid Biochem 1983; 18:437-440.
172. McGuire JS, Tomkins GM. The effects of thyroxine administration on the enzymic reduction of Δ^4 3-ketosteroids. J Biol Chem 1959; 234:791–794.
173. Voice MW, Seckl JR, Edwards CRW, et al. 11β-Hydroxysteroid dehydrogenase type 1 expression in 2S FAZA hepatoma cells is hormonally regulated: a model system for the study of hepatic glucocorticoid metabolism. Biochem J 1996; 317:621–625.
174. Moore JS, Monson JP, Kaltsas G, et al. Modulation of 11β-hydroxysteroid dehydrogenase isozymes by growth hormone and insulin-like growth factor: in vivo and in vitro studies. J Clin Endocrinol Metab 1999; 84:4172–4177.
175. Yamada S, Iwai K. Induction of hepatic cortisol-6-hydroxylase by rifampicin. Lancet 1976; 2:366–367.
176. Werk EEJ, MacGee J, Sholiton LJ. Effect of diphenylhydantoin on cortisol metabolism in man. J Clin Invest 1964; 43:1824–1835.
177. Whitworth JA, Stewart PM, Burt D, et al. The kidney is the major site of cortisone production in man. Clin Endocrinol (Oxf) 1989; 31:355–361.
178. Kyriazopoulou V, Parparousi O, Vagenakis AG. Rifampicin-induced adrenal crisis in addisonian patients receiving corticosteroid replacement therapy. J Clin Endocrinol Metab 1984; 59: 1204–1206.
179. Morris DJ, Brem AS. Metabolic derivatives of aldosterone. Am J Physiol 1987; 252:F365–F373.
180. Stalmans W, Laloux M. Glucocorticoids and hepatic glycogen metabolism. In Baxter JD, Rousseau GG (eds). Glucocorticoid Hormone Action. New York, Springer-Verlag, 1979, pp 518–533.
181. Exton JH. Regulation of gluconeogenesis by glucocorticoids. In Baxter JD, Rousseau GG (eds). Glucocorticoid Hormone Action. New York, Springer-Verlag, 1979, pp 535–546.
182. Magnuson MA, Quinn PG, Granner DK. Multihormonal regulation of phosphoenolpyruvate carboxykinase–chloramphenicol acetyltransferase fusion genes: insulin's effects oppose those of cAMP and dexamethasone. J Biol Chem 1987; 262:14917–14920.
183. Olefsky JM. Effect of dexamethasone on insulin binding, glucose transport, and glucose oxidation of isolated rat adipocytes. J Clin Invest 1975; 56:1499–1508.
184. Fain JH. Inhibition of glucose transport in fat cells and activation of lipolysis by glucocorticoids. In Baxter JD, Rousseau GG (eds). Glucocorticoid Hormone Action. New York, Springer-Verlag, 1979, pp 547–560.
185. Hauner H, Entenmann G, Wabitisch M, et al. Promoting effects of glucocorticoids on the differentiation of human adipocyte precursor cells cultured in a chemically defined medium. J Clin Invest 1989; 84:1663–1670.
186. Rebuffe-Scrive M, Krotkiewski M, Elfverson J, Bjorntorp P. Muscle and adipose morphology and metabolism in Cushing's syndrome. J Clin Endocrinol Metab 1988; 67:1122–1128.
187. Bronnegard M, Arner P, Hellstrom L, et al. Glucocorticoid receptor messenger ribonucleic acid in different regions of human adipose tissue. Endocrinology 1990; 127:1689–1696.
188. Bujalska IJ, Kumar S, Stewart PM. Does central obesity reflect "Cushing's disease of the omentum"? Lancet 1997; 349:1210–1213.
189. Leibovich SJ, Ross R. The role of the macrophage in wound repair: a study with hydrocortisone and antimacrophage serum. Am J Pathol 1975; 78:71–100.
190. Canalis E. Clinical review 83: mechanisms of glucocorticoid action in bone: implications to glucocorticoid-induced osteoporosis. J Clin Endocrinol Metab 1996; 81:3441–3447.
191. Manolagas SC. Birth and death of bone cells: basic regulatory mechanisms and implications for the pathogenesis and treatment of osteoporosis. Endocr Rev 2000; 21:115–137.
192. Van Staa TP, Leufkens HGM, Abenhaim L, et al. Use of oral corticosteroids in the United Kingdom. Q J Med 2000; 93:105–111.
193. Adler RA, Rosen CJ. Glucocorticoids and osteoporosis. Endocrinol Metab Clin North Am 1994; 23:641–670.
194. Wajchenberg BL, Pereira VG, Kieffer J, et al. Effect of dexamethasone on calcium metabolism and ^{47}Ca kinetics in normal subjects. Acta Endocrinol (Copenh) 1969; 61:173–192.
195. Laake H. The action of corticosteroids on the renal absorption of calcium. Acta Endocrinol (Copenh) 1960; 34:60–64.
196. Fraser R, Davies DL, Connell JMC. Hormones and hypertension. Clin Endocrinol (Oxf) 1989; 31:701–746.
197. Grunfeld J-P, Eloy L. Glucocorticoids modulate vascular reactivity in the rat. Hypertension 1987; 10:608—618.
198. Saruta T, Suzuki H, Handa M, et al. Multiple factors contribute to the pathogenesis of hypertension in Cushing's syndrome. J Clin Endocrinol Metab 1986; 62:275-279.
199. Stockigt JR, Hewett MJ, Topliss DJ, et al. Renin and renin substrate in primary adrenal insufficiency: contrasting effects of

glucocorticoid and mineralocorticoid deficiency. Am J Med 1979; 66:915–922.
200. Marver D. Evidence of corticosteroid action along the nephron. Am J Physiol 1984; 246:F111–F123.
201. Raff H. Glucocorticoid inhibition of neurohypophysial vasopressin secretion. Am J Physiol 1987; 252:R635–R644.
202. Slessor A. Studies concerning the mechanism of water retention in Addison's disease and in hypopituitarism. J Clin Endocrinol Metab 1951; 11:700–723.
203. Yu DTY, Clements PJ, Paulus HE, et al. Human lymphocyte subpopulations: effect of corticosteroids. J Clin Invest 1974; 53: 565–571.
204. Cidlowski JA, King KL, Evans-Storms RB, et al. The biochemistry and molecular biology of glucocorticoid-induced apoptosis in the immune system. Recent Prog Horm Res 1996; 51:457–491.
205. Scheinman RI, Cogswell PC, Lofquist AK, et al. Role of transcriptional activation of IκBα in mediation of immunosuppression by glucocorticoids. Science 1995; 270:283–286.
206. Auphan N, DiDonato JA, Rosette C, et al. Immunosuppression by glucocorticoids: inhibition of NF-κB activity through induction of IκB synthesis. Science 1995; 270:286–290.
207. Barnes PJ. Anti-inflammatory action of glucocorticoids: molecular mechanisms. Clin Sci 1998; 94:557–572.
208. Peers SH, Flowers RJ. The role of lipocortin in corticosteroid actions. Am Rev Respir Dis 1990; 141:S18-S21.
209. O'Connor TM, O'Halloran DJ, Shanahan F. The stress response and the hypothalamic-pituitary-adrenal axis: from molecule to melancholia. Q J Med 2000; 93:323–333.
210. McEwen BS, deKloet ER, Rostene W. Adrenal steroid receptors and action in the central nervous system. Physiol Rev 1986; 66: 1121–1188.
211. Salpolsky RM, Krey LC, McEwen BS. Prolonged glucocorticoid exposure reduces hippocampal neuron number: implications for aging. J Neurosci 1985; 5:1222–1227.
212. Clark AF. Steroids, ocular hypertension, and glaucoma. J Glaucoma 1995; 4:354–369.
213. Wordinger RJ, Clark AF. Effect of glucocorticoids on the trabecular meshwork: towards a better understanding of glaucoma. Prog Retin Eye Res 1999; 18:629–667.
214. Messer J, Reitman D, Sacks HS, et al. Association of adrenocorticosteroid therapy and peptic-ulcer disease. N Engl J Med 1983; 309:21–24.
215. Pressley L, Funder JW. Glucocorticoid and mineralocorticoid receptors in gut mucosa. Endocrinology 1975; 97:588–596.
216. Martial JA, Baxter JD, Goodman HM, Seeburg PH. Regulation of growth hormone messenger RNA by thyroid and glucocorticoid hormones. Proc Natl Acad Sci USA 1977; 74:1816–1820.
217. Blodget FM, Burgin L, Iezzou D, et al. Effects of prolonged cortisone therapy on the statural growth, skeletal maturation, and metabolic status of children. N Engl J Med 1956; 254:636–641.
218. Strickland AL, Underwood LE, Voina SJ. Growth retardation in Cushing's syndrome. Am J Dis Child 1972; 123:207–213.
219. Iannuzzi DM, Ertsey R, Ballard PL. Biphasic glucocorticoid regulation of pulmonary SP-A: characterization of inhibitory process. Am J Physiol 1993; 264:L236–L244.
220. Ballard PL, Ertsey R, Gonzales LW, et al. Transcriptional regulation of human pulmonary surfactant proteins SP-B and SP-C by glucocorticoids. Am J Respir Cell Mol Biol 1996; 14:599–607.
221. Wurtman RJ, Axelrod J. Control of enzymatic synthesis of adrenaline in the adrenal medulla by adrenal cortical steroids. J Biol Chem 1966; 241:2301–2305.
222. Christy NP. Principles of systemic corticosteroid therapy in nonendocrine disease. In Bardin CW (ed). Current Therapy in Endocrinology and Metabolism, 3rd ed. New York, BC Decker, 1988, pp 104–111.
223. Meikle AW, Weed JA, Tyler FH. Kinetics and interconversion of prednisolone and prednisone studied with new radioimmunoassays. J Clin Endocrinol Metab 1975; 41:717–721.
224. Fried J, Sabo EF. Synthesis of 17α-hydroxycortisone and its 9α-halo derivatives from 11-epi-17α-hydroxycorticosterone. J Am Chem Soc 1953; 75:2273–2274.
225. Dluhy RG, Newmark SR, Lauler DP, et al. Pharmacology and chemistry of adrenal glucocorticoids. In Azarnoff DL (ed). Steroid Therapy. Philadelphia, WB Saunders, 1975, pp 1–14.
226. Axelrod L. Glucocorticoid therapy. Medicine (Baltimore) 1976; 55:39–65.
227. Loprinzi CL, Jensen MD, Jiang N-S, et al. Effect of megestrol acetate on the human pituitary-adrenal axis. Mayo Clin Proc 1992; 67:1160–1162.
228. Danowski TS, Bonessi JV, Sabeh G, et al. Probabilities of pituitary-adrenal responsiveness after steroid therapy. Ann Intern Med 1964; 61:11–26.
229. Christy NP. Corticosteroid withdrawal. In Bardin CW (ed). Current Therapy in Endocrinology and Metabolism, 3rd ed. New York, BC Decker, 1988, pp 113–120.
230. Kane K, Emery P, Sheppard MC, Stewart PM. The insulin tolerance test versus the short Synacthen test in assessing the hypothalamo-pituitary-adrenal axis in patients on long-term glucocorticoid therapy. Q J Med 1995; 88:263–267.
231. Fauci AS. Alternate-day corticosteroid therapy. Am J Med 1978; 64:729–731.
232. Graber AL, Ney RL, Nicholson WE, et al. Natural history of pituitary-adrenal recovery following long-term suppression with corticosteroids. J Clin Endocrinol Metab 1965; 25:11–16.
233. Dixon RB, Christy NP. On the various forms of the corticosteroid withdrawal syndrome. Am J Med 1980; 68:224–230.
234. Byyny RL. Withdrawal from glucocorticoid therapy. N Engl J Med 1976; 295:30–32.
235. Christy NP. Iatrogenic Cushing's syndrome. In Christy NP (ed). The Human Adrenal Cortex. New York, Harper & Row, 1979, pp 395–425.
236. Walters W, Wilder RM, Kepler EJ. The suprarenal cortical syndrome with presentation of ten cases. Ann Surg 1934; 100:670–688.
237. Meador CK, Liddle GW, Island DP, et al. Cause of Cushing's syndrome in patients with tumors arising from "nonendocrine" tissue. J Clin Endocrinol Metab 1962; 22:693–703.
238. Orth DN. Ectopic hormone production. In Felig P, Baxter JD, Broadus AE, et al (eds). Endocrinology and Metabolism, 2nd ed. New York, McGraw-Hill, 1987, pp 1692–1735.
239. Ross EJ, Linch DC. Cushing's syndrome–killing disease: discriminatory value of signs and symptoms aiding early diagnosis. Lancet 1982; 2:646–649.
240. Wajchenberg BL, Bosco A, Marone MM, et al. Estimation of body fat and lean tissue distribution by dual energy X-ray absorptiometry and abdominal body fat evaluation by computed tomography in Cushing's disease. J Clin Endocrinol Metab 1995; 80: 2791–2794.
241. Lado Abeal J, Rodriguez Arnao J, Newell Price JD, et al. Menstrual abnormalities in women with Cushing's disease are correlated with hypercortisolemia rather than raised circulating androgen levels. J Clin Endocrinol Metab 1998; 83:3083–3088.
242. Chrousos GP, Torphy DJ, Gold PW. Interactions between the hypothalamic-pituitary-adrenal axis and the female reproductive system: clinical implications. Ann Intern Med 1998; 129:229–240.
243. Luton PJ, Thiebolt P, Valcke JC, et al. Reversible gonadotropin deficiency in male Cushing's disease. J Clin Endocrinol Metab 1977; 45:488–495.
244. Jeffcoate WJ, Silverstone JT, Edwards CRW, et al. Psychiatric manifestations of Cushing's syndrome: response to lowering of plasma cortisol. Q J Med 1979; 48:465-472.
245. Cohen SI. Cushing's syndrome: a psychiatric study of 29 patients. Br J Psychiatry 1980; 136:120–124.
246. Starkman MN, Schteingart DE. Neuropsychiatric manifestations of patients with Cushing's syndrome: relationship to cortisol and adrenocorticotropic levels. Arch Intern Med 1981; 141:215–219.
247. Dorn LD, Burgess ES, Dubbert B, et al. Psychopathology in patients with endogenous Cushing's syndrome: "atypical" or melancholic features. Clin Endocrinol (Oxf) 1995; 43:433–442.
248. Friess E, Wiedemann K, Steiger A, et al. The hypothalamic-pituitary-adrenocortical system and sleep in man. Adv Neuroimmunol 1995; 5:111–125.
249. Friedman TC, Garcia-Borreguero D, Hardwick D, et al. Decreased delta-sleep and plasma delta-sleep–inducing peptide in patients with Cushing syndrome. Neuroendocrinology 1994; 60: 626–634.
250. Ferguson JK, Donald RA, Weston TS, et al. Skin thickness in patients with acromegaly and Cushing's syndrome and response to treatment. Clin Endocrinol (Oxf) 1983; 18:347–353.
251. Urbanic RC, George JM. Cushing's disease: 18 years' experience. Medicine (Baltimore) 1981; 60:14–24.

252. Pleasure DE, Engel WK. Atrophy of skeletal muscle in patients with Cushing's syndrome. Arch Neurol 1970; 22:118–125.
253. Dale DC, Petersdorf RG. Corticosteroids and infectious diseases. Med Clin North Am 1973; 57:1277–1287.
254. Graham BS, Tucker WS Jr. Opportunistic infections in endogenous Cushing's syndrome. Ann Intern Med 1984; 101:334–338.
255. Hill AT, Stewart PM, Hughes EA, Mcleod DT. Cushing's disease and tuberculosis. Respir Med 1998; 92:604–605.
256. Taskinen MR, Nikkila EA, Pelkonen R, et al. Plasma lipoproteins, lipolytic enzymes, and very low density lipoprotein triglyceride turnover in Cushing's syndrome. J Clin Endocrinol Metab 1983; 57:619–626.
257. Christy NP, Laragh JH. Pathogenesis of hypokalemic alkalosis in Cushing's syndrome. N Engl J Med 1961; 265:1083.
258. Ulick S, Wang JZ, Blumenfeld JD, et al. Cortisol inactivation overload: a mechanism of mineralocorticoid hypertension in the ectopic adrenocorticotropin syndrome. J Clin Endocrinol Metab 1992; 74:963–967.
259. Stewart PM, Walker BR, Holder G, et al. 11β-Hydroxysteroid dehydrogenase activity in Cushing's syndrome: explaining the mineralocorticoid excess state of the ectopic ACTH syndrome. J Clin Endocrinol Metab 1995; 80:3617–3620.
260. Benker G, Raida M, Olbricht T, et al. TSH secretion in Cushing's syndrome: relation to glucocorticoid excess, diabetes, goiter and the "sick euthyroid syndrome." Clin Endocrinol (Oxf) 1990; 33:777–786.
261. Saketos M, Sharma N, Santoro NF. Suppression of the hypothalamo-pituitary-ovarian axis in normal women by glucocorticoids. Biol Reprod 1993; 49:1270–1276.
262. Sayegh F, Weigelin E. Intraocular pressure in Cushing's syndrome. Ophthalmic Res 1975; 7:390–394.
263. Panzer SW, Patrinely JR, Wilson HK. Exophthalmos and iatrogenic Cushing's syndrome. Ophthal Plast Reconstr Surg 1994; 10:278–282.
264. Bouzas EA, Mastorakos G, Friedman G, et al. Posterior subcapsular cataract in endogenous Cushing syndrome: an uncommon manifestation. Invest Ophthalmol Vis Sci 1993; 34:3497–3500.
265. Biller BMK. Pathogenesis of pituitary Cushing's syndrome: pituitary versus hypothalamic. Endocrinol Metab Clin North Am 1994; 23:547–554.
266. Boyar RM, Witkin M, Carruth A, et al. Circadian cortisol secretory rhythms in Cushing's disease. J Clin Endocrinol Metab 1979; 48:760–765.
267. Krieger DT, Glick SM. Growth hormone and cortisol responsiveness in Cushing's syndrome: relation to a possible central nervous system etiology. Am J Med 1972; 52:25–40.
268. Kling MA, Roy A, Doran AR, et al. Cerebrospinal fluid immunoreactive corticotropin-releasing hormone and adrenocorticotropin secretion in Cushing's disease and major depression: potential clinical implications. J Clin Endocrinol Metab 1991; 72:260–271.
269. Krieger DT, Amorosa L, Linick F. Cyproheptadine-induced remission of Cushing's disease. N Engl J Med 1975;293:893–896.
270. Lamberts SWJ, Klijn JGM, DeQuijada M, et al. The mechanism of the suppressive action of bromocriptine on adrenocorticotropin secretion in patients with Cushing's disease and Nelson's syndrome. J Clin Endocrinol Metab 1980; 51:307–311.
271. Guilhaume B, Bertagna X, Thomsen M, et al. Transsphenoidal pituitary surgery for the treatment of Cushing's disease: results in 64 patients and long term follow-up studies. J Clin Endocrinol Metab 1988; 66:1056–1064.
272. Bochicchio D, Losa M, Buchfelder M, et al. Factors influencing the immediate and late outcome of Cushing's disease treated by transsphenoidal surgery: a retrospective study by the European Cushing's Disease Survey Group. J Clin Endocrinol Metab 1995; 80:3114–3120.
273. Fitzgerald PA, Aron DC, Findling JW, et al. Cushing's disease: transient secondary adrenal insufficiency after selective removal of pituitary microadenomas. Evidence for a pituitary origin. J Clin Endocrinol Metab 1982; 54:413–422.
274. Gicquel C, Le Bouc Y, Luton J-P, et al. Monoclonality of corticotroph macroadenomas in Cushing's disease. J Clin Endocrinol Metab 1992; 75:472–475.
275. Biller BMK, Alexander JM, Zervas NT, et al. Clonal origins of adrenocorticotropin-secreting pituitary tissue in Cushing's disease. J Clin Endocrinol Metab 1992; 75:1303–1309.
276. Tonner D, Belding P, Moore SA, et al. Intracranial dissemination of an ACTH secreting pituitary neoplasm: a case report and review of the literature. J Endocrinol Invest 1992; 15:387–391.
277. Krieger DT. Physiopathology of Cushing's disease. Endocr Rev 1983; 4:22–43.
278. Van Cauter E, Refetoff S. Evidence for two subtypes of Cushing's disease based on the analysis of episodic cortisol secretion. N Engl J Med 1985; 312:1343–1349.
279. Liddle GW. Tests of pituitary-adrenal suppressibility in the diagnosis of Cushing's syndrome. J Clin Endocrinol Metab 1960; 20: 1539–1560.
280. Liu JH, Kazer RR, Rasmussen DD. Characterization of the twenty-four hour secretion patterns of adrenocorticotropin and cortisol in normal women and patients with Cushing's disease. J Clin Endocrinol Metab 1987; 64:1027–1035.
281. Stewart PM, Penn R, Gibson R, et al. Hypothalamic abnormalities in patients with pituitary-dependent Cushing's syndrome. Clin Endocrinol (Oxf) 1992; 36:453–458.
282. Jex RK, van Heerden JA, Carpenter PC, et al. Ectopic ACTH syndrome, diagnostic and therapeutic aspects. Am J Surg 1985; 149:276–282.
283. Howlett TA, Drury PL, Perry L, et al. Diagnosis and management of ACTH-dependent Cushing's syndrome: comparison of the features in ectopic and pituitary ACTH production. Clin Endocrinol (Oxf) 1986; 24:699—713.
284. Imura H, Matsukura S, Yamamoto H, et al. Studies on ectopic ACTH producing tumours: clinical and biochemical features in 30 cases. Cancer 1975; 35:1430–1437.
285. Findling JW, Tyrrell JB. Occult ectopic secretion of corticotropin. Arch Intern Med 1986; 146:929–933.
286. Limper AH, Carpenter PC, Scheithauer B, et al. The Cushing syndrome induced by bronchial carcinoid tumours. Ann Intern Med 1992; 117:209–214.
287. Odell WD. Bronchial and thymic carcinoids and the ectopic ACTH syndrome. Ann Thorac Surg 1991; 50:5–6.
288. Odell WD. Ectopic ACTH secretion: a misnomer. Endocrinol Metab Clin North Am 1991; 20:371–379.
289. Kohler PC, Trump DL. Ectopic hormone syndromes. Cancer Invest 1986; 4:543–554.
290. White A, Clark AJL. The cellular and molecular basis of the ectopic ACTH syndrome. Clin Endocrinol (Oxf) 1993; 39:131–141.
291. Dichek HL, Nieman LK, Oldfield EH, et al. A comparison of the standard high dose dexamethasone suppression test for the differential diagnosis of adrenocorticotropin dependent Cushing's syndrome. J Clin Endocrinol Metab 1994; 78:418–422.
292. Gaitan D, DeBold CR, Turney MK, et al. Glucocorticoid receptor structure and function in an adrenocorticotropin-secreting small cell lung cancer. Mol Endocrinol 1995; 9:1193–1201.
293. Ray DW, Littlewood AC, Clark AJL, et al. Human small cell lung cancer cell lines expressing the proopiomelanocortin gene have aberrant glucocorticoid receptor function. J Clin Invest 1994; 93:1625–1630.
294. Ray DW, Davies JRE, White A, Clark AJL. Glucocorticoid receptor structure and function in glucocorticoid-resistant small cell lung carcinoma cells. Cancer Res 1996; 56:3276–3280.
295. Carey RM, Varma SK, Drake CR Jr, et al. Ectopic secretion of corticotropin-releasing factor as a cause of Cushing's syndrome: a clinical, morphologic, and biochemical study. N Engl J Med 1984; 311:13–20.
296. Schteingart DE, Lloyd RV, Akil H, et al. Cushing's syndrome secondary to ectopic corticotropin-releasing hormone–adrenocorticotropin secretion. J Clin Endocrinol Metab 1986; 63:770–775.
297. Zarate A, Kovacs K, Flores M, et al. ACTH and CRF-producing bronchial carcinoid associated with Cushing's syndrome. Clin Endocrinol (Oxf) 1986; 24:523–529.
298. Jessop DS, Cunnah D, Millar JG, et al. A phaeochromocytoma presenting with Cushing's syndrome associated with increased concentrations of circulating corticotrophin-releasing factor. J Endocrinol 1987; 113:133–138.
299. O'Brien T, Young WF Jr, Davila DG, et al. Cushing's syndrome associated with ectopic production of corticotrophin-releasing hormone, corticotrophin and vasopressin by a phaeochromocytoma. Clin Endocrinol (Oxf) 1992; 37:460–467.
300. Puchner MJ, Ludecke DK, Valdueza JM, et al. Cushing's disease in a child caused by a corticotropin-releasing hormone–secreting intrasellar gangliocytoma associated with an adrenocorticotropic

hormone-secreting pituitary adenoma. Neurosurgery 1993; 33: 920–925.
301. Preeyasombat C, Sirikulchayanonta V, Mahachokelertwattana P, et al. Cushing's syndrome caused by Ewing's sarcoma secreting corticotropin releasing factor-like peptide. Am J Dis Child 1992; 146:1103–1105.
302. Muller OA, Von Werder K. Ectopic production of ACTH and corticotropin-releasing hormone (CRH). J Steroid Biochem Mol Biol 1992; 43:403–408.
303. Howlett TA, Price J, Hale AC, et al. Pituitary ACTH dependent Cushing's syndrome due to ectopic production of a bombesin-like peptide by a medullary carcinoma of the thyroid. Clin Endocrinol (Oxf) 1985; 22:91–101.
304. Smals AGH, Pieters GFFM, van Haelst UJG, et al. Macronodular adrenocortical hyperplasia in long-standing Cushing's disease. J Clin Endocrinol Metab 1984; 58:25–31.
305. Doppman JL, Miller DL, Dwyer AJ, et al. Macronodular adrenal hyperplasia in Cushing disease. Radiology 1988; 166:347–352.
306. Aron DC, Findling JW, Fitzgerald PA, et al. Pituitary ACTH dependency of nodular adrenal hyperplasia in Cushing's syndrome: report of two cases and review of the literature. Am J Med 1981; 71:302–306.
307. Hermus AR, Pieters GF, Smals AG, et al. Transition from pituitary-dependent to adrenal-dependent Cushing's syndrome. N Engl J Med 1988; 318:966–970.
308. Fish HR, Sobel DO, Miegel CA. Macronodular adrenal hyperplasia with hypothalamic-pituitary-adrenal suppression by ultrahigh dose dexamethasone. Clin Neuropharmacol 1986; 9:303–308.
309. Hutter AM Jr, Kayhoe DE. Adrenal cortical carcinoma: clinical features of 138 patients. Am J Med 1966; 41:572–580.
310. Bertagna C, Orth DN. Clinical and laboratory findings and results of therapy in 58 patients with adrenocortical tumors admitted to a single medical center (1951 to 1978). Am J Med 1981; 71:855–875.
311. Luton J-P, Cerdas S, Billaud L, et al. Clinical features of adrenocortical carcinoma, prognostic factors, and the effect of mitotane therapy. N Engl J Med 1990; 322:1195–1201.
312. Kasperlik-Zaluska AA, Migdalska BM, Zgliczynski S, et al. Adrenocortical carcinoma: a clinical study and treatment results of 52 patients. Cancer 1995; 75:2587–2591.
313. Larsen JL, Cathey WJ, Odell WD. Primary adrenocortical nodular dysplasia, a distinct subtype of Cushing's syndrome: case report and review of the literature. Am J Med 1986; 80:976–984.
314. Young WF Jr, Carney JA, Musa BU, et al. Familial Cushing's syndrome due to primary pigmented nodular adrenocortical disease: reinvestigation 50 years later. N Engl J Med 1989; 321: 1659–1664.
315. Doppman JL, Travis WD, Nieman L, et al. Cushing syndrome due to primary pigmented nodular adrenocortical disease: findings at CT and MR imaging. Radiology 1989; 172:415–420.
316. Carney JA, Gordon H, Carpenter PC, et al. The complex of myxomas, spotty pigmentation, and endocrine overactivity. Medicine (Baltimore) 1985; 64:270–283.
317. Carney JA, Young WF Jr. Primary pigmented nodular adrenocortical disease and its associated conditions. Endocrinologist 1992; 2:6–21.
318. Stratakis CA, Carney JA, Lin JP, et al. Carney complex, a familial multiple neoplasia and lentiginosis syndrome: analysis of 11 kindreds and linkage to the short arm of chromosome 2. J Clin Invest 1996; 97:699–705.
319. Casey M, Mah C, Merliss AD, et al. Identification of a novel genetic locus for familial cardiac myxomas and Carney complex. Circulation 1998; 98:2560–2566.
320. Kirschner LS, Carney JA, Pack SD, et al. Mutations of the gene encoding the protein kinase A type I-alpha regulatory subunit in patients with the Carney complex. Nat Genet 2000; 26:89–92.
321. Casey M, Vaughan CJ, He J, et al. Mutations in the protein kinase A R1alpha regulatory subunit cause familial cardiac myxomas and Carney complex. J Clin Invest 2000; 106:R31–R38. Erratum in J Clin Invest 2001; 107:235.
322. Yoshimoto M, Nakayama M, Baba T, et al. A case of neonatal McCune-Albright syndrome with Cushing's syndrome and hyperthyroidism. Acta Paediatr Scand 1991; 80:984–987.
323. Weinstein LS, Shenker A, Gejman PV, et al. Activating mutations of the stimulatory G protein in McCune-Albright syndrome. N Engl J Med 1991; 325:1688–1695.
324. Findlay JC, Sheeler LR, Engeland WC, et al. Familial adrenocorticotropin-independent Cushing's syndrome with bilateral macronodular adrenal hyperplasia. J Clin Endocrinol Metab 1993; 76:189–191.
325. Malchoff CD, MacGillivray D, Malchoff DM. Adrenocorticotropic hormone-independent adrenal hyperplasia. Endocrinologist 1996; 6:79–85.
326. Boston BA, Mandel S, LaFranchi S, et al. Activating mutation in the stimulatory guanine nucleotide-binding protein in an infant with Cushing's syndrome and nodular adrenal hyperplasia. J Clin Endocrinol Metab 1994; 79:890–893.
327. Lacroix A, Bolte E, Tremblay J, et al. Gastric inhibitory polypeptide-dependent cortisol hypersecretion: a new cause of Cushing's syndrome. N Engl J Med 1992; 327:974–980.
328. Reznik Y, Allali Zerah V, Chayvialle JA, et al. Food-dependent Cushing's syndrome mediated by aberrant adrenal sensitivity to gastric inhibitory polypeptide. N Engl J Med 1992; 327:981–986.
329. N'Diaye N, Hamet P, Tremblay J, et al. Asynchronous development of bilateral adrenal hyperplasia in gastric inhibitory polypeptide-dependent Cushing's syndrome. J Clin Endocrinol Metab 1999; 84:2616–2622.
330. Willenberg HS, Stratakis CA, Marx C, et al. Aberrant interleukin-1 receptors in a cortisol-secreting adrenal adenoma causing Cushing's syndrome. N Engl J Med 1998; 339:27–31.
331. Jordan RM, Ramos-Gabatin A, Kendall JW, et al. Dynamics of adrenocorticotropin (ACTH) secretion in cyclic Cushing's syndrome: evidence for more than one abnormal ACTH biorhythm. J Clin Endocrinol Metab 1982; 55:531–537.
332. Atkinson AB, Kennedy AL, Carson DJ, et al. Five cases of cyclical Cushing's syndrome. Br Med J 1985; 291:1453–1457.
333. Estopinan V, Varela C, Riobo P, et al. Ectopic Cushing's syndrome with periodic hormonogenesis: a case suggesting a pathogenetic mechanism. Postgrad Med J 1987; 63:887–889.
334. Stewart PM, Venn P, Heath DA, et al. Cyclical Cushing's syndrome. Br J Hosp Med 1992; 48:186–187.
335. Leinung MC, Zimmerman D. Cushing's disease in children. Endocrinol Metab Clin North Am 1994; 23:629–639.
336. Sheeler LR. Cushing's syndrome and pregnancy. Endocrinol Metab Clin North Am 1994; 23:619–627.
337. Close CF, Mann MC, Watts JF, et al. ACTH-independent Cushing's syndrome in pregnancy with spontaneous resolution after delivery: control of the hypercortisolism with metyrapone. Clin Endocrinol (Oxf) 1993; 39:375–379.
338. Wallace C, Toth EL, Lewanczuk RZ, Siminoski K. Pregnancy-induced Cushing's syndrome in multiple pregnancies. J Clin Endocrinol Metab 1996; 81:15–21.
339. Smalls AGH, Kloppenborg PWC, Njo KT, et al. Alcohol-induced cushingoid syndrome. Br Med J 1976; 2:1298.
340. Rees LH, Besser GM, Jeffcoate WJ, et al. Alcoholic pseudo-Cushing's. Lancet 1977; 1:726–728.
341. Kirkman S, Nelson DH. Alcohol-induced pseudo-Cushing's disease: a study of prevalence with review of the literature. Metabolism 1988; 37:390–394.
342. Stewart PM, Burra P, Shackleton CHL, et al. 11β-Hydroxysteroid dehydrogenase deficiency and glucocorticoid status in patients with alcoholic and non-alcoholic chronic liver disease. J Clin Endocrinol Metab 1993; 76:748–751.
343. Carroll BJ, Curtis GC, Mendels J. Neuroendocrine regulation in depression. II. Discrimination from depressed and nondepressed patients. Arch Gen Psychiatry 1976; 33:1051–1058.
344. Glass AR, Burman KD, Dahms WT, Boehm TM. Endocrine function in human obesity. Metabolism 1981; 30:89–104.
345. Ljung T, Andersson B, Bengtsson B-A, Björntorp P. Inhibition of cortisol secretion by dexamethasone in relation to body fat distribution: a dose-response study. Obes Res 1996; 4:277–282.
346. Streeteen DHP. Is hypothalamic-pituitary-adrenal hyperactivity important in the pathogenesis of excessive abdominal fat distribution? J Clin Endocrinol Metab 1993; 77:339–340.
347. Stewart PM, Boulton A, Kumar S, et al. Cortisol metabolism in human obesity: impaired cortisone-cortisol conversion in subjects with central obesity. J Clin Endocrinol Metab 1999; 84:1022–1027.
348. Andrew R, Phillip DIW, Walker BR. Obesity and gender influence cortisol secretion and metabolism in man. J Clin Endocrinol Metab 1998; 83:1806–1809.
349. Orth DN. Medical progress: Cushing's syndrome. N Engl J Med 1995; 332:791–803.

350. Newell-Price J, Trainer P, Besser M, Grossman A. The diagnosis and differential diagnosis of Cushing's syndrome and pseudo-Cushing's states. Endocr Rev 1998; 19:647–672.
351. Newell-Price J, Trainer P, Perry L, et al. A single sleeping midnight cortisol has 100% sensitivity for the diagnosis of Cushing's syndrome. Clin Endocrinol (Oxf) 1995; 43:545–550.
352. Vining RF, McGinley RA, Maksvytis JJ, et al. Salivary cortisol: a better measure of adrenal cortical function than serum cortisol. Ann Clin Biochem 1983; 20:329–335.
353. Laudat MH, Cerdas S, Fournier C, et al. Salivary cortisol measurement: a practical approach to assess pituitary-adrenal function. J Clin Endocrinol Metab 1988; 66:343–348.
354. Crapo L. Cushing's syndrome: a review of diagnostic tests. Metabolism 1979; 28:955–977.
355. Invitti C, Giraldi FP, Martin M, Cavagnini F. Diagnosis and management of Cushing's syndrome: results of an Italian multicentre study. J Clin Endocrinol Metab 1999; 84:440–448.
356. Nugent CA, Nichols T, Tyler FH. Diagnosis of Cushing's syndrome: single dose dexamethasone test. Arch Intern Med 1965; 116:172–176.
357. Cronin C, Igoe D, Duffy MJ, et al. The overnight dexamethasone test is a worthwhile screening procedure. Clin Endocrinol (Oxf) 1990; 33:27–33.
358. Montwill J, Igoe D, McKenna TJ. The overnight dexamethasone test is the procedure of choice in screening for Cushing's syndrome. Steroids 1994; 59:296–298.
359. Kennedy L, Atkinson AB, Johnston H, et al. Serum cortisol concentrations during low dose dexamethasone suppression test to screen for Cushing's syndrome. Br Med J 1984; 289:1188–1191.
360. Meikle AW. Dexamethasone suppression tests: usefulness of simultaneous measurement of plasma cortisol and dexamethasone. Clin Endocrinol (Oxf) 1982; 16:401–408.
361. Yanovski JA, Cutler GB Jr, Chrousos GP, et al. Corticotropin-releasing hormone stimulation following low-dose dexamethasone administration: a new test to distinguish Cushing's syndrome from pseudo-Cushing's states. JAMA 1993; 269:2232–2238.
362. Findling JW. Clinical application of a new immunoradiometric assay for ACTH. Endocrinologist 1992; 2:360-365.
363. Lindholm J. Endocrine function in patients with Cushing's disease before and after treatment. Clin Endocrinol (Oxf) 1992; 36: 151–159.
364. Tyrrell JB, Findling JW, Aron DC, et al. An overnight high-dose dexamethasone suppression test for rapid differential diagnosis of Cushing's syndrome. Ann Intern Med 1986; 104:180–186.
365. Biemond P, de Jong FH, Lamberts SWJ. Continuous dexamethasone infusion for seven hours in patients with the Cushing syndrome: a superior differential diagnostic test. Ann Intern Med 1990; 112:738–742.
366. Findling JW, Doppman JL. Biochemical and radiological diagnosis of Cushing's syndrome. Endocrinol Metab Clin North Am 1994; 23:511–537.
367. Avgerinos PC, Yanovski JA, Oldfield EH, et al. The metyrapone and dexamethasone suppression tests for the differential diagnosis of the adrenocorticotropin-dependent Cushing syndrome: a comparison. Ann Intern Med 1994; 121:318–327.
368. Trainer PJ, Faria M, Newell-Price J, et al. A comparison of the effects of human and ovine corticotropin-releasing hormone on the pituitary-adrenal axis. J Clin Endocrinol Metab 1995; 80: 412–417.
369. Orth DN, DeBold CR, DeCherney GS, et al. Pituitary microadenomas causing Cushing's disease respond to corticotropin-releasing factor. J Clin Endocrinol Metab 1982; 55:1017–1019.
370. Chrousos GP, Schulte HM, Oldfield EH, et al. The corticotropin-releasing factor stimulation test: an aid in the evaluation of patients with Cushing's syndrome. N Engl J Med 1984; 310:622–626.
371. Dickstein G, DeBold CR, Gaitan D, et al. Plasma corticotropin and cortisol responses to ovine corticotropin-releasing hormone (CRH), arginine vasopressin (AVP), CRH plus AVP, and CRH plus metyrapone in patients with Cushing's disease. J Clin Endocrinol Metab 1996; 81:2934–2941.
372. Nieman LK, Oldfield EH, Wesley R, et al. A simplified morning ovine corticotropin-releasing hormone stimulation test for the differential diagnosis of adrenocorticotropin-dependent Cushing's syndrome. J Clin Endocrinol Metab 1993; 77:1308–1312.
373. Newell-Price J, Perry L, Medbak S, et al. A combined test using desmopressin and corticotropin releasing hormone in the differential diagnosis of Cushing's syndrome. J Clin Endocrinol Metab 1997; 82:176–181.
374. Oldfield EH, Doppman LJ, Nieman LK, et al. Petrosal sinus sampling with and without corticotropin releasing hormone for the differential diagnosis of Cushing's syndrome. N Engl J Med 1991; 325:897–905.
375. Tabarin A, Greselle JF, San Galli F, et al. Usefulness of the corticotropin-releasing hormone test during bilateral inferior petrosal sinus sampling for the diagnosis of Cushing's disease. J Clin Endocrinol Metab 1991; 73:53–59.
376. Kaltsas GA, Giannulis MG, Newell Price JD, et al. A critical analysis of the value of simultaneous inferior petrosal sinus sampling in Cushing's disease and the occult ectopic adrenocorticotropin syndrome. J Clin Endocrinol Metab 1999; 84:487–492.
377. Saris SC, Patronas NJ, Doppman JL, et al. Cushing syndrome: pituitary CT scanning. Radiology 1987; 162:775–777.
378. Peck WW, Dillon WP, Norman D, et al. High-resolution MR imaging of pituitary microadenomas at 1.5 T: experience with Cushing disease. AJR 1989; 152:145–151.
379. Hall WA, Luciano MG, Doppman JL, et al. Pituitary magnetic resonance imaging in normal human volunteers: occult adenomas in the general population. Ann Intern Med 1994; 120:817–820.
380. Korobkin M, Francis IR. Adrenal imaging. Semin Ultrasound CT MR 1995; 16:317–330.
381. Miles JM, Wahner HW, Carpenter PC, et al. Adrenal scintiscanning with NP-59, a new radioiodinated cholesterol agent. Mayo Clin Proc 1979; 54:321–327.
382. de Herder WW, Krenning EP, Malchoff CD, et al. Somatostatin receptor scintigraphy: its value in tumor localization in patients with Cushing's syndrome caused by ectopic corticotropin or corticotropin-releasing hormone secretion. Am J Med 1994; 96:305–312.
383. Hoefnagel CA. Metaiodobenzylguanidine and somatostatin in oncology: role in the management of neural crest tumours. Eur J Nucl Med 1994; 21:561–581.
384. Valimaki M, Pelkonen R, Porkka L, et al. Long-term results of adrenal surgery in patients with Cushing's syndrome due to adrenocortical adenoma. Clin Endocrinol (Oxf) 1984; 20:229–236.
385. Gagner M, Lacroix A, Prinz RA, et al. Early experience with laparoscopic approach for adrenalectomy. Surgery 1993; 114: 1120-1124; discussion 1124–1125.
386. Wells SA, Merke DP, Cutler GB, et al. Therapeutic controversy: the role of laparoscopic adrenalectomy in adrenal disease. J Clin Endocrinol Metab 1998; 83:3041–3049.
387. Wilson CB, Tyrrell JB, Fitzgerald PA, et al. Cushing's disease and Nelson's syndrome. Clin Neurosurg 1980; 27:19–30.
388. Jenkins PJ, Trainer PJ, Plowman PN, et al. The long term outcome after adrenalectomy and prophylactic pituitary radiotherapy in adrenocorticotropin-dependent Cushing's syndrome. J Clin Endocrinol Metab 1995; 80:165–171.
389. Burch W. A survey of results with transsphenoidal surgery in Cushing's disease. N Engl J Med 1983; 308:103–104.
390. Trainer PJ, Lawrie HS, Verhelst J, et al. Transsphenoidal resection in Cushing's disease: undetectable serum cortisol as the definition of successful treatment. Clin Endocrinol (Oxf) 1993; 38: 73–78.
391. McCance DR, Besser M, Atkinson AB. Assessment of cure after transsphenoidal surgery for Cushing's disease. Clin Endocrinol (Oxf) 1996; 44:1–6.
392. Leinung MC, Kane LA, Scheithauer BW, et al. Long term follow-up of transsphenoidal surgery for the treatment of Cushing's disease in childhood. J Clin Endocrinol Metab 1995; 80:2475–2479.
393. Jennings AS, Liddle GW, Orth DN. Results of treating childhood Cushing's disease with pituitary irradiation. N Engl J Med 1977; 297:957–962.
394. Verhelst JA, Trainer PJ, Howlett TA, et al. Short and long-term responses to metyrapone in the medical management of 91 patients with Cushing's syndrome. Clin Endocrinol (Oxf) 1991; 35: 169–178.
395. Child DF, Burke CW, Burley DM, et al. Drug control of Cushing's syndrome: combined aminoglutethimide and metyrapone therapy. Acta Endocrinol (Copenh) 1976; 82:330–341.
396. Semple CG, Beastall GH, Gray CE, et al. Trilostane in the

management of Cushing's syndrome. Acta Endocrinol (Copenh) 1983; 102:107–110.
397. McCance DR, Hadden DR, Kennedy L, et al. Clinical experience with ketoconazole as a therapy for patients with Cushing's syndrome. Clin Endocrinol (Oxf) 1987; 27:593–599.
398. Plotz CM, Knowlton AI, Ragan C. The natural history of Cushing's syndrome. Am J Med 1952; 13:597–614.
399. Etxabe J, Vazquez JA. Morbidity and mortality in Cushing's disease: an epidemiological approach. Clin Endocrinol (Oxf) 1994; 40:479-484.
400. Colao A, Pivonello R, Spiezia S, et al. Persistence of increased cardiovascular risk factors in patients with Cushing's disease after five years of successful cure. J Clin Endocrinol Metab 1999; 84: 2664–2672.
401. Hermus AR, Smals AG, Swinkels LM, et al. Bone mineral density and bone turnover before and after surgical cure of Cushing's syndrome. J Clin Endocrinol Metab 1995; 80:2859–2865.
402. Vingerhoeds AC, Thijssen JH, Schwarz F. Spontaneous hypercortisolism without Cushing's syndrome. J Clin Endocrinol Metab 1976; 43:1128–1133.
403. Chrousos GP, Vingerhoeds AC, Brandon D, et al. Primary cortisol resistance in man: a glucocorticoid receptor disease. J Clin Invest 1982; 69:1261–1268.
404. Huizenga NATM, de Lange P, Koper JW, et al. Five patients with biochemical and/or clinical generalized glucocorticoid resistance without alterations in the glucocorticoid receptor gene. J Clin Endocrinol Metab 2000; 85:2076–2081.
405. Kong MF, Jeffcoate W. Eighty-six cases of Addison's disease. Clin Endocrinol (Oxf) 1994; 41:757–761.
406. Oelkers W. Adrenal insufficiency. N Engl J Med 1996; 335: 1206–1212.
407. Carey RM. The changing clinical spectrum of adrenal insufficiency. Ann Intern Med 1997; 127:1103–1105.
408. Zelissen PM, Bast EJ, Croughs RJ. Associated autoimmunity in Addison's disease. J Autoimmun 1995; 8:121–130.
409. Betterle C, Greggio NA, Volpato M. Clinical review 93: autoimmune polyglandular syndrome type 1. J Clin Endocrinol Metab 1998; 83:1049–1055.
410. Betterle C, Volpato M, Greggio NA, Presotto F. Type 2 polyglandular autoimmune disease (Schmidt's syndrome). J Pediatr Endocrinol Metab 1996; 9:113–123.
411. Ahonen P, Myllarniemi S, Sipila I, et al. Clinical variation of autoimmune polyendocrinopathy–candidiasis–ectodermal dystrophy (APECED) in a series of 68 patients. N Engl J Med 1990; 322:1829–1836.
412. Winqvist O, Gustafsson J, Rorsman F, et al. Two different cytochrome P450 enzymes are the adrenal antigens in autoimmune polyendocrine syndrome type I and Addison's disease. J Clin Invest 1993; 92:2377–2385.
413. Peterson P, Krohn KJ. Mapping of B cell epitopes on steroid 17α-hydroxylase, an autoantigen in autoimmune polyglandular syndrome type I. Clin Exp Immunol 1994; 98:104—109.
414. The Finnish-German APECED consortium. An autoimmune disease, APECED, caused by mutations in a novel gene featuring two PHD-type zinc-finger domains. Nat Genet 1997; 17:399–403.
415. Aaltonen J, Bjorses P. Cloning of the APECED gene provides new insight into human autoimmunity. Ann Med 1999; 31:111–116.
416. Song YH, Connor EL, Muir A, et al. Autoantibody epitope mapping of the 21-hydroxylase antigen in autoimmune Addison's disease. J Clin Endocrinol Metab 1994; 78:1108–1112.
417. Uibo R, Aavik E, Peterson P, et al. Autoantibodies to cytochrome P450 enzymes P450scc, P450c17, and P450c21 in autoimmune polyglandular disease types I and II and in isolated Addison's disease. J Clin Endocrinol Metab 1994; 78:323–328.
418. Yu L. DRB1*04 and DQ alleles: expression of 21-hydroxylase autoantibodies and risk of progression to Addison's disease. J Clin Endocrinol Metab 1999; 84:328–335.
419. Vita JA, Silverberg SJ, Goland RS, et al. Clinical clues to the cause of Addison's disease. Am J Med 1985; 78:461–466.
420. Piedrola G, Casado JL, Lopez E, et al. Clinical features of adrenal insufficiency in patients with acquired immunodeficiency syndrome. Clin Endocrinol (Oxf) 1996; 45:97–101.
421. Honour JW. HIV and adrenal function. Curr Opin Endocrinol Diabetes 1998; 5:162–167.
422. Norbiato G, Galli M, Righini V, et al. The syndrome of acquired glucocorticoid resistance in HIV infection. Baillieres Clin Endocrinol Metab 1994; 8:777–787.
423. Seidenwurm DJ, Elmer EB, Kaplan LM, et al. Metastases to the adrenal glands and the development of Addison's disease. Cancer 1984; 54:552–557.
424. Xarli VP, Steele AA, Davis PJ, et al. Adrenal hemorrhage in the adult. Medicine (Baltimore) 1978; 57:211–221.
425. Margaretten W, Nakai H, Landing BH. Septicemic adrenal hemorrhage. Am J Dis Child 1963; 105:346–351.
426. Reutins AT. Clinical and functional effects of mutations in the *DAX-1* gene in patients with adrenal hypoplasia congenita. J Clin Endocrinol Metab 1999; 84:504–511.
427. Lalli E, Sassone-Corsi P. DAX-1 and the adrenal cortex. Curr Opin Endocrinol Metab 1999; 6:185–190.
428. Taberin A, Achermann JC, Recan D, et al. A novel mutation in *DAX-1* causes delayed-onset adrenal insufficiency and incomplete hypogonadotrophic hypogonadism. J Clin Invest 2000; 105:321–328.
429. Achermann JC, Ito M, Hindmarsh PC, Jameson JL. A mutation in the gene encoding steroidogenic factor 1 causes YY sex reversal and adrenal failure. Nat Genet 1999; 22:125–126.
430. Scheuerle A, Greenberg F, McCabe ER. Dysmorphic features in patients with complex glycerol kinase deficiency. J Pediatr 1995; 126:764–767.
431. Moser HW, Moser AE, Singh I, et al. Adrenoleukodystrophy: survey of 303 cases. Biochemistry, diagnosis, and therapy. Ann Neurol 1984; 16:628–641.
432. Laureti S, Casucci G, Santeusanio F, et al. X-linked adrenoleukodystrophy is a frequent cause of idiopathic Addison's disease in young adult male patients. J Clin Endocrinol Metab 1996; 81: 470–474.
433. Mosser J, Douar A-M, Sarde C-O, et al. Putative X-linked adrenoleukodystrophy gene shares unexpected homology with ABC transporters. Nature 1993; 361:726–730.
434. Smith KD, Kemp S, Braiterman LT, et al. X-linked adrenoleukodystrophy: genes, mutations and phenotypes. Neurochem Res 1999; 24:521–535.
435. Shapiro E, Krivit W, Lockman L, et al. Long-term effect of bone-marrow transplantation for childhood-onset cerebral X-linked adrenoleukodystrophy. Lancet 2000; 356:713–718.
436. Huebner A, Elias LL, Clark AJL. ACTH resistance syndromes. J Paediatr Endocrinol Metab 1999; 12:277–293.
437. Heinrichs C, Tsigos C, Deschepper J, et al. Familial adrenocorticotropin unresponsiveness associated with alacrima and achalasia: biochemical and molecular studies in two siblings with clinical heterogeneity. Eur J Pediatr 1995; 154:191–196.
438. Handschug K, Sperling S, Yoon SJ, Hennig S, et al. Triple A syndrome is caused by mutations in AAAS, a new WD-repeat protein gene. Hum Mol Genet 2001; 10:283–290.
439. Stacpoole PW, Interlandi JW, Nicholson WE, et al. Isolated ACTH deficiency: a heterogenous disorder. Critical review and report of four new cases. Medicine (Baltimore) 1982; 61:13–24.
440. Nussey SS, Soo SC, Gibson S, et al. Isolated congenital ACTH deficiency: a cleavage enzyme defect? Clin Endocrinol (Oxf) 1993; 39:381–385.
441. O'Rahilly S, Gray H, Humphreys PJ, et al. Brief report: impaired processing of prohormones associated with abnormalities of glucose homeostasis and adrenal function. N Engl J Med 1995; 333: 1386–1390.
442. Krude H, Biebermann H, Luck W, et al. Severe early-onset obesity, adrenal insufficiency and red hair pigmentation caused by *POMC* mutations in humans. Nat Genet 1998; 19:155–157.
443. Yaswen L, Diehl N, Brennan MB, Hochgeschwender U. Obesity in the mouse model of pro-opiomelanocortin deficiency responds to peripheral melanocortin. Nat Med 1999; 5:1066–1070.
444. Burke CW. Adrenocortical insufficiency. Clin Endocrinol Metab 1985; 14:947–976.
445. Leigh H, Kramer SI. The psychiatric manifestations of endocrine disease. Adv Intern Med 1984; 29:413–445.
446. Artavia-Loria E, Chaussain JL, Bougneres PF, et al. Frequency of hypoglycemia in children with adrenal insufficiency. Acta Endocrinol Suppl (Copenh) 1986; 279:275–278.
447. Laczi F, Janaky T, Ivanyi T, et al. Osmoregulation of arginine-8-vasopressin secretion in primary hypothyroidism and in Addison's disease. Acta Endocrinol (Copenh) 1987; 114:389–395.

448. Muls E, Bouillon R, Boelaert J, et al. Etiology of hypercalcemia in a patient with Addison's disease. Calcif Tissue Int 1982; 34: 523–526.
449. Topliss DJ, White EL, Stockigt JR. Significance of thyrotropin excess in untreated primary adrenal insufficiency. J Clin Endocrinol Metab 1980; 50:52–55.
450. Hagg E, Asplund K, Lithner F. Value of basal plasma cortisol assays in the assessment of pituitary-adrenal insufficiency. Clin Endocrinol (Oxf) 1987; 26:221–226.
451. Lindholm J, Kehlet H. Re-evaluation of the clinical value of the 30 min ACTH test in assessing the hypothalamic-pituitary-adrenocortical function. Clin Endocrinol (Oxf) 1987; 26:53–69.
452. Clark PM, Neylon I, Raggatt PR, et al. Defining the normal cortisol response to the short Synacthen test: implications for the investigation of hypothalamic-pituitary disorders. Clin Endocrinol (Oxf) 1998; 49:287–292.
453. Oelkers W, Diederich S, Bahr V. Diagnosis and therapy surveillance in Addison's disease: rapid adrenocorticotropin (ACTH) test and measurement of plasma ACTH, renin activity, and aldosterone. J Clin Endocrinol Metab 1992; 75:259–264.
454. Ertuck E, Jaffe CA, Barkan AL. Evaluation of the integrity of the hypothalamo-pituitary adrenal axis by insulin hypoglycaemia test. J Clin Endocrinol Metab 1998; 83:2350–2354.
455. Stewart PM, Corrie J, Seckl JR, et al. A rational approach for assessing the hypothalamo-pituitary-adrenal axis. Lancet 1988; 1: 1208–1210.
456. Cunningham SK, Moore A, McKenna TJ. Normal cortisol response to corticotropin in patients with secondary adrenal failure. Arch Intern Med 1983; 143:2276–2279.
457. Streeten DHP, Anderson GH, Bonaventura MM. The potential for serious consequences from misinterpreting normal responses to the rapid adrenocorticotropin test. J Clin Endocrinol Metab 1996; 81:285–290.
458. Dickstein G, Shechner C, Nicholson WE, et al. Adrenocorticotropin stimulation test: effects of basal cortisol level, time of day, and suggested new sensitive low dose test. J Clin Endocrinol Metab 1991; 72:773–778.
459. Oelkers W. Dose-response aspects in the clinical assessment of the hypothalamo-pituitary adrenal axis and the low dose adrenocorticotropin test. Eur J Endocrinol 1996; 135:27–33.
460. Abdu TA, Elhadd TA, Neary R, Clayton RN. Comparison of the low dose short Synacthen test (1 microg), the conventional dose short Synacthen test (250 microg) and the insulin tolerance test for assessment of the hypothalamo-pituitary-adrenal axis in patients with pituitary disease. J Clin Endocrinol Metab 1999; 84: 838–843.
461. Jubiz W, Meikle AW, West CD, et al. Single dose metyrapone test. Arch Intern Med 1970; 125:472–474.
462. Schlaghecke R, Kornley E, Santen RT, Ridderskamp P. The effect of long-term glucocorticoid therapy on pituitary-adrenal responses to exogenous corticotropin-releasing hormone. N Engl J Med 1992; 326:226–230.
463. Esteban NV, Loughlin T, Yergey AL, et al. Daily cortisol production rate in man determined by stable isotope dilution/mass spectrometry. J Clin Endocrinol Metab 1991; 72:39–45.
464. Feek CM, Ratcliffe JG, Seth J, et al. Patterns of plasma cortisol and ACTH concentrations in patients with Addison's disease treated with conventional corticosteroid replacement. Clin Endocrinol (Oxf) 1981; 14:451–458.
465. Peacy SR. Glucocorticoid replacement therapy: are patients over treated and does it matter? Clin Endocrinol (Oxf) 1997; 46:255–261.
466. Howlett TA. An assessment of optimal hydrocortisone replacement therapy. Clin Endocrinol (Oxf) 1997; 46:263–268.
467. Fiad TM, Conway JD, Cunningham SK, McKenna TJ. The role of plasma renin activity in evaluating the adequacy of mineralocorticoid replacement in primary adrenal insufficiency. Clin Endocrinol (Oxf) 1996; 45:529–534.
468. Smith SJ, Markandu ND, Banks RA, et al. Evidence that patients with Addison's disease are undertreated with fludrocortisone. Lancet 1984; 1:11–14.
469. Arlt W, Callies F, van Vlijmen JC, et al. Dehydroepiandrosterone replacement in women with adrenal insufficiency. N Engl J Med 1999; 341:1013–1020.
470. Hunt PJ, Gurnell EM, Huppert FA, et al. Improvement in mood and fatigue after dehydroepiandrosterone replacement in Addison's disease in a randomized, double blind trial. J Clin Endocrinol Metab 2000; 85:4650–4656.
471. White PC, Speiser PW. Congenital adrenal hyperplasia due to 21-hydroxylase deficiency. Endocr Rev 2000; 21:245–291.
472. Urban MD, Lee PA, Migeon CJ. Adult height and fertility in men with congenital adrenal hyperplasia. N Engl J Med 1978; 299:1392–1396.
473. Klingensmith GJ, Garcia SC, Jones HW, et al. Glucocorticoid treatment of girls with congenital adrenal hyperplasia: effects on height, sexual maturation, and fertility. J Pediatr 1977; 90:996–1004.
474. Chrousos GP, Loriaux DL, Mann DL, et al. Late onset 21-hydroxylase deficiency mimicking idiopathic hirsutism or polycystic ovarian disease: an allelic variant of congenital virilizing adrenal hyperplasia. Ann Intern Med 1982; 96:143–148.
475. Speiser PW, Dupont B, Rubinstein P, et al. High frequency of nonclassical steroid 21-hydroxylase deficiency. Am J Hum Genet 1985; 37:650–667.
476. Azziz R, Dewailly D, Owerbach D. Nonclassic adrenal hyperplasia: current concepts. Clinical Review 56. J Clin Endocrinol Metab 1996; 78:810–815.
477. Rutgers JL, Young RH, Scully RE. The testicular "tumor" of the adrenogenital syndrome: a report of six cases and review of the literature on testicular masses in patients with adrenocortical disorders. Am J Surg Pathol 1988; 12:503–513.
478. Miller WL. Gene conversions, deletions, and polymorphisms in congenital adrenal hyperplasia. Am J Hum Genet 1988; 42:4–7.
479. Wilson RC, Mercado AB, Cheng KC, et al. Steroid 21-hydroxylase deficiency: genotype may not predict phenotype. J Clin Endocrinol Metab 1995; 80:2322–2329.
480. New MI, Lorenzen F, Lerner AJ, et al. Genotyping steroid 21-hydroxylase deficiency: hormonal reference data. J Clin Endocrinol Metab 1983; 57:320–326.
481. Forest MG, Betuel H, David M. Prenatal treatment in congenital adrenal hyperplasia due to 21-hydroxylase deficiency: update 88 of the French multicentric study. Endocr Res 1989; 15:277–301.
482. Seckl JR, Miller WL. How safe is long-term prenatal glucocorticoid treatment? JAMA 1997; 277:1077–1079.
483. Pang S, Clark AT, Freeman LC, et al. Maternal side effects of prenatal dexamethasone therapy for fetal congenital adrenal hyperplasia. J Clin Endocrinol Metab 1992; 75:249–253.
484. Mulaikal RM, Migeon CJ, Rock JA. Fertility rates in female patients with congenital adrenal hyperplasia due to 21-hydroxylase deficiency. N Engl J Med 1987; 316:178–182.
485. Meyer-Bahlburg HF. What causes low rates of child-bearing in congenital adrenal hyperplasia? J Clin Endocrinol Metab 1999; 84:1844–1847.
486. Rosler A, Levine LS, Schneider B, et al. The interrelationship of sodium balance, plasma renin activity, and ACTH in congenital adrenal hyperplasia. J Clin Endocrinol Metab 1977; 45:500–512.
487. Mirsky HA, Hines JH. Infertility in a man with 21-hydroxylase deficient congenital adrenal hyperplasia. J Urol 1989; 142:111–113.
488. White PC, Curnow KM, Pascoe L. Disorders of steroid 11β-hydroxylase isozymes. Endocr Rev 1994; 15:421–438.
489. Zachmann M, Tassinari D, Prader A. Clinical and biochemical variability of congenital adrenal hyperplasia due to 11β-hydroxylase deficiency: a study of 25 patients. J Clin Endocrinol Metab 1983; 56:222–229.
490. Rosler A, Leiberman E, Cohen T. High frequency of congenital adrenal hyperplasia (classic 11β-hydroxylase deficiency) among Jews from Morocco. Am J Med Genet 1992; 42:827–834.
491. Pang S, Levine LS, Lorenzen F, et al. Hormonal studies in obligate heterozygotes and siblings of patients with 11β-hydroxylase deficiency congenital adrenal hyperplasia. J Clin Endocrinol Metab 1980; 50:586–589.
492. Gabrilove JL, Sharma DC, Dorfman RI. Adrenocortical 11β-hydroxylase deficiency and virilism first manifest in an adult woman. N Engl J Med 1965; 272:1189–1194.
493. Simone G, Tommaselli AP, Rossi R, et al. Partial deficiency of adrenal 11-hydroxylase: a possible cause of primary hypertension. Hypertension 1985; 7:204–210.
494. Yanase T, Simpson ER, Waterman MR. 17α-Hydroxylase/17,20-lyase deficiency: from clinical investigation to molecular definition. Endocr Rev 1991; 12:91-108.
495. Biglieri EG. 17α-Hydroxylase deficiency: 1963–1966. J Clin Endocrinol Metab 1997; 82:48–50.

496. Winter JSD, Couch RM, Muller J, et al. Combined 17-hydroxylase and 17,20-desmolase deficiencies: evidence for synthesis of a defective cytochrome P450c17. J Clin Endocrinol Metab 1989; 68:309–316.
497. Zachmann M, Werder EA, Prader A. Two types of male pseudohermaphroditism due to 17,20-desmolase deficiency. J Clin Endocrinol Metab 1982; 55:487.
498. Peter M, Sippell WG, Wernze H. Diagnosis and treatment of 17-hydroxylase deficiency. J Steroid Biochem Mol Biol 1993; 45: 107–116.
499. Laflamme N, Leblanc J-F, Mailloux J, et al. Mutation R96W in cytochrome P450c17 gene causes combined 17α-hydroxylase/17-20-lyase deficiency in two French Canadian patients. J Clin Endocrinol Metab 1996; 81:264–268.
500. Yamaguchi H, Nakazato M, Miyazato M, et al. A 5′ splice site mutation in the cytochrome P450 steroid 17α-hydroxylase gene in 17α-hydroxylase deficiency. J Clin Endocrinol Metab 1997; 82: 1934–1938.
501. Rheaume E, Simard J, Morel Y, et al. Congenital adrenal hyperplasia due to point mutations in the type II 3β-hydroxysteroid dehydrogenase gene. Nat Genet 1992; 1:239–245.
502. Simard J, Rheaume E, Mebarki F, et al. Molecular basis of human 3β-hydroxysteroid dehydrogenase deficiency. J Steroid Biochem Mol Biol 1995; 53:127–138.
503. Pang S, Levine LS, Stoner E, et al. Nonsalt-losing congenital adrenal hyperplasia due to 3β-hydroxysteroid dehydrogenase deficiency with normal glomerulosa function. J Clin Endocrinol Metab 1983; 56:808–818.
504. Marui S, Castro M, Latronico AC, et al. Mutations in the type II 3β-hydroxysteroid dehydrogenase (*HSD3B2*) gene can cause premature pubarche in girls. Clin Endocrinol (Oxf) 2000; 52:67–75.
505. Pang S, Lerner AJ, Stoner E. Late-onset adrenal steroid 3β-hydroxysteroid dehydrogenase deficiency. I. A cause of hirsutism in pubertal and postpubertal women. J Clin Endocrinol Metab 1985; 60:428–439.
506. Bose HS, Sugawara T, Strauss JF III, et al. The pathophysiology and genetics of congenital lipoid adrenal hyperplasia. N Engl J Med 1996; 335:1870–1878.
507. Caron KM, Soo SC, Wetsel WC, et al. Targeted disruption of the mouse gene encoding steroidogenic acute regulatory protein provides insights into congenital adrenal hyperplasia. Proc Natl Acad Sci USA 1997; 94:11540-11545.
508. Nikkila H, Tannin GM, New MI, et al. Defects in the *HSD11* gene encoding 11 beta-hydroxysteroid dehydrogenase are not found in patients with apparent mineralocorticoid excess or 11-oxoreductase deficiency. J Clin Endocrinol Metab 1993; 77:687–691.
509. Suter SL, Baison-Lauber A, Shackleton C, Zachmann M. Apparent cortisone reductase (11-betaHSD1) deficiency: a rare cause of hyperandrogenemia and hypercortisolism. Proceedings of the 81st Annual Meeting of the Endocrine Society, 1999, P 3-334.
510. Taylor N, Bartlett WA, Dawson DJ. Cortisone reductase deficiency: evidence for a new inborn error in metabolism of adrenal steroids. J Endocrinol 1984; 102S:89.
511. Phillipov G, Palermo M, Shackleton CH. Apparent cortisone reductase deficiency: a unique form of hypercortisolism. J Clin Endocrinol Metab 1996; 81:3855–3860.
512. Savage MW, Barton RN, Doman TL, et al. Increased metabolic clearance of cortisol in corticosteroid 11-reductase deficiency. J Endocrinol 1991; 129S:219.
513. Nordenstrom A, Marcus C, Axelson M, et al. Failure of cortisone acetate treatment in congenital adrenal hyperplasia because of defective 11beta-hydroxysteroid dehydrogenase reductase activity. J Clin Endocrinol Metab 1999; 84:1210–1213.
514. Jamieson A, Wallace AM, Andrew R, et al. Apparent cortisone reductase deficiency: a functional defect in 11beta-hydroxysteroid dehydrogenase type 1. J Clin Endocrinol Metab 1999; 84:3570–3574.
515. Ulick S. Diagnosis and nomenclature of the disorders of the terminal portion of the aldosterone biosynthetic pathway. J Clin Endocrinol Metab 1976; 43:92–96.
516. Veldhuis JD, Melby JC. Isolated aldosterone deficiency in man: acquired and inborn errors in the biosynthesis or action of aldosterone. Endocr Rev 1986; 2:495–517.
517. Mitsuuchi Y, Kawamoto T, Miyahara K, et al. Congenitally defective aldosterone biosynthesis in humans: inactivation of the P-450C18 gene (*CYP11B2*) due to nucleotide deletion in CMO I deficient patients. Biochem Biophys Res Commun 1993; 190: 864–869.
518. Pascoe L, Curnow KM, Slutsker L, et al. Mutations in the human *CYP11B2* (aldosterone synthase) gene causing corticosterone methyloxidase II deficiency. Proc Natl Acad Sci USA 1992; 89: 4996–5000.
519. Speiser PW, Stoner E, New MI. Pseudohypoaldosteronism: a review and report of two new cases. Adv Exp Med Biol 1986; 196:173–195.
520. Kuhnle U, Nielsen MD, Tietze HU, et al. Pseudohypoaldosteronism in eight families: different forms of inheritance are evidence for various genetic defects. J Clin Endocrinol Metab 1990; 70:638–641.
521. Komesaroff PA, Verity K, Fuller PJ. Pseudohypoaldosteronism: molecular characterization of the mineralocorticoid receptor. J Clin Endocrinol Metab 1994; 79:27–31.
522. Chang SS, Grunder S, Hanukoglu A, et al. Mutations in subunits of the epithelial sodium channel cause salt wasting with hyperkalaemic acidosis, pseudohypoaldosteronism type 1. Nat Genet 1996; 12:248–253.
523. Klemm SA, Gordon RD, Tunny TJ, Thompson RE. The syndrome of hypertension and hyperkalaemia with normal GFR (Gordon's syndrome): is there increased proximal sodium reabsorption? Clin Invest Med 1991; 14:551–558.
524. Wilson FH, Disse-Nicodeme S, Choate KA, et al. Human hypertension caused by mutations in WNK kinases. Science 2001; 293: 1107–1112.
525. Schambelan M, Stockigt JR, Biglieri EG. Isolated hypoaldosteronism in adults: a renin-deficiency syndrome. N Engl J Med 1972; 287:573–578.
526. DeFronzo R. Hyperkalemia and hyporeninemic hypoaldosteronism. Kidney Int 1980; 17:118–134.
527. Sunderlin FS, Anderson GH, Streeten DHP, et al. The renin-angiotensin-aldosterone system in diabetic patients with hyperkalaemia. Diabetes 1981; 30:335–340.
528. Gicquel C, Le Bouc Y, Luton JP, Bertagna X. Pathogenesis and treatment of adrenocortical carcinoma. Curr Opin Endocrinol Diabetes 1998; 5:189–196.
529. Matzuk M, Finegold M, Mather J, et al. Development of cancer cachexia-like syndrome and adrenal tumors in inhibin-deficient mice. Proc Natl Acad Sci USA 1994; 91:8817–8821.
530. Gabrilove JL, Seman AT, Sabet R, et al. Virilizing adrenal adenoma with studies on the steroid content of the adrenal venous effluent and a review of the literature. Endocr Rev 1981; 2:462–470.
531. Kloos RT, Gross MD, Francis IR, et al. Incidentally discovered adrenal masses. Endocr Rev 1995; 16:460–484.
532. Rossi R, Tauchmanova L, Luciano A, et al. Subclinical Cushing's syndrome in patients with adrenal incidentaloma: clinical and biochemical features. J Clin Endocrinol Metab 2000; 85:1440–1448.
533. Flecchia D, Mazza E, Carlini M, et al. Reduced serum levels of dehydroepiandrosterone sulphate in adrenal incidentalomas: a marker of adrenocortical tumour. Clin Endocrinol (Oxf) 1995; 42:129–134.
534. Seppel T, Schlaghecke R. Augmented 17α-hydroxyprogesterone response to ACTH stimulation as evidence of decreased 21-hydroxylase activity in patients with incidentally discovered adrenal tumours ('incidentalomas'). Clin Endocrinol (Oxf) 1994; 41:445–451.
535. Latronico A, Chrousos GP. Extensive personal experience: adrenocortical tumours. J Clin Endocrinol Metab 1997; 82:1317-1324.

15 Endocrine Hypertension

Robert G. Dluhy, Jennifer E. Lawrence, and
Gordon H. Williams

Hypertension is a common disorder, occurring in approximately 20% of the United States population. The great majority of hypertensive subjects have the diagnosis of essential or primary hypertension.[1] Essential hypertension is a heritable syndrome reflecting a variety of pathophysiologic abnormalities that can lead, independently or together, to an elevated arterial blood pressure.[2] Although secondary causes exist in a smaller percentage (10%) of hypertensive subjects, they still represent a large number of patients.[3]

Broadly speaking, the secondary causes of hypertension can be divided into renal causes (e.g., parenchymal or renovascular disease) and endocrine causes. In some disorders, many cases can be diagnosed by an astute clinician because the signs and symptoms are often distinct (e.g., pheochromocytoma and Cushing's syndrome). In addition, hypertension refractory to antihypertensive treatment may prompt the physician to screen for secondary causes. The age and sex of the hypertensive patient may also be helpful in the diagnosis of disorders with the secondary etiologies. For example, fibromuscular hyperplasia and Cushing's syndrome are more commonly seen in younger females, whereas primary hypothyroidism most commonly occurs in older female patients. Finally, making a diagnosis of a secondary disorder is gratifying because it may lead to significant amelioration or in some instances cure of the elevated blood pressure.

PHYSIOLOGY OF THE SYMPATHOADRENAL SYSTEM AND PHEOCHROMOCYTOMA

The autonomic nervous system consists of the parasympathetic nervous system and the sympathoadrenal system. The neurotransmitter in the parasympathetic nervous system is primarily acetylcholine, and the neurotransmitters in the sympathoadrenal system include norepinephrine at sympathetic nerve endings in the periphery and central nervous system and epinephrine, which is secreted by the adrenal medulla into the systemic circulation. Another catecholamine, dopamine, acts primarily as a neurotransmitter in the central nervous system but is also secreted from peripheral sympathetic nerve endings. The sympathetic nervous system is under direct control of the central nervous system, allowing rapid onset of actions of short duration as a result of the abbreviated half-lives of catecholamines.

Structure and Organization of the Sympathoadrenal System

The sympathoadrenal system, which is composed of the ganglia of the sympathetic nervous system and the adrenal medulla, is embryologically derived from neural crest tissue.[4] The precursor sympathogonia differentiate into neuroblasts, ultimately giving rise to the paravertebral and preaortic ganglion cells. Sympathetic preganglionic axons arise in large part from cells located in the thoracolumbar spinal cord.[5, 6] These preganglionic sympathetic neurons in turn have synapses with descending tracks from neurons in the pons, medulla, and hypothalamus, allowing regulation of sympathetic activity by the brain (Fig. 15–1; see also Fig. 15–16). Thus, the limbic system and cortex can also regulate sympathetic activity by connections with central nuclei in the hypothalamus and medulla. In turn, these central nervous system neurons that influence sympathetic activity are regulated by a variety of factors including substrates (glucose) and hormones (corticotropin-releasing hormone).

The axons of the preganglionic neurons synapse with postganglionic cell bodies located in the paravertebral and preaor-

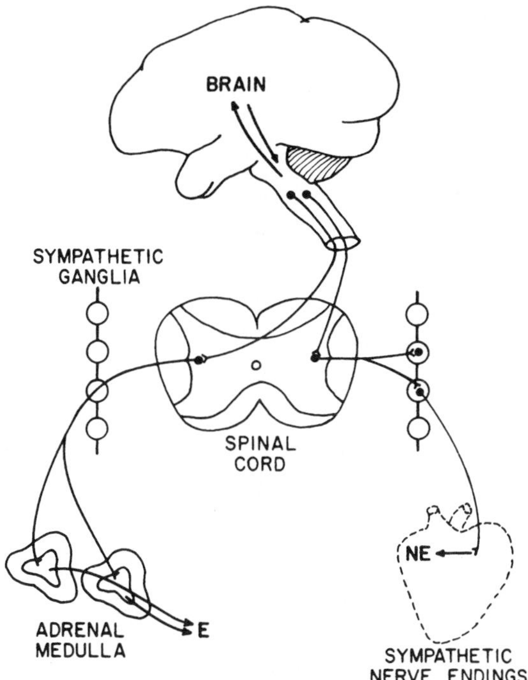

Figure 15–1. Organization of the sympathoadrenal system. Sympathetic preganglionic axons arise in large part from cells located in the thoracolumbar spinal cord. These preganglionic sympathetic neurons in turn have synapses with descending tracks from neurons in the pons, medulla, and hypothalamus, allowing regulation of sympathetic activity by the brain. In turn, these central nervous system neurons that influence sympathetic activity are regulated by a variety of factors, including substrates (glucose) and hormones (corticotropin-releasing hormone). (From Landsberg L, Young JB. Catecholamines and the adrenal medula. In Bondy PK, Rosenberg JE (eds). Metabolic Control and Disease, 8th ed. Philadelphia: WB Saunders, 1980:1621–1693.)

tic ganglia as well as neurons in the celiac and superior and inferior mesenteric ganglia (Fig. 15–2). Postganglionic axons from the cell bodies located in these ganglia in turn innervate the visceral organs. The splanchnic outflow of the lower thoracic and lumbar preganglionic axons also directly innervates the cells of the adrenal medulla (see Fig. 15–2). Acetylcholine is the neurotransmitter at the ganglionic synapses and at the adrenal medullary neurons. In different tissues, the postganglionic sympathetic innervation can be cholinergic or noradrenergic, or both. For example, at arteriolar synaptic clefts norepinephrine is released from postganglionic nerve terminals, and sweat glands have sympathetic cholinergic innervation. Adrenergic nerves also contain other mediators including the peptide substance P, neuropeptide Y, somatostatin, and chromogranin A.[7–10] These substances, which are released in peripheral and central adrenergic nerves, may have synergistic or direct actions with norepinephrine on effector cells. On the other hand, the adrenal medullary cells that secrete epinephrine into the systemic circulation are innervated by the splanchnic outflow of cholinergic preganglionic neurons.

The arterial blood supply to the adrenal gland is derived from the aorta (middle adrenal artery), the inferior phrenic artery, and the renal artery. Adrenal blood flow drains centrally toward the medulla, eventually forming a single adrenal vein, which drains into the renal vein on the left and into the vena cava on the right. Although the existence of a corticomedullary portal system remains controversial, it is likely that local high concentrations of glucocorticoids influence the biosynthesis of epinephrine by induction of the enzyme phenylethanolamine *N*-methyltransferase (PNMT).[11, 12]

Catecholamines

All naturally occurring catecholamines contain a catechol nucleus (Fig. 15–3). Epinephrine is synthesized and stored in the adrenal medulla and released into the systemic circulation. Norepinephrine is synthesized and stored at peripheral nerve endings. Dopamine acts primarily as a neurotransmitter in the central nervous system, although epinephrine and norepinephrine also act as central nervous system neurotransmitters.

Catecholamines act widely in the body and affect many cardiovascular and metabolic processes. Specific catecholamine receptors mediate the biologic actions of these compounds.[13, 14] The amount of endogenous catecholamines released at peripheral nerve endings and the plasma concentration of epinephrine are the main determinants of the physiologic responses to activation of the sympathetic nervous system. Identification of α-adrenergic and β-adrenergic receptors and their receptor subtypes (α_1, α_2, β_1, and β_2) in target tissue has led to an understanding of the physiologic responses to exogenous and endogenous administration of catecholamines.[15–17]

Moreover, the pharmacologic development of selective α- and β-adrenergic antagonists has added a wide range of treatments for a variety of clinical disorders. For example, β_2-agonists (terbutaline and albuterol), among their actions, can cause bronchial smooth muscle relaxation and are commonly prescribed in aerosol formulation for the treatment of bronchial asthma.[18, 19] On the other hand, β_1-antagonists (such as atenolol and metoprolol) are considered standard therapies for angina pectoris, hypertension, and cardiac arrhythmias. The α- and β-adrenergic receptors on cell surfaces reciprocally increase or decrease in response to the receptor-specific agonist concentration. Inhibition or stimulation of the intracellular adenylate cyclase (cyclic adenosine monophosphate [cAMP]) system mediates the majority of responses to receptor subtype–specific agonists.

Catecholamine Synthesis

Catecholamines are formed from the amino acid tyrosine by a process of hydroxylation and decarboxylation (see Fig. 15–3). This process of amine precursor uptake and decarboxylation (APUD) is a feature of neuroendocrine tissues that have a common origin. Most reactions occur in the cytoplasm except for hydroxylation of dopamine into norepinephrine, which occurs in the secretory vesicle.

The rate-limiting step in catecholamine biosynthesis is the conversion of tyrosine to 3,4-dihydroxyphenylalanine (dopa) by the enzyme tyrosine hydroxylase (TH).[20, 21] The reaction requires tyrosine as substrate and oxygen, iron (Fe^{2+}), and tetrahydrobiopterin as cofactors. Tyrosine hydroxylase is expressed only in neuronal tissues that synthesize catecholamines, and several factors regulate its activity. The intraneuronal or intracellular transport of tyrosine may be affected by other amino acids or drugs that compete for transport or act as competitive inhibitors of the transport system, such as α-methylparatyrosine. Increased intracellular levels of catechols downregulate the activity of the enzyme. As catechols are released from secretory granules in response to a stimulus, cytoplasmic catecholamines are depleted and the feedback inhibition of tyrosine hydroxylase is released. Four isoforms of tyrosine hydroxylase exist.[22] Transcription is stimulated by glucocorticoids, cAMP-dependent protein kinases, Ca^{2+}/phospholipid-dependent protein kinase, and Ca^{2+}/calmodulin-dependent protein kinase.[23, 24]

Aromatic L-amino acid decarboxylase (AADC) catalyzes the decarboxylation of dopa to dopamine, a process that can occur in any APUD tissue in which dopa is present. AADC is not specific for dopa. For example, decarboxylation of 5-hydroxytryptophan produces serotonin. Pyridoxal 5-phosphate is the cofactor required.

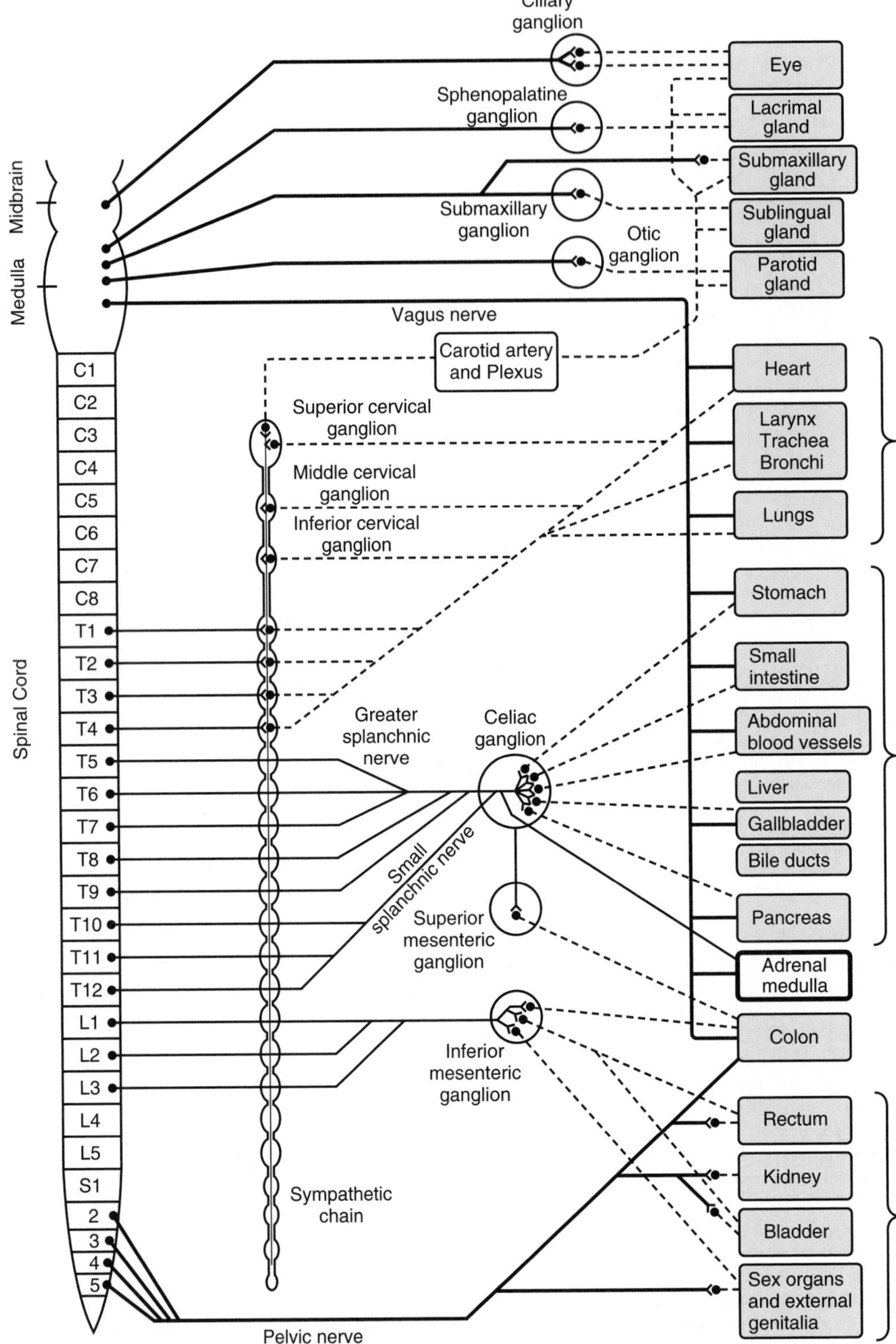

Figure 15–2. Sympathoadrenomedullary efferent autonomic pathways. The axons of the preganglionic neurons synapse with postganglionic cell bodies located in the paravertebral and preaortic ganglia as well as neurons in the celiac and superior and inferior mesenteric ganglia. Postganglionic axons from the cell bodies located in these ganglia in turn innervate the visceral organs. The splanchnic outflow of the lower thoracic and lumbar preganglionic axons also directly innervates the cells of the adrenal medulla.

Dopamine is actively transported into granulated vesicles to be hydroxylated to norepinephrine by the copper-containing enzyme dopamine β-hydroxylase (DBH). Oxygen is required, as is ascorbic acid, which acts as a cofactor and hydrogen donor. The enzyme is structurally similar to tyrosine hydroxylase and may share similar transcriptional regulatory elements, and both are stimulated by glucocorticoids and cAMP-dependent kinases.[25] These reactions occur in the synaptic vesicle of adrenergic neurons in the central nervous system, the peripheral nervous system, or the chromaffin cells of the adrenal

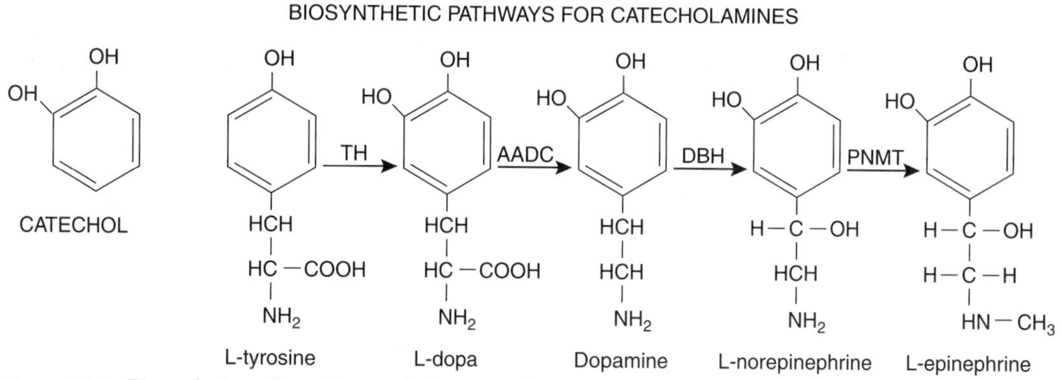

BIOSYNTHETIC PATHWAYS FOR CATECHOLAMINES

CATECHOL → L-tyrosine —TH→ L-dopa —AADC→ Dopamine —DBH→ L-norepinephrine —PNMT→ L-epinephrine

Figure 15–3. Biosynthetic pathway for catecholamines (*left to right*). All catecholamines contain the catechol nucleus. L-Tyrosine is converted to L-3,4-dihydroxyphenylalanine (L-dopa) in the rate-limiting step by tyrosine hydroxylase (TH). Aromatic L-amino acid decarboxylase (AADC) converts L-dopa to dopamine. Dopamine is hydroxylated to L-norepinephrine by dopamine β-hydroxylase (DBH). L-Norepinephrine is converted to L-epinephrine by phenylethanolamine *N*-methyltransferase (PNMT).

medulla. The major constituents of the granulated vesicle are dopamine β-hydroxylase (in either a membrane-bound or soluble form), ascorbic acid, chromogranin A, and adenosine triphosphate (ATP).[26] In the adrenal medulla, norepinephrine is released from the granule into the cytoplasm, where it combines with the cytosolic enzyme PNMT to produce epinephrine (see Fig. 15–3). Epinephrine is then transported back into another storage vesicle.

The N-methylation reaction by PNMT involves *S*-adenosylmethionine as the methyl donor as well as oxygen and magnesium. PNMT expression is regulated by the presence of glucocorticoids, which are in high concentration in the medulla through the corticomedullary portal system. Cholinergic stimulation through both nicotinic and muscarinic components affects transcriptional regulation of PNMT.[27, 28] Epinephrine produces a noncompetitive negative feedback inhibition of PNMT activity. PNMT expression occurs in other tissues, including the lung, pancreas, and kidney. In spite of peripheral conversion, the plasma concentration ratio of norepinephrine to epinephrine is almost 9:1. In normal adrenal medullary tissue, approximately 80% of the catecholamine released is epinephrine. In patients with Addison's disease who have diminished cortisol production, adrenal medullary epinephrine production is decreased.[29] Small adrenal pheochromocytomas tend to secrete predominantly epinephrine, whereas larger tumors often secrete predominantly norepinephrine.[30] Larger tumors may outgrow the corticomedullary blood supply, thus losing the exposure to high local concentrations of glucocorticoids that regulate the activity of PNMT.

Catecholamine Uptake and Release

Catecholamines are taken up into storage vesicles by active transport using an H^++-ATP–driven proton pump and carrier proteins, vesicular monoamine transporters (VMATs).[31] The ATP-driven pump maintains a steep electrical gradient. For every monoamine transported, ATP is hydrolyzed and two hydrogen ions are transported from the vesicle into the cytosol. Calcium is also maintained in high concentration within the vesicle.[32–34] Iodine 131–labeled metaiodobenzylguanidine (MIBG) appears to be imported by VMATs into the storage vesicles in the adrenal medulla, which makes imaging with MIBG useful for evaluation of pheochromocytomas.[35] Catecholamine uptake, as well as MIBG, is inhibited by reserpine.[36]

Acetylcholine originating from preganglionic sympathetic fibers stimulates nicotinic cholinergic receptors and causes depolarization of the adrenomedullary chromaffin cell. Depolarization leads to activation of voltage-gated Ca^{2+} channels resulting in exocytosis of secretory vesicle contents.[37] A Ca^{2+}-sensing receptor appears to be involved in the process of exocytosis.[38] During exocytosis, all of the granular contents are released into the extracellular space.

Catecholamine Metabolism

Metabolism of catecholamines occurs through two enzyme pathways (Fig. 15–4). Catechol-*O*-methyltransferase (COMT) is found primarily outside neuronal tissue and converts epinephrine to metanephrine and norepinephrine to normetanephrine by meta-*O*-methylation. *S*-Adenosylmethionine is used as the methyl donor, and Ca^{2+} is required.

Metanephrine and normetanephrine are oxidized by monoamine oxidase (MAO) to vanillylmandelic acid (VMA) by oxidative deamination. MAO may also oxidize epinephrine and norepinephrine to 3,4-dihydroxymandelic acid, which is then converted by COMT to VMA. MAO is located on the outer membrane of mitochondria. In the storage vesicle, norepinephrine is protected from metabolism by MAO. MAO action may play an important role in regulating the metabolism of norepinephrine and dopamine. Intravesical stores of norepinephrine increase when MAO is inhibited.[39]

Pheochromocytoma

Incidence and Importance

Pheochromocytomas are tumors of neuroectodermal origin arising from chromaffin cells. They are named for the dark staining reaction that is caused by the oxidation of intracellular catecholamine stores on exposure to dichromate salts. Although pheochromocytomas are a rare cause of hypertension, failure to recognize and treat a pheochromocytoma could prove a fatal oversight. Reportedly, less than 1% of patients who are evaluated for hypertension have pheochromocytomas, but this may be an underestimate. In one series, the incidence rate was calculated to be 0.8 per 100,000 person-years. In an autopsy series, approximately half of the pheochromocytomas were diagnosed at postmortem examination, demonstrating that this disorder is frequently not recognized.[40, 41]

Tumors that arise from chromaffin cells of the adrenal medulla are referred to as pheochromocytomas, and those that arise in paraganglia are termed paragangliomas or extra-adrenal pheochromocytomas. The paraganglia are collections of specialized neural crest cells that have migrated to their final

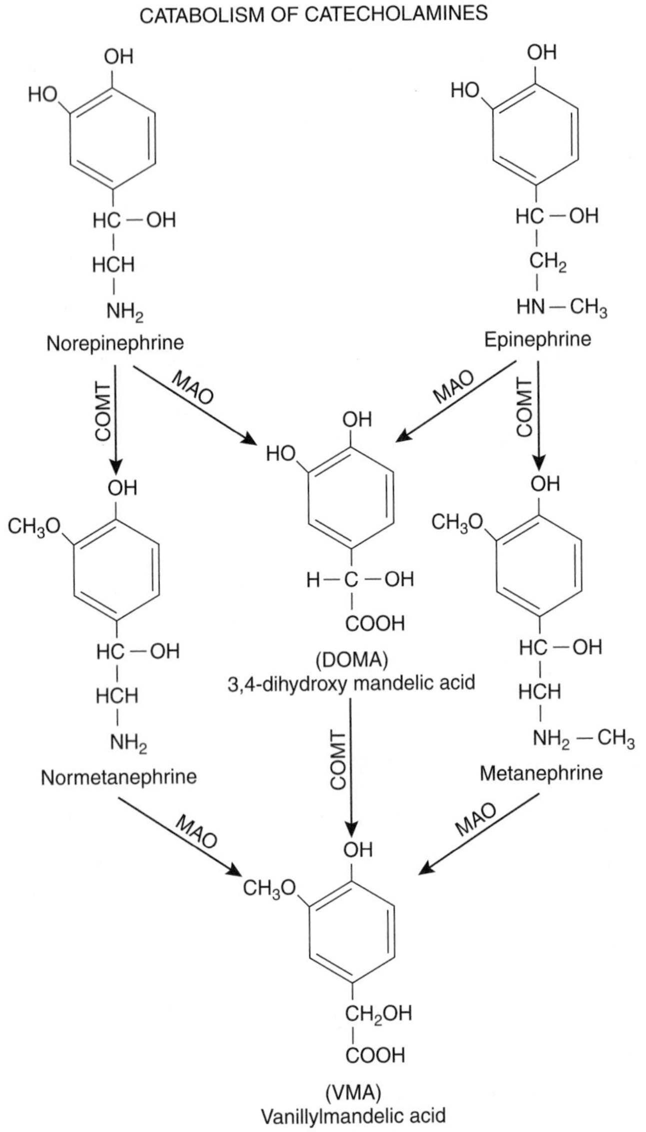

CATABOLISM OF CATECHOLAMINES

Figure 15–4. Catecholamine metabolism. Metabolism of catecholamines occurs through two enzyme pathways. Catechol-*O*-methyltransferase (COMT) converts epinephrine to metanephrine and converts norepinephrine to normetanephrine by meta-*O*-methylation. Metanephrine and normetanephrine are oxidized by monoamine oxidase (MAO) to vanillylmandelic acid (VMA) by oxidative deamination. MAO also may oxidize epinephrine and norepinephrine to dihydroxymandelic acid (DOMA), which is then converted by COMT to VMA.

destination throughout the body.[42] Tumors can arise from sympathetic ganglia located from the neck to the bladder as well as the carotid body, vagal body, mediastinum, aorta, organs of Zuckerkandl, and pelvis (the most common site) (see Fig. 15–2). It is commonly believed that the malignant potential is higher for extra-adrenal tumors than intra-adrenal tumors. However, some studies suggest that disease-free survival is similar for patients with extra-adrenal and intra-adrenal tumors.[43]

Clinical Manifestations

Hypertension is the most common clinical manifestation of pheochromocytoma and is present in 90% to 100% of patients. Sustained hypertension is seen in approximately half, paroxysmal hypertension in a third, and normal blood pressure in less than a fifth of patients.[44] In children, sustained hypertension occurs most frequently.

Patients with pheochromocytoma frequently present with paroxysmal episodes or spells that include the classic triad of severe headaches, palpitations, and diaphoresis.[45] These episodes may occur daily or as frequently as every few months. More than 90% of patients present with at least two of the three symptoms in the classic triad. The headaches are typically abrupt in onset, throbbing, and bilateral and diminish within an hour. The headaches may be associated with pallor or nausea, may be brief, or may persist over a week. The presence of palpitations, anxiety, or tremulousness may suggest the predominant secretion of epinephrine.[41, 46, 47] Less common symptoms include tremor, angina, nausea, Raynaud's phenomenon, livedo reticularis, and mass effect from the tumor.

Increased total peripheral resistance causes the hypertension in patients with pheochromocytoma, as in patients with essential hypertension. Heart rate is variably increased in patients with pheochromocytoma.[48–50] Normal cardiac output is maintained by a decreased stroke volume resulting from intravascular volume depletion.[51]

Lability of blood pressure is caused by a combination of the following: (1) episodic catecholamine release, (2) impaired sympathetic reflexes, and (3) unrecognized chronic volume depletion.[51] Altered sympathetic vascular regulation may underlie the orthostatic hypotension often seen in pheochromocytoma.[52] In rare cases of pheochromocytoma with predominant secretion of epinephrine, dopa, or dopamine, orthostatic hypotension may be the presenting symptom.[45] Patients with pheochromocytoma who are asymptomatic despite high circulating levels of catecholamines may have adrenergic receptor desensitization related to chronic stimulation.[53]

Other cardiovascular manifestations of pheochromocytomas include dilated cardiomyopathy[54] resulting from catecholamine excess or hypertrophic cardiomyopathy.[55] Both forms have been reported to be reversible with tumor resection. Myocarditis has also been described in patients with pheochromocytoma with a pathology characterized by infiltration of inflammatory cells, specifically perivascularly, and focal contraction band necrosis.[56]

Patients may also present with features of acute myocardial infarction including chest pain or electrocardiographic abnormalities including ST segment elevation or depression or inversion of T waves, or both.[46, 57] Other electrocardiographic manifestations of pheochromocytoma include left ventricular hypertrophy, sinus tachycardia, T-wave inversion, and rhythm disturbances such as supraventricular tachycardia or supraventricular ectopic beats.[51]

Hereditary Pheochromocytoma

The majority of pheochromocytomas are sporadic. However, approximately 10% or more occur in association with a familial disorder such as multiple endocrine neoplasia type 2A or 2B (MEN-2A or MEN-2B), von Hippel–Lindau (VHL) disease, or neurofibromatosis (see Chapter 36). The MEN-2 syndromes and VHL disease are inherited in an autosomal dominant pattern with age-related penetrance. MEN-2A (Sipple's syndrome) is characterized by pheochromocytoma, medullary carcinoma of the thyroid, and hyperparathyroidism. MEN-2B is characterized by pheochromocytoma, medullary carcinoma of the thyroid, and multiple mucosal neuromas, often in association with a marfanoid habitus. Germ line mutations of the *RET* proto-oncogene have been described in the MEN-2 syndromes, and the MEN-2A gene has been localized to chromosome 10q11.2.[58, 59] The mutation confers constitutive activation of the tyrosine kinase receptor leading to unregulated hyperplasia and increased susceptibility to malignant transformation.

The VHL disease phenotype includes pheochromocytoma,

cerebellar and retinal hemangioblastomas, renal carcinoma, and renal and pancreatic cysts. The VHL disease suppressor gene has been cloned to chromosome 3p25-p26.[60] A loss-of-function mutation leads to tumor formation with different kindreds demonstrating varied clinical manifestations related to different types of mutations. Missense mutations are thought to be more commonly associated with pheochromocytoma.[61, 62, 62a]

A low percentage (0.1% to 5.7%) of patients with von Recklinghausen's neurofibromatosis have pheochromocytoma.[63] However, a much higher percentage (50%) of pheochromocytoma is seen in such patients who have hypertension.[64] The majority of patients with von Recklinghausen's disease have solitary pheochromocytomas, whereas bilateral disease is often seen in other hereditary syndromes. Inactivating mutations in the neurofibromatosis F1 (*NF1*) gene, a tumor suppressor gene on chromosome 17 that encodes neurofibromin, lead to this disorder.[65]

Hereditary pheochromocytomas are typically intra-adrenal and bilateral. In one series, up to 83% of the patients with familial pheochromocytoma had bilateral tumors.[66] Patients with hereditary pheochromocytoma typically present at younger ages than those with sporadic pheochromocytoma. The mean age of diagnosis of familial pheochromocytoma was 38 ± 11 years, compared with 47 ± 16 years for patients with sporadic tumors.[66, 66a] Sporadic pheochromocytoma cases usually present with hypertension; in contrast, many cases of the familial syndrome are diagnosed earlier as a result of biochemical surveillance or genetic testing, often before hypertension is detected.[67]

The MEN-2 and VHL tumors make up most of the hereditary pheochromocytomas, but about 25% apparently sporadic patients may have germline mutations.[66a] It has been shown that MEN-2 tumors typically produce metanephrine, the metabolite of epinephrine, whereas tumors in patients with VHL disease produce normetanephrine, the metabolite of norepinephrine. These specific biochemical phenotypes demonstrate that unique mutation-dependent differential gene expression is probably involved in catecholamine synthesis. PNMT has been reported to be overexpressed in the MEN-2 tumors providing the epinephrine metabolism profile, whereas PNMT is underexpressed in VHL tumors providing the norepinephrine metabolism profile.[68]

MEN-2 pheochromocytomas also appear to have increased tyrosine hydroxylase activity, which accounts for the greater concentration of catecholamine metabolites measured and clinical symptoms seen in MEN-2 patients compared with VHL patients. Patients with MEN-2 typically demonstrate episodic symptoms of hypertension. On the other hand, a pattern of sustained hypertension is seen in VHL patients. Thus, the biochemical phenotypes in these syndromes appear to be associated with particular patterns of catecholamine synthesis and release. Measurement of plasma-free metanephrines has been used to distinguish between MEN-2 and VHL disease and to reveal the presence of pheochromocytoma prior to clinical symptoms with greater sensitivity and specificity than urine testing[68, 69] (see later).

Hereditary paragangliomas of the neck (glomus tumors) are associated with germ line mutations in a mitochondrial complex II gene, succinyl dehydrogenase subunit D (*SDHD*),[70] which encodes an enzyme that is involved in oxidative phosphorylation. Somatic and germ line mutations of the *SDHD* gene may also be associated with nonsyndromic, sporadic,[66a, 71] and familial pheochromocytoma.[72]

Diagnosis

Differential Diagnosis

Pheochromocytoma may be suspected when a crisis, the physiologic consequence of abrupt catecholamine release, is precipitated by factors such as exertion, trauma, certain drugs, anesthesia, surgery, or surgical manipulation of the tumor. Tricyclic antidepressants, droperidol, glucagon, metoclopramide, phenothiazines, and naloxone have all been reported to induce hypertensive episodes.[45, 46] Foods or beverages, such as certain aged cheeses or red wine that contain tyramine, may precipitate a crisis. The β-blockers may cause a paradoxical rise in blood pressure.

Several disorders may mimic the symptoms of pheochromocytoma and also cause elevations in catecholamines. Abrupt withdrawal from medications such as clonidine or from alcohol may produce such a picture. Cerebral events such as cerebral vasculitis, preeclampsia, subarachnoid hemorrhage, migraine, and intracranial lesions associated with increased intracranial pressure may mimic pheochromocytoma. Agents such as amphetamines, ephedrine, pseudoephedrine, isoproterenol, phenylpropanolamine, cocaine, phencyclidine (PCP), and lysergic acid diethylamide (LSD) also lead to excess catecholamine levels.

On the other hand, the symptoms of pheochromocytoma may be mistaken for those of panic attacks, hypoglycemic episodes, or accelerated hypertension of other etiologies. Lastly, disorders such as mastocytosis and the carcinoid syndrome, which are characterized by spells and episodic symptoms, may also mimic pheochromocytoma.[30, 47, 73] However, hypertensive crises, which often occur with pheochromocytoma, are notably absent in these disorders. In fact, episodic hypotension may occur with mastocytosis or the carcinoid syndrome as a result of peripheral vasodilation.

Indication for Screening

Because pheochromocytomas do not occur frequently, physicians must appreciate when screening for the disorder is appropriate. The following are reasonable indications for screening:

1. Hypertension with episodic features suggesting pheochromocytoma (the classic triad of headaches, palpitations, and diaphoresis)
2. Refractory hypertension
3. Prominent lability of blood pressure
4. Severe pressor response during anesthesia, surgery, or angiography
5. Unexplained hypotension during anesthesia, surgery, or pregnancy
6. Family history of pheochromocytoma or a familial disorder such as MEN-2, VHL disease, neurofibromatosis, or glomus tumors
7. Incidentally discovered adrenal masses
8. Idiopathic dilated cardiomyopathy

Biochemical Assessment

In pheochromocytoma, enzyme activity involved in synthesis of catecholamines is augmented and enzyme activity involved in catabolism is decreased. Because the catecholamine excess cannot be effectively stored, the hormones spill into the peripheral circulation. Biochemical measurement of excessive catecholamine production by the tumor confirms the diagnosis of pheochromocytoma (see later). However, because catecholamines are normally constitutively produced by the sympathoadrenal system, it is the magnitude of the elevation that is diagnostic of pheochromocytoma.

Basal Measurements

The diagnosis is made with the demonstration of elevated circulating or urinary catecholamines or metabolites (see Fig.

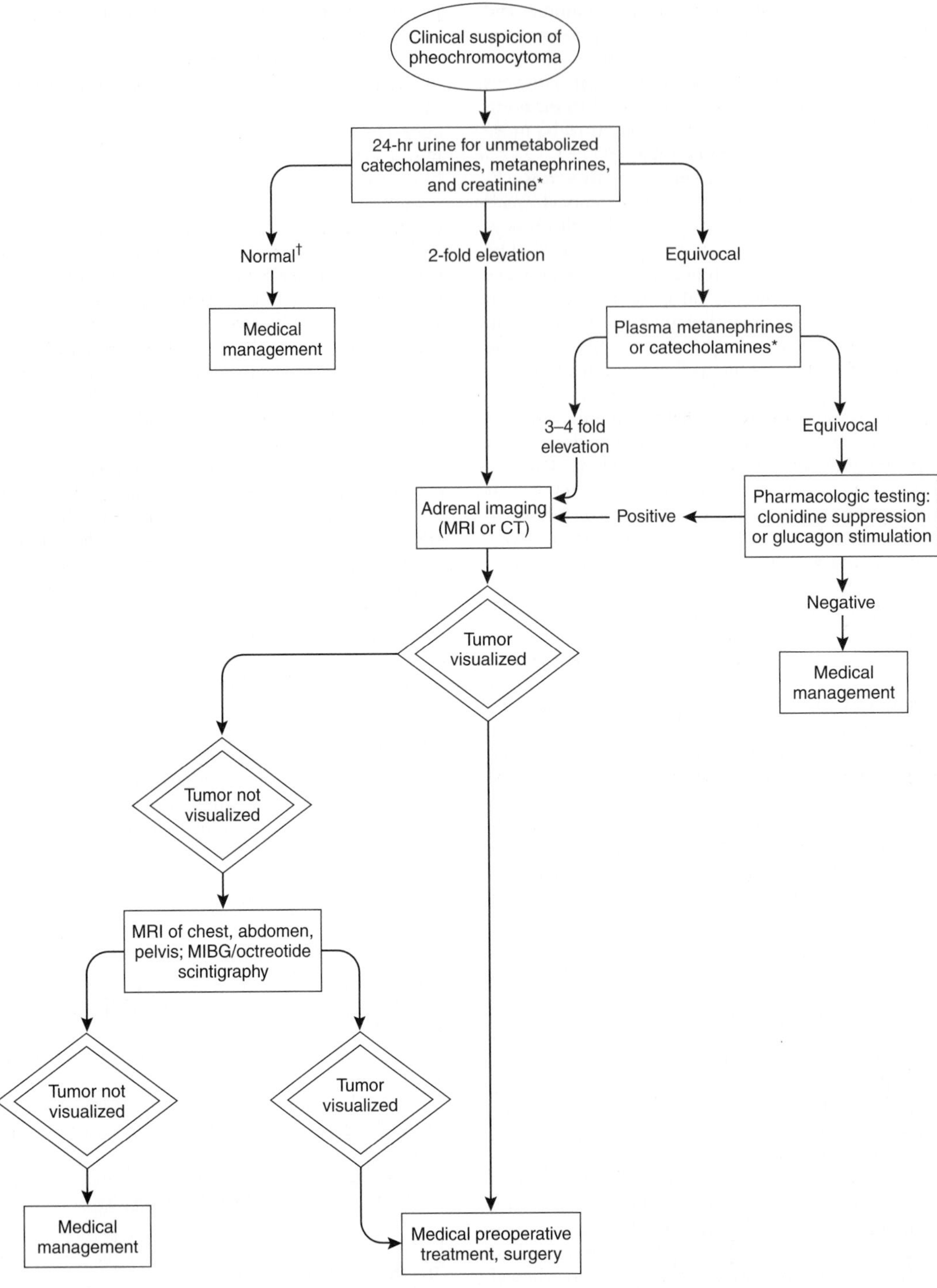

* In some institutions, plasma metanephrines are being used for the initial screening, especially in patients with hereditary syndromes. See text for details.

† Repeat 24-hour urine collection may be indicated during a hypertensive crisis or a paroxysm in a patient with episodic symptomatology.

Figure 15–5. Algorithm for diagnosis of pheochromocytoma. CT, computed tomography; MRI, magnetic resonance imaging.

15–3). Screening methods include (1) 24-hour urine collection for excretion of unmetabolized or so-called free catecholamines (epinephrine and norepinephrine) or catecholamine metabolites (metanephrine, normetanephrine, and vanillylmandelic acid) and (2) determination of plasma metanephrines and catecholamines (Fig. 15–5).

Pheochromocytomas are heterogeneous in hormone metabolism and secretion. Therefore, there is no one optimal test for screening and there is disagreement about the preferred test for diagnosis. For example, as catecholamines have short half-lives and are secreted episodically, a random plasma measurement may miss the peak catecholamine levels. On the other hand, plasma levels are particularly helpful when samples are collected during a paroxysm. Although the 24-hour urine collection has the advantage of integration of the catecholamine secretion over time, it is more cumbersome for patients and may yield a false-negative result if the collection is performed in absence of symptoms or hypertension in patients with episodic catecholamine secretion. The urinary metanephrine-to-creatinine ratio can be useful in compensating for overcollection (false-positives) or undercollection (false-negatives).[74] Overnight measurements of urine catecholamines have also been used to diagnose pheochromocytoma but involve an increased risk of both false-positive and false-negative results.[75]

In the initial evaluation of a patient suspected of having a pheochromocytoma, we recommend a 24-hour urine collection for free or unmetabolized catecholamines (epinephrine and norepinephrine), total metanephrines, and creatinine (see Fig. 15–5). Of the different metabolites that can be detected in a 24-hour urine collection, metanephrines are the most sensitive and specific.[74] There are less data concerning the appropriate use of plasma measurements. However, more experience with the measurement of plasma metanephrines is accruing, and it is considered by some to be a highly sensitive method for biochemical diagnosis, especially for hereditary pheochromocytoma (sensitivity 97%, specificity 96%).[76] Because pheochromocytomas secrete primarily metabolized catecholamines, plasma metanephrines may be more useful than plasma catecholamines.

Measurement of plasma-free metanephrines as opposed to the conjugated or sulfated forms is particularly helpful because free fraction levels result from the actions of COMT on tumor catecholamine production. As a result, plasma-free metanephrines may show larger increases above normal than plasma catecholamines in pheochromocytoma. On the other hand, although plasma metanephrines are highly sensitive in detecting pheochromocytoma, a high number of false-positives may occur, particularly in older patients. Accordingly, the sensitivities and specificities of urine and plasma biochemical tests remain under investigation. As a result, some centers advocate urine testing as the initial screening test whereas others suggest plasma-free metanephrine levels. It is important to remember that the current technology for measuring plasma metanephrines requires that the patient abstain from acetaminophen for 3 to 5 days before testing[77] (see Fig. 15–5).

Typically, a measurement of urinary catecholamines or metabolites that is two or three times above the upper limit of normal is considered diagnostic of pheochromocytoma. For example, the upper limit of normal for total urinary catecholamines is approximately 100 μg per 24 hours, and a measurement above 250 μg per 24 hours is obtained in most patients with pheochromocytoma. Urine collections should include measurement of urinary creatinine to verify the adequacy of collection. A strong acid (such as 6 N HCl) is added to a sealed container. The optimal system for plasma catecholamine determination includes having the patient fast overnight and lie comfortably in a supine position with a heparin lock inserted 20 to 30 minutes before collection for withdrawing the blood.

Certain precautions should be taken in interpreting catecholamine or metanephrine values. For example, iodinated contrast dyes can interfere with some biochemical measurements. Labetalol can give falsely elevated results when the following assays are employed: fluorometric methods of analysis used for catecholamine measurements, spectrophotometric methods used for metanephrine measurements, or radioenzymatic assays used for urinary-free catecholamine measurements.[78] Tricyclic antidepressants, prochlorperazine (Compazine), reserpine, clonidine, and clofibrate may interfere with urinary catecholamines and metabolite measurements.[79, 80] Such medications should be discontinued, preferably 2 weeks before collection. Blood pressure should be controlled with agents such as dihydropyridine calcium channel blockers that do not interfere with the assays.

To provide better resolution against interfering substances, many laboratories use a reverse-phase high-performance liquid chromatography method with electrochemical detection. Measurement of these compounds by mass spectroscopy, which eliminates the problem of interfering substances, and use of immunoassay techniques are future directions. Stresses associated with serious illnesses, such as myocardial infarction, cerebral vascular accidents, or congestive heart failure, cause elevation in catecholamine levels. In renal insufficiency, plasma and urinary levels may be falsely elevated and urinary collections should be expressed in milligrams of creatinine.[81] In these circumstances, other diagnostic tests including imaging modalities are required for evaluation.

Chromogranin A is a soluble protein stored and secreted with catecholamines in chromaffin tissue. This biochemical marker is not specific for pheochromocytoma, and elevations may be seen with other neuroendocrine tumors. Plasma chromogranin A levels are elevated in more than 80% of patients with pheochromocytomas.[82, 83] This assay is most often utilized in the postoperative surveillance of patients after resection of catecholamine-secreting tumors (see "Medical and Surgical Management"). Chronic renal failure is also associated with elevated chromogranin A levels.

Stimulation and Suppression Tests

The clonidine and glucagon tests are dynamic tests that are not routinely performed but are usually used when the suspicion of pheochromocytoma is high but the basal catecholamine levels are not diagnostic or are equivocal. Clonidine is a centrally acting α_2-adrenoceptor agonist that normally suppresses the release of catecholamines from neurons but does not affect the autonomous release of catecholamines from a neoplasm.[46, 84] In patients without pheochromocytoma, a decrease in basal plasma catecholamines by 50% or less than 3 nmol/L (500 pg/mL) is expected 2 to 3 hours after 0.3 mg of clonidine is administered.[46]

Provocative testing is utilized when clinical suspicion of pheochromocytoma is not supported by the biochemical testing. Patients with pheochromocytomas typically demonstrate a threefold increase in plasma catecholamine levels or a concentration greater than 12 nmol/L (2000 pg/mL) 2 minutes after administration of 1.0 mg of intravenous glucagon. The glucagon provocative test is considered highly specific but poorly sensitive, whereas the clonidine test is considered highly sensitive with poor specificity. If both tests are negative, the diagnosis of pheochromocytoma may be reasonably excluded.[46, 85]

Imaging Techniques

After the diagnosis of pheochromocytoma is confirmed by biochemical testing, imaging techniques are employed for tumor location. Localization techniques include magnetic resonance imaging (MRI), computed tomography (CT), and MIBG or octreotide scintigraphy. Pheochromocytomas are typically large tumors (2 to 5 cm in diameter) and may contain areas of hemorrhage or necrosis. Pheochromocytomas in hereditary syndromes tend to be bilateral and smaller.[86] The latter feature is probably related to early detection as the result of periodic surveillance.

Approximately 98% of pheochromocytomas are intra-abdominal, and 90% originate within the adrenal gland. How-

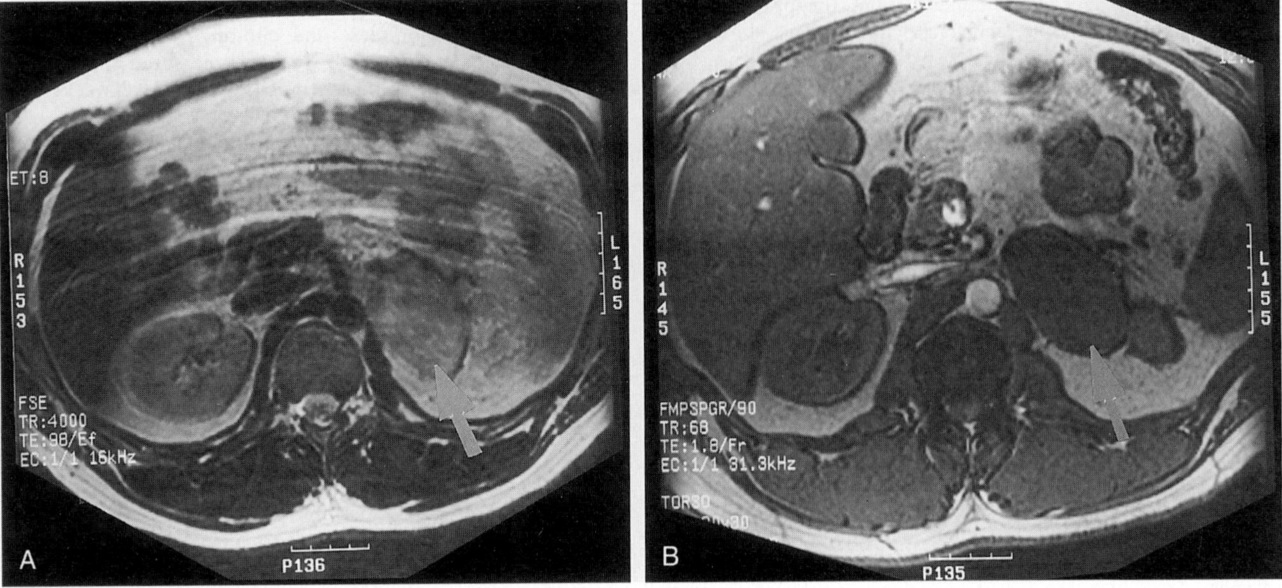

Figure 15–6. *A*, Axial in-phase gradient-echo image demonstrates left adrenal mass *(arrow)*. *B*, Axial image from the out-of-phase gradient-echo sequence demonstrates the left adrenal mass. In comparison to the in-phase image, no suppression of the adrenal mass is present. Suppression is the rule in lipid-containing cortical adenomas.

ever, pheochromocytomas may occur anywhere in the autonomic nervous system including the posterior mediastinum, pericardium, or bladder (see Fig. 15–2).

Because of their size, intra-adrenal tumors are usually easily imaged by either CT or MRI (Fig. 15–6). Although MRI may have greater specificity, CT has a sensitivity between 93% and 100%. Because of the tumor size, contrast agents are not required for visualization and, in fact, may precipitate a hypertensive crisis. With T2-weighted MRI, adrenal pheochromocytoma is usually three times as intense as liver. On T1-weighted images, the tumor is usually isointense with the liver. With gadolinium-diethylenetriaminepentaacetic acid (DTPA), the tumor appears hypervascular.[86] These general characteristics are not uniformly met, and rarely a pheochromocytoma is indistinguishable from other adrenal tumors. MRI is preferred for localization of paragangliomas, especially those located outside the abdomen, such as a posterior mediastinal or intracardiac tumor.

MIBG has chemical similarities to norepinephrine and is concentrated within intracellular storage granules of catecholamine-secreting tissues.[87] Radioiodinated MIBG is especially valuable for localization of pheochromocytomas of extra-adrenal origin and for confirmation of tumor resection in postoperative surveillance.[88] The sensitivity of MIBG is reported to be greater than 90% with a specificity of 100%.[87, 89] MIBG is labeled with ^{123}I or ^{131}I; the former isotope with gamma ray flux has fewer particulate emissions and may provide greater sensitivity. Thyroid uptake should be blocked by administration of iodide preparations 3 days before and 1 week after iodine-labeled MIBG is given. Medicines that could interfere with catecholamine metabolism, uptake, or release should be discontinued at least 72 hours before MIBG evaluation. For example, tricyclic antidepressants and phenylpropanolamine inhibit MIBG uptake; sympathomimetics (cocaine, labetalol, and reserpine) deplete the storage vesicle contents. Atypical antidepressants, phenothiazines and butyrophenones, which block adrenergic receptors, may also produce false-negative results.[90]

Somatostatin receptor scintigraphy is another localization technique because somatostatin receptors are normally expressed in adrenomedullary and paraganglionic tissues.[91] The receptor density is increased on pheochromocytoma tissue, which enables imaging with the somatostatin analogue octreotide. Octreotide, which binds to somatostatin receptor subtypes 2 and 5, is labeled with ^{111}In-DTPA. As with MIBG, octreotide scanning is best employed for detection of pheochromocytomas of extra-adrenal origin and of metastases from malignant pheochromocytoma.[92] Some malignant tumors down-regulate the expression of somastatin receptors. As a result, lack of uptake by octreotide may be a poor prognostic indicator in such patients.

In contrast to MIBG or octreotide scintigraphy, which requires 24 to 48 hours for optimal visualization, a promising new technology that can immediately image a pheochromocytoma is 6-[^{18}F]fluorodopamine positron emission tomography.[93] The uptake and retention of this radiopharmaceutical in chromaffin cells with subsequent imaging by emission scanning may provide a useful diagnostic test in patients with pheochromocytoma.

Finally, venous sampling has been utilized in the past to confirm or rule out the diagnosis of pheochromocytoma. The adrenal sampling effluent has a norepinephrine/epinephrine ratio less than 1. Higher ratios suggest the presence of pheochromocytoma.[94, 95]

Medical and Surgical Management

Preoperative Management

Surgical excision of a pheochromocytoma is the treatment of choice, but it involves a risk of morbidity as high as 40% and a risk of mortality of 2% to 4%.[73] Surgical outcomes have improved with preoperative treatment such as α-receptor blockade and volume expansion.[96] Volume expansion is initially achieved with a high-sodium diet (150 to 200 mEq/L [150 to 200 mmol/day]) unless contraindicated by congestive heart failure or renal insufficiency. Phenoxybenzamine, a noncompetitive α-blocker, has traditionally been used for preoperative preparation. Phenoxybenzamine is titrated to reduce blood pressure to normal levels or orthostasis, or both. The starting dose, 10 mg/day by mouth, is titrated upward every 2 days.

Most patients require 80 to 100 mg daily given in divided doses.

When α-blockade is established, β-blockade may be initiated if the patient is tachycardic or has arrhythmias. Without prior α-blockade, β-blockade alone can lead to unopposed α-receptor stimulation and further elevation of blood pressure. Because phenoxybenzamine blocks catecholamine binding to receptors, it minimizes the risk of a hypertensive crisis during intubation, during induction with anesthesia, or during exploration and tumor manipulation. A noncompetitive α-blocker is theoretically preferred to a competitive inhibitor because catecholamine levels, which can increase 500-fold, may overcome a competitive inhibitor.[96] However, complete α-blockade can mask the dramatic fall in blood pressure seen after tumor resection that signals to the surgeon that the pheochromocytoma is resected. Phenoxybenzamine may also lead to postoperative hypotension because of its prolonged half-life of 24 hours.[97]

Calcium channel blockers, in particular nicardipine from the dihydropyridine class, are increasingly popular. These agents improve intraoperative systemic vascular resistance by blunting catecholamine-mediated arterial vasoconstriction during tumor manipulation, and they have few side effects.[98, 99] The selective α_1 inhibitor doxazosin has been effective in preoperative management without causing tachycardia or other serious side effects.[100] The oral formulation of labetalol, with an α/β-blocking ratio of 1:3, may not be ideal for preparation for surgery because the α-blockade is weaker than that of phenoxybenzamine. As a result, additional vasodilators may be required intraoperatively in labetalol-pretreated subjects.[101] Finally, metyrosine, which inhibits catecholamine synthesis, has been used in combination with α-blockade for preoperative management.[102]

Tradition and experience have guided the length of preoperative therapy with volume expansion and α/β-blockade. Patients are typically treated for 10 to 14 days, although this time course has not been consistently associated with better operative and postoperative outcomes.[96] Unfortunately, there are no reliable features that predict a smooth surgical course. Thus, each patient must be evaluated on an individual basis when selecting antihypertensive medicines.

Surgical Management

The surgical approach is dictated by the clinical situation. In patients with familial pheochromocytoma, a transabdominal incision allows adequate visualization and bilateral adrenalectomy if required. The flank approach offers better exposure and reduced blood loss for the patient with a solitary tumor. Surgeons are gaining experience with laparoscopic adrenalectomy performed when the tumor is smaller than 6 cm.[103, 104] The patient with pheochromocytoma should be referred to a surgeon who has experience in the management of pheochromocytoma and who collaborates with an experienced anesthesiologist to establish a smooth team effort.

Intraoperative hypotension is managed initially with volume expansion and then with intravenous pressor agents if necessary. Postoperative hypoglycemia, which may be due to reactive hyperinsulinemia, should be anticipated and warrants routine screening of glucose monitoring in the early postoperative hours.[105] Surgical outcomes have been improved by intraoperative hemodynamic monitoring, the combination of fast-acting intravenous vasodilators and β-blockers (sodium nitroprusside and esmolol, respectively), and the use of intravenous vasoconstrictors (norepinephrine or epinephrine).

The following is an approach followed in our institution to prepare the patient for surgery. As soon as the diagnosis of pheochromocytoma is established, α-blockade is started and titrated upward (see earlier). Five days before surgery, if not earlier, a high-sodium (150 to 200 mEq/L [150 to 200 mmol]) diet is initiated; therapy with α-blockade is continued, and daily weights and vital signs are monitored. Admission for volume expansion with intravenous saline is considered, depending on the patient's status. One day before surgery, the patient is transferred to a monitored intensive care setting with intravenous arterial and Swan-Ganz catheters. Isotonic saline is administered to achieve a pulmonary capillary wedge pressure greater than 10 mm Hg. If systemic vascular resistance is elevated (>1000 dyne second/cm^5/m^2), intravenous sodium nitroprusside at 0.5 to 2 μg/kg per minute is initiated and increased as needed (500 to 1000 mg/minute may be required). On the day of surgery, the patient is given two separate intravenous lines, one for administration of pressors and the other for administration of vasodilators. Sodium nitroprusside, esmolol, epinephrine, and norepinephrine infusions are on standby in the event that they are required.

When surgery is performed, the catecholamine levels usually return to normal in approximately 2 weeks. If hypertension persists despite normal catecholamine levels and surgical etiologies such as inadvertent ligation of the renal artery are excluded, essential hypertension or hypertension secondary to renal damage may be the cause. In a series from the Mayo Clinic, 20% of patients who had postoperative hypertension were found to have essential hypertension.[45] Alternatively, the patient could harbor another pheochromocytoma or have metastatic disease. As a result, patients should be monitored indefinitely after surgical resection with annual biochemical screening and chromogranin A levels. Factors that predict recurrent pheochromocytoma include a hereditary pheochromocytoma syndrome, a low ratio of epinephrine to total catecholamines, and the presence of large, extra-adrenal or bilateral tumors.

Pregnancy

Management of pheochromocytoma in pregnancy is especially challenging. The mortality rate for mother and fetus is reported to be approximately 50%. Diagnosis before term improves these rates considerably.[106] Clinical symptoms are similar to those in nonpregnant individuals, but unique features can occur. For example, the gravid uterus may compress the pheochromocytoma, causing paroxysms in the supine position with normal blood pressure in the erect posture.

Pheochromocytomas may also be easily misdiagnosed as preeclampsia, especially later in pregnancy. The diagnosis is typically made by evaluation of the urinary collection of catecholamines and metanephrines. Methyldopa should be discontinued before collection because of interference in catecholamine measurements. MRI is the preferred imaging modality because there is no ionizing radiation, and MIBG is contraindicated. Surgery is typically performed before 20 to 24 weeks of gestation. Thereafter, medical therapy is attempted, depending on the maternal status, and cesarean section is planned followed by tumor resection.[107–109] Phenoxybenzamine has been used during pregnancy, but it does cross the placental barrier; as a result, calcium channel blockers may be preferable to control blood pressure.[110]

Malignant Pheochromocytoma

Malignant pheochromocytoma occurs in 3% to 13% of all cases. The 5-year survival rate is 23% to 44%, compared with 97% 5-year survival in benign pheochromocytoma.[45, 51, 111] These tumors typically grow slowly, and evidence of malignancy may not be seen for several years. Malignancy is defined by direct local invasion of sites that do not typically have chromaffin tissue. Malignant tumors most commonly metastasize to the lungs, bone, liver, or lymph nodes or may recur locally. Surgical removal or debulking is the treatment of choice.

After surgery, treatment goals are palliative to control the symptoms related to excess catecholamines. To achieve this end, α-blockade followed by β-blockade has most often been used (as discussed earlier). However, use of other antihypertensive treatments, such as dihydropyridine calcium channel blockers, is increasing. Unfortunately, the response to chemotherapeutic agents has been disappointing, but they may be tried in combination with antihypertensive treatment. Chemotherapeutic agents such as vincristine, cyclophosphamide, and dacarbazine have been used, often in combination.[112] Although the response rate is suboptimal, the experience with high-specific-activity ^{131}I-labeled MIBG is increasing, sometimes in combination with chemotherapy[113] External beam radiation has been attempted for palliation of bone metastases. Tumor embolization is another approach when surgery is not possible.[114]

RENIN-ANGIOTENSIN-ALDOSTERONE AXIS

Several different mechanisms can lead to an increase in blood pressure in patients with essential hypertension and are similar to the mechanisms that cause an increase in blood pressure in individuals with secondary forms. A leading candidate for one of these mechanisms is a derangement in the renin-angiotensin system.[115]

Components

Components of the renin-angiotensin system are shown in Figure 15–7.[116]

Renin

Renin is an enzyme produced in a number of cells in the body, principally in the juxtaglomerular apparatus of the kidney.[117] In tissues that produce renin, it is stored in granules and released in response to specific secretagogues. It is a member of the aspartyl proteinase family of enzymes and is synthesized as a pre-proprotein. In humans, the gene that encodes renin is located on the short arm of chromosome 1 (1q32–1q42). In the rat the gene is located on chromosome 13, and in the mouse it is located on chromosome 1[118, 119] (the mouse has two renin genes). In each species, the nucleotide sequence is approximately 12 kb, with 10 exons and 9 introns. The transcription product is a 1.5-kb messenger ribonucleic acid, and the initial protein consists of 340 amino acids, of which the first 43 are a prosegment cleaved to produce the active enzyme.

Renin is termed a *double-domain* enzyme because the N-terminal and C-terminal halves are similar.[118] Each domain contains a single aspartic acid residue critical for its catalytic activity. The three-dimensional structure of the enzyme has been characterized. A number of factors can regulate the transcription of the renin gene; consensus elements are present in the 5′-flanking region of the gene, including those for cAMP and a number of steroid receptors (estrogen, progesterone, and glucocorticoids).[118, 119]

Angiotensinogen

Angiotensinogen is the only known substrate for renin and is catabolized to angiotensin peptides. The interaction between enzyme and substrate appears to be species specific because minor structural variations in the substrate render it relatively inactive in different species.[120] Human angiotensinogen belongs to the serpin superfamily of proteins and is encoded by a gene on chromosome 1q42.3 near the renin gene.[121] The angiotensinogen gene consists of five exons and four introns and is approximately 13 kb long. The transcript encodes a protein of 485 amino acids, 33 of which constitute a presegment that is cleaved after secretion. Angiotensin I is composed of the first 10-amino-acid sequence following the presegment. The 5′ promoter region has consensus sequences for control by glucocorticoids, estrogens, and cytokines.[122, 123]

Angiotensin-Converting Enzyme

Angiotensin-converting enzyme (ACE), a second enzyme involved in the final production of angiotensin II (see Fig. 15–7), is a dipeptidyl carboxyl zinc metallopeptidase usually found bound to cell membranes.[124] It is also present in intra-

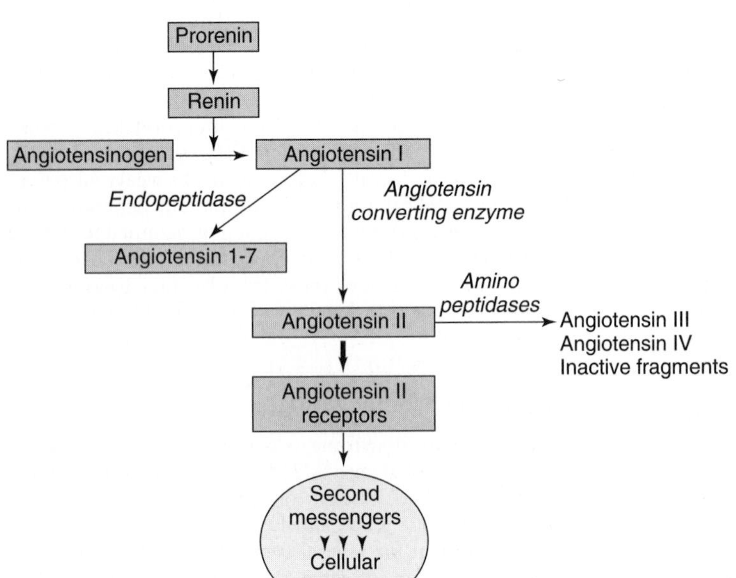

Figure 15–7. Components of the renin-angiotensin system. (Redrawn from Williams GH, Chao J, Chao L. Kidney hormones. In Conn PM, Melmed S [eds]. Endocrinology: Basic and Clinical Principles. Totowa, NJ, Humana Press, 1997, pp 393–404.)

Table 15–1. Amino Acid Composition of Angiotensin Peptides

AI	Asp-Arg-Val-Tyr-Ile-His-Pro-Phe-His-Leu
AII	Asp-Arg-Val-Tyr-Ile-His-Pro-Phe
A1-7	Asp-Arg-Val-Tyr-Ile-His-Pro
AIII	Arg-Val-Tyr-Ile-His-Pro-Phe
AIV	Val-Tyr-Ile-His-Pro-Phe

A, angiotensin.

cellular granules in certain tissues that produce angiotensin II. Its molecular weight is considerably greater than that of renin and it consists of two homologous domains, suggesting that there are two active sites in each molecule. In humans, the ACE gene is located on chromosome 17q23 and consists of 26 exons and 25 introns. Two molecular forms of ACE are products of a single gene but have separate promoter regions. One product is a somatic, or endothelial, ACE that consists of 1306 amino acids, and the second is a germinal ACE with a promoter region upstream from the 13th exon.[125]

Angiotensin Receptors

In humans, the two primary forms of the angiotensin receptor are termed AT_1 and AT_2.[126] A single gene on chromosome 3 encodes the angiotensin receptor in humans; rats have two genes. The 5′-flanking region contains three putative glucocorticoid response elements. The receptor has seven transmembrane regions, with a disulfide bridge linking the first and fourth extracellular segments. The principal signaling mechanism involved in the AT_1 receptor operates through a G_q protein–mediated activation of phospholipase C.[127] However, some data suggest a linkage to protein tyrosine kinase.[128–130] The AT_2 receptor gene has three exons and two introns and a seven-transmembrane-domain structure.[129, 130]

Angiotensin Peptides

At least four angiotensin-like peptides have biologic activity (Table 15–1).[131, 132] The action of renin on angiotensinogen produces angiotensin I, a decapeptide that does not appear to have biologic activity. Angiotensin II is formed by cleavage of the two carboxyl-terminal peptides by ACE[117] and has full biologic activity. Amino peptidase A can remove the amino-terminal aspartic acid to produce the heptapeptide, angiotensin III. Angiotensin II and angiotensin III have equivalent efficacy in promoting aldosterone secretion and modifying renal blood flow. However, angiotensin III has less pressor activity. Amino peptidase B can cleave an additional amino acid from angiotensin III to form angiotensin IV (angiotensin 3–8).[132] The function of this peptide is not clear, but it may be involved in the regulation of cerebral circulation and may produce vasodilation rather than vasoconstriction. A fourth biologically active compound is produced from angiotensin I by the action of a propyl endopeptidase to form angiotensin 1–7,[133] whose function is unclear.

Functions of Angiotensin II

The effects of the renin-angiotensin system can be mediated by local paracrine effects or through endocrine action.[117, 134] The endocrine system primarily involves renin from the juxtaglomerular apparatus of the kidney and angiotensinogen from the liver. In the circulation, the concentrations of each are such that variations in the angiotensinogen levels can modify angiotensin I generation. The half-life in the circulation of angiotensin II is short (probably less than a minute). Although circulating levels of angiotensin II are in the picomolar range, its affinity for its receptor is in the nanomolar range, suggesting that some angiotensin II effects may actually be mediated not by the circulating peptide but by its local generation.

Elements of the renin-angiotensin system are present in the adrenal, the kidneys, the heart, and the brain.[134] For example, the adrenal glomerulosa cells contain the proteins needed to produce and secrete angiotensin II.[135] Other tissues contain one or more components of the renin-angiotensin system and require other cells or circulating components, or both, to generate angiotensin II. For example, fat cells synthesize angiotensinogen but not renin or ACE, but they can generate angiotensin II locally.[136] An increasing body of evidence suggests that many of the functions of angiotensin II are mediated by these paracrine effects. In some tissues, such as the heart, the angiotensin II may be generated by a nonrenin system—the chymase system.

Angiotensin II functions through the AT_1 receptor to maintain normal extracellular volume and blood pressure in five ways[117]: (1) constriction of vascular smooth muscle, thereby increasing blood pressure and reducing renal blood flow; (2) release of norepinephrine and epinephrine from the adrenal medulla; (3) enhancement of the activity of the sympathetic nervous system by increasing central sympathetic outflow, thereby increasing norepinephrine discharge from sympathetic nerve terminals; (4) promotion of the release of vasopressin; and (5) increasing aldosterone secretion.

Other functions of angiotensin II mediated through the AT_1 receptor include (1) central nervous system effects, including modification of thirst or the sense of well-being, or both; (2) modification of the release of corticotropin from the pituitary gland; (3) possible effects on placental and ovarian function; (4) activation of plasminogen activator inhibitor type 1, thereby contributing to the coagulation cascade[137, 138]; and (5) modification of growth of the heart, kidneys, and vascular smooth muscle.[139, 140]

In many respects, the action of angiotensin II through the AT_2 receptor antagonizes its effects through the AT_1 receptor. Thus, AT_2-mediated effects include vasodilatation, renal sodium loss, and apoptosis (thereby antagonizing the growth-promoting effects of AT_1 receptor activation). AT_2 receptors are highly expressed in fetal compared with adult tissue unless the adult tissue is damaged.[141]

Functions of Aldosterone

Aldosterone's classical functions are twofold: regulation of extracellular volume and control of potassium homeostasis.[142] These effects are mediated by binding to the mineralocorticoid receptor in the cytosol of epithelial cells, principally in the renal collecting duct. Transport to the nucleus and binding to specific binding domains on targeted genes lead to their increased expression. Although not all the genes have been identified, serum and glucocorticoid-induced kinase appears to be a key intermediary.[143–145] Its increased expression leads to modification of the apical sodium channel and the basal lateral Na^+,K^+-adenosine triphosphatase (ATPase), resulting in increased sodium ion transport across the cell membrane (see Chapter 14). Glucocorticoids and mineralocorticoids bind equally to the mineralocorticoid receptor. Specificity of action is provided in many tissues by the presence of a glucocorticoid-degrading enzyme, 11β-hydroxysteroid dehydrogenase, which prevents glucocorticoids from interacting with the receptor (see Chapter 14).

A second protective mechanism for untoward mineralocorticoid action is "escape" from its renal sodium-retaining effect. This usual occurs within 3 to 5 days of continued administration. Several mechanisms contribute to this escape, including

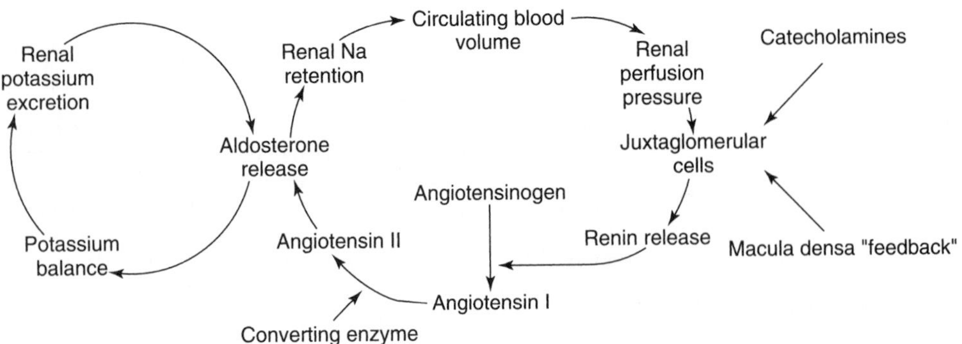

Figure 15–8. Renin-angiotensin-aldosterone and potassium-aldosterone negative feedback loops. Aldosterone production is determined by input from each loop. (Redrawn from Williams GH, Dluhy RG. Diseases of the adrenal cortex. In Braunwald E, Fauci AD, Kasper D, et al [eds]. Harrison's Principles of Internal Medicine, 15th ed. New York, McGraw-Hill, 2001, p 2087.)

renal hemodynamic factors and an increase in atrial natriuretic peptide.

In addition to these classical genomic actions, mediated by aldosterone binding to cytosolic receptors, an increasing body of data suggests that mineralocorticoids have acute, nongenomic actions secondary to activation of an unidentified cell surface receptor. This action involves a G protein signaling pathway and probably a modification of the sodium-hydrogen exchange activity. In both epithelial and nonepithelial cells (e.g., myocytes and leukocytes) this effect has been demonstrated.[146–149]

There are additional nonclassical effects of aldosterone primarily on nonepithelial cells. These actions, although probably genomic and therefore mediated by activation of the cytosolic mineralocorticoid receptor, do not include modification of sodium-potassium balance. Aldosterone-mediated actions include the expression of several collagen genes; genes controlling tissue growth factors, such as transforming growth factor β, and plasminogen activator inhibitor type 1; or genes mediating inflammation. The resultant actions lead to microangiopathy, necrosis (acutely), and fibrosis in a variety of tissues, such as heart, the vasculature, and kidney. Increased levels of aldosterone are not necessary to cause this damage. Rather, an imbalance between the volume or sodium balance state and the level of aldosterone appears to be the critical factor.[150–158]

Regulation

Renin

The release of renin into the circulation from the kidneys is controlled by four factors: (1) the macula densa, a specialized group of distal convoluted tubular cells that function as chemoreceptors for monitoring the sodium and chloride loads present in the distal tubule; (2) juxtaglomerular cells acting as miniature pressure transducers that sense renal perfusion pressure; (3) the sympathetic nervous system, which modifies the release of renin, particularly in response to upright posture in humans; and (4) humoral factors including potassium, angiotensin II, and atrial natriuretic peptides. The tissue renin-angiotensin systems are not necessarily regulated in the same manner as the circulating renin-angiotensin system.[119, 159, 160] For example, a high potassium intake reduces renal renin release and increases adrenal renin secretion.

Aldosterone

The action of angiotensin II on aldosterone involves a negative feedback loop that also includes extracellular fluid volume (Fig. 15–8). The major function of this feedback loop is to modify sodium homeostasis and, secondarily, to regulate arterial pressure.[161, 162] Thus, sodium restriction activates the renin-angiotensin-aldosterone axis. The effects of angiotensin II on both the adrenal cortex and the renal vasculature promote renal sodium conservation. Conversely, with suppression of renin release and suppression of the level of circulating angiotensin, aldosterone secretion is reduced and renal blood flow is increased, thereby promoting sodium loss.

In addition to the usual internal regulation of this negative feedback loop, a secondary fine-tuning component is related to the level of dietary sodium intake.[161, 162] Most endocrine negative feedback loops are not particularly sensitive to environmental factors. In contrast, the renin-angiotensin-aldosterone loop is exquisitely sensitive to dietary sodium intake. Sodium excess enhances the renal and peripheral vasculature responsiveness and reduces the adrenal responsiveness to angiotensin II (Fig. 15–9). Sodium restriction has the opposite effect. Thus, sodium intake modifies, or modulates, target tissue responsiveness to angiotensin II, a fine tuning that appears to be critical to maintaining normal sodium homeostasis without modifying blood pressure, particularly chronically. The mechanism or mechanisms by which dietary sodium intake induces these changes in the adrenal is unclear, but in the vascular system the effects are a consequence of angiotensin II down-regulation of the target tissue responsiveness to its agonists.

ESSENTIAL HYPERTENSION

The renin-angiotensin system has a powerful influence on both vasoconstrictor activity and volume regulation. Thus, defects in its regulation could lead to a rise in blood pressure by either or both of these mechanisms. Two other hormonal systems are implicated in the pathogenesis of essential hypertension: insulin (either directly or mediated by selective insulin resistance) and the calcium regulating systems.

Role of the Renin-Angiotensin System in the Pathogenesis of Essential Hypertension

In the late 1960s and early 1970s, Laragh and colleagues[163] developed a classification of hypertension based on the level of circulating renin activity. By controlling dietary sodium and potassium intake, they classified patients into those whose values were low, normal, or high and used this information to define whether an individual case of hypertension was more volume-dependent or vasoconstrictor-dependent (Fig. 15–10). The model predicted that individuals with low plasma renin activity (PRA) levels would have a volume-sensitive form of hypertension and those with high plasma levels would have a vasoconstrictor form of hypertension. It was presumed that classifying patients in this manner would lead to a more rational treatment program.

However, several concerns have been raised. First, age mod-

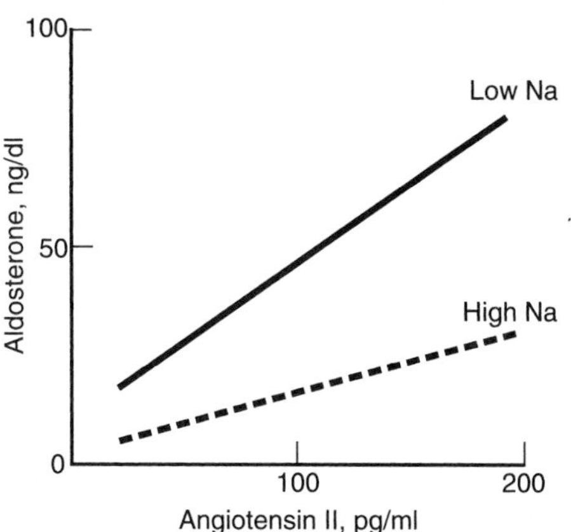

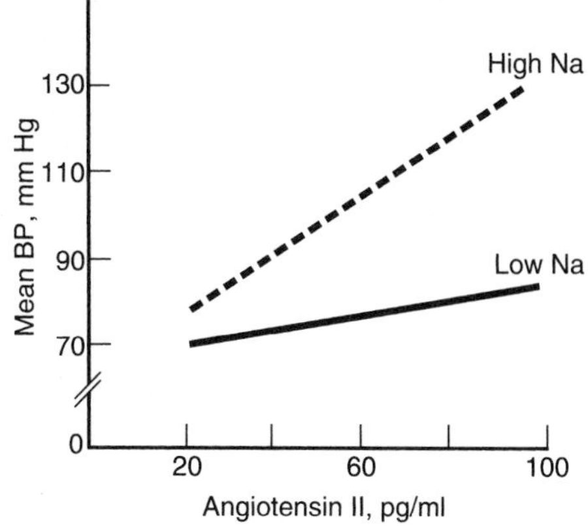

Figure 15–9. Modification of vascular and aldosterone response to angiotensin II by dietary salt intake. Sodium intake has a reciprocal influence on vascular and adrenal responses to angiotensin II. On a high salt intake the vascular response is enhanced while the adrenal response is suppressed. Sodium restriction has the opposite effect. (Redrawn from Williams GH, Hollenberg NK. "Sodium-sensitive" essential hypertension: emerging insights into pathogenesis and therapeutic implications. In Klahr S, Massry SG [eds]. Contemporary Nephrology. Vol 3. New York, Plenum Press, 1985, p 303, with permission.)

ifies the level of renin activity, older subjects having lower renin levels regardless of volume status. Second, race modifies the level of renin activity (whites, in general, have higher levels than blacks). Finally, in individuals who consume a relatively large amount of sodium (more than 175 mmol/day) low, normal, and high PRA levels are difficult to distinguish from each other. However, the concept of subclassification of hypertensive patients on the basis of the level of renin activity was useful in the development of better approaches to subclassifying patients.

HIGH RENIN (dry vasoconstriction)		LOW RENIN (wet vasoconstriction)
	PATHOPHYSIOLOGIC DIFFERENCES	
	Arterioles	
Higher	Peripheral resistance	High
High	Aldosterone	Low to High
Low	Plasma volume	High
Low	Cardiac output	High
High	Hematocrit	Low
High	Blood urea	Low
High	Blood viscosity	Low
Low	Tissue perfusion	High
Yes	Postural hypotension	No
	CLINICAL EXAMPLES	
High-renin essential hypertension		Low-renin essential hypertension
Renovascular and malignant hypertension		Primary aldosteronism
	VASCULAR SEQUELAE	
(+)	Stroke	(–)
(+)	Heart attack	(–)
(+)	Renal damage	(–)
(+)	Retinopathy-encephalopathy	(–)
	TREATMENTS	
(+)	Converting enzyme inhibitors	(–)
(+)	β-Blockers	(–)
(–)	Calcium channel blockers	(+)
(–)	Diuretics	(+)
(–)	α-Blockers	(+)

Figure 15–10. Relationship between the activity of the renin-angiotensin system and the mechanisms underlying the hypertension. (Redrawn from Laragh JH, Sealey JE, Niarchos AP, et al. The vasoconstrictor volume spectrum in normotension and in the pathogenesis of hypertension. Fed Proc 41:2415–2423, 1982.)

Pathophysiologic Mechanisms in Low-Renin Essential Hypertension

Several mechanisms are thought to cause volume expansion and suppress renin activity in some patients with essential hypertension.[164] Adrenal mechanisms may be involved in some subjects with low-renin hypertension because spironolactone (a mineralocorticoid antagonist) and aminoglutethimide (an inhibitor of steroid hormone biosynthesis) substantially reduce their blood pressure.[165, 166] Wisgerhof and Brown[167] reported that the adrenal response to angiotensin II is enhanced in some patients with low-renin essential hypertension and that the enhanced responsiveness alters the renin-angiotensin-aldosterone negative feedback loop, allowing restoration of normal sodium homeostasis with decreased PRA and angiotensin II levels.[168] However, with normal to high sodium intake, this enhanced adrenal response could result in a scenario in which aldosterone secretion would not be suppressed adequately, promoting sodium retention and an increase in blood pressure. The frequency of this abnormality is unclear because no population-based studies have been reported. However, even some patients with so-called normal renin essential hypertension appear to have a similar defect.[169]

Nonmodulating Hypertension: Salt Sensitivity and Normal to High Renin Levels

Some patients with normal or high renin levels have a peculiar form of salt-sensitive hypertension in which increased sodium intake fails to change the vascular and the adrenal response to angiotensin II.[170] These patients, termed *nonmodulators*, appear to be a subset of the essential hypertensive population, as documented by a bimodal distribution of several of their biochemical features.[171] Patients with these features have been reported from Argentina, Brazil, Japan, The Netherlands, France, Italy, and the United States.[172–174] In whites, between 25% and 30% of hypertensive subjects are nonmodulators, and in black hypertensives the frequency is likely to be greater.

Nonmodulators share several features with low-renin essential hypertensive patients: (1) they both have salt-sensitive hypertension, and (2) they tend to be older than the rest of the hypertensive population. However, nonmodulators have several features that are not similar to those of low-renin hypertension, including (1) fasting hyperinsulinemia, (2) a positive family history of hypertension and myocardial disease, (3) elevated levels of cholesterol and triglycerides, and (4) a decreased adrenal response to angiotensin II as assessed with a sodium-restricted intake. Finally, and perhaps most important, the characteristics associated with nonmodulation distribute in a bimodal fashion in the hypertensive population, suggesting a discrete subgroup.[171, 174–176]

In nonmodulators, target tissue responsiveness to angiotensin II does not change when sodium intake is modified. Two functional tests have been used to distinguish them from the rest of the hypertensive population. One measures the aldosterone response to an angiotensin II infusion of 3 ng/kg per minute with a low-salt (10 mEq) diet.[170, 171, 177] The other approach is to measure the renal blood flow response to the same dose of angiotensin II with a high-salt (200 mEq) diet.[170, 178] Unless the dietary sodium intake is precisely controlled, a hypertensive subject can be misclassified. The correlation between these two criteria is 70% to 80%.[171, 173] Thus, if feasible, the best approach is to require both criteria to be positive in defining a nonmodulator. Other characteristics of this subset include failure of renal blood flow to increase when dietary sodium intake is changed from low to high and an enhanced response of atrial natriuretic peptide to infused angiotensin II.[173, 179]

Nonmodulators appear to have an inherited form of hypertension, as evidenced by (1) bimodality of the distribution of the nonmodulating characteristic in the hypertensive population,[171] (2) the presence of the nonmodulating characteristic in normotensive subjects,[172] (3) a strong family history of hypertension in nonmodulators (approximately 80%, compared with about 30% for the rest of the hypertensive population),[176, 179] (4) familial aggregation of nonmodulating characteristics with hypertension,[180] and (5) the association of the nonmodulating phenotype with individuals who are homozygous for the angiotensinogen 235T genotype (Fig. 15–11).[181] Data also support the involvement of the ACE and aldosterone synthase (CYPllB2) genes. Nonmodulators are twice as likely as the rest of the hypertensive population to be homozygous for the angiotensinogen 235T genotype, four times as likely if they have both the angiotensinogen and ACE dd genotypes, and nearly six times as likely if they have the angiotensinogen, ACE, and CYP11B2-344T genotypes.

A defect in the renin-angiotensin system is likely to underlie nonmodulating hypertension. It is probably a defect in the local renal and adrenal renin-angiotensin systems, as evidenced by the following: (1) the previously cited genetic data involving genes of the renin-angiotensin-aldosterone system; (2) low renal blood flow with a high-sodium diet and a reduced renal vascular response to infused angiotensin II, suggesting inappropriately high local renal angiotensin II levels; (3) correction of the renal blood flow defect by administration of a converting enzyme inhibitor; and (4) correction of the nonmodulating adrenal defect by a converting enzyme inhibitor.[177–179]

The effect of sodium intake on blood pressure in nonmodulators has been extensively evaluated. Either short-term (3 days) or chronic (2 weeks) salt loading increases blood pressure in nonmodulators but not in other normal or high-renin hypertensive patients.[176, 179] The salt sensitivity of the hypertension is due to the tendency for nonmodulators to retain more of a salt load both acutely and chronically.[179] The abnormality in sodium handling is probably due to the alteration in renal hemodynamics with salt loading described previously[170, 178] and secondary to an inappropriately high local angiotensin II level. Support for this conclusion comes from correction of salt-sensitive hypertension in nonmodulators by converting enzyme inhibitors.

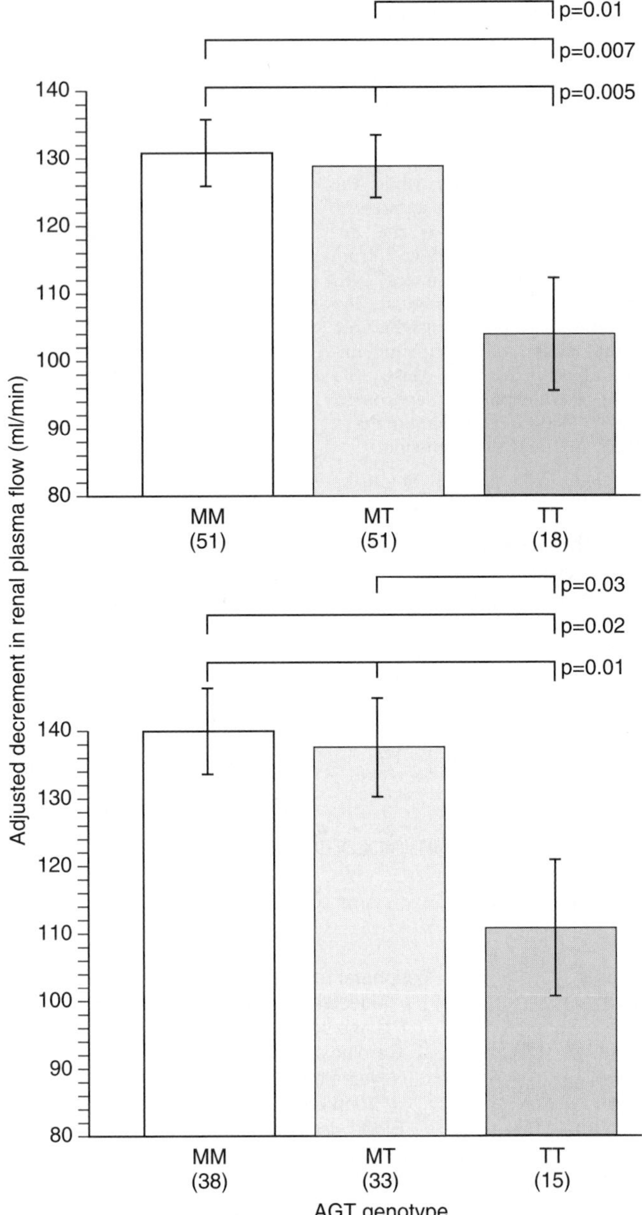

Figure 15–11. Effect of angiotensinogen genotype on renal blood flow responses to angiotensin II infusions. Subjects were classified according to their alleles at the 235 codon of the angiotensinogen gene as to whether they were homozygous for the wild type (MM), heterozygous (MT), or homozygous for the hypertensive-link (TT) alleles. The subjects with the TT235 genotype had a renal blood flow response to angiotensin II similar to that of nonmodulators. (Redrawn from Hopkins P, Lifton RP, Hollenberg NK, et al. Blunted renal vascular response to angiotensin II is associated with a common variant of the angiotensinogen gene and obesity. J Hypertens 1996; 14:199–207. Copyright 1996, Rapid Science Publishers.)

In summary, nonmodulators are a distinct subgroup of the essential hypertensive population and may constitute as much as 30% of that population. They have a sodium-sensitive form of hypertension, probably owing to a derangement of the local renin-angiotensin system in the kidney and the adrenal (Fig. 15–12). These patients also have insulin resistance, hypercholesterolemia, a family history positive for myocardial infarction,

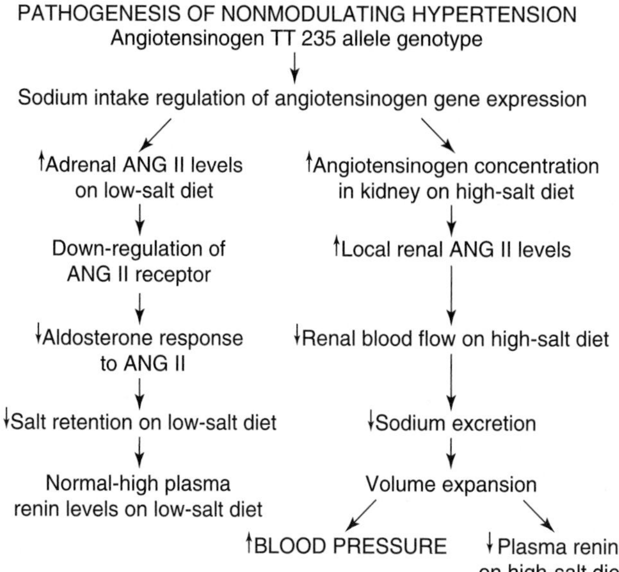

Figure 15–12. Pathogenesis of nonmodulating hypertension. ANG II, angiotensin II.

and an association with a specific allelic variant of the angiotensinogen gene. Finally, the defect appears to be correctable by the administration of converting enzyme inhibitors.

Insulin Resistance and Hypertension

Non–insulin-dependent diabetes mellitus (NIDDM), hypertension, and obesity are commonly associated, and the frequency of this association may be greater than their occurrence in the general population (see the review by Hopkins and colleagues[182]), suggesting a common etiology. In support of this possibility is the fact that insulin resistance and hypertension can coexist without obesity or other stigmata of NIDDM.[183, 184] There may be a genetic component of this interaction. For example, in whites of European descent there is a strong relation between insulin resistance and blood pressure, whereas in normotensive blacks or Pima Indians there is no such relationship (Fig. 15–13).[185] However, most hypertensive blacks are insulin resistant.

Causative Role of Insulin in Hypertension

Several mechanisms have been proposed to explain the insulin-resistant state, including abnormalities in insulin binding to its receptor, defects in glucose transport, changes in the signal transduction pathway within insulin-sensitive cells, and metabolic abnormalities in glycolysis, glucose oxidation, or gluca-

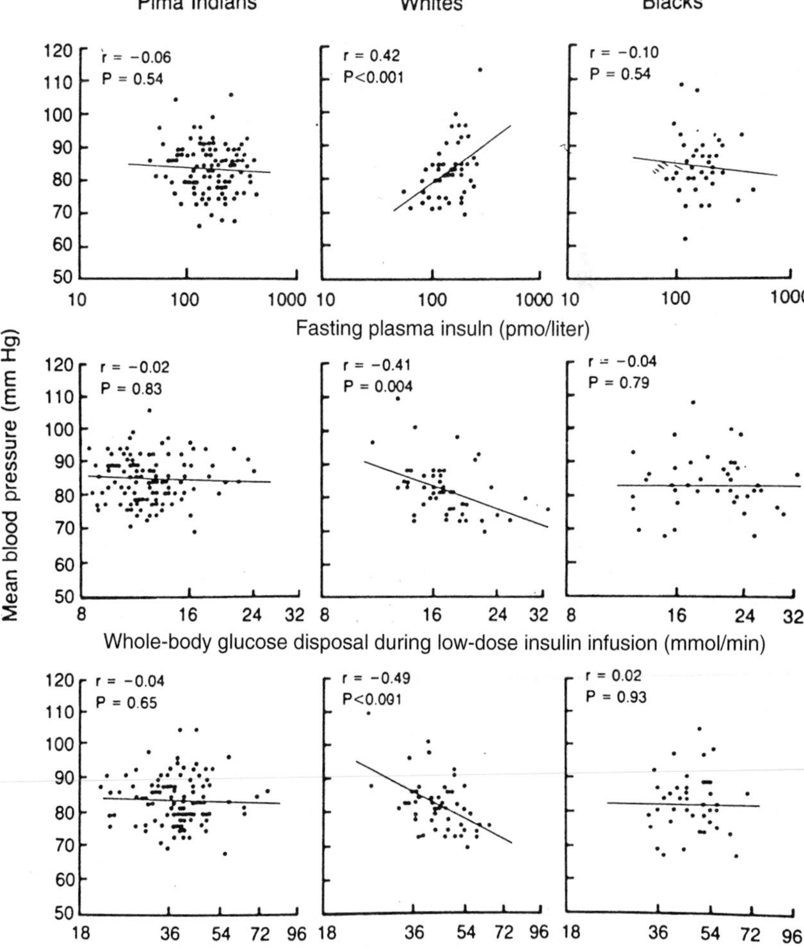

Figure 15–13. Relationship of arterial pressure to insulin resistance in normotensive ethnic subgroups. An index of insulin sensitivity, the glucose disposal rate, was determined with an insulin clamp and fasting insulin levels were measured in normotensive blacks, whites, and Pima Indians. There was a significant negative correlation between arterial blood pressure and glucose disposal rates in whites but not in the other subgroups. (From Saad MF, Lillioja S, Nyomba BL, et al. Racial differences in the relationship between arterial pressure and insulin resistance. N Engl J Med 1991; 324:733–739. Copyright 1991, Massachusetts Medical Society.)

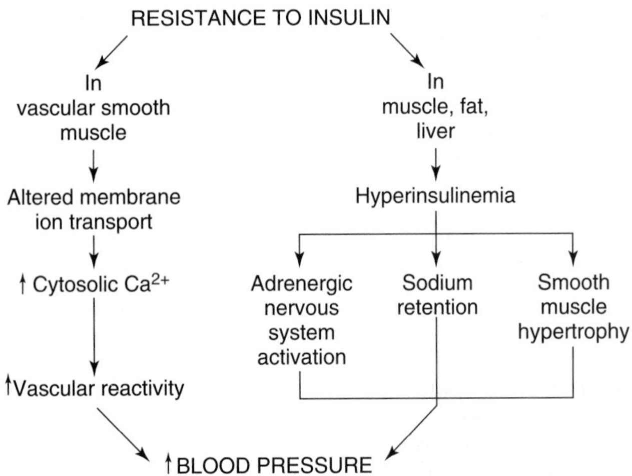

Figure 15–14. Mechanisms by which insulin resistance may produce hypertension.

gon synthesis. Yet little is known concerning the cause of insulin resistance in essential hypertension[182] (Fig. 15–14).

Several features are relevant. First, insulin resistance is common in essential hypertension whether defined by fasting or post–glucose load insulin levels or by euglycemic, hyperinsulinemic clamps.[186–188] Second, obesity cannot explain all cases of insulin resistance. Third, insulin directly stimulates the calcium pump in insulin-sensitive tissues and promotes calcium loss from the cell,[189] and raising cytosolic calcium levels in an adipocyte can induce insulin resistance.[190, 191] If a cell is resistant to insulin, the insulin-induced calcium loss from cells would be decreased, and in vascular smooth muscle cells the resultant increase in intracellular calcium would enhance responsiveness to vasoconstrictors and increase blood pressure.

Two other mechanisms have been proposed to explain the linkage between insulin resistance and hypertension: increased activity of the adrenergic nervous system[192] and increased renal sodium retention.[193] Underlying both these hypotheses is the assumption that insulin resistance in a hypertensive subject may be selective. Accordingly, insulin resistance in the skeletal muscle or liver, or both, would induce a rise in circulating insulin levels. However, there would be little, if any, resistance at the renal tubule or adrenergic nervous system. Finally, for the vasoconstrictor hypothesis to be correct, there would have to be an imbalance between insulin's direct vasodilator effect and the vasoconstriction induced by activation of the adrenergic nervous system.

A hyperinsulinemic response to glucose loading[194] and insulin resistance[195] has been described in salt-sensitive but not in salt-resistant normotensive subjects. This salt sensitivity also extends to metabolic abnormalities that are often associated with insulin resistance, such as increased levels of circulating low-density lipoprotein cholesterol in salt-sensitive hypertensives compared with salt-resistant hypertensives.[196] Thus, salt sensitivity of blood pressure is associated with lipid and glucose metabolic abnormalities and increased cardiovascular risk. Impaired insulin sensitivity[197] and hyperlipidemia[198] have been described in healthy volunteers with normal to high plasma renin levels compared with those with low renin levels. Thus, the data derived from these sources are inconsistent. Individuals who are salt-sensitive, as noted earlier, are likely to have low PRA. Yet salt-sensitive subjects as a group also have an increased risk of carbohydrate and lipid abnormalities.

In summary, insulin resistance occurs in some patients with essential hypertension who do not have obesity or NIDDM. Several lines of evidence suggest that insulin resistance per se or hyperinsulinemia, or both, could result in increased sodium reabsorption, enhanced vascular tone, and activation of the adrenergic nervous system. Alternatively, this state could be associated with abnormal regulation of the renin-angiotensin system. Environmental factors can exacerbate this defect. For example, if patients with insulin resistance gain weight or receive drugs that increase insulin resistance, such as diuretics or beta-blockers, the hypertension may be worsened. However, it is still unclear whether the insulin resistance is a marker for some other abnormality or a primary defect in these patients.

Calcium and Hypertension

In 1982 McCarron and co-workers[199] reported that dietary calcium intake in humans with hypertension was lower than in normotensive control subjects, and the inverse relation between blood pressure and calcium intake has been confirmed in epidemiologic studies.[200, 201] These studies also suggest an association between the level of calcium intake and the degree of sensitivity of the blood pressure to sodium intake. In part, this may not be surprising given the known relationship between the reabsorption of calcium and that of sodium by the proximal tubule of the kidney. Blood pressure, in part, may also correlate with magnesium intake, at least in women.[200] Indeed, the relative risk of developing hypertension was 0.65 when both magnesium (<200 mg/day) and calcium (<400 mg/day) intakes were lower. There appears to be a critical threshold for the effect of calcium intake on blood pressure, the effect not being evident unless calcium intake is less than 700 to 800 mg/day.[202] Thus, increasing calcium intake above this threshold may not modify blood pressure.

Clinical trials designed to evaluate the validity of these observational data have provided equivocal results. However, a meta-analysis of these trials suggests that high calcium intake causes a minimal reduction of blood pressure in the general population and a modest reduction in individuals who already have hypertension. In one meta-analysis[203] of results for 2412 subjects, high calcium intake reduced systolic blood pressure 1.33 mm Hg in the general population and 4.3 mm Hg in hypertensive patients. Hypertensive subjects also had a significant reduction in diastolic blood pressure (1.5 mm Hg). A second meta-analysis involving 1231 individuals did not demonstrate as large an effect.[204]

Pathophysiologic Mechanisms

The mechanisms responsible for the impact of calcium intake on blood pressure are uncertain. Some studies have shown that parathyroid hormone (PTH) levels, on average, are higher in hypertensive subjects compared with normal control subjects, suggesting a potential role for PTH in mediating hypertension. However, PTH levels in hypertensive patients are still within the normal range and are not inappropriate for the level of ionized calcium. Thus, it is unclear whether the elevated PTH causes an increase in blood pressure or is simply a reflection of a modest change in calcium homeostasis. Furthermore, when infused, PTH is a vasodilator,[205] and PTH inhibits contraction of vascular smooth muscle, presumably by inhibiting calcium entry.[206]

Pang and Lewanczuk[207] have suggested that there is a specific hypertensive factor from the parathyroid gland, distinct from PTH, that is increased in some patients with essential hypertension. Several studies in experimental hypertension suggest that the plasma level of the factor is elevated and that it can modify vascular smooth muscle function by increasing cytosolic calcium levels.[208] In some patients with hyperparathyroidism and hypertension, parathyroid hypertensive factor is said to be elevated and becomes undetectable after parathyroidectomy as blood pressure decreases.[209] However, only a single group has reported on the presence of such a factor.

PTH-related protein (PTHrP), a peptide with a structure similar to that of PTH but derived from a different gene, appears to share with PTH an ability to produce vasodilation. It has been suggested that a deficiency in PTHrP could lead to an elevated blood pressure, as this substance may be produced to counteract the effect of vasoconstrictors.[210]

Finally, the active metabolite of vitamin D (1,25-dihydroxy-cholecalciferol) increases calcium uptake in cardiac and vascular smooth muscle cells, induces vascular contractions, and exerts a myotrophic effect on vascular smooth muscle.[211] Patients with low-renin or salt-sensitive hypertension tend to have an increase in both PTH and 1,25-dihydroxycholecalciferol levels. With sodium loading, levels of both hormones increase further as the blood pressure increases. However, as with the changes in PTH levels, it is difficult to determine a cause-and-effect relationship. For example, the increase in 1,25-dihydroxycholecalciferol levels in these patients may be secondary to the higher PTH level because PTH stimulates 1α-hydroxylase activity.

In brief, epidemiologic and experimental evidence suggests that calcium and calcium-regulating hormones play a role in the control of vascular tone. Meta-analyses of clinical trials support a blood pressure–lowering effect of a high calcium intake, particularly in patients with essential hypertension. However, the mechanism or mechanisms involved and the relationship of the effects of calcium intake to the effects of sodium intake on blood pressure are still unclear. Finally, it is uncertain how many of these associations are primary versus secondary events.

Summary

Several lines of evidence suggest that many patients with essential hypertension have an endocrine basis for elevated blood pressure. Increased circulating hormone levels, changes in the responsiveness of target tissues to these hormones, and abnormalities in vascular tone can all contribute to the pathogenesis of the hypertension. Whether these endocrine abnormalities are primary or secondary events is unclear. Intriguingly, most do not fit the classical endocrine pattern for disease because hormonal overproduction is rare. Rather, there is a change in the response of target tissues to specific hormones, with associated adaptive responses probably the major contributor to the hypertensive process. Finally, a number of the abnormalities appear to have a major genetic component. This fact makes possible a more precise dissection of subgroups or phenotypes of hypertensive patients with the use of genetic markers.

RENIN-ANGIOTENSIN SYSTEM AND SECONDARY HYPERTENSION

In addition to its involvement in primary hypertension, the renin-angiotensin system is a major factor in the most common cause of secondary hypertension: renal disease. Indeed, many insights into the renin-angiotensin system have come from the study of patients with renal disease.

Renal Vascular Hypertension

Goldblatt and colleagues[212] described the pathologic role of excess renin production in the hypertension associated with constriction of a renal artery, and 4 years after their observations, a nephrectomy in a hypertensive patient with a small kidney led to correction of the hypertension.[213] Thus, renal vascular hypertension is defined as hypertension associated with either unilateral or bilateral ischemia. Unilateral renal vascular disease is likely to be the cause of elevated blood pressure in approximately 1% of the hypertensive population, and bilateral renal parenchymal disease is causative in another 2% to 4%.[214]

Table 15–2. Causes of Renal Vascular Hypertension

Atherosclerosis (65%–75%)
Fibromuscular dysplasia (25%–30%)
Miscellaneous (1%)
Extrinsic, e.g., hematoma, pheochromocytoma, fibrous band, retroperitoneal fibrosis
Intrinsic, e.g., emboli, arteritis, transplant rejection, Ask-Upmark kidney

It is important to distinguish between renal vascular disease and renal vascular hypertension. Perhaps 50% or more of subjects older than 60 years have renal vascular disease, only a minority of whom also have hypertension.[216] This discrepancy is not surprising when one considers Goldblatt's original experiment, which documented that the lumen of the renal artery needs to be reduced to less than 30% of its original size before hypertension develops. Documentation of a functional abnormality in association with a radiologically defined renal arterial lesion is a critical diagnostic maneuver before therapeutic intervention.

Blacks and patients with diabetes mellitus seem to have a lower frequency of renal vascular hypertension, even though in both groups the incidence of renal vascular disease is higher than in the nondiabetic white population.[214] Most patients with renal vascular disease have either atherosclerotic plaques or fibromuscular disease, and in 10% of the cases the lesion may not be in the main renal artery but in a segmental or branch artery (Table 15–2).

Pathophysiology

The initiating event in the hypertension in subjects with renal disease is a reduction in perfusion pressure to the affected kidney, which stimulates the release of renin.[117, 214, 215] The increased production of renin leads to increased angiotensin II levels and increased aldosterone secretion (secondary aldosteronism; see Fig. 15–8). As a consequence of the hyperaldosteronism, sodium is retained and potassium is lost. The combination of angiotensin II–induced vasoconstriction and sodium retention increases blood pressure and leads to a natriuresis through the contralateral kidney. The increased levels of renin, elevated blood pressure, and sodium retention all act in concert to suppress renin production from the contralateral kidney, an important feature in the diagnostic evaluation of these patients. With bilateral renal arterial disease, the vasculature to both kidneys is compromised. Thus, the ability of the kidneys to excrete sodium is reduced, a gradual volume expansion occurs, and circulating renin levels are suppressed.

In long-standing unilateral renal artery stenosis, the contralateral kidney may become damaged secondary to the elevated blood pressure.[217] Thus, the affected kidney is protected by the stenotic lesion and may ultimately suffer less damage, except for the ischemia induced by the stenosis. In these cases correction of the renal artery stenosis may not correct the elevated blood pressure, which can be sustained by the diffusely damaged contralateral kidney. Paradoxically, in this circumstance repair of the renal artery stenosis and removal of the contralateral kidney may normalize blood pressure.

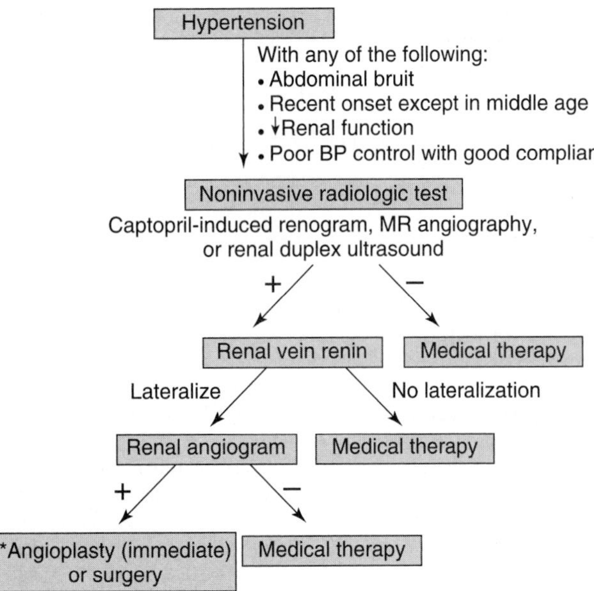

Figure 15–15. Diagnostic and therapeutic flow chart for evaluating patients for renovascular hypertension. BP, blood pressure; MR, magnetic resonance.* Stenting of renal arteries is commonly done following angioplasty.

Although renal vascular hypertension occurs in all age groups, the etiology varies. In individuals younger than 50 years, renal vascular hypertension is more common in women and is usually secondary to fibromuscular dysplasia of the renal artery. After the age of 50 it is more likely to be secondary to atherosclerosis and therefore more common in men. In addition to unilateral or bilateral vascular insufficiency, generalized renal ischemia can result from renal compression, such as in hydronephrosis. Initially the kidney is enlarged, but over time cortical atrophy develops.

Diagnosis

Renal vascular hypertension should be suspected in a normotensive individual of any age who has sudden onset of hypertension, in a known hypertensive subject with an acute acceleration of blood pressure, or in an individual younger than 30 years who has significant hypertension.[215] Other clinical features are suggestive of this condition (Fig. 15–15). In general, if the hypertension is mild to moderate (diastolic blood pressure ≤ 105 mm Hg) with an onset between ages 30 and 60 years, the probability of renal vascular hypertension is low. In these patients, a detailed search for renal vascular hypertension is probably not warranted.

The diagnosis of renal vascular hypertension rests on two criteria: (1) the identification of a significant arterial obstruction and (2) evidence of excess renin secretion by one or both kidneys.[218, 219] The following tests are particularly useful in patients with fibromuscular dysplasia whose hypertension is renin-dependent and often cured by revascularization. In elderly individuals with renal artery stenosis that is probably secondary to atherosclerosis, consideration of the therapeutic options may modify the extent of testing.

Noninvasive Testing

Gadolinium-Enhanced Magnetic Resonance Angiography

This procedure is useful for defining anatomic lesions of one or both renal arteries.[220] In some centers it is becoming the screening procedure of choice. Because gadolinium is not nephrotoxic, it may be particularly useful for individuals with renal insufficiency.[221, 222] The reported sensitivity (90% to 100%) and specificity (90% to 95%) are excellent for detecting a stenosis greater than 50%. Limitations of this technique include the requirement for breath holding, overestimation of stenosis, inadequate visualization of segmental and accessory renal arteries, low availability of MR angiography, and cost. With future development, rapid imaging techniques may permit the acquisition of hemodynamic data by visualization of the vascular phases.

Captopril Renography

This is a functional test. Captopril, a converting enzyme inhibitor, is administered 30 to 60 minutes before the renogram.[223, 224] This test takes advantage of the dependence of the hemodynamics of the renal vasculature on angiotensin II because both the efferent and afferent arterioles are highly sensitive to the vasoconstrictor actions of angiotensin II. Indeed, balanced constriction of these two vessels maintains a normal glomerular filtration rate with a variety of changes in renal blood flow, so-called renal autoregulation. An increase in angiotensin II levels secondary to unilateral stenosis of a renal artery leads to vasoconstriction of the afferent and efferent arterioles in both kidneys. Because of the stenotic lesion on the affected side, blood flow to the glomerulus, and therefore glomerular pressure, on this side is determined primarily by the structural lesion.

When a converting enzyme inhibitor (which reduces intrarenal angiotensin II levels) is given, angiotensin II–induced afferent arteriolar constriction is reduced in both kidneys. In the unaffected contralateral kidney there is a concomitant reduction in efferent arteriolar tone, an increase in blood flow, and no change in glomerular filtration rate. However, in the stenotic kidney, where perfusion of the glomeruli is restricted by the stenosis, a reduction in efferent arteriolar tone results in a fall in glomerular filtration rate and reduced uptake and delayed excretion of the isotopic tracer as assessed by the renogram. The sensitivity (80% to 90%) and specificity (65% to 80%) of the captopril renogram are somewhat less than those of the MR angiogram, particularly in patients with renal insufficiency.

Digital Subtraction Angiography

This procedure is used in some centers,[218, 225] but because of the cost and the need for arterial rather than venous injection, its role as a screening test is limited.

Renal Duplex Ultrasonography

This test provides both a functional (Doppler) and an anatomic (B-mode imaging) evaluation of the renal artery and renal perfusion.[226] Intrarenal ultrasonography measures the pulsatility index and blood flow acceleration during early systole. Its sensitivity (85% to 95%) and specificity (70% to 85%) fall between those of the captopril renogram and the MR angiogram. Although in theory this may be an ideal screening test, in practice its validity is dependent on the skills of the radiologist.[218, 219, 225, 227] Depending on operator availability, it is the procedure of choice in some centers.

Invasive Testing

The definitive test for a correctable renal vascular lesion is the combination of bilateral renal vein renin sampling and a selective renal arteriogram. As noted earlier, the renal arteriogram alone defines structural lesions but does not provide insight into their functional significance. Simultaneous bilateral renal vein renin measurement provides a valuable adjunct for predicting whether therapeutic intervention will modify the hypertension. When one kidney is ischemic and the other is normal, nearly all the circulating renin is produced by the affected side. As a result, the venous concentration of renin from the ischemic kidney is at least 1.5 times greater than that from the contralateral kidney. Theoretically, the renin concentration from the contralateral kidney should be the same as that in the peripheral circulation. Unfortunately, in many circumstances there is a varying degree of damage to the contralateral kidney, and therefore total suppression of renin from that kidney does not occur.

Some administer captopril before renal vein sampling to exaggerate the renin release from the stenotic side; all agents that suppress renin secretion, such as β-blockers, should be withheld before the study. If feasible, the patient should also have a low sodium intake to enhance renin release from the affected kidney. If these procedures are followed, approximately 80% of subjects with unilateral renin elevations that fulfill the preceding criteria have a beneficial response to therapeutic intervention.

Treatment

The treatment of choice in renal artery stenosis secondary to fibromuscular disease is renal angioplasty with or without insertion of a stent.[219, 228, 229] Lesions at the ostium of the renal artery often do not respond well to angioplasty alone, but the addition of a stent may improve the outcome. Surgical revascularization, previously the primary approach, is used less frequently in older adults with atherosclerotic lesions because the surgical risk is high in these individuals. The same reservation may apply to angioplasty or stenting, or both, in comparison with medical treatment.[230–232] Thus, surgery is usually reserved for individuals in whom angioplasty has proved unsuccessful.

Medical management to control blood pressure may be appropriate in elderly individuals, those who are not candidates for definitive corrective procedures, or those in whom these procedures have failed.[233] Converting enzyme inhibitors or an angiotensin II receptor antagonist would be the treatment of choice, given the pathophysiology of the disease. However, for the reasons outlined earlier, these agents may worsen ischemia in the affected kidney. Converting enzyme inhibitors should be used with great caution in individuals who may have bilateral renal artery disease or arterial disease in a solitary kidney because these agents may reduce the glomerular filtration rate, cause renal hypoxia, and precipitate renal failure. Finally, a more aggressive therapeutic approach to preserve renal function may require invasive techniques.[234]

Primary Reninism

Rarely, juxtaglomerular cell tumors of the kidney or ectopic tumors secrete renin.[235] Individuals with such tumors have typical features of renal vascular hypertension: hypertension, elevated renin levels, hypokalemia, and hyponatremia. Most, however, are young and have high circulating levels of renin in the blood and also severe hypertension at the time of diagnosis. When a mass lesion is discovered in the kidney, there is unilateral renin secretion but no evidence of renal artery stenosis. Radiologic evaluation with CT scanning is invaluable. Surgical removal of the tumor cures the hypertension and the hyperreninemia.

Renal Parenchymal Disease

A variety of conditions can cause hypertension associated with renal parenchymal disease, the most common of which are hypertension per se, diabetes mellitus, and autoimmune disease (e.g., systemic lupus erythematosus). In these patients there is the potential, depending on the level of sodium intake, for a shift from a vasoconstrictor (angiotensin II) form of hypertension to a volume-sensitive hypertension secondary to decreased capacity for renal sodium excretion. The local (intrarenal) renin-angiotensin system is activated to a variable degree in these subjects. This activation results in an elevation of hydraulic pressure in the glomeruli (so-called glomerular hypertension) secondary to the vasoconstrictor effect of angiotensin II on the efferent arteriole as noted earlier.[236] Chronic elevation of glomerular pressure leads to glomerular sclerosis and progressive loss of functioning nephron units.

The administration of converting enzyme inhibitors can slow the progression of renal damage in both diabetic and nondiabetic renal parenchymal disease.[237, 238] This effect appears to be an added action of converting enzyme inhibitors beyond their ability to lower systemic blood pressure, probably because they also selectively reduce renal glomerular pressure. Thus, agents that produce a decrease in systemic blood pressure equivalent to that accomplished by converting enzyme inhibitors do not afford the same degree of protection of renal function.

However, caution should be exercised in administering converting enzyme inhibitors to patients who may have an increased risk of bilateral renal artery stenosis. In such circumstances, instead of improvement, converting enzyme inhibitors would cause a sudden deterioration of renal function.[239] Interestingly, the renal protective actions of converting enzyme inhibitors work in advanced diabetic nephropathy, a condition usually associated with hyporeninemic hypoaldosteronism. Because of the possible further reduction of aldosterone production with converting enzyme inhibitors in such patients, frequent measurement of serum potassium levels is mandatory, with institution of appropriate measures to reduce potassium levels if hyperkalemia occurs (e.g., low-potassium diet, potassium-wasting diuretics). In some instances, the converting enzyme inhibitor may have to be discontinued.

Hypertension during Pregnancy

Pregnancy-induced hypertension (PIH), or gestational hypertension, is defined as de novo hypertension arising during the second half of pregnancy. The literature regarding the prevalence and pathophysiologic abnormalities in this disorder is clouded by studies that have often included pregnant patients with chronic hypertension. The classification of hypertensive disorders of pregnancy developed by the American College of Obstetricians and Gynecologists has been adopted by the National Institutes of Health[240]:

1. Chronic hypertension: blood pressure greater than 140/90 mm Hg before pregnancy or before the 20th week of pregnancy
2. Preeclampsia: a systolic blood pressure increase of at least 30 mm Hg or a diastolic blood pressure increase of at least 15 mm Hg over prepregnancy or early pregnancy values combined with proteinuria (≥300 mg per 24 hours) or edema, or both
3. Preeclampsia superimposed on chronic hypertension: the same criteria as for item 2 but occurring in women with preexisting hypertension
4. Transient hypertension: a blood pressure increase similar to that in preeclampsia but without proteinuria or edema

Preeclampsia may also progress to eclampsia, defined as the occurrence of convulsions. As viewed according to the preceding classification, PIH includes preeclampsia and transient hypertension of pregnancy. However, the prognosis for each is different. The preeclampsia form of PIH is self-limited and usually does not occur in subsequent pregnancies, whereas

Table 15–3. Pathophysiologic Changes in Preeclampsia Compared with Normal Pregnancy

Cardiovascular Measurements
Reduced circulating plasma volume
Increased systemic vascular resistance
Decreased cardiac index
Hormonal Indicators of Volume
Reduced circulating plasma renin activity (PRA), angiotensin II, and aldosterone
Enhanced angiotensin II pressor responsiveness
Increased levels of atrial natriuretic peptide (ANP)
Increased levels of digitalis-like factor (DLF)
Other Hormonal Alterations
Hyperinsulinemia and insulin resistance
Decreased prostacyclin and/or elevated thromboxane production

chronic hypertension commonly complicates all pregnancies. Significantly, preeclampsia increases both maternal and fetal morbidity and mortality.

Risk Factors for Pregnancy-Induced Hypertension

PIH arises in approximately 5% of nulliparous pregnant women, and the prevalence appears to be related to both environmental and genetic factors. For example, the prevalence of PIH is double in indigent, inner-city pregnant women. Other risk factors include nulliparity, low dietary calcium intake, multiple gestations, black race, chronic hypertension, increasing age, inherited and acquired coagulation disorders such as protein S and protein C deficiencies and antiphospholipid antibodies, and a history of a mother who had this syndrome.[241]

Pathophysiology

Pathophysiologic abnormalities in PIH should be divided into those in preeclampsia and those in transient hypertension of pregnancy. In normal pregnancy, plasma volume increases by 40%,[242] associated with a reduction in peripheral vascular resistance (40% to 80%) and a rise in cardiac output, renal blood flow, and glomerular filtration rate.[243] The renin-angiotensin-aldosterone system is activated despite the increase in plasma volume.[244] This activation is believed to be related to prostanoids, for example, prostacyclin and prostaglandin E_2; direct effects of estrogen; or an antinatriuretic action of progesterone.

A number of alterations have been reported in subjects with PIH, although many investigations do not clearly distinguish between patients with preeclampsia and those with transient hypertension of pregnancy. Table 15–3 presents the findings in preeclampsia compared with normotensive pregnancy. Plasma volume is reduced in preeclamptics,[245–247] and systemic vascular resistance is increased.[248, 249] Paradoxically, the hormonal markers of volume are consistent with a volume-expanded state: relative suppression of the renin-angiotensin-aldosterone system and increased levels of atrial natriuretic peptide[250–252] and digitalis-like factor.[253] This apparent paradox is unexplained unless these hormonal changes induce the volume changes or there is a misperception of extracellular fluid volume in this disorder. On the other hand, elevated levels of digitalis-like factor, an inhibitor of the Na^+,K^+-ATPase pump, could increase intracellular sodium levels, as reported in red blood cells in patients with PIH.[254] The role of digitalis-like factor is controversial, however, because of disparate findings for digoxin-like immunoreactivity versus measurement by bioassay, that is, inhibition of Na^+,K^+-ATPase.[255]

Enhanced maternal vascular reactivity is also seen in PIH with increased pressor sensitivity to infused angiotensin II even in normotensive phases of pregnancies, before patients progress to PIH. In contrast, in normal pregnancies pressor responsiveness to angiotensin II is blunted. One important hypothesis that could explain these observations includes decreased production of vasodilatory prostaglandins, such as prostaglandin E_1 and prostacyclin[256]; in fact, decreased prostacyclin production may precede the appearance of hypertension in PIH.[257] Others propose a relative increase in the vasoconstriction prostaglandin, thromboxane, and subnormal nitric oxide. Reported cation abnormalities include increased intracellular calcium and enhanced responses of intracellular calcium to vasopressin in platelets of patients with PIH.[258] These findings suggest that parallel changes might occur in vascular smooth muscle, where intracellular calcium is a major determinant of peripheral vascular resistance. It is unclear whether the abnormalities in PIH reflect initiating events or are secondary alterations that sustain the elevation of blood pressure.

One unifying hypothesis to explain PIH is uteroplacental hypoperfusion. Perhaps secondary to structural abnormalities in the spiral arteries supplying the uterus, uterine blood flow is impaired. Through unknown mechanisms, prostaglandin production is reduced and there is generalized endothelial damage (endothelin levels are elevated in PIH). Subsequently, platelet aggregation is enhanced, fibrin is deposited in the glomeruli, and proteinuria occurs. Although this is an attractive hypothesis, a number of links need to be established.

Treatment

There is little evidence that sodium restriction improves the outcome of pregnancy in women with PIH or is effective for prophylaxis against PIH.[259] On the other hand, some studies suggest that volume expansion may improve both blood pressure and outcome in preeclampsia.[260] It now appears that a moderate to liberal sodium diet should be recommended to pregnant women and that the diet should be adequate in calcium. Bed rest with lateral recumbency is commonly recommended for women with PIH and is believed to result in hemodynamic improvements, including increased renal and uterine blood flow and reduced peripheral vascular resistance with lowering of systemic blood pressure.

Low-dose aspirin (50 to 100 mg/day) may reduce the incidence of PIH, although the results of several large trials remain controversial. The rationale for low-dose aspirin is to restore the balance between vasodilator and vasoconstrictor prostaglandins (primarily by reducing thromboxane A_2 but without affecting prostacyclin levels).[261, 262] Antihypertensive agents are usually given when diastolic blood pressure exceeds 100 mm Hg. Traditional agents include methyldopa and hydralazine. α-Blockers, such as prazosin, and calcium channel blockers, primarily nifedipine, are being used with increased frequency because of their greater efficacy. These agents also appear to have acceptable safety profiles, although they have not been used as long as the traditional drugs. ACE inhibitors and angiotensin receptor antagonists are contraindicated in PIH because of adverse effects on kidney development in the fetus.

PRIMARY MINERALOCORTICOID EXCESS STATES

Primary mineralocorticoid excess states are characterized by suppressed PRA and hypokalemia and include primary aldos-

Table 15–4. Mineralocorticoid Excess States Associated with Low Plasma Renin Levels

Hypermineralocorticoidism
Primary aldosteronism
Aldosterone-producing adenoma (APA)
Idiopathic hyperplasia (idiopathic hyperaldosteronism)
Adrenocortical carcinoma
Glucocorticoid-remediable aldosteronism (GRA)
Congenital adrenal hyperplasia
11β-Hydroxylase deficiency
17α-Hydroxylase deficiency
Increased Mineralocorticoid Action
Apparent mineralocorticoid excess (AME)
Congenital
Licorice ingestion
Ectopic corticotropin production
Liddle's syndrome

teronism, deoxycorticosterone (DOC)-secreting tumors, and inherited diseases (Table 15–4).

Primary Aldosteronism

Primary aldosteronism, the cause of approximately 0.05% to 2.2% of all unselected cases of hypertension, was first described in 1955 by Conn[263] in conjunction with an aldosterone-producing adrenal adenoma (APA). Other etiologies include idiopathic bilateral hyperplasia (idiopathic hyperaldosteronism) and inherited entities. Its prevalence may be as high as 10% in hypertensive patients, depending on the study population and the criteria used. The prevalence of tumors remains fairly constant. However, the prevalence of bilateral hyperplasia can vary greatly.

Clinical Features

The clinical symptoms of primary aldosteronism are nonspecific and result from potassium depletion. Neuromuscular symptoms (weakness, periodic paralysis, cramps, or tetany), fatigue, and paresthesias are not uncommon; polyuria and nocturia probably result from a hypokalemia-induced renal concentrating defect. Despite the continuous high levels of aldosterone, patients rarely exhibit edema, presumably owing to escape, in which the sodium-retaining effects of chronic mineralocorticoid excess are lost. Intracellular potassium depletion can also impair insulin secretion and cause glucose intolerance or overt diabetes mellitus. Resetting of the osmostat can occur in primary aldosteronism, as evidenced by slightly higher than normal serum sodium levels.[264] This is a useful clinical point because there is a tendency for a reduced serum sodium level in states of secondary aldosteronism.

The hypertension associated with primary aldosteronism is usually moderate to severe with mean blood pressures (± standard deviation) of 184 ± 8/112 ± 16 mm Hg.[265] However, some patients have malignant hypertension, and others have normal or only mildly elevated blood pressure. Individuals with APA tend to have higher blood pressures than those with idiopathic hyperaldosteronism (IHA).[266] Patients with primary aldosteronism may be refractory to conventional antihypertensive agents and may experience severe hypokalemia after institution of potassium-wasting diuretics such as hydrochlorothiazide. Although it would be expected that the hypertension is related to volume expansion, measurements of extracellular sodium spaces in patients with APA are usually normal while peripheral resistance is increased.

End-organ damage with primary aldosteronism is variable. In general, the left ventricular hypertrophy is disproportionate to the level of blood pressure when compared with the situation in essential hypertension.[267] With removal of an aldosteronoma, its regression occurs even if blood pressure does not become normal. In addition, structural damage to the kidney, cerebral circulation, and retinal vasculature occurs more frequently than would be assumed on the basis of the duration and level of blood pressure. As many as 50% of patients with primary aldosteronism may have proteinuria, and renal failure may occur in as many as 15%. Thus, it is probable that, independent of aldosterone's effect on blood pressure, its excess production induces cardiovascular damage.

Mineralocorticoid excess states are associated with vascular remodeling that results in perivascular fibrosis and vascular wall thickening. Cardiac fibrosis has also been reported in postmortem studies of patients with adrenal adenoma with mineralocorticoid hypertension.[268] An excessive number of renal cysts has also been noted in association with hypokalemia and hyperaldosteronism (in as many as 60% of cases).[269] However, other studies reported a prevalence of renal cysts similar to that in the normal population.[266, 270]

Table 15–5. Causes of Primary Aldosteronism and Their Frequencies

Syndrome	Proportion of Cases
Aldosterone-producing adenoma, including renin-responsive adenoma	65%
Idiopathic hyperaldosteronism, including primary adrenal hyperplasia	30%–40%
Glucocorticoid-remediable aldosteronism (GRA)	1%–3%

Etiologies

Etiologies of primary aldosteronism are shown in Table 15–5.

Aldosterone-Producing Adenoma

The solitary APA is the most common cause of primary aldosteronism and accounts for approximately 65% of cases. These lesions are usually less than 2 cm in diameter, making them difficult to image. They are benign neoplasms and are surrounded by a well-defined capsule; microscopically, the most common cell type is a large, clear lipid-filled cell resembling a zona fasciculata cell.[271]

Idiopathic Hyperaldosteronism

Idiopathic hyperplasia (bilateral adrenal hyperplasia) is the cause of approximately 30% of cases of primary aldosteronism.[272] Microscopically, the glands show hyperplasia of the zona glomerulosa accompanied by adrenocortical nodules. The aldosterone excess in IHA is usually milder than in APA; as a result, the biochemical abnormalities such as hypokalemia and suppression of PRA are usually less severe than in APA.

Because the plasma aldosterone response to infused angiotensin II is exaggerated compared with that in normal individuals or patients with APA,[273] IHA has been hypothesized to represent a syndrome of enhanced responsiveness to angiotensin II. Others suggest that IHA is a form of essential hypertension representing one end of the distribution of aldosterone production in essential hypertension and is therefore related to low-renin essential hypertension, in which an enhanced aldosterone response to angiotensin II is seen (see earlier).

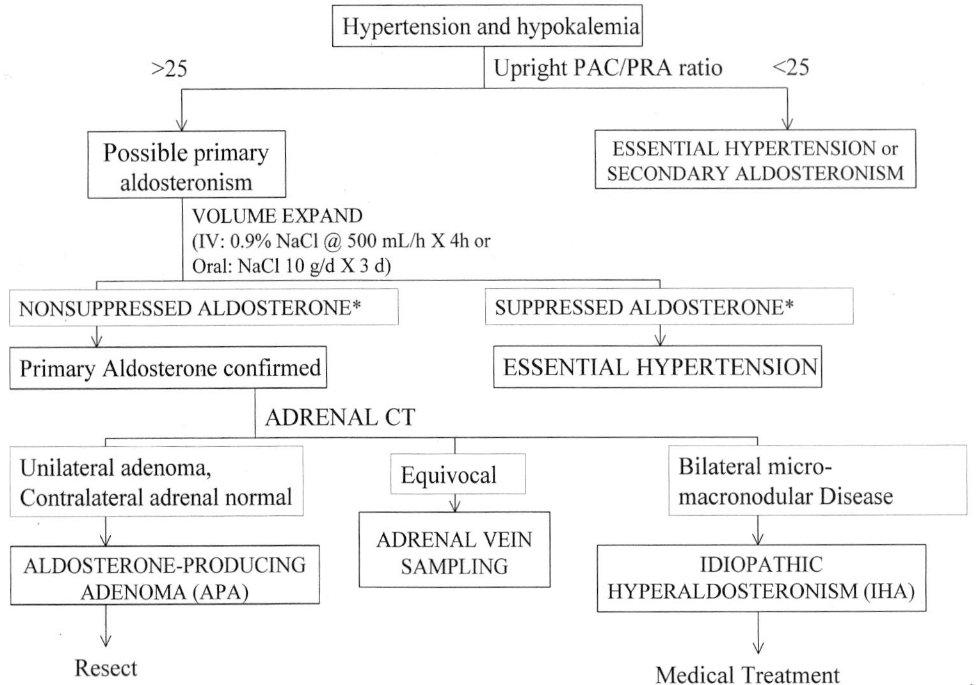

Figure 15–16. Diagnostic flow chart for evaluating the hypokalemic hypertensive patient. Differentiation of APA versus IHA. PRA, plasma renin activity; PAC, plasma aldosterone concentration; APA, aldosterone-producing adenoma; IHA, idiopathic hyperaldosteronism; CT, computed tomography. *Suppressed values: PAC < 280 pmol/L (< 10 ng/dL) following IV saline; aldosterone excretion rate 39 nmol/d (< 14 μg/d) after oral salt loading.

Adrenocortical Carcinoma

Adrenocortical carcinoma is an extremely rare cause of primary aldosteronism. In contrast to APAs, these tumors are usually large at the time of diagnosis (>6 cm).

Glucocorticoid-Remediable Aldosteronism (GRA)[274]

See later.

Regulation of Aldosterone Secretion

The renin-angiotensin system is suppressed in primary aldosteronism and does not contribute to the regulation of aldosterone production.[275] In this sense, aldosterone production is "autonomous." However, studies in patients with APA, for example, demonstrate that the adenomas are regulated by corticotropin and potassium. Thus, autonomy is defined by the failure of aldosterone production to respond to maneuvers that normally activate (upright posture) or suppress (sodium loading) the renin-angiotensin system. A variant form of APA has been described in which the adenomas are renin responsive (see later). Moreover, in IHA aldosterone production is usually responsive to stimuli that activate the renin-angiotensin system.[275] On the other hand, adrenal carcinomas are truly resistant to all secretagogues.

Diagnosis

Screening Tests

Spontaneous hypokalemia is commonly present. Some patients may have normal potassium levels, possibly because of self-selected dietary sodium restriction, because aldosterone-induced renal potassium wasting is diminished by decreased sodium delivery to the distal nephron. When potassium-wasting diuretics are given as antihypertensive agents, hypokalemia is more frequent and more severe. Serum potassium measurement is not a good screening test in GRA because many patients have normal potassium levels.[276]

PRA is suppressed in almost all patients (<1.0 ng/mL per hour [<0.8 nmol/L per hour]) and does not increase appropriately (>2 ng/mL per hour [>1.6 nmol/L per hour]) after dietary sodium restriction or after acute diuretic administration with furosemide followed by 90 to 120 minutes of upright posture.[277] Although a subset of patients with essential hypertension (25%) also have low PRA, documentation of a normal or high stimulated PRA level excludes primary aldosteronism.

Given the high prevalence of suppressed PRA levels in essential hypertension, documentation of a concomitant elevation of plasma aldosterone (PA) makes the diagnosis of primary aldosteronism more likely (Fig. 15–16). Thus, a PA/PRA ratio greater than 30 is suggestive and a ratio of 50 or more is virtually diagnostic of primary aldosteronism (when PRA is expressed as ng/mL per hour and PA as ng/dL).[266] To improve the accuracy of this test, salt intake should not be restricted and serum aldosterone levels should be greater than 500 pmol/L (>15 ng/dL). Because a number of drugs (ACE inhibitors, β-blockers, and spironolactone) alter PRA levels, such antihypertensives should be withdrawn for 2 to 4 weeks if possible (6 to 8 weeks for spironolactone) before determining the PA/PRA ratio. Hypokalemia reduces aldosterone levels, and diagnostic studies should be performed with patients in a potassium-repleted state. Specimens should be obtained after 2 hours of upright posture because stimulated ratios have been shown to have better diagnostic accuracy than supine values.[278]

The captopril test can also be used to diagnose primary aldosteronism.[279, 280] One protocol is to administer 50 mg orally at 9:00 AM; blood samples are obtained before and 90 minutes later. In normotensive individuals or essential hypertensives, acute inhibition of ACE decreases angiotensin-regulated aldosterone production. However, in primary aldosteronism aldosterone levels fail to decline because the renin-angiotensin system is suppressed and aldosterone production is autonomous. A postcaptopril aldosterone reduction of more than 20%, usually to less than 410 pmol/L (<15 ng/dL), is considered a normal response. Although the sensitivity of this test ranges from 90% to 100%, the specificity is significantly less (50% to 80%).

Diagnosis of Autonomous Aldosterone Production

Oral sodium loading for 3 days followed by a 24-hour urine collection for determination of aldosterone excretion can discriminate primary aldosteronism from essential hypertension with excellent sensitivity and specificity (96% and 93%, respectively).[281] A 24-hour urinary aldosterone excretion rate greater than 28 to 39 nmol/day (10 to 14 μg/day) in the presence of urinary sodium excretion greater than 250 mmol/day is considered diagnostic of primary aldosteronism.

Autonomous aldosterone production can also be demonstrated by acute intravascular volume expansion with isotonic saline. Isotonic saline is administered intravenously at a rate of 500 mL/hour for 4 to 6 hours. Postsaline plasma aldosterone levels greater than 280 pmol/L (>10 ng/dL)—a more stringent value of greater than 140 to 220 pmol/L (>5 to 8 ng/dL) has also been proposed[282, 283]—confirm the diagnosis of autonomous aldosterone production.

Differential Diagnosis

Hormonal Testing

Hormonal testing provides supportive data, especially if radiography fails to show a solitary tumor. The posture test is the most common study used in the differential diagnosis of primary aldosteronism. Samples are collected for PRA and plasma aldosterone when the subject is recumbent and after 2 to 4 hours of standing or walking. The response in normal subjects and those with essential hypertension is an increase in plasma aldosterone levels of at least 50% compared with recumbent levels. Before testing, hypokalemia should be corrected with oral potassium supplementation. The accuracy of the test is enhanced by simultaneous measurement of recumbent and upright cortisol levels.[284]

In patients with APA, aldosterone levels generally decline in parallel with the circadian secretion of cortisol, the so-called anomalous postural response.[285] This is because the renin-angiotensin system is suppressed in patients with APA, and therefore changes in posture do not stimulate increased production of aldosterone. In contrast, in IHA there is usually an increase in renin and aldosterone levels in response to assumption of the upright posture. The predictive value of the posture test in distinguishing between APA and IHA approaches 90%; however, the specificity of this test is reduced in variant forms of APA and IHA (see later). A postural decline in plasma aldosterone is also seen in GRA because aldosterone secretion is regulated solely by corticotropin in this disorder. Blood levels of 18-OH-corticosterone, an intermediate of the aldosterone biosynthetic pathway, are generally greater than 2800 nmol/mL (100 ng/dL) in subjects with APA, whereas patients with IHA have lower levels.[286]

Documentation of the unique hybrid 18-oxygenated cortisol compounds 18-oxocortisol and 18-OH-cortisol in a 24-hour urine collection can be used to make the diagnosis of GRA and also differentiate APA from IHA (see later).[287] In contrast to modest elevations in APA[287, 288] and normal levels in IHA, levels of these compounds are 10-fold above normal in GRA. A major drawback is the lack of general availability of assays for these compounds.

Radiologic Studies

Tomography using spiral CT techniques is the imaging modality of first choice. It is critical to make a biochemical diagnosis before imaging the adrenal because of the 2% to 10% incidence of nonfunctioning adrenal masses in CT studies of the abdomen.[290] The use of adrenal scintigraphy with NP-59 (^{131}I-6β-iodomethyl-19-norcholesterol) can differentiate APA from IHA because lateralization is seen in the former disorder. However, a lateralizing scan lacks specificity because it may also be seen with adrenal adenomas that do not produce aldosterone.

Adrenal venous sampling, which should be reserved for cases in which diagnostic imaging and biochemical studies are inconclusive, is the most sensitive means of differentiating APA from IHA. In most cases of APA, the ratio of the ipsilateral to the contralateral aldosterone concentration is greater than 10:1. This procedure is diagnostic in more than 95% of cases when catheterization of the right adrenal vein is successful. However, the incidence of unsuccessful procedures can be as high as 25%.[265] Furthermore, adrenal venous sampling is invasive and is associated with a small but significant risk of venous thrombosis, adrenal hemorrhage, or adrenal insufficiency.

Nonclassical Variants of Primary Aldosteronism

The aldosterone-producing renin-responsive adenoma (APRA) and primary adrenal hyperplasia are variants of primary aldosteronism[289, 290] that represent important exceptions in terms of both diagnosis and treatment. In contrast to findings in APA, the changes in plasma renin (features characteristically considered diagnostic of IHA) after upright posture in subjects with APRA cause an increase in aldosterone levels. Thus, in patients diagnosed with primary aldosteronism the importance of adrenal imaging in documenting a solitary lesion is emphasized by this unusual entity.

Primary unilateral adrenal hyperplasia is another variant form of primary aldosteronism.[290] The biochemical features resemble those in APA: no increase or a decline in aldosterone levels in response to upright posture and elevated levels of urinary 18-OH-cortisol and 18-oxocortisol. The syndrome can be ameliorated by unilateral adrenalectomy or a reduction in adrenal mass.

Therapy

Surgery is the treatment of choice for patients with APA, APRA, and primary adrenal hyperplasia. Cure rates (defined as blood pressure less than 140/90 without medications 6 to 12 months after surgery) vary between 35% and 50%.[266] All patients should receive medical treatment before surgery to control blood pressure and replete potassium stores (see later). Persistent postoperative hypertension may be related to the chronicity or severity of hypertension, the presence of end-organ changes, or concurrent essential hypertension. On the other hand, the hypertension in IHA responds poorly to bilateral adrenalectomy, although the potassium-wasting state is reversed. Pharmacologic treatment is the therapy of choice for IHA, for preoperative management of APA, or when the patient is not a surgical candidate.[291] A sodium-restricted diet (sodium < 2 g/day) is also prescribed in conjunction with pharmacologic treatment to minimize potassium wasting and lower the blood pressure.

Spironolactone, a competitive antagonist of aldosterone, has traditionally been the drug of first choice, with doses of 100 to 500 mg/day usually being required. Spironolactone also blocks testosterone biosynthesis and action, resulting in erectile dysfunction, decreased libido, and gynecomastia in men; menstrual irregularities are seen in women. Amiloride blocks the apical sodium channel in the distal nephron and is an alternative to spironolactone; it is given in divided doses starting at 5 mg twice daily with a maximal dose of 15 mg twice daily.

The sustained-release formulation of the calcium channel blocker nifedipine (dose range 30 to 90 mg/day) has also been used in the medical management of primary aldosteronism[292] because this compound inhibits aldosterone biosynthesis in vitro.[293] However, the antihypertensive response to this agent alone in primary aldosteronism is disappointing,[294] and nifedipine should be viewed as a second-line agent. ACE inhibitors and angiotensin II receptor antagonists may also have a role in the medical management of IHA because the response to angiotensin II may be exaggerated in this disorder.

Genetic Basis for Mineralocorticoid Excess States

Glucocorticoid-remediable aldosteronism (GRA) is the commonest heritable form of hyperaldosteronism.

In the following syndromes, the steroids responsible for the mineralocorticoid excess states include DOC and cortisol. As a result of the suppression of the renin-angiotensin system, the aldosterone levels are low—not elevated as in the previously described syndromes. Some forms of congenital adrenal hyperplasia have a mineralocorticoid component.

Other genetic causes include a mutation in enzymes not in the biosynthetic pathway or ion channels important in mediating or mimicking the action of aldosterone.

Hypermineralocorticoidism—Suppressed Plasma Renin Activity

Congenital Adrenal Hyperplasia

DOC excess is seen in several hypertensive forms of congenital adrenal hyperplasia or rarely in neoplasms (adenoma or carcinoma) that overproduce DOC. Congenital adrenal hyperplasia results from a deficiency in cortisol biosynthesis (see Chapter 14). Deficiencies in both 11β-hydroxylase (CYP11B) and 17α-hydroxylase (CYP17) are associated with hypertension and hypokalemia. In 11β-hydroxylase deficiency, the impaired conversion of 11-DOC to corticosterone results in accumulation of DOC, a potent mineralocorticoid. Virilization in females, usually recognizable in children, results from shunting into the androgen pathway. Blood levels of DOC, 11-deoxycortisol, and adrenal androgens are characteristically elevated. This form of congenital adrenal hyperplasia is more prevalent in Middle Eastern Moslems and Jews.

17α-Hydroxylase deficiency is characterized by hypogonadism, hypokalemia, and hypertension. As with 11β-hydroxylase deficiency, this disorder is a result of decreased production of cortisol with shunting into the unblocked mineralocorticoid pathway. Because 17α-hydroxylase is required for the biosynthesis of gonadal testosterone and estrogen, a defect in this enzyme in both sexes is associated with sexual immaturity, high gonadotropin levels, and low urinary 17-ketosteroid excretion. Females have primary amenorrhea and lack of development of secondary sexual characteristics. Males may have ambiguous external genitalia or a female phenotype (male pseudohermaphroditism). Blood levels of 17β-hydroxyprogesterone are low, and corticosterone and DOC levels are elevated.

The elevated blood pressure and hypokalemia in both syndromes result from elevated levels of DOC, a potent mineralocorticoid; excessive sodium retention and hypertension result and lead to suppression of PRA and low levels of aldosterone. The genetic lesions causing 11β-hydroxylase deficiency are in the gene that encodes CYP11B.[295] A large number of mutations in the *CYP17* gene can cause 17α-hydroxylase deficiency.[296, 297]

Glucocorticoid suppression with dexamethasone or prednisone restores normal levels of DOC and reverses the mineralocorticoid excess state in these adrenal hyperplasia syndromes. Caution must be exercised to avoid overdosing and induction of Cushing's syndrome.

Glucocorticoid-Remediable Aldosteronism

This syndrome is inherited in an autosomal dominant fashion and is probably responsible for fewer than 3% of cases of primary aldosteronism.[274] GRA is characterized by hypertension of early onset that is usually severe and refractory to conventional antihypertensive therapies.[298] Prospective screening of GRA pedigrees has revealed that many affected individuals are not hypokalemic.[276] The sine qua non of GRA is aldosterone production that is solely under the control of corticotropin.[299] As a result, the syndrome can be mitigated by exogenous glucocorticoid therapy.

GRA is caused by a chimeric gene duplication that results from unequal crossing over between the highly homologous 11β-hydroxylase (*CYP11B*) and aldosterone synthase (*CYP18*) genes.[300, 301] This chimeric gene contains the 3′ corticotropin-responsive portion of the promoter from the 11β-hydroxylase gene fused to the 5′ coding sequence of the aldosterone synthase gene. The result is ectopic expression of aldosterone synthase activity in the cortisol-producing zona fasciculata. Thus, mineralocorticoid production is regulated by corticotropin instead of the normal secretagogue, angiotensin II. This mutation results in overproduction of aldosterone and also the characteristic hybrid steroids 18-oxocortisol and 18-OH-cortisol, which can be measured in the urine to make the diagnosis.

Genetic Testing

The diagnosis of GRA was initially based on the family history and the clinical response to dexamethasone suppression. Subsequently, GRA was diagnosed by demonstrating markedly elevated levels of 18-oxocortisol and 18-OH-cortisol in a 24-hour urine collection. However, the discovery of the genetic basis of GRA by Lifton and co-workers[300, 301] made it possible to make a genetic diagnosis from a peripheral blood sample with the use of Southern blotting techniques. Genetic testing is a sensitive and specific means of diagnosing GRA and obviates the need to measure the urinary levels of 18-oxocortisol and 18-OH-cortisol or to perform dexamethasone suppression testing. Genetic analysis can be arranged by calling the International GRA Registry (617-732-5011). Because some individuals with GRA do not have hypokalemia and have only mild hypertension, other clues that may indicate the need for a genetic test include suppressed plasma renin levels and juvenile-onset hypertension, a history of early-onset hypertension in first-degree relatives, and a history of early hemorrhagic stroke in the subject or relative.[302]

Therapy

GRA is unique among the syndromes of primary aldosteronism in that the underlying pathophysiologic abnormality is the regulation of aldosterone production solely by corticotropin. As a result, glucocorticoid treatment usually reverses the syndrome. Of great importance is an awareness of the potential toxicity (Cushing's syndrome) of excessive doses of glucocorticoids, especially with the use of dexamethasone in children.[299] When a decision to use glucocorticoids is made, the smallest effective dose of shorter acting agents such as prednisone or hydrocortisone should be prescribed in relation to body surface area (hydrocortisone, 10 to 12 mg/m^2 per day). Target blood pressure in children should be guided by age-specific blood pressure percentiles.[303, 304] Children should be monitored by pediatricians with expertise in glucocorticoid therapy, with careful attention paid to preventing retardation of linear growth by overtreatment. Therapeutic alternatives in treating hypertension in GRA are mineralocorticoid antagonists, which also avoid the adverse effects of chronic glucocorticoid therapy. Amiloride and spironolactone are effective as monotherapies in most patients with GRA.[299]

Increased Mineralocorticoid Action—Low Plasma Renin Activity

Apparent Mineralocorticoid Excess

This syndrome is the result of impaired activity of the enzyme 11β-hydroxysteroid dehydrogenase (11β-HSD), which normally inactivates cortisol in the kidney by converting it to cortisone.[305] As a result of the enzyme deficiency, high levels of cortisol accumulate in the kidney. The characteristic abnormal urinary cortisol metabolite profile seen in apparent mineralocorticoid excess also reflects decreased 11β-HSD activity (ratio of cortisol to cortisone increased 10-fold compared with the normal ratio of approximately 1).[306, 307] As a result of elevated intrarenal levels, cortisol binds to mineralocorticoid receptors in the distal tubule, which are normally sites of aldosterone binding.

Underlying the pathogenesis of apparent mineralocorticoid excess is the nonselectivity of renal mineralocorticoid receptors, which in vitro bind cortisol with affinity equal to that of aldosterone.[308, 309] Thus, 11β-HSD normally excludes physiologic glucocorticoids from nonselective mineralocorticoid receptors by converting them to the inactive 11-keto compound, cortisone. 11β-HSD has bidirectional activity in different tissues, acting primarily as a reductase in the liver and a dehydrogenase in the kidney. These different activities are the consequence of two isoenzymes that are expressed in liver and kidney, respectively.[310, 311]

Decreased 11β-HSD activity may be hereditary or secondary to pharmacologic inhibition of enzyme activity by glycyrrhetinic acid, the active principle of licorice root and some chewing tobaccos. The hereditary form contains mutations in the gene coding for isoenzyme 2. The phenotype of patients with apparent mineralocorticoid excess includes hypertension, low PRA levels, hypokalemia, normal plasma cortisol levels, and low plasma aldosterone levels.

Treatment has been difficult, although some success has been achieved with use of a high-potency glucocorticoid to suppress endogenous cortisol production. Although the synthetic steroid can also bind to the mineralocorticoid receptor, its concentration is far less than that of the endogenous cortisol. Alternatively, the mineralocorticoid receptor antagonist spironolactone could be given. However, its antiandrogenic and progestational side effects limit its long-term use, particularly in children.

The mineralocorticoid excess state commonly seen in patients with the ectopic corticotropin syndrome is believed to be related to the high rates of cortisol production that cause a relative deficiency of 11β-HSD activity. However, DOC levels are high and could account for the hypokalemia in this disorder.

Liddle's Syndrome

This syndrome is inherited as an autosomal dominant disorder in which affected subjects present with hypertension, suppressed PRA, low aldosterone levels, and usually hypokalemia.[312] The hypokalemic state cannot be corrected by administration of the antimineralocorticoid spironolactone but is ameliorated by triamterene or amiloride, agents that block renal sodium reabsorption and potassium secretion by mineralocorticoid receptor–independent mechanisms. This disorder is caused by mutations in the subunits of the renal sodium epithelial channel.[313, 314] The amiloride-sensitive epithelial channel, considered the rate-limiting step for sodium absorption in the distal nephron, is composed of three subunits (α, β, γ); mutations have been found in two of these subunits.[313, 314] As a result of these mutations, constitutive activity of the epithelial channel leads to increased sodium absorption and volume expansion.

Hypermineralocorticoidism—High Plasma Renin Activity

Occasionally, hyperaldosteronism occurs without edema or hypertension (Bartter's and Gitelman's syndromes [Table 15–7]). Bartter's syndrome is usually characterized by severe hyperaldosteronism with hypokalemic alkalosis, substantial increases in PRA, hypercalciuria, no edema, normal blood pressure, and onset usually in childhood. The pathogenesis results from a defect in renal sodium or chloride conservation, or both. The hyperaldosteronism-induced hypokalemia can be accentuated by an additional defect in renal potassium conservation in some individuals. In many cases, Bartter's syndrome is caused by a mutation in the renal Na-K-2Cl cotransporter gene.

Gitelman's syndrome is an autosomal recessive trait also characterized by renal sodium wasting. As a result, as with Bartter's syndrome, there is activation of the renin-angiotensin-aldosterone system. Affected subjects therefore have low serum potassium and magnesium levels, high serum bicarbonate, and low blood pressure. In contrast to that in Bartter's syndrome, urinary calcium excretion is reduced. Gitelman's syndrome results from mutations that lead to loss of function of the renal thiazide-sensitive Na-Cl cotransporter.[315]

OTHER ENDOCRINE DISORDERS ASSOCIATED WITH HYPERTENSION

Glucocorticoid Excess (Cushing's Syndrome)

Cushing's syndrome, characterized by hypersecretion of cortisol, is associated with elevations in blood pressure in more than 80% of cases (see Chapter 14). Diastolic blood pressure exceeds 100 mm Hg in more than 50% of patients with endogenous Cushing's syndrome.[316] On the other hand, the incidence of hypertension is lower and more variable in patients treated with exogenous glucocorticoids. Nevertheless, hypertension and associated metabolic abnormalities (diabetes mellitus and hyperlipidemia) probably account for the atherosclerotic cardiovascular morbidity and mortality seen in spontaneous Cushing's syndrome.[317]

Mineralocorticoid production is usually normal in endogenous Cushing's syndrome. In Cushing's disease, commonly secondary to corticotropin hypersecretion from a pituitary microadenoma, aldosterone and renin levels are usually normal[318, 319] and DOC levels are normal or increased modestly.[320] On the other hand, in ectopic corticotropin syndrome, increased mineralocorticoid activity and hypokalemia are the rule as a result of elevated levels of DOC and mineralocorticoid effects of high levels of cortisol. In adrenal carcinomas, DOC and aldosterone may also be elevated. Thus, in adrenal carcinomas and in ectopic corticotropin secretion, mineralocorticoid production may contribute to the hypertension; in such situations, PRA is usually suppressed.[319, 321]

The elevation of blood pressure by cortisol and synthetic glucocorticoids (which have minimal mineralocorticoid activity) is mediated by multiple mechanisms. Glucocorticoids increase cardiac output[322] and activate the renin-angiotensin system by increasing the hepatic production of angiotensinogen.[319] Other actions of glucocorticoids include reduction of the synthesis of vasodilatory prostaglandins secondary to inhibition of phospholipase A_2, thus blocking the release of arachidonic acid from phospholipids. There is also evidence for reduction of the components of the kallikrein-kinin system[319] as well as enhanced pressor sensitivity to endogenous vasoconstrictors (epinephrine and angiotensin II).[322, 323] Glucocorticoids may also promote sodium influx into vascular smooth muscle cells.[324]

The screening for endogenous cortisol excess is accomplished by measuring the response of plasma cortisol to the 1-mg dexamethasone suppression test or by the measurement of elevated levels of free cortisol in a 24-hour urine collection. Further studies to determine the etiology of the cortisol excess state are outlined in Chapter 14.

Thyroid Disease

Hypothyroidism

Hypothyroidism may account for 1% to 2% of cases of diastolic hypertension in the general population (see Chapter 12). In a large series of patients screened for the secondary forms of hypertension by age, the prevalence of hypothyroidism was 3%.[325] In that study, hypothyroidism was thought to be a significant cause of secondary hypertension, especially in women older than 70 years. That hypothyroidism can actually cause hypertension was shown by Streeten and colleagues[326] in another study in which 32% of hypertensive hypothyroid patients had a fall in diastolic blood pressure to 90 mm Hg or less after replacement levothyroxine treatment and withdrawal of all hypertensive drugs. Postulated mechanisms for the elevation of blood pressure include extracellular volume expansion and elevation in systemic vascular resistance.

Hyperthyroidism

In contrast to the diastolic hypertension associated with hypothyroidism, hyperthyroidism usually causes elevated systolic blood pressure. Thyrotoxic patients usually have tachycardia, high cardiac output, increased stroke volume, and decreased peripheral vascular resistance[327, 328] (see Chapter 11). These hemodynamic alterations are usually ameliorated by β-blocker therapy. In elderly patients, atrial fibrillation may be the sole manifestation of thyrotoxicosis.

Acromegaly

Hypertension occurs in one third of patients with acromegaly (see Chapter 8), presumably owing to sodium retention with resultant extracellular volume expansion.[329] This retention of sodium, in the context of an increase in glomerular filtration rate and low PRA, is the consequence of uncharacterized antinatriuretic actions of growth hormone. Sodium retention is also a complication of exogenous administration of growth hormone. The prevalence of primary aldosteronism in acromegaly appears to be increased.[330] As previously discussed, in primary aldosteronism, plasma renin levels are suppressed and aldosterone levels are increased. In acromegaly, plasma renin levels also are suppressed owing to volume expansion but aldosterone levels are not increased.[331]

Hyperparathyroidism

In contrast to the overall incidence of 0.1% of primary hyperparathyroidism in the general population, this disorder occurs in approximately 1% of hypertensive patients (see Chapter 26). Conversely, approximately, 30% to 40% of individuals with hyperparathyroidism are hypertensive. The mechanisms are unclear because there is no direct correlation with the elevated PTH or calcium levels.[332, 333] Hypertension may or may not remit after successful parathyroidectomy.[334–337]

Table 15–6. Exogenous Causes of Secondary Hypertension

Mineralocorticoids (licorice and licorice-containing chewing tobacco; fludrocortisone)
Growth hormone
Glucocorticoids
Gonadal steroids
Oral contraceptives
Androgens
Sympathomimetic amines (amphetamines, cocaine)
Cyclosporine

Because the blood pressure response to correction of primary hyperparathyroidism is variable and hypertension is not a clear-cut manifestation of the hyperparathyroid state, hypertension is considered a minor criterion for recommending surgery to patients with mild asymptomatic primary hyperparathyroidism.[338] On the other hand, surgery may cause regression of myocardial hypertrophy in normotensive patients with hyperparathyroidism and may also reverse the increased mortality associated with hyperparathyroidism in subjects younger than 70 years.[339, 340] The hypertension associated with hyperparathyroidism can also result as a complication of hypercalcemia-induced renal impairment or when this disorder is part of a MEN syndrome that includes pheochromocytoma or primary aldosteronism.

Exogenous Treatments

Treatment with certain hormones or pharmacologic agents can elevate blood pressure (Table 15–6). Fludrocortisone, a potent mineralocorticoid used in the treatment of primary adrenal insufficiency, can cause hypertension when administered in supraphysiologic doses, as to patients with orthostatic hypotension, to cause volume expansion. Licorice and chewing tobacco abuse can result in hypokalemia, sodium and water retention, and blood pressure elevation, as noted earlier. The administration of growth hormone in pharmacologic doses to patients who have received transplants or to severely catabolic hospitalized subjects for its protein-sparing actions can raise blood pressure.

The hypertension associated with cyclosporine treatment appears to be related to renal vasospasm and secondary volume expansion. Glucocorticoid treatment in supraphysiologic doses for inflammatory and allergic disorders frequently elevates blood pressure, as noted earlier, but less commonly than in endogenous Cushing's syndrome. Oral contraceptive preparations containing higher dose estrogen-progesterone formulations are known to induce hypertension. It is not known whether current lower dose formulations cause hypertension. However, postmenopausal estrogen replacement therapy does not elevate blood pressure.[341] Androgens in pharmacologic doses can also produce volume expansion and arterial hypertension.[342]

Finally, as with the hypertension in pheochromocytoma, ingestion of sympathomimetic amines or substances that potentiate endogenous sympathetic nervous system activity (e.g., cocaine inhibits reuptake of catecholamines at adrenergic nerve endings) produces increased cardiac output, increased peripheral arteriolar vasoconstriction, and hypertension.

NORMOTENSIVE SYNDROMES

A diverse group of loss-of-function mutations in the sodium epithelial channel (ENaC), mineralocorticoid receptor (MR),

Table 15-7. Loss-of-Function Renal Salt-Wasting Syndromes

Disorder	Genes Mutated	Potassium Status*
Autosomal dominant pseudohypoaldosteronism type I (PHAI)	MR	Hyperkalemia*
Autosomal recessive (AR) PHAI	ENaC	Hyperkalemia
Gitelman's syndrome (AR)	Thiazide-sensitive Na–Cl cotransporter in DCT	Hypokalemia*
Bartter's syndrome (AR)	Ion transporters in thick ascending loop of Henle	Hypokalemia

*In all of these disorders aldosterone levels are markedly elevated as a result of activation of the renin–angiotensin system due to salt wasting, but in the PHAI syndromes increased mineralocorticoid action is blocked due to loss-of-function mutations of MR and ENaC.

Key: ENaC, sodium epithelial channel; MR, mineralocorticoid receptor; DCT, distal convoluted tubule; AR, autosomal recessive inheritance.

and renal tubule ion transporters result in sodium wasting and a tendency to hypotension unless compensated by a high sodium intake. In all these disorders, aldosterone levels are markedly elevated as a result of activation of the renin-angiotensin system owing to salt wasting. In the PHAI syndromes, increased mineralocorticoid action is blocked because of loss-of-function mutations of MR and ENaC. Accordingly, potassium levels will be low or elevated in each disorder depending on whether the mineralocorticoid action of the elevated aldosterone levels is expressed (Table 15–7).[343]

References

1. Williams GH. Hypertensive vascular disease. In Braunwald E, Fauci AS, Kasper D, et al (eds). Harrison's Principles of Internal Medicine, 15th ed. New York, McGraw-Hill, 2001, pp 1414–1429.
2. Williams GH, Hollenberg NK. Pathophysiology of essential hypertension. In Parmley WW, Chatterjee K (eds). Cardiology, vol 2. Philadelphia, JB Lippincott, 1990, pp 1–18.
3. Williams GH, Moore TJ. Hormonal aspects of hypertension. In DeGroot LJ, Besser M, Burger HG, et al (eds). Endocrinology, 3rd ed. Philadelphia, WB Saunders, 1994, pp 2917–2934.
4. LeDouarin NM, Smith J, LeLievre CS. From the neural crest to the ganglia of the peripheral nervous system. Annu Rev Physiol 1981; 43:653.
5. Gabella G. Structure of the Autonomic Nervous System. London, Chapman & Hall, 1976.
6. Cabot JB. Sympathetic preganglionic neurons: cytoarchitecture, ultrastructure and biophysical properties. In Loewy AD, Spyer K (eds). Central Regulation of Autonomic Functions. New York, Oxford University Press, 1990, pp 44–67.
7. Potter EK. Neuropeptide Y as an autonomic neurotransmitter. Pharmacol Ther 1988; 37:251–273.
8. Schwarzenbrunner U, Schmidle T, Obendorf D, et al. Sympathetic axons and nerve terminals: the protein composition of small and large dense-core and a third type of vesicles. Neuroscience 1990; 37:819–827.
9. Winkler H, Fischer-Colbrie R. The chromogranins A and B: the first 25 years and future perspectives. Neuroscience 1992; 49: 497–528.
10. Cryer PE, Wortsman J, Shah SD, et al. Plasma chromogranin A as a marker of sympathochromaffin activity in humans. Am J Physiol 1948; 153:586–600.
11. Axelrod J. Methylation reactions in the formation and metabolism of catecholamines and other biogenic amines. Pharmacol Rev 1966; 18:95.
12. Wurtman RJ, Axelrod J. Control of enzymatic synthesis of adrenaline in the adrenal medulla by adrenal cortical steroids. J Biol Chem 1966; 241:2301.
13. Lefkowitz RJ, Caron MG. Adrenergic receptors: models for the study of receptors coupled to guanine nucleotide regulatory proteins. J Biol Chem 1988; 263:4993–4996.
14. Ahlquist RP. A study of the adrenotropic receptors. Am J Physiol 1991; 260:E243–E246.
15. Milligan G, Svoboda P, Brown CM. Why are there so many adrenoceptor subtypes? Biochem Pharmacol 1994; 48:277–290.
16. Caron MG, Lefkowitz RJ. Catecholamine receptors: structure, function, and regulation. Recent Prog Horm Res 1993; 48:277–290.
17. Storsberg AD. Structural and functional diversity of β-adrenergic receptors. Ann NY Acad Sci 1995; 757:253–260.
18. Yang YT, McElligott MA. Multiple actions of β-adrenergic antagonists on skeletal muscle and adipose tissue. Biochem J 1989; 261:1–10.
19. Waller DG. β-Adrenoceptor partial agonists: a renaissance in cardiovascular therapy? Br J Clin Pharmacol 1990; 30:157–171.
20. Blaschko H. Catecholamine biosynthesis. Br Med Bull 1973; 29: 105.
21. Udenfriend S. Tyrosine hydroxylase. Pharmacol Rev 1966; 18:43.
22. Nagatsu T, Stjarne L. Catecholamine synthesis and release: overview. Adv Pharmacol 1998; 42:1–14.
23. Zigmond RE. Regulation of tyrosine hydroxylase by neuropeptides. Adv Pharmacol 1998; 42:21–25.
24. Vyas S, Biguet NF, Mallet J. Transcriptional and post-transcriptional regulation of tyrosine hydroxylase gene by protein kinase C. EMBO J 1990; 9:3707–3712.
25. Ishiguro H, Kim KT, Joh TH, et al. Neuron-specific expression of the human dopamine beta-hydroxylase gene requires both the cAMP-response element and a silencer region. J Biol Chem 1993; 268:17987–17994.
26. Winkler H, Westhead E. The molecular organization of adrenal chromaffin granules. Neuroscience 1980; 5:1803–1823.
27. Evinger MJ, Ernsberger P, Regunathan S, et al. A single transmitter regulates gene expression through two separate mechanisms: cholinergic regulation of phenylethanolamine *N*-methyltransferase mRNA via nicotinic and muscarinic pathways. J Neurosci 1994; 14:2106–2116.
28. Evinger MJ, Ernsberger P, Regunathan S, et al. Regulation of phenylethanolamine *N*-methyltransferase gene expression by imidazoline receptors in adrenal chromaffin cells. J Neurochem 1995; 65:988–997.
29. Bornstein SR, Breidert M, Ehrhart-Bornstein M, et al. Plasma catecholamines in patients with Addison's disease. Clin Endocrinol (Oxf) 1995; 42:215–218.
30. Bouloux PG, Fakeeh M. Investigation of phaeochromocytoma. Clin Endocrinol (Oxf) 1995; 43:657–664.
31. Schuldiner S, Shirvan A, Linial M. Vesicular neurotransmitter transporters: from bacteria to humans. Physiol Rev 1995; 75:369–392.
32. Johnson RG. Catecholamine transport and energy-linked function of chromaffin granules isolated from a human pheochromocytoma. Biochim Biophys Acta 1982; 716:366–376.
33. Johnson RG Jr. Accumulation of biological amines into chromaffin granules: a model for hormone and neurotransmitter transport. Physiol Rev 1988; 68:232–307.
34. Liu Y, Peter D, Roghani A, et al. A cDNA that suppresses MPP+ toxicity encodes a vesicular amine transporter. Cell 1992; 70:539–551.
35. Gasnier B, Roisin MP, Scherman D, et al. Uptake of metaiodobenzylguanidine by bovine chromaffin granule membranes. Mol Pharmacol 1986; 29:275–280.
36. Erickson JD, Eiden LE, Hoffman BJ. Expression cloning of a reserpine-sensitive vesicular monoamine transporter. Proc Natl Acad Sci USA 1992; 89:10993–10997.
37. Kibble AV, Burgoyne RD. Calmodulin increases the initial rate of exocytosis in adrenal chromaffin cells. Pflugers Arch 1996; 431:464–466.
38. McFerran BW, Graham ME, Burgoyne RD. Neuronal Ca^{2+} sensor 1, the mammalian homologue of frequenin, is expressed in chromaffin and PC12 cells and regulates neurosecretion from dense-core granules. J Biol Chem 1998; 273:22768–22772.
39. Eisenhofer G, Finberg JP. Different metabolism of norepinephrine and epinephrine by catechol-*O*-methyltransferase and mono-

amine oxidase in rats. J Pharmacol Exp Ther 1994; 268:1242–1251.
40. Beard CM, Sheps SG, Kurland LT, et al. Occurrence of pheochromocytoma in Rochester, Minnesota, 1950 through 1979. Mayo Clin Proc 1983; 58:802–804.
41. Sutton MG, Sheps SG, Lie JT. Prevalence of clinically unsuspected pheochromocytoma: review of a 50-year autopsy series. Mayo Clin Proc 1981; 56:354–360.
42. Whalen RK, Althausen AF, Daniels GH. Extra-adrenal pheochromocytoma. J Urol 1992; 147:1–10.
43. Pommier RF, Vetto JT, Billingsly K, et al. Comparison of adrenal and extra-adrenal pheochromocytomas. Surgery 1993; 114: 1160–1165.
44. Bravo EL. Evolving concepts in the pathophysiology, diagnosis, and treatment of pheochromocytoma. Endocr Rev 1994; 15:356–368.
45. Sheps SG, Jiang NS, Klee GG, et al. Recent developments in the diagnosis and treatment of pheochromocytoma. Mayo Clin Proc 1990; 65:88–95.
46. Bravo EL. Pheochromocytoma: new concepts and future trends. Kidney Int 1991; 40:544–556.
47. Manger WM, Gifford RW Jr. Pheochromocytoma: current diagnosis and management. Cleve Clin J Med 1993; 60:365–378.
48. Stein PK, Rottman JN, Hall AF, et al. Heart rate variability in a case of pheochromocytoma. Clin Auton Res 1996; 6:41–44.
49. Dabrowska B, Dabrowski A, Pruszczyk P, et al. Heart rate variability before sudden blood pressure elevations or complex cardiac arrhythmias in pheochromocytoma. J Hum Hypertens 1996; 10: 43–50.
50. Dabrowska B, Dabrowski A, Pruszczyk P, et al. Heart rate variability in pheochromocytoma. Am J Cardiol 1995; 76:1202–1204.
51. Gifford RW, Manger WM, Bravo EL. Pheochromocytoma. Endocrinol Metab Clin North Am 1994; 23:387–404.
52. Munakata M, Aihara A, Imai Y, et al. Altered sympathetic and vagal modulations of the cardiovascular system in patients with pheochromocytoma: their relations to orthostatic hypotension. Am J Hypertens 1999; 12:572–580.
53. Bravo E, Fouad-Tarazi F, Rossi G, et al. A reevaluation of the hemodynamics of pheochromocytoma. Hypertension 1990; 15: 1128–1131.
54. Gatzoulis KA, Tolis G, Theopistou, et al. Cardiomyopathy due to a pheochromocytoma: a reversible entity. Acta Cardiol 1998; 53:227–229.
55. Schuiki ER, Jenni R, Amann FW, et al. A reversible form of apical left ventricular hypertrophy associated with pheochromocytoma. J Am Soc Echocardiogr 1993; 6:327–331.
56. McManus BM, Fleury TA, Roberts WC. Fatal catecholamine crisis in pheochromocytoma: curable cause of cardiac arrest. Am Heart J 1981; 102:930–932.
57. Liao WB, Liu CF, Chiang CW, et al. Cardiovascular manifestations of pheochromocytoma. Am J Emerg Med 2000; 18:622–625.
58. Mulligan LM, Eng C, Healey CS, et al. Specific mutations of the *RET* proto-oncogene are related to disease phenotype in MEN 2A and FMTC. Nat Genet 1994; 6:70–74.
59. Donnis-Keller H, Dou S, Chi D, et al. Mutations in the *ret* proto-oncogene are associated with MEN 2A and FMTC. Hum Mol Genet 1993; 2:851–856.
60. Sims KB. Von Hippel–Lindau disease: gene to bedside. Curr Opin Neurol 2001; 14:695–703.
61. Garcia A, Matias-Guiu X, Cabezas R, et al. Molecular diagnosis of von Hippel–Lindau disease in a kindred with a predominance of familial pheochromocytoma. Clin Endocrinol (Oxf) 1997; 46: 359–363.
62. Friedrich CA. Genotype-phenotype correlation in von Hippel–Lindau syndrome. Hum Mol Genet 2001; 10:763–767.
62a. Bender BU, Gutsche M, Glasker S, et al. Differential genetic alterations in von Hippel–Lindau syndrome-associated and sporadic pheochromocytomas. J Clin Endocrinol Metab 2000; 85: 4568–4574.
63. Walther MM, Herring J, Enquist E. von Recklinghausen's disease and pheochromocytomas. J Urol 1999; 162:1582–1586.
64. Kalff V, Shapiro B, Lloyd R, et al. The spectrum of pheochromocytoma in hypertensive patients with neurofibromatosis. Arch Intern Med 1982; 142:2092–2098.
65. Colman SD, Wallace MR. Neurofibromatosis type 1. Eur J Cancer 1994; 30A:1974–1981.
66. Mulligan LM, Ponder BA. Genetic basis of endocrine disease: multiple endocrine neoplasia type 2. J Clin Endocrinol Metab 1995; 80:1989–1995.
66a. Neumann HP, Bausch B, McWhinney SR, et al. Germ-line mutations in nonsyndromic pheochromocytoma. N Engl J Med 2002; 346:1459–1466.
67. Pomares FJ, Canas R, Rodriguez JM, et al. Differences between sporadic and multiple endocrine neoplasia type 2A phaeochromocytoma. Clin Endocrinol (Oxf) 1998; 48:195–200.
68. Eisenhofer G, Walther MM, Huynh TT, et al. Pheochromocytomas in von Hippel–Lindau syndrome and multiple endocrine neoplasia type 2 display distinct biochemical and clinical phenotypes. J Clin Endocrinol Metab 2001; 86:1999–2008.
69. Eisenhofer G, Lenders JW, Linehan WM, et al. Plasma normetanephrine and metanephrine for detecting pheochromocytoma in von Hippel–Landau disease and multiple endocrine neoplasia type 2. N Engl J Med 1999; 340:1872–1879.
70. Baysal BE, Ferrell RE, Willett-Brozick JE, et al. Mutations in *SDHD*, a mitochondrial complex II gene, in hereditary paraganglioma. Science 2000; 287:848–851.
71. Gimm O, Armanios M, Dziema H, et al. Somatic and occult germline mutations in *SDHD*, a mitochondrial complex II gene, in non-familial pheochromocytomas. Cancer Res 2000; 60:6822–6825.
72. Astuti D, Douglas F, Lennard TWJ, et al. Germline *SDHD* mutation in familial phaeochromocytoma. Lancet 2001; 357: 1181–1182.
73. Werbel SS, Ober KP. Pheochromocytoma: update on diagnosis, localization, and management. Med Clin North Am 1995; 79: 131–153.
74. Heron E, Chatellier G, Billaud E, et al. The urinary metanephrine-to-creatinine ratio for the diagnosis of pheochromocytoma. Ann Intern Med 1996; 125:300–303.
75. Peaston RT, Lennard TW, Lai LC. Overnight excretion of urinary catecholamines and metabolites in the detection of pheochromocytoma. J Clin Endocrinol Metab 1996; 81:1378–1384.
76. Pacak K, Linehan WM, Eisenhofer G, et al. Recent advances in genetics, diagnosis, localization, and treatment of pheochromocytoma. Ann Intern Med 2001; 134:315–329.
77. Lenders JW, Keiser HR, Goldstein DS, et al. Plasma metanephrines in the diagnosis of pheochromocytoma. Ann Intern Med 1995; 123:101–109.
78. Feldman JM. Falsely elevated urinary excretion of catecholamines and metanephrines in patients receiving labetalol therapy. J Clin Pharmacol 1987; 27:288–292.
79. Young WF Jr. Pheochromocytoma and primary aldosteronism: diagnostic approaches. Endocrinol Metab Clin North Am 1997; 26:801–827.
80. Stein PP, Black HR. A simplified diagnostic approach to pheochromocytoma: a review of the literature and report of one institution's experience. Medicine (Baltimore) 1991; 70:46–66.
81. Juan D. Pheochromocytoma: clinical manifestations and diagnostic tests. Urology 1981; 17:1–12.
82. Hsiao RJ, Parmer RJ, Takiyyuddin MM, et al. Chromogranin A storage and secretion: sensitivity and specificity for the diagnosis of pheochromocytoma. Medicine (Baltimore) 1991; 70:33–45.
83. Stridsberg M, Husebye ES. Chromogranin A and chromogranin B are sensitive circulating markers for pheochromocytoma. Eur J Endocrinol 1997; 136:67–73.
84. Taylor HC, Mayes D, Anton AH. Clonidine suppression test for pheochromocytoma: examples of misleading results. J Clin Endocrinol Metab 1986; 63:238–242.
85. Grossman E, Goldstein DS, Hoffman A, Keiser HR. Glucagon and clonidine testing in the diagnosis of pheochromocytoma. Hypertension 1991; 17(6 Pt 1):733–741.
86. Korobkin M, Francis IR. Adrenal imaging. Semin Ultrasound CT MR 1995; 16:317–330.
87. Scott BA, Gatenby RA. Imaging advances in the diagnosis of endocrine neoplasia. Curr Opin Oncol 1998; 10:37–42.
88. Hanson MW, Feldman JM, Beam CA, et al. Iodine 131–labeled metaiodobenzylguanidine scintigraphy and biochemical analyses in suspected pheochromocytoma. Arch Intern Med 1991; 151: 1397–1402.
89. Lauriero F, Rubini G, D'Addabbo F, et al. I-131 MIBG scintigraphy of neuroectodermal tumors: comparison between I-131 MIBG and In-111 DTPA-octreotide. Clin Nucl Med 1995; 20: 243–249.

90. Bouloux PG, Fakeeh M. Investigation of phaeochromocytoma. Clin Endocrinol (Oxf) 1995; 43:657–664.
91. Kennedy JW, Dluhy RG. The biology and clinical relevance of somatostatin receptor scintigraphy in adrenal tumor management. Yale J Biol Med 1997; 70:565–575.
92. Tenenbaum F, Lumbroso J, Schlumberger M, et al. Comparison of radiolabeled octreotide and meta-iodobenzylguanidine (MIBG) scintigraphy in malignant pheochromocytoma. J Nucl Med 1995; 36:1–6.
93. Pacak K, Eisenhofer G, Carrasquillo JA, et al. 6-[^{18}F]Fluorodopamine positron emission tomographic (PET) scanning for diagnostic localization of pheochromocytoma. Hypertension 2001; 7:6–8.
94. Fonseca V, Bouloux PM. Phaeochromocytoma and paraganglioma. Baillieres Clin Endocrinol Metab 1993; 7:509–544.
95. Newbould EC, Ross GA, Dacie JE, et al. The use of venous catheterization in the diagnosis and localization of bilateral phaeochromocytomas. Clin Endocrinol (Oxf) 1991; 35:55–59.
96. Russell WJ, Metcalfe IR, Tonkin AL, et al. The preoperative management of phaeochromocytoma. Anaesth Intensive Care 1998; 26:196–200.
97. Gifford RW Jr, Manger WM, Bravo EL. Pheochromocytoma. Endocrinol Metab Clin North Am 1994; 23:387–404.
98. Colson P, Ryckwaert F, Ribstein J, et al. Haemodynamic heterogeneity and treatment with the calcium channel blocker nicardipine during phaeochromocytoma surgery. Acta Anaesthesiol Scand 1998; 42:1114–1119.
99. Ulchaker JC, Goldfarb DA, Bravo EL, et al. Successful outcomes in pheochromocytoma surgery in the modern era. J Urol 1999; 161:764–767.
100. Miura Y, Yoshinaga K. Doxazosin: a newly developed, selective alpha 1-inhibitor in the management of patients with pheochromocytoma. Am Heart J 1988; 116:1785–1789.
101. Russell WJ, Kaines AH, Hooper MJ, et al. Labetalol in the preoperative management of phaeochromocytoma. Anaesth Intensive Care 1982; 10:160–163.
102. Steinsapir J, Carr AA, Prisant LM, et al. Metyrosine and pheochromocytoma. Arch Intern Med 1997; 157:901–906.
103. Winfield HN, Hamilton BD, Bravo EL, et al. Laparoscopic adrenalectomy: the preferred choice? A comparison to open adrenalectomy. J Urol 1998; 160:325–329.
104. Suzuki K, Kageyama S, Ueda D, et al. Laparoscopic adrenalectomy: clinical experience with 12 cases. J Urol 1993; 150:1099–1102.
105. Reynolds C, Wilkins GE, Schmidt N, et al. Hyperinsulinism after removal of a pheochromocytoma. Can Med Assoc J 1983; 129:349–353.
106. Fudge TL, McKinnon WM, Geary WL. Current surgical management of pheochromocytoma during pregnancy. Arch Surg 1980; 115:1224–1225.
107. Harper MA, Murnaghan GA, Kennedy L, et al. Phaeochromocytoma in pregnancy: five cases and a review of the literature. Br J Obstet Gynaecol 1989; 96:594–606.
108. Almog B, Kupferminc MJ, Many A. Pheochromocytoma in pregnancy: a case report and review of the literature. Acta Obstet Gynecol Scand 2000; 79:709–711.
109. Demeure MJ, Carlsen B, Traul D, et al. Laparoscopic removal of a right adrenal pheochromocytoma in a pregnant woman. J Laparoendosc Adv Surg Tech A 1998; 8:315–319.
110. Stenstrom G, Swolin K. Pheochromocytoma in pregnancy: experience of treatment with phenoxybenzamine in three patients. Acta Obstet Gynecol Scand 1985; 64:357–361.
111. Plouin PF, Chatellier G, Fofol I, et al. Tumor recurrence and hypertension persistence after successful pheochromocytoma operation. Hypertension 1997; 29:1133–1139.
112. Averbuch SD, Steakley CS, Young RC, et al. Malignant pheochromocytoma: effective treatment with a combination of cyclophosphamide, vincristine and dacarbazine. Ann Intern Med 1988; 109:267–273.
113. Loh KC, Fitzgerald PA, Matthay KK. The treatment of malignant pheochromocytoma with iodine-131 metaiodobenzylguanidine (131I-MIBG): a comprehensive review of 116 reported patients. J Endocrinol Invest 1997; 20:648–658.
114. Timmis JB, Brown MJ, Allison DJ. Therapeutic embolization of phaeochromocytoma. Br J Radiol 1981; 54:420–422.
115. Conlin PR, Dluhy RG, Williams GH. Disorders of the renin-angiotensin-aldosterone system. In Schrier RW (ed). Renal and Electrolyte Disorders, 5th ed. Boston, Little, Brown, 1997, pp 349–392.
116. Williams GH, Chao J, Chao L. Kidney hormones: the kallikrein kinin and renin-angiotensin systems. In Conn PM, Melmed S (eds). Endocrinology: Basic and Clinical Principles. Totowa, NJ, Humana Press, 1997, pp 393–404.
117. Williams GH, Dluhy RG. Diseases of the adrenal cortex. In Braunwald E, Fauci AS, Kasper D, et al (eds). Harrison's Principles of Internal Medicine, 15th ed. New York, McGraw-Hill, 2001, pp 2084–2105.
118. Baxter JD, Dunkin K, Chu W, et al. Molecular biology of human renin gene. Recent Prog Horm Res 1991; 47:211–257.
119. Raizada MK, Phillips MI, Sumners C (eds). Cellular and Molecular Biology of the Renin-Angiotensin System. Boca Raton, FL, CRC Press, 1993.
120. Hate T, Takimoto E, Murakami K, et al. Comparative studies on species-specific reactivity between renin and angiotensinogen. Mol Cell Biochem 1994; 131:43–47.
121. Gaillard-Sanchez I, Mattei MG, Clauser E, et al. Assignment by in situ hybridization of angiotensinogen to chromosome band 1q42: the same region as human renin gene. Hum Genet 1990; 84:341–343.
122. Gaillard L, Clauser E, Corvol P. Structure of human angiotensinogen gene. DNA Seq 1989; 8:87–89.
123. Deschepper CF. Angiotensinogen: hormonal regulation and relative importance in the generation of angiotensin II. Kidney Int 1994; 46:1561–1563.
124. Bernstein KE, Shai SY, Howard T, et al. Structure and regulated expression of angiotensin-converting enzyme and the receptor for angiotensin II. Am J Kidney Dis 1993; 21(4 suppl 1):53–57.
125. Corvol P, Michaud A, Soubrier F, et al. Recent advances in knowledge of the structure and function of the angiotensin I converting enzyme. J Hypertens 1995; 13:S3–S10.
126. Timmermans PB, Wong PC, Chiu AT, et al. Angiotensin II receptors and angiotensin II receptor antagonists. Pharmacol Rev 1993; 45:205–251.
127. Shibata T, Suzuki C, Ohnishi J, et al. Identification of regions in the human angiotensin II receptor type 1 responsible for Gi and Gq coupling by mutagenesis study. Biochem Biophys Res Commun 1996; 218:383–389.
128. Schieffer B, Paxton WG, Marrero MB, et al. Importance of tyrosine phosphorylation in angiotensin II type 1 receptor signalling. Hypertension 1996; 27:476–480.
129. Tsuzuki S, Ichiki T, Nakakubo H, et al. Molecular cloning and expression of the gene encoding human angiotensin II type 2 receptor. Biochem Biophys Res Commun 1994; 200:1449–1454.
130. Nahmias C, Strosberg AD. The angiotensin AT_2 receptor: searching for signal-transduction pathways and physiological function. Trends Pharmacol Sci 1995; 16:223–225.
131. Wright JW, Harding JW. Brain angiotensin receptor subtypes AT_1, AT_2, and AT_4 and their functions. Regul Pept 1995; 59: 269–295.
132. Hall KL, Venkateswaran S, Hanesworth JM, et al. Characterization of a functional angiotensin IV receptor on coronary microvascular endothelial cells. Regul Pept 1995; 58:107–115.
133. Benter IF, Ferrario CM, Morris M, et al. Antihypertensive actions of angiotensin(1–7) in spontaneously hypertensive rats. Am J Physiol 1995; 269:H313–H319.
134. Paul M, Wagner J, Dzau VJ. Gene expression of the renin-angiotensin system in human tissues: quantitative analysis by the polymerase chain reaction. J Clin Invest 1993; 91:2058–2064.
135. Chiou CY, Williams GH, Kifor I. Study of the rat adrenal renin-angiotensin system at a cellular level. J Clin Invest 1995; 96: 1375–1381.
136. Harp JB, DiGirolamo M. Components of the renin-angiotensin system in adipose tissue: changes with maturation and adipose mass enlargement. J Gerontol A Biol Sci Med Sci 1995; 50:270–276.
137. Vaughan DE, Lazos SA, Tong K. Angiotensin II regulates the expression of plasminogen activator inhibitor-1 in cultured endothelial cells: a potential link between the renin-angiotensin system and thrombosis. J Clin Invest 1995; 95:995–1001.
138. Brown NJ, Agirbasli MA, Williams GH, et al. Effect of activation and inhibition of the renin-angiotensin system on plasma PAI-1. Hypertension 1998; 32:965–971.

139. Tian Y, Balla T, Baukal AJ, et al. Growth responses to angiotensin II in bovine adrenal glomerulosa cells. Am J Physiol 1995; 268:E135–E144.
140. Cox BE, Word RA, Rosenfeld CR. Angiotensin II receptor characteristics and subtype expression in uterine arteries and myometrium during pregnancy. Endocrinology 1996; 81:49–58.
141. Inagami T, et al. Molecular biology of angiotensin II receptors: an overview. J Hypertens 1994; 12:S83–S94.
142. Mortensen RM, Williams GH. Aldosterone action. In DeGroot LJ, Jameson JL, Burger HG, et al. Endocrinology, 4th ed. Philadelphia, WB Saunders, 2001, pp 1783–1790.
143. Chen SY, Bhargava A, Mastroberadino L, et al. Epithelial sodium channel regulated by aldosterone-induced protein sgk. Proc Natl Acad Sci USA 1999; 96:2514–2519.
144. Naray-Fejes-Toth A, Canessa C, Cleaveland ES, et al. SGK is an aldosterone-induced kinase in the renal collecting duct. J Biol Chem 1999; 274:16973–16978.
145. Bhargava A, Fullerton MJ, Myles K, et al. The serum and glucocorticoid-induced kinase is a physiological mediator of aldosterone action. Endocrinology 2001; 142:1587–1594.
146. Christ M, Klauss V, Pliml W, et al. Volumes and Na^+/H^+ antiporter activity of lymphocytes in patients with congestive heart failure. Clin Invest 1994; 72:985–991.
147. Wehling M, Neylon CB, Fullerton M, et al. Nongenomic effects of aldosterone on intracellular Ca^{2+} in vascular smooth muscle cells. Circ Res 1995; 76:973–979.
148. Gekle M, Silbernagl S, Wunsch S. Non-genomic action of the mineralocorticoid aldosterone on cytosolic sodium in cultured kidney cells. J Physiol (Lond) 1998; 25:117–123.
149. Benitah JP, Vassort G. Androsterone upregulates Ca^{2+} current in adult rat cardiomyocytes. Circ Res 1999; 85:1139–1145.
150. Brilla CG, Pick R, Tan LB, et al. Remodeling of the right and left ventricles in experimental hypertension. Circ Res 1990; 67: 1355–1364.
151. Brilla CG, Zhou G, Matsubara L, et al. Collagen metabolism in cultured adult rat cardiac fibroblasts: response to angiotensin II and aldosterone. J Mol Cell Cardiol 1994; 26:809–820.
152. Young M, Head G, Funder JW. Determinants of cardiac fibrosis in experimental hypermineralocorticoid states. Am J Physiol 1995; 269:E657–E662.
153. Schunkert H, Hense HW, Muscholl M, et al. Associations between circulating components of the renin-angiotensin-aldosterone system and left ventricular mass. Heart 1997; 77:24–31.
154. Pitt B, Zannad F, Remme WJ, et al. The effect of spironolactone on morbidity and mortality in patients with severe heart failure. Randomized Aldactone Evaluation Study Investigators. N Engl J Med 1999; 341:709–717.
155. Brown NJ, Kim KS, Chen YQ, et al. Synergistic effect of adrenal steroids and angiotensin II on plasminogen activator inhibitor-1 production. J Clin Endocrinol Metab 2000; 85:336–344.
156. Rocha R, Stier CT, Kifor I, et al. Aldosterone: a mediator of myocardial necrosis and renal arteriopathy. Endocrinology 2000; 141:3871–3878.
157. Martinez DV, Rocha R, Oestreicher E, et al. Cardiac damage prevention by eplereonone: comparison with low sodium diet or potassium loading. Hypertension 2002; 39 (part 2):641–618.
158. Rocha R, Williams GH. Rationale for the use of aldosterone antagonists in congestive heart failure. Drugs 2002; 62:723–731.
159. Vinson GP. The adrenal renin-angiotensin system. Adv Exp Med Biol 1995; 377:237–251.
160. Ganong WF. Reproduction and the renin-angiotensin system. Neurosci Biobehav Rev 1995; 19:241–250.
161. Hollenberg NK, Chenitz WR, Adams DF, et al. Reciprocal influence of salt intake on adrenal glomerulosa and renal vascular responses to angiotensin II in normal man. J Clin Invest 1974; 54:34–42.
162. Williams GH, Hollenberg NK. "Sodium sensitive" essential hypertension: emerging insights into pathogenesis and therapeutic implications. In Klahr S, Massry SG (eds). Contemporary Nephrology, 3rd ed. New York, Plenum, 1985, pp 303–331.
163. Laragh JH, Sealey JE, Niarchos AP, et al. The vasoconstrictor volume spectrum in normotension and in the pathogenesis of hypertension. Fed Proc 1982; 41:2415–2423.
164. Safar ME, London GM, Simon AC, et al. Volume factors, total exchangeable sodium, and potassium in hypertensive disease. In Genest J, Kuchel O, Hamet P, et al (eds). Hypertension: Pathophysiology and Treatment. New York, McGraw-Hill, 1983, pp 42–53.
165. Vaughan ED, Laragh JH, Gavras I, et al. Volume factor in low and normal renin essential hypertension: treatment with either spironolactone or chlorthalidone. Am J Cardiol 1973; 32:522–532.
166. Woods JW, Liddle GW, Michelakis AM, et al. Effect of an adrenal inhibitor in hypertensive patients with suppressed renin. Arch Intern Med 1969; 123:366–370.
167. Wisgerhof M, Brown RD. Increased adrenal sensitivity to angiotensin II in low renin essential hypertension. J Clin Invest 1979; 63:1456–1462.
168. Marks AD, Marks DB, Kanefsky TM, et al. Enhanced adrenal responsiveness to angiotensin II in patients with low renin essential hypertension. J Clin Endocrinol Metab 1979; 48:266–270.
169. Kisch ES, Dluhy RG, Williams GH. Enhanced aldosterone response to angiotensin II in human hypertension. Circ Res 1976; 38:502–505.
170. Shoback DM, Williams GH, Moore TJ, et al. Defect in the sodium-modulated tissue responsiveness to angiotensin II in essential hypertension. J Clin Invest 1983; 72:2115–2124.
171. Williams GH, Dluhy RG, Lifton RP, et al. Nonmodulation as an intermediate phenotype in essential hypertension. Hypertension 1992; 20:788–796.
172. Beretta-Piccoli C, Pusterla C, Stadler P, et al. Blunted aldosterone responsiveness to angiotensin II in normotensive subjects with familial predisposition to essential hypertension. J Hypertens 1988; 6:57–61.
173. Leonetti Luparini R, Ferri C, Santucci A, et al. Atrial natriuretic peptide in nonmodulating essential hypertension. Hypertension 1993; 21:803–809.
174. Hollenberg NK, Williams GH. Abnormal renal function, sodium-volume homeostasis and renin system behavior in normal-renin essential hypertension: the evolution of the nonmodulator concept. In Laragh JH, Brenner BM (eds). Hypertension: Pathophysiology, Diagnosis, and Management, 2nd edition. New York, Raven Press, 1995, pp 1837–1856.
175. Gaboury CL, Hollenberg NK, Hopkins PN, et al. Metabolic derangements in nonmodulating hypertension. Am J Hypertens 1995; 8:870–875.
176. Ferri C, Bellini C, Desideri G, et al. Relationship between insulin resistance and nonmodulation hypertension: linkage of metabolic abnormalities and cardiovascular risk. Diabetes 1999; 48: 1623–1630.
177. Taylor TT, Moore TJ, Hollenberg NK, et al. Converting enzyme inhibition corrects the altered adrenal response to angiotensin II in essential hypertension. Hypertension 1984; 6:92–99.
178. Redgrave JE, Rabinowe SL, Hollenberg NK, et al. Correction of abnormal renal blood flow response to angiotensin II by converting enzyme inhibition in essential hypertensives. J Clin Invest 1985; 75:1285–1290.
179. Hollenberg NK, Moore TJ, Shoback DM, et al. Abnormal renal sodium handling in essential hypertension: relation to failure of renal and adrenal modulation of responses to angiotensin II. Am J Med 1986; 81:412–418.
180. Lifton RP, Hopkins PN, Williams RR, et al. Evidence for heritability of nonmodulating essential hypertension. Hypertension 1989; 13:884–889.
181. Hopkins PN, Lifton RP, Hollenberg NK, et al. Blunted renal vascular response to angiotensin II is associated with a common variant of the angiotensinogen gene and obesity. J Hypertens 1996; 14:199–207.
182. Hopkins PN, Hunt SC, Wu LL, et al. Hypertension, dyslipidemia, and insulin resistance: links in a chain or spokes on a wheel? Curr Opin Metab 1996; 7:241–253.
183. DeFronzo RA, Ferrannini E. Insulin resistance: a multifaceted syndrome responsible for NIDDM, obesity, hypertension, dyslipidemia, and atherosclerotic cardiovascular disease. Diabetes Care 1991; 14:173–194.
184. Reaven GM, Hofman BB. Hypertension as a disease of carbohydrate and lipoprotein metabolism. Am J Med 1989; 8:S2–S6.
185. Saad MF, Lillioja S, Nyomba BL, et al. Racial differences in the relation between blood pressure and insulin resistance. N Engl J Med 1991; 324:733–739.
186. Modan M, Halkin H, Halmog S, et al. Hyperinsulinemia: a link between hypertension, obesity and glucose intolerance. J Clin Invest 1985; 75:809–816.

187. Ferrannini E, Buzzigoli G, Bonadonna R, et al. Insulin resistance in essential hypertension. N Engl J Med 1987; 317:350–357.
188. DeFronzo RA. Insulin resistance, hyperinsulinemia, and coronary artery disease: a complex metabolic web. J Cardiovasc Pharmacol 1992; 20:S1–S15.
189. Levy J, Gavin JR III, Hammerman MR, et al. Ca^{2+} + Mg^{2+} ATPase activity in kidney basolateral membrane in non insulin dependent diabetic rats: effect of insulin. Diabetes 1986; 35:899–905.
190. Draznin B, Lewis D, Houlder N, et al. Mechanism of insulin resistance induced by sustained levels of cytosolic free calcium in rat adipocytes. Endocrinology 1989; 125:2341–2349.
191. Draznin B, Sussman KE, Eckel RH, et al. Possible role of cytosolic free calcium concentrations in mediating insulin resistance of obesity and hyperinsulinemia. J Clin Invest 1988; 28:1848–1852.
192. Anderson EA, Hoffman RP, Balon TW, et al. Hyperinsulinemia produces both sympathetic neural activation and vasodilation in normal humans. J Clin Invest 1991; 84:2246–2252.
193. DeFronzo RA, Cooke CR, Adres R, et al. The effect of insulin on renal handling of sodium, potassium, calcium and phosphate in man. J Clin Invest 1975; 55:845–855.
194. Sharma AM, Rutland K, Spies KP, et al. Salt sensitivity in young normotensive subjects is associated with a hyperinsulinemic response to oral glucose. J Hypertens 1991; 9:329–335.
195. Sharma AM, Schorr U, Distler A. Insulin resistance in young, salt sensitive normotensive subjects. Hypertension 1993; 21:273–279.
196. Bigazzi R, Bianchi S, Baldari D, et al. Microalbuminuria in salt-sensitive patients: a marker for renal and cardiovascular risk factors. Hypertension 1994; 23:195–199.
197. Townsend RA, Zhao H. Plasma renin activity and insulin sensitivity in normotensive subjects. Am J Hypertens 1994; 7:894–898.
198. Egan BM, Stepniakowski K, Goodfriend TL. Renin and aldosterone are higher and the hyperlipidemic effect of salt restriction greater in subjects with risk factor clustering. Am J Hypertens 1994; 7:886–893.
199. McCarron DA, Morris CD, Cole C. Dietary calcium in human hypertension. Science 1982; 217:267–269.
200. Witteman JC, Willett WC, Stampfer MJ, et al. A prospective study of nutritional factors and hypertension among US women. Circulation 1989; 80:1320–1327.
201. McCarron DA, Morris CD, Henry HJ, et al. Blood pressure and nutrient intake in the United States. Science 1984; 224:1392–1398.
202. Morris CD, Reusser ME. Calcium intake and blood pressure: epidemiology revisited. Semin Nephrol 1995; 15:490–495.
203. Bucher HC, Cook RJ, Guyatt GH, et al. Effects of dietary calcium supplementation in blood pressure: a meta-analysis of randomized controlled trials. JAMA 1996; 275:1016–1022.
204. Allender PS, Cutler JA, Follmann D, et al. Dietary calcium and blood pressure: a meta-analysis of randomized clinical trials. Ann Intern Med 1996; 124:825–831.
205. Bukoski RD, Ishibashi K, Bian K. Vascular actions of the calcium regulating hormones. Semin Nephrol 1995; 15:536–549.
206. Wang R, Wu L, Karpinski E, et al. The changes in contractile status of single vascular smooth muscle cells and ventricular cells induced by bPTH(1–34). Life Sci 1993; 52:793–801.
207. Pang PKT, Lewanczuk RZ. Parathyroid origin of a new hypertensive factor in spontaneously hypertensive rats. Am J Hypertens 1989; 2:898–902.
208. Shan J, Benishin CG, Lewanczuk RZ, et al. Mechanism of the vascular action of parathyroid hypertensive factor. J Cardiovasc Pharmacol 1994; 23:S1–S8.
209. Lewanczuk RZ, Pang PKT. Expression of parathyroid hypertensive factor in hypertensive primary hyperparathyroid patients. Blood Press 1993; 2:22–27.
210. Takahashi K, Inoue D, Ando K, et al. Parathyroid hormone–related peptide as a locally produced vasorelaxant: regulation of its mRNA by hypertension in rats. Biochem Biophys Res Commun 1995; 208:447–455.
211. Ishibashi K, Evans A, Shingi T, et al. Differential expression and effect of calcitriol on myosin in the arterial tree. Am J Physiol 1995; 269:C443–C450.
212. Goldblatt H, Lynch J, Hanzel R. Studies on experimental hypertension. J Exp Med 1934; 59:347.
213. Leadbetter WF, Burkland CE. Hypertension in unilateral renal disease. J Urol 1938; 39:611.
214. Albers FJ. Clinical characteristics of atherosclerotic renovascular disease. Am J Kidney Dis 1994; 24:636–641.
215. Safian RD, Textor SC. Renal-artery stenosis. N Engl J Med 2001; 344:431–442.
216. Dustan HP, Humphries AW, deWolfe VG, et al. Normal arterial pressures in patients with renal artery stenosis. JAMA 1964; 187:1028.
217. Rimmer JM, Gennari FJ. Atherosclerotic renovascular disease and progressive renal failure. Ann Intern Med 1993; 118:712–719.
218. Canzanello VJ, Textor SC. Noninvasive diagnosis of renovascular disease. Mayo Clin Proc 1994; 69:1172–1181.
219. Johnson G. Renovascular hypertension: new diagnostic and therapeutic procedures. Scand J Urol Nephrol Suppl 1995; 170:1–78.
220. Soulez G, Oliva VL, Turpin S, et al. Imaging of renovascular hypertension: respective values of renal scintigraphy, renal Doppler US, and MR angiography. Radiographics 2000; 20:1355–1368.
221. Knopp MV, Floemer F, Schoenberg SO, et al. Non-invasive assessment of renal artery stenosis: current conclusions and future directions in magnetic resonance angiography. J Comput Assist Tomogr 1999; 23(suppl 1):S111–S117.
222. Bongers V, Bakker J, Beutler JJ, et al. Assessment of renal artery stenosis: comparison of captopril renography and gadolinium-enhanced breath-hold MR angiography. Clin Radiol 2000; 55:346–353.
223. Sfakianakis GN, Bourgoignie JJ, Georgiou M, et al. Diagnosis of renovascular hypertension with ACE inhibition scintigraphy. Radiol Clin North Am 1993; 31:831–848.
224. Nally JV Jr. Provocative captopril testing in the diagnosis of renovascular hypertension. Urol Clin North Am 1994; 21:227–234.
225. King BF Jr. Diagnostic imaging evaluation of renovascular hypertension. Abdom Imaging 1995; 20:395–405.
226. Johansson M, Jensen G, Aurell M, et al. Evaluation of duplex ultrasound and captopril renography for detection of renovascular hypertension. Kidney Int 2000; 58:774–782.
227. Nally VJ Jr, Olin JW, Lammert GK. Advances in noninvasive screening for renovascular disease. Cleve Clin J Med 1994; 61:328–336.
228. Ram CV, Clagett GP, Radford LR. Renovascular hypertension. Semin Nephrol 1995; 15:152–174.
229. Textor SC. Renovascular hypertension. Endocrinol Metab Clin North Am 1994; 23:235–253.
230. Van Jaarsveld BC, Krijnen P, Pieterman H, et al. The effect of balloon angioplasty on hypertension in atherosclerotic renal-artery stenosis. N Engl J Med 2000; 342:1007–1014.
231. Van de Ven PJ, Kaatee R, Beutler JJ, et al. Arterial stenting and balloon angioplasty in ostial atherosclerosis renovascular disease: a randomised trial. Lancet 1999; 353:282–286.
232. Plouin PF, Guery B, La Batide Alanore A. Atherosclerotic renal artery stenosis: surgery, percutaneous transluminal angioplasty, or medical therapy? Curr Hypertens Rep 2000; 2:482–489.
233. Rosenthal T. Drug therapy in renovascular hypertension. Drugs 1993; 45:895–909.
234. Morganti A. Renal angioplasty: better for treating hypertension or for rescuing renal function? J Hypertens 1999; 17(12 Pt 1):1659–1665.
235. Conn JW, Cohen EL, Lucas CP, et al. Primary reninism: hypertension, hyperreninemia, and secondary aldosteronism due to renin-producing juxtaglomerular cell tumors. Arch Intern Med 1972; 130:682–696.
236. Hollenberg NK, Raij L. Angiotensin-converting enzyme inhibition and renal protection: an assessment of implications for therapy. Arch Intern Med 1993; 153:2426–2435.
237. Lewis EJ, Hunsicker LG, Bain RP, et al. The effect of angiotensin-converting enzyme inhibition in diabetic nephropathy. The Collaborative Study Group. N Engl J Med 1993; 329:456–462.
238. Maschio C, Alberti D, Janin G, et al. Effect of the angiotensin-converting-enzyme inhibitor benazepril on the progression of chronic renal insufficiency. The Angiotensin-Converting-Enzyme Inhibition in Progressive Renal Insufficiency Study Group. N Engl J Med 1996; 334:939–945.
239. Kalra PA, Mamtora H, Holmes AM, et al. Renovascular disease and renal complications of angiotensin converting enzyme inhibitor therapy. Q J Med 1990; 77:1013–1018.

240. National High Blood Pressure Education Working Group report on high blood pressure in pregnancy. Am J Obstet Gynecol 1990; 163:1689–1712.
241. Guzick DS, Klein VR, Tyson JE, et al. Risk factors for the occurrence of pregnancy-induced hypertension. Clin Exp Hypertens 1987; B6:281–297.
242. de Swiet M. The physiology of normal pregnancy. In Rubin PC (ed). Hypertension in Pregnancy. Handbook of Hypertension, vol 10. Amsterdam, Elsevier, 1988, pp 1–9.
243. Chesley LC, Lindheimer MD. Renal hemodynamics and intravascular volume in normal and hypertensive pregnancy. In Rubin PC (ed). Hypertension in Pregnancy. Handbook of Hypertension, vol 10. Amsterdam, Elsevier, 1988,pp 38–65.
244. Graves SW, Moore TJ, Seely EW. Increased platelet angiotensin II receptor number in pregnancy-induced hypertension. Hypertension 1992; 20:627–632.
245. Chelsley LC. Plasma and red cell volumes during pregnancy. Am J Obstet Gynecol 1972; 112:440–450.
246. Hays PM, Cruikshank DP, Dunn LJ. Plasma volume determination in normal and preeclamptic pregnancies. Am J Obstet Gynecol 1985; 151:958–966.
247. Brown MA, Zammit VC, Mitar DM. Extracellular fluid volumes in pregnancy-induced hypertension. J Hypertens 1992; 10:61–68.
248. Groenendijk R, Trimbos MJ, Wallenburg HCS. Hemodynamics measurements in preeclampsia: preliminary observations. Am J Obstet Gynecol 1984; 150:232–236.
249. Wallenburg HCS. Hemodynamics in hypertensive pregnancy. In Rubin PC (ed). Hypertension in Pregnancy. Handbook of Hypertension, vol 10. Amsterdam, Elsevier, 1988, pp 66–101.
250. Seely EW, Williams GH, Graves SW. Markers of sodium and volume homeostasis in pregnancy-induced hypertension. J Clin Endocrinol Metab 1992; 74:150–156.
251. Miyamoto S, Shimokawa H, Sumioki H, et al. Physiologic role of endogenous human atrial natriuretic peptide in preeclamptic pregnancies. Am J Obstet Gynecol 1989; 160:155–159.
252. Lowe SA, Zammit VC, Mitar D, et al. Atrial natriuretic peptide and plasma volume in pregnancy-induced hypertension. Am J Hypertens 1991; 4:897–903.
253. Graves SW, Williams GH. Endogenous digitalis-like factors. Annu Rev Med 1987; 38:433–444.
254. Sowers JR, Zemel MB, Bronsteen RA, et al. Erythrocyte cation metabolism in preeclampsia. Am J Obstet Gynecol 1989; 161: 441–445.
255. Testa I, Rabini RA, Danieli G, et al. Abnormal membrane cation transport in pregnancy-induced hypertension. Scand J Clin Lab Invest 1988; 48:7–13.
256. Friedman SA. Preeclampsia: a review of the role of prostaglandins. Obstet Gynecol 1988; 71:122–137.
257. Fitzgerald DJ, Entman SS, Mulloy K, et al. Decreased prostacyclin biosynthesis preceding the clinical manifestation of pregnancy-induced hypertension. Circulation 1987; 75:956–963.
258. Zemel MB, Zemel PC, Berry S, et al. Altered platelet calcium metabolism as an early predictor of increased peripheral vascular resistance and preeclampsia in urban black women. N Engl J Med 1990; 323:434–438.
259. Bower D. The influence of dietary salt intake on preeclampsia. J Obstet Gynaecol Br Commonw 1964; 71:123–125.
260. Gallery EDM, Mitchell MDM, Redman CWG. Fall in blood pressure in response to volume expansion in pregnancy-associated hypertension (preeclampsia): why does it occur? J Hypertens 1984; 2:177–182.
261. Beaufils M, Uzan S, Donsimoni R, et al. Prevention of preeclampsia by early antiplatelet therapy. Lancet 1985; 1:840–842.
262. Schiff E, Peleg E, Goldenberg M, et al. The use of aspirin to prevent pregnancy-induced hypertension and lower the ratio of thromboxane A_2 to prostacyclin in relatively high risk pregnancies. N Engl J Med 1989; 321:351–356.
263. Conn JW. Presidential address: Part I. Painting background. Part II. Primary aldosteronism, a new clinical syndrome. J Lab Clin Med 1955; 45:3–17.
264. Gregoire JR. Adjustment of the osmostat in primary aldosteronism. Mayo Clin Proc 1994; 69:1108–1110.
265. Young WF Jr, Klee GG. Primary aldosteronism: diagnostic evaluation. Endocrinol Metab Clin North Am 1988; 17:367–395.
266. Blumenfeld JD, Sealey JE, Schlussel Y, et al. Diagnosis and treatment of primary hyperaldosteronism. Ann Intern Med 1994; 121: 877–885.
267. Shigematsu Y, Hamada M, Okayama H, et al. Left ventricular hypertrophy precedes other target-organ damage in primary aldosteronism. Hypertension 1997; 29:723–727.
268. Campbell SE, Diaz-Arias AA, Weber KT. Fibrosis of the human heart and systemic organs in adrenal adenoma. Blood Press 1992; 1:149–156.
269. Torres VE, Young WF Jr, Offord KP, et al. Association of hypokalemia, hypoaldosteronism, and renal cysts. N Engl J Med 1990; 322:345–351.
270. Hypokalemia, aldosteronism, and renal cysts (letter). N Engl J Med 1990; 323:29–31.
271. Ganguly A. Cellular origin of aldosteronomas. J Clin Invest 1992; 70:392–395.
272. Melby JC. Diagnosis of hyperaldosteronism. Endocrinol Metab Clin North Am 1991; 20:247–255.
273. Wisgerhof M, Brown RD, Hogan MJ, et al. The plasma aldosterone response to angiotensin II infusion in aldosterone-producing adenoma and idiopathic hyperaldosteronism. J Clin Endocrinol Metab 1981; 52:195–198.
274. Dluhy RG, Lifton RP. Glucocorticoid-remediable aldosteronism. Endocrinol Metab Clin North Am 1994; 23:285–297.
275. Ganguly A, Melada GA, Luetscher JA, et al. Control of plasma aldosterone in primary aldosteronism: distinction between adenoma and hyperplasia. J Clin Endocrinol Metab 1973; 37:765–775.
276. Rich GM, Ulick S, Cook S, et al. Glucocorticoid-remediable aldosteronism in a large kindred: clinical spectrum and diagnosis using a characteristic biochemical phenotype. Ann Intern Med 1992; 116:813–820.
277. Young WF Jr, Hogan MJ, Klee GG, et al. Primary aldosteronism: diagnosis and treatment. Mayo Clin Proc 1990; 65:96–110.
278. McKenna TJ, Sequeira SJ, Heffernan A, et al. Diagnosis under random conditions of AII disorders of the renin-angiotensin-aldosterone axis, including primary hyperaldosteronism. J Clin Endocrinol Metab 1991; 73:952–957.
279. Lyons DF, Kem DC, Brown RD, et al. Single dose captopril as a diagnostic test for primary aldosteronism. J Clin Endocrinol Metab 1983; 57:892–896.
280. Naomi S, Iwaoka T, Umeda T, et al. Clinical evaluation of the captopril screening test for primary aldosteronism. Jpn Heart J 1985; 26:549–556.
281. Bravo EL, Tarazi RC, Dustan HP, et al. The changing clinical spectrum of primary aldosteronism. Am J Med 1983; 74:641–651.
282. Holland OB, Brown H, Kuhnert L, et al. Further evaluation of saline infusion for the diagnosis of primary aldosteronism. Hypertension 1984; 6:717–723.
283. Kem DC, Weinberger MH, Mayes DM, et al. Saline suppression of plasma aldosterone in hypertension. Arch Intern Med 1971; 128:380–386.
284. Fontes RG, Kater CE, Biglieri EG, et al. Reassessment of the predictive value of the postural stimulation test in primary aldosteronism. Am J Hypertens 1991; 4:786–791.
285. Ganguly A, Dowdy AJ, Luetscher JA, et al. Anomalous postural response of plasma aldosterone concentration in patients with aldosterone-producing adrenal adenoma. J Clin Endocrinol Metab 1973; 36:401–404.
286. Fraser R, Lantos CP. 18-Hydroxycorticosterone: a review. J Steroid Biochem 1978; 9:273–286.
287. Ulick S, Blumenfield JD, Atlas SA, et al. The unique steroidogenesis of the aldosteronoma in the differential diagnosis of primary aldosteronism. J Clin Endocrinol Metab 1993; 76:873–878.
288. Chu MD, Ulick S. Isolation and identification of 18-hydroxycortisol from the urine of patients with primary aldosteronism. J Biol Chem 1982; 258:2218–2224.
289. Banks WA, Kastin AJ, Biglieri EG, et al. Primary adrenal hyperplasia: a new subset of primary aldosteronism. J Clin Endocrinol Metab 1984; 58:783–785.
290. Irony I, Kater CE, Biglieri EG, et al. Correctable subsets of primary aldosteronism: primary adrenal hyperplasia and renin responsive adenoma. Am J Hypertens 1990; 3:576–582.
291. Hsueth WA. New insights into the medical management of primary aldosteronism. Hypertension 1986; 8:76–82.
292. Nadler JL, Hseuth W, Horton R. Therapeutic effect of calcium channel blockade in primary aldosteronism. J Clin Endocrinol Metab 1985; 60:896–899.

293. Freed MI, Rastegar A, Bia MJ. Effects of calcium channel blockers on potassium homeostasis. Yale J Biol Med 1991; 64:177–186.
294. Bravo EL, Fouad FM, Tarazi RC. Calcium channel blockade with nifedipine in primary aldosteronism. Hypertension 1986; 8(suppl I):191–194.
295. White PC, Dupont J, New M, et al. A mutation in CYP11-1 (Arg-488—His) associated with steroid 11hydroxylase deficiency in Jews of Moroccan origin. J Clin Invest 1991; 87:1664–1667.
296. Biason A, Mantero F, Scaroni C, et al. Deletion within the CYP17 gene together with insertion of foreign DNA is the cause of combined complete 17α-hydroxylase/17,20-lyase deficiency in an Italian patient. Mol Endocrinol 1991; 5:2037–2045.
297. Fardella CE, Hum DW, Homoki J, et al. Point mutation of Arg440 to His in cytochrome P450c17 causes severe 17α-hydroxylase deficiency. J Clin Endocrinol Metab 1994; 79:160–164.
298. Dluhy RG, Anderson B, Harlin B, et al. Glucocorticoid-remediable aldosteronism is associated with severe hypertension in early childhood. J Pediatr 2001; 138:715–720.
299. Laidlaw JC. Dexamethasone-suppressible hyperaldosteronism: patients JS and LS 20 years later. In New MI, Borrelli P (eds). Dexamethasone-Suppressible Hyperaldosteronism. New York, Raven Press, 1986, pp 133–137.
300. Lifton RP, Dluhy RG, Powers M, et al. A chimaeric 11β-hydroxylase/aldosterone synthase gene causes glucocorticoid-remediable aldosteronism and human hypertension. Nature 1992; 355:262–265.
301. Lifton RP, Dluhy RG, Powers M, et al. Hereditary hypertension caused by chimaeric gene duplications and ectopic expression of aldosterone synthase. Nat Genet 1992; 2:66–74.
302. Litchfield WR, Anderson BF, Weiss RJ, et al. Intracranial aneurysm and hemorrhagic stroke in glucocorticoid-remediable aldosteronism. Hypertension 1998; 31(1 Pt 2):445–450.
303. Lieberman E. Pediatric hypertension: clinical perspective. Mayo Clin Proc 1994; 69:1098–1107.
304. Morgenstern BZ. Hypertension in pediatric patients: current issues. Mayo Clin Proc 1994; 69:1089–1097.
305. Funder JW. 11Hydroxysteroid dehydrogenase and the meaning of life. Mol Cell Endocrinol 1990; 68:C3–C5.
306. Stewart PM, Corrie JET, Shackleton CHL. Syndrome of apparent mineralocorticoid excess: a defect in the cortisol cortisone shuttle. J Clin Invest 1988; 82:340–349.
307. Stewart PM, Shackelton CHL, Edwards CRW. The cortisol cortisone shuttle and the genesis of hypertension. In Mantero F, Vecse P (eds). Corticosteroids and Peptide Hormones in Hypertension. New York, Raven Press, 1987, p 163.
308. Funder JW, Pearce PT, Smith R, et al. Mineralocorticoid action: target-tissue specificity is enzyme, not receptor, mediated. Science 1988; 242:583–585.
309. Arriza JL, Simerly RB, Swanson LW, et al. The neuronal mineralocorticoid receptor as a mediator of glucocorticoid response. Neuron 1988; 1:887–900.
310. Lakshmi V, Monder C. Purification and characterization of the corticosteroid 11β-dehydrogenase component of the rat liver 11β-hydroxysteroid dehydrogenase complex. Endocrinology 1988; 123:2390–2398.
311. Albiston A, Obeyesekere V, Smith R, et al. Cloning and tissue distribution of the human 11beta-hydroxysteroid dehydrogenase type II enzyme. Mol Cell Endocrinol 1994; 105:R11–R17.
312. Liddle GW, Blesdoe T, Coppage WS Jr. A familial renal disorder simulating primary aldosteronism but with negligible aldosterone secretion. Trans Assoc Am Physicians 1963; 76:199–213.
313. Shimkets RA, Warnock DG, Bositis CM, et al. Liddle's syndrome: heritable human hypertension caused by mutations in the subunit of the epithelial sodium channel. Cell 1994; 79:407–414.
314. Hansson JH, Nelson-Williams C, Suzuki H, et al. Hypertension caused by a truncated epithelial sodium channel subunit: genetic heterogeneity of Liddle syndrome. Nat Genet 1995; 11:76–82.
315. Simon DB, Nelson-Williams C, Gbia MJ, et al. Gitelman's variant of Bartter's syndrome, inherited hypokalaemic alkalosis, is caused by mutations in the thiazide-sensitive Na-Cl cotransporter. Nat Genet 1996; 12:24–30.
316. Ross EJ, Marshall-Jones P, Friedman M. Cushing's syndrome: diagnostic criteria. Q J Med 1966; 35:149.
317. Plotz CM, Knowlton AI, Ragan C. The natural history of Cushing's syndrome. Am J Med 1952; 13:597–614.
318. Gomez-Sanchez CE. Cushing's syndrome and hypertension. Hypertension 1986; 8:258–264.
319. Mantero F, Boscardo M. Glucocorticoid-dependent hypertension. J Steroid Biochem Mol Biol 1992; 43:409–413.
320. Cassar J, Loizou S, Kelly WF, et al. Deoxycorticosterone and aldosterone excretion in Cushing's syndrome. Metabolism 1980; 29:115–119.
321. Krakoff L, Nicolis G, Amsel B. Pathogenesis of hypertension in Cushing's syndrome. Am J Med 1975; 58:216–220.
322. Pirpiris M, Yeung S, Dewar E, et al. Hydrocortisone-induced hypertension in man: the role of cardiac output. Am J Hypertens 1993; 6:287–294.
323. Sato A, Suzuki H, Murakami M, et al. Glucocorticoid increases angiotensin II type I receptor and its gene expression. Hypertension 1994; 23:25–30.
324. Kornel L, Manisundaram B, Nelson W. Glucocorticoids regulate Na transport in vascular smooth muscle through the glucocorticoid receptor–mediated mechanism. Am J Hypertens 1993; 6: 736–744.
325. Anderson GH Jr, Blakeman N, Streeten DHP. The effect of age on prevalence of secondary forms of hypertension in 4429 consecutively referred patients. J Hypertens 1994; 12:609–615.
326. Streeten DHP, Anderson GH Jr, Howland T, et al. Effects of thyroid function on blood pressure: recognition of hypothyroid hypertension. Hypertension 1988; 11:78–83.
327. Klein I. Thyroid hormone and the cardiovascular system. Am J Med 1990; 88:631–637.
328. Woeber KA. Thyrotoxicosis and the heart. N Engl J Med 1992; 327:94–98.
329. Falkheden T, Sjögren B. Extracellular fluid volume and renal function in pituitary insufficiency and acromegaly. Acta Endocrinol (Copenh) 1964; 46:80–88.
330. Strauch G, Vallotton MB, Touitou Y, et al. The renin-angiotensin-aldosterone system in normotensive and hypertensive patients with acromegaly. N Engl J Med 1972; 287:795–799.
331. Cain JP, Williams GH, Dluhy RG. Plasma renin activity and aldosterone secretion in patients with acromegaly. J Clin Endocrinol Metab 1972; 34:73–81.
332. Pang PK, Benishin CG, Shan J, Lewanczuk RZ. PTH: The new parathyroid hypertensive factor. Blood Press 1994; 3:148–155.
333. Lind L, Wengle B, Wide L, et al. Hypertension in primary hyperparathyroidism: reduction of blood pressure by long-term treatment with vitamin D (alphacalcidol): double-blind, placebo-controlled study. Am J Hypertens 1988; 1:397–402.
334. Diamond TW, Botha JR, Wing J, et al. Parathyroid hypertension: a reversible disorder. Arch Intern Med 1986; 146:1709–1712.
335. Broulik PD, Horky K, Pacovsky V. Blood pressure in patients with primary hyperparathyroidism before and after parathyroidectomy. Exp Clin Endocrinol 1985; 86:346–352.
336. Jones DB, Jones JH, Lloyd HJ, et al. Changes in blood pressure and renal function after parathyroidectomy in primary hyperparathyroidism. Postgrad Med J 1983; 59:350–353.
337. Sancho JJ, Rouco J, Riera-Vida R, et al. Long-term effects of parathyroidectomy for primary hyperparathyroidism on arterial hypertension. World J Surg 1992; 16:732–736.
338. Consensus Development Conference Panel. Diagnosis and management of asymptomatic primary hyperparathyroidism: Consensus Development Conference Statement. Ann Intern Med 1991; 114:593–597.
339. Stefenelli T, Mayr H, Bergler-Klein J, et al. Primary hyperparathyroidism: incidence of cardiac abnormalities and partial reversibility after successful parathyroidectomy. Am J Med 1993; 95: 197–202.
340. Palmer M, Adami HO, Bergstrom R, et al. Survival and renal function in persons with untreated hypercalcemia: a population-based cohort study with 13 years of follow-up. Lancet 1987; 1: 59–62.
341. Knopp RH. The effect of postmenopausal estrogen therapy on the incidence of arteriosclerotic vascular disease. Obstet Gynecol 1988; 72:23S–30S.
342. Bretza JA, Novey HS, Vaziri ND, et al. Hypertension: a complication of danazol therapy. Arch Intern Med 1980; 140:1379–1380.
343. Lifton RP, Gharavi AG, Geller DS. Molecular mechanisms of human hypertension. Cell 2001; 104:545–556.

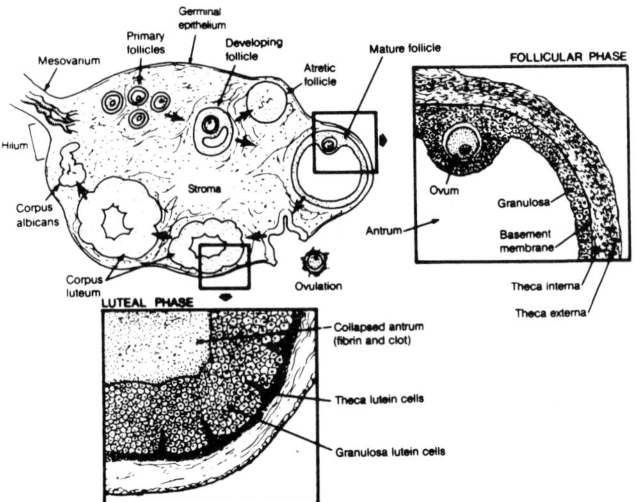

Figure 16–5. Functional anatomy and developmental changes in the adult ovary during an ovarian cycle. (From Carr BR, Wilson JD. Disorders of the ovary and female reproductive tract. In Braunwald E, Isselbacher KJ, Petersdorf RG, et al [eds]. Harrison's Principles of Internal Medicine, 11th ed. New York, McGraw-Hill, 1987, pp 1818-1837.)

16–5). One dominant follicle is recruited for ovulation during each cycle. The preovulatory follicle transforms into a corpus luteum after ovulation (see Fig. 16–5). In the absence of pregnancy, the corpus luteum regresses to become corpus albicans (see Fig. 16–5). The stromal tissue is composed of connective tissue and interstitial cells, which are derived from mesenchymal cells and have the ability to respond to LH or hCG with the production of androstenedione. The central medullary area of the ovary is derived largely from mesonephric cells.

Genetic Determinants of Ovarian Differentiation and Folliculogenesis

Ovarian differentiation and folliculogenesis depend on coordinate expression and interaction of a multitude of genes.[71] Targeted gene disruption or insertion in mice has made it possible to inquire about the function of specific genes in ovarian differentiation and folliculogenesis. Figure 16–6 summarizes the biologic roles of some of these genes.[71] Transgenic mice represent a first step in attempting to understand in vivo the various gene interactions that result in a functional ovary. Indeed, ovarian pathologic conditions in transgenic mice closely resemble disorders observed in mutant human homologues, as exemplified in cases involving the FSH-β subunit and FSH receptor. Many mouse models of ovarian pathologic conditions are available. In general, these can be divided into mice with prenatal ovarian failure with disordered gonad formation and diminished number of germ cells or absent germ cells and mice with postnatal ovarian failure as a result of defects at various stages of folliculogenesis (see Fig. 16–6).[71] These models should lead to the identification of genetic and molecular mechanisms responsible for the development and function of the human ovary.

Ontogeny of the Ovary

The Oocyte

The primordial germ cells are known to originate outside the embryo proper, from the endoderm of the yolk sac. At this site, they can be identified as early as the end of the third week of gestation by alkaline phosphatase staining.[72] Germ cells migrate to cross a remarkably long distance from the yolk sac to the genital ridge by ameboid movements with the aid of pseudopodia.[73] This long route of migration along the dorsal mesentery of the hindgut is interrupted only by the required lateral crossing of the coelomic angle at the level of the genital ridge (Fig. 16–7). Some chemotaxis is operational, but the precise cellular mechanisms underlying the guidance of germ cells to the genital ridge remain uncertain. Germ cells appear unable to persist outside the genital ridge, which may thus be viewed as the only region competent to sustain gonadal development. By the same token, germ cells play an indispensable role in the induction of gonadal development. In fact, no functional gonad is to be expected in the absence of germ cells.

On arrival at the genital ridge by the fifth week of gestation, the premeiotic germ cells are referred to as oogonia.[74] During the subsequent 2 weeks of intrauterine life (weeks 5 to 7 of gestation or the "indifferent" stage), the primordial gonadal structure constitutes no more than a bulge on the medial aspect of the urogenital ridge (see Fig. 16–7). This protuberance is created by proliferation of surface (coelomic) germinal epi-

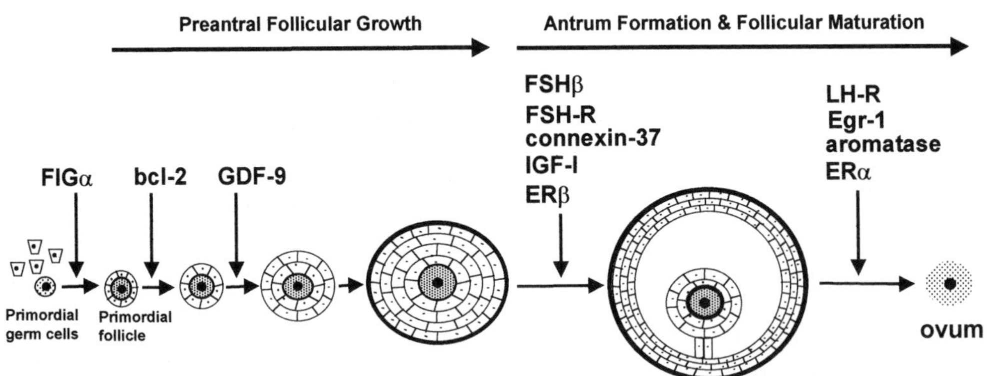

Figure 16–6. Diagram illustrating developmental stages at which certain murine genes affect oogenesis. Data from transgenic mice with disruption of various genes indicated critical roles of a number of genes during various phases of the follicular development. Preantral follicular growth is viewed to be gonadotropin-independent, whereas antrum formation and follicular maturation require action of follicle-stimulating hormone (FSH). bcl-2, β-cell leukemia/lymphoma-2; Egr-1, early growth response-1; ERα, estrogen receptor-α; ERβ, estrogen receptor-β; GDF-9, growth differentiation factor-9; FIGα, factor in the germ line-α; FSHβ, FSH β subunit; FSH-R, FSH receptor; IGF-I, insulin-like growth factor I, LH-R, luteinizing hormone receptor. (Modified from Simpson JL, Rajkovic A. Ovarian differentiation and gonadal failure. Am J Med Genet 1999; 89:186-200.)

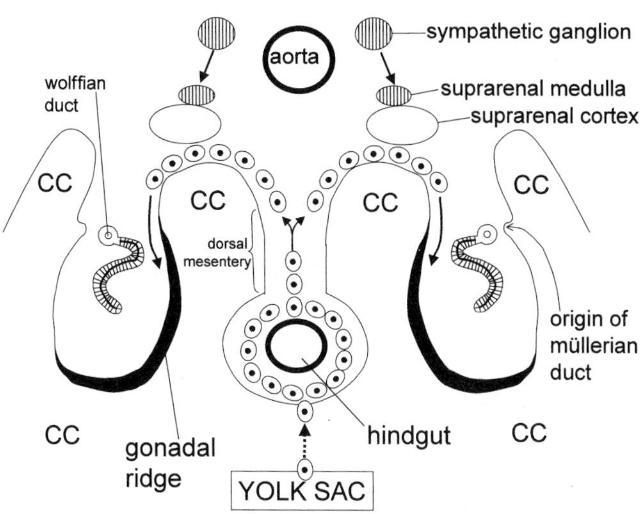

Figure 16–7. Transverse section of the caudal region of a 5-week embryo showing the location of gonadal ridges, the primordium of the adrenal glands, and the migration path of primordial germ cells. From the third week on, germ cells arising from the yolk sac cross the dorsal mesentery of the hindgut and migrate to the gonadal ridges. By the end of the fifth week, rapid division of primordial germ cells, gonadal epithelium, and mesenchyme starts the early gonad that differentiates subsequently to the ovary in a 46,XX fetus. CC, coelomic cavity. (Modified from Moore K. The Developing Human. Philadelphia, WB Saunders, 1983.)

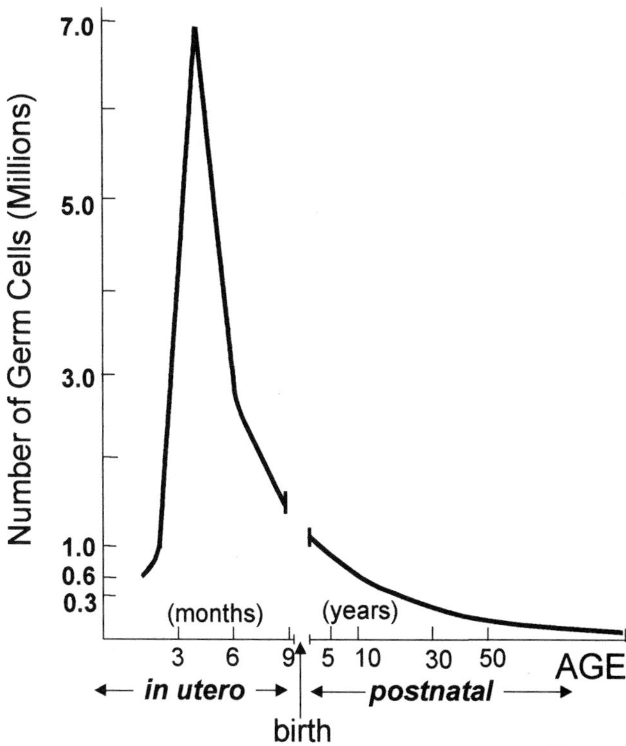

Figure 16–8. Age-dependent changes in germ cell number in the human ovary. The highest number of oocytes is found in the ovaries of a human fetus at midgestation. This number decreases sharply during the third trimester. After birth, the progressive decline in the number of ovarian follicles containing oocytes continues until complete depletion at the menopause. (From Baker TG. A quantitative and cytological study of germ cells in the human ovaries. Proc R Soc Biol Sci 1963; 158:417–433.)

thelium, by growth of the underlying mesenchyme, and by oogonial multiplication. The oogonia total 10,000 by about 6 to 7 weeks of intrauterine life. Because meiosis and oogonial atresia are not operational, the actual number of germ cells is dictated by mitotic division at this time.

It is during this indifferent phase that the gonadal cortex and medulla are first delineated. However, short of cytogenetic evidence, the precise sexual identity of the gonadal ridge cannot be ascertained at this point. Nevertheless, the absence of testicular development beyond 7 weeks of gestation is generally considered presumptive evidence of ovarian formation. Additional clues to the sexual identity of the gonad can be derived from the detection of oogonial meiosis at about 8 weeks of gestation because no comparable process is observed in the testis until puberty. The sexual identity of the gonadal ridge is histologically clear by 16 weeks of gestation, when the first primordial follicles can be visualized.

By about 8 weeks of intrauterine life, persistent mitosis increases the total number of oogonia to 600,000 (Fig. 16–8).[75] From this point on, the oogonial endowment is subject to three simultaneous ongoing processes: mitosis, meiosis, and oogonial atresia. Stated differently, the onset of oogonial meiosis and oogonial atresia is now superimposed on oogonial mitosis. As a result of the combined impact of these processes, that is, mitosis counterbalanced by meiosis and oogonial atresia, the number of germ cells peaks at 6 to 7 $\times$ 10^6 by 20 weeks of gestation (see Fig. 16–8). At this time, two thirds of the total germ cells are intrameiotic primary oocytes; the remaining third can still be viewed as oogonial. The midgestational peak and the postpeak decline are accounted for, if only in part, by the progressively decreasing rate of oogonial mitosis, a process destined to end entirely by about 7 months of intrauterine life. Equally relevant is the increasing rate of oogonial atresia, which peaks at about month 5 of gestation (see Fig. 16–8). During this period, regulation of the ovarian developmental process is complex and probably involves a diverse group of genes (see Fig. 16–7).[76, 77]

From midgestation onward, relentless and irreversible attrition progressively diminishes the germ cell endowment of the gonad.[78] Ultimately, some 50 years later, this is finally exhausted. For the most part, this is accomplished through follicular atresia rather than oogonial atresia, begins around month 6 of gestation, and continues throughout life (see Fig. 16–8). In contrast, oogonial atresia is destined to end at 7 months of intrauterine life as follicular atresia sets in. Follicular atresia has a profound effect on germ cell endowment, given that only 1 to 2 $\times$ 10^6 germ cells are present at birth (see Fig. 16–8).[79] Remarkably, this dramatic depletion of the germ cell mass occurs during a period as short as 20 weeks. No similar rate of depletion occurs earlier or subsequently. Consequently, newborn females enter life still far from realizing reproductive potential, having lost as much as 80% of their germ cell endowment. This decreases further to approximately 300,000 by the onset of puberty. Of these follicles, only 400 to 500 (i.e., less than 1% of the total) ovulate in the course of a reproductive life span.[80]

Between weeks 8 and 13 of fetal life, some of the oogonia depart from the mitotic cycle to enter the prophase of the first meiotic division. This change marks the conversion of these cells to primary oocytes well before actual follicle formation. Meiosis (beginning at about 8 weeks of gestation) provides temporary protection from oogonial atresia, thereby allowing the germ cells to invest themselves with granulosa cells and to form primordial follicles. Accordingly, oogonia that persist beyond the seventh month of gestation and have not entered meiosis are subject to oogonial atresia. Consequently, no oogonia are usually present at birth.

Once formed, the primary oocyte persists in prophase of the first meiotic division until the time of ovulation, when meiosis is resumed and the first polar body is formed and extruded

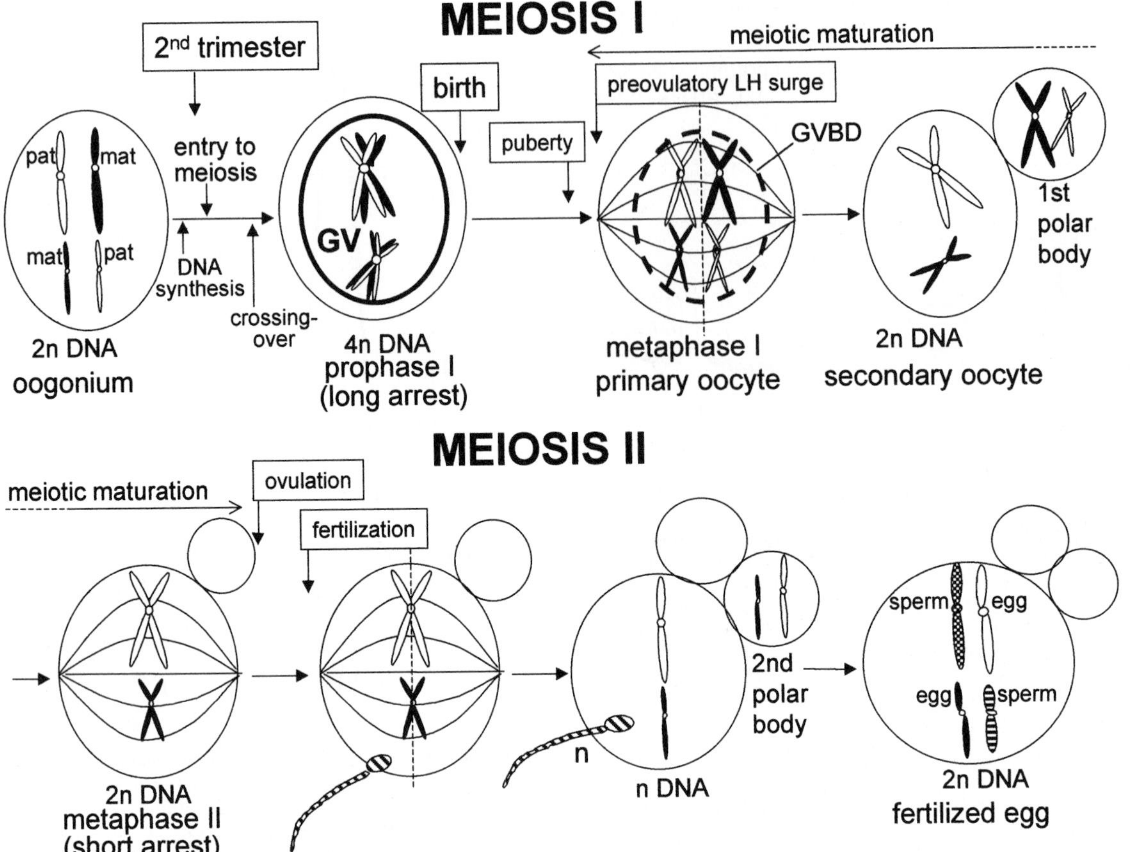

Figure 16–9. Meiotic cell division. Meiosis occurs exclusively in germ cells and serves two critical purposes: (1) generation of germ cells genetically distinct from the somatic cells and (2) generation of a mature egg with a reduction in the number of chromosomes from 46 to 23. Genetic recombination through crossing over of genes between homologous chromosomes and random assortment of (original) maternal and paternal chromosomes into daughter cells during the first meiotic division are responsible for the first function of meiosis, maintenance of genetic diversity. The second function is provided by a reduction in the number of chromosomes so that each daughter cell, or ovum, receives randomly one chromosome from each of the 23 pairs. During fertilization, the fusion of ovum and sperm, each of which has 23 chromosomes, produces a genetically novel individual with 46 chromosomes.

The chromosome marked as white in the oogonium (upper left corner) originates from the father of the fetus, whereas the black chromosome comes from the mother of the fetus. The random exchange of genes (alleles) between homologous chromosomes (crossing over) takes place before the meiotic arrest in the prophase I stage before birth. During postnatal life, these oocytes remain in meiotic arrest until puberty. In the developing oocyte in the graafian follicle, meiosis I is resumed immediately after the preovulatory luteinizing hormone (LH) surge during each ovulatory cycle. Meiotic maturation is defined as the period from the breakdown of the oocyte's nucleus (germinal vesicle, GV) until the oocyte reaches metaphase II (i.e., transition from oocyte to egg). A second and short meiotic arrest occurs at metaphase II until the oocyte is fertilized by a sperm. DNA, deoxyribonucleic acid; GVBD, germinal vesicle breakdown; mat, maternal; n, the amount of DNA material in haploid number (23) of chromosomes; pat, paternal.

(Fig. 16–9). Although the exact cellular mechanisms responsible for this meiotic arrest remain uncertain, it is generally presumed that a granulosa cell–derived putative meiosis inhibitor is in play. This hypothesis is based on the observation that denuded (granulosa-free) oocytes are capable of spontaneously completing meiotic maturation in vitro.

The primary oocyte is converted into a secondary oocyte by completion of the first meiotic metaphase and formation of the first polar body, before actual ovulation but after the LH surge. At ovulation, the secondary oocyte and the surrounding granulosa cells (cumulus oophorus) are extruded and enter the fallopian tube. If sperm penetration occurs, the secondary oocyte undergoes a second meiotic division, after which the second polar body is eliminated (see Fig. 16–9). Only germ cells undergo meiotic division, which serves two vital purposes through unique mechanisms. First, random genetic recombination that occurs during meiosis ensures the maintenance of maximal genetic diversity. Second, meiosis produces a fertilizable oocyte containing a haploid number (23) of chromosomes (see Fig. 16–9).

The Granulosa Cell Compartment

A basement lamina separates the oocyte and granulosa cells from the surrounding stromal cells.[81] Thus, the granulosa cells do not have direct access to the circulation (Fig. 16–10).

The avascular nature of the granulosa cell compartment necessitates contact between neighboring cells. Thus, the granulosa cells are interconnected by extensive intercellular gap junctions, which result in their coupling to yield an expanded, integrated, and functional syncytium (Fig. 16–11).[82–84] Gap junctions are composed of proteins called connexins. Con-

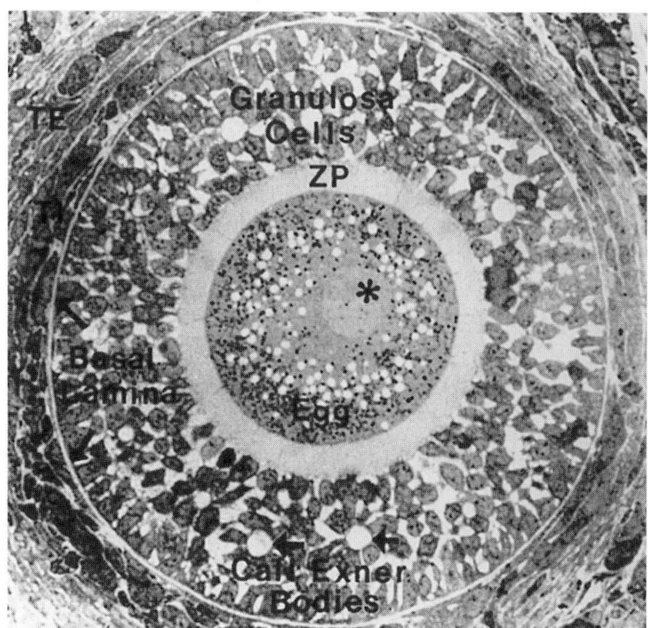

Figure 16–10. Photomicrograph of a section through a preantral follicle. The oocyte (in prophase I arrest) contains a large germinal vesicle (*) and a zona pellucida (ZP). Note that the granulosa cells are surrounded with a basal lamina and lack a vascular supply. Localized accumulations of fluid among granulosa cells appear as round structures and are termed Call-Exner bodies. These accumulations gradually increase in size, become confluent, and eventually give rise to the antrum. TE, theca externa. (From Erickson GF, Magoffin DA, Dyer CA, et al. The ovarian androgen producing cells: a review of structure/function relationships. Endocr Rev 1985; 6:371-399. Copyright © 1985 by The Endocrine Society.)

nexin-37 is present in gap junctions in follicles, and connexin-37–deficient mice lack graafian follicles, fail to ovulate, and develop inappropriate corpora lutea (see Fig. 16–6).[85] These specialized cell junctions may be important in metabolic exchange and in the transport of small molecules between neighboring granulosa cells. Moreover, the granulosa cells extend cytoplasmic processes that penetrate the zona pellucida to form gap junctions with the plasma membrane of the oocyte (see Fig. 16–11). In the connexin-37–deficient mice, the authors also found that oocyte development is arrested before meiotic competence.[85] Thus, gap junctions represent a crucial communication system that is needed for the tight control exerted by the cumulus granulosa cells on the resumption of meiosis by the enclosed primary oocyte.

The granulosa cells in the fully developed graafian follicle shortly before ovulation are stratified in a manner allowing the distinction of a number of populations of cells.[86, 87] The level of differentiation of these distinct populations of granulosa cells is not uniform.[88–91] The following types of granulosa cells have been identified:

1. The *membrana granulosa* is composed of mural and antral cells and represents the layer between basement membrane and the antrum filled with follicular fluid (Fig. 16–12). *Mural granulosa cells* constitute the outermost layer of the membrana granulosa and abut the basement layer. High intracellular levels of steroidogenic enzymes and LH receptors found in mural granulosa cells suggest that these cells account for the majority of steroidogenesis in the follicle.[86, 87] *Antral granulosa cells* of membrana granulosa (i.e., those closest to the antral cavity) seem to be steroidogenically and metabolically less active than mural granulosa cells.

2. The *cumulus oophorus* contains the egg and a surrounding mass of granulosa cells (see Fig. 16–12). At ovulation, the granulosa cell constituents of the cumulus oophorus are extruded with the egg, whereas the membrana granulosa becomes incorporated into the corpus luteum. The *cumulus granulosa cells* lack steroidogenic P450s and have a diminished content of LH receptors compared with the mural granulosa cells of the membrana granulosa.[88–91] Although the cumulus granulosa cells exhibit few markers of specialized function, they proliferate actively, thereby supplying the cells that will make up the membrana granulosa.

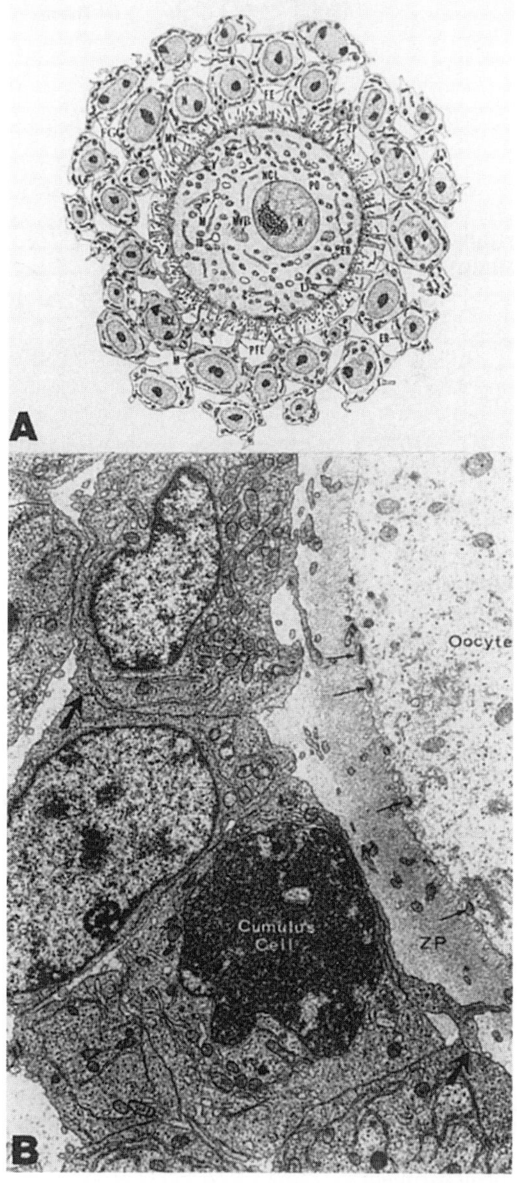

Figure 16–11. Structural relationship between the granulosa cell and the oocyte. *A*, Microvilli of an oocyte interdigitate with cytoplasmic extensions of granulosa cells, penetrating the zona pellucida. *B*, Note the penetration of the zona pellucida by cytoplasmic processes of granulosa cells. Small gap junctions *(thin arrows)* are observed between processes of the granulosa cell and the oocyte membrane. The *thick arrow* indicates a gap junction between granulosa cells. (From Erickson GF. An analysis of follicle development and ovum maturation. Semin Reprod Endocrinol 1986; 4:233, Thieme Medical Publishers, New York; with permission.)

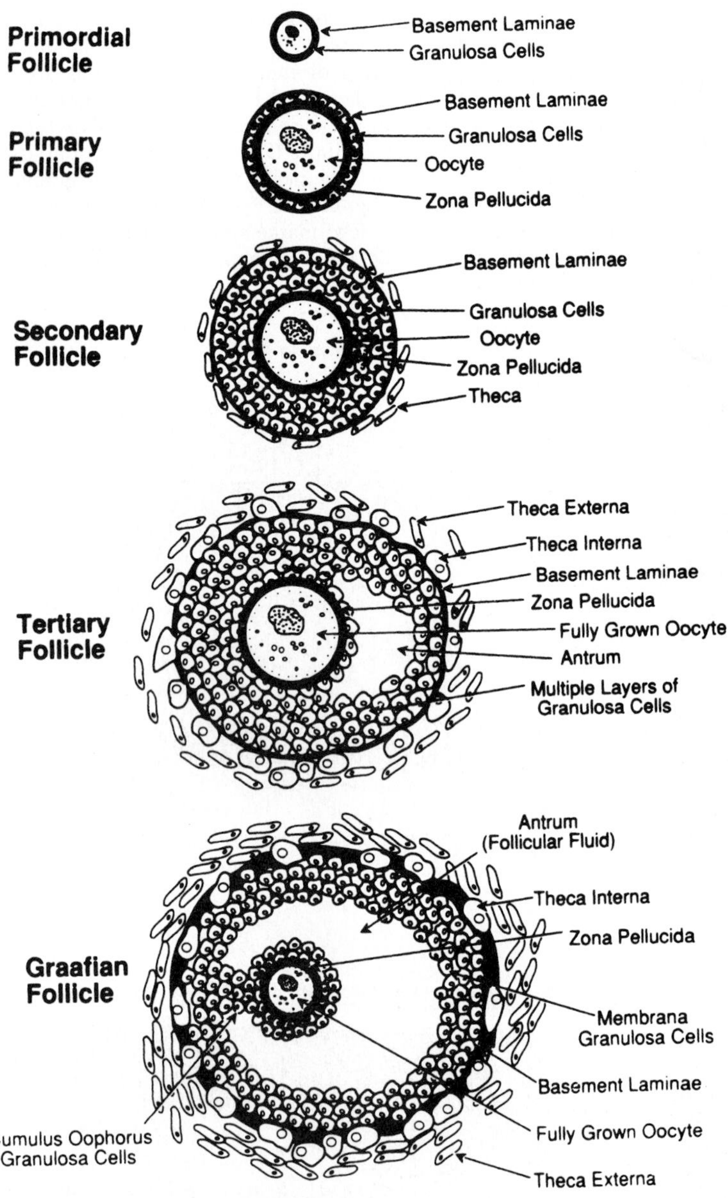

Figure 16–12. Developmental stages of the ovarian follicle. The primordial follicle is composed of a single layer of granulosa cells and a single immature oocyte arrested in the diplotene stage of the first meiotic division. The primordial follicle is separated from the surrounding stroma by a thin basal lamina (basement membrane). The oocyte and granulosa cells do not have a direct blood supply.

The first sign of follicular recruitment is cuboidal differentiation in the spindle-shaped cells inside the basal lamina, which thereafter undergo successive mitotic divisions to form a multilayered granulosa cell zone.The oocyte enlarges and secretes a glycoprotein-containing mucoid substance called the zona pellucida, which surrounds the oocyte and separates the granulosa cells from the oocyte. This structure is a primary follicle.

The secondary follicle is formed by further proliferation of granulosa cells and by the final phase of oocyte growth, in which the oocyte reaches 120 μm in diameter, coincident with proliferation of layers of cells immediately outside the basal lamina to constitute the theca.The portion of the theca adjacent to the basal lamina is termed the theca interna. Thecal cells that merge with the surrounding stroma are designated the theca externa. The secondary follicle acquires an independent blood supply consisting of one or more arterioles that terminate in a capillary bed at the basal lamina. Capillaries do not penetrate the basement membrane, and the granulosa and oocyte remain avascular.

The tertiary follicle is characterized by further hypertrophy of the theca and the appearance of a fluid-filled space among the granulosa cells, named the antrum.The fluid in the antrum consists of a plasma transudate and secretory products of granulosa cells, some of which (estrogens) are found there in strikingly higher concentrations than in peripheral blood.

The follicle rapidly increases in size under the influence of gonadotropins to form the mature or graafian follicle. In the graafian follicle, the granulosa and oocyte remain encased by the basal lamina and are devoid of direct vascularization. The antral fluid increases in volume, and the oocyte, surrounded by an accumulation of granulosa cells (the cumulus oophorus), occupies a polar, eccentric position within the follicle. The mature graafian follicle is ready to release the ovum by the process of ovulation. (Adapted from Erickson GF, Magoffin DA, Dyer CA. The ovarian androgen producing cells: a review of structure-function relations. Endocr Rev 1985; 6:371–379. Copyright © 1985 by The Endocrine Society.)

The Interstitial (Interfollicular) Compartment: Theca-Interstitial Cells

Ryan and Petro[92] demonstrated that the theca-interstitial cells produce C_{19}-steroids, which serve primarily as precursors for estrogen and androgen. Rice and colleagues[93, 94] noted the ability of the theca interna (see later) and interstitial tissue to undertake de novo synthesis of C_{19}-steroids (Fig. 16–13). The C_{19}-producing cells are located in the loose connective tissue of both the cortex and the medulla, arising in all likelihood from a population of unspecialized mesenchymal cells in the stromal compartment.[95]

The cells making up the theca-interstitial compartment are heterogeneous in nature. One contemporary view of the dynamic alterations characteristic of this ovarian compartment is that of Erickson and co-workers.[96] Four classes of interstitial cells have been identified:

1. *Primary interstitial cells.* Primary interstitial cells constitute a transient population of C_{19}-steroid–producing cells located in the medullary compartment of the fetal ovary.[97] Although apparent at about 12 weeks of gestation, these cells disappear by 20 weeks. Their function remains a mystery. Morphologically resembling fetal testicular Leydig cells, primary interstitial cells are functionally limited in terms of their steroidogenic capacity. Specifically, these cells appear to be incapable of de novo steroidogenesis, presumably owing to the lack of cholesterol side-chain cleavage activity. These cells are unresponsive to gonadotropic stimulation and could conceivably employ circulating steroidogenic precursors to yield androgens.

2. *Theca-interstitial cells.* Theca-interstitial cells represent the constant feature of all developing follicles (see Figs. 16–12 and 16–13). These cells are identified as theca interna, the stromal cell layer adjacent to the basal lamina around granulosa cells, and theca externa, a less well-defined layer of stromal cells that make up the outermost layer of the follicle (see later, Figs. 16–12 and 16–13). Theca-interstitial cells represent the main mature C_{19}-steroid–producing component of the follicle.

3. *Secondary interstitial cells.* Secondary interstitial cells represent hypertrophied theca interna remnants surviving follicular atresia. These cells settle in the region of the old follicle but otherwise remain functionally and structurally unchanged. The

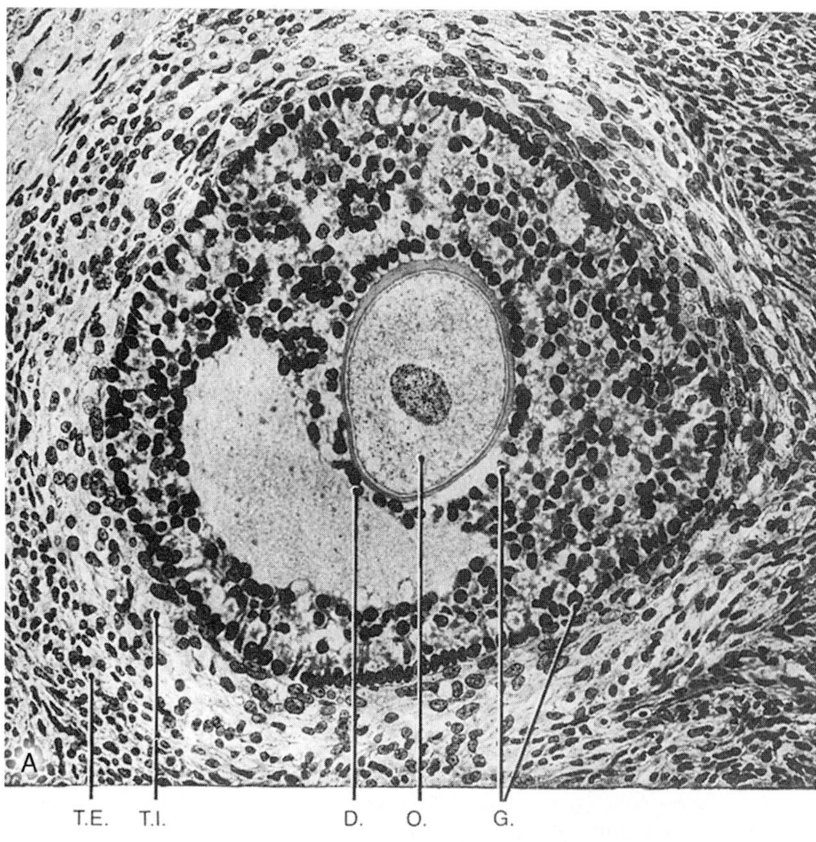

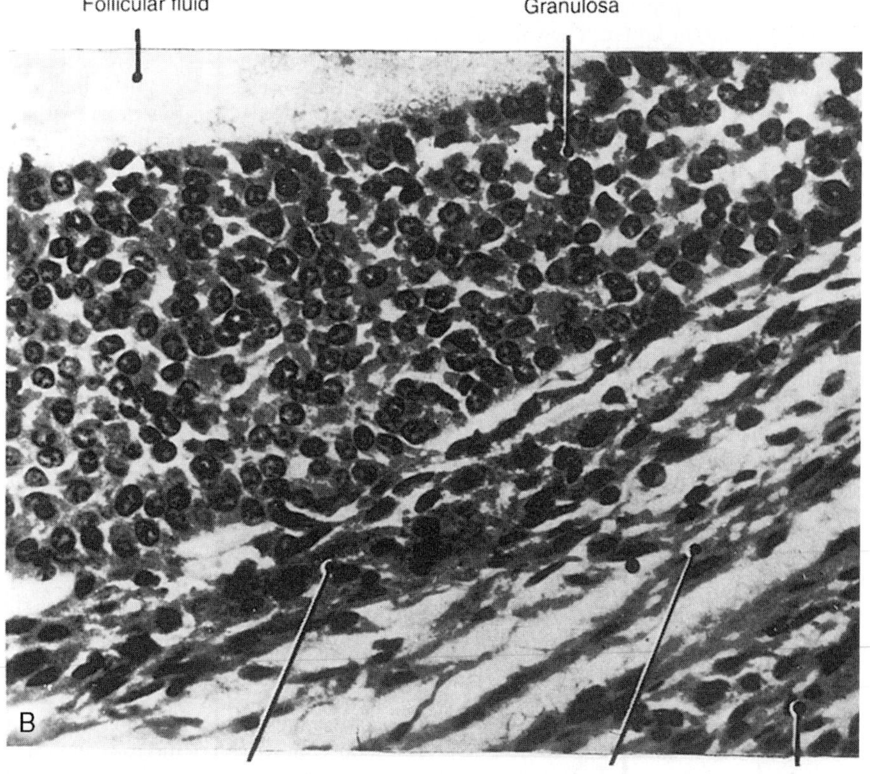

Figure 16–13. Histology of human graafian follicle. *A*, Cycle day 10 to 12 graafian follicle approaching maturity. D., discus proligerus (cumulus oophorus); G., granulosa cell layer; O., ovum; T.E., theca externa; T.I., theca interna. *B*, Section through the wall of a mature graafian follicle. (From Cunningham FG, Macdonald PC , Gant NF, et al. Pregnancy: overview and diagnosis; ovarian function and ovulation. In Williams Obstetrics, 19th ed. Stamford, Conn, Appleton & Lange, 1993, pp 11-55.)

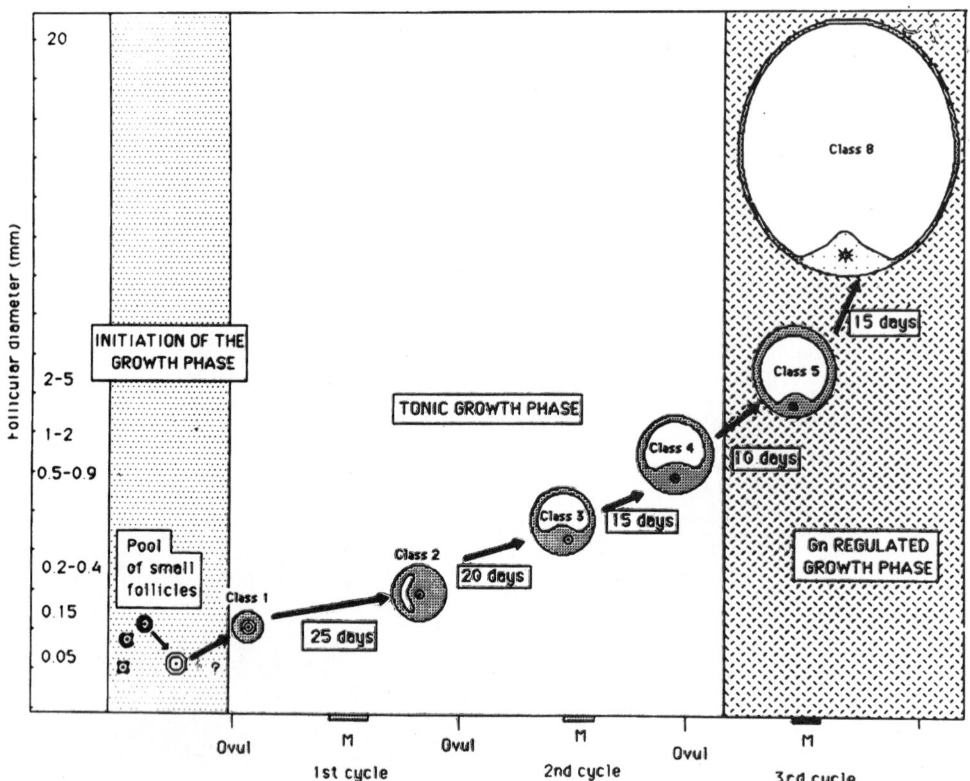

Figure 16–14. Complete follicular growth trajectory. Class 1 follicle is a secondary follicle with theca cells and is presumed to become responsive to gonadotropins. Although the tonic (early) stage of follicle development (class 1 to 4) is likely to be gonadotropin-dependent (albeit to a lesser extent), the final stages of follicular development (class 5 to 8) are the ones heavily dependent on gonadotropins. According to this view, late luteal phase, class 5 follicles constitute the cohort from which the follicle destined to ovulate in the following cycle is recruited. The exponential gonadotropin-dependent growth phase (class 5 to 8) takes place during the follicular phase of the cycle following the third menses from initiation of the growth phase. During this time, follicular selection and dominance are accomplished. The total duration of the process wherein a class 1 follicle is converted into preovulatory class 8 follicle is estimated to be 85 days and spans three ovulatory cycles. M, menses; Ovul, ovulation; Gn, gonadotropin. (Courtesy of A. Gougeon.)

secondary interstitial cells (unlike theca-interstitial cells) are the targets of noradrenergic innervation.

4. *Hilar interstitial cells.* Hilar interstitial cells are constituents of the ovarian hilum. They are large steroidogenic lutein-like cells with structural and functional characteristics indistinguishable from those of differentiated testicular Leydig cells. Both types of cells contain a unique hexagonal crystal lattice named after Reinke. Hilar cells are intimately associated with nonmyelinated sympathetic nerve fibers. The secretory function (i.e., androgen biosynthesis) of these cells is strongly suggested by their prominence at the time of puberty, during pregnancy, and around menopause.

Resident Ovarian White Blood Cells

Unlike the testicular seminiferous tubule, the ovary does not constitute an immunologically privileged site. Thus, resident ovarian mononuclear phagocytes (macrophages), lymphocytes, and polymorphonuclear granulocytes can be observed at various stages of the ovarian life cycle. For example, macrophages, but not other white blood cells, are known to constitute a major cellular component of the interstitial (i.e., interfollicular) ovarian compartment.[98] In part, these macrophages are present within the ovarian stroma near perifollicular capillaries. Lymphocytes and polymorphonuclear leukocytes, on the other hand, are observed in the follicle and corpus luteum in varying quantities during the follicular development, corpus luteum formation, and follicular atresia.[99–104]

The significance of the preceding observations may be that resident ovarian representatives of the white blood cell series constitute potential in situ modulators of ovarian function, acting through the local secretion of regulatory cytokines.[105] Because the flow of information is probably multidirectional, the same cells are probably targeted for steroidal and peptidergic input. Moreover, immune cells are endowed with steroidogenic capabilities that could, in their own right, affect steroid economy.[106, 107]

Follicles

The follicle represents the most important functional unit in the ovary with respect to germ cell development and steroid production. The follicles are embedded in loose connective tissue of the ovarian cortex and can be subdivided into two functional types: nongrowing (or primordial) and growing. The majority of follicles (90% to 95%) are nongrowing throughout reproductive life. Recruitment of a primordial follicle initiates dramatic changes in growth, structure, and function. The growing follicles are divided into four stages: primary, secondary, tertiary, and graafian (see Fig. 16–12). The first three stages of growth can occur in the absence of the pituitary and therefore appear to be controlled by intraovarian mechanisms (Fig. 16–14). The follicle destined to ovulate is recruited in the first few days of the current cycle.[108]

The early growth of follicles occurs over the time span of several preceding menstrual cycles, but the ovulatory follicle is one of a cohort recruited at the time of transition from the previous cycle's luteal phase and the current cycle's follicular phase (see Fig. 16–14).[109, 110] The total time to achieve preovulatory status is approximately 85 days (see Fig. 16–14).[109, 110] The majority of this period of development is FSH-independent.[111] Eventually, this cohort of follicles reaches a stage at which, unless recruited by FSH, the next step is atresia. Thus, a cohort of follicles measuring 2 to 5 mm is continuously available for a response to FSH (Fig. 16–15). The late luteal increase in FSH is the critical feature in rescuing this cohort of follicles from atresia, eventually allowing a dominant follicle to emerge and pursue a path to ovulation (see Fig. 16–15). In addition, maintenance of this increase in FSH for a critical duration of time is essential.[112]

Recruited primordial follicles either develop into dominant,

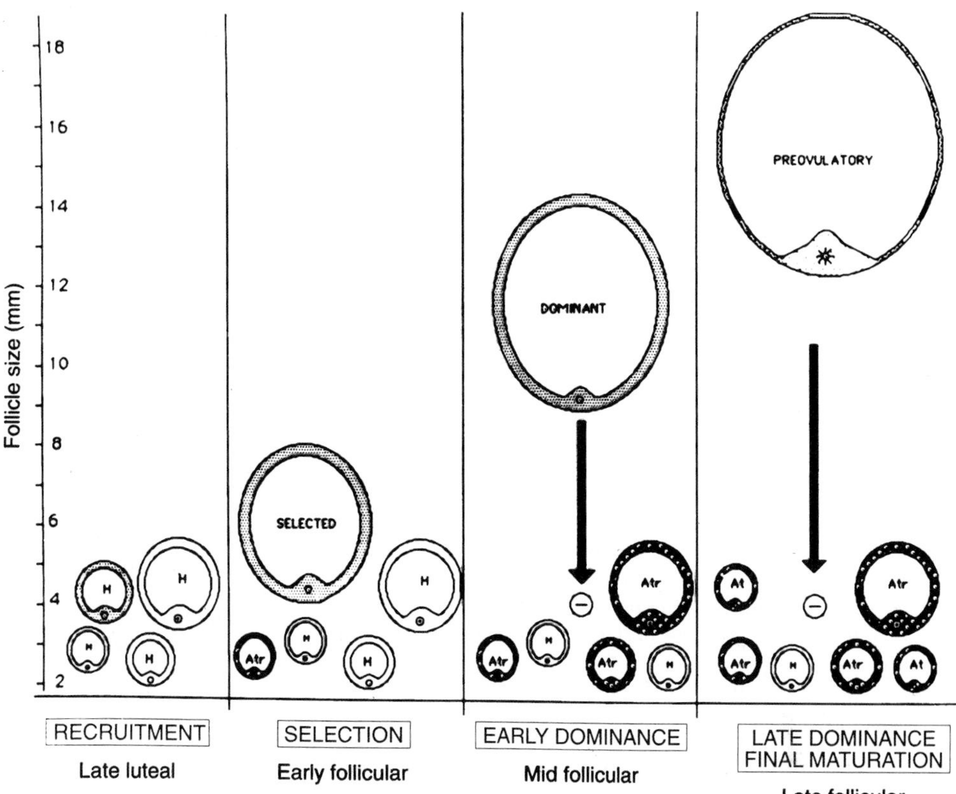

Figure 16–15. Gonadotropin-dependent (exponential) follicular growth phase: recruitment, selection, and the attainment of dominance. At and Atr, atretic follicle; H, healthy follicle. (Courtesy of A. Gougeon.)

mature graafian follicles destined to ovulate or degenerate as a result of atresia (see Fig. 16–15).[113] The average time for development of a selected follicle to the point of ovulation is 10 to 14 days (see Fig. 16–15).[114] If a follicle is not recruited, it goes through a process called atresia during which the oocyte and granulosa cells within the basal lamina die and are replaced by fibrous tissue. In contrast, the thecal cells outside the basal lamina do not die but dedifferentiate and return to the pool of cells consisting of ovarian interstitial or stromal cells.[70] The process of atresia is generally thought to result from lack of the hormones or growth factors that are formed by the mature dominant follicle through intrinsic intraovarian mechanisms. There is general agreement that atresia of follicles is due to apoptosis.[115] Apoptosis is an active and regulated process triggered by a cascade of caspase proteases that lead to characteristic fragmentation of DNA and blebbing of membranes.

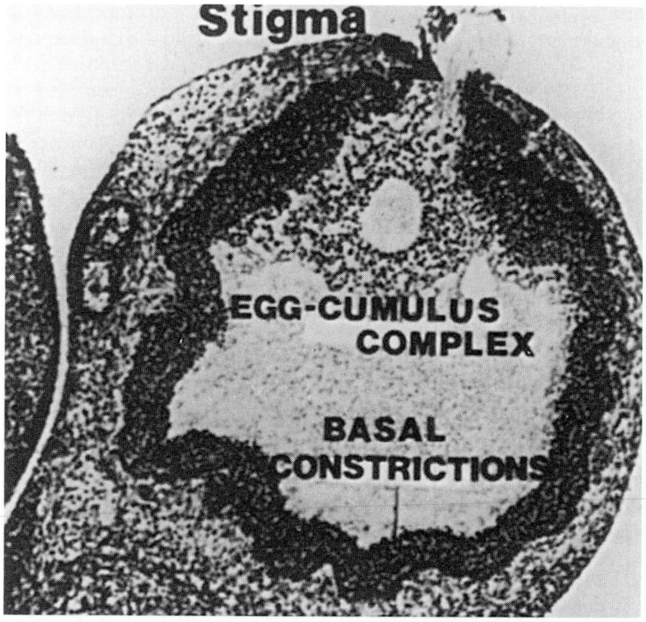

Figure 16–16. Ovulation of the cumulus-oocyte complex through the stigma. (From Erickson GF. An analysis of follicle development and ovum maturation. Semin Reprod Endocrinol 1986; 4:233, Thieme Medical Publishers, New York; with permission.)

Ovulation

There is a dramatic rise in circulating estradiol level as midcycle approaches (see later). This increase in estradiol is followed by a striking LH and to a lesser extent an FSH surge. This triggers the dominant follicle to ovulate. During each menstrual cycle, usually one follicle ovulates and gives rise to a corpus luteum. In the human, either LH or its surrogate hCG is essential to stimulate the rupture of the mature follicle. It was proposed that increased local prostaglandin biosynthesis in the follicle might mediate the ovulatory effect of LH.[116, 117]

Ovulation consists of rapid follicular enlargement followed by protrusion of the follicle from the surface of the ovarian cortex. This is followed by the rupture of the follicle and extrusion of an egg-cumulus complex into the peritoneal cavity (Fig. 16–16). Follicular rupture or ovulation occurs predictably 34 to 36 hours from the start of the LH surge. Elevation of a conical "stigma" on the surface of the protruding follicle precedes rupture (see Fig. 16–16). Rupture of this stigma is accompanied by a gentle rather than explosive expulsion of the ovum and antral fluid. The gonadotropin-dependent production of proteases acting locally on protein substrates in the basal lamina may play an important role in stigma formation and follicular rupture.[118, 119] In particular, plasminogen activator levels increase in the follicle before rupture.[120] Thus, plasminogen activator–mediated conversion of plasminogen to plasmin may contribute to the proteolytic digestion of the follicular wall, which is a prerequisite for follicular rupture.

Corpus Luteum

After ovulation, the dominant follicle reorganizes to become the corpus luteum (Fig. 16–17). After rupture of the follicle, capillaries and fibroblasts from the surrounding stroma proliferate and penetrate the basal lamina. This rapid vascularization of the corpus luteum may be guided by angiogenic factors, some of which are detected in the follicular fluid.[121] Vascular endothelial growth factor has been isolated from corpora lutea and has been postulated, along with basic fibroblast growth factor, to be a potential angiogenic agent in corpora lutea.[122, 123] Concurrently, the granulosa and theca cells undergo morphologic changes collectively referred to as luteinization. The granulosa cells become granulosa-lutein cells (large cells), and the theca cells are transformed into theca-lutein cells (small cells; see Fig. 16–17*B*).[124] The so-called K cells, scattered throughout the corpus luteum, are believed to be macrophages.[125]

The corpus luteum is the endocrine gland that serves as the major source of sex steroid hormones secreted by the ovary during the postovulatory phase of the cycle. The human corpus luteum secretes as much as 40 mg of progesterone per day during the midluteal phase of the ovarian cycle.[126] In view of the small size of the corpus luteum, it is the most active steroidogenic tissue in humans. An important aspect of corpus luteum formation is the penetration of the follicle basement membrane by blood vessels, which provides the granulosa-lutein cells with low-density lipoprotein (LDL).[120] As stated earlier, LDL cholesterol serves as the substrate for corpus luteum progesterone production.

A key regulator of steroidogenesis in the corpus luteum is LH. In humans, the LH receptor is maintained throughout the functional life span of corpora lutea and not down-regulated during the maternal recognition of pregnancy.[127] The rate-limiting step in LH-mediated progesterone formation in luteinized granulosa cells is the entry of cholesterol into the mitochondria, which is regulated by steroidogenic acute regulatory protein (StAR; see later).[128] Thus, the availability of LDL cholesterol and the StAR-mediated mitochondrial entry of cholesterol seem to be the two critical factors that account for the production of large amounts of progesterone in the corpus luteum.

The functional life span of the corpus luteum is normally 14 ± 2 days. Thereafter, the corpus luteum spontaneously regresses. It is replaced, unless pregnancy occurs, by an avascular scar referred to as the corpus albicans.

Factors that may regulate luteal life span include hormones such as hCG, maintenance of luteal vascularization, and immune cells.[129] There is little doubt about the central role of LH in the maintenance of corpus luteum function. Withdrawal of LH support in a variety of experimental circumstances has almost invariably resulted in luteal regression.[129] In pregnancy, however, the LH surrogate hCG, secreted by the gestational trophoblast, maintains the ability of the corpus luteum to elaborate progesterone; this stimulus helps to maintain the early gestation until the luteoplacental shift.[130] Accordingly, the corpus luteum doubles in size (compared with the prepregnancy size) during the first 6 weeks of gestation (see Fig. 16–17).[131] This increase is due to proliferation of connective tissues and blood vessels, along with hypertrophy of the luteinized granulosa and theca cells. This early hypertrophy is later followed by regression. The corpus luteum at term is only half the size of that during the menstrual cycle.

Hormones such as estrogens and prostaglandins have been suggested as important factors in the promotion of luteal demise.[132, 133] Immune factors may influence luteal life span because corpus luteal regression is associated with a progressive infiltration of lymphocytes and macrophages.[129]

Apoptosis may be the end-point mechanism by which human corpora lutea are deleted. Corpora lutea during the early luteal phase of the menstrual cycle and corpora lutea of early pregnancy show no evidence of apoptotic DNA fragmentation.[134] DNA fragmentation, on the other hand, is detected in midluteal and late luteal corpora.[134] Thus, it is hypothesized that apoptosis is a major mechanism for the demise of the corpus luteum. LH or hCG inhibits apoptosis in the corpus luteum. In the absence of these trophic factors, apoptosis ensues. The remaining corpus luteum is composed of dense connective tissue and is termed the *corpus albicans*.

Ovarian Follicle-Stimulating Hormone and Luteinizing Hormone Receptors

The FSH receptor is expressed exclusively by granulosa cells. The LH-hCG receptor is expressed primarily by the theca-interstitial cells of all follicles and by granulosa cells of large preovulatory follicles.

Granulosa cells in primary or secondary follicles that are in the early developmental stages before antrum formation (i.e., preantral follicles) primarily bind FSH but not LH.[135, 136] In these preantral follicles, the binding of LH and hCG is confined to theca-interstitial cells.[137] Granulosa cells in more mature tertiary follicles with an antrum appear capable of binding both LH and FSH.[136] Thus, FSH receptors are found in granulosa cells from follicles of all sizes, but LH receptors are found only in granulosa cells of large preovulatory follicles.[138–142] These observations are consistent with the concept that the acquisition of LH receptors on granulosa cells is under the influence of FSH.[143–145]

The receptors for the glycoprotein hormones have related structures (Fig. 16–18). The receptors belong to the large family of G protein–coupled receptors, whose members all have a transmembrane domain that consists of seven membrane-traversing α-helices connected by three extracellular and three intracellular loops (see Fig. 16–18). The glycoprotein hormone receptors form a separate subgroup within this large family by virtue of their large extracellular hormone-binding domain at the N-terminus. FSH binds to the FSH receptor, and LH and hCG both bind to the same LH receptor. Both LH and FSH receptor genes are located on chromosome 2 at the p21 region.[64] The relationship of the glycoprotein hormone receptors to the other G protein–coupled receptors is indicated by their sequence homology in the C-terminal half of the receptor. This domain, encoded by a single, last exon, contains the seven transmembrane segments and the G protein–coupling domain. The unusually large extracellular domain of the glycoprotein hormone receptors is encoded by the first 9 or 10 exons (Fig. 16–19).

Role of Follicle-Stimulating Hormone in Ovarian Function

As indicated by its name, FSH is the main promoter of follicular maturation. Given that FSH receptors have been exclusively localized to granulosa cells, it is generally presumed that FSH action in the ovary involves the granulosa cells. The ability of FSH to orchestrate follicular growth and differentiation depends on its ability to exert multiple actions concurrently.

Phenotypes of women with mutations that disrupt the function of the FSH-β subunit gene are in good agreement and demonstrate that FSH is necessary for normal follicular development, ovulation, and fertility.[64] Likewise, pubertal develop-

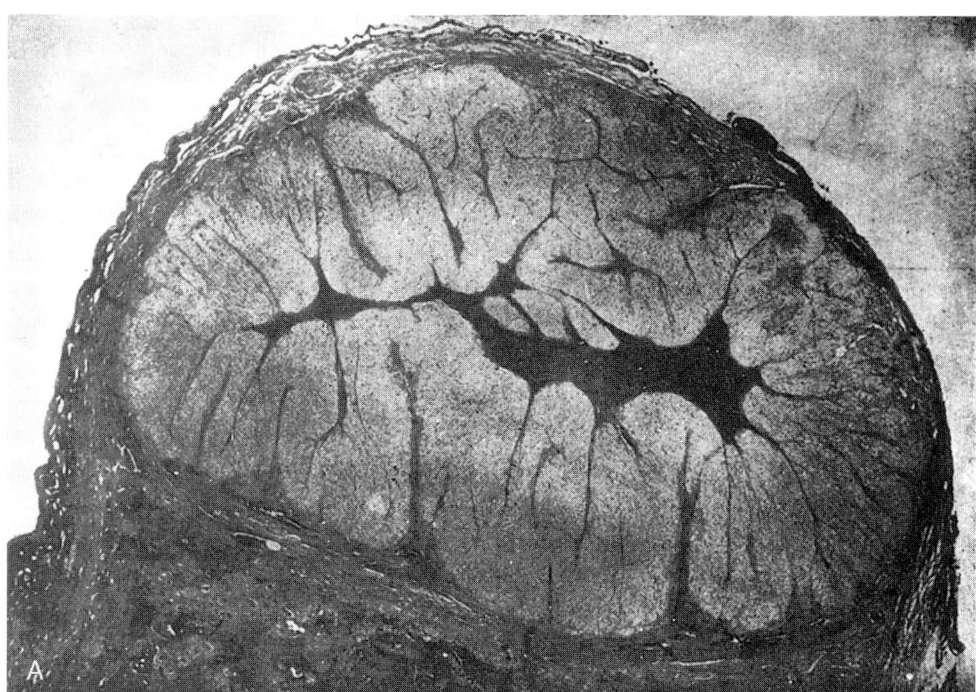

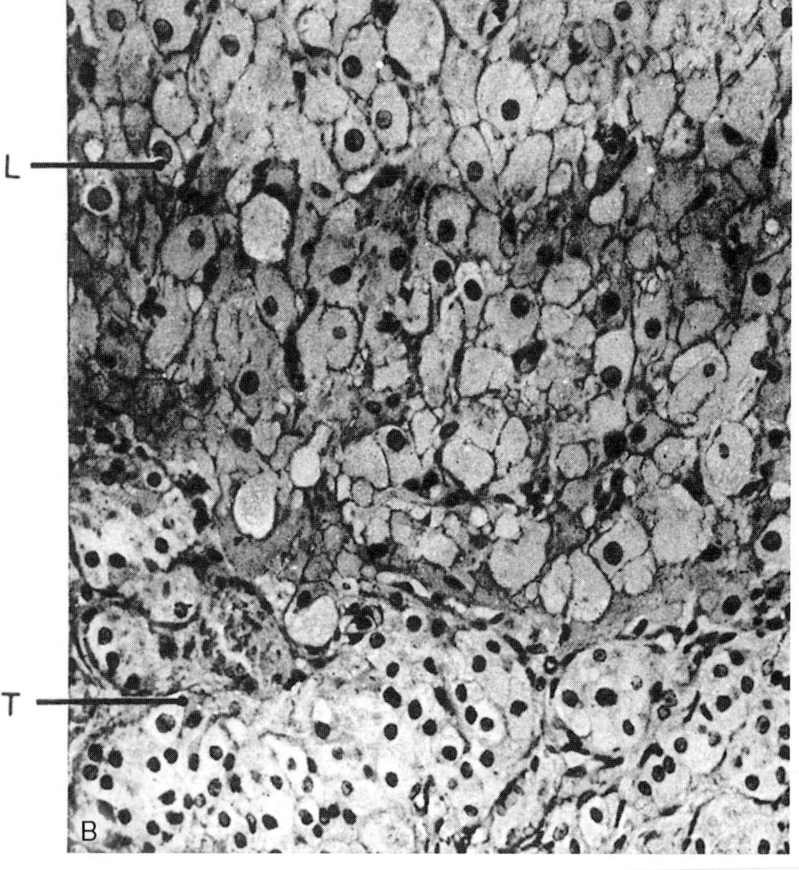

Figure 16–17. Corpus luteum of pregnancy. *A*, Lower power. *B*, High power. L, Granulosa lutein cells; T, theca lutein cells. (From Cunningham FG, MacDonald PC, Gant NF, et al. Pregnancy: overview and diagnosis; ovarian function and ovulation. In Williams Obstetrics, 19th ed. Stamford, Conn, Appleton & Lange, 1993, pp 11-55.)

ment is hampered in the absence of sufficient numbers of later stage follicles with the granulosa cells needed for adequate estrogen production. Treatment of at least one of these patients with exogenous FSH resulted in follicular maturation, ovulation, and normal pregnancy.[64] The presenting phenotype of FSH-β subunit deficiency is practically identical to that caused by inactivating mutations of the FSH receptor.[64] Women with FSH receptor mutations are clinically similar to patients with gonadal dysgenesis, with absent or poorly developed secondary sexual characteristics and high serum levels of FSH and LH. The notable difference was the presence of ovarian follicles in cases with FSH receptor mutation, consistent with the FSH independence of primordial follicle recruitment and early follicular growth and development. In contrast,

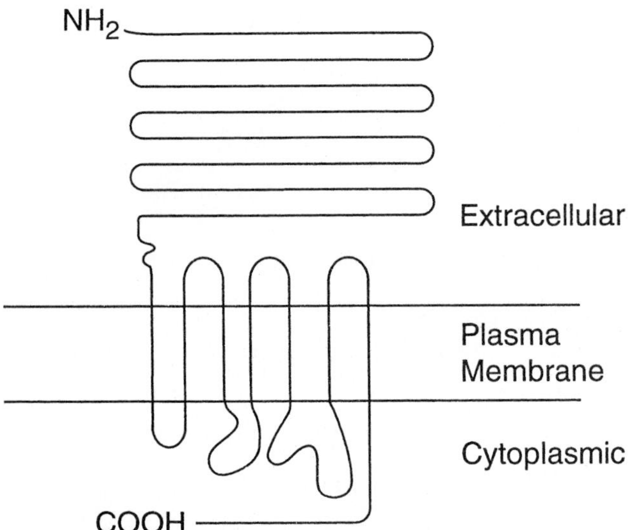

Figure 16–18. Gonadotropin receptor. The seven-transmembrane-domain, G protein–coupled receptors for luteinizing hormone and follicle-stimulating hormone located in the membranes of ovarian granulosa and theca cells typically have large extracellular domains. (From Bulun SE, Simpson ER, Mendelson CR. The molecular basis of hormone action. In Carr BR, Blackwell RE [eds]. Textbook of Reproductive Medicine, 2nd ed. Stamford, Conn, Appleton & Lange, 1998, pp 137–156.)

total absence of all follicles, including those in the primordial stage, was observed in the cases in which the FSH receptor mutation could not be detected.[64] Thus, the ovarian phenotype of FSH receptor deficiency is distinct from the common form of gonadal dysgenesis as found in Turner's syndrome with streak gonads and absence of growing follicles.[64]

In vivo rodent studies suggest that FSH is capable of increasing the number of its own receptors in the granulosa cell. Whereas estradiol by itself may be without effect on the distribution, number, or affinity of granulosa cell FSH receptors, estrogens have been shown to synergize with FSH to enhance the overall number of granulosa cell FSH receptors.[146] Consequently, changes in the production of estradiol by preantral follicles could increase their response to FSH through the regulation of granulosa cell-surface FSH receptors. This interaction between FSH and estradiol in follicular development has been well established in rodents. It appears that both estrogen receptor α (ERα) and ERβ may mediate the estrogenic effect on ovarian development and follicular maturation in mice.[147] On the other hand, it is not clear at this time whether a similar relationship exists in the human ovary. ERα is not detected in the human ovary in significant quantities. The demonstration of ERβ in the human ovary, however, suggests an interaction between FSH and estrogen in the regulation of normal follicle development and ovulation in women.[148]

One of the major actions of FSH is the induction of granulosa cell aromatase activity.[149, 150] Thus, little or no estrogen can be produced by FSH-unprimed granulosa cells even if they are supplied with aromatizable androgen precursors. On the other hand, treatment with FSH enhances the aromatization capability of granulosa cells, an effect related to enhancement of the granulosa cell aromatase content.[151–153]

Treatment with FSH has also been shown to induce LH receptors in granulosa cells.[154] The ability of FSH to induce LH receptors is augmented by the concomitant presence of estrogens.[155] Furthermore, progestins, androgens, and LH itself may also induce LH receptors. Once induced, the granulosa cell LH receptor requires the continued presence of FSH for its maintenance.

Circumstantial evidence, as deduced from studies of women with disrupting mutations of the genes that encode FSH and LH receptors and aromatase P450 (P450$_{arom}$), indicates that FSH action, but not estrogen or LH action, is essential for follicular growth in humans.[64, 156] In women with deficient LH action or estrogen biosynthesis, follicular growth and development up to the antral stage were observed, although these individuals were anovulatory.[64, 156] On the other hand, women with mutations of the FSH-β subunit or FSH receptor had only primordial follicles in their ovaries.[64] These data indicate that estrogen or LH is not critical for follicular development at least until the tertiary stage (see Figs. 16–12 and 16–14). It should be kept in mind, however, that FSH by itself is not sufficient to achieve normal follicular development and ovulation.

Role of Luteinizing Hormone in Ovarian Function

LH is essential for ovulation (follicular rupture) and the sustenance of corpus luteum function. In addition, LH plays other important roles in follicular function. First, it is likely that LH plays a major role in the promotion of theca-interstitial cell androgen production. Moreover, LH may well synergize with FSH in the more advanced phases of follicular development. Last, small and sustained increments in the circulating levels of LH are both necessary and sufficient to cause small antral follicles to grow and develop to the preovulatory stage.[157, 158]

It is presumed that LH acts on theca-interstitial cells of small follicles, where it promotes the biosynthesis of C_{19}-steroids.[159] The consequent increase in estrogen production is presumed to contribute to the growth and development of the follicles. Treatment with small doses of LH also presumably results in an increase in LH receptor content[160] as well as in induction of the key steroidogenic proteins such as StAR, side-chain cleavage P450 (P450$_{scc}$), 3β-hydroxysteroid dehydrogenase type II (3β-HSD-II), and 17 hydroxylase (P450$_{c17}$).

The role of LH action in human ovarian physiology was exemplified by the phenotype of a woman with a disrupting mutation of the LH receptor gene.[64] She presented with amenorrhea with normally developed secondary sexual characteristics, increased circulating FSH and LH levels, and low levels of estradiol and progesterone that were unresponsive to hCG treatment.[64] The ovary contained follicles that developed up to antral stage with a well-developed theca layer but no preovulatory follicles or corpora lutea. These observations collectively support the view that LH is essential for ovulation and sufficient estrogen production, whereas follicular development is initially autonomous and at later stages dependent on intact FSH action.

Ovarian Steroidogenesis

The preovulatory follicle secretes estradiol during the first half of the menstrual cycle, whereas the corpus luteum secretes both estradiol and progesterone during the second half of the cycle (Fig. 16–20). The production of these two biologically active steroids is orchestrated in the follicle and corpus luteum in a cell-specific manner under the control of LH and FSH.

The steroid hormone contents of the ovarian vein effluents and peripheral venous blood were compared to distinguish steroids secreted by the ovary from those secreted by the adrenal and from those produced by peripheral conversion of precursors.[161] These studies revealed that the ovaries secrete pregnenolone, progesterone, 17α-hydroxyprogesterone, dehydroepiandrosterone (DHEA), androstenedione, testosterone, estrone, and estradiol.[162, 163] Although such measurements provide insights into the steroidogenic pathways under study, they

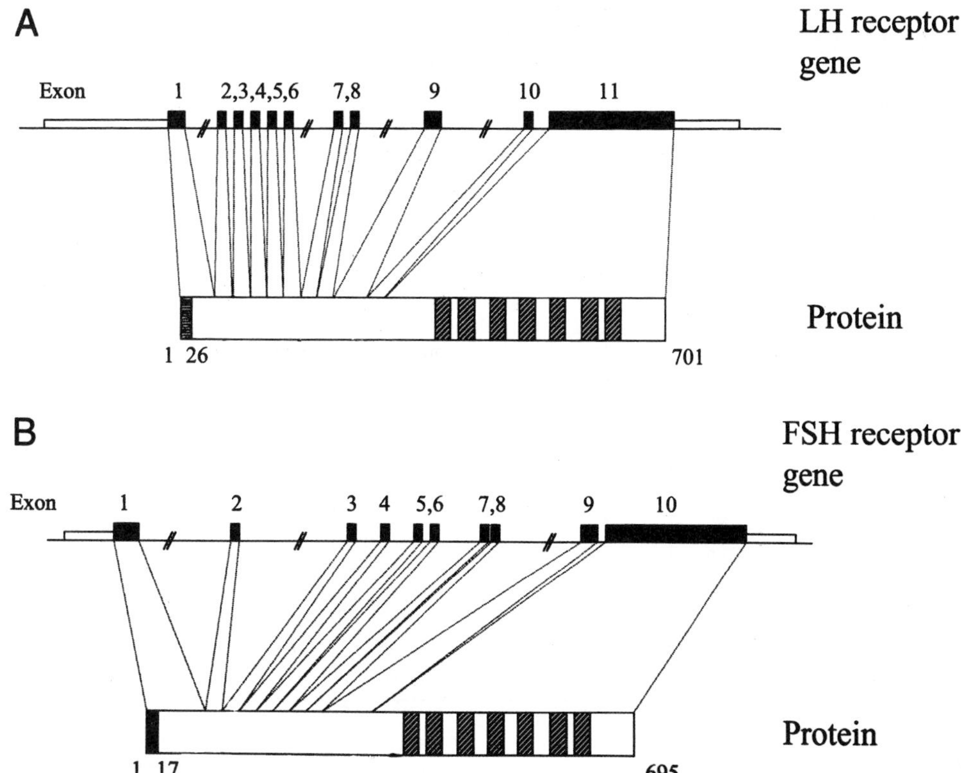

Figure 16–19. Schematic representation of the human gonadotropin receptor genes. The structure of the genes is depicted at the top of the drawings. The *open bars* indicate sections of the exons that encode untranslated regions of the messenger ribonucleic acid; the *closed bars* indicate the sequences that encode the protein. Both genes are at least 80 kb in size. The relation between the intron-exon structure of the gene and the domains on the protein is indicated by the lines connecting the gene to the protein. The *horizontally hatched* part of the protein indicates the signal peptide, and the *crosshatched bars* signify the seven segments of the transmembrane domain. The numbers below the protein indicate the start and end of the signal peptide and the length of the total protein product including the signal peptide. Note that the receptor genes are similar in structure with the exception of an additional exon in the luteinizing hormone (LH) receptor gene. Exon 1 encodes the signal peptide and a small part of the extracellular domain; the following eight or nine exons encode the rest of the extracellular domain, including the leucine-rich repeat motifs. In both receptor genes, the final exon is the largest and contains the information for the transmembrane signal transduction domain. FSH, follicle-stimulating hormone. (From Themmen APN, Huhtaniemi IT. Mutations of gonadotropins and gonadotropin receptors: elucidating the physiology and pathophysiology of pituitary-gonadal function. Endocr Rev 2000; 21:4551-583. Copyright © 2000 by The Endocrine Society.)

do not identify the specific ovarian cells involved. Studies using microdissected preovulatory follicles identified estrone and estradiol as the major steroid products (see Fig. 16–20). Progesterone and 17α-hydroxyprogesterone, on the other hand, proved to be the major products of the corpus luteum (see Fig. 16–20).[164, 165]

The biologically active ovarian steroids are estradiol and progesterone (Fig. 16–21). The major C_{19}-steroid product of the ovary, androstenedione, is not biologically active. Androstenedione, however, acts as a dual precursor and contributes to circulating levels of estrone and testosterone through conversion in extraglandular tissues such as adipose tissue and skin (see later).[166–169] It is likely that estrogenically weak estrone is further converted to the potent estrogen estradiol, and testosterone is converted to the much more potent androgen dihydrotestosterone (DHT) locally in target tissues such as brain, breast, prostate, and genital skin in order to exert potent biologic effects.[169] The presence of multiple proteins with overlapping enzymatic activities (i.e., 17β-HSD and 5α-reductase) that catalyze these conversions in a large number of human tissues is supportive of this idea.[170, 171]

The general steroidogenic pathway for the production of estrogens and androgens is depicted in Figure 16–21. There are three major categories of ovarian steroids, as follows.

C_{18}-Steroids

The naturally occurring estrogens are C_{18}-steroids characterized by the presence of an aromatic A ring, a phenolic hydroxyl group at C-3, and either a hydroxyl group (estradiol) or a ketone group (estrone) at C-17. Aromatase is the key enzyme for estrogen production in the ovary (see Fig. 16–21). The protein $P450_{arom}$ confers the specific activity of the aromatase enzyme complex. $P450_{arom}$ production in the ovarian granulosa cell is regulated primarily by FSH.[150] The principal and most potent estrogen secreted by the ovary is estradiol. Although estrone is also secreted by the ovary, another important source of estrone is extraglandular conversion of androstenedione in peripheral tissues.[172] Estriol (16-hydroxyestradiol) is the most abundant estrogen in urine and is produced by the metabolism of estrone and estradiol in extraovarian tissues. All C_{18}-steroids including estrone, estradiol, and estriol are commonly referred to as estrogens. It should be pointed out, however, that estrone and estriol are only weakly estrogenic and must be converted

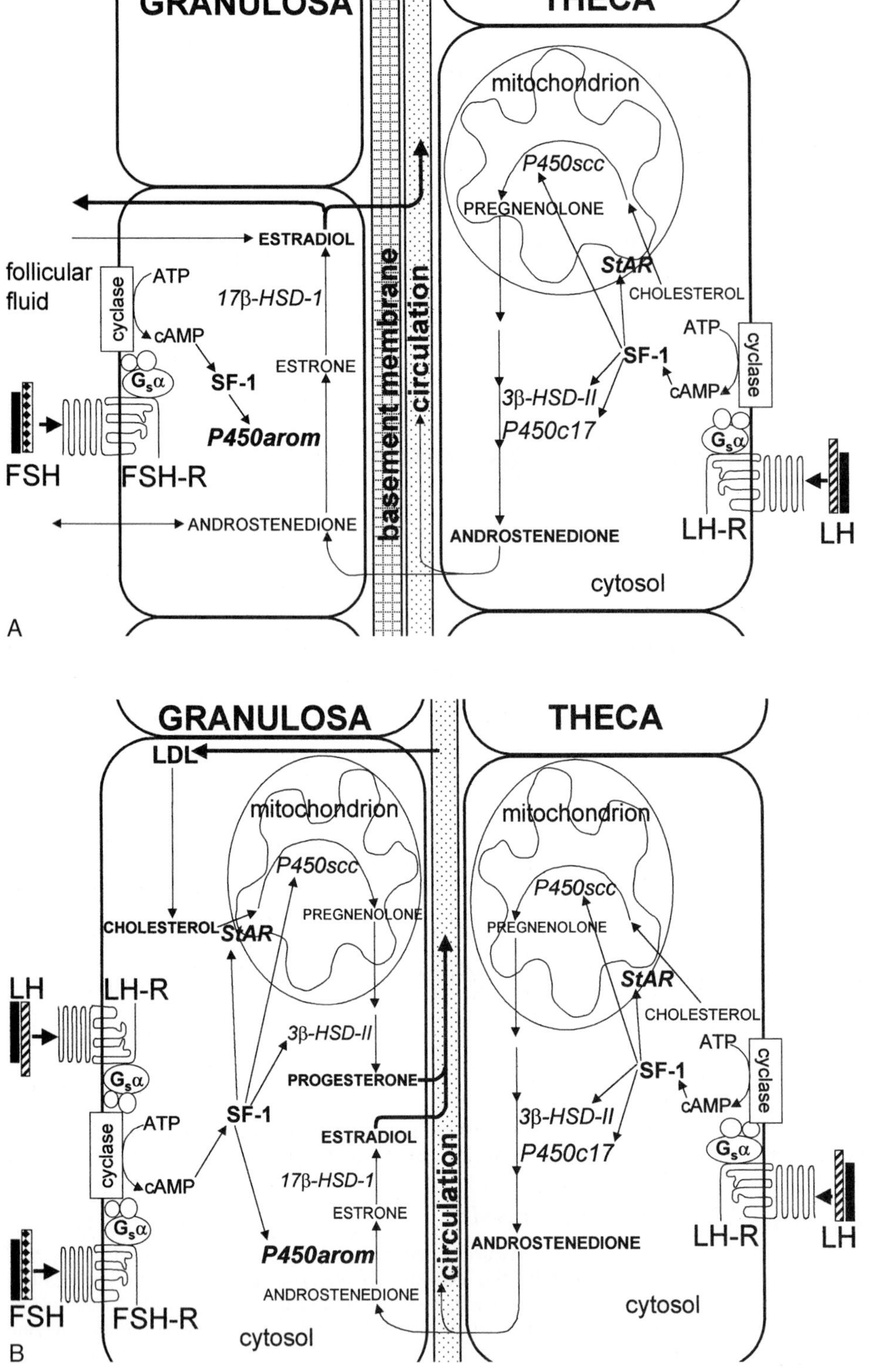

Figure 16–20. Two-cell hypothesis for ovarian steroidogenesis. *A*, The preovulatory follicle produces estradiol through a paracrine interaction between theca and granulosa cells. In response to stimulation with a gonadotropin, steroidogenic factor-1 (SF-1, a member of the orphan nuclear receptor family) acts as a master switch to initiate transcription of a series of steroidogenic genes in each cell type. Because granulosa cells do not have a direct connection to the circulation, aromatase (P450arom) in granulosa cells is dependent for substrate on androstenedione that diffuses from theca cells. Two critical steps in estradiol formation seem to be the entry of cholesterol into mitochondria facilitated by steroidogenic acute regulatory protein (StAR) in theca cells and the conversion of androstenedione to estrone catalyzed by P450arom in granulosa cells. *B*, In the corpus luteum, granulosa-lutein cells are heavily vascularized, which is critical for the entry of cholesterol into this cell type through primarily low-density lipoprotein receptors and for secretion of large amounts of progesterone into the circulation. The entry of cholesterol into mitochondria (by StAR) is likely to be the most critical steroidogenic step for progesterone formation in granulosa lutein cells. Androstenedione produced in theca-lutein cells serves as a substrate for estradiol produced in granulosa-lutein cells. Gonadotropins and the transcription factor SF-1 play key roles for important steroidogenic steps in both cell types. ATP, adenosine triphosphate; cAMP, cyclic adenosine monophosphate; FSH-R, follicle-stimulating hormone receptor; HSD, hydroxysteroid dehydrogenase; LH-R, luteinizing hormone receptor.

to estradiol to show full estrogenic action. There are at least seven enzymes in the 17β-HSD family with overlapping activities, which are capable of converting estrone to estradiol in the ovary and extraovarian tissues.[171]

Catechol estrogens are formed by hydroxylation of estrogens at the C-2 or C-4 position. The physiologic role of catechol estrogen, if any, is unclear. Low body weight and hyperthyroidism are associated with increased formation of catechol estrogens.[173] Estrone sulfate, formed by peripheral conversion of estradiol and estrone, is the most abundant estrogen in blood but is not physiologically active.[174] Estrone sulfate is presumed to serve as a reservoir for estrone formation in a number of tissues, including those that are targets of estrogen.[175] Estradiol regulates gonadotropin secretion and promotes development of the secondary sexual characteristics of women, uterine growth, thickening of the vaginal mucosa, thinning of the cervical mucus, and linear growth of the ductal system of the breast.

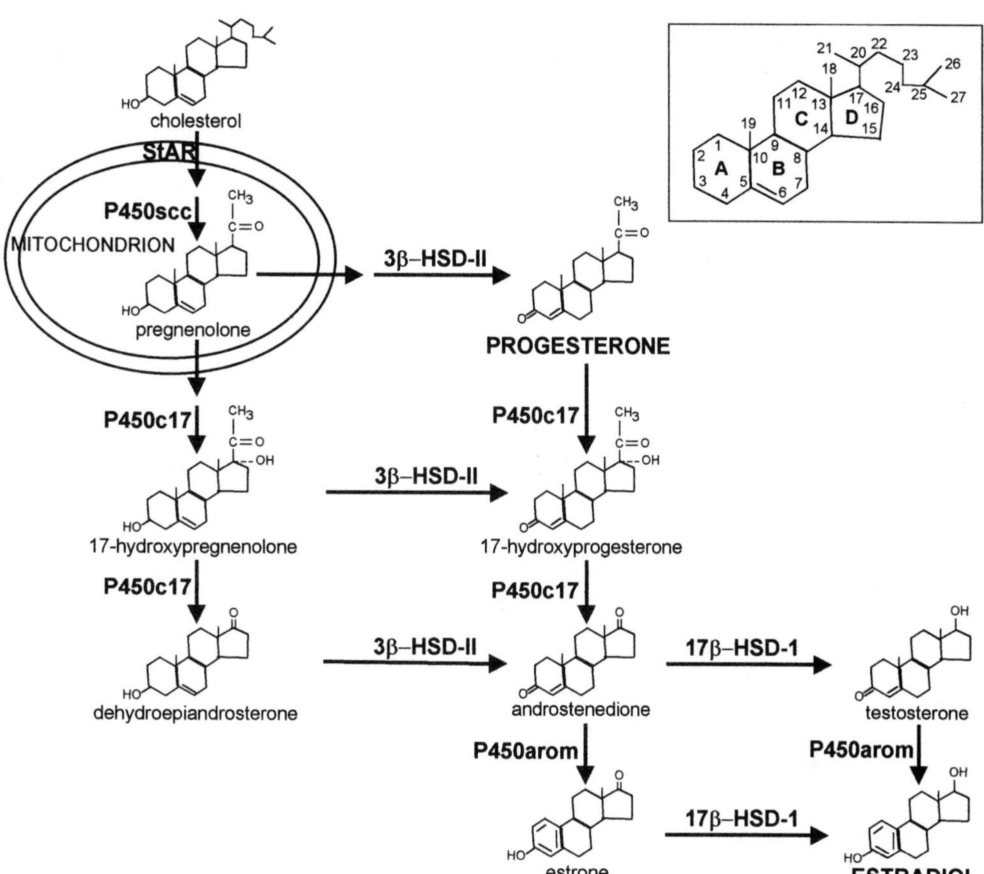

Figure 16–21. Steroidogenic pathway in the ovary. Biologically active steroids progesterone and estradiol are produced primarily in the ovary of a woman of reproductive age. Estradiol production requires the activity of six steroidogenic proteins including StAR and six enzymatic steps. P450c17, product of the CYP17 gene, catalyzes two enzymatic reactions. The four rings of the cholesterol molecule and its derivative steroids are identified by the first four letters in the alphabet, and the carbons are numbered in the sequence shown in the insert. 3β-HSD-II, 3β-hydroxysteroid dehydrogenase $\Delta^{5,4}$ isomerase type II; 17β-HSD-1, 17β-hydroxysteroid dehydrogenase type 1; P450arom, aromatase; P450c17, 17α-hydroxylase/17,20-lyase; StAR, steroidogenic acute regulatory protein.

C_{21}-Steroids

The principal progestogens are C_{21}-steroids and include pregnenolone, progesterone, and 17-hydroxyprogesterone (see Fig. 16–21). Pregnenolone is of primary importance in the ovary because of its key position as precursor of all steroid hormones. Progesterone is the principal secretory product of the corpus luteum and is responsible for the progestational effects (i.e., cell differentiation and induction of secretory activity in the endometrium of the estrogen-primed uterus). Progesterone is required for implantation of the fertilized ovum and maintenance of pregnancy. It also induces decidualization of the endometrium, inhibits uterine contractions, increases the viscosity of cervical mucus, promotes lateral (alveolar) development of the breast glands, and increases basal body temperature. On the other hand, 17-hydroxyprogesterone, also secreted by the corpus luteum, has little, if any, biologic activity.[174]

C_{19}-Steroids

The ovary secretes a variety of C_{19}-steriods, including DHEA, androstenedione, and testosterone (see Fig. 16–21). They are produced by the thecal cells and to a lesser degree by the ovarian stroma. The major C_{19}-steroid is androstenedione, part of which is secreted directly into plasma, with the remainder converted to estrogen by the granulosa cells. Androstenedione can be converted to estrogen or testosterone in the ovary and in extraglandular tissues. Only testosterone and DHT but not androstenedione are true androgens with the capacity of interacting with the androgen receptor (see later).

Steroids formed by the ovary, as well as other steroid-producing organs, are derived from cholesterol (see Fig. 16–21). There are several sources of cholesterol that can provide the ovary with substrate for steroidogenesis. These include (1) plasma lipoprotein cholesterol, (2) cholesterol synthesized de novo within the ovary, and (3) cholesterol from intracellular stores of cholesterol esters within lipid droplets. In the human ovary, LDL cholesterol is an important source of cholesterol utilized for steroidogenesis.[126] LH stimulates the activity of adenylate cyclase, increasing production of cyclic adenosine monophosphate (cAMP), which serves as a second messenger to increase LDL receptor mRNA and the binding and uptake of LDL cholesterol as well as the formation of cholesterol esters.[124, 126] LDL-derived cholesterol is particularly essential for normal levels of progesterone production in the granulosa lutein cells of the corpus luteum (see Fig. 16–20*B*).[126]

The first and rate-limiting step in the synthesis of all ovarian steroid hormones is the movement of cholesterol into the mitochondrion, which is regulated by StAR (see Fig. 16–21).[176] This movement is followed by conversion of cholesterol to pregnenolone, catalyzed by the mitochondrial enzyme complex consisting of $P450_{scc}$, adrenodoxin, and flavoprotein.[177] LH induces steroidogenesis by increasing intracellular cAMP, which increases the conversion of cholesterol to pregnenolone in two distinct ways: (1) acute regulation, over minutes, occurs through the phosphorylation of preexisting StAR and rapid synthesis of new StAR protein, and (2) chronic stimulation, within hours to days, occurs through the induction of $P450_{scc}$ expression and consequent increased steroidogenesis (see Fig. 16–20). StAR increases the flow of cholesterol to mitochondria, thus regulating substrate availability to whatever amount of $P450_{scc}$ is available on the inner mitochondrial membrane.[176] In the absence of StAR, only 14% of the maximal StAR-induced level of steroidogenesis persists as StAR-independent steroidogenesis.[176]

StAR expression in the preovulatory graafian follicle is limited primarily to the thecal cells (see Fig. 16–20).[178] The most important product of the thecal cell during the follicular phase is the estrogen precursor androstenedione, whose production is controlled primarily by StAR (see Fig. 16–20*B*). The biologically active steroid product of the ovary during the follicular phase is estradiol that arises from the granulosa cells located adjacent to theca cells (see Fig. 16–20*A*). The rate-limiting step for granulosa cell estradiol production is regulated by the FSH-dependent activity of the aromatase enzyme in a cyclic fashion (see Fig. 16–20).[150] During the luteal phase, cells of the corpus luteum, including granulosa lutein cells, also show intense StAR immunoreactivity with a patchy distribution (see Fig. 16–20*B*).[178] The delivery of cholesterol to the mitochondrial side-chain cleavage enzyme system in the corpus luteum is the rate-limiting step for progesterone biosynthesis and is regulated by StAR (see Fig. 16–20*B*).[128] Thus, estradiol production seems to be regulated primarily by StAR and $P450_{arom}$, whereas progesterone biosynthesis is under the control of StAR.

The ovarian granulosa, theca, and corpus luteum cells possess StAR plus five distinct proteins with specific enzyme activities for steroid hormone formation. These steroidogenic enzymes are $P450_{scc}$, 3β-HSD-II, $P450_{c17}$, $P450_{arom}$, and 17β-HSD-1.[150, 179, 180] These enzymes are responsible for the conversion of cholesterol to the two major biologically active products estradiol and progesterone.[181]

Steroidogenesis dependent on LH and FSH in both theca and granulosa cells is mediated by common signaling molecules including cAMP and the transcription factor steroidogenic factor-1 (SF-1) (see Fig. 16–20).[182, 183] SF-1 regulates the expression of genes that encode StAR, $P450_{scc}$, 3β-HSD-II, $P450_{c17}$, and $P450_{arom}$ (see Fig. 16–20). Thus, SF-1 can be regarded as a downstream master switch that orchestrates ovarian steroidogenesis.[183]

Summary of Updated Two-Cell Theory for Ovarian Steroidogenesis

The classical two-cell theory is supported by molecular findings in the following fashion. Ovarian steroidogenesis in the preovulatory follicle takes place through LH receptors on theca and FSH (possibly plus LH) receptors on granulosa cells (see Fig. 16–20). Cyclic AMP production and increased SF-1 binding to multiple steroidogenic promoters mediate LH action in theca cells. In particular, StAR is the primary regulator of production of androstenedione that subsequently diffuses into granulosa cells to serve as the estrogen precursor. In the preovulatory follicle, cholesterol in theca cells arises from circulating lipoproteins and de novo biosynthesis. FSH is responsible for follicular growth and also estrogen formation. FSH induces cAMP formation, increased SF-1 binding activity, and $P450_{arom}$ expression in preovulatory granulosa cells to give rise to estradiol formation primarily through aromatization of androstenedione (see Fig. 16–20).

In the corpus luteum, large deposits of cholesterol (i.e., the yellow color) arise primarily from circulating lipoproteins to support production of extremely high quantities of progesterone. Other key anatomic events in formation of the corpus luteum are the disruption of the basement membrane between the granulosa and theca and strikingly increased vascularization of granulosa lutein cells (see Fig. 16–17). Theca lutein cells possess LH receptors and produce androstenedione. Cyclic AMP, SF-1, and StAR induced by LH remain as the key regulators for biosynthesis of thecal androstenedione, which serves as the estrogen precursor in neighboring granulosa lutein cells.

The granulosa lutein cell of the corpus luteum is both anatomically and functionally different from its counterpart in the preovulatory follicle. First, these cells are luteinized and heavily vascularized and contain large quantities of cholesterol. Second, granulosa lutein cells contain high levels of LH receptors in addition to FSH receptors. Third, they produce large quantities of progesterone that is regulated primarily by LH and StAR. Granulosa lutein cells also aromatize androstenedione of thecal origin and eventually give rise to estradiol formation through FSH action and $P450_{arom}$. The common known mediators of LH and FSH in granulosa lutein cells are cAMP and increased SF-1 binding activity. Specific functions of these two gonadotropins (i.e., differentiation, growth, and progesterone formation versus estradiol formation) are probably determined by as yet unidentified modifying factors (see Fig. 16–20).

Peptide Hormones Produced by Ovary

The ovary produces a large number of peptides that can act in an intracrine, autocrine, paracrine, or endocrine fashion. These include numerous growth factors (e.g., insulin-like growth factors [IGFs]) and cytokines (e.g., interleukin-1β).

The group of peptides including inhibin, activin, and follistatin are produced in ovarian granulosa cells under the control of FSH (see Fig. 16–1). The production of inhibin and activin is not limited to the ovary. A number of other tissues, including the adrenal, pituitary, and placenta, synthesize these peptides. It has been well established that inhibin plays a major regulatory role in FSH production in the pituitary. Inhibin is a 32-kd glycoprotein composed of two subunits, α (18 kd) and β (12 kd), linked by disulfide bonds.[184] Structurally, inhibin is a heterodimer composed of a common α subunit but different β subunits, denoted β_A and β_B. The forms of inhibin, $\alpha\beta_A$ and $\alpha\beta_B$, are termed A and B, respectively. Although inhibin is produced by a number of tissues in the body, the majority is derived from the gonads. In the ovary, the source of inhibin is granulosa cells. The main role of inhibin, for which it was discovered and named, is to suppress FSH production in the pituitary (see Fig. 16–1).

Although both isoforms of inhibin seem to have similar biologic properties, their synthesis is regulated differently during the follicular and luteal phases. Inhibin B is secreted mainly during the early follicular phase, with levels decreasing in midfollicular phase and becoming undetectable after the LH surge.[185] Inhibin A levels are low during the first half of the follicular phase but increase gradually during midfollicular phase with a peak during the luteal phase. All three subunits are detected in small antral follicles by immunohistochemistry and in situ hybridization.[186–188] The α and β_A subunits are found in the dominant follicle and in the corpus luteum. All three subunits are expressed in response to gonadotropins or factors that increase intracellular cAMP.[189, 190] The mechanisms underlying the regulation of the different parts of the menstrual cycle by inhibin isoforms need further study for a fuller understanding.

Activin is structurally related to inhibin but may exert opposite actions. Activin contains two subunits that are identical to the β subunits of inhibins A and B. Thus, the three activin isoforms are activin A ($\beta_A\beta_A$), activin B ($\beta_B\beta_B$), and activin AB ($\beta_A\beta_B$). In the pituitary, activin stimulates the release of FSH. In the ovarian follicle, activin enhances FSH action.

Overview of the Hormonal Changes during the Ovarian Cycle

FSH secretion is suppressed by negative feedback of the ovarian hormones estrogen, inhibin, and progesterone during the early and midluteal phase. Upon the regression of the corpus luteum during the late luteal phase, however, the sharp decline in estrogen, inhibin, and progesterone abolishes this negative feedback (Fig. 16–22). This permits increased secre-

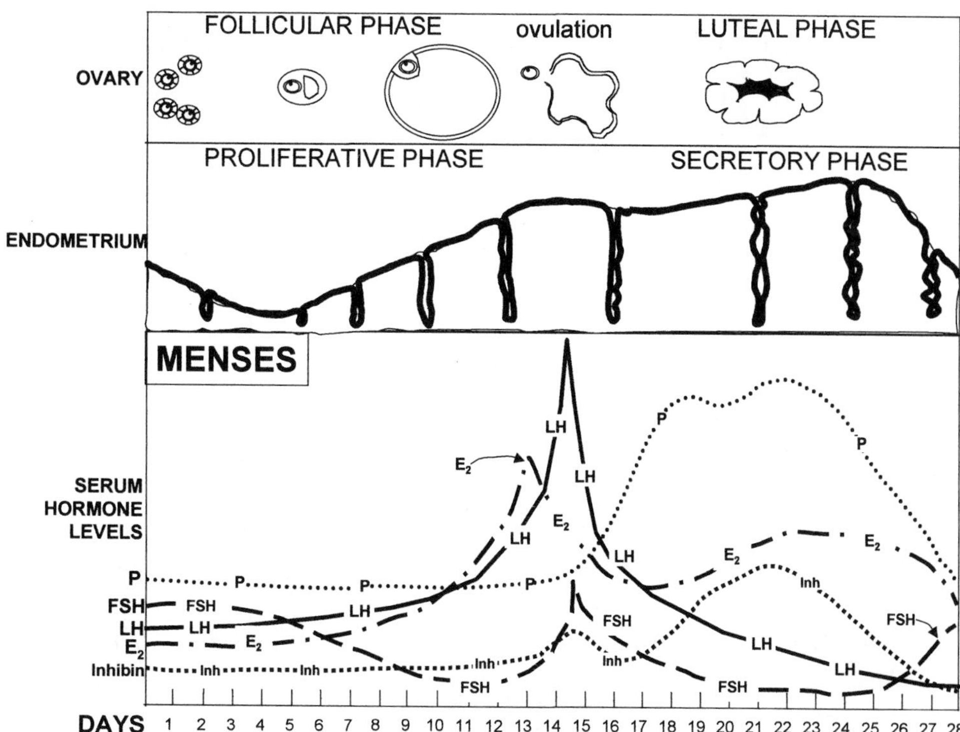

Figure 16–22. Changes in the ovarian follicle, endometrial thickness, and serum hormone levels during a 28-day menstrual cycle. Menses occur during the first few days of the cycle. E_2, estradiol; FSH, follicle-stimulating hormone; LH, luteinizing hormone; Inh, inhibin; P, progesterone.

tion of FSH just before and during menses. This initial increase in FSH is essential for follicle recruitment and growth and steroidogenesis (see Fig. 16–22). With continued growth of the follicle, autocrine and paracrine factors produced within the follicle maintain follicular sensitivity to FSH. Continuing and combined action of FSH and activin leads to the appearance of LH receptors on the granulosa cells, a prerequisite for ovulation and luteinization.

Ovulation is triggered by the rapid rise in circulating levels of estradiol. A positive feedback response at the level of the anterior pituitary and possibly at the hypothalamus results in the midcycle surge of LH necessary for expulsion of the egg and formation of the corpus luteum (see Fig. 16–22). A rise in progesterone follows ovulation along with a second rise in estradiol, producing the 14-day-long luteal phase characterized by low FSH and LH levels. The demise of the corpus luteum concomitant with a fall in hormone (progesterone, estradiol, and inhibin A) levels allows FSH to increase again toward the end of the luteal phase, thus initiating a new cycle (see Fig. 16–22). If pregnancy is established by the implantation of a blastocyst, however, the structural integrity and function (progesterone and estradiol production) of the corpus luteum are maintained by hCG that is secreted from the trophoblast. The hCG acts as a surrogate for LH on the corpus luteum.

In addition to FSH and LH, local factors (e.g., activin and inhibin) regulate follicular development and steroidogenesis. In the early follicular phase, activin produced by granulosa in immature follicles enhances the action of FSH on aromatase activity and FSH and LH receptor formation while simultaneously suppressing C_{19}-steroid formation in theca cells. In the late follicular phase, increased production of inhibin by the granulosa and decreased activin promote the synthesis of C_{19}-steroids in the theca layer in response to LH and local growth factors and cytokines to provide larger amounts of the precursor androstenedione for the production of estrone and ultimately estradiol in the granulosa cells (see Fig. 16–20).[185]

Both LH-mediated androstenedione production in theca cells and FSH-mediated estradiol production in granulosa cells are potentiated by IGFs.[191] The major endogenous IGF produced in the human ovarian follicle is IGF-II (versus IGF-I) in both granulosa and theca cells.[192] The actions of both IGF-I and IGF-II are mediated by IGF receptor type I in both cells. IGF receptor type I is structurally similar to the insulin receptor. Thus, it appears that gonadotropin-related IGF action in the ovary is regulated primarily by IGF-II and IGF receptor type I.[191]

In summary, ovulation is under the control of substances functioning as classical hormones (FSH, LH, estradiol, and inhibin) transmitting messages between the ovary and the hypothalamic-pituitary axis and paracrine and autocrine factors such as IGF-II, inhibin, and activin, which coordinate sequential activities within the follicle destined to ovulate. The negative feedback relationship between corpus luteum products (estradiol, progesterone, and inhibin) and FSH results in the critical initial rise in FSH immediately before and during menses, and the positive feedback relationship between estradiol and LH is responsible for the ovulatory stimulus (see Fig. 16–22). Within the ovary, IGF-II, inhibin, and activin modify follicular responses necessary for growth and function. These endocrine, paracrine, and autocrine factors undoubtedly represent only a portion of a complete picture. The causes of anovulation are diverse and may be related to defects in cell-surface receptors, intracellular elements of signal transduction, or cell-cell interactions.[193]

Extraovarian Steroidogenesis

Estradiol formation takes place in a number of tissues in the woman of reproductive age. These tissues may be placed in three categories: (1) the ovary, (2) peripheral tissues such as subcutaneous fat and skin, and (3) physiologic and pathologic target sites such as the hypothalamus, breast cancer cells, and the cells of endometriosis (Fig. 16–23).[169] The latter two sources of estrogen are particularly critical in anovulatory premenopausal and postmenopausal women. Although small quantities of estrogen are produced by an individual adipose or skin fibroblast in a continuous fashion, these cell types contribute to circulating estradiol levels because of their relative abun-

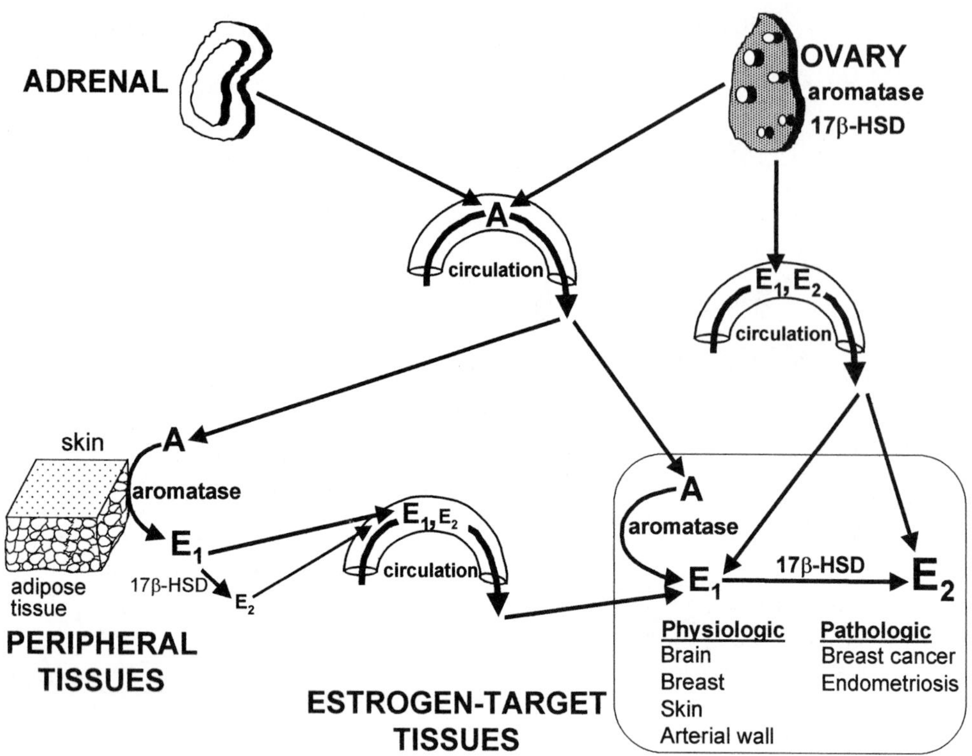

Figure 16–23. Estrogen biosynthesis in women. The biologically active estrogen estradiol (E_2) is produced in at least three major sites: (1) by direct secretion from the ovary in reproductive-age women; (2) by conversion of circulating androstenedione (A) of adrenal or ovarian origins, or both, to estrone (E_1) in peripheral tissues; and (3) by conversion of A to E_1 in estrogen target tissues. In the latter two instances, estrogenically weak E_1 is further converted to E_2 within the same tissue. The presence of the enzyme aromatase and 17β-hydroxysteroid dehydrogenase (17β-HSD) is critical for E_2 formation at these sites. E_2 formation by peripheral and local conversion is particularly important in postmenopausal women and in estrogen-dependent diseases such as breast cancer, endometriosis, and endometrial cancer.

dance (see Fig. 16–23).[169] This effect is more pronounced in obese women because of increased mass of the adipose tissue and skin.[166]

$P450_{arom}$ in adipose and skin fibroblasts is responsible for peripheral aromatization of androstenedione that arises from both the ovary and adrenal in premenopausal women and primarily from the adrenal in postmenopausal women (see Fig. 16–23). The product of this reaction, estrone, is only weakly estrogenic, however. Estrone is further converted to estrone sulfate, which serves as a reservoir for estrone in blood and other tissues.[175] Estrone (arising from androstenedione and estrone sulfate) is further converted to the biologically active estradiol in target tissues such as the endometrium and breast by a number of enzymatic proteins with overlapping reductive 17β-HSD activity (see Fig. 16–23).[171, 194, 195] It is likely that local $P450_{arom}$ expression in hypothalamus is critical for the regulation of gonadotropin secretion.[156] Finally, estrogen-dependent pathologic tissues such as those in breast cancer and endometriosis contain extremely high levels of $P450_{arom}$ that enhances tissue growth by increasing local estradiol concentrations (see Fig. 16–23).[196] Circulating androstenedione is the major substrate for aromatase activity in these physiologic and pathologic target tissues.[194, 196]

Significant quantities of circulating androstenedione can also be converted to testosterone in peripheral tissues (see later).[167] This is probably accomplished by the presence of multiple 17β-HSDs with overlapping reductive activities in peripheral tissues.[171] Androgenic action of testosterone is strikingly amplified by its conversion to DHT in peripheral and target tissues (e.g., skin and prostate). At least two distinct proteins encoded by two separate genes, 5α-reductase type 1 and type 2, catalyze the conversion of testosterone to DHT in the liver, prostate, and skin.[170] Local production of DHT in genital skin fibroblasts is critical for normal masculinization of external genitalia of male fetuses in utero.[170] DHT formation in the skin is also important in the etiology of hirsutism (see later).[197]

Endometrium

The endometrium is the mucosal lining of the uterine cavity. The decidua is the highly modified and specialized endometrium of pregnancy. From the evolutionary perspective, the human endometrium is highly developed to accommodate the hemochorioendothelial type of placentation, which requires the presence of spiral arteries (Fig. 16–24). Trophoblasts of the blastocyst invade spiral arteries during implantation and placentation in the establishment of uteroplacental vessels.

Spiral arteries of the human endometrium also confer another unique process termed menstruation. Menstruation is shedding of endometrial tissue with hemorrhage that is dependent upon sex steroid hormone–directed changes in blood flow in the spiral arteries. The presence of spiral arteries is essential for menstruation because only the human and a few other primates that have endometrial spiral arteries experience menstruation. With nonfertile but ovulatory ovarian cycles, menstruation affects desquamation of the endometrium. New endometrial growth and development must be initiated with each ovarian cycle, so that endometrial maturation corresponds rather precisely with the next opportunity for pregnancy. There seems to be a narrow window of endometrial receptivity to blastocyst implantation that corresponds to the period between days 20 and 24 during a 28-day menstrual cycle.[198, 199]

Functional Anatomy of the Endometrium

The endometrium can be divided morphologically into an upper two-thirds *functionalis* layer and a lower one-third *basalis* layer (see Fig. 16–24). The purpose of the functionalis layer is to prepare for the implantation of the blastocyst; therefore, it is the site of proliferation, secretion, and degeneration. The purpose of the basalis layer is to provide the regenerative endometrium following menstrual loss of the functionalis.[200] Major histologic components of the endometrium include (1) stromal cells that constitute the skeleton of the tissue, (2) a

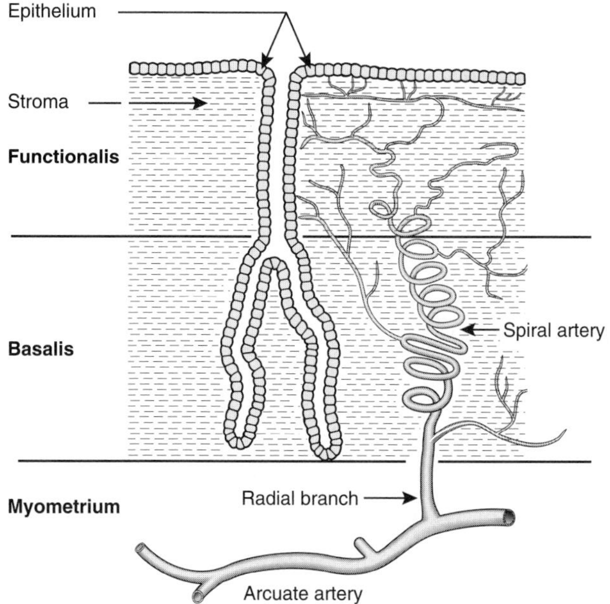

Figure 16–24. Functional anatomy of the endometrium. Endometrium is a multilayered mucosa specialized for implantation and support of pregnancy. A single, continuous layer of epithelial cells lines the surface of the stroma and penetrates the stroma with deep invaginations almost all the way down to the myometrium-endometrium junction. The entire thickness of the endometrium is penetrated by the spiral arteries and their capillaries. Spiral arteries originate from the radial branches of arcuate arteries, which in turn arise from uterine arteries. The superficial layer (functionalis) is shed during menstruation, whereas the permanent bottom layer (basalis) gives rise to the regeneration of endometrium after each menstruation. The striking changes in the spiral arteries (coiling, stasis, vasodilatation followed by intense vasoconstriction) are consistently observed before the onset of every menstruation episode. (Courtesy of Kristof Chwalisz.)

single layer of epithelial cells that lines the lumen of the endometrial cavity and invaginations of the stroma, (3) blood vessels, and (4) resident immune cells. The epithelial cells that line the rather deep invaginations of the stroma are also referred to as *glandular cells*. It should be noted, however, that these deep crypts represent simply extensions of the intracavitary lumen and are not true glands. These invaginations lined by epithelial cells extend from the surface of the functionalis layer (i.e., luminal epithelium) deep into the basalis level (the so-called glandular epithelium). Thus, after the functionalis layer is shed at the time of menstruation, the basalis that contains both epithelial and stromal cells can give rise to a new functionalis layer for the upcoming cycle (Fig. 16–25).

The cellular components of the functionalis layer undergo a striking progression during the menstrual cycle, whereas the basalis shows only modest alterations. The sequence of endometrial changes associated with an ovulatory cycle has been carefully studied by Noyes and colleagues[198] in the human and Markee[201, 202] and Bartelmez[203, 204] in the subhuman primate. The histologic changes that occur in the endometrium during the nonfertile but ovulatory menstrual cycle are summarized in Figure 16–26 as described originally by Noyes and co-workers.[198]

Hormone-Induced Morphologic Changes of the Endometrium

The cyclic changes in endometrial histology are faithfully reproduced during each ovulatory ovarian cycle. These sex steroid hormone–induced modifications can be summarized as follows. (1) During the preovulatory, or follicular, phase of the cycle, estradiol is secreted (principally by a single dominant follicle of one ovary) in increasing quantities until just before ovulation. (2) During the postovulatory, or luteal, phase of the cycle, progesterone is secreted by the corpus luteum in increasing amounts (up to 40 to 50 mg/day) until the midluteal

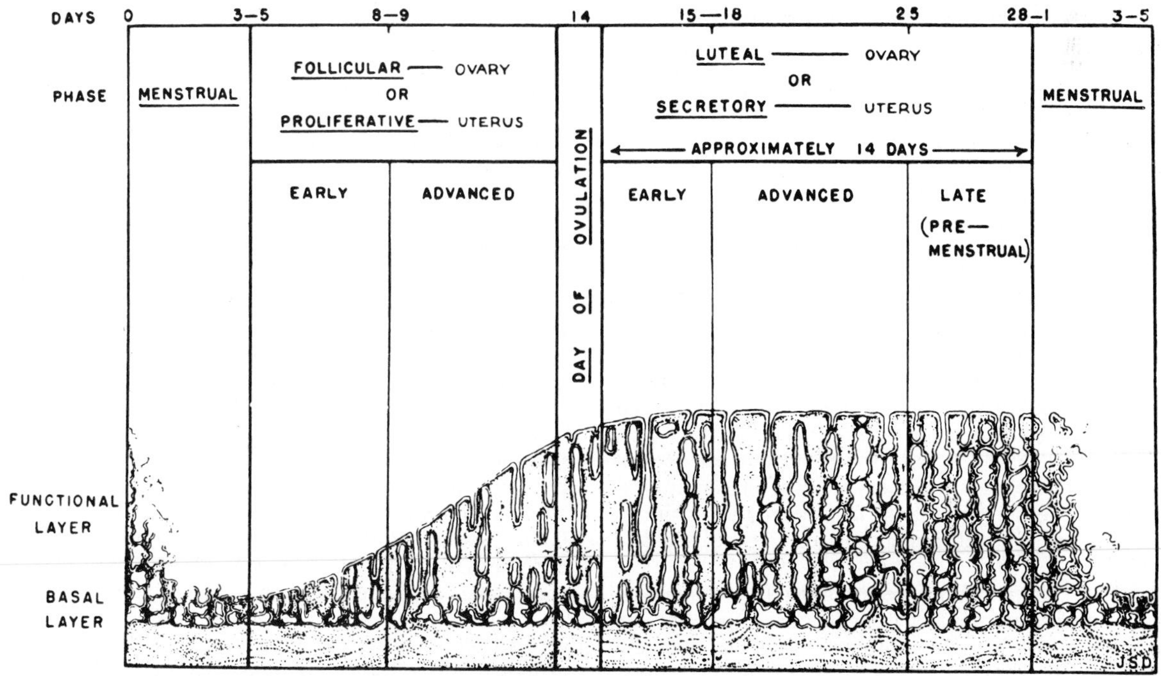

Figure 16–25. Cyclic changes in thickness and morphology of endometrium and the relation of these changes to those of the ovarian cycle. (From Cunningham FG, MacDonald PC, Gant NF, et al. The endometrium and decidua: menstruation and pregnancy. In Williams Obstetrics, 19th ed. Stamford, Conn, Appleton & Lange, 1993, pp 81–109.)

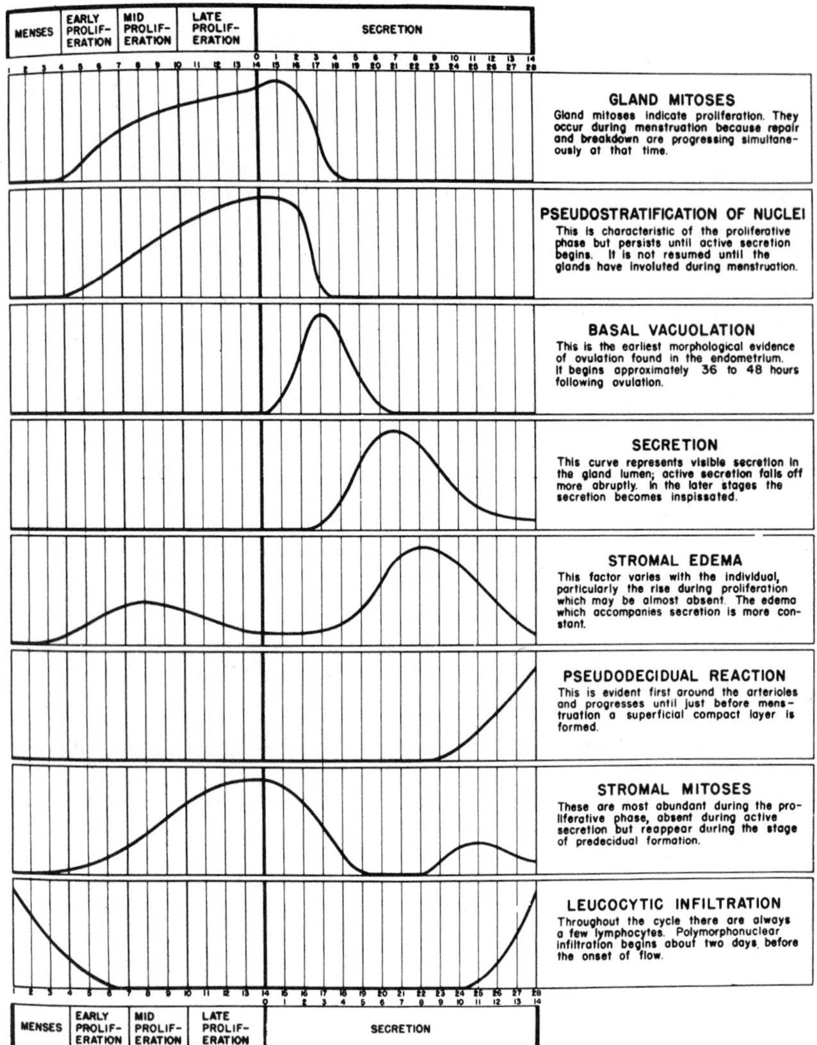

Figure 16–26. Dating the endometrium by morphology. (From Noyes RW, Hertig AW, Rock J. Dating the endometrial biopsy. Fertil Steril 1950; 1:3–25.)

phase. (3) Beginning about 7 to 8 days after ovulation, the rates of progesterone (and estrogen) secretion by the corpus luteum begin to decline and then diminish progressively before menstruation (see Fig. 16–22).

In response to these cyclic changes in the rates of ovarian sex steroid hormone secretion, there are five main stages of the corresponding endometrial cycle: (1) menstrual-postmenstrual *reepithelialization*; (2) *endometrial proliferation* in response to stimulation by estradiol; (3) abundant *epithelial secretion*, in response to the combined action of estradiol and progesterone; (4) *premenstrual ischemia*, the result of endometrial tissue volume involution, which causes stasis of blood in the spiral arteries; and (5) *menstruation*, which is preceded and accompanied by severe vasoconstriction of the endometrial spiral arteries and collapse and desquamation of all but the deepest layer of the endometrium. In the final analysis, menstruation is the consequence of the withdrawal of factors that maintain endometrial growth and differentiation (see Figs. 16–25 and 16–26).

Commonly, the initiation of menstruation is attributed to progesterone withdrawal. This concept was developed because the administration of estrogen to postmenopausal women and thence treatment or withdrawal with a progestin affect menstruation, even with continued estrogen treatment. Moreover, progesterone facilitates and permits decidualization of the endometrium and the maintenance of pregnancy, whereas progesterone withdrawal favors the initiation of menstruation, lactation, and parturition. There are probably multiple additional coordinated and interactive processes (other than progesterone withdrawal) that are operative and essential for the success of each of these events.

Both the preovulatory (follicular or proliferative) phase and the postovulatory (luteal or secretory) phase of the ovarian-endometrial cycles are customarily divided into early and late stages (see Fig. 16–22). The normal secretory phase of the endometrial (menstrual) cycle can be subdivided rather finely (almost day by day), by histologic criteria, from shortly after ovulation until the onset of menstruation. In fact, Noyes and other investigators[198] have provided an extremely detailed description of the histologic features of the secretory phase endometrium, which permit accurate dating during the luteal phase (see Fig. 16–26). Gynecologists use the histologic dating of the endometrial biopsies obtained during the luteal phase to evaluate ovulation, progesterone production, or the degree of biologic response of the endometrium to progesterone. Normal endometrial development is assumed when the histologic and chronologic endometrial dating agree within 2 days. When they differ by more than 2 days, the endometrium is considered to be out of phase. Out-of-phase endometrial tissue was proposed to be a cause of implantation failure giving rise to infertility. Understanding the limitations of this test is important, if infertility treatments are based on biopsy results, because the sensitivity and the specificity of the dating of endometrial biopsy for the evaluation of infertility are unknown.

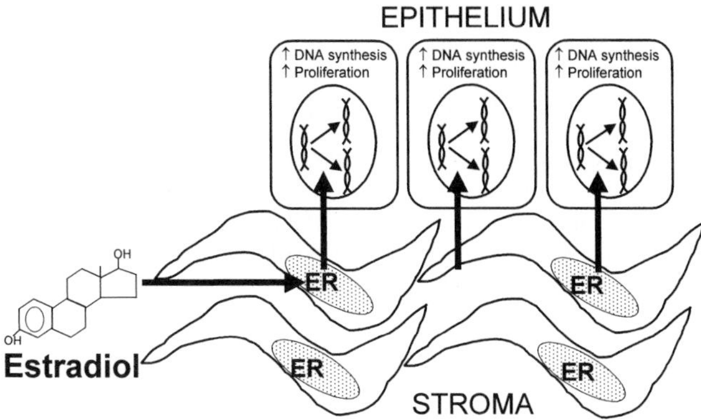

Figure 16–27. Critical epithelial effects of estrogen (e.g., deoxyribonucleic acid [DNA] synthesis, proliferation, and gene expression) are mediated primarily by estrogen receptor α (ER) in stromal cells in a paracrine manner in the endometrium.

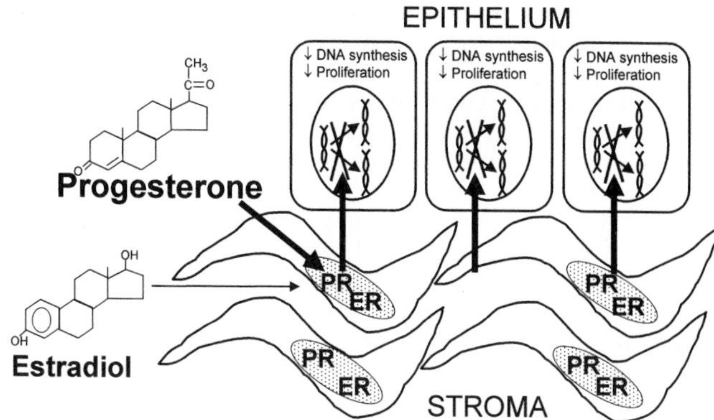

Figure 16–28. The antiestrogenic effects of progesterone on epithelial cells (e.g., decreased proliferation and enhanced differentiation) are mediated primarily by progesterone receptors (PRs) in stromal cells in a paracrine manner in the endometrium. DNA, deoxyribonucleic acid; ER, estrogen receptor α.

For example, one important disadvantage of this test is interobserver variation in histologic interpretation of biopsies.

Effects of Ovarian Steroids on Endometrium

Estradiol or synthetic estrogens cause a striking thickening of endometrial tissue. Both stromal and epithelial cells of the endometrium proliferate rapidly under the influence of estradiol. Estrogen increases mitotic activity and DNA synthesis in both cell types strikingly (Fig. 16–27). While promoting growth, estrogen also renders endometrial tissue responsive to progesterone by inducing the expression of progesterone receptors (PRs) in this tissue because progesterone action is dependent on previous or concurrent estrogen exposure of the endometrium.[205]

In contrast to the proliferative effects of estrogen, progesterone action primarily gives rise to the differentiation of the endometrium. For example, progesterone can inhibit and even reverse the proliferative action of estrogen on the functionalis layer (Fig. 16–28). Moreover, progesterone action prepares the endometrium for implantation of the embryo through differentiation of both epithelial and stromal cells. Progesterone induces the production and secretion of a glycogen-rich substance from the epithelial cells. Progesterone also causes an increase in the stromal cell cytoplasm, a process called *pseudodecidualization.*

Estrogen Action

Estradiol, the biologically potent, naturally occurring estrogen, which is secreted by the granulosa cells of the dominant ovarian follicle, acts to promote responses of the endometrium in a manner that is classical for steroid hormone action. Estradiol enters cells from blood by simple diffusion, but in estrogen-responsive cells, binding to the ER sequesters estradiol. ERs are proteins with high affinity for estradiol and other biologically active estrogens, that is, synthetic estrogens. The ER subtypes α and β are discussed in various chapters of this textbook. Although both ERα and ERβ are present in the endometrium, ERα seems to be the primary mediator of the estrogenic action in the endometrium.[206, 207] The estradiol-receptor complex, after transformational changes, is a transcriptional factor that becomes associated with the estrogen response elements of specific genes. This interaction brings about ER-specific initiation of gene transcription, which promotes the synthesis of specific mRNAs and thereafter the synthesis of specific proteins.[208] Among the many proteins synthesized in most estrogen-responsive cells are additional ERs, as well as PRs. Thus, estradiol acts in the endometrium and in other estrogen-responsive tissues to promote the perpetuation of estrogen action and to promote the responsiveness of that tissue to progesterone.

The endometrial epithelial cells are estrogen-responsive but probably do not replicate as a result of the direct action of estradiol on the epithelial cells. Replication of human endometrial epithelial cells in culture is not increased appreciably, if at all, when estrogen is added to the medium. Further, estrogen acts on mouse uterine stromal cells to promote the synthesis of epithelial cell growth factors (see Fig. 16–27).[209] These growth factors operate in a paracrine manner to cause increased DNA synthesis and replication in the adjacent epithelial cells. This type of paracrine arrangement may be the primary mechanism that mediates estrogen action in hormone-responsive tissues.

Progesterone Action

Progesterone also enters cells by diffusion and in responsive tissues becomes associated with PRs with high affinity for progesterone.[210] The two PR isoforms, PR-A and PR-B, are both present in the human endometrium.[211] Because PR-B but not PR-A levels in the endometrium are tightly regulated during the human menstrual cycle, PR-B is presumed to play a more important biologic role.[211] Commonly, the cellular content of PRs is dependent on previous estrogen action. The progesterone-PR complex also promotes gene transcription, but the response to progesterone is strikingly different from that evoked by the estradiol-ER complex.

Progesterone actions include a decrease in the synthesis of ER molecules.[212] This is one means by which progesterone (and synthetic progestins) attenuates estrogen action. Progesterone also acts to increase the rate of enzymatic inactivation of estradiol to estrone through an increase in the activity of an oxidative type 17β-HSD enzyme.[213] Progesterone-dependent transcription of a specific gene, namely 17β-HSD type 2, is responsible for this enzyme activity.[214] Progesterone also acts to increase sulfation of estrogens (estrogen sulfotransferase), another means of estrogen inactivation.[215] Therefore, progesterone acts as an antiestrogen in at least three ways: (1) by reducing the rate of synthesis of ERs, (2) by bringing about a decrease in the tissue levels of estradiol (through conversion to estrone), and (3) by enhancing estrogen inactivation through sulfation. As in the case of estrogen action in the uterus, tissue recombination experiments using uteri of PR knockout and normal mice demonstrated that many effects of progesterone on epithelial cells are also mediated in a paracrine fashion by PRs in stromal cells but not by those in epithelial cells (see Fig. 16–28).[216]

The most striking consequence of progesterone action is the differentiation of the endometrium. The histologic correlates of differentiation, stromal decidualization and epithelial secretion, are correlated with the presence of nuclear PRs and increased levels of circulating progesterone during the luteal phase.[210] Molecular correlates of progesterone action with respect to differentiation include increased production of lactoferrin and glycodelin in epithelial cells and prolactin and IGF binding protein 1 in stromal cells of the endometrium.

The Receptive Phase of the Endometrium for Implantation

Unless the ovum is fertilized within 24 hours of ovulation, it does not survive. Fertilization takes place in the ampullary (one third distal) portion of the oviduct. Over the next 2 days, the fertilized ovum remains unattached within the tubal lumen, utilizing tubal fluids and residual attached cumulus granulosa cells to sustain nutrition and energy for early cellular cleavage. After this stage, the solid ball of cells (morula), which is the embryo, leaves the oviduct and enters the uterine cavity. Fortunately, by this time endometrial secretions under the influence of luteal progesterone have filled the cavity and bathe the embryo in nutrients. This is the first of many neatly synchronized events that mark the conceptus-endometrial relationship. By 6 days after ovulation, the embryo (now a blastocyst) is ready to attach and implant. At this time, it finds an endometrial lining of sufficient depth, vascularity, and nutritional richness to sustain the important events of early placentation to follow. Just below the epithelial lining, a rich capillary plexus has been formed and is available for creation of the trophoblast–maternal blood interface. Later, the surrounding superficial portion of the functionalis zone, now occupying more and more of the endometrial cavity, provides a sturdy splint to retain endometrial architecture despite the invasive inroads of the burgeoning trophoblast.

Progesterone is essential for the maintenance of pregnancy. The blastocyst is dependent on progesterone produced by the corpus luteum at this time. The hCG that is secreted by the trophoblast prevents the regression of the corpus luteum by acting as a surrogate LH. This serves to maintain a continued supply of progesterone for the maintenance of pregnancy until the placental tissue itself starts to produce sufficient quantities of progesterone by 6 to 7 weeks after fertilization.

Studies in experimental and domestic animals have demonstrated that there must be synchronous development of the embryo and endometrium for normal implantation and development to occur.[217] In laboratory animals, there is a discrete window for implantation, which in some species lasts only a matter of hours.

The receptive phase of the endometrium is the temporal window of endometrial maturation during which the trophectoderm of the blastocyst can attach to the endometrial epithelial cells and subsequently proceed to invade the endometrial stroma.[198] In the study of human endometrial receptivity, a key question is the determination of the temporal window of implantation. Only factors expressed during this temporal window can be considered either markers or functional mediators of the receptive state.

The window of uterine receptivity can be inferred from what has been learned from transfer of embryos to uteri of women primed with exogenous estrogen and progesterone preparations (Fig. 16–29). There is a distinct window for embryo transfer leading to implantation, which spans endometrial cycle days 16 to 20. Presumably, the actual window of implan-

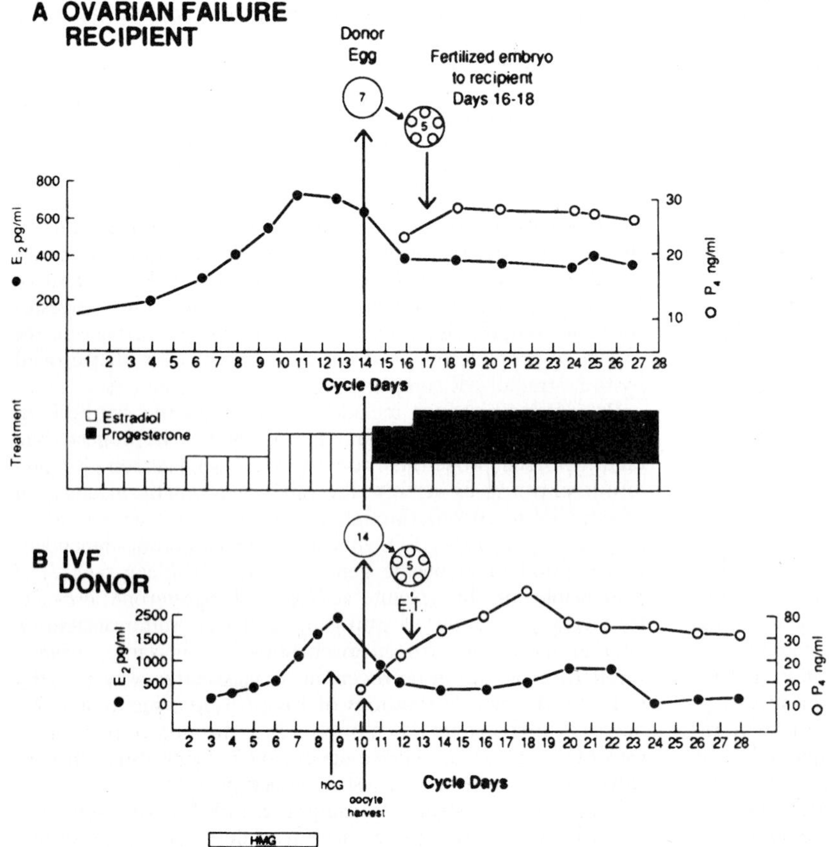

Figure 16–29. Diagrammatic representation of donation of excess oocytes by a woman undergoing in vitro fertilization (IVF) to a woman with ovarian failure treated with exogenous estrogen and progesterone. *A*, Woman with ovarian failure treated with increasing doses of estrogen during days 1 through 14 of the cycle. Exogenous progesterone was added to the estrogen treatment on days 15 through 28 and continued if pregnancy was diagnosed. Seven donor eggs were fertilized with sperm from the recipient's husband, and five embryos were transferred to the uterus on day 16 to 18. *B*, The IVF patient-donor was treated with human menopausal gonadotropin (hMG) until day 8, when human chorionic gonadotropin (hCG) was given, and oocytes were harvested 32 to 36 hours later. Half of the eggs were donated to the recipient, and the other half were fertilized with sperm from the donor's husband; the five fertilized eggs were transferred to the uterus of the IVF donor. Serum levels of E_2 (estradiol) and P_4 (progesterone) in both women are shown. To convert estradiol values to picomoles per liter, multiply by 3.671. To convert progesterone values to nanomoles per liter, multiply by 3.180. (Adapted from Rosenwaks Z. Donor eggs: their application in modern reproductive technologies. Fertil Steril 1987; 47:895–909.)

tation follows this window of transfer because embryos need to develop further from the four-cell to eight-cell stage to the blastocyst stage before initiation of attachment and frank invasion.

The window of implantation in the humans was estimated to be between days 20 and 24 of the cycle using serial measurements of serum hCG as a marker of initial embryonic-maternal interaction.[218] Thus, it appears that the window of implantation in the human is relatively wide (approximately 4 days). These observations agree with the earlier morphologic data from Hertig and colleagues.[219]

Mechanism of Menstruation

In the absence of pregnancy, failure of the appearance of hCG, despite otherwise appropriate tissue reactions, leads to the vasomotor changes associated with estrogen-progesterone withdrawal and menstrual desquamation. A program of endometrial remodeling is initiated; alterations in the extracellular matrix and infiltration of leukocytes lead to hypoxia-reperfusion injury and sloughing of the functionalis, followed by activation of hemostatic and regenerative processes. The main histologic features of the premenstrual phase are degradation of the stromal reticular network, stromal infiltration by polymorphonuclear and mononuclear leukocytes, and secretory exhaustion of the endometrial glands, whose epithelial cells now have basal nuclei (see Fig. 16–26). The endometrium shrinks preceding menstruation, in part as a result of diminished secretory activity and the catabolism of extracellular matrix.

The most prominent and final effect of progesterone and estrogen withdrawal is menstruation (see Fig. 16–25). The classical studies of Markee[220] suggested that an ischemic phase caused by vasoconstriction of the arterioles and coiled arteries precedes the onset of menstrual bleeding by 4 to 24 hours. Bleeding occurs after the arterioles and arteries relax, leading to hypoxia-reperfusion injury. The superficial endometrial layers are distended by the formation of hematomas, and fissures subsequently develop, leading to the detachment of tissue fragments. Lysis and fragmentation of cells and apoptosis are evident.[221] The menstrual efflux is composed of shed fragments of endometrium mixed with blood and liquefied by the fibrinolytic activity of the cellular debris (see Fig. 16–25). Clots of varying size may be present if blood flow is excessive.

Control of Endometrial Function Employing Synthetic Hormones

The fertility potential of a woman is primarily determined by the biologic quality of her oocytes, reflected in part by the capacity of the fertilized ovum to divide at an optimal rate and contain a normal chromosomal complement. This biologic quality of the oocyte declines sharply after the age of 35. The biologic potential of the endometrium for successful implantation, however, remains intact even at advanced ages.[222] Oocyte donation from a fertile woman and in vitro fertilization of these donor eggs with the recipient's male partner's sperm, followed by embryo transfer into the uterine cavity of the recipient woman who does not have functioning ovaries (e.g., premature ovarian failure), have been used successfully as a therapeutic strategy to treat infertility (see Fig. 16–29).[222, 223] This clinical application has provided unique opportunities to examine the hormonal requirements for endometrial maturation. A number of hormone replacement protocols have been proposed, and many pregnancies have resulted from donor oocytes in women with ovarian failure (see Fig. 16–29). The success of these procedures has averaged about 50% (pregnancy rate) per embryo transfer.

The degree of endometrial differentiation in response to exogenous hormones has been evaluated by histologic analysis of endometrial biopsy specimens. The epithelial elements exhibit delayed maturation early during progesterone administration on days 20 to 22, but catch up by day 26. Despite this apparent dyssynchrony, the pregnancy rate in these patients with donor oocytes is higher than in conventional in vitro fertilization.[223, 224]

The majority of infertility specialists currently use step-up administration of oral micronized estradiol in 2-, 4-, and 6-mg daily doses followed by 4 to 6 mg of estradiol combined with daily intramuscular progesterone (50 mg) to promote the secretory transformation. Serum estradiol levels in these subjects during the replacement "follicular" phase reach preovulatory peak levels of 800 to 1000 pg/mL. Intramuscular injection of 50 mg/day of progesterone in oil generates serum levels of progesterone greater than 10 ng/mL. The length of exposure to progesterone, but not absolute plasma progesterone concentrations achieved after adequate priming of the endometrium with estrogen, is a key factor for the development of uterine receptivity. Thus, the exogenous administration of only estradiol and progesterone is sufficient to prepare the endometrium for implantation in the absence of ovarian function. This observation further underscores the essential roles of these steroids in uterine physiology.

APPROACH TO THE WOMAN WITH REPRODUCTIVE DYSFUNCTION

Reproductive dysfunction in an adult woman is most often manifest by disruption of cyclic, predictable menses. Efficient diagnosis of the underlying disorder requires a thorough understanding of female reproductive physiology and pathology and an accurate history and physical examination. Without a critical analysis of clinical findings based on thorough knowledge of normal and abnormal reproductive function, the application of predetermined algorithms of laboratory testing causes unnecessary use of hormone measurements or imaging studies and delays diagnosis.

History

An essential tool for the evaluation of a woman with a reproductive disorder is a carefully recorded history. The history should be obtained from the patient with the aim of assessing the biologic effects of each of the various hormones. Recording the details of pubertal development as a reference for the onset of particular symptoms provides critical clues to the etiology of certain reproductive disorders. For example, anovulation manifest by irregular uterine bleeding associated with the polycystic ovary syndrome (PCOS) most often begins during the pubertal years.[225] The onset of gradually progressing hirsutism around puberty is suggestive of nonclassical adrenal hyperplasia or PCOS. In these cases, measurement of serum 17-hydroxyprogesterone may help to differentiate nonclassical adrenal hyperplasia from PCOS (see later). The appearance of hirsutism before puberty or several years after normal pubertal development should alert the clinician to the possibility of ovarian or adrenal neoplasms. The sudden (versus gradual) onset of hirsutism at any age or the presence of virilization should prompt the physician to rule out steroid-secreting ovarian or adrenal tumors. Most women with symptomatic endometriosis suffer from severe episodes of painful menses (dysmenorrhea), which start during pubertal years.

Evaluation of female reproductive function starts with a detailed history of the menses. For example, PCOS is extremely unlikely without a long-standing history of irregular periods since the menarche. By the same token, history of a period of cyclic, predictable menses before the onset of menstrual irregularities should draw attention to hypothalamic or other causes of anovulation. The current frequency, regularity, length, and quantity of uterine bleeding should be carefully recorded for several reasons. First, this information reflects tightly regulated interactions of several tissues, including the hypothalamus, pituitary, ovaries, and endometrium. Second, regular, predictable menses imply ovulation. Third, defining the type of menstrual irregularity may help with the diagnosis of the underlying etiology. For example, prolonged amenorrhea in a thin and estrogen-deficient woman suggests anovulation of hypothalamic etiology. Infrequent periods of varying duration and amount of blood loss in a well-estrogenized overweight woman, on the other hand, suggest a primary ovarian dysfunction such as PCOS. It should be kept in mind that anovulation in a thin but well-estrogenized woman may also be due to PCOS. Regular but heavy and prolonged menses with intermittent spotting may be due to uterine anatomic disorders such as adenomyosis or leiomyomas. Finally, neoplastic disorders of the endometrium including endometrial polyps, hyperplasia, or malignancies may be manifest by any pattern of irregular bleeding. The combination of vaginal ultrasonography and endometrial biopsy is extremely sensitive for the diagnosis of endometrial neoplasia.[226]

Disruption of cyclic and predictable menses is a common and alarming symptom that initially brings the patient to the clinician. After a careful evaluation of the menstrual symptoms, the clinician should identify other obvious symptoms of endocrine disorder underlying irregular periods. Pregnancy is the most common cause of amenorrhea (and possibly any other menstrual irregularity) in a woman of reproductive age. In a woman presenting with amenorrhea or any other menstrual irregularity, normal pregnancy, ectopic pregnancy or gestational trophoblastic disease must be excluded at the onset. Careful evaluation of any past reproductive history, as well as of the patient's sexual activity and contraceptive practices, can provide useful indications of the likelihood of pregnancy. Furthermore, the reproductive history may suggest the possibility of Sheehan's syndrome of postpartum pituitary necrosis if menses did not resume after a delivery complicated by significant hemorrhage.[227] In such instances, evidence of adrenal and thyroid insufficiency should be sought. A classical symptom of Sheehan's syndrome is the absence of lactation after delivery related to prolactin deficiency.

Amenorrhea is traditionally categorized as either primary (no history of menstruation) or secondary (cessation of menses after a variable time). The causes of primary amenorrhea are diverse and discussed extensively in Chapters 19 and 21. Although the distinction between primary and secondary amenorrhea is useful for identifying the mechanism of disease and differential diagnosis, the clinician should be aware that some disorders can initially present with either primary or secondary amenorrhea. For example, most women with gonadal dysgenesis have primary amenorrhea, but some patients have residual follicles and ovulate, and in these women with partial gonadal dysgenesis some menstruation and rare pregnancies may occur before the cessation of ovarian function.[228–230] Patients with PCOS usually have secondary amenorrhea but occasionally have primary amenorrhea.[231]

Secondary amenorrhea is most often due to chronic anovulation, which can be broadly categorized as (1) hypothalamic dysfunction, (2) galactorrhea-associated, (3) ovarian failure, (4) androgen excess, (5) chronic illness, and (6) primary uterine disease (e.g., intrauterine adhesion formation after a postpartum curettage). Establishing any association of secondary amenorrhea with various life events is extremely useful. Strenuous exercise is often associated with amenorrhea. Weight loss often precedes or accompanies secondary amenorrhea and has been suggested as evidence of hypothalamic dysfunction. An unusual dietary history may be suggestive of bulimia or anorexia nervosa. A history of dilatation and curettage, postpartum endometritis, or disseminated tuberculosis with absent to scant menses should suggest the possibility of intrauterine adhesion.[232] The presence of any signs or symptoms of estrogen deficiency, including painful intercourse, atrophic vagina, emotional lability, and vasomotor instability, should suggest anovulation of a central nature with low concentrations of circulating gonadotropins (hypogonadotropic hypogonadism) or ovarian failure with elevated gonadotropins (hypergonadotropic hypogonadism).

Galactorrhea in the absence of a recent history of pregnancy is suggestive of a host of diagnostic possibilities and is frequently a manifestation of excessive prolactin secretion, although it may be a result of increased sensitivity of breast tissue to the hormones necessary for milk production. This history frequently reveals drug ingestion as the cause. Various drugs (including several psychotropic agents and antihypertensive agents as well as oral contraceptives) have been implicated. Primary hypothyroidism may be associated with precocious puberty with galactorrhea in the child and with amenorrhea, galactorrhea, or both in the adult woman. A history of excessive nipple manipulation or chest wall disease should be elicited and may well be the cause of galactorrhea. Prolactinomas, the prolactin-secreting adenomas of the pituitary, are a common etiology of galactorrhea related to abnormally high serum levels of prolactin.

Physical Examination

The quantity and distribution of excessive hair growth should be considered in light of the familial history. Hypertrichosis—excessive growth of hair on the extremities, the head, and the back—must be distinguished from true hirsutism, which is the development of facial hair, chest hair, and a male escutcheon with or without signs of virilization in response to increased production of or sensitivity to biologically active androgens. Some degree of hypertrichosis is not uncommon in women of Mediterranean descent, whereas the occurrence of any facial hirsutism in the relatively hairless Asian woman may require thorough investigation. Hirsutism is best documented and quantified with the help of photographs. Virilization is characterized as thickening of voice, severe cystic acne, hair loss, increased muscle mass, and clitoromegaly and implies a more severe degree of androgen excess than that found with hirsutism. The syndrome of complete androgen insensitivity is characterized by sparse to absent pubic and axillary hair because of resistance to androgen.

A careful inspection of the breasts is essential for a thorough physical examination. Classification of the stage of breast development according to the method of Marshall and Tanner[233] is a convenient and valuable adjunct. Whether the breasts appear to have decreased in size recently (e.g., severe androgen excess), whether the areolae are well formed and pigmented (as they are in pregnancy), and whether a discharge (e.g., galactorrhea) can be expressed should be assessed.

A woman with PCOS who has never ovulated or taken a progestin-containing medication may have Tanner stage 4 breast development related to adequate estrogen production, whereas the progression to Tanner stage 5 requires exposure to progesterone through either ovulation or ingesting a progestin (e.g., administration of oral contraceptives). See Chapter 22 for a detailed description and hormonal basis of Tanner staging of breast development.

The vulva, vagina, and cervix also represent sensitive indicators of sex steroid action. Because sensitivity of the genital skin and mucosa to androgen decreases with time from the early stages of fetal development to adulthood, the extent of any virilization can be helpful in suggesting the timing of androgen exposure. The most profound androgenic effects, such as posterior labial fusion with or without formation of a penile urethra, are generally observed in patients exposed to androgens during the first trimester (12 weeks) of pregnancy. Such findings have been described in patients with virilizing congenital adrenal hyperplasia, true hermaphroditism, and drug-induced virilization. Significant postnatal clitoromegaly, on the other hand, requires marked hormonal stimulation and, in the absence of significant exogenous steroids, strongly implicates an androgen-secreting tumor. Measurement of the base of the clitoris versus its length is a more accurate method for the determination of androgen-dependent clitoral growth. A clitoral index, defined as the product of the sagittal and transverse diameters at the base, greater than 35 mm^2 falls outside the 95% confidence interval.

The vagina and uterine cervix are the most sensitive indicators of estrogen action. Under the influence of estrogen, the vaginal mucosa progresses during sexual maturation from a tissue with a shiny, bright red appearance with sparse, thin secretions to a dull, gray-pink rugated surface with copious, thick secretions. Well-estrogenized vaginal mucosa with stretchable cervical mucus (spinnbarkeit) may be indicative of the proliferative phase of the menstrual cycle in an ovulatory woman or extraovarian estrogen formation in an anovulatory woman with PCOS. The biologic activity of estrogen can also be quantified by vaginal cytology.

To summarize, irregular uterine bleeding is a common symptom that brings the woman with reproductive dysfunction to the physician's office. Various disorders of the hypothalamus, pituitary, ovaries, or uterus or other issues that affect reproductive function may be responsible for this alarming symptom. When pregnancy is ruled out, a detailed history and physical examination should be carefully recorded. In particular, the physician should pay attention to the salient features in the history and biologic indicators of hormone action at target tissues during the physical examination. An analysis of these findings most often leads to a tentative diagnosis. This diagnosis should then be confirmed with laboratory testing.

DISORDERS OF THE FEMALE REPRODUCTIVE SYSTEM

Chronic Anovulation

Chronic anovulation is one of the most common gynecologic problems encountered by the practitioner. These women may present with secondary amenorrhea, infrequent uterine bleeding (oligomenorrhea), or irregular episodes of excessive uterine bleeding. Infertility is an obvious consequence of chronic anovulation.

One group of anovulatory patients is estrogen-deficient. Common findings in this group include hypothalamic anovulation, galactorrhea-hyperprolactinemia (e.g., hypothyroidism, prolactinoma, nonfunctioning pituitary tumor), and premature ovarian failure in a woman of reproductive age. These patients are usually amenorrheic and deficient in estrogen. One serious consequence is bone loss giving rise to osteopenia and osteoporosis. If possible, the underlying cause should be corrected. Hormone replacement should be provided if ovulation cannot be restored.

Women with androgen excess constitute the second major group of anovulatory patients. A serious consequence of anovulation in this group is the greater risk for carcinoma of the endometrium because of unopposed action of estrogen formed continuously in extraovarian tissues. The most common disorder of the ovary associated with androgen excess and anovulation is PCOS. There is a new appreciation for the role of insulin resistance in this condition and for the clinical effects of insulin resistance and hyperandrogenism on the risks of developing cardiovascular disease and diabetes mellitus.[193] The clinician must recognize the long-term impact of PCOS and undertake therapeutic management of these anovulatory patients to avoid unwanted consequences. The clinician should also develop a plan with the patient to address long-term complications of unopposed estrogen formation associated with PCOS (e.g., endometrial neoplasia). Oral contraceptives or periodic progestin supplementation may be provided to prevent endometrial hyperplasia and cancer.

For practical purposes, the following five broad categories include the majority of the etiologic factors giving rise to chronic anovulation in a woman of reproductive age:

1. Hypothalamic anovulation.
2. Hyperprolactinemia.
3. Androgen excess.
4. Premature ovarian failure.
5. Chronic illness (e.g., hepatic or renal failure, acquired immunodeficiency syndrome).

There may be multiple mechanisms responsible for anovulation in chronic illness. Effective treatment of the primary illness may restore normal menses. Alternatively, anovulatory bleeding may be managed by exogenous hormones in these chronically ill patients as outlined further subsequently. The following are detailed descriptions of specific disorders that cause chronic anovulation in a reproductive-age woman.

Hypothalamic Anovulation

Production of LHRH in the neurons of the arcuate nucleus in the hypothalamus and its secretion into the portal vessels in the median eminence in a pulsatile fashion are responsible for the production and secretion of FSH and LH from the pituitary.[11] LHRH neurons depolarize and release LHRH at critical pulse frequencies of 60 to 200 minutes during specific phases of the menstrual cycle to increase or decrease secretion of FSH and LH.[14, 16] Variations in LHRH pulse frequency are achieved, at least partially, by gonadal steroid feedback. Local neuromodulators in the brain, including norepinephrine, dopamine, and β-endorphin, mediate the actions of gonadal steroids on the hypothalamus (see Fig. 16–4).[23] Any disorder of the central nervous system that interferes with this intricate process can thus cause anovulation. Some of these disorders may be demonstrated by defined genetic or anatomic evidence such as isolated gonadotropin deficiency (with or without anosmia), infection, suprasellar tumors (pituitary adenomas, craniopharyngioma), and head trauma.[11] These genetic and anatomic disorders affect the function of the hypothalamus, and some of them may be ruled out by history, physical examination, and imaging of the head (Table 16–3).

The most commonly observed form of hypothalamic anovulation, however, is not associated with a demonstrable neuroanatomic finding.[11] This common form is called functional hypothalamic anovulation because it is presumed to involve aberrant but reversible regulation of otherwise normal neuroendocrine pathways. Changes in lifestyle usually result in the return of normal ovulatory cycles. Functional hypothalamic anovulation may be associated with excessive exercise, abrupt weight loss, and emotional distress. It is hypothesized that these stress factors cause anovulation by affecting brain function and the LHRH pulse generator. Other causes of hypothalamic anovulation demonstrable by neuroanatomic or genetic evidence are relatively rare (see Table 16–3), and these are covered in detail in other chapters of this textbook (Chapters 8 and 24).

Functional Hypothalamic Anovulation

Anovulation of hypothalamic origin is characterized by estrogen deficiency and low levels of gonadotropins. No identifiable genetic or anatomic disorders are present in the majority of these patients. The concept of functional hypothalamic anovulation was first postulated 60 years ago as the failure of the hypothalamic-pituitary pathways to release LH from the anterior pituitary.[234] Since then, many clinical studies have confirmed this idea.[15, 235, 236] The data accumulated thus far suggest that the common underlying defect is an alteration in the pulsatile secretion of LHRH. Intriguingly, it has been shown in patients with this disorder that diverse etiologic factors such as malnutrition or caloric restriction, depression or psychogenic stress, excessive energy expenditure related to exercise, or combinations of these have preceded the onset of functional hypothalamic anovulation. Heightened awareness of diet and exercise and unrealistic expectations with respect to the body image of women have most likely contributed to the epidemic of this anovulatory disorder.

Diagnosis of Functional Hypothalamic Anovulation

Patients with functional hypothalamic anovulation most commonly present with secondary amenorrhea characterized by the absence of menstrual cycles for more than 6 months without evidence of an organic disorder. It should be emphasized once again that the diagnosis of hypothalamic anovulation is one of exclusion. There are many neuroanatomic or genetic disorders that can mimic functional hypothalamic anovulation (see Table 16–3). Thus, a careful and complete diagnostic evaluation is essential to make this diagnosis.

Women with functional hypothalamic anovulation usually present with a history of regular menses for a period of variable length after menarche. Thereafter, this period of normal ovulatory function (by history) is interrupted by anovulation usually manifest by secondary amenorrhea. It should be emphasized that women with functional hypothalamic anovulation may occasionally present with primary amenorrhea.

Women with functional hypothalamic anovulation are typically normal to thin in body weight, driven, and involved in high-stress occupations. The occupation of the patient (e.g., a ballerina or competitive athlete) may be an extremely important clue. A detailed interview may reveal a variety of emotional crises or stressful events (e.g., divorce, death of a friend) preceding the onset of amenorrhea. During the interview, additional environmental and interpersonal factors may become evident, including academic pressure, social maladjustment, and psychosexual problems. When evaluating the patient, one should take note of the current diet regimen, the use of any sedatives or hypnotics, and the rigorousness of the patient's exercise habits. Despite a careful interview, a history of stress, excessive physical exercise, or an eating disorder may not be readily revealed in some women with functional hypothalamic anovulation. These women usually do not complain of hot flashes, which, on the other hand, are commonly observed in ovarian failure.

The physician should exclude a possible hyperprolactinemic etiology (e.g., prolactinoma, hypothyroidism) and evidence of androgen excess (e.g., PCOS) during the physical examination. These women have normal secondary sexual characteristics. The pelvic examination usually shows a thinning vaginal mucosa accompanied by scant to absent cervical mucus with a normal to small uterus, all evidence of estrogen deficiency.

Table 16–3. Classification of Anovulation Caused by Disorders of the Hypothalamic-Pituitary Unit

Functional Hypothalamic Anovulation
Stress (psychogenic or physical)
Dieting
Vigorous exercise
Chronic illness (e.g., chronic liver or renal failure, AIDS)
Psychiatric-Medical Emergencies
Anorexia nervosa
Medications
Dopamine antagonists (e.g., haloperidol)
Opiates
Antihypertensives (e.g., methyldopa, reserpine)
Hypothyroidism
Anatomically or Genetically Defined Pathologies of the Hypothalamic-Pituitary Unit
Pituitary tumors
Prolactinoma
Clinically nonfunctioning adenoma
GH-secreting adenoma (acromegaly)
ACTH-secreting adenoma (Cushing's disease)
Other pituitary tumors (e.g., metastasis, meningioma)
Pituitary stalk section
Pituitary apoplexy (including Sheehan's syndrome)
Pituitary aneurysm
Infiltrative disease of the pituitary (e.g., lymphocytic hypophysitis, sarcoidosis, histiocytosis X, tuberculosis)
Empty sella syndrome
Isolated gonadotropin deficiency (including Kallmann's syndrome)
Tumors that affect hypothalamic function (e.g., metastasis, craniopharyngioma)
Infiltrative granulomatous disease of the hypothalamus (e.g., sarcoidosis, histiocytosis X, tuberculosis)
Head trauma
Irradiation to the head
CNS infection
Other

ACTH, adrenocorticotropic hormone; AIDS, acquired immunodeficiency syndrome; CNS, central nervous system; GH, growth hormone.

Signs of a well-estrogenized vagina and cervix observed during the physical examination make the diagnosis of hypothalamic anovulation unlikely.

Laboratory tests are obtained to exclude other causes of anovulation and secondary amenorrhea. LH and FSH levels should be obtained. Gonadotropin levels are usually lower than the normal values ordinarily found in the early follicular phase. TSH and prolactin levels are obtained to rule out hypothyroidism and hyperprolactinemia. The progestin challenge test (medroxyprogesterone acetate at 10 mg/day for 10 days) shows either a small spotting episode or absence of withdrawal uterine bleeding in most patients. This confirms that there is a scant or absent estrogenic effect on the endometrium because circulating estradiol levels are typically in the low or early follicular phase range. Measurement of the serum estradiol level is not necessary. Because a suprasellar or large pituitary tumor is in the differential diagnosis, a magnetic resonance imaging (MRI) scan of the head is necessary to rule this out. Imaging of the head is especially important if amenorrhea develops suddenly or is associated with a neurologic sign, both of which make the presence of a tumor more likely.

Pathophysiology of Functional Hypothalamic Anovulation

A key observation in functional hypothalamic anovulation is the absence of increased gonadotropin secretion despite the lack of inhibitory factors of ovarian origin, such as estradiol and inhibin. The secretory pattern of LH is abnormal. The causative factor in women with this type of anovulation is a slowdown in the frequency of pulsatile LHRH secretion.[15, 237, 238] Frequent peripheral blood samples were obtained from these patients to quantify the episodic secretion of LH, which provided an indirect assessment of endogenous LHRH secretion.[238]

There is considerable variability in the amplitude and frequency of the pulsatile LH secretion in functional hypothalamic anovulation. When the LH secretory patterns are compared with that of the follicular phase of the menstrual cycle, a characteristic abnormality in the LH pulse frequency and amplitude and on occasion a regression to a pronounced variability similar to what is seen in the prepubertal pattern are present.[15, 237] In severe cases, the frequency and amplitude of LH pulses are markedly reduced. These LH patterns also suggest that LHRH pulsatile secretion is not altered to the same degree in each individual. During the recovery phase of hypothalamic anovulation, a reversal of the LHRH-LH secretory pattern is often present, characterized by a sleep-associated increase in LH amplitude.

The response of the pituitary gland to LHRH with respect to production and release of gonadotropins is not impaired in functional hypothalamic anovulation. Intravenous pulsatile LHRH administration can restore normal levels of LH and FSH.[235, 239]

Norepinephrine, dopamine, and serotonin produced in the brain have been shown to modulate LHRH or LH release in animal studies.[240] Patients receiving medication that alters these neurotransmitters (e.g., sedatives, antidepressants, stimulants, and antipsychotics) have presented with abnormalities in their menstrual cycles. Thus, it can be noted as circumstantial evidence that disruptions of neural pathways can alter LHRH release in the human. From these observations, it appears that activation of the noradrenergic neurons principally stimulates release of LHRH,[241, 242] whereas dopaminergic and serotoninergic neurons can stimulate or inhibit LHRH-LH secretion.[240, 242, 243]

A number of neuropharmacologic agents have been used as probes to determine whether LHRH-LH secretion can be normalized. For example, metoclopramide blocks the action of dopamine.[244] A metoclopramide injection results in a prompt increase in LH secretion in patients with functional hypothalamic anovulation. These studies suggest enhanced dopaminergic activity in functional hypothalamic anovulation. It should be emphasized, however, that chronic administration of dopamine antagonists (e.g., haloperidol, metoclopramide) may also cause anovulation.

Another group of substances that have inhibitory influences on LHRH secretion are endogenous opioid peptides.[245, 246] Blockage of endogenous opiate receptors by the administration of naloxone, an opiate antagonist, to women with this disorder caused an increase in the frequency and amplitude of pulsatile LH release.[244, 247] Gonadotropin secretion resumes if the activity of the opiate receptor is blocked by long-term naloxone use in these anovulatory patients, and ovulatory function may even be regained in some cases.[248] These studies suggest that there is an overall increase in endogenous opiate activity, which can reduce pulsatile LHRH secretion in functional hypothalamic anovulation.

Reproductive function may be disrupted by chronic exposure to stress.[234, 236] In fact, activation of the pituitary-adrenocortical system is a common response in patients with chronic stress.[249] In functional hypothalamic anovulation, stressors such as exercise or emotional stress can chronically activate the hypothalamic-pituitary-adrenal axis. Daytime cortisol levels are markedly elevated, and the pituitary response to corticotropin-releasing hormone (CRH) is blunted.[239, 250] The stress response is associated with increased secretion of CRH, adrenocorticotropic hormone (ACTH), cortisol, prolactin, oxytocin, vasopressin, epinephrine, and norepinephrine.[251]

The association between emotional or physical stress and disruption of the reproductive function of the hypothalamus is complex and involves several mechanisms. In the animal model, CRH seems to be an important factor in the inhibition of LHRH pulsatility.[252–254] This inhibitory effect can be prevented by coadministration of a CRH antagonist or reversed by the opiate antagonist naloxone, which suggests that the action of CRH is mediated, in part, by activation of the opioidergic system. Moreover, ACTH administration blocks the pituitary response to LHRH at the pituitary level.[255–257] In addition, another stress hormone, oxytocin, can inhibit hypothalamic LHRH secretion.[246] In summary, overproduction of CRH and other stress-related hormones in the brain and activation of the pituitary-adrenocortical system by chronic stress seem to play causative roles in the inhibition of gonadotropin secretion in functional hypothalamic anovulation.

Hypothalamic Anovulation and Exercise

Regular vigorous exercise can lead to menstrual disturbances, a delay in menarche, luteal phase dysfunction, and secondary amenorrhea. Thirty percent of adolescent ballet dancers have problems with the progression of puberty. The mean age of menarche is delayed until 15. In fact, advancement of pubertal stages seems to coincide with times of prolonged rest or following recovery from an injury.[258–266] The intensity, length, and type of the sport determine the severity of the disease. Activities associated with an increased frequency of reproductive dysfunction are those that favor a lower body weight and include middle-distance and long-distance running, competitive swimming, gymnastics, and ballet dancing.[267]

Competitive athletes show endocrine abnormalities in the central nervous system consistent with those in other forms of functional hypothalamic anovulation. These include elevations on central CRH and β-endorphin levels.[268–270]

The management of exercise-related anovulation is dependent on the patient's choices and expectations. Side effects such as osteoporosis and delay of puberty must be discussed at length with the patient.[271] Decrease in exercise level and behavioral modification may be sufficient for the return of ovulatory function. Hormone replacement should be provided if sufficient results are not achieved. A low-dose oral contraceptive is a suitable option for women of reproductive age.

Hypothalamic Anovulation Associated with Eating Disorders

Two common eating disorders associated with hypothalamic dysfunction are anorexia and bulimia. In anorexia nervosa, there is an extreme loss of weight (weight decrease of greater than 25% of original body weight) and a distorted body image accompanied by a striking fear of obesity.[272] Bulimia is a related disorder characterized by alternating episodes of binge eating followed by periods of food restriction, self-induced vomiting, or excessive use of laxatives or diuretics.[273] About 90% to 95% of these patients are female. Most patients with eating disorders are white and are from middle-class or upper-middle-class families. The incidence of classical anorexia nervosa is about 1 per 100,000 in the general population.[274] Among high school and college female students, bulimia, however, is fairly common (2%).[275] The incidence of anorexia nervosa peaks twice during the teen years at ages 13 and 17. Bulimia usually begins at a later age, between 17 and 25 years. Anorexia nervosa has an extremely high mortality of 9% and is a true medical emergency. Death may be secondary to cardiac arrhythmia, which may be precipitated by diminished heart muscle mass and associated electrolyte abnormalities.[276, 277] These patients are also at increased risk for suicide.[278]

Gonadotropin secretion in anorexic women exhibits a prepubertal pattern that is similar to other forms of hypothalamic anovulation. Transitional patterns of LH secretion are seen when there are moderate degrees of weight recovery and there is a normal or supranormal response to LHRH. Anovulation can persist in up to 50% of anorexic patients even after achieving normal weight. Both anorexic and bulimic patients exhibit hyperactivation of the hypothalamus-pituitary system. Although the diurnal variation is maintained, there is a persistent hypersecretion of cortisol throughout the day.[279] Cushingoid features, however, are not present, in part because of mild hypercortisolemia and also a reduction of peripheral glucocorticoid receptors.[280] Levels of both CRH and β-endorphin are increased in the central nervous system.[281, 282]

In anorexia nervosa, basal metabolism is decreased because peripheral conversion of thyroxine (T_4) to biologically potent triiodothyronine (T_3) is decreased. Instead, T_4 is converted to reverse T_3, an inactive isoform. This alteration is also observed in severely ill patients and during starvation.[283] Anorexics also have partial diabetes insipidus and are unable to concentrate urine appropriately because of the impaired secretion of vasopressin.[284]

Both anorexia nervosa and bulimia are extremely difficult to treat. The most accepted approaches include individual psychotherapy, group therapy, and behavior modification.[263] Patients with eating disorders should have psychiatric consultation and follow-up. This helps with both the diagnosis and treatment. In patients who weigh less than 75% of their ideal body weight, immediate hospitalization and aggressive treatment are recommended. Chronic complications of anorexia nervosa include osteoporosis; other consequences are estrogen deficiency and generalized effects of malnutrition.[264] Hormone replacement in the form of an oral contraceptive should be provided until ovulatory function is achieved.

Treatment and Management of Functional Hypothalamic Anovulation

Treatment of chronic anovulation resulting from central nervous system–hypothalamic disorders should be directed at reversal of the primary cause (e.g., stress management, reduction of exercise, or correction of weight loss). The successful treatment of this disease state is underscored because these women are prone to the development of osteoporosis. For a considerable number of patients, spontaneous recovery of menstrual function takes place after a modification of lifestyle, psychological guidance, or accommodation to environmental stress.[236] Therefore, the initial treatment should be directed to a change in lifestyle and tailored to the individual patient. For individuals who remain amenorrheic, periodic assessment of reproductive status (every 4 to 6 months) is prudent.

If anovulation persists for more than 6 months or if reversal of the primary cause is not practical (e.g., professional athletes, ballerinas), a major concern is the long-term effect of hypoestrogenism, especially on bone metabolism. In addition to estrogen deficiency, IGF-I deficiency, hypercortisolism, or nutritional factors may all contribute to bone loss in this disorder.[285] Unfortunately, epidemiologic data on the risk of fractures and the benefits of hormone replacement are scant.[271, 286, 287] On the basis of studies of reproductive-age women who have been ovariectomized or who have undergone treatment with LHRH agonist for endometriosis, bone density would be expected to decrease significantly even within the first 6 months of amenorrhea. Because these patients are often reluctant to take medications, serial bone density studies of the lumbar spine and femur may be necessary to convince them of the necessity to begin estrogen replacement therapy.[288] If the patient is not at risk for thromboembolism and does not smoke cigarettes, a low-dose combination oral contraceptive is a reasonable replacement option. Alternatively, a combination of conjugated estrogens (0.625 mg) and medroxyprogesterone acetate (2.5 mg) daily may be administered to provide estrogenic support. The progestin (medroxyprogesterone acetate) is added solely to prevent endometrial hyperplasia.

If the patient desires ovulation in order to achieve pregnancy, the most physiologic approach is ovulation induction with pulsatile LHRH. This is currently the best physiologic means of induction because the cause of the anovulatory state is the decrease in endogenous LHRH secretion. Pulsatile intravenous LHRH, 5 μg every 90 minutes, was shown to be effective.[289, 290] Monitoring of serum estradiol levels or follicular development can be minimized because the ovarian follicular response and gonadotropin output mimic the natural menstrual cycle. In these patients, either continuation of pulsatile LHRH or human chorionic gonadotropin, 1500 units intramuscularly every 3 days for a total of four doses, can support the corpus luteum function. The intravenous LHRH treatment results in ovulation rates of approximately 90%, pregnancy rates up to 30%, and hyperstimulation rates of less than 1% per treatment cycle.[291] Because the intravenous LHRH pump is not a practical choice for many women, an alternative strategy is the use of subcutaneous recombinant FSH for the development of one to three follicles and the induction of ovulation with intramuscular hCG followed by luteal support using either intramuscular hCG or progesterone in oil.

Hyperprolactinemia

Prolactin and Reproductive Function

Structure and Function of Prolactin

Prolactin is secreted from the anterior pituitary and is essential for lactation. It is a 198-amino-acid polypeptide with a molecular mass of 22 kd. Its structure is remarkably similar to that of growth hormone.[292] The secondary structure is folded into a globular shape, and three disulfide bonds connect the folds. The amino acid sequences among prolactin, growth hormone, and human placental lactogen show an impressive degree of homology. Prolactin is produced in the lactotroph of the anterior pituitary. In the human pituitary, lactotrophs constitute 10% to 30% of the total pituitary cell mass and are located primarily in the posterior and lateral aspects of the adenohypophysis.

Regulation of Prolactin Secretion

A process that includes activation of a number of signaling pathways and gene transcription regulates prolactin synthesis and release. Prolactin is synthesized and packaged into secretory granules and is stored in the cytoplasm pending its release. On exposure to secretagogues, lactotrophs release prolactin from a readily releasable pool, and newly synthesized prolactin replenishes the releasable pool as well as a storage pool.[293] Dopamine, thyrotropin-releasing hormone (TRH), and estradiol were shown to regulate transcription of the prolactin gene.[294–296]

Dopamine is a well-characterized inhibitor of prolactin secretion.[297] Dopamine release is achieved through the portal vessels of the tuberoinfundibular dopaminergic system. Cell bodies of these neurons are located in the arcuate nucleus, and the axons extend to the median eminence. The biosynthesis and release of dopamine occur within the axonal terminals, which are adjacent to the portal capillaries. Thus, dopamine reaches the lactotroph by way of the portal circulation. Dopamine binds to its receptors on the lactotroph with resultant inhibition of prolactin secretion.[298] Dopamine concentrations are higher in the central portal vessels than in the lateral vessels.[298] The availability of lower amounts of circulating dopamine in the lateral aspects of the pituitary may account for the common presence of prolactinomas in the peripheral portions of the anterior pituitary.

In contrast to dopamine, TRH stimulates the release of pituitary prolactin.[299] TRH stimulates prolactin gene transcription within minutes because specific TRH receptors are present on the lactotroph. The result is an increase in mRNA accumulation in the cytoplasm and acute release of translated prolactin protein. Although the prolactin- and TSH-releasing actions of TRH are distinct, circulating levels of T_4 and T_3 influence prolactin release in response to TRH stimulation. Subnormal serum levels of T_3 and T_4, as in the case of primary hypothyroidism, increase TRH-induced prolactin release, whereas higher than normal serum levels of T_3 and T_4 inhibit prolactin mRNA accumulation and release of protein.[300] Unlike T_3, estradiol amplifies the stimulatory effects of TRH on prolactin release. Thus, a number of factors, including thyroid hormones, estradiol, and antithyroid medications, can modify the effects of TRH on prolactin release.

Estrogen stimulates the secretion of prolactin from the anterior pituitary in a dose- and time-dependent fashion. Administration of synthetic or natural estrogen increases blood prolactin levels in both premenopausal and postmenopausal women.[301, 302] Estrogen increases prolactin synthesis and release by direct stimulation of prolactin gene transcription, lactotroph proliferation, increased TRH receptors, and a decrease in dopaminergic activity.[303–306] The stimulatory effect of estrogen on prolactin secretion in vivo is usually subtle, as illustrated by mild increases in prolactin levels in women taking oral contraceptives.

Prolactin Action

The prolactin receptor belongs to the cytokine receptor superfamily that also includes the growth hormone receptor.[307] Growth hormone can bind to both the growth hormone receptor and the prolactin receptor.[308] Human prolactin, on the other hand, does not bind to the human growth hormone receptor. There are long and short isoforms of the prolactin receptor. Both isoforms can bind prolactin with high affinity and can stimulate prolactin-responsive cells to grow.[309] The functions of prolactin and growth hormone receptors are mediated, at least in part, by two families of signaling molecules: Janus kinases (JAKs) and signal transducers and activators of transcription (STATs).

The prolactin receptor is widely distributed, in some instances in the same tissue in which the ligand prolactin is also expressed. The receptor has been found in the hypothalamus, pituitary gland (both normal and neoplastic), gastrointestinal tract, prostate, bone, decidua, fetal membranes, and Leydig cells as well as in normal and neoplastic breast.[310] The expression of prolactin and its receptors in diverse tissues (pituitary gland, gastrointestinal tract, prostate, decidua, and the breast) is suggestive of the presence of autocrine and paracrine interactions in these tissues. Although a classical endocrine negative feedback cycle between prolactin of pituitary origin and its target tissues has not been described, these potential local mechanisms within target tissues may play important roles in the regulation of prolactin biosynthesis and action.

Hyperprolactinemia

Galactorrhea associated with hyperprolactinemia is one of the most common entities associated with chronic anovulation or secondary amenorrhea, or both. The impaired inhibition of prolactin secretion because of decreased dopamine production results in functional and secondary hyperprolactinemia, such as that caused by psychotropic medications. Another common cause of hyperprolactinemia is hypothyroidism associated with overproduction of TRH, which is a known inducer of prolactin secretion. The most common neuroanatomically demonstrable cause of hyperprolactinemia is a prolactin-secreting adenoma or prolactinoma. The processes that lead to the elevation of prolactin are numerous and can be found in Table 16–4.

Table 16–4. Causes of Hyperprolactinemia

Hypothalamic
Tumors that affect hypothalamic function
Metastasis
Craniopharyngioma
Glioma
Infiltrating granulomatous lesions
Sarcoidosis
Histiocytosis X
Tuberculosis
CNS infection
Irradiation
Head trauma
Pituitary
Pituitary tumors
Prolactinoma
Clinically nonfunctioning adenoma
GH-secreting adenoma (acromegaly)
ACTH-secreting adenoma (Cushing's disease)
Other pituitary tumors (e.g., metastasis, meningioma)
Pituitary stalk section
Pituitary aneurysm
Infiltrative disease of the pituitary
Lymphocytic hypophysitis
Sarcoidosis
Histiocytosis X
Tuberculosis
Empty sella syndrome
Hypothyroidism
Chronic illness
Renal failure
Liver failure
Ectopic secretion of prolactin
Bronchogenic carcinoma
Renal carcinoma
Neurogenic
Breast manipulation
Chest trauma
Chest or upper abdominal surgery
Herpes zoster infection
Medications causing inappropriate secretion of prolactin
Estrogen-containing medications (e.g., combination oral contraceptives)
Dopamine antagonists (e.g., phenothiazines, haloperidol)
Antihypertensives (reserpine, methyldopa)
Amphetamines, hallucinogens
Opiates
Cimetidine
Other
Idiopathic

ACTH, adrenocorticotropic hormone; CNS, central nervous system; GH, growth hormone.

Hyperprolactinemia Induced by Medications

A large number of medications impair dopaminergic inhibition of prolactin and give rise to hyperprolactinemia. The drugs that block synthesis, metabolism, reuptake, or receptor binding of dopamine reduce dopamine availability and result in the hypersecretion of prolactin (see Table 16–4). Conversely, drugs that enhance dopamine biosynthesis or dopamine agonists suppress the release of prolactin. Galactorrhea, therefore, is a relatively common complication in patients treated with phenothiazines, metoclopramide, reserpine, methyldopa, or similar agents.[311, 312] Menstrual irregularities or amenorrhea often develops in these patients, reflecting the importance of neurotransmitters and hyperprolactinemia in the regulation of LHRH secretion and impairment of ovarian function.

Hyperprolactinemia and Primary Hypothyroidism

Hyperprolactinemia and anovulation may be associated with primary hypothyroidism. Enlargement of the pituitary gland is frequently seen in long-standing primary hypothyroidism. A number of mechanisms may be involved. First, the clearance of prolactin tends to be decreased in hypothyroidism.[313] Second, patients with severe hypothyroidism may have elevated total and free estradiol levels, giving rise to increased prolactin production stimulated by excess free estrogen. The third, and possibly the most significant, mechanism involves the inhibitory effects of T_3 on TRH production and on TRH receptor expression. A decrease in T_3 feedback in hypothyroidism may induce an increase in hypothalamic TRH production and in the number of TRH receptors in the lactotroph. Increased TRH action on the lactotroph, in turn, may stimulate prolactin secretion.

Pituitary Prolactinoma

Prolactinomas are the most common hormone-producing pituitary tumors in women. Signs and symptoms include galactorrhea, anovulatory bleeding, amenorrhea, headache, and bitemporal hemianopsia. Prolactinomas are commonly classified as microadenomas for tumors less than 1 cm in diameter and macroadenomas for tumors larger than 1 cm. Macroadenomas are more likely to cause headaches and visual symptoms than microadenomas. Macroadenomas usually give rise to higher serum prolactin levels than microadenomas, although circulating prolactin levels associated with microadenomas and macroadenomas overlap extensively. Prolactin-secreting adenomas are almost always benign. Prolactin measurements and radiologic imaging lead to the diagnosis of these tumors. MRI is a suitable choice for imaging because it does not involve ionizing radiation and sensitivity is high. The lateral aspects of the pituitary represent the most common locations for prolactinomas.

Currently, the most common form of treatment is a dopamine agonist. Among these agents, bromocriptine has been the most commonly used drug. Tumor shrinkage is achieved in most cases. Prolactin levels return to normal; this usually results in the disappearance of headaches and galactorrhea, and the resumption of menses follows. Treatment must usually be continued indefinitely to maintain the euprolactinemic state. Treatment should be administered to amenorrheic women even if pregnancy is not the goal because osteopenia often occurs within 6 months of the amenorrhea because of the associated hypoestrogenemia.[314] The increase in parathyroid hormone–related protein (PTHrP) levels in hyperprolactinemic women may also contribute to bone loss.[315]

Side effects of bromocriptine are not uncommon and include syncope, nausea, and vomiting. A long-acting, parenteral form of bromocriptine decreases the incidence of side effects but is not yet approved for use in the United States. Selective D_2-type dopamine receptor agonists have become available. These include cabergoline and quinagolide.[316, 317] Both of these drugs have been shown useful in the treatment of bromocriptine-resistant tumors, in which there is decreased expression of the two D_2 dopamine receptor isoforms.[318] Cabergoline has a long half-life, requiring only twice-weekly dosing, and is approved for use in the United States; quinagolide requires daily administration and is not yet approved for use in the United States. The long half-life and decreased side effects of cabergoline have led to its increased use.

Treatment in the past was commonly transsphenoidal resection of these prolactin-secreting adenomas. There is, however, frequently a recurrence of hyperprolactinemia within 5 to 7 years after the surgery.[319] Thus, dopamine antagonists are the first line of therapy for both microadenomas and macroadenomas.

Continuation of bromocriptine therapy during pregnancy appears to be safe. If bromocriptine is stopped during pregnancy, however, clinically significant enlargement of prolactinomas is relatively uncommon. Approximately 6% of microadenomas and 30% of macroadenomas continue to grow during pregnancy.[320, 321] Eventually, the tumor may reach a size sufficient to cause headache and visual symptoms related to chiasmal compression. When visual symptoms become evident during pregnancy, resuming a dopamine agonist usually reduces the tumor mass and thus the visual symptoms. Transsphenoidal resection during pregnancy is rarely required when medical treatment is not sufficient to control visual disturbances and tumor growth. Pituitary apoplexy is an uncommon but serious complication of prolactinomas during pregnancy.

During pregnancy, serum prolactin levels cannot be used reliably to monitor the size of pituitary adenomas because the decidua (differentiated endometrial tissue under the unique hormonal influence of pregnancy) and normal prolactin-producing pituicytes are additional potential sources of serum prolactin. Therefore, central nervous system symptoms, such as subjective visual symptoms, and objective visual field examinations are used monthly to observe pregnant patients.

Hyperprolactinemia and Androgen Excess

Androgen excess and hirsutism were found in a significant number of patients with classical galactorrhea-anovulation syndromes in original reports.[322] This finding was verified by subsequent publications, which demonstrated that almost 40% of patients with pituitary adenomas and hyperprolactinemia had abnormal secretion and metabolism of androgen.[323–325] Hyperprolactinemia and ultrasound evidence of polycystic ovaries frequently overlap. Hirsutism was observed in 59% of hyperprolactinemic patients with polycystic-appearing ovaries and in 41% of hyperprolactinemic patients with normal-appearing ovaries on ultrasonography.[326]

Levels of testosterone and androgen precursors, namely dehydroepiandrosterone sulfate (DHEAS) and DHEA, are elevated, whereas testosterone-binding globulin (TeBG, see later) is reduced.[323–326] Reversal of these changes occurs after lowering the prolactin levels using oral bromocriptine. Furthermore, the levels of elevated androgen precursors are suppressed by dexamethasone, suggesting that hyperprolactinemia may exert a stimulatory action on adrenal C_{19}-steroid secretion.

Hyperprolactinemia and Bone Loss

Hyperprolactinemia is commonly associated with reduced bone mineral density.[314, 327, 328] Although hypoestrogenism can cause a decrease in bone mineral content, some euestrogenic patients have also been found to have reduced bone density. A direct action of prolactin on calcium mobilization may be a possible underlying mechanism. Prolactin has been shown to stimulate calcium mobilization from the bone independent of vitamin D and parathyroid hormone in the rat.[329] In addition, prolactin receptors are present in bone cells; thus, prolactin may directly act on the bone. Alternatively, prolactin-dependent increases in PTHrP levels in women with hyperprolactinemia may contribute to the osteoporotic effects of excessive prolactin.[315] Regardless of the mechanism, hyperprolactinemic patients are at risk for development of osteoporosis, and assessment of estrogen and bone mineral status is indicated. Prompt correction of hyperprolactinemia is the approach of choice. If hyperprolactinemia cannot be corrected, hormone replacement in the form of oral contraceptives is indicated.

Hyperprolactinemia and Hypothalamic Anovulation

Hyperprolactinemia is usually associated with anovulation, as exemplified by postpartum lactational amenorrhea and the galactorrhea-amenorrhea syndrome. Increased levels of prolactin inhibit the hypothalamic-pituitary-ovarian axis.[330] Both opioid peptides and hypothalamic dopamine regulate the pulsatile secretion of LHRH. Hyperprolactinemia inhibits LHRH activity by interacting with the hypothalamic dopaminergic and opioidergic systems through a short-loop feedback mechanism or by a direct effect on LHRH neurons, in which prolactin receptors are expressed.[330] Both possibilities are consistent with the observation that suppression of prolactin by the dopamine receptor antagonist bromocriptine restores ovulatory function.

Chronic Anovulation and Androgen Excess

Approach to the Patient with Androgen Excess

Two natural androgens are testosterone, which is transported to target tissue by the circulation, and DHT, which is produced primarily by target tissues. Increased levels of these androgens can lead to hirsutism, which is excessive androgenic hair growth, or to virilization, a more severe form of androgen excess. Hirsutism is defined as the presence of terminal (coarse) hair in locations at which hair is not commonly found in women. It includes facial hair on the cheek, above the upper lip, and on the chin (Fig. 16–30*A* and *B*). The presence of midline chest hair is also significant (Fig. 16–30*C*). In addition, a male escutcheon, hair on the inner aspects of the thighs, and midline lower back hair entering the intergluteal area are hair growth patterns compatible with androgen excess. A moderate amount of hair on the forearms and lower legs by itself may not be abnormal, although it may be viewed by the patient as undesirable and may be mistaken for hirsutism. Numerous scoring systems are available for quantifying hirsutism. One of the most detailed scales was proposed by Ferriman, Gallwey, and Lorenzo.[331] A practical and clinically useful means of quantifying hirsutism is recording the hair growth in detail using simple drawings and photographs. In particular, photographs are invaluable for documenting hirsutism accurately.

In contrast to hirsutism, virilization is a more severe form of androgen excess and implies significantly higher rates of testosterone production. Its manifestations include temporal balding, deepening of voice, decreased breast size, increased muscle mass, loss of female body contours, and clitoral enlargement (Fig. 16–31). Even if testosterone levels are moderately increased (<1.5 ng/mL), temporal balding and clitoromegaly may be observed over a long period of time (>1 year) in the presence of persistent androgen excess. A marked increase in androgen secretion, as may occur from production by neoplasms, however, leads to a more full-blown picture of virilization over a short duration of time (less than a few months).

Measurements of an enlarged clitoris may be used for the quantification of virilization. A clitoral length more than 10 mm is considered abnormal (see Fig. 16–31). Clitoral length is quite variable, however. An increase in clitoral diameter is a much more sensitive indicator of androgen action. Normal values for clitoral diameter are less than 7 mm at the base of the glans (see Fig. 16–31). The most accurate definition of clitoromegaly involves the use of the clitoral index (the product of the width and length of the glans clitoris). A clitoral index greater than 35 mm^2 is abnormal and correlates statistically with androgen excess.[332]

Origins of Androgens

Two natural C_{19}-steroids are capable of acting as androgens on target organs: testosterone and DHT. In this chapter, the use of the term androgen refers to either of these steroids. Testosterone in reproductive-age women is produced by two major mechanisms: (1) direct secretion by the ovary, accounting for roughly one third of testosterone production, and (2) conversion of the precursor androstenedione to testosterone in the peripheral (extragonadal) tissues, accounting for two thirds of testosterone production (Fig. 16–32).[333] These peripheral tissues include the skin and adipose tissue. Androstenedione, the direct precursor of testosterone, is produced in both the ovary and the adrenal. The C_{19}-steroids DHEAS and DHEA of adrenal origin and DHEA of ovarian origin indirectly contribute to testosterone formation by first being converted to androstenedione that is subsequently converted to testosterone (see Fig. 16–32).

Whereas testosterone is an androgen, DHEAS is a biologically inert steroid. Up to 20 mg of DHEAS is produced daily versus only 3 mg of androstenedione and 8 mg of DHEA per day. These C_{19}-steroids of adrenal origin (DHEAS, DHEA) exert their effects after conversion to the potent androgen testosterone (see Fig. 16–32). Only androstenedione can be converted directly to testosterone. The conversion rate of circulating androstenedione to testosterone in extragonadal tissues is about 5% in both men and women.[167]

Testosterone binds nuclear androgen receptors and activates androgen target genes. Testosterone, however, must be converted to an even more potent steroid, DHT, to exert full androgenic effects on target tissues such as hair follicles and external genitalia.[170, 197] For example, intense androgen action in sex skin fibroblasts requires receptor occupancy by DHT. This conversion is catalyzed by the enzyme 5α-reductase and takes place in the liver and within androgen target cells such as sex skin fibroblasts (i.e., intracrine effect). The protein products of two genes (5α-reductase type 1 and type 2) exhibit this enzymatic activity.[170] The androgenic potential of DHT with respect to hair growth and virilization of external genitalia is markedly higher than that of testosterone.

Androgen action in target tissues is determined at least in part by the level of local 5α-reductase activity and the androgen receptor content. Androgen receptors mediate androgenic action in critical target tissues (see Fig. 16–32).[197, 334] Local enzymes at target tissues other than 5α-reductase (e.g., aromatase and 17β-HSD or ketoreductase) also regulate androgen action by metabolizing testosterone to the androgenically inactive androstenedione or to estradiol, a potent estrogen. Thus, there appears to be a balance between the amplification of androgen action when DHT is formed and the reduction of androgenicity when inactive C_{19}-steroids or estradiol is formed from testosterone in target tissues and other extragonadal tissues. In particular, the metabolism of testosterone to DHT versus androstenedione-estradiol in these tissues is important with respect to androgen-dependent disorders (e.g., hirsutism, virilization) and estrogen-dependent disorders (e.g., malignancies of breast and endometrium).

Laboratory Evaluation of Androgen Action

Testosterone circulates in three forms: that which is bound to TeBG, the portion not bound to TeBG but rather loosely associated with albumin, and the fraction not bound by either

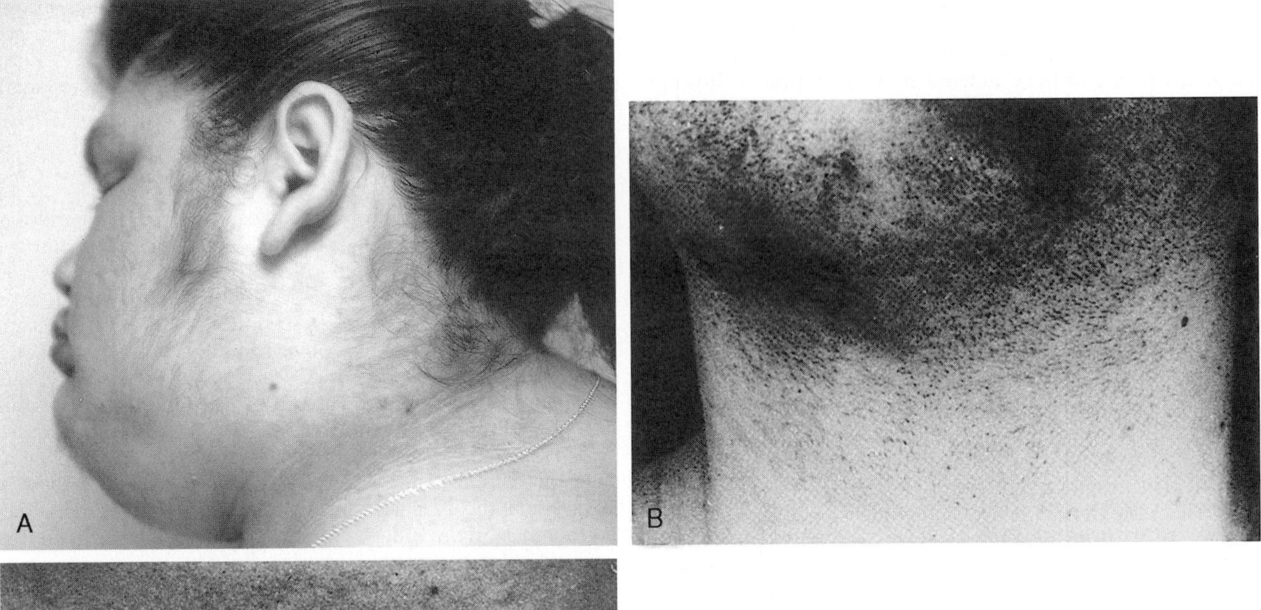

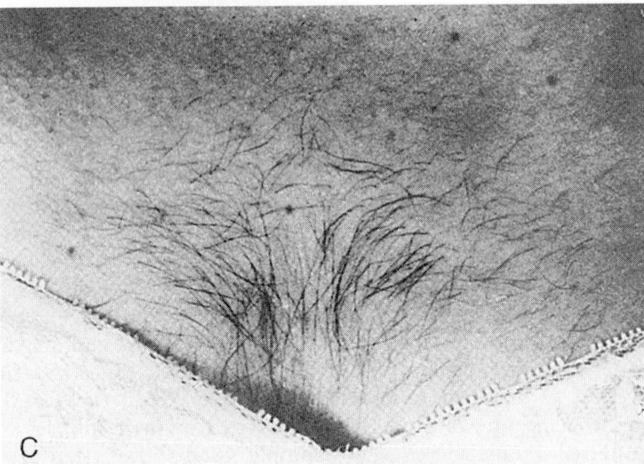

Figure 16–30. Hirsutism. *A*, Mild facial hirsutism. *B*, Severe facial hirsutism (chin), which requires regular shaving. *C*, Severe hirsutism on chest. (*B* and *C*, from Dunaif A, Hoffman AR, Scully RE, et al. The clinical, biochemical and ovarian morphologic features in women with acanthosis nigricans and masculinization. Obstet Gynecol 1985; 66:545–552.)

TeBG or albumin, that is, free or dialyzable testosterone.[335] Biologically active testosterone includes both the free and albumin-bound fractions.[335] Thus, the blood concentration of testosterone available to diffuse into target tissues is referred to as bioavailable or non–TeBG-bound testosterone.[335] The remainder is tightly bound to the protein TeBG.

TeBG is one of the primary regulators that determines the amounts of circulating bound and bioavailable testosterone available to act on target tissues. Conditions that decrease TeBG binding (e.g., androgen excess, obesity, acromegaly, hypothyroidism, and liver disease) also increase bioavailable testosterone, thus augmenting the effect of testosterone. TeBG

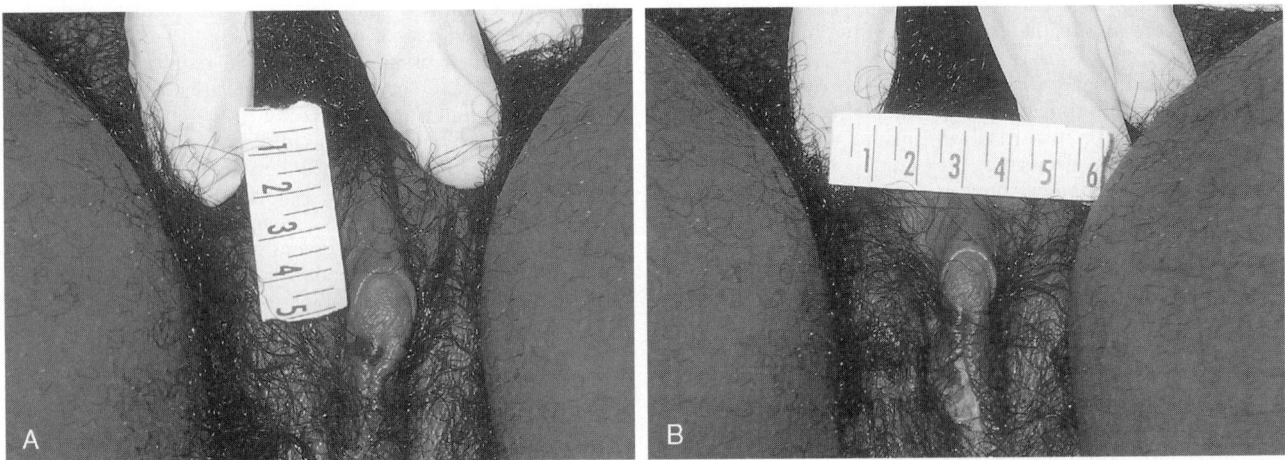

Figure 16–31. Severe clitoromegaly resulting from a testosterone-secreting ovarian tumor. *A*, The entire length of the clitoris is approximately 4 cm (normal < 1 cm). *B*, The transverse diameter of the clitoris measures 1.5 cm (normal < 0.7 cm).

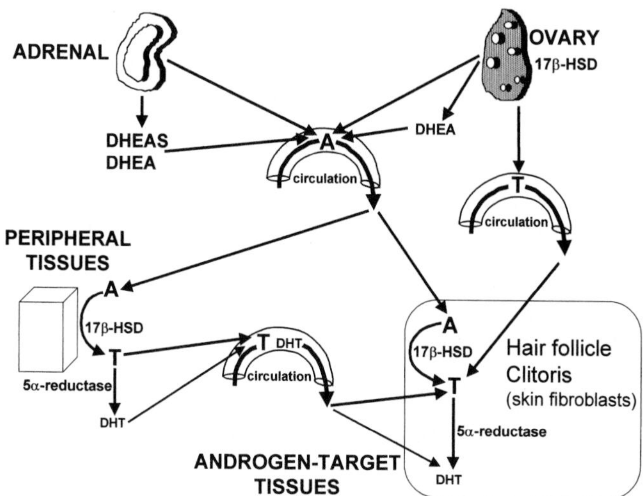

Figure 16–32. Androgen biosynthesis in women. There are two biologically active androgens, testosterone (T) and dihydrotestosterone (DHT). Depending on the menstrual cycle phase or postmenopausal status, 20% to 30% of T is secreted by the ovary. The rest of T production (blood) is accounted for by the conversion of circulating androstenedione (A) to T in various peripheral tissues. Both the adrenal and ovary contribute to circulating A directly or indirectly depending on the cycle phase, reproductive-age versus postmenopausal status, and chronologic age. Moreover, T may also be formed locally in androgen target tissues. Finally, T is converted to the more potent androgen DHT within the target tissues and cells. For example, local conversion of T to DHT in sex skin fibroblasts and hair follicles amplifies androgenic action for clitoral enlargement and hirsutism. DHEA, dehydroepiandrosterone; HSD, hydroxysteroid dehydrogenase.

also regulates the circulating amounts of bioavailable estradiol by binding a significant fraction of circulating estradiol. Hence, conditions that decrease TeBG levels also give rise to increased bioavailable (non–TeBG-bound) estradiol.

The measurement of non–TeBG-bound (bioavailable) forms of testosterone has been advocated in states of androgen excess to detect more accurately subtle forms of hirsutism.[335] Although the diagnostic yield of this measurement is clearly superior to that of total serum testosterone, the correlation between total and non–TeBG-bound testosterone is excellent and can frequently be predicted.[336] The purpose of measuring serum testosterone is to establish circulating androgen excess, to estimate the source of androgen production, and to detect extremely high values that might originate from an androgen-secreting neoplasm.

The normal serum levels of androgens and their precursors in women vary from laboratory to laboratory. Some approximate levels are as follows: testosterone, less then 0.6 ng/mL; free testosterone, less than 8 pg/mL; non–TeBG-bound testosterone (free + albumin-bound), less than 0.1 ng/mL; androstenedione, less than 3 ng/mL; DHEA, less than 9 ng/mL; DHEAS, less than 2.5 μg/mL; and DHT, less than 0.3 ng/mL. Androstenedione, DHEA, testosterone (total and free), and DHT fluctuate during the ovulatory cycle, and highest levels are found during the luteal phase because of increased secretion of these steroids or their precursors from the corpus luteum. Thus, steroid measurements should be obtained routinely during the early follicular phase, preferably at cycle day 3 (±1 day), so that these levels can be compared and interpreted more easily.

For practical purposes, measuring the levels of all of these C_{19}-steroids is not clinically necessary in the majority of patients presenting with androgen excess. The most useful initial test is a serum total testosterone level. An abnormal level in the presence of hirsutism or virilization may be associated with PCOS, hyperthecosis, nonclassical adrenal hyperplasia, or an androgen-secreting neoplasm. The majority of androgen-secreting tumors are of ovarian origin. The likelihood of a neoplasm correlates roughly with increasing testosterone levels. The following tests may be added on the basis of the clinical presentation: serum 17-hydroxyprogesterone (nonclassical adrenal hyperplasia), serum prolactin and TSH (mild androgen excess associated with hyperprolactinemia), serum FSH and LH (elevated LH/FSH ratio in PCOS), serum DHEAS (adrenal tumors), and imaging of ovaries and adrenals (PCOS, tumors).

Causes of Androgen Excess

A variety of disorders give rise to androgen excess. These include unusual causes such as iatrogenic or drug-induced androgen excess, congenital genital ambiguity (e.g., excessive in utero androgen formation in female pseudohermaphroditism), and conditions unique to pregnancy (luteoma of pregnancy and hyperreactio luteinalis). These uncommon causes and relatively more prevalent disorders associated with androgen excess are listed in Table 16–5. The term extra-ovarian steroid formation is used synonymously for extraglandular, extragonadal, or peripheral steroid formation in this text.

In most hyperandrogenic disorders, androgen originates from more than one source (see Fig. 16–32). For example, testosterone secretion is somewhat increased from the ovary in PCOS, but the bulk of testosterone comes from extraovarian conversion of significantly elevated circulating androstenedione of ovarian origin to testosterone. To add a further twist, patients with PCOS also show increased adrenal output of DHEAS, which (after peripheral conversion to DHEA that is further converted to androstenedione) contributes indirectly to extraovarian testosterone formation (see Fig. 16–32).

When androgen excess is associated with primary amenorrhea, abnormal in utero sexual differentiation should be strongly suspected. These disorders are covered in detail in Chapter 22. Furthermore, before embarking on a major work-up for hirsutism or virilization, the physician is well advised to rule out exogenous androgen use. It is best to ask the patient to list all prescriptions and over-the-counter medications that she takes on her own, including injections. This is usually more rewarding than simply asking the patient whether she takes any androgens. Medications that can cause hirsutism or

Table 16–5. Causes of Androgen Excess in a Reproductive-Age Woman

Ovarian
PCOS
Hyperthecosis (a severe PCOS variant)
Ovarian tumor (e.g., Sertoli-Leydig cell tumor)
Adrenal
Nonclassical adrenal hyperplasia
Cushing's syndrome
Glucocorticoid resistance
Adrenal tumor (e.g., adenoma, carcinoma)
Specific conditions of pregnancy
Luteoma of pregnancy
Hyperreactio luteinalis
Aromatase deficiency in fetus
Other
Hyperprolactinemia, hypothyroidism
Medications (danazol, testosterone, anabolizing agents)
Idiopathic hirsutism (normal serum testosterone in an ovulatory woman)

PCOS, polycystic ovary syndrome.

virilization are related to testosterone. These include anabolic steroids and similar compounds.

The most common identifiable cause of androgen excess is PCOS.[337] PCOS is discussed under a separate heading in this chapter. In this section, we first define some of the other disorders associated with hirsutism or virilization. This is followed by a simplified treatment strategy, which may be applied to the majority of hirsute patients within the categories PCOS, nonclassical adrenal hyperplasia, and idiopathic hirsutism.

Idiopathic Hirsutism

Excessive hair growth in the absence of demonstrable androgen excess in ovulatory women is also referred to as idiopathic or constitutional and occurs more frequently in certain ethnic populations, particularly in women of Mediterranean ancestry.[197] It is defined as hirsutism in conjunction with regular menstrual cycles and normal levels of serum testosterone. Idiopathic hirsutism is not associated with any sign of virilization. Its cause is not understood completely. It has been proposed that women with idiopathic hirsutism have significantly increased cutaneous 5α-reductase activity.[338] At this time, the presence or absence of such an association is not clear. Likewise, it is still unclear which of the 5α-reductase isoenzymes (type 1 or 2), if any, is predominant in the development of idiopathic hirsutism.[197]

Idiopathic hirsutism is diagnosed in women who have (1) hirsutism, (2) normal ovulatory function, and (3) normal total or free testosterone levels. Overall, more than 80% of women with cyclic predictable menses are ovulatory. Ovulatory function may be verified by a luteal phase day 7 progesterone level, which should be at least 5 ng/mL. Luteal phase day 7 corresponds to cycle day 17 for 24-day intervals, cycle day 21 for 28-day intervals, and cycle day 28 for 35-day intervals. The presence of oligo-ovulation or anovulation in hirsute women after the exclusion of related disorders (e.g., hypothyroidism, hyperprolactinemia, or nonclassical adrenal hyperplasia) is consistent with the diagnosis of PCOS.[197] Thyroid dysfunction and hyperprolactinemia should be excluded by the measurements of TSH and prolactin. The follicular phase basal 17-hydroxyprogesterone level should be measured to exclude 21-hydroxylase–deficient, nonclassical adrenal hyperplasia. The use of exogenous androgens should also be excluded. In summary, the diagnosis of idiopathic hirsutism is one of exclusion, in which ovulatory dysfunction, elevated circulating testosterone, and other causes of androgen excess are ruled out.

Androgen-Secreting Tumors of the Ovary and Adrenal

The majority of androgen-secreting tumors arise from the ovary. These ovarian tumors secrete large quantities of testosterone or its precursor androstenedione. They include Sertoli-Leydig cell tumors, hilus cell tumors, lipoid cell tumors, and, infrequently, granulosa-theca tumors. Steroidogenically inert ovarian neoplasms such as epithelial cystadenomas or cystadenocarcinomas may produce factors that stimulate steroidogenesis in adjacent non-neoplastic ovarian stroma and induce production of sufficient amounts of androgen precursors such as androstenedione. Approximately 5% of androstenedione is converted to testosterone in extraovarian tissues to give rise ultimately to androgen excess (see Fig. 16–32).

Sertoli-Leydig cell tumors, which account for less than 1% of all solid ovarian tumors, tend to occur during the second to fourth decades of life, whereas hilus cell tumors occur more frequently in postmenopausal women. By the time the signs and symptoms of androgen excess cause the patient to seek medical assistance, Sertoli-Leydig cell tumors are usually so large that they are readily palpable on pelvic examination, whereas hilus cell tumors are still small. In women with either type of tumor, serum testosterone is markedly elevated. Granulosa-theca tumors primarily produce estradiol but may occasionally produce testosterone.

Rapidly progressing symptoms of androgen excess suggest the presence of an androgen-producing tumor unless proved otherwise. This rapid progression is typical of both ovarian and adrenal androgen-producing tumors. The progression is usually from defeminizing signs (loss of female body contour, decrease in breast size) to the androgenic signs. As the tumor continues to grow, more and more testosterone is produced, resulting in rapidly worsening hirsutism and progressive virilization. With all ovarian tumors, serum testosterone is characteristically elevated. This may be mediated by two mechanisms: (1) production and secretion of testosterone directly by the tumor[339] or (2) secretion of large quantities of androstenedione that is converted to testosterone in extragonadal tissues. The testosterone levels produced by certain ovarian tumors (e.g., the Sertoli-Leydig cell tumor) may be suppressed using an LHRH agonist.[340] Therefore, use of an LHRH agonist cannot be relied upon to distinguish a neoplasm from another functional state.

In interpreting testosterone levels, the clinician should first be familiar with the normal ranges of the clinical laboratory used. A value of three times the upper normal range (or > 2 ng/mL) is suggestive of a neoplasm, particularly if the clinical history supports this diagnosis. It should be kept in mind that lower serum testosterone levels may occasionally be observed in association with virilizing ovarian tumors. When an androgen-secreting tumor is suspected, a measurement of androstenedione is also clinically useful. A severely elevated level of androstenedione is also consistent with an ovarian or adrenal tumor. When an elevated level of testosterone is found and confirmed by clinical history, meticulously performed transvaginal ultrasonography should be able to detect the ovarian tumor. Transvaginal ultrasonography is the most sensitive method for the detection of an ovarian tumor.

In contrast to testosterone-secreting tumors of the ovary, testosterone-secreting tumors of the adrenal are extremely rare.[341] The cells of testosterone-producing adrenal tumors may resemble ovarian hilus cells, which are analogous to Leydig cells. These tumor cells produce testosterone and may be stimulated by both LH and hCG. Thus, in patients with testosterone-producing adrenal adenomas, testosterone secretion usually decreases after LH suppression and increases after hCG stimulation.

Virilizing adrenal tumors commonly secrete large quantities of DHEAS, DHEA, and androstenedione, whereas testosterone is usually produced by extraovarian conversion of these precursors. Levels of serum DHEAS are highly elevated in most virilizing adrenal tumors.[342] When DHEAS levels exceed 8 μg/mL, a scan by either computed tomography or MRI should be ordered unless the history is more suggestive of PCOS (long-standing history of symptoms and no virilization). In the latter case, a functional abnormality of the adrenal is likely to be present: either an enzymatic defect, such as congenital adrenal hyperplasia, or an unexplained hyperfunctional state that is commonly associated with PCOS.[343] Under these circumstances, the scan can be deferred until further investigation has been carried out.

Levels of a variety of adrenal steroids including corticosteroids may be elevated in various combinations in the presence of an adrenal tumor. Thus, it is not possible to describe a particular pattern of hormones that defines an adrenal tumor.[342, 343] In general, high levels of serum DHEAS ($>$8 μg/mL) are suggestive of an adrenal tumor. Testosterone-secreting adrenal tumors are extremely rare.[341] Virilizing ovarian tumors, on the other hand, are encountered much more frequently than those of an adrenal origin. If the presentation is compatible with an androgen-secreting tumor and the ovaries are normal by transvaginal ultrasonography, the adrenals should be evaluated next by imaging.

Testosterone levels three times the upper normal range (or > 2 ng/mL) and DHEAS levels higher than 8 μg/mL have been used as guidelines to investigate further whether neoplasms of the ovary or adrenal are the sources of androgen excess. It should be emphasized that these numbers are provided only as guidelines and not as rules. The following exceptions to these guidelines must be pointed out. First, because tumors secrete androgens episodically, more than one value may be required to detect a significantly elevated level.[344] Second, other precursor steroids are often elevated as well (particularly androstenedione), and their measurement should be considered. Finally, the tumors may give rise to milder elevations of DHEAS and testosterone levels. In particular, even mild elevations in a postmenopausal woman are highly suspicious of an androgen-secreting tumor.[345] By the same token, severely elevated serum testosterone levels (three times the upper normal range or > 2 ng/mL) may be observed in women with severe ovarian hyperthecosis (a severe variant of PCOS) in the absence of a tumor.

Virilization of recent onset and short duration should warrant further investigation, even if testosterone and DHEAS are mildly elevated. With improvements in scanning techniques—vaginal ultrasonography for the ovary; abdominal ultrasonography, computed tomography, and MRI for the adrenal—the diagnosis of even a small (ovarian or adrenal) tumor may be made. However, if no neoplasm can be localized, imaging of the ovary or adrenal after intravenous administration of radiolabeled iodomethylnorcholesterol (NP-59), which detects active steroid-producing tumors, has proved useful.[346] These diagnostic studies should be pursued aggressively before the surgical exploration of a suspected tumor.

Non-Neoplastic Adrenal Disorders and Androgen Excess

A number of adrenal disorders, such as classical congenital adrenal hyperplasia, Cushing's syndrome, and glucocorticoid resistance, give rise to androgen excess related to overproduction of testosterone precursors from the adrenal. These disorders are discussed in other chapters. Here, we discuss nonclassical adrenal hyperplasia.

The debate regarding the diagnosis and prevalence of nonclassical adrenal hyperplasia still continues, although the disorder clearly exists. Other terms that have been used to describe this syndrome include late-onset, adult-onset, attenuated, incomplete, and cryptic adrenal hyperplasia. This form of adrenal hyperplasia is caused by a partial deficiency in 21-hydroxylase activity. Although deficiencies in 11β-hydroxylase and 3β-HSD may result in the disorder, defects in 21-hydroxylase account for more than 90% of cases.[347]

The clinical presentation is almost identical to that of patients with PCOS.[348] The prevalence of this disorder varies according to ethnic background, and the prevalence reported by different investigators has varied widely. The characteristic presentation consists of anovulatory uterine bleeding and progressive hirsutism of pubertal onset. These individuals are born with normal genitalia, do not exhibit salt wasting, and are symptom-free until puberty. Patients of northern European ancestry have a low frequency of this disorder, whereas Ashkenazi Jews, Hispanics, and patients of central European ancestry have a much higher prevalence.[349] Therefore, it is recommended that high-risk ethnic groups be screened.

Screening may first be carried out by obtaining an 8:00 AM serum 17-hydroxyprogesterone level in an anovulatory patient on any day. Although the majority of women with nonclassical adrenal hyperplasia are anovulatory, some women with this disorder present with regular periods and hirsutism of pubertal onset or with only unexplained infertility.[347] If nonclassical adrenal hyperplasia is suspected in an ovulatory patient on the basis of clinical presentation, an 8:00 AM serum 17-hydroxyprogesterone level should be obtained during the follicular phase because 17-hydroxyprogesterone levels are higher in the luteal phase versus the proliferative phase in affected or disease-free ovulatory women.[347] A level less than 2 ng/mL effectively rules out this diagnosis.[347]

The diagnosis of nonclassical adrenal hyperplasia can be made if the basal 17-hydroxyprogesterone level is higher than 8 ng/mL. No further testing is required in these cases. Values between 2 and 8 ng/mL are considered increased but not diagnostic of nonclassical adrenal hyperplasia. For example, disease-free women or patients with PCOS may also have basal 17-hydroxyprogesterone levels in this indeterminate range.[347] The only way to distinguish nonclassical adrenal hyperplasia from PCOS under these circumstances is with an ACTH stimulation test.[347] A rise of 17-hydroxyprogesterone to at least 10 ng/mL 60 minutes after intravenous injection of ACTH has been considered diagnostic of nonclassical adrenal hyperplasia.[350] It should be noted, however, that a higher basal 17-hydroxprogesterone level within the 2 to 8 ng/mL range is associated with a higher likelihood of nonclassical adrenal hyperplasia. For example, an 8:00 AM 17-hydroxyprogesterone level higher than 4 ng/mL had a sensitivity of 90% for the diagnosis of nonclassical adrenal hyperplasia.[347]

In a patient with androgen excess who belongs to an ethnic group in which there is high prevalence, a baseline 17-hydroxyprogesterone level should be measured at 8:00 AM. In addition, the following patients should have a screening baseline 17-hydroxyprogesterone level obtained: patients with premature pubarche, those with androgen excess of early pubertal onset, women with progressive hirsutism or virilization, and patients with strong family histories of severe androgen excess.[351]

Laboratory Testing to Aid the Differential Diagnosis of Androgen Excess

A number of algorithms exist for the differential diagnosis of anovulation associated with hirsutism or virilization, or both. Salient clinical features are of paramount importance to guide laboratory testing. The most important features include the onset and severity of the signs and the rapidity with which they progress. Rapidly progressing severe androgen excess implies an androgen-secreting tumor until proved otherwise. The possibility of a tumor is further underscored in a postmenopausal woman or in a reproductive-age woman with a recent history of cyclic, predictable periods. Ovarian hyperthecosis, a severe variant of PCOS, also gives rise to severe androgen excess that may progress rapidly, especially at the time of expected puberty. Androgen excess emerging at the time of puberty may be indicative of PCOS or nonclassical adrenal hyperplasia.

The most useful initial test to evaluate androgen excess is serum total testosterone (Table 16–6). Testosterone levels in most normal ovulatory women are below 0.6 ng/mL, although the value may vary from laboratory to laboratory. Women with idiopathic hirsutism have cyclic menses and normal testosterone levels. No further testing for androgen excess is required in this group.

If the testosterone level is elevated in an anovulatory woman, serum TSH and prolactin should be obtained next to rule out anovulation associated with hyperprolactinemia. Ultrasonography of the ovaries is also helpful at this time to assess the presence or absence of an ovarian tumor or polycystic

Table 16–6. Laboratory Tests for the Differential Diagnosis of Androgen Excess

Initial Testing
Total testosterone
Prolactin
TSH
Further Testing Based on Clinical Presentation*
17-Hydroxyprogesterone (8:00 AM)
17-Hydroxyprogesterone 60 min after intravenous ACTH
Cortisol (8:00 AM) after 1 mg dexamethasone at midnight
DHEAS
Androstenedione
Imaging of ovaries (transvaginal ultrasonography)
Imaging of adrenals (abdominal ultrasonography, CT scan, MRI)
Nuclear imaging after intravenous administration of radiolabeled cholesterol

*See text.

ACTH, adrenocorticotropic hormone; CT, computed tomography; DHEAS, dehydroepiandrosterone sulfate; MRI, magnetic resonance imaging; TSH, thyroid-stimulating hormone.

ovaries. If the ethnic background of the patient (Ashkenazi Jews, Hispanics, and those of central European ancestry), onset of hirsutism (puberty), or family history is suggestive of nonclassical adrenal hyperplasia, a baseline serum 17-hydroxyprogesterone level should be obtained at 8:00 AM. Rare etiologies of androgen excess include an adrenal tumor, Cushing's syndrome, and glucocorticoid resistance. A serum DHEAS level and adrenal imaging are required to assess the presence or absence of an adrenal tumor. A computed tomographic scan, MRI scan, or abdominal ultrasonography may be used to assess the adrenals, depending on the expertise of the local radiology laboratory. A screening test for Cushing's syndrome and glucocorticoid resistance may be performed to explore rare adrenal causes of androgen excess (see Chapter 14).[352]

Most women with chronic anovulation and mild to moderate hirsutism of pubertal onset fall into the category of PCOS. These women have high normal or elevated testosterone levels and no other laboratory abnormalities. When other diagnoses are ruled out either by laboratory testing or on clinical grounds, a diagnosis of PCOS can be made.

Treatment of Hirsutism

Therapy for androgen excess should be directed toward its specific cause and at suppression of abnormal androgen secretion. Specific treatments for hirsutism and virilization would be indicated for the following conditions: ovarian and adrenal tumors, hyperthecosis, Cushing's syndrome, and adrenal hyperplasia. Neoplasms warrant surgical intervention and are not discussed in greater detail. Suppression with an LHRH analogue may be tried initially for ovarian hyperthecosis. Unfortunately, bilateral oophorectomy is inevitable to control androgen excess arising from hyperthecosis in the majority of patients (see later). Patients with adrenal disease are treated specifically. For Cushing's syndrome, treatment is according to the source of hypercortisolism. For nonclassical adrenal hyperplasia, glucocorticoid replacement should be implemented as for adrenal insufficiency. When treating androgen excess associated with nonclassical adrenal hyperplasia, an antiandrogen (e.g., spironolactone) in combination with an oral contraceptive or a glucocorticoid may be used. The doses of glucocorticoids needed to suppress the adrenal, however, can often cause symptoms and signs of glucocorticoid excess during long-term treatment. Thus, a combination oral contraceptive plus spironolactone should be favored to treat androgen excess if the patient responds to this treatment with decreased hirsutism. Greater details of glucocorticoid therapy may be found in Chapters 14 and 22.

The general treatment of androgen excess is directed toward the prevention of abnormal hair growth and virilization. For practical purposes, the same approach is used for androgen excess associated with idiopathic hirsutism, PCOS, and nonclassical adrenal hyperplasia. The existing hair follicles and manifestations of virilization (e.g., thickening of voice, clitoromegaly, temporal balding) remain even after the elimination of excessive androgen production. Therefore, terminal hair should be removed by mechanical methods (e.g. electrolysis) at least 3 months after androgen suppression is achieved. Patients with clitoromegaly may be referred to a urologist for clitoral reduction surgery after the source of virilization is effectively eliminated. The following medications are available for the treatment of androgen excess and hirsutism.

Oral Contraceptives

Oral contraceptives reduce circulating testosterone and androgen precursors by suppression of LH and stimulation of TeBG levels and, thereby, reduce hirsutism in hyperandrogenic patients.[197] Oral contraceptives decrease circulating androgen in patients with PCOS and synergize with the effects of antiandrogens. It is possible that oral contraceptives may further improve the results of antiandrogen therapy in idiopathic hirsutism. It is advisable to use an oral contraceptive containing either 30 or 35 μg of ethinyl estradiol to achieve effective suppression of LH.[197]

Spironolactone

The most common androgen blocker used for the treatment of hirsutism in the United States is spironolactone, an aldosterone antagonist structurally related to progestins. Spironolactone is effective for abnormal hair growth associated with PCOS or idiopathic hirsutism.

Because spironolactone acts through mechanisms different from that of oral contraceptives, the overall effectiveness is improved by combining these two medications, even in patients with idiopathic hirsutism. Apart from the inhibition of steroidogenesis and acting as an androgen antagonist, spironolactone has a significant effect in inhibiting 5α-reductase activity.[197, 353] Basic and several clinical studies clearly point to the efficacy of spironolactone for hyperandrogenism and suggest that the principal effect is related to its peripheral blocking ability.[197]

Doses of spironolactone have varied in clinical studies from 50 to 400 mg daily. Although doses of 100 mg/day are generally effective for the treatment of hirsutism, higher doses (200 to 300 mg/day) may be preferable in extremely hirsute or markedly obese women.[197, 353] Thus, it is recommended to start with 100 mg/day and gradually increase the dose by 25 mg/day increments every 3 months up to 200 mg/day on the basis of the response. This approach may be helpful to minimize side effects such as gastritis, dry skin, and anovulation.

In patients with normal renal function, hyperkalemia is almost never seen. Hypotension is rare except in older women. Monitoring, however, is imperative for electrolytes and blood pressure within the first 2 weeks at each dose level. Adjustments in dose should be made only after 3 to 6 months, as with other antiandrogens, to account for the slow changes in the hair cycle. Patients usually note an initial transient diuretic effect. Some women with normal cycles complain of menstrual irregularity with spironolactone. The latter complaint is remedied by either a downward dose adjustment or the addition of an oral contraceptive. The mechanism for abnormal bleeding is unclear. In women with oligomenorrhea, such as those with PCOS, resumption of normal menses may occur. In part, this may be due to an alteration in levels of circulating androgens, although LH levels have only occasionally been noted to decrease.[354] Another important consideration is the potential in utero feminizing effect of this antiandrogen on the genitalia of a 46,XY fetus. Thus, effective contraception should always be provided in women taking spironolactone.

Cyproterone Acetate

Cyproterone acetate is a 17-hydroxyprogesterone acetate derivative with strong progestagenic properties. Cyproterone acetate acts as an antiandrogen by competing with DHT and testosterone for binding to the androgen receptor. There is also some evidence that cyproterone acetate and ethinyl estradiol in combination can inhibit 5α-reductase activity in skin.[355] Cyproterone acetate is currently not available in the United States but has been used in other countries. The drug is mostly administered in doses of 50 to 100 mg from days 5 through 15 of the treatment cycle. Because of its slow metabolism, it is administered early in the treatment cycle, whereas ethinyl estradiol, when added, is usually used at 50-μg doses between days 5 and 26. This regimen is needed for menstrual control and is usually referred to as the reverse sequential regimen. Cyproterone acetate in doses of 50 to 100 mg/day, combined with ethinyl estradiol at 30 to 35 μg/day, is as effective as the combination of spironolactone, 100 mg/day, and an oral contraceptive in the treatment of hirsutism.[197] In smaller doses (2 mg), cyproterone acetate has been administered as an oral contraceptive in daily combination with 50 or 35 μg of ethinyl estradiol. This regimen is primarily suited for individuals with a milder form of hyperandrogenism.[197]

Finasteride

Finasteride inhibits 5α-reductase activity and has been used primarily for the treatment of prostatic hyperplasia.[356] It can also be used in the treatment of hirsutism.[357, 358] At a dose of 5 mg/day, a significant improvement of hirsutism is observed after 6 months of therapy, without significant side effects. In hirsute women, the decline in circulating DHT levels is small and cannot be used to monitor therapy. Although this treatment regimen increases testosterone levels, TeBG levels remain unaffected.[357]

Finasteride primarily inhibits 5α-reductase type 2. As hirsutism results from a combination of effects of type 1 and type 2, this agent is only partially effective. Although prolonged experience with finasteride is lacking, one of the potential advantages of this agent appears to be its benign side-effect profile. One study showed efficacy with 1 year of hirsutism treatment.[359] It was also reported that finasteride is less effective than spironolactone with respect to the reduction of hirsutism.[197] Nevertheless, finasteride represents a useful option for treating women with hirsutism at a dose of 5 mg/day for prolonged periods because of its benign side-effect profile and good tolerance by patients.

Flutamide

Flutamide is a potent antiandrogen used in the treatment of prostate cancer.[360] It has been shown to be effective in the treatment of hirsutism.[361–364] Nevertheless, occasional severe hepatotoxicity makes this drug unsuitable for the indication of hirsutism.[365]

Summary

The preceding medications may be effective when administered as individual treatments. Patients with the most common form of hirsutism (i.e., PCOS) are often initially treated with a combination of two agents, one that suppresses the ovary (e.g., oral contraceptive) and another agent that suppresses the extraovarian (peripheral) action of androgens (e.g., spironolactone). Thus, an oral contraceptive containing 30 to 35 μg of ethinyl estradiol combined with spironolactone, 100 mg/day, is the initial treatment of choice. Even in women with idiopathic hirsutism, the addition of an oral contraceptive to the antiandrogen spironolactone can improve efficacy and prevent abnormal bleeding. For women with only minor complaints of hirsutism, the use of an oral contraceptive alone may be an appropriate first approach.

Because the growth phase of body hairs lasts 3 to 6 months, one should not expect a response before 6 months from the onset of the treatment. Objective means should be used to assess changes in hair growth. Scoring systems and evaluation of anagen hair shafts are difficult; taking photographs is the simplest and most objective tool. Patients are often unaware that change is indeed taking place unless there is some objective measurement. Pictures of face and selected midline body areas before and during therapy are especially useful for the encouragement of the patient and compliance with the treatment.

Suppression of androgen production and action only inhibits new hair growth. Thus, existing coarse hair should be removed mechanically. Plucking, waxing, and shaving are ineffective for hair removal and cause irritation, folliculitis, and ingrown hairs. Electrolysis is still the method of choice. Laser epilation is relatively new and needs further evaluation.[197]

The majority of patients with PCOS and idiopathic hirsutism respond to this treatment within 1 year. Patients should be encouraged to continue treatment for at least 2 years. After this, depending on the wishes and clinical responses of patients, therapy can be stopped and the patient reevaluated. Many patients require continuous treatment for the suppression of hirsutism.

The Polycystic Ovary Syndrome

PCOS is the most common form of chronic anovulation associated with androgen excess, perhaps occurring in 5% to 10% of reproductive-age women.[193] The diagnosis of PCOS is made by excluding other hyperandrogenic disorders (e.g., nonclassical adrenal hyperplasia, androgen-secreting tumors, and hyperprolactinemia) in women with chronic anovulation and androgen excess.[337]

During the reproductive years, PCOS is associated with important reproductive morbidity including infertility, irregular uterine bleeding, and increased pregnancy loss.[337] The endometrium of the patient with PCOS must be evaluated by biopsy because long-term unopposed estrogen stimulation leaves these patients at increased risk for endometrial cancer.[337] PCOS is also associated with increased metabolic and cardiovascular risk factors.[366] These risks are linked to insulin resistance and compounded by the common occurrence of obesity, although insulin resistance is also present in nonobese women with PCOS.[193]

PCOS is now viewed as a heterogeneous disorder of multifactorial etiology. PCOS risk is significantly increased with a positive family history of chronic anovulation and androgen excess, and this complex disorder may be inherited in a polygenic fashion.[367, 368]

Historical Perspective

In their pioneering studies, Stein and Leventhal[369] described an association between the presence of bilateral polycystic ovaries and signs of amenorrhea, oligomenorrhea, hirsutism, and obesity (Fig. 16–33). At the time, these signs were strictly adhered to in the diagnosis of what was then known as Stein-

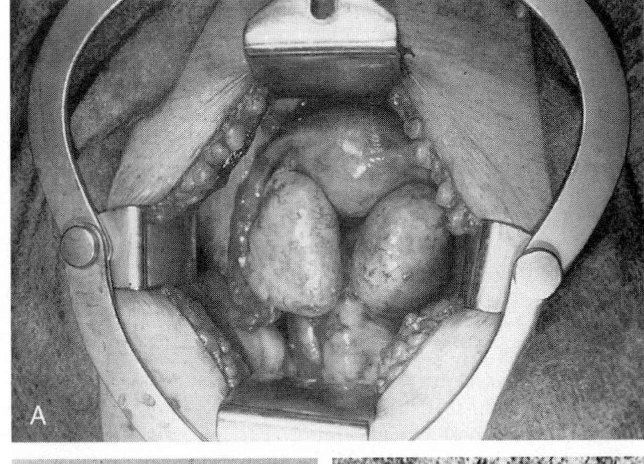

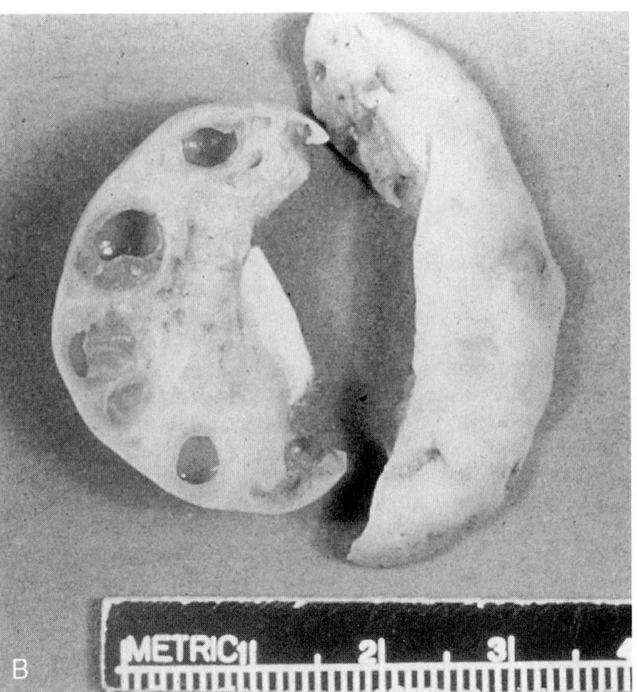

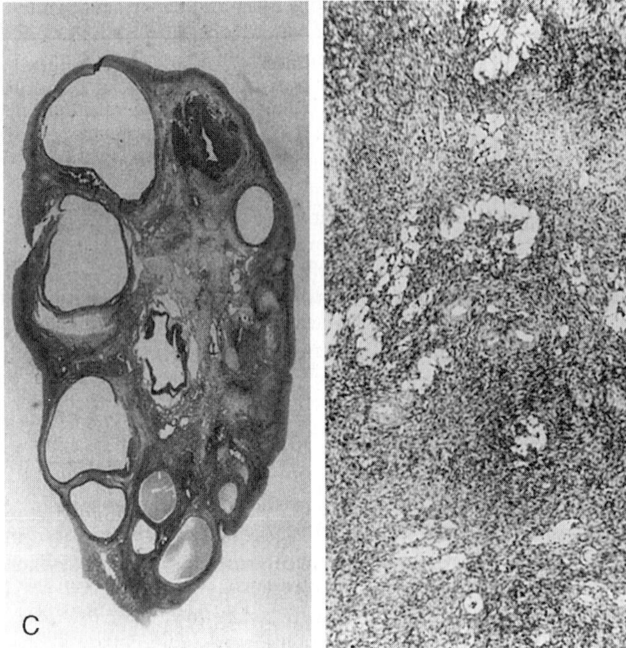

Figure 16–33. Polycystic ovaries. *A*, Operative findings of classical enlarged polycystic ovaries. The uterus is located adjacent to the two enlarged ovaries. *B*, Sectioned polycystic ovary with numerous follicles. *C*, Histologic section of a polycystic ovary with multiple subcapsular follicular cysts and stromal hypertrophy (low power, *left*). At higher power (× 100), islands of luteinized theca cells are visible in the stroma (*right*). This morphologic change is called stromal hyperthecosis and appears to be directly correlated with circulating insulin levels. (*C*, From Dunaif A. Insulin resistance and the polycystic ovary syndrome: mechanism and implications for pathogenesis. Endocr Rev 1997; 18:774–800. Copyright © 1997 by The Endocrine Society.)

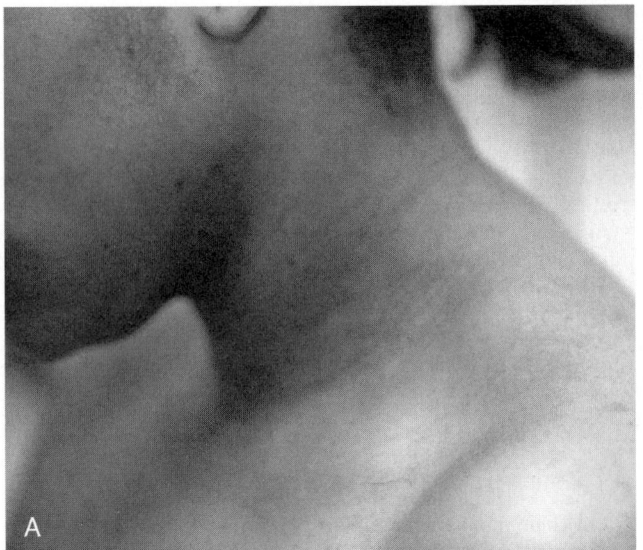

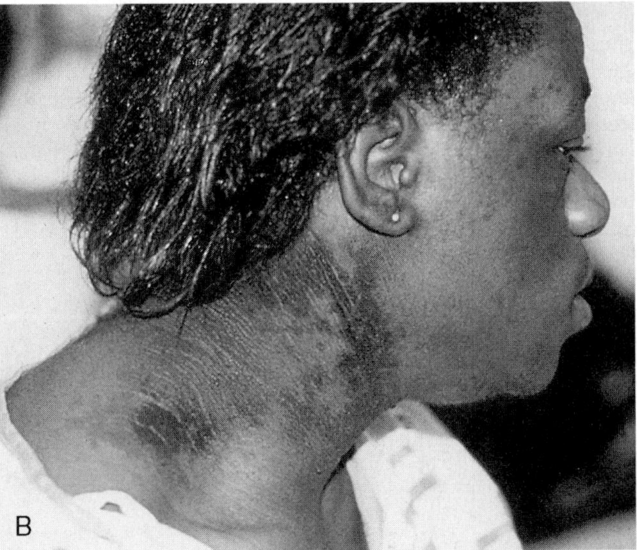

Figure 16–34. Acanthosis nigricans. *A*, Moderate acanthosis nigricans (darkening and thickening of skin) at the lateral lower fold of the neck. Note facial hirsutism (sideburns) in the same patient. *B*, Severe acanthosis nigricans in another patient with severe insulin resistance. (See also Color Plate.) (*B*, courtesy of Dr. R. Ann Word.)

Leventhal syndrome. These investigators also reported the results of bilateral wedge resection of the ovaries, removing at least one half of each ovary as a therapy for PCOS. Most of their patients resumed menses and achieved pregnancy after ovarian wedge resection. They postulated that removing the thickened capsule of the ovary would restore normal ovulation by allowing the follicles to reach the surface of the ovary (see Fig. 16–33). The exact mechanism responsible for the therapeutic effect of removing or destroying part of the ovarian tissue is still not well understood.

On the basis of Stein and Leventhal's work, a primary ovarian defect was inferred, and the disorder was commonly referred to as polycystic ovarian disease. Subsequent clinical, morphologic, hormonal, and metabolic studies have uncovered multiple underlying pathologies (see later). The term polycystic ovary syndrome was introduced to reflect the heterogeneity of this disorder.

One of the most significant discoveries regarding the pathophysiology of PCOS was the demonstration of a unique form of insulin resistance and associated hyperinsulinemia.[193] For the first time, Burghen and co-workers reported this finding in 1980.[370] The presence of insulin resistance in PCOS has since been confirmed by a number of groups worldwide.[193]

Diagnosis of Polycystic Ovary Syndrome and Laboratory Testing

One of the most prominent features of PCOS is the history of ovulatory dysfunction (amenorrhea, oligomenorrhea, or other forms of irregular uterine bleeding) of pubertal onset. Thus, a clear history of cyclic predictable menses of menarchal onset makes the diagnosis of PCOS unlikely. Acquired insulin resistance associated with significant weight gain or an unknown cause, however, may occasionally induce the clinical picture of PCOS in a woman with a history of previously normal ovulatory function. Hirsutism may develop prepubertally or during adolescence, or it may be absent until the third decade of life. Seborrhea, acne, and alopecia are other common clinical signs of androgen excess. In extreme cases of ovarian hyperthecosis (a severe variant of PCOS), clitoromegaly may be observed. Nonetheless, rapid progression of androgenic symptoms and virilization are rare in ordinary PCOS. Some women may never have signs of androgen excess because of genetic differences in target tissue sensitivity to androgens.[197] Infertility related to the anovulation may be the only presenting symptom.

During the physical examination, it is essential to search for and document signs of androgen excess (hirsutism or virilization or both), insulin resistance (acanthosis nigricans), and the presence of unopposed estrogen action (well-rugated vagina and stretchable clear cervical mucus) to support the diagnosis of PCOS (Fig. 16–34). It should be noted that none of these signs are specific for PCOS and may be associated with any of the conditions listed under the differential diagnosis of PCOS (Table 16–7).

The currently recommended diagnostic criteria for PCOS are androgen excess and ovulatory dysfunction with the exclusion of other causes of androgen excess such as nonclassical adrenal hyperplasia (21-hydroxylase deficiency), hyperprolactinemia (with or without hypothyroidism), or androgen-secreting neoplasms (Table 16–8).[337] The exclusion of hyperprolactinemia, hypothyroidism, nonclassical adrenal hyperplasia, and tumors requires a careful history and physical examination as well as laboratory testing as detailed previously (see Table 16–6). Cushing's syndrome and glucocorticoid resistance may give rise to androgen excess and anovulation after a period of normal ovulatory function in teens. An 8:00 AM cortisol level after dexamethasone (1 mg) administration at midnight is a useful screening test for both conditions. Cushing's syndrome may be recognized by its typical signs, whereas 8:00 AM and 4 PM cortisol levels are essential to suspect the diagnosis of glucocorticoid resistance.[352] Glucocorticoid resistance is characterized by preserved diurnal rhythm despite significantly elevated cortisol, ACTH, and adrenal C_{19}-steroid levels and absence of cushingoid symptoms and signs.[352]

As emphasized earlier, elevated total testosterone is the most direct evidence for androgen excess. Varying levels of testosterone are present in women with PCOS. Rarely, serum testosterone levels higher than 2 ng/mL may be encountered in association with the most severe form of PCOS, ovarian hyperthecosis. Overall, it is much more common to observe high normal levels or borderline elevations of testosterone in women with PCOS.

Prolactin and TSH should be obtained routinely to rule out mild androgen excess and anovulation that may be associated with hyperprolactinemia. If basal LH levels are used as a marker for PCOS, a significant number of patients slip through the cracks because they do not all manifest elevated LH levels or increased LH/FSH ratios. This issue prompted a National Institute of Child Health and Human Development–sponsored consensus conference on diagnostic criteria for PCOS in 1990 and the recommendation that LH and the LH/FSH ratio are not required for the diagnosis of PCOS.[371] The heterogeneity of LH values in PCOS may be caused by the pulsatile nature of LH secretion and negative effects of obesity on LH levels. Thus, an elevated LH/FSH ratio is supportive of the diagnosis of PCOS and may be useful in differentiating mild cases of nonobese PCOS without prominent androgen excess from hypothalamic anovulation. Failure to exhibit an elevated LH level, however, is of no diagnostic value.

By definition, nonclassical adrenal hyperplasia is not manifest as congenital virilization of external genitalia. Hyperandrogenic symptoms most commonly appear peripubertally or postpubertally. A 17-hydroxyprogesterone level at 8:00 AM is essential to rule out 21-hydroxylase–deficient nonclassical adrenal hyperplasia.[347] The majority of symptomatic patients with nonclassical adrenal hyperplasia are anovulatory and can be tested on any day at 8:00 AM. In an occasional ovulatory woman with androgen excess and suspected nonclassical adrenal hyperplasia, the 17-hydroxyprogesterone level should be obtained during the follicular phase to maximize specificity.[347] A basal 17-hydroxyprogesterone level less than 2 ng/mL effec-

Table 16–8. Criteria for Clinical Diagnosis of Polycystic Ovary Syndrome

Androgen excess with or without skin manifestations
Irregular uterine bleeding (anovulation or oligo-ovulation)
Absence of other causes of androgen excess (e.g., nonclassical adrenal hyperplasia, Cushing's syndrome, glucocorticoid resistance or ovarian or adrenal tumor)
(Demonstration of polycystic ovaries on ultrasonography is a common feature that is not essential for diagnosis)

Table 16–7. Differential Diagnosis of Polycystic Ovary Syndrome

Idiopathic hirsutism
Hyperprolactinemia, hypothyroidism
Nonclassical adrenal hyperplasia
Ovarian tumors
Adrenal tumors
Cushing's syndrome
Glucocorticoid resistance
Other rare causes of androgen excess

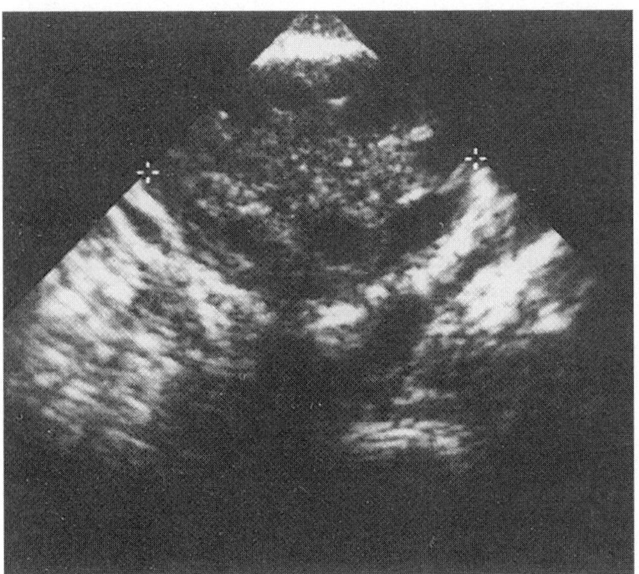

Figure 16–35. Transvaginal ultrasound image of a polycystic ovary. Note multiple midsized follicles in the periphery and increased solid area in the middle. (From Franks S. Medical progress: polycystic ovary syndrome. N Engl J Med 1995; 333:853–861.)

tively rules out nonclassical adrenal hyperplasia.[347] Patients with (proliferative phase 8:00 AM) 17-hydroxyprogesterone levels higher than 2 ng/mL should undergo an ACTH stimulation test. A 17-hydroxyprogesterone level higher than 10 ng/mL at 60 minutes after intravenous injection of ACTH is diagnostic of nonclassical adrenal hyperplasia. Please refer to Chapters 11 and 19 for details of the ACTH stimulation test. A screening test for Cushing's syndrome or glucocorticoid resistance should be performed as clinically indicated (see Chapters 14 and 22).

Serum DHEAS levels may be increased (up to 8 μg/mL) in about 50% of anovulatory women with PCOS. DHEAS originates almost exclusively from the adrenal.[372, 373] The etiology of adrenal hyperactivity in PCOS is not known. Obtaining a DHEAS level routinely in a patient with PCOS is not recommended because it does not change the diagnosis or management. On the other hand, if an adrenal tumor is suspected, a DHEAS level should be obtained. DHEAS levels above 8 μg/mL may be associated with steroidogenically active adrenal tumors, and imaging is then indicated.

The use of ultrasonography in the diagnosis of PCOS must be tempered by an awareness of the broad spectrum of women with ultrasonographic findings characteristic of polycystic ovaries. The typical polycystic-appearing ovary emerges in a nonspecific fashion when a state of anovulation persists for any length of time (Fig. 16–35). Whether diagnosis is by ultrasonography or by the traditional clinical and biochemical criteria, a cross-section of all anovulatory women at any point in time reveals that approximately 75% have polycystic-appearing ovaries as determined by ultrasonography.[374, 375] As there are numerous causes of anovulation, there are also numerous reasons for polycystic ovaries. A similar clinical picture and ovarian condition can reflect any of the dysfunctional states discussed previously. In other words, the polycystic-appearing ovary is the result of a functional derangement but not a specific central or local defect.

The application of rigid endocrine or clinical criteria for the diagnosis of PCOS results in a focused portion of the broad clinical spectrum of PCOS. This particularly applies to diagnosing PCOS with the use of ultrasonography. Criteria include an increase in the number of follicles and their frequent necklace-like arrangement, accompanied by an increase in ovarian volume related to stromal increase (see Fig. 16–35). From 8% to 25% of normal women demonstrate ultrasonographic findings typical of polycystic ovaries.[376–379] Even 14% of women taking oral contraceptives have been found to have this ultrasonographic picture.[377] Thus, ultrasonography is not a tool of choice and its use as a diagnostic aid is not of value. Magnetic resonance studies further confirm the unreliability of the imaging finding (i.e., the polycystic ovary) that was once presumed to be diagnostic of this condition.[380]

Biochemical evidence of insulin resistance or glucose intolerance is also not necessary for the diagnosis of PCOS. Glucose intolerance should nonetheless be investigated. Therefore, plasma glucose levels should be measured after a 75-g glucose load as a screen for glucose intolerance.

Women with PCOS commonly present with irregular uterine bleeding in the form of infrequent periods (oligomenorrhea) or amenorrhea. It is not necessary to document anovulation by ultrasonography, progesterone levels, or otherwise, especially if menstrual cycles are irregular with periods of amenorrhea. To confirm the diagnosis of chronic anovulation and unopposed estrogen exposure, most clinicians perform a progestin challenge test after a negative urine pregnancy test. Because endometrium is exposed to estradiol chronically in PCOS, these women respond to a challenge with a progestin (e.g., medroxyprogesterone acetate 10 mg/day orally for 10 days) by uterine bleeding within a few days after the last pill of progestin. The reasons for lack of uterine bleeding after a progestin challenge include pregnancy, insufficient prior estrogen exposure of the endometrium, or an anatomic defect. If uterine bleeding does not follow progestin challenge, pregnancy should be ruled out again along with other causes of chronic anovulation as described in this chapter. An anatomic defect such as intrauterine adhesions may be ruled out with a hysterosalpingogram or hysteroscopy.

Finally, during the initial work-up, it is advisable to obtain an endometrial biopsy specimen using a plastic minisuction cannula (e.g., Pipelle) in the physician's office. If chronic anovulation persists, endometrial biopsies should be repeated periodically. Response to oral contraceptives or periodic progestin treatment with predictable withdrawal bleeding episodes is reassuring, and these patients with predictable bleeding patterns do not need endometrial sampling during these treatments. In untreated patients, the risk of endometrial hyperplasia and malignancy is significantly increased even in young women with PCOS because of unopposed estrogen exposure.

Gonadotropin Production in Polycystic Ovary Syndrome

Women with PCOS have higher mean concentrations of LH but low or low-normal levels of FSH compared with levels found in normal women in the early follicular phase.[381, 382] The elevated LH levels are partly due to increased sensitivity of the pituitary to LHRH stimulation manifest by increases in LH pulse frequency and, in particular, LH pulse amplitude.[383–385] Interestingly, an increased level of LH bioactivity accompanies high levels of LH in women with PCOS.[384, 386]

The elevated LH levels in PCOS are presumed to be primarily due to accelerated LHRH-LH pulsatile activity.[385] Central opioid tone appears to be suppressed because the pattern of LH secretion does not change in response to naloxone.[387] Indeed, the enhanced pulsatile secretion of LHRH has been attributed to a reduction in hypothalamic opioid inhibition caused by the chronic absence of progesterone.[238, 388] An increase in amplitude and frequency of LH secretion also correlates with the steady-state levels of circulating estrogen.[389]

In obese women with PCOS, LH levels are not increased. The increase in LH pulse frequency is characteristic of the

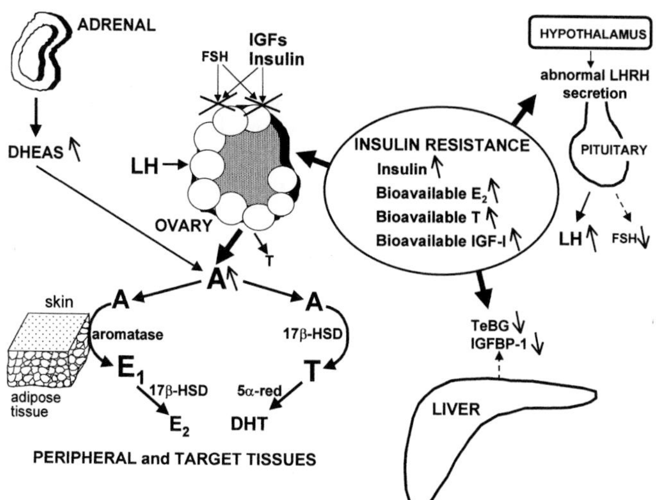

Figure 16-36. Pathologic mechanisms in polycystic ovary syndrome (PCOS). A deficient in vivo response of the ovarian follicle to physiologic quantities of follicle-stimulating hormone (FSH), possibly because of an impaired interaction between signaling pathways associated with FSH and insulin-like growth factors (IGFs) or insulin, may be an important defect in PCOS. This ovarian defect may be the key event responsible for anovulation in PCOS. Insulin resistance associated with increased circulating and tissue levels of insulin and bioavailable estradiol (E_2), testosterone (T), and IGF-I gives rise to abnormal hormone production in a number of tissues. Oversecretion of luteinizing hormone (LH) and decreased output of FSH by the pituitary, decreased production of testosterone-binding globulin (TeBG) and IGF-binding protein 1 (IGFBP-1) in the liver, increased adrenal secretion of dehydroepiandrosterone sulfate (DHEAS), and increased ovarian secretion of androstenedione (A) all contribute to the vicious circle that maintains anovulation and androgen excess in PCOS. Excessive amounts of E_2 and T arise primarily from the conversion of A in peripheral and target tissues. 17β-HSD, 17β-hydroxysteroid dehydrogenase; 5α-red, 5α-reductase.

anovulatory state regardless of the body fat content.[390] LH pulse amplitude, however, is comparatively normal in overweight women with PCOS, whereas it is increased in nonobese women with PCOS.[391, 392] The overall LH reduction in obese women with PCOS may also be due to factors other than changes in LH pulse amplitude.[393, 394] It should be noted again that a low LH value does not rule out the diagnosis of PCOS, whereas a high LH/FSH ratio is supportive of this diagnosis in an anovulatory woman.

Steroid Production in Polycystic Ovary Syndrome

Ovulatory cycles are characterized by cyclic fluctuating hormone levels that regulate ovulation and menses (see Fig. 16–22). Anovulation in women with PCOS, on the other hand, is associated with steady-state levels of gonadotropins and ovarian steroids. In patients with persistent anovulation, the average daily production of estrogen and androgens is both increased and dependent on LH stimulation (Fig. 16–36).[386, 395] This is reflected in higher circulating levels of testosterone, androstenedione, DHEA, DHEAS, 17-hydroxyprogesterone, and estrone.[396–399] Testosterone, androstenedione, and DHEA are secreted directly by the ovary, whereas DHEAS, elevated in about 50% of anovulatory women with PCOS, is almost exclusively an adrenal contribution.[372, 373] Circulating levels of androstenedione, secreted by polycystic ovaries, are particularly high (see Fig. 16–36).[398]

Estrone arises primarily from peripheral aromatization of androstenedione and, in part, from ovarian secretion (Fig. 16–37).[396] Estrone itself is not a potent estrogen but can be viewed as a precursor that must be converted to estradiol to exert full estrogenic action. The presence of a number of 17β-HSD isoenzymes with overlapping activities that catalyze the conversion of estrone to estradiol in peripheral (extraovarian) tissues is, in part, responsible for maintaining estradiol production in women with PCOS.[171, 396] Increased androstenedione leads to a detectable increase in circulating levels of estradiol in women with PCOS compared with estradiol levels measured during the first few days of an ovulatory cycle. This occurs through aromatase and 17β-HSD activities in extraovarian tissues such as skin and subcutaneous adipose tissue. Also, local conversion of estrone to estradiol is an important physiologic process for certain estrogen target tissues such as disease-free breast and genital skin. Finally, local conversion can also promote the growth of pathologic estrogen-dependent tissues such as breast cancer and endometriosis (see Fig. 16–37).[169, 171, 400, 401]

Overall, androstenedione of ovarian origin is the most strikingly elevated steroid in PCOS.[398] Androstenedione is not biologically active but serves as a dual precursor for both androgen (testosterone that is further converted to the biologically far stronger androgen DHT) and estrogen (estrone that is further converted to biologically active estradiol in target tissues) (see Fig. 16–37).[166, 167] Estradiol is an extremely potent steroid. Biologically effective circulating levels of estradiol are measured using units of pg/mL or pmol/L, whereas biologically effective levels of testosterone are measured in units of ng/mL or nmol/L and circulate at 10 to 100 times the physiologic levels of estradiol. Thus, even small rates of conversion of androstenedione to estrone may have a significant biologic impact, whereas markedly elevated production of androstenedione is required to produce significant amounts of testosterone and manifestations of androgen excess (see Fig. 16–37). Because such elevated production of androstenedione does occur in PCOS, extraovarian production of testosterone is biologically significant in this disease. In contrast, in postmenopausal women, who have much lower levels of androstenedione, ex-

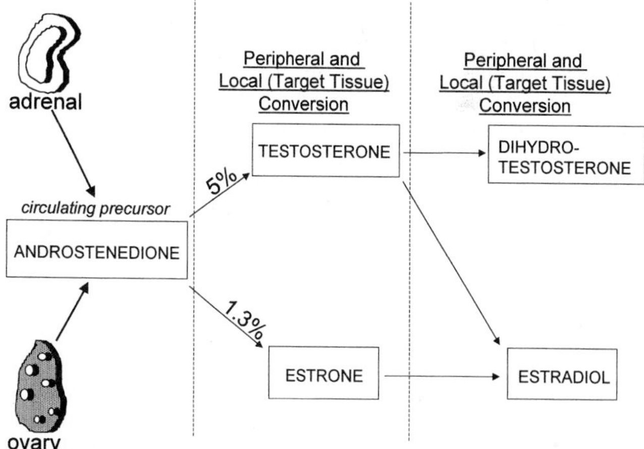

Figure 16-37. Extraovarian conversion of androstenedione to androgen and estrogen. Androstenedione of adrenal or ovarian origin, or both, acts as a dual precursor for androgen and estrogen. Five percent of circulating androstenedione is converted to circulating testosterone, whereas 1.3% of circulating androstenedione is converted to circulating estrone in peripheral tissues. Testosterone and estrone are further converted to biologically potent steroids, dihydrotestosterone and estradiol, in peripheral and target tissues. Biologically active amounts of estradiol in serum are measured in pg/mL (pmol/L), whereas biologically active levels of testosterone in serum are measured in ng/mL (nmol/L). Thus, 1.3% conversion of normal quantities of androstenedione to estrone may have a critical biologic impact in settings such as postmenopausal endometrial or breast cancer. Furthermore, significant androgen excess is observed in conditions with abnormally increased androstenedione formation (e.g., polycystic ovary syndrome).

traovarian production of testosterone is less important. On the other hand, relatively small quantities of estrone (and estradiol) produced primarily by peripheral aromatization of androstenedione have a biologic impact in men and postmenopausal women.[166]

Production of Testosterone-Binding Globulin in Polycystic Ovary Syndrome

TeBG binds both testosterone and estradiol and thus decreases the biologic activities of these critical steroids. In PCOS, there is an increase in the net production of androgen and estrogen. Increased estrogenic and androgenic effects in PCOS, however, are also due to a decrease in TeBG concentration giving rise to increased free or biologically active quantities of both estradiol and testosterone (see Fig. 16–36). The levels of TeBG are controlled by a balance of hormonal influences on its synthesis in the liver. Testosterone and insulin inhibit, whereas estrogen and T_4 stimulate, TeBG formation.[402] In anovulatory women with PCOS, circulating levels of TeBG are reduced approximately 50%; this may be a hepatic response to increased circulating levels of testosterone and insulin (see Fig. 16–36).[402] Circulating free estradiol and testosterone levels are increased because of the significant decrease in TeBG in patients with PCOS.

Thus, three mechanisms contribute to the presence of increased quantities of biologically available estradiol in PCOS: (1) increased production of estradiol from estrone in peripheral (extraovarian) tissues giving rise to increased levels of circulating estradiol,[396–398, 403] (2) increased biologically available circulating estradiol because of decreased TeBG, and (3) local conversion of estrone to estradiol at target tissues.[400] The last local mechanism is likely to be physiologically significant in estrogen targets such as the breast that proliferates in response to estrogen and in the central nervous system, which produces LHRH and gonadotropins under feedback regulation by estrogen (see Fig. 16–36).

In addition to giving rise to increased biologically available estradiol, decreased serum TeBG causes elevations in biologically available free testosterone levels. In turn, testosterone decreases serum TeBG levels, giving rise to a vicious feedback circle favoring low TeBG and high bioavailable testosterone levels (see Fig. 16–36). Insulin directly decreases serum TeBG concentrations in women with PCOS independent of any action of sex steroids.[402] Thus, insulin increases free testosterone in PCOS by two separate mechanisms: (1) by increasing ovarian secretion of testosterone precursors (e.g., androstenedione) and (2) by suppressing TeBG.[402]

Follicular Fate in Polycystic Ovary Syndrome

Under the influence of relatively low but constant levels of FSH, follicular growth is continuously stimulated, but not to the point of full maturation and ovulation.[404] Despite the fact that full growth potential is not realized, the follicular life span may extend several months in the form of multiple follicular cysts. Most of these follicles in polycystic ovaries are 2 to 10 mm in diameter, whereas some can be as large as 15 mm. Hyperplastic theca cells, often luteinized in response to the high LH levels, surround these follicles (see Fig. 16–33). The accumulation of follicles arrested at various stages of development allows increased and relatively constant production of steroids in response to steady-state levels of gonadotropins.

These follicles are also subject to atresia and are replaced by new follicles of similar limited growth potential. A steady state of stromal cell turnover contributes to the stromal compartment of the ovary, and it is sustained by tissue derived from follicular atresia. A degenerating granulosa compartment, leaving the theca cells to contribute to the stromal compartment of the ovary, accompanies atresia (see Fig. 16–33). This functioning stromal tissue secretes significant amounts of androstenedione under the influence of increased LH. Androstenedione is not a biologically active steroid but acts as a double precursor (see Fig. 16–37). Androstenedione is converted to both estrogen (estrone that is further converted to estradiol) and testosterone in extraovarian tissues. In turn, elevated testosterone suppresses TeBG synthesis, resulting in elevated free testosterone and free estradiol levels. The elevation in free testosterone further decreases TeBG. From the point of view of steroidogenesis and steroid action, the PCOS is the result of a complex vicious circle that includes a number of positive and negative feedback mechanisms (see Fig. 16–36).

Persistent anovulation and chronically elevated levels of LH give rise to the underdeveloped granulosa and hyperplastic and active, luteinized theca seen histologically in the ovaries of patients with PCOS (see Fig. 16–33). Cultured granulosa cells obtained from the small follicles of polycystic ovaries produce negligible amounts of estradiol but show a dramatic increase in estrogen production when FSH or IGF-I is added to the culture medium. Moreover, when FSH and IGF-I were added together in vitro, they synergized to increase estrogen biosynthesis in granulosa cells from polycystic ovaries.[154, 405]

These findings suggest an in vivo resistance to FSH action in PCOS, possibly related to the pathologic absence of an interaction between FSH- and IGF-related signaling pathways (see Fig. 16–36). Induction of ovulation in PCOS is achieved, therefore, by increasing FSH levels to overcome the block at the granulosa cell level. Two currently popular treatments, oral clomiphene citrate and injectable recombinant FSH, aim to provide increased levels of endogenous or exogenous FSH to overcome this in vivo defect. Granulosa cells develop and grow in response to FSH and produce estradiol; this increase in estradiol production precedes the resumption of ovulation. In fact, the polycystic ovary often overreacts to pharmacologic levels of FSH by the recruitment of a large number of developing follicles at once, occasionally giving rise to the ovarian hyperstimulation syndrome.[406, 407]

Ovarian Hyperthecosis

Ovarian hyperthecosis is a severe variant of PCOS. The term refers to significantly increased stromal tissue with luteinized theca-like cells scattered throughout large sheets of fibroblast-like cells. Both clinical and histologic findings represent an exaggerated version of PCOS.[408] This diagnosis can be made on clinical grounds; an ovarian biopsy is not necessary except to rule out an ovarian tumor.

Increased androgen production leads to the clinical picture of more intense androgenization. The higher testosterone levels may also lower LH levels by blocking estrogen action at the hypothalamic-pituitary level.[393, 394] Hyperthecosis seems to be an exaggerated version of the same process that gives rise to chronic ovulation in PCOS. A correlation exists between the severity of hyperthecosis and the degree of insulin resistance.[394] And in turn, because insulin and IGF-I stimulate proliferation of thecal interstitial cells, hyperinsulinemia may be an important pathophysiologic factor in the etiology of hyperthecosis.[409]

It is not uncommon to encounter markedly high levels of testosterone, even above 2 ng/mL, in ovarian hyperthecosis. Virilization is common. These patients usually do not ovulate in response to clomiphene or recombinant FSH. It is usually difficult to suppress testosterone production even using an LHRH agonist. Bilateral oophorectomy should be used as the last resort but, unfortunately, may be necessary to control testosterone production in a significant portion of these patients.

Genetics of Polycystic Ovary Syndrome

The strong trend of PCOS to aggregate in families is suggestive of an underlying genetic basis.[410–412] It was previously emphasized that PCOS is of a multifactorial nature and that a similar pathology emerges from diverse mechanisms. These features are strongly suggestive of a polygenic pattern of inheritance. Efforts are ongoing to understand the genetic basis of PCOS. At least one group of patients with this condition has been described who inherited the disorder by means of X-linked dominant transmission. There was a twofold higher incidence of hirsutism and oligomenorrhea with paternal transmission but with marked variability of phenotypic expression.[413] On the other hand, studies of large families were suggestive of inheritance in an autosomal dominant fashion, with premature balding as the phenotype in males.[414, 415] In addition, the strong link between hyperinsulinemia and hyperandrogenism suggests that the stimulatory effect of insulin on ovarian androgen production is influenced by a genetic predisposition. In fact, women with hyperandrogenism, anovulation, and polycystic ovaries have a higher incidence of female relatives with hyperinsulinemia and male relatives with baldness.[416] Finally, familial aggregation of increased serum testosterone levels in PCOS suggests that androgen excess per se is a genetic trait. Genetic linkage studies are under way to identify individual gene defects that may be responsible for PCOS.[367]

Insulin Resistance and Polycystic Ovary Syndrome

Insulin resistance is a major factor in the pathogenesis of non–insulin-dependent diabetes mellitus (NIDDM). The term insulin resistance can be defined as impaired whole-body insulin-mediated glucose disposal, as determined using techniques such as the hyperinsulinemic glucose clamp technique.[193] Insulin resistance is defined clinically as the inability of a known quantity of exogenous or endogenous insulin to increase glucose uptake and utilization in an individual as much as it does in a normal population. Insulin resistance is frequently observed in both lean and obese women with PCOS. More severe degrees of insulin resistance or impaired glucose tolerance, however, are more common in obese women with PCOS.[193]

The association between a disorder of carbohydrate metabolism and androgen excess was first described in 1921 by Archard and Thiers[417] and was called the "diabetes of bearded women." Since then, the association between PCOS and insulin resistance or impaired glucose tolerance has been well recognized.[193] This clinical association of insulin resistance and anovulatory hyperandrogenism is commonly found throughout the world and among different ethnic groups.[418, 419] In addition, androgen excess and insulin resistance are often associated with acanthosis nigricans.[420] Acanthosis nigricans is a gray-brown velvety discoloration and increased thickness of the skin, usually at the neck, groin, axillae, and under the breasts, and is a marker for insulin resistance (see Fig. 16–34). Hyperkeratosis and papillomatosis are the histologic characteristics of acanthosis nigricans. The presence of acanthosis nigricans in hyperandrogenic women is dependent on the presence and severity of hyperinsulinemia and insulin resistance.[421] The mechanism responsible for the development of acanthosis nigricans is uncertain. This abnormal growth response of the skin may be mediated through receptors for various growth factors, including those for insulin and IGF-I. Acanthosis nigricans is not specific for insulin resistance because it can be observed in the absence of insulin resistance or androgen excess.

Insulin resistance is characterized by an impaired glucose response to a specific amount of insulin.[422] In many of these patients, normal glucose levels are maintained at the expense of increased circulating insulin to overcome the underlying defect. More severe forms of insulin resistance in PCOS range from impaired glucose tolerance to frank NIDDM. Resistance to insulin-stimulated glucose uptake is a relatively common phenomenon in the general population, sometimes referred to as syndrome X.[422] The fundamental abnormality leading to the manifestations that make up syndrome X is resistance to insulin-mediated glucose uptake in muscle and increased lipolysis giving rise to elevated circulating free fatty acid levels.[423] These individuals also have dyslipidemia, hypertension, and increased risk of developing cardiovascular disease. Not surprisingly, the incidences of dyslipidemia and cardiovascular risk are also increased significantly in women with PCOS.[424, 425] The incidence of hypertension increases significantly after the menopause in women with a history of PCOS.[193] Thus, there is probably a significant clinical and pathologic overlap between syndrome X and PCOS. The extent of this overlap is not known at this time.

The clinical presentation of patients with insulin resistance depends on the ability of the pancreas to compensate for the target tissue resistance to insulin. During the first stages of the development of this condition, compensation is effective, and the only metabolic abnormality is hyperinsulinemia. In many patients, the beta cells of the pancreas eventually fail to meet the challenge, and declining insulin levels lead to impaired glucose tolerance and eventually frank diabetes mellitus. In fact, beta cell dysfunction is demonstrable in women with PCOS before the onset of glucose intolerance.[426]

Studies of well-characterized causes of hyperinsulinemia and androgen excess have illuminated various mechanisms of insulin resistance. Factors such as a decrease in insulin binding related to autoantibodies to insulin receptors, postreceptor defects, and a decrease in insulin receptor sites in target tissues are all involved in insulin resistance.[427, 428] These rare syndromes, however, are found in an extremely small portion of women with anovulation, androgen excess, and insulin resistance, leaving the majority of PCOS patients without any demonstrable abnormalities in the number or quality of receptors or antibody formation. The exact nature of insulin resistance in the great majority of women with PCOS is not well understood.

In order to understand the molecular defect underlying insulin resistance in PCOS, Dunaif and co-workers[193, 429] studied the differences between skin fibroblasts from women with and without PCOS with respect to insulin-dependent signal transduction. The fibroblasts of women with PCOS showed no change in insulin binding or receptor affinity. In half of the women with PCOS, however, a postreceptor defect was observed.[193, 429] This defect is characterized by increased basal insulin receptor serine phosphorylation and a decrease in insulin-dependent tyrosine phosphorylation of the insulin receptor.[193, 429] These abnormal patterns of phosphorylation of specific residues of the insulin receptor might represent a molecular mechanism responsible for the insulin resistance, anovulation, and androgen excess of PCOS.[193, 429] The cause of this abnormal phosphorylation pattern and consequences for insulin action are important topics for future study.

Role of Obesity in Insulin Resistance and Anovulation

Increased waist-to-hip ratio compounded by significantly increased body mass index is called android obesity because this type of adipose tissue distribution is observed more commonly in men. Overweight women with anovulatory androgen excess commonly have this particular body fat distribution.[430–432] Android obesity is the result of fat deposited in the abdominal wall and visceral mesenteric locations. This fat is more sensitive to catecholamines, less sensitive to insulin, and more active metabolically. Android obesity is associated with insulin resistance, glucose intolerance, diabetes mellitus, and an increase in androgen production rate resulting in decreased levels of TeBG and increased levels of free testosterone and estradiol.[430–432] Not surprisingly, android obesity is associated significantly with cardiovascular risk factors, including hypertension and dyslipidemia. It is also important to emphasize that android obesity has been tied to a notable increase in the risk of breast cancer, with a poor prognosis.[433, 434] No direct association, however, has been reported between PCOS and breast cancer risk.[435]

Although the combination of insulin resistance and androgen excess is often observed in obese women overall, women with android-type obesity appear to be at a significantly higher risk for insulin resistance and androgen excess. However, insulin resistance and androgen excess are not confined to obese anovulatory women but also occur in nonobese anovulatory women.[390] Although obesity by itself causes insulin resistance, the combination of insulin resistance and androgen excess is a specific feature of PCOS. Not surprisingly, the combination of obesity and PCOS is associated with more severe degrees of insulin resistance than those found in nonobese women with PCOS.[390, 436, 437] Android-type obesity, in contrast to general obesity, is a much more specific risk factor for PCOS.

Diagnosis of Insulin Resistance

In everyday clinical practice, the biochemical diagnosis of insulin resistance in an individual patient has not been standardized and is extremely complex. First, a quarter of the normal population has fasting and glucose-stimulated insulin levels that overlap those of insulin-resistant individuals[193, 429] because of great variability of insulin sensitivity in normal subjects. Second, clinically available measures of insulin action, such as fasting or glucose-stimulated insulin levels, do not correlate well with more detailed measurements of insulin sensitivity in research settings.

In view of these constraints, it is reasonable to consider all women with PCOS at risk for insulin resistance and the associated abnormalities of the insulin resistance syndrome (syndrome X)—dyslipidemia, hypertension, and cardiovascular disease. A lipid profile should be obtained in all cases of PCOS. Especially obese women with PCOS should have fasting glucose levels and glucose levels 2 hours after a 75-g glucose load as a screen for glucose intolerance. The clinician should encourage the patient to take every possible measure (e.g., weight reduction and exercise) to reduce insulin resistance.

Use of Antidiabetic Drugs to Treat Anovulation and Androgen Excess

A logical approach to the management of PCOS includes the use of medications that improve insulin sensitivity in target tissues, thus achieving reductions in insulin secretion and stability of glucose tolerance. Oral agents employed in the treatment of diabetes mellitus, such as metformin and troglitazone, have been used to induce ovulation and decrease circulating androgen in anovulatory women with PCOS. The biguanide metformin improves insulin sensitivity, but the primary effect is a significant reduction in gluconeogenesis, thus decreasing hepatic glucose production.

Metformin at a dose of 500 mg three times a day reduced hyperinsulinemia, basal and stimulated LH levels, and free testosterone concentrations in overweight women with PCOS.[438–440] A significant number of these anovulatory women ovulated and achieved pregnancy.[441, 442] The addition of metformin to clomiphene citrate resulted in a remarkable improvement in the ovulation rate in obese women with PCOS.[443] The improvements in ovulation and androgen levels in this study might in part result from the weight loss that often accompanies the use of metformin.[444] Investigators of subsequent published studies, however, concluded that in both lean and obese anovulatory women, metformin treatment reduced hyperinsulinemia and androgen excess independent of changes in body weight.[443, 445, 446] Metformin is thus a promising medication for reduction of cardiovascular risk and induction of ovulation in women with PCOS. The benign side-effect profile of this medication also makes it an attractive choice.

The thiazolidinediones are pharmacologic ligands for the nuclear receptor peroxisome proliferator–activated receptor γ (PPARγ). A member of this family, troglitazone, at a dose of 400 mg/day, markedly improves insulin action and insulin secretion through improved peripheral glucose utilization and beta cell function without weight changes. Troglitazone decreased insulin, LH, and testosterone levels and increased circulating TeBG.[447, 448] Resumption of ovulation in obese women has been reported with the use of troglitazone.[447, 448] However, troglitazone, the first thiazolidinedione approved by the Food and Drug Administration in the United States, proved to be hepatotoxic and was withdrawn from the market after the report of several dozens of deaths and cases of severe hepatic failure requiring liver transplantation. The safety and therapeutic potential of new thiazolidinediones are currently being tested in PCOS.[449]

Management of Long-Term Deleterious Effects of Polycystic Ovary Syndrome

The long-term consequences of PCOS include irregular uterine bleeding, anovulatory infertility, androgen excess (hirsutism or virilization or both), chronically elevated free estrogen associated with an increased risk of endometrial cancer, and insulin resistance associated with an increased risk of cardiovascular disease and diabetes mellitus. Therefore, treatment must encompass the following: aid in achieving a healthy lifestyle and normal body weight, protection of the endometrium from unopposed estrogen effects, and a reduction in testosterone levels.

If the patient desires pregnancy, she is a candidate for the medical induction of ovulation. When pregnancy is achieved, patients with polycystic ovaries appear to have an increased risk of spontaneous miscarriage.[450–452] This increased risk may be related to elevated levels of LH that may produce an adverse environment for the oocyte and the endometrium. Therefore, LH levels should be suppressed with oral contraceptives before inducing ovulation. This suppression can be achieved in most patients with PCOS by the use of an oral contraceptive for 4 to 6 weeks before ovulation induction with clomiphene citrate or recombinant FSH.

If the patient does not wish to become pregnant, therapy is directed toward the interruption of unopposed effect of estrogen on the endometrium. Nonfluctuating levels of unopposed estradiol in the absence of progesterone cause irregular uterine bleeding, amenorrhea, and infertility and increase the risk of endometrial cancer. Anovulatory women with PCOS may have endometrial cancer even in their early 20s.[453–455] Therefore, endometrial biopsy should be performed periodically in untreated women with PCOS regardless of age. The uterine bleeding pattern should not influence the decision to perform an endometrial biopsy. The presence of amenorrhea does not rule out endometrial hyperplasia. The critical factor that determines the risk of endometrial neoplasia is the duration of anovulation and exposure to unopposed estradiol. Long-term treatment with a progestin or oral contraceptive significantly decreases the risk of endometrial cancer.

One of the simplest and most effective ways to administer a progestin in the long term is to use an oral contraceptive. Also, oral contraceptives provide two more benefits: reduction of androgen excess and contraception. Oral contraceptive pills reduce circulating androgen levels through suppression of circulating LH and stimulation of TeBG levels and have been shown to reduce hirsutism in hyperandrogenic patients.[197]

A concern regarding possible insulin-desensitizing effects of oral contraceptives has been raised.[193] Older oral contraceptives cause increased insulin resistance because of the high estrogen component.[456] Long-term follow-up studies, however, have failed to detect any increase in the incidence of diabetes mellitus in past or current users of high-dose pills.[457, 458] In fact, more recent studies demonstrated that new oral contraceptives induced either no change or a significant decrease in insulin resistance in women with PCOS. The oral contraceptives that did not induce insulin resistance in women with PCOS contained an ethinyl estradiol dose of 30 μg or less and desogestrel, norgestimate, or gestodene as the progestin component.[459, 460] Furthermore, past users of oral contraceptives have no increased cardiovascular risk.[461, 462] Low-dose oral contraceptives have also been administered to women with gestational diabetes or insulin-dependent diabetes mellitus without an adverse impact.[463–466] Low-dose oral contraceptives have not increased the risk of retinopathy or nephropathy in diabetic patients, nor has there been any deterioration of lipid or biochemical markers.[463–466] It should be emphasized again that the major contributing factor to hyperinsulinemia and insulin resistance in PCOS is obesity.[390, 436] In summary, oral contraceptive treatment for anovulatory and hyperinsulinemic women with androgen excess does not increase cardiovascular risk.

For the patient who does not complain of hirsutism but is anovulatory and has irregular bleeding, treatment with a single progestin may be attempted as an alternative to oral contraceptives. Progestin therapy is directed toward interruption of the chronic exposure of endometrium to unopposed effects of estrogen. Medroxyprogesterone acetate, 10 mg daily for the first 10 days of every month, can be administered to ensure withdrawal bleeding and prevent endometrial hyperplasia. This treatment does not decrease androgen excess, nor does it provide contraception. Because new oral contraceptives (with an ethinyl estradiol content of 30 μg or less and a new progestin) suppress androgen excess of ovarian origin, provide contraception, protect the endometrium, and do not increase insulin resistance, a new low-dose oral contraceptive is the treatment of choice for nonsmokers with PCOS. An oral contraceptive together with the antiandrogen spirolactone, 100 mg/day, is the recommended starting treatment for a hirsute woman with PCOS. The dose of spironolactone can be increased in increments to suppress hair growth as previously described in this section.

Treatment with an oral contraceptive (plus or minus spironolactone) may not be effective in androgen suppression in severe cases of PCOS. In these patients resistant to oral contraceptives, suppression of the ovary with an LHRH agonist may be required. Because glucocorticoids increase insulin resistance, they should be used with caution in patients with hyperinsulinemia. Spironolactone does not affect insulin sensitivity in anovulatory women and can be used safely without causing adverse effects on carbohydrate or lipid metabolism.[467, 468]

The clinician must counsel women with PCOS regarding their increased risk of future diabetes mellitus. The age of onset of non–insulin-dependent diabetes is significantly earlier in these women than in the general population.[366] Women with PCOS are more likely to experience gestational diabetes.[469] Long-term follow-up studies have shown a significantly increased risk for the development of frank diabetes mellitus in anovulatory patients with PCOS.[193] It is therefore important to monitor glucose tolerance with periodic glucose levels after fasting and after a 75-g glucose load.

Because insulin resistance contributes to the abnormal lipid profile and increased cardiovascular risk in women with PCOS, weight loss is a high priority for patients who are overweight.[470, 471] Both insulin resistance and androgen excess can be reduced with a weight reduction of at least 5%.[472–475] Significant weight loss also resulted in ovulation and pregnancy in a number of patients with PCOS.[476, 477] Therefore, long-term nutritional counseling and an emphasis on lifestyle changes are essential components of the long-term management of PCOS.

The place of insulin sensitizers, such as metformin and thiazolidinediones, in the treatment of PCOS remains to be determined by data from future clinical trials. When one takes into account the design of how this treatment should work, the potential for its preventive benefits is impressive. Preliminary findings suggest that thiazolidinediones are a potent group of medications that restore ovulation by reducing insulin resistance and androgen excess.[447, 448] Unfortunately, troglitazone, the first compound approved by the Food and Drug Administration in the United States, proved to be hepatotoxic and was withdrawn from the market after the report of a small but significant number of liver failures and deaths. The most important factor determining the extent of use of new thiazolidinediones in PCOS will be their side-effect profiles (e.g., liver toxicity and teratogenesis). By contrast, the majority of publications on metformin show no serious side effects or teratogenicity. Metformin does seem to improve metabolic abnormalities and restore ovulation.[443, 445] Further studies are in progress to determine the roles of these antidiabetics as therapeutic agents in PCOS.

In long-term follow-up of women with PCOS, android obesity and hyperinsulinemia persisted during the postmenopausal years.[478] Thus, postmenopausal women who have previously been anovulatory, hyperandrogenic, and hyperinsulinemic are at risk for cardiovascular disease and diabetes mellitus. Aggressive preventive health care interventions that lower cardiovascular risk and other unfavorable consequences of PCOS are appropriate.[193, 337]

Genetic counseling is of paramount importance for the families of patients with PCOS. A growing body of evidence suggests that up to half of first-degree relatives and sisters may be affected by PCOS or at least by androgen excess in the presence of regular menses.[368] These individuals may be at higher than average risk for cardiovascular disease and may benefit from preventive measures that reduce this risk.

Ovulation Induction in Polycystic Ovary Syndrome

Clomiphene Citrate. To induce ovulation in PCOS, FSH levels are increased through the use of, for example, clomiphene citrate or by injection of recombinant FSH. Presumably, pharmacologic levels of FSH overcome the ovarian defect responsible for anovulation in PCOS.

Clomiphene citrate is a nonsteroidal ovulation-inducing ER ligand with mixed agonistic-antagonistic properties.[479] Acting as an antiestrogen, clomiphene citrate is thought to displace endogenous estrogen from hypothalamic ERs, thereby removing the negative feedback effect exerted by endogenous estrogens. The resultant change in pulsatile LHRH release is thought to normalize the release of pituitary FSH and LH, followed by follicular recruitment and selection, assertion of dominance, and, ultimately, ovulation.[479]

Clomiphene citrate treatment can be started at any time in an amenorrheic and anovulatory patient provided that a pregnancy test is performed beforehand. Alternatively, uterine

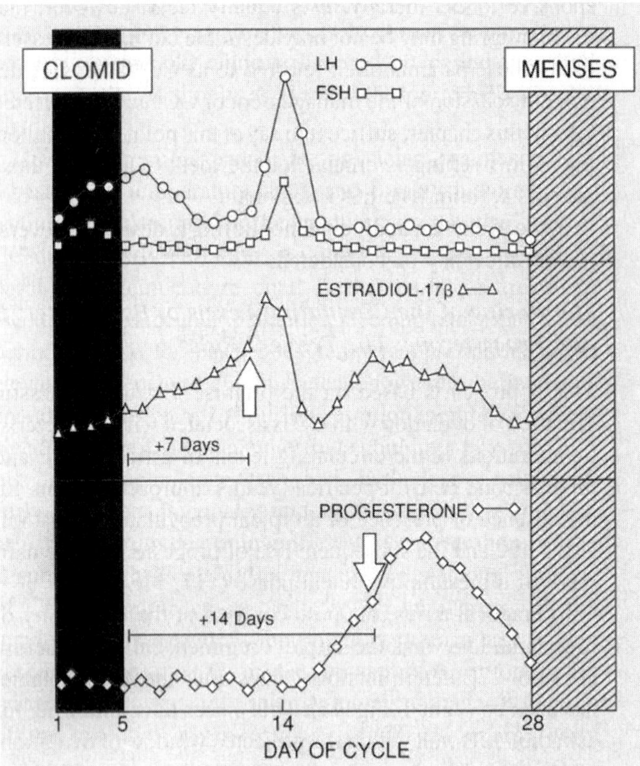

Figure 16–38. Hormonal monitoring in clomiphene citrate–initiated ovulation: use of the triple-7 regimen. Please see text. (From Adashi EY. Clomiphene citrate-initiated ovulation: a clinical update. Semin Reprod Endocrinol 1986; 4:255–276.)

bleeding may be induced after a 21-day treatment with an oral contraceptive or 10-day treatment with medroxyprogesterone acetate (10 mg/day). Clomiphene citrate at 50 mg/day is started orally on day 3, 4, or 5 of the cycle and continued for 5 days. Over the past 20 some years, we have used a practical approach termed triple-7 in order to monitor indicators of ovulation after the administration of clomiphene citrate.[479] The protocol is depicted in Figure 16–38. This approach is timed favorably to detect the preovulatory surge of serum estradiol 7 days after the last clomiphene citrate dose (arrow pointing up) and a serum progesterone level 14 days after the last clomiphene citrate dose (arrow pointing down) in order to document ovulation. A repeated office visit is scheduled 7 days after the progesterone determination, that is, 21 days after the last clomiphene citrate dose (see Fig. 16–38).[479] The patient should be encouraged to have intercourse every other day during the 10-day period following the last clomiphene citrate dose. Alternatively, measurement of urinary LH to detect an LH surge can be used to time intercourse.

If ovulation does not occur after the first course of therapy with clomiphene citrate at 50 mg/day, a second course of 100 mg daily for 5 days may be started. Lack of response at doses of 150 to 200 mg daily for 5 days should be an indication for a change of treatment. Most patients destined to conceive do so with the starting dose of clomiphene citrate (50 mg/day for 5 days). Most clomiphene citrate–initiated conceptions are likely to occur within the first six ovulatory cycles.[479] The incidence rate for multiple gestation in clomiphene citrate–induced pregnancies is 7.9%, of which 6.9% are twins.[479]

Letrozole. The aromatase inhibitor letrozole has been used as an experimental medication to induce ovulation.[480] The mechanism of action appears to be similar to that of clomiphene citrate. Oral administration of letrozole (2.5 mg/day on days 3 to 7 after uterine bleeding) is effective for ovulation induction in anovulatory infertility. Ovulation induction by an aromatase inhibitor is presumed to be mediated by estrogen deficiency induced at the level of the hypothalamus.[156, 480] Letrozole appears to avoid the unfavorable effects on the endometrium frequently seen with the use of antiestrogens (e.g., clomiphene citrate) for ovulation induction. Clinical data regarding this experimental treatment are extremely scarce at the moment.

Conventional-Dose Gonadotropin Therapy. For women who do not ovulate in response to clomiphene citrate, recombinant FSH is administered subcutaneously at a starting dose of two ampules (equivalent to 150 IU of FSH), starting on day 3 of spontaneous or progestin-induced uterine bleeding and increasing by 75 IU at 3- to 7-day intervals until serum estradiol concentrations begin to increase. The dose is then maintained until follicular rupture, which is induced by intramuscular administration of hCG (10,000 IU). Follicular growth is monitored by transvaginal ultrasonography and blood estradiol levels, which serve as biochemical markers for the granulosa cell mass in the growing follicle.[481] Three important complications of gonadotropin therapy in PCOS are significantly increased rates of multiple pregnancies, severe ovarian hyperstimulation syndrome, and spontaneous miscarriage.[481]

Low-Dose Gonadotropin Therapy. Conventional-dose gonadotropin therapy causes two important complications: (1) an alarming number of multiple pregnancies (range, 14% to 50% of treatment cycles) and (2) a significantly increased risk of severe ovarian hyperstimulation syndrome (range, 1.3% to 9.4% of treatment cycles).[481] Low-dose FSH regimens for induction of ovulation for women with PCOS have succeeded in reducing the rate of multiple pregnancies to as low as 6% in some series.[407] The low-dose regimen also practically eliminated the complication of severe ovarian hyperstimulation syndrome.[407] This has been achieved by reaching, but not exceeding, the threshold level of FSH, starting with a daily dose of

75 IU for 14 days and using small incremental dose increases when necessary. This regimen induces the development of a single follicle in 70% of cycles. Conception rates are comparable to those achieved with conventional therapy. The miscarriage rate remains somewhat higher than that after spontaneous conceptions (20% to 25%). The treatment time for the low-dose regimen is significantly longer than that required for conventional gonadotropin treatment. New data obtained using recombinant FSH for a low-dose regimen, rather than urinary gonadotropins, suggest that treatment time may be shortened.[482]

Premature Ovarian Failure

Premature ovarian failure, which is defined as early depletion of ovarian follicles before the age of 40, is a state of hypergonadotropic hypogonadism. These patients present with amenorrhea or oligomenorrhea. They go through a normal puberty and a variable period of cyclic menses followed by oligomenorrhea and amenorrhea. Therefore, premature ovarian failure should always be included in the differential diagnosis of chronic anovulation. History and physical examination may reveal menstrual irregularity or secondary amenorrhea accompanied by symptoms and signs of estrogen deficiency, such as hot flashes and urogenital atrophy. Elevated FSH levels (above the 95% confidence limits of the midcycle gonadotropin peak of the normal menstrual cycle, i.e., > 40 IU/L) on at least two occasions confirm the diagnosis.[483]

On average, the menopause occurs at the age of 50 years, with 1% of women continuing to menstruate beyond the age of 60 years and another 1% whose menopause occurs before 40 years. Thus, premature menopause or ovarian failure has been arbitrarily defined as the cessation of menses before 40 years of age.[484] In most cases, the etiology of premature ovarian failure is not clear. The patient may be counseled that the disorder is probably a genetic one causing ovarian follicles to disappear at a rate faster than normal. Specific sex chromosome anomalies may be identified in a subset of patients presenting with premature ovarian failure.[485] Among these, 45,X and 47,XXY are the most common, followed by mosaicism involving various combinations.[486]

The underlying ovarian defect may be manifest at varying ages, depending on the number of functional follicles left in the ovaries. The different symptoms may be regarded as phases in the process of perimenopausal change regardless of the actual age of the patient. If loss of follicles occurs rapidly before puberty, primary amenorrhea and lack of secondary sexual development ensue. The degree to which the adult phenotype develops and when the secondary amenorrhea actually occurs depend on whether follicle loss took place during or after puberty. In cases of primary amenorrhea associated with sexual infantilism, the ovarian remnants exist as streaks, and transvaginal ultrasonography usually cannot detect any ovaries.

Premature ovarian failure can be due to an autoimmune process, as this condition is frequently detected in association with autoimmune polyendocrine syndromes.[487] Other causes of premature failure can be related to the sudden destruction of the follicles through factors such as chemotherapy, radiation, or infections such as mumps oophoritis. The effect of radiation is dependent upon age and the x-ray dose.[488, 489] Steroid levels begin to fall and gonadotropins rise within 2 weeks after radiation of the ovaries. Young women exposed to radiation are less likely to have permanent ovarian failure because of the higher number of oocytes present at younger ages. When the radiation field excludes the pelvis or the ovaries are transposed out of the pelvis by laparoscopic surgery before radiation, there is no risk of premature ovarian failure.[490, 491] Most chemotherapeutic agents used for the eradication of malignancies are toxic to the ovaries and cause ovarian failure.[492] Resumption of menses and pregnancy have been reported after radiotherapy or chemotherapy.[493] By the same token, premature ovarian failure may occur years after chemotherapy or radiotherapy.[476]

Finally, single gene defects may give rise to ovarian failure. These include mutations of FSH and LH receptors and galactosemia.[494, 495] Mutations of galactose-1-phosphate uridyltransferase, for example, can lead to ovarian failure because of the accumulation of galactose-1-phosphate at toxic levels.[496]

Diagnosis and Management of Premature Ovarian Failure

Premature ovarian failure should be suspected in a woman who is younger than 40 years who presents with amenorrhea, oligomenorrhea, or another form of menstrual irregularity. Menopausal serum FSH levels (40 IU/L) on at least two occasions are sufficient for the diagnosis of premature ovarian failure. Thus, these young women can be diagnosed with ovarian failure and infertility if gonadotropin levels are repeatedly elevated. There are, however, a number of case reports of pregnancies in affected women occurring during hormone replacement therapy.[497–500] A randomized trial of hormone replacement in this setting showed that folliculogenesis occurred often but was less frequently followed by ovulation and even less frequently by pregnancy (up to 14%); estrogen therapy did not improve the rate of folliculogenesis, ovulation, or pregnancy.[483] Therefore, the clinician should inform patients diagnosed with premature ovarian failure that there is a small but significant likelihood of spontaneous pregnancy in the future. Women desirous of achieving pregnancy are still best served by assisted reproductive technology employing donor oocytes because the probability of spontaneous pregnancy is low. Use of donor oocytes followed by in vitro fertilization with the partner's sperm and intrauterine embryo transfer after synchronization of the recipient patient's endometrium with the donor's cycle using exogenous estrogen and progesterone are offered to the patient who wishes to carry a pregnancy in her uterus (see Fig. 16–29). This approach offers an excellent chance of pregnancy (>50% per donor oocyte–in vitro fertilization cycle).

Patients with premature ovarian failure are at increased risk for having an abnormal complement of chromosomes.[485] The risk of having an abnormal karyotype increases with decreasing age of onset of the ovarian failure. A chromosomal analysis is recommended for some of these patients because of increased risk of a gonadal tumor associated with the presence of a Y chromosome.[501] The arbitrarily chosen age group for chromosomal analysis includes women 30 years of age or younger because it is extraordinarily rare to encounter a gonadal tumor in patients with premature ovarian failure after the age of 30.[502, 503]

The presence of mosaicism including a Y chromosome has been associated with a high incidence of gonadal tumors.[501] These malignant tumors arise from germ cells and include gonadoblastomas, dysgerminomas, yolk sac tumors, and choriocarcinoma. In particular, the presence of secondary virilization in these patients with karyotypic abnormalities and premature ovarian failure significantly increases the risk of a dysontogenetic gonadal tumor. The precise risk of a tumor in various subsets of these patients is not well known because a significant number of women carrying a Y chromosome do not have symptoms of virilization. The frequency of Y-chromosome material determined by polymerase chain reaction is high in Turner's syndrome (12.2%), but the occurrence of a gonadal tumor among these Y-positive patients seems to be as low as 7% to 10%.[504]

Table 16–9. Laboratory Evaluation of Premature Ovarian Failure

FSH (to establish the diagnosis of premature ovarian failure)
Karyotype (< 30 yr of age or sexual infantilism)
Cortisol after ACTH stimulation (adrenal insufficiency)
TSH (hypothyroidism)
Glucose (fasting and 2 hr after 75-g glucose load, diabetes mellitus)
Calcium and phosphorus (hypoparathyroidism)
Sedimentation rate, complete blood count with differential, antinuclear antibody, rheumatoid factor (autoimmune disease)
Pregnenolone (to evaluate 17-hydroxylase deficiency in sexually infantile women)
Galactose-1-phosphate (galactosemia)

ACTH, adrenocorticotropic hormone; FSH, follicle-stimulating hormone; TSH, thyroid-stimulating hormone.

Premature ovarian failure may also occur as an isolated autoimmune disorder or in association with hypothyroidism, diabetes mellitus, hypoadrenalism, hypoparathyroidism, or systemic lupus erythematosus.[505] Therefore, the tests listed in Table 16–9 should be performed every few years because premature ovarian failure can be part of an autoimmune polyendocrine syndrome.[487] Thyroid and adrenal insufficiency and diabetes mellitus are the endocrine disorders most frequently associated with premature ovarian failure. It should be noted, however, that overall it is fairly rare to encounter any endocrine disorder associated with premature ovarian failure.[506]

Treatment of premature ovarian failure should be directed toward its specific cause, if this is possible. In most cases, however, it is not possible to identify a specific etiology if there are no karyotypic anomalies. If the patient desires pregnancy, she should be offered ovum donation and in vitro fertilization using her partner's sperm (see Fig. 16–29). If pregnancy is not desired, she should be treated with an oral contraceptive or with estrogen and progestin replacement. Estrogen therapy promotes and maintains secondary sexual characteristics and prevents premature osteoporosis.

Differential Diagnosis and Management of Anovulatory Uterine Bleeding

Acyclic production of estrogen during anovulatory cycles gives rise to irregular shedding of the endometrium. These bleeding manifestations of anovulatory cycles in the absence of uterine pathology or systemic illness are commonly referred to as dysfunctional uterine bleeding. Anovulatory uterine bleeding is the most common cause of chronic menstrual irregularities and is a diagnosis of exclusion. Pregnancy, uterine leiomyomas, endometrial polyps, and adenomyosis should be ruled out as anatomic causes of irregular uterine bleeding. Malignancies of the vagina, cervix, endometrium, myometrium, fallopian tubes, and ovaries should also be ruled out before a diagnosis of anovulatory uterine bleeding is made. Finally, coagulation abnormalities should be excluded.

Anovulatory uterine bleeding can be managed without surgical intervention by either restoring ovulation or mimicking the ovulatory hormonal profile by providing exogenous steroids. The rationale for using exogenous steroids is based on the knowledge of predictable responses of the endometrium to estrogen and progesterone. Physiologic responses of the endometrium to natural ovarian steroids have been uncovered by observing the gross and microscopic changes in the endometrium during thousands of normal ovulatory cycles in humans and other primates.[198, 201–204] The pharmacologic application of exogenous estrogens and progestins in women with anovulatory bleeding aims to correct the production of local tissue factors, which mediate physiologic steroid action, and thus reverse the excessive and prolonged flow typical of anovulatory cycles.

Clinical management of irregular uterine bleeding with exogenous hormones is a time-honored method and is also of diagnostic value. Failure to control vaginal bleeding with hormonal therapy, despite appropriate application and utilization, makes the diagnosis of anovulatory uterine bleeding considerably less likely. In this case, attention is directed to an anatomic pathologic entity within the reproductive axis as the cause of abnormal bleeding.

Heavy but regular menstrual bleeding (hypermenorrhea) can be encountered in ovulatory women. It may be due to anatomic causes such as a leiomyoma impinging on the endometrial cavity or the diffuse and pathologic presence of benign endometrial glands in the myometrium (adenomyosis). In the absence of a specific pathologic cause, however, it is presumed that hypermenorrhea reflects subtle disturbances in the endometrial tissue mechanism. In essentially all cases, evaluation and treatment are identical to the approach detailed in this section.

Characteristics of Normal Menses

Normal menstruation takes place about 14 days after each ovulation episode as a consequence of postovulatory estrogen-progesterone withdrawal. The quantity and duration of bleeding are quite reproducible. This predictability leads many women to expect a certain characteristic flow pattern. Any slight deviations, such as plus or minus 1 day in duration or minor deviation from expected tampon utilization, are causes for major concern in the patient. Most women of reproductive age can predict the timing of their flows so accurately that even some instances of minor variability may require reassurance by the clinician. Although variability of menstrual cycles is a common feature during teenage years and the perimenopausal transition, the characteristics of menstrual bleeding do not undergo appreciable change between ages 20 and 40.[507]

For ovulatory women, the changes in the length of menstrual cycles over the period of reproductive age are predictable. Between menarche and age 20, the cycle length for most ovulatory women is relatively longer. Between 20 and 40, there is increased regularity as cycles shorten. In the 40s, cycles begin to lengthen again. The highest incidence of anovulatory cycles occurs before age 20 and after age 40.[508, 509] In this age group, the average length of a cycle is between 25 and 28 days. Among ovulatory women, the frequency of a cycle less than 21 days long or a cycle greater than 35 days is extremely rare (less than 2%).[510] Overall, most women have cycles that last from 24 to 35 days (Fig. 16–39).[507] Between ages 40 and 50, menstrual cycle length increases and anovulation becomes more prevalent.[511]

The average postovulatory bleeding lasts from 4 to 6 days. The normal volume of menstrual blood loss is 30 mL. More than 80 mL is considered abnormal. Most of the blood loss occurs during the first 3 days of a period, so excessive flow may exist without prolongation of flow.[512, 513]

During an ovulatory cycle, the duration from the ovulation to menses is relatively constant and averages 14 days (see Fig. 16–22). Greater variability in the length of proliferative phase, however, produces a distribution in the duration of a menstrual cycle. Menstrual bleeding more often than every 24 days or less often than every 35 days requires evaluation.[507, 511] Flow that lasts 7 or more days also requires evaluation. A flow that totals more than 80 mL per month usually leads to anemia and should be treated.[514, 515] In clinical practice, however, it is quite difficult to quantify menstrual flow because evaluation and treatment are based solely on the patient's perceptions regarding the duration, amount, and timing of her menstrual bleed-

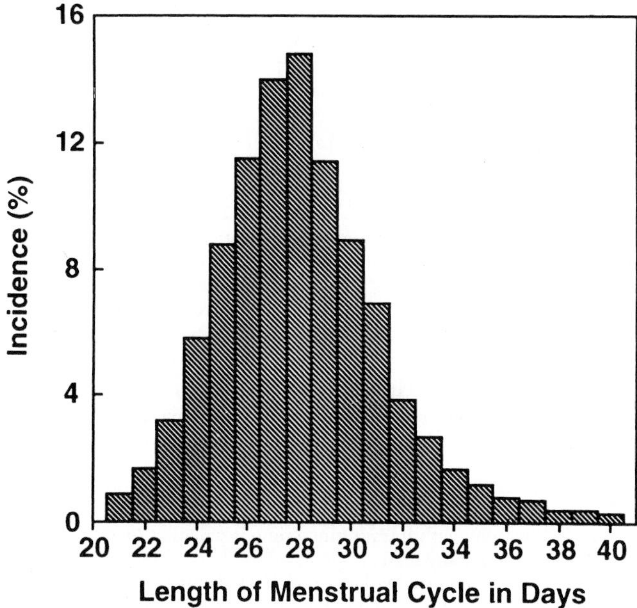

Figure 16–39. Variation of the duration of the menstrual cycle in women with regular cycles. (From Cunningham FG, MacDonald PC, Gant NF, et al. The endometrium and decidua: menstruation and pregnancy. In Williams Obstetrics, 19th ed. Stamford, Conn, Appleton & Lange, 1993, pp 81-109.)

ing. Despite this difficulty in quantifying menstrual blood loss, the clinician should evaluate the cause of excessive uterine bleeding. Anemia should be ruled out by a complete blood count.[516] A low hemoglobin value accompanied by microcytic and hypochromic red blood cells suggests excessive blood loss during menses. These patients should be provided with iron supplementation. The likely presence of coagulation defects, uterine leiomyomas, or adenomyosis underlying prolonged menses should also be evaluated in anemic patients through a meticulous history and physical examination followed by relevant laboratory tests.

Terminology Describing Abnormal Uterine Bleeding

Oligomenorrhea is defined as intervals between episodes of uterine bleeding greater than 35 days, and the term *polymenorrhea* is used to describe intervals less than 24 days. *Hypermenorrhea* refers to regular intervals (24 to 35 days) but excessive flow or duration of bleeding, or both. *Hypomenorrhea* refers to diminution of the flow or shortening of the duration of regular menses, or both.

Uterine Bleeding in Response to Steroid Hormones

Estrogen Withdrawal Bleeding. Uterine bleeding follows acute cessation of estrogen support to the endometrium. Thus, this type of uterine bleeding can occur after bilateral oophorectomy, radiation of mature follicles, or administration of estrogen to a castrate and then discontinuation of therapy. Similarly, the bleeding that occurs after castration can be delayed by concomitant estrogen therapy. Flow occurs on discontinuation of exogenous estrogen. Thus, estrogen withdrawal by itself (in the absence of progesterone) almost invariably causes uterine bleeding.

Estrogen Breakthrough Bleeding. Chronic exposure to varying quantities of estrogen stimulates the growth of endometrium continuously in the absence of progesterone, as in the case of excessive extragonadal estrogen production in PCOS. After a certain point, the amount of estrogen produced in extraovarian tissue remains insufficient to maintain structural support for the endometrium. This gives rise to unpredictable episodes of shedding of the surface endometrium. Relatively low doses of estrogen yield intermittent spotting that may be prolonged but is generally light in quantity of flow. On the other hand, high levels of estrogen and sustained availability lead to prolonged periods of amenorrhea followed by acute, often profuse episodes of bleeding with excessive loss of blood.

Progesterone Withdrawal Bleeding. The typical progesterone withdrawal bleeding occurs after ovulation in the absence of pregnancy. Removal of the corpus luteum is another example that leads to endometrial desquamation. Pharmacologically, a similar event can be achieved by administration and discontinuation of progesterone or a synthetic progestin. Progesterone withdrawal bleeding occurs only if the endometrium is initially primed by endogenous or exogenous estrogen. If estrogen therapy is continued as progesterone is withdrawn, the progesterone withdrawal bleeding still occurs. Only if estrogen levels are increased markedly is progesterone withdrawal bleeding delayed.[517] Thus, progesterone withdrawal bleeding is quite predictable in the presence of previous or concomitant estrogen exposure.

Progestin Breakthrough Bleeding. This is a pharmacologic phenomenon that occurs in the presence of an unfavorably high ratio of progestin to estrogen. In the absence of sufficient estrogen, continuous progestin therapy leads to intermittent bleeding of variable duration, similar to the low-dose estrogen breakthrough bleeding noted previously. This type of bleeding is associated with the combination oral contraceptives that contain low-dose estrogen and the long-acting progestin-only contraceptive methods such as Norplant and Depo-Provera.[518] Progestin breakthrough bleeding is highly unpredictable and characterized by extensive variability between women.

Causes of Irregular Uterine Bleeding

Pregnancy and its complications represent one of the most common causes of irregular uterine bleeding (Table 16–10). Pregnancy should be ruled out by a urine test in any woman of reproductive age presenting with irregular bleeding (Table 16–11).

As pointed out earlier, anovulatory uterine bleeding arising from responses of the endometrium to inappropriate production of ovarian steroids has also been called dysfunctional uterine bleeding because treatments that restore ovulatory function potentially reverse the irregular bleeding pattern. Common examples of anovulatory bleeding include those associated with exercise-related anovulation, hyperprolactinemia, hypothyroidism, or PCOS.[519] In these cases, either restoring ovulatory menses by correction of the underlying disorder or use of exogenous hormones can achieve predictable uterine bleeding. On the other hand, various pathologic entities of the genital tract (ovaries, uterus, vagina, or vulva) or a coagulation abnormality may also cause deviation from normal menses (see Table 16–10).

Anovulatory uterine bleeding is a diagnosis of exclusion for the following reasons. Vulvar, vaginal, or uterine malignancies can give rise to irregular bleeding. Moreover, an estrogen- or androgen-secreting ovarian tumor may cause abnormal uterine bleeding (see Table 16–10). Pregnancy and pregnancy-related problems such as ectopic pregnancy or spontaneous miscarriage are extremely common causes of abnormal uterine bleeding. In fact, the most common cause of disruption of a normal menstrual pattern is pregnancy or a complication of pregnancy.

Table 16–10. Causes of Irregular Uterine Bleeding

Complications of Pregnancy
Threatened miscarriage
Incomplete miscarriage
Ectopic pregnancy

Anovulation
Physiologic
  Uncomplicated pregnancy (amenorrhea)
  Pubertal (postmenarchal) anovulation
  Premenopausal anovulation
Medications (e.g., oral contraceptives, LHRH agonists, danazol)
Hypothalamic (frequently presents as amenorrhea)
  Functional (e.g., diet, exercise, stress)
  Anatomic (e.g., tumor, granulomatous disease, infection)
  Medications
  Other
Hyperprolactinemia, other pituitary disorders
  Prolactinoma
  Other pituitary tumors, granulomatous disease
  Hypothyroidism
  Medications
  Other
Androgen excess
  PCOS, hyperthecosis
  Ovarian tumor (e.g., Sertoli-Leydig cell tumor)
  Nonclassical adrenal hyperplasia
  Cushing's syndrome
  Glucocorticoid resistance
  Adrenal tumor (e.g., adenoma, carcinoma)
  Medications (e.g., testosterone, danazol)
  Other
Premature ovarian failure (frequently presents as amenorrhea)
Chronic illness
  Liver failure
  Renal failure
  AIDS
Other

Anatomic Defects Affecting the Uterus
Uterine leiomyomas
Endometrial polyps
Adenomyosis (usually presents as hypermenorrhea)
Intrauterine adhesions (usually presents as amenorrhea)
Endometritis
Endometrial hyperplasia, cancer
  Chronic estrogen exposure (e.g., PCOS, medication, liver failure)
  Estrogen-secreting ovarian tumor (e.g., granulosa cell tumor)
Advanced cervical cancer
Other

Coagulation Defects (Usually Present as Hypermenorrhea)
Von Willebrand's disease
Factor XI deficiency
Other

Extrauterine Genital Bleeding (May Mimic Uterine Bleeding)
Vaginitis
Genital trauma
Foreign body
Vaginal neoplasia
Vulvar neoplasia
Other

AIDS, acquired immunodeficiency syndrome; LHRH, luteinizing hormone–releasing hormone; PCOS, polycystic ovary syndrome.

Another common cause of irregular uterine bleeding is observed in oral contraceptive users in the form of progestin breakthrough bleeding. Progestin breakthrough bleeding during postmenopausal hormone replacement is also common (see later). Patients may be using other hormonal medications unknowingly with an impact on the endometrium. For example, the use of ginseng, an herbal root, has been associated with estrogenic activity and abnormal bleeding.[520] Although uterine bleeding is a common benign side effect of various long-term hormonal treatments, the clinician should always be convinced that no other pathology is present. Anatomically demonstrable pathologies of the menstrual outflow tract include endometrial hyperplasia and cancer, endometrial polyps, leiomyomata uteri, adenomyosis, and endometritis. Irregular, serious bleeding may also be associated with chronic illness, such as renal failure, liver failure, and acquired immunodeficiency syndrome. Finally, careful examination is worthwhile to discover genital injury or a foreign object (see Table 16–10).

Table 16–11. Diagnostic Tests to Evaluate Irregular Uterine Bleeding

Commonly Used Tests
Urine hCG test
Serum hCG level (incomplete miscarriage, ectopic pregnancy)
Transvaginal pelvic ultrasonography (intrauterine or ectopic pregnancy, uterine leiomyoma, endometrial polyp or neoplasia, ovarian tumor)
Serum FSH, LH (anovulation; ovarian failure)
Serum prolactin, TSH (anovulation; hyperprolactinemia)
Complete blood count, PT, PTT (coagulation defect)
Liver and renal functions, HIV (anovulation; chronic disease)
Endometrial biopsy (endometrial disease; polyp, neoplasia, endometritis)

Less Commonly Used Tests
Evaluation for PCOS, ovarian or adrenal tumor, nonclassical adrenal hyperplasia, Cushing's syndrome and glucocorticoid resistance (androgen excess)
Head CT or MRI scan (hypothalamic anovulation, hyperprolactinemia)
Pelvic MRI scan (adenomyosis, uterine leiomyoma)
Hysterosonography with intrauterine saline installation (endometrial polyp, uterine leiomyoma)
Hysteroscopy (endometrial polyp, uterine leiomyoma)
Dilatation and curettage (endometrial disease not diagnosed by ultrasonography or biopsy)

CT, computed tomography; FSH, follicle-stimulating hormone; hCG, human chorionic gonadotropin; HIV, human immunodeficiency virus; LH, luteinizing hormone; MRI, magnetic resonance imaging; PCOS, polycystic ovary syndrome; PT, prothrombin time; PTT, partial thromboplastin time; TSH, thyroid-stimulating hormone.

At puberty, the most common cause of irregular uterine bleeding is anovulation. Approximately 20% of these adolescents with excessive irregular uterine bleeding, however, have a coagulation defect.[521, 522] Among all women of reproductive age with hypermenorrhea, the prevalence of a coagulation disorder was reported to be 17%. Von Willebrand's disease was the most common defect, and factor XI deficiency was the second common diagnosis. Bleeding secondary to a coagulation defect is usually a heavy flow with regular, cyclic menses (hypermenorrhea), and the same pattern can be seen in patients being treated with anticoagulants.[523] Bleeding disorders are usually associated with hypermenorrhea since menarche and a history of bleeding with surgery or trauma. Hypermenorrhea may be the only sign of an inherited bleeding disorder.[524]

Early pregnancy or its complications should always be ruled out first by a sensitive urine hCG measurement in any reproductive-age women presenting with irregular bleeding (see Table 16–11). Threatened or incomplete miscarriage and ectopic pregnancy are extremely common causes of irregular uterine bleeding. Other tests should be ordered if necessary on the basis of the initial clinical evaluation. These include tests to evaluate anovulatory disorders of various etiologies (see Table 16–11). In patients with a history of prolonged heavy menses (hypermenorrhea) of pubertal origin, coagulation studies (e.g., prothrombin time, partial thromboplastin time, and bleeding time) and a complete blood count should be obtained.

Pelvic ultrasonography through a vaginal probe is an extremely useful test for the evaluation of normal or abnormal pregnancy, uterine leiomyomas, endometrial neoplasia, and ovarian tumors (see Table 16–11). Other imaging studies may be used judiciously to rule out pathologies of the hypothalamus, pituitary, or adrenal (see earlier). Of note is the use of pelvic MRI to rule out adenomyosis, a uterine disorder characterized by the abnormal presence of diffuse endometrial tissue in the myometrial layer (see Table 16–11). Advanced adenomyosis is associated with diffuse enlargement of the uterus, hypermenorrhea, and anemia.

Endometrial histology should be determined by an endometrial biopsy performed in the physician's office in patients at risk for the development of endometrial hyperplasia or cancer (e.g., PCOS, liver failure, obesity, diabetes mellitus, hormone replacement). A benign endometrial polyp or a uterine leiomyoma protruding into the uterine cavity can be diagnosed by hysterosonography using intrauterine saline installation or hysteroscopy. Hysterosonography and hysteroscopy are not appropriate tests to evaluate endometrial hyperplasia or cancer because these procedures may cause dissemination of malignant cells. If malignancy is suspected, it should be ruled out by an office endometrial biopsy (see Table 16–11). Occasionally, an office endometrial biopsy cannot be performed or is not diagnostic of endometrial neoplasia. In these rare instances, endometrial curettage under anesthesia is performed for a reliable tissue diagnosis.

We should underscore again that a careful history and physical examination eliminate the need for most of these diagnostic tests. A useful question to ask oneself before ordering a certain diagnostic study is whether that particular test will alter the ultimate clinical management.

Management of Anovulatory Uterine Bleeding

The terms *dysfunctional uterine bleeding* and *anovulatory bleeding* are used interchangeably and denote inappropriate stimulation of the endometrium during dysfunctional states of the reproductive system. If ovulatory function can be restored, anovulatory bleeding usually gives way to cyclic predictable periods. Because restoring ovulatory function may not be possible or practical in a large number of these women, exogenous estrogen and progestin are administered for a number of purposes. The indications for hormonal treatment of uterine bleeding include the need to stop acute uterine bleeding, to maintain predictable bleeding episodes, or to prevent endometrial hyperplasia. A number of hormonal treatments are used to stop anovulatory uterine bleeding and to induce predictable bleeding episodes. We should reemphasize that anovulatory uterine bleeding is a diagnosis of exclusion. Various anatomically demonstrable pathologies of the genital tract as listed in Table 16–10 should be ruled out before administration of the following regimens.

Oral Contraceptives

Use of combination oral contraceptives in an acute or chronic fashion is the most common treatment for irregular uterine bleeding. The estrogen component of the combination pill stabilizes the endometrial tissue and stops shedding within hours and decreases ovarian secretion of sex steroids by suppression of gonadotropins within several days. The progestin component of the pill directly affects endometrial tissue to decrease shedding over days and potentiates ovarian suppression induced by estrogen. The progestin (in the presence of estrogen) induces differentiation of the endometrial tissue into a stable form termed pseudodecidua. Typically, a monophasic oral contraceptive preparation that contains 30 or 35 μg of ethinyl estradiol is preferred. Triphasic oral contraceptives or those with less than 30 μg of ethinyl estradiol are not suitable for the treatment of excessive anovulatory uterine bleeding. A combination oral contraceptive in high doses (two or three pills a day) can be used for short intervals (weeks) to treat an acute episode of excessive uterine bleeding. A usual dose (one pill per day) may be administered for years to manage chronic anovulatory bleeding associated with PCOS or hyperprolactinemia.

Oral Contraceptives and Acute Excessive Uterine Bleeding Associated with Anemia

Unopposed estrogen exposure in women with anovulatory uterine bleeding is commonly associated with chronic endometrial buildup and heavy bleeding episodes. Therapy is administered as one pill twice a day for 1 week. In obese women, the oral contraceptive may be given three times a day. This therapy is maintained despite cessation of flow within 2 days. If flow does not abate, other diagnostic possibilities (polyps, incomplete abortion, and neoplasia) should be reevaluated. In case of anovulatory bleeding, the flow does diminish rapidly within 2 days after the beginning of high-dose (one pill two or three times a day) oral contraceptive treatment. Specific causes of anovulation and possible coagulation disorders are evaluated during the following few days. At this time, the physician also considers whether blood replacement or initiation of iron therapy is necessary. The high-dose estrogen-progestin combination has produced the structural rigidity intrinsic to the compact pseudodecidual reaction for the moment. Continued random breakdown of formerly fragile tissue is avoided and blood loss stopped. A large quantity of tissue, however, remains to react to estrogen-progestin withdrawal. The patient must be warned to anticipate a heavy flow with severely cramping flow a few days after stopping this therapy. The patient should also be warned of possible nausea that may be caused by high-dose oral contraceptive treatment.

At the end of a week of high-dose oral contraceptive treatment, the pill is stopped temporarily. A heavy flow usually starts within a few days. On the third day of this withdrawal bleeding, a regular dose of combination oral contraceptive medication (one pill a day) is started. This is repeated for several 3-week treatments interrupted by 1-week withdrawal intervals. A decrease in volume with each successive cycle is expected. Oral contraceptives reduce menstrual flow by more than half in most women.[525]

Early application of the estrogen-progestin combination limits growth and allows orderly regression of excessive endometrial height to normal levels. Because oral contraceptives do not treat the underlying cause of anovulation but provide symptomatic relief by directly affecting the endometrium, cessation of oral contraceptives results in the return of erratic uterine bleeding. Regardless of the requirement for contraception, oral contraceptives represent the best choice for hormonal management of heavy anovulatory bleeding and should be offered as long-term management.

Oral Contraceptives and Chronic Irregular Uterine Bleeding

PCOS is a common form of anovulation associated with chronic steady-state levels of unopposed estrogen that may give rise to endometrial hyperplasia and cancer (see earlier). Hypothalamic anovulation and hyperprolactinemia, on the other hand, are associated with low estrogen levels, insufficient to prevent bone loss. A combination oral contraceptive is a suitable long-term treatment for both forms of chronic anovulation.

Oral contraceptives represent the most suitable long-term symptomatic management option for any kind of anovulatory uterine bleeding, including oligomenorrhea. Before the administration of an oral contraceptive, pregnancy should be ruled out. For this purpose, one pill per day is ordinarily administered for 3-week periods interrupted by 1-week hormone-free intervals. Withdrawal bleeding is expected during the hormone-free interval. The progestin component serves to prevent endometrial hyperplasia associated with steady-state unopposed estrogen exposure in PCOS (see earlier). In cases of anovulation associated with hypoestrogenism (e.g., hypothalamic anovulation, hyperprolactinemia), on the other hand, the estrogen component of the pill provides sufficient replacement to prevent bone loss. The risk of thromboembolism, stroke, or myocardial infarction associated with long-term administration is extremely low in current nonsmokers and in the absence of a history of thromboembolism. Provided that an oral contraceptive controls the abnormal uterine bleeding effectively, a chronically anovulatory woman can continue this regimen until the menopause.

Synthetic Progestins

Synthetic progestins enhance endometrial differentiation and antagonize proliferative effects of estrogen on the endometrium (see Fig. 16–28).[213, 215, 526] The effects of progestins or natural progesterone include limitation of estrogen-induced endometrial growth and prevention of endometrial hyperplasia. The absence of naturally synthesized progesterone in anovulatory states is the rationale for administering a progestin.

The most common indication for long-term cyclic progestin administration is to prevent endometrial malignancy in a patient with PCOS and unopposed chronic estrogen exposure of the endometrium. A combination oral contraceptive is the treatment of choice in these cases. If the patient cannot use an oral contraceptive for some reason (e.g., history of thromboembolism), a progestin can be administered in a cyclic fashion to prevent endometrial hyperplasia. Before the administration of a progestin (or oral contraceptive), pregnancy should be ruled out. In the treatment of oligomenorrhea associated with PCOS, orderly limited withdrawal bleeding can be accomplished by administration of a progestin such as medroxyprogesterone acetate, 10 mg/day for at least 10 days every 2 months. Alternatively, norethindrone acetate at 5 mg/day or megestrol acetate at 20 mg/day may be administered for 10 days every 2 months. Absence of withdrawal bleeding requires further work-up.

In the treatment of excessive uterine bleeding (hypermenorrhea or polymenorrhea), these progestins at higher daily doses (medroxyprogesterone acetate 20 mg/day, norethindrone acetate 10 mg/day, or megestrol acetate 40 mg/day) are prescribed for 2 weeks to induce predecidual stromal changes in the endometrium. A heavy progestin withdrawal flow usually follows within 3 days after the last dose. Thereafter, repeated progestin treatment (medroxyprogesterone acetate 10 mg/day, norethindrone acetate 5 mg/day, or megestrol acetate 20 mg/day) is offered cyclically for at least the first 10 days of every other month to ensure therapeutic effect. Failure of progestin to correct irregular bleeding requires diagnostic reevaluation such as endometrial biopsy. On the other hand, predictable withdrawal bleeding within several days after each cycle of progestin administration suggests the absence of endometrial malignancy.

High-Dose Estrogen for Acute Excessive Uterine Bleeding

As already outlined, an oral contraceptive given two or three times a day is the treatment of choice to stop heavy anovulatory bleeding. A high-dose oral contraceptive regimen should be offered to women with heavy uterine bleeding plus or minus asymptomatic anemia after an anatomically demonstrable pathology of the genital tract has been ruled out (see Table 16–10). On the other hand, a patient with acute and severe anovulatory bleeding accompanied by symptomatic anemia represents a medical emergency. These patients should be hospitalized immediately and offered a blood transfusion. When genital tract pathology has been ruled by history, physical examination, and pelvic ultrasonography, intravenously administered high-dose estrogen is the treatment of choice to stop life-threatening bleeding. A well-established regimen is 25 mg of conjugated estrogen administered intravenously every 4 hours until bleeding markedly slows down or for at least 24 hours.[527] Estrogen most likely acts on the capillaries to induce clotting.[528] Before intravenous estrogen treatment is discontinued, an oral contraceptive pill is started three times a day. Oral contraceptive treatment is continued as described previously.

Because high-dose estrogen is a risk factor for thromboembolism, taking two or three oral contraceptives per day for a week or large doses of intravenous conjugated estrogens for 24 hours should also be regarded as significant risks. There are no data available, however, to evaluate any risk associated with this type of acute use of hormonal therapy for such short intervals. The physician and patient should make a decision regarding high-dose hormone therapy after considering its risks and benefits. Alternative treatment options may be offered to patients with significant risk factors. In women with a past episode of idiopathic venous thromboembolism or a strong family history, exposure to high doses of estrogen should be avoided. High-dose hormone treatment should also be avoided in women with severe chronic illness such as liver failure or renal failure. One alternative for these patients is dilatation and curettage, followed by an oral contraceptive at one pill per day until the uterine bleeding is under control.

Luteinizing Hormone–Releasing Hormone Analogues for Excessive Anovulatory Uterine Bleeding

LHRH analogues (see Table 16–1) may be given to women with excessive anovulatory bleeding or hypermenorrhea related to severe chronic illness such as liver failure or coagulation disorders. It should be pointed out that monthly depot injections of LHRH agonists are not effective for acute excessive uterine bleeding and may increase uterine bleeding for the first 2 weeks. LHRH antagonists, on the other hand, down-regulate FSH and LH without a delay and achieve amenorrhea more rapidly. Depot formulations of LHRH antagonists, however, are not available at present. Long-term side effects of LHRH analogues including osteoporosis make this an undesirable choice for long-term therapy. If long-term treatment with LHRH analogues is chosen, a combination of 0.625 mg of conjugated estrogens and 2.5 mg of medroxyprogesterone acetate daily should be added back when excessive anovulatory bleeding is controlled. This add-back regimen is usually sufficient to prevent osteoporosis and does not ordinarily worsen the uterine bleeding.

Hormone-Dependent Benign Gynecologic Disorders

Endometriosis

Endometriosis is defined as the presence of endometrium-like tissue outside the uterine cavity, most often on the peritoneal surfaces of the pelvis and the ovaries. It is one of the most common causes of infertility and chronic pelvic pain and affects 1 in 10 women in the reproductive age group.[529] The incidence increases to 30% in patients with infertility and to 45% in patients with chronic pelvic pain.[530]

Reliable diagnosis of endometriosis can be made only by direct visualization of these peritoneal lesions by laparoscopy or laparotomy. As in other common chronic diseases such as diabetes mellitus and asthma, endometriosis is inherited in a polygenic manner.[529] Relatives of women with this disease have a sevenfold increase in the incidence of endometriosis compared with relatives of control subjects.[529] Sampson proposed the most widely accepted mechanism for the development of endometriosis on pelvic peritoneal surfaces as the implantation of endometrial tissue on the peritoneum through retrograde menstruation.[529] Because retrograde menstruation occurs in more than 90% of all women, endometriosis may be caused by genetic defects that favor survival and establishment of endometrial tissue in menstrual debris on the peritoneum.[401]

Endometriosis and normal endometrial tissues respond to estrogen and progesterone with similar histologic changes.[401] Estrogen favors the growth of endometriosis, whereas progesterone may limit this mitogenic action of estrogen. Some endometriotic implants undergo atrophy in response to prolonged oral contraceptive therapy just as the normal endometrium does, the so-called pregnancy state. Yet, endometriotic tissue does not respond to progestins or native progesterone as predictably as normal endometrium does.[401] Endometriotic tissue in ectopic locations such as the peritoneum or ovary is strikingly different from the eutopic endometrium within the uterus with respect to production of cytokines and prostaglandins, steroid biosynthesis and metabolism, steroid receptor content, and clinical response to progestins.[195, 401, 530]

Although current hormonal therapy for infertility associated with endometriosis is not of proven value, it is somewhat successful for pelvic pain associated with endometriosis.[529] The duration of relief provided by medical (hormonal) treatment, however, is relatively short.[531] Various agents used are comparable in terms of efficacy. Most current medical treatments were designed to decrease estrogen secretion by the ovaries (e.g., LHRH agonists, oral contraceptives, danazol and progestins) or to antagonize the effects of estrogen on endometriotic implants (e.g., oral contraceptives, danazol and progestins). A possible alternative mechanism of action of the androgenic steroid danazol or a progestin is a direct antiproliferative effect on endometriotic tissue.

Many patients and physicians do not favor danazol because of its anabolic and androgenic side effects of weight gain and muscle cramps and occasional irreversible virilization (e.g., clitoromegaly and voice changes).[532] In fact, up to 50% of patients with endometriosis fail to complete 6 months of treatment with danazol.[533] The rest of the hormonal agents—oral contraceptives, progestins, and LHRH agonists—show comparable efficacy for the control of endometriosis-associated pain.[530, 534, 535] A 6-month course using any one of these agents results in a significant reduction of pain in more than 50% of patients.[530, 534, 535] Induction of pain relief with a continuously administered oral contraceptive or progestin takes longer than with an LHRH agonist. There is, however, a high incidence of persistence of the disease after all of these medical therapies.[531] Six months after completion of a 6-month course of treatment with a progestin, oral contraceptive, or LHRH agonist, moderate to severe pain symptoms recurred in 50% of initial responders.[535] The recurrence rate of pain in the rest of the patients was approximately 5% to 20% per year during a 5-year follow-up.[531] A 6-month course of LHRH agonist treatment is currently the most popular regimen. The most serious side effect of the LHRH agonist treatment for endometriosis is bone loss related to estrogen deficiency, and oral estrogen-progestin preparations or bisphosphonates are usually added back to minimize bone loss.[32]

We are still far from the cure of endometriosis, and current treatments are not satisfactory for effective control of pain. The radical treatment is the removal of both ovaries, and even this was not found to be effective in a number of cases of postmenopausal endometriosis.[536] New strategies are needed to offer women with endometriosis a reasonable chance to live without suffering from chronic pelvic pain for decades. There are two important caveats, which are not addressed by the LHRH agonist treatment. First, large quantities of estrogen can be produced locally within the endometriotic cells. This represents an intracrine mechanism of estrogen action, in contrast to ovarian secretion, which is an endocrine means of supplying this steroid to target tissues (see Fig. 16–23).[536, 401] Second, estradiol produced in peripheral tissue sites (e.g., adipose tissue and skin fibroblasts) may give rise to pathologically significant circulating levels of estradiol in a subset of women.[401] LHRH agonists do not inhibit peripheral estrogen formation or local estrogen production within the estrogen-responsive lesion. As a further twist, endometriosis is resistant to selective effects of progesterone and currently used progestins.[401] Thus, aromatase inhibitors and selective progesterone response modulators are candidate therapeutic agents for endometriosis. Preliminary evidence suggests that unusually aggressive endometriotic lesions resistant to other therapy can be treated successfully with aromatase inhibitors.[401, 536] There are a number of ongoing trials investigating the use of aromatase inhibitors and selective progesterone receptor modulators in the treatment of endometriosis.

Uterine Leiomyomas

Uterine leiomyomas originate from the myometrium and are the most common solid tumor of the pelvis.[537] Leiomyomas are responsible for over 200,000 hysterectomies per year in the United States. They are almost invariably benign and represent clonal expansion of individual myometrial cells. Leiomyomas can cause a variety of symptoms including irregular and excessive uterine bleeding, pressure sensation in the lower abdomen, pain during intercourse, pelvic pain, recurrent pregnancy loss, infertility, and compression of adjacent pelvic organs, or they may be totally asymptomatic. The prevalence rate of uterine leiomyomas is estimated to be 25% to 30%.[537] Leiomyomas are more common in black women and have a polygenic inheritance pattern. Diagnosis can be made by abdominal and transvaginal ultrasonography. Transvaginal ultrasonography is a sensitive method for determining the size, number, and location of uterine leiomyomas.

Uterine leiomyomas appear during the reproductive years and regress after menopause, indicating their ovarian steroid–dependent growth potential. The role of steroids or other growth factors in the initiation and growth of these tumors, however, is not well understood. The neoplastic transformation of myometrium to leiomyoma probably involves somatic mutations of normal myometrium and the complex interactions of sex steroids and growth factors.[538] Traditionally, estrogen has been considered the major promoter of myoma growth. More recent biochemical, histologic, and clinical evidence suggests an important role for progesterone in the growth of uterine leiomyomas. Biochemical and clinical studies suggest that progesterone and progestins, acting through the PR, might enhance proliferative activity in leiomyomas.[538]

The therapeutic choices depend on the goals of therapy, with hysterectomy most often used for definitive treatment and myomectomy when preservation of childbearing is desired.[539] Intracavitary and submucous leiomyomas can be removed by hysteroscopic resection. Laparoscopic myomectomy is now technically possible but apparently involves an increased risk of uterine rupture during pregnancy. The overall recurrence rate after myomectomy varies widely (10% to 50%). Although LHRH agonist–induced hypogonadism can reduce the overall volume of the uterus containing leiomyomas and tumor vascularity, the severe side effects and prompt recurrences make LHRH agonists useful only for short-term goals such as reducing anemia related to uterine bleeding or decreased tumor vascularity before hysteroscopic resection.[539]

MANAGEMENT OF THE MENOPAUSE

Consequences of the Menopause

The Climacteric

The menopause is the permanent cessation of menses as a result of the irreversible loss of a number of ovarian functions, including ovulation and estrogen production. The climacteric is a critical period of life during which striking endocrinologic, somatic, and psychologic alterations occur in the transition to the menopause. The climacteric is also referred to as the perimenopause. The climacteric encompasses the change from ovulatory cycles to cessation of menses and is marked by irregularity of menstrual bleeding.

The most sensitive clinical indication of the climacteric is the progressively increasing occurrence of menstrual irregularities. The menstrual cycle for most ovulatory women lasts from 24 to 35 days, whereas approximately 20% of all reproductive-age women experience irregular cycles.[507] When women are in their 40s, anovulation becomes more prevalent; prior to anovulation, the menstrual cycle length increases, beginning several years before menopause.[511] The median age for the onset of the climacteric transition is 47.5 years.[540] Regardless of the age of its onset, the menopause (cessation of menses) is consistently preceded by a period of prolonged cycle intervals.[541] Elevated circulating FSH marks this menstrual cycle change before menopause and is accompanied by decreased inhibin levels, normal levels of LH, and slightly elevated levels of estradiol.[542–546] These changes in serum hormone levels reflect a decreasing ovarian follicular reserve and can be detected more reliably on day 2 or 3 of the menstrual cycle.

During the climacteric, serum estradiol levels do not begin to decline until less than a year before menopause.[546] The average circulating estradiol levels in perimenopausal women are estimated to be somewhat higher than those in younger women because of an increased follicular response to elevated FSH.[547] The decline in inhibin production by the follicle, allowing a rise in FSH, in the later reproductive years reflects diminishing follicular reserve and competence.[543, 544] Ovarian follicular output of inhibin begins to decrease after 30 years of age, and this decline becomes much more pronounced after age 40. These hormonal changes are parallel to a significant decrease in fecundity, which starts at age 35.

The climacteric is a transitional period during which postmenopausal levels of FSH can be observed despite continued menses, whereas LH levels still remain in the normal range. The perimenopausal woman is not beyond the realm of an unexpected pregnancy because there is occasional ovulation and functional corpus luteum formation. Thus, until complete cessation of menses is observed or FSH levels higher than 40 IU/L are measured on two separate occasions, some form of contraception should be recommended to prevent unwanted pregnancies.[545]

The climacteric represents an optimal period to evaluate the general health of the mature woman and introduce the measures to prepare her for striking physiologic changes that come with the menopause. The patient and her clinician should attempt to achieve several important aims during the climacteric. The long-term goal is to maintain an optimal quality of physical and social life. Another immediate objective is the detection of any major chronic disorders that occur with aging. Finally, the clinician should counsel the perimenopausal woman about the symptoms and long-term consequences of menopause. The benefits and risks of lifelong hormone replacement should be discussed at great length at this time.

The Menopause

The median age of the menopause is approximately 51.[548] The age of menopause is probably determined in part by genetic factors because mothers and daughters tend to experience menopause at the same age.[549–551] A number of environmental factors may modify the age of menopause. For example, current smoking is associated with an earlier menopause, whereas alcohol consumption delays menopause.[548] Oral contraceptive use does not affect the age of menopause.

The symptoms frequently seen and related to decreased estrogen production in menopause include irregular frequency of menses followed by amenorrhea, vasomotor instability manifest as hot flashes and sweats, urogenital atrophy giving rise to pain during intercourse and a variety of urinary symptoms, and consequences of osteoporosis and cardiovascular disease. The combination and the extent of these symptoms differ widely for each patient. Some patients experience multiple severe symptoms that may be disabling, whereas others have no symptoms or mild discomfort associated with the climacteric.

Biosynthesis of Estrogen and Other Steroids in the Postmenopausal Woman

No follicular units can be detected histologically in the ovaries after the menopause.[552] In reproductive-age women, the granulosa cell of the ovulatory follicle is the major source of inhibin and estradiol. In the absence of these factors that inhibit gonadotropin secretion, both FSH and LH levels increase sharply after menopause. These levels peak a few years after menopause and decrease gradually and slightly thereafter.[553, 554] The postmenopausal serum level of either gonadotropin may be more than 100 IU/L. FSH levels are usually higher than LH levels because LH is cleared from the blood strikingly more quickly and possibly because the low levels of inhibin in the menopause selectively lead to increased FSH secretion. Nevertheless, increased LH is a major factor that maintains significant quantities of androstenedione and testosterone secretion from the ovary, although the total production rates of both steroids decline after menopause.

The primary steroid products of the postmenopausal ovary are androstenedione and testosterone.[555] The average premenopausal rate of production of androstenedione of 3 mg/day is decreased by half to approximately 1.5 mg/day.[555] This decrease is primarily due to a substantial reduction in the ovarian contribution to the circulating androstenedione pool. Adrenal secretion accounts for most of the androstenedione production in the postmenopausal woman, with only a small amount secreted from the ovary.[556] Both DHEA and DHEAS originate almost exclusively from the adrenal and decline steadily with advancing age independent of the menopause. The serum levels of both DHEA and DHEAS after menopause are about one fourth of those in young adult women.[557]

Testosterone production is decreased by approximately one third after menopause.[555] Total testosterone production can be approximated by the sum of ovarian secretion and peripheral formation from androstenedione (see Fig. 16–32). In the premenopausal woman, significant amounts of testosterone are produced by reduction of androstenedione in extraovarian tissues. Because ovarian androstenedione secretion is substantially decreased after the menopause, the decrease in postmenopausal

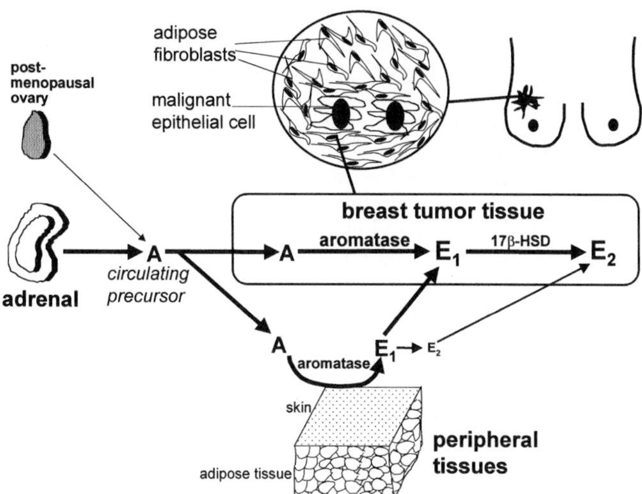

Figure 16–40. Tissue sources of estrogen in postmenopausal breast cancer. This figure exemplifies the important pathologic roles of extraovarian (peripheral) and local estrogen biosynthesis in an estrogen-dependent disease in postmenopausal women. The estrogen precursor androstenedione (A) originates primarily from the adrenal in the postmenopausal woman. Aromatase expression and enzyme activity in extraovarian tissues such as fat increase with advancing age. The aromatase activity in skin and subcutaneous adipose fibroblasts gives rise to formation of systemically available estrone (E_1) and to a smaller extent estradiol (E_2). The conversion of circulating A to E_1 in undifferentiated breast adipose fibroblasts compacted around malignant epithelial cells and subsequent conversion of E_1 to E_2 in malignant epithelial cells provide high tissue concentrations of E_2 for tumor growth. The clinical relevance of these findings is exemplified by the successful use of aromatase inhibitors to treat breast cancer.

testosterone production is accounted for, in large measure, by a decrease in the relative contribution of extraovarian sources.[555] With the disappearance of follicles and decreased estrogen, the elevated gonadotropins drive the remaining stromal tissue in the ovary to maintain testosterone secretion at levels observed during the premenopausal years. Thus, the contribution of the postmenopausal ovary to the total testosterone production is increased in the presence of seemingly unaltered ovarian secretion.[555]

The most dramatic endocrine alteration of the climacteric involves the decline in the circulating level and production rate of estradiol. The average menopausal level of circulating estradiol is less than 20 pg/mL. Both estradiol and estrone levels in postmenopausal women are usually slightly less than those in adult men. Circulating estradiol in postmenopausal women (and men) is derived from the peripheral conversion of androstenedione to estrone, which is, in turn, converted peripherally to estradiol (see Fig. 16–23).[403, 558, 559] The mean circulating level of estrone in postmenopausal women (37 pg/mL) is higher than that of estradiol. The average postmenopausal production rate of estrone is approximately 42 μg per 24 hours. After menopause, almost all estrone and estradiol are derived from the peripheral aromatization of androstenedione. Thus, there is a drastic change in the androgen-to-estrogen ratio because of the sharp decrease in estradiol levels and slightly reduced testosterone. The frequent onset of a mild hirsutism after menopause reflects this striking shift in the hormone ratio. During the postmenopausal years, DHEAS and DHEA levels continue to decline steadily with advancing age, whereas serum androstenedione, testosterone, estrone, and estradiol levels do not change significantly.[554, 558]

The aromatization of androstenedione to estrone in extraovarian tissues correlates positively with weight and advancing age (see Figs. 16–23 and 16–37).[168] Body weight correlates positively with the circulating levels of estrone and estradiol.[558] Because aromatase enzyme activity is present in significant quantities in adipose tissue, increased aromatization of androstenedione in overweight individuals may reflect the increased bulk of tissue containing the enzyme.[166] In addition, there is a twofold to fourfold increase in the specific activity of aromatase per cell with advancing age.[169] An increased overall number of adipose fibroblasts with aromatase activity and a decrease in the levels of TeBG cause an increased free estradiol level and contribute to the increased risk of endometrial cancer in obese women.[169] The production rate and circulating levels of estradiol after menopause are clearly insufficient to provide support for urogenital tissues and bone. Thus, osteoporosis and urogenital atrophy are some of the most dramatic and unwanted consequences of estradiol deficiency during the menopause.

Estrogen is also produced locally in pathologic tissues such as breast cancer through aromatase and reductive 17β-HSD (Fig. 16–40).[169, 196] In postmenopausal women, androstenedione of adrenal origin is the most important substrate for aromatase in tumor tissue.[169, 196] Estrone is produced primarily by aromatase that resides in undifferentiated adipose fibroblasts surrounding malignant epithelial cells (see Fig. 16–40).[169, 196] Estrone then diffuses into malignant epithelial cells that contain reductive 17β-HSD activity and is converted to biologically active estradiol (see Fig. 16–40).[194] Thus, paracrine interactions in breast tumor tissue serve to produce estradiol in malignant epithelial cells to give rise to an effect such as proliferation. The clinical relevance of these findings was exemplified by the successful use of aromatase inhibitors as both first-line and second-line endocrine treatments for postmenopausal breast cancer.[560]

Management of Postmenopausal Uterine Bleeding

Perimenopausal or postmenopausal bleeding can be due to hormone administration or excessive extraovarian estrogen formation. Irregular uterine bleeding is commonly observed during the perimenopausal transition as anovulatory cycles alternate with ovulatory cycles. Uterine bleeding after the menopause is less common if the patient is not receiving hormone replacement treatment (HRT). Obese patients are more likely to experience postmenopausal bleeding because of increased peripheral aromatization of adrenal androstenedione. Patients receiving a continuous combination regimen of HRT may experience unpredictable uterine bleeding (see later). The major objective in these circumstances is to rule out endometrial malignancy. This can be best achieved by tissue diagnosis through an office endometrial biopsy using a plastic cannula. Transvaginal ultrasonographic measurement of endometrial thickness may be used in postmenopausal women to avoid unnecessary biopsies.[226] A biopsy is required if an endometrial thickness greater than or equal to 5 mm is observed.

Before employing ultrasonography and endometrial biopsy to explore the etiology of bleeding that is assumed to arise from the intrauterine cavity, the clinician should rule out diseases of the vulva, vagina, and cervix as other potential causes of vaginal bleeding. Careful inspection of these organs and a normal cervical Pap smear within the past year are sufficient to rule out the vulva, vagina, and cervix as potential sources of bleeding. Postmenopausal uterine bleeding is the most common initial event that alerts the patient and her physician to the possibility of endometrial cancer. On the other hand, the causes of postmenopausal uterine bleeding are benign most of the time. Endometrial malignancy is encountered in patients with bleeding in only about 1% to 2% of postmenopausal endometrial biopsies.[561, 562] Approximately three quarters of these biopsies reveal either no pathology or an atrophic endometrium. Other histologic findings include hyperplasia (15%) and endometrial polyps (3%). Persistent unexplained uterine bleeding requires repeated evaluation, biopsy, hysteroscopy, or dilatation and curettage.

Unpredictable irregular uterine bleeding is observed in approximately 20% of postmenopausal women receiving a long-term (>1 year) continuous estrogen-progestin combination. This should also be evaluated appropriately with ultrasonography or biopsy, or both (see later).[226]

Hot Flash

The most frequent and striking symptom in the climacteric is the hot flash. The hot flash typically occurs at the time of transition from perimenopause to postmenopause, that is, the climacteric. The flash is also a major symptom of the postmenopause and can last up to 5 years after menopause.[563] More than four fifths of postmenopausal women experience hot flashes within 3 months after the cessation of ovarian function, whether natural or surgical in origin. Of these women, more than three fourths have them for more than 1 year and approximately half for up to 5 years.[563] Hot flashes lessen in frequency and intensity with advancing age, unlike other sequelae of the menopause, which progress with time.

A hot flash is a subjective sensation of intense warmth of the upper body, which typically lasts for 4 minutes but may range in duration from 30 seconds to 5 minutes. It may follow a prodrome of palpitations or headache and is frequently accompanied by weakness, faintness, or vertigo. This episode usually ends in profuse sweating and a cold sensation. The frequency may vary from extremely rare to recurring every few minutes. At night, flashes are more frequent and severe enough to awaken a woman from sleep. They are also more intense during times of stress. In a cool environment, hot flashes are fewer, less intense, and shorter in duration than in a warm environment.[564]

The hot flash results from a sudden reduction of estrogen levels rather than from hypoestrogenism itself. Therefore, regardless of the cause of menopause, natural, surgical, or estrogen withdrawal caused by a long-acting LHRH agonist, hot flashes are associated with an acute and significant drop in estrogen level.

The consistent association between the onset of flashes and acute estrogen withdrawal is also supported by the effectiveness of estrogen therapy and the absence of flashes in prolonged hypoestrogenic states, such as gonadal dysgenesis. Hypogonadal women experience hot flashes only after estrogen is administered and withdrawn.[565] Not all hot flashes, however, are due to estrogen deficiency. Sudden episodes of sweating and flash may be due to catecholamine- or histamine-secreting tumors (e.g., pheochromocytoma, carcinoid), hyperthyroidism, or chronic infection (e.g., tuberculosis). The hot flash may also be psychosomatic in origin and not due to estrogen withdrawal. Under these circumstances of doubt, the clinician should obtain a serum FSH level to confirm the climacteric or menopause before initiating hormone replacement. Obese women tend to be less troubled by hot flashes. Asymptomatic women are found to have significantly increased weight compared with severely symptomatic women, even when matched for age, ovarian status, and years since menopause.[566] The lower frequency and intensity of hot flashes in obese women may result from the elevated circulating free estradiol concentrations.[567]

Urogenital Atrophy

The urogenital sinus gives rise to the development of the lower vagina, vulva, and urethra during embryonic development, and these tissues are estrogen-dependent. The decrease in estrogen at menopause causes the vaginal walls to become pale because of diminished vascularity and to thin down to only three to four cell layers. The vaginal epithelial cells in postmenopausal women contain less glycogen, which prior to menopause was metabolized by lactobacilli to create an acidic pH, thereby protecting the vagina from bacterial overgrowth. Loss of this protective mechanism leaves the thin, friable tissue vulnerable to infection and ulceration. The vagina also loses its rugae and becomes shorter and inelastic. Postmenopausal women may complain of symptoms secondary to vaginal dryness, such as pain during intercourse, vaginal discharge, burning, itching, or bleeding. Genitourinary atrophy leads to a variety of symptoms that affect the ease and quality of living.

Urethritis with dysuria, stress urinary incontinence, and urinary frequency are further results of mucosal thinning of the urethra and bladder. Intravaginal estrogen treatment can effectively alleviate recurrent urinary tract infections and vaginal symptoms in the postmenopausal patient.[568] Oral estrogen replacement also rapidly reverses vaginal atrophy and urethral symptoms caused by estrogen deficiency.

Cognitive Function and Estrogen

Although Alzheimer's disease affects both men and women, studies in many different populations show that 1.5 to 3 times as many women as men suffer from this disease.[569] For women with this disease, one needs to consider behavioral and cognitive problems, therapeutic issues, and other gender-related risks. One obvious consideration is a possible link between estrogen deficiency and the increased incidence of Alzheimer's disease in postmenopausal women.[570] A number of studies have been published regarding the association of estrogen with cognition in women with or without Alzheimer's disease. Treatment of women free of Alzheimer's disease with hormone replacement for signs and symptoms of menopause led to improvements in verbal memory, vigilance, reasoning, and motor speed but no enhancement of other cognitive functions.[571] A meta-analysis of observational studies suggested that HRT was associated with a decreased incidence of dementia.[571] However, possible biases and lack of control for potential confounders limit interpretation of these studies.[571] Two small but randomized studies regarding the effects of short-term estrogen treatment on cognition in women with Alzheimer's disease produced conflicting data.[572, 573] Thus, future large randomized trials should target the potential benefits of HRT in improving cognition in women with menopausal symptoms as well as in the prevention and treatment of Alzheimer's disease. The ongoing large trial called the Women's Health Initiative may provide some answers in several years.

Cardiovascular Disease

It has long been suggested that estrogen protects against atherosclerosis because the incidence of cardiovascular disease is lower in women than in men in all age groups. The gender gap is widest during the premenopausal years.[574–576] For example, myocardial infarction is six times less common in premenopausal women than in men of the same age.[577, 578] This discrepancy has been attributed, in part, to the effects of estrogen.

During reproductive life, women have lower LDL cholesterol than men, although these levels gradually increase with advancing age and rise rapidly after menopause.[574–576] In contrast, despite consistently higher high-density lipoprotein (HDL) cholesterol levels in women than men throughout adulthood, this discrepancy persists after the menopause. HDL cholesterol becomes higher after puberty in girls but does not change greatly at menopause. The increases in LDL and total cholesterol levels at menopause are partially reversible with estrogen treatment.[579] Therefore, the increased myocardial infarction rate after menopause may be a function of rising LDL cholesterol levels that seem to be related to decreased estrogen levels.[574–576] Although HDL cholesterol levels do not decrease significantly in postmenopausal women, replacement with oral estrogen increases HDL cholesterol levels significantly; this may contribute to the cardioprotective effect of HRT.[580]

A strong correlation suggestive of a cause-and-effect relationship has been established between cholesterol levels and coronary heart disease in postmenopausal women.[581, 582] Postmenopausal women with elevated total cholesterol levels have a significantly increased risk of coronary heart disease compared with women with low levels.[581, 582] This risk is more pronounced in the first two decades after the menopause. The association becomes less pronounced with advancing age.[583] In both men and women, an HDL cholesterol level is the most specific determinant of coronary heart disease.[581, 582, 584] High levels of HDL cholesterol are protective, whereas a low level is a strong predictor of increased cardiovascular risk. Therefore, monitoring HDL cholesterol as well as total and LDL cholesterol levels is important in determining cardiovascular risk in postmenopausal women.[585]

Replacement with estrogen decreases LDL and increases HDL cholesterol levels in postmenopausal women.[580] Although estrogen also increases triglyceride levels, the impact of this effect on the cardiovascular system is unknown. If a progestin is added, the beneficial effects of estrogen may diminish. Overall, postmenopausal estrogen replacement with or without added progestin produces a favorable lipid profile.[586] These favorable biochemical effects may provide some protection against cardiovascular risk. Many trials including a large, randomized study demonstrated a favorable impact on cardiovascular risk factors in women taking estrogen as well as a combination of estrogen and progestin.[587] Moreover, the great majority of studies investigating coronary or cerebrovascular disease as an outcome concluded that postmenopausal use of estrogens protected against cardiovascular disease, although these studies have been observational rather than randomized and blinded trials.[533] Thus, the opinion of the medical community in general was that exogenous estrogen given in postmenopausal replacement doses decreased cardiovascular risk for all women.

A later randomized study of estrogen-progestin users with preexisting coronary disease (Heart and Estrogen/progestin Replacement Study, or HERS) showed an early increase in mortality.[588] Consequently, in 1999 the American College of Cardiology and American Heart Association revised their guidelines for providing HRT to patients with a history of acute myocardial infarction.[588, 589] The authors of HERS concluded that, over an average follow-up of 4 years, treatment with oral conjugated equine estrogen plus medroxyprogesterone acetate did not reduce the overall rate of coronary heart disease events in postmenopausal women with established coronary disease.[588, 589] HRT, however, was associated with small but statistically significant increases in the risks of deep venous thrombosis and pulmonary embolism.[590] No significant effect of HRT on the risk of stroke was detected in these postmenopausal women with coronary disease.[591] HRT in HERS also resulted in a marginally significant increase in the risk of symptomatic gallbladder disease and biliary tract surgery.[592] It was recommended that hormone replacement therapy should not be initiated solely for prevention of cardiovascular disease in postmenopausal women with preexisting coronary heart disease but can be continued in patients with cardiovascular disease already receiving HRT for other reasons.[588, 589]

Another randomized trial showed that estradiol does not reduce mortality or the recurrence of stroke in postmenopausal women with preexisting cerebrovascular disease.[593] Thus, HRT should not be prescribed for the secondary prevention of cerebrovascular disease.[593]

Recent findings from the Women's Health Initiative reinforce and expand the concerns raised by these randomized trials. In the Women's Health Initiative, more than 16,000 women with intact uteri were randomized to receive either placebo or conjugated estrogens 0.625 mg and medroxyprogesterone 2.5 mg daily. The study was terminated early, after an average of 5.2 years of therapy, because of a small but definite increase in the number of cases of invasive breast cancer and a negative global index of risks and benefits.[593a] Absolute excess risks per 10,000 person-years attributable to HRT were 7 more coronary heart disease events, 8 more strokes, 8 more pulmonary embolism events, and 8 more invasive breast cancers, while risk reductions were 6 fewer colon cancers and 5 fewer hip fractures. A significant decrease in vertebral fractures was also reported. It should also be noted that this study was not designed to investigate some potentially important benefits of HRT, including prevention of urogenital atrophy and improved sexual and cognitive functions. In summary, both the HERS trial and the Women's Health Initiative have failed to find any of the cardiovascular benefits predicted by earlier observational studies.

Postmenopausal Osteoporosis

Osteopenia and osteoporosis are extremely common in elderly postmenopausal women. Osteopenia indicates low bone mass measured by densitometry, whereas the term osteoporosis implies severely decreased bone mass associated with a significantly increased risk for fractures. The most frequent sites of fracture are the vertebral bodies, distal radius, and femoral neck. Osteoporosis has become a global health issue. It is currently at epidemic proportions in the United States, affecting over 20 million people.[594] The majority of osteoporotic patients are postmenopausal women.

Osteoporosis in postmenopausal women is a function of both advancing age and estrogen deficiency. Seventy-five percent or more of the bone loss in women during the first 15 years after menopause is attributed to estrogen deficiency rather than to aging itself.[595, 596] For the first 20 years after the cessation of ovarian estrogen secretion, postmenopausal osteoporosis accounts for a 50% reduction in trabecular bone and 30% loss of cortical bone.[595, 596] Vertebral bone is especially vulnerable because the trabecular bone of the vertebral bodies is metabolically very active and decreases dramatically in response to estrogen deficiency. Vertebral bone mass is already significantly decreased in perimenopausal and early postmenopausal women who have rising FSH and decreasing estrogen levels, whereas bone loss from the radius is not detected until at least a year after the menopause.[597]

The risk of fracture depends on two factors: the peak bone mass achieved at maturity (at approximately age 30) and the subsequent rate of bone loss. An accelerated rate of bone loss after menopause strongly predicts an increased risk of fracture. The combination of low premenopausal bone mass and accelerated loss of bone after menopause is additive, and these individuals are at the highest risk of fracture. An increased rate of average bone loss during menopause is an indicator of lower endogenous estrogen levels because postmenopausal bone loss is considerably slower in women with increased adipose tissue mass and thus elevated circulating estrogen.[169]

It has been shown conclusively by numerous studies that hormone replacement started at the climacteric prevents postmenopausal bone loss.[598] Hormone replacement started at any age in a postmenopausal woman has potential beneficial effects by at least preventing additional bone loss. It should be noted, however, that the incidence of fractures or rate of height loss was not reduced during a 4-year follow-up in women starting

HRT at a mean age of 66.7 (± 6.7) years.[257] More recently, in the part of the Women's Health Initiative discussed above, a decreased number of hip and vertebral fractures were noted in the group of postmenopausal women receiving estrogen/progestin[593a]; this important evidence was the first from randomized trials suggesting that estrogen prevents fractures.

Postmenopausal Hormone Replacement

The most common current practice is to treat all women disturbed by the symptoms of hormone deprivation (hot flashes and urogenital atrophy) with estrogen and to use long-term hormonal prophylaxis against osteoporosis and cardiovascular disease on the basis of an informed decision by the patient. Patients who have undergone a hysterectomy can be given estrogen therapy alone. A progestin is added to estrogen in the postmenopausal woman with a uterus in order to prevent endometrial hyperplasia or cancer. The recent findings from the Women's Health Initiative trial[593a] are too new to allow prediction of how the negative findings from this trial will affect practice. Modest increases in breast cancer, coronary heart disease, and stroke were balanced by modest decreases in fractures and colon cancer. How individual patients and physicians will balance the immediate and common benefits in the treatment of hot flashes and urogenital atrophy against the predominantly negative long-term consequences that affect a modest fraction of patients (at least over 5 years) remains to be determined. It should be noted that the part of the Women's Health Initiative involving the use of estrogen without progestin to treat women after hysterectomy has not been halted; those results will become available in 2005. The decision for using long-term hormone replacement should be made by the patient based on accurate information. The primary role of the physician is to provide scientific information to a patient, using understandable language.[598] This is not an easy task, given the complexity of the existing data and occasionally opposite opinions.[598]

Estrogens and progestins used for postmenopausal hormone replacement are among the most commonly prescribed medications in the United States. Currently, 46% of women who have experienced a natural menopause and 71% of women who have had bilateral oophorectomy report having used postmenopausal HRT.[599] The average duration of use in the United States as of 1992 was 6.6 years, but only 20% of users had maintained treatment for at least 5 years. Emphasizing the education of the patient and primary care physician on the basis of appropriate interpretation of epidemiologic studies and clinical trials will ensure appropriate use of long-term postmenopausal HRT.

Target Groups for Hormone Replacement

In women with gonadal dysgenesis and surgical menopause, the duration of estrogen deprivation is prolonged. Estrogen replacement is recommended for these patients for the reduction of hot flashes and for long-term prophylaxis against cardiovascular disease, osteoporosis, and target organ atrophy. A low-dose contraceptive may be offered to nonsmoking women until the age of 45. After this age, doses of estrogen equivalent to 0.625 mg of conjugated estrogens may be more appropriate because of a sharp age-related increase in risk for thromboembolic events. The physician should recommend a continuous estrogen-progestin combination to those with a uterus and an estrogen-only regimen to women without a uterus.

During the climacteric, hot flashes can be suppressed with an estrogen-progestin combination. Because bone loss related to estrogen deprivation also begins during this period, starting hormone replacement therapy during the climacteric is of paramount importance for minimizing osteoporosis.[600] In climacteric women, unexplained uterine bleeding should be evaluated with an endometrial biopsy before the start of hormone replacement.

The lifelong use of hormone therapy after menopause is dependent on the informed decision of the woman based on balanced and evidence-based advice provided by her physician. The benefits of hormone replacement with respect to bone metabolism, cognitive function, urogenital health, and sexual function are substantial and for many women outweigh the increased breast cancer and cardiovascular disease risk.[601, 602]

Estrogen Preparations and Beneficial Dose of Estrogen

The amount of estrogen that is optimally effective in maintaining the spine and femoral neck bone mass is equivalent to 0.625 mg/day of conjugated estrogens.[601] The effective doses of oral estrogen that reduce the incidence of fracture are 0.625 mg/day of conjugated estrogens and 1.25 mg/day of estrone sulfate.[601, 603, 604] Also, transdermal estradiol delivered at a rate of 0.1 mg/day was reported to reduce fracture risk.[605, 606] Transdermal estradiol at a dose of 0.05 mg/day is also presumed to lower fracture risk based on equivalent doses of various preparations that provide similar average circulating estradiol levels.[607, 608] Oral intake of 0.625 mg of conjugated estrogen, 1.25 mg of estrone sulfate, or 1 mg of micronized estradiol results in similar average serum levels of estrogens: estradiol, 30 to 40 pg/mL, and estrone, 150 to 250 pg/mL.[609, 610] Transdermal administration of estradiol with patches releasing 0.05 mg/day gave rise to similar average serum estradiol (30 to 40 pg/mL) but much lower estrone (40 pg/mL).[611–613]

Short-term cardiovascular or hemodynamic effects of estrogen vary according to blood estrogen levels. Improvements in left ventricular contraction and function are associated with levels achieved by 0.625 mg of oral conjugated estrogens.[614–616] Extremely high estradiol levels achieved with large doses of estrogen, on the other hand, decrease left ventricular function and aortic blood flow.[617] The beneficial effect of postmenopausal estrogen in preventing the hyperinsulinemia associated with aging is present with a dose of 0.625 mg of conjugated estrogens but lost with a dose of 1.25 mg.[618]

The effect of estrogen on arterial thrombosis is also dose-related. For example, oral contraceptives with high doses of estrogen significantly increase the risks of myocardial infarction and stroke, especially in smokers. Numerous studies suggest that doses of conjugated estrogens greater than 0.625 mg are, in fact, not as beneficial in terms of cardiovascular disease and mortality. However, the number of patients receiving these high doses was not large enough to achieve statistical significance.[619–621] Thus, it is imperative to achieve and maintain the lowest beneficial levels of circulating estradiol and avoid higher levels associated with unfavorable hemodynamic effects or thrombosis.

Estrogen-Progestin Regimens

The addition of a progestin, either cyclically or continuously, to concomitant estrogen replacement reduces the risk of estrogen-induced endometrial hyperplasia or carcinoma but poses additional problems.[618] These problems include regular withdrawal bleeding in up to 90% of women treated with cyclic therapy and irregular spotting in 20% of women treated with continuous estrogen plus progestin. Furthermore, progestins appear to reduce the beneficial effects of estrogen on HDL and LDL cholesterol and possibly cardiovascular risk.[618]

A time-honored sequential regimen involves oral administra-

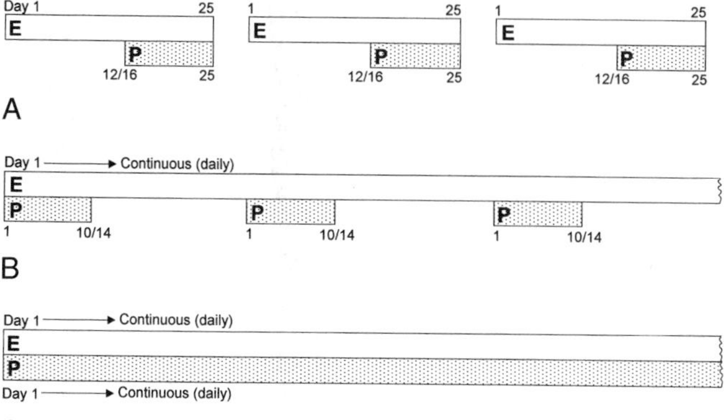

Figure 16–41. Regimens of hormone replacement therapy (HRT). Estrogen (E) is replaced in a postmenopausal woman to prevent osteoporosis, urogenital atrophy, and hot flashes. In the postmenopausal woman with a uterus, a progestin (P) is added to estrogen to prevent endometrial hyperplasia and cancer. E and P can be administered in a number of ways. *A* and *B*, The postmenopausal women receiving hormone replacement have predictable withdrawal bleeding episodes after each P course. *C*, These women take E and P together continuously. After a year of continuous combination therapy, the rate of unpredictable breakthrough spotting is 20%.

tion of 0.625 mg of conjugated estrogens or the equivalent doses of a variety of available products from day 1 to 25 of each month (Fig. 16–41). A daily dose of 10 mg of medroxyprogesterone acetate is added from day 12 to 25 or from day 16 to 25. Withdrawal bleeding is expected on or after day 26 of each month. Another common cyclic regimen involves continuous oral administration of 0.625 mg of conjugated estrogens or the equivalent daily dose (see Fig. 16–41). A daily dose of 5 to 10 mg of medroxyprogesterone acetate is added for the first 10 to 14 days of every month. One-year randomized trial data indicate that the 5-mg dose protects the endometrium as well as the 10-mg dose.[622] Progestin withdrawal bleeding occurs in 90% of women with a sequential or cyclic regimen.[587, 623] These regimens can also cause adverse symptoms related to the relatively high daily doses of progestin, such as breast tenderness, bloating, fluid retention, and depression. Thus, the lowest possible dose of a progestin is recommended.

The continuous combined method of treatment, on the other hand, has the potential benefit of reduced bleeding and amenorrhea but is occasionally complicated by breakthrough bleeding (see Fig. 16–41).[587, 623] In this regimen, a combination of 0.625 mg of conjugated estrogens and 2.5 mg of medroxyprogesterone acetate is given orally every day. The continuous combination regimen is simple, convenient, and associated with a higher incidence of amenorrhea in 80% of patients after at least 6 months of use. The rest of the patients continue to experience some degree of unpredictable spotting. Thus, overall compliance is much better in users of the continuous combination regimen. Moreover, the lower daily dose of medroxyprogesterone acetate is associated with a lower incidence of breast tenderness with this regimen. Other estrogen-progestin combinations are also available for similar continuous use.

Most postmenopausal women stop HRT within several years after the initiation of therapy because hot flashes decrease significantly or disappear at this time. Upon the cessation of HRT that had lasted several years, hot flashes usually do not return or are less severe than during the climacteric. Consequently, long-term compliance with HRT remains poor.[624, 625] The fear of malignancy and irregular uterine bleeding are two major factors that stop women from continuing HRT indefinitely.[626] The current data on breast cancer are indicative of a slightly increased risk for both estrogen-only and estrogen plus progestin regimens.[624, 625] The addition of a progestin to the estrogen-only regimen, on the other hand, has effectively prevented endometrial cancer.[622] Irregular uterine bleeding is another major reason for discontinuation of HRT. The incidence of persistent uterine bleeding with the traditional sequential regimen can be as high as 90%, which deters women from taking lifelong hormone replacement. By switching to the continuous combination regimen, this bleeding can be reduced to a 20% incidence of spotting with long-term (>1 year) use. Thus, more clinicians start women with the continuous combination treatment with the hope of improving compliance for long-term use (see Fig. 16–41).

Selective Estrogen Receptor Modulators as Hormone Replacement

Selective estrogen receptor modulators are compounds that act like estrogen in some target tissues but antagonize estrogenic effects in others.[627] One of the first selective estrogen receptor modulators was tamoxifen, for which estrogen-like agonist activity on bone was observed to occur simultaneously with estrogen antagonist activity on the breast.[628] An unwanted effect of tamoxifen is its estrogen-like action on the endometrium. Second-generation compounds have since been developed, most notably raloxifene, which has estrogen-like actions on bone, lipids, and the coagulation system; estrogen antagonist effects on the breast; and no detectable action in the endometrium.[629]

In randomized placebo-controlled studies involving postmenopausal women or patients with osteoporosis, raloxifene at 60 to 150 mg/day was effective in increasing bone mineral density over 12 to 36 months.[629] Raloxifene also decreased the risk of vertebral fractures. Raloxifene is similar to placebo in its endometrial effects and similar to estrogen in causing a twofold to threefold increase in the risk of venous thromboembolism.[630] Raloxifene lowers total and LDL cholesterol. HDL cholesterol and triglycerides are virtually unaffected.[84] The propensity of raloxifene to cause hot flashes precludes its use in women with vasomotor symptoms. On the other hand, the lack of stimulatory effects on the endometrium and the reduction in the incidence of invasive breast cancer indicate that raloxifene is an alternative to estrogen-progestin preparations for the management of postmenopausal osteoporosis, especially for patients reluctant to use estrogen. It should be emphasized that, at this time, postmenopausal hormone replacement with estrogen remains the "gold standard" for health benefits with respect to bone, cardiovascular system, urogenital organs, and possibly the central nervous system.

Management of Breakthrough Bleeding during Postmenopausal Hormone Replacement

Approximately 90% of women receiving estrogen plus cyclic administration of a progestin have monthly progestin withdrawal bleeding in a predictable fashion, whereas continuous combined estrogen-progestin therapy causes breakthrough bleeding in approximately 40% of women during the first 6 months. (The rest of the women with a continuous combination regimen are amenorrheic.) The pattern of vaginal bleeding in the continuous regimen is unpredictable and causes anxiety in most patients. Fortunately, the incidence of breakthrough bleeding with the continuous combined regimen decreases to 20% after 1 year of treatment.[587, 623, 631] Breakthrough bleeding with the combined continuous regimen remains the most important reason for discontinuance of this therapy. Most patients find it unacceptable and prefer to switch to a cyclic progestin regimen or discontinue hormone replacement altogether. There is no effective pharmacologic method to manage the breakthrough bleeding associated with continuous combined estrogen-progestin regimens. One can only reassure the patient that the bleeding is likely to subside within a year from the start of HRT. If breakthrough bleeding continues beyond a year, the regimen should be changed to daily estrogen plus cyclic progestin monthly for 10 days.

HRT can be started in the amenorrheic postmenopausal patient at any time. Perimenopausal women with oligomenorrhea, hot flashes, or other associated symptoms should also be given HRT. In the oligomenorrheic patient, a hormone replacement regimen can be initiated on day 3 of one of the infrequent menses. If the candidate for hormone replacement does not have irregular uterine bleeding, it is not essential to perform endometrial biopsies routinely before beginning treatment. Studies indicate that asymptomatic postmenopausal women rarely have endometrial abnormalities.[631–633] Pretreatment biopsies using a thin plastic biopsy cannula in the office may be limited to patients at higher risk for endometrial hyperplasia (e.g., unpredictable uterine bleeding, history of PCOS or chronic anovulation, obesity, liver disease, and diabetes mellitus).

Giving a woman a combined estrogen-progestin regimen does not preclude the development of endometrial cancer.[634] It is, therefore, necessary to rule out endometrial malignancy in women receiving HRT who are experiencing irregular uterine bleeding. The important task is to differentiate breakthrough bleeding from bleeding induced by hyperplasia or cancer. Because breakthrough bleeding is extremely common, a large number of biopsies would have to be performed to detect a rare case of endometrial abnormality during HRT. In order to decrease the number of endometrial biopsies, a screening method using transvaginal ultrasonography has been introduced.[226] The thickness of the postmenopausal endometrium as measured by transvaginal ultrasonography in postmenopausal women correlates with the presence or absence of pathology.[226] Patients receiving either a cyclic or daily combination hormone replacement regimen who have an endometrial thickness less than 5 mm can be managed conservatively.[635–637] An endometrial thickness equal to or greater than 5 mm requires biopsy. Following this algorithm, it is estimated that 50% to 75% of bleeding patients receiving HRT and evaluated by ultrasonography require biopsy.[226]

Side Effects of Postmenopausal Hormone Replacement

Deep Venous Thrombosis. It has been debated whether continuous combination hormone replacement using conjugated estrogens (0.625 mg/day) plus medroxyprogesterone acetate (2.5 mg/day) increases the risk of venous thromboembolism.[638–643] A recent randomized clinical trial has shown that this regimen of HRT significantly increases the risks of deep venous thrombosis and pulmonary embolism, although these increases were modest.[593a] Even if the relative risk is significantly increased, the actual risk remains extremely low because of the low frequency of this event in the general population.

Hyperlipidemia. This rare side effect is observed in patients with severe familial hypertriglyceridemia. An oral estrogen regimen can hasten severe hypertriglyceridemia or pancreatitis in women with severely elevated triglyceride levels.[644] Therefore, estrogen replacement is a relative contraindication in women with substantially increased triglyceride levels.

Gallbladder Disease. There is a minimally increased risk of gallbladder disease with estrogen use during the menopause.[645] There is a marginally significant increase in the risk of cholecystectomy in past and current users of HRT.[646, 647] Preexisting gallbladder disease is a relative contraindication for estrogen replacement.

Breast Cancer. Breast tissue is a major target for estrogen, and most breast tumors are estrogen-responsive. A number of case-control and cohort studies concluded that 5 or more years of current use of postmenopausal HRT is associated with a slight increase in the risk of breast cancer, a risk that is less than that associated with postmenopausal obesity or daily alcohol consumption.[648, 649] Many observational studies, however, have failed to develop evidence that long-term postmenopausal HRT increases the risk of breast cancer.[648, 649] Moreover, none of the epidemiologic studies found an increased risk of breast cancer associated with less than 5 years of use or past use of postmenopausal HRT.[649] The addition of a progestin to the treatment regimen slightly increased the risk observed in estrogen-only users.[649] In this context, the recent findings from the Women's Health Initiative support and extend the previous work, in that the combined use of estrogen and progestin led to a statistically significant increase in invasive breast cancer over the 5.2 years of the study.[593a] Because breast cancer was uncommon in this group of postmenopausal women, this increase represented an absolute increase of 8 cases per 10,000 women receiving hormone replacement.

Epidemiologic data indicate that a positive family history of breast cancer should not be a contraindication to postmenopausal estrogen use. Moreover, postmenopausal women in whom the cancer develops during HRT have a reduced risk of dying from breast cancer.[649] This reduced risk may be due to an increased rate of early detection and development of less aggressive tumors in association with HRT. In conclusion, there may be a minimally increased real risk of developing breast cancer in long-term HRT users. This risk, however, is extremely small compared with the clear-cut benefits of estrogen such as osteoporosis prevention and urogenital tissue support.

Hormone Replacement Therapy after a Diagnosis of Breast Cancer. HRT is typically withheld from women with breast cancer because of concerns that estrogen may stimulate recurrence. Surprisingly, a number of relatively small studies showed either unaltered or lower risks of recurrence and mortality in women who used HRT after a diagnosis of breast cancer compared with nonusers.[650, 651] HRT in most of these small studies was started after at least a 5-year disease-free interval.[650, 651] On the basis of these insufficient but encouraging data, a decision to provide HRT is dependent on the choice of the individual patient. In these patients, tamoxifen or raloxifene represents a viable alternative to estrogen replacement for long-term prophylaxis against osteoporosis.

References

1. Matsuo H, Baba Y, Nair R, et al. Structure of the porcine LH- and FSH-releasing hormone: I. The proposed amino acid sequence. Biochem Biophys Res Commun 1971; 43:1334–1339.
2. Barry J, Barette B. Immunofluorescence study of LRF neurons in primates. Cell Tissue Res 1975; 164:163–178.
3. Seeburg P, Adelman J. Characterization of cDNA for precursor of human luteinizing hormone releasing hormone. Nature 1984; 311:666–668.
4. Seeburg P, Mason A, Stewart T, et al. The mammalian GnRH gene and its pivotal role in reproduction. Recent Prog Horm Res 1987; 43:69–98.
5. Hayflick J, Adelman J, Seeburg P. The complete nucleotide sequence of the human gonadotropin-releasing hormone gene. Nucleic Acids Res 1989; 17:6403–6404.
6. Nikolics K, Mason A, Szonyi E, et al. A prolactin-inhibiting factor within the precursor for human gonadotropin-releasing hormone. Nature 1985; 316:511–517.

7. Ackland J, Nikolics K, Seeburg P, et al. Molecular forms of gonadotropin-releasing hormone associated peptide (GAP): changes within the rat hypothalamus and release from hypothalamic cells in vitro. Neuroendocrinology 1988; 48:376–386.
8. Ronnekleiv O, Naylor B, Bond C, et al. Combined immunohistochemistry for gonadotropin-releasing hormone (GnRH) and pro-GnRH, and in situ hybridization for GnRH messenger ribonucleic acid in rat brain. Mol Endocrinol 1989; 3:363–371.
9. Ronnekleiv O, Adelman J, Weber E. Immunohistochemical demonstration of pro-GnRH and GnRH in the preoptic-basal hypothalamus of the primate. Neuroendocrinology 1987; 45:518–521.
10. Bick D, Franco B, Sherin R, et al. Brief report: intragenic deletion of the *KALIG-1* gene in Kallmann's syndrome. N Engl J Med 1992; 326:1752–1755.
11. Knobil E. The neuroendocrine control of the menstrual cycle. Recent Prog Horm Res 1980; 36:53–88.
12. Van Vugt D, Diefenbach W, Ferin M. Gonadotropin-releasing hormone pulses in third ventricular cerebrospinal fluid of ovariectomized rhesus monkeys: correlation with luteinizing hormone pulses. Endocrinology 1985; 117:1550–1558.
13. Gross K, Matsumoto A, Southworth M, et al. Evidence for decreased luteinizing hormone–releasing hormone frequency in men with selective elevations of follicle-stimulating hormone. J Clin Endocrinol Metab 1985; 59:197–202.
14. Haisenleder D, Dalkin A, Ortolano G, et al. A pulsatile gonadotropin-releasing hormone stimulus is required to increase transcription of the gonadotropin subunit genes: evidence for differential regulation of transcription by pulse frequency in vivo. Endocrinology 1991; 128:509–517.
15. Reame N, Sauder S, Case G, et al. Pulsatile gonadotropin secretion in women with hypothalamic amenorrhea: evidence that reduced frequency of gonadotropin secretion is the mechanism of persistent anovulation. J Clin Endocrinol Metab 1985; 61:851–858.
16. Filicori M, Santoro N, Merriam G, et al. Characterization of the physiologic pattern of episodic gonadotropin secretion throughout the human menstrual cycle. J Clin Endocrinol Metab 1986; 62:1136–1144.
17. Wildt L, Hausler A, Marshall G, et al. Frequency and amplitude of gonadotropin-releasing hormone stimulation and gonadotropin secretion in the rhesus monkey. Endocrinology 1981; 109:376–385.
18. Wildt L, Hutchison J, Marshall G, et al. On the site of action of progesterone in the blockade of the estradiol-induced gonadotropin discharge in the rhesus monkey. Endocrinology 1981; 109: 1293–1294.
19. Herbison A. Noradrenergic regulation of cyclic GnRH secretion. Rev Reprod 1997; 2:1–6.
20. Gindoff P, Ferin M. Brain opioid peptides and menstrual cyclicity. Semin Reprod Endocrinol 1987; 5:125.
21. Rabinovici J, Rothman P, Monroe S, et al. Endocrine effects and pharmacokinetic characteristics of a potent new gonadotropin-releasing hormone antagonist (Ganirelix) with minimal histamine-releasing properties: studies in postmenopausal women. J Clin Endocrinol Metab 1992; 75:1220–1225.
22. Shoupe D, Montz F, Lobo R. The effects of estrogen and progestin on endogenous opioid activity in oophorectomized women. J Clin Endocrinol Metab 1985; 60:178–183.
23. Goodman R, Parfitt D, Evans N, et al. Endogenous opioid peptides control the amplitude and shape of gonadotropin-releasing hormone pulses in the ewe. Endocrinology 1995; 136:2412–2420.
24. Wildt L, Leyendecker G, Sir-Petermann T, et al. Treatment with naltrexone in hypothalamic ovarian failure: induction of ovulation and pregnancy. Hum Reprod 1993; 8:350–358.
25. Hadelsman D, Swerdloff R. Pharmacokinetics of gonadotropin-releasing hormone and its analogs. Endocr Rev 1986; 7:95–105.
26. Galbiati M, Zanisi M, Messi E. Transforming growth factor β and astrocytic conditioned medium influence luteinizing hormone–releasing hormone gene expression in the hypothalamic cell line GTI. Endocrinology 1996; 137:5605–5609.
27. Karten M, Ribier J. Gonadotropin-releasing hormone analog design. Structure-function studies toward the development of agonists and antagonists: rationale and perspective. Endocr Rev 1986; 7:44–66.
28. Lemay A, Maheux R, Faure N, et al. Reversible hypogonadism induced by a luteinizing hormone–releasing hormone (LHRH) agonist (buserelin) as a new therapeutic approach for endometriosis. Fertil Steril 1984; 41:863–871.
29. Carr B, Breslau N, Givens C, et al. Oral contraceptive pills, gonadotropin-releasing hormone agonists, or use in combination for treatment of hirsutism: a clinical research center study. J Clin Endocrinol Metab 1995; 80:1169–1178.
30. Cann C, Martin M, Genant H, et al. Decreased spinal mineral content in amenorrheic women. JAMA 1984; 251:626–629.
31. Matta W, Shaw R, Hesp R, Evans R. Reversible trabecular bone density loss following induced hypo-oestrogenism with the GnRH analogue buserelin in premenopausal women. Clin Endocrinol (Oxf) 1988; 29:45–51.
32. Surrey E. Add-back therapy and gonadotropin-releasing hormone agonists in the treatment of patients with endometriosis: can a consensus be reached? Add-Back Consensus Working Group. Fertil Steril 1999; 71:420–424.
33. Cetel N, Rivier J, Vale W, Yen S. The dynamics of gonadotropin inhibition in women induced by an antagonistic analog of gonadotropin-releasing hormone. J Clin Endocrinol Metab 1983; 57: 62–65.
34. Pavlou S, Debold C, Island D, et al. Single subcutaneous doses of a luteinizing hormone–releasing hormone antagonist suppress serum gonadotropin and testosterone levels in normal men [published erratum appears in J Clin Endocrinol Metab 1986; 63:940]. J Clin Endocrinol Metab 1986; 63:303–308.
35. Mortola J, Sathanandan M, Pavlou S, et al. Suppression of bioactive and immunoreactive follicle-stimulating hormone and luteinizing hormone levels by a potent gonadotropin-releasing hormone antagonist: pharmacodynamic studies. Fertil Steril 1989; 51:957–963.
36. Pavlou S, Wakefield G, Schlechter N, et al. Mode of suppression of pituitary and gonadal function after acute or prolonged administration of a luteinizing hormone–releasing hormone antagonist in normal men. J Clin Endocrinol Metab 1989; 68:446–454.
37. Edelstein M, Gordon K, Williams R, et al. Single dose long-term suppression of testosterone secretion by a gonadotropin-releasing hormone antagonist (Antide) in male monkeys. Contraception 1990; 42:209–214.
38. Behre H, Kliesch S, Puhse G, et al. High loading and low maintenance doses of a gonadotropin-releasing hormone antagonist effectively suppress serum luteinizing hormone, follicle-stimulating hormone, and testosterone in normal men. J Clin Endocrinol Metab 1997; 82:1403–1408.
39. Fujimoto V, Monroe S, Nelson L, et al. Dose-related suppression of serum luteinizing hormone in women by a potent new gonadotropin-releasing hormone antagonist (Ganirelix) administered by intranasal spray. Fertil Steril 1997; 67:469–473.
40. Pavlou S, Wakefield G, Schlechter N, et al. Mode of suppression of pituitary and gonadal function after acute or prolonged administration of a luteinizing hormone–releasing hormone antagonist in normal men. J Clin Endocrinol Metab 1987; 64:931–936.
41. Andreyko J, Monroe S, Marshall L, et al. Concordant suppression of serum immunoreactive luteinizing hormone (LH), follicle-stimulating hormone, a subunit, bioactive LH, and testosterone in postmenopausal women by a potent gonadotropin releasing hormone antagonist (detirelix). J Clin Endocrinol Metab 1992; 74:399–405.
42. Childs G, Hyde C, Naor Z, et al. Heterogeneous luteinizing hormone and follicle-stimulating hormone storage patterns in subtypes of gonadotropes separated by centrifugal elutriation. Endocrinology 1983; 113:2120–2128.
43. Childs G. Division of labor among gonadotropes. Vitam Horm 1995; 50:215–286.
44. Childs G. Functional ultrastructure of gonadotropes: a review. Curr Top Neuroendocrinol 1986; 7:49–97.
45. Clayton R. Gonadotropin-releasing hormone: its actions and receptors. Endocr Rev 1989; 120:11–19.
46. Conn P. The molecular basis of gonadotropin-releasing hormone action. Endocr Rev 1986; 7:3–10.
47. Marian J, Cooper R, Conn P. Regulation of the rat pituitary gonadotropin-releasing hormone receptor. Mol Pharmacol 1981; 19:399–405.
48. Loymaye E, Catt K. Homologous regulation of gonadotropin-releasing hormone receptors in cultured pituitary cells. Science 1982; 215:983–985.
49. Katt J, Duncan J, Herbon L, et al. The frequency of gonadotropin-releasing hormone stimulation determines the number of pituitary gonadotropin-releasing hormone receptors. Endocrinology 1985; 116:2113–2115.

50. Kaiser U, Jakubowiak A, Steinberger A. Regulation of rat pituitary gonadotropin-releasing hormone receptor mRNA levels in vivo and in vitro. Endocrinology 1993; 133:931–934.
51. Clayton R, Catt K. Gonadotropin-releasing hormone receptors: characterization, physiological regulation, and relation to reproductive function. Endocr Rev 1981; 2:186–209.
52. Bauer-Dantoin A, Weiss J, Jameson J. Roles of estrogen, progesterone, and gonadotropin-releasing hormone (GnRH) in the control of pituitary GnRH receptor gene expression at the time of the preovulatory gonadotropin surges. Endocrinology 1995; 136: 1014–1019.
53. Yasin M, Dalkin A, Haisenleder D, et al. Gonadotropin-releasing hormone (GnRH) pulse pattern regulates GnRH receptor gene expression: augmentation by estradiol. Endocrinology 1995; 136: 1559–1564.
54. Moretto M, Lopez F, Negro-Vilar A. Nitric oxide regulates luteinizing hormone–releasing hormone secretion. Endocrinology 1993; 133:2399–2402.
55. Moore R. Organization and function of a CNS circadian oscillator: the suprachiasmatic hypothalamic nucleus. Fed Proc 1983; 42:2783–2789.
56. Weindl A. Neuroendocrine aspects of circumventricular organs. In Ganong WF, Martini L (eds). Frontiers in Neuroendocrinology. New York, Oxford University Press, 1973, pp 3–32.
57. Naor Z, Harris D, Shacham S. Mechanism of GnRH receptor signaling: combinatorial cross-talk of Ca^{2+} and protein kinase C. Front Neuroendocrinol 1998; 19:1–19.
58. Gharib S, Wierman M, Shupnik J. Molecular biology of the pituitary gonadotropins. Endocr Rev 1990; 11:177–199.
59. Talmadge K, Vamvakopoulos N, Fiddes J. Evolution of the genes for the beta subunits of human chorionic gonadotropin and luteinizing hormone. Nature 1984; 307:37–40.
60. Jameson J, Becker C, Lindell C. Human follicle-stimulating hormone β-subunit gene encodes multiple messenger ribonucleic acids. Mol Endocrinol 1988; 2:806–815.
61. Jameson J, Chin W, Hollenberg A. The gene encoding the β-subunit of rat luteinizing hormone. J Biol Chem 1984; 259: 15474–15480.
62. Naylor S, Chin W, Goodman H. Chromosome assignments of genes encoding the alpha and beta subunits of glycoprotein hormones in man and mouse. Somat Cell Genet 1983; 9:757–770.
63. Chin W. Glycoprotein hormone genes. In Habener JF (ed). Genes Encoding Hormones and Regulatory Peptides. Clifton, NJ, Humana Press, 1986, pp 137–172.
64. Themmen A, Huhtaniemi I. Mutations of gonadotropins and gonadotropin receptors: elucidating the physiology and pathophysiology of pituitary-gonadal function. Endocr Rev 2000; 21:551–583.
65. Shupnik M. Gonadotropin gene modulation by steroids and gonadotropin-releasing hormone. Biol Reprod 1996; 54:279–286.
66. Abbud R, Ameduri R, Rao J, et al. Chronic hypersecretion of luteinizing hormone in transgenic mice selectively alters responsiveness of the alpha-subunit gene to gonadotropin-releasing hormone and estrogens. Mol Endocrinol 1999; 13:1449–1459.
67. Beitins I, Derfel R, O'Loughlin K, et al. Immunoreactive luteinizing hormone, follicle stimulating hormone and their subunits in human urine following gel filtration. J Clin Endocrinol Metab 1977; 44:149–159.
68. DeLeeuw R, Mulders J, Voortman G, et al. Structure-function relationship of recombinant follicle stimulating hormone (Puregon). Mol Hum Reprod 1996; 2:361–369.
69. Woodburne R. Essentials of Human Anatomy. New York, Oxford University Press, 1965, pp 527–528.
70. Mossman H, Duke K. Comparative Morphology of the Mammalian Ovary. Madison, Wis, University of Wisconsin Press, 1973.
71. Simpson J, Rajkovic A. Ovarian differentiation and gonadal failure. Am J Med Genet 1999; 89:186–200.
72. Baker T. A quantitative and cytological study of germ cells in human ovaries. Proc R Soc Biol 1963; 158:417–433.
73. Witschi E. Migration of the germ cells of human embryos from the yolk sac to the primitive gonadal folds. Contrib Embryol 1948; 32:67.
74. Baker T, Franchi L. The fine structure of oogonia and oocytes in human ovaries. J Cell Sci 1967; 2:213–224.
75. Ohno S, Klinger H, Atkin N. Human oogenesis. Cytogenetics 1962; 1:42.
76. Shifren J, Osathanondh R, Yeh J. Human fetal ovaries and uteri: developmental expression of genes encoding the insulin, insulin-like growth factor-I, and insulin-like growth factor II receptors. Fertil Steril 1993; 59:1036–1040.
77. Bennett R, Osathanondh R, Yeh J. Immunohistochemical localization of transforming growth factor-α, epidermal growth factor (EGF), and EGF receptor in the human fetal ovary. J Clin Endocrinol Metab 1996; 81:3073–3076.
78. Peters H. Intrauterine gonadal development. Fertil Steril 1976; 27:493–500.
79. Himelstein-Braw R, Byskov A, Peters H, Faber M. Follicular atresia in the infant human ovary. J Reprod Fertil 1976; 46:55–59.
80. Franchi L, Mandl A, Zuckermann S. The development of the ovary and the process of oogenesis. The Ovary. London, Academic Press, 1962, pp 1–88.
81. Weakly B. Electron microscopy of the oocyte and granulosa cells in the developing ovarian follicles of the golden hamster. J Anat 1966; 100:503–534.
82. Albertini D, Anderson E. The appearance and structure of intercellular connections during the ontogeny of the rabbit ovarian follicle with particular reference to gap junctions. J Cell Biol 1974; 63:234–250.
83. Amsterdam A, Joseph S, Liebermann M, Lindner H. Organization of intramembrane particles in freeze-cleaved gap junctions of rat graafian follicles: optical diffraction analysis. J Cell Sci 1976; 21:93–105.
84. Amsterdam A, Knecht M, Catt K. Hormonal regulation of cytodifferentiation and intercellular communication in cultured granulosa cells. Proc Natl Acad Sci USA 1981; 78:3000–3004.
85. Simon A, Goodenough D, Li E, et al. Female infertility in mice lacking connexin 37. Nature 1997; 385:525–529.
86. Zoller L, Weisz J. Identification of cytochrome P-450, and its distribution in the membrana granulosa of the preovulatory follicle using quantitative cytochemistry. Endocrinology 1979; 103: 310–313.
87. Zoller L, Weisz J. A quantitative cytochemical study of glucose-6-phosphate dehydrogenase and delta 5-3β-hydroxysteroid dehydrogenase activity in the membrana granulosa of the ovulable type of follicle of the rat. Histochemistry 1979; 62:125–135.
88. Channing C, Bae I, Stone S, et al. Porcine granulosa and cumulus cell properties: LH/hCG receptors, ability to secrete progesterone and ability to respond to LH. Mol Cell Endocrinol 1981; 22:359–370.
89. Hillensjo T, Magnusson C, Svensson U, et al. Effect of LH and FSH on progesterone synthesis in cultured rat cumulus cells. Endocrinology 1981; 108:1920–1924.
90. Lawrence T, Dekel M, Beers W. Binding of human chorionic gonadotropin by rat cumuli, oophori and granulosa cells: a comparative study. Endocrinology 1980; 106:1114–1118.
91. Magnusson C, Billig H, Eneroth P, et al. Comparison between the progestin secretion responsiveness to gonadotropins of rat cumulus and mural granulosa cells in vitro. Acta Endocrinol (Copenh) 1982; 101:611–616.
92. Ryan K, Petro Z. Steroid biosynthesis by human ovarian granulosa and thecal cells. J Clin Endocrinol Metab 1966; 26:46–52.
93. Rice B, Savard K. Steroid hormone formation in the human ovary. IV. Ovarian stromal compartment; formation of radioactive steroids from acetate-1-^{14}C and action of gonadotropins. J Clin Endocrinol Metab 1966; 26:593–609.
94. Savard K, Marsh J, Rice B. Gonadotropins and ovarian steroidogenesis. Recent Prog Horm Res 1965; 21:285.
95. Mossman H, Koering M, Ferry D. Cyclic changes of interstitial gland tissue of the human ovary. Am J Anat 1964; 115:235.
96. Erickson G, Magoffin D, Dyer C, et al. The ovarian androgen producing cells: a review of structure/function relationships. Endocr Rev 1985; 6:371–399.
97. Gondos B, Hobel C. Interstitial cells in the human fetal ovary. Endocrinology 1973; 93:736–739.
98. Hume D, Halpin D, Charlton H, et al. The mononuclear phagocyte system of the mouse defined by immunohistochemical localization of antigen F4/80: macrophages of endocrine organs. Proc Natl Acad Sci USA 1984; 81:4174–4177.
99. Parr E. Histological examination of the rat ovarian follicle wall prior to ovulation. Biol Reprod 1974; 11:483–503.
100. Nakamura Y, Smith M, Krishna A, et al. Increased number of mast cells in the dominant follicle of the cow: relationships

among luteal, stromal, and hilar regions. Biol Reprod 1987; 37: 546–549.
101. Krishna A, Terranova P. Alterations in mast cell degranulation and ovarian histamine in the proestrous hamster. Biol Reprod 1985; 32:1211–1217.
102. Krishna A, Terranova P, Matteri R, et al. Histamine and increased ovarian blood flow mediate LH-induced superovulation in the cyclic hamster. J Reprod Fertil 1986; 76:23–29.
103. Seow W, Thong Y, Waters M, et al. Isolation of a chemotactic protein for neutrophils from human ovarian follicular fluid. Int Arch Allergy Appl Immunol 1988; 86:331–336.
104. Cavender J, Murdoch W. Morphological studies of the microcirculatory system of periovulatory ovine follicles. Biol Reprod 1988; 39:989–997.
105. Takemura R, Werb Z. Secretory products of macrophages and their physiological functions. Am J Physiol 1984; 246:C1–C9.
106. Reynolds H, Nathan P, Srivastava L, et al. Release of estradiol from fetal bovine serum by rat thymus, spleen, kidney, lung and lung macrophage cultures. Endocrinology 1982; 110:2213–2215.
107. Milewich L, Chen G, Lyons C, et al. Metabolism of androstenedione by guinea-pig peritoneal macrophages: synthesis of testosterone and 5α-reduced metabolites. J Steroid Biochem 1982; 17: 61–65.
108. Mais V, Kazer R, Cetel N, et al. The dependency of folliculogenesis and corpus luteum function on pulsatile gonadotropin secretion in cycling women using a gonadotropin-releasing hormone antagonist as a probe. J Clin Endocrinol Metab 1986; 62:1250–1255.
109. Gougeon A. Dynamics of follicular growth in the human: a model from preliminary results. Hum Reprod 1986; 1:81–87.
110. Gougeon A. Regulation of ovarian follicular development in primates: facts and hypotheses. Endocr Rev 1996; 17:121–155.
111. Oktay K, Newton H, Mullan J, et al. Development of human primordial follicles to antral stages in SCID/hpg mice stimulated with follicle stimulating hormone. Hum Reprod 1998; 13:1133–1138.
112. Schipper I, Hop W, Fauser B. The follicle-stimulating hormone (FSH) threshold/window concept examined by different interventions with exogenous FSH during the follicular phase of the normal menstrual cycle: duration, rather than magnitude, of FSH increase affects follicle development. J Clin Endocrinol Metab 1998; 83:1292–1298.
113. Peters H, McNaty K. The Ovary. Berkeley, University of California Press, 1980.
114. Santen R, Paulsen C. Hypogonadotropic eunuchoidism II: gonadal responsiveness to exogenous gonadotropin. J Clin Endocrinol Metab 1973; 36:55–63.
115. Tilly J, Kowalski K, Johnson A. Involvement of apoptosis in ovarian follicular atresia and postovulatory regression. Endocrinology 1991; 129:2799–2801.
116. Bauminger S, Lindner H. Periovulatory changes in ovarian prostaglandin formation and their hormonal control in the rat. Prostaglandins 1975; 9:737–751.
117. Tsafriri A, Lindner H, Zor U, et al. Physiological role of prostaglandins in the induction of ovulation. Prostaglandins 1972; 2:1–10.
118. Espey L. Ovarian proteolytic enzymes and ovulation. Biol Reprod 1974; 10:216–235.
119. Bjersing L, Cajander S. Ovulation and the mechanism of follicle rupture. IV. Ultrastructure of membrana granulosa of rabbit graafian follicles prior to induced ovulation. Cell Tissue Res 1974; 153:1–14.
120. Beers W, Strickland S, Reich E. Ovarian plasminogen activator: relationship to ovulation and hormonal regulation. Cell 1975; 6: 387–394.
121. Frederick J, Shimanuki T, DiZerega G. Initiation of angiogenesis by human follicular fluid. Science 1984; 224:389–390.
122. Kamat B, Brown L, Manseau E, et al. Expression of vascular permeability factor/vascular endothelial growth factor by human granulosa and theca lutein cells: role in corpus luteum development. Am J Pathol 1995; 146:157–165.
123. Redmer D, Dai Y, Li J, et al. Characterization of expression of vascular endothelial growth factor (VEGF) in the ovine corpus luteum. J Reprod Fertil 1996; 108:157–165.
124. Ohara A, Mori T, Taii S, et al. Functional differentiation in steroidogenesis of two types of luteal cells isolated from mature human corpora lutea of menstrual cycle. J Clin Endocrinol Metab 1987; 65:1192–1200.
125. Gillim S, Christensen A, McLennon C. Fine structure of the human menstrual corpus luteum at its stage of maximum secretory activity. Am J Anat 1970; 126:409–415.
126. Carr B, MacDonald P, Simpson E. The role of lipoproteins in the regulation of progesterone secretion by the human corpus luteum. Fertil Steril 1982; 38:303–311.
127. Duncan W, McNeilly A, Fraser H, et al. Luteinizing hormone receptor in the human corpus luteum: lack of down-regulation during maternal recognition of pregnancy. Hum Reprod 1996; 11:2291–2297.
128. Strauss JF 3rd, Christenson L, Devoto L, Martinez F. Providing progesterone for pregnancy: control of cholesterol flux to the side-chain cleavage system. J Reprod Fertil Suppl 2000; 55:3–12.
129. Bukovsky A, Caudle M, Keenan J, et al. Is corpus luteum an immune-mediated event? Localization of immune system components and luteinizing hormone receptor in human corpora lutea. Biol Reprod 1996; 53:1373–1384.
130. Casper R, Yen S. Induction of luteolysis in the human with a long acting analog of luteinizing hormone–releasing factor. Science 1979; 205:408–410.
131. Gillman J, Stein H. The human corpus luteum of pregnancy. Surg Gynecol Obstet 1941; 72:129.
132. Schoonmaker J, Victery W, Karsch F. A receptive period for estradiol-induced luteolysis in the rhesus monkey. Endocrinology 1981; 108:1874–1877.
133. O'Grady J, Kohorn E, Glass R, et al. Inhibition of progesterone synthesis in vitro by prostaglandin $F_{2\alpha}$. J Reprod Fertil 1972; 30: 153–156.
134. Shikone T, Yamoto M, Kokawa K, et al. Apoptosis of human corpora lutea during cyclic luteal regression and early pregnancy. J Clin Endocrinol Metab 1996; 81:2376–2380.
135. Midgley AJ. Autoradiographic analysis of gonadotropin binding to rat ovarian tissue secretions. Adv Exp Med Biol 1973; 36:365–378.
136. Amsterdam A, Koch Y, Lieberman M, et al. Distribution of binding sites for human chorionic gonadotropin in the preovulatory follicle of the rat. J Cell Biol 1975; 67:894–900.
137. Bortolussi M, Marini G, Dal Lago A. Autoradiographic studies of the distribution of LH (hCG) receptors in the ovary of untreated and gonadotropin-primed immature rats. Cell Tissue Res 1977; 183:329–342.
138. Nimrod A, Erickson G, Ryan K. A specific FSH receptor in rat granulosa cells: properties of binding in vitro. Endocrinology 1976; 98:56–64.
139. Nimrod A, Bedrak E, Lamprecht S. Appearance of LH-receptors and LH-stimulatable cyclic AMP accumulation in granulosa cells during follicular maturation in the rat ovary. Biochem Biophys Res Commun 1977; 78:977–984.
140. Kammerman S, Canfield RE, Kolena J, et al. The binding of iodinated hCG to porcine granulosa cells. Endocrinology 1972; 91:65–74.
141. Channing C, Kammerman S. Binding of gonadotropins to ovarian cells. Biol Reprod 1974; 10:179–198.
142. Jaaskelainen K, Markkanen S, Rajaniemi H. Internalization of receptor-bound human chorionic gonadotropin in preovulatory rat granulosa cells in vivo. Acta Endocrinol (Copenh) 1983; 103: 406–412.
143. Uilenbroek J, Richards J. Ovarian follicular development during the rat estrous cycle: gonadotropin receptors and follicular responsiveness. Biol Reprod 1979; 20:1159–1165.
144. Zeleznik A, Midgley A, Reichert L. Granulosa cell maturation in the rat; increased binding of human chorionic gonadotropin following treatment with follicle-stimulating hormone in vivo. Endocrinology 1974; 95:818–825.
145. Zeleznik A, Keyes P, Menon K, et al. Development-dependent responses of ovarian follicles to FSH and hCG. Am J Physiol 1977; 233:E229–E234.
146. Richards J, Ireland J, Rao M, et al. Ovarian follicular development in the rat: hormone receptor regulation by estradiol, follicle-stimulating hormone and luteinizing hormone. Endocrinology 1976; 99:1562–1570.
147. Couse J, Hewitt S, Bunch D, et al. Postnatal sex reversal of the ovaries in mice lacking estrogen receptors alpha and beta. Science 1999; 286:2328–2331.

148. Brandenberger A, Tee M, Jaffe R. Estrogen receptor alpha (ER-alpha) and beta (ER-beta) mRNAs in normal ovary, ovarian serous cystadenocarcinoma and ovarian cancer cell lines: down-regulation of ER-beta in neoplastic tissues. J Clin Endocrinol Metab 1998; 83:1025–1028.
149. Dorrington J, Moon Y, Armstrong D. Estradiol-17β biosynthesis in cultured granulosa cells from hypophysectomized immature rats: stimulation by follicle-stimulating hormone. Endocrinology 1975; 97:1328–1331.
150. Simpson ER, Mahendroo MS, Means GD, et al. Aromatase cytochrome P450, the enzyme responsible for estrogen biosynthesis. Endocr Rev 1994; 15:342–355.
151. Armstrong D, Papkoff H. Stimulation of aromatization of exogenous and endogenous androgens in ovaries of hypophysectomized rat in vivo by follicle-stimulating hormone. Endocrinology 1976; 99:1144–1151.
152. Moon Y, Tsang B, Simpson W, et al. Estradiol-17β biosynthesis in cultured granulosa and theca cells of human ovarian follicles: stimulation by follicle-stimulating hormone. Clin Endocrinol Metab 1978; 47:263–267.
153. Moon Y, Dorrington J, Armstrong D. Stimulatory action of follicle-stimulating hormone on estradiol-17β secretion by hypophysectomized rat ovaries in organ culture. Endocrinology 1975; 97: 244–247.
154. Erickson G, Hsueh A, Quigley M, et al. Functional studies of aromatase activity in human granulosa cells from normal and polycystic ovaries. J Clin Endocrinol Metab 1979; 49:514–519.
155. Rani C, Salhanick A, Armstrong D. Follicle-stimulating hormone induction of luteinizing hormone receptor in cultured rat granulosa cells: an examination of the need for steroids in the induction process. Endocrinology 1981; 108:1379–1385.
156. Bulun S. Aromatase deficiency and estrogen resistance: from molecular genetics to clinic. Semin Reprod Med 2000; 18:31–39.
157. Richards J, Jongssen J, Kersey K. Evidence that changes in tonic luteinizing hormone secretion determine the growth of preovulatory follicles in the rat. Endocrinology 1980; 107:641–648.
158. Richards J, Bogvich K. Effects of human chorionic gonadotropin and progesterone on follicular development in the immature rat. Endocrinology 1982; 111:1429–1438.
159. Bogvich K, Richards J. Androgen biosynthesis in developing ovarian follicle: evidence that luteinizing hormone regulates theca 17α-hydroxylase and C17-20 lyase activity. Endocrinology 1982; 111:1201–1208.
160. Ireland J, Richards J. A previously undescribed role for luteinizing hormone (LH:hCG) on follicular cell differentiation. Endocrinology 1978; 102:1458–1465.
161. Barlow J, Emerson K, Saxena B. Estradiol production after ovariectomy for carcinoma of the breast. N Engl J Med 1969; 28: 633–637.
162. Baird D, Burger P, Heavon-Jones G, et al. The site of secretion of androstenedione in non-pregnant women. J Endocrinol 1974; 63:201–212.
163. Baird D, Fraser I. Concentration of estrone and estradiol-17β in follicular fluid and ovarian venous blood of women. Clin Endocrinol (Oxf) 1969; 4:171.
164. Tsang B, Armstrong D, Whitfield J. Steroid biosynthesis by isolated human ovarian follicular cells in vitro. J Clin Endocrinol Metab 1980; 51:1407–1411.
165. McNatty K, Makris A, DeGrazia C, et al. The production of progesterone, androgens, and estrogens by granulosa cells, thecal tissue, and stromal tissue from human ovaries in vitro. J Clin Endocrinol Metab 1979; 49:687–689.
166. Hemsell D, Grodin J, Brenner P, et al. Plasma precursors of estrogen. II. Correlation of the extent of conversion of plasma androstenedione to estrone with age. J Clin Endocrinol Metab 1974; 38:476–479.
167. Pang S, Softner B, Sweeney W. Hirsutism, polycystic ovarian disease, and ovarian 17-ketosteroid reductase deficiency. N Engl J Med 1987; 316:1295–1301.
168. Bulun S, Simpson E. Competitive reverse transcription–polymerase chain reaction analysis indicates that levels of aromatase cytochrome P450 transcripts in adipose tissue of buttocks, thighs, and abdomen of women increase with advancing age. J Clin Endocrinol Metab 1994; 78:428–432.
169. Bulun S, Zeitoun K, Sasano H, et al. Aromatase in aging women. Semin Reprod Endocrinol 1999; 17:349–358.
170. Mahendroo M, Russell D. Male and female isoenzymes of steroid 5alpha-reductase. Rev Reprod 1999; 4:179–183.
171. Peltoketo H, Luu-The V, Simard J, et al. 17β- Hydroxysteroid dehydrogenase (HSD)/17-ketosteroid reductase (KSR) family; nomenclature and main characteristics of the 17HSD/KSR enzymes. J Mol Endocrinol 1999; 23:1–11.
172. Siiteri P, MacDonald P. Role of extraglandular estrogen in human endocrinology. In Greep RO, Astwood EB (eds). Handbook of Physiology. Sect 7: Endocrinology, vol II, Female Reproductive System. Washington, DC, American Physiological Society, 1973, pp 615–630.
173. Merriam G, Lipsett M. Catechol Estrogens. New York, Raven Press, 1983.
174. Lipsett M. Steroid hormones. In Yen SSC, Jaffe RB (eds). Reproductive Endocrinology, 2nd ed. Philadelphia, WB Saunders, 1986, pp 140–153.
175. Hemsell D, Edman C, Marks J, et al. Massive extraglandular aromatization of plasma androstenedione resulting in feminization of a prepubertal boy. J Clin Invest 1977; 60:455–464.
176. Miller W, Strauss JR. Molecular pathology and mechanism of action of the steroidogenic acute regulatory protein, StAR. J Steroid Biochem Mol Biol 1999; 69:131–141.
177. Juengel J, Garverick H, Johnson A, et al. Apoptosis during luteal cell regression in cattle. Endocrinology 1993; 132:249–254.
178. Pollack S, Furth E, Kallen C, et al. Localization of the steroidogenic acute regulatory protein in human tissues. J Clin Endocrinol Metab 1997; 82:243–251.
179. Waterman M, Simpson E. Regulation of steroid hydroxylase gene expression is multifactorial in nature. Recent Prog Horm Res 1989; 45:533–566.
180. Isomaa VV, Ghersevich S, Maentausta O, et al. Steroid biosynthetic enzymes: 17beta-hydroxysteroid dehydrogenase. Ann Med 1993; 25:91–97.
181. Ying S. Inhibins, activins, and follistatins: gonadal proteins modulating the secretion of follicle-stimulating hormone. Endocr Rev 1988; 9:267–293.
182. Leers-Sucheta S, Morohashi K, Mason J, et al. Synergistic activation of the human type II 3beta-hydroxysteroid dehydrogenase/ delta5-delta4 isomerase promoter by the transcription factor steroidogenic factor-1/adrenal 4-binding protein and phorbol ester. J Biol Chem 1997; 272:7960–7967.
183. Hanley N, Ikeda Y, Luo X, et al. Steroidogenic factor 1 (SF-1) is essential for ovarian development and function. Mol Cell Endocrinol 2000; 163:27–32.
184. Burger H, Farnsworth P, Findlay J, et al. Aspects of current and future inhibin research. Reprod Fertil Dev 1995; 7:997–1002.
185. Groome N, Illingworth P, O'Brien M, et al. Measurement of dimeric inhibin B throughout the human menstrual cycle. J Clin Endocrinol Metab 1996; 81:1401–1405.
186. Jaatinen T, Penttila T, Kaipia A, et al. Expression of inhibin alpha, beta A and beta B messenger ribonucleic acids in the normal human ovary and in polycystic ovarian syndrome. J Endocrinol 1994; 143:127–137.
187. Roberts V, Barth S, el-Roeiy A, et al. Expression of inhibin/ activin subunits and follistatin messenger ribonucleic acids and proteins in ovarian follicles and the corpus luteum during the human menstrual cycle. J Clin Endocrinol Metab 1993; 77:1402–1410.
188. Roberts V, Barth S, el-Roeiy A, et al. Expression of inhibin/ activin system messenger ribonucleic acids and proteins in ovarian follicles from women with polycystic ovarian syndrome. J Clin Endocrinol Metab 1994; 79:1434–1439.
189. Aloi J, Dalkin A, Schwartz N, et al. Ovarian inhibin subunit gene expression: regulation by gonadotropins and estradiol. Endocrinology 1995; 136:1227–1232.
190. Eramaa M, Tuuri T, Hilden K, et al. Regulation of inhibin alpha- and beta A-subunit messenger ribonucleic acid levels by chorionic gonadotropin and recombinant follicle-stimulating hormone in cultured human granulosa-luteal cells. J Clin Endocrinol Metab 1994; 79:1670–1677.
191. Adashi E. The IGF family and folliculogenesis. J Reprod Immunol 1998; 39:13–19.
192. Voutilainen R, Franks S, Mason H, Martikainen H. Expression of insulin-like growth factor (IGF), IGF-binding protein, and IGF receptor messenger ribonucleic acids in normal and polycystic ovaries. J Clin Endocrinol Metab 1996; 81:1003–1008.

193. Dunaif A. Insulin resistance and the polycystic ovary syndrome: mechanism and implications for pathogenesis. Endocr Rev 1997; 18:774–800.
194. Sasano H, Frost A, Saitoh R, et al. Aromatase and 17beta-hydroxysteroid dehydrogenase type 1 in human breast carcinoma. J Clin Endocrinol Metab 1996; 81:4042–4046.
195. Zeitoun K, Takayama K, Sasano H, et al. Deficient 17beta-hydroxysteroid dehydrogenase type 2 expression in endometriosis: failure to metabolize estradiol-17alpha. J Clin Endocrinol Metab 1998; 83:4474–4480.
196. Bulun SE, Noble LS, Takayama K, et al. Endocrine disorders associated with inappropriately high aromatase expression. J Steroid Biochem Mol Biol 1997; 61:133–139.
197. Azziz R, Carmina E, Sawaya M. Idiopathic hirsutism. Endocr Rev 2000; 21:347–362.
198. Noyes R, Hertia A, Rock J. Dating the endometrial biopsy. Fertil Steril 1950; 1:3.
199. Psychoyos A. Uterine receptivity for nidation. Ann NY Acad Sci 1986; 476:36–42.
200. Wynn R. Histology and ultrastructure of the human endometrium. In Wynn RM (ed): Biology of the Uterus. New York, Plenum, 1977, pp 341–376.
201. Markee J. Menstruation in intraocular endometrial transplants in the rhesus monkey. Contrib Embryol 1940; 28:219.
202. Markee J. Morphological basis for menstrual bleeding: relation of regression to the initiation of bleeding. Bull NY Acad Med 1948; 24:253.
203. Bartelmez G. The form and the function of the uterine blood vessels in the rhesus monkey. Carnegie Inst Contrib Embryol 1957; 36:153.
204. Bartlemez G. The phases of the menstrual cycle and their interpretation in terms of the pregnancy cycle. Am J Obstet Gynecol 1957; 74:931.
205. Eckert R, Katzenellenbogen B. Human endometrial cells in primary tissue culture: modulation of the progesterone receptor level by natural and synthetic estrogens in vitro. J Clin Endocrinol Metab 1981; 52:699–708.
206. Matsuzaki S, Fukaya T, Suzuki T, et al. Oestrogen receptor alpha and beta mRNA expression in human endometrium throughout the menstrual cycle. Mol Hum Reprod 1999; 5:559–564.
207. Cooke P, Buchanan D, Lubahn D, et al. Mechanism of estrogen action: lessons from the estrogen receptor-alpha knockout mouse. Biol Reprod 1998; 59:470–475.
208. Katzenellenbogen B. Estrogen receptors: bioactivities and interactions with cell signaling pathways. Biol Reprod 1996; 54:287–293.
209. Cooke P, Buchanan D, Young P, et al. Stromal estrogen receptors mediate mitogenic effects of estradiol on uterine epithelium. Proc Natl Acad Sci USA 1997; 94:6535–6540.
210. Lessey BA, Killam AP, Metzger DA, et al. Immunohistochemical analysis of human uterine estrogen and progesterone receptors throughout the menstrual cycle. J Clin Endocrinol Metab 1988; 67:334–340.
211. Attia G, Zeitoun K, Edwards D, et al. Progesterone receptor isoform A but not B is expressed in endometriosis. J Clin Endocrinol Metab 2000; 85:2897–2902.
212. Tseng L, Gurpide E. Effects of progestins on estradiol receptor levels in human endometrium. J Clin Endocrinol Metab 1975; 41:402–404.
213. Tseng L, Gurpide E. Induction of human endometrial estradiol dehydrogenase by progestins. Endocrinology 1975; 97:825–833.
214. Casey M, MacDonald P, Andersson S. 17β-Hydroxysteroid dehydrogenase type 2: chromosomal assignment and progestin regulation of gene expression in human endometrium. J Clin Invest 1994; 94:2135–2141.
215. Tseng L, Liu H. Stimulation of acylsulfotransferase activity by progestin in human endometrium in vitro. J Clin Endocrinol Metab 1981; 53:418–421.
216. Kurita T, Young P, Brody J, et al. Stromal progesterone receptors mediate the inhibitory effects of progesterone on estrogen-induced uterine epithelial cell deoxyribonucleic acid synthesis. Endocrinology 1998; 139:4708–4713.
217. Pope W. A cause of embryonic loss. Biol Reprod 1988; 39:999–1003.
218. Bergh P, Navot D. The impact of embryonic development and endometrial maturity of the timing of implantation. Fertil Steril 1992; 58:537–542.
219. Hertig A, Rock J, Adams E. A description of 34 human ova within the first 17 days of development. Am J Anat 1956; 98:435.
220. Markee J. Menstruation in intraocular endometrial transplants in the rhesus monkey. Contrib Embryol 1940; 28:219.
221. Kokawa K, Shikone T, Nakano R. Apoptosis in the human uterine endometrium during the menstrual cycle. J Clin Endocrinol Metab 1996; 81:4144–4147.
222. Sauer M, Paulson R, Lobo R. Reversing the natural decline in human fertility: an extended clinical trial of oocyte donation to women of advanced reproductive age. JAMA 1992; 268:1275–1279.
223. Rosenwaks Z. Donor eggs: their application in modern reproductive technologies. Fertil Steril 1987; 47:895–909.
224. Sauer M, Paulson R. Oocyte and embryo donation. Curr Opin Obstet Gynecol 1995; 7:193–198.
225. Yen S. The polycystic ovary syndrome. Clin Endocrinol (Oxf) 1980; 12:177–207.
226. Langer R, Pierce JJ, O'Hanlan K, et al. Transvaginal ultrasonography compared with endometrial biopsy for the detection of endometrial disease. Postmenopausal Estrogen/Progestin Interventions Trial. N Engl J Med 1997; 337:1839–1840.
227. Sheehan H. The recognition of chronic hypopituitarism resulting from postpartum pituitary necrosis. Am J Obstet Gynecol 1971; 111:852–854.
228. Simpson J, Christakos A, Horwith M, et al. Gonadal dysgenesis in individuals with apparently normal chromosomal complements: tabulation of cases and compilation of genetic data. Birth Defects 1971; 8:215–228.
229. Rosen G, Kaplan B, Lobo R. Menstrual function and hirsutism in patients with gonadal dysgenesis. Obstet Gynecol 1988; 71:677–680.
230. Hague W, Adams J, Reeders S, et al. 45,X Turner's syndrome in association with polycystic ovaries: case report. Br J Obstet Gynaecol 1989; 96:613–618.
231. Yen S. Chronic Anovulation Caused by Peripheral Endocrine Disorders. In Yen SCC, Jaffe RB (eds). Reproductive Endocrinology, 3rd ed. Philadelphia, WB Saunders, 1991.
232. Asherman J. Amenorrhea traumatica (atretica). J Obstet Gynaecol Br Emp 1948; 55:23.
233. Marshall W, Tanner J. Variations in patterns of pubertal changes in girls. Arch Dis Child 1969; 44:291–303.
234. Klinefelter HJ, Albright F, Griswold G. Experience with a quantitative test for normal or decreased amounts of follicle-stimulating hormone in urine in endocrinological diagnosis. J Clin Endocrinol Metab 1943; 3:529.
235. Yen S, Rebar R, VandenBerg G, Judd H. Hypothalamic amenorrhea and hypogonadotropism: responses to synthetic LRF. J Clin Endocrinol Metab 1973; 36:811–816.
236. Lachelin G, Yen S. Hypothalamic chronic anovulation. Am J Obstet Gynecol 1978; 130:825–831.
237. Khoury K, Reame N, Kelch R, et al. Diurnal patterns of pulsatile luteinizing hormone secretion in hypothalamic amenorrhea: reproducibility and responses to opiate blockade and an alpha2-adrenergic agonist. J Clin Endocrinol Metab 1987; 64:755–762.
238. Berga S, Mortola J, Gierton L, et al. Neuroendocrine aberrations in women with functional hypothalamic amenorrhea. J Clin Endocrinol Metab 1989; 68:301–308.
239. Loucks A, Mortola J, Girton L, et al. Alterations in the hypothalamic-pituitary-ovarian and the hypothalamic-pituitary-adrenal axes in athletic women. J Clin Endocrinol Metab 1989; 68:402–411.
240. Kalra S, Kalra P. Neural regulation of luteinizing hormone secretion in the rat. Endocr Rev 1983; 4:311–351.
241. Wilson R, Kesner J, Kaufman J, et al. Central electrophysiologic correlates of pulsatile luteinizing hormone releasing hormone "pulse generator" in the rhesus monkey. Neuroendocrinology 1984; 39:256–260.
242. Kalra S. Catecholamine involvement in preovulatory LH release: reassessment of the role of epinephrine. Neuroendocrinology 1985; 40:139–144.
243. Rasmussen D. The interaction between mediobasohypothalamic dopaminergic and endorphinergic neuronal systems as a key regulator of reproduction: an hypothesis. J Endocrinol Invest 1991; 14:323–352.
244. Quigley M, Sheehan K, Casper R, et al Evidence for increased dopaminergic and opioid activity in patients with hypothalamic

hypogonadotropic amenorrhea. J Clin Endocrinol Metab 1980; 50:949–954.
245. Ropert J, Quigley M, Yen S. Endogenous opiates modulate pulsatile luteinizing hormone release in humans. J Clin Endocrinol Metab 1981; 52:583–585.
246. Gambacciani M, Yen SS, Rasmussen DD. GnRH release from the mediobasal hypothalamus: in vitro inhibition by corticotropin-releasing factor. Neuroendocrinology 1986; 43:533–536.
247. Yen S, Quigley M, Reid R, et al. Neuroendocrinology of opioid peptides and their role in the control of gonadotropin and prolactin secretion. Am J Obstet Gynecol 1985; 152:485–493.
248. Genazzani A, Petraglia F, Gastaldi M, et al. Naltrexone treatment restores menstrual cycles in patients with weight loss–related amenorrhea. Fertil Steril 1995; 64:951–956.
249. Selye H. The stress syndrome. Nature 1936; 138:32.
250. Suh B, Liu J, Berga S, et al. Hypercortisolism in patients with functional hypothalamic amenorrhea. J Clin Endocrinol Metab 1988; 66:733–739.
251. Gibbs D. Dissociation of oxytocin, vasopressin, and corticotropin secretion during different types of stress. Life Sci 1984; 35:487–491.
252. Palumbo A, Yeh J. Apoptosis as a basic mechanism in the ovarian cycle: follicular atresia and luteal regression. J Soc Gynecol Invest 1995; 2:565–573.
253. Xiao E, Luckhaus J, Niemann W, et al. Acute inhibition of gonadotropin secretion by corticotropin-releasing hormone in the primate: are the adrenal glands involved? Endocrinology 1989; 124:1632–1637.
254. Rivier C, Vale W. Influence of corticotropin-releasing factor on reproductive function in the rat. Endocrinology 1984; 114:914–921.
255. Matteri R, Moberg G, Watson J. Adrenocorticotropin-induced changes in ovine pituitary gonadotropin secretion in vitro. Endocrinology 1986; 118:2091–2096.
256. Kamel F, Kubajak C. Modulation of gonadotropin secretion by corticosterone: interaction with gonadal steroids and mechanism of action. Endocrinology 1987; 121:561–568.
257. Cauley J, Black D, Barrett-Connor E, et al. Effects of hormone replacement therapy on clinical fractures and height loss: the Heart and Estrogen/Progestin Replacement Study (HERS). Am J Med 2001; 110:442–450.
258. Baranowska B, Rozbicka G, Jeske W, et al. The role of endogenous opiates in the mechanism of inhibited luteinizing hormone (LH) secretion in women with anorexia nervosa: the effect of naloxone in LH, follicle-stimulating hormone, prolactin, and beta-endorphin secretion. J Clin Endocrinol Metab 1984; 59: 412–416.
259. Grandison L, Guidotti A. Stimulation of food intake by muscimol and beta endorphin. Neuropharmacology 1977; 16:533–536.
260. Atkinson R. Naloxone decreased food intake in obese humans. J Clin Endocrinol Metab 1982; 55:196–198.
261. Morley J, Levine A. Stress-induced eating is mediated through endogenous opiates. Science 1980; 209:1259–1261.
262. Garner D, Bemis K. A cognitive-behavioral approach to anorexia nervosa. Cognit Ther Res 1982; 6:123.
263. Fairburn C. A cognitive behavioral approach to the treatment of bulimia. Psychol Med 1981; 11:707–711.
264. Rigotti N, Neer R, Skates SJ, et al. The clinical course of osteoporosis in anorexia nervosa: a longitudinal study of cortical bone mass. JAMA 1991; 265:1133–1138.
265. Frisch R, Wyshak G, Vincent L. Delayed menarche and amenorrhea in ballet dancers. N Engl J Med 1980; 303:17–19.
266. Frisch R, Gotz-Webergen A, McArthur J, et al. Delayed menarche and amenorrhea of college athletes in relation to age of onset of training. JAMA 1981; 246:1559–1563.
267. Sanborn C, Martin B, Wagner W. Is athletic amenorrhea specific to runners? Am J Obstet Gynecol 1982; 143:859–861.
268. Rivier C, Rivier J, Vale W. Stress-induced inhibition of reproductive functions: role of endogenous corticotropin-releasing factor. Science 1986; 231:607–609.
269. Howlett T, Tomlin S, Ngahfoong L, et al. Release of beta-endorphin and met-enkephalin during exercise in normal women: response to training. Br Med J (Clin Res Ed) 1984; 288:1950–1952.
270. Laatikainen T, Virtanen T, Apter D. Plasma immunoreactive beta-endorphin in exercise-associated amenorrhea. Am J Obstet Gynecol 1986; 154:94–97.
271. Drinkwater B, Nilson K, Chesnut CH 3rd, et al. Bone mineral content of amenorrheic and eumenorrheic athletes. N Engl J Med 1984; 311:277–281.
272. Vigersky R, Loriaux D, Andersen A, et al. Anorexia nervosa: behavioral and hypothalamic aspects. Clin Endocrinol Metab 1976; 5:517–535.
273. Pyle R, Mitchell J, Eckert E, et al. The incidence of bulimia in freshman college students. Int J Eat Disord 1983; 2:75.
274. Willis J, Grossman S. Epidemiology of anorexia nervosa in a defined region of Switzerland. Am J Psychiatry 1983; 140:564–567.
275. Schotte D, Stunkard M. Bulimia vs bulimic behaviors on a college campus. JAMA 1987; 258:1213–1215.
276. Schwartz D, Thompson M. Do anorectics get well? Current research and future needs. Am J Psychiatry 1981; 138:319–323.
277. Patton G. Mortality in eating disorders. Psychol Med 1988; 18: 947–951.
278. Swift W. The long-term outcome of early onset anorexia nervosa: a critical review. J Am Acad Child Psychiatry 1982; 21:38–46.
279. Boyar R, Hellman L, Roffwarg H, et al. Cortisol secretion and metabolism in anorexia nervosa. N Engl J Med 1977; 296:190–193.
280. Kontula K, Anderson L, Huttumen M, et al. Reduced level of cellular glucocorticoid receptors in patients with anorexia nervosa. Horm Metab Res 1982; 14:619–620.
281. Gold P, Gwirtsman H, Avgerinos P, et al. Abnormal hypothalamic-pituitary-adrenal function in anorexia nervosa. N Engl J Med 1986; 314:1335–1342.
282. Kaye W, Gwirtsman H, George D, et al. Elevated cerebrospinal fluid levels of immunoreactive corticotropin-releasing hormone in anorexia nervosa: relation to state of nutrition, adrenal function and intensity of depression. J Clin Endocrinol Metab 1987; 64: 203–208.
283. Moshang TJ, Utiger R. Low triiodothyronine euthyroidism in anorexia nervosa. In Vigersky RS (ed). Anorexia Nervosa. New York, Raven Press, 1977, pp 263–270.
284. Gold P, Kaye W, Robertson G, et al. Abnormalities in plasma and cerebrospinal fluid arginine vasopressin in patients with anorexia nervosa. N Engl J Med 1983; 308:1117–1123.
285. Soyka L, Grinspoon S, Levitsky L, et al. The effects of anorexia nervosa on bone metabolism in female adolescents. J Clin Endocrinol Metab 1999; 84:4489–4496.
286. Prior J, Vigna Y, Schechter M, et al. Spinal bone loss and ovulatory disturbances. N Engl J Med 1990; 323:1221–1227.
287. Drinkwater B, Nilson K, Ott S, et al. Bone mineral density after resumption of menses in amenorrheic athletes. JAMA 1986; 256: 380–382.
288. Rupich R. New techniques in bone imaging for determination of bone density. Semin Reprod Endocrinol 1992; 10:27.
289. Liu J, Yen S. The use of gonadotropin-releasing hormone for the induction of ovulation. Clin Obstet Gynecol 1984; 27:975–982.
290. Martin K, Santoro N, Hall J, et al. Management of ovulatory disorders with pulsatile gonadotropin-releasing hormone. J Clin Endocrinol Metab 1990; 71:1081A–1081G.
291. Santoro N, Elzahr D. Pulsatile gonadotropin-releasing hormone therapy for ovulatory disorders. Clin Obstet Gynecol 1993; 36: 727–736.
292. Niall H. The chemistry of prolactin. In Jaffe RB (ed). Prolactin. New York, Elsevier North-Holland, 1981, p 1.
293. Stachura M, Tyler J, Kent P. Pituitary immediate release pools of growth hormone and prolactin are preferentially refilled by new rather than stored hormone. Endocrinology 1989; 124:444–449.
294. Day R, Mauer R. The distal enhancer region of the rat prolactin gene contains elements conferring response to multiple hormones. Mol Endocrinol 1989; 3:3–9.
295. Murdoch G, Waterman M, Evans R, Rosenfeld M. Molecular mechanisms of phorbol ester, thyrotropin-releasing hormone and growth factor stimulation of prolactin gene transcription. J Biol Chem 1985; 260:11852–11858.
296. Waterman M, Adler S, Nelson C, et al. A single domain of the estrogen receptor confers deoxyribonucleic acid binding and transcriptional activation of the prolactin gene. Mol Endocrinol 1988; 2:14–21.
297. MacLeod R, Kimura H, Login I. Inhibition of prolactin secretion

of dopamine and piribedil (ET-495). In Pecile A (ed). Growth Hormone and Related Peptides. New York, Elsevier North-Holland, 1976, p 443.
298. Gibbs D, Neill J. Dopamine levels in hypophysial stalk blood in the rat are sufficient to inhibit prolactin secretion in vivo. Endocrinology 1978; 102:1895–1900.
299. Sassin J, Frantz A, Weitzman E, Kapen S. Human prolactin: 24-hour pattern with increased release during sleep. Science 1972; 177:1205–1207.
300. Suginami H, Hamada K, Yano K, et al. Ovulation induction with bromocriptine in normoprolactinemic anovulatory women. J Clin Endocrinol Metab 1986; 62:899–903.
301. Liddle G, Island D, Meador C. Normal and abnormal regulation of corticotropin secretion in man. Recent Prog Horm Res 1962; 18:125.
302. Chang R, Mandel F, Lu JK, et al. Enhanced disparity of gonadotropin secretion by estrone in women with polycystic ovarian disease. J Clin Endocrinol Metab 1982; 54:490–494.
303. Watters J, Chun T, Kim Y, et al. Estrogen modulation of prolactin gene expression requires an intact mitogen-activated protein kinase signal transduction pathway in cultured rat pituitary cells. Mol Endocrinol 2000; 14:1872–1881.
304. Chrousos G, Loriaus D, Mann D, et al. Late-onset 21-hydroxylase deficiency mimicking idiopathic hirsutism or polycystic ovarian disease. Ann Intern Med 1982; 96:143–148.
305. New M, Lorenzen F, Lerner A, et al. Genotyping steroid 21-hydroxylase deficiency: hormonal reference data. J Clin Endocrinol Metab 1983; 31:320–326.
306. Moses A, Streeten D. Differentiation of polyuric states by measurement of responses to changes in plasma osmolality induced by hypertonic saline infusions. Am J Med 1967; 42:368–377.
307. Boutin J, Edery M, Shirota M, et al. Identification of a cDNA encoding a long form of prolactin receptor in human hepatoma and breast cancer cells. Mol Endocrinol 1989; 3:1455–1461.
308. Somers W, Ultsch M, De Vas A, et al. The x-ray structure of a growth hormone–prolactin receptor complex. Nature 1994; 372: 478–481.
309. Das R, Vonderhaar B. Transduction of prolactin's (PRL) growth signal through both long and short forms of the PRL receptor. Mol Endocrinol 1995; 9:1750–1759.
310. Weiss-Messer E, Ber R, Barkey R. Prolactin and MA-10 Leydig cell steroidogenesis: biphasic effects of prolactin and signal transduction. Endocrinology 1996; 137:5509–5518.
311. Healy D, Burger H. Sustained elevation of serum prolactin by metoclopramide: clinical model of idiopathic hyperprolactinemia. J Clin Endocrinol 1978; 46:709–714.
312. Kauppila A, Leinonen P, Vikho R, et al. Metoclopramide induced hyperprolactinemia impairs ovarian follicle maturation and corpus luteum function in women. J Clin Endocrinol Metab 1982; 54:955–960.
313. Cooper D, Ridgway E, Kliman B, et al. Metabolic clearance and production rates of prolactin in man. J Clin Invest 1979; 64: 1669–1680.
314. Schlechte J, Sherman B, Martin R. Bone density in amenorrheic women with and without hyperprolactinemia. J Clin Endocrinol Metab 1983; 56:1120–1123.
315. Kovacs C, Chik C. Hyperprolactinemia caused by lactation and pituitary adenomas is associated with altered serum calcium, phosphate, parathyroid hormone (PTH), and PTH-related peptide levels. J Clin Endocrinol Metab 1995; 80:3036–3042.
316. Rasmussen C, Bergh T, Wide L, Brownell J. Long term treatment with a new non-ergot long-acting dopamine agonist, CV 205–502, in women with hyperprolactinemia. Clin Endocrinol (Oxf) 1988; 29:271–279.
317. Morange I, Barlier A, Pellegrini I, et al. Prolactinomas resistant to bromocriptine: long-term efficacy of quinagolide and outcome of pregnancy. Eur J Endocrinol 1996; 135:413–420.
318. Caccavelli L, Feron F, Morange I, et al. Decreased expression of the two D_2 dopamine receptor isoforms in bromocriptine-resistant prolactinomas. Neuroendocrinology 1994; 60:314–322.
319. Feigenbaum S, Downey D, Wilson C, Jaffe RB. Transsphenoidal pituitary resection for preoperative diagnosis of prolactin-secreting pituitary adenoma in women: long term follow-up. J Clin Endocrinol Metab 1996; 81:1711–1719.
320. Molitch M. Pregnancy and the hyperprolactinemic woman. N Engl J Med 1985; 312:1364–1370.
321. Gemzell C, Wang C. Outcome of pregnancy in women with pituitary adenoma. Fertil Steril 1979; 31:363–372.
322. Forbes A, Hanneman P, Griswold G, et al. Syndrome characterized by galactorrhea, amenorrhea, and low urinary FSH: comparison with acromegaly and normal lactation. J Clin Endocrinol Metab 1954; 14:265.
323. Vermeulen A, Ando S. Prolactin and adrenal androgen secretion. Clin Endocrinol (Oxf) 1978; 8:295–303.
324. Glickman S, Rosenfield R, Bergenstal R, et al. Multiple androgenic abnormalities, including elevated free testosterone, in hyperprolactinemic women. J Clin Endocrinol Metab 1982; 55:251–257.
325. Lobo R, Kletzy O. Normalization of androgen and sex hormone–binding globulin levels after treatment of hyperprolactinemic women. J Clin Endocrinol Metab 1982; 55:251.
326. Isik A, Gulekli B, Zorlu C, et al. Endocrinological and clinical analysis of hyperprolactinemic patients with and without ultrasonically diagnosed polycystic ovarian changes. Gynecol Obstet Invest 1997; 43:183–185.
327. Klibanski A, Neer R, Beitins I, et al. Decreased bone density in hyperprolactinemic women. N Engl J Med 1981; 303:1511–1514.
328. Koppelmann M, Kurtz D, Morrish A, et al. Vertebral body bone mineral content in hyperprolactinemic women. J Clin Endocrinol Metab 1984; 59:1050–1053.
329. Pahuja D, DeLuca H. Stimulation of intestinal calcium transport and bone calcium mobilization by prolactin in vitamin D–deficient rats. Science 1981; 214:1038–1039.
330. Milenkovic L, D'Angelo D, Kelly P, Weiner RI. Inhibition of gonadotropin hormone–releasing hormone release by prolactin from GT1 neuronal cell lines through prolactin receptors. Proc Natl Acad Sci USA 1994; 91:1244–1247.
331. Hatch R, Rosenfield R, Kim M, et al. Hirsutism: implications, etiology, and management. Am J Obstet Gynecol 1981; 140:815–830.
332. Tagatz G, Kopher R, Nagel T, et al. The clitoral index: a bioassay of androgenic stimulation. Obstet Gynecol 1979; 54: 562–564.
333. Bardin C, Lipsett M. Testosterone and androstenedione blood production rates in normal women and women with idiopathic hirsutism or polycystic ovaries. J Clin Invest 1967; 46:891–902.
334. Mowszowicz I, Melanitou E, Doukani A, et al. Androgen binding capacity and 5α-reductase activity in pubic skin fibroblasts from hirsute patients. J Clin Endocrinol Metab 1983; 56:1209–1213.
335. Cumming D, Vickovic M, Wall S, et al. Defects in pulsatile LH release in normal menstruating runners. J Clin Endocrinol Metab 1985; 60:810–812.
336. Schwartz U, Moltz L, Brotherton J, et al. The diagnostic value of plasma free testosterone in non-tumorous and tumorous hyperandrogenism. Fertil Steril 1983; 40:66–72.
337. Lobo R, Carmina E. The importance of diagnosing the polycystic ovary syndrome. Ann Intern Med 2000; 132:989–993.
338. Paulson R, Serafini P, Catalino J, et al. Measurements of $3\alpha,17\beta$-androstenediol glucuronide in serum and urine and the correlation with skin 5α-reductase activity. Fertil Steril 1986; 46:222–226.
339. Barbieri R, Gao X. Presence of 17 beta-hydroxysteroid dehydrogenase type 3 messenger ribonucleic acid transcript in an ovarian Sertoli-Leydig cell tumor. Fertil Steril 1997; 68:534–537.
340. Kennedy L, Traub A, Atkinson A, et al. Short-term administration of gonadotropin-releasing hormone analog to a patient with testosterone-secreting tumor. J Clin Endocrinol Metab 1987; 64: 1320–1322.
341. Brown J, Fishman L. Biosynthesis and metabolism of steroid hormones by human adrenal carcinomas. Braz J Med Biol Res 2000; 33:1235–1244.
342. Derksen J, Nagesser S, Meinders A, et al. Identification of virilizing adrenal tumors in hirsute women. N Engl J Med 1994; 331: 968–973.
343. O'Driscoll J, Mamtora H, Higginson J, et al. A prospective study of the prevalence of clear-cut endocrine disorders and polycystic ovaries in 350 patients presenting with hirsutism or androgenic alopecia. Clin Endocrinol (Oxf) 1994; 41:231–236.
344. Friedman C, Schmidt G, Kim M, et al. Serum testosterone concentrations in the evaluation of androgen-producing tumors. Am J Obstet Gynecol 1985; 153:44–49.
345. Surrey E, de Ziegler D, Gambone J, et al. Preoperative localization of androgen-secreting tumors: clinical, endocrinologic, and

442. Diamanti-Kandarakis E, Kouli C, Tsianateli T, Bergiele A. Therapeutic effects of metformin on insulin resistance and hyperandrogenism in polycystic ovary syndrome. Eur J Endocrinol 1998; 138:269–274.
443. Nestler J, Jakubowicz D, Evans W, et al. Effects of metformin on spontaneous and clomiphene-induced ovulation in the polycystic ovary syndrome. N Engl J Med 1998; 338:1876–1880.
444. Crave J, Fimbel S, LeJeune H, et al. Effects of diet and metformin administration on sex hormone–binding globulin, androgens, and insulin in hirsute and obese women. J Clin Endocrinol Metab 1995; 80:2057–2062.
445. Nestler J, Jakubowicz D. Lean women with polycystic ovary syndrome respond to insulin reduction with decreases in ovarian P450c 17a activity and serum androgens. J Clin Endocrinol Metab 1997; 82:4075–4079.
446. Moghetti P, Castello R, Negri C, et al. Metformin effects on clinical features, endocrine and metabolic profiles, and insulin sensitivity in polycystic ovary syndrome: a randomized, double-blind, placebo-controlled 6-month trial, followed by open, long-term clinical evaluation. J Clin Endocrinol Metab 2000; 85:139–146.
447. Dunaif A, Scott D, Finegood D, et al. The insulin-sensitizing agent troglitazone improves metabolic and reproductive abnormalities in the polycystic ovary syndrome. J Clin Endocrinol Metab 1996; 81:3299–3306.
448. Ehrmann D, Schneider D, Sobel B, et al. Troglitazone improves defects in insulin action, insulin secretion, ovarian steroidogenesis, and fibrolysis in women with polycystic ovary syndrome. J Clin Endocrinol Metab 1997; 82:2108–2116.
449. Iuorno M, Nestler J. Insulin-lowering drugs in polycystic ovary syndrome. Obstet Gynecol Clin North Am 2001; 28:153–164.
450. Saagle M, Bishop K, Ridley N, et al. Recurrent early miscarriage and polycystic ovaries. Br Med J 1988; 297:1027–1028.
451. Regan L, Owen E, Jacobs H. Hypersecretion of luteinizing hormone, infertility and miscarriage. Lancet 1990; 336:1141–1144.
452. Tulppala M, Stenman U-H, Cacciatore B, et al. Polycystic ovaries and levels of gonadotrophins and androgens in recurrent miscarriage: prospective study in 50 women. Br J Obstet Gynaecol 1993; 100:348–352.
453. Formigli L, Formigli G, Roccio C. Donation of fertilized uterine ova to infertile women. Fertil Steril 1988; 47:162–165.
454. Dockety M, Lovelady S, Faust G. Carcinoma of the corpus uteri in young women. Am J Obstet Gynecol 1991; 61:966.
455. Gitsch G, Hanzal E, Jensen D, et al. Endometrial cancer in premenopausal women 45 years and younger. Obstet Gynecol 1995; 85:504–508.
456. Godsland I, Crook D. Update on the metabolic effects of steroidal contraceptives and their relationship to cardiovascular disease risk. Am J Obstet Gynecol 1994; 170:1528–1536.
457. Duffy T, Ray R. Oral contraceptive use: prospective follow-up of women with suspected glucose intolerance. Contraception 1984; 30:197–208.
458. Hannaford P, Kay C. Oral contraceptives and diabetes mellitus. Br Med J 1989; 299:1315–1316.
459. Petersen K, Christiansen E, Madsbad S, et al. Metabolic and fibrinolytic response to changed insulin sensitivity in users of oral contraceptives. Contraception 1999; 60:337–344.
460. Escobar-Morreale H, Lasuncion M, Sancho J. Treatment of hirsutism with ethinyl estradiol–desogestrel contraceptive pills has beneficial effects on the lipid profile and improves insulin sensitivity. Fertil Steril 2000; 74:816–819.
461. Stampfer M, Willett W, Colditz G, et al. Past use of oral contraceptives and cardiovascular disease: a meta-analysis in the context of the Nurses' Health Study. Am J Obstet Gynecol 1990; 163: 285–291.
462. Colditz GA. Oral contraceptive use and mortality during 12 years of follow-up: the Nurses' Health Study. Ann Intern Med 1994; 120:821–826.
463. Kjos S, Shoupe D, Douyan S, et al. Effect of low-dose oral contraceptives on carbohydrate and lipid metabolism in women with recent gestational diabetes: results of a controlled, randomized, prospective study. Am J Obstet Gynecol 1990; 163:1822–1827.
464. Kjos S, Peters R, Xiang A, et al. Contraception and the risk of type 2 diabetes in Latino women with prior gestational diabetes. JAMA 1998; 280:533–538.
465. Garg S, Chase H, Marshall G, et al. Oral contraceptives and renal and retinal complications in young women with insulin-dependent diabetes mellitus. JAMA 1994; 271:1099–1102.
466. Petersen K, Skouby S, Sidelmann J, et al. Effects of contraceptive steroids on cardiovascular risk factors in women with insulin-dependent diabetes mellitus. Am J Obstet Gynecol 1994; 171: 400–405.
467. Ramsay L, Yeo W, Jackson P. Influence of diuretics, calcium antagonists, and alpha-blockers on insulin sensitivity and glucose tolerance in hypertensive patients. J Cardiovasc Phys 1992; 20S: S49–S53.
468. Diamanti-Kandarakis E, Mitrakou A, Hennes M, et al. Insulin sensitivity and antiandrogenic therapy in women with polycystic ovary syndrome. Metabolism 1995; 44:525–531.
469. Lanzone A, Fulghesus A, Cucinelli F, et al. Preconceptional and gestational evaluation of insulin secretion in patients with polycystic ovary syndrome. Hum Reprod 1996; 11:2382–2386.
470. Wild R, Alaupovic P, Parker I. Lipid and apolipoprotein abnormalities in hirsute women: the association with insulin resistance. Am J Obstet Gynecol 1992; 166:1191–1196.
471. Slowinska-Srzednicka J, Zgliczynski S, Wierzbicki M, et al. The role of hyperinsulinemia in the development of lipid disturbances in non-obese and obese women with the polycystic ovary syndrome. J Endocrinol Invest 1991; 14:569–575.
472. Kiddy D, Hamilton-Fairley D, Bush A, et al. Improvement of endocrine and ovarian function during dietary treatment of obese women with polycystic ovary syndrome. Clin Endocrinol (Oxf) 1992; 36:105–111.
473. Guzick D, Wing R, Smith D, et al. Endocrine consequences of weight loss in obese, hyperandrogenic anovulatory women. Fertil Steril 1994; 61:598–604.
474. Andersen P, Selifeflot I, Abdelnoor M, et al. Increased insulin sensitivity and fibrinolytic capacity after dietary intervention in obese women with polycystic ovary syndrome. Metabolism 1995; 44:611–616.
475. Jakubowicz D, Nestler J. 17 alpha-Hydroxyprogesterone responses to leuprolide and serum androgens in obese women with and without polycystic ovary syndrome after dietary weight loss. J Clin Endocrinol Metab 1997; 82:556–560.
476. Clark A, Ledger W, Galletly C, et al. Weight loss results in significant improvement in pregnancy and ovulation rates in anovulatory obese women. Hum Reprod 1995; 10:2705–2712.
477. Hollmann M, Runnebaum B, Gerhard I. Effects of weight loss on the hormonal profile in obese, infertile women. Hum Reprod 1996; 11:1884–1891.
478. Dahlgren E, Johansson S, Lindstedt G, et al. Women with polycystic ovary syndrome wedge resected in 1956 to 1965: a long term follow-up focusing on natural history and circulating hormones. Fertil Steril 1992; 57:505–513.
479. Adashi E. Clomiphene citrate–initiated ovulation: a clinical update. Semin Reprod Endocrinol 1986; 4:255–276.
480. Mitwally M, Casper R. Use of an aromatase inhibitor for induction of ovulation in patients with an inadequate response to clomiphene citrate. Fertil Steril 2001; 75:305–309.
481. Hamilton-Fairley D, Franks S. Common problems in induction of ovulation. Baillieres Clin Obstet Gynaecol 1990; 4:609–625.
482. Marci R, Senn A, Dessole S, et al. A low-dose stimulation protocol using highly purified follicle-stimulating hormone can lead to high pregnancy rates in in vitro fertilization patients with polycystic ovaries who are at risk of a high ovarian response to gonadotropins. Fertil Steril 2001; 75:1131–1135.
483. Taylor A, Adams J, Mulder J, et al. A randomized, controlled trial of estradiol replacement therapy in women with hypergonadotropic amenorrhea. J Clin Endocrinol Metab 1996; 81:3615–3621.
484. Conway G. Premature ovarian failure. Br Med Bull 2000; 56: 643–649.
485. Dewald G, Spurbeck J. Sex chromosome anomalies associated with premature gonadal failure. Semin Reprod Endocrinol 1983; 1:79.
486. Devi A, Metzger D, Luciano A, Benn PA. 45,X/46,XX mosaicism in patients with idiopathic premature ovarian failure. Fertil Steril 1998; 70:89–93.
487. Myhre A, Halonen M, Eskelin P, et al. Autoimmune polyendocrine syndrome type 1 (APS I) in Norway. Clin Endocrinol (Oxf) 2001; 54:211–217.

488. Gradishar W, Schilsky R. Ovarian function following radiation and chemotherapy. Semin Oncol 1989; 16:425–436.
489. Wallace W, Shalet SM, Crowne E, et al. Ovarian failure following abdominal irradiation in childhood natural history and prognosis. Clin Oncol 1989; 1:75–79.
490. Madsen B, Giudice L, Donaldson S. Radiation-induced premature menopause: a misconception. Int J Radiat Oncol Biol Phys 1995; 32:1461–1464.
491. Morice P, Thiam-Ba R, Castaigne D, et al. Fertility results after ovarian transposition for pelvic malignancies treated by external irradiation or brachytherapy. Hum Reprod 1998; 13:660–663.
492. Bines J, Oleske D, Cobleigh M. Ovarian function in premenopausal women treated with adjuvant chemotherapy for breast cancer. J Clin Oncol 1996; 14:1718–1729.
493. Byrne J, Mulvihill J, Myers M, et al. Effects of treatment on fertility in long-term survivors of childhood cancer. N Engl J Med 1987; 317:1315–1321.
494. Aittomaki K. The genetics of XX gonadal dysgenesis. Am J Hum Genet 1994; 58:844–851.
495. Toledo S, Brunner H, Kraaij R, et al. An inactivating mutation of the luteinizing hormone receptor causes amenorrhea in a 46,XX female. J Clin Endocrinol Metab 1996; 81:3850–3854.
496. Guerrero N, Singh R, Manatunga A, et al. Risk factors for premature ovarian failure in females with galactosemia. J Pediatr 2000; 137:833–841.
497. Rebar R, Connolly H. Clinical features of young women with hypergonadotropic amenorrhea. Fertil Steril 1990; 53:804–810.
498. Aiman J, Smentck C. Premature ovarian failure. Obstet Gynecol 1985; 66:9–14.
499. Nelson L, Anasti J, Kimzey L, et al. Development of luteinized graafian follicles in patients with karyotypically normal spontaneous premature ovarian failure. J Clin Endocrinol Metab 1994; 79: 1470–1475.
500. Laml T, Huber J, Albrecht A, et al. Unexpected pregnancy during hormone-replacement therapy in a woman with elevated follicle-stimulating hormone levels and amenorrhea. Gynecol Endocrinol 1999; 13:89–92.
501. Giltay J, Ausems M, van Seumeren I, et al. Short stature as the only presenting feature in a patient with isodicentric (Y)(q11.23) and gonadoblastoma: a clinical and molecular cytogenic study. Eur J Pediatr 2001; 160:154–158.
502. Manuel M, Katayama K, Jones JH. The age of occurrence of gonadal tumors in intersex patients with a Y chromosome. Am J Obstet Gynecol 1976; 124:293–300.
503. Troche V, Hernandez E. Neoplasia arising in dysgenetic gonads. Obstet Gynecol Surv 1986; 41:74–79.
504. Gravhold C, Fedder J, Naeraa R, et al. Occurrence of gonadoblastoma in females with Turner syndrome and Y chromosome material: a population study. J Clin Endocrinol Metab 2000; 85: 3199–3202.
505. Nelson L. Autoimmune ovarian failure: comparing the mouse model and the human disease. J Soc Gynecol Invest 2001; 8(1 suppl):S55–S57.
506. Wheatcroft N, Salat C, Milford-Ward A, et al. Identification of ovarian antibodies by immunofluorescence, enzyme-linked immunosorbent assay or immunoblotting in premature ovarian failure. Hum Reprod 1997; 12:2617–2622.
507. Belsey E, Pinol A. Menstrual bleeding patterns in untreated women. Task Force on Long-Acting Systemic Agents for Fertility Regulation. Contraception 1997; 55:57–65.
508. Collett M, Wertenberger G, Fiske V. The effect of age upon the pattern of the menstrual cycle. Fertil Steril 1954; 5:437.
509. Chiazze LJ, Brayer F, Macisco JJ, et al. The length and variability of the human menstrual cycle. JAMA 1968; 203:377–380.
510. Munster K, Schmidt L, Helm P. Length and variation in the menstrual cycle: a cross-sectional study from a Danish county. Br J Obstet Gynaecol 1992; 99:422–429.
511. Treloar A, Boynton R, Borghild G, et al. Variation of the human menstrual cycle through reproductive life. Int J Fertil 1967; 12: 77–126.
512. Rybo G. Menstrual blood loss in relation to parity and menstrual pattern. Acta Obstet Gynecol Scand 1966; 45(suppl 7):1–23.
513. Haynes P, Hodgson H, Anerson A, et al. Measurement of menstrual blood loss in patients complaining of menorrhagia. Br J Obstet Gynaecol 1977; 84:763–768.
514. Higham J, O'Brien P, Shaw R. Assessment of menstrual blood loss using a pictorial chart. Br J Obstet Gynaecol 1990; 97:734–739.
515. Cohen B, Gibor J. Anemia and menstrual blood loss. Obstet Gynecol Surv 1980; 35:597–618.
516. Fraser I, McCarron G, Markham R. A preliminary study of factors influencing perception of menstrual blood loss volume. Am J Obstet Gynecol 1984; 149:788–793.
517. de Ziegler D, Bergeron C, Cornel C, et al. Effects of luteal estradiol on the secretory transformation of human endometrium and plasma gonadotropins. J Clin Endocrinol Metab 1992; 74: 322–331.
518. Belsey E. Vaginal bleeding patterns among women using one natural and eight hormonal methods of contraception. Contraception 1988; 38:181–206.
519. Wilansky D, Greisman B. Early hypothyroidism in patients with menorrhagia. Am J Obstet Gynecol 1989; 160:673–677.
520. Hopkins M, Androff L, Benninghoff A. Ginseng face cream and unexplained vaginal bleeding. Am J Obstet Gynecol 1988; 159: 1121–1122.
521. Claessens E, Cowell C. Acute adolescent menorrhagia. Am J Obstet Gynecol 1981; 139:277–280.
522. Smith Y, Quint E, Hertzberg R. Menorrhagia in adolescents requiring hospitalization. J Pediatr Adolesc Gynecol 1998; 11:13–15.
523. van Eijkeren M, Christiaens G, Haspels A, et al. Measured menstrual blood loss in women with a bleeding disorder or using oral anticoagulant therapy. Am J Obstet Gynecol 1990; 161:1261–1263.
524. Edlund M, Blomback M, von Schoultz B, et al. On the value of menorrhagia as a predictor for coagulation disorders. Am J Hematol 1996; 53:234–238.
525. Nilsson L, Rybo G. Treatment of menorrhagia. Am J Obstet Gynecol 1971; 110:713–720.
526. Kirkland J, Murthy L, Stancel G. Progesterone inhibits the estrogen-induced expression of c-fos messenger ribonucleic acid in the uterus. Endocrinology 1992; 130:3223–3230.
527. DeVore G, Owens O, Kase N. Use of intravenous Premarin in the treatment of dysfunctional uterine bleeding: a double-blind randomized control study. Obstet Gynecol 1982; 59:285–291.
528. Livio M, Mannucci P, Vigano G, et al. Conjugated estrogens for the management of bleeding associated with renal failure. N Engl J Med 1986; 315:731–735.
529. Olive D, Schwartz L. Endometriosis. N Engl J Med 1993; 328: 1759–1769.
530. Vercellini P, Cortesi I, Crosignani P. Progestins for symptomatic endometriosis: a critical analysis of the evidence. Fertil Steril 1997; 68:393–401.
531. Waller K, Shaw R. Gonadotropin-releasing hormone analogues for the treatment of endometriosis: long-term follow-up. Fertil Steril 1993; 59:511–515.
532. Shaw R. An open randomized comparative study of the effect of goserelin depot and danazol in the treatment of endometriosis. Zoladex Endometriosis Study Team. Fertil Steril 1992; 58:265–272.
533. A decision tree for the use of estrogen replacement therapy or hormone replacement therapy in postmenopausal women: consensus opinion of The North American Menopause Society. Menopause 2000; 7:76–86.
534. Vercellini P, Trespidi L, Colombo A, et al. A gonadotropin-releasing hormone agonist versus a low-dose oral contraceptive for pelvic pain associated with endometriosis. Fertil Steril 1993; 60:75–79.
535. Gestrinone Italian Study Group. Gestrinone versus a gonadotropin-releasing hormone agonist for the treatment of pelvic pain associated with endometriosis: a multicenter, randomized, double-blind study. Fertil Steril 1996; 66:911–919.
536. Takayama K, Zeitoun K, Gunby R, et al. Treatment of severe postmenopausal endometriosis with an aromatase inhibitor. Fertil Steril 1998; 69:709–723.
537. Stewart E. Uterine fibroids. Lancet 2001; 357:293–298.
538. Maruo T, Matsuo H, Samoto T, et al. Effects of progesterone on uterine leiomyoma growth and apoptosis. Steroids 2000; 65:585–592.
539. Haney A. Clinical decision making regarding leiomyomata: what we need in the next millennium. Environ Health Perspect 2000; 108(suppl):835–839.

540. McKinlay S, Brambilla D, Posner J. The normal menopause transition. Maturitas 1992; 14:103–115.
541. den Tonkelaar I, te Velde E, Looman C. Menstrual cycle length preceding menopause in relation to age at menopause. Maturitas 1998; 29:115–123.
542. Buckler H, Evans A, Mamlora H, et al. Gonadotropin, steroid and inhibin levels in women with incipient ovarian failure during anovulatory and ovulatory 'rebound' cycles. J Clin Endocrinol Metab 1991; 72:116–124.
543. MacNaughton J, Bangah M, McCloud P, et al. Age-related changes in follicle stimulating hormone, luteinizing hormone, oestradiol and immunoreactive inhibin in women of reproductive age. Clin Endocrinol (Oxf) 1992; 36:339–345.
544. Hee J, MacNaughton J, Bangah M, et al. Perimenopausal patterns of gonadotrophins, immunoreactive inhibin, oestradiol and progesterone. Maturitas 1993; 18:9–20.
545. Metcalf M, Livesay J. Gonadotropin excretion in fertile women: effect of age and the onset of the menopausal transition. J Endocrinol 1985; 10:357–362.
546. Rannevik G, Jeppsson S, Johnell O, et al. A longitudinal study of the perimenopausal transition: altered profiles of steroid and pituitary hormones, SHBG and bone mineral density. Maturitas 1995; 21:103–113.
547. Santoro N, Brown J, Adel T, et al. Characterization of reproductive hormonal dynamics in the perimenopause. J Clin Endocrinol Metab 1996; 81:1495–1501.
548. McKinlay S, Bigano N, McKinlay J. Smoking and age at menopause. Ann Intern Med 1985; 103:350–356.
549. Torgerson D, Avenell A, Russell I, et al. Factors associated with onset of menopause in women aged 45–49. Maturitas 1994; 19: 83–92.
550. Torgerson D, Thomas R, Campbell M, et al. Alcohol consumption and age of maternal menopause are associated with menopause onset. Maturitas 1997; 26:21–25.
551. Cramer D, Xu H, Harlow B. Family history as a predictor of early menopause. Fertil Steril 1995; 64:740–745.
552. Gosden R. Follicular status at menopause. Hum Reprod 1987; 2: 617–621.
553. Chakravarti S, Collins W, Forecast J, et al. Hormonal profiles after the menopause. Br Med J 1976; 2:784–787.
554. Jiroutek M, Chan M-H, Johnston C, et al. Changes in reproductive hormones and sex hormone–binding globulin in a group of postmenopausal women measured over 10 years. Menopause 1998; 5:90–94.
555. Adashi E. The climacteric ovary as a functional gonadotropin-driven androgen-producing gland. Fertil Steril 1994; 62:20–27.
556. Grodin J, Siiteri P, McDonald P. Source of estrogen production in postmenopausal women. J Clin Endocrinol Metab 1963; 36: 207.
557. Labrie F, Belanger A, Cusan L, et al. Marked decline in serum concentrations of adrenal C19 sex steroid precursors and conjugated androgen metabolites during aging. J Clin Endocrinol Metab 1997; 82:2396–2402.
558. Meldrum D, Davidson B, Tataryn I, et al. Changes in circulating steroids with aging in postmenopausal women. Obstet Gynecol 1981; 57:624–628.
559. Judd H, Judd G, Lucas W, et al. Endocrine function of the postmenopausal ovary: concentration of androgens and estrogens in ovarian and peripheral vein blood. J Clin Endocrinol Metab 1974; 39:1020–1024.
560. Bonneterre J, Buzdar A, Nabholtz J, et al. Anastrozole is superior to tamoxifen as first-line therapy in hormone receptor positive advanced breast carcinoma. Cancer 2001; 92:2247–2258.
561. Einerth Y. Vacuum curettage by the Vabra method: a simple procedure for endometrial diagnosis. Acta Obstet Gynecol Scand 1982; 61:373–376.
562. Feldman S, Shapter A, Welch W, et al. Two-year follow-up of 263 patients with post/perimenopausal vaginal bleeding and negative initial biopsy. Gynecol Oncol 1994; 55:56–59.
563. Oldenhave A, Jaszmann L, Haspels A, et al. Impact of climacteric on well-being. Am J Obstet Gynecol 1993; 168:772–780.
564. Kronnenberg F, Barnard R. Modulation of menopausal hot flashes by ambient temperature. J Therm Biol 1992; 17:43.
565. Yen S. The biology of menopause. J Reprod Med 1977; 18:287–296.
566. Erlik Y, Meldrum D, Judd H. Estrogen levels in postmenopausal women with hot flushes. Obstet Gynecol 1982; 59:403–407.
567. Davidson B, Gambone J, Lagasse L. Free estradiol in postmenopausal women with and without endometrial cancer. J Clin Endometrial Metab 1981; 52:404–408.
568. Raz R, Stamm W. A controlled trial of intravaginal estradiol in postmenopausal women with recurrent urinary tract infection. N Engl J Med 1993; 329:753–756.
569. Barrett A. Probable Alzheimer's disease: gender-related issues. J Gend Specif Med 1999; 2:55–60.
570. Geerlings M, Ruitenberg A, Witteman J, et al. Reproductive period and risk of dementia in postmenopausal women. JAMA 2001; 285:1475–1481.
571. LeBlanc E, Janowsky J, Chan B, et al. Hormone replacement therapy and cognition: systematic review and meta-analysis. JAMA 2001; 285:1489–1499.
572. Henderson V, Paganini-Hill A, Miller B, et al. Estrogen for Alzheimer's disease in women: a randomized, double-blind, placebo-controlled trial. Neurology 2000; 54:295–301.
573. Asthana S, Baker L, Craft S, et al. High-dose estradiol improves cognition for women with AD: results of a randomized study. Neurology 2001; 57:605–612.
574. Matthews K, Meilahn E, Kuller L, et al. Menopause and risk factors for coronary heart disease. N Engl J Med 1989; 321:641–646.
575. Campos H, McNamara J, Wilson P, et al. Differences in low density lipoprotein subfractions and apolipoproteins in premenopausal and postmenopausal women. J Clin Endocrinol Metab 1988; 67:30–35.
576. Stevenson J, Crook D, Godsland I. Influence of age and menopause on serum lipids and lipoproteins in healthy women. Atherosclerosis 1993; 98:83–90.
577. van Beresteijn E, Korevaar J, Huijbregts P, et al. Perimenopausal increase in serum cholesterol: a 10-year longitudinal study. Am J Epidemiol 1993; 137:383–392.
578. Matthews K, Wing R, Kuller L, et al. Influence of the perimenopause on cardiovascular risk factors and symptoms of middle-aged healthy women. Arch Intern Med 1994; 154:2349–2355.
579. Bruschi F, Meschia M, Soma M, et al. Lipoprotein(a) and other lipids after oophorectomy and estrogen replacement therapy. Obstet Gynecol 1996; 88:950–954.
580. Walsh B, Schiff I, Rosner B, et al. Effects of postmenopausal estrogen replacement on the concentrations and metabolism of plasma lipoproteins. N Engl J Med 1991; 325:1196–1204.
581. Brunner D, Weisbort J, Meshulam N, et al. Relation of serum total cholesterol and high-density lipoprotein cholesterol percentage to the incidence of definite coronary events: twenty-year follow-up of the Donolo–Tel Aviv Prospective Coronary Artery Disease Study. Am J Cardiol 1987; 59:1271–1276.
582. Jacobs JD, Mebane I, Bangdiwala S, et al. High density lipoprotein cholesterol as a predictor of cardiovascular disease mortality in men and women: the follow-up study of the Lipid Research Clinics Prevalence Study. Am J Epidemiol 1990; 131:32–47.
583. Hulley S, Newman T. Cholesterol in the elderly: is it important? JAMA 1994; 272:1372–1374.
584. Kannel W. Metabolic risk factors for coronary heart disease in women: perspective from the Framingham Study. Am Heart J 1987; 114:413–419.
585. Downs J, Clearfield M, Weis S, et al. Primary prevention of acute coronary events with lovastatin in men and women with average cholesterol levels: results of AFCAPS/TexCAPS. JAMA 1998; 279:1615–1622.
586. Espeland M, Marcovina S, Miller V, et al. Effect of postmenopausal hormone therapy on lipoprotein(a) concentration. PEPI Investigators. Postmenopausal Estrogen/Progestin Interventions. Circulation 1998; 97:979–986.
587. The Writing Group for the PEPI Trial. Effects of estrogen or estrogen/progestin regimens on heart disease risk factors in postmenopausal women: the Postmenopausal Estrogen/Progestin Interventions (PEPI) trial. JAMA 1995; 273:199–208.
588. Hulley S, Grady D, Bush T, et al. Randomized trial of estrogen plus progestin for secondary prevention of coronary heart disease in postmenopausal women. JAMA 1998; 280:605–613.
589. Spinler S, Hilleman D, Cheng J, et al. New recommendations from the 1999 American College of Cardiology/American Heart Association acute myocardial infarction guidelines. Ann Pharmacother 2001; 35:589–617.
590. Grady D, Wenger N, Herrington D, et al. Postmenopausal hor-

mone therapy increases risk for venous thromboembolic disease. The Heart and Estrogen/progestin Replacement Study. Ann Intern Med 2000; 132:689–696.

591. Simon J, Hsia J, Cauley J, et al. Postmenopausal hormone therapy and risk of stroke: the Heart and Estrogen-progestin Replacement Study (HERS). Circulation 2001; 103:620–622.
592. Simon J, Hunninghake D, Agarwal S, et al. Effect of estrogen plus progestin on risk for biliary tract surgery in postmenopausal women with coronary artery disease. The Heart and Estrogen/progestin Replacement Study. Ann Intern Med 2001; 135:493–501.
593. Viscoli C, Brass L, Kernan W, et al. A clinical trial of estrogen-replacement therapy after ischemic stroke. N Engl J Med 2001; 345:1243–1249.
593a. Writing Group for the Women's Health Initiative. Risks and benefits of estrogen plus progestin in healthy postmenopausal women. JAMA 2002; 288:321–333.
594. Dempster D, Lindsay R. Pathogenesis of osteoporosis. Lancet 1993; 341:797–801.
595. Richelson L, Wahner H, Melton L III, et al. Relative contributions of aging and estrogen deficiency to postmenopausal bone loss. N Engl J Med 1984; 311:1273–1275.
596. Nilas L, Christiansen C. Bone mass and its relationship to age and the menopause. J Clin Endocrinol Metab 1987; 65:697–702.
597. Johnston JC, Hui S, Witt R, et al. Early menopausal changes in bone mass and sex steroids. J Clin Endocrinol Metab 1985; 61: 905–911.
598. Christiansen C. Hormone replacement therapy and osteoporosis. Maturitas 1996; 23(suppl):S71–S76.
599. Brett K, Madans J. Use of postmenopausal hormone replacement therapy: estimates from a nationally representative cohort study. Am J Epidemiol 1997; 145:536–545.
600. Riis B, Hansen M, Jensen A, et al. Low bone mass and fast rate of bone loss at menopause: equal risk factors for future fracture: a 15-year follow-up study. Bone 1996; 19:9–12.
601. Lindsay R, Hart D, Clark D. The minimum effective dose of estrogen for postmenopausal bone loss. Obstet Gynecol 1984; 63: 759–763.
602. Genant H, Baylink D, Gallagher J. Estrogens in the prevention of osteoporosis in postmenopausal women. Am J Obstet Gynecol 1989; 161:1842–1846.
603. Doren M, Samsioe G. Prevention of postmenopausal osteoporosis with oestrogen replacement therapy and associated compounds: update on clinical trials since 1995. Hum Reprod Update 2000; 6:419–426.
604. Maxim P, Ettinger B, Spitalny G. Fracture protection provided by long-term estrogen treatment. Osteoporos Int 1995; 5:23–29.
605. Lufkin E, Wahner H, O'Fallon W, et al. Treatment of postmenopausal osteoporosis with transdermal estrogen. Ann Intern Med 1992; 117:1–9.
606. Balfour J, McTavish D. Transdermal estradiol: a review of its pharmacological profile, and therapeutic potential in the prevention of postmenopausal osteoporosis. Drugs Aging 1992; 2:487–507.
607. Alexandersen P, Riis B, Christiansen C. Monofluorophosphate combined with hormone replacement therapy induces a synergistic effect on bone mass by dissociating bone formation and resorption in postmenopausal women: a randomized study. J Clin Endocrinol Metab 1999; 84:3013–3020.
608. Hillard T, Whitcroft S, Marsh M, et al. Long-term effects of transdermal and oral hormone replacement therapy on postmenopausal bone loss. Osteoporos Int 1994; 4:341–348.
609. O'Connell M. Pharmacokinetic and pharmacologic variation between different estrogen products. J Clin Pharmacol 1995; 35: 18S–24S.
610. Reginster J, Sarlet N, Deroisy R, et al. Minimal levels of serum estradiol prevent post-menopausal bone loss. Calcif Tissue Int 1998; 51:340–343.
611. Scott RJ, Ross B, Anderson C, et al. Pharmacokinetics of percutaneous estradiol: a crossover study using a gel and a transdermal system in comparison with oral micronized estradiol. Obstet Gynecol 1991; 77:758–764.
612. Steingold K, Laufer L, Chetkowski R, et al. Treatment of hot flashes with transdermal estradiol administration. J Clin Endocrinol Metab 1985; 61:627–632.
613. Setnikar I, Rovati L, Vens-Cappell B, et al. Pharmacokinetics of estradiol and estrone during application of a new 7-day estradiol transdermal patch with active matrix. Arzneimittelforschung 1998; 48:275–285.
614. Pines A, Fishman E, Ayalon D, et al. Long-term effects of hormone replacement therapy on Doppler-derived parameters of aortic flow in postmenopausal women. Chest 1992; 102:1496–1498.
615. Pines A, Fisman E, Averbuch M, et al. The long-term effects of transdermal estradiol on left ventricular function and dimensions. Eur J Menopause 1995; 2:22.
616. Pines A, Fisman E, Shapira I, et al. Exercise echocardiography in postmenopausal hormone users with mild hypertension. Am J Cardiol 1996; 78:1385–1389.
617. Pines A, Fisman E, Drory Y, et al. The effects of sublingual estradiol on left ventricular action at rest and exercise in postmenopausal women: an echocardiographic assessment. Menopause 1998; 5:79–85.
618. Lindheim S, Presser S, Kitkoff E, et al. A possible bimodal effect of estrogen on insulin sensitivity in postmenopausal women and the attenuating effect of added progestin. Fertil Steril 1993; 60: 664–667.
619. Stampfer M, Colditz G, Willett W, et al. Postmenopausal estrogen therapy and cardiovascular disease: ten-year follow-up from the Nurse's Health Study. N Engl J Med 1991; 325:756–762.
620. Henderson B, Paganini-Hill A, Ross R. Decreased mortality in users of estrogen replacement therapy. Arch Intern Med 1991; 151:75–78.
621. Ettinger B, Friedman G, Bush T, et al. Reduced mortality associated with long-term postmenopausal estrogen therapy. Obstet Gynecol 1996; 87:6–12.
622. Woodruff J, Pickar J. Incidence of endometrial hyperplasia in postmenopausal women taking conjugated estrogens (Premarin) with medroxyprogesterone acetate or conjugated estrogens alone. The Menopause Study Group. Am J Obstet Gynecol 1994; 170: 1213–1223.
623. Archer D, Pickar J, Bottiglioni F. Bleeding patterns in postmenopausal women taking continuous combined or sequential regimens of conjugated estrogens with medroxyprogesterone acetate. Menopause Study Group. Obstet Gynecol 1994; 83:686–692.
624. Speroff T, Dawson N, Speroff L, et al. A risk-benefit analysis of elective bilateral oophorectomy: effect of change in compliance with estrogen therapy on outcome. Am J Obstet Gynecol 1991; 164:165–174.
625. Berman R, Epstein R, Lydick E. Compliance of women in taking estrogen replacement therapy. J Womens Health 1996; 213.
626. Ravnikar V. Compliance with hormonal therapy. Am J Obstet Gynecol 1987; 156:1332–1334.
627. Dardes R, Jordan V. Novel agents to modulate oestrogen action. Br Med Bull 2000; 56:773–786.
628. Diez J. Skeletal effects of selective oestrogen receptor modulators (SERMs). Hum Reprod Update 2000; 6:255–258.
629. Clemett D, Spencer C. Raloxifene: a review of its use in postmenopausal osteoporosis. Drugs 2000; 60:379–411.
630. Burger H. Selective oestrogen receptor modulators. Horm Res 2000; 53(suppl):25–29.
631. Nand S, Webster M, Baber R, et al. Bleeding pattern and endometrial changes during continuous combined hormone replacement. Obstet Gynecol 1998; 91:678–684.
632. Archer D, McIntyre-Seltman K, Wilborn W, et al. Endometrial morphology in asymptomatic postmenopausal women. Am J Obstet Gynecol 1991; 165:317–320.
633. Korhonen M, Symons J, Hyde B, et al. Histologic classification and pathologic findings for endometrial biopsy specimens obtained from 2964 perimenopausal and postmenopausal women undergoing screening for continuous hormones as replacement therapy (CHART 2 Study). Am J Obstet Gynecol 1997; 176: 377–380.
634. McGonigle K, Karlan B, Barabuto D, et al. Development of endometrial cancer in women on estrogen and progestin hormone replacement therapy. Gynecol Oncol 1994; 55:126–132.
635. Karlsson B, Granberg S, Wikland M, et al. Transvaginal ultrasonography of the endometrium in women with postmenopausal bleeding: a Nordic multicenter study. Am J Obstet Gynecol 1995; 172:1488–1494.
636. Bakos O, Smith P, Heimer G. Transvaginal ultrasonography for identifying endometrial pathology in postmenopausal women. Maturitas 1995; 20:181–189.

637. Granberg S, Ylosstalo P, Wikland M, et al. Endometrial sonographic and histologic findings in women with and without hormonal replacement therapy suffering from postmenopausal bleeding. Maturitas 1997; 27:35–40.
638. Grodstein F, Stampfer M, Goldhaber S, et al. Prospective study of exogenous hormones and risk of pulmonary embolism in women. Lancet 1996; 348:983–987.
639. Daly E, Vesey M, Hawkins M, et al. Risk of venous thromboembolism in users of hormone replacement therapy. Lancet 1996; 348:977–980.
640. Jick H, Derby L, Myers M, et al. Risk of hospital admission for idiopathic venous thromboembolism among users of postmenopausal oestrogens. Lancet 1996; 348:981–983.
641. Varas-Lorenzo C, Garcia-Rodriguez L, Cattaruzzi C, et al. Hormone replacement therapy and the risk of hospitalization for venous thromboembolism: a population-based study in Southern Europe. Am J Epidemiol 1998; 147:387–390.
642. Gutthann S, Rodriguez L, Castellsague J, et al. Hormone replacement therapy and risk of venous thromboembolism: population based case-control study. Br Med J 1997; 314:796–800.
643. Cummings S, Norton L, Eckert S, et al. Raloxifene reduces the risk of breast cancer and may decrease the risk of endometrial cancer in postmenopausal women: two-year findings from the Multiple Outcomes of Raloxifene Evaluation (MORE) trial. http:/www.asco.org/, 1998.
644. Glueck C, Lang J, Hamer T, et al. Severe hypertriglyceridemia and pancreatitis when estrogen replacement therapy is given to hypertriglyceridemic women. J Lab Clin Med 1994; 123:59–64.
645. Grodstein F, Colditz G, Stampfer M. Postmenopausal hormone use and cholecystectomy in a large prospective study. Obstet Gynecol 1994; 83:5–11.
646. Petitti D, Sidney S, Perlamn J. Increased risk of cholecystectomy in users of supplemental estrogen. Gastroenterology 1988; 94:91–95.
647. LaVecchia C, Negri E, D'Avanzo B, et al. Oral contraceptives and noncontraceptive oestrogens in the risk of gallstone disease requiring surgery. J Epidemiol Community Health 1992; 46:234–236.
648. Koukoulis G. Hormone replacement therapy and breast cancer risk. Ann NY Acad Sci 2000; 900:422–428.
649. Santen R, Pinkerton J, McCartney C, Petroni G. Risk of breast cancer with progestins in combination with estrogen as hormone replacement therapy. J Clin Endocrinol Metab 2001; 86:16–23.
650. Col N, Hirota L, Orr R, et al. Hormone replacement therapy after breast cancer: a systematic review and quantitative assessment of risk. J Clin Oncol 2001; 19:2357–2363.
651. O'Meara E, Rossing M, Daling J, et al. Hormone replacement therapy with a diagnosis of breast cancer in relation to occurrence and mortality. J Natl Cancer Inst 2001; 93:754–762.

17 Fertility Control: Current Approaches and Global Aspects

Michael Kafrissen and Eli Adashi

GLOBAL ASPECTS OF FERTILITY CONTROL

Regulation of human fertility encompasses social, legal, and health care measures, including the employment of medical technologies and procedures that result in limiting the number of offspring. This can be achieved by spacing the birth of individual children in the sense of family planning or by terminating procreation when the desired family size has been achieved. The aim of fertility control is to achieve a family or population size that is compatible with a reasonable quality of life and is culturally and economically supported.

Growth of the Human Population

History and Current Status

The explosion of the world population is a relatively recent phenomenon (Fig. 17–1). By AD 1, 200 million people lived on this planet. By 1650, more than 1600 years later, this number had increased to 500 million. Thereafter, the population-doubling time became progressively shorter. By 1850, the human population numbered 1 billion, and within 80 years, in 1930, the population reached 2 billion. In 2000 the world population crossed the 6 billion milestone, and the growth continues.[1, 2]

Consequences of Overpopulation: From Malthus to Ehrlich

During the industrial revolution, Thomas Malthus, an English political economist, noticed the soaring population of the British Isles, a geographic area with limited arable land, and concluded that the human population would outrun the available food supplies. Between 1798 and 1816, Malthus published a series of essays in which he predicted that a collision of population growth and lack of world food supplies would result in worldwide disasters such as famines, epidemics, and wars. Malthus believed that strict limits on reproduction were essential to the betterment of humankind.[3]

In 1968, at a time when humankind experienced the most prominent population increase (see Fig. 17–1), Paul Ehrlich, a biologist at Stanford University, brought the issue of overpopulation to the public consciousness in his disquisition *The Population Bomb*. Ehrlich pointed out the negative effects of population growth on the environment, nonrenewable natural resources, and general economic progress.[4, 5]

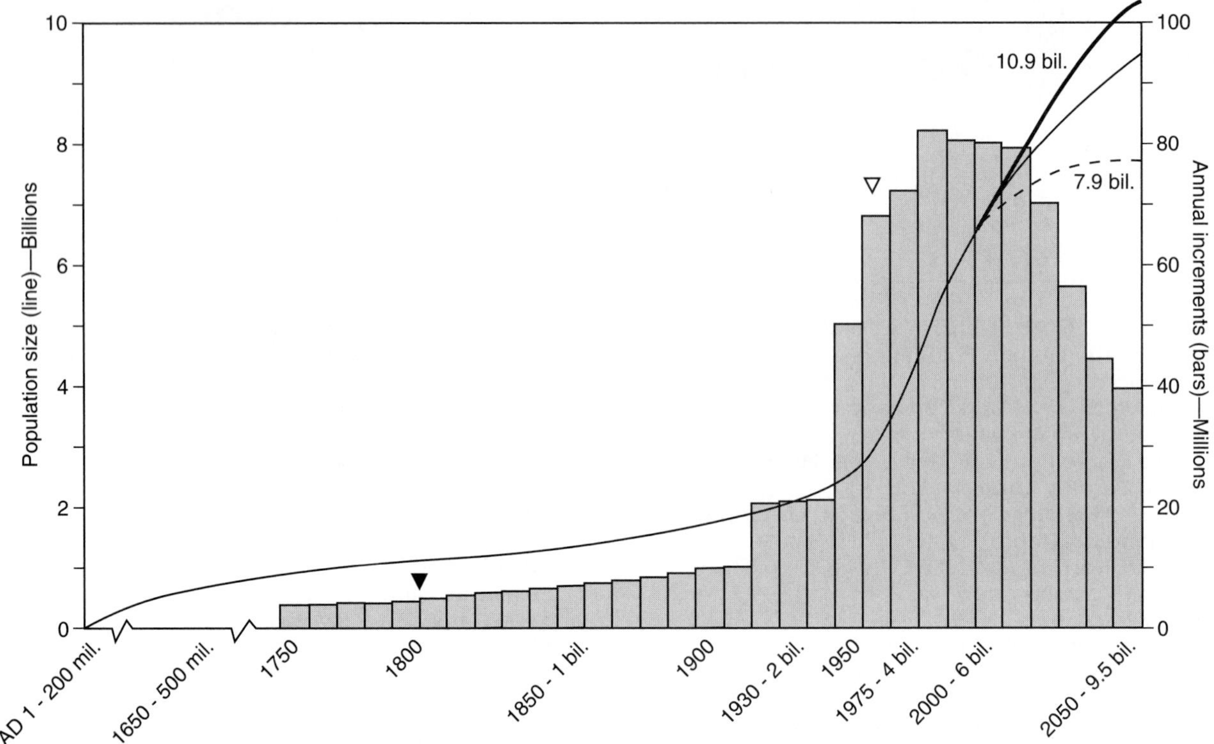

Figure 17-1. The growth of the world population (billion) and increments by decades (million). (▼) Publication of Malthus' essay on population. Since then, the world population has increased six times. (▽) Publication of Paul Ehrlich's *The Population Bomb*. Since then, the world population has increased from 4 billion to 6 billion. (Modified from Raleigh VS. Trends in world population: how will the millennium compare with the past? Hum Reprod Update 1999; 5:500.)

Coping with the Population Growth

Human ingenuity has largely disproved the predictions of both Malthus and Ehrlich. The extraordinary demographic history of the 20th century that occurred without global malthusian disasters can be explained mainly by two phenomena: innovations in agriculture and advances in medicine.[6–8]

Agriculture: From the Neolithic to the Green Revolution

Historically, the phases in which the growth of the world population took an upward trend have coincided with improvement in agricultural techniques. In the Neolithic era, humans started to grow food supplies and this transition from hunting and gathering resulted in the first substantial population growth. However, further agricultural progress was slow, and so was the population growth.

Not until the 18th and 19th centuries were more advanced agricultural methods applied. The industrialization of agriculture dates only from the beginning of the 20th century, when the farm tractor, introduced in Iowa in 1901, led to mechanization of the farmer's work. Further improvements, known collectively as the *green revolution*, followed. They included the use of chemical fertilizers, herbicides, and insecticides; the development of hybrid grains; and, more recently, the genetic manipulation of rice and grains. Farmers in the United States planted hybrid seeds and increased yields of grains by one third in only one decade, between 1930 and 1940.[6, 8] During the first 35 years of the green revolution, global grain production doubled.

Famine, which historically has been a worldwide and perennial problem, became much less of a threat in the 20th century. Although the last 100 years have seen devastating famines in numerous areas of the world and millions of undernourished people have died, the demographic impact of these famines was relatively local and short-term. Famines are endemic on the Indian subcontinent, for example, but its population increased from 300,000 in the year 1900 to 1.3 billion in 2001. Despite predictions that the world population would outstrip food production, food production has risen a full 16% above population growth.[9] Today, there are fewer hungry people than ever before in history. In 1996, the number of hungry people of the world was 17%, whereas in 1970, 25 years earlier, 35% of the world's people fit in the "hungry" classification.[9]

The increased productivity of industrialized agriculture has demographic consequences. Currently, 2% of the world's farmers, most of them in developed and rapidly developing countries, produce one fourth of the world's food. The reduced need for workers has liberated the industrial farmer from the pressure to have a large family. By contrast, traditional farmers, mostly in the underdeveloped countries, still feel the need to secure the necessary agricultural workforce through having more children.[6, 8]

The success of industrial farming, however, came at a price. The expansion of arable land disturbed the balance of the ecosystem. For example, deforestation and reduction of natural pastures led to droughts and floods in certain areas. During the next 50 years, the growing global population will require further advances in agricultural production to ensure a sufficient, secure, and equitable food supply. To control—and pos-

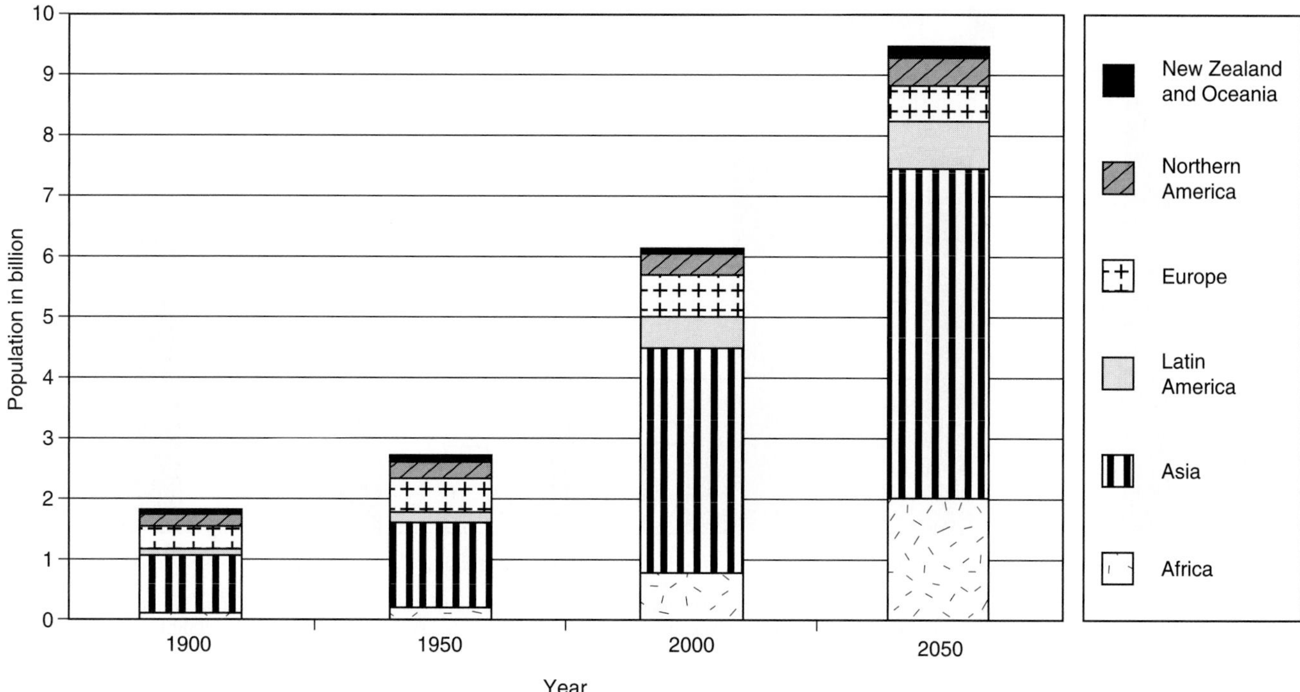

Figure 17–2. The population growth in individual continents. (From United Nations Population Division. World Population Prospects: The 2000 Revision. New York, United Nations, 2000.)

sibly reverse—the environmental impacts of agricultural expansion, intensive scientific efforts must be implemented along with regulatory, technologic, and policy changes.[10, 11]

Medicine: From Art to Science

During the 20th century, major advances in the practice of medicine and the application of preventive medicine increased worldwide population survival rates. A number of factors contributed to enhanced survival: an increase in the number of infants born alive, a decrease in infant and child mortality, and the containment of the spread of major epidemics. In the developed countries, the perinatal mortality rate fell from 225 per 1000 live births to under 20 per 1000. In the less developed countries, the perinatal mortality rate also decreased, but the disparity between underdeveloped and some industrialized nations was staggering. In 1988, the perinatal mortality was 5 per 1000 for Japan but it was 118 per 1000 for Bangladesh.[8]

Globally, life expectancy increased from approximately 30 years at the beginning of the 20th century to 47 years in the middle of the century and 65 years by the end of the century. It is projected that by the year 2050, life expectancy will be 76 years. The current 180,000 living centenarians—most of them in Europe, Japan, China, and the United States—best attest to the improved health conditions of humankind.

The kinds of epidemics that decimated populations in the past have become less of a peril. Historians estimate that in the 1350s, in medieval England, the epidemic of plague—known as the "black death"—reduced the total English population by 20% and decreased life expectancy to under 18 years.[7] The acquired immunodeficiency syndrome (AIDS), a modern-day parallel to a medieval plague, has taken its toll mainly in Africa, where 28 million of the 36 million AIDS-afflicted people live. Nevertheless, even in the sub-Saharan nations, where the incidence of AIDS is as high as 30% and life expectancy has been reduced to 37.2 years, the population continues to expand, although at a slower rate than before the outbreak of the epidemic. However, in some countries of sub-Saharan Africa, notably in South Africa and Zimbabwe, a negative growth rate is expected.[1]

In summary, malthusian predictions of global catastrophes caused by overpopulation did not materialize. However, the balance of a steadily growing population and potential technologic limitations on resources remains precarious.

Population Projections

Current projections for the growth of the world population by the middle of the 21st century vary from 7.9 billion to 10.9 billion (see Fig. 17–1).[1, 2] With respect to individual continents, Asia will remain the most populous. The most significant growth is expected to occur in Africa, with the population rising from the current 900 million to 2 billion. Notable population growth is also projected for countries in both North America and Latin America. The United States will probably be the only industrialized nation with a population increase. The population of Europe is expected to decrease (Fig. 17–2).[1] However, there is a broader question related to the world population growth, namely what is the optimal number of people the world can support? In 1994, a serious attempt to answer this question was made at the International Conference on Population and Development, now known as the Cairo Conference. The conference forecasted a world population of 10 billion in 2050 and recommended holding the population at that level.[12, 13]

The Future of the World Population

Medical progress has affected human demographics by another innovation: the development of effective means of preventing pregnancy. Introduced in the 1960s when the population was increasing, modern contraception was immediately recognized as a potential instrument for large-scale family planning.[6]

Indeed, available demographic data show that since the 1980s, population growth rates, along with fertility rates, have

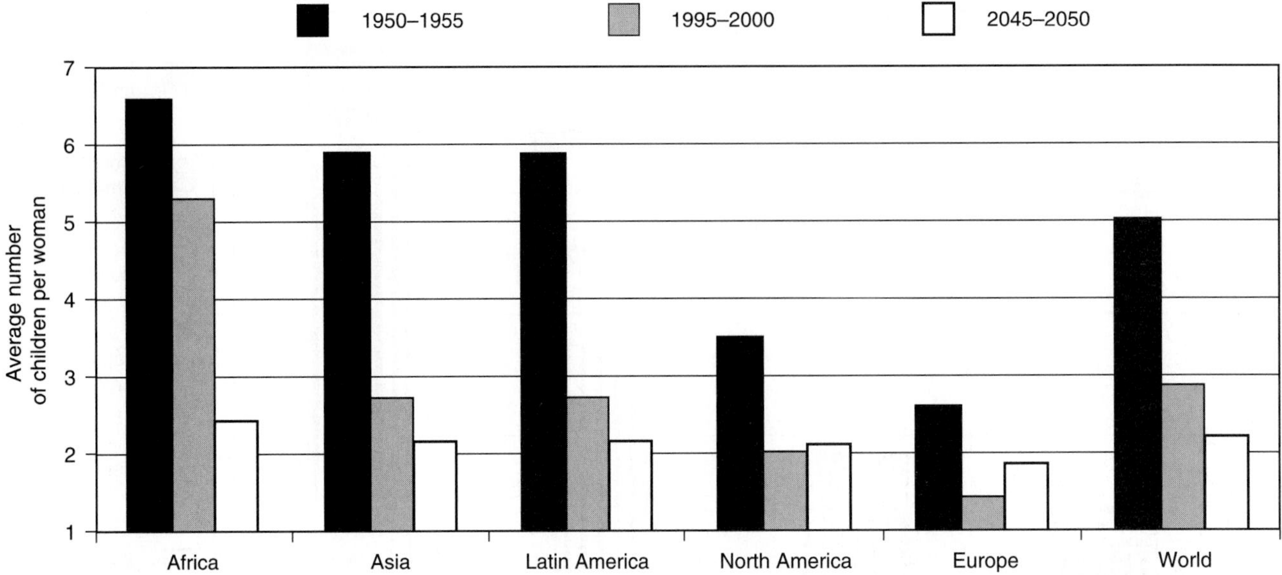

Figure 17–3. Birth rates from 1950 to 2000 and projections for the first half of the 21st century. (From United Nations Population Division. World Population Prospects: The 2000 Revision. New York, United Nations, 2000.)

been falling (Fig. 17–3; see Fig. 17–1). This signifies a tapering off of the most rapid phase of world population growth. However, the data also show that the momentum of growth will persist into the middle of this century, when the world population is projected to be 10 billion.

The goal of holding the world population at 10 billion can be accomplished if the fertility rate is limited to an average of 2.1 children per woman, the essential replacement rate; this can be achieved by effective fertility control.[14]

The Role of Family Planning

Historically, most societies rewarded families for having children by reducing their tax burden and giving awards to mothers of numerous children. In the second half of the last century, however, certain societies, pressured by overpopulation, installed strong disincentives for families that had more than a prescribed number of children. In China, for example, a family that has more than the allowable one child is castigated. In Singapore, a highly developed but crowded country, the acceptable number of children for a family used to be determined, among other things, by the parents' educational level. In other cultural environments, the government resorted to positive incentives by providing gifts to individuals who underwent voluntary sterilization. Coercive methods of family planning have been criticized and are globally unacceptable.[15]

Modern family planning must respect the freedom of reproductive choices, free access to family planning facilities, and availability of up-to-date methods of fertility control. Individual families as well as entire nations must be educated to comprehend that effective family planning makes good social and economic sense. Currently available data show that the decrease of birth rates is inversely proportional to the percentage of the population practicing contraception. The data also show that nations enjoying the highest living standards—or those striving to overcome economic hurdles—have the lowest birth rates. Examples of the latter are the countries of the former Eastern European bloc (Fig. 17–4).

Effective fertility control can be achieved only when the society supports it. Initially, after their introduction in the 1960s, modern methods of human fertility control were accessible only to the affluent. Today, in the milieu of globalization, contraception has become a matter of governmental policy in many nations. It is also of primary concern to global organizations such as the World Health Organization (WHO) and the United Nations Educational, Scientific, and Cultural Organization as well as private institutions such as the Population Council and the Alan Guttmacher Institute of Family Planning.

The Role of the Physician and Other Health Care Givers in Fertility Control

Health care givers in nearly all specialties have become increasingly involved in issues of fertility control. Practitioners ranging from pediatricians who care for teenage girls to internists who care for premenopausal women are frequently asked to provide contraceptive advice.

The role of medical specialists in reproductive health care is also undergoing a transition. Two major challenges have arisen. The first is a result of the existing and widening cultural diversification in developed countries, where physicians frequently face problems that not only challenge their medical skills but also test their ability to deal with the family planning needs of communities with diverse ethnic, cultural, and religious backgrounds. The second challenge has to be met by all those working in reproductive health care and family planning: the increasing emphasis on state-of-the-art medical practice. There is a global need for the rapid incorporation of appropriate technologies into daily clinical practice, substantially increasing the quality of rational medical care, worldwide.[16]

The individual methods and technologies of fertility control are discussed in the following sections of this chapter.

Methods of Fertility Control: Efficacy, Continuation of Use, Changing Trends

When making a recommendation to a candidate for contraception, three aspects of each method have to be examined: efficacy, tolerability, and whether the method is suitable for temporary or permanent cessation of procreation.

Table 17–1 lists the principal methods of fertility control currently available and indicates their contraceptive efficacy as

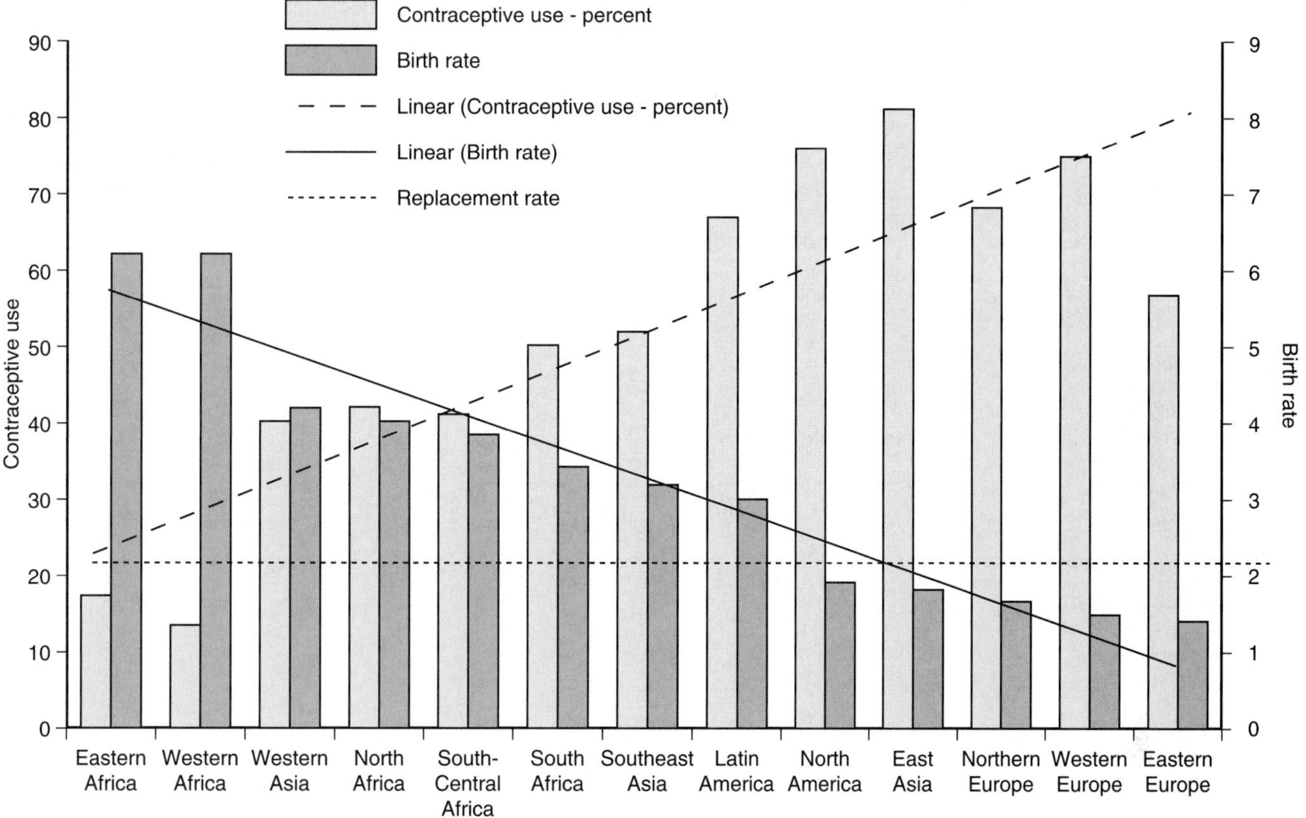

Figure 17-4. The decrease of the birth rate is inversely proportional to the percentage of the population practicing contraception and positively related to the standard of living. (Modified from Potts M. The unmet need for family planning. Sci Am 2000; 282[1]:69.)

well as the average time patients adhere to an individual method.[17–19] The estimates of contraceptive failure during "perfect" use are derived from studies conducted for research and registration purposes; they include volunteers—a self-selected group—who are highly motivated to adhere to the study protocol. Therefore, the results are more favorable than those obtained during "typical" use, that is, use in the general population. Data on the efficacy for typical use are generated by the National Surveys of Family Growth, among others.[20]

Efficacy and Continuation

If the outcome was left to chance—that is, no method of fertility control was practiced—85 of 100 women of reproductive age would become pregnant within a year. Surgical sterilization, for both men and women, remains one of the most effective methods of contraception, although it is not failure proof. The small proportion of early failures may be associated with suboptimal surgical techniques, such as mistaking other anatomic structures for the fallopian tube or vas deferens; insufficient electrocoagulation when this method is used in women; or unprotected early intercourse after vasectomy while live spermatozoa are still present in the part of vas deferens that is distal to the interruption. Late failures, between the 3rd and 10th years after surgery, also occur and are discussed in the section on sterilization. The major advantage of surgical sterilization is that it is permanent and can be a welcome solution to parents with large families. Chemical sterilization of women aims at producing tubal occlusion by injection of a substance (e.g., quinacrine) into the junction between the tube and the uterus. Data from a large study conducted in Vietnam show that this method is inferior to surgical sterilization.[21, 22]

Among the hormonal contraceptive methods, long-acting approaches such as implants, injectables, and copper- or hormone-containing intrauterine devices (IUDs) achieve a higher level of efficacy than oral contraceptives (OCs) that require a daily conscientious action by the user. According to revised data of 1995,[20] the failure rates of OC formulations are higher than previously thought. Emergency postcoital contraception, when properly used, is also effective; however, it is recommended only as an emergency provision.

Hormonal methods of fertility control also encompass nonsurgical termination of pregnancy by pharmacologic means ("contragestion"). Mifepristone and prostaglandins administered not later than the seventh week of pregnancy achieve complete abortion in a high proportion of cases. The procedure is less effective when employed after the seventh week of pregnancy.

The efficacy of IUDs has been improved by incorporating either progesterone or a synthetic progestogen, levonorgestrel. The copper IUD has staged an impressive revival, principally outside the United States. Its efficacy and safety have been improved and are now comparable to those of hormonal contraception. Copper- and progestin-bearing IUDs are likely to continue to grow in popularity.

Other methods of fertility control are less effective. For the barrier methods, there is a large discrepancy between the efficacy of ideal use and that of typical use. With the cervical cap and the vaginal sponge, failure rates are high even with perfect use. The same applies to the "natural" methods of fertility control. They rely, one way or another, on prediction or detection of ovulation and require continuous watchfulness and motivation of both partners. Therefore, their efficacy does not compare favorably with that of the hormonal or intrauterine

Table 17–1. Fertility Control Methods: Failure Rates and Continuation of Use (United States Data)

Method	Percent Pregnant during First Year of Use: Estimates 1987 and 1990,* All Methods — Perfect use	Typical	Estimates 1995,† Reversible Methods	Continuation after First Year of Use* (%)
Chance	85	85	85	?
Sterilization				
Male	0.1	0.2		100
Female	0.2	0.4	ND	100
Surgical				
Chemical (quinacrine)‡				
Women <35 y		13.0		?
Women ≥35 y		7.0		?
Hormonal contraception, emergency contraception, and contragestion				
Combination pill	0.1	5.0	8.0	78
Progestagen-only pill	0.5	5.0		81
Norplant	0.05	0.05	2.0	85
Depo-Provera	0.3	0.3	3.0	70
Emergency contraception—hormonal	0.1	3.0	ND	ND
Contragestion—pharmacologic abortion	1.0–5.0 (up to 7 wk)	9.0 (> 7 wk)	ND	ND
Intrauterine devices (IUDs)				
IUD-progesterone T	1.5	2.0		80
IUD-levonorgestrel 20	0.1	0.1	ND	81
IUD-T 380 (copper)	0.6	0.8		78
Barrier methods				
Condom				
Male	3.0	14.0	14.0	63
Female	5.0	21.0	ND	56
Diaphragm	6.0	20.0	18.0	58
Cervical cap				
Parous women	26.0	40.0	12.0	42
Nulliparous women	9.0	20.0		56
Sponge				
Parous women	20.0	40.0		42
Nulliparous women	9.0	20.0	ND	56
Spermicides	6.0	26.0	26.0	40
Withdrawal	4.0	19.0	24.0	?
Periodic abstinence§				63
Calendar	9.0	?		
Ovulation method	3.0	?	21.0	
Postovulation	1.0	?		
Symptothermal[d]	2.0	?		
Lactational amenorrhea provides an effective but temporary method of contraception				

*Data from references 17, 18, 19.
†New estimates of contraceptive failure according to correction for abortion underreporting, from 1995 National Survey of Family Growth.[20]
‡Data on quinacrine sterilization from reference 21.
§Periodic abstinence methods. *Calendar:* The woman records the length of 6 to 12 cycles and determines the beginning of the fertile period by subtracting 18 days from the shortest cycle. The end of the fertile period is estimated by subtracting 11 days from the longest cycle. *Ovulation method*: Women are taught to recognize the character of the cervical mucus during the fertile period. Sexual abstinence begins on the day when the mucus becomes clear, slippery, and stretchy (usually a few days before ovulation). At the peak of the fertile period, the mucus stretches between the finger and thumb to the maximum (spinnbarkeit). Intercourse is resumed on the third or fourth day after the peak mucus. *Symptothermal method:* Cervical mucus (ovulation) method supplemented by calendar in the preovulatory phase and basal body temperature in the postovulatory phase. *Postovulatory method*: Ovulation is estimated by the basal body temperature or cervical mucus methods; unprotected intercourse is allowed 3 to 4 days thereafter. *Note*: Sophisticated electronic devices are currently available to estimate ovulation more precisely, some of them measuring the estrogen and luteinizing hormone concentrations in urine.
ND, no data.

methods. Lactational amenorrhea affords protection against pregnancy; however, breakthrough ovulations do occur, particularly when breast-feeding is not exclusive and is interrupted by other types of baby nourishment.

Women frequently discontinue the use of contraception. Overall, 31% of women discontinue use of reversible contraceptives for a method-related reason within 6 months of use; 44% do so within 12 months. However, 68% of women overall resume use of a method within 1 month and 76% do so within 3 months. High rates of method-related discontinuations reflect dissatisfaction with available methods or management, or both.[23]

Trends in Fertility Control in the United States

In the third quarter of the last century, the use of fertility control methods in the United States underwent a major change (Table 17–2).[24, 25]

Among women, hormonal contraception has remained the most popular method. Two events positively influenced the employment of hormonal methods: the advent of hormonal implants and the approval of medroxyprogesterone acetate (MPA) depot injections for contraception.

As physicians became versatile in laparoscopic surgeries, the

Table 17–2. Trend in Contraceptive Use by Women 15 to 44 Years of Age in the United States, 1973 to 1995 (Percent Users)

Method	1973*	1982†	1988†	1995†
Sterilization	23.5	34.1	39.2	38.6
Female	12.3	23.2	27.5	27.7
Male	11.2	10.9	11.7	10.9
Hormonal methods	36.1	28.0	30.7	31.2
Pill	36.1	28.0	30.7	26.9
Implant	NA	NA	NA	1.3
Injectable	NA	NA	NA	3.0
Intrauterine device	9.6	7.1	2.0	0.8
Diaphragm	3.4	8.1	5.7	1.9
Male condom	13.5	12.0	14.6	20.4
Foam	5.0	2.4	1.1	0.4
Periodic abstinence	4.0	3.9	2.3	2.3
Withdrawal	2.1	2.0	2.2	3.0
Other‡	2.7	2.5	2.1	1.3

*Data from Ford K. Contraceptive utilization among currently married women 15–44 years of age: United States, 1973. Mon Vital Stat 1976; 25/7 (suppl): 1–15.

†Data from Piccino LJ, Mosher WD. Trends in contraceptive use in the United States: 1982–1995. Fam Plann Perspect 1998; 30:4–10, 46.

‡Other includes douche, sponge, jelly or cream alone, and other methods.

NA, not applicable.

frequency of female sterilization jumped from 12% in 1973 to 23% in 1982; 1995 brought a further increase to nearly 30%. The proportion of male sterilization remained stable at 11%.

The condom now ranks as the third method of choice. Between 1982 and 1995, the frequency of its use rose from 12% to 27%, most markedly among unmarried women in the age group 15 to 29 years. Fear of human immunodeficiency virus (HIV) and other sexually transmitted diseases (STDs) impelled this shift.

Possibly the most dramatic change in the use of contraceptive methods was the virtual abandonment of IUDs in the United States. This was triggered by the Dalkon Shield episode ending in 1973—the occurrence of excess pelvic infection in women using the device. Another negative factor was the recall of the “copper 7” IUD from the market in 1986 because of putative infertility of women who had discontinued its use. A newly designed copper IUD has surfaced, although U.S. physicians are still more hesitant to prescribe it than their colleagues outside the United States. Uptake of the hormone-bearing IUD is similarly slow.

Contraceptive foams alone are used rarely; currently, manufacturers and physicians recommend that they be used simultaneously with barrier methods.

Table 17–3. Fertility Control in the Developing World (Percent Users), Trend 1980–1993

Method	1980	1993
Female sterilization	24	39
Intrauterine device	32	26
Pill	13	11
Male sterilization	13	8
Injectables	0	4
Vaginal	0	0.3
Condom	5	4
Traditional	12	9

From Bongaarts J, Johansson E. Future trends in contraception in the developing world: prevalence and method mix. Stud Fam Plan 2002; 32:24.

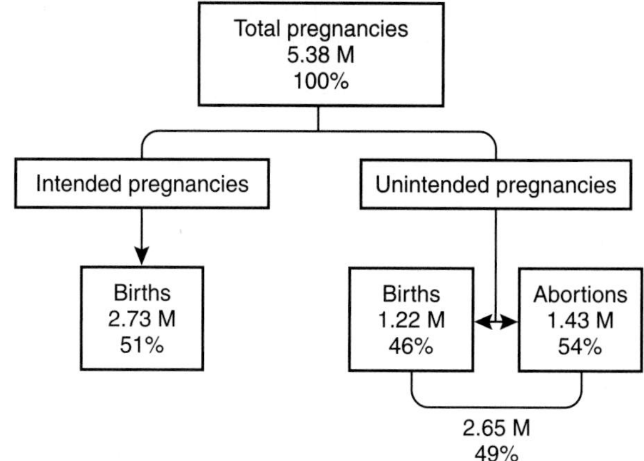

Figure 17–5. Intended and unintended pregnancies in the United States, 1994. (Data adapted from Henshaw SK. Unintended pregnancy in the United States. Fam Plann Perspect 1998; 30:24–29, 46.)

Trends in Fertility Control Methods in the Developing World

Surgical female sterilization is the most frequently used method of effective fertility control in the developing countries (Table 17–3).[26] The biggest difference between the United States and developing countries is the high use of IUDs; use by approximately 30% of women in developing countries makes IUD insertion the second most frequent method of contraception. Hormonal contraception ranks third, possibly because of its high cost and problems with access. In Sri Lanka, for instance, some women buy only five pills at a time because their financial situation does not allow them to acquire a full month’s supply.[14]

Contraceptive Failures

Given the length of time that most women practice a reversible method of fertility control, experiencing at least one contraceptive failure is likely. By sheer statistical probability, failure can happen even if the most effective methods are used perfectly. Between the ages of 16 to 30, a hormonal contraception user has a more than 50% chance of becoming pregnant. During a lifetime of use of reversible methods, the typical woman experiences 1.8 contraceptive failures. This applies particularly when the health status of a woman prohibits the use of a highly effective method, such as the pill, and the couple has to resort to methods that have fewer adverse effects but may also be less effective.[27, 28]

A National Survey of Family Growth analyzed the outcome of unplanned pregnancies in the United States that occurred despite contraception between 1994 and 1995.[28, 29] The analysis took into account the total number of births and therapeutic abortions in the year 1994. Miscarriages were excluded from analysis because it was difficult to calculate the proportion of women who did not plan the pregnancy. For purposes of the analysis, the authors assumed that all therapeutic abortions resulted from unintended pregnancies.

In 1994, there were 5.38 million pregnancies in the United States; of those, 2.73 million (51%) were intended and resulted in births of live children (Fig. 17–5). A full 2.65 million (49%) pregnancies were unintended; of those, 1.22 million or 46% resulted in births and 1.43 million or 54% ended as therapeutic abortions. Alternatively, of the total 3.95 million births (100%), the majority of 2.75 million or 70% were intended and 1.22 million or 30% were unintended.

The survey further revealed that 48% of women from 15 to

Table 17–4. Contraceptive Antecedents to Medical Abortion, 1994–1995: Percentage Distribution of Abortion Patients by Contraceptive Method Used at Time of Conception

Method	All Abortion Patients, Total 9985 (100%)		Patients Who Were Using Contraception at Time of Conception (58% of Total)
Long-acting methods			
Sterilization	0.2	0.9	1.5
Implant	0.1		
Intrauterine device	0.1		
Injectable	0.5		
Pill	11.7		20.3
Male condom	32.4		56.6
Withdrawal	5.9		10.3
Other*	6.4		11.3
No contraception	42.5		NA
Total	100.0		100.0

*Female condom, diaphragm, sponge, foam, suppository, periodic abstinence.
NA, not applicable.
From Henshaw SK, Kost K. Abortion patients in 1994–1995: characteristics and contraceptive use. Fam Plann Perspect 1998; 28:140–147, 158.

44 years of age had had one or more unintended pregnancies, either an unplanned birth or an abortion, or both. The percentage increased with age to a high of 60% among women in the age group 35 to 39 years.

The information on the use of contraceptive methods at the time when an unplanned pregnancy was conceived and later resulted in therapeutic abortion is based on a representative subset of 9985 patients who had abortions (Table 17–4). Of these, 42.5% did not use any contraception at the time of conception and 57.5% practiced some method of fertility control. The male condom was most frequently associated with contraceptive failure. More than half of the women who resorted to abortion reported the use of condoms.[29]

Among women who experienced contraceptive failure, 76% of those younger than 18 years preferred the condom. However, only 46% of women older than 30 years used this method. Pill use peaked at 25% among women aged 20 to 29 and decreased to 16% after the age of 30. On the other hand, the use of methods classified as other (see Table 17–4) rose from 1% in the age group younger than 18 years to 24% in the age group 30 years or older.

The Need for Future Improvements

The high discontinuation rate, the number of unintended pregnancies, and the number of abortions testify to the fact that present reproductive health care is still deficient in providing adequate fertility control options to all women. The health care system alone cannot be blamed for the large number of unplanned pregnancies. Patients frequently choose methods of low efficacy, the primary example being the use of the male condom. When effective methods are recommended, they are frequently applied incorrectly or their use is interrupted, even if it is resumed later on.

These problems can be partially remedied by appropriate information about the available contraceptive choices and by intensive counseling adjusted to the level of the individual patient. Informing the general public about new findings and advances in reproductive health care has been largely facilitated by access to electronic sources of information; the medical profession should take full advantage of this progress.

The proportion of women who did not use any contraception at the time of an unplanned conception is disturbing. This problem could be partially addressed by the development of a highly effective postcoital method. An alternative solution would be implementation of an effective system that would make the presently available postcoital contraceptives promptly accessible. Finally, there must be renewed interest in improving present methods and designing new effective and safe approaches to fertility control.

TECHNOLOGIES OF FERTILITY CONTROL

Hormonal Contraception

Development of Hormonal Contraceptives

The knowledge that estrogens and progestagens can inhibit ovulation has been the foundation of the modern hormonal methods of contraception. In 1940, for the first time, Sturgis and Albright[30] achieved inhibition of ovulation in women by estrogens in order to relieve dysmenorrhea.

The foundation of modern contraception was laid in Manhattan in 1950 at a lengthy conference. Among the participants were Gregory Pincus, director of the Worcester Foundation, and a small group of fertility control advocates including Margaret Sanger, the founder of the Planned Parenthood movement. The conference ended by granting Pincus seed money of $2100 to initiate his research on hormonal contraception.[31] In 1953, working with a Boston gynecologist, John Rock, Pincus started to test oral progesterone for ovulation inhibition. In 1956, Pincus' group of scientists and physicians published results of the first successful contraceptive clinical trial, which took place in Puerto Rico using a synthetic progestagen, norethynodrel, provided by the G.D. Searle company.[32] Norethynodrel, however, was not the first orally active progestagen. This priority belongs to norethindrone, synthesized in 1951, which became the lead compound in the development of clinically important oral progestagens.[33, 34]

Starting in the 1930s, chemists searched for orally active steroids. In 1938, a group at the Schering Corporation in Berlin, Germany, developed the first orally active steroidal estrogen by attaching the ethinyl group ($\cdots C \equiv CH$) to the 17th carbon of the estradiol molecule (Fig. 17–6 and Fig. 17–8).[35] Ethinylestradiol still constitutes the estrogenic component of nearly all combined OCs. The development of orally active progestagens was triggered by the discovery that when the C-19 methyl group of testosterone is split off, the resulting molecule loses androgenicity and acquires progestagenic properties. In 1951, Carl Djerassi, leading a team of chemists in Mexico City, reasoned that attaching the ethinyl group ($\cdots C \equiv CH$) to the 17th carbon of the nortestosterone molecule would greatly enhance its progestagenic activity and make the compound orally active (Figs. 17–7 and 17–8). Djerassi and colleagues produced 17α-ethinyl-19-nortestosterone.[36] The compound, known by its generic names *norethindrone* and in Europe *norethisterone* (commonly abbreviated NET), had 10 times the activity of natural progesterone when orally administered. To this day, norethindrone has remained the progestagenic component of many combined OCs (Table 17–6). In a parallel development, manipulation of the progesterone molecule produced a group of orally highly active progestagens, such as medroxyprogesterone acetate (MPA) (Provera) (see Fig. 17–10 later).

Originally, hormonal contraception included only the pill, that is, an orally active combination of an estrogen and a progestagen. The pill offered several advantages over other available contraceptive methods. For the first time, its high

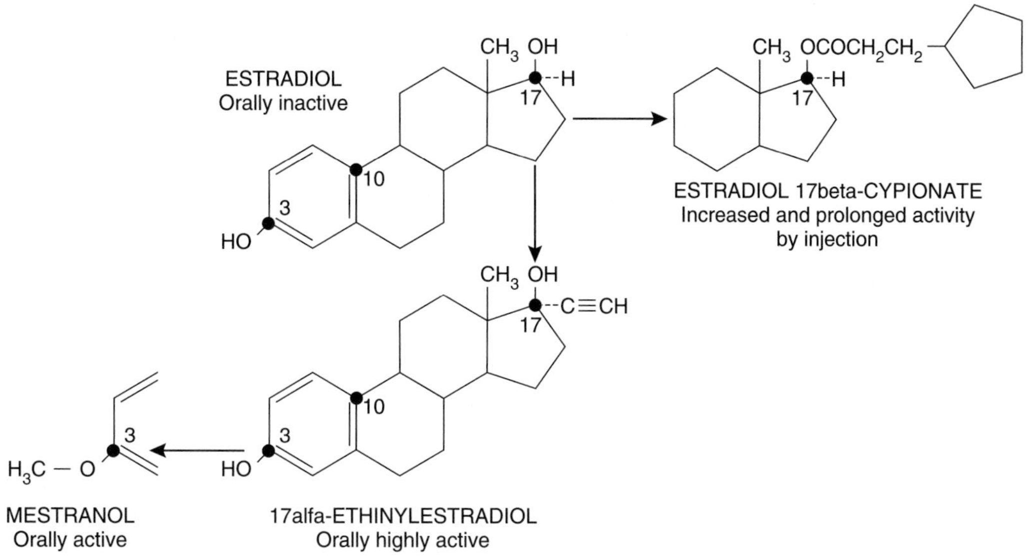

Figure 17–6. Attachment of the ethinyl group to C-17 of estradiol creates an orally highly active estrogen, ethinylestradiol (EE). Mestranol has a methyl group on C-3 of EE. Mestranol is a prohormone because it must be metabolically converted to EE to be able to bind to estrogen receptors. Modification of the estradiol molecule on C-17 provides long-acting 17β-cypionate, used in injectable preparations. For numbering of the steroid molecule, see Figure 17–8.

efficacy brought confidence in a contraceptive method and freedom from the fear of pregnancy. It produced only temporary and reversible infertility; therefore, it was ideal for family planning. Because the method was not linked to coitus, the spontaneity of the sexual act could be preserved. The pill has become popular among women in both developed and developing countries, and today 10 million women in the United States and 60 million women worldwide adhere to this method.

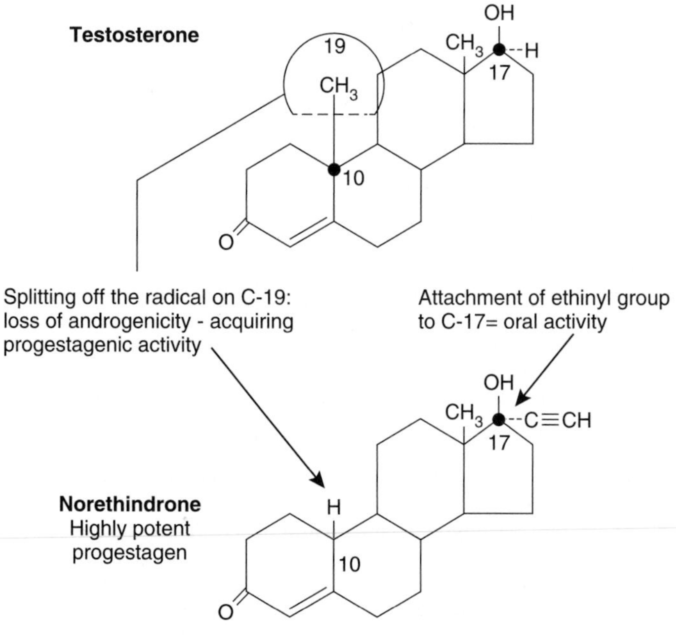

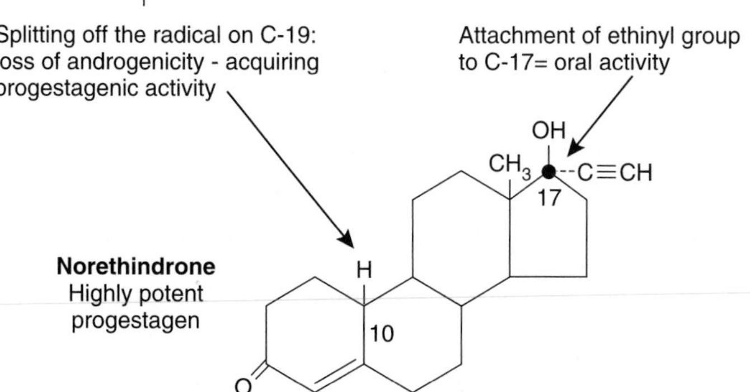

Figure 17–7. Development of norethindrone from testosterone. Splitting off the C-19 radical from the testosterone molecule changes this androgen to a progestagen. Attachment of the ethinyl group to C-17 enhances the progestagenic activity of the compound and makes it orally active. For numbering of the steroid molecule, see Figure 17–8.

However, use of the pill requires a conscious daily action on the part of the user, and it has been postulated that missing pills could be the reason for the discrepancy between pregnancy rates during perfect and typical use (see Table 17–1). To close this gap, long-term methods of hormonal contraception have been invented that require only one or a limited number of actions on the part of the user. Hormonal implants, depot injections, and hormonal IUDs are examples of such long-term methods with high efficacy during typical use.

Unintended pregnancies can result from failure of contraceptives or from exposure to an unplanned sexual contact. Such events necessitate short-term preventive steps. Two important developments took place in this direction: emergency post-coital contraception and the use of antiprogestagenic steroids for contragestion.

Hormonal Contraceptives in Clinical Use

The hormonal contraceptives available today can be categorized by the way they are administered and by the duration of their action (see Table 17–5).

Oral Contraception

Steroidal Components

In the following paragraphs we describe the pharmacologic and biologic properties of the two hormonal components of OCs, the estrogens and the progestagens.

Contraceptive Estrogens

Structure and Function

In the combined estrogen-progestagen OCs, one type of estrogen prevails, 17α-ethinylestradiol. A limited number of OC preparations contain a derivative of ethinylestradiol, mestranol.

The ethinyl group protects ethinylestradiol and mestranol (MEE) from oxidation and conversion into less active estrogens such as estriol. Mestranol is a prodrug that does not bind

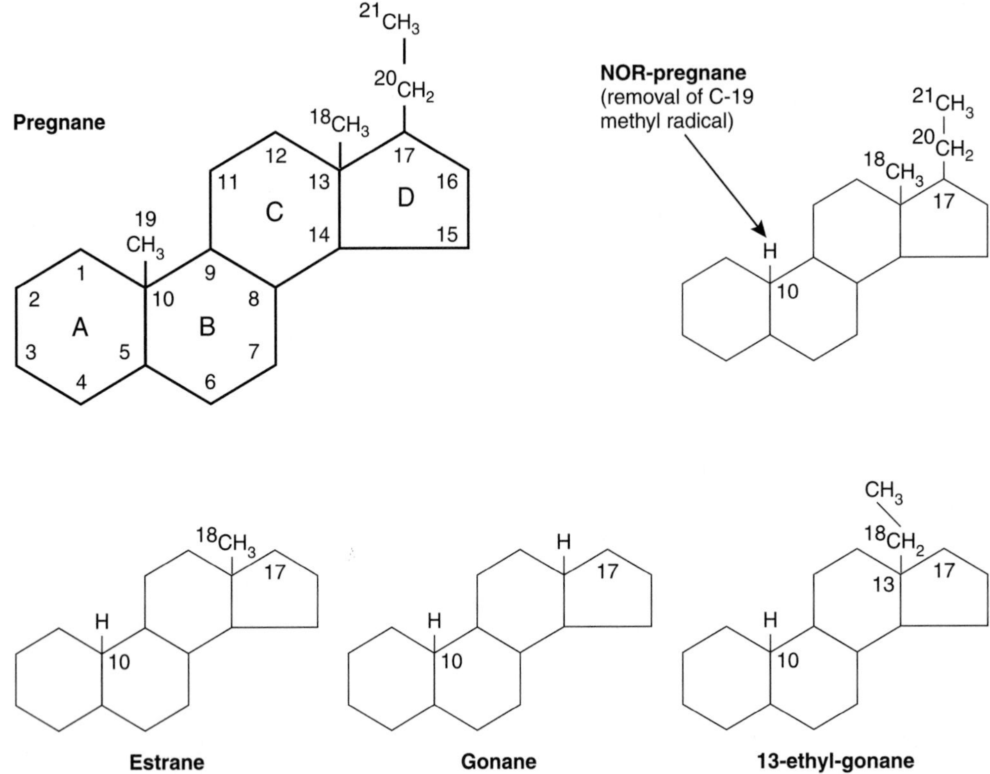

Figure 17–8. Contraceptive progestagens are derived from three skeleton structures, pregnane, estrane, and gonane (see details in the text). The pregnane molecule shows the numbering system of contraceptive steroids.

to estrogen receptors and has to be converted into ethinylestradiol in order to become biologically active. MEE has been replaced by ethinylestradiol in virtually all OCs worldwide.

Pharmacokinetics and Metabolism

After ingestion, ethinylestradiol is rapidly absorbed from the gastrointestinal tract. The time to the maximum ethinylestradiol concentration in plasma (T_{max}) is 1 to 2 hours and the elimination half-life is wide, ranging from about 9 to 27 hours. In the intestine and in the liver, ethinylestradiol is readily conjugated with sulfuric and glucuronic acids and undergoes enterohepatic circulation. Intestinal bacteria possessing the appropriate enzymes can hydrolyze ethinylestradiol sulfates, and some of the deconjugated estrogen is reabsorbed. One could speculate that the use of oral antibiotics that affect intestinal flora may influence blood levels of ethinylestradiol; so far, clinical proof of this assumption is lacking. The pharmacokinetics and metabolism of mestranol are similar to those of ethinylestradiol except that T_{max} is longer than might have been expected because mestranol has to be converted to ethinylestradiol.[37]

Individual subjects vary considerably in the amount of absorbed ethinylestradiol and the circulating concentrations of ethinylestradiol as well as in the elimination time. Intrasubject variations can also be prominent. These variations may explain why adverse effects and contraceptive failures occur in only certain individuals and why the same woman can experience side effects during some treatment cycles but remains symptom-free during others. The basis of the intersubject and intrasubject variations has not been explained satisfactorily.

As we are witnessing another wave of reduction of the ethinylestradiol content in the combination pills to 20 μg, bioavailability becomes an issue. As these and ever lower doses of ethinylestradiol become more common, we must be certain to provide OCs in formulations that deliver the digested amounts of steroids at appropriate concentrations for the individual user.

Contraceptive Progestagens

In contrast to estrogen synthesis, the synthesis of progestagens has been prolific. The reasons for this dichotomy are several. Because ethinylestradiol exhibited potent oral activity and was not protected by patents, there was little incentive to search for other OC estrogens. New progestagens were synthesized in order to secure proprietary rights for the developers of OCs. Also, synthesis of new compounds was prompted by the desire to produce a highly effective progestagen that would minimize the dose of the progestagen in the OC combination and thus reduce the incidence of progestagen-related adverse events. Currently, about a dozen progestagens are being used clinically in established contraceptive preparations and several compounds are in various stages of preclinical and clinical testing.

According to the classical definition, progestagens transform the estrogen-primed endometrium into a secretory one and support the development and maintenance of pregnancy. The advent of molecular biology has defined progestagens as compounds that bind to and activate progesterone receptors within the target cells. However, binding to progesterone receptors does not preclude the progestagen molecule binding with other receptors or expressing effects other than progestagenic effects, or both. For example, norethindrone, under certain circumstances, can stimulate the proliferation of the atrophic endometrium.[38, 39] Besides being a potent progestagen, cypro-

Table 17–5. Hormonal Contraceptives in Clinical Use

Oral contraception (see details in Table 17–6)
 Cyclic estrogen-progestagen combinations
 Continuous progestagen-only oral contraception
Long-acting preparations
 Injectable preparations
  Progestagen-only preparations
   Depot–medroxyprogesterone acetate, 150 mg, q3mo, IM
   Norethindrone enanthate, 200 mg, q2mo, IM (not used in the United States)
  Estrogen-progestagen combination injectables
   Medroxyprogesterone acetate, 25 mg + estradiol cypionate, 5 mg, q28 ± 5d, IM
 Hormonal subdermal implants (see Table 17–12)
  Norplant: 6 capsules with total amount of 216 mg of levonorgestrel
  Norplant II (Jadelle): 2 rods with total amount of 150 mg of levonorgestrel
 Hormonal intrauterine systems
  Progestasert: T-shaped; vertical arm releases progesterone, ~65 μg/d
  Mirena (levonorgestrel-20): T-shaped; vertical arm releases levonorgestrel, ~15 μg/d
 Vaginal rings releasing contraceptive hormones—NuvaRing approved in 2001
 Transdermal patch releasing contraceptive hormones
  Ortho EVRA: 20 cm² patch, delivers 150 μg norelgestromin, 20 μg/d ethinylestradiol
Emergency methods of fertility control
 Postcoital hormonal contraception
  a. 1 mg norgestrel and 100 μg ethinylestradiol within 72 h of unprotected intercourse, repeated after 12 h
  b. 0.75 mg levonorgestrel within 72 h of unprotected intercourse, repeated after 12 h
 Contragestion
  Mifepristone, 200–600 mg, orally, followed by 400–800 μg misopristol orally

terone acetate is a recognized antiandrogen in both men and women.[40]

Classification of Contraceptive Progestagens

Contraceptive progestagens have been classified in various ways, for example, according to the amount of ethinylestradiol with which they are combined, the type of progestagen they contain, and the time when they became available for clinical use.

According to the chemical structure of the steroids, the classification of contraceptive progestagens presented recognizes three basic groups, *pregnanes, estranes*, and *gonanes* (Fig. 17–9; see Fig. 17–8). Certain compounds—norpregnanes, drospirenone, and dienogest—combine structural elements of other progestagens or chemical groups. They are designated as hybrid progestagens. Their structural and biologic characteristics are discussed in the section "Hybrid Progestagens."

The structures of pregnane, estrane, and gonane and the numbering of the steroid molecule are given in Figure 17–8.

Structure and Function of Contraceptive Progestagens

Pregnanes

Pregnanes can be divided into three subgroups. The first consists of derivatives of 17α-hydroxyprogesterone acetate, which has been developed by an intricate manipulation of the progesterone molecule (Fig. 17–10). The C-6 and C-17 positions are of key importance for progestagenic activity. Chemical manipulations at C-17 profoundly change the function of the molecule.[41] Thus, progesterone loses its biologic activity with the introduction of an α-hydroxyl group at C-17. Esterification of this group not only restores the progestational activity but also renders the resulting substance—17α-hydroxypro-

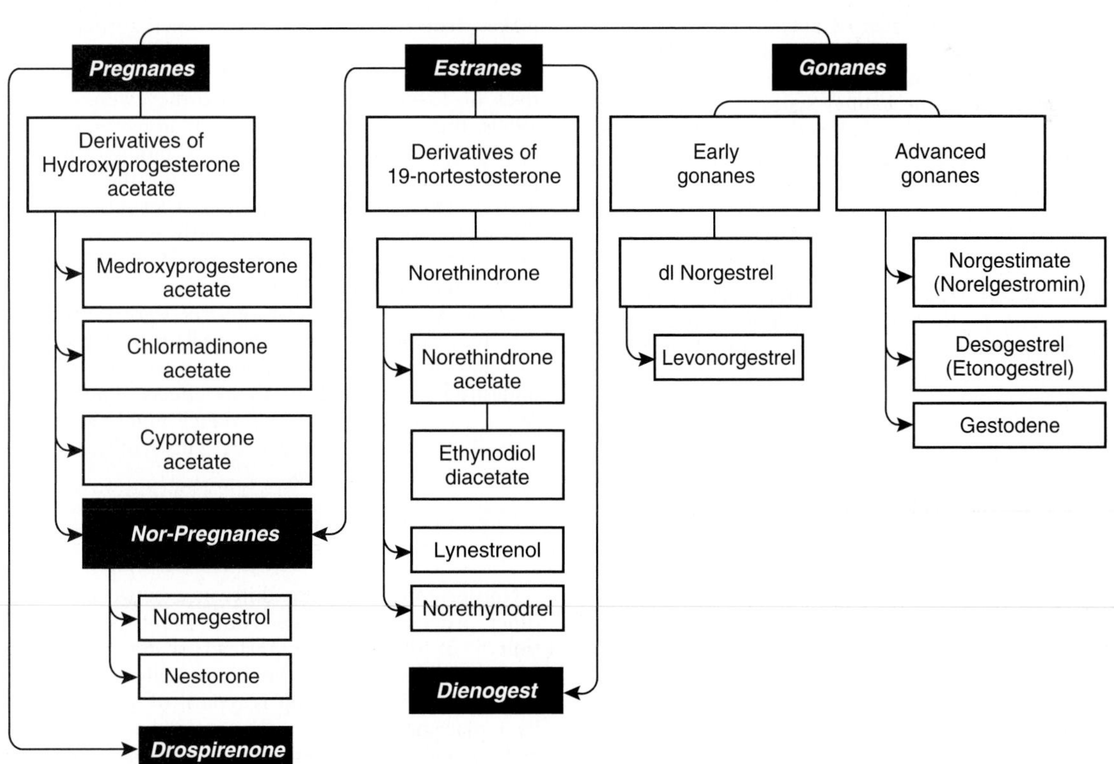

Figure 17–9. Classification of contraceptive steroids. Hybrid progestagens are in gray boxes. In parentheses are the active progestagenic metabolites of norgestimate and desogestrel.

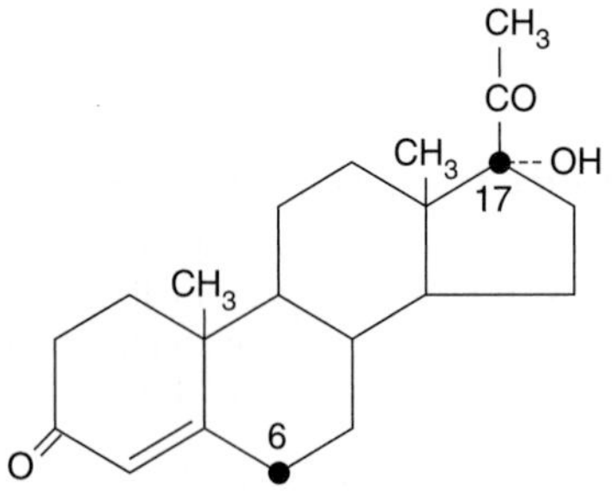

17alpha-hydroxyprogesterone
Inactive

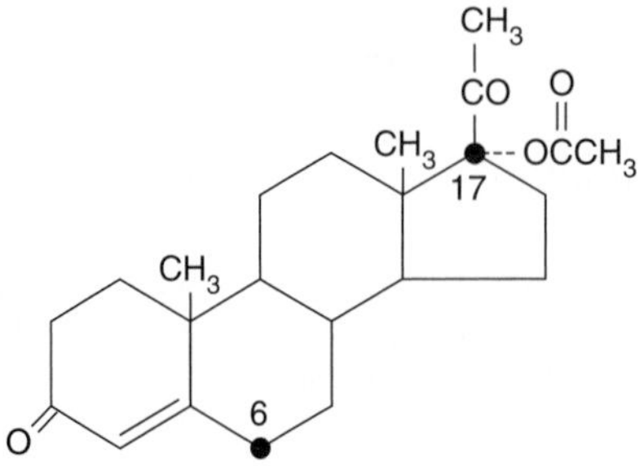

17alpha-hydroxyprogesterone acetate
Weak progestagen

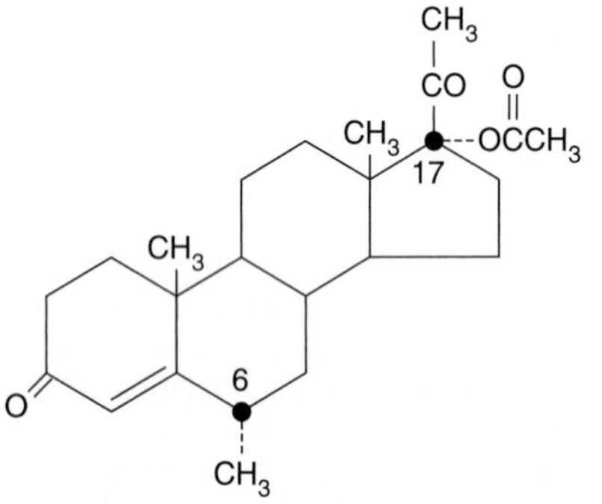

Medroxyprogesterone acetate (MPA)
Highly potent progestagen–orally active

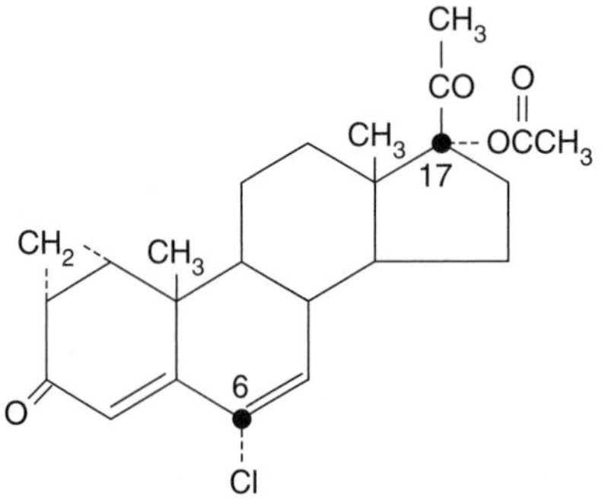

Cyproterone acetate
Progestagen, antiandrogen

Figure 17–10. Progestagens derived from progesterone. Progesterone loses its activity when a hydroxyl group is attached to C-17. Formation of an acetate restores the progestational activity, which is further enhanced by manipulations at C-6. Derivatives of hydroxyprogesterone acetate are potent progestagens as well as antiandrogens.

gesterone acetate—orally active. This became the starting point for the synthesis of a number of potent pregnanes, made so mainly by modifications at C-6. Examples are MPA and acetates of megestrol, chlormadinone, and cyproterone. The last two are not available in the United States (see Fig. 17–10).

The pregnane group also includes the hybrid progestagens—*norpregnanes* and *drospirenone*. They are discussed in a later section.

Estranes

The estrane structure lacks the C-19 angular methyl radical between rings A and B. Removal of a radical from a certain position in the molecule is abbreviated in chemical shorthand as NOR, that is, "no radical." Removal of the C-19 methyl radical from the testosterone molecule changed this androgen into a progestagen; moreover, attachment of the ethinyl group (···C≡CH) to the 17th carbon made the compound more potent and orally active (see Figs. 17–7 and 17–8) These chemical reactions led to the synthesis of *norethindrone*, the first orally highly active progestagen, which enabled the development of oral contraception. All estranes are 19-norsteroids.[41]

Figure 17–11 shows the structural formulas of norethindrone and its four derivatives, which must be metabolically converted into norethindrone in order to become biologically active.[37]

Gonanes

The *gonane* structure lacks both the C-18 and the C-19 angular methyl radicals. However, all gonane progestagens bear an ethyl group between rings C and D at C-13 (Figs. 17–12 and 17–13; see Fig. 17–8). This chemical modification makes them more active progestational agents than estranes.

Early Gonanes. *dl*-Norgestrel and levonorgestrel are derivatives of 13-ethylgonane. Because they were developed in the 1960s, they are categorized as early gonanes. Only the *l*-isomer of *dl*-norgestrel, levonorgestrel, is biologically active. As expected, levonorgestrel exhibited twice the potency of *dl*-norgestrel. The successful separation of levonorgestrel enabled the development of OC regimens with an extremely low amount of progestagen, and levonorgestrel soon replaced all *dl*-norgestrel–containing OC preparations.

dl-Norgestrel and levonorgestrel were synthesized in order to acquire a more potent progestagen than norethindrone, but they also increased the compound's androgenic properties with undesired clinical and metabolic effects. Thus, the next task of the steroid chemist was to produce highly active progestagens without the androgenic effects. The synthesis of the later gonanes met this challenge.

Later Gonanes. Three progestagens belong to this family, norgestimate, desogestrel, and gestodene (see Fig. 17–13).

Norgestimate. The key difference between norgestimate and other progestagens is the oxime group (-C=N-OH) in position 3 of the molecule instead of the keto group (C=O). Norgestimate is solely the biologically active *levo* form. Because the C-3 keto group is typical of androgenic compounds, its replacement by the oxime may contribute to the reduced androgenicity of norgestimate as compared with levonorgestrel.

Desogestrel. This advanced gonane is interesting in that its progestagenic activity has been increased by substitution on C-

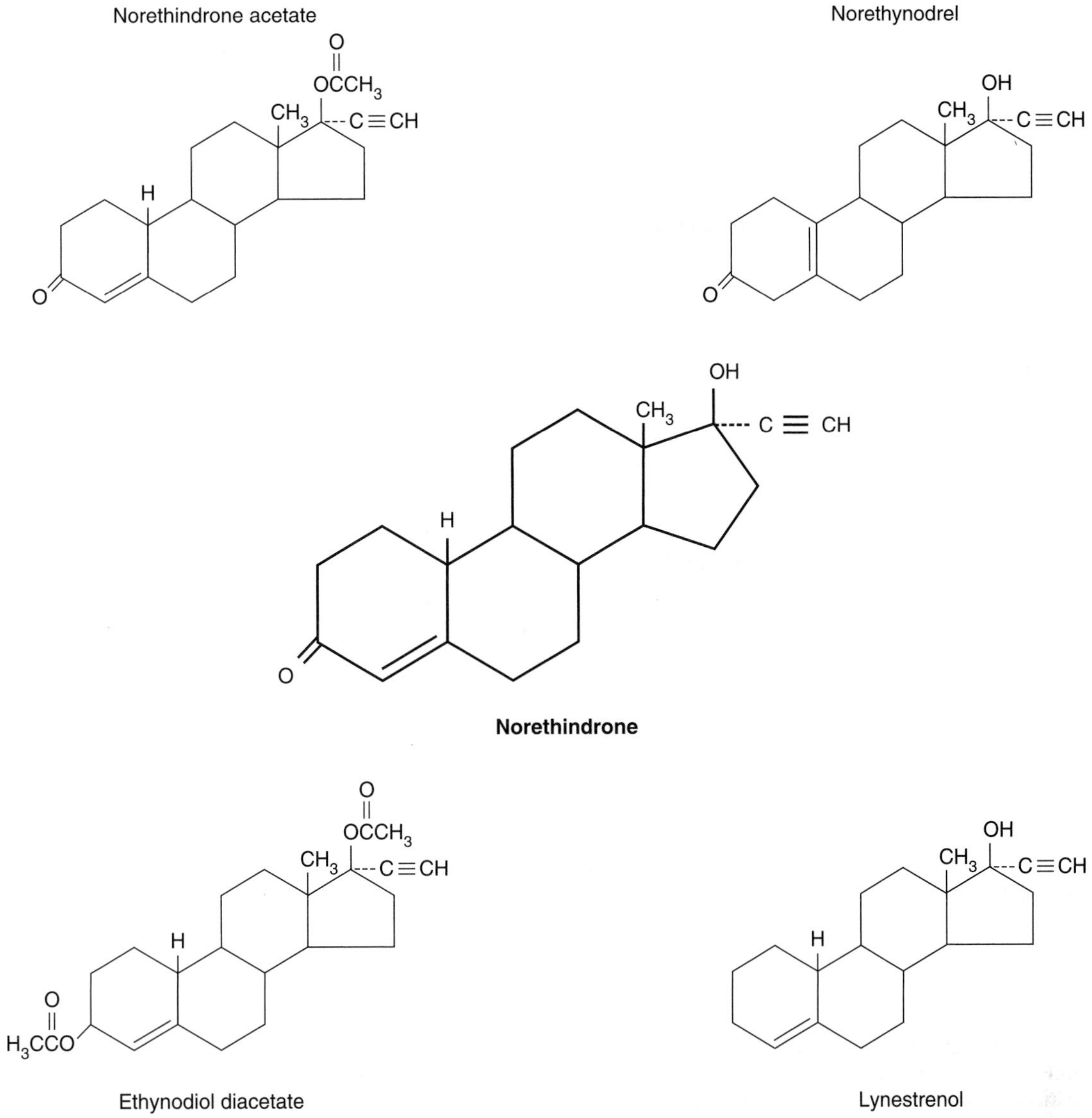

Norethindrone acetate

Norethynodrel

Norethindrone

Ethynodiol diacetate

Lynestrenol

Figure 17–11. Norethindrone (NET) and its derivatives. In order to become biologically active, the individual derivatives must be converted into NET.

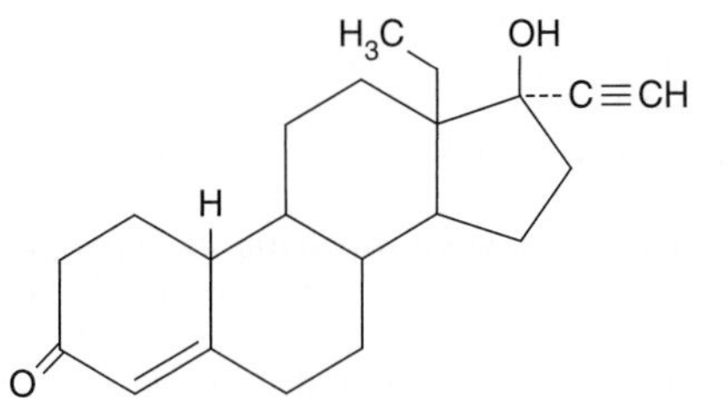

LEVONORGESTREL
l (-) enantiomer

NORGESTREL
d,l - mixture composed of above structure
and its mirror image

Figure 17–12. Early gonanes: levonorgestrel and norgestrel.

11. Manipulations at C-11 give the steroid molecule the ability to bind to the progesterone, glucocorticoid, and mineralocorticoid receptors. The intensity of the binding depends on the structure of the substituting groups.

Gestodene. Gestodene differs from norgestrel in a single feature, namely the double bond between C-15 and C-16. This seemingly simple change has a profound effect on the configuration of the molecule, principally on the spatial arrangement of the D ring and C-17. One can speculate that these changes affect the conformation of the molecule in a way that affects its binding to hormone receptors. In vitro studies have shown that gestodene binds to the heme of the P450 enzymes that inactivate estrogens, with consequent increased concentrations of these hormones.[42] The clinical relevance of this finding is unknown.

Some Aspects of the Clinical Pharmacology of Contraceptive Progestagens

The orally active contraceptive progestagens are rapidly absorbed from the digestive tract and are transported to the liver

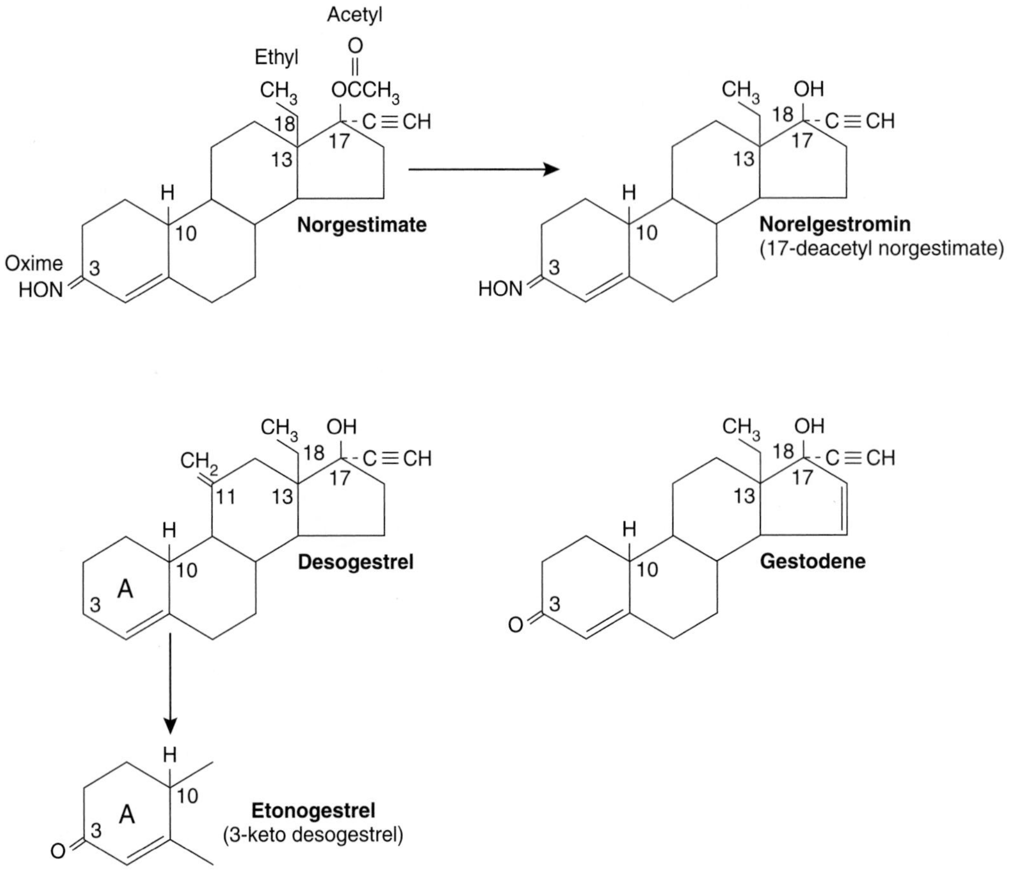

Figure 17–13. Progestagens of the advanced gonane group. Norgestimate and desogestrel are prohormones, metabolically converted into the active progestagenic substances, norelgestromin and etonogestrel, respectively. Gestodene is active without metabolic conversion.

through the portal circulation. Thereafter, they enter the general circulation, where they form a hormonal pool. In the general circulation, progestagens are present either in the free form or bound to albumins or to the sex hormone–binding globulin (SHBG), or both. Only the free form reaches receptors in the respective target tissues and becomes biologically active. Progestagens can easily be released from the steroid-albumin complex; the bond with SHBG is firmer.

During first-pass liver metabolism, progestagens can be structurally modified with consequent changes of their biologic activity. Glucuronidation and sulfuration of progestagens facilitate their excretion by the kidneys. A variable fraction of progestagens is excreted in the feces. During first-pass liver metabolism, progestagens act on hepatocytes in ways that can alter their metabolism (see later).

The pharmacologic properties of progestagens determine their clinical use. Progestagens of the pregnane series can bind strongly to progestagenic as well as to androgenic receptors and can act as antiestrogens. Oral MPA is used for treatment of various gynecologic disorders, for example, for the management of dysfunctional uterine bleeding, and in the menopause. The compound has been developed as the first injectable long-term contraceptive. In the past, medroxyprogesterone and other pregnane derivatives were proscribed for contraceptive use in the United States because preclinical toxicology had shown an accelerated development of benign and malignant breast nodules in beagle dogs—a breed that suffers spontaneously from a high incidence of breast tumors, including carcinoma. Extensive clinical trials conducted by the WHO have lifted the cloud of potential carcinogenicity hanging over MPA, and it is used as an injectable contraceptive globally.[43]

The accelerated growth of breast nodules in beagle dogs was not observed in toxicologic studies with progestagens of the estrane and gonane series. The reasons for this difference in animal carcinogenic potential of pregnanes versus estranes and gonanes have not been adequately elucidated. It is noteworthy that long-term toxicologic studies in monkeys have not shown the formation of any type of breast nodules. In monkeys, spontaneous breast carcinoma is unknown, and the induction of hormone-associated breast pathology would have been particularly important.

Of the other pregnanes, acetates of chlormadinone, cyproterone, and megestrol are used in OCs in some countries outside the United States. They are also used for management of breast, endometrial, and prostatic carcinomas. Because they are also highly effective antiandrogens, they have been part of the management of benign prostatic hypertrophy, prostatic carcinoma, precocious puberty, and certain hyperandrogenic symptoms in women.

In the estrane series, the four derivatives of norethindrone are rapidly converted to norethindrone. Within 30 minutes after ingestion of any of the derivatives, only norethindrone can be detected in the general circulation.

The earliest OCs contained norethindrone and norethynodrel, originally combined with up to 150 μg of ethinylestradiol. Today, OCs containing more than 50 μg of ethinylestradiol are considered "high-dose" estrogen preparations and have been removed from the OC market in the United States.

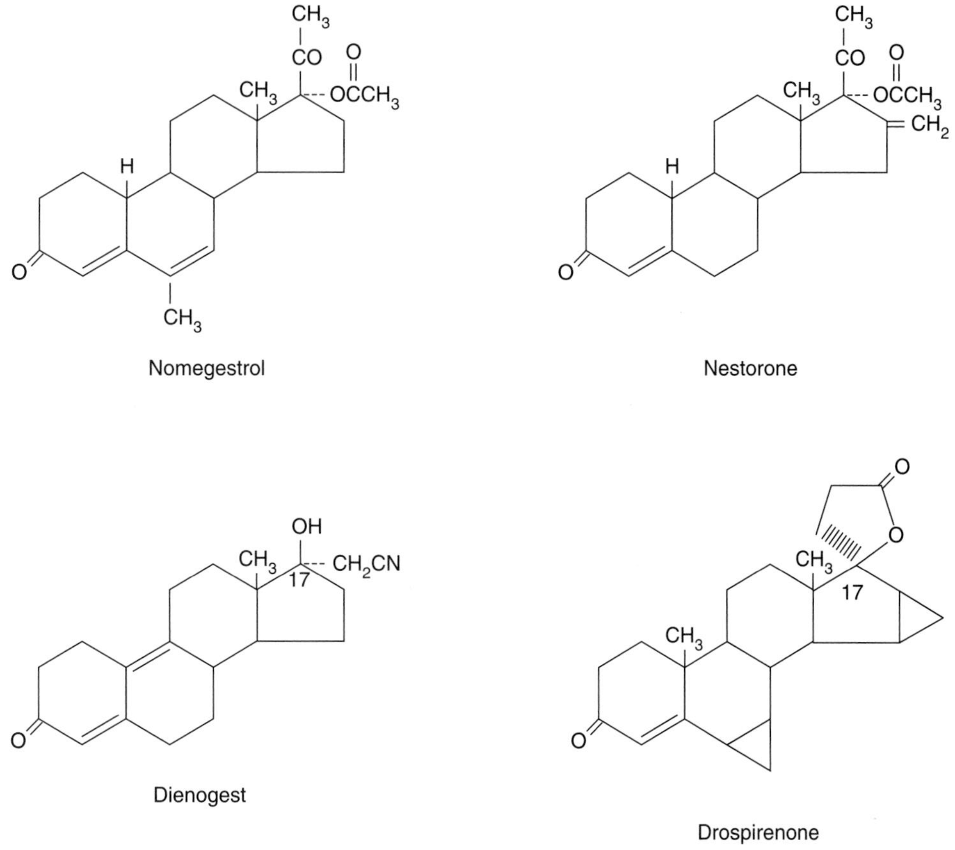

Nomegestrol

Nestorone

Dienogest

Drospirenone

Figure 17–14. Hybrid progestagens: norpregnanes nomegestrol and nestorone, dienogest, and drospirenone. Drospirenone is a spironolactone derivative.

"Mid-dose" estrogen preparations contain 50 μg of ethinylestradiol, and "low-dose" preparations contain less than 50 μg of ethinylestradiol. Currently, the low-dose OCs are recommended; the mid-dose preparations are recommended only exceptionally.

The early gonanes, norgestrel and levonorgestrel, display certain unique features.[44, 45] The time required for the circulating levels of levonorgestrel to decline by 50% is about 15 hours, and for norethindrone it is about 7 hours. The difference in the elimination time is one of the reasons that contraceptive doses of levonorgestrel can be lower than those of norethindrone. Norgestrel and levonorgestrel are strong progestagens with antiestrogenic properties; however, they also show some androgenicity. Levonorgestrel also decreases the plasma concentration of SHBG by 50% and, in combined OCs, suppresses the estrogen-induced formation of SHBG. Consequently, less SHBG is available for binding testosterone. A combined OC composed of 150 μg of levonorgestrel and 30 μg of ethinylestradiol increases the levels of SHBG only slightly—about 20% from baseline. In contrast, women using norgestimate or desogestrel-ethinylestradiol OCs have a threefold increase in circulating levels of SHBG, which results in a 50% decrease of free testosterone.

Compounds of the late gonane series, norgestimate and desogestrel, are metabolized extensively (see Fig. 17–13). After ingestion, norgestimate is rapidly converted into norelgestromin and desogestrel is converted into etonogestrel. These metabolites account for the biologic activity of the parent compounds. Norelgestromin has been synthesized as a specific hormone for the contraceptive patch, and etonogestrel is used in silastic implants for contraception.[46]

Gestodene is the only compound of the gonane series that is not rapidly metabolized. It is a highly potent progestagen; however, at the time of this writing the compound has not been approved for clinical use in the United States.

Hybrid Progestagens

19-Norpregnanes

The 19-norpregnanes are a cross between the pregnanes and estranes. These compounds are derived from 17α- hydroxyprogesterone acetate but lack the C-19 methyl radical and in that respect are related to estranes (Fig. 17–14). *Nomegestrol*, an important member of this series, is currently being investigated as a contraceptive implant.[47]

Nestorone is another 19-norpregnane of the 17α-acetoxyprogesterone series, which has a methylene group on C-16. In receptor assays, nestorone had progestational effects equal to or better than those of levonorgestrel without estrogenic, androgenic, and anabolic activities.[48] However, nestorone binds to glucocorticoid receptors. Nestorone has low oral but high parenteral progestational activity. Therefore, the Population Council is studying nestorone as a contraceptive in subdermal implants, vaginal rings, and transdermal formulations. The compound may be suitable for nursing mothers because of its low oral bioavailability.

Other Hybrid Progestagens

Dienogest is a new addition to the estranes. In this compound, the cyanomethyl group (···$CH_2C{\equiv}N$) has replaced the

C-17 ethinyl group (···C≡CH) (see Fig. 17–14). Dienogest is 100% orally available. Some evidence suggests that the compound lacks androgenic activity and produces less glucocorticoid antagonism than mifepristone.

The compound suppresses endometrial growth and is being tested in the management of endometriosis. The antigonadotropic activity of dienogest is relatively low, mandating the use of 2 mg in combination with 30 μg of ethinylestradiol in a 21-day cyclic regimen.[49]

Drospirenone. An addition to contraceptive progestagens has been *drospirenone*. It is a progestagen derived from spironolactone, a potent steroid with antimineralocorticoid activity, which also has progestagenic properties. Drospirenone is a relatively weak progestagen; a daily dose for a contraceptive regimen is 3 mg combined with 30 μg of ethinylestradiol. The compound has antiandrogenic and antimineralocorticoid properties and causes potassium retention. Therefore, it should not be taken by patients with kidney, liver, or adrenal gland disease or with other drugs that increase potassium concentrations in the circulation. Such drugs include nonsteroidal anti-inflammatory drugs, potassium-sparing diuretics (spironolactone and others), potassium supplementation, angiotensin-converting enzyme inhibitors, angiotensin II receptor antagonists, and heparin.[50]

Progestagenic Potency, Androgenicity, and Comparative Metabolic Effects of Oral Contraception

Multiple Steroid Actions

Significant determinants of the biologic activity of a steroid include its bioavailability to the target tissues and its affinity for relevant receptors. The multifaceted nature of the steroid molecule is illustrated by its capacity to bind to several different receptors and activate them to various degrees.[51, 52] The final biologic activity depends on the proportion of activated receptors—progestagenic, estrogenic, androgenic, and glucocorticoid—in the target tissue. Most contraceptive progestagens, besides binding strongly to progesterone receptors, also bind to a lesser extent to androgen receptors. Moreover, some progestagens bind to glucocorticoid receptors.

Progestagenic and Androgenic Activity

It is difficult to establish the relative progestagenic and androgenic potency of progestagens because systematic testing of all progestagens by one method has not been performed. Different progestagens have been tested by different methods. The relative binding affinities of progesterone and gonanes for rabbit uterine progestagen receptors are shown in Figure 17–15. The binding affinity of norgestimate and its 17-deacetylated metabolite (norelgestromin) was similar to that of progesterone; levonorgestrel was about five times and gestodene and 3-ketodesogestrel were about nine times more active than progesterone.

The relative binding activities of progesterone and gonane progestagens for rat prostatic androgen receptors are depicted in Figure 17–16. Norgestimate and norelgestromin, which have the same progestagenic activity as progesterone, display low androgenic activity. Levonorgestrel, a 5 times more potent progestagen than progesterone, has 44 times higher androgenic activity than progesterone. Although 3-ketodesogestrel and gestodene are more active progestagens than levonorgestrel, they have less androgenic activity than levonorgestrel. In this assay, the androgenic activity of dihydrotestosterone is 200-fold greater than that of progesterone (not shown in Fig. 17–16). The androgenic activity of levonorgestrel is one fourth the activity of dihydrotestosterone.

Biologic tests of androgenicity were conducted on castrated rats, the end point being the weight increase of the prostatic gland. In this assay, the androgenic potency of testosterone equals 100%; that of levonorgestrel is 15% and that of norethindrone is only 1.6%. Medroxyprogesterone and chlormadinone acetates displayed no androgenic action in this test.[53]

Non–Receptor-Mediated Action

In skin and some other tissues, testosterone is a prohormone and becomes biologically active only after conversion into *dihydrotestosterone* by 5α-reductase. In vitro experiments have demonstrated that norgestimate and desogestrel inhibit the action of 5α-reductase.[54] This may partially explain the beneficial effects of these progestagens in the management of androgenic skin lesions such as acne.

Metabolic Actions of Progestagens

Lipid Metabolism

Important differences exist among progestagens in their effect on lipid metabolism, particularly on the cardioprotective lipoproteins. Estrogens increase total cholesterol, but they also increase the high-density lipoprotein (HDL) fraction and decrease the low-density lipoprotein (LDL) fraction of cholesterol. Progestagens exert an antagonistic effect on these positive actions of estrogens by various mechanisms, including an increase in the activity of hepatic lipase, which degrades HDL. There are quantitative differences among individual progestagens, however, and the net metabolic effect depends on an intricate interplay between the two components of the combined contraceptives, the type and dose of the progestagen, and the treatment regimen, whether it is monophasic or triphasic. In general, the higher the androgenic properties of a progestagen, the more pronounced are the negative effects on cardioprotective lipoproteins.

Because norethindrone and estrane progestagens are derived from testosterone, and testosterone is part of the chemical name of the compounds, it is sometimes assumed that norethindrone and its analogues have androgenic properties. In doses and combinations used in current clinical practice, norethindrone and its analogues do not exhibit substantial clinical or metabolic androgenic effects. A monophasic combination OC (0.5 μg of norethindrone plus 35 μg of ethinylestradiol per day) has been associated with a 10% increase of HDL and a 10% decrease of LDL.[55]

With respect to gonanes, levonorgestrel increases LDL only slightly but reduces HDL significantly. Norgestimate, a later gonane, significantly elevates HDL with a nonsignificant effect on LDL (Fig. 17–17).[55, 56]

Protein Binding

Natural and synthetic sex steroid hormones enter the target cells by passive diffusion. The capacity of sex steroids to reach receptors in these target cells is modulated by SHBG and other proteins, such as albumins. Natural sex steroids and some synthetic progestagens bind to SHBG with higher affinity and specificity than they bind to albumin.[57, 58] As long as a sex steroid is bound to SHBG, it cannot affect its biologic action, which is accomplished by the free or non–SHBG-bound fraction of the steroid. The binding of sex steroids to albumin is less tight, and albumin-bound steroids are more readily available to target cells, ensuring a rapid pharmacologic response.

Estrogens stimulate hepatocytes to produce SHBG, and androgens and some progestagens interfere with this action. Depending on their composition, OCs are associated with increased formation of SHBG and reduced levels of free

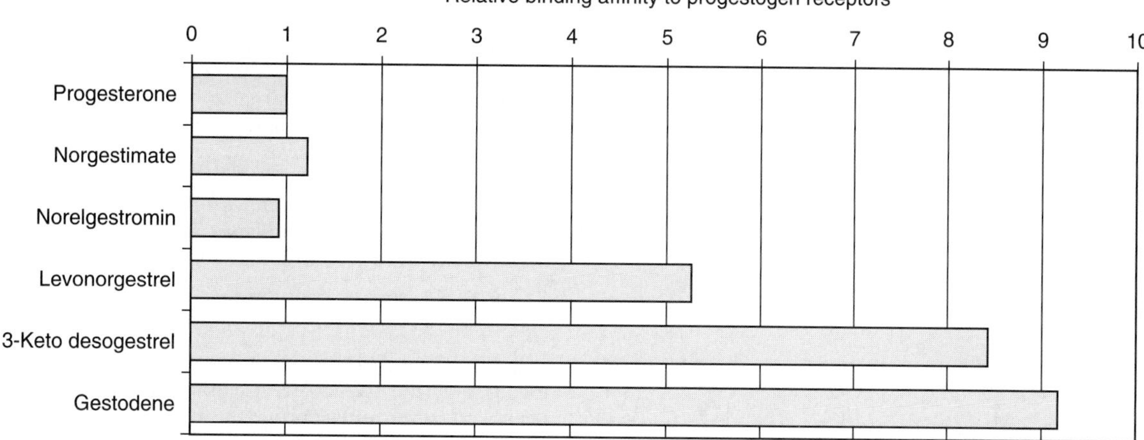

Figure 17-15. Relative binding affinities of contraceptive progestagens for progesterone receptors. The assay measures displacement of ^{3}H-labeled R5020 from progestagen receptors isolated from the rabbit uterus. The [^{3}H]R5020 is a radiolabeled synthetic progestagen used in in vitro studies. (Data from Phillips A, Demarest K, Hahn DW, et al. Progestational and androgenic receptor binding affinities and in vivo activities of norgestimate and other progestins. Contraception 1990; 41:399.)

testosterone. For example, OCs with desogestrel and norgestimate do not interfere with the estrogen-stimulated formation of SHBG, and free testosterone levels are reduced. These changes are thought to confer clinical benefits in certain hyperandrogenic conditions in women.[59]

Progestagens may also compete for SHBG binding sites and indirectly increase the concentration of free estradiol and testosterone in plasma.[60] The binding affinity of norgestrel for SHBG is relatively high. Desogestrel binding to SHBG is much less tight, and the affinity of norgestimate and its main metabolite, norelgestromin, for SHBG is practically nil.

Insulin and Carbohydrate Metabolism

The original high-dose OCs were associated with insulin resistance and glucose intolerance. Glucose tolerance tests showed a significant increase of blood glucose and insulin after 1 year of OC use.[61] It was initially thought that these changes in glucose tolerance were related to the estrogenic component of the pill. However, after tests of estrogens alone, even in high doses, demonstrated no such negative effects, it was found that high doses of many progestagens can impair carbohydrate metabolism. With the advent of low-dose OCs, the effect of contraceptive hormones on carbohydrate metabolism has been minimized.[55, 56, 61-64]

Mechanism of Contraceptive Action

Originally, it was assumed that the contraceptive action of combined steroid hormones primarily involved inhibition of the pituitary gonadotropins with consequent blocking of ovulation. This is certainly the case with the combined estrogen-progestagen OC.[65] However, blood levels of progesterone and pituitary gonadotropins indicated that during progestagen-only contraception, ovulatory function has been preserved during many cycles. Therefore, other mechanisms of contraceptive action were explored. Among these were changes in the consistency and increases in the thickness of the cervical mucus that impair the ability of the sperm to penetrate it. Low doses

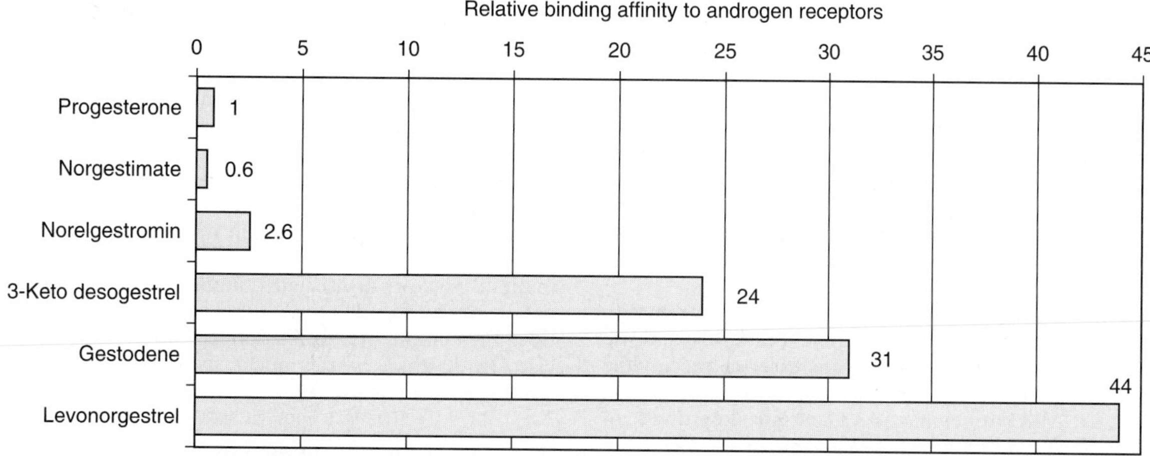

Figure 17-16. Relative binding affinity of contraceptive progestagens for androgen receptors. The assay measures displacement of ^{3}H-labeled dihydrotestosterone from rat prostatic androgen receptors. (Data from Phillips A, Demarest K, Hahn DW, et al. Progestational and androgenic receptor binding affinities and in vivo activities of norgestimate and other progestins. Contraception 1990; 41:399.)

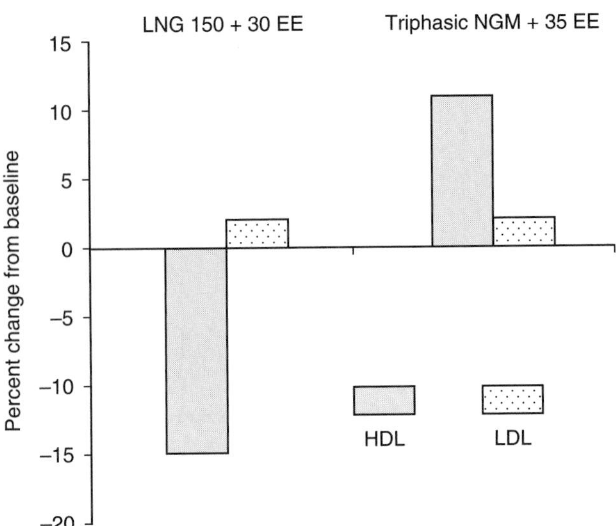

Figure 17–17. Contrasting effects of oral contraceptives containing levonorgestrel (LNG) and norgestimate (NGM) on high-density and low-density lipoproteins (HDL and LDL). (Modified from Henzl M. Norgestimate: from the laboratory to three clinical indications. J Reprod Med 2001; 46:647–661.)

of progestagens also alter the function of the endometrium, leading to an intrauterine milieu hostile to pregnancy.[66]

Oral Contraceptive Treatment Regimens

Combined Oral Contraception: Cyclic Estrogen-Progestagen Combinations

In this method both hormonal components are given in a cyclic fashion, usually from the 5th through the 25th day of the menstrual cycle. With most of the currently used preparations, a 7-day placebo period follows the 21-day hormonal treatment so that women do not need to keep track of when to start a new cycle of contraceptive pills. There is growing interest in developing combined oral contraception (COC) for continuous use to avoid monthly withdrawal bleeding.

Since the inception of COC, the developmental trend aimed at reduction of the amounts of hormonal components in the combination to a level that would make the pill safer and still provide high contraceptive protection and cycle control.

The current COC preparations can be classified according to the amount of ethinylestradiol in the daily dose: (1) 20 μg of estrogen, the lowest dose used in the United States; (2) more than 20 μg to less than 50 μg, the dose most frequently recommended today; and (3) 50 μg, a dose that is rarely recommended. Preparations with an estrogen content greater than 50 μg/day have been removed from the market in the United States. A further distinction is made according to whether the dosage regimen is monophasic, biphasic, or triphasic.

The monophasic dosage regimens consist of contraceptive steroids given in a fixed estrogen-progestagen combination from the 1st through the 21st day of treatment.

With the biphasic preparations, the daily dose of ethinylestradiol is usually constant throughout the entire 21 days of use but the initially low progestagen dose increases at the middle of the cycle, from day 11 on. A special case of biphasic dosage is a preparation (Mircette) employing a constant dose of 20 μg of ethinylestradiol combined with 150 μg of desogestrel given from day 1 through 21. This is followed by 2 days of placebo and then 5 days of ethinylestradiol at 10 μg/day.

In the triphasic treatment regimens, the daily doses of one or both steroidal components are modified three times during the treatment period. The individual dosage regimens for OC are listed in Table 17–6.

The development of the biphasic and triphasic treatment regimens was motivated by the desire to mimic the hormonal events of the normal menstrual cycle and to decrease the total load of contraceptive steroids per month. These dosage modifications have contributed to the variety of OC choices. Rigorous comparative studies have not been conducted to show whether the phasic regimens offer any clinically meaningful advantages over the monophasic schedules. However, similar performance at lower hormonal doses has theoretical appeal.

The Sequential Method

In this method, estrogens were given in a fixed dose throughout the 21-day treatment period; however, progestagens were given only during the last 5 to 9 days. The use of this regimen was discontinued in the United States in the 1970s because of concerns that repeated exposure of the endometrium to unopposed estrogens may induce atypical hyperplasia. The method is mentioned here because it is described in earlier literature.

Continuous Progestagen-Only Oral Contraception

The continuous progestagen-only method, known as the *minipill*, was developed to eliminate the estrogens entirely from OC preparations. The preparations currently available in the United States contain norethindrone, 350 μg/day; norgestrel, 75 μg/day; and levonorgestrel, 30 μg/day. Outside the United States, preparations with other progestagens are available: lynestrenol, 500 μg/day; ethynodiol diacetate, 500 μg/day; and desogestrel, 75 μg/day. The pregnancy rate for a typical user is higher than with the estrogen-progestagen OC, and the cycle control is less satisfactory.

The method is well suited for breast-feeding mothers. The amounts of progestagen that are excreted into the milk of breast-feeding mothers are negligibly low and do not affect the quantity and the composition of the milk. The combination of the ovulation-suppressive effect of prolactin and the contraceptive effects of the progestagen-only pill offers excellent protection from pregnancy. Another group of women who could benefit from this method are women around the age of 40 with naturally decreased fecundity. Good candidates for progestagen-only contraception are women who do not tolerate estrogens and who reject the use of an IUD.

Some preparations using the continuous progestagen-only method (minipill) have been associated with ectopic pregnancy. For this reason, when pregnancy occurs, all efforts must be made to rule out ectopic pregnancy. The physician must be attentive to complaints of pelvic pain by users of the progestin-only method; sometimes the diagnosis of ectopic pregnancy is delayed because symptoms of ectopic pregnancy such as irregular uterine bleeding, prolonged cycles, and amenorrhea resemble typical side effects.

The decreased efficacy of the minipill compared with combined OCs is probably due to its mechanism of action. The minipill does not consistently inhibit ovulation (about 40% of cycles are ovulatory); thus, other mechanisms become operative. Prevention of fertilization is largely due to changes in viscosity of the cervical mucus in addition to other changes that are inhospitable to impregnation of the ovum.

Benefits of Oral Contraception

Physicians, patients, and the general public have been made well aware of adverse effects of hormonal contraception. Data obtained over the last two decades brought evidence that the

Table 17–6. Oral Contraceptives Used in the United States

Manufacturer Brand Name Number/Doses	Product Type	Progestagen	Estrogen* (μg)
Berlex			
Levlen	Combination	0.15 mg levonorgestrel	30
Tri-Levlen	Combination, triphasic		
6		0.05 mg levonorgestrel	30
5		0.075 mg levonorgestrel	40
10		0.125 mg levonorgestrel	30
Yasmin	Combination	3.0 mg drospirenone	30
Bristol-Myers Squibb			
Ovcon-35	Combination	0.4 mg norethindrone	35
Ovcon-50	Combination	1.0 mg levonorgestrel	50
Organon			
Desogen	Combination	0.15 mg desogestrel	35
Mircette	Biphasic, special combination		
21		0.15 mg desogestrel	20
5		–	10
Cyclessa	Combination, triphasic		
7		0.1 mg desogestrel	25
7		0.125 mg desogestrel	25
7		0.15 mg desogestrel	25
Ortho-MacNeil Pharmaceutical			
Micronor	Progestagen-only	0.35 mg norethindrone	
Modicon	Combination	0.50 mg norethindrone	35
Ortho-Cept	Combination	0.15 mg desogestrel	30
Ortho-Cyclen	Combination	0.25 mg norgestimate	35
Ortho-Novum 1/35	Combination	1.0 mg norethindrone	35
Ortho-Novum 1/50	Combination	1.0 mg norethindrone	50†
Ortho-Novum	Combination, triphasic		
7		0.5 mg norethindrone	35
7		0.75 mg norethindrone	35
7		1.0 mg norethindrone	35
Ortho-Novum	Combination, biphasic		
10		0.5 mg norethindrone	35
11		1.0 mg norethindrone	35
Ortho-Tricyclen	Combination, triphasic		
7		0.180 mg norgestimate	35
7		0.215 mg norgestimate	35
7		0.250 mg norgestimate	35
Parke-Davis			
Estrostep	Combination, triphasic		
5		1.0 mg norethindrone acetate	20
7		1.0 mg norethindrone acetate	30
9		1.0 mg norethindrone acetate	35
Loestrin 1/20	Combination	1.0 mg norethindrone acetate	20
Loestrin 1.5/30	Combination	1.5 mg norethindrone acetate	30
Norlestrin 1/50	Combination	1.0 mg norethindrone acetate	50
Norlestrin 2.5/50	Combination	2.5 mg norethindrone acetate	50
Watson Laboratories			
Brevicon	Combination	0.5 mg norethindrone	35
Norinyl 1 + 35	Combination	1.0 mg norethindrone	35
Norinyl 1 + 50	Combination	1.0 mg norethindrone	50
Nor-Q.D.	Progestagen-only	0.35 mg norethindrone	
Tri-Norinyl	Combination, triphasic		
7		0.5 mg norethindrone	35
9		1.0 mg norethindrone	35
5		0.5 mg norethindrone	35
Searle			
Demulen 1/35	Combination	1.0 mg ethynodiol diacetate	35
Demulen 1/50	Combination	1.0 mg ethynodiol diacetate	50
Wyeth-Ayerst			
Alesse	Combination	0.100 mg levonorgestrel	20
Lo/Ovral	Combination	0.300 mg levonorgestrel	30
Nordette	Combination	0.150 mg levonorgestrel	30
Ovral	Combination	0.500 mg norgestrel	50
Ovrette	Progestagen-only	0.075 mg norgestrel	

Table continued on following page

Table 17–6. Oral Contraceptives Used in the United States *Continued*

Manufacturer Brand Name Number/Doses	Product Type	Progestagen	Estrogen* (μg)
Triphasil	Combination, triphasic		
6		0.050 mg levonorgestrel	30
5		0.075 mg levonorgestrel	40
10		0.125 mg levonorgestrel	30

*Ethinylestradiol unless noted otherwise.
†Mestranol.
Adapted and updated from Mishell DR. Contraception. In Yen SSC, Jaffe RB, Barbieri RT (eds). Reproductive Endocrinology, 4th ed. Philadelphia, WB Saunders, 1999, pp 676–708.

use of hormonal contraception has also been associated with numerous and not insignificant beneficial effects in addition to contraception.

These *noncontraceptive* benefits can be conveniently divided into those *affecting the reproductive tract* and *nonreproductive* benefits (Table 17–7).

Noncontraceptive Reproductive Benefits of Oral Contraception

Endometrial and Ovarian Carcinoma

The most impressive noncontraceptive benefit of hormonal contraception is the decreased incidence of endometrial and ovarian carcinomas. In the United States, endometrial carcinoma is the most common pelvic cancer in women. Current estimates indicate that 36,000 new cases are diagnosed yearly with a death rate of 6500. The 5-year survival rate is 83% when it is diagnosed early; more advanced cases have a survival rate of 65%. For the most part endometrial carcinoma affects women past reproductive age, although younger women are not immune to the disease.

The decreased risk is related to the length of use of OCs. A decrease is evident after only 1 year of use; women who have been practicing hormonal contraception for 4 years or more have risk reduced by more than 50%. It is important to note that hormonal contraception offers long-term protection and that the residual protective effects persist for 20 years or longer. It is also important that the protective effect has been associated with the use of all OCs for which data have been gathered. Data on progestagen-only contraception and preparations with 20 μg of ethinylestradiol are not yet available, but it is likely that they would offer the same protection as the other preparations.

The mechanism of the protective effect on the endometrium most likely involves the direct antiestrogenic effects of the progestagen component of the OCs. Estrogens stimulate synthesis of both estrogen and progestagen receptors, and progestagens inhibit this synthesis. Part of the antiestrogenic effect of progestagens may also involve the stimulation of estradiol 17β-hydrolases in the endometrial cell and accelerated conversion of estradiol to estrone, a less potent estrogen than estradiol.[67] Consequently, the proliferation of the endometrial epithelium, both endometrial glands and stroma, proceeds at a reduced rate with less mitotic activity.

With an estimated 26,700 new cases per year, ovarian carcinoma occurs less frequently than endometrial carcinoma; however, it is more deadly. With 14,800 deaths per year, ovarian cancer is the fourth leading cause of death from cancer, after lung, breast, and colon and rectal carcinomas. The 5-year survival rate is less than 45% after the diagnosis has been established. The protective effect of hormonal contraception is evident with only 3 to 6 months of use. It becomes highly significant after 7 years of use (relative risk 0.2 to 0.4), and the residual protective effect extends at least 10 to 15 years after termination of use.[68]

Hormonal contraception reduces the risk of functional ovarian cysts by 60%. This can be important because functional ovarian cysts are the fourth leading reason for hospitalization of women in the United States, with 160,000 admissions per year. We can speculate that the decreased relative risk of both ovarian carcinoma and functional ovarian cysts is probably due to inhibition of monthly proliferation of the graafian follicles.[69] Ovarian suppression associated with low-dose OCs is less pronounced than with higher dose OCs.[70]

Each year, more than 1 million women in the United States experience an episode of pelvic inflammatory disease (PID). Epidemiologic data suggest that women taking OCs have a reduced risk of being hospitalized for PID, but further work is needed to assess the effects of OCs on the incidence of PID.[71, 72]

With respect to ectopic pregnancy, studies from the early

Table 17–7. Noncontraceptive Health Benefits of Hormonal Contraception

Condition	Relative Risk (Risk for Nonusers = 1)
A. Reduced Risk of Morbidity	
Endometrial carcinoma	
Years of use	
1	0.8
2	0.6
≥4	0.4
Overall	0.5
Ovarian carcinoma*	
Years of use	
>3	0.5
≥7	0.2–0.4
Overall	0.3
Ovarian cysts	0.4
Pelvic inflammatory disease	0.1
Ectopic pregnancy	0.1
Benign breast tumors	0.5
B. Reduced Risk and Improvement of Quality of Life	
Dysmenorrhea	0.4
Menorrhagia	0.5
Anemia	0.6
Premenstrual syndrome	0.7
Irregular menses	0.7

*Residual protective effect lasts for 10 to 15 years after termination of use.

1990s showed that the incidence rate of ectopic pregnancy per 1000 woman-years is 3.0 for women who do not practice contraception at all. The incidence rate is reduced to 0.005 in women using combination OCs. In women using a Cu-T IUD or the levonorgestrel-containing implant Norplant and in women who have undergone tubal sterilization, the incidence rate is still low (0.2 to 0.3).[73, 74]

Uterine Leiomyomas

High doses of norethindrone only, or norethindrone given simultaneously with gonadotropin-releasing hormone (GnRH) agonists, can achieve reduction of the size of leiomyomas. Because leiomyoma is the most frequently encountered tumor of the female genital tract, there has been great interest in determining whether OCs protect against the occurrence of this tumor. The question has been addressed by several studies that provided opposing results, and the problem remains unresolved. At least, there does not appear to be an increased risk.[75]

Endometriosis

OCs have been recommended for mild forms of endometriosis. However, well-designed studies proving a substantive effect are lacking. OCs may protect against the occurrence of endometriosis,[76] and some clinicians use OCs as a follow-up for the prevention of recurrence of endometriosis after a completed course of GnRH agonists.

Other Reproductive Noncontraceptive Benefits

Table 17–7 also shows the beneficial effect of OCs on conditions that are not always serious but negatively affect the quality of life. Such conditions include dysmenorrhea, mittelschmerz, menorrhagia and irregular menses, premenstrual syndrome, and iron deficiency anemia. The beneficial effects are achieved by suppression of ovulation and by influencing the endometrium.

Nonreproductive Benefits of Oral Contraception

Management of Hyperandrogenism

OCs have been used in the management of hyperandrogenic conditions such as acne, seborrhea, and hirsutism. Triphasic norgestimate-ethinylestradiol regimens and three other OC combinations of ethinylestradiol with norethindrone acetate, levonorgestrel, or desogestrel[77–80] have been shown in randomized, blinded, placebo-controlled trials to be effective in the treatment of acne. The efficacy of other OCs has also been supported by studies conducted under less rigorous protocols.[81, 82] For example, a single-blind randomized study demonstrated alleviation of acne by treatment with a pregnane type of progestagen, chlormadinone acetate, combined with ethinylestradiol.[83]

Several modes of action have been considered to explain the efficacy of OCs in hyperandrogenism. OCs can suppress production of ovarian androgens by inhibiting pituitary gonadotropins. An increase of circulating levels of SHBG is associated with a decrease of bioavailable testosterone, and inhibition of 5α-reductase in the skin tissues can also contribute to this antiandrogenic effect.

Medical treatment of hirsutism with OCs is more difficult. In addition to a number of supportive case series reports, two well-controlled clinical trials using OCs with or without GnRH agonists have been reported.[84, 85] The first one employed a randomized, double-blind, placebo-controlled study design. Neither the OC Norinyl 1/35 (1 mg of norethindrone plus 35 μg of ethinylestradiol) nor placebo had a beneficial effect on hirsutism. In the second study, which was investigator-blind but not placebo-controlled, the contraceptive Demulen (1 mg of ethynodiol diacetate plus 35 μg of ethinylestradiol) had no effect on hirsutism. However, OC complements GnRH agonist analogues in the management of hirsutism. In these two studies, only the combination of OC and a GnRH agonist had a clinically and statistically significant beneficial effect on hirsutism.

Bone Mineral Density

Well-designed studies demonstrate that the use of OCs increases bone mineral density so that users enter menopause with higher bone mass than nonusers, by 12% on the average. This beneficial effect depends on the duration of OC use; the greatest protection is afforded to women who use OCs for 10 years or more. The ultimate question, whether previous OC users suffer fewer bone fractures during menopause than nonusers, has been addressed by a large case-control study. The results have shown a 25% reduction in hip fractures in previous users of OCs.[86, 87]

Rheumatoid Arthritis

The relationship between OC use and rheumatoid arthritis has been of interest in countries where this disease affects larger segments of the population. A case-control study from Holland reported 60% protection in ever-users of OCs.[88] Other studies and meta-analyses of various clinical trials have not provided an unequivocal conclusion.[89]

Colorectal Cancer

Several studies employing epidemiologic methodology have provided evidence that OCs afford about 50% protection from colorectal cancer and that this effect is directly proportional to the duration of OC use. The subject remains controversial because other clinical observations failed to confirm the protective effect. The mechanism by which OCs would exert a protective effect against colorectal cancer is not clear.[90, 91]

Adverse Events Associated with the Use of Oral Contraception

The frequency of adverse events associated with oral contraception has decreased continuously since hormonal contraception was first introduced for general clinical use. There are several reasons for this favorable development. The amount of estrogens in the pill has been gradually reduced since estrogens were identified as the culprit in the most severe adverse events, principally cardiovascular and cerebrovascular complications. This reduction was paralleled by decreases in the daily doses of the progestagenic component of OC. In addition, candidates for OCs are being selected more carefully as risk factors for potential complications have been identified, notably smoking among women older than 35. Researchers realized that more frequent follow-up of new OC users could detect early signs and symptoms of complications. For example, measurements of blood pressure before therapy and during the first 3 months of OC use identify individuals predisposed to hypertension. Finally, physicians defined appropriate contraceptive options for patients with medical problems.

Most Commonly Reported Adverse Events

The use of hormonal contraception is associated with a number of less serious adverse events that are nonetheless important because they constitute reasons for discontinuation.

Breakthrough Bleeding. This event can be expected in 10% to 30% of women during the first 3 months of use of hormonal contraception; thereafter, it is much less frequent. Depending on its intensity and duration, it can be handled by reassuring the patient or by short-term administration of a supplementary estrogen such as micronized estradiol.

Amenorrhea. Amenorrhea, that is, lack of bleeding during the active pill-free period, is always a cause for anxiety because of the possibility of pregnancy. Pregnancy should be ruled out by a sensitive urine or blood pregnancy test. If pregnancy is ruled out and the patient is comfortable with amenorrhea, she may resume the same OC. Alternatively, she may be switched to another OC, usually with more estrogen dominance. Sometimes supplementation by estrogens is recommended. Repeated episodes of amenorrhea can be bothersome and irritating, and it is sometimes best to recommend another method of contraception. A positive pregnancy test should alert the physician to the unlikely but critical possibility of an ectopic pregnancy.

Other Adverse Effects. One study compared two groups of patients, randomly assigned to receive either a tricyclic combination of ethinylestradiol and norgestimate (Ortho Tri-Cyclen) or a placebo. Symptoms that are usually attributed to the use of OCs, such as common headaches, nausea, breast tension and tenderness, weight gain, and mood change, were assessed before and during treatment. The difference in the incidence of side effects between the two groups was not statistically significant. Only the higher incidence of breast tenderness and mood change in the OC group approached significance ($P = .07$).[92]

Women who discontinue OC use conceive later than women practicing nonhormonal methods of contraception. "Postpill amenorrhea" develops in ≤1% of users.

Caution. Despite the reassuring reports with respect to adverse events, the prescribing physician must be aware that certain conditions warrant caution or constitute a frank contraindication to hormonal contraception. These conditions are discussed in the sections "Contraindications" and "Contraception for Women with Health Problems."

Cardiovascular and Cerebrovascular Adverse Events

From the inception of their clinical use in the 1960s, OCs have been associated with cardiovascular and cerebrovascular complications, namely idiopathic venous thromboembolism (VTE), stroke, and myocardial infarction (MI). These adverse events merit reevaluation in the light of epidemiologic studies that were prompted by the introduction of low-dose OCs into clinical practice.[93]

Venous Thromboembolism

The Role of Estrogens. Since the first reports of VTE in OC users, clinicians suspected that the noxious agent is the estrogenic component of the combination pill. A dose-response relationship between the estrogen dose and VTE was demonstrated in an epidemiologic study of 234,218 women between 1980 and 1986, when both high-dose and low-dose estrogen pills were being prescribed. The highest incidence of VTE, 10 per 10,000 woman-years, occurred among women who used OCs with an ethinylestradiol content of more than 50 μg/day. With preparations containing the medium dose of ethinylestradiol, 50 μg/day, the incidence of VTE decreased to 7 per 10,000 woman-years; with pills having an ethinylestradiol content less than 50 μg/day, the rate of VTE decreased to 4.2 events per 10,000 woman-years. The difference between the incidence of VTE at 50 μg/day ethinylestradiol and the incidence at less than 50 μg/day ethinylestradiol was statistically significant.[93]

Table 17–8. Relative Risk of Idiopathic Venous Thromboembolism in Pregnancy and during the Use of Contraceptive Hormones

Population	Relative Risk Estimates	95% Confidence Interval
Unexposed	1	
Emergency contraception*	0	
Hormone replacement therapy	2.3	0.4–15.0
Progestagen-only contraception	2.4	0.8–6.5
Levonorgestrel-containing oral contraceptives (second generation)	3.4	0.8–13.7
Third generation oral contraceptives (gestodene, desogestrel)	8.0	2.1–29.9
Progestogens for menstrual disorders	5.3	1.5–18.7
Pregnant, postpartum	12.3	4.6–36.4

*Vasilakis C, Jick SS, Jick H. The risk of venous thromboembolism in users of post-coital contraceptive pills. Contraception. 1999; 59:79–83.

Modified from Vasilakis C, Jick H, del Mar Melero-Montez M. Risk of idiopathic venous thromboembolism in users of progestagens alone. Lancet 1999; 354: 1610–1611.

A subsequent study analyzed idiopathic VTE in a cohort of 74,086 women during the 5-year period from 1993 to 1997.[94] In this epidemiologic study, the relative risk of VTE was defined for pregnancy, various forms of oral contraception including combination OC and the progestagen-only method, therapeutic use of progestagens, and hormonal replacement therapy. The results are summarized in Table 17–8, to which we have added an analysis of the relative risk of VTE associated with emergency contraception.[95] The highest risk of VTE is associated with pregnancy—13 times higher than in nonpregnant women. Emergency contraception is not associated with a substantive risk. There is a slight but nonsignificant association between progestagen-only contraception and VTE, the relative risk being 2.4 with a 95% confidence interval (CI) of 0.8 to 6.5. A similar association has been reported for women using hormonal replacement therapy, the relative risk being 2.3 (CI 0.4 to 15.0). With the therapeutic use of progestagens for menstrual disorders, the relative risk for development of VTE rose to 5.3 (CI 1.5 to 18.7). The daily doses in progestagen-only contraception are normally less than 0.5 mg, whereas the therapeutic doses range from 5.0 to 30.0 mg/day.

An ongoing controversy involves reports that the risk of VTE associated with combination OCs containing desogestrel and gestodene is more than twice that for OCs with norgestrel and norethindrone (3.4 versus 8.0). This finding merits a discussion of the role of progestagens in the genesis of VTE.

The Role of Progestagens. In 1995, several independent clinical epidemiologic studies presented evidence that OCs containing desogestrel and gestodene are associated with double the risk of nonfatal VTE compared with earlier OCs containing norethindrone or levonorgestrel.[96–98] The results were surprising because thrombotic phenomena have not been conventionally associated with the progestagenic component of OCs. The data were immediately questioned, and the relationship of the various progestagens to VTE became controversial. However, a study analyzing OC use for the 7-year period between 1993 and 1999 confirmed that the risk for development of

VTE of women using OCs containing desogestrel and gestodene is twice that of women using OCs with levonorgestrel.[99] The controversy concerning the third-generation pills containing gestodene and desogestrel continued into 2001, when a meta-analysis established a 1.7-fold risk for third-generation versus second-generation pills.[100]

Norgestimate has not been included in these analyses. An analysis based on postmarketing surveillance of adverse events associated with the use of COCs containing desogestrel and norgestimate showed a threefold to fourfold excess of reported cases of deep vein thrombosis in desogestrel users compared with norgestimate users. Both compounds were launched at approximately the same time, but the estimated number of distributed pill cycles was markedly higher for norgestimate.[101] It is important to note that all low-dose OCs are safer than older high-dose products and that all current products are much safer than pregnancy vis-à-vis VTE.

Venous Thromboembolism and Coagulation Factors. Studies of the effects of hormonal contraceptive agents on blood coagulation factors reveal that OCs increase the synthesis of globulins in the liver, including many clotting factors. Consequently, circulating concentrations of many clotting factors are affected but not to a clinically significant level. Most frequently affected are fibrinogen and factors dependent on vitamin K (prothrombin and factors VII, IX, and X) and factor XII. At the same time, a decrease in the levels of antithrombin III, an anticoagulation factor, was noted. Despite the fact that these changes had occurred in virtually all OC users tested, VTE remains a rare event.

In discussing these findings, several issues have to be taken into account. Even under physiologic conditions, concentrations of the clotting factors are excessive in the circulation of healthy women, in some cases reaching 200% of the "normal" values. For hemostasis, however, only a fraction of this activity is needed. The coagulation factors are proenzymes that are present in the circulation in their inactive form. Damage to the blood vessel must occur to activate the coagulation cascade. With respect to antithrombin III, the OC-induced decrease is about 10%, far short of the profound reduction needed to form a clot.[102]

Changes in blood coagulation depend on the dose of estrogen. The decrease of the ethinylestradiol content to below 50 μg/day, common in current OC preparations, has considerably limited the changes in blood coagulation factors that were observed in OCs with a higher ethinylestradiol content.[103]

Venous Thromboembolism and Leiden Factor V. During the normal coagulation process, protein C and its cofactor S prevent hypercoagulation by inhibiting the activity of coagulation factors V and VII. The Leiden mutation, a genetic mutation of factor V consisting of an alteration of a single amino acid, makes factor V resistant to the action of protein C. The Leiden mutation of factor V occurs in 5% of the U.S. white population and is less frequent in black and Hispanic women. Its presence predisposes the carrier to VTE (Table 17–9).

In women of reproductive age, the rate of VTE increases to 5.7 VTE events per 10,000 woman-years, and in OC users the increase amounts to 28.5 events per 10,000 woman-years. The identification of the Leiden factor V mutation is the first instance in which increased VTE events in OC users could be linked to a concrete defect in a coagulation cascade. However, screening for the Leiden mutation would be impractical because examination of 1 million potential OC users would detect only 50 women at risk. In addition, 62,000 women would have false-positive results.[104, 105]

Physicians generally consider a personal history of venous thrombosis an absolute contraindication to the use of OCs.

Table 17–9. Oral Contraception and Factor V Leiden: Risk of Idiopathic Venous Thromboembolism

Population	Relative Risk	Incidence per 10,000 Woman-Years
Controls	1	0.8
Oral contraception only	3.8	3.0
Factor V Leiden mutation	7.9	5.7
Factor V Leiden mutation—oral contraceptive users	34.7	28.5

Modified from Vandenbroucke JP, Koster T, Briet E, et al. Increased risk of venous thrombosis in oral-contraceptive users who are carriers of factor V Leiden mutation. Lancet 1994; 344:1453–1457; Vandenbroucke JP, van der Meer FJ, Helmerhorst FM, Rosendaal FR. Factor V Leiden: should we screen oral contraceptive users and pregnant women? BMJ 1996; 313:1127–1130.

Screening for factor V Leiden may be justified in women with a strong family history of venous thrombosis. The presence of superficial varicose veins that are not a consequence of previous venous thrombosis is not a contraindication to the use of oral contraception.[106]

In conclusion, although significant strides have been made in accumulating knowledge about VTE and OCs, the phenomenon remains as enigmatic as before. Reducing the dose of ethinylestradiol in the combination pill to less than 50 μg/day, along with other preventive measures, has substantially lowered the risk of VTE although it has not been eliminated entirely. There are no substantive data supporting increased safety for products containing 20 μg versus 30 to 35 μg despite the logical appeal. In-depth molecular biologic research is needed to understand VTE and pave the road to its rational prevention.

Stroke and Oral Contraception

Stroke has been recognized as one of the serious complications of OC use, although its incidence has been rare. In 1976, Vessey and Doll[107] reported 41 to 45 strokes per 100,000 woman-years in OC users, a fourfold to fivefold increase over the rate of stroke in nonusers. Later studies had more reassuring outcomes. In 1996, a large epidemiologic study demonstrated that women using OCs with a low estrogen content (<50 μg of ethinylestradiol) are not at increased risk for stroke.[108] The published findings were based on investigations of a large California health organization, Kaiser Permanente, and included an analysis of 1.1 million women, 14 to 40 years of age, who were observed during the 5 years 1991 to 1994 for a total of 3.6 million woman-years. During this time period, 408 women suffered a proven stroke. This confirms the fact that stroke occurs rarely in young women, with an incidence rate of only 11.3 cases per 100,000 woman-years. With respect to OCs, 94% of the women studied used daily preparations with low estrogen content (<50 μg) and none of them took preparations with a daily dose of estrogen higher than 50 μg.

Table 17–10 compares the risk of stroke in current OC users with the risk in never-users and past OC users. If the risk for never-users and past OC users equals 1.0, then for current users of low-estrogen OCs the relative risk of ischemic stroke equals 1.18 (95% CI 0.54 to 2.59) and that of hemorrhagic stroke equals 1.14 (CI 0.60 to 2.15). There is no statistically significant difference among these risk estimates. Thus, we can conclude that low-estrogen OC does not appreciably

Table 17–10. Relative Risk of Stroke in Women Using Low-Estrogen Oral Contraception (<50 μg Ethinylestradiol)*

Investigated Risk Factors	Relative Risk of Stroke (95% Confidence Interval)	
	Ischemic	Hemorrhagic
Use of oral contraception		
Never or past users only	1.00	1.00
Current users	1.18 (0.54–2.59)	1.14 (0.60–2.16)
Current users plus smoking	0.74 (0.17–3.25)	3.64 (0.95–13.87)
Health status and lifestyle		
Hypertension	7.78 (3.51–17.31)	4.64 (2.14–10.06)
Diabetes	7.15 (3.17–16.13)	2.5 (0.62–0.08)
>3 Drinks per week	1.93 (0.87–4.29)	2.02 (1.06–3.85)

*The low-estrogen oral contraceptive contains ethinylestradiol at a dose of less than 50 μg.

From Petitti DB, Sidney S, Bernstein A, et al. Stroke in users of low-dose oral contraception. N Engl J Med 1996; 335:8.

Table 17–11. Myocardial Infarction: Effects of Oral Contraception, Health Status, and Lifestyle

Investigated Factors	Relative Risk	95% Confidence Interval
Oral Contraception		
No oral contraception	1.00	1.00
Combination oral contraceptive		
All users	1.40	0.78–2.52
Norgestrel	1.10	0.52–2.30
Gestodene, desogestrel	1.96	0.87–4.39
Progestogens only	1.48	0.60–3.65
Health Status and Lifestyle		
Cardinal health risk factors*	5.80	4.38–7.67
Ever smoked	6.88	5.05–9.36
Alcohol intake 1 d/wk	0.6	0.45–0.80
Exercise ≥1 h/wk	0.45	0.32–0.64

*Smoking, hypertension, diabetes mellitus, angina pectoris, hyperlipidemia, family history of myocardial infarction.

Modified from Dunn N, Thorogood M, Faragher B, et al. Oral Contraceptives and myocardial infarction: results of MICA case-control study. BMJ 1999: 318: 1579–1584.

increase the risk of either ischemic or hemorrhagic stroke for nonsmokers.

The report has further confirmed the negative effects of smoking and simultaneous use of OCs; smoking increases the risk of hemorrhagic stroke to 3.64. This may be due to the damage that smoking inflicts upon endothelial cells secreting agents that direct vasodilatation during increased demands on the cardiovascular system. Other conditions that increase the risk of stroke include diabetes, hypertension, and excessive use of alcohol.

The use of low-estrogen OCs contributed to the favorable results of the study. Moreover, study participants were carefully chosen with regard to identified risk factors before recommending a contraceptive method.

Myocardial Infarction and Oral Contraception

MI in women of childbearing age is rare: 0.05 per 1000 women-years. For that reason, studies investigating MI in OC users must be very large in order to show any relationship.

Between 1997 and 1999, three important studies addressed this issue. A multicenter study organized by the WHO found a 5-fold increased risk of MI in current users of OC in Europe but only a 2.6-fold increase in women who had their blood pressure checked before prescription of an OC.[109] When a subset of patients from England was analyzed, the odds ratio was 2.10 (CI 0.63 to 7.07); in other countries the odds ratio was much higher, possibly indicating different practices in selecting patients for OC. Another international study pointed out that any risk of MI is confined to women with known cardiovascular risk factors.[110]

The third study was a case-control study conducted in 1993 to 1995. A group of 448 women of childbearing age, all of whom had suffered an incident of MI, was matched with 1728 control subjects without a history of MI. It is important to note that during the time period of the analysis, OCs with an ethinylestradiol content of less than 50 μg, combined with norgestrel or levonorgestrel as well as with norgestimate, desogestrel, and gestodene, were already in clinical use. This study had sufficient power to examine the effects of OCs with different progestagens on the incidence of MI.[111]

The study has shown that the risk of MI in OC users is not increased and that there is no difference between OCs with an ethinylestradiol content less than 50 μg combined with norgestrel and levonorgestrel or with norgestimate, desogestrel, and gestodene. Progestagen-only contraception was found to have no effect on the genesis of MI. The study confirmed the high risk of MI associated with hypertension, diabetes, hyperlipidemia, angina, diabetes mellitus, and smoking. Of these, the highest risk factor was smoking. On the other hand, modest alcohol intake (once a week) and physical exercise for 1 hour or more per week were found to be beneficial (Table 17–11). These study conclusions were strengthened by the observation that of women younger than 45 years who suffered MI, 87% were not taking OCs but most of them had one or more known cardiovascular risk factors.

Oral Contraception and Smoking

Perhaps in no other condition have the adverse effects of smoking been so well defined as in oral contraception. Cardiovascular and cerebrovascular complications of OC use have been recognized since the early surveillance studies that also pointed out the negative effects of smoking.[112, 113] Whereas the probability of developing these complications has been minimized for nonsmokers by reducing the amount of estrogens, smoking OC users are still exposed to a considerable risk of MI and stroke.

A long-term follow-up of women by the Royal College of General Practitioners contributed considerably to our understanding of the relation between OC, smoking, and MI. In 1998, data for 10,073 women were evaluated to determine whether changes in smoking habits have an effect on the risk estimates for MI.[114] When the information on smoking supplied by the women at their entrance into the study was taken into consideration, the relative risk of MI was 3.6 (95% CI 2.2 to 5.9). However, during the study, 53% of women who had ever smoked regularly stopped smoking and only 4.5% of nonsmokers started smoking. Therefore, the authors performed another analysis in which they took into consideration the smoking status of the women at the occurrence of MI. As expected, women who continued smoking throughout the study were at a much higher risk for MI than those who did not smoke at the occurrence of the event. The relative risk for smokers was 5.1 (95% CI 3.0 to 8.7).

The increased risk of smokers for MI has also been underscored in the Myocardial Infarction Causality case-control study conducted between 1993 and 1995 in the United Kingdom. Odds ratios for risk of MI in smokers versus nonsmokers showed a strong dose response, from 2.47 (95% CI 1.12 to 5.45) in smokers of 1 to 5 cigarettes per day to 74.6 (95% CI 33.0 to 169.0) in smokers of ≥40 cigarettes per day.[115] The relative risk of MI for all users of combination OCs was at 1.40 (95% CI 0.78 to 2.52), but the relative risk for women who ever smoked was significantly higher, 6.88 (95% CI 5.05 to 9.36).[111, 115]

The association of stroke, OCs, and smoking is not as strong as that for MI, although an increased risk of stroke for smokers using OCs was demonstrated in epidemiologic as well as case-control studies.

The landmark epidemiologic study by Petitti and colleagues in 1996[108] showed that for young women smokers in the United States using OCs with less than 50 μg of ethinylestradiol, the risk of hemorrhagic stroke is three times higher than for nonsmokers. In this study, smoking did not increase the risk of ischemic stroke.

Two WHO collaborative studies in 1996 evaluated the effect of smoking in a case-control design. With respect to hemorrhagic stroke in women of all ages, the odds ratios for current OC users who were also current cigarette smokers were greater than 3. For female smokers younger than 35 years of age, the odds ratios were 2.6 in Europe and developing countries; for female smokers older than 35 years the odds ratios were 3.9 for Europe and 5.4 for developing countries.[116] With respect to ischemic stroke, the WHO collaborative study showed that the OC-associated odds ratios were higher among current smokers in Europe (7.2 smokers versus 2.1 nonsmokers) as well as in developing countries (4.8 smokers versus 2.6 nonsmokers), suggesting a synergistic effect of both factors.[117]

Currently, mechanisms by which smoking exerts its negative effects are being investigated. Attention is focused on nicotine's interference with endothelial cells, principally with their ability to secrete vasodilating substances and to regenerate.[118]

The data presented indicate that OCs can be safely prescribed to women of all ages as long as they do not smoke and have no other risk factor. OCs can be prescribed to smokers younger than 35 years, but after this age limit OCs must be avoided unless the women stop smoking. For patients of any age, smoking cessation may be the single most effective preventive action any health care provider can recommend. Women seeking contraceptive advice must be thoroughly questioned about their smoking history, and the dangers of smoking must be clearly delineated.

Neoplastic Changes

The relationship between contraceptive hormones and neoplastic growth has been of concern, and the subject has been evaluated in several excellent reviews.[119–121] Several epidemiologic studies and meta-analyses have drawn attention to this important issue.

Breast Carcinoma

Breast cancer is a frightening malignancy. In the United States, 182,000 new cases are detected annually. It is the most common carcinoma in women, and with 46,000 deaths a year it is the second most lethal cancer in women. Because of fear of breast cancer, many women do not start OCs or may discontinue their use.

Fortunately, a recent study has convincingly demonstrated that present or past use of oral contraceptives is not associated with an increased risk of breast cancer.[122, 122a] This clinical trial was a population-based case-control study conducted under an extremely rigorous protocol.[122b] The "cases"—4575 women newly diagnosed with breast cancer during July 1994 through April 1998, were matched and compared to 4682 control women without breast carcinoma. The probands were 35–64 years of age, a period of life during which breast cancer strikes most frequently. The study enrolled both Caucasian as well as African Americans and was conducted in five regions of the United States. Among current OC users the relative risk of breast cancer was 1.0 (95% confidence interval 0.8 to 1.3); for former users the risk was 0.9 (95% confidence interval 0.8 to 1.0). The study has also failed to detect any significant association between the risk of breast cancer and the amount of estrogen in the combination, duration of OC use, the initiation of use during adolescence, the race of the probands, or family history of breast cancer.

An earlier study from 1996[122c] was a meta-analysis of 54 small studies conducted over a period of 25 years. However, the study had the disadvantages of a meta-analysis, for example, non-uniform study designs and protocols, different quality of study conduct and analyses, and follow-up. The study showed only a slightly increased risk of breast carcinoma among current OC users and a gradual decline of the risk during the postpill period, until the risk completely disappeared 10 years after stopping the pill.

The cancers diagnosed in women who had used combined OCs were less advanced clinically than those diagnosed in women who had never used OCs. For ever-users of OCs compared with never-users, the relative risk for tumors spreading beyond the breast was 0.88 (CI 0.81 to 0.95; $P = .002$). Moreover, the positive association between OC use and localized breast cancer extends for up to 20 years after stopping the pill.[122c] Why breast cancer in OC users is less advanced than in nonusers has not been explained.

Whether women with a family history of breast cancer are at a higher risk for the disease while using OCs was analyzed in more detail in another case-control study. Study participants included 394 sisters and daughters and 3002 granddaughters and nieces of 436 families of breast cancer probands. OC use was associated with an increased risk of breast cancer among daughters and sisters (relative risk 3.3; CI 1.6 to 6.7) but not among granddaughters and nieces.[123] Other studies have been consistent with regard to family history as an OC risk factor. The study underscores the importance of obtaining a thorough family history not only before prescribing OCs but for women in general.

Cervical Carcinoma and Oral Contraception

In the United States, 12,800 cases of invasive cervical cancer are diagnosed annually and 4800 women die from this disease. Cervical cancer used to be the most frequently diagnosed malignancy in women in the United States. Over the last 30 to 40 years, its incidence has been declining, most likely as a result of early treatment of precursor lesions. Today, it has assumed the fifth place among the most frequently encountered cancers in women. Nevertheless, concerns about its association with the use of OCs remain.

Squamous Cell Cervical Carcinoma

Epidemiologic studies of the relation between oral contraception and squamous cell carcinoma of the uterine cervix originate from the late 1980s and early 1990s. No association between cervical carcinoma and OCs was found during the first 5 years of use, but the incidence of cervical carcinoma doubled at and after 10 years of use.[124–126]

Cervical Adenocarcinoma

Cervical adenocarcinoma arises from the columnar epithelium of the endocervical canal and constitutes 10% to 15% of

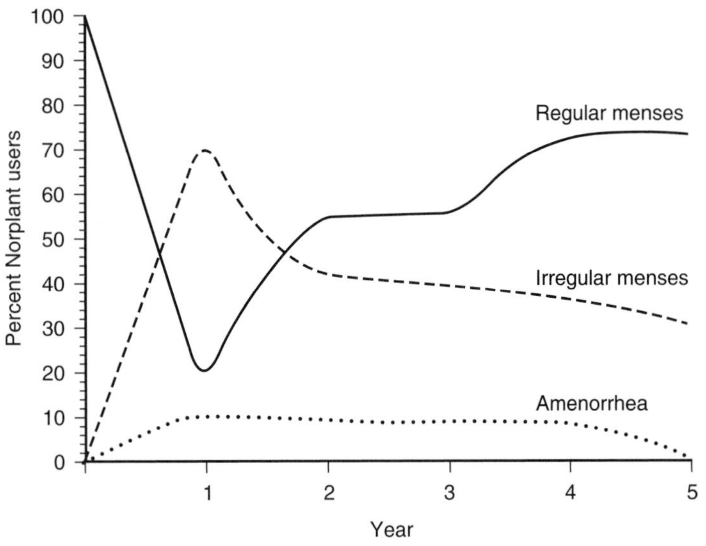

Figure 17–18. Menstrual patterns during 5 years of using contraceptive hormonal implant with levonorgestrel. (From Speroff L, Darney PD. A clinical guide for contraception, 3rd ed. Philadelphia: Lippincott Williams & Wilkins, 2001.)

Efficacy and Properties of Individual Steroids

The contraceptive efficacy of Norplant is high. Extensive data show pregnancy rates of less than 0.5 per 100 woman-years even after 5 years of use. Bleeding irregularities may be a problem, particularly during the first year of use (Fig. 17–18). The contraceptive efficacy of Implanon, the system using etonogestrel, is also impressively high; no pregnancies were reported during more than 53,000 cycles of use. This high efficacy is probably related to ovulation suppression throughout the projected time of effective use; only during the last 6 months of use has an occasional ovulation been observed. The system is designed for 3 years of protection.

So far, data on the nestorone implant have shown high contraceptive efficacy, with only one pregnancy during 4000 cycles of use. Nestorone is a unique steroid that is not orally active because of rapid disintegration in the alimentary tract. Therefore, the implant is especially well suited for breast-feeding mothers.[54, 137, 138]

Return to Fertility

After removal of the implant, ovulatory cycles occur promptly with rapid return of fertility. This is the main difference between the implant and MPA depot injections (Depo-Provera), in which residual deposits release the compound for a prolonged period after treatment has been discontinued, thus delaying pregnancy.

Table 17–13. Advantages and Disadvantages of Hormonal Implants

Advantages	Disadvantages
No estrogen	Minor surgery needed for initiation and termination of method
Long-term use not necessitating repeated effort on the part of the patient	Dependence on trained health care personnel to insert and remove the implants
Efficacy independent of compliance	High prevalence of endometrial bleeding irregularities
Exposure to progestagen lower than with the pill or injectables	High costs if discontinued early
In spite of menstrual irregularities, total blood loss is decreased	

Adverse Events and Continuation Rates

During the first year after implantation, the major complaint has been irregular uterine bleeding, which caused some patients to discontinue the method. During later months of use, amenorrhea becomes more prominent (Fig. 17–18). Despite these complications, the continuation rate after the first year has been close to 80% and after 5 years it has been 35% to 70%.

Because in some cases Norplant capsules were difficult to insert and even more difficult to remove, formation of scar tissue could not be avoided. The ensuing medical-legal problems and diminished demand led to voluntary withdrawal of the preparation from some markets, notably in Great Britain.

In conclusion, the advantages and disadvantages of hormonal implants are summarized in Table 17–13.

Injectable Progestagen-Only Preparations

The progestagens most widely used in long-acting injectable preparations are MPA, under the name Depo-Provera, and norethindrone enanthate, which is not available in the United States.

Depot Medroxyprogesterone Acetate

Depot MPA is an aqueous suspension on microcrystals of the hormone. A dose of 150 mg is injected every 3 months intramuscularly, preferably deep into the gluteal or deltoidal muscle. There is at least a 2-week safety margin after the prescribed 90 days when a new injection should be administered. A 300-mg dose is given every 6 months. The efficacy of depot MPA is high; the pregnancy rate is $\leq$0.5 per 100 woman-years for 12 months of use. This result presumes that women are able to obtain their injection at appropriate intervals.

Norethindrone Enanthate

Norethindrone enanthate is given intramuscularly in a dose of 200 mg. The first two injections should be given at 60-day intervals ($\pm$5 days), followed by injections every 12 weeks or 84 $\pm$ 7 days. The contraceptive efficacy of norethindrone enanthate is high, usually less than 1 pregnancy per 100 woman-years.

Long-acting injectable preparations are usually administered within the first 5 days of the menstrual cycle; when given later, a backup method—usually a barrier contraceptive—should be used for the first 14 days after dosing.

The main disadvantages of progestagen-only contraception are bleeding irregularities including metrorrhagia and amenorrhea. Another disadvantage is the delayed return to fertility; women do not become pregnant until about 6 months after they have discontinued treatment. Appropriate pretherapy counseling reduces requests for discontinuation. Depot MPA has been associated with decreased circulating levels of estradiol and a small and reversible decrease of bone mineral density.[139] This finding is still debated, particularly with regard to use of depot MPA as a contraceptive method for teenage women.

Monthly Injectable Combination Contraception

To circumvent the disadvantages of progestagen-only contraception, monthly combination injectable contraception has been developed. Injection of 25 mg of MPA combined with 5 mg of estradiol cypionate—a long-acting derivative of estradiol (see Fig. 17–6)—is performed within the first 5 days of the menstrual cycle and repeated every 28 ± 5 days. This method presents several improvements over the progestagen-only injectables for women who may use estrogen. Improvements include regular cyclic bleeding and, after discontinuation of this method, prompt resumption of fertility as with combination OC. Unlike use of OC, monthly injectable combination contraception does not require daily actions on the part of the users; however, the user must return to the health care practitioner every month to receive the injection. This presents a certain disadvantage compared with an injection of depot MPA or norethindrone enanthate every 3 months. However, the combination injections provide a high degree of protection; the reported pregnancy rate is 0.1 per 100 woman-years for women who return for injection at appropriate intervals.[140]

Contraceptive Vaginal Rings

Contraceptive vaginal rings use another route of administration of contraceptive steroids. Vaginal mucosa has been found to absorb steroid hormones in amounts that are sufficient for contraception. In the United States, Mishell's group[141] has devoted considerable effort to the development of hormone-releasing vaginal rings since the late 1960s.

The current vaginal contraceptive rings are of the core design, in which the steroid is formulated into silicone rods that are placed within polysiloxane tubing. The release rate is directly proportional to the surface of the silicone core and inversely proportional to the thickness of the polysiloxane tubing.

The vaginal ring system was studied for progestagen-only contraception using two strategies: intermittent application, with monthly removal and reinsertion of the device, or continuous use for 3 months, after which the ring is exchanged. Nearly all available progestagens have been tested in the vaginal rings.

Other clinical studies were conducted with vaginal rings containing an estrogen-progestagen combination.[142,143] In 2001, the Food and Drug Administration (FDA) approved the use of a vaginal ring releasing etonogestrel and ethinylestradiol over 21 days (NuvaRing, Organon, West Orange, New Jersey).

Transdermal Contraceptive Patch

Skin has been recognized as an excellent tissue for delivery of drugs. Hormonal patches for menopausal women were developed many years ago and have been well accepted.

The development of the contraceptive hormonal patch was motivated, in part, by the need to increase the compliance of patients who do not wish to take the pill daily. At present, only one contraceptive patch is available: Ortho EVRA. The patch is about 4 cm in diameter (20 cm^2), and it is designed to deliver 150 μg of norelgestromin and 20 μg of ethinylestradiol daily for 7 days. Effectiveness and compliance have been comparable to those of a triphasic OC regimen in clinical studies. Like monophasic OCs, the patch may one day be explored as a continuous versus cyclic method.[144]

EMERGENCY METHODS OF FERTILITY CONTROL

Hormonal Method

Despite the wide availability of birth control methods, many women become pregnant unintentionally. In the United States, this number reaches an annual total of close to 3.5 million pregnancies; of these, over 1 million end in abortion. The following situations may lead to unintended pregnancies:

1. Unprotected intercourse.
2. Intercourse during failure or inadequate use of a barrier contraceptive method, such as a slipped or broken condom; incorrectly inserted, dislodged, or expulsed diaphragm, cervical cap, or IUD; incorrectly placed female condom.
3. Intercourse after having missed progestagen-only contraceptive pills at any time of the cycle or after having missed combined contraceptive pills, in particular at the beginning or at the end of the pack, so that the pill-free interval is more than 7 days.
4. Unprotected intercourse or improper contraception shortly after a vasectomy when viable sperm are still in the vas deferens distal to the ligation (see "Vasectomy").

The need for emergency contraception, popularly known as the "morning-after pill," had already been perceived in the development of hormonal contraceptive methods. Morris and van Wagenen[145] coined the term "interception" and conducted early studies with diethylstilbestrol. Although diethylstilbestrol successfully prevented unintended pregnancy, it was quickly abandoned because of unacceptable adverse effects such as nausea, vomiting, and metrorrhagia.

More successful was the Yuzpe method, named after the Canadian gynecologist who invented it. The method consists of taking two tablets, each containing 0.5 mg of norgestrel combined with 50 μg of ethinylestradiol. This dose of 1 mg norgestrel and 100 μg ethinylestradiol must be repeated after 12 hours. Under ideal circumstances, the first dose should be taken within 72 hours of unprotected intercourse.[146]

In order to eliminate the estrogen-related adverse events of the combination pills, emergency contraception with a progestagen only has been developed. The treatment regimen consists of taking two doses of 0.75 mg of levonorgestrel 12 hours apart. As with the Yuzpe method, the dosing must start within 72 hours after the unprotected intercourse. The protective effect of the regimen gradually decreases when the pills are started later than 72 hours after unprotected intercourse.[147]

Successful clinical studies have been conducted with mifepristone in twice-daily doses of 5.0 and 25 mg. Compared with the methods described previously, mifepristone (see "Contra-

Table 17–14. Emergency Hormonal Contraception: Dosing and Most Commonly Reported Side Effects*

	Side effects (%)	
Dosing	**Nausea**	**Vomiting**
0.01 mg ethinylestradiol plus		
1.00 mg *dl*-norgestrel × 2	50	20
0.75 mg levonorgestrel × 2	20	6
5.00 mg × 2 mifepristone	17	2
25.00 mg × 2 mifepristone	Delay of menses	

*The first dose of the hormones must be taken 72 hours after intercourse at the latest. The second dose follows in 12 hours.

gestion") at the lower dose is associated with somewhat decreased side effects, principally vomiting, and the higher dose is associated with postponement of menses (Table 17–14).[148]

The mechanism of action has not been completely elucidated. The hormonal intervention may affect the timing of ovulation—mostly postponement—and produce an out-of-phase endometrium. The administered hormones may interfere with fertilization by affecting the ovum or the transport of sperm, or both.

The emergency contraception just described provides about 98% protection from an exposure to pregnancy risk when taken as prescribed. One of the major disadvantages of emergency contraception is not the method itself but its availability. Two states, Washington and California, have initiated a pilot program in which selected pharmacies following a strict protocol can distribute the morning-after pill directly to women who ask for it. Similar programs are being prepared in Oregon and Alaska.

When resorting to emergency contraception, patients are advised to take certain precautions that are specific for this kind of contraception. Along with combined estrogen-progestagen emergency pills, the patients may be given an antiemetic drug to minimize the adverse gastrointestinal events. After taking emergency hormones, ovulation and the following menstruation may be delayed. Patients should be advised to schedule an examination if menstrual bleeding does not occur within 3 weeks after the treatment. Patients should also be instructed to start to use a regular method of contraception. The use of emergency contraception as a primary method must be discouraged because of its side effects, including cycle and ovulation irregularities, and its relative unreliability with cumulative failure rates if used as the routine method.

Intrauterine Device as an Emergency Contraceptive

An IUD inserted 5 to 7 days after unprotected intercourse can provide an effective means of emergency fertility control. The method is contraindicated if an STD is present or suspected. Consequently, it is not suitable after rape, after coerced intercourse, or for women with multiple partners. In addition, the presence or a history of PID and suspected ectopic pregnancy are important contraindications to the method. The mechanism of IUD emergency contraception has not been defined.[149] Also, unlike hormonal methods that are FDA approved, the IUD approach is not currently an approved method for emergency contraception.

Contragestion

The attempts to terminate early pregnancy by pharmacologic means have culminated in the development of a hormonal method for which the name *contragestion* has been suggested. The key hormone is mifepristone, a synthetic derivative of norethindrone, characterized by a complex structure (dimethylaminophenyl group) attached to C-11 (Fig. 17–19). It is recognized that manipulation of the C-11 position of the steroid molecule leads to compounds with glucocorticoid activity as well as to compounds with an increased capacity to bind to progesterone receptors. Desogestrel, a C-11–substituted steroid, is a potent progestagen. The modification on C-11 of mifepristone gives the molecule a unique ability to compete for specific binding sites on progesterone receptors. In fact, mifepristone has twice as much affinity for progesterone receptors as progesterone itself but without exercising any progestagenic activity. Thus, mifepristone is a true progesterone antagonist. Mifepristone also binds to glucocorticoid receptors. However, in order to exercise any antiglucocorticoid activity, the amounts must be larger than those needed for its antiprogestagenic action.

It has been assumed that brief interruption of progesterone action leads to irreversible damage to the decidualized endometrium and interferes with nidation and the development of the early conceptus. Progesterone has a quieting effect on myometrial contractility. By antagonizing progesterone, mifepristone releases the myometrium from the suppressive action of progesterone, and myometrial activity intensifies. However, complete expulsion of the conceptus follows in only 40% of cases. Prostaglandins are potent stimulators of myometrial contractions, but when administered by themselves, they were able to terminate pregnancy in only 20% of the cases. With the availability of orally active prostaglandins, it was logical to combine the effect of an antiprogestagen with a prostaglandin. With administration before the 49th day of pregnancy, the success rate of achieving complete abortion has been 92% to 98%.

Most experience with contragestion has been in England, France, and China. The treatment regimens consist of a single dose of mifepristone, 200 to 600 mg orally. Thirty-six to 48 hours thereafter, the women return to the clinic to receive an oral dose of 400 to 800 μg of misoprostol, a synthetic analogue of the natural prostaglandin E_1.

Prostaglandin vaginal suppositories can also be used. Prostaglandins of the prostaglandin E_1 series exert a dilatory effect on the uterine cervix, and it is possible that placing the prostaglandin suppository close to the cervix facilitates this effect. A large, well-designed study has proved that vaginal misoprostol is highly effective in achieving complete abortion; however, the study did not compare vaginal and oral dosing directly.[150]

Because approximately 50% of women expel the conceptus within 4 hours and an additional 11% do so during the fifth

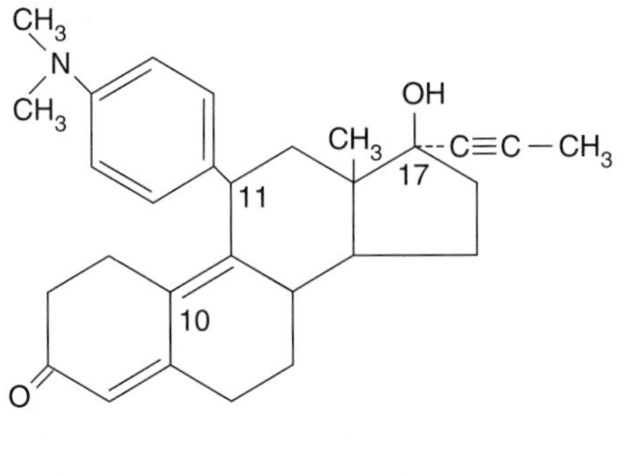

Mifepristone (RU 486)

Figure 17–19. The structure of mifepristone. The major modification of the 19-nor steroid molecule is on C-11.

hour after the administration of misoprostol, women should be under observation at the clinic for up to 5 hours. If they do not expel the conceptus and there are no medical reasons for further observation or intervention, the woman is allowed to complete the abortion at home. She is scheduled for a follow-up examination within the next 14 days and instructed to notify the clinic if she experiences excessive uterine bleeding or other medical complication or if no bleeding occurs. Within 24 hours after receiving misoprostol, 75% of women expel the conceptus completely.

In the United States, a large study was conducted under the auspices of the Population Council.[151] A total of 2015 women, ≤49 to 63 days pregnant, were enrolled. Of these, 92% achieved complete termination of pregnancy when the hormones were given on or before the 49th day of pregnancy. With more advanced gestation, the success rate decreased substantially. Complete abortion occurred in 83% of women pregnant 50 to 56 days and in 77% of women pregnant 57 to 63 days. Overall, for 85% of the 2015 patients, the treatment resulted in complete abortion. This percentage would probably be close to the success rate of the method in "real-life" situations, when the selection of suitable patients is less strict than under tightly controlled research conditions.

After dosing, the patients bleed for a median of 13 to 15 days. Although uterine bleeding is expected after pregnancy interruption, this bleeding was the main source of complaints and complications. Some of the complications required surgical intervention, intravenous administration of fluids, and, infrequently, blood transfusions. Other reported adverse events included uterine cramping, abdominal pain, nausea and vomiting, diarrhea, dizziness, and headaches. In some patients, endometritis was reported.

Mifepristone has been approved for general clinical use in the United States and is available under the name Mifeprex. Women seeking abortion should be counseled about the details of all options. Surgical intervention remains most common in the United States.

INTRAUTERINE DEVICES

Currently, there are three types of IUDs: nonmedicated, copper, and hormone-releasing intrauterine systems. Only the latter two are available in the United States.

The first modern IUD was designed by E. Gräfenberg, a German physician, in the 1920s. It was a pliable ring of coiled silver wire, 18 mm in diameter, inserted into the uterus after cervical dilation. This basic design has been modified over the years in various parts of the world, and stainless steel has replaced silver. With the advent of plastic materials with memory, new forms and shapes of IUDs were invented in order to increase efficacy, make the insertion easier, and facilitate the IUD's removal when needed.[152]

Today, the WHO does not recommend the use of inert IUDs because copper IUDs and the hormone-releasing intrauterine systems are more effective and safer.

In the United States, IUDs have declined in popularity because of problems with the Dalkon Shield. This IUD was designed to cover a large area of the uterine cavity because it was speculated that the contraceptive efficacy of IUDs was directly related to the area of contact with the endometrium. However, the use of this device became associated with an increased risk of PID, and the Dalkon Shield was withdrawn from the market in 1974. It is believed that the reason for the increased incidence of PID was the *multifilament* tailstring, which facilitated proliferation of bacteria between the mashes of the string and ascension of infection into the uterine cavity. Current IUDs are equipped with a monofilament tailstring, and no substantive increased risk of PID has been associated with this appendage.

The first copper-bearing IUD was devised by the Chilean scientist Jaime Zipper, who studied the antifertility properties of copper.[152] The first marketed copper IUD was the copper 7 IUD, based on Zipper's studies. It was distributed by the G.D. Searle company until 1986, when it was withdrawn from the market because of putative infertility of women who discontinued its use.

The modern copper IUDs are represented by Paragard T380. The IUD has a T-shaped polyethylene body with a copper wire wound around the vertical arm of the T; each of the transverse arms carries a copper sleeve. The exposed areas of copper are 380 mm^2, hence the name. This IUD is designed for 10-year protection against pregnancy. However, it is likely that the duration of efficacy is years longer. The pregnancy rate under controlled conditions is 0.7% and 0.3% for the first and the second year, respectively.[153]

In Europe, a frameless copper IUD is being developed. The protective duration is 5 years (Fig. 17–20) This IUD consists of a string with six copper beads covering a surface area of 330 mm^2. The string is anchored in the fundal myometrium. This kind of IUD is recommended for women who experience difficulties, principally uterine cramping, with other IUDs. However, users of this frameless IUD must be alert to the possibility of "silent" expulsion.[154]

The first hormone-releasing intrauterine system was the Progestasert (1971). It is a T-shaped device with a drug reservoir in the vertical arm of the T containing progesterone in silicone oil. A vinyl membrane controls the rate of release—approximately 65 μg of progesterone per day. The pregnancy rate for Progestasert is about 2 per 100 woman-years.[152] In addition, it must be replaced annually.

Another hormone-releasing IUD uses levonorgestrel (LNG). The LNG-20 or Mirena is also a T-shaped device with a sleeve on the vertical arm, which is a reservoir for a total of 52 mg of levonorgestrel. The hormone is released into the uterine cavity at a daily rate of 15 μg (calculated from in vitro release). The reported pregnancy rate for perfect use is 0.2% for the first year. It is intended for 5-year use.[155]

Management Issues with Intrauterine Devices

Pregnancy and Continuation Rates

The modern copper and hormone-releasing IUDs are among the most effective means of reversible contraception. With long-term use the yearly pregnancy rate is less than 0.5%, and the cumulative pregnancy rate of 2.2% over a 12-year period rivals the 10-year pregnancy rate of tubal ligation (1.9%).[156, 157] The continuation rate of IUDs is the highest among all reversible methods of fertility control—80% after the first year of use. The 5-year continuation rate is 40% among women using the copper IUD and 33% among women fitted with the levonorgestrel-releasing device.[158–160]

The use of IUDs is associated with a number of issues that must be considered in management. These include adverse events such as uterine perforation, changes in the uterine bleeding pattern, cramping, and PID. The relationship between IUD use and pregnancy, both intrauterine and ectopic, is addressed separately.

Medical therapy for Wilson's disease has been increasingly successful with the result that many affected women enter the reproductive age and need contraceptive counseling. Concerns have been expressed that copper ions released from the copper IUD may reach the general circulation and precipitate symptoms of the disease. In healthy women wearing copper IUDs,

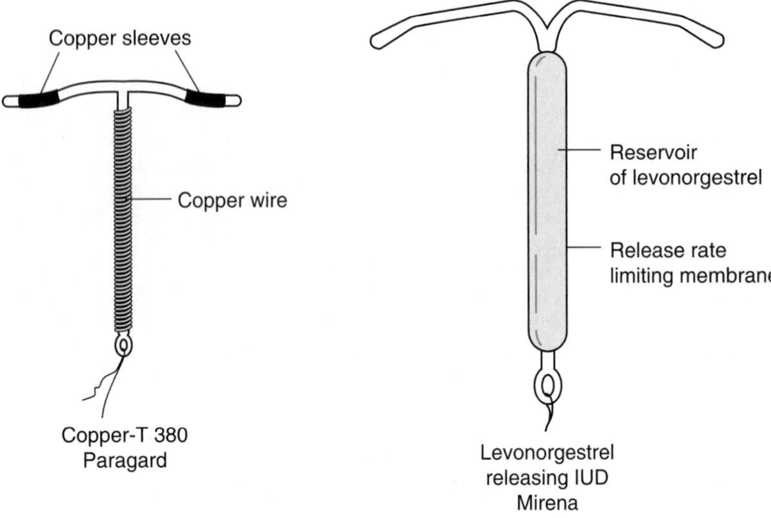

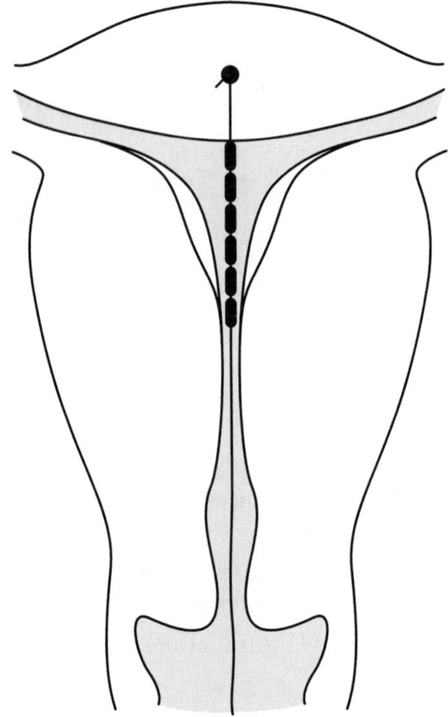

Figure 17–20. Types of intrauterine devices (IUDs). The copper T380 and the levonorgestrel-releasing IUD are clinically used in the United States. The frameless copper IUD is available in Europe.

circulating concentrations of copper and ceruloplasmin have not been elevated even after 12 to 24 months of use. The amount of copper released from the IUD has been calculated as 14 to 29 μg/day, which constitutes only about 1% to 2% of the dietary intake of copper. In Wilson's disease, serum ceruloplasmin levels are decreased and free serum copper concentrations are increased, although total copper levels can be within normal limits or low.[161–165] It seems unlikely that wearing a copper IUD could affect circulating copper levels in Wilson's disease. This condition is rare, 1 in 200,000; thus, it has been difficult to generate data on contraceptive practices of the affected women. However, because Wilson's disease is a serious condition and numerous contraceptive options exist, the lack of substantive safety data relegates copper-bearing IUDs to a bottom-tier choice for women with this condition.

Uterine Perforation

The rate of uterine perforations is low, 0.6 per 1000 insertions. With the progestagen-containing IUD, it is 1.1 per 1000 insertions.[156]

Expulsion

The spontaneous expulsion rate for modern IUDs, including the copper T380 and levonorgestrel-releasing systems, is 5%

to 6% during the first year and 1% to 2% per year during the subsequent years of use. Primiparas, secundiparas, and women 15 to 24 years of age have a higher rate of expulsions than women who are older or have had more than two pregnancies, or both.[156]

Changes in Uterine Bleeding

The copper T380 is removed for uterine bleeding and cramping in 12% of users during the first year and 2% to 4% during subsequent years. The levonorgestrel-releasing system usually decreases uterine bleeding, and this phenomenon can be utilized therapeutically in patients with menorrhagia or adenomyosis and can prevent proliferative endometrial changes in patients undergoing long-term tamoxifen treatment.[166] On the other hand, patients using the levonorgestrel-releasing system complain of a higher incidence of amenorrhea, and removal of the device for this side effect is the main reason for the lower continuation rate compared with the copper T380 IUD. In both cases, proper counseling enhances continuation.

Pelvic Inflammatory Disease

The risk of IUD users for PID is inversely related to the time since insertion. A large WHO study concluded that the risk of PID is increased during the first 20 days after IUD insertion; beyond this time period, PID is an infrequent event.[157, 167] This finding may be related to bacteriologic evidence showing bacterial contamination of the uterus at insertion of the IUD. Women scheduled for hysterectomy had an IUD inserted 24 hours before the surgery. Upon culture of the uterine contents, bacterial contamination was frequently found. It is even more significant that 30 days after IUD insertion, the uterine contents were sterile.[168]

The development of PID also depends on the lifestyle of the women receiving the IUD. Women who are at minimal or no risk of exposure to sexually transmitted infections are less likely to experience PID than those who are. This is true with or without an IUD. As with other effective methods, an IUD user who is at risk for STDs should use a barrier method as well. In order to prevent PID, the use of prophylactic antibiotics is sometimes recommended. However, large clinical trials have shown that with copper IUDs the rate of salpingitis is 1 per 1000, regardless of whether prophylactic antibiotics were given. In general, in the United States, prophylaxis is not routinely recommended.[157]

A direct comparison of levonorgestrel-releasing systems and copper IUDs demonstrated a low PID rate over a 7-year period with both IUDs and no significant difference between the two types.[169] A large multicenter European study showed that after 36 months, the cumulative discontinuation rates for PID were 0.5% and 2.0% for the levonorgestrel and copper IUDs, respectively ($P < .02$); after 60 months, the corresponding rates were 0.8% and 2.2%.[170]

Tubal infertility is closely related to the problem of PID. Conflicting results have been reported; however, a thorough review of the question concluded that fair evidence indicates no important effect of IUD use on infertility.[157]

Pregnancy and Intrauterine Devices

Intrauterine Pregnancy

Pregnancy with an IUD in situ frequently leads to spontaneous abortion and, rarely, sepsis. Physicians recommend removal of the IUD when pregnancy has been diagnosed. There is no evidence that the risk of malformations is increased in infants born to women with an IUD in situ.

Ectopic Pregnancy

Studies with the modern copper and levonorgestrel-releasing IUDs have demonstrated a low incidence of ectopic pregnancy. For users fitted with IUDs releasing copper from a 200-mm^2 surface, the estimated rate of ectopic pregnancy was four tenths that of nonusers of contraception; the rate of ectopic pregnancy with devices releasing copper from a 350-mm^2 surface was one tenth of that of nonusers of contraception. With the hormonal IUD releasing 20 μg of levonorgestrel daily, the ectopic pregnancy rate was also one tenth of the rate for nonusers.[73, 154] These studies dispel the worries of physicians and women about ectopic pregnancy with respect to the modern copper and levonorgestrel IUDs. It can be concluded that the modern IUDs reduce the risk of both uterine and ectopic pregnancy.

Selection of Candidates and Contraindications for Intrauterine Devices

Selection

As with any contraceptive method, contraceptive protection, acceptable adverse events, and continuation of use of IUDs depend on the proper selection of candidates. PID is best prevented by selecting candidates at low risk for PID and excluding the presence of PID during the preinsertion examination. Clinically manifest vaginal and cervical infection should be identified and treated, and bacteriologic examination of the cervix should be carried out when possible. The appropriate IUD candidate is a parous woman at low risk for sexually transmitted infection. IUDs are well suited for women who cannot use or do not desire hormonal contraception.[156, 157] It is a particularly important option for women considering surgical sterilization. A decade of easily reversible contraception may suit many women. Because the association between IUDs and PID is limited to the 3 weeks after insertion, it is prudent to observe the patient for symptoms of PID.

Contraindications

Insertion of an IUD is contraindicated when a pregnancy is suspected or confirmed and during an acute episode of PID. Caution should be exercised for women with a history of PID, undiagnosed uterine bleeding, enlarged or distorted uterus, confirmed or suspected uterine or cervical malignancy, untreated acute cervicitis or vaginitis, multiple sexual partners, and the presence of genital actinomycosis. Patients (and providers) sometimes have a sketchy memory; therefore, the presence of a previously inserted IUD must be excluded.

Noncontraceptive Benefits and Advantages and Shortcomings of Intrauterine Devices

The possible role of IUDs in carcinogenesis has been addressed in several population-based studies. Two well-conducted case-control studies have provided reassurance that IUDs do not increase the risk of endometrial cancer and suggested a possible protective effect, even in women older than 55 years, an age group with an increased risk of endometrial cancer.[171, 172] Two other case-control studies have shown a straightforward protective effect. The relative risk of developing an endometrial carcinoma was 0.51 and 0.61 in these two respective studies, with a 95% CI of 0.3 to 0.8.[173, 174] IUD use has no effect on the development of cervical carcinoma or breast tumors. An extended nonmedical benefit of IUDs is their low life-use cost. When used in the long term, they are the least expensive contraceptive agents.

Table 17–15 summarizes advantages and disadvantages of IUDs and shows that benefits outweigh shortcomings of intrauterine contraception.

Mechanism of Action

At least two studies have demonstrated that IUDs exert their contraceptive action before fertilization occurs.

An especially intriguing finding came from studies with volunteers wearing copper IUDs. Over several cycles, blood samples were examined for human chorionic gonadotropin (hCG) by extremely sensitive methods from day 10 of the cycle until the onset of menses. Concentrations of hCG were not elevated in any subject with an IUD. In the control group of women who wished to become pregnant, two showed an increase of hCG during the critical period of the luteal phase and this "chemical" pregnancy was later confirmed by obstetric examination.[175] A similar study involving women with nonmedicated IUDs showed essentially the same result.[176] Further, failed attempts to retrieve fertilized ova support prevention of fertilization as the mechanism of action.

Several modes of contraceptive action of IUDs have been suggested. After insertion, IUDs incite a foreign body reaction in the uterine cavity, which includes rapid invasion of leukocytes and increased production of prostaglandins. The changed environment in the uterine cavity impairs the viability of the sperm and inhibits its motility. This reaction is particularly well expressed with the copper IUDs. The levonorgestrel IUDs inhibit endometrial growth and induce changes in the cervical mucus that make sperm penetration difficult. However, the contraceptive action of IUDs has not been clarified.

Table 17–15. Advantages and Shortcomings of Intrauterine Devices

Advantages	Disadvantages
Easiness of application, low costs	Transient increased risk of pelvic inflammatory disease
High protection against pregnancy	Expulsion
Highest continuation rate of all reversible methods	Uterine perforation
Immediately reversible	
Suitable for breast-feeding mothers	Candidates must be carefully examined for factors predisposing to the development of pelvic inflammatory disease
Protection against endometrial cancer	
No increased risk of cervical and breast cancer	Close follow-up during the first 3–4 wk after insertion is needed
Levonorgestrel-releasing IUDs control excessive uterine bleeding	Amenorrhea associated with levonorgestrel-releasing IUD causes discontinuation of use

IUD, intrauterine device.

BARRIER METHODS

The Male Condom

The male condom is important not only as a contraceptive device but also as one that reduces the risk of both HIV and HPV infection, the latter being associated with condylomata acuminata and cervical cancer. Modern condoms were originally made of rubber, but since a liquid latex process was introduced in the 1930s, the bulk of the world's condom supply has been made of latex. The production process was gradually mechanized, which lowered the cost substantially. The condom is one of the least expensive contraceptive methods and is the best protection against the spread of sexually transmitted infection.

Condoms can also be made of polyurethane and silicone rubber as well as of lamb intestines. The "natural skin" condoms do not protect against the viral STDs.

The production standard requires that the thickness of a condom does not exceed 0.03 to 0.08 mm, and there are strict quality control safeguards against leakage and breakage. For example, FDA regulations require that randomly selected condoms from the production run be filled with 300 mL of water and inspected for leaks. In Britain, the condom is required to hold 3 L of water without breaking.

Latex can be weakened by oil-based lubricants and by various vaginal ointments or creams. Instructions for the use of vaginal antifungal preparations contain a warning that women should not rely on condoms for protection against pregnancy and STDs while using such preparations. Condoms made of polyurethane are not harmed by oil-based lubricants, but their breakage rate is significantly higher than that of latex condoms.[177, 178] The surface of some types of condoms can be coated with an appropriate lubricant or spermicide, or both, to improve acceptability and efficacy.

The Female Condom

The female condom is much less frequently used than the male condom. The female condom is a polyurethane sheath 15 cm in length and 7 cm in diameter. A flexible ring is attached to its open end, and a loose removable ring inside the condom facilitates the insertion of the device into the vagina. The advantages of the female condom over the male condom are that the method is controlled by the woman and it is independent of the immediate sexual act. The female condom can be placed into the vagina several hours before intercourse takes place.[179]

The Diaphragm

Diaphragms are made of latex in the form of a thin dome mounted on a ring containing a flat or spiral spring. The sizes vary in diameter from 45 to 105 mm in steps of 2.5 to 5.0 mm. In determining the correct size of diaphragm, the distance between the posterior aspect of the symphysis pubis and the posterior fornix of the vagina is assessed. A correctly fitted diaphragm occupies this space with the dome covering the cervix. The diaphragm should always be applied with a spermicidal cream or jelly and should be left in place for a minimum 6 hours after intercourse. After removal, the diaphragm should be washed and dried but no talcum powder should be applied.

Used consistently, the diaphragm has a low failure rate: 2% to 3%. This low failure rate is rarely achieved; in fact, rates of 20 to 30 pregnancies per 100 woman-years have been reported. The high failure rate results from poor motivation, inconsistency of use, poor fit of the diaphragm because the anatomy of the genitalia has changed (e.g., after delivery), incorrect insertion, slippage during intercourse, defects in the latex, and reluctance of users to apply the spermicide because it is "messy." A diaphragm should not be prescribed if there is an evident uterine prolapse, poor vaginal tonus, or a marked cystocele. After delivery, fitting of a diaphragm should be delayed at least a few weeks to allow rebuilding of muscular tone.

Clinicians speculate that diaphragms may reduce the risk of cervical gonorrhea, PID, and possibly cervical and endocervical malignancies. However, data on these subjects are not as supportive as those for the male condom. On the other hand, an increased incidence of urinary tract infection has been observed among diaphragm users. A few cases of toxic shock syndrome have been reported in cases in which the diaphragm was left in situ for 24 hours or longer.[180]

In conclusion, a diaphragm with a spermicide is an inexpensive way to prevent pregnancy, and it is an excellent choice for women who do not wish to use one of the more effective methods, have infrequent intercourse, and are compliant. Such women are more inclined to use the method consistently, and consistency of use is the key to barrier success.

The Cervical Cap

In the United states, one type of cervical cap has been approved for general use. The Prentif cap is made of soft rubber, and a firm round rim is affixed to the open end. When successfully inserted, the rim fits around the cervix close to the vaginal fornices.

The efficacy is about the same as that of a diaphragm at best and can be ensured by filling the cup with a spermicide. For nulliparous women, the failure rate is 20% for typical use and 9% for perfect use. For parous women, the failure rate is higher, 40% for typical use and 26% for perfect use. The cap can stay in place for 48 hours irrespective of the frequency of intercourse during that time. The earliest time for removal of the cervical cap is 8 hours after intercourse. The major problems with the cap are difficulties with insertion and with proper fitting and the possibility of displacement.[181] Also, some women find it difficult to remove.

NATURAL FAMILY PLANNING

Natural family planning restricts intercourse to the "safe period," that is, the period of "physiologic sterility" in each menstrual cycle. Assuming that ova are available for fertilization for only 24 hours and that spermatozoa remain highly viable for 48 hours, theoretically, there would be only 3 days in each cycle during which conception is possible. To identify the days of possible conception and decide which days are safe is difficult given the less than perfect regularity of the menstrual cycle. The calendar method is based on the expectation that ovulation takes place 12 to 16 days prior to the next menstruation. In this "rhythm" method, the woman records the length of 6 or preferably 12 cycles and determines the beginning of the fertile period by subtracting 18 days from the shortest period. Then she estimates the end of the fertile period by subtracting 11 days from the longest cycle.

Women practicing the cervical mucus method are instructed to observe the changes of the cervical mucus throughout the cycle and recognize the characteristics of the mucus during the fertile period. The symptothermal method combines the cervical mucus method with measurements of basal body temperature. With this method, abstinence begins on the day when mucus becomes clear, slippery, and stretchy (spinnbarkeit); this usually happens a few days before ovulation. Intercourse is resumed on the third or fourth day after the basal body temperature shifts to the luteal phase pattern.

There are various modifications of these three methods, and instruments have been designed to facilitate monitoring the safe period. The failure rate, when the methods are correctly practiced, can be as low as 2% to 3%. However, typical failure rates can be 20% or more.

The high typical failure rate for natural family planning results from several factors. The method depends on keeping meticulous records of menstrual cycles for 6 to 12 months in order to determine the safe period. This may be difficult for the busy modern woman. A less controllable reason is the unpredictable duration of the follicular phase of the menstrual cycle and consequently of the entire cycle. If the differences between the cycle lengths exceed 10 days, natural birth control should not be practiced.

In addition, in some individuals, emotional or physical stress can postpone the time of ovulation, creating the possibility that intercourse, based on previous calculations, may take place during the "unsafe" period. Although the efficacy of the rhythm method can be improved by daily measurements of basal body temperature, this too can be complicated because not all basal body temperature curves can pinpoint the occurrence of ovulation. Self-examination of cervical mucus can be somewhat awkward and the results even more difficult to interpret.[182, 183]

All in all, natural family planning requires alertness on the part of the woman and a high level of motivation, cooperation, and discipline in both partners. It also requires a clear understanding that pregnancy is a distinct possibility.

STERILIZATION

Female Sterilization

Female sterilization involves occluding or dividing the fallopian tubes. The approach of choice is laparoscopy as an outpatient procedure. Minilaparotomy or a full laparotomy is usually performed when complications are anticipated with laparoscopy, for example, when a patient has extensive adhesions after previous surgeries, after PID, and post partum.

The procedure is usually done using general anesthesia. Local anesthesia with sedation is also common. After proper insertion of the laparoscope into the abdominal cavity under visual control, the fallopian tube is grasped by an instrument approximately 1 to 2 cm from the isthmus, and electrocoagulation is performed to the extent of 2 to 3 cm. The tubes can also be occluded by insertion of clips or a silastic ring. A loop of the fallopian tube is pushed through a dilated ring, which is then allowed to contract, thus providing tight occlusion of the tube.

When sterilization is done through minilaparotomy or laparotomy, most surgeons prefer the simple Pomeroy procedure or partial tubectomy. A loop of the tube is formed by grasping the tube with a forceps and ligating the loop about 1 to 2 cm below the apex of the loop. The segment of the tube that forms the loop is then dissected, and the open ends of tube may be electrocoagulated. A vaginal approach to tubal ligation has also been developed.

Efficacy

All methods of tubal sterilization are highly effective in reducing the risk of pregnancy. The pregnancy rate after tubal sterilization is 0.1% during the first year after the procedure, although the rates vary by procedure. The long-term pregnancy rates are higher. In the United States, a Collaborative Review of Sterilization Group observed 10,685 women for 8 to 14 years after tubal sterilization and identified 143 failures, with pregnancies occurring later than 2 years after the procedure. The cumulative 10-year probability of pregnancy was 18.5 per 1000 procedures irrespective of which method was used. The most effective methods were partial postpartum salpingectomy and laparoscopic unipolar coagulation, with 7.5 pregnancies per 1000 procedures. The clip was associated with 36.5 pregnancies per 1000 procedures. An overall cumulative probability of ectopic pregnancies was calculated as 7.5 per 1000 procedures.[184]

Women sterilized at young age had the highest risk of pregnancy, most likely because they were being exposed to the possibility of recanalization or fistulization of the tubes for a longer period of time.

Complications

The most serious complications are those associated with bowel or blood vessel damage. The *post-tubal sterilization syndrome* includes a number of symptoms that women frequently ascribe to the procedure, such as premenstrual tension, dysmenorrhea, and emotional and psychosexual problems. The attributable reality of this syndrome is controversial. The length of the menstrual cycle is not influenced by tubal sterilization.

Manifestations of regret are more common in younger women. A functional *reanastomosis* may be difficult to achieve; however, success rates up to 70% have been reported. As discussed previously, the long-duration IUD and other methods should be discussed as alternatives to surgical sterilization.

Chemical Sterilization

Cyanoacrylates and quinacrine, a resin-like substance, have been evaluated as tubal occlusive materials. Neither has yet succeeded. For example, quinacrine causes local inflammation, fibrosis, and occlusion of the intramural segment of the tube. The method had been used on a large scale in India, where it was banned because of the associated high rate of pregnancies and complications. Data from Vietnam indicate a pregnancy rate of 13% for women younger than 35 years of age and 7% for women older than 35 years, higher occurrence of ectopic pregnancy, and PID.[21, 22]

Male Surgical Sterilization

Vasectomy

This procedure is done mostly using local anesthesia. The vas is palpated through the skin of the upper scrotum and exposed through a small incision. The vas is ligated at two sites, and the part between the two ligations is then surgically severed or excised. The vas may also be occluded by diathermy or by a clip.

Efficacy

It is important to convey to the patient that vasectomy is not immediately effective. It may take several weeks before all the sperm that remains in the distal part of the vas is ejaculated. An alternative method of contraception must be used until azoospermia is achieved, usually after 12 weeks or 20 ejaculations. In about 2% of cases, vasectomy is not successful and must be redone if sperm is present in the seminal fluid for several months. Rarely, spontaneous late reanastomosis can occur up to 10 years after vasectomy. Pregnancy that occurs such a long time after the procedure is a sensitive issue because questions of paternity may arise, and it must be handled judiciously.

Complications

Complications of vasectomy are rare and consist mostly of local infection and hematoma. Antisperm antibodies develop in about 50% of men, but there is no evidence that this is associated with any pathologic condition.[185]

SURGICAL ABORTION

Surgical abortion should not be a primary method of fertility control, although in some countries it is practiced as such. It is estimated that, worldwide, 50 million abortions are performed annually, 20 million of these illegally.

In the United States, after legalization of therapeutic interruption of pregnancy, the number of abortions rose from 16.3 per 1000 women in 1973 to 29.3 per 1000 in 1980. Thereafter, the rate of therapeutic abortions declined steadily to 22.2 per 1000 women in 1997. In that year, 1.33 million abortions were performed. Statistics also indicated that the majority (52%) of those undergoing abortion were younger than 25 years and 29% were teenagers.

In the United States, therapeutic abortions are performed by suction curettage under local or light general anesthesia. The mortality associated with therapeutic abortion is exceedingly low at 1 in 530,000 if performed within the first 8 weeks of pregnancy. This rate increases to 1 per 17,000 at 16 to 20 weeks and 1 per 6000 at 21 weeks of gestation. The overall mortality rate associated with abortion is 0.8 per 100,000 legal abortions. The maternal mortality rate at childbirth is 10 per 100,000 births, and that associated with ectopic pregnancy is 50 per 100,000 cases. The risk of nonfatal complications is less than 1%. These complications include pelvic infection, hemorrhage requiring a blood transfusion, and unintended major surgery.

The majority of abortions, 57%, are performed during gestations of less than 6 to 8 weeks duration. Thirty three percent of women have abortions between weeks 9 and 12, and 12% have abortions later than 15 weeks. Approximately 50% of women having an abortion later than 15 weeks indicate that the delay was caused by problems of finding abortion facilities and having the procedure done. Teenagers are more inclined to delay abortion than older women.[186–188]

DISCUSSING CONTRACEPTIVE CHOICES WITH THE PATIENT

Before recommending a specific method of contraception, the health status of the woman and her personal circumstances must be thoroughly evaluated. Crucial in the contraceptive decision-making process is whether the woman wishes to preserve her fertility or has attained her reproductive goals and is ready for permanent cessation of childbearing. The contraceptive choice is further influenced by the age of the patient, her smoking habits, her weight, and the presence or a history of health problems such as cardiovascular and cerebrovascular diseases and diabetes mellitus.

The initial visit and the yearly follow-up examinations are an opportunity to conduct a complete physical examination, take Pap smears, check for the presence of vaginal and sexually transmitted infections, and perform breast examinations. Mammography may be recommended, depending on the findings, the age of the woman, and her family history of breast disease. It is also prudent to check the lipid profile and blood sugar. The physician should discourage smoking, particularly if the contraceptive choice is hormonal.

Sexually active women frequently need protection not only against pregnancy but also against STDs, particularly in regions with a high prevalence of HIV and AIDS, chlamydia, gonorrhea, and syphilis infections. Dual protection, such as oral contraception along with the use of a condom, may be recommended, depending on the individual circumstances of the woman. Hormonal contraception for teenagers may be started after menarche. At the other end of the spectrum, women who have completed their families may choose an IUD or surgical sterilization. The important watchword is individualization of choice among all appropriate methods.

Lactation provides protection against pregnancy only if the woman is exclusively breast-feeding, but even such women can experience breakthrough ovulations, particularly after the 10th postpartum week. As long as a woman is breast-feeding, combination hormonal contraceptives should be avoided because they suppress production of breast milk. If breast-feeding is interrupted by bottle feeding, the risk of breakthrough ovulations increases significantly. For lactating women, progestagen-only contraception is an excellent choice irrespective of whether they breast-feed exclusively or supplement breast-feeding by bottle feeding. Low-dose progestagen-only contraception does not affect the composition and quantity of breast milk and can be started immediately after delivery.

In nonlactating women, uterine bleeding followed by ovulation usually occurs after the sixth week of the puerperium but can happen earlier. Therefore, nonlactating women should not delay contraception for more than 2 to 3 weeks. Combination OCs have not been recommended before the third week after delivery because of concern that they could compound the naturally increased risk of postpartum thromboembolism. In nonlactating women, a progestagen-only OC or an effective nonhormonal contraceptive method, such as an IUD, can be started immediately post partum.

After an uncomplicated spontaneous or induced abortion, women can start OCs on the same day. Provided there are no contraindications, an IUD can be inserted at the conclusion of the procedure.

Women who have achieved their desired family size should be offered surgical sterilization or an appropriate reversible method, such as a copper IUD.

It is good clinical practice to schedule women for a follow-up examination within 3 months after starting contraception. At that time, the physician determines whether the patient practices contraception correctly and inquires about possible adverse effects, such as chest pain, shortness of breath, edema, headaches, blurred vision, and depression. If the findings are satisfactory, the patient typically moves to an annual visit schedule.

An important part of recommending a contraceptive method is counseling about expected adverse events and pointing out those that are transient and benign versus those that require medical attention. Factual and balanced information about adverse events frequently averts discontinuation of the contraceptive method by the patient but can also facilitate therapeutic intervention if required.

CONTRACEPTION FOR WOMEN WITH HEALTH PROBLEMS

Recommending an adequate contraceptive method to women with health problems is always a challenge. In women with compromised health, both pregnancy and contraception could bring about a deterioration of the underlying disease. The risks of contraception versus the risks of pregnancy must be carefully weighed. Extensive and sensitive counseling by health personnel is especially important for women with medical problems because erroneous information can further imperil their health. Support of the partner can also be a positive influence on the success of a contraceptive method.

Both physician and patient must collaborate fully in making a decision concerning which contraceptive method to use. The seriousness of the disease in question must first be evaluated. When there are reasons to believe that pregnancy would permanently worsen the patient's health or be fatal for her, sterilization of one of the partners should be discussed. When pregnancy would substantially impair the patient's health but would not be life-threatening, long-term methods with high efficacy and safety could be recommended, for example, copper or levonorgestrel-containing IUDs or hormonal methods when not contraindicated. Certain diseases do not impose major safety risks with respect to pregnancy. Should that be the case, patients who express the desire to preserve their fertility may use a wide range of methods according to preference and clinical compatibility. Before prescribing, the physician should take a thorough inventory of the patient's medications because certain preparations decrease the effectiveness of hormonal contraception.

Contraceptive Choices in Individual Diseases

Cardiovascular Disease

For a patient with any heart disease, a copper IUD may be the method of first choice because of its high efficacy and lack of systemic effects. The insertion of the IUD should be covered by antibiotics if the patient is at risk for bacterial endocarditis. Patients who receive anticoagulation therapy can be fitted with a levonorgestrel IUD; the progestagen released suppresses the growth of the endometrium. Combination OCs should not be recommended if the patient is currently suffering from or indicates a personal history of MI, congestive heart failure, stroke, uncontrolled hypertension, or thromboembolism. Women with varicose veins can use OCs. Uncomplicated valvular heart disease, including mitral valve prolapse, is not a contraindication to hormonal contraception. If valvular disease is complicated by pulmonary hypertension, atrial fibrillation, subacute bacterial endocarditis, and signs and symptoms of cardiac congestion, combination OCs must be avoided.

For those with a number of heart conditions, progestagen-only contraception can be used in the form of pills, injections, and subdermal implants. These conditions include a history of thrombophlebitis, valvular heart disease (uncomplicated and complicated), and controlled hypertension with systolic blood pressure ≤140 mm/≤90 mm Hg. A history of ischemic heart disease or stroke does not preclude the use of progestagen-only contraception, but it should be used only if other options are not available or acceptable to the patient and if the patient can be properly monitored. In the United States, the product label of progestagen-only contraceptives is as restrictive as that for combination OCs. However, international guidelines permit a wider range of indications for progestagen-only contraception.[189]

Diabetes Mellitus

In diabetes mellitus, the frequency and severity of vascular complications increase with age and in pregnancy. Diabetic patients should be advised of these possibilities and counseled on early family planning decisions. Effective contraception is critical for the health of diabetic patients. The contraceptive method of first choice should be the copper IUD, which is suited for patients with uncomplicated as well as with complicated diabetes mellitus.

The American College of Obstetricians and Gynecologists developed guidelines recommending that use of combined OCs be limited to nonsmoking, otherwise healthy women with diabetes who are younger than 35 years and show no evidence of hypertension, nephropathy, retinopathy, or other vascular diseases.[190]

Combined OCs do not impair the course of either type 1 or type 2 diabetes. The critical question of whether OCs increase the risk of early diabetic renal or retinal complications, or both, has been explored in a retrospective case-control study of two matched groups of patients with type 1, insulin-dependent diabetes mellitus. The study group patients took OCs for at least 1 year; the control group consisted of never-users of OCs. During the observation period, markers of diabetic renal damage and results of eye examinations were not significantly different in the two groups; the longitudinal hemoglobin A_{1c} values were similar for both study and control subjects. The study indicates that the use of OCs by young women with insulin-dependent diabetes mellitus does not pose an additional risk for the development of early diabetic retinopathy or nephropathy.[191] A prospective cohort study of 98,000 women nurses found no increased risk of type 2 diabetes when subjects were taking OCs.[192] A history of gestational diabetes does not preclude the use of hormonal contraception. If the health status and desire of the patient indicate, sterilization should be considered.

Liver Disease

The interaction between the liver and contraceptive hormones is manifold. In experimental animals, conditions resembling peliosis hepatis can be induced by estrogens, and the possibility of liver adenomas in OC users has been considered. The incidence of these tumors is rare, 1 to 3 per 1 million women per year, and the risk attributable to oral contraception is difficult to assess. An increased risk for development of primary hepatocellular carcinoma in OC users has not been proved. In patients with impaired liver function, contraceptive steroids may not be efficiently metabolized, and such patients may have increased circulating levels of these hormones. The clinical import of these biochemical changes is uncertain. Gallbladder disease has been linked to oral contraception, but epidemiologic evidence has not been consistent.

A copper IUD should be considered the method of first choice for patients with liver problems. As stated in the section "Contraindications," the use of combined hormonal contraception should be avoided in patients with active liver disease, severe cirrhosis, and liver tumors or even a history of liver tumor. Under close supervision, patients with compensated cirrhosis can use progestagen-only contraception. There are no restrictions for the use of any type of contraception for carriers of hepatitis viruses.[189]

Human Immunodeficiency Virus Infection

HIV-positive women have shown less inclination to procreate than healthy women, irrespective of their socioeconomic status and background. Sexually active HIV-infected women who desire contraception should practice procedures that are highly effective in preventing an unintended pregnancy and at the same time protect them from acquiring another STD and prevent transmission of the HIV infection to the woman's sexual partner. These objectives are best achieved by the dual-protection technique, with which the HIV-infected woman uses an effective contraceptive method (OC, medicated IUD, possibly tubal sterilization) and she or her male partner uses a condom.

HIV-positive women who want to become pregnant or are already pregnant should be counseled on the availability of treatment and prevention of vertical transmission of the infection from mother to infant.[193]

Patients with Compromised Mental Health

Patients with reduced or limited mental abilities have a right to a safe sexual life. This has to be balanced with the right of caregivers, for whom a pregnant mentally ill patient can cause substantial distress. Also, one has to take into account a patient's need for adequate parental care. For all these reasons, the choice of contraception is crucial. Before the choice is made, several questions must be answered. Is the patient competent enough to decide upon the right form of contraception? Is she able to use a method consistently and correctly? Are bleeding and hygiene manageable? In no case must the patient be forced to use a particular method; rather, she or her legal guardian must give legal consent. If sterilization is indicated, the decision should be made by the patient or her legal guardian, or both, with a team of experts including a psychiatrist, a social worker, and a lawyer in accord with local regulations.[194]

Other Diseases

Hormonal contraception is not contraindicated for patients with epilepsy; however, one has to bear in mind that antiepileptic drugs may decrease the effects of contraceptive hormones. Similarly, rifampin decreases the effects of hormonal contraceptives in patients with tuberculosis. In both conditions, the choice of appropriate contraception should be individualized. For example, some women who take antiepileptic medication do well with a relatively higher dose OC. On the other hand, drugs used for the treatment of malaria do not affect contraceptive hormones, and oral contraception is not contraindicated in patients with malaria.

A coincidence of migraine and stroke has been recognized in several epidemiologic studies. A large-scale prospective epidemiologic study in the United States followed up 12,220 subjects between the years 1971 and 1984 and was published in 1997.[195] The results of the study strengthened previous evidence regarding a nonrandom association of migraine and severe nonspecific headaches with a significantly increased risk of stroke, particularly among young women. In women younger than 45 years, all cases of stroke occurred in OC users. However, the study was conducted during a period when use of low-dose OCs was not common. This probably also applies to a case-control study examining the risk of ischemic stroke in young women with migraine. In this study, stroke was strongly associated with migraine with aura (odds ratio 6.2) as well as without aura (odds ratio 3.0). OCs increased the risk of ischemic stroke to 13.9.[196] Another study estimated the odds ratio in migrainoid women using COC as 16.9.[197]

Contraindications to the use of combined hormonal contraception are migraines with aura, migraines without aura if they are unusually severe or last more than 72 hours, migraines treated with ergot preparations, and all types of migraines when other risk factors for stroke are present. These contraindications are included in the British practice guidelines.[198] The American College of Obstetrics and Gynecology[199] recommends methods other than OCs for women with migraines. This prudent approach to combined OCs is warranted because an array of reliable nonhormonal methods is available today. Progestagen-only oral contraception can be tried in patients with simple migraines.

Patients with concomitant diseases who want and need contraception require special care and possibly more frequent follow-up. With the present availability of a wide variety of contraceptives, no health-compromised patient needs to be without protection from pregnancy.

THE FUTURE OF FAMILY PLANNING: NEEDS AND RESEARCH

Family planning in the second part of the 20th century was a remarkable success; almost 60% of couples of reproductive age now use contraception, and the fertility rate worldwide decreased nearly to the replacement level (see Fig. 17–3). Is this a reason for satisfaction? The number of unwanted pregnancies, over 2.5 million in the United States alone and 50 million worldwide, sends us the message that there is ample room for improvement.

Human Immunodeficiency Virus–Acquired Immunodeficiency Syndrome

Today's major medical problem is HIV infection and AIDS. With respect to reproductive health care, the research challenge is to develop a reliable microbicidal-spermicidal agent that will simultaneously protect against the two dangerous viral infections, HIV and HPV. Another research task is to design ways to prevent the transmission of the HIV infection from mother to fetus. Finally, prevention of pregnancy in women with HIV-AIDS requires education of infected women with regard to an effective method of fertility control and provision of suitable means—including financial—to do so.

The statistics of the HIV-AIDS epidemic are chilling: HIV-AIDS affects 16 million women and 1.4 million children younger than 15 years worldwide. The yearly death toll for women is 1.3 million and for children younger than 15 years is 500,000.[200] To protect women from HIV-AIDS and to prevent transmission of the infection to infants is an urgent task.

Expanding Contraceptive Choices

There are several goals at the heart of expanding contraceptive choices that include tailoring contraception to the individual needs of the woman or the couple and designing new delivery systems for existing hormones. A meaningful contribution has been the successful completion of clinical trials with a contraceptive patch and the current research on vaginal rings releasing contraceptive hormones. These and other parenteral delivery systems for contraceptive steroids have been described in the appropriate section of this chapter.

With respect to the development of new nonhormonal methods of fertility control, most of the current efforts involve modifications of previous designs.

Departure from 1-Month to 3-Month Regimen

Traditionally, OC treatment was designed for 1-month use. However, a number of women perceive monthly withdrawal bleedings as a nuisance and would prefer to reduce the number of bleeding episodes and symptoms accompanying such episodes. For many years, physicians have prescribed continuous combined OCs to avoid withdrawal bleeding. Currently, a 3-month regimen of ethinylestradiol and levonorgestrel is being investigated in the United States. The effect on the endometrium and evolution of endometrial hyperproliferation at the end of the 3-month dosing period must be investigated and defined.[201]

Contraception for Nursing Women

There is still a need for additional contraceptive options for breast-feeding women. Although lactation reduces fertility substantially, unpredictable breakthrough ovulations do occur, particularly when breast-feeding is not exclusive or is irregular. Pilot studies with breast-feeding women have shown that small amounts of estradiol delivered by transdermal patches significantly reduce pituitary gonadotropins more than in untreated breast-feeding women. The growth of ovarian follicles was also significantly suppressed in the treated women.[202] Before this information can be translated into a practical contraceptive method for lactating women, many questions must be answered, including the long-term effects of low doses of estrogen on the mother, the transfer of estrogen into the breast milk, and possible effects on the infant. For now, barrier and progestagen-only methods remain most reasonable.

Immunocontraception

Since 1975, a WHO research program has devoted considerable effort to developing an anti-hCG antibody that would protect women from pregnancy for 6 to 12 months. Although the research has yielded an impressive amount of basic scientific data, human application had to be discontinued because of unexpected adverse events. New immunologic leads are being pursued. Antisperm vaccines, antiovum vaccines, and anti-GnRH vaccines are also being contemplated but have not crossed from the laboratory into the clinic.[203]

Developing a Male Contraceptive

After years of trying various approaches, the only effective and well-tolerated methods of male contraception are vasectomy and the condom. Attempts have been made to develop systemic male contraception using the same principles as in female contraception, that is, blocking the pituitary gonadotropins in order to reduce sperm production in the testes to the point at which the man becomes infertile. Testosterone enanthate alone suppresses pituitary gonadotropins and interferes with spermatogenesis.[204] Combination of this androgen with a GnRH agonist or a GnRH antagonist achieved an impressive reduction of spermatogenesis without affecting the sexual function of the men studied.[205]

The addition of a progestagen to testosterone has been associated with more rapid and effective suppression of spermatogenesis than with testosterone alone. Therefore, considerable research efforts have been directed toward testing combinations of testosterone with contraceptive progestagens, including levonorgestrel, cyproterone acetate, MPA, norethindrone enanthate, and desogestrel.[206–212] The major disadvantage of testosterone is its conversion to dihydrotestosterone and the consequent stimulation of the prostate gland. The negative effect of testosterone on lipid metabolism is also of concern. Although treatments with testosterone alone and in combination with either GnRH agonists and antagonists or with various progestagens have contributed substantially to our knowledge of spermatogenesis and its suppression, a practical method of male contraception has not been developed.

However, one approach is promising. The Population Council is conducting clinical testing with steroid hormones of the 19-nortestosterone series, notably with 7α-methyl-19-nortestosterone. The 7α-methyl group protects the compound from conversion to dihydrotestosterone; therefore, its effects on the prostate gland are limited. However, 7α-methyl-19-

nortestosterone is 10 times more potent in suppressing pituitary gonadotropins. Because of its lack of oral bioavailability, the compound has been formulated in a subdermal implant.

Human studies have progressed to initial clinical pharmacology testing. One-month dose-response studies have identified the daily amount of 7α-methyl-19-nortestosterone that successfully suppresses both luteinizing hormone and follicle-stimulating hormone, and studies of the effect of 7α-methyl-19-nortestosterone on spermatogenesis in humans are in progress.[213]

The Future

In the search for a new method of male contraception, it might be necessary to depart from the traditional hormonal approach and look for potential leads in the molecular regulation of sperm biology. One approach would be to interfere with sperm capacitation in the epididymis. Maturation of the sperm surface composition is critical for fertilization of the egg, and any disruption can impede sperm progress through the cells and carbohydrate matrix of the cumulus oophorus and the glycoproteins of the zona pellucida. Decapacitated sperm may attach to the surface of the cumulus but fail to penetrate it.

During epididymal transit, the sperm undergoes maturation, a series of processes that have been only partially elucidated. Incomplete sperm maturation within the epididymis could explain the failure of sperm binding to the zona pellucida in unsuccessful human in vitro fertilizations. A group of newly discovered proteins (HE2 β and HE2 γ) that are synthesized in the epididymis and secreted into that tubule might interact with sperm and affect their maturation. If the role of these epididymis-specific proteins in sperm maturation is confirmed and defined, they could be a source of potential contraceptive targets. This approach is an attempt to apply the lessons of molecular cell biology in the clinic.[214]

With respect to hormonal contraception for women, the trend has been to introduce new types of progestagens with minimal metabolic impact and a specific action on the endometrium. Is there really a need for new progestagens? Progestagens of the advanced gonane series, such as norgestimate and desogestrel, already have no negative effects on the metabolism of lipids, proteins, and insulin, and they may be the answer to the quest for a progestagen with minimal metabolic action.

With respect to estrogens, we are still using a compound synthesized in biochemically prehistoric times—in 1938. Perhaps we should start looking for a selective estrogen receptor modulator that suppresses the pituitary gland with no or little effect on the endometrium, no effect on the blood clotting mechanisms, and no potential for thromboembolism. To date, no product is available that meets these criteria.

The development of new contraceptive modalities depends on close cooperation between three institutions: academia, government agencies, and the pharmaceutical industry. This is true for the development of any drug, but it is perhaps more important for the development of contraceptives because contraceptive research involves a number of public health issues and, in many instances, financial support for reproductive research depends on public opinion and attitudes.

References

1. United Nations Population Division. World Population Prospects: The 2000 Revision. New York, United Nations, 2000.
2. Raleigh VS. Trends in world population: how will the millennium compare with the past? Hum Reprod Update 1999; 5:500.
3. Malthus T. An Essay on the Principle of Population. London, J. Johnson, in St. Paul's churchyard, 1798. Rendered into HTML format by Ed Stephan, August 10, 1997.
4. Ehrlich PR. The Population Bomb. New York, Ballantine Books, 1968.
5. Martin LG. Six billion and counting. Harvard Int Rev 2000; Fall: 1 (updated January 2001).
6. Rudel HW, Kincl FA, Henzl MR. Birth Control. Contraception and Abortion. New York, Macmillan, 1973.
7. Davies N. Europe: A History. New York, Oxford University Press, 1996.
8. Roberts JM. Twentieth Century. The History of the World 1901–2000. New York, Viking, 1999.
9. McGovern G. The Third Freedom: Ending Hunger in Our Time. New York, Simon & Schuster, 2001.
10. Tilman D, Fargione J, Wolff B, et al. Forecasting agriculturally driven global environmental change. Science 2001; 292:291.
11. Conquest R. Reflections on a Ravaged Century. New York, Norton, 2000.
12. Potts M. Making Cairo work. Lancet 1999; 353:315.
13. Potts M. The population policy pendulum: needs to settle near the middle and acknowledge the importance of numbers. BMJ 1999; 319:933.
14. Potts M. The unmet need for family planning. Sci Am 2000; 282(1):69.
15. Campbell MM. Schools of thought: an analysis of interest groups influential in international population policy. Popul Environ 1998; 19:487.
16. Glasier A, Gebbie A (eds). Handbook of Family Planning and Reproductive Healthcare, 4th ed. New York, Churchill Livingstone, 2000, pp VII–VIII.
17. Trussell J, Kost K. Contraceptive failure in the United States: a critical review of the literature. Stud Fam Plann 1987;18:237.
18. Trussell J, Hatcher HA, Cates W, et al. Contraceptive failure in the United States: an update. Stud Fam Plann 1990;21:51.
19. Trussell J. Contraceptive efficacy. In Hatcher RA, Trussell J, Stewart F, et al (eds). Contraceptive Technology, 17th ed. New York, Irvington, 1998.
20. Fu H, Darroch JE, Haas T, et al. Contraceptive failure rates: new estimates from the 1995 National Survey of Family Growth. Fam Plann Perspect 1999; 30:56.
21. Sokal D, Hieu DT, Weiner DH, et al. Long term follow-up after quinacrine sterilization in Vietnam. Part I. Interim efficacy analysis. Fertil Steril 2000; 74:1084.
22. Sokal D, Hieu DT, Weiner DH, et al. Long term follow-up after quinacrine sterilization in Vietnam. Part II. Interim safety analysis. Fertil Steril 2000; 74:1092.
23. Trussell J, Vaughan B. Contraceptive failure, method related discontinuation and resumption of use: results from the 1995 National Survey of Family Growth. Fam Plann Perspect 1999; 31: 64–72, 93.
24. Ford K. Contraceptive utilization among currently married women 15–44 years of age: United States, 1973. Mon Vital Stat 1976; 25/7(suppl):1.
25. Piccino LJ, Mosher WD. Trends in contraceptive use in the United States: 1982–1995. Fam Plann Perspect 1998; 30:4–10, 46.
26. Bongaarts J, Johansson E. Future trends in contraceptive prevalence and method mix in the developing world. Stud Fam Plan 2002; 33:24.
27. Ellertson C. Contraceptive choice. In Glasier A, Gebbie A (eds). Handbook of Family Planning and Reproductive Healthcare, 4th ed. New York, Churchill Livingstone, 2000, pp 1–22.
28. Henshaw SK. Unintended pregnancy in the United States. Fam Plann Perspect 1998; 30:24–29, 46.
29. Henshaw SK, Kost K. Abortion patients in 1994–1995: characteristics and contraceptive use. Fam Plann Perspect 1998; 28: 140–147, 158.
30. Sturgis SH, Albright R. Mechanism of estrin therapy in the relief of dysmenorrhea. Endocrinology 1940; 26:68.
31. Maisel AQ. The Hormone Quest. New York, Random House, 1965.
32. Pincus G. The Control of Fertility. New York, Academic Press, 1956.
33. Marks LV. Sexual Chemistry: A History of the Contraceptive Pill. New Haven, Conn, Yale University Press, 2001.
34. Djerassi C. This Man's Pill. Reflections on the 50th Birthday of the Pill. New York, Oxford University Press, 2001.
35. Inhoffen HH, Hohlweg W. Neue per os wirksame weibliche Keimdruesenhormonderivate. Naturwissenschaften 1938; 26:96.

36. Djerassi D, Miramontes L, Rosenkranz G. 17alpha-Ethynyl-19-nortestosterone. American Chemical Society Meeting, 1952, abstract 18J.
37. Goldzieher JW. Pharmacology of contraceptive steroids. In Shoupe D, Haseltine FP (eds). Contraception. New York, Springer-Verlag, 1993, pp 17–24.
38. Henzl MR, Jirasek JE, Horsky J, et al. Proliferative effect of 17alpha-ethinyl, 19-nortestosterone. Arch Gynaekol 1963; 199: 335.
39. Oropeza MV, Campos MG, Lemus AE, et al. Estrogenic actions of norethisterone and its A-ring reduced metabolites: induction of in vitro uterine sensitivity to serotonin. Arch Med Res 1994; 25: 307.
40. Neumann F. The antiandrogen cyproterone acetate: discovery, chemistry, basic pharmacology, clinical use and tool in basic research. Exp Clin Endocrinol 1994; 102:1.
41. Henzl MR. Synthetic sex steroids. In Adashi EY, Rock JA, Rosenwaks Z (eds). Reproductive Endocrinology, Surgery, and Technology. New York, Lippincott-Raven, 1996, pp 585–604.
42. Kuhl H. Comparative pharmacology of newer progestogens. Drugs 1996; 51:188.
43. WHO collaborative study on neoplasia and steroid contraceptives. Breast cancer and depot-medroxyprogesterone acetate: a multinational study. Lancet 1991; 338:833.
44. Fotherby K. Levonorgestrel: clinical pharmacokinetics. Clin Pharmacokinet 1995; 28:203.
45. Fotherby K. Potency and pharmacokinetics of gestagens. Contraception 1990; 41:533.
46. McGuire JL, Phillips A, Hahn DW, et al. Pharmacological and pharmacokinetic characteristics of norgestimate and its metabolites. Am J Obstet Gynecol 1990; 163:2127.
47. Coutinho EM, de Souza JC, Athayde C, et al. Multicenter clinical trial on the efficacy and acceptability of a single contraceptive implant of nomegestrol acetate, Uniplant. Contraception 1996; 53:121.
48. Kumar N, Koide SS, Tsong YY, et al. Nestorone: a progestin with a unique pharmacological profile. Steroids 2000; 65:629.
49. Oettel M, Breitbarth H, Graeser T, et al. The pharmacological profile of dienogest. Proceedings of the 5th Congress of the European Society of Contraception, 17–20 June 1998, Prague. Eur J Contracept Reprod Health Care 1998; 3(suppl 1):76.
50. Anonymous. Yasmin. A Factsheet. Wayne, NJ, Berlex Laboratories, May 2001.
51. Edgren RA, Elton RL. Estrogen antagonism: effect of steroidal spironolactones on estrogen induced uterine growth in mice. Proc Exp Biol Med 1960; 104:665.
52. Henzl MR. Safety of modern oral contraceptives. Lancet 1996; 347:257.
53. Phillips A, Demarest K, Hahn DW, et al. Progestational and androgenic receptor binding affinities and in vivo activities of norgestimate and other progestins. Contraception 1990; 41:399.
54. Rabe T, Kowald A, Ortmann J, et al. Inhibition of skin 5α-reductase by oral contraceptive progestins in vitro. Gynecol Endocrinol 2000; 14:223.
55. Godsland IF, Crook D, Simpson R, et al. The effects of different formulations of oral contraceptive agents on lipid and carbohydrate metabolism. N Engl J Med 1990; 323:1375.
56. Burkman RT Jr, Kafrissen ME, Olson W, et al. Lipid and carbohydrate effects of a new triphasic oral contraceptive containing norgestimate. Acta Obstet Gynecol Scand Suppl 1992; 156:5.
57. Hammond GL. Determinants of steroid hormone bioavailability. Biochem Soc Trans 1997; 25:577.
58. Phillips A, Hahn DW, McGuire JL. Relative binding affinity of norgestimate and other progestins for human sex hormone–binding globulin. Steroids 1990; 55:373.
59. Redmond GP, Olson WH, Lippman JS, et al. Norgestimate and ethinylestradiol in the treatment of acne vulgaris: a randomized, placebo-controlled trial. Obstet Gynecol 1997; 89:615.
60. Stumpf PG, Nakamura RM, Mishell DR Jr. Changes in physiologically free circulating estradiol and testosterone during exposure to levonorgestrel. J Clin Endocrinol Metab 1981; 52:138–143.
61. Spellacy WN. Oral contraceptives effect on glucose metabolism. In Shoupe D, Haseltine FP (eds). Contraception. New York, Springer Verlag, 1993, pp 25–33.
62. Cibula D, Sindelka J, Skrha J, et al. Insulin sensitivity during treatment of PCOS women with oral contraceptives containing norgestimate. Book of Abstracts, p 76 (FC2.30.01). XVI FIGO World Congress of Gynecology and Obstetrics, September 3–8, 2000, Washington, DC.
63. Petersen KR, Christiansen E, Madsbad S, et al. Metabolic and fibrinolytic response to changed insulin sensitivity in users of oral contraceptives. Contraception 1999; 60:337.
64. Godsland IF. The influence of female sex hormones on glucose metabolism and insulin action. J Intern Med 1996; 240(suppl 738):1.
65. Mishell DR Jr, Kletzky OA, Brenner PF, et al. The effect of contraceptive steroids on hypothalamic pituitary function. Am J Obstet Gynecol 1977; 180:S302.
66. Moghisi KS, Syner FN, McBride LC: Contraceptive mechanism of microdose norethindrone. Obstet Gynecol 1973; 4:585.
67. Centers for Disease Control, National Institute of Child Health and Human Development. Combination oral contraceptive use and the risk of endometrial cancer. JAMA 1987; 257:796.
68. The reduction in risk of ovarian cancer associated with oral contraceptive use: the Cancer and Steroid Hormone Study of the Centers for Disease Control and the National Institute of Child Health and Human Development. N Engl J Med 1987; 316:650.
69. Grimes DA, Hughes JM. Use of multiphasic oral contraceptives and hospitalizations of women with functional ovarian cysts in the United States. Obstet Gynecol 1989; 73:1037.
70. Holt VL, Daling JR, McKnight B, et al. Functional ovarian cysts in relation to the use of monophasic and triphasic oral contraceptives. Obstet Gynecol 1992; 79:529.
71. Eschenbach DA, Harnisch JP, Holmes KK. Pathogenesis of acute pelvic inflammatory disease: role of contraception and other risk factors. Am J Obstet Gynecol 1977; 128:838.
72. Panser LA, Phipps WR. Type of oral contraceptive in relation to acute initial episodes of pelvic inflammatory disease. Contraception 1991; 43:91.
73. Sivin I. Dose- and age-dependent ectopic pregnancy risks with intrauterine contraception. Obstet Gynecol 1991; 78:291.
74. Franks AL, Beral V, Cates W Jr, et al. Contraception and ectopic pregnancy risk. Am J Obstet Gynecol 1990; 163:1120.
75. Burkman RT. Management of the fibroid uterus. Adv Obstet Gynecol 1996; 3:103.
76. Sangi-Haghpeykar H, Poindexter AN III. Epidemiology of endometriosis among parous women. Obstet Gynecol 1995; 85:983.
77. Lucky AW, Henderson TA, Olson WH, et al. Effectiveness of norgestimate and ethinylestradiol in treating moderate acne vulgaris. J Am Acad Dermatol 1997; 37:746.
78. Thiboutot D, Archer DF, Lemay A, et al. A randomized, controlled trial of a low-dose contraceptive containing 20 mcg of ethinylestradiol and 100 mcg of levonorgestrel for acne treatment. Fertil Steril 2001; 76:461.
79. Gilliam M, Elam G, Maloney JM, et al. Acne treatment with a low-dose oral contraceptive. Obstet Gynecol 2001; 97(4 suppl 1): S9.
80. Katz HI, Kempers S, Akin MD, et al. Effect of a desogestrel-containing oral contraceptive on the skin. Eur J Contracept Reprod Health Care 2000; 5:248.
81. Thorneycroft IH, Stanczyk FZ, Bradshaw KD, et al. Effect of low-dose oral contraceptives on androgenic markers and acne. Contraception 1999; 60:255.
82. Palatsi R, Hirvensalo E, Liukko P, et al. Serum total and unbound testosterone and sex hormone binding globulin (SHBG) in female acne patients treated with two different oral contraceptives. Acta Derm Venereol 1984; 64:517.
83. Worret I, Arp W, Zahradnik HP, et al. Acne resolution rates: results of a single-blind, randomized, controlled, parallel phase III trial with EE/CMA (Belara®) and EE/LNG (Microgynon). Dermatology 2001; 203:38.
84. Heiner JS, Greendale GA, Kawakami AK, et al. Comparison of a gonadotropin-releasing hormone agonist and a low dose oral contraceptive given alone or together in the treatment of hirsutism. J Clin Endocrinol Metab 1995; 80:3412.
85. Azziz R, Ochoa TM, Bradley EL Jr, et al. Leuprolide and estrogen versus oral contraceptive pills for the treatment of hirsutism: a prospective randomized study. J Clin Endocrinol Metab 1995; 80:3406.
86. Kleerekopper M, Brienza RS, Schultz LR. Oral contraceptive use may protect against low bone mass. Arch Intern Med 1991; 151: 1971.

87. Michaelsson K, Baron JA, Farahmand BY, et al. Oral contraceptive use and risk of hip fracture: a case-control study. Lancet 1999; 353:1481.
88. Hazes JMW, Dijkmans BAC, Vandenbroucke JP, et al. Reduction of the risk of rheumatoid arthritis among women who take oral contraceptives. Arthritis Rheum 1990; 33:173.
89. Pladeval-Vila M, Delclos GL, Varas C, et al. Controversy of oral contraceptives and risk of rheumatoid arthritis: meta-analysis of conflicting studies and review of conflicting meta-analyses with special emphasis on analysis of heterogeneity. Am J Epidemiol 1996; 144:1.
90. Martinez ME, Grodstein E, Giovannucci E, et al. A prospective study of reproductive factors, oral contraceptive use, and risk of colorectal cancer. Cancer Epidemiol Biomarkers Prev 1997; 6:1.
91. Franceschi S, La Vecchia CL. Oral contraceptives and colorectal tumors: a review of epidemiological studies. Contraception 1998; 58:335.
92. Redmond G, Godwin AJ, Olson W, et al. Use of placebo controls in an oral contraceptive trial: methodological issues and adverse event incidence. Contraception 1999; 60:81.
93. Gerstman BB, Piper JM, Tomita DK, et al. Oral contraceptive estrogen dose and the risk of deep venous thromboembolic disease. Am J Epidemiol 1991; 133:32.
94. Vasilakis C, Jick H, del Mar Melero-Montez M. Risk of idiopathic venous thromboembolism in users of progestogens alone. Lancet 1999; 354:1610.
95. Vasilakis C, Jick SS, Jick H. The risk of venous thromboembolism in users of post-coital contraceptive pills. Contraception 1999; 59:79–83.
96. World Health Organization Collaborative Study of Cardiovascular Disease and Steroid Hormone Contraception. Venous thromboembolic disease and combined oral contraceptives: results of international multicentre case-control study. Lancet 1995; 346: 1575.
97. World Health Organization Collaborative Study of Cardiovascular Disease and Steroid Hormone Contraception. Effect of different progestogens in low oestrogen oral contraceptives on venous thromboembolic disease. Lancet 1995; 346:1582.
98. Jick H, Jick SS, Gurewich V, et al. Risk of idiopathic cardiovascular death and nonfatal venous thromboembolism in women using oral contraceptives with differing progestagen components. Lancet 1995; 346:1589.
99. Jick H, Kaye JA, Vasilakis-Scaramozza C, et al. Risk of venous thromboembolism among users of third generation oral contraceptives compared with users of oral contraceptives with levonorgestrel before and after 1995: cohort and case-control analysis. BMJ 2000; 321:1190.
100. Kemmeren JM, Algra A, Grobbee DE. Third generation oral contraceptives and risk of venous thrombosis: meta-analysis. BMJ 2001; 323:131
101. Lippman JS, Shangold GA. A review of post-marketing safety and surveillance data for oral contraceptives containing norgestimate and ethinylestradiol. Int J Fertil 1997; 42:230.
102. Notelovitz M. Oral contraceptives: effect on hemostasis. In Shoupe D, Haseltine FP (eds). Contraception. New York, Springer Verlag, 1993, pp 42–59.
103. Winkler UH. Blood coagulation and oral contraceptives: a critical review. Contraception 1998; 57:203.
104. Vandenbroucke JP, Koster T, Briet E, et al. Increased risk of venous thrombosis in oral-contraceptive users who are carriers of factor V Leiden mutation. Lancet 1994; 344:1453–1457.
105. Vandenbroucke JP, van der Meer FJ, Helmerhorst FM, et al. Factor V Leiden: should we screen oral contraceptive users and pregnant women? BMJ 1996; 313:1127–1130.
106. Vandenbroucke JP, Rosing J, Bloemenkamp KWM, et al. Oral contraceptives and the risk of venous thrombosis. N Engl J Med 2001; 344:1527.
107. Vessey MP, Doll R. Is the "pill" safe enough to continue using? In Shatt RV, Baird DT (eds). Contraceptives of the Future. London, The Royal Society, 1976.
108. Petitti DB, Sidney S, Bernstein A, et al. Stroke in users of low-dose oral contraception. N Engl J Med 1996; 335:8.
109. World Health Organization. Collaborative study of cardiovascular disease and steroid hormone contraception. Lancet 1997; 349: 1202.
110. Lewis MA, Heinemann LAJ, Spitzer WO, et al. On behalf of Trans-National Research Group on Oral Contraceptives and the Health of Young Women. The use of oral contraceptives and the occurrence of acute myocardial infarction in young women. Contraception 1997; 56:129.
111. Dunn N, Thorogood M, Faragher B, et al. Oral contraceptives and myocardial infarction: results of MICA case-control study. BMJ 1999; 318:1579.
112. Tietze CH. New estimates of mortality associated with fertility control. Fam Plann Perspect 1977; 9:74.
113. Jain AK. Mortality risk associated with the use of oral contraceptives. Stud Fam Plann 1977; 8:50.
114. Owen-Smith V, Hannaford PC, Warskyj M, et al. Effects of changes in smoking status on risk estimates for myocardial infarction among women recruited for the Royal College of General Practitioners' Oral Contraception Study in the UK. J Epidemiol Community Health 1998; 52:420.
115. Dunn N, Faragher B, Thorogood M, et al. Risk of myocardial infarction in young female smokers. Heart 1999; 82:581.
116. WHO Collaborative Study of Cardiovascular Disease and Steroid Hormone Contraception. Haemorrhagic stroke, overall stroke risk, and combined oral contraceptives: results of an international, multicentre, case-control study. Lancet 1996; 348:505.
117. WHO Collaborative Study of Cardiovascular Disease and Steroid Hormone Contraception. Ischaemic stroke and combined oral contraceptives: results of an international, multicentre, case-control study. Lancet 1996; 348:498.
118. Raij L, DeMaster EG, Jaimes EA. Cigarette smoke–induced endothelium dysfunction: role of superoxide anion. J Hypertens 2001, 19:891.
119. Edgren RA. Oral contraceptive and cancer. Int J Fertil 1991; 36(suppl 3):37.
120. Committee on the Relationship between Oral Contraceptives and Breast Cancer. Oral Contraceptives and Breast Cancer. Washington, DC, National Academy Press, 1991.
121. Fraser IS. Forty years of combined oral contraception: the evolution of a revolution. Med J Aust 2000; 173:541
122. Marchbanks PA, McDonald JA, Wilson HG, et al. Oral contraceptives and the risk of breast cancer. N Engl J Med 2002; 346: 2025.
122a. Davidson NE, Helzlsouer KJ, et al. Good news about oral contraceptives. N Engl J Med 2002; 346:2078
122b. Marchbanks PA, McDonald JA, Wilson HG, et al. The NICHD Women's Contraceptive and Reproductive Experiences Study: methods and operational results. Ann Epidemiol 2002, 12: 213.
122c. Collaborative Group on Hormonal Factors and Breast Cancer. Breast cancer and hormonal contraceptives: Collaborative reanalysis of individual data on 53 297 women with breast cancer and 100 239 women without breast cancer from 54 epidemiological studies. Lancet 1996; 347:1713.
123. Grabrick D, Hartmann LC, Cerhan JR, et al. Risk of breast cancer with oral contraceptive use in women with a family history of breast cancer. JAMA 2000; 284:1791.
124. Schlesselman JJ. Oral contraceptives in relation to cancer of the breast and reproductive tract: an epidemiological review. Br J Fam Plann 1989; 15(suppl):23.
125. Parazzini F, La Vecchia C. Epidemiology of adenocarcinoma of the cervix. Gynecol Oncol 1990; 39:40.
126. Kjaer SK, Brinton LA. Adenocarcinomas of the uterine cervix: the epidemiology of an increasing problem. Epidemiol Rev 1993; 15:486.
127. Ursin G, Peters RK, Henderson BE, et al. Oral contraceptive use and adenocarcinoma of cervix. Lancet 1994; 344:1390.
128. Thomas DB, Ray RM. Oral contraceptives and invasive adenocarcinomas and adenosquamous carcinomas of the uterine cervix. The World Health Organization Collaborative Study of Neoplasia and Steroid Contraceptives. Am J Epidemiol 1996; 144:281.
129. Brinton LA, Reeves WC, Brenes MM, et al. Oral contraceptive use and risk of invasive cervical cancer. Int J Epidemiol 1990; 19: 4.
130. Lacey JV, Brinton LA, Abbas FM. Oral contraceptives as risk factors for cervical adenocarcinomas and squamous cell carcinomas. Cancer Epidemiol Biomarkers Prev 1999; 8:1079.
131. Mishell DR Jr. Contraception. N Engl J Med 1989; 320:77.
132. Beral V, Hermon C, Kay C, et al. Mortality associated with oral contraceptive use: 25 year follow up of 46 000 women from

Royal College of General Practitioners' oral contraception study. BMJ 1999; 318:96.
133. Skegg DCG. Oral contraception and health: long term study of mortality shows no overall effect in a developed country. BMJ 1999; 318:69.
134. Szoka PR, Edgren RA. Drug interactions with oral contraceptives: compilation and analysis of an adverse experience report database. Fertil Steril 1988; 49(suppl):31S.
135. Fraser IS. Progestogen only contraception. In Glasier A, Gebbie A (eds). Handbook of Family Planning and Reproductive Healthcare, 4th ed. New York, Churchill Livingstone, 2000, pp 77–103.
136. Segal SJ, Alvarez-Sanchez F, Brache V, et al. Norplant implants: the mechanism of contraceptive action. Fertil Steril 1991; 56:273.
137. Coutinho EM, Athayde C, Dantas C, et al. Use of a single implant of elcometrine (ST-1435), a nonorally active progestin, as a long acting contraceptive for postpartum nursing women. Contraception 1999; 59:115.
138. Faundes A, Alvarez F, Brache V, et al. Correlation of endocrine profiles with bleeding patterns during use of Nestorone contraceptive implants. Hum Reprod 1999; 14:3013.
139. Petitti DB, Piaggio G, Mehta S, et al, for the WHO study of hormonal contraception and bone health. Steroid hormone contraception and bone mineral density: a cross sectional study in an international population. Obstet Gynecol 2000; 97:736.
140. Kaunitz AM. Injectable long-acting contraceptives. Clin Obstet Gynecol 2001; 44:73.
141. Mishell DR Jr, Talas M, Parlow AF, et al. Contraception by means of a Silastic vaginal ring impregnated with medroxyprogesterone acetate. Am J Obstet Gynecol 1970; 107:100.
142. Brache V, Alvarez-Sanchez F, Faundes A, et al. Progestin only contraceptive rings. Steroids 2000; 65:687.
143. Ballagh SA. Vaginal ring hormone delivery systems in contraception and menopause. Clin Obstet Gynecol 2001; 44:106.
144. Audet M-C, Moreau M, Koltun WD, et al, for the Ortho EVRA study group. Evaluation of contraceptive efficacy and cycle control of transdermal contraceptive patch vs an oral contraceptive. JAMA 2001: 285:2347.
145. Morris JM, van Wagenen G. Interception: the use of postovulatory estrogens to prevent implantation. Am J Obstet Gynecol 1973; 115:101.
146. Yuzpe AA, Smith PR, Rademaker AW. A multicenter clinical investigation employing ethinyl estradiol combined with levonorgestrel as a post-coital contraceptive agent. Fertil Steril 1982; 37: 508.
147. Task Force on Postovulatory Methods of Fertility Regulation. Randomized controlled trial of levonorgestrel versus the Yuzpe regimen of combined oral contraceptives for emergency contraception. Lancet 1998; 352:428.
148. Task Force on Postovulatory Methods of Fertility Regulation. Comparison of three single doses of mifepristone as emergency contraception: a randomized trial. Lancet 1999; 353:697.
149. Glasier A. Drug therapy: emergency post-coital contraception. N Engl J Med 1997; 337:105.
150. Schaff EA, Fielding SL, Westhoff C, et al. Vaginal misoprostol administered 1, 2, or 3 days after mifepristone for early medical abortion: a randomized trial. JAMA 2000; 284:1948.
151. Spitz IM, Bardin CW, Benton L, et al. Early pregnancy termination with mifepristone and misoprostol in the United States. N Engl J Med 1998; 338:1241.
152. Henzl MR. Intrauterine devices. In Rudel HW, Kincl FA, Henzl MR (eds). Birth Control: Contraception and Abortion. New York, Macmillan, 1973, pp 154–185.
153. United Nations Development Programme. Long-term reversible contraception: two years of experience with the TCu 380A and TCu 220C. Contraception 1997; 56:341.
154. Wildemeersch SD, Batar I, Webb A, et al. GyneFIX. The frameless intrauterine contraceptive implant: an update for interval, emergency, and postabortal contraception. Br J Fam Plann 1999; 24:149.
155. French RS, Cowan FM, Mansour D, et al. Levonorgestrel-releasing (20 microgram/day) intrauterine systems (Mirena) compared with other methods of reversible contraceptives. BJOG 2000; 107:1218.
156. Pasquale S. Clinical experience with today's IUDs. Obstet Gynecol Surv 1996; 51:25S.
157. Grimes DA. Intrauterine device and upper-genital tract infection. Lancet 2000; 356:1013.
158. Sivin I, Mahgoub S, McCarthy T, et al. Long-term contraception with the levonorgestrel 20 mcg/day (LNG 20) and the copper T 380Ag intrauterine devices: a five-year randomized study. Contraception 1990; 42:361.
159. Sivin I, Stern J, International Committee for Contraception Research. Health during prolonged use of levonorgestrel 20 microgram/day and the copper TCu 380 Ag intrauterine contraceptive device. Fertil Steril 1994; 61:70.
160. Ronnerdag M, Odlind M. Health effects of long-term use of the intrauterine levonorgestrel-releasing system: a follow-up study over 12 years of continuous use. Acta Obstet Gynecol Scand 1999; 78:716.
161. Hagenfeldt K. Intrauterine contraception with the copper-T device. Contraception 1972; 6:37.
162. Prema K, Lakshmi BA, Babu S. Serum copper in long-term users of copper intrauterine devices. Fertil Steril 1980; 34:32.
163. Fahmy K, Ghoneim M, Eisa I, et al. Serum and endometrial copper, zinc, iron and cobalt with inert and copper-containing IUCDs. Contraception 1993; 47:483.
164. Rodrigues da Cunha AC, Dorea JG, Cantuaria AA. Intrauterine device and maternal copper metabolism during lactation. Contraception 2001; 63:37.
165. Bunke H, Cario WR, Schneider M. Variations in the composition of breast milk in Wilson's disease. Kinderarztl Prax 1989; 57:89.
166. Gardner FJ, Konje JC, Abrams KR, et al. Endometrial protection from tamoxifen-stimulated changes by a levonorgestrel-releasing intrauterine system: a randomized controlled trial. Lancet 2000; 356:1711.
167. Farley TM, Rosenberg MJ, Rowe PJ, et al. Intrauterine devices and pelvic inflammatory disease: an international perspective. Lancet 1992; 339:785.
168. Mishell DR Jr, Bell JH, Good RG. The intrauterine device: a bacteriological study of the endometrial cavity Am J Obstet Gynecol 1966; 96:119.
169. Sivin I, Stern J, Coutinho E, et al. Prolonged intrauterine contraception: a seven-year randomized study of the levonorgestrel 20 mcg/day (LNG 20) and the copper T380 Ag IUDs. Contraception 1991; 44:473.
170. Andersson K, Odlind V, Rybo G. Levonorgestrel releasing and copper releasing (Nova-T) IUDs during 5 years of use: a randomized comparative trial. Contraception 1994; 49:56.
171. Rosenblatt KA, Thomas DB. Intrauterine devices and endometrial cancer. The WHO Collaborative Study of Neoplasia and Steroid Contraceptives. Contraception 1996; 54:328.
172. Sturgeon SR, Brinton LA, Berman ML, et al. Intrauterine device use and endometrial cancer risk. Int J Epidemiol 1997; 26:496.
173. Castellsague X, Thompson WD, Dubrow R. Intra-uterine contraception and the risk of endometrial cancer. Int J Cancer 1993; 54:911.
174. Hill DA, Weiss NS, Voigt LF, et al. Endometrial cancer in relation to intra-uterine device use. Int J Cancer 1997; 70:278.
175. Segal SJ, Alvarez-Sanchez F, Adejuwon CA, et al. Absence of chorionic gonadotropin in sera of women who use intrauterine devices. Fertil Steril 1985; 44:214.
176. Wilcoz AJ, Weinberg CR, Armstrong EG, et al. Urinary human chorionic gonadotropin among intrauterine device users: detection with a highly specific and sensitive assay. Fertil Steril 1987; 47:265.
177. Rosenberg MJ, Waugh MS. Latex condom breakage and slippage in a controlled clinical trial. Contraception 1997; 56:17.
178. Frezieres RG, Walsh TL, Nelson AL, et al. Evaluation of the efficacy of a polyurethane condom: results from a randomized, controlled clinical trial. Fam Plann Perspect 1999; 31:81.
179. Farr G, Gabelnick H, Sturgen K, et al. Contraceptive efficacy and acceptability of the female condom. Am J Public Health 1994; 84:1960.
180. Centers for Disease Control. Toxic shock syndrome. United States 1970–1982. MMWR Morb Mortal Wkly Rep 1982; 31: 307.
181. Stewart F. Vaginal barriers: the diaphragm, contraceptive sponge, cervical cap, and female condom. In Hatcher RA, Trussell J, Stewart F (eds). Contraceptive Technology, 17th ed. New York, Ardent Media, 1998.
182. Wilcox AJ, Weinberg CR, Baird DD. Timing of sexual intercourse in relation to ovulation: effects on the probability of con-

ception, survival of the pregnancy, and sex of the baby. N Engl J Med 1995; 333:1517.
183. Speroff L, Darney PD. Periodic abstinence. In Speroff L, Darney PD (eds). A Clinical Guide for Contraception, 3rd ed. Philadelphia, Lippincott Williams & Wilkins, 2001, pp 297–307.
184. Peterson HB, Xia Z, Hughes J, et al. The risk of pregnancy after tubal sterilization: findings from the U.S. Collaborative Review of Sterilization. Am J Obstet Gynecol 1996; 174:1161.
185. Glasier A. Sterilization. In Glasier A, Gebbie A (eds). Handbook of Family Planning and Reproductive Healthcare, 4th ed. New York, Churchill Livingstone, 2000, pp 177–194.
186. National Center for Health Statistics. Health, United States, 1994. Hyattsville, Md, Public Health Service, 1995.
187. Robinson BA. Abortion: facts and opinions. Updated January 2001. http://www.religioustolerance.org/abo-fact.htm#data. Accessed May 21, 2001.
188. The Alan Guttmacher Institute. Induced abortion worldwide (5/99). http://www.agi-usa.org/pubs/fb 0599.html. Accessed May 21, 2001.
189. International Medical Advisory Panel (IMAP). Statement on contraception for women with medical disorders. IPPF Med Bull 1999; 33/5:1–3.
190. ACOG Practice Bulletin. The use of hormonal contraception in women with coexisting medical conditions. No 18, July 2000. Int J Gynaecol Obstet 2001; 75:93-106.
191. Garg SK, Chase HP, Marshall GA, et al. Oral contraceptives and renal and retinal complications in young women with insulin-dependent diabetes mellitus. JAMA 1994; 271:1099.
192. Chasan-Taber L, Willett WC, Stampfer MJ, et al. A prospective study of oral contraceptives and NIDDM among US women. Diabetes Care 1997; 20:330.
193. Cates W Jr. Use of contraception by HIV-infected women. IPPF Med Bull 2001; 35/1:1–2.
194. Anonymous. IMAP statement on contraception for women with medical conditions. IPPF Medical Bulletin 1999; 33(5):1–3.
195. Merikangas KR, Fenton BT, Cheng SH, et al. Association between migraine and stroke in a large-scale epidemiological study of the United States. Arch Neurol 1997; 54:362.
196. Tzourio C, Tehindrazanarivelo A, Iglesias S, et al. Case-control study of migraine and risk of ischaemic stroke in young women. BMJ 1995; 310:830.
197. Chang LC, Donaghy M, Poulter N, et al. Migraine and stroke in young women: case-control study. BMJ 1999; 318:13.
198. MacGregor EA, Guillebaud J. Combined oral contraceptives, migraine and ischaemic stroke. Clinical and Scientific Committee of the Faculty of Family Planning and Reproductive Health Care, and the Family Planning Association. Br J Fam Plann 1998; 24(2):55–60.
199. MacGregor EA, de Lignieres B. The place of combined oral contraceptives in contraception. Cephalagia 2000; 20:157–163.
200. World HIV/AIDS statistics. April 6, 2001. http://www.avert. org/worldstats.htm. Accessed May 23, 2001.
201. Archer DF. New contraceptive options. Clin Obstet Gynecol 2001; 44:122.
202. Perheentupa A, Critchley HOD, Illingworth PJ, et al. Enhanced sensitivity to steroid-negative feedback during breast-feeding: low dose estradiol (transdermal estradiol supplementation) suppresses gonadotropins and ovarian activity assessed by inhibin B. J Clin Endocrinol Metab 2000; 85:4280.
203. United Nations Development Programme. Reproductive Health Research at WHO: A New Beginning. Biennial Report 1998–1999. Geneva, World Health Organization, 2000.
204. WHO task force on methods for the regulation of male fertility. Contraceptive efficacy of testosterone-induced azoospermia and oligozoospermia in normal men. Fertil Steril 1996; 65:821.
205. Swerdloff RS, Bagatell CJ, Wang C, et al. Suppression of spermatogenesis in man induced by Nal-Glu gonadotropin-releasing hormone antagonist and testosterone enanthate (TE) is maintained by TE alone. J Clin Endocrinol Metab 1998; 83:3527.
206. Buchter D, von Eckardstein S, von Eckardstein A, et al. Clinical trial of transdermal testosterone and oral levonorgestrel for male contraception. J Clin Endocrinol Metab 1999; 84:1244.
207. Bebb RA, Anawalt BD, Christensen RB, et al. Combined administration of levonorgestrel and testosterone induces more rapid and effective suppression of spermatogenesis than testosterone alone: a promising male contraceptive approach. J Clin Endocrinol Metab 1996; 81:757–762.
208. Meriggiola MC, Bremner WJ, Paulsen CA, et al. A combined regimen of cyproterone acetate and testosterone enanthate as a potentially highly effective male contraceptive. J Clin Endocrinol Metab 1996; 81:3018–3023.
209. Handelsman DJ, Conway AJ, Howe CJ, et al. Establishing the minimum effective dose and additive effects of depot progestin in suppression of human spermatogenesis by a testosterone depot. J Clin Endocrinol Metab 1996; 81:4113–4121.
210. Kamischke A, Venherm S, Ploger D, et al. Intramuscular testosterone undecanoate and norethisterone enanthate in a clinical trial for male contraception. J Clin Endocrinol Metab 2001; 86: 303–309.
211. Wu FC, Balasubramanian R, Mulders TM, Coelingh-Bennink HJ. Oral progestogen combined with testosterone as a potential male contraceptive: additive effects between desogestrel and testosterone enanthate in suppression of spermatogenesis, pituitary-testicular axis, and lipid metabolism. J Clin Endocrinol Metab 1999; 84:112–122.
212. Hair WM, Kitteridge K, O'Connor DB, Wu FC. A novel male contraceptive pill-patch combination: oral desogestrel and transdermal testosterone in the suppression of spermatogenesis in normal men. J Clin Endocrinol Metab 2001; 86:5201–5209.
213. Sundaram K, Kumar N. 7α-Methyl-19-nortestosterone (MENT): the optimal androgen for male contraception and replacement therapy. Int J Androl 2000; 23(suppl 2):13.
214. Hamil KG, Sivashanmugam P, Richardson RT, et al. HE2 beta and HE2 gamma, new members of an epididymis-specific family of androgen-regulated proteins in the human. Endocrinology 2000; 141:1245.

18 Disorders of the Testes and the Male Reproductive Tract

James E. Griffin and Jean D. Wilson

The testes produce sperm and the hormones that regulate male sexual life; both functions are controlled by the hypothalamic-pituitary system. The pathways for hormone formation and the regulatory control of the testes are similar to those in the ovaries and the adrenal glands, and all steroid hormones work by similar mechanisms. However, the major steroid hormone of the testes, testosterone, has few direct actions; instead, it serves as a circulating prohormone (or precursor) for formation of 5α-reduced androgens and estrogens, metabolites that mediate most androgen actions.

The regulation of testicular hormone production and the mechanisms of hormone action are similar at all stages of life, but the physiologic effects of these hormones differ at different times of life—for example, inducing formation of the male urogenital tract during embryogenesis and promoting sexual maturation at the time of puberty. As a result, abnormal testicular function causes different consequences depending on when it develops, from early gestation to old age.

DEVELOPMENT OF THE TESTES

Embryogenesis

Testicular differentiation is controlled by genes on the Y chromosome.[1] The short arm of the Y is invariable in size, whereas in normal men the long arm can vary considerably in length. The short arm contains genes responsible for testicular development, and additional Y-encoded genes are essential for spermatogenesis. The short arm of the Y chromosome is composed of two distinct regions.[2] The so-called pairing segment on the distal end of the short arm is homologous to a region on the end of the short arm of the X chromosome and is responsible for the pairing between the X and Y that is essential for correct segregation of the sex chromosomes during meiosis. Recombination can occur between the shared regions of the X and the Y. Genes and sequences in this region of the X chromosome fail to exhibit typical X linkage, and the pattern of inheritance of such genes is termed *pseudoautosomal*.[1]

The region of the short arm of the Y chromosome between the pairing segment and the centromere encodes genes that do not recombine with the X chromosome, including the *SRY* (*s*ex-determining *r*egion *Y* chromosome) gene responsible for testis determination. The *SRY* gene is Y-chromosome specific, conserved among mammals, and expressed principally in the testes,[3] and female mice carrying an *SRY* transgene develop into phenotypic males with testes.[4] *SRY* encodes a protein of the HMG (high-mobility group) box type[5] that probably acts to influence chromatin structure, and other genes in the sex determination cascade, including the steroidogenic factor 1 gene *(SF1)*, Wilms' tumor–related gene *(WT1)*, the dosage-sensitive sex reversal–adrenal hypoplasia congenita gene *(DAX1)*, and the SRY-related genes HMG-box 3 *(SOX3)* and HMG-box 9 *(SOX9)*[6, 7] (Fig. 18–1). Mutations in *WT1*, *SF1*, *SRY* or any of the downstream genes under its control can impair testicular development (see Chapter 22).

Testes contain three principal cell types:

1. *Germ cells*, derived from primitive ectodermal cells of the inner cell mass (initially identifiable in the yolk sac).
2. *Supporting cells*, derived from the coelomic epithelium of the gonadal ridge that differentiate into the Sertoli cells in the testis (or granulosa cells in the ovary).
3. *Stromal (interstitial) cells*, derived from the mesenchyme of the gonadal ridge that differentiate into Leydig cells.

The primordial germ cells express specific cell markers[8] and are recognizable in the 4.5-day-old human blastocyst.[7] Before day 23 of human gestation, these cells are located in the dorsal and caudal portions of the yolk sac entoderm (Fig. 18–2*A*). They then migrate by ameboid movement from the gut endoderm through the mesentery to reach the genital ridge (see

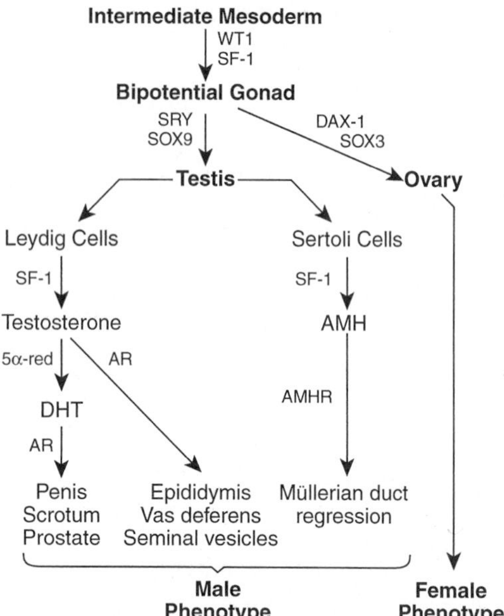

Figure 18–1. Schematic diagram of sexual differentiation beginning with formation of the bipotential gonads from intermediate mesoderm, differentiation of the testes and ovaries from the bipotential gonads, and formation of the sexual phenotypes. The genes known to be involved and their presumed sites of action are indicated. 5α-red, steroid 5α-reductase 2; AMH, antimüllerian hormone; AMHR, antimüllerian hormone receptor; AR, androgen receptor; DAX-1, dosage-sensitive sex reversal–adrenal hypoplasia congenital gene; DHT, dihydrotestosterone; SF-1, steroidogenic factor 1; SOX3, SRY-related gene HMG–box 3; SOX9, SRY-related gene HMG–box 9; SRY, sex-determining region of the Y chromosome; WT1, Wilms' tumor–related gene 1.

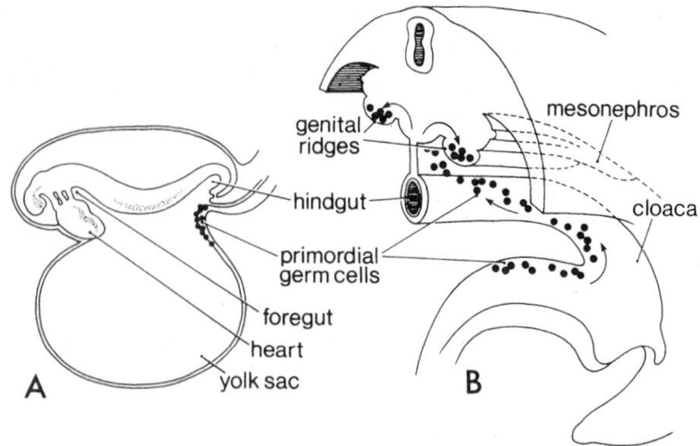

Figure 18–2. Germ cells. *A*, Schematic drawing of a 3-week-old embryo showing the site of origin of germ cells in the wall of the yolk sac. *B*, Migration path of primordial germ cells along the wall of the yolk sac and along the dorsal mesentery into the genital ridge. (From George FW, Wilson JD. Embryology of the genital tract. In Walsh PC, Gittes RF, Perlmutter AD, et al [eds]. Campbell's Urology, 5th ed. Philadelphia, WB Saunders, 1986, pp 1804–1818.)

Fig. 18–2*B*). The forces that control the migration are unknown, but the germ cells replicate during migration so that more cells reach the genital ridge than were present in the yolk sac.[9] On reaching the genital ridge the germ cells, together with adhering epithelial cells, infiltrate the underlying mesenchyme. This process is identical in male and female embryos and culminates by 5 to 6 weeks of gestation in the formation of the genital blastema containing the three basic cell types. Primordial germ cells that fail to reach the genital ridge degenerate or differentiate into other cell types and may serve as the progenitors of extragonadal germ cell tumors in later life.[10]

Sexual dimorphism of the gonad begins between 6 and 7 weeks of gestation with the development of seminiferous cords in the fetal testis. By contrast, histologic differentiation of the fetal ovary is not apparent until the sixth month of gestation, when granulosa cells organize around the dividing oocytes to form the primary ovarian follicle.[11] The somatic cells of the gonad can undergo partial organization into ovary or testis as specified by the sex chromosomes even if the germ cells are prevented from migrating to the genital ridge, suggesting that some determinants for gonadal development are inherent in the cells of the genital ridge.[12]

Testicular Descent

Histologic development of the testes is largely complete by the end of the third month of gestation, whereas testicular descent from the abdominal cavity to the scrotum occurs later[13] (Fig. 18–3). Between 10 and 15 weeks of human gestation, the testes remain anchored to the future inguinal canal by the caudal ligament of the testis, the gubernaculum, whereas the ovary moves cranially.[13] Simultaneously, the cranial suspensory ligament that anchors the testes to the posterior abdominal wall regresses. The gonadal positions in the two sexes deviate further after 25 weeks of gestation, when the gubernaculum descends into the scrotum and begins to degenerate as it is hollowed out by a diverticulum of the peritoneum, the processus vaginalis.

The actual descent of the testis through the processus vaginalis into the scrotum occurs as intra-abdominal pressure increases as a consequence of the closure of the umbilical cord, descent being completed between 7 months of gestation and shortly after birth. Continued development of the abdominal musculature causes closure of the inguinal rings and obliteration of the processus vaginalis. Conditions that impair development of intra-abdominal pressure, such as congenital defects in the abdominal musculature, are associated with cryptorchidism.[14]

The genetic and endocrine factors that control testicular

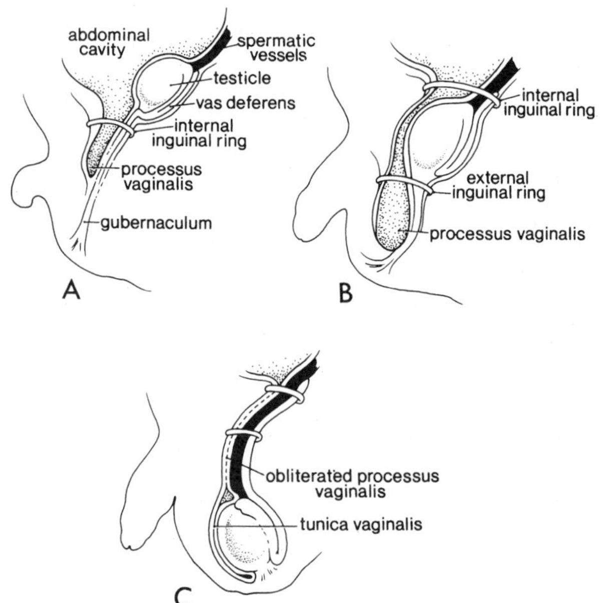

Figure 18–3. Descent of the testis. (From George FW, Wilson JD. Embryology of the genital tract. In Walsh PC, Gittes RF, Perlmutter AD, et al [eds]. Campbell's Urology, 5th ed. Philadelphia, WB Saunders, 1986, pp 1804–1818.)

descent are now understood in large part.[15] The role of *androgens* has been established by two types of evidence: (1) dihydrotestosterone promotes testicular descent in rats, and (2) the position of the testes in 46,XY subjects with mutations that impair the androgen receptor correlates with the severity of impairment of receptor function.[16] Thus, androgen action may involve the formation, enlargement, or degeneration of the processus vaginalis or the gubernaculum. Androgens may also enhance the release of calcitonin gene–related peptide, from the genitofemoral nerve, which in turn may promote descent.[13]

Antimüllerian hormone (AMH) (also called müllerian-inhibiting substance and müllerian duct inhibitor) may also play a role in testicular descent, possibly in the contraction of the gubernaculum. The testes in some men with persistent müllerian duct syndrome are located high in the retroperitoneal space[17, 18] as a result of impaired formation or action of AMH. The *INSL3 gene* (also designated Ley I-L and relaxin-like factor, *RLF*), a member of the insulin-like superfamily, controls development of the gubernaculum, and mice with targeted disruption of *INSL3* have bilateral cryptorchidism with freely moving intra-abdominal testes.[19, 20] Diethylstilbestrol-induced cryptorchidism in mice is also associated with failure of gubernaculum development and impairment of expression of *INSL3*.[21] A similar phenotype, namely long gubernacular cords and intra-abdominal testes, results from targeted disruption of the homeobox gene *HOXA-10*.[22]

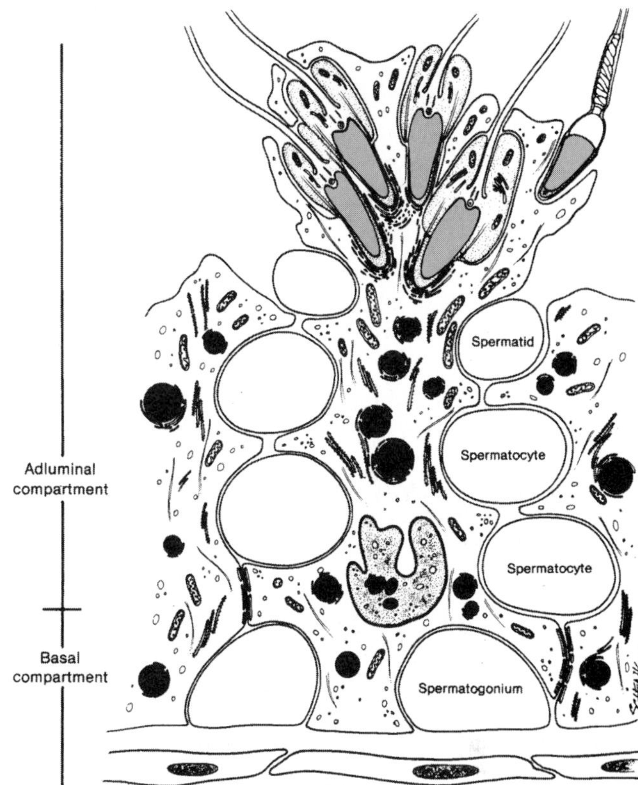

Figure 18–4. Diagram of the Sertoli cell showing the relation between Sertoli cell cytoplasm and developing spermatocytes.

STRUCTURAL ORGANIZATION OF THE TESTES

The testes contain a network of tubules for the production and transport of sperm to the excretory-ejaculatory ducts and a system of interstitial or Leydig cells that synthesize androgens.[23] The functional complexity of the tissue is illustrated in Figure 18–4. Spermatogenic tubules are composed of germ cells and Sertoli cells. Tight junctions between the Sertoli cells separate the spermatogonia from the primary spermatocytes and form a diffusion barrier that divides the testis into two functional compartments—*basal* and *adluminal*. The barrier between these two compartments has limited permeability to macromolecules, analogous to the blood-brain barrier and other epithelial barriers. The basal compartment consists of the Leydig cells, the boundary tissue of the tubule including peritubular myoid cells, and the outer layers of the spermatogenic tubules that contain the spermatogonia. The adluminal compartment consists of the inner two thirds of the tubules, including primary spermatocytes and cells in more advanced stages of spermatogenesis.

The structure and function of the Sertoli cell are closely linked (see Fig. 18–4).[23] The base of the cell is adjacent to the outer basement membrane of the spermatogenic tubule, whereas the inner portion consists of an arborized cytoplasm containing large gaps or lacunae, analogous to the branches of a tree. The mechanism by which the spermatogonia pass through the tight junctional complexes between the Sertoli cells as spermatogenesis commences is not known, but the arborized cytoplasm of the Sertoli cell encompasses the differentiating spermatocytes and spermatids so that spermatogenesis takes place within the Sertoli cell cytoplasm network. Sertoli cells synthesize hormones such as AMH, inhibin, activin, and prodynorphin as well as factors essential for spermatogenesis such as transferrin.[24]

The lipid droplets responsible for the foamy appearance of Leydig cell cytoplasm are composed largely of esterified cholesterol, derived in part from circulating lipoproteins and in part from locally synthesized cholesterol.[25] The esterified cholesterol serves as a reservoir of substrate for testosterone synthesis. After hydrolysis of cholesterol ester, free cholesterol moves to mitochondria under the control of the *steroidogenic acute regulatory (StAR) protein*, where the initial reaction in testosterone biosynthesis takes place, namely side-chain cleavage of cholesterol to pregnenolone.[26] Pregnenolone in turn is converted to testosterone in the endoplasmic reticulum. The amount of testosterone stored in the Leydig cell is small because newly synthesized testosterone diffuses promptly into the testicular venous blood.[27]

PHYSIOLOGY OF TESTICULAR FUNCTION

Hypothalamic-Pituitary-Testicular Axis

Hypothalamic Hormones

The hypothalamus is connected to the pituitary gland both by a portal vascular system and by neural pathways (Fig. 18–5). The portal vascular system provides a mechanism for the delivery of releasing hormones from the brain to the pituitary gland, the major system by which the brain controls anterior pituitary function. Reverse flow through this hypophyseal-portal circulation may also allow pituitary hormones to reach the brain by a more direct path than through the general circulation.[28] The preoptic area and the medial basal region of the hypothalamus (particularly the arcuate nucleus) contain important centers for control of gonadotropin secretion. Peptidergic neurons in this region secrete gonadotropin-releasing hormone (GnRH), also called luteinizing hormone–releasing

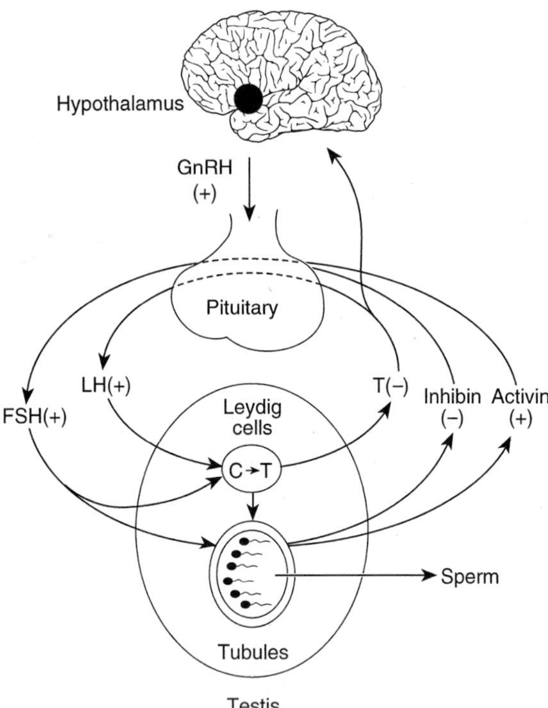

Figure 18–5. The hypothalamic-pituitary-testicular axis. C, cholesterol; FSH, follicle-stimulating hormone; GnRH, gonadotropin-releasing hormone; LH, luteinizing hormone; T, testosterone. (From Griffin JE, Wilson JD. Disorders of the testes. In Braunwald E, Fauci AS, Kasper DL, et al [eds]. Harrison's Principles of Internal Medicine, 15th ed. New York, McGraw-Hill, 2001, pp 2143–2154.)

hormone (LHRH), in a pulsatile fashion.[29] Neurons from other regions of the brain terminate in this area and influence both the frequency and the amplitude of GnRH secretory pulses through catecholamine-related, dopamine-related, and endorphin-related mechanisms.

GnRH is a decapeptide that is widely distributed in the central nervous system (CNS) and other tissues. However, a physiologic role has not been established for the hormone in sites other than the pituitary. The metabolic clearance rate of GnRH averages about 800 L/m^2 body surface area per day.[30] Increased excretion in urine of immunoreactive GnRH metabolites coincides with pubertal development in boys, and in adult men GnRH levels in urine correlate with those of luteinizing hormone (LH) and follicle-stimulating hormone (FSH).[31]

Pituitary Hormones

LH and FSH are the primary pituitary hormones that regulate testicular function. These hormones were named on the basis of their ovarian effects before their roles in testicular function were recognized. LH and FSH are secreted by the same basophilic cells in the pituitary. Like thyrotropin (or thyroid-stimulating hormone) and human chorionic gonadotropin (hCG), LH and FSH are glycoproteins composed of two polypeptide chains designated α and β. The α subunits of the four hormones are identical; the individual immunologic and functional characteristics of the hormones are determined by unique β subunits.[32] Both subunits are required for full biologic activity.

The structures of the β subunits of LH and hCG are similar except that the carboxyl end of hCGβ contains an additional 30 amino acids and additional carbohydrate residues. The disappearance of exogenous LH from blood is described by two linear exponentials with half-times of 40 and 120 minutes, and the metabolic clearance rate is approximately 25 mL/minute.[33] Only a small fraction of secreted LH appears in the urine. Because of the increased glycosylation of hCG, its half-life is longer.[34] The turnover of FSH is also slower, the metabolic clearance rate being about 14 mL/minute,[35] and the disappearance of FSH from blood is described by two exponentials with half-times of 4 and 70 hours, respectively.[36]

Mechanism of Action of Gonadotropin-Releasing Hormone and Gonadotropins

GnRH interacts with high-affinity cell-surface receptors coupled to G proteins on the plasma membrane of pituitary gonadotrophs. The acute administration of GnRH stimulates the release of both LH and FSH by a mechanism involving calcium or phosphoinositides as second messengers.[37] GnRH probably also acts long-term to enhance gonadotropin synthesis. The amounts of LH and FSH released in response to GnRH depend on age and hormonal status. In monkeys, the gonadotroph response to GnRH reaches a peak in the first few months of life and then declines and remains low until the onset of puberty, when it again increases to attain an adult response.[38] Before puberty, the secretion of FSH in response to GnRH is greater than that of LH. Slow-frequency GnRH pulses favor FSH secretion, whereas frequent pulses favor LH secretion.[39] In some species, GnRH effects can be demonstrated in testes, but GnRH does not appear to have a direct effect on the human Leydig cell.[40]

The LH receptor on the plasma membrane of Leydig cells is a member of the superfamily of G protein–coupled, seven-transmembrane domain receptors.[41] The binding of LH to the receptor activates signal transduction by both the adenylate cyclase–cyclic adenosine monophosphate (cAMP) and phospholipase C–inositol 1,4,5-triphosphate systems (see Chapter 5). The intracellular loops of the receptor form contact sites for interaction with G proteins. In the testis, receptor activation is coupled primarily to G_s proteins, leading to stimulation of adenylate cyclase and formation of cAMP, which binds to the regulatory subunit of a protein kinase and causes dissociation of the regulatory subunit and activation of the catalytic subunit. The activated protein kinase operates through unidentified steps to stimulate the synthesis of the enzymes of testosterone biosynthesis.[42] The signal is terminated by endocytosis and degradation of the LH-receptor complex.[43]

In the intact testis and in cultured Leydig cells, the number of LH receptors decreases after administration of LH or hCG.[43] The loss in receptor number is dose-dependent, reaches a nadir 24 hours after LH administration, is associated with a decrease in LH receptor messenger ribonucleic acid (mRNA), and returns to control levels within several days.[43] This down-regulation of receptor number is associated with decreased responsiveness (desensitization) to subsequent LH administration. Desensitization cannot be solely the result of the decrease in receptor number and appears to result in part from inhibition of some postreceptor event because cAMP is ineffective in reversing desensitization.[44] Whatever the mechanism, the diminished response of the Leydig cell to LH after administration of LH is a critical component of the regulation of testosterone production.

The primary site of action of FSH is the basal aspect of the plasma membrane of Sertoli cells, where the hormone binds to the FSH receptor, also a member of the G protein–coupled, seven-transmembrane domain receptor family.[45] The second messenger is cAMP, which is also linked to the activation of protein kinase and stimulation of the synthesis of proteins such as androgen-binding protein and the aromatase that converts testosterone to estradiol.[46] The precise role of FSH in the control of spermatogenesis remains uncertain and may vary among species (see later).

FSH plays an indirect role in androgen biosynthesis by inducing maturation of Leydig cells during development, possibly a consequence of the release of a paracrine factor by Sertoli cells,[47] but FSH does not play a major role in the control of Leydig cell function in adults.[48] Like LH and other peptide hormones, FSH regulates the number of its own receptors, but the physiologic significance of this phenomenon is unclear.

Regulation of Secretion of Gonadotropin-Releasing Hormone and Gonadotropins

Episodic secretion of GnRH into the hypophyseal-portal system[49] causes episodic secretion of both immunoreactive and bioactive LH.[50] In adult men, LH secretory pulses occur at a frequency of 8 to 14 per 24 hours and vary in magnitude. Pulsatile secretion of FSH is temporally coupled to that of LH but is lower in amplitude.[51]

LH secretion is under negative-feedback control by gonadal steroids at the level of the hypothalamus and the pituitary gland (see Fig. 18–5). Both testosterone and estradiol can effect this inhibition. Testosterone can be converted to estradiol in the brain and pituitary gland, but the two hormones are thought to act independently in the CNS.[52–56] One major effect of androgen in the CNS is to slow the hypothalamic pulse generator and consequently decrease the frequency of LH pulsatile release.

Endogenous opiates have a role in the negative-feedback actions of androgen and estrogen on pulsatile LH secretion in men. Furthermore, in monkeys with hypothalamic lesions that abolished endogenous GnRH release and in whom normal pulsatile secretion of LH was mimicked by chronic intermittent intravenous GnRH administration, bilateral orchidectomy caused minor elevations of plasma LH levels, whereas castration of monkeys with an intact hypothalamus given similar pulses of GnRH was followed by a marked rise in LH levels, indicating that LH is controlled by the negative feedback of gonadal steroids at the hypothalamic level.[57] Acute infusions of estradiol also lowered LH levels associated with an increased frequency and a decreased amplitude of the LH pulses.[52]

The fact that dihydrotestosterone, which cannot be converted to estrogen, exerts a negative-feedback control on LH secretion indicates that testosterone does not require aromatization to inhibit LH secretion.[52] Testosterone also appears to have a negative-feedback action on LH secretion directly at the pituitary level because administration of exogenous testosterone to GnRH-deficient men who were given pulsatile LHRH infusions caused a decrease in mean plasma LH levels and in LH pulse amplitude.[58] Hyperprolactinemia suppressed LH secretion, probably by inhibiting the pulsatile secretion of GnRH.[59]

The negative-feedback control of FSH secretion involves peptide and steroid hormones from the testes. Serum FSH concentrations increase in proportion to the loss of germinal elements in the testis, whereas LH levels change little. *Inhibin*, a peptide secreted by Sertoli cells that inhibits pituitary FSH secretion, is a heterodimer consisting of a 20-kd α subunit and a 15-kd β subunit. The β subunit occurs in two forms, so that there are two inhibins—*inhibin A* and *inhibin B*—each 31 kd in size. Inhibin B is thought to be the physiologically important hormone in men.[60] FSH stimulates inhibin production, and both FSH and androgen are involved in normal inhibin production.[61] Dimers of the β subunit of inhibin (termed *activin*) stimulate FSH release, and the pituitary protein *follistatin* binds and inactivates activin.

Testosterone and estradiol also influence FSH secretion.[62] In castrated rats treated with subphysiologic amounts of testosterone but physiologic amounts of estradiol, plasma FSH levels increase to the castration range but LH concentrations are normal. Indeed, alterations in the ratio of testosterone to estradiol can alter plasma FSH levels.[62] In addition, varying the pattern of GnRH administration to hypogonadotropic men so that the same total dose was administered but with less frequent pulses caused selective increases in FSH levels.[63]

In the rhesus monkey with a hypophyseotropic clamp, administration of inhibin maintained FSH levels in the precastration range when episodic gonadotropin secretion was maintained by intermittent GnRH infusion.[64] Thus, the suppression of FSH secretion by inhibin does not require the action of testosterone and must take place at the level of the pituitary gland.

Androgen Physiology

Testosterone Synthesis and Secretion

The pathways of testosterone synthesis are illustrated in Figures 18–6 and 18–7. As stated earlier, the precursor steroid cholesterol can either be synthesized de novo or derived from the plasma pool by receptor-mediated endocytosis of low-density lipoprotein (LDL), and both sources are important in the human Leydig cell.[65]

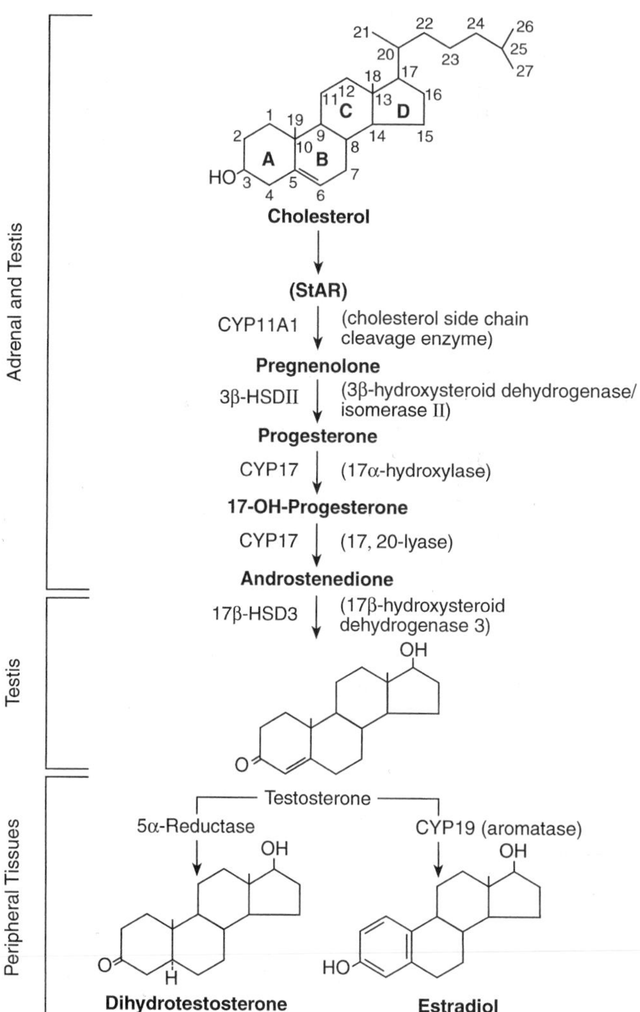

Figure 18–6. Pathway of testosterone formation in the testis and the conversion of testosterone to active metabolites in peripheral tissues. StAR, steroidogenic acute regulatory protein. (Revised from Griffin JE, Wilson JD. Disorders of the testes. In Braunwald E, Fauci AS, Kasper DL, et al [eds]. Harrison's Principles of Internal Medicine, 15th ed. New York, McGraw-Hill, 2001, pp 2143–2154.)

The hormonal requirements for the initiation of spermatogenesis in maturing animals differ from those for maintenance in adults or for reinitiation after hypophysectomy. After hypophysectomy in the adult male, spermatogenesis can be restored by treatment with FSH (human menopausal gonadotropin [hMG]) plus hCG. After spermatogenesis is restored, it can usually be maintained by hCG treatment alone.[151] The latter phenomenon, together with the finding that in otherwise normal subjects with suppressed FSH activity spermatogenesis can be restored by LH alone,[155] suggests that FSH is essential for initiation but not maintenance of spermatogenesis. However, FSH may be necessary for quantitatively normal sperm production in men,[156] and a hypophysectomized man with an activating mutation of the FSH receptor had sustained spermatogenesis.[157]

Fertilization

Fertilization normally takes place within the fallopian tube, and spermatozoa usually require a period in the female genital tract before they can fertilize. This functional change, termed *capacitation*, is believed to consist of at least two components: (1) enhancement of the rate of flagellar beat with acceleration of sperm movement and (2) development of the capacity to undergo an acrosome reaction and consequently allow the plasma membrane of the sperm to fuse with the ovum.[158]

The time required for optimal capacitation of normal sperm can vary from 2 hours to more than 6 hours.[159] Whether capacitation is an absolute requirement in the human or serves only to enhance fertilizing capabilities is not known. Because fertilization can take place in vitro when sperm and eggs are combined with no preincubation, the minimal time required for some spermatozoa to undergo capacitation must be short.[159]

Capacitation appears to involve a change in the intracellular concentration or metabolism of calcium or cAMP.[160] The acrosome reaction may also involve calcium.[158] Neither the fallopian tube nor the egg itself appears to be essential for the acrosome reaction, which begins as a fusion between the acrosomal membrane and the overlying plasmalemma and is followed by calcium influx into the sperm. Subsequently, the acrosome fragments and disappears. The acrosome is derived from lysosomes, and its disintegration causes release of hydrolytic enzymes and proteases.

The fact that the acrosome reaction is followed within a few hours by a loss of sperm motility means that variability in the timing of capacitation in a sperm population relative to the moment of insemination increases the chance of successful fertilization. Ordinarily, about a fifth of motile spermatozoa recovered from the oviduct at variable times after insemination have undergone the reaction. The net effect of the enhanced motility and the acrosome reaction is that sperm acquire the capacity to penetrate the formidable vestments of the ovum.[158]

One consequence of the sequential acceleration of motility and initiation of the acrosome reaction is that sperm transport to the site of fertilization in the fallopian tube is a culling process. Only a small number of the millions of sperm that are ejaculated reach the site of fertilization. The features that distinguish spermatozoa that reach the ampulla and fertilize the egg are not known, but these sperm are presumed to exhibit the fastest motility and the most delayed initiation of the acrosome reaction.

Understanding of the mechanism of sperm penetration is based largely on studies of fertilization of human eggs in vitro, a situation that may not be identical to the phenomenon in intact humans.[161] Ovulated eggs are surrounded by layers of cumulus cells embedded in a matrix of hyaluronic acid. The mechanism by which spermatozoa tunnel through the cumulus is not known. Possibly, hyaluronidase is released by the degenerating acrosome, and the mechanical agitation of the flagellum may disperse the cumulus cells. Under in vitro conditions, prior disposal of the cumulus with hyaluronidase is necessary to allow penetration of the zona pellucida and hence to permit fertilization by the sperm.

Phases of Normal Testicular Function

The phases of normal testicular function can be delineated in terms of the plasma testosterone concentration (Fig. 18–14). In the male embryo, the production of testosterone by the testes begins to rise at the end of the second month of gestation and shortly thereafter reaches a maximal value that is maintained until late in gestation and then decreases.[162, 163] At the time of birth, the plasma testosterone level is only slightly higher in males than in females.[164, 165] Shortly afterward, the plasma testosterone level again commences to rise in the male infant and remains elevated for approximately 3 months, falling to low levels by 1 year.[164, 165] The plasma level then remains low (but higher in boys than in girls) until the onset of puberty, when it again increases in boys and reaches adult levels by about age 17.[166]

Plasma levels remain more or less constant in the adult until middle age and then gradually decline during the later decades of life.[167, 168] Sperm production takes place after puberty. The physiologic events during these various periods differ, as do

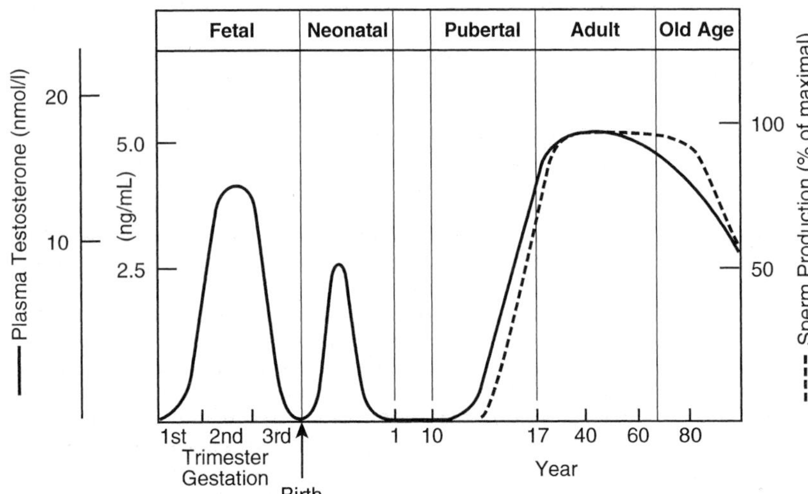

Figure 18–14. Schematic diagram of the different phases of male sexual function during life as indicated by mean plasma testosterone level and sperm production at different ages. (From Griffin JE, Wilson JD. The testis. In Bondy PK, Rosenberg LE [eds]. Metabolic Control and Disease, 8th ed. Philadelphia, WB Saunders, 1980, pp 1535–1578.)

the consequences of testicular derangements at different stages of life.

Embryonic Male Sexual Differentiation

The process of sexual differentiation is described in Chapter 22. In brief, the embryos of both sexes develop in an identical fashion until the seventh week of gestation. Thereafter, the anatomic development and the physiologic development diverge, with formation of the male or female phenotypes.

As formulated by Jost,[169] normal sexual development in the mammalian embryo depends on three sequential processes. The first involves the establishment of genetic sex, which is defined by the sex chromosome constitution established at the time of conception. The heterogametic sex (XY) in mammals is male, whereas the homogametic sex (XX) is female. In the second phase, the sex chromosomes determine whether the indifferent gonad differentiates into a testis in the male or an ovary in the female. The third step involves the translation of gonadal sex into phenotypic sex and is the direct consequence of the type of gonad formed; that is, testicular secretions determine that the urogenital tract and external genitalia will be male in character.

The internal genitalia in the two sexes are derived from the wolffian and müllerian ducts that exist side by side in early embryos of both sexes.[170] The wolffian ducts serve as the excretory ducts of the mesonephric kidney and are physically attached to the indifferent gonad, whereas the müllerian duct has no continuity with the gonad. In the male, the wolffian ducts give rise to the epididymis, vasa deferentia, seminal vesicles, and ejaculatory ducts and the müllerian ducts disappear. In the female, the fallopian tubes, uterus, and upper vagina are derived from the müllerian ducts and the wolffian ducts disappear.

The external genitalia and the urethra in the two sexes develop from common anlagen: the urogenital sinus and the genital tubercle, folds, and swelling. The urogenital sinus gives rise to the prostate and prostatic urethra in the male and to the lower portion of the vagina and urethra in the female. The genital tubercle becomes the glans penis in the male and the clitoris in the female. The urogenital swelling becomes the scrotum or the labia majora, and the genital folds develop into the shaft of the penis or the labia minora.

In the absence of the testis, as in the normal female or in the male embryo castrated before the onset of phenotypic differentiation, the development of phenotypic sex proceeds along female lines.[169] Thus, masculinization of the fetus requires the action of testicular hormones, whereas the female phenotype develops in the absence of gonadal secretions. Under ordinary circumstances, chromosomal sex, gonadal sex, and phenotypic sex are concordant; that is, chromosomal sex determines gonadal sex and gonadal sex in turn determines phenotypic sex, without deviation from the chromosomal program.

Control over the formation of the male phenotype is vested in the action of three hormones.[170] Two of the three, AMH and testosterone, are secretory products of the fetal testis. AMH, a glycoprotein hormone of the embryonic testis, acts ipsilaterally in the male embryo to suppress the müllerian ducts and consequently prevents development of the uterus and fallopian tubes.[171] Testosterone converts the wolffian ducts into the epididymides, vasa deferentia, and seminal vesicles and is also the precursor for the third fetal hormone, dihydrotestosterone.[170] The latter hormone, which is formed within the urogenital sinus and lower urogenital tract from circulating testosterone, acts in the urogenital sinus to induce formation of the male urethra and prostate and in the genital tubercle, swelling, and folds to cause the midline fusion, elongation, and enlargement that eventuate in the male external genitalia.[172]

Thus, androgens function during fetal life to induce the formation of the accessory organs of male reproduction. Testosterone and dihydrotestosterone act through the same receptor mechanism during embryogenesis and in the adult[172] (see Fig. 18–10). The formation of the male phenotype is largely completed by 12 to 15 weeks of gestation, but at the time of completion of the male urethra, the external genitalia in the two sexes do not differ in size.[170] Descent of the testes and differential growth of the external genitalia in the male take place largely during the second half of gestation.

The control of testosterone formation by the embryonic testis is incompletely understood. By the 13th week of human gestation, testosterone secretion appears to be regulated by LH from the fetal pituitary gland or by placental hCG in the fetal circulation, or by both.[173] The decrease in testosterone synthesis late in gestation correlates both with a decline in the number of LH-hCG receptors in the testis[174] and with a decrease in the level of hCG and LH in the fetal circulation.[173] Castration of the male rhesus monkey during late gestation results in a further decrease in plasma testosterone and elevation of plasma gonadotropins.[175] Anencephaly and other forms of congenital hypopituitarism cause the syndrome of microphallus.[176] Taken together, these findings indicate that testosterone production during the second half of gestation is regulated by LH or hCG and that LH production itself is under negative-feedback control by testosterone.

The mechanism by which testosterone production is controlled between gestational weeks 8 and 12, when male phenotypic development takes place in the human embryo, is not clear. In the rabbit embryo, testosterone production during the analogous phase of male development appears to be independent of gonadotropin, but for technical reasons this phase of embryonic development in human gestation has not been adequately examined. The fact that most male infants with anencephaly, congenital hypopituitarism, or both have normal male urethras suggests either that androgen synthesis during early gestation is independent of gonadotropins or that chorionic gonadotropin, which apparently is not present in the rabbit, acts as a fail-safe mechanism to guarantee normal male development in the absence of LH from the fetal pituitary gland.[176] However, the fact that loss-of-function mutations of the LH receptor gene cause impairment of the virilization of the male external genitalia (but not of the wolffian ducts) indicates that LH or hCG plays a role in early androgen synthesis.[177]

In addition to their role in male phenotypic development, androgens secreted during fetal or neonatal life (or both) exert at least two types of effects on the CNS in some species: regulation of the hypothalamic-pituitary system and control of diverse sexually dimorphic behavior patterns.[178] Androgens are presumed to act in brain through the same receptor as in the urogenital tract and other androgen target tissues. Social imprinting also plays a critical role in sex-specific behavior in some species. Male sexual development, apart from spermatogenesis, is remarkably complete during embryogenesis. For example, male infants have periodic erections during the later phases of gestation, which indicates that the complex neurogenic pathways that regulate this process have developed by that time.

The extent to which androgen action in the human CNS influences human sexual behavior has not been established. There is no evidence for permanent imprinting by fetal androgens on the hypothalamic control of gonadotropin production in the human, and it is not established whether gonadal hormones have any direct effect on gender identity or gender behavior apart from their role in anatomic development of the sexual phenotype. Nevertheless, both androgens and cultural factors probably play important roles in the development of characteristic male behavior.[178] Therefore, in making clinical decisions about sex assignment in subjects with ambiguous genitalia, it is important to undertake a thorough diagnostic evaluation and appropriate therapeutic intervention as early as possible, preferably in the newborn nursery, to ensure that the culture of peripheral blood leukocytes or of tissue fibroblasts in medium containing an agent such as phytohemagglutinin that induces the cells to divide. A spindle poison such as colchicine, which arrests mitosis at metaphase, is added; the cells are harvested and stained; and the number and histologic characteristics of the chromosomes are assessed in several cells. This technique is valuable for establishing the exact chromosome complement, the presence of mosaicism, the presence of structural chromosome alterations, and the sex chromosome composition. The study of multiple tissues may be necessary to establish chromosome mosaicism. In a given tissue, 20 cells must be examined to exclude with 95% confidence a mosaicism of 15% or greater.

Estrogenic Function

History and Physical Examination

Gynecomastia (enlargement of the male breast), the most consistent feature of feminizing states in men, is the consequence of proliferation of glandular tissue. The physician should seek the presence of gynecomastia by examining the patient while he is in the sitting position; the fingers are used to grasp the glandular tissue. Palpation with the flat part of the hand while the patient is supine may result in failure to detect early or minimal breast enlargement. In obese men, it is important to try to detect the edge of the rim of glandular tissue that separates it from the adipose tissue of the chest wall. Ultrasonography or mammography may be useful in separating true gynecomastia from lipomastia.

Plasma Estrogens

As discussed earlier, most estradiol and estrone in normal men are formed by extraglandular aromatization of circulating androgens. As assessed by immunoassay, plasma estradiol is usually less than 180 pmol/L (50 pg/mL) in normal men and plasma estrone is somewhat higher but usually less than 300 pmol/L (80 pg/mL). A recombinant cell bioassay has been developed to measure estradiol at low levels.[244]

ABNORMALITIES OF ANDROGEN METABOLISM AND TESTICULAR FUNCTION

Abnormalities of testicular function have different consequences, depending on the phase of sexual life in which they are first manifested. Although there are problems inherent in all classifications and although some assignments are arbitrary, such a categorization of testicular diseases has a sound physiologic rationale. For example, although Klinefelter's syndrome is a disorder of chromosomal sex, it is usually diagnosed in individuals when manifestations become apparent after the time of expected puberty. Although such limitations must be recognized, disorders of the testes can be classified as abnormalities of fetal development, puberty, adult life, and senescence.

Fetal Life

Abnormalities of Male Sexual Differentiation

Disturbances in sexual differentiation can arise from a variety of mechanisms:

1. Environmental insult, as in the ingestion of a virilizing drug during pregnancy.
2. Nonfamilial aberrations of the sex chromosomes, as in 45,X/46,XY chromosomal mosaicism.
3. Developmental birth defects of multifactorial origin, as in most cases of hypospadias.
4. Hereditary disorders resulting from single-gene mutations, as in the testicular feminization syndrome.

The disorders of sexual differentiation and their management are described in Chapter 22, but because 46,XX men and men with Klinefelter's syndrome ordinarily present with problems of undervirilization or infertility, they are also discussed in this chapter.

Cryptorchidism

Descent of the testes is essential to normal function because spermatogenesis requires the lower temperature that is present in the scrotum. Failure can occur at any site in the normal pathway of descent, from high in the abdomen to the scrotum itself. The implications and sequelae of cryptorchidism differ, depending on the site at which descent ceases.[245] A large portion of the literature in this field is difficult to interpret because of imprecise definitions. Cryptorchidism can be defined as a testis that is not 4 cm or more below the pubic tubercle in an infant of normal size and subclassified, depending on the location of the maldescended testis, as follows:

1. The *intra-abdominal testis* (10%) cannot be felt. It is usually located just above the internal inguinal ring. Infants with bilateral intra-abdominal testes can be distinguished from female pseudohermaphrodites by assessment of the chromosomal karyotype and from boys with bilateral anorchia by demonstrating that the plasma testosterone level increases after administration of hCG. Unilateral intra-abdominal testes must be separated from the syndrome of mixed gonadal dysgenesis, in which a testis is present on one side and an intra-abdominal streak gonad is present on the other.
2. The *canalicular testis* (20%) has traversed the internal inguinal ring and is present in the inguinal canal; it may move intermittently between the canal and the upper scrotum. Such testes are small or would not be able to pass the external inguinal ring. When the testis is in the canal, the aponeurosis of the external oblique muscle forms such a firm barrier that the testis can rarely be palpated.
3. The *high scrotal testis* (40%) is farther along the pathway of descent but does not reach the bottom of the scrotum. It is characteristically smaller than its normal partner and has a limited range of motion so that it can retract into the groin but not past the internal ring. Retraction may make accurate diagnosis and classification difficult.
4. The *obstructed testis* (30%) is a fourth category in which failure of descent appears to be due to a physical barrier formed by a cord of fascia between the inguinal pouch and the inlet of the scrotum.

Another category is the *ectopic testis*. On rare occasions, the testis may deviate from its normal pathway of descent and become ectopic in location.[246] The five most frequent sites of ectopia are the perineum, the femoral canal, the superficial inguinal pouch, the suprapubic area, and the opposite scrotum. Testicular ectopia is believed to be caused by an abnormality of the gubernaculum.[247] In most situations, the higher the location of the testis or the more extreme the ectopia, the more difficult surgical repair becomes.

About 3% of full-term male infants have at least one cryptorchid testis at birth. Completion of descent usually occurs during the first few weeks after birth so that the incidence of cryptorchidism at 6 to 9 months and in adult men is about

0.7% to 0.8%. Accurate diagnosis and classification may require careful, repeated observations by a single observer to be certain that a normally (or partially) descended testis has not retracted into the groin. The concept that spontaneous descent can occur after a few months of age is a misconception that arose because of the failure to recognize that many normal testes are retractile in young boys and that elicitation of the cremasteric reflex can cause at least partial retraction of fully descended testes in three fourths of boys. The incidence of retraction declines with age, and it rarely occurs after midpuberty.

It is important to appreciate that a testis in the superficial inguinal pouch may be a temporarily retracted normal testis, a temporarily retracted high scrotal testis, a transiently palpable canalicular testis, or an obstructed testis and that differentiation among these possibilities is not always simple.

Pathogenesis

The cause of testicular maldescent is not well understood. The cryptorchid testis functions poorly in regard to both androgen secretion and spermatogenesis, but it is not always clear whether the testis functions poorly because of maldescent or fails to descend completely because it was abnormal to begin with. Maldescent of the testis occurs with increased frequency in many congenital defects, including virtually all disorders that impair virilization or prevent development of normal intra-abdominal pressure. Although maldescent is common in individuals with severe impairment of the androgen receptor, mutations of the androgen receptor gene are rare in boys with isolated cryptorchidism.[248] Likewise, defects of the gubernaculum are common in cryptorchid testes,[249] but mutations of the *INSL 3* gene have not been detected in men with idiopathic cryptorchidism.[250]

In some instances, a clear relation exists between maldescent and malfunction of the testis. For example, in the obstructed testis, in which a physical barrier prevents descent,[247] and in syndromes in which intra-abdominal pressure is inadequate because the abdominal muscles are absent or incomplete, such as the prune-belly syndrome,[14] inadequate testicular function in later life is the consequence of impeded descent. Conversely, in all series testes appear to have been abnormal from the first, and it is reasonable to assume that the defect in these instances plays a causal role in the maldescent.

As many as half of boys with a unilateral nonpalpable testis and a contralateral descended testis have an absent *(vanishing)* testis rather than a cryptorchid testis.[251] The diagnosis of vanishing testis is suggested when compensatory testicular hypertrophy causes the contralateral descended testis to be larger than the mean for the age.[252] Cryptorchid testes can sometimes be identified by magnetic resonance imaging or ultrasonography[246] but definitive diagnosis may require laparoscopy.[253]

Sequelae

About 10% of testicular tumors arise in an undescended testis, whereas cryptorchidism is present in fewer than 1% of adult men.[247] Thus, malignancy is more likely to develop in an undescended testis than in a fully descended one. The greatest risk of malignancy is associated with intra-abdominal testes. Such malignancies commonly involve the germ cells, most commonly seminomas or embryonal cell carcinomas. Surgical correction of cryptorchidism does not remove this risk because malignancy may develop in a previously cryptorchid testis many years after orchiopexy. Moreover, the contralateral normally descended scrotal testis is the site of development of malignancy in approximately a fifth of tumors associated with unilateral cryptorchidism.

The frequency of malignancy in cryptorchid testes should not be exaggerated because the chance of tumor development in any individual with cryptorchidism is low, but lifelong follow-up is required. Each cryptorchid testis should be surgically placed in a site that allows ready examination, and if this is not possible the cryptorchid testis should be removed. Periodic examination of the testes should be mandatory in the routine care of men with a history of cryptorchidism.[247] In unilateral cryptorchidism, regardless of whether surgical correction has been undertaken, overall androgen production and levels are generally normal, presumably because malfunction of one testis can be compensated by the other testis.[254]

Although as many as 60% of men in whom bilateral cryptorchidism was corrected in childhood can father children,[255] cryptorchidism is associated with defective spermatogenesis. Mean sperm density is lower in adult men after surgical repair of cryptorchid testes in childhood,[254] and spermatogenesis can also be decreased in the normally descended testis in men in whom one testis is cryptorchid. Basal FSH levels and FSH responsiveness to GnRH are higher on average in such men.[254] Considered together, these types of evidence support the concept that testicular malfunction, as evidenced by impaired spermatogenesis, is a major factor in maldescent.

Management

Cryptorchidism should be treated by surgical or medical means, or both, and although correction may not prevent all sequelae, it is generally believed that correction should be undertaken before age 5 years. In the case of intra-abdominal testes (unilateral or bilateral), the issue is to exclude vanishing testes as the cause and bring intra-abdominal testes into the scrotum, where they can be monitored by physical examination. Measurement of levels of serum inhibin B[179] and AMH[256] may be useful in distinguishing bilateral intra-abdominal testes from vanishing testes. The testes that cannot be brought into the scrotum should be removed. Likewise, obstructed testes must be treated surgically.

The unresolved issue concerns the role of medical therapy in boys with canicular or high scrotal testes; in relatively large randomized trials, treatment of such boys with hCG, GnRH, or both agents in seriatim was said to cause descent of the testes into a normal position in about a fifth of cases.[257] However, the stimulation of apoptosis of germ cells by hCG and GnRH may have long-term deleterious consequences.[258–260] Apoptosis is increased 1 month after hCG treatment but returns to normal subsequently.[258] In one study, however, the level of apoptosis in the original testicular biopsy correlated many years later negatively with testis volume and positively with serum FSH levels, whereas sperm density was not affected.[259] Treatment of cryptorchid boys with GnRH or hCG before orchiopexy caused a similar decrease in germ cells per tubule.[260] Whether any hormonal treatment of cryptorchidism affects subsequent fertility is not known.

Neonatal Life

It is not clear whether abnormality in the neonatal surge in testosterone secretion results in pathologic consequences in humans. As mentioned earlier, however, temporary inhibition of the pituitary-testicular axis in the neonatal primate is associated with impaired testicular function at puberty.[181]

Puberty

The central issue in dealing with disorders of puberty in both sexes is separating subjects with true absence or precocity of pubertal development from those at the extreme limits of normal variation. Normal puberty in the male is variable in onset, duration, and sequence of events. The spectrum of normal puberty and the disorders of puberty are discussed in detail in Chapter 24. (Feminizing states in prepubertal and pubertal boys can result from either absolute or relative increases in estrogen levels, as discussed later.) However, partial impairments of puberty may not be recognized until adulthood, as in Klinefelter's syndrome (see Chapter 22), in some androgen resistance syndromes in men (see Chapter 22), and in isolated gonadotropin deficiency (see Chapter 24).

Adulthood

Adult abnormalities of testicular function can be due to hypothalamic-pituitary defects, testicular disorders, or abnormalities in sperm transport (Table 18–3). Most such abnormalities are associated with underandrogenization and infertility, but some exhibit isolated infertility. Even partial defects in Leydig cell function can cause infertility because spermatogenesis requires androgen action. Therefore, although the evaluation of infertility differs from that of the underandrogenized man, it is essential to exclude the presence of subtle Leydig cell dysfunction in every man with infertility.

Certain factors or conditions (e.g., hyperprolactinemia, radiation, cyclophosphamide administration, environmental toxins, autoimmunity, paraplegia, androgen resistance) can cause either isolated infertility or a combined defect in testicular function (see Table 18–3). In addition to the manifestations of androgen deficiency described earlier in relation to assessment of Leydig cell function, testosterone deficiency can cause osteoporosis[261, 262] and mild elevations of serum total and LDL cholesterol and triglyceride levels.[263]

Table 18–3. Adult Abnormalities of Testicular Function

Infertility with Undervirilization	Infertility with Normal Virilization
Hypothalamic-Pituitary	
Fasting, critical illness	Isolated FSH deficiency
Isolated gonadotropin deficiency	Congenital adrenal hyperplasia
Adrenal hypoplasia congenita	Androgen administration
GnRH receptor mutations	
LHβ/FSHβ mutations	
Cushing's syndrome	
Hyperprolactinemia	
Hemochromatosis	
Panhypopituitarism	
Testicular	
Developmental and structural defects	
LH receptor mutations	Germinal cell aplasia
Klinefelter's syndrome	AZF mutations of Y chromosome
XX male syndrome	FSH receptor mutations
	Cryptorchidism
	Varicocele
	Immotile cilia syndrome
Acquired defects	
Viral orchitis	*Mycoplasma* infections
Trauma	
Radiation	Radiation
Drugs (e.g., spironolactone, alcohol, ketoconazole, cyclophosphamide)	Drugs (e.g., cyclophosphamide, sulfasalazine)
Environmental toxins	Environmental toxins
Autoimmumity	Autoimmunity
Granulomatous disease	
Defects associated with systemic disease	
Liver disease	Febrile illness
Renal failure	Celiac disease
Sickle cell disease	
Immunologic disease (HIV, rheumatoid arthritis)	
Neurologic disease (myotonic dystrophy, paraplegia, spinobulbar muscular atrophy)	Neurologic disease (paraplegia)
Androgen resistance	
Undervirilized man	Infertile man
Sperm Transport	
	Obstruction of epididymis/vas deferens (cystic fibrosis, congenital absence, vasectomy, diethylstilbestrol exposure)

AZF, azoospermia factor; FSH, follicle-stimulating hormone; GnRH, gonadotropin-releasing hormone; HIV, human immunodeficiency virus.

Infertility with Impaired Virilization

Hypothalamic and Pituitary Disorders

Disorders of the hypothalamus and pituitary gland can impair secretion of gonadotropins and cause secondary decreases in androgen production and spermatogenesis, either as an isolated defect or as part of more complex pituitary insufficiency (see Chapter 8). Thus, destructive lesions of the hypothalamus and pituitary gland such as infarction, pituitary macroadenomas, metastatic or suprasellar tumors, infections, granulomatous processes, or radiation injury can cause *panhypopituitarism* and lead to a secondary testicular defect. Likewise, isolated, functional impairment of hypothalamic GnRH secretion can occur with fasting or critical illness.[264–266]

Congenital isolated gonadotropin deficiency occurs in both sporadic and familial forms.[267, 268] The incidence of the disorder is not established, but in most centers it is second only to Klinefelter's syndrome as a cause of hypogonadism in men. The disorder was originally described by Kallmann as a familial syndrome associated with anosmia and can be manifest in childhood as microphallus or cryptorchidism. Male urethral development is usually complete. Because most penile growth occurs during the latter two thirds of gestation, the presence of microphallus in this disorder has been interpreted as evidence for a role of pituitary gonadotropin in regulating testosterone production during the later portion of gestation. Growth in childhood is normal although bone age is usually retarded.

Most affected individuals are identified because of failure to undergo puberty. Some individuals, particularly familial cases, have associated defects such as cleft lip or palate, or both; hearing defect; colorblindness; and eye movement abnormalities.[269] Less severely affected individuals have only partial defects in the production of FSH or LH. A variant in which Leydig cell function is impaired despite testes of normal or near-normal size was originally known as the fertile eunuch syndrome, which is even harder to separate from delayed puberty than is the typical disorder.[270] Isolated gonadotropin deficiency of all types is less common in women than in men.[267]

The underlying defect is in the pulsatile release of gonadotropins.[267] The most common pattern is total absence of detectable LH pulses associated with profound impairment of pubertal maturation. Other individuals exhibit a developmental arrest pattern with nocturnal pulses similar to those of early puberty and some testicular growth. Alternatively, the defect appears to impair LH pulse amplitude or pulse frequency. Consequently, the disorder encompasses a spectrum of defects in LH secretion.

The underlying defect in most patients is at the hypothalamic level; short-term administration of GnRH causes an increase in plasma LH and FSH levels in about half of individuals, and GnRH treatment for 5 days or longer increases plasma gonadotropin levels to the normal range in most men with isolated gonadotropin deficiency but not in individuals with panhypopituitarism.[271] The more severe the deficiency, the longer GnRH must be administered to correct gonadotropin secretion.[272]

Isolated gonadotropin deficiency can be inherited as an autosomal dominant, autosomal recessive, or X-linked trait. The X-linked form with anosmia is the best characterized. The neurons that secrete GnRH originate in the olfactory placode of the fetus and migrate into the brain with the olfactory, terminalis, and vomeronasal nerves. A defect in the *KAL* gene in the X-linked disorder impairs the migration of these nerves and thus causes GnRH deficiency, the olfactory disturbance, and hypoplasia of the olfactory bulbs. The genetic locus has been assigned to Xp23.3, and the gene encodes a protein, anosmin, that has homology to neural cell adhesion molecules.[273] In a study of 104 individuals with isolated gonadotropin deficiency, Oliveira and colleagues[274] identified *KAL* mutations in 3 of 21 familial and in 4 of 39 sporadic cases but in no instance in the absence of anosmia and concluded that the majority of mutations do not involve *KAL*.

In the presence of olfactory disturbances, other midline defects, a positive family history, or a combination of these factors, the diagnosis of the *KAL* disorder is not difficult to establish either in an infant with microphallus or in an undervirilized adult. In men with anosmia or hyposomia, defects of the rhinencephalon may be demonstrated by magnetic resonance imaging.[267] In older individuals without midline abnormalities or anosmia and with uninformative family histories, the diagnosis can be made (after the presence of a pituitary tumor is excluded) by documenting a normal acute response to GnRH administration after a week of GnRH treatment. This approach is rarely followed in practice. In the middle teen years, separation of individuals with hypogonadotropic hypogonadism from those with delayed puberty may require prolonged observation (see Chapter 24).

Additional mutations that cause gonadotropin deficiency encompass a variety of different mechanisms. One involves a mutation on the X chromosome that causes the X-linked form of *adrenal hypoplasia congenita* in which adrenal insufficiency is associated with hypogonadotropic hypogonadism and which is due to mutations or deletions of the *DAX1* gene (see earlier), which encodes a member of the nuclear hormone receptor family of transcription regulatory factors that are expressed in the hypothalamus, pituitary gland, adrenal glands, and gonads.[268, 275] The fact that the response of LH to GnRH is variable suggests underlying defects in both the hypothalamus and pituitary gland.[276]

One individual with adrenal hypoplasia congenita virilized in response to hCG, but 3 years of combination therapy with hCG and hMG did not induce spermatogenesis.[277] The adrenal insufficiency is manifested during infancy, and the hypogonadotropic hypogonadism is recognized at the time of expected puberty, although rarely both may be incomplete or late in onset.[278]

Mutations in the *GnRH receptor* can cause an autosomal recessive form of congenital isolated gonadotropin deficiency unassociated with anosmia.[279] The phenotype is variable, even within a given family, with some patients having partial responses to GnRH and partial hypogonadism. One family exhibited a decrease in the amplitude of LH pulses.[279]

A functional form of hypogonadotropic hypogonadism has been described in a family with a mutation in the *LH β gene*.[280] The proband did not undergo spontaneous puberty and had low plasma testosterone and elevated immunoreactive LH levels, but testosterone levels increased after administration of exogenous LH and hCG. A missense mutation in the LH β gene impaired binding of LH to the LH receptor. Heterozygous male carriers for the mutation may have low testosterone levels and impaired fertility.

Similarly, a partial deletion of the coding sequence of the *FSH β gene* caused a truncation of the molecule and hypogonadism in one man.[281] Serum FSH was undetectable, and LH levels were elevated despite the low testosterone level, suggesting that the absence of FSH impaired Leydig cell function.

Hypogonadotropic hypogonadism also occurs in the *Prader-Willi syndrome* (obesity, short stature, mental retardation, and hypotonia) caused by partial deletions or uniparental disomy of chromosome 15.[282, 283]

Three forms of therapy have been used for hypogonadotropic hypogonadism:

1. Androgen replacement to virilize.
2. Gonadotropin therapy to induce fertility.
3. Intermittent administration of GnRH analogues (except in patients with mutations in the GnRH receptor gene).

In the infant or the young child with microphallus, administration of testosterone for limited periods (3 months) may cause enlargement of the penis to the normal range without affecting linear growth or causing other significant virilization.[284] In the older child or the adult, long-acting testosterone esters are administered parenterally, as with other forms of hypogonadism (see later). As in other forms of androgen deficiency, the closer to the time of onset of normal puberty that replacement therapy is begun, the more effective the promotion of normal virilization.

Administration of hCG over the long term also causes serum testosterone levels to increase to normal adult male levels.[285] In men with severe (prepubertal) hypogonadotropic hypogonadism, however, the induction of fertility usually requires the administration of FSH, in the form of human menopausal gonadotropin, in addition to hCG.[286] The response to gonadotropin therapy is not influenced by prior testosterone therapy but is a function of the initial testis size, men with testes less than 4 mL in volume responding less favorably.[287] Once a normal sperm count is achieved, it may be maintained by use of hCG or, occasionally, by testosterone esters. In rare cases of partial defects in gonadotropin secretion, spermatogenesis can be promoted by testosterone therapy alone.[267] The long-term administration of GnRH in a pulsatile manner to men with hypogonadotropic hypogonadism results in normal plasma testosterone levels, normal pulsatile secretion of LH, normal mean levels of plasma LH and FSH, and, in most, mature sperm in the ejaculate.[267]

Acquired isolated gonadotropin deficiency can be caused by pathologic states that impair the hypothalamus or pituitary secondarily. For example, elevated plasma cortisol levels, as in *Cushing's syndrome*, can depress LH secretion independently of a space-occupying lesion of the pituitary.[266] Likewise, chronic administration of exogenous glucocorticoids can lower testosterone levels by inhibiting GnRH secretion.[266]

Hyperprolactinemia associated with both pituitary microadenomas and macroadenomas also causes secondary testicular dysfunction. Macroadenomas may cause hyperprolactinemia either because of direct secretion by prolactinomas or because of interference with the delivery of inhibitory hormones from the hypothalamus to the pituitary gland by the mass effect of a nonsecretory tumor. Hypogonadism can result from hyperprolactinemia itself, destruction of the normal pituitary gland, or a combination of these effects. Prolactin excess by itself can cause underandrogenization, infertility, and impotence, probably by impairing GnRH release. Administration of low doses of bromocriptine to men with microadenomas caused an initial increase in plasma LH level and a subsequent increase in serum testosterone level.[288] The preferred treatment is bromocriptine or cabergoline (see Chapter 8).

Hemochromatosis causes iron deposition in the pituitary gland and testes, and about half of affected men have hypogonadism, usually accompanied by testicular atrophy. Abnormal testicular function in this disorder may result in part from the associated liver disease, but most testicular dysfunction is due to hypogonadotropic hypogonadism.[266] The pituitary nature of the hypogonadism was recognized because of the lack of response of LH to GnRH administration and the normal response of plasma testosterone to hCG. A primary testicular abnormality may also occur.[266] Acquired transfusional iron overload can cause similar abnormalities of the pituitary-testicular axis.[289] In both states, reduction of iron stores may result in recovery of gonadotropin secretion.

Hypothalamic or pituitary injury can occur after head trauma even in the absence of fracture, and the most common manifestation is deficiency of gonadotropins and human growth hormone, although multiple deficiencies can be present. Clinical evidence of hormone deficiency may be apparent immediately after injury or not until years later.[290]

In conditions in which testosterone levels are decreased despite normal LH levels, the mechanism is less clear. Men with massive obesity have decreased SHBG levels and decreased levels of total and bioavailable testosterone that return toward normal with weight loss.[291] For example, in men with a body mass index greater than 40, free testosterone levels, LH, and LH pulse amplitude are decreased, implying malfunction of the hypothalamic-pituitary system.[292] Obesity may be the cause of decreased testosterone levels in the pickwickian syndrome.[293] Men with temporal lobe seizures may also have hormonal findings consistent with hypogonadotropic hypogonadism.[294] Finally, acquired hypogonadotropic hypogonadism may be idiopathic.[295, 296]

Testicular Disorders

Abnormalities of testicular function in the adult can be grouped into developmental and structural defects of the testes, acquired testicular defects, abnormalities associated with systemic or neurologic diseases, and androgen resistance.

Developmental and Structural Defects

LH Receptor Mutations. Inactivating mutations *of the LH receptor gene* cause variable defects in testosterone formation.[297] The more severe defects in LH receptor function result in an autosomal recessive form of male pseudohermaphroditism in which 46,XY individuals have a female phenotype, a blind-ending vagina, and inguinal testes with absence of Leydig cells (Leydig cell hypoplasia) (see also Chapter 22). Less severe impairments of LH receptor function are associated with variable defects, including a male phenotype and microphallus. Testosterone levels are low in the presence of elevated gonadotropins. In most subjects, the phenotypic defects correlate with both the basal level of the LH receptor and the response of plasma testosterone to hCG,[298] but in one individual with a male phenotype associated with a deletion of exon 10 of the LH receptor gene, serum testosterone levels increased after treatment with hCG.[299]

Klinefelter's Syndrome. The most common developmental defect of the testis is *Klinefelter's syndrome* (see also Chapter 22).[300] The disorder is characterized by small, firm testes; various degrees of impaired sexual maturation; azoospermia; gynecomastia; and elevated gonadotropin levels. The underlying defect is the presence of an extra X chromosome, the usual chromosomal karyotype being either 47,XXY (classic form) or 46,XY/47,XXY (mosaic form). The incidence is approximately 1 in 500 males.

Table 18–4. Characteristics of Patients with Classic Versus Mosaic Klinefelter's Syndrome*

Characteristic	47,XXY (%)	47,XY/47,XXY (%)
Abnormal testicular histologic features	100	94†
Decreased length of testis	99	73†
Azoospermia	93	50†
Decreased testosterone level	79	33
Decreased facial hair	77	64†
Increased gonadotropin level	75	33
Decreased sexual function	68	56
Gynecomastia	55	33†
Decreased axillary hair	49	46
Decreased length of penis	41	21

*Table based on 519 47,XXY patients and 51 46,XY/47,XXY patients.
†Significantly different at $P < .05$ or better.
Data from Gordon DL, Krmpotic E, Thomas W, et al. Pathologic testicular findings in Klinefelter's syndrome. 47,XXY vs. 46,XY-47, XXY. Arch Intern Med 1972; 130:720–729.

Prepubertal boys with Klinefelter's syndrome have small testes with a decreased number of spermatogonia but are endocrinologically normal; the diagnosis at this age may be made on the basis of the cognitive features (see later). The diagnosis is usually made after the time of expected puberty because of gynecomastia or underandrogenization and later by infertility (Table 18–4). Damage to the seminiferous tubules and azoospermia are consistent features of the 47,XXY variety. The small, firm testes are usually less than 2 cm in length and less than 4 mL in volume. Histologic changes in the testes include hyalinization of the tubules, absence of spermatogenesis, and an apparent increase in the number of Leydig cells (see Fig. 18–17 *C*).

Mean body height is increased because of a longer lower body segment; the presence of this feature before puberty suggests that it is not secondary to androgen deficiency but is probably related to the underlying chromosomal abnormality. Gynecomastia occurs in about 85% of affected individuals, develops during adolescence, is usually bilateral and painless, and may become disfiguring.

Klinefelter's syndrome can cause learning disabilities and poor impulse control. These tendencies may explain the increased frequency of the disorder among men in mental and penal institutions. Indeed, although many men with the disorder have above average or superior intelligence, poor school performance is common, with decreased verbal scores and a higher incidence of dyslexia and attention-deficit disorder.[301]

The risk of breast cancer is increased, presumably because of the presence of gynecomastia,[302, 303] and there is an increased prevalence of extragonadal germ cell tumors in the mediastinum and brain.[304, 305] Autoimmune disorders appear to be more common, perhaps related to the altered levels of gonadal hormones.[300] Varicose veins, venous stasis ulcers, and thromboembolic disease are also more common. Levels of plasminogen activator inhibitor 1 were reported to be elevated in subjects with Klinefelter's syndrome with leg ulcers but not in those without leg ulcers.[306] Forty percent of men with Klinefelter's syndrome have taurodontism, an abnormality of the dental pulp that predisposes to early tooth decay.[300] Most have a male psychosexual orientation and function sexually as men. The syndrome may go undiagnosed in the majority of affected men, even as adults.[307]

46,XY/47,XXY mosaicism is the cause of about one fourth of cases of Klinefelter's syndrome, as estimated by chromosomal karyotypes of peripheral blood leukocytes.[308] The true prevalence may be underestimated because chromosomal mosaicism can be present in the testes in individuals in whom the chromosomal karyotype of peripheral leukocytes is normal. As summarized in Table 18–4, the manifestations of the mosaic form are usually less severe, and the testes may be normal in size. The endocrine abnormalities are also less severe, and gynecomastia and azoospermia are less common, with occasional men being fertile. Additional karyotypic varieties of Klinefelter's syndrome have been described (see Chapter 22).

The 47,XXY form of Klinefelter's syndrome is due to meiotic nondisjunction of the chromosomes during gametogenesis. About 40% of the responsible meiotic nondisjunction occur in the father and 60% occur in the mother. Advanced maternal age is a predisposing factor in the latter cases.[300] In contrast, mitotic nondisjunction after fertilization of the zygote causes the mosaic form and can arise in either a 46,XY zygote or a 47,XXY zygote.

Characteristic endocrine changes include elevation of plasma FSH and LH levels. FSH shows the best discrimination, and little overlap occurs with normal individuals, a consequence of the consistent damage to the seminiferous tubules. In the late teens, the plasma testosterone level may be normal. By the middle 20s, the plasma testosterone level averages half the normal value, but the range is broad and overlaps the normal range.[300] Mean plasma estradiol levels are elevated, and SHBG levels are about twice normal.[309] The net result is a variable degree of feminization and insufficient androgenization.

The feminization, including development of gynecomastia, is thought to depend on the ratio of circulating estrogen to androgen (see later). Before puberty, plasma gonadotropin levels and the response to GnRH are normal, but by the time of expected puberty plasma gonadotropins and the response to GnRH are elevated.[310] Older men with untreated Klinefelter's syndrome may have an enlarged or an abnormal sella turcica, presumably secondary to impairment of gonadal steroid feedback and gonadotrope hyperplasia.[311]

Optimally, affected boys should be identified in childhood to allow treatment of the testosterone deficiency early before it has an effect on BMD and to prevent adverse psychological effects of incomplete sexual maturation. The commencement of testosterone replacement before age 20 results in a normal BMD, whereas institution of therapy in older individuals does not enhance BMD.[312] Androgen replacement has no effect on fertility but has the same general benefits as in other forms of male hypogonadism.[313] Plasma LH levels usually return to normal with therapy, sometimes after many months.[314] Men with rare spermatozoa in the ejaculate or with spermatids or more advanced stages of spermatogenesis on biopsy may achieve fertility with in vitro fertilization using ICSI (see later). However, as many of 15% of the sperm produced by men with the disorder contain a 24,XY chromosome composition, which may result in an increased incidence of the disorder in offspring.[315]

XX Male Syndrome. The *XX male syndrome*, a variant of Klinefelter's syndrome, occurs in about 1 in 20,000 male births.[308, 316] The testes are small and firm, generally less than 2 cm long; gynecomastia is usual; the penis is normal to small in size; and azoospermia and hyalinization of the seminiferous tubules are present. Affected individuals have male psychosexual identification and absence of female internal genitalia. The mean plasma testosterone level is low, and levels of plasma estradiol and gonadotropins are high.[317] The phenotype differs from that of Klinefelter's syndrome in that the average height is less than that of normal men, the incidence of cognitive impairment is not increased, and hypospadias or ambiguous genitalia may be present.

Four theories were proposed to explain male development in the absence of a Y chromosome: (1) mosaicism in some tissues for a Y-chromosome–containing cell line, (2) a gain-of-function mutation for some autosomal gene, (3) deletion or inactivation of some gene or genes that normally suppress testicular development, and (4) interchange of a portion of the Y chromosome with the X chromosome.[318] Evidence has now been obtained for the presence of mechanisms 1, 2, and 4 in men with this disorder. Y-chromosome sequences are detectable in approximately 80% of 46,XX men and are usually located in the distal region of the X chromosome.[319, 320] Thus, the etiology in most XX males is analogous to that in the *sxr* mouse, in which a fragment of the Y chromosome has been translocated to the X chromosome.[321] Mosaicism involving an intact Y chromosome was present in 1% of the cells in one individual.[319]

The other third of 46,XX men are Y-negative and lack sequences for *SRY*. The Y-negative group is more likely to have ambiguity of the external genitalia, whereas the Y-positive group has the Klinefelter phenotype.[318–320] The translated region of the Y can be quite small and involve only the *SRY* gene itself. The *SRY*-negative variant is sometimes familial and may occur in families with true hermaphroditism, suggesting that these disorders are due to variable manifestations of the same genetic defect.[322] Such a defect could either be autosomal or X-linked. One 46,XX male had a duplication of the *SOX9* gene (a downstream gene involved in *SRY*-mediated testicular differentiation), indicating an autosomal mechanism.[322]

In one *SRY*-positive man with genital ambiguity, the presence of a duplication of the *SOX9* gene, a downstream target of *SRY* in testicular differentiation, indicated autosomal inheritance.[323] Most *SRY*-positive 46,XX males do not have genital ambiguity, and in one *SRY*-positive man with genital ambiguity more than 90% of the of the Y*p* fragment containing *SRY* was located on the inactive X chromosome in blood lymphocytes.[324] In parallel studies of a 46,XX man with no ambiguity, the Y*p* fragment was located predominately in the active X chromosome.[324] These findings document the complexity and heterogeneity of the disorder. The management is similar to that for Klinefelter's syndrome.

Acquired Defects

Mumps. The most common cause of acquired testicular failure in the adult is *viral orchitis*. Mumps virus is most frequent, but echovirus, lymphocytic choriomeningitis virus, and group B arboviruses also cause orchitis. The disorder is due to invasion of the tissue by the virus rather than to indirect effects of infection. Orchitis is common in mumps, occurring in as many as a fourth of adult men with the disease.[325] In about two thirds of cases it is unilateral. It usually develops 4 to 8 days after the onset of parotitis but occasionally precedes it.

After the acute inflammatory phase, the testis gradually decreases in size, although swelling can persist for months. The testis may return to normal size and function or undergo atrophy. The atrophy results from both the direct effects of the virus and ischemia caused by pressure and edema within the taut tunica albuginea.

The histologic features of the atrophic testis include progressive tubular sclerosis and hyalinization.[325] The degree of atrophy is not necessarily proportional to the severity of the orchitis. It is usually apparent within 1 to 6 months after the orchitis subsides, but the full extent of damage may not be evident for many years. Atrophy occurs in approximately a third of men with orchitis and is bilateral in about a tenth. The hormonal changes associated with gynecomastia related to mumps orchitis include normal estrogen and decreased testosterone production.[326]

The frequency with which mumps results in infertility is not known. Almost 50% of men with unilateral mumps orchitis have sperm densities of less than 10 million/mL in the first 3 months, but the sperm count returns to normal within 1 to 2 years in about 75%.[325] In contrast, semen parameters return to normal in less than a third of men with bilateral orchitis.

The initial treatment is bed rest and scrotal support. If pain is severe, administration of prednisone can reduce swelling and pain. Glucocorticoid therapy does not appear to have a beneficial effect on the return of the sperm count to normal.[325] In one study, treatment with interferon α shortened the duration of symptoms and prevented atrophy.[327]

Trauma. Trauma is second to viral orchitis as a cause of testicular atrophy in the adult. The exposed position of the testis in the scrotum renders it uniquely susceptible to both thermal and physical damage. In a prospective study, testicular atrophy occurred in half of men after blunt trauma to the scrotum.[328]

Radiation. Both spermatogenesis and testosterone production are sensitive to radiation; impaired secretion of testosterone appears to result from decreased testicular blood flow.[329] The incidence of radiation-associated damage to Leydig cells is directly related to the dosage and inversely related to age at treatment.[330] Most prepubertal boys have normal plasma testosterone levels and normal pubertal maturation after receiving 12 Gy of radiation to the testes, but the presence of an increased LH level in some suggests that compensatory changes are involved in the achievement of normal testosterone levels. In most prepubertal boys, radiation doses greater than 20 Gy cause permanent testosterone deficiency.[330] In contrast, radiation doses above 30 Gy cause testosterone deficiency in only half of adolescent boys and young adults. (Also see "Infertility with Normal Virilization.")

Drugs. Drugs can cause underandrogenization and infertility in several ways: direct inhibition of testosterone synthesis, blockade of the peripheral actions of androgen, and enhancement of estrogen levels. In addition, agents such as propranolol and guanethidine can impair erectile function in men whose hypothalamic-pituitary-testicular axis is normal.[266]

Two drugs that in high doses block testosterone synthesis are *spironolactone* and *cyproterone*, both of which interfere with the late reactions in testosterone biosynthesis. Spironolactone appears to impair CYP17 activity.[331] Plasma testosterone levels do not change appreciably, however, during usual therapeutic regimens.

The antifungal agent *ketoconazole* blocks testosterone synthesis, also by inhibiting CYP17 activity.[332] The decrease in testosterone after a single dose of ketoconazole is transient, with the nadir occurring within 4 to 8 hours and testosterone returning to baseline within 24 hours as ketoconazole levels fall. However, with doses of ketoconazole greater than 400 mg/day, depression of plasma testosterone levels may be sustained. Impairment of libido is common in men with epilepsy, partly as a consequence of medication.[333]

Enzyme-inducing antiepileptic drugs such as *phenytoin* and *carbamazepine* lower bioavailable testosterone, raise plasma SHBG and LH levels, and decrease the metabolic clearance of testosterone.[334] The effect is more pronounced with multiple-drug regimens.[333] Valproic acid does not appear to have as severe an adverse effect in this regard.[266]

Independent of its effects on the liver, *ethanol* ingestion reduces testosterone levels acutely and chronically,[335] the result of inhibition of testosterone synthesis.[336] The inhibition of steroidogenesis appears to occur at the 3β-HSD reaction as the result of a decrease in the concentration or availability of the pyridine nucleotide cofactors for the reaction, an effect probably mediated by the ethanol metabolite acetaldehyde.[337] The fact that ethanol lowers testosterone levels without causing appropriate elevations of plasma LH suggests that hypothalamic-pituitary function is also impaired.[335] Ethanol can also impair spermatogenesis.[338]

Antineoplastic and chemotherapeutic agents, especially *cyclophosphamide*, commonly induce infertility (see later). *Combination chemotherapy* for acute leukemia, Hodgkin's disease, and other malignancies may also impair Leydig cell function.[339] This toxic effect on the Leydig cell seems to be produced primarily by *alkylating agents*. Treatment with alkylating agents during the prepubertal years does not interfere with testicular function in later life, but elevated LH levels develop in many men after treatment, implying the presence of subclinical Leydig cell dysfunction.[330] Treatment of adult men with alkylating agents does not alter LH or testosterone levels.[339] High-dose interleukin-2 therapy for metastatic cancer causes a transient reduction in serum testosterone levels.[340]

Plasma testosterone levels may be low in men ingesting large amounts of *marijuana*, *heroin*, or *methadone*.[341, 342] Plasma LH is usually normal, suggesting combined hypothalamic-pituitary and testicular defects. Hyperprolactinemia may contribute to the lowering of testosterone levels.[266]

Elevated plasma estradiol and decreased plasma testosterone levels may occur in men taking *digitalis* preparations, the mechanism being unclear.[266] Drugs can interfere with gonadotropin production either as the result of a direct inhibition[343, 344] (as in *medroxyprogesterone acetate* administration) or as a secondary consequence of enhanced prolactin secretion (as with *phenothiazine* therapy).[345] Medroxyprogesterone may also impair testosterone secretion at the testicular level.[346]

Several drugs inhibit androgen action by competition at the receptor level. Although *spironolactone* can inhibit testosterone synthesis, in the usual dosage regimens it acts primarily by antagonizing the binding of androgen to the androgen receptor, which leads to gynecomastia and impotence.[331]

Cyproterone also acts as an androgen antagonist. The most commonly administered androgen antagonist is *cimetidine*.[347, 348] Gynecomastia can occur in men who are treated with the drug, and decreased sperm density and elevated basal testosterone levels are accompanied by impairment of the LH response to GnRH.

Ranitidine appears to be a less potent antiandrogen.[348] *Omeprazole* can also cause gynecomastia and impotence.[349]

Environmental Toxins. Prolonged exposure to *lead* results in direct testicular toxicity and an impaired pituitary response of plasma LH.[350]

Autoimmune Disorders. Testicular failure can occur as part of a generalized *autoimmune disorder* in which multiple primary endocrine deficiencies coexist and circulating antibodies to the basement membrane of the testes are present (see Chapter 37).[351, 352]

Granulomatous Disease. The testes can also be involved in granulomatous disease. Testicular atrophy occurs in 10% to 20% of men with *lepromatous leprosy* as the result of invasion of the tissue (and in some instances of paratesticular structures as well) by the bacilli. The result is a decreased plasma testosterone level and elevated plasma LH and FSH levels.[353] Destruction of the testis is less common with other systemic granulomatous diseases.

Defects Associated with Systemic Diseases

Abnormalities of the hypothalamic-pituitary-testicular axis occur in a number of systemic diseases. Given the chronic ill health and generalized wasting that may coexist, it is often difficult to distinguish specific effects of the underlying condition (e.g., renal failure) from those of malnutrition. The inflammatory cytokines interleukin-1β, tumor necrosis factor α, and interleukin-6 lower testosterone and have variable effects on plasma LH levels.[266, 354–356] In in vitro preparations, these agents inhibited several steroidogenic enzymes and StAR protein.[354, 355]

Renal Failure. About 50% of men undergoing dialysis for renal failure experience decreased libido and impotence associated with impairments in both spermatogenesis and testosterone biosynthesis. The defect in spermatogenesis varies from partial to total destruction of the germ cells.[357] The decrease in plasma testosterone and increase in plasma LH and FSH levels indicate a defect at the testicular level.[266] Plasma testosterone production rates are decreased, and the response of plasma testosterone to hCG is subnormal.[357] After dialysis, plasma testosterone levels and testosterone production rates improve but usually not to the normal range.[266]

Hyperprolactinemia occurs in 25% of men who undergo long-term dialysis.[357] In contrast, successful renal transplantation results in a return of testosterone and prolactin levels to normal and a slight decrease in LH and FSH levels.[266] Most men experience improved sexual function after transplantation, and half have sperm densities of more than 10 million/mL.[358]

Hepatic Disease. *Cirrhosis* of the liver can impair testicular function apart from the direct toxic effects of ethanol. Gynecomastia and testicular atrophy occur in half of men with cirrhosis, and 75% of men with hepatic cirrhosis are impotent. Decreased spermatogenesis and peritubular fibrosis are present in about 50% of patients. Plasma estradiol levels are usually elevated, and plasma testosterone levels are decreased.[266] The net result is a ratio in serum of unbound estradiol to unbound testosterone that is about 10 times normal. Levels of SHBG are about twice normal. The metabolic clearance and production rates of testosterone are decreased, and estradiol production is increased.

Extraglandular conversion of androgens, primarily adrenal androgens, to estradiol and estrone is increased about threefold, presumably because of decreased hepatic extraction of androgens. Basal levels of LH and FSH range from normal to moderately elevated. In men with low testosterone levels pulsatile LH secretion is impaired, implying a defect at the hypothalamic-pituitary level, whereas dynamic tests of the pituitary-testicular axis and hCG responsiveness tests point to a testicular defect.

Gonadotropin levels decrease as liver function fails.[266] The reason for abnormal testicular and hypothalamic-pituitary function is uncertain. Elevated estrogen levels can cause both defects. Testosterone therapy has been tried.[266, 359] Although estradiol levels increase (in correlation with the severity of the cirrhosis) after administration of testosterone enanthate, the estrogen/androgen ratio may become normal[359] and gynecomastia may regress.[266] Men with alcoholic cirrhosis may experience spontaneous recovery of sexual function with abstinence from alcohol despite persistent liver abnormalities. Men with alcoholic cirrhosis and testicular atrophy, however, are less likely to experience improvement in sexual function with abstinence from alcohol. Sexual function and testosterone levels are also decreased in men with other forms of liver disease.[266] The hormonal abnormalities in the pituitary-testicular axis can be reversed by liver transplantation.

Sickle Cell Anemia. Sexual maturation can be impaired in boys with sickle cell anemia.[266] Furthermore, in adult men with sickle cell anemia, secondary sexual characteristics are subnormal in most and testicular atrophy occurs in about a third.[360] Testicular biopsy in two men revealed maturation arrest of spermatogenesis. The defect may be either testicular or hypothalamic.

Chronic Illness. Abnormal Leydig cell function, frequently accompanied by decreased sperm counts, occurs in a many systemic diseases including *protein-calorie malnutrition*,[266] advanced *Hodgkin's disease* and *cancer* before chemotherapy,[266] *cystic fibrosis*,[361] *chronic pulmonary disease*,[266] and *amyloidosis*.[362] Such disorders usually cause a low plasma testosterone level and either a normal or slightly increased plasma LH level, suggesting combined hypothalamic-pituitary and testicular defects. The low plasma testosterone level is not the result of plasma factors that inhibit its binding to SHBG and hence is not analogous to that in the euthyroid sick syndrome (see Chapter 10). Indeed, because mean plasma SHBG levels are elevated, bioavailable testosterone may be lower than total testosterone. These changes in testosterone and LH may be nonspecific effects of illness because similar changes occur after *surgery*, *myocardial infarction*, and *severe burns*.[266]

Thyrotoxicosis. The changes in the hypothalamic-pituitary-testicular axis in thyrotoxicosis may be secondary to increased estrogen levels and include decreased sperm count and semen volume, increased plasma total testosterone level, and normal levels of unbound testosterone.[266] The testosterone response to hCG is blunted, and basal LH levels are increased.

Immune Disorders. Immune disease may cause testicular dysfunction, and primary or secondary hypogonadism is common in men with *acquired immunodeficiency syndrome* (AIDS), about half of whom have low testosterone levels with normal or appropriately increased plasma LH.[266] Although the disease may involve the testes directly, the hormonal changes suggest a nonspecific response to systemic illness and perhaps the toxic effects of immune cytokines. Many HIV-positive men who progress to AIDS have a transient state of increased LH and normal testosterone levels before testosterone levels become low. Serum SHBG levels are increased in HIV-positive men independent of CD4 count,[363] but bioavailable testosterone levels decrease progressively as CD4 counts decline.[364] Levels of bioavailable testosterone decline in men with AIDS before wasting occurs.[365]

The current practice is to provide androgen replacement in men with AIDS when testosterone deficiency becomes manifest. Testosterone replacement in such men results in an increase in lean body mass,[366, 367] improved quality of life,[366, 368] and increased muscle strength.[369]

Men with *rheumatoid arthritis* may have low serum testosterone, particularly during disease flares and while they are receiving glucocorticoids.[370] In contrast, testosterone levels are usually normal in men with long-standing, stable rheumatoid arthritis.

Neurologic Disease. Neurologic disease can cause testicular abnormalities. Men with *myotonic dystrophy* usually have small testes, low plasma testosterone levels, and elevated plasma LH and FSH levels.[371] *Spinobulbar muscular atrophy* (Kennedy's syndrome) is a form of adult-onset degenerative motor neuropathy associated with gynecomastia, testicular atrophy, a hormonal profile suggestive of androgen resistance (see later), and an expansion of the homopolymeric glutamine repeat region in the amino-terminal end of the androgen receptor gene.[132]

Although the effects are variable, *spinal cord lesions* that cause quadriplegia or paraplegia initially cause diminished plasma testosterone levels that usually return toward normal, but semen parameters may be permanently abnormal.[266, 372] Some paralyzed men retain the capacity to have erections and ejaculate, depending on the extent of involvement of the lumbosacral spinal cord.[373]

Men with trisomy 21 *(Down's syndrome)* have impairment of both germinal and Leydig cell function and elevation of FSH and LH levels.[374]

Androgen Resistance

Partial androgen resistance can cause underandrogenization and infertility in men with normal external genitalia. In such men, androgen resistance is manifested by increased testosterone production, elevated plasma LH levels in some, and abnormal androgen receptors in cultured genital skin fibroblasts.[375] The presence of elevated testosterone or LH levels, or both, is not a reliable predictor of which men have a receptor defect. Testicular biopsy reveals maturation arrests or germinal cell aplasia similar to that shown in Figure 18–16*D* and *E*. In some families, affected men have had gynecomastia and undervirilization but, in some, preserved fertility.[375–377] Point mutations have been identified in the androgen receptor in men with the isolated infertility and undervirilized, fertile male phenotypes (see Chapter 22).[117, 376, 377]

Infertility with Normal Virilization

Isolated infertility with normal Leydig cell function is caused by a separate group of disorders. Isolated infertility can be due to defects in the hypothalamic-pituitary system, the testis, or the sperm transport system (see Table 18–3).

Hypothalamic-Pituitary Disorders

Isolated FSH deficiency has been reported in men in whom virilization and plasma LH and plasma testosterone levels were normal but plasma FSH levels were persistently low.[378, 379] Plasma FSH levels in such men may increase[378] or remain undetectable[379] after GnRH administration. One man with no FSH response to GnRH had a point mutation in the FSH β gene.[379] In some men with chronic untreated or undertreated *congenital adrenal hyperplasia* related to CYP21 deficiency, suppression of gonadotropin secretion by adrenal androgens causes infertility.[380] This diagnosis is suggested by the presence of small testes, normal to elevated levels of testosterone, and suppressed levels of gonadotropins and is confirmed by finding elevated plasma levels of 17-hydroxyprogesterone and androstenedione (see Chapters 14 and 22).

When androgens are administered in pharmacologic doses to normal men, gonadotropins are suppressed and about 50% of the men have azoospermia (see Chapter 17). Although men who present with isolated infertility are unlikely to be receiving testosterone replacement therapy, the use of androgens by weight-lifters and body-builders is common. Self-prescribed regimens may include parenteral testosterone esters and a variety of oral and parenteral substituted androgens, often termed *anabolic steroids* (see later). Supraphysiologic androgen administration can cause reversible azoospermia in normal men.[266, 381]

Testicular Disorders

Developmental and Structural Defects

Germinal Cell Defects. Also known as the *Sertoli cell–only syndrome*, germinal cell aplasia is a poorly understood defect of the testis. The disorder encompasses histologic features that can have several causes, one of which may be a single-gene defect. Other men with typical histologic and clinical features have a history of viral orchitis, cryptorchidism,[382] alcoholism,[383] or androgen resistance.[376] Testicular biopsy reveals complete absence of germinal elements (see Fig. 18–16*E*). The clinical features include azoospermia, normal virilization, absence of gynecomastia, normal to small testes, and normal chromosomal complement. Plasma testosterone and LH values are usually normal, and plasma FSH values are high.

The concept of germinal cell aplasia became even more complex with the recognition that one or more Y chromosome determinants other than the *SRY* gene are essential for spermatogenesis.[384] Some men have a deletion of the long arm of the Y chromosome that includes an azoospermia factor (AZF) that maps to Yq11.23.[385] As many as 18% of men with azoospermia (occasionally severe oligospermia) have chromosome microdeletions in this region.[386] Testicular histology varies from germinal cell aplasia to maturation arrest, and the plasma FSH is elevated.

Candidate genes for AZF have been identified by positional cloning; the first is a family of genes termed Y-located RNA recognition motif *(YRRM)* genes[387] that encode RNA-binding proteins. The *YRRM* genes are expressed in germ cells, but the fact that multiple genes exist in this family makes it hard to assess their function.

The second AZF candidate, termed *DAZ* (*d*eleted in *az*oospermia), also encodes a testis-specific RNA recognition motif.[388] In one study, microdeletions in the AZF region were present in a third of men with idiopathic azoospermia and a fourth of men with oligospermia of unknown origin.[389] These microdeletions include the *DAZ* and *YRRM* regions and additional sequences.[389] Microdeletions were present in 7% of 46,XY men with known causes of infertility.[390]

A mutation in the *FSH receptor* gene in several Finnish families is associated with variable defects in spermatogenesis and infertility.[391]

Histologic findings in men with azoospermia include hypospermatogenesis or spermatogenic arrest (see Fig. 18–16*F*). Familial male infertility with hypospermatogenesis or maturation arrest can be inherited as X-linked[392] or autosomal recessive traits.[393] In most men, however, the family history is uninformative[393] and the cause of infertility is unknown. In both familial and sporadic cases, meiosis is defective.

Cryptorchidism. Unilateral cryptorchidism, even when corrected before puberty, is associated with abnormal semen in many individuals (see earlier). This finding suggests that the testicular abnormality is bilateral even in unilateral cryptorchidism.

Varicocele. Varicocele is believed to be the most common treatable cause of male infertility, possibly of causative importance in a third of infertile men.[394] Varicocele is caused by retrograde flow of blood into the internal spermatic vein and results in a progressive, often palpable, dilation of the peritesticular pampiniform plexus of veins. It is thought to be due to incompetence of the valve between the internal spermatic vein and the renal vein and is more common (85%) on the left. The incidence of varicocele is about 10% to 15% in the general population and 20% to 40% in men with infertility. The findings on semen analysis are usually nonspecific, but sperm density is often decreased with medium or large varicoceles.[395]

Most men with varicocele are fertile and have no detectable abnormality of the hypothalamic-pituitary-testicular axis. The leading theory concerning the adverse effect is that varicocele leads to an increased scrotal (and testicular) temperature, and the elevated scrotal surface temperatures in men with both unilateral and bilateral varicoceles can improve after surgical repair.[396] The testis on the side of the varicocele may be small.[397] Men with varicocele can also have unrelated causes of infertility.[398] Of men with varicocele and sperm counts less than 5 million/mL, about a fifth have microdeletions in the Y chromosome.[398]

On average, semen quality improves after surgical repair of varicoceles, but the effect on fertility is inconsistent in that impregnation rates after varicocele repair are probably less than 50%. In one large study of almost 1000 men there was an association between subsequent fertility and preoperative sperm density, and the men with preoperative sperm densities greater than 10 million/mL had a 70% impregnation rate after repair.[399]

Immotile Cilia Syndrome. The immotile cilia syndrome is a hereditary disorder characterized by defective motility of the cilia in the airways and elsewhere in the body and either immotile or poorly motile sperm.[150] The disorder is usually inherited as an autosomal recessive trait. In the airways, defective cilia cause chronic sinusitis and bronchiectasis and the immotile sperm cannot fertilize. *Kartagener's syndrome* is a subcategory of the syndrome and is associated with situs inversus.

The structural abnormalities that impair motility of cilia can be defined by electron microscopy and include missing or abnormally short dynein arms, short spokes with no central sheath, missing central microtubules, and displacement of one of the microtubule doublets. Cilia from epithelia and sperm from the same individual usually exhibit the same defects, but some mutations can apparently result in immotile sperm without impairment of cilia in the lung.[400] In evaluating sperm for structural abnormalities, the physician should take care to examine a number of axonemes and to confirm the structural defect because axonemal structure can vary in normal respiratory cilia and sperm. The infertility should be treatable, at least theoretically, by empirical methods (see later).

Acquired Defects

***Mycoplasma* Infection.** A role for *Mycoplasma (Ureaplasma urealyticum)* in infertility is inferred because infections are common in women whose infertility is associated with a "male factor," suggesting that genital tract mycoplasma infection may cause male infertility.[401] Eradication of the infection improves the pregnancy rate despite the fact that the severity of mycoplasma infection in men does not correlate with any specific alteration in sperm density or morphology.[402] Other evidence suggests that the presence of mycoplasma in the lower urogenital tract may represent silent colonization rather than infection.[403]

Radiation. Radiation can cause isolated infertility, with damage sometimes being demonstrable after only 0.15 Gy (15 rad). Doses higher than 1 Gy (100 rad) can cause extreme oligospermia or azoospermia, and higher doses decrease sperm counts and damage spermatids. A return to baseline sperm density takes 9 to 18 months after doses of 1 Gy (100 rad) or less, 30 months for doses of 2 to 3 Gy (200 to 300 rad), and 5 years or more for doses of 4 to 6 Gy (400 to 600 rad).[404] Fractionated radiation may have a more profound effect on the testes than single doses.[405]

Permanent infertility can occur after radiation for malignant lymphoma of the abdomen despite shielding of the testes.[406] Administration of radioactive iodine to men for thyroid cancer can also impair spermatogenesis and elevate plasma FSH levels; recovery occurs in about 2 years.[407] Prior suppression of testicular function by administration of testosterone or GnRH, or both, does not protect the testes from radiotherapy (or cytotoxic drugs).[408]

Drugs. The principal drugs that cause isolated infertility are *alkylating agents* such as *cyclophosphamide*.[409] Spermatocytes and spermatogonia may disappear completely, causing the picture of germinal cell aplasia with only Sertoli cells lining the tubular lumen. Serum FSH levels can increase fivefold and serve as a marker for germ cell loss; levels of inhibin B decline.[410] Serum LH and testosterone levels usually remain within normal limits. Cessation of cyclophosphamide therapy is followed by return of spermatogenesis within 3 years in about half of azoospermic men.[411] *Vinblastine*, *doxorubicin*, *procarbazine*, and *cisplatin* are also toxic to the germinal epithelium.

Combination regimens such as *mechlorethamine*, *vincristine*, *procarbazine*, and *prednisone* (*MOPP*) have an even more profound impact on spermatogenesis.[409] The combination of *doxorubicin*, *bleomycin*, *vinblastine*, and *dacarbazine* is less toxic than MOPP.[412] Combination chemotherapy that includes cyclophosphamide or procarbazine causes postpubertal azoospermia in about half of prepubertal boys,[413] whereas *etoposide* in combination chemotherapy causes less toxicity.[414]

Chemotherapy-induced azoospermia after treatment with vinblastine, bleomycin, and cisplatin for testicular cancer is usually reversible within 2 years of stopping treatment[415]; cisplatin is thought to be the primary mediator of the toxicity.[416]

Sulfasalazine and *methotrexate* can also cause oligospermia and infertility.[417, 418]

Environmental Toxins. Because of the potential toxicity of physical and chemical agents, the occupational and recreational history should be carefully evaluated in all men with infertility. Known *environmental toxins* include chemicals such as the nematocide *dibromochloropropane* and related compounds, *ethylene glycol*, *cadmium*, *lead*, and *organic chloride* compounds.[419] In a large meta-analysis of studies of normal men, sperm density was said to have declined from 113 million/mL in 1940 to 66 million/mL in 1990.[420] This report has subsequently been confirmed[421] and refuted (reviewed in reference 419). Environmental toxins that might act as estrogens or antiandrogens have been proposed as the cause. Cigarette smoking may also contribute to decreasing sperm density.[419]

Autoimmunity. Although autoimmunity may cause combined underandrogenization and infertility, the usual manifestation is isolated infertility, and antibodies to the basement membrane of the seminiferous tubules or to the sperm themselves may be responsible. Antisperm antibodies of the immunoglobulin A (IgA) class may prevent the penetration of cervical mucus by sperm.[422] IgG and IgA antibodies may impair the acrosome reaction and the binding of sperm to the zona pellucida of the oocyte.

Therapy usually involves in vitro fertilization (see later). Development of antisperm antibodies is not always a primary phenomenon because the antibodies have been identified in men with both bilateral and unilateral obstruction of the vas deferens[423] and after vasectomy.

Defects Associated with Systemic Diseases

Temporary impairment of semen quality, particularly decreased sperm density, is common after *acute febrile illness*. This is one reason that several semen analyses must be obtained in the work-up for men with infertility to be confident that true basal parameters have been determined (see earlier).

Men with *celiac disease* have a distinct testicular abnormality—namely, endocrine features typical of androgen resistance with elevated plasma testosterone and LH levels.[424–426] Improvement in gluten enteropathy may reverse the androgen resistance–like state.[424–426]

As discussed earlier, *spinal cord injury* is commonly associated with isolated infertility.[266]

Androgen Resistance

Androgen resistance may cause infertility without underandrogenization (see earlier).[117] It was originally thought on the basis of functional studies that androgen receptor defects might account for 10% to 20% of idiopathic azoospermia or severe oligospermia,[427, 428] but loss-of-function mutations in the androgen receptor gene are present in only about 2% of such men.[429–431] Expansion of the CAG repeat sequence in the N-terminal region of the androgen receptor (see earlier) appears to be more common in men with azoospermia or severe oligospermia.[432, 433]

Impairment of Sperm Transport

Disorders of sperm transport may cause as much as 6% of male infertility.[394] Such disorders can be unilateral or bilateral, congenital or acquired. Infertility in men with unilateral obstruction may be due to antisperm antibodies.[423] Obstructive azoospermia at the level of the epididymis also occurs in association with *chronic infections of the paranasal sinuses and lungs.*[434] In *polycystic kidney disease*, dilated cysts of the seminal vesicles may obstruct semen transport.[435] *Tuberculosis*, *leprosy*, and *gonorrhea* can obstruct the ejaculatory system, and sperm transport can be obstructed by deep *midline müllerian cysts.*[436]

Congenital defects of the vas deferens can cause azoospermia or oligospermia in sons of women given *diethylstilbestrol during pregnancy.*[437] Congenital bilateral absence of the vas deferens is common in men with *cystic fibrosis*, and mutations in the gene responsible, the transmembrane conductor regulator *(CFTR)* gene, can cause bilateral absence of the vas deferens without other manifestations of the disease.[438] Congenital unilateral absence of the vas deferens may be an incomplete form of the bilateral disorder.[438, 439] Thus, congenital absence of the vas deferens and cystic fibrosis are variable manifestations of mutations of the same gene.

Idiopathic Infertility

In large series, known causes were identified for only about 60% of cases of infertility in males, with the remainder classified as *idiopathic* (Table 18–5).[394, 440] Because at best only about half of infertile men with a varicocele achieve fertility after surgical repair, it is likely that even a larger fraction of infertile men have idiopathic infertility. Some may have androgen resistance, and as many as a fifth may have disorders involving the *AZF* gene (see earlier). Others have oligospermia or azoospermia with normal plasma LH and testosterone but elevated FSH levels in the absence of cryptorchidism, radiation, or drug exposure.

Studies of such men indicate that isolated FSH elevation may be associated with a decreased GnRH pulse frequency[441] and that FSH levels may be corrected with pulsatile GnRH therapy.[442, 443] Men with oligospermia and normal FSH levels may also have altered pulsatile secretion of gonadotropins and testosterone,[444] and testosterone production rates are said to be low in selected infertile men with isolated FSH elevations and normal total serum testosterone.[445] Whether these abnormalities are of causative significance is unknown.

A subset of men with severe idiopathic oligospermia associated with a decreased ratio of serum testosterone to estradiol have shown an increase in sperm density after treatment with an aromatase inhibitor.[446] Testicular biopsies of men with idiopathic infertility have shown increased apoptosis associated with maturation arrest and hypospermatogenesis,[447, 448] decreased expression of the c-*kit* receptor,[448] and increased mutations consistent with abnormal DNA repair mechanisms.[449]

Table 18–5. Relative Frequency of Causes and Associated Conditions in Men Who Present with Infertility

Cause or Condition	% in Study of Greenberg et al.[394] (n = 425)	% in Study of Baker et al.[440] (n = 1041)
Hypogonadotropic hypogonadism	0.9	0.6
Klinefelter's syndrome	1.6	1.9
Cryptorchidism	6.1	6.4
Varicocele	37.4	40.3
Immotile sperm	0.5	0.6
Viral orchitis	1.9	1.6
Radiation-chemotherapy	—	0.5
Obstruction of epididymis or vas deferens	6.1	4.1
Androgen resistance	—	0.1
Coital disorders	4.0	0.5
Idiopathic disorders	41.5*	43.4†

*Includes miscellaneous semen abnormalities, 10.2%, and undiagnosed primary testicular failure, 5.9.%

†Includes possible obstruction, 4.5%.

Management of Infertility

The management of infertility is usually unsatisfactory because the number of potentially correctable causes is small (see Table 18–5). When appropriate, however, associated hormonal disorders and coexisting medical conditions may be treated and offending drugs can be discontinued.

Although claims of success have been made for a variety of empirical therapies for infertility with oligospermia, most such claims fail to take into account the spontaneous fertility rate in untreated oligospermic men (~25% in 1 year).[240] The fact that treatment-independent pregnancy occurs in all forms of human infertility (male and female factors) makes it necessary for all therapies to be evaluated by randomized clinical trials.[450] When several forms of empirical therapy—including testosterone rebound, nonaromatizable androgen (mesterolone), gonadotropin, antiestrogen (clomiphene), antibiotics, bromocriptine, varicocele repair, artificial insemination, and no therapy—were compared in one large retrospective analysis of oligospermic men, none were effective.[451]

In Vitro Fertilization

The only effective empirical therapy for male infertility is in vitro fertilization. Standard techniques of in vitro fertilization require about 500,000 motile sperm/mL of ejaculate. Although the fertilizing capacity of sperm from men with abnormal sperm parameters is diminished, conventional techniques can result in 10% or more live births per attempt in men with mild to moderate abnormalities.[452] Such rates are threefold to fivefold higher than natural impregnation rates in such men. However, standard in vitro fertilization is ineffective in men with more severe defects in spermatogenesis. In the Melbourne experience, fertilization rates were low in men with severe oligospermia, poor motility, and increased numbers of abnormal forms.[453]

Intracytoplasmic Sperm Injection

Better results have been obtained with the development of intracytoplasmic sperm injection (ICSI)—namely, fertility rates of 50% or more using poor quality semen, including decreased sperm number, impaired motility, increased abnormal forms, and combined defects.[454] In men with obstructive azoospermia in whom sperm must be aspirated from the epididymis, fertilization rates are nearly normal.

In the past, men with nonobstructive azoospermia, typically with elevated plasma FSH levels, were not treatable. Such patients include men with maturation arrest, postcryptorchidism tubular atrophy, mumps orchitis, and Klinefelter's syndrome. However, when minute amounts of sperm could be identified by testicular biopsy, fertilization and impregnation have been achieved with rare spermatozoa or spermatids retrieved from such biopsy specimens using ICSI.[454] ICSI should not be undertaken until men with abnormal semen undergo a complete work-up so that hypogonadotropic hypogonadism or some other treatable condition is not missed. Furthermore, ICSI may increase the chances of transmitting the father's disorder to offspring, as has been reported in men with Klinefelter's syndrome and men with *AZF* mutations.[455, 456]

Old Age

The role of the decrease in total and bioavailable testosterone and the increase in estradiol in the decline of male sexual function with aging is not clear (see the following). However, this changing hormonal milieu may be involved in the pathogenesis of breast enlargement in elderly men and in the development of prostatic hyperplasia.

Prostatic Hyperplasia

Enlargement of the prostate to the extent that it obstructs urethral outflow is common in elderly men.[457, 458] The gland weighs a few grams at birth, and at puberty androgen-mediated growth causes the prostate to reach the adult size of about 20 g by age 20. This growth is accompanied by transformation of the cuboidal epithelium of the acini to a columnar, secretory epithelium and by initiation of secretion of the prostatic component of the ejaculate. The weight of the gland remains stable for about 25 years.

Beginning in the fifth decade of life, a hyperplastic phase of prostatic growth ensues in most men. The second growth phase, unlike the earlier growth, which involves the gland diffusely, typically begins in the periurethral region as a localized proliferation of glandular and stromal elements. The hyperplasia may remain limited in scope, but in many men growth continues and eventually compresses the remaining normal portion of the prostate. The progressive increase in gland size can cause lower urinary tract symptoms and urinary obstruction, but the correlation between symptoms and anatomic changes can be unpredictable. On the one hand, hyperplasia primarily of the periurethral region can obstruct urine outflow in the absence of gross prostatic enlargement; on the other hand, men with gross enlargement of the gland can be asymptomatic.

The second growth spurt, like the growth at puberty, requires a functioning testis. Dihydrotestosterone formed within the prostate from testosterone mediates the embryonic development, pubertal growth, and hyperplastic growth of the prostate.[459] Administration to animals of a 5α-reductase inhibitor to block dihydrotestosterone formation caused involution of the prostate despite elevation of testosterone levels within the gland.[460, 461] Furthermore, although plasma testosterone may decline with age, the level of dihydrotestosterone in the hyperplastic gland either remains constant or increases.[462]

Prostatic hyperplasia also occurs in the aging male dog, and most research on its pathogenesis has been done in that species. Administration to the castrated dog of androgens that cause an increase in the prostatic dihydrotestosterone level caused prostatic enlargement comparable to that seen in the naturally occurring disorder.[463] Estrogen acts synergistically with dihydrotestosterone to enhance prostatic growth in the dog[463] because estrogen increases the amount of androgen receptor in the tissue.[459] Thus, two hormones participate in the development of prostatic hyperplasia in the dog; dihydrotestosterone is responsible for prostate growth, and estradiol enhances dihydrotestosterone action.

Three types of evidence suggest that dihydrotestosterone and estradiol are also involved in human prostatic hyperplasia:

1. Either surgical or pharmacologic castration causes a decrease in the size of the hyperplastic prostate gland,[464, 465] indicating that continuing androgen action is essential to maintain the hyperplastic state.
2. Inhibition of prostatic 5α-reductase with agents such as finasteride causes a profound decrease in prostatic dihydrotestosterone levels[466] and a 20% to 30% decrease in prostate volume after 3 to 6 months of therapy. This effect is maintained for up to 4 years and is associated with few side effects.[467]
3. There is a temporal relation between the development of prostatic hyperplasia and the increase in plasma estradiol with age, but a causal relation between estradiol and human prostatic hyperplasia has not been established.[468]

Demonstration that hormones play a role in prostatic hyperplasia does not necessarily provide insight into its pathogenesis because their action could be permissive rather than causal, and the reason that the disorder varies so markedly in its manifestations is unclear. Similarly, the therapeutic role of 5α-reductase inhibitors is not established because there is a strong placebo effect on urinary symptoms, there is no clear-cut relation between symptoms and urine flow, and the natural history of the disorder—particularly how to predict which subset of men will develop significant obstruction—is not understood. As a consequence, although a variety of minimally invasive or medical therapies are now available, the indications for surgical or medical management, compared with watchful waiting, are sometimes unclear.[457, 458, 469]

Prostatic Cancer

The endocrine aspects of prostatic cancer are discussed in Chapter 39.

Disorders of All Ages

Testicular Tumors

Tumors of the testes occur with an incidence of 2 to 3 per 100,000 men per year in the United States and account for about 1% of cancer deaths in men.[470] The incidence in most Western countries has risen since the 1930s, particularly in adults,[471] but mortality rates have declined.[471, 472] The frequency shows a trimodal curve, with peaks in childhood (embryonal carcinomas and teratocarcinomas), young adulthood, and old age (seminomas). The incidence in blacks is a sixth or less that in whites, but overall the tumors are the second most common malignancy (after leukemia) in men between ages 20 and 35 years. The tumors are commonly bilateral (either simultaneous or sequential, e.g., a seminoma developing in one testis many years after the removal of the other).[473]

Occurrence is familial in 1% to 2% of cases.[474] The presence of an isochromosome of the short arm of chromosome 12 is characteristic of germ cell tumors of all subtypes.[475]

Several factors predispose to testicular malignancy. Men with cryptorchidism have a fivefold increased risk of development of such tumors, men with intra-abdominal testes being more at risk than those with high inguinal testes,[476] so that in one series 10 of 131 men with testicular cancer had antecedent maldescent.[477] Three fourths of tumors associated with maldescent are seminomas, the remainder being other germ cell tumors.

Early orchiopexy facilitates detection, but whether it reduces the incidence of tumor development is not clear.[478] Testicular malignancy may be more frequent in individuals with abnormal sexual development (i.e., 45,X/46,XY mixed gonadal dysgenesis or 46,XY testicular feminization) than with other forms of testicular maldescent.[479] Occupational exposure to extremely high or low temperature can increase the risk.[480] Estrogen administration to pregnant women may be a predisposing factor in male offspring,[477] and Down's syndrome,[481] Klinefelter's syndrome,[482] and HIV infection[483] are associated with an increased incidence.

Table 18–6. Classification of Testicular Tumors

I. Germ cell tumors (95%)
  A. Single-cell–type tumors (60%)
    1. Seminomas
    2. Yolk sac tumors (embryonal cell tumors)
    3. Teratomas
    4. Choriocarcinoma
  B. Combination tumors (40%)
II. Tumors of gonadal stroma (1–2%)
  A. Leydig cell
  B. Sertoli cell
  C. Primitive gonadal structures
III. Gonadoblastomas
  A. Germ cell + stroma cell

Data from Mostofi FK. Pathology of germ cell tumors of testis: a progress report. Cancer 1980; 45:1735–1754.

Most testicular tumors in men with congenital adrenal hyperplasia related to steroid 21-hydroxylase (CYP21) deficiency consist of adrenal cell rests, are dependent on corticotropin for growth and secretion, and occur in men who are inadequately treated and hence have elevated plasma corticotropin levels.[484] However, the tumors can be difficult to separate histologically from interstitial cell tumors.

Diagnosis

Most testicular cancers produce local symptoms, but delay in making a diagnosis is common because of oversights by both physicians and patients. Testicular cancers usually occur before age 45, and men should be educated about the need to seek prompt medical advice for any change in a previously normal testis, including enlargement, pain or a feeling of heaviness, swelling, or other unusual findings.[485] Pain occurs in half of affected men, and to reduce delay physicians should consider any testicular mass to be a tumor until proved otherwise and to obtain surgical consultation if symptoms and signs persist.[486]

Classification

The most widely used classification is that of Mostofi[487] (Table 18–6) and is based on the cell type from which the tumor originates.

Germ Cell Tumors

Germ cell tumors are the most common types.

Seminomas are characterized by large cells with clear cytoplasm in a delicate fibrovascular stroma infiltrated with lymphocytes; the granulomatous reaction around the tumor can be so intense as to suggest a graft-versus-host reaction.[488] These tumors account for at least half of all testicular neoplasms and can be subdivided into *spermatocytic seminomas*, which occur in older men and are associated with a 90% to 95% 5-year survival, and *anaplastic seminomas*, which have a poor prognosis.

Embryonal carcinomas are the most common testicular tumors in boys, resemble embryonal carcinomas of the ovary, and are associated with 5-year survivals of about 70% in infants and 25% in adults.

Choriocarcinomas contain syncytiotrophoblastic cells and usually occur in the second and third decades of life; the prognosis is poor.

Teratomas contain at least two germ cell layers and may be either benign or malignant; they are second in frequency to embryonal carcinomas in childhood and are unusual in adults.

Tumors that contain combinations of germ cell types account for 40% of germ cell tumors; the biology of such tumors is determined by the least differentiated (most malignant) element. Of mixed tumors that contain cells of germinal and stromal origin, perhaps the most distinctive is the *gonadoblastoma*, which consists of germ cells, sex cords, and, usually, Leydig cells.[489] Gonadoblastomas usually occur in dysgenetic testes containing a Y chromosome and synthesize androgen.

Germ cell tumors of all types can also originate in extragonadal sites, including the mediastinum[490] and the brain.[491] These extragonadal tumors are presumed to arise from aberrant migration of germ cells early in embryogenesis; from some common precursor stem cell line that normally gives rise to germ cells, thymus, and pineal gland; or from migration of transformed gonadal germ cells.[492]

Testicular germ cell tumors usually occur as a nodule or painless swelling of the testis but may be identified as the result of metastases or because of the peripheral manifestations of hCG secretion by the tumor. After diagnosis, the tumors are staged either by surgical exploration or by computed tomographic scanning or magnetic resonance imaging. Stage I is limited to the testes, stage II involves metastases to infradiaphragmatic lymph nodes but not beyond, stage III involves supradiaphragmatic lymph nodes, and stage IV involves extralymphatic metastases.

Germinomas can secrete several distinct tumor cell markers into plasma, including hCG and its β subunit, α-fetoprotein, lactate dehydrogenase, carcinoembryonic antigen, and placental alkaline phosphatase.[493] Virtually all germ cell tumors synthesize hCG and its subunits, but the hormone is secreted in large amounts only by some nonseminoma germ cell tumors (choriocarcinomas, teratocarcinomas, and yolk sac tumors).[494] α-Fetoprotein is a marker of tumors containing yolk sac elements, and teratomas can secrete carcinoembryonic antigen.[495] An elevated level of one of these tumor markers in the plasma of a patient whose tumor has been classified as a pure seminoma usually indicates that the tumor is actually a combination tumor. These markers are particularly useful for following the response to therapy.[493] Secreted hCG may be endocrinologically active and cause enhanced formation of testosterone[496] and, more important, of estradiol[497] by the testes. The net result can be a feminizing syndrome and inhibition of the secretion of LH and FSH by the pituitary (see later).[498]

The treatment of germ cell tumors constitutes a major triumph of cancer therapy. Appropriate therapeutic strategies include debulking of the tumor mass, resection of involved lymph nodes, administration of chemotherapy (usually combinations of cisplatin, vinblastine, etoposide, and bleomycin), radiation, and monitoring of tumor cell markers.[499] The cure rates for patients with seminomas are approximately 90% for stage I disease, and individuals with stage III nonseminoma tumors, which were previously uniformly lethal, now have good survival rates.[500]

Because young men with germ cell tumors may have infertility related to castration, radiation, chemotherapy, or a combination, cryopreservation of semen before treatment has been advocated as a means of preserving fertility,[501] but many men have adequate sperm production after chemotherapy.[502] Treatment is associated with a small risk of recurrence and the development of secondary solid tumors and leukemia[503] and with the late sequelae of chemotherapy such as nephrotoxicity and neurotoxicity.[504]

Stromal Cell Tumors

Stromal tumors *(Leydig cell tumors, Sertoli cell tumors)* account for 1% to 2% of testicular tumors, and both cell types may coexist within the same tumor. Rarely, adrenal rest tumors occur in the testes.[505] As would be expected, Leydig cell tumors commonly secrete testosterone and thus may cause virilization in prepubertal boys (precocious pseudopuberty); many of the tumors secrete estradiol as well and cause mixed signs of feminization and virilization during the prepubertal years and feminizing signs in adult men. The hormones from such tumors can suppress levels of endogenous gonadotropins and testosterone and can cause azoospermia and decreased size of the contralateral testis.[506] Because the tumors may be so small as to be recognized only by ultrasonography, documenting that the testis is the site of increased estrogen production may require selective catheterization of the testicular veins.

Sertoli cell tumors show a bimodal age distribution, most patients being younger than 1 year or between ages 20 and 45 years. The tumors are frequently bilateral and familial (usually as a component of the Peutz-Jeghers syndrome).[507, 508] Gynecomastia occurs in about 25% of patients, and estrogen secretion can impair spermatogenesis and cause shrinkage of the contralateral testis. Leydig cell hyperplasia can occur in the area around the tumor, implying either that the tumor is of mixed cell origin or that Sertoli cells secrete some factor that stimulates Leydig cell development.[509] Complete cure and regression of feminizing signs usually follow surgical resection. Approximately 10% of stromal tumors are malignant.[510]

Rete Testis Tumors

Adenocarcinoma of the rete testis is rare but tends to be highly malignant.[511]

Summary

Testicular tumors can enhance production of estradiol and testosterone by more than one mechanism. When tumors produce steroid hormones autonomously, plasma gonadotropin levels and androgen secretion by uninvolved portions of the testes are depressed, and azoospermia is common. When hCG is secreted by the tumor, production of estradiol and testosterone is increased in unaffected areas of the testes, and azoospermia is uncommon. Furthermore, occasional choriocarcinomas that cannot synthesize steroids de novo nevertheless convert circulating androgens to estrogens. When hormones are formed directly or indirectly by the tumors, the response varies depending on the pattern of hormones produced and the age of the subject.

ABNORMALITIES IN ESTROGEN METABOLISM

Gynecomastia

Administration of large amounts of estrogen to men, as for carcinoma of the prostate or in preparation for sex change surgery, causes a variety of side effects, including fluid retention and congestive heart failure, hypertension, electrocardiographic changes, myocardial infarction, and thromboembolic disease.[512] At lower levels, as can occur with estrogen-secreting testicular tumors, estrogen excess suppresses gonadotropin secretion, secondarily impairs testosterone production, and inhibits spermatogenesis. However, the most common manifestation of estrogen excess in men is gynecomastia (breast enlargement).

Sexual dimorphism in breast development at the time of puberty is due to the ovarian secretion of estrogen, and estrogen excess at any stage of life can cause breast enlargement in men. In the absence of a progestagen, the breast acini and lobules do not undergo complete female development,[513] probably explaining why galactorrhea is unusual in men.

Clinical Features

At the clinical level, gynecomastia is complicated by problems of definition. The common view has been that any palpable breast tissue in men is abnormal except for three situations: transient gynecomastia of the newborn, pubertal gynecomastia, and gynecomastia that occasionally occurs in elderly men.[514] However, this view was challenged by Nuttall[515] and Niewoehner and Nuttall,[516] who reported that 36% of normal adult men and two thirds of hospitalized men have palpable breast tissue. The prevalence may have increased because of some unrecognized cause.

A confounding problem is that it can be difficult to distinguish enlargement of breast tissue from lipomastia, in which enlargement is caused by adipose tissue.[517] True gynecomastia can be separated from lipomastia by mammography[518] or sonography.[519] Autopsy data are not of much help in establishing the frequency of gynecomastia because they do not provide information about what fraction of gynecomastia—active or inactive—is theoretically palpable.[520] For the purposes of this discussion, breast enlargement in men (other than in the three so-called physiologic states) may be indicative of an underlying endocrinopathy and deserves at least a limited evaluation.

Histopathology and Etiology

Gynecomastia is frequently asymmetrical, and unilateral gynecomastia can be temporary in that one breast may enlarge months or years before the other. The process begins with proliferation of the stroma and the duct system, which elongates, buds, and duplicates. With time, progressive fibrosis and hyalinization are accompanied by regression of epithelial cells so that the ducts decrease in number.[521] On correction of the cause, resolution involves reduction in size and cell content of the epithelia followed by gradual disappearance of the ducts, leaving hyaline bands that may persist or eventually disappear.

Gynecomastia is generally viewed as the consequence of absolute or relative estrogen excess,[522] and it can be classified as either *physiologic* or *pathologic* (Table 18–7).

Physiologic Gynecomastia

During three phases of male life, breast enlargement can be a normal finding.

Gynecomastia in the Newborn

Enlargement of the breast in the newborn is probably due to maternal or placental estrogens, or both. The swelling may or may not be associated with milk production and usually disappears in a few weeks but can persist longer.[523]

Adolescent Gynecomastia

Transient enlargement of the breast occurs in about 40% of adolescent boys.[524] The median age at onset is 14 years, the breasts may be asymmetrical and tender, and by age 20 only a small number of men have palpable vestiges of gynecomastia. The most severe disorder, termed *pubertal macromastia* (breast tissue > 4 cm), may persist into adulthood and is more commonly associated with an underlying endocrinopathy.[525]

The cause of pubertal breast enlargement is uncertain. Plasma estradiol levels in boys normally reach the adult range before plasma testosterone,[526] and average plasma estradiol levels are higher in boys with gynecomastia.[527] As a result, the

Table 18–7. Classification of Endocrine Gynecomastia

Physiologic Gynecomastia
- Gynecomastia in the newborn
- Adolescent gynecomastia
- Gynecomastia of aging

Pathologic Gynecomastia
- Relative estrogen excess
  - Congenital defects
    - Congenital anorchia
    - Klinefelter's syndrome
    - Androgen resistance (testicular feminization and Reifenstein's syndrome)
    - Defects in testosterone synthesis
  - Secondary testicular failure (viral orchitis, trauma, castration, neurologic and granulomatous diseases, renal failure)
- Increased estrogen production
  - Increased testicular estrogen secretion
    - Testicular tumors
    - Bronchogenic carcinoma and other tumors producing hCG
    - True hermaphroditism
  - Increased substrate for extraglandular aromatase
    - Adrenal disease
    - Liver disease
    - Starvation
    - Thyrotoxicosis
  - Increase in extraglandular aromatase
- Drugs
  - Estrogens or drugs that act like estrogens (diethylstilbestrol, estrogen-containing cosmetics, birth control pills, digitalis, estrogen-contaminated foods, phytoestrogens)
  - Drugs that enhance endogenous estrogen formation (gonadotropins, clomiphene)
  - Drugs that inhibit testosterone synthesis and/or action (ketoconazole, metronidazole, cimetidine, etomidate, alkylating agents, cisplatin, flutamide, spironolactone)
  - Drugs that act by unknown mechanisms (busulfan, isoniazid, methyldopa, calcium channel–blocking agents, captopril, tricyclic antidepressants, penicillamine, diazepam, marijuana, heroin)

Idiopathic Gynecomastia

hCG, human chorionic gonadotropin.

plasma ratios of estradiol to testosterone and of estrone to adrenal androgens tend to be high in boys with pubertal gynecomastia.[528] Local formation of estrogen within the breast may also play a role in the gynecomastia of puberty.[529]

Gynecomastia of Aging

Gynecomastia can occur in otherwise healthy elderly men, but because gynecomastia can also be due to underlying pathology, the diagnosis of involutional gynecomastia is one of exclusion. Approximately 40% of elderly men at autopsy have true gynecomastia,[514] and the prevalence is approximately 70% in hospitalized men aged 50 to 69 years.[516] Because many older men take medications and have concurrent disorders, gynecomastia of aging, if it exists, may be caused by coexisting medical problems rather than by age itself.

Changes in estrogen and androgen metabolism in men older than 70 years include decreases in mean levels of total and bioavailable plasma testosterone, elevation of plasma SHBG, increase in the rate of peripheral aromatization, decrease in the ratio of androgen to estrogen, increase in levels of plasma LH and FSH, and blunting or loss of the circadian rhythm of plasma testosterone levels (see earlier). Such changes may cause a sufficient alteration of the ratio of testosterone to estradiol to induce breast enlargement in the absence of disease.

Pathologic Gynecomastia

Pathologic gynecomastia can be due to a relative (as in testosterone deficiency) or absolute increase in estrogen formation (as in Leydig cell tumors), to drugs, or to unknown causes.

Relative Estrogen Excess

Failure of testosterone synthesis or action causes elevated plasma gonadotropin levels, and relative estrogen excess ensues because of the extraglandular aromatization of adrenal androgens and on occasion a secondary increase in testicular estrogen secretion (see Fig. 18–18*A*).

Congenital Defects

Congenital Anorchia. Congenital anorchia is a rare, often familial disorder in which the testes are missing in phenotypically normal 46,XY males (see Chapter 22). Affected individuals are thought to have bilateral cryptorchidism at birth, but no testes are located on surgical exploration of the abdomen. Because testicular hormones are necessary for male phenotypic development and because the penis is normal in this disorder, it is believed that testes are present and function normally until late in embryonic life and then regress for unknown reasons. Approximately half of anorchid men develop gynecomastia.

In some anorchid men, Leydig cells secrete small amounts of testosterone into the circulation even if testes cannot be found at surgery.[530] Other men with congenital anorchia have profound testosterone deficiency and a small amount of estradiol formed by the indirect pathway androstenedione → estrone → estradiol in extraglandular tissues.[531] These findings imply that the critical factor for feminization is not the absolute level of estrogen but rather some ratio of testosterone to estradiol. Androgen appears to block estrogen action by competing with estradiol for binding to the estrogen receptor.[532]

Klinefelter's Syndrome. Approximately half of nonmosaic and a third of mosaic men with Klinefelter's syndrome have gynecomastia after the expected time of puberty.[300] Plasma FSH and LH levels are high, and the average plasma testosterone level is half normal, although some have normal testosterone levels. Variations in plasma levels of testosterone and estradiol are associated with variable degrees of androgenization and feminization in the disorder.[309]

The causes of elevated plasma estradiol are complex.[533, 534] Early in adolescence, plasma testosterone is usually in the normal male range as the result of elevated plasma LH, which also causes enhanced estradiol secretion by the testes. Testicular function becomes progressively impaired with time, so that after age 15 years, serum testosterone and estrogen levels begin to decline[310] and the end stage resembles anorchia (see earlier). Diminished estrogen clearance may further increase estrogen/androgen ratios.

Androgen Resistance (Testicular Feminization and Reifenstein's Syndrome). Hereditary defects in the X-linked gene that encodes the androgen receptor cause a spectrum of syndromes of incomplete virilization in 46,XY men who have testes and male testosterone levels but who are resistant to their own and to exogenous androgens (see Chapter 22). In the most severe form, affected individuals are phenotypic women with testicular feminization. If the impairment of receptor function is less complete, the phenotype is that of men with Reifenstein's syndrome (hypospadias and gynecomastia) or men with undervirilization or infertility, or both.[117]

Women with complete testicular feminization and men with Reifenstein's syndrome have normal or elevated production

A. DEFICIENT TESTOSTERONE FORMATION

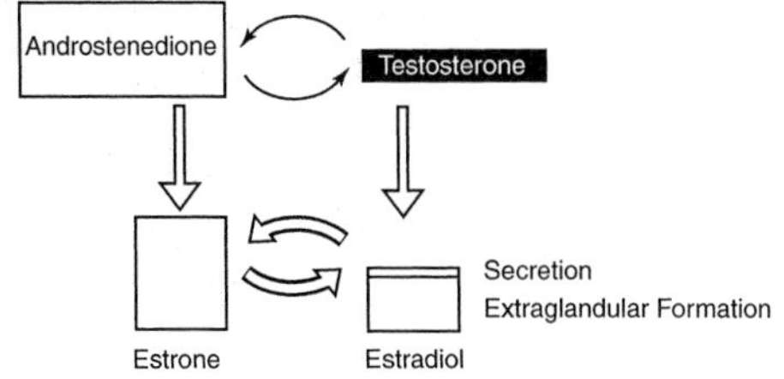

Examples: Congenital anorchia
Defects in testosterone synthesis
Testicular failure

B. INCREASED ESTROGEN SECRETION

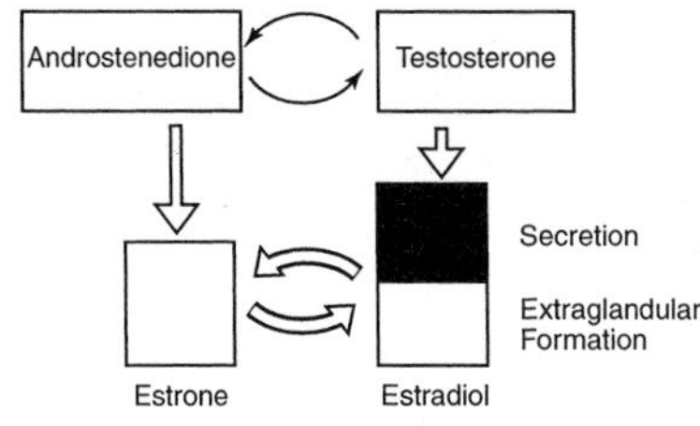

Examples: Leydig cell and Sertoli cell tumors
True hermaphroditism
HCG-secreting tumors

C. INCREASED EXTRAGLANDULAR ESTROGEN FORMATION – INCREASED SUBSTRATE

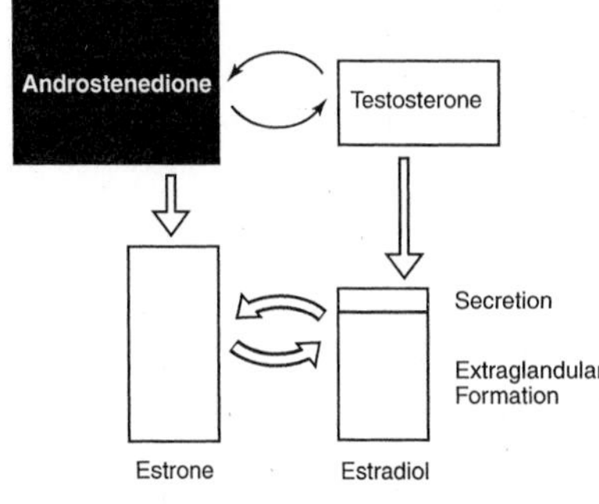

Examples: Adrenal tumors
Congenital adrenal hyperplasia
17β-HSD 3 deficiency

D. INCREASED EXTRAGLANDULAR ESTROGEN FORMATION – INCREASED AROMATASE ENZYME

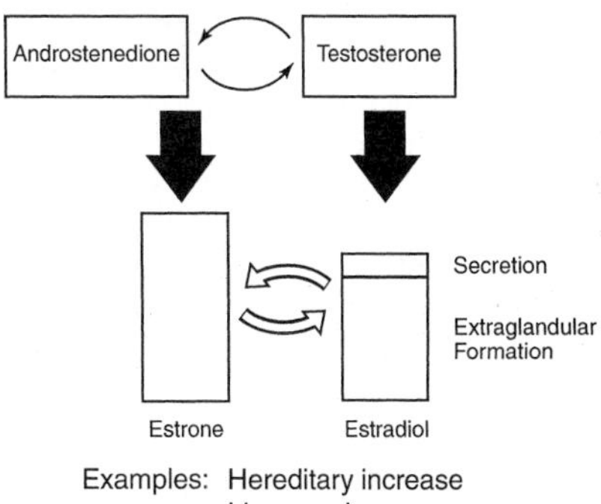

Examples: Hereditary increase
Liver carcinoma
Obesity

Figure 18–18. Four different patterns of abnormal androgen-estrogen dynamics can result in the development of gynecomastia. The altered component in each pattern is highlighted in *black*, and specific examples of each type of abnormality are listed at the *bottom* of each panel. Details of normal androgen-estrogen dynamics are shown in Figure 18–8. HCG, human chorionic gonadotropin; HSD, hydroxysteroid dehydrogenase.

rates for testosterone and estradiol, presumably because of increased secretion by the testes in response to elevated plasma gonadotropin levels (Fig. 18–18*B*).[117] FSH and LH levels are elevated because of resistance at the hypothalamic-pituitary level to negative-feedback control by testosterone. However, there is no direct relation between the rates of estrogen secretion in these disorders and the degree of feminization that results, probably because the degree of feminization is influenced by other factors such as the severity of the androgen resistance and the variable elevation of plasma androgen levels.

Defects in Testosterone Synthesis. Five inherited defects impair testosterone synthesis and prevent normal virilization of the male embryo (see Chapter 22). Each of the defects involves a critical biochemical step in the conversion of cholesterol to testosterone. The completeness of the defects and the severity of clinical manifestations vary, but gynecomastia is common in two of the disorders, 3β-HSDII deficiency and 17β-HSDIII deficiency.

Feminization in these disorders can arise from more than one mechanism. For example, normal or low levels of plasma estrogen can cause feminization in the presence of diminished androgen production,[535] analogous to the situation in congenital anorchia. Alternatively, estrogen production may be increased because of increased availability for extragonadal aromatization of steroids such as androstenedione that accumulate proximal to the enzymatic block.[536] Partial deficiency of 17β-HSDIII and late-onset 3β-HSDII deficiency are rare causes of gynecomastia in otherwise phenotypically normal men.

Testicular Failure

Viral orchitis is the most common cause of testicular failure after puberty, and mumps is the most frequent etiology (see earlier). In men with gynecomastia and bilateral testicular atrophy related to orchitis, testosterone production is severely impaired, whereas production of estradiol and estrone is normal, arising almost entirely from extraglandular sources[326] (Fig. 18–18*A*).

The second most common cause of acquired testicular atrophy in the adult is *trauma*, and gynecomastia can result.[537] Trauma to the testes can be associated with elevated levels of plasma estradiol many years later.[537] *Neurologic disease*, including *myotonic dystrophy* and *spinal cord injury*, can also cause testicular atrophy.[538] Testicular atrophy, decreased plasma testosterone levels, elevated gonadotropin levels, and gynecomastia are also common in *leprosy*.[539]

Gynecomastia is present in approximately half of men undergoing hemodialysis for *renal failure*.[357, 540] Plasma LH and FSH levels are elevated, the plasma testosterone level is low, and plasma prolactin levels are elevated. Estradiol levels may also be high (see earlier).

Increased Estrogen Production

Estrogen production in men can increase because of (1) increased testicular secretion, (2) increased availability of substrate for extraglandular formation, or (3) increased activity of extraglandular aromatase itself.

Increased Testicular Estrogen Secretion (see Fig. 18–18*B*)

Testicular Tumors. Testicular tumors can feminize in three ways.

First, germinal cell tumors (*embryonal carcinomas, choriocarcinomas, teratomas,* and rarely *seminomas*) can produce hCG or fragments of hCG, which can act in uninvolved areas of the testes to stimulate the synthesis of estradiol and testosterone,[494] which in turn suppress plasma LH and FSH.

Second, stromal cell tumors (*Leydig* and *Sertoli cell tumors*) can secrete testosterone and estradiol autonomously. About 20% of men with Leydig cell tumors have gynecomastia,[541] and gynecomastia may be even more common with Sertoli cell tumors.[498, 509, 542] Feminization can occur before such tumors are detectable by physical examination, but even small tumors can usually be identified by ultrasonography.[543, 544] Similarly, in choriocarcinomas[545] and in hepatocellular carcinomas,[546] aromatase in the tumor tissue can convert circulating adrenal and testicular androgens to estrogens.

Third, some Sertoli cell tumors stimulate adjacent Leydig cells to secrete androgens that serve as substrate for aromatase in the tumor cells.[547] (See earlier for discussion of diagnosis and management of testicular tumors.)

Bronchogenic Carcinoma. Lung cancer can cause an increase in hCG levels in plasma, and gynecomastia in this condition correlates with the amount of estradiol secreted by the testes.[548] Indeed, hCG secretion by any tumor, such as by *transitional cell tumors* of the urinary tract, can cause feminization.[549]

True Hermaphroditism. In true hermaphroditism (see Chapter 22), both the ovarian and the testicular components of the gonads are endocrinologically active and cause a mixed pattern of feminization and virilization at puberty.[550] Gynecomastia is due to gonadal estrogen secretion (see Fig. 18–18*B*), presumably by the ovarian elements of the ovotestes.[550]

Increased Substrate for Peripheral Aromatase (see Fig. 18–18*C*)

Adrenal Disease. In *feminizing adrenal carcinoma,* estrogen production is usually due to massive increases in the levels of the adrenal androgens androstenedione and DHEA, which serve as substrates for extraglandular aromatization. In rare instances, adrenal tumors secrete estrogen.[551, 552] Feminization in boys with *congenital adrenal hyperplasia* (as in CYP21 or CYP11A2 deficiency) is usually the consequence of increased production of androstenedione by the adrenal glands and hence of increased substrate for peripheral aromatase.[553, 554] In some instances, decreased testosterone levels may play a role in the gynecomastia.[555] Increased androstenedione is also the usual cause of feminization in men with *17β-HSDIII deficiency.*[536]

Androgen Administration. Administration of testosterone to children commonly causes gynecomastia, correlating with an increase in estrogens, whereas replacement with conventional doses in adult men increases plasma estradiol but rarely causes gynecomastia.[556] In contrast, testosterone administration to men with impaired liver function can cause profound increases in plasma estrogen levels. In addition, administration of supraphysiologic amounts of aromatizable androgens can increase estradiol levels as much as sevenfold in normal men,[557] and gynecomastia is common in users of anabolic steroids.[558, 559] In probing patients' histories for possible causes of gynecomastia, it should be remembered that some androgens are not aromatizable or are weak substrates for the enzyme (see the following).

Liver Disease. Liver disease is a common cause of feminization. Gynecomastia is thought to be largely a result of overproduction of estrogen. However, the liver is not the direct source of the estrogens, which are mainly due to decreased hepatic catabolism of androstenedione and the consequent increased availability of androstenedione for extrasplanchnic aromatization.[560] In carcinoma of the liver, feminization can be the consequence of increased aromatase activity in the tumor itself.[561]

Starvation. Gynecomastia was common in American prisoners of war during World War II.[562] About a third of the cases occurred during refeeding after release, other instances were associated with temporary improvements in the food supply during imprisonment, and most regressed within a few months. The pathophysiology of starvation gynecomastia may be similar to that with liver disease (see earlier).

Thyrotoxicosis. Thyrotoxicosis can cause gynecomastia.[563] Elevation of plasma estradiol levels is probably due to increased androstenedione production rates and increased formation of estrogen in extraglandular sites.[564, 565]

Increase in Extraglandular Aromatase (see Fig. 18–18*D*)

Increased activity of aromatase enzymes in peripheral tissues[566–568] can increase estrogen production as much as 50-fold,[566] and in at least one family the trait appeared to be inherited in an autosomal dominant pattern through three generations, being manifested in females by precocious puberty and macromastia and in males by gynecomastia.[568] A characteristic feature is that the onset of gynecomastia correlates with the onset of adrenarche and occurs before the time of normal puberty. A similar trait is present in the Sebright bantam chicken, in which an autosomal dominant gene increases extraglandular aromatization more than 100-fold.[569]

Drugs

Drugs can cause gynecomastia by direct action as estrogens, by enhancement of testicular production of estrogens, by inhibition of testosterone synthesis or action, or by unknown mechanisms.

Estrogens and Estrogen Mimetics

Estrogens given to men in any form can cause gynecomastia, as in the treatment of prostatic cancer with diethylstilbestrol[570] and of transsexual men with estrogens.[571] Young men and boys are particularly sensitive to estrogens, and gynecomastia can develop as a result of industrial exposure or dermal ointments containing estrogens.[572] Identifying the source may require a high index of suspicion, as in the case of a barber who massaged the scalps of customers with ointment containing estrogen,[573] factory workers who manufacture oral contraceptives,[574] children of workers in a diethylstilbestrol manufacturing plant who absorbed the drug from the clothing of their fathers,[575] and offspring of women who use topical estrogen preparations.[576] Sufficient estrogen to induce gynecomastia can be absorbed by men during sexual intercourse with partners who use vaginal creams containing estrogen.[577] In the United States, no federal regulations cover estrogens in cosmetics, and estradiol levels may be as high as 18 ng/g in creams and 50 mg/dL in lotions.[578]

Epidemics of gynecomastia among children have resulted from the ingestion of milk or meat from estrogen-treated cows,[579] raising the possibility that long-term exposure to small amounts of estrogens may be a cause of idiopathic gynecomastia. Sources may include meat and dairy products from animals treated with estrogens other than diethylstilbestrol,[580] endogenous estrogens in animal tissues,[581] or plant or fungal estrogens in foods.[582]

About 10% of men given digitalis for a year had gynecomastia[583]; however, abnormal liver function is common in such men, and gynecomastia is said to correlate better with congestive heart failure than with administration of digitalis.[584] Nevertheless, digitalis preparations associated with gynecomastia also have estrogenic effects on the vaginal epithelium in postmenopausal women.[585] Digitalis binds to the estrogen receptor and may act as a direct estrogen agonist.[586]

Drugs That Enhance Endogenous Estrogen Formation

Administration of hCG can cause gynecomastia as a consequence of increased estradiol secretion by the testes.[587] Clomiphene citrate (both an estrogen agonist and antagonist) has been used to treat gynecomastia in boys, but paradoxically it can cause gynecomastia on withdrawal, presumably by increasing LH secretion and consequently increasing estradiol secretion by the testes.[588]

Drugs That Inhibit Testosterone Synthesis or Action

The antifungal drug ketoconazole and other imidazoles block steroid hormone synthesis.[589] The inhibition of steroid synthesis by ketoconazole is transient, and plasma testosterone values return to normal after blood levels of the drug fall. Gynecomastia occurs only if the drug causes prolonged lowering of plasma androgen levels.[590] Gynecomastia is presumably due to altered ratios of estradiol to testosterone.[591]

Antineoplastic agents can cause long-term impairment of testosterone synthesis, presumably through toxic effects on Leydig cells; such damage may occur when the therapy is for systemic neoplasms (e.g., alkylating agents for Hodgkin's disease) or for testicular cancers.[592] The cause of gynecomastia has not been elucidated, but it may be due to elevated plasma gonadotropin levels secondary to testicular damage and enhancement of testicular estrogen synthesis.[592]

Gynecomastia is common in men treated with spironolactone.[593] At low doses, the drug prevents the binding of androgen to its receptor, and at high dose it inhibits testosterone synthesis.[331, 594]

Antiandrogens, including *cyproterone*, *flutamide*, *zanoterone*, and *bicalutamide*, inhibit testosterone binding to the receptor and can cause gynecomastia.[595–598] Gynecomastia is a common side effect of treatment with *cimetidine*,[599] which also blocks the binding of androgen to the androgen receptor and may inhibit the catabolism of estradiol.[600] Gynecomastia is less common in subjects receiving ranitidine. Suggestive evidence for induction of gynecomastia by an environmental antiandrogen has come from studies of an epidemic of temporary gynecomastia that affected Haitian refugees in five detention centers in the United States in 1981.[601] The delousing agent used in these centers binds to the androgen receptor and acts as an antiandrogen in rats.[602] All antiandrogens are believed to impair the feedback control of gonadotropin production and cause elevation of plasma LH, which in turn increases estradiol secretion from the testes.

Drugs That Act by Unknown Mechanisms

A variety of drugs cause gynecomastia by unknown mechanisms. For example, gynecomastia occurred in boys and in men given human growth hormone.[603, 604] Many drugs are associated with gynecomastia with a frequency that is probably not coincidental; these include busulfan, calcium channel–blocking agents, angiotensin-converting enzyme inhibitors, diazepam, isoniazid, methyldopa, omeprazole, penicillamine, tricyclic antidepressants, and a variety of antiviral agents, particularly protease inhibitors used for the treatment of HIV.[605–612] Some of these agents may act by altering liver function. Both marijuana and heroin are suspected causes of gynecomastia, but a direct causal relation has not been established.[613, 614]

Idiopathic Gynecomastia

In all published series, 50% or more of subjects evaluated for gynecomastia did not have an endocrine or drug cause identifiable at autopsy[615] or by laboratory evaluation.[616] If one adds the instances in which the designated cause is tenuous, the idiopathic category may account for 75% of cases. It is not known whether men with idiopathic gynecomastia are in fact normal (as proposed by Nuttall[515]), whether a feminizing factor had been transiently present but had disappeared at the time of evaluation, whether the gynecomastia is due to long-term exposure to small amounts of one or more environmental estrogens or antiandrogens, or whether the gynecomastia is the consequence of subtle, unrecognized endocrine disease.

The extent to which minor endocrine disorders are not recognized with current methodologies is uncertain. The fact that gynecomastia can develop as the result of subtle environmental exposure to estrogens or antiandrogens (as described earlier) raises the possibility that a large fraction of idiopathic gynecomastia may be the consequence of unrecognized exposure to endocrine disruptors.[602] The critical clinical point is that, whatever the cause, the diagnosis of idiopathic gynecomastia carries no known import related to health.

Lack of Role of Prolactin in Gynecomastia

Plasma prolactin levels are usually normal in men with gynecomastia of diverse causes, and men who have prolonged elevation in plasma prolactin secondary to use of psychotropic drugs do not commonly have gynecomastia.[617, 618] Consequently, prolactin is not believed to play a direct role in the disorder. This conclusion is in keeping with the fact that prolactin is not a growth hormone for the breast. Furthermore, when gynecomastia develops in men with prolactin-secreting tumors of the pituitary gland and high plasma prolactin levels or in men taking psychotropic agents, the gynecomastia is probably the consequence of secondary testicular failure as a result either of the effects of the tumor mass or of inhibition of LH secretion by prolactin.

Diagnosis

The dilemma is to distinguish men with significant endocrine disease from those with idiopathic gynecomastia. In general, only men with symptomatic gynecomastia are evaluated; however, if there is a question about whether the gynecomastia is real, the issue is best solved by mammography or ultrasonography.[518, 519]

Most of the known causes of gynecomastia can be identified by a work-up that includes the following:

1. A careful drug history that encompasses potential environmental and indirect exposures to endocrine substances.
2. A detailed physical examination including the testes (the finding of small testes bilaterally suggests testicular insufficiency, and asymmetrical testes raise the possibility of testicular tumors).
3. Evaluation of liver function.
4. A limited endocrine work-up, including (a) measurement of plasma DHEAS or urinary 17-ketosteroids (usually elevated in adrenal feminizing states), (b) measurement of plasma estradiol (helpful if elevated but usually normal), (c) assessment of plasma hCGβ (sometimes elevated with testicular tumors), and (d) measurement of plasma LH and testosterone.*

If these parameters are normal, as is frequently the case, the usual recourse is to observe the patient without treatment. If the symptoms persist or worsen and if the enlargement is progressive, a more extensive evaluation may have to be undertaken.

Treatment

The difficulty in treating gynecomastia is inherent in its natural history. If the feminizing process persists for a long period, the initial glandular hyperplasia is replaced by progressive fibrosis and hyalinization that do not regress after the source of excess estrogen is corrected.[522] Consequently, surgery remains the mainstay of therapy and is frequently indicated for psychological and cosmetic reasons. Such surgery is usually accomplished through a circumareolar approach.[619]

Medical management is most successful when it is addressed to gynecomastia of recent onset or to prevention of its development. Testosterone administration has inconsistent effects in Klinefelter's syndrome but can cause dramatic improvement in other forms of testicular failure (e.g., anorchia, viral orchitis).

Several drugs have been tried for gynecomastia, including the antiestrogens tamoxifen[620] and clomiphene,[621] the aromatase inhibitor testolactone,[622] and danazol,[623] a weak androgen that inhibits gonadotropin secretion. In one study, tamoxifen was about twice as effective in treating idiopathic gynecomastia as danazol[624]; in another study, tamoxifen was uniformly effective in treating the gynecomastia induced by antiandrogen treatment in men with prostatic carcinoma.[625] Treatment with dihydrotestosterone (which cannot be aromatized to estrogen) was also reported to provide symptomatic improvement.[626]

Perhaps the most effective therapy for gynecomastia is to prevent its development by radiating the breasts before the institution of estrogen therapy in men with prostatic carcinoma[627] or of antiandrogen therapy in male sex offenders.[628] This therapy is about 90% effective, and the complication rate is low.

Impairment of Estrogen Formation or Action

The study of men with single-gene mutations that impair estrogen formation or action has provided insight into the role of estrogen in male physiology.[138, 629] These forms of estrogen deficiency are rare, but the fact that the phenotypes in the two disorders are similar establishes the importance of this role.

Aromatase Deficiency

Aromatase deficiency is the consequence of autosomal recessive loss-of-function mutations in the CYP19 gene.[56, 630] In the two reported men with this disorder, childhood development was considered normal but skeletal growth continued into the 20s despite pubertal maturation and resulted in tall stature. This growth pattern was associated with failure of epiphyseal closure, marked delay in bone age, and osteopenia.

One man had undetectable estrogen in plasma and elevated levels of testosterone, dihydrotestosterone, and gonadotropins; testicular volume was normal, and semen analysis was declined.[56] The other affected man was evaluated because of tall stature, infertility, and skeletal pain associated with severe osteopenia; the testicular volume was 8 mL bilaterally, the sperm density was very low with many immotile sperm, and testicular biopsy revealed a maturation arrest at the spermatocyte stage.[630] The etiology of the infertility in the latter patient was not clear because a brother was infertile in the presence of a normal CYP19 gene, suggesting that the infertility in this family may be due to some other disorder. The man responded dramatically to estradiol therapy with an increase in bone density to the normal range, resolution of bone pain, and lowering of elevated levels of total and LDL cholesterol and triglycerides.[630]

These men had different homozygous missense mutations in the CYP19 gene that caused single amino acid substitutions and resulted in the formation of mutant enzymes with 0.2% to 0.4% of the activity of normal enzyme.[56, 630]

Estrogen Receptor α Deficiency

An autosomal recessive, loss-of-function mutation in the estrogen receptor α gene has been described in a man with tall stature, unfused epiphyses, osteopenia, and acanthosis nigricans.[55] Virilization was normal, and he had a normal level of plasma testosterone. Plasma levels of estradiol, estrone, FSH, and LH were elevated, and semen analysis revealed a normal sperm density but decreased sperm motility. Serum lipoprotein levels were normal, but the presence of hyperinsulinemia and impaired glucose tolerance indicated insulin resistance. He did not respond to treatment with high-dose, transdermal estradiol sufficient to raise the plasma free estradiol 10-fold above normal, as indicated by no change in plasma gonadotropins or in bone density after 6 months. He was homozygous for a missense mutation in exon 2 of the estrogen receptor α gene that resulted in a premature termination codon and hence precluded the formation of functional receptor.

In summary, the evidence from these rare disorders of estrogen formation and action indicates that estrogen plays a major role in controlling skeletal maturation and both the accrual and maintenance of bone mass in men. In both conditions, there was no pubertal spurt in growth; growth was instead steady and continued in association with failure of epiphyseal closure. Despite testosterone levels that were normal or increased, gonadotropin levels were elevated. These findings are in accord with studies of aromatase inhibitors, which indicate that estrogens are important for feedback control of gonadotropin secretion at the level of the pituitary and the hypothalamus.[631] Abnormalities of carbohydrate and lipid metabolism in these patients appear to be inconsistent. The fact that gender identity and gender role behavior are male in both conditions indicates that estrogen does not play a critical role on these parameters.[629]

*High LH and normal or low testosterone levels suggest testicular insufficiency; low LH and low testosterone levels suggest hypopituitarism, estrogen secretion from a tumor, or an exogenous source of estrogen; and high LH and high testosterone levels suggest androgen resistance).

HORMONAL THERAPY

Androgen Therapy

When administered by mouth, testosterone is absorbed into the portal blood and degraded by the liver so that only a small fraction reaches the systemic circulation. Parenterally injected testosterone is also rapidly absorbed and degraded. As a consequence, effective androgen therapy requires either administration of testosterone in a slowly absorbed form (transdermal or micronized oral preparations) or administration of chemically modified analogues. Such chemical alterations either retard absorption or catabolism to maintain effective blood levels or enhance the androgenic potency of each molecule so that physiologic effects can be achieved at a lower plasma level of drug.

Three general types of modification of testosterone are clinically useful:

1. Esterification of the 17β-hydroxyl group (type A).
2. Alkylation at the 17α position (type B).
3. Modification of the A, B, or C rings, particularly substitutions at the 1, 2, 9, and 11 carbons (type C) (Fig. 18–19).

Most agents actually contain combinations of ring structure alterations and either 17α alkylation or esterification of the 17β-hydroxyl group.

Esterification of testosterone with various carboxylic acids decreases the polarity of the steroid, makes it more soluble in the fat vehicles that are used for injection, and hence slows release of the injected steroid into the circulation.[632] The esters of 19-nortestosterone have particularly slow release and turnover rates.[381] The longer the carbon chain in the ester, the more fat soluble the steroid becomes and hence the more prolonged the action. For example, testosterone propionate must be injected daily, whereas testosterone cypionate and testosterone enanthate can be administered every 2 or 3 weeks.[633] Even more slowly hydrolyzed esters are under investigation, such as testosterone buciclate, which is administered every 12 weeks,[634] and testosterone undecanoate, which is administered every 6 weeks.[635] Testosterone cypionate or enanthate was for many years the treatment of choice for male hypogonadism.

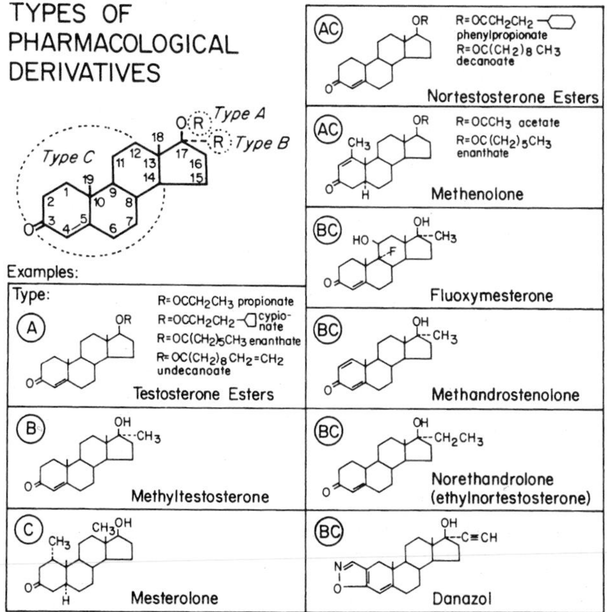

Figure 18–19. Types of androgen preparations available for clinical use. Type A derivatives are esterified in the 17β position. Type B steroids have alkyl substitutions in the 17α position. Type C derivatives involve a variety of alterations of ring structure that enhance activity, impede catabolism, or influence both functions. Most androgen preparations involve combinations of type AC or type BC changes.

Although testosterone esters can be detected in plasma, they must be hydrolyzed before the hormone acts so that the effectiveness of therapy can be monitored by assaying the plasma level of testosterone after administration. Most esters must be injected, but two—methenolone acetate and testosterone undecanoate—can be administered by mouth. Testosterone undecanoate is absorbed through the lymphatic system into the systemic circulation, and physiologic blood levels of testosterone can be achieved at doses of approximately 120 mg/day.[636] Because of rapid turnover, testosterone undecanoate must be administered two to three times a day.[637] The reason for the oral effectiveness of methenolone acetate (and of mesterolone) is not entirely clear.[638]

The use of transdermal testosterone formulations makes it possible to sustain serum testosterone levels in the normal male range while avoiding the necessity for parenteral administration. These formulations include a scrotal patch, two nonscrotal patches, and a gel. The scrotal patch Testoderm is designed to deliver either 4 or 6 mg of testosterone over 24 hours and takes advantage of the fact that absorption across the scrotal skin is efficient in the absence of permeation enhancers.[639] After application in the morning, serum levels peak in 2 to 3 hours and are maintained throughout the day.

The nonscrotal patches, Androderm and Testoderm TTS, differ in recommended application sites and times to peak serum levels, but both provide physiologic testosterone levels throughout the day.[640–642] Androderm, available in 2.5- and 5-mg doses, is applied at bedtime; peak levels are achieved in 8 hours, and the application site must be rotated to avoid skin irritation. Testoderm TTS delivers 5 mg of testosterone from a larger surface area, is applied in the morning, results in a maximal serum level in 2 to 3 hours, and appears to cause minimal skin irritation.[641] In a randomized comparative study, Androderm therapy did not cause the temporary supraphysiologic levels of estradiol and of total and bioavailable testosterone that occur after injections of testosterone enanthate.[642] The transdermal preparation resulted in more normal testosterone levels, less frequent suppression of plasma LH, and less frequent elevation of plasma hemoglobin levels.[642]

A transdermal 1% testosterone gel has been developed for the application of 50 to 100 mg of testosterone to the shoulders or abdomen each morning, the usual dose being 50 mg.[643, 644] The absorption of testosterone appears to be largely independent of the surface area to which it is applied, and steady-state serum levels are achieved within a few days. The hands must be washed carefully after each application to avoid inadvertent transmission of the hormone, but the application site should not be washed for 6 hours to maintain absorption efficiency. Application site skin-to-skin transfer may occur with close physical contact. In comparison with the 5-mg nonscrotal patch, 50 mg of testosterone gel causes somewhat higher serum testosterone levels.[644]

Administration of a 5-mg preparation of testosterone cyclodextrin sublingually three times a day also results in normal plasma testosterone levels in hypogonadal men.[645] 17α-Alkylated androgens, such as methyltestosterone and methandrostenolone, are effective by mouth because alkylated steroids are absorbed into the portal circulation, are slowly catabolized by the liver, and reach the systemic circulation in effective amounts. For this reason, 17α-methyl or 17α-ethyl substitution is present in most orally active androgens. Because 17α-alkylated androgens are believed to act within the cell as such (i.e., the alkyl groups are not removed), because assays are not routinely available for monitoring blood levels, and because they can cause abnormal liver function, these steroids have a limited role in medicine.[646]

Other alterations of the ring structure either alter the metabolism or enhance the potency of a given molecule. For example, the potency of fluoxymesterone, 19-nortestosterone, and 1-methyl–substituted steroids may be enhanced because they are poor precursors for estrogen formation in extraglandular tissues.[647] Similarly, 19-nortestosterone is a more potent androgen than testosterone because its more planar ring structure, like that of dihydrotestosterone, fits more tightly into the binding site of the androgen receptor.[648] 7α-Methyl-19-nortestosterone cannot be 5α-reduced and may be useful when androgen replacement is needed with minimal effects on the prostate.[649, 650]

As with 17α-alkylated steroids, androgens with ring alterations are not converted to testosterone in vivo, and specific assays for each must be used to monitor blood levels. One orally effective androgen, mesterolone, is neither esterified nor alkylated in the 17α position and cannot be aromatized to estrogens in peripheral tissues. Consequently, effective androgen replacement can be achieved by oral administration without causing abnormalities of liver function; unfortunately, the steroid is ineffective in regulating gonadotropin secretion and consequently is a poor agent for routine androgen replacement therapy.[638]

The subcutaneous implantation of testosterone-filled silicone elastomer (Silastic) capsules results in slow release of hormone into plasma for long periods,[651] but this mode is impractical because of the large size of such capsules. When large amounts of testosterone are given by mouth in microparticulate form (200 to 400 mg/day), physiologic blood levels can be achieved, but the preparation has to be taken several times a day[652] and these doses induce hepatic drug-metabolizing enzymes, the long-term effects of which are uncertain.[653]

Androgens for Normal Men

When the plasma testosterone level is raised above the normal range, both the basal levels of LH and FSH and the peak levels after GnRH administration are diminished. As a consequence, the testicular volume is decreased about 20%, sperm production is uniformly decreased by 90% or more, and the volume of the ejaculate remains unchanged.[654, 655] Acne is common, and the serum estradiol level increases twofold.[654]

Administration of usual replacement doses of testosterone enanthate (100 mg/week) to normal men caused significant decreases in truncal and total body fat and increases in BMD in the spine,[656, 657] effects that are probably the consequence of the temporary increases in testosterone levels above the normal range after the injections. Administration of six times this dose (600 mg/week) of testosterone enanthate to normal men caused an increase in fat-free body mass, triceps and quadriceps muscle size, and muscle strength.[658, 659]

In a similar study, there was no change in levels of prostate-specific antigen (PSA).[660] In a dose-response study in healthy young men, testosterone enanthate caused increases in fat-free body mass, muscle strength, and hemoglobin levels and decreases in fat mass and HDL cholesterol levels, beginning with a dose that was just above replacement levels (125 mg/week).[661] Sexual function, visual-spatial cognition, mood, and PSA levels did not change at any dose.[661]

Androgens for Hypogonadal Men

The aim of androgen therapy in hypogonadal men is to restore or normalize male secondary sexual characteristics (beard, body hair, external genitalia) and male sexual behavior and to promote normal male somatic development (hemoglobin, voice, muscle mass, nitrogen balance, and epiphyseal closure). Because a reliable assay for plasma testosterone is widely available for monitoring therapy, the treatment of androgen deficiency is straightforward and almost universally successful. The parenteral administration of a long-acting testosterone ester, such as 100 to 300 mg of testosterone enanthate at 1- to 3-week intervals, results in a sustained increase in plasma testosterone concentration to the normal male range or slightly above.[314, 633, 642] The usual replacement regimen is 200 mg every 2 weeks.[633] Similar effects are obtained with the transcutaneous administration of testosterone.[640, 642, 644]

Such regimens usually reduce the plasma LH level (if elevated) and maintain serum testosterone within the normal range.[633] Serum testosterone should be measured after 4 to 6 weeks of therapy to assess adequacy of dosage; the trough level is measured in men receiving intramuscular testosterone, and midmorning levels are assessed in men receiving transdermal formulations. If the hypogonadism is primary and of long duration (as in Klinefelter's syndrome), suppression of the plasma LH value to the normal range may not occur for many weeks, if at all.[314] In postpubertal testicular failure, even of many years' duration, resumption of normal sexual activity is usual after adequate replacement, primarily because of increased libido[662] and increased frequency of erections.[663]

Androgen therapy does not restore spermatogenesis in hypogonadal states, but the volume of the ejaculate, derived largely from the prostate and seminal vesicles, and other secondary sexual characteristics return to normal. Treatment of hypogonadal men with testosterone results in growth of the prostate to the same degree as that of age-matched controls.[664] Testosterone replacement in such men can cause dramatic changes in body composition, strength, and BMD, although maximal effects may not be seen for as long as 2 years.[665–670] Improvement in BMD involves both trabecular and cortical bone and is independent of the age at which replacement is started.[670]

In men of all ages in whom hypogonadism develops before expected puberty (such as in hypogonadotropic hypogonadism), it is appropriate to bring plasma testosterone into the adult range slowly. When therapy is begun at the time of expected puberty, the normal events of male puberty proceed in the usual fashion. If therapy is delayed until after the time of usual puberty, the degree of virilization is variable, but many such men undergo a late but relatively complete anatomic and functional male maturation (Fig. 18–20). Intermittent androgen therapy is sometimes given to prepubertal hypogonadal boys with microphallus to stimulate penile growth[183, 284] (also see Chapter 22), and such therapy does not appear to have an adverse effect on final penile size.[671] If patients are monitored closely and androgen is given for only short periods, such therapy also probably has no effect on somatic growth.

In boys of pubertal age with either isolated hypogonadotropic hypogonadism or primary testicular deficiency, the initial administration of small doses of testosterone esters followed by a gradual increase to doses of 100 to 150 mg/m^2 of body surface area per month results in a normal pubertal growth spurt.[672] Penile growth, deepening of the voice, and appearance of other secondary sexual characteristics usually commence during the first year of treatment. Puberty in normal boys extends over several years, and treatment that is designed to replicate normal development cannot shorten the process greatly (see Chapter 24).

The usual practice in hypogonadal boys is to institute androgen therapy between the ages 12 and 14 years, depending on their subjective need for sexual development. Testosterone exerts its full action only in the presence of a balanced hormonal environment and particularly in the presence of adequate levels of growth hormone. Consequently, hypogonadal boys with coexisting growth hormone deficiency have a dimin-

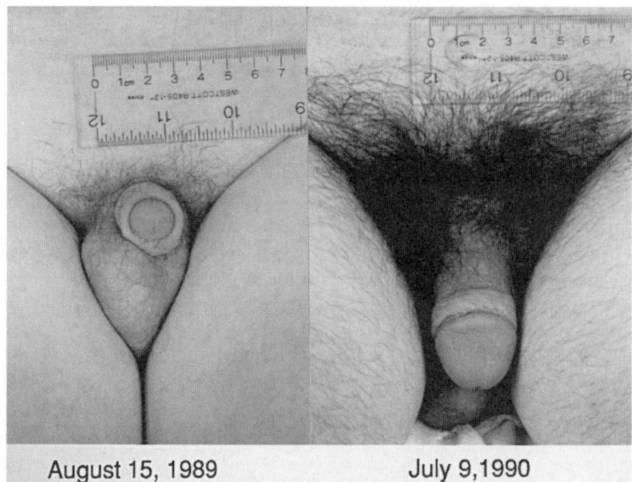

Figure 18–20. Effect on penile size of 200 mg of testosterone cypionate intramuscularly every 2 weeks for 11 months in a previously untreated 22-year-old man with microphallus caused by hypogonadotropic hypogonadism. (From Griffin JE, Wilson JD. Disorders of sexual differentiation. In Walsh PC, Retik AB, Stamey TA, et al [eds]. Campbell's Urology, 6th ed. Philadelphia, WB Saunders, 1992, pp 1509–1542.)

ished response to androgens in regard to both growth and the development of secondary sexual characteristics unless growth hormone is given simultaneously.[672, 673] As noted earlier, the promotion of growth by testosterone is the consequence of enhanced secretion of growth hormone and IGF-I.[199, 674]

The presence of prostate or breast cancer is a contraindication to androgen therapy, and men older than 50 should be screened for preexisting prostate cancer by digital rectal examination and measurement of the serum PSA level. Indeed, in men with severe hypogonadism, biopsy can reveal occult prostate cancers in which PSA levels are not elevated because of androgen deficiency.[675] Consequently, older men should have a repeated digital rectal examination and PSA measurement within 2 to 3 months of initiation of testosterone therapy and at 6- to 12-month intervals thereafter.

Androgen replacement does not cause an increase in prostate size or PSA level above that of age-matched men,[664] and benign prostatic hyperplasia is not a contraindication to androgen replacement. However, switching androgen replacement from testosterone esters to transdermal testosterone causes lowering of PSA levels,[676] suggesting that more physiologic levels of testosterone provide less stimulation to the prostate. The presence of polycythemia or obstructive sleep apnea may be a relative contraindication to testosterone therapy (see "Toxic Side Effects" following).

Androgens for Healthy Older Men with Decreased Bioavailable Testosterone Levels

Because many of the changes in body composition, libido, and erectile function with aging also occur with male hypogonadism, androgen administration has been evaluated in healthy older men. The criterion for inclusion in such studies is a low level of total testosterone or of bioavailable (non–SHBG-bound) testosterone.

In one study of older men with a total serum testosterone less than 14 nmol/L (<420 ng/dL), administration of testosterone enanthate at 100 mg/week returned plasma testosterone levels to normal, increased lean body mass and hemoglobin levels, and decreased total and LDL cholesterol levels.[677] In another study of men with low levels of bioavailable testosterone, treatment with testosterone enanthate at 200 mg every 2 weeks increased muscle strength and hemoglobin levels without increasing PSA levels.[678]

In a larger, long-term placebo-controlled study of older men, the use of a testosterone patch increased BMD significantly in the men with low levels of total testosterone but had minimal effects in men with normal levels of total testosterone.[679, 680] Lean body mass and hemoglobin levels were increased and fat mass was decreased in all men receiving testosterone. The PSA levels increased by 0.5 ng/mL and then were stable after 6 months.

Although these studies suggest that such treatment is beneficial in men with low plasma testosterone, many questions are still unanswered.[681] For example, it will be necessary to perform long-term studies to be certain that the risk-to-benefit ratio is favorable before such treatment can be recommended routinely.

Use of Androgens for Purposes Other Than Replacement Therapy

Administration of testosterone to hypogonadal men has systemic effects in addition to those on the male urogenital tract, including reduction in the urinary excretion of nitrogen, sodium, potassium, and chloride and induction of weight gain. A major component of androgen-induced weight gain and nitrogen retention involves an increase in skeletal and muscle mass. In several species, including humans, the skeletal muscles that support the forelimbs, namely the muscles of the pectoral and shoulder region, show the greatest response, but most muscles probably respond to androgen administration. Such muscles enlarge because of formation of new myofilaments along the myofibrils and because of division of the enlarging myofibrils; the net consequence is an increase in the diameter of muscle fibers and fibrils.[682]

The effects of androgens on muscle and the urogenital tract are not due to different actions of the same hormone but represent the same action in different tissues. It is theoretically possible that a steroid might be devised that would be taken up by or retained selectively by muscle,[683] but no anabolic hormone devoid of androgenic effects has been found. Indeed, all anabolic agents tested in humans so far are also androgens and in appropriate doses could be used for androgen replacement. Androgens have been tried in a variety of clinical situations other than hypogonadism with the hope that improvement in nitrogen balance and muscle development could outweigh any deleterious side effects.

Attempts to Improve Nitrogen Balance in Catabolic States

After injury, infection, or surgery, the breakdown of body protein is accelerated, and as a consequence excess nitrogen is excreted in the urine. During the recovery phase, nitrogen deficits are replaced. Anabolic steroids can improve the nitrogen balance during the first few days after relatively minor operations in well-nourished individuals,[684] but the decrease in nitrogen loss is minimal and does not appear to be of therapeutic benefit. Likewise, any effect of androgens on weight in undernourished, debilitated, or elderly men is complicated by the fact that many such men, including some men with AIDS, also have secondary testosterone deficiency (see earlier).[685]

There is no convincing evidence that testosterone supplementation improves strength or outcome in wasting disorders in the absence of androgen deficiency.[686] Androgens are also of no proven value in the management of nitrogen accumulation in chronic renal failure.

Androgens and Athletic Performance

The use of androgens by athletes who believe that athletic performance will be improved constitutes a widespread form of drug abuse. Weight-lifters and body-builders began to use them in the 1950s, and the practice spread to all levels of athletic competition from high school to professional. Several lines of evidence suggest that androgens may have a beneficial effect on strength:

1. In a meta-analysis of 16 studies in athletes, Elashoff and colleagues[687] concluded that androgen administration to trained athletes results in about 5% improvement in strength.
2. Forbes[688] deduced that administration of a total dose of about 20 g of exogenous androgen causes an increase of about 18 kg of lean body mass.
3. Griggs and colleagues[689] reported that large amounts of testosterone increase muscle protein synthesis and muscle mass in normal men.
4. Bhasin and co-workers[658] showed that pharmacologic amounts of testosterone esters increase lean body mass, muscle size, and strength.

Considered together, these studies support the views of athletes and their trainers that such agents are effective in adult male athletes. Although controlled studies have not been carried out in women and boys, it is clear on the basis of uncontrolled studies in the German Democratic Republic that the agents are even more effective in these groups.[690]

Unfortunately, the side effects of the drugs are also more striking in women and children. The doses of androgens taken by athletes are often 10 to 100 times ordinary replacement doses. At these doses, androgens may promote anabolism by functioning as antagonists to the catabolic effects of glucocorticoids and hence promote nitrogen retention independent of the androgen receptor.

The question of efficacy, interesting though it may be, is independent of the side effects of the drugs. Because many athletes take oral agents such as nandrolone phenpropionate and stanozolol along with testosterone esters by injection, the potential toxic side effects are formidable.

Stimulation of Erythropoiesis

The difference in the hematocrit between men and women is the result of enhancement of erythropoietin formation and erythropoiesis by testosterone. After castration of men, red blood cell mass decreases 10%, red blood cell diameter decreases 40%, and osmotic fragility increases. Occasionally, the resulting anemia may be severe. In normal men given pharmacologic doses of testosterone esters, the average increase in hemoglobin is about 10 g/L (1 g/dL).[654] As a consequence, androgens have been used in the treatment of refractory anemia.[691]

The mechanism by which androgens stimulate erythropoietin formation by the kidneys involves the same receptor mechanism that has been documented for other androgen actions, and all androgens have the capacity to enhance erythropoiesis. In humans, some erythropoietin is synthesized outside the kidneys, and the presence of renal tissue is not an absolute requirement for stimulation of erythropoiesis by androgens.[691, 692] Androgen has been given to treat anemias associated with bone marrow failure but has been used infrequently since erythropoietin became available for therapy.

Occasional dramatic increases in hemoglobin level occur after administration of androgens to individuals with bone marrow failure.[693, 694] In unselected patients who were treated with androgens, approximately 50% appeared to respond.[693] Improvement appears to be more common when the bone marrow is hypoplastic or when there is myelofibrosis than when the marrow is hypercellular. Furthermore, in a prospective randomized trial of androgen therapy in patients with aplastic anemia, the use of oral androgens at high dosages (1 mg/kg body weight per day) was associated with hematologic improvement and increased survival, primarily in the less severe cases.[695]

Androgens have also been used for the anemia of renal failure. Androgen-induced increases in erythropoietin and hemoglobin levels are less marked in the anephric state, as would be expected if the beneficial effect were due to increased erythropoietin formation.[696] In most studies, androgen therapy increased the hemoglobin level (10 to 50 g/L [1 to 5 g/dL]) and red blood cell volume (325 to 350 mL), provided that dialysis was adequate and stores of iron and folate were normal.[697, 698] Whether the benefits of such treatment outweigh the potential adverse effects is unclear,[699] and the use of androgens for this purpose has largely been replaced by erythropoietin therapy.

Hereditary Angioneurotic Edema

In this autosomal dominant disorder, the serum inhibitor of the first component of complement is nonfunctional or absent and unopposed activation of the complement cascade generates factors that enhance the permeability of vessels and produce attacks of angioedema. A variety of 17α-alkylated steroids can increase the activity of the inhibitor in serum and restore the complement components that are depleted secondarily in the disorder.[700–702] Orally active androgens are effective, and steroids such as danazol that are weak androgens appear to be as effective as or more effective than potent androgens.

The response in men and women appears to be the same. Because 17α-alkylated androgens (but not testosterone or testosterone esters) cause elevations of several plasma glycoproteins, including haptoglobin, protein-bound sialic acid, plasminogen, and the inhibitor of the first component of complement,[703, 704] the beneficial effect of oral androgens in this disorder is probably the result of the side effect of 17α-alkylated steroids on liver function rather than androgen action per se. No reports of the effect of testosterone esters in angioneurotic edema have been published.

Short Stature

Androgens have been used in the management of growth retardation of various causes other than pituitary insufficiency. Their administration before the epiphyses close accelerates linear growth, and the mean height age may be advanced more than skeletal age.[705, 706] Administration of androgens for short periods (6 months or less) has no permanent effects on hypothalamic-pituitary or gonadal maturation. The acceleration of growth may be due to increased levels of plasma growth hormone,[707] but such treatment does not appear to increase final height.[708] Indeed, such therapy in short children before the age of 9 years may actually have a deleterious effect on adult height.[706]

Carcinoma of the Breast

See Chapter 39.

Side Effects of Androgens

Some side effects of androgens are due to physiologic actions of the hormones (through the androgen receptor) but in an inappropriate setting. For example, the virilizing actions are desirable in hypogonadal men but undesirable in women and young boys. In some older hypogonadal men, androgen therapy may cause previously unrecognized prostate cancer to become clinically apparent.[709] Other side effects are the results of actions of androgen metabolites, and because different androgens are metabolized differently, the side effects vary. Testosterone can be metabolized to estrogens and can have feminizing as well as virilizing effects, whereas 5α-reduced androgens such as dihydrotestosterone cannot be converted to estrogens and consequently do not have feminizing effects.

Normal people vary in the frequency of side effects, just as there is variability in the degree of virilization of males at puberty. There are also age differences in the occurrence of some side effects. For example, androgens in children may cause premature closure of the epiphyses, may induce gynecomastia, or may produce virilization, even when used in small amounts and for limited periods. The incidence of side effects may also be increased by coexisting clinical conditions. Hepatoma may occur more frequently after androgen treatment of individuals with Fanconi's anemia, sodium retention is worse in patients with congestive heart failure, and feminizing side effects are more prominent in men with hepatic cirrhosis.

A physiologic effect of androgen administration is an increase in the hematocrit, and some men develop polycythemia with such treatment.[710, 711] In one retrospective study, three of nine older men with high hematocrit values had cerebrovascular events after discontinuation of testosterone therapy.[710]

In a randomized study, significant increases in hematocrit values were more common in men given testosterone esters than a testosterone patch and the increase in hematocrit was related to age, bioavailable testosterone levels, and estradiol levels.[642]

Virilizing Side Effects

All androgens involve the risk of virilizing women and children of both sexes.[690, 712, 713] Coarsening of the voice, hirsutism, and menstrual irregularities are common. If treatment is discontinued as soon as these effects are noticed, the manifestations may slowly subside. With prolonged treatment, male-pattern baldness, hirsutism, coarsening of the voice and enlargement of the cricoid cartilage, and hypertrophy of the clitoris become largely irreversible.

Feminizing Side Effects

The feminizing side effects of androgens are poorly understood. Testosterone can be converted (aromatized) in peripheral tissues to estradiol. Although the conversion of all androgen analogues to estrogens has not been documented, it is presumed that most, if not all, C_{19} steroids with a Δ^4,3-keto configuration can be converted to estrogens and that feminization is the effect of estrogenic metabolites of the parent steroids. Administration of testosterone esters to men increases plasma estrogen levels.[654] The most common manifestation of feminization, development of gynecomastia, is unpredictable and in adult men usually occurs only after high-dose androgen therapy. However, in children given androgens, gynecomastia is common (see earlier).

Toxic Side Effects

Some degree of sodium retention is a common consequence of androgen therapy.[654] The amount of retained sodium is usually minor but can cause edema in the presence of underlying heart disease or renal failure.[696]

17α-Alkylated androgens impair liver function as evidenced by elevation of plasma alkaline phosphatase and conjugated bilirubin levels during therapy.[714] Such changes are rare in men given parenteral testosterone esters.[715] The predominant effect on hepatic function appears to be at the site of transport of metabolites from hepatocyte into bile. The clinical consequences of abnormal liver function probably depend on the previous integrity of the liver, but jaundice can occur in the absence of preexisting liver disease because of a hypersensitivity reaction. The changes in liver function induced by 17α-alkylated drugs include increases in a variety of plasma proteins[703, 704] and decreased conjugation of adrenal steroids.[716]

The most serious complications of oral androgen use are development of peliosis hepatis (blood-filled cysts in the liver) and hepatoma. These disorders are more common in patients with aplastic anemia[717, 718] but also occur in persons given oral androgens for other reasons, including hypogonadism.[719–721] Although they are usually benign and regress after discontinuation of the drugs, the tumors may undergo malignant transformation.[722]

Occasional hyperlipidemia has been reported with oral androgens.[723] All androgens including testosterone cause decreases in serum HDL cholesterol levels,[724, 725] and testosterone is the major cause of the differences in serum levels of HDL between men and women.[726] 17α-Alkylated androgens may cause a further suppression of HDL and raise LDL levels,[727] but replacement with physiologic levels of testosterone in hypogonadal men does not suppress HDL cholesterol below levels seen in normal men.[728] Sleep apnea has been reported in occasional men given pharmacologic amounts of testosterone esters,[729] possibly the consequence of increased collapse of the upper airways during sleep.[730] Obese men at risk for sleep apnea should be monitored for related symptoms when receiving testosterone therapy. Priapism has occurred in men treated with testosterone enanthate.[731]

Gonadotropin Therapy

Gonadotropin treatment can establish or restore fertility in men who have gonadotropin deficiency either as an isolated disorder or as a part of more extensive anterior pituitary failure. Because men with hypogonadotropic hypogonadism may become resistant to gonadotropins after long-term treatment (presumably as the result of the development of neutralizing antibodies), the customary strategy is to treat such individuals initially with testosterone esters as described earlier and to reserve gonadotropin therapy until fertility is desired.[732] Prior androgen therapy does not impair subsequent gonadotropin induction of spermatogenesis in men with hypogonadotropic hypogonadism.[733]

Two gonadotropin preparations are available: hMG and hCG. The usual preparation of hMG (menotropins), purified from the urine of postmenopausal women, contains 75 IU of FSH and 75 IU of LH per vial. There are several sources of hCG, which is available in vials containing 5000 to 20,000 IU. The hCG is devoid of FSH activity and resembles LH in its ability to stimulate Leydig cells. Because of the expense of hMG, treatment is usually begun with hCG alone, and hMG is added later to stimulate the FSH-dependent stages of spermatid development.

A high ratio of LH to FSH activity and a long duration of treatment are necessary to bring about the maturation of prepubertal testes.[734] In hypophysectomized adult men with long-term suppression of spermatogenesis, it is not predictable whether administration of preparations with both FSH and LH activities is necessary to initiate spermatogenesis. However, after spermatogenesis has been restored in hypophysectomized patients or initiated in hypogonadotropic hypogonadal men by combined therapy, sperm production can usually be maintained by hCG alone.

In men with hypogonadotropic hypogonadism, the dose of hCG required to maintain a normal plasma testosterone level varies from 1000 to 6000 IU/week. Most regimens for the induction of spermatogenesis involve starting with doses of 2000 IU three times or more a week until most of the clinical parameters, including normal male plasma testosterone values, indicate an optimal effect. During initial treatment, the testis volume may reach only 8 mL. Then hMG is added, with as little as 12.5 IU of FSH being required three times a week to complete the development of spermatogenesis and cause further growth of the testes. Optimal spermatogenesis may require treatment for 12 to 24 months.[734]

In most men with hypogonadotropic hypogonadism and no history of cryptorchidism, such a regimen brings sperm counts to the fertile range[735]; for those in whom sperm production is not sufficient for fertility, in vitro fertilization may be successful.[736] The addition of hMG may not be necessary in individuals with partial hypogonadotropic hypogonadism who presumably have some endogenous FSH secretion. Anti-hCG antibodies may develop after long-term hCG treatment, but development of resistance to the action of the hormone is less common.[737]

Recombinant human FSH (rhFSH) is similarly successful in inducing puberty and spermatogenesis in gonadotropin-deficient adolescent and adult men[738, 739] but is ineffective in the treatment of idiopathic infertility.[740]

Treatment with hCG has been used to attempt to promote permanent descent of inguinal testes into the scrotum. Although there are discrepancies among studies because of varying definitions of cryptorchidism, such therapy appears to be successful in about a fifth of patients and makes it possible to identify unambiguously the cryptorchid boys who should be treated surgically[257] (see earlier). Such therapy is associated with a variety of virilizing and feminizing side effects in boys because of enhancement of the testicular production of estradiol and testosterone (see Chapter 24).

Gonadotropin-Releasing Hormone Therapy

GnRH agonists can produce diametrically opposite effects depending on the mode of administration. When given in a pulsatile fashion to mimic physiologic secretory patterns, such therapy enhances gonadotropin secretion. In contrast, the tonic administration of the same agonist inhibits gonadotropin secretion and causes a physiologic (reversible) castration[741, 742] (see discussion of antiandrogens later). In addition, antagonists have been designed that have no agonist action, regardless of the pattern of administration.[742]

Agonistic effects are of benefit in hypogonadotropic hypogonadism and cryptorchidism. Because the most common cause of isolated gonadotropin deficiency is defective synthesis or release of GnRH, this agent is the most physiologic treatment of the disorder. In such individuals, the long-term pulsatile administration of GnRH through a portable infusion pump induces normal pubertal development. Normal levels of plasma testosterone, LH, and FSH can be attained with small doses of gonadorelin administered subcutaneously every 90 to 120 minutes.[743, 744]

Pulsatile GnRH therapy does not appear to have advantages over gonadotropin therapy in men with hypogonadotropic hypogonadism.[734, 745] GnRH and its analogues have also been used to treat boys with cryptorchidism. The success (or failure) rates for descent of inguinal testes in boys so treated appear to be comparable to those achieved with gonadotropins (see earlier).[746]

Antiandrogens and 5α-Reductase Inhibitors

Agents that block the synthesis or action of androgens are used for treatment of hyperplasia and carcinoma of the prostate, acne, male-pattern baldness, virilizing syndromes in women, precocious puberty in boys, and male sex offenders.

Inhibitors of Testosterone Synthesis

The most effective inhibitor of testosterone synthesis is either *GnRH* itself or a GnRH agonist or antagonist (see Chapter 8 for details). These agents cause a decline in the plasma levels of LH and testosterone and induce a pharmacologic (and reversible) castration. Such therapy provides a medical alternative to castration for producing androgen deprivation in men with prostatic cancer and produces fewer deleterious side effects than estrogen therapy.[747]

In individuals with prostatic carcinoma, such agents are usually administered in conjunction with androgen receptor antagonists, which block the action of androgens of adrenal origin, to produce total androgen deprivation.[747] In contrast, monotherapy with GnRH analogues is effective in individuals with precocious puberty,[748] some men with paraphilias,[749] and selected men with prostatic hyperplasia.[750] These agents are administered parenterally. The frequency of administration and dosage vary with the agent, but long-acting agents such as depot leuprolide acetate are effective when given at monthly intervals in doses of 7.5 mg.[747] Vasomotor symptoms characteristic of the castrated state are common and may be severe; management of the latter symptoms is frequently unsuccessful, but they may respond to megestrol acetate.[751]

The progestagen *medroxyprogesterone acetate* inhibits testosterone biosynthesis by at least two mechanisms; at low concentrations it inhibits synthesis directly, and at higher concentrations it inhibits LH secretion.[752] Dosages of 400 mg/week by parenteral injection induce a pharmacologic castration and have been used successfully in some men with paraphilia.[753]

Antifungal agents of the imidazole class, such as *ketoconazole* and *liarozole*, secondarily block cytochrome P450 enzymes in steroid hormone biosynthesis, effects that have been used to induce androgen deprivation in some patients with prostate cancer.[754] Gastrointestinal side effects, short duration of action, and inhibition of the biosynthesis of adrenal steroids limit the usefulness of these agents.

Spironolactone, an aldosterone antagonist (see Chapters 14 and 15), is also a weak inhibitor of the binding of androgen to the androgen receptor and impairs androgen biosynthesis. In some women with hirsutism, the drug decreases the growth rate and mean diameter of facial hair[755]; because it may cause menstrual irregularity, it is commonly given together with an oral contraceptive.[756] In efficacy studies, spironolactone was about as effective as finasteride in improving hirsutism scores.[757]

5α-Reductase Inhibitors

Because the conversion of testosterone to dihydrotestosterone is essential for certain androgen actions, inhibition of steroid 5α-reductase selectively blocks androgen action in the tissues (e.g., prostate, certain hair follicles) in which continuing production of dihydrotestosterone is essential. The azasteroid *finasteride* is an orally active inhibitor that preferentially blocks steroid 5α-reductase 2 but may also inhibit enzyme 1.[758] At ordinary dosages, the agent causes a profound decline in dihydrotestosterone levels in serum and prostate but has little if any effect on serum testosterone or LH levels. It also has no significant effect on potency or libido.[759]

In men with prostatic hyperplasia, finasteride at a dosage of 5 mg/day causes a consistent decrease in prostate size and improvement in urine flow and symptoms in a third, and thus provides an alternative to surgery in men with moderate disease manifestations.[760, 761] Finasteride is also effective at a dose of 1 mg/day for male-pattern baldness.[762] Additional 5α-reductase inhibitors, including agents specific for the individual isozymes, are under development.

Androgen Receptor Antagonists

Several anilide derivatives block the binding of androgen to its receptor. *Bicalutamide*, a nonsteroidal antiandrogen that blocks binding of dihydrotestosterone to the androgen receptor, is devoid of other hormonal activity and has a half-life that allows once-daily oral dosing. Bicalutamide appears to have a low incidence of adverse effects.[763] *Flutamide*, given at doses of 750 mg/day, is converted in vivo to 2-hydroxyflutamide, a potent antiandrogen, but because of rapid turnover must be administered three times daily.[764] *Nilutamide* has similar effects at doses of 300 mg/day.[765]

In normal men, all three agents block the inhibitory feedback of androgen on LH production and result in an increase in the frequency of LH secretory bursts and hence an increase in serum LH and testosterone. The rise in serum testosterone serves to limit the antiandrogenic effectiveness. Consequently, they are most useful in inhibiting androgen action in castrated men, in men in whom LH is inhibited (e.g., in men receiving GnRH agonists), or in women (in whom LH production is not under androgenic control). The principal use is for treatment of prostatic cancer, usually in conjunction with GnRH blockade or estrogen.[747]

In men with advanced prostate cancer, bicalutamide and flutamide, each used in combination with a GnRH analogue, have similar effects.[766] Flutamide has also been used for the treatment of hirsutism in women.[757] If the agent crossed the placenta, it would be expected to cause male pseudohermaphroditism in male embryos and consequently should always be given to women in conjunction with an oral contraceptive. Flutamide can cause diarrhea and hepatotoxicity, and nilutamide is associated with side effects similar to those seen with disulfiram (Antabuse) and visual disturbances.

The progestagen *cyproterone acetate* is an androgen antagonist that also suppresses the secretion of gonadotropins and thus interferes with testosterone production.[767] The principal effect is believed to be competition with dihydrotestosterone for binding to the androgen receptor.[768] In castrated animals, dosages about five times that of testosterone blocked androgenic responses by about 50% and with larger dosages the antagonism was almost complete.[767] The administration of cyproterone acetate at 100 mg/day to normal men caused a 50% decrease in serum levels of LH and FSH and a 75% decrease in serum testosterone.[768] The agent has been used for the treatment of acne, male-pattern baldness, and hirsutism and virilizing syndromes in women[767] and to induce chemical castration in men with paraphilias.[769] The agent has orphan drug status in the United States. The fact that it can cross the placenta and induce male pseudohermaphroditism in male embryos[767] and that its use has been associated with severe liver damage, including development of hepatocellular carcinoma,[770] limits its usefulness.

Aromatase Inhibitors and Antiestrogens

Aromatase Inhibitors

Second-generation aromatase inhibitors that are both selective and potent include letrozole and anastrozole, both of which are orally active and can be administered once daily.[771] At a dose of 1 mg/day, anastrozole lowered plasma estradiol in men by about half and caused reciprocal increases in plasma LH and testosterone levels,[631, 772] and letrozole had similar effects in male monkeys.[773]

Although not approved for these indications, such agents may be useful in the treatment of familial testitoxicosis in boys,[774] selected cases of gynecomastia,[775] and the aromatase excess syndrome.[568] Potential adverse effects include asthenia, nausea and vomiting, and headache.[776]

Estrogen Receptor Antagonists

(see Chapter 39)

Of the two estrogen receptors identified, current antagonists were designed to block the α receptor, and it is assumed that dual or selective β-receptor antagonists would have different consequences. Tamoxifen at a dose of 20 mg/day was reported to provide resolution in about 75% of cases of idiopathic gynecomastia,[624] and 16 of 18 men with mastalgia or gynecomastia associated with spironolactone therapy for hepatic cirrhosis improved significantly with a dose of 20 mg of tamoxifen twice a day.[777] Similar beneficial effects of tamoxifen have been reported in flutamide-induced gynecomastia[778] and in the gynecomastia that follows castration or leuprolide therapy.[779] A variety of side effects have been reported, including development of fatty liver.[780]

References

1. Vogel F, Motulsky AG. Human Genetics: Problems and Approaches. Berlin, Springer-Verlag, 1997, pp 29–44.
2. Burgoyne PS. Mammalian X and Y crossover. Nature 1986; 320: 170–172.
3. Sinclair AH, Berta P, Palmer MS, et al. A gene from the human sex-determining region encodes a protein with homology to a conserved DNA-binding motif. Nature 1990; 346:240–244.
4. Koopman P, Gubbay J, Vivian N, et al. Male development of chromosomally female mice transgenic for *Sry*. Nature 1991; 351: 117–121.
5. Clepet C, Schafer AJ, Sinclair AH, et al. The human *SRY* transcript. Hum Mol Genet 1993; 2:2007–2012.
6. Graves JA. Evolution of the mammalian Y chromosome and sex-determining genes. J Exp Zool 1998; 281:472–481.
7. Parker KL, Shedl A, Schimmer BP. Gene interactions in gonadal development. Annu Rev Physiol 1999; 61:417–433.
8. Castrillon DH, Quade BJ, Wang TY, et al. The human *VASA* gene is specifically expressed in the germ cell lineage. Proc Natl Acad Sci USA 2000; 97:9585–9590.
9. Mintz B, Russell ES. Gene-induced embryological modification of primordial germ cells in the mouse. J Exp Zool 1957; 134: 207–230.
10. Friedman NB, Van de Velde RL. Germ cell tumors in man, pleiotropic mice, and continuity of germplasm and somatoplasm. Hum Pathol 1981; 12:772–776.
11. Gillman J. The development of the gonads in man, with a consideration of the role of fetal endocrines and the histogenesis of ovarian tumors. Carnegie Contrib Embryol Carnegie Inst Wash 1948; 32:83–131.
12. McCarrey JR, Abbott UK. Chick gonad differentiation following excision of primordial germ cells. Dev Biol 1978; 66:256–265.
13. Hutson JM, Hasthorpe S, Heyns CF. Anatomical and functional aspects of testicular descent and cryptorchidism. Endocr Rev 1997; 18:259–280.
14. Burke EC, Shin MH, Kelalis PP. Prune belly syndrome: clinical findings and survival. Am J Dis Child 1969; 117:668–671.
15. Frey HL, Rajfer J. Role of the gubernaculum and intraabdominal pressure in the process of testicular descent. J Urol 1984; 131: 575–579.
16. Barthold JS, Kumasi-Rivers K, Upadhyay J, et al. Testicular position in the androgen insensitivity syndrome: implications for the role of androgens in testicular descent. J Urol 2000; 164:497–501.
17. Guerrier D, Tran D, Vanderwinden JM, et al. The persistent

müllerian duct syndrome: a molecular approach. J Clin Endocrinol Metab 1989; 68:46–52.
18. Josso N, Picard J-Y, Imbeaud S, et al. Clinical aspects and molecular genetics of the persistent müllerian duct syndrome. Clin Endocrinol (Oxf) 1997; 47:137–144.
19. Zimmermann S, Steding G, Emmen JM, et al. Targeted disruption of the *Insl3* gene causes bilateral cryptorchidism. Mol Endocrinol 1999; 13:681–691.
20. Nef S, Parada LF. Cryptorchidism in mice mutant for *Insl3*. Nat Genet 1999; 22:295–297.
21. Emmen JM, McLuskey A, Adham IM, et al. Involvement of insulin-like factor 3 (Insl3) in diethylstilbestrol-induced cryptorchidism. Endocrinology 2000; 141:846–849.
22. Rijli FM, Matyas R, Pellegrini M, et al. Cryptorchidism and homeotic transformation of spinal nerves and vertebrae in Hoxa-10 mutant mice. Proc Natl Acad Sci USA 1995; 92:8185–8189.
23. Fawcett DW. Ultrastructure and function of the Sertoli cell. In Greep RO, Astwood EB (eds). Handbook of Physiology, sect 7: Endocrinology, vol V. Male Reproductive System. Washington, DC, American Physiological Society, 1975, pp 21–55.
24. Griswold MD. The central role of Sertoli cells in spermatogenesis. Semin Cell Dev Biol 1998; 9:411–416.
25. Saez JM. Leydig cells: endocrine, paracrine, and autocrine regulation. Endocr Rev 1994; 15:574–626.
26. Stocco DM, Clark BJ. Regulation of the acute production of steroids in steroidogenic cells. Endocr Rev 1996; 17:221–244.
27. Maddocks S, Hargreave TB, Reddie K, et al. Intratesticular hormone levels and the route of secretion of hormones from the testis of the rat, guinea pig, monkey and human. Int J Androl 1993; 16:272–278.
28. Oliver C, Mical RS, Porter JC. Hypothalamic-pituitary vasculature: evidence for retrograde blood flow in the pituitary stalk. Endocrinology 1977; 101:598–604.
29. Silverman AJ, Krey LC, Zimmerman EA. A comparative study of the luteinizing hormone releasing hormone (LHRH) neuronal networks in mammals. Biol Reprod 1979; 20:98–110.
30. Huseman CA, Kelch RP. Gonadotropin responses and metabolism of synthetic gonadotropin-releasing hormone (GnRH) during constant infusion of GnRH in men and boys with delayed adolescence. J Clin Endocrinol Metab 1978; 47:1325–1331.
31. Bourguignon J-P, Hoyoux C, Reuter A, et al. Urinary excretion of immunoreactive luteinizing hormone–releasing hormone–like material and gonadotropins at different stages of life. J Clin Endocrinol Metab 1979; 48:78–84.
32. Vaitukaitis JL, Ross GD, Braunstein GD, et al. Gonadotropins and their subunits: basic and clinical studies. Recent Prog Horm Res 1976; 32:289–331.
33. Veldhuis JD, Fraioli F, Rogol AD, et al. Metabolic clearance of biologically active luteinizing hormone in man. J Clin Invest 1986; 77:1122–1128.
34. VanHall EV, Vaitukaitis JL, Ross GT, et al. Effects of progressive desialylation on the rate of disappearance of immunoreactive hCG from plasma in rats. Endocrinology 1971; 89:11–15.
35. Coble YD Jr, Kohler PO, Cargille CM, et al. Production rates and metabolic clearance rates of human follicle-stimulating hormone in premenopausal and postmenopausal women. J Clin Invest 1969; 48:359–363.
36. Yen SSC, Llerena LA, Pearson OH, et al. Disappearance rates of endogenous follicle-stimulating hormone in serum following surgical hypophysectomy in man. J Clin Endocrinol 1970; 30:325–329.
37. Hawes BE, Conn PM. Assessment of the role of G proteins and inositol phosphate production in the action of gonadotropin-releasing hormone. Clin Chem 1993; 39:325–332.
38. Huhtaniemi IT, Koritnik DR, Korenbrot CC, et al. Stimulation of pituitary-testicular function with gonadotropin-releasing hormone in fetal and infant monkeys. Endocrinology 1979; 105:109–114.
39. Marshall JC, Griffin ML. The role of changing pulse frequency in the regulation of ovulation. Hum Reprod 1993; 8(Suppl 2):56–61.
40. Rajfer J, Sikka SC, Swerdloff RS. Lack of a direct effect of gonadotropin hormone–releasing hormone agonist on human testicular steroidogenesis. J Clin Endocrinol Metab 1987; 64:62–67.
41. Dufau ML. The luteinizing hormone receptor. Annu Rev Physiol 1998; 60:461–496.
42. Payne AH, Youngblood GL. Regulation of expression of steroidogenic enzymes in Leydig cells. Biol Reprod 1995; 52:217–225.
43. LaPolt PS, Jia XC, Sincich C, et al. Ligand-induced down-regulation of testicular and ovarian luteinizing hormone (LH) receptors is preceded by tissue-specific inhibition of alternatively processed LH receptor transcripts. Mol Endocrinol 1991; 5:397–403.
44. West AP, Cooke BA. The LH receptor cytoplasmic tail is required for desensitization of LH action but not cyclic AMP production. Biochem Soc Trans 1992; 20:320S.
45. Wahlstrom T, Huhtaniemi I, Hovatta O, et al. Localization of luteinizing hormone, follicle-stimulating hormone, prolactin, and their receptors in human and rat testis using immunohistochemistry and radioreceptor assay. J Clin Endocrinol Metab 1983; 57: 825–830.
46. Means AR, Fakunding JL, Huckins C, et al. Follicle-stimulating hormone, the Sertoli cell, and spermatogenesis. Recent Prog Horm Res 1976; 32:477–527.
47. Levalle O, Zylbersztein C, Aszpis S, et al. Recombinant human follicle-stimulating hormone administration increases testosterone production in men, possibly by a Sertoli cell–secreted nonsteroid factor. J Clin Endocrinol Metab 1998; 83:3973–3976.
48. Young J, Couzinet B, Chanson P, et al. Effects of human recombinant luteinizing hormone and follicle-stimulating hormone in patients with acquired hypogonadotropic hypogonadism: study of Sertoli and Leydig cell secretions and interactions. J Clin Endocrinol Metab 2000; 85:3239–3244.
49. Neill JD, Patton JM, Dailey RA, et al. Luteinizing hormone releasing hormone (LHRH) in pituitary stalk blood of rhesus monkeys: relationship to level of LH release. Endocrinology 1977; 101:430–434.
50. Dufau ML, Veldhuis JD, Fraioli F, et al. Mode of secretion of bioactive luteinizing hormone in man. J Clin Endocrinol Metab 1983; 57:993–1000.
51. Veldhuis JD, King JC, Urban RJ, et al. Operating characteristics of the male hypothalamo-pituitary-gonadal axis: pulsatile release of testosterone and follicle-stimulating hormone and their temporal coupling with luteinizing hormone. J Clin Endocrinol Metab 1987; 65:929–941.
52. Santen RJ. Is aromatization of testosterone to estradiol required for inhibition of luteinizing hormone secretion in men? J Clin Invest 1975; 56:1555–1563.
53. Winters SJ, Troen P. Evidence for a role of endogenous estrogen in the hypothalamic control of gonadotropin secretion in men. J Clin Endocrinol Metab 1985; 61:842–845.
54. Lacroix A, McKenna TJ, Rabinowitz D. Sex steroid modulation of gonadotropins in normal men and in androgen insensitivity syndrome. J Clin Endocrinol Metab 1979; 48:235–240.
55. Smith EP, Boyd J, Frank GR, et al. Estrogen resistance caused by a mutation in the estrogen-receptor gene in a man. N Engl J Med 1994; 331:1056–1061.
56. Morishima A, Grumbach MM, Simpson ER, et al. Aromatase deficiency in male and female siblings caused by a novel mutation and the physiological role of estrogens. J Clin Endocrinol Metab 1995; 80:3689–3698.
57. Plant TM, Dubey AK. Evidence from the rhesus monkey *(Macaca mulatta)* for the view that negative feedback control of luteinizing hormone secretion by the testis is mediated by deceleration of hypothalamic gonadotropin-releasing hormone pulse frequency. Endocrinology 1984; 115:2145–2153.
58. Sheckter CB, Matsumoto AM, Bremner WJ. Testosterone administration inhibits gonadotropin secretion by an effect directly on the human pituitary. J Clin Endocrinol Metab 1989; 68:397–401.
59. Nieschlag E, Behre HM. Andrology: Male Reproductive Health and Dysfunction. Berlin, Springer-Verlag, 1997, p 127.
60. Anawalt BD, Begg RA, Matsumoto AM, et al. Serum inhibin B levels reflect Sertoli cell function in normal men and men with testicular dysfunction. J Clin Endocrinol Metab 1996; 81:3341–3345.
61. McLachlan RI, Matsumoto AM, Burger HG, et al. Relative roles of follicle-stimulating hormone and luteinizing hormone in the control of inhibin secretion in normal men. J Clin Invest 1988; 82:880–884.
62. Sherins RJ, Patterson AP, Brightwell D, et al. Alteration in the plasma testosterone:estradiol ratio: an alternative to the inhibin hypothesis. Ann NY Acad Sci 1982; 383:295–306.

63. Gross KM, Matsumoto AM, Bremner WJ. Differential control of luteinizing hormone and follicle-stimulating hormone secretion by luteinizing hormone–releasing hormone pulse frequency in man. J Clin Endocrinol Metab 1987; 64:675–680.
64. Majumdar SS, Mikuma N, Ishwad PC, et al. Replacement with recombinant human inhibin immediately after orchidectomy in the hypophysiotropically clamped male rhesus monkey (*Macaca mulatta*) maintains follicle-stimulating hormone (FSH) secretion and FSH beta messenger ribonucleic acid levels at precastration values. Endocrinology 1995; 136:1969–1977.
65. Carr BR, Parker CR Jr, Ohashi M, et al. Regulation of human fetal testicular secretion of testosterone: low-density lipoprotein-cholesterol and cholesterol synthesized de novo as steroid precursor. Am J Obstet Gynecol 1983; 146:241–247.
66. Auchus RJ, Lee TC, Miller WL. Cytochrome b5 augments the 17,20-lyase activity of human P450c17 without direct electron transfer. J Biol Chem 1998; 273:3158–3165.
67. Miller WL. Molecular biology of steroid hormone synthesis. Endocr Rev 1988; 9:295–318.
68. Hammond GL, Ruokonen A, Kontturi M, et al. The simultaneous radioimmunoassay of seven steroids in human spermatic and peripheral venous blood. J Clin Endocrinol Metab 1977; 45: 16–24.
69. George FW, Carr BR, Noble JF, Wilson JD. 5α-Reduced androgens in the human fetal testis. J Clin Endocrinol Metab 1987; 64: 628–630.
70. Morse HC, Horike N, Rowley MJ, et al. Testosterone concentrations in testes of normal men: effects of testosterone propionate administration. J Clin Endocrinol Metab 1973; 37:882–886.
71. Mendelson C, Dufau ML, Catt KJ. Gonadotropin binding and stimulation of cyclic adenosine 3′,5′-monophosphate and testosterone production in isolated Leydig cells. J Biol Chem 1975; 250:8818–8823.
72. Huhtaniemi I, Bolton N, Leinonen P, et al. Testicular luteinizing hormone receptor content and in vitro stimulation of cyclic adenosine 3′,5′-monophosphate and steroid production: a comparison between man and rat. J Clin Endocrinol Metab 1982; 55:882–889.
73. Cigorraga SB, Sorrell S, Bator J, et al. Estrogen dependence of a gonadotropin-induced steroidogenic lesion in rat testicular Leydig cells. J Clin Invest 1980; 65:699–705.
74. Payne AH, Quinn PG, Rani CS. Regulation of microsomal cytochrome P-450 enzymes and testosterone production in Leydig cells. Recent Prog Horm Res 1985; 41:153–197.
75. Hales DB, Sha L, Payne AH. Testosterone inhibits cAMP-induced de novo synthesis of Leydig cell cytochrome P-$450_{17\alpha}$ by an androgen receptor–mediated mechanism. J Biol Chem 1987; 262:11200–11206.
76. Padron RS, Wischusen J, Hudson B, et al. Prolonged biphasic response of plasma testosterone to single intramuscular injections of human chorionic gonadotropin. J Clin Endocrinol Metab 1980; 50:1100–1104.
77. Smals AGH, Pieters GFFM, Lozekott DC, et al. Dissociated responses of plasma testosterone and 17-hydroxyprogesterone to single or repeated human chorionic gonadotropin administration in normal men. J Clin Endocrinol Metab 1980; 50:190–193.
78. Matsumoto AM, Paulsen CA, Hopper BR, et al. Human chorionic gonadotropin and testicular function: stimulation of testosterone, testosterone precursors, and sperm production despite high estradiol levels. J Clin Endocrinol Metab 1983; 56:720–728.
79. Ahokoski O, Virtanen A, Huupponen R, et al. Biological day-to-day variation and daytime changes of testosterone, follitropin, lutropin, and oestradiol-17β in healthy men. Clin Chem Lab Med 1998; 36:485–491.
80. Bridges NA, Hindmarsh PC, Pringle PJ, et al. The relationship between endogenous testosterone and gonadotrophin secretion. Clin Endocrinol (Oxf) 1993; 38:373–378.
81. Bartke A. Pituitary-testis relationship: role of prolactin in the regulation of testicular function. In Hubinont PO (ed). Progress in Reproductive Biology, vol 1. Basel, S Karger, 1976, pp 136–152.
82. Gnessi L, Fabbri A, Spera G. Gonadal peptides as mediators of development and functional control of the testis: an integrated system with hormones and local environment. Endocr Rev 1997; 18:541–609.
83. Schlatt S, Meinhardt A, Nieschlag E. Paracrine regulation of cellular interactions in the testis: factors in search of a function. Eur J Endocrinol 1997; 137:107–117.
84. Saez JM. Leydig cells: endocrine, paracrine, and autocrine regulation. Endocr Rev 1994; 16:574–626.
85. Hammond GL, Underhill DA, Smith CL, et al. The cDNA-deduced primary structure of human sex hormone–binding globulin and location of its steroid-binding domain. FEBS Lett 1987; 215:100–104.
86. Cornelisse MM, Bennett PE, Christiansen M, et al. Sex hormone binding globulin phenotypes: their detection and distribution in healthy adults and in different clinical conditions. Clin Chim Acta 1994; 225:115–121.
87. Fortunati N. Sex hormone–binding globulin: not only a transport protein. What news is around the corner? J Endocrinol Invest 1999; 22:223–234.
88. Dunn JF, Nisula BC, Rodbard D. Transport of steroid hormones: binding of 21 endogenous steroids to both testosterone-binding globulin and corticosteroid-binding globulin in human plasma. J Clin Endocrinol Metab 1981; 53:58–68.
89. Pardridge WM. Serum bioavailability of sex steroid hormones. Clin Endocrinol Metab 1986; 15:259–278.
90. Rosner W, Hryb DJ, Khan MS, et al. Sex hormone–binding globulin: binding to cell membranes and generation of a second messenger. J Androl 1992; 13:101–106.
91. Plymate SR, Leonard JM, Paulsen CA, et al. Sex hormone–binding globulin changes with androgen replacement. J Clin Endocrinol Metab 1983; 57:645–648.
92. Pardridge WM. Transport of protein-bound hormone into tissues in vivo. Endocr Rev 1981; 2:103–123.
93. Moore RJ, Gazak JM, Wilson JD. Regulation of cytoplasmic dihydrotestosterone binding in dog prostate by 17β-estradiol. J Clin Invest 1979; 63:351–357.
94. Wilson JD, Aiman J, MacDonald PC. The pathogenesis of gynecomastia. Adv Intern Med 1980; 25:1–32.
95. MacDonald PC, Madden JD, Brenner PF, et al. Origin of estrogen in normal men and in women with testicular feminization. J Clin Endocrinol Metab 1979; 49:905–916.
96. Ito T, Horton R. The source of plasma dihydrotestosterone in man. J Clin Invest 1971; 50:1621–1627.
97. Bruchovsky N, Wilson JD. The conversion of testosterone to 5α-androstan-17β-ol-3-one by rat prostate in vivo and in vitro. J Biol Chem 1968; 243:2012–2021.
98. Anderson KM, Liao S. Selective retention of dihydrotestosterone by prostatic nuclei. Nature 1968; 219:277–279.
99. Dorfman RI, Shipley RA. Androgens: Biochemistry, Physiology, and Clinical Significance. New York, John Wiley & Sons, 1956.
100. Thigpen AE, Davis DL, Milatovich A, et al. Molecular genetics of steroid 5α-reductase 2 deficiency. J Clin Invest 1992; 90:799–809.
101. Wilson JD, Griffin JE, Russell DW. Steroid 5α-reductase 2 deficiency. Endocr Rev 1993; 14:577–593.
102. Moore RJ, Wilson JD. Steroid 5α-reductase in cultured human fibroblasts: biochemical and genetic evidence for two enzyme activities. J Biol Chem 1976; 251:5895–5900.
103. Russell DW, Wilson JD. Steroid 5α-reductase: two genes/two enzymes. Annu Rev Biochem 1994; 63:25–61.
104. George FW, Peterson K. 5α-Dihydrotestosterone formation is necessary for embryogenesis of the rat prostate. Endocrinology 1988; 122:1159–1164.
105. George FW, Russell DW, Wilson JD. Feed-forward control of prostate growth: dihydrotestosterone induces expression of its own biosynthetic enzyme, steroid 5α-reductase. Proc Natl Acad Sci USA 1991; 88:8044–8047.
106. Kato R, Onoda K, Omori Y. Mechanism of thyroxine-induced increase in steroid Δ^4-reductase activity in male rats. Endocrinol Jpn 1970; 17:215–219.
107. Horton R, Pasupuletti V, Antonipillai I. Androgen induction of steroid 5α-reductase may be mediated via insulin-like growth factor-I. Endocrinology 1993; 133:447–451.
108. Wilson JD, Lasnitzki I. Dihydrotestosterone formation in fetal tissues of the rabbit and rat. Endocrinology 1971; 89:659–668.
109. Bayne EK, Flanagan J, Einstein M, et al. Immunohistochemical localization of types 1 and 2 5α-reductase in human scalp. Br J Dermatol 1999; 141:481–491.
110. Frederiksen DW, Wilson JD. Partial characterization of the nuclear reduced nicotinamide adenine dinucleotide phosphate: Δ^4-3-

ketosteroid 5α-oxidoreductase of rat prostate. J Biol Chem 1971; 246:2584–2593.
111. Corbin CJ, Graham-Lorence S, McPhaul MJ, et al. Isolation of a full-length cDNA insert encoding human aromatase system cytochrome P-450 and its expression in nonsteroidogenic cells. Proc Natl Acad Sci USA 1988; 85:8948–8952.
112. Mahendroo MS, Mendelson CR, Simpson ER. Tissue-specific and hormonally controlled alternative promoters regulate aromatase cytochrome P450 gene expression in human adipose tissue. J Biol Chem 1993; 268:19463–19470.
113. Brooks RV. Androgens. Clin Endocrinol Metab 1975; 4:503–520.
114. Scheller A, Hughes E, Golden KL, Robins DM. Multiple receptor domains interact to permit, or restrict, androgen-specific gene activation. J Biol Chem 1998; 273:24216–24222.
115. Evans RM. The steroid and thyroid hormone receptor superfamily. Science 1988; 240:889–895.
116. George FW, Wilson JD. Sex determination and differentiation. In Knobil E, Neill JD (eds). The Physiology of Reproduction, 2nd ed. New York, Raven Press, 1994, pp 3–28.
117. Griffin JE, McPhaul MJ, Russell DW, Wilson JD. The androgen resistance syndromes: steroid 5α-reductase 2 deficiency, testicular feminization, and related disorders. In Scriver CR, Beaudet AL, Sly WS, Valle D (eds). The Metabolic and Molecular Basis of Disease, 8th ed. New York, McGraw-Hill, 2001, pp 4117–4146.
118. Payne AH, Kawano A, Jaffe RB. Formation of dihydrotestosterone and other 5α-reduced metabolites by isolated seminiferous tubules and suspensions of interstitial cells in a human testis. J Clin Endocrinol Metab 1973; 37:448–453.
119. Price P, Wass JAH, Griffin JE, et al. High dose androgen therapy in male pseudohermaphroditism due to 5α-reductase deficiency and disorders of the androgen receptor. J Clin Invest 1984; 74:1496–1508.
120. Wilson EM, French FS. Binding properties of androgen receptors: evidence for identical receptors in rat testes, epididymis, and prostate. J Biol Chem 1976; 251:5620–5629.
121. Snochowski M, Dahlberg E, Gustafsson J-A. Characterization and quantification of the androgen and glucocorticoid receptors in cytosol from rat skeletal muscle. Eur J Biochem 1980; 111: 603–616.
122. McGill HC Jr, Anselmo VC, Buchanan JM, et al. The heart is a target organ for androgen. Science 1980; 207:775–777.
123. McCormick PD, Razel AJ, Spelsberg TC, et al. Evidence for an androgen receptor in the human placenta. Am J Obstet Gynecol 1981; 140:8–13.
124. Tsai Y-H, Sanborn BM, Steinberger A, et al. Sertoli cell chromatin acceptor sites for androgen-receptor complexes. J Steroid Biochem 1980; 13:711–718.
125. Verhoeven G. Androgen receptor in cultured interstitial cells derived from immature rat testis. J Steroid Biochem 1980; 13:469–474.
126. Grino PB, Griffin JE, Wilson JD. Testosterone at high concentrations interacts with the human androgen receptor similarly to dihydrotestosterone. Endocrinology 1990; 126:1165–1172.
127. Migeon BR, Brown TR, Axelman J, et al. Studies of the locus for androgen receptor: localization on the human X chromosome and evidence for homology with the tfm locus in the mouse. Proc Natl Acad Sci USA 1981; 78:6339–6343.
128. Lubahn DB, Joseph DR, Sullivan PM, et al. Cloning of human androgen receptor complementary DNA and localization to the X chromosome. Science 1988; 240:327–330.
129. Chang C, Kokontis CJ, Liao S. Molecular cloning of human and rat complementary DNA encoding androgen receptors. Science 1988; 240:324–326.
130. Trapman J, Klaassen P, Kuiper GGJM, et al. Cloning, structure and expression of a cDNA encoding the human androgen receptor. Biochem Biophys Res Commun 1988; 153:241–248.
131. Edwards A, Hammond HA, Jin L, et al. Genetic variation of five trimeric and tetrameric tandem repeat loci in four human populations. Genomics 1992; 12:241–245.
132. Pinsky L, Beitel LK, Trifiro MA. Spinobulbar muscular atrophy. In Scriver CR, Beaudet Al, Sly WS, Valle D (eds). The Metabolic and Molecular Basis of Inherited Disease, 8th ed. New York, McGraw-Hill, 2001, pp 4147–4157.
133. Kovacs WJ, Griffin JE, Weaver DD, et al. A mutation that causes lability of the androgen receptor under conditions that normally promote transformation to the DNA-binding state. J Clin Invest 1984; 73:1095–1104.
134. Deslypere J-P, Young M, Wilson JD, et al. Testosterone and 5α-dihydrotestosterone interact differently with the androgen receptor to enhance transcription of the *MMTV-CAT* reporter gene. Mol Cell Endocrinol 1992; 88:15–22.
135. Zhou ZX, Wong CI, Sar M, et al. The androgen receptor: an overview. Recent Prog Horm Res 1994; 49:249–274.
136. Rundlett SE, Miesfeld RL. Quantitative differences in androgen and glucocorticoid receptor DNA binding properties contribute to receptor-selective transcriptional regulation. Mol Cell Endocrinol 1995; 109:1–10.
137. Roehrborn CG, Lange JL, George FW, et al. Changes in amount and intracellular distribution of androgen receptor in human foreskin as a function of age. J Clin Invest 1987; 79:44–47.
138. Grumbach MM, Auchus RJ. Estrogen: consequences and implications of human mutations in synthesis and action. J Clin Endocrinol Metab 1999; 84:4677–4694.
139. Hess RA, Bunick D, Lee K-H, et al. A role for oestrogens in the male reproductive system. Nat Genet 1997; 390:509–511.
140. Grootegoed JA, Siep M, Baarends WM. Molecular and cellular mechanisms in spermatogenesis. Ballieres Clin Endocrinol Metab 2000; 14:331–343.
141. McLachlan RI. The endocrine control of spermatogenesis. Ballieres Clin Endocrinol Metab 2000; 14:345–362.
142. Johnson L, Petty CS, Neaves WB. Further quantification of human spermatogenesis: germ cell loss during postprophase of meiosis and its relationship to daily sperm production. Biol Reprod 1983; 29:207–215.
143. Clermont Y. The cycle of the seminiferous epithelium in man. Am J Anat 1963; 112:35–45.
144. Johnson L. A new approach to study the architectural arrangement of spermatogenic stages revealed little evidence of a partial wave along the length of human seminiferous tubules. J Androl 1994; 15:435–441.
145. Fawcett DW. The Cell, 2nd ed. Philadelphia, WB Saunders, 1981, pp 604–617.
146. Heller CG, Clermont Y. Spermatogenesis in man: an estimate of its duration. Science 1963; 140:184–186.
147. Rowley MJ, Teshima F, Heller CG. Duration of transit of spermatozoa through the human male ductular system. Fertil Steril 1970; 21:390–396.
148. Hinrichsen MJ, Blaquier JA. Evidence supporting the existence of sperm maturation in the human epididymis. J Reprod Fertil 1980; 60:291–294.
149. Gibbons BH. Studies on the mechanism of flagellar movement. In Fawcett DW, Bedford JM (eds). The Spermatozoon. Baltimore, Urban & Schwarzenberg, 1979, pp 91–97.
150. Afzelius BA, Mossberg B. Immotile-cilia syndrome (primary ciliary dyskinesia), including Kartagener syndrome. In Scriver CR, Beaudet AL, Sly WS, Valle D (eds). The Metabolic and Molecular Bases of Inherited Disease, 7th ed. New York, McGraw-Hill, 1995, pp 3943–3954.
151. Setchell BP. Regulation of spermatogenesis and possible sites for contraceptive action. In Jeffcoate SL, Sandler M (eds). Progress Towards a Male Contraceptive. New York, John Wiley & Sons, 1982, pp 1–18.
152. Zirkin BR. Spermatogenesis: its regulation by testosterone and FSH. Semin Cell Dev Biol 1998; 9:417–421.
153. Bremner WJ, Millar MR, Sharpe RM, et al. Immunohistochemical localization of androgen receptors in the rat testis: evidence for stage-dependent expression and regulation by androgens. Endocrinology 1994; 135:1227–1234.
154. Lyon MF, Glenister PH, Lamoreux ML. Normal spermatozoa from androgen-resistant germ cells of chimeric mice and the role of androgen in spermatogenesis. Nature 1975; 258:620–622.
155. Matsumoto AM, Paulsen CA, Bremner WJ. Stimulation of sperm production by human luteinizing hormone in gonadotropin-suppressed normal men. J Clin Endocrinol Metab 1984; 59:882–887.
156. Matsumoto AM, Karpas AE, Bremner WJ. Chronic human chorionic gonadotropin administration in normal men: evidence that follicle-stimulating hormone is necessary for the maintenance of quantitatively normal spermatogenesis in man. J Clin Endocrinol Metab 1986; 62:1184–1192.
157. Gromoll J, Simoni M, Nieschlag E. An activating mutation of the follicle-stimulating hormone receptor autonomously sustains spermatogenesis in a hypophysectomized man. J Clin Endocrinol Metab 1996; 81:1367–1370.

158. Tarin JJ, Trounson AO. Inducers of the acrosome reaction. Reprod Fertil Dev 1994; 6:33–35.
159. Perreault SD, Rogers BJ. Capacitation pattern of human spermatozoa. Fertil Steril 1982; 38:258–260.
160. Gorus FK, Finsy R, Pipeleers DG. Effect of temperature, nutrients, calcium, and cAMP on motility of human spermatozoa. Am J Physiol 1982; 242:C304–C311.
161. Yanagimachi R. Mammalian fertilization. In Knobil E, Neill JD (eds). The Physiology of Reproduction, 2nd ed. New York, Raven Press, 1994, pp 189–318.
162. Siiteri PK, Wilson JD. Testosterone formation and metabolism during male sexual differentiation in the human embryo. J Clin Endocrinol Metab 1974; 38:113–125.
163. Reyes FI, Bordoditsky RS, Winter JSD, et al. Studies on human sexual development. II: Fetal and maternal serum gonadotropin and sex steroid concentrations. J Clin Endocrinol Metab 1974; 38:612–617.
164. Forest MG, Cathiard AM. Pattern of plasma testosterone and Δ^4-androstenedione in normal newborns: evidence for testicular activity at birth. J Clin Endocrinol Metab 1975; 41:977–984.
165. Winter JSD, Hughes IA, Reyes FI, et al. Pituitary-gonadal relations in infancy. 2: Patterns of serum gonadal steroid concentrations in man from birth to two years of age. J Clin Endocrinol Metab 1976; 42:679–686.
166. August GP, Grumbach MM, Crapo L, et al. Hormonal changes in puberty. III: Correlation of plasma testosterone, LH, FSH, testicular size, and bone age with male pubertal development. J Clin Endocrinol Metab 1972; 34:319–326.
167. Bremner WJ, Vitiello MV, Prinz PM. Loss of circadian rhythmicity in blood testosterone levels with aging in normal men. J Clin Endocrinol Metab 1983; 56:1278–1281.
168. Davidson JM, Chen JJ, Crapo L, et al. Hormonal changes and sexual function in aging men. J Clin Endocrinol Metab 1983; 57: 71–77.
169. Jost A. A new look at the mechanism controlling sex differentiation in mammals. Johns Hopkins Med J 1972; 130:38–53.
170. George FW, Wilson JD. Embryology of the genital tract. In Walsh PC, Retik AB, Stamey TA, et al (eds). Campbell's Urology, 6th ed. Philadelphia, WB Saunders, 1992, PP 1496–1508.
171. Donahoe PK, Cate RL, MacLaughlin DT, et al. Müllerian inhibiting substance: gene structure and mechanism of action of a fetal regressor. Recent Prog Horm Res 1987; 43:431–468.
172. George FW, Noble JF. Androgen receptors are similar in fetal and in adult rabbits. Endocrinology 1984; 115:1451–1458.
173. Kaplan SL, Grumbach MM. The ontogenesis of human foetal hormones. II: Luteinizing hormone (LH) and follicle stimulating hormone (FSH). Acta Endocrinol (Copenh) 1976; 81:808–829.
174. Molsberry RL, Carr BR, Mendelson CR, et al. Human chorionic gonadotropin binding to human fetal testis as a function of gestational age. J Clin Endocrinol Metab 1982; 55:791–794.
175. Ellinwood WE, Baughman WL, Resko JA. The effects of gonadectomy and testosterone treatment on luteinizing hormone secretion in fetal rhesus monkeys. Endocrinology 1982; 110:183–189.
176. Zondek LH, Zondek T. Observations on the testis in anencephaly with special reference to the Leydig cells. Biol Neonate 1965; 8:329–347.
177. Chan W-Y. Molecular, genetic, biochemical, and clinical implications of gonadotropin receptor mutations. Mol Genet Metab 1998; 63:75–84.
178. Wilson JD. Gonadal hormones and sexual behavior. In Besser GM, Martini L (eds). Clinical Neuroendocrinology, Vol II. New York, Academic Press, 1982, pp 1–29.
179. Andersson AM, Toppari J, Haavisto AM, et al. Longitudinal reproductive hormone profiles in infants: peak of inhibin B levels in infant boys exceeds levels in adult men. J Clin Endocrinol Metab 1998; 83:675–681.
180. De Moor P, Verhoeven G, Heyns W. Permanent effects of fetal and neonatal testosterone secretion on steroid metabolism and binding. Differentiation 1973; 1:241–253.
181. Mann DR, Gould KG, Collins DC, et al. Blockade of neonatal activation of the pituitary-testicular axis: effect on peripubertal luteinizing hormone and testosterone secretion and on testicular development in male monkeys. J Clin Endocrinol Metab 1989; 68:600–607.
182. Reiter EO, Grumbach MM, Kaplan SL, et al. The response of pituitary gonadotropes to synthetic LRF in children with glucocorticoid-treated congenital adrenal hyperplasia: lack of effect of intrauterine and neonatal androgen excess. J Clin Endocrinol Metab 1975; 40:318–325.
183. Guthrie RD, Smith DW, Graham CB. Testosterone treatment for micropenis during early childhood. J Pediatr 1973; 83:247–252.
184. Ducharme JR, Collu R. Pubertal development: normal, precocious and delayed. Clin Endocrinol Metab 1982; 11:57–87.
185. Winter JSD, Faiman C. Serum gonadotropin concentrations in agonadal children and adults. J Clin Endocrinol Metab 1972; 35: 561–564.
186. Jakacki RI, Kelch RP, Sauder SE, et al. Pulsatile secretion of luteinizing hormone in children. J Clin Endocrinol Metab 1982; 55:453–458.
187. Boyar RM, Rosenfeld RS, Kapen S, et al. Human puberty: simultaneous augmented secretion of luteinizing hormone and testosterone during sleep. J Clin Invest 1974; 54:609–618.
188. Lucky AW, Rich BH, Rosenfield RL, et al. LH bioactivity increases more than immunoreactivity during puberty. J Pediatr 1980; 97:205–213.
189. Parra A, Cervantes C, Sanchez M, et al. The relationship of plasma gonadotrophins and androgen concentrations to body growth in boys. Acta Endocrinol (Copenh) 1981; 98:137–147.
190. Katz SH, Hediger ML, Zemel BS, et al. Adrenal androgens, body fat and advanced skeletal age in puberty: new evidence for the relations of adrenarche and gonadarche in males. Hum Biol 1985; 57:401–413.
191. Mantzoros CS, Flier JS, Rogol AD. A longitudinal assessment of hormonal and physical alterations during normal puberty in boys. V. Rising leptin levels may signal the onset of puberty. J Clin Endocrinol Metab 1997; 82:1066–1070.
192. Andersson A-M, Juul A, Petersen JH, et al. Serum inhibin B in healthy pubertal and adolescent boys: relation to age, stage of puberty, and follicle-stimulating hormone, luteinizing hormone, testosterone, and estradiol levels. J Clin Endocrinol Metab 1007; 82:3976–3981.
193. Nielsen CT, Skakkebaek NE, Richardson DW, et al. Onset of the release of spermatozoa (spermarche) in boys in relation to age, testicular growth, pubic hair, and height. J Clin Endocrinol Metab 1986; 62:532–535.
194. Scow RO, Hagan SN. Effect of testosterone propionate on myosin, collagen and other protein fractions in striated muscle of gonadectomized rats. Endocrinology 1957; 60:273–276.
195. Hamilton JB. The role of testicular secretions as indicated by the effects of castration in man and by studies of pathological conditions and the short lifespan associated with maleness. Recent Prog Horm Res 1948; 3:257–322.
196. Finkelstein JS, Klibanski A, Neer RM, et al. Osteoporosis in men with idiopathic hypogonadotropic hypogonadism. Ann Intern Med 1987; 106:354–361.
197. Kirkland RT, Keenan BS, Probstfield JL, et al. Decrease in plasma high-density lipoprotein cholesterol levels at puberty in boys with delayed adolescence: correlation with plasma testosterone levels. JAMA 1987; 257:502–507.
198. Mauras N, Blizzard RM, Link K, et al. Augmentation of growth hormone secretion during puberty: evidence for a pulse amplitude–modulated phenomenon. J Clin Endocrinol Metab 1987; 64:596–601.
199. Merimee TJ, Zapf J, Hewlett B, et al. Insulin-like growth factors in pygmies: the role of puberty in determining final stature. N Engl J Med 1987; 316:906–911.
200. Marshall WA, Tanner JM. Variations in the pattern of pubertal changes in boys. Arch Dis Child 1970; 45:13–23.
201. Lee PA, Jaffe RB, Midgley AR Jr. Serum gonadotropin, testosterone and prolactin concentrations throughout puberty in boys: a longitudinal study. J Clin Endocrinol Metab 1974; 39:664–672.
202. Schonfeld WA. Primary and secondary sexual characteristics: study of their development in males from birth through maturity, with biometric study of penis and testes. Am J Dis Child 1943; 65:535–549.
203. Harlan WR, Grillo GP, Cornoni-Huntley J, et al. Secondary sex characteristics of boys 12 to 17 years of age: the U.S. Health Examination Survey. J Pediatr 1979; 95:293–297.
204. Zachmann M, Prader A, Kind HP, et al. Testicular volume during adolescence: cross-sectional and longitudinal studies. Helv Paediatr Acta 1974; 29:61–72.

205. Karling P, Hammar M, Varenhorst E. Prevalence and duration of hot flushes after surgical or medical castration in men with prostatic carcinoma. J Urol 1994; 152:1170–1173.
206. Wilson JD, Roehrborn C. Long-term consequences of castration in men: lessons from the Skoptzy and the eunuchs of the Chinese and Ottoman courts. J Clin Endocrinol Metab 1999; 84:4324–4331.
207. Harrison RG. Effect of temperature on the mammalian testis. In Greep RO, Astwood EB (eds). Handbook of Physiology, sect 7: Endocrinology, vol V. Male Reproductive System. Washington, DC, American Physiological Society, 1975, pp 219–223.
208. Bremner WJ, Vitiello MV, Prinz PN. Loss of circadian rhythmicity in blood testosterone with aging in normal men. J Clin Endocrinol Metab 1983; 56:1278–1281.
209. Nankin HR, Calkins JH. Decreased bioavailable testosterone in aging normal and impotent men. J Clin Endocrinol Metab 1986; 63:1418–1420.
210. Tenover JS, Matsumoto AM, Plymate SR, et al. The effects of aging in normal men on bioavailable testosterone and luteinizing hormone secretion: response to clomiphene citrate. J Clin Endocrinol Metab 1987; 65:1118–1126.
211. Gray A, Feldman HA, McKinley JB, et al. Age, disease, and changing sex hormone levels in middle-aged men: results of the Massachusetts Male Aging Study. J Clin Endocrinol Metab 1991; 73:1016–1025.
212. Krithivas K, Yuragalevitch SM, Mohr BA, et al. Evidence that the CAG repeat in the androgen receptor gene is associated with the age-related decline in serum androgen levels in men. J Endocrinol 1999; 162:137–142.
213. Leifke E, Gorenol V, Wichers C, et al. Age-related changes of serum sex hormones, insulin-like growth factor-1 and sex-hormone binding globulin levels in men: cross-sectional data from a healthy male cohort. Clin Endocrinol (Oxf) 2000; 53:689–695.
214. Rolf C, Behre HM, Nieschlag E. Reproductive parameters of older men compared to younger men of infertile couples. Int J Androl 1996; 19:135–142.
215. Neaves WH, Johnson L, Petty CS. Seminiferous tubules and daily sperm production in older adult men with varied numbers of Leydig cells. Biol Reprod 1987; 36:301–308.
216. Mahmoud AM, Goemaere S, De Bacquer D, et al. Serum inhibin B levels in community-dwelling elderly men. Clin Endocrinol (Oxf) 2000; 53:141–147.
217. Morley JE, Kaiser FE, Perry HM III, et al. Longitudinal changes in testosterone, luteinizing hormone, and follicle-stimulating hormone in healthy older men. Metabolism 1997; 46:410–413.
218. Deslypere JP, Kaufman JM, Vermeulen T, et al. Influence of age on pulsatile luteinizing hormone release and responsiveness of the gonadotrophs to sex hormone feedback in men. J Clin Endocrinol Metab 1987; 64:68–73.
219. Urban RJ, Veldhuis JD, Blizzard RM, et al. Attenuated release of biologically active luteinizing hormone in healthy aging men. J Clin Invest 1988; 81:1020–1029.
220. Tenover JS, Dahl KD, Hsueh AJW, et al. Serum bioactive and immunoreactive follicle-stimulating hormone levels and the response to clomiphene in healthy young and elderly men. J Clin Endocrinol Metab 1987; 64:1103–1107.
221. Winters SJ, Atkinson L. Serum LH concentrations in hypogonadal men during transdermal testosterone replacement through scrotal skin: further evidence that ageing enhances testosterone negative feedback. Clin Endocrinol (Oxf) 1997; 47:317–322.
222. Veldhuis JD, Iranmanesh A, Godschalk M, Mulligan T. Older men manifest multifold synchrony disruption of reproductive neurohormone outflow. J Clin Endocrinol Metab 2000; 85:1477–1486.
223. Mulligan T, Iranmanesh A, Kerzner R, et al. Two-week pulsatile gonadotropin releasing hormone infusion unmasks dual (hypothalamic and Leydig cell) defects in the healthy aging male gonadotropic axis. Eur J Endocrinol 1999; 141:257–266.
224. Van den Beld AW, de Jong FH, Grobbee DE, et al. Measures of bioavailable serum testosterone and estradiol and their relationship with muscle strength, bone density, and body composition in elderly men. J Clin Endocrinol Metab 2000; 85:3276–3282.
225. Falahati-Nini A, Riggs BL, Atkinson EJ, et al. Relative contributions of testosterone and estrogen in regulating bone resorption and formation in normal elderly men. J Clin Invest 2000; 106: 1553–1560.
226. Barrett-Connor E, Von Muhlen DG, Kritz-Silverstein D. Bioavailable testosterone and depressed mood in older men: the Rancho Bernardo study. J Clin Endocrinol Metab 1999; 84:573–577.
227. Barrett-Connor E, Goodman-Gruen D, Patay B. Endogenous sex hormones and cognitive function in older men. J Clin Endocrinol Metab 1999; 84:3681–3685.
228. Wang C, Alexander G, Berman N, et al. Testosterone replacement therapy improves mood in hypogonadal men: a clinical research center study. J Clin Endocrinol Metab 1996; 81:3578–3583.
229. Katznelson L, Finkelstein JS, Schoenfeld DA, et al. Increase in bone density and lean body mass during testosterone administration in men with acquired hypogonadism. J Clin Endocrinol Metab 1996; 81:4358–4365.
230. Spratt DI, O'Dea LSL, Schoenfeld D, et al. Neuroendocrine-gonadal axis in men: frequent sampling of LH, FSH, and testosterone. Am J Physiol 1988; 254:E658–E666.
231. Vermeulen A, Verdonck G. Representativeness of a single point plasma testosterone level for the long term hormonal milieu in men. J Clin Endocrinol Metab 1992; 74:939–942.
232. Winters SJ, Kelley DE, Goodpaster B. The analog free testosterone assay: are the results clinically useful? Clin Chem 1998; 44: 2178–2182.
233. Cooke RR, McIntosh RP, McIntosh JGA, et al. Serum forms of testosterone in men after an hCG stimulation: relative increase in non–protein bound forms. Clin Endocrinol (Oxf) 1990; 32:165–175.
234. Vermeulen A, Verdonck L, Kaufman JM. A critical evaluation of simple methods for the estimation of free testosterone in serum. J Clin Endocrinol Metab 1999; 84:3666–3672.
235. Walsh PC, Curry N, Mills RC, et al. Plasma androgen response to hCG stimulation in prepubertal boys with hypospadias and cryptorchidism. J Clin Endocrinol Metab 1976; 42:52–59.
236. Wollesen F, Swerdloff RS, Odell WD. LH and FSH responses to luteinizing-releasing hormone in normal, adult, human males. Metabolism 1976; 28:845–863.
237. Synder PJ, Rudenstein RS, Gardner DF, et al. Repetitive infusion of gonadotropin-releasing hormone distinguishes hypothalamic from pituitary hypogonadism. J Clin Endocrinol Metab 1979; 48: 864–868.
238. Diamond JM. Variation in human testis size. Nature 1986; 320: 488–489.
239. Taskinen S, Taavitsainen M, Wikstrom S. Measurement of testicular volume: comparison of 3 different methods. J Urol 1996; 155:930–933.
240. Sherins RJ, Brightwell D, Sternthal PM. Longitudinal analysis of semen of fertile and infertile men. In Troen P, Nankin HR (eds). The Testis in Normal and Infertile Men. New York, Raven Press, 1977, pp 473–488.
241. Wilton LJ, Teichtahl H, Temple-Smith PD, et al. Structural heterogeneity of the axonemes of respiratory cilia and sperm flagella in normal men. J Clin Invest 1985; 75:825–831.
242. Kim ED, Gilbaugh JH, Patel VP, et al. Testis biopsies frequently demonstrate sperm in men with azoospermia and significantly elevated follicle-stimulating hormone levels. J Urol 1997; 157: 144–146.
243. Craft I, Tsirigotis M, Courtauld E, et al. Testicular needle aspiration as an alternative to biopsy for assessment of spermatogenesis. Hum Reprod 1997; 12:1483–1487.
244. Klein KO, Baron J, Colli MJ, et al. Estrogen levels in childhood determined by an ultrasensitive recombinant cell bioassay. J Clin Invest 1994; 94:2475–2480.
245. Toppari J, Kaleva M. Maldescendus testis. Horm Res 1999; 51: 261–269.
246. Gill B, Kogan S. Cryptorchidism: current concepts. Pediatr Clin North Am 1997; 44:1211–1227.
247. Rafjer J. Congenital anomalies of the testes. In Walsh PC, Retik AB, Stamey TA, et al (eds). Campbell's Urology, 6th ed. Philadelphia, WB Saunders, 1992, pp 1543–1562.
248. Wiener JS, Marcelli M, Gonzales ET Jr, et al. Androgen receptor gene alterations are not associated with isolated cryptorchidism. J Urol 1998; 160:863–865.
249. Favorito LA, Sampaio FJ, Javaroni V, et al. Proximal insertion of gubernaculum testis in normal human fetuses and in boys with cryptorchidism. J Urol 2000; 164:792–794.
250. Krausz C, Quintana-Murci L, Fellous M, et al. Absence of muta-

tions involving the *INSL3* gene in human idiopathic cryptorchidism. Mol Hum Reprod 2000; 6:298–302.
251. Cortes D, Thorup JM, Lenz K, et al. Laparoscopy in 100 consecutive patients with 128 impalpable testes. Br J Urol 1995; 75: 281–287.
252. Huff DS, Snyder HM III, Hadziselimovic F, et al. An absent testis is associated with contralateral testicular hypertrophy. J Urol 1992; 148:627–628.
253. Lindgren BW, Darby EC, Faiella L, et al. Laparoscopic orchiopexy: procedure of choice for the nonpalpable testis? J Urol 1998; 159:2132–2135.
254. Lipshultz LI, Caminos-Torres R, Greenspan CS, et al. Testicular function after orchiopexy for unilaterally undescended testis. N Engl J Med 1976; 295:15–18.
255. Lee PA, O'Leary LA, Songer NJ, et al. Paternity after bilateral cryptorchidism: a controlled study. Arch Pediatr Adolesc Med 1997; 151:260–263.
256. Lee MM, Donahoe PK, Silverman BL, et al. Measurements of serum müllerian inhibiting substance in the evaluation of children with nonpalpable gonads. N Engl J Med 1997; 336:1480–1486.
257. Pyorala S, Huttunen N-P, Uhari M. A review and meta-analysis of hormonal treatment of cryptorchidism. J Clin Endocrinol Metab 1995; 80:2795–2799.
258. Heiskanen P, Billig H, Toppari J. Apoptotic cell death in the normal and cryptorchid human testis: the effect of human chorionic gonadotropin on testicular cell survival. Pediatr Res 1996; 40:351–356.
259. Dunkel L, Taskinen S, Hovatta O, et al. Germ cell apoptosis after treatment of cryptorchidism with human chorionic gonadotropin is associated with impaired reproductive function in the adult. J Clin Invest 1997; 100:2341–2346.
260. Cortes D, Thorup J, Visfeldt J. Hormonal treatment may harm the germ cells in 1 to 3-year-old boys with cryptorchidism. J Urol 2000; 163:1290–1292.
261. Finkelstein JS, Klibanski A, Neer RM, et al. Osteoporosis in men with idiopathic hypogonadotropic hypogonadism. Ann Intern Med 1987; 106:354–361.
262. Greenspan SL, Oppenheim DS, Klibanski A. Importance of gonadal steroids to bone mass in men with hyperprolactinemic hypogonadism. Ann Intern Med 1989; 110:526–531.
263. Oppenheim DS, Greenspan SL, Zervas NT, et al. Elevated serum lipids in hypogonadal men with and without hyperprolactinemia. Ann Intern Med 1989; 111:288–292.
264. Aloi JA, Bergendahl M, Iranmanesh A, Veldhuis JD. Pulsatile intravenous gonadotropin-releasing hormone administration averts fasting-induced hypogonadotropism and hypoandrogenemia in healthy, normal weight men. J Clin Endocrinol Metab 1997; 82:1543–1548.
265. Woolf PD, Hamill RW, McDonald JV, et al. Transient hypogonadotropic hypogonadism caused by critical illness. J Clin Endocrinol Metab 1985; 60:444–450.
266. Baker HWG. Reproductive effects of nontesticular illness. Endocrinol Metab Clin North Am 1998; 27:831–850.
267. Hayes FJ, Seminara SB, Crowley WF. Hypogonadotropic hypogonadism. Endocrinol Metab Clin North Am 1998; 27:739–763.
268. Seminara SB, Hayes FJ, Crowley WF Jr. Gonadotropin-releasing hormone deficiency in the human: pathophysiological and genetic considerations. Endocr Rev 1998; 19:521–539.
269. Waldstreicher J, Seminara SB, Jameson JL, et al. The genetic and clinical heterogeneity of gonadotropin-releasing hormone deficiency in the human. J Clin Endocrinol Metab 1996; 81:4388–4395.
270. Smals AGH, Kloppenborg PWC, Van Haelst UJG, et al. Fertile eunuch syndrome versus classic hypogonadotrophic hypogonadism. Acta Endocrinol (Copenh) 1978; 87:389–399.
271. Reitano JF, Caminos-Torres R, Snyder PJ. Serum LH and FSH responses to the repetitive administration of gonadotropin-releasing hormone in patients with idiopathic hypogonadotropic hypogonadism. J Clin Endocrinol Metab 1975; 41:1035–1042.
272. Barkan AL, Reame NE, Kelch RP, et al. Idiopathic hypogonadotropic hypogonadism in men: dependence of the hormone responses to gonadotropin-releasing hormone (GnRH) on the magnitude of the endogenous GnRH secretory defect. J Clin Endocrinol Metab 1985; 61:1118–1125.
273. Franco B, Guilo S, Pragliola A, et al. A gene deleted in Kallmann's syndrome shares homology with neural cell adhesion and axonal path-finding molecules. Nature 1991; 353:529–536.
274. Oliveira LMB, Seminara SB, Beranova M, et al. The importance of autosomal genes in Kallmann syndrome: genotype-phenotype correlations and neuroendocrine characteristics. J Clin Endocrinol Metab 2001; 86:1532–1538.
275. McCabe ERB. Adrenal hypoplasias and aplasias. In Scriver CR, Beaudet AL, Sly WS, Valle D (eds). The Metabolic and Molecular Bases of Inherited Disease, 8th ed. New York, McGraw Hill, 2001, pp 4263–4274.
276. Habiby RL, Boepple P, Nachtigall L, et al. Adrenal hypoplasia congenita with hypogonadotropic hypogonadism: evidence that *DAX-1* mutations lead to combined hypothalamic and pituitary defects in gonadotropin production. J Clin Invest 1996; 98:1055–1062.
277. Seminara SB, Achermann JC, Genel M, et al. X-linked adrenal hypoplasia congenita: a mutation in *DAX1* expands the phenotypic spectrum in males and females. J Clin Endocrinol Metab 1999; 84:4501–4509.
278. Tabarin A, Achermann JC, Recan D, et al. A novel mutation in *DAX1* causes delayed-onset adrenal insufficiency and incomplete hypogonadotropic hypogonadism. J Clin Invest 2000; 105:321–328.
279. Beranova M, Oliveira LMB, Bedecarrats GY, et al. Prevalence, phenotypic spectrum, and modes of inheritance of gonadotropin-releasing hormone receptor mutations in idiopathic hypogonadotropic hypogonadism. J Clin Endocrinol Metab 2001; 86:1580–1588.
280. Weiss J, Axelrod L, Whitcomb RW, et al. Hypogonadism caused by a single amino acid substitution in the β subunit of luteinizing hormone. N Engl J Med 1992; 326:179–183.
281. Philip M, Arbelle JE, Segev Y, Parvari R. Male hypogonadism due to a mutation in the gene for the β-subunit of follicle-stimulating hormone. N Engl J Med 1998; 338:1729–1732.
282. Nicholls RD. Genomic imprinting and uniparenteral disomy in Angelman and Prader-Willi syndromes: a review. Am J Med Genet 1993; 46:16–25.
283. Nagai T, Mori M. Prader-Willi syndrome, diabetes mellitus and hypogonadism. Biomed Pharmacother 1999; 53:452–454.
284. Burstein S, Grumbach MM, Kaplan SL. Early determination of androgen-responsiveness is important in the management of microphallus. Lancet 1979; 2:983–986.
285. Wang C, Paulsen CA, Hopper BR, et al. Acute steroidogenic responsiveness to human luteinizing hormone in hypogonadotropic hypogonadism. J Clin Endocrinol Metab 1980; 51:1269–1273.
286. Finkel DM, Phillips JL, Snyder PJ. Stimulation of spermatogenesis by gonadotropins in men with hypogonadotropic hypogonadism. N Engl J Med 1985; 313:651–655.
287. Burris AS, Rodbard HW, Winters SJ, et al. Gonadotropin therapy in men with isolated hypogonadotropic hypogonadism: the response to human chorionic gonadotropin is predicted by initial testicular size. J Clin Endocrinol Metab 1986; 66:1144–1151.
288. Davis JL. Lowering prolactin level in a hyperprolactinemic man: responses of luteinizing hormone, follicle-stimulating hormone, and testosterone. Arch Intern Med 1982; 142:146–148.
289. Schafer AI, Cheron RG, Dluhy R, et al. Clinical consequence of acquired transfusional iron overload in adults. N Engl J Med 1981; 304:319–324.
290. Edwards OM, Clark JDA. Post-traumatic hypopituitarism: six cases and a review of the literature. Medicine (Baltimore) 1986; 65:281–290.
291. Strain GW, Zumoff B, Miller LK, et al. Effect of massive weight loss on hypothalamic-pituitary-gonadal function in obese men. J Clin Endocrinol Metab 1988; 66:1019–1023.
292. Giagulli VA, Kaufman JM, Vermeulen A. Pathogenesis of the decreased androgen levels in obese men. J Clin Endocrinol Metab 1994; 79:997–1000.
293. Semple PA, Graham A, Malcolm Y, et al. Hypoxia, depression of testosterone, and impotence in pickwickian syndrome reversed by weight reduction. Br Med J 1984; 29:801–802.
294. Herzog AG, Seibel MM, Schomer DL, et al. Reproductive endocrine disorders in men with partial seizures of temporal lobe origin. Arch Neurol 1986; 43:347–350.
295. Cunningham GR. Idiopathic post-pubertal LH deficiency. Clin Res 1983; 31:896A.
296. Nachtigall LB, Boepple PA, Pralong FP, Crowley WF Jr. Adult-onset idiopathic hypogonadotropic hypogonadism: a treatable form of male infertility. N Engl J Med 1997; 336:410–415.

297. Themmen APN, Martens JWM, Brunner HG. Activating and inactivating mutations in LH receptors. Mol Cell Endocrinol 1998; 145:137–142.
298. Martens JWM, Verhoef-Post M, Abelin N, et al. A homozygous mutation in the luteinizing hormone receptor causes partial Leydig cell hypoplasia: correlation between receptor activity and phenotype. Mol Endocrinol 1998; 12:775–784.
299. Gromoll J, Eiholzer U, Nieschlag E, Simoni M. Male hypogonadism caused by homozygous deletion of exon 10 of the luteinizing hormone (LH) receptor: differential action of human chorionic gonadotropin and LH. J Clin Endocrinol Metab 2000; 85:2281–2286.
300. Smyth CM, Bremmer WJ. Klinefelter syndrome. Arch Intern Med 1998; 158:1309–1314.
301. Rovet J, Netley C, Keenan M, et al. The psychoeducational profile of boys with Klinefelter syndrome. J Learn Disabilities 1996; 29:180–196.
302. Sasco AJ, Lowenfels AB, Pasker-de Jong P. Review article: epidemiology of male breast cancer. A meta-analysis of published case-control studies and discussion of selected aetiological factors. Int J Cancer 1993; 53:538–549.
303. Hultborn R, Hanson C, Kopf I, et al. Prevalence of Klinefelter's syndrome in male breast cancer patients. Anticancer Res 1997; 17:4293–4298.
304. Hasle H, Mellembaard A, Nielsen J, Hansen J. Cancer incidence in men with Klinefelter syndrome. Br J Cancer 1995; 71:416–420.
305. Prall JA, McGavran L, Greffe BS, Partington MD. Intracranial malignant germ cell tumor and the Klinefelter syndrome. Pediatr Neurosurg 1995; 23:219–224.
306. Zollner TM, Veraart JCJM, Wolter M, et al. Leg ulcers in Klinefelter's syndrome: further evidence for an involvement of plasminogen activator inhibitor-1. Br J Dermatol 1997; 136:341–344.
307. Abramsky L, Chapple J. 47,XXY (Klinefelter syndrome) and 47,XYY: estimated rates of and indication for postnatal diagnosis with implications for prenatal counseling. Prenat Diagn 1997; 17: 363–368.
308. Nielsen J, Wohlert M. Chromosome abnormalities found among 34910 newborn children: results from a 13-year incidence study in Arhus, Denmark. Hum Genet 1991; 87:81–83.
309. Wang C, Baker HWG, Burger HG, et al. Hormonal studies in Klinefelter's syndrome. Clin Endocrinol (Oxf) 1975; 4:399–411.
310. Salbenblatt JA, Bender BG, Puck MH, et al. Pituitary-gonadal function in Klinefelter syndrome before and during puberty. Pediatr Res 1985; 19:82–86.
311. Samaan NA, Stepanas AV, Danziger J, et al. Reactive pituitary abnormalities in patients with Klinefelter's and Turner's syndromes. Arch Intern Med 1979; 139:198–201.
312. Kubler A, Schulz G, Cordes U, et al. The influence of testosterone substitution on bone mineral density in patients with Klinefelter's syndrome. Exp Clin Endocrinol 1992; 100:129–132.
313. Nielsen J, Pelsen B, Sorensen K. Follow-up of 30 Klinefelter males treated with testosterone. Clin Genet 1988; 33:262–269.
314. Caminos-Torres R, Ma L, Snyder PJ. Testosterone-induced inhibition of the LH and FSH responses to gonadotropin-releasing hormone occurs slowly. J Clin Endocrinol Metab 1977; 44:1142–1153.
315. Foresta C, Galeazzi C, Bettella A, et al. High incidence of sperm sex chromosomes aneuploidies in two patients with Klinefelter's syndrome. J Clin Endocrinol Metab 1998; 83:203–205.
316. de la Chapelle A, Hastbocka J, Korhonen T, Maenpaa J. The etiology of XX sex reversal. Reprod Nutr Dev Suppl 1990; 1: 39S–49S.
317. Schweikert HU, Weissbach L, Leyendecker G, et al. Clinical, endocrinological, and cytological characterization of two 46,XX males. J Clin Endocrinol Metab 1982; 54:745–752.
318. Ferguson-Smith MA, Cooke A, Affara NA, et al. Genotype-phenotype correlations in XX males and their bearing on current theories of sex determination. Hum Genet 1990; 84:198–202.
319. Fechner PY, Marcantonio SM, Jaswaney V, et al. The role of the sex-determining region Y gene in the etiology of 46,XX maleness. J Clin Endocrinol Metab 1993; 76:690–695.
320. Boucekkine C, Toublanc JE, Abbas N, et al. Clinical and anatomical spectrum in XX sex reversed patients: relationship to the presence of Y-specific DNA sequences. Clin Endocrinol (Oxf) 1994; 40:733–742.
321. Mardon G, Mosher R, Disteche CM, et al. Duplication, deletion, and polymorphism in the sex-determining region of the mouse Y chromosome. Science 1989; 243:78–80.
322. Sarafoglou K, Ostrer H. Familial sex reversal: a review. J Clin Endocrinol Metab 2000; 85:483–493.
323. Huang B, Wang S, Ning Y, et al. Autosomal XX sex reversal caused by duplication of *SOX9*. Am J Med Genet 1999; 87:349–353.
324. Kusz K, Kotecki M, Wojda A, et al. Incomplete masculinization of XX subjects carrying the *SRY* gene on an inactive X chromosome. J Med Genet 1999; 36:452–456.
325. Manson AL. Mumps orchitis. Urology 1990; 36: 355–358.
326. Aiman J, Brenner PF, MacDonald PC. Androgen and estrogen production in elderly men with gynecomastia and testicular atrophy after mumps orchitis. J Clin Endocrinol Metab 1980; 50: 380–386.
327. Ku JH, Kim YH, Jeon YS, Lee NK. The preventive effect of systemic treatment with interferon-α2B for infertility from mumps orchitis. BJU Int 1999; 84:839–842.
328. Cross JJ, Berman LH, Elliott PG, Irving S. Scrotal trauma: a cause of testicular atrophy. Clin Radiol 1999; 54:317–320.
329. Wang J, Galil KAA, Setchell BP. Changes in testicular blood flow and testosterone production during aspermatogenesis after irradiation. J Endocrinol 1983; 98:35–46.
330. Sklar C. Reproductive physiology and treatment-related loss of sex hormone production. Med Pediatr Oncol 1999; 33:2–8.
331. Loriaux DL, Menard R, Taylor A, et al. Spironolactone and endocrine dysfunction. Ann Intern Med 1976; 85:630–636.
332. Rajfer J, Sikka SC, Rivera F, et al. Mechanism of inhibition of human testicular steroidogenesis by oral ketoconazole. J Clin Endocrinol Metab 1986; 63:1193–1198.
333. Brunet M, Rodamilans M, Martinez-Osaba MJ, et al. Effects of long-term antiepileptic therapy on the catabolism of testosterone. Pharmacol Toxicol 1995; 76:371–375.
334. Wheeler MJ, Toone BK, Dannatt A, et al. Metabolic clearance rate of testosterone in male epileptic patients on anti-convulsant therapy. J Endocrinol 1991; 129:465–468.
335. Cicero TJ. Alcohol-induced deficits in the hypothalamic-pituitary–luteinizing hormone axis in the male. Alcohol Clin Exp Res 1982; 6:207–215.
336. Van Thiel DH, Gavaler JS, Lester R, et al. Alcohol-induced testicular atrophy: an experimental model for hypogonadism occurring in chronic alcoholic men. Gastroenterology 1975; 69: 326–332.
337. Van Thiel DH, Cobb CF, Herman GB, et al. An examination of various mechanisms for ethanol-induced testicular injury: studies utilizing the isolated perfused rat testes. Endocrinology 1981; 109:2009–2015.
338. Pajarinen JT, Karhunen PJ. Spermatogenic arrest and 'Sertoli cell-only' syndrome: common alcohol-induced disorders of the human testis. Int J Androl 1994; 17:292–299.
339. Chapman RM, Rees LH, Sutcliff SB, et al. Cyclical combination chemotherapy and gonadal function. Lancet 1979; 1:285–289.
340. Meikle AW, Cardoso de Sousa JC, Ward JH, et al. Reduction of testosterone synthesis after high dose interleukin-2 therapy of metastatic cancer. J Clin Endocrinol Metab 1991; 73:931–935.
341. Kolodny RC, Masters WH, Kolodner RM, et al. Depression of plasma testosterone levels after chronic intensive marihuana use. N Engl J Med 1974; 290:872–874.
342. Wang C, Chan V, Yeung RTT. The effect of heroin addiction on pituitary-testicular function. Clin Endocrinol (Oxf) 1978; 9: 455–461.
343. Hong CY, Chaput de Saintonge DM, Turner P. Δ^9-Tetrahydrocannabinol inhibits human sperm motility. J Pharm Pharmacol 1981; 33:746–747.
344. Blumer D, Migeon C. Hormone and hormonal agents in the treatment of aggression. J Nerv Ment Dis 1975; 160:127–137.
345. Rinieris P, Hatzimanolis J, Markianos M, Stefanis C. Effects of 4 weeks treatment with chlorpromazine and/or trihexyphenidyl on the pituitary-gonadal axis in male paranoid schizophrenics. Eur Arch Psychiatry Neurol Sci 1988; 237:189–193.
346. Rosenthal SM, Grumbach MM. Gonadotropin-independent familial sexual precocity with premature Leydig and germinal cell maturation (familial testotoxicosis): effects of a potent luteinizing hormone–releasing factor agonist and medroxyprogesterone acetate therapy in four cases. J Clin Endocrinol Metab 1983; 57: 571–579.

347. Van Thiel DH, Gavaler JS, Smith WI Jr, et al. Hypothalamic-pituitary-gonadal dysfunction in men using cimetidine. N Engl J Med 1979; 300:1012–1015.
348. Peden NR, Boyd EJS, Browning MCK, et al. Effects of two histamine H2-receptor blocking drugs on basal levels of gonadotrophins, prolactin, testosterone and oestradiol-17β during treatment of duodenal ulcer in male patients. Acta Endocrinol (Copenh) 1981; 96:564–568.
349. Lindquist M, Edwards IR. Endocrine adverse effects of omeprazole. Br Med J 1992; 305:451–452.
350. Ng TP, Goh HH, Ng YL, et al. Male endocrine function in workers with moderate exposure to lead. Br J Ind Med 1991; 48: 485–491.
351. Murthy GG, Peress NS, Khan SA. Demonstration of antibodies to testicular basement membrane by immunofluorescence in a patient with multiple primary endocrine deficiencies. J Clin Endocrinol Metab 1976; 42:637–641.
352. Elder M, Maclaren N, Riley W. Gonadal autoantibodies in patients with hypogonadism and/or Addison's disease. J Clin Endocrinol Metab 1981; 52:1137–1142.
353. Saporta L, Yuksel A. Androgenic status in patients with lepromatous leprosy. Br J Urol 1994; 74:221–224.
354. Lin T, Wang D, Nagpal ML, et al. Interleukin-1 inhibits cholesterol side-chain cleavage cytochrome P450 expression in primary cultures of Leydig cells. Endocrinology 1991; 129:1305–1311.
355. Maduit C, Gasnier F, Rey C, et al. Tumor necrosis factor-α inhibits Leydig cell steroidogenesis through a decrease in steroidogenic acute regulatory protein expression. Endocrinology 1998; 139:2863–2868.
356. Tsigos C, Papanicolaou DA, Kyrou I, et al. Dose-dependent effects of recombinant human interleukin-6 on the pituitary-testicular axis. J Interferon Cytokine Res 1999; 19:1271–1276.
357. Holdsworth S, Atkins RC, de Kretser D. The pituitary-testicular axis in men with chronic renal failure. N Engl J Med 1977; 296: 1245–1249.
358. Holdsworth SR, de Kretser DM, Atkins RC. A comparison of hemodialysis and transplantation in reversing the uremic disturbance of male reproductive function. Clin Nephrol 1978; 10:146–150.
359. Kley HK, Strohmeyer G, Kruskemper HL. Effect of testosterone application on hormone concentrations of androgens and estrogens in male patients with cirrhosis of the liver. Gastroenterology 1979; 76:235–241.
360. Abbasi AA, Prasad AS, Ortega J, et al. Gonadal function abnormalities in sickle cell anemia: studies in adult male patients. Ann Intern Med 1976; 85:601–605.
361. Landon C, Rosenfeld RG. Short stature and pubertal delay in male adolescents with cystic fibrosis: androgen treatment. Am J Dis Child 1984; 138:388–391.
362. Handelsman DJ, Yue DK, Turtle JR. Hypogonadism and massive testicular infiltration due to amyloidosis. J Urol 1983; 129:610–612.
363. Salehian B, Jacobson D, Swerdloff RS, et al. Testicular pathologic changes and the pituitary-testicular axis during human immunodeficiency virus infection. Endocr Pract 1999; 5:1–9.
364. Laudat A, Blum L, Guechot J, et al. Changes in systemic gonadal and adrenal steroids in asymptomatic human immunodeficiency virus–infected men: relationship with the CD4 cell counts. Eur J Endocrinol 1995; 133:418–424.
365. Dobs AS, Few WL III, Blackman MR, et al. Serum hormones in human immunodeficiency virus–associated wasting. J Clin Endocrinol Metab 1996; 81:4198–4112.
366. Grinspoon S, Corcoran C, Askari H, et al. Effects of androgen administration in men with the AIDS wasting syndrome: a randomized, double-blind, placebo-controlled trial. Ann Intern Med 1998; 129:18–26.
367. Grinspoon S, Corcoran C, Anderson E, et al. Sustained anabolic effects of long-term androgen administration in men with AIDS wasting. Clin Infect Dis 1999; 28:6344–636.
368. Grinspoon S, Corcoran C, Stanley T, et al. Effects of hypogonadism and testosterone administration on depression indices in HIV-infected men. J Clin Endocrinol Metab 2000; 85:60–65.
369. Bhasin S, Storer TW, Javanbakht M, et al. Testosterone replacement and resistance exercise in HIV-infected men with weight loss and low testosterone levels. JAMA 2000; 283:763–770.
370. Martens HF, Sheets PK, Tenover JS, et al. Decreased testosterone levels in men with rheumatoid arthritis: effect of low dose prednisone therapy. J Rheumatol 1994; 21:1427–1431.
371. Vazquez JA, Pinies JA, Martul P, et al. Hypothalamic-pituitary-testicular function in 70 patients with myotonic dystrophy. J Endocrinol Invest 1990; 13:375–379.
372. Claus-Walker J, Scurry M, Carter RE, et al. Steady state hormonal secretion in traumatic quadriplegia. J Clin Endocrinol Metab 1977; 44:530–535.
373. Piera JB. The establishment of a prognosis for genito-sexual function in the paraplegic and tetraplegic male. Paraplegia 1973; 10:271–278.
374. Hasen J, Boyar RM, Shapiro LR. Gonadal function in trisomy 21. Horm Res 1980; 12:345–350.
375. Aiman J, Griffin JE, Gazak JM, et al. Androgen insensitivity as a cause of infertility in otherwise normal men. N Engl J Med 1979; 330:223–227.
376. Yong EL, Ng SC, Roy AC, et al. Pregnancy after hormonal correction of severe spermatogenic defect due to mutation in androgen receptor gene. Lancet 1994; 344:826–827.
377. Giwercman A, Kledal T, Schwartz M, et al. Preserved male fertility despite decreased androgen sensitivity caused by a mutation in the ligand-binding domain of the androgen receptor gene. J Clin Endocrinol Metab 2000; 85:2253–2259.
378. Mozaffarian GA, Higley M, Paulsen CA. Clinical studies in an adult male patient with 'isolated follicle stimulating hormone (FSH) deficiency.' J Androl 1983; 4:393–398.
379. Lindstedt G, Nystrom E, Matthews C, et al. Follitropin (FSH) deficiency in an infertile male due to FSHβ gene mutation: a syndrome of normal puberty and virilization but underdeveloped testicles with azoospermia, low FSH but high lutropin and normal serum testosterone concentrations. Clin Chem Lab Med 1998; 36:663–665.
380. Bonaccorsi AC, Adler I, Figueiredo JG. Male infertility due to congenital adrenal hyperplasia: testicular biopsy findings, hormonal evaluation, and therapeutic results in three patients. Fertil Steril 1987; 47:664–670.
381. Schurmeyer T, Belkien L, Knuth UA, et al. Reversible azoospermia induced by the anabolic steroid 19-nortestosterone. Lancet 1984; 1:417–420.
382. Rothman CM, Sims CA, Stotts CL. Sertoli cell only syndrome 1982. Fertil Steril 1982; 38:388–390.
383. Pajarinen JT, Karhunen PJ. Spermatogenic arrest and 'Sertoli cell–only' syndrome: common alcohol-induced disorders of the human testis. Int J Androl 1994; 17:292–299.
384. Tiepolo L, Zuffardi O. Localization of factors controlling spermatogenesis in the nonfluorescent portion of the human Y chromosome long arm. Hum Genet 1976; 34:119–124.
385. Chandley AC, Cooke HJ. Human male fertility: Y-linked genes and spermatogenesis. Hum Mol Genet 1994; 3:1449–1452.
386. Najmabadi H, Huant V, Yen P, et al. Substantial prevalence of microdeletions of the Y-chromosome in infertile men with idiopathic azoospermia and oligozoospermia detected using a sequence-tagged site-based mapping strategy. J Clin Endocrinol Metab 1996; 81:1347–1352.
387. Ma K, Inglis JD, Sharkey A, et al. A Y chromosome gene family with RNA-binding protein homology: candidates for the azoospermia factor AZF controlling human spermatogenesis. Cell 1993; 75:1287–1295.
388. Reijo R, Lee T-Y, Alagappan R, et al. Diverse spermatogenic defects in humans caused by Y chromosome deletions encompassing a novel RNA-binding protein gene. Nat Genet 1995; 10: 383–393.
389. Foresta C, Ferlin A, Garolla A, et al. Y-chromosome deletions in idiopathic severe testiculopathies. J Clin Endocrinol Metab 1997; 82:1075–1080.
390. Krausz C, Quintana-Murci L, Barbaux S, et al. A high frequency of Y chromosome deletions in males with nonidiopathic infertility. J Clin Endocrinol Metab 1999; 84:3606–3612.
391. Tapanainen JS, Vaskiuvuo T, Aittomaki K, Huhtaniemi IT. Inactivating FSH receptor mutations and gonadal dysfunction. Mol Cell Endocrinol 1998; 145:129–135.
392. Chaganti RSK, German J. Human male infertility, probably genetically determined, due to defective meiosis and spermatogenic arrest. Am J Hum Genet 1979; 31:634–641.
393. Chaganti RSK, Jhanwar SC, German J. Genetically determined asynapsis, spermatogenic degeneration, and infertility in men. Am J Hum Genet 1980; 32:833–848.

394. Greenberg SH, Lipshultz LI, Wein AJ. Experience with 425 subfertile male patients. J Urol 1978; 119:507–510.
395. Fariss BL, Fenner DK, Plymate SR, et al. Seminal characteristics in the presence of a varicocele as compared with those of expectant fathers and prevasectomy men. Fertil Steril 1981; 35:325–327.
396. Wright EJ, Young GP, Goldstein M. Reduction in testicular temperature after varicocelectomy in infertile men. Urology 1997; 50:257–259.
397. Zini A, Buckspan M, Berardinucci D, Jarvi K. Loss of left testicular volume in men with clinical left varicocele: correlation with grade of varicocele. Arch Androl 1998; 41:37–41.
398. Moro E, Marin P, Rossi A, et al. Y chromosome microdeletions in infertile men with varicocele. Mol Cell Endocrinol 2000; 161: 67–71.
399. Dubin L, Amelar RD. Varicocelectomy: 986 cases in a twelve-year study. Urology 1977; 10:446–449.
400. Pedersen H, Hammen R. Ultrastructure of human spermatozoa with complete subcellular derangement. Arch Androl 1982; 9: 251–259.
401. Cassell GH, Younger JB, Brown MB, et al. Microbiologic study of infertile women at the time of diagnostic laparoscopy. N Engl J Med 1983; 308:502–505.
402. Toth A, Lesser ML, Brooks C, Labriola D. Subsequent pregnancies among 161 couples treated for T-mycoplasma genital-tract infection. N Engl J Med 1983; 308:505–507.
403. Pannekoek Y, Trum JW, Bleker OP, et al. Cytokine concentrations in seminal plasma from subfertile men are not indicative of the presence of *Ureaplasma urealyticum* or *Mycoplasma hominis* in the lower genital tract. J Med Microbiol 2000; 49:697–700.
404. Hahn EW, Feingold SM, Nisce L. Aspermia and recovery of spermatogenesis in cancer patients following incidental gonadal irradiation during treatment: a progress report. Radiology 1976; 119:223–225.
405. Shapiro E, Kinsella TJ, Makuch RW, et al. Effects of fractionated irradiation on endocrine aspects of testicular function. J Clin Oncol 1985; 3:1232–1239.
406. Asbjornsen G, Molne K, Klepp O, et al. Testicular function after radiotherapy to inverted 'Y' field for malignant lymphoma. Scand J Haematol 1976; 17:96–100.
407. Handelsman DJ, Turtle JR. Testicular damage after radioactive iodine (I-131) therapy for thyroid cancer. Clin Endocrinol (Oxf) 1983; 18:465–472.
408. Howell SJ, Shalet SM. Pharmacological protection of the gonads. Med Pediatr Oncol 1999; 33:41–45.
409. Schilsky RL, Sherins RJ. Gonadal dysfunction. In DeVita VT Jr, Hellman S, Rosenberg SA (eds). Cancer: Principles and Practice of Oncology, vol 2. Philadelphia, JB Lippincott, 1985, pp 2032–2039.
410. Wallace EM, Groome NP, Riley SC, et al. Effects of chemotherapy-induced testicular damage on inhibin, gonadotropin and testosterone secretion: a prospective longitudinal study. J Clin Endocrinol Metab 1997; 82:3111–3115.
411. Buchanan JD, Fairley KF, Barrie JU. Return of spermatogenesis after stopping cyclophosphamide therapy. Lancet 1975; 2:156–157.
412. Santoro A, Viviani S, Zucali R, et al. Comparative results and toxicity of MOPP vs ABVD combined with radiotherapy in PS IIB, III Hodgkin's disease (abstract). Proc Am Soc Clin Oncol 1983; 2:223.
413. Mustieles C, Munoz A, Alonso M, et al. Male gonadal function after chemotherapy in survivors of childhood malignancy. Med Pediatr Oncol 1995; 24:347–351.
414. Gerres L, Bramswig JH, Schlegel W, et al. The effects of etoposide on testicular function in boys treated for Hodgkin's disease. Cancer 1998; 83:2217–2222.
415. Drasga RE, Einhorn LH, Williams SD, et al. Fertility after chemotherapy for testicular cancer. J Clin Oncol 1983; 1:179–183.
416. Trimmer EE, Zamble DB, Lippard SJ, Essigmann JM. Human testis-determining factor SRY binds to the major DNA adduct of cisplatin and a putative target sequence with comparable affinities. Biochemistry 1998; 37:352–362.
417. Birnie GG, McLeod TIF, Watkinson G. Incidence of sulphasalazine-induced male infertility. Gut 1981; 22:452–455.
418. Morris LF, Harrod MJ, Menter MA, et al. Methotrexate and reproduction in men: case report and recommendations. J Am Acad Dermatol 1993; 29:913–916.
419. Brinkworth MH, Handelsman DJ. Environmental influences on male reproductive health. In Nieschlag E, Behre HM (eds). Andrology, 2nd ed. Berlin: Springer-Verlag, 2000, pp 254–270.
420. Carlsen E, Giwercman A, Keiding N, et al. Evidence for decreasing quality of semen during past 50 years. Br Med J 1992; 305: 609–613.
421. Auger J, Kunstmann JM, Czyglik F, et al. Decline in semen quality among fertile men in Paris during the past 20 years. N Engl J Med 1995; 332: 281–285.
422. Hjort T. Antisperm antibodies and infertility: an unsolvable question? Hum Reprod 1999; 14:2423–2426.
423. Hendry WF, Parslow JM, Stedronska J, et al. The diagnosis of unilateral testicular obstruction in subfertile males. Br J Urol 1982; 54:774–779.
424. Green JRB, Goble HL, Edwards CRW, et al. Reversible insensitivity to androgens in men with untreated gluten enteropathy. Lancet 1977; 1:280–282.
425. Farthing MJG, Edwards CRW, Rees LH, et al. Male gonadal function in coeliac disease. 1: Sexual dysfunction, infertility, and semen quality. Gut 1982; 23:608–614.
426. Farthing MJG, Rees LH, Boylan LM, et al. Male gonadal function in coeliac disease. 2: Sex hormones. Gut 1983; 24:127–135.
427. Aiman J, Griffin JE. The frequency of androgen receptor deficiency in infertile men. J Clin Endocrinol Metab 1982; 54:725–732.
428. Morrow AF, Gyorki S, Warne GL, et al. Variable androgen receptor levels in infertile men. J Clin Endocrinol Metab 1987; 64:1115–1121.
429. Wang Q, Ghadessy FJ, Yong EL. Analysis of the transactivation domain of the androgen receptor in patients with male infertility. Clin Genet 1998; 54:185–192.
430. Wang Q, Ghadessy FJ, Trounson A, et al. Azoospermia associated with a mutation in the ligand-binding domain of an androgen receptor displaying normal ligand binding, but defective *trans*-activation. J Clin Endocrinol Metab 1998; 83:4303–4309.
431. Hiort O, Holterhus P-M, Horter T, et al. Significance of mutations in the androgen receptor gene in males with idiopathic infertility. J Clin Endocrinol Metab 2000; 85:2810–2815.
432. Tut TG, Ghadessy FJ, Trifiro MA, et al. Long polyglutamine tracts in the androgen receptor are associated with reduced *trans*-activation, impaired sperm production, and male infertility. J Clin Endocrinol Metab 1997; 82:3777–3782.
433. Yoshida K-I, Yano M, Chiba K, et al. CAG repeat length in the androgen receptor gene is enhanced in patients with idiopathic azoospermia. Urology 1999; 54:1078–1081.
434. de Kretser DM, Huidobro C, Southwick GJ, Temple-Smith PD. The role of the epididymis in human infertility. J Reprod Fertil Suppl 1998; 53:271–275.
435. Van der Linden EFH, Bartelink AKM, Ike BW, et al. Polycystic kidney disease and infertility. Fertil Steril 1995; 64:202–203.
436. Sharlip ID. Obstructive azoospermia or oligozoospermia due to müllerian duct cyst. Fertil Steril 1983; 39:435–436.
437. Gill WB, Schumacher FGB, Bibbo M. Pathological semen and anatomical abnormalities of the genital tract in human male subjects exposed to diethylstilbestrol in utero. J Urol 1977; 117:477–480.
438. Chillon M, Casals T, Mercier B, et al. Mutations in the cystic fibrosis gene in patients with congenital absence of the vas deferens. N Engl J Med 1995; 332:1475–1480.
439. Mak V, Zielenski J, Tsui L-C, et al. Proportion of cystic fibrosis gene mutations not detected by routine testing in men with obstructive azoospermia. JAMA 1999; 281:2217–2224.
440. Baker HWG, Burger HG, de Kretser DM, et al. Relative incidence of etiological disorders in male infertility. In Santen RJ, Swerdloff RS (eds). Male Reproductive Dysfunction: Diagnosis and Management of Hypogonadism, Infertility and Impotence. New York, Marcel Dekker, 1986, pp 341–372.
441. Gross KM, Matsumoto AM, Southworth MB, et al. Evidence for decreased luteinizing hormone–releasing hormone pulse frequency in men with selective elevations of follicle-stimulating hormone. J Clin Endocrinol Metab 1985; 60:197–202.
442. Gross KM, Matsumoto AM, Berger RE, et al. Increased frequency of pulsatile luteinizing hormone–releasing hormone administration selectively decreases follicle-stimulating hormone

levels in men with idiopathic azoospermia. Fertil Steril 1986; 45: 392–396.
443. Honigl W, Knuth UA, Nieschlag E. Selective reduction of elevated FSH levels in infertile men by pulsatile LHRH treatment. Clin Endocrinol (Oxf) 1986; 24:177–182.
444. Reyes-Fuentes A, Chavarria ME, Carrera A, et al. Alterations in pulsatile luteinizing hormone and follicle-stimulating hormone secretion in idiopathic oligoasthenospermic men: assessment by deconvolution analysis. A clinical research center study. J Clin Endocrinol Metab 1996; 81:524–529.
445. Booth JD, Merriam GR, Clark RV, et al. Evidence for Leydig cell dysfunction in infertile men with a selective increase in plasma follicle-stimulating hormone. J Clin Endocrinol Metab 1987; 64:1194–1198.
446. Pavlovich CP, King P, Goldstein M, Schlegel PN. Evidence of a treatable endocrinopathy in infertile men. J Urol 2001; 165:837–841.
447. Lin WW, Lamb DJ, Wheeler TM, et al. In situ end-labeling of human testicular tissue demonstrates increased apoptosis in conditions of abnormal spermatogenesis. Fertil Steril 1997; 68:1065–1069.
448. Feng HL, Sandlow JI, Sparks AE, et al. Decreased expression of the c-kit receptor is associated with increased apoptosis in subfertile human testes. Fertil Steril 1999; 71:85–89.
449. Nudell D, Castillo M, Turek PJ, Pera RR. Increased frequency of mutations in DNA from infertile men with meiotic arrest. Hum Reprod 2000; 15:1289–1294.
450. Collins JA, Wrixon W, Janes LB, et al. Treatment-independent pregnancy among infertile couples. N Engl J Med 1983; 309: 1201–1205.
451. Baker HWG. Male infertility of undetermined etiology. In Krieger DT, Bardin CW (eds). Current Therapy in Endocrinology 1983–1984. Philadelphia, BC Decker, 1983, pp 366–371.
452. Bhasin S, de Kretser DM, Baker HWG. Pathophysiology and natural history of male infertility. J Clin Endocrinol Metab 1994; 79:1525–1529.
453. Baker HWG, Liu DY, Bourne H, et al. Diagnosis of sperm defects in selecting patients for assisted fertilization. Hum Reprod 1993; 8:1779–1780.
454. Schlegel PN, Girardi SK. In vitro fertilization for male factor infertility. J Clin Endocrinol Metab 1997; 82:709–716.
455. Page DC, Silber S, Brown LG. Men with infertility caused by AZFc deletion can produce sons by intracytoplasmic sperm injection but are likely to transmit the deletion and infertility. Hum Reprod 1999; 14:1722–1726.
456. Reubinoff BE, Abeliovich D, Werner M, et al. A birth in nonmosaic Klinefelter's syndrome after testicular fine needle aspiration, intracytoplasmic sperm injection and preimplantation genetic diagnosis. Hum Reprod 1998; 13:1887–1892.
457. McConnell JD. Epidemiology, etiology, pathophysiology, and diagnosis of benign prostatic hyperplasia. In Walsh PC, Retik AB, Vaughan ED Jr, Wein AF (eds). Campbell's Urology, 7th ed. Philadelphia, WB Saunders, 1998, pp 1429–1452.
458. Lepor H. Natural history, evaluation, and nonsurgical management of benign prostatic hyperplasia. In Walsh PC, Retik AB, Vaughan ED Jr, Wein AF (eds). Campbell's Urology, 7th ed. Philadelphia, WB Saunders, 1998, pp 1453–1477.
459. Wilson JD. The pathogenesis of benign prostatic hyperplasia. Am J Med 1980; 68:745–756.
460. Wenderoth UK, George FW, Wilson JD. The effect of a 5α-reductase inhibitor on androgen-mediated growth of the dog prostate. Endocrinology 1983; 113:569–573.
461. Brooks JR, Berman C, Glitzer MS, et al. Effect of a new 5α-reductase inhibitor on size, histological characteristics and androgen concentrations of the canine prostate. Prostate 1982; 3:35–44.
462. Hammond GL. Endogenous steroid levels in the human prostate from birth to old age: a comparison of normal and diseased tissues. J Endocrinol 1978; 78:7–19.
463. Walsh PC, Wilson JD. The induction of prostatic hypertrophy in the dog with androstanediol. J Clin Invest 1976; 57:1093–1097.
464. Schroder FH. Medical treatment of benign prostatic hyperplasia: the effect of surgical or medical castration. Prog Clin Biol Res 1994; 386:191–196.
465. Peters CA, Walsh PC. The effect of nafarelin acetate, a luteinizing hormone–releasing hormone agonist, on benign prostatic hyperplasia. N Engl J Med 1987; 317:599–604.
466. McConnell JD, Wilson JD, George FW, et al. Finasteride, an inhibitor of 5α-reductase, suppresses prostatic dihydrotestosterone in men with benign prostatic hyperplasia. J Clin Endocrinol Metab 1992; 74:505–508.
467. Stoner E. Three-year safety and efficacy data on the use of finasteride in the treatment of benign prostatic hyperplasia. Urology 1994; 43:284–292.
468. Farnsworth WE. Estrogen in the etiopathogenesis of BPH. Prostate 1999; 41:263–274.
469. Barry M, Roehrborn C. Management of benign prostatic hyperplasia. Annu Rev Med 1997; 48:177–189.
470. Richie JP. Neoplasms of the testis. In Walsh PC, Gittes RF, Perlmutter AD, et al (eds). Campbell's Urology, 6th ed. Philadelphia, WB Saunders, 1992, pp 1222–1263.
471. Ekbom A, Akre O. Increasing incidence of testicular cancer: birth cohort effects. APMIS 1998; 106:225–231.
472. Moller H, Jorgensen N, Forman D. Trends in incidence of testicular cancer in boys and adolescent men. Int J Cancer 1995; 61: 761–764.
473. Lefevre RE, Levin HS, Banowsky LH, et al. Bilateral testicular tumors of germ cell origin. J Urol 1975; 114:556–559.
474. Dieckmann KP, Pichlmeier U. The prevalence of familial testicular cancer: an analysis of two patient populations and a review of the literature. Cancer 1997; 80:1954–1960.
475. Dean RC, Moul JW. New tumor markers of testis cancer. Urol Clin North Am 1998; 25:365–373.
476. Fonger JD, Filler RM, Rider WD, et al. Testicular tumors in maldescended testes. Can J Surg 1981; 24:353–355.
477. Henderson BE, Benton B, Jing J, et al. Risk factors for cancer of the testis in young men. Int J Cancer 1979; 23:598–602.
478. Raina V, Shukla NK, Gupta NP, et al. Germ cell tumours in uncorrected cryptorchid testis at Institute Rotary Cancer Hospital, New Delhi. Br J Cancer 1995; 71:380–382.
479. Simpson JL, Photopulos G. The relationship of neoplasia to disorders of abnormal sexual differentiation. Birth Defects Orig Art Ser 1976; 12:15–50.
480. Zhang ZF, Vena JE, Zielezny M, et al. Occupational exposure to extreme temperature and risk of testicular cancer. Arch Environ Health 1995; 50:13–18.
481. Dieckmann KP, Rube C, Henke RP. Association of Down's syndrome and testicular cancer. J Urol 1997; 157:1701–1704.
482. Carroll PR, Morse J, Koduru PPK, et al. Testicular germ cell tumor in patient with Klinefelter syndrome. Urology 1988; 31: 72–74.
483. Buzelin F, Karam G, Moreau A, et al. Testicular tumor and the acquired immunodeficiency syndrome. Eur Urol 1994; 26:71–76.
484. Srikanth MS, West BR, Ishitani M, et al. Benign testicular tumors in children with congenital adrenal hyperplasia. J Pediatr Surg 1992; 27:639–641.
485. Turner D. Testicular cancer and the value of self-examination. Nurs Times 1995; 91:30–31.
486. Bosl GJ, Vogelzang NJ, Goldman A, et al. Impact of delay in diagnosis on clinical stage of testicular cancer. Lancet 1981; 2: 970–973.
487. Mostofi FK. Pathology of germ cell tumors of testis: a progress report. Cancer 1980; 45:1735–1754.
488. Marshall AHE, Dayan AD. An immune reaction in man against seminomas, dysgerminomas, pinealomas, and the mediastinal tumours of similar histological appearance? Lancet 1964; 2:1102–1104.
489. Scully RE. Gonadoblastoma: a review of 74 cases. Cancer 1970; 25:1340–1356.
490. Bush SE, Martinez A, Bagshaw MA. Primary mediastinal seminoma. Cancer 1981; 48:1877–1882.
491. Kasper CS, Schneider NR, Childers JH, et al. Suprasellar germinoma: unresolved problems in diagnosis, pathogenesis, and management. Am J Med 1983; 75:705–711.
492. Chaganti RS, Houldsworth J. The cytogenetic theory of the pathogenesis of human adult male germ tumors. APMIS 1998; 106:80–83.
493. Anonymous. Tumour markers in germ cell cancer: EGTM recommendations. Anticancer Res 1999; 19:2785–2820.
494. Cochran JS, Walsh PC, Porter JC, et al. The endocrinology of human chorionic gonadotropin-secreting testicular tumors: new methods in diagnosis. J Urol 1975; 114:549–555.
495. Szymendera JJ, Zborzil J, Sikorowa L, et al. Value of five tumor

markers (AFP, CEA, hCG, hPL, and SP1) in diagnosis and staging of testicular germ cell tumors. Oncology 1981; 38:222–229.

496. Fung LC, Honey RJ, Gardiner GW. Testicular seminoma presenting with features of androgen excess. Urology 1994; 44:927–929.
497. Aiginger P, Kolbe H, Kuhbock J, et al. The endocrinology of testicular germinal cell tumors. Acta Endocrinol (Copenh) 1981; 97:419–426.
498. Reznik Y, Rieu M, Kuhn JM, et al. Luteinizing hormone regulation by sex steroids in men with germinal and Leydig cell tumours. Clin Endocrinol (Oxf) 1993; 38:487–493.
499. Ellis M, Sikora K. The current management of testicular cancer. Br J Urol 1987; 59:2–9.
500. Lawton AJ, Mead GM. Staging and prognostic factors in testicular cancer. Semin Surg Oncol 1999; 17:223–229.
501. Reed E, Sanger WG, Armitage JO. Results of semen cryopreservation in young men with testicular carcinoma and lymphoma. J Clin Oncol 1986; 4:537–539.
502. Fossa SD, Lehne G, Heimdal K, et al. Clinical and biochemical long-term toxicity after low-stage testicular cancer. Oncology 1995; 52:300–305.
503. Bokemeyer C, Schmoll HJ. Treatment of testicular cancer and the development of secondary malignancies. J Clin Oncol 1995; 13:283–292.
504. Grossfeld GD, Small EJ. Long-term side effects of treatment for testis cancer. Urol Clin North Am 1998; 25:503–515.
505. Freeman DA. Steroid hormone–producing tumors in man. Endocr Rev 1986; 7:204–220.
506. Masumori N, Kumamoto Y, Itoh N, et al. Leydig cell tumor: a case report with reference to its endocrinological features. Eur Urol 1993; 24:302–304.
507. Niewenhuis JC, Wolf MC, Kass EJ. Bilateral asynchronous Sertoli cell tumor in a boy with the Peutz-Jeghers syndrome. J Urol 1994; 152:1246–1248.
508. Dreyer L, Jacyk WK, du Plessis DJ. Bilateral large-cell calcifying Sertoli cell tumor of the testes with Peutz-Jeghers syndrome: a case report. Pediatr Dermatol 1994; 11:335–337.
509. Gabrilove JL, Freiberg EK, Leiter E, et al. Feminizing and nonfeminizing Sertoli cell tumors. J Urol 1980; 124:757–767.
510. Nogales FF, Andujar M, Zulauga A, et al. Malignant large cell calcifying Sertoli cell tumor of the testis. J Urol 1995; 153:1935–1937.
511. Stein JP, Freeman JA, Esrig D, et al. Papillary adenocarcinoma of the rete testis: a case report and review of the literature. Urology 1994; 44:588–594.
512. de Voogt HJ, Smith PH, Pavone-Macaluso M, et al. Cardiovascular side effects of diethylstilbestrol, cyproterone acetate, medroxyprogesterone acetate, and estramustine phosphate used for the treatment of prostate cancer: results from European Organization for Research on Treatment of Cancer trials 30761 and 30762. J Urol 1986; 135:303–307.
513. Kanhai RC, Hage JJ, van Diest PJ, et al. Short-term and long-term histologic effects of castration and estrogen treatment on breast tissue of 14 male-to-female transsexuals in comparison with two chemically castrated men. Am J Surg Pathol 2000; 24: 74–80.
514. Williams MJ. Gynecomastia: its incidence, recognition and host characterization in 447 autopsy cases. Am J Med 1963; 34:103–112.
515. Nuttall FQ. Gynecomastia as a physical finding in normal men. J Clin Endocrinol Metab 1979; 48:338–340.
516. Niewoehner CB, Nuttall FQ. Gynecomastia in a hospitalized male population. Am J Med 1984; 77:633–638.
517. Georgiadis E, Papandreou L, Evangelopoulou C, et al. Incidence of gynaecomastia in 954 young males and its relationship to somatometric parameters. Ann Hum Biol 1994; 21:579–587.
518. Chantra PK, So GJ, Wollman JS, et al. Mammography of the male breast. AJR 1995; 164:853–858.
519. Jackson VP, Gilmore RL. Male breast carcinoma and gynecomastia: comparison of mammography with sonography. Radiology 1986; 149:533–536.
520. Andersen JA, Gram JB. Male breast at autopsy. Acta Pathol Microbiol Immunol Scand [A] 1982; 90:191–197.
521. Bannayan GA, Hajdu SI. Gynecomastia: clinicopathologic study of 351 cases. Am J Clin Pathol 1972; 57:431–437.
522. Gabrilove JL. Some recent advances in virilizing and feminizing syndromes and hirsutism. Mt Sinai J Med 1974; 41:636–654.
523. McKiernan JF, Hudd D. Breast development in the newborn. Arch Dis Child 1981; 56:525–529.
524. Nydick M, Bustos J, Dale JD Jr, et al. Gynecomastia in adolescent boys. JAMA 1961; 178:449–454.
525. Sher ES, Migeon CJ, Berkovitz GD. Evaluation of boys with marked breast development at puberty. Clin Pediatr (Phila) 1998; 37:367–371.
526. Lee PA. The relationship of concentrations of serum hormones to pubertal gynecomastia. J Pediatr 1975; 86:212–215.
527. LaFranchi SH, Parlow AF, Lippe BM, et al. Pubertal gynecomastia and transient elevation of serum estradiol level. Am J Dis Child 1975; 129:927–931.
528. Moore DC, Schlaepfer LV, Paunier L, et al. Hormonal changes during puberty: V. Transient pubertal gynecomastia: abnormal androgen-estrogen ratios. J Clin Endocrinol Metab 1984; 58: 492–499.
529. Bulard J, Mowszkowicz I, Schaison G. Increased aromatase activity in pubic skin fibroblasts from patients with isolated gynecomastia. J Clin Endocrinol Metab 1987; 64:618–623.
530. Kirschner MA, Jacobs JB, Fraley EE. Bilateral anorchia with persistent testosterone production. N Engl J Med 1970; 289:240–244.
531. Edman CD, Winters AJ, Porter JC, et al. Embryonic testicular regression: a clinical spectrum of XY agonadal individuals. Obstet Gynecol 1977; 49:209–217.
532. Casey RW, Wilson JD. Antiestrogenic action of dihydrotestosterone in mouse breast: competition with estradiol for binding to the estrogen receptor. J Clin Invest 1984; 74:2272–2278.
533. Aiman J, Hemsell DL, Brenner PF, et al. Origin of estrogen in adolescents with Klinefelter syndrome and gynecomastia (abstract). J Androl 1981; 2:6.
534. Gabrilove JL, Freiberg EK, Nichols GL. Testicular function in Klinefelter's syndrome. J Urol 1980; 124:825–826.
535. Martin F, Perheentupa J, Adlercreutz H. Plasma and urinary androgens and oestrogens in a pubertal boy with 3β-hydroxysteroid dehydrogenase deficiency. J Steroid Biochem 1980; 13:197–201.
536. Imperato-McGinley J, Peterson RE, Stoller R, et al. Male pseudohermaphroditism secondary to 17β-hydroxysteroid dehydrogenase deficiency: gender role change with puberty. J Clin Endocrinol Metab 1979; 49:391–395.
537. Nolten WE, Viosca SP, Korenman SG, et al. Association of elevated estradiol with remote testicular trauma in young fertile men. Fertil Steril 1994; 62:143–149.
538. Heruti RJ, Dankner R, Berezin M, et al. Gynecomastia following spinal cord disorder. Arch Phys Med Rehabil 1997; 78:534–537.
539. Kannan V, Vijaya G. Endocrine testicular functions in leprosy. Horm Metab Res 1984; 16:146–150.
540. Nagel TC, Freinkel N, Bell RH, et al. Gynecomastia, prolactin, and other peptide hormones in patients undergoing chronic hemodialysis. J Clin Endocrinol Metab 1973; 36:428–432.
541. Xciarra A, Casale P, Di Nocola S, et al. Hormonal profile of patients with Leydig cell tumors: a urologic cause of gynecomastia. Minerva Urol Nefrol 1998; 50:225–231.
542. Gabrilove JL, Nicholis GL, Mitty HA, et al. Feminizing interstitial cell tumor of the testis: personal observations and a review of the literature. Cancer 1975; 38:1184–1202.
543. Mellor SG, McCutchan JDS. Gynaecomastia and occult Leydig cell tumour of the testis. Br J Urol 1989; 63:420–422.
544. Kuhn JM, Mahoudeau JA, Billaud L, et al. Evaluation of diagnostic criteria for Leydig cell tumours in adult men revealed by gynaecomastia. Clin Endocrinol (Oxf) 1987; 26:407–416.
545. Whitcomb RW, Schimke RN, Kyner JL, et al. Endocrine studies in a male patient with choriocarcinoma and gynecomastia. Am J Med 1986; 81:917–920.
546. Agarwal VR, Takayama K, Van Wuk JJ, et al. Molecular basis of severe gynecomastia associated with aromatase expression in a fibrolamellar hepatocellular carcinoma. J Clin Endocrinol Metab 1998; 83:1797–1800.
547. Berensztein E, Belgorosky A, de Davila MT, et al. Testicular steroid biosynthesis in a boy with a large calcifying Sertoli cell tumor producing prepubertal gynecomastia. Steroids 1995; 50: 220–225.
548. Forst T, Beyer J, Cordes U, et al. Gynaecomastia in a patient with hCG producing giant cell carcinoma of the lung: case report. Exp Clin Endocrinol Diabetes 1995; 103:28–32.

549. Wurzel RS, Yamase HT, Nieh PT. Ectopic production of human chorionic gonadotropin by poorly differentiated transitional cell tumors of the urinary tract. J Urol 1987; 137:502–504.
550. Aiman J, Hemsell DL, MacDonald PC. Production and origin of estrogen in two true hermaphrodites. Am J Obstet Gynecol 1978; 132:401–409.
551. Desai MB, Kapadia SN. Feminizing adrenocortical tumors in male patients: adenoma versus carcinoma. J Urol 1988; 139:101–103.
552. Sayed A, Stock JL, Liepman MK, et al. Feminization as a result of both peripheral conversion of androgens and direct estrogen production from an adrenocortical carcinoma. J Endocrinol Invest 1994; 17:275–278.
553. Kadair RG, Block MB, Katz FH, et al. 'Masked' 21-hydroxylase deficiency of the adrenal presenting with gynecomastia and bilateral testicular masses. Am J Med 1977; 62:278–282.
554. Gabrilove JL, Nicolis GL, Sohval AR. Non-tumorous feminizing adrenogenital syndrome in the male subject. J Urol 1973; 110: 710–713.
555. Frank-Raue K, Raue F, Korth-Schutz S, et al. Clinical features and diagnosis of mild 3β-hydroxysteroid dehydrogenase deficiency in men. Dtsch Med Wochenschr 1989; 114:331–334.
556. Cunningham GR, Silverman VE, Thornby J, et al. The potential for an androgen male contraceptive. J Clin Endocrinol Metab 1979; 49:520–526.
557. Alen M, Reinila M, Vihko R. Response of serum hormones to androgen administration in power athletes. Med Sci Sports Exerc 1985; 17:354–359.
558. Evans NA. Gym and toxic: a profile of 100 male steroid users. Br J Sports Med 1997; 31:54–58.
559. Korkia P, Stimson GV. Indications of prevalence, practice and effects of anabolic steroid use in Great Britain. Int J Sports Med 1997; 18:557–562.
560. Gordon GG, Olivo J, Rafii F, et al. Conversion of androgens to estrogens in cirrhosis of the liver. J Clin Endocrinol Metab 1975; 40:1018–1026.
561. Kew MC, Kirschner MA, Abrahams GE, et al. Mechanism of feminization in primary liver cancer. N Engl J Med 1977; 296: 1084–1088.
562. Zurbiran S, Gomez-Mont F. Endocrine disturbances in chronic human malnutrition. Vitam Horm 1953; 11:97–132.
563. Becker KL, Winnacker JL, Matthews MJ, et al. Gynecomastia and hyperthyroidism: an endocrine and histological investigation. J Clin Endocrinol Metab 1968; 28:227–285.
564. Chopra IJ, Tulchinsky D. States of estrogen-androgen balance in hyperthyroid men with Graves' disease. J Clin Endocrinol Metab 1974; 38:269–277.
565. Southren AL, Olivo J, Gordon GG, et al. The conversion of androgens to estrogens in hyperthyroidism. J Clin Endocrinol Metab 1974; 38:207–214.
566. Hemsell DL, Edman CD, Marks JF, et al. Massive extraglandular aromatization of plasma androstenedione resulting in feminization of a prepubertal boy. J Clin Invest 1977; 60:455–464.
567. Berkowitz GD, Gerami A, Brown TR, et al. Familial gynecomastia with increased extraglandular aromatization of plasma carbon 19-steroid. J Clin Invest 1985; 75:1763–1769.
568. Stratakis CA, Vottero A, Brodie A, et al. The aromatase excess syndrome is associated with feminization of both sexes and autosomal dominant transmission of aberrant P450 aromatase gene transcription. J Clin Endocrinol Metab 1998; 83:1348–1357.
569. Wilson JD, Leshin M, George FW. The Sebright bantam chicken and the genetic control of extraglandular aromatase. Endocr Rev 1987; 8:363–376.
570. Hendrickson DA, Anderson WR. Diethylstilbestrol therapy: gynecomastia. JAMA 1970; 213:468.
571. Orentreich N, Durr NP. Mammogenesis in transsexuals. J Invest Dermatol 1974; 63:142–146.
572. Halperin DK, Sizoneko PC. Prepubertal gynecomastia following topical inunction of estrogen-containing ointment. Helv Paediatr Acta 1983; 38:361–366.
573. Cimorra FA, Gonzalez-Peirona E, Ferrandez A. Percutaneous oestrogen-induced gynaecomastia: a case report. Br J Plast Surg 1982; 35:209–210.
574. Landolt R, Murset G. Premature signs of puberty as late sequelae of unintentional estrogen administration. Schweiz Med Wochenschr 1968; 98:638–641.
575. Pacynski A, Budzynska A, Przylecki S. Hiperestrogenizm v pracownikow Zakladow farmaceutyczaych I ich dzieci jako choroba zawodowa. Endokrynol Pol 1971; 22:149–154.
576. Felner EI, White PC. Prepubertal gynecomastia: indirect exposure to estrogen cream. Pediatrics 2000; 105:E55.
577. DeRaimondo CV, Roach AC, Meador CK. Gynecomastia from exposure to vaginal estrogen cream. N Engl J Med 1980; 302: 1089–1090.
578. Abramowicz M. Estrogens in cosmetics. Med Lett 1985; 27:54–55.
579. Kimball AM, Hammadeh R, Mahmood RAH, et al. Gynaecomastia among children in Bahrain. Lancet 1981; 1:671–672.
580. Sundlof SF, Strickland C. Zearenone and zeranol: potential residue problems in livestock. Vet Hum Toxicol 1986; 28:242–250.
581. Henricks DM, Gray SL, Hoover JLB. Residue levels of endogenous estrogens in beef tissues. J Anim Sci 1983; 57:247–255.
582. Adlercreutz CH, Goldin BR, Gorbach SL, et al. Soybean phytoestrogen intake and cancer risk. J Nutr 1995; 125(3 Suppl): 757S–770S.
583. LeWinn EB. Gynecomastia during digitalis therapy. N Engl J Med 1953; 248:316–320.
584. Murray NP, Daly MJ. Gynaecomastia and heart failure: adverse drug reaction or disease process? J Clin Pharm Ther 1991; 16: 275–279.
585. Navab A, Koss LG, Ladue JS. Estrogen-like activity of digitalis: its effect on the squamous epithelium of the female genital tract. JAMA 1965; 194:30–32.
586. Rifka SM, Pita JC, Vigersky RA, et al. Interaction of digitalis and spironolactone with human sex steroid receptors. J Clin Endocrinol Metab 1977; 46:338–344.
587. Maddock WO, Nelson WO. The effects of chorionic gonadotropin in adult men: increased estrogen and 17-ketosteroid excretion, gynecomastia, Leydig cell stimulation and seminiferous tubule damage. J Clin Endocrinol Metab 1997; 46:338–344.
588. Lee PA. The occurrence of gynecomastia upon withdrawal of clomiphene citrate treatment for idiopathic oligospermia. Fertil Steril 1980; 34:285–286.
589. Feldman D. Ketoconazole and other imidazole derivatives as inhibitors of steroidogenesis. Endocr Rev 1986; 7:409–420.
590. Fagan TC, Johnson DG, Grosso DS. Metronidazole-induced gynecomastia. JAMA 1985; 254:3217.
591. Pont A, Goldman ES, Sugar AM, et al. Ketoconazole-induced increase in estradiol-testosterone ratio. Arch Intern Med 1985; 145:1429–1431.
592. Saeter G, Fossa DK, Norman N. Gynaecomastia following cytotoxic therapy for testicular cancer. Br J Urol 1987; 59:348–352.
593. Pitt B, Zannad F, Remme WJ, et al. The effect of spironolactone on morbidity and mortality in patients with severe heart failure. N Engl J Med 1999; 341:709–717.
594. De Gasparo M, Whitebread SE, Preiswerk G, et al. Antialdosterones: incidence and prevention of sexual side effects. J Steroid Biochem 1989; 32:223–227.
595. Geller J, Vazakas G, Fruchtman B, et al. The effect of cyproterone acetate on advanced carcinoma of the prostate. Surg Gynecol Obstet 1968; 127:748–758.
596. Caine M, Perlberg S, Gordon R. The treatment of benign prostatic hypertrophy with flutamide (SCH 13521): a placebo controlled study. J Urol 1975; 114:564–568.
597. Berger BM, Naadimuthu A, Boddy A, et al. The effect of zanoterone, a steroidal androgen receptor antagonist, in men with benign prostatic hyperplasia: the Zanoterone Study Group. J Urol 1995; 154:1060–1064.
598. Verhelst J, Denis L, Van Vliet P, et al. Endocrine profiles during administration of the new non-steroidal anti-androgen Casodex in prostate cancer. Clin Endocrinol (Oxf) 1994; 41:525–530.
599. Rodriguez LAG, Jick H. Risk of gynaecomastia associated with cimetidine, omeprazole, and other antiulcer drugs. Br Med J 1994;308:503–506.
600. Galbraith RA, Michnovicz JJ. The effects of cimetidine on the oxidative metabolism of estradiol. N Engl J Med 1989; 321:269–274.
601. Gynecomastia in Haitians: Puerto Rico, Florida, Texas, New York. MMWR Morb Mortal Wkly Rep 1982; 31:205–206.
602. Brody SA, Winters J, Down MA, et al. An epidemic of gynecomastia among Haitian refugees: possible exposure to anti-androgen. Endocr Soc Abstr 1983; 724.

603. Malozowski S, Stadel BV. Prepubertal gynecomastia during growth hormone therapy. J Pediatr 1995; 126:659–661.
604. Cohn L, Feller AG, Draper MW, et al. Carpal tunnel syndrome and gynaecomastia during growth hormone treatment of elderly men with low circulating IGFI concentrations. Clin Endocrinol (Oxf) 1993; 39:417–425.
605. Markusse HM, Meyboom RHB. Gynaecomastia associated with captopril. Br Med J 1988; 296:1262–1263.
606. Tanner LA, Bosco LA. Gynecomastia associated with calcium channel blocker therapy. Arch Intern Med 1988; 148:379–380.
607. Bergman D, Futterweit W, Segal R, et al. Increased oestradiol in diazepam related gynaecomastia. Lancet 1981; 1:1225–1226.
608. Reid DM, Martynoga AG, Nuki G. Reversible gynecomastia associated with D-penicillamine in a man with rheumatoid arthritis. Br Med J 1982; 285:1083–1084.
609. Lindquist M, Edwards IR. Endocrine adverse effects of omeprazole. Br Med J 1992; 305:451–452.
610. Boyd IW. Gynaecomastia in association with calcium antagonists. Med J Aust 1994; 161:328.
611. Llop R, Gomez-Farran F, Figueras A, et al. Gynecomastia associated with enalapril and diazepam. Ann Pharmacother 1994; 28: 671–672.
612. Peyriere H, Mauboussin JM, Rouanet I, et al. Report of gynecomastia in five male patients during antiretroviral therapy for HIV infection. AIDS 1999; 13:2167–2169.
613. Harmon JW, Aliapoulios MA. Marijuana-induced gynecomastia: clinical and laboratory experience. Surg Forum 1974; 25:423–425.
614. Cicero TJ, Bell RD, Wiest WG, et al. Function of the male sex organs in heroin and methadone users. N Engl J Med 1975; 292: 882–887.
615. Bannayan GA, Hajdu SI. Gynecomastia: clinicopathologic study of 351 cases. Am J Clin Pathol 1972; 57:431–437.
616. McFadyen IJ, Bolton AE, Camerson EHD, et al. Gonadal-pituitary hormone levels in gynaecomastia. Clin Endocrinol (Oxf) 1980; 13:77–86.
617. Turkington RW. Serum prolactin levels in patients with gynecomastia. J Clin Endocrinol Metab 1972;32:64–68.
618. Large DM, Anderson DC, Laing I. Twenty-four hour profiles of serum prolactin during male puberty with and without gynaecomastia. Clin Endocrinol (Oxf) 1980; 12:293–302.
619. Saad MN, Kay S. The circumareolar incision: a useful incision for gynaecomastia. Ann R Coll Surg Engl 1984; 66:35–40.
620. Parker LN, Gray DR, Lai MK, et al. Treatment of gynecomastia with tamoxifen: a double-blind crossover study. Metabolism 1986; 35:705–708.
621. Plourde PV, Kulin HE, Santner SJ. Clomiphene in the treatment of adolescent gynecomastia. Am J Dis Child 1983; 137:1080–1082.
622. Zachmann M, Eiholzer U, Mritano M, et al. Treatment of pubertal gynaecomastia with testolactone. Acta Endocrinol (Copenh) 1980; 95:77–180.
623. Buckle R. Danazol in the treatment of gynaecomastia. Drugs 1980; 19:356–361.
624. Ting AC, Chow LW, Leung YF. Comparison of tamoxifen with danazol in the management of idiopathic gynecomastia. Am Surg 2000; 66:38–40.
625. Staiman VR, Lowe FC. Tamoxifen for flutamide/finasteride-induced gynecomastia. Urology 1997; 50:929–933.
626. Kuhn JM, Roca R, Laudat MH, et al. Studies on the treatment of idiopathic gynecomastia with percutaneous dihydrotestosterone. Clin Endocrinol (Oxf) 1983; 19:513–520.
627. Fass D, Steinfeld A, Brown J, et al. Radiotherapeutic prophylaxis of estrogen-induced gynecomastia: a study of late sequelae. Int J Radiat Oncol Biol Phys 1986; 12:407–408.
628. Eriksson T, Eriksson M. Irradiation therapy prevents gynecomastia in sex offenders treated with antiandrogens. J Clin Psychiatry 1998; 59:432–433.
629. Simpson ER. Genetic mutations resulting in estrogen deficiency in the male. Mol Cell Endocrinol 1998; 145:55–59.
630. Carani C, Qin K, Simoni M, et al. Effect of testosterone and estradiol in a man with aromatase deficiency. N Engl J Med 1997; 337:91–95.
631. Hayes FJ, Seminara SB, Decruz S, et al. Aromatase inhibition in the human male reveals a hypothalamic site of estrogen feedback. J Clin Endocrinol Metab 2000; 85:3027–3035.
632. Honrath WL, Wolff A, Meli A. The influence of the amount of solvent (sesame oil) on the degree and duration of action of subcutaneously administered testosterone and its propionate. Steroids 1963; 2:425–428.
633. Snyder PJ, Lawrence DA. Treatment of male hypogonadism with testosterone enanthate. J Clin Endocrinol Metab 1980; 51:1335–1339
634. Behre HM, Nieschlag E. Testosterone buciclate (20 Aet-1) in hypogonadal men: pharmacokinetics and pharmacodynamics of the new long-acting androgen ester. J Clin Endocrinol Metab 1992; 75:1204–1210.
635. Nieschlag E, Buchter D, von Eckardstein S, et al. Repeated intramuscular injections of testosterone undecanoate for substitution therapy in hypogonadal men. Clin Endocrinol (Oxf) 1999; 51:757–763.
636. Gooren LJ. A ten-year safety study of the oral androgen testosterone undecanoate. J Androl 1994; 15:212–215.
637. Schurmeyer TH, Wickings EJ, Freischem CW, et al. Saliva and serum testosterone following oral testosterone undecanoate administration in normal and hypogonadal men. Acta Endocrinol (Copenh) 1983; 102:456–462.
638. Luisi M, Franchi F. Double-blind group comparative study of testosterone undecanoate and mesterolone in hypogonadal male patients. J Endocrinol Invest 1980; 3:305–308.
639. Place VA, Atkinson L, Prather DA, et al. Transdermal testosterone replacement through genital skin. In Nieschlag S, Behre HM (eds). Testosterone: Action, Deficiency, Substitution. Berlin, Springer-Verlag, 1990, pp 165–180.
640. Meikle AW, Arver S, Dobs AS, et al. Pharmacokinetics and metabolism of permeation-enhanced testosterone transdermal system in hypogonadal men: influence of application site—a clinical research center study. J Clin Endocrinol Metab 1996; 81:1832–1840.
641. Jordan WP, Atkinson LE, Lai C. Comparison of the skin irritation potential of two testosterone transdermal systems: an investigational system and a marketed product. Clin Ther 1998; 20: 80–87.
642. Dobs AS, Meikle AW, Arver S, et al. Pharmacokinetics, efficacy, and safety of a permeation-enhanced testosterone transdermal system in comparison with bi-weekly injections of testosterone enanthate for the treatment of hypogonadal men. J Clin Endocrinol Metab 1999; 84:3469–3478.
643. Wang C, Berman N, Longstreth JA, et al. Pharmacokinetics of transdermal testosterone gel in hypogonadal men: application of gel at one site versus four sites: a general clinical research center study. J Clin Endocrinol Metab 2000; 85:964–969.
644. Swerdloff RS, Wang C, Cunningham G, et al. Long-term pharmacokinetics of transdermal testosterone gel in hypogonadal men. J Clin Endocrinol Metab 2000; 85:4500–4510.
645. Salehian B, Wang C, Alexander G, et al. Pharmacokinetics, bioefficacy, and safety of sublingual testosterone cyclodextrin in hypogonadal men: comparison to testosterone enanthate: a clinical research center study. J Clin Endocrinol Metab 1995; 80: 3567–3575.
646. Alkalay D, Khemani L, Bartlett MF. Spectrophotofluorometric determination of methyltestosterone in plasma or serum. J Pharm Sci 1972; 61:1746–1749.
647. Doerr P, Pirke KM. Regulation of plasma oestrogens in normal adult males. Acta Endocrinol (Copenh) 1974; 75:617–624.
648. Liao S, Liang T, Fang S, et al. Steroid structure and androgenic activity: specificity involved in the receptor binding and nuclear retention of various androgens. J Biol Chem 1973; 248:6154–6162.
649. Cummings DE, Kumar N, Bardin CW, et al. Prostate-sparing effects in primates of the potent androgen 7α-methyl-19-nortestosterone: a potential alternative to testosterone for androgen replacement and male contraception. J Clin Endocrinol Metab 1998; 83:4212–4219.
650. Anderson RA, Martin CW, Kung AWC, et al. 7α-Methyl-19-nortestosterone maintains sexual behavior and mood in hypogonadal men. J Clin Endocrinol Metab 1999; 84:3556–3562.
651. Marberger H. Hormonal therapy with steroid-filled Silastic rubber implants. Br J Urol 1976; 48:153–154.
652. Fogh M, Corker CS, McLean H, et al. Serum-testosterone during oral administration of testosterone in hypogonadal men and transsexual women. Acta Endocrinol (Copenh) 1978; 87:643–649.

653. Johnsen SG, Kampmann JP, Bennett EP, et al. Enzyme induction by oral testosterone. Clin Pharmacol Ther 1976; 20:233–237.
654. Amory JK, Bremner WJ. The use of testosterone as a male contraceptive. Ballieres Clin Endocrinol Metab 1998; 12:471–484.
655. Palacios A, McClure RD, Campfield A, et al. Effect of testosterone enanthate on testis size. J Urol 1981; 126:46–48.
656. Herbst KL, Anawalt B, Amory J, et al. Testosterone administration to normal men changes body composition from fat to lean without changing body weight. Endocr Soc Abstr 2000; 82:656.
657. Amory JK, Bremner WJ, Herbst KL, et al. Testosterone rapidly increases vertebral bone mineral density in eugonadal men. Endocr Soc Abstr 2000; 82:657.
658. Bhasin S, Storer TW, Berman N, et al. The effects of supraphysiologic doses of testosterone on muscle size and strength in normal men. N Engl J Med 1996; 335:1–7.
659. Tricker R, Casaburi R, Storer TW, et al. The effects of supraphysiological doses of testosterone on angry behavior in healthy eugonadal men: a clinical research center study. J Clin Endocrinol Metab 1996; 81:3754–3758.
660. Cooper CS, MacIndoe JH, Perry PJ, et al. The effect of exogenous testosterone on total and free prostate specific antigen levels in healthy young men. J Urol 1996; 156:438–442.
661. Bhasin S, Woodhouse L, Casaburi R, et al. Testosterone dose-response relationships in healthy young men. Am J Physiol Endocrinol Metab 2001; 281:E1172–E1181.
662. Kwan M, Greenleaf WJ, Mann J, et al. The nature of androgen action on male sexuality: a combined laboratory self-report study on hypogonadal men. J Clin Endocrinol Metab 1983; 57:557–562.
663. Greenstein A, Plymate SR, Katz PG. Visually stimulated erection in castrated men. J Urol 1995; 153:650–652.
664. Behre HM, Bohmeyer J, Nieschlag E. Prostate volume in testosterone-treated and untreated hypogonadal men in comparison to age-matched normal controls. Clin Endocrinol (Oxf) 1994; 40: 341–349.
665. Brodsky IG, Balagopal P, Nair KS. Effects of testosterone replacement on muscle mass and muscle protein synthesis in hypogonadal men: a clinical research center study. J Clin Endocrinol Metab 1996; 81:3469–3475.
666. Bhasin S, Storer TW, Berman N, et al. Testosterone replacement increases fat-free mass and muscle size in hypogonadal men. J Clin Endocrinol Metab 1997; 82:407–413.
667. Snyder PJ, Peachey H, Berlin JA, et al. Effects of testosterone replacement in hypogonadal men. J Clin Endocrinol Metab 2000; 85:2670–2677.
668. Want C, Eyre DR, Clark R, et al. Sublingual testosterone replacement improves muscle mass and strength, decreases bone resorption, and increases bone formation markers in hypogonadal men: a clinical research center study. J Clin Endocrinol Metab 1996; 81:3654–3662.
669. Wang C, Swerdloff RS, Iranmanesh A, et al. Transdermal testosterone gel improves sexual function, mood, muscle strength, and body composition parameters in hypogonadal men. J Clin Endocrinol Metab 2000; 85:2839–2853.
670. Leifke E, Korner H-C, Link TM, et al. Effects of testosterone replacement therapy on cortical and trabecular bone mineral density, vertebral body area and paraspinal muscle area in hypogonadal men. Eur J Endocrinol 1998; 138:51–58.
671. Bin-Abbas B, Conte FA, Grumbach MM, Kaplan SL. Congenital hypogonadotropic hypogonadism and micropenis: effect of testosterone treatment on adult penile size. J Pediatr 1999; 134:579–583.
672. Zachmann M, Prader A. Anabolic and androgenic effect of testosterone in sexually immature boys and its dependency on growth hormone. J Clin Endocrinol 1970; 30:85–95.
673. Tanner JM, Whitehouse RH, Hughes PCR, et al. Relative importance of growth hormone and sex steroids for the growth at puberty of trunk length, limb length, and muscle width in growth hormone–deficient children. J Pediatr 1976; 89:1000–1008.
674. Parker MW, Johanson AJ, Rogol AD, et al. Effect of testosterone on somatomedin-C concentrations in prepubertal boys. J Clin Endocrinol Metab 1984; 58:87–90.
675. Morgentaler A, Brunning CO III, DeWolf WC. Occult prostate cancer in men with low serum testosterone levels. JAMA 1996; 276:1904–1906.
676. Meikle AW, Arver S, Dobs AS, et al. Prostate size in hypogonadal men treated with a nonscrotal permeation-enhanced testosterone transdermal system. Urology 1997; 49:191–196.
677. Tenover JS. Effects of testosterone supplementation in the aging male. J Clin Endocrinol Metab 1992; 75:1092–1098.
678. Sih R, Morley JE, Kaiser FE, et al. Testosterone replacement in older hypogonadal men: a 12-month randomized controlled trial. J Clin Endocrinol Metab 1997; 82:1661–1667.
679. Snyder PJ, Peachey H, Hannoush P, et al. Effect of testosterone treatment on bone mineral density in men over 65 years of age. J Clin Endocrinol Metab 1999; 84:1966–1972.
680. Snyder PJ, Peachey H, Hannoush P, et al. Effect of testosterone treatment on body composition and muscle strength in men over 65 years of age. J Clin Endocrinol Metab 1999; 84:2647–2653.
681. Bhasin S, Bagatell CJ, Bremner WJ, et al. Issues in testosterone replacement in older men. J Clin Endocrinol Metab 1998; 83: 3435–3448.
682. Venable JH. Morphology of the cells of normal, testosterone-deprived and testosterone-stimulated levator ani muscles. Am J Anat 1966; 119:271–301.
683. Toth M. Relative androgenic and myotropic activity plots of 19-nortestosterone. J Steroid Biochem 1981; 14:1085–1090.
684. Tweedle D, Walton C, Johnston IDA. The effect of an anabolic steroid on postoperative nitrogen balance. Br J Clin Pract 1972; 27:130–132.
685. Rabkin JG, Rabkin R, Wagner G. Testosterone replacement therapy in HIV illness. Gen Hosp Psychiatry 1995; 17:37–42.
686. Bross R, Casaburi R, Storer TW, Bhasin S. Androgen effects on body composition and muscle function: implications for the use of androgens as anabolic agents in sarcopenic states. Ballieres Clin Endocrinol Metab 1998; 12:365–378.
687. Elashoff JD, Jacknow AD, Shain SG, et al. Effects of anabolic-androgenic steroids on muscular strength. Ann Intern Med 1991; 115:387–393.
688. Forbes GB. The effect of anabolic steroids on lean body mass: the dose response curve. Metabolism 1985; 34:571–573.
689. Griggs RC, Kingston W, Jozefowicz RF, et al. Effects of testosterone on muscle mass and muscle protein synthesis. J Appl Physiol 1989; 66:498–503.
690. Franke WW, Berendonk B. Hormonal doping and androgenization of athletes: a secret program of the German Democratic Republic government. Clin Chem 1997; 43:1262–1279.
691. Shahidi NT. Androgens and erythropoiesis. N Engl J Med 1973; 289: 72–80.
692. Evens RP, Amerson AB. Androgens and erythropoiesis. J Clin Pharmacol 1974; 14:94–101.
693. Hengstum V, Steenbergen J, Haanen C. Clinical course in 28 unselected patients with aplastic anaemia treated with anabolic steroids. Br J Haematol 1979; 41:323–333.
694. Najean Y. Long-term follow-up in patients with aplastic anemia: a study of 137 androgen-treated patients surviving more than two years. Am J Med 1981; 71:543–551.
695. French Cooperative Group for the Study of Aplastic and Refractory Anaemias. Androgen therapy in aplastic anaemia: a comparative study of high and low doses and of 4 different androgens. Scand J Haematol 1986; 36:346–352.
696. Mirand EA, Murphy GP. Erythropoietin activity in anephric humans given prolonged androgen treatment. J Surg Oncol 1971; 3: 59–65.
697. Hendler ED, Goffinet JA, Ross S, et al. Controlled study of androgen therapy in anemia of patients on maintenance hemodialysis. N Engl J Med 1974; 291:1046–1051.
698. Cattran DC, Fenton SSA, Wilson DR, et al. A controlled trial of nandrolone decanoate in the treatment of uremic anemia. Kidney Int 1977; 12:430–437.
699. Besa EC. Hematologic effects of androgens revisited: an alternative therapy in various hematologic conditions. Semin Hematol 1994; 31:134–145.
700. Rosse WF, Logue GL, Silberman HR. The effect of synthetic androgens in hereditary angioneurotic edema: alteration of C1 inhibitor and C4 levels. Trans Assoc Am Physicians 1976; 89: 122–132.
701. Gelford JA, Sherins RJ, Alling DW, et al. Treatment of hereditary angioedema with danazol: reversal of clinical and biochemical abnormalities. N Engl J Med 1976; 295:1444–1448.
702. Agostoni A, Cicardi M, Cugno M, et al. Clinical problems in the

C1-inhibitor deficient patient. Behring Inst Mitt 1993; 93:306–312.

703. Barbosa J, Seal US, Doe RP. Effects of anabolic steroids on haptoglobin, orosomucoid, plasminogen, fibrinogen, transferrin, ceruloplasmin, α_1-antitrypsin, β-glucuronidase and total serum proteins. J Clin Endocrinol 1971; 33:388–398.
704. Carl-Bertil L, Rannevik G. A comparison of plasma protein changes induced by danazol, pregnancy, and estrogens. J Clin Endocrinol Metab 1979; 49:719–725.
705. Limbeck GA, Ruvalcaba RHA, Mahoney CP, et al. Studies on anabolic steroids. IV: the effects of oxandrolone on height and skeletal maturation in uncomplicated growth retardation. Clin Pharmacol Ther 1971; 12:798–805.
706. Bettman HK, Goldman HS, Abramowicz M, et al. Oxandrolone treatment of short stature: effect on predicted mature height. J Pediatr 1971; 79:1018–1023.
707. Clayton PE, Shalet SM, Price DA, et al. Growth and growth hormone responses to oxandrolone in boys with constitutional delay of growth and puberty (CDGP). Clin Endocrinol (Oxf) 1988; 29:123–130.
708. Adan L, Souberbielle JC, Brauner R. Management of the short stature due to pubertal delay in boys. J Clin Endocrinol Metab 1994; 78:478–482.
709. Jackson JA, Waxman J, Spiekerman AM. Prostatic complications of testosterone replacement therapy. Arch Intern Med 1989; 149: 2365–2366.
710. Krauss DJ, Taub HA, Lantinga LJ, et al. Risks of blood volume changes in hypogonadal men treated with testosterone enanthate for erectile impotence. J Urol 1991; 146:1566–1670.
711. Hajjar RR, Kaiser FE, Morley JE. Outcomes of long-term testosterone replacement in older hypogonadal males: a retrospective analysis. J Clin Endocrinol Metab 1997; 82:3793–3796.
712. Fruehan HE, Frawley TH. Current use of anabolic steroids. JAMA 1963; 184:527–532.
713. Fyrand O, Fiskaadal HJ, Trygstad O. Acne in pubertal boys undergoing treatment with androgens. Acta Derm Venereol 1992; 72:148–149.
714. deLorimier AA, Gordan GS, Lowe RC, et al. Methyltestosterone, related steroids, and liver function. Arch Intern Med 1965; 116: 289–294.
715. Yoshida EM, Erb SR, Scudamore CH, et al. Severe cholestasis and jaundice secondary to an esterified testosterone, a non-C17 alkylated anabolic steroid. J Clin Gastroenterol 1994; 18:268–270.
716. Muller AF, Valatlan M, Manning EL. Effet de la 17-ethyl-19-nor-testosterone sur la sécrétion du cortisol. Helv Med Acta 1960; 27:678–682.
717. Shapiro P, Ikeda RM, Ruebner BH, et al. Multiple hepatic tumors and peliosis hepatis in Fanconi's anemia treated with androgens. Am J Dis Child 1977; 131:1104–1106.
718. McDonald EC, Speicher CE. Peliosis hepatis associated with administration of oxymetholone. JAMA 1978; 240:243–244.
719. Hernandez-Nieto L, Bruguera M, Bombi JA, et al. Benign liver-cell adenoma associated with long-term administration of an androgenic-anabolic steroid (methandienone). Cancer 1977; 40: 1761–1764.
720. Boyd PR, Mark GJ. Multiple hepatic adenomas and a hepatocellular carcinoma in a man on oral methyl testosterone for eleven years. Cancer 1977; 40:1765–1770.
721. Coombes GB, Reiser J, Paradinas EJ, et al. An androgen-associated hepatic adenoma in a trans-sexual. Br J Surg 1978; 65:869–870.
722. Balazs M. Primary hepatocellular tumours during long-term androgenic steroid therapy: a light and electron microscopic study of 11 cases with emphasis on microvasculature of the tumours. Acta Morphol Hung 1991; 39:201–216.
723. Shephard RJ, Killinger D, Fried T. Response to sustained use of anabolic steroid. Br J Sports Med 1977; 11:170–173.
724. Thompson PD, Cullinane EM, Sady SP, et al. Contrasting effects of testosterone and stanozolol on serum lipoprotein levels. JAMA 1989; 261:1165–1168.
725. Zmuda JM, Fahrenbach MC, Younkin BT, et al. The effect of testosterone aromatization on high-density lipoprotein cholesterol level and postheparin lipolytic activity. Metabolism 1993; 42:446–450.
726. Asscheman H, Gooren LJ, Megens JA, et al. Serum testosterone level is the major determinant of the male-female differences in serum levels of high-density lipoprotein (HDL) cholesterol and HDL2 cholesterol. Metabolism 1994; 43:935–939.
727. Bagatell CJ, Bremner WJ. Androgen and progestagen effects on plasma lipids. Prog Cardiovasc Dis 1995; 38:255–271.
728. Dobs AS, Bachorik PS, Arver S, et al. Interrelationships among lipoprotein levels, sex hormones, anthropometric parameters, and age in hypogonadal men treated for 1 year with a permeation-enhanced testosterone transdermal system. J Clin Endocrinol Metab 2001; 86:1026–1033.
729. Matsumoto AM, Sandblom RE, Schoene RB, et al. Testosterone replacement in hypogonadal men: effects on obstructive sleep apnea, respiratory drives, and sleep. Clin Endocrinol (Oxf) 1985; 22:713–721.
730. Cistulli PA, Grunstein RR, Sullivan CE. Effect of testosterone administration on upper airway collapsibility during sleep. Am J Respir Crit Care Med 1994; 149:530–532.
731. Zelissen PMJ, Stricker BHC. Severe priapism as a complication of testosterone substitution therapy. Am J Med 1988; 85:273–274.
732. Sokol RZ, McClure RD, Peterson M, et al. Gonadotropin therapy failure secondary to human chorionic gonadotropin–induced antibodies. J Clin Endocrinol Metab 1981; 52:929–933.
733. Burger HG, de Kretser DM, Hudson B, et al. Effects of preceding androgen therapy on testicular response to human pituitary gonadotropin in hypogonadotropic hypogonadism: a study of three patients. Fertil Steril 1981; 35:64–68.
734. Butcher D, Behre HM, Kliesch S, Nieschlag E. Pulsatile GnRH or human chorionic gonadotropin/human menopausal gonadotropin as effective treatment for men with hypogonadotropic hypogonadism. Eur J Endocrinol 1998; 139:298–303.
735. Kirk JM, Savage MO, Grant DB, et al. Gonadal function and response to human chorionic and menopausal gonadotrophin therapy in male patients with idiopathic hypogonadotrophic hypogonadism. Clin Endocrinol (Oxf) 1994; 41:57–63.
736. van de Berk D, Wijnberg M, van Dop PA. Initiation of spermatogenesis and successful in vitro fertilization in an infertile male with panhypopituitarism: superiority of pulsatile LH-RH over gonadotrophins? A case report. Eur J Obstet Gynecol Reprod Biol 1991; 40:153–157.
737. Claustrat B, David L, Faure A, et al. Development of antihuman chorionic gonadotropin antibodies in patients with hypogonadotropic hypogonadism: a study of four patients. J Clin Endocrinol Metab 1983; 57:1041–1047.
738. Barrio R, De Luis D, Alonzo M, et al. Induction of puberty with human chorionic gonadotropin and follicle-stimulating hormone in adolescent males with hypogonadotropic hypogonadism. Fertil Steril 1999; 71:244–248.
739. Liu PY, Turner L, Rushford D, et al. Efficacy and safety of recombinant human follicle stimulating hormone (Gonal-F) with urinary human chorionic gonadotrophin for induction of spermatogenesis and fertility in gonadotrophin-deficient men. Hum Reprod 1999; 14:1540–1545.
740. Kamischke A, Gehre HM, Bergmann M, et al. Recombinant human follicle stimulating hormone for treatment of male idiopathic infertility: a randomized double-blind, placebo-controlled, clinical trial. Hum Reprod 1998; 13:596–603.
741. Peters CA, Walsh PC. The effect of nafarelin acetate, a luteinizing hormone–releasing hormone agonist, on benign prostatic hyperplasia. N Engl J Med 1987; 317:599–604.
742. Vickery BH. Comparison of the potential for therapeutic utilities with gonadotropin-releasing hormone agonists and antagonists. Endocr Rev 1986; 7:115–124.
743. Santoro N, Filicori M, Crowley WF Jr. Hypogonadotropic disorders in men and women: diagnosis and therapy with pulsatile gonadotropin-releasing hormone. Endocr Rev 1986; 7:11–23.
744. Delemarre-Van de Wall HA. Induction of testicular growth and spermatogenesis by pulsatile, intravenous administration of gonadotrophin-releasing hormone in patients with hypogonadotrophic hypogonadism. Clin Endocrinol (Oxf) 1993; 38:473–480.
745. Schopohl J. Pulsatile gonadotrophin releasing hormone versus gonadotrophin treatment of hypothalamic hypogonadism in males. Hum Reprod 1993; 8(Suppl 2):175–179.
746. Cacciari E, Frejaville E, Becca A. Treatment of cryptorchidism by intranasal synthetic LH-RH and its analogue D-Ser(TBU)6-LHRH-EA10. Eur J Pediatr 1982; 139:280–284.

747. Crawford ED, DeAntoni EP. Current status of combined androgen blockade: optimal therapy for advanced prostate cancer. J Clin Endocrinol Metab 1995; 80:1062–1066.
748. Carel JC, Lahlou N, Guazzarotti L, et al. Treatment of central precocious puberty with depot leuprorelin: French Leuprorelin Trial Group. Eur J Endocrinol 1995; 132:699–704.
749. Richer M, Crismon ML. Pharmacotherapy of sexual offenders. Ann Pharmacother 1993; 27:316–320.
750. Gonzalez-Barcena D, Vadillo-Buenfil M, Gomez-Orta F, et al. Responses to the antagonistic analog of LH-RH (SB-75, Cetrorelix) in patients with benign prostatic hyperplasia and prostatic cancer. Prostate 1994; 24:84–92.
751. Loprinzi CL, Michalak JC, Quella SK, et al. Megestrol acetate for the prevention of hot flashes. N Engl J Med 1994; 331:347–352.
752. Barbieri RL, Ryan KJ. Direct effects of medroxyprogesterone acetate (MPA) and megestrol acetate (MGA) on rat testicular steroidogenesis. Acta Endocrinol (Copenh) 1980; 94:419–425.
753. Meyer WJ, Walker PA, Emory LE, et al. Physical, metabolic, and hormonal effects on men of long-term therapy with medroxyprogesterone acetate. Fertil Steril 1985; 43:102–109.
754. Mahler C, Verhelst J, Denis L. Ketoconazole and liarozole in the treatment of advanced prostatic cancer. Cancer 1993; 71(Suppl 3):1068–1073.
755. Dorrington-Ware P, McCartney ACE, Holland S, et al. The effect of spironolactone on hirsutism and female androgen metabolism. Clin Endocrinol (Oxf) 1985; 23:161–167.
756. Helfer EL, Miller JL, Rose LI. Side effects of spironolactone therapy in women. J Clin Endocrinol Metab 1988; 40:208–211.
757. Cusan L, Dupont A, Gomez J-L, et al. Comparison of flutamide and spironolactone in the treatment of hirsutism: a randomized controlled trial. Fertil Steril 1994; 61:281–287.
758. Bartsch G, Rittmaster RS, Klocker H. Dihydrotestosterone and the concept of 5α-reductase inhibition in human benign prostatic hyperplasia. Eur Urol 2000; 37:367–380.
759. Cunningham GR, Hirshkowitz M. Inhibition of steroid 5α-reductase with finasteride: sleep-related erections, potency, and libido in healthy men. J Clin Endocrinol Metab 1995; 80:1934–1940.
760. Stoner E. The clinical effects of a 5α-reductase inhibitor, finasteride, on benign prostatic hyperplasia: the Finasteride Study Group. J Urol 1992; 147:1298–1302.
761. Ekman P. A risk-benefit assessment of treatment with finasteride on benign prostatic hyperplasia. Drug Saf 1998; 18:161–170.
762. Hogan DJ, Chamberlain M. Male pattern baldness. South Med J 2000; 93:657–662.
763. Iversen P. Update of monotherapy trials with the new anti-androgen, Casodex (ICI 176,334). Eur Urol 1994; 26(Suppl 1):5–9.
764. Neri RO. Antiandrogens. Adv Sex Horm 1976; 2:233–262.
765. Dose EJ, Holdsworth MT. Nilutamide: an antiandrogen for the treatment of prostate cancer. Ann Pharmacother 1997; 31:65–75.
766. Schellhammer P, Sharifi R, Block N, et al. A controlled trial of bicalutamide versus flutamide, each in combination with luteinizing hormone–releasing hormone analogue therapy, in patients with advanced prostate cancer: Casodex Combination Study Group. Urology 1995; 45:745–752.
767. Neumann F. The antiandrogen cyproterone acetate: discovery, chemistry, basic pharmacology, clinical use and tool in basic research. Exp Clin Endocrinol 1994; 102:1–32.
768. Knuth UA, Hano R, Nieschlag E. Effect of flutamide or cyproterone acetate on pituitary and testicular hormones in normal men. J Clin Endocrinol Metab 1984; 59:963–969.
769. Bradford JM, Pawlak A. Double-blind placebo crossover study of cyproterone acetate in the treatment of the paraphilias. Arch Sex Behav 1993; 22:383–402.
770. Watanabe S, Yamasaki S, Tanae A, et al. Three cases of hepatocellular carcinoma among cyproterone users. Lancet 1994; 344: 1567–1568.
771. Johnston JO. Aromatase inhibitors. Crit Rev Biochem Mol Biol 1998; 33:375–405.
772. Mauras N, O'Brien KO, Klein KO, Hayes V. Estrogen suppression in males: metabolic effects. J Clin Endocrinol Metab 2000; 85:2370–2377.
773. Shetty G, Krishnamurthy H, Krishnamurthy HN, et al. Effect of estrogen deprivation on the reproductive physiology of male and female primates. J Steroid Biochem Mol Biol 1997; 61:157–166.
774. Feuillan P, Merke D, Leschek EW, Cutler GB Jr. Use of aromatase inhibitors in precocious puberty. Endocr Relat Cancer 1999; 6:303–306.
775. Braunstein GD. Aromatase and gynecomastia. Endocr Relat Cancer 1999; 6:315–324.
776. Goss PE. Risks versus benefits in the clinical application of aromatase inhibitors. Endocr Relat Cancer 1999; 6:325–332.
777. Li CP, Lee FY, Hwang SJ, et al. Treatment of mastalgia with tamoxifen in male patients with liver cirrhosis: a randomized crossover study. Am J Gastroenterol 2000; 95:1051–1055.
778. Staiman VR, Lowe FC. Tamoxifen for flutamide/finasteride-induced gynecomastia. Urology 1997; 50:929–933.
779. Serels S, Melman A. Tamoxifen as treatment for gynecomastia and mastodynia resulting from hormonal deprivation. J Urol 1998; 159:1309.
780. Murata Y, Ogawa Y, Saibara T, et al. Unrecognized hepatic steatosis and non-alcoholic steatohepatitis in adjuvant tamoxifen for breast cancer patients. Oncol Rep 2000; 7:1299–1304.

19 Sexual Dysfunction in Men and Women

Shalender Bhasin, Jennifer Berman,
Laura Berman, and Wayne J. G. Hellstrom

Erectile dysfunction (ED), previously referred to as *impotence*, is the inability of the male to attain or maintain a penile erection sufficient for satisfactory sexual intercourse. *Sexual dysfunction* is a more general term that also includes libidinal, orgasmic, and ejaculatory dysfunction in addition to the inability to attain or maintain penile erection.[1]

MALE SEXUAL DYSFUNCTION

PREVALENCE AND INCIDENCE RATES

The best data on the prevalence of ED in men have emerged from two cross-sectional studies that have used probability sampling techniques, namely the *Massachusetts Male Aging Study* (MMAS)[2–4] and the *National Health and Social Life Survey* (NHSLS).[5, 6] The MMAS was a cross-sectional, community-based random sample epidemiologic survey in which 1709 men in the greater Boston area, 40 to 70 years of age, were first surveyed between 1987 and 1989.[2, 3] Of these, 847 men were resurveyed between 1995 and 1997.[3] This survey revealed that 52% of men between the ages 40 and 70 were affected by ED to some degree; 17.2% of surveyed men reported minimal ED, 25.2% moderate ED, and 9.6% complete ED.

The NHSLS was a national probability survey of English-speaking Americans, 18 to 59 years of age living in the United States in 1992.[5, 6] In this survey, 7% of men between 18 to 29 years of age, 9% between 30 and 39 years of age, 11% between 40 and 45 years, and 18% between 50 and 59 years reported ED, based on self-reports of difficulty in obtaining or maintaining erections.

These two landmark studies and data from several other

studies suggest ED is a common problem affecting 20 to 30 million men in the United States alone.[1, 4] The prevalence of ED increases with age; it affects fewer than 10% of men younger than 45 years of age but 75% of men older than 80 years of age.[2] Men with other medical problems, such as hypertension, diabetes, cardiovascular disease, and end-stage renal disease, have a significantly higher prevalence of ED compared with healthy men.[1, 2]

There is a paucity of longitudinal data on the annual incidence rates of ED in men. Most of the available information has been derived from two studies. In the MMAS, of the 1297 men 40 to 70 years of age who were originally surveyed in 1987 to 1989, follow-up information was gathered from 847 men between 1995 and 1997. In this study, the crude incidence rate of ED in white men in the Boston area was 25.9 cases per thousand man-years. The incidence rates increased from 12.4 cases per thousand man-years for men aged 40 to 49 years to 29.8 cases per thousand man-years for men aged 50 to 59 years, and 46.4 per thousand man-years for men aged 60 to 69 years.

In another study, incidence rates were derived from a survey of 3250 men, 6 to 83 years of age, seen at a preventive medicine clinic between 1987 and 1991. This study found the incidence rates of ED to be fewer than 3 cases per 1000 man-years among men younger than 45 years of age and 52 cases per thousand man-years among men 65 years of age or older. On the basis of these two studies, it is estimated that there are 600,000 to 700,000 new cases of ED each year in the United States alone.

REGULATION OF MALE SEXUAL FUNCTION AND PHYSIOLOGY OF PENILE ERECTION

Sexual function is a complex, multicomponent biologic process that comprises central mechanisms for regulation of libido and arousability as well as local mechanisms for the generation of penile tumescence, rigidity, orgasm, and ejaculation. Androgen-deficient men have decreased overall sexual activity but can achieve normal erections in response to visual erotic stimuli.[7-12] These observations have led to the prevalent dogma that libido is testosterone-dependent and that the local mechanisms for penile erection are androgen-independent. There is emerging evidence that testosterone is a regulator of nitric oxide synthase (NOS) activity in the cavernosal smooth muscle.[13] Therefore, it is possible that physiologically normal testosterone concentrations might be required for optimal penile rigidity. Orgasm and ejaculation are not androgen-dependent and can occur without a full penile erection.

Normal penile erection requires coordinated involvement of intact central and peripheral nervous systems and the corpora cavernosa and spongiosa as well as a normal arterial blood supply and venous drainage (Fig. 19–1).[14-18] The cavernosal arteries and their branches (the helicine arteries) provide blood flow to the penis.[18] Helicine arteries deliver blood into the cavernosal sinuses. Dilatation of the helicine arteries increases the blood flow and pressure in the cavernosal sinuses.[14, 15] Relaxation of the cavernosal smooth muscle that surrounds the cavernosal sinuses along with increased blood flow results in pooling of blood in the cavernosal spaces and penile engorgement. The expanding corpora cavernosa compress the venules against the rigid tunica albuginea, restricting the venous outflow from the cavernosal spaces. This facilitates entrapment of blood in the cavernosal sinuses and achievement of a rigid erection.[14]

The erectile state of the penis is determined by the tone of the corporal smooth muscle cells.[19] When the cavernosal smooth muscle cells are relaxed, the tone is low and the penis is engorged with blood and erect. Conversely, when the cavernosal smooth muscle tone is high, the penis is flaccid. The smooth muscle tone in the corpora cavernosa is maintained by agonist-stimulated release of intracellular calcium into the cytoplasm and influx of calcium through membrane channels (Fig. 19–2*A*). An increase in intracellular calcium through its binding to calmodulin activates myosin light chain kinase, resulting in phosphorylation of myosin light chain, actin-myosin interactions, and muscle contraction. The transmembrane and intracellular calcium flux in the cavernosal smooth muscle cells is regulated by a number of cellular processes and signaling molecules such as potassium ion (K^+) flux through potassium channels, connexin 43–derived gap junctions, norepinephrine, prostaglandin E_1, (PGE_1) and nitric oxide (NO) (see Fig. 19–2).

Movement of K^+ across the membrane determines the membrane potential of the cavernosal smooth muscle cells; at least four subtypes of potassium channels mediate this K^+ efflux.[19] The adjacent smooth muscle cells are interconnected in a syncytium through connexin 43–derived gap junctions.[20-23] Therefore, changes in K^+ channel activity in one myocyte affect the membrane potential of adjacent cells, resulting in rapid transmission of electrical and biochemical signaling throughout the syncytium (Fig. 19–2*B*).[20-23]

The vascular smooth muscle contraction in the corpora cavernosa is regulated by the noradrenergic pathway. Norepinephrine binds to adrenergic receptors, resulting in generation of diacylglycerol and inositol triphosphate (IP_3). Diacylglycerol activates protein kinase C, which in turn can inhibit K^+ channels, whereas IP_3 increases intracellular calcium and calcium influx through the membrane. The net increase in intracellular calcium promotes actin-myosin interaction, resulting in smooth muscle contraction.

PGE_1 activation of its receptor results in generation of cyclic adenosine monophosphate (cAMP), which activates protein kinase A (PKA). Activated PKA stimulates K^+ channels, resulting in K^+ efflux from the cell. In addition, PKA-mediated processes also result in a net decrease in intracellular calcium, favoring smooth muscle cell relaxation. Nitric oxide, through stimulation of synthesis of intracellular cyclic guanosine monophosphate (cGMP), also decreases intracellular calcium and K^+ efflux.

The relaxation of the cavernosal smooth muscle trabeculae is under the regulation of the autonomic nervous system.[14-18, 24, 25] A number of cholinergic, adrenergic, and noradrenergic, noncholinergic (NANC) mediators regulate cavernosal smooth muscle relaxation. The NANC mediators include vasoactive intestinal peptide (VIP), calcitonin gene-related peptide (CGRP), and nitric oxide. Nitric oxide is derived from the nerve terminals innervating the corpora cavernosa, the endothelial lining of penile arteries and cavernosal sinuses,[14-18, 24, 25] and is an important biochemical regulator of cavernosal smooth muscle relaxation. Nitric oxide also induces arterial dilatation. The actions of nitric oxide on the cavernosal smooth muscle and the arterial blood flow are mediated through the activation of guanyl cyclase and production of cyclic GMP.[14-18, 24-26] The latter acts as an intracellular second messenger and causes smooth muscle relaxation by lowering intracellular calcium.[18]

A class of enzymes, called *cyclic nucleotide phosphodiesterases*, degrades cGMP into an inactive form, GMP. Researchers have now identified at least 11 different isoforms of cyclic nucleotide phosphodiesterases. These isoforms are widely distributed throughout the body; the predominant isoform of this enzyme in the cavernosal smooth muscle is cyclic nucleotide phosphodiesterase type 5 (PDE5).[14, 16, 18] Hydrolysis of cGMP by this enzyme results in reversal of the smooth muscle relaxation and

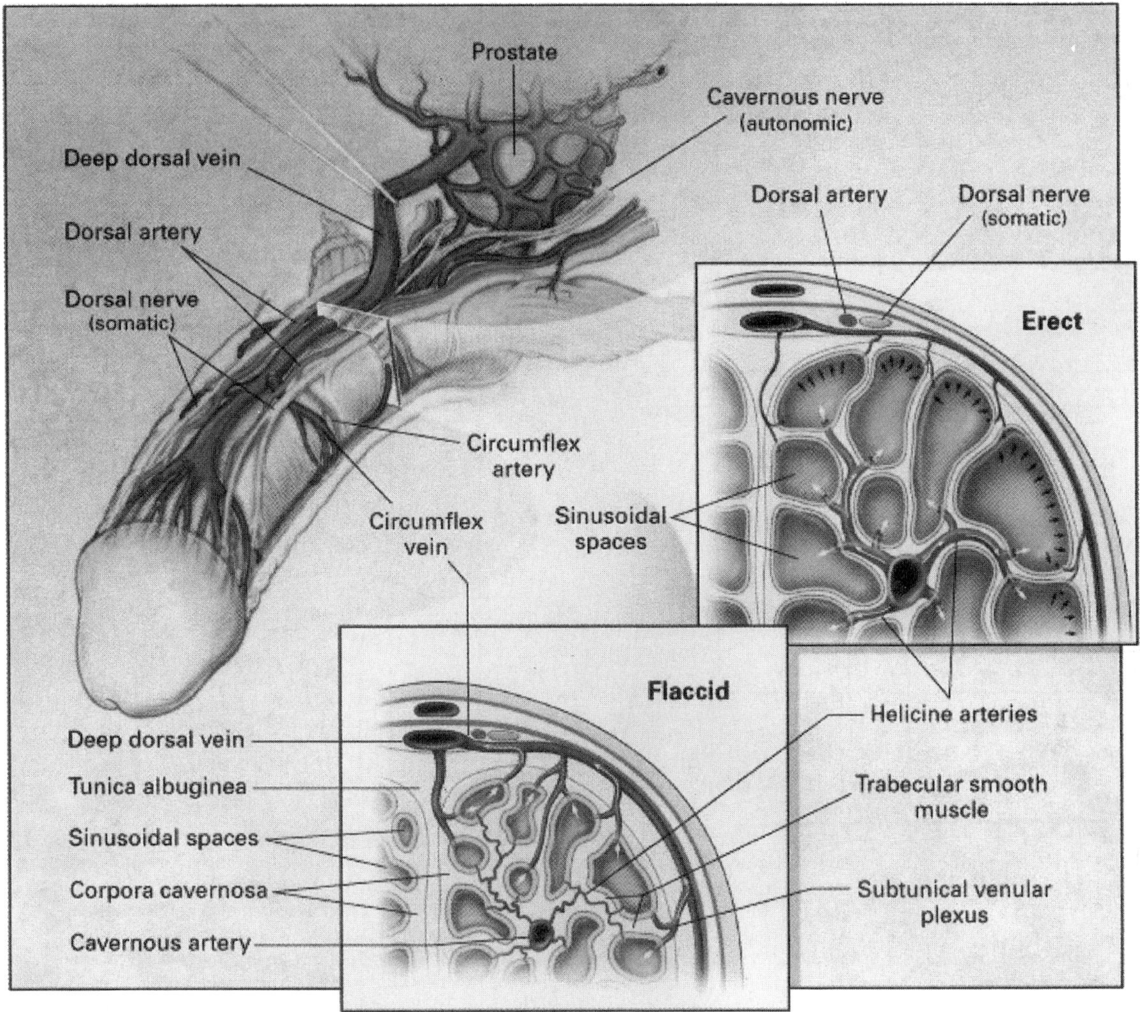

Figure 19–1. Anatomy and mechanism of penile erection. The corpora cavernosa are made up of trabecular spaces that are surrounded by cavernosal smooth muscle. Helicine arteries provide the arterial supply to the cavernosal spaces. The dorsal nerve provides the sensory innervation to the penis. During erection, the relaxation of the trabecular smooth muscle and the increased blood flow result in engorgement of the sinusoidal spaces in the corpora cavernosa. The expansion of the sinusoids compresses the venous return against the tunica albuginea, resulting in entrapment of blood. This imparts rigidity to the tumescent penis. (Adapted from Lue T. Erectile dysfunction. N Engl J Med 2000; 342:1802–1813.)

reversal of penile erection. Sildenafil (Viagra, Pfizer) is a potent and selective inhibitor of type 5 PDE activity that prevents breakdown of cGMP and thereby enhances penile erection.[27]

PHYSIOLOGIC, LIFESTYLE, AND PSYCHOSOCIAL CORRELATES AND RISK FACTORS FOR ERECTILE DYSFUNCTION

Epidemiologic studies indicate that the best predictors of the risk of ED are age, a history of diabetes mellitus, hypertension, medication use, and cardiovascular disease. Advancing age is an important risk factor for ED in men: fewer than 10% of men below age 40 years and more than 50% of men older than age 70 years are anticipated to be affected by ED. In both studies mentioned earlier (MMAS and NHSLS), the prevalence of ED increased with each decade of life.

Among the chronic diseases associated with ED, diabetes mellitus is the most important risk factor. In the MMAS, the age-adjusted risk for development of complete ED was three times higher in men with history of treated diabetes mellitus than in men without such a history. Of men with diabetes mellitus, 50% are expected to experience ED at some time during the course of their illness. In the MMAS, treated heart disease, treated hypertension, and hyperlipidemia were associated with significantly increased risk of ED. Among men with treated heart disease and hypertension, the probability of ED was more than two times greater for smokers than for nonsmokers. Smoking also increases the risk of ED in men taking medications for cardiovascular diseases. Cardiovascular disorders, including hypertension, stroke, coronary artery disease, and peripheral vascular disease, are all associated with increased risk of ED.

Several reviews have emphasized the relationship of prescription medications and the occurrence of ED. In the MMAS, the use of antihypertensive agents, cardiac medication,

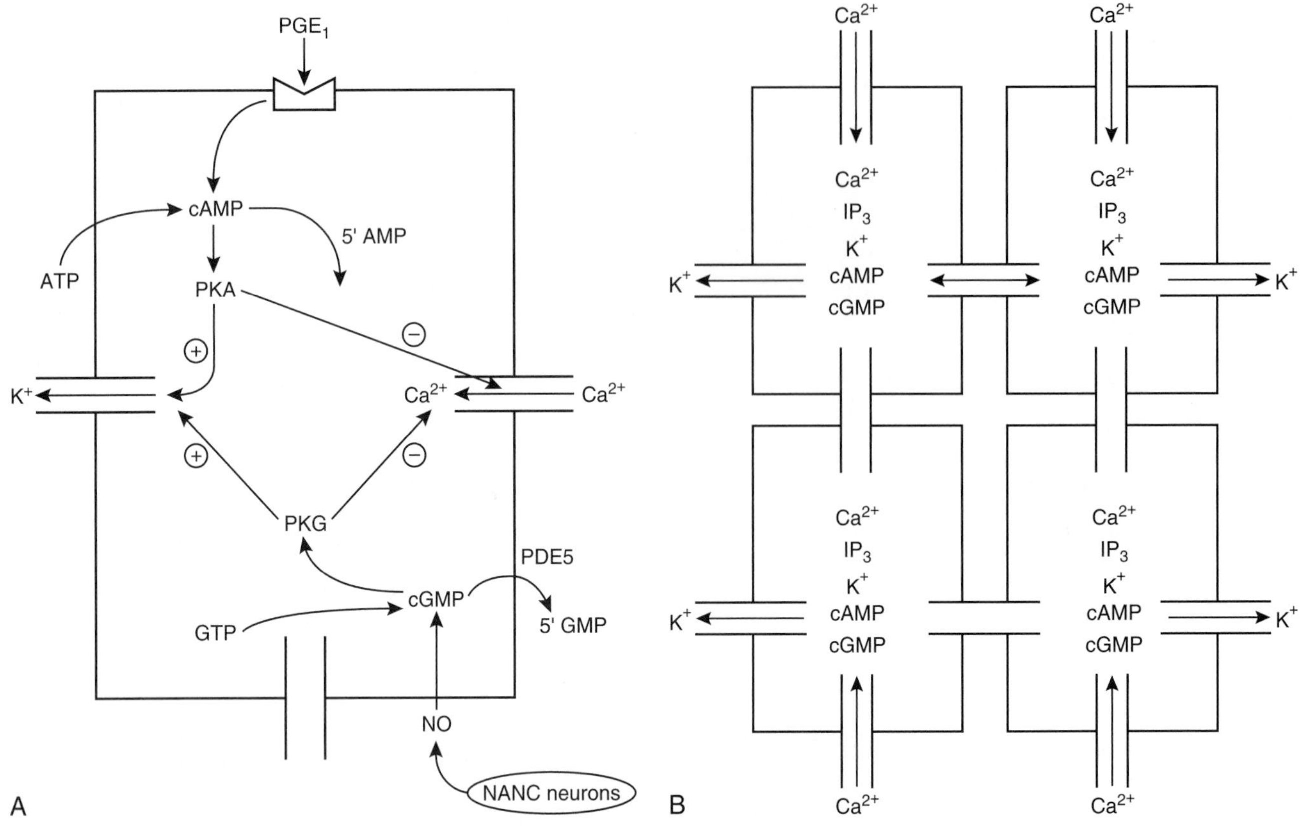

Figure 19–2. Biochemical mechanisms of penile smooth muscle relaxation.

A, Relaxation of the cavernosal smooth muscle is regulated by intracellular cyclic adenosine monophosphate (cAMP) and cyclic guanidine monophosphate (cGMP). The intracellular second messengers, by activation of specific protein kinases, cause sequestration of intracellular calcium (Ca^{2+}), closure of calcium channels, and opening of potassium (K^+) channels. This results in a net decrease in intracellular calcium, causing smooth muscle relaxation. Nitric oxide, released by noradrenergic, noncholinergic nerve endings (NANC), stimulates guanyl cyclase. By inhibiting phosphodiesterase type 5 (PDE5), sildenafil increases the amount of intracellular cGMP. Prostaglandin E_1 (PGE_1) stimulates generation of cAMP. Papaverine inhibits PDE_2, PDE_3, and PDE_4 and thereby increases the amount of intracellular cAMP. AMP, adenosine monophosphate; GTP, guanosine triphosphate; IP_3, inositol 1,4,5-triphosphate; NO, nitric oxide; PKA, protein kinase A; PKG, cGMP-specific protein kinase.

B, Interconnection of cavernosal smooth muscle cells in the penis. The smooth muscle cells in the corpora cavernosa are interconnected through connexin 43–derived gap junctions. Therefore, alterations in action potential and potassium channel activity in any myocyte affect the adjacent myocytes.

(*A* and *B*, Adapted and redrawn from Melman A, Christ GJ. Integrative erectile biology: the effects of age and disease on gap junctions and ion channels and their potential value to the treatment of erectile dysfunction. Urol Clin North Am 2001; 28:28:217–231.)

and oral hypoglycemic drugs was associated with an increased risk of ED. Thiazide diuretics and psychotropic drugs used in the treatment of depression may be the most common drugs associated with ED, simply because of the high prevalence of their use. A variety of drugs, however, including almost all antihypertensive agents, digoxin, histamine-2 receptor antagonists, anticholinergics, cytotoxic agents, and androgen antagonists, have been implicated in the pathophysiology of ED.

PATIENT EVALUATION

History

The diagnostic work-up of the patient with ED should start with an evaluation of general health (Table 19–1).[16, 28] The general medical history should be directed at identifying etiologic factors as well as factors that might affect the selection and response to therapy. The presence of diabetes mellitus, coronary artery disease, peripheral vascular disease, and hypertension may suggest a vascular cause. A history of stroke, spinal cord or back injury, multiple sclerosis, or dementia may point to a neurologic disorder. Also relevant is any history of pelvic trauma, prostate surgery, or priapism.

The social history must include ascertainment of recreational drug abuse—particularly tobacco, use of cocaine, marijuana and alcohol. Information about medications, particularly antihypertensive agents, antiandrogens, antidepressants, and antipsychotic drugs is important because almost 25% of all cases of impotence can be attributed to medications. Psychiatric illnesses (e.g., depression, psychosis) or drugs used to treat these disorders may be associated with sexual dysfunction.

A detailed sexual history, including the nature of relationships, partner expectations, situational erectile failure, performance anxiety, and marital discord, needs to be elicited (see Table 19–1).[16, 28] It is important to distinguish between an inability to achieve erection, changes in sexual desire, failure to achieve orgasm and ejaculation, and dissatisfaction with the sexual relationship. The physician should inquire about the onset, quality, and duration of erections and the presence of nocturnal and early morning erections.

Table 19–1. Diagnostic Evaluation of Erectile Dysfunction

History
1. Ascertain psychosexual history of:
   a. The strength of marital relationship and marital discord
   b. Depression
   c. Stress
   d. Performance anxiety
2. Ascertain etiologic factors, such as:
   a. The presence of diabetes mellitus, hypertension, end-stage renal disease, peripheral vascular disease
   b. History of spinal cord injury, stroke, or Alzheimer's disease
   c. Prostate or pelvic surgery
   d. Pelvic injury
   e. Concomitant medications, such as antihypertensive, antidepressant, and antipsychotic agents; antiandrogens, such as flutamide, bicalutamide, cyproterone acetate, and cimetidine; and inhibitors of androgen production, such as ketoconazole and GnRH agonists
   f. The use of recreational drugs such as alcohol, cocaine, opiates, and tobacco
3. Ascertain factors that might affect choice of therapy and the patient's response to it, such as:
   a. Coexisting coronary artery disease and its symptoms and severity
   b. The use of nitrates for angina
   c. Exercise tolerance
   d. The use of vasodilators for hypertension or congestive heart failure

Physical Examination
1. Ascertain signs of androgen deficiency, such as loss of secondary sex characteristics, eunuchoidal proportions, small testicular volume, or breast enlargement
2. Exclude neurologic findings of spinal cord lesion, previous stroke, or peripheral neuropathy; genital and perineal sensation
3. Palpate femoral and pedal pulses, and exclude evidence of lower extremity ischemia
4. Perform penile examination to exclude Peyronie's disease

Laboratory Evaluation
1. Brachial penile blood pressure index
2. Intracavernosal injection of vasodilator
3. Duplex Doppler ultrasonography
4. Pelvic arteriography
5. Cavernosography

Physical Examination

A directed physical examination should assess secondary sex characteristics, the presence or absence of breast enlargement, and testicular volume. An evaluation of femoral and pedal pulses can provide clues to the presence of peripheral vascular disease (see Table 19–1). The neurologic examination focuses on the presence of motor weakness, perineal sensation, anal sphincter tone, and bulbocavernosus reflex. The examination of the penis notes any unusual curvature, palpable plaques, or superficial lesions.

Self-Reporting Questionnaires

Over the last decade, there has been a general shift in most male sexual dysfunction clinics away from expensive, time-consuming, and invasive techniques (e.g., dynamic infusion cavernosometry, penile duplex Doppler ultrasonography, and Rigiscan studies) toward the use of simple, noninvasive, self-reporting questionnaires. These questionnaires have been found to be of value because many men with ED, for a variety of reasons, do not voluntarily come forward to their physicians and state their sexual complaints. Many men with ED feel embarrassed, whereas others consider ED an inevitable concomitant of the aging process. Some physicians themselves feel uncomfortable while discussing issues of such personal nature; this creates an atmosphere that is not conducive to effective communication. These self-reporting questionnaires can help break the ice and facilitate communication. These instruments are widely available and easy to complete, and they can complement or enhance the work-up of sexual dysfunction.

The *International Index of Erectile Function* (IIEF) is a multidimensional scale consisting of 15 questions that address relevant domains of male sexual function.[29] The IIEF has been validated in several languages, used in many multinational clinical trials, and has been found to have adequate sensitivity and specificity for detecting treatment-related changes, including response to oral erectogenic agents in men with ED.

Considerable effort has been invested in the development of abbreviated questionnaires that take less time than the IIEF but more concisely address similar aspects of male sexuality (e.g., *Sexual Health Inventory for Men Questionnaire* [SHIM]).[30]

Laboratory Tests

The diagnostic evaluation of a man with ED starts with general health evaluation. This may include measurements of hemoglobin, white blood cells, blood glucose, aspartate transaminase (AST), alanine transaminase (ALT), bilirubin, alkaline phosphatase, blood urea nitrogen (BUN), and creatinine.

Measurement of serum total testosterone concentrations can help detect androgen deficiency. Although there is no consensus on this issue, it is important to exclude androgen deficiency in men presenting with ED because this deficiency may be a manifestation of serious underlying illness, such as a pituitary tumor or human immunodeficiency virus (HIV) infection. In addition, testosterone replacement is desirable in men with androgen deficiency not only for restoration of sexual function but also for maintaining bone mineral density, muscle mass and protein metabolism, and a sense of well-being.

If the history, physical examination, and ED questionnaire do not identify any obvious medical concerns warranting further work-up, a more cost-effective approach for a busy practitioner is to prescribe a trial of oral medication (e.g., sildenafil) if there are no contraindications (e.g., nitrate use). See algorithm A.

Evaluation of Penile Vasculature and Blood Flow

Several tests are available to assess the integrity of penile vasculature and blood flow.[16, 28] Of these, the *penile brachial blood pressure index* is a simple and specific, but not a very sensitive, indicator of vascular insufficiency.[31–34] It is of historical interest but is rarely used today.

Intracavernosal injection of a vasoactive agent such as PGE_1 can be used as both a diagnostic and potential therapeutic modality.[16, 28] This procedure can show whether the patient will respond to this therapeutic modality and can facilitate patient education about the procedure and its potential side effects. Failure to respond to intracavernosal injection sometimes suggests vascular insufficiency or a venous leak that might need further evaluation and treatment.

Most men with ED do not need duplex color sonography, cavernosography, or pelvic angiography.[16, 28] These procedures should be reserved for patients in whom the results of these tests would alter the management or prognosis and only by physicians with considerable experience in their use. For instance, angiography may be useful in a young man with arterial insufficiency associated with pelvic trauma. Similarly, suspicion of congenital or traumatic venous leak in a young man presenting with ED would justify cavernosography. In each instance, confirmation of the vascular lesion might lead to consideration of surgery. Duplex ultrasonography can provide a noninvasive evaluation of vascular function.[16]

Nocturnal Penile Tumescence

Although recording of formal nocturnal penile tumescence (NPT) in a sleep laboratory for successive nights can help differentiate organic from psychogenic impotence, this test is expensive and labor-intensive and is not required in most men with ED. In most cases, formal NPT studies are reserved for medical-legal documentation.

The introduction of portable Rigiscan devices in 1985 has provided clinicians with a reliable means of continuously monitoring penile tumescence and rigidity at home. The patient wears this multicomponent device at bedtime for two to three nights. Two wire–gauge loops are placed around the base and tip of the penis to record changes in penile circumference and rigidity. Data are stored and then downloaded via a software program that allows for sophisticated interpretation.

NPT testing is not needed for most men with ED. It is recommended only for patients with a high clinical suspicion of psychogenic ED or situational problems or to document preoperatively poor penile rigidity. For most cases, a careful history eliciting nighttime or early morning erections provides a reasonable correlation with formal NPT and Rigiscan studies.[35]

Diagnostic Tests to Exclude Androgen Deficiency and Hypothalamic-Pituitary Lesions

There is considerable debate about the usefulness and cost-effectiveness of hormonal evaluation and the extent to which androgen deficiency should be investigated in men presenting with ED. Of all men with ED, 8% to 10% have low testosterone levels; the prevalence of androgen deficiency increases with advancing age.[9, 36–41] The prevalence of low testosterone levels is not significantly different in men who present with ED and in an age-matched population.[36, 39] Urologic studies report that in 6% to 8% of men with ED there is an endocrine basis to the condition. These data are consistent with the proposal that ED and androgen deficiency are two common but independently distributed disorders.[39]

Yet, it is important to exclude androgen deficiency in this patient population.[42] Androgen deficiency is a correctable cause of sexual dysfunction, and some men with ED and low testosterone levels do respond to testosterone replacement. Hypogonadism can have additional deleterious effects on the patient's health; for instance, hypogonadism might contribute to osteoporosis, loss of muscle mass and function, and increased risk of disability, falls, and fracture. In addition, in cross-sectional epidemiologic studies, low testosterone levels are associated with increased risk of midsegment obesity,[43, 44] insulin resistance,[45, 46] type 2 diabetes mellitus,[45, 46] and coronary artery disease[47]; however, we do not know whether testosterone replacement can reduce visceral fat and improve insulin sensitivity and cardiovascular risk in middle-aged men with midsegment obesity. Regardless of the presence of sexual dysfunction, androgen deficiency should be corrected by appropriate hormone replacement therapy. Further, androgen deficiency may be a manifestation of a serious underlying disease, such as HIV infection or a hypothalamic-pituitary space-occupying lesion.

In large studies,[36, 37, 40] only a small fraction of men with ED and low testosterone levels have been found to have space-occupying lesions of the hypothalamic-pituitary region. In one large survey, all of the hypothalamic-pituitary lesions were found in men with serum testosterone levels below 150 ng/dL.[40] Therefore, the cost-effectiveness of the diagnostic work-up to rule out an underlying lesion of the hypothalamic-pituitary region can be increased by limiting the work-up to men with serum testosterone levels less than 150 ng/dL.

TREATMENT

The selection of the therapeutic modality should be based on the underlying etiology, the patient's preference (goal-directed approach), the nature and strength of relationship with the man's sexual partner, and the absence or presence of underlying cardiovascular disease and other co-morbid conditions.[16, 28] In current practice, it is common to employ a step approach that first utilizes minimally invasive therapies that are easy to use and produce fewer adverse effects and then progresses to more invasive therapies that may require injections in some circumstances or surgical interventions after the first-line choices have been exhausted (Table 19–2). The physician needs to discuss the risks, benefits, and alternatives of all the diagnostic procedures and therapies with the couple.

It is intuitive that, in the execution of good medical practice, all associated medical disorders need to be optimized. In men with diabetes mellitus, efforts to optimize glycemic control are instituted, although improving glycemic control may not necessarily improve sexual function. In men with hypertension, control of blood pressure is optimized, and, if possible, the therapeutic regimen may need to be modified to discontinue antihypertensive drugs that impair sexual function. This strategy is not always possible because almost all antihypertensive agents have been associated with sexual dysfunction; the frequency of this adverse event is less with angiotensin-converting enzyme (ACE) inhibitors than with other agents.

All patients with ED can benefit from psychosexual counseling.[16, 28] Unfortunately, many couples are reluctant to pursue this avenue. When there is latent marital discord, the sensitive and astute clinician should direct affected couples appropriately.

First Line Therapies

Psychosexual Counseling

Counseling can be of benefit in both psychogenic and organic causes of sexual dysfunction (see Table 19–2). It can help decrease performance anxiety and increase the patient's ability to cope with the problem. Involving the partner in the counseling process can help dispel misperceptions about the problem, decrease stress, enhance intimacy and ability to talk about sex, and increase the chances of successful outcome of therapy. Counseling sessions are also helpful in uncovering conflicts in relationships, psychiatric problems, alcohol and drug abuse, and significant misperceptions about sex. Although psychobehavioral therapy has been claimed to relieve depression and anxiety, there is a striking paucity of outcome data on the effectiveness of this therapeutic modality.

Table 19–2. A Stepwise Approach to Treatment of Erectile Dysfunction

1. All patients and their sexual partners can benefit from and should receive psychosexual counseling.
2. First-line therapies
   a. Sildenafil citrate
   b. Vacuum constriction devices
3. Second-line therapies
   a. Intracavernosal injection of alprostadil
   b. Intracavernosal injections of other vasoactive amines
4. Third-line therapies
   a. Penile prosthesis
   b. Vascular surgery

Sildenafil

Sildenafil (Viagra) is the first effective oral agent for the treatment of ED. It was introduced to the United States market in March 1998, and since that time millions of tablets have been dispensed. Sildenafil is a selective type 5 PDE inhibitor that is a safe and effective first-line, oral treatment for ED (Tables 19–3 and 19–4).[27, 48–54]

Mechanism of Action

Sildenafil blocks the hydrolysis of cGMP induced by nitric oxide.[48–50] Therefore, sildenafil action requires an intact nitric oxide response as well as constitutive synthesis of cGMP by the smooth muscle cells of the corpora cavernosa. By selectively inhibiting cGMP catabolism in the cavernosal smooth-muscle cells, sildenafil restores the natural erectile response to sexual stimulation but, importantly, does not produce an erection in the absence of sexual stimulation. The fidelity of the nitric oxide production pathway and sexual stimulation are both necessary requirements for sildenafil to induce an erection.

Efficacy

The efficacy of sildenafil was demonstrated in a randomized dose-response study[26] in which 532 men with organic, psychogenic, or mixed ED were randomized to receive placebo or 25, 50, or 100 mg of sildenafil for 24 weeks. In this dose-response study,[26] patients taking sildenafil performed better in terms of increased rigidity, frequency of vaginal penetration, and maintenance of erection. Increasing doses of sildenafil were associated with higher mean scores for the questions assessing frequency of penetration and maintenance of erections after sexual penetration.

In a follow-up dose escalation study,[27] 329 men were randomly assigned to receive placebo or 50 mg of sildenafil for 12 weeks. At each follow-up, the dose of sildenafil was increased or decreased by 50%, depending on the therapeutic response or side effects. Sixty-four percent of attempts at intercourse were successful for the men receiving sildenafil, compared with 22% of men receiving placebo. The mean number of successful attempts per month was 5.9 for men receiving sildenafil and 1.5 for men receiving placebo. The mean scores for orgasms, intercourse satisfaction, and overall satisfaction domain were also significantly higher in the sildenafil group compared with the placebo group.[27]

Table 19–3. Recommendations for the Use of Sildenafil by Men with Cardiac Disease (American College of Cardiology and American Heart Association)

1. Sildenafil (Viagra) is absolutely contraindicated in men taking long-acting or short-acting nitrate drugs on a regular basis.
2. If the patient has stable coronary artery disease, is not taking long-acting nitrates, and uses short-acting nitrates only infrequently, the use of sildenafil should be guided by careful consideration of risks.
3. All men taking nitrates should be warned about the risks of the potential interaction between nitrates and sildenafil. The patients should also be warned that concurrent recreational use of inhaled nitrates or "poppers" may result in marked hypotension that may be serious or even fatal.
4. Sildenafil is contraindicated within 24 hours of ingestion of any form of nitrate.
5. In men with preexisting coronary artery disease, the physician should assess the risks of inducing cardiac ischemia during sexual activity before prescribing sildenafil. This assessment may include a stress test.
6. Men who are taking a combination antihypertensive medication should be warned about the possibility of sildenafil-induced hypotension. This is of particular concern in men with congestive heart failure who have borderline low blood volume or who are receiving complex regimens that include vasodilators or diuretics.

From Cheitlin MD, Hutter AM Jr, Brindis RG, et al. Use of sildenafil (Viagra) in patients with cardiovascular disease: Technology and Practice Executive Committee [erratum appears in Circulation 1999; 100:2389]. Circulation 1999; 99:168–177.

Table 19–4. Common Adverse Events Associated with the Use of Sildenafil in men with Erectile Dysfunction*

Adverse Event	Sildenafil	Placebo
Headache	16%	4%
Flushing	10%	1%
Dyspepsia	7%	2%
Rate of discontinuation	2.5%	2.3%

*Morales and colleagues reviewed the safety and tolerability data on 4274 men with erectile dysfunction from a series of placebo-controlled and open-label studies of sildenafil (see Ref. 55, Int J Impot Res 1998; 10:69–73). Most adverse effects were reported to be mild to moderate in intensity and transient (see Ref. 55). In other studies, associated visual disturbances resulting in blue-green color-tinged vision, increased light perception, and blurred vision, and myalgias have also been reported (see Cheitlin et al, Ref 60).

In a separate randomized clinical trial,[49] 268 men with diabetes mellitus and ED received either placebo or sildenafil for 12 weeks. Fifty-six percent of men receiving sildenafil reported improved erections compared with 10% of those receiving placebo ($P < .001$). The rate of men reporting at least one successful attempt at intercourse was 61% for the sildenafil group versus 22% for the placebo group. The study demonstrated that sildenafil was an effective treatment for ED in patients with diabetes mellitus.[49]

Sildenafil is also effective in men with ED due to a variety of other causes, including spinal cord injury and postradical prostatectomy.[52, 53] In general, baseline sexual function correlated positively with response to sildenafil, and patients with diabetes mellitus or previous prostate surgery responded less well than patients with psychogenic or vasculogenic ED.[53] Because there is no baseline characteristic that predicts the likelihood of failure to respond to sildenafil therapy, a therapeutic trial of sildenafil is warranted in all patients except in those in whom it is contraindicated.[53]

Adverse Effects Associated with Sildenafil Therapy

In clinical trials, the adverse effects that have been reported with greater frequency in sildenafil-treated men than placebo-treated men include headache, flushing, dyspepsia, respiratory tract disorders, and visual disturbances (see Table 19–4).[55] Sildenafil does not affect semen characteristics.[56] No cases of priapism were noted in any of the pivotal clinical trials.

Hemodynamic Effects of Sildenafil Citrate

In postmarketing surveillance, several instances of myocardial infarction and sudden death were reported in men using sildenafil.[57–61] Forty-four of the 130 deaths reported by the U.S. Food and Drug Administration, from March to November 1998, occurred in temporal relation to the ingestion of sildenafil[57–61]; 16 of these deaths occurred in individuals who were taking nitrates. Because most men presenting with ED also have high prevalence of cardiovascular risk factors, it is unclear whether these events were causally related to the ingestion of sildenafil, underlying heart disease, or both.[60]

Third-Line Therapy: The Penile Prosthesis

In the early part of the 20th century, the treatment of ED was virtually nonexistent. It was the introduction of the semirigid and inflatable penile prostheses in the early 1970s that initiated the great strides that have been made in recent years in the treatment of ED. To some, penile prostheses are considered invasive and costly, but for many patients with advanced organic disease who are unresponsive to any contemporary form of therapy, have significant structural disorders of the penis (e.g., Peyronie's disease), or have suffered corporal loss from cancer or traumatic injury, prostheses remain a highly effective and predictable method for restoring erectile function.

Implantation surgery usually takes less than an hour and in most cases can be done as an outpatient procedure with general or regional anesthesia. Recent studies have reported that more than 80% of patients and 70% of partners are pleased with their prosthesis and the togetherness that it brings to their relationship.[90, 91]

Penile implants are paired supports that are placed one in each of the two erectile bodies. There are two basic types: (1) hydraulic or fluid-filled (inflatable) implants and (2) semirigid implants, which are bendable but always remain firm in the penis.

With a number of recent modifications incorporating newer materials and designs, the chance of mechanical malfunction is only 5% to 10% in the first 10 years. Penile prostheses have a higher reliability rate than any other mechanical device implanted in the human body. The most feared complication by surgeons with prosthesis implantation is infection, which occurs in 1% to 3% of cases, but this can be higher in revision surgery, especially in diabetic patients.

Oral Therapeutic Agents under Development

It has been clearly established, in North America at least, that the preferred route of administration for an ED treatment is by mouth. The huge success of sildenafil attests to the demand for an effective oral erectogenic agent. Research and development in this field by other pharmaceutical enterprises has introduced a number of new PDE type 5 inhibitors with supposedly increased potency and fewer side effects.

PDEs have a ubiquitous presence in the human body. PDE type 5 inhibitors are recognized to enhance the effects of sexual stimulation through nitric oxide increases in cGMP in the penis. Besides acting in the corpus cavernosum of the penis, PDE type 5 inhibition is active in skeletal muscle, vascular smooth muscle, platelets, and visceral smooth muscle. It is the PDE type 5 inhibition cross-reacting in other tissues that causes most of the recognized side effects (e.g., headache, gastroesophageal reflux, muscle cramps, visual acuity changes).

The efficacy and side effects of PDE inhibitors are a function of pharmacologic specificity and bioavailability. Vardenafil (Bayer) and Cialis (Lilly-ICOS) are two new PDE type 5 inhibitors with better tissue specificity and pharmacokinetic profiles than sildenafil and are in advanced stages of clinical development (Table 19–6). Because of their reported increased selectivity, overall efficacy, and decreased number of adverse effects in Phase II and III studies, they show clinical promise. Their availability in the United States market is anticipated.

The PDE type 5 inhibitors are recognized to act as peripheral conditioners (i.e., enhance a local pathway to cause an erection). Another exciting area of research are drugs that initiate erections by actions directed within the central nervous system. Apomorphine SL (TAP Pharmaceuticals, Inc.) is an aporphine (not an opiate) that acts as a dopaminergic agonist.

Table 19–6. Specificity of Phosphodiesterase (PDE) Type 5 Inhibitors

Isoenzyme	Distribution	IC_{50} (nM) Sildenafil	Cialis	Vardenafil
PDE Type 5	Corpus cavernosum platelets, skeletal muscle, vascular and visceral smooth muscle	3.5	0.94	0.7
PDE Type 6	Retina	34	730	157

IC_{50} is the concentration of a given agent to inhibit 50% of a given phosphodiesterase.

It is effective centrally at picomolar concentrations and has actions on the paraventricular and supraoptic nuclei of the midbrain. It has been reformulated for sublingual absorption with an onset of action within 15 to 20 minutes. Adverse effects include nausea, vomiting, and, rarely, syncope. Ongoing clinical research studies and experience from Europe since its approval in June 2001 may bring it to the United States in the near future.

Another central initiator of erection in early development is α-melanocyte-stimulating hormone (melanotan-II). It not only has dopaminergic agonist activity but also has beneficial effects on libido.

In a double-blind, placebo-controlled crossover study, there was significant improvement in Rigiscan events, penile rigidity, and sexual desire in 10 patients with documented ED risk factors who were taking melanotan-II compared to those taking placebo. Nausea was the most common adverse event.[92]

Gene Therapy and Erectile Dysfunction

Gene therapy can be defined as the introduction of genetic material (ribonucleic acid [RNA] or deoxyribonucleic acid [DNA]) into an appropriate cell type, thus altering gene expression of that cell in order to produce a therapeutic effect.[93] The goal of gene therapy for ED is to introduce novel genetic material into an appropriate cell in an attempt to restore normal cellular and physiologic function.

Gene therapy has been proposed as a viable treatment option for diseases that have a vascular origin, such as arteriosclerosis, congestive heart failure, and pulmonary hypertension.[93–96] This, by biologic extension, suggests that gene therapy may also be employed to treat vascular diseases of the penis; ED in most cases is a manifestation of vascular disease.

One advantage of applying gene therapy for the treatment of ED is the easily accessible external location of the penis.[97, 98] Hence, a tourniquet can be placed around the base of the penis and the desired gene can be administered directly into the corpora cavernosa without entering the systemic circulation. Further, in the penis only a small number of cells need to be transfected because smooth muscle cells of the corpus cavernosum are interconnected by gap junctions that allow second messenger molecules and ions to be transferred to a number of interconnected smooth muscle cells, thus causing physiologically relevant changes in erectile function.[98] Moreover, the vascular smooth muscle cells of the penis have a relatively low turnover rate, thus allowing a desired gene to be expressed for long periods of time.

The concept of gene therapy for ED treatment focuses on preventing cavernosal tissue degradation and increasing cavernosal smooth muscle tone. Smooth muscle relaxation is the necessary step for achieving a normal erection. Therefore, molecules, enzymes, or growth factors that influence the signal transduction pathway of corporal smooth muscle relaxation represent potential targets for ED gene therapy. Nitric oxide has been recognized to be the principal mediator of penile erection.[99] However, other diverse mediators, such as the prostaglandins, VIP, and CGRP, play a role in erectile physiology.

Garban and associates first demonstrated that gene therapy could be performed in the penis by using naked complementary DNA (cDNA) encoding the penile inducible NOS gene, leading to physiologic benefit in the aging rat.[100] Christ and colleagues later showed that injection of hSlo cDNA, which encodes the human smooth muscle maxi-K^+ channel, into the rat corpora cavernosa can increase gap junction formation and enhance erectile responses to nerve stimulation in the aged rat.[101] More recently, Bivalacqua and colleagues used an adenoviral gene transfer approach in which an adenoviral construct encoding the eNOS and CGRP genes were shown to reverse age-related ED in rats.[95, 96, 102–104]

In these studies, cytomegalovirus and Rous sarcoma adenoviruses were utilized, and both eNOS and CGRP expression were sustained for at least 1 month in the corpora cavernosa of the rat penis. Five days after transfection with the Ad-CMVeNOS or AdRSVeNOS viruses, aged rats had significant increases in erectile function, as determined by cavernosal nerve stimulation and pharmacologic injection with the endothelium-dependent vasodilator acetylcholine and the type 5 PDE inhibitors zaprinast and sildenafil.[95, 102, 103]

Lue and colleagues demonstrated that intracavernous injection of adeno-associated virus brain–derived neurotrophic factor could improve erectile function after cavernosal nerve injury.[16, 17, 17a] This neurotrophic factor purportedly restored neuronal NOS in the major pelvic ganglion, thus enhancing the recovery of erectile function after bilateral cavernous nerve injury. These early but innovative studies provide evidence that in vivo gene transfer can have beneficial physiologic effects on penile erection; this approach still requires a significant amount of basic research before in vivo gene therapy techniques can be applied to humans.

FEMALE SEXUAL DYSFUNCTION

Female sexual dysfunction is a multicausal and multidimensional medical problem that adversely affects physical health and emotional well-being. There has been a conspicuous paucity of basic science research on female sexuality. Thus, our knowledge and understanding of the anatomy and physiology of normal female sexual response and the pathophysiology of female sexual dysfunction are limited. On the basis of our understanding of the physiology of the male erectile response, recent advances in technology, and heightened interest in women's health, the study of female sexual function and dysfunction is evolving.

PREVALENCE AND INCIDENCE RATES

Sexual dysfunction in women is age-related, progressive, and highly prevalent, affecting 30% to 50% of American women.[6, 105] In the National Health and Social Life Survey, which included 1749 women,[106, 107] 43% of adult women had complaints of sexual dysfunction. Although this study had a large sample size, with minority representation, and used modern probability sampling, it was limited by its cross-sectional design. In addition, the NHSLS did not include women over age 60 years and did not make any adjustment for menopausal status or medical risk factors.

Another study that surveyed 448 women over 60 years of age demonstrated that two thirds of these women were sexually inactive, 12% of married women had difficulty with intercourse, and 14% experienced pain with intercourse. Sexual activity was strongly correlated with marital status.[106] Women over age 60 years were less likely to have sex if their partners were in poor health and if they had feelings of low self-worth.[107]

The incidence rates of sexual dysfunction in women are not known. The same disease processes and risk factors that are associated with ED in men such as aging, hypertension, cigarette smoking, and hypercholesterolemia, are also associated with sexual dysfunction in women.[108, 109]

PHYSIOLOGY OF THE FEMALE SEXUAL RESPONSE CYCLE

Masters and Johnson first characterized the female sexual response as consisting of four successive phases: excitement, plateau, orgasm, and resolution.[110] During sexual arousal, the clitoris and the labia minora become engorged with blood and vaginal and clitoral length and diameter increase. These authors observed that the labia minora increase in diameter by two to three times during sexual excitement and consequently become everted, exposing their inner surface.

Kaplan proposed the aspect of "desire," and the three-phase model, consisting of desire, arousal, and orgasm. In this model, desire is the factor that incites the overall response cycle.[111] This three-phase model is the basis for the *Diagnostic and Statistical Manual (DSM IV)* definitions of female sexual dysfunction, and the recent reclassification system proposed by the American Foundation of Urologic Disease (AFUD) Consensus Panel in October 1998.[112]

Others have suggested that sexual function should be viewed as a circuit, with four main domains: libido, arousal, orgasm, and satisfaction. Each of these four domains may overlap and feed back negatively or positively upon the other three domains.[113]

PELVIC ANATOMY IN WOMEN

An understanding of female pelvic anatomy and physiology is essential for the evaluation and treatment of female sexual dysfunction. Although the female pelvis is composed of a continuum of organs interrelated in structure and function, it is helpful to group the pelvic organs into two categories: the *external* and *internal* genitalia.

The organs of the external genitalia are collectively known as the vulva, which is bound anteriorly by the symphysis pubis, posteriorly by the anal sphincter and laterally by the ischial tuberosities. The vulva consists of the labia, interlabial space, clitoris and vestibular bulbs.

The internal genitalia consist of the vagina, uterus, fallopian tubes, and ovaries.

Vagina

The vagina is a midline cylindrical organ that connects the uterus with the external genitalia. It usually measures 7 to 15 cm in length, depending on the position of the uterus. It can easily dilate and expand for intercourse and childbirth. Anteriorly, two pleats of sensitive tissue, the *labia minora* (inner lips), surround the opening of the vagina and are protected by the larger folds known as the *labia majora* (outer lips). The labia minora enclose an area called the vestibule, which contains the clitoris, the urethral opening and vaginal opening. The portion of the labia minora that covers the clitoris is known as the prepuce, or clitoral hood.

The wall of the vagina consists of three layers: (1) an inner aglandular mucous membrane epithelium; (2) an intermediary, richly supplied, vascular muscularis layer; and (3) an outer adventitial supportive mesh. Vaginal mucosa is a mucous type, stratified, nonkeratinized, squamous cell epithelium that undergoes hormone-related cyclical changes during the menstrual cycle. The middle muscularis layer is highly infiltrated with smooth muscle and an extensive tree of blood vessels, which engorges during sexual arousal. The surrounding outer fibrosa layer provides structural support to the vagina.

The vagina has many rugae, which are necessary for distensibility of the organ and are more prominent in the lower third of the vagina. Smaller ridges increase frictional tension during intercourse.[114, 115]

Blood Supply to the Vagina

The vascular system of the vagina consists of an extensive anastomotic network of blood vessels throughout its length. The main arterial supply to the vagina arises from vaginal branches of the uterine arteries, pudendal arteries (vaginal branches), and ovarian arteries.

Innervation of the Vagina

The autonomic innervation of the vagina originates from two separate plexuses: the superior hypogastric and the pelvic. Sympathetic fibers originate in the lateral gray column of T11-L2 and form the hypogastric plexuses. Parasympathetic fibers originate in the intermediolateral cell column of S2-S4 and synapse in the pelvic plexus. Sympathetic and parasympathetic nerve fibers leave the pelvic plexus and travel within the uterosacral and cardinal ligaments, along with the vessels, to supply the proximal two thirds of the vagina and the corporal bodies of the clitoris.

Somatic motor fibers originate from the anterior horns of sacral cord levels S2-S4 and travel within the pudendal nerve to innervate the bulbocavernosus and ischiocavernosus muscles. Sensory fibers innervating the introitus and perineum travel within the perineal and posterior labial nerves to the pudendal nerve (Fig. 19–3).[114, 115]

Immunohistochemical studies have revealed an abundance of nerve fibers in the distal vagina, as compared with the more proximal part. This area of increased innervation, which plays an important role in sexual function, can be damaged during performance of bladder suspension procedures and vaginal hysterectomies.

Physiologic Changes in the Vagina during Sexual Arousal

During sexual arousal, genital vasocongestion occurs as a result of increased blood flow. The vaginal canal is lubricated by secretions from uterine glands, and by a transudate that originates from the subepithelial vascular bed. This is passively transported through the intraepithelial spaces, which are sometimes referred to as "intercellular channels." Engorgement of the vaginal wall raises pressure inside the capillaries and increases the transudation of plasma through the vaginal epithelium.[116] This vaginal lubricative plasma flows through the epithelium onto the surface of the vagina, initially forming sweat-like droplets that coalesce to form a lubricative film that covers the vaginal wall.

Additional moistening during intercourse comes from secretions of the paired, greater vestibular or Bartholin's glands, although some believe that these glands have a more primal function of emitting an odoriferous fluid to attract the male. In addition to its lubrication, the vagina lengthens and dilates during sexual arousal as a result of relaxation of the smooth muscle in its wall. In human and animal models, sexual stimulation results in increased vaginal blood flow and decreased vaginal luminal pressure.[117]

Clitoris

The clitoris is an erectile organ similar to the penis and arises from the same embryologic structure, the genital tubercle. It is composed of three parts: the outermost glans or head, the middle *corpus* or body, and the innermost *crura*. The glans and body of the clitoris are 2 to 4 cm long, and the crura are 9 to 11 cm.[114, 115] The clitoris consists of fused midline erectile bodies (corpora cavernosa) that give rise to bilateral crura. The glans clitoris is visible as it emerges from the labia minora. The labia minora bifurcate to form the upper prepuce anteriorly and the lower frenulum posteriorly.

Each corpus cavernosum is ensheathed by a thick, fibrous connective tissue structure, the tunica albuginea, that covers the lacunar sinusoids, which are surrounded by a trabecula of vascular smooth muscle and collagen fibers. The two separate crura of the clitoris, formed from the separation of the most proximal parts of the corpora in the perineum, attach bilaterally to the undersurface of the pubis along the ischiopubic rami.

The main arterial supply to the clitoris is via the iliohypogastric-pudendal arterial bed (Fig. 19–3*A* and *B*). With sexual stimulation, increased blood flow to the clitoral cavernosal arteries results in increased clitoral intracavernosus pressure and tumescence and protrusion of the glans. Studies show that, unlike the penis, the clitoris lacks a subalbugineal layer between the erectile tissue and the tunica albuginea layer. In the male, this layer possesses a rich venous plexus that, during sexual excitement, expands against the tunica albuginea, reducing venous outflow and making the penis rigid. The absence of this venous plexus in the clitoris allows this organ to achieve tumescence, but not rigidity, during sexual arousal.

Duplex ultrasound of the clitoris reveals that during sexual simulation the clitoris increases in length and diameter and blood flow almost doubles.[117]

Vestibular Bulb

The vestibular bulbs are 3-cm-long, paired structures that lie along the sides of the vaginal orifice, directly beneath the skin of the labia minora (Fig. 19–3*A* and *B*). Although they are homologous to the corpus spongiosum of the penis and are composed of vascular smooth muscle, they are distinct, in that they are separated from the clitoris, urethra, and vestibule of the vagina. Recent cadaver dissections reveal that in young premenopausal women, the bulbs lie on the superficial aspect of the vaginal wall and do not form the core of the labia minora. Furthermore, there are considerable age-related variations in the dimensions of the erectile tissue between young premenopausal specimens and older, postmenopausal specimens.[118]

The main arterial supply to the vestibular bulbs is via bulbar, inferior perineal, and posterior labial branches of the internal pudendal artery (see Fig. 19–3).

The somatic sensory innervation of the labia minora travels via the perineal and posterior labial branches of the pudendal nerve. Autonomic innervation consists of sympathetic and parasympathetic fibers that travel with the vessels to reach the vestibular bulb.

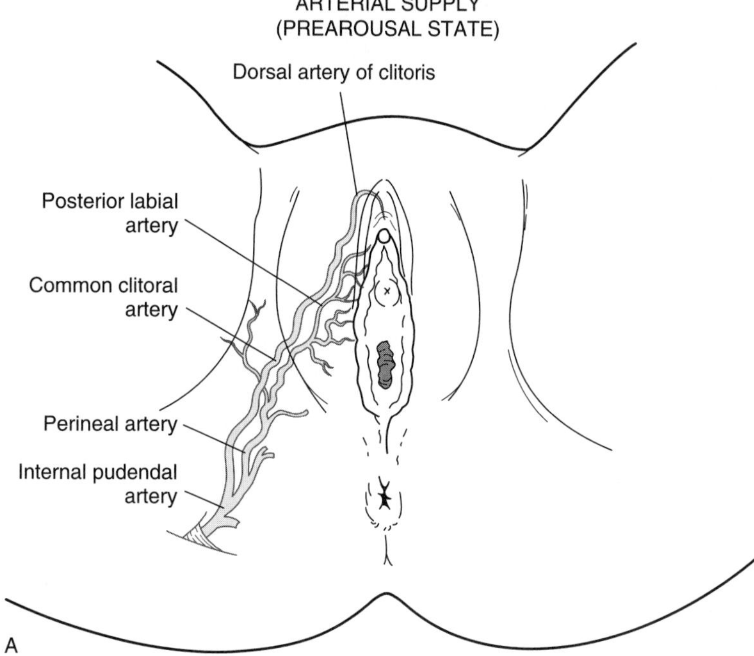

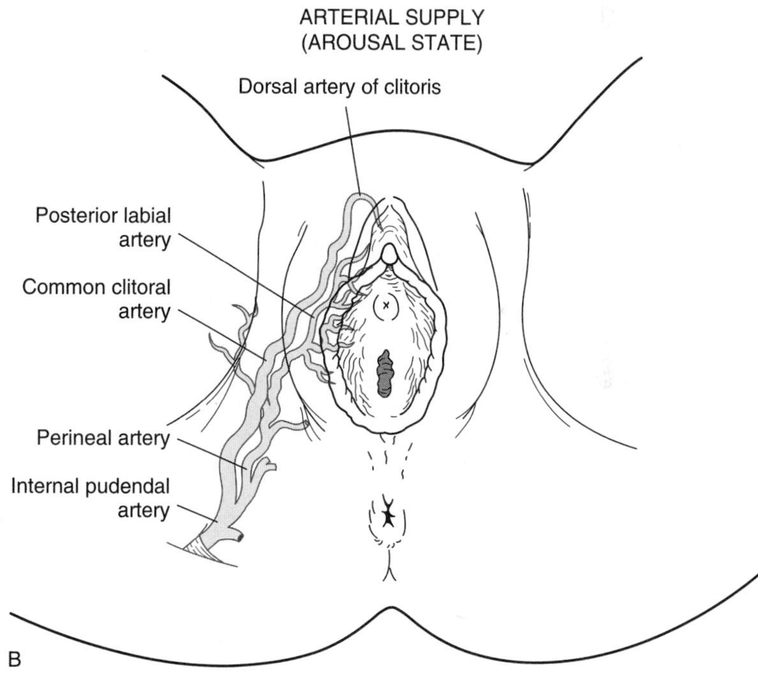

Figure 19–3. Arterial supply of the perineum and clitoris in prearousal *(A)* and arousal *(B)* states.

In the labia minora, blood flow increases during sexual stimulation, particularly to the vestibular bulbs. This causes a twofold to threefold increase in diameter and eversion of the labia with exposure of its inner surface.

Uterus

The uterine and cervical glands secrete mucus during sexual arousal to lubricate the vagina. Uterine and other pelvic surgical procedures can have a significant impact on female sexual response and function. The innervation of the uterus is closely proximate to the bladder and vagina, and pelvic dissection, as it is currently performed, can adversely affect a woman's later sexual health by damaging the uterine innervation. Surgical menopause brought on by hysterectomy and oophorectomy affects sexual function by multiple mechanisms. Even hysterectomy alone, without the removal of the ovaries, can result in sexual dysfunction.[119] Symptoms that women commonly experience postoperatively after hysterectomy include decreased desire, decreased arousal, decreased genital sensation, and orgasmic dysfunction.

The anatomic and physiologic basis for sexual dysfunction after hysterectomy is poorly understood. Understanding of female neurovascular anatomy is limited but vital to the understanding of normal sexual arousal and function. The sexual dysfunction symptoms women experience after hysterectomy are probably the result of nerve or vascular injuries as well as the loss of ovarian estrogens and androgens. Removal of the uterus and ligation of the arterial supply at the uterine pedicles can result in ovarian atrophy as well as fibrosis of vaginal wall and clitoral cavernosal smooth muscle. Disruption of the pelvic autonomic and cervical plexuses as well as the uterosacral and cardinal ligaments, which are associated with autonomic nerve fibers, results in difficulties in genital arousal and orgasm. This is an area of current focus and research, and in the future, perhaps women will be offered nerve-sparing pelvic procedures similar to those now routinely performed in men.

Pelvic Floor Muscles

The pelvic floor is a collection of tissues that span the opening within the bony pelvis. In addition to supporting the abdominal and pelvic organs and maintaining continence of urine and stool, the pelvic floor allows for intercourse and parturition. The pelvic floor musculature—in particular, the pelvic diaphragm that is formed by the *levator ani* muscles, the urogenital diaphragm, and the perineal membrane—is important for pelvic support. The perineal membrane that consists of the ischiocavernosus, bulbocavernosus, and superficial transverse perineal muscles is closely related to the vestibular bulbs and clitoris and plays a role in sexual response. These muscles, when voluntarily contracted, can intensify orgasm of both the female and her male partner.

The *levator ani muscle* has two different parts, the pubococcygeus and the iliococcygeus. These muscles can be palpated during pelvic examination as a distinct ridge just above the hymenal ring along each lateral wall of the pelvis. The function of this group of muscles is to pull the rectum, vagina, and urethra anteriorly toward the pubic bones to compress the lumens closed. Nonvoluntary pelvic floor spasm associated with vaginal penetration, or even examination with a speculum, is referred to as vaginismus. This disorder prevents sexual intercourse and is associated with dyspareunia and other sexual pain disorders. If the opposite problem exists, consisting of laxity and hypotonia of the pelvic floor musculature due to aging, menopause, or childbirth, for instance, symptoms of vaginal hypoanesthesia, coital anorgasmia, as well as incontinence during sexual intercourse or orgasm can develop. Women with pelvic floor disorders often have coexisting urologic and sexual dysfunction complaints. As a result of this overlap, all women who present with voiding dysfunction should be questioned about their sexual function as well.

NEUROGENIC MEDIATORS OF FEMALE SEXUAL RESPONSE

Within the central nervous system, the medial preoptic, anterior hypothalamic region and related limbic-hippocampal structures are responsible for sexual arousal. Upon activation, these centers transmit electrical signals through the parasympathetic and sympathetic nervous system. The neurogenic mechanisms modulating vaginal and clitoral smooth muscle tone, and vaginal and clitoral vascular smooth muscle relaxation are currently under investigation.

Noradrenergic, Noncholingeric (NANC)–Mediated Responses

Immunohistochemical studies in human vaginal tissues have shown the presence of nerve fibers containing neuropeptide Y (NPY), VIP, NOS, CGRP and substance P.[120] Preliminary studies suggest that VIP and nitric oxide are involved in modulating vaginal relaxation and secretory processes. In the clitoris, nitric oxide has been identified in human tissue and is thought to be the primary mediator of clitoral and labial engorgement.[121] Organ bath analysis of rabbit clitoral cavernosal smooth muscle strips demonstrates enhanced relaxation in response to sodium nitroprusside and L-arginine (both nitric oxide donors), which supports this hypothesis (Berman et al, unpublished data). Recently, PDE type 5, the enzyme responsible for degradation of cGMP, has been isolated in human clitoral, vestibular bulb, and vaginal smooth muscle culture and is inhibited by sildenafil citrate.[121] Human and rabbit vaginal smooth muscle cells, treated with the nitric oxide donor sodium nitroprusside, in the presence of sildenafil have enhanced intracellular cGMP synthesis and accumulation. PGE_1 and forskolin also produce a marked increase in intracellular cGMP.[122]

In organ bath studies, sildenafil causes dose-dependent relaxation of female rabbit clitoral and vaginal smooth muscle strips (Berman), further suggesting a role for nitric oxide as a mediator of clitoral cavernosal and vaginal wall smooth muscle relaxation. The exact identity of the relaxant NANC neurotransmitter, however, remains unclear. VIP is a NANC neurotransmitter that, like nitric oxide, may play a role in enhancing vaginal blood flow, lubrication, and secretions. The vagina is heavily innervated with VIP-immunoreactive nerve fibers in close relation to the epithelium and blood vessels.[123] In organ bath studies, VIP also causes dose-dependent relaxation of rabbit clitoral cavernosal and vaginal smooth muscle tissue, suggesting a similar role for endogenous VIP as a NANC neurotransmitter in clitoral and vaginal tissues (Berman et al, unpublished data).

$Alpha_1$-Adrenergic and $Alpha_2$-Adrenergic Responses

In men, adrenergic receptors exist in the brain centers and are associated with penile erection, libido, and ejaculation. Agents that affect these receptors have been extensively studied and used in the treatment of male ED. α-Adrenergic agonists such as norepinephrine activate sympathetic nerve terminals, resulting in contraction of penile trabecular smooth muscle and detumescence. In addition, α_2 agonists cause similar responses. Activation of α_2 receptors results in a decrease in intracellular adenosine 3′5′-monophosphate concentrations and in potent contraction in blood vessels. α-Adrenergic mediators also appear to play a physiologic role in female sexual arousal.[124]

Preliminary organ chamber experiments using rabbit vaginal tissue suggest that adrenergic mechanisms modulate smooth muscle tone. Exogenous norepinephrine (α_1 and α_2 agonist) causes dose-dependent contraction of vaginal smooth muscle and α_1 (prazosin and tamsulosin) and α_2 (delequamine) selective antagonists inhibit the contraction (Berman et al, unpublished data). These observations suggest that adrenergic nerves mediate contractile response. Furthermore, there appears to be a difference in the quality of the contractile responses in upper and lower vaginal segments, which is consistent with their different innervation and embryologic origin.

HORMONAL REGULATION: THE ROLES OF ESTROGEN AND TESTOSTERONE

Estrogen

Estrogen plays a significant role in regulating female sexual function. Estradiol affects cells throughout the peripheral and central nervous systems and influences nerve transmission. A decline in serum estrogen levels results in thinning of vaginal mucosal epithelium and atrophy of vaginal wall smooth muscle. Decreased estrogen levels also result in a less acidic environment in the vaginal canal. These changes, associated with estrogen deficiency, can predispose women to vaginal infections, urinary tract infections, incontinence, and sexual dysfunction.[125]

In animal models, estradiol administration results in expanded touch receptor zones along the distribution of the pudendal nerve, suggesting that estrogen affects sensory thresholds. In postmenopausal women, estrogen replacement restores clitoral and vaginal vibration and pressure thresholds to levels close to those of premenopausal women.[125] Estrogens also have vasoprotective and vasodilatory effects, which result in increased vaginal, clitoral, and urethral arterial flow, resulting in maintenance of the female sexual response by preventing atherosclerotic compromise to pelvic arteries and arterioles.[126]

With menopause and the decline in circulating estrogen levels, a majority of women experience some degree of change in sexual function. Common sexual complaints include loss of desire, decreased frequency of sexual activity, painful intercourse, diminished sexual responsiveness, difficulty achieving orgasm, and decreased genital sensation. Masters and Johnson first published their findings of the physiologic changes occurring in menopausal women that related to sexual function in 1966.[110] We have since learned that symptoms related to alterations in genital sensation and blood flow are, in part, secondary to declining estrogen levels and that there is a direct correlation between the presence of sexual complaints and levels of estradiol below 50 pg/mL.[125, 126] Some of the symptoms associated with menopause, such as vaginal dryness and diminished genital sensation, improve with estrogen replacement. However, some postmenopausal women continue to experience lack of sexual interest, fantasy and satisfaction, flat mood, and diminished well-being despite appropriate estrogen replacement; these symptoms are often attributed to androgen deficiency. As discussed later, it remains unclear whether physiologic testosterone replacement can improve sexual function in older women or whether this symptom complex is even due to androgen deficiency.

Estrogen also plays a role in regulating vaginal and clitoral NOS expression, the enzyme responsible for the production of nitric oxide. Aging and surgical castration result in decreased vaginal and clitoral NOS expression and apoptosis of vaginal wall smooth muscle and mucosal epithelium. Estrogen replacement restores vaginal mucosal health, increases vaginal NOS expression, and decreases vaginal mucosal cell death.[127] These findings suggest that medications such as sildenafil, which mediate vascular and nonvascular smooth muscle relaxation via nitric oxide, may have a potential role in the treatment of female sexual dysfunction, in particular that associated with sexual arousal disorder.

Testosterone

The role of androgen deficiency in the pathophysiology of female sexual dysfunction remains controversial. Most commercial assays for the measurement of total and free testosterone levels were developed to measure the much higher circulating concentrations in men; these assays lack the sensitivity and precision required to measure the low levels prevalent in androgen-deficient women.[128] Because of the paucity of normative data on serum total and free testosterone concentrations in healthy, menstruating women,[128] there is no consensus on the thresholds that can be used to define androgen deficiency in women. Until recently, the available testosterone formulations were designed to deliver the much higher dose required in hypogonadal men. However, two new formulations, the testosterone transdermal matrix patch for women and the testosterone gel are now undergoing phase 1 and phase 2 studies.[129, 130]

There is agreement that androgens, by acting within the brain, influence sexual behavior, although a woman's libido is also determined by environmental, emotional, cultural, and hormonal factors.[131–133] The effects of androgens in the brain are mediated, in part, directly through the androgen receptor and through aromatization of testosterone to estradiol. Androgen receptors have been identified in the cortex, pituitary, hypothalamus, preoptic region, thalamus, amygdala, and brain stem. In addition, both testosterone and estrogen have been shown to exert nongenomic effects in the central nervous system.

Testosterone might have additional effects on the genitalia in women. Androgen receptors have been reported in the vaginal wall, leading to speculation that testosterone might induce vaginal smooth muscle relaxation.[134] We do not know whether NOS activity in the clitoris is under testosterone regulation as it is in the cavernosal smooth muscle in the penis.

CLASSIFICATIONS AND DEFINITIONS OF FEMALE SEXUAL DYSFUNCTION (1998)

The Sexual Function Health Council of the American Foundation for Urologic Disease convened the AFUD Consensus Panel, an interdisciplinary conference panel, consisting of a multinational group of experts in female sexual dysfunction. The panel included specialists from many relevant disciplines, including endocrinology, family medicine, gynecology, nursing, pharmacology, physiology, psychiatry, psychology, rehabilitation medicine, and urology. The panel's objective was to evaluate and revise existing definitions and classifications of female sexual dysfunction. Specifically, medical risk factors and etiologic mechanisms of female sexual dysfunction were incorporated with the preexisting psychologically based definitions to generate an updated, unified classification system.[135]

The AFUD Consensus Panel classified female sexual dysfunction into several categories, described next (Table 19–7).

Hypoactive Sexual Desire Disorder

Hypoactive sexual desire disorder refers to the persistent or recurring deficiency (or absence) of sexual fantasies or thoughts and/or desire for or receptivity to sexual activity that causes personal distress. This disorder may result from psychological or emotional factors or may be secondary to physiologic problems (e.g., hormone deficiency) and medical or surgical interventions. Any disruption of the female hormonal milieu caused

Table 19–7. AFUD Classification of Female Sexual Dysfunction

1. Hypoactive Sexual Desire Disorder
2. Sexual Aversion Disorder
3. Sexual Arousal Disorder
4. Orgasmic Disorder
5. Sexual Pain Disorders
   a. Dyspareunia
   b. Vaginismus
   c. Other Sexual Pain Disorders

In 1998, the Sexual Function Health Council of the American Foundation for Urologic Disease convened a consensus panel that proposed a new classification for female sexual dysfunction. (see text for definitions).

hormone [FSH], total testosterone). Increased FSH levels can help document ovarian failure and menopausal status and can aid in differentiating primary ovarian dysfunction from disorders of the hypothalamus and pituitary gland. Measurements of LH levels in women do not add a great deal of information to that obtained from FSH measurements but can provide confirmatory data. Total testosterone levels, measured by an assay that has adequate sensitivity and precision, are needed to determine whether sexual dysfunction is due to androgen deficiency.

Estradiol levels vary greatly in women, depending on the phase of the menstrual cycle; very low levels can confirm ovarian failure but provide little additional information beyond what can be inferred from menstrual history and FSH levels. In women with hypogonadotropic hypogonadism, measurement of serum prolactin and a magnetic resonance imaging (MRI) study of the hypothalamic pituitary region may be needed to exclude the presence of a space-occupying lesion. In addition, these patients may need evaluation of other pituitary hormones to exclude deficiencies of other trophic hormones.

It is important to exclude systemic illness and medical conditions that disrupt the hypothalamic-pituitary axis such as HIV infection, end-stage renal disease, chronic obstructive lung disease, menopause, prior chemotherapy or bilateral salpingo-oophorectomy. Complete blood counts and a chemistry panel should be part of the general health evaluation. Medications that adversely affect sexual function should be addressed and changed if possible (Table 19–8).

Evaluating the female sexual response in the clinical setting both validates the patient's problem and potentially aids in diagnosis of organic disease, such as vascular insufficiency, a hormonal abnormality, or a neurologic disorder. Current investigations seek to define ranges of normal and the possible relevance to therapeutics for the following parameters:

1. Genital blood flow (clitoral, labial, urethral, and vaginal peak systolic velocities and end-diastolic velocities can be measured with duplex Doppler ultrasound).
2. Vaginal lubrication, as reflected by pH.
3. Vaginal compliance and elasticity (pressure-volume changes).
4. Genital sensation and vibration perception thresholds.

Psychosocial and Psychosexual Assessment

In addition to the medical evaluations, all patients should be evaluated for emotional and relational issues. This includes the context in which the patient experiences her sexuality, her self-esteem and body image, and her ability to communicate her sexual needs with her partner. This is an integral component of the female sexual function evaluation. Emotional and/or relational issues should be addressed before treatment and, certainly, before treatment efficacy is determined. If ongoing therapy is desired or required, it should also be provided.

Several instruments are available for assessment of self-reported sexual function, in particular sexual arousal. These self-report measures can be useful in clinical screening of patients and in clinical trials.

The *Brief Index of Sexual Function Inventory* (BISF-W), for example, is a validated 21-item self-reported listing of sexual interest, activity, satisfaction, and preference and discriminates between depressed, sexually dysfunctional, and healthy patients.[149] The BISF-W is sensitive to the effects of androgen replacement in oophorectomized women.[150]

The *Female Sexual Function Index* has also been used in clinical studies and practice.[151] Its self-report measures have been found to have a high degree of reliability and validity. This instrument can discriminate between women with sexual dysfunction and age-matched controls.

Table 19–8. Medications That Adversely Affect Sexual Function (Desire, Arousal, and Orgasm)

1. *Antihypertensive agents*
   Clonidine, guanethidine, reserpine, propranolol, prazosin, spironolactone, thiazide diuretics, beta blockers, calcium channel blockers
2. *Antidepressants*
   Imipramine, amitryptiline, clomipramine, amoxapine, monoamine oxidase inhibitors, lithium carbonate
3. *Selective serotonin reuptake inhibitors* (SSRIs)
   Fluoxetine, sertraline, paroxetine, venlafaxine
4. *Anxiolytics/sedative-hypnotics*
   Diazepam, alprazolam
5. *Neuroleptics*
   Phenothiazines, butyrophenones, thioridazine, chlorpromazine, chlorprothixene, fluphenazine
6. *Anticonvulsants*
   Phenobarbital, tegretol, primidone, phenytoin
7. *Antiulcer drugs*
   Cimetidine
8. *Anticancer drugs*
   Procarbazine, busulfan, chlorambucil, cyclophosphamide, tamoxifen, raloxifen

Daily diaries and sexual event logs have also been used in clinical trials. Subjective sexual response data reflect the personal experience of the patient, an important variable to evaluate because the ultimate goal is to enhance the personal sexual experience of the woman. Intervention is not considered successful unless the woman is able to experience sexual arousal, pleasure, and satisfaction. Thus, it is important to determine whether physiologic changes or improvement in blood flow translate into a better sexual experience.

TREATMENT

Treatment of female sexual dysfunction is gradually evolving as more clinical and basic research studies are targeting this problem. Medical management remains in the early experimental phases. Most treatment modalities being used by patients and physicians are based on empirical observations and are neither supported by rigorous clinical trial data nor approved by the U.S. Food and Drug Administration. Although it is premature to make general evidence-based recommendations for the treatment of female sexual dysfunction, it is important to recognize that not all female sexual complaints are psychological and that there are potential therapeutic options that might be useful in individual patients.

Estrogen Therapy

Estrogen replacement therapy is often indicated in menopausal women (either spontaneous or surgical). Aside from relieving hot flashes and preventing osteoporosis,[152, 153] estrogen therapy probably results in improved clitoral sensitivity and in decreased pain and burning during intercourse. Although cross-sectional epidemiologic studies had previously reported lower prevalence of cardiovascular disease among estrogen users, a recent randomized placebo-controlled trial was unable to demonstrate beneficial effects of estrogen replacement in secondary prevention of heart disease in postmenopausal women.[154, 155]

The role of estrogen replacement in the primary and secondary prevention of heart disease in women remains unclear and is the focus of ongoing investigation.[155, 156] In women with established heart disease, estrogen replacement has not been shown to improve cardiovascular outcomes. In the HERS study, event rates were higher in women given estrogen replacement than in women given placebo.[154] In menopausal women or in oophorectomized women, local or topical estrogen application relieves symptoms of vaginal dryness, burning, and urinary frequency and urgency.[125, 126, 157] A vaginal estradiol ring (Estring) delivers low-dose estrogen locally and may benefit breast cancer patients and other women who are unable to take oral or transdermal estrogen.

Androgen Formulations

Testosterone supplementation is associated with increased well-being, energy, and appetite and with improved somatic and psychological scores in surgically menopausal women.[131, 141, 158] In one study, such women, who were given supraphysiologic doses of testosterone enanthate by intramuscular injection alone or in combination with estrogen, experienced a greater increase in sexual desire, fantasies, and arousal than women who received estrogen alone.[131] In another study, combined administration of testosterone and estradiol implants increased sexual activity, satisfaction, pleasure, and frequency of orgasm more than estrogen implants alone.[158] The dose of testosterone used in each of these studies was supraphysiologic.

A later study[150] evaluated the effects of physiologic testosterone replacement in women who had undergone hysterectomy and oophorectomy and who were receiving stable estrogen replacement (at least 0.625 mg of conjugated equine estrogen daily orally). These women were randomized to receive either placebo patches or testosterone patches designed to achieve nominal delivery of either 150 μg (one active and one placebo patch) or 300 μg (two active patches) of transdermal testosterone daily for 12 weeks each. The highest dose of testosterone resulted in a mean serum free testosterone slightly above the physiologic range and significantly increased scores for frequency of sexual activity, pleasure, and orgasm. It also increased sexual fantasies, masturbation, and positive well-being.

Objectively, testosterone supplementation has been reported to increase vaginal vasocongestion, as measured by vaginal plethysmography during exposure to a potent visual stimulus in a small number of women with hypothalamic amenorrhea.[159, 160] Dehydroepiandrosterone (DHEA) replacement of 50 mg/day for 4 months in women with adrenal insufficiency increased sexuality and well-being.[161] It is unclear whether these effects were secondary to direct effect of DHEA on the brain or to an indirect effect via an increase in androgen synthesis. In contrast, a cross-sectional study of perimenopausal women did not show correlation between sexual function and androgen levels. Although pharmacologic doses of testosterone undoubtedly improve overall sexual function, we do not know whether physiologic testosterone replacement can produce clinically meaningful changes in health-related outcomes.

All androgens carry the risk of inducing virilization in women. Early reversible manifestations include acne, oiliness of skin, hirsutism, and menstrual irregularities. Long-term side effects such as male-pattern baldness, hirsutism, voice changes, and hypertrophy of the clitoris are largely irreversible. There is also evidence that testosterone supplementation in supraphysiologic doses decreases high-density-lipoprotein (HDL) cholesterol levels. Women with history of breast cancer should not be prescribed testosterone because testosterone is converted to estrogen by the aromatase enzyme. Surprisingly, the reported prevalence of virilizing side effects, even with the use of supraphysiologic doses of testosterone in surgically menopausal women, has been relatively low.[131, 141, 150, 158, 162–164]

17α-Methyltestosterone is commonly used in combination with estrogen in menopausal women for sexual dysfunction.[145, 163] There are conflicting reports regarding the benefit of methyltestosterone for treatment of inhibited desire or vaginismus in premenopausal women. The suggested dose of methyltestosterone for premenopausal and postmenopausal women ranges from 0.25 to 1.25 mg/day. The dose should be adjusted according to symptoms, free testosterone levels, and cholesterol, triglyceride HDL levels, and liver function tests. The potential side effects include weight gain, clitoral enlargement, increased facial hair, and hypercholesterolemia. The pharmacokinetics and clinical efficacy of this formulation have not been rigorously studied.

Two novel testosterone formulations are currently in early phases of clinical development. A transdermal matrix testosterone delivery system (patch) for women that is applied twice a week is being investigated.[129] Each patch provides a nominal delivery of 150 μg of testosterone daily.[129, 130, 165] Thus, two patches applied simultaneously twice a week can achieve a daily delivery of 300 μg of testosterone, approximating the daily production rates of testosterone in healthy women.[150] The skin tolerability of the patch is excellent.[129, 150] Initial pharmacokinetic studies have demonstrated that each 150-μg patch increases serum total testosterone concentrations by 25 to 30 ng/dL on average in healthy menstruating women and in surgically postmenopausal women.[129, 130] A testosterone gel for women is in initial stages of development. Each milligram of testosterone applied to the nongenital skin can increase serum testosterone concentration by 7 to 8 ng/dL.

Data from clinical trials thus agree that supraphysiologic doses of testosterone improve several aspects of sexual function in oophorectomized women with sexual dysfunction; however, we do not know whether physiologic testosterone that raises serum testosterone levels from low normal to high end of the normal range in women can produce clinically meaningful improvements in sexual function in postmenopausal women.

Sildenafil

Functioning as a selective type 5 (cGMP-specific) PDE inhibitor, this medication decreases the catabolism of cGMP, the second messenger in nitric oxide–mediated relaxation of clitoral and vaginal smooth muscle. Sildenafil may prove useful alone or perhaps in combination with other vasoactive substances for treatment of female sexual dysfunction. Phase II clinical studies assessing safety and efficacy of this medication for use in women are now in progress. Two studies have demonstrated that sildenafil is successful in treating female sexual dysfunction associated with aging and menopause and secondary to SSRI use.[137, 166]

Therapeutic Agents under Development

A number of drugs that have previously been used for the treatment of ED in men are now being investigated in women with sexual dysfunction. In the absence of efficacy data from randomized clinical trials, it is premature to make general recommendations about their use at this time.

L-Arginine functions as a precursor to the formation of nitric oxide, which mediates the relaxation of vascular and nonvascular smooth muscle. Although L-arginine has not been tested in clinical trials in women, preliminary studies in men appear promising. A combination of L-arginine and yohimbine (an α_2-adrenergic blocker) is currently being investigated for use in women.

An intraurethral formulation of PGE_1, absorbed via the mucosa (MUSE), is now available for male patients. A similar application of PGE_1, delivered intravaginally, is under investigation for use in women.

Currently available in an oral preparation, phentolamine functions as a nonspecific α-adrenergic blocker and causes vascular smooth muscle relaxation. A pilot study in menopausal women with sexual dysfunction demonstrated enhanced vaginal blood flow and subjective arousal with the medication.[167]

Apomorphine is a short-acting dopamine agonist that facilitates erectile responses in both normal men and men with ED. This drug is being tested in women with sexual dysfunction.

SUMMARY

The ideal approach to female sexual dysfunction is a collaborative effort between therapists and physicians and should include a complete medical and psychosocial evaluation as well as inclusion of the partner or spouse in the evaluation and treatment process. Although there are significant anatomic and embryologic parallels between men and women, the multifaceted nature of female sexual dysfunction is distinct from that of the male. The context in which a woman experiences her sexuality is equally, if not more, important than the physiologic outcome she experiences, and these issues need to be determined before beginning medical therapy or attempting to determine treatment efficacies. Even in women with identifiable organic disease, there are often psychosocial, emotional, or relational factors that contribute to sexual dysfunction. For this reason, a comprehensive approach, addressing both psychological as well as physiologic factors is instrumental to the evaluation of female patients with sexual complaints.

Whether sildenafil or other vasoactive agents are demonstrated to be effective in women with arousal disorder remains to be seen. There is a pressing need for more clinical and basic science research. Until more definitive efficacy data from randomized clinical trials become available, the treatment of women with sexual dysfunction should be individualized and preceded by a discussion of the uncertainty about beneficial effects and the potential for known and unknown adverse effects of drug therapy.

References

1. Benet AE, Melman A. The epidemiology of erectile dysfunction. Urol Clin North Am 1995; 22:699–709.
2. Feldman HA, Goldstein I, Hatzichristou DG, et al. Impotence and its medical and psychosocial correlates: results of the Massachusetts Male Aging Study. J Urol 1994; 151:54–61.
3. Johannes CB, Araujo AB, Feldman HA, et al. Incidence of erectile dysfunction in men 40 to 69 years old: longitudinal results from the Massachusetts male aging study. J Urol 2000; 163:460–463.
4. Lewis RW. Epidemiology of erectile dysfunction. Urol Clin North Am 2001; 28:209–16, vii.
5. Laumann EO, Paik A, Rosen RC. The epidemiology of erectile dysfunction: results from the National Health and Social Life Survey. Int J Impot Res 1999; 11 Suppl 1:S60–S64.
6. Laumann EO, Paik A, Rosen RC. Sexual dysfunction in the United States: prevalence and predictors. JAMA 1999; 281:537–544.
7. Carani C, Granata AR, Bancroft J, Marrama P. The effects of testosterone replacement on nocturnal penile tumescence and rigidity and erectile response to visual erotic stimuli in hypogonadal men. Psychoneuroendocrinology 1995; 20:743–753.
8. Cunningham GR, Hirshkowitz M, Korenman SG, Karacan I. Testosterone replacement therapy and sleep-related erections in hypogonadal men. J Clin Endocrinol Metab 1990; 70:792–797.
9. Carani C, Zini D, Baldini A, et al. Effects of androgen treatment in impotent men with normal and low levels of free testosterone. Arch Sex Behav 1990; 19:223–234.
10. Davidson JM, Camargo CA, Smith ER. Effects of androgen on sexual behavior in hypogonadal men. J Clin Endocrinol Metab 1979; 48:955–958.
11. Kwan M, Greenleaf WJ, Mann J, et al. The nature of androgen action on male sexuality: a combined laboratory/self-report study on hypogonadal men. J Clin Endocrinol Metab 1983; 57:557–562.
12. Salmimies P, Kockott G, Pirke KM, et al. Effects of testosterone replacement on sexual behavior in hypogonadal men. Arch Sex Behav 1982; 11:345–353.
13. Lugg JA, Rajfer J, Gonzalez-Cadavid NF. Dihydrotestosterone is the active androgen in the maintenance of nitric oxide–mediated penile erection in the rat. Endocrinology 1995; 136:1495–1501.
14. Andersson KE, Wagner G. Physiology of penile erection. Physiol Rev 1995; 75:191–236.
15. Christ GJ. The penis as a vascular organ: the importance of corporal smooth muscle tone in the control of erection. Urol Clin North Am 1995; 22:727–745.
16. Lue TF. Erectile dysfunction. N Engl J Med 2000; 342:1802–1813.
17. Lue TF, Tanagho EA. Hemodynamics of erection. In Tanagho EA, Lue TF, McClure RD (eds). Contemporary Management of Impotence and Infertility. Baltimore, Williams & Wilkins, 1988, pp 28–38.
17a. Bakircioglu ME, Lin CS, Fan P, et al. The effect of adeno-associated virus mediated brain derived neurotrophic factor in an animal model of neurogenic impotence. J Urol 2001; 165:2103–2109.
18. Naylor AM. Endogenous neurotransmitters mediating penile erection. Br J Urol 1998; 81:424–431.
19. Melman A, Christ GJ. Integrative erectile biology: the effects of age and disease on gap junctions and ion channels and their potential value to the treatment of erectile dysfunction. Urol Clin North Am 2001; 28:217–231, vii.
20. Christ GJ, Moreno AP, Melman A, Spray DC. Gap junction–mediated intercellular diffusion of Ca^{2+} in cultured human corporal smooth muscle cells. Am J Physiol 1992; 263:C373–C383.
21. Moreno AP, Campos de Carvalho AC, Christ G, et al. Gap junctions between human corpus cavernosum smooth muscle cells: gating properties and unitary conductance. Am J Physiol 1993; 264:C80–C92.
22. Campos de Carvalho AC, Roy C, Moreno AP, et al. Gap junctions formed of connexin 43 are found between smooth muscle cells of human corpus cavernosum. J Urol 1993; 149:1568–1575.
23. Tsai H, Werber J, Davia MO, et al. Reduced connexin 43 expression in high grade, human prostatic adenocarcinoma cells. Biochem Biophys Res Commun 1996; 227:64–69.
24. Rajfer J, Aronson WJ, Bush PA, et al. Nitric oxide as a mediator of relaxation of the corpus cavernosum in response to nonadrenergic, noncholinergic neurotransmission. N Engl J Med 1992; 326:90–94.
25. McDonald LJ, Murad F. Nitric oxide and cyclic GMP signaling. Proc Soc Exp Biol Med 1996; 211:1–6.
26. Nehra A, Barrett DM, Moreland RB. Pharmacotherapeutic advances in the treatment of erectile dysfunction. Mayo Clin Proc 1999; 74:709–721.
27. Goldstein I, Lue TF, Padma-Nathan H, et al. Oral sildenafil in the treatment of erectile dysfunction. Sildenafil Study Group. [Erratum in N Engl J Med 1998; 339:59]. N Engl J Med 1998; 338:1397–1404.
28. Conference NC. Consensus Development Panel on Impotence. JAMA 1993; 270:83–90.
29. Cappelleri JC, Rosen RC, Smith MD, et al. Diagnostic evaluation of the erectile function domain of the International Index of Erectile Function. Urology 1999; 54:346–351.
30. Rosen RC, Cappelleri JC, Smith MD, et al. Development and evaluation of an abridged, 5-item version of the International Index of Erectile Function (IIEF-5) as a diagnostic tool for erectile dysfunction. Int J Impot Res 1999; 11:319–326.
31. Ruutu ML, Virtanen JM, Lindstrom BL, Alfthan OS. The value of basic investigations in the diagnosis of impotence. Scand J Urol Nephrol 1987; 21:261–265.
32. Takasaki N, Kotani T, Miyazaki S, Saitou S. [Measurement of penile brachial index (PBI) in patients with impotence]. Hinyokika Kiyo 1989; 35:1365–1368.
33. Aitchison M, Aitchison J, Carter R. Is the penile brachial index a reproducible and useful measurement? Br J Urol 1990; 66:202–204.
34. Mueller SC, Wallenberg-Pachaly H, Voges GE, Schild HH. Comparison of selective internal iliac pharmaco-angiography, pe-

nile brachial index and duplex sonography with pulsed Doppler analysis for the evaluation of vasculogenic (arteriogenic) impotence. J Urol 1990; 143:928–932.
35. Brock G. Tumescence monitoring devices: past and present. In Handbook of Sexual Dysfunction 1999:65–69.
36. Korenman SG, Morley JE, Mooradian AD, et al. Secondary hypogonadism in older men: its relation to impotence. J Clin Endocrinol Metab 1990; 71:963–969.
37. Buvat J, Lemaire A. Endocrine screening in 1,022 men with erectile dysfunction: clinical significance and cost-effective strategy. J Urol 1997; 158:1764–1767.
38. Carani C, Bancroft J, Granata A, et al. Testosterone and erectile function, nocturnal penile tumescence and rigidity, and erectile response to visual erotic stimuli in hypogonadal and eugonadal men. Psychoneuroendocrinology 1992; 17:647–654.
39. Kaiser FE, Viosca SP, Morley JE, et al. Impotence and aging: clinical and hormonal factors. J Am Geriatr Soc 1988; 36:511–519.
40. Citron JT, Ettinger B, Rubinoff H, et al. Prevalence of hypothalamic-pituitary imaging abnormalities in impotent men with secondary hypogonadism. J Urol 1996; 155:529–533.
41. Morales A, Johnston B, Heaton JP, Lundie M. Testosterone supplementation for hypogonadal impotence: assessment of biochemical measures and therapeutic outcomes. J Urol 1997; 157: 849–854.
42. Hajjar RR, Kaiser FE, Morley JE. Outcomes of long-term testosterone replacement in older hypogonadal males: a retrospective analysis. J Clin Endocrinol Metab 1997; 82:3793–3796.
43. Khaw KT, Barrett-Connor E. Lower endogenous androgens predict central adiposity in men. Ann Epidemiol 1992; 2:675–682.
44. Seidell JC, Bjorntorp P, Sjostrom L, et al. Visceral fat accumulation in men is positively associated with insulin, glucose, and C-peptide levels but negatively with testosterone levels. Metabolism 1990; 39:897–901.
45. Haffner SM. Sex hormone-binding protein, hyperinsulinemia, insulin resistance and noninsulin-dependent diabetes. Horm Res 1996; 45:233–237.
46. Haffner SM, Shaten J, Stern MP, et al. Low levels of sex hormone–binding globulin and testosterone predict the development of non–insulin-dependent diabetes mellitus in men. Multiple Risk Factor Intervention Trial (MRFIT Research Group). Am J Epidemiol 1996; 143:889–897.
47. Alexandersen P, Haarbo J, Christiansen C. The relationship of natural androgens to coronary heart disease in males: a review. Atherosclerosis 1996; 125:1–13.
48. Goldstein I. A 36-week, open label, non-comparative study to assess the long-term safety of sildenafil citrate (Viagra) in patients with erectile dysfunction. Int J Clin Pract Suppl 1999; 102:8–9.
49. Rendell MS, Rajfer J, Wicker PA, Smith MD. Sildenafil for treatment of erectile dysfunction in men with diabetes: a randomized controlled trial. Sildenafil Diabetes Study Group. JAMA 1999; 281:421–426.
50. Boolell M, Allen MJ, Ballard SA, et al. Sildenafil: an orally active type 5 cyclic GMP-specific phosphodiesterase inhibitor for the treatment of penile erectile dysfunction. Int J Impot Res 1996; 8: 47–52.
51. Moreland RB, Goldstein I, Traish A. Sildenafil, a novel inhibitor of phosphodiesterase type 5 in human corpus cavernosum smooth muscle cells. Life Sci 1998; 62:PL309–PL318.
52. Giuliano F, Hultling C, el Masry WS, et al. Randomized trial of sildenafil for the treatment of erectile dysfunction in spinal cord injury. Sildenafil Study Group. Ann Neurol 1999; 46:15–21.
53. Jarow JP, Burnett AL, Geringer AM. Clinical efficacy of sildenafil citrate based on etiology and response to prior treatment J Urol 1999; 162:722–725.
54. Dinsmore WW, Hodges M, Hargreaves C, et al. Sildenafil citrate (Viagra) in erectile dysfunction: near normalization in men with broad-spectrum erectile dysfunction compared with age-matched healthy control subjects [erratum appears in Urology 1999; 53:1072]. Urology 1999; 53:800–805.
55. Morales A, Gingell C, Collins M, et al. Clinical safety of oral sildenafil citrate (Viagra) in the treatment of erectile dysfunction. Int J Impot Res 1998; 10:69–73.
56. Aversa A, Mazzilli F, Rossi T, et al. Effects of sildenafil (Viagra) administration on seminal parameters and postejaculatory refractory time in normal males. Hum Reprod 2000; 15:131–134.
57. Feenstra J, Drie-Pierik RJ, Lacle CF, Stricker BH. Acute myocardial infarction associated with sildenafil (letter). Lancet 1998; 352:957–958.
58. Zusman RM, Morales A, Glasser DB, Osterloh IH. Overall cardiovascular profile of sildenafil citrate. Am J Cardiol 1999; 83: 35C–44C.
59. Arora RR, Timoney M, Melilli L. Acute myocardial infarction after the use of sildenafil (letter). N Engl J Med 1999; 341:700.
60. Cheitlin MD, Hutter AM Jr, Brindis RG, et al. Use of sildenafil (Viagra) in patients with cardiovascular disease: Technology and Practice Executive Committee [erratum appears in Circulation 1999; 100:2389]. Circulation 1999; 99:168–177.
61. Muller JE, Mittleman A, Maclure M, et al. Triggering myocardial infarction by sexual activity: low absolute risk and prevention by regular physical exertion—determinants of Myocardial Infarction Onset Study Investigators. JAMA 1996; 275:1405–1409.
62. Herrmann HC, Chang G, Klugherz BD, Mahoney PD. Hemodynamic effects of sildenafil in men with severe coronary artery disease. N Engl J Med 2000; 342:1622–1626.
63. Padma-Nathan H, Steers WD, Wicker PA. Efficacy and safety of oral sildenafil in the treatment of erectile dysfunction: a double-blind, placebo-controlled study of 329 patients. Sildenafil Study Group. Int J Clin Pract 1998; 52:375–379.
64. Goldenberg MM. Safety and efficacy of sildenafil citrate in the treatment of male erectile dysfunction. Clin Ther 1998; 20:1033–1048.
65. Conti CR, Pepine CJ, Sweeney M. Efficacy and safety of sildenafil citrate in the treatment of erectile dysfunction in patients with ischemic heart disease. Am J Cardiol 1999; 83:29C–34C.
66. Osterloh IH, Collins M, Wicker P, Wagner G. Sildenafil citrate (Viagra): overall safety profile in 18 double-blind, placebo-controlled, clinical trials. Int J Clin Pract Suppl 1999; 102:3–5.
67. Young J. Sildenafil citrate (Viagra) in the treatment of erectile dysfunction: a 12-week, flexible-dose study to assess efficacy and safety. Int J Clin Pract Suppl 1999; 102:6–7.
68. Kloner RA. Cardiovascular risk and sildenafil. Am J Cardiol 2000; 86:57F–61F.
69. McMahon CG, Samali R, Johnson H. Efficacy, safety and patient acceptance of sildenafil citrate as treatment for erectile dysfunction. J Urol 2000; 164:1192–1196.
70. McGarvey MR. Tough choices: the cost-effectiveness of sildenafil (editorial). Ann Intern Med 2000; 132:994–995.
71. Smith KJ, Roberts MS. The cost-effectiveness of sildenafil. Ann Intern Med 2000; 132:933–937.
72. Tan HL. Economic cost of male erectile dysfunction using a decision analytic model: for a hypothetical managed-care plan of 100,000 members. Pharmacoeconomics 2000; 17:77–107.
73. Witherington R. Vacuum devices for the impotent. J Sex Marital Ther 1991; 17:69–80.
74. Lewis JH, Sidi AA, Reddy PK. A way to help your patients who use vacuum devices. Contemp Urol 1991; 3:15–21.
75. Lewis RW, Witherington R. External vacuum therapy for erectile dysfunction: use and results. World J Urol 1997; 15:78–82.
76. Ganem JP, Lucey DT, Janosko EO, Carson CC. Unusual complications of the vacuum erection device. Urology 1998; 51:627–631.
77. Morales A. Nonsurgical management options in impotence. Hosp Pract (Off Ed) 1993; 28:15–20, 23.
78. Bagatell CJ, Heiman JR, Rivier JE, Bremner WJ. Effects of endogenous testosterone and estradiol on sexual behavior in normal young men [erratum appears in J Clin Endocrinol Metab 1994; 78:1520]. J Clin Endocrinol Metab 1994; 78:711–716.
79. Skakkebaek NE, Bancroft J, Davidson DW, Warner P. Androgen replacement with oral testosterone undecanoate in hypogonadal men: a double blind controlled study. Clin Endocrinol (Oxf) 1981; 14:49–61.
80. McClure RD, Oses R, Ernest ML. Hypogonadal impotence treated by transdermal testosterone. Urology 1991; 37:224–228.
81. Nankin HR, Lin T, Osterman J. Chronic testosterone cypionate therapy in men with secondary impotence. Fertil Steril 1986; 46: 300–307.
82. Arver S, Dobs AS, Meikle AW, et al. Improvement of sexual function in testosterone-deficient men treated for 1 year with a permeation enhanced testosterone transdermal system. J Urol 1996; 155:1604–1608.
83. Buena F, Swerdloff RS, Steiner BS, et al. Sexual function does

not change when serum testosterone levels are pharmacologically varied within the normal male range. Fertil Steril 1993; 59:1118–1123.
84. Bhasin S, Fielder T, Peacock N, et al. Dissociating antifertility effects of GnRH-antagonist from its adverse effects on mating behavior in male rats. Am J Physiol 1988; 254:E84–E91.
85. Fielder TJ, Peacock NR, McGivern RF, et al. Testosterone dose-dependency of sexual and nonsexual behaviors in the gonadotropin-releasing hormone antagonist-treated male rat. J Androl 1989; 10:167–173.
86. Jain P, Rademaker AW, McVary KT. Testosterone supplementation for erectile dysfunction: results of a meta-analysis. J Urol 2000; 164:371–375.
87. Engelhardt PF, Plas E, Hubner WA, Pfluger H. Comparison of intraurethral liposomal and intracavernosal prostaglandin E_1 in the management of erectile dysfunction. Br J Urol 1998; 81:441–444.
88. Kim ED, McVary KT. Topical prostaglandin E_1 for the treatment of erectile dysfunction. J Urol 1995; 153:1828–1830.
89. Peterson CA, Bennett AH, Hellstrom WJ, et al. Erectile response to transurethral alprostadil, prazosin and alprostadil-prazosin combinations. J Urol 1998; 159:1523–1527.
90. Carson CC, Mulcahy JJ, Govier FE. Efficacy, safety and patient satisfaction outcomes of the AMS 700CX inflatable penile prosthesis: results of a long-term multicenter study. AMS 700CX Study Group. J Urol 2000; 164:376–380.
91. Wilson SK, Cleves MA, Delk JR 2nd. Comparison of mechanical reliability of original and enhanced Mentor Alpha I penile prosthesis. J Urol 1999; 162:715–718.
92. Wessells H, Gralnek D, Dorr R, et al. Effect of an α-melanocyte-stimulating hormone analog on penile erection and sexual desire in men with organic erectile dysfunction. Urology 2000; 56:641–646.
93. Nabel EG, Pompil VJ, Plantz GE, Nabel GJ. Gene transfer and vascular disease. Cardiovasc Res 1994; 28:445–455.
94. Heistad DD, Faraci FM. Gene therapy for cerebral vascular disease. Stroke 1996; 27:1688–1693.
95. Champion HC, Bivalacqua TJ, Hyman AL, et al. Gene transfer of endothelial nitric oxide synthase to the penis augments erectile responses in the aged rat. Proc Natl Acad Sci USA 1999; 96: 11648–11652.
96. Champion HC, Bivalacqua TJ, Toyoda K, et al. In vivo gene transfer of prepro-calcitonin gene-related peptide to the lung attenuates chronic hypoxia-induced pulmonary hypertension in the mouse. Circulation 2000; 101:923–930.
97. Bivalacqua TJ, Hellstrom WJ. Potential application of gene therapy for the treatment of erectile dysfunction. J Androl 2001; 22: 183–190.
98. Christ GJ, Melman A. The application of gene therapy to the treatment of erectile dysfunction. Int J Impot Res 1998; 10:111–112.
99. Burnett AL, Lowenstein CJ, Bredt DS, et al. Nitric oxide: a physiologic mediator of penile erection. Science 1992; 257:401–403.
100. Garban H, Marquez D, Magee T, et al. Cloning of rat and human inducible penile nitric oxide synthase: application for gene therapy of erectile dysfunction. Biol Reprod 1997; 56:954–963.
101. Christ GJ, Rehman J, Day N, et al. Intracorporal injection of hSlo cDNA in rats produces physiologically relevant alterations in penile function. Am J Physiol 1998; 275:H600–608.
102. Bivalacqua TJ, Champion HC, Mehta YS, et al. Adenoviral gene transfer of endothelial nitric oxide synthase (eNOS) to the penis improves age-related erectile dysfunction in the rat. Int J Impot Res 2000; 12 Suppl 3:S8–S17.
103. Champion HC, Bivalacqua TJ, D'Souza FM, et al. Gene transfer of endothelial nitric oxide synthase to the lung of the mouse in vivo: effect on agonist-induced and flow-mediated vascular responses. Circ Res 1999; 84:1422–1432.
104. Bivalacqua TJ, Rajasekaran M, Champion HC, et al. The influence of castration on pharmacologically induced penile erection in the cat. J Androl 1998; 19:551–557.
105. Spector IP, Carey MP. Incidence and prevalence of the sexual dysfunctions: a critical review of the empirical literature. Arch Sex Behav 1990; 19:389–408.
106. Diokno AC, Brown MB, Herzog AR. Sexual function in the elderly. Arch Intern Med 1990; 150:197–200.
107. Mooradian AD, Greiff V. Sexuality in older women. Arch Intern Med 1990; 150:1033–1038.
108. Hsueh WA. Sexual dysfunction with aging and systemic hypertension. Am J Cardiol 1988; 61:18H–23H.
109. Scott RS, Hsueh GS. A clinical study of the effects of galvanic vaginal muscle stimulation in urinary stress incontinence and sexual dysfunction. Am J Obstet Gynecol 1979; 135:663–665.
110. Masters EH, Johnson V. Human Sexual Response. Boston, Little, Brown, 1966.
111. Kaplan H. The New Sex Therapy. London, Balliere Tindall, 1974.
112. Berman JR, Berman L, Goldstein I. Female sexual dysfunction: incidence, pathophysiology, evaluation, and treatment options. Urology 1999; 54:385–391.
113. Graziottin A. Libido: The biological scenario. Maturitas 2000; 34(suppl)1:9–16.
114. Sjoberg I. The vagina: morphological, functional and ecological aspects. Acta Obstet Gynecol Scand 1992; 71:84–85.
115. Weber AM, Walters MD, Schover LR, Mitchinson A. Vaginal anatomy and sexual function. Obstet Gynecol 1995; 86:946–949.
116. Levin RJ. The physiology of sexual function in women. Clin Obstet Gynaecol 1980; 7:213–252.
117. Park K, Goldstein I, Andry C, et al. Vasculogenic female sexual dysfunction: the hemodynamic basis for vaginal engorgement insufficiency and clitoral erectile insufficiency. Int J Impot Res 1997; 9:27–37.
118. O'Connell HE, Hutson JM, Anderson CR, Plenter RJ. Anatomical relationship between urethra and clitoris. J Urol 1998; 159: 1892–1897.
119. Carlson KJ. Outcomes of hysterectomy. Clin Obstet Gynecol 1997; 40:939–946.
120. Hoyle CH, Stones RW, Robson T, et al. Innervation of vasculature and microvasculature of the human vagina by NOS and neuropeptide-containing nerves. J Anat 1996; 188:633–644.
121. Park K, Moreland RB, Goldstein I, Atala A, Traish A. Sildenafil inhibits phosphodiesterase type 5 in human clitoral corpus cavernosum smooth muscle. Biochem Biophys Res Commun 1998; 249:612–617.
122. Traish A, Moreland RB, Huang YH, et al. Development of human and rabbit vaginal smooth muscle cell cultures: effects of vasoactive agents on intracellular levels of cyclic nucleotides. Mol Cell Biol Res Commun 1999; 2:131–137.
123. Helm G, Ottesen B, Fahrenkrug J, et al. Vasoactive intestinal polypeptide (VIP) in the human female reproductive tract: distribution and motor effects. Biol Reprod 1981; 25:227–234.
124. Meston CM, Heiman JR. Ephedrine-activated physiological sexual arousal in women. Arch Gen Psychiatry 1998; 55:652–656.
125. Sarrell P. Sexuality and menopause. Obstet Gynecol 1990; 75: 26S.
126. Sarrel PM. Ovarian hormones and vaginal blood flow: using laser Doppler velocimetry to measure effects in a clinical trial of post-menopausal women. Int J Impot Res 1998; 10 Suppl 2:S91–S93; discussion, S98–S101.
127. Berman JR, McCarthy MM, Kyprianou N. Effect of estrogen withdrawal on nitric oxide synthase expression and apoptosis in the rat vagina. Urology 1998; 51:650–656.
128. Sinha-Hikim I, Arver S, Beall G, et al. The use of a sensitive equilibrium dialysis method for the measurement of free testosterone levels in healthy, cycling women and in human immunodeficiency virus–infected women [erratum appears in J Clin Endocrinol Metab 1998; 83:2959]. J Clin Endocrinol Metab 1998; 83:1312–1318.
129. Javanbakht M, Singh AB, Mazer NA, et al. Pharmacokinetics of a novel testosterone matrix transdermal system in healthy, premenopausal women and women infected with the human immunodeficiency virus. J Clin Endocrinol Metab 2000; 85:2395–2401.
130. Mazer NA. New clinical applications of transdermal testosterone delivery in men and women. J Control Release 2000; 65:303–315.
131. Sherwin BB, Gelfand MM, Brender W. Androgen enhances sexual motivation in females: a prospective, crossover study of sex steroid administration in the surgical menopause. Psychosom Med 1985; 47:339–351.
132. Rako S. Testosterone supplemental therapy after hysterectomy with or without concomitant oophorectomy: estrogen alone is not enough. J Womens Health Gend Based Med 2000; 9:917–923.

133. Rako S. Testosterone deficiency: a key factor in the increased cardiovascular risk to women following hysterectomy or with natural aging? J Womens Health 1998; 7:825–829.
134. Sadeghi-Nejad H, Moreland RB, Traish AM, et al. Preliminary report on the development and characterization of rabbit clitoral smooth muscle cell culture. Int J Impot Res 1998; 10:165–169.
135. Basson R, Berman J, Burnett A, et al. Report of the international consensus development conference on female sexual dysfunction: definitions and classifications. J Urol 2000; 163:888–893.
136. Tarcan T, Park K, Goldstein I, et al. Histomorphometric analysis of age-related structural changes in human clitoral cavernosal tissue. J Urol 1999; 161:940–944.
137. Berman JR, Berman LA, Lin H, et al. Effect of sildenafil on subjective and physiologic parameters of the female sexual response in women with sexual arousal disorder. J Sex Marital Ther 2001; 27:411–420.
138. Goldstein I, Berman JR. Vasculogenic female sexual dysfunction: vaginal engorgement and clitoral erectile insufficiency syndromes. Int J Impot Res 1998; 10 Suppl 2:S84–S90; discussion, S98–S101.
139. Sipski ML, Alexander CJ, Rosen RC. Orgasm in women with spinal cord injuries: a laboratory-based assessment. Arch Phys Med Rehabil 1995; 76:1097–102.
140. Rozenman D, Janssen E. Sexual function after hysterectomy. Jama 2000; 283:2238–2239.
141. Davis S. Androgen replacement in women: a commentary. J Clin Endocrinol Metab 1999; 84:1886–1891.
142. Burger HG, Dudley EC, Hopper JL, et al. The endocrinology of the menopausal transition: a cross-sectional study of a population-based sample. J Clin Endocrinol Metab 1995; 80:3537–3545.
143. Dennerstein L, Dudley EC, Hopper JL, Burger H. Sexuality, hormones and the menopausal transition. Maturitas 1997; 26:83–93.
144. Dennerstein L, Dudley E, Burger H. Well-being and the menopausal transition. J Psychosom Obstet Gynaecol 1997; 18:95–101.
145. Simon J, Klaiber E, Wiita B, et al. Differential effects of estrogen-androgen and estrogen-only therapy on vasomotor symptoms, gonadotropin secretion, and endogenous androgen bioavailability in postmenopausal women. Menopause 1999; 6:138–146.
146. Rosen RC, Lane RM, Menza M. Effects of SSRIs on sexual function: a critical review. J Clin Psychopharmacol 1999; 19:67–85.
147. Berman JR, Goldstein I. Sildenafil in postmenopausal women with sexual dysfunction. Urology 1999; 54:578–579.
148. Nurnberg HG, Hensley PL, Lauriello J, et al. Sildenafil for women patients with antidepressant-induced sexual dysfunction. Psychiatr Serv 1999; 50:1076–1078.
149. Mazer NA, Leiblum SR, Rosen RC. The brief index of sexual functioning for women (BISF-W): a new scoring algorithm and comparison of normative and surgically menopausal populations. Menopause 2000; 7:350–363.
150. Shifren JL, Braunstein GD, Simon JA, et al. Transdermal testosterone treatment in women with impaired sexual function after oophorectomy. N Engl J Med 2000; 343:682–688.
151. Rosen R, Brown C, Heiman J, et al. The Female Sexual Function Index (FSFI): a multidimensional self-report instrument for the assessment of female sexual function. J Sex Marital Ther 2000; 26:191–208.
152. Seeman E. Osteoporosis: trials and tribulations. Am J Med 1997; 103:74S–87S; discussion, 87S–89S.
153. Raisz LG. The osteoporosis revolution. Ann Intern Med 1997; 126:458–462.
154. Hulley S, Grady D, Bush T, et al. Randomized trial of estrogen plus progestin for secondary prevention of coronary heart disease in postmenopausal women. Heart and Estrogen/progestin Replacement Study (HERS) Research Group. JAMA 1998; 280: 605–613.
155. Herrington DM, Reboussin DM, Brosnihan KB, et al. Effects of estrogen replacement on the progression of coronary-artery atherosclerosis. N Engl J Med 2000; 343:522–529.
156. Mosca L, Barrett-Connor E, Wenger NK, et al. Design and methods of the Raloxifene Use for The Heart (RUTH) study. Am J Cardiol 2001; 88:392–395.
157. Shifren JL, Nahum R, Mazer NA. Incidence of sexual dysfunction in surgically menopausal women. Menopause 1998; 5:189–190.
158. Davis SR, McCloud P, Strauss BJ, Burger H. Testosterone enhances estradiol's effects on postmenopausal bone density and sexuality. Maturitas 1995; 21:227–236.
159. Heiman JR, Rowland DL, Hatch JP, Gladue BA. Psychophysiological and endocrine responses to sexual arousal in women. Arch Sex Behav 1991; 20:171–186.
160. Tutten A, Laan E, Panhuysen G, et al. Discrepancies between genital responses and subjective sexual function during testosterone substitution in women with hypothalamic amenorrhea. Psychosom Med 1996; 58:234–241.
161. Arlt W, Callies F, van Vlijmen JC, et al. Dehydroepiandrosterone replacement in women with adrenal insufficiency. N Engl J Med 1999; 341:1013–1020.
162. Sherwin BB, Gelfand MM. Effects of parenteral administration of estrogen and androgen on plasma hormone levels and hot flushes in the surgical menopause. Am J Obstet Gynecol 1984; 148:552–557.
163. Sarrel P, Dobay B, Wiita B. Estrogen and estrogen-androgen replacement in postmenopausal women dissatisfied with estrogen-only therapy: sexual behavior and neuroendocrine responses. J Reprod Med 1998; 43:847–856.
164. Watts NB, Notelovitz M, Timmons MC, A, et al. Comparison of oral estrogens and estrogens plus androgen on bone mineral density, menopausal symptoms, and lipid-lipoprotein profiles in surgical menopause. Obstet Gynecol 1995; 85:529–537.
165. Simon JA, Mazer NA, Wekselman K. Safety profile: transdermal testosterone treatment of women after oophorectomy. Obstet Gynecol 2001; 97:S10–S11.
166. Gupta S, Droney T, Masand P, Ashton AK. SSRI-induced sexual dysfunction treated with sildenafil. Depress Anxiety 1999; 9:180–182.
167. Rosen RC, Phillips NA, Gendrano NC 3rd, Ferguson DM. Oral phentolamine and female sexual arousal disorder: a pilot study. J Sex Marital Ther 1999; 25:137–144.

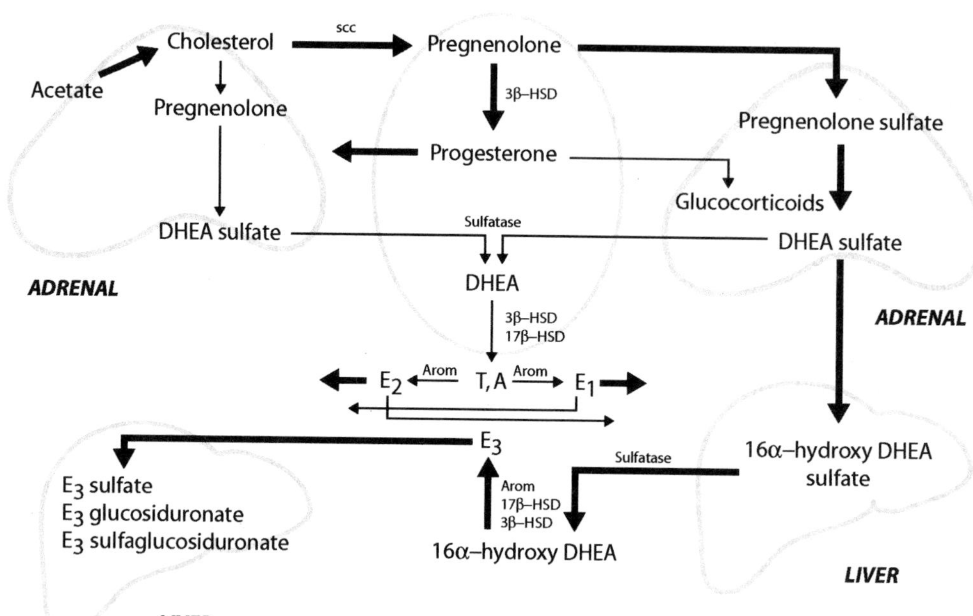

Figure 20–3. Steroidogenesis in the maternal-fetal-placental unit. SCC, cholesterol side-chain cleavage enzyme; DHEA, dehydroepiandrosterone; HSD, hydroxysteroid dehydrogenase; AROM, aromatase-enzyme complex.

gesterone to estrogen. Pregnenolone produced in the placenta enters the fetal compartment, where it is taken up by the fetal zone of the adrenal cortex, which also synthesizes pregnenolone from fetal LDL cholesterol. Pregnenolone is conjugated with sulfate by fetal steroid sulfotransferase in the fetal liver and adrenals to form pregnenolone sulfate and is converted in the fetal adrenals to 17α-hydroxy-pregnenolone sulfate and then DHEAS by 17α-hydroxylase and 17,20-lyase (CYP17) activities.[113]

The DHEAS enters the fetal circulation and undergoes hydroxylation in the fetal liver to form 16α-hydroxy-DHEAS, which is converted to 16α-DHEA in the placenta through the action of placental sulfatase. Further metabolism in the trophoblast by 3β-HSD-I, 17β-hydroxysteroid dehydrogenase (17β-HSD), and aromatase (CYP19) leads to the generation of estriol, which is quantitatively the major estrogen in the maternal circulation during pregnancy. The maternal liver actively conjugates estriol with glucosiduronate and sulfate, which are excreted into the urine. Approximately 90% of the estriol present in the maternal serum and urine is derived from fetal precursors, and therefore measurement of estriol levels in serum or urine serves as an index of fetal well-being.[113]

DHEAS from both the fetus and mother is also taken up by the placenta and converted to estradiol by the actions of sulfatase, 3β-HSD-I, 17β-HSD, and aromatase or to estrone by sulfatase, 3β-HSD-I, and aromatase. An estrogen unique to pregnancy, estetrol, is generated by 15α-hydroxylation of 16α-DHEAS in the fetal adrenal followed by enzymatic conversion by placental sulfatase, 3β-HSD-I, 17β-HSD, and aromatase.[114]

During pregnancy, estrogens have several actions.[102] They accomplish the following[102, 115–117]:

1. Enhance receptor-mediated uptake of LDL cholesterol, which is important for normal placental steroid production.
2. Increase uteroplacental blood flow.
3. Increase endometrial prostaglandin synthesis.
4. Prepare the breasts for lactation.

However, estrogen action does not appear to be essential in maintaining pregnancy because a fetus with deletion of the gene encoding placental sulfatase cannot remove the sulfate moiety from 16α-hydroxy-DHEAS and therefore has maternal estrogen levels approaching only about 10% of normal.[118] Similarly, pregnancies complicated by fetal aromatase deficiency may continue to term, again suggesting that the high concentrations of estrogens found in normal pregnancy are not necessary.[119]

Protein Hormones

Human Chorionic Gonadotropin

Chemistry

Human chorionic gonadotropin (hCG) is a glycoprotein composed of two dissimilar subunits, α and β, which are noncovalently linked through hydrophobic bonding. This molecule shares structural homology with the other glycoprotein hormones, human luteinizing hormone (hLH), hFSH, and hTSH. These hormones have α subunits that contain the same sequence of 92 amino acids and differ only in their carbohydrate composition; the β subunits differ in both amino acid and carbohydrate structure and are responsible for the biologic and immunologic specificity of the heterodimeric (intact) hormones. The 22,200-dalton β subunit of hCG is composed of 145 amino acids. Approximately 80% of the first 115 amino acids are homologous to those in the β subunit of hLH. hCG has an additional 24 amino acids on its carboxyl-terminal end that enhance its biologic activity.

Both subunits of hCG contain two oligosaccharide chains attached to asparagine residues through N-glycosidic linkages, and the β subunit contains in addition four O-serine–linked oligosaccharide units in the carboxyl-terminal peptide. The carbohydrate composition of hCG contains microheterogeneity and affects hormone clearance and biologic activity. The tertiary structure of hCG is determined by the carbohydrate composition and multiple disulfide bonds within each subunit. The α subunit contains five disulfide bonds; the β subunit has six. In each of the subunits, three of the disulfide bonds form a cystine knot, similar to that found in PDGF-β and transforming growth factor β (TGF-β).[120, 121]

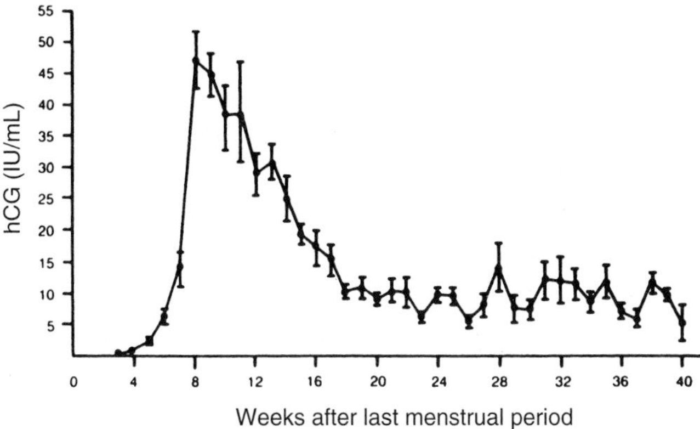

Figure 20–4. Mean (±SE) maternal serum human chorionic gonadotropin (hCG) levels throughout normal pregnancy. (From Braunstein GD, Rasor J, Danzer H, et al. Serum human chorionic gonadotropin levels throughout normal pregnancy. Am J Obstet Gynecol 1976; 126: 678.)

Biosynthesis

The single α subunit gene, located on chromosome 6, is actively expressed in both the cytotrophoblast and syncytiotrophoblast. In contrast, the β subunit is encoded by a cluster of six genes located on chromosome 19 in proximity to the hLH-β gene.[122] Three of the hCG-β genes are actively transcribed during pregnancy, primarily in the syncytiotrophoblast, which thus has the ability to synthesize and secrete free subunits and intact hCG. After synthesis of the protein core, each subunit is glycosylated, undergoes further post-translational modification through trimming of the carbohydrate, and then combines to form intact hCG.[120, 123, 124]

Secretion of hCG differs from that of many of the other placental proteins, whose secretory pattern parallels that of the trophoblastic mass. hCG is first detected in maternal serum 6 to 9 days after conception.[5] The levels rise in a logarithmic fashion, peaking 8 to 10 weeks after the last menstrual period, followed by a decline to a nadir at 18 weeks, with subsequent levels remaining constant until delivery[125] (Fig. 20–4). The placenta also secretes free subunits. During the first 13 weeks of pregnancy, relatively more β subunit is synthesized than α subunit, and throughout the remainder of pregnancy the opposite occurs.[126] In addition, a hyperglycosylated form of α subunit *(big α)* that is unable to combine with free β subunit is secreted into the maternal serum.

The physiologic factors that regulate hCG secretion in vivo are unknown. Much of the data concerning factors that stimulate or inhibit hCG synthesis and secretion has been derived from in vitro studies and is difficult to extrapolate to the in vivo situation. There is strong circumstantial evidence that GnRH, synthesized in both the cytotrophoblast and syncytiotrophoblast, may be an important factor in hCG secretion. This peptide is identical to hypothalamic GnRH and stimulates placental hCG production both in vitro and in vivo,[120, 127] whereas GnRH antagonists decrease basal hCG secretion.[128]

Immunohistochemical staining for GnRH in placental tissue is highest at 8 weeks of gestation and lower afterward,[129] roughly paralleling the pattern of hCG production, as do the circulating levels of GnRH measured in maternal serum.[130] In addition, the placenta contains GnRH receptors.[131] Placental GnRH release is stimulated by cyclic adenosine monophosphate (cAMP), prostaglandin E_2, prostaglandin F_2, epinephrine, epidermal growth factor, insulin, and vasoactive intestinal peptide (VIP), factors also noted to increase hCG secretion in vitro.[122, 132, 133]

Two other peptides synthesized by the cytotrophoblast, activin and inhibin, also modulate GnRH and hCG secretion; activin increases both, and inhibin inhibits the action of GnRH on the syncytiotrophoblast.[50] Increases in hCG production have also been found after trophoblast exposure to FGF, calcium, glucocorticoids, and phorbol esters.[122, 132, 133] Decreased production occurs with TGF-β, follistatin, and progesterone.[50, 122, 133] The decidua may also influence hCG production through paracrine mechanisms. Decidual interleukin-1 stimulates hCG secretion in cultured trophoblasts,[134] while decidual prolactin and an 8- to 10-kd decidual protein inhibit hCG production.[135, 136]

Finally, hCG may autoregulate its own production to some extent. hCG receptors are present on the surface of trophoblastic cells, and the addition of hCG to placental cells in culture stimulates cAMP production as well as proliferation and differentiation of the cytotrophoblasts into syncytiotrophoblasts.[137, 138] Both hCG mRNA and hCG production are stimulated by analogues of cAMP or agents that activate adenylate cyclase, probably through a protein kinase.[132, 139, 140] Thus, the net effect of an increase in syncytiotrophoblast mass and cAMP would be enhancement of hCG secretion.

The placenta is not the only site of hCG synthesis. Immunoreactive hCG has been found by immunocytochemistry or by immunoassay of extracts of a wide variety of normal tissues, including spermatozoa, testes, endometrium, kidney, liver, colon, gastric tissue, lung, spleen, heart, fibroblast, brain, and pituitary gland,[141–143] and the hormone has been shown to be synthesized in some fetal tissues.[144] The pituitary gland appears to be the major source of hCG or an hCG-like material present in nonpregnant individuals. Immunoactive and bioactive hCG has been partially purified from pituitary glands; the material is secreted in vitro by fetal pituitary cells and is shown by immunocytochemistry to be present in gonadotroph-type cells that do not contain hLH or human FSH.[141, 143, 145, 146]

Immunoreactive hCG has been measured in sera from normal, nonpregnant individuals, with the highest concentrations found in postmenopausal women.[147–150] In postmenopausal women, this material is secreted in a pulsatile fashion in parallel with hLH pulses, and during the normal menstrual cycle the immunoreactive hCG shows a midcycle peak concomitant with the hLH peak.[148, 150] In both men and postmenopausal women, GnRH stimulates secretion of the hormone, whereas its secretion is inhibited by oral contraceptives in women and by a GnRH agonist in agonadal men.[148–150]

Both gestational and nongestational trophoblastic tumors secrete hCG and its free subunits. The sources of hCG secretion in nongestational trophoblastic neoplasms are the syncytiotrophoblastic cells and in seminomas are the trophoblastic giant cells.[151] In many instances, the tumors produce incomplete forms of hCG or its subunits, and differences in carbohydrate content from the hCG in pregnancy have been especially apparent. A wide variety of nontrophoblastic tumors also secrete hCG, although the predominant moiety appears to be the free β subunit of hCG.[151, 152]

Metabolism

After it is secreted, hCG exhibits a biexponential clearance from the circulation with a fast half-time ($T_{1/2}$) of 6 hours and a slow $T_{1/2}$ of close to 36 hours. In contrast, the free β subunit has a 41-minute fast $T_{1/2}$ and a slow $T_{1/2}$ of 4 hours, and the free α subunit has a 13-minute fast $T_{1/2}$ and a 76-minute slow $T_{1/2}$.[153] Approximately 22% of the intact hormone appears in the urine unchanged; the rest undergoes metabolic degradation (Fig. 20–5). One of the early steps is proteolytic cleavage ("nicking") of the β subunit at Val^{44}-Leu^{45} and Gly^{47}-Val^{48}. Human leukocyte elastase, present in macrophages and leukocytes, appears to be responsible for some of the nicking of the β subunit.[153]

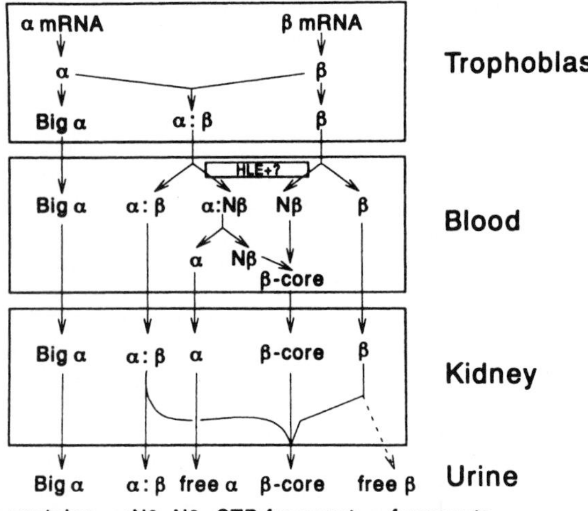

Figure 20–5. Proposed pathways for metabolism of human chorionic gonadotropin. α:β, intact hCG; α:Nβ, hCG with nicked β subunit; Nβ, free nicked β subunit; CTP fragment, carboxy-terminal fragment; mRNA, messenger RNA. (From Braunstein GD. Physiologic functions of human chorionic gonadotropin during pregnancy. In Mochizuki M, Hussa R [eds]. Placental Protein Hormones. Amsterdam, Elsevier Science, 1988, p 33.)

Nicked hCG is unstable and dissociates into free α subunit and nicked free β subunit. The latter is further metabolized, primarily in the kidney, to produce the β-core fragment, which is composed of the β subunit amino acids 6 to 40 disulfide bridged to amino acids 55 to 92, trimmed of a portion of carbohydrate, and has a molecular mass of 10,479 daltons.[153] This fragment is the major form of immunoreactive hCG present in the urine in pregnancy.[154] In normal pregnancy, the urine also contains variable quantities of the hyperglycosylated form of α subunit, free α subunit, free β subunit, nicked hCG, nicked free β subunit, carboxyl-terminal fragments of the β subunit, and fragments of the α subunit.[153]

Physiologic Functions

Most, if not all, of the physiologic functions of hCG occur after interaction of the hormone with the hLH-hCG receptor. The receptor gene is located on chromosome 2 and encodes for a G protein–coupled receptor with seven hydrophobic transmembrane domains and a large extracellular amino terminus that binds to hCG (and hLH). The receptor is part of superfamily of receptors, including those for hFSH, hTSH, AVP, VIP, PTH, and receptors for a variety of biogenic amines and neurotransmitters.[155] The hCG-receptor interaction results in increased cAMP production and, in some tissues, increased phosphoinositide turnover.[155]

Because of the close structural homology of the hLH-hCG receptor with the other glycoprotein hormone receptors, hCG may interact with the hTSH and hFSH receptors and thus has weak intrinsic hTSH and hFSH biologic activity. As previously noted, the hTSH-like activity of hCG is clinically manifested during normal pregnancy by the reciprocal decrease in maternal hTSH at the time of the hCG peak between 8 and 12 weeks after the last menstrual period. It is especially important in patients with hydatidiform moles and other forms of trophoblastic disease in which hCG levels may exceed 100,000 IU/L and result in clinical thyrotoxicosis[52, 53] (see Fig. 20–1).

One of the major functions of hCG during pregnancy is the "rescue" of the corpus luteum during the conception cycle.[109] During a menstrual cycle without conception, progesterone concentrations in the serum increase for the first 6 to 7 days of the luteal phase, followed by a 3- to 4-day plateau and then a decrease resulting in shedding of the endometrial lining. After conception and implantation, the corpus luteum continues to secrete progesterone and 17-hydroxyprogesterone for another 4 to 6 weeks. The maternal serum progesterone and 17-hydroxyprogestetrone concentrations then decrease, indicating a marked diminution in corpus luteum function.[156] The fall in 17-hydroxyprogesterone concentrations continues, but the drop in progesterone levels is only transient. This marks the transition from dependence on ovarian progesterone production to placental progesterone secretion (the luteal-placental shift). As previously noted, luteectomy during the first 50 days after the last menstrual period is associated with a decline in progesterone levels and expulsion of the products of conception. After a therapeutic abortion, progesterone levels also drop rapidly.

Thus, the fetal-placental unit is responsible for the signal to maintain the corpus luteum. The data supporting the idea that hCG is that physiologic signal include the following[109]:

1. The presence of hLH-hCG receptors on the corpus luteum.
2. The early production of hCG by the implanting trophoblast.
3. The dose-dependent increase in cAMP, progesterone, and estradiol from luteal cells cultured in vitro after exposure to hCG.
4. The parallel rise of progesterone and hCG in early pregnancy.
5. The enhanced progesterone secretion and prolongation of the menstrual cycle in nonpregnant women given exogenous hCG during their luteal phase.

The inability of hCG to prolong the life of the corpus luteum of pregnancy beyond the sixth to eighth week of pregnancy appears to be due to homologous desensitization of the adenylate cyclase system and the inhibitory effects of the high estrogen levels on progesterone synthesis through inhibition of 3β-hydroxysteroid dehydrogenase and $\Delta^{5\text{-}4}$-isomerase in the corpus luteum.

Another physiologic role for hCG is in the differentiation of fetal male genitalia through stimulation of the hLH-hCG receptors on the fetal testicular Leydig cells during the period when differentiation of wolffian duct structures and development of the external genitalia occur. The maximum testosterone production per unit weight of the testes coincides with the maximum binding of ^{125}I-labeled hCG to the fetal testicular receptors at 10 to 12 weeks of development, and fetal Leydig cells produce cAMP and testosterone in vitro after exposure to hCG. The hCG concentrations in fetal serum parallel the fetal testicular testosterone levels at a time when the amount of fetal pituitary hLH is not sufficient to stimulate the testosterone production.[157]

There are several other possible actions of hCG during normal pregnancy. In vitro, hCG stimulates the differentiation of cytotrophoblast to syncytiotrophoblast and hence may play an important paracrine role in regulating syncytiotrophoblast mass and production of trophoblast hormones.[136, 137, 158] Additional data supporting this autoregulatory effect of hCG include the in vitro stimulation of placental synthesis of cAMP, activation of glycogen phosphorylase, and incorporation of radiolabeled galactose and leucine into placental proteins upon exposure to hCG.[157] The fetal zone of the adrenal releases DHEAS in response to hCG exposure in vitro, and therefore hCG may have adrenocorticotropic activities in concert with fetal pituitary ACTH and placental ACTH.[157]

It has also been suggested that hCG plays a role in the immunosuppression that occurs during pregnancy. Many early studies on this topic were hampered by the use of impure preparations of hCG or the presence of preservatives such as phenol that may alter the end-points of the test systems used to define immunosuppression. In addition, the immunosuppressive effects may be due to gonadal steroid secretion in response to the hCG in the in vivo models used in some of the studies.[15, 159] Relaxin secretion from the corpus luteum is stimulated by hCG both in vivo and in vitro.[160]

Finally, the decrease in osmotic threshold for thirst and AVP release during pregnancy is clearly related to hCG.[65] Whether this decrease is due to a direct effect of hCG or an indirect effect through stimulation of gonadal steroids or interaction with hLH-hCG receptors present in vascular smooth muscle is unclear.[161]

Gestational Trophoblastic Disease

Gestational trophoblastic disease (GTD) includes complete and partial hydatidiform moles, choriocarcinoma, and placental-site trophoblastic tumor.[162] Complete molar pregnancy is the most common variety, occurring in 1 to 2 in 1000 pregnancies. Patients usually present with vaginal bleeding, a uterus that is larger than expected for the duration of pregnancy, anemia, and excessive vomiting. Pathologically, trophoblast hyperplasia, marked edema of the chorionic villi, and absence of fetal tissues are observed. In contrast, partial moles demonstrate focal trophoblast hyperplasia and villous swelling and often have fetal tissues with congenital malformations. Approximately 20% of patients with complete moles develop persistent trophoblastic disease, whereas only 2% to 4% of patients develop persistent disease after partial molar pregnancy. Persistent trophoblastic disease also can occur after a normal term pregnancy as well as pregnancies that end in spontaneous or induced abortion.

Choriocarcinoma is the most aggressive malignant form of persistent trophoblastic disease and may involve complications from local uterine disease, such as bleeding and rupture of the uterus, or from the effects of metastases, especially those involving the liver, lungs, and brain. The least common form of GTD is placental-site trophoblastic tumor, which is derived from the intermediate trophoblast and is often associated with vaginal bleeding and amenorrhea.[163]

All of these neoplasms secrete hCG, free β subunit, and often additional forms of these molecules. With the exception of placental-site trophoblastic tumor, which secretes relatively low amounts of hCG, the serum and urine concentrations of hCG roughly parallel the tumor burden and also provide prognostic information. Thus, hCG measurements in concert with clinical and radiologic findings, especially vaginal ultrasonography findings, are useful for making the diagnosis of GTD.

Hydatidiform moles are initially treated with uterine dilatation and evacuation with or without adjunctive single-agent chemotherapy with methotrexate or actinomycin D. Approximately 90% of patients with low-risk, persistent trophoblastic disease are cured by single-agent chemotherapy; 75% of patients with high-risk, metastatic disease are cured by multiagent chemotherapy, including etoposide, methotrexate, actinomycin D, cyclophosphamide, and vincristine. Serial hCG measurements are invaluable for monitoring as they accurately reflect the effect of therapy on the tumor.[162]

Human Placental Lactogen

Also called chorionic somatomammotropin, hPL is a single-chain, nonglycosylated polypeptide composed of 191 amino acid residues and two disulfide bridges, with a molecular mass of 21,600 daltons.[39] It is closely related chemically and biologically to both GH (85% amino acid homology) and prolactin (13% amino acid homology).[40] The hGH-hPL gene cluster is located on the long arm of chromosome 17 and consists of five genes—one coding for pituitary hGH (hGH-N), one for placental hGH (hGH-V), and three for placental hPL (hPL-L, hPL-A, and hPL-B, of which only hPL-A and hPL-B are transcribed).[44]

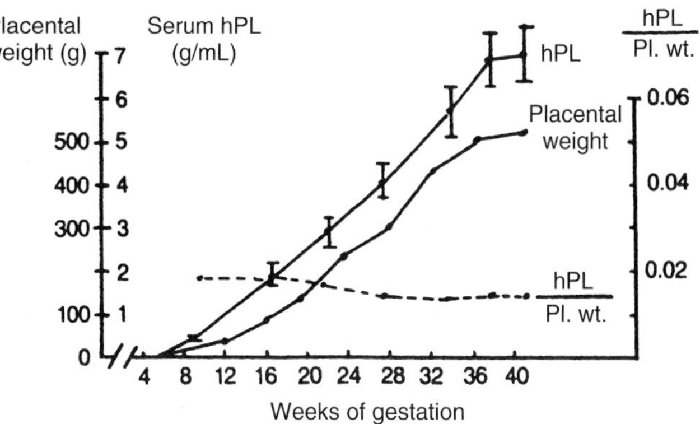

Figure 20–6. Placental weight (Pl. wt.) and maternal serum concentrations of human placental lactogen (hPL) during pregnancy. (From Selenkow HA, Saxena BN, Dana CL. Measurement and pathophysiologic significance of human placental lactogen. In Pecile A, Finzi C [eds]. The Feto-Placental Unit. Amsterdam, Excerpta Medica, 1969, p 340.)

hPL is synthesized and secreted by the syncytiotrophoblast and is detected in maternal serum between 20 and 40 days of gestation.[40] The maternal serum levels rise rapidly and peak at 34 weeks, followed by a plateau[17, 164] (Fig. 20–6). Both the serum concentrations and placental hPL mRNA concentrations are closely correlated with placental weight and syncytiotrophoblastic mass.[17, 164, 165] The maternal serum concentrations at term average between 6 and 7 μg/mL; at that time, on the basis of the 9- to 15-minute $T_{1/2}$ of disappearance from the circulation, the placental production rate of hPL is in excess of 1 g/day.[166] The fetal serum levels are 1/50 to 1/100 of the maternal levels.[167]

The physiologic in vivo regulation of hPL synthesis and secretion, other than the constitutive production related to placental mass, is unknown. Several studies have examined the possible role of nutrients in hPL secretion in pregnant women. Neither acute hyperglycemia nor hypoglycemia appeared to alter the hPL concentrations, although prolonged glucose infusions decreased and prolonged fasting increased the concentrations.[168–174] Arginine infusions, dexamethasone administration, and changes in plasma free fatty acid levels did not affect the maternal hPL concentrations.[175, 176] Glucose, estrogens, glucocorticoids, prostaglandins, epinephrine, oxytocin, TRH, GnRH, and L-dopa have been examined in in vitro systems and found to be without consistent effects.[177–182]

Angiotensin II, IGF-I, phospholipase A_2, arachidonic acid, and epidermal growth factor stimulated hPL release in vitro.[183–185] Epidermal growth factor probably enhances production through promotion of cytotrophoblast-to-syncytiotrophoblast differentiation.[183] Apolipoprotein AI also stimulated hPL synthesis and release through cAMP-dependent and arachidonic acid–dependent pathways.[40, 186–189] Because changes in the maternal plasma apolipoprotein AI concentrations parallel those of hPL during pregnancy, it is likely that this apoprotein, alone and as part of circulating HDL, is important in the secretion of hPL.[187]

hPL has a number of biologic activities that are qualitatively similar to those of hGH and prolactin and can bind to both the hGH and prolactin receptors.[190] In various bioassay systems, hPL had weak somatotropic and lactogenic effects.[191–193] It appears to be a major regulator of IGF-I production, and during pregnancy, hPL concentrations are correlated with those of IGF-I.[40, 45, 194] HPL also affects the metabolism of maternal nutrients. It stimulates pancreatic islet insulin secretion, both directly and after carbohydrate administration,[168, 195, 196] and is a diabetogenic factor during pregnancy through its promotion of insulin resistance. It enhances lipolysis, leading to a rise in free fatty acids, which may in part be responsible for the insulin resistance.[197]

The various biologic activities of hPL have led to the hypothesis that the role of hPL during pregnancy is to provide the fetus with a constant supply of glucose and amino acids.[168] The hPL-stimulated lipolysis allows the mother to utilize free fatty acids for energy during fasting, allowing glucose, amino acids, and ketone bodies to cross the placenta for use by the fetus. In addition, hPL has actions in the fetus, promoting amino acid uptake by muscle and stimulating protein production, IGF-I production, and glycogen synthesis.[194]

Despite the proposed importance of hPL in maternal and fetal metabolic homeostasis during pregnancy, its absence does not appear to impair pregnancy. Deficient or absent hPL production related to gene defects has been described in several women who experienced normal pregnancies and delivered normal infants.[198–200]

Placental Growth Hormone

Placental GH, hGH-V, is synthesized and secreted by the syncytiotrophoblast.[40] Alternate splicing of the hGH-V gene results in two nonglycosylated isoforms with molecular masses of 22 and 26 kd.[42, 167] The 22-kd variant may also be glycosylated and circulate as a 26-kd protein.[167] HGH-V is detected in the maternal plasma from 10 weeks of gestation and peaks during the third trimester[40, 42, 201] (Fig. 20–7).

HGH-V has somatotropic activity and stimulates IGF-I production, and the increase in IGF-I concentrations may in turn be responsible for the suppression of maternal pituitary hGH secretion[194, 201–203] (see Fig. 20–7). Unlike pituitary hGH, hGH-V is not secreted in a pulsatile fashion, nor is it released from the trophoblast by growth hormone–releasing hormone (GHRH), but it is inhibited by glucose.[204] It has been estimated that at term, 85% of the GH biologic activity in maternal serum is due to hGH-V, 12% to hPL, and only 3% to pituitary hGH.[205] Within 48 hours of delivery, pituitary hGH secretion returns to normal.

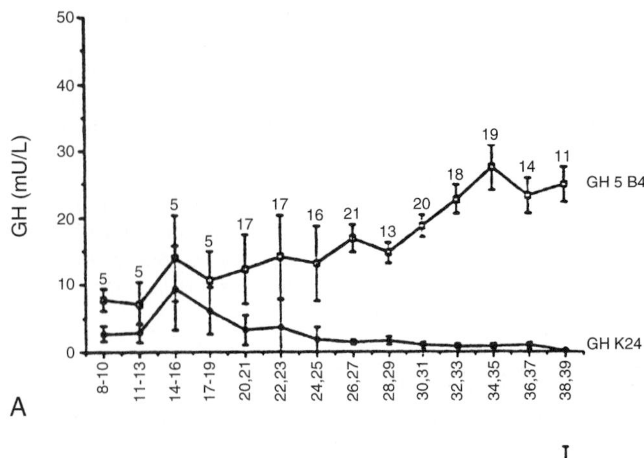

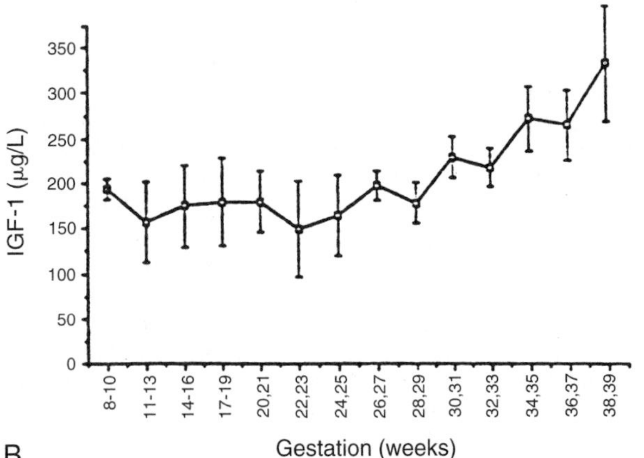

Figure 20–7. Mean (± standard error) of plasma human growth hormone (hGH) *(A)* and insulin-like growth factor-1 (IGF-1) *(B)* levels throughout pregnancy. The number of individual assays of growth hormone (GH) and IGF-1 at each gestational stage is indicated in *A* on top of vertical bars. GH 5 B4 indicates placental GH (hGH-V); GH K24 indicates pituitary GH. (From Mirlesse V, Frankenne F, Alsat E, et al. Placental growth hormone levels in normal pregnancy and in pregnancies with intrauterine growth retardation. Pediatr Res 1993; 34:39.)

Human Chorionic Corticotropin

The syncytiotrophoblast synthesizes an ACTH-like peptide, human chorionic corticotropin (hCC), as well as several proopiomelanocortin-derived peptides, including β-lipotropin, β-endorphin, and α-melanocyte-stimulating hormone.[55, 58, 62, 206–209] The maternal serum concentrations of ACTH increase as pregnancy progresses, and the elevation of free cortisol levels during pregnancy may be related in part to both placental hCC and pituitary ACTH production.[206]

HCC secretion is stimulated by CRH, which is probably the most important factor regulating the local production of the peptide through paracrine or autocrine mechanisms, or both, because it is also produced by both the cytotrophoblast and the syncytiotrophoblast.[210] Unlike the situation with the pituitary, glucocorticoids and oxytocin also stimulate hCC release from placental cultures.[60, 208] Indeed, the resistance of maternal plasma ACTH concentrations to suppression after glucocorticoid administration may reflect the placental hCC contribution to the total pool of circulating immunoreactive ACTH.[61]

Hypothalamic Peptides

Gonadotropin-Releasing Hormone

Both the cytotrophoblast and the syncytiotrophoblast synthesize and secrete GnRH, which has the same chemical structure and biologic activity as hypothalamic GnRH.[127, 129, 211–213] Although the GnRH mRNA levels in the placenta are similar throughout gestation, the highest concentrations of the peptide in the placenta and serum are found during the first trimester and correlate with the mass of the cytotrophoblast and peak hCG concentrations.[129, 214]

In vitro, GnRH production by placental explants or purified trophoblasts is stimulated by prostaglandins, epinephrine, activin, insulin, epidermal growth factor, VIP, estradiol, and estriol, and secretion is reduced by inhibin, progesterone, and κ-opiate and μ-opiate agonists.[133, 215, 216] The syncytiotrophoblast contains low-affinity GnRH receptors, whose concentrations parallel the hCG secretory pattern.[131, 217]

Because GnRH stimulates hCG secretion by placental explants and purified trophoblast cells in vitro, with the response of early to midtrimester placentas being greater than that of term trophoblast, it is reasonable to conclude that GnRH is an important autocrine or paracrine regulator of hCG secretion.[133, 215, 218] The hCG-stimulatory effect of GnRH can be blocked by administration of a GnRH antagonist.[128]

Corticotropin-Releasing Hormone

Both the cytotrophoblast and the syncytiotrophoblast synthesize and secrete a 41-amino-acid peptide that is identical to hypothalamic CRH.[56, 219, 220] CRH mRNA is first detected in trophoblast at 7 weeks of gestation. The levels remaining low during the first 30 weeks of pregnancy but rise 20-fold during the final 5 weeks, a pattern that is parallel to the rise of CRH content in the placenta and concentrations in maternal plasma.[220–225] In maternal plasma, CRH circulates bound to a 37-kd protein that is synthesized by the placenta, liver, and brain and that reduces the biologic activity of the CRH.[224–226]

In vitro, placental CRF production is stimulated by prostaglandins (E_2 and $F_{2\alpha}$), norepinephrine, acetylcholine, oxytocin, neuropeptide Y, AVP, angiotensin II, and interleukin-1.[133, 227, 228] Glucocorticoids have been shown to increase both CRH mRNA and peptide, whereas in the hypothalamus suppression is found.[60, 227] CRH secretion is reduced by progesterone and nitric oxide donors.[227, 229] The placenta contains CRH binding sites, and the addition of CRH to cultured placental cells results in a dose-dependent increase in hCC, β-endorphin, and α-melanocyte-stimulating hormone secretion.[208, 230] Thus, it is likely that CRH has an autocrine or paracrine effect in the placenta.

Whether CRH has a physiologic effect on the maternal pituitary secretion of ACTH is unclear; the circulating CRH may be biologically inactive because of the binding protein. However, just before parturition, the binding protein concentration decreases by approximately 50% and the CRH levels rise.[57, 226] At this time, CRH stimulates the synthesis and release of prostaglandins from the decidua, amnion, and chorion, which enhances cervical ripening.[231] The myometrium contains CRH receptors, and CRH may increase myometrial contractility.[232] Thus, CRH may have a role in initiating and promoting parturition.[57] CRH may also stimulate the fetal pituitary production of ACTH, which, in turn, may lead to increased fetal adrenal DHEA production and ultimately estriol synthesis by the fetoplacental unit.[219]

Other Peptides

A peptide with properties of TRH that is not identical to hypothalamic TRH has been identified in the placenta[233, 234] It is capable of stimulating the release of hTSH in vitro and in vivo.[211, 235] It has unknown physiologic significance because there is no convincing evidence that a chorionic thyrotropin exists, and hCG appears to be the major trophoblastic thyrotropin-like substance.

Immunoreactive somatostatin has been identified in the cytotrophoblast in first-trimester placentas.[236–238] The levels decrease as pregnancy advances.[236, 237] This pattern has led to the speculation that somatostatin inhibits hPL production and that the loss of inhibition allows the placenta to secrete increasing quantities of hPL.[237] The finding of somatostatin receptors in the placenta adds some indirect support to this hypothesis.[238] However, somatostatin does not inhibit hPL (or hGH-V) production by placental cells exposed to the peptide in vitro.[238]

A substance with GHRH-like activity has been found in the placenta.[239] However, because exposure of placental cells to hypothalamic GHRH does not result in stimulation of hPL or hGH-V secretion, it is unlikely that human placental GHRH is physiologically important.

Several other neuropeptides have been found in the placenta, usually through immunohistochemical techniques. These include methionine enkephalin,[240, 241] leucine enkephalin,[241] dynorphin,[241, 242] neuropeptide Y,[243] and oxytocin.[244] The physiologic functions of these placental peptides are unknown. It has been suggested that dynorphin may have a role in the paracrine regulation of hPL release through its binding to placental κ-opiate receptors.[241, 242] Neuropeptide Y and oxytocin stimulate the secretion of CRH from placental cells in culture.[133]

Growth Factors

Many growth factors, growth factor–binding proteins, and growth factor receptors have been identified in the placenta. These include IGF-I, IGF-II, relaxin, epidermal growth factor, PDGF, nerve growth factor, FGF, TGF-β, inhibin, activin, and folliculostatin.[50, 133, 160, 245] As reviewed earlier, a number of these factors have been implicated in the autocrine or paracrine regulation of placental hormone synthesis and release and placental angiogenesis, and they may have important actions in fetal development. In addition to the placenta, the human endometrium is a rich source of growth factors, cytokines, and vasoactive neuropeptides that are important for uteroplacental function.[9, 246]

References

1. Wilcox AJ, Weinberg CR, O'Connor JF, et al. Incidence of early loss of pregnancy. N Engl J Med 1988; 319:189.
2. Braunstein GD, Karow WG, Gentry WD, et al. Subclinical spontaneous abortion. Obstet Gynecol 1977; 50(1 Suppl):41s.
3. Norwitz ER, Schust DJ, Fisher JJ. Mechanisms of disease: implantation and the survival of early pregnancy. N Engl J Med 2001; 345:1400.
4. Enders AC. Trophoblast-uterine interactions in the first days of implantation: models for the study of implantation events in the human. Semin Reprod Med 2000; 18:255.
5. Braunstein GD, Grodin JM, Vaitukaitis J, et al. Secretory rates of human chorionic gonadotropin by normal trophoblast. Am J Obstet Gynecol 1973; 115:447.
6. Kimber SJ. Molecular interactions at the maternal-embryonic interface during the early phase of implantation. Semin Reprod Med 2000; 18:237.
7. Cross JC, Werb Z, Fisher SJ. Implantation and the placenta: key pieces of the development puzzle. Science 1994; 266:1508.
8. Greiss FC Jr, Anderson SG, Still JG. Uterine pressure-flow relationships during early gestation. Am J Obstet Gynecol 1976; 126: 799.
9. Tabibzadeh S. Human endometrium: an active site of cytokine production and action. Endocr Rev 1991; 12:272.
10. Armant DR, Wang J, Liu Z. Intracellular signaling in the developing blastocyst as a consequence of the maternal-embryonic dialogue. Semin Reprod Med 2000; 18:273.
11. Gordon JD, Shifren JL, Foulk RA, et al. Angiogenesis in the human female reproductive tract. Obstet Gynecol Surv 1995; 50: 688.
12. Usuki K, Norberg L, Larsson E, et al. Localization of platelet-derived endothelial cell growth factor in human placenta and purification of an alternatively processed form. Cell Regul 1990; 1:577.
13. Sharkey AM, Charnock-Jones DS, Boocock CA, et al. Expression of mRNA for vascular endothelial growth factor in human placenta. J Reprod Fertil 1993; 99:609.
14. Fisher DA. Endocrinology of fetal development. In Wilson JD, Foster DW, Kronengberg HM, Larsen PR (eds). Williams Textbook of Endocrinology. Philadelphia, WB Saunders, 1998, p 1273.
15. Siiteri PK, Febres F, Clemens LE, et al. Progesterone and maintenance of pregnancy: is progesterone nature's immunosuppressant? Ann NY Acad Sci 1977; 286:384.
16. Schmidt CM, Orr HT. Maternal/fetal interactions: the role of the MHC class I molecule HLA-G. Crit Rev Immunol 1993; 13: 207.
17. Braunstein GD, Rasor JL, Engvall E, et al. Interrelationships of human chorionic gonadotropin, human placental lactogen, and pregnancy-specific beta 1-glycoprotein throughout normal human gestation. Am J Obstet Gynecol 1980; 138:1205.
18. Hytten FE. Weight gain in pregnancy. In Hytten FE, Chamberlain G (eds). Clinical Physiology in Obstetrics. Oxford, Blackwell, 1991, p 173.
19. Edman CD, Toofanian A, MacDonald PC, et al. Placental clearance rate of maternal plasma androstenedione through placental estradiol formation: an indirect method of assessing uteroplacental blood flow. Am J Obstet Gynecol 1981; 141:1029.

119. Shozu M, Akasofu K, Harada T, et al. A new cause of female pseudohermaphroditism: placental aromatase deficiency. J Clin Endocrinol Metab 1991; 72:560.
120. Ren SG, Braunstein GD. Human chorionic gonadotropin. Semin Reprod Endocrinol 1992; 10:95.
121. Sturgeon CM, McAllister EJ. Analysis of hCG: clinical applications and assay requirements. Ann Clin Biochem 1998; 35:460.
122. Jameson JL, Hollenberg AN. Regulation of chorionic gonadotropin gene expression. Endocr Rev 1993; 14:203.
123. Muyan M, Boime I. Secretion of chorionic gonadotropin from human trophoblasts. Placenta 1997; 18:237.
124. Iles RK, Chard T. Molecular insights into the structure and function of human chorionic gonadotrophin. J Mol Endocrinol 1993; 10:217.
125. Braunstein GD, Rasor J, Danzer H, et al. Serum human chorionic gonadotropin levels throughout normal pregnancy. Am J Obstet Gynecol 1976; 126:678.
126. Ozturk M, Bellet D, Manil L, et al. Physiological studies of human chorionic gonadotropin (hCG), alpha hCG, and beta hCG as measured by specific monoclonal immunoradiometric assays. Endocrinology 1987; 120:549.
127. Khodr GS, Siler-Khodr TM. Placental luteinizing hormone–releasing factor and its synthesis. Science 1980; 207:315.
128. Siler-Khodr TM, Khodr GS, Vickery BH, et al. Inhibition of hCG, alpha hCG and progesterone release from human placental tissue in vitro by a GnRH antagonist. Life Sci 1983; 32:2741.
129. Miyake A, Sakumoto T, Aono T, et al. Changes in luteinizing hormone–releasing hormone in human placenta throughout pregnancy. Obstet Gynecol 1982; 60:444.
130. Siler-Khodr TM, Khodr GS, Valenzuela G. Immunoreactive gonadotropin-releasing hormone level in maternal circulation throughout pregnancy. Am J Obstet Gynecol 1984; 150:376.
131. Currie AJ, Fraser HM, Sharpe RM. Human placental receptors for luteinizing hormone releasing hormone. Biochem Biophys Res Commun 1981; 99:332.
132. Ringler GE, Strauss JF III. In vitro systems for the study of human placental endocrine function. Endocr Rev 1990; 11:105.
133. Petraglia F, Santuz M, Florio P, et al. Paracrine regulation of human placenta: control of hormonogenesis. J Reprod Immunol 1998; 39:221.
134. Masuhiro K, Matsuzaki N, Nishino E, et al. Trophoblast-derived interleukin-1 (IL-1) stimulates the release of human chorionic gonadotropin by activating IL-6 and IL-6-receptor system in first trimester human trophoblasts. J Clin Endocrinol Metab 1991; 72: 594.
135. Yuen BH, Moon YS, Shin DH. Inhibition of human chorionic gonadotropin production by prolactin from term human trophoblast. Am J Obstet Gynecol 1986; 154:336.
136. Ren SG, Braunstein GD. Decidua produces a protein that inhibits choriogonadotrophin release from human trophoblasts. J Clin Invest 1991; 87:326.
137. Menon KM, Jaffe RB. Chorionic gonadotropin sensitive adenylate cyclase in human term placenta. J Clin Endocrinol Metab 1973; 36:1104.
138. Shi QJ, Lei ZM, Rao CV, et al. Novel role of human chorionic gonadotropin in differentiation of human cytotrophoblasts. Endocrinology 1993; 132:1387.
139. Jameson JL, Jaffe RC, Gleason SL, et al. Transcriptional regulation of chorionic gonadotropin alpha- and beta-subunit gene expression by 8-bromo-adenosine 3′,5′-monophosphate. Endocrinology 1986; 119:2560.
140. Cemerikic-Jekic B, Pavlovic-Hournac M. Modification of protein kinase pattern in human placentae during gestation. Placenta 1984; 5:443.
141. Braunstein GD, Kamdar V, Rasor J, et al. Widespread distribution of a chorionic gonadotropin–like substance in normal human tissues. J Clin Endocrinol Metab 1979; 49:917.
142. Braunstein GD, Rasor J, McCready J, et al. Varying bioactive to immunoactive ratios of the human chorionic gonadotropin–like substance present in normal human tissues. J Clin Endocrinol Metab 1984; 58:170.
143. Odell WD, Griffin J, Sawitzke A. Chorionic gonadotropin secretion in normal, nonpregnant humans. Trends Endocrinol Metab 1990; 1:418.
144. McGregor WG, Kuhn RW, Jaffe RB. Biologically active chorionic gonadotropin: synthesis by the human fetus. Science 1983; 220:306.
145. Odell WD, Griffin J, Bashey HM, et al. Secretion of chorionic gonadotropin by cultured human pituitary cells. J Clin Endocrinol Metab 1990; 71:1318.
146. Hammond E, Griffin J, Odell WD. A chorionic gonadotropin–secreting human pituitary cell. J Clin Endocrinol Metab 1991; 72:747.
147. Borkowski A, Muquardt C. Human chorionic gonadotropin in the plasma of normal, nonpregnant subjects. N Engl J Med 1979; 301:298.
148. Odell WD, Griffin J. Pulsatile secretion of human chorionic gonadotropin in normal adults. N Engl J Med 1987; 317:1688.
149. Stenman UH, Alfthan H, Ranta T, et al. Serum levels of human chorionic gonadotropin in nonpregnant women and men are modulated by gonadotropin-releasing hormone and sex steroids. J Clin Endocrinol Metab 1987; 64:730.
150. Odell WD, Griffin J. Pulsatile secretion of chorionic gonadotropin during the normal menstrual cycle. J Clin Endocrinol Metab 1989; 69:528.
151. Braunstein GD. Placental proteins as tumor markers. In Herberman RB, Mercer DW (eds). Immunodiagnosis of Cancer. New York, Marcel Dekker, 1991, p 673.
152. Bidart JM, Bellet D. Human chorionic gonadotropin: molecular forms, detection, and clinical implications. Trends Endocrinol Metab 1993; 4:285.
153. Braunstein GD. Beta core fragment: structure, production, metabolism, and clinical utility. In Lustbader JW, Puett D, Ruddon RW (eds). Glycoprotein Hormones. New York, Springer-Verlag, 1994, p 293.
154. Kato Y, Braunstein GD. Beta-core fragment is a major form of immunoreactive urinary chorionic gonadotropin in human pregnancy. J Clin Endocrinol Metab 1988; 66:1197.
155. Hsueh AJW, La Polt PS. Molecular basis of gonadotropin receptor regulation. Trends Endocrinol Metab 1992; 3:164.
156. Yoshimi T, Strott CA, Marshall JR, et al. Corpus luteum function in early pregnancy. J Clin Endocrinol Metab 1969; 29:225.
157. Braunstein GD. Physiologic functions of human chorionic gonadotropin during pregnancy. In Mochizuki M, Hussa R (eds). Placental Protein Hormones. Amsterdam, Elsevier Science Publishers, 1988, p 33.
158. North RA, Whitehead R, Larkins RG. Stimulation by human chorionic gonadotropin of prostaglandin synthesis by early human placental tissue. J Clin Endocrinol Metab 1991; 73:60.
159. Nisula B, Bartocci A. Choriogonadotropin and immunity: a reevaluation. Ann Endocrinol 1984; 45:315.
160. Bryant-Greenwood GD, Schwabe C. Human relaxins: chemistry and biology. Endocr Rev 1994; 15:5.
161. Rodway MR, Rao CV. A novel perspective on the role of human chorionic gonadotropin during pregnancy and in the gestational trophoblastic disease. Early Pregnancy 1995; 1:176.
162. Schorge JO, Goldstein DP, Bernstein MR, Berkowitz RS. Recent advances in gestational trophoblastic disease. J Reprod Med 2000; 45: 692.
163. Chang Y-L, Chang T-C, Hsueh S, et al. Prognostic factors and treatment for placental site trophoblastic tumor—report of 3 cases and analysis of 88 cases. Gynecol Oncol 1999; 73:216.
164. Selenkow HA, Saxena BN, Dana CL. Measurement and pathophysiologic significance of human placental lactogen. In Pecile A, Finzi C (eds). The Feto-Placental Unit. Amsterdam, Excerpta Medica, 1969, p 340.
165. Hoshina M, Boothby M, Boime I. Cytological localization of chorionic gonadotropin alpha and placental lactogen mRNAs during development of the human placenta. J Cell Biol 1982; 93: 190.
166. Kaplan SL, Gurpide E, Sciarra JJ, et al. Metabolic clearance rate and production rate of chorionic growth hormone-prolactin in late pregnancy. J Clin Endocrinol Metab 1968; 28:1450.
167. Barrera-Saldana HA. Growth hormone and placental lactogen: biology, medicine and biotechnology. Gene 1998; 211:11.
168. Grumbach MM, Kaplan SL, Sciarra JJ, et al. Chorionic growth hormone-prolactin (CGP): secretion, disposition, biologic activity in man, and postulated function as the 'growth hormone' of the 2d half of pregnancy. Ann NY Acad Sci 1968; 148:501.
169. Ajabor LN, Yen SS. Effect of sustained hyperglycemia on the levels of human chorionic somatomammotropin in mid-pregnancy. Am J Obstet Gynecol 1972; 112:908.
170. Burt RL, Leake N, Rhyne L. Human placental lactogen and insulin blood glucose homeostasis. Obstet Gynecol 1970; 36:233.

171. Tyson JE, Austin KL, Farinholt JW. Prolonged nutritional deprivation in pregnancy: changes in human chorionic somatomammotropin and growth hormone secretion. Am J Obstet Gynecol 1971; 109:1080.
172. Kim YJ, Felig P. Plasma chorionic somatomammotropin levels during starvation in midpregnancy. J Clin Endocrinol Metab 1971; 32:864.
173. Spellacy WN, Buhi WC, Schram JD, et al. Control of human chorionic somatomammotropin levels during pregnancy. Obstet Gynecol 1971; 37:567.
174. Gaspard U, Sandront H, Luyckx A. Glucose-insulin interaction and the modulation of human placental lactogen (HPL) secretion during pregnancy. J Obstet Gynaecol Br Commonw 1974; 81: 201.
175. Morris HH, Vinik AI, Mulvihal M. Effects of acute alterations in maternal free fatty acid concentration on human chorionic somatomammotropin secretion. Am J Obstet Gynecol 1974; 119:224.
176. Ylikorkala O, Kauppila A. Effect of dexamethasone on serum levels of human placental lactogen during the last trimester of pregnancy. J Obstet Gynaecol Br Commonw 1974; 81:368.
177. Suwa S, Friesen H. Biosynthesis of human placental proteins and human placental lactogen (HPL) in vitro. II. Dynamic studies of normal term placentas. Endocrinology 1969; 85:1037.
178. Desole E, Springolo E, Dichiari F, et al. Human placental lactogen production in vitro 1. Dynamic studies of normal term placentas after stimulation with 17-beta-oestradiol. In Salvadori B (ed). Therapy of Feto-Placental Insufficiency. Berlin, Springer Verlag, 1973, p 313.
179. Niven PA, Buhi WC, Spellacy WN. The effect of intravenous oestrogen injections on plasma human placental lactogen levels. J Obstet Gynaecol Br Commonw 1974; 81:466.
180. Belleville F, Lasbennes A, Nabet P, et al. Study of compounds capable of intervening in the in vitro regulation of the secretion of chorionic somatomammotropin by placenta in culture. C R Seances Soc Biol Fil 1974; 168:1057.
181. Handwerger S, Barrett J, Tyrey L, et al. Differential effect of cyclic adenosine monophosphate on the secretion of human placental lactogen and human chorionic gonadotropin. J Clin Endocrinol Metab 1973; 36:1268.
182. Hershman JM, Kojima A, Friesen HG. Effect of thyrotropin-releasing hormone on human pituitary thyrotropin, prolactin, placental lactogen, and chorionic thyrotropin. J Clin Endocrinol Metab 1973; 36:497.
183. Wilson EA, Jawad MJ, Vernon MW. Effect of epidermal growth factor on hormone secretion by term placenta in organ culture. Am J Obstet Gynecol 1984; 149:579.
184. Petit A, Guillon G, Tence M, et al. Angiotensin II stimulates both inositol phosphate production and human placental lactogen release from human trophoblastic cells. J Clin Endocrinol Metab 1989; 69:280.
185. Bhaumick B, Dawson EP, Bala RM. The effects of insulin-like growth factor-I and insulin on placental lactogen production by human term placental explants. Biochem Biophys Res Commun 1987; 144:674.
186. Handwerger S, Quarfordt S, Barrett J, et al. Apolipoproteins AI, AII, and CI stimulate placental lactogen release from human placental tissue. A novel action of high density lipoprotein apolipoproteins. J Clin Invest 1987; 79:625.
187. Desoye G, Schweditsch MO, Pfeiffer KP, et al. Correlation of hormones with lipid and lipoprotein levels during normal pregnancy and postpartum. J Clin Endocrinol Metab 1987; 64:704.
188. Rosing U, Samsioe G, Olund A, et al. Serum levels of apolipoprotein A-I, A-II and HDL-cholesterol in second half of normal pregnancy and in pregnancy complicated by pre-eclampsia. Horm Metab Res 1989; 21:376.
189. Wu YQ, Jorgensen EV, Handwerger S. High density lipoproteins stimulate placental lactogen release and adenosine 3′,5′-monophosphate (cAMP) production in human trophoblast cells: evidence for cAMP as a second messenger in human placental lactogen release. Endocrinology 1988; 123:1879.
190. Lesniak MA, Gorden P, Roth J. Reactivity of non-primate growth hormones and prolactins with human growth hormone receptors on cultured human lymphocytes. J Clin Endocrinol Metab 1977; 44:838.
191. Arezzini C, De Gori V, Tarli P, Neri P. Weight increase of body and lymphatic tissues in dwarf mice treated with human chorionic somatomammotropin (HCS). Exp Biol Med 1972; 141: 98.
192. Kaplan SL, Grumbach MM. Studies of a human and simian placental hormone with growth hormone–like and prolactin-like activities. J Clin Endocrinol Metab 1964; 24:80.
193. Marakawa S, Raben MS. Effect of growth hormone and placental lactogen on DNA synthesis in rat costal cartilage and adipose tissue. Endocrinology 1968; 83:645.
194. Handwerger S, Freemark M. The roles of placental growth hormone and placental lactogen in the regulation of human fetal growth and development. J Ped Endocrinol Metab 2000; 13:343.
195. Martin JM, Friesen H. Effect of human placental lactogen on the isolated islets of Langerhans in vitro. Endocrinology 1969; 84: 619.
196. Sorenson RL, Brelje TC. Adaptation of islets of Langerhans to pregnancy: beta-cell growth, enhanced insulin secretion and the role of lactogenic hormones. Horm Metab Res 1997; 29:301.
197. Grumbach MM, Kaplan SL, Abrams CL, et al. Plasma free fatty acid response to the administration of chorionic 'growth hormone-prolactin.' J Clin Endocrinol Metab 1966; 26:478.
198. Nielsen PV, Pedersen H, Kampmann EM. Absence of human placental lactogen in an otherwise uneventful pregnancy. Am J Obstet Gynecol 1979; 135:322.
199. Sideri M, De Virgiliis G, Guidobono F, et al. Immunologically undetectable human placental lactogen in a normal pregnancy. Br J Obstet Gynaecol 1983; 90:771.
200. Parks JS, Nielsen PV, Sexton LA, et al. An effect of gene dosage on production of human chorionic somatomammotropin. J Clin Endocrinol Metab 1985; 60:994.
201. Mirlesse V, Frankenne F, Alsat E, et al. Placental growth hormone levels in normal pregnancy and in pregnancies with intrauterine growth retardation. Pediatr Res 1993; 34:39.
202. Caufriez A, Frankenne F, Englert Y, et al. Placental growth hormone as a potential regulator of maternal IGF-I during human pregnancy. Am J Physiol 1990; 258:E1014.
203. MacLeod JN, Worsley I, Ray J, et al. Human growth hormone-variant is a biologically active somatogen and lactogen. Endocrinology 1991; 128:1298.
204. Eriksson L, Frankenne F, Eden S, et al. Growth hormone 24-h serum profiles during pregnancy—lack of pulsatility for the secretion of the placental variant. Br J Obstet Gynaecol 1989; 96: 949.
205. Petraglia F, Florio P, Nappi C, et al. Peptide signaling in human placenta and membranes: autocrine, paracrine, and endocrine mechanisms. Endocr Rev 1996; 17:156.
206. Rees LH, Burke CW, Chard T, et al. Possible placental origin of ACTH in normal human pregnancy. Nature 1975; 254:620.
207. Odagiri E, Sherrell BJ, Mount CD, et al. Human placental immunoreactive corticotropin, lipotropin, and beta-endorphin: evidence for a common precursor. Proc Natl Acad Sci USA 1979; 76:2027.
208. Margioris AN, Grino M, Protos P, et al. Corticotropin-releasing hormone and oxytocin stimulate the release of placental proopiomelanocortin peptides. J Clin Endocrinol Metab 1988; 66:922.
209. Laatikainen T, Saijonmaa O, Salminen K, et al. Localization and concentrations of beta-endorphin and beta-lipotrophin in human placenta. Placenta 1987; 8:381.
210. Riley SC, Walton JC, Herlick JM, et al. The localization and distribution of corticotropin-releasing hormone in the human placenta and fetal membranes throughout gestation. J Clin Endocrinol Metab 1991; 72:1001.
211. Gibbons JM Jr, Mitnick M, Chieffo V. In vitro biosynthesis of TSH- and LH-releasing factors by the human placenta. Am J Obstet Gynecol 1975; 121:127.
212. Lee JN, Seppala M, Chard T. Characterization of placental luteinizing hormone–releasing factor–like material. Acta Endocrinol 1981; 96:394.
213. Kelly AC, Rodgers A, Dong KW, et al. Gonadotropin-releasing hormone and chorionic gonadotropin gene expression in human placental development. DNA Cell Biol 1991; 10:411.
214. Lin LS, Roberts VJ, Yen SS. Expression of human gonadotropin-releasing hormone receptor gene in the placenta and its functional relationship to human chorionic gonadotropin secretion. J Clin Endocrinol Metab 1995; 80:580.
215. Petraglia F, Lim AT, Vale W. Adenosine 3′,5′-monophosphate, prostaglandins, and epinephrine stimulate the secretion of immu-

noreactive gonadotropin-releasing hormone from cultured human placental cells. J Clin Endocrinol Metab 1987; 65:1020.
216. Petraglia F, Vaughan J, Vale W. Steroid hormones modulate the release of immunoreactive gonadotropin-releasing hormone from cultured human placental cells. J Clin Endocrinol Metab 1990; 70:1173.
217. Iwashita M, Evans MI, Catt KJ. Characterization of a gonadotropin-releasing hormone receptor site in term placenta and chorionic villi. J Clin Endocrinol Metab 1986; 62:127.
218. Butzow R. Luteinizing hormone releasing factor increases release of human chorionic gonadotropin in isolated cell columns of normal and malignant trophoblasts. Int J Cancer 1985; 29:9.
219. Majzoub JA, Karalis KP. Placental corticotropin-releasing hormone: function and regulation. Am J Obstet Gynecol 1999; 180: S242.
220. Reis FM, Fadalti M, Florio P, et al. Putative role of placental corticotropin-releasing factor in the mechanisms of human parturition. J Soc Gynecol Invest 1999; 6:109.
221. Shibasaki T, Odagiri E, Shizume K, et al. Corticotropin-releasing factor–like activity in human placental extracts. J Clin Endocrinol Metab 1982; 55:384.
222. Sasaki A, Liotta AS, Luckey MM, et al. Immunoreactive corticotropin-releasing factor is present in human maternal plasma during the third trimester of pregnancy. J Clin Endocrinol Metab 1984; 59:812.
223. Laatikainen T, Virtanen T, Raisanen I, et al. Immunoreactive corticotropin-releasing factor and corticotropin during pregnancy, labor and puerperium. Neuropeptides 1987; 10:343.
224. Mastorakos G, Ilias I. Maternal hypothalamic-pituitary-adrenal axis in pregnancy and the postpartum period. Ann NY Acad Sci 2000; 900:95.
225. Saeed BO, Weightman DR, Self CH. Characterization of corticotropin-releasing hormone binding sites in the human placenta. J Recept Signal Transduct Res 1997; 17:647.
226. Petraglia F, Florio P, Gallo R, et al. Corticotropin-releasing factor–binding protein: origins and possible functions. Horm Res 1996; 45:187.
227. Petraglia F, Sutton S, Vale W. Neurotransmitters and peptides modulate the release of immunoreactive corticotropin-releasing factor from cultured human placental cells. Am Obstet Gynecol 1989; 160:247.
228. Florio P, Lombardo M, Gallo R, et al. Activin A, corticotropin-releasing factor and prostaglandin F2 alpha increase immunoreactive oxytocin release from cultured human placental cells. Placenta 1996; 17:307.
229. Ni X, Chan EC, Fitter JT, et al. Nitric oxide inhibits corticotropin-releasing hormone exocytosis but not synthesis by cultured human trophoblasts. J Clin Endocrinol Metab 1997; 82:4171.
230. Petraglia F, Giardino L, Coukos G, et al. Corticotropin-releasing factor and parturition: plasma and amniotic fluid levels and placental binding sites. Obstet Gynecol 1990; 75:784.
231. Jones SA, Challis JR. Local stimulation of prostaglandin production by corticotropin-releasing hormone in human fetal membranes and placenta. Biochem Biophys Res Commun 1989; 159: 192.
232. Majzoub JA, McGregor JA, Lockwood CJ, et al. A central theory of preterm and term labor: putative role for corticotropin-releasing hormone. Am J Obstet Gynecol 1999; 180(Suppl):232.
233. Youngblood WW, Humm J, Lipton MA, et al. Thyrotropin-releasing hormone–like bioactivity in placenta: evidence for the existence of substances other than Pyroglu-His-Pro-NH2 (TRH) capable of stimulating pituitary thyrotropin release. Endocrinology 1980; 106:541.
234. Bajoria R, Babawale M. Ontogeny of endogenous secretion of immunoreactive-thyrotropin releasing hormone by the human placenta. J Clin Endocrinol Metab 1998; 83:4148.
235. Shambaugh G III, Kubek M, Wilber JF. Thyrotropin-releasing hormone activity in the human placenta. J Clin Endocrinol Metab 1979; 48:483.
236. Kumasaka T, Nishi N, Yaoi Y, et al. Demonstration of immunoreactive somatostatin-like substance in villi and decidua in early pregnancy. Am J Obstet Gynecol 1979; 134:39.
237. Watkins WB, Yen SS. Somatostatin in cytotrophoblast of the immature human placenta: localization by immunoperoxidase cytochemistry. J Clin Endocrinol Metab 1980; 50:969.
238. Caron P, Buscail L, Beckers A, et al. Expression of somatostatin receptor SST4 in human placenta and absence of octreotide effect on human placental growth hormone concentration during pregnancy. J Clin Endocrinol Metab 1997; 82:3771.
239. Berry SA, Srivastava CH, Rubin LR, et al. Growth hormone–releasing hormone–like messenger ribonucleic acid and immunoreactive peptide are present in human testis and placenta. J Clin Endocrinol Metab 1992; 75:281.
240. Sastry BV, Barnwell SL, Tayeb OS, et al. Occurrence of methionine enkephalin in human placental villus. Biochem Pharmacol 1980; 29:475.
241. Ahmed MS, Cemerikie B, Agbas A. Properties and functions of human placental opioid system. Life Sci 1992; 50:83.
242. Lemaire S, Valette A, Chouinard L. Purification and identification of multiple forms of dynorphin in human placenta. Neuropeptides 1983; 3:181.
243. Petraglia F, Calza L, Giardino L, et al. Identification of immunoreactive neuropeptide-gamma in human placenta: localization, secretion, and binding sites. Endocrinology 1989; 124:2016.
244. Fields PA, Eldridge RK, Fuchs AR, et al. Human placental and bovine corpora luteal oxytocin. Endocrinology 1983; 112:1544.
245. Prager D, Weber MM, Herman-Bonert V. Placental growth factors and releasing/inhibiting peptides. Semin Reprod Endocrinol 1992; 10:83.
246. Graf AH, Hutter W, Hacker GW, et al. Localization and distribution of vasoactive neuropeptides n the human placenta. Placenta 1996; 17:413.

21 Endocrinology of Fetal Development

Delbert A. Fisher

The unfolding of our understanding of mammalian pregnancy and fetal development represents one of the dramatic chapters of scientific progress during the past half-century, but we are only beginning to understand the complex genetic, growth factor, and hormonal interactions involved in implantation, placentation, embryonic and fetal development, parturition, and fetal adaptation to extrauterine life. An array of homeobox genes program embryogenesis and fetal development in concert with autocrine, paracrine, and endocrine networks of chemicals, hormones, and growth factors that provide the cellular communication coordinating maternal-placental-fetal interactions and fetal maturation. An important concept that has emerged is that the fetal-placental endocrine milieu is unique and the insights from studies of endocrine and growth factor systems of mature species are not directly applicable to the fetal environment.

Unique features of the placental-fetal endocrine environment (Table 21–1) include the growing spectrum of placental hormones and growth factors and a variety of transient fetal endocrine adaptations to the intrauterine environment. The fetal adrenal cortex, the para-aortic chromaffin system including the paired organs of Zuckerkandl, and the intermediate lobe of the pituitary are prominent among these. Vasotocin, the parent neurohypophyseal hormone in submammalian species, is expressed transiently during fetal life, and calcitonin, a largely vestigial hormone in adult mammals, plays a significant role in fetal calcium and bone metabolism.

In addition, the active adrenal glucocorticoid, cortisol, and the major thyroid hormone, thyroxine (T_4), are largely inactive during much of fetal life because of the preferential synthesis of inactive moieties. Hormones and growth factors that play prominent roles in the fetus include catecholamines, parathyroid hormone–related protein (PTHrP), antimüllerian hormone, insulin-like growth factor II (IGF-II), transforming growth factor α (TGF-α), and the neuroregulins. In the perinatal period, cortisol serves to modulate the functional adaptations requisite for extrauterine survival. In addition, hormonal imprinting during the fetal-perinatal period conditions the adult functional characteristics of selected endocrine systems.

This chapter reviews the current status of our understanding of the fetal-placental endocrine and growth factor milieu, maturation of the fetal endocrine systems, and adaptations of the fetal endocrine system to extrauterine life.

PLACENTA

The fetal milieu depends on a functioning placenta, which develops in parallel with the fertilized ovum.[1-5] By 6 to 7 days after conception, the blastocyst consists of an outer layer of trophoblast cells and an inner cell mass destined to become the embryo. The trophoblast cells have implanted in the endometrium and within 10 days have developed two distinct layers, an inner cytotrophoblast layer and an outer layer of continuous cytoplasm, the syncytiotrophoblast, which forms the early fetal-maternal interface. Pockets of cytotrophoblast cells in the mature placenta serve as a reservoir of stem cells for continuing syncytiotrophoblast development.

The predominantly syncytiotrophoblastic placenta grows progressively throughout gestation. As the placenta develops, the chorionic villi containing the fetal capillaries extend into the maternal lakes of blood within the maternal decidua. Within the villi three layers of fetal tissue separate the fetal circulation from the maternal circulation: the cytotrophoblast-syncytiotrophoblast layer, the fetal mesenchyme layer of extraembryonic connective tissue, and the fetal capillary endothelium. The syncytiotrophoblast is the major site of diffusion between the maternal lakes of blood in the placenta and the fetal capillaries (Fig. 21–1).

Table 21–1. Features of the Fetal Endocrine Environment

Placental Hormone Production
Estrogens
Progesterone
Polypeptide hormones
Neuropeptides
Growth factors
Unique Fetal Endocrine Systems
Fetal adrenal cortex
Para-aortic chromaffin system
Intermediate lobe of the pituitary
Prominent Fetal Hormones or Metabolites
Vasotocin
Calcitonin
Cortisone
Reverse triiodothyronine (rT_3)
Sulfated iodothyronines
Ectopic neuropeptides
Fetal Endocrine System Adaptations
Adrenal-placental interactions
Testicular control of male phenotypic differentiation
Developmentally regulated growth factor control of fetal growth
Neuropeptides and fetal water metabolism
Parathyroid glands and placental calcium transport
Catecholamine and vasopressin responses to hypoxia
Cortisol programming for extrauterine exposure
Catecholamine and cortisol control of extrauterine adaptation
Perinatal hormonal imprinting

Placental Hormone Transfer

The placenta regulates maternal-fetal molecular exchange, and thin areas of the syncytiotrophoblast adjacent to the fetal capillaries seem to be specialized for this function (see Fig. 21–1).[1, 5, 6] However, the fetal endocrine milieu is largely independent of maternal hormones because the placenta is impermeable to most peptide hormones.

There are two major routes for the transfer of molecules across the placenta: an *extracellular* route through fluid-filled intercellular channels and a *transcellular* route. The rate of extracellular diffusion is related to the luminal diameter of the intercellular or paracellular channels and to the molecular weight (molecular radius or size) and lipid solubility or hydrophilicity of the transferred molecule. The placenta is more permeable to lipid-soluble molecules, and the permeability for both lipid-soluble and lipid-insoluble molecules decreases with increasing molecular weight.[6, 7] The transfer or diffusion of L-glucose is believed to be accomplished by extracellular diffusion.

The placental transfer of a number of hormones is summarized in Table 21–2.[1, 8] The differences in placental structure among species have a limited influence on placental hormone transfer, and data derived from some animal and primate species are included. Hormones larger than 0.7 to 1.2 kd have little or no access to the fetal compartment. The exception is immunoglobulin G, which is actively transported from mother to fetus during the latter half of gestation.[9]

Placental cell membranes contain a variety of receptors for polypeptide hormones and growth factors, including insulin, the IGFs, and epidermal growth factor (EGF).[10, 11] These receptors bind and in some instances degrade their respective ligands but do not facilitate placental transfer.

Hormones that traverse the placenta by the transcellular route and are metabolized en route include cortisol, estradiol, thyroid hormones, and catecholamines.[12–16] The placental cells contain an active 11β-hydroxysteroid dehydrogenase (11β–HSD) that catalyzes the conversion of most of the cortisol to inactive cortisone.[13, 15] Placental 17β-hydroxysteroid dehydrogenase is considered to prevent passage of excessive estrogens to the fetus by catalyzing inactivation of estradiol to estrone.[15] Placental tissue also contains an iodothyronine inner ring monodeiodinase, which deiodinates most of the T_4 to inactive reverse triiodothyronine (rT_3) and converts active 3,5,3′-triio-

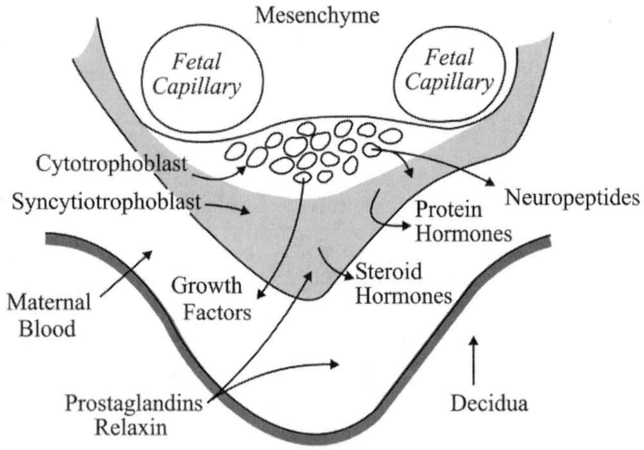

Figure 21–1. Diagrammatic representation of a chorionic villus extending into the maternal blood lake and showing fetal capillaries in the fetal mesenchyme. The villus is sheathed by the syncytiotrophoblast. The residual sparse areas of cytotrophoblast provide cells to renew and maintain the syncytiotrophoblast layer. The villus is surrounded by maternal blood in the maternal intervillous space. The placenta serves as an important endocrine organ. Hormones are produced by cytotrophoblast and syncytiotrophoblast cells. Neuropeptides appear to modulate syncytiotrophoblast production of placental protein hormones, and decidual prostaglandins and cytotrophoblast growth factors may participate in regulation of syncytiotrophoblast steroid hormone production. See text for details.

Table 21–2. Placental Transfer of Hormones

Hormone	Approximate Molecular Size (daltons)	Placental Transfer
Catecholamine	180	Yes
Melatonin	230	Yes
Steroid hormones	350	Yes
Vitamin D	350	Yes
Thyrotropin-releasing hormone (TRH)	360	Yes
Thyroid hormones	800	Limited
Oxytocin (OT)	1,000	No
Vasopressin	1,100	No
Luteinizing hormone–releasing hormone (LHRH)	1,200	Yes
Atrial natriuretic hormone	3,080	No
Calcitonin (CT)	3,400	No
Glucagon	3,600	No
Corticotropin	4,500	No
Corticotropin-releasing hormone (CRH)	4,800	No
Insulin	6,000	No
Parathyroid hormone (PTH)	9,000	No
Growth hormone (GH)	22,000	No
Thyrotropin	27,000	No
Luteinizing hormone (LH)	30,000	No
Erythropoietin	30,400	No
Renin	40,000	No

dothyronine (T_3) to inactive diiodothyronine.[14, 17] Catecholamine-degrading enzymes in placental tissue include both monoamine oxidase and catechol *O*-methyltransferase,[12, 18] and both metanephrine and dihydroxymandelic acid metabolites of catecholamines are present in placental homogenates.

Placental Hormone Production

The placenta functions as a major endocrine organ, providing a secondary source of hypothalamic, pituitary, adrenal, and gonadal hormones and growth factors (Table 21–3).[1, 5, 8, 19] The syncytiotrophoblast manufactures steroid and protein hormones; after the eighth week of pregnancy, it is the most active fetal or maternal endocrine organ. The steroid hormones are produced from both fetal and maternal substrates. The protein hormones are synthesized in the rough endoplasmic reticulum of the syncytiotrophoblast from amino acids of maternal origin. Secretion is predominantly into the maternal circulation, but significant amounts reach the fetal compartment. The cytotrophoblast produces a variety of neuropeptides and growth factors, and decidual tissue is a major source of prostaglandins and relaxin.

The network of peptides expressed by the placenta provides an autocrine-paracrine system regulating the fetal-maternal unit.[1, 5, 19] Local placental control systems resemble a miniature hypothalamic–pituitary–target organ network. Maternal and fetal hormones in the placental circulation may also regulate placental hormone production.[1, 5, 19] In addition to the local effects, a number of placental hormones are involved in modulation of maternal and fetal homeostasis during pregnancy (see Fig. 21–1).

Placental Estrogen

The human placenta near term secretes large amounts of estrogens, including estrone, estradiol, and estriol.[5, 20, 21] Excretion rates of these steroids during the latter third of pregnancy are approximately 2, 1, and 30 to 40 mg/day, respectively, whereas total estrogen production in nonpregnant women is less than 1 mg/day. This production is due to the combined effects of the fetal adrenal gland and the placenta, first characterized by Diczfalusy[22] as the human fetoplacental unit. Most of the estrogen is secreted into the maternal circulation, but fetal concentrations and levels in amniotic fluid are high.

The major substrates for placental estrogen synthesis are dehydroepiandrosterone (DHEA) and androstenedione. These relatively inactive adrenal steroids are derived from both fetal and maternal adrenal glands. The fetal zone of the adrenal cortex is deficient in an enzyme with 3β-hydroxysteroid dehydrogenase (3β–HSD) and $\Delta^{4,5}$ isomerase activities but has high steroid sulfokinase activity.[20, 23] Thus, the conversion of pregnenolone to progesterone is limited and the major product of fetal adrenal steroidogenesis is DHEA sulfate (DHEAS), which is transported to the liver for 16-hydroxylation. DHEAS and 16-hydroxy-DHEAS are hydrolyzed in the placenta by steroid sulfatase and converted to androstenedione and 16-hydroxyandrostenedione, respectively. Androstenedione in turn is a substrate for placental estrone biosynthesis; 16-hydroxyandrostenedione is the major substrate for placental estriol synthesis.

The features of the fetoplacental unit are summarized in Figure 21–2. The rate of placental estrogen biosynthesis is a function of placental mass and the amount of C_{19}-steroid production by the fetal adrenal gland.

Estrogens, acting through a factor or factors other than the level of progesterone, play a critical role in the maintenance of primate pregnancy.[21, 24] They support placental progesterone synthesis by stimulating placental low-density lipoprotein (LDL) cholesterol uptake and cholesterol side-chain cleavage enzyme (CYP11A1) activity. Estrogens also augment maternal

Table 21–3. Hormones and Growth Factors Produced by the Placenta

Cytotrophoblast	Syncytiotrophoblast
Corticotropin-releasing hormone (CRH)	*Estrogens*
Growth hormone-releasing hormone (GRH)	Estradiol
Gonadotropin-releasing hormone (GnRH)	Estriol
Thyrotropin-releasing hormone (TRH)	Estrone
Somatostatin (SRIF)	Progesterone
Inhibin	Placental growth hormone
Activin	Chorionic gonadotropin
Neuropeptide Y	Chorionic somatomammotropin
Enkephalins	CRH
Dynorphin	Leptin
Atrial natriuretic hormone	Urocortin
Parathyroid hormone–related protein (PTHrP)	***Decidua***
Leptin	Prolactins
Vascular endothelial growth Factor (VEGF)	Relaxin
Insulin-like growth factor I (IGF-I)	Prostaglandins
IGF-II	Renin
Erythropoietin	IGF binding protein
Renin	
Relaxin	

SRIF, somatotropin release-inhibiting factor.

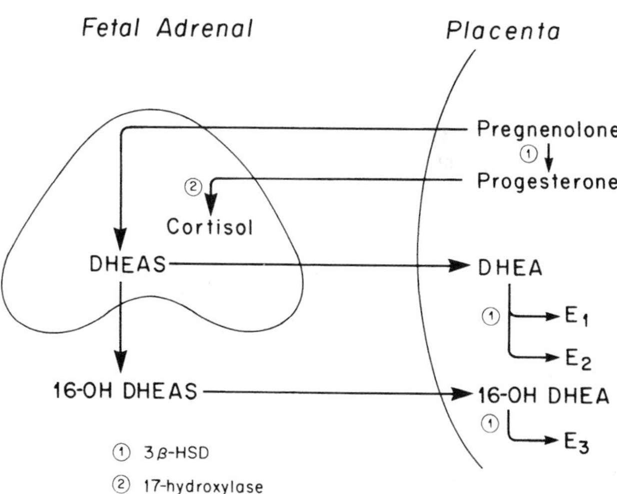

Figure 21–2. Diagrammatic representation of the fetoplacental unit composed of the fetal adrenal cortex and the placenta. The placenta is deficient in 17-hydroxylase activity and cannot synthesize estrogens from progesterone. The fetal adrenal cortex has low 3β–hydroxysteroid dehydrogenase (3β–HSD) and $\Delta^{4,5}$ isomerase activity and cannot synthesize progesterone. Sulfokinase activity is high in fetal adrenal tissue, and steroid sulfatase activity is high in placental tissue. Thus, the placenta produces progesterone, which is predominantly converted to dehydroepiandrosterone (DHEA) by the fetal adrenal cortex; the DHEA can be sulfated to form DHEA sulfate (DHEAS). Part of this is 16-hydroxylated by the fetal liver, and both DHEA and DHEAS are used by the placenta as substrates for estrone (E_1) and estradiol (E_2) synthesis, respectively. Placental sulfatase converts DHEAS and 16-hydroxy-DHEAS to DHEA and 17-hydroxy-DHEA. The 16-hydroxy-DHEA is used for estriol (E_3) synthesis. See text and references for details.

blood volume and uteroplacental blood flow, promote uterine growth and placental neovascularization, stimulate production of albumin and globulins in the maternal liver, and promote mammary growth.[21] In conditions associated with decreased placental estrogen production (placental sulfatase deficiency, placental aromatase deficiency, fetal anencephaly), both estrogen production and estrogen levels may be reduced 80% to 90% but placental progesterone production and fetal development are normal.[21] Thus, in normal pregnancy there is a considerable excess of estrogen production relative to the levels necessary for estrogen receptor–mediated effects.

Placental Progesterone

During normal pregnancy, there is a marked and progressive increase in progesterone production. The maternal corpus luteum is the major source of plasma progesterone during the first 5 to 6 weeks of gestation; after 12 weeks, the placenta is the major source.[5, 20, 23] The principal substrate for placental progesterone synthesis is circulating maternal LDL and very-low-density lipoprotein (VLDL) cholesterol; de novo placental synthesis of cholesterol from acetate is limited. Placental progesterone production is largely independent of the maternal pituitary or adrenal glands, and fetal death in utero has little acute effect on maternal progesterone levels. Progesterone production is regulated by the number of LDL receptors and thus placental mass.

The major factor in control of placental progesterone production appears to be the expression of steroidogenic enzymes, including CYP11A1 and 3β–HSD, in cytotrophoblast cells.[25] The type I 3β–HSD enzyme is expressed in placenta, whereas type II activity is expressed in adrenal and gonadal tissues. Expression of messenger ribonucleic acid (mRNA) for all the placental steroidogenic enzymes is stimulated by cyclic adenosine monophosphate (cAMP), which appears to be produced constitutively in mature cytotrophoblast cells. There is some evidence that endogenous steroids may modulate placental progesterone production.

The production of progesterone is approximately 200 mg/day during the third trimester, a value some 10-fold higher than that during the midluteal phase of the normal menstrual cycle; 90% of this amount is secreted into the maternal circulation.[20, 25] Progesterone acts on the uterine musculature to maintain a state of quiescence and inhibits maternal cell-mediated immune responses to foreign (fetal) antigens. Despite the predominant secretion of progesterone into the maternal circulation, fetal blood progesterone levels are twofold to threefold higher than maternal values because of lower metabolic clearance of progesterone by the fetus.[20] The significance of this progesterone to the fetus is not clear.

Placental Polypeptide Hormone

The placenta produces several pituitary-like hormones. The most abundant are human chorionic gonadotropin (hCG) and human placental lactogen (hPL), also called human chorionic somatomammotropin.[5, 26] hCG is a glycoprotein of 36 to 40 kd with structural, biologic, and immunologic similarities to the pituitary gonadotropins and thyrotropin (also called thyroid-stimulating hormone [TSH]); hCG also has weak thyrotropic hormone–like activity. hPL is a 191-amino-acid protein with 96% homology to human growth hormone (hGH). It has 3% or less of the growth-promoting bioactivity of hGH and equivalent prolactin (PRL)-like effects. hCG is secreted predominantly during the first half of gestation, and hPL is secreted mainly during the second half.

The control of the synthesis and secretion of these placental hormones is not well understood,[26] but hormone secretion is related to placental mass and continues in the absence of the fetus. Luteinizing hormone–releasing hormone (LHRH, also called chorionic gonadotropin-releasing hormone), EGF, activin, and hCG increase hCG synthesis in placental tissue in vitro, whereas inhibin and progesterone suppress synthesis.[25, 26]

It is likely that hCG plays a role in the maintenance of the corpus luteum early in pregnancy as well as stimulation of the fetal testes and stimulation of placental progesterone production.[25, 26] hCG has weak thyrotropin-like activity; there is less than 0.5 mU of thyrotropin per unit of hCG, and hCG produces minimal, but sometimes significant, thyroidal hyperactivity and hyperthyroidism during normal pregnancy.[27] hPL has weak hGH-like and PRL-like bioactivities and may exert an anti-insulin effect on maternal carbohydrate and lipid metabolism, thereby increasing maternal glucose and amino acid levels and augmenting maternal-to-fetal substrate flow.[25] In addition, hPL appears to be an important stimulus of fetal growth.

The same gene is responsible for the β subunit expressed in the placenta for hCG and in the pituitary for production of luteinizing hormone (LH), follicle-stimulating hormone (FSH), and thyrotropin.[28] There is also a single gene for the β subunit of LH, whereas there are seven genes or pseudogenes, or both, for the hCG β subunit. These hCG and LH β genes have similar structures, and it appears that the hCG gene arose from the LH β gene and that the hCG β gene family is early in the process of evolution of pseudogenes.[27, 29]

The PRL, hGH, and hPL genes are also closely related.[25, 30, 31] The PRL gene is presumed to be the ancestral gene; hGH evolved nearly 400 million years ago, whereas hPL evolved within the last 10 million years. The hGH gene cluster includes five similar gene loci, two for hGH and three for hPL; these loci have 93% sequence homology in mRNA and probably evolved by repeated duplication over time.[25, 31] Only two of the hPL sequences are expressed in the placenta, and they produce identical hPL molecules. Placental tissue also expresses pituitary PRL and one of the hGH genes *(hGHV)*, and placental hGH may contribute to the maternal hGH-like effects mediated by somatomedins during pregnancy.[32, 33]

The human placenta synthesizes a pro-opiomelanocortin (POMC) and contains the POMC-derived peptides corticotropin (adrenocorticotropic hormone [ACTH] or adrenocorticotropin), α–lipotropin and β-lipotropin, β-endorphin, α-melanocyte-stimulating hormone (α–MSH), and three forms of endorphin.[5, 25] Corticotropin-releasing hormone (CRH) is also produced by the placenta, and CRH stimulates corticotropin production from perfused human placental fragments, suggesting a possible paracrine role for placental CRH in modulating corticotropin production in the placenta.[34] Glucocorticoids, however, have no effect on placental CRH or corticotropin release, and oxytocin (OT) stimulates placental POMC release but has no effect on pituitary release of corticotropin.[35]

Compared with corticotropin, β-endorphin and α-MSH are released from placenta in larger amounts. Thus, control and processing of placental POMC are different than in the anterior pituitary.[34] The increased plasma levels of POMC-derived peptides in pregnant women and the resistance of maternal plasma corticotropin to glucocorticoid suppression in pregnancy suggest that the placenta may be involved in regulation of the maternal pituitary-adrenal axis during pregnancy.[5]

Inhibin and activin are produced by placental tissue.[36, 37] The mRNAs for inhibin subunits (α, β_A, and β_B) are present in the placenta, and inhibin A ($\alpha\beta_A$) and activin A ($\beta_A\beta_A$) are produced throughout pregnancy. Inhibin and activin A levels in maternal serum increase progressively during pregnancy and decrease rapidly after delivery. Immunoreactive and bioactive inhibins are also present in umbilical cord serum and amniotic fluid; umbilical artery and vein concentrations are similar and lower than maternal values.

Activin A is present in cord serum only at term, whereas activin B is present in fetal blood and amniotic fluid before birth; activin B is largely absent from maternal serum. The role of these hormones during pregnancy is not clear. Inhibin production in placenta is stimulated by hCG, FSH, EGF, and prostaglandins. Inhibin suppresses hCG production, whereas activin can stimulate growth hormone–releasing hormone (GHRH), LHRH, progesterone, and prostaglandin production by placental cells in culture.[36, 38] A paracrine role for these hormones in the placenta is suggested.

Renin activity is present in homogenates and in cultured explants of placenta and has been localized in chorionic tissue by immunohistochemical assay.[39] The amino acid composition and NH_2-terminal sequence of chorionic renin are identical to those of kidney renin. Renin mRNA is present in the chorion throughout pregnancy; no mRNA has been detected in decidua, amnion, or myometrium. Placental renin mRNA concentrations at term are about 10% of kidney levels, and the total placental renin mRNA level is approximately 20% of the kidney content. Angiotensinogen mRNA is restricted to the spiral arteries and has not been detected in placental tissue.[39]

Functional angiotensin II receptors (AT_2) are present in skeletal muscle and connective tissue of the rat embryo in late gestation.[40] In fetal skin fibroblasts, these receptors are coupled to membrane phospholipid turnover and mediate increases in cellular inositol phosphate and cytosolic calcium concentrations. Moreover, injection of angiotensin II into 18-day-old rat fetuses increased amino acid incorporation into skin protein.[40] These observations suggest a role for angiotensin II in fetal growth, and placental renin may play a role in the production of fetal angiotensin II.

The placenta produces a parathyroid hormone (PTH)–like bioactivity that is similar in composition to the PTHrP produced by tumors associated with hypercalcemia.[41–43] The PTHrP-PTH receptor is also widely expressed in the human ureteroplacental unit. Localization of the receptor in smooth muscle reflects the ability of PTHrP to relax both uterine and vascular smooth muscle.[41] PTHrP regulates placental calcium transport in sheep, and targeted disruption of the PTHrP gene in mice results in skeletal malformations and perinatal death.[41, 44] Calcitonin mRNA and a calcitonin-like immunoreactivity are also present in the rat placenta.[45] The significance of these proteins is discussed later under the heading "Parathyroid Hormone/Calcitonin System."

Leptin, a 167-amino-acid protein secreted from adipose tissue, is also produced by the placenta.[46–49] Leptin protein was demonstrated in the cytoplasm of syncytiotrophoblast cells as well as amnion cells and is widely distributed in murine fetal tissues. Serum leptin levels are relatively high in cord blood and show a significant correlation with adiposity at birth.[49] A role for leptin in fetal growth has been postulated.[46]

Placental Neuropeptide

The human placenta contains and produces LHRH, thyrotropin-releasing hormone (TRH), somatostatin (also called somatotropin release–inhibiting factor), CRH, and GHRH.[1, 5, 19] LHRH is produced in the cytotrophoblast and can bind to receptors in the syncytiotrophoblast. Because synthetic LHRH increases in vitro production of hCG and perhaps of progesterone, estrone, estradiol, and estriol from placental explants, endogenous chorionic LHRH may have a paracrine role in the regulation of placental hCG and steroid hormone production.

Placental TRH immunoreactivity and chromatographic characteristics are similar to those of synthetic TRH, and bioactivity has been demonstrated.[5, 8, 19] Sheep placental TRH levels vary with the thyroid status of the fetus, increasing with hypothyroidism and decreasing after administration of T_3 to the fetus.[50] These data suggest that regulation of placental *TRH* gene transcription resembles that of hypothalamic TRH.

Immunoreactive chorionic somatostatin, like LHRH, is localized in the cytotrophoblast.[5, 8, 19] The finding that the somatostatin-containing cells in the placenta disappear as pregnancy progresses and that hPL production increases progressively during the second half of gestation led to the speculation that chorionic somatostatin may exert negative paracrine control on the production of hPL by the syncytiotrophoblast.

Immunoreactive CRH has been identified in human and sheep placental extracts and in third-trimester plasma.[1, 5, 19] It is not detected in plasma of pregnant women during the first or second trimesters and disappears post partum. CRH mRNA is present in full-term human placental tissue, and immunoreactive CRH, with chromatographic characteristics similar to those of synthetic CRH, is produced by placental fragments in vitro. The lack of correlation of maternal plasma corticotropin or cortisol and CRH levels has suggested that placental CRH is not primarily involved in maternal pituitary corticotropin regulation. However, maternal plasma CRH levels correlate with gestational age, which suggests a relationship to placental function. Moreover, studies in the baboon, which resembles the human with regard to CRH metabolism during pregnancy, have shown a blunted maternal pituitary corticotropin response to CRH after CRH infusion.[51] These studies support a role of placental CRH in modulating maternal pituitary and adrenal function during pregnancy.

In contrast to the negative-feedback effect of glucocorticoid on hypothalamic CRH production, glucocorticoid stimulates placental CRH mRNA and CRH production.[52, 53] This observation and the parallel increases in placental CRH and CRH mRNA concentrations during the last 5 weeks of pregnancy suggest that the increase in fetal glucocorticoid production near term may stimulate placental CRH and POMC production and may further augment prenatal fetal cortisol production and parturition.[5, 51]

Immunoreactive GHRH and biologically active GHRH are present in rat placenta.[54] Two forms of GHRH activity were identified by high-performance liquid chromatography, one eluting identically with synthetic GHRH and one similar to the methionine sulfoxide analogue. By analogy with other placental releasing factors, chorionic GHRH may be involved in paracrine control of hPL or placental hGH production. Plasma GHRH levels, like CRH concentrations, are elevated during the third trimester of human gestation, correlate with gestational age and hPL concentrations, and become undetectable 3 days post partum.[55] A relationship to placental function seems likely.

The placenta also produces a variety of neurotransmitter and transcription factor molecules that may have roles in the regulation of placental neuropeptide and polypeptide hormone secretion. These include catecholamines, prostaglandins, pituitary factor-1 (Pit-1), and neuropeptide Y.[5, 55, 56] Neuropeptide Y stimulates CRH production, and Pit1 stimulates hPL and hGH gene transcription in placental tissue in vitro.[56, 57] Prostaglandins and catecholamines stimulate CRH and LHRH secretion in vitro.[5, 53, 58]

Placental Growth Factor

Human placental tissue contains both IGF-I and IGF-II mRNA species,[59, 60] and translation of placental RNA in vitro results in the production of a 14-kd protein that is immunoprecipitable with IGF-I antiserum.[58] Term placental explants also produce a 24-kd immunoprecipitable IGF-I–like protein.[58] The IGF-II complementary deoxyribonucleic acid (cDNA) isolated from human placenta has a 5′-untranslated region different from that produced in human liver, and IGF-II mRNA in placenta may differ from that in liver or kidney.[60] Only one IGF-II gene is present in the human genome, and there may be unique tissue-specific and developmental alteration of somatomedins by human placental tissue. The role of placental somatomedins and control of their production remain to be characterized. Placental cells possess IGF-I receptors by the sixth week of gestation, and placental IGF-I may have an autocrine or a paracrine role in placental growth.[59]

Nerve growth factor β (NGF-β) from human placenta is similar in molecular weight, chromatographic properties, and biologic (neurite-promoting) activity to mouse salivary gland NGF-β.[61, 62] Human placental NGF does not cross-react, however, with antisera to mouse NGF-β. The significance of placental NGF with regard to fetal development is not clear.

EGF and TGF-α mRNAs and proteins have been demonstrated in pools of placental tissue from early, middle, and late gestation.[63, 64] Placental levels of TGF-α protein are relatively high throughout gestation (90 to 180 ng/mg protein), whereas EGF values are low (3 to 9 ng/mg protein).[63] The placenta is richly endowed with receptors that bind both EGF and TGF-α.[64, 65] TGF-α mRNA is localized in the maternal decidua early in gestation in the mouse and is present in fetal tissues.[66, 67] EGF induces differentiation of human trophoblast to syncytiotrophoblast, and this differentiation is associated with increased production of hCG and hPL.[68] These studies have suggested that TGF-α or EGF, or both, may influence placental maturation and function.

Transforming growth factor β has been purified from human placenta, and precursor mRNA is present in placental tissue.[69] In addition, placental growth factor, PTHrP, platelet-derived growth factor, vascular endothelial growth factor, endothelin-1, tumor necrosis factor α, oncomedullin, erythropoietin, and several colony-stimulating factors and receptors have been demonstrated in placental tissue and conditioned media.[1, 5, 8, 70–73] These factors are also postulated to have autocrine-paracrine roles in placental growth and function.

ECTOPIC FETAL HORMONE PRODUCTION

Ectopic Fetal Polypeptide Hormone

Kidney, liver, and testes from 16- to 20-week-old human fetuses produce immunoreactive and bioactive hCG in vitro.[74] Kidney tissue produces nearly half as much hCG (per milligram of protein) as placenta; liver activity is lower. Corticotropin-like immunoreactivity is present in relatively high concentrations in neonatal rat pancreas and kidney.[75] This material is presumably derived from a POMC parent molecule.

Extraneural Fetal Neuropeptide

Hypothalamic neuropeptides are present in a variety of adult tissues, particularly in the pancreas and gut.[76–82] In the fetus, hypothalamic neuropeptides are also present in the gut and tissues derived from it. High concentrations of TRH and somatostatin immunoreactivity have been reported in neonatal rat pancreas and gastrointestinal tract tissues, whereas hypothalamic concentrations of these immunoreactive substances are low.[83–86] These neuropeptides have immunoreactive and chromatographic properties similar to those of the synthetic hypothalamic peptides. Other peptides cleaved from pre-pro-TRH are present in perinatal rat pancreas.[87] In addition, encephalectomy does not alter the circulating TRH levels in the neonatal rat, whereas significant reductions are produced by pancreatectomy. TRH production by monolayer cultures of fetal rat pancreatic cells is stimulated by serotonin and inhibited by carbachol; catecholamines, γ-aminobutyric acid, and histamine have no effect.[88] Specific neurotransmitter control has been postulated. In the sheep fetus, thyroid hormones modulate pancreatic and gut TRH concentrations, which suggests thyroid hormone control of extrahypothalamic *TRH* gene transcription or translation in the fetus.[50]

TRH and somatostatin are present in the human neonatal pancreas[89, 90] and in blood of the human newborn.[50, 91, 92] It seems likely that both hormones are derived mostly from extrahypothalamic sources.[88, 92] The presence of TRH at high concentrations in fetal ovine blood and the control of fetal pancreatic, placental, and blood TRH levels by thyroid hormones suggest a role for extrahypothalamic TRH in the control of fetal pituitary thyrotropin secretion before the near-term maturation of hypothalamic TRH.[50] Infusion of TRH into the fetal sheep also evoked behavioral arousal, caused increased body and eye movements, and stimulated fetal breathing.[93] The role of extraneural somatostatin in the fetus is undefined.

There is a general tendency toward hypersecretion of fetal pituitary hormones during the last half of gestation, and pituitary hormones found at high levels in cord blood from aborted human fetuses and premature human infants include hGH, thyrotropin, corticotropin, β-endorphin, β-lipotropin, LH, and FSH.[94, 95] Development of hypothalamic-pituitary control is complex, involving maturational events in the cortex and midbrain, the hypothalamus and hypothalamic-pituitary portal vascular system, peripheral endocrine systems, and the placenta itself, including hormone, growth factor, and neuropeptide production. The fetal pituitary hyperfunction appears to be related more to relatively delayed maturation of the central nervous system and hypothalamic control with unrestrained secretion of stimulating hypothalamic hormones than to the action of placental neuropeptides.[95, 96]

FETAL ENDOCRINE SYSTEMS

Anterior Pituitary and Target Organs

Development

The human fetal forebrain is identifiable by 3 weeks of gestation, the diencephalon and telencephalon by 5 weeks. Rathke's pouch, the buccal precursor of the anterior pituitary gland, separates from the primitive pharyngeal stomodeum by 5 weeks of gestation.[5, 8, 95] The neural components of the transducer system (the hypothalamus, the pituitary stalk, and the posterior pituitary) are largely developed by 7 weeks of gestation, and the bony floor of the sella turcica is present by this time, separating the adenohypophysis from the primitive gut. Capillaries develop within the proliferating anterior pituitary mesenchymal tissue around Rathke's pouch and the diencephalon by 8 weeks of gestation, and intact hypothalamic-pituitary portal vessels are present by 12 to 17 weeks.[5, 8, 95] Maturation of the pituitary portal vascular system continues, and the system becomes functionally intact during the period of histologic differentiation of the hypothalamus and development of the portal vascular extension into hypothalamic tissue; this maturation process extends to 30 to 35 weeks of gestation.

The hypothalamic cell condensations, which represent the hypothalamic nuclei, and the interconnecting fiber tracts are demonstrable histologically by 15 to 18 weeks of gestation.[5, 8, 95] Hypothalamic cells and diencephalic fiber tracts for the hypothalamic neuropeptides somatostatin, CRH, GHRH, and LHRH are also visible by this time. Concentrations of dopamine, TRH, LHRH, and somatostatin are significant in hypothalamic tissue by 10 to 14 weeks of gestation. Specialized anterior pituitary cell types, including lactotropes, somatotropes, corticotropes, thyrotropes, and gonadotropes, can be

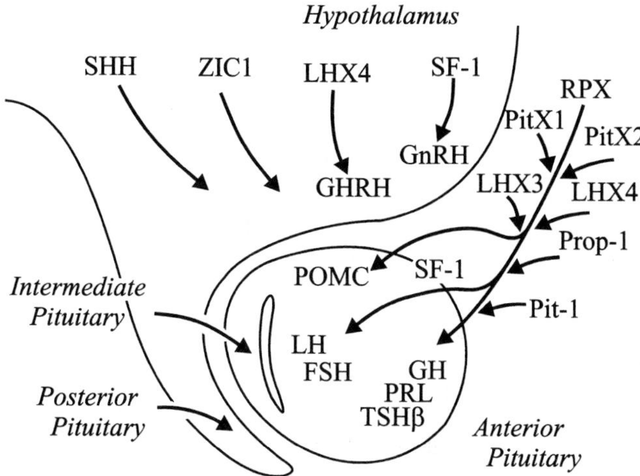

Figure 21–3. Cartoon illustrating the homeobox genes programming hypothalamic and pituitary embryogenesis and function. *SHH* and *ZIC2* are the sonic hedgehog and *Drosophila* odd-paired homologues, mutations of which have been shown to cause human holoprosencephaly. *RPX* is the Rathke's pouch homeobox gene involved in anterior pituitary gland embryogenesis. *LHX3* and *LHX4* are LIM class homeodomain transcription factors also essential for normal pituitary embryogenesis. *PROP1* and *PIT1* defects in mice and humans lead to growth hormone (GH), prolactin (PRL), and thyroid-stimulating hormone (TSH) deficiency. FSH, follicle-stimulating hormone; LH, luteinizing hormone; POMC, pro-opiomelanocortin. See text for details.

recognized in the anterior pituitary between 7 and 16 weeks of gestation. Anterior pituitary hormones (including hGH, PRL, thyrotropin, LH, FSH, and corticotropin) are detectable by radioimmunoassay between 10 and 17 weeks of gestation. Thus, the anatomy and biosynthetic mechanisms that make up the hypothalamic-pituitary neuroendocrine transducer appear to be functional by 12 to 17 weeks of gestation in humans.

This embryogenic process is regulated by a series of homeodomain proteins or transcription factors that have been characterized by mutation analysis, gene transfection, and gene knockout studies.[97–100] Mutations of the homeobox genes sonic hedgehog *(SHH)* and *ZIC2* have been identified in patients with familial and sporadic holoprosencephaly. *HESX1* homeobox gene mutations have been shown in siblings with septo-optic dysplasia in association with midline brain defects and pituitary hypoplasia.[99] Other genes involved in hypothalamic development include *SF1* and *LHX4*. Early pituitary homeodomain factors include the Rathke pouch homeobox gene (*RPX*), *LHX3*, and *LHX4*. The later factors *PROP1* and *PIT1* program development and function of the pituitary cells producing GH, TSH, and PRL. Mutations in *PROP1* and *PIT1* have been described in patients with familial hypopituitarism and are fully addressed in Chapter 8[5, 8, 95, 101] (Fig. 21–3).

Human Fetal Pituitary Growth Hormone and Prolactin

The human fetal pituitary gland can synthesize and secrete hGH by 8 to 10 weeks of gestation.[94, 95] Pituitary hGH content increases from about 1 nmol (20 ng) at 10 weeks to 45 nmol (1000 ng) at 16 weeks of gestation. Fetal plasma hGH levels in cord blood samples are in the range 1 to 4 nmol/L during the first trimester and increase to a mean peak of approximately 6 nmol/L at midgestation. Plasma hGH levels fall progressively during the second half of gestation to a mean value of 1.5 nmol/L at term.[95] Pituitary hGH mRNA and hGH content generally parallel the increase in plasma hGH concentration between 16 and 24 weeks of gestation.[102] This pattern of ontogenesis of plasma hGH reflects a progressive maturation of hypothalamic-pituitary and forebrain function. The responses of plasma hGH to somatostatin and GHRH and to insulin and arginine are mature at term in human infants.[94, 95] Plasma hGH levels are low in anencephalic infants.

The high plasma hGH concentrations at midgestation after the development of the pituitary portal vascular system may reflect unrestrained secretion.[95] Studies of 9- to 16-week-old human fetal pituitary cells in culture have shown a predominant response to GHRH and a limited effect of somatostatin, which suggests that the inhibitory action of somatostatin develops later in gestation.[103] This interpretation has been substantiated by in vivo studies in the sheep fetus, which have shown a failure of somatostatin to inhibit GHRH-stimulated GH release early in the third trimester and maturation of the inhibitory effect of somatostatin near term.[104] Thus, a predominant GHRH enhancement and limited somatostatin inhibition of hGH secretion at midgestation are presumably associated with a limited capacity for inhibition of hGH release by somatomedin feedback. In addition, there may be unrestrained hGH secretion at the pituitary cell level or immaturity of limbic and forebrain inhibitory circuitry that modulates hypothalamic function, or both.[95] Whatever the mechanisms, control of hGH secretion matures progressively during the last half of gestation and the early weeks of postnatal life so that mature responses to sleep, glucose, and L-dopa are present by 3 months of age.

The ontogenesis of fetal plasma PRL differs significantly from that of hGH (Fig. 21–4); levels are low until 25 to 30

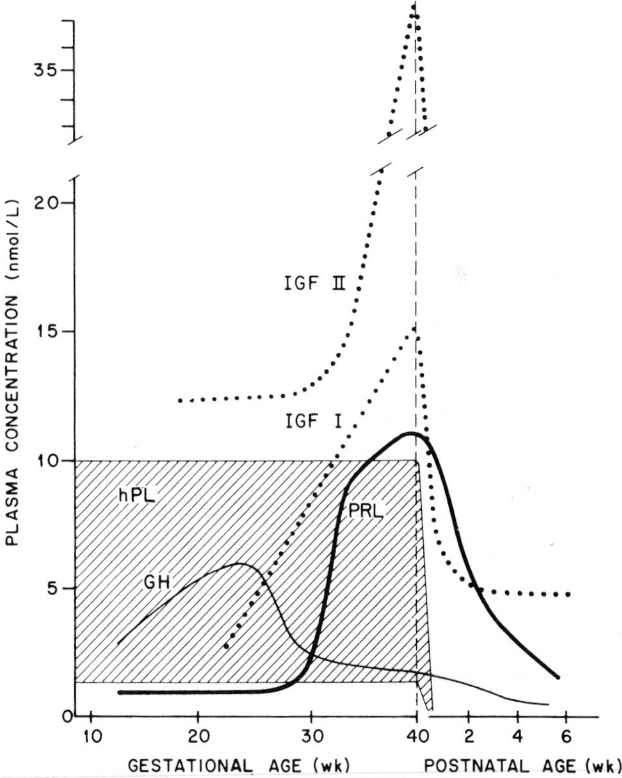

Figure 21–4. Patterns of change of fetal plasma human placental lactogen (hPL), growth hormone (GH), prolactin (PRL), insulin-like growth factor I (IGF I), and insulin-like growth factor II (IGF II) during gestation and in the neonatal period. The range of fetal plasma hPL concentrations is shown as the *hatched area*. (Data from Bennett A, Wilson DM, Liu R, et al. J Clin Endocrinol Metab 1983; 57:609–612; Kaplan SL, Grumbach MM, Aubert ML. Recent Prog Horm Res 1976; 32:161–243; Bala RM, Lopatka J, Leung A, et al. Clin Endocrinol Metab 1981; 52:508–512.)

weeks of gestation and increase to a mean peak value of approximately 11 nmol/L at term.[95] Pituitary PRL content increases progressively from 12 to 15 weeks, and in vitro fetal pituitary cells from midgestation fetuses show limited autonomous PRL secretion, although PRL release increases in response to TRH and decreases in response to dopamine.[94] Brain and hypothalamic control of PRL matures late in gestation and during the first months of extrauterine life.[94, 95] Estrogen stimulates PRL synthesis and release by pituitary cells, and the marked increase in fetal plasma PRL concentration in the last trimester parallels the increase in fetal plasma estrogen levels, although lagging by several weeks.[94, 95] Anencephalic fetuses have plasma PRL concentrations in the normal or low-normal range.[95] These data support a role for estrogen in stimulating fetal PRL release. The fetal sheep exhibits a similar pattern of fetal plasma PRL levels, indicating that maturation and integration of brain and hypothalamic mechanisms modulating PRL release develop late in gestation and in the postnatal period, accounting for the delayed postnatal fall in plasma PRL level in the neonate of this species.[95]

The somatomedins IGF-I and IGF-II are important factors in fetal growth. The mRNA and protein for both factors are present early in gestation in essentially all fetal tissues.[95] IGF-II transcripts are more abundant than those of IGF-I and are predominant in fibroblasts and mesenchymal tissues.[105] Receptors for the IGFs are also widespread in fetal tissues. Studies of transgenic mice with null mutations of the genes encoding IGF-I, IGF-II, or the IGF-I receptor have defined the role of the somatomedins; the birth weight of the embryos lacking IGF-I or IGF-II was 60% of that of the control mice.[106] When both genes were inactive birth weight was reduced another 30%, and mice lacking IGF-I receptor had birth weights averaging 45% of control values.[106]

Postnatally, GH acts through receptors in liver and other tissues to stimulate production of IGF-I and, to a lesser degree, IGF-II. Prenatally, in contrast, GH receptor mRNA levels and receptor binding are low in fetal liver, although receptor mRNA is present in other fetal tissues.[95] The growth of anencephalic fetuses is nearly normal, however, suggesting that factors other than GH stimulate fetal somatomedin production. Nutritional factors are known to play a role.[106, 107] PRL receptors are present in most fetal tissues during the first trimester of gestation, and it is likely that lactogenic hormones have a significant role in organ and tissue development early in gestation.[108, 109] The coordinate increase in fetal adipose tissue and adipose tissue PRL receptors PRLR1 and PRLR2 suggests that PRL may play a role in growth and maturation of fetal adipose tissue later in gestation.[110] PRL also plays a role in fetal skeletal maturation.[109] Ovine placental lactogen stimulates glycogen synthesis in fetal ovine liver, and hPL stimulates amino acid transport, DNA synthesis, and IGF-I production in human fetal fibroblasts and muscle cells. GH and PRL have little activity in these tissues.

Fetal Pituitary-Adrenal System

The primordium of the adrenal gland can be recognized just cephalad of the developing mesonephros by 3 to 4 weeks of gestation.[111, 112] The fetal adrenal is composed of three functional zones. The fetal zone expresses CYP17 (p450c17), the enzyme necessary for production of the C_{19} androgens DHEA and DHEAS. A transitional zone expresses CYP17 and 3β-hydroxysteroid dehydrogenase/isomerase (3β−HSD) enzymes for cortisol production. The outer definitive zone, which produces mineralocorticoids, expresses 3β−HSD but not CYP17. The large eosinophilic cells of the fetal zone are well differentiated by 9 to 12 weeks of gestation and are capable of active steroidogenesis. The fetal adrenal gland grows rapidly and progressively in mass; the combined glandular weight is approximately 8 g at term, when the fetal zone makes up about 80% of the mass of the gland.[111, 112]

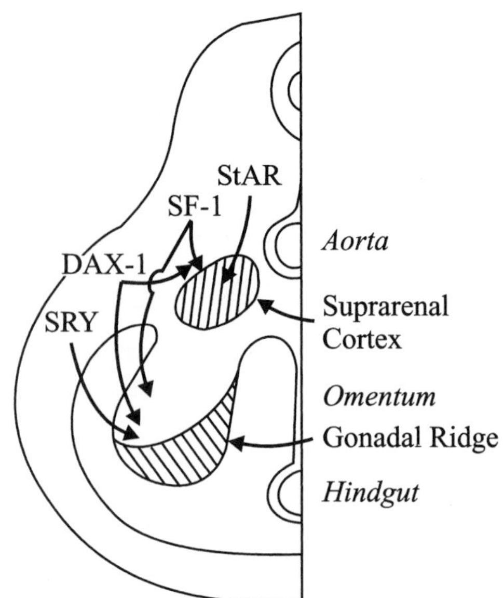

Figure 21–5. Hemi-cross-section of a 5-week human embryo with location of the adrenal primordia (suprarenal cortices) and gonadal ridges. The homeobox genes programming adrenal and gonadal embryogenesis are indicated. *SF1* (steroidogenic factor 1) is involved in testicular and ovarian development, whereas *SRY* is the single critical regulator of testicular embryogenesis. Inactivation of the *DAX1* gene leads to adrenal hypoplasia. The steroidogenic acute regulatory protein (StAR) is the rate-limiting factor for adrenal steroidogenesis. See text for details.

The fetal zone of the adrenal gland also has relatively high steroid sulfotransferase activity, and because of the low 3β−HSD and high sulfotransferase activities, the major steroid products of the fetal adrenal are DHEA, DHEAS, pregnenolone sulfate, several $\Delta^5$3β-hydroxysteroids, and limited amounts of $\Delta^5$3-ketosteroids, including cortisol and aldosterone.[111, 112] The definitive zone contributes only a small fraction of total fetal adrenal steroid output. Cholesterol, the major substrate for fetal adrenal steroidogenesis, is derived from circulating LDL and from de novo adrenal synthesis[113]; LDL cholesterol, largely of fetal liver and testicular origin, contributes 70% of the total. The fetal zone contains more LDL binding sites and manifests a greater rate of de novo cholesterol synthesis than does the definitive zone, in keeping with its greater steroidogenic activity.[113]

Development of the fetal adrenal cortex is under control of several genes and growth factors. The genes include those coding for the orphan nuclear receptors SF-1 (steroidogenic factor-1) and DAX-1 (dosage-sensitive sex reversal, adrenal hypoplasia congenita, X-chromosome factor) (Fig. 21–5).[114] These genes show coordinate expression in adrenal cortex, testis, ovary, hypothalamus, and pituitary tissues. SF-1 gene knockout mice manifest adrenal and gonadal agenesis, gonadotropin deficiency, and absence of the hypothalamic ventromedial nucleus.[115] Inactivating DAX-1 gene mutations are associated with adrenal hypoplasia and gonadotropin deficiency.[115] The steroidogenic acute regulatory protein (StAR) is a rate-limiting factor in adrenal steroidogenesis. StAR knockout mice manifest glucocorticoid and mineralocorticoid deficiency and female genitalia in XY animals.[116] In humans, inactivating StAR mutations cause adrenal hyperplasia and adrenal hormone insufficiency.[116]

Fetal adrenal transitional zone development is ACTH-dependent.[117] Proliferation of both the fetal and definitive zones

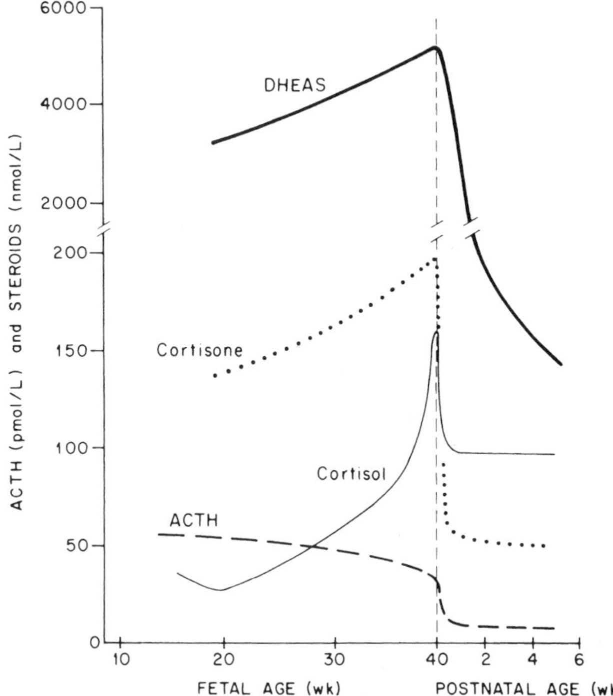

Figure 21–6. Patterns of change of fetal plasma adrenocorticotropic hormone (ACTH), cortisol, cortisone, and dehydroepiandrosterone sulfate (DHEAS) during gestation and in the neonatal period. The trend of average values is shown for each hormone in nanomoles per liter. Note the broken scale for DHEAS. (Data from Winters AJ, Oliver C, Colston C, et al. J Clin Endocrinol Metab 1974; 39:269–273; Murphy BEP. Am J Obstet Gynecol 1982; 144:276–282; Beitins IZ, Bayard F, Ances FIG, et al. Pediatr Res 1973; 7:509–513; Winter JSD. In Polin RA, Fox WW [eds]. Neonatal and Fetal Medicine. Philadelphia, WB Saunders, 1992, pp 1829–1841.)

is stimulated by fibroblast growth factor and EGF, and the fetal adrenal expresses high levels of IGF-II mRNA and protein, which are responsive to ACTH.[5] Moreover, IGF-II augments ACTH-stimulated expression of CYP11A1 (p450scc), CYP17, and 3βHSD and stimulates cortisol and DHEA-S production in fetal adrenal cortical cells, suggesting a role in adrenal regulation during fetal and postnatal life.[5] The pattern of enzyme maturation in the fetal adrenal suggests that cortisol production does not occur de novo from cholesterol until 30 weeks of gestation.[5]

The major control of fetal adrenal function is mediated by fetal pituitary ACTH. Maternal levels of CRH are elevated during the last trimester of gestation and reach values of 0.5 to 1 nmol/L at term; normal values in nonpregnant women are less than 0.01 nmol/L.[118] This CRH is bioactive and levels correlate with maternal cortisol concentrations, suggesting that CRH plays a role in stimulating maternal corticotropin release. Fetal plasma CRH levels at term, however, are approximately 0.03 nmol/L and, relative to the presumably high levels in pituitary portal blood, probably have little role in modulating fetal corticotropin release. Midgestation fetal plasma corticotropin concentrations average about 55 pmol/L (250 pg/mL), levels that maximally stimulate fetal adrenal steroidogenesis, and concentrations are higher throughout gestation than in postnatal life, although they fall near term (Fig. 21–6).[5, 111]

Thus, the fetal adrenal cortex is maximally stimulated by pituitary corticotropin and produces large quantities of DHEA and pregnenolone and their sulfate conjugates. Much of the DHEA is converted to 16-hydroxy-DHEAS by the fetal adrenal and fetal liver. As already discussed, DHEA serves as a substrate for placental estrone and estradiol production; 16-hydroxy-DHEA undergoes metabolism to estriol in the placenta. In the anencephalic fetus, placental estrogen production is reduced to about 10% of normal.[5, 111] An important factor in fetal adrenal function appears to be substrate inhibition of 3β–HSD activity by placental estrogens and intracellular adrenal steroids.[111] Near term the fetal cortisol production rate in blood, per unit body weight, is similar to that in the adult.[119] About two thirds of fetal cortisol is derived from the fetal adrenal glands, and one third is derived from placental transfer.[112] Both fetal adrenal cortisol and placental estradiol regulate hepatic synthesis of cholesterol in the fetus.

The corticotropin feedback control system matures progressively during the second half of gestation and the early neonatal period. Dexamethasone can suppress the human fetal pituitary-adrenal axis at term but not at 18 to 20 weeks of gestation.[111, 112] In the fetal sheep, hypothalamic and pituitary glucocorticoid receptors are present at midgestation and corticotropin suppressibility can be demonstrated by the midpoint of the third trimester of gestation.[96, 120] The number of glucocorticoid receptors in the pituitary gland increases at term at the time of increasing glucocorticoid levels, suggesting that some process in the fetus allows the normal autoregulation of glucocorticoid receptors to be overridden at term.[96]

Adrenal hormone receptors, including *glucocorticoid receptors* (GRs) and *mineralocorticoid receptors* (MRs), are members of the nuclear receptor superfamily of steroid hormone, thyroid hormone, vitamin D, and retinoid receptors.[121] GRs are present in most body tissues by the second trimester and play an important role in fetal development. Mice lacking GR receptor function manifest enlarged and disorganized adrenal cortices, adrenal medullary atrophy, lung hypoplasia, and defective gluconeogenesis.[121, 122] They appear normal at birth but do not survive without treatment.

Fetal cortisol is converted to cortisone through an 11β–HSD in fetal tissues, and levels of circulating cortisone in the fetus at midgestation are fourfold to fivefold higher than cortisol concentrations (see Fig. 21–6). Cortisone is a relatively inactive glucocorticoid, and this metabolism protects the anabolic milieu of the fetus because cortisol can retard both placental and fetal growth.[123] GRs are present at birth and are probably present at midgestation in most tissues, including placenta, lung, brain, liver, and gut.[96, 111, 124] As term approaches, selected fetal tissues including liver and lung express 11-ketosteroid reductase activity that promotes local conversion of cortisone to cortisol.[111] Cortisol serves as an important stimulus to prepare the fetus for extrauterine survival. The increase in fetal cortisol concentration occurs during the last 10 weeks of gestation and is the result of increased cortisol secretion and decreased conversion of cortisol to cortisone.[111] This increase in fetal cortisol production has an important role in the maturation of several fetal systems or functions that are critical to extrauterine survival[111, 125] (see "Transition to Extrauterine Life").

The human fetal adrenal gland is capable of aldosterone secretion near term, and fetal plasma aldosterone concentrations in infants who are born by cesarean section are threefold to fourfold higher than maternal levels.[111, 126] Vaginal delivery and maternal salt restriction increase levels in both mother and infant. The increased aldosterone levels in the fetus are due to increased fetal adrenal secretion and persist during the first year of extrauterine life.[127] However, there is a poor correlation between plasma renin activity (PRA) and aldosterone levels in cord blood.[128] Aldosterone secretion is low in the midgestation human fetal adrenal and is unresponsive to the secretagogues that are known to modulate aldosterone production in the adult. In sheep, fetal aldosterone becomes responsive to PRA and angiotensin II in the neonatal period.[129] In this species, in which late fetal aldosterone levels are also high compared with adult levels, furosemide stimulates PRA but not aldosterone during the third trimester; the aldosterone response to furosemide (and PRA) is delayed until the neonatal period.[129, 130] This situation also appears to be the case in the human fetus and neonate.

MRs are present in fetal tissues from 12 to 16 weeks of gestation.[131] MR immunoreactivity is detectable in fetal kidney, skin, hair follicles, trachea and bronchioles, esophagus, stomach, small intestine, colon, and pancreatic exocrine ducts.[131] The role of MRs in these fetal tissues remains unclear. MR knockout mice appear normal at birth but demonstrate defects in mineralocorticoid and renin-angiotensin system functions in the postnatal period.[132]

Angiotensin II levels in the sheep fetus are similar to maternal values, and blockade of fetal production with angiotensin-converting enzyme inhibitors decreases the fetal glomerular filtration rate.[130] Two subtypes of angiotensin receptors, AT_1 and AT_2, are detectable in various tissues early in fetal development.[133] AT_1 receptor mRNA expression in the fetal sheep kidney is low early in gestation, increases in the latter third of pregnancy, and decreases postnatally; AT_2 mRNA levels, in contrast, are high at midgestation and decrease during the third trimester.[133] These changes are believed to reflect growth factor–mediated changes in cells that contain AT in various tissues. Hormonal factors modulate fetal renal AT gene expression in sheep; angiotensin II suppresses both AT_1 and AT_2, and cortisol increases AT_1 gene expression.[133]

The role of the fetal renin-angiotensin system is not clear; rather than modulating renal sodium excretion through aldosterone, it may maintain renal excretion of salt and water into amniotic fluid to prevent oligohydramnios.[130] This renal effect is presumably mediated by modulation of arterial pressure. The mechanism for the high aldosterone levels in the fetal and neonatal periods remains unclear. Because plasma atrial natriuretic factor concentrations are high in the fetus, the increased PRA and aldosterone levels are not due to relative atrial natriuretic factor deficiency.[134]

Aldosterone affects renal sodium excretion in the fetal sheep and in premature infants.[111, 126, 129] Despite the fact that the newborn human kidney is relatively unresponsive to exogenous aldosterone, manifestations of mineralocorticoid deficiency in the newborn term infant can occur as a result of aldosterone deficiency or competition for binding to renal MRs by other steroids such as 17-hydroxyprogesterone.[111] Relatively reduced glomerular filtration in the newborn limits sodium loss initially, but by 1 week of age aldosterone deficiency produces the characteristic manifestations of hyponatremia, hyperkalemia, and volume depletion.

Fetal Pituitary Thyroid System

The thyroid gland is a derivative of the primitive buccopharyngeal cavity and develops from contributions of two anlagen, a midline thickening of the pharyngeal floor (median anlage) and paired caudal extensions of the fourth pharyngobranchial pouches (lateral anlagen).[135, 136] These structures are discernible by 16 to 17 days of gestation, and by 24 days the median anlage develops a thin, flasklike diverticulum extending from the floor of the buccal cavity to the fourth branchial arch. By 50 days of gestation, the median and lateral anlagen have fused and the buccal stalk has ruptured. During this period the thyroid gland migrates caudally to its definitive location in the anterior neck. By 70 days of gestation, colloid is visible histologically and thyroglobulin synthesis and iodide accumulation can be demonstrated within the gland. During the final follicular phase of development, colloid spaces increase in size and there is progressive cell growth and accumulation of thyroid hormones. At 12 weeks of gestation the fetal thyroid gland weighs about 80 mg, and at term it weighs 1 to 1.5 g.

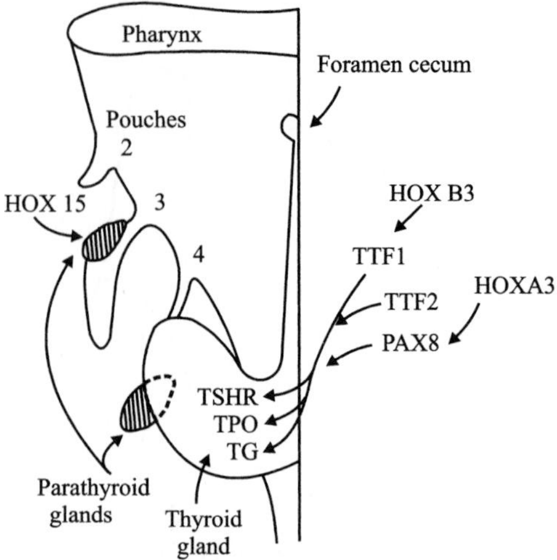

Figure 21–7. Cartoon showing the homeobox genes programming development of the thyroid and parathyroid glands. *HOXB3* may be responsible for activation of thyroid transcription factor 1 (TTF1) during early embryogenesis, with *TTF2* and *PAX8* involved in a synergistic cascade programming thyroid gland embryogenesis. These factors are also involved in thyroid follicular cell function, promoting thyroglobulin (TG), thyroid peroxidase (TPO), and thyroid-stimulating hormone receptor (TSHR) gene transcription. *HOX15* gene knockout in mice causes parathyroid gland aplasia. See text for details.

The parathyroid glands develop between 5 and 12 weeks of gestation from the third and fourth pharyngeal pouches. The third pouches encounter the migrating thyroid anlage, and the parathyroid anlagen are carried caudally with the thyroid gland, finally coming to rest at the lower poles of the thyroid lobes as the inferior parathyroid glands. The fourth pouches encounter the thyroid anlage later and come to rest at the upper poles of the thyroid lobes as the superior parathyroid glands. The individual parathyroid glands increase in diameter from less than 0.1 mm at 14 weeks of gestation to 1 to 2 mm at birth. The fifth pouches contribute paired ultimobranchial bodies that are incorporated into the developing thyroid gland as the parafollicular or C cells that secrete calcitonin.

Four or more homeobox genes are involved in thyroid and parathyroid gland embryogenesis. These include the genes for thyroid transcription factors 1 and 2 (*TTF1*, *TTF2*) and *PAX8*[137–139] (Fig. 21–7). *TTF2* gene knockout in mice results in thyroid dysgenesis and cleft palate. *TTF1* knockout produces pulmonary hypoplasia and thyroid agenesis. Inactivating *PAX8* mutations produce thyroid hypoplasia and renal anomalies. *TTF1* knockout also produces parafollicular C-cell aplasia. The *HOX* genes appear to be important in the expression of *TTF1* and *PAX8*. *HOX15* gene disruption in mice results in parathyroid gland aplasia.[140] *TTF2* and *PAX8* gene mutations have been identified in 2% of patients with familial thyroid dysgenesis and congenital hypothyroidism.[137, 138] However, most cases of congenital hypothyroidism occur sporadically, and the pathogenesis in these cases remains unclear.

During the first half of gestation, before the onset of significant fetal thyroid hormone production, fetal T_4 is derived from maternal-fetal-placental transfer. T_4 is detectable in human coelomic fluid at levels of 0.5 to 2 nmol/L between 6 and 11 weeks of gestation, before the onset of fetal thyroid function.[141] At term, serum T_4 levels in the athyroid fetus range from 30 to 70 nmol/L (2.3 to 5.4 μg/dL).[142] Isotopic equilibrium studies with pregnant rats at term suggest that 15% to 20% of the T_4 in fetal tissues is of maternal origin.[143]

Pituitary and plasma thyrotropin (TSH) concentrations begin to increase during the second trimester in the human fetus, about the time that pituitary portal vascular continuity devel-

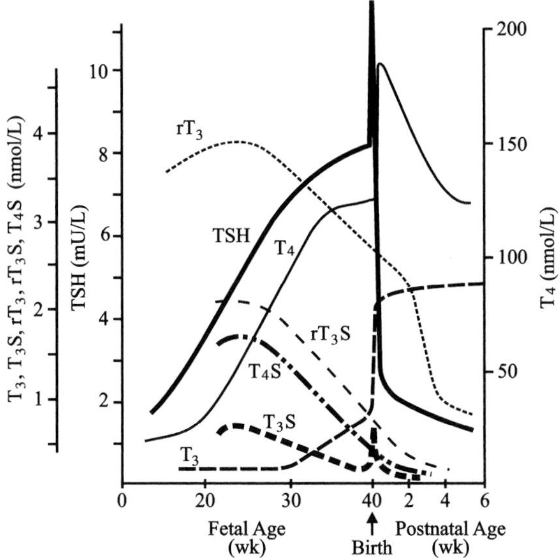

Figure 21–8. Patterns of change of fetal plasma thyroid-stimulating hormone (TSH), thyroxine (T_4), triiodothyronine (T_3), reverse T_3 (rT_3), and iodothyronine sulfate (T_4S, rT_3S, and T_3S) levels during gestation and in the neonatal period. The patterns for T_4S and rT_3S are based on limited 30-week data. (Data from Fisher DA, Klein AH. N Engl J Med 1981; 304:702–712; Santini F, Chiovato L, Ghirri P, et al. J Clin Endocrinol Metab 1999; 84:493–498; Burrow GN, Fisher DA, Larsen PR. N Engl J Med 1994; 331:1072–1078.)

ops (Fig. 21–8).[144, 145] Plasma thyrotropin levels increase progressively during the last half of gestation. Plasma T_4-binding globulin and total T_4 concentrations increase progressively from low levels at 16 to 18 weeks of gestation to maximal levels at 35 to 40 weeks. Free T_4 levels also increase as a consequence of the increase in T_4 production.

The increases in plasma TSH and T_4 levels during the third trimester reflect a progressive maturation of hypothalamic pituitary control and of thyroid gland responsiveness to TSH. Pituitary TSH secretion is responsive to TRH early in the third trimester. Premature infants born at 26 to 28 weeks of gestation respond to exogenous TRH with an increase in plasma TSH concentration comparable to that in adults.[146] Moreover, injection of T_4 into the amniotic fluid 24 hours before elective cesarean section increases fetal plasma T_4 and decreases thyrotropin levels, which indicates negative-feedback control of thyrotropin. Hypothalamic-pituitary-thyroid control matures during an interval corresponding to the third trimester and early neonatal period of human development.[144, 147] This maturation includes coordinate maturation of hypothalamic TRH secretion, pituitary TRH sensitivity, thyrotropin negative-feedback control, and thyroid follicular cell responsiveness to TSH.

The period of parallel increases in fetal TSH and free T_4 levels during the latter half of gestation is followed by the sequential TSH and free T_4 surges in the early neonatal period and a final slow equilibration of the TSH/free T_4 ratio to adult values during infancy and childhood.[136, 147] The mean TSH/free T_4 ratio (mU/L/ng/dL) progresses from a value of 15 at midgestation to 2.8 in early infancy and 0.97 in adults.[147] Functionally, the fetus progresses from a state of both primary (thyroidal) and tertiary (hypothalamic) hypothyroidism at midgestation through a state of mild tertiary hypothyroidism during the final weeks in utero to a fully mature hypothalamic-pituitary-thyroid axis by 2 months postnatally.

The adult thyroid follicular cell can modify iodine transport or uptake with changes in dietary iodine intake, independent of variations in serum thyrotropin levels.[148–150] Before 36 to 40 weeks of gestation, the thyroid gland lacks this autoregulatory mechanism and is susceptible to iodine-induced inhibition of thyroid hormone synthesis.[136, 149] The fetal thyroid follicular cell, when exposed to high circulating levels of iodide, is unable to reduce iodide trapping and prevent the high intracellular iodide concentrations that produce the blockade of hormone synthesis referred to as the Wolff-Chaikoff effect. Failure of the immature thyroid to exhibit autoregulation is probably due to failure of down-regulation of thyroid cell membrane sodium-iodide symporter units, which may be related to the absence or reduced iodination of an 8- to 10-kd protein in the thyroid follicular cell.[148, 149] In addition to maturation of autoregulation, thyroidal responsiveness to thyrotropin increases during the last trimester.[136]

The metabolism of thyroid hormones occurs through a progressive series of monodeiodinations.[144, 151] Several enzymes act on the iodines in the outer (phenolic) ring or the inner (tyrosyl) ring of the diiodothyronine molecule. Most of the circulating, biologically active T_3 in adults is derived by outer-ring monodeiodination of T_4 in liver and other nonthyroidal tissues; biologically inactive rT_3 derives from inner-ring deiodination of T_4 in peripheral tissues. Three iodothyronine monodeiodinase subtypes have been characterized. Type I, an outer-ring monodeiodinase in liver and kidney, is a high-Michaelis-constant (K_m) enzyme inhibited by propylthiouracil and stimulated by thyroid hormone. This enzyme also has inner-ring deiodinative activity and catalyzes the conversion of rT_3 to 3,3′-diiodothyronine. Type II outer-ring monodeiodinase in brain, pituitary, and brown adipose tissue is a low-K_m enzyme insensitive to propylthiouracil and inhibited by thyroid hormone. Type III monodeiodinase in liver, heart, skin, and placenta is responsible for inner-ring deiodination of T_4 to rT_3 and of T_3 to diiodothyronine. The type I monodeiodinase is largely responsible for production of T_3 that escapes from the cells into the circulation, whereas the type II enzyme is responsible for production of local T_3 in brain, pituitary, and brown adipose tissue. rT_3 also diffuses out of most tissues to appear in plasma.

The type III enzyme is expressed in most fetal tissues and in the placenta early in gestation and is responsible for production of the high levels of fetal plasma rT_3, which peak at midgestation in the range of 3 to 4 nmol/L (200 to 300 ng/dL).[136, 144] The persistence of elevated plasma levels of rT_3 in the neonate for several weeks after birth indicates that significant amounts of circulating rT_3 are produced by fetal tissues rather than by the placenta.

There is little conversion of T_4 to circulating T_3 in the midgestation human fetus; plasma T_3 levels are low (<0.2 nmol/L [<15 ng/dL]) until 30 weeks of gestation, after which the mean value increases to 0.7 nmol/L (50 ng/dL) at term (Fig. 21–9).[144, 145] Sulfation is active in fetal tissues, and the predominant thyroid hormone metabolites in the fetus are iodothyronine sulfates.[144, 152] In the last third of gestation in fetal sheep, the mean plasma production rates for T_4 and metabolites are T_4 = 40, T_4 sulfate (T_4S) = 10, rT_3 = 5, rT_3S = 12, T_3 = 2, and T_3S = 2 μg/kg body weight per day. All are biologically inactive except for T_3 and perhaps T_3S so that 90% of the T_4 metabolites in the fetus are biologically inactive.[152] The sulfated metabolites accumulate in fetal serum as a result of the low type I monodeiodinase activity in fetal tissues and because the sulfated iodothyronines are not substrates for type III monodeiodinase.[144, 152]

The production rate of T_3 increases progressively between 30 weeks of gestation and term because of maturation of type I monodeiodinase activity in the liver and other tissues and because of decreasing type III monodeiodinase activity in placenta.[136, 153, 154] In the fetal sheep, hepatic type I monodeiodinase activity increases progressively during the last trimester.[155] Type II monodeiodinase activity is present in the brain at

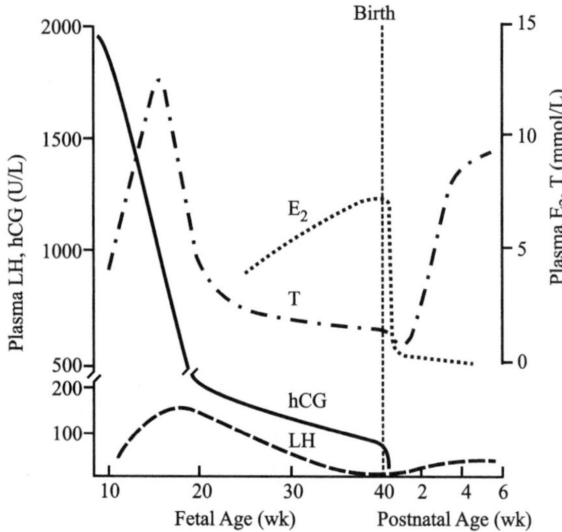

Figure 21–9. Patterns of change of plasma levels of human chorionic gonadotropin (hCG), luteinizing hormone (LH), testosterone (T), and estradiol (E_2) in a male fetus during gestation and in the neonatal period. (Data from Reyes FI, Boroditsky RS, Winter JS, et al. J Clin Endocrinol Metab 1974; 38:612–617; Kaplan SL Grumbach MM, Aubert ML. Recent Prog Horm Res 1976; 32:161–243; Winter JS, Faiman C, Hobson WC, et al. J Clin Endocrinol Metab 1975; 40:545–551; Forest MG, Cathiard AM. J Clin Endocrinol Metab 1975; 41: 977–980; and Penny R, Parlow AF, Frasier SD. Pediatrics 1979; 64: 604–608.)

midgestation and helps guarantee adequate brain T_3 in the sheep, a species in which brain maturation depends on thyroid hormone during the second half of gestation.[155]

Two genes code for the thyroid hormone receptors TRα and TRβ, members of the steroid, retinoid, vitamin D family of nuclear transcription factors. Alternative splicing of expressed mRNA species leads to production of several TR isoforms. The major isoforms, TRα1, TRα2, TRβ1, and TRβ2, are developmentally regulated and are present in characteristic concentration ratios in various adult tissues.[156] In human fetal brain, low levels of nuclear T_3 binding have been detected at 10 weeks of gestation, with higher levels at 16 to 18 weeks. Liver, heart, and lung receptor binding has also been identified at 16 to 18 weeks.[136]

Human fetal growth is the net result of a complex interplay of genetic, hormonal, and growth factor effects, which are independent of thyroid hormone.[136] Bone maturation of the hypothyroid infant, however, is delayed in 50% to 60% of cases and fontanelle closure is often delayed. Serum TSH concentrations are characteristically elevated. Congenitally hypothyroid infants with marked hypothyroxinemia may manifest prolonged jaundice, lethargy, feeding difficulties, umbilical hernia, or macroglossia, but the classical signs and symptoms of congenital hypothyroidism, including myxedema, metabolic derangements, growth retardation, and irreversible mental and neurologic dysfunction, accrue progressively during the early months and years of life. The relative lack of signs and symptoms in the athyroid fetus and infant is probably related to the effects of transplacentally acquired maternal T_4, which at term provides an estimated 20% of fetal thyroid hormone turnover. Developmental regulation of T_3-mediated transcriptional events in various organs and tissues and tissue-specific regulation of deiodinase activity are additional mechanisms.[156]

However, thyroid hormone is essential for normal central nervous system maturation. It regulates a diverse array of processes, including neurogenesis and neural cell migration, neuronal differentiation, dendritic and axonal growth, synaptogenesis, gliogenesis, myelination, and neurotransmitter enzyme synthesis. The most subtle effect of thyroid hormone on fetal brain development is observed in pregnancies associated with maternal hypothyroxinemia.[157] Even subclinical maternal hypothyroidism has been associated with 5- to 10-point I.Q. deficits in the offspring.[157]

The molecular mechanisms by which thyroid hormone mediates these central nervous system effects remain unclear. Aside from a hearing impairment, TRβ knockout mice exhibited neither morphologic or functional abnormalities of brain development nor significant differences in mRNA levels of a number of T_3-dependent cerebellar genes.[136, 158] No gross defects in behavior or in myelination have been reported to date in TRα knockout mice.[158] Thus, the major thyroid hormone effects on brain maturation are probably mediated by pathways common to both TR genes.[158]

Fetal Pituitary-Gonadal Axis

The mammalian gonad is derived from two tissue anlagen, the primordial germ cells of the yolk sac wall and somatic, stromal cells that migrate from the primitive mesonephros.[159, 160] By 4 to 5 weeks of gestation, the germ cells have begun their migration from the yolk sac and the gonadal ridge has appeared as a derivative of the mesonephros. The germ cells are incorporated into the developing gonadal ridge during the sixth week, when the primitive gonad is composed of a surface epithelium, primitive gonadal cords continuous with the epithelium, and a dense cellular mass referred to as the gonadal blastema.[159]

Embryogenesis of the gonads is programmed by genes coding for the male sexual determinant SRY as well as SF-1 and DAX-1.[161, 162] SRY is the single critical regulator of male gonadal differentiation[163] (see Fig. 21–5). SF-1 is also required for testicular and ovarian development and mediates müllerian-inhibiting hormone gene expression and gonadotropin production.[161] SF-1 and DAX-1 are orphan receptors of the steroid-thyroid hormone family of nuclear receptors and appear to interact as heterodimers coordinately involved in the regulation of target genes in the adrenal glands and in hypothalamic gonadotroph cells and the ventromedial hypothalamic nucleus.[161, 162] The hierarchic pathway or pathways for these genes' programming events and the full menu of downstream gene targets remain to be defined. The net result, however, is the highly organized pattern of gonadal development and phenotypic sexual differentiation. Fetal pituitary gonadotropins are not required for gonadal development or sexual differentiation; LH or FSH receptor knockout mice are born phenotypically normal.[164]

Male gonadal differentiation begins at 7 weeks of gestation with organization of the gonadal blastema into interstitium and germ cell–containing testicular cords. The primitive cords lose their connections with the epithelium, primitive Sertoli cells and spermatogonia become visible within the cords, and the epithelium differentiates to form the tunica albuginea.[159] Leydig cells derived from the undifferentiated interstitium are visible by the end of the eighth week of gestation and are capable of androgen synthesis at this time. By 14 weeks of gestation these cells make up as much as 50% of the cell mass, but as the tubules develop they account for a smaller percentage of the tissue. The fetal testes grow from approximately 20 mg at 14 weeks of gestation to 800 mg at birth; at 5 to 6 months they descend into the inguinal canal in association with the epididymis and the ductus deferens.[159] Targeted disruption of the *INS13* gene in mice impairs gubernaculum development and leads to bilateral cryptorchidism.[165]

In females, differentiation of ovaries begins during the seventh week of gestation. The gonadal blastema differentiates into interstitium and medullary cords containing the primitive germ cells now referred to as oogonia. The cords degenerate and cortical layers of surface epithelium, containing individual small oogonia, appear. By 11 to 12 weeks of gestation clusters of dividing oogonia are surrounded by cord cells within the cortex; the medulla at this time consists largely of connective tissue.[159] At 12 weeks of gestation, primitive granulosa cells begin to replicate and many of the large oogonia in the deepest layers of the cortex enter their first meiotic division; other oogonia degenerate. Maturation continues toward the superficial layers through the ninth month, by which time all the surviving oogonia have undergone the first meiotic division to become primary oocytes. Primordial follicles are present by 5 months of gestation, and during the seventh month stroma-derived thecal cells develop around the primordial follicles as they mature to primary follicles. This process continues after birth, again progressing toward the superficial layers. Each fetal ovary weighs about 15 mg at 14 weeks of gestation and 300 to 350 mg at birth.[159]

In the male, the development of Leydig cells leads to an increase in fetal testosterone production between gestational weeks 10 and 20[159, 160] (see Fig. 21–9). In vitro studies in the rat have shown that hCG binding to fetal testis cells does not down-regulate LH receptors. If this is true in vivo, continuous exposure of the Leydig cell to hCG would not desensitize the fetal testis and would allow the maintenance of augmented testosterone production during development. Fetal LH may contribute to fetal Leydig cell function, but quantitatively hCG is the predominant gonadotropin. Testosterone itself, acting through the androgen receptor, stimulates differentiation of the primitive mesonephric ducts into bilateral ductus deferens, epididymides, seminal vesicles, and ejaculatory ducts. Dihydrotestosterone stimulates male differentiation of the urogenital sinus and external genitalia, including differentiation of the prostate, growth of the genital tubercle to form a phallus, and fusion of the urogenital folds to form the penile urethra. Dihydrotestosterone is formed from testosterone by the 5α-reductase enzyme within the urogenital sinus and urogenital tubercle and acts through the same androgen receptor that mediates the action of testosterone in the wolffian ducts.

The fetal testis also produces antimüllerian hormone (AMH), which causes dedifferentiation of the müllerian duct system in the male fetus.[166, 167] AMH is a glycoprotein with a monomer molecular size of approximately 72 kd and multimer sizes ranging from 145 to 235 kd. It is produced by testicular Sertoli cells and reaches the müllerian ducts largely by diffusion; duct regression in vitro requires a 24- to 36-hour exposure to AMH, which is synthesized early in gestation, production peaking at the time of müllerian duct regression. Biosynthesis continues throughout gestation and decreases after birth. *AMH* gene expression is activated by the *SRY* gene.[164] AMH also has autocrine and paracrine effects on testicular steroidogenic function during fetal life.[167]

Male phenotypic differentiation is mediated by testicular testosterone and AMH and occurs between 8 and 14 weeks of gestation. In the female fetus the müllerian duct system differentiates in the absence of AMH, the mesonephric ducts fail to develop in the absence of testosterone, and the undifferentiated urogenital sinus and external genitalia mature into female structures.

Estrogen effects are mediated by cognate receptors, members of the large family of steroid and thyroid hormone, vitamin D, and retinoid receptors.[168] Two receptors, ERα and ERβ have been identified with 96% and 58% homology in the DNA-binding and ligand-binding domains, respectively.[168] Expression profiles of mRNAs of both receptors, products of separate genes, have been characterized in the 16- to 23-week human fetus. One or both receptor mRNAs are present in most tissues. ERβ message is predominant, particularly in testis, ovary, spleen, thymus, adrenal, brain, kidney, and skin. ERα message is prominent in uterus with relatively low levels in most other tissues.[168]

The significance of estrogen receptors in fetal development remains unclear. Knockout of the ERα gene in mice did not impair fetal development, but adult females were infertile with hypoplastic uteri and polycystic ovaries and adult males manifested decreased fertility.[169] ERβ knockout mice also developed normally and female adults were fertile with normal sexual behavior; adult males reproduced normally but had prostate and bladder hyperplasia.[170] It is known that estrogens regulate DHEA production in the baboon and human fetal adrenal.[21, 168] Studies of mice with knockout of both ERα and ERβ functions should further clarify the role of these receptors in fetal development.

Gonadal hormones also control gonadotropin production in the brain that results in cyclic ovarian function and normal function of the testes.[171, 172] Testosterone administration to neonatal female rats produces permanent inhibition of cyclic hypothalamic control through local aromatization to estradiol and estrogen receptor binding. In primates and humans, estrogens seem to be more effective in this regard. However, there is no evidence for permanent programming in the primate, and there appear to be no major tissue biochemical differences between the sexes in utero to account for sexual dimorphic behavioral or gonadotropic programming.[172] Thus, the mechanisms for these effects are not yet clear in the primate and human fetus.

Intermediate Lobe of the Pituitary

The intermediate lobe of the pituitary gland is prominent in both the human and the sheep fetus.[173, 174] Intermediate lobe cells begin to disappear near term and are virtually absent in the adult human pituitary, although the intermediate lobe in the adult of some lower species is anatomically and functionally distinct.[173] The major secretory products of the intermediate lobe are α-MSH and β-endorphin derived from cleavage of the POMC molecule. Cleavage of POMC in the anterior lobe results predominantly in corticotropin and β-lipotropin formation.

In rhesus monkeys and humans, the fetal pituitary contains high concentrations of compounds resembling α-MSH and corticotropin-like intermediate lobe peptide[175]; α-MSH levels in the human fetus decrease with increasing fetal age.[95] The circulating levels of both β-endorphin and β-lipotropin are high in the fetal lamb, and the ratio of β-endorphin to β-lipotropin increases during hypoxic stimulation of the anterior pituitary.[95] Because hypoxia provokes corticotropin release and β-lipotropin production from the anterior pituitary, these data have been interpreted to suggest that basal β-endorphin levels in the fetus originate in the intermediate lobe.[92] α-MSH and corticotropin-like intermediate lobe peptide may play a role in fetal adrenal activation, and α-MSH may play a role in fetal growth.[176, 177] However, these effects are probably minor; the processing of pituitary POMC in the human fetus by the end of the second trimester is similar to that in the adult,[178] but the role of these intermediate lobe peptides in the fetus remains obscure.

Posterior Pituitary

The fetal neurohypophysis is well developed by 10 to 12 weeks of gestation and contains both arginine vasopressin (AVP, also called antidiuretic hormone) and OT.[179, 180] In addition, arginine vasotocin (AVT), the parent neurohypophyseal hormone in submammalian vertebrates, is present in the fetal pituitary and pineal glands and in adult pineal glands from several mammalian species, including humans.[181] AVT is present in the pituitary during fetal life and disappears in the neonatal period. In adult mammals, instillation of AVT into cerebrospinal fluid inhibits gonadotropin and corticotropin release, stimulates PRL release by the anterior pituitary, and induces sleep; however, its physiologic importance in these regards remains unclear. The role of AVT in the fetal pineal gland is unknown.

In the fetal sheep, the baseline fetal plasma AVP concentrations are similar to maternal levels after midgestation. During the last trimester of gestation, fetal hypothalamic and pituitary responsiveness to both volume and osmolar stimuli for AVP secretion are well developed and AVP exerts antidiuretic effects on the fetal kidney.[179, 180] Baseline plasma levels of AVT in fetal sheep during the last trimester approximate values for AVP and OT.[181] Presumably this AVT is derived from the posterior pituitary, but the stimuli for AVT secretion in the fetus are not defined. The neurohypophyseal peptides are synthesized as large precursor molecules (neurophysins) and processed to bioactive amidated peptides.[182] Enzymatic processing involves progressive cleavage of carboxyl terminal–extended peptides producing sequentially (for OT) OT-glycine-lysine-arginine (OTGKR), OTGK, OTG, and OT. Similar progressive processing yields AVPG and AVP from the AVP neurophysin. Enzymatic processing of neurophysins matures progressively in the fetus so that early in gestation fetal plasma contains relatively large concentrations of the extended peptides. For OT, the ratio of OT extended peptides to OT in fetal sheep serum is approximately 35 : 1 early in gestation and 3 : 1 late in gestation.[182]

In the fetus, AVP appears to function as a stress-responsive hormone. Perhaps the major potential stress for the fetus is hypoxia, and the response of AVP to hypoxia is increased compared with the maternal response and with the fetal AVP responses to osmolar stimuli.[180, 183–186] Plasma AVP concentrations in human cord blood are elevated in association with intrauterine bradycardia and meconium passage.[183] The vasopressor action of AVP may be important in the maintenance of fetal circulatory homeostasis during hemorrhage and hypoxia; AVP has a limited effect on fetoplacental blood flow.[180, 185] Fetal hypoxia is also a major stimulus for catecholamine release. There is little information on interaction between AVP and catecholamines during fetal hypoxia, but both fetal hypoxia and AVP stimulate anterior pituitary function.[185] A role for AVP as a CRH is established in the adult, and the ovine fetal pituitary responds separately and synergistically to AVP and CRH early in the third trimester.[187] The role of AVP in controlling fetal corticotropin release seems to decrease with gestational age. It is not known whether AVT functions as a fetal CRH.

OT receptors have been demonstrated in human fetal membranes at term, and AVP receptors have been found in renal medullary membranes of newborn sheep.[188–190] Both AVP and AVT evoke antidiuretic actions in the sheep fetus during the last third of gestation, and both hormones act to conserve water for the fetus by inhibiting fluid loss into amniotic fluid through the lungs and kidneys.[179, 180] Aquaporin-1, aquaporin-2, and aquaporin-3 water channel receptors are present in the human fetal and newborn kidney, and the ability of the newborn infant to regulate free water clearance in response to volume and osmolar stimuli has been demonstrated.[191, 192] Whether AVT exerts its effects through AVP receptors or separate fetal AVT receptors is not clear. Maximal concentrating capacity by the fetal kidney is limited to about 600 mmol/L. This limitation is due not to inadequate AVP stimulation but rather to inherent immaturity of the renal tubules.

Fetal Autonomic Nervous System

The primordia of the sympathetic trunk ganglia are visible in the human fetus by 6 to 7 weeks of gestation. The preaortic sympathetic primordia at this time are composed of primitive sympathetic neurons and chromaffin cells, which condense into chains of cell masses along the abdominal aorta. By 10 to 12 weeks of gestation the paired adrenal masses are well developed. In addition, numerous extramedullary paraganglia (derived from preaortic condensations of sympathetic neurons and chromaffin cells) are scattered throughout the abdominal and pelvic sympathetic plexuses.[193] Each of these extramedullary paraganglia may reach a maximal diameter of 2 to 3 mm by 28 to 30 weeks of gestation. The largest of the paraganglia, the organs of Zuckerkandl near the origin of the inferior mesenteric arteries, enlarge to 10 to 15 mm in length at term. After birth, the paraganglia gradually atrophy and disappear by 2 to 3 years of age. With increasing gestational age there is progressive growth of the adrenal medullae, increasing catecholamine content of the adrenal medullae, and progressive maturation of medullary functional capacity. Histologically, the adrenal medullae are somewhat immature at birth, but by the age of 1 they resemble the adult glands.

Both chromaffin and sympathetic nerve cells are derived from common neuroectodermal stem cells, and both respond to NGF.[194] Sympathetic nervous system development is NGF-dependent, and injections of NGF antiserum into neonatal rats lead to degeneration of immature chromaffin cells, sympathetic cells, and pheochromoblasts. Whether NGF and other growth factors are involved in the transient life span and function of the paraganglia in the human fetus and neonate remains to be clarified. The role of placental NGF in maturation of the fetal autonomic nervous system is also unclear.

Catecholamines are present in the para-aortic chromaffin tissue by 10 to 15 weeks of gestation, and concentrations increase until term. The predominant catecholamine is norepinephrine (NE), presumably because of low activity of phenylethanolamine *N*-methyltransferase in para-aortic chromaffin tissue. This enzyme, which catalyzes the methylation of NE to epinephrine, appears to be activated by the high levels of cortisol that diffuse into the adrenal medulla from the adrenal cortex; in contrast, cortisol levels in extramedullary chromaffin tissue are low.[193–195]

In fetal mammals, the chromaffin cells of the adrenal medulla can respond directly to asphyxia, long before splanchnic innervation develops, by secreting NE; the noninnervated para-aortic tissue responds similarly.[196] In the fetal sheep, a similar developmental transition occurs between days 120 and 135 of the 150-day gestation.[193–195] The central nervous system responds to stimuli that evoke sympathetic nervous system responses before the adrenomedullary splanchnic innervation, but the adrenal medulla is relatively unresponsive to such stimuli. The transition is heralded by an adrenomedullary response to hypoglycemia mediated by the central nervous system.[188] This response is present in developing sheep, monkeys, and human fetuses during the third trimester of gestation.[197–199] Central and adrenal enkephalins are also involved in fetal autonomic nervous system function, and pretreatment with naloxone potentiates and methadone inhibits the catecholamine response to hypoxia.[193, 195]

Basal plasma epinephrine, NE, and dopamine levels during the last third of gestation decrease as term approaches.[200] The metabolic clearance rate of epinephrine increases with gestational age, whereas the production rate remains unchanged,[201] indicating that the decreasing basal catecholamine levels that occur with fetal age are due to maturation of clearance mechanisms. The fetal sheep responds to maternal exercise or hypoxia with increased catecholamine levels.[202] The human neonate responds to parturition with an increase in plasma epinephrine and NE concentrations, and these responses are augmented by hypoxia and acidosis.[193–195] In the newborn infant catecholamine secretion also increases after cold exposure and hypoglycemia.[195, 199]

Catecholamines are critical for fetal cardiovascular function and fetal survival. Gene knockout studies in mice targeting either tyrosine hydroxylase or dopamine β-hydroxylase produced fetal catecholamine deficiency and midgestation fetal death in 90% of the mutant embryos.[203, 204] In addition, fetal catecholamines are the major stress hormones in the fetus.[195, 197, 198] The fetal adrenal and the para-aortic chromaffin masses discharge large amounts of catecholamines directly into the circulation in response to fetal hypoxia.[195] Moreover, the defense against fetal hypoxia involves catecholamine actions mediated through cardiac α-receptors that are unique to immature animals. α-Adrenergic receptors predominate in immature cardiac tissue and gradually decline in number as β-adrenergic receptors increase with maturation. Chromaffin tissue in the fetus is also innervated by opiate receptors and contains relatively large amounts of opiate peptides that appear to be co-secreted with the catecholamines.[195] The extent to which these peptides or pituitary endorphins are involved in modulating fetal catecholamine secretion remains unclear.

Parathyroid Hormone/Calcitonin System

Parathyroid gland development from the third and fourth pharyngeal pouches proceeds in synchrony with thyroid embryogenesis[135, 136] (see Fig. 21–8). Disruption of the *HOX15* gene in mice resulted in parathyroid gland aplasia, indicating that this gene functions as part of the gene cascade programming normal thyroid-parathyroid gland development.[140] Both endocrine systems are functional during the second and third trimesters.

Studies in fetal sheep and monkey and measurements in human preterm and term infants indicate that high concentrations of fetal calcium (averaging 2.75 to 3 mmol/L in the last trimester) are maintained by active placental transport from maternal blood.[205, 206] The transport of calcium occurs across the syncytiotrophoblast, which contains a calcium-binding protein that buffers intracellular calcium ions as they are transported across the syncytial cell to the basement membrane. An adenosine triphosphate–dependent calcium pump transports the calcium across the cell membrane to the fetal circulation.[206] The placental calcium pump is stimulated by a midmolecule portion of the PTHrP secreted by the fetal parathyroid gland and by the placenta, where it may exert a paracrine effect.[206–208] The placenta is impermeable to PTH, PTHrP, and calcitonin, but 25-hydroxyvitamin D and 1,25-dihydroxyvitamin D are transported across the placenta and free vitamin D levels in fetal blood are similar to or higher than maternal values.[205, 206]

Thyroparathyroidectomy in the fetal sheep caused a rapid decrease in fetal plasma calcium concentration and a loss of the placental calcium gradient.[206] In mice, knockout of the gene for PTHrP abolished the maternal-fetal calcium gradient and placental transport of calcium was reduced.[206, 209] Placental calcium transport in these models was restored by the midmolecule fragment of PTHrP (amino acids 67 to 86) but not by PTH or PTHrP fragments 1 to 34, which activate the PTH/PTHrP receptor.[208, 209] Thus, a second, as yet unidentified PTHrP receptor recognizing the PTHrP 38 to 94 ligand appears to be involved in placental calcium pump activation.[206]

Other factors are also involved in maintenance of fetal serum calcium levels because knockout of the mouse gene for PTH-PTHrP also results in hypocalcemia in the presence of normal or increased placental calcium transport.[206, 208] PTH and PTHrP, through the PTH-PTHrP receptor, presumably modulate fetal skeletal calcium flux, calcium excretion through the fetal kidney, and perhaps reabsorption of calcium from amniotic fluid. PTHrP has a major role in fetal bone development and metabolism as well as fetal calcium homeostasis. PTHrP knockout mice displayed increased ossification of the basal portion of the skull, long bones, vertebral bodies, and pelvic bones and mineralization of the normally cartilaginous portions of the ribs and sternum; as a result of the cartilaginous mineralization, the animals died of asphyxiation in the early neonatal period.[206, 209]

Fetal nephrectomy also reduces fetal calcium concentrations, and the hypocalcemia can be prevented by administration of 1,25-dihydroxyvitamin D, $1,25(OH)_2D$.[206] Moreover, infusion into the sheep fetus of antibody to $1,25(OH)_2D$ reduced the placental calcium gradient.[206] Thus, fetal PTHrP and PTH appear to stimulate fetal renal $1,25(OH)_2D$ production, which acts to enhance maternal-fetal transport of calcium by the placenta. The fetal kidney can synthesize $1,25(OH)_2D$ via 1-hydroxylation of 25-hydroxycholecalciterol, and the placenta contains both $1,25(OH)_2D$ receptors and a vitamin D–dependent calcium-binding protein. In the sheep fetus, the endogenous production rate of $1,25(OH)_2D$ during the last third of gestation was six times greater than that in the mother.[210] The metabolic clearance of $1,25(OH)_2D$ was also higher in the fetus than in the mother.

The fetal parathyroid-placental axis promotes maternal-fetal transfer of bone mineral and accretion of fetal bone mineral. The high blood levels of calcitonin in the fetus, probably resulting from the chronic stimulation by fetal hypercalcemia, are thought to contribute to the fetal bone mineral accretion.[205, 206] A prominent effect of calcitonin is to inhibit bone resorption, and the high fetal serum calcium concentrations coupled with high circulating calcitonin promote bone mineral anabolism.[205] Calcitonin has been called a vestigial hormone because of its limited role in postnatal calcium regulation, but it may have an important role in the fetus. Placental calcitonin production may contribute to the calcitonin in fetal plasma, but the persistence of high plasma levels in neonatal plasma argues for predominant fetal production. Also, $1,25(OH)_2D$ or $24,25(OH)_2D$ may play a role in fetal cartilage growth and bone mineral accretion.[211] These concepts are summarized in Figure 21–10.

Endocrine Pancreas: Insulin and Glucagon

Embryogenesis of the pancreas is mediated by a series of homeobox genes, including *IDX1*, *ISL1*, *PAX4*, and *PAX6*.[212] *IDX1* gene knockout in the mouse results in pancreatic agenesis, *ISL1* knockout leads to islet cell agenesis, and *PAX4* or *PAX6* knockout results in beta cell or alpha cell agenesis or hypogenesis, respectively. The $\beta 2$/neuroD gene knockout in the mouse leads to marked beta cell dysplasia and hypoplasia and early death from diabetes.[212] These factors and perhaps others farther downstream program the orderly maturation of pancreatic development and function (Fig. 21–11).

The fetal pancreas is identifiable by 4 weeks of gestation, and alpha and beta cells can be recognized by 8 to 9 weeks. Insulin, glucagon, somatostatin, and pancreatic polypeptide are measurable by 8 to 10 weeks of gestation.[8, 213] Alpha cells are more numerous than beta cells in the early fetal pancreas and reach a relative peak at midgestation; beta cells increase throughout the second half of gestation so that by term the ratio of alpha cells to beta cells is approximately 1:1.[213, 214] The insulin content of the pancreas increases from less than 3.6 pmol/g (0.5 U/g) at 7 to 10 weeks to 30 pmol/g (4 U/g) at 16 to 25 weeks of gestation and 93 pmol/g (13 U/g) near term; the concentration in the adult pancreas is approximately 14 pmol/g (2 U/g).[213]

Although the fetal beta cell is functional by 14 to 24 weeks of gestation, secretion of insulin by the fetal pancreas is low.

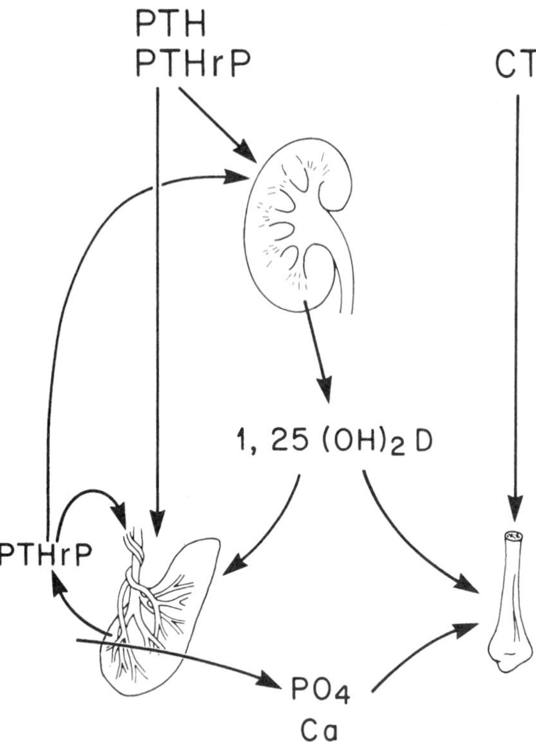

Figure 21–10. Proposed actions of parathyroid hormone (PTH), PTH-related protein (PTHrP), and calcitonin (CT) in the fetus. PTHrP and perhaps PTH from the parathyroid glands and PTHrP from the placenta act on the placenta to promote calcium (Ca) and phosphate (PO_4) transport from the maternal to the fetal circulation to maintain the relative fetal hypercalcemia and the high rate of fetal bone formation during the last half of gestation. PTHrP also acts on the kidney to promote 1-hydroxylation of 25-hydroxycholecalciferol to 1,25-dihydroxyvitamin D, 1,25(OH)2D, which augments placental calcium transport and promotes fetal bone growth. High fetal CT levels tend to promote bone accretion. See text for details.

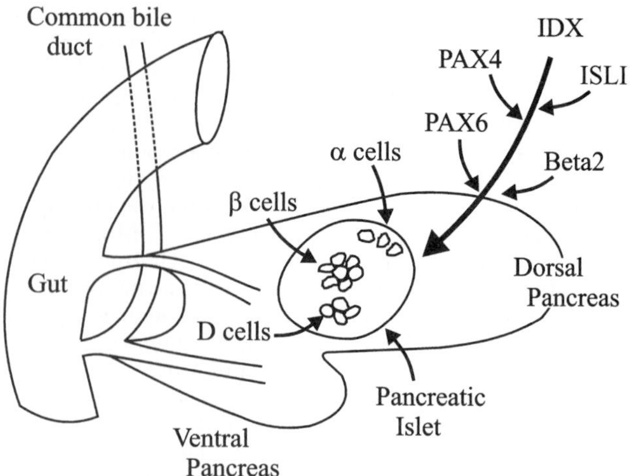

Figure 21–11. Cartoon showing the homeobox genes programming development of the pancreas. *IDX1* gene knockout in the mouse leads to pancreatic agenesis, whereas *ISL1* knockout produces islet cell agenesis. Knockout of *PAX4* and *PAX6* leads to beta cell or alpha cell agenesis or hypogenesis; *Beta2* gene disruption also produces beta cell hypoplasia. See text and Koshimizu et al. J Clin Endocrinol Metab 1895; 61:78–82.[92]

Insulin release from the fetal rat pancreas in vitro in response to glucose or pyruvate is minimal but can be stimulated by leucine, arginine, tolbutamide, or potassium chloride, indicating that parts of the secretory mechanism are functional in the fetus.[213, 215] Insulin secretion in adult islets is mediated by two or more mechanisms, including stimulation of the adenylate cyclase system with production of cAMP and inhibition of potassium efflux, which leads to depolarization of the cell membrane and opening of voltage-dependent calcium channels.[215] The former mechanism, although suppressed in the fetal islets, can be augmented by theophylline, but calcium channel activation does not occur in fetal islets in response to initiators of insulin release that cause depolarization of adult islet cells. The infusion of glucose or arginine in pregnant women before hysterotomy fails to provoke fetal insulin secretion at midgestation or near term, and plasma insulin levels in the late human fetus are relatively unresponsive to high glucose concentrations before the onset of labor.

Similar observations have been made in the monkey. In this species, neither glucose nor arginine stimulated fetal insulin release near term but glucagon evoked prompt insulin secretion.[213] Late in gestation in the ovine fetus, epinephrine inhibited insulin release through a receptor pathway.[213] In the anencephalic human fetus, the endocrine pancreas develops normally if maternal carbohydrate metabolism is not impaired, but beta cell hypertrophy and hyperplasia do not occur in the anencephalic fetus or in decapitated fetal rabbits exposed to chronic hyperglycemia. This lack of beta cell response to hyperglycemia may be the result of GH deficiency because GH stimulates insulin gene expression and may play a permissive role in beta cell hyperplasia and hypertrophy.[216]

Pancreatic glucagon concentrations are relatively high in fetal plasma and increase progressively with fetal age.[213, 214] The fetal pancreatic glucagon content at midgestation is approximately 6 $\mu g/g$, compared with an adult level of 2 $\mu g/g$. As is true for insulin, the capacity for glucagon secretion is blunted in the fetus. Hyperglycemia does not suppress fetal plasma glucagon levels in rats, monkeys, or sheep, and acute hypoglycemia does not evoke glucagon secretion in the rat fetus. Amino acids, which are important secretagogues for insulin and glucagon in the adult, probably have little role in modulating insulin and glucagon secretion in the preterm fetus. However, infusion of alanine into women at term increased both maternal and cord blood glucagon levels, indicating a fetal glucagon response to amino acids in the term fetus. Catecholamines also evoked glucagon release in the near-term ovine fetus.[213]

Thus, the fetal pancreatic islet cells, although histologically mature and capable of hormone synthesis and hyperplasia, are relatively immature functionally at birth with regard to the capacity to secrete both insulin and glucagon. The rapid maturation of responsiveness to glucose in the neonatal period in both premature and mature infants suggests that this blunted state may be a secondary result of the relatively stable fetal serum glucose levels maintained by placental transfer of maternal glucose rather than a primary, temporally fixed maturation process. The blunted capacity for insulin and glucagon secretion has been related to a deficient capacity of the fetal pancreatic islet cells to generate cAMP or a rapid destruction of cAMP by phosphodiesterase, or both.[213]

Insulin and glucagon are normally not necessary for substrate metabolism in the fetus.[214] Glucose is obtained by placental transfer through facilitated diffusion. The fetal respiratory quotient is approximately 1, which suggests that glucose is the primary energy substrate for the fetus. Other substrates such as amino acids and lactate may also be utilized in the human as in the sheep fetus. However, at least early in gestation, hepatic metabolism and substrate utilization appear to be independent of insulin and to be modulated in an autoregulatory fashion by glucose.[213] In addition, the constant supply of glucose normally precludes the necessity for endogenous gluconeogenesis, and gluconeogenic enzyme activities are low in the fetal liver.

Glycogen storage in the fetus is modulated by fetal glucocorticoids and probably by placental hPL. Fetal insulin plays a role near term, when insulin also has the capacity to increase fetal glucose uptake and lipogenesis.[213, 214] Insulin receptors are present on most fetal cells in higher numbers than on adult cells; moreover, hyperinsulinemia fails to down-regulate fetal insulin receptors.[213] Fetal hepatic glucagon receptors, in contrast, are reduced in number, and fetal liver is relatively resistant to the glycemic effect of glucagon. These conditions tend to potentiate the fetal anabolic milieu during the period of rapid growth in the last trimester of gestation.

NEUTRALIZATION OF HORMONE ACTIONS IN THE FETUS

After the period of embryogenesis, the fetal milieu is programmed to optimize body growth and organ development through an array of generalized and specialized growth factors (see "Fetal Growth"). These function in a stable metabolic environment with substrate supply maintained by the placenta. The endocrine-metabolic systems characterizing the extrauterine environment are programmed to maintain metabolic stability in a changing external environment with intermittent substrate provision. Hormonal systems in the fetus are programmed to maintain anabolism with minimal hormonal perturbation. Thus, production of catabolic and thermogenic hormones is limited and the effects of the hormones altering metabolic substrate supply and distribution pathways are muted.

Limitation of Hormone Secretion

The human fetal pancreas is functional during the second trimester, but secretion of insulin in response to glucose or pyruvate is minimal until the neonatal period.[213, 215] Glucagon secretion is also blunted, although fetal blood glucagon levels are relatively high.[213] Fetal islet hyperplasia and increased insulin secretion occur in response to chronic hyperglycemia as in the infant of the diabetic mother, and insulin release can be stimulated by acute fetal infusions of leucine, arginine, or tolbutamide.[213, 214] Moreover, responsiveness of both insulin and glucagon secretion to glucose develops rapidly in the neonatal period.[213] It is not clear whether the limited fetal islet cell responsiveness is due to the relatively stable fetal serum glucose levels or a temporally fixed maturation process (for details, see "Endocrine Pancreas: Insulin and Glucagon").

Production of Inactive Metabolites

Throughout the latter part of gestation, cortisol is metabolized in fetal tissues to inactive cortisone through an 11β–HSD. The placenta is permeable to steroid hormones including cortisol. During midgestation, placental 11β–HSD activity is low and cortisol is transferred to the fetus. Placental 11β–HSD activity increases during the second half of pregnancy under the control of placental estrogens, and enzyme activity near term is high.[5, 21] Thus, maternal-fetal cortisol transfer decreases progressively. In addition, although many adult tissues can convert cortisone to cortisol, conversion is limited during most of fetal life. Consequently, most of the cortisol that crosses the placenta or is produced by the fetus is inactivated to cortisone by the placenta or by fetal tissues.

Table 21–4. Neutralization of Hormone Actions in the Fetus*

Production of Inactive Metabolites	
Active Hormone	*Inactive Metabolites*
Cortisol	Cortisone
Thyroxine (T_4)	rT_3, T_4S, rT_3S
Triiodothyronine (T_3)	T_3S, T_2
Delayed Expression or Neutralization of Receptors	
Active Hormone	*Receptor*
Growth hormone (GH)	GHR
Thyroid hormone	TRα, TRβ
Catecholamines	βAR
Estrogens	ER
Glucagon	GR
Limited Hormone Secretion	
Active Hormone	*Secretory Cell*
Insulin	Islet cell β
Glucagon	Islet cell α

*See text for details.
RT$_3$, reverse T$_3$; T$_4$S, T$_4$ sulfate.

Levels of cortisone in fetal plasma exceed those of cortisol by threefold to fourfold until after 30 weeks of gestation (see Fig. 21–5). Teleologically, this would help preserve the anabolic and growth-promoting milieu of the fetus and minimize premature maturational and parturitional effects of cortisol. After 30 weeks, the ratio of cortisol to cortisone in fetal tissues and plasma increases as a result of increased fetal secretion and decreased conversion of cortisol to cortisone within the placenta and fetal tissues.[20, 21] Cortisol has important maturational action on several fetal tissues near term (see later under "Transition to Extrauterine Life").

Fetal thyroid hormone metabolism is characterized by conversion of active thyroid hormones to inactive rT_3 and inactive sulfated iodothyronines and by limited receptor and postreceptor responsiveness to thyroid hormone in selected tissues.[144, 152] The placenta contains an iodothyronine inner-ring monodeiodinase that catalyzes conversion of maternal T_4 to rT_3. In addition, the fetal sheep liver and kidney, in contrast to the adult liver and kidney, manifest low levels of iodothyronine type I outer-ring monodeiodinase activity so that conversion of T_4 to active T_3 is limited and large amounts of inactive iodothyronine sulfoconjugates accumulate.[144, 150, 155] As a consequence, plasma T_3 levels in the fetus remain low until the last few weeks of gestation (see Fig. 21–9). Selected fetal tissues (brain, brown adipose tissue) have active iodothyronine, type II, outer-ring monodeiodinase activities that contribute to local tissue T_3 concentrations; local T_3 is important in development, particularly in the hypothyroid fetus.[144, 217] Near term and in the neonatal period in the human fetus, the dramatic increase in plasma T_3 levels, and presumably T_3 production, heralds the onset of thyroid hormone actions on growth and development and on metabolism (Table 21–4).

Neutralization of Receptor Response

Selected ovine fetal tissues seem relatively unresponsive to thyroid hormones. Fetal ovine liver and kidney thermogenesis (as evidenced by oxygen consumption, Na^+,K^+-adenosine triphosphatase activity, and mitochondrial α-glycerophosphate activity) is unresponsive to exogenous T_3 during the third trimester, and thyroid hormone responsiveness in a number of tissues (cardiac, hepatic, renal, and skin) develops only during the perinatal period.[218] β-Adrenergic receptor binding in heart and lung of the ovine fetus is unresponsive to T_3 late in the third trimester but increases in response to T_3 in the neonatal period.[136, 218] In rodent species, in which development at birth is comparable to human fetal development at midgestation, pituitary GH concentrations become responsive to thyroid hormone only during the first weeks of extrauterine life.[219] Mouse submandibular gland EGF and NGF levels become responsive to thyroid hormone during the second week of life, as do urine and kidney EGF concentrations and hepatic EGF receptor levels.[220–221] Mouse skin EGF levels and EGF receptors are responsive during the first neonatal week.[222–223]

Thus, despite the presence of nuclear T_3 receptors in significant concentrations in developing rat and sheep, many thyroid hormone actions in these species are delayed.[224] The mechanism of this delayed thyroid hormone responsiveness is not clear; suppressor nuclear proteins may block gene expression in response to thyroid hormones during fetal development, and the levels of these suppressor proteins may determine the onset and degree of action of thyroid hormones during development.[156]

The effect of the high circulating concentrations of GH in the fetus is also limited. Fetal somatic growth is only partially GH-dependent; indeed, the GH-deficient fetus has little or no growth retardation.[95] The paucity of fetal GH effects is probably due to delayed maturation of GH receptors or postreceptor mechanisms. In animals such as sheep, hepatic GH receptor binding appears only during the neonatal period.[95, 108, 109] Receptor deficiency may also be a factor in the limited PRL bioactivity in the fetus near term.[109]

There is less information on fetal hormone responsiveness in other systems. β-Adrenergic receptor binding in heart and lung of the sheep fetus is relatively low near term and increases in the neonatal period in response to thyroid hormones.[218] Moreover, premature lambs have an augmented plasma catecholamine surge at birth but have a relatively mild increase in plasma free fatty acid levels, which suggests reduced catecholamine responsiveness.[225] The high levels of progesterone and estrogens in fetal blood also seem to have limited effects in the fetus. Progesterone receptors are present in low concentration in fetal guinea pig kidney, lung, and uterus at midgestation and increase progressively until term.[226] Estrogen receptors appear in neonatal rat uterus, oviduct, cervix, and vagina during the first 10 days of extrauterine life, and both ERα and ERβ mRNAs are present in human fetal tissues during the second trimester.[168, 227] The human neonate often manifests mild breast enlargement at birth, and vaginal estrogenation may be evident in female infants at birth. Estrogen effects otherwise appear limited (see Table 21–4).

FETAL GROWTH

Insulin-like Growth Factors

The somatomedins are involved in regulation of uterine and placental growth during pregnancy and in early embryonic and fetal development. IGF-I, EGF, and estrogens are mitogens for endometrial stromal cells, and the endometrial contents of IGF-I and IGF-I mRNA are high at implantation and during early embryogenesis in the sow.[228] Uterine IGF-I and IGF-I mRNA levels decrease progressively with advancing gestation.[228] Placental tissue also contains IGF-I and IGF-II mRNAs, significant concentrations of the respective proteins, and IGF-I receptors.[59, 60] Autocrine and paracrine roles for the IGFs in uterine and placental tissues are postulated. IGF-I and insulin are produced by embryonic tissues during the prepancreatic stage of mouse development, and both factors stimulate growth of embryonic mouse cells.[229]

Immunoreactive IGF-I is present in most fetal tissues including brain, and fetal growth is regulated by the somatomedins.[230–233] Transgenic mice with inactivating mutations of IGF-I, IGF-II, or IGF-I receptor have reduced birth weights, organ hypoplasia, and delayed bone development.[230, 231] Animals deficient in IGF-I receptor and some mice deficient in IGF-I die at birth; mice deficient in IGF-II survive and have near-normal postnatal growth, whereas surviving IGF-I–deficient animals have deficient postnatal growth. IGF-I and IGF-II mRNAs are localized in mesenchymal and fibroblast-like cells in interstitial and perivascular connective tissues and surrounding capsular tissues.[234] In addition, immunoreactive IGF-I is produced by in vitro explant cultures of fetal mouse tissues, and fibroblasts cultured from fetal rat lung and skin synthesize both IGFs.[234] These findings are consistent with a predominantly paracrine mode of action for these growth factors in the fetus.

Somatomedin-binding proteins are present as early as 5 weeks of gestation, and prenatally, as postnatally, somatomedins circulate associated with binding proteins.[106, 235] Thus, during fetal and postnatal life, plasma concentrations of somatomedins are relatively high compared with tissue concentrations. In the fetus, IGF-II levels are higher than those of IGF-I, in contrast to these levels in children and adults. Fetal levels of both peptides at term are 30% to 50% of adult levels. In most studies, cord blood IGF-I concentrations correlate with birth size.[235] In spite of the fetal growth-enhancing effects of IGF-II, IGF-II levels are only weakly related to size at birth, largely because of the inhibiting effect of soluble IGF-II receptor (IGF2R).[236] Soluble IGF2R is derived through proteolytic cleavage of the transmembrane region of the receptor in many tissues. Somatomedin receptors have been identified as early as 5 weeks of gestation and are widespread in fetal tissues.[235] IGF-I stimulates glycogenesis in cultured fetal rat hepatocytes and induces formation of myotubes in cultured myoblasts. IGF-II is active in cultured muscle and neonatal rat astroglial cells. Insulin receptors are increased in fetal cells and are resistant to down-regulation; no similar data are available for the IGF-I receptor.

As discussed earlier, GH receptors are relatively deficient and receptors for hPL predominate in fetal tissues.[108, 109] Moreover, hPL stimulates IGF-I production and augments amino acid transport and DNA synthesis in human fetal fibroblasts and muscle cells. In addition, nutrition influences somatomedins in developing mammals. IGF-I levels fell in suckling rats deprived of milk,[235] and IGF-I and IGF-II levels were reduced in fetuses of protein-starved pregnant rats and placentally restricted sheep.[107, 237] The low IGF-II levels in the protein-starved rats were reversed by hPL.[237] There is no evidence that thyroid hormones modulate GH or somatomedin levels in the mammalian fetus but, as mentioned earlier, glucocorticoids can inhibit fetal growth, presumably by inhibiting somatomedin action.

These data support the view that the somatomedins are important in embryonic and fetal growth and that in the fetus they are regulated, at least in part, by hPL and by nutritional substrate derived transplacentally. The high levels of IGF-II in fetal rat serum, the high levels of IGF-II mRNA in fetal tissues, and the presence of a truncated form of IGF-I in human fetal brain tissue suggest unique developmental actions of these peptides[235, 237] (Table 21–5).

Insulin

Insulin has been proposed to act as a fetal growth factor. Infants born to women with diabetes mellitus may have hyperinsulinemia associated with increased birth weight.[238] Most of this increased weight is accounted for by body fat; there is little increase in body length, but some organomegaly may

Table 21–5. Growth Factors and Fetal Growth*

Tissues Affected	Growth Factors
Neural tissue	BNF, NT3, NGF
	Neuregulin, TGF-α, EGF
	IGF-I, IGF-II
Ectodermal derivatives	TGF-α, EGF, PDGF
	IGF-II, IGF-I
Mesodermal derivatives	IGF-II, IGF-I
	TGF-α, EGF, FGF family, Insulin, PDGF
Endodermal derivatives	IGF-II, IGF-I
	TGF-α, EGF, FGF
Hematopoietic tissues	HGF, EGF, PDGF
	Colony-stimulating factors
Specialized tissues	
Adipose tissue	Insulin
Skeletal tissue	PTHrP, IGF-I, IGF-II
	Calcitonin

*This listing will be expanded and more detailed as knockout and other information develops.

BNF, brain-derived neurotropic factor; EGF, epidermal growth factor; FGF, fibroblast growth factor; HGF, hematopoietic growth factor; IGF-II, insulin-like growth factor; NGF, nerve growth factor; NT3, neurotropin 3; PDGF, platelet-derived growth factor; PTHrP, parathyroid hormone–related protein; TGF-α, transforming growth factor α.

occur. Infants with hyperinsulinemia caused by nesidioblastosis or the Beckwith-Wiedemann syndrome may also have increased somatic growth in utero. Conversely, the human fetus with pancreatic agenesis is small and has decreased muscle bulk and little or no adipose tissue.[238] Homozygosity for a null mutation of the insulin receptor gene in fetal mice led to early neonatal death with hyperglycemia and ketonemia; the pups, however, had a normal birth weight.[239] These and other studies suggest that insulin may act as a fetal growth factor by promoting growth or hypertrophy of selected tissues. In clinical conditions associated with fetal hyperinsulinemia, insulin may act through insulin receptors (in adipose and liver tissues) or through type I IGF-I receptors. Insulin may also have a role in regulating IGF-I release.[238]

Epidermal Growth Factor–Transforming Growth Factor α System

The EGF/TGF-α system has been characterized in considerable detail.[240–245] EGF is a 6-kd peptide product of a large 1207-amino-acid precursor molecule and acts through a 170-kd membrane receptor glycoprotein. This receptor, like the somatomedin receptor, has intrinsic tyrosine kinase activity, and tyrosine kinase–mediated autophosphorylation is a critical event in EGF signal transduction. TGF-α, which has 35% amino acid homology with murine EGF and 44% homology with human EGF, also acts through the EGF receptor system.[240, 241] Several additional family members have been characterized, including amphiregulin, heparin-binding EGF, betacellulin, and neuregulins.[241–243] Three additional receptors are referred to as ErbB2, ErbB3, and ErbB4 in animals; the human receptors are referred to as human EGF receptor (HER) 2, 3, and 4.[241, 244] All were characterized in malignant tissues, where they function as oncogenes, and all are widely distributed in normal mammalian tissues.

EGF is a potent mitogen for ectodermal and mesodermal cells in tissue and organ culture.[240–241] These cells include keratinocytes derived from skin and conjunctival and pharyngeal tissues, corneal endothelial cells, vascular smooth muscle cells, chondrocytes, fibroblasts, liver cells, thyroid follicular cells, granulosa cells, and mammary gland cells. In adult humans, EGF is present in highest concentrations in sweat glands, salivary glands, Brunner's (duodenal) glands, stomach, pancreas, bone marrow, prostate, kidney, and endocrine glands (pituitary, adrenal, and thyroid). High concentrations of EGF are also present in urine.[240]

The roles of EGF and TGF-α in humans are incompletely understood. In rodents and sheep, EGF provokes precocious eyelid opening and tooth eruption in neonatal animals; stimulates lung maturation; promotes palatal development in organ culture; stimulates gastrointestinal maturation; evokes secretion of pituitary hormones including GH, PRL, and corticotropin; and stimulates secretion of chorionic gonadotropin and placental lactogen by the placenta.[240, 242, 246] Both EGF and TGF-α compete for binding to the EGF receptor, and both factors accelerate eye opening and tooth eruption in the neonatal rodent, presumably through interaction with the same "EGF" receptor.[240]

EGF and pre-pro-EGF mRNA are present in most tissues in the postnatal rodent and most adult mouse tissues, but mRNA levels are highest in salivary glands and kidneys. EGF and pre-pro-EGF mRNA levels are absent or low in the fetal rodent, and levels remain low in mouse tissues during the early neonatal period.[240] Nonetheless, the EGF receptor knockout mouse exhibits epithelial immaturity and multiorgan failure with early death.[242] Tissue concentrations of both EGF and EGF mRNA increase in the mouse during the first 2 months of postnatal life; indeed, levels of EGF in the salivary glands increase several thousandfold between 3 weeks and 3 months of age. Mouse urinary levels increase 200-fold, and kidney concentrations increase 10-fold between 1 week and 2 months of age. EGF concentrations in mouse ocular tissues increase 100-fold during the first week of life.[240] Liver EGF concentrations increase more slowly, as do serum levels, and there is a high degree of correlation between serum and liver EGF levels in the developing mouse.[240] Thus, the production of EGF in the rodent is accelerated during the early neonatal period, and it is during this time that most hormone-stimulated growth and development occur.

There are few data on tissue TGF-α concentrations in developing mammals.[240, 247] Immunoreactive TGF-α concentrations are measurable at relatively high levels in lung and brain tissues at 20 days of gestation in the rat and show minimal changes through day 50 postnatally.[247] Liver, which also has high TGF-α levels at 20 days of gestation, shows a progressive reduction in concentrations postnatally to nadir values in the young adult. Kidney tissue has low concentrations of TGF-α in late gestation, and levels increase progressively during the first 2 months of postnatal life. Thus, the ontogenic pattern of TGF-α is tissue specific; most late fetal tissues studied contain TGF-α, and levels persist or increase in most tissues through the period of growth and development.[247]

EGF plays an important role in pregnancy and fetal development. Maternal salivary gland and plasma EGF concentrations in the mouse increase fourfold to fivefold during pregnancy.[248] Removal of the salivary glands prevents the increase in plasma EGF; moreover, salivary gland removal reduces the number of mice completing term pregnancy (by 50%), decreases the percentage of live pups, and decreases the crown-rump length of fetuses delivered.[248] Administration of EGF antiserum to pregnant mice without salivary glands further increases the abortion rate, whereas administration of EGF improves pregnancy outcome.[248] These observations suggest an important role of EGF in pregnancy in the mouse. Because maternal EGF is too large a molecule to traverse the placental barrier, an effect on maternal metabolism and an effect on the placenta are likely.[248] The placenta is richly endowed with EGF receptors, and placental tissue binds and degrades EGF to constituent amino acids.[240]

EGF receptors are present in embryonal and fetal tissues, and EGF stimulates protein synthesis during the morula-blastocyst transition and in postimplantation mouse embryo tissue.[240] In vitro, EGF stimulates differentiation of the inner cell mass during early embryonic development.[249] However, EGF and EGF precursor mRNA levels are absent or present at low levels in selected fetal mouse tissues.[240] Low levels are also present in submandibular gland and kidney during the early neonatal period. Fetal mouse and human tissues have high levels of TGF-α, suggesting that this factor may be the ligand for the fetal EGF receptor.[250] TGF-α is produced by the maternal decidua during the first half of gestation in rodents, and pro–TGF-α mRNA is present in decidua. Decidual pro–TGF-α mRNA levels peak at 8 days of gestation (term = 21 days) and decline through day 15, when the decidua is being absorbed. EGF receptors are present in decidua, and TGF-α may stimulate proliferation of decidual tissue and enhance decidual PRL production.

Inactivation of the gene encoding the EGF receptor in mice led to fetal or neonatal death of homozygous fetuses.[242] The receptor-deficient animals manifested impaired epithelial development in several organs, including skin, lungs, and gastrointestinal tract. Further evidence for a role of EGF in early mammalian development has come from studies of the effect of the administration of EGF antiserum to neonatal mice.[251] EGF antiserum delayed eye and ear opening, delayed tooth eruption, accelerated hair growth, and reduced weight gain during the first 30 days of life.

The factors that control EGF and TGF-α production are incompletely understood. The increases in EGF concentration in tissues, blood, and urine of the neonatal rodent correlate with and may be conditioned by the increases in thyroidal and gonadal hormone levels.[240] EGF concentrations in the mouse submandibular gland are increased by thyroid hormones and testosterone. Thyroid hormones increase EGF concentrations in skin, ocular tissue, kidney, and urine in the developing mouse and up-regulate EGF gene expression and the production of pro-EGF in rat kidney; thyroid hormones also increase EGF receptor levels in developing mouse skin and liver.[221, 223, 240, 252] Urinary EGF excretion is highly correlated with serum thyroid hormone concentrations in premature and term human infants.[253] GH increases urinary EGF concentrations in the neonatal mouse, and estrogens increase EGF and EGF mRNA levels in mouse uterus.[240] Testosterone stimulates EGF and EGF mRNA levels in submandibular gland and increases EGF receptor levels in prostatic tissue.[240, 254] Thus, EGF may mediate growth and developmental actions of a variety of hormones in selected tissues (see Table 21–5). There is little information about the regulation of TGF-α production postnatally or prenatally. Amphiregulin binds to and stimulates EGF receptor and HER2 in human epithelial cells and has been localized to breast and colonic epithelium.[255]

Considerable evidence suggests a role for the EGF family of growth factors in mammalian central nervous system development.[240] EGF, TGF-α, neuregulins, and the EGF receptors are widely distributed in the nervous system.[240, 256–260] EGF promotes proliferation of astroglial cells, acts as an astroglial differentiation factor, and enhances survival and outgrowth of selected neuronal cells.[256, 257] Transgenic mice with a deficiency of neuregulin, ErbB2, ErbB3, or ErbB4 die in utero with cardiac anomalies and developmental anomalies of the hindbrain, midbrain, and ventral forebrain[244, 245, 258, 259] (see Table 21–5).

Nerve Growth Factor

NGF is a 13-kd protein that is present at high concentrations in mouse salivary gland and at low concentrations in many adult tissues.[241] It is also produced by human placental tissue. It is the original member of an expanding family of neurotropic growth factors that now include brain-derived neurotropic factor, neurotropin 3, and two less well characterized factors and involving two receptors, NGF and NGF2 (or Trk).[241, 261–264]

NGF binds to high-affinity plasma membrane receptors and is internalized and transported to subcellular organelles, including the nucleus, in neurons of the peripheral nervous system. It promotes neurite outgrowth and enhances tyrosine hydroxylase and dopamine β-hydroxylase activities in developing sympathetic neurons. NGF acts on undifferentiated sympathetic cell precursors to evoke both hyperplastic and hypertrophic effects[241, 261] and plays a permissive role in stimulating the development of immature autonomic neurons along either a sympathetic or a cholinergic pathway.[261]

The injection of NGF in neonatal mice causes a marked increase in the volume of the superior cervical ganglia and increases in RNA polymerase, ornithine decarboxylase, and tyrosine hydroxylase activities. This growth factor also increases the nerve supply of body organs. Likewise, injection of NGF antiserum during early neonatal life results in a decrease in the size of the superior cervical ganglia, reduction in tyrosine hydroxylase activity, and permanent sympathectomy.[261] Maternal NGF autoantibodies in rats and rabbits impair autonomic nervous system development in utero.[262, 265] This impairment affects sympathetic and dorsal root ganglia and autonomic innervation of peripheral organs. NGF is produced by neonatal mouse astroglial cells in tissue culture, is present in developing mouse brain tissue, and, with brain-derived neurotropic factor and neurotropin 3, plays an important role in brain development.[263, 264, 266, 267]

Thyroid hormones and testosterone modulate postnatal NGF levels in the submandibular gland of the mouse. Thyroid hormones increase NGF, neurotropin 3, and brain-derived neurotropic factor mRNA levels in adult rat brain.[268]

Other Factors

Additional growth factors are involved in fetal growth and development, including hematopoietic growth factors, platelet-derived growth factors, fibroblast growth factors, vascular endothelial growth factor, and members of the TGF-β family.[241, 269–271]

Hematopoietic growth factors are also active in the fetus during development[272–275]; erythropoietin in the fetal sheep is produced by the liver rather than the kidney and erythropoietin gene expression in fetal sheep is regulated by glucocorticoids.[274] A switch to kidney production occurs after parturition.[275, 276] Postnatally, thyroid hormones, testosterone, and hypoxia modulate erythropoietin production.

Platelet-derived growth factor (PDGF) represents a family of homodimers and heterodimers of PDGF-A and PDGF-B chains derived from two gene loci.[270] Two PDGF receptors have been characterized, PDGFα and PDGFβ. The genes for PDGF and its receptors are expressed in many tissues. PDGF-A gene inactivation in mice led to defects in lung, skin, intestine, testes, and brain resulting in early postnatal death.[270] PDGF-B gene inactivation led to microvessel disruption and leakage with hemorrhage and edema and intrauterine death.[270]

The fibroblast growth factor (FGF) family of heparin-binding growth factors now includes 17 members with diverse effects on development, angiogenesis, wound healing, and other biologic systems.[241, 277] These effects are mediated by ligand-activated tyrosine protein kinase receptors (FGFRs) transcribed from four related genes. Several receptor isoforms are products of alternative RNA splicing.[241, 277]

Targeted disruptions of FGF and FGFR genes in mice have

defined critical roles in development.[241, 277–279] FGF3-deficient mice show tail and inner ear defects. Knockout of the *FGF4* gene is lethal, leading to early death. Knockout of the *FGFR1* gene also leads to early fetal death. *FGF10* knockout mice die at birth because of pulmonary agenesis. FGF4, FGF8, FGF9, FGF10, or FGF17 deficiency is associated with limb deformities. FGF8 deficiency leads to abnormal left-right axis patterning. In mice, *FGFR3* knockout results in chondrocyte hypertrophy and increased bone length.[241]

In humans, a variety of gain-of-function FGFR mutations are associated with chondrodysplasias and craniosynostosis syndromes.[241] FGF, like EGF, stimulates the production of hCG from a choriocarcinoma cell line.[280] These observations and the fact that the placenta contains FGF, NGF, TGF-α, TGF-β, IGF-I, and IGF-II suggest that the placenta may play an important role in modulating fetal growth (see Table 21–5).

TRANSITION TO EXTRAUTERINE LIFE

The transition to extrauterine life involves abrupt delivery from the protected intrauterine environment and succor by the placenta to the relatively hostile extrauterine environment. The neonate must initiate air breathing and defend against hypothermia, hypoglycemia, and hypocalcemia as the placental supply of energy and nutritional substrate is removed. Both the adrenal cortex and the autonomic nervous system, including the para-aortic chromaffin system, are essential for extrauterine adaptation. Longer term transition requires adaptation to an environment of intermittent nutrient supply and transient substrate deficiency and requires maturation of the secretory control mechanisms for the PTH-calcitonin system and the endocrine pancreas.

Cortisol Surge

In most mammals, a cortisol surge occurs near term and is mediated by increased cortisol production by the fetal adrenal and a decreased rate of conversion of cortisol to cortisone. Pepe and Albrecht[21] have proposed that the preterm fetal cortisol surge is due to the progressive stimulation by estrogens of placental 11β–HSD activity and the subsequent increase in placental conversion of cortisol to cortisone. The resulting decrease in maternal-to-fetal cortisol transfer results in stimulation of fetal CRH and corticotropin secretion through the negative-feedback control loop. The concomitant estrogen-stimulated increase in 11β–HSD activity in fetal tissues potentiates the relative fetal cortisol deficiency and the CRH-corticotropin response.[21] Placental CRH may also potentiate the fetal adrenal activation.

The cortisol surge augments surfactant synthesis in lung tissue; increases lung liquid reabsorption; increases adrenomedullary phenylethanolamine *N*-methyltransferase activity, which in turn increases methylation of NE to epinephrine; increases hepatic iodothyronine outer-ring monodeiodinase activity and hence increases conversion of T_4 to T_3; decreases sensitivity of the ductus arteriosus to prostaglandins, which facilitates ductus closure; induces maturation of several enzymes and transport processes of the small intestine; and stimulates maturation of hepatic enzymes[8, 125, 281] (Fig. 21–12). In some cases, these events involve increased synthesis of specific proteins or enzymes. In other instances, such as the action on the ductus arteriosus, the mechanism remains obscure.

Secondary effects of cortisol also promote extrauterine adaptations. The increased T_3 levels stimulate β-adrenergic receptor binding, potentiate surfactant synthesis in lung tissue, and increase the sensitivity of brown adipose tissue to NE. The significance of prenatal cortisol is demonstrated by the effects of gene-targeted CRH or glucocorticoid receptor deficiency in mice; the progeny of homozygous CRH-deficient or glucocorticoid receptor–deficient animals die in the first 12 hours with lung dysplasia and surfactant deficiency.[282, 283]

Catecholamine Surge

Parturition also evokes a dramatic catecholamine surge in the newborn, resulting in extraordinarily high levels of NE, epinephrine, and dopamine in cord blood.[193] As indicated earlier, plasma NE concentrations exceed epinephrine levels because of peripheral and adrenomedullary and para-aortic catecholamine release. Cord blood NE levels of 15 nmol/L (2500 pg/mL) and epinephrine levels of 2 nmol/L (370 pg/mL) are common after spontaneous delivery of term infants.[193] Levels of 25 nmol/L (4200 pg/mL) of NE and 35 nmol/L (640 pg/mL) of epinephrine are common in cord blood of premature infants. These changes evoke critical cardiovascular adaptations, including increased blood pressure and increased cardiac inotropic effects; increased glucagon secretion; decreased insulin secretion; increased thermogenesis in brown adipose tissue and increased plasma free fatty acid levels; and pulmonary adaptation, including mobilization of pulmonary fluid and increased surfactant release.[193, 195, 281]

Thermogenesis in Neonatal Brown Adipose Tissue

Brown adipose tissue is the major site of thermogenesis in the newborn and is especially prominent in the mammalian fetus. The largest accumulations of brown adipose tissue envelop the kidneys and adrenal glands, and smaller amounts surround the blood vessels of the mediastinum and neck.[284] The mass of brown adipose tissue peaks at the time of birth and gradually decreases during the early weeks of life. Surgical removal of this tissue leads to neonatal hypothermia. NE, through β-adrenergic receptors, stimulates thermogenesis by brown adipose tissue, and optimal responsiveness of this tissue to NE is dependent on thyroid hormone.[284, 285]

Brown adipose tissue is rich in mitochondria containing a unique 32-kd protein (thermogenin) that uncouples oxidation and phosphorylation of adenosine diphosphate, reduces adenosine triphosphate production, and consequently enhances thermogenesis.[284, 286] Thermogenin is T_3-dependent, and brown adipose tissue contains a 5′-monoiodothyronine deiodinase that synthesizes T_3 locally from T_4.[284, 286]

Full maturation of catecholamine-stimulated cellular respiration in brown adipose tissue occurs before delivery in the ovine fetus and requires thyroid hormone.[284, 286–288] Fetal thyroidectomy in this species leads to marked hypothermia, with low plasma free fatty acid levels and increased plasma epinephrine concentrations.[286] In vitro, basal brown adipose tissue thermogenesis and NE-stimulated and dibutyryl cAMP–stimulated thermogenesis are decreased by fetal thyroidectomy.

The rapid onset of thermogenesis in brown adipose tissue is essential for survival in newborn infants. Catecholamine release is the stimulus for brown adipose tissue thermogenesis in the early neonatal period, and responsiveness to catecholamines is markedly increased by cutting of the umbilical cord.[285] Fetal hypoxia and placental inhibitors, including prostaglandin E_2 and adenosine, appear to inhibit brown adipose tissue thermogenesis in utero.[285] Cord cutting, neonatal cooling, catecholamine stimulation, and augmented conversion of T_4 to T_3 in brown adipose tissue in the neonatal period are the essential features that mediate and condition newborn thermogenesis.

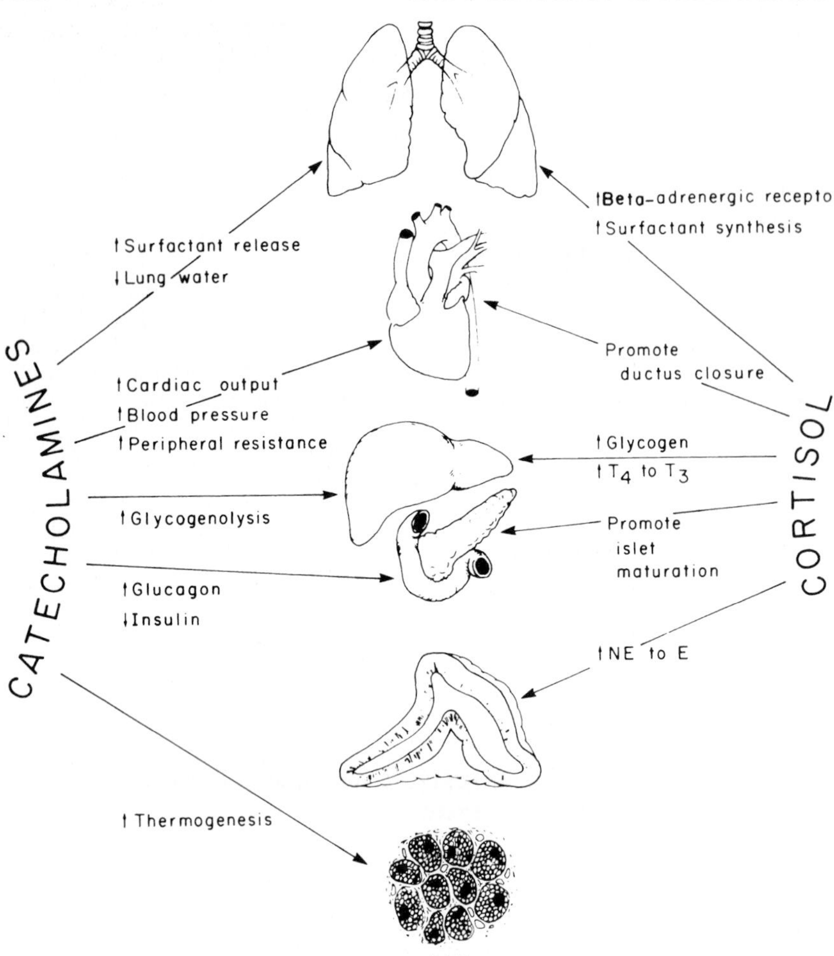

Figure 21–12. Actions of cortisol and catecholamines during fetal adaptation to the extrauterine environment. The prenatal cortisol surge acts to promote functional maturation of several organ systems as indicated. The neonatal catecholamine surge triggers or potentiates a number of the extrauterine cardiopulmonary and metabolic functional adaptations that are critical to extrauterine survival. See text for details. BAT, brown adipose tissue; E, epinephrine; NE, norepinephrine; T3, triiodothyronine; T4, thyroxine.

Calcium Homeostasis

The neonate must adjust rapidly from a *high-calcium* environment regulated by PTHrP and calcitonin to a *low-calcium* environment that requires regulation by PTH and vitamin D. With removal of the placenta in term infants, plasma total calcium concentration falls and reaches a nadir of approximately 2.3 mmol/L (9 mg/dL),[206] and the ionized calcium concentration reaches a low level of about 1.2 mmol/L (4.8 mg/dL) by 24 hours of life.[289] Plasma PTH levels are relatively low in the neonatal period and are minimally responsive to hypocalcemia during the first 2 to 3 days of life.

Calcitonin concentrations are high in cord blood (~2000 ng/L), increase further during the early neonatal period, and remain high for several days after birth.[206, 290] The relatively obtunded PTH response and the high calcitonin levels lead to a 2- to 3-day period of transient neonatal hypocalcemia.[290, 291] Inhibition of calcitonin secretion and stimulation of PTH secretion gradually result in increased serum calcium levels in the neonate. The disappearance of PTHrP in the neonatal lamb is approximately coincident with the time of restoration of calcium levels to the adult range.[206] The mechanism of transition from PTHrP to PTH secretion by the neonatal parathyroid glands is not clear.

Calcium homeostasis is also affected in the human newborn period by the low level of glomerular filtration that persists for several days.[290, 291] In addition, renal responsiveness to PTH is reduced in the first few days of life. These factors limit phosphate excretion and predispose the neonate to hyperphosphatemia, particularly if the diet includes high-phosphate milk such as unmodified cow's milk. Premature infants tend to have lower PTH and higher calcitonin levels and more immature kidney function; in these infants, neonatal hypocalcemia may be more marked and prolonged and the incidence of symptomatic hypocalcemia is higher. Birth asphyxia also predisposes the neonate to hypocalcemia.[291] Infants born to mothers with hypercalcemia related to hyperparathyroidism have a high incidence of symptomatic hypocalcemia. These infants have a more marked suppression of parathyroid function and a longer period of transient hypoparathyroidism in the neonatal period. PTH secretion and calcium homeostasis usually return to normal in 1 to 2 weeks in full-term infants and within 2 to 3 weeks in the small premature infant.

Glucose Homeostasis

The abrupt withdrawal of the placental glucose supply leads to a prompt fall in plasma glucose in the term neonate.[213, 214, 292] The low glucose and high catecholamine levels stimulate glucagon secretion, and the plasma glucagon level peaks within 2 hours after birth.[213, 214, 292] Plasma insulin levels are low at birth and tend to fall further with hypoglycemia. The early glucagon response is short-lived; however, levels remain at about 100 ng/L for the first 12 to 24 hours, and the glucagon/insulin ratio is high enough to stabilize glucose levels in the range 2.8 to 4 mmol/L (50 to 70 mg/dL) during this period.

The early glucagon and catecholamine surges deplete hepatic glycogen stores so that the return of plasma glucose levels to normal after 12 to 18 hours requires maturation of hepatic gluconeogenesis under the stimulus of a high plasma glucagon/insulin ratio.[214, 292] Glucagon secretion gradually increases during the early hours after birth, especially with protein feeding, which stimulates gut glucagon release and pancreatic glucagon secretion.[213, 214, 292] Premature infants have more severe and prolonged hypoglycemia because of reduced glycogen stores and impaired hepatic gluconeogenesis. Infants born to diabetic mothers have more severe neonatal hypoglycemia because of relative hyperinsulinism. In the healthy term infant, glucose homeostasis is achieved within 5 to 7 days of life; in premature infants, 1 to 2 weeks may be required.

Other Hormonal Adaptations

Delivery of the placenta results in decreases in fetal blood levels of estrogens, progesterone, hCG, and hPL. The fall in estrogen levels presumably removes the major stimulus to fetal PRL release, and PRL levels decrease within several weeks. The relatively delayed fall may be due to lactotrope hyperplasia in the fetal pituitary or to delayed maturation of hypothalamic dopamine secretion. The gradual fall of hGH levels during the early weeks of life is due to delayed maturation of hypothalamic-pituitary and feedback control of hGH release.[95] In the neonatal primate are concomitant decreases in plasma GH levels and GH responsiveness to exogenous GHRH.[293] The mechanisms remain unclear. Changes in secretion or in pituitary sensitivity to GHRH or somatostatin, or both, may be involved. Somatomedin levels fall to infantile values within a few days, presumably because of the removal of placental hPL and placental somatomedin production (see Fig. 21–5).

In male infants (see Fig. 21–11), after a transient fall in testosterone levels as the hCG stimulus abates, pituitary LH secretion rebounds and there is a secondary surge of plasma testosterone that persists at significant levels for several weeks.[95, 294, 295] This surge is mediated by hypothalamic LHRH, and blockade of neonatal activation of the pituitary-testicular axis with an LHRH agonist in neonatal monkeys ablated the neonatal increments in LH and testosterone.[295] Such a blockade also resulted in subnormal increments in plasma LH and testosterone levels and subnormal testicular enlargement at puberty in these animals, which suggests that neonatal LHRH release with pituitary-testicular activation may be critical for normal sexual maturation of male primates.[295] In females, a transient, secondary surge in FSH may transiently elevate estrogen levels.

Delivery results in a reversal of the high fetal cortisone/cortisol ratio, and plasma cortisol concentrations are higher in the neonate despite relatively lower plasma corticotropin concentrations (see Fig. 21–7). Presumably, this increase is due to decreased inhibition of adrenal 3β–HSD by estrogen and perhaps to removal of a placental CRH action on fetal pituitary corticotropin release. Plasma DHEAS and DHEA levels fall as the fetal adrenal atrophies.

The increase in serum thyrotropin levels during the early minutes after birth is due to cooling of the neonate in the extrauterine environment.[136, 144] The thyrotropin surge peaks at 30 minutes at a concentration of about 70 mU/L (see Fig. 21–9). This peak evokes increased secretion of T_4 and T_3 by the thyroid gland. In addition, increased conversion of T_4 to T_3 by liver and other tissues maintains the T_3 level in the extrauterine range of 1.6 to 3.4 nmol/L (105 to 220 ng/dL). The reequilibration of thyrotropin levels to the normal extrauterine range is probably due to the readjustment of prevailing serum T_3 levels and to maturation of feedback control of thyrotropin by thyroid hormones during the early weeks of life.[136, 147] Production of rT_3 by fetal and neonatal tissues abates by 3 to 4 weeks of age, at which time serum rT_3 reaches adult levels.

IMPRINTING OF DEVELOPING ENDOCRINE SYSTEMS

Data for several mammalian species indicate that hormonal imprinting or programming occurs during a critical fetal or perinatal period of development. In the female rodent, transient neonatal androgen administration masculinized the pattern of hypothalamic control of LHRH secretion and pituitary gonadotropin secretion, masculinized adult behavior and adult sexual activity, permanently altered the pattern of GH secretion, increased longitudinal bone growth and body weight, and masculinized the pattern of hepatic steroid metabolism.[296, 297] Prenatal androgens program the timing of neuroendocrine puberty in sheep; the higher the dose of prenatal testosterone, the earlier the initiation of the pubertal LH rise.[298] Estrogen administration to pregnant rats during the last third of gestation produced cryptorchid male offspring and may permanently suppress spermatogenesis in adult males.[299]

Perinatal estrogen administration to the developing female rodent produced long-term effects including persistent vaginal cornification, hyperplastic vaginal lesions, and cervicovaginal cancer; synthetic nonsteroidal estrogen (diethylstilbestrol) had similar effects.[300–302] Chronic hyperprolactinemia also occurred, presumably secondary to the low-level continuous estrogen secretion in these anovulatory animals.[300] Prenatal or neonatal diethylstilbestrol in the hamster predisposed to hyperplastic and neoplastic uterine lesions. In these exposed animals uterine levels of c-Jun, c-Fos, c-Myc, BAX, and Bcl-x were markedly increased in luminal and glandular epithelial cells, whereas Bcl-2 levels were decreased.[301] Glucocorticoids are essential for many aspects of normal brain development. Rodents and primates exposed to excess levels of glucocorticoid in utero exhibited hyperactivity of the hypothalamic-pituitary-adrenal axis.[303] Behavioral alterations after glucocorticoid exposure have also been documented in rodent species.

Transient levothyroxine administration to neonatal rodents led to growth retardation, delayed puberty, decreased adult pituitary weight, decreased pituitary TRH concentrations, low serum thyrotropin levels, and decreased thyrotropin responsiveness to propylthiouracil challenge.[304, 305] Adult adrenal function and EGF metabolism were also altered.[306] Administration of insulin or alloxan to neonatal rats produced permanent alteration of glucose tolerance,[307] and a single dose of vasopressin to the neonatal rat permanently enhanced the adult response to vasopressin.[308] Neonatal catecholamine administration altered the response of adult rat vascular tissue to NE.[302] Fetal exposure to high maternal glucocorticoid levels in the rat inhibited fetal growth and led to subsequent hypertension in the offspring.[309]

There is less information about hormonal imprinting in primates and humans. Blockade of LHRH in neonatal monkeys with an LHRH agonist resulted in obtundation of plasma LH and testosterone levels and decreased testicular size at puberty.[295] Diethylstilbestrol administration to pregnant women increased the prevalence of vaginal adenocarcinoma in female offspring during the second and third decades of life.[310] Congenital hypothyroidism in human infants may be associated with alteration of the set-point for feedback control of thyrotropin release so that serum thyrotropin levels remain inappropriately elevated after return of serum T_4 levels to normal with treatment.[311]

A growing literature now supports the concept of fetal programming of cardiovascular disease. It is now clear that intrauterine growth retardation with low birth weight for gestational age is associated with an increased risk of hypertension, insulin resistance and diabetes, and coronary heart disease.[312–314] The mechanisms are not yet clear, but permanent prenatal changes of fetal endocrine and growth factor homeostasis seem to be involved. These include IGF metabolism, insulin secretion and action, kidney growth and structure, the renin-angiotensin system, and the hypothalamic-pituitary-adrenal axis.[312–314] These permanent changes also lead to reduced fetal growth and raised blood pressure in the next generation.[315] The evidence also suggests that the polycystic ovary syndrome in women may be conditioned by excessive androgen exposure during fetal life.[316, 317]

The mechanisms for imprinting remain obscure. Neonatal administration of testosterone or glucocorticoid can have permanent effects on brain structure.[297, 303] The effects in some instances may be transmitted to subsequent generations.[304, 307, 315] A functional overlap of hormone-mediated imprinting may also occur; the administration of both thyrotropin and FSH to the rodent neonate altered the adult response to thyrotropin, and neonatal OT or vasopressin exposure can alter the adult response to vasopressin.[304, 308] Hormonal imprinting is also demonstrable in cell lines and in unicellular organisms, in which a single exposure to a hormone can produce persistent alteration of the hormonal response characteristics.[302]

These observations suggest that hormone imprinting or programming may be due to plasticity of the hormone system during a critical period of maturation. Gene expression and nuclear receptors or plasma membrane receptors, or both, may be involved.[303] Prohormone processing may also be involved; in newborn rat intermediate pituitary lobe cells, in vitro treatment with dexamethasone decreased production of α-MSH and increased production of corticotropin-related peptides.[318] Whatever the mechanisms, the developing endocrine systems have significant plasticity, and the maturation of endocrine control systems can be influenced by alterations in the prevailing hormone concentrations.

SUMMARY

The foregoing review summarizes current understanding of the intrauterine endocrine milieu and highlights progress in this challenging frontier of medicine. This progress has set the stage for fetal endocrine disease diagnosis, therapy of fetal endocrine and metabolic disorders, management of disorders of fetal growth, and diagnosis and management of perinatal or neonatal endocrine dysfunction. In addition, understanding of developmental endocrinology is increasingly relevant to management strategies for premature infants and infants and children with fetal growth retardation and for our understanding of the pathogenesis of adult endocrine and metabolic diseases.

We are now entering the era of direct access to and management of the intrauterine environment with provision of medical and surgical fetal therapy, entailing both potential advantages and risks.[319, 320] With expansion of the application and scope of amniotic fluid and fetal cell sampling and the advent of fetal visualization and intrauterine fetal blood sampling, direct access for fetal diagnosis is now possible.[145, 321–323] Women are treated with glucocorticoids to stimulate fetal lung maturation.[324] Intrauterine diagnosis and treatment of fetal adrenal and thyroid disorders have become the standard of care.[325–327] Intravenous nutritional supplementation of fetal sheep can prevent some forms of growth retardation, and chronic fetal therapy through indwelling pumps is feasible in animal fetuses.[328] These approaches, coupled with increasing availability of synthetic hormones and growth factor agonists and antagonists, facilitate direct fetal endocrine therapy. In addition, intrauterine stem cell transplantation has been successful in the correction of congenital hematologic disease; the fetus in early gestation is a favorable recipient of cellular therapy, and fetal cell transplantation may be applicable to therapy for selected endocrine and metabolic diseases.[329]

References

1. Petraglia F, Santuz M, Florio P, et al. Paracrine regulation of human placenta: control of hormonogenesis. J Reprod Immunol 1998; 39:221–233.
2. Tamaka TS, Jaradat SA, Lim MK, et al. Genome-wide expression profiling of the mid-gestation placenta and embryo using a 15,000 mouse developmental cDNA microarray. Proc Natl Acad Sci USA 2000; 97:9127–9132.
3. Albrecht ED, Pepe GJ. Central integrative role of oestrogen in modulating the communication between the placenta and fetus that results in primate fetal-placental development. Placenta 1999; 20:129–139.
4. Chard T. Proteins of the human placenta: some general concepts. In Grudzinskas JG, Seppala M (eds). Pregnancy Proteins. New York, Academic Press, 1982, pp 3–21.
5. Jaffe RB, Neuroendocrine-metabolic regulation of pregnancy, In Yen SSC, Jaffe RB, Barbieri RL (eds). Reproductive Endocrinology, 4th ed. Philadelphia, WB Saunders, 1999, pp 757-784.
6. Leach L, Firth JA. Advances in understanding permeability in fetal capillaries of the human placenta: a review of the organization of the endothelial paracellular clefts and their junctional complexes. Reprod Fertil Dev 1995; 7:1451–1456.
7. Sibley CP, Boyd RDH. Mechanisms of transfer across the human placenta. In Polin RA, Fox WW (eds). Fetal and Neonatal Physiology, 2nd ed. Philadelphia, WB Saunders, 1998, pp 77–89.
8. Fisher DA. Fetal and neonatal endocrinology. In DeGroot LJ, Jameson JL (eds). Endocrinology, 4th ed. Philadelphia, WB Saunders, 2000, pp 2400–2411.
9. Palfi M, Selbing A. Placental transport of maternal immunoglobulin G. Am J Reprod Immunol 1998; 39:24–26.
10. Blay J, Hollenberg MD. The nature and function of the polypeptide growth factor receptors in the human placenta. J Dev Physiol 1989; 12:237–248.
11. Jones CJP, Hartmann M, Desoye G. Ultrastructural localization of insulin receptors in human placenta. Am J Reprod Immunol 1993; 30:136–145.
12. Sodha RJ, Proegler M, Schneider H. Transfer and metabolism of norepinephrine studied from maternal to fetal and fetal to maternal sides in the in vitro perfused human placental life. Am J Obstet Gynecol 1984; 148:474–481.
13. Benediktsson R, Calder A, Edwards CRW, Seckl JR. Placental 11β-hydroxysteroid dehydrogenase: a key regulator of fetal glucocorticoid exposure. Clin Endocrinol (Oxf) 1997; 46:161–166.
14. Krysin E, Brzezinska-Slebodzinska E, Slebodzinski AB. Divergent deiodination of thyroid hormones in the separated parts of the fetal and maternal placenta in pigs. J Endocrinol 1997; 155:295–303.
15. Murphy BEP. Cortisol and cortisone in human fetal development. J Steroid Biochem 1979; 11:509–513.
16. Takeyama J, Sasano H, Suzuki T, et al. 17β-Hydroxysteroid dehydrogenase types 1 and 2 in human placenta: an immunohistochemical study with correlation to placental development. J Clin Endocrinol Metab 1998; 83:3710–3715.
17. Roti E, Gnudi A, Braverman LE. The placental transport, synthesis and metabolism of hormones and drugs which affect thyroid function. Endocr Rev 1983; 4:131–149.
18. Iisalo E, Castren O. The enzymatic inactivation of noradrenaline in human placental tissue. Ann Med Exp Biol Fenn 1967; 45: 253–257.
19. Siler-Khodr TM. Endocrine and paracrine function of the human placenta, In Polin RA, Fox WW (eds). Fetal and Neonatal Physiology, 2nd ed. Philadelphia, WB Saunders, 1998, pp 89–102.
20. Albrecht ED, Pepe GJ. Placental steroid hormone biosynthesis in primate pregnancy. Endocr Rev 1990; 11:124–150.
21. Pepe GJ, Albrecht ED. Actions of placental and fetal adrenal steroid hormones in primate pregnancy. Endocr Rev 1995; 16: 608–648.
22. Diczfalusy E. Endocrine functions of the human fetoplacental unit. Fed Proc 1964; 23:791–798.
23. Falcone T, Little AB. Placental synthesis of steroid hormones. In

Tulchinsky D, Little AB (eds). Maternal-Fetal Endocrinology, 2nd ed. Philadelphia, WB Saunders, 1994, pp 2–14.
24. Albrecht ED, Aberdeen GW, Pepe GJ. The role of estrogen in the maintenance of primate pregnancy. Am J Obstet Gynecol 2000; 182:432–438.
25. Perry S, Strauss JF III. Placental hormones. In DeGroot LJ, Jameson JL (eds). Endocrinology, 4th ed. Philadelphia, WB Saunders, 2000, pp 2379–2390.
26. Falcone T, Little AB. Placental polypeptides. In Tulchinsky D, Little AB (eds). Maternal-Fetal Endocrinology, 2nd ed. Philadelphia, WB Saunders, 1994, pp 15–32.
27. Yoshimura M, Hershman JM. Thyrotropic action of human chorionic gonadotropin. Thyroid 1995; 5:425–434.
28. Miller WL, Eberhardt NL. Structure and evolution of the growth hormone gene family. Endocr Rev 1983; 4:97–130.
29. Barsh GS, Seeburg PH, Gelinas RE. The human growth hormone gene family: structure and evolution of the chromosomal locus. Nucleic Acids Res 1983; 11:3939–3985.
30. Walker WH, Fitzpatrick AL, Barrera-Saldana HA, et al. The human placental lactogen genes: structure, function, evolution, and transcriptional regulation. Endocr Rev 1991; 12:316–328.
31. MacLeod JN, Lee AK, Liebhaber A, et al. Developmental control and alternative splicing of the placentally expressed transcripts from the human growth hormone gene cluster. J Biol Chem 1992; 267:14219–14226.
32. Boguszewski CL, Svensson PA, Jansson T, et al. Cloning of two novel growth hormone transcripts expressed in human placenta. J Clin Endocrinol Metab 1998; 83:2878–2885.
33. Golander A, Hurley T, Barrett J, et al. Prolactin synthesis by human chorion-decidual tissue: a possible source of prolactin in the amniotic fluid. Science 1978; 202:311–313.
34. Grino M, Chrousos GP, Margioris AN. The corticotropin releasing hormone gene is expressed in human placenta. Biochem Biophys Res Commun 1987; 148:1208–1214.
35. Margioris AN, Grino M, Protos P, et al. Corticotropin releasing hormone and oxytocin stimulate the release of placental proopiomelanocortin peptides. J Clin Endocrinol Metab 1988; 66:922–926.
36. Qu J, Thomas K. Inhibin and activin production in human placenta. Endocr Rev 1995; 16:485–507.
37. Petraglia F. Inhibin, activin and follistatin in the human placenta: a new family of regulatory proteins. Placenta 1997; 18:3–8.
38. Yamaguchi M, Endo H, Tasaka K, et al. Mouse growth hormone releasing factor secretion is activated by inhibin and inhibited by activin in placenta. Biol Reprod 1995; 16:368–372.
39. Poisner AM. The human placental renin-angiotensin system. Front Neuroendocrinol 1998; 19:232–252.
40. Millan MA, Carvallo P, Izumi SI, et al. Novel sites of expression of functional angiotensin II receptors in the late gestation fetus. Science 1989; 244:1340–1342.
41. Ferguson JE, Seaner RM, Bruns DE, et al. Expression and specific immunolocalization of the human parathyroid hormone/parathyroid hormone–related protein receptor in the uteroplacental unit. Am J Obstet Gynecol 1998; 179:321–329.
42. Curtis NE, Thomas RJ, Gillespie MT, et al. Parathyroid hormone related protein (PTHrP) mRNA splicing and parathyroid hormone/PTHrP receptor mRNA expression in human placenta and fetal membranes. J Mol Endocrinol 1998; 21:225–234.
43. Ferguson JE, Gorman JV, Bruns DE, et al. Abundant expression of parathyroid hormone related protein in human amnion and its association with labor. Proc Natl Acad Sci USA 1992; 89:8384–8388.
44. Karaplis AC, Luz A, Glowacki J, et al. Lethal skeletal dysplasia from targeted disruption of the parathyroid hormone–related peptide gene. Genes Dev 1994; 8:277–289.
45. Jousset V, Legendre B, Besnard P, et al. Calcitonin-like immunoreactivity and calcitonin gene expression in the placenta and in the mammary gland of the rat. Acta Endocrinol 1988; 119:443–451.
46. Hoggard N, Hunter L, Duncan JS, et al. Leptin and leptin receptor mRNA and protein expression in the murine fetus and placenta. Proc Natl Acad Sci USA 1997; 94:11073–11078.
47. Masuzaki H, Ogawa Y, Sagawa N, et al. Nonadipose tissue production of leptin: leptin as a novel placenta-derived hormone in humans. Nat Med 1997; 3:1029–1033.
48. Senaris R, Garcia-Caballero T, Casabiell X, et al. Synthesis of leptin in human placenta. Endocrinology 1997; 138:4501–4504.
49. Hassink SG, deLancey E, Sheslow DV, et al. Placental leptin: an important new growth factor in intrauterine and neonatal development. Pediatrics 1997; 100:1–6.
50. Polk DH, Reviczky AL, Lam RW, Fisher DA. Thyrotropin releasing hormone in the ovine fetus: ontogeny and effect of thyroid hormone. Am J Physiol 1991; 23:E53–E58.
51. Goland RS, Stark RI, Wardlaw SL. Response to corticotropin-releasing hormone during pregnancy in the baboon. J Clin Endocrinol Metab 1990; 70:925–929.
52. Robinson BG, Emanuel RL, Frim DM, et al. Glucocorticoid stimulates expression of corticotropin-releasing hormone gene in human placenta. Proc Natl Acad Sci USA 1988; 85:5244–5248.
53. Frim DM, Emanuel RL, Robinson BG, et al. Characterization and gestational regulation of corticotropin releasing hormone messenger RNA in human placenta. J Clin Invest 1988; 82:287–292.
54. Baird A, Wehrenberg WB, Bohlen P, et al. Immunoreactive and biologically active growth hormone releasing factor in rat placenta. Endocrinology 1985; 117:1598–1601.
55. Jeske W, Soszynski P, Rogozinski W, et al. Plasma GHRH, CRH, ACTH, β–endorphin, human placental lactogen, GH, and cortisol concentrations at the third trimester of pregnancy. Acta Endocrinol 1989; 120:785–789.
56. Bamberger AM, Bamberger CM, Pu LP, et al. Expression of pit1 messenger RNA and protein in the human placenta. J Clin Endocrinol Metab 1995; 80:2021–2026.
57. Petraglia F, Calza L, Giardino L, et al. Identification of neuropeptide Y in human placenta: localization, secretion and binding sites. Endocrinology 1989; 124:2016–2022.
58. Petraglia F, Lim ATW, Vale W. Adenosine 3′,5′-monophosphate, prostaglandins, and epinephrine stimulate the secretion of immunoreactive gonadotropin-releasing hormone from cultured human placental tissue. J Clin Endocrinol Metab 1987; 65:1020–1025.
59. Mills NC, D'Ercole AJ, Underwood LE, et al. Synthesis of somatomedin C/insulin-like growth factor I by human placenta. Mol Biol Rep 1986; 11:231–236.
60. Shen SJ, Daimon M, Wang CY, et al. Isolation of an insulin-like growth factor II cDNA with a unique 5′ untranslated region from human placenta. Proc Natl Acad Sci USA 1988; 85:1947–1951.
61. Goldstein LD, Reynolds CP, Perez Polo JR. Isolation of human nerve growth factor from placental tissue. Neurochem Res 1978; 3:185–193.
62. Walker P, Weichsel ME Jr, Fisher DA. Human nerve growth factor: lack of immunoreactivity with mouse nerve growth factor. Life Sci 1980; 26:195–200.
63. Bissonnette F, Cook C, Geoghegan T, et al. Transforming growth factor and epidermal growth factor messenger ribonucleic acid and protein levels in human placentas from early, mid and late gestation. Am J Obstet Gynecol 1992; 166:192–199.
64. Hofmann GEJ, Drews MR, Scott RT Jr, et al. Epidermal growth factor and its receptor in human implantation trophoblast: immunohistochemical evidence for autocrine/paracrine function. J Clin Endocrinol Metab 1992; 74:981–988.
65. Hock RA, Hollenberg MD. Characterization of the receptor for epidermal growth factor–urogastrone in human placental membranes. J Biol Chem 1980; 255:10731–10736.
66. Han VKM, Hunter ES III, Pratt RM, et al. Expression of rat transforming growth factor alpha mRNA during development occurs predominantly in the maternal decidua. Mol Cell Biol 1987; 7:2335–2343.
67. Freemark M, Comer M. Epidermal growth factor (EGF)–like transforming growth factor (TGF) activity and EGF receptors in ovine fetal tissues: possible role for TGF in ovine fetal development. Pediatr Res 1987; 22:609–615.
68. Morrish DW, Bhardwaj D, Dabbagh LK, et al. Epidermal growth factor induces differentiation and secretion of human chorionic gonadotropin and placental lactogen in normal human placenta. J Clin Endocrinol Metab 1987; 65:1282–1290.
69. Frolick CA, Dart LL, Meyers CA, et al. Purification and initial characterization of a type β transforming growth factor from human placenta. Proc Natl Acad Sci USA 1983; 80:3676–3680.
70. Cheung CY, Singh M, Ebaugh E, et al. Vascular endothelial growth factor gene expression in ovine placenta and fetal membranes. Am J Obstet Gynecol 1995; 173:753–759.

71. Horwitz MJ, Clarke MR, Kanbour-Shakir A, et al. Developmental expression and anatomical localization of endothelin-1 messenger ribonucleic acid and immunoreactivity in the rat placenta: a Northern analysis and immunohistochemical study. J Lab Clin Med 1995; 125:713–718.
72. Yang Y, Yelavarthi KK, Chen HL, et al. Molecular, biochemical and functional characteristics of tumor necrosis factor-α produced by human placental cytotrophoblastic cells. J Immunol 1993; 150: 5614–5624.
73. Saito S, Fukunaga R, Ichijo M, et al. Expression of granulocyte colony-stimulating factor and its receptor at the fetomaternal interface in murine and human pregnancy. Growth Factors 1994; 10:135–143.
74. Goldsmith PC, McGregor WG, Raymoure WJ, et al. Cellular localization of chorionic gonadotropin in human fetal liver and kidney. J Clin Endocrinol Metab 1983; 57:654–661.
75. Kapcala LP. Immunoassayable adrenocorticotropin in peripheral organs: concentrations during early development. Life Sci 1985; 37:2283–2290.
76. Martino E, Lernmark A, Seo H, et al. High concentration of thyrotropin releasing hormone in pancreatic islets. Proc Natl Acad Sci USA 1978; 75:4265–4267.
77. Pekary AE, Meyer NV, Vaillant C, et al. Thyrotropin releasing hormone and a homologous peptide in the male rat reproductive system. Biochem Biophys Res Commun 1980; 95:993–1000.
78. Suda T, Tomori N, Tozawa F, et al. Distribution and characterization of immunoreactive corticotropin-releasing factor in human tissues. J Clin Endocrinol Metab 1984; 59:861–866.
79. Petrusz P, Merchenthaler I, Maderdrut JL, et al. Corticotropin-releasing factor (CRF)–like immunoreactivity in the vertebrate endocrine pancreas. Proc Natl Acad Sci USA 1983; 80:1721–1725.
80. Nieuwenhuyzen Kruseman AC, Linton EA, Ackland J, et al. Heterogeneous immunocytochemical reactivities of CRF-41–like material in the human hypothalamus, pituitary and gastrointestinal tract. Neuroendocrinology 1984; 38:212–216.
81. Thompson RC, Seasholtz AF, Herbert E. Rat corticotropin releasing hormone gene: sequence and tissue specific expression. Mol Endocrinol 1987; 1:363–370.
82. Shibaski T, Kiyosawa Y, Masuda A, et al. Distribution of growth hormone releasing hormone–like immunoreactivity in human tissue extracts. J Clin Endocrinol Metab 1984; 59:263–268.
83. Koivusalo F, Leppaluoto J. High TRH immunoreactivity in purified pancreatic extracts of fetal and newborn rats. Life Sci 1979; 24:1655–1658.
84. Engler P, Scanlon MF, Jackson IMD. Thyrotropin releasing hormone in the systemic circulation of the neonatal rat is derived from the pancreas and other extraneural tissues. J Clin Invest 1981; 67:800–808.
85. McIntosh N, Pictet RL, Kaplan SL, et al. The developmental pattern of somatostatin in the embryonic and fetal rat pancreas. Endocrinology 1977; 101:825–829.
86. Koshimizu T. The development of pancreatic and gastrointestinal somatostatin-like immunoreactivity and its relationship to feeding in neonatal rats. Endocrinology 1983; 112:911–916.
87. Wu P, Jackson IMD. Identification, characterization and localization of thyrotropin releasing hormone precursor peptides in perinatal rat pancreas. Regul Pept 1988; 22:347–360.
88. Lamberton P, Wu P, Jackson IMD. Thyrotropin releasing hormone release from rat pancreas is stimulated by serotonin but inhibited by carbachol. Endocrinology 1985; 117:1834–1838.
89. Rahier J, Wallon J, Henquin JC. Abundance of somatostatin cells in the human neonatal pancreas. Diabetologia 1980; 18:251–254.
90. Leduque P, Aratan-Spire S, Czernichow P, et al. Ontogenesis of thyrotropin-releasing hormone in the human fetal pancreas. J Clin Invest 1986; 78:1028–1034.
91. Saito H, Saito S, Sano T, et al. Fetal and maternal plasma levels of immunoreactive somatostatin at delivery: evidence for its increase in the umbilical artery and its arteriovenous gradient in the fetoplacental circulation. J Clin Endocrinol Metab 1983; 56: 567–571.
92. Koshimizu T, Ohyama Y, Yokota Y, et al. Peripheral plasma concentrations of somatostatin-like immunoreactivity in newborns and infants. J Clin Endocrinol Metab 1985; 61:78–82.
93. Umans JG, Umans HR, Szeto HH. Effects of thyrotropin releasing hormone in the fetal lamb. Am J Obstet Gynecol 1986; 155: 1266–1271.
94. Mulchahey JJ, DiBlasio AM, Martin MC, et al. Hormone production and peptide regulation of the human fetal pituitary gland. Endocr Rev 1987; 8:406–425.
95. Grumbach MM, Gluckman PD. The human fetal hypothalamus and pituitary gland: the maturation of neuroendocrine mechanisms controlling secretion of fetal pituitary growth hormone, prolactin, gonadotropins, adrenocorticotropin-related peptides and thyrotropin. In Tulchinsky D, Little AB (eds). Maternal-Fetal Endocrinology, 2nd ed. Philadelphia, WB Saunders, 1994, pp 193–261.
96. Yang K, Jones SA, Challis JRG. Changes in glucocorticoid receptor number in the hypothalamus of the sheep fetus with gestational age and after adrenocorticotropin treatment. Endocrinology 1990; 126:11–17.
97. Roessler E, Belloni E, Gaudenz K, et al. Mutations in the human Sonic Hedgehog gene cause holoprosencephaly. Nat Genet 1996; 14:357–360.
98. Brown SA, Warburton D, Brown LY, et al. Holoprosencephaly due to mutation in ZIC1, a homologue of *Drosophila* odd-paired. Nat Genet 1998; 20:180–183.
99. Dattani MT, Martinez-Barbera JP, Thomas PQ, et al. *HESX1* a novel homeobox gene implicated in septo-optic dysplasia (Abstract 06). Horm Res 1998; 8(Suppl 3).
100. Millis PE. Transcription factors in pituitary gland development and their clinical impact on phenotype. Horm Res 2000; 54:107–119.
101. Wu W, Cogan JD, Pfaffle RM, et al. Mutations in PROP-1 cause familial combined pituitary hormone deficiency. Nat Genet 1998; 18:147–149.
102. Suganuma N, Seo H, Yamamoto N, et al. The ontogeny of growth hormone in the human fetal pituitary. Am J Obstet Gynecol 1989; 160:729–733.
103. Goodyear CG, Sellen JM, Fuks M, et al. Regulation of growth hormone secretion from human fetal pituitaries, interactions between growth hormone releasing factor and somatostatin. Reprod Nutr Dev 1987; 27:461–470.
104. de Zegher F, Daaboul J, Grumbach MM, et al. Hormone ontogeny in the ovine fetus and neonate. XXII: The effect of somatostatin on the growth hormone (GH) response to GH-releasing factor. Endocrinology 1989; 124:1114–1117.
105. D'Ercole AJ. Growth factors and development. In Polin RA, Fox WW (eds). Fetal and Neonatal Physiology. Philadelphia, WB Saunders, 1992, pp 1820–1828.
106. Clemmons DR. Insulin-like growth factor-1 and its binding proteins. In DeGroot LJ, Jameson JL (eds). Endocrinology, 4th ed. Philadelphia, WB Saunders, 2001, pp 439–460.
107. Kind KL, Owens JA, Robinson JS, et al. Effect of restriction of placental growth on expression of IGFs in fetal sheep: relationship to fetal growth, circulating IGFs and binding proteins. J Endocrinol 1995; 146:23–34.
108. Freemark M, Driscoll P, Maaskant R, et al. Ontogenesis of prolactin receptors in the human fetus in early gestation. J Clin Invest 1997; 99:1107–1117.
109. Clement-Lacroix P, Ormandy C, Lepescheux L, et al. Osteoblasts are a new target for prolactin analysis of bone formation in prolactin receptor knockout mice. Endocrinology 1999; 140: 3404–3410.
110. Symonds ME, Phillips ID, Anthony RV, et al. Prolactin receptor gene expression and fetal adipose tissue. J Neuroendocrinol 1998; 10:885–890.
111. Winter JSD. Fetal and neonatal adrenocortical physiology. In Polin RA, Fox WW (eds). Maternal-Fetal Endocrinology. Philadelphia, WB Saunders, 1998, pp 2447–2459.
112. Pepe GJ, Albrecht ED. Regulation of the primate fetal adrenal cortex. Endocr Rev 1990; 11:151–176.
113. Carr BR, Simpson ER. De novo synthesis of cholesterol by human fetal adrenal gland. Endocrinology 1981; 108:2154–2162.
114. Ikeda Y, Swain A, Weber TH, et al. Steroidogenic factor 1 and DAX-1 localize in multiple cell lineages: potential links in endocrine development. Mol Endocrinol 1996; 10:1261–1272.
115. Muscatelli F, Strom TM, Walker AP, et al. Mutations in the DAX-1 gene give rise to both X-linked adrenal hypoplasia and congenital and hypogonadotropic hypogonadism. Nature 1994; 372:672–676.
116. Miller WL. Steroid hormone biosynthesis and actions in the materno-feto-placental unit. Clin Perinatol 1998; 25:799–817.

214. Girard J. Control of fetal and neonatal glucose metabolism by pancreatic hormones. Baillieres Clin Endocrinol Metab 1989; 3: 817–836.

215. Ammon HP, Glocker C, Waldner RG, et al. Insulin release from pancreatic islets of fetal rats mediated by leucine, b-BCH, tolbutamide, glibenclamide, arginine, potassium chloride, and theophylline does not require stimulation of Ca^{2+} net uptake. Cell Calcium 1989; 10:441–450.

216. Formby B, Ullrich A, Coussens L, et al. Growth hormone stimulates insulin gene expression in cultured human fetal pancreatic islets. J Clin Endocrinol Metab 1988; 66:1075–1079.

217. Ruiz de Ona C, Obregon MJ, Escobar del Rey F, et al. Developmental changes in rat brain 5′-deiodinase and thyroid hormones during the fetal period: the effects of fetal hypothyroidism and maternal thyroid hormones. Pediatr Res 1988; 24:588–594.

218. Polk DH, Cheromcha D, Reviczky A, et al. Nuclear thyroid hormone receptors: ontogeny and thyroid hormone effects in sheep. Am J Physiol 1989; 256:E543–E549.

219. Coulombe P, Ruel J, Dussault JH. Effects of neonatal hypo- and hyperthyroidism on pituitary growth hormone content in the rat. Endocrinology 1980; 107:2027–2033.

220. Lakshmanan J, Perheentupa J, Macaso T, et al. Acquisition of urine, kidney and submandibular gland epidermal growth factor responsiveness to thyroxine administration in neonatal mice. Acta Endocrinol 1985; 109:511–516.

221. Alm J, Scott SM, Fisher DA. Epidermal growth factor receptor ontogeny in mice with congenital hypothyroidism. J Dev Physiol 1986; 8:377–385.

222. Hoath SB, Lakshmanan J, Fisher DA. Thyroid hormone effects on skin and hepatic epidermal growth factor concentrations in neonatal and adult mice. Biol Neonate 1984; 45:49–52.

223. Hoath SB, Lakshmanan J, Fisher DA. Epidermal growth factor binding to neonatal mouse skin explants and membrane preparations: effect of triiodothyronine. Pediatr Res 1985; 19:277–280.

224. Perez Castillo A, Bernal J, Ferriero B, et al. The early ontogenesis of thyroid hormone receptor in the rat fetus. Endocrinology 1985; 117:2457–2461.

225. Padbury JF, Lam RW, Newnham JP, et al. Neonatal adaptation: greater neurosympathetic system activity in preterm than full term sheep at birth. Am J Physiol 1985; 248:E443–E449.

226. Pasqualini JR, Sumida C, Gelly C, et al. Progesterone receptors in the fetal uterus and ovary of the guinea pig: evolution during fetal development and induction and stimulation in estradiol-primed animals. J Steroid Biochem 1976; 7:1031–1038.

227. Yamashita S, Newbold RR, McLachlan JA, et al. Developmental pattern of estrogen receptor expression in female mouse genital tracts. Endocrinology 1989; 125:2888–2896.

228. Simmen FA, Simmon RCM, Letcher LR, et al. IGFs in pregnancy: developmental expression in uterus and mammary glanc and paracrine actions during embryonic and neonatal growth. Ir LeRoith D, Raizada MK (eds). Molecular and Cellular Biology o Insulin-Like Growth Factors and Their Receptors. New York Plenum, 1989, pp 195–208.

229. Spaventi R, Antica M, Pavelic K. Insulin and insulin-like growtl factor I (IGF I) in early mouse embryogenesis. Developmen 1990; 108:491–495.

230. De Chiara TM, Efstradiadis A, Robertson EJ. A growth defi ciency phenotype in heterozygous mice carrying an insulin lik growth factor II gene disrupted by targeting. Nature 1990; 34 78–80.

231. Liu JKP, Baker J, Perkins AS, et al. Mice carrying null mutatior of the genes encoding insulin-like growth factor I and type I IG receptor. Cell 1993; 75:59–72.

232. Baker J, Liu JP, Robertson EJ, et al. Role of insulin-like grow factors in embryonic and postnatal growth. Cell 1993; 75:73–82

233. Lee KH, Calikoglu AS, Ye P, D'Ercole J. Insulin-like grow factor-1 (IGF-1) ameliorates and IGF binding protein-1 (IGFB 1) exacerbates the effects of undernutrition on brain growth du ing early postnatal life: studies in IGF-I and IGFBP-I transger mice. Pediatr Res 1999; 45:331–336.

234. Han VKM, D'Ercole AJ, Lund PK. Cellular localization of sy thesis of somatomedin (insulin-like growth factor) messeng RNA in the human fetus. Science 1987; 236:193–197.

235. D'Ercole AJ, Applewhite GT, Underwood LE. Evidence tl somatomedins are synthesized by multiple tissues in the fet Dev Biol 1980; 75:315–328.

117. Leavitt MG, Albrecht EO, Pepe GJ. Development of the baboon fetal adrenal gland: regulation of the ontogenesis of the definitive and transitional zones by adrenocorticotropin. J Clin Endocrinol Metab 1999; 84:3831–3835.

118. Goland RS, Wardlow SL, Blum M, et al. Biologically active corticotropin-releasing hormone in maternal and fetal plasma during pregnancy. Am J Obstet Gynecol 1988; 159:884–890.

119. Beitins IZ, Bayard F, Ances FIG, et al. The metabolic clearance rate, blood production, interconversion and transplacental passage of cortisol and cortisone in pregnancy near term. Pediatr Res 1973; 7:509–519.

120. Rose JC, Turner CS, Ray DeW, et al. Evidence that cortisol inhibits basal adrenocorticotropin secretion in the sheep fetus by 0.70 gestation. Endocrinology 1988; 123:1307–1313.

121. Baulieu EE, Mester J, Redeuilh G. Nuclear receptor superfamily. In DeGroot LJ, Jameson JL (eds). Endocrinology, 4th ed. Philadelphia, WB Saunders, 2000, pp 123–141.

122. Cole TJ, Blendy JA, Monaghan AD, et al. Targeted disruption of the glucocorticoid receptor gene blocks adrenergic chromaffin development and severely retards lung maturation. Genes Dev 1995; 9:1608–1625.

123. Johnson JW, Mitzner W, Beck JC, et al. Long term effects of betamethasone in fetal development. Am J Obstet Gynecol 1981; 141:1053–1064.

124. Pavlik A, Buresova M. The neonatal cerebellum: the highest level of glucocorticoid receptors in the brain. Dev Brain Res 1984; 12: 13–20.

125. Liggins GC. The role of cortisol in preparing the fetus for birth. Reprod Fertil Dev 1994; 6:141–150.

126. Beitins IZ, Bayard F, Levitsky L, et al. Plasma aldosterone concentrations at delivery and during the newborn period. J Clin Invest 1972; 51:386–394.

127. Beitins IZ, Graham GG, Kowarski A, et al. Adrenal function in normal infants and in marasmus and kwashiorkor: plasma aldosterone concentration and aldosterone secretion rate. J Pediatr 1974; 84:444–451.

128. Katz FH, Beck P, Makowski EL. The renin-aldosterone system in mother and fetus at term. Am J Obstet Gynecol 1974; 118:51–55.

129. Siegel SR, Fisher DA. Ontogeny of the renin-angiotensin-aldosterone system in the fetal and newborn lamb. Pediatr Res 1980; 14:99–102.

130. Lumbers ER. Functions of the renin-angiotensin system during development. Clin Exp Pharmacol Physiol 1995; 22:499–505.

131. Berger S, Bleich M, Schmid N, et al. Mineralocorticoid receptor knockout mice: pathophysiology of Na^{+} metabolism. Proc Natl Acad Sci USA 1998; 95:9424–9429.

132. Hirasawa G, Sasano H, Suzuki T, et al. 11β-Hydroxysteroid dehydrogenase type 2 and mineralocorticoid receptor in human fetal development. J Clin Endocrinol Metab 1999; 84:1453–1458.

133. Robillard JE, Page WV, Matthews MS, et al. Differential gene expression and regulation of renal angiotensin II receptor subtypes (AT1 and AT2) during fetal life in sheep. Pediatr Res 1995; 38:896–904.

134. Ito Y, Matsumoto T, Ohbu K, et al. Concentrations of human atrial natriuretic peptide in the cord blood and the plasma of the newborn. Acta Paediatr Scand 1988; 77:76–78.

135. Pintar JE. Normal development of the hypothalamic-pituitary-thyroid axis. In Braverman LE, Utiger RD (eds). The Thyroid, 8th ed. Philadelphia, JB Lippincott, 2000, pp 7–19.

136. Fisher DA, Brown RS. Thyroid physiology in the perinatal period and during childhood. In Braverman LE, Utiger RD (eds). The Thyroid, 8th ed. Philadelphia, JB Lippincott, 2000, pp 961–972.

137. Missero C, Cobellis G, DeFelice M, DiLauro R. Molecular events involved in differentiation of thyroid follicular cells. Mol Cell Endocrinol 1998; 140:37–43.

138. Kambe F, Seo H. Thyroid specific transcription factors. Endocr J 1997; 44:775–784.

139. Guazzi S, Lonigro R, Pintonello L, et al. The thyroid transcription factor-1 gene is a candidate target for regulation by HOX proteins. EMBO J 1994; 13:3339–3347.

140. Chisaka O, Capecchi MR. Regionally restricted developmental defects resulting from targeted disruption of the mouse homeobox gene hox-1.5. Nature 1991; 350:473–479.

141. Contempre B, Jauniaux E, Calvo R, et al. Detection of thyroid hormones in human embryonic cavities during the first trimester of pregnancy. J Clin Endocrinol Metab 1993; 77:1719–1722.

142. Vulsma T, Gons MH, de Vijlder JJ. Maternal-fetal transfer of thyroxine in congenital hypothyroidism due to a total organification defect or thyroid agenesis. N Engl J Med 1989; 321:13–16.

143. Morreale De Escobar G, Calvo R, Obregon MJ, et al. Contribution of maternal thyroxine to fetal thyroxine pools in normal rats near term. Endocrinology 1990; 126:2765–2767.

144. Burrow GN, Fisher DA, Larsen PR. Maternal and fetal thyroid function. N Engl J Med 1994; 331:1072–1078.

145. Thorpe Beeston JG, Nicolaides KH, McGregor AM. Fetal thyroid function. Thyroid 1992; 2:207–217.

146. Roti E. Regulation of thyroid stimulating hormone (TSH) secretion in the fetus and neonate. J Endocrinol Invest 1988; 11:145–158.

147. Fisher DA, Nelson JC, Carlton EI, Wilcox RB. Maturation of human hypothalamic-pituitary-thyroid function and control. Thyroid 2000; 10:229–234.

148. Eng PHK, Cardona GR, Fang SL, et al. Escape from the acute Wolff-Chaikoff effect is associated with a decrease in thyroid sodium/iodide symporter messenger ribonucleic acid and protein. Endocrinology 1999; 140:3404–3410.

149. Sherwin JR. Development of regulatory mechanisms in the thyroid: failure of iodide to suppress iodide transport activity. Proc Soc Exp Biol Med 1982; 169:458–462.

150. Spitzweg C, Heufelder AE, Morris JC. Thyroid iodide transport. Thyroid 2000; 10:321–330.

151. Leonard JL, Koehrle J. Intracellular pathways of iodothyronine metabolism. In Braverman LE, Utiger RD (eds). The Thyroid, 8th ed. Philadelphia, JB Lippincott, 2000, pp 136–173.

152. Polk DH, Reviczky A, Wu SY, et al. Metabolism of sulfoconjugated thyroid hormone derivatives in developing sheep. Am J Physiol 1994; 266:E892–E896.

153. Santini F, Chiovato L, Ghirri P, et al. Serum iodothyronines in the human fetus and newborn: evidence for an important role of placenta in fetal thyroid hormone homeostasis. J Clin Endocrinol Metab 1999; 84:493–498.

154. Richard K, Hume R, Kaptein E, et al. Ontogeny of iodothyronine deiodinases in human liver. J Clin Endocrinol Metab 1998; 83:2868–2874.

155. Polk DH, Wu WY, Wright C, et al. Ontogeny of thyroid hormone effect on tissue 5′-monodeiodinase activity in fetal sheep. Am J Physiol 1988; 254:E337–E341.

156. Anderson GW, Mariash CN, Oppenheimer JH. Molecular actions of thyroid hormone. In Braverman LE, Utiger RD (eds). The Thyroid, 8th ed. Philadelphia, JB Lippincott, 2000, pp 174–195.

157. Morreale De Escobar G, Obregon MJ, Escabor Del Rey F. Is neuropsychological development related to maternal hypothyroidism or to maternal hypothyroxinemia? J Clin Endocrinol Metab 2000; 85:3975–3987.

158. Forrest D, Vennstrom B. Functions of thyroid hormone receptors in mice. Thyroid 2000; 10:41–52.

159. Pelliniemi LJ, Dym M. The fetal gonad and sexual differentiation. In Tulchinsky D, Little AB (eds). Maternal-Fetal Endocrinology, 2nd ed. Philadelphia, WB Saunders, 1994, pp 298–320.

160. Ray R, Picard JY. Embryology and endocrinology of genital development. Baillieres Clin Endocrinol Metab 1998; 12:17–33.

161. Ikida Y, Swain A, Weber TH, et al. Steroidogenic factor 1 and DAX-1 localize in multiple cell lineages: potential links in endocrine development. Mol Endocrinol 1996; 10:1261–1272.

162. Swain A, Zanaria E, Hacker A, et al. Mouse DAX-1 expression is consistent with a role in both adrenal development and sex determination. Nat Genet 1996; 12:404–409.

163. Haqq CM, King CY, Ukiyama E, et al. Molecular basis of mammalian sexual determination: activation of müllerian inhibiting substance gene expression by SRY. Science 1994; 266:1494–1500.

164. Zang FP, Poutanen M, Wilbertz J, Huhtaniemi L. Normal prenatal but arrested postnatal sexual development of luteinizing hormone receptor knockout (LURKO) mice. Mol Endocrinol 2001; 15:172–183.

165. Zimmerman S, Steding G, Emmen JMA, et al. Targeted disruption of the *Ins13* gene causes bilateral cryptorchidism. Mol Endocrinol 1999; 13:681–691.

166. Josso N. Antimüllerian hormone and intersex states. Trends Endocrinol 1991; 2:227–233.

167. Roviller Fabre V, Carmona S, Abou Merhi A, et al. Effect of anti-müllerian hormone on Sertoli and Leydig cell functions in fetal and immature rats. Endocrinology 1998; 139:1213–1220.
168. Brandenberger AW, Tee MK, Lee JY, et al. Tissue distribution of estrogen receptors alpha (ERα) and beta (ERβ) mRNA in the midgestation human fetus. J Clin Endocrinol Metab 1997; 82: 3509–3512.
169. Korach KS, Couse JF, Curtis SW, et al. Estrogen receptor gene disruption: molecular characterization and experimental and clinical phenotypes. Recent Prog Horm Res 1996; 51:159–188.
170. Krege JH, Hadgin JB, Couse JF, et al. Generation and reproductive phenotypes of mice lacking estrogen receptor β. Proc Natl Acad Sci USA 1998; 95:15677–15682.
171. Naftolin F, Brawer JB. The effect of estrogens on hypothalamic structure and function. Am J Obstet Gynecol 1978; 132:758–765.
172. Sholl SA, Goy RW, Kim KL. 5α–Reductase, aromatase, and androgen receptor levels in the monkey brain during fetal development. Endocrinology 1989; 124:627–634.
173. Visser M, Swaab DF. Life span changes in the presence of alpha-melanocyte-stimulating-hormone-containing cells in the human pituitary. J Dev Physiol 1979; 1:161–178.
174. Perry RA, Mulvogue HM, McMillen IC, et al. Immunohistochemical localization of ACTH in the adult and fetal sheep pituitary. J Dev Physiol 1985; 7:397–404.
175. Silman RE, Holland T, Chard T, et al. The ACTH family tree of the rhesus monkey changes with development. Nature 1978; 276:526–528.
176. Glickman JA, Carson GD, Challis JRG. Differential effects o[f] synthetic adrenocorticotropin and melanocyte stimulating hormone on adrenal formation in human and sheep fetus. Endocrinology 1979; 104:34–39.
177. Swaab DF, Martin JT. Functions of alpha melanotropin an[d] other opiomelanocortin peptides in labour, intrauterine growt[h] and brain development. Ciba Found Symp 1981; 81:196–217.
178. Facchinetti F, Storchi AR, Petraglia F, et al. Ontogeny of pitui[-] tary β–endorphin and related peptides in the human embryo an[d] fetus. Am J Obstet Gynecol 1987; 156:735–739.
179. Leake RD, Fisher DA. Ontogeny of vasopressin in man. In Czer[-] nichow P, Robinson AG (eds). Diabetes Insipidus in Man. Fron[-] tiers in Hormone Research, vol 13. Basel, S Karger, 1985, p[p] 42–51.
180. Leake RD. The fetal-maternal neurohypophysial system. In Poli[n] RA, Fox WW (eds). Fetal and Neonatal Physiology, 2nd e[d.] Philadelphia, WB Saunders, 1998, pp 2442–2446.
181. Ervin MG, Leake RD, Ross MG, et al. Arginine vasotocin i[n] ovine maternal and fetal blood, fetal urine, and amniotic fluid. [J] Clin Invest 1985; 75:1696–1701.
182. Morris M, Castro M, Rose JC. Alterations in prohormone pro[c-] essing during early development in the fetal sheep. Am J Physi[ol] 1992; 263:R738–R740.
183. Zhao X, Nijland MJM, Ervin G, Ross MG. Regulation of hyp[o-] thalamic arginine vasopressin content in fetal sheep: effect [of] acute tonicity alterations and fetal maturation. Am J Obst[et] Gynecol 1998; 179:899–905.
184. DeVane GW, Porter JC. An apparent stress-induced release [of] arginine vasopressin by human neonates. J Clin Endocrinol M[e-] tab 1980; 51:1412–1416.
185. Matthews SG, Challis JRG. Regulation of CRH and AVP mRN[A] in the developing ovine hypothalamus: effects of stress and gluc[o-] corticoids. Am J Physiol 1995; 268:E1096–E1107.
186. Irion GL, Mack CE, Clark KE. Fetal hemodynamic and fetop[la-] cental vascular response to exogenous arginine vasopressin. A[m J] Obstet Gynecol 1990; 162:1115–1120.
187. Brooks AN, White A. Activation of pituitary adrenal function [in] fetal sheep by corticotrophin-releasing factor and arginine va[so-] pressin. J Endocrinol 1990; 124:27–35.
188. Benedetto MT, DeCicco F, Rossiello F, et al. Oxytocin recep[tors] in human fetal membranes at term and during labor. J Ster[oid] Biochem 1990; 35:205–208.
189. Tribollet E, Charpak S, Schmidt A, et al. Appearance and tr[an-] sient expression of oxytocin receptors in fetal, infant and peri[pu-] bertal rat brain studied by autoradiography and electrophysiol[ogy.] J Neurosci 1989; 9:1764–1773.
190. Ervin MG, Miller SJ, Ramseyer LJ, et al. Renal arginine v[aso-] pressin receptors in newborn and adult sheep. Clin Res 1990; 170A.

EGF receptor levels in regions of adult rat brain. Mol Brain Res 1992; 16:316–322.
261. Gospodarowicz D. Epidermal and nerve growth factors in mammalian development. Annu Rev Physiol 1981; 43:251–263.
262. Gorin PD, Johnson EM. Effects of exposure to nerve growth factor antibodies on the developing nervous system of the rat, an experimental autoimmune approach. Dev Biol 1980; 80:313–323.
263. Sendtner M, Holtmann B, Kolbeck R, et al. Brain derived neurotrophic factor prevents the death of motoneurons in newborn rats after nerve section. Nature 1992; 360:757–759.
264. Yan Q, Elliott J, Snider WD. Brain derived neurotrophic factor rescues spinal motor neurons from axotomy-induced cell death. Nature 1992; 360:753–755.
265. Padbury JF, Lam RW, Polk DH, et al. Autoimmune sympathectomy in fetal rabbits. J Dev Physiol 1986; 8:369–376.
266. Tarris RH, Weichsel ME Jr, Fisher DA. Synthesis and secretion of a nerve growth stimulating factor by neonatal mouse astrocyte cells in vitro. Pediatr Res 1986; 20:367–372.
267. Lakshmanan J, Weichsel ME Jr, Tarris R, et al. Nerve growth factor in developing mouse cerebral cortical synaptosomes: measurement by competitive radioimmunoassay and bioassay. Pediatr Res 1986; 20:391–397.
268. Giordano T, Pan JB, Casuto D, et al. Thyroid hormone regulation of NGF, NT3 and BDNF RNA in the adult rat brain. Mol Brain Res 1992; 16:239–245.
269. Bonyada M, Rusholme SAB, Cousins FM, et al. Mapping of a major genetic modifier of embryonic lethality in TGFβ1 knockout mice. Nat Genet 1997; 15:207–211.
270. Betsholtz C. Functions of platelet-derived growth factor and its receptors deduced from gene inactivation in mice. J Clin Ligand Assay 2000; 23:206–213.
271. Kitamoto Y, Tokunaga H, Tomito K. Vascular endothelial growth factor is an essential molecule for mouse kidney development: glomerulogenesis and nephrogenesis. J Clin Invest 1997; 99:2351–2357.
272. Sieff CA. Hematopoietic growth factors. J Clin Invest 1987; 79: 1549–1557.
273. Dame JB, Christensen RD, Juul SA. The distribution of granulocyte-macrophage colony-stimulating factor and its receptor in the developing human fetus. Pediatr Res 1999; 46:358–366.
274. Lim GB, Dodic M, Earnest L, et al. Regulation of erythropoietin gene expression in fetal sheep by glucocorticoids. Endocrinology 1996; 137:1658–1663.
275. Zanjani ED, Ascensau JL, McGlave PB. Studies on the liver to kidney switch of erythropoietin production. J Clin Invest 1981; 67:1183–1188.
276. Moritz KM, Lim GB, Wintour EM. Developmental regulation of erythropoietin and erythropoiesis. Am J Physiol 1997; 273: R1829–R1844.
277. Szebenyi G, Fallon JF. Fibroblast growth factors as multifunctional signalling factors. Int Rev Cytol 1999; 185:45-106.
278. Lewandoski M, Sun X, Martin GR. Fgf8 signalling from the AER is essential for normal limb development. Nat Genet 2000; 26:460–463.
279. Sekine K, Ohuchi H, Fujiwara M, et al. Fgf10 is essential for limb and lung development. Nat Genet 1999; 21:138–141.
280. Oberbauer AM, Linkhart TA, Mohan S, et al. Fibroblast growth factor enhances human chorionic gonadotropin synthesis independent of mitogenic stimulation in Jar choriocarcinoma cells. Endocrinology 1988; 123:2696–2700.
281. Wallace MJ, Hooper SB, Harding R. Effects of elevated fetal cortisol concentrations on the volume, secretion, and reabsorption of lung liquid. Am J Physiol 1995; 269:R881–R887.
282. Muglia L, Jacobson L, Dikkes P, et al. Corticotropin-releasing hormone deficiency reveals major fetal but not adult glucocorticoid need. Nature 1995; 373:427–432.
283. Cole TJ, Blendy JA, Monaghan P, et al. Targeted disruption of the glucocorticoid receptor gene blocks adrenergic chromaffin cell development and severely retards lung maturation. Genes Dev 1995; 9:1608–1621.
284. Polk DH. Thyroid hormone effects on neonatal thermogenesis. Semin Perinatol 1988; 12:151–156.
285. Gunn TR, Gluckman PD. Perinatal thermogenesis. Early Hum Dev 1995; 42:169–183.
286. Obregon MJ, Pitamber R, Jacobsson A, et al. Euthyroid status is essential for the perinatal increase in thermogenin mRNA in brown adipose tissue of rat pups. Biochem Biophys Res Commun 1987; 148:9–14.
287. Polk DH, Padbury JF, Callegari CC, et al. Effect of fetal thyroidectomy on newborn thermogenesis in lambs. Pediatr Res 1987; 21:453–457.
288. Fisher DA, Polk DH, Wu SY. Fetal thyroid metabolism: a pluralistic system. Thyroid 1994; 4:367–371.
289. Longhead JL, Minouni F, Tsang RC. Serum ionized calcium concentrations in normal neonates. Am J Dis Child 1988; 142: 516–518.
290. Venkataraman PS, Tsang RC, Chen IW, et al. Pathogenesis of early neonatal hypocalcemia: studies of serum calcitonin, gastrin and plasma glucagon. J Pediatr 1987; 110:599–603.
291. Mimoumi F, Tsang RC. Perinatal mineral metabolism. In Tulchinsky D, Little AB (eds). Maternal-Fetal Endocrinology, 2nd ed. Philadelphia, WB Saunders, 1994, pp 402–417.
292. Menon RK, Sperling MA. Carbohydrate metabolism. Semin Perinatol 1988; 12:157–162.
293. Wheeler MD, Styne DM. Longitudinal changes in growth hormone response to growth hormone–releasing hormone in neonatal rhesus monkeys. Pediatr Res 1990; 28:15–18.
294. Penny R, Parlow AF, Frasier O. Testosterone and estradiol concentrations in paired maternal and cord sera and their correlation with the concentration of chorionic gonadotropin. Pediatrics 1979; 64:604–608.
295. Mann DR, Gould KG, Collins DC, et al. Blockade of neonatal activation of the pituitary-testicular axis: effect on peripubertal luteinizing hormone and testosterone secretion and on testicular development in male monkeys. J Clin Endocrinol Metab 1989; 68:600–607.
296. Dohler KD. The special case of hormonal imprinting: the neonatal influence on sex. Experientia 1986; 42:759–769.
297. Resko JA, Roselli CE. Prenatal hormones organize sex differences in the neuroendocrine reproductive system: observations on guinea pigs and nonhuman primates. Cell Mol Neurobiol 1997; 17:627–648.
298. Kosut SS, Wood RI, Herbosa-Encaracion C, Foster DL. Prenatal androgens time neuroendocrine puberty in the sheep: effect of testosterone dose. Endocrinology 1997; 138:1072–1077.
299. Grocock CA, Charlton HM, Pike MC. Role of fetal pituitary in cryptorchidism induced by exogenous maternal oestrogen during pregnancy in mice. J Reprod Fertil 1988; 83:295–300.
300. Bern HA, Talamentes FJ Jr. Neonatal mouse models and their relation to disease in the human female. In Herbst AL, Bern HA (eds). Developmental Effects of Diethylstilbestrol (DES) in Pregnancy. New York, Thieme-Stratton, 1981, pp 129–147.
301. Zheng X, Hendry WJ III. Neonatal diethylstilbestrol treatment alters the estrogen-regulated expression of both cell proliferation and apoptosis-related proto-oncogene (c-*jun*, c-*fos*, c-*myc*, *bax*, *bcl-2*, and *bcl-x*) in the hamster uterus. Cell Growth Differ 1997; 8: 425–434.
302. Csaba G. Receptor ontogeny and hormonal imprinting. Experientia 1986; 42:750–759.
303. Mathews SG. Antenatal glucocorticoids and programming of the developing CNS. Pediatr Res 2000; 47:291–300.
304. Martin SM, Moberg GP. Effects of early neonatal thyroxine treatment on development of the thyroid and adrenal axes in rats. Life Sci 1981; 29:1683–1688.
305. Walker P, Courtin F. Transient neonatal hyperthyroidism results in hypothyroidism in the adult rat. Endocrinology 1985; 116: 2246–2250.
306. Alm J, Lakshmanan J, Hoath S, et al. Neonatal hyperthyroidism alters hepatic epidermal growth factor receptor ontogeny in mice. Pediatr Res 1988; 23:557–560.
307. Csaba G, Inczefi Gonda A, Dobozy O. Hereditary transmission in the F_1 generation of hormonal imprinting (receptor memory) induced in rats by neonatal exposure to insulin. Acta Physiol Hung 1984; 63:93–99.
308. Csaba G, Ronai A, Laszlo V, et al. Amplification of hormone receptors by neonatal oxytocin and vasopressin treatment. Horm Metab Res 1980; 12:28–31.
309. Benediktsson R, Lindsay RD, Noble J, et al. Glucocorticoid exposure in utero: new model for adult hypertension. Lancet 1993; 341:339–341.
310. Herbst AL. The epidemiology of vaginal and cervical clear cell adenocarcinoma. In Herbst AL, Bern HA (eds). Developmental

Effects of Diethylstilbestrol (DES) in Pregnancy. New York, Thieme-Stratton, 1981, pp 63–70.
311. Fisher DA, Schoen EJ, LaFranchi S, et al. The hypothalamic-pituitary-thyroid negative feedback control axis in children with treated congenital hypothyroidism. J Clin Endocrinol Metab 2000; 85:2722–2727.
312. Osmond C, Barker DJP. Fetal, infant, and childhood growth are predictors of coronary heart disease, diabetes and hypertension in adult men and women. Environ Health Perspect 2000; 108:545–553.
313. Jaquet D, Gaboriau A, Czernichow P, Levy-Marchal C. Insulin resistance early in adulthood in subjects born with intrauterine growth retardation. J Clin Endocrinol Metab 2000; 85:1401–1406.
314. Terauchi Y, Kubota N, Tamemoto H, et al. Insulin effect during embryogenesis determines fetal growth: a possible molecular link between birth weight and susceptibility to type 2 diabetes. Diabetes 2000; 49:82–86.
315. Barker DJP, Shiell AW, Barker ME, Law CM. Growth in utero and blood pressure levels in the next generation. J Hypertens 2000; 18:843–846.
316. Nilsson C, Niklasson M, Ericksson E, et al. Imprinting of female offspring with testosterone results in insulin resistance and changes in body fat distribution at adult age in rats. J Clin Invest 1998; 101:74–78.
317. Eisner JR, Domesic DA, Kemnitz JW, Abbott DH. Timing of prenatal androgen excess determines differential impairment in insulin secretion and action in adult female rhesus monkeys. J Clin Endocrinol Metab 2000; 85:1206–1210.
318. Sato SM, Mains RE. Plasticity in the adrenocorticotropin-related peptides produced by primary cultures of neonatal rat pituitary. Endocrinology 1988; 122:68–77.
319. Evans MI, Adzick MS, Johnson MP, et al. Fetal therapy 1994. Curr Opin Obstet Gynecol 1994; 6:58–64.
320. Flake AW. Fetal therapy: medical and surgical approaches. In Creasy RK, Resnik R (eds). Maternal-Fetal Medicine, 4th ed. Philadelphia, WB Saunders, 1999, pp 365–377.
321. Donner C, Vermeylen D, Kirkpatrick C, et al. Management of the growth-restricted fetus: the role of noninvasive tests and fetal blood sampling. Obstet Gynecol 1995; 85:965–970.
322. Manning FA. General principles and applications of ultrasonography, In Creasy RK, Resnik R (eds). Maternal-Fetal Medicine, 4th ed. Philadelphia, WB Saunders, 1999, pp 169–206.
323. Harman CR. Percutaneous fetal blood sampling. In Creasy RK, Resnik R (eds). Maternal-Fetal Medicine, 4th ed. Philadelphia, WB Saunders, 1999, pp 341–361.
324. Jobe AH. Fetal lung development, tests for maturation, induction of maturation and treatment. In Creasy RK, Resnik R (eds). Maternal-Fetal Medicine, 4th ed. Philadelphia, WB Saunders, 1999, pp 404–422.
325. Abuhamad AZ, Fisher DA, Warsof SL, et al. Antenatal diagnosis and treatment of goitrous hypothyroidism: case review and review of the literature. Ultrasound Obstet Gynecol 1995; 6:368–371.
326. Garmer PR. Management of congenital adrenal hyperplasia during pregnancy. Endocr Pract 1996; 2:397–405.
327. Wallace C, Couch R, Ginsberg J. Fetal thyrotoxicosis: a case report and recommendations for prediction, diagnosis, and treatment. Thyroid 1995; 5:125–128.
328. Charlton V, Johengen M. Fetal intravenous nutritional supplementation ameliorates the development of embolization-induced growth retardation in sheep. Pediatr Res 1987; 22:55–61.
329. Flake AW, Zanjani ED. In utero hematopoietic stem cell transplantation. JAMA 1997; 278:932–937.

whether ovaries are present or not. Thus, the sexual dimorphism in phenotype in placental mammals is mediated by the fetal testis and its dual hormonal secretions and not by the ovary (Table 22–1). When testicular secretions are present, male differentiation takes place despite a fetal environment in which the concentration of circulating estrogens and progestogens is high.

Abnormalities of sexual development can be classified into two broad categories: (1) disorders of sex determination, which most often are caused by sex chromosome or gene abnormalities that affect gonadogenesis, and (2) disorders of sex differentiation, which usually are caused by a genetic defect and less often by adverse factors in the intrauterine environment. Before the genetic control of sex determination and gonadogenesis are discussed, a description of aspects of cytogenetics that are important to understanding abnormalities of sex determination is presented.

Chromosomal Sex and X and Y Chromosomes

A systematized array of metaphase chromosomes from a single cell is known as a *karyotype*.[28] The meaning of this term is usually extended to imply that the chromosomal pattern in that cell typifies all the diploid cells of that individual or even of that species, although this is by no means always true. The 22 autosomes and two sex chromosomes (i.e., two X chromosomes or an X and a Y) are arranged and serially numbered according to size. The X chromosomes resemble the larger autosomes in the medium-sized group with submedian centromeres (group 6 to 12). The Y chromosome resembles the short acrocentric autosomes in chromosomes 21 and 22 (Fig. 22–1).[28]

Each of the pairs of chromosomes can be identified with chromosome banding and painting techniques.[28–30] The pattern of DNA replication in human chromosomes can be studied by pulse labeling cell cultures with tritiated thymidine and preparing autoradiographs of the chromosomal spreads[31, 32] or by using the bromodeoxyuridine dye technique. One of the two X chromosomes in the female replicates late during DNA synthesis in the cell cycle,[31, 32] and this X chromosome gives rise to the distinctive X chromatin or Barr body seen in female somatic cells (see later discussion).

Chromosome banding techniques differentially stain chromosome segments. Caspersson and associates[33, 34] introduced a fluorescent staining method referred to as the Q staining method, in which substances such as quinacrine mustard or quinacrine hydrochloride are used to give a distinctive banding pattern (Q bands) for each chromosome (Fig. 22–2). The distal portion of the Y chromosome fluoresces intensely. Pardue and Gall[35] subsequently reported a Giemsa staining technique that preferentially stains the centromeric regions of the chromosome; the areas of constitutive (centromeric) heterochromatin are known as C bands. The Giemsa staining technique[36] has been modified by use of a multitude of pretreatment procedures on fixed metaphase chromosomes (e.g., hypertonic saline, sodium hydroxide, variation of pH, temperature, cation concentration, proteolytic enzymes), which produce Giemsa-stained bands that are identical (with minor exceptions) to the Q bands described by Caspersson and associates; this method yields permanent preparations for conventional light microscopy (see Fig. 22–2), and the resulting bands are designated G bands. Reverse (R) banding is a Giemsa staining method that produces a pattern of chromosome banding that is the reverse of either the Q or G bands. The structural components of the chromosome that give rise to the banding patterns are uncertain, but the differential distribution of base composition and the state of condensation of the chromatin appear to be involved. The Q bands result from binding of quinacrine stains to adenine- and thymine-rich (AT-rich) regions of DNA, whereas guanine- and cytosine-rich (G-C-rich) regions of the chromosome quench the fluorescence. The G bands appear to be a consequence of differential binding of dye to nonhistone protein overlying the AT-rich regions.

High-resolution chromosome banding and painting techniques provide precise methods for identification of each chromosome and analysis of chromosome abnormalities, including chromosome rearrangements (see Fig. 22–2). A standard nomenclature for identification and designation of individual

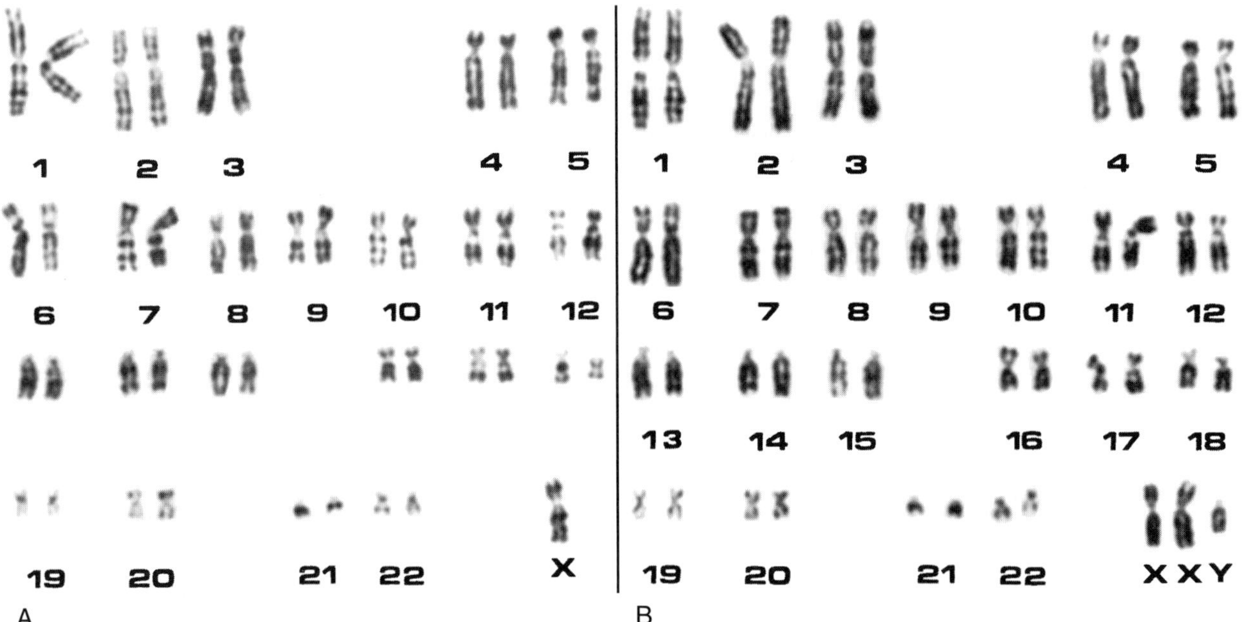

Figure 22–1. Typical G-banded karyotypes of patients with abnormal gonadal differentiation. *A*, The 45,X karyotype of a patient with streak gonads, short stature, and physical stigmata of Turner's syndrome. *B*, The 47,XXY karyotype of a phenotypic male with seminiferous tubule dysgenesis (chromatin-positive Klinefelter's syndrome).

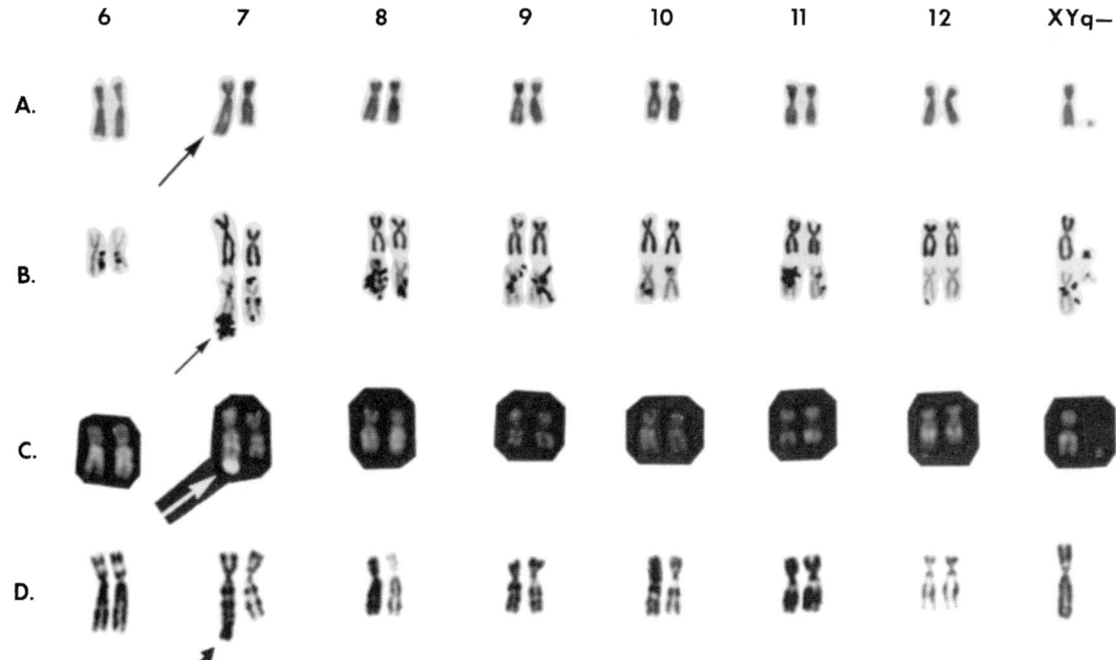

Figure 22–2. A partial karyotype of C group (chromosome numbers 6 to 12) and X and Y in a patient with a 46,X,t(Y;7)(q11;q36) karyotype. Standard Giemsa staining, autoradiography, fluorescent (Q), and Giemsa (G) banding techniques were used to identify the chromosome anomaly. *A*, The standard staining technique for karyotype analysis revealed an enlarged C group chromosome and a deleted G group chromosome. *B*, Autoradiography after incubation of lymphocyte culture with tritiated thymidine showed a late-labeling segment on the distal arms of the C chromosome and absence of a late-labeling segment on the deleted long arm of the presumptive Y. *C*, Quinacrine hydrochloride staining and fluorescence microscopy demonstrated a translocation of the brightly fluorescent segment of the long arm of the Y chromosome to the long arm of chromosome 7. *D*, Giemsa banding confirmed that the C group chromosome involved in the translocation was chromosome 7.

chromosomes, chromosome regions and bands, and structurally altered chromosomes is embodied in the report of the 1995 International System for Human Cytogenetics Nomenclature.[28] Table 22–2 summarizes the nomenclature applied to sex chromosome anomalies.

The identification of normal and structurally abnormal chromosomes, of supernumerary chromosomes, and of specific DNA sequences and genes (chromosome microdissection) has been revolutionized by the development of fluorescence in situ hybridization (FISH), the labeling of normal or abnormal DNA with fluorescent dyes,[37] so-called chromosome painting. With the use of special cameras (multiplex FISH) or Fourier spectroscopy (spectral karyotyping), a variety of fluorophores, and computer programs, the karyotype of normal and complex chromosome spreads can be determined rapidly (Fig. 22–3).[29, 30, 38–40]

Mechanisms of Chromosome Anomalies

Chromosome errors can arise from faulty replication of the germ cells during spermatogenesis or oogenesis or from faulty mitotic division of cells in the zygote after fertilization.

Aneuploidy

Aneuploid cells contain a total number of chromosomes different from that characteristic of the species. One mechanism producing aneuploidy is nondisjunction, which can occur during either mitotic or meiotic division.[41, 42] Nondisjunction is characterized by failure of either of a pair of sister chromatids or members of a pair of homologous chromosomes to separate during anaphase. As a result, one daughter cell receives an extra chromosome and the other is one short (Fig. 22–4). Aneuploidy can also be caused by anaphase lag, in which there is a simple loss of a chromosome from one or both of the two daughter cells, presumably because of failure of one chromosome to become properly oriented at the equatorial plate during metaphase. If both chromatids are lost, both daughter cell lines lack this chromosome. If only one member of the chromatid pair is lost, the descendants of one daughter cell are normal, and those of the other are one chromosome short (see Fig. 22–4). Nondisjunction in the oocyte increases with advanced maternal age[41–43]; an abnormality in reciprocal recombination in the fetus manifested as a compromised exchange configuration predisposes to missegregation during the completion of meiosis I (less frequently of meiosis II) immediately before ovulation 10 to 40 years later.[42, 44, 45]

Mosaicism

Mosaicism is the presence in an individual of two or more cell lines that differ in chromosomal constitution but originate from a single zygote. This condition can arise only from errors in mitosis after fertilization has occurred, but embryos with abnormal chromosomal makeup are prone to further errors of replication. Mosaicism is more common than first supposed, and many of the seeming paradoxes between genotype and phenotype are attributable to studies in which mosaicism was not rigorously excluded.[46] The difficulty in detecting or, especially, in excluding sex chromosome mosaicism cytogenetically was formidable in the past, but recombinant DNA techniques provide more specific and more accurate detection.[47] The use of X and Y DNA probes and chromosome- and locus-specific FISH analysis together with the polymerase chain reaction

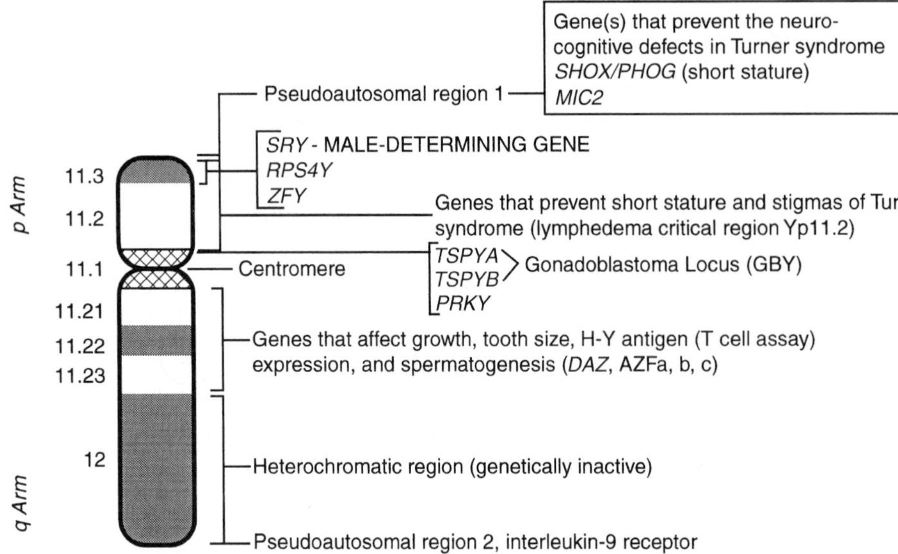

Figure 22–7. Diagram of a G-banded Y chromosome. Y-linked genes are shown. *SHOX/PHOG*, *s*hort stature/*p*seudoautosomal *h*omeob*o*x-containing *o*steogenic gene on the X; *MIC2*, a cell-surface antigen recognized by the monoclonal antibody 12E7; *SRY*, sex-determining region Y; *RPS4Y*, ribosome protein S4Y; *ZFY*, zinc finger Y; *TSPYA*, *TSPYB*, testes-specific protein Y; *PRKY*, a member of the cyclic adenosine monophosphate–dependent serine threonine protein kinase gene family, homologous to *PRKX*. *DAZ*, deleted in azoospermia; *AZF*, azoospermific factor.

The finding of a 47,XXY sex chromosome constitution in men with Klinefelter's syndrome and only a single X chromosome in women with the syndrome of gonadal dysgenesis (Turner's syndrome) provided convincing evidence that the Y chromosome carries a male-determining gene that can induce testicular development even in the presence of two or more X chromosomes. The presence of a Y chromosome drives testicular differentiation even in individuals with a 49,XXXXY sex chromosome constitution, whereas testicular differentiation does not occur in 45,X individuals. In addition, the Y chromosome is essential to spermatogenesis. In subsequent work the testis-determining gene, *SRY*, was localized to the short arm of the Y chromosome.

The human Y chromosome, which is composed of the remnants of a conserved region and, predominantly, of a single autosomal region addition estimated to have occurred 80 to 130 million years ago,[49–51] represents about 2% of the human genome DNA and is approximately 60 Mb in length. A total of 33 genes on the Y chromosome are known, including 10 genes in pseudoautosomal region 1 (PAR1) and 4 genes in PAR2; the Y chromosome is unique because it contains few active genes and a large heterochromatic segment on the distal long arm. It contains genes that influence stature (*GCY*, growth controlling gene(s) on Yq[52]) in addition to a gene affecting growth located in the PAR1 of the Y and X chromosomes. XYY boys have a mean final height of about 188 cm, more than 13 cm taller than their fathers.[53] Phenotypic females with a 46,X der(X) karyotype having three doses of *SHOX/PHOG* are tall, as are XXY patients.[54] Whether the increased stature in XYY patients is related solely to the extra dose of the pseudoautosomal *SHOX/PHOG* gene or to additional Y-borne genes is not known.

The length of the human Y chromosome varies as much as threefold in normal men. The length and morphology of the Y are heritable, are relatively constant in first-degree male relatives, and exhibit ethnic variation. Most of this variation is in the length of the long arm and in particular in the length of its distal, heterochromatic, brilliantly fluorescent segment in Q-stained preparations (Fig. 22–8; see also Fig. 22–7). This polymorphism in the size of the fluorescent portion and even loss of part of the distal nonfluorescent portion of the long arm are consistent with normal male sex differentiation and are not associated with known phenotypic effects; consequently, it is likely that a large segment of the long arm of the Y chromosome is not engaged in gene transcription. The long arm of the Y chromosome contains highly repetitious Y chromosome–specific and non–Y chromosome–specific sequences of DNA. The euchromatic short arm and the proximal portion of the long arm of the human Y chromosome make up about 0.5% of the diploid genome (XY + 44 autosomes).

The euchromatic portion of the Y chromosome[55] contains two regions, a Y-specific segment and regions at the distal ends of the short and long arms—the so-called pseudoautosomal regions (PARs)—that are homologous to the distal ends of the short and the long arms, respectively, of the X chromosome. The X and Y chromosomes pair and recombine obligately only along these small segments at the distal ends during meiosis. They form chiasmata, thereby maintaining sequence homology and allowing for the proper distribution of sex chromosomes to the daughter cells. This process is critical to sex determination. Genes on the distal short and long arms of the X and Y chromosomes are paired and are not subject to dosage compensation (i.e., gene inactivation); hence, they are expressed like autosomal genes rather than X-linked genes, leading to the PAR designation (see Fig. 22–7).

At least 10 genes are located on the PAR1 of the short arm of the X and Y chromosomes.[55–57] The short arm PAR (PAR1) is about 2.6 Mb in length, the boundaries being demarcated distally by the telomeres of the X and Y chromosomes and proximally by the Alu repeat sequence on the Y chromosome. The PARs of the X and Y chromosomes are 99% homologous distal to the Alu sequence. Distally on the short arm PAR is *PGPL*, which encodes a putative guanosine triphosphate (GTP)–binding protein; next is *SHOX/PHOG*, then *CSF2RA*, which encodes the α-subunit of the granulocyte colony-stimulating factor receptor.[55] Proximal to *CSF2RA* is *IL3RA* (encoding the α-subunit for the IL3A receptor), followed by *ANT3* (adenine nucleotide translocase), *ASMTL* (ASMT-like), and *ASMT* (acetyl serotonin methyl transferase), *XE7* (X-escape inactivation, function unknown), *TRAMP* (sequence homology with transposases suggests involvement in transposition), and *MIC2* at the PAR boundary. *PBDX* is the XG blood group gene, and its homologue on the Y chromosome is an expressed pseudogene of XH.[56–57]

The congruence between short stature and deletions of either Xp or Yp[58] suggested that a gene for stature was present in the distal 700 kb of the PAR1 because patients with only a single copy of this region have short stature. A gene from this 700-kb distal PAR region of Xp and Yp (PAR1), called *PHOG* (*p*seudoautosomal *h*omeob*o*x-containing *o*steogenic *g*ene), is ex-

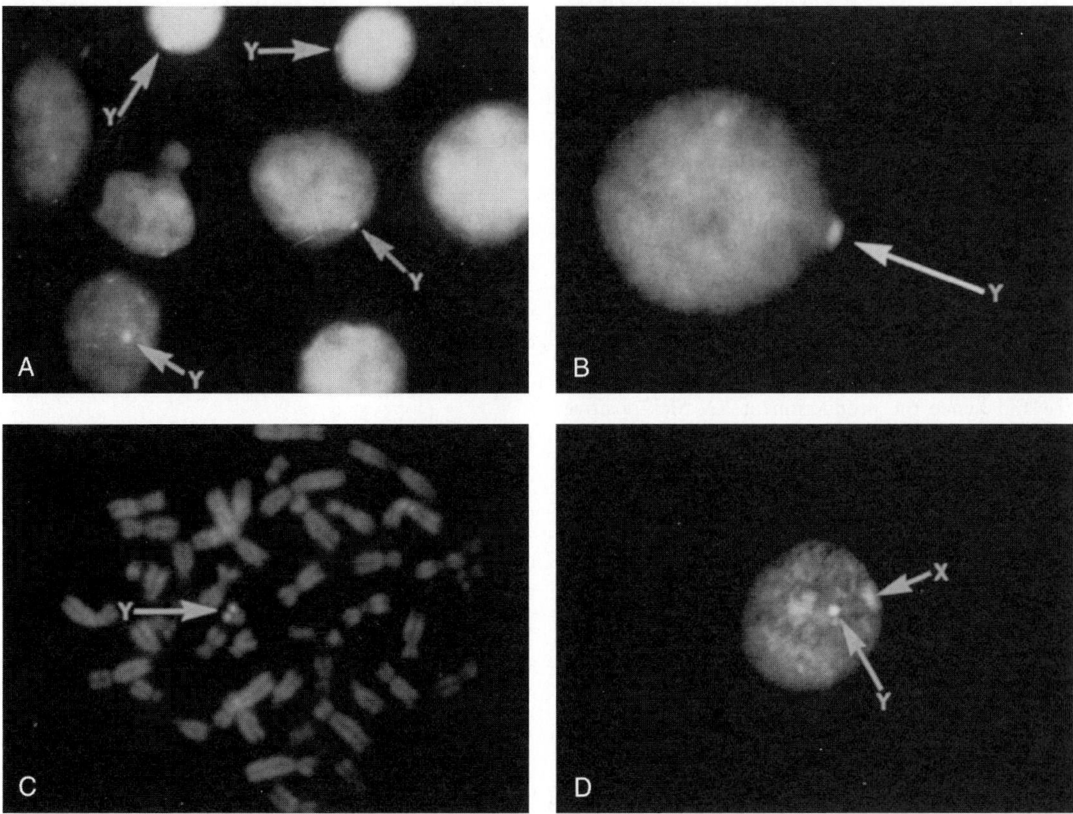

Figure 22–8. *A*, Q staining and fluorescence microscopy of interphase cells from a normal male, illustrating typical Y bodies. *B*, An enlarged photograph of one cell, showing a fluorescent Y body at the periphery of the nucleus. *C*, Metaphase chromosomes from a normal male, illustrating the brightly fluorescent distal segment of the long arm of the Y chromosome. *D*, An interphase nucleus in a buccal smear of a patient with a 47,XXY karyotype. A brightly fluorescent Y body and an X chromatin body (which exhibits much weaker fluorescence) were identified by Q staining and fluorescence microscopy.

pressed mainly in osteogenic cells and bone marrow stromal fibroblasts[59] and encodes a transcription regulatory factor. Its location in the distal PAR, the nature of its predicted protein, and its expression in bone made deletions of this gene a strong candidate for the gene responsible for the short stature in patients with the syndrome of gonadal dysgenesis (Turner's syndrome).[59] An identical gene was cloned from a 170-kb critical segment of PAR1 and termed *SHOX* (*s*hort stature *h*omeo*box*-containing gene).[58] This homeobox gene, *SHOX (PHOG)*, is alternatively spliced and encodes proteins of 292 and 225 amino acids.[58] It is expressed on both the inactive and active X chromosome as well as the Y chromosome[58, 59]; the SHOX protein acts as a cell-type specific transcriptional activator with an exclusive nuclear localization in the cell.[60]

The association of short stature with *SHOX/PHOG* haploinsufficiency in patients with Xp−, Yp−, in short otherwise "normal" males, and in patients with Leri-Weill syndrome and its expression in developing limbs and the first and second pharyngeal pouches suggested that it is involved in mesomelic short stature as well as the skeletal anomalies of Turner's syndrome.[54, 58–62] Homozygous loss of *SHOX/PHOG* causes Langer's type of severe mesomelic dwarfism.[63] Analysis of 32 Leri-Weill patients from 18 families revealed *SHOX/PHOG* deletions in only 10 of the 18 families, suggesting multiple genetic causes of Leri-Weill syndrome.[64] The phenotypic variation in patients with *SHOX/PHOG* heterozygous deletions or mutations (i.e., short normal male → Turner syndrome stigmata → Leri-Weill syndrome) is not understood.

A second PAR is found on the distal long arms of the X and Y chromosomes.[65] This region is 330 kb long and recombines during meiosis at a 2% rate, much slower than the Xp/Yp pseudoautosomal region combines but six times greater than average for X-specific DNA.[66] The proximal 295 kb contain two genes *SYBLI* (synaptobrevin-like 1), a gene that may be involved in synaptic signaling, and *HSPRY3* (human sprouty 3), a putative intracellular modulator of fibroblast growth factor (FGF) and FGF receptor tyrosinase activity, which antagonizes *Ras*-dependent mitogen-activated protein (*ras*/MAP) kinase signaling.[55] Unlike genes on PAR1, these genes are inactivated on both the inactive X and the Y chromosome.[66] The distal 35 kb of PAR2 contains two genes that are not inactivated: *IL9R*, the interleukin-9 receptor, and *CXY orf1*, a gene of unknown function, located 5 kb from the Xq telomere.[66]

The second region of the euchromatic portion of the Y chromosome, the so-called sex-specific region present only in the male, extends from the proximal boundary of the PAR to the heterochromatic portion of the long arm of the chromosome. Deletion analyses of the Y chromosome in 46,XX males and 46,XY females indicate that the segment just proximal to the PAR on the short arm of the Y chromosome carries a gene or genes critical to testicular organogenesis and subsequent male sex differentiation. A 35-kb region immediately adjacent to the PAR boundary contains a gene termed *SRY* (*s*ex-determining *r*egion *Y*).[4, 12, 67, 68] This gene encodes a testis-specific transcript that exhibits structural homology to two DNA-binding proteins: Mc, a mating-type protein of the fission yeast *Schizosaccharomyces pombe*, and HMG1 and HMG2, so-called nuclear high-mobility-group proteins.[68] Proximal to *SRY* is a gene for ribosomal protein subunit-4 *(RPS4Y)*, one of many housekeeping proteins that are encoded in slightly different forms by the Y chromosome and its homologue on the long arm of the X chromosome *(RPS4X)*.[55] On the short arm of the Y chromosome proximal to *RPS4Y* is a gene that encodes for a protein that has 13 CysCys/HisHis zinc fingers and both an acidic and a basic domain and that has been termed *ZFY* (*z*inc *f*inger *Y*).[69] By analogy to similar zinc finger proteins, such as *Xenopus* transcription factor IIIA, the protein is thought to bind to DNA in a sequence-specific manner and to regulate transcription. Among other genes on the short arm of the Y chromosome are *PRKY* (*pr*otein *k*inase *Y*), *TSPY* (*t*estis-*s*pecific *p*rotein, *Y* encoded), and *AMELY* (amelogenin), the gene that encodes the major extracellular matrix enamel protein in the developing tooth bud.[55]

PRKY has a homologous site on the X chromosome *(PRKX)*, which allows for illegitimate recombination between the X and Y chromosome and hence the production of XX *SRY*-positive males.[70] *TSPY* is present as a multicopy gene on the Y chromosome. *TSPY* may function as an oncogene responsible for gonadoblastoma formation in dysgenetic gonads.[71] Its repetitive units map to the GBY (gonadoblastoma) critical regions on the Y chromosome.[71, 72]

The euchromatic portion of the long arm of the Y chromosome can be divided into three regions: AZFa, AZFb, and AZFc for azoospermic factors a, b, and c.[73] These three nonoverlapping regions contain genes that when deleted result in infertility.[74, 75] AZFa is the region proximal to the centromere of the Y chromosome and it encompasses four genes: *USP9Y*, a ubiquitin-specific protease that encodes an H-Y antigen epitope, *DBY* (*d*ead *b*ox, *Y*), *UTY* (*u*biquitous *t*etratricopeptide repeat motif *Y*), and *TB4Y* (*t*hymosin *B4*, *Y* isoform).[55] AZFb contains five genes, prominent among which are *SMCY* (*s*elected *m*ouse *c*DNA, *Y*), which encodes two H-Y antigen epitopes[39] and *RBMY* (*R*NA-*b*inding *m*otif, *Y*) a gene with a putative role in spermatogenesis.[55] AZFc at the distal end of the euchromatic region has a five-gene cluster at its boundary, the most prominent of which is *DAZ* (*d*eleted in *az*oospermia), an RNA-binding protein.[55] Deletions in *DAZ* and one or more members of the *RBMY* family as well as *USP9Y* and *DBY* are a common cause of spermatogenic failure.[75] Deletions of AZFc including the *DAZ* gene family result in azoospermia more frequently than a deletion involving AZFa and AZFb.[75–77] Other genes postulated to reside on the Y chromosome but not yet cloned include genes affecting height, on the long arm pericentromeric region GCY,[78] as well as genes preventing the stigmata of the syndrome of gonadal dysgenesis, on the short arm, and genes affecting spermatogenesis.[79]

Y Chromatin (Y Body)

The fluorescent end of the human Y chromosome in metaphase, when stained with the fluorochrome quinacrine hydrochloride or its mustard derivative, is visualized as a small, brightly fluorescent body (Y body) in a high proportion of diploid interphase nuclei of cells from male buccal mucosal smears, lymphocytes, and polymorphonuclear leukocytes in peripheral blood cells, hair root sheath cells, and cells grown in culture. In 46,XY males, a single Y body, sometimes bipartite in structure, is present in interphase nuclei (see Fig. 22–8), whereas two Y bodies are detectable in nuclei in 47,XYY and 48,XXYY males (Table 22–3). In a small percentage of normal males (<0.05%), a small Y chromosome is present that lacks all or most of the distal fluorescent segment and a Y body is absent in somatic nuclei. By using FISH for Y chromosome and X chromosome satellite DNA analysis the sex chromosomes can be identified in interphase cells. *SRY* and other single copy genes are identifiable in interphase cells by FISH or primed in situ labeling (PRINS).[80]

Q-stained X chromatin bodies have been observed in cultured female fibroblasts and certain other female tissues, but the intensity of fluorescence of the X body is less, and the size is three to five times larger than that of the Y body (see Fig. 22–8). In sum, more than 30 genes and gene families are currently identified on the Y chromosome.[55, 75, 81]

Table 22–3. Sex Chromosome Complement Correlated with X Chromatin and Y Bodies in Somatic Interphase Nuclei*

Sex Chromosomes	Maximal Number in Diploid Somatic Nuclei: X Bodies	Y Bodies
45,X	0	0
46,XX	1	0
46,XY	0	1
47,XXX	2	0
47,XXY	1	1
47,XYY	0	2
48,XXXX	3	0
48,XXXY	2	1
48,XXYY	1	2
49,XXXXX	4	0
49,XXXXY	3	1
49,XXXYY	2	2

*Maximal number of X chromatin bodies in diploid somatic nuclei is one less than the number of Xs, whereas maximal number of Y fluorescent bodies is equivalent to the number of Ys in the chromosome constitution.

They are subclassified as follows:

1. Pseudoautosomal genes with identical sequences on X and Y (e.g., *IL9R* and *MIC2*).
2. Those located on the X-Y homologous regions of the nonrecombining region of Y (NRY); these genes are ubiquitously expressed and include *DBY* and *UTY*.
3. Genes that are Y specific and expressed only in the testis (e.g., *DAZ, USPY*).

Although *SRY* is Y specific, it does not fit this classification in view of its different pattern of expression and its single copy nature. Surprisingly, nearly half of all genes involved in early stages of spermatogenesis are X linked, a specialty role of the X chromosome in sperm production that emerged as it evolved from an ancestral autosome.[50, 83]

Biologic Functions of the X Chromosome

The biologic functions of the X chromosome are more complex than those of the Y chromosome. The X chromosome consists of about 160 Mb; landmark DNA sequences (sequence-tagged sites) have been determined over the entire X chromosome. A large number of genes on one of the two X chromosomes of the female undergo X inactivation, a gene-silencing mechanism activated in early embryonic development, to balance the expression of X-linked genes between males and females (see later). Genes on the X chromosome have a critical influence on sex determination in both the female and the male and on the differentiation of the somatic sex structures in the male. More than 300 gene loci unrelated to sex development are known to be X linked.[3, 15, 16]

The organization of the X chromosome resembles that of the Y chromosome in that it has both a pseudoautosomal region (PAR) on its distal short arm (PAR1), homologous to that on the Y chromosome (Xp22.36pter), an X-specific region, and a PAR on the long arm (PAR2) (Fig. 22–9).[65] PAR1 of the Xp is the locus for at least 11 genes *(PGPL, CSF2RA, SHOX/PHOG, IL3RA, ANT3, ASMT, XE7, TRAMP, MIC2,*

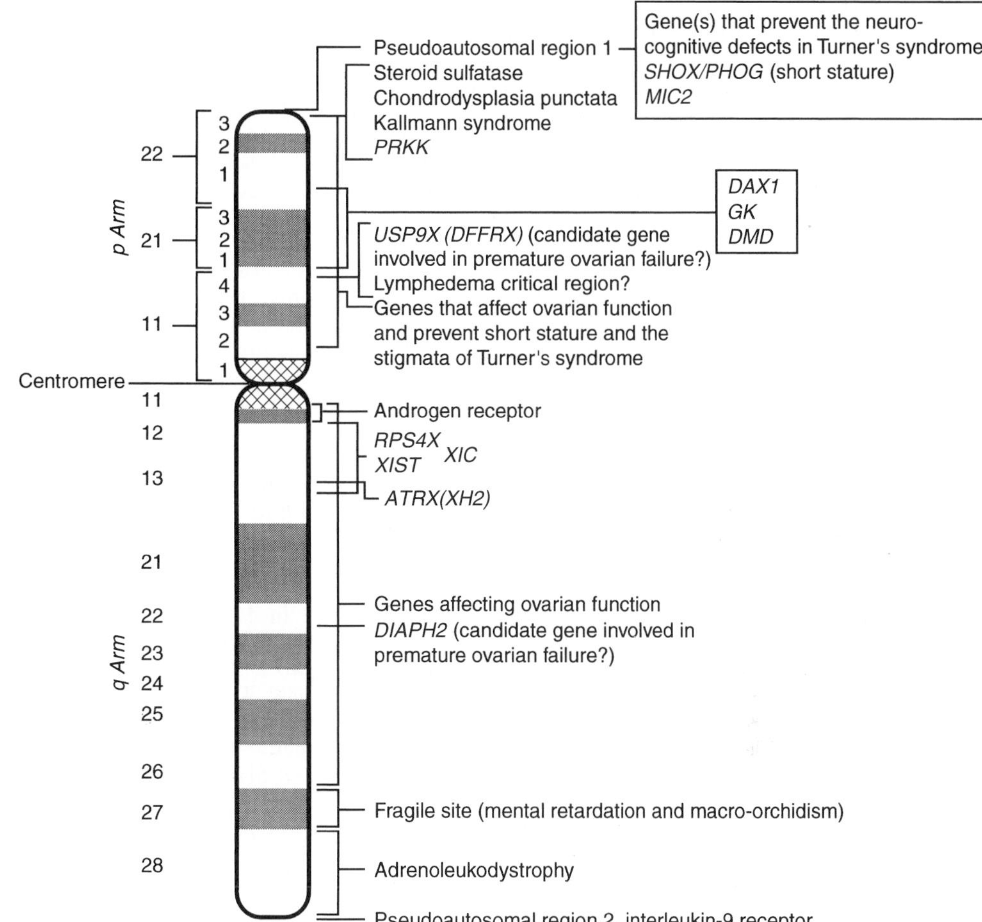

Figure 22–9. Diagram of a G-banded X chromosome. Selected X-linked genes are shown. *SHOX/PHOG*, *s*hort stature/*p*seudoautosomal *h*omeob*ox*-containing *o*steogenic gene; *MIC2*, a cell-surface antigen recognized by monoclonal antibody 12E7; *PRKX*, a member of the cyclic adenosine monophosphate–dependent serine threonine protein kinase gene family. Illegitimate X-Y interchange occurs frequently between *PRKX* and *PRKY*. *DAX1*, dosage-sensitive sex reversal congenital adrenal hypoplasia critical region on the X chromosome-1; *GK*, glycerol kinase; *DMD*, Duchenne's muscular dystrophy; *USP9X*, human X-linked homologue of the *DFFRX* (*Drosophila* fat facets–related X gene); *RPS4X*, ribosomal protein S4X; *Xist*, Xi specific transcripts; *XIC*, X-inactivation center; *ATRX*, α-thalassemia, X-linked mental retardation; *DIAP2*, human homologue of the *Drosophila* diaphanous gene, mutations of which affect oogenesis and spermatogenesis.

and *PBDX*), and a gene deletion results in the neurocognitive defects seen in Turner's syndrome. The locus of the *PBDX* gene (the XG blood group gene) is unusual in that it appears to span the PAR boundary on the X chromosome.[84] Immediately proximal to the boundary of the PAR are the loci for many genes, including those for chondrodysplasia punctata and steroid sulfatase *(STS)*,[85] the gene encoding the amelogenin enamel protein in the developing tooth bud,[86] and the locus for the zinc finger X gene *(ZFX)*,[87] which cross-hybridizes with DNA probes of the *ZFY* gene. Because the ZFX protein has 13 zinc fingers with 97% amino acid sequence homology to ZFY, it appears that both these zinc finger proteins may bind to the same nucleic acid sequences. Genes in the area of the X chromosome immediately proximal to the PAR (i.e., *XG [PBDX], STS, KAL1, ZFX*) escape X inactivation.[85] Other genes are postulated to reside in this region, including a gene or genes that prevent many of the somatic abnormalities found in the syndrome of gonadal dysgenesis.[46, 79, 88] Proximal to this region are genes that are not homologous to sequences on the Y chromosome and are subject to dosage compensation by X inactivation on all X chromosomes in excess of one.

Several genes that play a role in sex determination and differentiation are present on the short arm of the X chromosome. These include the Kallmann syndrome gene, *KAL1*, deletion or mutation of which results in anosmia and hypogonadotropic hypogonadism.[89] *KAL1* maps about 1.5 Mb proximal to *STS* on Xp22.3 and encodes a protein, anosmin, that is critical for the migration of the luteinizing hormone–releasing hormone (LHRH) neurosecretory neurons from the olfactory placode to the hypothalamus.[89] Proximal to the genes for Duchenne muscular dystrophy *(DMD)* and glycerol kinase (*GK*) in the Xp21 region is a locus that contains two overlapping regions, *AHC* (*a*drenal *h*ypoplasia *c*ongenita) and *DSS* (*d*osage-sensitive *s*ex *r*eversal). A gene, *DAX1* (*DSS/AHC* critical region on the *X* chromosome), has been cloned from this region.[90] Deletions and mutations in the *DAX1* gene are associated in the male with adrenal hypoplasia and hypogonadotropic hypogonadism.[91] Duplication of the *DAX1* gene in the XY human (and rodent) results in testicular dysgenesis and lack of or incomplete masculinization of the internal and external genitalia.[92, 93] Duplications in 46,XX females, however, do not affect ovarian function.[92] In contrast, deletions of the *DAX1* gene have no effect on testicular determination and differentiation and subsequent in utero masculinization of 46,XY individuals. More proximal on the short arm, a lymphedema critical region has been proposed to reside in Xp11.4.[79, 94]

Two X chromosomes are required in the human for normal ovarian differentiation and follicular maturation: 45,X individuals have bilateral streak gonads. Studies of patients with deletions of the X chromosome indicate that loci on both the short and long arms of the X chromosome are involved in ovarian differentiation and maturation.[79, 95]

The long arm of the X chromosome contains a large number of genes that are subject to X inactivation and are responsible for a wide variety of X-linked traits. The gene for the androgen receptor protein is located in the paracentromeric region of the long arm of the X.[96] The *RPS4X* gene is also located in this region and is subject to X inactivation. This region also contains the X-inactivation center, XIC, the site around which the X chromosome condenses to form the sex chromatin body and from which X inactivation spreads.[97] (See X Chromatin and Gene Expression.)

X Chromatin (X or Barr Body)

Whereas the Y chromosome is one of the smallest human chromosomes and is mainly concerned with testis organogenesis, the X chromosome is the eighth longest and contains about 5% of the total DNA content of the haploid genome (X + 22 autosomes). Furthermore, the X chromosome contains genes that encode functions involving every system in the body. Because females have twice as much of this genetic material in their cells as males, the biologic differences between the sexes should be far greater than is the case. Theories proposed to explain this paradox are an outgrowth of Barr's pioneering observations of the X chromatin body in somatic cells of females.

In 1949 Barr and Bertram described the presence of a stainable chromatin mass at the periphery of the nucleus in resting ganglion cells of female but not of male cats. This distinguishing characteristic of the female sex is present in most mammalian cells and can be used as a cytologic means of assessing the number of X chromosomes in humans (reviewed in reference 280) (Fig. 22–10; see Table 22–3).

The X chromatin body is usually planoconvex, with the flattened side in apposition to the inner surface of the nuclear membrane; in some nuclei it has a bipartite structure. It is about 1 μm in diameter and stains positively for DNA. In certain tissues, such as amniotic membrane, almost every interphase nucleus is chromatin positive. In buccal mucosal smears (the most commonly used preparation for determining the X chromatin pattern), the proportion of X chromatin–positive nuclei in females may be lower than in other somatic tissues, but in most studies these nuclei are detected in no less than 20% of all nuclei.

In polymorphonuclear leukocytes in females, 1% to 15% of neutrophils (mean, 2.5%) have a drumstick-shaped, dense chromatin accessory nuclear appendage not found in normal males (see Fig. 22–10*D*). These appendages have the same significance as X chromatin in other somatic tissues.

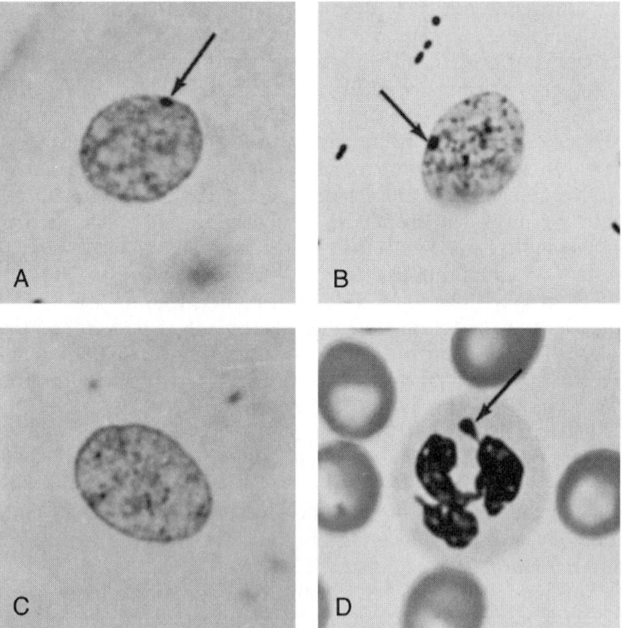

Figure 22–10. *A* and *B*, Photomicrographs showing the X chromatin body (Barr body, *arrow*) in the nucleus of buccal mucosal cells from a normal female (thionine stain, ×2000). Such cells are found in about 25% of well-preserved nuclei. *C*, A buccal mucosal cell from a normal male, illustrating absence of this body (thionine stain, ×2000). *D*, A typical "drumstick" nuclear appendage *(arrow)* found in a variable proportion of leukocytes of female subjects.

In patients with more than one X chromosome, the maximal number of X chromatin bodies in any diploid nucleus is one less than the total number of X chromosomes. In 47,XXX females or 48,XXXY males, for example, at most two Barr bodies are present in diploid nuclei, whereas 46,XY and 45,X individuals are X chromatin negative[31, 280] (see Table 22–3). Abnormalities in shape and size of the X chromatin body can often be correlated with structural abnormalities of the X chromosome. The X chromatin body is small in females with one normal X and one deleted X chromosome (46,XXp−) and in those with one ring X chromosome (46,XXr). A large X body is associated with a long arm isochromosome (Xqi). When an X is structurally abnormal, the aberrant X chromosome replicates late and gives rise to the X chromatin (except when the structurally abnormal X is an X-autosome translocation).

X Chromatin and Gene Expression

In 1959 Ohno and co-workers reported the first evidence that X chromatin (the Barr body) arises from only one of the two X chromosomes in the interphase nuclei of female somatic cells. The staining characteristics of such nuclei arise from the fact that a portion of one X chromosome is highly condensed (heteropyknotic); the other X, like the autosomes, is extended and filamentous.[98] This difference in staining quality betokens a striking difference in the functional roles of the two X chromosomes. By studying the sequence of incorporation of tritiated thymidine into replicating chromosomes, Grumbach and colleagues[31, 32] showed that the X chromosome that gives rise to X chromatin completes DNA synthesis later than any other chromosome and that the maximal number of X chromatin bodies in a single diploid nucleus is equal to the number of late-replicating X chromosomes (Fig. 22–11). These observations and the incisive genetic studies of Lyon, Beutler, and others led to the concept that only one X chromosome in each cell is genetically active during interphase, the other X chromosome being heterochromatinized and genetically inactive for most functions.[31, 32, 99, 100] We do not refer here to constitutive heterochromatin but rather to facultative heterochromatin-euchromatic (active) chromosome regions silenced by transformation into a heterochromatin (or inactive) form.[101, 102]

The change in state (inactivation)[31, 101, 103, 104] of one X chromosome in each female cell occurs during the late blastocyst stage, between the 12th and the 18th day in the human embryo. X inactivation is a multistep process that leads to stable and epigenetic silencing of genes on all X chromosomes in excess of one X. It involves (1) counting (ascertainment of X-autosome location and inactivation of all X chromosomes in excess of 1); (2) random selection of which X chromosome, either the maternal or paternal X to inactivate; and (3) silencing—the initiation, establishment, and maintenance of X-inactivation.[99, 100, 105] The female germ cells beyond the stage of oogonia are the only cell lines known to be exempted from heterochromatinization and inactivation,[103] a finding in keeping with the requirement for a second X chromosome for normal ovarian differentiation. Both X chromosomes in mouse oocytes are active and code for the X-linked genes for glucose-6-phosphate dehydrogenase and hypoxanthine-guanine phosphoribosyltransferase.[104] This observation has been confirmed in human fetal and postnatal oocytes.[101] In each somatic cell, however, either the maternally or the paternally derived X chromosome is usually randomly inactivated. Once this transformation is accomplished, the inactive state of that particular X chromosome is transmitted to all descendants of that cell.

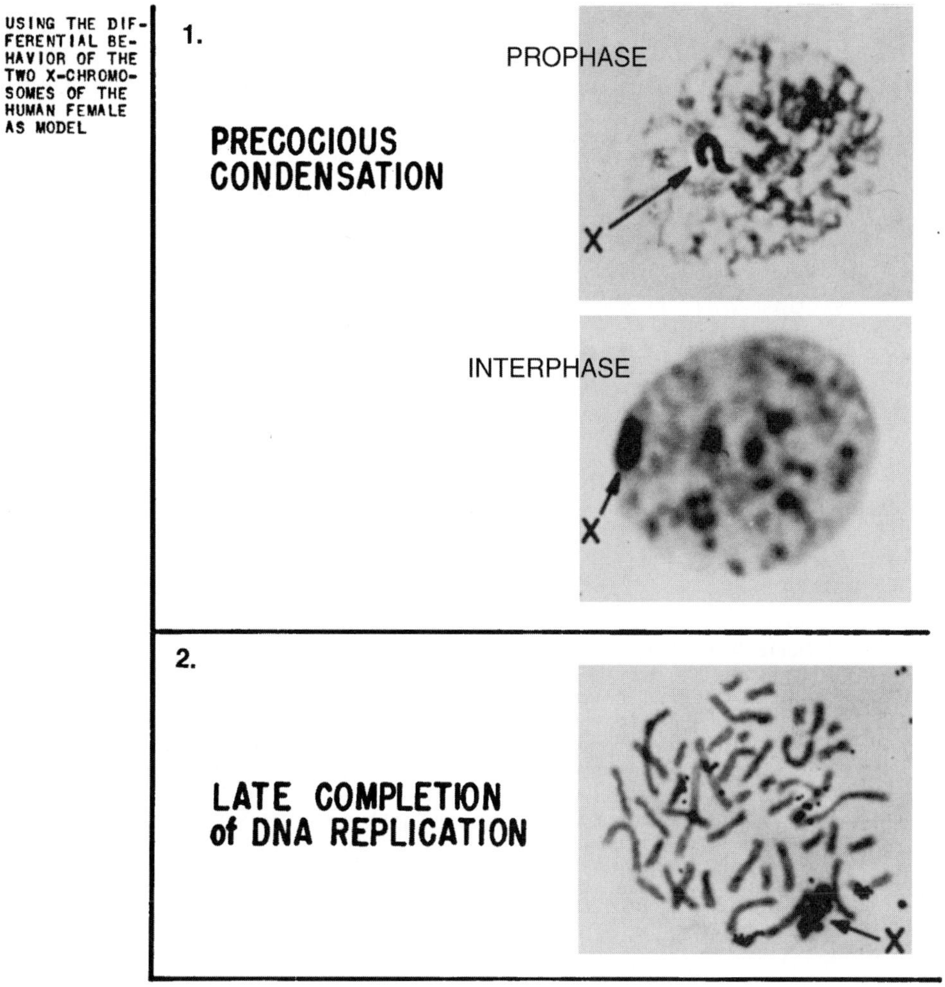

USING THE DIFFERENTIAL BEHAVIOR OF THE TWO X-CHROMOSOMES OF THE HUMAN FEMALE AS MODEL

1. PRECOCIOUS CONDENSATION

PROPHASE

X

INTERPHASE

X

2. LATE COMPLETION of DNA REPLICATION

X

Figure 22–11. Characteristics of heterochromatin formation as exemplified by differential behavior of the two X chromosomes of the female in somatic cells. *1,* Precocious condensation of a large part of one of the two X chromosomes in prophase and formation of the X chromatin body in interphase nuclei. *2,* Delayed replication of DNA in one of the X chromosomes (*arrow* indicates silver grains overlying one X chromosome in the autoradiogram of metaphase chromosomes from a normal female exposed to tritiated thymidine late in the synthetic period). With some exceptions (PAR region, etc.) gene activity on the heterochromatic late-replicating X chromosome is silenced or modified. (From Grumbach MM. On the significance of sex chromatin. In Second International Conference on Congenital Malformations. New York, International Medical Congress, 1964, pp 62–67.)

This control system functions as an epigenetic mechanism of dosage compensation by which each female somatic cell functions virtually as if it had only one active X chromosome.[99, 100, 101, 106–108] The female, in effect, has only a little more active genetic material than does the male. This hypothesis is commonly referred to as the "Lyon hypothesis"[108a] (or the "inactive X theory," or the "fixed differentiation hypothesis of X chromosome behavior") (Fig. 22–12). Although inactivation of structurally normal X chromosomes in individuals with more than one X chromosome in their genome is usually random, instances of skewed inactivation are well documented.[109–111] XX individuals heterozygous for X-linked immunodeficiencies and mental retardation disorders, Lesch-Nyhan syndrome, or adrenoleukodystrophy may appear to have nonrandom activation of their X chromosomes owing to postinactivation selection (i.e., in vivo selection against those cells in which the normal allele is inactivated in tissues where the gene product is required).[109, 110] Skewed inactivation of the X chromosome has been reported in families with X-linked diseases and in monozygotic twins discordant for an X-linked disease.[109] If inactivation occurs normally as a random event in a small number of cells, 10% of "normal females" may show an 80:20 proportion of inactivated X chromosomes from one parent and even manifest symptoms of an X-linked mutant allele. Skewed inactivation also occurs in patients with a structurally abnormal X chromosome: the structurally abnormal X chromosome is inactivated, unless it is a part of an X-autosome translocation, in which case the X-autosome translocation will always be active, probably as the result of cell selection. A skewed pattern of X inactivation also has been described in a multigenerational study, suggesting that this character is controlled in some families by one or more X-linked genes.[112]

The fact that normal females function as genetic mosaics insofar as X-linked traits are concerned has been documented in the mouse and in humans. For example, Davidson and associates[112a] demonstrated two populations of cells in females heterozygous for a mutant form of the X-linked gene for glucose-6-phosphate dehydrogenase (see Fig. 22–12). Inactivation of all X chromosomes in excess of one also explains the relatively minor phenotypic changes in women with more than two X chromosomes (Fig. 22–13). By contrast, trisomy for an autosome as small as chromosome 21, as in Down's syndrome, is usually associated with profound effects. Biochemical analysis of DNA methylation of active and inactive X chromosomes and studies with 5-azacytidine (which impairs methylation of cytosine) suggest that DNA methylation plays an important role in the maintenance of X chromosome inactivation, late replication, and sex chromatin formation.[99, 113–115] DNA methylation differs in the two X chromosomes. The double-stranded palindromic cytosine-guanine dinucleotide clusters, the so-called CpG islands, commonly found at the 5′ end of genes, are methylated mainly in genes on the inactive X chromosome. The methylated cytosine residues serve to maintain the suppressed transcriptional activity and relative resistance to nuclease. The chromatin of the inactive X contains more unacetylated histones (histones H3 and H4) than the chromatin of the active X chromosome does.[116] Histones function as DNA-packaging proteins; the DNA helix is wrapped around core

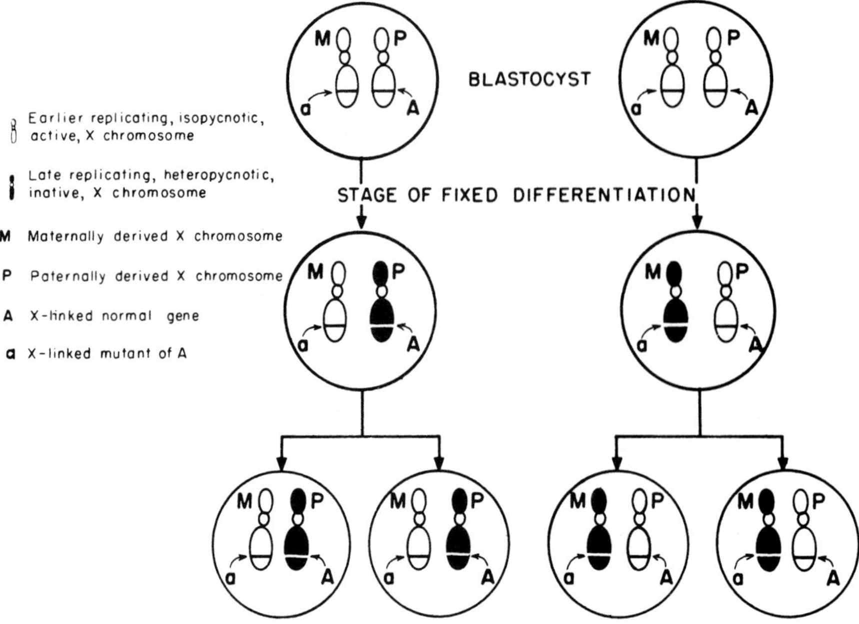

Figure 22–12. Diagram of the fixed differentiation or Lyon hypothesis of X chromosome behavior in somatic cells of the human female. At the late blastocyst stage (the time when X chromatin can first be identified), one of the two X chromosomes becomes heterochromatinized in each cell and gives rise to an X chromatin body; it is by chance in each cell whether this differentiation involves a maternally derived X (M) or a paternally derived X (P). Once differentiation has occurred, this characteristic is fixed in succeeding generations of somatic cells. Most of the genes on the heterochromatic portion of an X chromosome are suppressed or inactivated, thus serving as a means of "dosage compensation" for the greater number of X-linked genes in the female than in the male. This mechanism has an important bearing on expressivity and penetrance of an X-linked mutant gene in a heterozygous female. In the diagram, the maternally derived X carries a mutant gene (a) that is expressed only in cells in which this X is the isopyknotic, euchromatic active X (white X^M). Although the heterochromatinized X *(black X)* in this diagram is represented as wholly inactive, some loci on the heterochromatinized X do remain active and exert genetic effects. The female germ cell line beyond the oogonia stage is exempted from heterochromatinization.

histone protein. In addition, a core histone 2A variant, macro histone H2A1, is enriched on the inactive X chromosome.[117, 118] Furthermore, methylation of X-chromosomal histone H3 lysine 9 is an early event in X inactivation.[101, 119, 120] Underacetylated and methylated histones bind more tightly to nearby DNA and inhibit transcription of DNA to RNA, resulting in transcriptional silencing and down-regulation of gene expression. Acetylation, a common requisite for the activation of gene expression, is mediated by histone acetyl transferase A, encoded by the *HATA* gene.[121]

In contrast to the mouse, human X chromosome inactivation does not involve the entire chromosome. The heteropyknotic X in the human female is only segmentally inactive in terms of transcriptional activity[122]; early studies of the heterochromatin-

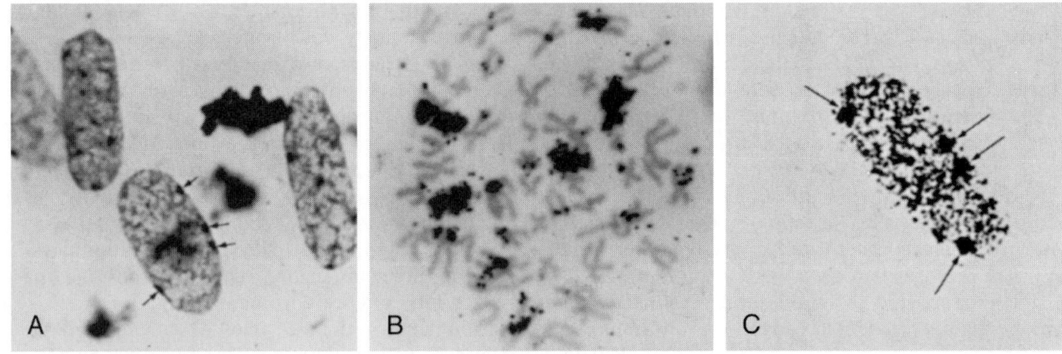

Figure 22–13. Diploid somatic cells from a girl with a 49,XXXX karyotype. *A*, Four X chromatin bodies *(arrows)* in an interphase nucleus from a culture of skin fibroblasts. *B*, Autoradiogram of metaphase chromosomes, illustrating four areas of high grain density overlying four of the five X chromosomes. *C*, An autoradiogram of an interphase nucleus in a culture of skin fibroblasts; four peripheral "hot" areas *(arrows)* of high grain density overlie four X chromatin bodies and provide direct evidence that each X chromatin body is derived from one late-labeling X chromosome. (Modified from Grumbach MM, Morishima A, Taylor JA. Human sex chromosome abnormalities in relation to DNA replication and heterochromatization. Proc Natl Acad Sci USA 1963; 49:581–589; and Grumbach MM. On the significance of sex chromatin. In Second International Congress on Congenital Malformations. New York: International Medical Congress, 1964, pp. 62–67.)

ized X chromosome suggest that about 21% of genes on Xp escape inactivation in contrast to about 3% of genes on Xq. Genes on the PAR of the short and long arm as well as genes scattered along the short and long arms of the heteropyknotic X chromosome escape inactivation.[122] Individuals with a 45,X or 47,XXY constitution, for example, have abnormalities both in gonadal development and in somatic features unrelated to sex. Furthermore, as noted previously, the gene for the red blood cell antigen Xg *(PBDX)*, the *STS* gene, and the *ZFX* genes escape inactivation and are active on both X chromosomes in the female; these genes have been mapped to the distal part of the short arm of the X,[85, 87] outside the PAR1. Two genes, *XIST* (*Xi*-*s*pecific *t*ranscripts)[123] and *RPS4*,[124] which are located on the proximal long arm of the X chromosome, escape inactivation on the heteropyknotic X chromosome. Inactivation of the X chromosome is mediated by a *cis*-acting region of the X chromosome, the XIC (X-inactivating center), from which inactivation spreads along the X. The *XIST* gene, discovered by Willard and his colleagues, is an essential component of the XIC, at Xq13.[100, 125–127]

XIST is a unique gene in that its product, a noncoding RNA, is expressed in high levels only on the inactive X chromosome.[100, 127, 128] Its expression correlates with the inactivation of the X chromosome in female somatic cells and with meiosis in spermatogonia.[100, 127, 129–131] The XIST allele is turned off on the active X; hence, its lack of expression on an X chromosome indicates that the genes encoded by that X chromosome are transcriptionally active. Human and mouse *XIST/Xist* genes encode a long noncoding RNA transcript that is retained in the nucleus "coating" the inactive X chromosome and initiating the gene silencing process.[100] Knockout of the *Xist* gene in embryonic stem cells prevents X inactivation in *cis*, whereas deletions of 65 kb of DNA at the 3′ end of *Xist* (mouse homologue) result in that chromosome always being inactivated.[105, 131] In the mouse the gene-silencing function of *Xist* is lost with deletion of a conserved repeat sequence at the 5′ end, but this mutant *Xist* continued to exhibit chromatin association and spreading.[126] Additionally, the insertion of ectopic copies of *Xist* into autosomes of murine stem cells results in the molecular and heterochromatic features of X inactivation, including *Xist* RNA association in *cis*, gene inactivation, late replication, and a decrease in histone H4 acetylation.[130, 131] *XIST* apparently is not required for maintenance of X inactivation.[132] The silent *Xist* gene on the active X chromosome is fully methylated at its 5′ end.[127] In the mouse placenta, X inactivation is imprinted—the paternal X chromosome is inactivated. A mouse *Xist* antisense gene, *Tsix*, is located 15 kb downstream of Xist and extends across the *Xist* locus on the opposite strand.[133] *Tsix* is thought to play a role in the repression of the maternal Xist allele in the mouse.[134, 135] However, the suppression of *Xist* by *cis*-acting *Tsix*, which prevents the initiation of X inactivation, does not account for random selection of the X.[136]

Lee and co-workers searched for a *trans*-acting factor involved in X-chromosome choice in the mouse. They found a candidate, *trans*-acting molecule, the ubiquitous chromatin insulator and transcription regulator CTCF, which has 11 zinc fingers.[137] However, Percec and associates using chemical mutagenesis detected two genetically different autosomal dominant mutations (not involving CTCF) that affect X chromosome choice in the early embryo. They designated these mutations X-inactivation autosomal factors 1 and 2.[138]

Migeon and co-workers have identified the human homologue of *Tsix*, *TSIX* on the X chromosome.[139] However, unlike *Tsix*, *TSIX* RNA is truncated at the 5′ end, does not cover the *XIST* promoter, and does not have a CpG island, which is critical for the function of *Tsix*.[139] These differences have led Migeon to question the function of *TSIX* in X-chromosome inactivation in humans. Its apparent lack of functionality may explain the discrepancy in X-chromosome imprinting in the human placenta between the human[139, 140] and rodent and creates uncertainty about the role of the human *TSIX* gene in X chromosome choice. The progress over the past decade in illuminating the epigenetic mechanism of X inactivation is remarkable.

Some patients with a 45,X/46X, "tiny" ring X chromosome karyotype differ in phenotype from other patients with gonadal dysgenesis with a ring X chromosome in their genome.[141] These tiny ring X chromosomes do not express *XIST*, have histone H4 acetylation at a level consistent with that found on an active X chromosome, and contain genes that are active.[141] These tiny ring X chromosomes that lack the *XIST* gene do not undergo X inactivation; as a consequence, the phenotype in affected patients results from functional disomy caused by lack of dosage compensation.[141] In general, patients with small ring X chromosomes have a greater incidence of mental retardation than those with other forms of Turner's syndrome.[141] Other congenital malformations such as syndactyly and abnormal facies are common.[142]

Genes and Testicular Organogenesis

The genetic sex of the zygote is established by fertilization of a normal ovum by an X- or Y-bearing sperm, and the mechanisms involved in the translation of genetic sex into a testis or an ovary are understood in broad terms. From the early days of human chromosome analysis, compelling evidence was obtained for the regulation of testicular gonadogenesis by a gene (or genes) on the Y chromosome. Indeed, sex determination is essentially testis determination. The short arm of the Y chromosome contains a gene *(SRY)* that controls testis determination and, hence, maleness. The gene acts in a dominant fashion and leads to differentiation of the bipotential gonad as a testis. Several hypotheses were proposed to explain testicular morphogenesis (Fig. 22–14). H-Y antigen and *ZFY* were proposed as the sex determinators, but that proposal was discarded.[143–145] Reports beginning in 1988 have provided compelling evidence that the *SRY* gene is the master gene that controls male sex determination.

H-Y Antigen

In 1955 Eichwald and Silmser discovered in males of a highly inbred strain of mice the H-Y antigen, a male-specific cell membrane component encoded by the Y chromosome that causes rejection by female mice of skin grafts from male donors of the same strain. Antibodies to H-Y antigen were identified serologically in male-grafted female mice by Goldberg and associates in 1971 and were utilized for measurement of H-Y antigen. Initial reports suggested that H-Y antigen was a good candidate for the testicular determining factor (TDF) on the Y chromosome, but the lack of reproducibility of the H-Y antigen assay led to increasing skepticism about its role in testicular determination. Finally, it was demonstrated that the gene for H-Y antigen is located on the long arm of the Y chromosome, separate and distinct from the gene for male sex determination.[143]

ZFY Gene

In 1987 Page and associates proposed that the sex-determining function of the Y chromosome is located within a 140-kb segment of the short arm of the Y chromosome (see Fig. 22–14). A gene in this region encodes a protein with 13 CysCys/HisHis zinc fingers at the carboxyl terminus (and a basic and acidic region at the amino terminus).[144] By analogy to *Xenopus* transcription factor IIIA, it was suggested by Page that this

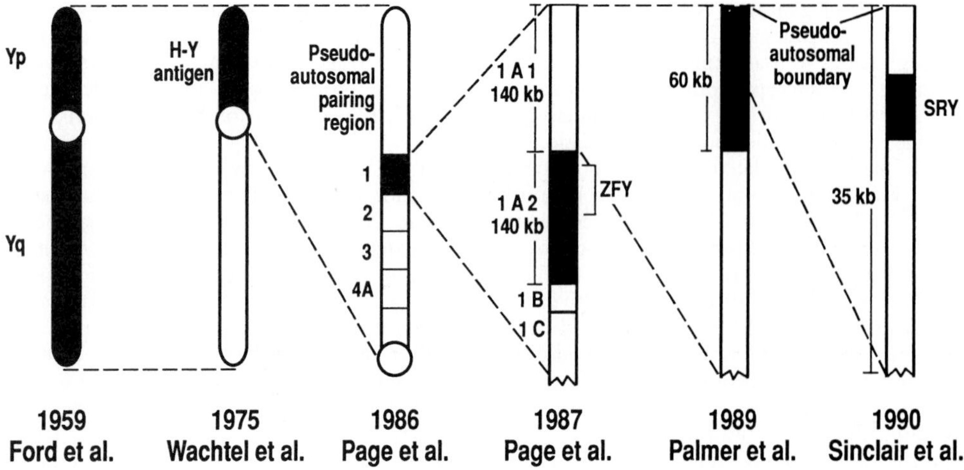

Figure 22–14. Diagram of the historical search for the testis-determining factor. The shaded area on the Y chromosome is the region to which this factor has been localized. ZFY, zinc finger Y; SRY, sex-determining region Y; numbers 1 to 4A indicate arbitrary deletion segments on the Y chromosome. (Modified from McLaren A. What makes a man a man? Reprinted by permission from Nature, vol. 346, pp. 216–217. © 1990 Macmillan Magazines Ltd.)

protein binds to DNA and/or RNA in a sequence-specific manner and regulates transcription and that this zinc finger protein, ZFY, is the primary sex-determining signal on the Y chromosome. A sequence homologous to ZFY is present on the X chromosome (ZFX) in the Xp21.2-p22.1 region.[87] The latter finding initially suggested that X inactivation (dosage compensation) might play a role in sex determination, but ZFX escapes inactivation, so X-chromosome inactivation cannot play a role in this process.[87] Convincing evidence has shown that *ZFY* is not the testis-determining gene. Furthermore, in metatherian species (marsupials), sex determination is Y dependent even though ZFY-related sequences are not located on the X and Y chromosomes of these animals but rather on autosomes.[145]

SRY Gene

The long quest for the testes-determining factor (TDF) finally met with success with the identification of the *SRY* gene. In 1989, Palmer and co-workers described three 46,XX males and one true hermaphrodite, the sibling of one of the 46,XX males.[67] They were all ZFY negative, in spite of evidence for a Y-to-X chromosome exchange as the mechanism of their XX karyotype in the presence of testes with male sex differentiation.[67] The fragment of Y chromosome translocated to the X chromosome in these patients involved sequences that were distal to the ZFY locus on the short arm of the Y chromosome. This demonstration of testes in patients with a Y fragment but no ZFY sequences, along with studies in marsupials[145] and mice, doomed the hypothesis that ZFY was the TDF on the Y chromosome.[146] The Y-to-X exchange in these four patients involved Y-specific sequences located within 35 kb of the boundary of the PAR on the short arm of the Y chromosome (Fig. 22–15).[67] A 2.1-kb clone, pY53.3, was identified in this region within 8 kb of the PAR boundary.[147] This probe detected male sequences in a wide variety of eutherian mammals.[147]

Studies in mice established that *Sry* (the mouse homologue of the human *SRY* gene) is the TDF. *Sry* is present in the Sxr,XX mouse, a "male" mouse that has the smallest piece of Y chromosome known to code for testicular determination and differentiation translocated to the X chromosome.[147] *Sry* is absent in the XY fertile "female" mouse, which has an 11-kb deletion involving the testes-determining region.[148, 149] Further studies in the mouse model demonstrated that *Sry* is expressed in the embryonic genital ridge for only a brief period, from 10.5 to 12.5 days after coitus and 24 hours before the genital ridge differentiates into a testis.[150] *Sry* expression is limited to pre-Sertoli cells in the genital ridge; in contrast, *Sry* in the adult testes is expressed in the germ cells.[151] The function of *Sry* transcripts in the adult mouse testes is unknown, because the transcripts are circular and are not associated with polyribosomes; they appear not to be translated into a protein.[151] Definitive proof that *Sry* was the TDF came from the demonstration that 46,XX mice with a transgene that contains a 14-kb piece of the Y chromosome including *Sry* differentiate as males with testes.[152] In the first series of animals, one 46,XX progeny that expressed the transfected *Sry* gene was a well-differentiated 46,XX male that exhibited appropriate male sexual mating behavior.[152] Histologic examination of the testes revealed normal somatic elements, absent spermatogenesis, and degenerating germ cells.[152, 153] The two other mice were 46,XX females; one was able to transmit the *Sry* transgene to her progeny, resulting in the generation of 46,XX males; 46,XX hermaphrodites; and 46,XX females.[153] That the *Sry* transgene produced sex reversal in only 25% of transfected embryos may be attributable to the incorporation of the transgene into a region of the genome where it is either not expressed, expressed at a low level, or expressed late in relation to gonadal determination and differentiation.[153] Nevertheless, this critical transgene experiment proved conclusively that *Sry* is the only gene on the Y chromosome necessary for testes determination and differentiation and that *Sry* is the TDF gene. In addition, these studies indicated that Y-borne genes other than *Sry* are involved in the regulation of spermatogenesis.

Evidence in the human from sex-reversed 46,XX males and 46,XY females confirms the conclusion that *SRY* is the TDF. In humans, an aberrant Y-to-X interchange during paternal spermatogenesis can transfer Y-specific loci to the X chromosome, and 80% of 46,XX males have a variable amount of the Y chromosome translocated to the X.[154] All these patients are *SRY* positive.[111] Between 30% to 40% of Xp/Yp interchanges occur between Xp22.3 (*PRKX* gene) and a region on the Y chromosome (*PRKY* gene) proximal to the *SRY* gene.[70] The *PRKX/PRKY* genes are 94% homologous, are oriented in the same direction, and encode proteins with an adenosine triphosphate (ATP)–binding domain and a catalytic domain.[70] The reciprocal translocation (i.e., Xp22.3→ Yp31) results in 46,XY females who are SRY negative.[70] In general, *SRY*-negative 46,XX males have an increased prevalence of ambiguity of the external genitalia and siblings with true hermaphroditism.[154] The familial occurrence of 46,XX males and 46,XX true hermaphrodites who are *SRY* negative suggests the constitutative activation or inactivation of an X-linked or autosomal downstream gene (or genes) in the sex determination and differentiation cascade that is normally regulated by *SRY*.

Fifteen to 20 percent of females with the complete form of 46,XY gonadal dysgenesis have inactivating mutations in the

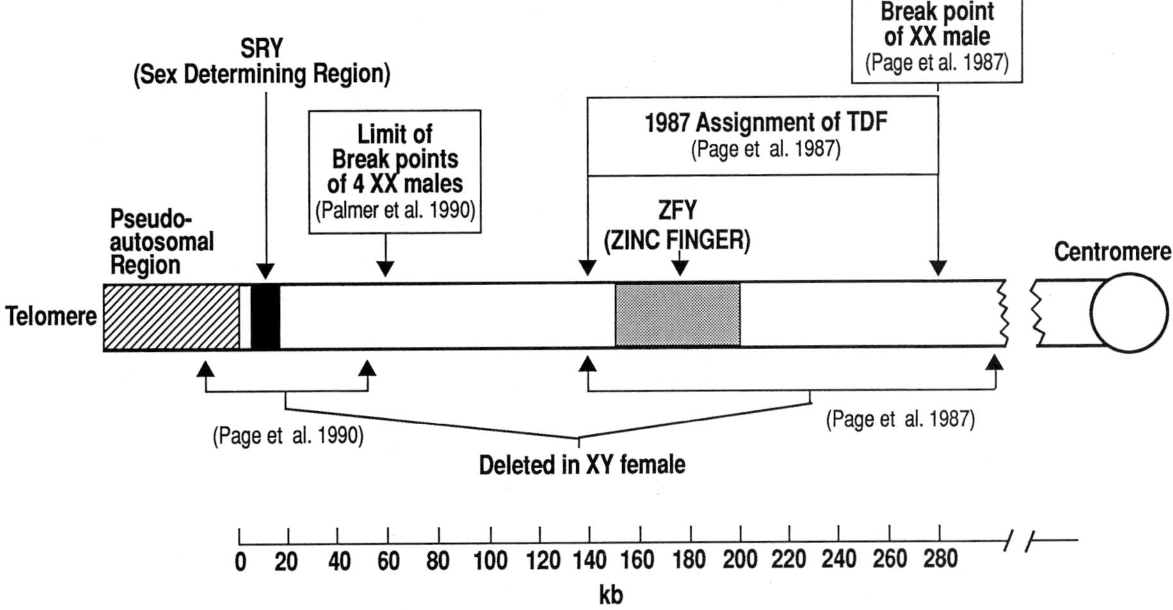

Figure 22–15. Localization of the putative sex-determining region, *SRY*, on the short arm of the Y chromosome. The zinc finger locus *ZFY* (the suggested site of the testis-determining factor in 1987) is shown, as well as the break points observed in four 46,XX males described by Palmer and co-workers. The break points of one 46,XX male and one 46,XY female studied by Page and colleagues are also indicated. Note that the 46,XY female has a noncontinuous deletion that involves both *ZFY* and *SRY*. (From Page DC, Fisher EMC, McGillivray B, et al: Additional deletion in the sex-determining region of the human Y chromosome resolves the paradox of Xt[y;22] female. Nature 1990; 346: 279–281.)

single exon *SRY* gene, an architectural transcription factor.[70, 154] Most of the mutations occur in the DNA-binding domain of the SRY protein (Fig. 22–16), the high-mobility-group (HMG) box that appears to act as a transcription factor and has the capacity of binding to and bending DNA.[154] Rare mutations in the 5′ and 3′ flanking regions in patients have led to complete and partial gonadal dysgenesis, respectively.[155–158] The HMG box contains two nuclear localization signals [NLS]) that bind calmodulin and importin B.[22, 159] Mutations in these nuclear localization signal domains in the HMG box of *SRY* result in failure to transport the SRY protein into the nucleus and result in consequent XY gonadal dysgenesis.[160] The evidence in the mouse and in humans with sex reversal strongly support the critical role of *SRY* in sex determination and male sex differentiation.

The human *SRY* gene contains no introns and produces a 900-base-pair transcript[161] that encodes a protein of 204 residues with three domains: an amino-terminal domain, a central DNA-binding domain consisting of a single HMG box, and a carboxyl-terminal domain.[68] In humans it is expressed in 46,XY gonads coincident with sex cord formation and it persists (unlike the brief expression of *Sry* in the embryonic mouse Sertoli cell) until at least 18 weeks of gestation in fetal Sertoli cells[162] as well as adult Sertoli and germ cells. Comparison of nucleotide sequences of the *SRY* gene from different species indicates that only the HMG box is conserved.[163] The HMG box is about an 80-amino acid residue domain that is similar to the DNA-binding domain of over 100 genes. A family of genes referred to as *SOX* (SRY-like HMG b*ox*) genes, exists in which the HMG region exhibits more than 60% sequence homology with that of *SRY*.[164] The SRY protein binds specifically to the linear consensus DNA sequence 5′-A/T)AACAAT(A/T)-3′ and nonspecifically to cruciform (four-way junction) DNA.[165, 166] The SRY/HMG protein is made up of three helices and amino- and carboxyl-terminal domains.[167, 168] The HMG box has an "L" or boomerang shape and presents a concave surface to the DNA for sequence-specific binding.[168–170] DNA binding occurs in the minor groove of the DNA and results in a bend of 40 to 70 degrees from linearity in the DNA, conforming to the shape of the HMG box.[168, 169] Additional conformational changes in the DNA include helix unwinding and minor groove expansion.[168, 170] The carboxyl terminus of SRY contains a 7-amino acid that can bind PDZ (P_{SD-95}, Disc large, Z_{0-1}) domains in the nuclear protein SiP1 (SRY-interacting protein 1).[171] A 41-residue deletion in the carboxyl terminus of SRY resulted in XY gonadal dysgenesis.[158] Furthermore, phos-

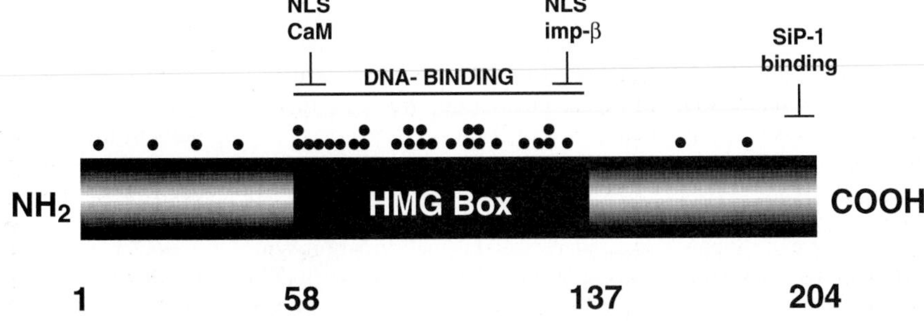

Figure 22–16. Diagram of the human SRY protein. The HMG box is an 80 amino acid DNA-binding domain with two nuclear localization signals at either end: CaM, calmodulin and imp β, importen β. The last seven amino acids of SRY can bind to either of the PDZ domains found in SRY-interacting protein 1 (SIP-1). The *solid circles* indicate selected mutations reported in the SRY protein affecting testicular differentiation and consequent male development.

phorylation of serine motifs in the amino-terminal region of the human SRY protein affects SRY DNA binding and subsequent transcriptional activity in vitro).[172]

SRY has no recognizable *trans*-activation domain. The control of gene expression by SRY may be mediated by the conformational changes in DNA that result in the approximation of distant regulatory elements of the transcriptional apparatus, thereby allowing them to interact with one another. Analysis of mutations in the HMG box in women with 46,XY gonadal dysgenesis suggests that the spatial rearrangements (bending) in DNA produced by the HMG-domain protein are critical to its activity, as is its binding.[173] Induction of a structural bend in the DNA helix may allow the interaction of other spatially dependent proteins with the DNA.[168] Mutations in the SRY HMG box that affect binding, bending, or nuclear transport of SRY and as yet undefined mechanisms can result in the loss of transcriptional activity.[160, 173] The transcriptional activity of *SRY* has been demonstrated in vitro with the use of FOS-related antigen-1 promoter constructs.[174] However, neither the upstream regulatory genes nor the downstream targets of *SRY* have been ascertained. The consensus sequence (A/T)AACAAT(A/T) is ubiquitous in the human genome, occurring at more than 105 sites, which makes it difficult to ascribe specificity to the interaction of *SRY* with a specific gene based solely on the presence of the consensus sequence in its promoter. The target gene is expressed in pre-Sertoli cells in temporal relationship to SRY protein and is directly transactivated by it. Because of the lack of an apparent strict relation between the absence of *SRY* and testicular development in some 46,XX males and 46,XX true hermaphrodites, McElreavey and associates[175] proposed that the main function of SRY is to repress a putative gene termed "Z" that itself represses differentiation of the testis. At least four cellular roles for SRY protein have been defined.[7] They include (1) the induction of Sertoli cell differentiation,[176] (2) the migration of mesonephric cells into the genital ridge,[177] (3) the proliferation of cells in the genital ridge,[178] and (4) male-specific vasculature with recruitment of a large number of endothelial cells from the mesonephros.[179] However, as noted previously, in spite of more than 10 years of research on the *SRY* gene,[6, 7, 180] as yet we remain uncertain of its upstream regulators or its downstream target genes. The strongest contenders are the downstream autosomal gene *SOX9* (see later) and upstream *WT1* (+*KTS* isoform).[180, 181] In sum, the evolutionary conserved HMG domain of SRY protein seems the only component essential for function. The only candidate downstream gene for *SRY*, at present, is the activation of *SOX9*.[22, 180] Finally, Graves has challenged the conventional wisdom that the *SRY* is the ultimate and all-powerful male determiner. She points out that *SRY* is an "ephemeral gene" recruited recently from a transcription factor possibly involved in brain development, is younger than the Y chromosome, and whose structure and function in evolutionary terms has evolved relatively rapidly. Graves estimates that the human Y chromosome and its *SRY* gene might only last another 5 to 10 million years![182]

Autosomal and X Chromosomal Genes

Other genes on autosomes and the X chromosome participate in the testis determination dosage-sensitive combinatorial network of complex interactions (Table 22–4). These still incompletely understood, regulatory interactions are more than a linear cascade.

SOX9

Campomelic dysplasia is a severe skeletal malformation syndrome associated with an increased prevalence (75%) of 46,XY gonadal dysgenesis and consequent male to female sex reversal.[183–185] The campomelic dysplasia and sex reversal locus has been mapped to 17q24.3-25.1, and a gene designated as *SOX9* has been cloned from this locus.[183–185] *SOX9* belongs to a family of HMG domain protein transcription factors related to the "testis determining factor" *SRY* that share very similar HMG box DNA-binding attributes.[186, 187] *SOX9*, in contrast to *SRY*, has an intron and a well-defined transcriptional *trans*-activation domain—the carboxyl-terminal 108 amino acids.[187–188] Similar to *SRY*, *SOX9* has nuclear localization signal sequences at either end of the HMG box that when mutated can reduce nuclear importation and result in campomelic dysplasia and XY sex reversal.[189] *SOX9* is expressed in the kidney, central nervous system, pancreas, chondrogenic precursor cells, and Sertoli cells of the testes.[184–189] The *SOX9* protein HMG box, about 70% homologous to the *SRY* HMG box, binds to a specific sequence, 5′-AGAACAATGG-3′,[166] in the minor groove of DNA, resulting in unwinding and bending of the DNA in a manner similar to other SOX proteins.[168, 190] Furthermore, *SOX9* binds to the 6-base-pair DNA sequences ATGAAT and CACAAT found in the chondrocyte specific enhancer of the first intron of the human type II collagen gene *(COL2A1)*, activating this gene and inducing chondrogenesis.[191] A heterozygous mutation in the *SOX9* gene can result in campomelic dysplasia in the absence of sex reversal in 46,XY individuals; chondrogenesis seems more sensitive to *SOX9* gene dosage than sex determination (Fig. 22–17). A mouse with haploinsufficiency of *SOX9* had defective cartilage development and premature mineralization of cartilage, a phenocopy of the severe skeletal manifestations in patients with campomelic dysplasia.[192] Notably, haploinsufficiency in the mouse did not result in XY sex reversal; the testes in the affected males were normal. Other features such as micrognathia, cleft palate, respiratory distress, and neonatal death are similar to those in the affected human.[192]

Whereas mutations in the *SRY* gene occur predominantly in the HMG box, they occur throughout the *SOX9* gene (see Fig. 22–17). Mutations resulting in campomelic dysplasia and/or XY sex reversal include splice acceptor/donor changes, missense, nonsense, translocation, and frameshift mutations.[185] The two major classes of mutations causing campomelic dysplasia and/or XY sex reversal are amino acid substitutions in the HMG domain and truncations or frameshifts that affect the carboxyl-terminal (*trans*-activation) domain of *SOX9*.[189]

SOX9 plays a critical role in the sex-determination pathway in all eutherian vertebrates.[22, 185] It is sexually dimorphically expressed; *SOX9* is up-regulated in the testis-determining pathway shortly after *SRY* is expressed in the mouse as well as human.[162, 193, 194] *SOX9* and *SRY* are both expressed in Sertoli cell precursors and Sertoli cells.[162, 194] Expression of *SOX9* is restricted to the nuclei of Sertoli cells after 6.5 weeks of gestation in the human male embryo, whereas its expression remains cytosolic in the XX embryonal gonads.[195] In the XX embryo, *SOX9* is not expressed in the mouse ovary; in the human a low level of expression is described after 7 weeks of gestation.[62, 194] *SOX9* may be the only critical gene needed downstream of *SRY* for male sex determination; for example, duplication of *Sox9* in XX mice and *SOX9* in humans, and the *Od* sex mutation in mice (which up-regulates *Sox9* expression), both result in XX female to male sex reversal.[196–198] *SOX9* in concert with *SF1*, *WT1*, and *GATA4* through combinatorial protein-protein and protein-DNA complex interactions activates antimüllerian hormone (AMH) transcription, which results in müllerian duct expression in 46,XY male mice.[195]

DAX1/DSS

46,XY individuals with duplications of the Xp21 region of the short arm of the X chromosome have dysgenetic gonads and male-to-female sex reversal.[92] The presence of two active

Table 22–4. Genes Involved in Human Gonadogenesis

Gene	Encodes	Human Gene Locus	Human Phenotype	Mouse Phenotype
WT1	Transcription factor	11p13	Heterozygous mutation in exons encoding zinc finger motifs: Denys-Drash syndrome (male pseudohermaphrodite) Heterozygous mutation in splice site junction with loss of +KTS isoform: Frasier syndrome (XY gonadal dysgenesis) Deletion: WAGR syndrome (XY, ambiguous genitalia, aniridia, etc.)	Null: no kidneys or gonads
SF1	Orphan nuclear receptor Transcription factor	9q33	Heterozygous missense mutation: XY sex reversal with adrenal insufficiency XX: adrenal insufficiency, normal ovaries Homozygous missense mutation: XY sex reversal with adrenal insufficiency; familial heterozygotes not affected	Null: no adrenals or gonads
SRY	Transcription factor	Yp11.3	Mutation: XY gonadal dysgenesis Translocation: to X → XX male	Mutation: XY fertile female Translocation: to X or autosome → XX male
SOX9	Transcription factor	17q24	Haploinsufficiency: XY male pseudohermaphrodite (~70%), campomelic dysplasia Duplication: XX male	Conditional (gonad) *Sox9* transgenic: XX male Insertional mutation: XX male Null mutation: XY male pseudohermaphrodite, campomelic dysplasia
DMRT1	Transcription factor	9p24.3	Deletion of 9p24.3→pter haploinsufficiency: XY male pseudohermaphrodite, anomalies, mental retardation XX females have variable ovarian function	Null: normal male sex differentiation Phenotype: postnatal loss of germ cells and Sertoli cells "vanishing testes"
DAX1	Orphan nuclear receptor Transcription repressor	Xp21.3	Mutation: XY (normal testis differentiation), adrenal hypoplasia, hypogonadotropic hypogonadism Duplication: XY male pseudohermaphrodite	XY null: infertile male XX null: ovaries Transgenic XY: female
WNT4	Signaling molecule	1p35	Duplication: XY male pseudohermaphrodite	Null: XX mouse lacks müllerian ducts, masculinization of female gonad → androgen secretion by "gonads," results in wolffian ducts but female external genitalia, loss of oocytes
ATRX (XH2)	Helicase	Xq13.3	Deletions and mutations: male pseudohermaphrodite, α-thalassemia, mental retardation	ND*
10q−	?	10q25-qter	Male pseudohermaphrodite, multiple congenital anomalies syndrome	ND*
FOXL2	Transcription factor	3q23	Mutations: blepharophimosis/ptosis/epicanthus inversus (BPES) syndrome BPES type 1: premature ovarian failure Affected males are fertile	Deletion of 1q43 in the goat (homologous to 3q23 in humans) affects *FOXL2* and *PIST1* causing the polled intersex syndrome (lack of horns and XX sex reversal)
DHH	Signaling molecule	12q13.1	Homozygous missense mutation (ATG → ACG) in one patient with 46,XY partial gonadal dysgenesis and minifascicular neuropathy External genitalia female, streak on one side with hemi-tube, hypoplastic testes on other side	Null mutations, two phenotypes, 7.5% males, 92.5% females Testes from feminized XY mice lacked adult Leydig cells

*ND, not described in the mouse. Not described in the human but identified in the mouse: *Lim1*, *Lhx9*, *Emx2*, *M33* (all transcription factors), *Fgf-9*, *Vanin*, and *Nexin*.

copies of the *DAX1* gene at this dosage-sensitive sex reversal locus (DSS) impairs testicular differentiation despite a normal-functioning *SRY* gene. The smallest Xp21 duplication found in an XY sex-reversed patient is a 160-kb region of Xp21 that contains the *DAX1* gene. Deletions or intragenic mutations in the *DAX1* gene cause X-linked cytomegalic congenital adrenal hypoplasia and hypogonadotropic hypogonadism.[90, 91, 199] *DAX1*, an orphan nuclear receptor,[90] is a transcriptional regulator. The gene consists of two exons separated by an intron.[90] The encoded protein has 410 amino acids and is composed of a

uncertain. In two 46,XX femal
Ogata and co-workers found ev
nesis.[251] Accordingly, *DMRT1* l
the indifferent gonad and hap
spectrum of gonadal dysfunctior

Chromosome 10q

Terminal deletions of chrom
frequently associated with urog
hypoplasia, cryptorchidism, mic
tic labia major, and, rarely, co
candidate gene on distal 10q
though suspected clinically, has

ATRX

The α-thalassemia mental
X-linked disorder characterized
semia, severe mental retardatio
tal anomalies, including genit
fected 46,XY individuals.[255] Th
XNP) is located at Xq13.3, sp
exons, and undergoes X inacti
encodes two alternatively spli
expressed in the embryonic te
of the ATRX protein contains
portion has the ATPase and
boxyl-terminal region a "P"
regulation and a "Q" box is th
interaction.[255] The spectrum o
undescended testes to hyposp
degrees of XY sex reversal.[255]
lead to truncation of ATRX w
region (the helicase domain) u
ities.[255] The spectrum of genit
cended testes to hypospadias,
of XY sex reversal.[255] Mutatio
truncation of ATRX with loss
(the helicase domain) usually
Affected 46,XY individuals v
have streak gonads, and abse
The absence of müllerian duc
of testes was interrupted afte
tion of Sertoli cells downstre
cient expression of AMH to
ducts.[258] Ion and co-workers
in *ATRX* that resulted in a p
associated with XY gonadal
and mental retardation simila
mia mental retardation syndr
thalassemia.[259]

Other Genes Involved in Gon and Differentiation

Lhx (Lim) 1 and 9 are men
genes involved in developme
proteins are characterized by
cated in the amino-terminal
a DNA-binding homeobox d
logue of human *LIM1*, is
gonadal development.[260–262]
termediate mesoderm and ne
gous for targeted deletions
gonads, and anterior head s
not as yet been described in
of gonadal agenesis or dysg
normalities.

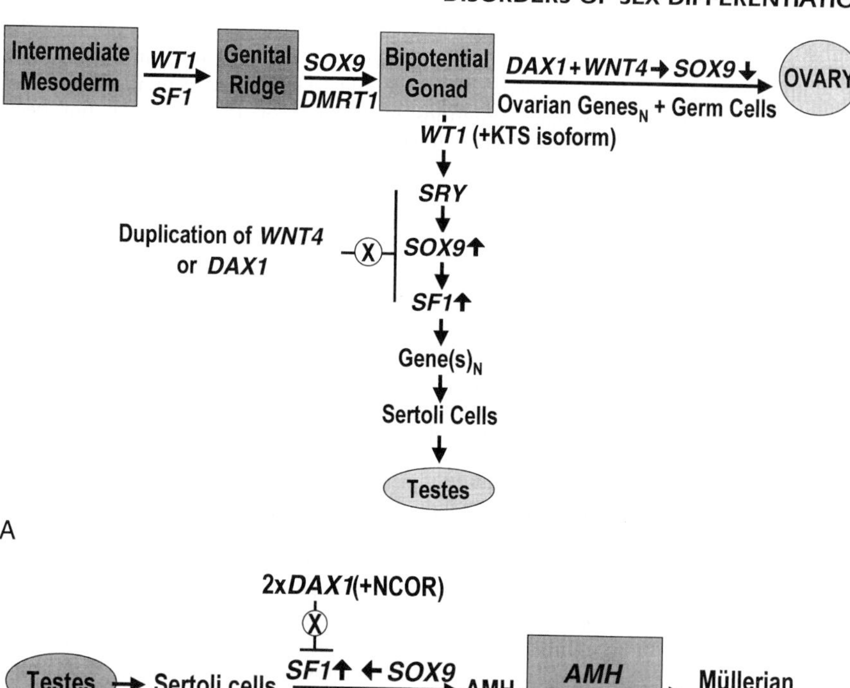

Figure 22–19. A and B, Hypothetical linear cascade and network of genes involved in human sex determination and differentiation (refer to manuscript for genes described in the mouse). *WT1*, Wilms' tumor suppressor gene; *SF1*, steroidogenic factor 1; *DAX1*, dosage-sensitive sex reversal adrenal hypoplasia critical region on the X gene 1; *SOX9*, autosomal gene containing *SRY*-like *HMG* box; *SRY*, sex-determining region Y; *DMRT1*, double sex, mab3-related transcription factor 1; *WNT4*, a member of the vertebrate homolog family of the *Drosophila* segment polarity gene, "wingless"; *AMH*, antimüllerian hormone; GATA4, transcription factor.

ation usually disappear, although they may persist outside the gonad and give rise to germ cell neoplasms.[302]

Spermatogenesis

During early testicular differentiation the primordial germ cells become distributed throughout the primitive seminiferous tubules as progenitors of spermatogonia. A series of mitotic divisions occurs, followed thereafter by inhibition of entry into meiotic prophase presumably by a putative local factor secreted by Sertoli cells until the transient postnatal increase in mitosis, and later the initiation of full spermatogenesis late in the prepubescent period. Furthermore, it appears that both male and female germ cells are programmed to enter meiosis unless they are inhibited by a putative signal from the testicular somatic cells.[307, 308] With the onset of puberty, the basement membrane of the spermatogenic tubule becomes lined by proliferating spermatogonia that arise by the mitotic division of prespermatogonia.[307, 308] A glial cell line neutrophilic factor (GDNF) secreted by Sertoli cells appears to play a role in the proliferation and differentiation of spermatogonia.[309] The spermatogonia in turn give rise by mitotic division to primary spermatocytes, which enter meiosis at puberty.

The formation of haploid secondary spermatocytes from the euploid primary spermatocytes is accomplished by the special form of cell division termed *meiosis.* Whereas in mitotic division both daughter cells receive duplicates of each of the 46 parental chromosomes, in the first meiotic division each daughter cell receives only 23 chromosomes, one from each of the homologous pairs (Fig. 22–20). Thus, half of the secondary spermatocytes contains 22 autosomes and an X chromosome, and the other half contains 22 autosomes and a Y chromosome. Each haploid daughter cell receives by random chance either the maternally or the paternally derived chromosomes of each homologous pair, but not both. This process ensures great diversity in the genetic composition of the gametes, because by independent assortment and recombination of the 23 pairs of paternal and maternal chromosomes it is possible to obtain 2^{22} different kinds of gametes. This is not the only mechanism for ensuring genetic variation, however, because the special nature of the prophase during this reduction division facilitates exchanges of DNA (crossover) between homologous chromosomes. The details of this complex process are described in standard genetics texts. Secondary spermatocytes give rise to spermatids by a second meiotic division, but this division is more analogous to mitosis than to the first meiotic division, because daughter cells are again produced by a longitudinal split of the two chromatid filaments constituting each of the unpaired chromosomes (see Fig. 22–20); the haploid number is not altered.

Spermatids do not undergo further division but rather develop into spermatozoa by metamorphosis. Germ cells in the

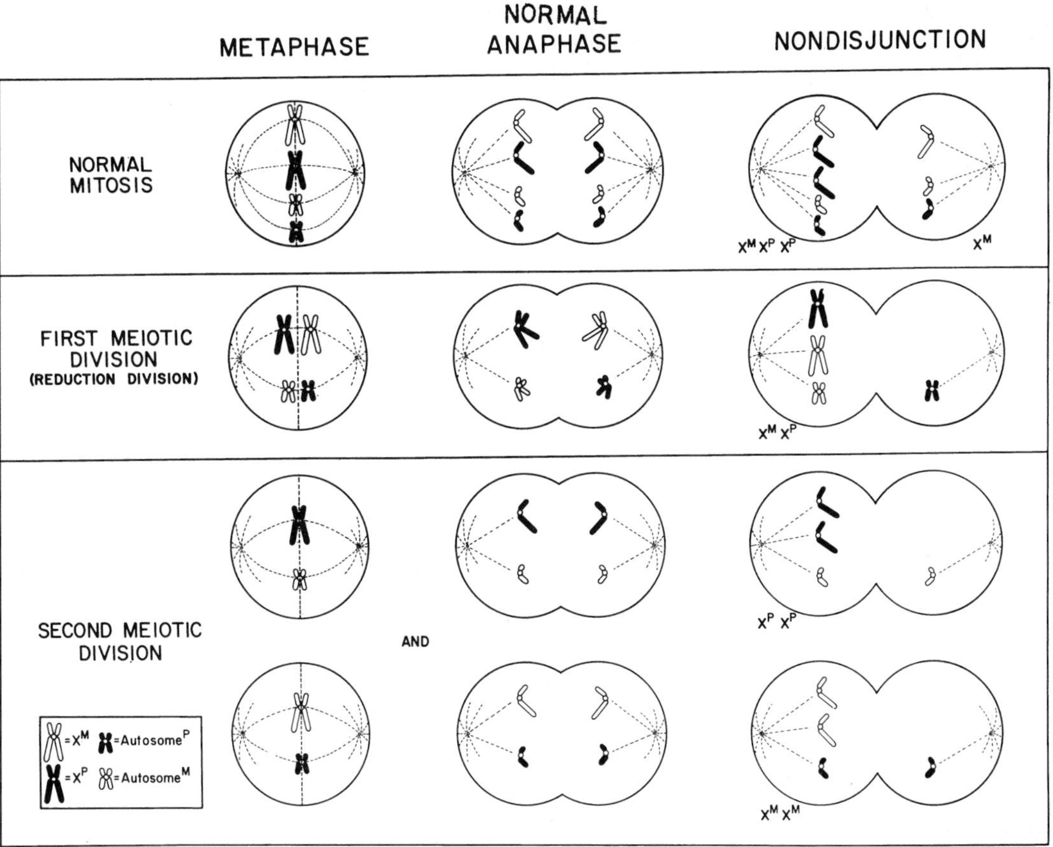

Figure 22–20. Types of cell division. A female somatic cell undergoing mitosis is represented. At the metaphase plate are two X chromosomes and two homologous autosomes of group 21 to 22. Division occurs through the centromere, giving rise to two daughter cells of identical chromosomal composition. Replication of each arm into two chromatids takes place while the chromosomes are extended and before the next metaphase. The first meiotic division involves pairing of homologous chromosomes. The centromere does not divide in this cell division. It is by chance whether the maternal (X^M) or paternal (X^P) member of each pair goes to the respective daughter cells. During the complex prophase of first meiotic division *(not shown)*, multiple chiasmata are formed between the chromosomes of each pair, facilitating exchanges of chromosomal segments (crossing over) between them. During the second meiotic division, the centromere again divides, giving rise to daughter cells identical to the parent cell. This division more nearly resembles mitosis than the first meiotic division. Nondisjunction can take place in mitosis or in the first or second meiotic division; representative examples are illustrated.

adult male are continually being renewed and undergoing maturation. Heller and Clermont[310] estimated that the complete cycle in adult males from spermatogonium to mature sperm requires 74 ± 5 days.

The X chromosome undergoes inactivation in pachytene spermatocytes during meiosis.[308] The condensed sex chromosomes form a sex vesicle or XY body. XY pairing must occur during normal meiosis,[311] and X inactivation may be involved in the heterochromatinization of those regions of the X chromosome that are similar to but not homologous to regions on the Y chromosome.

Oogenesis

Female germ cells pursue a different course. During ovarian differentiation, the primary germ cells undergo vigorous mitotic replication and successive differentiation into oogonia. When mitotic division ceases and the cells enter meiosis, they are then termed *oocytes.* Meiotic oocytes are critical for differentiation of pre-follicular cells into follicular cells. The absence or loss of meiotic oocytes leads to degeneration of the pre-follicular cells. The period of oogonial proliferation results in a peak population of about 6 million to 7 million germ cells in the two ovaries at 5 months' gestational age, including oogonia, oocytes in various stages of prophase, and degenerating oocytes.[312, 313] Oocytes degenerate at different stages of meiosis. Only 5% of the peak number of germ cells in the fetal ovary reach the diplotene stage.[312] Formation of oogonia from primary germ cells ceases by the seventh month of gestation. Some oocytes remain in undifferentiated nests, whereas others form primordial follicles. A primordial follicle is formed when presumptive granulosa cells surround the diplotene (meiotic) oocyte and an intact basal lamina encloses this unit. If the oocyte is not enclosed in a follicle, it degenerates. The number of primordial follicles in the ovary is maximal at birth, and the number thereafter diminishes. In the germ cells that survive, the oocyte is arrested at late prophase of the first meiotic division (diplotene state). Oocytes remain in the prophase of the first meiotic division from fetal life until puberty when some unknown stimulus allows them to progress and eventually ovulation occurs.[299] Before ovulation, the first polar body is extruded, thus completing the first meiotic division. The haploid secondary oocyte immediately begins a second meiotic division but remains in metaphase and does not extrude the second polar body until the ovum is penetrated by a sperm. The triploidy that is common in spontaneously aborted fetuses may be caused either by failure of extrusion of the second polar body (polygyny) or by double fertilization (polyspermy).

The long life span of female germ cells, in contrast to those of the male, may explain the increased prevalence of certain chromosomal anomalies with advanced maternal age (see section on aneuploidy).

Differentiation of the Testis and the Ovary

The gonads of both sexes develop from anlagen located on the medioventral border of the urogenital ridge, adjacent to the kidney and the primitive adrenal (Fig. 22–21).[314] Until the 12-mm stage (approximately 42 days of gestation), the gonads of the male and female are indistinguishable on morphologic grounds and could potentially differentiate either as testes or as ovaries. The close ontogenic and anatomic relation between gonadal and adrenal cells at this early stage is noteworthy, because, as differentiation proceeds, nests of adrenal cells frequently separate with the gonad and are found as adrenal rests in the hilum of the mature ovary or testis. Such rests may become a problem in patients with long-standing untreated congenital adrenal hyperplasia (CAH). Adrenal cell rests in testes, for example, may enlarge under persistent corticotropin (ACTH, adrenocorticotropin) stimulation and be mistaken for testicular tumors or true testicular enlargement (see Chap. 24).

The primitive undifferentiated gonad is made up of four cell lineages, germ cells, connective tissue cells, steroid-producing cells, and supporting cells. They are derived from proliferation of the mesodermal coelomic epithelium, the mesenchymal cell mass in the urogenital ridge, mesonephric elements,[1, 7, 177, 179, 315] and the large alkaline phosphatase-containing primordial germ cells that have migrated from the posterior endoderm of the yolk sac through the mesenchyme of the mesentery to the gonad.[305, 316] According to Witschi and co-workers,[317] the number of migrating germ cells in the human embryo is 700 to 1300, and by the eighth week of embryogenesis about 600,000 germ cells are present, which later become either oogonia or spermatogonia. Lack of germ cells is incompatible with ovarian differentiation but does not prevent testicular morphogenesis. However, in the mouse, genes such as the steel *(S1)* gene, which encodes a peptide growth factor (SCF, stem cell factor), the proto-oncogene c-*kit* (also known as white spotting *[W]*), which encodes a tyrosine kinase receptor in the plasma cell membrane (a receptor for S1), and cadherins affect the proliferation, mobility, and migration of primordial germ cells to the urogenital ridge.[316, 318] SCF, in its transmembrane second form, is expressed in human Sertoli cells and acts as an adhesion protein, binding germ cells.[318] The precursor of the Sertoli cell of the testis and its counterpart in the ovary, the granulosa cell, originate from the coelomic epithelium.[7, 319]

There is a striking sexual dimorphism in the timing of gonadal differentiation. Under the influence of the testis-determining genes, testis organization begins at about 45 days of gestation (6 to 7 wk); the testis develops more rapidly than the ovary.[320] The ovary does not emerge from the indifferent stage until 3 months of gestation, when the earliest sign appears: the beginning of meiosis, as evidenced by the maturation of oogonia into oocytes.[321]

Testis

In the past it was believed that the testis is derived primarily from the medullary portion of the primitive gonad and the ovary from the cortical portion. According to this concept, the testis and ovary are not strictly homologous. Witschi and co-workers[317, 327] suggested that in genetic males the medullary portion secretes an inductor substance that stimulates development of seminiferous tubules and inhibits cortical development; conversely, the cortex of genetic females, the coelomic epithelium, was thought to secrete an inductor substance that inhibits testicular development and results in ovarian dominance. The proposal was that the differentiation of the primordial gonad was regionalized.

Jost and co-workers,[322, 323] Jirasek,[5] and van Wagenen and Simpson,[321] among others, called into question the histologic descriptions of gonadal differentiation that served as the basis for these theories. After careful examination of early embryos, Jost[322] and Jirasek[5] concluded that it is not possible to identify primary sex cords as such before the 15-mm stage and that the primitive gonad is truly bipotential. At about 45 days morphologic sex dimorphism is evident in the intermediate mesoderm of the genital ridge when epithelial cords derived from the coelomic epithelium, the gonadal blastema including stromal cells of mesonephric origin, and the primordial germ cells, antecedents of the seminiferous tubules, are apparent in the male. The onset of testicular differentiation is marked by the *SRY*-dependent differentiation of the Sertoli cell, the first cell type to differentiate, and by the subsequent incorporation of the germ cells into the primitive seminiferous cords, when proliferation of the germ cells is suppressed and differentiation is arrested at the primitive spermatogonial stage. The XY gonadal somatic cells essentially block the bipotential primordial germ cell (pre-spermatogonia) from advancing to meiotic prophase (a cardinal feature of oocyte differentiation) and promote their spermatogenetic differentiation.[324]

While the somatic cells of the primordial gonad are bipotential, *SRY* expression directs the delaminated and proliferating somatic cells derived from the coelomic epithelium to differentiate into Sertoli cells—the first cell to differentiate (whether Sertoli cells are derived as well from other progenitors) is not yet resolved. The differentiation of Sertoli cells drives development of the testis. This *SRY*-directed process includes proliferation of the somatic cells, which is more rapid and extensive in the XY gonad than the XX gonad[178, 325, 326]; migration of stromal mesonephric cells and endothelial cells from the adjacent mesonephros into the gonad, which occurs only in XY gonads and is dependent on the expression of SRY[328–331]; testis cord development and Sertoli cell differentiation, the initiation of which in the mouse, appears to be dependent on the migration of mesonephric cells. The latter include the progenitors of Leydig cells and peritubular myoid cells; and the differentiation of a testis-specific vasculature.[328, 330, 332] The stromal cells migrating from the mesonephros have the capacity to differentiate into peritubular myoid cells that surround the developing testis cords and to contribute along with the coelomic epithelium to the differentiation of Leydig cells and the testis-specific architecture. In sum, the developing testis is composed of (1) germ cells, the progenitors of future spermatogonia that migrated into the genital ridge from an extragonadal source; (2) Sertoli cells derived from the coelomic epithelium, which with their envelopment of the primordial germ cells leads to the formation of testicular cords containing (3) peritubular myoid cells of mesonephric origin that surround the testicular cords; and (4) the interstitial Leydig cells, which originate from the mesonephros and coelomic epithelium.[330, 333] This construct is largely derived from lineage tracing, studies in the mouse embryo by Capel and associates that included the use of differentiation and proliferation markers, and in the human, from ultrastructural studies of the early fetal gonad.[334]

Burgoyne and associates[335–337] proposed from studies of XX:XY chimeric mice that the *Sry* gene acts autonomously to induce Sertoli cell differentiation, which then mediates further testicular differentiation. After testicular differentiation occurs (at 43 to 50 days' gestational age),[5] the male fetus can also be recognized by beginning regression of the primitive müllerian

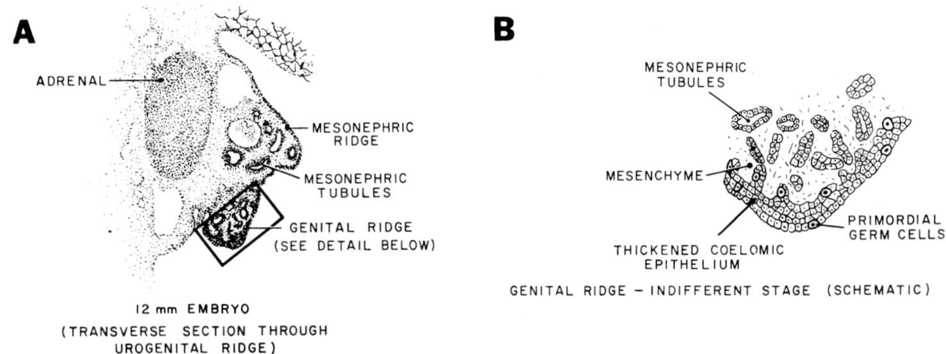

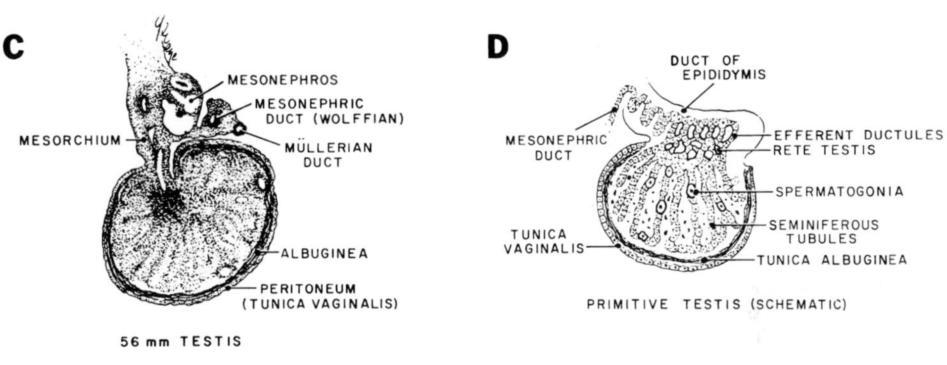

Figure 22–21. Anatomic and schematic representations of gonadal differentiation. *A* and *B*, Transverse section through the urogenital ridge at the stage of the indifferent gonad. Note the proximity of a large fetal adrenal to the hilar portion of gonad. *C* and *D*, Transverse section through the fetal testis at 56-mm stage. *E* and *F*, Transverse section through the fetal ovary at 60-mm stage. In ovarian development, coelomic epithelium continues to proliferate for a much longer period. (Modified from Arey LB. Developmental Anatomy, 7th ed. Philadelphia, WB Saunders, 1965; and Witschi E. Development of Vertebrates. Philadelphia, WB Saunders, 1956.)

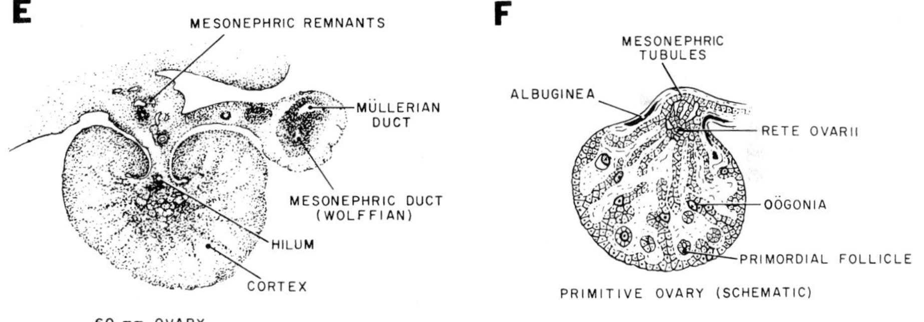

ducts (30-mm stage, about 60 days' gestation) and by differentiation of male external genitalia (45-mm stage, 65 to 77 days' gestation).

An early endocrine function of the fetal testis is the secretion by the Sertoli cells of AMH,[338] a homodimeric glycoprotein that functions as a paracrine secretion; it passes by diffusion to the paired müllerian ducts and induces their dissolution by apoptosis.[339] The versatile Sertoli cell also secretes inhibin, nurtures the germ cells, expresses stem cell factor, synthesizes an androgen-binding protein, and prevents meiosis. Both fetal Sertoli and germ cells exhibit apoptosis as well as proliferation during gestation.[340]

Leydig cells are first found in 32- to 35-mm fetuses (about 60 days' gestation). After differentiation of the primitive testicular cords, they rapidly proliferate during the third month and the first half of the fourth month[5, 323, 333, 341]; during this period the interstitial spaces between the seminiferous tubules are crowded with Leydig cells. The onset of testosterone biosynthesis occurs at about 9 weeks.[342–344] Human chorionic gonadotropin/luteinizing hormone (hCG/LH) receptors are present on fetal Leydig cells by 10 to 12 weeks of gestation,[345–346] an observation that suggests that the initial secretion of testosterone is independent of hCG and fetal LH.[19] The Leydig cells secrete testosterone, the regulator of male differentiation of the wolffian ducts, urogenital sinus, and external genitalia. The plasma concentration of testosterone in the male fetus correlates with the biosynthetic activity of the fetal testes.[342, 347] Peak concentrations in the fetal circulation (7 to 21 nmol/L [200 to 600 ng/dL]), values comparable to those in the adult male,[348, 349] are reached by about 16 weeks of gestation. Between 16 and 20 weeks of gestation the testosterone level falls to about 3.5 nmol/L (100 ng/dL); after 24 weeks the plasma level of testosterone is low (in the early pubertal range). Testosterone in amniotic fluid shows a similar pattern.[350] Clinical as well as biochemical data indicate that hCG secreted by the syncytiotrophoblast stimulates testosterone secretion during the critical period of male sex differentiation,[345, 349] but whether testosterone synthesis at its onset is hCG dependent is unclear.[351] The question of whether hCG is required to initiate testosterone secretion in the human is complicated further by the presence of hCG-like material in the fetal testis.[352] The pattern of testosterone secretion early in gestation follows that of hCG.[19, 349, 353] The number of Leydig cells decreases after 18 weeks, by apoptosis[340] and by dedifferentiation, and few cells show Leydig cell characteristics in the interstitium of the testis at birth. However, a low level of testosterone secretion is maintained after 15 weeks of gestation under the control of fetal pituitary LH and hCG.[19, 349, 353] Fetal pituitary gonadotropins are essential for the continued growth and function of the fetal testis after the early period of sex differentiation.[19, 353] Fetal pituitary LH is necessary for the normal growth of the differentiated penis and scrotum during the latter half of gestation and for the descent of the testes.[19, 353] The male fetus with anencephaly or congenital hypopituitarism often has hypoplastic male external genitalia and undescended testes containing a decreased number of Leydig cells.[19] Fetal Leydig cells differ from adult Leydig cells in their morphology, their regulatory mechanisms, and their lack of desensitization to high doses of hCG and LH.[19, 333, 354, 355]

Figure 22–22 correlates the pattern of testosterone, hCG, and fetal pituitary FSH and LH concentrations during gestation with the histologic changes in the fetal testis. In sum, organogenesis of the testis involves successive differentiation of the Sertoli cell and the seminiferous cords with envelopment of the extragonadally derived germ cells by Sertoli cells, development of the tunica albuginea, appearance of Leydig cells, and differentiation of the mesonephric tubules into the ductuli efferentes, which connect the seminiferous tubules and rete network with the epididymis to provide the pathway for sperm transport into the ejaculatory duct system.

Ovary

In the absence of testis-determining genes, the gonadal primordium has an inherent tendency to develop as an ovary, provided that germ cells are present and survive. The indifferent stage persists in the female fetus weeks after testis organogenesis begins. There is, however, continued proliferation of the coelomic epithelium and primordial germ cells, which gradually enlarge and become oogonia. Despite the discordance in the histologic appearance of the primordial testis and ovary, George and Wilson[356] noted the simultaneous development at 8 weeks of gestation of the capacity of the fetal testis to synthesize testosterone and of the fetal "ovary" to synthesize estradiol when incubated with C_{21}-steroid precursors. In contrast to the fetal adrenal gland, the gonads of both male and female fetuses have steroid 3β-hydroxysteroid dehydrogenase 2 (3β-HSD) activity at this stage; however, the activity of this enzyme is more than 50-fold greater in the fetal testis.[356] Testosterone is synthesized by the fetal Leydig cell, but the site of the meager synthesis of estradiol in the primordial ovary is not known. Gondos and Hobel[357] identified interstitial cells in the ovarian primordium at about 12 weeks of gestation that have the ultrastructural characteristics of steroidogenic cells and that may be a site of estrogen synthesis. The human fetus is bathed in estrogens of placental origin, but the fetal ovary does not contribute significantly to circulating estrogens, which in the fetus are almost exclusively of placental origin. The ovary has no documented role in differentiation of the female genital tract.[358]

During the ninth week the rete ovarii arise from the hilar mesonephric tubules and infiltrate the gonad as a syncytium of tubules and cords. At about the 11th to 12th week (80-mm stage), long after differentiation of the testis in the male fetus, germ cells in the ovary begin to enter meiotic prophase, which characterizes the transition of oogonia into oocytes and marks the onset of ovarian differentiation.[324, 359] The oogonia in the central part of the ovary are the first to come in contact with the rete ovarii and the first to enter meiosis but not beyond the diplotene phase. According to Byskov, the rete secretes a meiosis-inducing substance; meiosis activity sterol (MAS), a precursor of cholesterol, is suggested as the factor initiating meiosis in the fetal ovary.[360, 361] The initial stages of ovarian gonadogenesis and the formation of primordial follicles do not involve placental or fetal pituitary gonadotropins or their receptors (see reference 19). After the diplotene stage, the first meiotic division stops and the chromosomes enter a resting stage until meiosis is completed just before ovulation in the adult. The formation of primordial follicles (in which the oocyte is enveloped by a single layer of flat granulosa cells that share a common lineage with Sertoli cells) reaches a maximum during the 20th to the 25th week of gestation. In contrast to the fetal testis, FSH and LH/hCG receptors are not detected in the human fetal ovary between 8 and 16 weeks' gestation; the fetal ovary becomes responsive to FSH stimulation later in gestation (see reference 19). The genetic regulation of early folliculogenesis has been clarified. During this period the plasma level of fetal pituitary FSH attains its peaks[19, 349, 353] and the first primary follicles are formed (Fig. 22–23). By the 20th to the 25th week the gonad has the morphologic characteristics of a definitive ovary. As discussed earlier, the maximal number of germ cells decreases from a peak of 6 to 7 million to 2 million at term. In the late anencephalic female fetus, the ovaries are small and have a decreased number and hypoplasia of primary follicles, whereas the hilar cells seem to be similar in anencephalic and normal fetuses, suggesting that the hilar cells differentiate independently of the effect of pituitary gonadotropins.[19, 349] The growth, development, and maintenance of follicles appear to be regulated in late gestation by fetal pituitary gonadotropins, mainly FSH.

The sequence and timing of events in gonadal organogenesis and their relation to the differentiation of male and female somatic sexual characteristics are shown in Figure 22–24.

Differentiation of the Genital Ducts

At the seventh week of intrauterine life, the fetus is equipped with both male and female genital ducts derived from the mesonephros. The müllerian ducts serve as the anlagen of the uterus and fallopian tubes, whereas the mesonephric or wolffian ducts have the potential to differentiate further into the epididymis, vas deferens (ejaculatory ducts of the male), and seminal vesicles. During the third fetal month, either the müllerian or wolffian ducts complete their development, and involution occurs simultaneously in the opposite structures (Fig. 22–25).

Jost[362, 363] demonstrated that secretions from the fetal testis play a decisive role in determining the direction of genital duct development. In the presence of functional testes, the müllerian structures involute and undergo programmed cell death and the wolffian ducts complete their development; in the absence of testes, the wolffian ducts do not develop and the müllerian structures differentiate (Fig. 22–26). The regression of the müllerian ducts and the stabilization and differentiation of the wolffian ducts are mediated by different secretions of the fetal testes: the glycoprotein AMH secreted by the fetal Sertoli cells, and the steroid testosterone synthesized by the fetal Leydig cells.

Female development is not contingent on the presence of an ovary, because development of the uterus and tubes occurs if no gonad is present. However, the müllerian duct (paramesonephric duct) fails to differentiate in the absence of the mesonephric ducts, which serve as the anlage for both the male urogenital tract and the metanephros (primordial kidney); and

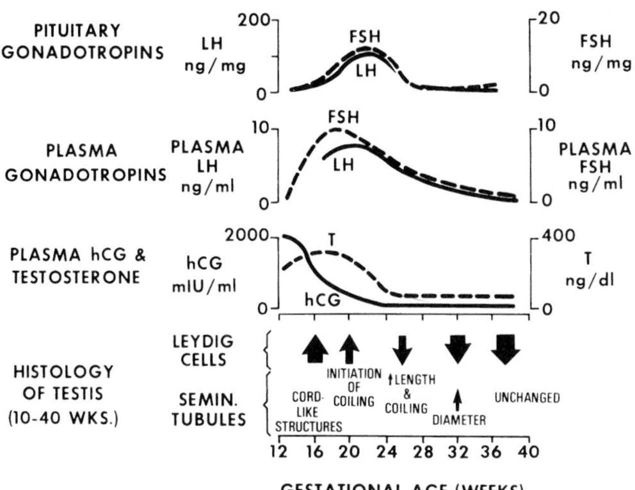

Figure 22–22. Comparison of the pattern of change of serum testosterone and human chorionic gonadotropin (hCG) and serum and pituitary luteinizing hormone (LH) (LER960) and follicle-stimulating hormone (FSH) (LER869) in the human male fetus during gestation with morphologic changes in the fetal testis. (Adapted from Kaplan SL, Grumbach MM. Pituitary and placental gonadotropins and sex steroids in the human and subhuman primate fetus. Clin Endocrinol Metab 1978; 7:487–511.)

therefore renal aplasia is commonly associated with hypoplasia of the fallopian tubes and uterus and vaginal agenesis.

The influence of the fetal testis on duct development is exerted locally and unilaterally; if one testis is removed at an early stage of development, the oviduct develops normally on that side but müllerian regression occurs on the side of the intact testis.[363]

Systemic administration of androgen to an early embryo does not cause regression of müllerian structures. Even when large amounts of androgen are implanted locally in the gonadal region of female fetuses, the müllerian ducts do not atrophy, although the differentiation of the wolffian ducts is stimulated.[362, 363] On the other hand, if a testis is grafted onto an ovary, müllerian regression and wolffian stimulation occur on that side (see Fig. 22–26). For these reasons, Jost proposed that the fetal testis secretes a müllerian duct–inhibiting substance that is distinct from ordinary androgens.

Jost and co-workers[1] and Josso and associates[339] studied the influence of the fetal testis on müllerian duct inhibition in organ culture. Direct contact between the testis and the müllerian anlage was not necessary to bring about this inhibition. By separating the testis from the müllerian ducts with dialysis membranes, they concluded that the material secreted from the testis was a protein and not a steroid. They also demonstrated that the human fetal testis, regardless of age, inhibits the müllerian ducts of 14.5-day-old fetal rats in similar organ culture studies and that AMH activity is present in human testes until 8 to 10 years of age.[364, 365] Using bovine fetal testes in which tubules and interstitial tissue were isolated and assayed separately, they showed that AMH activity is derived from the Sertoli cell, with peak levels occurring at the time of müllerian duct regression (9 to 12 weeks).[339, 365] Thereafter, the levels remain high until birth, after which a steady decline occurs until the pubertal period.[339, 365] The decline (but not disappearance) in AMH levels observed at puberty in males has been attributed to various factors that include testosterone secretion, meiotic entry, and terminal maturation of the Sertoli cells.[366] AMH is present in the ovarian follicle and is synthesized and secreted by the granulosa cells, but only after birth; whereas plasma concentrations are low in childhood, they increase at puberty.[364, 365] Elevated serum levels of AMH occur in patients with granulosa cell tumors.[367] AMH secretion by the postnatal ovary does not affect the fallopian tubes and the uterus, because they are apparently insensitive to AMH after 9 to 12 weeks of gestation, the period during which müllerian duct regression usually occurs.[368, 369]

In the freemartin the fetal ovary and the müllerian structures are exposed to AMH before the refractory period. AMH secreted by the fetal Sertoli cells of the male twin passes by means of placental vascular anastomoses to the female twin and results in müllerian regression, ovarian inhibition with loss of germ cells, tunica albuginea formation, and development of seminiferous tubule-like cords.[370, 371] Studies show that transgenic female mice that persistently express the human AMH gene resemble the bovine freemartin.[372, 373] The AMH transgenic female mice lack müllerian derivatives, and at birth the ovaries have fewer germ cells than normal. During the first 2 weeks of life germ cells are lost, and the somatic cells become organized into seminiferous tubule-like structures that do not persist to adulthood.[372] In the transgenic male mice, sex differentiation is usually normal, although some males, those that express the highest AMH levels, have incomplete virilization of the external genitalia, incomplete wolffian duct development, and undescended testes secondary to the effect of AMH on Leydig cell maturation and steroid synthesis.[373, 375] The relevance of these studies to normal sex differentiation is unclear, because the levels of AMH and its continuous secretion are different from those in the normal mouse fetus. Gene knockout of Amh (murine antimüllerian hormone) produced normal

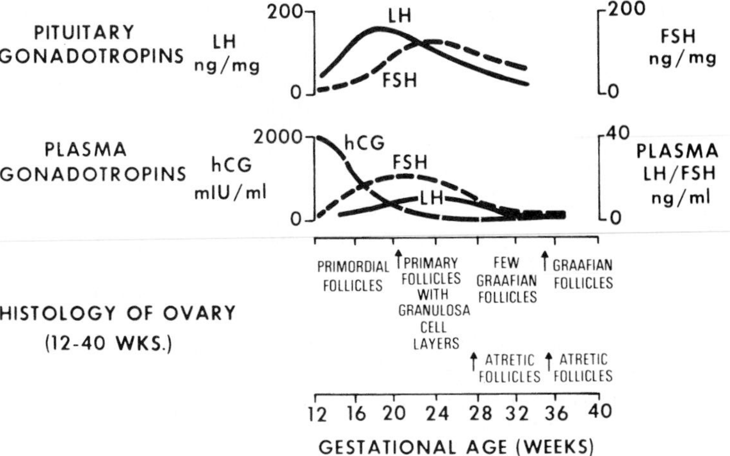

Figure 22–23. Comparison of the pattern of serum follicle-stimulating hormone (FSH), luteinizing hormone (LH), and human chorionic gonadotropin and pituitary FSH and LH in the human female fetus during gestation with the developmental histology of the fetal ovary. (Adapted from Kaplan SL, Grumbach MM. Pituitary and placental gonadotropins and sex steroids in the human and subhuman primate fetus. Clin Endocrinol Metab 1978; 7:487–511.)

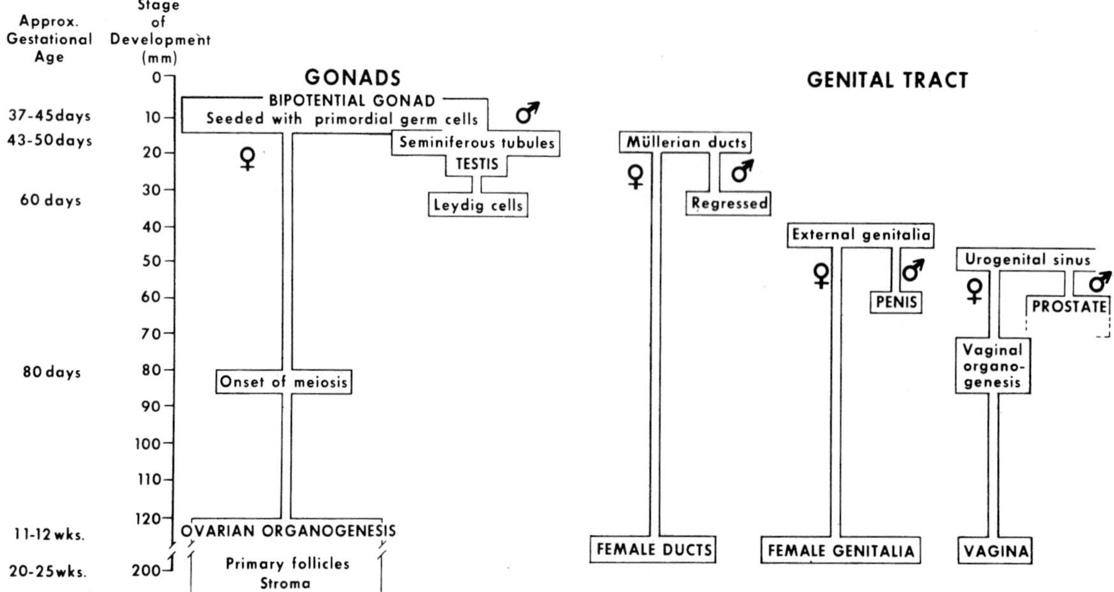

Figure 22–24. The sequence of sexual differentiation in the human fetus. The sequence as schematically depicted here emphasizes that testicular development in the male fetus precedes all other forms of sexual dimorphism. There is an inherent propensity of the gonads, genital ducts, and external genitalia to feminize, whereas masculinization requires Y chromosome–mediated (SRY) differentiation of the fetal testes. (Modified from Jost A. Hormonal factors in the sex differentiation of the mammalian foetus. Philos Trans R Soc Lond [Biol] 1970; 259:119–130.)

female mice with normal müllerian duct derivatives that were fertile, indicating that AMH is not required for normal ovarian function, at least in mice.[369, 373] The Amh-deficient males, as expected, had persistence of the müllerian derivatives.[369, 373] Ninety percent of the Amh-deficient mice were infertile because of interference by the müllerian duct derivatives with the passage of sperm from the epididymis and vas deferens to the urethra. The testes showed normal spermatogenesis but marked Leydig cell hypoplasia, suggesting that AMH may affect Leydig cell proliferation.[369, 373, 374]

The mechanism of action of AMH includes proteinase activated programmed cell death.[338] It causes a gradient of cranial to caudal regression of müllerian ducts during a critically short period of 9 to 12 weeks in the human[373] and thus cancels differentiation of the uterus, fallopian tubes, and upper vagina. A similarly expressed gradient of AMH type II receptors mediates AMH action on the mesenchyme but not the epithelium of the müllerian ducts (Fig. 22–27).[376, 378, 379]

AMH, a member of the transforming growth factor-β (TGF-β) family, as characteristic of this family, signals through receptor complexes composed of two related serine/threonine kinase transmembrane receptors.[377] One, MIS (müllerian-inhibiting substance) type II expressed only in the mesenchyme surrounding the müllerian duct, provides the specificity for

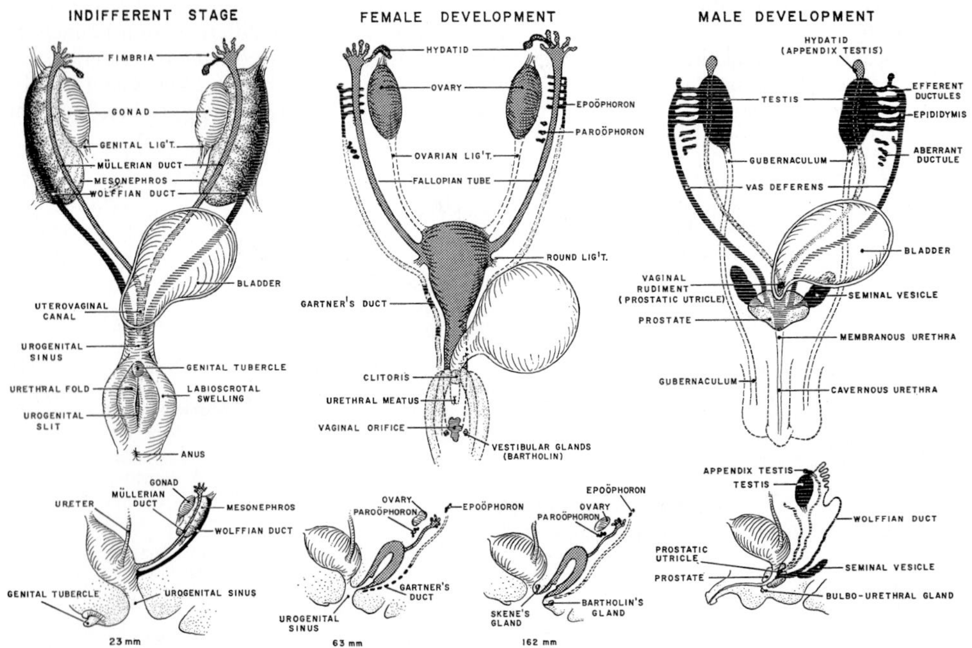

Figure 22–25. Embryonic differentiation of male and female genital ducts from wolffian and müllerian primordia. *Left*, An indifferent stage showing large mesonephric body. *Middle*, Female ducts. Remnants of mesonephros and wolffian ducts are now termed the *epoöphoron*, *paroöphoron*, and *Gartner duct*. *Right*, Male ducts before descent into scrotum. The only müllerian remnant is the testicular appendix. Prostatic utricle (vagina masculina) is derived from urogenital sinus. (Modified from Corning HK. Lehrbuch der Entwicklungsgeschichte des Menschen. Munich, JF Bergmann, 1921; and Wilkins L. The Diagnosis and Treatment of Endocrine Disorders in Childhood and Adolescence, 3rd ed. 1965. Courtesy of Charles C Thomas, Publisher, Springfield, IL.)

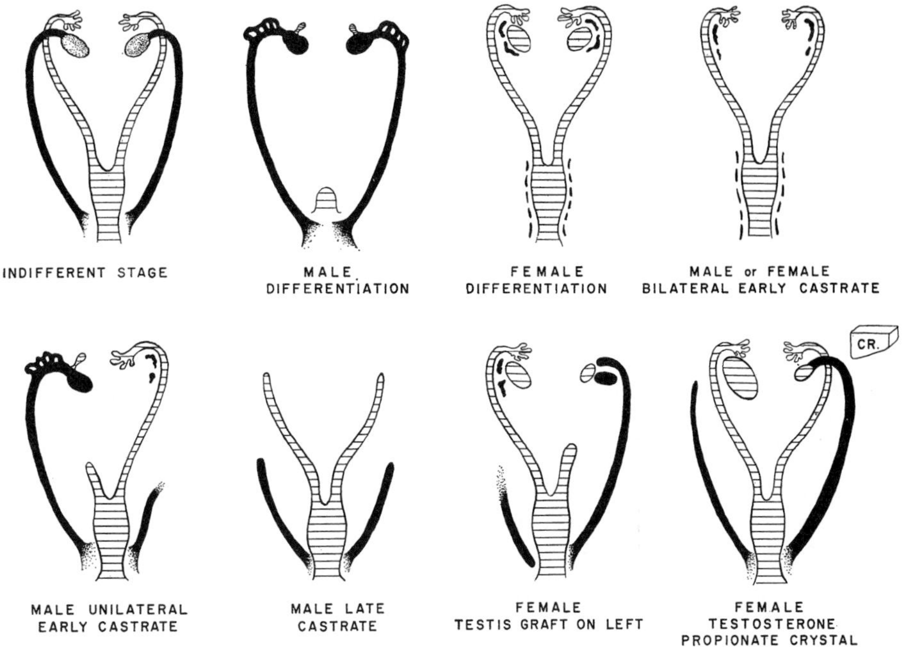

INDIFFERENT STAGE

MALE DIFFERENTIATION

FEMALE DIFFERENTIATION

MALE or FEMALE BILATERAL EARLY CASTRATE

CR.

MALE UNILATERAL EARLY CASTRATE

MALE LATE CASTRATE

FEMALE TESTIS GRAFT ON LEFT

FEMALE TESTOSTERONE PROPIONATE CRYSTAL

Figure 22–26. A schematic summary of Jost's experiments with rabbit embryos. The fetal testis plays a decisive role in determining the differentiation of the genital ducts. Testosterone stimulates wolffian development but fails to effect involution of müllerian structures. (Data from Jost A. Embryonic sexual differentiation [morphology, physiology, abnormalities]. In Jones HW, Scott WW [eds]. Hermaphroditism, Genital Anomalies and Related Endocrine Disorders, 2nd ed. Baltimore, Williams & Wilkins, 1971, p 16.)

AMH signaling; the other heteromere, ALK2, is expressed not only in the müllerian duct mesenchyme but, more ubiquitously.[378, 379] AMH acting through its heteromeric receptor activates a bone morphogenic protein–like pathway.[378, 379] A similarly expressed gradient of AMH type II receptors mediates, along with ALK2, AMH action on the mesenchyme surrounding the müllerian ducts, but not the duct epithelium. This suggests a paracrine signal arising from the müllerian duct mesenchyme induces a factor(s) that activates programmed cell death resulting in apoptosis. One such paracrine signal has been identified, a member of the matrix metalloproteinase family, MMP2, which when activated by AMH signaling induces regression of the müllerian duct.[338] Physiologic roles for AMH in males after regression of the müllerian ducts and in adult females are yet to be defined.

AMH is a dimeric glycoprotein composed of identical subunits linked by disulfide bonds.[339, 364, 368, 369] The monomer has a molecular mass of 72 kd, and the multimer ranges from 145 to 235 kd.[339, 364] The carboxyl-terminal domain exhibits marked homology with TGF-β and the beta chain of inhibin and activin.[380] The gene for AMH is 275 base-pairs long, contains five exons, and is located on the short arm of chromosome 19 band 19p13.3.[380, 381] The 3′ part of the number 5 exon codes for the bioactive part of the protein, which is the

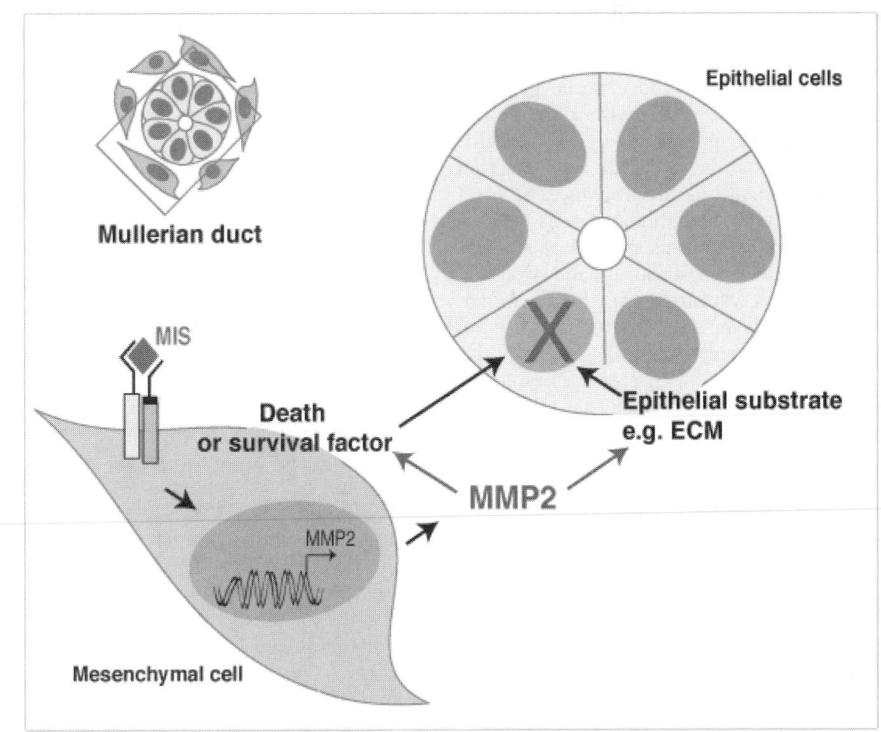

Figure 22–27. Mechanism of action of antimüllerian hormone (AMH/MIS). AMH/MIS binds to the ubiquitous AMH type I (ALK2) and the müllerian duct–specific AMH type II receptor, forming a heterodimer that induces signaling through the SMAD pathway and binding to DNA, resulting in the production of MMP2, matrix metalloprotein 2 in the müllerian duct mesenchyme. Pro MMP2 is secreted into the extracellular space, where it is activated by a membrane based metalloproteinase. Apoptosis (cell death) may occur as a result of activation of a death factor or inactivation of a survival factor. An alternate hypothesis is that MMP2 acts to cleanse the epithelial cell basement membrane. (Redrawn from Roberts LM, Visser JA, Ingraham HA. Involvement of a matrix metalloproteinase in MIS-induced cell death during urogenital development. Development 2002; 129:1487–1496).

only part of the protein similar to other TGF-β members.[374] AMH is expressed only in the gonad. It is cleaved from its prohormone by specific protein convertases to its bioactive form within the fetal testis and at its target site.[382] Presently, data show that AMH transcription is initiated by *SOX9* with up-regulation being mediated by *SF1*, *WT1*, and *GATA4*.[374]

The gene for the MIS type II receptor is localized to 12q13 and consists of 11 exons spanning 8.5 kb[383]; the ubiquitous ALK2 receptor gene maps to 2q23-q24, and encodes a 509-amino acid transmembrane protein consisting of a ligand-binding cysteine-rich extracellular domain, a transmembrane domain, and an intracellular domain with serine threonine specificity.[384]

Studies of humans with various forms of intersex have confirmed that regression of the müllerian ducts is the primary effect of AMH in the human male.[364] In patients with rudimentary gonads, the uterus and fallopian tubes develop normally regardless of the chromosomal sex. In true hermaphrodites who have a testis on one side and an ovary on the other, regression of the müllerian ducts is most marked on the side of the testis. Similarly, müllerian derivatives are absent in 46,XY women with the androgen resistance (insensitivity) syndrome, a disorder characterized by unresponsiveness of tissues to the action of androgens. Conversely, early intrauterine exposure of human female fetuses to high levels of androgens (as in CAH) fails to hinder normal development of the uterus and fallopian tubes.

Although müllerian involution is not androgen dependent, the differentiation of primitive wolffian ducts into the epididymides, vas deferens, and seminal vesicles requires testosterone and the androgen receptor.[385, 386] Mice, rats, and dogs treated with cyproterone acetate (an agent that blocks androgen action) and androgen-resistant XY humans and animals show the expected regression of the müllerian ducts, but structures derived from wolffian ducts generally remain vestigial.[387] Jost[1] showed that the implantation of a crystal of testosterone adjacent to the fetal rabbit ovary stimulates differentiation of male ducts on that side and to a lesser extent on the contralateral side; similar results were obtained by grafting a fetal testis adjacent to the ovary (see Fig. 22–26).

The lateralization of these effects suggests that higher local concentrations of androgen are required for male duct stimulation than for masculinization of the external genitalia and derivatives of the urogenital sinus. Unlike the masculinization of the urogenital sinus and external genitalia, in which testosterone reaches these target tissues systemically through the circulation (a classic endocrine effect), local diffusion of testosterone from the testis may be involved in stabilization and differentiation of wolffian duct derivatives. The local effect of a hormone from one cell on neighboring cells resulting from local dissemination is referred to as a *paracrine* action.

During differentiation of the wolffian ducts to form the epididymides, vasa deferentia, and seminal vesicles, the wolffian ducts lack the enzyme 5α-reductase, which converts testosterone to dihydrotestosterone (DHT).[342] Experimental data and studies in humans with steroid 5α-reductase type-2 deficiency provide additional evidence that testosterone (not DHT) mediates the differentiation of the wolffian ducts. This is in striking contrast to the urogenital sinus and genital tubercle, which express steroid 5α-reductase-2 even before the testis has developed the capacity to synthesize testosterone.[388] DHT mediates the masculinization of the urogenital sinus (including formation of the prostate) and external genitalia. Despite this difference in the action of testosterone and DHT on the primordia of the genital tract, the androgen receptor, at least in the rabbit fetus, is the same in the wolffian duct and in the anlage of the urogenital sinus and external genitalia.[389]

In patients with ambiguous genitalia, male genital ducts are well differentiated only in those who have functional testes and androgen receptors. Females with CAH do not display wolffian duct differentiation even though their external genitalia may be highly virilized in utero. Patients with asymmetric gonadal differentiation likewise have asymmetric male duct development that correlates with the degree of testicular differentiation on that side.

If the critical role of the testis in male duct development is to provide a high local concentration of testosterone, male duct development would be expected to be deficient, even though testes are present, in patients with severe defects in steroid biosynthesis (e.g., deficiency of steroidogenic acute regulatory protein [StAR]) and in XY patients whose tissues are unresponsive to testosterone (complete androgen resistance syndrome). The epididymides and vasa deferentia of these patients are generally underdeveloped. However, wolffian duct remnants (and sometimes fully developed duct derivatives) are observed with 17β-hydroxysteroid dehydrogenase 3 deficiency, Leydig cell hypoplasia (hCG/LH unresponsiveness) and, indeed, in some patients with complete androgen resistance. During sex differentiation, testosterone and AMH effect their morphogenetic actions on the underlying mesenchymal cells rather than directly affecting the epithelial cells.[374–377] Action of the hormone-stimulated mesenchyme on the epithelial cells mediates the morphogenesis of the male ducts and retrogression of the müllerian ducts[376, 377, 390]; members of the fibroblast growth factor (FGF) family produced by mesenchymal cells may be important mediators of mesenchymal-epithelial interactions by androgen.[391] Furthermore, from animal studies, EGF and GH may also play a role in stabilizing wolffian duct development.[392, 393]

Differentiation of the External Genitalia and Urogenital Sinus

Origin of the External Genitalia

At the eighth fetal week the external genitalia of both sexes are identical and have the capacity to differentiate in either direction.[280, 423] They consist of a urogenital slit bounded by paired urethral folds and, more laterally, by labioscrotal swellings. The urogenital slit is surmounted by a genital tubercle[395] consisting of corpora cavernosa and glans (Fig. 22–28). The mucosa-lined urethral folds may remain separate, in which case they are called labia minora, or they may fuse to form a corpus spongiosum enclosing a phallic urethra. The fleshy labioscrotal swellings may remain separate to form labia majora or fuse in the midline to form a scrotum and the ventral epidermal covering of the penis. The distinction between a clitoris and a penis is based primarily on size and whether the labia minora fuse to form a corpus spongiosum. The clitoris has two corporeal bodies that are analogous to but smaller than those of the penis. Baskin and colleagues describe in detail the neural innervation and the extensive, pudendal nerve–derived neurovascular network of the fetal clitoris through three-dimensional computer reconstructions.[396] This study has an important bearing on the preservation of sensation and function in the design of clitoral reconstructive surgery.

By the 50-mm crown-rump stage, male and female fetuses can be distinguished by inspection of the external genitalia; in the male, the urethral folds have fused completely in the midline to form the cavernous urethra and corpus spongiosum by 12 to 14 weeks of gestation.[396–398] Penile length in the male increases linearly, at about 0.7 mm/wk, from 10 weeks to normal term; a 12-fold increase occurs from 0.3 cm at 10 weeks to 3.5 cm at term, a rate of growth about 3.5 times that of the clitoris.[399] The mean stretched length of the penis in full-term infants is 3.5 $\pm$ 0.7 cm (SD) and the diameter is 1.1 $\pm$ 0.2 cm (SD).[399] The clitoral size in full-term infants is similar in several studies.[400, 401] The mean clitoral length is

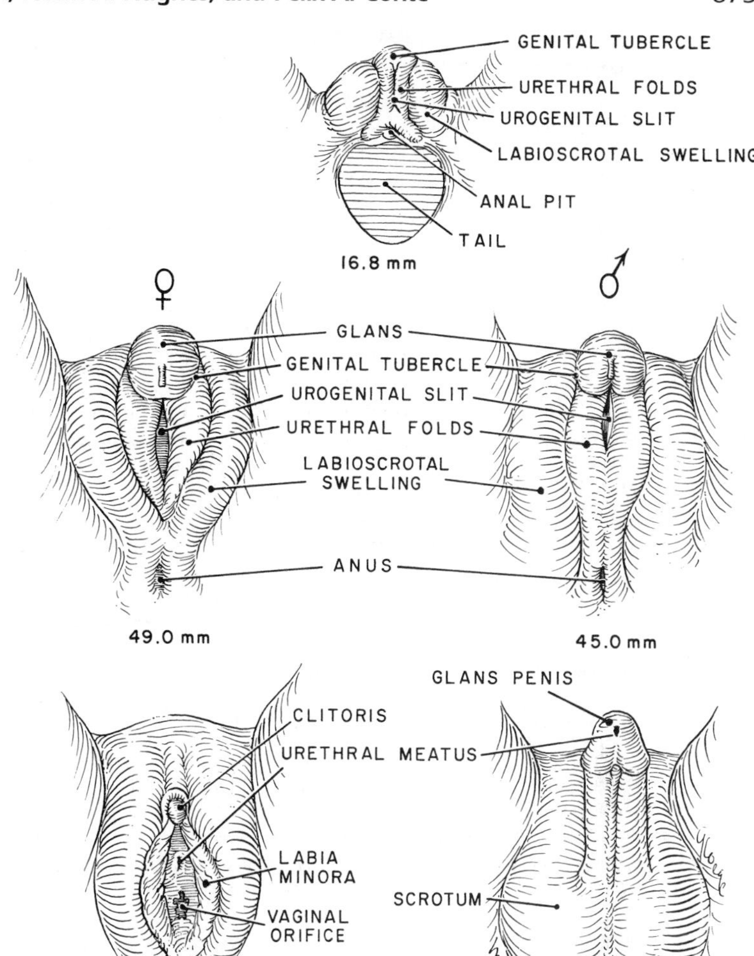

Figure 22–28. Differentiation of male and female external genitalia from indifferent primordia. Male development occurs only in the presence of androgenic stimulation during the first 12 fetal weeks. (Adapted from Spaulding MH. The development of the external genitalia in the human embryo. Contrib Embryol Carnegie Inst 1921; 13:69–88.)

0.40 ± 0.012 cm (SD), and the width is 0.033 ± 0.078 cm (SD).[400] In contrast, in normal women the mean length of the clitoris is 1.6 ± 0.4 cm (SD); the length of the glans clitoris is 0.51 ± 0.14 cm (SD) and its width is 0.34 ± 0.10 cm (SD); the clitoral index (glans length × glans width) is 1.85 ± 0.95 cm^2 (SD).[402]

Origin of the Vagina

The urogenital sinus separates from a common cloaca in early fetal life.[403] There is disagreement about the relative contribution of the müllerian duct and the urogenital sinus to the vagina, but the contact and interaction of the fused müllerian ducts with the urogenital sinus is essential for normal development of the vagina.[404, 405] In normal female development, proliferation of the vesicovaginal septum pushes the vaginal orifice posteriorly so that it acquires a separate external opening; thus no urogenital sinus, as such, is preserved. The lower vagina probably originates from the urogenital sinus. Uroplakins are membrane proteins specific to the urothelial plaque. Examination of human female fetuses of 9 to 18 weeks of gestation showed expression of uroplakins in the urothelium of the urogenital sinus, including the part that evaginates to form the sinovaginal bulbs.[406] In male development, the vaginal pouch is usually obliterated when the müllerian ducts are resorbed, although a vestigial blind vaginal pouch known as the prostatic utricle can sometimes be demonstrated; it is the site of prostate formation later in development.

The prostate gland and bulbourethral glands of Cowper in the male are outgrowths of the urogenital sinus; their differentiation is mediated by DHT and requires the presence of androgen receptors. In the female, the paraurethral glands of Skene and the vestibular glands of Bartholin have homologous origins (Table 22–5).

Mechanism of Androgen Action

The effects of testosterone are varied and tissue specific and reflect the sum of its action and the actions of its conversion products, DHT and estradiol (Fig. 22–29).[407–409] Testosterone enters the cell by diffusion. It can be 5α-reduced to DHT or aromatized to estradiol. Subsequently, testosterone and DHT bind to a high-affinity androgen receptor; this receptor has a greater binding affinity for DHT than for testosterone, and the DHT-receptor complex also is more stable. The androgen receptor is encoded by a gene located between the centromere and Xq13 on the X chromosome[96] and is present in androgen-sensitive target tissues of both males and females. The androgen receptor, a ligand-activated transcriptional factor, is a phosphoprotein and a member of a family of regulatory proteins that includes the nuclear receptors for other steroid hormones and for vitamin D, thyroid hormone, retinoic acid, 9-

Table 22–5. Homologies Between Male and Female Sexual Structures

Male Derivative	Primordial Structure	Female Derivative
	Gonad	
	Indifferent gonad derived from	
Sertoli cells	Coelomic epithelium	Granulosa cells
Leydig cells	Mesenchymal cell mass	Theca cells
Rete testes	Mesonephric elements	Interstitial cells
Septa and tunica albuginea		Rete ovarii
Tunica vaginalis		
Spermatogonia→sperm	Primordial germ cells	Oogonia→ova
	Genital Ducts	
Ductuli efferentes	Mesonephric tubules	Epoöphoron
Aberrant ductules		Paroöphoron
Epididymis	Mesonephric (wolffian) ducts	Gartner ducts
Vas deferens		
Seminal vesicles		
Ejaculatory ducts		
Appendix testis (hydatid)	Müllerian ducts	Fallopian tubes
		Uterus
		Upper vagina
	External Genitalia	
Penis	Genital tubercle	Clitoris
Corpora cavernosa		Corpora cavernosa
Glans penis		Glans clitoris
Corpus spongiosum (enclosing penile urethra)	Urethral folds	Labia minora
Scrotum and ventral epidermis of penis	Labioscrotal swellings	Labia majora
Prostrate	Urogenital sinus	Paraurethral glands (of Skene)
Bulbourethral glands (of Cowper)		Bartholin glands
Prostatic utricle (vagina masculina)		Vagina (lower)

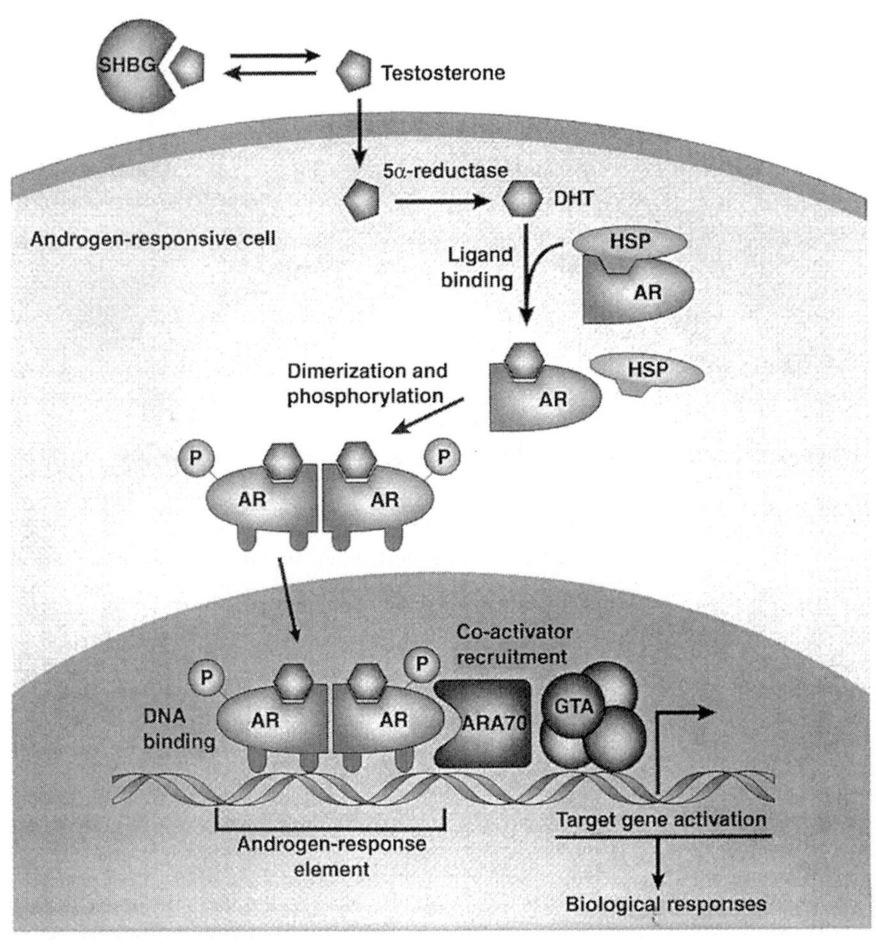

Figure 22–29. Scheme of androgen action. A small fraction of blood testosterone is in the free or unbound form; the major component of circulating testosterone is bound to sex hormone–binding globulin and albumin. Testosterone entering the cell is converted by 5α-reductase 1 or 2 to dihydrotestosterone (DHT) and by aromatase to estradiol (not shown). When DHT binds to the androgen receptor (AR), heat shock proteins (HSP) dissociate from the AR. The AR with its ligand (DHT or T) dimerizes, undergoes phosphorylation, and binds to androgen response elements on the promoter region of target genes. Coactivators (e.g., ARA70) and corepressors bind to the AR complex augmenting or inhibiting its interaction with the general transcription apparatus (GTA). Activation of target genes leads to an array of biological responses (including, e.g., in the prostate synthesis of prostate-specific antigen [PSA]). In addition, testosterone has nongenomic actions. (Redrawn from Feldman BJ, Feldman D. The development of androgen-independent prostate cancer. Nature Rev Cancer 2001; 1:34–45.)

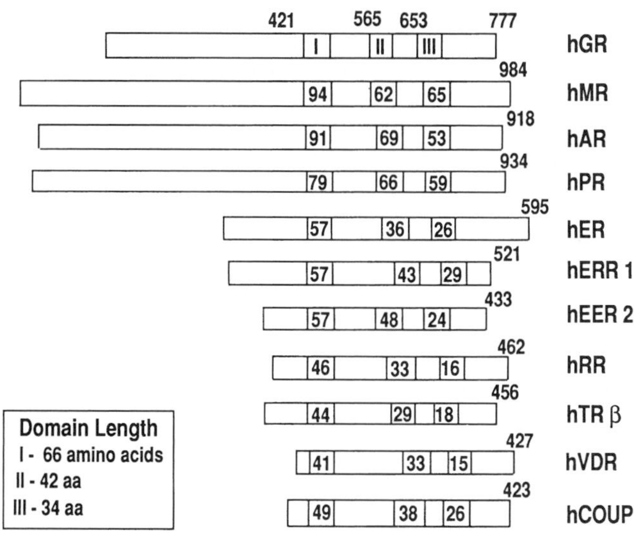

Figure 22-30. Linear representations of the steroid/thyroid hormone receptor superfamily are shown to illustrate sequence homology. hGR is the glucocorticoid receptor; hMR, the mineralocorticoid receptor; hAR, the androgen receptor; hPR, the progesterone receptor; hER, the estrogen receptor; hERR 1 and hERR 2, estrogen-related receptors; hRR, the retinoic acid receptor; hTRβ, the thyroid hormone receptor; hVDR, the vitamin D receptor; and hCOUP, the chicken ovalbumin upstream promotor. The DNA-binding site (region I) and the hormone-binding regions (II and III) are shown. (From O'Malley B. The steroid receptor superfamily: more excitement predicted in the future. Mol Endocrinol 1990; 4:363–369. © by The Endocrine Society.)

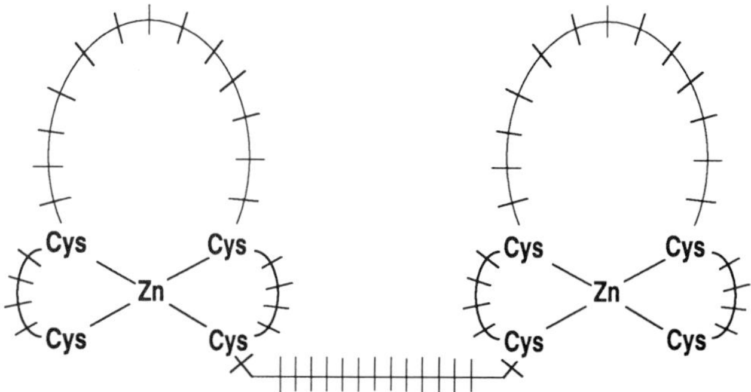

Figure 22-31. Type II zinc fingers. +++ indicates the amino acid skeleton of the zinc fingers, which specifies DNA binding in a sequence-specific manner.

cis-retinoic acid, ecdysone, and a group of orphan receptors, the ligands for which are unknown[407] (Fig. 22–30; see also Chapter 4). These nuclear receptors have in common three domains: (1) an amino-terminal domain thought to be involved in gene transcription; (2) a central DNA-binding domain that contains two zinc fingers (see Fig. 22–30), of which one has information for sequence-specific binding to DNA and the other is thought to stabilize binding of the receptor to DNA (Fig. 22–31); and (3) a carboxyl-terminal signal-receiving domain that binds the ligand (androgen).[407–410] Between the DNA and androgen-binding domains is a hinge domain. The degree of homology among the receptors in this family is highest in the DNA-binding domain and second highest in the ligand-binding domain.[407] The amino-terminal domains of these receptors show little homology. This domain contains an activation function (AF-1) region, which, at least in the case of the androgen receptor, is autonomously involved in gene *trans*-activation.[408, 411] The androgen receptor also has a unique amino-terminal polymorphic glutamine region as a result of a variable number of CAG repeats. The CAG repeat length has a direct influence on transcriptional efficiency.[412] Hyperexpansion of the CAG repeats causes spinal bulbar muscular trophy (Kennedy's disease).[413] A second activation function (AF-2) resides in the carboxyl terminus and mediates heat shock protein interactions, dimerization, nuclear localization signaling, and ligand binding.

In the absence of ligand, steroid hormone receptors (but not the thyroid hormone receptor) are complexed to chaperone proteins that are heat shock proteins and form large receptor complexes.[407, 408] Ligand binding causes a conformational change in the receptor, additional phosphorylation of serine residues located in the amino-terminal *trans*-activation domain,[411] dissociation of the receptor from heat shock proteins, and "activation" of the receptor.[407, 408] The monomeric activated steroid-receptor complex is smaller (<4S) than the unactivated complex (>8S). The steroid-receptor complex dimerizes and binds to palindromic steroid-responsive elements in genomic DNA that are upstream from CAAT and TATA boxes.[407, 408, 410] The AF regions interact with an intermediary group of proteins termed co-regulators to form protein-protein interactions in a ligand-dependent manner to either increase (co-activator) or decrease (co-repressor) gene transcription.[414–416] The multiprotein complex includes co-regulators such as CBP, SRC-1, and ARA70, the last one believed to be a protein more specifically associated with the androgen receptor.[417] Co-regulators appear to act as a physical bridge to link nuclear receptor transcription factors to the general transcriptional machinery,[416] such as RNA polymerase.

RNA polymerase and other transcription factors and co-activators are recruited to initiate transcription of the steroid response gene at a point 19 to 27 kb downstream of the TATA box.

The mechanism of *trans*-activational transcription is ill understood but the ligand-dependent AF-2 region is located within one of the α-helices (H12) of the ligand-binding domain that binds to receptor-interacting motifs, LXXLL, in co-regulators (L is leucine, X is any amino acid).[414–420] The crystal structures of several nuclear receptor ligand-binding domains, including most recently the androgen receptor, have been characterized.[421] They have in common 12 α-helices in the form of a sandwich fold. The most carboxyl terminus is helix 12, which becomes realigned by closing like a lid to form a hydrophobic pocket in the presence of ligand; thus the ligand is internalized and does not reside on the surface of the androgen receptor. Much information has been gained about structural and functional key roles for residues in the androgen receptor by the study of a range of mutations that cause androgen resistance (see later). After transcription and processing of the mRNA, the RNA moves to the cytoplasm, where it is translated by cytoplasmic ribosomes and results in synthesis of new proteins and hence androgenic effects. Despite an abundance of biologic actions of androgens ranging from male sex differentiation to muscle growth, erythropoiesis and skeletal development, little is known about the target genes that mediate these effects. Known androgen-responsive genes are the prostate-specific proteins, probasin and prostate-specific antigen.[422] However, the myriad of androgen-responsive genes that must be developmentally regulated during male fetal sex differentiation remain to be identified and characterized.

It is thought that testosterone and DHT have different roles. The testosterone-receptor complex modulates the secretion of LH by the hypothalamic-pituitary unit and affects the stabilization of the wolffian ducts, whereas the DHT-receptor complex acts in the fetus to promote masculinization of the urogenital sinus and external genitalia of the fetus and acts at puberty to induce maturation of secondary sex characteristics.[408] A defect in any of the essential steps in the action of

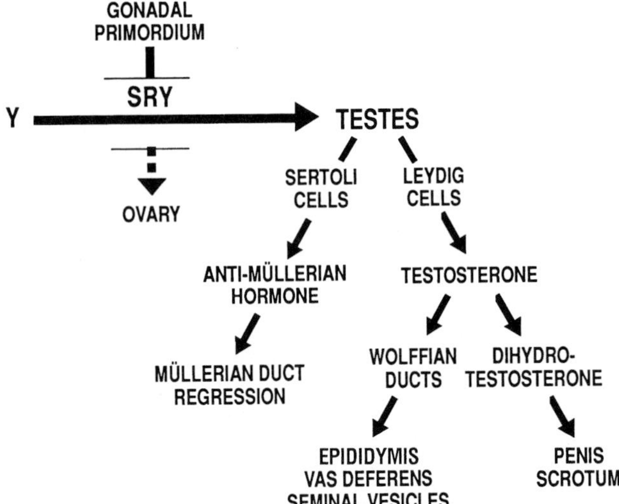

Figure 22–32. A simplified scheme of male sex differentiation. (Modified from Grumbach MM. Genetic mechanisms of sex development. In Vallet HL, Porter IH [eds]. Genetic Mechanisms of Sexual Development. New York, Academic, 1979, pp 33–73.)

androgen in a male fetus impairs masculinization of the urogenital sinus and external genitalia (Fig. 22–32).

Role of Androgens in the Differentiation of the External Genitalia and Urogenital Sinus

The induction of male differentiation of the external genitalia and urogenital sinus is affected by DHT, the 5α-reduced metabolite of testosterone. Testosterone is the prohormone that is delivered through the blood stream to these target tissues, which are rich in the enzyme 5α-reductase and can readily convert testosterone to DHT, even before the fetal testis acquires the capacity to secrete testosterone.[388] DHT binds to the androgen receptor and initiates the events that lead to androgen action. As in the case of the genital ducts, there is an inherent tendency for the external genitalia and urogenital sinus to feminize in the absence of fetal gonadal androgen secretions. Complete male differentiation of the external genitalia and urogenital sinus occurs only if the androgenic stimulus is received during the critical period of development (8 to 12 weeks) in fetal life.[423] DHT stimulates growth of the genital tubercle and induces fusion of the urethral folds and labioscrotal swellings.[11] It also induces differentiation of the prostate[11, 418] and inhibits growth of the vesicovaginal septum, thereby preventing the development of the vagina.[423] These morphogenetic effects of androgen seem to be mediated by the mesenchyme of these tissues and not by the overlying epithelium.[380]

After about the 12th week, when the vagina has separated from the urogenital sinus, fusion of the labioscrotal folds and urethral groove cannot occur, even with an intense androgenic stimulus.[423] The pattern of expression of the androgen receptor explicates, at least in part, why androgen exposure that begins after about the 12th to 13th week of gestation in the female fetus no longer has the capacity to masculinize the urogenital sinus and its derivatives.[406] Androgen receptors, which are expressed as early as the 9th week of gestation, are absent or greatly diminished by the 14th week in the urothelium of the urogenital sinus and the lower vaginal epithelium as well as in the surrounding stroma.[406] However, androgen receptors persist in the clitoris; androgenic stimulation can cause clitoral hypertrophy at any time during fetal life or after birth.

The male fetus with steroid 5α-reductase-2 deficiency and impaired conversion of testosterone to DHT has defective masculinization of the external genitalia and urogenital sinus, including absence or hypoplasia of the prostate. The failure of testosterone to masculinize the fetal external genitalia has been ascribed primarily to inability of the target tissues to form DHT. The growth of the external genitalia at puberty in patients with steroid 5α-reductase-2 deficiency is attributed to the postnatal expression of the isozyme 5α-reductase-1.

Whereas in some species fetal pituitary gonadotropins are required to sustain the secretion of testosterone by the fetal testes, in humans, placental hCG stimulates fetal Leydig cell development and function; human fetal pituitary LH plays a role only after differentiation of the external genitalia is already advanced. This probably explains why the external genitalia of male infants with anencephaly or fetal hypopituitarism and pituitary gonadotropin deficiency usually differentiate normally but remain small. Incomplete fusion of the labial folds and retention of the vaginal pouch in male infants may therefore be caused by deficient androgen secretion or by failure of the target tissues to respond to androgenic stimulation. Conversely, if female infants are subjected in utero to androgenic stimulation from some gonadal or extragonadal source, the external genitalia can masculinize, ranging from clitoral hypertrophy to the formation of a normal-appearing penis. Thus, similar external abnormalities can be produced in the male by androgen deficiency (or failure of the target tissues to respond) and in the female by exposure to androgen from some pathologic source in the fetus or mother.

Endocrine and Paracrine Control Mechanisms in Sex Differentiation

The regulation of sex differentiation by chemical messengers involves two types of control mechanisms. One is the classic endocrine mechanism: a cell, usually in a discrete endocrine gland, secretes a hormone into the blood stream, where it is transported to a distant target tissue to regulate or induce differentiation. Testosterone is a striking example of an endocrine secretion; testosterone secreted by the fetal Leydig cell is delivered through the circulation to the anlagen of the external genitalia and urogenital sinus. Similarly, hCG synthesized by the syncytiotrophoblast acts on the Leydig cell to stimulate testosterone secretion.

The second type of regulation in sex differentiation is paracrine control. This local and more primitive regulatory mechanism involves the dissemination of a hormone from its site of synthesis to its target cells by local diffusion through the extracellular space. Examples of this delivery system for chemical messengers are the action of AMH on the müllerian duct and the action of testosterone on the wolffian duct (in this instance testosterone is a paracrine secretion).

Hormonal Sex Differentiation

Sex differentiation is not complete until the secondary sexual characteristics have matured, fertility is attained, and the ultimate goal, reproduction, becomes possible (Fig. 22–33). These developments occur during puberty. In the past, puberty was regarded as a de novo event because of the dramatic changes brought about by the maturation of the gonads and the increased secretion of gonadal steroids. However, the development of gonadal function is actually a continuum extending from the differentiation of the gonad and the ontogeny of the hypothalamic-pituitary-gonadal system in the fetus, through puberty, to the attainment of full sexual maturation and fertility. Puberty is not an isolated event but rather a critical stage in a sequence of complex maturational changes. The hypotha-

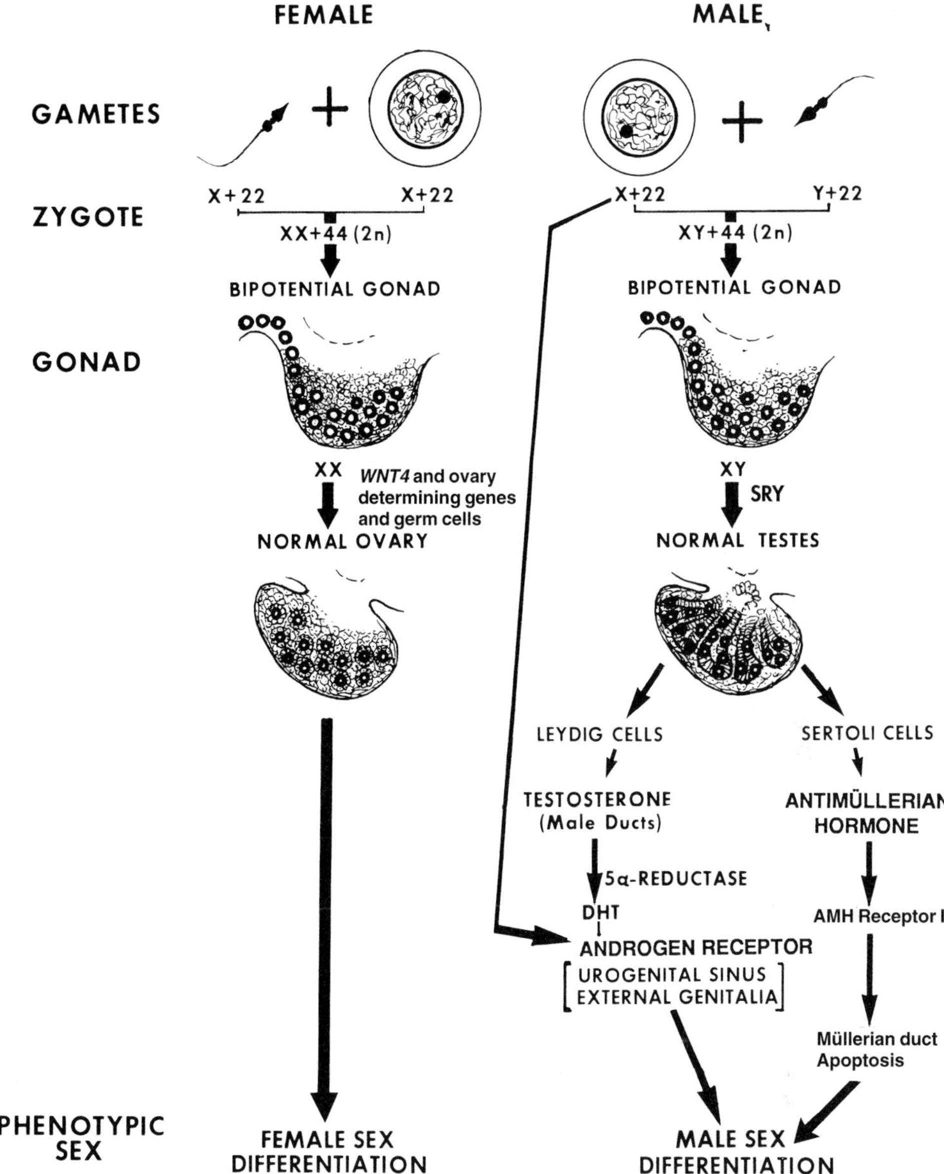

Figure 22–33. Diagram of human sex determination and differentiation. Intrinsic or extrinsic factors adversely affecting any stage of these processes can lead to anomalies of sex (see text). (Modified from Grumbach MM. The reproductive system. Anatomic and physiologic conditions. In Cooke RE (ed). The Biologic Basis of Pediatric Practice. New York, McGraw-Hill, 1967, pp 1058–1082.)

lamic-pituitary unit (including the pulsatile secretion of hypothalamic LHRH and of FSH and LH) functions in the fetus, is suppressed to a low level of activity for about a decade during childhood, and is reactivated at the onset of puberty.[424] The hormonal changes and the neuroendocrinology of puberty, including adrenarche and gonadarche, are reviewed in Chapter 24.

Sex Differentiation in the Hypothalamus

Although the control of gonadal function in both sexes is mediated by both FSH and LH, the secretory patterns of the gonadotropins differ in males and females. The male pituitary characteristically secretes both FSH and LH in a pulsatile but relatively constant and sustained manner, whereas in the mature female the pulsatile secretion of FSH and LH is cyclic and is characterized by a preovulatory gonadotropin surge that leads to ovulation.

In 1936, Pfeiffer[425] reported that the rat pituitary becomes differentiated during the early postnatal period according to the nature of the gonads, but the cyclic secretory pattern characteristic of the female pituitary is not an innate property of the pituitary itself. The pituitary of a male animal, when grafted under the hypothalamus of an adult female, is fully able to sustain the rhythm of repeated estrous cycles. When the male pituitary is grafted elsewhere in the recipient, ovulation fails to occur. Therefore, the hypothalamus or higher neural centers function differently in the two sexes.[426–429, 431–440] In the rat, mouse, hamster, guinea pig, and sheep there is an inherent tendency to a female hypothalamic-hypophyseal pattern of gonadotropin release, and this pattern is converted to a male pattern if the newborn animal is exposed to androgens or estrogens during the neonatal period[427–429]; in the guinea pig and sheep the androgen must be administered prenatally.

Once the male pattern is imprinted on "sex centers" in the hypothalamus (usually by testicular androgens aromatized to estrogen in the central nervous system), the potential for cyclic activity of pituitary gonadotropins is irrevocably lost. In the rat, the critical period is the first 10 days of life; the administration of as little as 1 μg of testosterone to female rats during this period causes structural changes in the hypothalamus,[429] permanent infertility because gonadotropin secretion at maturity is sustained rather than cyclic, and failure of ovulation.

and function of the developing central nervous system, are the *sole determining factor* in the evolution of male gender identity. We do not know if there is a critical period for masculinization of the fetal brain as is the case in the guinea pig. And quantitative, even grossly qualitative, aspects of the magnitude of androgen exposure and the variation in the central nervous system response leading to masculinization of the brain are not known. Rather, the complex, still poorly understood interaction of nature (androgens and genes) and nurture (primarily socialization, parental interaction and reinforcement, and self experience) results in genetic identity. That no one factor has proven to be an invariant determiner is a manifestation of the plasticity and complexity of the process and of the variation of biologic and psychosocial factors, even the dominance of one over the other in a given individual. For example, *SRY* and *ZFY* are expressed in the male brain, but yet XY individuals with complete androgen resistance (well represented by those with a deletion or null mutation of the X-linked gene encoding the androgen receptor) exhibit female gender identity. Female pseudohermaphrodites with virilizing CAH exhibit varying degrees of fetal androgen effects on the brain, but the vast majority express female gender identity, especially those in whom glucocorticoid treatment has suppressed the postnatal androgen excess. The few studies of ablatio penis discussed earlier, and the studies of Reiner and associates in XY patients with cloacal exstrophy orchidectomized in the neonatal period and assigned a female sex of rearing, support the critical role of the secretion of testosterone by the normal fetal testes in masculinizing the brain. However, even in these rare disorders some affected XY individuals had a female gender identity whereas others had a strong male gender identity.[488] In addition, the outcomes of genital surgical techniques, once quite discouraging, have greatly advanced, including the repair of severe hypospadias often at a single stage and feminizing genitoplasty of the masculinized external genitalia of female pseudohermaphrodites.[506–508]

Our understanding of the complexity of determinants of gender identity and gender role behavior has advanced remarkably in recent years. But there are large gaps in our knowledge and understanding; particularly limiting is the lack of long-term follow-up into adulthood of intersex individuals treated in the past two to three decades, which leaves little room for dogma.

CLASSIFICATION OF ERRORS IN SEX DIFFERENTIATION

In the past, individuals with hermaphroditism were classified according to their gonadal morphology. In the terminology of Klebs, a *true hermaphrodite* is a person who possesses both ovarian and testicular tissue. A *male pseudohermaphrodite* is one whose gonads are exclusively testes but whose genital ducts or external genitalia, or both, exhibit the phenotype of a female or incompletely differentiated male. A *female pseudohermaphrodite* is a person with ovaries whose external genitalia exhibit some masculine characteristics. We have classified errors in sex differentiation by a modification and expansion of this broad framework and have attempted to blend etiologic mechanisms and clinical entities into a simplified rational classification (Table 22–7). The clinical and etiologic heterogeneity of syndromes with similar anatomic findings merits emphasis. The format of this edition thus maintains the traditional pseudohermaphroditism terminology, which is useful clinically for diagnostic algorithms. In discussing intersexuality with patients and parents it is important to refer to the masculinized female and the undermasculinized male.

Table 22–7. Classification of Anomalous Sexual Development

I. Disorders of Gonadal Differentiation
  A. Seminiferous tubule dysgenesis (Klinefelter syndrome)
  B. Syndrome of gonadal dysgenesis and its variants (Turner syndrome)
  C. Complete and incomplete forms of XX and XY gonadal dysgenesis
  D. True hermaphroditism
II. Female Pseudohermaphroditism
  A. Androgen-induced
    1. Congenital virilizing adrenal hyperplasia
    2. CYP19 ($P450_{arom}$) aromatase deficiency
    3. Glucocorticoid receptor gene mutation
    4. Androgens and synthetic progestagens transferred from maternal circulation
  B. Other teratologic factors (non–androgen-induced) associated with malformations of intestine and urinary tract
III. Male Pseudohermaphroditism
  A. Testicular unresponsiveness to hCG and LH (Leydig cell agenesis or hypoplasia due to hCG/LH receptor defect)
  B. Inborn errors of testosterone biosynthesis
    1. Enzyme deficits affecting synthesis of both corticosteroids and testosterone (variants of congenital adrenal hyperplasia)
      a. StAR deficiency (congenital lipoid adrenal hyperplasia)
      b. Side-chain ($P450_{scc}$) cleavage deficiency heterozygote
      c. 3β-Hydroxysteroid dehydrogenase/$\Delta^{4,5}$-isomerase type 2 (3β-HSD-2) deficiency
      d. CYP17 ($P450_{c17}$ [17α-hydroxylase/17,20 lyase]) deficiency
      e. Smith-Lemli-Opitz syndrome: 7-dehydrocholesterol reductase deficiency
    2. Enzyme defects primarily affecting testosterone biosynthesis by the testes
      a. CYP17 ($P450_{c17}$ [17,20 lyase]) deficiency
      b. 17β-Hydroxysteroid dehydrogenase type 3 (17β-HSD 3) deficiency
  C. Defects in androgen-dependent target tissues
    1. End-organ resistance to androgenic hormones
      a. Syndrome of complete androgen resistance and its variants (testicular feminization and its variant forms)
      b. Syndrome of incomplete androgen resistance and its variants (Reifenstein's syndrome)
      c. Androgen resistance in phenotypically normal males (infertile and fertile)
    2. Defects in testosterone metabolism by peripheral tissues; 5α-reductase-2 (SRD5A2) deficiency (pseudovaginal perineoscrotal hypospadias)
  D. Dysgenetic male pseudohermaphroditism
    1. XY gonadal dysgenesis (incomplete)
    2. XO/XY mosaicism, structurally abnormal Y chromosome, *SRY* mutation
    3. Denys-Drash syndrome (*WT1* mutation)
    4. Frasier syndrome (mutation of *WT1* splice site junction mutation-deleting KTS)
    5. WAGR syndrome (*WT1* deletion)
    6. Campomelic dysplasia (*SOX9* mutation)
    7. *SFI* mutation
    8. *DAX1* (duplication)
    9. *WNT4* (duplication)
    10. $9p^-$ (*DMRT1* deletion)
    11. $10q^-$
    12. ATRX syndrome (*XH2* mutation)
    13. Testicular regression syndrome
  E. Defects in synthesis, secretion, or response to antimüllerian hormone: persistent müllerian duct syndrome (female genital ducts in otherwise normal men; herniae uteri inguinale)
  F. Maternal ingestion of progestagens
  G. Environmental chemicals (endocrine disrupters)
IV. Unclassified Forms of Abnormal Sexual Development
  A. In males
    1. Hypospadias
    2. Ambiguous external genitalia in XY males with multiple congenital anomalies
  B. In females, absence or anomalous development of the vagina, uterus, and uterine tubes (Rokitansky-Küster syndrome)

Disorders of Gonadal Differentiation and Sex Chromosome Anomalies

Not all patients with anomalies of sex chromosomes have abnormal gonads; conversely, congenital defects in gonadal differentiation are not always caused by chromosomal errors. The association is so frequent, however, that these topics are inseparable. Exceptions to this association are of special importance in defining the genetic and chromosomal determinants of gonadogenesis (see Table 22–4).

Seminiferous Tubule Dysgenesis: Klinefelter's Syndrome and Its Variants

47,XXY Seminiferous Tubule Dysgenesis (Typical Klinefelter's Syndrome)

Seminiferous tubule dysgenesis is a common cause of primary hypogonadism and male infertility (Table 22–8). This syndrome, as defined by Klinefelter and associates,[509] usually becomes manifest first during adolescence as gynecomastia, a variable degree of androgen deficiency, small atrophic testes with hyalinization of the seminiferous tubules, aggregation of Leydig cells, aspermatogenesis, and increased plasma gonadotropins, especially plasma FSH.[280]

In 1956, several groups found that a high proportion of patients with this syndrome are X chromatin positive despite their phenotypic male appearance. In 1959, Jacobs and Strong[510] and Ford and co-workers[511] first reported a 47,XXY sex chromosome constitution in patients with this disorder, explaining the positive sex chromatin pattern. Various other sex chromosome compositions, including mosaicism, were described subsequently. Virtually all these variants have in common the presence of at least two X chromosomes and a Y chromosome, except for the rare group that has a 46,XX sex chromosome complement by karyotype analysis of multiple tissues.

The differentiation of testes and lack of ovarian differentiation in patients with 47,XXY and, more strikingly, in those with 49,XXXXY complements indicate that a single Y chromosome and the expression of the testis-determining gene *(SRY)* are sufficient to bring about testis organogenesis and male sex differentiation in the presence of as many as four X chromosomes.

Clinical Features.[280, 512–515] In the postpubertal patient, the only constant clinical features are a male phenotype, small testes (<3 cm in length, and often <1.5 cm), and azoospermia (Fig. 22–34). Gynecomastia is common. Undescended testes are more than threefold as frequent as in normal boys. Prepubertal studies indicate that children with a 47,XXY karyotype, as a group, have lower birth weights; smaller mean head circumference; a slightly increased incidence of congenital anomalies, especially clinodactyly; height percentiles that increase with age; a lower verbal I.Q. than normal boys; and delayed emotional development and poor motor control and muscle tone.[514–518] Impairment in verbal I.Q. is slight (10 to 20 points), and the mean I.Q. falls between 85 and 90, with a wide range of variation.[517–521] Most boys with Klinefelter's syndrome require help in reading and spelling.[522, 523] Severe retardation is uncommon. One study of 13 47,XXY males monitored from birth through adolescence noted a mean I.Q. 21 points lower than that of a matched control group.[522] Despite neurocognitive difficulties including reading and writing, 12 of 13 graduated from high school and 4 attended college. In general, lack of motor skills hindered participation in competitive sports; 3 of 13 were successful in achieving personal goals and in their family relationships. The families of these 3 boys were among the most stable and supportive of the study group. Most patients with Klinefelter's syndrome do not have behavioral disorders,[520] and, in spite of verbal deficits, adult men with Klinefelter's syndrome are not significantly different as a group from other hypogonadal males or even normal controls as far as education, employment, socioeconomic status, social adjustment, and criminal behavior are concerned.[524]

Table 22–8. Clinical Features of Klinefelter's Syndrome

Karyotype:	47,XXY
Inheritance:	Sporadic; associated with advanced maternal age; nondisjunction during first or second meiotic division in either parent (67% maternal, 33% paternal); mitotic nondisjunction
Genitalia:	Male
Wolffian duct derivatives:	Normal
Müllerian duct derivatives:	Absent
Gonads:	Small, firm testes; seminiferous tubule dysgenesis; azoospermia; Leydig cell hyperplasia
Habitus:	Poor to normal virilization at puberty: gynecomastia; disproportionately long legs
Hormone profile:	Testosterone levels variable but usually decreased; increased levels of plasma LH and FSH postpubertally

FSH, follicle-stimulating hormone; LH, luteinizing hormone.

Patients with a 47,XXY karyotype tend to be taller (mean height 180 cm compared with 174 cm for their normal adult brothers[525]) than average because of disproportionate length of the legs.[519, 525] This finding is present before clinical signs of puberty are evident and may not be accompanied by a proportional increase in arm span. The prepubertal onset suggests that disproportionate leg length is not related to androgen deficiency or delayed epiphyseal closure. Androgen deficiency after the age of puberty augments the prepubertal deviation in skeletal proportions.[525] XXY individuals have three pseudoautosomal *SHOX* genes (one in each X chromosome and one on the Y chromosome).

Prepubertally, the basal plasma concentration of FSH and LH and the response to LHRH are within the normal range for age.[526–528] The timing and onset of secondary sexual characteristics and puberty were reported as normal in one study[528] and as delayed in another.[529] With the onset of puberty, testicular histology becomes abnormal and testosterone synthesis is impaired. In postpubertal patients the plasma concentrations of testosterone[528] tend to be low, the levels of plasma estradiol are normal or increased, and the gonadotropin levels are elevated. Testosterone responses to hCG appear to be normal in childhood and early adolescence and blunted in adulthood.[528] Potency is usually diminished in the adult, and Leydig cell reserve is impaired, as reflected by a subnormal increase in the concentration of serum testosterone after administration of hCG and an increased concentration of LH in plasma.[530] The testosterone production rate, levels of total and free testosterone, and rates of metabolic clearance of testosterone and estradiol tend to be low, whereas plasma estradiol levels are normal or elevated.[512, 531] Gynecomastia and signs of androgen deficiency, such as diminished facial and body hair, a female escutcheon, a small phallus, poor muscular development, and a further increase in the disproportion between leg and body length, usually become evident during or after puberty. The testicular failure in Klinefelter's syndrome appears to progress with age. Gynecomastia, which occurs in about 90% of patients, is considered to be secondary to an increased ratio of serum estradiol to testosterone[528] (see also Chapter 18).

Associated Abnormalities. Abnormalities in thyroid function include a diminished thyroid response to thyrotropin, de-

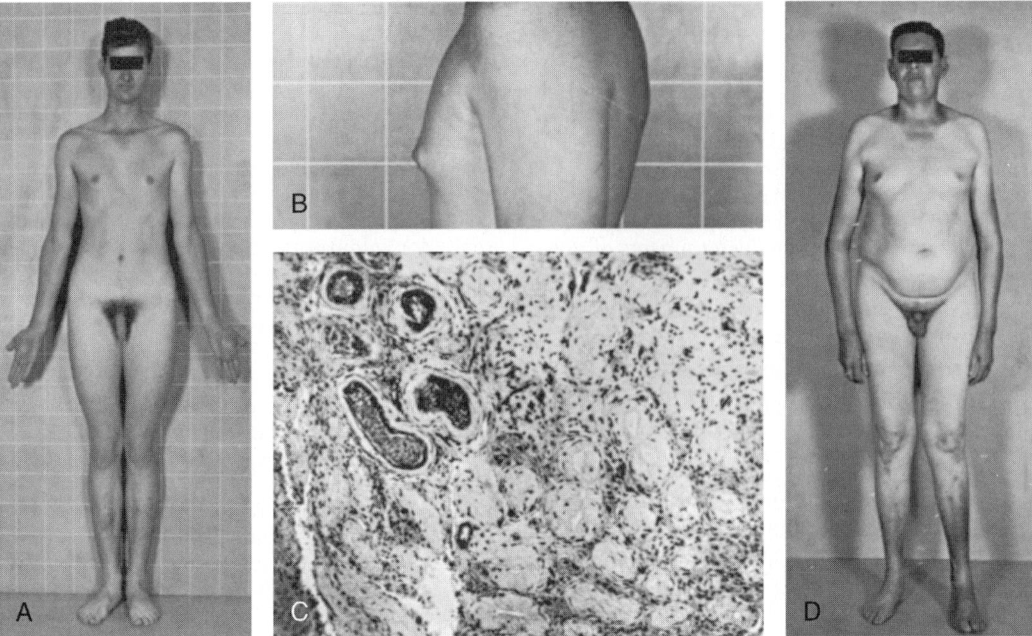

Figure 22–34. *A*, A 19-year-old phenotypic male with chromatin-positive seminiferous tubule dysgenesis (Klinefelter's syndrome). The karyotype was 47,XXY, gonadotropin levels were elevated, and testosterone levels were low normal. Note normal virilization with long legs and gynecomastia (*B, C*). The testes were small and firm and measured 1.8 × 0.9 cm. Testicular biopsy revealed a severe degree of hyalinization of the seminiferous tubules and clumping of Leydig cells. *D*, A 48-year-old male with 47,XXY Klinefelter's syndrome with severe leg varicosities.

creased uptake of radioactive iodine, and a subnormal increase in serum thyrotropin concentration after administration of thyrotropin-releasing hormone.[532] Clinically significant thyroid disease is uncommon. Approximately 10% of men with Klinefelter's syndrome have antibodies to thyroglobulin.[515]

The frequency of diabetes mellitus is increased. Nielsen[533] reported that 19% had impaired glucose tolerance and that 8% had overt diabetes. The prevalence of diabetes mellitus was also increased in the parents. The patients with diabetes mellitus were usually younger than 50 years of age, and the type II diabetes was usually mild. Insulin resistance with secondary hyperinsulinemia may be the cause of glucose intolerance.[534]

47,XXY patients with gynecomastia have an increased predisposition to cancer of the breast. In a survey of 187 males with breast cancer, 8 patients with chromatin-positive seminiferous tubule dysgenesis were detected, about 18 times the expected prevalence.[535] Whether this increased incidence is solely the consequence of the gynecomastia is unclear (see Chapter 17). Further, whereas male breast cancer is rare, a Swedish study of Klinefelter patients concluded that there is a 50-fold increased risk of developing breast cancer relative to normal males.[536] Infiltrating ductal carcinoma is the most common histologic type.[537] Even though a study of 696 men with Klinefelter's syndrome did not report an overall increase in cancer incidence,[538] the prevalence of germ cell tumors (particularly in the mediastinum) that secrete hCG and cause LHRH-independent sexual precocity is increased.[539–541] Twenty to 50 percent of boys 8 years of age or older with primary mediastinal germ cell tumors have Klinefelter's syndrome.[541, 542] The latter diagnosis is suggested by the association of prepubertal-size testes with sexual precocity. Routine screening is not indicated, given an estimated incidence of germ cell tumors of 1.5 per 1000 persons with Klinefelter's syndrome[541] but the diagnosis of Kleinfelter's syndrome should be considered in all boys with a germ cell tumor at any site (see Chap. 24).

A British study of mortality and cancer incidence in 646 patients with Klinefelter's syndrome showed that mortality was increased from diabetes, cardiovascular and respiratory disease, as well as lung and breast cancer.[542]

About 25% of adults with Klinefelter's syndrome have osteoporosis,[543] but it is uncommon in patients on testosterone replacement. Chronic pulmonary disease and varicose veins with stasis ulcers may also be more prevalent in adults. Patients with both androgen resistance and a 47,XXY karyotype have been reported.[544] These patients had female or ambiguous male genitalia and some clinical features of the 47,XXY karyotype. This combined defect is probably caused by fertilization of an oocyte containing two X chromosomes, each bearing a defect in the X-linked gene coding for the androgen receptor (e.g., uniparental disomy for the X chromosome), by a normal sperm containing a Y chromosome. Similarly, a null mutation, which causes intrauterine death in males usually with X-linked dominant incontinentia pigmenti, is associated with survival in affected XXY patients.[545]

Several males with 46,XY plus a marker chromosome have been reported. In these patients, the marker found was a small ring X chromosome that did not express *XIST* and hence was not inactivated. The abnormal dosage of X-active chromosome genes caused developmental delay and dysmorphic features.[546]

Frequency. Surveys of the prevalence of 47,XXY fetuses by karyotype analysis of unselected newborns indicate an incidence of about 1 per 800 to 1000 males, the most common human chromosomal abnormality. No racial or geographic predilection has been observed.[547]

Testicular Lesions. Klinefelter's syndrome accounts for 10% to 20% of men attending a male infertility clinic. Changes in the histologic structure of the testis become more marked with age in 47,XXY individuals.[548] A limited number of studies of fetal testes have been reported, and the findings are variable. Grumbach and associates[549] reported normal histology for the testes of a 1700-g chromatin-positive premature infant, as was similarly reported in a 49,XXXXY 21-week fetus,[550] but exami-

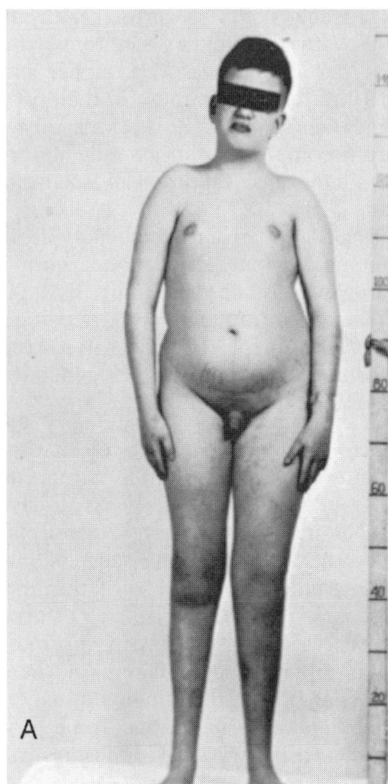

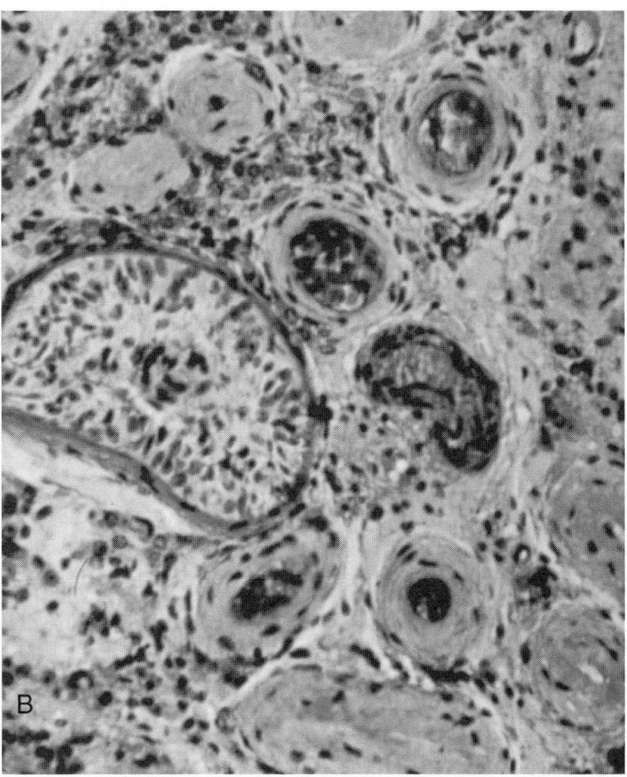

Figure 22–35. *A*, An 8½-year-old boy with a 48,XXXY chromosome constitution, mental retardation, precocious sexual development, and accelerated growth. The appearance of pubic hair was noted at age 6. By 8 years, acne, a deep voice, tall stature, and axillary hair were present. Height was 148 ± 2.9 cm, weight was 47.7 ± 3.9 kg, span was 140 cm, and upper segment/lower segment ratio was 0.87. Testes measured 2.1 × 1.3 cm. Note the long legs, prognathism, small hands and feet, gynecomastia, and secondary sexual characteristics. His I.Q. was 62. The urinary 17-ketosteroid level was 3.2 mg/day and urinary gonadotropin levels were elevated. Bone age was 13.5 years. Roentgenogram of chest was normal. The buccal smear contained nuclei with a maximum of two X chromatin bodies. Karyotype of cells derived from skin and blood was 48,XXXY. *B*, Testicular biopsy showed hyalinized tubules and clumping of Leydig cells; germ cells were absent. The findings suggest that true precocious puberty, with stimulation of juvenile testes by pituitary gonadotropin, led to premature appearance of typical histologic changes of seminiferous tubule dysgenesis. (Courtesy of M. M. Grumbach and A. Morishima, unpublished data.)

nation of several other affected fetuses suggested that the germinal epithelium was deficient and that germ cells were heterotopic[551]; these observations indicate that the histology of the fetal testes varies. In three infants aged 3 to 12 months with a 47,XXY karyotype, spermatogonia were decreased.[552] In later childhood, testicular biopsies have revealed small tubules with progressive reduction in spermatogonia.[553] In considering the testicular lesion, it seems that a normal or near-normal complement of germ cells is present early in fetal life. During late gestation and early infancy, a drastic loss of spermatogonia ensues, possibly because of an exaggeration of the normal apoptosis of spermatogonia in the neonatal period. In addition, excessive germ cell loss could result from defective maturation[554] or failure of the germ cells to migrate to the periphery of the tubule and align in opposition to the basement membrane. An experimental XXY mouse model has been established.[555] The histology of the testes in adult mice is consistent with the human syndrome. Progressive loss of germ cells in XXY mice was observed by 10 days after birth.

With the approach of adolescence, even before pubertal signs are well advanced, the actions of pituitary gonadotropins on the intrinsically defective testis induce progressive hyalinization of the seminiferous tubules and pseudoadenomatous clumping of Leydig cells. Despite this clumping, the mean volume of Leydig cells usually is normal.[555] After pubescence, the testes are characterized by small dysgenetic tubules with arrested development, fibrosis, and hyalinization. The result is testes that are small in size and firm in consistency. Peritubular elastic tissue is usually absent or diminished.[315, 320] That gonadotropin secretion plays a direct or indirect role in the progressive degeneration of the testes was suggested in a 7-year-old 48,XXXY boy with true precocious puberty and elevated urinary gonadotropin levels. Unlike the relatively normal testicular architecture in most boys of this age with Klinefelter's syndrome, the testes of this boy exhibited extensive hyalinization and fibrosis of the tubules and clumping of Leydig cells (Fig. 22–35). Conversely, 47,XXY patients with gonadotropin deficiency do not exhibit the typical changes in testicular histology.

Hyalinization of the tubules is usually extensive but varies in degree from patient to patient and even between the testes of the same patient. The fibrosis tends to progress with age, and in some older patients few tubules can be identified. Conversely, in some patients the tubules are lined by Sertoli cells, tubular fibrosis is relatively slight, and the histologic appearance resembles that of germinal cell aplasia. Rarely, spermatogenesis is found in isolated tubules. This finding could represent hidden mosaicism in the gonad or possibly mitotic nondisjunction or anaphase lag in germ cells giving rise to 46,XY cells that would then go on to spermatogenesis. There have been sporadic reports of paternity; most fertile individuals proved to have sex chromosome mosaicism, and in others acceptable documentation of paternity was not provided. Fertile patients with 46,XY/47,XXY mosaicism often lack features that

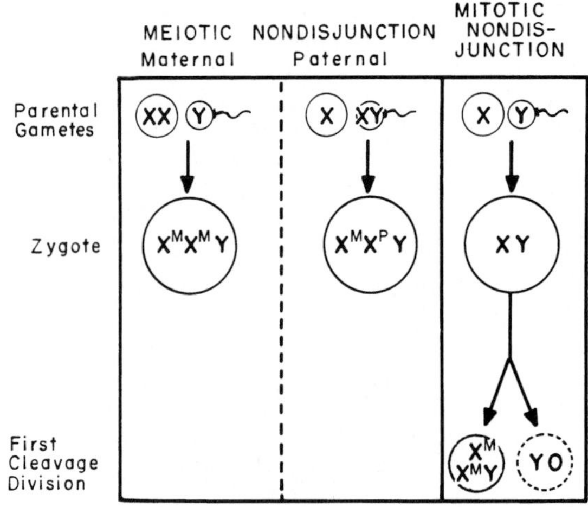

Figure 22–36. Origin of the 47,XXY karyotype. Superscripts M and P designate, respectively, maternal and paternal X chromosomes. The *dashed circle* indicates a nonviable cell line. (From Grumbach MM. The testes. In Beeson PB, McDermott W [eds]. Cecil Loeb Textbook of Medicine, 13th ed. Philadelphia, WB Saunders, 1971, pp 1804–1818.)

distinguish them from patients with typical Klinefelter's syndrome. Analyses of sperm chromosomes from a 46,XY/47,XXY male showed that 1% of sperm had a 24,XY haplotype, which suggests that some 47,XXY cells can undergo meiosis and form XY-bearing spermatozoa.[556] The technique of intracytoplasmic sperm injection (ICSI) has been used with some success for achieving fertility, including the birth of twins.[557, 558] However, there is a risk of trisomy 21 in offspring of patients with Klinefelter's syndrome.[559]

Origin of 47,XXY Constitution. 47,XXY males may develop through nondisjunction of the sex chromosomes during either the first or second meiotic division in either parent[41–43] or, less commonly, through mitotic nondisjunction in the zygote at the time of or after fertilization (see Figs. 22–4 and 22–20). Fertilization of a 46,XX ovum by a Y-bearing sperm or of an X ovum by a 46,XY-bearing sperm would yield a 47,XXY zygote. Mitotic nondisjunction of the sex chromosomes in a 46,XY zygote could yield a 47,XXY and a 45,Y daughter cell (Fig. 22–36). Because the 45,Y cell line is nonviable, only the 47,XXY cell line would survive.

These abnormalities of meiosis almost always occur in parents with normal sex chromosome constitution. However, Rosenkranz[560] described two 47,XXY patients whose mothers were, respectively, 47,XXX and 46,XX/47,XXX mosaic. Whether a 47,XXY karyotype is derived more frequently than previously suspected from a polysomic X constitution in the mother remains to be determined.

In a study of 47,XXY males, Jacobs and colleagues[561] found that the XXY constitution resulted from paternal nondisjunction in the first meiotic division in 53% of the patients, from maternal nondisjunction during the first meiotic division in 34%, and from maternal nondisjunction during the second meiotic division in 9%. Three percent of cases appeared to be related to postzygotic mitotic nondisjunction. Ferguson-Smith and colleagues[562] and others reported a positive association with advanced maternal age in 47,XXY patients, although this association is less marked than in trisomy 21. The association with advanced maternal age correlates with first meiotic division errors.[44, 45, 561] Some studies in X^MX^PY individuals indicate that paternal nondisjunction does not depend on age,[561–563] a finding reminiscent of that in patients with autosomal trisomy. Nevertheless, the prevalence of XY, YY, and XX disomy in human sperm appears to be increased in older men.[564] Furthermore, in a study of the sperm of healthy men who were fathers of boys with Klinefelter's syndrome, the frequency of XY sperm (7.5 per 10,000) was 31% higher among fathers in their 40s and 100% higher for those in their 50s.[565]

Rarely, Klinefelter's syndrome is associated with a supernumerary X chromosome that is structurally abnormal, for example, an X-autosome translocation or an isochromosome for the long arm of the X.

Among a small, rare group of phenotypic females with a 42,XXY karyotype, six (one set of monozygotic twins) had the complete androgen resistance syndrome. Both X chromosomes harbored a deleted or mutant gene encoding the androgen receptor. One 47,XXY fertile woman had a structurally abnormal Y chromosome devoid of the *SRY* gene attributable to an illegitimate X-Y interchange.[565a]

Etiologic Factors. An important factor in the origin of the 47,XXY chromosome constitution is advanced maternal age and maternal nondisjunction.[43, 561–563] As discussed previously, the maternal age effect in chromosome abnormalities may be a consequence of the long diplotene stage of human ova. Oocytes remain suspended in prophase of the first meiotic division from birth to ovulation, which may not occur for decades. The defective segregation of the two X chromosomes could be caused, at least in part, by reduction of the length of the chiasma as the length of the diplotene stage increases (see section on aneuploidy). As in the syndrome of gonadal dysgenesis, the prevalence of twinning in sibships of 47,XXY individuals may be increased.

Genetic factors that predispose to nondisjunction have been demonstrated in lower species. Although chromosome abnormalities are usually sporadic, families have been reported in which leukemia and various chromosome abnormalities have occurred in siblings and relatives. In addition, patients with more than one form of trisomy seem to occur more frequently than expected by chance alone. A role for radiation, viruses, environmental toxins, folate deficiency, or autoimmunity as a predisposing factor has not been established.

Diagnosis and Treatment. The diagnosis of Klinefelter's syndrome in the postpubertal male is suggested by the typical phenotype and hormonal changes and confirmed by the finding of a 47,XXY karyotype or a variant sex chromosome complement in blood, skin, or gonads. Treatment should be directed toward androgen replacement therapy when there is evidence of androgen deficiency. In general, parenteral androgens are more effective in inducing virilization and are safer than oral preparations (see also Chapters 18 and 24). Hepatic tumors and abnormalities in liver function have been associated with chronic administration of oral androgens that have substitutions at the 17α-position (e.g., a methyl group), but such abnormalities are not a problem with testosterone ester preparations such as propionate or enanthate or the testosterone dermal patch. Testosterone enanthate in oil, 200 mg intramuscularly every 2 to 3 weeks, is recommended for full replacement therapy, but it is wise to begin therapy at a lower dose (e.g., 50 mg intramuscularly every 4 weeks) to avoid rapid virilization and bone maturation, especially in adolescent males. The testosterone dermal patch is a useful, but more expensive, therapeutic approach. In general, conspicuous and long-standing gynecomastia does not diminish as a result of androgen replacement. However, in some patients, especially those with less striking gynecomastia, regression can occur with androgen replacement therapy. Severe or psychologically disturbing gynecomastia is corrected by reduction mammoplasty or by liposuction.

The diagnosis of Klinefelter's syndrome should be suspected in prepubertal patients with one or more of the following: (1) long legs, (2) smaller than normal prepubertal testes and/or penis, (3) learning disorders, and (4) developmental delay in speech and language. Similarly, based on the outcome of cytogenetic surveys of newborns, it is recommended that all boys with undescended testes or a micropenis or who have gynecomastia should have a karyotype performed. Many of these features are amenable to therapy, so early detection and intervention may be beneficial. Nielsen and Pelsen[524] suggested that prepubertally diagnosed patients with Klinefelter's syndrome should be offered therapy with testosterone at 11 to 12 years of age to initiate puberty and to prevent the physical and psychological complications of hypogonadism. We have employed a regimen that begins replacement therapy with 50 mg of testosterone enanthate in oil intramuscularly each month at a bone age of 12 years.[566] When the bone age has advanced to 14 years, the dose may be increased to 100 mg intramuscularly monthly. After several years of treatment at these doses, a height is usually attained that is appropriate for genetic height potential of the individual and pubertal progression is usually adequate. When full masculinization is desired, an adult replacement dose of 200 mg every 2 weeks or 300 mg every 3 weeks may be given.

Variant Forms of Klinefelter's Syndrome

46,XY/47,XXY Mosaicism. 46,XY/47,XXY mosaicism is the second most common karyotype in chromatin-positive men. The presence of a normal XY cell line in these patients can modify the clinical expression of the 47,XXY cell line. In general, these patients manifest a lesser degree of gynecomastia, androgen deficiency, and testicular pathology. As a group they are older (mean age, 45 years) at the time of diagnosis than 47,XXY patients. Decreased libido and potency may not appear until the fourth or fifth decade. At the time of diagnosis, serum FSH levels are elevated and serum testosterone concentrations often are in the normal male range. Secondary sexual characteristics are more normal than those of patients with 47,XXY karyotypes, and seminiferous tubules exhibit spermatogenesis more commonly than in 47,XXY patients.[513] Some patients with 46,XY/47,XXY mosaicism are fertile.[513]

The diagnosis of 46,XY/47,XXY mosaicism is established by the finding of at least 5% XY cells in blood, skin, or gonads in which the second cell line is 47,XXY. 46,XY/47,XXY mosaicism may result from nondisjunction or anaphase lag in a 47,XXY zygote.

48,XXYY. Individuals with a 48,XXYY karyotype have the typical findings of Klinefelter's syndrome and often exhibit additional features. They constitute about 3% of chromatin-positive males and most are mentally retarded, although this may in part relate to ascertainment bias, because a significant proportion of cases are detected in screening mental and psychiatric hospitals. The 48,XXYY karyotype is usually associated with tall stature (the mean height of 26 patients was 181 cm), disproportionately long lower extremities, gynecomastia, delinquent behavior, and unusual dermatoglyphic patterns. Peripheral vascular disease, especially varicose veins and stasis dermatitis, has been observed. Secondary sexual characteristics are poorly developed, and testicular histology is similar to that of 47,XXY patients. The sex chromatin pattern is indistinguishable from that of the 47,XXY groups; however, two fluorescent Y bodies are present in a high proportion of somatic nuclei.

To have two Y chromosomes, nondisjunction must occur in paternal meiosis. In two informative matings the Xg blood groups indicated that the father contributed an X as well as two Y chromosomes, suggesting that an X ovum was fertilized by an XYY sperm (arising from successive nondisjunction in the first and second meiotic divisions). The 48,XXYY karyotype in a patient whose mother was 47,XXX[567] could have arisen by the fertilization of an XX ovum by a YY sperm.

48,XXXY and 49,XXXYY. All reported patients with a 48,XXXY karyotype have moderate to severe mental retardation, normal to tall stature, facial dysmorphology, small testes, and signs of androgen deficiency.[568] With the increase in the number of X chromosomes, the severity and frequency of somatic anomalies such as short neck, epicanthal folds, radioulnar synostosis, and clinodactyly increase. Mental retardation, somatic anomalies, and small testes also occur in 49,XXXYY patients.[569]

49,XXXXY. The 49,XXXXY karyotype has been reported in more than 100 patients since the first report by Fraccaro and colleagues in 1960.[570] The diagnosis may be suspected from the clinical features. Mental deficiency can vary from moderate to profound. Phenotypic features include (1) skeletal abnormalities, especially radioulnar synostosis, genu valgum, pes cavus, and clinodactyly, and (2) hypoplastic external genitalia with a small penis, underdeveloped scrotum, and very small and frequently undescended testes; external genitalia may be ambiguous because of hypospadias, bifid scrotum, hypoplastic phallus, and cryptorchidism.[569, 571, 572] Fifteen to 20% of patients have cardiac defects, the most common of which is patent ductus arteriosus.[569] In adults, androgen deficiency is severe and gynecomastia is absent. In contrast to other males with multiple X chromosomes in their constitution, most affected patients are short.[569] Before puberty, the testes often contain hypoplastic seminiferous tubules. Other anomalies include congenital heart disease, cleft palate, strabismus, and microcephaly. The face may have a characteristic appearance, with a Down's syndrome–like slant of the eyes, epicanthal folds, hypertelorism, strabismus, and a wide nose.[571, 572] Sarto and co-workers[573] suggested that the phenotypic abnormalities noted in patients with aneuploidy involving supernumerary X chromosomes result from an effect of non-inactivated genes on the X chromosomes and/or asynchronous replication of the supernumerary X chromosomes, so that more than one X chromosome is active in cells. Analyses of the parental origin of sex chromosome polysomies indicate that the extra sex chromosomes are always derived from one parent, probably by successive nondisjunction during the first and second meiotic divisions of either paternal or maternal gametogenesis.[574]

46,XX Males. A 46,XX karyotype is present in about 1 of every 20,000 phenotypic males.[154, 575] These patients have a male phenotype and psychosocial orientation and are similar clinically and endocrinologically to individuals with classic Klinefelter's syndrome except for minor differences. Postpubertally, as in Klinefelter's syndrome, they have varying degrees of testosterone deficiency, gynecomastia, and small testes with azoospermia.[576, 577] Testosterone production is usually decreased, as is the response to hCG.[576] Both basal and LHRH-induced FSH and LH levels are increased.[576, 577] There is a 10% incidence of hypospadias that is attributed to a deficiency of testosterone formation by the fetal Leydig cells. 46,XX males with genital abnormalities usually lack evidence of SRY DNA in their genome and manifest a greater prevalence and degree of gynecomastia than 46,XX men in whom a Y-to-X translocation is present.[577, 578] Compared with males with a 47,XXY karyotype, 46,XX males have a lower frequency of intellectual and psychosocial problems; they are shorter (mean height, 168 cm) than 47,XXY or normal males; they have smaller tooth crowns (Y-linked gene) than normal males; and, in contrast to 47,XXY individuals, they usually have normal skeletal proportions.[154, 577–579]

The histology of the testes is similar to that in 47,XXY males; seminiferous tubules are decreased in size and number, germinal cells usually are absent, and peritubular and interstitial fibrosis occurs. The Leydig cells appear hyperplastic. In some patients the morphology of the testes is similar to that in germinal cell aplasia or intermediate between it and the morphology in Klinefelter's syndrome. In contrast to 47,XXY patients, maternal age is not increased.

The paradoxical finding of males with a 46,XX karyotype has fascinated investigators and led to an expansion of the understanding of the genes that control sex determination. Several theories have been advanced to explain this type of sex reversal: (1) loss of a Y chromosome early in embryogenesis, (2) cryptic sex chromosome mosaicism in a 46,XX male with an undetected and/or circumscribed cell line containing a Y chromosome,[580] (3) translocation between a Y chromosome and an X chromosome or autosome resulting in the presence of the testis-determining gene (or genes) on an X chromosome or autosome,[581] and (4) a mutation involving either an autosomal or X-linked gene in the pathway to testis differentiation.[578, 582] Studies involving X- and Y-linked marker genes,[583] cytogenetic observations,[584, 585] and direct molecular genetic analyses[154, 585–593] suggest that 80% to 90% of 46,XX males result from an anomalous Y-to-X translocation during meiosis.

As discussed earlier, the X and Y chromosomes have a homologous region on the distal short arms, the PAR1. The homology of this region and the proper segregation of sex chromosomes are maintained by an obligate crossover within the region at meiotic pairing. The *SRY* gene is located just proximal to the boundary of the PAR.[147, 154] 46,XX males can arise from a balanced aberrant nonhomologous interchange between Yp and Xp that includes the sex-determining locus[154, 591] (Fig. 22–37) or from aberrant unequal nonhomologous exchange resulting in an X chromosome that has part of its PAR as well as the sex-determining region of the Y and its PAR[592, 594] (see Fig. 22–37*B*). Such 46,XX patients have had three copies of the pseudoautosomal gene *MIC2*. The resulting Y chromosome in both the anomalous balanced and unbalanced exchanges lacks the testis-determining region of the Y chromosome and hence could give rise to a 46,XY phenotypic female with XY gonadal dysgenesis.[154, 595, 596] The Y-to-X translocation in *SRY*-positive 46,XX males is heterogeneous, involving most of the short arm in approximately 40% of cases but as little as the *SRY* sequence and the PAR.[154, 597] A novel protein kinase gene on the Y chromosome, *PRKY*, its homologous partner on the X chromosome, *PRKX*, both located proximal to the pseudoautosomal region (PAR1), are the site of the translocation breakpoint in about one third of *SRY*-positive 46,XX males.[598] In general, the greater amount of Y material present, the more virilized the phenotype.[154, 597] Illegitimate Y-to-X recombinations can also occur in homologous segments of the X and Y chromosome that are outside the PAR[597] (see Fig. 22–37). Three patients with 47,XXX karyotypes and male sex differentiation have been reported.[593, 598] All three were Y chromosome positive. Two of the three had two maternal X chromosomes, and the third had two paternal X chromosomes. These findings suggest that both anomalous Y-to-X exchange and maternal or paternal nondisjunction occurred in these patients.[597]

Approximately 20% of 46,XX males are *SRY* negative.[154, 597] These males have a much higher prevalence of genital ambiguity, such as micropenis, hypospadias, and undescended testes than those who are *SRY* positive.[154, 597, 599–601] SRY-negative (Y DNA-negative) 46,XX males have been reported in several familial cohorts associated with true hermaphroditism.[591, 599–604] These observations are consistent with the origin of a small proportion of 46,XX males as a consequence of a mutation in a downstream autosomal or X-linked gene (or genes) involved in the testis-determining cascade (see Fig. 22–19). They also suggest that 46,XX males and 46,XX true hermaphrodites may arise by similar pathogenetic mechanisms. In sum, the 46,XX male syndrome arises mainly as a result of a Y-to-X translocation; other possible mechanisms include mutation in an X chromosomal or autosomal gene and cryptic mosaicism that involves a Y-bearing cell line in at least the Sertoli cells.

Syndrome of Gonadal Dysgenesis: Turner's Syndrome and Its Variants

In 1938 Turner described seven phenotypic women with short stature, sexual infantilism, webbing of the neck, and cubitus valgus. Studies of this syndrome and its variants have made a major contribution to the evolution of current concepts of sex differentiation. (For reviews, see references 46 and 605 to 613.)

In the early 1940s Albright and colleagues and Varney and associates found that the excretion of urinary gonadotropin was increased in affected adolescents and adults. Wilkins and Fleischmann soon thereafter described the gonads as bilateral, pale "streaks" of connective tissue situated in the mesosalpinges and devoid of any germ cells. Wilkins proposed, in light of Jost's fetal castration experiments in the rabbit, that some of these functionally agonadal patients might be genetic males, because fetal castration of either sex invariably leads to a female phenotype. The discovery in 1954 that many of these patients, contrary to their phenotype, were X chromatin negative seemed initially to confirm that hypothesis,[280] but after techniques became available for analysis of the chromosome constitution Ford and co-workers[614] reported that the sex chromosome constitution in a 14-year-old phenotypic female with this syndrome was 45,X rather than 46,XY. Work in many laboratories thereafter defined more precisely the chromosomal basis of this and related disorders.

The absence of a second sex chromosome (X chromosome monosomy with haploinsufficiency) is associated with five cardinal features: female phenotype, short stature, sexual infantilism owing to rudimentary gonads, a variety of associated somatic abnormalities, and embryonic lethality. These features may be modified by the presence of lesser degrees of sex chromosome deficiency. It is therefore useful to consider the syndrome of gonadal dysgenesis and its variants as a continuum of features ranging from those of the typical 45,X phenotype to that of a normal female or male. The functional importance of chromosomal additions to the basic 45,X pattern can be deduced from the extent to which they modify toward normal, in at least some cases, the short stature, sexual infantilism, and somatic anomalies that typify the 45,X patient.

Partial sex chromosome monosomy (haploinsufficiency) may be attributed to a structurally abnormal second sex chromosome (X or Y), sex chromosome mosaicism involving a 45,X cell line, or both. Even though the modified clinical forms are almost invariably associated with partial sex chromosome monosomy, the contrary is not necessarily true; partial sex chromosome monosomies can cause the typical clinical picture found in 45,X patients.

Typical 45,X Gonadal Dysgenesis (Turner's Syndrome)[88, 154, 605–613]

In patients with the cardinal features of sex chromosome monosomy, the X chromatin pattern is negative in about 60%; most of these patients have a 45,X sex chromosome constitution (Table 22–9). Significant variability occurs in expression of the somatic anomalies associated with sex chromosome monosomy (Fig. 22–38).

Clinical Aspects. The typical patient (see Fig. 22–38) is often recognizable by the distinctive facies, in which micrognathia; epicanthal folds; prominent, low-set, rotated and/or deformed ears; a fish-like mouth with a narrow, high-arched palate; ptosis; and strabismus are present with varying degrees of frequency. The chest is usually square and shield-like with microthelia and inverted nipples. The areolae appear to be widely spaced. The neck is short and broad, and the hairline in back is low. Webbing of the neck is present in 25% to 40%, and

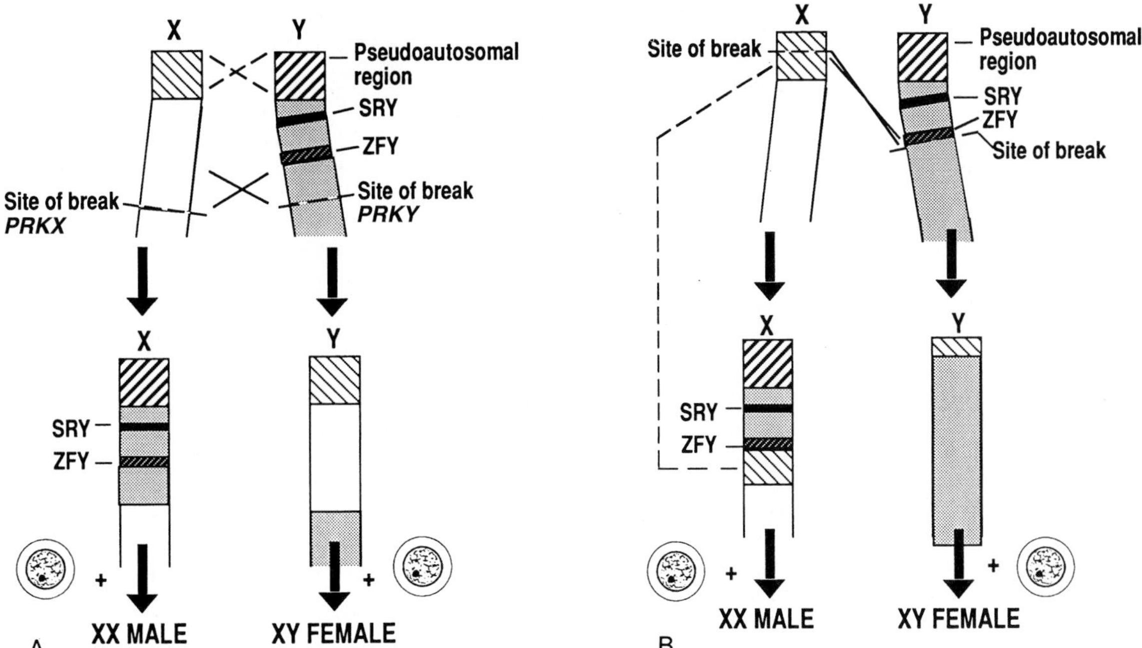

Figure 22–37. Diagram of the short arms of the X and Y chromosomes during meiotic pairing. *A*, A crossover *(dashed lines)* usually occurs between the pseudoautosomal regions of the X and Y chromosomes. Anomalous but equal crossovers *(solid lines)* can occur that result in an X chromosome with the sex-determining region (SRY) and a Y chromosome deficient in the SRY. It is estimated to occur at the *PRKX* and *PRKY* locus in 40% of *SRY*+XX males. Zygotes with these sex chromosomes will become XX males or XY females as indicated. *B*, Anomalous unequal crossovers *(solid lines)* during male meiosis can result in an X chromosome with an *SRY* gene as well as the pseudoautosomal regions of both the X and Y chromosomes. SRY, sex-determining region Y; ZFY, zinc finger Y.

coarctation of the aorta occurs in 10% to 20%. Those with coarctation usually also have webbing of the neck. Additional anomalies include congenital lymphedema of the feet and hands (30%) (Fig. 22–39) or puffiness of the dorsum of the fingers; short fourth metacarpals (50%); renal abnormalities (40%); high-arched palate; various skeletal anomalies, including cubitus valgus, Madelung's deformity of the wrist, genu valgum, and scoliosis[610]; increased number of pigmented nevi; tendency to keloid formation; abnormal nails; recurrent otitis media, which may result in conductive hearing loss (as well as progressive sensorineural loss of hearing); unexplained hypertension[614]; and, rarely, gastrointestinal bleeding secondary to intestinal telangiectasia, hemangiomatoses, or dilated veins.[610] Money and others have reported that impairments of directional sense and space-form recognition, visual-motor coordination, and motor learning are common; this perceptual disability results in a lower mean performance I.Q. than in the general population and is evidence of diffuse or multifocal cerebral dysfunction,[615, 616] whereas verbal ability (including comprehension and vocabulary) is normal. In general, patients with gonadal dysgenesis do not tend to differ from siblings in overall intelligence[617, 618]; however, mental retardation (I.Q. < 70) may be more common than the 1% to 3% incidence reported in the general population.[619–621] Gender identity and sexual attitudes are feminine. Girls with gonadal dysgenesis are generally more immature and distractable and have less self-esteem, poorer peer relations, and more difficulty at school than peers.[53, 621, 622] Skuse and associates described poorer adjustment and "social cognition" in 45,X^M (X^M, maternally derived X chromosome) than in 45,X^P (X^P, paternally derived X chromosome) individuals with Turner's syndrome. This difference was attributed to genomic imprinting, the silencing of some gene on the maternal X chromosome located in the pericentric region of the short arm or on the long arm of the X chromosome.[623, 624] This putative gene, which apparently escapes inactivation, is the first imprinted gene proposed for the human X chromosome. Further studies of parental origin of the X chromosome in Turner's syndrome are helping to elucidate behavioral phenotypes for a number of neurodevelopmental aspects.[623–626]

As adults, women with gonadal dysgenesis exhibit more conservative sexual attitudes and a more negative body image.[612, 613, 627] Lack of ovarian function (including infertility), rather than height, was the major concern of adult women with the syndrome of gonadal dysgenesis in one study.[628] Severe psychopathic manifestations are uncommon. In general, most women with gonadal dysgenesis are independent, self-sufficient, and sexually active.[619] One study of 63 women with Turner's syndrome reported normal psychological well-being but more difficulties in establishing social and partner relationships compared with the general population.[629]

Table 22–9. Clinical Features of 45,X Gonadal Dysgenesis (Turner's Syndrome)

Karyotype:	45,X
Inheritance:	Sporadic; meiotic or mitotic nondisjunction
Genitalia:	Female
Wolffian duct derivatives:	Absent
Müllerian duct derivatives:	Normal female
Gonads:	Streak
Habitus:	Short stature; sexual infantilism at puberty; somatic stigmata
Hormone profile:	Increased plasma LH and FSH concentrations; decreased plasma estradiol levels

LH, luteinizing hormone; FSH; follicle-stimulating hormone

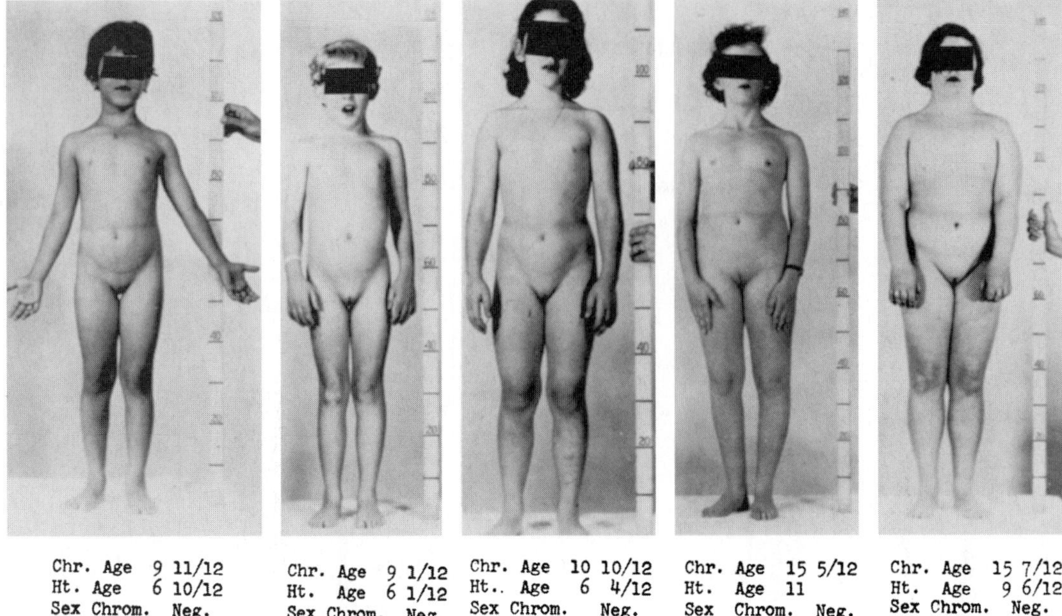

Figure 22–38. Variation in physical appearance in five patients with the typical form of the syndrome of gonadal dysgenesis. All of these patients had a 45,X karyotype, and all had differences between height age and chronologic age of 3 years or more. (Modified from Grumbach MM. Some considerations of the pathogenesis and classification of anomalies of sex in man. In Astwood EB [ed]. Clinical Endocrinology. New York, Grune & Stratton, 1960, pp 407–436.)

The risk of anorexia nervosa and inflammatory bowel disease may be increased.[611]

The eponym Bonnevie-Ullrich syndrome has been applied to phenotypic female infants with lymphedema of the distal extremities and loose folds of skin over the back of the neck in addition to the typical features of gonadal dysgenesis (Fig. 22–40). In the neonate, pleural effusions and ascites that clear spontaneously are not uncommon,[630] and pericardial effusion has been reported. The serous effusions and the lymphedema are attributable to hypoplasia and other defects of the lymphatic system.[631, 632] 45,X abortuses commonly exhibit generalized edema and a large hygroma of the neck.[633, 634] Postnatally, the latter abnormality results in webbing of the neck. These findings can be detected by prenatal ultrasonography.[633] Shephard and Fantel[632] suggested that the severe edema that occurs secondary to hypoalbuminemia and lymphatic duct hypoplasia in 45,X fetuses is responsible for many of the malformations involving the ears, hairline, neck, nipples, nails, and kidneys. The increased incidence of congenital heart disease associated with webbed neck, especially coarctation of the aorta (40%), has led to the suggestion that lymphatic obstruction is involved in the pathogenesis of both types of deformation.[635, 636]

The prevalence of cardiovascular abnormalities has varied from 20% to 50%. In a Danish study of 179 patients, 26% had cardiovascular malformations.[637] Coarctation of the aorta was the most common, occurring in 10% of patients, primarily those with a 45,X karyotype. The prevalence of bicuspid aortic valves in Turner syndrome determined by echocardiography has ranged from 9% to 34%.[610, 637, 638] Bicuspid aortic valves carry an increased risk for subacute bacterial endocarditis and tend to evolve with age into stenotic and/or insufficient aortic valves.[610, 637] An increased incidence of mitral valve prolapse has been reported in patients with gonadal dysgenesis.[610] Other studies have reported an increased incidence of partial anomalous venous drainage[638] and hypoplastic left heart syndrome.[639] On echocardiography, 8% to 29% of patients with the syndrome of gonadal dysgenesis have aortic root dilatation,[640, 641] and rupture from aortic dilatation has been reported in more than 20 patients.[641] Therefore, all patients with Turner's syndrome should have a thorough baseline cardiac evaluation, including an echocardiogram or magnetic resonance imaging study or both in infancy and again at adolescence.[642, 643] Patients with increased risk factors for dissection and rupture (e.g., those with coarctation, hypertension, and aortic root dilatation) require yearly follow-up and therapeutic measures to decrease the risk of dissection.[613] Pregnancy (after in vitro fertilization) carries an increased risk of fatal aortic dissection.[644] Patients with a bicuspid aortic valve should be given prophylactic antibiotic therapy before surgery or dental procedures, to prevent subacute bacterial endocarditis.

The most common renal abnormalities are rotation of the kidney, horseshoe kidney, duplication of the renal pelvis and ureter, and hydronephrosis secondary to ureteropelvic obstruction. Complete absence of the kidney and gross renal ectopia in 7 of 141 patients was reported by Lippe and associates.[645] Malformation of the kidneys and upper collecting system including an abnormal vascular supply are so common that intravenous urography, a renal sonogram or renography should be obtained routinely at the time of diagnosis.

Skeletal maturation is normal or slightly delayed in childhood and lags further in adolescence as a result of gonadal steroid deficiency. In most cases, the skeleton exhibits localized areas of rarefaction (fish-net appearance), especially of the hands, feet, elbows, and upper femurs.[646, 647] Prepubertal girls with gonadal dysgenesis have normal bone density for height and age but decreased density at the wrist for bone age and body mass index.[648] The risk of wrist fractures is increased.[648] Bechtold and colleagues, using quantitative computed tomography of the forearm and human growth hormone (hGH) in estrogen-treated adolescent and young adult patients, detected low total volumetric bone mineral density owing to decreased cortical thickness and suggested bone strength may be inadequate for the relatively high body weight.[649] Patients not treated with estrogen often develop a severe form of the postmenopausal type of osteoporosis and may develop fractures

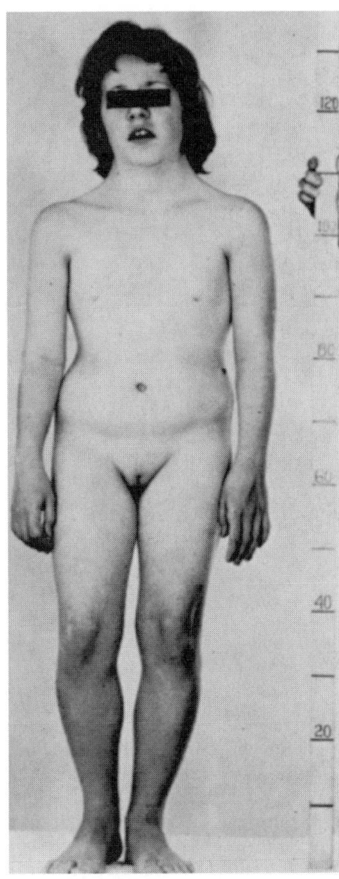

Figure 22–39. A patient aged 14 years, 10 months with the typical form of the syndrome of gonadal dysgenesis. The X chromatin pattern was negative and the karyotype was 45,X. She was short (height, 134.5 cm; height age, 9 years, 5 months), was sexually infantile except for the appearance of sparse pubic hair, and exhibited characteristic stigmata of the syndrome: a short webbed neck, shield-like chest with widely separated nipples, bilateral short fourth metacarpals, puffiness over dorsum of fingers, cubitus valgus, and an increased number of pigmented nevi. The facies were characteristic and the ears low set. The bone age was 13.5 years. Plasma gonadotropin levels were elevated. Vaginal smears and urocytogram showed an immature pattern in which cornified squamous cells were absent. With estrogen therapy, female secondary sexual characteristics were induced; cyclic estrogen administration resulted in periodic estrogen-withdrawal bleeding.

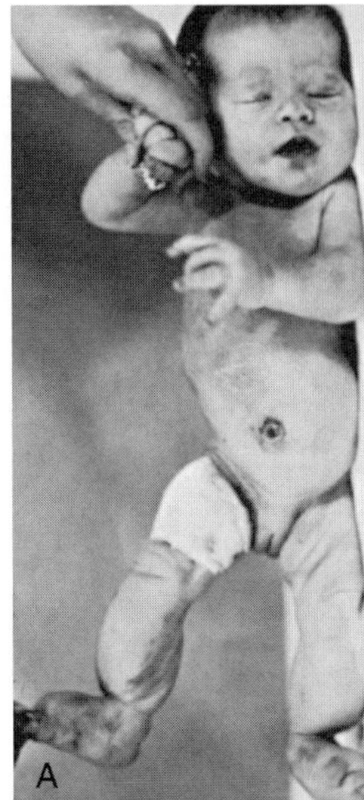

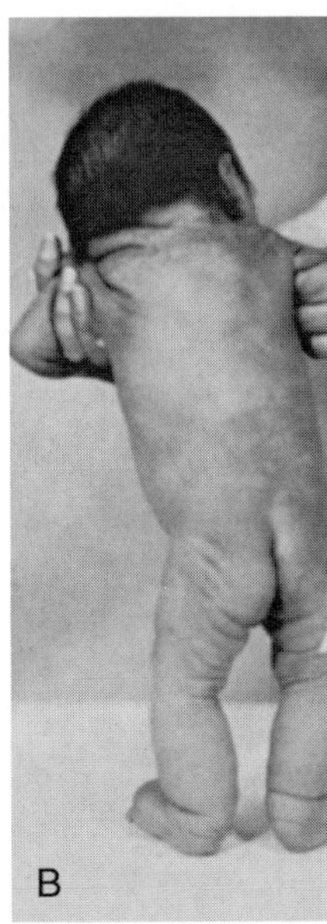

Figure 22–40. *A* and *B*, An infant with the syndrome of gonadal dysgenesis (karyotype 45,X) and associated lymphedema of extremities. The term *Bonnevie-Ullrich syndrome* is applied when this characteristic swelling of the feet or hands or both is associated with other features of gonadal dysgenesis. (From Grumbach MM. Chromosomal sex and the prepubertal diagnosis of gonadal dysgenesis. Reproduced by permission of Pediatrics 20:740. Copyright 1957.)

and vertebral collapse. Lanes and associates reported in young women with Turner's syndrome the failure to obtain normal peak bone mass despite estrogen replacement therapy begun in adolescence.[650] Osteochondrosis-like changes of the spine, vertebral hypoplasia, and scoliosis are common.[646, 647]

In addition to the metacarpal sign (shortening of the fourth metacarpal), Kosowicz described a carpal sign characterized by a more acute angular configuration of the proximal row of carpal bones. Madelung's or "bayonet" deformity of the wrist, a feature of the Leri-Weill syndrome caused by haploinsufficiency of the *SHOX* gene,[61] is present in about 10% of patients. Cubitus valgus (an increased carrying angle) occurs in half, is a consequence of a developmental abnormality of the trochlear head, and develops after birth. The knee may show deformities of the medial tibial and femoral condyles with obliquely tipped tibial epiphyses and medial projections of the tibial metaphyses that can result in genu valgum.[610] The pelvis tends to have a male-type inlet. Midface hypoplasia is common. The growth of the temporal bone, condylar cartilage, and spheno-occipital synchondrosis is abnormal.[610] Scoliosis is present in approximately 10% of patients, secondary either to hemivertebrae, leg-length inequality, or idiopathic causes, and requires monitoring.[610] Gonadotropic hyperplasia may cause enlargement of the sella turcica, especially in untreated adults with hypergonadotropic hypogonadism. An "empty sella" was noted on computed tomographic (CT) scan in two of our patients.

Short Stature. Short stature is an invariant feature in 45,X individuals and may be evident in utero. Intrauterine growth retardation is common, and the average birth weight (2.83 ± 0.57 kg) and length (48.2 ± 3.2 cm) are 1 standard deviation (SD) below the mean value for normal infants of comparable gestational age[651, 652]; the growth retardation is evident by the middle of the second trimester of gestation and affects all long bones.[653] The mean final height of patients in different series ranged from 142 to 147 cm.[651, 652, 654–656] In a survey of 12 European countries, a total of 661 patients were found, 51% of whom were 45,X and had a mean final height of 144.3 ± 6.7 cm; none had received estrogen therapy before the age of 14 years.[657] The ratio of sitting to standing height is frequently increased by late childhood and reflects the greater retardation in growth of the legs.[610, 658] Growth curves specific for Turner's syndrome are available, including growth curves for some nationalities (Fig. 22–41).[659]

Postnatal growth failure is evident from early infancy. By age 3 years, the mean deficit in height is −3.0 ± 1.5 SD.[660] By a bone age of 9 years the difference in mean height between patients and normal individuals (16 cm) is close to the difference at maturity (20 cm).[652] Hence, there is little additional loss of height relative to normal individuals after a bone age of 9 years despite the lack of a pubertal growth spurt[653] (see Fig. 22–41). This may be a result of prolongation of growth as a consequence of the effect of estrogen deficiency on bone maturation. Although final height in untreated patients may not be achieved until late in the second decade of life, there is no major gain in height after the age of 16 years.[657] Final height correlates with birth weight and target height.

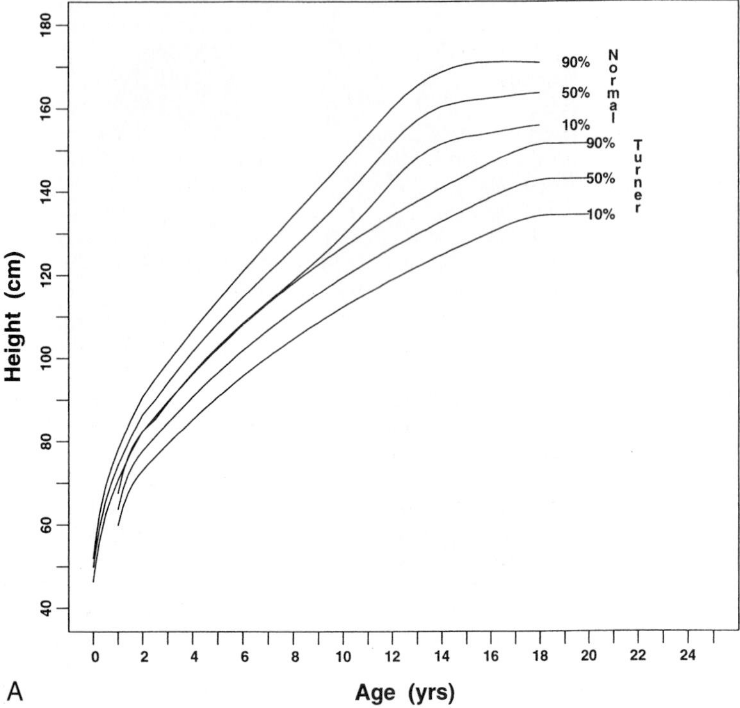

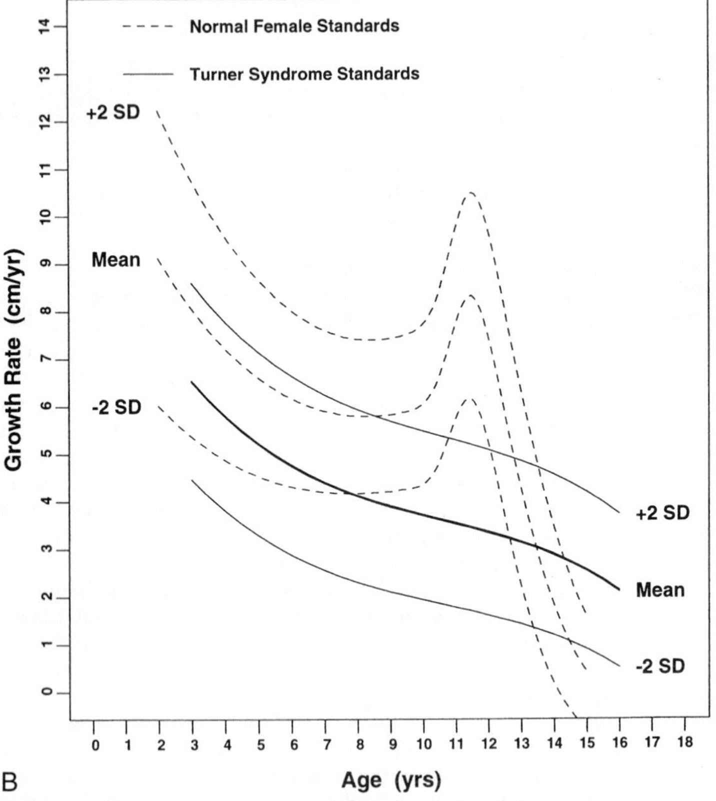

Figure 22–41. *A*, The mean height (50th percentile) in untreated patients with gonadal dysgenesis (mainly 45,X karyotype), compared with the growth curve of normal females. *B*, The mean height velocity in patients with gonadal dysgenesis and in normal females. Data derived from various sources. Note the lack of a pubertal growth spurt. (*B*, Courtesy of J. Frame and K. Attie, Genentech, Inc.)

The short stature is not attributable to a deficiency of growth hormone, insulin-like growth factor I (IGF-I, also called somatomedin-C), IGF-II,[661] or adrenal or gonadal steroids[662] (see Chapter 23). Decreased amplitude and frequency of growth hormone pulses have been reported after 8 years of age.[663] Likewise, IGF-I levels that are normal up to 10 years of age are low thereafter[661]; however, administration of either estrogen[661] or growth hormone induces a rise in the concentration of plasma IGF-I. The changes in growth hormone secretory dynamics and IGF-I concentrations after 8 to 10 years of age are probably secondary to the lack of the estrogen-induced rise in plasma growth hormone concentration and IGF-I levels at puberty. The cause of the progressive growth failure is attributable, at least in part, to the missing PAR1 gene, *PHOG* or *SHOX*, on the absent or structurally abnormal second sex chromosome.[662]

Sexual Infantilism. The genital tract and external genitalia in this syndrome are female in character but immature. Located in the mesosalpinges parallel to the fallopian tubes are long, attenuated, pale, fibrous streaks of connective tissue. Typically, these streak-like or spindle-shaped structures consist of fibrous stroma arranged in whorls similar to those in ovarian stroma, but they lack primordial follicles. Vestigial medullary elements and rudimentary mesonephric tubules like those found in the primitive genital ridge are common at the hilus. After puberty, aggregates of epithelioid cells resembling Leydig or hilus cells are present in variable quantity. Ultrasonography of the pelvis or MRI commonly detects the small uterus and streak gonads.

Singh and Carr[631] studied the gonadal ridges of eight spontaneously aborted embryos and fetuses ranging in gestational age from 5 weeks to 4 months. Primordial germ cells were observed in all eight specimens. Until the third month of gestation, no appreciable differences were noted between these gonads and those from 46,XX fetuses; after that, connective tissue stroma increased and formation of follicles was impaired, suggesting that primordial germ cells seed the 45,X gonad, that many degenerate during oocyte formation and folliculogenesis, and that surviving oocytes undergo accelerated apoptosis.[663] Jirasek[664] reported that oocytes in patients with a 45,X karyotype degenerate shortly after formation of the primary follicle, possibly because the surrounding follicular cell layer is incomplete. Two active X chromosomes appear to be required for the normal development of human oogonia and oocytes. Follicles are common in the gonadal streaks of 45,X infants at birth but are uncommon by late childhood and adolescence. Nevertheless, spontaneous puberty, menses, and fertility can occur in putative 45,X patients.

Longitudinal studies of both basal and LHRH-evoked gonadotropin secretion demonstrate a lack of feedback inhibition of the hypothalamic-pituitary axis by the dysgenetic gonads in infants and young children with gonadal dysgenesis.[665, 666] In 58 patients aged 2 days to 20 years, plasma FSH levels were elevated in those aged 2 days to 4 years and decreased to high normal values between 5 and 10 years of age (Fig. 22–42). After 10 years, the plasma FSH level rose again into the castrate range.[665] Therefore, the pattern of plasma FSH concentration followed a diphasic curve similar to but higher than that in normal infants and children. The pattern of change in LH levels was comparable, but the concentrations were one third to one tenth those of FSH. LHRH-induced LH and FSH responses exhibited a diphasic pattern with age, similar to those of basal levels.[666] In patients younger than 5 years of age, both the mean basal levels and the rise in gonadotropin levels induced by administration of LHRH were increased. Between ages 5 and 10 years, basal levels of FSH and LH and LHRH-evoked responses were less than those of younger patients with gonadal dysgenesis (see Fig. 22–42). In some patients between ages 6 and 10 years, both FSH and LH concentrations and the LHRH-induced gonadotropin responses were comparable to those in normal children. After age 11 years a striking rise in basal and readily releasable LH and FSH levels was observed. Therefore, between the ages of 5 and 10 years, basal and LHRH-elicited gonadotropin responses may not reflect the functional status of the gonads in all patients with gonadal dysgenesis.

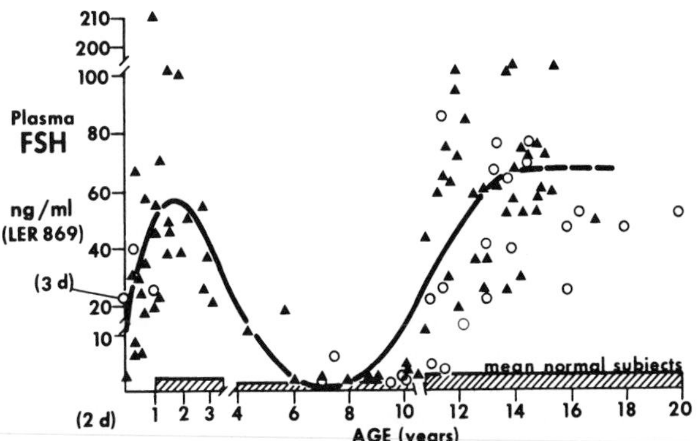

Figure 22–42. The pattern of plasma follicle-stimulating hormone (FSH) concentration in relation to age in 58 patients with the syndrome of gonadal dysgenesis. ▲, patients with 45,X karyotype; ○, patients with structural abnormalities of the X chromosome and mosaics. The *hatched* area shows the mean to the lower limits of the assay for FSH values in normal females. (From Conte FA, Grumbach MM, Kaplan SL. A diphasic pattern of gonadotropin secretion in patients with the syndrome of gonadal dysgenesis. J Clin Endocrinol Metab 40: 670–674, 1975. © The Endocrine Society.)

Although streak gonads are the rule in 45,X gonadal dysgenesis, exceptions have been documented. Primary follicles have been described in the gonadal ridges of some 45,X individuals at adolescence, and this correlates with the rare occurrence of menarche and a variable but attenuated period of regular menses. On ultrasonography, 30% of a series of 32 45,X females had nonstreak gonads.[667] In this study, 3 of the 32 patients had breast development but had not menstruated.[667] This number correlates with previous data suggesting that 5% to 10% of patients with gonadal dysgenesis have a sufficient number of ovarian follicles (>10^4) at adolescence to initiate breast development.[668] Conceptions have been documented despite extensive karyotypic studies revealing only a 45,X cell line in multiple tissues.[669–671] In a large study of Turner's syndrome patients older than 12 years, including, in addition to 45,X patients, those with X chromosome mosaicism and structural abnormalities, spontaneous pubertal development occurred in 16%, including menarche at a mean age of 13 years.[672] Regular menses occurred 9 years post menarche in just over one third of this group. The presence of a second X chromosome was much more evident in those with spontaneous puberty. The figure for spontaneous pregnancy appears to be 3% to 5%.[672, 673] In addition to variability in the rate of follicular atresia, another possible explanation for the presence of oogonia in 45,X individuals is that a certain number of 45,X germ cells may undergo mitotic nondisjunction with the formation of 46,XX oogonia.[674] This process normally occurs in the female creeping vole and serves as a sex-determining mechanism in this species. Alternatively, some fertile 45,X patients may be unrecognized sex chromosome mosaics. Women with a 45,X cell line have increased fetal wastage and an increased number of chromosomally abnormal liveborn infants, including those with gonadal dysgenesis or Down's syndrome.[671, 675–677]

Adrenarche in patients with gonadal dysgenesis is associated with a normal rise in adrenal androgen production in childhood but sparse pubic and axillary hair. Before the age of 10 years, the plasma concentration of adrenal androgens is normal,[678] but levels of dehydroepiandrosterone (DHEA), testosterone, and androstenedione are lower than normal after age 15, reflecting absence of the gonadal contribution.[679] Adrenarche occurs independently of gonadarche.[678]

Rarely, enlargement of the clitoris may be present at birth or develop at puberty. Secretion of androgens by "Leydig cells" in the gonadal streak is a possible cause, as is the presence of a cryptic Y cell line.

Males with a 45,X karyotype have a Y to X chromosome or a Y-autosome translocation involving variable segments of the euchromatic (sex-determining) region of the Y chromosome.[680–685] Translocations have been reported involving the short arm of chromosomes 5, 14, 15, and 18 and the X chromosome.[680–685] Most patients have had either minor or major anomalies not usually associated with the syndrome of gonadal dysgenesis, such as the cri-du-chat syndrome. These additional anomalies are no doubt related to the autosome involved in the translocation and to the degree of deletion involved.

Incidence in Abortuses, Newborns, and Twins. The incidence of gonadal dysgenesis is approximately 1 per 2000 live female births,[686, 687] and approximately 50% of the patients have a 45,X karyotype. There is, in addition, a considerable loss of 45,X embryos and fetuses.[688] About 7% of spontaneous abortuses have a 45,X constitution.[688] It is estimated that the frequency of 45,X zygotes is 2%, probably the most common chromosome anomaly in humans but fewer than 1% of 45,X conceptuses survive to term.[689] Hook and Warburton[690] have analyzed chromosome karyotypes in embryonic and fetal deaths and demonstrated a significant disparity between the 45,X karyotype and those with mosaicism and/or an isochromosome for the long arm of the X chromosome (Xqi). They postulated a "fetoprotective" effect of more than one dose of some locus or loci on the long arm of the X chromosome.[690]

Associated Disorders.[613, 691] Turner's syndrome carries a threefold increase in mortality and a reduction in life expectancy of 6 to 13 years; it is less in 45,X patients than in non-45,X Turner syndrome.[692]

The incidence of autoimmune disorders is increased; the most prevalent is autoimmune thyroiditis and Graves' disease, which occurs in 15% to 30%.[613] The prevalence of thyroid antibodies and hypothyroidism (or hyperthyroidism) increases during childhood and adolescence[693, 694] and in adulthood may approach 50% of patients (a 10-fold relative risk).[691] Early diagnosis may be facilitated by monitoring levels of thyroid antibody and basal thyroid-stimulating hormone with the use of sensitive assays. Basal and thyrotropin-releasing hormone–induced concentrations of prolactin may be elevated in euthyroid patients with gonadal dysgenesis. Prevalences of rheumatoid and psoriatic arthritis and inflammatory bowel disease are increased in patients with a 45,X karyotype.[613, 695]

Carbohydrate intolerance with mild insulin resistance is common, especially after age 16 years and may become worse with obesity or during treatment with growth hormone or oxandrolone.[696, 697] The risk of type 2 diabetes mellitus is increased fourfold and that of type 1, onefold.[691] Mean cholesterol levels may be elevated after 11 years of age, independent of age and body mass index.[698]

The prevalence of chronic liver disease is increased; Gravhold and co-workers[691] report a relative risk of 5.7 for cirrhosis; 44% of women had an elevated concentration of serum liver enzymes.[613] The risk of developing Crohn's disease and ulcerative colitis is increased and the inflammatory bowel disease is often severe.[613]

As discussed earlier, congenital renal anomalies are common (about ninefold greater than the general population) and the risk of the obstructive uropathy and pyelonephritis is greatly increased. In addition, vascular malformations involving the kidney are more prevalent.

During childhood, problematic otitis media is common and may result in conductive hearing loss.[699] Abnormalities in the growth of the temporal bone, condylar cartilage, and spheno-occipital synchondrosis result in an abnormality in the positioning of the external auditory meatus and the relation of the middle ear to the eustachian tube in patients with the syndrome of gonadal dysgenesis.[699] These changes, along with abnormalities in the shape of the palate, are thought to be responsible for the increased incidence of otitis media. Sensorineural deafness is present in about two thirds of adult patients.[700] The frequent episodes of otitis media and the sensorineural hearing loss are independent variables in gonadal dysgenesis; the sensorineural hearing loss may be related to loss of genes on the X chromosome responsible for the gonadal dysgenesis phenotype.[701]

In a Danish study, Turner's syndrome women had a fivefold increased risk of developing cancer of the colon and rectum.[691] As noted previously, the prevalence of anorexia nervosa is increased; its onset usually coincides with the initiation of estrogen treatment.

Origin of 45,X Constitution and Phenotype. A 45,X chromosome constitution (see Figs. 22–1*A* and 22–4) may be a consequence of nondisjunction[42] or chromosome loss during gametogenesis in either parent that results in a sperm or ovum lacking a sex chromosome. Although errors of mitosis in a normal zygote often lead to mosaicism, a purely 45,X constitution may arise at the first cleavage division from anaphase lag with loss of a sex chromosome or, less likely, from mitotic nondisjunction with failure of the complementary 47,XXX or 47,XYY cell line to survive (see Fig. 22–4). Loss of one X or Y chromosome between fertilization and the first cleavage division may be a frequent but not the only cause of a 45,X embryo.[42]

Several lines of evidence support the hypothesis of a mitotic error (as well as meiotic errors) in this syndrome: (1) the lack of association with advanced maternal age, in contrast to XXY Klinefelter's syndrome (indeed the incidence of 45,X conceptuses is increased in teenage pregnancies)[702, 703]; (2) the prevalence of sex chromosome mosaicism; (3) the increased frequency of twinning in sibships with a 45,X individual[704]; and (4) the occurrence of a 46,XY monozygotic cotwin of a 45,X individual.[705]

Family studies of X-linked traits (e.g., color blindness, Xg blood group) indicate that loss of the paternally derived X chromosome is more common than would be expected with random loss of either the maternally or the paternally derived X chromosome; in informative pedigrees, 77% of 45,X individuals have loss of the paternal sex chromosome (45,X^M), and 23% have loss of the maternal X chromosome (45,X^P). Similar findings have been obtained with the use of molecular cytogenetic analysis.[706, 707]

The deviation in parental origin of the retained X chromosome[713] raised the possibility that retention of the maternal X chromosome might play a role in survival in addition to affecting the phenotype through "imprinting."[708] However, the percentage of aborted fetuses with a 45,X^M karyotype is the same as in liveborn infants.[709, 710] Therefore, imprinting does not appear to affect fetal survival in 45,X individuals. Although some studies showed no effect of imprinting on phenotype,[711] 45,X^M patients appear to have an increased prevalence of cardiovascular anomalies and webbed neck; furthermore, the height in 45,X^M correlates more strongly with maternal height than with midparental height.[712] A putative imprinted gene on the maternal X chromosome,[623] which affects social cognition, is discussed earlier in the section on clinical aspects.

The very high embryonic and fetal mortality of 45,X conceptuses, as opposed to those with 45,X/46,XX or 45,X/46,XY mosaicism or a structurally abnormal X chromosome, raised the possibility that all liveborn individuals with the gonadal dysgenesis syndrome are mosaics.[714] This hypothesis has not been supported by cytogenetic data[715] or by molecular analysis with X chromosome probes.[716, 717] However, the possibility of prenatal mosaicism and nonrandom loss of structurally abnormal sex chromosomes postnatally has not been ruled out. Molecular analysis with the use of Y-specific probes has been inconclusive.[47] From 0% to 33% of patients with gonadal dysgenesis whose karyotype is other than 45,X/46,XY have a low percentage of Y chromosome material.[47, 718] Chu and colleagues[47] studied 87 patients with the use of multiple Y chromosome probes and found 3.4% to be positive for low-percentage mosaicism for all or part of the Y chromosome. The similar results obtained by Binder and colleagues[719] indicate a low level of Y chromosome mosaicism in 45,X and chromatin-positive individuals with gonadal dysgenesis. The significance of low-percentage mosaicism for Y chromosome material and its relation to gonadal differentiation and the risk of malignancy are still to be determined. Cryptic Y chromosome identification by sensitive PCR techniques may, however, not show concordance between clinical signs of hyperandrogenism and molecular studies on gonad material. In such Y-negative gonads there is hilus cell hyperplasia. The routine screening of all Turner's syndrome patients for the presence of *SRY* is not recommended.

The classic gonadal dysgenesis phenotype is usually associated with absence of all or a proximal portion of the short arm of the X or Y chromosome. The haploinsufficiency of genes in these loci that are not inactivated is postulated to cause the phenotype. Page and co-workers suggested that the genes that encode ribosome protein S4X *(RPS4X)*, and its homologue on the Y chromosome *(RPS4Y)*, are candidate genes.[124] However, the location of this gene on the long arm of the X chromosome and the fact that it is expressed in patients with 46,XXp− and 46X,Xqi karyotypes make it an unlikely candidate.[720] Zinn and associates using both cytogenetic and molecular analyses found evidence of a critical region, Xp11.2-p22.1, that included loci for short stature (in addition to the more distal *SHOX* gene), gonadal failure, high arched palate, and thyroid autoimmunity.[721]

Ogata and Matsuo[54] postulated that the gonadal dysgenesis phenotype is multifactorial in origin. According to their construct, the phenotype is related to (1) quantitative loss or alteration of euchromatic or noninactivated genes (haploinsufficiency), leading to global nonspecific developmental defects; (2) haploinsufficiency of pseudoautosomal and/or Y-specific growth genes and lymphogenic genes, resulting in short stature and the "deformative" stigmata; and (3) oocyte loss and gonadal dysgenesis from impaired or failed chromosome pairing during meiotic prophase.[54, 722]

The underlying cause of this sex chromosome abnormality is not known. An increased frequency of thyroid autoimmunity in patients with the syndrome of gonadal dysgenesis and in their parents suggests that the genetic predisposition to develop autoantibodies in one or both parents is associated with an increased prevalence of the 45,X constitution and other chromosome abnormalities in the offspring. Infants with the syndrome of gonadal dysgenesis have been born after artificial insemination and in vitro fertilization.[723] Familial occurrence of 45,X gonadal dysgenesis is rare.

Diagnosis and Treatment.[613] Phenotypic females with the following features should have a karyotype analysis: (1) short stature (>2.5 SD below the mean height value for age), (2) somatic stigmata associated with gonadal dysgenesis, and (3) delayed adolescence with increased plasma or urinary gonadotropin levels. Although determination of the X chromatin pattern (Barr body) is a rapid method of screening, karyotype analysis is the definitive procedure. The concentration of plasma FSH and inhibins is useful in assessing the functional status of the gonads.

Even though many severely affected 45,X individuals with prominent dysmorphic features (lymphedema, loose folds of skin over the back of the neck) or coarctation of the aorta are recognized at birth or early infancy, the diagnosis in the less severely affected may be delayed until childhood when short stature is evident or until the age of puberty when secondary sex characteristics fail to appear. It is important to obtain a karyotype on all girls with unexplained short stature especially those with even subtle dysmorphic features of the syndrome of gonadal dysgenesis. Savendahl and Davenport found that (excluding those in whom the diagnosis was made in infancy) overall delay in diagnosis was 7.7 years.[724] Early diagnosis is important for more optimal long-term management, treatment, and counseling, including, if appropriate and with informed parental consent, the use of recombinant hGH treatment before the child falls below −2.0 SD in height, to achieve better growth in childhood and potentially normal adult stature.

Table 22–10. Suggested Follow-up of Adults with Syndrome of Gonadal Dysgenesis (Turner's Syndrome)

Baseline	Annual	3–5 Yearly
Karyotype	Physical examination (e.g., BMI, blood pressure, CVS)	Echocardiography Bone densitometry
Renal and pelvic ultrasound	Thyroid function	Audiogram
Echocardiography	Fasting lipids	
Thyroid autoantibodies	Fasting blood glucose	
Gonadotropins	Liver function	
	Renal function	

BMI, Body mass index; CVS, cardiovascular system.
From Elsheikh M, Dunger DB, Conway GS, Wass JA. Turner's syndrome in adulthood. Endocr Rev 2002; 23:120–140.

The following studies should be done in women when the diagnosis of the syndrome of gonadal dysgenesis is made: an intravenous pyelogram or ultrasonographic examination to exclude a renal anomaly; an echocardiogram or MRI study to assess cardiovascular function; periodic hearing examination and evaluation of thyroid function and thyroid antibodies; regular measurements of plasma glucose levels after adolescence; and monitoring for scoliosis and bone density in late adolescence and adulthood for evidence of osteopenia.[725] Guidelines for the diagnosis and management for Turner's syndrome in childhood and adulthood have been updated following an international consensus workshop[726] and reviewed by Elsheikh and co-workers.[613] There is particular emphasis on long-term monitoring for cardiovascular disease (including hypertension, aortic dilatation and the risk of aortic dissection),[613, 727] regular screening for thyroid dysfunction, recognition of hearing impairment which worsens in adult life and early planning for any request for assisted conception. Table 22–10 presents the suggested follow-up of adults with Turner's syndrome.[613]

Therapy is directed toward augmenting stature, correcting somatic anomalies, inducing secondary sexual characteristics and menses, and counseling. As noted, the short stature in gonadal dysgenesis is not related to a deficiency of growth hormone, insulin-like growth factors, thyroid hormone, or adrenal or gonadal steroids. However, administration of pharmacologic doses of biosynthetic hGH increases growth rate and augments final height by a mean of 5 to 10 cm.[659, 728–731] The heterogeneity in response appears to be related to the chronologic age at the start of therapy, the duration of therapy, the dose and frequency of growth hormone administration, the use of oxandrolone and/or estrogen, the growth standards used, the height of the parents, and the growth hormone peak elicited by pharmacologic stimuli.[659, 728–734] Rosenfeld and co-workers have the longest and most extensive study.[728, 735] Starting in 1983, 70 patients between the ages of 4.7 and 12.4 years with normal growth hormone responses to provocative stimuli were studied.[728] They were randomly assigned to (1) a control group for 1 year; (2) the anabolic steroid oxandrolone at a dose of 0.125 mg/kg by mouth daily; (3) growth hormone 0.125 mg/kg subcutaneously three times per week; or (4) a combination of oxandrolone and growth hormone. After 12 to

24 months, all groups except the growth hormone alone group were placed on combination therapy; however, the oxandrolone dose was lowered to 0.0625 mg/kg because of signs of virilization. After 3 years, most patients received daily growth hormone rather than thrice weekly; however, the dose of 0.375 mg/kg per week was unchanged. The mean height in patients who completed therapy was 151.7 cm, for a net mean gain of 9 cm over projected height and historical controls. Long-term studies now indicate that when growth hormone treatment alone is started early enough, most girls will benefit and some will achieve normal final height.[735–738] Attaining a final height of 150 cm is now a realistic target.[738] It is important to individualize the dose of growth hormone depending on the patient's growth response to the usual dose (0.375 mg/kg per week in six or seven divided doses). Growth hormone treatment should be considered when the patient's height falls below −2.0 SD on the growth curve for normal girls.

Growth hormone therapy is approved by the U.S. Food and Drug Administration for the treatment of patients with Turner's syndrome, and it was approved earlier in Japan and many Western European countries. It is prudent to discuss growth hormone therapy with the parents and patients, including its efficacy and side effects, in all patients with gonadal dysgenesis whose height is more than 2.0 SD below the mean value for age, especially those whose growth rate is less than 5 cm/yr. Studies are in progress to evaluate the effects of initiating growth hormone therapy at 5 to 6 years of age before the growth deficit is severe. Growth hormone therapy is usually continued until the growth rate falls to less than 2 cm/yr or the bone age exceeds 15 years. Supraphysiologic doses of growth hormone induced insulin resistance but not hyperglycemia; the increased insulin values returned to the normal range when growth hormone treatment was discontinued.[739]

Estrogen therapy has commonly been deferred until age 15 or later on the assumption that treatment at an earlier age leads to rapid skeletal maturation and diminished height. This premise was based largely on the fact that pharmacologic doses of estrogens can accelerate bone maturation and lead to premature epiphyseal fusion without a proportionate increase in height. Studies in patients with aromatase deficiency and in a patient with a mutation in the estrogen receptor indicate that estrogen rather than androgen is the principal gonadal hormone involved in bone maturation and fusion and bone mineral accretion.[358, 740, 741] We examined the effect of early low dose, conjugated estrogen therapy on linear growth, bone age, and the development of secondary sexual characteristics in a group of patients with gonadal dysgenesis.[654] Low-dose conjugated estrogens (9 μg/kg body weight per day) or ethinyl estradiol (141 ng/kg body weight per day) was given to 21 patients with the syndrome of gonadal dysgenesis who had a mean age of 13 years and mean bone age of 10.7 years. Growth rate was transiently accelerated but declined to below the pretherapy rate after 12 months of therapy. The final height of the patients treated with low-dose estrogen was not different from that of control nontreated patients or that of a group of six girls with Turner's syndrome in whom normal ovarian function was present and spontaneous puberty ensued. Hence, no increase or decrease in mean final height was noted in our study. However, girls who received estrogen with a bone age of less than 11 years were shorter than the girls who began low-dose estrogen therapy after a bone age of 11 years.[654] Similar results have been obtained subsequently in other studies.[743, 744] Initially it is important to use the lowest dose of an estrogen preparation (including an estradiol patch)[745] that gradually will induce pubertal development.

Serious psychological effects are frequently associated with a prolonged delay in the treatment of sexual infantilism.[746] The institution of low-dose, conjugated estrogen, synthetic estrogen therapy or transdermal estradiol patch[745] alone at approximately 13 years of age (bone age >11 years) elicits a brief growth spurt without inordinate advancement of skeletal maturation or reduction in final height and induces the development of secondary sexual characteristics at an age comparable to that of normal peers, thereby obviating the undesirable psychological consequences and deficient bone mineralization of a prolonged delay in sexual maturation. Studies in which growth hormone treatment was combined with early estrogen therapy (i.e., in patients younger than 12 years of age) indicate a shorter final height than in patients who received growth hormone treatment and "late" estrogen substitution therapy.[747] The number of years of growth hormone therapy before estrogen therapy is a critical factor in predicting height gained, and hence the time of initiation of estrogen therapy in the growth hormone–treated patient has an important influence on final height.[747] Earlier introduction of growth hormone therapy or the use of higher doses of growth hormone or both to induce normal or near-normal height for age[738, 748] permits the initiation of estrogen therapy by about 13 years of age, an important psychologic consideration. Therefore, in the treatment of girls with Turner's syndrome, the goal of increased adult stature must be balanced against the desire for sexual maturation in each individual patient.

Estrogen replacement therapy may improve certain neuropsychologic deficits (nonverbal processing speed, motor function, and memory).[749, 750] However, the neurocognitive deficits in adult women with Turner's syndrome were not altered significantly by estrogen replacement.[751]

A number of instances of endometrial carcinoma have been reported in patients with gonadal dysgenesis.[752] The evidence suggests that estrogens, especially when unopposed by progesterone, can produce a progression of histologic changes from endometrial hyperplasia to invasive carcinoma (see also Chapter 16). To clarify the relation between estrogen therapy and endometrial pathology in gonadal dysgenesis, Rosenwaks and colleagues[753a] studied 41 patients receiving estrogen replacement therapy. Increased risk of abnormal endometrial histology correlated with (1) a lifetime dosage of conjugated estrogens of more than 2500 mg, (2) more than 7 years of estrogen therapy, and (3) a daily dose of conjugated estrogens greater than 1.25 mg. Progestagens can modify the effect of estrogens on endometrial histology. It is therefore prudent to treat patients with gonadal dysgenesis with low-dose cyclic estrogen replacement therapy, with progestagen added at the end of each cycle. Further studies are necessary to assess the optimal dose of estrogen that reduces the risk of endometrial carcinoma while concurrently preventing osteoporosis.

Rarely, patients with a 45,X karyotype and no cytogenetic evidence of Y chromosome material develop gonadoblastomas.[754] However, a study employing multiple Y-specific DNA probes indicates that 3.4% of apparent 45,X patients have Y chromosomal material present.[47] These 45,X patients may be at risk for gonadoblastoma formation. Most patients with a 45,X karyotype have little or no risk of neoplastic transformation of the streak gonads.

Replacement Therapy. We routinely initiate therapy (depending on the height) at about 13 years of age with 0.3 mg of conjugated estrogen or 5 μg of ethinyl estradiol by mouth or very low dose transdermal 17β-estradiol.[745] The oral dose is gradually increased over the next 2 to 3 years to 0.6 to 1.25 mg of conjugated estrogens or 10 μg of ethinyl estradiol daily for the first 21 days of the month. The patient is maintained on the minimal dose of estrogen needed to maintain secondary sexual characteristics, permit withdrawal bleeding, and prevent osteopenia. Medroxyprogesterone acetate, 5 to 10 mg/day, is given from the 10th through the 21st day of the month to ensure more physiologic menses and to reduce the risks of endometrial and breast cancer. There is only limited clinical experience on the use of transdermal estradiol patch in adolescent girls, but with this approach (while more expensive) the natural estradiol reaches the systemic circulation directly without first undergoing metabolism by the intestine and liver.[745] The common late adolescent and adult oral dose of estrogen replacement therapy often fails to increase to normal the size of the uterus (especially an adult fundal-cervical ratio as assessed by pelvic ultrasonography).[746] The attainment of a mature heart-shaped uterine configuration is important only if the patient elects to become pregnant by oocyte donation and in vitro fertilization.[747]

An important part of the management is the education of the patient and family.[748] A frank discussion with the parents of the pathophysiology of the condition is appropriate when the diagnosis is made and reinforced at later sessions. Thereafter, the child should be given as much information about her condition as she can comprehend to allay any false fears or anxieties. An honest assessment of reproductive function based on clinical findings as well as hormone levels should be given to the patient when appropriate. Advances in in vitro fertilization and embryo transplantation make pregnancy possible for these patients, but the miscarriage rate is high[749] and the risk of aortic rupture is increased during pregnancy. The importance of medical and psychosocial management throughout life in patients with the syndrome of gonadal dysgenesis must be emphasized. Social and psychosocial support from the parents and the physician usually results in a well-adjusted woman.

Partial Sex Chromosome Monosomy and Clinical Variants of the Syndrome of Gonadal Dysgenesis

Partial sex chromosome monosomy may or may not modify the expression of the classic 45,X phenotype.[46, 749a] Forty to 50 percent of patients with the typical syndrome of gonadal dysgenesis are X chromatin positive. This group usually has a structurally abnormal X chromosome or sex chromosome mosaicism involving a 45,X cell line. Chromatin-positive and chromatin-negative variants of gonadal dysgenesis are discussed here in relation to the more usual types of sex chromosome aberrations with which they may be associated. The diagram in Figure 22–43 shows the variable effect of partial sex chromosome monosomy (haploinsufficiency) on the typical features of the syndrome.

In patients with sex chromosome mosaicism, the ratio in each gonad of 45,X primordial germ cells and blastemal components to those with a normal 46,XX or 46,XY constitution is probably the major determinant of whether the ultimate gonadal structure is a streak, a dysgenetic or hypoplastic ovary or testis, or a relatively normal gonad.[46, 88, 154, 749] The weight of evidence supports the idea that, after migration into the primitive gonad, primordial germ cells that bear a 45,X constitution degenerate more rapidly, quite likely by apoptosis, than do 46,XX cells, resulting in a streak, hypoplastic, or normal ovary.[79] Similarly, if the gonadal blastemal components, in particular the Sertoli cells, do not contain an appropriate number of 46,XY cells, testicular development does not take place[750] (Fig. 22–44).

The quantitative relation between 45,X cells and those with a 46,XX or 46,XY pattern in peripheral tissues may also be responsible for the variable effect of mosaicism on stature and associated somatic stigmata.[46]

In patients with a single cell line (euploid) containing a structurally abnormal sex chromosome, the somatic and gonadal consequences appear to be related to the nature and degree of the short or long arm deficiency of the second X or Y chromosome. Table 22–11 summarizes the correlation between structural abnormalities of the X and Y chromosomes and the clinical manifestations. The use of deletion mapping of the human sex chromosomes to clarify the relation of phenotype to karyotype has limitations. Structural abnormalities are often associated with mosaicism because of loss of the structurally abnormal sex chromosome from the stem cell line. Furthermore, structural rearrangements of chromosomes are complex. However, the advent of chromosome banding and molecular genetic techniques has facilitated the analysis of structurally abnormal sex chromosomes. At present, the data suggest that (1) ovarian determinants are located on both the long and short arms of the X chromosome and that patients with short arm deletions proximal to band Xp21 or long arm deletions proximal to band Xq25 usually have streak gonads and sexual infantilism[79, 95, 154, 749, 750]; and (2) the short arm of the X chromosome (and to a lesser extent the long arm) contains loci that, if deleted, result in short stature and the somatic stigmata of the syndrome of gonadal dysgenesis (see section on biologic functions of the X chromosome and Y chromosome).[79, 95, 154, 749, 750]

X Chromatin–Positive Variants of Gonadal Dysgenesis

45,X/46,XX, 45,X/47,XXX, and 45,X/46,XX/47,XXX Mosaicism. 45,X/46,XX mosaicism is the most common finding in patients with chromatin-positive gonadal dysgenesis and is second in frequency only to 45,X; the mosaic karyotype arises through loss of one X chromosome in a 46,XX conceptus.[46, 754a] Patients with this form of mosaicism usually exhibit fewer of the associated somatic anomalies, are not invariably short, may menstruate, and may even be fertile. One gonad may be of the streak type, and the contralateral gonad may be either a hypoplastic or a normal ovary; alternatively, both ovaries may be either normal or hypoplastic. During a family survey for a leukocyte anomaly, a normal grandmother with 45,X/46,XX/47,XXX mosaicism was discovered fortuitously. Some appreciation of the variable clinical features may be gleaned from nine patients with these forms of mosaicism studied by Morishima and Grumbach.[46] All had normal female external genitalia. Of seven who attained pubertal age, four developed some female secondary sexual characteristics, and two menstruated regularly. One of the two has had three pregnancies. In some, no important somatic abnormalities were detected, and two were of normal stature. One of the 45,X/46,XX patients had a webbed neck, coarctation of the aorta, and other gonadal dysgenesis stigmata but was of normal stature and menstruated regularly. A 12-year-old 45,X/46,XX/47,XXX patient had primary hypothyroidism and autoimmune thyroiditis.

46,XXqi and 45,X/46,XXqi. Patients with the Xqi structural abnormality (isochromosome for the long arm of the X) have an X chromosome that consists primarily of two long arms (Xq) and lacks a short arm (Xp); it arises mainly as a consequence of a break in sequence in the proximal short arm and not by centromere misdivision[48] (Fig. 22–45) and occurs in about 15% of Turner's syndrome individuals (about 1 in 13,000 female live births). The Xqi chromosomes may be either monocentric or dicentric X.[754a, 754b] In a review of 89 cases, 29 were monocentric. Of these, only 5 of 17 were associated with mosaicism for a 45,X cell line.[753] In contrast, 49 of 60 patients with a dicentric isochromosome had a 45,X cell line. Dicentric X isochromosomes are more unstable than monocentric forms and probably result more frequently in sex chromosome mosaicism through loss of the heteromorphic dicentric X chromosome. In 14 patients studied with molecular biologic techniques, Xp markers were found in three dicentric Xqi chromosomes and in three monocentric Xqi chromosomes.[754] In five instances the Xqi was paternally derived. Isochromosome for the long arm of the X is the most common form of structural rearrangement of the X chromosome.

Patients with a long arm X isochromosome are invariably

Table 22–16. Summary of Clinical Findings in 14 Patients with the Syndrome of Webbed Neck, Ptosis, Hypogonadism, Congenital Heart Disease, and Short Stature

Clinical Characteristics	No. Males	No. Females
Short stature (>2 SD below mean)	2/2	8/12
Typical facies	2/2	12/12
Triangular shape of face	2/2	7/12
Prominent brow	2/2	12/12
Hypertelorism	2/2	12/12
Epicanthus	2/2	9/12
Antimongoloid palpebral slant	2/2	10/12
Ptosis	2/2	12/12
Depressed nasal bridge	1/2	2/12
Broad apex nasi	2/2	11/12
Low-set and/or malformed ears	2/2	8/12
High-arched palate	2/2	8/12
Neck		
Short	2/2	10/12
Webbing	2/2	10/12
Low hairline	2/2	10/12
Chest		
Shield-like	1/2	11/12
Wide-spaced nipples	2/2	11/11
Pectus excavatum	2/2	5/12
Cardiac abnormalities	2/2	11/12
Pulmonic stenosis (PS)	2/2	5/10
PS and ventricular septal defect	0/2	1/10
Atrial septal defect (ASD)	2/2	6/10
ASD with anomalous pulmonary venous return	0/2	1/10
Endocardial cushion defect (ECD)	0/2	2/10
ECD + patent ductus arteriosus and mitral insufficiency	0/2	1/10
Both PS and ASD	2/2	3/10
Patent ductus arteriosus (PDA)	0/2	2/10
Undiagnosed heart disease	0/2	2/10
Incompletely evaluated	0/2	2/12
Extremities		
Cubitus valgus	2/2	9/12
Gracile fingers	1/2	8/12
Short stubby fingers	1/2	2/12
Lymphedema	0/2	3/12
Dystrophic nails	2/2	2/12
Shortened fourth metacarpal(s)	0/2	3/12
Clinodactyly of fifth finger(s)	1/2	2/12
Palmar simian crease	1/2	1/12
Undescended testes	2/2	—
Delayed puberty	1/1	3/3
Skeletal retardation	2/2	8/10
Mental development		
Retarded	2/2	4/12
Borderline	0/2	5/12
Normal	0/2	3/12
Intrauterine growth retardation	1/2	4/12
Renal collecting system		
Normal	2/2	7/8
Abnormal	0/2	1/8
Normal karyotype	2/2	12/12

factor XI deficiency. The chromosome constitution is normal, and gonadal differentiation is appropriate for the phenotypic and chromosomal sex. Cryptorchidism is common in males, and the testes may be hypoplastic and exhibit germinal aplasia. Puberty is delayed, and androgen deficiency is not uncommon. However, 50% of affected males have normal testicular function, including fertility in the absence of cryptorchidism. Affected females have functioning ovaries and, although the onset of puberty may be delayed, female secondary sexual characteristics eventually emerge.

Noonan's syndrome has an incidence of 1 in 1000 to 1 in 2500 live births and about 50% of cases are sporadic.[845] Familial clusters are usually consistent with autosomal dominant inheritance in this genetically heterogeneous disorder.[851] Linkage analysis in a large Dutch kindred suggested location of a gene for Noonan's syndrome on the long arm of chromosome 12 (12q24).[851] Missense mutations in *PTPN11,* the gene encoding the nonreceptor protein tyrosine-2 phosphatase (SHP-2) that contains two Src homology-2 (SH2) domains, is a cause of Noonan's syndrome, accounting for about 50% of affected individuals. A gain of function arising from excess SHP-2 activity is postulated as the disease mechanism.[852, 853] The abnormality of gonadal function and the higher incidence of congenital heart disease in males may play a part in the apparently higher maternal transmission of the mutant gene.

The diagnosis is based on the constellation of stigmata, the most prominent of which are short stature, webbed neck, pectus excavatum, ptosis, and right-sided congenital heart disease in a patient with a normal sex chromosome constitution. The differential diagnosis of this syndrome is extensive and includes structural abnormalities of the Y chromosome (especially those involving the short arm), 45,X/46,XY mosaicism, and dysmorphic syndromes secondary to hydantoin, primidone, or alcohol exposure during gestation.[568] At puberty, affected males may require testosterone replacement therapy. Mean final height tends to follow the lower limits of the growth curve; mean adult height was 162.5 cm in men and 152.7 cm in women according to Ranke and co-workers.[854] A United Kingdom study of the effect of recombinant hGH therapy found an initial improvement in height velocity but only a small increment in final height; no adverse effects in patients with hypertrophic cardiomyopathy were noted.[855, 856]

True Hermaphroditism

The diagnosis of true hermaphroditism requires the presence of both ovarian (containing follicles) and testicular tissue in either the same or opposite gonads.[857–859] Failure to adhere to this definition has led to considerable confusion. Gonadal stroma arranged in whorls, similar to those found in the ovary but lacking oocytes, should not be considered sufficient evidence to designate the rudimentary gonad as an ovary. Similarly, if testicular tissue is present in the contralateral gonad, we do not consider the presence of a few oocytes in a streak gonad to be adequate evidence for the diagnosis of true hermaphroditism. Because rare female-type germ cells may be found in patients with 45,X gonadal dysgenesis, it is of little value from the clinical, cytogenetic, embryologic, or nosologic standpoint to classify as true hermaphrodites the 45,X/46,XY mosaics or individuals with 46,XY complete gonadal dysgenesis in whom a dysgenetic gonad contains rare oocytes.[780] Similarly, the status of the internal and external genitalia, which invariably exhibit some degree of ambisexual development, should not be used as a criterion for classification of an individual as a true hermaphrodite. This uncommon type of intersex is relatively more prevalent in South African blacks.[859, 869]

Classification

True hermaphroditism is uncommon but has been reported in more than 400 individuals.[859–862] Patients with this syndrome may be subclassified according to the type and location of the gonads.

Lateral. A testis is present on one side, and an ovary is present on the other in about 20% of patients.[859–862] The ovary is frequently found on the left side.[859, 862]

Bilateral. Both testicular and ovarian tissue are present bilaterally, usually as ovotestes, in about 30% of patients.[859–863]

Unilateral. Testicular and ovarian tissue is present on one side and a testis or ovary is found on the other side in slightly less than one half of cases.[859–863] A testis or ovotestis may be

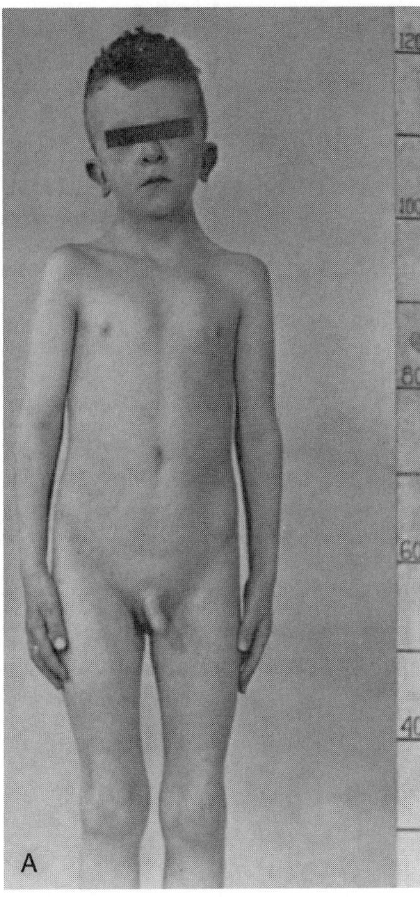

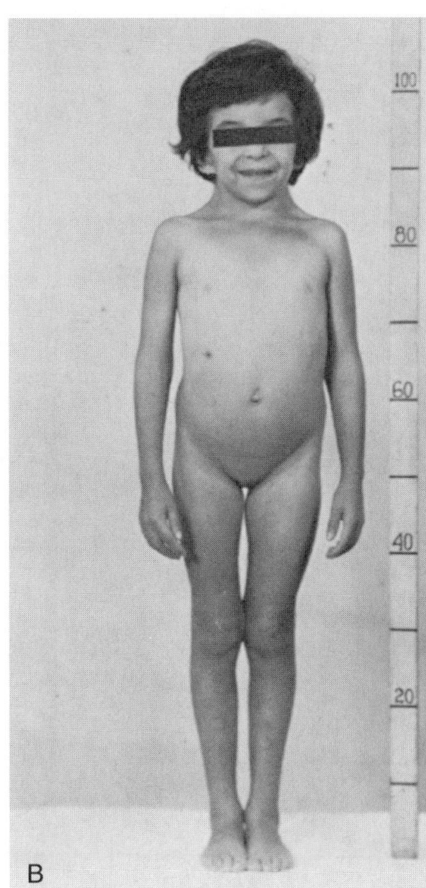

Figure 22–51. Phenotypic male and female with syndrome of webbed neck, ptosis, congenital heart disease, short stature, and hypogonadism (pseudo-Turner's syndrome, Noonan's syndrome). *A*, A boy, aged 9 years, 7 months, exhibited characteristic abnormalities: triangular facies, prominent brow, hypertelorism, ptosis, antimongoloid slant of palpebral fissures, broad apex nasi, low-set ears, webbed neck, pectus excavatum, pulmonic stenosis and atrial septal defect, short stature (−3.5 SD), bilateral undescended testes, and high-grade mental retardation. At age 18, he was 154.0 cm in height (height age: 12 years, 5 months); the boy had Leydig cell hypofunction. Biopsy of testes showed germinal aplasia. (From Grumbach MM, Barr ML. Cytologic tests of chromosomal sex in relation to sexual anomalies in man. Recent Prog Horm Res 1958; 14:255–334.) *B*, An 8-year-old girl with similar features. Height was 106.2 cm (height age: 4 years, 4 months). Pulmonic stenosis was present, and the karyotype was 46,XX.

situated along the normal pathway of descent of a testis, but an ovary is almost invariably in its normal position. A testis or ovotestis is more common on the right side.[559, 862] The asymmetric distribution of gonadal tissue has been attributed to an early differential growth advantage of the embryonic testis.[864]

Clinical Features

The differentiation of the genital tract and the development of secondary sexual characteristics are variable (Table 22–17; Fig. 22–52). The external genitalia may simulate those of either a male or a female, or they may be ambiguous; most of the patients are reared as males because of the size of the phallus and because of social factors.[859, 860] Almost all have hypospadias, which varies in extent from perineal to penile, and incomplete fusion of the labioscrotal folds. The labioscrotal folds are asymmetric in half of the patients, with the right side more predominant.[860] In rare cases a penile urethra is present. Cryptorchidism is common, but at least one gonad is usually palpable in the labioscrotal fold or in the inguinal region.[861] An inguinal hernia, which may contain a gonad or uterus, is present in about one half of the cases, and a vagina and a uterus are present in most patients; the uterus may be underdeveloped (hemiuterus), rudimentary, or absent.[860, 861] The differentiation of the genital ducts usually follows that of the gonads. The ovotestis is the most common gonad in true hermaphrodites, followed by the ovary and, least commonly, the testis.[860–862, 865–869] In patients with a testis on one side and an ovary on the other, the development of the homolateral duct is usually consistent with that of the gonad, despite the varied appearance of the external genitalia. Most patients with an ovotestis have predominantly female development of the genital ducts. The relation between gonadal structure and differentiation of the genital tract in true hermaphroditism provides additional evidence for the local action of AMH secreted by the Sertoli cells of the embryonic and fetal testes.

Breast development is common during puberty in true hermaphrodites, and menses occur in more than half of the patients. Periodic hematuria associated with menstruation is a late clue to the diagnosis. Spermatogenesis is rare; seminiferous tubules in an ovotestis or testes are abnormal in most cases, and interstitial fibrosis of the testes is common.[861, 862] Ovulation is not uncommon, and pregnancy and childbirth can occur in patients with a 46,XX karyotype,[867, 870, 871] whereas only one 46,XY true hermaphrodite has been reported to have fathered a child.[872]

Few studies of hypothalamic-pituitary-gonadal function have been carried out in true hermaphrodites. Whereas an ovary or

Table 22–17. Clinical Features of True Hermaphroditism

Karyotype:	46,XX (most common), 46,XX/46,XY, or 46,XY (rare)
Inheritance:	Familial cases (autosomal recessive, autosomal dominant transmission) rare
Genitalia:	Ambiguous; cryptorchidism frequent; ovotestis possibly located in labioscrotal fold
Wolffian duct derivatives: Müllerian duct derivatives:	Duct differentiation after that of the homolateral gonad
Gonad:	Testis, ovary, or ovotestis
Habitus:	Breast development and virilization common at puberty
Molecular studies:	Approximately 10% of 46,XX true hermaphrodites are *SRY* positive

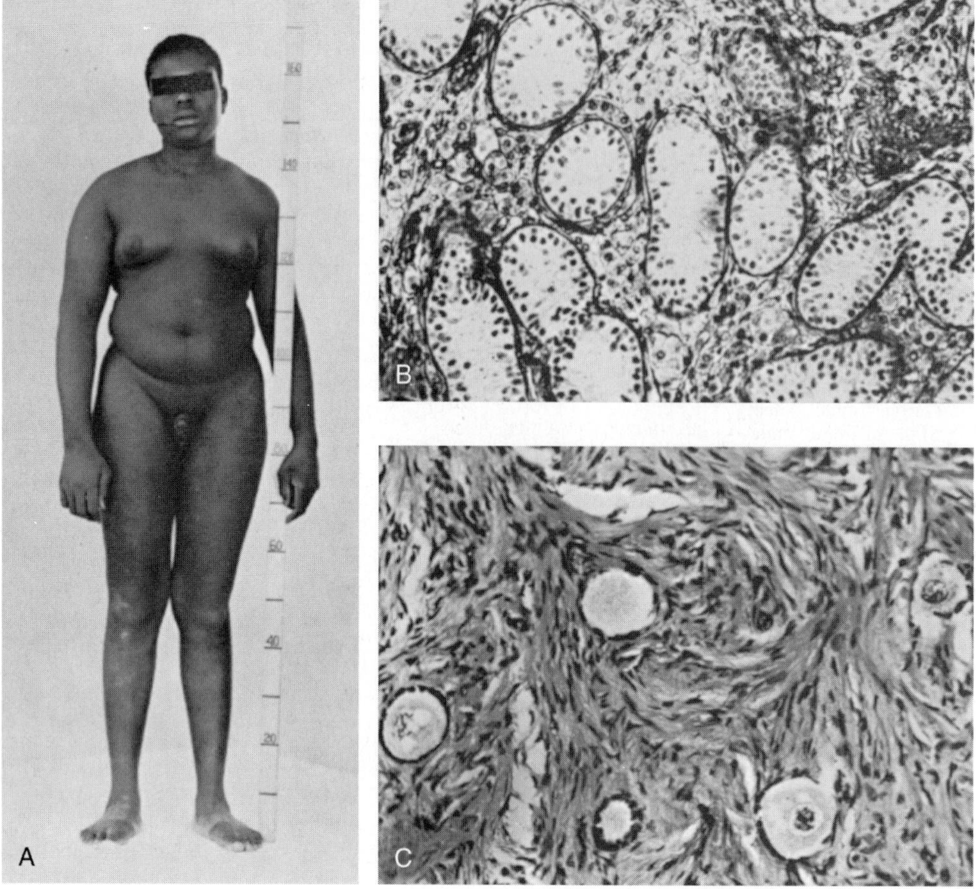

Figure 22–52. *A*, A 17-year-old true hermaphrodite with bilateral scrotal ovotestes and a 46,XX sex chromosome constitution in cultures of peripheral blood and skin, perineal hypospadias (partially repaired in photograph), moderate bilateral gynecomastia and pubic hair (recently shaved in picture), sparse axillary hair, a high-pitched voice, and absent facial hair. Height was 168 cm. Urinary 17-ketosteroid level was 1.3 mg/day; urinary gonadotropin levels were elevated. A male type of urethra, bilateral scrotal fallopian tubes and ovotestes, and rudimentary bicornuate uterus and vagina attached to the posterior urethra were seen at operation. The photomicrographs show histopathology of the ovarian and testicular portion of one ovotestis. *B*, Immature seminiferous tubules lined with Sertoli cells and spermatogonia and Leydig cells. *C*, Ova and follicles. (From Grumbach MM, Barr ML. Cytologic tests of chromosomal sex in relation to sexual anomalies in man. Recent Prog Horm Res 1958; 14:255–334.)

ovarian portion of an ovotestis may function normally, the testis or testicular component of the ovotestis is usually abnormal.[861, 873] The cyclic pattern of FSH and LH secretion can be similar to that in normal women.[872] As in other men with gynecomastia, a low ratio of testosterone to estradiol, caused by enhanced secretion of estradiol by the ovotestis and/or testes, plays a role in the breast development that is seen frequently in postpubertal true hermaphrodites.[874]

Chromosomal Findings

By far the most common karyotype found in true hermaphrodites is 46,XX, followed by 46,XX/46,XY chimerism, mosaicism, and, rarely, 46,XY (7%).[860–862, 865, 866]

Origins of True Hermaphroditism

True hermaphroditism could result from sex chromosome mosaicism (apparent or cryptic), chimerism, Y-to-autosome or Y-to-X chromosome translocation,[600, 601, 875–877] or mutation of either X-linked or autosomal genes involved in sex determination.[602] Most 46,XX true hermaphrodites (~85%) are *SRY* negative in leukocyte DNA.[878–880] However, by the use of molecular genetic and histochemical techniques for the *SRY* gene and the SRY protein, *SRY* gene expression and protein has been detected in the ovotestes of XX true hermaphrodites in whom leukocytes and fibroblast DNA were negative for SRY.[861, 881–883] In six XX hermaphrodites in whom the peripheral karyotype was SRY negative, all eight ovotestes exhibited low levels of expression of the *SRY* gene and SRY protein was detected mainly in Sertoli and germ cells.[883] These observations suggest cryptic mosaicism or chimerism of a Y-bearing cell may be more common in XX (*SRY*−) true hermaphrodites than previously thought.

The gene (or genes) responsible for XX (*SRY*−) true hermaphroditism has not yet been identified; however, it is probably a downstream gene in the sex determination pathway that, when mutated, allows for testicular differentiation. That Y sequence–negative 46,XX males and 46,XX true hermaphrodites can occur in the same pedigree is well documented.[278, 602, 604, 880] Kuhnle and associates,[602] for example, studied a pedigree with two 46,XX true hermaphrodites and a 46,XX male who were first cousins. The three patients were negative for Y sequences, including *PABY* (*p*seudo*a*utosomal *b*oundary *Y*), *SRY*, and *ZFY*. The pattern of inheritance of 46,XX true hermaphroditism and 46,XX maleness was compatible with an autosomal dominant or an X-linked dominant mode of transmission with variable expression.[602] In the case of a putative X-linked gene mutation, it has been postulated that random inactivation would result in true hermaphroditism and nonrandom inactivation would lead to an XX male.[881] However, no evidence for nonrandom X-inactivation in SRY-negative 46,XX males has been reported. Because of the postulated role of a gene on the X chromosome as a cause of true hermaphroditism, Spurdle and colleagues[883b] carried out a detailed DNA analysis of the X chromosome in a study of sixteen 46,XX *SRY*-negative true hermaphrodites and found no evidence of uniparental disomy of the X chromosome.[882] Sarafoglou and Ostrer[604] reviewed the familial cases of true hermaphroditism and pedigrees in which both true hermaphroditism and XX maleness have occurred. An *SRY*-X translocation was detected in one pedigree, but in the other affected families an X-linked gene, a sex-limited autosomal dominant gene, or an autosomal recessive gene could have fit the mode of inheritance.

A small number of "Y-positive" 46,XX true hermaphrodites have been reported in kindreds with 46,XX males.[604, 883] It has been postulated that inactivation of the X chromosome bearing the Y chromosome translocation could lead to inactivation of the *SRY* gene by the spread of inactivation into the translocated segment. However, in one *SRY*-positive 46,XX true hermaphrodite, the translocated X was randomly inactivated; on the other hand, nonrandom inactivation of the X chromosome bearing the Y translocation was found in another *SRY*-positive 46,XX male.[883] Accordingly, in some instances X inactivation may play a role in the gonadal phenotype of 46,XX *SRY*-positive males.

Sex chromosome mosaicism arises from mitotic or meiotic errors. In contrast, 46,XX/46,XY chimerism is usually a consequence of double fertilization or, possibly, fusion of two normally fertilized ova.[884] Chimeric individuals have two distinct populations of cells, each of which has a different genetic origin (in contrast to mosaicism). Study of 46,XX/46,XY chimeras provides evidence for the fertilization of a binucleate ovum by two sperms, one bearing an X and the other a Y.[885, 886] Not all patients with whole-body chimerism have true hermaphroditism. One 46,XX/46,XY patient was a phenotypic male without true hermaphroditism; a likely mechanism for the chimerism in this case, based on the blood group studies and other findings, is fusion of two zygotes or fertilization of an ovum and its polar body. The experiments of Tarkowski[887] with XX and XY mouse blastocytes demonstrated that random fusion of two blastocytes seldom produces 46,XX/46,XY true hermaphroditism; fused mouse blastocysts usually develop testes rather than ovaries or ovotestes. A 46,XY true hermaphrodite, the least common form,[875] had an apparently normal Y chromosome and *SRY* gene. However, DNA analysis of the "ovotestes" uncovered mosaicism for a normal *SRY* gene and a mutated *SRY* gene with a nonconservative amino acid substitution.[875] This suggested that a postzygotic gonadal mutation in *SRY* resulted in ovotestes and, thus, true hermaphroditism. It may be that all 46,XY true hermaphrodites are cryptic gonadal mosaics for an *SRY* mutation or another gene mutation in the gonadal differentiation cascade, or they may harbor a 46,XX cell line. Rare familial cases of putative XY true hermaphroditism have been reported in the past; however, these have not been studied with newer cytogenetic or molecular biologic techniques.[888]

Diagnosis and Therapy

The diagnosis of true hermaphroditism should be considered in all patients with ambiguous genitalia. A 46,XX/46,XY karyotype in a patient with ambiguous external genitalia strongly suggests the diagnosis, and a 46,XX or 46,XY karyotype does not exclude the diagnosis. The finding of a gonad in the labioscrotal fold (especially on the right side) with a lobulated bipolar consistency compatible with an ovotestis is suggestive. Pelvic ultrasonography and especially MRI are useful in visualizing the internal genitalia and assessing gonadal structure. In one study, 11 of 12 46,XX true hermaphrodites examined before 6 months of age had basal plasma testosterone levels greater than 40 ng/dL (upper range of normal in females of this age, 15 ng/dL), suggesting the presence of Leydig cells.[861] All children examined after 6 months of age in the same study had basal testosterone levels lower than 15 ng/dL; however, administration of hCG induced testosterone responses that were greater than 40 ng/dL.[861] Therefore, both basal testosterone values in infants younger than 6 months of age and hCG-induced testosterone responses are useful for ascertaining the presence of Leydig cells. Plasma, inhibin B (before puberty), and AMH levels are detectable in true hermaphrodites with functional Sertoli cells.[365] The estradiol response to repetitive injections of human menopausal gonadotropins (hMG) has been proposed as a reliable indicator of ovarian tissue.[888] We prefer the use of recombinant hFSH. Similarly, the determination of inhibin A is useful for the detection of ovarian follicles before 4 months of age or after 10 years of age. If all other forms of pseudohermaphroditism have been ruled out, the diagnosis of true hermaphroditism should be confirmed by the demonstration of both ovarian and testicular tissues histologically.

The management is contingent on the age at diagnosis and assessment of the functional capacity of the internal and external genitalia. In infants in whom gender identity has not already been established, either a male or female assignment of sex can be made. However, in 46,XX true hermaphrodites we believe that, except for patients who have a well-developed phallic structure and who lack a uterus or possess a vestigial one, a female sex assignment is prudent because ovarian tissue is usually functional, pregnancy has been documented, and surgical reconstruction of the external genitalia has led to a satisfactory functional result.[861, 867] The risk of malignant transformation in the ovarian tissue of 46,XX true hermaphrodites is unknown.[889] If a male gender role is assigned, all müllerian and ovarian structures should be removed. The testis or testicular component of an ovotestis is usually dysgenetic, and the risk of neoplasm is increased. The prevalence of gonadoblastoma and/or germinoma arising in the testicular tissue of 46,XX true hermaphrodites has been estimated at 3% to 4%.[859, 861] Accordingly, in 46,XX true hermaphrodites raised as males we recommend removal of dysgenetic testes or testicular tissue, the insertion of prosthetic testes, and hormone replacement at puberty. In 46,XX/46,XY chimeras and 46,XY true hermaphrodites, especially when a testis is present on one side and an ovary on the contralateral side and the size of the phallus is adequate, one should weigh the alternative of retaining a histologically normal-appearing testis in the scrotum and raising the patient as a male, even though the risk of gonadal malignancy may be increased, especially if evidence of carcinoma in situ is found on histologic examination. In true hermaphrodites reared as females, all testicular tissue should be removed. Postoperative assessment of the plasma testosterone response to hCG is useful to ascertain the persistence of Leydig cells as well as determination of either plasma AMH or inhibin B, markers of retained testicular tissue. In older patients, gender identity is the major consideration; usually it conforms to the sex of rearing. The discordant gonad and dysgenetic gonadal tissue should be removed, and plastic repair of the external genitalia should be carried out. Appropriate gonadal hormone replacement therapy is recommended at the age of puberty.

Gonadal Neoplasms in Dysgenetic Gonads

The prevalence of gonadal neoplasms is increased in patients with certain types of dysgenetic gonads, in particular all those with a Y-bearing cell line.[904–909] Germinoma (dysgerminoma, seminoma), teratoma, and gonadoblastoma have been found. Cryptorchid testes, even when not associated with intersexuality, are also associated with an increased risk of malignancy. The probability that cryptorchid testes will undergo malignant degeneration is difficult to assess, but it is at least 10 times greater than the probability for normally descended testes.[907, 908] Approximately 7% of males with testicular neoplasms have been or are cryptorchid at the time of diagnosis.[908] In addition, in one third of patients with cryptorchidism who develop carcinoma of the testis, the neoplasm occurs after orchiopexy; in patients with unilateral cryptorchidism, 25% of tumors were located in the contralateral descended testes.[907, 908] CIS is a premalignant lesion of the testes.[786, 787, 910, 911] It is characterized by germ cells that are larger than normal spermatogenia, have clumped chromatin, are highly aneuploid, and are positive for placental alkaline phosphatase.[910, 911] CIS, also called intratubular germ cell neoplasm (IGCN), is commonly seen adjacent to germ cell tumors in adults.[910] However, it is not found adjacent to tumors before puberty, and the cells differ morphologically from those in postpubertal males. The natural history of CIS in prepubertal patients remains to be determined.[910] About 50% of postpubertal patients with CIS develop germ cell tumors within 5 years of diagnosis; it has been suggested that, with time, the incidence may approach 100%.[910] CIS is thought to originate from primordial germ cells. It occurs in 2% to 4% of males with cryptorchidism, in 25% of XY individuals with ambiguous genitalia, in individuals with dysgenetic testes and an XY cell line (XY gonadal dysgenesis, XO/XY mosaicism), and in the syndrome of androgen resistance.[910] Localized low-dose radiotherapy to the testis will eradicate CIS and germ cells but preserves Leydig cells. The progression from CIS to invasive germ cell tumors appears to correlate with expression of cyclins and cyclin-dependent kinase inhibitors.[913]

Gonadal neoplasms are uncommon in patients with 47,XXY seminiferous tubule dysgenesis, but a small number of patients have gonadal or extragonadal germ cell tumors.[538, 908, 912, 914] Similarly, gonadal tumors are rare in the streak gonads of 45,X patients and in 45,X mosaics with a normal or structurally abnormal X chromosome in the second cell line. Gonadoblastoma and dysgerminoma,[908, 915–917] mucinous cystadenoma,[918] and a hilus cell tumor with signs of virilization have been reported in gonadal dysgenesis.[919, 920] However, these patients have not been studied for a low percentage of Y chromosome mosaicism by molecular analyses.[47]

Gonadoblastomas are usually composed of three elements; large germ cells, sex cord derivatives (Sertoli-granulosa cells), and stromal elements (theca cells, Leydig cells). They are found almost exclusively in patients who have a 46,XY cell line. They may be microscopic or large, especially if overgrown by other germ cell elements, and often are calcified. A comprehensive review of gonadoblastoma was published by Scully[906] (see Fig. 22–50). In 27 of 74 patients, a tumor was present in both gonads. Thirty patients were younger than 15 years of age when the tumor was diagnosed, and 10 were younger than 10 years. A third of these tumors were detected incidentally on histologic examination of dysgenetic gonads removed for other indications. In patients in whom chromosomal studies were carried out, the predominant karyotypes were 45,X/46,XY and 46,XY. Although 80% of 46,XY patients are reared as females, most display some degree of clitoromegaly or hirsutism; rarely, the tumors secrete enough estrogen to induce breast development (see Fig. 22–50). Pure gonadoblastomas can be regarded as germ cell tumors in situ and as such do not metastasize.[907, 908] In half the cases, however, the germ cells infiltrate the stroma of the tumor to form a seminoma.[921, 922] Gonadoblastomas are also associated with more highly malignant germ cell tumors such as endodermal sinus tumors, embryonal carcinoma, and choriocarcinoma (10%).[907, 923] There is an increased risk of gonadal tumors (gonadoblastoma and/or germinoma) in patients with 46,XY gonadal dysgenesis and particularly in familial cases.[923] The strikingly disparate propensity for neoplastic transformation in the streak or dysgenetic gonads of patients with 46,XY gonadal dysgenesis in contrast to 46,XX gonadal dysgenesis must be emphasized. The gonadoblastoma locus *(GBY)* has been mapped to a critical interval on the short arm and adjacent centromeric region of the Y chromosome.[71, 72, 924] Five functional genes have been identified in this region as possible candidates for the cancer-predisposing locus. *TSPY*, one of the encoded proteins, is preferentially expressed in the germ cells of gonadoblastoma specimens.[71, 924]

In view of the well-documented malignant potential of dysgenetic gonads, the question of prophylactic gonadectomy merits serious attention. The neoplasms are infrequent in childhood,[905, 922] but the risk rises appreciably in young adults.[905, 908] High gonadotropin levels may play a role in their growth, and substitution therapy with gonadal steroids may afford some protection. A prudent course is to advise laparotomy or laparoscopy and removal of the dysgenetic gonads of all patients with 46,XY gonadal dysgenesis (complete and incomplete forms) and of all patients with the syndrome of gonadal dysgenesis who have a cell line with a normal or a structurally abnormal Y chromosome or who have Y chromosomal material as determined by molecular genetic studies. Exceptions to this rule occur in patients who are 45,X/46,XY mosaics with normal male genitalia, histologically normal testes, and normal gonadotropin levels and in patients with 45,X/46,XY mosaicism with ambiguous genitalia who have been assigned a male gender role and in whom a histologically normal gonad is located in the scrotum. However, the fact that a gonad is located in the scrotum or labial folds and is palpable does not guarantee against a disastrous result, because seminomas can metastasize at an early stage, before a local mass is obvious. Hence, it is prudent to sample these testes postpubertally to ascertain the presence of CIS (a premalignant lesion).[786] Patients with 45,X gonadal dysgenesis who have no suggestion of clitoromegaly are not at risk. The incidence of gonadal tumors in patients with other X chromosome abnormalities, such as 45,X/46,XX, 46,XXr, 46,XXp−, and 46,XXq−, is low; however, these patients should be examined at regular intervals and, if indicated, monitored by ultrasonography of the pelvis for signs of gonadal or uterine neoplasm.

Sex Chromosome Abnormalities Unassociated with Gonadal Defects

The addition of one or more sex chromosomes to the genome has a deleterious effect on cognitive function. The following five sex chromosome abnormalities are not accompanied by a typical gonadal defect but are frequently associated with mental retardation.

47,XXX

This common chromosome abnormality has the frequency of about 1 per 1000 female newborns. The prevalence of 47,XXX individuals in institutions for the mentally retarded is 4.3 per 1000,[890] suggesting an increased risk for severe mental retardation. 47,XXX females have reduced general intelligence and low scores on tests of attention, concept formation, spatial thinking, verbal fluency, and academic skills.[522, 891, 892] XXX individuals demonstrated less overall psychosocial adaptation and a greater degree of psychological disturbance, compared with patients with Klinefelter's syndrome or gonadal dysgenesis.[522] Although some have delayed menarche or premature ovarian failure, most 47,XXX females have normal ovarian function. 47,XXX females can rarely give birth to 47,XXY sons,[567] and the prevalence of congenital malformations is increased in the progeny of 47,XXX women.[893] Subtle clinical features in infants ascertained by karyotype analysis include the following: a tendency to low birth weight, decreased head circumference, advanced mean parental age, an increased incidence of clinodactyly, normal postnatal growth patterns, an increased risk of speech and language problems, and a lower mean I.Q. than the siblings or a control group.[522, 892] The extra X chromosome is of maternal origin in most instances, arising mainly from nondisjunction during the first or second meiotic divisions.[894]

The diagnosis of 47,XXX can be confirmed by the finding of two sex chromatin bodies in interphase cells and by the demonstration of a 47,XXX karyotype through the use of appropriate banding techniques. Because of the increased risk in the offspring of a sex chromosome abnormality (47,XXY and 47,XXX) and congenital malformations, prenatal counseling and amniocentesis should be considered in 47,XXX females who become pregnant.

48,XXXX

This rare anomaly[569, 895, 896] is associated with considerable phenotype heterogeneity, making identification by clinical means difficult. The most constant feature is a variable degree of mental retardation affecting speech.[896] Ovarian function is usually normal. Average adult height is 169 cm; the prevalence of skeletal anomalies, such as clinodactyly and radioulnar synostosis, is increased.[569] The diagnosis is suggested by finding three sex chromatin bodies in 6% to 9% of somatic nuclei and is confirmed by karyotype analysis.

49,XXXXX[569, 897]

The rare penta-X syndrome is invariably associated with severe prenatal and postnatal growth delay and mental retardation. Other stigmata include microcephaly, hypertelorism, epicanthal folds, up-slanted palpebral fissures, depressed nasal bridge, abnormal dentition, a short neck, congenital heart disease, clinodactyly, overlapping toes, and joint laxity. The external genitalia and gonadal function are usually normal; however, fertility is still to be documented.[569] A proportion of interphase nuclei contain four X chromatin bodies and four late replicating X chromosomes[31] (Fig. 22–13).

47,XYY

The first subject reported by Sandberg and associates[898] was an essentially normal fertile man of average intelligence who was detected only because he had a daughter with Down's syndrome. However, surveys in penal institutions suggested an increase in prevalence of this anomaly, especially in tall prisoners, and gave rise to an undeserved stereotype that has been modified by later studies.[899–901] Among 43 47,XYY boys 1 to 12 years of age, ascertained by routine karyotype analysis in the newborn period, no clear-cut 47,XYY syndrome emerged in childhood.[514] No major deviations could be attributed to an extra Y chromosome, with the possible exception of a skew to the left in I.Q. scores, although full-scale I.Q. scores ranged from 80 to 140.[520] In general, 47,XYY patients tend to be easily distractible and hyperactive and to have low tolerance of frustration.[520] The prevalence of antisocial and other behavioral difficulties is increased.[53] 47,XYY is a common sex chromosome abnormality, occurring in 1 per 1000 male births; it is the only aneuploidy not selected against before birth. Among the features are tall stature,[53] nodulocystic acne, and skeletal anomalies such as radioulnar synostosis. Sexual development is usually normal, and the rare reports of hypospadias in 47,XYY patients may be coincidental. The diagnosis should be suspected in hyperactive tall men with nodulocystic acne and can be confirmed by demonstration of two fluorescent Y bodies in somatic interphase nuclei or by karyotype analysis. The additional Y chromosome most commonly arises by nondisjunction at meiosis II.[902]

48,XYYY

The variable phenotypes associated with this rare karyotype include multiple somatic abnormalities and mental retardation.[903] The diagnosis is confirmed by finding three fluorescent Y bodies in interphase nuclei or by karyotype analysis.

Sex Differentiation Genes

The genes known to be involved in sex differentiation are listed in Table 22–18.

Female Pseudohermaphroditism

Female pseudohermaphroditism (Table 22–19) is the easiest of the sexual anomalies to comprehend, because the ovaries and müllerian derivatives are normal and anatomic abnormality is limited to the external urogenital sinus and genitalia. Because in the absence of testes there is an inherent tendency for the external genitalia to feminize, a female fetus is masculinized only if exposed to androgens. The degree of fetal masculinization is determined by the stage of differentiation at the time of exposure. Once the vagina has separated from the urogenital sinus (at about the 12th fetal week), androgens cause only clitoral hypertrophy[423] (Fig. 22–53). Even with severe masculinization of the external genitalia, the uterus and fallopian tubes are normal, because regression of the primordia for these structures, the müllerian ducts, requires secretion of AMH by fetal testes, and this action cannot be mimicked by androgens. Although the presence of virilized genitalia usually provides prima facie evidence of an androgenic influence during gestation, ambiguous genitalia, superficially resembling those produced by androgen, are an occasional feature of other, more generalized teratologic malformations.

Congenital Adrenal Hyperplasia

CAH[925–929] accounts for most of the cases of female pseudohermaphroditism and approximately half of all patients with ambiguous external genitalia.

Biochemical Variants of Congenital Adrenal Hyperplasia

Mutations in five genes, four that encode biosynthetic enzymes for steroid hormone synthesis (*CYP21*, *CYP17*, *CYP11B1*, *CYP11A1*, and *HSD3B2*) and one that encodes the intracellular cholesterol transport protein (StAR, steroid acute regulatory protein), can cause CAH, each resulting in distinctive biochemical consequences and clinical features[925–929] (Fig. 22–54; see Chapter 14). All (but the rare CYP11A1 heterozygous mutation) are transmitted as autosomal recessive traits. The common denominator in all six biochemical defects is impaired cortisol secretion, which results in hypersecretion of corticotropin-releasing hormone (CRH) and corticotropin and consequent hyperplasia of the adrenal cortex. Only deficiencies of 21-hydroxylase (CYP21) and 11β-hydroxylase (CYP11B1), however, are predominantly virilizing disorders. In patients with "classic" forms of these two enzymatic defects, the most striking abnormality of the sexual phenotype is masculinization of the female fetus because of overproduction of adrenal an-

Table 22–18. Genes Involved in Sex Differentiation

Gene	Encodes	Human Locus	Human Phenotype (Mutation or Deletion)	Mouse Phenotype
AMH	Antimüllerian hormone; member of TGF-β family: causes regression of müllerian ducts	19p13.3	46XY: Persistent müllerian duct syndrome, cryptorchidism, type 1	KO: Persistent müllerian ducts, Leydig cell hyperplasia Transgenic: females without müllerian ducts. Most males normal. Males with highest expression of AMH → ambiguous genitalia, impaired wolffian duct development, undescended testes
AMH type 2 receptor (interacts with type 1 receptor)	Serine/threonine kinase: type II receptor for TGF-β related proteins	12q13	46,XY: Persistent müllerian duct syndrome, type II	KO: Persistent müllerian duct syndrome
hCGβ	Beta-subunit of hCG	19q13.32	Not reported; presumably lethal	NA
hCG/LH receptor	Receptor	2p21	46XY: male pseudohermaphrodite	KO: Males normal at birth; postnatal arrest in sexual development Females: underdeveloped external genitalia
StAR (steroidogenic acute regulatory protein)	StAR mediates transport of cholesterol from outer mitochondrial membrane to inner; not expressed in human placenta	8p11.2	46,XY: male pseudohermaphrodite with adrenal and gonadal steroid deficiency 46,XX: adrenal insufficiency, progressive postpubertal gonadal failure	KO: Mouse phenotype same as human
CYP11A1 (P450scc)	Enzyme that catalyzes conversion of cholesterol to pregnenolone	15q23–24	46,XY: heterozygote, male pseudohermaphrodite, late-onset adrenal insufficiency	KO: (phenotype in the rabbit same as human, lethal)
HSD3B2	Enzyme that catalyzes conversion of C_{21}- and C_{19}- Δ^5-steroids to Δ^4-steroids by the gonads and adrenals	1p13	46,XY: Severe deficiency—male pseudohermaphrodite with adrenal insufficiency 46,XX: ± clitoromegaly with adrenal insufficiency Milder mutation: as above without clinical aldosterone or glucocorticoid deficiency	NA
AR	Androgen receptor	Xq11–12	46,XY: female → ambiguous → "normal" male genitalia with small penis. Fertility documented in some with normal male external genitalia. Sexual hair: none → sparse → normal; absent müllerian ducts, normal wolffian ducts; cryptorchidism ± in those with ambiguous genitalia; testes: normally developed 46,XX: clinically normal	Same as human
SRD5A2 (5α-reductase-2)	Enzyme that catalyzes 5α-reduction of testosterone to dihydrotestosterone in gonads during sex differentiation and postpubertally	2p23	46,XY: male pseudohermaphrodite; pseudovaginal perineoscrotal hypospadias; normal wolffian ducts; virilization at puberty 46,XX: no clinical manifestation	KO: 5α-reductase 1 and 2 XY: no clinical abnormalities KO: 5α-reductase 1 XX: impaired cervical ripening, defective parturition
CYP19 (P450arom)	Enzyme that converts C_{19}-steroids to C_{18}-estrogens in the placenta (protecting the female fetus from masculinization), gonads, extraglandular tissues	15q21	46,XX: female pseudohermaphrodite virilization at puberty, tall stature, no female secondary sexual characteristics, ovarian cysts, osteoporosis 46,XY: normal male differentiation, tall stature, osteoporosis, elevated gonadotropins, lack of epiphyseal fusion, macro-orchidism	KO: normal sex differentiation

Table 22–18. Genes Involved in Sex Differentiation *Continued*

Gene	Encodes	Human Locus	Human Phenotype (Mutation or Deletion)	Mouse Phenotype
HSD3B1	Enzyme that catalyzes conversion of C_{21} and C_{19}-Δ^5-steroids to Δ^4-steroids in extra-adrenal and extragonadal tissues	1p13	Not reported, presumably lethal, 3βHSD1 is expressed in placenta	NA
CYP17 (P450c17)	Enzyme that catalyzes the 17α-hydroxylation of Δ^5-pregnenolone and progesterone and the scission of C_{21}, 17-OH steroids, primarily 17-OH pregnenolone to dehydroepiandrosterone by the adrenal and gonad	10q24-25	46,XY: male pseudohermaphrodite with hypertension (17-hydroxylase deficiency) 46,XX: normal differentiation with hypertension and primary gonadal failure (17-hydroxylase deficiency) 17,20 lyase defect: 46,XY male pseudohermaphrodite 46,XX: not reported; probably normal female with primary ovarian failure	NA
CYP21 (CYP21A2; P450c21)	Enzyme that catalyzes the 21-hydroxylation of 17-hydroxyprogesterone to 11-deoxycortisone and 21-hydroxylation of progesterone to deoxycorticosterone	6p21-3	Severe: 46,XX—female pseudohermaphrodite with adrenal insufficiency (cortisol and aldosterone deficiency) 46,XY: sexual precocity (macrogenitosomia praecox), adrenal insufficiency Non-salt loser: as above but no clinical evidence of aldosterone or cortisol deficiency Late onset: 46,XX and 46,XY—premature pubarche with progressive virilization; no clinical evidence of cortisol/aldosterone deficiency	KO: normal genitalia, adrenal insufficiency
CYP11B1 (P450c11)	Enzyme that catalyzes the 11-hydroxylation of deoxycortisol to cortisol	8q21-22	46,XX: female pseudohermaphrodite with hypertension 46,XY: sexual precocity (macrogenitosomia praecox) with hypertension	NA
HSD17B3	Enzyme that converts androstenedione to testosterone in the testis	9q22	46,XY: male pseudohermaphrodite with virilization and ± gynecomastia at puberty 46,XX: no clinical manifestations	NA
DHCR7	Enzyme (3β-hydroxysteroid Δ^7-reductase) that catalyzes the conversion of 7-dehydrocholesterol	11q12-13	Smith-Lemli-Opitz syndrome: mental retardation, dysmorphic facies, cleft palate, 2nd-3rd toe syndactyly, ± adrenal insufficiency 46,XY: ambiguous genitalia, hypospadias type II Severe lethal form of Smith-Lemli-Opitz syndrome	KO: resembles severe form of Smith-Lemli-Opitz syndrome, craniofacial anomalies, intrauterine growth retardation, death in first day of life secondary to poor suckling reflex
WNT7A			Not reported in the human	XY: persistence of the müllerian ducts due to lack of AMH receptor XX: lead to abnormal development of the müllerian ducts and uterus resulting in infertility
WNT5A			Not reported in the human	XY: absence of the phallus XX: lack of external genitalia

KO, Knockout; AMH, antimüllerian hormone; hCG, human chorionic gonadotropin; TGF-β, transforming growth factor-beta.

Table 22–19. Classification of Female Pseudohermaphroditism

I. Androgen-Induced
  A. Fetal source
    1. Congenital adrenal hyperplasia
      a. Virilism only, defective adrenal 21-hydroxylation (CYP21)
      b. Virilism with salt-losing syndrome, defective adrenal 21-hydroxylation (CYP21)
      c. Virilism with hypertension, defective adrenal 11β-hydroxylation (CYP11B1)
      d. Virilism with adrenal insufficiency, deficient 3β-HSD 2 (HSD3B 2)
    2. P450 aromatase (CYP19) deficiency
    3. Glucocorticoid receptor gene mutation
  B. Maternal source
    1. Iatrogenic
      a. Testosterone and related steroids
      b. Certain synthetic oral progestagens and rarely diethylstilbestrol
    2. Virilizing ovarian or adrenal tumor
    3. Virilizing luteoma of pregnancy
    4. Congenital virilizing adrenal hyperplasia in mother*
  C. Undetermined source
    1. ?Virilizing luteoma of pregnancy
II. Non–Androgen-Induced Disturbances in Differentiation of Urogenital Structures

*In pregnant patients whose disease is poorly controlled or who are noncompliant, especially during the first trimester.

drogens and androgen precursors. Affected males have no abnormalities of the genitalia. These autosomal recessive disorders of steroid biosynthesis, of which more than 90% are caused by 21-hydroxylase deficiency, are discussed in this section as causes of female pseudohermaphroditism.

Patients with 3β-HSD, CYP17, CYP11A1, or StAR deficiencies have defects that not only block cortisol synthesis but also impair the production of gonadal steroids by the gonads and by the adrenal glands. Affected males have varying degrees of male pseudohermaphroditism because of deficient testosterone production by the fetal Leydig cells, whereas affected females may or may not exhibit virilization. If present, virilization in females is much less severe than in CYP21 and CYP11B1 deficiencies. These forms of CAH in the male are discussed in the section on male pseudohermaphroditism. Administration to the pregnant rat of selective synthetic inhibitors of the enzymes involved in adrenal and testicular steroid biogenesis produced abnormalities of sex differentiation in the offspring that are the counterparts of CAH in humans and served to clarify the role of steroidogenic enzymes in the control of fetal sex differentiation.[930]

CYP21 (21-Hydroxylase) Deficiency

Simple Virilizing Form of CYP21 Deficiency. Deficiency of CYP21 (CYP21A2; cytochrome $P450_{c21}$), the most common cause of ambiguous genitalia in infants, is inherited (as are the other forms) as an autosomal recessive trait. The simple virilizing form of CYP21 deficiency has an incidence of about 1 per 50,000 persons and accounts for approximately 25% of subjects with CYP21 deficiency[931] (Table 22–20).

The abnormality in adrenal biosynthesis in patients with the simple virilizing form of CYP21 deficiency is primarily defective hydroxylation at C21 of progesterone and 17-hydroxyprogesterone in the adrenal gland, which results in increased production of progesterone and 17-hydroxyprogesterone and impaired synthesis of cortisol.[925–929, 931] As a consequence of defective cortisol synthesis, hypersecretion of corticotropin causes hyperpigmentation and stimulation of the adrenals to produce excessive amounts of cortisol precursors, including androgen precursors, proximal to the block in the biosynthetic pathway. Hence, in affected patients the concentrations of plasma 17-hydroxyprogesterone and 21-deoxycortisol are increased, as are the plasma levels of androstenedione, testosterone, and, to a lesser extent, progesterone and 17α-hydroxypregnenolone. Postnatally, metabolites of these steroids are excreted as urinary 17-ketosteroids, pregnanetriol, and 11-ketopregnanetriol. Prenatally, excess adrenal androgen synthesis in the fetus, which exceeds in the first trimester the capacity of placental aromatase to convert C_{19}-steroids to estrogens,[358, 932] results in elevated circulating testosterone levels. Before the 12th week of gestation, high fetal androgen levels lead to a varying degree of labioscrotal fusion and clitoral enlargement in the affected female fetus; exposure to androgen after week 12 causes isolated clitoromegaly.[423] (See Role of Androgens in the Differentiation of the External Genitalia and Urogenital Sinus.) Exposure to excess androgens in the male during gestation can result in subtle penile enlargement (e.g., testotoxicosis, virilizing adrenal hyperplasia).

The genitalia of females with the virilizing forms of CAH (CYP21 and CYP11B1) may exhibit a spectrum of masculinization from simple enlargement of the clitoris to complete labioscrotal fusion with a penile urethra (see Fig. 22–53).[933] In severe cases the urogenital sinus is usually preserved and serves as a common outlet for both the urethra and vagina. The hypersecretion of androgens and androgen precursors begins weeks before the 12th week of gestation, especially in patients

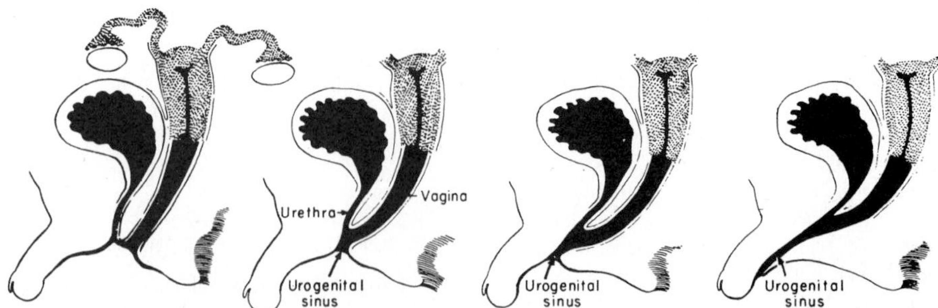

Figure 22–53. Female pseudohermaphroditism induced by prenatal exposure to androgens. Exposure after 12th fetal week leads only to clitoral hypertrophy *(diagram on left)*. Exposure at progressively earlier stages of differentiation *(depicted from left to right in drawings)* leads to retention of the urogenital sinus and labioscrotal fusion. If exposure occurs sufficiently early, the labia fuse to form a penile urethra. (From Grumbach MM, Ducharme JR. The effects of androgens on fetal sexual development: androgen-induced female pseudohermaphroditism. Fertil Steril 1960; 11:157–180. Reproduced with permission of the publisher. © The American Fertility Society.)

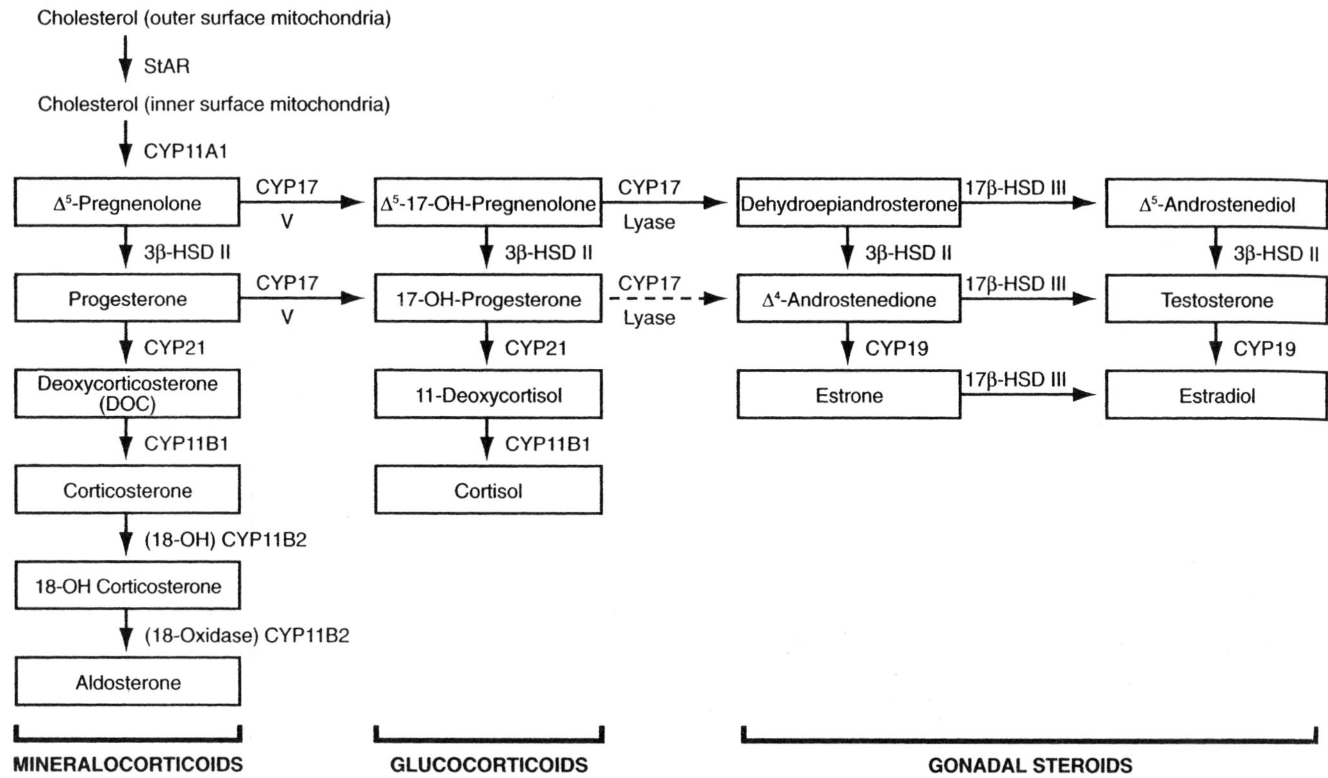

Figure 22–54. Diagram of the steroid biosynthetic pathways and the biosynthetic defects that result in congenital adrenal hyperplasia. The defect in patients with "lipoid adrenal hyperplasia" is not (except for one reported case) in the CYP11A1 (cholesterol side-chain cleavage) enzyme but in StAR, the steroidogenic acute regulatory protein. This protein is involved in the transport of cholesterol from the outer mitochondrial membrane to the inner membrane where the CYP11A1 enzyme is located. CYP11B1 (11β-hydroxylase) catalyzes 11-hydroxylation of deoxycorticosterone and 11-deoxycortisol primarily. CYP17 (17α-hydroxylase/17,20-lyase) catalyzes both 17-hydroxylation and splitting of the 17,20 bond, but for the latter it has preferential Δ^5-17,20-lyase activity (see text). CYP19 (aromatase) catalyzes the conversion of androstenedione to estrone and testosterone to estradiol. CYP11B2 (aldosterone synthetase) catalyzes the conversion of corticosterone to aldosterone. 3β-HSD I and 3β-HSD II, 3β-hydroxysteroid dehydrogenase/$\Delta^{4,5}$-isomerase types I and II; CYP21 (P450$_{c21}$), 21-hydroxylase; 17β-HSD 3, 17β-hydroxysteroid dehydrogenase type 3. In the human, deletion of or a homozygous null mutation of *CYP11A1* (P450$_{scc}$) is probably lethal in utero but a heterogeneous mutation caused congenital lipoid adrenal hyperplasia (see text).

who manifest more than simple clitoromegaly. In addition to the traditional pathway, Auchus has raised the possibility that 5α-reduced C_{21}-steroids such as 17α-hydroxyallopregnanolone may be an important substrate for conversion to dihydrotestosterone by peripheral tissues. The uterus and fallopian tubes (müllerian structures) and the ovaries are normally formed, except in rare cases. Wolffian duct development is consistently absent regardless of the degree of virilization of the external genitalia in affected females. Thus, internal genital morphogenesis corresponds to gonadal sex in both affected females and males.

Postnatally, secretion of testosterone by the adrenal gland and conversion of androstenedione to testosterone in peripheral tissues result in continued virilization of the untreated patient. In the simple virilizing form of CYP21 deficiency, the 21-hydroxylation of C_{21} 17-hydroxysteroids and 17-deoxysteroids is primarily impaired.[925, 931, 935] However, even in patients with "mild," late-onset CYP21 deficiency the 21-hydroxylation of mineralocorticoids is defective, as evidenced by elevated plasma 21-deoxycorticosterone levels after corticotropin stimulation.[935] Untreated patients with simple virilizing CYP21 deficiency usually, but not always, have normal plasma renin levels and normal aldosterone secretion rates.[936] In untreated patients, increased androgen production leads to the early appearance of pubic hair, acne, clitoromegaly (or penile enlargement in the male), increased muscular development, other signs of virilization, rapid growth during childhood, and disproportionate increase in the rate of skeletal maturation, which results in premature closure of the epiphyses and short stature in adolescence and adulthood.[925, 937]

CYP21 Deficiency with Salt Loss. In patients with severe CYP21 deficiency, both virilization and salt loss can occur. This variant, which occurs in about 75% of patients with classic CYP21 deficiency (1 in 15,000 live births),[938–940] is caused by a severe or complete defect in adrenal 21-hydroxylation that leads to impaired cortisol (adrenal fasciculata) and aldosterone (adrenal glomerulosa) secretion[925, 927–929, 931] and increased plasma renin. Electrolyte and fluid losses due to aldosterone deficiency cause hyponatremia, hyperkalemia, acidosis, dehydration, vascular collapse, and, if untreated, death.[98] About 50% of patients have the first salt-losing adrenal crisis at between 6 and 14 days of age; it is infrequent before that time. However, plasma potassium concentrations may be elevated before 6 days of age. Hypoglycemia may be an early manifestation of adrenal insufficiency. Less frequently, the "crisis" occurs as late as 6 to 12 weeks of age, usually in association with a concomitant stress. Masculinization of the external genitalia and urogenital sinus in affected females tends to be more severe in complete CYP21 deficiency than in sim-

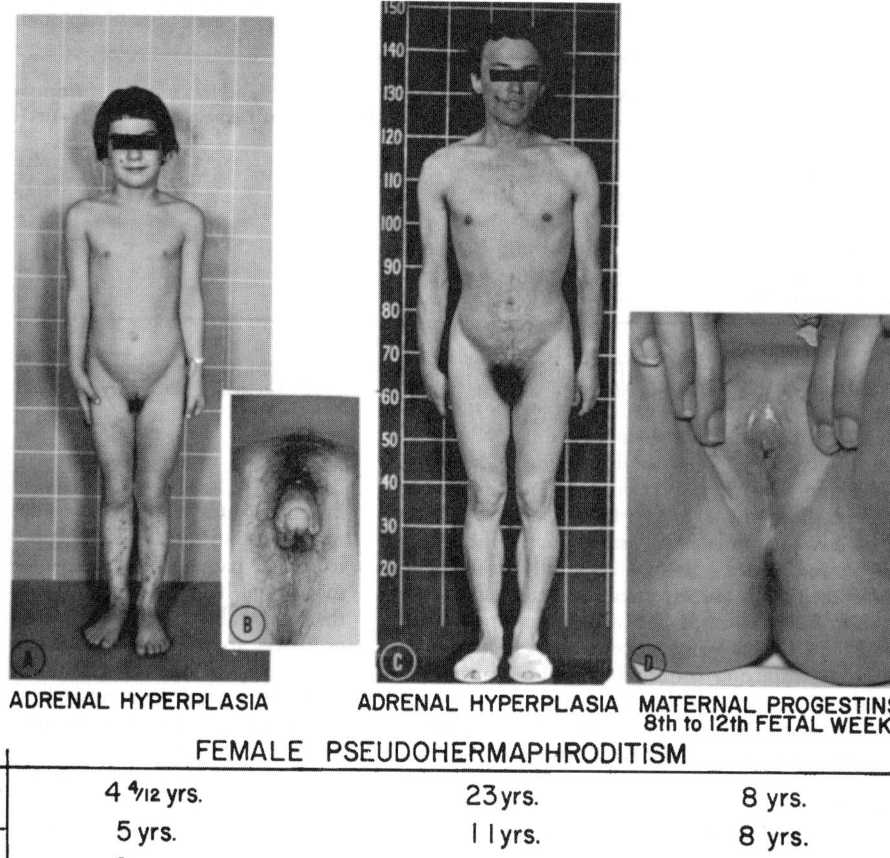

	ADRENAL HYPERPLASIA	ADRENAL HYPERPLASIA	MATERNAL PROGESTINS 8th to 12th FETAL WEEK
AGE	4 4/12 yrs.	23 yrs.	8 yrs.
HT. AGE	5 yrs.	11 yrs.	8 yrs.
BONE AGE	9 yrs.	ADULT	8 1/2 yrs.
17 K.S.	6.0 mgm / 24 hrs.	50 mgm / 24 hrs	1.8 mgm / 24 hrs.
Pregnanetriol	13.6 mgm / 24 hrs.	—	<0.5 mgm / 24 hrs.

Figure 22–60. *A* and *B*, An untreated girl with the non–salt-losing form of congenital adrenal hyperplasia. Androgens caused disproportionate acceleration of bone maturation compared with stature. *C*, Virilized adult female with non–salt-losing adrenal hyperplasia. The patient had a deep voice, shaved daily, and wore a toupee for baldness. After treatment with cortisone, her 17-ketosteroid levels fell to normal values, her breasts enlarged, she underwent a normal menarche, and hair regrew on her head. Note short stature and short extremities. *D*, Female pseudohermaphroditism caused by maternal ingestion of an oral progestational compound from the 8th to 12th week of pregnancy. Labioscrotal fusion is sufficient to obscure the vaginal orifice and create a urogenital sinus. Clitoris is enlarged. There is no progressive virilizing tendency. (*C*, from Wilkins L. The Diagnosis and Treatment of Endocrine Disorders in Childhood and Adolescence, 3rd ed. Springfield, IL, Charles C Thomas, 1965.)

adrenal rests can be reversed when glucocorticoid therapy is reinitiated.[994] In some patients, surgical ablation of enlarged adrenal rests has been indicated.[1007] Adrenal rests can be detected by ultrasonography in 30% to 50% of men with classic CAH, particularly the salt-losing form.

Noncompliant patients are at increased risk for adrenal adenoma or carcinoma[1009] and adrenal incidentalomas, which may occur in more than 70% of affected adults, including those with the nonclassic form of CAH and even heterozygotes.[1010]

It is recommended that all patients receive treatment throughout life with a glucocorticoid and, if indicated, a mineralocorticoid (Fig. 22–60; Table 22–21).

With the improved fertility rate with modern medical and surgical management of affected females, one can look forward to an increased number of successful pregnancies. When possible, these patients should be managed in a tertiary center with the facilities, personnel, and experience to care for high-risk pregnancies. It is important to use glucocorticoids that are metabolized by placental 11β-hydroxysteroid dehydrogenase II (e.g., hydrocortisone, prednisone, prednisolone, not dexamethasone). Table 22–22 contains guidelines for the care of women with classic CAH during pregnancy and delivery.[1001]

Genital surgery should not be undertaken until the parents provide informed consent after disclosure and thorough review of clinical status; issues surrounding the need for and the type of surgery, the experience and skill of the surgical team, and the surgery to be undertaken; and the options. Emerging clinical evidence suggests that the recommended time of genitoplasty is at age 2 to 6 months, especially for infants with a high proximal junction of the vagina and urethra.[507, 508, 1011, 1012] Clitoroplasty is the procedure of choice, not clitoridectomy,[507, 1013–1015] and it merits thorough consideration. If clitoroplasty is undertaken, it is essential, as indicated by long-term outcome studies,[1012, 1014] to preserve the neurovascular bundle, the glans, and surrounding skin.[396, 507, 508, 1014, 1015] In a retrospective study of cosmetic and anatomic outcomes in a selected group of women (which included those with CAH) who had feminizing genital surgery in childhood, nearly half had a poor cosmetic result and nearly all the patients needed further treatment for tampon use or intercourse.[1016] The time of revision of the vaginoplasty in adolescence is the decision of the patient and, if undertaken before 18 years of age, the patient and the family. The patient and parents must be reassured that with appropriate treatment and compliance the child will grow and

Table 22–22. Suggested Guidelines for the Management of Women with Classic Congenital Adrenal Hyperplasia Owing to 21-Hydroxylase Deficiency during Pregnancy and Delivery

Gestational Management

Adrenal Steroid Replacement and Adrenal Androgen Suppression

- Use a glucocorticoid that is metabolized by placental 11β-hydroxysteroid dehydrogenase-II (e.g., hydrocortisone, cortisone acetate, prednisone, methylprednisolone).
- Assess clinical status, serum electrolytes, and serum androgen levels regularly to determine the need for increased glucocorticoid and/or mineralocorticoid therapy. Excessive nausea, salt craving, and poor weight gain suggest adrenal steroid insufficiency. In select cases, measurement of plasma renin activity may be helpful.
- Serum testosterone and free testosterone levels should be measured every 6 weeks in the first trimester and every 6 to 8 weeks thereafter. Target free testosterone levels to the high normal range for pregnancy; however, management must be individualized for each patient. Avoid inducing cushingoid effects from too high a dose of glucocorticoids.
- Fetal gender determination by ultrasonography may be helpful in guiding treatment goals, because maternal androgen excess will have minimal effects on the male fetus.

Labor and Delivery

Stress Dose Glucocorticoid Therapy

- A soluble hydrocortisone ester (up to 50–100 mg IV every 8 hr) should be given at the initiation of active labor and continued until after delivery, followed by a rapid taper to previous maintenance doses.

Cesarean versus Vaginal Delivery

- Android pelvic characteristics may increase the risk for cephalopelvic disproportion.
- Elective cesarean section should be considered in all patients, especially those who have had reconstructive genital surgery.

Evaluation of the Infant

- Examine the infant for ambiguous genitalia. Female pseudohermaphroditism may be a consequence of either maternal hyperandrogenism or, if the father is a carrier, fetal 21-hydroxylase deficiency* (Male infants may have enlarged external genitalia.)
- If the external genitalia are ambiguous, appropriate laboratory studies in the infant should be carried out to exclude 21-hydroxylase deficiency.

*In an affected mother with 21-hydroxylase deficiency, we estimate the risk of having an affected female infant with fetal congenital adrenal hyperplasia to be approximately 1 in 240 based on an estimated 1 in 60 incidence for heterozygous individuals (see text for further details).

Adapted from Lo JC, Schwitzgebel VM, Tyrrell JB, et al. Normal female infants born of mothers with classic congenital hyperplasia due to 21-hydroxylase deficiency. J Clin Endocrinol Metab 1999; 84:930–936.

develop into a normal, functional adult. Fertility in males and feminization, menstruation, and fertility in females can be expected in the adequately treated patient. Psychological guidance and support and continuity of care are essential components of long-term management.[482, 505]

Two websites that provide highly useful, top-drawer information and guidelines for families are ⟨www.rch.unimelb.edu.au/index-ext.html⟩ and ⟨www.hopkinsmedicine.org/pediatricendocrinology/patient.html⟩.

Experimental Surgical and Medical Approaches to Treatment. For more than five decades, administration of exogenous glucocorticoids, as first shown by Lawson Wilkins in 1950, has been the keystone, along with mineralocorticoid replacement therapy, in the treatment of the virilizing forms of CAH (historical review).[985] Even though the combined regimen protects severely affected patients from adrenal crises and death, it frequently fails to adequately suppress the increased secretion of corticotropin despite supraphysiologic doses of glucocorticoids. On the other hand, glucocorticoid overdosage leads to cushingoid features that include impaired growth, excessive weight gain, and subnormal bone mineralization. Glucocorticoid doses insufficient to suppress adrenal androgens effectively are associated with progressive virilization and disproportionate advancement in skeletal maturation with premature epiphyseal closure. An effective intermediate dose cannot consistently be achieved in some patients, especially those with the severest form of CAH associated with null mutations. Adolescents and adults with this disorder who have been treated from infancy are being assessed currently in many clinics, and despite the improvement in survival, the overall results, even with acceptable compliance with the treatment, are disappointing in terms of growth, obesity, bone mineral density, and, in women, fertility, especially in those with severe CYP21 deficiency.[1017, 1018] These considerations have led to a reassessment of therapy and the proposal to test and assess surgical and novel medical treatments.[1017, 1019, 1020]

Adrenalectomy by laparoscopy is increasingly being used in a small number of centers for females with null *CYP21* gene mutations, on the basis that physiologic glucocorticoid and mineralocorticoid substitution therapy may be easier in the absence of ACTH-induced hypersecretion of abnormal amounts of androgens and estrogens and their precursors.[1017–1020] This still controversial procedure is now safely undertaken by laparoscopy and normal menses, and body composition can be restored in poorly controlled adult females.[1020, 1021] Recurrence of virilization has been reported after adrenalectomy in females, the source of androgens being ovarian or ectopic adrenal tissue.[1019, 1022]

A second experimental approach involves the use of pharmacologic agents to improve skeletal growth.[1019, 1020a, 1020b, 1020c] Trials are in progress to study the effects of third-generation aromatase inhibitors to reduce the conversion of androgens to estrogens in conjunction with an antiandrogen. The usefulness of aromatase inhibitors such as letrozole or anastrozole to block estrogen production in the periphery was suggested by the finding of delayed skeletal maturation in a man with estrogen resistance[1023] and in men and women with severe generalized aromatase (CYP19) deficiency,[358, 741, 1024] indicating a critical role for estrogen in epiphyseal maturation and fusion. Pharmacologic blockade of estrogen production and androgen action may make it possible to reduce the dose of glucocorticoid to a physiologic level. A 2-year interim analysis of a study of children with CAH given testolactone (a weak aromatase inhibitor) and flutamide (an antiandrogen) showed a reduction in the dose of hydrocortisone (8.6 mg/m^2 per day versus 13.5 mg in treated and control groups, respectively) and improved short-term growth and skeletal maturation.[1020b, 1020c] The long-term outcome of this approach and the safety of such polypharmacy for the treatment of CAH will require careful evaluation and monitoring. Experience with LHRH agonists in true precocious puberty has led to a trial in a small cohort of short CAH patients of treatment with hGH with or without an LHRH agonist; this approach improved growth velocity, and predicted final height[1025] and long-term data are awaited with interest.[1025]

Other potential future therapies may involve the application of corticotropin-releasing factor (CRF or CRH) receptor antagonists that already are showing promising results in the treatment of psychiatric disorders.[1020a] Because receptors for CRF are widely expressed, the challenge will be to use antagonists selective for the role of CRF in pituitary-adrenal function.

The management of single gene disorders such as CAH has the potential to benefit from the advances in gene therapy. Restoration of normal adrenal steroidogenesis was reported in homozygous 21-hydroxylase–deficient mice given intra-adrenal injections of an adenoviral vector encoding the genomic sequence of human CYP21.[1026] There are clearly issues to resolve not only about efficient, safe, stable, tissue-specific gene delivery systems but also about the practicalities of serial intra-adrenal injections in patients with CAH. Nevertheless, the adrenal may be a "privileged site" for gene therapy.

CYP11B1 (11β-Hydroxylase) Deficiency: Virilization with Hypertension[925, 927, 928, 1027-1030]

Cytochrome $P450_{c11}$ is located on the mitochondrial inner membrane. It serves as a terminal oxidase of an electron transport chain that includes adrenodoxin reductase and adrenodoxin. There are two distinct 11β-hydroxylase enzymes, CYP11B1 ($P450_{c11\beta}$) and CYP11B2 ($P450_{c11AS}$), encoded by two genes located in tandem at 8q21-22.[1031, 1032] The genes contain nine exons and are 93% identical.[1031] *CYP11B1* encodes 11β-hydroxylase, which converts 11-deoxycorticosterone to corticosterone and 11-deoxycortisol to cortisol,[1029] whereas *CYP11B2* encodes the enzyme aldosterone synthetase, which catalyzes the conversion of deoxycorticosterone to corticosterone and corticosterone to aldosterone. CYP11B1 has little 18-hydroxylation and 18-oxidation activity.[1029, 1030] *CYP11B1* is expressed in the zona fasciculata and is primarily under the influence of corticotropin, whereas *CYP11B2* is expressed in the zona glomerulosa and is under the control of angiotensin II and potassium.

CAH resulting from CYP11B1 deficiency was first described by Eberlein and Bongiovanni[1027] and accounts for 5% to 8% of patients with CAH, occurring in about 1 of 100,000 births of European extraction.[1029, 1030] However, there is an increased incidence of 11β-hydroxylase deficiency among Sephardic Jews from Morocco (1 in 5,000 to 1 in 7,000) and Arabs.[1033] In its classic form, CYP11B1 deficiency impairs conversion of 11-deoxycortisol to cortisol and of deoxycorticosterone (DOC, a mineralocorticoid) to corticosterone in the zona fasciculata of the adrenal gland, resulting in accumulation of these steroid precursors.[1030, 1034] The cortisol deficiency results in increased corticotropin secretion and leads to increased secretion of 11-deoxycortisol, DOC, corticosterone, and androgen by the adrenal gland. Hypertension, a hallmark of 11β-hydroxylase deficiency, occurs in approximately two thirds of patients, sometimes as early as the first few years of life.[1028] Hypertension is presumably a consequence of the excess DOC secretion, with resultant salt and water retention, and volume expansion. Classically, plasma renin activity levels are low (low renin hypertension); hypokalemia is uncommon.[1028, 1030] The presence of hypertension does not always correlate with the plasma concentration of DOC,[1029, 1030] and, contrariwise, transient salt loss has been reported in rare infants with apparent classic 11β-hydroxylase deficiency.[1035, 1036]

Excess androgen secretion in utero by the stimulated fetal adrenal gland masculinizes the external genitalia of the female fetus and causes female pseudohermaphroditism. Postnatally, untreated males and females experience progressive virilization and rapid somatic growth and skeletal maturation. Prepubertal gynecomastia can occur in untreated patients and regresses with glucocorticoid therapy.[1030]

Putative mild, late-onset, and even cryptic forms of 11β-hydroxylase deficiency have been reported.[1030, 1037-1039] These patients are born with normal genitalia and develop signs and symptoms of androgen excess in childhood, at adolescence, or as adults, but they usually do not manifest hypertension.

Molecular Genetics. Over 31 mutations in the *CYP11B1* gene have been reported associated with 11β-hydroxylase deficiency (Fig. 22-61).[1030, 1040, 1041] Most are substitutions with a small number of deletions or insertions. There appears to be some clustering in exons 6 to 8 of the gene mutations.[1030, 1040-1042] In Moroccan Jews, all affected patients are homozygous for the same mutation, Arg448His, consistent with a founder effect.[1043] This mutation is also found in other ethnic groups.[1041] Another mutation, Arg448Cys, occurs in codon 448, suggesting that this codon is a "hot spot" for mutations.[1041] Although *CYP11B1* and *CYP11B2* are closely linked homologues, both genes are functional, and gene conversions are not a cause of impaired enzyme activity.[1030] As with 21-hydroxylase deficiency, the nonsense mutations (i.e., those resulting in less enzymatic activity) would be expected to result in the more severe phenotypic manifestations. However, as in 21-hydroxylase deficiency, heterogeneity in phenotypic manifestations with the same genotype can occur.[1037]

Mutations in the CYP11B2 gene impair the conversion of DOC to aldosterone and result in hyponatremia, hyperkalemia, and failure to thrive but do not impair sex differentiation or gonadal function.[1044-1047] Two forms exist: so-called corticosterone methyl oxidase I (CMOI) deficiency, a defect in the 18-hydroxylation of corticosterone; and corticosterone methyl oxidase II (CMOII) deficiency, a defect in the 18-oxidation of 18-hydroxycorticosterone to aldosterone. Neither of these mutations affects cortisol synthesis or results in excess androgen secretion. Glucocorticoid-suppressible hyperaldosteronism and hypertension result from the fusion of the 5′ end of the *CYP11B1* gene and the 3′ end of the *CYP11B2* gene; as a consequence of this mutation, synthesis of aldosterone in the zona fasciculata is mediated by corticotropin.[1029, 1030, 1048] There is no defect in 11β-hydroxylation of deoxycortisol; hence, virilization does not occur.

Diagnosis. The diagnosis of 11β-hydroxylase deficiency is made by detecting elevated basal or corticotropin-induced 11-

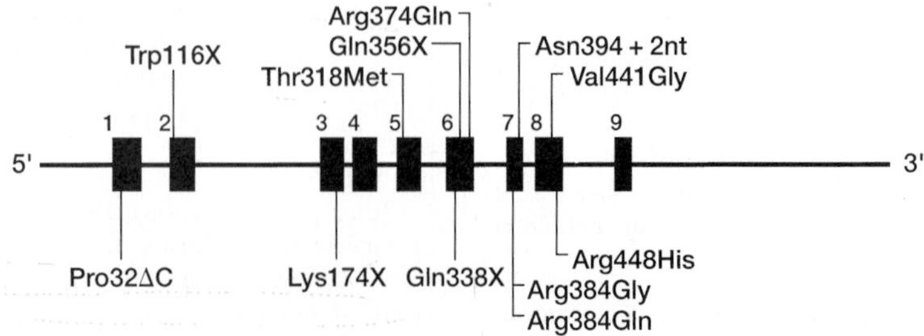

Figure 22-61. Diagram of the *CYP11B1* ($P450_{c11\beta}$) gene with representative mutations causing 11β-hydroxylase deficiency. The exons are the numbered black boxes. Missense mutations causing amino acid substitutions in the enzyme are indicated by the three-letter abbreviation for the wild-type amino acid, followed by the amino acid number in the enzyme and then by the three-letter abbreviation for the substituted amino acid. X indicates a nonsense (stop) mutation; Pro32ΔC indicates the deletion of a cytosine in the proline 32 codon, causing a frameshift; Asn394 + 2nt designates the addition of two nucleotides in the asparagine 394 codon, causing a frameshift. Mutations in *CYP11B1* are distinct from those in *CYP11B2* ($P450_{AS}$).

deoxycortisol, DOC, and corticosterone levels in plasma or measurement of tetrahydrometabolites in urine.[1030] The diagnosis should be suspected in patients who have levels of these steroids that are at least threefold higher than the 95th percentile for age.[1049] The increased secretion of the mineralocorticoid DOC produces salt and water retention and consequently results in the suppression of plasma renin activity and aldosterone. Heterozygotes for CYP11B1 deficiency do not differ from normal individuals in the response of 11-deoxycortisol, DOC, or corticosterone to the administration of corticotropin.[1050] The disorder can be detected prenatally,[1050–1052] and the masculinization of the external genitalia of affected female fetuses can be prevented by prenatal dexamethasone treatment.[1030]

Treatment. The treatment of CYP11B1 deficiency is similar to that of the non–salt-losing form of CYP21 deficiency. Cortisol suppresses corticotropin secretion and, as a consequence, corrects the increased secretion of adrenal androgens and DOC. Replacement therapy usually arrests virilization and alleviates the hypertension. However, in patients with longstanding hypertension, adjunctive therapy with antihypertensive agents may be necessary to control the hypertension. The principles concerning surgical repair of the external genitalia are similar to those relating to CAH caused by 21-hydroxylase deficiency.

3β-Hydroxysteroid Dehydrogenase/$\Delta^{4,5}$-Isomerase Deficiency[925, 928, 929, 1053, 1054]

3β-Hydroxysteroid dehydrogenase/$\Delta^{4,5}$-isomerase (3β-HSD) catalyzes the conversion of 3β-hydroxysteroids, such as Δ^5-pregnenolone, Δ^5-17-hydroxypregnenolone, DHEA, and androstenediol, into Δ^4-3-ketosteroids, such as progesterone, 17-hydroxyprogesterone, androstenedione, and testosterone, respectively. This enzyme, which is critical in the biosynthesis of progesterone, aldosterone, cortisol, estrogens, and testosterone,[1055] is expressed in the placenta, adrenals, testes, and ovaries and in peripheral tissues such as skin, adipose tissue, breast, lung, liver, and brain.[1053, 1056] There are two genes located in the chromosome 1p13.1 region that encode two different 3β-HSD isozymes.[1057] These genes, called 3β-HSD type 1 *(HSD3B1)* and 3β-HSD type 2 *(HSD3B2)*, consist of four exons and three introns and are 93% homologous.[1053, 1054, 1058, 1059] The *HSD3B1* gene is expressed predominantly in skin, mammary gland, and placenta, whereas the *HSD3B2* gene is expressed almost exclusively in the adrenal gland, testes, and ovary.[1059] Mutations in the *HSD3B2* gene are found in patients with 3β-HSD deficiency.[1054, 1060–1062] Inheritance of 3β-HSD deficiency, like that of other forms of CAH, is autosomal recessive; the presence of two defective alleles is necessary to manifest the biochemical and clinical phenotype. 3β-HSD deficiency was first described by Bongiovanni in 1962.[1063] Complete deficiency of 3β-HSD results in almost complete impairment of conversion of Δ^5-3β-hydroxysteroids to Δ^4,3-ketosteroids and thereby impairs synthesis of aldosterone and cortisol in the adrenals and of testosterone and estradiol in the gonads. In addition to cortisol and aldosterone deficiency in the neonatal period, affected females have none to slight to moderate clitoral enlargement and affected males have varying degrees of male pseudohermaphroditism with incomplete masculinization of the external genitalia. The mild virilization in affected females occurs not as a direct androgenic effect of the excess DHEA but as a result of its conversion, as well as that of other Δ^5-3β-hydroxy C_{19}-steroids, to testosterone by the 3β-HSD type I isozyme in the placenta and in the peripheral tissues of the fetus. This conversion, coupled with the limited capacity of the placenta to aromatize androgens to estrogens early in gestation,[358, 932] can lead to an increase in circulating androgens in the female fetus and in a minority of patients to modest clitoromegaly. As in CYP21 deficiency, there is considerable phenotypic heterogeneity. A non–salt-wasting form of 3β-HSD type II deficiency, caused by less severe defects in enzyme synthesis,[1061, 1062, 1064–1066] and a putative nonclassic, late-onset form have been described.[927, 1062, 1067] As in CYP21 deficiency, various mutations can result in phenotypic heterogeneity.[1062, 1066, 1067]

In general, patients with the classic form of 3β-HSD deficiency, including salt wasting, are homozygotes or compound heterozygotes for point mutations, including nonsense, frameshift, and missense mutations in *HSD3B2* that essentially abolish 3β-HSD activity (null mutations) in the adrenals and gonads (Fig. 22–62).[1054, 1062, 1063] More than 29 different mutations are now described. Patients with the non–salt-losing form of 3β-HSD deficiency are homozygotes or compound heterozygotes principally for missense mutations that result in 1% to 10% of the normal activity of the enzyme in assays in transfected cultured cells (see Fig. 22–57).[1054, 1062] As in CYP21 deficiency, minimal enzymatic activity apparently is sufficient for aldosterone synthesis and the prevention of salt wasting. Except for the one female patient who had an Ala82Thr mutation associated with premature pubarche, no mutation has been detected in either the *HSD3B1* or the *HSD3B2* gene in the females reported with premature pubarche and/or hirsutism and putative late onset or nonclassic 3β-HSD deficiency.[927, 1054, 1066, 1068]

After many years of speculation about the existence of and the laboratory criteria for the diagnosis of a less severe or nonclassic variant of 3β-HSD deficiency, the issue has been clarified by the studies of Pang and her associates.[1069] The HSD3B2 genotype was studied in 55 patients (including girls with premature pubarche) suspected of this mild variant. The patients with or lacking deleterious homozygous or compound heterozygous mutations had a variety of plasma Δ^5-17α-hydroxypregnenolone and the Δ^5 C_{19}- and C_{21}-steroids determined before and after an intravenous bolus of ACTH across the age span. The most useful hormonal determinations were the effect of ACTH on plasma Δ^5-17α-hydroxypregnenolone/cortisol ratio after ACTH. In the patients with *HSD3B2* mutations the mean SD above the values obtained in individuals who lacked mutations varied from +5 SD in infants to +221 SD in adults. This study has simplified the hormonal work-up for individuals suspected of having mild 3β-HSD deficiency.[1069]

The fact that the peripheral 3β-HSD type I enzyme has a 10-fold higher affinity for substrate than the 3β-HSD type II enzyme could facilitate Δ^4-steroid synthesis from lower concentrations of Δ^5-precursors. Mutations in the *HSD3B1* gene have not yet been reported and may be lethal, because the *HSD3B1* gene is expressed in the placenta and is probably essential for placental progesterone synthesis. Three human 3β-HSD pseudogenes have been identified.[1062]

Diagnosis. The plasma levels of 17-hydroxypregnenolone, DHEA and its sulfate (DHEAS), and other C_{21}- and C_{19}-steroids with a Δ^5-3β-hydroxy configuration are elevated in affected patients. Of note, the plasma concentration of 17-hydroxyprogesterone may be increased as a result of peripheral conversion of Δ^5-17-hydroxypregnenolone to 17-hydroxyprogesterone by the type I enzyme. However, after an intravenous bolus of ACTH the plasma concentration of Δ^5-17-hydroxypregnenolone and the plasma Δ^5-17-hydroxypregnenolone/cortisol ratio are strikingly elevated in patients with 3β-HSD deficiency.[1062, 1069] The excretion of urinary 17-ketosteroids, especially DHEAS and 16-hydroxy DHEAS, is elevated. Suppression of the increased plasma and urinary levels of C_{19}- and C_{21}-3β-hydroxysteroids by glucocorticoids distinguishes 3β-HSD deficiency from a virilizing adrenal tumor. Therapy is similar to that for patients with CYP21 deficiency. The risk of death from adrenal insufficiency is high in infants with the severe form of this disorder.

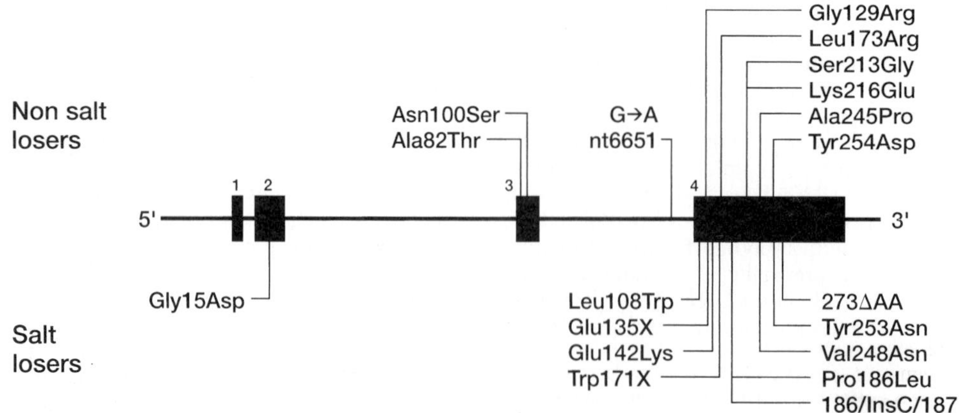

Figure 22–62. Diagram of the 3β-hydroxysteroid dehydrogenase type 2 *(HSD3B2)* gene with selected mutations that result in 3β-HSD deficiency. The numbered solid boxes indicate the exons. Missense mutations causing amino acid substitutions in the enzyme are indicated by the three-letter abbreviation for the wild-type amino acid, followed by the amino acid number in the enzyme and then the three-letter abbreviation for the substituted amino acid. X indicates a nonsense (stop) mutation. G→A, nt6651 is a guanine-to-adenine transition at nucleotide 6651 in intron 3 that creates a new splice junction. 186/InsC/187 is a single-nucleotide cytosine insertion after codon 186 (proline) that changes the reading frame and causes an aberrant 16-amino-acid sequence before a stop codon. 273ΔAA is a deletion of two adenines in codon 273 (AAA), which encodes lysine. This deletion causes a frameshift resulting in a premature termination at residue 279 and results in a truncated protein 94 amino acids shorter than the wild type. Mutations with less than 1% 3β-HSD activity are indicated below the gene and cause salt loss. Missense and splicing mutations, indicated above the gene, result in 2% to 4.7% enzymatic activity and are associated with the non–salt-losing phenotype.

CYP17 (17α-Hydroxylase/17,20-Lyase) Deficiency: Male Pseudohermaphroditism, Sexual Infantilism, Hypertension, and Hypokalemic Alkalosis

A single microsomal enzyme, CYP17 ($P450_{c17}$), catalyzes (1) the 17α-hydroxylation of pregnenolone and progesterone (17α-hydroxylase activity) and (2) the side-chain cleavage of 17-hydroxypregnenolone to DHEA and, much less effectively in the human, the conversion of 17-hydroxyprogesterone to androstenedione (17,20-lyase activity) in both the adrenal gland and the gonads.[1070, 1071] The $P450_{c17}$ system has a central role in human steroidogenesis; it is referred to as the qualitative regulator of steroidogenesis.[1072] In contrast to the rat and the pig, the human and bovine $P450_{c17}$ enzymes preferentially convert 17-hydroxypregnenolone to DHEA (Δ^5-17,20-lyase activity)[1073] and have very poor Δ^4-17,20-lyase activity[1074]; the human Δ^5-17,20-lyase is about 50 times more efficient than the Δ^4-17,20-lyase.[1075] This enzyme also has significant 16α-hydroxylase activity. The enzyme is bound to the smooth endoplasmic reticulum where it accepts electrons from a specific flavoprotein, NADPH–P450 oxidoreductase. The gene *CYP17*, which encodes the enzyme, is approximately 13 kb long, contains eight exons, is located on chromosome 10 at 10q24q25,[1071, 1076, 1077] and is expressed in the adrenals and gonads, but not in the placenta or in ovarian granulosa cells.

Two types of enzymatic deficiency causing this rare form of CAH have been reported: (1) combined deficiency of 17α-hydroxylase and 17,20-lyase; and (2) isolated 17,20-lyase deficiency. The combined form is most common (discussed in the section on male pseudohermaphroditism). However, rare patients with putative isolated 17,20-lyase deficiency have been described.[1072] Women with 17,20-lyase deficiency would be expected to have sexual infantilism with lack of adrenarche and elevated gonadotropins at puberty resulting from an inability to synthesize both androgens and estrogens in the adrenals and gonads. In contrast to 17α-hydroxylase deficiency, there should be no defect in cortisol synthesis and no mineralocorticoid (DOC) excess and hypertension.[1078] Studies on a patient with combined 17α-hydroxylase and 17,20-lyase deficiency demonstrated another defect: the absence of 16-ene-synthetase activity, which resulted in impaired conversion of pregnenolone to a C_{19}-steroid sex pheromone precursor and suggests that CYP17 affects 16-ene-synthetase activity in the gonads.[1079]

17α-Hydroxylase deficiency is a rare autosomal recessive disorder that occurs in approximately 1 in 50,000 individuals. More than 130 cases have been reported. It was initially reported by Biglieri and colleagues in 46,XX females who had low renin hypertension, hypokalemia, and sexual infantilism.[1080] Subsequently, this defect was described in 46,XY male infants, children, and adults with pseudohermaphroditism.[1072, 1081–1087] A defect in 17α-hydroxylation in both the adrenal cortex and gonads results in impaired synthesis of 17-hydroxyprogesterone and 17-hydroxypregnenolone and thus of cortisol, androgens, and estrogens. Decreased cortisol synthesis causes increased corticotropin secretion, which results in excessive secretion of 17-deoxysteroids by the adrenal cortex, including the mineralocorticoid DOC, corticosterone, and 18-hydroxycorticosterone. Excess DOC secretion leads to hypertension, hypokalemic alkalosis, suppression of the renin-angiotensin system, and, secondarily, diminished aldosterone synthesis and secretion in most reported patients. Corticosterone is a weak glucocorticoid; the high plasma concentrations in this disorder prevent the signs and symptoms of cortisol deficiency and modulate the secretion of corticotropin.[1088]

The phenotypic manifestations are a consequence of the biochemical defects in adrenal and gonadal steroid biosynthesis. 17α-Hydroxylase deficiency is usually recognized at the time of expected puberty in the female because of the presence of hypertension and/or hypokalemia associated with hypergonadotropic hypogonadism (and, in the male, pseudohermaphroditism).[1081] Affected 46,XX females have normal female internal and external genital tracts, but the ovaries cannot secrete estrogens at puberty, resulting in sexual infantilism and hypogonadism with elevated plasma FSH and LH levels. In addition, the lack of adrenal and ovarian androgens can result in little or no growth of pubic and axillary hair. In affected 46,XX individuals the ovaries have a high proportion of atretic follicles and some ovaries contain an increased number of enlarged follicular cysts. (For manifestations in 46,XY males, see

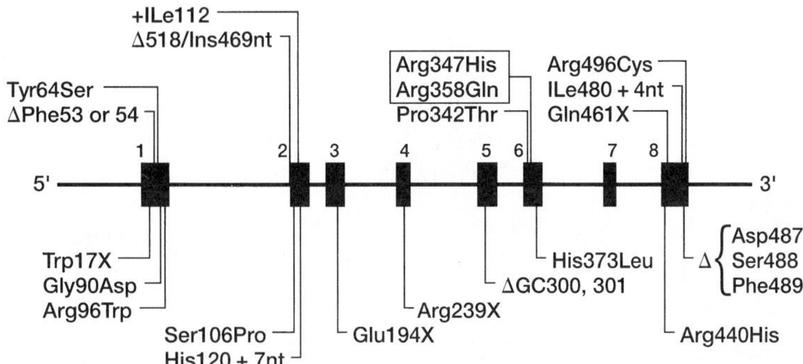

Figure 22–63. Diagram of selected mutations in the *CYP17* gene (17α-hydroxylase/17,20-lyase deficiency). The exons are the numbered black boxes. Missense mutations causing amino acid substitutions in the enzyme are indicated by the three-letter abbreviation for the wild-type amino acid, followed by the amino acid number in the enzyme and the three-letter abbreviation for the substituted amino acid. X indicates a nonsense (stop) mutation. ΔPhe53 or 54 is a deletion of phenylalanine at codon 53 or 54. Δ518/Ins469nt is a deletion of 518 nucleotides and an insertion of 469 nucleotides. His120 + 7nt is a seven-nucleotide duplication at codon 120 (histidine). +ILe112 is a duplication of isoleucine at codon 112. ΔGC300,301 is a deletion of two nucleotides, guanine and cytosine, at codon 300 and 301. ILe480 + 4nt is a four-nucleotide duplication (cytosine-adenine-thymidine-cytosine) at codon 480. ΔAsp487, Ser488, Phe489 indicates a deletion of aspartic acid (codon 487), serine (codon 488), and phenylalanine (codon 489). All of these mutations cause 17α-hydroxylase deficiency. Missense mutations at codons 347 and 358 *(indicated by the box)* have been associated with "isolated" 17,20-lyase deficiency.

the section on male pseudohermaphroditism.) In patients with mild defects in CYP17, hypertension may not be present and aldosterone secretion may be normal[1081, 1082] or even elevated.[1087] Ten to 15 percent of reported patients are neither hypertensive nor hypotensive.[1087] Corticosterone levels, which are usually 50- to 100-fold higher than normal, provide adequate glucocorticoid effects and prevent symptoms of cortisol deficiency.

The *CYP17* gene has been studied in many patients, and more than 22 different mutations have been identified in its coding region (Fig. 22–63).[1072, 1073, 1080–1091] Complete absence of 17α-hydroxylase/17,20-lyase activity has resulted from a variety of mutations, including single base-pair changes resulting in missense mutations, duplications, deletions, and premature translational termination.[1072, 1073, 1089, 1090] These mutations, except for one reported in Mennonite kindreds and one in Micronesian patients, appear to be random.[1073, 1089] The most common mutation is the four base-pair duplication in exon 8, shared by Mennonites and individuals in the Friesland region of the Netherlands, which is attributed to a founder effect originating in Friesland.[1091] The mutations in the *CYP17* gene that result in complete loss of 17α-hydroxylase activity provide strong evidence that only one enzyme has 17α-hydroxylase activity.

Patients with partial combined deficiencies of both activities have been analyzed.[1089, 1092, 1093] 46,XX females with homozygous deletions of the phenylalanine codon at amino acid 53 or 54 in exon 1 had regular menses.[1089] This mild mutation in *CYP17* did result in increased levels of DOC and/or corticosterone in blood, as well as suppressed plasma renin activity.[1092] A 46,XY male with this same mutation had only hypospadias and cryptorchidism.[1093] Another 46,XY male with ambiguous genitalia was a compound heterozygote with a stop codon (TGA) at amino acid position 239 in exon 4 (a null mutation) on one allele and a missense mutation on the other allele that changes a proline to threonine at amino acid 342 (Pro342Thr) in exon 6.[1089] This patient had 20% of normal 17α-hydroxylase activity in transfected cells.[1089, 1092] Analysis of these patients suggests that 5% of normal activity in a 46,XX female is sufficient to allow estrogen production with normal secondary sexual characteristics and irregular menses,[1089, 1092] whereas more than 25% of normal activity appears to be necessary to achieve normal virilization of the external genitalia of affected 46,XY males.[1089, 1092]

Diagnosis. 17α-Hydroxylase/17,20-lyase deficiency should be considered in all patients with ambiguous genitalia and hypergonadotropic hypogonadism and in all phenotypic females with or without sexual infantilism, including absent adrenarche, who have hypertension and hypokalemic alkalosis. Elevated levels of 17-deoxy-C_{21}-steroids such as progesterone, pregnenolone, DOC, and corticosterone in plasma and increased urinary excretion of their metabolites establish the diagnosis. The basal plasma concentrations of DOC, corticosterone, 18-hydroxycorticosterone, and 18-hydroxy-DOC and their response to a corticotropin challenge can be used to discriminate among homozygous, heterozygous, and unaffected individuals.[1094, 1095]

Glucocorticoid therapy for 21-hydroxylase deficiency suppresses DOC and corticosterone secretion. With suppression of the excess circulating mineralocorticoids, the blood pressure and serum potassium level return to normal. At puberty, both affected males and affected females usually require gonadal steroid replacement.

StAR Deficiency (Congenital Lipoid Adrenal Hyperplasia): Male Pseudohermaphroditism, Sexual Infantilism, and Adrenal Insufficiency

This autosomal recessive form of CAH is associated with severe glucocorticoid and mineralocorticoid deficiency, in which no C_{18}-, C_{19}-, or C_{21}-steroids are elaborated by the adrenal glands or gonads because of failure to convert cholesterol to pregnenolone.[1113, 1114] This disorder is the most severe genetic defect in steroidogenesis.[1096–1098, 1112–1114] Affected males have female external genitalia with a blind vaginal pouch and absent müllerian derivatives. Females with this disorder have normal internal and external genital differentiation. Clinical manifestations of adrenal insufficiency, including hyponatremia, hypokalemia, acidosis, dehydration, and hypoglycemia, usually become apparent in the first few weeks of life, but survival for months without therapy has been described.[1099, 1100, 1108, 1112] Hyperpigmentation is common, and respiratory distress occurs in about one fourth of neonates. On ultrasonography, CT, or MRI, markedly enlarged, lipid-laden adrenals displace the kidneys downward.

Most of the more than 80 patients with StAR deficiency are of Japanese and Korean origin[1097–1112]; it is second to CYP21 deficiency in prevalence in Japan and Korea. There is an unexplained 3:1 male/female sex ratio.[1101] Many affected individuals

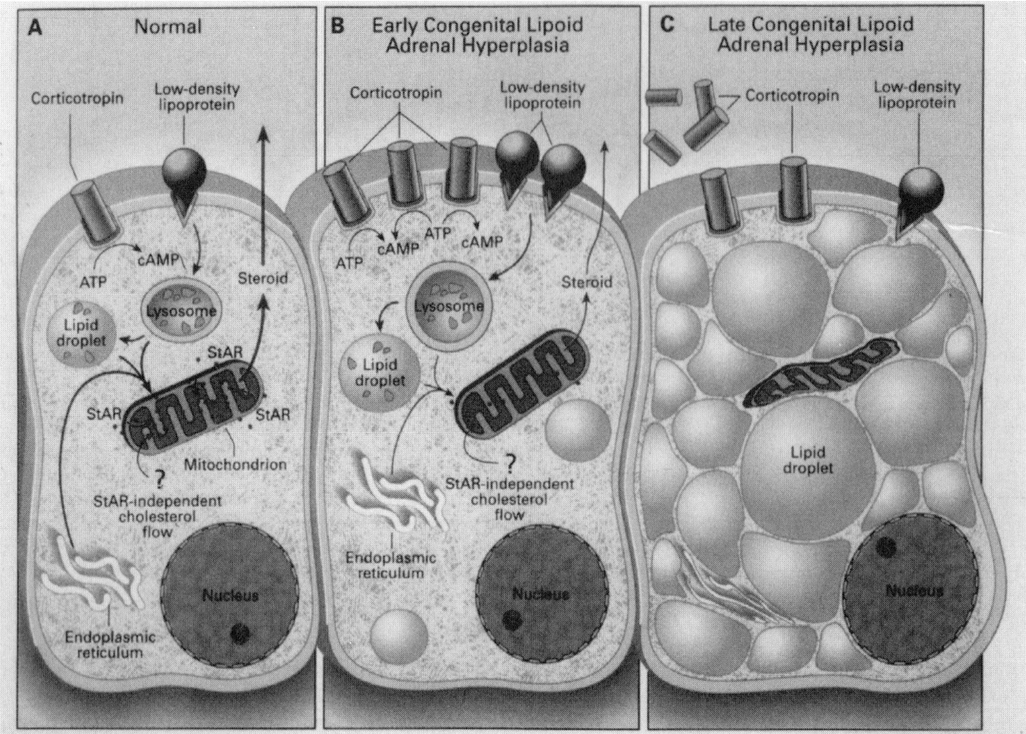

Figure 22–64. Model of the steroid-synthesizing cell (adrenal/gonadal) showing conversion of cholesterol to steroids (see Color Plates). *A*, Cholesterol from low-density lipoprotein, from cholesterol esters stored in lipid droplets, and from endogenous synthesis in the endoplasmic reticulum is transported from the outer mitochondrial membrane to the inner membrane. This transport, which is a rate-limiting step in steroid synthesis, is facilitated by StAR (steroidogenic acute regulatory protein) as well as by other, StAR-independent mechanisms. In the mitochondria, steroid synthesis then ensues as a result of the conversion of cholesterol to Δ^5-pregnenolone by the enzyme CYP11A1 ($P450_{scc}$). *B*, In patients with congenital lipoid adrenal hyperplasia, a mutation in the gene encoding StAR results in little or no activity of the mutant StAR, causing greatly diminished cholesterol transport into the mitochondria. Low levels of steroidogenesis via mechanisms independent of StAR can occur; however, increased ACTH (LH/FSH) secretion results in cholesterol accumulation in the cells as lipid droplets. *C*, Continued stimulation and resultant accumulation of cholesterol causes engorgement of these cells, with both mechanical and chemical perturbation of the cell function. Females with congenital lipoid adrenal hyperplasia feminize at puberty and menstruate but have progressive hypergonadotropic hypogonadism. It has been hypothesized by Bose and co-workers that this occurs because the follicular cells are relatively quiescent in utero and before puberty; hence, they are undamaged. At the beginning of each cycle, they are recruited, and a small amount of estradiol can be produced as a result of StAR-independent mechanisms. This can occur until the follicular cells are engorged and rendered nonfunctional. (From Bose HS, Sujiwara T, Strauss JF III, Miller WL. The pathophysiology and genetics of congenital lipoid adrenal hyperplasia. N Engl J Med 1996; 335:1870–1878. Copyright 1996, Massachusetts Medical Society. All rights reserved.) (See text.)

die in infancy (approximately one third survive with replacement therapy); we have cared for one patient for more than 30 years.[1101]

In contrast to the severe fetal and postnatal testosterone deficiency in affected 46,XY individuals, surviving affected 46,XX females can enter puberty and menstruate; they later develop polycystic ovaries and progressive ovarian failure.[1099, 1112] The prolonged survival described in a few patients before the onset of adrenal insufficiency and the puberty and menses described in females have been perplexing.[1099] As proposed by Bose, two separate events seem responsible for these phenomena.[1099] The first event is the loss of steroid hormone synthesis, which is dependent on StAR in steroid-producing cells.[1099] The second event is the accumulation of cholesterol, which cannot be converted to pregnenolone by the cell. Eventually this accumulation engorges the cell and results in disruption of the structural and functional integrity of the cell.[1099] It is assumed that the functional activity of the cell in question mediates the time course to functional and structural disruption. Hence, postnatal survival for a period of time may reflect the relatively low level of activity of the definitive adrenal glands prenatally. Postnatally, the zona glomerulosa and fasciculata can make a limited amount of steroids independent of StAR until they become engorged and dysfunctional.[1099] The ovaries, in contrast to the testes, remain relatively quiescent through fetal life and childhood. At puberty, estrogen synthesis independent of StAR can occur, leading to feminization and menses.[1099, 1109, 1110] Progressive gonadal failure due to cholesterol engorgement of steroidogenic cells then results (Fig. 22–64; see also Color Plates).[1099, 1109, 1110] In support of the two-hit hypothesis, no surviving XY patient has had evidence of testicular function at the expected age of puberty. All patients are markedly pigmented. The StAR knockout mouse has a similar phenotype to patients with congenital lipoid adrenal hyperplasia, consistent with the two-hit hypothesis model.[1110a]

The transfer of cholesterol from the outer to the inner mitochondrial membrane is the rate-limiting step in acute or rapid steroid synthesis.[1113, 1114, 1118–1122] A 30-kd mitochondrial protein in adrenal cells rapidly increases in response to corticotropin stimulation and is inhibited by cyclohexamide; it is

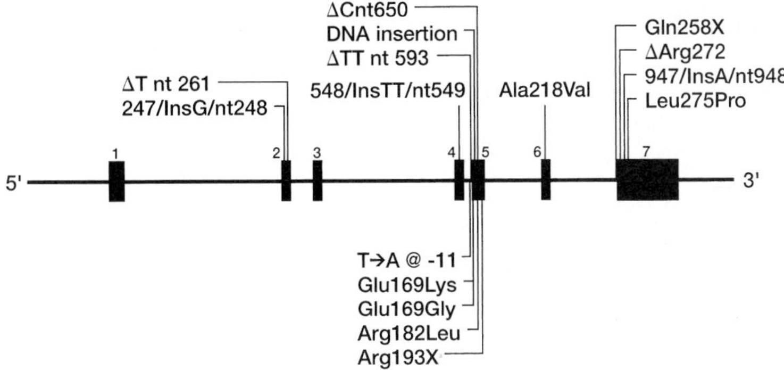

Figure 22–65. Diagram of the selected mutations identified in the StAR gene associated with congenital lipoid adrenal hyperplasia. Nucleotide (nt) and amino acid numbers are given according to the cDNA sequence. Missense mutations causing amino acid substitutions are indicated by the three-letter abbreviation for the wild-type amino acid, followed by the amino acid number in the protein and the three-letter abbreviation for the substituted amino acid. X indicates a nonsense (stop) mutation. 247/InsG/nt248 is an insertion of a guanine causing a frameshift between nucleotides 247 and 248. ΔT nt261 is a deletion of a thymidine at nucleotide 261. 548/InsTT/nt549 is an insertion of two thymidines in exon 4 between nucleotides 548 and 549, causing a frameshift. ΔTT nt593 is a deletion of two thymidines at nucleotide 593, causing a frameshift. ΔCnt650 is a deletion of a cytosine at nucleotide 650, causing a frameshift. T→A @ − 11 is a thymidine-to-adenine transition minus 11 nucleotides (5′) from the intron 4/exon 5 junction. 947/InsA/nt948 is the insertion of an adenine between nucleotides 947 and 948, which results in a frameshift. (Data from Bose H, Sugawara T, Stauss JF, Miller WL. The pathophysiology and genetics of congenital lipoid adrenal hyperplasia. N Engl J Med 1996; 335:1870–1878.)

also present in the gonads.[1114, 1120–1122] The cDNA for this factor has been cloned, and the protein transcript for this gene was named the *s*teroidogenic *a*cute *r*egulatory (StAR) protein.[1120, 1121] As with other steroid hormone hydroxylases, the StAR gene is transcriptionally regulated by SF1.[1122] The stimulation of StAR by corticotropin and by LH is mediated through a cyclic adenosine monophosphate (AMP)/protein kinase A–dependent pathway and involves the phosphorylation of the StAR protein.[1112, 1122] The stimulation of cholesterol transport by StAR from the outer to the inner mitochondrial membrane, the site of the cholesterol side-chain cleavage complex, apparently does not require the import of StAR across the mitochondrial membrane.[1123] Human StAR is encoded by a gene on chromosome 8p11.2 and is expressed in the adrenal gland and gonad, but not in the placenta or the central nervous system.[1108, 1114, 1121, 1122, 1124, 1125] Fifty-seven patients with congenital lipoid adrenal hyperplasia (studied from 10 countries) had mutations in the gene encoding StAR (Fig. 22–65).[1099, 1112, 1115] In 80% of affected alleles from affected Japanese and Korean individuals, a Gln258Stop mutation was detected, whereas an Arg182Leu mutation was present in 78% of alleles from affected Arabs.[800] Study of congenital lipoid adrenal hyperplasia provided the decisive evidence of the critical role of StAR in steroid hormone biosynthesis in humans. Unlike *CYP11A1*, the gene encoding the StAR protein is not expressed in the human placenta, and mutations in StAR do not impair progesterone synthesis by the placenta.

In patients with StAR deficiency, little or no C_{18}-, C_{19}-, and C_{21}-steroids are detectable in plasma or urine, even after corticotropin stimulation. In 46,XX females the differential diagnosis includes congenital adrenal hyperplasia. Demonstration of greatly enlarged adrenals in StAR deficiency by imaging techniques readily differentiates these two entities, although one patient with a frameshift mutation had unexpected small adrenal glands on imaging.[1115] Affected males are raised as females, and their functionless testes are removed to reduce the risk of malignant transformation and for cosmetic reasons. Therapy requires replacement with glucocorticoids and mineralocorticoids and the addition of estrogen when gonadal failure ensues.

In obligate heterozygotes with a StAR mutation, unlike heterozygotes with other forms of CAH, steroid responses to corticotropin are normal.[1107] Prenatal diagnosis of StAR deficiency was successfully demonstrated in a family with two previously affected children.[1107] Amniotic fluid levels of progesterone and pregnenolone were 30% and 50% of normal, respectively, but the concentrations of steroids such as 17-hydroxyprogesterone, cortisol, DHEA, androstenedione, and estradiol were low or undetectable.[1107] Absent fetal steroidogenesis and subsequent failure to synthesize fetal adrenal precursors for transformation to estrogens by the placenta result in low maternal plasma and urine estriol values.

The clinical manifestations of each form of CAH are summarized in Table 22–23.

Congenital Lipoid Adrenal Hyperplasia Caused by a Heterozygous Mutation in CYP11A1 ($P450_{scc}$). Initially it was thought that congenital lipoid hyperplasia was caused by a mutation in *CYP11A1* ($P450_{scc}$), the gene encoding the cholesterol side-chain cleavage enzyme, until studies of the StAR protein were performed.[1103, 1104, 1106] A homozygous *CYP11A1* gene deletion has been discovered in the rabbit, which causes congenital lipoid adrenal hyperplasia in this species.[1116] It was thought that because side-chain cleavage of cholesterol in the primate is essential for the placental synthesis of progesterone and therefore the maintenance of pregnancy, mutations in the gene encoding the CYP11A1 enzyme may be incompatible with sustained human pregnancy. (In the rabbit the corpus luteum, not the placenta, is the source of progesterone.) However, a late-onset form of congenital lipoid adrenal hyperplasia has now been reported in a 46,XY phenotypic female with isolated clitoromegaly and symptomatic but mild adrenal insufficiency (sex reversal) associated with a heterozygous two amino acid in-frame insertion mutation in the *CYP11A1* gene.[1117] There was no dominant negative effect of this mutation in a functional enzyme assay so a form of haploinsufficiency may lead to a later onset of adrenal failure mechanistically similar to the two-hit model of StAR deficiency. Unlike patients with mutations in both alleles of the StAR gene, the $P450_{scc}$ haploinsufficient patient had a later age at onset of the adrenal insufficiency and did not exhibit the characteristic large adrenal glands.

Table 22–23. Clinical Manifestations of Various Types of Congenital Adrenal Hyperplasia

Gene	*StAR*‡		*HSD3B2*		*CYP17*		*CYP11B1*		*CYP 21*	
Enzymatic defect	(no defect)		3β-HSD 2		P-450$_{c17}$ (17α-Hydroxylase)		P-450$_{c11}$ (11β-Hydroxylase)		P-450$_{c21}$ (21α-Hydroxylase)	
Chromosomal sex	XX	XY	XX	XY	XX	XY	XX	XY	XX	XY
External genitalia	Female	Female	Female (clitoromegaly)	Ambiguous	Female	Female or ambiguous	Ambiguous	Male	Ambiguous	Male
Postnatal virilization	–*	–†	±	Mild to moderate	–	±	+		+	
Addisonian crises	+		±		–		–		+ in 80%	
Hypertension	–		–		+		±		–	

*At puberty, female secondary sex characteristics develop, followed by ovarian failure.
†Sexual infantalism at puberty.
‡StAR mutations impair transport of cholesterol to the inner mitochondrial membrane and thus by substrate deprivation impair steroid biogenesis; the disorder leads as well to storage of lipid in the cells of the adrenal and gonad—congenital lipoid adrenal hyperplasia.

Placental Aromatase Deficiency

Aromatase (CYP19, cytochrome P450$_{arom}$, formerly estrogen synthetase) catalyzes the conversion of testosterone to estradiol and androstenedione to estrone in many tissues, including the gonads, placenta, brain, liver, and adipose tissue.[1126] Placental aromatase deficiency causes female pseudohermaphroditism. Only one *CYP19* gene has been isolated; its tissue-specific expression is mediated by tissue-specific promoters using alternative promoter choice, but the protein translated is the same in all tissues.[1126]

Description of female pseudohermaphroditism occurring in five 46,XX females as a result of autosomal recessive inheritance of mutations in the *CYP19* gene illustrates the critical role that this enzyme plays in protecting the fetus from excess androgen exposure in utero.[358, 932, 1127–1131] The placenta lacks CYP17 enzymatic activity and thus cannot convert C$_{21}$-steroids such as progesterone to C$_{19}$-steroids and thereafter to estrogens.[1132] During gestation, large quantities of DHEAS are produced in the fetal adrenal gland and by the maternal adrenal. DHEAS is 16α-hydroxylated in the fetal adrenal and liver. 16α-Hydroxy-DHEAS from the fetus and DHEAS from the fetus and mother are transferred to the placental unit, where the sulfate moiety is cleaved by placental sulfatase. These steroids can then be converted to androstenedione and 16α-hydroxyandrostenedione by 3β-HSD type I $\Delta^{4,5}$-isomerase, to testosterone and 16α-hydroxytestosterone by 17β-HSD, and to estrogens (mainly estriol from 16α-hydroxy-DHEA) by placental aromatase (Fig. 22–66). Androstenedione and 16α-hydroxyandrostenedione may be directly aromatized to estrogens.[1133] In the absence of aromatase, estrogen cannot be synthesized by the placenta, and large quantities of placental testosterone and androstenedione are transferred to the fetal and maternal circulation, resulting in masculinization of the urogenital sinus and of the genital tubercle of the female fetus and virilization of the mother during pregnancy. Putative CYP19 deficiency has been described in the spotted hyena, which provides, in part, an explanation for the strikingly masculinized external genitalia and aggressive behavior of the female spotted hyena.[358, 1134]

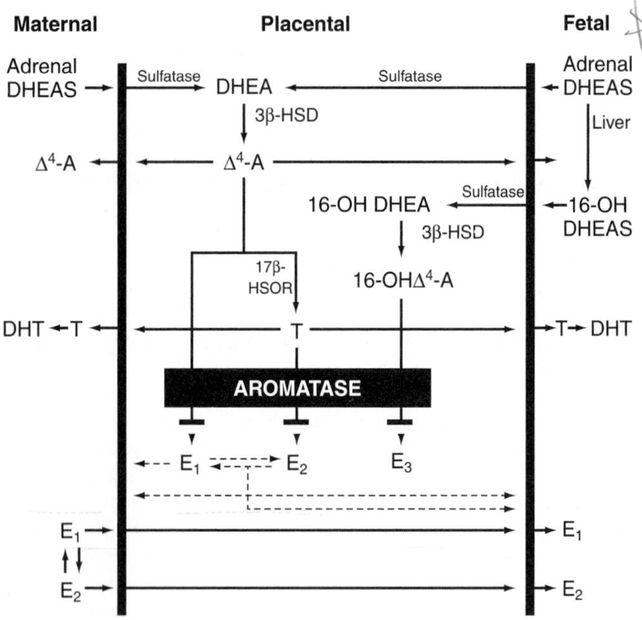

Figure 22–66. The biosynthetic defects in converting C$_{19}$-steroids (androgens, androgen precursors) to C$_{18}$-steroids (estrogens) in the CYP19 (P450$_{arom}$)-deficient fetal placental unit. 3β-HSD, 3β-hydroxysteroid dehydrogenase/$\Delta^{4,5}$-isomerase; 17β-HSD, 17β-hydroxysteroid dehydrogenase; DHEA, dehydroepiandrosterone; DHEAS, DHEA sulfate; DHT, dihydrotestosterone; T, testosterone; Δ^4-A, androstenedione; E$_1$, estrone; E$_2$, estradiol; E$_3$, estriol. (Modified and redrawn from Conte FA, Grumbach MM, Ito Y, et al. A syndrome of female pseudohermaphrodism, hypergonadotropic hypogonadism, and multicystic ovaries associated with missense mutations in the gene encoding aromatase (P450$_{arom}$). J Clin Endocrinol Metab 1994; 78:1287–1292. © 1994, The Endocrine Society.)

Affected females are born with clitoromegaly, varying degrees of posterior fusion, scrotalization of the labioscrotal folds, and, in some infants with a urogenital sinus, a single

Table 22–24. Clinical Features of CYP19 (P450$_{arom}$) Deficiency in the Female

Karyotype:	46,XX
Inheritance:	Autosomal recessive
Maternal history:	Virilization of mother during pregnancy
Genitalia:	Ambiguous or female with clitoriomegaly
Wolffian duct derivatives:	Absent
Müllerian duct derivatives:	Present
Gonads:	Ovaries: multicystic in infancy and postpubertally
Habitus:	Tall stature and virilization at puberty Severe estrogen deficiency with increased plasma gonadotropins in infancy and at puberty Polycystic ovaries Increased plasma androstenedione and testosterone Delayed bone age; osteoporosis Normal psychosocial orientation Response to estrogen therapy

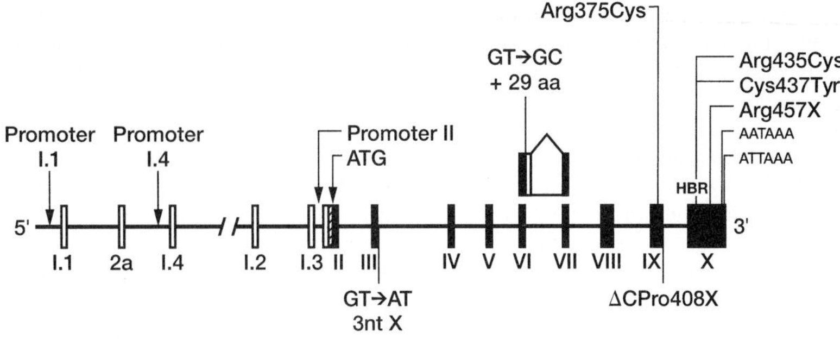

Figure 22–67. Diagram of the *CYP19* ($P450_{arom}$) gene and selected mutations causing aromatase deficiency. The numbered black boxes represent translated exons. The septum in the open box in exon II represents the 3′ acceptor splice junction for the untranslated exons. The multiple alternate promoters and the untranslated exons *(open boxes)* are indicated. Missense mutations causing amino acid substitutions in the enzyme are indicated by the three-letter abbreviation for the wild-type amino acid, followed by the amino acid number in the enzyme and the three-letter abbreviation for the substituted amino acid. X indicates a nonsense (stop) mutation. GT→AT 3nt X is a guanine-to-adenine transition at the splice junction between exon 3 and intron 3, resulting in a stop codon (X) three nucleotides downstream (3′). GT→GC + 29 aa is a thymidine-to-cytosine transition at the splice junction between exon 6 and intron 6, giving rise to a 29-amino-acid insert in the protein. ΔCPro408X, a deletion of a cytosine occurring in codon 408 (proline), results in a frameshift and a stop codon 111 nucleotides (37 amino acids) downstream (3N). HBR, heme-binding region. (Modified from Morishima A, Grumbach MM, Simpson ER, et al. Aromatase deficiency in male and female siblings caused by a novel mutation and the physiological role of estrogens. J Clin Endocrinol Metab 1995; 80:3689–3698. © 1995, The Endocrine Society.)

perineal orifice (Table 22–24). Müllerian structures are normal.[358, 932, 1024, 1129–1131] During infancy, basal and LHRH-induced FSH and LH are elevated.[932] The histology of the ovaries in infancy is normal, but under increased FSH stimulation in the absence of ovarian CYP19, multiple enlarged follicular cysts develop. At puberty affected females have hypergonadotropic hypogonadism, fail to develop female secondary sexual characteristics, and exhibit progressive virilization.[358, 932, 1024] Plasma androstenedione and testosterone are elevated, and estrone and estradiol levels are low or unmeasurable.[358, 932, 1024] The ovaries enlarge and develop multiple cysts at puberty; in one affected female, polycystic ovaries were detected in infancy. The hypergonadotropism and the multiple ovarian cysts respond to estrogen replacement therapy.

All three postpubertal patients had tall stature, delayed bone maturation and epiphyseal fusion, and osteopenia, suggesting that estrogens are essential for the prevention of osteoporosis in males and females and for normal skeletal maturation and proportions (but not for linear growth in men).[358, 741, 932, 1024]

The affected 2 adult men had normal sex differentiation and pubertal maturation with macro-orchidism (in one male) and elevated concentrations of FSH, LH, and testosterone in plasma.[358, 1024] They also had osteoporosis, hyperinsulinemia, and abnormal plasma lipids, similar to the findings in a tall man with a null mutation in the estrogen receptor.[1023] These observations suggest that estrogens as well as testosterone and inhibin play a role in the regulation of gonadotropin secretion in males and females and that estrogen deficiency in males can be associated with insulin resistance and hyperinsulinemia and an abnormal plasma lipid profile.[358, 1024]

The finding of apparently normal psychosexual development in the three aromatase-deficient adolescent or adult patients and in the man with an estrogen receptor defect suggests that estrogen does not play a critical role in sex differentiation of the human brain, as has been reported in nonprimate mammals.[358, 1024, 1135, 1136] The detection of severe defects in critical regions of the gene encoding CYP19 that lead to generalized aromatase deficiency is strong evidence that survival of the conceptus can occur in the absence of estrogen synthesis by the implanting blastocyst, the fetus, and the fetal compartment of the placenta.[358, 922, 1024]

Analysis of the *CYP19* gene in nine affected individuals has revealed 10 different mutations (Fig. 22–67) (Table 22–25). The patient of Shozu and colleagues was homozygous for a

Table 22–25. Mutations of CYP19: Relation between Aromatase Activity in In Vitro Expression Systems and Virilization of the Mother

Study	Sex of Affected Child	Genetic Defect	Activity (% of Normal)	Mother
Kanazawa, 1992	F	Splice junction defect (exon VI)	0.3	Virilized
San Francisco, 1993	F	Arg435Cys	1.1	Not virilized
		Cys437Tyr (exon X)	0	
New York, 1995 (sibs)	F&M	Arg375Cys (exon IX)	0.2	Virilized
Lyon, 1996	F	Arg457X (exon X)	"0"*	Virilized
Bern, 1997	F	Exon III (splice site)	"0"*	Virilized
		Pro408X	"0"*	
Modena, 1997	M	Arg365Gln (exon IX)	0.4	?
Bonn, 1998	F	Val370Met (exon IX)	ND*	Virilized
Bern, 1999	M	C base deletion → frameshift → stop codon (exon V)	0	Virilized

From Grumbach MM, Auchus RJ. Estrogen: Consequences and implications of human mutations in synthesis and action. J Clin Endocrinol Metab 1999; 84:4677–4694.

*Presumed lack of activity because of stop codon.

ND, not determined.

point mutation (GT → GC) in the consensus 5′ splice acceptor sequence in the gene. This mutation resulted in a CYP19 protein with a 29-amino acid insert and less than 0.3% of normal enzyme activity.[1127] A second patient was a compound heterozygote with two missense mutations.[1128] Assay of the expressed mutated proteins showed that one allele had 1.1% of the activity of the wild-type CYP19, whereas the other had no activity.[1128] The male and female siblings reported by Morishima and associates were both homozygous for a single base change that resulted in an amino acid substitution.[1024] Expression of this mutant cDNA showed that it had 0.2% of the wild-type aromatase activity. The patient of Mullis and coworkers had a cytosine deletion in one allele (codon 408, proline) that corresponds to the consensus aromatic region of the enzyme.[1129] This mutation results in a frameshift causing a stop codon 37 amino acids downstream.[1129] The other allele, inherited from the father, had a guanine-to-thymidine (G6T) transversion at the splice junction between exon 3 and intron 3.[1129] Both mutations resulted in a complete lack of enzymatic activity.[1129] Another patient described from France had a homozygous mutation that resulted in a stop codon (Arg457X) in exon 10 of the *CYP19* gene.[1130] The affected female from Bonn had a homozygous mutation in exon 9. The affected male infant from Bern had 1 base-pair C deletion in exon 5 causing a frameshift and homozygous null mutation.[1131] As in other patients, this mutation occurs in the critical heme-binding region of the aromatase enzyme.[358, 1024, 1126]

The diagnosis of CYP19 deficiency should be suspected in female pseudohermaphrodites in whom CAH has been excluded. The presence of elevated concentrations of androstenedione and testosterone of gonadal origin and elevated plasma gonadotropin levels can be observed even in infancy. Prenatal diagnosis of CYP19 deficiency is possible. Signs of an affected female or male fetus include unexplained maternal virilization during pregnancy, which was observed in five of the six pregnancies with affected infants (see Table 22–24), and the detection of increased maternal levels of Δ^4-androstenedione, testosterone, and DHT and low levels of plasma estriol and urinary estriol. Homozygous or heterozygous null mutations are usually associated with striking virilization of the mother.[358, 1131]

The absence of maternal virilization in the one patient reported may result from the fact that this patient, unlike the others reported, had 1.1% activity of Arg435Cys mutation, which may have allowed for some degree of aromatization in the placenta during gestation and therefore lower levels of maternal androgens.[358, 1128] Amniotic fluid concentrations of androstenedione and testosterone are high, and those of estrone, estradiol, and estriol are low.

Glucocorticoid Receptor Gene Mutation

Autosomal dominant forms of glucocorticoid resistance, a rare disorder, are a consequence of a heterozygous mutation in the gene encoding the glucocorticoid receptor, usually in the ligand-binding domain of this transcription factor. End-organ insensitivity to glucocorticoids in the heterozygote is heterogeneous in its manifestations but characteristically there is excess ACTH secretion, with elevated cortisol levels without Cushing syndrome and usually with few symptoms. Nevertheless, the hypersecretion of ACTH increases adrenal steroidogenesis and can lead not only to increased cortisol secretion but also to increased mineralocorticoids (as a consequence, hypertension and hypokalemia may occur) and androgen precursors.[1138, 1139, 1140, 1141] The latter steroids can produce acne, hirsutism, adolescent hyperandrogenism, menstrual abnormalities in the female,[1140] and sexual precocity in the male.[1141]

A Brazilian girl has been reported who had female pseudohermaphroditism owing to a novel homozygous inactivating mutation in the glucocorticoid receptor gene. Born of consanguineous clinically unaffected parents, she had a large clitoris, posterior labioscrotal fusion, and a urogenital sinus. When she was 9 years of age, studies showed low renin hypertension and hypokalemia with increased plasma DOC and corticosterone, high concentrations of plasma ACTH and cortisol, and impaired suppression of plasma cortisol during a dexamethasone test. Consistent with her advanced bone age and progressive virilization, the concentrations of plasma testosterone, androstenedione, and 17-hydroxyprogesterone were elevated. Molecular analysis identified a homozygous Val571Ala mutation involving the ligand-binding region. Mutant receptors had less than one sixth the binding affinity and one tenth to one fiftieth of the *trans*-activation activity of the wild-type receptor. After repair of the hypokalemia, high-dose dexamethasone therapy (6 mg/day) led to impressive clinical improvement.[1142]

Maternal Androgens and Progestagens

Masculinization of the external genitalia of female infants has been observed after maternal ingestion of testosterone or synthetic progestational agents during the first trimester of pregnancy[423, 1143–1145] (see Fig. 22–60). If the exposure occurs after the 12th week of gestation, the labioscrotal folds do not fuse, although the clitoris may enlarge.[423, 1143] Severe masculinization of the external genitalia of a female fetus may be caused, for example, by methyltestosterone in dosages as low as 3 mg daily, even though androgenic effects are not noticeable in the mother.[423] Placenta aromatase may be unable to efficiently aromatize synthetic androgens such as methyltestosterone.

Because progesterone itself is only slightly active when administered orally, various synthetic derivatives that may be taken orally were prescribed in the past for women with habitual or threatened abortion. Most of these progestagens are 19-nortestosterone derivatives; they are intrinsically androgenic to some degree and can cause virilization of female fetuses in experimental animals. Principal among the offenders have been norethindrone and ethisterone and, less commonly, norethynodrel and the C_{21}-steroid medroxyprogesterone acetate.[1143, 1145] Ishizuka and co-workers[1146] reported some degree of masculinization of the external genitalia in 2.75% of female infants whose mothers received synthetic progestagens of various types during pregnancy. This consequence of synthetic progestagen administration to the pregnant female is dose and time dependent.

Danazol, the 2,3-disoxazole derivative of 17α-ethinyltestosterone, a progestagen, is used for the treatment of endometriosis. Danazol crosses the placenta and can cause virilization of the external genitalia of the fetus in a manner similar to other androgenic compounds.[1147] Several instances of female pseudohermaphroditism are believed to be the consequence of maternal ingestion of danazol.[1147–1149]

In four cases of female pseudohermaphroditism, the mothers received only stilbestrol in large doses.[1150] The mechanism of masculinization is unknown but may be related to inhibition of 3β-HSD by stilbestrol or its metabolites.

Masculinization of the female fetus occurs on occasion if the mother has a virilizing ovarian tumor (usually arrhenoblastoma or Krukenberg's tumor) or adrenal tumor, a virilizing form of CAH, or virilization of some other cause during pregnancy.[423, 1144, 1151–1153] An increasing number of women with CAH are becoming pregnant as a result of improved treatment and it is reassuring to note that female offspring of such pregnancies are not virilized (with a single exception), despite higher than usual maternal testosterone levels.[1001, 1153, 1154] Luteoma of pregnancy, an ovarian pseudotumor composed of hyperplastic luteinized thecal cells that regress after delivery, has been associated with masculinization of the external genitalia of female infants, especially in the presence of maternal virilization.[1155, 1156] Ovarian lutein cysts in pregnancy (hyperreactio luteinalis), considered by some to be a cystic form of luteoma, are less frequently associated with maternal virilization and only rarely with fetal masculinization.[1157, 1158] Placental aromatization of androgens such as testosterone and androstenedione protects the mother and the female fetus from virilization[358, 932, 1158] unless the placental CYP19 ($P450_{arom}$) activity is insufficient for the androgen steroid load or unless the synthetic androgen is not a substrate for CYP19.

Some of the rare cases of female pseudohermaphroditism of undetermined origin may have resulted from a luteoma of pregnancy that regressed spontaneously after delivery or an undiagnosed placental aromatase deficiency.[932, 1024] In these patients a history of maternal ingestion of androgenic steroids is lacking and the postpartum course of the mother is inconsistent with a virilizing neoplasm, but the clinical features are most compatible with fetal exposure to androgens. The absence of virilism in the mother does not exclude a maternal source of androgen in these children, because the amounts of androgen required to masculinize the external genitalia of a female fetus may be less than those required to cause overt manifestations in the mother.

Female pseudohermaphroditism caused by the transfer of androgenic steroids from the mother to the fetus is the most easily treated of all types of ambisexual development. No hormone therapy is necessary, postnatal virilism does not occur, and female secondary sexual characteristics can be expected to emerge at the usual age of adolescence. Surgical correction of the external genitalia in infancy or childhood is rarely indicated.

Malformations of the Intestine and the Urinary Tract (Non–Androgen-Induced Female Pseudohermaphroditism)

Genital abnormalities are frequently associated with imperforate anus, renal agenesis or dysplasia, and other congenital malformations of the lower intestine and urinary tract.[1159–1162, 1162a] Carpentier and Potter reviewed the findings in such infants and suggested the term "nonspecific female pseudohermaphroditism."[1161] Some of these anomalies are incompatible with life. Renal failure, often accompanied by pyelonephritis, is common and may confuse the clinical picture with that of adrenal insufficiency. In contrast to other forms of female pseudohermaphroditism, the female müllerian derivatives may also be malformed. The findings in these patients may be bizarre; persistence of a primitive cloaca, imperforate anus, and fistulae are not infrequent. The pathogenesis of these anomalies is different from that of other types of ambisexual development and should be considered in the context of other forms of developmental field defects. Familial occurrence of nonadrenal female pseudohermaphroditism with multiple anomalies has been reported.[1161] Clitoromegaly may sometimes be the presenting feature of neurofibromatosis and may be more common in this neurologic disorder than is realized.[1163] The clitoris is richly innervated, and biopsies have confirmed the presence of neuromas when clitoromegaly occurs with neurofibromatosis. Surgical excision is not curative because of the tendency for recurrence of the neuromas.

Male Pseudohermaphroditism

Male pseudohermaphroditism is a heterogeneous condition in which the gonads are exclusively testes but the genital ducts and/or external genitalia are incompletely masculinized. The clinical spectrum varies from individuals with female external genitalia to those with mild impairment of masculinization of the external genitalia, as represented by hypospadias, cryptorchidism, and minimal ambiguity of the external genitalia.

With the advances in the knowledge of pathogenesis, systems of nomenclature based on eponyms and phenotype have become less important. There are at least six major etiologic categories of male pseudohermaphroditism, with many subtypes, all of which are associated with incomplete masculinization of the fetal genital tract and/or incomplete regression of the müllerian ducts.

In this section, forms of male pseudohermaphroditism in 46,XY individuals with relatively normal embryonic differentiation of the testes are discussed. In such patients, defective male development must be ascribed to a more specific failure of the fetal testes to overcome the inherent tendency toward feminization of the somatic sex structures. This failure may stem either from a secretory failure of the testes during the critical period of sex differentiation or from a failure of target tissues to respond normally to androgen stimulation or to AMH. Table 22–26 reflects an attempt to classify the many forms of male pseudohermaphroditism on the basis of cause, insofar as that is known.

The ability of the testes to virilize at adolescence is in many ways a recapitulation of their capacity to masculinize the external genitalia in utero. The greater the development of the phallus in an infant, the greater likelihood that male secondary sexual characteristics will emerge at the time of expected puberty. Individuals with ambiguous genitalia may remain eunuchoid, exhibit mild virilism, or develop breast enlargement and other female secondary sexual characteristics. Those with an external female phenotype usually either feminize or remain sexually infantile. These are only approximate guides, however, and the development of male sexual characteristics at adolescence may occur, especially in patients with partial androgen resistance, 17β-hydroxysteroid dehydrogenase-3 deficiency, or 5α-reductase-2 deficiency.

Male pseudohermaphroditism can result from (1) testicular unresponsiveness to hCG and LH and consequent Leydig cell aplasia or hypoplasia; (2) a specific enzyme defect in testosterone biosynthesis; (3) familial end-organ resistance to androgen caused by abnormalities in the cytosolic receptor for testosterone and DHT or by an enzyme defect in the intracellular metabolism of testosterone; (4) aberrations in testicular organogenesis (dysgenetic male pseudohermaphroditism); (5) defective synthesis, secretion, or response to AMH; (6) administration of progestagens during pregnancy; and (7) putative environmental exposures. Apart from dysgenetic male pseudohermaphroditism and the persistent müllerian duct syndrome, all other forms of male pseudohermaphroditism are characterized by the absence of müllerian duct derivatives. Except for some variants of dysgenetic male pseudohermaphroditism and the maternal ingestion of progestagens, virtually all forms of male pseudohermaphroditism are familial and characterized by genetic heterogeneity. No doubt many subtypes will be defined and characterized by molecular, genetic, and biochemical techniques. Although dysgenetic male pseudohermaphroditism—the group of disorders associated with defective organogenesis of the testes—has already been discussed, it is included under male pseudohermaphroditism because this category of intersexuality must be considered by the clinician in the differential diagnosis of male pseudohermaphroditism. In Table 22–4 and Figure 22–15 genes implicated in sex determination (gonadogenesis) are shown; Table 22–19 lists genes involved in sex differentiation.

Defects in Testosterone Biosynthesis and Metabolism

Testicular Unresponsiveness to hCG and LH, LH/hCG Resistance (Leydig Cell Agenesis or Hypoplasia)

The production of testosterone by fetal Leydig cells is critical to male sexual differentiation of the wolffian ducts and the

Table 22–26. Classification of Male Pseudohermaphroditism

I. *Male Pseudohermaphroditism*
  A. Testicular unresponsiveness to hCG and LH (Leydig cell agenesis or hypoplasia due to hCG/LH receptor defect)
  B. Inborn errors of testosterone biosynthesis
    1. Enzyme deficits affecting synthesis of both corticosteroids and testosterone (variants of congenital adrenal hyperplasia)
      a. StAR deficiency (congenital lipoid adrenal hyperplasia)
      b. Side-chain (P450scc) cleavage deficiency heterozygote
      c. 3β-Hydroxysteroid dehydrogenase/$\Delta^{4,5}$-isomerase type II (3β-HSD II) deficiency
      d. CYP17 ($P450_{c17}$ [17α-hydroxylase/17,20-lyase]) deficiency
      e. Smith-Lemli-Opitz syndrome: 7-dehydrocholesterol reductase deficiency
    2. Enzyme defects primarily affecting testosterone biosynthesis by the testes
      a. CYP17 ($P450_{c17}$ [17,20 lyase]) deficiency
      b. 17β-Hydroxysteroid dehydrogenase type 3 (17β-HSD 3) deficiency
  C. Defects in androgen-dependent target tissues
    1. End-organ resistance to androgenic hormones
      a. Syndrome of complete androgen resistance and its variants (testicular feminization and its variant forms)
      b. Syndrome of incomplete androgen resistance and its variants (Reifenstein's syndrome)
      c. Androgen resistance in phenotypically normal males (infertile and fertile)
    2. Defects in testosterone metabolism by peripheral tissues; 5α-reductase-2 (SRD5A2) deficiency (pseudovaginal perineoscrotal hypospadias)
  D. Dysgenetic male pseudohermaphroditism
    1. XY gonadal dysgenesis (incomplete)
    2. XO/XY mosaicism, structurally abnormal Y chromosome, SRY mutation
    3. Denys-Drash syndrome (*WT1* mutation)
    4. Frasier syndrome (mutation of *WT1* splice site junction mutation-deleting KTS)
    5. WAGR syndrome (*WT1* deletion)
    6. Campomelic dysplasia (*SOX9* mutation)
    7. *SFI* mutation
    8. *DAX1* (duplication)
    9. *WNT4* (duplication)
    10. 9p$^-$ (*DMRT1* deletion)
    11. 10q$^-$
    12. ATRX syndrome (*XH2* mutation)
    13. Testicular regression syndrome
  E. Defects in synthesis, secretion, or response to antimüllerian hormone: persistent müllerian duct syndrome (female genital ducts in otherwise normal men; herniae uteri inguinale)
  F. Maternal ingestion of progestagens
  G. Environmental chemicals (endocrine disrupters)

II. *Unclassified Forms of Abnormal Sexual Development*
  A. In males
    1. Hypospadias
    2. Ambiguous external genitalia in XY males with multiple congenital anomalies
  B. In females, absence or anomalous development of the vagina, uterus, and uterine tubes (Rokitansky-Küster syndrome)

hCG, human chorionic gonadotropin; LH, luteinizing hormone.

external genitalia. Leydig cell unresponsiveness to hCG/LH can result in male pseudohermaphroditism (Fig. 22–68) with Leydig cell agenesis or hypoplasia[1164–1174] (Table 22–27).

Phenotypically, the external genitalia vary, from those of a normal-appearing female to those of a male with micropenis and hypoplastic external genitalia.[1172–1174] Müllerian derivatives are absent in all patients; rudimentary wolffian derivatives (vas deferens, epididymis) have been present in some of the most severely affected patients despite the presence of female external genitalia.[1165, 1166] Basal FSH and LH concentrations and

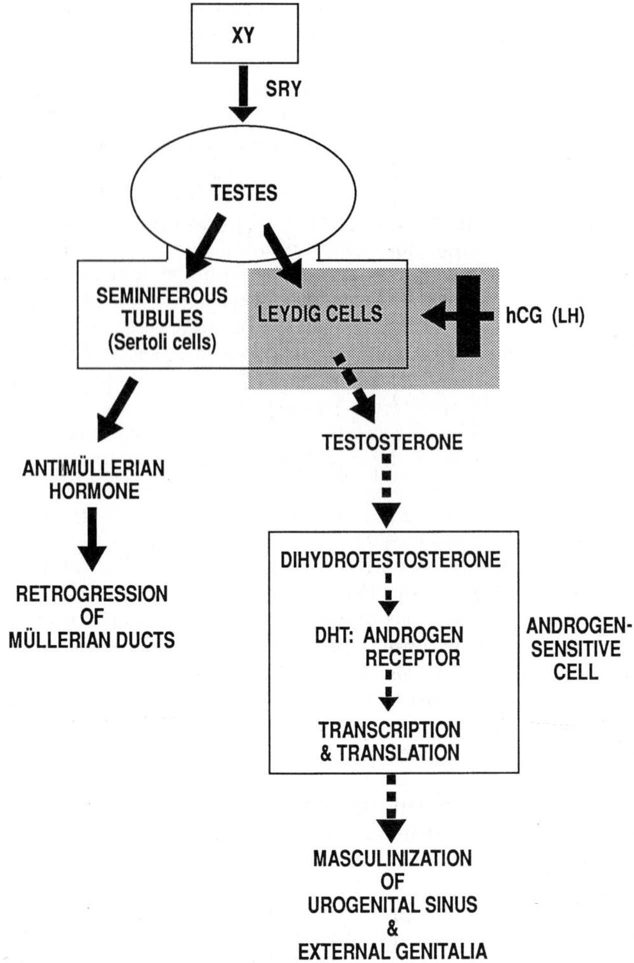

Figure 22–68. hCG/LH resistance. Diagram of male sex determination and differentiation showing a defect in the hCG/LH receptor that causes Leydig cell unresponsiveness to hCG (LH) and results in male pseudohermaphroditism. *Solid bar* delineates defect, and *stippled area* designates general site of defect. *Dashed lines* indicate that subsequent processes may be completely or partially affected.

Table 22–27. Clinical Features of Testicular Unresponsiveness to hCG/LH (Leydig Cell Aplasia or Hypoplasia)

Karyotype:	46,XY
Inheritance:	Autosomal recessive; homogeneous, compound heterozygous mutations in the LH/hCG receptor gene
Genitalia:	Female → ambiguous male → hypoplastic male
Wolffian duct derivatives:	Absent → hypoplastic → male
Müllerian duct derivatives:	Absent
Gonads:	Small undescended testes with absent or decreased number of Leydig cells → descended of normal size (with ↓ no. of Leydig cells)
Habitus:	Lack of or poor virilization at puberty
Hormone profile:	Increased gonadotropins postpubertally, decreased testosterone levels with decreased or absent response to hCG stimulation, decreased or normal binding of hCG/LH by Leydig cell depending on mutation

hCG, human chorionic gonadotropin; LH, luteinizing hormone.

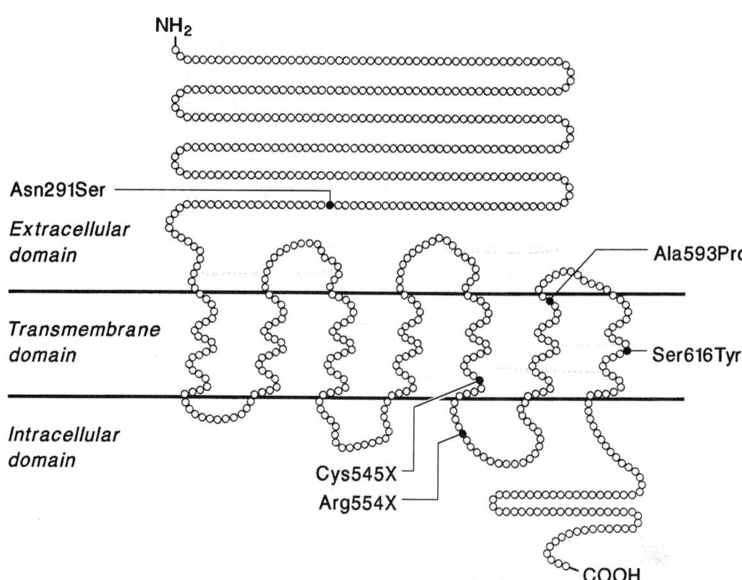

Figure 22–69. Diagram of the LH/hCG receptor with its seven transmembrane alpha helices and selected mutations that cause male pseudohermaphroditism. The *open circles* represent the amino acid residues on the LH/hCG receptor protein. The *solid circles* indicate the amino acid substitutions in patients with male pseudohermaphroditism. The mutations are indicated by the three-letter abbreviation of the wild-type amino acid, followed by the position number of the amino acid in the protein and the three-letter abbreviation for the substituted amino acid or the letter X, which indicates a nonsense (stop) mutation leading to an inactive, truncated receptor.

LHRH-evoked responses are elevated in postpubertal patients.[1172] Plasma levels of 17-hydroxyprogesterone, androstenedione, and testosterone are low, and stimulation with hCG elicits little or no increase. Plasma LH levels decrease after testosterone administration.[1167]

The undescended testes in the severe form are small, but not dysgenetic, and undergo progressive degenerative changes. On histologic examination, the testes lack distinct Leydig cells in prepubertal patients. Postpubertal patients have absent or decreased numbers of Leydig cells without Reinke's crystalloids, the normal-appearing Sertoli cells, and discrete seminiferous tubules with spermatogenic arrest are responsible for size of the testes.[1165–1167, 1173] In five patients in whom the LH receptor was studied, there was absent or diminished binding of labeled hCG and LH to Leydig cells.[1168, 1169] Familial studies indicate autosomal recessive transmission.[1173] The counterpart to this disorder described in the rat is termed the *vestigial testis syndrome* and is apparently caused by an LH-receptor defect.[1176]

Kremer and associates studied two 46,XY siblings who had female external genitalia and hypergonadotropic hypogonadism.[1177] Plasma levels of testosterone and its precursors were low, and hCG elicited no response. Leydig cells were sparse in the testes. Both siblings had a homozygous missense mutation, Ala593Pro, in the sixth transmembrane domain of the gene encoding the LH receptor (Fig. 22–69). In vitro, this mutated receptor binds hCG normally but does not evoke an increase in cyclic AMP or testosterone synthesis.[1177] A sibship reported by Latronico and colleagues contained four affected individuals, three 46,XY females with Leydig cell hypoplasia and hypergonadotropic hypogonadism, and a sexually mature 46,XX female with elevated plasma LH levels and amenorrhea.[1178] All four siblings were homozygous for an Arg554Stop (null) mutation within the third cytosolic loop of the LH receptor, which resulted in a truncated receptor protein incapable of transducing the LH signal.[1178] A 6-year-old 46,XY male with a micropenis, descended testes, and no testosterone response to the administration of hCG had a homozygous mutation (Ser616Tyr) in the seventh *trans*-membrane domain of the LH receptor gene. The mutant receptor did not bind hCG.[1178] Homozygous mutations in eight 46,XY males analyzed resulted in fetal and postnatal testosterone deficiency and a spectrum in appearance of the external genitalia extending from female external genitalia to a micropenis and in hypergonadotropic hypogonadism.[1178] Wu and associates described a compound heterozygous loss of function mutation with a nonsense mutation (Cys545X) in exon 11 of the LH receptor in one allele and a 33 base-pair insertion in exon 1 on the other allele in two 46,XY females with Leydig cell hypoplasia and LH/hCG resistance.[1179] In 10 patients with clinical features of Leydig cell hypoplasia, only 2 patients had mutations in the coding region of the LH/hCG receptor, which suggests that mutations may occur in other regions of the gene or a mutation in other Leydig cell–specific genes may produce the same phenotype.[1180] For example, in the mouse Desert hedgehog (DHH) a signaling protein and its receptor Patched 1 (Ptch 1) are critical factors in the differentiation of fetal Leydig cells in the mouse but do not affect cell migration from the mesonephros nor the contribution of interstitial cells from the coelomic epithelium.[271] An XY Dhh-null mouse bred on a mixed strain background exhibited severely impaired fetal Leydig cell differentiation and female external genitalia.[271, 274] A homozygous mutation in *DHH* was reported in a 46,XY male pseudohermaphrodite with partial gonadal dysgenesis and polyneuropathy.[276] These observations support the genetic heterogeneity of the syndrome and the importance of searching for genes involved in Leydig cell differentiation and function. Null mutations of the LH receptor in 46,XX females do not prevent normal development of female secondary sexual characteristics at puberty, but affected women have high plasma concentrations of LH, normal FSH levels, primary or secondary amenorrhea, and ovaries that varied from normal to enlarged and multicystic.[1178, 1181, 1182]

In patients with testicular unresponsiveness to hCG/LH, fetal testosterone deficiency impairs masculinization of the external genitalia, but müllerian duct regression is complete because the secretion of AMH by the fetal Sertoli cells is intact. Of interest is the paradoxical finding of wolffian derivatives, which are testosterone dependent, in some patients with no or minimal masculinization of the external genitalia (only posterior labial fusion). One explanation, supported by the variation in masculinization of the external genitalia, is that the defect in the hCG/LH receptor is of variable severity. A second, more likely possibility is that during the early fetal period, sufficient testosterone may have been secreted locally and autonomously[351]—independently of circulating hCG—to induce male duct development, but the concentration of testosterone in the fetal circulation was too low to evoke normal male differentiation of the external genitalia and urogenital sinus. hCG is necessary to sustain Leydig cell differentiation and growth and testosterone secretion by the fetal testes, at least by about the 10th week of gestation, but, as discussed previously, it may not be essential for initiation of these functions at week 8. Variation in the magnitude of hCG/LH resistance of the undifferentiated embryonic and fetal Leydig cells would result in variable degrees of fetal testosterone deficiency and thus a variable degree of failure to develop normal male external genitalia.

Therapy depends on the age at diagnosis and the degree of virilization. In the severe form of testicular unresponsiveness to hCG/LH with female external genitalia, sex assignment is usually female. The gonads are removed, and estrogen replacement therapy is instituted at the time of expected puberty. In the less extreme forms with predominantly male external genitalia, testosterone therapy augments phallic development and virilizes the patient at puberty.

In the human male fetus, deficient fetal pituitary gonadotropin secretion associated with anencephaly, hypothalamic hypopituitarism, and isolated gonadotropin deficiency (including Kallmann syndrome) is not associated with ambiguous external genitalia (with one possible exception[1183]), although undescended testes, hypoplasia of the scrotum, and microphallus are common. These clinical observations are consistent with the important role of hCG in testosterone secretion by the human fetal testis during the critical period of male sex differentiation; fetal pituitary FSH and LH are not required for normal differentiation of testes or male external genitalia but do play a role in their growth during the last half of gestation.

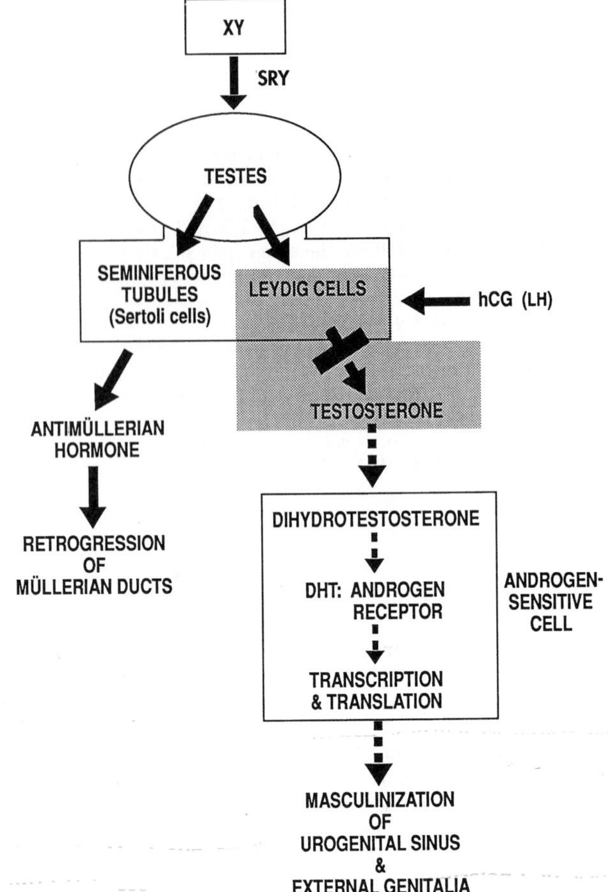

Figure 22–70. Diagram of male sex determination and differentiation showing the consequences of an enzymatic block in biosynthesis of testosterone that results in male pseudohermaphroditism. *Solid bar* indicates defect (see legend for Figure 22–63).

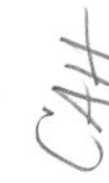

Enzyme Defects of Testosterone Biosynthesis Affecting Both Adrenal Steroid and Testosterone Biosynthesis (Variants of Congenital Adrenal Hyperplasia)

Enzyme defects common to adrenal and testicular biosynthesis include 3β-HSD, CYP17, cholesterol side-chain cleavage, as well as abnormalities in the intracellular steroid transport protein, StAR. These have already been reviewed in the section on CAH. Some additional features are described for the 17,20-lyase variant of CYP17 deficiency in view of the primary effect on testicular steroid biosynthesis and, hence, male pseudohermaphroditism.

Defects in testosterone biosynthesis (Fig. 22–70) have been described, one at each of the enzymatic steps required for the conversion of cholesterol to testosterone[1096] (Fig. 22–71). Three of the defects (3β-HSD, CYP17, CYP11A1 [$P450_{scc}$]) involve enzymes, and the third, StAR, a protein that affects both glucocorticoid and gonadal steroid biosynthesis; these errors in steroid biosynthesis are discussed, in part, in the section on CAH. A fourth defect involves the biosynthesis of cholesterol (7α-cholesterol reductase deficiency) and results in multisystem metabolic malformation syndrome.

StAR Deficiency (Congenital Lipoid Adrenal Hyperplasia)

Infants with this defect (Table 22–28; see previous discussion in the section on CAH) present with severe adrenal insufficiency and accumulation of lipid in the cells of both the adrenal cortex and the gonads. The second most common form of CAH in Japan (the Gln258X mutation was found in over 80% of Japanese patients studied) and Korea, it is rare in the United States and Europe.[1184, 1185] Affected males have female external genitalia with a blind vaginal pouch and hypoplastic male genital ducts but no uterus or fallopian tubes; the genitalia of affected females are normal. In males, the testes may be abdominal, inguinal, or in the labia. All reported patients are diffusely pigmented; glucocorticoid and mineralocorticoid insufficiency is severe; and adrenal crises in infancy can lead to death if untreated. However, three male pseudohermaphrodites survived the perinatal period without therapy and presented at 6 weeks, 12 weeks, and 10 months of age[1100, 1101, 1186] (see discussion of StAR and its mutations in the section on female pseudohermaphroditism). The patient reported by Hauffa and co-workers[1101] (and in the previous editions of this chapter) is more than 35 years old and well maintained on glucocorticoid and mineralocorticoid replacement therapy. Sexual hair is absent unless small doses of testosterone are given; female secondary sexual characteristics are induced by estrogen replacement. As described in the section on CAH, no secondary sexual characteristics (either male or female) develop at the age of puberty in affected males, in contrast to females with this disorder.[1099, 1109, 1110] Pedigree analysis of families and DNA analysis of affected patients and parents indicate autosomal recessive transmission.[1099, 1109, 1110] The male/female ratio in this disorder appears to be 3:1.[1099] The unusual ratio of affected patients is yet to be explained and may represent, at least in part, ascertainment bias. The molecular genetics of StAR deficiency are illustrated in Figure 22–65.[1099, 1112, 1114]

The diagnosis of StAR deficiency should be suspected in patients with male pseudohermaphroditism, including all phenotypic female infants with evidence of adrenal insufficiency. The diagnosis can be confirmed by documentation of low or absent mineralocorticoids, glucocorticoids, and gonadal steroids and their metabolites in plasma and urine and an absent steroid response to corticotropin and hCG administration. The adrenals are large and lipid laden and displace the kidneys caudad on ultrasonography, CT, or MRI; the enlargement can

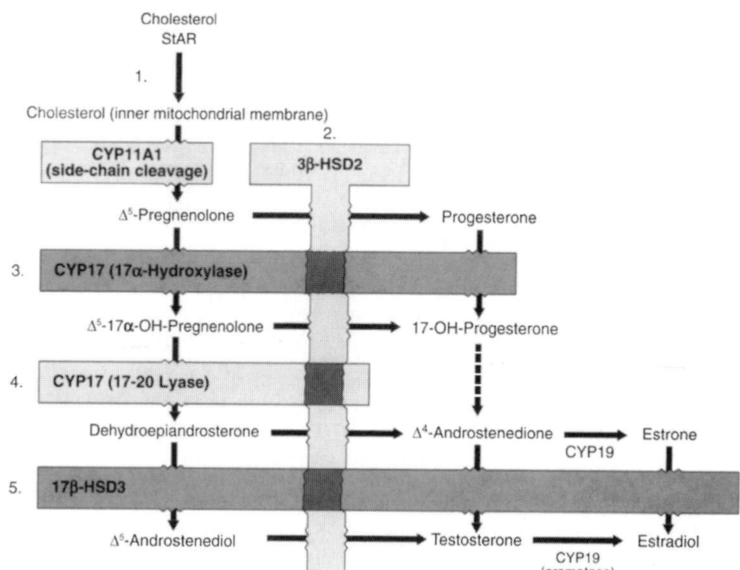

Figure 22–71. Defects in the biosynthetic pathway for testosterone. Five defects cause male pseudohermaphroditism in affected males (1 to 5). Even though all blocks affect both gonadal and adrenocortical steroidogenesis, only those at steps 1, 2, and 3 are associated with major abnormalities in biosynthesis of glucocorticoids and mineralocorticoids. StAR mutations impair transport of cholesterol to the inner mitochondrial membrane, the site of CYP11A1. In the human, null mutations in CYP11A1 are probably lethal in utero (see text). CYP17 (17α-hydroxylase/17,20-lyase) primarily catalyzes the scission of 17-hydroxypregnenolone to dehydroepiandrosterone. Only minimal conversion of 17-hydroxyprogesterone to androstenedione occurs normally. Therefore, synthesis of gonadal steroids is mainly through the Δ^5-pathway.

persist for months after glucocorticoid therapy. Therapy requires replacement doses of glucocorticoid and mineralocorticoid from the time of diagnosis. All affected 46,XY males have been reared as females. Estrogen replacement therapy to induce female sexual characteristics at puberty and low-dose testosterone treatment to elicit development of sexual hair are indicated; prophylactic orchidectomy is appropriate.[1187, 1188]

Congenital Lipoid Adrenal Hyperplasia due to Haploinsufficiency of Cholesterol Cleavage Enzyme (P450$_{scc}$; CYP11a). P450$_{scc}$ is the enzyme that converts cholesterol to pregnenolone, the first step in steroidogenesis. As noted in the section on CAH and female pseudohermaphroditism, null mutations in both alleles of this gene would lead to failure of placental production of progesterone, which in the human (unlike, for example, the rabbit) would be incompatible with continued gestation beyond the 8th to 10th week. Tajima and his associates described a hyperpigmented 4-year-old XY male pseudohermaphrodite with mild virilization of the external genitalia as evidenced by clitoromegaly but no labial fusion, with a blind vaginal pouch, who had had bilateral inguinal testes removed.[1117] It was not until age 4 years that she experienced life-threatening adrenal insufficiency with a low concentration of plasma cortisol, a high plasma ACTH and plasma renin activity, but normal concentrations of serum sodium and potassium.

Table 22–28. Clinical Features of StAR Deficiency in 46,XY Males

Karyotype:	46,XY
Inheritance:	Autosomal recessive*
Genitalia:	Female
Wolffian duct derivatives:	Absent → hypoplastic
Müllerian duct derivatives:	Absent
Gonads:	Testes
Habitus:	Severe adrenal insufficiency in infancy, no virilization at puberty
Hormone profile:	Decreased or absent glucocorticoids, mineralocorticoids, and gonadal steroids in plasma and urine; increased plasma LH and FSH; increased plasma renin

*46,XY male with heterozygous mutation of P450$_{scc-}$. Genitalia: Clitoromegaly separate vaginal and urethral openings, no labial fusion, no müllerian ducts, childhood onset of adrenal insufficiency.

LH, luteinizing hormone; FSH, follicle-stimulating hormone.

Haploinsufficiency. A heterozygous mutation in the *CYP11A1* gene—an in-frame insertion of Gly and Asp between Asp 271 and Val 272—was identified that lacked P450$_{scc}$ enzymatic activity.[1189] The suggestion that the P450 haploinsufficiency eventually led to a late-onset type of congenital lipoid hyperplasia is consistent with the two-stage model of pathogenesis proposed for StAR deficiency.[1099] The discrepancy between the compromised function of the fetal testes and the resultant male pseudohermaphroditism and the relatively late onset of symptomatic adrenal insufficiency is incompletely understood. In contrast to the absent müllerian duct derivatives in this patient, the male pseudohermaphrodite with adrenal insufficiency caused by haploinsufficiency of the *SF1* gene due to Gly35Glu mutation had a uterus[237] as did the male pseudohermaphrodite with a homozygous mutation (arg92Gln).[240]

3β-Hydroxysteroid Dehydrogenase/$\Delta^{4,5}$-Isomerase 2 Deficiency

This rare autosomal recessive disorder is a consequence of mutations in *HSD3B2*, the gene encoding the 3β-HSD/$\Delta^{4,5}$-isomerase type 2 isozyme, which is expressed mainly in the adrenals and gonads. This enzyme catalyzes a crucial step in the biosynthesis of all steroid hormones, the conversion of Δ^5- to Δ^4-steroids. The type 1 isozyme is expressed predominantly in the placenta and in peripheral tissues (e.g., skin, breast), has 93% homology in structure with the type II isozyme, is about five times as active, and is closely linked to the type II isozyme (both are encoded by genes on chromosome 1p13).[1053–1059] The type 1 isozyme is not associated with CAH, and mutations in the coding region of type I are probably lethal because they prevent or compromise progesterone synthesis by the placenta and, hence, survival of the fetus.

Males with 3β-HSD 2 deficiency have CAH associated with male pseudohermaphroditism with or without adrenal insufficiency (salt loss) (Table 22–29). The external genitalia in males are usually ambiguous, with a small phallic structure, second- or third-degree hypospadias, partial fusion of the labia, a urogenital sinus, and a blind vaginal pouch; rarely, the external genitalia are female in appearance.[1054, 1062, 1190–1194]

Wolffian duct differentiation is normal. The testes are usually in the scrotum or lower inguinal region, and, as with other blocks in testosterone biosynthesis and defects in androgen action, müllerian structures are absent (Fig. 22–72).

Table 22–29. Clinical Features of 3β-Hydroxysteroid Dehydrogenase II Deficiency in 46,XY Males

Karyotype:	46,XY
Inheritance:	Autosomal recessive, mutations in *3βHSD2* gene
Genitalia:	Ambiguous; hypospadiac male
Wolffian duct derivatives:	Normal
Müllerian duct derivatives:	Absent
Gonads:	Testes
Habitus:	Severe adrenal insufficiency in infancy; poor virilization at puberty with gynecomastia. Mild form: no mineralocorticoid deficiency, premature adrenarche → mild virilization
Hormone profile:	Increased concentrations of Δ^5 C_{21}- and C_{19}- steroids (e.g., 17-hydroxypregnenolone, DHEA, and their sulfates) in urine and plasma; increased 17-hydroxypregnenolone and 17-hydroxypregnenolone/cortisol ratio response to corticotropin; 17-hydroxypregnenolone and DHEA suppressible by dexamethasone

DHEA, dehydroepiandrosterone.

Newborns with severe deficiencies of the 3β-HSD II (e.g., null mutations) have severe CAH and exhibit signs or symptoms of both glucocorticoid and mineralocorticoid deficiency after the first 5 to 7 days of life. In those infants with severe deficiency of the enzyme, adrenal insufficiency may result in death if the diagnosis is missed and therapy is delayed.[1063] 46,XY males with partial deficiency of 3β-HSD II are not salt losers; the mutant gene in these cases encodes an enzyme with 2% to 10% of residual 3β-HSD II enzymatic activity in the adrenals and gonads, as assessed in intact transfected cells.[1054, 1195] This amount of enzymatic activity is apparently sufficient to prevent salt wasting and adequate for aldosterone synthesis but not enough to provide sufficient fetal testosterone to virilize the external genitalia.[1062]

Gynecomastia can occur at puberty in both affected males and affected females,[1054, 1191] presumably by peripheral conversions of Δ^5-C_{19}-steroids to Δ^4-C_{19}-steroids by the 3β-HSD 1 isozyme expressed principally in peripheral tissues and the subsequent aromatization of androgens to estrogens. Menses in treated females and fertility in males have been been reported.[1060, 1065] A 46,XY male had a null mutation in the *HSD3B2* gene caused by a premature stop codon (Try171X) in one allele and a frameshift in the other allele.[1060, 1192] This patient, who had male pseudohermaphroditism and adrenal insufficiency requiring replacement therapy for survival, virilized at puberty and developed gynecomastia and was sufficiently fertile to father two children[1060, 1065]; paternity was confirmed in one child by DNA analysis.[1060] The source of the 3β-HSD enzymatic activity to enable the synthesis of sufficient testosterone to facilitate spermatogenesis was undetermined. However, the 3β-HSD 1 enzyme in peripheral tissues and in small amounts in the testes is a likely candidate.[1060, 1194]

Simard and co-workers reviewed the molecular genetics of 3β-HSD 2 deficiency in 17 patients, 10 of whom were salt losers[1054]; they described eight different point mutations in the 10 latter patients. All of the mutations led to profound impairment of enzymatic activity (to <1%)[1054]; they were nonsense, missense, and frameshift mutations that clustered in the fourth exon of the gene (see Fig. 22–62). Seven different mutations were found in patients from six families with the so-called non–salt-losing form of 3β-HSD deficiency (see Fig. 22–62).[1054] All were missense mutations except for one mutation that produced a splice error.[1054, 1196] These mutations resulted in 1% to 10% of the wild-type 3β-HSD enzymatic activity in transfected cells.[1054, 1196] Additional studies of the molecular genetics and enzymatic activity of the mutant genes are reported.[1062, 1197, 1198] No mutations in either *HSD3B1* or *HSD3B2* have been found in patients with the putative "late onset," "attenuated," or nonclassic form of 3β-HSD deficiency.[1068, 1195, 1199]

Mendonca and colleagues described four patients in two families with an arginine-to-threonine substitution at amino acid 82 (Arg82Thr) in the *HSD3B2*.[1066] Two males in one family were pseudohermaphrodites with differing degrees of mild salt loss. A 46,XX phenotypic female sibling homozygous for the same mutation had normal breast development, normal menses, and no evidence of androgen excess. Analysis of plasma and urinary steroids showed biochemical evidence of 3β-HSD deficiency, as manifested by increased production of Δ^5-steroids. In contrast, an unrelated 46,XX female from another family with the same mutation had acne and premature pubarche as well as elevated plasma 17-hydroxypregnenolone and DHEA levels.[1066] Hence, as in patients with 21-hydroxylase deficiency, the same mutations may be "cryptic" in some individuals and cause severe symptoms in others.

The diagnosis of 3β-HSD 2 deficiency should be suspected in all 46,XY males with ambiguous genitalia and adrenal insufficiency. The hormonal characteristics are increased levels of Δ^5-3β-hydroxy C_{21}- and C_{19}-steroids (e.g., 17-hydroxypregnenolone and DHEA and their sulfates) and their metabolites in plasma and urine and striking increases in ACTH stimulated Δ^5-17-hydroxypregnenolone (>50 SD above controls) and Δ^5-17-hydroxypregnenolone to cortisol ratios (>30 SD above controls). However, the diagnosis in early infancy can be confounded by the elevated concentrations of Δ^5-3β-hydroxy C_{21}- and C_{19}-steroids normally seen in premature and full-term in-

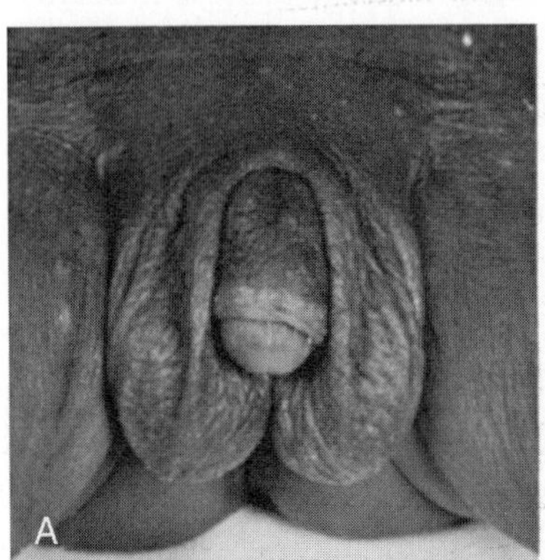

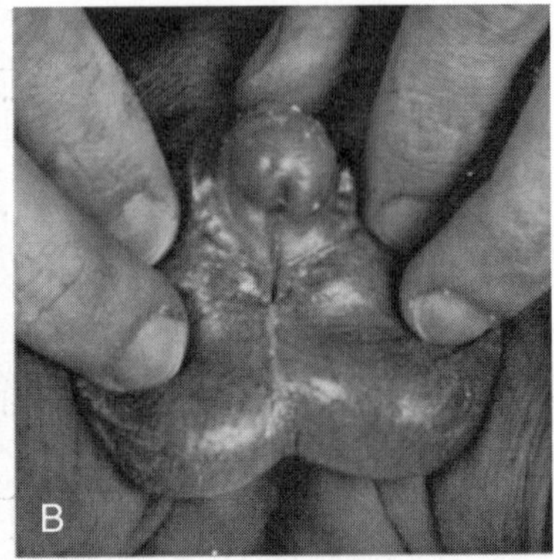

Figure 22–72. *A* and *B*, Genitalia of male infant with congenital adrenal hyperplasia resulting from 3β-HSD 2 deficiency. The boy was admitted at 9 days of age in a salt-losing crisis and died at 3 months of unexplained muscular paralysis. Paresis, resembling that of Werdnig-Hoffmann syndrome, became progressively more severe even though adrenal replacement therapy was adequate and blood electrolytes were normal. Biochemical findings revealed a severe block in the conversion of Δ^5-3β-hydroxysteroids to Δ^4-3-ketosteroids.

Table 22–30. Clinical Features of CYP17 Mutations with Both 17α-Hydroxylase and 17,20-Lyase Deficiencies in 46,XY Males

Karyotype:	46,XY
Inheritance:	Autosomal recessive; *CYP17* ($P450_{c17}$) gene mutations
Genitalia:	Female → ambiguous → hypospadiac male; blind vaginal pouch
Wolffian duct derivatives:	Absent → hypoplastic
Müllerian duct derivatives:	Absent
Gonads:	Testes
Habitus:	Absent or poor virilization at puberty, gynecomastia
Hormone and metabolic profile:	Decreased plasma testosterone; increased plasma LH and FSH levels; increased plasma deoxycorticosterone, corticosterone, and progesterone concentrations; decreased plasma renin activity
	Low renin hypertension with hypokalemic alkalosis

LH, luteinizing hormone; FSH, follicle-stimulating hormone.

fants during the first few weeks of life and by the peripheral conversion of Δ^5-3β-hydroxysteroids to Δ^4-3β-ketosteroids by the type I enzyme in peripheral tissues. Newborn males with severe 3β-HSD II deficiency can have elevated levels of 17-hydroxyprogesterone in infancy secondary to the peripheral conversion of 17-hydroxypregnenolone to 17-hydroxyprogesterone[1195, 1200] by the type I isozyme. However, in these patients the ratio of basal plasma 17-hydroxypregnenolone to 17-hydroxyprogesterone is high and is exaggerated by administration of corticotropin, consistent with adrenal and gonadal deficiency of 3β-HSD II. Therefore, in infancy, it is important to interpret the increased concentrations of Δ^5-3β-hydroxysteroids in relation to normal values for age and to determine the ratios of Δ^5- to Δ^4-steroids.[1044] Therapy involves replacement of glucocorticoids and mineralocorticoids (if necessary), as in salt-wasting patients with CYP21 deficiency.

CYP17 (17α-Hydroxylase/17,20-Lyase) Deficiency

17α-Hydroxylase/17,20 lyase deficiency (due to mutations in a single gene, *CYP17*) is a defect that impairs both adrenal and gonadal steroidogenesis but not mineralocorticoid steroidogenesis (Table 22–30; see previous discussion in the section on CAH). The phenotype of 46,XY males with 17α-hydroxylase deficiency varies from that of an individual with normal-appearing female external genitalia and a blind vaginal pouch to (rarely) that of a male with hypospadias and a small phallus.[1073, 1081, 1084–1087, 1089, 1092, 1201, 1202] The magnitude of the impaired masculinization in the male fetus correlates with the severity of the block in 17α-hydroxylation and the magnitude of the consequent impairment in fetal testosterone synthesis.[1073, 1087, 1092] A male with a homozygous deletion of the phenylalanine codon (TTC) at amino acids 53 or 54 of exon 1 of the *CYP17* gene had mild hypospadias and cryptorchidism.[1092] Analysis of the 17α-hydroxylase and 17,20-lyase activity of this mutant protein showed less than 23% and 5% activity, respectively, compared with the wild-type enzyme.[1092] Hence, it appears that more than 25% of normal enzymatic activity is necessary for normal fetal masculinization of the external genitalia.[1089, 1092] The testes may be intra-abdominal, in the inguinal canal, or in the labioscrotal folds. Inguinal hernias are commonly present. In one affected 46,XY patient, no gonads were found at laparotomy.[1203] Müllerian structures are absent, and wolffian derivatives are usually hypoplastic. Bone age is retarded during childhood and can lead to tall stature. Excessive secretion of DOC and corticosterone, the consequence of the failure of 17α-hydroxylation of the C_{21}-steroids, usually leads to hypertension, hypokalemia, and alkalosis. The adrenal zona fasciculata is the source of the increased plasma concentration of DOC, corticosterone, 18-hydroxy-DOC, and 18-hydroxycorticosterone.[1094] Salt and water retention, volume expansion, and hypertension suppress renin and, consequently, aldosterone secretion in the classic form (although aldosterone concentrations are normal or elevated in some patients).[1202] This process is reversible with cortisol therapy. Because gonadal sex steroid secretion is low, severely affected patients fail to develop secondary sexual characteristics, including pubic and axillary hair. Plasma and urinary FSH and LH levels are increased. One patient with a partial deficiency of 17α-hydroxylase activity developed prominent gynecomastia and incomplete male secondary sexual characteristics at the expected time of puberty.[1204] As previously discussed in the section on CAH, mutations in the *CYP17* gene (see Fig. 22–63) that are associated with less than 25% of normal 17α-hydroxylase activity in intact transfected cells result in female (complete deficiency) or ambiguous genitalia in affected 46,XY males, whereas activity equal to at least 25% of that of the normal enzyme is associated with normal male genitalia.[1072, 1089, 1092, 1204]

The diagnosis of 17α-hydroxylase deficiency should be suspected in male pseudohermaphrodites, including 46,XY phenotypic females, who have hyporeninemic hypertension and hypokalemic alkalosis. Plasma concentrations of corticotropin, DOC, corticosterone, and progesterone are high, and those of aldosterone, 17α-hydroxyprogesterone, cortisol, and gonadal steroids are low. Replacement therapy with physiologic doses of glucocorticoids suppresses DOC and corticosterone secretion and causes return of serum potassium levels, blood pressure, and plasma renin and aldosterone levels to normal. At puberty, appropriate gonadal steroid replacement therapy is indicated, and gonadectomy should be performed in 46,XY patients who have been assigned a female sex of rearing.

Smith-Lemli-Opitz Syndrome (7-Dehydrocholesterol Reductase Deficiency

The Smith-Lemli-Opitz syndrome has a broad phenotypic spectrum[1205–1207] but typically includes microcephaly, mental retardation, ptosis, upturned nose, micrognathia, polydactyly, syndactyly of toes, severe hypospadias, micropenis, and growth failure. The abnormalities of the external genitalia in 71% of XY patients vary from hypospadias to complete failure of masculinization, resulting in a female phenotype. It has now been established that the syndrome is caused by a deficiency of 7-dehydrocholesterol reductase (sterol Δ7-reductase, DHCR7), the phylogenetically conserved sterol-sensing domain–containing enzyme required for the last step in the biosynthetic pathway from acetate to cholesterol biosynthesis (Fig. 22–73).[1208] This is the first characterized metabolic malformation syndrome; the defect in cholesterol metabolism acts as a multisystem teratogen perhaps related in part to defective signaling of Hedgehog proteins.[1209] The diagnosis is confirmed biochemically by demonstrating low plasma levels of cholesterol and elevated levels of 7-dehydrocholesterol[585]; the plasma cholesterol concentration correlates negatively with severity. The gene encoding this enzyme *(DHCR7)* maps to 11q12–13[1210] and more than 70 different mutations have now been described.[1211, 1212] The syndrome appears to be most common in white Europeans, with an incidence of 1 in 20,000 to 1 in 30,000 births based on case ascertainment. The prevalence of the syndrome is an indication for obtaining a serum cholesterol level in a suspected male pseudohermaphrodite. Screening for the most common mutation, a splice acceptor site mutation, 1V58–¹G-C, suggests an incidence of between 1 in

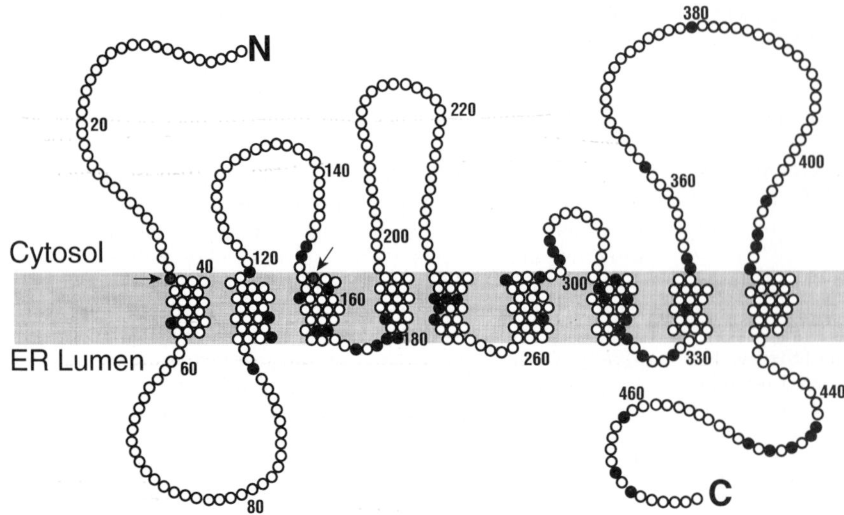

Figure 22–73. The topology of Δ-5-sterol reductase. Dark circles designate amino acid substitutions due to missense mutations in *DHCR7*. The two arrows indicate site of stop codons. (From Witsch-Baumgartner M, Loffler J, Utermann G. Mutations in the human *DHCR7* gene. Hum Mutat 2001; 17:172–182.)

7,000 and 1 in 13,400 with a carrier rate as high as 1 in 30.[1213] The difference in incidence figures may be caused by fetal loss, undiagnosed neonatal deaths or, perhaps, missed mild cases. Ambiguity of the external genitalia is common in XY individuals, and, in the severely affected XY individual, ambiguity of the external genitalia usually is associated with polydactyly and cleft palate. Testis development is apparently normal, and normal, elevated, or low concentrations of plasma testosterone have been described in affected male infants with intact hypothalamic-pituitary gonadotropin function.[840, 1214–1218] The severe impairment of cholesterol metabolism affects intracellular cholesterol and the sterol composition of plasma membranes. Surprisingly, in at least some XY infants, testosterone biosynthesis seems intact.[1215–1217] Two XY infants with female external genitalia had adrenal insufficiency.[1218] A defect in 5α-reductase-2 activity and resistance to the action of fetal androgens are suggested possibilities for the explication of the impaired masculinization of the external genitalia, but the mechanism is uncertain. However, Shackleton and co-workers found 5,7-diene and 5,8(9)-diene homologues of normal urinary C_{21}- and C_{19}-steroid in two newborn phenotypic female XY infants with the syndrome,[1219] which raises the issue of the cross-reactivity of unsaturated "androstenes" in the testosterone radioimmunoassay, for example, and the androgenic activity of these homologues of normal C_{19}- steroids. One XY newborn with female external genitalia had intra-abdominal epididymides and deferent ducts and a uterus suggesting impaired action or synthesis of AMH despite the effect of testosterone on wolffian duct differentiation.[840] A mouse model of the Smith-Lemli-Opitz syndrome has been created by disruption of the *DHCR7* gene. This shows the typical biochemical profile, growth retardation, craniofacial anomalies, but no genital abnormalities.[1220]

Clinical trials are underway with dietary cholesterol supplementation in this cholesterol deficiency disorder.

The Smith-Lemli-Opitz syndrome is another cause of a low concentration of maternal serum unconjugated estriol and of urinary estriol; more specifically, determination of urinary dehydroestriol and dehydropregnanetriol is a noninvasive approach to prenatal diagnosis.[1221] In addition, the amniotic fluid of affected fetuses has a high ratio of 7-dehydrocholesterol (μg/mL) to cholesterol (mg/dL).[1222]

Table 22–31. Clinical Features of CYP17 Mutations with Only 17,20-Lyase Deficiency in 46,XY Males

Karyotype:	46,XY
Inheritance:	Autosomal recessive—certain mutations in *CYP17 ($P450_{c17}$)* gene (Arg347His; Arg 358Gln)
Genitalia:	Female → male with perineal hypospadias → hypoplastic male; blind vaginal pouch
Wolffian duct derivatives:	Rudimentary → normal
Müllerian duct derivatives:	Absent
Gonads:	Testes
Habitus:	Normal stature; sexual infantilism; ± gynecomastia
Hormone profile:	Decreased plasma testosterone, androstenedione, dehydroepiandrosterone (DHEA), and estradiol concentrations; abnormal increase in plasma 17-hydroxyprogesterone and 17-hydroxypregnenolone and increased ratio of 17-hydroxy C_{21}-deoxysteroids to C_{19}-steroids (DHEA, Δ^4-androstenedione) after hCG stimulation test; plasma LH and FSH elevated

Enzyme Defects Primarily Affecting Testosterone Biosynthesis by the Testes

CYP17 (Isolated 17,20-Lyase) Deficiency (Table 22–31)

The 17α-hydroxylation of pregnenolone and progesterone and the conversion of the C_{21}-steroids 17-hydroxypregnenolone and 17-hydroxyprogesterone to the C_{19}-steroids DHEA and androstenedione are mediated by a single microsomal enzyme encoded by the *CYP17* gene located on chromosome 10q24–25.[1070–1077] In the adrenal gland, CYP17 catalyzes 17α-hydroxylation in the biosynthesis of glucocorticoids, and in both the adrenal and the gonad it catalyzes the 17α-hydroxylation of C_{21}-steroids and the subsequent conversion of 17-hydroxypregnenolone and 17-hydroxyprogesterone to the C_{19}-steroids DHEA and androstenedione (17,20-lyase activity). The Δ^5-17,20-lyase activity of CYP17 is much greater in the human than its Δ^4-17,20-lyase activity.[1074] Little or no Δ^4-17,20-lyase activity can be demonstrated in the human testis or in cultured human theca cells[1074]; the conversion of 17α-hydroxypregnenolone to DHEA is about 50 times more efficient than the conversion of 17α-hydroxyprogesterone to androstenedione.[1074, 1223] The control of 17,20-lyase activity in the adrenal appears to be independent of that in the gonad; adrenal 17,20-lyase activity is age dependent, as illustrated by adrenarche. Data suggest that the ratio of 17α-hydroxylase to 17,20-lyase activity of the CYP17 enzyme is a function of the molar ratio of its electron transfer (redox) partners P450 oxidoreductase and of cytochrome b5.[1223–1225] Increasing the amount of either NADPH-P450 reductase or cytochrome b_5 increases the activity of 17,20-lyase severalfold.[1223–1226] Furthermore, the CYP17 enzyme undergoes post-translational modification through phosphorylation of serine and threonine residues by cyclic AMP–dependent protein kinase A.[1227] Phosphorylation of the enzyme increases 17,20-lyase activity, and dephosphorylation reduces or eliminates it.[1225, 1227] Both these mechanisms appear to play a role in control of 17,20-lyase activity in the adrenal and gonads.

There have been about 18 case reports of putative isolated 17,20-lyase deficiency,[1073, 1089] despite the fact that one gene encodes a single enzyme with both 17α-hydroxylase and 17,20-lyase activities. Isolated 17,20-lyase deficiency, however, is exceedingly rare; there are only two patients in whom the diagnosis has been established unequivocably by demonstration of the mutation and detailed functional and structural studies.[934, 1075, 1228, 1229]

Zachmann and colleagues[1230] initially reported two first cousins with a familial form of male pseudohermaphroditism ascribed to a partial deficiency of 17,20-lyase in both the adrenals and testes. The patients had ambiguous genitalia, inguinal or intra-abdominal testes, and a 46,XY sex chromosome constitution. Both cousins had severe hypospadias with a male-type urethra and male duct development. Only urinary steroids were examined. A sample of testicular tissue from one cousin studied in vitro exhibited a defect in the conversion of C_{21}-steroids to testosterone (C_{19}-steroids). Subsequent studies of the cousins at ages 12 and 13 years disclosed a putative partial defect in the conversion of Δ^5 and Δ^4 C_{21}-steroids to C_{19}-steroids.[1231] Analysis of the *CYP17* gene in one cousin detected compound heterozygosity with two different mutant alleles. Transfection studies indicated combined 17α-hydroxylase and 17,20-lyase deficiencies despite the clinical findings.[1232] Further study of the steroid pattern in this patient revealed that although 17α-hydroxylase activity had been putatively normal in childhood and adolescence, it was decreased in adulthood.[1231]

Two Brazilian male pseudohermaphrodites are described from consanguineous marriages with presumed isolated 17,20-lyase deficiency.[1228, 1233] Both had 46,XY karyotypes, microphallus, perineal hypospadias, bifid scrotum, a blind vaginal pouch, and cryptorchidism. Basal LH and FSH concentrations were elevated in the postpubertal case, and testosterone levels were low. The administration of hCG resulted in a marked rise in plasma 17-hydroxyprogesterone with a paucity of response in DHEA, androstenedione, and testosterone, consistent with isolated 17,20-lyase deficiency. Molecular modeling and site-directed mutagenesis indicated that the Arg347Ala mutation selectively ablates 17,20-lyase activity in the rat[1234] or human enzyme while leaving 17α-hydroxylase activation intact.[1225, 1235] Analyses of CYP17 in these patients showed one to be homozygous for an Arg347His mutation and the other to have an Arg358Gln mutation (see Fig. 22–63).[1228] These two mutations are located in the redox partner binding site of the CYP17 enzyme and therefore cause a decrease in 17,20-lyase activity by reducing electron transfer.[1225] These are the first patients with "isolated" 17,20-lyase deficiency defined by molecular analyses and the first example of prediction of the specific location for a mutation by site-directed mutagenesis and modeling.[1072, 1075, 1225, 1228, 1229] The role of redox partners in the regulation of 17,20-lyase is illustrated by a description of a male pseudohermaphrodite with congenital methemoglobinemia due to a mutation in cytochrome b5.[1233]

Depending on the degree of impairment in 17,20-lyase activity and its effect on fetal testosterone production during gestation, the external appearance may vary from female to ambiguous to hypoplastic male. The testes may be intra-abdominal, in the inguinal region, or in the scrotum. As with other defects in testosterone synthesis, wolffian duct derivatives are either hypoplastic or normal, depending on the severity of the testosterone deficiency, and müllerian duct derivatives are absent. Gynecomastia can occur at the age of puberty.[1228] In the 46,XX females, putative isolated 17,20-lyase deficiency leads to failure of pubertal development and elevated gonadotropin levels.[1236]

The diagnosis of 17,20-lyase deficiency should be considered in male pseudohermaphrodites with absent müllerian derivatives and in 46,XX females who have no abnormality in glucocorticoid or mineralocorticoid synthesis but fail to develop secondary sexual characteristics at the expected time of puberty and have elevated concentrations of FSH and LH. In prepubertal male pseudohermaphrodites, 17,20-lyase deficiency must be distinguished from the partial form of androgen resistance, 5α-reductase-2 deficiency, and 17β-HSD type 3 deficiency.

In the prepubertal patient, both corticotropin and hCG stimulation may be useful in unmasking the defect. Prenatal diagnosis is possible by the measurement of amniotic fluid C_{21}- and C_{19}-steroids[1237] and by DNA analysis. The age at diagnosis and the degree of masculinization of the external genitalia are important determinants of the sex of rearing. Gonadal steroid replacement therapy usually is necessary in both sexes at puberty. Gonadectomy is recommended in 46,XY patients raised as females.

17β-Hydroxysteroid Dehydrogenase 3 Deficiency

The 17β-HSD reaction in the human is mediated by six known isozymes[1238] that catalyze the reduction of androstenedione, DHEA, and estrone to testosterone, Δ^5-androstenediol, and estradiol, respectively, as well as the reverse reaction. The type 1 (17β-HSD 1) isozyme, a member of the short-chain alcohol dehydrogenase family, is cytosolic, is expressed at highest levels in the ovary and placenta, and primarily interconverts estrone and estradiol; its gene is located on chromosome 17q21.[1238–1240] A second gene, located on chromosome 16q24, encodes the 17β-HSD 2 isozyme,[1239, 1241] which is expressed in placental liver and endometrial microsomes and primarily oxidizes (inactivates) both androgens and estrogens.[1239, 1242] The 17β-HSD 3, a microsomal enzyme, utilizes NADPH as a cofactor[1239, 1243]; it is encoded by a gene on chromosome 9q22 that is 23% homologous to the genes for 17β-HSD 1 and 17β-HSD 2 and is expressed primarily in the testes, where it favors the reduction of androstenedione to testosterone; male pseudohermaphroditism is a consequence of mutations in the gene encoding 17β-HSD 3.[1239, 1243] 17β-HSD 4 encodes a low activity 17β-estradiol dehydrogenase (E_2 to E_1) and is expressed in multiple tissues. 17β-HSD 5 is encoded by a gene on chromosome 10p14–15 and favors the reduction of androstenedione to testosterone and of DHEA to androst-5-ene-3β,17β–diol in peripheral tissues and the ovary.[1238] 17β-HSD 7 is expressed in the placenta, mammary gland, and kidney and efficiently catalyzes the conversion of E_1 to E_2.

Male pseudohermaphroditism caused by 17β-HSD 3 deficiency (also called 17β-hydroxysteroid oxidoreductase or 17-ketosteroid reductase) was first reported by Saez and colleagues[1244, 1245] (Table 22–32). Many patients have been described, including a cohort of 68 subjects from a highly inbred population in the Gaza Strip.[1246, 1247] Except for a few 46,XY individuals with ambiguous genitalia at birth,[1248–1250] most affected 46,XY males have predominantly female external genitalia, testes (usually located in the inguinal canal), male wolffian duct derivatives (epididymides, vas deferens, seminal vesicles, and ejaculatory ducts), and a blind vaginal pouch.[1239, 1243, 1250] Because of unambiguous female genitalia at birth, such individuals are usually assigned a female sex, raised

Table 22–32. Clinical Features of 17β-Hydroxysteroid Dehydrogenase Type 3 Deficiency in 46,XY Males

Karyotype:	46,XY
Inheritance:	Autosomal recessive; mutations in *HSD17B3* gene
Genitalia:	Female → ambiguous; blind vaginal pouch
Wolffian duct derivatives:	Hypoplastic
Müllerian duct derivatives:	Absent
Gonads:	Testes (usually undesended)
Habitus:	Virilization at puberty (phallus enlargement, deepening of voice, and development of facial and body hair); gynecomastia variable
Hormone profile:	Increased plasma estrone and androstenedione; decreased ratio of plasma testosterone/androstenedione and estradiol/estrone after hCG stimulation test; increased plasma FSH and LH levels

hCG, human chorionic gonadotropin; FSH, follicle-stimulating hormone; LH, luteinizing hormone

as females, and in some cases mistakenly assumed to have the complete androgen resistance syndrome. However, at the age of puberty, gonadotropin levels and plasma concentrations of androstenedione, estrone, and testosterone increase. The levels of testosterone in some cases approach the normal male range, and some virilization invariably ensues[1239, 1250–1253, 1263]; the pubertal increase in testosterone is most often derived from extraglandular conversion from androstenedione presumably by 17β-HSD 5 mainly or in patients with partial 17β-HSD 3 deficiency directly from the testes. In the patients from the Gaza Strip described by Rösler, the phallus, although bound down by chordee, reached lengths of 4 to 8 cm.[1246, 1247] Deepening of the voice, male body hair distribution, and increased muscle mass ensue. Gynecomastia is a variable most likely related to the severity of the enzymatic defect and the ratio of androgens to estrogens.[1250, 1254, 1263] Estrogens are derived from the conversion of androstenedione by aromatase in extraglandular tissue and the action of the 17β-HSD 1 or 17β-HSD 2 isoenzymes. The striking virilization at puberty is in sharp contrast to the impaired masculinization of the external genitalia in utero. Like patients with 5α-reductase-2 deficiency, some patients, especially those from the Gaza Strip, have changed their gender role from female to male at puberty.[1246, 1247, 1253, 1263] Studies in our patients and in others indicate that the principal source of plasma testosterone in patients with a severe defect in 17β-HSD 3 is extraglandular conversion rather than direct testicular secretion.[1250] In two patients studied in San Francisco, testicular vein sampling indicated that androstenedione levels were markedly increased, whereas testosterone secretion was estimated at 0.05 and 0.2 mg/day, as opposed to about 4 mg/day in adult males. Although 17β-HSD 3 activity appears to be completely deficient in infancy, a progressive rise occurs in plasma testosterone from puberty to adulthood.[1250, 1256–1258, 1263] This apparent "recovery" of 17β-HSD 3 enzymatic activity is undoubtedly a result of the increase with puberty in gonadotropin and androstenedione secretion as well as the extragonadal activity of the other 17β-HSD isozymes in converting androstenedione to testosterone.[1250, 1263] However, the patients described from the Gaza Strip had a less severe enzyme block, with 15% to 20% of normal 17β-HSD 3 activity and evidence of synthesis of testosterone by the testes at the expected time of puberty.[1243, 1250]

Analyses of 17 patients with classic 17β-HSD 3 deficiency, including 4 from San Francisco, revealed 14 mutations in the *HSD17B3* gene.[1239, 1243, 1250] Twelve patients had homozygous mutations, 4 were compound heterozygotes, and 1 was a presumed heterozygote[1239, 1243, 1250] (see Fig. 22–74). The mutations included a frameshift, 3 splice site abnormalities, and 10 missense mutations. Expression of 8 of the 9 missense mutations revealed complete absence of 17β-HSD 3 enzymatic activity.[1250] The Arg80Gln missense mutation in the Gaza Strip Arab patients resulted in an enzyme with partial activity.[1243, 1250]

Only mutations in the *HSD17B3* gene that encodes the testis-specific enzyme cause male pseudohermaphroditism. The gene is located on chromosome 9q22 and is composed of 11 exons.[1243] Of 20 mutations described in affected patients, 16 are missense, 3 are splice junction, and 1 is an in-frame mutation[1239, 1243, 1250, 1259, 1260, 1263] (Fig. 22–74). Some patients are compound heterozygotes. Expression studies of the mutant enzymes in heterologous cells generally show complete absence of activity in the conversion of androstenedione to testosterone compared with the normal enzyme. The mutation that is predominant in the Arab population (Arg80Gln)[1258] and has also been described in a European patient does demonstrate activity when studied in vitro (as noted earlier). Another mutation,

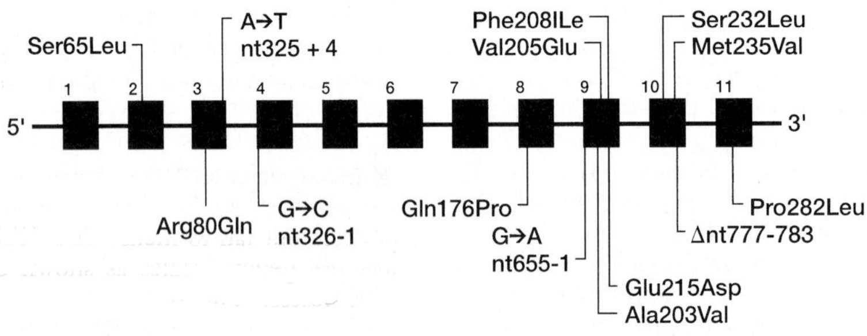

Figure 22–74. Diagram of the gene encoding 17β-hydroxysteroid dehydrogenase type 3 with selected mutations reported to cause 17β-HSD deficiency. The exons are the numbered black boxes. Missense mutations causing amino acid substitutions in the enzyme are indicated by the three-letter abbreviation for the wild-type amino acid, followed by the amino acid number in the enzyme and the three-letter abbreviation for the substituted amino acid. nt325 + 4 is a splice junction mutation, a transition of adenine (A) to thymidine (T), located four nucleotides downstream (3′) of the boundary between exon 3 and intron 3; nucleotide 325 is the closest base pair in the exon to the mutation. nt326 − 1 is a splice junction mutation, a transition of guanine (G) to cytosine (C), located one nucleotide upstream (5′) of the boundary between intron 3 and exon 4. nt665 − 1 is a splice junction mutation, a transition of guanine (G) to adenine (A), located one nucleotide upstream (5′) of the splice junction between intron 8 and exon 9. Δnt777-783 indicates a deletion of nucleotides 777 to 783 in the gene. (Redrawn from Andersson S, Geissler WM, Wu L, et al. Molecular genetics and pathophysiology of 17β-hydroxysteroid dehydrogenase 3 deficiency. J Clin Endocrinol Metab 1996; 81:130–136. © 1996, The Endocrine Society.)

Ala56Thr, on kinetic analysis showed a 20-fold decrease in NADPH cofactor affinity and a 6-fold decrease in affinity for the androstenedione substrate.

The presence of wolffian duct derivatives in these patients with homozygous mutations of the 17β-HSD 3 isoenzyme that result in complete absence of enzymatic activity is unexplained.[1250] Andersson and colleagues[1239] suggested that because the androgen receptor in the wolffian duct appears to be identical to the mature androgen receptor,[1261] there must be an alternate pathway for testosterone synthesis by 17β-HSD in utero to induce wolffian duct stabilization.

The diagnosis of 17β-HSD 3 deficiency should be considered in (1) male pseudohermaphrodites who have no abnormality in adrenal steroid biosynthesis, absent müllerian ducts, and normal wolffian duct structures and (2) male pseudohermaphrodites who virilize at puberty either with or without gynecomastia. The absence of müllerian duct derivatives generally distinguishes patients with defective testosterone biosynthesis or androgen resistance from those with dysgenetic male pseudohermaphroditism. In the prepubertal or young adolescent patient, basal androstenedione and estrone levels may not be elevated for age. However, at any age the defect in testosterone biosynthesis can be demonstrated best by a prolonged hCG stimulation test.[1246, 1263] In response to hCG, there is a disproportionate rise in plasma androstenedione and estrone levels, compared with testosterone and estradiol concentrations.[1233, 1246, 1257, 1262, 1263] The ratio of plasma testosterone to androstenedione concentrations after hCG stimulation usually well distinguishes androgen insensitivity from 17β-HSD3 deficiency. A ratio less than 0.8 is typically found in 17β-HSD deficiency; although similarly low ratios can be encountered in testicular dysgenesis, the absolute amount of plasma C_{18} and C_{19} steroids after the administration of hCG is strikingly different.

Little or no 17β-HSD 3 is expressed in the human ovary.[1238] Women with homozygous or compound heterozygous mutations of 17β-HSD 3 are asymptomatic.[1078, 1258, 1283] A putative late-onset form of 17β-HSD deficiency causing gynecomastia and hypogonadism in males has been reported[1264] but has not been confirmed by DNA analyses of the coding sequence of the *HSD17B3* gene.[1239]

In the past, in patients reared as females treatment involved castration followed by estrogen substitution therapy at puberty, but this approach needs to be reexamined, especially in view of the dramatic advances in neonatal diagnosis and DNA analysis. Patients with ambiguous genitalia in whom 17β-HSD3 deficiency is detected in infancy should probably be reared as a male; testosterone therapy to augment phallic size and genitoplasty are indicated in infancy. As noted previously, male pseudohermaphroditism caused by 17β-HSD 3 deficiency is relatively common among Arabs of the Gaza Strip.[1247, 1258] The natural history in this isolate is virilization at puberty; furthermore, a change in gender role behavior from female to male is the rule. Because of this, Gross and colleagues[1262] proposed that these patients should be given male gender assignment at diagnosis. They described seven young affected 46,XY males with female external genitalia who after biochemical confirmation were treated with testosterone enanthate, 25 to 50 mg each month for 3 months. Most patients received two or three courses of testosterone therapy, which resulted in an increase in phallic length into the normal range for age.[1262] First-stage genitoplasty was then undertaken when the patients were between 2 and 3 years of age. Ten of the 11 children treated in this way were reported to have a "pleasing appearance" of their external genitalia with a penile length within 1 SD of the normal mean value.[1265] Cosmetic and functional results in adolescents were also reported to be "encouraging"; however, the results of this treatment in adults were "poor."[1265]

In the study from Brazil,[1263] psychological assessment was carried out by psychologists over a 13-year period. Seven of 10 affected XY individuals raised as females chose to maintain a female gender identity; 3 changed to a male social sex, and 2 additional affected individuals who were not available for evaluation also changed to a male role. Five of 12 XY individuals with 17β-HSD 3 deficiency in these two families elected to change from a female assigned sex to male. As Wilson[484] has emphasized, whereas androgens are a major factor in the determination of gender role, only some of the affected males reared as females changed their gender identity to male, even from the same sibship, an indication of the complexities involved and the role of other determinants.

When the patient is reared as a male, testosterone replacement therapy at the age of puberty is necessary to achieve full masculinization and to prevent, at least in some, the appearance of gynecomastia. A plausible explanation for the absence of spermatogenesis in these patients, aside from cryptorchidism, is the low concentration of testosterone in the testis. In patients raised as males with retained gonads, cryptorchidism and elevated gonadotropin levels (postpubertally) may increase the risk for testicular neoplasm.

Defects in Androgen-Dependent Target Tissues

A defect at any step in the mechanism of action of androgens on their target cells (see Fig. 22–29)—5α-reduction of testosterone, binding of DHT to the receptor, nuclear localization of the steroid receptor complex to hormone response elements on DNA and subsequent transcription, or translation—can lead to impaired androgen action and result in male pseudohermaphroditism. Two major forms have been identified: end-organ resistance to androgenic hormones (androgen receptor defects) and errors in testosterone metabolism in target tissues (5α-reductase deficiency).

End-Organ Resistance to Androgens (Androgen Receptor Defects)[408, 1266–1269]

The spectrum of phenotypes in 46,XY individuals with resistance to androgens varies from patients with normal female external genitalia through those with genital ambiguity to those with a normal male phenotype who have a small phallus and are fertile. The syndromes of androgen insensitivity are a paradigm of clinical disorders resulting from resistance to the action of normal or increased circulating concentrations of a hormone.[1270]

Complete Androgen Insensitivity Syndrome and Its Variants (Androgen Resistance, Testicular Feminization, Feminizing Testes). The term "testicular feminization," coined by Morris[1271] but no longer used, was applied to a highly distinctive X-linked disorder[280] in which affected males are phenotypic females and develop female secondary sexual characteristics at puberty but fail to menstruate (Table 22–33). Affected individuals are genetic males as shown by the 46,XY karyotype and have testes. The prevalence of this disorder is estimated at between 1 in 20,000 and 1 in 60,000 live male births.[1272, 1273] The syndromes of androgen insensitivity represent the most common identifiable cause of male pseudohermaphroditism. Phenotypically, these patients have unambiguous female external genitalia; hypoplastic labia majora; a blind vaginal pouch; absent or, rarely, vestigial müllerian structures (uterus and tubes); testes located in the labia, the inguinal canal, or the abdomen; and absent or vestigial wolffian derivatives[280, 408, 1274–1276] (Fig. 22–75). Histologically, the testes are difficult to distinguish from normal before puberty.[280] After puberty, there are Sertoli-cell only seminiferous tubules within nodules, spermatogonia are sparse, and spermatogenesis is absent. The Ley-

Table 22–33. Clinical Features of Complete Androgen Resistance

Karyotype:	46,XY
Inheritance:	X-linked recessive; mutations in *AR* gene
Genitalia:	Female with blind vaginal pouch
Wolffian duct derivatives:	Usually absent; less commonly, rudimentary or hypoplastic
Müllerian duct derivatives:	Absent or vestigial
Gonads:	Testes
Habitus:	Scant or absent pubic and axillary hair; breast development and female habitus at puberty; primary amenorrhea ("hairless woman")
Hormone and metabolic profile:	Increased plasma LH and testosterone concentration; increased estradiol (for men); FSH levels often normal or slightly increased
	Resistance to androgenic and metabolic effects of testosterone
Androgen receptor studies:	Genetic heterogeneity; mutations can lead to low or undetectable amount of normal receptor (receptor-negative), unstable receptor (thermolabile, partial receptor deficiency), or the receptor-positive form

LH, luteinizing hormone; FSH, follicle-stimulating hormone.

dig cells are hyperplastic and tend to form adenomatous clumps.[1277–1279] The testes are predisposed to malignant transformation.[1272, 1275] Carcinoma in situ and seminoma have been reported, especially in patients with the partial form of androgen insensitivity.[911, 1266] The overall risk of a testicular neoplasm in the affected adult has been estimated at 4%[908] to 9%[1275]; however, the risk appears to be significantly less in those younger than 20 years of age.[908]

At birth and in childhood the diagnosis should be suspected in phenotypic females with an inguinal hernia (particularly if bilateral) and a testis-like mass in the inguinal region or in the labia. It has been estimated that 1% to 2% of phenotypic females with inguinal hernias have the syndrome.[1280] Nevertheless, it is debatable whether a routine karyotype should be performed in all female infants with inguinal hernias. At adolescence, female secondary sexual characteristics develop and include normal breasts and female body habitus but no menses. Pubic and axillary hair is usually sparse and is completely lacking in about one third of patients. This was the case in a family with complete deletion of the androgen receptor, representing the null phenotype of this syndrome. The presence of sparse pubic hair has been attributed to a partial form of the syndrome, but some clitoromegaly is generally a constituent of this severe variant of the syndrome. Adult stature is generally between the average for normal males and females.[1281] In the study by Marcus and colleagues of 28 women, the average height of 174 cm compared with the average height of adult American women of 162.3 cm; however, 30% of the adult women with complete androgen resistance exceeded 180 cm.[1281, 1282]

Pathophysiology and Hormone Profile

The Androgen Receptor

In 1950 Wilkins first suggested that failure of androgenization of the male fetus and the development of female rather than male secondary sexual characteristics at puberty could be explained by end-organ unresponsiveness to androgen based on lack of virilization with 50 mg of methyltestosterone administered daily (Fig. 22–76). Studies by subsequent workers supported this contention by failing to demonstrate a clinical or metabolic response to testosterone administration in patients with the complete form of this syndrome.[408, 1292] This X-linked

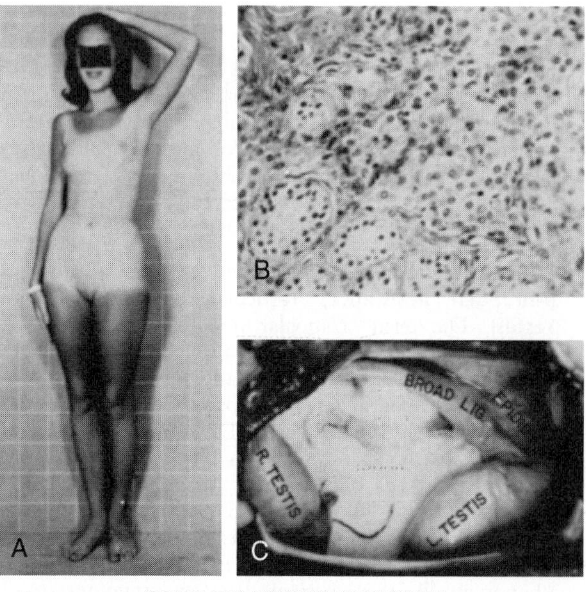

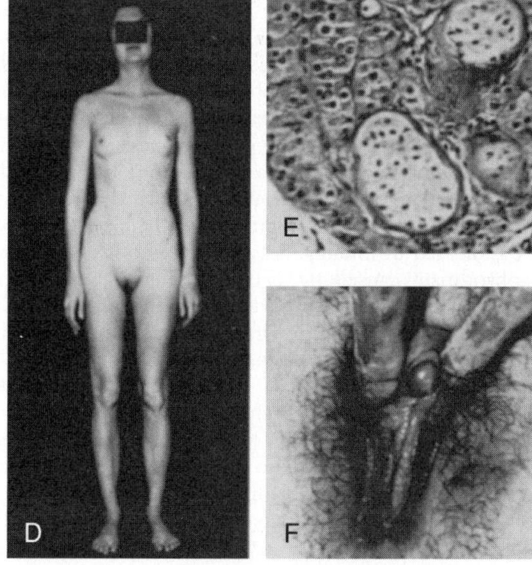

COMPLETE FORM OF SYNDROME VARIANT FORM OF SYNDROME

Figure 22–75. The syndrome of complete androgen resistance and its "variant" form. *A*, A 17-year-old patient with the complete syndrome. This phenotypic female was chromatin negative, had a 46,XY karyotype, and had total absence of sexual hair with female secondary sexual characteristics. A small vagina ended blindly. *B*, The testes exhibited Leydig cell hyperplasia and seminiferous tubules that lacked germinal elements. *C*, At laparotomy, abdominal testes, rudimentary wolffian structures, and no müllerian structures were found. *D*, The variant form of syndrome in a 25-year-old female. Sexual hair was present, although sparse. *E*, The testes exhibited Leydig cell hyperplasia. *F*, The clitoris was hypertrophied, but there was no labial fusion. A shallow vagina ended blindly. At laparotomy, hypoplastic wolffian structures and absent müllerian structures were noted.

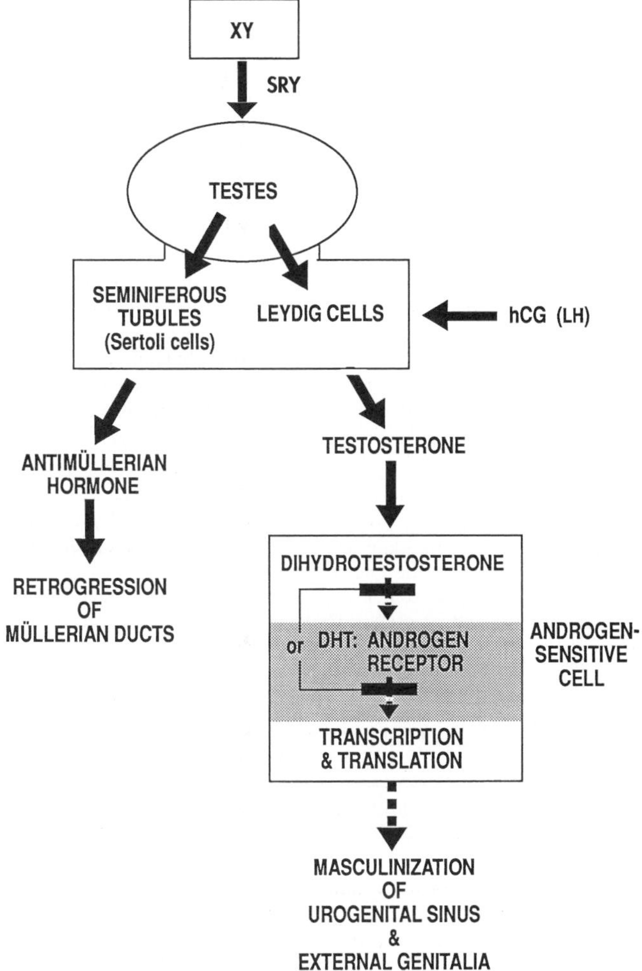

Figure 22–76. Diagram of male pseudohermaphroditism caused by complete or partial androgen resistance illustrating defects in the androgen receptor that result in absent or reduced binding of DHT or impaired function of the ligand-bound receptor.

disorder has been described in several mammalian species, including the mouse, rat, bull, and chimpanzee.[1293]

Studies in two animal models, the tfm mouse and rat,[1176, 1293–1295] suggested that the primary defect is a deficient number of androgen receptors for DHT and testosterone. An undetectable or low amount of androgen receptor activity was subsequently demonstrated in cultured fibroblasts from the genital skin of karyotypic males with the syndrome.[1296] These observations were amply confirmed by others.[408, 1297, 1298] The lack of androgen binding in genital skin fibroblasts from patients with this disorder provided an explanation for the observed failure of androgen action.

Extensive studies of the parameters of androgen binding in genital skin fibroblasts using DHT and synthetic androgens showed a range of quantitative and qualitative defects.[408, 1299] Typically, there was absent specific androgen binding in patients with the complete androgen insensitivity. In contrast, there was detectable binding in the partial form of the syndrome, but this was qualitatively abnormal as based on characteristics such as decreased binding affinity, thermolability of binding, and increased dissociation kinetics. In some instances, there was curiously normal or increased androgen binding that was only adequately explained once the androgen receptor had been cloned[1300, 1301] (see later). Knowledge of the functional domains of the androgen receptor protein as a result of characterizing the androgen receptor gene led to a more functional interpretation of androgen-binding results. The lack of strict correlation between phenotype and receptor binding, as well as the apparently normal binding found in patients with androgen resistance, was clarified by studies of the molecular biology of the androgen receptor and of mutations in the gene encoding the receptor.[408]

Molecular Biology of the Androgen Receptor (see Hormonal Sex Differentiation)

The androgen receptor gene is located at Xq11-q12, comprises eight exons, and encodes a 110- to 114-kd protein that varies in length from 910 to 919 amino acids[1274, 1303] (Fig. 22–77; see also Fig. 22–29). In common with other nuclear receptors, the androgen receptor comprises three functional domains involved in transcriptional regulation, DNA, and ligand binding.[409, 416, 1304–1308]

A large number of androgen receptor gene mutations have been described in patients with androgen insensitivity,[408, 1274, 1309, 1310] and they are recorded on an international database (see http://www.mcgill.ca/androgendb/) (Fig. 22–78). About 400 mutations distributed throughout the gene are now described. The vast majority are missense/nonsense nucleotide substitutions located predominantly in exons encoding the hormone-binding domain. There are also examples of splice site intronic mutations, small deletions and insertions, and, rarely, complete deletions of the gene. Mental retardation was an associated fea-

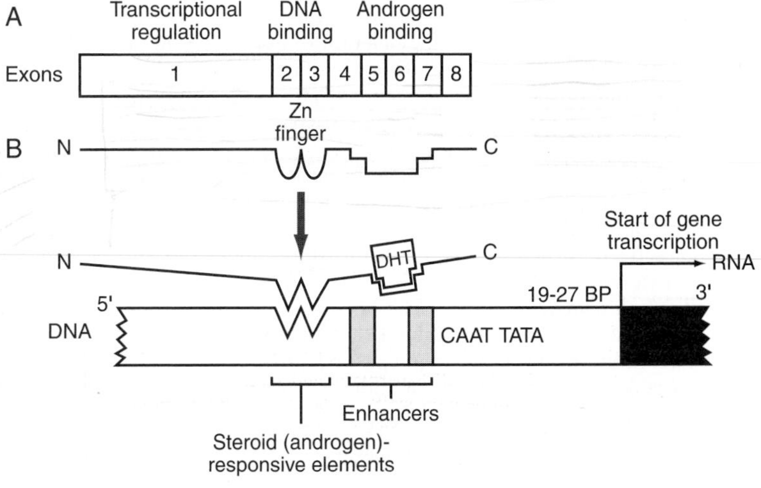

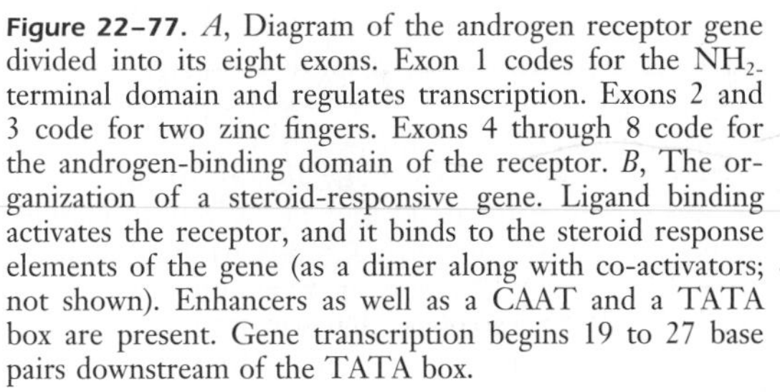
Figure 22–77. *A*, Diagram of the androgen receptor gene divided into its eight exons. Exon 1 codes for the NH_2-terminal domain and regulates transcription. Exons 2 and 3 code for two zinc fingers. Exons 4 through 8 code for the androgen-binding domain of the receptor. *B*, The organization of a steroid-responsive gene. Ligand binding activates the receptor, and it binds to the steroid response elements of the gene (as a dimer along with co-activators; not shown). Enhancers as well as a CAAT and a TATA box are present. Gene transcription begins 19 to 27 base pairs downstream of the TATA box.

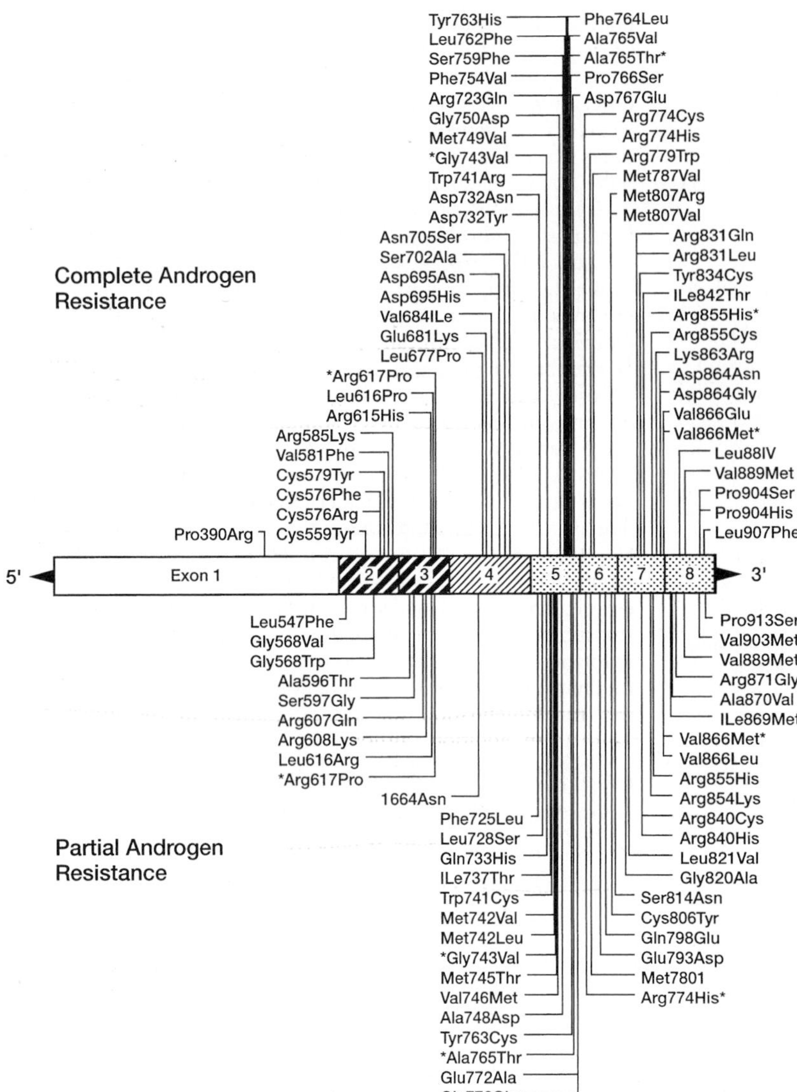

Figure 22–78. Diagram of the androgen receptor gene (AR) with missense mutations that cause complete androgen resistance (CAR) and partial androgen resistance (PAR). Asterisks indicate mutations that have been found to cause both complete and partial androgen resistance. Each mutation is indicated by the three-letter abbreviation for the wild-type amino acid, followed by the position number of the amino acid in the protein and the three-letter abbreviation for the substituted amino acid. Exon 1 *(open box)* regulates transcription. Exons 2 and 3 *(heavy diagonal lines)* encode the DNA-binding region of the androgen receptor. Part of exon 4 *(thin diagonal lines)* encodes the "hinge region" of the androgen receptor, which contains a nuclear localization signal. The 3′ end of exon 4 through exon 8 *(stippled)* encodes the ligand (androgen)-binding region. A mutational hot spot is located in exon 5 and can cause both CAR and PAR. Not shown are nonsense, frameshift, and splice junction mutations and deletions that can cause either CAR or PAR. (Redrawn from Quigley CA, De Bellis A, Marschke KB, et al. Androgen receptor defects: historical, clinical and molecular perspectives. Endocr Rev 1995; 16:271–321. © 1995, The Endocrine Society.)

ture in two such unrelated patients with complete androgen insensitivity.[1311] In general, mutations that severely affect protein structure and function result in the complete phenotype whereas the partial forms of the syndrome are invariably associated with missense mutations. The results of androgen-binding studies in genital skin fibroblasts can now be interpreted more meaningfully in relation to mutation type. For example, two sisters with complete androgen insensitivity and increased androgen binding had an in-frame deletion of exon 3 encoding one of the zinc fingers in the DNA-binding domain. This ablated the function of the androgen receptor as a transcription factor but left the hormone-binding domain intact.[1312, 1313] Proof that a nucleotide substitution is the cause of resistance to androgens is based on experiments in vitro to re-create the mutant receptor in heterologous cells and analyze function using an appropriate reporter gene.[1314–1316] These studies have led indirectly to structure-function information about the androgen receptor in the absence, until recently, of data from crystallographic analysis.[1317–1319] The hormone-binding domain is highly homologous to that of the progesterone receptor.

The relationship between genotype and phenotype can be quite variable in the syndromes of androgen insensitivity, particularly in the partial forms (see Fig. 22–78). This can also be the case within families harboring the same mutation. These observations are consistent with the influence of epistatic factors, apart from the derangement of the gene encoding the androgen receptor, that affect the phenotypic manifestations in these families.[1320–1322] For the complete form, this phenotype is consistent within families for a given mutation. Even so, there is evidence of somatic mosaicism in a number of patients who usually have partial insensitivity to androgens.[1323] Some expression of the wild-type receptor will have a variable effect on androgen action. The de novo mutation rate may be as high as 30%, a figure typical for X-linked recessive disorders.[1324]

The role of co-regulator protein dysfunction in androgen action may be relevant in some forms of androgen insensitivity. Targeted disruption of the mouse *Src1* gene leads to partial resistance to sex steroids and thyroid hormone.[439] This coactivator is one component of the large multi-protein complex that interacts with nuclear transcription factors. ARA 70 cofactor, which appears to bind relatively specifically to the androgen receptor, was screened for mutations in a group of patients with the phenotype of partial androgen insensitivity, but no abnormalities were found.[1325] Seldom is a mutation of the androgen receptor gene not found in the complete form of androgen insensitivity. A Japanese patient with the syndrome was reported to have a normal gene on sequencing and absence of a specific co-activator for the androgen receptor that was present in normal genital skin fibroblasts.[1326] The protein is yet to be characterized, but the case illustrates the possibility of some hormone resistance syndromes being caused by disorders in nuclear co-regulators.[1327]

Germ line mutations have been reported in male breast cancer[1328, 1329]; the mutations affected adjacent arginine residues in the second zinc finger part of the DNA-binding domain in all three reported patients. Somatic mutations are described in prostate cancer, a disease that is androgen dependent in its initial stages. A common mutation is Thr877Ala, which is also found in the human prostate LNCaP cell line.[1330] A unique inactivating somatic mutation (Tyr619Cys) has been identified that is transcriptionally inactive and appears to sequester the SRC1 co-activator protein, a pathophysiologic feature analogous to what occurs as a result of the increased triplet repeats in Kennedy's disease.[1331]

Hormone Profile

The hormone profile is similar in all variants of androgen insensitivity but is best characterized in the complete form. The hallmark at puberty and in the adult is an elevated concentration of plasma LH and testosterone in the absence of virilization.

However, plasma LH and testosterone levels were strikingly low in 9 of 10 neonates with the complete form of androgen resistance at 30 and 60 days of age as was the LH response to the administration of LHRH. In contrast, 5 similarly studied neonates with partial androgen resistance had plasma testosterone levels in the high normal range and exhibited a normal neonatal LH surge. The suggestion is that the normal postnatal range of testosterone and LH in male infants is abolished or attenuated by the lack of or very functionally defective androgen receptors in the hypothalamus whereas the less functionally defective androgen receptor abnormalities in the partial androgen resistance syndrome are sufficient for the expression of the characteristic surge.[1332]

The pattern of LH and testosterone at puberty and in the adult is much the same in the partial form of the syndrome. Indeed, elevated LH in the face of normal to increased adult male-related testosterone concentrations in men with reduced sperm counts may be a marker of mild androgen insensitivity secondary to an androgen receptor gene mutation.[1333, 1334] Estradiol levels are elevated, both as a direct effect of testicular secretion and peripheral aromatization of androgens to estrogens.[1335, 1336] Feminization takes place at puberty amplified by estrogen action unopposed by androgens. Plasma FSH concentrations are generally within the normal range. When gonadectomy is performed, there is a further elevation of plasma LH and a rise in FSH concentration that suggests that both estradiol and inhibin play a role in the negative feedback of gonadotropins in patients with androgen resistance.[1337]

Sex hormone–binding globulin (SHBG) levels are higher in adult females compared with males as a result of an estrogen effect. SHBG levels are in the female range in androgen insensitivity. The lack of SHBG response to the rise in testosterone concentrations after hCG stimulation has been proposed as a useful biochemical screen for androgen insensitivity before puberty.[1338] Furthermore, the anabolic-androgenic steroid stanozolol fails to suppress SHBG levels in complete androgen insensitive patients, whereas there was an intermediate response in patients with the partial form as compared with normal male controls.[1339] However, this bioassay is not useful in newborns because of the normal decrease in the concentration of SHBG in the neonate. Few confirmatory data have been published in older patients; an increased plasma level of AMH may be a marker of androgen resistance during the first year of life and after the onset of puberty.[1340, 1341]

Diagnosis. The diagnosis in the complete form of androgen insensitivity is relatively straightforward and can usually be established on clinical grounds.[280] This is particularly so when there is a positive family history. It is not unusual to establish a history of an older "sister" having had surgery to repair bilateral inguinal herniae. The main differential in infancy is 17β-HSD 3 deficiency and Leydig cell hypoplasia (LH/hCG resistance), hence the recommendation to perform an hCG stimulation test. Later the differential is mainly with complete XY gonadal dysgenesis, where typically there is absent or poor breast development and the retention of müllerian structures.

The *partial form of the syndrome* is much more of a diagnostic challenge; the disorders that can give rise to a similar phenotype have already been discussed. As yet there is no readily available, clinically practical, in vivo or in vitro assay of the *trans*-activational capacity of the androgen receptor[1342]; but new approaches are promising.[1343] It is mandatory to assess the androgen response to hCG stimulation, ensuring that androstenedione, testosterone, and DHT concentrations are measured in plasma. There is sometimes a response in growth of the phallus after the hCG stimulation test, particularly if prolonged. Furthermore, a short course of testosterone injections is recommended as a diagnostic test.[1344, 1575] However, a response does not necessarily exclude partial androgen insensitivity because it is now known from *trans*-activation studies of mutant receptors in vitro that certain androgen receptor gene mutations are compatible with male sex of rearing.[1345–1347] The phallic response to testosterone is an important assessment in the recommendation for sex assignment in the affected infant.[1515] In addition, although the phallic response has been used as a predictive test of androgen responsiveness and future phallic growth, in some cases the results have been equivocal and a neonatal response has not invariably been followed by a response to testosterone at puberty.[1344]

Management. The sex of rearing is female in the complete form of androgen insensitivity, and the gonads need to be removed, owing to a later risk of malignancy. The testes may be left in place (especially if they are not located in the labia major) until late adolescence to provide a natural source of estrogen. The patient may then elect to undergo orchidectomy, having undergone spontaneous pubertal feminization. Using laparoscopy it is feasible to repair an inguinal hernia in childhood without removing the testis(es). The status of the intra-abdominal testis(es) can be monitored by periodic (every 2 to 4 years) sonography or MRI scans of the pelvis. There is also the question of a modest decrease in bone mineralization in patients with complete androgen insensitivity, although the risk does not seem to be related to when gonadectomy is performed.[1282] The limited data available on bone mineral density in partial androgen insensitivity indicate less of a deficit in bone mineralization.[1282]

A potential surgical problem in the complete form of androgen insensitivity is the shortened vagina. There are numerous techniques described to re-fashion a vagina, and the details are beyond the scope of this chapter. Most patients do not require surgery if graded vaginal dilators are used on a regular basis in adolescence. Estrogen treatment is required after gonadectomy; a transdermal patch is widely used but is expensive.[745] It is generally thought that the lack of a uterus precludes the necessity for concomitant treatment with a progestagen. Outcome studies indicate that psychosexual development and sexual function are generally satisfactory in adult life.[1349] The practice of not disclosing full information to the patient about the nature of her medical condition is no longer acceptable. The authors recommend that with consent of the parents and the establishment of an appropriate psychosocial support system, the diagnosis, pathophysiology, quality of life issues be disclosed to the patient in an age-appropriate manner, step-by-step, throughout childhood and adolescence. The patient needs to be counseled and repeatedly assured of her potential to lead a life as a woman, except for fertility, including marriage if she so desires and adoptive parenthood. In North America, the United Kingdom, and Australia, androgen insensitivity support groups with websites are available and are active in educating women with the disorder as well as physicians. If disclosure is not done in childhood and adolescence, issues surrounding disclosure in the adult need to be explored by experienced clinicians with great discretion, perceptiveness, and sensitivity, and in our view on a need-to-know basis. A potentially painful if not disastrous scenario is one in which the adult patient inadvertently discovers the diagnosis. Carrier detection for genetic counseling purposes is often requested and can be undertaken once the gene mutation within a family has been identified. The polymorphic CAG repeat sequence in exon 1 is useful to analyze segregation of the two X chromosomes in a carrier female.[1350] Furthermore, this linked marker can be useful to exclude the possibility of partial androgen insensitivity in familial hypospadias of unknown cause.

Management of partial androgen insensitivity syndrome is complicated by the major issue of predicting the likely response to androgens at puberty. The disorder is no different to other causes of severe undermasculinization (e.g., in 45X/46,XY karyotype) where decisions are often based on the response of the penis to a course of intramuscular testosterone. The surgical issues concerning creating a functional phallus, which in the past had been an important consideration, are no longer compelling in light of the remarkable advances in the surgical correction of severe degrees of hypospadias.[397, 505] There is evidence that male sex of rearing is increasingly chosen despite severe undermasculinization at birth. Some patients respond at least partially to high-dose androgen therapy.[1364, 1365] Outcome studies are sparse, but studies of males with micropenis reported heterosexual orientation and normal male sexual function in the majority.[1351, 1352] If the parents select a female sex assignment, it is necessary to inform them that a variable degree of masculinization as well as feminization will occur at puberty. In patients in whom the assigned female sex and their gender identity are congruent, orchidectomy is usually advisable by early puberty.

Partial (Incomplete) Form of Androgen Resistance and Its Variants (Reifenstein's Syndrome)

A heterogeneous group of 46,XY individuals have partial androgen resistance[408, 1266] (see Table 22–34; see also Fig. 22–79). The external genitalia range from perineoscrotal hypospadias with cryptorchidism and micropenis to clitoromegaly with partial labial fusion. The patients described in the past by Lubs, Gilbert, Dreyfus, Reifenstein, Rosewater, Walker, and their associates quite likely had partial androgen resistance.[408, 1266, 1283, 1284] The variable degree of masculinization of affected males within and between kinships is well illustrated by one family studied by Wilson and colleagues.[1285] Eleven males were affected; two had a relatively mild defect in masculinization of the external genitalia (small penis and bifid scrotum), eight had perineal hypospadias, and one had hypospadias, a urogenital sinus with a blind vaginal pouch, and an absent vas deferens. All lacked müllerian structures. In contrast, families with the complete form of androgen resistance exhibit little variability in expression of the mutant gene. The most common presentation in infancy is that of an apparent male with third-degree hypospadias (the urethral orifice located at the base of the phallus), a small penis, and, often, cryptorchidism. Müllerian duct derivatives are absent; wolffian duct derivatives are usually present but hypoplastic. At puberty, pubic and axillary hair and gynecomastia usually develop, male secondary sexual characteristics are incompletely developed, and the testes remain small and exhibit azoospermia because of germinal cell arrest beyond the primary spermatocyte stage. Less severely affected men may exhibit a bifid scrotum, infertility, and poor virilization at puberty. More severely affected males may have ambiguous genitalia, a blind vaginal pouch, and poorly developed wolffian structures. As in other patients with androgen insensitivity, the concentrations of plasma LH and testosterone are elevated and the high LH levels are resistant to suppression by exogenous androgens. Estradiol and testosterone production rates are increased. However, the degree of feminization at puberty, despite elevated estradiol secretion, is less than in the complete form of androgen resistance (see Fig. 22–79).

Table 22–34. Clinical Features of Partial Androgen Resistance

Karyotype:	46,XY
Inheritance:	X-linked recessive; mutations in *AR* gene
External genitalia:	Ambiguous with blind vaginal pouch → hypoplastic male → normal male with infertility → normal fertile male
Wolffian duct derivatives:	Rudimentary → hypoplastic → normal
Müllerian duct derivatives:	Absent
Gonads:	Testes (usually undesended)
Habitus:	Decreased to normal axillary and pubic hair, beard growth, and body hair; gynecomastia common at puberty
Hormone and metabolic profile:	Increased plasma LH and testosterone concentrations; increased estradiol (for men); FSH levels may be normal or slightly increased
	Partial resistance to androgenic and metabolic effects of testosterone
Androgen receptor studies:	Genetic heterogeneity; partial deficiency of normal receptor; mutations lead to qualitatively abnormal receptor

LH, luteinizing hormone; FSH, follicle-stimulating hormone.

Androgen Resistance in Infertile Men

Analysis of a large kindred with Reifenstein's syndrome (partial androgen resistance syndrome) led to the detection of two phenotypically normal males who were infertile and lacked the clinical features of androgen resistance. These infertile males could not be distinguished endocrinologically or by androgen receptor studies from their more severely affected relatives.[408, 1356] Subsequently, Aiman and co-workers[1357] reported infertility in three unrelated men with uninformative family histories and a quantitative deficiency of the androgen receptor. Two of the men had a normal adult male phenotype; one had slight gynecomastia, decreased body hair, and a modest reduction in testicular size. All were infertile and had severe oligospermia or azoospermia. The significant hormonal findings were normal or elevated serum concentrations of testosterone in the presence of high plasma concentrations of LH. Two of the three men had increased blood production rates for testosterone, androstenedione, and estradiol. The decreased amount of androgen receptor in genital skin fibroblasts was consistent with a quantitative deficiency of the androgen receptor. Further studies suggested the existence of both quantitative and qualitative abnormalities in the androgen receptor in infertile males.[1357] To estimate the frequency of androgen receptor abnormalities in men with idiopathic infertility, Aiman and Grif-

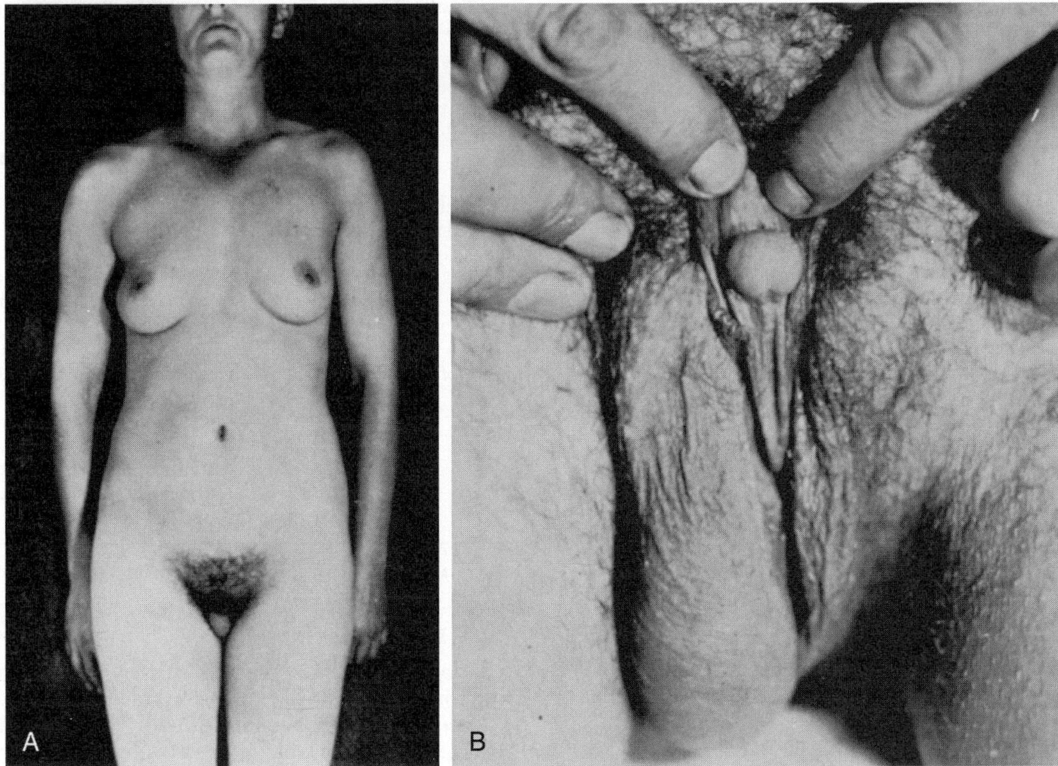

Figure 22–79. A patient with partial androgen resistance (Reifenstein's syndrome). Both the patient and his brother had hypospadias, poor masculinization, and marked gynecomastia. Both had a normal 46,XY karyotype, normal wolffian duct derivatives, and no müllerian structures. (Reproduced, with permission, from Bowen P, Lee CSN, Migeon CJ, et al. Hereditary male pseudohermaphroditism with hypogonadism, hypospadias, and gynecomastia [Reifenstein's syndrome]. Ann Intern Med 1965; 62:252–270. Courtesy of Dr. E. C. Reifenstein, Jr.)

fin[1358] studied 28 unrelated, phenotypically normal men with idiopathic azoospermia or oligospermia. Using genital skin fibroblasts, they observed a partial deficiency of the receptor in 9 (40%) of 22 of the azoospermic or oligospermic subjects.[1358] In contrast to previously studied patients with androgen resistance, six of nine infertile men had normal levels of plasma LH and testosterone, and the plasma production rate of testosterone was elevated in only two of six.[1358] Other studies have detected subtle defects in the androgen receptor in some subfertile men.[1333, 1359–1361]

Androgen Resistance in Fertile Men

It was postulated that infertility in otherwise normal men was the most consistent and most subtle clinical manifestation of quantitative and qualitative defects in the androgen receptor.[408, 1358, 1359] However, families have now been described that include men with normal male genitalia, postpubertal gynecomastia, and poor virilization in spite of elevated plasma testosterone levels.[1290, 1362] Studies of the androgen receptor in affected individuals detected several qualitative abnormalities, including receptor instability, failure of up-regulation, increased dissociation of receptor-synthetic androgen complexes, and thermal instability.[1290, 1362] Molecular analysis of the *AR* gene in one cohort revealed a single nucleotide substitution in the androgen-binding domain, a leucine to phenylalanine change at amino acid 789 (Leu789Phe).[1290] Expression of the mutant gene in transfected cells demonstrated a decrease in *trans*-activational activity with this substitution compatible to that seen in this mild form of androgen resistance. Hence, subtle undervirilization (phallus length, 5 to 6 cm in two patients) with or without gynecomastia, rather than infertility, may represent the extreme of the phenotypic spectrum of subtle defects in androgen receptor function.[1290, 1361, 1362]

Defects in Testosterone Metabolism by Peripheral Tissues: Steroid 5α-Reductase Type 2 Deficiency (Male Pseudohermaphroditism with Virilization at Puberty)

In 1961, Nowakowski and Lenz[1366] described a familial type of male pseudohermaphroditism, which they called "pseudovaginal perineoscrotal hypospadias," that was transmitted as an autosomal recessive trait.[1367] The patients resemble those with other forms of male pseudohermaphroditism by having a 46,XY karyotype, normally differentiated testes, male internal ducts, and ambiguous external genitalia. At puberty, striking but selective signs of masculinization appear.

In 1974, Walsh and associates[1368] and Imperato-McGinley and colleagues[1369–1371] reported a defect in the conversion of testosterone to its 5α-reduced metabolite DHT in patients with this syndrome (Fig. 22–80). Imperato-McGinley described a genetic isolate from villages in the southwestern part of the Dominican Republic. The classic features (Table 22–35) of this form of male pseudohermaphroditism in infancy include a clitoris-like, hypospadiac phallus bound in chordee of variable degree, a bifid scrotum, and a urogenital sinus that opens on the perineum. A blind vaginal pouch opens either into the urogenital sinus or onto the perineum behind the urethral orifice. The testes are well differentiated and are located in the inguinal canal or the labioscrotal folds. No müllerian structures are present. The wolffian structures (epididymis, vas deferens,

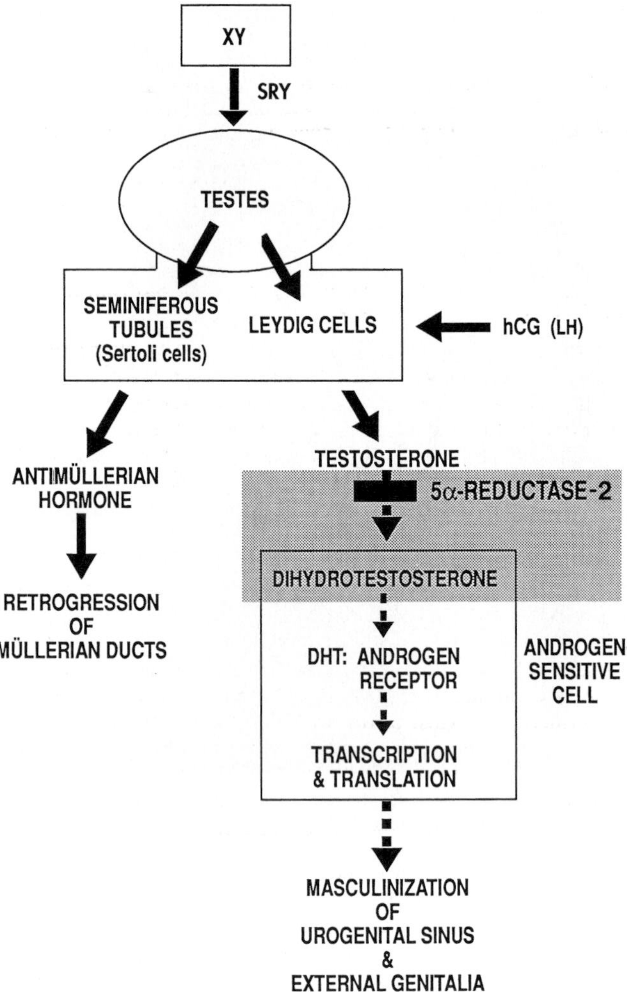

Figure 22–80. Diagram of male pseudohermaphroditism resulting from 5α-reductase deficiency.

Table 22–35. Clinical Features of 5α-Reductase-2 Deficiency

Karyotype:	46,XY
Inheritance:	Autosomal recessive; mutations in *SRD5A2* gene
Genitalia:	Usually ambiguous with small, hypospadiac phallus; blind vaginal pouch → hypoplastic male
Wolffian duct derivatives:	Normal
Müllerian duct derivatives:	Absent
Gonads:	Normal testes
Habitus:	Partial virilization at puberty without gynecomastia; decreased facial and body hair, no temporal hair recession; prostate not palpable
Hormone profile:	Decreased ratio of $5\alpha/5\beta$ C_{21}- and C_{19}-steroids in urine; increased plasma testosterone/dihydrotestosterone (T/DHT) ratio before and after hCG stimulation; modest increase in plasma LH and decreased conversion of T to DHT in vivo

hCG, human chorionic gonadotropin; LH, luteinizing hormone.

and seminal vesicle) are well differentiated; the ejaculatory ducts usually terminate in the blind vaginal pouch. If a vaginal pouch is not present, the wolffian ducts terminate on the perineum next to the urethra. The prostate is hypoplastic. At puberty, plasma testosterone levels increase into the adult male range, whereas DHT levels remain disproportionately low but measurable. Affected males virilize to a variable degree without gynecomastia: the voice deepens; muscle mass increases; the phallus, although bound in chordee of variable severity, enlarges to 4 to 8 cm in length; libido ensues; and penile erections occur.[408, 1372] The bifid scrotum becomes rugated and pigmented, and the testes enlarge and descend into the labioscrotal folds. However, none of the postpubertal affected males have acne, more than sparse facial or body hair, temporal hair recession, or enlargement of the prostate, nor do they develop gynecomastia. Histologic examination of the adult testes in affected males shows Leydig cell hyperplasia and decreased spermatogenesis.[1373, 1374] In general, spermatogenesis is either absent or profoundly impaired, which appears to be due to the cryptorchidism.[1373, 1374] Semen analyses of nine patients with 5α-reductase-2 deficiency from the Dominican cohort revealed normal sperm concentration, total count, and mobility in one patient with hypospadias and bilaterally descended testes and in a second patient after hypospadias repair.[1374] Semen volume and viscosity were abnormal in all nine patients. The finding of a normal sperm count and concentration in a male with 5α-reductase-2 deficiency suggests that DHT, in contrast to testosterone, does not play a major role in spermatogenesis.[1374, 1375] Three male siblings in a Swedish family affected with 5α-reductase deficiency had successful hypospadias repair in infancy and two brothers were demonstrably fertile.[1376] All were compound heterozygotes for mutations in the *SRD5A2* gene.

As with other forms of male pseudohermaphroditism, phenotypic variability has been described both within and between cohorts.[408, 1377] Approximately 55% of patients have had a pseudovagina; the rest have a urogenital sinus, a hypospadiac phallus, or even a microphallus with a penile urethra.[1377–1380] Eighteen of 19 46,XY patients with 5α-reductase-2 deficiency from the Dominican cohort who were raised "unambiguously" as females changed their gender identity and gender role behavior to male after the onset of puberty (Fig. 22–81).[492] Similar observations were reported in 19 of 40 families with 5α-reductase-2 deficiency, as well as in male pseudohermaphrodites with 17β-HSD 3 deficiency or XO/XY mosaicism.[408, 484, 1381, 1382] This phenomenon appears to be particularly prevalent, although not exclusively so, in 46,XY male pseudohermaphrodites whose gonads are retained and who produce testosterone that results in masculinization at puberty.[484, 1382] An isolated case of 5α-reductase deficiency was reported where the child was raised as a girl but on virilization at puberty the gender was changed to male.[1383] The parents were first cousins of Pakistani origin. These patients raise provocative questions about the effect of sex of rearing, social and cultural factors, and of learning and prenatal androgen exposure on the brain and Y-bearing genes on psychosexual development. A genetic isolate of individuals from New Guinea deficient in 5α-reductase-2 was described by Herdt and Davidson.[497] As in the Dominican cohort, a third category of sex was identified in this cultural isolate, the so-called Turnim man. However, sex reversal at puberty has not been as common in this cultural isolate as in others, where the sex reversal appears to be in part a consequence of social and cultural pressure rather than solely a sex hormone effect on behavior.[497] Another cluster of cases has been described from Southern Lebanon.[1381] Again, affected individuals were unambiguously female at birth and remained so until puberty, when there was a change in gender role.

Females homozygous for 5α-reductase-2 deficiency are phenotypically normal and undergo normal pubertal maturation

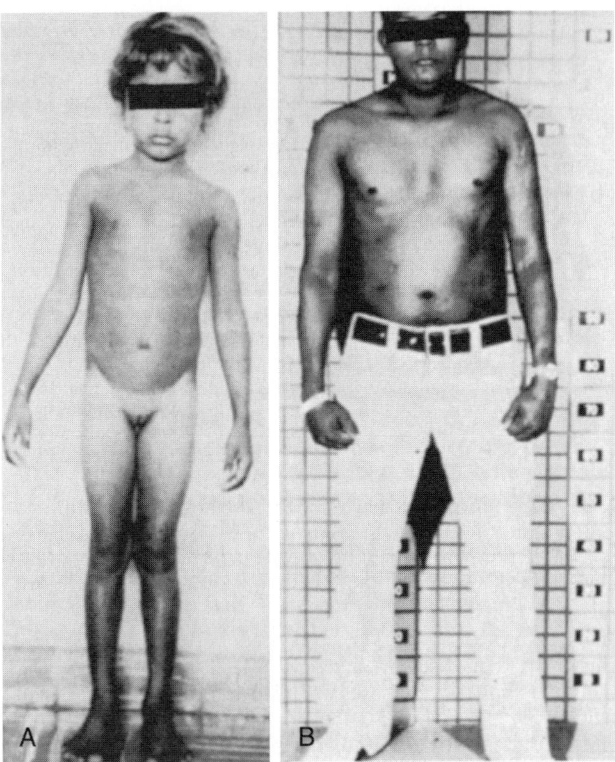

Figure 22–81. *A*, A prepubertal 46,XY child with 5α-reductase-2 deficiency who was raised as a female. *B*, A postpubertal male with 5α-reductase-2 deficiency who has virilized and changed gender role behavior. (From Peterson RE, Imperato-McGinley J, Gautier T, et al. Male pseudohermaphroditism due to 5α-steroid deficiency. Am J Med 1977; 62:170–191.)

except for delayed menarche.[1377, 1381, 1383, 1384] They have an absence of hair on the arms and legs and decreased axillary and pubic hair, which suggests an important effect of DHT on the growth of body hair.[1384] Fertility is normal, and two of the three homozygous females studied in the Dominican kindred gave birth to nonidentical twins, which suggests a role for DHT in the regulation of ovarian follicular maturation[1384]; the human ovary has 5α-reductase-2 activity.

In infancy and childhood, patients with 5α-reductase-2 deficiency have normal to elevated plasma concentrations of testosterone and decreased levels of DHT after the administration of hCG.[408, 1368, 1385] In affected postpubertal patients, the testosterone/DHT ratio in peripheral blood is increased from 12 ± 3.1 (mean ± SD) to 35 to 84.[1385] Postpubertally, plasma LH levels are either normal or slightly elevated; plasma FSH levels are elevated in about 50% of patients.[408] Studies of estrogen and androgen synthesis demonstrate normal male androgen and estrogen production; this explains the lack of gynecomastia postpubertally in these patients, compared with patients with partial androgen resistance.[408] Additional biochemical features of 5α-reductase-2 deficiency are a diminished ratio of urinary 5α to 5β-reduced C_{19}- and C_{21}-steroids. Analysis of 5α-reduced C_{21}-steroid urinary products can be a useful diagnostic test if the gonads have already been removed. Deficient or abnormal 5α-reductase-2 activity in fibroblasts cultured from genital skin[408] is typically seen, but the range of activity in normal individuals is very wide and varies between cell passage number. This is no longer used for diagnosis now that molecular studies of the *SRD5A2* gene are possible. Heterozygotes for 5α-reductase-2 deficiency have no clinical manifestations and have intermediate ratios of urinary 5α-reduced to 5β-reduced C_{19}-steroids (e.g., androsterone/etiocholanolone).[408]

Genetics. The disorder is transmitted as an autosomal recessive trait. There are two steroid 5α-reductase enzymes.[408, 1386–1388] Both isozymes, which share 50% homology, are located in microsomes and catalyze the NADPH-dependent conversion of testosterone to the more androgenic DHT.[1388] Steroid 5α-reductase-1 is encoded by a gene located on chromosome 5p15[1387]; the gene, *SRD5A1*, has five exons and four introns and encodes a protein with a neutral to basic pH optimum.[1388] It is expressed at birth in the liver and nongenital skin.[1388, 1389] Although the expression of the type 1 enzyme persists in the liver throughout postnatal life,[1388] its expression decreases in skin to unmeasurable levels after 2 to 3 years of age and remains low until puberty, when it is again present in nongenital skin, especially the sebaceous glands of the scalp.[1388] No mutations in the type 1 gene have as yet been described. Targeted disruption of the *SRD5A1* gene in XX mice causes a defect in parturition that is caused by impaired cervical ripening.[1390]

Steroid 5α-reductase-2 is encoded by the *SRD5A2* gene on chromosome 2p23, which, like the type 1 gene, contains five exons and encodes a 254-amino acid protein.[1387, 1388] The type 2 isozyme has a lower Michaelis constant (K_m) for testosterone than does the type 1 isozyme; steroid 5α-reductase-2 has an acidic pH optimum and is more sensitive to inhibition by finasteride.[408, 1388] Most of the 5α-reductase activity in the early fetus is caused by the type 2 enzyme.[1389] It is expressed in the primordia of the prostate and external genitalia before their differentiation,[1389] but it is not expressed in the embryonic wolffian duct until after the differentiation of the epididymides, vas deferens, and seminal vesicles, which are induced by testosterone and not by DHT.[342] Similar observations were found in the human male reproductive tract based on immunohistochemistry.[1391]

Type 2 expression increases in liver and nongenital skin at birth.[1389] It persists in the liver throughout life but diminishes to unmeasurable levels in nongenital skin after 3 years of age. A pseudogene has been mapped to the long arm of the X chromosome at band q24-qter.[1392]

Steroid 5α-reductase-2 deficiency is inherited as an autosomal recessive trait and is genetically heterogeneous and more than 30 mutations have been detected in the gene (Fig. 22–82).[408, 1372, 1377, 1380, 1381, 1393, 1394] Most are missense mutations and distributed throughout the coding region of the gene. In general, mutations involving the 3′ end of the gene and the carboxyl terminus of the enzyme are associated with a decrease in the affinity for the cofactor NADPH, whereas mutations that affect the binding of testosterone involve exons that encode either the NH_2 or COOH-terminal ends of the enzyme.[408, 1388] About 35% of the mutation-positive cases are compound heterozygotes and there are relative "hot spots" in exons 4 and 5.

Consanguinity has been described in approximately 40% of patients.[408, 1387] The occurrence of the disorder in three genetic isolates in the Dominican Republic (Arg246Trp), the Sambia tribe of the New Guinea highlands (deletion of the *SRD5A2* gene),[1395] Southern Lebanon (Leu55Gin), and cohorts in Turkey is probably the result of a "founder effect."[408] The severity of undermasculinization does not appear to be closely related to the type of mutation, especially in nongenetic isolates. The phenotypes resulting from either *17βHSD 3* or 5α-reductase-2 deficiency are very similar. Consequently, the report of mutations in both *HSD17B3* and *SRD5A2* in a large isolated Turkish kindred with male pseudohermaphroditism is noteworthy.[1396] The results of molecular analysis were complex, with some members homozygous for the *SRD5A2* mutation but

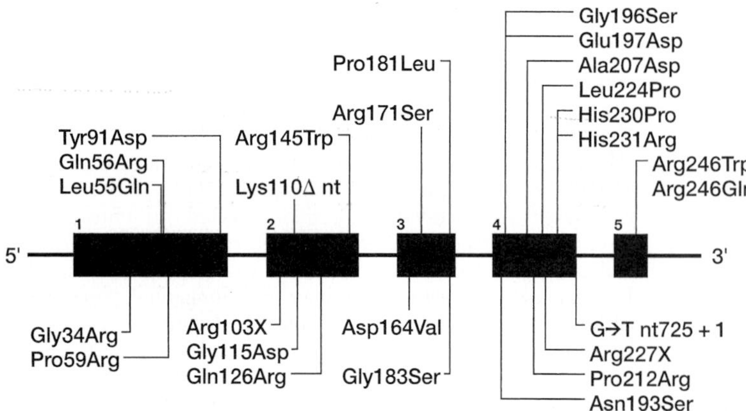

Figure 22–82. Diagram of the gene encoding 5α-reductase-2 with representative mutations causing 5α-reductase-2 deficiency. The exons are the numbered black boxes. Missense mutations causing amino acid substitutions in the enzyme are indicated by the three-letter abbreviation for the wild-type amino acid, followed by the position number of the amino acid in the enzyme and the three-letter abbreviation for the substituted amino acid. X indicates a nonsense (stop) mutation. G→T nt725 + 1 is a splice junction mutation of guanine (G) to thymidine (T) one nucleotide downstream of the boundary between exon 4 and intron 4. Nucleotide 725 is the closest nucleotide in the exon to the mutation. A cohort of patients from New Guinea has been described with complete deletion of the 5α-reductase-2 gene. (Redrawn from Wilson JD, Griffin JE, Russell DW. Steroid 5α-reductase deficiency. Endocr Rev 1993; 14:577–593. © 1993, The Endocrine Society.)

heterozygous for the *HSD17B3* mutation, and vice versa for other affected family members. There was some phenotypic distinction as judged by the presence of mild gynecomastia if an individual was homozygous for the *HSD17B3* mutation. There is evidence that 5α-reductase-2 deficiency may result from uniparental disomy (UPD). This is based on a report of two unrelated patients with the enzyme deficiency whose parents were heterozygous carriers for two different but identical mutations in the two families (Glu197Asp and Pro212Arg).[1397] One patient was a compound heterozygote for the two mutations, but the other was a homozygote for the paternal mutation (Glu197Asp). The reduction to homozygosity for this mutation suggested not only the first example of 5α-reductase deficiency resulting from UPD but also the first case of paternal (as opposed to maternal) UPD involving chromosome 2.

The finding of two 5α-reductase genes with different tissue distributions and different temporal expressions has clarified the nature of the pubertal masculinization in this disorder, which contrasts to the failure of masculinization of the external genitalia during embryogenesis. Even patients with a deletion of the *SRD5A2* gene (null genotypes) have measurable levels of DHT at puberty, which is attributed to the conversion of testosterone to DHT in peripheral tissues by the expression of the type 1 enzyme in nongenital skin and liver at puberty. The masculinization at puberty can result from the increased plasma DHT levels as well as the chronic effect of adult levels of testosterone on the androgen receptor.

Diagnosis. The diagnosis of 5α-reductase-2 deficiency can be difficult, especially before the age of puberty. It should be suspected in all prepubertal male pseudohermaphrodites, especially those with perineoscrotal hypospadias with or without a blind vaginal pouch, in males with hypospadias or microphallus or both, and in male pseudohermaphrodites who virilize at puberty without evidence of gynecomastia. Virilization at puberty and the absence of gynecomastia in male pseudohermaphrodites are not unique to 5α-reductase-2 deficiency. For example, patients with 17β-HSD 3 deficiency or partial androgen resistance may present in this manner, but they can be distinguished biochemically or by DNA analysis from patients with 5α-reductase-2 deficiency. The diagnosis of 5α-reductase-2 deficiency can be confirmed prepubertally and postpubertally by demonstration of an abnormally high testosterone/DHT ratio in peripheral blood before and/or after hCG administration.[1378, 1379, 1385, 1398–1400] The testosterone/DHT ratio under basal conditions in postpubertal affected males is 35 to 84, whereas the ratio in normal men is 12 ± 3.1. In normal male infants, when there is active testicular steroidogenesis, the testosterone/DHT ratio ranges from 1.7 to 17 (mean ± SD, 4.9 ± 2.9).[1385] In view of the low levels of testosterone and DHT in prepubertal males, it is usually necessary to administer hCG (1500 U/m^2 intramuscularly every 24 hours three times) to demonstrate the defect. Patients with 5α-reductase-2 deficiency have high testosterone/DHT ratios after hCG administration. Similarly, the ratio of 5α- to 5β-metabolites of testosterone and of tetrahydrocortisol (THF) to allotetrahydrocortisol (5α-THF) in urine is a marker both prepubertally and postpubertally of 5α-reductase-2 deficiency.[1378, 1379, 1400] Using both basal and hCG-induced increases in testosterone level and urinary analyses of 5α- and 5β-steroid metabolites, Imperato-McGinley and co-workers detected 5α-reductase-2 deficiency in three infants between the ages of 1 and 3 months.[1401] Mutations in the *SRD5A2* gene have been reported rarely in boys with isolated hypospadias.[1402] Two of the mutations (Ala49Thr and Leu113Val) have not been reported in patients with typical 5α-reductase deficiency. A positive family history of hypospadias was not necessarily a pointer to a mutation being more likely.

Early diagnosis of 5α-reductase-2 deficiency is important because of its bearing on the assignment of sex in the affected infant. Although the majority of missense mutations in the *SRD5A2* gene are associated with less than 0.4% of normal activity, mutations with 3% to 15% residual activity have been reported in 46,XY individuals with sufficient masculinization of the external genitalia at birth to be assigned a male gender.[1399, 1400] Masculinization in utero and the plasma testosterone/DHT ratio in early infancy correlate with the degree of residual 5α-reductase-2 activity.[1399] The natural history of patients with this deficiency—that is, the propensity in some patients for change to male gender role behavior and for virilization at puberty—makes male assignment of neonatally diagnosed patients the recommendation of choice, especially in affected individuals with ambiguous or hypoplastic male genitalia.[1378, 1383, 1399]

Therapy with DHT should increase phallic length into the normal range for age and enable repair of hypospadias. Carpenter and co-workers[1403] described a 9-month-old infant with 5α-reductase-2-deficiency who had been assigned a male gender at birth. The genitalia exhibited penoscrotal hypospadias with a phallus 1.9 cm in length and bound down in chordee. Therapy was instituted with DHT, 25 mg/day (2% by weight in a cold cream base), applied to the patient's abdomen. Four months of therapy resulted in an increase of stretched phallus length from 1.8 to 3.8 cm. No advancement in bone maturation was noted. Hypospadias repair was undertaken, and a second course of DHT was given without consequence.[1403] Two affected siblings with very small phalluses and a bifid scrotum containing palpable gonads were treated with topic DHT cream applied to the external genitalia.[1378] There was significant phallic growth in both siblings, which also aided subsequent hypospadias corrective surgery.[1378] In adults with 5α-reductase-2 deficiency, supraphysiologic doses of testoster-

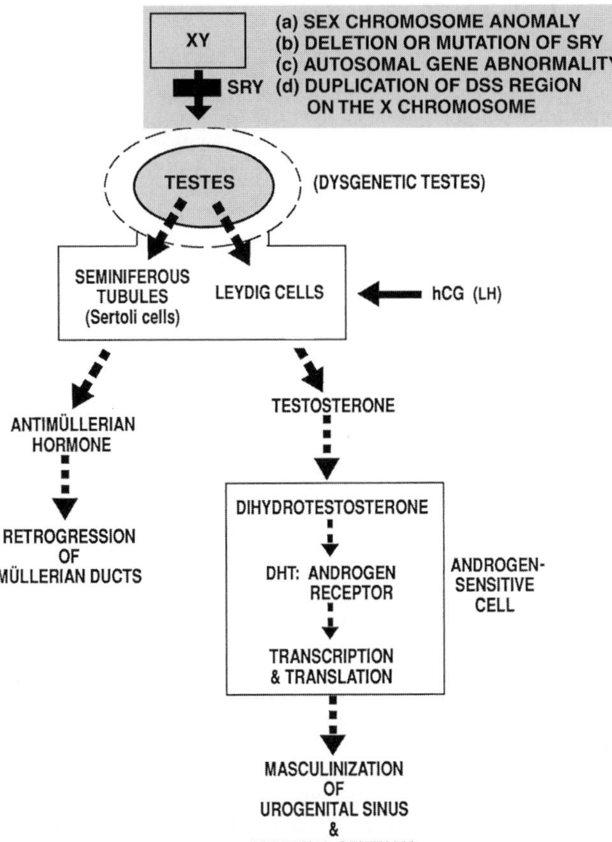

Figure 22–83. Diagram of the pathogenesis of dysgenetic male pseudohermaphroditism. This condition can result from a sex chromosome anomaly or from a mutant gene in the male sex determination or differentiation cascade. The degree of masculinization is dependent on the functional ability of the dysgenetic gonads to produce antimüllerian hormone and testosterone.

one have resulted in normal DHT levels and partial masculinization[1364]; the conversion to DHT is mediated by the type 1 5α-reductase isozyme. However, Mendonca and colleagues[1377] report that treatment of late adolescents or adults with high doses of testosterone and/or DHT induced an increase in phallic size that remained more than 2 SD below the normal mean and usually did not exceed 5 cm. Should the patient inadvertently be assigned a female sex role or the parents elect to rear the infant or child as a female, we suggest that female genitoplasty and orchidectomy not be performed until the age of puberty and only with the consent of the adolescent as well as the parents.

Dysgenetic Male Pseudohermaphroditism (Ambiguous Genitalia Resulting from Dysgenetic Gonads)

Ambiguous development of the genital ducts, urogenital sinus, and external genitalia occurs in patients with dysgenetic gonads. They usually present with evidence of AMH deficiency as well as androgen deficiency and therefore have müllerian duct derivatives and ambiguous external genitalia. Mutations and deletions of any and all of the genes involved in the testes determination and differentiation cascade (see Fig. 22–19 and Table 22–4 and earlier section on sex determination) have been implicated in the etiology of dysgenetic male pseudohermaphroditism. The differential diagnosis encompasses a spectrum of abnormalities of the Y chromosome as well as

Table 22–36. Clinical Features of DAX1 Duplication in 46,XY Males

Karyotype:	46,XY dup Xp21
Inheritance:	X-linked → duplication of *DAX1* gene
Genitalia:	Female → ambiguous (rare)
Wolffian duct derivatives:	Absent → hypoplastic (rare)
Müllerian duct derivatives:	Normal → hypoplastic (rare)
Gonads:	Ovaries → hypoplastic testes (rare)
Habitus:	No somatic abnormalities associated with *DAX1*. Duplications including segments contiguous to *DAX1* may be associated with delayed psychomotor developmental and growth and dysplastic facies
Hormone profile:	Consistent with functional integrity of gonad

mosaicism involving a 45,X chromosome cell line and a cell line with Y chromosome DNA, which we have classified as "abnormalities of gonadal differentiation" (see sections on X-chromatin–negative variants of the syndrome of gonadal dysgenesis and familial and sporadic XY gonadal dysgenesis). These patients, all of whom have in common a defect in testes differentiation, can present with the clinical syndrome of "dysgenetic male pseudohermaphroditism"[1404] (Fig. 22–83).

Certain abnormalities of the X chromosome or an autosome are associated with dysgenetic male pseudohermaphroditism (see Fig. 22–19 and Table 22–4). Duplications of the Xp21.3 region that contains the *DAX1* gene can cause dysgenetic male pseudohermaphroditism as well as other extragenital anomalies and mental retardation (Table 22–36).[92, 199, 202] Mutations in *DAX1* cause X-linked congenital adrenal hypoplasia and hypogonadotropic hypogonadism. *DAX1* encodes a protein with three and one-half repeats of a motif that may be a DNA-binding domain.[90] The gene is expressed in the ovaries, testes, hypothalamus, and pituitary gland[1405] and has a steroidogenic factor (SF1) response element in its promoter.[199, 1406] Mutations in *DAX1* in XY males have no apparent effect on either the differentiation of the testes or male differentiation of the external genitalia; DNA analysis of 46,XY phenotypic females has failed to detect an abnormality in the *DAX1* gene.[90] Deletion of DAX1 does not impair testicular determination and differentiation, but duplications of the DAX1 region impair testicular differentiation in 46,XY individuals. This observation has led to the suggestion that *DAX1* may function as a repressor of male differentiation[92, 93, 201, 1407] in the human as well as the mouse.[1408] However, a duplication of the *DAX1* gene alone (not the Xp21.3 region) has not yet been described, in the human, in contrast to the mouse. Furthermore, it has been proposed that *SRY* may act as a repressor of *DAX1* in the testis differentiation cascade (hence, *DAX1* is a candidate for the putative testis repressor gene *Z*).[93, 201, 825]

46,XY dysgenetic male pseudohermaphroditism has been associated with mental retardation and thalassemia, the "ATRX syndrome."[1409] Mutations in a gene called *XH2*, located at Xq13.3, that encodes a DNA helicase are described in patients with an atypical form of this syndrome.[259] Terminal deletions at chromosome 10q (10q26-qter) and at 9p24-pter are associated with dysgenetic male pseudohermaphroditism and dysmorphic features.[242–252, 826] The putative gene on the long arm of chromosome 10 autosomes involved in testes development has not been ascertained.[252–254] However, accumulating evidence suggests that haploinsufficiency of a gene related to double sex in *Drosophila*, *DMRT1*, in chromosome 9p24.3 leads to defective testis differentiation.[243, 248, 1410, 1411]

Anomalies of the urinary tract are common in patients with abnormalities of genital differentiation.[1412] Less common is the association of dysgenetic male pseudohermaphroditism with

Table 22–37. Clinical Features of Denys-Drash Syndrome in 46,XY Males*

Karyotype:	46,XY
Inheritance:	Autosomal dominant: heterozygous mutations in exon 9 of the *WT1* gene on 11p13
Genitalia:	Phenotypic female (40%) → ambiguous genitalia → hypoplastic male
Wolffian duct derivatives:	Absent → hypoplastic
Müllerian duct derivatives:	Present → hypoplastic
Gonads:	Streak → dysgenetic testes
Other features:	Renal failure in first year of life due to focal or diffuse mesangial sclerosis. Wilms' tumor in the first decade of life (~75%); gonadoblastoma (~5%)
Hormone profile:	Elevated LH, FSH levels; decreased testosterone values

*Denys-Drash syndrome and Frasier's syndrome may be variants of the same underlying syndrome.

LH, luteinizing hormone; FSH, follicle-stimulating hormone.

Table 22–38. Clinical Features of Frasier Syndrome in 46,XY Males*

Karyotype:	46,XY
Inheritance:	Autosomal dominant: mutation in splice donor site in intron 9 of the *WT1* gene on 11p13 affecting the inclusion of 3 amino acids (KTS) and thus altering the normal balance of ± KTS isoforms.
Genitalia:	Female (hypospadiac male with cryptorchidism, rare)
Wolffian duct derivatives:	Absent (hypoplastic, rare)
Müllerian duct derivatives:	Present → hypoplastic
Gonads:	Streak → dysgenetic → hypoplastic testes
Other features:	Late-onset renal disease from focal and segmental sclerosis of the kidney; increased incidence of gonadal tumors, especially gonadoblastoma; Wilms' tumor rare (~4%)
Hormone profile:	Elevated plasma LH, FSH levels

*Frasier's syndrome and Denys-Drash syndrome may be variants of the same underlying syndrome.

LH, luteinizing hormone; FSH, follicle-stimulating hormone.

congenital or early-onset renal disease (diffuse mesangial sclerosis) and the development of Wilms' tumor in the first decade (i.e., the Denys-Drash syndrome)[215, 1413] or with the childhood onset of renal disease and gonadal tumors (the Frasier syndrome).[1414, 1415]

XY individuals with Denys-Drash syndrome usually present in the newborn period with ambiguous genitalia, although both normal male and normal female genitalia have been reported (Table 22–37).[208, 1413] The karyotype is 46,XY, albeit affected 46,XX females with renal disease and normal genitalia have been reported. Gonadal development in males varies from streak gonads to dysgenetic testes. The differentiation of the müllerian ducts varies depending on the functional status of the Sertoli cells of the gonads. Diffuse mesangial sclerosis, leading to renal failure, is seen on renal biopsy.[1413] Wilms' tumor occurs in the first decade of life, and 4% of patients with Denys-Drash syndrome develop a gonadoblastoma.[1413] Frasier and associates described a pair of 46,XY monozygotic twins with streak gonads and gonadoblastoma, one of whom developed renal failure[1414]; these patients appear to represent a component of the spectrum of the Denys-Drash syndrome (Table 22–38).[219, 1415] DNA analysis of patients with Denys-Drash syndrome has revealed heterozygous mutations of the Wilms' tumor suppressor gene *(WT1)* located on 11p13.[203–205, 215] The *WT1* gene encodes a transcription factor with four CysCys/HisHis zinc fingers[203, 205] that is expressed in the fetal kidney, gonad, and genital ridge.[204] Heterozygous mutations, mostly missense mutations, are most common in exon 9 of the *WT1* gene, with Arg394Trp being the most frequent in patients with Denys-Drash syndrome.[205, 208, 215, 216] The majority of *WT1* mutations in Denys-Drash syndrome are de novo and appear to act as dominant negative mutations.[205, 208, 216, 1418]

The Frasier syndrome, a variant of the Denys-Drash syndrome, is characterized in XY individuals by XY complete gonadal dysgenesis, with streak gonads resulting in female external and internal genital structures, late-onset glomerulopathy, focal glomerular sclerosis with renal failure occurring in the second decade, and predisposition to the development of a gonadoblastoma rather than Wilms' tumor. The syndrome is associated with a heterozygous mutation in the *WT1* gene at the donor splice site of intron 9.[206, 207, 217, 218] The mutation leads to a reversal in the ratio +KTS/−KTS (lysine, threonine, serine) isoforms from 2/1 to 1/2 in the WT1 proteins that compromises the normal function of *WT1*. The Denys-Drash syndrome and the Frasier syndrome are now regarded as interrelated disorders of the *WT1* gene and two extremes of a spectrum of clinical features rather than separate disease entities.[219, 1419] (See section on sex differentiation.)

Heterozygous deletions of *WT1* and contiguous genes produce the WAGR syndrome (*W*ilms' tumor, *a*niridia [absence or malformation of the iris], *g*enitourinary abnormalities, and mental *r*etardation).[1420] The genitourinary anomalies in the WAGR syndrome include renal agenesis, horseshoe kidney, urethral atresia, hypospadias, and cryptorchidism,[1420] and they are usually less severe than those observed in the Denys-Drash syndrome. (A mutation or deletion of *WT1* has not been found in *SRY*-positive patients with dysgenetic gonads who do not have evidence of renal disease.[1421])

Heterozygous mutations of the autosomal *SOX9* gene cause campomelic dysplasia, often a lethal skeletal malformation, in which three fourths of affected 46,XY patients have dysgenetic male pseudohermaphroditism (Table 22–39; see also Fig. 22–

Table 22–39. Clinical Features of *SOX9* Deficiency in 46,XY Males

Karyotype:	46,XY
Inheritance:	Autosomal dominant: heterozygous loss of function mutations in the *SOX9* coding region on chromosome 17q24.3–17q25.1 or break points with translocation 50 kb or more 5′ to the *SOX9* gene
Genitalia:	Female → ambiguous (70% of XY) → normal male
Wolffian duct derivatives:	Absent → hypoplastic → present
Müllerian duct derivatives:	Normal → hypoplastic → absent
Gonads:	Testes → dysgenetic testes → ovotestes → ovaries (rare)
Habitus:	Campomelic dysplasia, usually lethal bony dysplasia associated with male-to-female sex reversal in two thirds of affected males; testes in one third with male external genitalia Prominent features of campomelic dysplasia: bowing of femora and tibiae, hypoplastic scapulae, 11 pairs of ribs, pelvic malformations, clubfeet, cleft palate, micrognathia, etc.

17).[1422, 1423] The disorder has an incidence of 0.05 to 1.6 per 10,000 live births.[1423–1425] Manifestations include bowed long bones, hypoplastic scapula, a deformed pelvis, 11 pairs of ribs, a small thoracic cage, cleft palate, macrocephaly, micrognathia, hypertelorism, and a variety of cardiac and renal defects.[1423] Death from respiratory distress usually occurs in the neonatal period, but long-term survival has been reported.[1422, 1423] The external genitalia of affected 46,XY males varies from that of normal males with descended testes through ambiguous genitalia to female external genitalia, depending on the functional status of the fetal gonads.[1422, 1423, 1426] Affected 46,XX females have normal external genitalia and apparently normal ovaries.[1423] Histologic examination of the gonads from 46,XY patients with ambiguous or female external genitalia showed varying degrees of testicular dysgenesis extending to streak gonads with primordial follicles.[1422, 1423, 1426]

Tommerup and co-workers[183] mapped the sex-reversal locus associated with campomelic dysplasia to 17q24.3q25.1 from studies of three patients with balanced de novo reciprocal translocations. The break point in these patients was distal to the growth hormone locus and proximal to the thymidine locus on 17q.[183, 1427] Because the murine gene *Sox9* had been localized to a region in the murine genome that is homologous to 17q and this gene is expressed in skeletal tissue, the corresponding human gene *SOX9* was considered to be a candidate for campomelic dysplasia.[1428] Subsequently, missense, nonsense, frameshift, and splice junction mutations were detected in the *SOX9* gene in patients with campomelic dysplasia with or without gonadal dysgenesis.[183–185, 837] However, no correlation between the mutations and the gonadal phenotype (sex reversal) has been found.[1429] In one family, the same *SOX9* mutation resulted in siblings with campomelic dysplasia as a result of a germline mosaicism for a *SOX9* mutation in the father.[1430] However, the gonadal phenotype varied in the two 46,XY males from dysgenetic gonads to "normal" ovaries, and the affected 46,XX female had "normal" ovaries.[1430] In all patients studied, the mutation has been identified in only one *SOX9* allele (heterozygous), which suggests that both the campomelic dysplasia and sex reversal are caused by haploinsufficiency of the *SOX9* gene.[184, 1426] The absence of sex reversal in approximately one fourth of 46,XY individuals with campomelic dysplasia and in patients with translocations that involve break points in 17q more than 130 kb from the *SOX9* gene in which no mutations have been found is unexplained.

The *SOX9* gene has three exons and two introns,[184, 185] the first of the *SOX* genes to have introns,[184, 185] and encodes a 509-residue protein that localizes to the nucleus and contains an HMG box with 71% homology to that of the SRY protein.[22, 188] The HMG box binds to the same DNA motif CAACAAAGC as other HMG transcription factors and *trans*-activates transcription of a downstream target gene or genes.[22, 188, 190] The *trans*-activation function of *SOX9* appears to reside in the carboxyl-terminal domain of the protein.[22, 188, 190] *SOX9* is expressed in the developing gonad, rete testis, and seminiferous tubule and in the mesenchyme that gives rise to skeletal tissue.[193, 194, 837, 839] During chondrogenesis *SOX9* is co-expressed with *COL2A1*, the gene that encodes type II collagen[1431]; the SOX9 protein binds to regulatory gene sequences in the *COL2A1* gene and regulates its expression.[1432] It is apparent from the study of patients with campomelic dysplasia that *SOX9* is an integral part of testicular development cascade.

SF1

Steroidogenic factor 1 (SF1, or Ad4BP, adrenal 4 binding protein), a zinc finger "orphan" nuclear receptor,[225, 226, 230, 1433] is a member of the steroid hormone/thyroid hormone receptor superfamily of transcription regulatory factors. SF1 is encoded by a gene on chromosome 9q33[223] and binds to a DNA motif consisting of an estrogen receptor half-site, AGGTCA, and to nucleotides 5′ to this half-site (see Fig. 22–18).[226, 230, 1434] The presence of this motif in the promoters of CYP steroid hydroxylase genes, as well as in in vivo expression studies, suggests that SF1 is a key regulator of CYP steroidogenic enzymes in the adrenals and gonads.[225, 226, 230, 1433, 1435] However, in the placenta the expression of *CYP11A1* ($P450_{scc}$) and other CYP steroidogenic genes occurs in the absence of expression of the *SF1* gene,[1436] as is the case in the central nervous system where neurosteroids are produced locally.[1436] The *SF1* gene is critical to the in vivo expression of AMH and the β-subunit of LH.[230, 231, 375, 1437]

Sf1 and the embryonal long terminal repeat binding protein (ELP, a protein that suppresses expression of Moloney murine leukemia virus in mouse undifferentiated embryonal carcinoma cells) are isoforms transcribed from the same gene by alternative promoter usage and splicing.[226, 230, 231] Sf1/ELP is the mouse homologue of *Drosophila* FTZF1, a transcription factor that regulates the fushi-tarazu gene.[226, 230, 1438] "Knockout" of the *Sf1* gene in mice causes complete absence of the adrenals and gonads.[229] All male and female knockout mice die of presumed adrenal insufficiency in the neonatal period.[229] The external genitalia are female in both XX and XY mice, müllerian duct derivatives are normally developed, and the ventromedial nucleus of the hypothalamus is aplastic or hypoplastic.[1439] The expression of *Sf1* in the developing gonad is sexually dimorphic. At 12.5 days of embryonic development, when the bipotential gonad develops into an ovary or testis in the mouse and before expression of the CYP steroidogenic genes, *Sf1* expression persists in the Leydig and Sertoli cells of the testes but is extinguished in the primordial ovary.[229]

In Sf1 knockout mice the genital ridges developed normally until 10.5 days after coitus and thereafter underwent apoptosis.[229] Therefore, Sf1 appears to play a critical role in the development of the adrenals, ovaries, testes, hypothalamus, and gonadotropes and in modulation of AMH and CYP steroidogenic enzymes. As discussed previously, SF1 deficiency in three humans has been shown to cause severe adrenal insufficiency with impairment of testicular determination. Whether it affects ovarian determination is still to be determined (Table 22–40). Patients with 9p− syndrome and putative haploinsufficiency of DMRT1 also manifest male pseudohermaphroditism, as discussed previously (Table 22–41).

Vanishing Testes Syndrome (Embryonic Testicular Regression Syndrome)

Various terms (XY gonadal dysgenesis, XY gonadal agenesis, rudimentary testis syndrome, congenital anorchia) have been used to describe the spectrum of genital anomalies resulting from cessation of testicular function during the middle phase of male sex differentiation, between 8 and 14 weeks of gestation. We first used the term *vanishing testes syndrome* for this form of male pseudohermaphroditism in 1957 because the genitalia in these cases suggested that the testes functioned initially and then "vanished" (for obscure reasons) at some time during the process of male sex differentiation.[280] These patients have a 46,XY karyotype. Gonadal elements are absent, and differentiation of the genital ducts, urogenital sinus, and external genitalia is variable. At one end of the spectrum is the group of 46,XY individuals with female external and internal genitalia in whom the deficiency of embryonic testicular function presumably occurred before 8 weeks of gestation.[1442] These individuals have either no gonads (46,XY agonadism) or streak gonads.[1442] Loss of function of the fetal testes at 8 to 10 weeks of gestation would lead to ambiguous genitalia and variable development of the genital ducts, from complete absence of both müllerian and wolffian ducts to partial development of

Table 22–40. Clinical Features of *SF1* Deficiency in 46,XY Males*

Karyotype:	46,XY
Inheritance:	Autosomal dominant: de novo heterozygous Gly35Glu mutation of *SF1* gene on chromosome 9q33 Autosomal recessive due to homozygous Arg92Gln mutation (heterozygote normal)
Genitalia:	Female
Müllerian duct derivatives:	Normal
Gonads:	Absent
Wolffian duct derivatives:	Absent
Habitus:	No pubic or axillary hair or breast development; increased pigmentation
Hormone and metabolic profile:	Absent adrenals; primary adrenal insufficiency in infancy. No sex steroid secretion.
GnRH:	In the XY phenotypic female with a heterozygous *SF1* mutation, at age 10 years: LH 1.2 → 8.8 mIU/mL FSH 17.8 → 38 mIU/mL No testosterone response to hCG

*One 46,XX female reported with Arg255Leu heterozygous mutation; adrenal insufficiency; normal female genitalia; ? normal ovaries.

LH, luteinizing hormone; FSH, follicle-stimulating hormone; hCG, human chorionic gonadotropin.

Table 22–41. Clinical Features of 9p− Syndrome in 46,XY Males

Karyotype:	46,XY
Inheritance:	Heterozygous deletion of 9p24.3 → 9-pter (distal short arm). The 5′ end of *DMRT1* is within 30 kb of the break point defining the minimal deletion causing sex reversal
Genitalia:	Female → ambiguous → male (rare)
Wolffian duct derivatives:	Absent → hypoplastic
Müllerian duct derivatives:	Present → hypoplastic → absent (rare)
Gonads:	Absent → dysgenetic → hypoplastic testes
Habitus:	Short stature (variable), mental retardation, microcephaly, trigonencephaly
Hormone profile:	Hypergonadotropic hypogonadism

either, a constellation referred to by some as the *XY gonadal agenesis syndrome*.[1443–1445] Loss of testicular function after the critical phase of male differentiation (12 to 14 weeks) results in anorchia, a syndrome characterized by normal male differentiation both internally and externally but no gonadal tissue. The presence of normal male genitalia and absence of müllerian duct derivatives implies that fetal testicular function was normal before its loss. Sporadic and familial forms of unilateral and bilateral anorchia, including monozygotic twins concordant and discordant for anorchia, have been described.[1446–1448] Fetal testicular insufficiency and incomplete regression of the fetal testes after 12 to 14 weeks would be expected to produce a syndrome similar to that described by Bergada and colleagues,[1449–1451] that is, small, rudimentary testes with microphallus and male ejaculatory ducts.

The nature of the underlying defect, which in some cases leads to absence or regression of genital ducts as well as testes and in some cases other congenital anomalies, is not known.[1452, 1453] Several sibships with multiple affected individuals have been described. Josso and Briard[1454] reported on two siblings, one of whom was a normally differentiated male with microphallus and anorchia. The other sibling had a 46,XY karyotype but was raised as a female. She had a normal clitoris, fused labioscrotal folds, a single perineal opening that led into a urogenital sinus, and a vagina. At laparotomy, absent gonads with coexistent müllerian and wolffian structures were found. This patient's phenotype was compatible with a diagnosis of XY gonadal agenesis. Despite the absent gonads, the patients had distinct phenotypic differences in the internal and external genitalia. The coexistence of so-called XY gonadal agenesis and anorchia in the same sibship suggests that the disorders are related and are caused by embryonic testicular regression occurring at different stages of male development in utero; the familial cases support the operation of a rare, mutant gene in at least some patients with this syndrome. All eight boys with bilateral congenital anorchia confirmed at surgical exploration were *SRY* positive.[1455]

The diagnosis of "true" anorchia (in contrast to the testicular regression syndrome with ambiguous external genitalia) can be suspected in normally differentiated males with bilateral cryptorchidism, elevated gonadotropin levels, and low plasma AMH and inhibin levels. It is infrequently familial. We have demonstrated a diphasic childhood pattern of gonadotropin levels in anorchic males similar to that seen in females with the syndrome of gonadal dysgenesis.[1456] In particular, plasma FSH levels are elevated in infancy, decrease into the normal range in middle childhood, and rise into the agonadal range after age 9 to 10 years. LHRH-induced increases in plasma FSH and LH concentrations are elevated throughout infancy and childhood. Hence, the LHRH test may be helpful diagnostically in middle childhood, when basal gonadotropin levels are normal or near normal. It has been proposed that the finding of elevated plasma FSH levels in conjunction with lack of a plasma testosterone response to hCG (1500 U/m^2 intramuscularly every 48 hours × 7) establishes the diagnosis of anorchia and obviates the need for laparotomy.[1457] This approach has been called into question by the finding of testes at laparotomy in two prepubertal males in whom no testosterone response to hCG was elicited.[1458] Immunoassay of plasma AMH in infancy and childhood is a useful additional test to assess for the presence of a testis; the concentration of plasma AMH in anorchia is very low, as is the determination in plasma of another Sertoli cell secretion, inhibin B[365, 1459–1461]; indeed, the concentration of plasma inhibin B highly correlates with the testosterone response to hCG[1461] and may well substitute for the hCG test, and it is more cost effective. Furthermore, CT or MRI, ultrasonography, and laparoscopy are useful procedures for evaluation of the patient with suspected anorchia. We have deferred laparoscopic exploration of males with presumed "true" anorchia (phenotypic males with nonpalpable testes, elevated gonadotropin levels, and no rise in the plasma concentration of testosterone in response to hCG) until the time of insertion of prosthetic testes. The typical findings at laparoscopy are a nubbin of testicular tissue adfixed to spermatic vessels exiting the internal inguinal ring. No recognizable testicular elements are evident in the nubbin.[1462–1463] The true vanishing testis syndrome typified by normal male genital development has been attributed to a prenatal torsion event. An interesting case study described antenatal ultrasound findings of a male fetus with a left hydrocele and a normal right testis but at birth the right testis was nonpalpable.[1464] At surgical exploration, there was torsion of the spermatic cord on the left side and a normal testis, whereas on the right side the spermatic cord ended in a nubbin of tissue. It was postulated that there was bilateral antenatal torsion but the vanishing testis syndrome was not bilateral because the left hydrocele had a protective effect on the vascular supply during the antenatal testicular torsion. The vanishing testis syndrome can be unilateral, occurring after descent but before fixation of the tunica vaginalis to the scrotal wall.[1465]

Defects in Synthesis, Secretion, or Response to Antimüllerian Hormone

Persistent Müllerian Duct Syndrome (Female Ducts in Otherwise Normal Men; Herniae Uteri Inguinale)

AMH/MIS, a 148-kd glycoprotein homodimer, is secreted by the Sertoli cells of the testes beginning with differentiation of the fetal seminiferous tubules and continuing until pubertal maturation. AMH is not secreted by the fetal ovary,[364] but postnatally (see section on sex differentiation) it is expressed in the granulosa cells of antral and preantral ovarian follicles.[364, 368, 369] AMH, a member of the TGF-β superfamily of growth and differentiation factors,[364, 380, 1466] is processed intracellularly and secreted in its mature, bioactive form.[382, 1467] It binds to the AMH type II serine/threonine kinase receptor[369, 379, 380] located in the mesenchyme surrounding the müllerian ducts before 8 weeks of gestation (when the müllerian ducts respond to AMH), causing epithelial-mesenchymal interaction, apoptosis of the müllerian duct epithelium, and regression of the müllerian duct.[338, 364, 376, 1468] Studies in the bovine freemartin and in transgenic mice overexpressing AMH indicate that AMH can cause regression of germ cells in the ovary and reorganization of the ovary into cord-like seminiferous tubules and can inhibit CYP19 activity.[364, 372, 373] Five of 21 transgenic male mice that chronically expressed human AMH exhibited mammary gland development, arrested wolffian duct differentiation, and undescended testes.[372, 373] These observations suggest that high levels of AMH can impair Leydig cell function and steroidogenesis in the testes.[373] AMH levels are measurable in the normal male in plasma until pubertal maturation.[364]

AMH is encoded by a 2.75-kb gene containing five exons in the region of chromosome 19p13.3.[381] The gene has an upstream regulatory element, the estrogen response element, half-site AGGTCA type, to which SF1 binds to regulate AMH secretion.[230, 1437]

The AMH/MIS receptor, a serine/threonine kinase with a single transmembrane domain, is a member of the family of type II receptors for TGF-β–related proteins (see Fig. 22–27).[369, 383, 1468, 1469] The AMH type II receptor binds ligand but requires the ubiquitous type I receptor for signal transduction.[338, 368, 377–379]

The AMH II receptor is encoded by a gene that contains 11 exons.[1466, 1469] Exons 1 to 3 code for the signal sequence and the extracellular domain of the AMH receptor, exon 4 codes for the transmembrane domain, and exons 5 through 11 code for the intracellular serine/threonine domain.[1466, 1469] In addition to the mesenchyme surrounding the fetal müllerian ducts (but not the epithelial cells), this receptor is expressed in adult granulosa and Sertoli cells, which suggests a possible autocrine action of AMH in these cells.[1469]

A distinctive disorder, persistent müllerian duct syndrome (PMDS), has been described in which 46,XY men and boys have well-developed testes, normal male ducts and external genitalia, and müllerian duct derivatives[364, 1470–1472] (Fig. 22–84). The diagnosis often is not made until a fallopian tube and uterus are encountered in patients undergoing inguinal hernia repair, orchiopexy, or abdominal surgery. Because of the trend for early surgical repair of an inguinal hernia or undescended testis, more cases are detected in infancy.[1473] There are two anatomic forms. In the more prevalent form, there is a hernia containing a partially descended or scrotal testis and the ipsilateral tube and uterus are in the hernia.[1472] In some instances the contralateral testis and tube are present in the hernial sac as well. The presence of transverse testicular ectopia should suggest PMDS.[1472] In the second form, the uterus, tubes, and testes are in the pelvis.

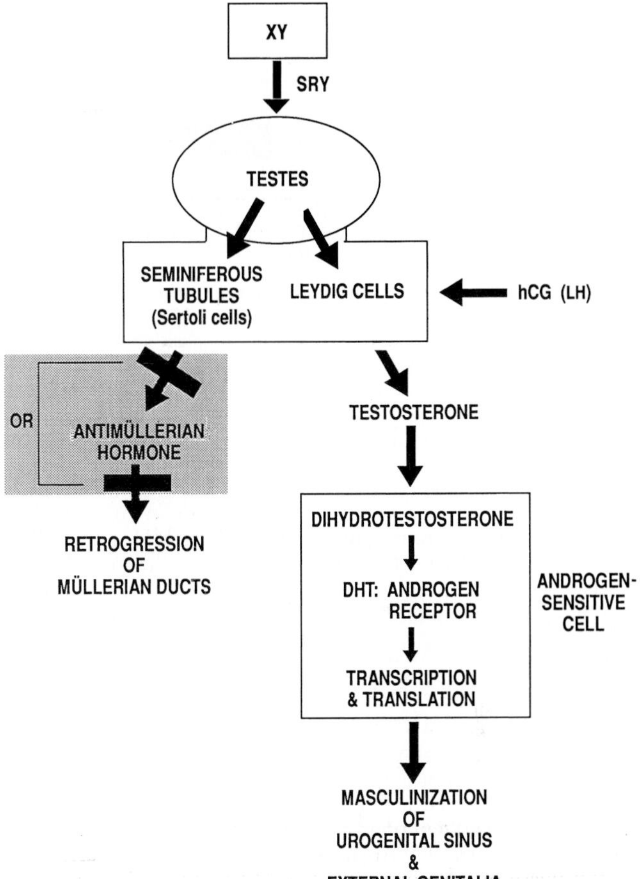

Figure 22–84. Diagram of the pathogenesis of the persistent müllerian duct syndrome.

PMDS is a heterogeneous condition that is inherited in a sex-limited autosomal recessive manner. Females homozygous for null mutations in the *AMH* gene have normal müllerian ducts, external genitalia, and ovarian function, including fertility.[1474] Therefore *AMH* does not appear to play a critical role in ovarian differentiation or formation.

The retention of müllerian structures in normally differentiated males can result from failure of the testes to synthesize or secrete AMH or from a defect in the response of the duct to AMH because of an AMH receptor defect or possibly an abnormality in the timing or secretion of the hormone.[1475, 1476] Mutations in the *AMH* gene can lead to absence of AMH as a cause of PMDS (Fig. 22–85).[364, 1469, 1474, 1477] *AMH* mutations are most common in Mediterranean and Arab countries with high rates of consanguinity, and most familial mutations are homozygous; on the other hand, mutations in the gene encoding the AMH type II receptor (AMHR-II) are more common in France and Northern Europe and are often heterozygous mutations.[1478–1480]

In an extensive study of 69 families with PMDS, 28 mutations in the *AMH* gene were detected in 31 families (see Fig. 22–85).[1474, 1478, 1481] Both homozygous and compound heterozygous mutations were found in affected families,[1474] including splicing, missense, nonsense, and deletion mutations affecting the whole gene but mainly exon 1 and the 3′ half of exon 5.[1474, 1478, 1481] In 27 families, deleterious mutations in the type II AMH receptor were detected, including deletion, missense, and nonsense mutations[1478] (Fig. 22–86). The most common mutation was a 27-base pair deletion in exon 10, which was found on at least one allele in 10 out of 16 families and stands

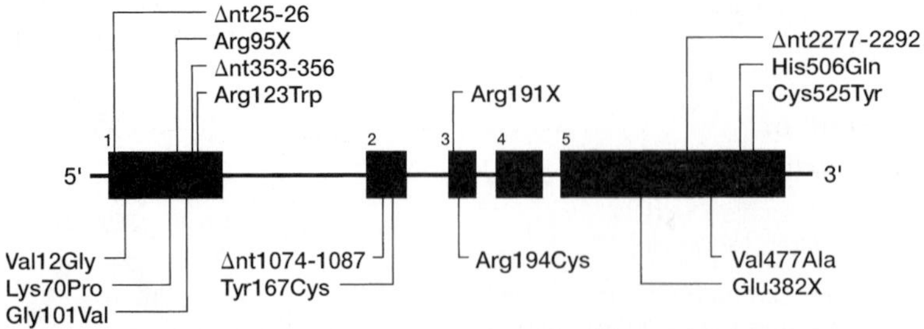

Figure 22–85. Diagram of the mutations in the antimüllerian hormone gene that cause the persistent müllerian duct syndrome. Exons are the black numbered boxes. Mutations are indicated by the three-letter abbreviation for the wild-type amino acid, followed by the position number of the amino acid in the protein and the three-letter abbreviation for the substituted amino acid or X for a nonsense (stop) mutation. Δnt25–26 is a deletion of nucleotides 25 and 26; Δnt353-356, Δnt1074-1087, and Δnt2277-2292 indicate similar deletions of the respective nucleotides. (Redrawn from Imbeaud S, Carré Eusebe D, Rey R, et al. Molecular genetics of the persistent müllerian duct syndrome: a study of 19 families. Hum Mol Genet 1994; 3:125–131. By permission of Oxford University Press.)

in contrast to the diverse mutations in the AMH gene.[1478] In 11 families (16% of the total number), no abnormality in AMH or AMH receptor genes was detected. Patients with PMDS caused by mutations of the AMH gene have low or undetectable levels of serum AMH; in contrast, AMH concentrations are high normal or elevated in patients with mutations of the AMH receptor.[1481, 1482]

Treatment of PMDS is directed toward an attempt to ensure fertility in males, a difficult issue because of the anatomic findings. Testicular differentiation and function are normal in these patients, but an increased prevalence of testicular degeneration has been described, which is probably secondary to torsion of the testes.[1483] Anatomic abnormalities of the epididymis and the vas deferens are common. Infertility may result from late orchiopexy or from mechanical problems associated with entrapment of the vas deferens in the müllerian derivatives, which is usually present.[364, 1473] Early orchiopexy, proximal salpingectomy (leaving the epididymis attached to the fimbrae of the fallopian tube), dissection of the vas deferens from the lateral walls of the uterus, and a complete hysterectomy are recommended as a useful surgical approach.[1472, 1473] Despite these recommendations, men with high pelvic testes rarely have successful orchiopexy, and many of these individuals are androgen deficient.

Maternal Ingestion of Progestagens and Estrogens

Progestagens and synthetic estrogens, alone or in combination, have been implicated as rare causes of male pseudohermaphroditism. Courrier and Jost[1484] in 1942 demonstrated an antiandrogen effect on the male fetus induced by a synthetic progestagen, ethisterone. Neumann and colleagues[387] observed that relatively high doses of progesterone or of synthetic progestagens impaired urethral groove fusion in fetal male rats. Aarskog[1485] reported on 130 patients with hypospadias who were studied retrospectively. A history of maternal ingestion of oral progestagens in early pregnancy was obtained in 11 cases. In 6, the agent was administered for threatened abortion, and in 5 the progestagen in combination with estrogens was given as a pregnancy test. Hypospadias occurred anywhere from the glans to the base of the penile shaft; the location correlated with the week of gestation in which therapy was initiated. Other studies have also suggested an association between progestagens and hypospadias,[1486, 1487] although this relation has been questioned.[1488]

Aarskog postulated that maternal progestagens may inhibit testosterone synthesis by the fetal testes or impair the reduction of testosterone to DHT at the target tissue and thereby

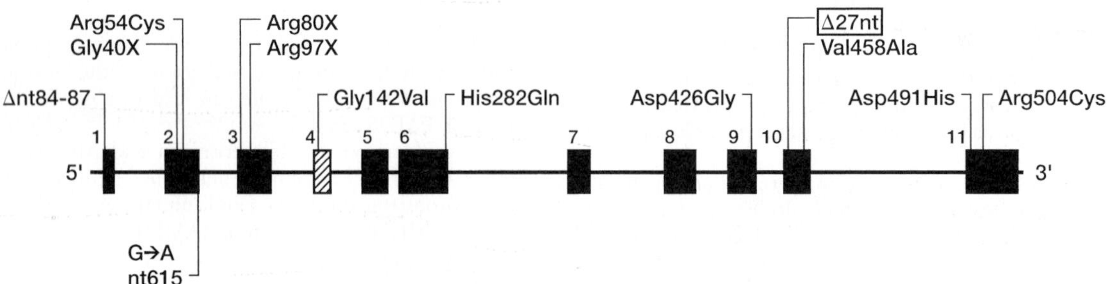

Figure 22–86. Diagram of selected mutations in the gene for the AMH receptor type II. Black numbered boxes are exons. Exons 1 to 3 encode the extracellular domain of the receptor. Exon 4 *(diagonal lines)* encodes the transmembrane domain, and exons 5 through 11 encode the intracytoplasmic domain. Mutations are indicated by the three-letter abbreviation for the wild-type amino acid, followed by the position number of the amino acid in the receptor protein and the three-letter abbreviation for the substituted amino acid or X for a nonsense (stop) mutation. Δnt84–87 designates a deletion/insertion at nucleotides 84–87. G→A nt615 is a guanine-to-adenine transition at nucleotide 615, which is at the splice site between exon 2 and intron 2. Δ27nt *(open box)* is a 27-nucleotide deletion, the most common mutation causing the AMH-positive form of the persistent müllerian duct syndrome, a mutation present in 25% of the patients studied with this form. (Redrawn from Imbeaud S, Belville C, Messike-Zeitoun L, et al. A 27 base-pair deletion of the antimüllerian type II receptor gene is the most common cause of the persistent müllerian duct syndrome. Hum Mol Genet 1996; 5:1269–1277. By permission of Oxford University Press.)

lead to failure of urethral groove fusion and hypospadias. Some progestagens can inhibit 5α-reductase activity in vitro.[1489] Inhibition of this enzymatic activity at an early fetal stage (e.g., through placental transfer of drugs given to the mother) could impair masculinization of the male external genitalia. Alternatively, progestagens may bind to androgen receptors and impair androgen action.

Kaplan[1490] described male pseudohermaphroditism in a boy whose mother received large doses of diethylstilbestrol during early pregnancy. However, no additional reports of this association have appeared. Because of the report of Herbst linking maternal diethylstilbestrol therapy during pregnancy with vaginal and cervical adenocarcinoma in daughters, abnormalities in the genital tract have been sought in males.[1491] Increased incidences of meatal stenosis, epididymal cysts, hypoplastic testes, and abnormal semen have been observed, but hypospadias has not been reported.[1492, 1493]

Environmental Chemicals

An increase in the prevalence of disorders of the development and function of the male reproductive system, especially hypospadias and cryptorchidism, and in some European countries a fall in the sperm count and a rise in cancer of the testis, has occurred during the past 50 years.[1494–1496] Some investigators have speculated that the increase in reproductive abnormalities observed in human males is related to an increase in the exposure in utero to exogenous estrogenic chemicals, so-called environmental estrogens, in the maternal diet, either as a natural occurrence or as a result of chemical contamination.[1494] Administration of diethylstilbestrol or the putative environmental estrogen, 4-octylphenol, to pregnant rats resulted in decreased expression of CYP17 mRNA and protein in Leydig cells of XY male offspring.[1497, 1498] Suppression of CYP17 may play a role in the putative adverse effect of environmental estrogens on fetal masculinization. The dichlorodiphenyltrichloroethane (DDT) metabolite *p,p'*DDE (1,1-dicloro2,2-*bis*-(*p*-chlorophenyl) ethylene), unlike DDT itself, has little ability to bind to the estrogen receptor,[1499] but it binds to the androgen receptor and inhibits androgen action in the developing urogenital tract of rodents.[1499] Further studies on the levels and risks of natural and environmental estrogens and antiandrogens in humans are necessary before the putative increased prevalence of certain abnormalities of the reproductive tract can be attributed to these agents as well as their putative role in the pathogenesis of the testicular dysgenesis syndrome.[1496]

Unclassified Forms of Abnormal Sexual Development

Extraordinary advances in the understanding of male pseudohermaphroditism and its heterogeneity have been made since the first edition of this textbook. The major subgroups are now defined, and genetic defects in testosterone biosynthesis, androgen action, and testis organogenesis are recognized. Nonetheless, some forms of male pseudohermaphroditism are not readily categorized, and their pathogenesis is obscure. A collaborative French study[1499a] underscores the lacunae in our current ability to establish an etiologic diagnosis. Sixty-seven patients with ambiguous external genitalia and testicular tissue or a 46,XY karyotype or both had an extensive workup including detailed clinical examinations and extensive hormonal and molecular genetic studies. A definitive diagnosis was made in 32 patients (48%) who had a form of dysgenetic male pseudohermaphroditism, true hermaphroditism, partial androgen insensitivity syndrome, or 17β-HSD 3 deficiency. In 35 patients (52%) an etiologic diagnosis was not established and the documented male pseudohermaphroditism was unexplained; this group had an increased prevalence of intrauterine growth retardation and somatic malformations. Complications at conception or early in pregnancy and impaired prenatal growth are common in unexplained male pseudohermaphroditism[1499b]; a striking discordance in birth weight and length in a pair of monozygotic 46,XY twins was described. The unaffected male twin was of normal birth size.[1499c]

Other Sexual Abnormalities in Males

Hypospadias

Hypospadias, which may be defined as incomplete fusion of the penile urethra,[1559] is one of the common congenital anomalies. It has an estimated incidence of 4 to 8 per 1000 male births.[1368, 1495, 1500] As noted previously, the rate appears to have doubled in some countries in the 1970s and 1980s.[1494] Analysis of the family histories of patients with hypospadias revealed an increase in the occurrence of hypospadias in males in the pedigrees.[1501, 1502] This finding suggested a multifactorial mode of inheritance in some cases; the cause in most instances is unknown.[1502]

On theoretical grounds, incomplete masculinization of the external genitalia implies either subnormal Leydig cell function in utero, a mild degree of androgen resistance or of 5α-reductase-2 deficiency, or a transient, functional, timing-related abnormality in the availability or action of DHT on the primordia of the external genitalia. Environmental agents with antiandrogen effects in animals may have an as yet undocumented role in the apparent increase in prevalence of hypospadias.[1494, 1503]

Aarskog carried out a careful prospective study of 100 consecutive patients with hypospadias without other somatic anomalies, most of which were referred from a surgery clinic.[1504] One patient was a genetic female with virilizing CAH, five had sex chromosome abnormalities, one had the incomplete form of 46,XY gonadal dysgenesis, and nine were from pregnancies in which the mother had taken synthetic progestational agents during the first trimester.[1504] Thus, in 15% of the patients a pathogenetic mechanism was found or suspected. Both maternal cocaine use and environmental estrogens and antiandrogens have also been implicated in the development of hypospadias.[1494, 1495, 1505] Even though androgen receptor defects have been suggested to play a significant role in the origin of hypospadias,[1506–1508] androgen receptor defects are a rare cause of isolated hypospadias.[1509, 1510]

Hypospadias is a feature of many malformation syndromes, such as the Opitz syndrome.[1511] The cardinal manifestations of this syndrome are widely spaced eyes and hypospadias. This disorder is genetically heterogeneous; an X-linked form involves a locus at Xp22, and an autosomal form involves a locus at 22q11.2.[1511] Hypospadias is also a feature of the hand-foot-genital syndrome in males.[1512] Limb anomalies include short first metacarpals, short distal phalanges of the thumbs, and a short great toe.[1512] A mutation in the *HOXA13* gene was detected in a pedigree with this syndrome.[1512]

The mildest and most common form of hypospadias is glandular or coronal and occurs in about 85% of cases; with surgical repair, these boys, at least in middle childhood, are not at risk for the development of "gender-atypical" behavior.[1513] Even though rare cases have been reported of 5α-reductase deficiency and androgen receptor defects with isolated, simple hypospadias, extensive endocrine and cytogenetic evaluation of the otherwise normal male with glandular hypospadias and no somatic anomalies is not warranted. More severe hypospadias with or without cryptorchidism and somatic anomalies is an indication for complete evaluation, including karyotype analysis, hCG stimulation studies, and visualization of the genitourinary tract.[1513a]

Cryptorchidism

Undescended testes, the most common urogenital abnormality in malformation syndromes, is associated with more than 40 syndromes. Although normal testes may fail to descend into the scrotum because of coincidental anatomic abnormalities, in many instances cryptorchidism is caused by a defective testis. Fetal pituitary gonadotropin deficiency, either partial or complete, may play a role in some instances of cryptorchidism as well as microphallus.[1514–1516] Cryptorchidism and its management are considered in greater detail in Chapter 18 and in several reviews.[1517–1520]

Ambiguous Genitalia in 46,XY Males with Multiple Anomalies

The presence of ambiguous genitalia is associated with many malformation syndromes.[568] In malformation syndromes such as the Aarskog and Opitz syndromes, the genital anomaly is of diagnostic significance.

Other reports of rare causes of male pseudohermaphroditism include a patient with a putative "biologically inactive" but immunologically reactive LH and a group of familial cases in which a defect was postulated in fetal Leydig cell maturation with inadequate fetal testosterone production and impaired differentiation of germinal elements.[1520a] The latter patients had ambiguous genitalia at birth but normal virilization at puberty and may represent examples of SRD5A2 deficiency, 17β-HSD 3 deficiency, or partial androgen resistance.

Other Sexual Abnormalities in Females

The association of congenital absence of the vagina with abnormal or absent müllerian structures has been recognized for more than 100 years[1521, 1522] and is usually known as the Mayer-Rokitansky-Küster-Hauser syndrome. Congenital absence of the vagina occurs in 1 in 5000 female births.[1521] It was the second most common cause of primary amenorrhea in a series of 538 patients reviewed by Ross and van de Wiele.[1523] The principal features of the syndrome are primary amenorrhea in 46,XX females with well-developed female secondary sexual characteristics, an absent or hypoplastic vagina, and müllerian derivatives that vary from a normal uterus to bicornuate cords to absence of the uterus. Ovarian function is usually normal, and patients exhibit cyclic gonadotropin secretion with ovulation.[1524] Renal and skeletal anomalies may be present.[1526] Hearing loss, both conductive and sensorineural, occurs in 25% of patients with the Mayer-Rokitansky-Küster-Hauser syndrome.[1522] Clitoromegaly is not a feature and that distinguishes it from the adrenal and nonadrenal forms of female pseudohermaphroditism; the 46,XX karyotype and normal plasma gonadal steroid values differentiate this disorder from androgen insensitivity. Familial aggregates of women with anomalous müllerian differentiation may be explained by multifactorial inheritance.[1526]

It has been suggested that patients with skeletal and renal anomalies should be considered as a separate group, the GRES (genital-renal-ear-skeletal syndrome).[1527, 1528] The association of uterine anomalies with malformations of the extremities is well described.[1512, 1529, 1530] The association of absence of the uterus and the upper part of the vagina, renal anomalies, and cervical somite dysplasia (Klippel-Feil syndrome) has been called the MURCS association (müllerian duct aplasia, renal agenesis/ectopia, and cervical somite dysplasia).[1531] Ultrasonography and CT and MRI scans are useful for determining the presence of a uterus and its structure. Hematocolpos is a preventable complication if surgical reconstruction is begun before puberty is advanced.[1532–1535]

If the vagina is too small for sexual intercourse, nonsurgical or surgical correction should be undertaken at an appropriate age. Vaginal lubrication, orgasm, and coitus have been reported to be satisfactory in adults who have had successful vaginal reconstruction.[1534, 1536]

MANAGEMENT OF PATIENTS EXHIBITING AMBISEXUAL DEVELOPMENT

The advances in the management of patients with intersexuality have undergone a dramatic change over the past 50 years. A major deficiency in promoting guidelines for the modern management of intersexuality is the lack of critical outcome data or the selective nature of the available data. A background for these changes is the dramatic shift in our society's attitude toward sexuality—it has come out of the closet and discarded many formerly deeply embedded Victorian attitudes. Before 1953, when one of us became committed to the clinical, scientific, and management aspects of intersex, these patients were largely managed by surgeons and urologists. Some were paternalistic authoritarians who had little tolerance for anyone questioning their empirical decisions—the sex of the gonad was a cardinal criterion for determination of assigned sex. The mantra was "It's an anatomical anomaly, fix it or cut it out."

A sea change in this approach began with Lawson Wilkins and his associates at the Harriet Lane Home of Johns Hopkins Hospital in the early 1950s. This was the beginning of group decision making by an evolving team that initially was composed of Dr. Howard Jones, a gynecologic surgeon; Drs. Joan and John Hampson, child and adult psychiatrists; John Money, a psychologist newly arrived from Boston, Wilkins and his fellows Judson Van Wyk and Melvin M. Grumbach, George Clayton, and Alfred Bongiovanni, a young faculty member in the group and the director of the pediatric endocrine laboratory. Social workers provided important family care skills. After the departure of the Hampsons for the University of Washington in the late 1950s and Lawson Wilkins' death in 1964, Money's extended studies led him to propose the gender socialization hypothesis of gender identity later referred to by his disciples as the "optimal-gender policy." The notion was that "sex of assignment and rearing were consistently and conspicuously a more reliable prognosticator" of the gender identity of an intersex patient than the chromosomal sex, gonadal sex, hormonal sex, the sex of the internal genital organs, or the degree of ambiguity of the external genitalia.[491, 496, 504] Money and his associates stressed the importance of a decision about the sex of assignment in infancy.

Beginning in 1959 with the report by Phoenix and Young of "masculinization" of the female guinea pig brain by prenatal administration of testosterone, mounting evidence, at first a trickle[460] but later virtually a torrent of experimental and behavioral studies, indicated the effect of androgens on sex dimorphic behavior.[10] Further concern had arisen about the recommendations that infants with micropenis but normally found external genitalia and testes be assigned a female sex.[1352] Furthermore, the Intersex Society of North America raised important issues about the management of intersexuality. The article by John Colapinto in *Rolling Stone* and his later book, *As Nature Made Him: The Boy Who Was Raised as a Girl*,[489] served to accelerate the re-examination of the clinical care of the intersex patient. This reassessment was led by psychologists, psychiatrists, and pediatric endocrinologists, as well

Table 22–42. Management of Ambiguous Genitalia

Get help! Team approach: pediatrician, endocrinologist, child mental health expert, social worker, and surgeon.

- Arrive at a (prompt) definitive diagnosis if possible
- Inform the parents of your diagnosis: the natural history of the disorder, prognosis, and the therapeutic options. Full disclosure!!
- Consider the parents' level of understanding, cultural background, and religious views in order to allow them to come to a decision on the "sex" of their child and to provide truly "informed consent."

as a number of informed pediatric surgeons and urologists.[461, 482, 1537–1545, 1561] The Winter 1998 (Vol. 9, No. 4) issue of the *Journal of Clinical Ethics* was devoted to "Intersexuality."[1562] In a historical perspective on hermaphroditism, Dreger has emphasized how ingrained are our attitudes about "gender normality" but it also exemplifies how much our attitudes have changed.[1546]

Considerations Governing Choice of Sex for Rearing

With early, carefully weighed assignment of sex for rearing and appropriate continued management with an emphasis on continuity of care, individuals with ambiguities of the genitalia have the potential to lead well-adjusted lives and ultimately a satisfactory sex life. To obtain this favorable result, it is incumbent on the physician to make a correct diagnosis as early as possible and to provide the parents with pros and cons of sex assignment so that they may acquire sufficient knowledge to arrive at an informed decision on the sex for rearing. Lucid, simple, comprehensive discussions with the parents, taking into account their anxieties, religious views, social mores, cultural factors,[1540] and level of understanding, are critical for an appropriate gender assignment. The detection of genital ambiguity in a newborn infant can be seen as an urgent neonatal psychosocial necessity, beginning with how the parents are informed about the genital ambiguity. Once the sex for rearing is assigned, the gender role is reinforced by the use of whatever appropriate surgical, hormonal, and psychological measures are indicated.

Studies of patients reared in a sex discordant with their chromosomal sex, gonadal sex, hormonal sex, and even external genital organs have shown that no one parameter is an infallible basis on which to assign sex for rearing. A large body of evidence supports the masculinizing effect of exposure of the female as well as the male fetus to androgens; however, the magnitude of this influence cannot be predicted with certainty in the individual case. In intersex patients the degree of masculinization of the external genitalia does not correlate strongly with that of the central nervous system. The physician should consider the modern surgical advances in genital repair,[507] including repair of hypospadias,[506] and the use of exogenous testosterone in the treatment of androgen-sensitive microphallus.[1352, 1515] In some cultures, the social, cultural, and economic benefits of a male gender are more compelling than phallic adequacy and are a prevailing, if not the most important, factor in the parental decision on the sex of rearing (Table 22–42).[1540, 1547]

The hormonal sex expected at maturity and the increasing possibility of fertility with advances in assisted reproduction technology are of importance. With the exception of female pseudohermaphrodites and true hermaphrodites reared as females, ambiguities of the external genitalia are caused by lesions that severely compromise but do not eliminate the possibility of fertility in view of the advances of modern reproductive techniques. A major goal in intersex patients should be the possibility of achieving cosmetic and functionally normal external genitalia by surgical and endocrinologic means. In considering a decision to recommend a male sex of rearing, emphasis should be placed on the size of the shaft and glans and its potential for growth. All phenotypic males with micropenis (stretched penis length < 2.5 cm at birth) should be given a trial of testosterone enanthate in oil, 25 to 50 mg intramuscularly monthly for three doses, to ascertain the potential of the phallus for further growth before a decision on sex of rearing is made.[1515] Failure of the phallus to lengthen significantly (mean response, 2.0 ± 0.6 cm) raises the possibility of inadequate growth of the phallus in later childhood and at puberty. The parents should be made aware of the difficulties in making a dogmatic recommendation with the limited data on outcome. Principles governing the differential diagnosis and the surgical, hormonal, and psychological management of patients with genital ambiguity are treated more extensively in the following sections.

Differential Diagnosis of Ambisexual Development in Infancy

Abnormalities of sex differentiation should be suspected not only in infants with ambiguous genitalia (Fig. 22–87) but also in apparent females with inguinal masses, inguinal hernias, or slight clitoral enlargement. Apparent males with cryptorchidism, hypospadias, or unusually small genitalia or gonads likewise deserve close scrutiny. Sufficient investigation should be carried out in the newborn period to ascertain, if at all possible, an etiologic diagnosis to permit an informal decision by the parents on the assignment of sex. A karyotype or FISH analysis of sex chromosomes is an imperative first step in all such newborns (Fig. 22–88).

Infants with a 46,XX Karyotype

All infants with sexual ambiguity and a 46,XX karyotype should receive sufficient study in the neonatal period to differentiate the various forms of female pseudohermaphroditism (Table 22–18) from true hermaphroditism and the rare XX male.

Congenital Adrenal Hyperplasia

Female pseudohermaphrodites with virilizing CAH are reared as females in most cultures (Table 22–43). If female pseudohermaphroditism is secondary to CAH (primarily CYP21 deficiency), plasma levels of 17-hydroxyprogesterone and androstenedione and excretion of urinary 17-ketosteroids should be markedly elevated. A plasma 17-hydroxyprogesterone level higher than 90 nmol/L (3000 ng/dL) in an infant with ambiguous genitalia who is 24 hours of age or older is virtually diagnostic of 21-hydroxylase deficiency. However, premature and stressed infants may have elevated plasma 17-hydroprogesterone levels for 4 to 5 days. The diagnosis of CAH is sometimes difficult in the newborn period and may require multiple steroid determinations and the use of an intravenous bolus of ACTH to stimulate plasma 17-hydroxyprogesterone for the detection of 21-hydroxylase deficiency and 11-deoxycortisol for 11-hydroxylase deficiency. Any infant with ambiguous external genitalia who fails to thrive or who develops vomiting, dehydration, and signs of hypoglycemia during the first few weeks of life should be suspected of having a severe salt-losing form of CAH. If such an infant has hyperkalemia associated with acidosis and hyponatremia, the diagnosis is virtually assured, and vigorous therapy with hydrocortisone, salt, and mineralocorticoids should be instituted on an urgent

1. History: family history, pregnancy (hormones, virilization inspection)
   Palpation of inguinal region and labioscrotal folds; rectal examination
   Karyotype analysis
   Initial studies: plasma 17-hydroxyprogesterone, androstenedione, dehydroepiandrosterone, testosterone, & dihydrotestosterone
   Serum electrolytes
   Sonogram or MRI of kidneys, ureters & pelvic contents
   Provisional Dx

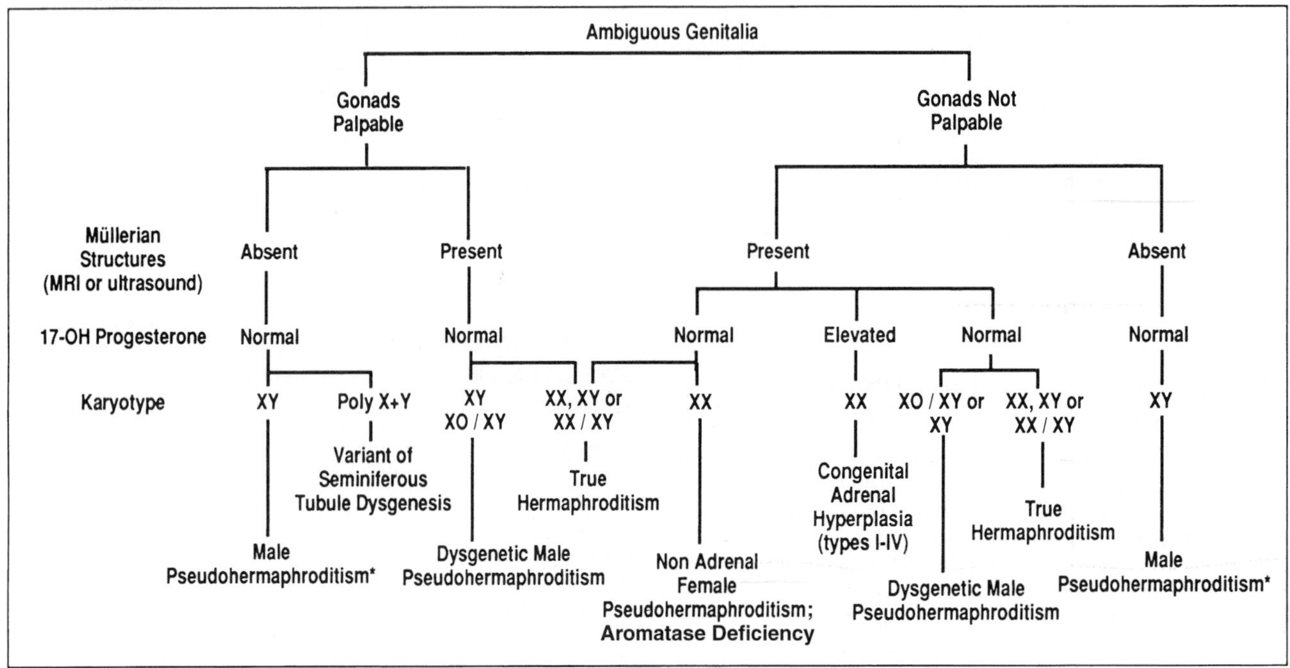

2. "Vaginogram" (urogenital sinogram): selected cases
   Endoscopy, laparotomy, gonadal biopsy: restricted to male pseudohermaphrodites, true hermaphrodites, and selected instances of nonadrenal female pseudohermaphroditism

*Plasma 17-hydroxyprogesterone levels may be modestly elevated in patients with **CYP11** (Type III), 3β-hydroxysteroid dehydrogenase deficiency (Type IV) and are "low" in patients with **CYP17** (Type V) and **CYP11A1** deficiency (Type VI)

Figure 22–87. Steps in the diagnosis of intersexuality in infancy and childhood. Step 1 involves initial work-up and provisional diagnosis. Step 2 is used in selected cases.

basis to prevent collapse and sudden death. Once the diagnosis of adrenal hyperplasia is established, glucocorticoid therapy should be instituted and continued for life.

Other Forms of Female Pseudohermaphroditism

A small proportion of 46,XX female pseudohermaphrodites have aromatase (CYP19) deficiency. A history of virilization of the mother during pregnancy and elevated levels of androgens, androgen precursors, and FSH and unmeasurable levels of estrone and estradiol are diagnostic. 46,XX infants may be presumed to have non–androgen-induced female pseudohermaphroditism if adrenal hyperplasia, aromatase deficiency, and a glucocorticoid receptor defect have been excluded and if there is a reliable history of the mother receiving androgens or progestational hormones during pregnancy or of the mother developing some virilizing tendency during pregnancy. These latter children require no further hormonal medication during childhood and feminize normally at adolescence. Non–androgen-induced female pseudohermaphroditism is associated with gross anomalies of the lower intestine and/or urinary tract. Such children should be studied for the presence of pyelonephritis and anomalies in other systems. Patients with female pseudohermaphroditism usually have a normal uterus and fallopian tubes with ovaries in the normal location. For this reason, the diagnosis should be viewed with suspicion if there is an inguinal hernia or if gonad-like masses are palpable in the groin. Such masses are frequently testes. The presence of a uterus can often be detected in the newborn period by digital examination via the rectum; however, the use of pelvic ultrasonography is now routine because it is more informative and less stressful. If there is uncertainty, MRI of the pelvis is useful.

True Hermaphroditism

Most patients with true hermaphroditism have a 46,XX karyotype, and it may be difficult to distinguish some of them from patients with the rare nonadrenal causes of female pseudohermaphroditism. True hermaphrodites, however, often have gonads located in the labia or inguinal canals; a bipartite gonad is highly suggestive of ovotestes. In true hermaphrodites the assignment of sex should be deferred until the nature of the internal genital structures and gonads can be determined by ultrasonography, MRI, urethroscopy, or radiologic study with contrast media and, if necessary, laparoscopy. Most 46,XX true hermaphrodites are raised as females. Not infrequently, the heterologous gonadal tissue can be removed. It is important to emphasize the risk of malignant degeneration of the dysgenetic testicular tissue that is retained. In general, assignment of female sex and an attempt to preserve an ovary or

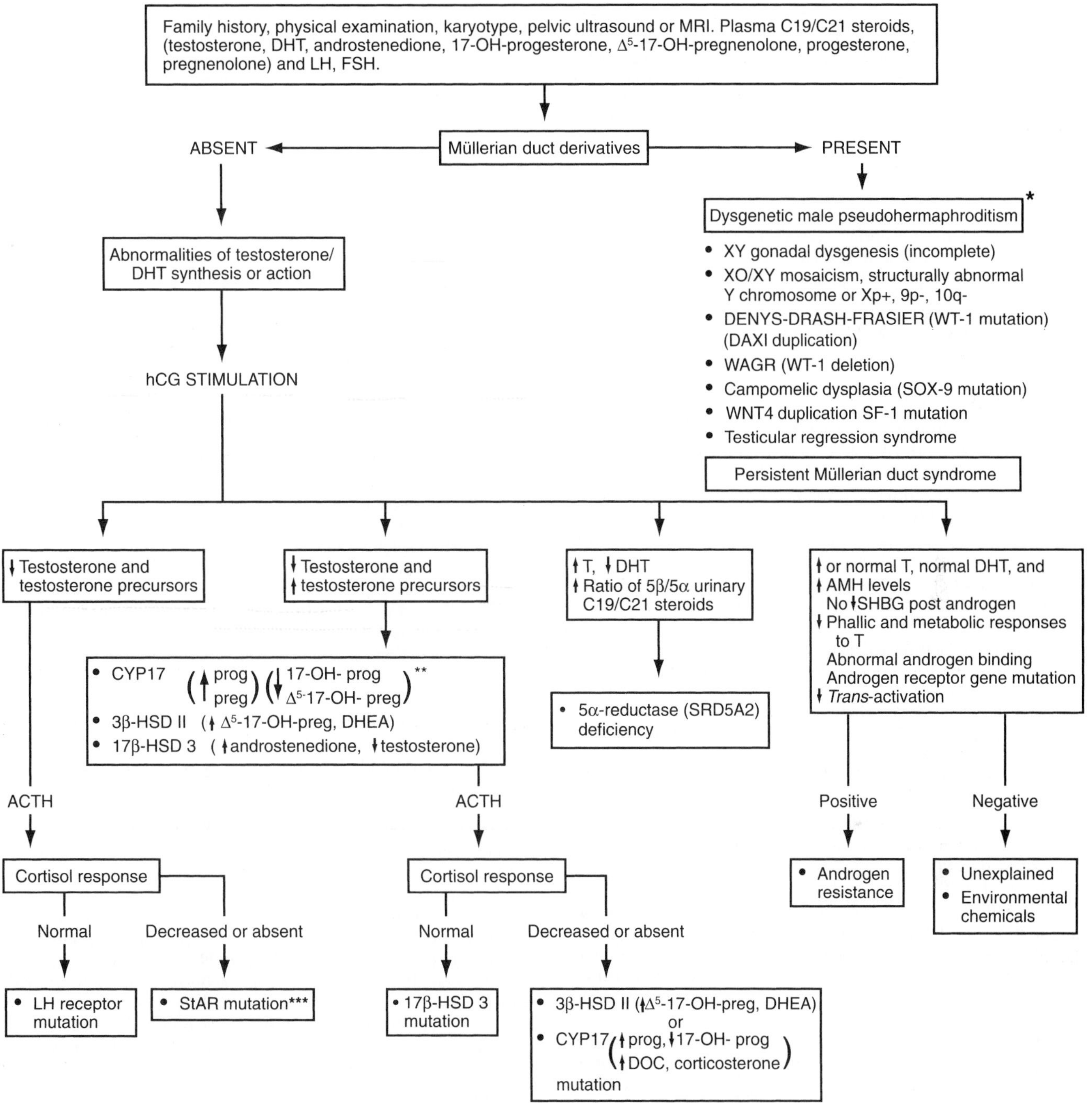

Figure 22–88. Steps in the differential diagnosis of male pseudohermaphroditism.

*Patients with dysgenetic male pseudohermaphroditism may manifest varying degrees of testicular dysgenesis with either complete or partial testosterone/DHT and/or AMH deficiency.Therefore, not all patients may manifest either ambiguous genitalia or the presence of müllerian ducts.

**CYP17 ($P450_{c17}$) catalyzes the 17-hydroxylation of progesterone and pregnenolone to 17-hydroxyprogesterone and Δ^5-17-hydroxypregnenolone as well as the scission (lyase) of 17-hydroxypregnenolone to DHEA. Patients with 17,20-lyase deficiency have elevated levels of 17-hydroxyprogesterone and Δ^5-17-hydroxypregnenolone in relation to androstenedione and DHEA either before or after hCG stimulation.

***The StAR (*s*teroidogenic *a*cute *r*egulatory) protein is involved in the transport of cholesterol from the outer to the inner mitochondrial membrane where the enzyme CYP11A1($P450_{scc}$) resides. Patients with a mutation in the gene for this protein have a markedly diminished ability to convert cholesterol to Δ^5-pregnenolone, although their CYP11A1 enzymatic activity is intact. They manifest congenital lipoid adrenal hyperplasia. WAGR, Wilms tumor, aniridia, genital anomalies, and mental retardation; SF1, steroidogenic factor-1; CYP17, 17α-hydroxylase/17,20-lyase; 3β-HSD II, 3β-hydroxysteroid dehydrogenase/Δ^5-isomerase; 17β-HSD 3, 17β-hydroxysteroid dehydrogenase (oxidoreductase) type 3; T, testosterone; DHT, dihydrotestosterone; AMH, antimüllerian hormone; SHBG, sex hormone-binding globulin; DHEA, dehydroepiandrosterone.

Table 22–43. Management of 46,XX Female Pseudohermaphrodite with Congenital Adrenal Hyperplasia

- Raise as females.
- Severely masculinized affected infants with a penile urethra (Prader V) present a management dilemma if unrecognized in infancy.
- When the diagnosis is made in infancy, a female sex assignment is indicated. Consideration of a sex change (male to female) in childhood or later mandates extensive consultation and discussion and an informed decision by parents.

Table 22–44. Management of True Hermaphrodite

- Most are raised as females with preservation of ovarian component.
- When external genitalia are well masculinized and in the rare 46,XY variant, some parents select male sex of rearing.

ovarian tissue are appropriate except in those rare true hermaphrodites who have a 46,XY karyotype, no uterus, and adequate phallic development (Table 22–44).

Infants with a 46,XY Karyotype

Male pseudohermaphroditism is a heterogeneous group of disorders in which ambiguous genitalia result from either androgen deficiency or androgen resistance during the critical period of sex differentiation (see Fig. 22–88) (Table 22–45). The existence of both complete and partial defects in androgen biosynthesis, metabolism, and action; the occurrence of more than one gene encoding a protein with the same enzymatic activity but with different tissue specificities or developmental expression (e.g., 3β-HSD, 17β-HSD, 5α-reductase); and the presence of different phenotypes in some patients with the same molecular genetic defect confound the clinical picture and the predictions about the natural history of these disorders.

A great effort should be made to establish an etiologic diagnosis, because this may have an important bearing on subsequent management, including family counseling. A detailed family history with construction of a pedigree is important, because many sexual abnormalities are hereditary and because this type of historical information is not always volunteered. For example, a history of aunts who have never menstruated or of an inguinal hernia or labial mass in a phenotypic female first-degree relative may suggest the diagnosis of androgen resistance. The mother should also be asked about signs of virilization during pregnancy and drugs or hormones that she may have taken during the early part of pregnancy.

Studies during the newborn period should always include an examination of the karyotype. A sufficient number of metaphase plates should be examined to reduce the possibility of overlooking mosaicism. The morphology of the sex chromosome and the autosomes should be determined and selective FISH analysis carried out.

Pelvic ultrasonography or MRI, radiographic contrast studies of the urogenital sinus, and fiberoptic endoscopic examination may aid in this initial evaluation. Laparoscopy or laporotomy is rarely indicated in the neonatal period except in infants suspected of having true hermaphroditism. Before an informal decision about sex assignment is made by the parents it is important to evaluate fully karyotypic studies, the pattern of plasma gonadal steroids before and after hCG stimulation, and other measures to identify a specific type of male pseudohermaphroditism.

Urinary steroids and plasma androgens should be measured before and after administration of corticotropin (0.15 to 0.25 mg intravenously) and hCG (1500 U/m^2 intramuscularly daily $\times$ 3 doses or every 48 hours $\times$ 7) to ascertain whether the patient has a block in testosterone synthesis or 5α-reductase deficiency.[1548] The testosterone response to hCG may result in measurable phallic enlargement. Therefore, in addition to providing objective information about the functional capacity of the Leydig cells to secrete testosterone, the test may also provide evidence for the capacity of androgen-sensitive target tissues to respond to androgens. In the patient with male pseudohermaphroditism and no evidence of a testosterone biosynthetic error, 5α-reductase-2 deficiency, or dysgenetic male pseudohermaphroditism, clinical or metabolic evidence of testosterone responsiveness should be assessed before a sex assignment is made.

Male infants with congenital hypopituitarism or isolated hypogondotrophic hypogonadism frequently have micropenis and unilateral or bilateral cryptorchidism, and this diagnosis should be excluded by appropriate studies of pituitary function before considering sex reassignment.[1352, 1516, 1549] It is our view that all male infants with micropenis should be given a trial of testosterone parenterally before a conclusion is made that the phallus lacks the capacity for growth.[1352, 1515] Administration of a dose of 25 mg (100 mg/m^2) of testosterone enanthate intramuscularly once a month for 3 months in the newborn should provide an adequate androgen stimulus to make this assessment.[1515] Rarely, this treatment may cause a slight advancement of the skeletal age, but this consideration is trivial when weighed against the momentous question of deciding the future sex of rearing. It is also important to assess penis size periodically and to repeat the course of testosterone therapy to maintain phallus size within the normal range for age. It has been suggested by inference from studies in rats that early exposure of the penis to androgens in childhood may result in a significant reduction in adult phallic size.[1550] However, data obtained by us and others suggest that early exposure to androgens does not cause a decrease in the developmentally programmed, final penile length.[1551]

In many patients, a precise etiologic diagnosis and appropriate sex assignment can be made on the basis of the criteria just stated. In the rare patient with no evidence of defective testosterone synthesis, end-organ unresponsiveness to androgen, or testicular dysgenesis, true hermaphroditism should be considered. In these patients the demonstration of both ovarian and testicular tissue at laparoscopy establishes the diagnosis.

All of the findings (anatomic, karyotypic, genetic, and hormonal), along with the natural history of the specific disorder and the possibilities for surgical reconstruction and normal sexual function, need to be discussed with the parents. Their informed consent, understanding, and cooperation are critical to a successful gender assignment. Once the parental decision is made to rear the infant as a boy or as a girl, it is important to support the parents and patient in reinforcing this decision and to obtain mental health counseling. It is critical to assist the parents in addressing uncertainties and doubts that may arise during follow-up visits.

Table 22–45. Management of 46,XY Male Pseudohermaphrodite

- Administer testosterone enanthate 25 mg intramuscularly monthly $\times$ 3: "normal" response $>$ 0.9 cm increase in phallic length
- Raise 46,XY male pseudohermaphrodites as males except those with:
  - Complete androgen insensitivity syndrome. The dilemma presented by partial androgen insensitivity syndrome
  - Completely female genitalia (?)
  - Compelling reasons for sex assignment as female, including parents' informed decision

Reassignment of Sex After the Newborn Period

Children may be assigned an inappropriate sex because of errors in diagnosis or ignorance of the principles that should properly determine this choice. In such cases, the knotty decision to change the sex of rearing or to leave matters undisturbed depends largely on the age of the child and the degree to which the gender identity has been established. Money has stated that a change in the sex of rearing is feasible until the age of 18 months and is sometimes successful until 30 months,[462, 491] but thereafter, in our culture, serious and sometimes complex psychiatric and social consequences may be encountered. This concept has been challenged. Nevertheless, change of gender assignment in children should be undertaken after 18 months only after a review of alternatives and with the provision of close supervision and long-term counseling of the patient, parents, and siblings.

Before, at, or during adolescence, the patient may reach the decision that he or she has been reared in the wrong sex and may request assistance in changing his or her sex of assignment. If there are sufficient grounds for this belief, the request should be considered seriously and honored. Some patients may have serious psychological disturbances, and both psychiatric and legal counsel should be sought.[1197]

Reconstructive Surgery

Because the presence of ambiguous external genitalia is likely to reinforce doubt about the sexual identity of the infant or child, it is desirable to initiate reconstructive surgery as early as is medically and surgically feasible. The functional result, rather than the cosmetic, is paramount. It is highly desirable that surgery on the external genitalia be initiated before 6 months of age when practicable.[507, 508, 923, 1012, 1553, 1554]

The management of clitoromegaly in female pseudohermaphrodites and in male pseudohermaphrodites reared as females has been controversial. Two different operative approaches have been used: clitoral recession, first reported by Lattimer in 1961 to replace the then widely used clitorectomy,[1013, 1555] and clitoroplasty.[396, 507, 508, 1015] Clitoridectomy[857, 1556] has long been abandoned as a mutilating procedure. Documentation of the role of the clitoris as an erotic organ in women[1557] makes it clear that clitoridectomy must be avoided. Clitoral recession has significant drawbacks mainly because of painful clitoral erections.[1013] Clitoroplasty, as recommended by Donahoe,[507] Rink,[508] Hutson,[1015] and Baskin[396] requires excision of the shaft and corpora with retention of the glans. This procedure and modifications of it[1012] are used most widely at present. Long-term data are still necessary to evaluate the efficacy of this procedure with respect to appearance and sexual function.

The extent of the initial repair of the urogenital sinus and vagina depends in large part on the skill and experience of the surgeon. These are not procedures that should be undertaken by surgeons or urologists who have not had training and experience with these techniques and are not part of a team of professionals that address clinical issues. Even when the initial repair has been done in the past by an experienced surgeon, it has not been uncommon for patients who have had vaginoplasties performed at age 18 months or earlier to require secondary operations because of stenosis of the introitus.[1554] We believe that reconstruction of a vagina in male pseudohermaphrodites reared as females and in female pseudohermaphrodites can be deferred until adolescence or until requested by the patient. A small vaginal pouch often can be enlarged by daily manipulations with a suitable mold.[1559] Even if the vagina remains too shallow for satisfactory coitus, manual dilatation makes it easier to carry out subsequent surgical correction.

Table 22–46. Removal of the Gonads

- Retain histologically normal and functional scrotal testes in 45,X/46,XY male pseudohermaphrodites.
- Follow closely. Consider biopsy postpubertally to detect carcinoma in situ and perform periodic ultrasonography of testes.
- Complete androgen insensitivity: testes may be retained until after puberty.
- Partial androgen insensitivity or biosynthetic defects: if female sex of rearing is selected by parents, we recommend gonadal removal before puberty to prevent virilization.

A male with hypospadias no longer requires multiple procedures to create a phallic urethra. In recent years, new surgical techniques have reduced the number of operations and the length of hospitalization and have increased the success rate and parental expectations for "normality" in both the short and the long term.[506] Circumcision should be avoided to preserve as much tissue as possible. Laparoscopy can be undertaken (if necessary) simultaneously with the initial operation. It is often desirable to insert prosthetic testes to give the scrotum dependency and to improve cosmetic appearance. These may be changed to adult-sized prostheses in adolescence.

Removal of the Gonads

A high incidence of gonadal tumors in patients with certain forms of gonadal dysgenesis and dysgenetic male pseudohermaphroditism especially makes it mandatory that an evaluation of this risk be given priority in deciding whether and when the gonads should be removed. Although the incidence of gonadoblastomas and germinomas (seminomas or dysgerminomas) increases near the normal time of adolescence, tumors are sometimes discovered during the first decade. Because temporizing serves no useful purpose and may expose the child to hormone secretions inappropriate to the chosen sex for rearing, it is advisable to proceed with gonadectomy concurrently with the initial repair of the external genitalia in patients who are at high risk, especially in the instance of intra-abdominal rudimentary testes. We are evaluating the use of MRI of the pelvis every 1 to 2 years to screen for gonadal neoplasms in children at risk.

Although prevalence of gonadal tumors has been reported to be as high as 9% in patients with the androgen resistance syndrome based on studies over three decades ago, some patients who developed tumors may have had atypical forms of gonadal dysgenesis; a modern survey is not available. The prevalence of gonadal malignancy before age 25 years in patients with androgen resistance appears to be relatively low. If the patient has a hernia and surgical repair is indicated, we recommend gonadectomy at that time to avoid a second operation. Otherwise, in the patient with complete androgen resistance, the undescended testes may be left in situ until after puberty. Thereafter, a frank and open discussion with the patient of the pathophysiology of androgen resistance and an assessment of the risk of gonadal malignancy needs to be undertaken to obtain informed consent for gonadectomy (Table 22–46).

There is a risk of some degree of virilization at the time of puberty in patients with the partial form of androgen resistance and in those with other forms of male pseudohermaphroditism with retained testes in whom a female sex for rearing has been assigned. In these cases, gonadectomy before puberty has been advanced and should be considered and discussed with the patient and parents. In some male pseudohermaphrodites who are raised as males, at least partial development of male secondary sexual characteristics will occur at the expected time of puberty. Provided the testes are not dysgenetic and are sufficiently descended to permit palpation, it is reasonable to leave the testes in situ. Such patients should be carefully examined at regular intervals for the presence of a tumor. MRI, ultrasonography, and examination of testicular biopsy specimens are useful in the early diagnosis of CIS and testicular neoplasm.[1560]

Hormone substitution therapy in hypogonadal patients should be prescribed in such a way that secondary sexual characteristics emerge appropriately in both timing and sequence. The goal of therapy should be to approximate normal adolescent development as closely as possible.

In females, including patients with the syndrome of gonadal dysgenesis, estrogenic hormone substitution therapy is initiated with low oral doses of estrogen (0.3 mg conjugated estrogens or 5 μg ethinyl estradiol daily) or a transdermal estradiol patch.[745] Breast enlargement and growth of the uterus frequently occur within 3 months. Usually, cyclic therapy with estrogen and an oral progestagen is begun after 6 to 12 months of estrogen therapy or sooner if breakthrough bleeding occurs (see section on treatment of gonadal dysgenesis).

Development of male secondary sexual characteristics is usually better with repository injections of testosterone or a transdermal testosterone patch than with oral preparations. Few data are available on the use of dermal testosterone therapy in childhood or adolescence. Many oral synthetic androgens have the added disadvantage of predisposing to biliary stasis, jaundice, and hepatic tumors. Rapid virilization is usually inadvisable, and it is preferable to promote virilization gradually over many months in a manner similar to that in normal boys. The effect of gonadal steroids on skeletal maturation is dose related, whereas the effect on linear growth is less so. The relation between attained stature and skeletal maturation at the inception of therapy and the dose of androgen prescribed determine the ultimate effect of this therapy on adult height. An initial intramuscular dose of 50 mg of testosterone enanthate or other long-acting testosterone ester may be given monthly, beginning at age 12 to 13 years. Thereafter, the dose should be increased gradually over 3 to 4 years to the adult replacement dose of 200 mg every 2 weeks, usually reaching the adult level after a bone age of 17 years has been attained (see Table 22–45). In selected patients we have used the transdermal testosterone patch; initially the 2.5-mg patch is applied overnight for 8 hours. Subsequently the length of application is gradually increased to 24 hours.

Psychological Management

The newborn with ambiguous genitalia presents a clinical, social, and psychological challenge.[1561] Initially, in infants with ambiguous genitalia it is best for the physician to admit uncertainty regarding the "true sex" of the child and to urge the parents not to immediately assign a name and send out birth announcements. The filing of the birth certificate with the name should be delayed until a definite gender assignment and name has been given to the child. Clinical, cytogenetic, hormonal, and radiologic evaluation should be undertaken expeditiously. Thereafter, clearly presented, comprehensive, and informative discussions with the parents should ensue with all members of the team (i.e., endocrinologist, infant's physician, geneticist, surgeon, mental health specialist, social worker) present, if possible. This discussion should take into account the anxieties, religious views, social mores, cultural background, and level of understanding of the parents to make the best gender assignment for the infant and to obtain informed consent for the decision from the parents. A simple explanation of the normal process of sexual differentiation with appropriate illustrative material is useful because it lays the groundwork for the concept that all fetuses are bipotential initially and that sex differentiation is a complex process that may not be completed in utero. An analogy to other so-called birth defects (e.g., cleft lip, congenital heart disease) is accurate, easily understood, and less psychologically threatening. It should be stated clearly that the anatomic abnormalities can be surgically repaired by an experienced surgeon, that hormone replacement can be given if necessary, and that psychological support is available (Table 22–47). Continuing follow-up by the team members should address any questions that arise during infancy and childhood. In this age of "freedom of information," it is prudent to discuss in an age-appropriate manner and in progressive stages all aspects of the diagnosis, pathophysiology, management, and treatment of the ambiguous genitalia with the patient as soon as his or her level of increased understanding allows for this.

Table 22–47. Management of Ambiguous Genitalia

- Hormone therapy at puberty if necessary.
- Progressive, step-by-step, age-appropriate discussion of diagnosis, pathophysiology, gender, and potential for fertility with the patient from childhood through adolescence, as well as with the parents. Secrecy is unwarranted and counterproductive.
- Involve the patient in decisions about surgery and sex hormone replacement therapy.
- Provide continuing psychosocial and endocrinologic support to the patient and the family.
- Long-term follow-up data on the outcome of modern management needs to be a high priority.

The implications of these observations for the management of intersex are debated in a series of published papers in the *Journal of Clinical Ethics*.[1552]

References

1. Jost A, Vigier B, Prepin J, et al. Studies on sex differentiation in mammals. Recent Prog Horm Res 1973; 29:1–41.
2. Austin CR, Edwards RG. Mechanisms of Sex Differentiation in Animals and Man. London: Academic Press, 1981.
3. Hamosh A, Scott AF, Amberger J, Valle D, McKusick VA. Online Mendelian Inheritance in Man (OMIM). Hum Mutat 2000; 15:57–61.
4. Swain A, Lovell-Badge R. Mammalian sex determination: a molecular drama. Genes Dev 1999; 13:755–767.
5. Jirasek JE. Development of the Genital System and Male Pseudohermaphroditism. Baltimore: Johns Hopkins University Press, 1971.
6. Capel B. Sex in the 90s: SRY and the switch to the male pathway. Annu Rev Physiol 1998; 60: 497–523.
7. Capel B. The battle of the sexes. Mech Dev 2000; 92:89–103.
8. McLaren A, Ferguson-Smith MA (eds). Sex determination in mouse and man. Philos Trans R Soc Lond B Biol Sci 1988; 322:1–157.
9. McLaren A. Germ cells and germ cell sex. Philos Trans R Soc Lond B Biol Sci 1995; 350:229–233.
10. Wizemann TM, Pardue ML (eds). Exploring the Biological Contributions to Human Health: Does Sex Matter? Committee on Understanding the Biology of Sex and Gender Differences, Institute of Medicine. Washington, DC: National Academy Press, 2001.
11. Wilson JD, George FW, Renfree MB. The endocrine role in mammalian sexual differentiation. Recent Prog Horm Res 1995; 50:349–364.
12. Koopman P. The genetics and biology of vertebrate sex determination. Cell 2001; 105:843–847.
13. Byskov AG, Hryer PE. Embryology of mammalian gonads and ducts. In: Knobil E, Neill JD, eds. The Physiology of Reproduction. 2nd ed. New York: Raven Press, 1994: 487–540.
14. Hughes IA (ed). Sexual differentiation. Bailliere's Clin Endocrinol Metab, London 1998; 12: 1–198.
15. Lander ES, Linton LM, Birren B, et al. Initial sequencing and analysis of the human genome. Nature 2001; 409:860–921.

16. Venter JC, Adams MD, Myers EW, et al. The sequence of the human genome. Science 2001; 291:1304–1351.
17. Pinsky L, Erickson RP, Schimke RN (eds.). Genetic Disorders of Human Sexual Development. Oxford University Press, 1999.
18. Veitia RA, Salas-Cortes L, Ottolenghi C, et al. Testis determination in mammals: more questions than answers. Mol Cell Endocrinol 2001; 179:3–16.
19. Grumbach MM, Gluckman PD. The human fetal hypothalamus and pituitary gland: the maturation of neuroendocrine mechanisms controlling the secretion of fetal pituitary growth hormone, prolactin, gonadotropins, adrenocorticotropin-related peptides and thyrotropin. In: Tulchinsky D, Little AB, eds. Maternal-Fetal Endocrinology. 2nd ed. Philadelphia: WB Saunders, 1994: 193–261.
20. Vaiman D, Pailhoux E. Mammalian sex reversal and intersexuality: deciphering the sex-determination cascade. Trends Genet 2000; 16:488–494.
21. Parker KL, Schimmer BP. Steroidogenic factor 1: a key determinant of endocrine development and function. Endocr Rev 1997; 18:361–377.
21a. Parker KL, Schimmer BP, Schedl A. Genes essential for early events in gonadal development. Cell Mol Life Sci 1999; 55:831–838.
22. Clarkson MJ, Harley VR. Sex with two SOX on: SRY and SOX9 in testis development. Trends Endocrinol Metab 2002; 13:106–111.
23. Pask A, Marshall Graves JA. Sex chromosomes and sex-determining genes: insights from marsupials and monotremes. Cell Mol Life Sci 1999; 55:864–875.
24. Parkhurst SM, Meneely PM. Sex determination and dosage compensation: lessons from flies and worms. Science 1994; 264: 924–932.
24a. Vincent S, Perkins LA, Perrimon N. Doublesex surprises. Cell 2001; 106:399–402.
25. Western PS, Sinclair AH. Sex, genes, and heat: triggers of diversity. J Exp Zool 2001; 290:624–631.
26. Marshall Graves JA, Shetty S. Sex from W to Z: evolution of vertebrate sex chromosomes and sex determining genes. J Exp Zool 2001; 290:449–462.
27. Moreno-Mendoza N, Harley VR, Merchant-Larios H. Temperature regulates SOX9 expression in cultured gonads of *Lepidochelys olivacea*, a species with temperature sex determination. Dev Biol 2001; 229:319–326.
28. Mittelman F, ed. International System for Human Cytogenetics Nomenclature. Basel, Switzerland: S Karger, 1995.
29. Henegariu O, Heerema NA, Bray-Ward P, Ward DC. Colour-changing karyotyping: an alternative to M-FISH/SKY. Nat Genet 1999; 23:263–264.
30. Niimura Y, Gojobori T. *In silico* chromosome staining: reconstruction of Giemsa bands from the whole human genome sequence. Proc Natl Acad Sci USA 2002; 99:797–802.
31. Grumbach MM, Morishima A, Taylor JH. Human sex chromosome abnormalities in relation to DNA replication and heterochromatinization. Proc Natl Acad Sci USA 1963; 49:581–589.
32. Morishima A, Grumbach MM, Taylor JH. Asynchronous duplication of human chromosomes and the origin of sex chromatin. Proc Natl Acad Sci USA 1962; 48:756–763.
33. Caspersson T, Zech L, Johansson C, et al. Identification of human chromosomes by DNA binding fluorescent agents. Chromosoma 1970; 30:215–217.
34. Caspersson T, Zech L. Chromosome identification by fluorescence. Hosp Pract 1972; 7:51–62.
35. Pardue ML, Gall JG. Chromosomal localization of mouse satellite DNA. Science 1970; 168:1356–1358.
36. Pearson P. The use of new staining techniques for human chromosome identification. J Med Genet 1972; 9:264–275.
37. Speicher MR, Ward DC. The coloring of cytogenetics. Nat Med 1996; 2:1046–1048.
38. LeBeau MM. One FISH, two FISH, red FISH, blue FISH. Nat Genet 1996; 12:341–344.
39. Schrock E, du Manoir S, Veldman T, et al. Multicolor spectral karyotyping of human chromosomes. Science 1996; 273:494–497.
40. Fauth C, Speicher MR. Classifying by colors: FISH-based genome analysis. Cytogenet Cell Genet 2001; 93:1–10.
41. Hassold T, Abruzzo M, Adkins K, Griffin D, Merrill M, Millie E, Saker D, Shen J, Zaragoza M. Human aneuploidy: incidence, origin, and etiology. Environ Mol Mutagen 1996; 28:167–175.
42. Hassold T, Hunt P. To err (meiotically) is human: the genesis of human aneuploidy. Nat Rev Genet 2001; 2:280–291.
43. Abruzzo MA, Hassold TJ. Etiology of nondisjunction in humans. Environ Mol Mutagen 1995; 25(Suppl 26):38–47.
44. Lamb NE, Freeman SB, SavageAustin A, et al. Susceptible chiasmate configurations of chromosome 21 predispose to nondisjunction in both maternal meiosis I and meiosis II. Nat Genet 1996; 14:400–405.
45. Dailey T, Dale B, Cohen J, et al. Association between nondisjunction and maternal age in meiosisII human oocytes. Am J Hum Genet 1996; 59:176–184.
46. Morishima A, Grumbach MM. The interrelationship of sex chromosome constitution and phenotype in the syndrome of gonadal dysgenesis and its variants. Ann N Y Acad Sci 1968; 155:695–715.
47. Chu CE, Connor JM, Donaldson MDC, et al. Detection of Y mosaicism in patients with Turner's syndrome. J Med Genet 1995; 32:578–580.
48. Wolff DJ, Miller AP, Van Dyke DL, et al. Molecular definition of breakpoints associated with human Xq isochromosomes: implications for mechanisms of formation. Am J Hum Genet 1996; 58:154–160.
49. Lahn BT, Page DC. Retroposition of autosomal mRNA yielded testis-specific gene family on human Y chromosome. Nat Genet 1999; 21:429–433.
50. Marshall Graves JA. Human Y chromosome, sex determination, and spermatogenesis—a feminist view. Biol Reprod 2000; 63: 667–676.
51. Waters PD, Duffy B, Frost CJ, Delbridge ML, Graves JAM. The human Y chromosome derives largely from a single autosomal region added to the sex chromosomes 80–130 million years ago. Cytogenet Cell Genet 2001; 92:74–79.
52. Kirsch S, Weiss B, De Rosa M, Ogata T, Lombardi G, Rappold GA. FISH deletion mapping defines a single location for the Y chromosome stature gene, GCY.
53. Ratcliffe SG. The psychological and psychiatric consequences of sex chromosome abnormalities in children, based on population studies. In: Poustka F, ed. Basic Approaches to Genetic and Molecular Biological, Developmental Psychiatry. Berlin: Quintessenz, 1994: 99–122.
54. Ogata T, Matsuo N, Nishimura G. SHOX haploinsufficiency and overdosage: impact of gonadal function status. J Med Genet 2001; 38:1–6.
55. Quintana-Murci L, Krausz C, McElreavey K. The human Y chromosome: function, evolution and disease. Forensic Sci Int 2001; 118:169–181.
56. Weller PA, Critcher R, Goodfellow PN, German J, Ellis NA. The human Y chromosome homologue of XG: transcription of a naturally truncated gene. Hum Mol Genet 1995; 4:859–868.
57. Vogt PH, Affara N, Davey P, Hammer M, Jobling MA, Lau YF, Mitchell M, Schempp W, Tyler-Smith C, Williams G, Yen P, Rappold GA. Report of the Third International Workshop on Y Chromosome Mapping 1997. Heidelberg, Germany, April 13–16, 1997. Cytogenet Cell Genet 1997; 79:1–20.
58. Rao E, Weiss B, Takami M, et al. Pseudoautosomal deletions encompassing a novel homeobox gene cause growth failure in idiopathic short stature and Turner syndrome. Nature Genet 1997; 16:54–62.
59. Ellison JW, Wardak Z, Young MF, et al. *PHOG:* a candidate gene for involvement in the short stature of Turner syndrome. Hum Mol Genet 1997; 6:1341–1347.
60. Rao E, Blaschke RJ, Marchini A, Niesler B, Burnett M, Rappold GA. The Leri-Weill and Turner syndrome homeobox gene SHOX encodes a cell-type specific transcriptional activator. Hum Mol Genet 2001; 10:3083–3091.
61. Clement-Jones M, Schiller S, Rao E, et al. The short stature homeobox gene SHOX is involved in skeletal abnormalities in Turner syndrome. Hum Mol Genet 2000; 9:695–702.
62. Belin V, Cusin V, Viot G, et al. SHOX mutations in dyschondrosteosis (Leri-Weill syndrome). Nat Genet 1998; 19:67–69.
63. Shears DJ, Vassal HJ, Goodman FR, et al. Mutation and deletion of the pseudoautosomal gene SHOX cause Leri-Weill dyschondrosteosis.
64. Schiller S, Spranger S, Schechinger B, et al. Phenotypic varia-

356. George FW, Wilson JD. The regulation of androgen and estrogen formation in fetal gonads. Ann Biol Anim Biochim Biophys 1979; 19(4B):1297–1306.
357. Gondos B, Hobel CJ. Interstitial cells in the human fetal ovary. Endocrinology 1973; 93:736–739.
358. Grumbach MM, Auchus RJ. Estrogen: consequences and implications of human mutations in synthesis and action. J Clin Endocrinol Metab 1999; 84:4677–4694.
359. Epifano O, Dean J. Genetic control of early folliculogenesis in mice. Trends Endocrinol Metab 2002; 13:169–173.
360. Byskov AG, Baltsen M, Andersen CY. Meiosis-activating sterols: background, discovery, and possible use. J Mol Med 1998; 76: 818–823.
361. Byskov AG, Andersen CY, Leonardsen L, Baltsen M. Meiosis activating sterols (MAS) and fertility in mammals and man. J Exp Zool 1999; 285:237–242.
362. Jost A. Problems of fetal endocrinology: the gonadal and hypophyseal hormones. Recent Prog Horm Res 1953; 8:379–418.
363. Jost A. Embryonic sexual differentiation (morphology, physiology, abnormalities). In: Jones HW Jr, Scott WW, eds. Hermaphroditism, Genital Anomalies and Related Endocrine Disorders. Baltimore: Williams & Wilkins, 1971:16–64.
364. Josso N, Cate RL, Picard JY, et al. Anti-müllerian hormone: the Jost factor. Recent Prog Horm Res 1993; 48:1–59.
365. Josso N, Legeai L, Forest M, et al. An enzyme linked immunoassay for antimüllerian hormone: a new tool for the evaluation of testicular function in infants and children. J Clin Endocrinol Metab 1990; 70:23–27.
366. Rajpert-De Meyts E, Jorgensen N, Graem N, Muller J, Cate RL, Skakkebaek NE. Expression of anti-Müllerian hormone during normal and pathological gonadal development: association with differentiation of Sertoli and granulosa cells. J Clin Endocrinol Metab 1999; 84:3836–3844.
367. Gustafson ML, Lee MM, Scully RC, et al. Müllerian inhibiting substance as a marker for ovarian sex-cord tumor. N Engl J Med 1992; 326:466–471.
368. Teixeira J, Maheswaran S, Donahoe PK. Müllerian inhibiting substance: an instructive developmental hormone with diagnostic and possible therapeutic applications. Endocr Rev 2001; 22:657–674.
369. Josso N, di Clemente N, Gouedard L. Anti-Müllerian hormone and its receptors. Mol Cell Endocrinol 2001; 179:25–32.
370. Vigier B, Tran D, Legeai L, et al. Origin of anti-müllerian hormone in bovine freemartin fetuses. J Reprod Fertil 1984; 70: 473–479.
371. Vigier B, Watrin F, Magre S, et al. Purified bovine AMH induces a characteristic freemartin effect in fetal rat prospective ovaries exposed to it in vitro. Development 1987; 100:43–55.
372. Behringer RR, Cate RL, Froelick GJ. Abnormal sexual development in transgenic mice chronically expressing müllerian inhibitory substance. Nature 1990; 345:167–170.
373. Behringer RR. The in vivo roles of Müllerian-inhibiting substance. Curr Top Dev Biol 1994; 29:171–187.
374. Behringer RR, Finegold MJ, Cate RL. Müllerian-inhibiting substance function during mammalian sexual development. Cell 1994; 79:415–425.
375. Ingraham HA, Hirokawa Y, Roberts LM, Mellon SH, McGee E, Nachtigal MW, Visser JA. Autocrine and paracrine Müllerian inhibiting substance hormone signaling in reproduction. Recent Prog Horm Res 2000; 55:53–67.
376. Tsuji M, Shima H, Yonemura CY, et al. Effect of human recombinant müllerian inhibiting substance on isolated epithelial and mesenchymal cells during müllerian duct regression in the rat. Endocrinology 1992; 131:1481–1488.
377. Massague J. TGF-beta signaling: receptors, transducers, and Mad proteins. Cell 1996; 85:947–950.
378. Visser JA, Olaso R, Verhoef-Post M, et al. The serine/threonine transmembrane receptor ALK2 mediates Müllerian inhibiting substance signaling. Mol Endocrinol 2001; 15:936–945.
379. Clarke TR, Hoshiya Y, Yi SE, et al. Müllerian inhibiting substance signaling uses a bone morphogenetic protein (BMP)-like pathway mediated by ALK2 and induces SMAD6 expression. Mol Endocrinol 2001; 15:946–959.
380. Donahoe PK, Cate RL, MacLaughlin DT, et al. Müllerian inhibiting substance: gene structure and mechanism of action of a fetal regressor. Recent Prog Horm Res 1987; 43:431–467.
381. Cohen-Haguenauer O, Picard JY, Mattei MG, et al. Mapping of the gene for anti-müllerian hormone to the short arm of human chromosome 19. Cytogenet Cell Genet 1987; 44:2–6.
382. Nachtigal MW, Ingraham HA. Bioactivation of müllerian inhibiting substance during gonadal development by a kex2/subtilisinlike endoprotease. Proc Natl Acad Sci USA 1996; 93:7711–7716.
383. di Clemente N, Wilson C, Faure E, Boussin L, Carmillo P, Tizard R, Picard JY, Vigier B, Josso N, Cate R. Cloning, expression, and alternative splicing of the receptor for anti-Müllerian hormone. Mol Endocrinol 1994; 8:1006–1020.
384. Attisano L, Carcamo J, Ventura F, Weis FM, Massague J, Wrana JL. Identification of human activin and TGF beta type I receptors that form heteromeric kinase complexes with type II receptors. Cell 1993; 75:671–680.
385. Wilson JD, Lasnitzki I. Dihydrotestosterone formation in fetal tissues of rabbit and rat. Endocrinology 1971; 89:659–668.
386. Wilson JD. Testosterone uptake by the urogenital tract of the rabbit embryo. Endocrinology 1973; 92:1192–1199.
387. Neumann F, von Berswordt-Wallrabe R, Elger W, et al. Aspects of androgen-dependent events as studied by antiandrogens. Recent Prog Horm Res 1970; 26:337–410.
388. Wilson JD, Siiteri PK. Developmental pattern of testosterone synthesis in the fetal gonad of the rabbit. Endocrinology 1973; 92:1182–1191.
389. Krongrad A, Wilson JD, McPhaul MJ. Cloning and partial sequence of the rabbit androgen receptor: expression in fetal urogenital tissues. J Androl 1995; 16:209–212.
390. Cunha GR, Chung LWK, Shannon JM, et al. Stromal-epithelial interactions in sex differentiation. Biol Reprod 1980; 22:19–42.
391. Alarid ET, Rubin JS, Young P, et al. Keratinocyte growth factor functions in epithelial induction during seminal vesicle development. Proc Natl Acad Sci USA 1994; 91:1074–1078.
392. Gupta C. The role of epidermal growth factor receptor (EGFR) in male reproductive tract differentiation: stimulation of EGFR expression and inhibition of Wolffian duct differentiation with anti-EGFR antibody. Endocrinology 1996; 137:905–910.
393. Nguyen AP, Chandorkar A, Gupta C. The role of growth hormone in fetal mouse reproductive tract differentiation. Endocrinology 1996; 137:3659–3666.
394. Wilson JD, Griffin JE, George FW, et al. The role of gonadal steroids in sexual differentiation. Recent Prog Horm Res 1981; 37:1–39.
395. Haraguchi R, Suzuki K, Murakami R, et al. Molecular analysis of external genitalia formation: the role of fibroblast growth factor (Fgf) genes during genital tubercle formation. Development 2000; 127:2471–2479.
396. Baskin LS, Erol A, Li YW, Liu WH, Kurzrock E, Cunha GR. Anatomical studies of the human clitoris. J Urol 1999; 162: 1015–1020.
397. Baskin LS. Hypospadias and urethral development. J Urol 2000; 163:951–956.
398. Kim S, Liu W, Cunha GR, Russell DW, Huang H, Shapiro E, Baskin LS. Expression of the androgen receptor and 5 alpha-reductase type 2 in the developing human fetal penis and urethra. Cell Tissue Res 2002; 307:145–153.
399. Feldman KW, Smith DW. Fetal phallic growth and penile standards for newborn male infants. J Pediatr 1975; 86:395–398.
400. Oberfield SE, Mondok A, Shahrivar F, Klein JF, Levine LS. Clitoral size in full-term infants. Am J Perinatol 1989; 6:453–454.
401. Sane K, Pescovitz OH. The clitoral index: a determination of clitoral size in normal girls and in girls with abnormal sexual development. J Pediatr 1992; 120:264–266.
402. Verkauf BS, Von Thron J, O'Brien WF. Clitoral size in normal women. Obstet Gynecol 1992; 80:41–44.
403. O'Rahilly R. The development of the vagina in the human. Birth Defects 1977; 13:123.
404. Forsberg JG. Origin of vaginal epithelium. Obstet Gynecol 1965; 25:787–791.
405. Cunha GR. The dual origin of vaginal epithelium. Am J Anat 1975; 143:387–392.
406. Shapiro E, Huang HY, Wu XR. Uroplakin and androgen receptor expression in the human fetal genital tract: insights into the development of the vagina. J Urol 2000; 164:1048–1051.
407. Tsai MJ, O'Malley BW. Molecular mechanisms of action of

steroid/thyroid receptor superfamily members. Ann Rev Biochem 1994; 63:451–486.
408. Griffin JE, McPhaul MJ, Russell DW, Wilson JD. The androgen resistance syndromes: steroid 5α-reductase 2 deficiency, testicular feminization, and related disorders. In: Scriver CR, Beaudet AL, Sly WS, et al, eds. The Metabolic and Molecular Basis of Inherited Disease. 8th ed. New York: McGraw Hill, 2001: 4117–4146.
409. O'Malley B. The steroid receptor superfamily: more excitement predicted in the future. Mol Endocrinol 1990; 4:363–369.
410. Liao S, Konkontis J, Tetsujun S, et al. Androgen receptors: structures, mutations, antibodies and cellular dynamics. J Steroid Biochem 1989; 34:41–51.
411. Kuiper GGJM, Brinkman AO. Phosphotryptic peptide analysis of the human androgen receptor: deletion of a hormone induced phosphopeptide. Biochemistry 1995; 34:1851–1857.
412. Chamberlain NL, Driver ED, Miesfeld RL. The length and location of CAG trinucleotide repeats in the androgen receptor N-terminal domain affect transactivation function. Nucleic Acids Res 1994; 22:3181–3186.
413. McEwan IJ. Structural and functional alterations in the androgen receptor in spinal bulbar muscular atrophy. Biochem Soc Trans 2001; 29:222–227.
414. McKenna NJ, Lanz RB, O'Malley BW. Nuclear receptor coregulators: cellular and molecular biology. Endocr Rev 1999; 20: 321–344.
415. Robyr D, Wolffe AP, Wahli W. Nuclear hormone receptor coregulators in action: diversity for shared tasks. Mol Endocrinol 2000 14: 329–347.
416. McKenna NJ, O'Malley BW. Combinatorial control of gene expression by nuclear receptors and coregulators. Cell 2002; 108:465–74.
417. Heinlein CA, Chang C. Androgen receptor (AR) coregulators: an overview. Endocr Rev 2002; 23:175–200.
418. Yeh S, Chang C. Cloning and characterization of a specific coactivator, ARA70, for the androgen receptor in human prostate cells. Proc Natl Acad Sci USA 1996; 93:5517–5521.
419. Moras D, Gronemeyer H. The nuclear receptor ligand-binding domain: structure and function. Curr Opin Cell Biol 1998; 10: 384–391.
420. Poujol N, Wurtz JM, Tahiri B, et al. Specific recognition of androgens by their nuclear receptor. A structure-function study. J Biol Chem 2000; 275:24022–24031.
421. Sack JS, Kish KF, Wang C, et al. Crystallographic structures of the ligand-binding domains of the androgen receptor and its T877A mutant complexed with the natural agonist dihydrotestosterone. Proc Natl Acad Sci USA 2001; 98:4904–4909.
422. Rennie PS, Bruchovsky N, Leco KJ, Sheppard PC, McQueen SA, Cheng H, Snoek R, Hamel A, Bock ME, MacDonald BS, et al. Characterization of two cis-acting DNA elements involved in the androgen regulation of the probasin gene. Mol Endocrinol 1993; 7:23–36.
423. Grumbach MM, Ducharme JR. The effects of androgens on fetal sexual development: androgen-induced female pseudohermaphrodism. Fertil Steril 1960; 11:157–180.
424. Grumbach MM, Kaplan SL. The neuroendocrinology of human puberty: an ontogenic perspective. In: Grumbach MM, Sizonenko PC, Aubert ML, eds. Control of the Onset of Puberty. Baltimore: Williams & Wilkins, 1990: 1B68.
425. Pfeiffer CA. Sexual differences of the hypophyses and their determination by the gonads. Am J Anat 1936; 58:195–225.
426. Harris GW. Sex hormones, brain development and brain function. Endocrinology 1964; 75:627–648.
427. Gorski RA, Jacobson CD. Sexual differentiation of the brain. In: Kogan SJ, Hafez ESE, eds. Pediatric Andrology. The Hague: Martinus Nijhoff, 1981: 109–134.
428. Gorski RA. Sexual differentiation of the endocrine brain and its control. In: Motta M, ed. Brain Endocrinology. 2nd ed. New York: Raven Press, 1991: 71–104.
429. Raisman G, Field PM. Sexual dimorphism in the neuropil of the preoptic area of the rat and its dependence on neonatal androgen. Brain Res 1973; 54:1–29.
430. Reiter EO, Grumbach MM, Kaplan SL, et al. The response of pituitary gonadotropins to synthetic LRF in children with glucocorticoid-treated congenital adrenal hyperplasia. J Clin Endocrinol Metab 1975; 40:318–325.
431. Gorski RA. Gonadal hormones and the organization of brain structure and function. In: Magnusson D, ed. The Lifespan Development of Individuals—Behavioral, Neurobiological, and Psychosocial Perspectives. Cambridge: Cambridge University Press, 1996: 315–340.
432. Goy RW, McEwen BS. Sexual Differentiation of the Brain. Cambridge, MA: MIT Press, 1980.
433. Bleier R, Byne W, Siggelkow I. Cytoarchitectonic sexual dimorphisms of the medial preoptic and anterior hypothalamic areas in guinea pig, rat, hamster, and mouse. J Comp Neurol 1982; 212:118–130.
434. Breedlove SM. Sexual dimorphism in the vertebrate nervous system. J Neurosci 1992; 12:4133–4142.
435. Madeira MD, Lieberman AR. Sexual dimorphism in the mammalian limbic system. Prog Neurobiol 1995; 45:275–333.
436. Madeira MD, Leal S, Paula-Barbosa MM. Stereological evaluation and Golgi study of the sexual dimorphisms in the volume, cell numbers, and cell size in the medial preoptic nucleus of the rat. J Neurocytol 1999; 28:131–148.
437. Lisciotto CA, Morrell JI. Sex differences in the distribution and projections of testosterone target neurons in the medial preoptic area and the bed nucleus of the stria terminalis of rats. Horm Behav 1994; 28:492–502.
438. Leal S, Andrade JP, Paula-Barbosa MM, Madeira MD. Arcuate nucleus of the hypothalamus: Effects of age and sex. J Comp Neurol 1998; 401:65–88.
439. Matsumoto A, Sekine Y, Murakami S, Arai Y. Sexual differentiation of neuronal circuitry in the hypothalamus. In: Matsumoto A, ed. Sexual Differentiation of the Brain. New York: CRC, 2000:203–227.
440. Simerly RB. Organization and regulation of sexually dimorphic neuroendocrine pathways. Behav Brain Res 1998; 92:195–203.
441. Allen LS, Hines M, Shryne JE, Gorski RA. Two sexually dimorphic cell groups in the human brain. J Neurosci 1989; 9: 497–506.
442. Allen LS, Gorski RA. Sexual dimorphism of the anterior commissure and massa intermedia of the human brain. J Comp Neurol 1991; 312:97–104.
443. Swaab DF, Fliers E. A sexually dimorphic nucleus in the human brain. Science 1985; 228:1112–1115.
444. Giedd JN, Castellanos FX, Rajapakse JC, et al. Sexual dimorphism of the developing human brain. Prog Neuropsychopharmacol Biol Psychiatry 1997; 21:1185–1201.
445. Hofman MA, Swaab DF. The sexually dimorphic nucleus of the preoptic area in the human brain: A comparative morphometric study. J Anat 1989; 164:55–72.
446. Voigt J, Pakkenberg H. Brain weight of Danish children. A forensic material. Acta Anat (Basel) 1983; 116:290–301.
447. de Lacoste MC, Holloway RL, Woodward DJ. Sex differences in the fetal human corpus callosum. Hum Neurobiol 1986; 5: 93–96.
448. Pakkenberg B, Gundersen HJ. Neocortical neuron number in humans: Effect of sex and age. J Comp Neurol 1997; 384:312–320.
449. Hofman MA, Fliers E, Goudsmit E, Swaab DF. Morphometric analysis of the suprachiasmatic and paraventricular nuclei in the human brain: Sex differences and age-dependent changes. J Anat 1988; 160:127–143.
450. Pfaff DW, Arnold AP, Etgen Am, Fahrbach SE, Rubin RT, eds. Hormones, Brain, and Behavior. San Diego: Academic Press, 2002. [A 5-volume comprehensive compendium of the state-of-the-art across species lines that includes reviews of research in human and non-human primates.]
451. Sizonenko PC, Schindler AM, Kohlberg IJ, et al. Gonadotrophins, testosterone and oestrogen levels in relation to ovarian morphology in 11-hydroxylase deficiency. Acta Endocrinol 1972; 71:539–550.
452. Karsch FJ, Dierschke DJ, Knobil E. Sexual differentiation of pituitary function: apparent difference between primates and rodents. Science 1973; 179:484–486.
453. Barbarino A, De Marinis L, Lafuentl G, et al. Presence of positive feedback between oestrogen and LH in patients with Klinefelter's syndrome, and Sertoli cellonly syndrome. Clin Endocrinol 1979; 10:235–242.
454. Hofman MA, Swaab DF. Sexual dimorphism of the human brain: myth and reality. Exp Clin Endocrinol 1991; 98:161–170.
455. Swaab DF, Hofman MA. Sexual differentiation of the human

hypothalamus in relation to gender and sexual orientation. Trends Neurosci 1995; 18:264–270.
456. Pilgrim C, Hutchison JB. Developmental regulation of sex differences in the brain: can the role of gonadal steroids be redefined? Neuroscience 1994; 60:843–855.
457. Mayer A, Lahr G, Swaab DF, Pilgrim C, Reisert I. The Y-chromosomal genes SRY and ZFY are transcribed in adult human brain. Neurogenetics 1998; 1:281–288.
458. Swaab DF, Chung WC, Kruijver FP, Hofman MA, Ishunina TA. Structural and functional sex differences in the human hypothalamus. Horm Behav 2001; 40:93–98.
459. Xu J, Qiu Y, DeMayo FJ, Tsai SY, Tsai MJ, O'Malley BW. Partial hormone resistance in mice with disruption of the steroid receptor coactivator-1 (SRC-1) gene. Science 1998; 279: 1922–1925.
460. Phoenix CH, Goy RW, Gerall AA, Young WC. Organizing action of prenatally administered testosterone proprionate on the tissues mediating mating behavior in the female guinea pig. Endocrinology 1959; 65:369–382.
461. Zucker KJ. Intersexuality and gender identity differentiation. Annu Rev Sex Res 1999; 10:1–69.
462. Money J. Sex Errors of the Body and Related Syndromes: A Guide to Counseling Children, Adolescents and Their Families. 2nd ed. Baltimore: Paul H Brookes, 1994.
463. Stoller RJ. A further contribution to the study of gender identity. Int J Psychoanal 1968; 49:364–369.
464. Ehrhardt AA, Meyer-Bahlburg HFL. Effects of prenatal sex hormones on gender-related behavior. Science 1981; 211:1312–1318.
465. Pardridge WM, Gorski RA, Lippe BM, et al. Androgens and sexual behavior. Ann Intern Med 1982; 96:488–501.
466. MacLusky NJ, Naftolin F. Sexual differentiation of the central nervous system. Science 1981; 211:1294–1303.
467. Diamond M. A critical evaluation of the ontogeny of human sexual behavior. Q Rev Biol 1965; 40:147–175.
468. Cooke B, Hegstrom CD, Villeneuve LS, Breedlove SM. Sexual differentiation of the vertebrate brain: principles and mechanisms. Front Neuroendocrinol 1998; 19:323–362.
469. McEwen BS. Permanence of brain sex differences and structural plasticity of the adult brain. Proc Natl Acad Sci USA 1999 Jun 22; 96:7128–7130.
470. MacLusky NJ, Naftolin F. Sexual differentiation of the central nervous system. Science 1981; 211:1294–1303.
471. McEwen BS. Neural gonadal steroid actions. Science 1981; 211: 1303–1311.
472. Olsen KL. Androgen-insensitive rats are defeminized by their testes. Nature 1979; 279:238–239.
473. Zhou JN, Hofman MA, Gooren LJ, et al. A sex difference in the human brain and its relation to transsexuality. Nature 1995; 378: 68–70.
474. Kruijver FPM, Zhou J-N, Pool CW, et al. Male-to-female transsexuals have female neuron numbers in a limbic nucleus. J Clin Endocrinol Metab 2001; 85:2034–2041.
475. Vega-Matuszczyk JV, Larsson K. Sexual preference and feminine and masculine sexual behavior of male rats prenatally exposed to anti-androgen or anti-estrogen. Horm Behav 1995; 29: 191–206.
476. Geschwind N, Galaburda AM. Cerebral lateralization: biological mechanisms, association and pathology. II. A hypothesis and a program for research. Arch Neurol 1985; 42:521–522.
477. Nass R, Baker S, Speiser P, et al. Hormones and handedness: left handed bias in female congenital adrenal hyperplasia patients. Neurology 1987; 37:711–715.
478. Wisniewski AB. Sexually-dimorphic patterns of cortical asymmetry, and the role for sex steroid hormones in determining cortical patterns of lateralization. Psychoneuroendocrinology 1998; 23:519–547.
479. Berenbaum SA, Duck SC, Bryk K. Behavioral effects of prenatal versus postnatal androgen excess in children with 21-hydroxylase-deficient congenital adrenal hyperplasia. J Clin Endocrinol Metab 2000; 85:727–733.
480. Berenbaum SA. Cognitive function in congenital adrenal hyperplasia. Endocrinol Metab Clin North Am 2001; 30:173–192.
481. Meyer-Bahlburg HFL. Hormones and psychosexual differentiation: implications for the management of intersexuality, homosexuality and transsexuality. Clin Endocrinol Metab 1982; 11: 681–701.
482. Meyer-Bahlburg HL. Gender and sexuality in classic congenital adrenal hyperplasia. Endocrinol Metab Clin North Am 2001; 30:155–172.
483. Wilson JD. The role of androgens in male gender role behavior. Endocr Rev 1999; 20:726–737.
484. Wilson JD. Androgens, androgen receptors, and male gender role behavior. Horm Behav 2001; 40:358–366.
485. Berenbaum SA. How hormones affect behavioral and neural development. Developmental Neuropsychology 1998; 14:175–196.
486. Money J, Ehrhardt AA. Man and Woman, Boy and Girl: The Differentiation and Dimorphism of Gender Identity from Conception to Maturity. Baltimore: Johns Hopkins University Press, 1972.
487. Diamond M, Sigmundson K. Sex reassignment at birth. Arch Pediatr Adol Med 1997; 151:248–304.
488. Reiner W. Outcomes in gender assignment: cloacal exstrophy. In Grumbach M, Chair: "Neonatal Management of Genital Ambiguity." Symposium presented at Annual Meeting of the Lawson Wilkins Pediatric Endocrine Society, Boston, May 2000.
489. Colapinto J. As Nature Made Him: The Boy Who Was Raised As A Girl. New York: Harper Collins, 2000. [See also Colapinto J. The true story of John/Joan. Rolling Stone 1997 (December 11):54–73, 92–96.]
490. Bradley SJ, Oliver GD, Chernick AB. Zucker KJ. Experiment of nurture: Ablatio penis at 2 months, sex reassignment at 7 months, and a psychosexual follow-up in young adulthood. Pediatrics 1998; 102(1):e9.
491. Money J, Hampson JG, Hampson JL. An examination of some basic sexual concepts: The evidence of human hermaphroditism. Johns Hopkins Med J 1955; 97:301–319.
492. Imperato-McGinley JL, Peterson RE, Gautier T et al. Androgens and the evolution of male-gender identity among male pseudohermaphrodites with 5α-reductase deficiency. N Engl J Med 1979; 300:1233–1237.
493. Money J, Hampson JG, Hampson JL. Hermaphroditism: Recommendations concerning assignment of sex, change of sex, and psychologic management. Johns Hopkins Med J 1955; 97:284–300.
494. Ehrhardt AA, Meyer-Bahlburg HFL. Effects of prenatal sex hormones on gender-related behavior. Science 1981; 211:1312–1318.
495. Ehrhardt AA, Epstein R, Money J. Fetal androgens and female gender identity in the early-treated adrenogenital syndrome. Johns Hopkins Med J 1968; 122:160–167.
496. Simerly RB. Wires for reproduction: Organization and development of sexually dimorphic circuits in the mammalian forebrain. Annu Rev Neurosci 2002; 25:507–536.
497. Herdt GH, Davidson J. The Sambia "Turnim-Man": Sociocultural and clinical aspects of gender formation in male pseudohermaphrodites with 5-alpha-reductase deficiency in Papua, New Guinea. Arch Sex Behav 1988; 17:33–56.
497a. Gajdusek DC. Urgent opportunistic observations. The study of changing, transient and disappearing phenomena of medical interest in disrupted human communities. In: Health and Disease in Tribal Societies, CIBA Symposium 49 (New Series). Amsterdam: Elsevier/Excerpta Medica, 1997:89–94.
498. Wallen K. Nature needs nurture: the interaction of hormonal and social influences on the development of behavioral sex differences in rhesus monkeys. Horm Behav 1996; 30:364–378.
499. Money J. Determinants of human gender identity/role. In: Money J, Musaph H, eds. Handbook of Sexology. Amsterdam: Elsevier, 1977:57–79.
500. Money J, Schwartz M, Lewis VG. Adult erotosexual status and fetal hormonal masculinization and demasculinization: 46,XX congenital virilizing adrenal hyperplasia and 46,XY androgeninsensitivity compared. Psychoneuroendocrinology 1984; 9:405–414.
501. Dittmann RW, Kappes ME, Kappes MH. Sexual behavior in adolescent and adult females with congenital adrenal hyperplasia. Psychoneuroendocrinology 1992; 17:153–170.
502. Kuhnle U, Bullinger M, Schwarz HP. The quality of life in adult female patients with congenital adrenal hyperplasia: A comprehensive study of the impact of genital malformations and chronic disease on female patients' life. Eur J Pediatr 1995; 154: 708–716.

503. Meyer-Bahlburg HL. What causes low rates of childbearing in congenital adrenal hyperplasia? J Clin Endocrinol Metab 1999; 84:1844–1847.
504. Money J, Hampson JG, Hampson JL. Imprinting and the establishment of gender role. Arch Neurol Psych 1957; 77:333–336.
505. Zucker KJ, Bradley SJ, Oliver G, Blake J, Fleming S, Hood J. Psychosexual development of women with congenital adrenal hyperplasia. Horm Behav 1996; 30:300–318.
506. Baskin L. Hypospadias: a critical analysis of cosmetic outcomes using photography. BJU Int 2001; 87:534–539.
507. Schnitzer JJ, Donahoe PK. Surgical treatment of congenital adrenal hyperplasia. Endocrinol Metab Clin North Am 2001; 30: 137–154.
508. Rink RC, Adams MC. Feminizing genitoplasty: state of the art. World J Urol 1998; 16:212–218.
509. Klinefelter HF Jr, Reifenstein EC Jr, Albright F. Syndrome characterized by gynecomastia, aspermatogenesis without a Leydigism and increased excretion of follicle-stimulating hormone. J Clin Endocrinol 1942; 2:615–627.
510. Jacobs PA, Strong JA. A case of human intersexuality having a possible XXY sex-determining mechanism. Nature 1959; 83: 302–303.
511. Ford CE, Jones KW, Miller OH, et al. The chromosomes in a patient showing both mongolism and the Klinefelter syndrome. Lancet 1959; 1:709–710.
512. Hsueh WA, Hsu TH, Federman DD. Endocrine features of Klinefelter's syndrome. Medicine (Baltimore) 1978; 57:447–461.
513. Leonard JM, Paulsen CA, Ospina LF, et al. The classification of Klinefelter's syndrome. In: Vallet HL, Porter IH, eds. Genetic Mechanisms of Sexual Development. New York: Academic Press, 1978:407–423.
514. Robinson A, Lubs HA, Bergsma D. Summary of clinical findings: profiles of children with 47,XXY, 47,XXX and 47,XYY karyotypes. Birth Defects 1979; 15:261–281.
515. Amory JK, Anawalt BD, Paulsen CA, Bremner WJ. Klinefelter's syndrome. Lancet 2000; 356:333–335.
516. Mandokim W, Gavla SS, Hofman RP, et al. A review of Klinefelter syndrome in children and adolescents. J Am Acad Child Adolesc Psychiatry 1991; 30:167B172.
517. Ratcliffe SG, Bancroft J, Axworthy D, et al. Klinefelter's syndrome in adolescence. Arch Dis Child 1982; 57:6–12.
518. Schwartz ID, Root AW. The Klinefelter syndrome of testicular dysgenesis. Endocrinol Metabol Clin North Am 1991; 20:153–163.
519. Stewart DA, Netley CT, Park E. Summary of clinical findings of children with 47,XXY, 47,XYY and 47,XXX karyotypes. Birth Defects 1982; 18:1–5.
520. Robinson A, Bender BG, Linden MG. Summary of clinical findings in children and young adults with sex chromosome anomalies. In: Evans JA, Hamerton JL, Robinson A, eds. Birth Defect Original Article Series. Vol 26. New York: Wiley-Liss, 1991; 26:225–228.
521. Graham JM Jr, Bashir AS, Stark RE, et al. Oral and written language abilities of XXY boys: implications for anticipatory guidance. Pediatrics 1988; 81:795–806.
522. Bender B, Harmon RJ, Linden MG, Robinson A. Psychosocial adaptation of 39 adolescents with sex chromosome abnormalities. Pediatrics 1995; 96:302–308.
523. Geschwind DH, Boone KB, Miller BL, Swerdloff RS. Neurobehavioral phenotype of Klinefelter syndrome. Ment Retard Dev Disabil Res Rev 2000; 6:107–116.
524. Nielsen J, Pelsen B. Followup 20 years later of 34 Klinefelter males with karyotype 47,XXY and 16 hypogonadal males with karyotype 46,XY. Hum Genet 1987; 77:188–192.
525. Schibler D, Brook CGD, Kind HP, et al. Growth and body proportions in 54 boys and men with Klinefelter's syndrome. Helv Paediatr Acta 1974; 29:325–333.
526. Illig R, Tolkdorf M, Murset G, et al. LH and FSH responses to synthetic LHRH in children and adolescents with Turner's and Klinefelter's syndrome. Helv Paediatr Acta 1975; 30:221–231.
527. Ratcliffe SG. The sexual development of boys with the chromosome constitution 47,XXY (Klinefelter's syndrome). Clin Endocrinol Metab 1982; 11:703–716.
528. Salenblatt JA, Bender BG, Puck MH, et al. Pituitary-gonadal function in Klinefelter syndrome before and during puberty. Pediatr Res 1985; 19:82–86.
529. Sorenson K. Klinefelter's Syndrome in Childhood, Adolescence and Youth: A Genetic, Clinical, Developmental, Psychiatric and Psychological Study. Lancaster, UK: Parthenon, 1988.
530. Smals AHG, Kloppenberg WC, Bernard TJ. Effect of short and long term human chorionic gonadotropin (hCG) administration on plasma testosterone levels in Klinefelter's syndrome. Acta Endocrinol 1974; 77:753–764.
531. Wang C, Baker HWG, Burger HG, et al. Hormonal studies in Klinefelter syndrome. Clin Endocrinol 1975; 4:399–411.
532. Smals AHG, Kloppenborg PWC, Lequin RL, et al. The pituitary-thyroid axis in Klinefelter's syndrome. Acta Endocrinol 1977; 84:72–79.
533. Nielsen J. Diabetes mellitus in patients with aneuploid chromosome aberrations and in their parents. Humangenetik 1972; 16: 165–170.
534. Geffner ME, Kaplan SA, Bersche N, et al. Insulin resistance in Klinefelter syndrome. J Pediatr Endocrinol 1987; 2:173–177.
535. Harnden DG, Maclean N, Langlands AO. Carcinoma of the breast and Klinefelter's syndrome. J Med Genet 1971; 8:460–461.
536. Hultborn R, Hanson C, Kopf I, et al. Prevalence of Klinefelter's syndrome in male breast cancer patients. Anticancer Res 1997; 17:4293–4297.
537. Sanchez AG, Villanueva AG, Redoudo C. Lobular carcinoma of the breast in a patient with Klinefelter syndrome: a case with bilateral, synchronous, histologically different breast tumors. Cancer 1986; 57:1180–1183.
538. Hasle H, Mellemgaard A, Nielsen J, et al. Cancer incidence in men with Klinefelter syndrome. Br J Cancer 1995; 71:416–420.
539. Chaussain JL, Lemerle J, Roger M, et al. Klinefelter syndrome, tumor and sexual precocity. J Pediatr 1980; 97:607–609.
540. Nichols CR, Heerema NA, Palmer C, et al. Klinefelter syndrome associated with mediastinal germ cell neoplasms. J Clin Oncol 1987; 5:1290–1294.
541. Derenoncourt AN, Castro-Magana M, Jones KL. Mediastinal teratoma and precocious puberty in a boy with mosaic Klinefelter syndrome. Am J Med Genet 1995; 55:38–42.
542. Schneider DT, Schuster AE, Fritsch MK, et al. Genetic analysis of mediastinal nonseminomatous germ cell tumors in children and adolescents. Genes Chromosomes Cancer 2002; 34:115–125.
543. Horowitz M, Wishart JM, O'Loughlin PD, et al. Osteoporosis and Klinefelter's syndrome. Clin Endocrinol 1992; 36:113–118.
544. Uehara S, Tamura M, Nata M, Kanetake J, Hashiyada M, Terada Y, Yaegashi N, Funato T, Yajima A. Complete androgen insensitivity in a 47,XXY patient with uniparental disomy for the X chromosome. Am J Med Genet 1999; 86:107–111.
545. Kenwrick S; The International IP Consortium. Survival of male patients with incontinentia pigmenti carrying a lethal mutation can be explained by somatic mosaicism or Klinefelter syndrome. Am J Hum Genet 2001; 69:1210–1217.
546. Rauch A, Pfeiffer RA, Trautmann U, et al. A study of ten small supernumerary (marker) chromosomes identified by fluorescence in situ hybridization (FISH). Clin Genet 1992; 42:84–90.
547. Hook EB, Hamerton JG. The frequency of chromosome abnormalities detected in consecutive newborn studies: difference between studies. Results by sex and severity of phenotypic involvement. In: Hook EB, Porter IH, eds. Population Cytogenetics Studies in Humans. New York: Academic Press 1977: 63–79.
548. Rutgers JL, Scully RE. Pathology of the testis in intersex syndromes. Semin Diagn Pathol 1987; 4:275–291.
549. Grumbach MM, Blanc WA, Engle ET. Sex chromatin pattern in seminiferous tubule dysgenesis and other testicular disorders: relationship to true hermaphrodism and to Klinefelter's syndrome. J Clin Endocrinol Metab 1957; 17:703–736.
550. Fryns JP, Moerman PL, Kleczkowska A. Normal testicular histology in a midtrimester 49,XXXXY fetus. Clin Genet 1995; 47: 331 (letter).
551. Citoler P, Aechter J. Histology of testis in XXY fetuses. In: Murken JD, Stengel-Rutkowski S, Schwinger E, eds. Prenatal Diagnosis: Proceedings of the 3rd European Conference on Prenatal Diagnosis of Genetic Disorders. Stuttgart: Ferdinand Enke, 1979: 336–337.
552. Mikano K, Aguercif M, Hazeghi P, et al. Chromatin-positive Klinefelter syndrome. Fertil Steril 1968; 19:731–739.
553. Ferguson-Smith MA. The prepubertal testicular lesions in chro-

matin positive Klinefelter's syndrome (primarily microorchidism) as seen in mentally handicapped children. Lancet 1959; 1:219–222.

554. Ohno S. Control of meiotic processes. In: Troen P, Nankin HR, eds. The Testis in Normal and Infertile Men. New York: Raven Press, 1977: 1–33.
555. Ahmad KN, Dykes JRW, Ferguson-Smith MA, et al. Leydig cell volume in chromatin positive Klinefelter's syndrome. J Clin Endocrinol Metab 1971; 33:517–520.
556. Cozzi J, Chevret S, Rousseaux S, et al. Achievement of meiosis in XXY germ cells: study of 543 sperm karyotypes from an XY/XXY mosaic patient. Hum Genet 1994; 93:32–34.
557. Ron-El R, Strassberger D, Gelman-Kohan S, et al. A 47,XXY fetus conceived after ICSI of spermatozoa from a patient with non-mosaic Klinefelter's syndrome: case report. Hum Reprod 2000; 15:1804–1806.
558. Nordas F, De Vincentiis S, Olmedo, et al. Birth of twin males with normal karyotpye after intracytoplasmic sperm injection with use of testicular spermatozoa from a nonmosaic patient with Klinefelter's syndrome. Fertil Steril 1999; 71:1149–1152.
559. Hennebicq S, Pelletier R, Bergues U, et al. Risk of trisomy 21 in offspring of patients with Klinefelter's syndrome. Lancet 2001; 357:2104–2105.
560. Rosenkranz VW. Klinefelter Syndrom bei Kindern von Frauen mit Geschlechtschromosomen Anomalien. Helv Paediatr Acta 1965; 20:359–368.
561. Jacobs PA, Hassold TJ, Whittington E, et al. Klinefelter's syndrome: an analysis of the origin of the additional sex chromosome using molecular probes. Ann Hum Genet 1988; 52:147–151.
562. Ferguson-Smith MA, Mack WS, Ellis PM, et al. Parental age and the source of the X chromosomes in XXY Klinefelter's syndrome. Lancet 1964; 1:46.
563. Carothers AD, Filippi G. Klinefelter's syndrome in Sardinia and Scotland: comparative studies of parenteral age and other aetiological factors in 47,XXY. Hum Genet 1988; 81:71–75.
564. Griffin DK, Abruzzo MA, Millie EA, et al. Nondisjunction in human sperm: evidence for an effect of increasing paternal age. Hum Mol Genet 1995; 4:2227–2232.
565. Lowe X, Eskenazi B, Nelson DO, Kidd S, Alme A, Wyrobek AJ. Frequency of XY sperm increases with age in fathers of boys with Klinefelter syndrome. Am J Hum Genet 2001; 69:1046–1054.
565a. Röttger S, Schiebel K, Senger G, et al. An SRY-negative 47,XXY mother and daughter. Cytogenet Cell Genet 2000; 91: 204–207.
566. Van Dop C, Burstein S, Conte FA, et al. Isolated gonadotropin deficiency in boys: clinical characteristics and growth. J Pediatr 1987; 111:684–692.
567. Zizka J, Balicek P. XXYY son of a triple X mother. Humangenetik 1975; 26:159–160.
568. Jones KL. Smith's Recognizable Patterns of Human Malformation. 5th ed. Philadelphia: WB Saunders, 1997.
569. Linden MG, Bender BG, Robinson A. Sex chromosome tetrasomy and pentasomy. Pediatrics 1995; 96:672–682.
570. Fraccaro M, Kaljser K, Lindsten J. A child with 49 chromosomes. Lancet 1960; 2:899–902.
571. Curts LM, Scheppers-Tijdink G, Wiegers A, et al. The 49,XXXXY syndrome: clinical and psychological findings in five patients. J Intellect Disabil Res 1990; 34:277–282.
572. Borghgraeff M, Fryns JP, Smeets E, et al. The 49,XXXXY syndrome: clinical and psychologic followup data. Clin Genet 1988; 33:429–434.
573. Sarto GE, Otto PG, Kuhn EM, et al. What causes the abnormal phenotype in a 49,XXXXY male? Hum Genet 1987; 76:1–4.
574. Leal CA, Belmont JW, Nachtman R, et al. Parental origin of the extra chromosomes in polysomy X. Hum Genet 1994; 94: 423–426.
575. de la Chapelle A. The etiology of maleness in XX men. Hum Genet 1981; 58:105–116.
576. Perez-Palacios G, Medina M, Ullao-Aguirre, et al. Gonadotropin dynamics in XX males. J Clin Endocrinol Metab 1981; 53: 254–257.
577. Boucekkine C, Toublanc JE, Abbas N, et al. Clinical and anatomical spectrum in XX sex reversed patients: relationship to the presence of Y specific DNA sequences. Clin Endocrinol 1994; 40:733–742.
578. Ferguson-Smith MA, Cooke A, Affara NA, et al. Genotype-phenotype correlations in XX males and their bearing on current theories of sex determination. Hum Genet 1990; 84:198–202.
579. Ferguson-Smith MA, Affara NA. Accidental XY recombination and the aetiology of XX males and true hermaphroditism. Philos Trans R Soc Lond B Biol Sci 1988; 322:133–144.
580. Miro R, Cabellin MR, Marsini S, et al. Mosaicism in XX males. Hum Genet 1978; 45:103–106.
581. Ferguson-Smith MA. XY chromosomal interchange in the aetiology of true hermaphroditism and XX Klinefelter's syndrome. Lancet 1966; 2:475–476.
582. de la Chapelle A, Koo GC, Wachtel SS. Recessive sex-determining genes in human XX male syndrome. Cell 1978; 15:837–842.
583. de la Chapelle A, Tippett PA, Wetterstrand G, et al. Genetic evidence of XY interchange in a human XX male. Nature 1984; 307:170–171.
584. Evans HJ, Buckton KE, Spowart G, et al. Heteromorphic X chromosomes in 46,XX males: evidence for the involvement of XY interchange. Hum Genet 1979; 49:11–31.
585. Magenis RE, Casanova M, Fellous M, et al. Further cytologic evidence of XpYp translocation in XX males using in situ hybridization with Y derived probe. Hum Genet 1987; 75:228–233.
586. Guellaen G, Casanova M, Bishop C, et al. Human XX males with Y single-copy DNA fragments. Nature 1984; 307:172–173.
587. Muller U, La Lande M, Donlon T, et al. Moderately repeated sequences for the short arm of the human Y chromosome are present in XX males and reduced in copy number in an XY female. Nucleic Acids Res 1986; 14:1325–1340.
588. Affara NA, Ferguson-Smith MA, Tolmie J, et al. Variable transfer of Y specific sequences in XX males. Nucleic Acids Res 1986; 14:5375–5387.
589. Andersson M, Page DC, de la Chapelle A. Chromosome Y-specific DNA is transferred to the short arm of X chromosome in human XX males. Science 1986; 223:786–788.
590. Buckle VJ, Boyd Y, Fraser N, et al. Localization of Y chromosome sequences in normal and XX males. J Med Genet 1987; 24:197–203.
591. Petit C, de la Chapelle A, Levilliers J, et al. An abnormal XY interchange accounts for most but not all cases of human XX maleness. Cell 1987; 49:595–602.
592. Rouyer F, Simmler MC, Page DC, et al. A sex chromosome rearrangement in a human XX male caused by AluAlu recombination. Cell 1987; 51:417–425.
593. Muller U, Latt SA, Donlon T. Y specific DNA sequences in male patients with 46,XX and 47,XXX karyotypes. Am J Med Genet 1987; 28:393–401.
594. Stalvey JRD, Durbin EJ, Erickson RP. Sex vesicle "entrapment": translocation or nonhomologous recombination of misaligned Yp and Xp as alternative mechanisms for abnormal inheritance of the sex-determining region. Am J Med Genet 1989; 32:564–572.
595. Disteche CM, Casanova M, Saal M, et al. Small deletions of the short arm of the Y chromosome in 46,XY females. Proc Natl Acad Sci USA 1986; 83:7841–7844.
596. Page DC, Fisher EMC, McGillivray B, et al. Additional deletion in sex determining region of human Y chromosome resolves paradox of X,t(Y:22) female. Nature 1990; 346:279–281.
597. Weil D, Wang I, Dietrich A, et al. Highly homologous loci on the X and Y chromosomes are hotspots for ectopic recombinations leading to XX maleness. Nat Genet 1994; 7:414–419.
598. Schiebel K, Winkelmann M, Mertz A, Xu X, Page DC, Weil D, Petit C, Rappold GA. Abnormal XY interchange between a novel isolated protein kinase gene, PRKY, and its homologue, PRKX, accounts for one third of all (Y+)XX males and (Y−)XY females. Hum Mol Genet 1997; 6:1985–1989.
599. Turner B, Fechner PY, Fuqua JS, et al. Combined Leydig cell and Sertoli cell dysfunction in 46,XX males lacking the sex determining region Y gene. Am J Med Genet 1995; 57:440–443.
600. Skordis NA, Stetka DG, MacGillivray MH, et al. Familial 46,XX males coexisting with familial 46,XX true hermaphrodites in same pedigree. J Pediatr 1987; 110:224–248.

601. Pereira ET, Cabral de Almeida JC, Gunha A, et al. Use of probes for ZFY, SRY, and the Y pseudoautosomal boundary in XX males, XX true hermaphrodites and an XY female. J Med Genet 1991; 28:591–595.
602. Kuhnle U, Schwarz HP, Lōrs U, et al. Familial true hermaphroditism: paternal and maternal transmission of true hermaphroditism (46,XX) and XX maleness in the absence of Ychromosomal sequences. Hum Genet 1993; 92:571–576.
603. Ramos ES, Moreira-Filho CA, Vicente YA, Llorach-Velludo MA, Tucci S Jr, Duarte MH, Araujo AG, Martelli L. SRY-negative true hermaphrodites and an XX male in two generations of the same family. Hum Genet 1996 May;97(5):596–598.
604. Sarafoglou K, Ostrer H. Familial sex reversal: a review. J Clin Endocrinol Metab 2000; 85:483–493.
605. Engel E, Forbes AP. Cytogenetic and clinical findings in 48 patients with congenitally defective or absent ovaries. Medicine (Baltimore) 1965; 44:135–165.
606. Hall JG, Sybert VP, Williamson RA, et al. Turner's syndrome. West J Med 1982; 137:32–44.
607. Palmer CG, Reichman A. Chromosomal and clinical findings in 110 females with Turner syndrome. Hum Genet 1976; 35:35–49.
608. Rosenfeld R, Grumbach MM, eds. Turner Syndrome. New York: Marcel Dekker, 1990.
609. Hibi I, Takano K. Basic and Clinical Approach to Turner Syndrome. Amsterdam: Elsevier Science Publishers BV, 1993.
610. Lippe BM. Turner syndrome. In: Sperling M, ed. Pediatric Endocrinology. Philadelphia: WB Saunders, 1996: 384–421.
611. Albertsson-Wikland K, Ranke MB (eds). Turner Syndrome in a Life Span Perspective: Research and Clinical Aspects. Amsterdam: Elsevier Science BV, 1995.
612. Saenger P, Pasquino AM, eds. Optimizing Health Care for Turner Patients in the 21st Century. Amsterdam: Elsevier, 2000.
613. Elsheikh M, Dunger DB, Conway GS, Wass JA. Turner's syndrome in adulthood. Endocr Rev 2002; 23:120–140.
614. Ford CE, Jones KW, Polani PE, et al. A sex chromosome anomaly in a case of gonadal dysgenesis (Turner's syndrome). Lancet 1979; 1:711–713.
614a. Virdis R, Cantu MC, Ghizzoni L, et al. Blood pressure behavior and control in Turner syndrome. Clin Exp Hypertens 1986; 8:787–791.
615. Money J, Alexander D, Ehrhardt A. Visual constructional deficit in Turner's syndrome. J Pediatr 1966; 69:126–127.
616. Bender B, Puck M, Sallenblatt J, et al. Cognitive development of unselected girls with complete and partial X monosomy. Pediatrics 1984; 73:175–182.
617. Garron DC. Intelligence among persons with Turner's syndrome. Behav Genet 1977; 7:105–127.
618. Downey JI, Ehrhardt AA. The long-term behavior of patients with Turner syndrome: an update. In: Rosenfeld RG, Grumbach MM, eds. Turner Syndrome. New York: Marcel Dekker, 1990: 483–490.
619. Sybert VP. The adult patient with Turner syndrome. In: Albertsson-Wikland K, Ranke M, eds. Turner Syndrome in a Life Span Perspective: Research and Clinical Aspects. Amsterdam: Elsevier Science BV, 1995, pp 205–218.
620. Swillen A, Fryns JP, Kleczkowska A, et al. Intelligence, behavior and psychosocial development in Turner syndrome: A cross sectioned study of 50 preadolescent and adolescent girls (4–20 years). Genet Couns 1993; 4:7–18.
621. Ratcliffe S. Long term outcome in children of sex chromosome abnormalities. Arch Dis Child 1999; 80:192–195.
622. McCauley E, Ross JL, Kushner H, Cutler G Jr. Self-esteem and behavior in girls with Turner syndrome. J Dev Behav Pediatr 1995; 16:82–88.
623. Skuse DH, James RS, Bishop DVM, et al. Evidence from Turner's syndrome of an unprinted X-linked locus affecting cognitive function. Nature 1997; 387:705–708.
624. Skuse DH. Behavioural phenotypes: what do they teach us? Arch Dis Child 2000; 82:222–225.
625. Bishop DV, Cunning E, Elgar K, et al. Distinctive patterns of memory function in subgroups of females with Turner syndrome: evidence for imprinted loci on the X-chromosome affecting neurodevelopment. Neuropsychologia 2000; 38:712–721.
626. Skuse DH. Imprinting the X-chromosome, and the male brain: Explaining sex differences in the liability to autism. Pediatr Res 2000; 47:9–16.
627. Pavlidis K, McCauley E, Sybert VP. Psychosocial and sexual functioning in women with Turner syndrome. Clin Genet 1995; 47:85–89.
628. Sylven L, Magnusson C, Hagenfeldt K, von Schoultz B. Life with Turner's syndrome: a psychosocial report from 22 middle-aged women. Acta Endocrinol 1993; 129:188–194.
629. Boman UW, Bryman I, Halling K, et al. Women with Turner syndrome: psychological well-being, self-rated health and social life. J Psychsom Obstet Gynaecol 2001; 22: 113–122
630. Gordon RR, O'Neill EM. Turner's infantile phenotype. Br Med J 1969; 1:483–485.
631. Singh RF, Carr DH. The anatomy and histology of XO human embryos and fetuses. Anat Rec 1966; 155:369–384.
632. Shephard TH, Fantel AG. Pathogenesis of congenital defects associated with Turner's syndrome: the role of hypoalbuminemia and edema. Acta Endocrinol 1986; 113(Suppl 279):440–447.
633. van der Putte SCJ. Lymphatic malformation in human fetuses: a study of fetuses with Turner's syndrome or status Bonnevie-Ullrich. Virchows Arch [A] 1977; 376:233–246.
634. Boyd PA, Anthony M, Mannning N, et al. Antenatal diagnosis of cystic hygroma or nuchal pad: Report of 92 cases with follow up survivors. Arch Dis Child Fetal Neonatal Ed 1996; 74:F38-F42.
635. Clark EB. Web neck and congenital heart defects: a pathogenic association in 45,XO Turner syndrome? Teratology 1984; 29: 355–361.
636. Lacro RV, Jones KL, Benirschke K. Coarctation of the aorta in Turner syndrome: a pathologic study of fetuses with nuchal cystic hygromas, hydrops fetalis, and female genitalia. Pediatrics 1988; 81:445–451.
637. Grtzsche CO, Krag-Olsen B, Nielsen J, et al. Prevalence of cardiovascular malformations and association with karyotypes in Turner's syndrome. Arch Dis Child 1994; 71:433–436.
638. Miller MJ, Geffner ME, Lippe BM, et al. Echocardiography reveals a high incidence of bicuspid aortic valve in Turner syndrome. J Pediatr 1983; 102:47–50.
639. Van Egmond H, Orye E, Praet M, et al. Hypoplastic left heart syndrome and the 45,X karyotype. Br Heart J 1988; 60:69–71.
640. Allen DB, Hendrichs A, Levy JM. Aortic dilatation in Turner syndrome. J Pediatr 1986; 109:302–305.
641. Lin AE, Lippe BM, Geffner ME, et al. Aortic dilation, dissection, and rupture in patients with Turner syndrome. J Pediatr 1986; 109:820–826.
642. Saenger P. Clinical review 48: The current status of diagnosis and therapeutic intervention in Turner's syndrome. J Clin Endocrinol Metab 1993; 77:297–301.
643. American Academy of Pediatrics. Health supervision for children with Turner syndrome. Pediatrics 1995; 96:1166–1173.
644. Garvey P, Elovitz M, Landsberger EJ. Aortic dissection and myocardial infarction in a pregnant patient with Turner syndrome. Obstet Gynecol 1998; 91(5 Pt 2):864.
645. Lippe B, Geffner ME, Dietrich RB, et al. Renal malformations in patients with Turner syndrome: imaging in 141 patients. Pediatrics 1988; 82:852–856.
646. Lubin MB, Gruber HE, Rimoin DL, et al. Skeletal abnormalities in the Turner syndrome. In: Rosenfeld RG, Grumbach MM, eds. Turner Syndrome. New York: Marcel Dekker, 1989: 281–291.
647. Prager L, Steinbach HL, Moskowitz P, et al. Roentgenographic abnormalities in phenotypic females with gonadal dysgenesis: a comparison of chromatin positive patients and chromatin negative patients. Am J Roentgenol Radium Ther Nucl Med 1968; 104:899–910.
648. Ross JL, Meyerson L, Feuillan PP, et al. Normal bone density of the wrist and spine and increased wrist fractures in girls with Turner's syndrome. J Clin Endocrinol Metab 1991; 73:355–359.
649. Bechtold S, Rauch F, Noelle V, et al. Musculoskeletal analyses of the forearm in young women with Turner syndrome: a study using peripheral quantitative computed tomography. J Clin Endocrinol Metab 2001; 86:5819–5823.
650. Lanes R, Gunczler P, Esaa S, Martinis R, Villaroel O, Weisinger JR. Decreased bone mass despite long-term estrogen re-

746. Ehrhardt AA. Behavioral effects of estrogen in the human female. Pediatrics 1978; 62:1166–1170.
746a. Paterson WF, Hollman AS, Donaldson MD. Poor uterine development in Turner syndrome with oral oestrogen therapy. Clin Endocrinol (Oxf) 2002; 56:359–365.
747. Chernausek SD, Attie KM, Cara JF, Rosenfeld RG, Frane J. Growth hormone therapy of Turner syndrome: the impact of age of estrogen replacement on final height. Genentech, Inc., Collaborative Study Group. J Clin Endocrinol Metab 2000; 85: 2439–2445.
748. Reiter EO, Blethen SL, Baptista J, Price L. Early initiation of growth hormone treatment allows age-appropriate estrogen use in Turner's syndrome. J Clin Endocrinol Metab 2001; 86:1936–1941.
749. Abir R, Fisch B, Nahum R, Orvieto R, Nitke S, Ben Rafael Z. Turner's syndrome and fertility: current status and possible putative prospects. Hum Reprod Update 2001; 7:603–610.
749a. Ross JL, Roeltgen D, Feuillan P, Kushner H, Cutler GB Jr. Effects of estrogen on nonverbal processing speed and motor function in girls with Turner's syndrome. J Clin Endocrinol Metab 1998; 83:3198–3204.
749b. Ferguson-Smith MA. Genotype-phenotype correlations in individuals with disorders of sex determination and development including Turner's syndrome. Semin Devel Biol 1991; 2:265–276.
750. Ross JL, Roeltgen D, Feuillan P, Kushner H, Cutler GB Jr. Use of estrogen in young girls with Turner syndrome: effects on memory. Neurology 2000; 54:164–170.
751. Ross JL, Stefanatos GA, Kushner H, Zinn A, Bondy C, Roeltgen D. Persistent cognitive deficits in adult women with Turner syndrome. Neurology 2002; 58:218–225.
751a. Leonova J, Hanson C. A study of 45,X/46,XX mosaicism in Turner syndrome females: a novel primer pair for the (CAG)n repeat within the androgen receptor gene. Hereditas 1999; 131: 87–92.
752. Levine LS. Treatment of Turner's syndrome with estrogen. Pediatrics 1979; 62:1178–1183.
753. Rosenwaks Z, Urban MD, Wentz AC, et al. Endometrial pathology and its relation to estrogen therapy in patients with hypogonadism. Pediatrics 1979; 62:1184–1188.
754. Fujita H, Tanigawa Y, Yoshida Y, et al. Cytological findings of 10 cases of i(Xq) and one with dic(X). Hum Genet 1977; 39: 147–155.
754a. Lorda-Sanchez I, Binkert F, Maechler H, Schinzel A. A molecular study of X isochromosomes: parental origin, centromeric structure, and mechanisms of formation. Am J Hum Genet 1991; 49:1034–1040.
754b. Otto PG, Vianna-Morgante AM, Otto PA, et al. The Turner phenotype and the different types of human X isochromosome. Hum Genet 1981; 57:159–164.
755. Stafford TM, Palmer CG, Cleary RE. Gonadal dysgenesis with isochromosome X and menstruation. Am J Obstet Gynecol 1973; 116:886.
756. de Kerdanet, Lucas J, Lemee F, Lecornu M. Turner's syndrome with X-isochromosome and Hashimoto's thyroiditis. Clin Endocrinol 1994; 41:673–676.
757. Dewald GW. Isodicentric X chromosomes in humans: origin, segregation behavior, and replication band patterns. In: Sandberg AA, ed. Cytogenetics of the Mammalian X Chromosome. Part A: Basic Mechanisms of X Chromosome Behavior. New York: Alan R Liss, 1983: 405–426.
758. Turner C, Dennis NR, Skuse DH, Jacobs PA. Seven ring (X) chromosomes lacking the XIST locus, six with an unexpectedly mild phenotype. Hum Genet 2000; 106:93–100.
759. Dallapiccola B, Bruni L, Boscherini B, et al. Segregation of an X ring chromosome in two generations. J Med Genet 1980; 17: 306–308.
760. Migeon BR, Ausems M, Giltay J, et al. Severe phenotypes associated with inactive ring X chromosomes. Am J Med Genet 2000; 93:52–57.
761. Grompe M, Rao N, Elder FF, et al. 45,X/46,X + r(X) can have a distinct phenotype different from Ullrich-Turner syndrome. Am J Med Genet 1992; 42:39–43.
762. Callen DF, Eyre HJ, Dolman G, et al. Molecular cytogenetic characterization of a small ring X chromosome in a Turner patient and in a male patient with congenital abnormalities: role of X inactivation. J Med Genet 1995; 32:113–116.
763. Callen DF, Eyre HJ, Dolman G, et al. Molecular cytogenetic characterization of a small ring X chromosome in a Turner patient and in a male patient with congenital abnormalities: role of X inactivation. J Med Genet 1995; 32:113–116.
764. Crolla JA, Llerena JC Jr. A mosaic 45,X/46,X,r(?) karyotype investigated with X and Y centromere-specific probes using a non autoradiographic in situ hybridization technique. Hum Genet 1988; 81:81–84.
765. Disteche C. The use of DNA probes to characterize sex chromosome anomalies. In: Rosenfeld RG, Grumbach MM, eds. Turner Syndrome in a Life Span Perspective: Research and Clinical Aspects. New York: Marcel Dekker, 1990: 37–54.
766. Herva R, Kaluzewski B, de la Chapelle A. Inherited interstitial del(Xp) with minimal consequences: with a note on the location of genes controlling phenotypic features. Am J Med Genet 1979; 3:43–58.
767. Kalousek D, Schiffrin A, Berguer AM, et al. Partial short arm deletions of the X chromosome and spontaneous pubertal development in girls with short stature. J Pediatr 1979; 94:891–894.
768. Fryns JP, Petit P, Van den Berghe H. The various phenotypes in Xp deletion: observation in eleven patients. Hum Genet 1981; 57:385–387.
769. Wilson MG, Modebe O, Towner JW, et al. Ullrich-Turner syndrome associated with interstitial deletion of Xp11.4-p22.31. Am J Med Genet 1983; 14:567–576.
770. James RS, Coppin B, Dalton P, et al. A study of females with deletions of the short arm of the X chromosome. Hum Genet 1998; 102:507–516.
771. Fraccaro M, Maraschio P, Pasquali F, et al. Women heterozygous for deficiency of the (p21-pter) region of the X chromosome are fertile. Hum Genet 1977; 39:283–292.
772. Leichtman DA, Schmickel RD, Gelehrter TD, et al. Familial Turner syndrome. Ann Intern Med 1978; 89:473–476.
773. Wandstrat AE, Conroy JM, Zurcher VL, et al. Molecular and cytogenetic analysis of familial Xp deletions. Am J Med Genet 2000; 94:163–169.
774. Geerkens C, Just W, Vogel W. Deletions of Xq and growth deficit: a review. Am J Med Genet 1994; 50:105–113.
775. Maraschio P, Tupler R, Barbierato L, et al. An analysis of Xq deletions. Hum Genet 1996; 97:375–381.
776. Mirzayants GG, Baranovskaya LI. XX translocation in a patient with gonadal dysgenesis and the problem of phenotypic-karyotypic correlations. Hum Genet 1978; 40:249–257.
777. Madan K. Balanced structural changes involving the human X: effect on sexual phenotype. Hum Genet 1983; 63:216–221.
778. Schmidt M, Du Sart D. Functional disomies of the X chromosome influence the cell selection and hence X inactivation pattern in females with balanced X-autosome translocation: a review of 122 cases. Am J Med Genet 1992; 42:161–169.
779. Zah W, Kalderon HE, Tucci JR. Mixed gonadal dysgenesis. Acta Endocrinol 1975; 79(Suppl 197):3–39.
780. Akin JW, Tho SPT, McDonough PG. Reconsidering the difference between mixed gonadal dysgenesis and true hermaphroditism. Adolesc Pediatr Gynecol 1993; 6:102–104.
781. Robboy SJ, Miller T, Donahoe PK, et al. Dysgenesis of testicular and streak gonads in the syndrome of mixed gonadal dysgenesis: perspective derived from clinico-pathologic analysis of 21 cases. Hum Pathol 1982; 13:700–716.
782. Wheeler M, Peakman D, Robinson A, et al. 45X/46XY mosaicism: contrast of prenatal and postnatal diagnosis. Am J Med Genet 1988; 29:565–571.
782a. Rosenberg C, Frota-Pessoa O, Vianna-Morgante AM, et al. Phenotypic spectrum of 45X,46XY individuals. Am J Med Genet 1987; 27:553–559.
783. Chang HJ, Clark RD, Bachman H. The phenotype of 45,X/46,XY mosaicism: an analysis of 92 prenatally diagnosed cases. Am J Med Genet 1990; 46:156–168.
784. Hsu LYF. Phenotype/karyotype correlations of Y chromosome aneuploidy with emphasis on structural aberrations in postnatally diagnosed cases. Am J Med Genet 1994; 53:108–140.
785. Bonaventura L, Roth LM, Cleary RE. The Sertoli cell in mixed gonadal dysgenesis. Obstet Gynecol 1979; 53:324–329.
786. Müller J, Skakkebaek NE, Ritzen M, et al. Carcinoma in situ of the testis in children with 45,X/46,XY gonadal dysgenesis. J Pediatr 1985; 106:431–436.
787. Müller J, Ritzen EM, Ivarsson SA, Rajpert-De Meyts E, Norja-

vaara E, Skakkebaek NE. Management of males with 45,X/46,XY gonadal dysgenesis. Horm Res 1999; 52:11–14.
788. Gravholt CH, Fedder J, Naeraa RW, et al. Occurrence of gonadoblastoma in females with Turner syndrome and Y chromosome material—a population study. J Clin Endocrinol Metab 2000; 85:3199–3202.
789. Caspersson TA, Hulten M, Jonasson J, et al. Translocation causing nonfluorescent Y chromosomes in human XO/XY mosaicism. Hereditas 1971; 68:317–324.
790. Kluzewski B, Jokineu A, Hortling H, et al. A theory explaining the abnormality in 45,X/46,XY mosaicism with nonfluorescent Y chromosome: presentation of 3 cases. Ann Genet 1978; 21:5–11.
791. Madan K, Gooren L, Shoemaker J. Three cases of sex chromosome mosaicism with a nonfluorescent Y. Hum Genet 1979; 46:295–304.
792. Magenis E, Donlon T. Nonfluorescent Y chromosomes: cytologic evidence of origin. Hum Genet 1982; 60:133–138.
793. Weckworth PF, Johnson HW, Pantzer JT, et al. Dicentric Y chromosome and mixed dysgenesis. J Urol 1988; 139:91–94.
794. Sugarman ID, Crolla JA, Malone PS. Mixed gonadal dysgenesis and cell line differentiation: case presentation and literature review. Clin Genet 1994; 46:313–315.
795. Canto P, de la Chesnaye E, Lopez M, Cervantes A, Chavez B, Vilchis F, Reyes E, Ulloa-Aguirre A, Kofman-Alfaro S, Mendez JP. A mutation in the 5′ non-high mobility group box region of the SRY gene in patients with Turner syndrome and Y mosaicism. J Clin Endocrinol Metab 2000; 85:1908–1911.
796. Borer JG, Ntti VW, Glassberg KI. Mixed gonadal dysgenesis and dysgenetic male pseudohermaphroditism. J Urol 1995; 153:1267–1273.
797. Yanagisawa S. Structural abnormalities of the Y chromosome and abnormal external genitalia. Hum Genet 1980; 53:183–188.
798. Reijo R, Lee TY, Salo P, et al. Diverse spermatogenic defects in humans caused by Y chromosome deletions encompassing a novel RNA-binding protein gene. Nat Genet 1995; 10:383–393.
799. Najmabadi H, Huang V, Yen P, et al. Substantial prevalence of microdeletions of the Y chromosome in infertile men with idiopathic azoospermia and oligospermia detected using a sequence-tagged site based mapping strategy. J Clin Endocrinol Metab 1996; 81:347–352.
800. Pryor JL, Kent-First M, Muallem A, et al. Microdeletions in the Y chromosome of infertile males. N Engl J Med 1997; 336:534–539.
801. Cooke HJ, Elliott DJ. RNA-binding proteins and human male infertility. Trends Genet 1997; 13:87–89.
802. Bernstein R. X:Y chromosome translocations and their manifestations. In: Sandberg AA, ed. Progress and Topics in Cytogenetics, the Y Chromosome. New York: Alan R Liss, 1985: 171–206.
803. Harnden DG, Stewart JSS. The chromosomes in a case of pure gonadal dysgenesis. Br Med J 1959; 2:1285–1287.
804. Nazareth HR de S, Farah LMS, Cunha AJB, et al. Pure gonadal dysgenesis (type XX): report on a family with four affected sibs. Hum Genet 1977; 37:117–120.
805. McDonough PG, Byrd JR, Tho PT, et al. Phenotypic and cytogenetic findings in eighty-two patients with ovarian failure: changing trends. Fertil Steril 1977; 28:638–641.
806. Judd HL, Scully RE, Atkins L, et al. Pure gonadal dysgenesis with progressive hirsutism: demonstration of testosterone production by gonadal streaks. N Engl J Med 1970; 282:881–885.
807. Aittomaki K. The genetics of XX gonadal dysgenesis. Am J Hum Genet 1994; 54:844–851.
808. Heufelder AE. Gonads in trouble: follicle-stimulating hormone receptor gene mutation as a cause of inherited streak ovaries. Eur J Endocrinol 1996; 134:296–297.
809. Aittomaki K, Herva R, Stenman UH, et al. Clinical features of primary ovarian failure caused by a point mutation in the follicle-stimulating hormone receptor gene. J Clin Endocrinol Metab 1995; 81:3722–3726.
810. Tapanainen JS, Aittomaki K, Min J, et al. Men homozygous for an inactivating mutation of the follicle stimulating hormone (FSH) receptor gene present variable suppression of spermatogenesis and fertility. Nat Genet 1997; 15:205–206.
811. Pallister PD, Opitz JM. The Perrault syndrome: autosomal recessive ovarian dysgenesis with facultative, non-sex-limited sensorineural deafness. Am J Med Genet 1979; 4:239–246.
812. Nishi Y, Hamamoto K, Kajiyama M, et al. The Perrault syndrome: clinical report and review. Am J Med Genet 1988; 31:623–629.
813. Hamet P, Kuchel O, Nowaczynski W, et al. Hypertension with adrenal, genital, renal defects, and deafness. Arch Intern Med 1973; 131:563–569.
814. Skre H, Bassoe HH, Berg K, et al. Cerebellar ataxia and hypergonadotropic hypogonadism in two kindreds: chance occurrence, pleiotropism or linkage? Clin Genet 1976; 9:234–244.
815. Nicolino M, Bost M, David M, et al. Familial blepharophenosis: an uncommon marker of ovarian dysgenesis. J Pediatr Endocrinol Metab 1995; 8:127–133.
816. Amati P, Gasparini P, Zlotogora J, et al. A gene for premature ovarian failure associated with eyelid malformation maps to chromosome 3q22-q23. Am J Hum Genet 1996; 58:1089–1092.
817. Crisponi L, Deiana M, Loi A, et al. The putative forkhead transcription factor FOXL2 is mutated in blepharophimosis/ptosis/epicanthus inversus syndrome. Nat Genet 2001; 27:159–166.
818. De Baere E, Dixon MJ, Small KW, et al. Spectrum of FOXL2 gene mutations in blepharophimosis-ptosis-epicanthus inversus (BPES) families demonstrates a genotype–phenotype correlation. Hum Mol Genet 2001; 10:1591–1600.
819. Kennerknecht I, Sorgo W, Oberhoffer R, et al. Familial occurrence of agonadism and multiple internal malformations in phenotypically normal girls with 46,XY and 46,XX karyotypes, respectively: a new autosomal recessive syndrome. Am J Med Genet 1993; 47:1166–1170.
820. Mendonca BB, Barbosa AS, Arnhold IJP, et al. Gonadal dysgenesis in XX and XY sisters: evidence for the involvement of an autosomal gene. Am J Med Genet 1994; 52:39–43.
821. Swyer GIM. Male pseudohermaphrodism: a hitherto undescribed form. Br Med J 1955; 2:709–712.
822. Warner BA, Monsaert RP, Stumpf PG, et al. 46,XY gonadal dysgenesis: is oncogenesis related to HY antigen phenotype or breast development? Hum Genet 1985; 69:79–85.
823. Schmitt-Ney M, Thiele H, Kaltwasser P, et al. Two novel SRY missense mutations reducing DNA binding identified in XY females and their mosaic fathers. Am J Hum Genet 1995; 56:862–869.
824. Blagowidow N, Page DC, Huff D, et al. Ullrich-Turner syndrome in an XY female fetus with deletion of the sex determining portion of the Y chromosome. Am J Med Genet 1989; 34:159–162.
825. McElreavey K, Vilain E, Abbas N, et al. A regulatory cascade hypothesis for mammalian sex determination: SRY represses a negative regulator of male development. Proc Natl Acad Sci USA 1993; 90:3368–3372.
826. Bennett CP, Docherty Z, Robb A, et al. Deletion 9p and sex reversal. J Med Genet 1993; 30:518–520.
827. Hawkins JR, Taylor A, Goodfellow PN, et al. Evidence for increased prevalence of SRY mutations in XY females with complete rather than partial gonadal dysgenesis. Am J Hum Genet 1992; 51:979–984.
828. McElreavey K, Vilain E, Abbas N, et al. XY sex reversal associated with a deletion 5′ to the SRY "HMG box" in the testis-determining region. Proc Natl Acad Sci USA 1992; 89:11016–11020.
829. Nasrin N, Buggs C, Kong XF, et al. DNA-binding properties of the product of the testes-determining gene and related protein. Nature 1991; 354:317–320.
830. Harley VR, Jackson DI, Hextall PJ, et al. DNA binding activity of recombinant SRY from normal males and XY females. Science 1992; 255:453–456.
831. Jager RJ, Harley VR, Pfeifter RA, et al. A familial mutation in the testis-determining gene SRY shared by both sexes. Hum Genet 1992; 90:350–355.
832. Poulat F, Soullier S, Goze C, et al. Description and functional implications of a novel mutation in the sex-determining gene SRY. Hum Mutat 1994; 3:200–204.
833. Chemke J, Carmichael R, Stewart JM, et al. Familial XY gonadal dysgenesis. J Med Genet 1970; 7:105–111.
834. Vilain E, McElreavey K, Jaubert F, et al. Familial case with sequence variant in the testis-determining region associated with two sex phenotypes. Am J Hum Genet 1992; 50:1008–1011.
835. Scherer G, Shempp W, Bacchichetti C, et al. Duplication of an Xp segment that includes the ZFX locus causes sex inversion in man. Hum Genet 1989; 81:291–294.

1187. Korsch E, Peter M, Hiort O, Sippell WG, Ure BM, Hauffa BP, Bergmann M. Gonadal histology with testicular carcinoma in situ in a 15-year-old 46,XY female patient with a premature termination in the steroidogenic acute regulatory protein causing congenital lipoid adrenal hyperplasia. J Clin Endocrinol Metab 1999; 84:1628–1632.

1188. Aya M, Ogata T, Sakaguchi A, Sato S, Matsuo N. Testicular histopathology in congenital lipoid adrenal hyperplasia: a light and electron microscopic study. Horm Res 1997; 47:121–125.

1189. Tajima T, Fujieda K, Kouda N, et al. Heterozygous mutation in the cholesterol side chain cleavage enzyme (P450scc) gene in a patient with 46, XY sex reversal and adrenal insufficiency. J Clin Endocrinol Metab 2001; 86: 3820–3825.

1190. Mendonca BB, Bloise W, Arnhold IJP, et al. Male pseudohermaphroditism due to nonsalt losing 3-beta-hydroxysteroid dehydrogenase deficiency: gender role change and absence of gynecomastia at puberty. J Steroid Biochem 1987; 28:669–675.

1191. Parks GA, Bermudez JA, Anast CS, et al. Pubertal boy with the 3-beta-hydroxysteroid dehydrogenase defect. J Clin Endocrinol Metab 1971; 33:269–278.

1192. Schneider G, Genel M, Bongiovanni AM, et al. Persistent testicular Δ^5-isomerase-3-beta-hydroxysteroid dehydrogenase (Δ^5-3-beta-HSD) deficiency in the Δ^5-3-beta-HSD form of congenital adrenal hyperplasia. J Clin Invest 1975; 55:681–690.

1193. Simard J, Rheaume E, Sanchez R, et al. Molecular basis of congenital adrenal hyperplasia due to 3 beta-hydroxysteroid dehydrogenase deficiency. Mol Endocrinol 1993; 7:716–728.

1194. Sanchez R, Mebarki F, Rheaume E, et al. Functional characterization of the novel L108W and P186L mutations detected in the type II 3 beta-hydroxysteroid dehydrogenase gene of a male pseudohermaphrodite with congenital adrenal hyperplasia. Hum Mol Genet 1994; 3:1639–1645.

1195. Morel Y, Mebarki F, Rheaume E, et al. Structure-function relationship of 3 beta-hydroxysteroid dehydrogenase: contribution made by molecular genetics of 3 beta-hydroxysteroid dehydrogenase deficiency. Steroids 1997; 62:176–184.

1196. Russell AJ, Wallace AM, Forest MG, et al. Mutation in the human gene for 3-beta-hydroxysteroid dehydrogenase type II leading to male pseudohermaphroditism without salt loss. J Mol Endocrinol 1994; 12:225–237.

1197. Moisan AM, Ricketts ML, Tardy V, et al. New insight into the molecular basis of 3-beta-hydroxysteroid dehydrogenase deficiency: identification of eight mutations in the HSD3B2 gene eleven patients from seven new families and comparison of the functional properties of twenty-five mutant enzymes. J Clin Endocrinol Metab 1999; 84:4410–4425.

1198. Alos N, Moisan AM, Ward L, Desrochers M, Legault L, Leboeuf G, Van Vliet G, Simard J. A novel A10E homozygous mutation in the HSD3B2 gene causing severe salt-wasting 3-beta-hydroxysteroid dehydrogenase deficiency in 46,XX and 46,XY French-Canadians: evaluation of gonadal function after puberty. J Clin Endocrinol Metab 2000; 85:1968–1974.

1199. Zerah M, Rheaume E, Mani P, et al. No evidence of mutations in the genes for type I and type II 3 beta-hydroxysteroid dehydrogenase (3 beta-HSD) in nonclassical 3 beta-HSD deficiency. J Clin Endocrinol Metab 1994; 79: 1811–1817.

1200. Cara JF, Moshang T Jr, Bongiovanni AM, et al. Elevated 17-hydroxyprogesterone and testosterone in a newborn with 3 beta-hydroxysteroid dehydrogenase deficiency. N Engl J Med 1985; 313:618–621.

1201. Jones HW Jr, Lee PA, Rock JA, et al. A genetic male patient with 17 alpha-hydroxylase deficiency. Obstet Gynecol 1982; 59: 254–259.

1202. Peter M, Sippell WG, Wernze H. Diagnosis and treatment of 17 hydroxylase deficiency. J Steroid Biochem Mol Biol 1993; 45: 107–116.

1203. Tvedegaard M, Frederiksen V, Olgaard K, et al. Two cases of 17 alpha-hydroxylase deficiency: one combined with complete gonadal agenesis. Acta Endocrinol 1981; 98:267–273.

1204. Ahlgren R, Yanase T, Simpson ER, et al. Compound heterozygous mutations (Arg 239 6 stop, Pro 342 6 Thr) in the CYP17 (P450 17-alpha) gene lead to ambiguous external genitalia in a male with partial combined 17 alpha-hydroxylase/17,20 lyase deficiency. J Clin Endocrinol Metab 1992; 74:667–672.

1205. Cunniff C, Kratz LE, Moser A, Natowicz MR, Kelley RI. Clinical and biochemical spectrum of patients with RSH/Smith-Lemli-Opitz syndrome and abnormal cholesterol metabolism. Am J Med Genet 1997; 68:263–269.

1206. Opitz JM. RSH (so-called Smith-Lemli-Opitz) syndrome. Curr Opin Pediatr 1999; 11:353–362.

1207. Kelley RI, Hennekam RCM. The Smith-Lemli-Opitz syndrome. J Med Genet 2000; 37:321–335.

1208. Tint GS, Salen G, Batta AK, et al. Correlation of severity and outcome with plasma sterol levels in variants of the Smith-Lemli-Opitz syndrome. J Pediatr 1995; 127:82–87.

1209. Kelley RI. RSH/Smith-Lemli-Opitz syndrome: mutations and metabolic morphogenesis. Am J Hum Genet 1998; 63:322–326.

1210. Fitzky BU, Witsch-Baumgartner M, Erdel M, Lee JN, Paik YK, Glossmann H, Utermann G, Moebius FF. Mutations in the Δ7-sterol reductase gene in patients with the Smith-Lemli-Opitz syndrome. Proc Natl Acad Sci USA 1998; 95:8181–8186.

1211. Yu H, Lee MH, Starck L, Elias ER, Irons M, Salen G, Patel SB, Tint GS. Spectrum of delta(7)-dehydrocholesterol reductase mutations in patients with the Smith-Lemli-Opitz (RSH) syndrome. Hum Mol Genet 2000; 9:1385–1391. [Erratum in: Hum Mol Genet 2000; 9:1903.]

1212. Witsch-Baumgartner M, Loeffler J, et al. Mutations in the human DHCR7 gene. Hum Mutat 2001; 17:172–182.

1213. Witsch-Baumgartner M, Ciara E, Loffler J, et al. Frequency gradients of DHCR7 mutations in patients with Smith-Lemli-Opitz syndrome in Europe: evidence for different origins of common mutations. Eur J Hum Genet 2001; 9:45–50.

1214. Greene C, Pitts W, Rosenfeld R, Luzzatti L. Smith-Lemli-Opitz syndrome in two 46,XY infants with female external genitalia. Clin Genet 1984; 25:366–372.

1215. Lachman MF, Wright Y, Whiteman DA, Herson V, Greenstein RM. Brief clinical report: a 46,XY phenotypic female with Smith-Lemli-Opitz syndrome. Clin Genet 1991; 39:136–141.

1216. Pankau R, Partsch CJ, Funda J, Sippell WG. Hypothalamic-pituitary-gonadal function in two infants with Smith-Lemli-Opitz syndrome. Am J Med Genet 1992; 43:513–516.

1217. Berensztein E, Torrado M, Belgorosky A, Rivarola M. Smith-Lemli-Opitz syndrome: in vivo and in vitro study of testicular function in a prepubertal patient with ambiguous genitalia. Acta Paediatr 1999; 88:1229–1232.

1218. Andersson HC, Frentz J, Martinez JE, Tuck-Muller CM, Bellizaire J. Adrenal insufficiency in Smith-Lemli-Opitz syndrome. Am J Med Genet 1999; 82:382–384.

1219. Shackleton CH, Roitman E, Kelley R. Neonatal urinary steroids in Smith-Lemli-Opitz syndrome associated with 7-dehydrocholesterol reductase deficiency. Steroids 1999; 64:481–490.

1220. Wassif CA, Zhu P, Kratz L, et al. Biochemical, phenotypic and neurophysiological characterization of a genetic mouse model of RSH/Smith-Lemli-Opitz syndrome. Hum Mol Genet 2001; 15: 555–564.

1221. Shackleton CH, Roitman E, Kratz L, Kelley R. Dehydro-oestriol and dehydropregnanetriol are candidate analytes for prenatal diagnosis of Smith-Lemli-Opitz syndrome. Prenat Diagn 2001; 21:207–212.

1222. Bradley LA, Palomaki GE, Knight GJ, et al. Levels of unconjugated estriol and other maternal serum markers in pregnancies with Smith-Lemli-Opitz (RSH) syndrome fetuses. Am J Med Genet 1999; 82:355–358.

1223. Auchus RJ, Lee TC, Miller WL. Cytochrome b5 augments the 17,20-lyase activity of human P450c17 without direct electron transfer. J Biol Chem 1998; 273:3158–3165.

1224. Yanagibashi K, Hall PF. Role of electron transport in the regulation of the lyase activity of C21 side chain cleavage P450 from porcine adrenal and testicular microsomes. J Biol Chem 1986; 261:8429–8433.

1225. Miller WL, Auchus RJ, Geller DH. The regulation of 17,20 lyase activity. Steroids 1997; 62:133–142.

1226. Katagiri M, Kagawa N, Waterman MR. The role of cytochrome b_5 in the biosynthesis of androgens by human $P450_{c17}$. Arch Biochem Biophys 1995; 317:343–347.

1227. Zhang LH, Rodriguez H, Ohno S, Miller WL. Serine phosphorylation of human P450c17 increases 17,20-lyase activity: implications for adrenarche and the polycystic ovary syndrome. Proc Natl Acad Sci USA 1995; 92:10619–10623.

1228. Geller DH, Auchus RJ, Mendonca BB, et al. The genetic and functional basis of isolated 17,20 lyase deficiency. Nat Genet 1997; 17:201–205.

1229. Geller DH, Auchus RJ, Miller WL. P450c17 mutations R347H and R358Q selectively disrupt 17,20-lyase activity by disrupting interactions with P450 oxidoreductase and cytochrome b5. Mol Endocrinol 1999; 13:167–175.
1230. Zachmann M, Vollmin JA, Hamilton W, et al. Steroid 17,20 desmolase deficiency: a new cause of male pseudohermaphroditism. Clin Endocrinol 1972; 1:369–385.
1231. Zachmann M, Kempkin B, Manella B, Navarro E. Conversion from pure 17,20 desmolase to combined 17,20 desmolase/17 alpha hydroxylase deficiency with age. Acta Endocrinol 1992; 127:97–99.
1232. Yanase T, Waterman MR, Zachmann M, et al. Molecular basis of apparent isolated 17,20 lyase deficiency: compound heterozygous mutations in the Cterminal region (Arg(496)6Cys, Gln(461)6Stop) actually cause combined 17 alpha-hydroxylase/ 17,20 lyase deficiency. Biochem Biophys Acta 1992; 1139:275–279.
1233. Auchus RJ. The genetics, pathophysiology, and management of human deficiencies of P450c17. Endocrinol Metab Clin North Am 2001; 30:101–119.
1234. Kitamura M, Buczbo E, Dufau ML. Dissociation of hydroxylase and lyase activities by site-directed mutagenesis of the rat $P450_{17\alpha}$. Mol Endocrinol 1991; 5:1373–1380.
1235. Lin D, Zhang LH, Chiao E, Miller WL. Modeling and mutagenesis of the active site of human P450c17. Mol Endocrinol 1994; 8:392–402.
1236. Larrea F, Lisker R, Banuelos R, et al. Hypergonadotropic hypogonadism in an XX female subject due to 17,20-desmolase deficiency. Acta Endocrinol 1983; 103:400–405.
1237. Forest MG. Familial male pseudohermaphroditism due to 17,20 desmolase deficiency. I. In vivo endocrine studies. J Clin Endocrinol Metab 1980; 50:826–833.
1238. Labrie F, Luu-The V, Lin SX, Simard J, Labrie C. Role of 17 beta-hydroxysteroid dehydrogenases in sex steroid formation in peripheral intracrine tissues. Trends Endocrinol Metab 2000; 11:421–427.
1239. Andersson S, Russell DW, Wilson J. 17-beta-hydroxysteroid dehydrogenase 3 deficiency. Trends Endocrinol 1996; 7:121–125.
1240. Luu The V, Labrie C, Zhao HF, et al. Characterization of cDNAs for human estradiol 17-beta-dehydrogenase and assignment of one gene to chromosome 17: evidence for two mRNA species with distinct 5′-termini in human placenta. Mol Endocrinol 1989; 3:1301–1309.
1241. Wu L, Einstein M, Geissler WM, et al. Expression cloning and characterization of human 17-beta-hydroxysteroid dehydrogenase type 2, a microsomal enzyme possessing 20 alpha-hydroxysteroid dehydrogenase activity. J Biol Chem 1993; 268:12964–12969.
1242. Casey ML, MacDonald PC, Andersson S. 17-beta-hydroxysteroid dehydrogenase type 2: chromosomal assignment and progestin regulation of gene expression in human endometrium. J Clin Invest 1994; 94:2135–2141.
1243. Geissler WM, Davis DL, Wu L, et al. Male pseudohermaphroditism caused by mutations of testicular 17-beta-hydroxysteroid dehydrogenase 3. Nat Genet 1994; 7:34–39.
1244. Saez JM, de Peretti E, Morera AM, et al. Familial male pseudohermaphroditism with gynecomastia due to a testicular 17-ketosteroid reductase defect. I. In vivo studies. J Clin Endocrinol Metab 1971; 32:604–610.
1245. Saez JM, Morera AM, de Peretti E, Bertand J. Further in vivo studies in male pseudohermaphroditism with gynecomastia due to a testicular 17-ketosteroid reductase defect (compared to a case of testicular feminization). J Clin Endocrinol Metab 1972; 34:598–600.
1246. Rosler A, Kohn G. Male pseudohermaphroditism due to 17 beta-hydroxysteroid dehydrogenase deficiency: studies on the natural history of the defect and effect of androgens on gender role. J Steroid Biochem 1983; 19:663–674.
1247. Rosler A. Steroid 17 beta-hydroxysteroid dehydrogenase deficiency in man: an inherited form of male pseudohermaphroditism. J Steroid Biochem Mol Biol 1992; 43:989–1002.
1248. Dumic M, Plavsic V, Fattorini I, et al. Absent spermatogenesis despite early bilateral orchiopexy in 17 ketoreductase deficiency. Horm Res 1985; 22:100–106.
1249. Ulloa-Aguirre A, Bassol S, Poo J, et al. Endrocine and biochemical studies in a 46,XY phenotypically male infant with 17-ketosteroid reductase deficiency. J Clin Endocrinol Metab 1985; 60:639–643.
1250. Andersson S, Geissler WM, Wu L, et al. Molecular genetics and pathophysiology of 17 beta-hydroxysteroid dehydrogenase 3 deficiency. J Clin Endocrinol Metab 1996; 81:130–136.
1251. Givens JR, Wiser WL, Summitt RL, et al. Familial male pseudohermaphroditism without gynecomastia due to deficient testicular 17-ketosteroid reductase activity. N Engl J Med 1974; 291:938–944.
1252. Pittaway DE, Andersen RN, Givens JR. Deficient 17 beta-hydroxysteroid oxidoreductase activity in testes from a male pseudohermaphrodite. J Clin Endocrinol Metab 1976; 43:457–461.
1253. Imperato-McGinley J, Peterson RE, Stoller R, et al. Male pseudohermaphroditism secondary to 17-hydroxysteroid dehydrogenase deficiency: gender role change with puberty. J Clin Endocrinol Metab 1979; 49:391–395.
1254. Millan M, Audi L, Martinez-Mora J, et al. 17-Ketosteroid reductase deficiency in an adult patient without gynecomastia but with female psychosocial orientation. Acta Endocrinol 1983; 102:633–640.
1255. Akesode FA, Meyer WJ, Migeon CJ. Male pseudohermaphroditism with gynecomastia due to testicular 17-ketosteroid reductase deficiency. Clin Endocrinol 1977; 7:443–452.
1256. Rosler A, Belanger A, Labrie F. Mechanisms of androgen production in male pseudohermaphroditism due to 17 beta-hydroxysteroid dehydrogenase deficiency. J Clin Endocrinol Metab 1992; 75:773–778.
1257. Eckstein B, Cohen S, Farkas S, R'sler A. The nature of the defect in familial male pseudohermaphroditism in Arabs of the Gaza. J Clin Endocrinol Metab 1994; 64:477–485.
1258. Rosler A, Silverstein S, Abeliovich D. A (R80Q) mutation in 17 beta-hydroxysteroid dehydrogenase type 3 gene among Arabs of Israel is associated with pseudohermaphroditism in males and normal asymptomatic females. J Clin Endocrinol Metab 1996; 81:1827–1831.
1259. Boehmer AL, Brinkmann AO, Sandkuijl LA, et al. 17-Beta-hydroxysteroid dehydrogenase-3 deficiency: diagnosis, phenotypic variability, population genetics, and worldwide distribution of ancient and de novo mutations. J Clin Endocrinol Metab 1999; 84:4713–4721.
1260. Moghrabi N, Hughes IA, Dunaif A, Andersson S. Deleterious missense mutations and silent polymorphism in the human 17-beta-hydroxysteroid dehydrogenase 3 gene (HSD17B3). J Clin Endocrinol Metab 1998; 83:2855–2860.
1261. Bentvelsen FM, McPhaul MJ, Wilson JD, George FW. The androgen receptor of the urogenital tract of the fetal rat is regulated by androgen. Mol Cell Endocrinol 1994; 105:21–26.
1262. Gross DJ, Landau H, Kohn G, et al. Male pseudohermaphroditism due to 17 beta-hydroxysteroid dehydrogenase deficiency: gender assignment in early infancy. Acta Endocrinol 1986; 112: 238–246.
1263. Mendonca BB, Inacio M, Arnhold IJ, et al. Male pseudohermaphroditism due to 17 beta-hydroxysteroid dehydrogenase 3 deficiency. Diagnosis, psychological evaluation, and management. Medicine 2000; 79:299–309.
1264. Castro-Magana M, Angulo M, Uy J. Male hypogonadism with gynecomastia caused by late onset deficiency of testicular 17-ketosteroid reductase. N Engl J Med 1993; 328:1297–1301.
1265. Farkas A, Rosler A, et al. Ten years experience with masculinizing genitoplasty in male pseudohermaphroditism due to 17 beta-hydroxysteroid dehydrogenase deficiency. Eur J Pediatr 1993; 152(Suppl 2):S88-S90.
1266. Quigley C, De Bellis A, Marschke KB, et al. Androgen receptor defects: historical, clinical, and molecular perspectives. Endocr Rev 1995; 16:271–321.
1267. Patterson MN, McPhaul MJ, Hughes IA. Androgen insensitivity syndrome. Baillieres Clin Endocrinol Metab 1994; 8:379–404.
1268. MacLean HE, Warne GL, Zajac JD. Defects of androgen receptor function: from sex reversal to motor neurone disease. Mol Cell Endocrinol 1995; 112:133–141.
1269. Gottlieb B, Pinsky L, Beitel LK, et al. Androgen insensitivity. Am J Med Genet 1999; 89: 210–217.
1270. Brantley K, Gao T, McPhaul MJ. Genetic alterations of androgen receptor function. In: Jameson JL ed. Hormone Resistance Syndromes. Totowa, NJ: Humana Press, 1999: 209–232.
1271. Morris JM, Mahesh VB. Further observations on the syndrome,

1458. Bartone FF, Huseman CA, Maizels M, et al. Pitfalls in using human chorionic gonadotropin (hCG) stimulation test to diagnose anorchia. J Urol 1984; 132:563–567.
1459. Dunkel L, Sümes MA, Bremner WJ. Reduced inhibin and elevated gonadotropin levels in early pubertal boys with testicular defects. Pediatr Res 1993; 33:514–518.
1460. Byrd W, Bennett MJ, Carr BR, Dong Y, Wians F, Rainey W. Regulation of biologically active dimeric inhibin A and B from infancy to adulthood in the male. J Clin Endocrinol Metab 1998; 83:2849–2854.
1461. Kubini K, Zachmann M, Albers N, Hiort O, Bettendorf M, Wolfle J, Bidlingmaier F, Klingmuller D. Basal inhibin B and the testosterone response to human chorionic gonadotropin correlate in prepubertal boys. J Clin Endocrinol Metab 2000; 85: 134–138.
1462. Cendron M, Schned AR, Ellsworth PI. Histological evaluation of the testicular nubbin in the vanishing testis syndrome. J Urol 1998; 160: 1161–1162.
1463. Spires SE, Woolums CS, Pulito AR, et al. Testicular regression syndrome: a clinical and pathologic study of 11 cases. Arch Pathol Lab Med 2000; 124: 694–698.
1464. Gong M, Geary ES, Shortcliffe LM. Testicular torsion with contralateral vanishing testis. Urology 1996; 48:306–307.
1465. Belman AB, Rushton HG. Is the vanished testis always a scrotal event? BJU Int 2001; 87: 480–483.
1466. Cate RL, Mattaliano RJ, Hession C, et al. Isolation of the bovine and human genes for müllerian inhibiting substance and expression of the human gene in animal cells. Cell 1986; 45: 685–689.
1467. MacLaughlin DT, Epstein J, Donahoe PK. Bioassay, purification, cloning, and expression of müllerian inhibiting substance. Methods in Enzymology 1991; 198:358–369.
1468. Baarends WM, van Helmond MJ, Post M, et al. A novel member of the transmembrane serine/threonine kinase receptor family is specifically expressed in the gonads and in mesenchymal cells adjacent to the müllerian duct. Development 1994; 120: 189–197.
1469. Josso N, diClemente N. Serine/threonine kinase receptors and ligands. Curr Opin Genet Dev 1997; 7:371–377.
1470. Brook CGD, Wagner H, Zachmann M, et al. Familial occurrence of persistent müllerian structures in otherwise normal males. Br Med J 1973; 1:771–773.
1471. Josso N, Fekete C, Cachin O, et al. Persistence of müllerian ducts in male pseudohermaphroditism, and its relationship to cryptorchidism. Clin Endocrinol 1983; 19:247–258.
1472. Guerrier D, Tran D, Vanderwinden JM, et al. The persistent müllerian duct syndrome: a molecular approach. J Clin Endocrinol Metab 1989; 68:46–52.
1473. Loeff D, Imbeaud S, Reyes HM, et al. Surgical and genetic aspects of persistent müllerian duct syndrome. J Pediatr Surg 1994; 29:61–65.
1474. Imbeaud S, Carre-Eusebe D, Rey R, Belville C, Josso N, Picard JY. Molecular genetics of the persistent mullerian duct syndrome: a study of 19 families. Hum Mol Genet 1994; 3:125–131.
1475. Taguchi O, Cunha GR, Lawrence WD, et al. Timing and irreversibility of müllerian duct inhibition in the embryonic reproductive tract of the human male. Dev Biol 1984; 106:394–398.
1476. Fuqua JS, Sher ES, Perlman EJ, et al. Abnormal gonadal differentiation in two subjects with ambiguous genitalia, Müllerian structures, and normally developed testes: evidence for a defect in gonadal ridge development. Hum Genet 1996; 97:506–511.
1477. Knebelmann B, Boussin L, Guerrier D, et al. Anti-Müllerian hormone Bruxelles: a nonsense mutation associated with the persistent Müllerian duct syndrome. Proc Natl Acad Sci USA 1991; 88:3767–3771.
1478. Imbeaud S, Belville C, Messika-Zeitoun L, et al. A 27 base pair deletion of the antimüllerian type II receptor gene is the most common cause of the persistent müllerian duct syndrome. Hum Mol Genet 1996; 5:1269–1277.
1479. Imbeaud S, Carre-Eusebe D, Rey R, et al. Molecular genetics of the persistent müllerian duct syndrome: a study of 19 families. Hum Mol Genet 1994; 3:125–131.
1480. Messika-Zeitoun L, Gouedard L, Belville C, et al. Autosomal recessive segregation of a truncating mutation of anti-Mullerian type II receptor in a family affected by the persistent Mullerian duct syndrome contrasts with its dominant negative activity in vitro. J Clin Endocrinol Metab 2001; 86:4390–4397.
1481. Belville C, Josso N, Picard JY. Persistence of Müllerian derivatives in males. Am J Med Genet 1999; 89:218–223.
1482. Imbeaud S, Faure E, Lamarre I, et al. Insensitivity to antimüllerian hormone due to a mutation in the human antimüllerian hormone receptor. Nat Genet 1995; 11:382–388.
1483. Imbeaud S, Rey R, Berta P, Chaussain JL, Wit JM, et al. Testicular degeneration in three patients with the persistent mullerian duct syndrome. Eur J Pediatr 1995; 154:187–190.
1484. Courrier R, Jost A. Intersexualité totale provoqué par la pregneninolone au cours de la grossesse. C R Soc Biol (Paris) 1942; 136:395–396.
1485. Aarskog D. Maternal progestins as a possible cause of hypospadias. N Engl J Med 1979; 300:75–78.
1486. Sweet RA, Schrott HG, Kurland R, et al. Study of the incidence of hypospadias in Rochester, Minnesota, 1940–1970, and a case control comparison of possible etiologic factors. Mayo Clin Proc 1974; 49:52–58.
1487. Lorber CA, Cassidy SB, Engel E. Is there an embryofetal exogenous sex steroid exposure syndrome (EFESSES)? Fertil Steril 1979; 31:21–24.
1488. Czezel A, Toth J. Correlation between the birth prevalence of hypospadias and parental subfertility. Teratology 1990; 41:167–172.
1489. Voight W, Hsia SL. Further studies on testosterone 5-alpha-reductase of human skin: structural features of steroid inhibitors. J Biol Chem 1973; 248:4280–4285.
1490. Kaplan NM. Male pseudohermaphrodism: report of a case, with observations on pathogenesis. N Engl J Med 1959; 261:641–644.
1491. Henderson BE, Benton B, Cosgrove M, et al. Urogenital tract abnormalities in sons of women treated with diethylstilbestrol. Pediatrics 1976; 58:505–507.
1492. Driscoll SG, Taylor SH. Effects of prenatal maternal estrogen on the male urogenital system. Obstet Gynecol 1980; 56:537–542.
1493. Penny R. The effect of DES on male offspring. West J Med 1982; 136:329–330.
1494. Sharpe RM, Skakkebaek NE. Are oestrogens involved in falling sperm counts and disorders of the male reproductive tract? Lancet 1993; 341:1392–1395.
1495. Paulozzi LJ, Erickson JD, Jackson RJ. Hypospadias trends in two US surveillance systems. Pediatrics 1997; 100:831–834.
1496. Skakkebaek NE, Rajpert-De Meyts E, Main KM. Testicular dysgenesis syndrome: an increasingly common developmental disorder with environmental aspects. Hum Reprod 2001; 16: 972–978.
1497. Majdic G, Sharpe RM, O'Shaughnessy, et al. Expression of cytochrome P450 17α-hydroxylase/17,20 lyase in fetal rat testes is reduced by maternal exposure to exogenous estrogens. Endocrinology 1996; 137:1063–1070.
1498. McLachlan JA, Newbold RR, Burow ME, Li SF. From malformations to molecular mechanisms in the male: three decades of research on endocrine disrupters. APMIS 2001; 109:263–272.
1499. Kelce WR, Stone CR, Laws SC, et al. Persistent DDT metabolite *p,p*NDDE is a potent androgen receptor antagonist. Nature 1995; 375:581–585.
1499a. Morel Y, Rey R, Teinturier C, Nicolino M, et al. Aetiological diagnosis of male sex ambiguity: A collaborative study. Eur J Pediatr 2002; 161:49–59.
1499b. Francois I, van Helvoirt M, de Zegher F. Male pseudohermaphroditism related to complications at conception, in early pregnancy or in prenatal growth. Horm Res 1999; 51:91–95.
1499c. Mendonca BB, Billerbeck AE, de Zegher F. Nongenetic male pseudohermaphroditism and reduced prenatal growth. N Engl J Med 2001; 345:1135.
1499d. Baskin LS, Erol A, Jegatheesan P, Li Y, Liu W, Cunha GR. Urethral seam formation and hypospadias. Cell Tissue Res 2001; 305:379–387.
1500. Belman AB. Hypospadias and other urethral abnormalities. In: Kelalis PP, King LR, Belman AB, eds. Clinical Pediatric Urology. 3rd ed, Vol 1. Philadelphia: WB Saunders, 1992:619–663.
1501. Bauer SB, Relik AB, Colodny AA. Genetic aspects of hypospadias. Urol Clin North Am 1981; 8:559.
1502. Harris EL, Beaty TH. Segregation analysis of hypospadias: a

reanalysis of published pedigree data. Am J Med Genet 1993; 45:420–425.
1503. Baskin LS, Himes K, Colborn T. Hypospadias and endocrine disruption: is there a connection? Environ Health Perspect 2001; 109:1175–1183.
1504. Aarskog D. Clinical and cytogenetic studies in hypospadias. Acta Paediatr Scand 1970; 203(Suppl):1–62.
1505. Bauer SB, Relik AB, Colodny AA. Genetic aspects of hypospadias. Urol Clin North Am 1981; 8:559.
1506. Svensson J, Snochowski M. Androgen receptor levels in preputial skin from boys with hypospadias. J Clin Endocrinol Metab 1979; 49:340–345.
1507. Warne GL, Gyorski S, Risibridger GP, et al. Fibroblast studies on clinical androgen insensitivity. J Steroid Biochem 1983; 18: 583–586.
1508. Keenan BS, McNeel RL, Gonzales ET. Abnormality of intracellular 5α-dihydrotestosterone binding in simple hypospadias: studies on equilibrium steroid binding in sonicates of genital skin fibroblasts. Pediatr Res 1984; 18:216–220.
1509. Allera A, Herbst MA, Griffin JE, et al. Mutations of the androgen receptor coding sequence are infrequent in patients with isolated hypospadias. J Clin Endocrinol Metab 1995; 80:2697–2699.
1510. Sutherland RW, Wiener JS, Hicks JP, et al. Androgen receptor gene mutations are rarely associated with isolated penile hypospadias. J Urol 1996; 156:828–831.
1511. Robin NH, Feldman GJ, Aronson AL, et al. Opitz syndrome is genetically heterogenous with one locus on Xp22, and a second locus on 22q11.2. Nat Genet 1995; 11:459–461.
1512. Mortlock DP, Innis JW. Mutation of HOXA13 in hand-foot-genital syndrome. Nat Genet 1997; 15:179–180.
1513. Sandberg DE, Meyer-Bahlburg HFL, Yager TJ, et al. Gender development in boys born with hypospadias. Psychoneuroendocrinology 1995; 20:693–709.
1513a. Kaefer M, Diamond D, Hendren WH, et al. The incidence of intersexuality in children with cryptorchidism and hypospadias: stratification based on gonadal palpability and meatal position. J Urol 1999; 162:1003–1007.
1514. Walsh PC, Wilson JD, Allen TD, et al. Clinical and endocrinological evaluation of patients with congenital microphallus. J Urol 1978; 120:90–95.
1515. Burstein S, Grumbach MM, Kaplan SL. Early determination of androgen-responsiveness is important in the management of microphallus. Lancet 1979; 2:983–986.
1516. Lovinger RD, Kaplan SL, Grumbach MM. Congenital hypopituitarism associated with neonatal hypoglycemia and microphallus: four cases secondary to hypothalamic hormone deficiencies. J Pediatr 1975; 87:1171–1181.
1517. Rozanski TA, Bloom DA. The undescended testis: theory and management. Urol Clin North Am 1995; 22:107–118.
1518. Hadziselimovic F. Cryptorchidism: the disease and its management. Acta Urol Belg 1995; 63:83–88.
1519. Lee PA. Consequence of cryptorchidism: relationship to etiology and treatment. Curr Probl Pediatr 1995; 25:232–236.
1520. Cortes D, Thorup JM, Beck BL. Quantitative histology of germ cells in the undescended testes of human fetuses, neonates and infants. J Urol 1995; 154:1188–1192.
1520a. Meyer WJ III, Keenan BS, De Lacorda L, et al. Familial male pseudohermaphrodism with normal Leydig cell function at puberty. J Clin Endocrinol Metab 1978; 49:593–603.
1521. Griffin JE, Edwards C, Madden JD, et al. Congenital absence of the vagina: the Mayer-Rokitansky-Küster-Hauser syndrome. Ann Intern Med 1976; 85:224–236.
1522. Neinstein LS, Castle G. Congenital absence of the vagina. Am J Dis Child 1983; 137:671.
1523. Ross GT, van de Wiele RL. The ovaries. In: Williams RH, ed. Textbook of Endocrinology. 5th ed. Philadelphia: WB Saunders, 1974: 368–422.
1524. Fraser ID, Baird DT, Hobson BM, et al. Cyclical ovarian function in women with congenital absence of the uterus and vagina. J Clin Endocrinol Metab 1973; 36:634–637.
1525. Strubbe EH, Cremers CW, Dikkers FG, Willemsen WN. Hearing loss and the Mayer-Rokitansky-Khster-Hauser syndrome. Am J Otol 1994; 15:431–436.
1526. Simpson JL. Genetics of the female reproductive ducts. Am J Med Genet 1999; 89:224–239.
1527. Strubbe EH, Cremers CW, Willemsen WN, et al. The Mayer-Rokitansky-Khster-Hauser (MRKH) syndrome without and with associated features: two separate entities? Clin Dysmorphol 1994; 3:192–199.
1528. Strubbe EH, Lemmens JA, Thijn CJ, et al. Spinal abnormalities and the atypical form of the Mayer-Rokitansky-Kuster-Hauser syndrome. Skeletal Radiol 1992; 21:459–462.
1529. Pinsky L. A community of human malformation syndromes involving the müllerian ducts, distal extremities, urinary tract and ears. Teratology 1974; 9:65–79.
1530. Michels VV, Caskey TC. Müllerian aplasia with hypoplastic thumbs: two case reports. Int J Gynaecol Obstet 1979; 17:6–10.
1531. Duncan PA, Shapiro LR, Stangel JJ, et al. The MURCS association: müllerian duct aplasia, renal aplasia, and cervico-thoracic somite dysplasia. J Pediatr 1979; 95:399–402.
1532. Haskins JL, Gysler M, Cowell CA. Anatomical amenorrhea: the problems of congenital vaginal agenesis and its surgical correction. Pediatr Clin North Am 1981; 28:345–354.
1533. Fliegner JR, Pepperell RJ. Management of vaginal agenesis with a functioning uterus: is hysterectomy advisable? Aust N Z J Obstet Gynecol 1994; 34:467–470.
1534. Hendren WH, Atala A. Use of bowel for vaginal reconstruction. J Urol 1994; 152:752–755.
1535. Hensle TW, Reiley EA. Vaginal replacement in children and young adults. J Urol 1998; 159:1035–1038.
1536. Hecker BR, McGuire LS. Psychosocial function in women treated for vaginal agenesis. Am J Obstet Gynecol 1977; 129: 543–547.
1537. Meyer-Bahlburg HF. Gender assignment and reassignment in 46,XY pseudohermaphroditism and related conditions. J Clin Endocrinol Metab 1999; 84:3455–3458.
1538. Reiner W. To be male or female–that is the question. Arch Pediatr Adolesc Med 1997; 151:224–225.
1539. Bradley SJ, Oliver GD, Chernick AB, Zucker KJ. Experiment of nurture: ablatio penis at 2 months, sex reassignment at 7 months, and a psychosexual follow-up in young adulthood. Pediatrics 1998; 102:e9 (E91–E95).
1540. Kuhnle U, Krahl W. The impact of culture on sex assignment and gender development in intersex patients. Perspect Biol Med 2002; 45:85–103.
1541. Warne GL, Zajac JD. Disorders of sexual differentiation. Endocrinol Metab Clin North Am 1998; 27:945–967.
1542. Zucker KJ. Intersexuality and gender identity differentiation. J Pediatr Adolesc Gynecol 2002; 15:3–13.
1543. Dittmann RW. Ambiguous genitalia, gender-identity problems, and sex reassignment. J Sex Marital Ther 1998; 24:255–271.
1544. Lee PA. Should we change our approach to ambiguous genitalia? Endocrinologist 2001; 11:118–123.
1545. Daaboul J, Frader J. Ethics and the management of the patient with intersex: a middle way. J Pediatr Endocrinol Metab 2001; 14:1575–1583.
1546. Dreger AD. Hermaphrodites and the Medical Invention of Sex. Cambridge: Harvard University, 1998.
1547. Taha SA. Male pseudohermaphroditism: factors determining the gender of rearing in Saudi Arabia. Urology 1994; 43:370–374.
1548. Forest MG. Pattern of the response of testosterone and its precursors to human chorionic gonadotropin stimulation in relation to age in infants and children. J Clin Endocrinol Metab 1979; 49:132–137.
1549. Aaronson IA. Micropenis: medical and surgical implications. J Urol 1994; 152:4–14.
1550. McMahon DR, Kramer SA, Husmann DA. Micropenis: does early treatment with testosterone do more harm than good? J Urol 1995; 154:825–829.
1551. Sutherland RS, Kogan BA, Baskin LS, et al. The effect of prepubertal androgen exposure on adult penile length. J Urol 1996; 156:783–787.
1552. Howe EG, Dreger AD, Groveman SA, et al. Special Issue: Intersexuality. J Clin Ethics 1998; 9:337–430.
1553. Lim YJ, Batch JA, Warne GL. Adrenal 21-hydroxylase deficiency in childhood: 25 years' experience. J Paediatr Child Health 1995; 31:222–227.
1554. Krege S, Walz KH, Hauffa BP, Korner I, Rubben H. Long-term follow-up of female patients with congenital adrenal hyperplasia from 21-hydroxylase deficiency, with special emphasis on the results of vaginoplasty. BJU Int 2000; 86:253–259.

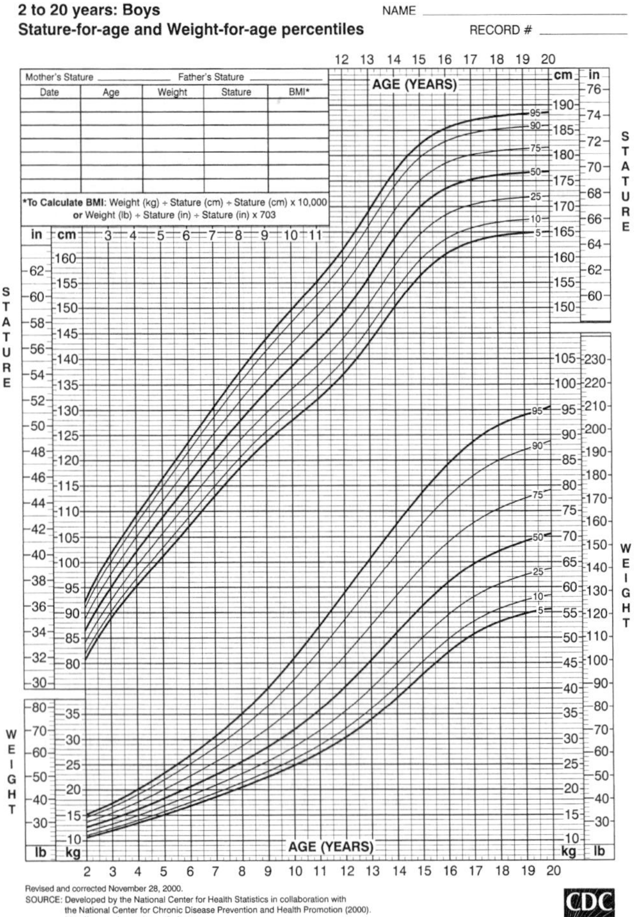

Figure 23–10. Stature-for-age and weight-for-age percentiles for boys (2 to 20 years). Developed by the National Center for Health Statistics in collaboration with the National Center for Chronic Disease Prevention and Health Promotion (2000). *http://www.cdc.gov/growthcharts*

velopment,[37] was developed by Bayley and Pinneau[42] and relies on bone age, height, and a semiquantitative allowance for chronologic age (Table 23–1). The system of Tanner and colleagues[38, 43] employs height; bone age; chronologic age; height and bone age increments during puberty in the previous year; and menarchal status. Roche and associates[44] employ the combination of height, bone age, chronologic age, midparental height, and weight. Further, attempts have been made to calculate final height predictions without requiring the use of skeletal age[45, 46] by using multiple regression analyses with available data such as height, weight, birth measurements, and midparental stature. All of these systems are, by nature, empirical and are not absolute predictors. The more advanced the bone age, the greater the accuracy of the adult height prediction because a more advanced bone age places a patient closer to final height.

All methods of predicting adult height are based on data from normal children, and none has been documented to be accurate in children with growth abnormalities. For this kind of precision, it would be necessary to develop disease-specific (e.g., achondroplasia, Turner's syndrome) atlases of skeletal maturation.

Parental Target Height

Because genetic factors are important determinants of growth and height potential, it is useful to assess a patient's stature relative to that of siblings and parents. Tanner and associates developed a growth chart modifying the heights of children, aged 2 to 9 years, by the midparental height.[47] Further, the child's predicted adult height (see earlier) may be related to a *parental target height*, or the mean parental height with the addition or subtraction of 6.5 cm for boys and girls, respectively. The two standard deviation (2 SD) range for this calculated parental target height is about ± 10 cm, so that calculated target heights, like predicted adult heights, are approximations.

Recent statistical reassessment shows a tendency for regression to the mean of the children's height as related to the midparental target height.[48] Failure to realize this may lead to inappropriately using short parental height as an explanation for marked short stature in a child. Nevertheless, when a child's growth pattern clearly deviates from that of parents or siblings, the possibility of underlying pathology should be considered. Although it is certainly important to measure the heights of parents and siblings, rather than accept their statural claims, one must recall as well that it is not always possible to know the heights of the true biologic parents.

ENDOCRINE REGULATION OF GROWTH

The Pituitary Gland

The concept of the pituitary as a "master gland," controlling the endocrine activities of the body, has been replaced by recognition of the importance of the brain and, particularly, the hypothalamus in regulating hormonal production and secretion. Nevertheless, the pituitary gland is central to understanding the regulation of growth.

Embryologically, the pituitary gland is formed from two distinct sources[49]: Rathke's pouch, a diverticulum of the primitive oral cavity (stomodeal ectoderm), gives rise to the adenohypophysis. The neurohypophysis (posterior pituitary) originates in the neural ectoderm of the floor of the forebrain, which also develops into the third ventricle. The adenohypophysis normally constitutes 80% of the weight of the pituitary and consists of anterior, intermediate, and infundibular lobes. In humans, the anterior lobe is the largest component and houses the most hormone-producing cells.

Rathke's pouch, the origin of the adenohypophysis, can be identified in the 3-mm embryo during the 3rd week of pregnancy. GH-producing cells can be found in the adenohypophysis by 9 weeks of gestation.[50] Vascular connections between the anterior lobe of the pituitary and the hypothalamus develop about this time,[51, 52] although hormone production can occur in the pituitary in the absence of connections with the hypothalamus. Somatotrophs can frequently be demonstrated in the pituitary in anencephalic newborns.[53] Nevertheless, the initiation of development of the anterior pituitary is probably dependent on responsiveness of the oral ectoderm to inducing factors from the ventral diencephalon (Fig. 23–14).[54–60]

A complex orchestration of temporally sequenced and geographically restricted expression of multiple extracellular signaling peptides and intracellular transcription factors regulates this developmental process.[60–62] The developing pituitary gland and hypothalamus are in close anatomic juxtaposition, and their embryonic development is likely to be codependent. Some of the diencephalic factors that have been identified to be critical in formation and patterning of Rathke's pouch, which, in the mouse, is initiated on embryonic day 8 (e8) are bone morphogenetic proteins 4 and 2 (BMP-4/2), Wnt5a, and fibroblast growth factor 8 (FGF-8).[54, 60, 63] The dorsal neuro-

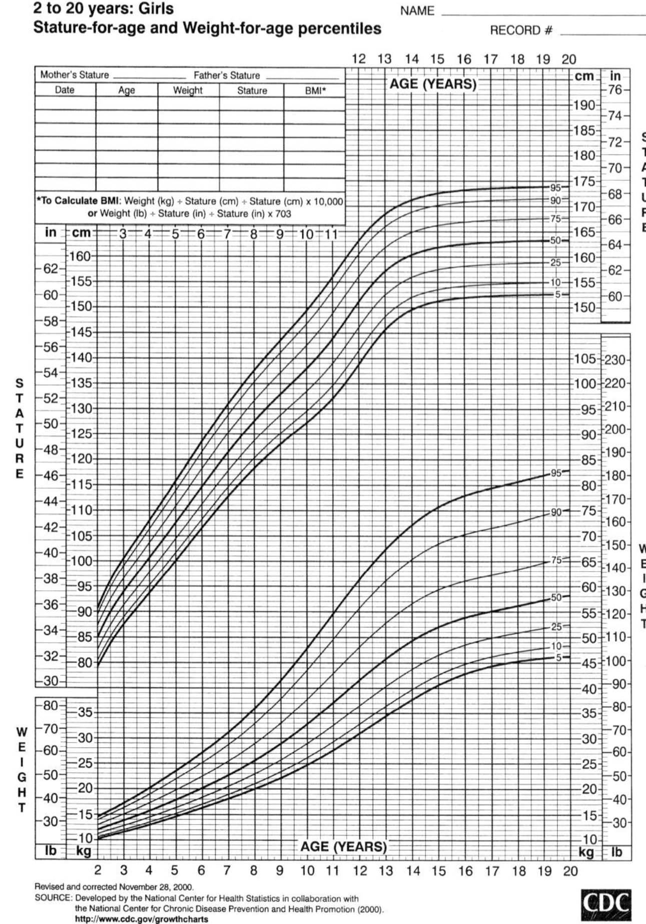

Figure 23–11. Stature-for-age and weight-for-age percentiles for girls (2 to 20 years). Developed by the National Center for Health Statistics in collaboration with the National Center for Chronic Disease Prevention and Health Promotion (2000). *http://www.cdc.gov/growthcharts*

epithelial signal, BMP-4, is needed for "organ commitment" of the pituitary, whereas a BMP-2 (ventral) and FGF-8 (dorsal) gradient determines pituitary cell phenotypes (i.e., gonadotrophs and the Pit-1–dependent lines, somatotrophs, lactotrophs, and thyrotrophs [ventral] and melanotrophs and corticotrophs [dorsal]).[54, 55, 57, 60] It seems that reciprocal interaction of at least two transcription factors, Pit-1 and GATA-2, are important in implementing the cell-determination signals of BMP-2 and FGF-8.[54, 61]

Explant studies in the mouse have demonstrated that if Rathke's pouch is removed from the oral ectoderm on e10.5 and incubated in appropriate culture medium, differentiation of each of the pituitary cell types continues, indicating that by that point, organogenesis of the anterior pituitary is no longer dependent on hypothalamic signals,[60] although such signals may remain critically involved in pituitary hormone production.

A number of pituitary-specific transcription factors are involved in the determination of pituitary cell lineages and cell-specific expression of anterior pituitary hormones[57, 58, 60, 64–66] To date, defects in several homeodomain transcription factors shown to be involved in human anterior pituitary development and differentiation have now been associated with various combinations of pituitary hormone deficiencies (see Fig. 23–14 and Table 23–5). Because additional gene defects have been implicated in abnormal murine pituitary development, it seems likely that the number of human genetic defects will expand.

In the adult, the mean pituitary size is 13 × 9 × 6 mm.[67] The mean weight is 600 mg (range, 400 to 900 mg), is slightly greater in women than in men, and increases during pregnancy.[68] In the newborn, pituitary weight averages about 100 mg. Normally, the pituitary resides in the sella turcica, immediately above and partially surrounded by the sphenoid bone. The volume of the sella turcica is a good index of pituitary size and may be reduced in the child with pituitary hypoplasia[69] or increased in some with *PROP1* defects (see Table 23–5). The anatomic proximity between the optic chiasm and the pituitary is important because hypoplasia of the optic chiasm may occur together with hypothalamic/pituitary dysfunction in the syndrome of septo-optic dysplasia.[70] Children with congenital blindness or nystagmus should be monitored carefully for hypopituitarism, and suprasellar growth of a pituitary tumor may initially manifest with visual complaints or evidence of decreases in peripheral vision.

The existence of a portal circulatory system within the pituitary gland is critical for normal pituitary function. The blood supply of the pituitary is shown in Figure 23–15.[51, 52] Hypothalamic peptides, produced in neurons that terminate in the infundibulum, enter the primary plexus of the hypophyseal portal circulation and are transported via the hypophyseal portal veins to the capillaries of the anterior pituitary. This portal system thus provides a means of communication between the neurons of the hypothalamus and the anterior pituitary.

Growth Hormone

Chemistry

Human GH is produced as a single chain, 191–amino acid, 22-kd protein (Fig. 23–16).[71, 72] It is not glycosylated, but it does contain two intramolecular disulfide bonds. GH shares sequence homology with prolactin, chorionic somatomammotropin (CS) (placental lactogen), and a 22-kd GH variant (GH-V) secreted only by the placenta[73] that differs from pituitary GH by 13 amino acids. The genes for these proteins have probably evolved from a common ancestral gene, even though the genes are located on different chromosomes (chromosome 6 for prolactin, chromosome 17 for GH).[74] The genes for GH, prolactin, and placental lactogen share a common structural organization, with four introns separating five exons. In fact, the GH subfamily contains five members, whose genes are located on a 78-kb section of chromosome 17; the 5′ to 3′ order of the genes are GH, a CS pseudogene, CS-A, GH-V, and CS-B.[75]

Normally, about 75% of GH produced by the pituitary is of the mature, 22-kd form. Alternative splicing of the second codon results in deletion of amino acids 32 to 46, yielding a 20-kd form, which normally accounts for 5% to 10% of pituitary GH.[74, 76] The remainder of pituitary GH includes desamidated and *N*-acetylated forms and various GH oligomers.

Secretion

The pulsatile pattern characteristic of GH secretion largely reflects the interplay of two hypothalamic regulatory peptides, growth hormone–releasing hormone (GHRH)[77, 78] and somatostatin (somatotropin release–inhibiting factor [SRIF]),[79] with presumed modulation by putative other GH-releasing factors.[80] GHRH activity is species-specific, presumably reflecting the specificity of binding to a G protein–related receptor on the pituitary somatotrophs. Regulation of GH production by GHRH is mediated largely at the level of transcription and is enhanced by increases in intracellular cyclic adenine monophosphate (cAMP) levels.

The GHRH receptor is a member of the G protein–coupled receptor family B-III, also called the *secretin family*, and has partial sequence identity with receptors for vasoactive in-

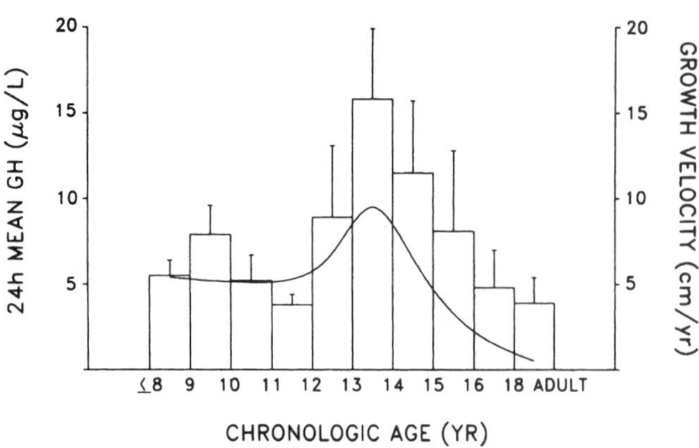

Figure 23–17. Relation between 24-hour (24h) mean growth hormone (GH) levels and age in boys and men. *Bars* represent values for the 24-hour mean (± SE) levels of GH (left axis) from 60 24-hour GH profiles of healthy boys and men subdivided according to chronologic age. An idealized growth velocity curve reproduced from the 50th percentile values for whole-year height velocity of North American boys (9) is superimposed. (From Martha PM Jr, Rogol AD, Veldhuis JD, et al. Alterations in the pulsatile properties of circulating growth hormone concentrations during puberty in boys. J Clin Endocrinol Metab 1989; 69:563–570.)

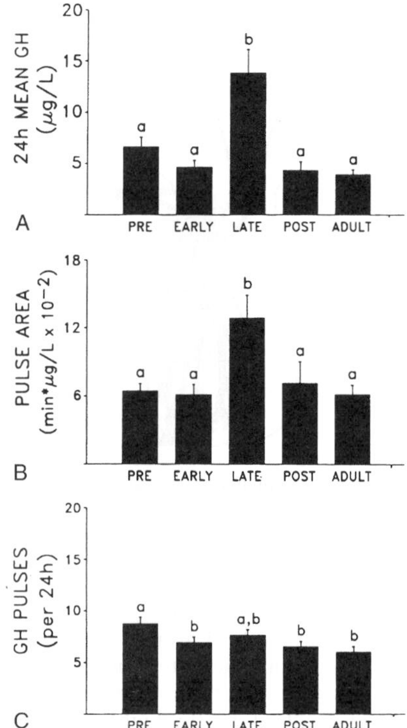

Figure 23–18. *A*, The mean (± SE) 24-hour (24h) levels of growth hormone (GH) for groups of normal boys at varied stages of pubertal maturation. *B*, The mean (± SE) area under the GH concentration versus time curve for individual GH pulses, as identified by the Cluster pulse detection algorithm. *C*, The number of GH pulses (± SE), as detected by the Cluster algorithm, in the 24-hour GH concentration profiles for boys in each of the pubertal study groups. *Note:* The mean 24-hour GH concentration changes are largely mediated by changes in the amount of GH secreted per pulse rather than the frequency of pulses. In each panel, *bars* bearing the same letter are statistically indistinguishable. (From Martha PM Jr, Rogol AD, Veldhuis JD, et al. Alterations in the pulsatile properties of circulating growth hormone concentrations during puberty in boys. J Clin Endocrinol Metab 1989; 69:563–570.)

entropy, and cosine regression analysis, Veldhuis and associates[136, 167] carefully evaluated intensive GH sampling data, derived from measurements in sensitive GH assays, in prepubertal and pubertal boys and girls. In addition to the amplified secretory burst mass originating from jointly increased GH pulse amplitude and duration, they found that sex steroids selectively affected facets of GH neurosecretory control; estrogen increases basal GH secretion rate and irregularity of GH release patterns, whereas testosterone stimulates greater GH secretory burst mass and IGF-I concentrations.

Obesity is characterized by markedly decreased GH production, reflected by nearly a marked decrease in number of GH secretory bursts and of half-life duration.[159, 170] Obesity in childhood and adolescence, similarly, is characterized by decreased GH production but normal IGF and increased GHBP levels and often increased linear growth.[170] The hyperinsulinism associated with obesity causes lowered IGF-binding protein (IGFBP)-1 and, perhaps, higher free IGF-I levels.[171] Endogenous GH secretion and levels achieved during provocative tests in these obese subjects[165] approximate the diagnostic range of GHD. Fasting increases both the number and amplitude of GH secretory bursts, presumably reflecting decreased somatostatin secretion and enhanced GHRH release while lowering GHBP concentrations. Rapid changes in levels of IGFBPs in response to altered nutrition and changes of insulin levels may modify the effect of IGF-I on its negative feedback and effector sites.[123, 170] Body mass also influences GH production in normal prepubertal and pubertal children and adults.[127, 134, 172]

Growth Hormone Receptor/Growth Hormone–Binding Protein

Leung and colleagues[173] cloned both the rabbit and human complementary DNAs (cDNAs) for the GHR. Each contains an open reading frame of 638 amino acids and encodes a mature receptor of 620 amino acids and a predicted molecular

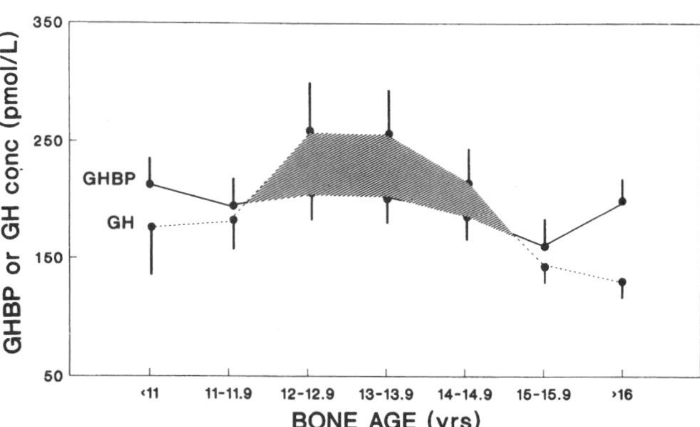

Figure 23–19. Levels of growth hormone (GH) and growth hormone–binding protein (GHBP) measured in normal pubertal boys throughout adolescence. GHBP levels do not significantly change during puberty, but there is a significant increment of GH production and, therefore, of GH levels during this same time. These data suggest that there may be greater amounts of "free GH" during this period, leading to greater production of insulin-like growth factor I. (Data from Martha PM Jr, et al. J Clin Endocrinol Metab 1989; 69:563–570; and Martha PM Jr, et al. J Clin Endocrinol Metab 1991; 73:175–181.)

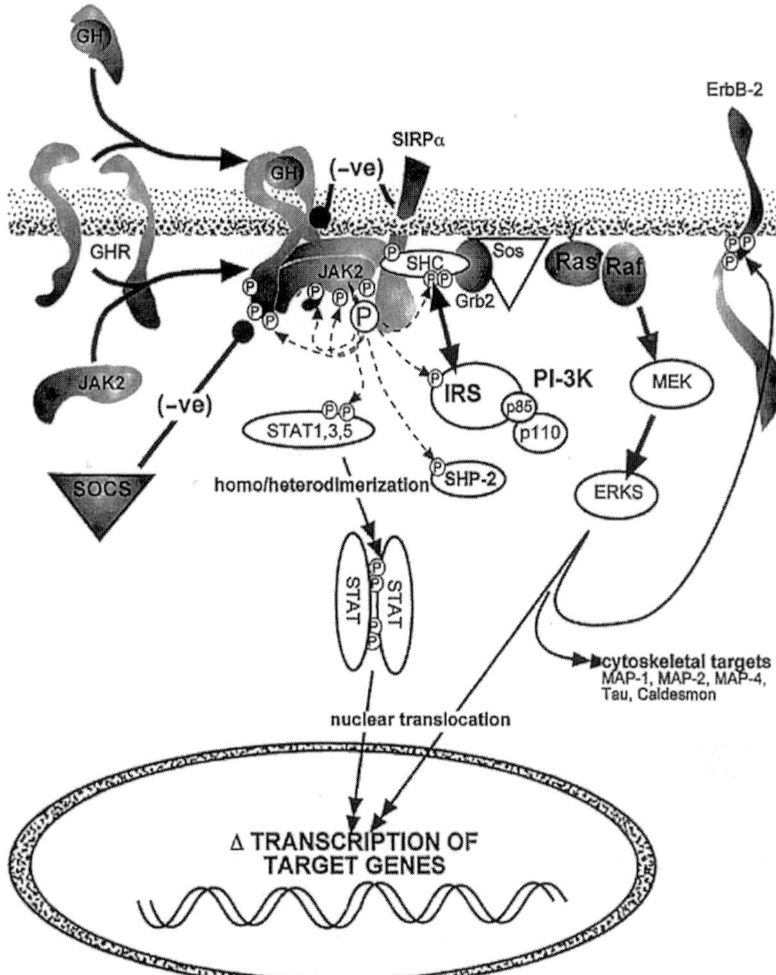

Figure 23–20. A model depicting intracellular signaling intermediates induced by binding of growth hormone (GH) with the GH receptor (GHR). ERKS, extracellular signal-regulated kinase; Grb, growth factor receptor–binding protein; JAK, Janus kinase; IRS, insulin receptor substrate; MAP, mitogen-activated protein kinase; MEK, MAPK-ERK kinase; PKC, protein kinase C; SHP-2, protein tyrosine phosphatase; SOCS, suppressors of cytokine signaling; STAT, signal transducer and activator of transcription. (From Le Roith D, Bondy C, Yakar S, et al. The somatomedin hypothesis. Endocr Rev 2001; 22:53–74. © The Endocrine Society.)

weight of 70 kd before glycosylation. There are three domains: (1) an extracellular, hormone-binding domain, (2) a single membrane-spanning domain, and (3) a cytoplasmic domain.

In humans, the most important circulating GH-binding protein appears to be derived from proteolytic cleavage of the extracellular domain of the receptor.[174] In the mouse[175, 176] and rat,[177] however, there are multiple transcripts for the GHR; the larger, 3.4 to 4.8 kb, transcript codes for the intact receptor and the 1.2 to 1.9 kb transcript codes for the soluble GHBP.

The coding and 3′ untranslated regions of the human GHR are encoded by nine exons, numbered 2 to 10.[178, 179] The gene for the human GHR is located on chromosome 5p13.1-p12, where it spans more than 87 kb.[180] The GHR shows sequence homology with the prolactin receptor and with receptors for interleukin (IL)-2, IL-3, IL-4, IL-6, and IL-7, as well as receptors for erythropoietin, granulocyte-macrophage colony-stimulating factor (GM-CSF), and interferon.[178] The GHR is a member of the class 1 hematopoietic cytokine family.[181] Examination of the crystal structure of the GH/GHR complex revealed that the complex consists of one molecule of GH bound to two GHR molecules, indicating a GH-induced receptor dimerization, which is necessary for GH action.[182]

After binding to its receptor, GH stimulates phosphorylation of a protein with an apparent molecular weight ratio of 120 kd.[183] Although it was originally suspected that the GHR might be capable of autophosphorylation, it is now apparent that the major tyrosine-phosphorylated protein is associated with the receptor rather than being the receptor itself. JAK2 has been recently identified as the critical GHR–associated tyrosine kinase.[184] The presumed sequence of steps in GH action is shown in Figure 23–20:

1. Binding of GH to the membrane-associated GHR.
2. Sequential dimerization of the GHR through binding to each of two specific sites on GH.
3. Interaction of the GHR with JAK2.
4. Tyrosine phosphorylation of both JAK2 and the GHR.
5. Changes in cytoplasmic and nuclear protein phosphorylation and dephosphorylation.
6. Stimulation of target gene transcription.

GH-dependent and JAK2-dependent phosphorylation and activation have been demonstrated for many cytoplasmic signaling molecules that, after forming homodimers or heterodimers, translocate into the nucleus, bind DNA, and activate transcription.[185–187] How all of these seemingly redundant pathways interact to mediate the various anabolic and metabolic actions of GH remains to be elucidated.

The major GHBP in human plasma binds GH with high specificity and affinity but with relatively low capacity, because about 45% of circulating GH is bound.[153, 188–191] The GHBP is, in essence, the extracellular domain of the GHR and has an apparent molecular weight ratio of approximately 55 kd. An additional GHBP, not related to the GHR, binds approximately 5% to 10% of circulating GH with lower affinity.[153, 191] GHBP prolongs the half-life of GH, presumably by impairing its glomerular filtration, and modulates its binding to the GHR. In general, GHBP levels reflect GHR levels and activity; that is, low levels are associated with states of *growth hormone insensitivity* (GHI).[153, 191] In the rapidly growing child, however, levels of GHBP are quite low.[192, 193] Initial assays for GHBP involved incubation of serum with [^{125}I]-GH and separation of bound from free radioligand.[153] Carlsson and coworkers[194] have developed a ligand-mediated immunofunctional assay for measurement of GHBP.

Levels of GHBP are low in early life, rise through childhood, and plateau during the pubertal years and adulthood.[152, 191–193] Once puberty is reached, levels are usually constant for a given individual.[152] Impaired nutrition, diabetes mellitus, hypothyroidism, chronic liver disease, and a spectrum of inherited abnormalities of the GHR are associated with low levels of GHBP, whereas obesity, refeeding, early pregnancy, and estrogen treatment can cause elevated levels of GHBP.[153, 191]

A direct correlation exists between GHBP levels and body mass index.[195] Serum GHBP levels correlate inversely with 24-hour GH production[152]; this reciprocal relationship between GH production and GHBP in normal subjects—and in subjects with idiopathic short stature (ISS)[196, 197]—may result from adjustments of GH secretion to accommodate GHR levels that may be genetically determined or modulated by environmental factors such as nutritional status.[195, 198] Assays of serum levels of GHBP are useful in identifying subjects with GH insensitivity due to genetic abnormalities of the GHR.[199, 200] Patients with GHI due to nonreceptor abnormalities, defects of the intracellular domain of the GHR, or inability of the receptor to dimerize may, however, have normal serum levels of GHBP.[169, 201–203]

Inhibition of GH signaling by several members of the GH-inducible suppressors of cytokine signaling (SOCS) family has been reported.[204] The importance of SOCS proteins in controlling growth is demonstrated by the finding of gigantism in SOCS-2 knockout mice.[205] Endotoxin and proinflammatory cytokines, such as IL-1β and tumor necrosis factor α (TNF-α), which can also induce SOCS proteins,[206] produce GHI. SOCS-3 induced by IL-1β and TNF-α or by endotoxin in vivo may play a role in the GHI induced by sepsis.[207] Critically ill patients with septic shock treated with GH had increased mortality,[208] possibly related to induction of GHI in specific tissues as a consequence of endotoxinemia and cytokinemia.

Growth Hormone Actions

According to the somatomedin hypothesis, the anabolic actions of GH are mediated through the IGF peptides.[209, 210] Although this theory is largely true, GH is also capable of inducing effects that are independent of IGF activity. Indeed, the actions of GH and IGF are, on occasion, contradictory, as evident in the diabetogenic actions of GH[211, 212] and the glucose-lowering activity of IGFs. Green and colleagues[213] have attempted to resolve some of these differences in a *dual-effector model*, in which GH stimulates precursor cells, such as prechondrocytes, to differentiate. When differentiated cells or neighboring cells then secrete IGFs, these peptides act as mitogens and stimulate clonal expansion. This hypothesis is based on the ability of IGF peptides to work not only as hormones that are transported through the blood but also as paracrine or autocrine growth factors.

GH has a variety of metabolic actions, some of which appear to be independent of IGF production, such as enhancement of lipolysis,[214] stimulation of amino acid transport in diaphragm[215] and heart,[216] and enhancement of hepatic protein synthesis. Thus, there are multiple sites of GH action, and it is often not entirely clear which of these actions are mediated through the IGF system and which might represent IGF-independent effects of GH.[217] These sites of action include the following:

1. *Epiphysis:* stimulation of epiphyseal growth.
2. *Bone:* stimulation of osteoclast differentiation and activity, stimulation of osteoblast activity, and increase of bone mass by endochondral bone formation.
3. *Adipose tissue:* acute insulin-like effects, followed by increased lipolysis, inhibition of lipoprotein lipase, stimulation of hormone-sensitive lipase, decreased glucose transport, and decreased lipogenesis.
4. *Muscle:* increased amino acid transport, increased nitrogen retention, increased lean tissue, and increased energy expenditure.

The concept of IGF-independent actions of GH is supported by in vivo studies, in which IGF-I cannot duplicate all of the effects of GH, such as nitrogen retention and insulin resistance.[218] The administration of GH for 1 to 3 weeks to calorically restricted normal or obese men results in significant nitrogen retention, although this effect does not persist with prolonged therapy.[219] The effects of GH in normal human aging[220] and in catabolic states[221] are subjects of active investigation.

Insulin-Like Growth Factors

Historical Background

The IGFs (or somatomedins) are a family of peptides that are, in part, GH-dependent and that mediate many of the anabolic and mitogenic actions of GH. Originally identified in 1957 by their ability to stimulate [^{35}S] sulfate incorporation into rat cartilage and termed *sulfation factor*,[209] concurrent investigations indicated that only a component of the insulin-like activity of normal serum could be blocked by the addition of anti-insulin antibodies. The remaining activity, termed *nonsuppressible insulin-like activity* (NSILA), was subsequently demonstrated to contain two soluble, low-molecular-weight (7-kd) forms, named NSILA-I and NSILA-II.[222, 223] A third line of investigation arose from studies by Dulak and Temin[224] on the mitogenic nature of bovine serum; the mitogenic factor was termed *multiplication-stimulating activity* (MSA) and shares metabolic and mitogenic activities with both sulfation factor and NSILA.

In 1972, the restrictive labels of *sulfation factor* and *NSILA* were replaced by the term *somatomedin*.[225] The following criteria for a somatomedin were established:

1. The concentration in serum must be GH-dependent.
2. The factor must possess insulin-like activity in extraskeletal tissues.
3. The factor must promote the incorporation of sulfate into cartilage.
4. The factor must stimulate DNA synthesis and cell multiplication.

Purification yielded two somatomedin peptides: a basic peptide (somatomedin-C) and a neutral peptide (somatomedin-A).[226, 227] In 1978, Rinderknecht and Humbel[228, 229] isolated two active somatomedins from human plasma, and after demonstrating a striking structural resemblance to proinsulin, renamed them *insulin-like growth factors* (IGFs).

IGF Structure and Molecular Biology

IGF-I, a basic peptide of 70 amino acids, correlates with somatomedin-C, and IGF-II is a slightly acidic peptide of 67 amino acids. The two peptides share 45 of 73 possible amino acid positions and have approximately 50% amino acid homology to insulin.[210, 228, 229] Like insulin, both IGFs have A and B chains connected by disulfide bonds. The connecting C-peptide region is 12 amino acids long for IGF-I and 8 amino acids for IGF-II, bearing no homology with the C-peptide region of proinsulin. IGF-I and IGF-II also differ from proinsulin in possessing carboxy-terminal extensions, or D-peptides, of 8 and 6 amino acids, respectively. This structural similarity explains the ability of both IGFs to bind to the insulin receptor and of insulin to bind to the type I IGF receptor (see later). On the other hand, structural differences probably also explain the failure of insulin to bind with high affinity to the IGFBPs (see later).

IGF Variants

There are several variants of the two IGF peptides. Rinderknecht and Humbel[229] reported that up to one fourth of the IGF-II isolated from human plasma lacked the *N*-terminal alanine. Jansen and colleagues[230] demonstrated that an IGF-II cDNA isolated from a human liver library predicted an IGF-II variant in which Ser[29] was replaced by Arg-Leu-Pro-Gly, and Zumstein and associates[231] identified this variant peptide subsequently in human plasma. Zumstein and associates isolated a 10-kd IGF-II variant from human plasma that contains a 21-residue carboxy extension, representing a portion of the E domain of pro-IGF-II (see later). In one peptide fragment isolated, Ser[33] was replaced by Cys-Gly-Asp. A 25-kd IGF-II variant was isolated by Gowan and colleagues, presumably representing a carboxyl-terminal extension.[232]

The significance of "big" IGF-II forms is still uncertain. In general, these variants appear capable of binding to IGF and insulin receptors and to IGFBPs and can participate in formation of the 150-kd IGF/IGFBP-3/acid-labile subunit (ALS) ternary complex. Big IGF-II can be produced by mesenchymal tumors and can cause non–islet-cell tumor hypoglycemia (NICTH).

Daughaday and co-workers[233] described a patient with a leiomyosarcoma and recurrent hypoglycemia, in whom 70% of serum IGF-II was in higher-molecular-weight forms. Removal of the tumor eliminated big IGF-II from the serum and corrected the hypoglycemia. The presence of big IGF-II in NICTH has been confirmed in multiple laboratories, but it is unclear why hypoglycemia occurs in the face of normal *total* serum IGF-II levels.

Zapf[234] has proposed that NICTH occurs when secretion of big IGF-II results in suppression of GH, insulin, and 7-kd IGF-II, leading to decreased production of IGF-I, IGFBP-3, and the ALS and increased production of IGFBP-2. This leads to a shift in the distribution of IGF-II from the 150-kd ternary complex to the 40- to 50-kd molecular-weight complex, composed of IGFBP-3, IGFBP-2, and a number of other low-molecular-weight IGFBPs. It is presumed that this results in increased bioavailability of IGF-II to target tissues, enhanced glucose consumption, and decreased hepatic glucose production.

Big forms of IGF-I have not been as thoroughly documented as with IGF-II. Powell and associates,[235] however, have reported that IGF-I forms with an apparent molecular weight ratio as high as 19 kd may be found in uremic serum. Large molecular forms of IGF-I have also been identified in conditioned media of human fibroblast cell lines.

Two IGF-I precursor molecules have been identified.[210] The first 134 amino acids of each are identical, comprising the signal peptide (48 amino acids), the mature IGF-I molecule (70 amino acids), and the first 16 amino acids of the E domain of the precursor. IGF-IA has additional 19 amino acids, and IGF-IB has additional 61 amino acids (total 195 residues). Alternative splicing of the *IGF-I* gene presumably generates the two mRNAs. The primary IGF-II translation product in human, rat, and mouse contains 180 amino acids, including a 24-residue signal peptide, the 67–amino acid mature IGF-II sequence, and a carboxyl-terminal E peptide of 89 amino acids.

The *IGF-I* Gene

The IGF genes (Fig. 23–21) are expressed differently in the embryo, fetus, child, and adult.[210, 236–238] Single large genes encode both IGF-I and IGF-II. The human *IGF-I* gene is located on the long arm of chromosome 12,[239, 240] and it contains at least six exons. Exons 1 and 2 encode alternative signal peptides, probably each containing several transcription start sites. Exons 3 and 4 encode the remaining signal peptide, the remainder of the mature IGF-I molecule, and part of the trailer peptide (E peptide). Exons 5 and 6 encode, alternatively, used segments of the trailer peptide (resulting in the IGF-IA and IGF-IB forms) and 3′ untranslated sequences with multiple different polyadenylation sites. The wide diversity of IGF-I mRNAs thus reflects the following:

1. Multiple leader exons and transcription start sites.
2. Alternative splicing of exons 5 or 6.
3. Multiple polyadenylation sites in exon 6.

The *IGF-II* Gene

The human *IGF-II* gene (Fig. 23–22) is located on the short arm of chromosome 11[239–241] adjacent to the insulin gene and spans 35 kb of genomic DNA, containing 9 exons. Exons 1 to 6 encode 5′ untranslated RNA; exon 7 encodes the signal peptide and most of the mature protein; and exon 8 encodes the carboxy-terminal portion of the protein and part of the trailer peptide, whose coding is completed in exon 9.

Thus, multiple mRNA species exist for both IGF-I and IGF-II, allowing for tissue-specific expression of specific transcripts and for developmental and hormonal regulation. The mechanisms involved in the regulation of IGF gene expression include the existence of multiple promoters, heterogeneous transcription initiation within each of the promoters, alternative splicing of various exons, differential RNA polyadenylation, and variable mRNA stability. Translation of *IGF-I* genes may also be under complex control.

Regulation of IGF Gene Expression

GH appears to be the primary regulator of *IGF-I* gene transcription, which begins as early as 30 minutes after intraperitoneal injection of GH into hypophysectomized rats.[242] Transcriptional activation by GH affects both IGF-I promoters equivalently, resulting in a 20-fold rise in IGF-I mRNA. This coordinated, rapid induction of all IGF-I mRNA species coincides with induction of Spi 2.1 gene by GH, although the relationship between these two processes is still not clear.[242] Furthermore, there may be tissue-to-tissue variability in GH-induced expression of IGF-I mRNA.[243] Other factors that influence *IGF-I* gene expression include estrogen, which stimulates IGF-I mRNA expression in the uterus but inhibits GH-stimulated IGF-I transcription in the liver.[244] The pubertal rise in serum IGF-I levels reflects the effect of gonadal steroids on IGF-I transcription, some of which results from the pubertal rise in GH secretion and some of which is due to a direct effect of gonadal steroids on IGF synthesis or secretion, because a pubertal rise in serum IGF levels is also observed in patients with GHI.

The factors involved in the regulation of *IGF-II* gene expression are less clear.[245] In humans and rats, *IGF-II* gene expression is high in fetal life and has been detected as early as the blastocyst stage in mice.[246] Serum levels of IGF-II are high in midgestation in pregnant rabbits.[247] Fetal tissues generally

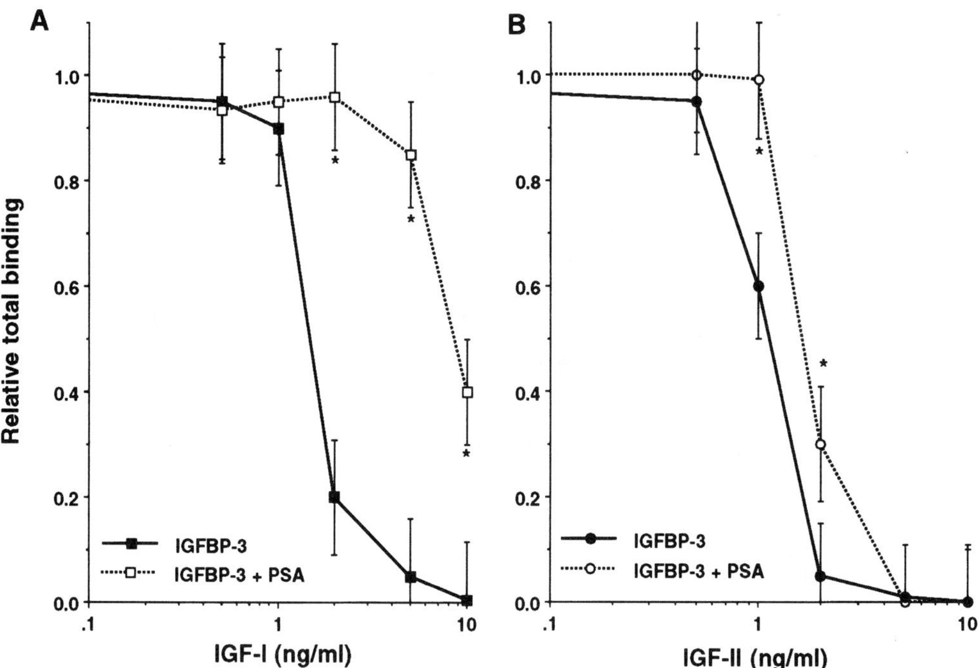

Figure 23–32. The effect of insulin-like growth factor–binding protein 3 (IGFBP-3) proteolysis by prostate-specific antigen (PSA) on IGFBP-3 affinity for IGF-I *(A)* and IGF-II *(B)*. (From Cohen P, Peehl DM, Graves HC, Rosenfeld RG. Biological effects of prostate-specific antigen as an insulin-like growth factor–binding protein-3 protease. J Endocrinol 1994; 142:407–415.)

variety of body fluids and cell culture media[409, 410, 412, 413, 415] and are postulated to play a role in altering IGF availability by lowering the affinities of IGFBPs for their ligand, thereby increasing the availability of IGFs to cell membrane receptors (see earlier).[414, 432]

Under certain conditions, the IGFBPs potentiate IGF action. In human and bovine fibroblasts, DNA synthesis and α-aminoisobutyric acid transport are potentiated when cells are preincubated with IGFBP-3, whereas IGFBP-3 is inhibitory if added at the same time as IGF-I.[433, 434] These observations have suggested that cell association of IGFBP-3 during preincubation is essential for its IGF-potentiating effect, perhaps allowing IGFBP-3 to serve as a reservoir for IGFs and bringing the ligand into closer proximity to the type 1 IGF receptors. This cell surface association of IGFBP-3 may involve interaction with heparin and heparin sulfate proteoglycans on the cell membrane or specific IGFBP-3 receptors.[396]

IGF-Independent Actions of IGF-Binding Proteins

The IGFBPs are bioactive molecules that, in addition to binding IGF, have a variety of IGF-independent functions. These include growth inhibition in some cell types,[435] growth stimulation in other tissues,[436] direct induction of apoptosis,[437] and modulation of the effects of other non-IGF growth factors. These effects of IGFBPs are mediated by binding to their own receptors. The IGFBP signaling pathways are currently being unraveled and involve interaction of IGFBPs with nuclear retinoid receptors as well as with other molecules on the cell surface and in the cytoplasm.[438]

IGFBP-3, itself, appears to have intrinsic inhibitory effects on cells, independent of its interaction with IGF. Villaudy and co-workers[439] found that the stimulation of DNA synthesis by basic FGF is inhibited by simultaneous treatment with IGFBP-3, even in the presence of levels of insulin, suggesting that sequestration of IGF peptides from type 1 IGF receptors is not the only means whereby IGFBP-3 inhibits cell growth. IGFBP-3 is also more effective than immunoneutralization of IGF-I in inhibiting serum-stimulated DNA synthesis, and IGFBP-3 inhibits FSH-stimulated DNA synthesis in cultured ovarian granulosa cells, with or without added IGF.[440] Under the same conditions, IGFBP-2 is less inhibitory, despite its higher affinity for IGF peptides. Expression of a transfected human IGFBP-3 cDNA in mouse fibroblasts inhibits both IGF-stimulated and insulin-stimulated cell proliferation (Fig. 23–35).[401] Similar studies in fibroblasts derived from mouse embryos homozygous for a targeted disruption of the type 1 IGF receptor again demonstrated inhibition with overexpression of IGFBP-3.[441] These studies strongly support an IGF-independent action for IGFBP-3 (Fig. 23–36).

IGFBP-3 binds with high affinity to the surface of various cell types, including human breast cancer cells and rat chondrocytes, and inhibits monolayer growth of these cells in an IGF-independent manner (Fig. 23–37).[396, 442, 443] Furthermore, transcriptional regulation of IGFBP-3 expression may be the mechanism for the inhibition of breast cancer cell growth by both transforming growth factor 2 (TGF-2) and retinoic acid (Fig. 23–38).[444–447] Reduction of IGFBP-3 production through the use of IGFBP-3 antisense oligodeoxynucleotides decreases the inhibitory effects of both TGF-2 and retinoic acid, suggesting that IGFBP-3 production may be a common pathway for multiple hormones and growth factors involved in the modulation of cell growth.[444] For example, estrogen inhibits expression and secretion of IGFBP-3, whereas antiestrogens stimulate production of IGFBP-3 in estrogen receptor–positive human breast cancer cells.[448] Similarly, the mitogenic action of epidermal growth factor (EGF) in human cervical epithelial cells is associated with inhibition of IGFBP-3 expression, and the inhibitory effect of retinoic acid is accompanied by increased IGFBP-3 expression.[449] Regulation of *IGFBP-3* gene expression plays a role in signaling by p53, a potent tumor suppressor protein.[450]

The presence of cell membrane proteins or receptors that specifically bind IGFBP-3 provides a potential mechanism for IGF-independent growth inhibitory actions of IGFBP-3 (Fig. 23–39).[396] IGFBP-3 may inhibit cell growth both by sequestering IGF ligands (IGF-dependent action of IGFBP-3) and also by binding to the cell surface (IGF-independent action of IGFBP-3). IGFBP-3 proteases may not only degrade intact

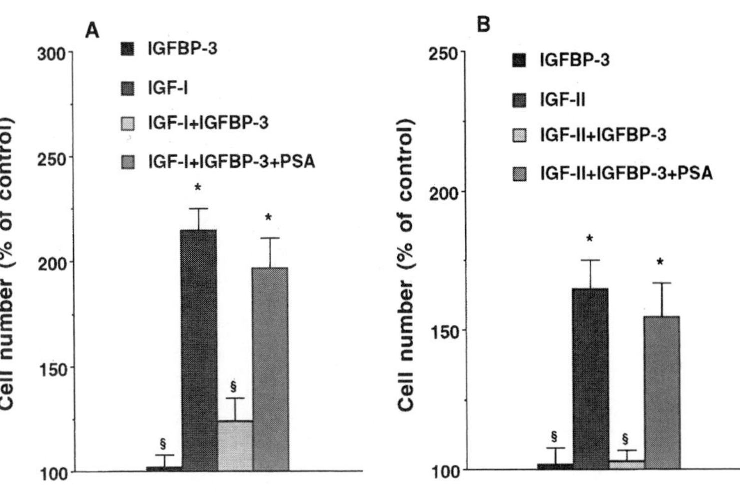

Figure 23–33. The effect of insulin-like growth factor–binding protein 3 (IGFBP-3) proteolysis by prostate-specific antigen (PSA) on the ability of IGFBP-3 to inhibit IGF-I *(A)* and IGF-II *(B)* action. (From Cohen P, Peehl DM, Graves HC, Rosenfeld RG. Biological effects of prostate-specific antigen as an insulin-like growth factor–binding protein-3 protease. J Endocrinol 1994; 142:407–415.)

IGFBP-3 to forms with lower affinities for IGFs but also generate IGFBP-3 fragments with enhanced affinity for cell surface IGFBP-3–interacting proteins or receptors. A proteolytic fragment of IGFBP-3 that fails to bind IGFs still retains its ability to inhibit cell proliferation.[451]

Characteristics of IGF-Binding Proteins 1 to 6

IGF-Binding Protein 1

IGFBP-1 was the first of the IGFBPs to be purified and to have its cDNA cloned.[452] The protein was actually identified and purified from several different tissues, including amniotic fluid[453] and Hep G2 conditioned media,[454] placental membranes (placental protein 12),[455] and endometrium (pregnancy-associated α_1-globulin).[456] Its gene is 5.2 kb long, located on the short arm of chromosome 7, and composed of four exons.[457] The mature protein is 30 kd and is nonglycosylated. mRNA for IGFBP-1 is strongly expressed in decidua (although not in placental trophoblasts), liver, and kidney.

IGFBP-1 may be involved in reproductive functions, including endometrial cycling,[458] oocyte maturation,[459] and fetal growth.[429, 460] It is the major IGFBP in fetal serum in early gestation, reaching levels as high as 3000 μg/L by the second trimester. Levels of IGFBP-1 in newborn serum are inversely correlated with birth weight, consistent with an inhibitory role on fetal IGF action.

IGFBP-1 also appears to have an important metabolic role, because its gene expression is enhanced in catabolic states,[314, 461, 462] and serum levels undergo diurnal variation.[463] Insulin suppresses and glucocorticoids enhance IGFBP-1 mRNA levels.[461, 464] The acute modulation of serum IGFBP-1 levels may regulate the free fraction of circulating IGF peptides.[461, 463] For example, administration of IGFBP-1 transiently reduces the glucose-lowering capability of IGF-I in rats.[465]

Although most in vitro studies are consistent with an inhibitory effect of IGFBP-1 on IGF actions, presumably reflecting interference with IGF ligand-receptor interactions,[388] IGFBP-1 potentiates IGF effects in certain cell systems,[466] possibly as the result of the binding of IGFBP-1 to cell membranes through its Arg-Gly-Asp (RGD) sequence; RGD is an integrin receptor recognition sequence that presumably allows IGFBP-1 to associate with the $\alpha_5\beta_1$ integrin (fibronectin) receptor.[393] The ability of IGFBP-1 to inhibit or potentiate IGF action may depend on post-translational modifications of IGFBP-1, such as phosphorylation, which appears to enhance IGFBP-1 affinity for IGF-I and thereby inhibit IGF action.[467]

IGF-Binding Protein 2

The *IGFBP-2* gene is located on the long arm of chromosome 2.[468, 469] A single 1.6-kb mRNA yields a mature protein of approximately 34 kd. Like IGFBP-1, IGFBP-2 is highly expressed in fetal tissues, particularly in the CNS.[470] IGFBP-2 is also similar to IGFBP-1 in its lack of *N*-glycosylation and in the presence of an RGD sequence, perhaps allowing cell association and potentiation of IGF action.[471] Nevertheless, knockout of the *IGFBP-2* gene[472] or overexpression of *IGFBP-1* in transgenic mice[473] appears to have little effect on phenotype, possibly reflecting "redundancy" in the IGF*BP* system, in which one *IGFBP* can compensate for loss of another.

The existence of a low-molecular-weight IGFBP in cerebrospinal fluid was inferred from studies demonstrating a 34-kd IGFBP that did not react with antibodies to IGFBP-1 (or IGFBP-3).[474] This IGFBP appeared to be consistent with a previous observation of CSF IGFBPs with preferential affinity for IGF-II.[475]

IGFBP-2 is expressed in secretory endometrium and endometrial tumors[458] and is the major IGFBP in seminal fluid and in the conditioned media of prostatic epithelial cells.[476] Interestingly, *IGFBP-2* gene expression is markedly reduced in prostatic stromal cells from patients with benign prostatic hyperplasia, suggesting that IGFBP-2 may inhibit stromal growth.[477] Serum levels of IGFBP-2 are frequently elevated in patients with prostatic carcinoma.[478]

IGF-Binding Protein 3

The *IGFBP-3* gene is located on chromosome 7 in proximity to the gene for IGFBP-1.[479] It contains four exons homologous to those of IGFBP-1 and IGFBP-2 and a fifth exon, consisting of 3′ untranslated sequences. In all human tissues studied to date, a single 2.6-kb mRNA has been observed, whereas an additional 1.7-kb mRNA species suggests alternative splicing in baboons.[480] mRNA levels are high in liver, but IGFBP-3 appears to be synthesized in hepatic endothelia (portal venous and sinusoidal) and Kupffer cells, whereas ALS is synthesized in hepatocytes.[481, 482]

IGFBP-3 is GH-dependent, due to either a direct GH effect or regulation by IGF. IGF-I administration to hypophysectomized rats increases serum levels of IGFBP-3.[421–423] On the other hand, IGF-I treatment of patients with GHI does not alter serum IGFBP-3 levels,[120, 393, 409] whereas GH treatment of GH-deficient patients does increase serum levels. Whether these observations mean that GH has a direct effect on IGFBP-3 or reflect GH regulation of ALS and ternary complex formation is unclear.

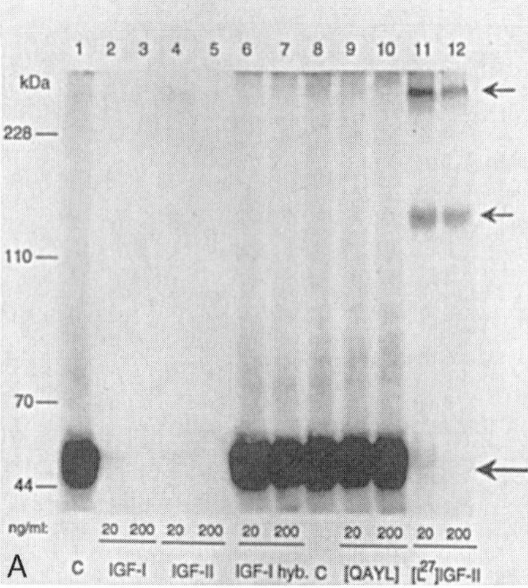

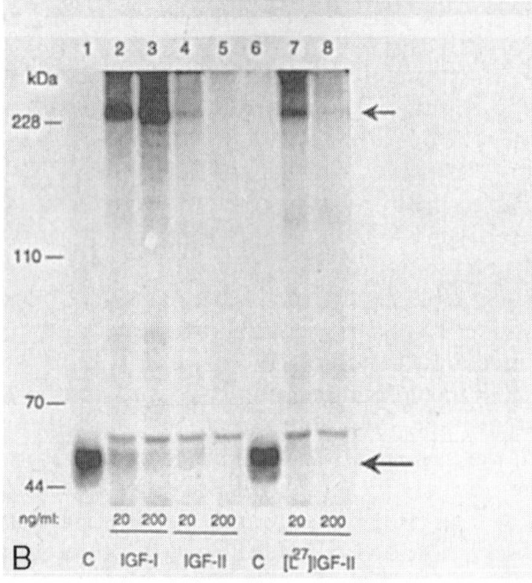

Figure 23–34. Affinity cross-linking of [125I]IGF-I *(A)* and [125I]IGF-II *(B)* to membranes from Hs578T breast cancer cells. In the absence of unlabeled insulin-like growth factor (IGF) peptide (lane 1), IGF was predominantly bound to 40- to 45-kd IGFBP-3; no type I or type II IGF receptors were observed. Iodinated IGF was readily displaceable by unlabeled IGF-I or IGF-II (lanes 2 to 5) but not by unlabeled IGF-I/insulin hybrid molecule (lanes 6 and 7) or by an IGF analogue with decreased affinity for IGF-binding proteins (QAYL, lanes 9 and 10 in *A*). However, addition of [Leu27] IGF-II, which has decreased affinity for the type I IGF receptor (lanes 11 and 12 in *A* and lanes 7 and 8 in *B*), resulted in "unmasking" of the 130-kd α subunit of the type I IGF receptor *(A)* and the 250-kd type II IGF receptor. (From Oh Y, Muller HL, Lamson G, Rosenfeld RG. Insulin-like growth factor [IGF]-independent action of IGF–binding protein 3 in hs578T human breast cancer cells: cell surface binding and growth inhibition. J Biol Chem 1993; 268:14964–14971.)

The mature IGFBP-3 protein has a molecular weight of approximately 29 kd; however, because it is *N*-glycosylated, it normally migrates as a doublet-triplet of 40 to 46 kd. Glycosylation does not appear to alter its affinity for IGF-I or -II.[483] IGFBP-3 also undergoes serine phosphorylation of IGFBP-3, although its physiologic significance is uncertain.[484] Perhaps the most significant post-translational modification of IGFBP-3 is proteolysis (see earlier). Discrepancies between immunoblot analyses and radioimmunoassays for IGFBP-3 reflect the altered affinity of IGFBP-3 fragments for IGF ligands, although some proteolytic fragments of IGFBP-3 are capable of ternary complex formation.[411] In pregnancy serum the predominant form of IGFBP-3 is a glycosylated 29-kd fragment. A similar-sized IGFBP-3 fragment is present in serum from patients who are postsurgical or catabolic[485] and from patients with non–insulin-dependent diabetes mellitus (non-IDDM).[486]

IGFBP-3 is the predominant IGFBP in adult serum, where it carries approximately 75% of the total IGF, primarily as part of the 150-kd ternary complex. Serum levels are reduced in patients with GHD or GHI, conditions in which assays for serum IGFBP-3 have important diagnostic value (see later).

IGFBP-3 associates with cell membranes. Affinity cross-linking studies employing [125I]IGF-I and a human breast cancer cell line have demonstrated no binding to the type 1 IGF receptor but rather to membrane-associated 45-kd IGFBP-3 (see Fig. 23–34). When IGF analogues with selective affinity for IGFBPs were added, a typical 135-kd α subunit of the type 1 IGF receptor was uncovered, demonstrating that membrane-associated IGFBP-3, with its high affinity for IGF peptides, normally "masks" the IGF receptors. Oh and associates[444] demonstrated that the binding of IGFBP-3 to cell membrane proteins was specific, cation-dependent, and of high affinity. Whether these proteins constitute genuine *IGFBP-3 receptors* remains to be demonstrated, although they may mediate IGF-independent actions of IGFBP-3. Alternatively, IGFBP-3 may associate with heparin-containing proteoglycans both in the extracellular matrix and in the cell membrane, because both IGFBP-3 and IGFBP-5 contain heparin-binding consensus sequences in their COOH termini.[487] However, treatment of cell monolayers with heparinase or chondroitinase has only minor effect on IGFBP-3 binding.

Like other IGFBPs, IGFBP-3 inhibits IGF action, especially when the binding protein is present in excess. Presumably, inhibition of IGF action by IGFBP-3 reflects a sequestering of IGF peptides away from the type 1 receptor. Proteolysis of IGFBP-3, resulting in a decrease in affinity for IGF ligands, decreases the inhibitory effects of the binding protein.

IGF-Binding Protein 4

The *IGFBP-4* gene, located on chromosome 17, contains four exons.[488] A single 2.6-kb mRNA has been identified with high expression in liver. The protein is the smallest of the IGFBPs with 237 amino acids in humans, including 20 cysteines and one *N*-linked glycosylation site. In immunoblots of most biologic fluids, IGFBP-4 is a 24/28-kd doublet; deglycosylation eliminates the 28-kd band.[489] IGFBP-4 appears to interact with connective tissues,[490] but there is no evidence of membrane association, consistent with a primary role for IGFBP-4 as a soluble, extracellular IGFBP.

IGFBP-4 was initially isolated on the basis of its ability to inhibit IGF-stimulated cell proliferation in bone,[491] and there is no evidence for any IGF-potentiating effects. The inhibitory effects of IGFBP-4 are reduced by proteolysis of the protein, much as has been observed with IGFBP-3 degradation. IGFBP-4 proteases are produced by a wide variety of cells, including neuroblastoma,[492] smooth muscle,[493] fibroblasts,[494] osteoblasts,[495] and prostatic epithelium.[496] Activation of IGFBP-4 proteolysis occurs in the presence of IGF-I or IGF-II, presumably reflecting a conformational change in IGFBP-4 resulting from IGF occupancy.[497, 498] The clinical use of IGFBP-4 measurements is minor.[499]

IGF-Binding Protein 5

Complementary DNAs for IGFBP-5 have been isolated and sequenced from rat ovary and human placenta and from a human osteosarcoma.[391, 500] The gene is located on chromosome 5 and contains four exons. A single 6.0-kb mRNA is expressed in a wide variety of tissues, particularly in kidney. Mature IGFBP-5 is produced as a 252–amino acid protein with no *N*-linked glycosylation sites but with one *O*-linked glycosylation site.[501]

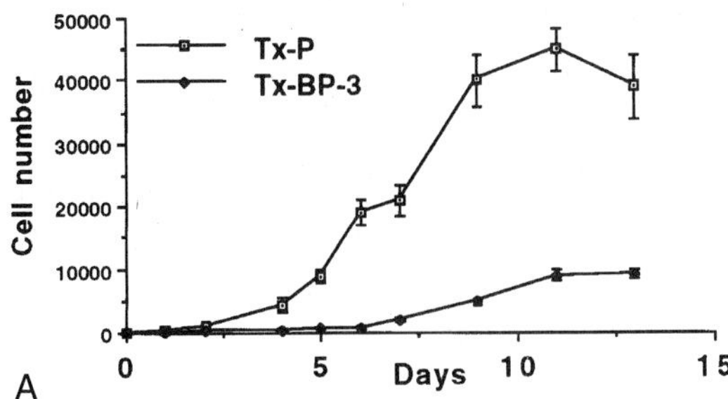

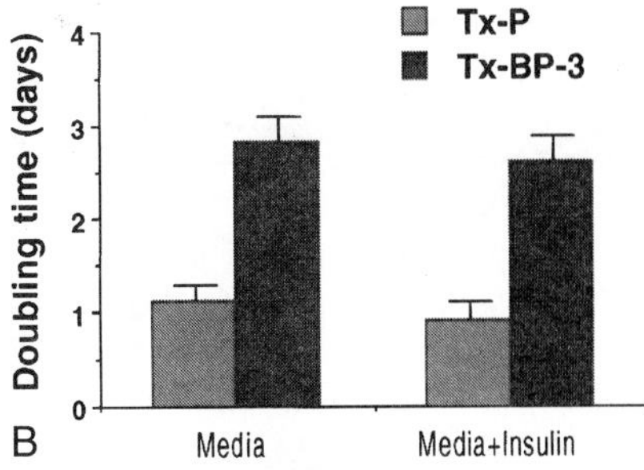

Figure 23–35. Effect of transfection of Balb/c fibroblasts with a human insulin-like growth factor–binding protein 3 (IGFBP-3) complementary DNA (cDNA) (Tx-BP-3) or with the control plasmid (Tx-P) on cell growth. Transfection with the IGFBP-3 cDNA resulted in a decreased cell proliferation *(A)* and increased cell doubling time *(B)*. The latter effect could not be overcome with insulin, supporting the concept that the inhibitory effects of IGFBP-3 are IGF independent. (From Cohen P, Lamson G, Okajima T, Rosenfeld RG. Transfection of the human insulin-like growth factor–binding protein 3 gene into Balb/c fibroblasts inhibits cellular growth. Mol Endocrinol 1993; 7:380–386. © The Endocrine Society.)

The addition of excess IGFBP-5 to human osteosarcoma cells inhibits IGF-I–stimulated DNA and glycogen synthesis.[502] However, when IGFBP-5 adheres to fibroblast extracellular matrix, it potentiates the growth-stimulatory effects of IGF on DNA synthesis.[503] The affinity of IGFBP-5 for IGF-I is reduced approximately sevenfold when the binding protein is associated with extracellular matrix, providing a potential mechanism for release of IGFs to cell surface receptors. Association of IGFBP-5 with extracellular matrix also appears to protect it from proteolysis.[504] Addition of IGFBP-5 to conditioned medium from fibroblasts results in proteolysis to a 21-kd fragment that does not potentiate IGF action, whereas the deposition of IGFBP-5 in extracellular matrix of fibroblasts makes it relatively resistant to degradation. Andress and Birnbaum[505] purified a 23-kd IGFBP-5 fragment from U-2 osteosarcoma cells that has reduced affinity for IGFs but enhances IGF-I–stimulated mitogenesis. The 23-kd IGFBP-5 fragment stimulates mitogenesis in an IGF-independent manner, presumably by binding to a specific "receptor" on the cell membrane.

Unlike proteolysis of IGFBP-4, which is enhanced by addition of IGFs, degradation of IGFBP-5 is inhibited by the binding of IGF peptides.[46, 415, 501] Proteolysis of IGFBP-5 results in the formation of 16- to 23-kd fragments demonstrated on immunoblots. Degradation of IGFBP-5 may have particular importance in the regulation of granulosa cell activity. In healthy ovarian follicles, neither IGFBP-4 nor IGFBP-5 is expressed, whereas both binding proteins are expressed in atretic follicles, thereby providing a mechanism for intrafollicular regulation of IGF action.[506, 507] Furthermore, FSH enhances IGF action in the ovary and stimulates IGFBP-5 proteolysis.[415]

IGFBP-5 and IGFBP-4 also appear to be major IGFBPs in bone, where, in addition to inhibiting IGF actions, IGFBP-5 may promote IGF-receptor interactions. Thus, depending on the conditions, IGFBP-5 can either inhibit or potentiate IGF actions.

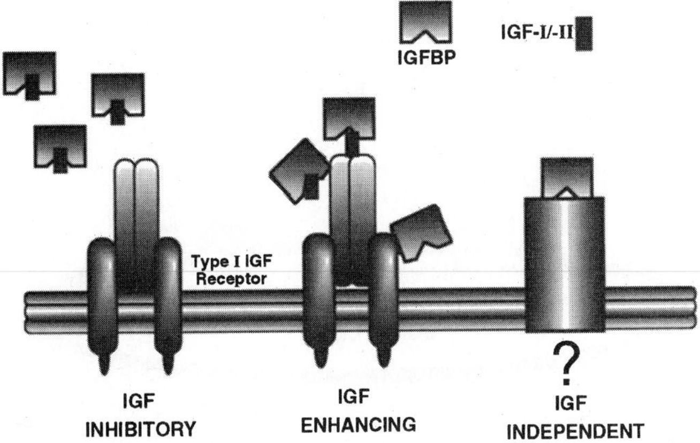

Figure 23–36. Theoretical mechanisms of cellular insulin-like growth factor–binding protein (IGFBP) actions.

IGF-Binding Protein 6

The human *IGFBP-6* gene is located on chromosome 12 and contains four exons. IGFBP-6 transcripts include a major 1.3-kb mRNA and a minor 2.2-kb transcript.[508] The mature peptide contains 216 amino acids and has a molecular mass of approximately 23 kd, although it may migrate at a higher molecular weight on SDS gels, presumably reflecting *O*-glycosylation.[509] Although IGFBP-6 binds both IGF-I and IGF-II, it has a significantly greater affinity for IGF-II.[510] IGFBP-6 is found in relatively high levels in cerebrospinal fluid, as is also the case for IGFBP-2, which also binds IGF-II with selectively high affinity. IGFBP-6 may also have a role in regulating ovarian activity, perhaps by functioning as an antigonadotropin.[511]

Radioimmunoassays for the IGF-Binding Proteins

Specific radioimmunoassays have been developed for IGFBP-1,[512–514] IGFBP-2,[478] IGFBP-3,[411, 515, 516] IGFBP-4,[517] IGFBP-5, and IGFBP-6. Measurement of IGFBP-3 appears to have the greatest clinical value because it is GH-dependent (Fig. 23–40). Blum and colleagues[516] have suggested that immunoassay of serum levels of IGFBP-3 may be superior to IGF-I assays in the diagnosis of GHD, because normal levels of IGF-I are so low in young children and many "normal" short children have low levels of IGF-I. Because IGFBP-3 determinations reflect the levels of both IGF-I and IGF-II, their age dependency is not nearly as striking as that of IGF-I; even in young children normal levels are higher than 500 μg/L. The use of IGFBP assays in the evaluation of IGF deficiency and GHD is discussed later. Measurement of IGFBP levels in biologic fluids may be useful for evaluation of malignancies or other pathologic states where the IGFBP levels may be altered.

Gonadal Steroids

Although androgens and estrogens do not contribute substantially to normal growth before puberty, the adolescent rise

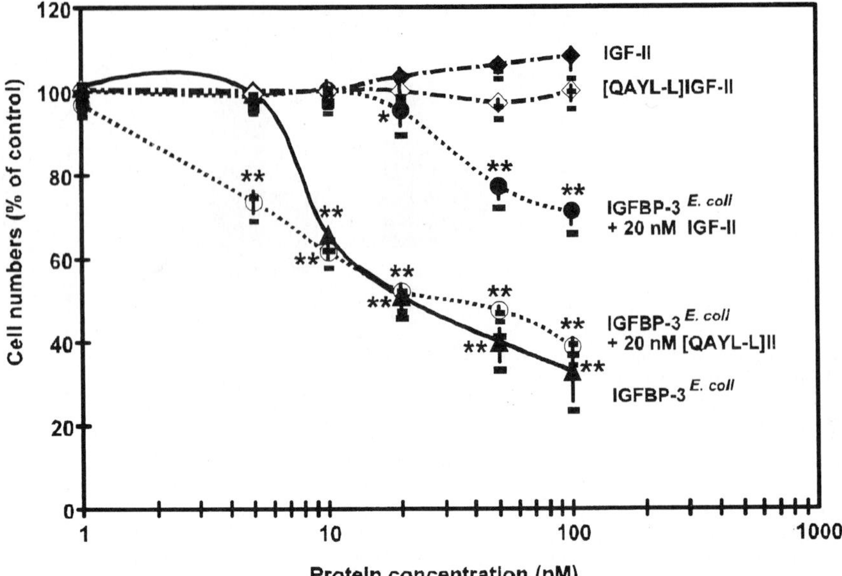

Figure 23–37. Inhibition of Hs578T breast cancer cell growth by insulin-like growth factor–binding protein 3 (IGFBP-3) is IGF independent. Recombinant IGFBP-3 from *Escherichia coli* results in decreased cell number and cannot be overcome by the addition of an IGF analogue with normal affinity for IGF receptors but decreased affinity for IGFPB-3 (QAYL-Leu-IGF-II). On the other hand, IGF-II, which itself does not stimulate cell proliferation in Hs578T cells, partially releases cells from the growth-inhibitory effects of IGFBP-3, presumably by causing dissociation of IGFBP-3 from the cell membrane. (From Oh Y, Muller HL, Lamson G, Rosenfeld RG. Insulin-like growth factor [IGF]-independent action of IGF-binding protein 3 in Hs578T human breast cancer cells. J Biol Chem 1993; 268: 14964–14971.)

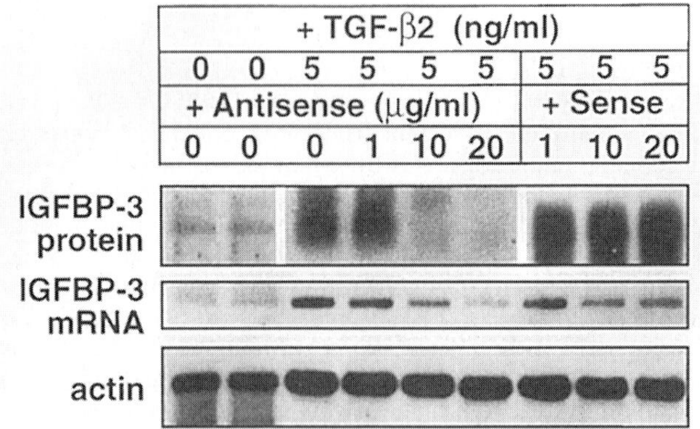

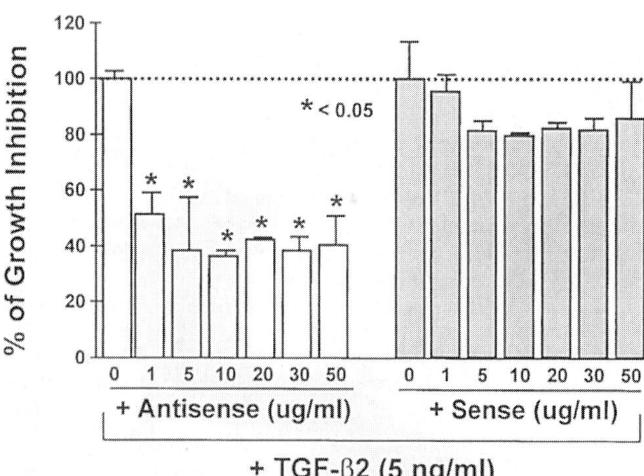

Figure 23–38. Transforming growth factor β_2 (TGF-β2) inhibits Hs578T cell growth by transcriptional regulation of insulin-like growth factor–binding protein 3 (IGFBP-3). Reduction in IGFBP-3 messenger RNA (mRNA) and protein levels through the use of an IGFBP-3 antisense oligodeoxynucleotide resulted in significant reduction in the growth inhibitory actions of TGF-β2. (From Oh Y, Muller HL, Ng L, Rosenfeld RG. TGF-β2–induced cell growth inhibition in human breast cancer cells is mediated through IGFBP-3 action. J Biol Chem 1995; 270:13589–13592.)

in serum gonadal steroid levels is an important part of the pubertal growth spurt. States of androgen or estrogen excess prior to epiphyseal fusion cause rapid linear growth and skeletal maturation. Thus, just as growth deceleration requires evaluation, growth acceleration can be as abnormal and may be a sign of precocious puberty or virilizing congenital adrenal hyperplasia.

A GH-replete state is obligatory for a normal growth response to gonadal steroids, and children with GHD do not have a normal growth response to either endogenous or exogenous androgens. Gonadal steroids work, in part, by enhancing GH secretion and also stimulate IGF-I production directly, as evidenced by the rise in serum IGF-I levels and pubertal growth spurt in children with mutations of the GHR.[169]

Both androgens and estrogens increase skeletal maturation. It is likely that androgens primarily act in this regard after conversion to estrogens by aromatase in extraglandular tissues but may also have independent action.[518] Indeed, mutation of the estrogen receptor in a man was associated with tall stature and open epiphyses,[32] and similar findings occur in patients with mutations of the gene encoding the aromatase enzyme.[33, 34] In addition, women with an estrogen receptor variant have increased height,[519] whereas estrogen receptor polymorphisms, but not serum estradiol levels, are related to bone density and height in males.[520]

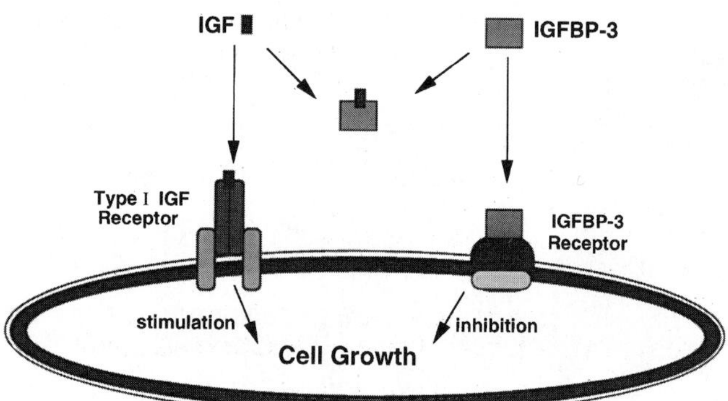

Figure 23–39. Schematic diagram of insulin-like growth factor (IGF)-independent and IGF-dependent actions of IGF-binding protein 3 (IGFBP-3), the latter being mediated through a putative membrane-associated IGFBP-3 receptor.

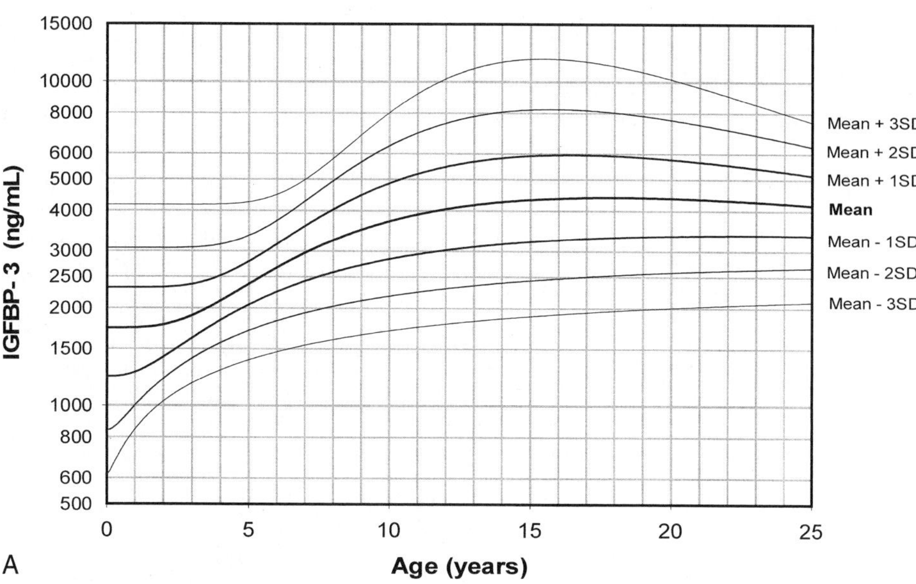

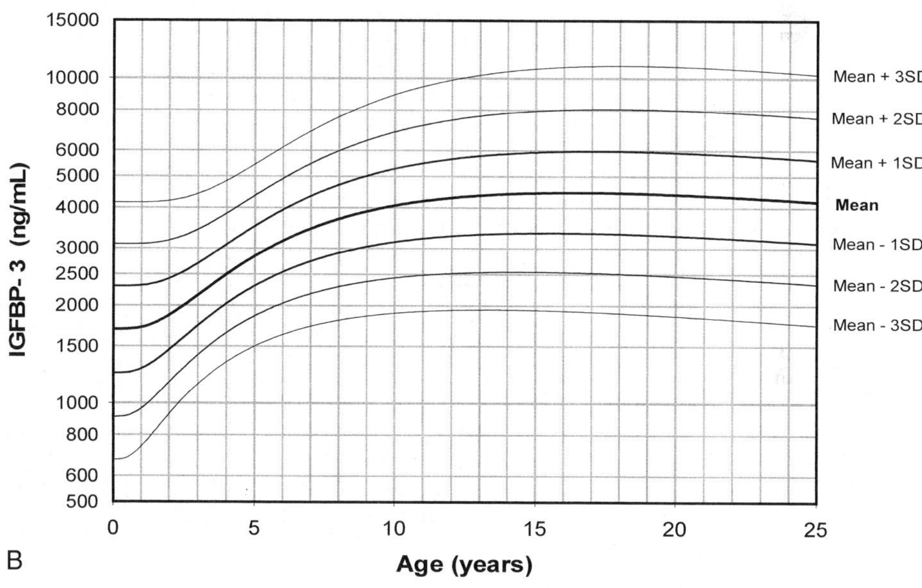

Figure 23–40. Normal serum levels of insulin-like growth factor–binding protein 3 (IGFBP-3) (micrograms per milliliter) by age for males *(A)* and females *(B)*. The *lines* represent the mean ± 3 SD. (Data courtesy of Diagnostic Systems Laboratories, Inc., Webster, Texas.)

Skeletal development, in terms of bone mass accretion, is an important pubertal phenomenon and is largely mediated by estrogen action.[521–524] A longitudinal analysis of pubertal calcium accretion found that approximately 26% of adult calcium is laid down during the two adolescent years of maximal growth.[525] More than 90% of skeletal mass is present by 18 years of age,[526, 527] and estrogens appear to regulate the timing of the growth spurt, stabilization of bone modeling, and endosteal mineral apposition.[521, 528]

Rubin[30] described a schema by which early and mid puberty are a time of linear growth, increased bone mineral content, and mineral density (a reflection of bone growth, perhaps largely mediated by the GH-estrogen synergism). It appears that pubertal males have stronger bones than females, perhaps due to greater bone deposition on the periosteal surface in contrast with increased bone on the endocortical surface in females.[529] Late puberty is characterized by bone maturation (epiphyseal closure) and increased volumetric density (true bone mineral density that is not size based), which are apparently mediated more clearly by estrogen. Late menarche and delayed puberty appear to be risk factors for later osteopenia,[530] but some data exist to suggest that low bone mass may already be present prepubertally in these individuals.[531] Independent and synergistic effects of gonadal steroids, GH, and IGF-I contribute to the attainment of peak bone mass in adults.[30, 31, 521, 528, 532, 533]

Thyroid Hormone

Thyroid hormone is a major contributor to postnatal growth, although, like GH, it is of relatively little importance to growth of the fetus. Hypothyroidism postnatally can cause profound growth failure and virtual arrest of skeletal maturation. In addition to a direct effect on epiphyseal cartilage, thyroid hormones appear to have a permissive effect on GH

Table 23–2. Classification of Growth Retardation

I. Primary Growth Abnormalities
- A. Osteochondrodysplasias
- B. Chromosomal abnormalities
- C. Intrauterine growth retardation

II. Secondary Growth Disorders
- A. Malnutrition
- B. Chronic disease
- C. Endocrine disorders
  1. Hypothyroidism
  2. Cushing's syndrome
  3. Pseudohypoparathyroidism
  4. Rickets
     a. Vitamin D–resistant rickets
  5. IGF deficiency
     a. GHD due to hypothalamic dysfunction
     b. GHD due to pituitary GH deficiency
     c. GH resistance
        (1) Primary GH insensitivity
        (2) Secondary GH insensitivity
     d. Primary defects of IGF synthesis
     e. Primary defects of IGF transport and clearance
     f. IGF insensitivity
        (1) Defects of the type 1 IGF receptor
        (2) Postreceptor defects

III. Idiopathic Short Stature
- A. Genetic short stature
- B. Constitutional delay of growth and maturation
- C. Heterozygous defects of the GH receptor

GH, growth hormone; GHD, growth hormone deficiency; IGF, insulin-like growth factor.

secretion. Patients with hypothyroidism have decreased spontaneous GH secretion and blunted responses to GH provocative tests. Treatment with thyroid hormone results in rapid "catch-up" (accelerated) growth, which is typically accompanied by marked skeletal maturation, potentially causing overly rapid epiphyseal fusion and compromise of adult height.

GROWTH RETARDATION

A classification of growth retardation is shown in Table 23–2. Growth disorders are subdivided into these categories:

1. *Primary growth abnormalities*, in which the defect(s) appears to be intrinsic to the growth plate.
2. *Secondary growth disorders*, or growth failure resulting from chronic disease or endocrine disorders (the newly introduced category of "IGF deficiency" can result from GHRH deficiency, GHD, or GH or IGF insensitivity).
3. *ISS*, including variants of normal *(constitutional delay of growth and maturation* [CDGM] and genetic short stature), heterozygous mutations of the *GH receptor gene* (*GHR* gene, a variant of GHI) and as yet unclarified mutations throughout the growth-related genome.

PRIMARY GROWTH ABNORMALITIES

Osteochondrodysplasias

The osteochondrodysplasias encompass a heterogeneous group of disorders characterized by intrinsic abnormalities of cartilage or bone, or both.[534, 535] These conditions share the following features:

1. Genetic transmission.
2. Abnormalities in the size and shape of bones of the limbs, spine, and/or skull.
3. Radiologic abnormalities of the bones (generally).

More than 100 osteochondrodysplastic conditions have been identified to date on the basis of physical features and radiologic characteristics, and biochemical, molecular, and genetic studies of these conditions will undoubtedly lead to the recognition of additional types. An international classification for the osteochondrodysplasias, developed in 1970[536] and revised in 1978[537] and 1992,[534] is summarized in Table 23–3. Of note, the category of dysostosis has been dropped from the classification, which focuses on developmental disorders of bone and cartilage.

Diagnosis of osteochondrodysplasias can be difficult. Although the underlying molecular and biochemical defects have been identified in many of these conditions, clinical and radiologic evaluation remain central to the diagnosis. Frequently, the clinical features are characteristic, and the diagnosis can be made at birth or even prenatally by ultrasonography. The family history is critical, although many cases are due to fresh mutations, as is generally the case in the classical autosomal dominant achondroplasia and hypochondroplasia. Measurement of body proportions should include arm span, sitting height, upper and lower body segments, and head circumference. Clinical and radiologic evaluation should be used to determine whether involvement is of the long bones, skull, and vertebrae and whether abnormalities are primarily at the epiphyses, metaphyses, or diaphyses.

Two of the more common osteochondrodysplasias are achondroplasia and hypochondroplasia.[538]

Table 23–3. Classification of Osteochondrodysplasias

I. Defects of the Tubular (and Flat) Bones and/or Axial Skeleton
- A. Achondroplasia group
- B. Achondrogenesis
- C. Spondylodysplastic group (perinatally lethal)
- D. Metatropic dysplasia group
- E. Short rib dysplasia group (with/without polydactyly)
- F. Atelosteogenesis/diastrophic dysplasia group
- G. Kniest-Stickler dysplasia group
- H. Spondyloepiphyseal dysplasia congenita group
- I. Other spondylo epi-(meta)-physeal dysplasias
- J. Dysostosis multiplex group
- K. Spondylometaphyseal dysplasias
- L. Epiphyseal dysplasias
- M. Chondrodysplasia punctata (stippled epiphyses) group
- N. Metaphyseal dysplasias
- O. Brachyrachia (short spine dysplasia)
- P. Mesomelic dysplasias
- Q. Acro/acro-mesomelic dysplasias
- R. Dysplasias with significant (but not exclusive) membranous bone involvement
- S. Bent bone dysplasia group
- T. Multiple dislocations with dysplasias
- U. Osteodysplastic primordial dwarfism group
- V. Dysplasias with increased bone density
- W. Dysplasias with defective mineralization
- X. Dysplasias with increased bone density

II. Disorganized Development of Cartilaginous and Fibrous Components of the Skeleton

III. Idiopathic Osteolyses

Achondroplasia

Achondroplasia is the most common of the osteochondrodysplasias, with a frequency of about 1:26,000. Although transmitted as an autosomal dominant disorder, 80% to 90% of cases appear to be due to new mutations. Achondroplasia is due to a mutation in a transmembranous domain of the gene for FGF receptor 3 (FGF-R3)[539, 540] located on the short arm of chromosome 4(4p16.3).[539, 541–543]

Most cases identified to date are caused by activating mutations at a "hot spot" at nucleotide 1138 (codon380, gly380arg) of the *FGF-R3* gene,[538–540, 544, 545] and because these mutations create new recognition sites for restriction enzymes, they can be easily diagnosed. The mutation rate reported at this site indicates that it may be the most mutable gene in the human genome.[544, 545] The homogeneity of mutation in achondroplasia probably explains the minimal heterogeneity in its phenotype. Infants homozygous for this condition have severe disease, typically dying in infancy from respiratory insufficiency due to the small thorax. Diminished growth velocity is present from infancy, although short stature may not be evident until after 2 years of age. Mean adult heights in males and females are 130 and 120 cm, respectively.[546] Growth curves for achondroplasia have been developed and are of value in following patients.[26]

With increasing age, the diagnosis of achondroplasia becomes easier because these patients have characteristic abnormalities of the skeleton, including megalocephaly, low nasal bridge, lumbar lordosis, short trident hand, and rhizomelia (shortness of the proximal legs and arms) with skin redundancy. Radiologic findings include small, cuboid-shaped vertebral bodies with short pedicles and progressive narrowing of the lumbar interpedicular distance. The iliac wings are small, with narrow sciatic notches. The small foramen magnum may lead to hydrocephalus, and spinal cord and/or root compression may result from kyphosis, stenosis of the spinal canal, or disc lesions.[547, 548] GH secretion in these children is comparable to that in normal children.[549]

In a mouse with an equivalent *FGF-R3* mutation showing many features of human achondroplasia, there is ligand-independent dimerization and phosphorylation of *FGF-R3* with activation of STAT proteins and up-regulation of cell cycle inhibition.[550] Additionally, such mutant mice also exhibit down-regulation of expression of the Indian hedgehog and *PTHrP* receptor genes, which are also involved in bone formation.[551] As a result of the overexpression of this receptor activity, there is abnormal chondrogenesis and osteogenesis during endochondral ossification.

Hypochondroplasia

Hypochondroplasia is an autosomal dominant disorder, previously described as a "mild form" of achondroplasia, that frequently results from a mutation (Asn540Lys) in the *FGF-R3* gene.[538, 552–554] The two disorders do not occur in the same family.[555] About 70% of affected individuals are heterozygous for a mutation in the *FGF-R3* gene, but locus heterogeneity exists as other unidentified mutations cause a similar pheotype.[538, 556] Mullis and co-workers, using restriction enzyme analysis, suggested that the *IGF-I* gene may be a candidate gene for hypochondroplasia,[557] but other molecular abnormalities are likely to be found.

The facial features of achondroplasia are absent, and both the short stature and rhizomelia are less pronounced. Adult heights typically are in the 120- to 150-cm range. In contrast with achondroplasia, poor growth may not be evident until after 2 years of age, but stature then deviates progressively from normal. Occasionally, the disproportionate short stature is not apparent until adulthood. Outward bowing of the legs may be accompanied by genu varum. Lumbar interpedicular distances diminish between L1 and L5, and, as with achondroplasia, there may be flaring of the pelvis and narrow sciatic notches. The diagnosis is exceedingly difficult to make in young children. Mild variants of the syndrome may not be clinically distinguishable from normal, and radiologic studies should be performed if a question arises.

Chromosomal Abnormalities

Abnormalities of autosomes or sex chromosomes may cause growth retardation, frequently associated with somatic abnormalities and mental retardation, as in deletion of chromosome 5 or trisomy 18 or 13. Such abnormalities, however, may be subtle, and the diagnosis of Turner's syndrome must be considered in any girl with unexplained short stature. In many cases, the precise cause of growth failure is not clear because the genetic defects do not affect known components of the GH-IGF system. The chromosomal lesion may directly influence normal tissue growth and development or, indirectly, modulate local responsivity to IGF.

Down's Syndrome

Trisomy 21, or Down's syndrome, is probably the most common chromosomal disorder associated with growth retardation, affecting approximately 1 in 600 live births. On average, newborns with Down's syndrome have birth weights 500 g below normal and are 2 to 3 cm shorter. Growth failure continues postnatally and is typically associated with delayed skeletal maturation and a delayed and incomplete pubertal growth spurt. Adult heights range from 135 to 170 cm in men and 127 to 158 cm in women.[27] The cause of growth failure in Down's syndrome and in other autosomal defects is unknown.

Attempts to find underlying hormonal explanations for growth retardation have been unsuccessful, even though hypothyroidism due to Hashimoto's thyroiditis is more common than normal in Down's syndrome and should be sought. Marginal levels of GH secretion and low serum levels of IGF-I have been reported in Down's syndrome,[558–561] and exogenous GH may be efficacious in the short term.[562–566] It is more likely, however, that the growth failure reflects a generalized biochemical abnormality of the epiphyseal growth plate.

Gonadal Dysgenesis

In girls with gonadal dysgenesis (Turner's syndrome), short stature is the single most common feature, occurring more frequently than delayed puberty, cubitus valgus, or webbing of the neck.[567–569] In large series of such individuals, short stature occurs in 95% to 100% of girls with a 45,X karyotype (see Chapter 22).[570–572] Several distinct phases of growth have been identified in girls with Turner's syndrome[573–575]:

1. Mild intrauterine growth retardation (IUGR), with mean birth weights and lengths of 2800 g and 48.3 cm, respectively.
2. Slow growth during infancy falling to −3 SDS by 3 years of age.
3. Delayed onset of the "childhood phase" of growth[14, 15, 575] and progressive decline in height velocity from 3 years of age until approximately 14 years of age, resulting in further deviation from normal height percentiles.
4. A prolonged adolescent growth phase, characterized by a partial return toward normal height, followed by delayed epiphyseal fusion.

Mean adult heights in the United States and Europe range from 142.0 to 146.8 cm (lower in Asia). There are important genetic and ethnic influences on growth in these girls. Parental height correlates well with final patient height,[576, 577] and a cross-cultural study in 15 countries demonstrated a strong correlation (r = 0.91) between final height in Turner's syndrome and in the normal population with an approximate 20-cm deficit.[570]

The cause of growth failure in Turner's syndrome remains unclear. Girls have a skeletal dysplasia and are haploinsufficient for the *SHOX* gene (short stature homeobox-containing gene) located in the pseudoautosomal region of the short arm of the X chromosome.[578] Mutations and deletions of this gene are associated with poor height growth and several syndromes of skeletal dysplasia including Madelung's deformity, which is also seen in Turner's syndrome.[578–580] The incidence of IUGR is much greater in girls lacking two copies of the *SHOX* gene (46% versus 7%).[581]

Most patients have normal GH and IGF levels during childhood; reports of low GH or IGF levels in adolescents with Turner's syndrome are likely due to low serum levels of gonadal steroids.[582] Growth impairment is evident prior to the period when activity of the GH-IGF axis is decreased. Nevertheless, GH therapy is capable of both accelerating short-term growth and increasing adult height.[572, 583, 584] This diagnosis must be considered in all girls with unexplained growth failure and especially in girls who are short for family but are growing between the 5th and 10th percentiles in the first decade of life. Nonetheless, a recent study found that the mean age at diagnosis lagged 5.3 years behind the age at which patients with Turner's syndrome fell below the 5th percentile,[585] where its frequency is approximately 1/100. Such data affirm the need for vigorous assessment of all girls who are either absolutely short or relatively small for family heights.

Table 23–4. Causes of Intrauterine Growth Retardation

I. Intrinsic Fetal Abnormalities
- A. Chromosomal disorders
- B. Syndromes associated with primary growth failure
  1. Russell-Silver syndrome
  2. Seckel's syndrome
  3. Noonan's syndrome
  4. Progeria
  5. Cockayne's syndrome
  6. Bloom's syndrome
  7. Prader-Willi syndrome
  8. Rubenstein-Taybi syndrome
- C. Congenital infections
- D. Congenital anomalies

II. Placental Abnormalities
- A. Abnormal implantation of the placenta
- B. Placental vascular insufficiency; infarction
- C. Vascular malformations

III. Maternal Disorders
- A. Malnutrition
- B. Constraints on uterine growth
- C. Vascular disorders
  1. Hypertension
  2. Toxemia
  3. Severe diabetes mellitus
- D. Uterine malformations
- E. Drug ingestion
  1. Tobacco
  2. Alcohol
  3. Narcotics

18q Deletions

Deletion of the long arm of chromosome 18 has an estimated prevalence of 1 in 40,000 live births. In a review of 50 cases, 64% of children (mean age 5.8 ± 4.5 years) had heights greater than 2 SD below the mean, with only 6% greater than 0 SDS.[586] Fifteen percent had serum IGF-I concentrations, and 9% had IGFBP-3 concentrations below −2 SD. Seventy-two percent of children had reduced GH responses to provocative testing, although such testing was not always rigorous. Clinical trials of GH therapy in such cases are currently in progress.

Intrauterine Growth Retardation

Infants with IUGR comprise a heterogeneous group with birth weight and/or length below the 3rd or 10th percentile for gestational age, depending on the study.[587–591] They may also be referred to as small-for-gestational-age (SGA) infants, in contrast with those who are appropriate for gestational age (AGA). The importance of this distinction, in addition to a number of issues influencing neonatal morbidity, is in the prediction of later growth: Most AGA low-birth-weight infants experience catch-up growth during the first 2 years of life, in contrast with the slower, attenuated growth of SGA infants who may have persistent height deficits throughout childhood and adolescence.[589–592] First-trimester growth failure has been closely associated with low birth weight and low-birth-weight percentile.[593] The earlier in gestation that fetal growth is impaired, the less likely that complete recapture of lost growth will occur.

IUGR can arise from abnormalities in the fetus, the placenta, or the mother (Table 23–4). Factors affecting fetal growth include nutrition provided by the maternal-placental system, alterations of fetal IGF production, and as yet unclarified genes. Although it is understandable why uterine constraint or twin pregnancies might result in limited fetal growth, the reason for abnormal fetal growth in most cases of IUGR is unclear.

The implications of IUGR may extend beyond fetal life. Although most SGA infants exhibit catch-up growth by 2 years of age, a large subgroup remains small. In a retrospective study of 47 individuals who had IUGR, 23 men had an adult height of 162 cm and 24 women had an adult height of 148 cm.[594] Larger studies[589–591] demonstrated that SGA children had a fivefold to sevenfold greater chance of short stature than AGA children did. Ten percent to 15% of SGA infants will have short stature, and this group makes up as much as 20% of all short children. In a study of a more severely affected neonatal intensive care unit SGA population, 27% had not yet achieved catch-up by 6 years of age.[595] Final adult height is −0.8 to −0.9 SDS, which is a mean deficit of 3.6 to 4 cm when adjusted for family stature.[590] The endocrinologic mechanisms of the poor growth are varied but may include abnormalities of GH production and secretory patterns[589] and insensitivity to GH and IGF-I action.[596]

The childhood and adolescent endocrine disorders associated with the SGA children include premature adrenarche, insulin resistance, functional ovarian hyperandrogenism, and an attenuated pubertal growth spurt.[589, 597] Furthermore, SGA infants have an increased risk of hypertension, maturity-onset diabetes mellitus, and cardiovascular disease later in life.[598–600] Not all of these problems appear to occur in those IUGR babies who do not have catch-up growth, although insulin resistance has been described.[601] Whether IUGR is *causally* related to these disorders or is a symptom of an underlying inborn metabolic disorder is not yet known.

Intrinsic Fetal Factors

In contrast with the role of the endocrine system in postnatal growth, intrauterine growth is less dependent on fetal pituitary hormones.[602, 603] Athyreotic and agonadal infants are of normal length and weight at birth. Pituitary GH is synthesized and secreted by the latter half of the first trimester, with midgestational levels peaking at 150 μg/L and then falling to around 30 μg/L at term.[141] Because the anencephalic fetus is normal in size, the pituitary was thought to be unnecessary for fetal growth.[604, 605] However, documentation of birth size of rats and humans with congenital GHD[606–609] and of human newborns with mutations of the GH or GHR genes[169] indicate that GH from the fetal pituitary makes a small contribution to birth size. Infants with neonatal GHD are around −0.5 to −1.5 SD below the mean in length and are heavy for this length.[607–609]

These observations should not be interpreted to mean that the IGF axis is unimportant in fetal growth. Gene knockout studies show that causing elimination of paracrine/autocrine production of IGF-I, and IGF-II, as well as of the type 1 IGF receptor, impairs fetal growth, although placenta size is normal.[259, 260, 277, 610] Circulating IGF-I levels in fetal and cord blood correlate with fetal size and are reduced in IUGR, especially in situations associated with decreased growth velocity.[150, 306, 611–614]

Similar data suggestive of marked GHI are found in the first week of life following severe fetal malnutrition.[615] The molar ratio of IGF-II to the IGF-II receptor was also found to be related to birth and placenta weight.[616] The initial case of a deletion of the *IGF-I* gene had profound intrauterine growth failure.[270, 617] The implication of that report is that local tissue production of IGF-I is critical for intrauterine growth and that its regulation is largely GH independent. Human umbilical cord lymphocytes have increased numbers of IGF receptors,[618] and mRNAs for both IGF-I and -II are abundant in fetal tissues.[619, 620] Exogenous IGF-I administration increases neonatal growth rate and protein and fat accretion in pigs with IUGR.[621] Hepatic levels of GHR mRNA and of GHR are low,[141, 622, 623] perhaps explaining the modest impact of GH on IGF production and linear growth. In neonates with IUGR, GH levels are elevated,[624] and exogenous GH treatment has little or no effect on growth, body composition, or energy expenditure,[625, 626] further supporting a state of relative insensitivity to GH at this developmental stage. With defects of the GHR, neonatal IGF levels are low,[141] suggesting a role for GH in regulating IGF production. Similarly, IGFBPs are identifiable in serum and other biologic fluids in the fetus and newborn.[429] However, serum levels of IGFBP-3 and ALS, the major serum carriers of IGF peptides in the adult, are low in the fetus and newborn. Thus, the components of the IGF system are apparently regulated directly by glucose levels or indirectly by fetal insulin secretion, with less impact of GH levels.[611, 627, 628]

The role of insulin production in fetal growth is demonstrated by somatic overgrowth of the hyperinsulinemic infants of mothers with diabetes and of infants with the syndrome of persistent neonatal hyperinsulinemic hypoglycemia (nesidioblastosis).[587, 629, 630] In contrast, infants with pancreatic agenesis or with abnormalities of the insulin receptor in the "leprechaun" syndrome are SGA.[587] Further, the inverse relationship of insulin and IGFBP-1 levels and the finding that fetal IGFBP-1 levels are elevated in IUGR[628] support an important role for insulin in fetal growth regulation. In addition to these well-characterized endocrine profiles, cord blood cortisol levels are inversely related to IGF-I and directly to IGFBP-3 concentrations.[614] In infants with IUGR, a close correlation ($r = -0.54$) was observed between cord blood cortisol levels and length growth during the first 3 months of life. This is a period during which substantial catch-up growth occurs in some, but clearly not all, IUGR infants.[589]

Infants with IUGR exhibiting poor postnatal growth, particularly when the abnormalities are intrinsic to the fetus, have frequently been categorized as having "primordial growth failure." Several syndromes are briefly noted in the following sections.

Russell-Silver Syndrome

Russell-Silver syndrome (RSS) is a condition that was independently described by Russell[631] and by Silver and associates.[632] Although this syndrome is probably due to a heterogeneous group of disorders, the common findings include IUGR, postnatal growth failure, congenital hemihypertrophy, and small, triangular facies.[633–636] Nonspecific findings include clinodactyly, precocious puberty, delayed closure of the fontanels, and delayed bone age.[633–635] Adults are short, with final heights about −4 SD below the mean.[634, 636] Endogenous GH secretion in prepubertal children with RSS is similar to that in other short IUGR children and less than in AGA short children.[589, 637]

Because no genetic or biochemical basis for this disorder has been identified, RSS is often used incorrectly as a designation for IUGR of unknown etiology. Maternal uniparental disomy of chromosome 7 exists in 7% to 10% of cases.[63, 638–640] Candidate genes in chromosome region 7p11-13, such as those for IGFBP-1, IGFBP-3, and EGF-R, all show biallelic expression, but a growth suppression gene, *GRB10*, which binds to the insulin and IGF-I receptors and replicates asynchronously, remains a candidate gene for overexpression.[640, 641] Paternally expressed imprinted genes at 7q32, PEG/MEST, and g2-COP are other candidates.[639, 642, 643]

Seckel's Syndrome

Originally described by Mann and Russell in 1959,[644] the condition most commonly termed Seckel's syndrome is also known as *Seckel's bird-headed dwarfism*.[645] The syndrome is an autosomal recessive disorder characterized by IUGR and severe postnatal growth failure, combined with microcephaly, prominent nose, and micrognathia. Final height is typically 90 to 110 cm, with moderate to severe mental retardation. The nature of the underlying defect is unknown, although the gene defect may be at 3q22.1-q24.[646]

Noonan's Syndrome

Although Noonan's syndrome shares certain phenotypic features with Turner's syndrome, the two disorders are clearly distinct.[647, 648] In Noonan's syndrome, the sex chromosomes are normal and transmission is apparently autosomal dominant; neither the gene locus nor product has been identified, although linkage with chromosome 12 has been demonstrated. Both males and females may be affected, which may explain the misleading terms *Turner-like syndrome* and *male Turner's syndrome*.

Affected individuals typically have webbing of the neck, a low posterior hairline, ptosis, cubitus valgus, and malformed ears. Cardiac abnormalities are primarily right-sided (pulmonary valve) rather than the left-sided lesions (aorta, aortic valve) characteristic of Turner's syndrome.

Although birth weight is generally within the normal range, mean growth in length and weight is below the 3rd percentile through much of childhood with a falling height velocity not dissimilar to that seen in Turner's syndrome except for the late and attenuated pubertal increments.[649, 650] GH secretory abnormalities do not account for the short stature, although endogenous GH production may be reduced somewhat.[651, 652] Microphallus and cryptorchidism are common, and puberty may be delayed or incomplete. Mental retardation of variable degrees is present in approximately 25% to 50% of patients.

ten ameliorates growth retardation and can be associated with an accelerated catch-up phase.[848, 853]

The use of spacer devices and effective nebulizer solutions may permit use of inhaled glucocorticoids in young children without growth impairment.[523, 855, 856] Clearly, however, sufficient glucocorticoid delivered by any route can diminish growth and impede the function of the adrenal gland.[857] Nonetheless, judicious utilization of inhaled glucocorticoid results in normal adult height despite long-term exposure and an initial decrement of linear growth velocity.[858] Indeed, examination of near adult heights of Swedish men with asthma demonstrated an improvement in the mean difference between "severe" asthmatics and normal controls in the era of inhaled corticosteroid use.[859] Overall, normal adult height is usually achieved.[860, 861]

Bronchopulmonary dysplasia (BPD), a sequela of hyaline membrane disease and prematurity, is characterized by an incidence as high as 35% in very-low-birth-weight infants (<1500 g).[862] The use of dexamethasone in the neonatal treatment of BPD causes a transient cessation of growth[863] and has engendered long-term concern for neurodevelopment and somatic growth.[864] Growth in surviving infants is poor through early childhood,[865–867] but the defect generally disappears by 8 years of age.[868–870] Long-term hypoxemia, poor nutrition, chronic pulmonary infections, and reactive airway disease are responsible for the poor early growth.

In patients with cystic fibrosis (CF), chronic pulmonary infection with bronchiectasis, pancreatic insufficiency with exocrine and endocrine inadequacy, malabsorption, and malnutrition[694, 871–876] all contribute to decreased growth and late sexual maturation. In 17,857 patients with CF, mean height was at the 21st percentile and mean weight was at the 9th percentile.[877] Early impairment of height and weight growth and retardation of skeletal maturation may progress or plateau during middle childhood years but become most marked in the preadolescent period when growth and maturational changes are delayed.[871, 877–880]

The degree of growth retardation is related most closely to the severity and variability of the pulmonary disease rather than to pancreatic dysfunction.[694, 873, 874] The degree of steatorrhea does not correlate well with growth impairment, although improved nutrition programs enhance the overall clinical picture.[875, 876] Adult heights in surviving patients with CF approach the normal range.[694] Endocrine abnormalities, such as failure of both alpha and beta islet cells with decreased glucagon and insulin production do not seem to influence prepubertal growth patterns in children with CF. The incidence of diabetes mellitus increases as patients live past the second decade.[877] Alterations of vitamin D metabolism, although potentially affecting skeletal mineralization, do not diminish growth.[881] Delayed sexual maturation in which GnRH administration evokes a prepubertal pattern of pituitary gonadotropin secretion in adolescent patients is similar to that in CDGM.[879, 880] The GH-IGF axis shows evidence for acquired GHI with lowered mean IGF-I and elevated GH levels.[882]

GH treatment of prepubertal children with CF for 1 year resulted in an anabolic effect with greater growth velocity and nitrogen retention and increased protein and decreased fat stores.[883, 884] Pulmonary function improved in most patients. A 4-year longitudinal study using the National Cystic Fibrosis Foundation Registry found that improved nutrition status and growth were associated with a slower age-related decrement of pulmonary function.[885]

Chronic Inflammation and Infection

Poor growth is a characteristic feature of chronic inflammatory disease and recurrent serious infection. We have discussed impaired growth associated with disorders such as Crohn's disease, CF, and asthma in which inflammatory processes may be significant. De Benedetti and co-workers,[886] studying juvenile rheumatoid arthritis in humans and a transgenic murine model expressing excessive IL-6, demonstrated an IL-6–mediated decrease in IGF-I production to be a credible mechanism by which chronic inflammatory disease could lead to poor growth. The close relationship of the GHR to that of multiple cytokines[181] makes this an interesting hypothesis. A complex cascade of cytokines, as part of the inflammatory response to acute and chronic infection, can impact the endocrine system at many levels,[887, 888] impairing mineral and nutrient metabolism and the growth and remodeling of bone.[889]

Exposure to human immunodeficiency virus (HIV) in children and adolescents occurs through perinatal transmission, blood transfusions, drug usage and sexual contact, most commonly via perinatal transmission from HIV-infected mothers. Growth failure is a cardinal feature of childhood *acquired immunodeficiency syndrome* (AIDS).[890–895] Mean length and weight measurements during early childhood years are at or below −1 SD below the mean, but weight-for-height data may be normal[893, 895] in contrast with the "wasting" syndrome described in adult patients with AIDS.[896, 897]

In a drug treatment study of 88 HIV-infected children (mean age, 3.1 years), more than 90% were below the 50th percentile for both height and weight. Only 44% of this group survived 4 years after initiation of the study.

Height or growth velocity is not a useful predictive indicator for survival.[893] In hemophiliac boys with HIV growth impairment, delayed pubertal onset and progression, and lower skeletal age were common.[894] Despite this delayed pubertal maturation, serum testosterone levels were not significantly decreased. In many developing countries, chronic infestation with parasites (e.g., schistosomiasis, hookworm, roundworm) contributes to nutritional debilitation and growth failure.[898]

Endocrine Disorders

Hypothyroidism

Growth may be retarded in children with hypothyroidism, but the development of newborn screening programs for congenital hypothyroidism has resulted in more prompt diagnosis and treatment of such newborns (~1/4100 live births). Growth in appropriately treated infants and children with congenital hypothyroidism is normal for age,[899, 900] so that skeletal maturation approximates chronologic age.[900] These data do demonstrate the essential role of T_4 in linear growth during the first year of life.[901] Pubertal growth and maturation and final adult height are normal in well-treated congenital hypothyroidism.[902]

Many features of adult myxedema are present in children with hypothyroidism. The most prominent manifestation of acquired hypothyroidism is growth failure, which may be profound.[903] In acquired hypothyroidism, growth retardation may take several years to become clinically evident; once present, however, it is typically severe and progressive. The poor growth is more apparent in height than in weight gain, so those children tend to be overweight for height.

Rivkees and associates[903] reported a mean 4.2-year delay between slowing of growth and the diagnosis of hypothyroidism. At diagnosis, girls were 4.04 SD below and boys 3.15 SD below mean heights for age. (This is one of several situations in which the diagnosis of short stature is later in girls than in boys.) Body proportion is immature, with an increased upper body to lower body segment ratio. Skeletal age is usually markedly delayed. Although chronic hypothyroidism is usually associated with delayed puberty, precocious puberty and premature menarche can occur in hypothyroid children (see Chapter 24).

The diagnosis of primary hypothyroidism is usually straightforward. Serum levels of T_4 are reduced, and thyrotropin levels are elevated. The presence of antithyroid antibodies (usually thyroperoxidase antibodies) is consistent with a diagnosis of Hashimoto's thyroiditis, the most common cause of acquired childhood hypothyroidism in the United States. Isolated secondary or tertiary hypothyroidism, due to thyrotropin or thyrotropin-releasing hormone (TRH) deficiency, respectively, is a rare cause of hypothyroidism.

Replacement therapy results in rapid catch-up growth. Nevertheless, accelerated growth may not restore full growth potential because rapid skeletal maturation is rapid during the first 18 months of treatment.

In one study of profoundly hypothyroid children, those treated at a mean chronologic age of 11 years had adult heights approximately −2 SD below the mean, final heights that were lower than midparental and predicted adult heights.[903] The deficit in adult stature correlated with the duration of hypothyroidism before initiation of treatment.

In a separate study of hypothyroid children treated at a mean age of 9 years and with a 3-year delay of bone age,[904] mean height SDS for bone age fell from +0.59 to −0.55 in girls and from +1.6 to −0.87 in boys. Catch-up growth may be particularly compromised when therapy is initiated near puberty.[905]

On the basis of these studies, it may be appropriate to use lower than usual replacement dosages of levothyroxine and to consider a pharmacologic delay of puberty and epiphyseal fusion.

Cushing's Syndrome

Glucocorticoid excess impairs skeletal growth,[906, 907] interferes with normal bone metabolism by inhibiting osteoblastic activity, and enhances bone resorption,[908–910] effects related to the duration of steroid excess,[911] regardless of whether Cushing's syndrome is due to ACTH hypersecretion, adrenal tumor, or glucocorticoid administration. The effects of glucocorticoids are probably at the level of the epiphysis[778, 780, 781, 912] because GH secretion and serum concentrations of IGF peptides and IGFBPs are usually normal.[910, 913]

GH treatment cannot completely overcome the growth-inhibiting effects of excess glucocorticoids, although short-term GH or IGF-I administration can diminish many of the catabolic effects.[221, 909, 914] Linear growth in children receiving glucocorticoids falls during GH therapy if the exogenous prednisone dose is greater than 0.35 mg/kg per day.[910, 915] The "toxic" effects of glucocorticoids on the epiphysis may persist, in part, after correction of chronic glucocorticoid excess, and patients frequently do not attain target heights.[916, 917] The longer the duration and the greater the intensity of glucocorticoid excess, the less likely is catch-up growth to be completed. Therefore, exposure to excess glucocorticoids should be limited as much as the underlying condition allows, frequently by the use of alternate-day therapy.[848, 853, 915, 918]

Adrenal tumors secreting large amounts of glucocorticoids can produce excess androgen, which may mask growth-inhibitory effects of glucocorticoids. In addition, Cushing's syndrome in children may not cause all the clinical signs and symptoms associated with the disorder in adults and may present with growth arrest. However, Cushing's syndrome is an unlikely diagnosis in children with obesity, because exogenous obesity is associated with normal or even accelerated skeletal growth and growth deceleration is generally evident by the time other signs of Cushing's syndrome appear (Fig. 23–43). In a series of 10 children and adolescents treated for Cushing's disease with surgery and cranial radiation, mean final height was −1.36 SDS. Post-therapy GHD was common, and GH replacement contributed to a positive change of the difference between height and target height from diagnosis to final height (−1.72 to −0.93).[919, 920]

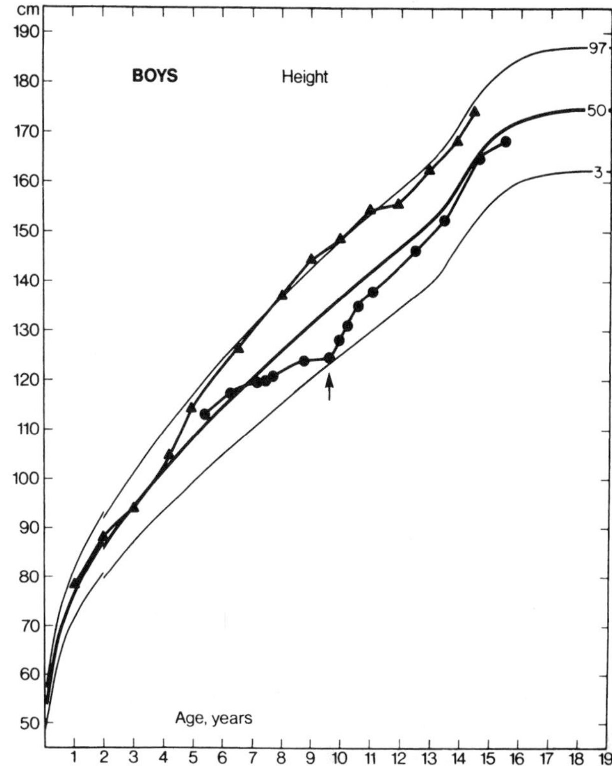

Figure 23–43. Growth curves of two boys with obesity. The boy depicted by the *circles* had cortisol excess related to Cushing's disease. An onset of rapid weight gain was associated with a decrease in linear growth velocity at 7 years of age. The diagnosis was established, and an adrenalectomy *(arrow)* was performed at the age of 9½ years, with an almost immediate increase in growth rate and striking catch-up. The boy whose growth is depicted by *triangles* had exogenous obesity. At the age of 9½ years, his weight was approximately the same as that of the patient with Cushing's disease, but his height was at the 97th percentile, reflecting the enhancement of linear growth in this individual with exogenous obesity.

Pseudohypoparathyroidism

Pseudohypoparathyroidism (detailed in Chapter 26) is mentioned here because growth failure is a common feature.[921] This condition typically combines growth failure, characteristic dysmorphic features, and hypocalcemia and hyperphosphatemia secondary to end-organ resistance to parathyroid hormone. Affected children are short and have truncal obesity with short metacarpals, subcutaneous calcifications, round facies, and mental retardation.

Rickets

In the past, hypovitaminosis D was a major cause of short stature often associated with other causes of growth failure, such as malnutrition, prematurity, malabsorption, hepatic disease, or chronic renal failure (see Chapter 27). In isolated vitamin D deficiency, breast-fed infants typically have poor exposure to sunlight and are not nutritionally supplemented with vitamin D. Characteristic skeletal manifestations of rickets include frontal bossing, craniotabes, rachitic rosary, and bowing of the legs. Such children usually begin to synthesize $1{,}25(OH)_2D$ as they become older, broaden their diet, and have increased exposure to sunlight with amelioration of the transient early decrease of linear growth velocity.

The association of vitamin D receptor gene polymorphism with birth length, growth rate, adult stature, and bone mineral

Table 23–5. Genetic Defects of the GH-IGF Axis Resulting in Insulin-like Growth Factor Deficiency

Mutant Gene	Inheritance	Phenotype	References	Murine Homologue	Reference
GHD Due to Hypothalamic-Pituitary Dysfunction: Developmental Abnormalities					
HESX1	AR	Septo-optic dysplasia; variable involvement of pituitary hormones	987, 988	*Hesx1/Rpx*	64, 987, 990
PROP1	AR	GH, PRL, TSH, LH, FSH deficiencies; Variable degree of ACTH deficiency	1097, 1098	*Prop1* (Ames mouse)	1097, 1098
POU1F1 (Pit-1)	AR, AD	GH, PRL deficiency; variable degree of TSH deficiency	971, 1151, 1119, 1124	*Pit1/Ghf1* (Snell and Jackson mouse)	1118
RIEG	AD	Rieger syndrome; IGHD	532, 1126	*Rieg Pitx2*	1127, 1128
IGHD					
GHRHR	AR	IGHD, type IB form of IGHD	1131–1134	*Ghrhr* (little mouse)	1114, 1116, 1137–1139
GH1	AR	Type IA form of IGHD	971, 140	*Gh* (spontaneous dwarf rat)	1584
	AR	Type IB form of IGHD	971, 1096, 1120		
	AD	Type II form of IGHD	971, 1096, 1120		
	X-linked	Type III form of IGHD; hypogamma-globulinemia	1148		
	AD	Bioinactive GH molecule	1151, 1152		
GHI					
GHR				Ghr	267
Extracellular domain	AR, AD	IGF-I deficiency, decreased or normal GHBP	169, 1178, 1179		
Transmembrane domain	AR	IGF-I deficiency; normal or increased GHBP	203, 1185		
Intracellular domain	AD	IGF-I deficiency; normal or increased GHBP	1186, 1187		
Primary Defects of IGF Synthesis					
IGFI	AR	IGF-I deficiency; IUGR and postnatal growth failure	270	IgfI	277

ACTH, adrenocorticotropic hormone; AD, autosomal dominant; AR, autosomal recessive; FSH, follicle-stimulating hormone; GH, growth hormone; GHBP, GH-binding protein; GHD, GH deficiency; GHI, GH insensitivity; GHR, GH receptor; GHRH, GH-releasing hormone; GHRHR, GHRH receptor; IGF, insulin-like growth factor; IGHD, isolated GHD; LH, luteinizing hormone; PRL, prolactin; TSH, thyrotropin (thyroid-stimulating hormone).

density[922–926] further emphasizes the importance of vitamin D in normal growth. Additionally, vitamin D and estrogen receptor genotypes appear to interactively affect infant growth, especially in males.[924, 927] The presence of high-affinity binding sites for the vitamin D receptor DNA–binding domain in the GH promoter suggests that the vitamin D receptor may actually modulate GH expression.[928]

Vitamin D–Resistant (Hypophosphatemic) Rickets

Vitamin D–resistant (hypophosphatemic) rickets is an X-linked dominant disorder that is due to decreased renal tubular reabsorption of phosphate related to mutations in the phosphate-regulating endopeptidase gene (*PHEX*, Xp22.1) (see Chapter 27). The features are usually more severe in boys and include short stature, prominent bowing of the legs, and (sometimes) rachitic signs.[929] The metabolic and skeletal abnormalities cannot be overcome by vitamin D therapy alone, hence the name *vitamin D–resistant rickets*.

Treatment requires oral phosphate replacement, but such therapy may result in poor calcium absorption from the intestine. The addition of calcitriol to oral phosphate increases intestinal phosphate absorption and prevents hypocalcemia and secondary hyperparathyroidism. Such combined therapy does improve the rickets but does not necessarily correct growth.[930–932] There is no clear association between endogenous GH secretion, IGF-I, or phosphate levels and height in this disorder.[933–935] Nevertheless, GH therapy, in eight trials including 83 patients, has resulted in an enhancement of skeletal growth and improvement in bone mineral density.[936–938] In 14 of these patients, treatment for 4 to 5 years resulted in a height gain of up to 1.2 SDS.

IGF-I Deficiency

Because IGF-I is a major mediator of skeletal growth, its deficiency can result in severe growth failure. Causes of IGF-I deficiency include:

1. Central hypothalamic-pituitary dysfunction with failure of pituitary GH production (i.e., hypopituitarism or GHD). It may be impossible to discriminate between hypothalamic and pituitary dysfunction if both organs have the same pathologic process.
2. Primary or secondary GH insensitivity (GHI).

We use the term *insulin-like growth factor I* (IGF-I) *deficiency syndrome* to describe the generic condition, whether caused by GHD, dysfunction, or insensitivity, to illustrate this unifying concept.

It is not always possible to discriminate completely between hypothalamic and pituitary dysfunction because both organs may be involved in the same pathologic process. In addition, as described earlier, embryonic development of the hypothalamus and pituitary appears to be codependent. A number of factors produced in the developing ventral diencephalon function as molecular signals for initial formation and development of Rathke's pouch; subsequent differentiation of each of the vari-

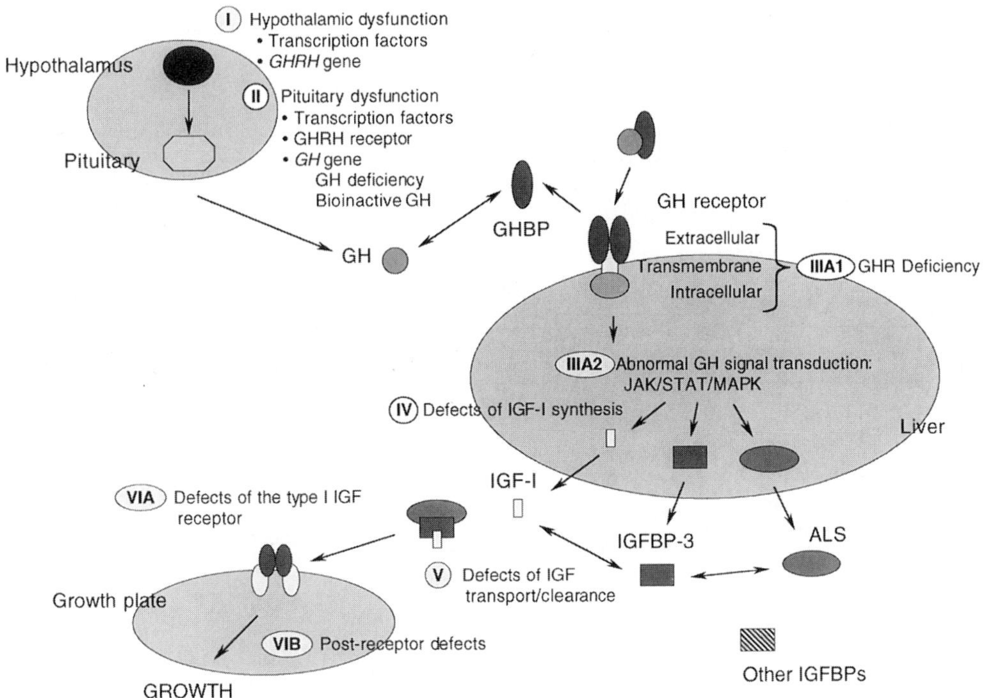

Figure 23–44. The hypothalamic-pituitary-IGF axis: sites of established and hypothetical defects. The established defects are shown as Roman numerals in the gray-shaded circles or ovals, and the hypothetical defects are shown in the white circles or ovals. ALS, acid-labile subunit; GH, growth hormone; GHBP, GH-binding protein; GHRH, GH-releasing hormone; IGF, insulin-like growth factor; IGFBP, IGF-binding protein; JAK, Janus kinase; MAPK, mitogen-activated protein kinase; STAT, signal transducer and activator of transcription. (From Lopez-Bermejo A, Buckway CK, Rosenfeld RG: Genetic defects of the growth hormone–insulin-like growth factor axis. Trends Endocrinol 2000; 11:43.)

ous anterior pituitary cell types appears to be primarily regulated by a strict temporal and spatial pattern of pituitary transcription factors. It is somewhat of a semantic issue as to whether to label some of the molecular defects either "hypothalamic" or "pituitary"; nevertheless, some arbitrary classification decisions have been made in the following discussions. Table 23–5 presents our current classification of molecular defects of the GH-IGF axis, whereas the sites of defined and likely sites of genetic defects are shown in Figure 23–44. The murine homologues of these gene defects are also listed in Table 23–5.

A potential system for analysis of the known and potential genetic errors in patients with IGF deficiency syndrome is shown in Figure 23–45. It is to be anticipated that significant development will be made in our understanding of these defects over the next few years and that this classification will require frequent updating and modification.

Clinical Features

IGF-I deficiency due to hypothalamic dysfunction with abnormalities of GHRH, endogenous GHS or SRIF synthesis or secretion, primary or secondary decreased pituitary GH production, or GHI share a common phenotype. The similarity among these patients emphasizes the role of IGF-I in mediating most of the anabolic and growth-promoting actions of GH. This point is further supported by the capability of IGF-I therapy to correct growth in children with mutations of the GHR gene. Accordingly, the typical clinical features of severe IGF deficiency are shared by all of these conditions. If GH or IGF deficiency is acquired, clinical signs and symptoms appear at a later age.

Birth size is normal or near normal in most children with IGF-I deficiency but low in severe congenital GHD and GHI and in the single case of a deletion of the *IGF-I* gene.[270] Typically, birth length and weight are within 10% of normal, and severe IUGR is *not* part of typical IGF deficiency but is present in infants with profound IGF deficiency, confirming the critical role of IGF-I in intrauterine growth. Infants with early-onset GHD may have birth lengths of around 2 SD below the mean.[607–609, 939]

Although at least 50% of infants diagnosed before 2 years of age have birth lengths more than 2 SD below the mean (both in isolated GH and in multiple pituitary hormone deficiencies), mean birth weight is about −1 SD, lending an appearance of relative adiposity, even in the neonatal period.[608] These data further support an intrauterine role of the GH-IGF system in growth regulation along with the high frequency of abnormalities of the hypothalamic-pituitary area defined by magnetic resonance imaging (MRI).[141, 940, 941] Anatomic abnormalities include dysgenesis of the pituitary stalk, ectopic placement of the posterior pituitary inferior to the median eminence, and diminished volume of the anterior pituitary (Fig. 23–46).[942–948] There is high frequency of breech deliveries and perinatal asphyxia.[141, 607–609, 949–951] Neonatal morbidity can include hypoglycemia and prolonged jaundice with direct hyperbilirubinemia due to cholestasis and giant cell hepatitis.[952, 953] When GHD is combined with deficiency of ACTH and thyrotropin, hypoglycemia may be severe. The combination of GHD with gonadotropin deficiency can cause microphallus, cryptorchidism, and hypoplasia of the scrotum.[954] GHD (or GHI) should, therefore, be considered in the differential diagnosis of neonatal hypoglycemia and of microphallus/cryptorchidism.

Postnatal growth is abnormal in severe congenital IGF deficiency (Fig. 23–47). Most surveys of GHD and GHI indicate that growth failure can occur during the first months of

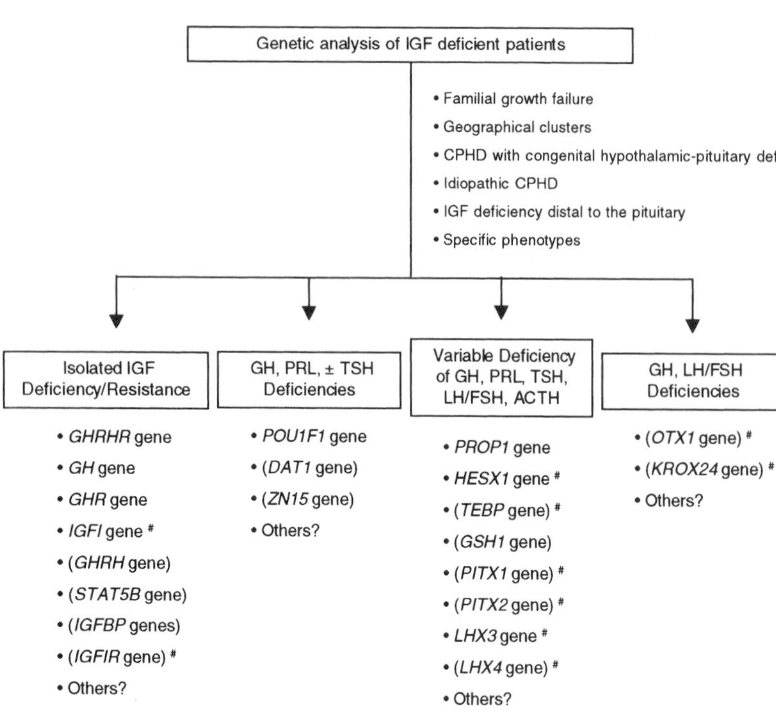

Figure 23–45. Decision tree for the investigation of genetic defects in patients with IGF deficiency. Hypothetical genetic defects are presented in parentheses. In those defects shown with a # sign, abnormalities in other organs and structures besides the hypothalamus-pituitary-IGF axis are expected to occur as a result of these genetic defects. ACTH, adrenocorticotropic hormone; CPHD, combined pituitary hormone deficiencies; FSH, follicle-stimulating hormone; GH, growth hormone; GHR, GH receptor; GHRHR, GH-releasing hormone receptor; IGF, insulin-like growth factor; IGFIR, IGF-I receptor; LH, luteinizing hormone; PRL, prolactin; STAT5, signal transducer and activator of transcription 5; TSH, thyrotropin (thyroid-stimulating hormone). (From Lopez-Bermejo A, Buckway CK, Rosenfeld RG: Genetic defects of the growth hormone–insulin-like growth factor axis. Trends Endocrinol 2000; 11:43.)

life.[607–609, 949] By 6 to 12 months of age, the growth rate is definitely slow and deviates from the normal growth curve, with lengths 3 to 4 SD below the mean. This stresses the importance of normal IGF-I production and action in the neonatal period and early childhood. We emphasize that the single most important clinical manifestation of IGF deficiency of all causes is growth failure, and careful documentation of growth rates is critical to making the correct diagnosis. Deviation from the normal growth curve should always be a cause of concern; between 2 years of age and the onset of puberty, growth deceleration (or acceleration) must *always* be considered pathologic.

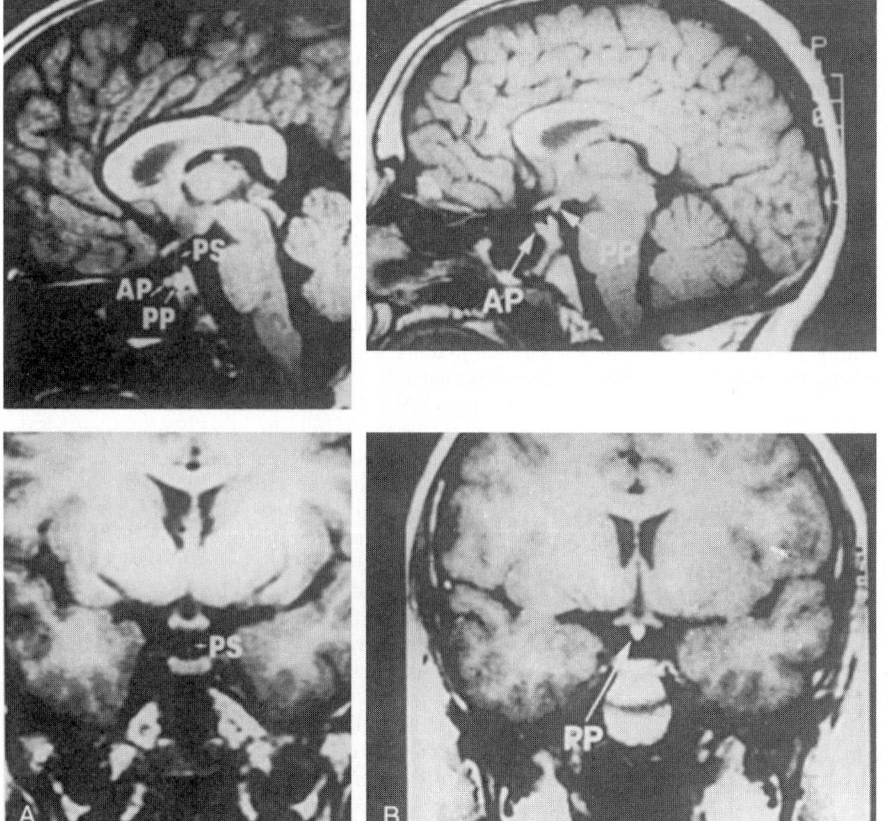

Figure 23–46. Magnetic resonance image of infundibular dysgenesis. *A*, T1-weighted sagittal and coronal images of the hypothalamic-pituitary area in a normal 8-year-old girl. The anterior pituitary (AP) and posterior pituitary (PP) lobes and the pituitary stalk (PS) are marked. *B*, T1-weighted sagittal and coronal images of the hypothalamic-pituitary area of a 17-year-old boy with isolated human growth hormone deficiency. The anterior pituitary (AP) lobe is hypoplastic, the posterior pituitary (PP) lobe is ectopic, and the pituitary stalk is absent. (From Root AW, Martinez CR. Magnetic resonance imaging in patients with hypopituitarism. Trends Endocrinol Metab 1992; 3:283–287.)

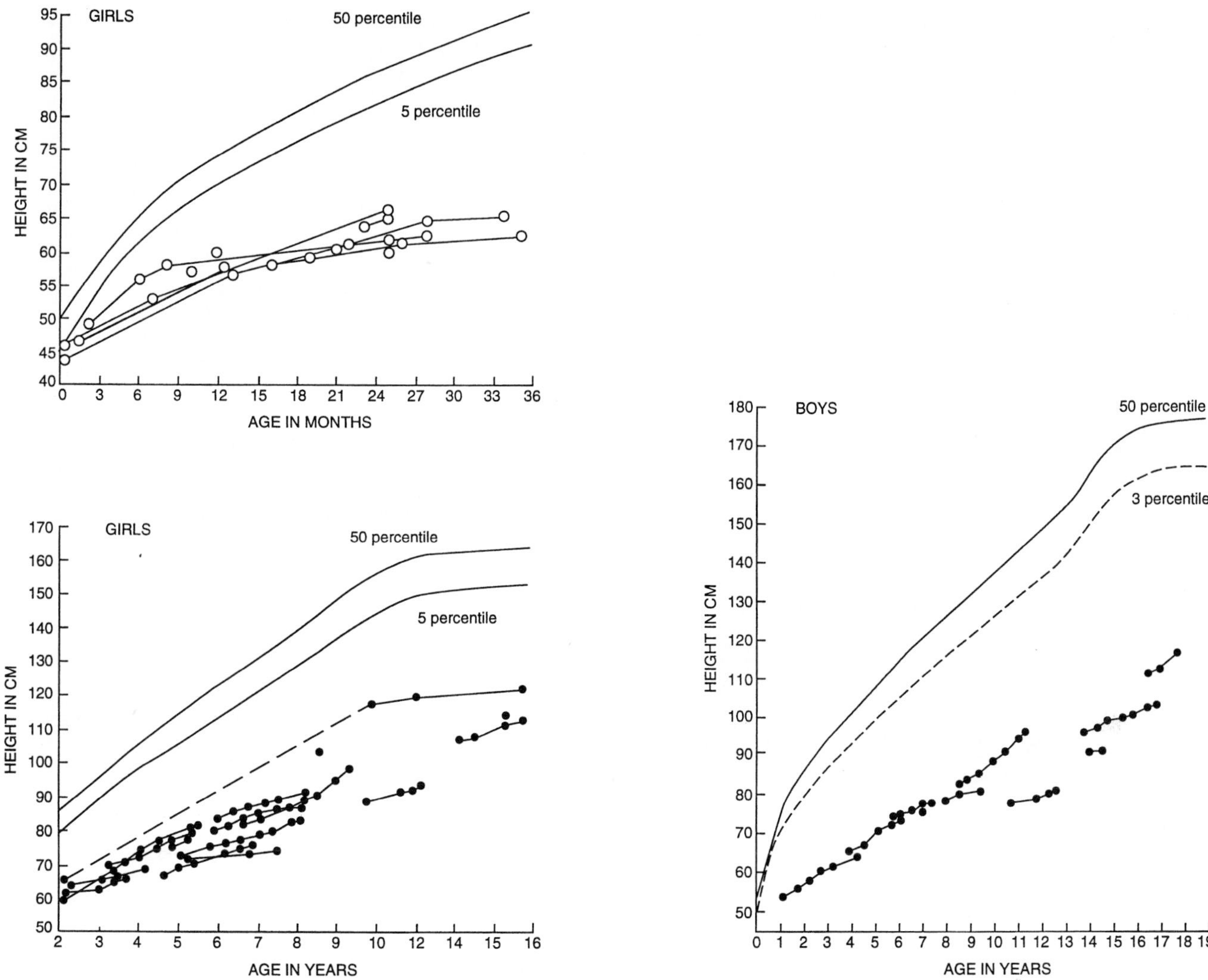

Figure 23–47. Height measurements for Ecuadorian children with insulin-like growth factor deficiency resulting from growth hormone insensitivity. (From Rosenfeld RG, Rosenbloom AL, Guevara-Aguirre J. Growth hormone [GH] resistance due to primary GH receptor deficiency. Endocr Rev 1994; 15:369–390. © The Endocrine Society.)

Skeletal proportions tend to be relatively normal but correlate better with bone age than with chronologic age. Skeletal age may be delayed to less than 60% of the chronologic age but in the absence of hypothyroidism is similar to the height age.[949] In acquired GHD, as from a CNS tumor that causes increased intracranial pressure, bone age may approximate the chronologic age; delayed skeletal maturation, therefore, should not be required for the diagnosis of GHD.

Assessment of volumetric bone mineral density reveals decreased mineralization beyond that dependent on small size.[955] Weight-to-height ratios tend to be increased, and fat distribution is often "infantile" or "doll-like" in pattern. Musculature is poor, especially in infancy and can cause delay in gross motor development and lead to the erroneous impression of mental retardation in an immature-appearing child. Facial bone growth may be particularly retarded, with an underdeveloped nasal bridge and frontal bossing (Fig. 23–48). Fontanel closure is often delayed, but the overall growth of the skull is normal, leading to cephalofacial disproportion and the appearance of hydrocephalus. The voice is infantile because of hypoplasia of the larynx. Hair growth is sparse and thin, especially during early life; nail growth is also slow. Even with normal gonadotropin production, the penis is small and puberty is usually delayed.

Final height data in patients with untreated GHD are not plentiful. Wit and colleagues[956–959] summarized data from 22 untreated men and 14 women with severe isolated GHD with a mean final height SDS of −4.7. In 19 patients with multiple pituitary hormone deficiencies, thus lacking in gonadal steroids, mean final height was −3.1 SDS.[959]

Etiology

Two surveys of nearly 63,000 GH-treated patients, in databases managed by Pharmacia (Pharmacia International Growth Database [KIGS]) and Genentech (National Collaborative Growth Study [NCGS]), cared for by pediatric endocrinologists throughout the world include more than half of the internationally treated patients.[960, 961] The patients are diverse and include subjects with GHD and with Turner's syndrome and miscellaneous other disorders. About 59% of the total group (~37,000 patients) had GHD (as defined by a stimulated GH level of < 10 μg/L) of whom 78% had "idiopathic" GHD and 22% had "acquired" or "organic" (neoplasms, trauma, inflammation, miscellaneous) causes of GHD. The latter group includes patients with congenital (developmental) GHD-associated syndromes. The organic/acquired group is probably underestimated because many of the patients classified as idio-

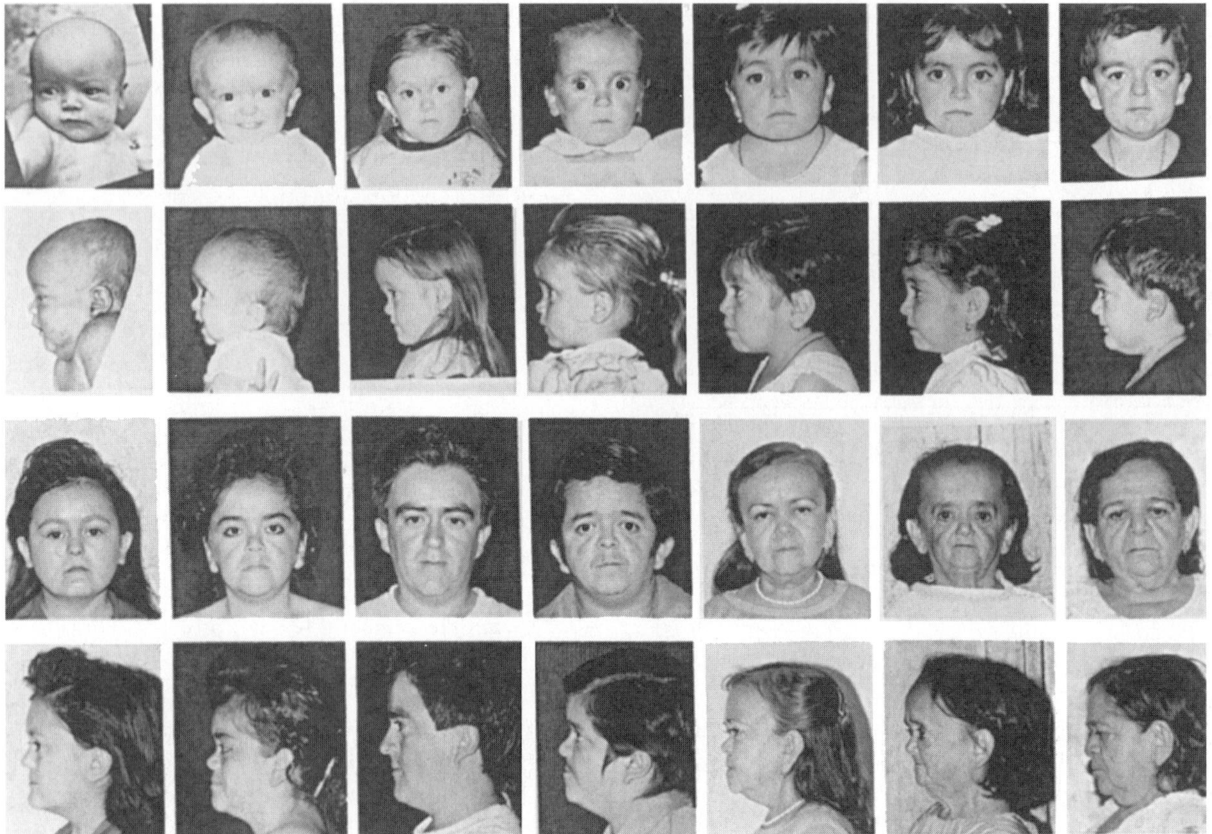

Figure 23–48. Facial appearance of Ecuadorian patients with insulin-like growth factor deficiency due to growth hormone insensitivity. (From Rosenfeld RG, Rosenbloom AL, Guevara-Aguirre J. Growth hormone [GH] resistance due to primary GH receptor deficiency. Endocr Rev 1994; 15:369–390. © The Endocrine Society; photography by A. L. Rosenbloom, M.D.)

pathic had not had definitive imaging assessments of the hypothalamic-pituitary region and possibly have congenital structural abnormalities.

With the availability of synthetic IGF-I for treatment of patients with inherited abnormalities of the GHR, approximately 200 patients with primary GHI have been identified. This is an exceedingly small number of subjects, even with the addition of the potentially larger group of individuals with heterozygous abnormalities of the GHR.[962, 963] In contrast, patients with secondary GHI, including those with malnutrition or chronic systemic disease, must be considered as potentially a huge number, on a worldwide basis.

An incidence of GHD of 1:60,000 live births has been reported from the United Kingdom,[964] and a survey of Scottish schoolchildren indicated prevalence as high as 1:4000.[965] The best estimate in the United States population is approximately 1:3480.[966] It is likely, however, that childhood GHD is an *overdiagnosed condition*. In particular, the diagnosis of acquired, idiopathic, isolated GHD should always be suspect. Although one might argue that (1) destructive or inflammatory lesions of the hypothalamus or pituitary may affect only GH secretion *or* (2) isolated GHD due to a mild mutation or deletion of the GHRH receptor gene or GH gene may appear late *or* (3) *combined pituitary hormone deficiencies* (CPHDs) may first present with what appears to be isolated GHD, such circumstances appear to be rare. In the absence of anatomic abnormalities evident on imaging studies, or biochemical evidence of CPHD, the diagnosis of acquired, isolated, idiopathic GHD demands careful and thorough documentation, with greater skepticism as children approach adolescence. The entity of partial, transient GH insufficiency related to sex steroid deficiency in delayed puberty is particularly confounding.

Central: Hypothalamic-Pituitary Abnormalities

Many of the disorders that affect hypothalamic regulation of GH synthesis and secretion also have a direct impact on pituitary function. Consequently, it is not always possible to definitively establish the primacy of hypothalamic or pituitary dysfunction, hence the term *idiopathic*. Nevertheless, congenital (developmental) or functional abnormalities of the hypothalamus account for most idiopathic cases of hypopituitarism, and many such cases of GHD prove to have a molecular basis. Acquired structural damage to this area (such as from neoplasm and trauma) causes about 25% of GHD cases.

Hypothalamic Dysfunction: Genetic Abnormalities. Hypothalamic factors involved in regulating GH synthesis and secretion include, but may not be limited to, GHRH,[77, 78] GHSs, endogenous GH-releasing peptides such as ghrelin,[102, 104] PACAP,[110, 967] galanin,[968] and somatostatin.[79] Mutations of the genes encoding these or other hypothalamic peptides may explain some cases of IGF deficiency due to hypothalamic dysfunction. To date, however, mutations of the genes encoding GHRH have not been identified.[969–971] Targeted disruption of the murine homeobox gene *T/ebp*, expressed in the ventral diencephalon but not in Rathke's pouch or in the pituitary during embryogenesis, results in early ablation of the pituitary primordium.[59]

A *Gsh-1* homeobox gene, expressed in varied parts of the developing murine CNS,[84] plays an important role in pituitary development because mutant strains have impaired production of GHRH with anterior pituitary hypoplasia and GHD.[85] The broad impact of defects of this gene on hypothalamic releasing factors may be similar to mutations of the *Pit-1* gene because deficiencies of prolactin and LH also occur.[85] Deletions of the murine dopamine transporter (DAT) result in increased dopaminergic tone, anterior pituitary hypoplasia, and dwarfism.[972] This suggests an important role for hypothalamic dopamine in pituitary development.

Congenital Malformations Involving the Hypothalamus. Hypothalamic dysfunction from congenital malformations of the brain or hypothalamus is a common cause of hypopituitarism. As noted earlier, patients with early diagnosed congenital GHD frequently have an abnormal pituitary stalk, ectopia of the posterior pituitary, and hypoplasia of the anterior pituitary. Anencephaly results in a pituitary gland that is small or abnormally formed and is frequently ectopic.[141, 973, 974] Despite the loss of hypothalamic regulation, somatotrophs differentiate and proliferate diminished overall mass.[53]

During intrauterine life, serum GH and IGF-I levels are 30% to 50% of the normal range,[150] and pituitary GH content at birth is about 15% to 20% of normal,[141, 150] with similarly low neonatal plasma GH levels.[142, 975, 976] Holoprosencephaly, due to abnormal midline development of the embryonic forebrain, is typically associated with hypothalamic insufficiency[977, 978] and caused by at least two heterozygous mutations.[112, 979] Chromosomal-mediated abnormalities of PACAP and PACAP-R expression may be associated with some cases.[111] Facial dysmorphism of holoprosencephaly ranges from cyclopia to hypertelorism, accompanied by absence of the nasal septum, midline clefts of the palate or lip, and sometimes a single central incisor. GHD may be accompanied by other pituitary hormone insufficiencies. The incidence of GHD is increased in cases of simple clefts of the lip and/or palate alone[980, 981] and children with cleft palates who grow abnormally require further evaluation.

In its complete form, the syndrome of septo-optic dysplasia combines hypoplasia or absence of the optic chiasm or optic nerves, agenesis or hypoplasia of the septum pellucidum or corpus callosum, and hypothalamic insufficiency.[982–984] The extent of the anatomic and functional abnormalities can vary but generally are in parallel to each other.[982, 983] GHD can occur by itself or in combination with deficiencies of thyrotropin, ACTH, and gonadotropins. About 50% of children with severe anatomic defects have hypopituitarism,[141, 985] and the diagnosis should be considered in any child with growth failure associated with pendular or rotatory nystagmus or impaired vision and a small optic nerve disc. In some patients, hypoplastic or interrupted pituitary stalks and ectopic posterior pituitary placement have been identified by MRI.[141, 984, 986] It is not clear whether this disorder is inherited, but there is an increased incidence in offspring of young mothers and in firstborn children.

Mutations of *HESX1*, a paired-like homeodomain gene, expressed early in pituitary and forebrain development, are associated with familial forms of septo-optic dysplasia.[987, 988] Three of 228 patients with a broad spectrum of congenital pituitary defects ranging from pituitary hypoplasia and septo-optic dysplasia were found to have heterozygous mutations of the *HESX1* gene.[989] Transgenic mice lacking this gene exhibit a variety of anterior midline CNS defects (e.g., abnormalities of the corpus callosum and septum pellucidum and microphthalmia) and pituitary dysplasia.[64, 987, 990]

In most patients, so-called idiopathic hypopituitarism or GHD is due to abnormalities of synthesis or secretion of the hypothalamic hypophysiotropic factors.[99–101] In a number of reports, idiopathic GHD is associated with MRI findings of an ectopic neurohypophysis, pituitary stalk dysgenesis, and hypoplasia or aplasia of the anterior pituitary.[941–948, 991–993]

In multiple series involving 397 children with isolated GHD or with CPHDs, 54% had the characteristic MRI findings; 93% of CPHD patients were abnormal in contrast with 32% of patients with isolated GHD.[944–948, 992, 993]

Abrahams and co-workers[942] studied 35 patients with idiopathic GHD and found that those with MRI abnormalities could be divided into two groups: (1) 43% had an ectopic neurohypophysis (neurohypophysis located near the median eminence), absent infundibulum, and absence of the normal posterior pituitary bright spot; and (2) 43% had a small anterior pituitary, either as an isolated finding or combined with an ectopic neurohypophysis. Overall, those patients with the most striking abnormalities of the hypothalamic-pituitary region, largely those with CPHD, had the smallest anterior pituitary glands.[947, 993] Patients with more severe deficiencies of GH have greater frequency of significant morphologic abnormalities.[994, 995]

Although the increased incidence of breech presentation and birth trauma with neonatal asphyxia in congenital idiopathic hypopituitarism has led some to suggest an etiologic role for these occurrences,[943, 992] the syndrome of pituitary stalk dysgenesis with congenital hypopituitarism is probably due to abnormal development, and the perinatal difficulties are likely the consequence rather than the cause of the abnormalities. Findings of a similar MRI appearance in patients with septo-optic dysplasia,[141, 984] in association with type I Arnold-Chiari syndrome and syringomyelia[141, 949, 993] and perhaps also in holoprosencephaly[141] and the occurrence of micropenis with this syndrome,[141, 607–609, 954] all support the concept that congenital hypopituitarism is a genetic or developmental malformation, not a birth injury.

A single report of an apparent autosomal dominant mutation of early brain development with infundibular dysgenesis associated with GHD supports the primary nature of the anomaly.[996] Further indirect evidence in studies[997] of isolated, complete anterior pituitary aplasia indicates that hypothalamic hypopituitarism and breech delivery are consequences of congenital midline brain defects, although perinatal residua of breech delivery may exacerbate ischemic damage to the hypothalamic-pituitary unit.

The MRI findings described earlier for patients with an early diagnosis of hypopituitarism are also found in children diagnosed at a later age. Most of these children have hypothalamic dysfunction as the cause of diminished pituitary hormone secretion. In the older group, as in the infants, structural, acquired hypothalamic, stalk, or pituitary abnormalities must be considered.

Patients with myelomeningocele with long-term survival have growth failure, decreased bone mineral density, and pubertal abnormalities.[998–1000] Diminished growth is due to maldevelopment of the vertebral-skeletal system and to diverse midline CNS developmental anomalies such as hydrocephalus and Arnold-Chiari malformation. Many have hypothalamic-pituitary dysfunction including GHD and precocious puberty.[998, 999] GH treatment does improve growth in these patients, although most of the growth is in the trunk and arms.[998, 1001, 1002] In children with shunted hydrocephalus, nearly two thirds have endocrine abnormalities.[1003, 1004] As a group, prepubertal patients were about 1 SDS below control populations and had a higher body mass index. Sixteen (30%) of 54 patients had inadequate GH production–associated lower

Table 23–9. Key History and Physical Examination Findings in Growth Hormone Deficiency (Growth Hormone Research Society)*

In the neonate, hypoglycemia, prolonged jaundice, microphallus or traumatic delivery
Cranial radiation
Head trauma or central nervous system infection
Consanguinity and/or an affected family member
Craniofacial midline abnormalities
Severe short stature (< −3 SD)
Height < −2 SD and a height velocity over 1 year < −1 SD
A decrease in height SD of >0.5 over 1 year in children >2 years of age
A height velocity < −2 SD over 1 year
A height velocity >1.5 SD below the mean sustained over 2 years
Signs indicative of an intracranial lesion
Signs of multiple pituitary hormone deficiency
Neonatal symptoms and signs of growth hormone deficiency

See Growth Hormone Research Society. Consensus guidelines for the diagnosis and treatment of growth hormone (GH) deficiency in childhood and adolescence: summary statement of the GH Research Society. J Clin Endocrinol Metab 2000; 85:3990–3993.

ation for GHD permits concomitant assessment of ACTH/cortisol secretion during insulin-induced hypoglycemia.

The diagnosis of GHD in a newborn is especially challenging. The presence of micropenis in a male newborn should always lead to an evaluation of the GH-IGF axis. A GH level must be measured in the presence of neonatal hypoglycemia occurring in the absence of a metabolic disorder, such as hyperammonemia or carnitine deficiency syndromes. A level below 20 mg/L in a polyclonal radioimmunoassay suggests GHD. The use of standard GH stimulation tests, except for the glucagon test, is not recommended in neonates. Normative data are not available for stimulated serum GH levels, but a cut-off of 25 ng/mL is probably appropriate and stimulated values lower than 20 ng/mL certainly should raise suspicion. MRI is essential when the diagnosis is suspected, and useful clinical information defining developmental abnormalities of the hypothalamic-pituitary area may be available sooner than GH assay data. An IGFBP-3 level is of value for the diagnosis of neonatal GHD, but IGF-I levels are rarely helpful.[1261] In fact, serum IGFBP-3 should be performed as the test of choice in suspected neonatal GHD.

In summary, a child should be considered a candidate for GH therapy if he or she meets one of these auxologic criteria, supported by biochemical evidence of GHD based on sex steroid–primed provocative tests or evidence of IGF deficiency based on measurement of IGF-I and IGFBP-3 concentrations. Such patients should also undergo MRI studies of the hypothalamus-pituitary and assessment of other pituitary hormone deficiencies. It is understood that this approach will result in GH treatment of some children with idiopathic, isolated GHD or IGF deficiency and that such cases require careful monitoring of both pituitary status and responsiveness to GH treatment. The latter can be assessed relative to recently developed predictive models[1262, 1263] and the diagnosis of GHD reconsidered in the child with idiopathic, isolated GHD, normal MRI findings, and a subnormal clinical response to GH.

Diagnosis of IGF Deficiency Syndrome: Growth Hormone Insensitivity

The combination of decreased serum levels of IGF-I, IGF-II, and IGFBP-3 plus increased serum levels of GH suggests a diagnosis of GHI.[169] The possibility of GHR deficiency is supported by a family history consistent with autosomal recessive transmission. Savage and associates[1257, 1264] devised a scoring system for evaluating short children for the diagnosis of GHR deficiency, based on five parameters:

1. Basal serum GH higher than 10 μ/L (~5 μg/L).
2. Serum IGF-I below 50 μg/L.
3. Height SDS below −3.
4. Serum GHBP less than 10%, based on binding of (^{125}I)GH.
5. A rise in serum IGF-I levels after GH administration of less than twofold the intra-assay variation (~10%).

Blum and colleagues[1265] proposed that these criteria could be strengthened by:

1. Evaluating GH secretory profiles, rather than isolated basal levels.
2. Employing an age-dependent range and the 0.1 percentile as the cut-off level for evaluation of serum IGF-I concentrations.
3. Using highly sensitive IGF-I immunoassays and defining a failed GH response as the inability to increase serum IGF-I levels by at least 15 μg/L.
4. Measuring both basal and GH-stimulated IGFBP-3 levels.

These criteria fit well with the population of patients with GHR deficiency in Ecuador, but that is a homogeneous population with severe GHI.[169, 1256] The applicability of these criteria elsewhere remains to be evaluated. An important biochemical marker is the response of IGF-I (and, possibly, IGFBP-3) to GH stimulation. Normal ranges and age-defined responses of serum IGF-I levels have not been established.[1266, 1267]

Decreased serum levels of GHBP suggest the diagnosis of GHR deficiency, but some individuals with GHR deficiency have normal serum concentrations of GHBP.[169, 202, 203] Such cases represent mutations in the dimerization site or in the intracellular domain of the receptor or abnormalities of postreceptor signal transduction mechanisms. On the other hand, polymorphisms of the *GHR* gene, without associated reductions in levels of IGF-I or IGFBP-3, should not be considered examples of GHI. At this point, definitive diagnosis of GHI requires (1) the classic phenotype, (2) decreased serum levels of IGF-I and IGFBP-3, and (3) identification of an abnormality of the *GHR* gene.

Idiopathic Short Stature

Many children and early adolescents are short (<3rd percentile), with slowed linear growth velocity (<25th percentile). They may have delayed skeletal maturation and an impaired or attenuated pubertal growth spurt, with or without a family history manifesting some or all of these clinical features, and have no chronic illnesses or apparent endocrinopathies. Such children usually have normal GH secretory dynamics, although provocative test results may be blunted under some circumstances; GH-dependent peptides are lower than expected on a chronologic, although usually not skeletal, age basis; treatment with exogenous GH usually augments linear growth.

Such children are usually considered to have variants of normal growth and achieve a final adult height within the range considered acceptable for the family. In most of these children, the cause of the slowed childhood growth and commonly delayed pubertal spurt has not been established. Because this is the largest group of short children, continuing efforts are under way to develop a rational categorization and the means of distinguishing between these children from children with an abnormality of the GH-IGF axis. Several groups of patients, including those with CDGM, genetic or familial short stature, and heterozygous abnormalities of the GHR, are described later. Additional causes of ISS will likely be identified at each level of the hypothalamic-pituitary-IGF axis.[963]

Constitutional Delay of Growth and Maturation

The term *constitutional delay*[1268–1271] describes children with a normal variant of maturational tempo; characterized by short stature but relatively normal growth rates during childhood; delayed puberty with a late and attenuated pubertal growth spurt; and attainment of normal adult height. Most children with constitutional delay begin to deviate from the normal growth curve during the early years of life, and they are at or slightly below the 5th percentile for height by age 2 years.[1272] During middle childhood years, height SDS may gradually drift lower, but this does not appear to affect adult height outcome.[1273] Final height, although usually within the normal population range, is often in the lower part of the parental height target zone,[1274–1276] with few patients exceeding that target height. The predicted final height, especially when the skeletal age is extremely delayed, is greater than that usually achieved.[1277–1279]

The delayed growth spurt may adversely affect growth of the spine and mineralization of the vertebrae, which is not overcome when the pubertal growth acceleration finally occurs, thus limiting the final height.[1278, 1280] The osteopenia reported in men with a history of delayed puberty[1280] may be due to a profound alteration of normal pubertal bone mineral accretion or to a prepubertal and continuing deficit in bone mass that is an intrinsic part of CDGM.[530, 531]

GH secretion may be decreased with transient partial GHD at the time of the delayed pubertal growth spurt, apparently the consequence of inadequate production of gonadal steroids.[132, 1094, 1281, 1282] Such children would be expected to have delayed skeletal ages, normal or slightly low serum IGF-I but usually normal IGFBP-3 levels for skeletal age, and normal GH provocative tests (if pretreated with gonadal steroids). Overnight GH secretion is generally normal in these children when control groups are carefully matched.[1076] By definition, children with pure CDGM should have bone ages sufficiently delayed to result in normal predicted adult heights (>163 cm in males and >150 cm in females) (Table 23–10), although the correlation between predicted and final height is imperfect and must be viewed with caution.[1277–1279] When CDGM occurs in the context of familial short stature (see later), however, children may experience both a delayed adolescent growth spurt *and* a short final height.

As stated earlier, some have attributed the diminished growth in the peripubertal period in CDGM to a transient GHD or to a "lazy" pituitary, a concept that is probably due to the inadequacies of GH testing, especially to the failure to pretreat patients with a brief course of gonadal steroids.[132, 1230] Low serum levels of IGF-I and IGFBP-3 or a poor GH response to provocative testing (after priming with gonadal steroids) should mandate an investigation for underlying pathology, such as intracranial tumors.

Table 23–10. Criteria for Presumptive Diagnosis of Constitutional Delay of Growth and Maturation

1. No history of systemic illness
2. Normal nutrition
3. Normal physical examination, including body proportions
4. Normal thyroid and GH levels
5. Normal CBC, sedimentation rate, electrolytes, BUN
6. Height at or below the 3rd percentile, but with annual growth rate above the 5th percentile for age
7. Delayed puberty
   a. *Males*: failure to achieve Tanner G2 stage by age 13.8 years or P2 by 15.6 years
   b. *Females*: failure to achieve Tanner B2 stage by age 13.3 years
8. Delayed bone age
9. Normal predicted adult height
   a. *Males*: >163 cm (64 inches)
   b. *Females*: >150 cm (59 inches)

BUN, blood urea nitrogen; CBC, complete blood count; GH, growth hormone.

Genetic (Familial) Short Stature

The control of growth in childhood and the final height attained are polygenic in nature. For this reason, familial height affects an individual's growth, and evaluation of a specific growth pattern must be placed in the context of familial growth and stature. Formulas have been developed for determination of parental target height, and growth curves that relate a child's height to parental height are available.[47] As a general rule, a child who is growing at a rate that is inconsistent with that of siblings or parents warrants further evaluation.

Furthermore, many organic diseases characterized by growth retardation are genetically transmitted. This list includes multiple causes, such as GHI due to mutations of the *GHR* gene, *GH* gene deletions, mutations of the *PROP1* or *POUF1* gene, pseudohypoparathyroidism, diabetes mellitus, and some forms of hypothyroidism. Inherited nonendocrine diseases characterized by short stature include osteochondrodysplasias (see earlier), dysmorphic syndromes associated with IUGR (see earlier), inborn errors of metabolism, renal disease, and thalassemia (see later). Identifying short stature as inherited thus does not, by itself, relieve the physician of responsibility for determining the underlying cause of growth failure.

Nonetheless, a constellation of clinical findings describes a normal variant referred to as *genetic short stature* (GSS) (or familial short stature) that differs from the syndrome of CDGM discussed earlier. In GSS, childhood growth is at or below the 5th percentile but the velocity is generally normal. The onset and progression of puberty are normal or even slightly early and more rapid than normal, so that skeletal age is concordant with chronologic age. Parental height is short (both parents are often below the 10th percentile), and pubertal maturation is normal. Final heights in patients with GSS are short and in the target zone for the family.[1276] The GH-IGF system is normal, but exogenous GH therapy during middle childhood years may increase linear growth velocity substantially without disproportionate augmentation of skeletal maturation. Whether long-term GH treatment enhances final height outcome, however, is not clear.

Heterozygous Mutations of the Growth Hormone Receptor

The level of the GHR may be genetically determined, although modulated by such factors as nutritional status; GH production appears to be inversely related to GHR/GHBP levels.[195, 198] Accordingly, GHBP levels have been assessed in subjects with ISS.[196, 197, 1283] Serum levels of GHBP in 90% of children with ISS are lower than the normal mean, 20% being below the normal range, especially a subgroup with low IGF-I and higher mean 12-hour levels of GH.[196, 197] Such data raise the possibility that an abnormality of GHR content or structure might impair GH action.

The inverse relationship of GHBP levels to GH production is consistent with this hypothesis.[152] In a small group of patients with growth failure, low levels of IGF-I, and poor response to exogenous GH, heterozygous GHR mutations were present in 28%.[962] In contrast with the rarity of homozygous GHR mutations in GHR, heterozygosity is more common and may be a frequent cause of short stature.[963, 1189] In heterozygotes, protein from the mutant allele may disrupt the normal dimerization that occurs when GH interacts with its receptor, leading to diminished GH action and growth impairment.

The IGF-I/IGFBP-3 generation test following 4 days of GH administration may reveal individual patients with findings of low basal and provoked peptides and modestly elevated GH levels that might represent partial GHI.[1284, 1285] Biochemical confirmation of insensitivity is mandatory in such cases.

TREATMENT OF GROWTH RETARDATION

When growth failure is the result of a chronic underlying disease, such as renal failure, CF, or malabsorption, therapy must be directed at treatment of the underlying condition. Although growth acceleration may occur in such children with GH or IGF-I therapy, complete catch-up requires correction of the primary medical problem. If treatment of the underlying condition involves glucocorticoids, growth failure may be profound and is unlikely to be correctable until steroids are reduced or discontinued.

Correction of growth failure associated with chronic hypothyroidism requires appropriate thyroid replacement. As discussed earlier, thyroid therapy causes dramatic catch-up growth but also markedly accelerates skeletal maturation, potentially limiting adult height. More gradual thyroid replacement or the use of gonadotropin inhibitors to delay puberty, or both, may be necessary to obtain maximal final height.

Treatment of Constitutional Delay

CDGM is a normal variant, with (by definition) potential for a normal (although delayed) pubertal maturation and a normal (albeit diminished for target zone) adult height. Most subjects can be managed by careful evaluation to rule out other causes of abnormal growth and delayed puberty combined with appropriate explanation and counseling. The skeletal age and Bayley-Pinneau table are often helpful in explaining the potential for normal growth to the patient and parents. A family history of constitutional delay is also a source of reassurance. On occasion, however, the stigmata of short stature and delayed maturation may be psychologically disabling for the preadolescent or teenager.

Some adolescents with delayed puberty have poor self-images and limited social involvement.[1286] In such patients and in some in whom pubertal delay is predicted on the basis of the overall clinical picture, there is a role for the judicious use of short-term gonadal steroids.

Two aspects of this syndrome are addressed by androgen treatment: *short stature*, especially in boys between ages 10 and 14, and *delayed puberty* after age 14 years. In the younger group, in whom CDGM is apparent, the orally administered, synthetic androgen, oxandrolone, has been used extensively.[1287] In several controlled studies,[1288–1293] oxandrolone therapy for 3 months to 4 years increased linear growth velocity of 3 to 5 cm/year without adverse affects or decreasing either actual[1293–1295] or predicted[1290, 1294, 1296] final height. The growth-promoting effects of oxandrolone appear related to its androgenic and anabolic effects rather than to augmentation of the GH-IGF axis.[1297, 1298] Currently recommended treatment is 0.1 mg/kg orally per day. In older boys, in whom delayed pubertal maturation is unbearable and anxiety-provoking, testosterone enanthate has been administered intramuscularly with success.[1287, 1288, 1299] Criteria for therapy of such adolescents should include:

1. A minimal age of 14 years.
2. Height below the 3rd percentile.
3. Prepubertal or early Tanner G2 stage with a early morning serum testosterone lower than 3.5 nmol/L (<1 ng/mL).
4. A poor self-image that does not respond to reassurance alone.

Therapy consists of intramuscular testosterone enanthate, 50 to 200 mg every 3 to 4 weeks, for a total of four to six injections.[1286, 1300] Patients typically show early secondary sex characteristics by the fourth injection and grow an average of 10 cm in the ensuing year. Despite attempts to choose subjects carefully for treatment programs in CDGM, a spectrum of activation of the reproductive system is inevitable; growth responses to short courses of therapy are best in the boys who have early pubertal gonadotropin secretory patterns.[1301] Testosterone enhances growth velocity by direct actions and increases GH production.[13, 132, 163–166] Brief testosterone regimens do not cause overly rapid skeletal maturation, compromise adult height, or suppress pubertal maturation.[1302] It is important to emphasize to the patient that he is normal, that therapy is short-term and designed to provide some pubertal development earlier than he would on his own, and that treatment will not increase adult height. In such situations, the combination of short-term androgen therapy, reassurance, and counseling helps the boys with constitutional delay to cope with a difficult adolescence.

The availability of several new forms of testosterone, which are approved for adults with hypogonadism, provides adolescents with an opportunity for a choice among different androgen replacement therapies. Although effectiveness of these preparations has not been demonstrated in children with constitutional delay, we have personal experience with their successful use, finding an equivalent response to that obtained with testosterone injections. Testosterone gel is painless and easy to apply and has proven popular since its release.[1303] Testosterone patches also avoid the need for injections, but they work best when applied to the scrotum and are often accompanied by complaints of itching.[1304] The dosing of these alternative forms of therapy in children and adolescents has not yet been established. In view of the important role of estrogen in the process of skeletal maturation, aromatase inhibitors might be used in conjunction with androgen therapy to prevent an acceleration of bone age and further enhance final adult height.[1305]

Patients must be reevaluated to ensure that they enter "true" puberty. One year after testosterone treatment, boys should have testicular enlargement and a serum testosterone in the pubertal range. If this is not the case, the diagnosis of hypothalamic-pituitary insufficiency or hypogonadotropic hypogonadism should be considered. Although the diagnosis of constitutional growth delay remains most likely in such patients, some eventually prove to be gonadotropin-deficient, especially if they are still prepubertal late in adolescence.

Referrals for constitutional delay are more common in boys than girls, undoubtedly reflecting our cultural values. When constitutional delay is a problem in girls, short-term estrogen therapy can be employed, but the advancement of bone is a greater hazard at doses that enhance growth velocity and sexual maturation. The use of GH in patients with constitutional delay is discussed in the following sections.

Treatment of Growth Hormone Deficiency

Nomenclature and Potency Estimation

The nomenclature for the various biosynthetic GH preparations reflects the source and the chemical composition of the product. *Somatropin* refers to GH of the same amino acid sequence as that in naturally occurring human GH. Somatropin from human pituitary glands is abbreviated GH or pit-GH; recombinant-origin somatropin is termed *recombinant GH* (rGH). *Somatrem*, abbreviated met-rGH, refers to the methionine derivative of rGH. Although the latter preparation is a more antigenic preparation, that propensity is not clinically relevant; despite the presence of anti-GH antibodies, growth responses to met-rGH are similar to those seen in patients treated with rGH.[1306, 1307] We refer to these biosynthetic preparations as GH in the subsequent discussions.

The biopotency of commercially available biosynthetic GH preparations, expressed as International Units per milligram of the new WHO rGH reference reagent 88/624 for somatropin, is 3 IU/mg.[1308] It was necessary to standardize the early GH preparations by bioassay because of variable production techniques (such as extraction and column purification). The most common bioassays have been the hypophysectomized rat weight gain assay, the tibial width assay, and the more sensitive Nb2 rat lymphoma proliferation assay.[1308–1311] With the availability of purified and essentially equivalent rGH products, the requirement for bioassays has become an FDA requisite to substantiate biologic activity rather than to assess potential differences between preparations. It is likely that the bioassays will be replaced by in vitro binding assays using GHRs or GHBP derived from molecular techniques.[1308]

Historical Perspective

Because untreated patients with IGF deficiency syndrome have profound short stature (averaging nearly −5 SDS[956–959]), the clinical urgency to use GH therapy as soon as it was available has been apparent.[1220] The action of GH is highly species-specific, and humans do not respond to animal-derived GH.[1312–1317] Unlike most other hormones, the only GH that is biologically active in humans is primate GH. For many years, human cadaver pituitary glands were the only practical source of primate GH for treatment of GHD, and more than 27,000 children with GHD worldwide were treated with pit-GH.[1318] The limited supplies of pit-GH, low doses, and interrupted treatment regimens resulted in incomplete growth increments; usually therapy was discontinued in boys whose height reached 5 feet, 5 inches in height and in girls who reached 5 feet in height. Nonetheless, this treatment did increase linear growth and in many patients enhanced final adult height. The dose-response relationship and the relation of age to GH response were recognized during this period.[1319]

Distribution of pit-GH was halted in the United States and most of Europe in 1985 because of concern about a causal relationship with Creutzfeldt-Jakob disease (CJD), a rare and fatal spongiform encephalopathy that had been previously reported to be capable of iatrogenic transmission through human tissue.[1320, 1321] In North America and Europe, the incidence of this disorder is approximately 1 case per million in the general population; it is exceedingly rare before age 50 years. To date, more than 100 young adults who had received human cadaver pituitary products have been identified as cases of CJD, with the sad likelihood that all will die of the disease.[1322–1324] In patients in the United States, the onset of CJD was 14 to 33 years after starting treatment, whereas the large cohort of French patients had a median incubation period approximately 5 years shorter.[1324] Vigilant surveillance for this dreadful complication continues.

Fortunately, by the time the risks of pituitary-derived GH were discovered, rGH was being tested for safety and efficacy.[1306, 1325, 1326] The original rGH included an N-terminal methionine, added as a start signal for transcription (met-rGH). This preparation mimicked pit-GH in regard to both anabolic and metabolic actions. Subsequent rGH preparations do not contain the additional methionine. rGH has universally replaced pit-GH as the treatment for children with GHD.

Treatment Regimens

The recommended therapy–starting dose of GH in GHD is 0.18 to 0.35 mg/kg of body weight per week, administered in seven daily doses, with the mean dose in the United States being 0.3 mg/kg per week.[1327] Alternative regimens include a 6-day/week or 3-day/week schedule, with the same weekly dosage, but they are not as successful. In general, the growth response to GH is a function of the log-dose given, so that increasing dosages further enhance growth velocities,[1262, 1318, 1319] but daily dosing may be the most important treatment parameter.[1328] Either subcutaneous or intramuscular administration has equivalent growth-promoting activity[1329]; the former is now used almost exclusively. GH is available in several vehicles, and multiple systems are now available for administering GH (Table 23–11).

The standard preparation is lyophilized GH that is highly water-soluble, so that it may be brought into solution with a small volume of diluent. An aqueous solution is ready to use and has 28-day stability. A sustained-release preparation of GH with protein integrity in a poly(lactide-coglycolide) polymer that is biocompatible and biodegradable permits once-monthly or twice-monthly treatments.[1330] The pharmacokinetics of this system show an early release of GH and then a sustained release over 12 to 28 days. Average exposure to GH and IGF-I following administration of current treatment regimens of depot GH is approximately half that of daily GH therapy. Either reconstituted or liquid GH is administered in insulin syringes with ultrafine needles that are almost pain-free in skilled hands. Pen devices with internal reconstitution of the GH are frequently used because of ease, accuracy, and "hidden" needles. Needle-free, jet injector systems are available and do yield a normal serum immunoreactive and bioactive GH profile.[1331] The sustained-release GH is administered through a short, larger-bore needle, but the injection pain is balanced against the low frequency of treatments. At this time, all of the GH preparations yield comparable short-term growth outcomes, except long-acting GH, in which mean first year growth rates are about 2 cm lower per year.[1330]

GH treatment should be continued after growth ceases, because GH has other important metabolic effects, including support of normal gonadal function[1332] and attainment of normal adult bone mineral density.[1333, 1334] A report from the Drug and Therapeutics committee of the Lawson Wilkins Pediatric Endocrine Society summarized the society's views on the use of GH in children with diverse syndromes of short stature.[1335]

Growth responses to exogenous GH vary, depending on the frequency of administration, dosage, age (greater absolute gain in a younger child, though not necessarily of growth velocity SDS), weight, and GHR amount, as assessed by serum GHBP levels.[195, 198, 1336] On this general regimen, nonetheless, the typ-

Table 23–11. New Modalities for Treatment of Growth Hormone Deficiency

Liquid formulations
Pen-type delivery devices
Needle-less devices
Oral secretagogues
Long-acting GH formulations
GH-releasing hormone
Inhaled GH delivery systems

GH, growth hormone.

200. Baumann G, Shaw MA, Winter RJ. Absence of plasma growth hormone–binding protein in Laron-type dwarfism. J Clin Endocrinol Metab 1987; 65:814–816.
201. Buchanan CR, Maheshwari HG, Norman MR, et al. Laron-type dwarfism with apparently normal high-affinity serum growth hormone–binding protein. Clin Endocrinol (Oxf) 1991; 35:179–185.
202. Douquesnoy P, Sobrier ML, Duriez B. A single amino acid substitution in the exoplasmic domain of the human growth hormone (GH) receptor confers familial GH resistance (Laron syndrome) with positive GH-binding activity by abolishing receptor homodimerization. EMBO J 1994; 13:1386–1395.
203. Woods KA, Fraser NC, Postel-Vinay MC, et al. A homozygous splice site mutation affecting the intracellular domain of the growth hormone (GH) receptor resulting in Laron syndrome with elevated GH-binding protein. J Clin Endocrinol Metab 1996; 81:1686–1690.
204. Hansen JA, Londberg K, Hilton DJ, et al. Mechanism of inhibition of growth hormone receptor signaling by suppressor of cytokine signaling proteins. Mol Endocrinol 1999; 13:1832–1843.
205. Metcalf D, Greenhalgh CJ, Viney E, et al. Gigantism in mice lacking supressor cytokine signalling-2. Nature 2000; 405:1069–1073.
206. Colson A, Le Cam A, Maiter D, et al. Potentiation of growth hormone–induced liver suppressors of cytokine signaling messenger ribonucleic acid by cytokines. Endocrinology 2000; 141: 3687–3695.
207. Mao Y, Ling PR, Fitzgibbons TP, et al. Endotoxin-induced inhibition of growth hormone signaling in rat liver in vivo. Endocrinology 1999; 140:5505–5515.
208. Takala J, Ruokonen E, Webster NR, et al. Increased mortality associated with growth hormone treatment in critically ill adults. N Engl J Med 1999; 341:785–792.
209. Salmon WD Jr, Daughaday WH. A hormonally controlled serum factor which stimulates sulfate incorporation by cartilage in vitro. J Lab Clin Med 1957; 49:825–836.
210. Daughaday WH, Rotwein P. Insulin-like growth factors I and II: peptide, messenger ribonucleic acid and gene structures, serum and tissue concentrations. Endocr Rev 1989; 10:68–91.
211. Sherwin RS, Schulman GA, Hendler R, et al. Effect of growth hormone on oral glucose tolerance and circulating metabolic rules in man. Diabetologia 1983; 24:155–161.
212. Rosenfeld RG, Wilson DM, Dollar LA, et al. Both human pituitary growth hormone and recombinant DNA–derived human growth hormone cause insulin resistance at a postreceptor level. J Clin Endocrinol Metab 1982; 54:1033–1038.
213. Green H, Morikawa M, Nixon T. A dual-effector theory of growth hormone action. Differentiation 1985; 29:195–198.
214. Gerich JE, Lorenzi M, Bier DM, et al. Effects of physiologic levels of glucagon and growth hormone on human carbohydrate and lipid metabolism: studies involving administration of exogenous hormone during suppression of endogenous hormone secretion with somatostatin. J Clin Invest 1976; 57:875–884.
215. Kostyo JL, Hotchkiss J, Knobil E. Stimulation of amino acid transport in isolated diaphragm by growth hormone added in vitro. Science 1959; 130:1653–1656.
216. Hjalmarson, A, Isaksson O, Ahmen K. Effects of growth hormone and insulin on amino acid transport in perfused rat heart. Am J Physiol 1969; 217:1795–1802.
217. Carrel AL, Allen DB. Effects of growth hormone on body composition and bone metabolism. Endocrine 2000; 12:163–172.
218. Griffin EE, Miller LL. Effects of hypophysectomy of liver donor on net synthesis of specific plasma proteins by the isolated perfused rat liver: modulation of synthesis of albumin, fibrinogen, $alpha_1$-acid glycoprotein, $alpha_2$ (acute-phase)-globulin, and haptoglobin by insulin, cortisol, triiodothyronine, and growth hormone. J Biol Chem 1974; 249:5062–5069.
219. Snyder DK, Clemmons DR, Underwood LE. Treatment of obese, diet-restricted subjects with growth hormone for 11 weeks: effects on anabolism, lipolysis, and body composition. J Clin Endocrinol Metab 1988; 67:54–61.
220. Rudman D, Feller AG, Nagraj HS, et al. Effects of human growth hormone in men over 60 years old. N Engl J Med 1990; 323:1–6.
221. Horber FF, Haymond MV. Human growth hormone prevents the protein catabolic side effects of prednisone in humans. J Clin Invest 1990; 86:265–272.
222. Burgi H, Muller WA, Humbel RE, et al. Non-suppressible insulin-like activity of human serum. I. Physicochemical properties, extraction, and partial purification. Biochem Biophys Acta 1966; 121:349–359.
223. Froesch ER, Zapf J, Meuli C, et al. Biological properties of NSILA-S. Adv Metab Disord 1975; 8:211–235.
224. Dulak NC, Temin HM. A partially purified polypeptide fraction from rat liver cell conditioned medium with multiplication-stimulating activity for embryo fibroblasts. J Cell Physiol 1973; 81: 153–160.
225. Daughaday WH, Hall K, Raben MS, et al. Somatomedin: proposed designation for sulphation factor. Nature 1972; 235:107.
226. Hall K, Takano K, Fryklund L, Sievertsson H. Somatomedins. Adv Metab Disord 1975; 8:19–46.
227. Van Wyk JJ, Underwood LE, Hintz RL, et al. The somatomedins: a family of insulin-like hormones under growth hormone control. Recent Prog Horm Res 1974; 30:259–318.
228. Rinderknecht E, Humbel RE. The amino acid sequence of human insulin-like growth factor I and its structural homology with proinsulin. J Biol Chem 1978; 253:2769–2776.
229. Rinderknecht E, Humbel RE. Primary structure of human insulin-like growth factor II. FEBS Lett 1978; 89:283–286.
230. Jansen M, Van Schaik SM, Van Tol H, et al. Nucleotide sequence of cDNAs encoding precursors of human insulin-like growth factor II (IGF-II) and an IGF-II variant. FEBS Lett 1985; 179:243
231. Zumstein PP, Luthi C, Humbel RE. Amino acid sequence of a variant pro-form of insulin-like growth factor II. Proc Natl Acad Sci USA 1985; 82:3169
232. Gowan LK, Hampton B, Hill DJ, et al. Purification and characterization of a unique high-molecular-weight form of insulin-like growth factor II. Endocrinology 1987; 121:449–458.
233. Daughaday WH, Emaneule MA, Brooks MH, et al. Insulin-like growth factor II synthesis and secretion by a leiomyosarcoma with associated hypoglycemia. N Engl J Med 1988; 319:1434–1440.
234. Zapf J. Insulin-like growth factor–binding proteins and tumor hypoglycemia. Trends Endocrinol Metab 1995; 6:37–42.
235. Powell DR, Lee PDK, Chang D, et al. Antiserum developed for the E-peptide region of insulin-like growth factor IA prohormone recognizes a serum protein by both immunoblot and radioimmunoassay. J Clin Endocrinol Metab 1987; 65:868
236. Sussenbach JS. The gene structure of the insulin-like growth factor family. Prog Growth Factor Res 1989; 1:33–48.
237. Lund PK, Moats-Staats BM, Hynes MA, et al. Somatomedin-C/insulin-like growth factor-I and insulin-like growth factor-II mRNAs in rat fetal and adult tissues. J Biol Chem 1986; 261: 14539–14544.
238. Brown AL, Graham DE, Nissley SP, et al. Developmental regulation of insulin-like growth factor II mRNA in different rat tissues. J Biol Chem 1986; 261:13144–13150.
239. Brissenden JE, Ullrich A, Francke U. Human chromosomal mapping of genes for insulin-like growth factors I and II and epidermal growth factor. Nature 1984; 310:781–784.
240. Tricoli JV, Rall LB, Scott J, et al. Localization of insulin-like growth factor genes to human chromosomes 11 and 12. Nature 1984; 310:784–785.
241. Bell GI, Gerhard DS, Fong NM, et al. Isolation of the human insulin-like growth factor genes: insulin-like growth factor II and insulin genes are contiguous. Proc Natl Acad Sci USA 1985; 82:6450–6454.
242. Yoon JB, Berry SA, Seelig S, Towle HC. An inducible nuclear factor binds to a growth hormone–regulated gene. J Biol Chem 1990; 265:19947–19954.
243. Lowe WL Jr, Roberts CT Jr, Lasky SR, LeRoith D. Differential expression of alternative 5′ untranslated regions in mRNAs encoding rat insulin-like growth factor I. Proc Natl Acad Sci USA 1987; 84:8946–8950.
244. Murphy LJ, Friesen HG. Differential effects of estrogen and growth hormone on uterine and hepatic insulin-like growth factor I gene expression in the ovariectomized hypophysectomized rat. Endocrinology 1988; 122:325–332.
245. Holthuizen PE, Rodenburg RJT, Scheper W, Sussenbach JS. Regulation of IGF-II gene expression and post-transcriptional

processing of IGF-II mRNAs. In Baxter RC, Gluckman PD, Rosenfeld RG (eds). The Insulin-Like Growth Factors and Their Regulatory Proteins. Amsterdam, Elsevier Science, 1994, pp 43–53.
246. Rappolee DA, Sturm KS, Behrendtsen O, et al. Insulin-like growth factor II acts through an endogenous growth pathway regulated by imprinting in early mouse embryos. Genes Dev 1992; 6:939–952.
247. Nason KS, Binder ND, Labarta JI, et al. IGF-II and IGF-binding proteins increase dramatically during rabbit pregnancy. J Endocrinol 1996; 148:121–130.
248. Stylianopoulou F, Herbert J, Soares MB, Efstratiadis A. Expression of the insulin-like growth factor II gene in the choroid plexus and the leptomeninges of the adult rat central nervous system. Cell Biol 1988; 85:141–145.
249. Reeve AE, Eccles MR, Wilkins RJ, et al. Expression of insulin-like growth factor II transcripts in Wilms' tumour. Nature 1985; 317:258–260.
250. Ogawa O, Eccles MR, Szeto J, et al. Relaxation of insulin-like growth factor II gene imprinting implicated in Wilms' tumor. Nature 1993; 362:749–751.
251. Zhan S, Shapiro D, Zhang L, et al. Concordant loss of imprinting of the human insulin-like growth factor II gene promoters in cancer. J Biol Chem 1995; 270:27983–27986.
252. El-Badry OM, Helman LJ, Chatten J, et al. Insulin-like growth factor II–mediated proliferation of human neuroblastoma. J Clin Invest 1991; 87:648–657.
253. Haselbacher GK, Irminger JC, Zapf J, et al. Insulin-like growth factor in human adrenal pheochromocytomas and Wilms' tumors: expression of the mRNA and protein level. Proc Natl Acad Sci USA 1987; 84:1104–1106.
254. Rainier S, Johnson LA, Dobry CJ, et al. Relaxation of imprinted genes in human cancer. Nature 1993; 362:747–749.
255. Tricoli JV, Rall LB, Karakousis CP, et al. Enhanced levels of insulin-like growth factor messenger RNA in human colon carcinomas and liposarcomas. Cancer Res 1986; 46:6169–6173.
256. Werner H, Roberts CT Jr, LeRoith D. Transcriptional repression of the IGF-II and IGF-I receptor genes by tumor suppressor WT1: implications for normal kidney development and Wilms' tumor. In Baxter RC, Gluckman PD, Rosenfeld RG (eds). The Insulin-Like Growth Factors and Their Regulatory Proteins. Amsterdam, Elsevier Science, 1994, pp 107–115.
257. Mahar ER, Reik W. Beckwith-Wiedemann syndrome: imprinting in clusters revisited. J Clin Invest 2000; 105:247–252.
258. Ohlsson R, Nystrom A, Pfeifer-Ohlsson S, et al. IGF2 is parentally imprinted during human embryogenesis and in the Beckwith-Wiedemann syndrome. Nature Genet 1993; 4:94–97.
259. DeChiara TM, Efstratiadis A, Robertson EJ. A growth-deficiency phenotype in heterozygous mice carrying an insulin-like growth factor II gene disrupted by targeting. Nature 1990; 345: 78–80.
260. Baker J, Liu JP, Robertson EJ, Efstratiadis A. Role of insulin-like growth factors in embryonic and postnatal growth. Cell 1993; 75:73–82.
261. Giannoukakis N, Deal C, Paquette J, et al. Parental genomic imprinting of the human IGF2 gene. Nature Genet 1993; 4:98–100.
262. Deal CL. Parental genomic imprinting. Curr Opin Pediatr 1995; 7:445–458.
263. Mutter GL, Stewart CL, Chaponot ML, Pomponio RL. Oppositely imprinted genes H19 and insulin-like growth factor 2 are coexpressed in human androgenetic trophoblast. Am J Hum Genet 1993; 53:1096–1102.
264. Steenman MJC, Rainier S, Dobry CJ, et al. Loss of imprinting of IGF2 is linked to reduced expression and abnormal methylation of H19 in Wilms' tumor patients. Nat Genet 1994; 7:433–438.
265. Barlow DP, Stoger R, Hermann BG, et al. The mouse insulin-like growth factor type-2 receptor is imprinted and closely linked to the Tme locus. Nature 1991; 349:84–87.
266. Estratiadias A. Genetics of mouse growth. Int J Dev Biol 1998; 42:955–976.
267. Zhou Y, Xu BC, Maheshawari HG, et al. A mammalian model for Laron syndrome produced by targeted disruption of the mouse growth hormone receptor/binding protein gene (the Laron mouse). Proc Nat Acad Sci USA 1997; 94:13215–13220.
268. Sims NA, Clement-Lacroix P, DaPonte F, et al. Bone homeostasis in growth hormone receptor-null mice is restored by IGF-I but independent of Stat5. J Clin Invest 2000; 106:1095–1103.
269. Lupu F, Terwilliger JD, Lee K, et al. Roles of growth hormone and insulin-like growth factor I in mouse postnatal growth. Dev Biol 2001; 229:141–162.
270. Woods KA, Camacho-Hubner C, Savage MO, Clark AJL. Intrauterine growth retardation and postnatal growth failure associated with deletion of the insulin-like growth factor I gene. N Engl J Med 1996; 335:1342–1349.
271. Sjogren K, Liu JL, Blad K, et al. Liver-derived insulin-like growth factor I (IGF-I) is the principal source of IGF-I in blood but is not required for postnatal body growth in mice. Proc Nat Acad Sci USA 1999; 96:7088–7092.
272. Yakar S, Liu JL, Stannard B, et al. Normal growth and development in the absence of hepatic insulin-like growth factor I. Proc Natl Acad Sci USA 1999; 96:7324–7329.
273. Le Roith D, Bondy C, Yakar S, et al. The somatomedin hypothesis: 2001. Endocrine Rev 2001; 22:53–74.
274. Butler AA, LeRoith D. Minireview: tissue-specific versus generalized gene targeting of the *IGF1* and *IGF1R* genes and their roles in insulin-like growth factor physiology. J Clin Endocrinol Metab 2001; 142:1685–1688.
275. Ueki I, Ooi GT, Tremblay ML, et al. Inactivation of the acid labile subunit gene in mice results in mild retardation of postnatal growth despite profound disruptions in the circulating insulin-like growth factor system. Proc Natl Acad Sci USA 2000; 97:6868–6873.
276. Le Roith D, Scavo L, Butler A. What is the role of circulating IGF-I? Trends Endocrinol Metab 2001; 12:48–52.
277. Liu JP, Baker J, Perkins AS, et al. Mice carrying null mutations of the genes encoding insulin-like growth factor I (Igf-1) and type 1 IGF receptor (Igf1r). Cell 1993; 75:73–82.
278. Lau MM, Stewart CE, Liu Z, et al. Loss of the imprinted IGF2/cation-independent mannose 6-phosphate receptor results in fetal overgrowth and perinatal lethality. Genes Dev 1994; 8: 2953–2963.
279. Nolan CM, Lawlor MA. Variable accumulation of insulin-like growth factor II in mouse tissues deficient in insulin-like growth factor II receptor. Int J Biochem Cell Biol 1999; 31:1421–1433.
280. Filson AJ, Louvi A, Efstratiadis A, Robertson EJ. Rescue of the T-associated maternal effect in mice carrying null mutations in *IGF-2* and *IGF2R*, two reciprocally imprinted genes. Development 1993; 118:731–736.
281. Hall K. Quantitative determination of the sulphation factor activity in human serum. Acta Endocrinol (Kbh) 1970; 63:338–350.
282. Phillips LS, Herington AC, Daughaday WH. Somatomedin stimulation of sulfate incorporation in porcine costal cartilage discs. Endocrinology 1974; 94:856–863.
283. Garland JT, Lottes ME, Kozak S, Daughaday WH. Stimulation of DNA synthesis in isolated chondrocytes by sulfation factor. Endocrinology 1972; 90:1086–1090.
284. Garland JT, Buchanan F. Stimulation of RNA and protein synthesis in isolated chondrocytes by human serum. J Clin Endocrinol Metab 1976; 43:842–846.
285. Meuli C, Froesch ER. Effects of insulin and of NSILA-S on the perfused rat heart: glucose uptake, lactate production, and efflux of 3-O-methyl glucose. Eur J Clin Invest 1975; 5:93–99.
286. Hall K, Takano K, Fryklund L. Radioreceptor assay for somatomedin A. J Clin Endocrinol Metab 1974; 39:973–976.
287. Van Wyk JJ, Underwood LE, Baseman JB, et al. Explorations of the insulin-like and growth-promoting properties of somatomedin C by membrane receptor assays. Adv Metab Disord 1975; 8: 128–150.
288. Zapf J, Kaufmann U, Eigenmann EJ, Froesch ER. Determination of nonsuppressible insulin-like activity in human serum by a sensitive protein-binding assay. Clin Chem 1977; 23:677–672.
289. Schalch DS, Heinrich UE, Koch JG, et al. Nonsuppressible insulin-like activity (NSILA): development of a new sensitive competitive protein–binding assay for determination of serum levels. J Clin Endocrinol Metab 1978; 46:664–671.
290. Furlanetto RW, Underwood LE, Van Wyk JJ, Handwerger S. Estimation of somatomedin-C levels in normals and patients with pituitary disease by radioimmunoassay. J Clin Invest 1977; 60:646–756.

291. Zapf J, Walter H, Froesch ER. Radioimmunological determination of insulin-like growth factors I and II in normal subjects and in patients with growth disorders and extrapancreatic tumor hypoglycemia. J Clin Invest 1981; 68:1321–1330.
292. Bala RM, Bhaumick B. Radioimmunoassay of a basic somatomedin: comparison of various assay techniques and somatomedin levels in various sera. J Clin Endocrinol Metab 1979; 49:770–777.
293. Baxter RC, Axiak S, Raison RL. Monoclonal antibody against human somatomedin-C/insulin-like growth factor I. J Clin Endocrinol Metab 1982; 54:474–476.
294. Rosenfeld RG, Wilson DM, Lee PDK, Hintz RL. Insulin-like growth factors I and II in the evaluation of growth retardation. J Pediatr 1986; 109:428–433.
295. Daughaday WH, Kapadia M, Mariz I. Serum somatomedin-binding proteins: physiologic significance and interference in radioligand assay. J Lab Clin Med 1986; 109:355–363.
296. Powell DR, Rosenfeld RG, Baker BK, et al. Serum somatomedin levels in adults with chronic renal failure: the importance of measuring insulin-like growth factor (IGF)-1 and -2 in acid chromatographed uremic serum. J Clin Endocrinol Metab 1986; 63:1186–1192.
297. Horner JM, Liu F, Hintz RL. Comparison of [^{125}I] somatomedin-A and [^{125}I] somatomedin C radioreceptor assays for somatomedin peptide content in whole and acid-chromatographed plasma. J Clin Endocrinol Metab 1978; 47:1287–1295.
298. Daughaday WH, Mariz IK, Blethen SL. Inhibition of access of bound somatomedin to membrane receptor and immunobinding sites: a comparison of radioreceptor and radioimmunoassay of somatomedin in native and acid-ethanol–extracted serum. J Clin Endocrinol Metab 1980; 51:781–788.
299. Blum WF, Ranke MB, Bierich JR. A specific radioimmunoassay for IGF-II: the interference of IGF-binding proteins can be blocked by excess IGF-I. Acta Endocrinol 1988; 118:374–380.
300. Bang P, Ericksson U, Sara V, et al. Comparison of acid ethanol extraction and acid gel filtration prior to IGF-I and IGF-II radioimmunoassays: improvement of determinations in acid ethanol extracts by the use of a truncated IGF-I as radioligand. Acta Endocrinol (Copenh) 1991; 124:620–629.
301. Khosravi MJ, Diamondi A, Mistry J, Lee PD. Noncompetitive ELISA for human serum insulin-like growth factor-I. Clin Chem 1996; 42:1147–1154.
302. Cohen P. Implications of IGF-I elevations in prostate cancer sera. J Natl Cancer Inst 1998; 12:876–879.
303. Quarmby V, Quan C, Ling C, et al. How much insulin-like growth factor I (IGF-I) circulates? Impact of standardization on IGF-I assay accuracy. J Clin Endocrinol Metab 2000; 83:1211–1216.
304. Bennett A, Wilson DM, Liu F, et al. Levels of insulin-like growth factor-I and -II in human cord blood. J Clin Endocrinol Metab 1983; 57:609–612.
305. Gluckman PD, Barrett-Johnson JJ, Butler JH, et al. Studies of insulin-like growth factor I and II by specific radioligand assays in umbilical cord blood. Clin Endocrinol (Oxf) 1983; 19:405–413.
306. Lassare C, Hardouin S, Daffos F, et al. Serum insulin-like growth factors and their binding proteins in the human fetus: relationships with growth in normal subjects and in subjects with intrauterine growth retardation. Pediatr Res 1991; 29:219–225.
307. Hall K, Hansson U, Lundin G, et al. Serum levels of somatomedins and somatomedin-binding protein in pregnant women with type I or gestational diabetes and their infants. J Clin Endocrinol Metab 1986; 63:1300–1305.
308. Luna AM, Wilson DM, Wibbelsman CJ, et al. Somatomedins in adolescence: a cross-sectional study of the effect of puberty on plasma insulin-like growth factor I and II levels. J Clin Endocrinol Metab 1983; 57:258–271.
309. Cara JF, Rosenfield RL, Furlanetto RW. A longitudinal study of the relationship of plasma somatomedin-C concentration to the pubertal growth spurt. Am J Dis Child 1987; 141:562–564.
310. Cuttler L, Van Vliet G, Conte FA, et al. Somatomedin-C levels in children and adolescents with gonadal dysgenesis: differences from age-matched normal females and effect of chronic estrogen replacement therapy. J Clin Endocrinol Metab 1985; 60:1087–1091.
311. Rosenfeld RG, Hintz RL, Johanson AJ, et al. Methionyl human growth hormone and oxandrolone in Turner syndrome: preliminary results of a prospective randomized trial. J Pediatr 1986; 109:936–940.
312. Copeland KC. Effects of acute high-dose and chronic low-dose estrogen on plasma somatomedin-C and growth in patients with Turner's syndrome. J Clin Endocrinol Metab 1988; 66:1278–1282.
313. Johanson AJ, Blizzard RM. Low somatomedin-C levels in older men rise in response to growth hormone administration. Johns Hopkins Med J 1981; 149:115–117.
314. Donovan SM, Oh Y, Pham H, Rosenfeld RG. Ontogeny of serum insulin-like growth factor binding proteins in the rat. Endocrinology 1989; 125:2621–2627.
315. Glasscock GF, Gelber SE, Lamson G, et al. Pituitary control of growth in the neonatal rat: effects of neonatal hypophysectomy on somatic and organ growth, serum insulin-like growth factors (IGF)-I and -II levels, and expression of IGF binding proteins. Endocrinology 1990; 127:1792–1803.
316. Moore DC, Ruvalcaba RHA, Smith EK, Kelley VC. Plasma somatomedin-C as a screening test for growth hormone deficiency in children and adolescents. Horm Res 1982; 16:49–55.
317. Reiter EO, Lovinger RD. The use of a comercially available somatomedin-C radioimmunoassay in patients with disorders of growth. J Pediatr 1981; 99:720–724.
318. Hintz RL, Clemmons DR, Underwood LE, Van Wyk JJ. Competitive binding of somatomedin to the insulin receptors of adipocytes, chondrocytes, and liver membranes. Proc Natl Acad Sci USA 1972; 69:2351–2353.
319. Megyesi K, Kahn CR, Roth J, et al. Insulin and non-suppressible insulin-like activity (NSILA-s): evidence for separate plasma membrane receptor sites. Biochem Biophys Res Commun 1974; 57:307–315.
320. Massague J, Czech MP. The subunit structures of two distinct receptors for insulin-like growth factors I and II and their relationship to the insulin receptor. J Biol Chem 1982; 257:5038–5045.
321. Kasuga M, Van Obberghen E, Nissley SP, Rechler MM. Demonstration of two subtypes of insulin-like growth factor receptors by affinity crosslinking. J Biol Chem 1981; 256:5305–5308.
322. Chernausek SD, Jacobs S, Van Wyk JJ. Structural similarities between receptors for somatomedin C and insulin: analysis by affinity labeling. Biochemistry 1981; 20:7345–7350.
323. Rosenfeld RG, Hintz RL. Somatomedin receptors: structure, function, and regulation. In Conn M (ed). The Receptors. New York, Academic Press, 1986, pp 281–329.
324. Oh Y, Muller H, Neely EK, et al. New concepts in insulin-like growth factor receptor physiology. Growth Reg 1993; 3:113–123.
325. LeRoith D, Werner H, Beitner-Johnson D, Roberts CT Jr. Molecular and cellular aspects of the insulin-like growth factor I receptor. Endocr Rev 1995; 16:143–163.
326. Ullrich A, Gray A, Tam AW, et al. Insulin-like growth factor I receptor primary structure: comparison with insulin receptor suggests structural determinants that define functional specificity. EMBO J 1986; 5:2503–2512.
327. Kato H, Faria TN, Stannard B, et al. Role of tyrosine kinase activity in signal transduction by the insulin-like growth factor-I (IGF-I) receptor. J Biol Chem 1993; 265:2655–2661.
328. Kato H, Faria TN, Stannard B, et al. Essential role of tyrosine residues 1131, 1135, and 1136 of the insulin-like growth factor-I (IGF-I) receptor in IGF-I action. Mol Endocrinol 1994; 8:40–50.
329. Yamaski H, Prager D, Gebremedhin S, Melmed S. Human insulin-like growth factor I receptor 950 tyrosine is required for somatotroph growth factor signal transduction. J Biol Chem 1992; 267:20953–20958.
330. Gronborg M, Wulff BS, Rasmussen JS, et al. Structure-function relationship of the insulin-like growth factor-I receptor tyrosine kinase. J Biol Chem 1993; 258:23435–23440.
331. Abbott AM, Bueno R, Pedrini MT, et al. Insulin-like growth factor I receptor gene structure. J Biol Chem 1992; 267:10759–10763.
332. Ullrich A, Bell JR, Chen EY, et al. Human insulin receptor and its relationship to the tyrosine kinase family of oncogenes. Nature 1985; 313:756–761.

333. Bondy CA, Werner H, Roberts CT Jr, LeRoith D. Cellular pattern of insulin-like growth factor-I (IGF-I) and type I IGF receptor gene expression in early oranogenesis: comparison with IGF-II gene expression. Mol Endocrinol 1990; 4:1386–1398.
334. Werner H, Woloschak M, Adamo M, et al. Developmental regulation of the rat insulin-like growth factor I receptor gene. Proc Natl Acad Sci USA 1989; 86:7451–7455.
335. Lowe WL Jr, Adamo M, Werner H, et al. Regulation by fasting of rat insulin-like growth factor I and its receptor: effects on gene expression and binding. J Clin Invest 1989; 84:619–626.
336. Frattali AL, Pessin JE. Relationship between alpha subunit ligand occupancy and beta subunit autophosphorylation in insulin/insulin-like growth factor-1 hybrid receptors. J Biol Chem 1993; 268:7393–7400.
337. Treadway JL, Morrison BD, Soos MA, et al. Transdominant inhibition of tyrosine kinase activity in mutant insulin/insulin-like growth factor I hybrid receptors. Proc Natl Acad Sci USA 1991; 88:214–218.
338. Shemer J, Adamo M, Wilson GL, et al. Insulin and insulin-like growth factor-I stimulate a common endogenous phosphoprotein substrate (pp185) in intact neuroblastoma cells. J Biol Chem 1987; 262:15476–15482.
339. Kuhne MR, Pawson T, Lienhard GE, Feng GS. The insulin receptor substrate-1 associates with the SH2-containing phosphotyrosine phosphatase Syp. J Biol Chem 1993; 268:11479–11481.
340. Skolnik EY, Batzer A, Li N, et al. The function of GRB2 in linking the insulin receptor to ras signaling pathways. Science 1993; 260:1953–1955.
341. Lee CH, Li W, Nishimura R, et al. Nck associates with the SH2 domain-docking protein IRS-1 in insulin-stimulated cells. Proc Natl Acad Sci USA 1993; 90:11713–11717.
342. Kadowaki T, Tanemoto H, Tobe K, et al. Insulin resistance and growth retardation in mice lacking insulin receptor substrate-1 and identification of insulin receptor substrate-2. Diabet Med 1996; 13:103–108.
343. Tsuruzoe K, Emkey R, Kriauciunas KM, et al. Insulin receptor substrate 3 (IRS-3) and IRS-4 impair IRS-1- and IRS-2-mediated signaling. Mol Cell Biol 2001; 21:26–38.
344. Sasaoka T, Rose DW, Juhn BH, et al. Evidence for a functional role of Shc proteins in mitogenic signaling induced by insulin, insulin-like growth factor-I, and epidermal growth factor. J Biol Chem 1994; 269:13689–13694.
345. Lamphere L, Leinhard GE. Components of signaling pathways for insulin and insulin-like growth factor-I in muscle myoblasts and myotubes. Endocrinology 1992; 131:2196–2202.
346. Oemar BS, Law NM, Rosenweig SA. Insulin-like growth factor-I induces tyrosyl phosphorylation of nuclear proteins. J Biol Chem 1991; 266:27241–27244.
347. Werner H, LeRoith D. The insulin-like growth factor-I receptor signaling pathways are important for tumorogenesis and inhibiiton of apoptosis. Crit Rev Oncol 1997; 8:71–92.
348. Chao MV. Growth factor signaling: where is the specificity? Cell 1992; 68:995–997.
349. Porcu P, Ferber A, Pietrzkowski Z, et al. The growth-stimulatory effect of Simian virus 40 T antigen requires the interaction of insulin-like growth factor I with its receptor. Mol Cell Biol 1992; 12:5069–5077.
350. Baserga R. The double life of the IGF-I receptor. Receptor 1992; 2:261–266.
351. Sell C, Rubini M, Rubin R, et al. Simian virus 40 large tumor antigen is unable to transform mouse embryonic fibroblasts lacking type I insulin-like growth factor receptor. Proc Natl Acad Sci USA 1993; 90:11217–11221.
352. Kaleko M, Rutter WJ, Miller AD. Overexpression of the human insulin-like growth factor I receptor promotes ligand-dependent neoplastic transformation. Mol Cell Biol 1990; 10:464–473.
353. Prager D, Li HL, Asa S, Melmed S. Dominant negative inhibition of tumorigenesis in vivo by human insulin-like growth factor I receptor mutant. Proc Natl Acad Sci USA 1994; 91:2181–2185.
354. Alexandrides TK, Chen JH, Bueno R, et al. Evidence for two insulin-like growth factor I receptors with distinct primary structure that are differentially expressed during development. Regul Pept 1993; 48:279–290.
355. Alexandrides TK, Smith RJ. A novel fetal insulin-like growth factor (IGF) I receptor: mechanism for increased IGF-I and insulin-stimulated tyrosine kinase activity in fetal muscle. J Biol Chem 1989; 264:12922–12930.
356. Garofalo RS, Rosen OM. Insulin and insulin-like growth factor I (IGF-I) receptors during central nervous system development: expression of two immunologically distinct IGF-I receptor beta subunits. Mol Cell Biol 1989; 9:2806–2817.
357. Tally M, Li CH, Hall K. IGF-2 stimulated growth mediated by the somatomedin type 2 receptor. Biochem Biophys Res Commun 1987; 148:811–816.
358. Minniti CP, Kohn EC, Grubb JH, et al. The insulin-like growth factor II (IGF-II)/mannose 6-phosphate receptor mediates IGF-II–induced motility in human rhabdomyosarcoma cells. J Biol Chem 1992; 267:9000–9004.
359. Nishimoto I, Murayama Y, Katada T, et al. Possible direct linkage of insulin-like growth factor-II receptor with guanine nucleotide–binding proteins. J Biol Chem 1989; 264:14029–14038.
360. Moxham CP, Duronio V, Jacobs S. Insulin-like growth factor I receptor beta subunit heterogeneity: evidence for hybrid tetramers composed of insulin-like growth factor I and insulin receptor heterodimers. J Biol Chem 1989; 264:13238–13244.
361. Soos MA, Siddle K. Immunological relationships between receptors for insulin and insulin-like growth factor I: evidence for structural heterogeneity of insulin-like growth factor I receptors involving hybrids with insulin receptors. Biochem J 1989; 263: 553–563.
362. Moxham CP, Jacobs S. Insulin/IGF-I receptor hybrids: a mechanism for increasing receptor diversity. J Cell Biochem 1992; 48:136–140.
363. Misra P, Hintz RL, Rosenfeld RG. Structural and immunological characterization of insulin-like growth factor II binding to IM-9 cells. J Clin Endocrinol Metab 1986; 63:1400–1405.
364. Soos MA, Field CE, Siddle K. Purified hybrid insulin/insulin-like growth factor-I, but not insulin, with high affinity. Biochem J 1993; 290:419–425.
365. Kasuya J, Paz B, Madduz BA, et al. Characterization of human placental insulin-like growth factor-I/insulin hybrid receptors by protein microsequencing and purification. Biochemistry 1993; 32:13531–13536.
366. Morgan DO, Edman JC, Strandring DN, et al. Insulin-like growth factor II receptor as a multifunctional binding protein. Nature 1987; 329:301–307.
367. MacDonald RG, Pfeffer SR, Coussens L, et al. A single receptor binds both insulin-like growth factor II and mannose-6-phosphate. Science 1988; 239:1134–1137.
368. Kornfeld S. Trafficking of lysosomal enzymes. FASEB J 1987; 1:462–468.
369. Rosenfeld RG, Conover CA, Hodges D, et al. Heterogeneity of insulin-like growth factor-I affinity for the insulin-like growth factor-II receptor: comparison of natural, synthetic, and recombinant DNA-derived insulin-like growth factor-I. Biochem Biophys Res Commun 1987; 143:195–205.
370. Beukers M, Oh Y, Zhang H, et al. [Leu27] insulin-like growth factor II is highly selective for the type II IGF receptor in binding, cross-linking, and thymidine incorporation. Endocrinology 1991; 128:1201–1203.
371. Furlanetto RW, DiCarlo JN, Wisehart C. The type II insulin-like growth factor receptor does not mediate deoxyribonucleic acid synthesis in human fibroblasts. J Clin Endocrinol Metab 1987; 64:1142–1149.
372. Mottola C, Czech MP. The type II insulin-like growth factor receptor does not mediate DNA synthesis in H-35 hepatoma cells. J Biol Chem 1984; 259:12705–12713.
373. Kiess W, Haskell JF, Lee L, et al. An antibody that blocks insulin-like growth factor (IGF) binding to the type II IGF receptor is neither an agonist nor an inhibitor of IGF-stimulated biologic response in L6 myoblasts. J Biol Chem 1987; 162: 12756–12761.
374. Adashi EY, Resnick CE, Rosenfeld RG. Insulin-like growth factor-I (IGF-I) hormonal action in cultured rat granulosa cells: mediation via type I but not type II IGF receptors. Endocrinology 1989; 126:216–222.
375. Canfield WM, Kornfeld S. The chicken liver cation-independent mannose-6-phosphate receptor lacks the high-affinity binding site for insulin-like growth factor II. J Biol Chem 1989; 264: 7100–7103.

sulin-dependent diabetes mellitus. Eur J Endocrinol 1995; 133: 440–444.

831. Munoz MT, Barrios V, Pozo J, Argente J. Insulin-like growth factor I, its binding proteins 1 and 3, and growth hormone-binding protein in children and adolescents with insulin-dependent diabetes mellitus: clinical implications. Pediatr Res 1996; 39:992–998.
832. Bereket A, Lang CH, Wilson TA. Alterations in the growth hormone–insulin-like growth factor axis in insulin-dependent diabetes mellitus. Horm Metab Res 1999; 31:172–181.
833. Dunger DB. Insulin and insulin-like growth factors in diabetes mellitus. Arch Dis Child 1995; 72:469–471.
834. Suikkari AM, Koivisto VA, Rutanen EM, et al. Insulin regulates the serum levels of low-molecular-weight insulin-like growth factor–binding protein. J Clin Endocrinol Metab 1988; 66:266–272.
835. Holly JMP, Biddlecomb RA, Dunger DB, et al. Circadian variation of GH-dependent IGF-binding protein in diabetes mellitus and its relation to insulin: a new role for insulin? Clin Endocrinol 1988; 29:667–677.
836. Batch JA, Baxter RC, Werther G. Abnormal regulation of insulin-like growth factor–binding proteins in adolescents with insulin-dependent diabetes mellitus. J Clin Endocrinol Metab 1991; 73:964–968.
837. Taylor AM, Dunger DB, Preece MA, et al. The growth hormone–independent insulin-like growth factor I–binding protein BP-28 is associated with serum insulin-like growth factor I inhibitory bioactivity in adolescent insulin-dependent diabetes mellitus. Clin Endocrinol (Oxf) 1990; 32:229–239.
838. Bereket A, Lang CH, Blethen SL, et al. Insulin-like growth factor–binding protein-3 proteolysis in children with insulin-dependent diabetes mellitus: a possible role for insulin in the regulation of IGFBP-3 protease activity. J Clin Endocrinol Metab 1995; 80:2282–2288.
839. Winter RJ, Phillips LS, Klein MN, et al. Somatomedin activity and diabetic control in children with insulin-dependent diabetes. Diabetes 1979; 28:952–954.
840. Jivani SKM, Rayner PHW. Does control influence the growth of diabetic children? Arch Dis Child 1973; 48:109–115.
841. Tattersall RB, Pyke DA. Growth in diabetic children: studies in identical twins. Lancet 1973; 2:1105–1109.
842. Clarson D, Daneman D, Ehrlich RM. The relation of metabolic control to growth and pubertal development in children with insulin-dependent diabetes. Diabetes Res 1985; 2:237–241.
843. Du Caju MVL, Rooman RP, Op De Beeck L. Longitudinal data on growth and final height in diabetic children. Pediatr Res 1995; 38:607–611.
844. Pitukcheewanont P, Alemzadeh R, Jacobs WR, et al. Does glycemic control affect growth velocity in children with insulin-dependent diabetes mellitus. Acta Diabetol 1995; 32:148–152.
845. Tamborlane WV, Hintz RL, Bergman M, et al. Insulin infusion pump treatment of diabetes: influence of improved metabolic control on plasma somatomedin levels. N Engl J Med 1981; 305:303–307.
846. Marsden D, Barshop BA, Capistrano-Estrada S, et al. Anabolic effect of human growth hormone: management of inherited disorders of catabolic pathways. Biochem Med Metab Biol 1994; 52:145–154.
847. Bain MD, Nussey SS, Jones M, Chalmers RA. Use of human somatotropin in the treatment of a patient with methylmalonic aciduria. Eur J Pediatr 1995; 154:850–852.
848. Russell G. Asthma and growth. Arch Dis Child 1993; 69:695–698.
849. Cohen MB, Abram LE. Growth patterns of allergic children. J Allergy 1948; 19:165–171.
850. Balfour-Lynn L. Growth and childhood asthma. Arch Dis Child 1986; 61:1049–1055.
851. Crowley S, Hindmarsh PC, Matthews DR, Brook CGD. Growth and the growth hormone axis in prepubertal children with asthma. J Pediatr 1995; 126:297–303.
852. Ninan TK, Russell G. Asthma, inhaled corticosteroid treatment, and growth. Arch Dis Child 1992; 67:703–705.
853. Nassif E, Weinberger M, Sherman B, Brown K. Extrapulmonary effects of maintenance corticosteroid therapy with alternate-day prednisolone and inhaled beclomethasone in children with chronic asthma. J Allergy Clin Immunol 1987; 80:518–528.
854. Falliers CJ, Tan LS, Szentivanyi J, et al. Childhood asthma and steroid therapy as influences on growth. Am J Dis Child 1963; 105:127–137.
855. Versano I, Volovitz B, Malik H, Amir Y. Safety of 1 year of treatment with budesonide in young children with asthma. J Allergy Clin Immunol 1990; 85:914–920.
856. Volovitz B, Amir J, Malik H, et al. Growth and pituitary-adrenal function in children with severe asthma treated with inhaled budesonide. N Engl J Med 1996; 329:1703–1708.
857. Todd G, Dunlop K, McNaboe J, et al. Growth and adrenal suppression in asthmatic children treated with high-dose fluticasone propionate. Lancet 1996; 348:27–29.
858. Agertoft L, Pedersen S. Effect of long-term treatment with inhaled budesonide on adult height in children with asthma. N Engl J Med 2000; 343:1064–1069.
859. Norjavaara E, de Verdier MG, Lindmark B. Reduced height in Swedish men with asthma at the age of conscription for military service. J Pediatr 2000; 137:25–29.
860. Martin AJ, McLennan LA, Landau LI, Phelan PD. The natural history of chlidhood asthma to adult life. BMJ 1980; 280:1397–1400.
861. Shohat M, Shohat T, Kedem R, et al. Childhood asthma and growth outcome. Arch Dis Child 1987; 62:63–65.
862. Avery ME, Tooley W, Keller J, et al. Is chronic lung disease in low-birth-weight infants preventable? A survey of eight centers. Pediatrics 1987; 79:26–30.
863. Gibson AT, Pearse RG, Wales JKH. Growth retardation after dexamethasone administration: assessment by knemometry. Arch Dis Child 1993; 69:505–509.
864. Finer NN, Craft A, Vaucher YE, et al. Postnatal steroids: Short-term gain, long-term pain? J Pediatr 2000; 137:9–13.
865. Kurzner SI, Garg M, Bautista D, et al. Growth failure in infants with bronchopulmonary dysplasia: nutrition and elevated resting metabolic expenditure. Pediatrics 1988; 81:379–384.
866. Yu V, Orgill A, Lim S, et al. Growth and development of very-low-birth-weight infants recovering from bronchopulmonary dysplasia. Arch Dis Child 1983; 58:791–794.
867. Meisels S, Plunkett J, Roloff D, et al. Growth and development of preterm infants with respiratory distress syndrome and bronchopulmonary dysplasia. Pediatrics 1986; 77:345–352.
868. Vrlenich LA, Bozynski MEA, Shyr Y, et al. The effect of bronchopulmonary dysplasia on growth at school age. Pediatrics 1995; 95:855–859.
869. Ross G, Lipper E, Auld P. Growth achievement of very-low-birth-weight premature children at school age. J Pediatr 1990; 117:307–309.
870. Robertson M, Etches P, Goldson E, Kyle J. Eight-year school performance, neurodevelopmental, and growth outcome of neonates with bronchopulmonary dysplasia: a comparative study. Pediatrics 1992; 89:365–372.
871. Landon C, Rosenfeld RG. Short stature and pubertal delay in male adolescents with cystic fibrosis. Am J Dis Child 1984; 138: 388–391.
872. Sproul A, Huang N. Growth patterns in children with cystic fibrosis. J Pediatr 1964; 65:664–676.
873. Lapey A, Kattwinkel J, DiSant'Agnese PA, Laster L. Steatorrhea and azotorrhea and their relation to growth and nutrition in adolescents and young adults with cystic fibrosis. J Pediatr 1974; 84:328–334.
874. Mearns M. Growth and development. In Hodson E, Norman A, Batten J (eds). Cystic Fibrosis. London, Baillieres Tindall, 1983, pp 183–196.
875. Shepherd RW, Holt TL, Thomas BJ, et al. Nutritional rehabilitation in cystic fibrosis: controlled studies of effects on nutritional growth retardation, body protein turnover, and course of pulmonary disease. J Pediatr 1986; 109:788–794.
876. Reiter EO, Gerstle RS. Cystic fibrosis in puberty and adolescence. In Lerner RM, Petersen AC, Brooks-Gunn J (eds). Encyclopedia of Adolescence. New York, Garland Publishing, 1991, pp 187–195.
877. FitzSimmons SC. The changing epidemiology of cystic fibrosis. J Pediatr 1993; 122:1–9.
878. Karlberg J, Kjellmer I, Kristiansson B. Linear growth in children wth cystic fibrosis: I. Birth to 8 years of age. Acta Paediatr Scand 1991; 80:508–514.
879. Reiter EO, Stern RC, Root AW. The reproductive system in

cystic fibrosis: I. Basal gonadotropin and sex steroid levels. Am J Dis Child 1981; 135:422–426.

880. Reiter EO, Stern RC, Root AW. The reproductive system in cystic fibrosis: II. Changes in gonadotrophins and sex steroids following LHRH. Clin Endocrinol (Oxf) 1982; 16:127–137.
881. Reiter EO, Brugman SM, Pike JW, et al. Vitamin D metabolites in adolescents and young adults with cystic fibrosis: effects of sun and season. J Pediatr 1985; 106:21–26.
882. Laursen EM, Juul A, Lanng S, et al. Diminished concentrations of insulin-like growth factor I in cystic fibrosis. Arch Dis Child 1995; 72:494–497.
883. Huseman CA, Columbo JL, Brooks MA, et al. Anabolic effect of biosynthetic growth hormone in cystic fibrosis. Pediatr Pulmonol 1996; 22:90–95.
884. Hardin DS, Stratton R, Kramer JC, et al. Growth hormone improves weight velocity and height velocity in prepubertal children with cystic fibrosis. Horm Metab Res 1998; 30:636–641.
885. Zemel BS, Jawad AF, FitzSimmons S, Stallings VA. Longitudinal relationship among growth, nutritional status, and pulmonary function in children with cystic fibrosis: analysis of the Cystic Fibrosis Foundation National CF Patient Registry. J Pediatr 2000; 137:374–380.
886. De Benedetti F, Alonzi T, Moretta A, et al. Interleukin 6 causes growth impairment in transgenic mice through a decrease in insulin-like growth factor-I. J Clin Invest 1997; 99:643–650.
887. McCann SM, Lyson K, Karanth S, et al. Role of cytokines in the endocrine system. Ann NY Acad Sci 1994; 741:50–63.
888. Vassilopoulou-Sellin R. Endocrine effects of cytokines. Oncology 1994; 8:43–50.
889. Skerry TM. The effects of the inflammatory response on bone growth. Eur J Clin Nutr 1994; 48(suppl 1):S190-S198.
890. Abrams EJ, Rogers MF. Pediatric HIV infection. Baillieres Clin Haematol 1991; 4:333–339.
891. McKinney RE, Robertson JWR, and the Duke Pediatric AIDS Clinical Trials Unit. Effect of human immunodeficiency virus infection on the growth of young children. J Pediatr 1993; 123: 579–582.
892. Saavedra JM, Henderson RA, Perman JA, et al. Longitudinal assessment of growth in children born to mothers with human immunodeficiency virus infection. Arch Pediatr Adolesc Med 1995; 149:497–502.
893. McKinney RE, Wilfert C, and the AIDS Clinical Trials Group Protocol 043 Study Group. Growth as a prognostic indicator in children with immunodeficiency virus infection treated with zidovudine. J Pediatr 1994; 125:728–733.
894. Gertner JM, Kaufman FR, Donfield SM, et al. Delayed somatic growth and pubertal development in human immunodeficiency virus–infected hemophiliac boys: hemophila growth and development study. J Pediatr 1994; 124:896–902.
895. Moye J, Rich KC, Kalish LA, et al. Natural history of somatic growth in infants born to women infected by human immunodeficiency virus. J Pediatr 1996; 128:58–69.
896. Grunfeld C. What causes wasting in AIDS? N Engl J Med 1995; 333:123–124.
897. Grunfeld C, Feingold KR. Metabolic disturbances and wasting in the acquired immunodeficiency syndrome. N Engl J Med 1992; 327:329–337.
898. Anonymous. Infections as deterrents of growth. Nutr Rev 1981; 39:328
899. Chiesa A, de Papendieck G, Keselman A, et al. Growth follow-up in 100 children with congenital hypothyroidism before and during treatment. J Pediatr Endocrinol 1994; 7:211–217.
900. Grant DB. Growth in early treated congenital hypothyroidism. Arch Dis Child 1994; 70:464–468.
901. Heyerdahl S, Ilicki A, Karlbarg J, et al. Linear growth in early-treated children with congenital hypothyroidism. Acta Paediatr 1997; 86:479–483.
902. Dickerman Z, De Vries L. Prepubertal and pubertal growth, timing and duration of puberty, and attained adult height in patients with congenital hypothyroidism (CH) detected by the neonatal screening programmed for CH: a longitudinal study. Clin Endocrinol (Oxf) 1997; 47:649–654.
903. Rivkees SA, Bode HH, Crawford JD. Long-term growth in juvenile acquired hypothyroidism. N Engl J Med 1988; 318: 599–602.
904. Pantsiouou S, Stanhope R, Urena M, et al. Growth prognosis and growth after menarche in primary hypothyroidism. Arch Dis Child 1991; 66:838–840.
905. Boersma B, Otten BJ, Stoelings GBA, Wit JM. Catch-up growth after prolonged hypothyroidism. Eur J Pediatr 1996; 155:362–367.
906. Magiakou MA, Mastorakos G, Oldfield EH, et al. Cushing's syndrome in children and adolescents: presentation, diagnosis, and therapy. N Engl J Med 1994; 331:629–636.
907. Lee PA, Weldon VV, Migeon CJ. Short stature as the only clinical sign of Cushing's syndrome. J Pediatr 1975; 86:89–91.
908. Reid IR. Pathogenesis and treatment of steroid osteoporosis. Clin Endocrinol (Oxf) 1989; 30:83–103.
909. Giustina A, Bussi AR, Jacobello C, Wehrenberg WB. Effects of recombinant human growth hormone (GH) on bone and intermediary metabolism in patients receiving chronic glucocorticoid treatment with suppressed endogenous GH response to GH-releasing hormone. J Clin Endocrinol Metab 1995; 80:122–129.
910. Allen DB, Goldberg BD. Stimulation of a collagen synthesis and linear growth by growth hormone in glucocorticoid-treated children. Pediatrics 1992; 89:416–421.
911. Schatz M, Dudl J, Zeiger RS, et al. Osteoporosis in corticosteroid-treated asthmatic patients: clinical correlates. Allergy Proc 1993; 14:341–345.
912. Luo J, Murphy LJ. Dexamethasone inhibits growth hormone induction of insulin-like growth factor-I (IGF-I) messenger ribonucleic acid (mRNA) in hypophysectomized rats and reduces IGF-I mRNA abundance in the intact rat. Endocrinology 1989; 125:165–171.
913. Magiakou MA, Mastorakos G, Gomez MT, et al. Suppressed spontaneous and stimulated growth hormone secretion in patients with Cushing's disease before and after surgical cure. J Clin Endocrinol Metab 1994; 78:131–137.
914. Mauras N, Beaufrere B. rhIGF-I enhances whole body protein anabolism and significantly diminishes the protein-catabolic effects of prednisone in humans without a diabetogenic effect. J Clin Endocrinol Metab 1995; 80:869–874.
915. Rivkees SA, Danon M, Herrin J. Prednisone dose limitation of growth hormone treatment of steroid-induced growth failure. J Pediatr 1994; 125:322–325.
916. Mosier HD, Smith FG, Schultz MA. Failure of catch-up growth after Cushing's syndrome in childhood. Am J Dis Child 1972; 124:251–253.
917. Leong GM, Mercado-Asis LB, Reynolds JC, et al. The effect of Cushing's disease on bone mineral density, body composition, growth, and puberty: a report of identical adolescent twin pair. J Clin Endorinol Metab 1996; 81:1905–1911.
918. Reimer LG, Morris HG, Ellis FE. Growth of asthmatic children during treatment with alternate day steroids. J Allergy Clin Immunol 1975; 55:224–231.
919. Lebrethon MC, Grossman AB, Afshar F, et al. Linear growth and final height after treatment for Cushing's disease in childhood. J Clin Endocrinol Metab 2000; 85:3262–3265.
920. Savage MO, Lienhardt A, Lebrethon MC, et al. Cushing's disease in childhood: presentation, investigation, treatment, and long-term outcome. Horm Res 2001; 55:24–30.
921. Schwindinger WF, Levine MA. Albright hereditary osteodystrophy. Endocrinologist 1994; 4:17–27.
922. Minamitani K, Takahashi Y, Minagawa M, et al. Difference in height associated with a translation start site poymorphism in the vitamin D receptor gene. Pediatr Res 1998; 44:628–632.
923. Lorentzon M, Lorentzon R, Nordstrom P. Vitamin D receptor gene polymorphism is associated with birth weigbht, growth to adolescence, and adult stature in healthy Caucasian men: a cross-sectional and longitudinal study. J Clin Endocrinol Metab 2000; 85:1666–1671.
924. Suarez F, Zeghoud F, Rossignol C, et al. Association between vitamin D receptor gene polymorphism and sex-dependent growth during the first two years of life. J Clin Endocrinol Metab 1997; 82:2966–2970.
925. Kanan RM, Varanasi SS, Francis RM, et al. Vitamin D receptor gene start codon polymorphism (Fokl) and bone mineral density in healthy male subjects. Clin Endocrinol (Oxf) 2000; 53:93–98.
926. Arai H, Miyamoto KI, Taketani Y, et al. A vitamin D receptor gene polymorphism translation initiation codon: effect on protein activity and relation to bone mineral density in Japanese women. J Bone Mineral Res 2012; 12:915–921.

loss-of-function mutations in the GPC3 gene. Hum Mol Genet 2000; 22:1321–1328.

1561. Tauber M, Pienkowski C, Rochiccioli P. Growth hormone secretion in children and adolescents with familial tall stature. Eur J Pediatr 1994; 153:311–316.
1562. Dickerman Z, Loewinger J, Laron Z. The pattern of growth in children with constitutional tall stature from birth to age 9 years: a longitudinal study. Acta Paediatr Scand 1984; 73:530–536.
1563. Josse EE, Temperli R, Mullis PE. Adult height in constitutionally tall stature: accuracy of five different height prediction methods. Arch Dis Child 1992; 67:1357–1362.
1564. Ignatius A, Lenko HL, Perheentupa J. Oestrogen treatment of tall girls: effect decreases with age. Acta Paediatr Scand 1991; 80:712–717.
1565. De Waal WJ, Greyn-Fokker MH, Stijnen TH, et al. Accuracy of final height prediction and effect of growth-reductive therapy in 362 constitutionally tall children. J Clin Endocrinol Metab 1996; 81:1206–1216.
1566. Bierich JR. Estrogen treatment of girls with constitutional tall stature. Pediatrics 1978; 62(suppl):1196–1201.
1567. Sorgo W, Scholler K, Heinze F, et al. Critical analysis of height reduction in oestrogen-treated tall girls. Eur J Pediatr 1984; 142:260–265.
1568. Trygstad O. Oestrogen treatment of adolescent tall girls: short-term side effects. Acta Endocrinol 1986; 113(suppl 279):170–173.
1569. Forbes GB. Nutrition and growth. J Pediatr 1977; 91:40.
1570. Spence HJ, Trias EP, Raiti S. Acromegaly in a 9 1/2-year-old boy. Am J Dis Child 1972; 123:504–506.
1571. AvRuskin TW, Sau K, Tang S, Juan C. Childhood acromegaly: successful therapy with conventional radiation and effects of chlorpromazine on growth hormone and prolactin secretion. J Clin Endocrinol Metab 1973; 37:380.
1572. DeMajo SF, Onativia A. Acromegaly and gigantism in a boy: comparison with three overgrown non-acromegalic children. Pediatrics 1960; 57:382
1573. Lefkowitz RJ. G proteins in medicine. N Engl J Med 1995; 332:186–187.
1574. Lightner ES, Winter JSD. Treatment of juvenile acromegaly with bromocriptine. J Pediatr 1981; 98:494–496.
1575. Geffner ME, Nagel RA, Dietrich RB, Kaplan SA. Treatment of acromegaly with a somatostatin analog in a patient with McCune-Albright syndrome. 1987; J Pediatr 3:740–743.
1576. Hoffman WH, Perrin JS, Halac E, et al. Acromegalic gigantism and tuberous sclerosis. J Pediatr 1978; 93:478
1577. Daughaday WH. Extreme gigantism: analysis of growth velocity and occurrence of severe peripheral neuropathy and neuropathic arthropathy (Charcot joints). N Engl J Med 1977; 297:1267–1269.
1578. Elis LLK, Huebner A, Metherell LA, et al. Tall stature in familial glucocorticoid deficiency. Clin Endocrinol (Oxf) 2000; 53:423–430.
1579. Ogata T, Kosho T, Wakui K, et al. Short stature homeobox-containing gene duplication on the der(X) chromosome in a female with 45X/46,Xder(X), gonadal dysgenesis, and tall stature. J Clin Endocrinol Metab 2000; 85:2927–2930.
1580. Ogata T, Matsuo N. Sex chromosome aberrations and stature: deduction of the principal factors involved in the determination of adult height. Hum Genet 1993; 91:551–562.
1581. Nakamura Y, Suehiro Y, Sugino N, et al. A case of 46,X, der(X)(pter q21::p21pter) with gonadal dysgenesis, tall stature, and endometriosis. Fertil Steril 2001; 75:1224–1225.
1582. Tanner JM, Whitehouse RH, Takaishi M. Standards from birth to maturity for height, weight, height velocity, and weight velocity: British children, 1965. Arch Dis Child 1966; 41:454–471.
1583. Post EM, Richman RA. A condensed table for predicting adult stature. J Pediatr 1981; 98:440–442.
1584. Takeuchi T, Suzuki H, Sakurai S, et al. Molecular mechanism of growth hormone (GH) deficiency in the sponmtaneous dwarf rat: detection of abnormal splicing of GH messenger ribonucleic acid by the polymerase chain reaction. Endocrinology 1990; 126:31–38.
1585. Dana K, Baptista J, Blethen SL. Updated National Collaborative Growth Study (NCGS) data. Personal communication, 2001.
1586. Tanner JM, Whitehouse RH. Clinical longitudinal standards for height, weight, height velocity, weight velocity, and the stages of puberty. Arch Dis Child 1976; 51:170–179.
1587. Rotwein P. Structure, evolution, expression, and regulation of insulin-like growth factors I and II. Growth Fact 1991; 5:3–18.
1588. Cohen P, Rosenfeld RG. The IGF axis. In Rosenbloom AL (ed). Human Growth Hormone: Basic and Scientific Aspects. Boca Raton, Fla, CRC Press, 1995, pp 279–285.

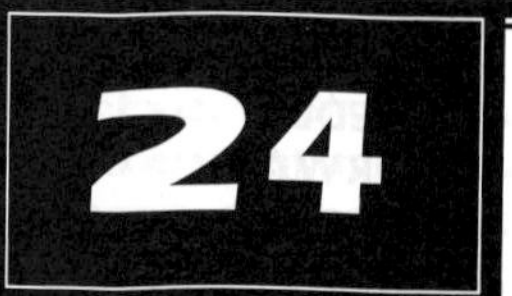

Puberty: Ontogeny, Neuroendocrinology, Physiology, and Disorders

Melvin M. Grumbach and Dennis M. Styne

Puberty should not be considered as a de novo event but rather as a phase in the continuum of the development of gonadal function and the ontogeny of the hypothalamic-pituitary-gonadal system in the fetus, through puberty, to the attainment of full sexual maturation and fertility. By puberty, secondary sexual characteristics appear and the adolescent growth spurt occurs, which result in the striking sexual dimorphism of mature individuals, fertility is achieved, and profound psychological effects ensue.[1] These changes are a consequence of stimulation of the gonads by pituitary gonadotropins and increase in gonadal steroid output. Adolescence, a term usually considered to relate to the psychosocial aspects of the teenage years, is accompanied by the onset of adult patterns of sociosexual and economic behavior.[2]

The human being is the most reproductively successful of mammals, and many anthropologists have attributed this success to the prolonged pattern of human growth and development[3, 4] and the delay in attaining full sexual maturity.[2, 5] The evolution of the human scheme of growth involves the development of two stages: a childhood stage and an adolescent stage that includes an adolescent or pubertal growth spurt (Fig. 24–1). Not even our closest biologic relative, the chimpanzee, which matures twice as rapidly as the human, unequivocally exhibits these two stages including the unique human adolescent growth spurt. (The estimated date for divergence of the chimpanzee and human lineages is 4 million to 5 million years ago.)

Evolution theorists proposed that a critical part of human success and of many biosocial characteristics emanates from the learning and practice of adult behaviors related to sex and childrearing, particularly provisioning children (not just infants) with food,[2] which is unique to humans. These include learning skills related to production of food, cooperative hunting, division of labor according to sex, sharing food, tool making, and adjusting to the social organization and cultural environment. Bogin, on the other hand, noting that tool making preceded the evolutionary development of adolescence, suggested that, in addition, the evolution and value of human childhood and adolescence and this unique pattern of growth and development have had a significant role in the comparatively striking reproductive advantage and success of the human being.[2, 5–7] Mayr[8] has called this process of selection "selection for reproductive success."

Historical evidence suggests that puberty occurs at an earlier age today than in the past, usually reflected by age of menarche, which is removed by several years from the first sign of secondary development in girls.[9–13] The average age of menarche in industrialized European countries has decreased 2 to 3 months per decade over the past 150 years, and in the United States the decrease has been approximately 2 to 3 months per decade in the last century[10–12, 14] (Fig. 24–2). However, this secular trend has slowed or ceased in "developed" countries such as the United States, Australia, and Western Europe (e.g., Britain and Holland) since approximately 1940, presumably because of improved socioeconomic status and health and the benefits of urbanization.[10–13, 15–17] The social class difference in

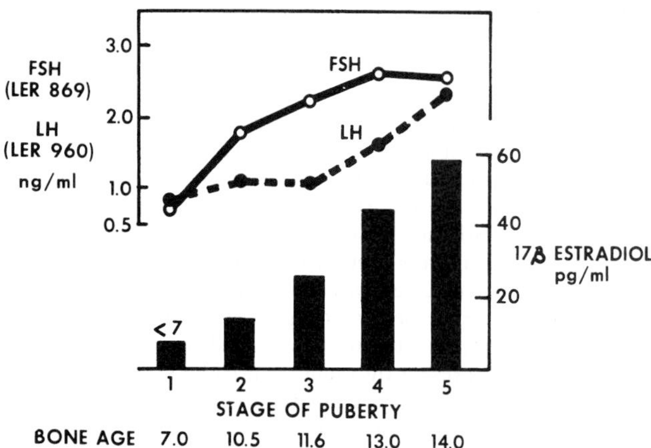

Figure 24–17. Mean plasma estradiol, follicle-stimulating hormone (FSH), and luteinizing hormone (LH) concentrations in prepubertal and pubertal females by pubertal stage of maturation (1 = prepubertal; 5 = menstruating adolescents) and the mean bone age for each stage. Single daytime values of gonadotropins have limited usefulness because of pulsatility of gonadotropin release and the increased amplitude of LH pulses during sleep through puberty. The gonadal steroid values, however, are useful in determining the stage of pubertal development. To convert FSH values (LER-869) to international units per liter, multiply by 8.4. To convert LH values (LER-960) to international units per liter, multiply by 3.8. To convert estradiol values to picomoles per liter, multiply by 3.671. (From Grumbach MM. Onset of puberty. In Berenberg SR [ed]. Puberty, Biologic and Social Components. Leiden, HE Stenfert Kroese, 1975, pp 1–21. Reprinted by permission of Kluwer Academic Publishers.)

stimulating gonadotropin or gonadal steroid secretion before puberty become effective with the onset of puberty[462]; thus, an amplification occurs in the hypothalamic-pituitary-gonadal axis with progression of puberty.[462, 482, 496] Whereas the LHRH test usually requires multiple sampling after the administration of LHRH, a single determination at 30, 45, or 60 minutes may suffice with the new, sensitive immunoradiometric assay, but only if a positive result is obtained.[499] Further, the use of an LHRH agonist (e.g., nafarelin) in a single dose with determination of serum gonadotropins and sex steroids can help to differentiate the pubertal from the prepubertal state.[500, 501]

The pattern of release of gonadotropins and testosterone was determined in boys at every stage of pubertal development by sampling serum every 20 minutes for 24 hours. Disorderly patterns of secretion of LH but not FSH were noted just before the onset of puberty, followed by increased orderliness in early puberty and then increased disorderliness again in later puberty. This suggests that a more integrated feedback system operates in early puberty, which is followed by less stability.[502]

Levels of biologically active LH as determined by rat or mouse interstitial cell assays and of biologically active FSH as assessed by rat Sertoli or granulosa cell assays have been compared with immunoreactive LH and FSH levels estimated by radioimmunoassay.[497, 503–508] Although discrepancies between serum bioactivity and immunoactivity of LH were reported earlier, more recent data indicate that a change in the bioactive/immunoactive ratio does not occur during puberty in boys or girls.[508]

Qualitative[509] as well as the well-defined quantitative changes occur in the pattern of FSH and LH in the pituitary gland, serum, and urine during development. The pattern of glycosylation of the α and the β subunits of the gonadotropins is influenced by maturation, LHRH secretion, and the action of gonadal steroids on the pituitary gonadotrophs. Variation in glycosylation that affects the size and charge of the hormone is the principal cause of the heterogeneity of FSH and LH and the large number of isoforms, which vary according to the more acidic or more basic charge.[510, 511] This pleomorphism has an important effect on biologic half-life and biologic activity and provides an additional mechanism of regulating the biologic activity of the gonadotropins.[497, 507, 510–515]

Although it has been difficult to characterize a diurnal variation of immunoreactive FSH secretion, secretion of bioactive FSH increases at night during sleep and is more resistant to testosterone-induced suppression than is immunoreactive LH.[497, 505]

Gonadal Steroids

Estrogen exerts different effects than testosterone, but only lately has it been appreciated that many actions on linear skeletal growth, skeletal maturation, and accretion of bone mass thought to be due to testosterone in the male are mainly attributable to its peripheral aromatization to estrogen.

Testosterone

The Leydig cells of the testes produce testosterone and, in lesser amounts, androstenedione, α5-androstenediol, dihydrotestosterone, and estradiol. In addition to direct secretion, a small amount of testosterone is derived from extraglandular conversion of androstenedione secreted by the testes and the adrenal.[516] Although testosterone induces development of a male body habitus and voice change, dihydrotestosterone derived by 5α reduction in the target cell is the major mediator of the development of the phallus and the prostate, temporal hair recession, and beard growth.[517] In the female, extraglandular conversion of ovarian and adrenal[510] androstenedione accounts for almost all of the circulating testosterone.

Prepubertal boys and girls have plasma testosterone concentrations less than 0.3 nmol/L (0.1 ng/mL)[467, 471, 477, 491, 518] except during the first 3 to 5 months of infancy in the male, when pubertal levels are found.[118, 519–521] Nighttime elevations of serum testosterone levels are detectable in the male by 5 years of age, before the onset of physical signs of puberty, and increase during early puberty after the appearance of sleep-entrained secretion of LH[467, 485, 522] and increased pituitary sensitivity to LHRH. There is a lag of about 60 minutes between the peak of LH and the increase in testosterone, presumably related to synthesis and secretion of the steroid.[467, 523] In the daytime, increases in testosterone levels are detectable at approximately 11 years in boys when the testis volume is at least 4 mL, with a consistent increase throughout puberty.[491, 518] The steepest increment in testosterone occurs between pubertal stages 2 and 3 in males (Fig. 24–18); testosterone concentrations can rise from 0.7 to 8 nmol/L (0.2 to 2.4 ng/mL) within 10 months.[518]

Normal values for testosterone and other androgen metabolites are described; measurements of the ratio of testosterone to its metabolites can be used to identify athletes using illicit androgen preparations.[524] Unfortunately, the ratio of testosterone to epitestosterone in the urine, which is used in this manner to evaluate "doping," may be elevated normally during the progression through puberty, casting doubts upon this testing procedure during puberty.

Free testosterone values are low or nondetectable until the age of normal pubertal development, at which time they rise in boys and girls.[525] A sensitive mammalian cell recombinant bioassay for androgen bioactivity strongly correlated with serum immunoreactive testosterone concentration but not with 5α-dihydrotestosterone, dehydroepiandrosterone, or androstenedione.[526]

Sex steroids can be measured in saliva (as can many other types of steroids) for screening purposes or for monitoring

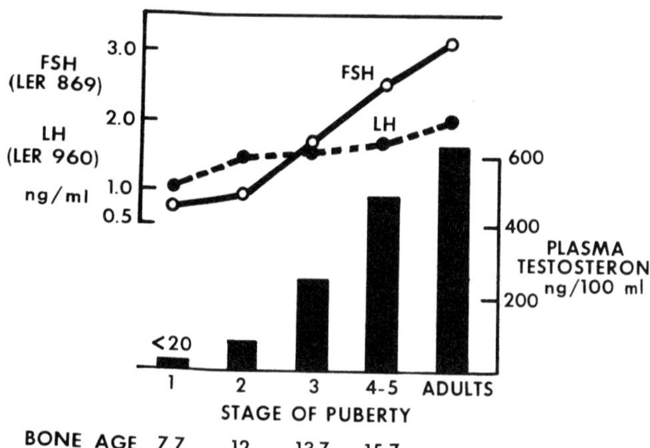

Figure 24–18. Mean plasma testosterone and gonadotropin levels in normal boys by stage of maturation (1 = prepubertal) and mean bone age for each stage. (See legend for Fig. 24–17.) To convert testosterone values to nanomoles per liter, multiply by 0.03467. (From Grumbach MM. Onset of puberty. In Berenberg SR [ed]. Puberty, Biologic and Social Components. Leiden, HE Stenfert Kroese, 1975, pp 1–21. Reprinted by permission of Kluwer Academic Publishers.)

therapy. Testosterone in saliva correlates well with serum levels of testosterone in normal subjects and in patients with chronic disease such as cystic fibrosis.[527, 528]

Estrogens

In the female, the major estrogen, estradiol, is principally secreted (90%) by the ovary; a small fraction of circulating estradiol arises from the extraglandular conversion of testosterone and androstenedione. In the male, approximately 75% of estradiol is derived from extraglandular aromatization of testosterone and (indirectly) androstenedione and 25% from testicular secretion.[516] Aromatase is absent or present in barely detectable amounts in prepubertal testes but maximal amounts appear in late puberty. In normal testes aromatase is predominantly present in the Leydig cells, but in testicular tumors of either Sertoli or Leydig cells, for example, associated with the Peutz-Jeghers syndrome, the Sertoli cells of the tumor express aromatase.[529, 530]

In the fetus and at term, levels of estrogen are high because of the conversion of fetal and maternal adrenal C_{19}-steroids to estrogen by the placenta. Plasma levels of estrogen drop precipitously in the first few days of life. Estrogen levels are so low in prepuberty that detection has been difficult with standard techniques, but a highly sensitive bioassay demonstrated measurable serum concentrations of estradiol in both boys and girls before puberty with higher estradiol concentrations in girls than boys.[221]

The mean concentration of serum estradiol equivalents in 21 prepubertal girls (7.7 ± 1.9 years) was 0.6 ± 0.6 (SD) pg/mL, significantly greater than the concentration (0.08 ± 0.2 pg/mL) found in 23 prepubertal boys (9.4 ± 2.0 years). The higher estrogen levels in girls may be an important factor in the more advanced levels of skeletal maturation in girls and play a part in their earlier onset of sexual maturation.[173] Subsequently, the plasma estradiol level rises steadily through the stages of puberty until maturity[492] and exhibits a diurnal rhythm[531] (see Fig. 24–17), when concentrations of about 500 pg/mL are reached in the follicular stage and about 200 pg/mL in the luteal phase; estrone levels rise early and reach a plateau by midpuberty.[492] The daily peak of estradiol in early pubertal girls occurs about 6 to 9 hours after the peak of serum LH detected during the night,[532] apparently related to the time necessary for ovarian synthesis of estradiol.

Table 24–14. Differences in the Timing of the Onset of Estrogen Synthesis in Girls and Boys

Girls
Follicle-stimulating hormone (FSH) from late fetal life through puberty stimulates aromatase and estrogen synthesis by the ovary.
Boys
FSH leads to enlargement of the testes, the earliest sign of puberty in the male; spermarche occurs early in puberty and spermaturia at a mean age of 13.3 years before the sharp rise in testosterone levels and peak height velocity.
Estrogen synthesis is not detectable in fetal or prepubertal Leydig cells and is at a very low level, until luteinizing hormone stimulates Leydig cell aromatase at late stage II to stage III of male secondary sexual maturation. Estradiol does not reach the level found in girls in early puberty who exhibit a pubertal growth spurt until at least midpuberty.

In all stages of puberty, boys have higher concentrations of estrone than estradiol, and levels of both estrogens are lower than those in girls at comparable stages.[467, 533] Boys have higher levels of estrone and estradiol in pubertal stage 5 than in stage 1. A new ultrasensitive estradiol assay demonstrated measurable serum estradiol equivalents in prepubertal boys with a rise through puberty until the pubertal growth spurt and a decrease thereafter.[173, 222, 223] Klein and co-workers[223] found a high correlation with peak growth velocity and the rise in estradiol concentration, which in boys occurred about 3 years after the onset of puberty. The mean estradiol level at peak growth velocity was similar in boys and girls at about 3 to 4 pg/mL (Table 24–14).

Adrenal Androgens

There is a progressive increase in plasma levels of Δ5-steroids, dehydroepiandrosterone (DHEA) and dehydroepiandrosterone sulfate (DHEAS), in both boys and girls beginning before age 8 (skeletal age of 6 to 8) and continuing through early adulthood (Table 24–15). The increase in the secretion of adrenal androgen and its precursors is known as adrenarche. Plasma DHEA has a diurnal rhythm similar to that of cortisol, but plasma DHEAS shows less variation and is a useful biochemical marker of adrenarche. The role of adrenarche in puberty is discussed later (see "Adrenal Androgens and Adrenarche").

Testosterone-Binding Globulin (Sex Steroid–Binding Globulin)

Between 97% and 99% of circulating testosterone and estradiol is reversibly bound to TeBG; only the free steroid is physiologically active.[134] TeBG is a glycoprotein of 90 to 100 kd, consists of heterogeneous monomers, and has one steroid binding site per dimeric molecule.[534] Prepubertal levels of TeBG are approximately equal in boys and girls, and a decrease in TeBG level occurs with advancing prepubertal age and the concomitant increase in the plasma gonadal steroid levels; at puberty there is a small decrease in TeBG levels in girls and, as a consequence of testosterone, a greater decrease in boys.[535–537] The rise in adrenal androgen levels at adrenarche may explain the early drop in TeBG levels, which allows more circulating free hormone at a given concentration of testosterone.[538] Although the plasma concentration of testosterone is 20 times greater in men than in women, the concentration of free testosterone is 40 times greater.[539–542] Boys with hypogonadotropic hypogonadism and patients with the androgen resistance syndrome show the same characteristic fall in TeBG levels at puberty, but values are intermediate between

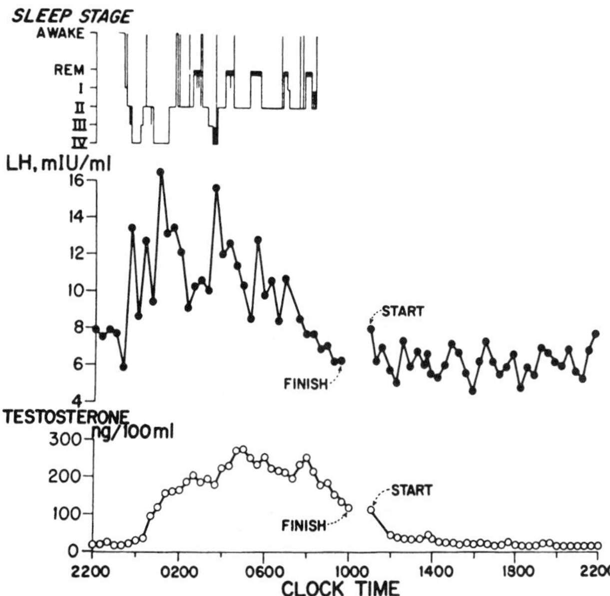

Figure 24–40. Plasma luteinizing hormone (LH) and testosterone sampled every 20 minutes in a 14-year-old boy in pubertal stage 2. The histogram displaying sleep stage sequence is depicted above the period of nocturnal sleep. Sleep stages are rapid eye movement (REM) with stages I to IV shown by depth of line graph. Plasma LH is expressed as mIU/mL. Plasma testosterone is expressed as nanograms per 100 mL. To convert LH values to international units per liter, multiply by 1.0. To convert testosterone values to nanomoles per liter, multiply by 0.03467. (From Boyar RM, Rosenfeld RS, Kapen S, et al. Human puberty: simultaneous augmented secretion of luteinizing hormone and testosterone during sleep. Reproduced from the Journal of Clinical Investigation, 1974, vol. 54, pp. 609–618 by copyright permission of the American Society for Clinical Investigation.)

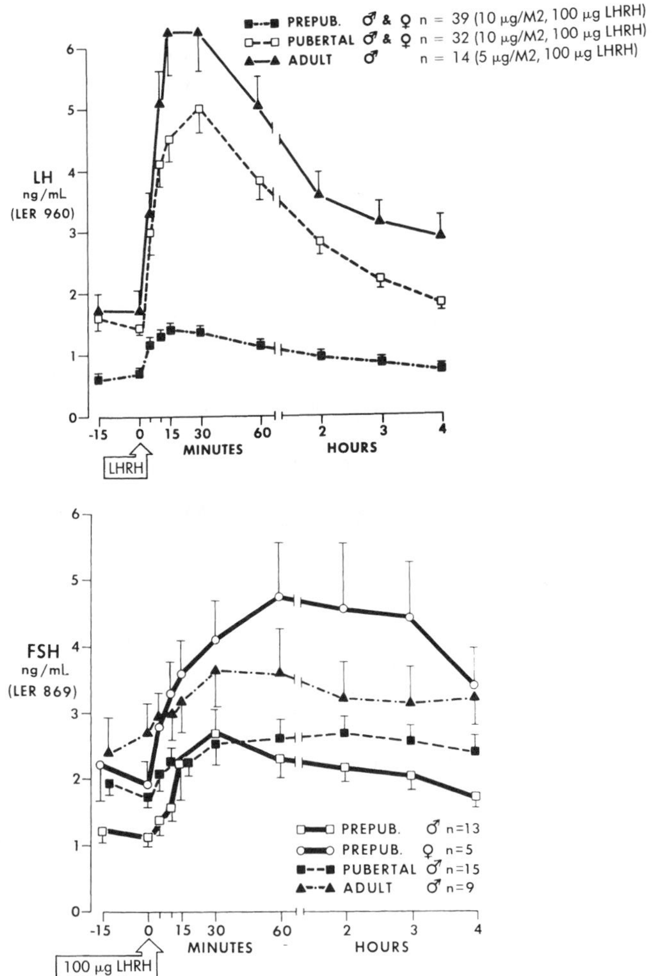

Figure 24–41. Changes in plasma luteinizing hormone (LH) *(top)* and follicle-stimulating hormone (FSH) *(bottom)* levels in prepubertal, pubertal, and adult individuals. Note the limited LH response in prepubertal children compared with that of pubertal and adult subjects. The FSH response to LH-releasing hormone (LHRH) is similar in prepubertal, pubertal, or adult males. In females, the FSH response is significantly greater than that of prepubertal, pubertal, or adult males. For conversion to SI units, see the legend of Figure 24–17. (Modified from Grumbach MM, Roth JC, Kaplan SL, et al. Hypothalamic pituitary regulation of puberty in man: evidence and concepts derived from clinical research. In Grumbach MM, Grave GD, Mayer FE [eds]. Control of the Onset of Puberty. New York, John Wiley & Sons, 1974, pp 115–166.)

idiopathic true precocious puberty in girls and in the occurrence of premature thelarche.[945] The available data are consistent with the hypothesis that less LHRH is required for FSH than for LH release. These findings also point out the difference between pituitary sensitivity and the actual secretory rate of FSH and LH.

The responses to LHRH in peripubertal children who do not yet exhibit physical signs of sexual maturation provide evidence that the self-priming effect[462] of endogenous LHRH augments pituitary responsiveness to exogenous LHRH and is an important factor in the increased gonadotropin secretion at puberty. This change in responsiveness of the gonadotrophs is apparently mediated by increased pulsatile secretion of LHRH[462, 463]; the increased LH response to synthetic LHRH is one of the earliest hormonal markers of puberty onset.

The degree of previous exposure of gonadotrophs to endogenous LHRH appears to affect both the magnitude and the quality of LH responses to a single intravenous dose of LHRH. Studies of the effects of acute and chronic administration of synthetic LHRH in hypergonadotropic hypogonadism, hypogonadotropic hypogonadism, constitutional delayed growth and adolescence, and idiopathic precocious puberty support this concept of self-priming.[462, 482, 484, 496, 722, 940, 946–950] The prepubertal pituitary gland has a smaller pool of releasable LH and decreased responsiveness to the acute administration of synthetic LHRH. With the approach of puberty, the derepression of the hypothalamic LHRH pulse generator and the increased pulsatile secretion of LHRH augment pituitary sensitivity to LHRH and enlarge the reserve of LH. The reason for the discordance in FSH and LH release prepubertally is not clear, but the frequency of LHRH pulses may be a factor.[677, 717, 723, 724, 951] In the adult rhesus monkey with ablative hypothalamic lesions that eliminate endogenous LHRH secretion, reduction of the frequency of exogenous LHRH pulses from one per hour to one every 3 hours increased the FSH/LH ratio.[723] Furthermore, inhibin and endogenous gonadal steroids may also affect this ratio through action on the hypothalamus, the pituitary gland, or both.

These observations and the previously discussed role of the intermittence of the LHRH signal to the gonadotrophs as an essential factor in the neural control of gonadotropin secretion have important implications for the induction of puberty. Pulsatile administration of LHRH to prepubertal monkeys promptly initiated puberty (and, in females, ovulatory menstrual cycles) and restored complete gonadal function in adult monkeys with hypothalamic lesions.[717, 718, 951–953] Similar studies in the human yielded comparable results in prepubertal children and in adults with hypothalamic hypogonadotropic hypogonadism.[724, 900, 935, 946–950, 954] These results provide further support for reactivation of the hypothalamic LHRH pulse generator as the first hormonal change in the onset of puberty.

Responsiveness of the gonads to gonadotropins also increases during puberty. For example, the augmented testosterone secretion in response to administration of hCG at puberty in boys[955] is probably a consequence of the priming effect of the increase in endogenous secretion of LH (in the presence of FSH)[956] on the Leydig cell.

Maturation of Positive Feedback Mechanism

In normal women, the midcycle surge in LH and FSH secretion is attributed to the positive feedback effect of an increased concentration of plasma estradiol for a sufficient length of time during the latter part of the follicular phase.[677, 943, 957] Estradiol has both negative and positive feedback effects on the hypothalamic-pituitary system. Although the suppressive effect is probably operative from late fetal life on, the positive action of endogenous (or exogenous) estradiol on gonadotropin release has not been demonstrated in normal prepubertal and early pubertal children.[462, 463, 958] Hence, acquisition of positive feedback, a requisite for ovulation, is a late maturational event in puberty and, from the present evidence, probably does not occur before midpuberty in normal girls.[462, 463, 958, 959]

Among the requirements for a positive feedback action of estradiol on gonadotropin release at puberty[462] are (1) ovarian follicles primed by FSH to secrete sufficient estradiol to reach and maintain a critical level in the circulation, (2) a pituitary gland that is sensitized to LHRH and contains a large enough pool of releasable LH to support an LH surge, and (3) controversial in the human but not in lower animals, sufficient LHRH stores for the LHRH neurosecretory neurons to respond with an acute increase in LHRH release in addition to the usual adult pattern of pulsatile LHRH secretion.

The main site of action of estradiol is at the level of the anterior pituitary, but estrogen has dual sites of action[960] including a negative as well as positive feedback action on the hypothalamus. Knobil and colleagues[961] have shown in the rhesus monkey that positive as well as negative feedback can occur in adult ovariectomized females in whom the medial basal hypothalamus is surgically disconnected from the remainder of the CNS. In monkeys with hypothalamic lesions, unvarying, intermittent LHRH administration leads to sufficient estradiol release from the ovary to induce an ovulatory LH surge in the absence of an increase in the dose of the LHRH pulses.[677, 953] Estradiol has a positive feedback effect directly on the pituitary gland in normal women, and prolonged administration of estradiol is accompanied by an augmented LH response to LHRH administration in women.[944] The fact that the major positive feedback action on the pituitary gland is demonstrable in the absence of an increase in pulsatile LHRH secretion suggests that the failure to elicit a positive feedback action with administration of estradiol to prepubertal girls could be related to the inadequate LHRH pulses or insufficient LH reserve, respectively, or both components.

That gonadotropin cyclicity[962, 963] and estradiol-induced positive feedback can be demonstrated by midpuberty and before menarche does not imply that the positive feedback loop is complete.[1, 462, 770, 958, 959] Indeed, the modulating effect of the pubertal ovary and its output of estradiol on the hypothalamic–pituitary gonadotropin unit may be insufficient to induce an ovulatory LH surge even when there is an adequate pituitary store of readily releasable LH and FSH. The ovary, because of lack of sufficient gonadotropin stimulation, decreased responsivity, or other local factors, does not secrete estradiol at a high level or long enough to induce an ovulatory LH surge. We visualize the process leading to ovulation as a gradual one in which the ovary (the Zeitgeber for ovulation[677]) and the hypothalamic–pituitary gonadotropin complex become progressively more integrated and synchronous until, finally, an ovary primed for ovulation secretes sufficient estradiol to induce an ovulatory LH surge.[770]

Studies of basal body temperature[962] and of plasma progesterone concentrations[133, 964] suggest that as many as 55% to 90% of cycles are anovulatory during the first 2 years after menarche and that the proportion decreases to less than 20% of cycles by 5 years after menarche. A cyclic surge of LH occurs during some anovulatory cycles in adolescence, but the mechanism of ovulation seems unstable and immature and does not appear to have attained the fine-tuning and synchronization requisite for maintenance of regular ovulatory cycles.

There is a rise in BMI, waist circumference, hip circumference, serum LH, androstenedione, testosterone, and DHEAS in the few years following menarche.[965]

Summary of Present Concept

Our present concept of the role of the hypothalamic-pituitary-gonadal system in the control of the onset of puberty is illustrated in Table 24–20. Clearly, the understanding of these complex maturational processes is incomplete. Puberty is not an immutable process; it can be arrested or even reversed. Environmental factors and certain disorders that affect the onset or progression of puberty mediate their effects by direct or indirect suppression of the hypothalamic LHRH pulse generator and its periodic oscillatory signal, LHRH. For example, strenuous physical conditioning in girls[966] (but not boys) and anorexia nervosa[967] can delay or arrest puberty or lead to the reversion of the hypothalamic-pituitary unit to a prepubertal state, depending on the magnitude of the functional LHRH insufficiency. With a decrease in physical activity in the former and with resumption of weight gain and attainment of sufficient body mass in the latter, the pubertal process is reactivated. In rare instances, true precocious puberty caused by an extrinsic mass lesion that impinges on the hypothalamus can be reversed by decompression or removal of the mass (a subarachnoid cyst, for example).[463, 871]

ADRENAL ANDROGENS AND ADRENARCHE

The adrenal component of pubertal maturation (the adrenarche) and the interactions between adrenal and gonadal hormones are poorly understood.[224, 968, 969] Speculation has focused on the mechanism of adrenarche, the fact that adrenarche occurs earlier than gonadarche (the maturation of the hypothalamic-pituitary-gonadal system), and the interaction between adrenal and gonadal hormones at puberty.

Nature and Regulation of Adrenal Androgens

The major adrenal androgen precursors secreted by the adrenal cortex are DHEA, DHEAS, and androstenedione; apparently, none of these C_{19}-steroids directly activate the androgen receptor. By extraglandular metabolism, the so-called adrenal androgens contribute to physiologically active testosterone and estradiol. In normal adult women, only androstenedione is an important precursor; DHEA and DHEAS contribute little to circulating testosterone and estradiol but can be converted locally to these steroids in some peripheral tissues.[172] However, scant information is available on the metabolism and kinetics

Pituitary Tumors

Pituitary adenomas are rare in childhood and adolescence as only 2% to 6% of all pituitary adenomas occur in this age group. In one study, 50% of pituitary adenomas occurring before adulthood were prolactinomas, 20% were GH-secreting adenomas, and 30% were chromophobe adenomas.[1058] Hyperprolactinemia related to microprolactinomas or macroprolactinomas of the pituitary is uncommon in childhood and adolescence and is a rare cause of delayed puberty in both boys and girls.[1059–1062] Among our patients, only 2 of 29 had delayed onset of puberty,[1062] although primary amenorrhea was the presenting symptom in 13 of 20 pubertal females. Galactorrhea may be absent by history but is often demonstrable by manual manipulation of the nipples (because serum prolactin may rise after manipulation of the nipples, samples should be obtained before examination or many hours later).

Transsphenoidal resection of microprolactinomas in children and adolescents was an effective treatment with an 89% cure rate.[1062] The dopamine agonist bromergocryptine is used by some as a method of decreasing serum prolactin concentrations and decreasing the size of the tumors[1063]; we use this approach in children and adolescents in whom resection of the adenoma is incomplete and to reduce the size of large macroprolactinomas before attempted surgical removal. Pubertal progression in affected boys and girls as well as normal menstrual function in girls usually follows the reduction in serum prolactin levels. In a series of prolactinomas in children and adolescents, there was a preponderance of microadenomas in girls and of macroadenomas in boys, and these larger tumors led to local symptoms related to their size

Other Central Nervous System Disorders Leading to Delayed Puberty

Langerhans' Cell Histiocytosis (Hand-Schüller-Christian Disease, or Histiocytosis X)

This disorder, now thought to be a clonal proliferative disorder of Langerhans' histiocytes or their precursors,[1064, 1065] is characterized by the infiltration of lipid-laden histiocytic cells or foam cells in the skin, viscera, and bone.[1066–1068] Diabetes insipidus, usually resulting from infiltration of the hypothalamus or the pituitary stalk or both, is the most common endocrine manifestation.[1069] However, GH deficiency and delayed puberty may occur.[1070, 1071] There may be visceral involvement including the lung, liver, and spleen. Other findings include cyst-like areas in flat bones of the skull, the ribs, the pelvis, and the scapula; in the long bones of the arms and legs; and in the dorsolumbar spine. Lesions of the mandible lead to the radiographic impression of "floating teeth" within rarefied bone and the clinical finding of absent or loose teeth. Infiltration of the orbit may lead to exophthalmos, and mastoid or temporal bone involvement may lead to chronic otitis media.[1072] Treatment with glucocorticoids, antineoplastic agents, and radiation is promising in terms of survival, but more than 50% of patients have late sequelae or progression.[1068, 1072–1074] The natural waxing and waning course of this disease makes evaluation of therapy difficult.[1075, 1076]

Postinfectious Inflammatory Lesions of the Central Nervous System, Vascular Abnormalities, and Head Trauma

These are unusual causes of hypogonadotropic hypogonadism. Rarely, tuberculous or sarcoid granulomas of the CNS are associated with delayed puberty.[1077] Hydrocephalus may cause delayed puberty that can be reversed with decompression,[1078, 1079] as can pressure from a subarachnoid cyst as noted earlier.

Radiation of the Head

Radiation of the head for treatment of CNS tumors, leukemia, or neoplasms of the head and the face may result in gradual onset of hypothalamic-pituitary failure.[1080] Although GH deficiency is the most common hormone disorder resulting from radiation, gonadotropin deficiency also occurs.[898, 1081] Decreased growth caused by GH deficiency with early onset of puberty can lead to a decrease in the final height of children with acute lymphocytic leukemia treated with CNS radiation.[1082] The advance in the age of onset of puberty is positively correlated with the age of diagnosis of the condition for which the radiation was given and positively correlated with BMI at diagnosis.[1083] Newer radiation treatment regimens using 18 Gy instead of 24 Gy may have less influence on advancing the age of menarche and may lead to less long-term morbidity.[1084, 1085] One study found that girls receiving 25 Gy of CNS irradiation after 7 years of age were more likely to have delayed puberty whereas in those treated earlier the onset of puberty was not affected, although they ultimately had diminished height[1086]; the later part of this study contrasts with the more frequently reported advance of puberty with radiation therapy as noted earlier.

Developmental Defects

Midline malformations of the head and the CNS are associated with a variety of endocrine deficiencies. Septo-optic or optic dysplasia is caused by abnormal development of the prosencephalon. The optic nerve is usually affected, leading to small, dysplastic, pale optic discs and pendular (evenly moving side to side) nystagmus; severely affected patients may be blind. The midline hypothalamic defect may lead to GH deficiency and diabetes insipidus and may be associated with deficient ACTH, TSH, and gonadotropin secretion; short stature and delayed puberty result, although true precocious puberty is an alternative outcome (see later).[1087] The septum pellucidum is often absent in association with optic hypoplasia or dysplasia, which is readily demonstrable by imaging techniques.[118, 1088] The pituitary gland may be hypoplastic, presumably because of the lack of hypothalamic stimulatory factors, and in some patients the neurohypophysis may have an ectopic location.[1089]

In our series, the syndrome is associated with decreased maternal age. A mutation in the *HESX1* gene is a rare cause of septo-optic dysplasia.[1090, 1091] Other developmental defects of the anterior pituitary gland associated with hypogonadotropic hypogonadism and other pituitary hormone deficiencies are caused by autosomal recessive mutations in homeobox genes encoding transcription factors involved in the early aspects of pituitary development. These include, in addition to *HESX1*, mutations in *LHX3*[1092] and *PROP1*.[1093, 1094] *PROP1* mutations, which cause GH and TSH deficiency, can be associated in affected males and females with delayed puberty or late onset of secondary hypogonadism in adulthood.[1094] In one study of 73 patients with "idiopathic" multiple pituitary hormone deficiencies, 35 had a mutation in *PROP1*.[1095] Less commonly ACTH deficiency is a feature of *PROP1* mutations.[1096] Other congenital midline defects ranging from complete dysraphism and holoprosencephaly to cleft palate or lip are also associated with hypothalamic-pituitary dysfunction.[1078] Homozygous mutations in the *LHX3* gene, which encodes a member of the LIM class of homeodomain proteins, are associated with multiple pituitary hormone deficiencies including LH and FSH and severe restriction of head rotation.[1092] Twenty cases of duplication of the hypophysis were reported with delayed puberty present in at least one.[1097] Individuals with myelomeningocele (myelodysplasia) have an increased frequency of endocrine abnormalities, including hypothalamic hypothyroidism, hyperprolactinemia, and elevated gonadotropin concentrations, and some patients demonstrate true precocious puberty.[1098, 1099]

Isolated Gonadotropin Deficiency

Isolated hypogonadal hypogonadism is characterized by selective deficiency of gonadotropins owing to a defect at the level of the hypothalamus involving the LHRH pulse generator or the gonadotrophs, or both, without an anatomic lesion (Tables 24–23 and 24–24).[950, 954, 1029, 1059, 1100–1103] As a consequence, signs of puberty fail to occur by age 14 years in boys and age 13 years in girls or the pubertal maturation is incomplete or transient. In boys, micropenis or undescended testes or both signs are evidence of a fetal testosterone deficiency. The heterogeneous disorders that lead to isolated hypogonadotropic hypogonadism are typically associated with a prepubertal concentration of gonadal sex steroid values (testosterone in boys; estradiol in girls) and low or normal gonadotropin levels. In the severe form, the concentration of gonadal sex steroids and gonadotropins is low, pulsatile secretion of LH is absent or virtually so, and the LH response to the administration of LHRH is deficient. The testes, if palpable, are small and the concentration of serum inhibin B and estimate of seminiferous tubule function are low.[1104, 1105]

Isolated gonadotropin deficiency may occur in families (about 20% to 30% of patients) or sporadically. The pattern of inheritance in affected families is that of an autosomal dominant, autosomal recessive, or X-linked recessive trait.[1106–1108] In contrast to patients with CNS tumors, who usually have associated GH deficiency and growth failure, and to patients with constitutional delay in growth and adolescence, who are short for chronologic age, patients with isolated gonadotropin deficiency are usually of appropriate height for their age (Fig. 24–48). Because their concentrations of gonadal steroids are too low for the epiphyses to fuse at the normal age, these patients develop increased arm span for height and decreased upper/lower ratios (eunuchoid body proportions) and, if untreated, usually become tall adults.[1109] An autosomal recessive form has been described in the mouse (*hyg/hyg*) in which there is a deletion of a part of the LHRH gene. The mutant RNA is incapable of generating functional LHRH.[1110]

Kallmann's Syndrome

This genetically heterogeneous syndrome (Table 24–25) is the most common form of isolated hypogonadotropic hypogonadism with delayed puberty in which anosmia or hyposmia resulting from agenesis or hypoplasia of the olfactory lobes or sulci, or both, is associated with LHRH deficiency.[1111, 1112] The prevalence in boys is about four times that in girls (Fig. 24–49). Although the extent of the defect in olfaction usually seems to correlate with the degree of LHRH deficiency, even in patients with complete anosmia the LHRH deficiency may be partial (the fertile eunuch syndrome).[1105, 1113] Rarely, affected men who had a severe delay in puberty may recover spontaneously, experience an increase in testicular size, and enter full puberty.[1114, 1115] The magnitude of the LHRH deficiency correlates with the size of the testes[1104] (Fig. 24–50). Affected individuals often do not notice impaired olfaction; testing with graded dilutions of pure scents is useful to discriminate the magnitude of the deficit in olfaction.[1116] Undescended testes and gynecomastia are common in this and all types of hypogonadotropic hypogonadism in boys.[1104] About one half of males with Kallmann's syndrome are born with a micropenis.[1117]

Associated defects inconsistently present are cleft lip, cleft palate, imperfect facial fusion, seizure disorders, short metacarpals, pes cavus, neurosensory hearing loss, cerebellar ataxia and nystagmus, ocular motor abnormalities,[1118] and, limited to the X-linked form, unilateral or rarely bilateral renal aplasia or dysplasia,[1119] and mirror movements of the upper extremities (synkinesia)[1111, 1120] (see Table 24–24). All of these structures and organs are sites of expression of the *KAL* gene in the human fetus[1121] (see Table 24–24).

Coronal and axial cranial MRI scans of the olfactory bulbs and sulci are useful as an ancillary approach to diagnosis,[1122 1123] especially in affected infants and children of prepubertal age.[1123] In a review of MRI findings in 64 individuals with Kallmann's syndrome, 56% had bilateral agenesis of the olfactory bulbs (in 2% the agenesis was unilateral) and 56% had absent or abnormal olfactory sulci bilaterally (in 17% the abnormality was unilateral).[1124] Altogether, in Kallmann's syndrome less than 10% have normal cranial MRI findings. Serum LH and FSH are indistinguishable from those in prepubertal children except for lack of or diminished nocturnal pulses of gonadotropin in patients with Kallmann's syndrome.[1125]

This syndrome is genetically heterogeneous and can be transmitted as an X-linked, autosomal dominant, or autosomal recessive trait. Only 14% of familial cases of Kallmann's syndrome and 11% of sporadic cases have mutations in the *KAL* gene on the X chromosome, but these cases are more likely to have complete absence of gonadotropin secretion pulses and have absence of migration of GnRH neurons to the hypothalamus.[1126] The autosomal pattern is more frequent in families in which there are both anosmic and hyposmic individuals as well as patients with normosmic findings.

Reports of affected males who were infertile suggested an X-linked mode of inheritance,[1111] and X linkage has been substantiated by gene mapping techniques in some patients. The Xp22.3 locus is the site of the *KAL1* gene, an X-linked gene that escapes X inactivation and maps 1.5 megabases proximal to the steroid sulfatase gene at the same locus. The *KAL1* gene encodes a 680-amino-acid glycoprotein, named anosmin-1, with characteristics of an extracellular neural adhesion molecule that could putatively function as a pathfinder in the guidance of LHRH neurons to the medial basal hypothalamus (see earlier discussion). The developmental distribution of anosmin-1 by immunostaining and by in situ hybridization with KAL1 mRNA in the human embryo and fetus provides evidence of its widespread distribution including the olfactory placode and forebrain by week 5 to 6.

Anosmin-1 is an extracellular matrix component, with the implication that its action is mainly local. The human embryonic and fetal tissues in which it has been detected include the mesonephros and metanephros, precartilaginous skeleton, inner ear, and cerebellum.[1127] Only the molecular genetics of the X-linked form is well established.[1128] A variety of deletions and mutations of the *KAL* gene have been described, including large and small (exon) deletions,[924, 1129, 1130] point mutations, and a variety of nonsense mutations leading to frameshift and premature stop codons.[924, 1124] A small proportion of familial cases in which X-linked inheritance is well documented apparently do not have a mutation in the coding region of the *KAL* gene; the defect in some of these patients may be located in the promoter region of the *KAL* gene.[1131] Contiguous gene

Table 24–23. Isolated Gonadotropin Deficiency

Males more commonly affected
Familial or sporadic
Height normal for age; tall adult height if untreated
Eunuchoid skeletal proportions
Delayed bone age
Small, often cryptorchid testes: Diameter <2.5 cm prepubertal size; phallus may be small
Normal adrenarche
Examine for anosmia or hyposmia (Kallmann's syndrome)
Look for associated malformations (facial, central nervous system, skeletal, renal)

Table 24–24. Isolated Gonadotropin Deficiency: Clinical Features in 20 Adolescent Boys

Classification	Age and Range* (yr)	Testicular Enlargement	Undescended Testes	Gynecomastia	Ocular Anomalies	Other Anomalies
Euosmic	3⁵⁄₁₂–20⁶⁄₁₂	3/10	3/10	2/10	3/10	6/10†
Anosmic or hyposmic	7–18	2/10	8/10	6/10	7/10	7/10‡
Total		5/20	11/20	8/20	10/20	13/20

*First evaluated at University of California, San Francisco, Pediatric Endocrine Clinic. All of the patients had delayed puberty; mean height was normal for age.
†Cohen syndrome (1); congenital adrenal hypoplasia (1).
‡Absent kidney (1); talipes, camptodactyly (1).

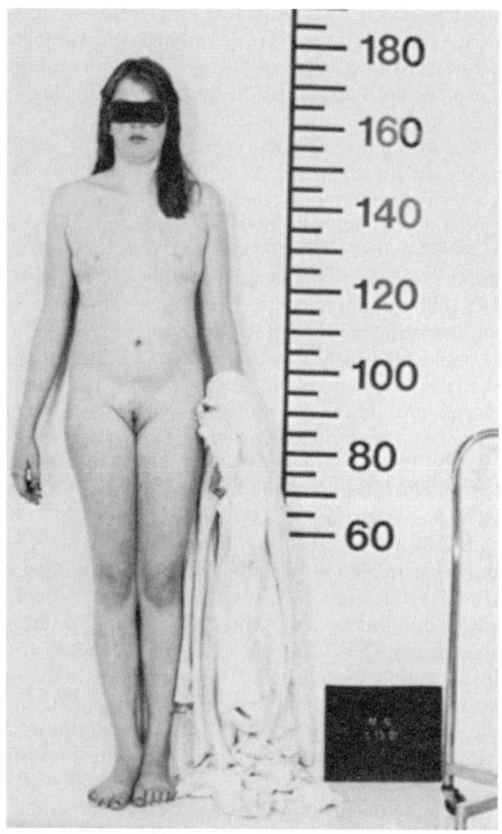

Figure 24–48. A girl 18 years, 8 months of age, with isolated gonadotropin deficiency (sexual infantilism and primary amenorrhea). Height was 173 cm (+1 SD), weight was 66.5 kg (+1 SD), and skeletal age was 13 years. Adrenarche with pubic hair development occurred at age 13½ years. At the time of the photograph, pubic hair was in stage 3 and there was slight breast and nipple development resulting from a previous short course of estrogen therapy. Immature labia minora and majora were noted, and no estrogen effect was present on the vaginal mucosa. Olfactory testing was normal. The plasma luteinizing hormone (LH) (LER-960) level after LH-releasing hormone (LHRH) administration rose from 0.5 to 1.8 ng/mL (a prepubertal response). Serum estradiol was undetectable. The dehydroepiandrosterone sulfate (DHEAS) level was 92 μg/dL (appropriate for pubic hair stage 2). Note the discrepancy between adrenarche and gonadarche. For conversion to SI units, see the legends of Figures 24–17 and 24–36. (From Styne DM, Grumbach MM. Puberty in the male and female: its physiology and disorders. In Yen SCC, Jaffe RB [eds]. Reproductive Endocrinology, 2nd ed. Philadelphia, WB Saunders, 1986, pp 313–384.)

deletions in this region of the X chromosome can lead to an association of Kallmann's syndrome with X-linked ichthyosis caused by steroid sulfatase deficiency, mental retardation, and chondroplasia punctata.[924, 1129]

Autosomal dominant inheritance of the phenotype is supported by some early studies,[1117, 1132] and this pattern of inheritance is further suggested by a report of an affected male who fathered an affected son after treatment with hCG.[1133] Apparent autosomal recessive inheritance characterizes other kindreds.[1134] Thus, the various forms of Kallmann's syndrome are due to heterogeneous mutations[1112, 1117, 1126, 1132, 1134] in which the phenotype can vary. For example, a 20-year-old man with the complete picture of Kallmann's syndrome had an identical twin brother (proved by genetic fingerprinting) with anosmia but a normal adult phenotype and normal plasma testosterone and gonadotropin concentrations.[1135]

In classical, X-linked Kallmann's syndrome, fetal LHRH neurosecretory neurons fail to migrate from the olfactory placode, where they arise, to the medial basal hypothalamus, where they constitute the LHRH pulse generator (see earlier discussion). The defect may be absolute or relative. The fetal LHRH-containing cells and neurites are arrested in their migration to the brain and end in a tangle around the cribriform plate and in the dural layers adjacent to the meninges beneath the forebrain.[734] As noted previously, in some patients this abnormality can be seen in cranial MRI scans[1123, 1136] (Fig.

Table 24–25. Features of Kallmann Syndrome

Clinical
- LHRH deficiency: absent or arrested puberty
- Anosmia or hyposmia
- In infancy: microphallus; cryptorchidism
- Normal stature and growth in childhood
- Normal adrenarche
- Eunuchoid proportions
- Associated midline defects (e.g., cleft lip, cleft palate, midline cranial anomalies)
- MRI: aplasia or hypoplasia of olfactory bulbs and/or sulci

Prevalence: approximately 1 in 7500 males, 1 in 50,000 females; one-tenth prevalence of Klinefelter's syndrome

Inheritance: sporadic and familial cases; genetic heterogeneity
- X linked
  - X-linked recessive (Kallmann et al.[1111])
  - X chromosome deletion: Xp22.3 (Ballabio et al.[1129])
- Autosomal
  - Dominant (sex limitation) (Santen and Paulsen[1132]; Merriam et al.[1133])
  - Recessive (White et al.[1134])

Anatomy: developmental field defect
- Aplasia or hypoplasia of olfactory bulb and sulcus
- Arrested migration of LHRH neurosecretory neurons from olfactory placode to medial basal hypothalamus

LHRH, luteinizing hormone–releasing hormone.

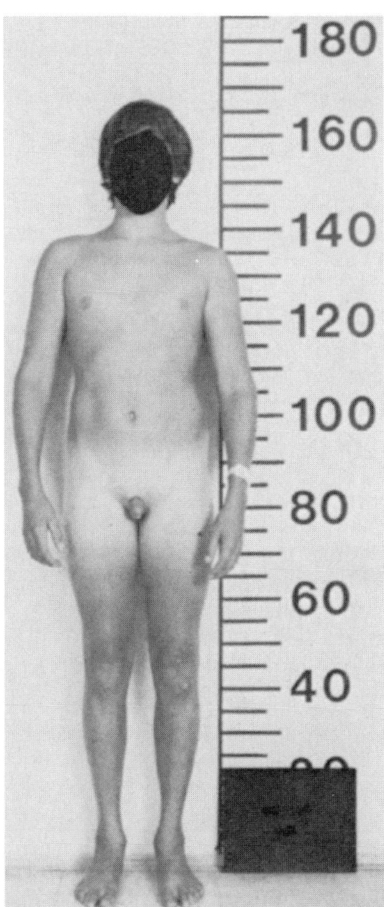

Figure 24–49. A boy of 15 years, 10 months, with isolated gonadotropin deficiency and anosmia (Kallmann's syndrome). He had undescended testes, but after administration of 10,000 U of human chorionic gonadotropin (hCG) the testes descended and were palpable in the scrotum. Height, 163.9 cm (−1.5 SD); the upper/lower body ratio was 0.86, which is eunuchoid. The phallus measured 6.3 × 1.8 cm, and the testes were 1.2 × 0.8 cm. The concentration of plasma luteinizing hormone (LH) was less than 0.3 ng/mL; of follicle-stimulating hormone (FSH), 1.2 ng/mL; of testosterone, 16 ng/dL. After 100 μg of LH-releasing hormone (LHRH) the plasma LH (LER-960) was 0.7 ng/mL and FSH (LER-869) 2.4 ng/mL. For conversion to SI units, see the legends of Figures 24–17 and 24–18. (From Styne DM, Grumbach MM. Puberty in the male and female: its physiology and disorders. In Yen SCC, Jaffe RB [eds]. Reproductive Endocrinology, 2nd ed. Philadelphia, WB Saunders, 1986, pp 313–384.)

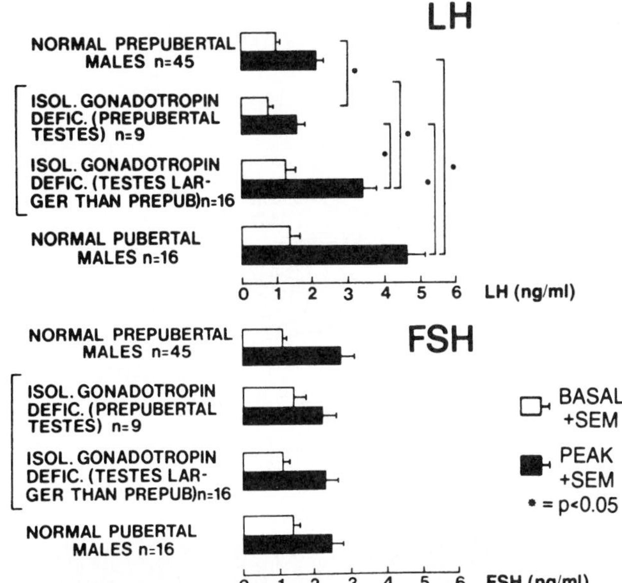

Figure 24–50. Serum luteinizing hormone (LH) and follicle-stimulating hormone (FSH) responses to the administration of LH-releasing hormone (LHRH) in 25 males with an isolated gonadotropin deficiency with or without anosmia, segregated according to whether the volume of the testes was prepubertal or greater than 2.5 cm³; testicular volume in those with testes greater than 2.5 cm³ were as large as 4 cm³. Basal and LHRH-stimulated gonadotropin levels after the intravenous injection of 100 μg LHRH (peak value) are shown. *$P < .05$. For conversion to SI units, see the legend of Figure 24–17. (From Van Dop C, Burstein S, Conte FA, et al. Isolated gonadotropin deficiency in boys: clinical characteristics and growth. J Pediatr 1987; 111: 684–692.)

24–51). Hence, Kallmann's syndrome can be considered a developmental malformation caused by a field defect.

Other Forms of Isolated Hypogonadotropic Hypogonadism

Hypogonadotropic hypogonadism may be transmitted by autosomal recessive inheritance with none of the other features of Kallmann's syndrome. Males with cerebellar ataxia and deficient gonadotropin production are reported in kindreds with X-linked inheritance (possibly a variant form of Kallmann's syndrome), and hypogonadotropic hypogonadism may be associated with the multiple lentigenes and basal cell nevus syndromes.

Luteinizing Hormone–Releasing Hormone Receptor Mutations

A mutation in the human LHRH gene itself has not been reported, in contrast to the mutation described in the *hyg/hyg* mouse.[1110] However, familial and sporadic patients have been reported with mutations in the gene encoding the GnRH receptor, the G protein–coupled seven transmembrane segments, which lead to various degrees of hypogonadotropic hypogonadism with normosmia.[1106, 1108, 1137–1142]

More than six families as well as sporadic patients have been described in this autosomal recessive disorder, with heterozygous or homozygous mutations in the LHRH receptor. Mutations are dispersed throughout the coding region of the gene. The clinical presentation is heterogeneous even within the same pedigree and especially in patients with compound heterozygous mutations. The patients may present with severe features of isolated hypogonadotropic hypogonadism, sexual infantilism, long-delayed puberty, relatively mild hypogonadism, and infertility. The clinical variants include the fertile eunuch variant and reversal in adulthood.[1143] The impairment of signal transmission by the mutant LHRH receptor is highly variable; in one affected woman, pulsatile LHRH treatment induced ovulation and made a successful pregnancy possible.[1144]

In all types of congenital gonadotropin deficiency, male patients are likely to manifest micropenis (penile length less than 2.5 cm at birth and in infancy) because of lack of fetal gonadotropin stimulation of fetal testes during the last half of gestation. Rarely, boys with congenital GH deficiency have micropenis even if gonadotropin function is normal.[1145] Infants and children with micropenis related to hypothalamic deficiencies may be treated with one or two 3-month courses of testosterone enanthate, 25 mg per month given intramuscularly, to enlarge the size of the penis.[1146] Although concern was raised that early testosterone therapy might not allow the attainment of a normal adult penile size, experience has proved otherwise.

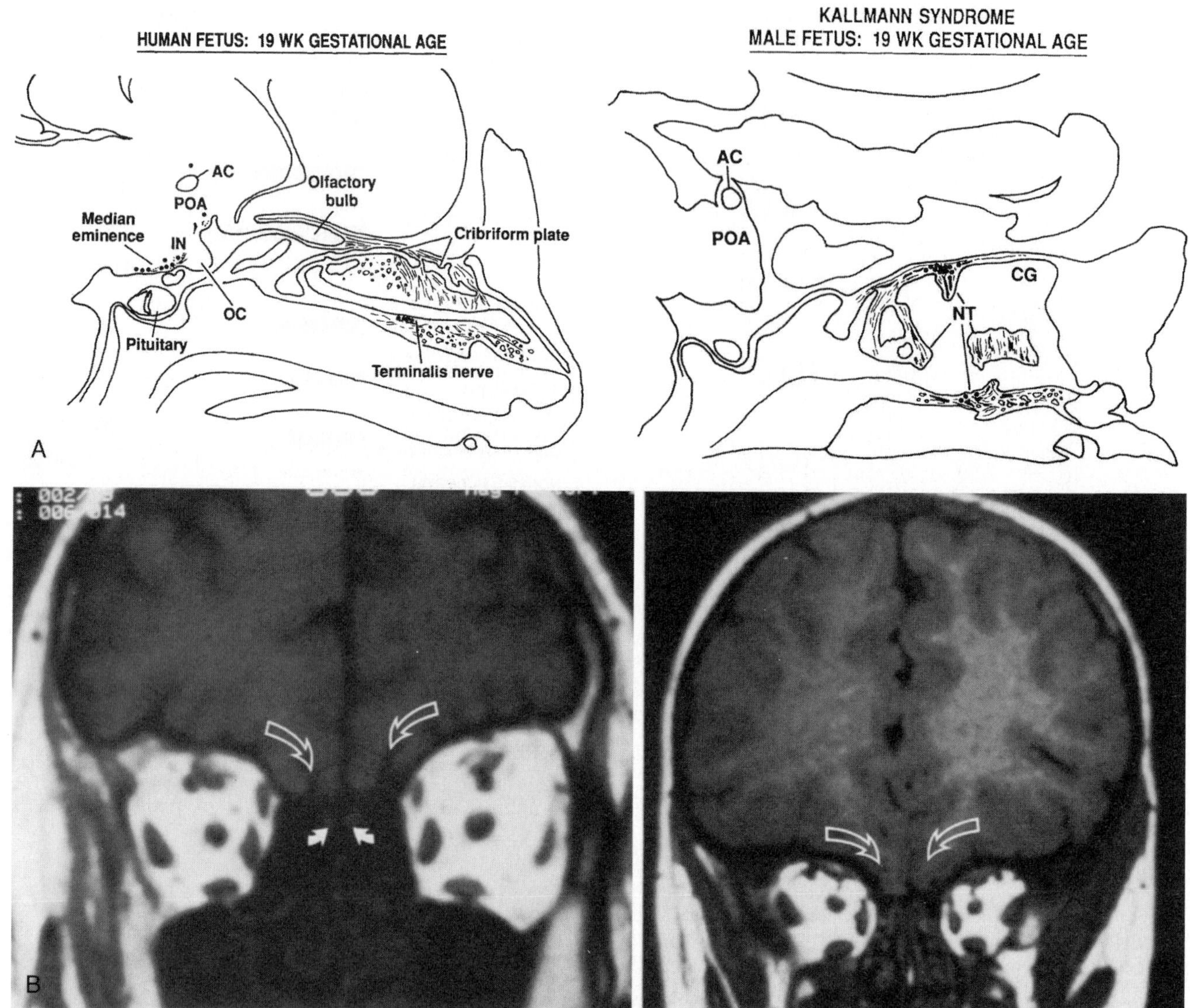

Figure 24–51. Comparison of the brain and nasal cavities of a normal 19-week-old male fetus *(upper left)* and those of a male fetus of similar age with Kallmann's syndrome caused by an X chromosome deletion at Xp22.3 *(upper right)*. In the normal fetal brain the luteinizing hormone–releasing hormone (LHRH) neurosecretory neurons *(black dots)* are located in the hypothalamic area including the medial basal hypothalamus; the anterior hypothalamic area; and, of interest regarding hypothalamic hamartoma as an ectopic LHRH pulse generator, the premammillary and retromammillary areas. A small cluster of LHRH neurons is present among the fibers of the terminalis nerve on the floor of the nasal septum. In the male fetus with Kallmann's syndrome, no LHRH neurons were detected in the hypothalamic region including the basal hypothalamus, median eminence, and preoptic area. The LHRH cells fail to migrate to and enter the brain from their origin in the nose; these cells end in a tangle beneath the forebrain on the dorsal surface of the cribriform plate and in the nasal cavity. AC, anterior commissure; CG, crista galli; IN, infundibular nucleus; NT, terminalis nerve; OC, optic chiasm; POA, preoptic area. (Adapted from Schwanzel-Fukuda M, Bick D, Pfaff DW. Luteinizing hormone–releasing hormone (LHRH)-expressing cells do not migrate normally in an inherited hypogonadal (Kallmann) mouse. Mol Brain Res 1989; 6:311–326.) Lower panels show magnetic resonance imaging scans of brain (coronal section, TI-weighted image). *Lower left,* Normal olfactory sulci *(open white arrows)* and bulbs *(small solid white arrows)* in a 15-year-old boy. *Lower right,* Absent olfactory sulci *(open white arrows)* and bulbs in a 17-year-old anosmic, sexually infantile boy with Kallmann's syndrome.

Further, the concern that the penis might not respond to androgens later in life if exposed to testosterone in childhood, a pattern noted in the rat, proved incorrect.[94] Thus, it is appropriate to treat male infants and children with micropenis related to gonadotropin or GH deficiency with short courses of androgens to enlarge the penis into the normal childhood range. It is not appropriate to reverse the sex of a male infant because of microphallus owing to such causes as fetal testosterone deficiency.

X-Linked Congenital Adrenal Hypoplasia and Hypogonadotropic Hypogonadism

This uncommon X-linked recessive disorder of adrenocortical organogenesis is due to a deletion or mutation in the *DAX1* gene (*d*osage-sensitive, sex reversal, *a*drenal hypoplasia congenita, *X* chromosome gene *1*).[1147–1151] The *DAX1* gene, a member of the nuclear receptor superfamily, encodes an orphan receptor that is a putative transcriptional repressor. The

DAX1 locus undergoes X inactivation. It maps to the *DSS* (*d*osage-*s*ensitive *s*ex reversal) locus (Xp21); a double dose of *DAX1* is associated with a female phenotype or ambiguous genitalia in 46,XY males.

DAX1 protein has a novel domain in the amino terminus that contains two putative unique zinc finger motifs, and the carboxyl terminus contains a conserved ligand-binding domain[1148, 1150] that binds deoxyribonucleic acid (DNA), localizes in the nucleus, and contains a transcriptional silencing domain that antagonizes the steroidogenic factor-1 (SF-1) *trans*-activation function.[1152, 1153] DAX1 has an SF-1 response element in the 5′promoter region.[1154, 1155] SF-1 is another orphan member of the nuclear hormone receptor superfamily; both DAX1 and SF-1 are expressed in the adrenals, gonads, pituitary, and hypothalamus,[1156] which raises the possibility of an important interaction between these two genes and their products.

Abnormalities of the *DAX1* gene are characterized by severe glucocorticoid, mineralocorticoid, and, at puberty, androgen deficiency.[1157–1161] A mature adrenal cortex is lacking and the abnormal structure of the adrenal cortex resembles that of the fetal zone made up of disorganized vacuolated cytomegalic cells.[1159, 1161–1163] In the majority of affected boys, the severe primary adrenal insufficiency with hyponatremia, hyperkalemia, acidosis, and hypoglycemia (failure to thrive, vomiting, poor feeding, dehydration, circulatory collapse, increased pigmentation) is lethal if untreated early in life.[1159, 1161] The concentration of plasma ACTH and plasma renin activity are high; plasma cortisol and aldosterone levels are low. Less commonly, the onset of symptomatic adrenal insufficiency is delayed into later childhood, an early sign of which is increased skin pigmentation.

In the infant male, signs of salt wasting are usually the most prominent feature but cortisol deficiency is present and detectable, and the adrenal insufficiency includes deficient secretion of the zona reticularis steroids, DHEA and its sulfoconjugate. The testes are undescended in less than half of the patients; micropenis is rare, but urogenital abnormalities and hearing loss are occasionally present. Most commonly, because of hypogonadotropic hypogonadism, signs of sexual maturation at the age of puberty are lacking, including absence of pubic and axillary hair and testicular enlargement; the concentrations of serum FSH, LH, and testosterone are low.[1157–1161] There are exceptions to this typical presentation, related in part to the nature of the *DAX1* mutation; for example, the adrenal dysfunction may be subtle and delayed puberty, owing to hypogonadotropic hypogonadism, the prominent clinical feature.[1164]

Boys who do not present with clinical evidence of adrenal insufficiency in infancy often have a more insidious onset during childhood.[1165, 1166] In rare instances, the adrenal insufficiency is not detected until adulthood and the hypogonadotropic hypogonadism is partial.[1167] In a pedigree in which two affected boys had a hemizygous *DAX1* nonsense mutation and neonatal onset of adrenal insufficiency, a maternal aunt who was homozygous for the mutation had sexual infantilism and primary amenorrhea but even after decades of follow-up maintained normal adrenal function. A maternal grandfather who carried the same mutation was asymptomatic.[1168] This pedigree again highlights the limitations and complexities of genotype and phenotype correlations.[1169] A survey of 106 individuals with various etiologies of pubertal delay or hypogonadotropic hypogonadism indicated that a mutation of *DAX1* is rare and most unlikely to be the cause in such cases unless there is a history of adrenal insufficiency.[1170]

For many years, the nature of the hypogonadotropic hypogonadism in this condition has been uncertain.[1158–1161] Two advances clarified this issue. First, as discussed subsequently, intragenic mutations in the *DAX1* gene[1148, 1149, 1171, 1172] indicate that the hypogonadotropic hypogonadism is an intrinsic characteristic of the disorder, a manifestation of the single gene mutation and not related to the involvement of a contiguous gene. Second, the *DAX1* gene is expressed not only in the adrenal cortex and testes (and weakly in the ovary)[1147, 1171] but also in the hypothalamus and pituitary.[1150, 1173] More commonly, there is evidence of both LHRH deficiency and an abnormality in the gonadotrophs, giving a mixed picture of both hypothalamic and intrinsic gonadotroph defects, but in some instances one or the other defect is primary, usually at the pituitary level.[1161] The pulsatile secretion of LH is absent or erratic; basal immunoreactive LH and FSH levels may be normal but the gonadotropins seem to lack bioactivity.[1174] Of interest, in affected male infants in whom hypothalamic–pituitary gonadotropin–testicular function was assessed at birth and in infancy (as late as 140 days), the serum concentration of testosterone was normal (i.e., elevated to pubertal levels), as was that of FSH and LH and there was the expected pubertal response to LHRH administration.[1166, 1175–1177] In addition to the glucocorticoid and mineralocorticoid deficiencies, the serum DHEAS levels were low. These observations suggest that, at least in some affected boys, the LHRH pulse generator–pituitary gonadotropin apparatus is intact and functional in infancy and early childhood and that the LHRH-gonadotroph defects are not manifest until later in childhood or the peripubertal period.

A tall 2-year-old boy with a *DAX1* mutation resulting in a frameshift and premature stop codon had as his first clinical manifestation penile enlargement and pubic hair that proved to be due to LHRH-independent sexual precocity. Serum testosterone values were in the early pubertal range; basal and LHRH-stimulated LH and FSH were prepubertal. The sexual precocity was not modified by LHRH agonist treatment; the LH receptor gene had a normal sequence. At age 3 years, he became progressively pigmented and cortisol and aldosterone deficiencies were documented as well as extremely high levels of plasma ACTH. On replacement therapy with cortisone acetate and 9α-fludrocortisone, the size of his testes decreased and the concentration of serum testosterone fell into the prepubertal range. The observations suggested that the exceedingly high circulating ACTH levels, possibly acting through the human melanocortin 1 receptor present in human Leydig cells, were the underlying cause of the increased steroidogenesis and testosterone secretion, which was reversed by glucocorticoid treatment. In addition, as DAX1 inhibits the SF-1 *trans*-activation, a regulator of steroidogenic genes, the loss of DAX1 inhibition of SF-1 transcriptional activity may also have had a role.[1178]

Data on seminiferous tubule function are limited. Azoospermia unresponsive to gonadotropin treatment was detected in a few affected men.[1167, 1179] Delayed puberty is a manifestation in some female carriers of a *DAX1* mutation.[1179]

In addition to a deletion of *DAX1*, most mutations in the gene are nonsense mutations and frameshifts; missense mutations with a change in a single amino acid are relatively uncommon.[1147, 1148, 1150, 1171, 1172, 1174] In a review of 86 patients reported to have intragenic mutations in *DAX1*, the most common were frameshift mutations (49%); nonsense mutations were described in 28% and missense mutations in 20%, almost all of which were located in the ligand-binding domain.[1180]

Contiguous gene syndromes are not uncommon in association with X-linked congenital adrenal hypoplasia, the gene of which maps to Xp21, distal to the glycerol kinase (*GK*) gene and the Duchenne muscular dystrophy (*DMD*) gene and proximal to the gene associated with mental retardation.[1181] Hence, a deletion of the adrenal hypoplasia congenita locus can include the *GK* and *DMD* genes if it extends toward the centromere or mental retardation with extension toward the telomere.

Isolated Luteinizing Hormone Deficiency

Isolated LH deficiency (the fertile eunuch syndrome) is associated with deficient testosterone production (which responds to administration of hCG) in the presence of variable spermatogenesis; in most instances, it is an incomplete form of isolated gonadotropin deficiency.[1182] The disorder may be idiopathic or secondary to a hypothalamic pituitary neoplasm.

Isolated Bioinactive Luteinizing Hormone

Rarely, isolated bioinactive LH is due to a mutation in the gene encoding the β LH subunit. The only known patient had a striking discrepancy between immunoactive and bioactive LH. A 17-year-old male with a history of delayed puberty with increased immunoreactive serum LH levels but no LH bioactivity and normal serum FSH concentrations had a homozygous mutation in exon 3 of the β LH subunit gene (glutamine 54 arginine). Biopsy of the testis showed absent Leydig cells and arrested spermatogenesis. Treatment with hCG increased testosterone secretion and spermatogenesis. The serum LH of the heterozygote mother exhibited only 50% of normal binding to the LH receptor.[1183] He had normal male sex differentiation, most likely because of the action of hCG during the second trimester and extending into the third trimester.

The patient had low testosterone concentrations; it is uncertain that he completely lacked LH bioactivity in late fetal life as he did not have micropenis, a common finding in male infants with congenital LHRH deficiency.[1184]

Isolated Follicle-Stimulating Hormone Deficiency

Mutations in the FSH β subunit, either homozygous or compound heterozygous, have been reported in three females and two males. The three affected women presented with delayed puberty, lack of breast development or poorly developed secondary sex characteristics, and primary amenorrhea but normal adrenarche. Immunoactive FSH was not detected in the serum; the LH concentration was elevated and serum estradiol was low. There are three female cases of disordered puberty with FSH β subunit mutations.[710, 1185–1188] Two of three women had a homozygous nonsense mutation in the FSH β subunit gene (Val 61 X) and the other was a compound heterozygote (Cys 51 Gly/Val 61 X).

Two affected men have been reported. Both had azoospermia; small, soft testes; and absence of serum FSH. In one man with normal puberty and LH and testosterone values, the missense mutation was a Cys 82 Arg substitution.[1189] The other man, with a nonsense mutation (Val 61 X), had delayed puberty, low testosterone and inhibin B, and high LH.[1190]

Two males with this mutation had a normal (or only slightly delayed) onset and progression of puberty, but because of abnormal Sertoli development, the testes were small and soft and there was azoospermia.[1189, 1190] A woman with a mutation in the prohormone convertase 1 (*PC1*) gene had extreme childhood obesity, hypocortisolemia, defects in conversion of proinsulin to insulin, and isolated hypogonadotropic hypogonadism.[1191]

Idiopathic Hypopituitary Dwarfism

Idiopathic hypopituitarism is usually caused by a deficiency of hypothalamic releasing factors (Fig. 24–52). In the untreated state, patients with deficient LHRH with rare exceptions have delayed puberty. In contrast, patients with isolated GH deficiency ultimately undergo spontaneous pubertal development, without exogenous gonadal steroids, when the bone age reaches the pubertal stage of 11 to 13 years.[211, 1192, 1193] Those who have associated gonadotropin deficiency do not undergo spontaneous puberty, even when the bone age advances to the pubertal stage during GH therapy.

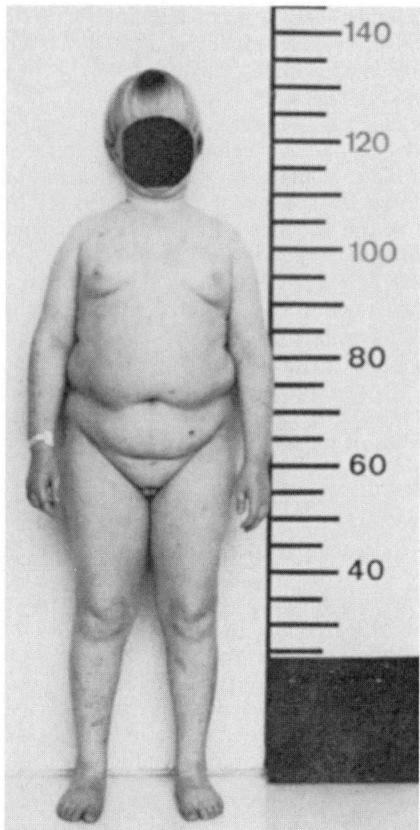

Figure 24–52. A 20-year-old male with idiopathic hypopituitary dwarfism and deficiencies of gonadotropins, thyrotropin, corticotropin, and growth hormone, who had a history of arrested hydrocephalus. Height, 129 cm (−8 SD); the phallus was 2 cm in length, and the testes measured 1.5 × 1 cm. He had received thyroid and glucocorticoid replacement. Basal luteinizing hormone (LH) was less than 0.2 ng/mL (LER-960), follicle-stimulating hormone (FSH) was 0.5 ng/mL (LER-869), and testosterone was less than 0.1 ng/mL. In response to 100 μg of LH-releasing hormone (LHRH), the plasma LH concentration increased slightly to 0.6 ng/mL, and there was no increase in plasma testosterone. The excretion of urinary 17-ketosteroids was 1.1 mg/24 hours. The bone age was 10 years, and the volume of the sella turcica was small on skull radiographs. For conversion to SI units, see the legends of Figures 24–17 and 24–18. (From Styne DM, Grumbach MM. Puberty in the male and female: its physiology and disorders. In Yen SCC, Jaffe RB [eds]. Reproductive Endocrinology, 2nd ed. Philadelphia, WB Saunders, 1986, pp 313–384.)

Common to many patients with idiopathic hypopituitary dwarfism is early onset of growth failure; late onset of diminished growth suggests the presence of a CNS tumor. There is an association between breech delivery, especially in males, perinatal distress, and idiopathic hypopituitarism,[118, 1192] and malformations of the pituitary stalk demonstrable by MRI are common in such patients.[118] The familial forms of multiple pituitary hormone deficiencies with either autosomal recessive or X-linked inheritance are less common.[211, 1093–1096, 1194–1196] The degree of hormone deficit and the age of onset of pituitary hormone deficiencies may vary within a single kindred with the same genetic defect.

The absence of GH and gonadotropins may allow long-term but slow growth to increase final height; the height at the onset of puberty and the height in relation to bone age determine the final height that is reached. One patient was reported to be taller than expected for the family after the diagnosis of panhypopituitarism was made at 25 years of age and treatment was given.[1197] Treatment with GH in prepubertal children with isolated GH deficiency can increase the rate of pubertal development. Alternatively, if GH treatment is instituted in children already in puberty who have a limited height potential, limitation of the amount of growth attained with GH treatment often results. In these instances, the use of LHRH agonists to suppress pubertal development in addition to the use of GH can increase final height.[1198] The judicious use of low-dose testosterone in affected boys of pubertal age with associated gonadotropin deficiency does not seem to impair growth achieved by GH replacement.[1199]

Miscellaneous Conditions

Prader-Willi Syndrome

This autosomal dominant syndrome—early-onset childhood hyperphagia; pathologic obesity and carbohydrate intolerance; infantile central hypotonia and lethargy; delayed onset and poor fetal activity; a tendency for intrauterine growth retardation; short stature by 15 years of age; small hands and feet; mild to moderate mental retardation; emotional instability including perseveration, obsessions, and compulsions; and characteristic facies with almond-shaped eyes, triangular mouth, and narrow bifrontal diameter—is associated with delayed puberty and hypogonadotropic hypogonadism caused by hypothalamic dysfunction. In spite of this, there is a tendency to early adrenarche.[1200–1205]

Affected boys often have micropenis and cryptorchidism. Weight reduction may lead to menarche in some females. Hence, severe obesity may play a role in the impaired puberty in some patients. Plasma GH responses to provocative stimuli and to sleep are usually low but may be normal. The assessment of GH secretion has been confounded by the obesity; it is often decreased in non–GH-deficient obese individuals.

The role of relative GH deficiency in this disorder is uncertain and controversial (see Eiholzer and colleagues[1206] for a contrary view). In the past, GH deficiency has been advocated to support the treatment of Prader-Willi syndrome with recombinant human GH (rhGH). This justification is no longer needed. In June 2000 the U.S. Food and Drug Administration (FDA) approved Prader-Willi syndrome as an indication for rhGH treatment in affected children without a requirement for assessing GH secretion; genetic testing is required to confirm the clinical diagnosis.

The decision to approve rhGH treatment was strongly influenced by long-term randomized control trials in Prader-Willi syndrome.[1207–1209] GH treatment decreases body fat and increases fat utilization, lean body mass, linear growth, and energy expenditure and there are possible improvements in physical strength and motor development. The recommended dose is 1.0 to 1.5 mg/m^2/day (0.03 to 0.05 mg/kg/day). The optimal dose, maintenance of positive clinical effects, optimal age for initiation of treatment, and frequency of adverse side effects including type 2 diabetes mellitus remain to be established.

A striking observation is the discovery that patients with Prader-Willi syndrome have 4- to 5-fold higher fasting concentrations of plasma ghrelin (the "hunger hormone") than in equivalently obese controls.[1451] Ghrelin, a novel enteric hormone secreted among other tissues by the stomach, increases food intake (a powerful orexigen), body weight, and growth hormone secretion. This finding raises the possibility of new pharmacologic and surgical approaches to treatment.

The ghrelin gene is widely expressed in human tissues, the highest level is in the fundus of the stomach[1504]; where its novel acylated peptide ghrelin is localized to X/A cells, a distinctive endocrine cell population in the oxyntic mucca.[2142a]

This distinct genetic disorder with a frequency of about 1 in 20,000, rarely familial (the recurrence risk depends on the type of genetic defect), is caused by abnormalities involving the long arm of chromosome 15 in the region q11-q13. Approximately 70% of Prader-Willi cases are caused by a paternal deletion of 15q11-q13 (commonly about 3 to 5 megabase pairs in size); 20% to 25% of cases have maternal uniparental disomy (either isodisomy or heterodisomy) in which both chromosomes 15 are derived from the mother, possibly by nondisjunction during maternal meiosis, and represent a striking example of genomic imprinting. In 2% to 5%, an imprinting center defect has been detected.[1204, 1210–1214] The lack of a functional paternal 15q11-q13 region, caused by any of a variety of genetic mechanisms,[1205, 1215] can result in the syndrome. One candidate imprinted gene, among several, that maps to this region, *SNRPN* (small nuclear ribonucleoprotein-associated polypeptide SmN) implicated in splicing pre-mRNA, is expressed in the brain including the hypothalamus and has been advanced as one explanation of the syndrome.[1216, 1217] Little is known about the fine structure of the brain in this syndrome. A study of the hypothalamic paraventricular nucleus described a decrease in the number of immunoreactive oxytocin-containing cells—"putative satiety" neurosecretory neurons.[1218]

Laurence-Moon and Burdet-Biedl Syndromes

The *Laurence-Moon syndrome*[1219, 1220] has frequently been incorrectly combined with the *Bardet-Biedl* syndrome although they are now regarded as distinct entities. Both are rare autosomal recessive traits and both combine retinitis pigmentosa and hypogonadism of various etiologies. Many of the Bardet-Biedl patients have developmental delay, as do all of the Laurence-Moon patients. The Laurence-Moon syndrome, however, is associated with spastic paraplegia, whereas the Bardet-Biedl syndrome involves postaxial polydactyly, onset of obesity usually in early infancy, renal dysplasia, and a relatively high prevalence among the Bedouin of the Middle East. Similar findings are present in the Biemond syndrome II with iris coloboma, hypogenitalism, obesity, polydactyly, and developmental delay, but it too is a distinct entity. The genetically and phenotypically heterogeneous Bardet-Biedl syndrome is linked to six loci that map to chromosomes 2, 3, 11, 15, 16, and 20; in most cases three mutant genes are required for a phenotype.[1222–1224]

Functional Gonadotropin Deficiencies

Severe systemic and chronic disorders and malnutrition are associated with delayed puberty or failure to progress through the stages of puberty. It is necessary to distinguish the effects of malnutrition, which can lead to functional hypogonadotropic hypogonadism, from the primary effects of the disease. For example, a group of malnourished rural children from Kenya had chronologic delay in pubertal development and excreted less urinary FSH and LH than well-nourished urban children of the same age. When the two groups were matched by pubertal stage rather than chronologic age, there was no longer a difference in gonadotropin excretion.[1221, 1225] A study of girls who had previously suffered from kwashiorkor demonstrated no delay in breast development or peak height velocity but a delay in pubic hair development and menarche.[795] In general, weight loss of any cause to less than 80% of ideal weight for height can lead to gonadotropin deficiency[780, 1226] and low serum leptin levels; weight regain usually restores hypothalamic-pituitary gonadal function over a variable period.[1227] If adequate nutrition and body weight are maintained in patients with regional enteritis or chronic pulmonary disease,[1228, 1229] gonadotropin secretion is usually adequate.

Cystic fibrosis also delays puberty, in large part through malnutrition.[1230, 1231] However, even with normal pubertal progression, boys with cystic fibrosis almost universally have oligospermia caused by obstruction of the spermatic ducts unrelated to their nutritional status.[1232] The greater prevalence of reproductive difficulties in male patients with cystic fibrosis than in female patients may be due to the greater prevalence of the cystic fibrosis transmembrane regulator (CFTR) in male reproductive tissues such as the epididymis and vas deferens and as a consequence more viscoid luminal contents, which ultimately damage the testes.[1233] In addition, epididymides may be deficient and the vas deferens absent. Normal ovaries do not express the CFTR, and endometrial tissue expresses it only after puberty with variable levels in cervical epithelium and fallopian tubes. Even though the CFTR gene and its protein are expressed in the human hypothalamus and in an immortalized mouse hypothalamic LHRH-secreting cell line, mutations in the CFTR gene do not appear to affect LH and FSH secretion.

Further, boys with cystic fibrosis have an autoimmunity to their sperm that appears at the time of puberty and the appearance of spermatogenesis.[1234] Boys with cystic fibrosis have antisperm immunoglobulin M (IgM) antibodies when prepubertal and IgA, IgM, and IgG antibodies during puberty; men with congenital absence of the vas deferens, for comparison, had IgM and IgG antisperm antibodies predominantly.[1234]

Jamaican boys and girls with sickle cell disease have a mean 1.4-year delay in the pubertal growth spurt and a 1.6-year delay in peak height velocity, although final height is comparable to that of normal adults; girls have a 2.3-year mean delay in the onset of menstruation.[1235] There is a similar delay in affected Brazilian boys and girls.[1236] Boys with sickle cell anemia often exhibit impaired Leydig cell function caused by ischemia of the testes, gonadotropin deficiency, or both factors.[1237]

Thalassemia carries the risk of hemochromatosis that causes multiple endocrine abnormalities. Delayed puberty with decreased gonadotropin secretion is the most common problem, with GH deficiency following in prevalence.[1241, 1242] Thalassemia major leads to abnormal sexual maturation in 65% to 80% of boys and 75% of girls, with a similar percentage of patients experiencing growth failure.[1238] The primary hypothyroidism prevalent in this condition is part of the problem, but hypogonadotropic hypogonadism is of importance in many.[1239] There may be additional complications of cytotoxic effects of the alkylating agents used to prepare patients for bone marrow transplantation.[1240]

Before the advent of subcutaneous chelation therapy (monitoring of serum ferritin), complete absence of pubertal development occurred in over 40% of patients with thalassemia[1243, 1244] because of transfusional iron and iron overload deposition in the pituitary and hypothalamus resulting in hypogonadotropic hypogonadism.[1242, 1245] The gonads can be stimulated by exogenous gonadotropins, and satisfactory sexual development including fertility can be promoted by the use of hCG and hFSH.[1246–1248, 1242] In poorly controlled cases, primary gonadal damage from iron deposition may be severe.[1249] Of note, deferoxamine therapy may cause skeletal dysplasia and compromise pubertal growth.

The Hemophilia Growth and Development Study observed more than 180 boys affected with acquired immunodeficiency syndrome (AIDS). Growth in stature was delayed, but weight for height was equal to that in normal boys. Remarkably, serum testosterone concentrations were not affected but bone age was delayed, as was the progression through the stages of puberty. As GH secretion is usually not affected in AIDS, the poor growth appeared more related to the delay in pubertal development.[1250]

Chronic gastrointestinal disease such as Crohn's disease is often accompanied by delayed puberty; therapy to restore nutrition, if successful, enables puberty to progress. The delayed puberty may allow a longer period of prepubertal growth that compensates to some degree for the poor growth noted earlier in this disorder. There is compromise of the pubertal growth spurt with active inflammatory bowel disease, especially if glucocorticoid therapy is necessary.[1251] Celiac disease decreases the growth rate in childhood and adolescence, but with appropriate dietary restrictions final adult height appears normal.[1252]

Chronic renal disease has been associated with delayed pubertal development[1253, 1254] and decreased pulsatile gonadotropin secretion related to a decrease in the mass of bioactive and immunoactive LH secreted rather than an alteration of the frequency; successful renal transplantation usually restores gonadotropin secretion.[1254, 1255] Patients with nephrotic syndrome have poor pubertal growth, poor secondary sexual development, and deficient gonadotropin secretion in a pattern resembling constitutional delay in puberty.[1256] Treatment of glomerulonephritis with alternate-day glucocorticoid therapy leads to a late, diminished but prolonged pubertal growth spurt that can result in a normal final height.[1257] Children with end-stage renal disease receiving renal or peritoneal dialysis are often delayed in reaching sequential pubertal stages and deficient in linear growth; this loss of growth leads to decreased final height despite the improved growth experienced after renal transplantation.[1258, 1259] Immunoreactive gonadotropin concentrations may be elevated, presumably because of impaired renal clearance, but the response to LHRH is blunted in severe renal impairment.[1260, 1261] TeBG is elevated in chronic renal failure and free testosterone is low.[1262] Although improved growth and pubertal development usually ensue after renal transplantation, the glucocorticoid treatment that follows transplantation presents its own problems. Survivors of renal transplantation who have immune suppression and alternate-day steroid treatment often have delayed onset of puberty and decreased pulsatility of GH and gonadotropins at night.[1256, 1263]

Advances in the treatment of leukemia have improved the prognosis. Children with early onset and long-term remission experience puberty at an appropriate age or with only slight delay, whereas patients with initial symptoms of leukemia in late childhood may have considerable delay of pubertal development.[1264]

The type of therapy for malignancy also influences the age of puberty; radiation to the head may cause hypogonadotropic hypogonadism or GH deficiency, or both, and radiation to the abdomen or pelvis and certain types of chemotherapy, especially if administered during puberty, may impair gonadal function and cause primary hypogonadism.[1265] Total-body irradiation for bone marrow transplantation may lead to a decrease in growth in the presence of normal GH secretion. Girls with leukemia treated with CNS radiation demonstrated a diminished pubertal growth spurt and diminished final height; this effect appears to be true whether 24 or 18 Gy is used at a later age, but the final height in boys was reduced only with the higher dose.[1266, 1267] Further, treatment with 24 Gy before the age of 6 years carries a high risk of short stature.[1268] Remarkably, chemotherapy combined with radiation therapy limited to the CNS carries a risk of short stature mainly related to decreased growth of the spine.[1269] However, patients treated with chemotherapy without radiation had a normal final height following a period of catch-up growth after the chemotherapy.[1270] Secondary malignancies, such as papillary thyroid carcinoma and pulmonary fibrosis, are additional risks with total-body radiation.[1271] A follow-up study of over 100 patients treated for acute lymphocytic leukemia before puberty indicated an incidence of obesity of over 45%, indicating the need for dietary counseling in such cases.[1272]

Hypothyroidism may delay the onset of puberty or menarche; treatment with levothyroxine reverses this pattern. There is likely to be a permanent loss of height if diagnosis is delayed; with thyroxine (T_4) replacement, growth may continue for a longer period after menarche than is the norm but the deficit in height is not regained.[1273] Poorly controlled diabetes mellitus can lead to poor growth, fatty infiltration of the liver, and sexual infantilism (Mauriac's syndrome),[1274, 1275] probably related to poor nutritional status; prepubertal children are most vulnerable to poor glycemic control, and pubertal subjects exhibit normal growth unless severe hyperglycemia occurs.[1276] The degree of control necessary to avoid these complications cannot be exactly quantified, but adolescents with even moderately poor control frequently manifest some degree of growth impairment and delayed puberty or irregular menses.[1277] Serum IGF-I is decreased in children and adolescents with poorly controlled diabetes mellitus regardless of pubertal stage.[1278]

Cushing's disease can be associated with delayed onset or arrest of gonadarche, which is usually corrected by transsphenoidal removal of an ACTH-secreting pituitary adenoma.[1279, 1280] The corticotroph adenoma is the most common prepubertal adenoma.[1281]

Anorexia nervosa, a common cause of gonadotropin deficiency in adolescence, is a functional disorder, apparently increasing in prevalence in girls but rare in boys, characterized by a distorted body image, obsessive fear of obesity, and food avoidance that can cause severe self-induced weight loss (to less than 85% of normal weight for age and height or BMI < 17.5 kg/m^2 after cessation of growth), primary or secondary amenorrhea, widespread endocrine disorders, and even death (specific diagnostic details are in the DSM-IV criteria of the American Psychiatric Association[1282]).[1283] Other common features include onset in middle adolescence,[1284] hyperactivity, defective thermoregulation with hypothermia and sensitivity to cold, constipation, bradycardia and hypotension, decreased basal metabolic rate, dry skin, fine downy hypertrichosis, peripheral edema, and parotid enlargement.[1285–1287] The clinician should be aware of the subclinical form. The pathogenesis is multifactorial and includes a genetic factor and a well-characterized psychological component.[1288, 1289] Anorexia nervosa may rarely occur in association with a primary psychiatric disorder.

It is important to rule out organic disease before the diagnosis of anorexia nervosa is assigned; one girl with a macroprolactinoma presented with signs consistent with anorexia nervosa.[1060] The prevalence of anorexia nervosa is increased in Turner's syndrome. Hypogonadotropic hypogonadism is documented in many patients with anorexia nervosa and, at least in part, is related to weight loss.[1285, 1287] However, unidentified factors may contribute to the amenorrhea of anorexia nervosa, especially when the onset of amenorrhea precedes the onset of severe weight loss. It is not uncommon for a patient with anorexia nervosa to be referred months after the onset of the condition; growth failure may be the first sign of anorexia nervosa, and this condition must be considered in the differential diagnosis of growth failure.[1290]

In anorexia nervosa, the concentrations of plasma FSH, LH, leptin, and estradiol and the excretion of urinary gonadotropins are characteristically low. In adult women, there may be a reversion to a circadian rhythm of LH secretion and to the sleep-associated increase in episodic LH secretion characteristic of puberty; in severe cases, the amplitude of the pulsatile episodes is diminished and resembles the pattern in prepubertal children.[1291] Similarly, the LH response to LHRH correlates with the severity of the weight loss.[1292, 1293] In patients who weigh less than 75% of the appropriate weight and have strikingly reduced BMI and percent body fat, there is either a blunted or an absent LH response to the administration of synthetic LHRH and undetectable or small LH pulses. Administration of intravenous LHRH at 90- to 120-minute intervals can stimulate the pituitary to produce LH pulses that are indistinguishable from the normal pubertal pattern.[1291] This response further supports the important role of functional LHRH deficiency in the amenorrhea of anorexia nervosa. Serum leptin levels are low, remarkably so with severe malnutrition consistent with the strikingly decreased mass of adipose tissue, and increase when weight is regained.[1294–1296] Other hormonal changes include an increased mean concentration of plasma GH and plasma cortisol; low levels of plasma IGF-I, DHEAS, and plasma triiodothyronine (T_3) with normal levels of T_4 (unless associated with the low-thyroxine syndrome) and TSH; a decreased rise in serum prolactin after the administration of thyrotropin-releasing hormone (TRH) or insulin-induced hypoglycemia[1297, 1298]; and a diminished capacity to concentrate urine.

The restoration of normal endocrine and metabolic function after weight gain suggests that many of these changes are secondary to starvation and severe weight loss; nevertheless, the amenorrhea may persist for months after weight gain, suggesting persistent hypothalamic dysfunction.[1299] Treatment of this disorder requires skillful management, understanding, patience, and psychiatric consultation.[1289] Various approaches have been used to increase the food intake. In view of the associated mortality, parenteral alimentation may be indicated in resistant patients with severe weight loss, especially in the presence of infection or an electrolyte imbalance.

Functional amenorrhea can also occur in women of normal weight but decreased percentage of body fat and is characterized by normal basal levels of gonadotropin and normal gonadotropin response to LHRH stimulation but lack of or an inadequate midcycle LH surge and a decrease in normal pulsatile secretion (amplitude or frequency or both) of gonadotropins.[1300, 1301] In addition, these patients have decreased leptin concentrations, quite likely because of subtle dysfunction of eating patterns and altered energy expenditure.[967] The consequences range in severity from severe estrogen deficiency to anovulation to a short luteal phase.

Bulimia nervosa is thought to be a variant of anorexia nervosa[1289, 1302]; it occurs in about 1.5% of young women. In this disorder the individual consumes large amounts of food, but food gorging is followed by induced vomiting.[1299] A hand lesion from the induced vomiting (Russell's sign) and an abnormal level of serum electrolytes are useful clinical markers. Abuse of laxatives, diet pills, and diuretics is frequent. Although weight loss is not frequent, amenorrhea is common.[1303] Bulimia is especially prevalent in high school and college women students. A history of childhood sexual abuse is more frequent than in unaffected adolescents.

Cessation of growth can occur in infants and young children with psychosocial dwarfism. Stressful social situations can also inhibit growth and physical pubertal development at adolescence.[1304]

Exercise, Hypo-Ovarianism, and Amenorrhea (the Female Athlete)

In the late 1970s, reports of amenorrhea in female long-distance runners and delayed menarche in other female athletes, including ballet dancers, figure skaters, and gymnasts, appeared.[1305] In 1992 the American College of Sports Medicine defined the female athletic triad of primary or secondary amenorrhea, disordered eating, and osteoporosis or osteopenia derived from the chronic lack of estrogen.[966] Although there are substantial endocrine effects of excessive athletic training in girls, elite prepubertal and pubertal athletes suffer relatively few physical injuries.[1319]

Increasing information strengthened the link between increased physical activity and abnormalities of puberty.[1305–1307] An incidence of 15% of bulimia, anorexia nervosa, or anorexia athletica was found in 603 Norwegian girls; the athletes most affected are those engaged in sports emphasizing weight.[1308] In healthy ballet dancers and female athletes, factors other than

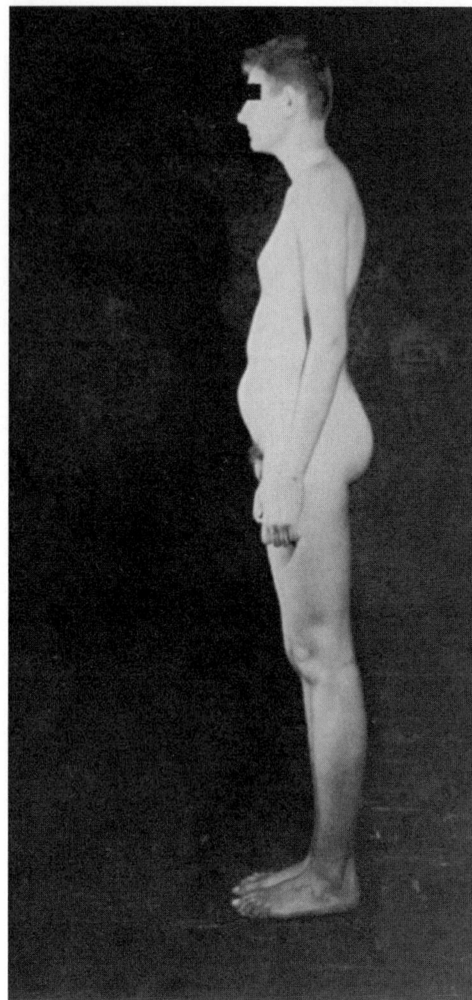
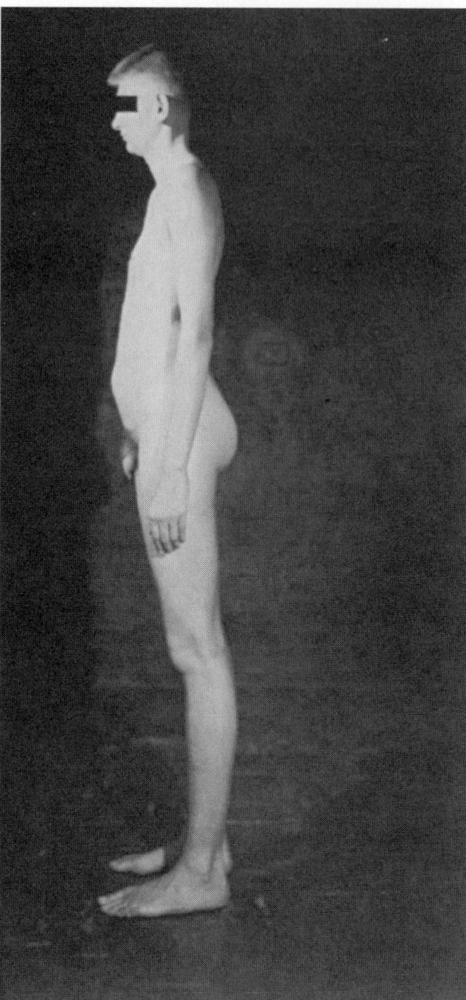

Figure 24–53. 47,XXY Klinefelter's syndrome in 17-year-old identical twins. At age 15 gynecomastia was noted. The twins had a eunuchoid habitus and poorly developed male secondary sexual characteristics. Both were 187 cm in height; arm spans were 187 cm and 189.5 cm; the voices were high-pitched; the testes measured 1.8 × 1.5 cm; penis length was 7.5 cm. Gynecomastia and signs of androgen deficiency were more evident in the twin on the left. Urinary gonadotropins, greater than 50 mU/24 hours. The testes exhibited extensive tubular fibrosis, small dysgenetic tubules, and clumping or pseudoadenomatous formation of Leydig cells; germ cells were rare. The microscopic appearance was typical of seminiferous tubule dysgenesis. (Patients are described in Grumbach MM, Barr ML. Cytologic tests of chromosome sex in relation to sexual anomalies in man. Recent Prog Horm Res 1958; 14:255–324.)

decreased body weight can impair pubertal progression and delay menarche through inhibition of the hypothalamic LHRH pulse generator.[786, 791–794, 1299, 1305, 1309] Indeed, there can be a 1.3- to 2-year delay in teenage girls who are elite gymnasts compared with nonathletes or with their mothers' age of menarche.[1310, 1311] Teenage ballet dancers are lighter, have less body fat than less physically active girls, and have a high incidence of delayed puberty and of primary and secondary amenorrhea. When the strenuous physical activity is interrupted (e.g., by injury), puberty advances, and menarche often occurs within a few months in those with amenorrhea, in some cases before a significant change in body composition or weight.[1299]

Female athletes of normal weight who have less fat and more muscle than nonathletic girls (e.g., ice skaters or swimmers) are also at risk for delayed puberty and for primary and secondary amenorrhea.[791, 1312] However, the mechanism is apparently different from that of the hypothalamic amenorrhea in runners and ballet dancers. In swimmers, menstrual cycles were frequently irregular and anovulatory rather than absent, and the plasma concentrations of DHEAS and LH were higher than normal, with normal plasma estrogen levels.[966, 1313] Both thinness and strenuous physical activity appear to act synergistically, but strenuous exercise training by itself may inhibit the LHRH pulse generator. The effect on pulsatile LHRH secretion may be mediated in part by endogenous opioidergic pathways involving β-endorphin, but the neuroendocrine factors that associate exercise and reproductive function are poorly defined. Even though gonadarche is retarded, adrenarche is not delayed.[791, 1312] Athletes who began strenuous training before menarche had a delay in menarcheal age.[786]

A prospective study of 22 gymnasts contrasted with 21 swimmers demonstrated decreased growth velocity, stunting in leg length growth, and decreased height prediction in the gymnasts, suggesting that heavy training in gymnastics starting before puberty and continuing through puberty leads to a decrease in ultimate height.[1314] Gymnasts, in contrast to nonathletic girls, had a significantly delayed age of menarche, had significantly less body fat, and were shorter and lighter. The gymnasts had a decreased growth spurt compared with the controls, and the final height of 6 of 21 studied was at least 3.5 to 7.5 cm shorter than expected according to parental height.[1315] These studies suggest that extensive training (10 to 12 hours per week) may be excessive for prepubertal girls. On the contrary, a study of 222 intensively trained adolescent girls and their mothers showed a positive correlation between the delayed menarche found in the girls and the age of menarche of their mothers.[1316] Likewise, another study of 96 girls demonstrated a relationship between the age of onset of puberty and menarche in athletes and their mothers; there is a relationship between the choice of sport and constitutional factors, according to these authors, with no indication that the sport causes changes in growth rate or height.[1317, 1318] These studies emphasize the role of genetic factors in the age of menarche, pubertal development, and growth rather than the role of energy expenditure. Thus, the biology of pubertal delay in female athletes remains controversial and uncertain.

Although men are less affected than women, males may also

be affected by rigorous physical training. Males may have decreased LH response to LHRH and decreased spontaneous LH pulse frequency and amplitude; the serum testosterone is normal or low.

Ballet dancers have a higher incidence of scoliosis than the general population and, as already noted, often have delayed puberty; idiopathic scoliosis in the general population has an association with a statistically earlier age of menarche (0.4 years earlier) and an early adolescent growth spurt.[1320] The strongest association with scoliosis is taller stature at the time of the pubertal growth spurt, which, in this study, occurred at an earlier than average age; this combination leads to only a slight increase in final height.[1321] Scoliosis usually develops during the pubertal growth spurt and occurs more often in girls with a more rapid pubertal growth spurt.[1321] Final height in familial constellations of scoliosis does not vary from the family norm.[1322]

Prolactin levels may be elevated in women athletes and could contribute to the delayed menarche found in this group.[1062, 1323]

Other Causes of Delayed Puberty

Marijuana use has been associated with gynecomastia[1324] and is a putative cause of pubertal delay.[1325]

Gaucher's disease caused delay in pubertal development in two of three patients in one study.[1326]

Girls with familial dysautonomia have delayed menarche and often a severe premenstrual syndrome.[1327] The condition is ultimately compatible with pregnancy.

Delayed Puberty and Mood

A prospective study of the intramuscular administration of long-acting testosterone preparations to boys with delayed puberty, aged 14 to 17 years, revealed an effect on mood.[1328] The boys were randomly assigned to a course of 200 mg of testosterone enanthate, administered intramuscularly four times at 3-week intervals, or to no treatment. At 1-year follow-up, all of the boys in the testosterone group exhibited excellent growth in stature; growth in the control subjects was significantly lower than that of the testosterone group. Both groups showed improved self-image, and the treated subjects also exhibited notable increases in both school-related and extracurricular social activity. Thus, a relatively brief course of testosterone enanthate had beneficial effects on growth and on inducing or advancing pubertal maturation that was related to improved social function over that achieved simply by the passing of 1 year.

In contrast, however, a study of psychological tests in boys and girls with delayed puberty of mixed causes, including constitutional delay, treated with periods of three doses of sex steroid alternating with no treatment,[1329] demonstrated only one significant treatment effect, namely an increase in withdrawn behavior problems during administration of low-dose estrogen in girls. There were no consistent sex differences. The authors concluded that the administered testosterone or estrogen had minimal effects on behavior problems or mood in adolescents (see earlier for the effects of this treatment schema on sexuality).

Hypergonadotropic Hypogonadism: Sexual Infantilism Caused by Primary Gonadal Disorders

Primary gonadal failure and the impaired secretion of gonadal steroids lead to decreased negative feedback and elevated LH and FSH levels. The most common forms of primary gonadal failure are associated with sex chromosome abnormalities and characteristic physical findings.[1330] Testicular or ovarian dysfunction as an isolated finding is less commonly a cause of pubertal hypergonadotropic hypogonadism. The study of the factors responsible for apoptosis or programmed cell death has shed light on the control of the degeneration of germ cells in the ovary and testes.[126]

Klinefelter's Syndrome (Syndrome of Seminiferous Tubular Dysgenesis) and Its Variants

Klinefelter's syndrome, or seminiferous tubular dysgenesis, and its variants occur in approximately 1 in 1000 males and are the most common forms of male hypogonadism (see Chapter 22).[1330, 1331] The invariable clinical features include small, firm testes (less than 3.5 cm in length), impaired spermatogenesis, and a male phenotype, usually with gynecomastia and eunuchoid proportions[1330] (Fig. 24–53). Elevated gonadotropin levels are found postpubertally; before the age of 12, gonadotropin concentrations are in the prepubertal range. Rarely, low gonadotropin concentrations occur when hypogonadotropic hypogonadism is associated with 47,XXY Klinefelter's syndrome.[1332]

Hyalinization and fibrosis of the seminiferous tubules and pseudoadenomatous changes of the Leydig cells develop after puberty; prepubertal testes show only subtle histologic changes, although the testes are small and the germ cell content is reduced. Prepubertally, the disproportionate length of the lower extremities and decreased upper/lower body ratio can identify patients without an increase in arm span.[1333] There is variation in Leydig cell function, but the plasma concentration of testosterone tends to be in the normal range until about age 14, after which age it may fail to rise to normal adult levels.[1334, 1335] The onset of puberty is usually not delayed, but impaired Leydig cell reserve and low testosterone levels may lead to slow progression or arrest of pubertal changes.

Testosterone replacement should be considered when the LH level rises above the normal range of values. Serum estradiol/testosterone ratios and TeBG levels are higher than those in normal males, which indicates an increased estrogen effect and decreased testosterone effect. These factors probably account, at least in part, for the gynecomastia characteristic of Klinefelter's syndrome during adolescence.[1335–1337] Testosterone administration does not appear to reduce the gynecomastia, but dihydrotestosterone[1338] and aromatase inhibitors or estrogen receptor antagonists may be effective. If the gynecomastia does not regress, a reduction mammoplasty is required. Tall stature for family size is common in this disorder because of the disproportionate growth of the legs.

Neurobehavioral abnormalities, primarily in language and frontal executive functions, are frequent, and some say universal, in Klinefelter's syndrome. These problems may be severe enough to lead to evaluation in childhood and the prepubertal recognition of the syndrome.

The global I.Q. in unselected populations of subjects with Klinefelter's syndrome is normal or near normal, but verbal I.Q. (VIQ), in contrast to that in Turner's syndrome, is usually lower than performance I.Q. (PIQ).[1339] As patients with clinical or psychological problems are referred more often for evaluation, some studies are skewed to suggest more significant deficits than are prevalent in an unselected population of XXY individuals.

Whereas younger patients with Klinefelter's syndrome have a VIQ that is less than their PIQ, there are older adults who have PIQ less than VIQ.[1340] It was suggested the PIQ drops in late puberty while VIQ remains stable.[1341] Further, prepubertal patients with Klinefelter's syndrome have reduced left hemisphere specialization for verbal tasks and enhanced right hemisphere specialization for nonverbal tasks. However, these abnormalities tended to normalize after puberty began, suggesting hemispheric reorganization during puberty.[1342] A reduced head circumference and reduced total finger ridge count in Klinefelter's syndrome are evidence of prenatal slowing of neural cell division and of development, a finding that may be related to impairment of verbal ability.[1343] Slowed development is suggested to reduce the growth of the left hemisphere while allowing more unrestrained growth of the right hemisphere before and soon after birth.[1344] Decreasing PIQ and improving VIQ are postulated to be related to the relatively low testosterone concentrations and relatively high estrogen concentrations characteristic of some patients with Klinefelter's syndrome during puberty, which is reflected as well in the development of gynecomastia. Estrogen is known to enhance verbal skills, and reduced androgen levels decrease visual-spatial function.[1345] However, the local aromatization of testosterone to estrogen that is not fully reflected in serum values of these hormones and the varying effect of testosterone and estrogen in Klinefelter's syndrome on physical features such as gynecomastia and habitus make detailed interpretation of these cognitive changes difficult.

Hypotheses have been advanced supporting the effect of prenatal testosterone on cerebral dominance and language and reading pathology,[1346] but such explanations are unlikely to explain the difficulties faced by patients with Klinefelter's syndrome as androgen deficiency is not apparent until puberty begins. Anecdotal clinical observation suggests that improvement in psychosocial and self-image problems occurs with testosterone administration, but convincing studies documenting these observations are not yet at hand.[1347] Although there is a growing feeling among parents that testosterone treatment in the early pubertal period improves language, reading, and behavior in boys with Klinefelter's syndrome, well-controlled studies supporting this contention are not available. One study did report better mood, less irritability, more energy and drive, less tiredness, more endurance and strength, less need for sleep, better concentration ability, and better relations with others during testosterone treatment of mid–20-year-old adults with Klinefelter's syndrome.[1348]

Affected individuals detected by karyotype analysis at birth and in screening studies had minimal impairment (10 to 20 points) in VIQ compared with control subjects and normal full-scale I.Q. Severe retardation is uncommon, although there is an increased prevalence of speech and learning disorders and adjustment problems in adolescence. Psychopathology is rare in most studies, and a 20-year follow-up of 47,XXY individuals showed little or no variation from nonaffected controls in employment, social status, mental or physical health, or criminality.[1349–1351]

Conditions associated with Klinefelter's syndrome include aortic valvular disease and ruptured berry aneurysms (six times the normal rate)[1352]; breast carcinoma (20 times the rate in normal men and one fifth that of women)[1353]; other malignancies such as acute leukemia, lymphoma, and germ cell tumors at any midline site[1349]; systemic lupus erythematosus[1354, 1355]; and osteoporosis.[1356] There is an increased risk of diabetes mellitus and thyroid disease. About 25% of men with Klinefelter's syndrome have osteoporosis.

About 20% of mediastinal germ cell tumors are associated with Klinefelter's syndrome, and they occur at a younger age than the mediastinal germ cell tumors that are not associated with Klinefelter's syndrome (average age 16 versus 27 years in one study).[1357, 1358] With rare exceptions, these germ cell tumors, which may be located in the midline anywhere from the CNS to the pelvis, secrete hCG and induce sexual precocity. Klinefelter's syndrome needs to be considered in boys with hCG-secreting germ cell tumors, especially if the tumor is located in the mediastinum or CNS[1359–1361] (see Chapter 22). There is an increased incidence of fatigue, varicose veins, and essential tremor.

Most patients have a 47,XXY chromosomal karyotype. The next most common variant is 46,XY/47,XXY; 48,XXYY and 48,XXXY karyotypes are found with lower frequency and are associated with a higher incidence of mental retardation and somatic anomalies. The rare 46,XX male has some features of Klinefelter's syndrome[1330] (see Chapter 22). The 49,XXXXY karyotype is associated with a specific syndrome characterized by severe mental deficiency, skeletal abnormalities (such as radioulnar synostosis), and hypoplastic external genitalia with a small penis and undescended testes.[1330]

Other Forms of Primary Testicular Failure

Survival of childhood cancer is increasing. Most cancer therapy affects testicular function and can lead to adult infertility.[1362, 1363] Chemotherapeutic agents used in the treatment of nephrotic syndrome or leukemia, such as cyclophosphamide or chlorambucil, have led to Sertoli cell, Leydig cell, and germ cell damage in prepubertal patients[1364]; these effects are sometimes reversible. Chemotherapy for childhood Hodgkin's disease, including chlorambucil, vinblastine, mechlorethamine (Mustargen), vincristine (Oncovin), procarbazine, and prednisone, may allow spontaneous progression through puberty, but both FSH and LH concentrations may be elevated and the inhibin B concentrations decreased during puberty, indicative of gonadal damage.[1365]

The basal serum FSH and the rise in LH and FSH after LHRH are correlated with the dose of cyclophosphamide.[1366–1368] Therapy for Hodgkin's disease with COPP and Mustargen, Oncovin, procarbazine, and prednisone (MOPP) can cause severe damage to germinal cells apparently without much effect on Leydig cells even if therapy occurred in the prepubertal period.[1369]

Serum FSH is often elevated and inhibin B levels are low in such patients treated with chemotherapy and basal LH is normal although LHRH-stimulated serum LH is elevated; thus, germinal cell damage is evident but Leydig cell function appears normal.[1370] In addition, doxorubicin (Adriamycin), bleomycin, vinblastine, and dacarbazine (ABVD) can cause germ cell depletion. Although some degree of gonadal maturation such as that noted during puberty was considered to be necessary before these drugs could cause gonadal damage, gonadal damage can occur earlier as a result of therapy in the prepubertal period but may not be demonstrable until the age of puberty.[1371, 1372]

Radiation of the gonads can cause primary testicular failure, usually resulting in azoospermia, although normal testosterone secretion may be associated with elevated LH and FSH values (compensated Leydig cell failure).[1373] Because they might be included in a radiation therapy field, the gonads must be shielded from the treatment, if possible. Doses of 0.35 Gy to the testes may lead to temporary aspermia, doses over 2 Gy lead to permanent aspermia, and doses over 15 Gy may cause Leydig cell dysfunction.[1374]

Sperm preservation is possible in a boy who will undergo chemotherapy or radiotherapy, although the patient's parents may express concern about the collection of sperm in teenagers by masturbation or electroejaculation.[1375] Cryopreservation of sperm in a sperm bank, as carried out for adult patients undergoing orchiectomy, is an option.[1376, 1377] For a prepubertal or early pubertal boy, standard sperm banking techniques may not be appropriate. However, testicular tissue can be preserved frozen, to be reimplanted later in the subject's own testis or be stimulated to mature for use in intracytoplasmic sperm injection.[1378, 1379] Other methods of preserving fertility years after treatment for childhood cancers are under consideration.[1375] Advances in germ cell preservation are promising, and unexpected developments will undoubtedly emerge over the next two decades.

Testicular Biosynthetic Defects

Male pseudohermaphrodism caused by 17α-hydroxylase/17,20-lyase ($P450_{c17}$) deficiency related to mutations in *CYP17* is associated with sexual infantilism and a female phenotype; the testosterone biosynthetic defect blocks the synthesis of testosterone and adrenal androgens, impairing masculinization at all stages of development (see Chapter 22). Associated cortisol deficiency and increased mineralocorticoid secretion in this condition lead to hypertension, decreased serum potassium levels, and metabolic alkalosis. Glucocorticoid replacement suppresses ACTH and mineralocorticoid excess and corrects the electrolyte abnormalities, but no sexual development occurs unless exogenous gonadal steroids are administered. Less severe deficiencies are associated with ambiguous genitalia; one case of delayed puberty in a phenotypic male was attributed to partial deficiency of 17,20-desmolase and 17-hydroxylase.[1380] *CYP17* mutations leading to isolated 17,20-lyase deficiency are quite rare.

A rare autosomal recessive condition is steroidogenic acute regulatory protein (StAR) deficiency in which the ability to produce C_{21}-, C_{19}-, and C_{18}-steroids is lost; severely affected patients have lipid-laden adrenal glands. The adrenal glands and gonads have a severe impairment of the conversion of cholesterol to pregnenolone.[1381]

The large adrenal glands may be visualized on sonographic, CT, or MRI scans. Death often occurs in infancy because of unrecognized glucocorticoid and mineralocorticoid deficiency. Affected individuals appear physically to be sexually infantile females, whether their karyotype is 46,XY or 46,XX; because of the absence of gonadal or adrenal androgen production, the affected XY phenotypic females do not develop secondary sexual characteristics including pubic hair.[1330] However, surprisingly, XX females even with a null mutation[1382, 1383] develop female sex characteristics at puberty, including pubic hair and multicystic ovaries, but have either primary or secondary amenorrhea. Apparently, in contrast to the fetal testis, the fetal ovary, which is insensitive to FSH and steroidogenically inactive, is undamaged in fetal life; it remains so until the onset of puberty, when, under FSH stimulation and the recruitment of ovarian follicles, the ovaries undergo progressive damage and cyst formation.

Luteinizing Hormone Resistance

Presumptive evidence of LH resistance caused by an LH receptor[1384] abnormality on the Leydig cell was reported in an 18-year-old boy with a male phenotype, no male secondary sexual development, gynecomastia, elevated plasma LH levels, and early pubertal plasma testosterone concentrations that did not increase after hCG administration; there was no elevation of testosterone precursor levels.[1385] The testes were prepubertal in size and had the microscopic appearance of normal prepubertal testes. Plasma membrane receptor preparations from the testes bound only half as much radiolabeled hCG as control testes.

This autosomal recessive disorder is due to a mutation in the gene encoding the G protein–coupled, seven-transmembrane LH/hCG cell receptor[710] in affected males (see Chapter 22); mutations causing a severe compromise in LH/hCG receptor function are associated with XY male pseudohermaphrodism. Another affected phenotypic male had a homozygous deletion of exon 10 of the LH receptor.[1386] This deletion causes incomplete loss of function of the LH receptor. Homozygous missense mutations, Ser 616 Tyr[1387] and Ile 625 Lys,[1388] are associated with micropenis (but not hypospadias) related to partial impairment of LH receptor function. The Ser 616 Tyr mutant receptor shows an interesting discordance: a poor response to LH but not to hCG.

Nephropathic cystinosis in boys leads to hypergonadotropic hypogonadism.[1389]

Anorchia and Cryptorchidism[1390–1392]

In the 46,XY male without palpable testes, it is important to determine whether any testicular tissue is present. The patient may have intra-abdominal testes, which carry an increased risk of malignant degeneration; anorchia (the "vanishing testes" syndrome), in which no testes are found at laparotomy; or retractile testes, a variation of normal.[764, 1330] The presence of a male phenotype and male internal ducts indicates that functioning fetal testes capable of secreting testosterone and AMH were present early during fetal life but degenerated thereafter.

Administration of 3000 U per m^2 hCG intramuscularly usually evokes an increased concentration of plasma testosterone after 72 hours when functional Leydig cells are present[1393]; lack of a rise in testosterone concentration, in conjunction with an increased plasma concentration of FSH and LH or an augmented gonadotropin response to LHRH,[1246] is evidence for the diagnosis of bilateral anorchia. Alternatively, measurement of AMH indicates the presence of testicular tissue in a range of suspected conditions in prepubertal boys, from presumed anorchia to male pseudohermaphrodism and true hermaphrodism.[581, 584] Serum inhibin B is a useful indicator of the presence of functional testicular tissue; values were correlated with the testosterone response to hCG administration, values less than 15 pg/mL indicating anorchia.[577]

Unilateral cryptorchidism versus the presence of a descended testes on one side and none on the other side presents a diagnostic dilemma. In most, but not all (90%),[1394] cases there is testicular compensatory hypertrophy of the descended testes if there is absence of the contralateral testes,[1395] probably because of elevation of FSH secretion. As the finding does not universally predict monorchia, laparoscopy is recommended in this condition.

Cryptorchid testes may descend into the scrotum during more prolonged treatment with hCG (3000 U/m^2 surface area intramuscularly every other day for six doses), intranasal LHRH, or a combination of hCG and LHRH treatment.[1396] Although such descent occurs in retractile testes, it can occur in true cryptorchid testes in which descent is not prevented by local anatomic factors. Normally, testicular descent has occurred by 1 year of age; although later descent is described, the incidence is low.[1390, 1391] Orchidopexy is recommended between 12 and 18 months of age in testes not expected to descend spontaneously.

Two critical steps in the maturation of germ cells are described in the prepubertal testis: (1) at 2 to 3 months of age, the gonocytes (primitive spermatogonia), the fetal stem cell pool, transform into the adult dark spermatogonia, the adult stem cell pool[1397] (possibly related to the surge in LH, FSH, and testosterone in early infancy); (2) at 4 to 5 years of age, the onset of meiosis and the appearance of primary spermatocytes occur.[1397] The identification of the gonocyte transformation has influenced recommendations concerning the timing of orchidopexy. Postpubertal orchidopexy is associated with a high (>85%) prevalence of azoospermia or oligospermia.[1398, 1399] In a study in Copenhagen, the risk of neoplasia was 5% in patients with an intra-abdominal testis, abnormalities of the external genitalia, or an abnormal sex chromosome karyotype compared with 10% (1185) in patients with cryptorchidism who lacked these characteristics.[1400] It has been surmised that cryptorchid testes, even if replaced in the scrotum, may never have normal spermatogenic function as a consequence of an early abnormality in germ cell maturation, vascular damage to the testicular circulation during orchidopexy, or an intrinsic testicular defect.[1391, 1401–1404] However, the phenomenon may have been based on a sample of boys who underwent orchidopexy later than is currently believed to be optimal. In a follow-up study of men with cryptorchidism who had an orchidopexy between 1955 and 1975, the paternity rate was 65% for men who had had bilateral cryptorchidism compared with 90% for the formerly unilateral cryptorchid and 93% for control men. The reduction in fertility was supported by semen and hormone analyses.[1392]

Successful fertilization by the use of intracytoplasmic injection of sperm extracted from the testes of cryptorchid men who had orchidopexy after puberty was reported.[1405–1408]

Early orchidopexy seems to reduce the risk of carcinoma of the testes,[1391, 1409] although dysgenetic testes, even if located in the scrotum, carry an increased risk of malignant transformation.[1330] Undescended testes remain at a higher temperature than descended testes and have a maturation arrest at the conversion of the gonocyte to the spermatogonia, which appears to direct the testes toward malignant degeneration.[1391] Estimates place the incidence of testicular carcinoma at 0.5 per 100,000 in boys with an increase of 6% per year in adolescents.[1410] Skakkebaek and co-workers[1411] expressed concern that adverse environmental factors may be important in the apparent increase in testis cancer, cryptorchidism, hypospadias, and low semen quality. A study of 794 men with testicular cancer in England reported that the increasing performance of orchidopexy before 10 years of age appears to have reduced the increased risk of testicular carcinoma associated with undescended testes.[1412] There is a small risk of carcinoma of the testes in prepuberty, but the absence of carcinoma in situ in prepuberty is not an assurance that carcinoma will not develop in adult life. Periodic sonography of the testis is recommended after the onset of puberty.[1413, 1414] At present, the earlier the orchidopexy is carried out, the better for ultimate function and reduced risk of malignant degeneration.[1401] One year is a useful age at which to consider orchidopexy for undescended testes because it is an age at which the likelihood of spontaneous descent lessens but the benefits to the testes of orchidopexy remain.

The risk of breast cancer is increased in men with a history of undescended testes, orchidopexy, orchitis, testicular injury, infertility, or any cause of delayed puberty. This risk is associated with the gynecomastia that occurs in these conditions.[1415]

Syndrome of Gonadal Dysgenesis and Its Variants (Turner's Syndrome)

See also Chapter 22.[1330, 1416–1421] The most common form of hypergonadotropic hypogonadism in the female is the syndrome of gonadal dysgenesis or Turner's syndrome and its variants, a sporadic disorder with an incidence of 1 per 2500 liveborn girls[1416, 1422, 1423] in which all (X chromosome monosomy with haploinsufficiency) or part of the second sex chromosome (partial sex chromosome monosomy) is absent. About 99% of 45,X conceptuses abort spontaneously and 1 in 15 spontaneous abortions has a 45,X karyotype.[1424, 1425] The 45,X karyotype is associated with female phenotype, short stature, sexual infantilism, various somatic abnormalities, and frequent fetal demise.

Sex chromosome mosaicism or structural abnormalities of an X or Y chromosome may modify the features of this syndrome, although about 40% of individuals with the five features noted previously have mosaicism or structural abnormalities of the X chromosome. Thus, we may view the syndrome of gonadal dysgenesis and its variants as a continuum ranging from the typical 45,X phenotype to a normal male or female phenotype.[1330] Comprehensive recommendations for the diagnosis and management of Turner's syndrome have been presented by an international committee.[1426]

45,X Turner's Syndrome

Short stature and sexual infantilism are invariable features of sex chromatin–negative 45,X gonadal dysgenesis or Turner's syndrome (Fig. 24–54) (also see Chapter 22). This karyotype is found in approximately 60% of cases of Turner's syndrome.[1330, 1425] The short stature is due to loss of a homeobox-containing gene located on the pseudoautosomal region (PAR 1) of the short arms of the X (Xp22) and Yp11.3 chromosomes,[1427, 1428] which encodes an osteogenic factor.[1428] The gene is called *SHOX* (short *s*tature *h*omeob*ox*-containing gene)[1427] or *PHOG* (*ps*eudoautosomal *h*omeobox *o*steogenic *g*ene).[1428] Because it is located on the pseudoautosomal region of the short arm of the X and Y chromosomes, it escapes X inactivation.

SHOX haploinsufficiency is responsible for, in addition to abnormal growth, mesomelic growth retardation and Madelung's deformity of the wrist (bilateral bowing of the radius with a dorsal subluxation of the distal ulna)[1429, 1430] in Leri-Weill dyschondrosteosis (*SHOX* haploinsufficiency). Langer mesomelic dysplasia, which includes severe dwarfism with striking hypoplasia or aplasia of the ulnar and fibula, is due to *SHOX* nullizygosity. *SHOX* haploinsufficiency appears to be responsible for −2.0 SD of the approximately −3.0 SD deficit in stature and the skeletal abnormalities in Turner's syndrome.[1431–1434] A patient with complete gonadal dysgenesis and tall stature had a 45,X/46X,der(X) and three doses of the *SHOX* gene because of the SHOX duplication on the der(X) chromosome.[1435]

Turner's syndrome may be recognized in the newborn period. 45,X abortuses have edema and large hygromas of the neck that may be seen with prenatal ultrasound studies; this lymphatic defect is the basis for the loose skinfolds that ultimately form the webbed neck (pterygium colli). Affected newborn infants may also have lymphedema of the extremities; the term Bonnevie-Ullrich syndrome has been applied to newborn infants with these features of Turner's syndrome. It is important to determine whether coarctation of the aorta or a bicuspid aortic valve or both are present because of the risk of hypertension and aortic rupture (see Chapter 22).

Features noted during childhood are spread to various locations in the body. Frequent features are distinct facies with micrognathia, "fishmouth" appearance, high-arched palate with dental abnormalities, epicanthal folds, ptosis, low-set or deformed ears, short neck with low hairline and webbing (pterygium colli), and recurrent otitis media often leading to impaired hearing; about 25% of affected adults require hearing aids.[1330, 1436, 1437]

A broad, shield-like chest leads to the appearance of wide-spaced nipples; the areolae are often hypoplastic. Skeletal defects include short fourth metacarpals and cubitus valgus (which may develop after birth), Madelung's deformity of the wrist (in about 7%), genu valgum, and scoliosis. The skin demonstrates extensive pigmented nevi, a tendency to keloid formation, and hypoplastic nails.[1330, 1438] Lymphatic obstruction leads not only to the infantile puffiness of extremities and pterygium colli but also to a distinctive shape of the ears. Cardiovascular anomalies include coarctation of the aorta in about 10% (40% have associated webbing of the neck), aortic stenosis, and bicuspid aortic valves; the latter individuals are at risk for a dissecting aortic aneurysm.[1439]

An echocardiogram of the cardiovascular system must be obtained. Prophylactic antibiotics are indicated if an anatomic abnormality is demonstrated. Abnormal pelvocaliceal collecting systems, abnormal position or alignment of the kidneys, and

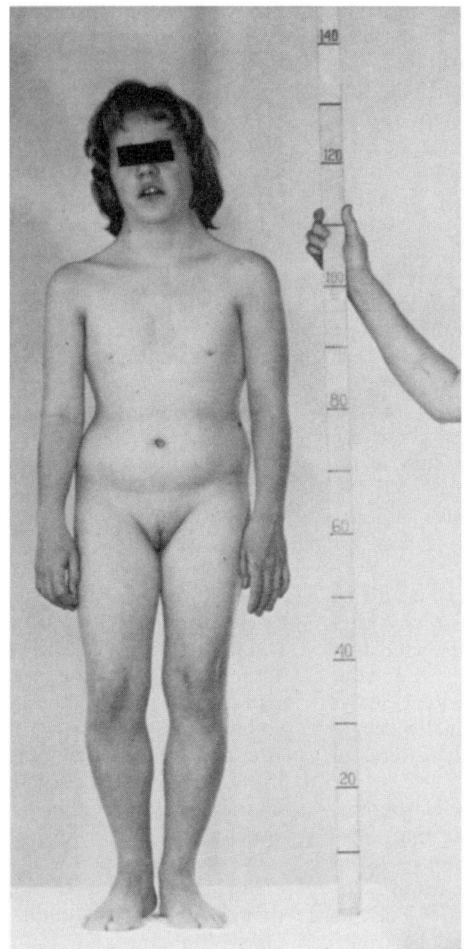

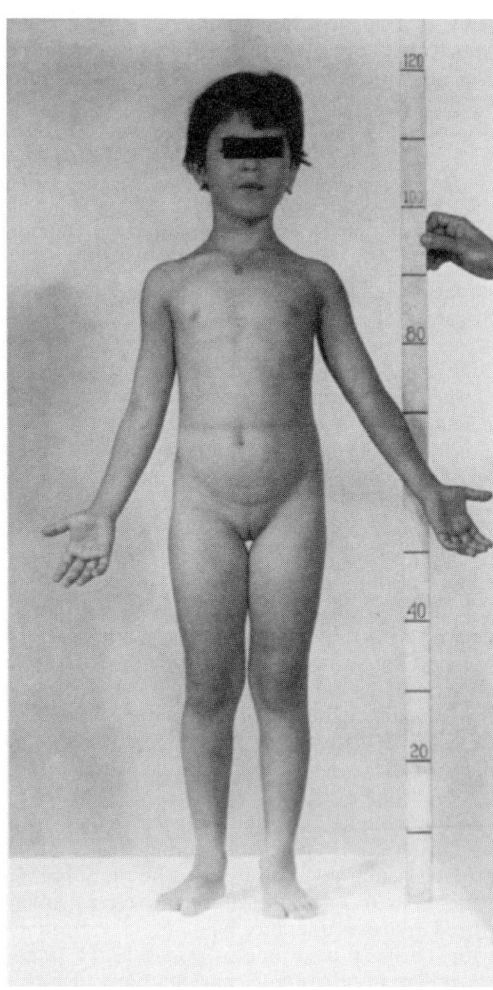

Figure 24–54. *Left,* A 14 10/12-year-old patient with the typical form of the syndrome of gonadal dysgenesis (Turner's syndrome). The X chromatin pattern was negative, and the karyotype was 45,X. She was short (height 134.5 cm; height age 9 5/12 years) and sexually infantile except for the appearance of sparse pubic hair, and exhibited characteristic stigmata of the syndrome: a short webbed neck, shield-like chest with widely separated nipples, bilateral metacarpal signs, puffiness over the dorsum of the fingers, cubitus valgus, increased number of pigmented nevi, characteristic facies, and low-set ears. The bone age was 13 6/12 years; urinary 17-ketosteroids 5.1 mg/day; urinary gonadotropin greater than 100 mU/day. Vaginal smears and the urocytogram showed an immature pattern in which cornified squamous cells were absent. With estrogen therapy, female secondary sexual characteristics were induced; the cyclic administration resulted in periodic estrogen withdrawal bleeding. *Right,* A 45,X, 9 11/12-year-old patient with Turner's syndrome. Apart from short stature (height 118 cm; age 6 10/12 years), increased pigmented nevi, and subtle changes in the fingers and toes, she had few somatic anomalies. In contrast to the patient at the left, the main clinical feature was short stature.

abnormal vascular supply to the kidney are encountered in 30% to 60% of patients, and recurrent urinary tract infections are not uncommon.[1440] Defects of the gastrointestinal system include intestinal telangiectasias and hemangiomatoses that rarely lead to massive gastrointestinal bleeding. Furthermore, the prevalence of inflammatory bowel disease, chronic liver disease, and colon cancer is increased.[1420, 1441–1444]

The uterus and fallopian tubes are infantile. Pelvic ultrasonography or MRI usually permits the detection of even a small uterus in these patients and commonly streak gonads. Autoimmune diseases, such as Hashimoto's thyroiditis (a 16-fold relative risk) and Graves' disease, are common,[1445] and an association with juvenile rheumatoid arthritis and psoriatic arthritis is described. Glucose intolerance resulting from increased insulin resistance is also common after the age of puberty; in some, this may be due to associated obesity. The risk of type 2 diabetes mellitus is increased.[1446]

Affected patients are usually small at birth because of intrauterine growth retardation with a mean deficit in length of 2.6 cm (−1.24 SD) and exhibit a slow childhood growth rate that results in a loss of about 8 to 9 cm (−3.0 SD) by age 3 years.[1456] This study, derived from longitudinal measurements on 47 full-term patients with Turner's syndrome, indicates that the first 3 years of life contribute a major part of the height deficit. Further, there is a decrease in growth rate at the time of expected puberty and failure to undergo a pubertal growth spurt.[1457–1459]

Individuals with Turner's syndrome in the United Kingdom and United States have a mean final height of approximately 142 to 143 cm,[1458] about 20 cm less than the average height of normal women; the adult stature of these patients correlates with midparental height and with the height of unaffected women of the same ethnic group.[1460, 1461] Their pattern of growth does not suggest that these individuals are GH-deficient.[1459] Rather, haploinsufficiency of the *SHOX* gene located in the pseudoautosomal region on the short arm of X and Y (see earlier) is estimated to contribute two thirds of the height deficit. It is postulated that a second gene on the short arm of X that does not undergo X inactivation contributes the other one third of the deficit.

Specific growth curves are available for plotting the growth of affected children.[1458, 1459] In a group of girls with Turner's syndrome and spontaneous puberty, height velocity was transiently higher during puberty than in girls with amenorrhea, but final adult height was not different (see Chap. 22). GH treatment is now approved by the FDA for Turner's syndrome to increase height. Trials of the effect of treatment with rhGH in children with Turner's syndrome began in 1983. It soon became apparent that hGH administration increased the rate of growth, and data are now available on final height including the results of some randomized dose-response trials from groups around the world.

The average height gain has varied from 4 to 16 cm.[1462–1464] This variability in gain in height is incompletely understood, but many factors have been implicated including the age of initiation of therapy, dose duration, age of beginning estrogen replacement (especially number of years from beginning hGH treatment), number of injections per week, compliance, and whether the last measured height represented final height.[1465–1468] The weekly dose of hGH is 0.375 mg/kg divided into seven daily doses. It is important to individualize the dose. The Dutch Advisory Group on Growth Hormone reported that a treatment regimen that gradually increased the dose 0.63 mg/kg per week elicited a 16.0 ± 4.1 cm increase in height. It is now apparent that the early initiation of hGH therapy (e.g., 2 to 8 years of age) and a mean duration of treatment of about 7 years can lead to the majority of treated patients achieving a final height greater than 150 cm; in the Dutch study, the mean final height was 162.3 ± 6.1 cm with the high-dose schedule.[1469] The timing of the introduction of estrogen can have an important effect on final height,[1470] but with an early age of initiation of GH therapy, low-dose estrogen can be introduced at an appropriate age (about age 13) without compromising adult height. At present, hGH treatment of patients with Turner's syndrome has been safe; untoward events are infrequent.

It is essential that the parents are fully informed about the pros and cons of hGH treatment and that the child is informed in an age-appropriate manner about the use of hGH. The long-term protocol is laborious and expensive and the treatment is invasive but, with the use of new devices for administration, minimally painful.

The age of diagnosis of Turner's syndrome continues to be delayed with the exception of newborns with the striking phenotype (Bonnevie-Ullrich syndrome). It is recommended that all girls of prepubertal age below −2.0 SD who have at least two somatic stigmata of the syndrome have a karyotype analysis; early diagnosis is of key importance for optimal management of the growth failure and detection of occult features of the syndrome.[1471]

Although glucose values do not change with GH therapy, insulin levels rise reversibly during treatment, indicating a degree of insulin resistance caused by the GH.[1472] About 50% of patients with Turner's syndrome have a tendency toward impaired glucose tolerance without GH treatment.[1473] Patients with Turner's syndrome as young as 11 years can have elevated serum cholesterol concentrations (before treatment with GH or estrogen).[1474]

As discussed earlier, the biphasic pattern of gonadotropin secretion in normal infancy and childhood (see Fig. 24–32) is exaggerated in Turner's syndrome. Thus, baseline gonadotropin concentrations and peak LH and FSH values after LHRH administration are above normal between birth and 4 years of age and again after age 10. Baseline values of FSH are 3 to 10 times higher than LH values. However, between ages 4 and 10, mean gonadotropin concentrations in this syndrome are similar to the mean values in normal girls (see Figs. 24–32, 24–33 and Fig. 24–34) and are lower than those before age 4 and after age 10.[872, 873]

The appearance of pubic hair is often delayed in the syndrome of gonadal dysgenesis, even though adrenarche, as assessed by the increase in concentration of plasma DHEAS, occurs at the normal age.[969] The pubic hair of affected individuals is sparse, but estrogen therapy increases the growth of pubic hair despite a lack of increase in adrenal androgen secretion.[1475] The streak gonads result in sexual infantilism; rarely, probably in about 10% of cases, puberty, menarche, and, even more rarely, pregnancy may occur.[1330]

In addition, as described earlier, skeletal abnormalities are a common feature and may affect areal BMD determinations. Most untreated children have a normal volumetric bone density (by phalangeal radiographic absorptiometry), in contrast to the less accurate areal BMD in patients with Turner's syndrome, compared with normal girls. Recent studies have not confirmed an increased prevalence of wrist fractures. In an hGH-treated group of girls in whom estrogen therapy was begun at 12 years of age, BMD SD scores were above the mean value.[1476] When peripheral quantitative CT, a state-of-the-art technique for assessing volumetric BMD, was used to determine volumetric BMD at two radial sites, a decrease in radial bone mass was found because of a reduction in cortical bone thickness (the endocortical bone surface) with a corresponding increase in bone marrow cross-sectional area, but trabecular volumetric BMD was normal.[1477] These reports reiterated the limitations of estimates of areal BMD by DEXA scans in contrast to volumetric BMD in Turner's syndrome.[1478] Human GH treatment in childhood appears to have a positive effect on BMD. Estrogen therapy is critical for the prevention and repair of osteoporosis. Although estrogen therapy is important in adolescents and adults, the optimal dose preparation and site of delivery for the prevention of osteoporosis are not known. Nor are data available on the usefulness or adverse effects of continuation of rhGH treatment after final height is achieved in adolescence.

The IQ is normal when verbal ability including comprehension and vocabulary is considered, but spatiotemporal processing, visuomotor coordination,[1447, 1448] and mathematical ability (particularly in geometry) may be impaired, leading to a decrease in the performance IQ[1446, 1449] The neurocognitive phenotype associated with Turner's syndrome maps to distal Xp.[1450]

Girls with Turner's syndrome have a normal VIQ but a discrepancy between VIQ and PIQ, with the latter about 1 SD below the mean value. This is opposite to the pattern found in Klinefelter's syndrome (see earlier). Turner's syndrome is associated with impaired visuoconstructional or visual-perceptual abilities in association with executive dysfunction and decreased attention span, which can lead to learning difficulties.[1479, 1480] In most studies visual-spatial abilities are impaired in girls with Turner's syndrome, but one study found no specific deficits in visual-spatial or tactile-spatial tasks.[1481]

Normal girls perform better on motor tasks as they get older, a trend that is not found in Turner's syndrome. Although one study found diminished lateralization of motor tasks,[1482] a later study found no difference in lateralization and performance of motor tasks in individuals with Turner's syndrome compared with control subjects; there was superior performance of the dominant or right hand in contrast to the nondominant or left hand.[1480]

Anatomic changes of the brain and neurocognitive changes occur in Turner's syndrome. There are consistent MRI abnormalities in the right parietal lobe and the occipital lobes that show decreased volumes in these areas implicated in visuospatial processing. Using positron emission tomography, Murphy and colleagues showed decreased glucose metabolism in the right parietal and occipital lobes.[421, 1483, 1484] These anatomic data relate to the difficulties in visual-spatial skills found in most studies of girls with Turner's syndrome because these problems are most closely linked to the right parietal region.[1485]

Girls with Turner's syndrome resemble normal girls in verbal and language skills, but there are frequently difficulties with memory and attention and decreased arithmetic skills, related to mistakes on operation and alignment processes,[1486] with girls with 45,X mosaicism associated with a 46,XX cell line, 45,X/46,XX, scoring closer to normal than those with other types of mosaicisms. However, girls with Turner's syndrome can score higher on reading achievement tests than predicted by I.Q. or age; this hyperliteracy is a strength in many girls with this disorder. Only 3.3% of girls with Turner's syndrome have mental retardation in the absence of a variant of the syndrome caused by a ring X chromosome.[1487]

Because most girls lack ovarian estrogen production and are treated during the teenage years with exogenous estrogen (hormone replacement therapy), Turner's syndrome provides an opportunity to determine the effects of estrogen on neurocognitive function. There appear to be estrogen-dependent and estrogen-independent tasks that are affected in Turner's syndrome. However, there is controversy about which are estrogen-dependent and which are not. For example, visual-spatial perceptual deficits appear to begin in childhood and persist into adult life unaffected by estrogen treatment according to some studies.[1488, 1489] However, another group of studies show that the effects of estrogen are dependent on dose and time, with untreated patients and those treated with high-dose or long-term therapy performing equally poorly.[1490]

Thus, girls with Turner's syndrome improve spontaneously in testing on visuospatial abilities from younger than 12 years to older than 15 years of age, and the older girls treated with estrogen for 3 to 24 months improved further. However, the ability of those treated with estrogen for more than 2 years decreased to that of untreated age-matched Turner's patients. A decrease in spatial abilities has been reported in normal girls going through puberty; it is suggested that this is another example of a biphasic effect of estrogen, with low levels, as in prepuberty, fostering spatial ability but higher levels, at the end of puberty and thereafter, suppressing such ability.[1490] Some motor-related skills and nonverbal processing were performed more rapidly in estrogen-treated girls with Turner's syndrome.[1491, 1492] Study of event-related potentials in preteen and post-teen girls with Turner's syndrome compared with age-matched controls demonstrated congenital and age-related abnormalities; age-related abnormalities are later ameliorated by estrogen treatment if started early enough.[1493]

The results of a double-blind study of estrogen versus placebo treatment for 1 to 3 years in 7- to 9-year-old girls with Turner's syndrome show direct effects of estrogen. These girls were part of a larger double-blind study to determine the effect of GH and estrogen on final height. GH therapy in Turner's syndrome led to an increased growth rate. In addition, the girls felt better about their attractiveness, intelligence, and popularity; they perceived that they experienced less teasing; and there was no effect on school performance with GH therapy.[1494] Girls with Turner's syndrome younger than 6 years did not perceive that they had a problem with height, but by 7 to 12 and especially 13 to 15 years, affected girls have a strong desire for GH therapy and even unrealistic expectations of what GH therapy might accomplish in terms of adult height.[1495] GH therapy improved self-esteem even if there remained a significant difference in height between Turner girls and RGW normal range. GH did not affect the nonverbal neuron-cognitive defects in Turner's syndrome,[1496] nor did it affect IQ or achievement scores.[1497]

Placebo-treated girls with Turner's syndrome performed less well than either control or estrogen-treated individuals with Turner's syndrome in recall of digit span backward and immediate and delayed recall of the children's word list, suggesting that estrogen replacement therapy improves verbal and nonverbal memory. This observation raises the possibility that a prepubertal deficit in estrogen may affect performance of these tasks as well as suggesting a potential role for low-dose estrogen replacement therapy in late prepubertal girls with Turner's syndrome.[1498] These results are similar to the improvement in short-term and long-term verbal memory found in postmenopausal or surgically castrated women treated with estrogen replacement therapy.[1499, 1500]

Treatment with estrogen for more than 4 years appeared to move the scores for girls with Turner's syndrome on self-esteem and psychological well-being toward normal control values as they reached 16 years of age, compared with a significant difference documented at 12 years of age. No such change occurred in the non–estrogen-treated group, suggesting that the estrogen effects caused the change rather than the passage of years.

Several mechanisms are proposed to explain these estrogen effects: (1) estrogen acts as a neuromodulator in a transient time frame, (2) estrogen alters synapse formation and remodeling in a permanent time frame, or (3) both mechanisms. Thus, estrogen may function as an organizational agent in the brain of the young but as a stabilizing agent in older individuals.

The increase in mental health problems documented in Turner's syndrome may be rooted in the increased peer ridicule experienced by girls with Turner's syndrome as opposed to a biologic abnormality. The teasing can by itself lead to decreased self-image and depression.[1501]

There is an increased risk of impaired social adjustment in Turner's syndrome.[1451, 1452] 45,X females with Turner's syndrome have higher ratings of social and attention problems and withdrawn behaviors than their own sisters.[1503] The risk is higher if the single X chromosome comes from the mother (X_m) rather than the father (X_p).[1452, 1453] Individuals with Turner's syndrome have difficulty in inferring affective intention from facial appearance. As an explanation for these phenomena, there appears to be a locus on the X chromosome on Xq or close to the centromere on Xp that escapes X inactivation and affects social cognition.[1452, 1495, 1505] This locus is apparently imprinted and not expressed from the maternally derived X chromosome.[1452] When the locus was inherited from the father, the 45,X individuals were significantly better adjusted, with superior verbal and higher order executive function skills, which mediate social interactions. If expressed only on the paternally derived X chromosome, the existence of this putative locus may explain, in part, why 46,XY males (whose single X chromosome is maternal) are more vulnerable to developmental disorders of language and social cognition, such as autism, than 46,XX females. Accordingly, in addition to haploinsufficiency and its consequences, sex chromosome imprinting appears to be a factor in the Turner syndrome phenotype.

In the first example of an imprinted gene on the X chromosome, the locus resides in the pericentric region of the short arm or on the long arm of the X chromosome. Skuse and coworkers[1452] postulated that this imprinted gene may play a role in male-female differences in social behavior and developmental disorders. It is useful to monitor the patient's progress in high school mathematics. Gender identity and sexual orientation are female.[1446] Although it has been generally accepted that these patients do well in their psychological development, consistent with the report of Skuse and associates,[1452] a study of 103 children with Turner's syndrome demonstrated a significant decrease in social competence score, an increase in total behavior problems, and social and attention problem scales with difficulty in schooling, in peer relationships, and in concentration as well as immaturity, hyperactivity, and nervousness; the origin of the X chromosome was not determined. Structural abnormalities of the X chromosome were associated with more behavior problems than a missing X chromosome or mosaicism of the X chromosomes.[1454] Hyperactive behavior usually improves after the age of puberty.[1448] Mental retardation and a "severe" phenotype are associated with a small ring X chromosome to undergo X inactivation resulting in X chromosome disomy for genes that undergo X inactivation.[1455]

The origin of the single X chromosome affects memory performance as well because those with a maternally derived X have increased verbal forgetting but normal nonverbal forgetting whereas those with a paternally derived X chromosome have the opposite pattern of problems.[1506]

Sex Chromatin–Positive Variants of the Syndrome of Gonadal Dysgenesis

Mosaicism of 45,X/46,XX, 45,X/47,XXX, or 45,X/46,XX/47,XXX chromosomes is associated with a chromatin-positive buccal smear and usually fewer manifestations of the syndrome of gonadal dysgenesis. Likewise, structural abnormalities of the X chromosome can be associated with fewer phenotypic features of the syndrome. Lack of genetic material on the long or the short arm of the second X chromosome can cause decreased gonadal function; loss of all or part of the short arm of the X leads to the physical findings of Turner's syndrome (see Chapter 22).[1330] Depending on the location and extent of the deletion on the short arm of the X chromosome, these patients are more likely to have modest pubertal growth and some spontaneous pubertal development.[1507]

Sex Chromatin–Negative Variants of Gonadal Dysgenesis

These variants include 45,X/46,XY mosaicism and structural abnormalities of the Y chromosome. Affected individuals vary in phenotype from that of classical gonadal dysgenesis to that of ambiguous genitalia to phenotypic males.[1330] Patients may present with short stature, delayed puberty, and a history of hypospadias repair.[1508] There is variable testicular differentiation, ranging from a streak gonad to functioning testes. Patients with mosaicism involving a Y cell line or abnormalities of the Y chromosome are at risk for neoplastic transformation of the dysgenetic testes. Gonadoblastomas, benign nonmetastasizing tumors, may arise within the gonad and produce either testosterone or estrogens; the neoplasm may become calcified sufficiently to be detected on an abdominal radiograph. Thus, the appearance of feminization or virilization in a patient with dysgenetic gonads and a Y cell line may indicate gonadoblastoma formation. Of greater significance is the increased prevalence of malignant germ cell tumors arising within the dysgenetic gonad or gonadoblastoma.[1509] Such tumors occur more often in postpubertal subjects and rarely in children.[1510] The management of gonads in patients with a Y cell line is discussed in Chapter 22.[1330]

46,XX and 46,XY Gonadal Dysgenesis

Pure gonadal dysgenesis refers to phenotypic females with sexual infantilism and a 46,XX or 46,XY karyotype without chromosomal abnormalities.[1330]

Familial and Sporadic 46,XX Gonadal Dysgenesis and Its Variants

The usual phenotype of 46,XX gonadal dysgenesis includes normal stature, sexual infantilism, bilateral streak gonad, normal female internal and external genitalia, and primary amenorrhea. The streak gonad occasionally produces estrogens or androgens, but malignant transformation is rare. Incomplete forms of this condition may result in hypoplastic ovaries that produce enough estrogen to cause some breast development and a few menstrual periods followed by secondary amenorrhea. This heterogeneous syndrome[1511] occurs sporadically or with autosomal recessive inheritance and in some instances is associated with other congenital malformations; some familial cases have been associated with sensorineural deafness (Perrault's syndrome)[1330] (see later).

Familial and Sporadic 46,XY Gonadal Dysgenesis and Its Variants

A phenotype that includes female genitalia with or without clitoral enlargement, normal or tall stature, bilateral streak gonads, normal müllerian structures, sexual infantilism, and a eunuchoid habitus is typical of 46,XY gonadal dysgenesis. About 15% of the patients have a deletion or mutation in the *SRY* gene. If the dysgenetic testes produce significant amounts of testosterone, slight clitoral enlargement may occur at birth and virilization may ensue at puberty. The incomplete form of 46,XY gonadal dysgenesis may involve any degree of ambiguity of the external genitalia and internal ducts. The risk of neoplastic transformation of the streak gonads or dysgenetic testes is increased, and gonadectomy is indicated.[1330] The disorder is usually transmitted as an X-linked or sex-limited autosomal dominant trait, less commonly as an autosomal recessive trait[1330] (see Chapter 22). A novel homozygous missense mutation in exon 1 of the desert hedgehog gene was reported in a patient with polyneuropathy associated with partial XY gonadal dysgenesis.[1512]

Other Causes of Primary Ovarian Failure

Primary ovarian failure is increasing in prevalence as a consequence of the long-term effects of cytotoxic chemotherapy and radiation as these agents prolong life in children and adolescents with cancer.[1363]

Radiation Therapy

Radiation therapy that includes the ovaries within the field can cause primary ovarian failure[1373]; a dose of 4 Gy to the ovaries leads to sterility in 30% of young women and 100% of older women.[1374] It is useful surgically to move the ovaries out of the radiation field; ovarian transposition before radiation therapy is compatible with normal menses, pubertal development, and pregnancy in most cases.[1513] The uterus may also be affected by radiation and may not expand normally during pregnancy. Careful endocrine follow-up of these children and adolescents is essential.

Chemotherapy

Successful treatment of childhood acute lymphoblastic leukemia is now commonplace. In a large study by Quigley and colleagues,[1514] after cytotoxic chemotherapy boys and girls had extensive germ cell damage as evidenced by increased FSH secretion and boys had decreased testicular size for the stage of puberty. The concentration of plasma inhibin B is usually decreased, a sensitive indicator of damage to the germinal epithelium,[1515] and the girls at puberty had evidence of a compensated decrease in ovarian follicular function. Quite likely as a result of cranial radiation, the mean age of menarche was advanced about 12 months despite the ovarian damage; puberty was not advanced in the boys. The type of chemotherapy is related to the effects on the gonads. Nitroso compounds (carmustine and lomustine) or procarbazine for the treatment of brain tumors has been linked to primary gonadal failure manifested by elevated plasma gonadotropin levels in boys and girls; the boys had small testes but were able to secrete adequate testosterone for their pubertal stage.[1371, 1516, 1517] Adjuvant chemotherapy for localized osteosarcoma in the prepubertal period is compatible with ovarian function and fertility.[1522]

Although it was previously thought that cancer therapy does not cause gonadal damage in prepubertal individuals, current evidence suggests otherwise.[1518, 1519] Prepubertal boys and girls treated with abdominal radiation for Wilms' tumor plus chemotherapy (dactinomycin, vincristine with Adriamycin, or cyclophosphamide in most) may experience gonadal damage, whereas those given chemotherapy alone usually do not.[1517] The ovary is less vulnerable to the effects of radiation and chemotherapy than the testis. The prevalence of ovarian damage does not appear to be high as fertility and regular menses are reported in a majority of females treated as children.[1520] Nevertheless, age at treatment has a significant role: treatment between 13 and 19 years of age was associated with a more than twofold increase in premature ovarian failure during the third decade.[1521] Attempts to protect the gonads by suppressing the pituitary-gonadal axis with gonadal steroids or LHRH agonists are ineffective.

Autoimmune Oophoritis

Premature menopause may occur at any age before the normal climacteric and has been reported in adolescent girls; cessation of ovarian function usually occurs as secondary amenorrhea. Autoimmune oophoritis can cause ovarian failure leading to primary amenorrhea, oligomenorrhea, arrest of puberty, and occasionally cystic enlargement of the ovaries.[1523–1527] Most often it is associated with other autoimmune endocrinopathies, especially autoimmune Addison's disease, in which it may precede the onset of adrenal insufficiency, but it rarely, if ever, occurs in isolated premature ovarian failure.[1523, 1527, 1528] Thirty-six percent of women with type I autoimmune polyglandular insufficiency, also known as APECED, a rare systemic autoimmune disorder (hypoparathyroidism, adrenal insufficiency, gonadal failure, diabetes mellitus, pernicious anemia, hypothyroidism, chronic hepatitis, mucocutaneous candidiasis, dystrophic nail hypoplasia, vitiligo, alopecia, keratinopathy, and intestinal malabsorption), exhibited ovarian failure before age 20, whereas only 4% of affected men had testicular failure by this age.[1525] This autosomal recessive disorder is due to more than 30 mutations in the *AIRE-1* gene.[1529]

Autoimmune oophoritis is present in more than 20% of patients with autoimmune adrenal insufficiency. Various autoantibodies have been detected in autoimmune oophoritis, including autoantibodies to cytochrome P450 steroidogenic enzymes[1523, 1527, 1528, 1530, 1531]; some are organ-specific, whereas others react with antigens in more than one tissue and more than one cell type.[1524] Glucocorticoid therapy may improve, at least temporarily, ovarian function.

Miscellaneous Causes of Ovarian Failure

Homozygous galactosemia is commonly associated with primary ovarian failure (from failure to develop puberty to primary or secondary amenorrhea and premature menopause), but puberty is usually normal in males and the risk of testicular dysfunction is low[1535]; compound heterozygotes have normal onset of puberty.[1535, 1536] Dietary restriction programs have not prevented the ovarian failure. Most cases are detected by newborn screening programs.[1537]

Dysplasia and Premature Ovarian Failure

A rare autosomal dominant disorder involving eyelid dysplasia and premature ovarian failure is due to haploinsufficiency of the *FOXL2* gene, a member of the winged helix–forkhead family of transcription factors.[1538] The eyelid abnormalities include small palpebral fissures, ptosis, and a small skinfold extending inward and upward from the lower lid (epicanthus inversus). The gene is expressed in the follicular cells and the mutations that lead to haploinsufficiency are associated with an increased rate of follicular atresia; the degree of ovarian failure is variable from primary amenorrhea to irregular menses and premature ovarian failure, ranging from normal-appearing ovaries on ultrasonography to streak gonads and on ovarian biopsy a variable number of primordial follicles.[1539] The infertility component of the syndrome is limited to the female.

Congenital disorders of glycosylation-1 (carbohydrate-deficient glycoprotein syndrome type I) constitute an autosomal recessive disorder associated with circulating glycoproteins deficient in their terminal carbohydrate moieties, including a wide range of glycoproteins, enzymes, binding proteins, and coagulation factors.[1540] A typical isoform pattern of serum transferrin on isoelectric focusing is used as a diagnostic test. The dominant clinical features are neurologic manifestations of involvement of the central and peripheral nervous system. Among the other organ systems affected is the pituitary-gonadal system.

The hypergonadotropic hypogonadism is more severe in females than males who virilize at puberty. There are two interesting aspects: both the ovary and the pituitary gland are affected. The affected girls have sexual infantilism; the ovaries are hypoplastic or atrophic. High serum FSH and LH levels exhibit normal electrophoretic isoform patterns but appear to have decreased but not absent FSH bioactivity in an FSH bioassay, and in the only three girls tested, a response to the administration of human menopausal gonadotropin was indicated by an increase in serum estradiol and, in one patient, ovarian follicular growth. These observations suggest an abnormality in both the FSH molecule and the ovary, in the latter case a defect in the configuration and activation of the FSH receptor itself and the binding of ligand or a postreceptor defect.[1541, 1542]

Resistant ovary is a heterogeneous cause of primary hypogonadism, a syndrome associated with elevated concentrations of plasma FSH and LH and ovaries that contain primordial follicles.[1532, 1533] The syndrome is usually idiopathic, but an increasing number of genetic abnormalities have been described in addition to the more common X-chromosomal defects.[1534]

Follicle-Stimulating Hormone Receptor Gene Mutations and Hypergonadotropic Hypogonadism.[710]

The FSH receptor is a member of the G protein–linked receptor seven-transmembrane superfamily; it has a large, extended extracellular ligand-binding domain.[1543, 1544] An autosomal recessive disorder related to a mutation in the extracellular ligand-binding domain of the FSH receptor in affected females in six Finnish families mainly from the north central region[1545] resulted in delayed (40%) or normal puberty but primary amenorrhea, elevated gonadotropins, and hypergonadotropic ovarian dysgenesis with arrest of ovarian follicular development at the primary follicle stage and continued atresia.[1545, 1546] The clinical features are quite similar to the findings in FSH-deficient mice generated by targeted disruption of the gene encoding the FSH β subunit.[1547] It is likely that this disorder is responsible for most cases of the resistant ovary syndrome. The FSH receptor gene maps to the short arm of chromosome 2 (2p16-p21) and contains nine small exons (1 to 9) that encode the extracellular ligand-binding domain and one large exon (10) that designates the remainder of the receptor including the seven transmembrane and the intracellular domains.[1543] The Finnish mutation, an alanine 1989 valine substitution, is in the extracellular domain.[1548] Expression of the mutation in transfected cells indicated a small FSH effect on cAMP production and a striking reduction of FSH-binding capacity but apparently normal binding affinity.[1548]

The FSH receptor mutation in the Finnish patients is not a null mutation. It remains to be determined whether the loss or complete inactivation of the FSH receptor leads to failure of puberty and sexual infantilism or to estrogen synthesis by the immature ovarian follicles described in the FSH β subunit knockout mouse.[1547] Affected males in these families are normally masculinized at puberty but tend to have small testes. They have a variable degree of spermatogenic insufficiency but not azoospermia, increased plasma concentrations of FSH and LH, decreased inhibin β levels, and normal plasma testosterone values.[1549]

These patients illustrate the striking sex difference in the effect of lack of FSH function on the ovary and testis. LH/hCG resistance related to mutations in the gene encoding the seven-transmembrane LH/hCG receptor is discussed in Chapter 22. In the affected XY individual, this autosomal recessive disorder leads to varying degrees of male pseudohermaphrodism as would be predicted, the mildest represented by isolated micropenis.[1387, 1388] Less severe mutations of the LH/hCG re-

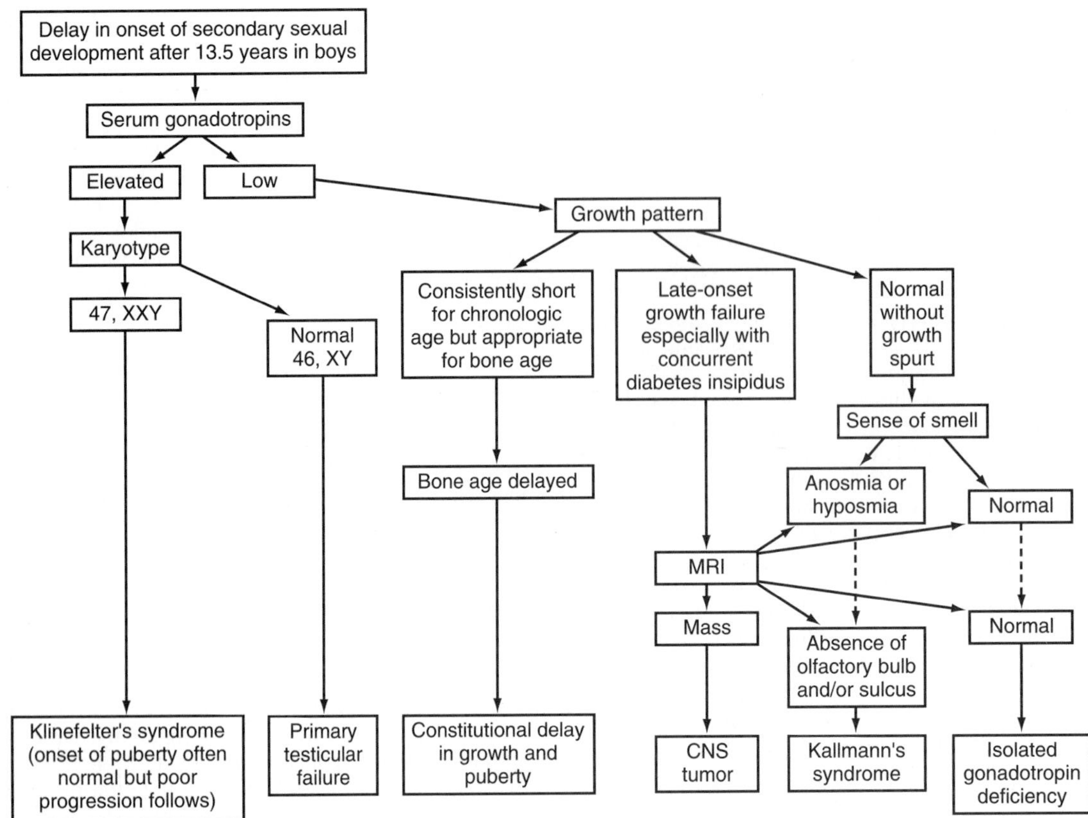

Figure 24–55. The evaluation of delayed puberty in boys.

ceptor could be associated with delayed puberty. In the affected female, on the other hand, LH/hCG resistance does not affect pubertal maturation but leads to amenorrhea with high serum LH levels but normal FSH and estradiol concentrations.[1550]

Polycystic Ovary Disease

Polycystic ovary disease or functional ovarian hyperandrogenism does not delay the onset of puberty but often delays menarche or causes menstrual abnormalities[1551–1553] (see Chapter 22).

Noonan's Syndrome (Pseudo-Turner's Syndrome, Ullrich's Syndrome)

Individuals with Noonan's syndrome (see Chapter 29) have webbed neck, ptosis, down-slanting palpebral fissures, low-set ears, short stature, cubitus valgus, and lymphedema, and hence this phenotype has been called pseudo-Turner's syndrome.[1330] Features that differentiate these individuals from those with Turner's syndrome include triangular facies, pectus excavatum, right-sided heart disease (e.g., pulmonic stenosis, often with valve dysplasia, or atrial septal defect), hypertrophic cardiomyopathy, varied blood clotting defects, and an increased incidence of mental retardation. Females with Noonan's syndrome have normal ovarian function. Males have normal differentiation of external genitalia but may have undescended testes; germinal aplasia or hypoplasia and impaired Leydig cell function may be present.[1554] Puberty may be delayed an average of 2 years.[1555] Stature is decreased, usually following the −2 SD curve; the pubertal growth spurt is often delayed or attenuated but final height is usually at the low limits of normal.[1556] Administration of hGH increased the growth rate, but long-term effects are not yet available.[1557]

Adult males with Noonan's syndrome are reported to have osteopenia, which has been attributed to estrogen deficiency because estrogen administration improves the decreased bone mineral content.[1558] Patients who have sufficient ovarian function to undergo spontaneous pubertal development and menarche have adequate BMD compared with those in whom puberty was induced by estrogen and who exhibited osteopenia despite hormone replacement.[1559] Noonan's syndrome is usually inherited as an autosomal dominant trait.[1330] A gene implicated in Noonan's syndrome has been localized to the long arm of chromosome 12 (12q 24.1).[1511] Mutations in PTPNII, the gene encoding the non-receptor protein tyrosine phosphatase SHP-2, which contains RE Src homology-2 (SH2) domains, account for about 50% of cases. The incidence is estimated as 1 in 1000 to 1 in 5000. One parent may have features of the syndrome in 40% to 60% of cases. About 50% of cases are thought to be the result of new mutations.

Frasier Syndrome

Chronic renal failure is combined with gonadal dysgenesis in the Frasier syndrome.[1560] This diagnosis should be considered in any phenotypic female with end-stage renal disease (related to focal segmental glomerulosclerosis) and sexual infantilism; the karyotype may be 46,XY or 46,XX.[1561]

Diagnosis of Delayed Puberty and Sexual Infantilism

See Figures 24–55 and 24–56 and Table 24–26. Signs of puberty have not yet appeared in 0.4% of normal boys by age

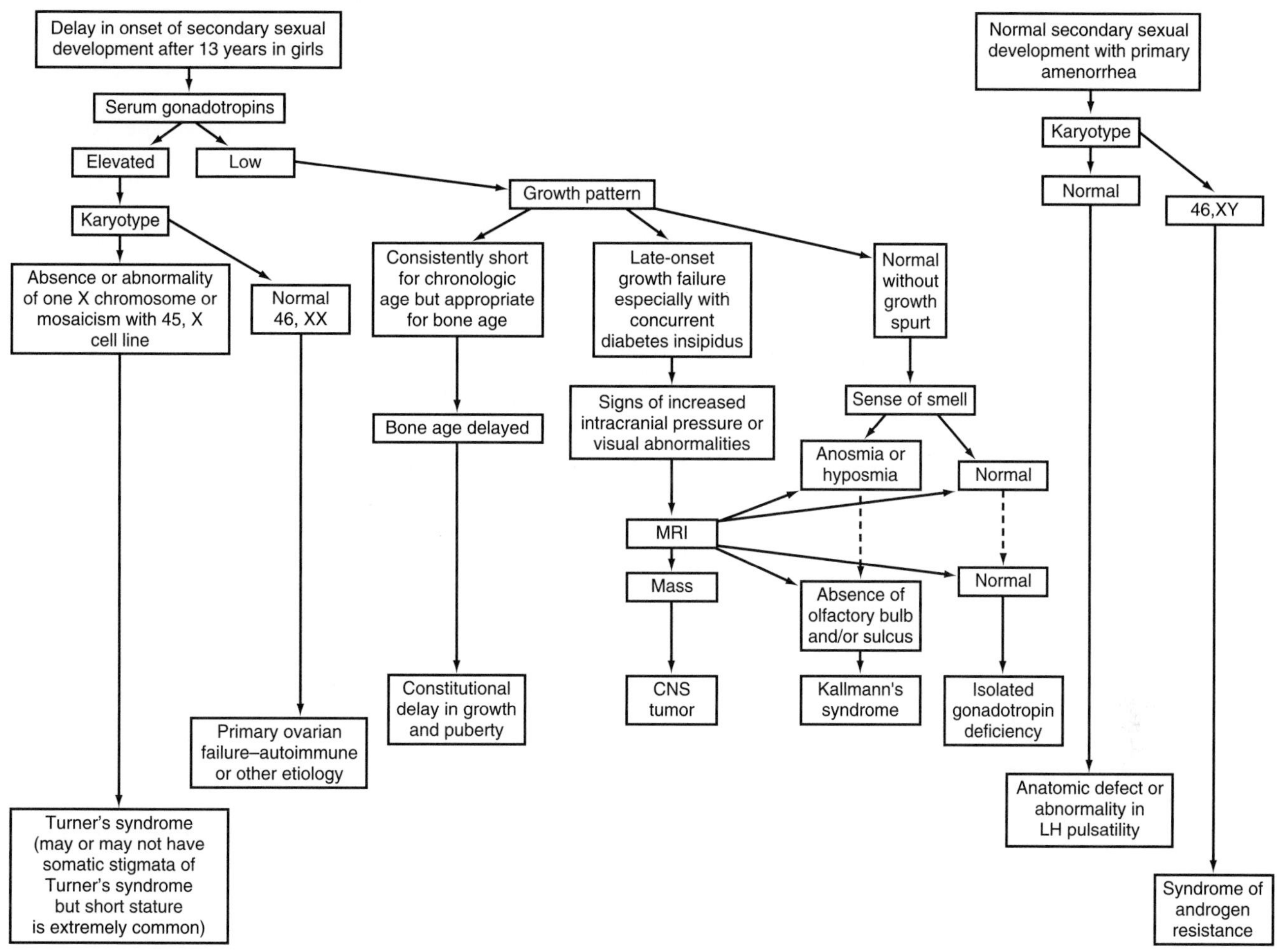

Figure 24–56. The evaluation of delayed puberty in girls.

15 and 0.4% of normal girls by age 13 in the United States according to data collected in the 1970s. Thus, when prepubertal girls present at age 12 or prepubertal boys present at age 14, the physician must make a clinical judgment concerning which represent variants of the norm and which require extensive evaluation and treatment. Lack of progression through the stages of puberty, even if the age at onset is normal, may also require evaluation; a boy who has not completed secondary sexual maturation within 4.5 years after onset of puberty or a girl who does not menstruate within 5 years after onset may have a hypothalamic, pituitary, or gonadal disorder.

The diagnosis of hypergonadotropic hypogonadism is readily established by elevation of random plasma LH and FSH concentrations. However, the differential diagnosis of hypogonadotropic hypogonadism versus constitutional delay in growth and adolescence is more difficult because of the overlap in physical and laboratory findings in the two conditions, including inability to differentiate between normal and low concentrations of serum gonadotropins (Table 24–27). No single test consistently makes this distinction. The majority of boys with pubertal delay have a self-limited variant in the tempo of growth and pubertal onset. The task of the physician is, on the one hand, to avoid a costly investigation of an essentially healthy boy while, on the other, identifying those who have an underlying disorder compromising the hypothalamic–pituitary gonadotropin–gonadal system.

Unfortunately, many patients with Kallmann's syndrome wait years for the correct diagnosis to be made even in the presence of classical findings[1562]; a high index of suspicion by the physician is important.

A presumptive diagnosis can usually be formed during the initial evaluation on the basis of the history and physical examination. Has puberty failed to occur or did it begin but fail to progress or regress? History taking must elicit all symptoms of chronic or intermittent illnesses and all details pertaining to growth and development as well as questioning about the patient's sense of smell. Disorders of pregnancy, abnormalities of labor and delivery, and birth trauma, if present in the patient's history, suggest that a congenital or neonatal event may be related to the delay in puberty. Poor linear growth and poor nutritional status during the neonatal period and childhood may reflect long-standing abnormalities of development. A growth chart is plotted to represent graphically the increase in stature and to assess growth velocity from birth. Late onset of growth failure usually indicates a serious condition requiring evaluation as soon as it is noted. Family history may reveal disorders of puberty or infertility, anosmia, or hyposmia in relatives as well as delay in the age of onset of puberty in parents or siblings. Recalled age of pubertal onset is relatively reliable in women[1563] but less often accurate in men. A history of consanguinity is important in the detection of autosomal recessive disorders.

The physical examination starts with determination of height and weight; the upper/lower segment ratio or sitting height is calculated, and the arm span is measured and compared with

Table 24–26. Differential Diagnostic Features of Delayed Puberty and Sexual Infantilism

Condition	Stature	Plasma Gonadotropins	LHRH Test LH Response	Plasma Gonadal Steroids	Plasma DHEAS	Karyotype	Olfaction
Constitutional delay in growth and adolescence	Short for chronologic age, usually appropriate for bone age	Prepubertal, later pubertal	Prepubertal, later pubertal	Low, later normal	Low for chronologic age, appropriate for bone age	Normal	Normal
Hypogonadotropic hypogonadism							
Isolated gonadotropin deficiency	Normal, absent pubertal growth spurt	Low	Prepubertal or no response	Low	Appropriate for chronologic age	Normal	Normal
Kallmann's syndrome	Normal, absent pubertal growth spurt	Low	Prepubertal or no response	Low	Appropriate for chronologic age	Normal	Anosmia or hyposmia
Idiopathic multiple pituitary hormone deficiencies	Short stature and poor growth since early childhood	Low	Prepubertal or no response	Low	Usually low	Normal	Normal
Hypothalamic-pituitary tumors	Late onset decrease in growth velocity	Low	Prepubertal or no response	Low	Normal or low for chronologic age	Normal	Normal
Primary gonadal failure							
Syndrome of gonadal dysgenesis (Turner's syndrome) and variants	Short stature since childhood	High	Hyper-response for age	Low	Normal for chronologic age	45,X or variant	Normal
Klinefelter's syndrome and variants	Normal to tall	High	Hyper-response at puberty	Low or normal	Normal for chronologic age	47,XXY or variant	Normal
Familial XX or XY gonadal dysgenesis	Normal	High	Hyper-response for age	Low	Normal for chronologic age	46,XX or 46,XY	Normal

the height. The height velocity should be documented over a period of at least 6 months, preferably 12 months. The signs of puberty are noted, and the stage of secondary sexual development is determined according to the standards presented earlier (see Figs. 24–3 to 24–5). Questionnaires utilizing pictures are sometimes used to allow children to determine their own stage of puberty. These techniques are commonly used in survey studies but do not replace the physical examination; results are reported to be accurate although there is a tendency to overestimate development early in puberty and underestimate late in puberty.[79, 1564] The length and width of the testes are measured or the volume is assessed using an orchidometer. The length and diameter of the stretched penis are determined in boys, and the diameter of glandular breast tissue and areolar size are noted in girls. The presence or absence of galactorrhea is defined. Obese boys often appear to have a small penis because of excessive adipose tissue surrounding the phallus; only when the fat is retracted can the full extent of phallic development be assessed. (This feature is among the most common causes of inappropriate referral for hypogonadism.) The extent of pubic and axillary hair is noted, as is the degree of acne. The possibility of cryptorchidism or retractile testes should be differentiated if no testes are palpated in the scrotum. Neurologic examination, including examination of the optic discs and visual fields by frontal confrontation perimetry and evaluation of olfaction, may reveal findings suggesting the presence of a CNS neoplasm or a developmental defect (Kallmann's syndrome). The stigmata of gonadal dysgenesis (Turner's syndrome) or the small testes and gynecomastia of Klinefelter's syndrome may suggest one of these diagnoses. Complete physical examination including the lungs, heart, kidney, and the gastrointestinal tract is also important in the search for a chronic disorder that may delay puberty.

Table 24–27. Endocrine Diagnosis of Constitutional Delayed Adolescence and Hypogonadotropic Hypogonadism

No single test reliably discriminates between the two diagnoses.
Onset of puberty in boys is indicated by
Testes > 2.5 cm in diameter
Serum testosterone concentration > 50 ng/dL
Pubertal LH response to LHRH bolus
Pubertal pattern of LH pulsatility

LH, luteinizing hormone; LHRH, LH-releasing hormone.

Laboratory studies (Table 24–28) include determination of plasma LH and FSH concentrations, measurement of the rise in LH level after LHRH administration, determination of testosterone concentrations in boys and estradiol levels in girls, and measurements of T_4 and prolactin concentrations in boys and girls if the clinical features warrant. It is important to use one of the few national endocrine laboratories for the determinations of the hormones of puberty because most local laboratories are interested only in differentiating normal, higher, adult values from inappropriately low levels and not the low concentrations characteristic of the early stage of pubertal development. For example, levels of estradiol below 15 pg/mL are not measured routinely or with confidence in many clinical laboratories despite the availability of methods and commercial kits to measure accurately values as low as 1.5 pg/mL.

Table 24–28. Endocrine and Imaging Studies in Delayed Adolescence

Initial assessment
Plasma testosterone or estradiol
Plasma FSH and LH
Plasma thyroxine (and prolactin)
Bone age and lateral skull roentgenograph
Test of olfaction
Follow-up studies
Karyotype (short, phenotypic females)
MRI with contrast enhancement
Pelvic ultrasonography (females)
LHRH test
hCG test (males)
Pattern of pulsatile LH secretion
Visual acuity and visual fields

FSH, follicle-stimulating hormone; hCG, human chorionic gonadotropin; LH, luteinizing hormone; MRI, magnetic resonance imaging.

Radiographic examination includes bone age determination and, if the diagnosis is at all consistent with a CNS lesion, an MRI of the brain with specific attention to the pituitary and hypothalamic area using contrast; only advanced pituitary tumors or significantly calcified craniopharyngiomas appear on lateral skull films, and, although a positive result is useful, a negative radiograph cannot rule out a CNS defect.[1565] In contrast to MRI scans, CT scanning can detect calcification. Ultrasound evaluation of the uterus and ovaries is not usually indicated initially in work-up of delayed puberty but provides useful information about the state of development of these structures.[127] Again, it is important that the ultrasonographer has experience with children and young adolescents. Regrettably, individuals with normal internal genital organs have been told that they lack a uterus or ovaries, or both, by ultrasonographers inexperienced with this age group. One study demonstrated streak gonads in 50% of a group of 70 patients with Turner's syndrome.[1566] Assessment of chromosomal karyotype should be considered in all short girls, even in the absence of somatic signs of Turner's syndrome and especially if puberty is delayed, and in boys with suspected Klinefelter stigmata or behavior.

A presumptive diagnosis of constitutional delay in growth and adolescence is made if the history and growth chart reveal a history of short stature but consistent growth rate for skeletal age (and no signs or symptoms of hypothalamic lesions), if the family history includes parents or siblings with delayed puberty, if the physical examination (including assessment of the olfactory threshold) is normal, if optic discs and visual fields are normal, and if the bone age is significantly delayed. In classical cases, an MRI scan of the hypothalamic-pituitary region may not be necessary. The rate of growth in these patients is usually appropriate for bone age; a decrease in growth velocity occurs in some normal children just before the appearance of secondary sexual characteristics and may awaken concerns if such a pattern occurs in these subjects. Further, in these individuals the onset at puberty correlates better with bone age than with chronologic age. Elevated concentrations of gonadotropins and gonadal steroids to early pubertal levels precede secondary sexual development by several months; thus, measurements of serum LH, FSH, estradiol, or testosterone levels may help in predicting future development. The third-generation LH assays are reported to be sufficiently sensitive to allow the determination of the onset of endocrine puberty with a single blood sample in most boys, but an LHRH test is still often performed. An increase in the concentration of LH of more than 7.5 IU/L (2 ng/mL LER-960) determined by conventional polyclonal radioimmunoassay after intravenous administration of 100 μg of LHRH usually precedes the first physical sign of sexual maturation by less than 1 year.

Clomiphene citrate, an antiestrogen with weak estrogenic effects, decreases secretion of gonadotropins in prepubertal patients but increases gonadotropin secretion in pubertal patients and in adults. However, we have not found administration of clomiphene citrate to be useful in the diagnosis of constitutional delay of growth and adolescence.

Various tests have been proposed for differentiating hypogonadotropic hypogonadism from constitutional delay in puberty. Trials assessing the prolactin response to TRH,[1567, 1568] chlorpromazine,[1569] metoclopramide,[1570] or domperidone[1571] for differential diagnosis either failed or gave inconsistent results.[1570, 1571] The combination of the prolactin response to metoclopramide and the gonadotropin response to LHRH has been suggested,[1572] as has the use of priming doses of LHRH with evaluation of the gonadotropin response to a subsequent dose of LHRH[1573–1575] or to a superactive LHRH agonist.[1576, 1577] The FSH response is higher in patients with hypothalamic-pituitary deficiencies who undergo pubertal development.[1578] A sensitive immunofluorometric assay for LH may help to distinguish between constitutional delay of growth and adolescence and hypogonadotropic hypogonadism better than the polyclonal LH radioimmunoassay.[1579] Urinary gonadotropin excretion is lower in hypogonadotropic patients than in delayed puberty, but this method of differential diagnosis may require years of observation before the difference is apparent.[1255] Although some methods are promising, their efficacy remains to be confirmed. There is a tendency for hypogonadotropic patients to undergo adrenarche at a normal age and to have a higher DHEAS concentration than those with constitutional delay in growth, and this pattern is helpful in the differential diagnosis.[969, 1580, 1581]

Measurement of 8 AM serum testosterone is proposed to be an accurate indication of impending pubertal development; a value greater than 0.7 nmol/L (20 ng/dL) predicts enlargement of testes to greater than 4 mL by 12 months in 77% of cases and by 15 months in 100% of cases, whereas of those with a value less than 0.7 nmol/L only 12% entered puberty in 12 months and only 25% entered puberty in 15 months. This technique may help predict spontaneous pubertal development but still requires considerable watching and waiting.[1582]

At present, there does not appear to be a practical and reliable endocrine test for indisputably differentiating between constitutional delay in growth and adolescence and hypogonadotropic hypogonadism. Watchful waiting remains the procedure of choice.

A typical patient with isolated gonadotropin deficiency is of average height for age and has eunuchoid proportions; low plasma concentrations of gonadal steroids, LH, and FSH; and no increase or a blunted response of LH after LHRH administration. The amplitude and usually the frequency of LH pulses are decreased when serial blood samples are studied over a 24-hour period. In some but not all forms of Kallmann's syndrome, the sense of smell is absent or impaired. However, differentiation of isolated gonadotropin deficiency in the absence of hyposmia or anosmia from constitutional delay in puberty may be difficult at initial study. Gonadotropin-deficient patients may be as short as those with constitutional delay in growth and adolescence, and concentrations of LH and FSH in hypogonadotropic hypogonadism may be indistinguishable from those of normal prepubertal children or children with constitutional delay. Sometimes years of observation are necessary to detect the appearance of spontaneous and progressive signs of secondary sexual development or to document rising concentrations of gonadotropins or gonadal steroids before the diagnosis is clear. In general, but not in all cases, absence of the first signs of sexual maturation or failure of a rise in gonadotropins or gonadal steroid levels by age 18 in the presence of a normal concentration of serum DHEAS for chronologic age supports the diagnosis of isolated gonadotropin deficiency.

Patients with deficiency of gonadotropins combined with deficiency of other pituitary hormones require careful evaluation for a CNS neoplasm. Visual field or optic disc abnormalities support the diagnosis of CNS tumor; even if these tests are normal, cranial MRI should be performed to evaluate the pituitary gland and stalk and the hypothalamic region. CT scans but especially MRI scans of the head are valuable in detecting mass lesions and developmental abnormalities of the hypothalamic-pituitary region.[1565, 1583]

Treatment of Delayed Puberty and Sexual Infantilism

Treatment of delayed puberty (Table 24–29) depends on the diagnosis and the nature of the disorder. Patients with constitutional delay in growth and adolescence ultimately have spontaneous onset and progression through puberty. Often, reassurance and continued observation to ensure that the expected sexual maturation occurs are sufficient. However, the stigma of appearing less mature than one's peers can cause psychological stress; such individuals may be unable to participate in the dating activities their friends are starting, smaller size may lead them to avoid participation in athletics, immature appearance may lead to ridicule especially in the locker room, and school work may suffer because of their poor self-image.[1584, 1585] Some children feel such intense peer pressure and low self-esteem that only the appearance of signs of puberty reassures them and enables them to participate in sports and social activities with their peers. Poor self-image in late-maturing boys may carry into adulthood even after normal puberty ensues.[1584, 1585] The growth retardation is often responsible for most of the stress rather than the delay in pubertal development itself.[1586]

For psychological reasons, in boys of age 14 or older who show no signs of puberty, a 4- to 6-month course of testosterone enanthate, cypionate, or cyclopropionate (50 to 100 mg intramuscularly every 4 weeks) may be helpful.[1587–1589] The low dose of testosterone enanthate is generally considered to be safe but can raise LDL and lower HDL cholesterol values as an expected effect.

Oral treatment with 2.5 mg of fluoxymesterone (Halotestin) for 6 to 60 months allows increased pubertal development without adverse effects on final height, although the necessity to take a daily dose may decrease compliance.[437] Low-dose oxandrolone (2.5 mg/day orally)[1590] is sometimes used as an oral alternative to intramuscular testosterone enanthate; this agent increases growth through androgenic effects reflected by suppression of LH and FSH but does not stimulate GH secretion as it is not aromatized to estrogen.[1591] The temporary increase in growth velocity found with oxandrolone does not affect final height.[1592–1594] Short-term treatment with fluoxymesterone (2.5 mg/day orally) was also reported to be a safe treatment that does not compromise adult height.[437] Testosterone undecanoate at 40 mg/day is likewise an effective but expensive treatment for those choosing oral therapy.[1595–1597] Transdermal testosterone may be applied as a daily patch or a gel, although experience with these forms of androgen is more limited than with the other forms. Preliminary experience suggests that overnight (approximately 8 to 9 hours) or every other night use of 2.5 mg is effective. Testosterone gel is being investigated as a daily topical preparation to advance pubertal development.

For girls of age 13 or older, a 3- to 4-month course of ethinylestradiol (5 μg/day orally) or conjugated estrogens (0.3 mg/day orally) may be used to initiate maturation of the secondary sexual characteristics without unduly advancing bone age or limiting final height.[1598, 1599]

A fourth-generation aromatase inhibitor, letrozole, administered along with testosterone in a randomized controlled trial in boys with constitutional delay in puberty and growth decreased the advancement in bone age, an effect that will presumably lead to a greater adult height[1600] by strikingly decreasing the synthesis of estradiol from testosterone. Estradiol[172] is the sex steroid that has the major effect on skeletal maturation. Letrozole does not block the virilizing effects of testosterone. This promising treatment is experimental; it may improve the decreased adult height in some boys with constitutional delay compared with their predicted genetic potential,[1011, 1012, 1014, 1015, 1601] a decrease that testosterone cannot overcome.

If, during the 3 to 6 months after discontinuing gonadal steroid therapy, spontaneous puberty does not ensue or the concentrations of plasma gonadotropins and plasma testosterone in boys or plasma estradiol in girls do not increase toward pubertal values, the treatment may be repeated. Usually, only one or two courses of therapy are necessary. When treatment is discontinued after bone age has advanced, for example, to 12 to 13 years in girls or 13 or 14 years in boys, patients with constitutional delay usually continue pubertal development on their own, whereas those with gonadotropin deficiency do not progress and may, in fact, regress.

Alleviating the underlying problem treats functional hypogonadotropic hypogonadism associated with chronic disease. Delayed puberty in this situation is usually a result of inadequate nutrition and low weight; when weight returns to normal values, puberty usually occurs spontaneously. Treatment with T_4 allows normal pubertal development in hypothyroid patients with delayed puberty.

Congenital or acquired gonadotropin deficiency as a result of a lesion or surgery requires replacement therapy with gonadal steroids at an age approximating the normal age of onset of puberty (Tables 24–30 and 24–31). An exception may occur when GH deficiency coexists with gonadotropin deficiency; if bone age advancement and epiphyseal fusion are brought about by testosterone or estradiol replacement before therapy with GH causes adequate linear growth, adult height is compromised. However, if puberty is not initiated early enough, the patient may well suffer psychological damage. It is generally advisable to initiate puberty in such patients with low-dose

Table 24–29. Management and Treatment of Delayed Puberty

Objectives
Determine site and etiology of abnormality
Induce and maintain secondary sexual characteristics
Induce pubertal growth spurt
Prevent the potential short-term and long-term psychological, personality, and social handicaps of delayed puberty
Ensure normal libido and potency
Attain fertility

Therapy
Concerned but not anxious or socially handicapped adolescent:
- Reassurance and follow-up (tincture of time)
- Repeat evaluation (including serum testosterone or estradiol) in 6 mo

Psychosocial handicaps, anxiety, highly concerned:
- Therapy for 4 mo with
- Boys: testosterone enanthate 100 mg intramuscularly every 4 wk at 14–14.5 yr of age, or overnight transdermal testosterone patch
- Girls: ethinyl estradiol 5–10 μg daily by mouth or conjugated estrogens 0.3 mg daily by mouth or overnight ethinyl estradiol patch at 13 yr of age
- No therapy for 4–6 mo; reevaluate status including serum testosterone or estradiol; if indicated repeat treatment regimen

Table 24–30. Hormonal Substitution Therapy in Boys with Hypogonadism

Goal: to approximate normal adolescent development *when diagnosis is established*
Initial therapy: at 13 yr of age, testosterone enanthate (or other long-acting testosterone ester) 50 mg intramuscularly every month for about 9 mo (6–12 mo)
Over the next 3 to 4 yr: gradually increase dose to adult replacement dose of 200 mg every 2–3 wk
Begin *replacement therapy in boys with suspected hypogonadotropic hypogonadism* by bone age ≤ 14 yr
To induce fertility at appropriate time: pulsatile LHRH or FSH and hCG therapy

Table 24–31. Hormonal Substitution Therapy in Girls with Hypogonadism

When diagnosis of hypogonadism is firmly established (e.g., girls with 45,X gonadal dysgenesis), begin hormonal substitution therapy at 12–13 yr of age
Goal: to approximate normal adolescent development
Initial therapy: ethinyl estradiol 5 μg by mouth or conjugated estrogen 0.3 mg (or less) by mouth daily for 4–6 mo
After 6 mo of therapy (or sooner if "breakthrough" bleeding occurs) begin cyclic therapy:
Estrogen: first 21 days of month
Progestagen: (e.g., medroxyprogesterone acetate 5 mg by mouth) 12th to 21st day of month
Gradually increase dose of estrogen over next 2–3 yr to conjugated estrogen 0.6–1.25 mg or ethinyl estradiol 10–20 μg daily for first 21 days of month
In hypogonadotropic hypogonadism: to induce ovulation at appropriate time: pulsatile LHRH or FSH and hCG therapy

gonadal steroids by age 14 in boys and age 13 in girls regardless of the definitive diagnosis of gonadotropin deficiency; thus, these children with GH deficiency would be treated similarly to those with isolated delayed puberty.

Patients with isolated GH deficiency may have a delayed onset of puberty; with GH administration, puberty usually occurs at an appropriate age but may progress faster than in normal individuals.[1602, 1603] A study of over 200 children with GH deficiency treated with hGH showed a correlation between the age of onset of induced puberty and final height in patients who were also gonadotropin-deficient, whereas those who underwent spontaneous puberty, which occurred earlier than the age of hormone-induced puberty in the gonadotropin-deficient children, had a lower final height; this supports the advisability of waiting to initiate puberty in GH- and gonadotropin-deficient subjects.[1604] Height at the onset of puberty is also correlated with final height in GH-deficient children.[1605] Clinical trials are in progress to determine the effects of artificially delaying puberty with an LHRH analogue to attempt to achieve a greater final height in patients with isolated GH deficiency treated with hGH[1606] (see earlier).

Micropenis resulting from fetal androgen deficiency caused by a primary testicular defect or gonadotropin deficiency[1607] can be successfully treated with small doses of testosterone enanthate (25 to 50 mg/month intramuscularly) administered for short periods during infancy[1146, 1607] (also see Chapter 22). Patients with isolated congenital GH deficiency occasionally have micropenis that may be successfully treated with GH replacement alone.[1608]

As discussed earlier, episodic administration of LHRH can elicit pulsatile LH and FSH release and gonadal stimulation in prepubertal children or hypogonadotropic patients.[946, 949, 950] Portable pumps have been used to administer LHRH in episodic fashion over prolonged periods. Pulsatile LHRH therapy can induce puberty and promote the development of secondary sexual characteristics and spermatogenesis in men[1609–1613] and ovulation in women[1614, 1615]; pregnancy has been achieved with this regimen in women with hypogonadotropic hypogonadism. A lower frequency of LHRH administration favors FSH secretion and a higher frequency favors LH secretion and, ultimately, has been associated with a PCOS-like picture.[1616] A comparison of two different frequencies of LHRH administration did not reveal a difference between an LH pulse given subcutaneously every 3 hours or every 45 minutes in the rapidity of onset of pubertal development or serum LH, FSH, or sex steroid concentrations; this indicates that the hypothalamic-pituitary-gonadal axis is sufficiently robust to accommodate various frequencies of LHRH secretion.[1617] The use of pulsatile LHRH administration is not practical for the routine induction of puberty in adolescent boys and girls with gonadotropin deficiency. Both hCG and human menopausal gonadotropin can be used as effective substitutes for recombinant human pituitary LH and FSH to produce full gonadal maturation, especially in those with pituitary pathology. But, again, this regimen is cumbersome and expensive.[1618] Thus, long-term gonadal steroid replacement therapy is the treatment of choice for hypothalamic or pituitary gonadotropin deficiency until fertility is achieved.[1619]

Hypergonadotropic hypogonadism is treated by replacement of testosterone in boys and estradiol in girls. For treatment of gonadal dysgenesis, estrogen therapy should be initiated when the patient is age 13 (bone age > 11 years) to allow secondary sexual development at an appropriate chronologic age. The Klinefelter syndrome is compatible with varying degrees of masculinization at puberty, but some patients require testosterone replacement. The concentrations of plasma testosterone and LH should be monitored every 6 months during puberty and yearly thereafter. If the LH level rises more than 2.5 SD above the mean value or the testosterone level decreases below the normal range for age, testosterone replacement therapy is indicated.

Patients receiving gonadal steroid replacement follow the same treatment regimen whether the diagnosis is hypogonadotropic hypogonadism or hypergonadotropic hypogonadism (see Tables 24–30 and 24–31). Various testosterone preparations with several routes of administration are available.[1620] Alkylated testosterone preparations are to be avoided because of the risk of peliosis hepatis (hemorrhagic liver cysts), which is not related to dose or duration of treatment; although regression is possible with discontinuation of testosterone treatment, progression to liver failure can occur.[1621, 1622] Males may receive testosterone enanthate, propionate, or cypionate, 50 to 100 mg every 4 weeks intramuscularly at the start; later the dosage is gradually increased to 200 to 300 mg every 2 to 3 weeks. Low-dose replacement therapy is appropriate until well into the pubertal growth spurt.[168]

Testosterone may be administered by cutaneous patch on scrotal skin or nonsexual skin to cause secondary sexual development in hypogonadal adolescents; patches may be given at night to recreate the diurnal variation of testosterone seen in early puberty. Physiologic values of serum testosterone are possible along with secondary sexual development.[1623, 1624] A teenage boy may be less likely to apply a patch daily, and biweekly or monthly injections may allow better compliance; nonetheless, we and others find that 2.5- and 5-mg dermal testosterone patches may be useful in motivated teenagers. New testosterone gel preparations, usually rubbed onto the forearms, are approved for adults and may be used in a similar manner. Testosterone ointment may be used as therapy for microphallus to enlarge the size of the phallus intentionally,[1625] but an infant coming in contact with the skin of an individual with testosterone gel (before it is absorbed into the intended subject's skin) runs the risk of unplanned testosterone effects.

Initially, girls 12 to 13 years of age are given ethinylestradiol, 5 μg/day orally, or conjugated estrogens, 0.3 mg/day by mouth, on the first 21 days of the month. The dose is gradually increased over the next 2 to 3 years to 10 μg of ethinylestradiol or 0.6 to 1.25 mg of conjugated estrogen for the first 21 days of the month. The maintenance dose should be the minimal amount to maintain secondary sexual characteristics, sustain withdrawal bleeding, and prevent osteoporosis. After breakthrough bleeding occurs, or no later than 6 months after the start of cyclic therapy, a progestagen (e.g., medroxyprogesterone acetate, 5 mg/day) is added on days 12 through 21 of the month. Undesirable effects are uncommon but may include weight gain, headache, nausea, peripheral edema, and mild hypertension. Application of portions of transdermal 17β-estradiol patches at night was shown to mimic levels of estrogen produced in early puberty and to bring about breast development slowly[1626]; other therapeutic schedules are possible.[1627–1630] As with testosterone, there must be care that the preparation is not placed in contact with young children or untoward estrogen effects may occur.

There is concern about the increased risk of endometrial and breast carcinoma in patients receiving chronic estrogen replacement therapy including patients with Turner's syndrome. This is not an issue in adolescents or young adults but is a consideration in older women. The use of progestational agents to antagonize the effect of estrogens reduces the risk of endometrial cancer, but knowledge of the optimal dose of estrogen and progesterone to enhance development without unduly increasing the risk of cancer must come from future studies. Estrogen replacement is important for its antiosteoporotic action on bone. Surprisingly, we lack controlled studies on optional sex steroid replacement regimens in adolescent women.

Patients with hypopituitarism may complain of sparse pubic hair growth or, in girls, total absence of pubic hair. Pubic hair thickens further in affected males with hCG treatment that adds the testicular contribution of testosterone to the exogenous testosterone therapy. GH therapy in males with GH and gonadotropin deficiency enhances the steroidogenic response of the testes to hCG administration.[1631] Further, adolescent or young adult women have been given low doses (25 mg) of long-acting intramuscular testosterone every 4 weeks to stimulate the growth of pubic hair without virilization.[1632]

The result of treatment with testosterone in boys with radiation-induced primary testicular failure is normal final height, although in a group of patients with concomitant spinal radiation, the upper/lower segment ratio was much reduced, indicating impaired spinal growth.[1633] The results of clinical trials of biosynthetic hGH therapy in Turner's syndrome indicate that an increase in growth rate with a substantial increase in final height into the lower range of the normal growth curves is possible, especially with a dose higher than used in GH deficiency (see more detailed earlier discussion in the section on Turner's syndrome).[1462–1465, 1634, 1635] There is some degree of improvement of the abnormal body proportions of Turner's syndrome with hGH treatment, but the disproportionate growth of the foot may dissuade some girls from continuing treatment to maximal benefit for height.[1469]

The addition of estrogen therapy at low doses has been reported either to exert no effect on adult height or to reduce the adult height obtained with GH therapy administered alone.[1634–1642] Indeed, the length of time of exposure to GH before estrogen treatment is said to be the major determinant of whether GH and estrogen treatment increased final height.[1643] However, it is postulated that if GH is started early enough (e.g., 2 to 8 years of age), estrogen therapy may be added at an age (~13 years) appropriate for the institution of puberty (see discussion in Turner's syndrome section).[1644] Counseling and a peer support group are exceedingly important components of the long-term management.[1603]

The bone density is decreased in Turner's syndrome, at least in part, because of hypogonadism at puberty, and this tendency becomes more severe with age in patients who discontinue or do not receive estrogen replacement therapy.[1645, 1646] Transdermal estrogen was shown to increase bone density in subjects with Turner's syndrome who have finished statural growth.[1647]

Sexual Precocity

Sexual precocity (Table 24–32) is defined as the appearance of any sign of secondary sexual maturation at an age more than 2.0 SD below the mean; in the past, the ages of 8 years in girls and 9 years in boys were considered the lower limits of the normal onset of puberty.[154, 1648] Present data detailed previously indicate that the limits in normal boys remain at 9 years but that the lower limit for white girls is 7 years and for black girls is 6 years, assuming that there is no sign or symptom of CNS disorders or other serious or chronic disease that might cause sexual precocious puberty. These guidelines are similar to those proposed by the Drug and Therapeutics and Executive Committees of the Lawson Wilkins Pediatric Endocrine Society.[100] The new data noted in the first section of this chapter show that breast development and pubic hair development may occur in girls as young as 6 years in substantial numbers, especially in black girls, leading to a need for careful evaluation and conservatism, even in these young years, in evaluating and treating girls with only minimal, relatively nonprogressive signs of sexual precocity.

If the sexual precocity results from premature reactivation of the hypothalamic LHRH pulse generator–pituitary gonadotropin–gonadal axis, the condition is called complete isosexual precocity or true or central precocious puberty and is LHRH-dependent. Pulsatile LH release has a pubertal pattern in this form, and the rise in the concentration of LH after LHRH administration is indistinguishable from the normal pubertal pattern of serum LH. If extrapituitary secretion of gonadotropins or secretion of gonadal steroids independent of pulsatile LHRH stimulation leads to virilization in boys or feminization in girls, the condition is termed incomplete isosexual precocity, pseudoprecocious puberty, or LHRH-independent sexual precocity. The production of excessive estrogens in males leads to inappropriate feminization, and the production of increased androgen levels in females leads to inappropriate virilization; these conditions are termed contrasexual precocity (also termed heterosexual precocity). Hence, the disorders that cause sexual precocity can be separated into those in which the increased secretion of gonadal steroids depends on LHRH stimulation of pituitary gonadotropins and those in which it is unrelated to activation of the hypothalamic LHRH pulse generator.

In all forms of sexual precocity, the increased gonadal steroid secretion increases height velocity, somatic development, and the rate of skeletal maturation and, because of premature epiphyseal fusion, can lead to the paradox of tall stature in childhood but short adult height. Data on the final height in true precocious puberty are scarce (see Table 24–32), but several studies of untreated females with idiopathic central precocious puberty demonstrated a mean final height of 151 to 155 cm.[871, 1649–1656] There are few reports of final height in boys with untreated precocious puberty[1649] (Table 24–33). In the boys followed to adult stature by Thamdrup,[1650] the mean height was 155.4 cm ± 8.3 (SD) and all were well below midparental height and far below the fathers' height.

Blood pressure matches that of height- and weight-related

normal subjects rather than age-matched normal persons; thus, elevated blood pressure for age in patients with sexual precocity may not indicate hypertension (blood pressure in normal children is best related to height rather than to age, and this is an extension of the concept). Serum alkaline phosphatase and IGF-I concentrations reflect the degree of sexual development rather than chronologic age.[391]

True or Central Precocious Puberty: Complete Isosexual Precocity (LHRH-Dependent Sexual Precocity)

In our series of over 200 patients with true precocious puberty,[871] girls had true precocious puberty five times more commonly than boys and the idiopathic form was eight times more common in girls than in boys (Table 24–34). Neurologic abnormalities occurred at least as often as idiopathic true precocious puberty in boys, whereas in girls neurologic lesions were a fifth as common as idiopathic disorders. Thus, it is essential to search for a neurologic etiology for true precocious puberty, especially in boys. In some cases, sexual precocity may be the only manifestation of a CNS tumor[871, 875, 1657, 1658] (Table 24–35).

Long-Term Follow-up of True Precocious Puberty

Pregnancy has occurred in patients with true or central precocious puberty as early as 5 years of age.[1659] Of course, such pregnancies are in fact the result of childhood sexual abuse of a child with true precocious puberty, a fact rarely reported by the sensational press. Fertility in later life is less well documented, but in our experience as well as that of others, normal pregnancies have occurred in women who had idiopathic true precocious puberty,[1659, 1660] a CNS abnormality triggering true precocious puberty,[871, 1654] or premature menarche. In the isosexual precocity of the McCune-Albright syndrome, there are also reports of adult fertility.[675, 1661, 1662]

Idiopathic True or Central Precocious Puberty

By common definition, 2.5% of normal children develop signs of puberty before the lower limits of normal. The Herman-Giddens study found that 27% of black and 7% of white girls have some manifestation of secondary sex development by 7 years of age. Thus, as stated previously, a useful definition of sexual precocity is onset before 6 years in black girls, before 7 years in white girls, and before 9 years in boys, assuming there

Table 24–32. Classification of Sexual Precocity

True Precocious Puberty or Complete Isosexual Precocity (LHRH-Dependent Sexual Precocity or Premature Activation of the Hypothalamic LHRH Pulse Generator)

- Idiopathic true precocious puberty
- CNS tumors
  - Optic glioma associated with neurofibromatosis type 1
  - Hypothalamic astrocytoma
- Other CNS disorders
  - Developmental abnormalities including hypothalamic hamartoma of the tuber cinereum
  - Encephalitis
  - Static encephalopathy
  - Brain abscess
  - Sarcoid or tubercular granuloma
  - Head trauma
  - Hydrocephalus
  - Arachnoid cyst
  - Myelomeningocele
  - Vascular lesion
  - Cranial irradiation
- True precocious puberty after late treatment of congenital virilizing adrenal hyperplasia or other previous chronic exposure to sex steroids

Incomplete Isosexual Precocity (Hypothalamic LHRH-Independent)

Males

- Gonadotropin-secreting tumors
  - hCG-secreting CNS tumors (e.g., chorioepitheliomas, germinoma, teratoma)
  - hCG-secreting tumors located outside the CNS (hepatoma, teratoma, choriocarcinoma)
- Increased androgen secretion by adrenal or testis
  - Congenital adrenal hyperplasia (CYP21 and CYP11B1 deficiencies)
  - Virilizing adrenal neoplasm
  - Leydig cell adenoma
  - Familial testotoxicosis (sex-limited autosomal dominant pituitary gonadotropin-independent precocious Leydig cell and germ cell maturation)
  - Cortisol resistance syndrome

Females

- Ovarian cyst
- Estrogen-secreting ovarian or adrenal neoplasm
- Peutz-Jeghers syndrome

In Both Sexes

- McCune-Albright syndrome
- Hypothyroidism
- Iatrogenic or exogenous sexual precocity (including inadvertent exposure to estrogens in food, drugs, or cosmetics)

Variations of Pubertal Development

- Premature thelarche
- Premature isolated menarche
- Premature adrenarche
- Adolescent gynecomastia in boys
- Macro-orchidism

Contrasexual Precocity

Feminization in Males

- Adrenal neoplasm
- Chorioepithelioma
- CYP11B1 deficiency
- Late-onset adrenal hyperplasia
- *Testicular neoplasm* (Peutz-Jeghers syndrome)
- Increased extraglandular conversion of circulating adrenal androgens to estrogen
- Iatrogenic (exposure to estrogens)

Virilization in Females

- Congenital adrenal hyperplasia
  - CYP21 deficiency
  - CYP11B1 deficiency
  - 3β-HSD deficiency
- Virilizing adrenal neoplasm (Cushing's syndrome)
- Virilizing ovarian neoplasm (e.g., arrhenoblastoma)
- Iatrogenic (exposure to androgens)
- Cortisol resistance syndrome
- Aromatase deficiency

LHRH, luteinizing hormone-releasing factor (GnRH); CNS, central nervous system; CYP21, 21-hydroxylase; CYP11B1, 11-hydroxylase; 3β-HSD, 3β-hydroxysteroid dehydrogenase 4,5-isomerase.

Modified from Grumbach MM. True or central precocious puberty. In Kreiger DT, Bordin CW, (eds). Current Therapy in Endocrinology and Metabolism, 1985–1986. Toronto, BC Decker, 1985, pp 4–8.

Table 24–33. Historical Controls of Untreated Children with True Precocious Puberty

Reference	No. of Patients (Women/Men)	Final Ht (cm)*	
		Women	Men
Thamdrup[1650]			
Sigurjonsdottir and	26/8	151.3 ± 8.8	155.4 ± 8.3
Hayles[1654]	40/11	152.7 ± 8.0	156.0 ± 7.3
Werder et al[1655]	4/0	150.9 ± 5.0	
Lee[1653]	15/0	155.3 ± 9.6	
UCSF	8/4	153.8 ± 6.8	159.6 ± 8.7
Total	93/23	152.7 ± 8.6	155.6 ± 7.7

*Mean ± 1 SD.

From Paul D, Conte FA, Grumbach MM, Kaplan SL. Long-term effect of gonadotropin-releasing hormone agonist therapy on final and near-final height in 26 children with true precocious puberty treated at a median age of less than 5 years. J Clin Endocrinol Metab 1995; 80:546–551.

is no sign or symptom of CNS or other serious disease. Although this definition is a useful guideline, a significant proportion of girls 6 to 8 years of age with idiopathic precocious puberty represent one end of the bell-shaped curve for normal puberty onset, as described at the beginning of the chapter, and are examples of early normal puberty, just as those with constitutional delay in growth and adolescence are healthy but late maturers who fall in the older age segment of the normal distribution.

The nature of the striking sex difference in the prevalence of idiopathic true precocious puberty (females >> males) in contrast to constitutional delay in growth and puberty (males >> females) is poorly understood. There may be a history of early maturation in the family; rarely, true precocious puberty is transmitted as an autosomal recessive trait in boys and girls.[871, 1663] A larger group of children, however, develop true precocious puberty with no familial tendency toward early maturation and no signs of organic disease; these children have idiopathic true precocious puberty. This condition, which may be manifest in infancy, is about nine times more common in girls than in boys (see Table 24–35) and is commonly associated with electroencephalographic abnormalities.[1664] The age at onset in girls in about 50% of cases is 6 to 7 years, in about 25% is 2 to 6 years, and in 18% is in infancy[871] (Fig. 24–57). Organic forms of true precocious puberty, especially if associated with hypothalamic hamartoma, have an earlier mean age of onset than the idiopathic form.[871, 889]

In boys (Fig. 24–58) the testes usually enlarge under gonadotropin stimulation before any other signs of puberty are

Table 24–34. Distribution by Sex of Children with Idiopathic and Neurogenic Precocious Puberty

Series	Idiopathic		Neurogenic	
	Male	Female	Male	Female
Thamdrup (1961)[1650]	4	34	7	11
Wilkins (1965)[675]	13	67	10	5
Sigurjonsdottir and Hayles (1968)[1654]	8	54	16	16
University of California, San Francisco (1981)*	13	121	26	45

*Unpublished.

Table 24–35. Etiology of True Precocious Puberty*

Etiology	Number and Sex
Idiopathic	121F, 13M
Other causes	
CNS-hypothalamic tumors including hamartomas	11F, 15M
Arachnoid cyst	2F, 1M
Hydrocephalus	6F, 1M
Head trauma (child abuse)	1F
Perinatal asphyxia, cerebral palsy	3F, 1M
Encephalitis or meningitis	3F, 1M
Sex chromosome abnormalities (47,XXY; 48,XXXY)	2M
Nonspecific seizure disorder or mental retardation	26F, 16M
Degenerative CNS disease	3M
Congenital virilizing adrenal hyperplasia with secondary true precocious puberty	3M

*Data from University of California, San Francisco, Pediatric Endocrine Clinic.

From Kaplan SL, Grumbach MM. Pathogenesis of sexual precocity. In Grumbach MM, Sizonenko PC, Aubert ML, (eds). Control of the Onset of Puberty. Baltimore, Williams & Wilkins, 1990, pp 620–660. © 1990, the Williams & Wilkins Co., Baltimore.

seen; in girls (see Fig. 24–57) an increase in the rate of growth, the appearance of breast development, enlargement of the labia minora, and maturational changes in the vaginal mucosa are the usual presenting signs, with variable manifestations of pubic hair depending on the age at onset. Progression of secondary sexual maturation is often more rapid than the normal pattern of pubertal maturation. A waxing and waning course of development may be encountered.[1665] The rapid growth is associated with the rise in estrogen synthesis and secretion and the increased GH secretion and elevation of serum IGF-I levels because of stimulation by estradiol.[172, 173, 192, 209] The ratio of bone age to chronologic age and the rise of IGF-I above normal values for age are predictive of outcome; more mildly affected children progress less rapidly and tend to maintain their target height.[1666] Patients with slowly progres-

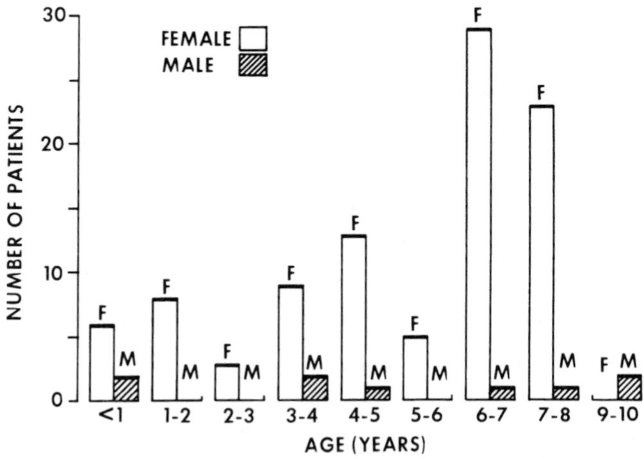

Figure 24–57. Age at onset of idiopathic true precocious puberty in 106 children. Open bars, female; hatched bars, male. At all ages, the frequency is greater in females than in males. The peak prevalence in girls is between ages 6 and 8 years. (From Kaplan SL, Grumbach MM. The neuroendocrinology of human puberty: an ontogenetic perspective. In Grumbach MM, Sizonenko PC, Aubert ML [eds]. Control of the Onset of Puberty. Baltimore, Williams & Wilkins, 1990, pp 1–68. © 1990, the Williams & Wilkins Co., Baltimore.)

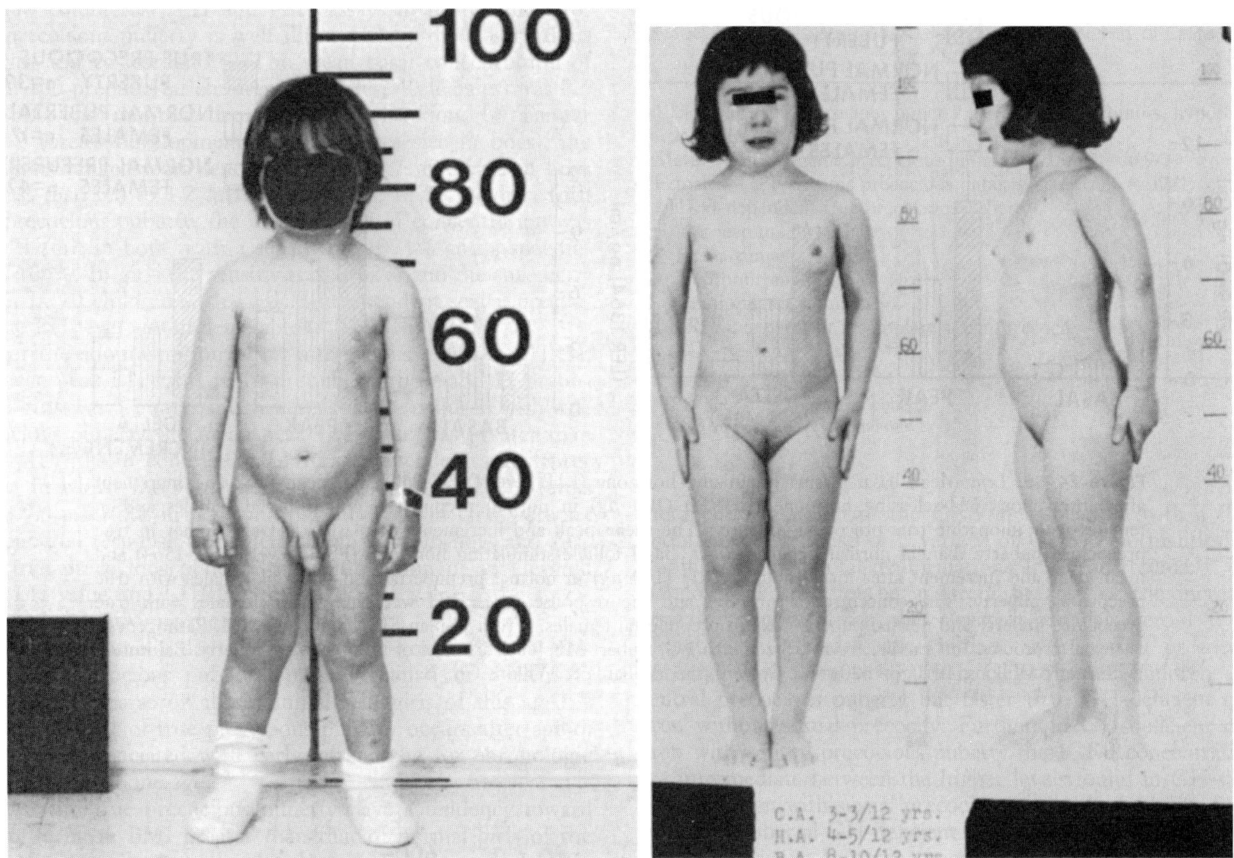

Figure 24–58. *Left,* A boy 2 years, 5 months of age with idiopathic precocious puberty. He had pubic hair and phallic and testicular enlargement by 10 months of age. At 1 year of age, his height was 86 cm (+4 SD); the phallus measured 10 × 3.5 cm, and the testes measured 2.5 × 1.5 cm. Plasma luteinizing hormone (LH) was 1.9 ng/mL (LER-960); follicle-stimulating hormone (FSH) 1.2 ng/mL (LER-869); and testosterone 416 ng/dL. After 100 μg of LH-releasing hormone (LHRH), the plasma LH increased to 8.4 ng/mL and FSH to 1.8 ng/mL, a pubertal response. When photographed, the patient had been treated with medroxyprogesterone acetate for 1.5 years. His height was 95.2 cm (+ 1 SD), the phallus was 6 × 3 cm, and the testes were 2.4 × 1.3 cm. Basal concentrations of LH (LER-960) were 0.9 ng/mL; FSH (LER-869) 0.8 ng/mL; and testosterone 7 ng/dL. After 100 μg of LHRH, LH concentrations rose to 2.3 ng/mL, whereas FSH concentrations did not change when he was on treatment with medroxyprogesterone acetate. For conversion to SI units, see the legends of Figures 24–17 and 24–18. (*Left,* From Styne DM, Grumbach MM. Puberty in the male and female: its physiology and disorders. In Yen SCC, Jaffe RB, [eds]. Reproductive Endocrinology, 2nd ed. Philadelphia, WB Saunders, 1986, pp 313–384.) *Right,* A 3 3/12-year-old girl with idiopathic true precocious puberty who had recurrent vaginal bleeding since 9 months of age. Height age, 4 5/12 years; bone age, 8 10/12 years.

sive or unsustained puberty have little or no loss of predicted final height[1665] and are characterized by the presence of normal or only slightly elevated estrogen and IGF-I concentrations.[1666] If height prediction is normal at the time of diagnosis rather than reduced, the patient does not require therapy.[1667–1669] Spermatogenesis in males and ovulation in females often occur, and fertility is possible.

The uterus and ovaries increase in size in true precocious puberty. The ovaries may also develop a multicystic appearance that may remain even after successful treatment with an LHRH agonist.[1670] True precocious puberty in females does not lead to premature menopause. However, in girls there is an increased risk for the development of carcinoma of the breast[36–39, 41] in adulthood. Psychosexual development[1671, 1672] is advanced only modestly in patients with sexual precocity (about 1½ years in girls with idiopathic true precocious puberty).[1673]

The pituitary gland undergoes hypertrophy in early infancy, puberty, and pregnancy and is increased in size on MRI in patients with central precocious puberty.[175, 1674, 1675] T1 images indicate a convex upper border of the pituitary gland in patients in normal or central precocious puberty, indicating the similarity in the physiologic changes of both conditions. Two sisters have been reported with the rare finding of pituitary gland hyperplasia (height greater than 1 cm) in central precocious puberty.[1676] Although empty sella may be associated with central precocious puberty, the empty sella syndrome is less frequently observed in patients with central precocious puberty than in patients with pituitary hypofunction. Although empty sella was found in 10% of children imaged for suspected hypothalamic-pituitary disorders including hypogonadotropic hypogonadism, the incidence in the general population is not known.[1677–1679]

The gonadotropin and gonadal steroid concentrations in plasma, the LH response to LHRH administration, and the amplitude and frequency of LH pulses are in the normal pubertal range[492, 940, 945] (Figs. 24–59 and 24–60; see Fig. 24–41). The new third-generation gonadotropin assays may allow the diagnosis of true precocious puberty by determination in a single serum sample for LH in the basal state or 40 minutes after a single subcutaneous dose of LHRH.[1680–1682] The notable improvement in the discriminatory power and specificity of

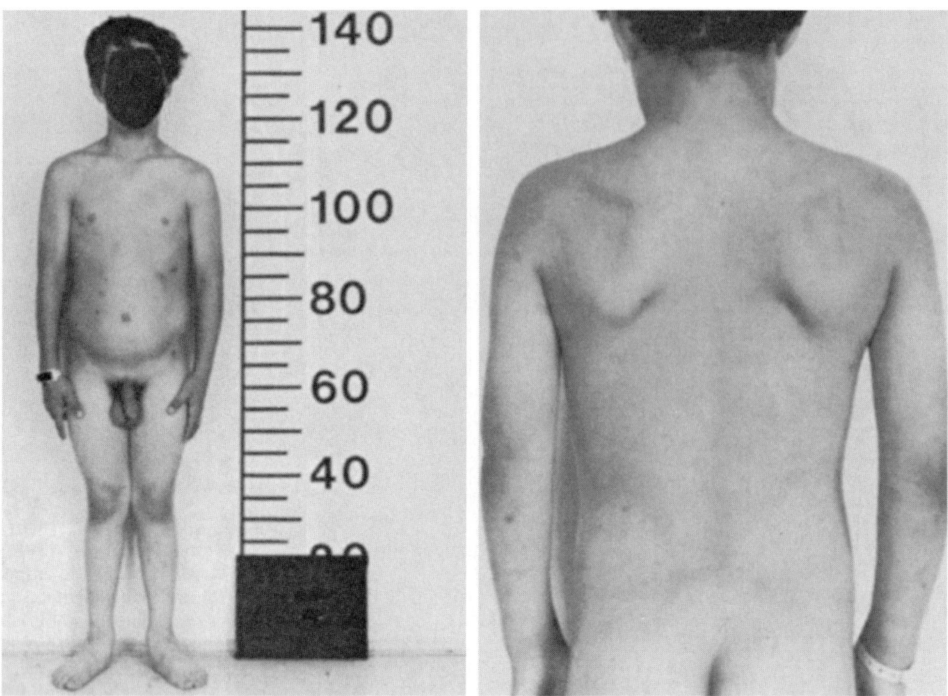

Figure 24–64. A boy of 8 years, 8 months with neurofibromatosis and precocious puberty, secondary to a hypothalamic glioma. He had tonic-clonic seizures at 2½ years and rapid growth starting at 4 years; an enlarged penis and testes and the presence of pubic hair were first noted at 7½ years. At this time, his height was 139.9 cm (+ 1.4 SD); the phallus was 9 × 3 cm; the right testis measured 5.5 × 3.2 cm and the left measured 5.4 × 2.9 cm. He had stage 3 pubic hair and 24 large café-au-lait spots. Computed tomographic scans and pneumoencephalography revealed a 1.5 × 2.5 cm hypothalamic mass, which was treated with radiation. The plasma concentration of luteinizing hormone (LH) was 0.5 ng/mL (LER-960); follicle-stimulating hormone (FSH) 0.4 ng/mL (LER-869); testosterone 221 ng/dL. After 100 μg of intravenous LH-releasing hormone (LHRH) the peak concentration of LH was 4.9 ng/mL, and that of FSH 1.4 ng/mL, a pubertal response. For conversion to SI units, see the legends of Figures 24–17 and 24–18. (From Styne DM, Grumbach MM. Puberty in the male and female: its physiology and disorders. In Yen SCC, Jaffe RB [eds]. Reproductive Endocrinology, 2nd ed. Philadelphia, WB Saunders, 1986, pp 313–384.)

hypertrophic and bulged through the diaphragm sellae,[933] which induced activation of the LHRH pulse generator through a mass effect and compromise of restraint mechanisms. More studies are needed to clarify this hypothesis in the human being.

Hamartomas of the tuber cinereum should not be approached surgically except in unusual circumstances. Although there are cases in which removal of a hypothalamic hamartoma has led to reversal of the pubertal process,[887, 1705, 1716] deaths have been reported after attempted operative removal.[887] Long-term follow-up of the hypothalamic hamartomas associated with true precocious puberty demonstrated lack of growth on monitoring with periodic CT or MRI scans.[889, 1686, 1717] The precocious sexual development can be controlled by treatment with LHRH agonist therapy.[1686, 1718, 1719] Accordingly, although some have advocated neurosurgical removal of these hamartomas,[1720, 1721] we do not recommend neurosurgical extirpation in the absence of strong evidence of growth of the mass or of an associated complication such as intractable seizures or hydrocephalus.[871, 875, 889, 1721–1723]

Central Nervous System Neoplasms

Sexual precocity may be the first manifestation of a hypothalamic tumor of any cell type when it arises in or impinges on the posterior hypothalamus. However, neurologic symptoms such as headaches and visual disturbances may develop, and children may have diabetes insipidus, hydrocephalus, or optic atrophy caused by an enlarging tumor.[871, 1654]

The location of CNS tumors causing true precocious puberty makes surgical removal difficult. A conservative approach calls for biopsy of the neoplasm and radiation therapy or chemotherapy or both, depending on the pathologic findings.

Other Central Nervous System Conditions

True precocious puberty may be secondary to encephalitis, static cerebral encephalopathy, hydrocephalus, brain abscess, or sarcoid granulomas or tuberculous granulomas of the hypothalamus, with or without tuberculous meningitis.[1080, 1724, 1725] Central precocious puberty can occur after severe head trauma[1726] (usually in girls), and it has been associated with the cerebral atrophy or focal encephalomalacia following cerebral edema complicating the treatment of severe diabetic ketoacidosis.[1727] Children with nontumor hydrocephalus, even if shunted, experience earlier pubertal development, and those who have not been adequately treated may develop true precocious puberty.[398, 871, 1724, 1728] Delayed puberty is an alternative outcome in a minority of affected children.[1079] The growth pattern of children with severe hydrocephalus often includes poor prepubertal growth and an early pubertal growth spurt leading to decreased final height.[1729]

Arachnoid cysts arising de novo, after infection, or after surgery can cause premature sexual development, possibly with associated GH deficiency.[463, 871, 1730] Head nodding, abnormal gait, and abnormalities of visual fields are reported in 30% to 40% of cases. Erosion or enlargement of the sella turcica into a J shape may occur. Decompression and extirpation of a suprasellar arachnoid cyst can reverse the sexual precocity[463, 1731, 1732] (see Fig. 24–36).

Neurofibromatosis type 1 (von Recklinghausen's disease) is associated with a propensity to develop the optic chiasmal tumors that are the most common[1733] but not the only[1734] cause for development of true precocious puberty in a child with neurofibromatosis. The prevalence of optic gliomas in neurofibromatosis type 1 is about 17%, most appearing in the first decade, but only about 20% to 30% become symptomatic; these tumors rarely progress in the years after diagnosis.[786, 1733, 1735, 1736] The tumor suppressor *NF1* gene located on the long arm of chromosome 17 (q11.2), which has a high mutation rate, encodes a 327-kd protein, neurofibromin, which is widely expressed, even though neurofibromatosis type 1 involves mainly tissues derived from the neural crest.[1737–1739] A wide variety of mutations of the gene have been reported, especially deletions and nonsense and truncating mutations distributed over the coding region of the *NF1* gene.[1736] In sporadic cases, the new mutation originates in the paternally derived *NF1* allele in the vast majority of instances, which suggests a role for genomic imprinting.[1740]

Neurofibromatosis type 1 is characterized by multiple pigmented areas and overgrowth of nerve sheaths and fibrous tissue elements (Fig. 24–64).[1055, 1056, 1741, 1742] Multiple café-au-lait spots are frequent and are smoother in outline than those of the McCune-Albright syndrome. The diagnosis is made if two or more of the following are observed: (1) six or more café-au-lait macules, the greatest diameter of which is more than 5 mm in prepubertal and more than 12.5 mm in postpubertal subjects; (2) two or more neurofibromas of any type or one plexiform neurofibroma; (3) freckling in the axilla or inguinal region; (4) optic glioma; (5) two or more iris Lisch nodules (ophthalmic hamartomas); (6) a distinctive osseous lesion such as sphenoid dysplasia or pseudoarthrosis; and (7) a first-degree relative with neurofibromatosis type 1 according to the preceding criteria.[1736, 1742, 1743]

Neurofibromas of the skin in neurofibromatosis may be subcutaneous sessile or deep plexiform masses in children; pedunculated lesions develop in later childhood. Internal neurofibromas cause most of the complications. Bone abnormalities such as cysts and pseudoarthrosis, hemihypertrophy, bowing, scoliosis, and skull and facial defects are common (20%); dumbbell-shaped tumors of spinal nerve roots may cause pain, sensory and motor dysfunction, and bone erosions; gliomas or neurofibromas of any part of the CNS, including the optic nerves and hypothalamus, may calcify. Lisch nodules of the iris are frequent, particularly in adults.[1736, 1743] Sarcomatous degeneration occurs in 5% to 15% of patients. Other neoplasms include CNS astrocytomas often involving the visual pathways, ependymomas, meningiomas, neurofibrosarcomas, rhabdomyosarcomas, and nonlymphocytic leukemias.[1744] Pheochromocytoma may develop in affected adults.

The clinical manifestations of neurofibromatosis include seizures, visual defects, and either delayed or true precocious puberty.[1741] Mental retardation occurs more often in this population but is usually not severe[1745]; there is also an increased incidence of psychiatric disease.[1746] Most affected children have some manifestations of the disease by 1 year of age.[1055, 1056, 1739, 1741, 1742] Screening MRI scans are recommended for early detection of CNS tumors.

Other CNS abnormalities associated with true precocious puberty but without demonstrable lesions on imaging study include epilepsy,[1664] laughing seizures,[1747] mental retardation, and the post-traumatic state.[1748] Septo-optic dysplasia (described earlier) may be associated not only with multiple pituitary hormone deficiencies and delayed puberty but also rarely with true precocious puberty.[1087, 1695, 1749] Thus, there may be coexisting deficiencies of some pituitary hormones and excessive secretion of others, including prolactin.[1750] Patients with myelomeningocele (myelodysplasia) have an increased prevalence of endocrine abnormalities, including hypothalamic hypothyroidism, hyperprolactinemia, and elevated gonadotropin concentrations, that in some patients are associated with true precocious puberty.[901, 1099]

True Precocious Puberty in Children Adopted from Developing Countries[1751]

An increased prevalence of true precocious puberty occurred in children (with established birth dates) from developing countries adopted after 3 years of age into families in Sweden and in children referred after kwashiorkor prior to 3 years of age,[1323, 1752] as well as in The Netherlands, France, and Italy.[1753] A hypothesis involving the primary role of recovery from nutritional deprivation has been challenged. In a retrospective study of true precocious puberty from Belgium, 28% (39 girls, 1 boy) were foreign children who had emigrated from developing countries. A toxicologic screen found a greatly elevated mean concentration of the organochlorine pesticide dichlorodiphenyltrichloroethane (DDT) derivative *p,p'*-dichlorodiphenyldichloroethylene (*p,p'*-DDE), which raised the possibility of a role of endocrine disrupters.[1753] The etiology is not established but may be related to the effects of undernutrition or its rapid repair during a sensitive time in development. In Sweden, the adopted Indian children had pubertal growth spurts similar to those of Swedish children, but the loss of height in childhood and the early puberty appeared to be responsible for a decrease in adult height.[1323, 1324, 1754] Use of a GnRH agonist in addition to GH treatment increased the final height of a group of affected children.[1755]

True Precocious Puberty after Virilizing Disorders

If a virilizing condition has been long-standing, correction of the virilization may be followed by development of true precocious puberty with activation of the hypothalamic–pituitary gonadotropin–gonadal system. This phenomenon, secondary true precocious puberty, occurred in boys and girls with congenital virilizing adrenal hyperplasia in whom glucocorticoid replacement therapy was begun after age 4 to 8 and who had an advanced bone age.[224, 675, 945, 1756] True precocious puberty has also been documented in children who received or were exposed to androgens or estrogens for long periods during early childhood for a variety of conditions.

Management of True Precocious Puberty

The objectives in the management and therapy of true precocious puberty are summarized in Table 24–38, which addresses the major psychosocial and clinical goals.[1722] (Psychosocial issues must be dealt with to provide optimal management for affected children.[1673]) Three principal agents have been used in the treatment of true precocious puberty whether idiopathic or neurologic: medroxyprogesterone acetate, cyproterone acetate, and superactive LHRH agonists.

Medroxyprogesterone and cyproterone reversed or arrested the progression of secondary sexual characteristics but had no apparent effect or a small effect on final height, especially in affected girls.[1330, 1653, 1655, 1656] This failure may be due in part to the disproportionate action of the small amount of circulating estradiol on skeletal growth relative to its effect on secondary sexual characteristics. In any event, in none of the early studies with medroxyprogesterone or cyproterone was the concentration of plasma estradiol in girls and of testosterone in boys

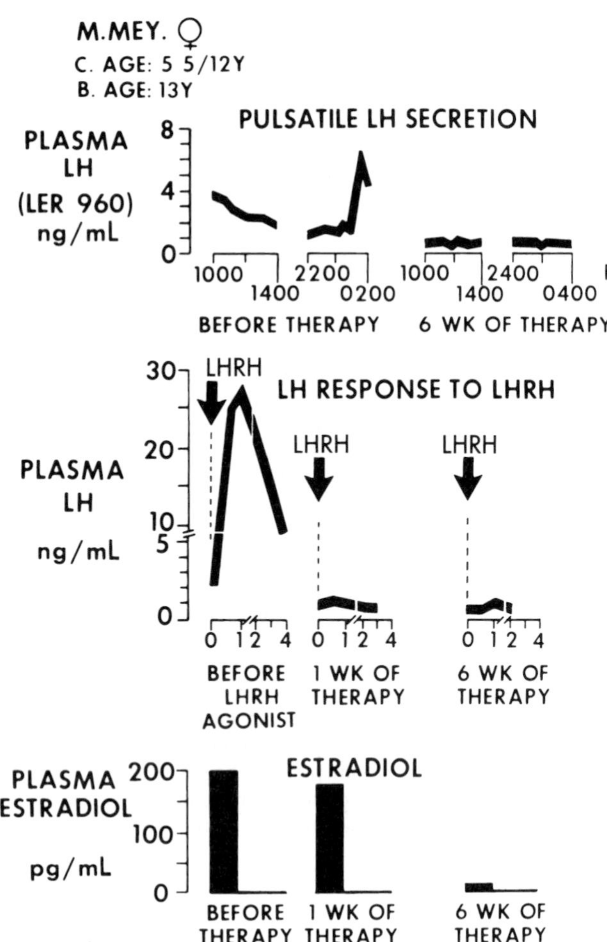

Figure 24–65. Effect of administration of the luteinizing hormone–releasing hormone (LHRH) agonist deslorelin (4 μg/kg/day subcutaneously) on pulsatile secretion of LH *(top)*, LH response to LHRH *(middle)*, and plasma concentration of estradiol *(bottom)* in a 5 1/12-year-old girl with idiopathic true precocious puberty. This patient, who had a bone age of 13 years when treatment was begun, has been administered deslorelin for 7 years. During this period, the estimated predicted final height increased by 15 cm. Surprisingly, the bone age advanced by only about 6 months on serial examinations for several years. For conversion to SI units, see the legend of Figure 24–17. (Modified from Grumbach MM, Kaplan SL. Recent advances in the diagnosis and management of sexual precocity. Acta Paediatr Jpn 1988; 30[suppl]:155–175.)

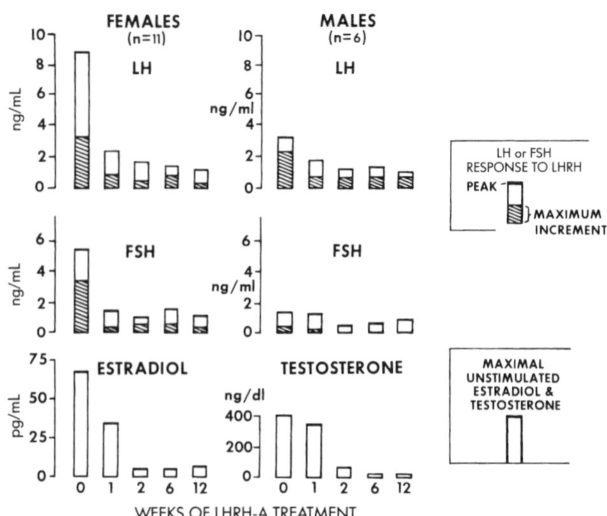

Figure 24–66. Deslorelin treatment (4 μg/kg/day subcutaneously) of girls and boys with true precocious puberty: effect during the first 12 weeks of treatment on the luteinizing hormone (LH) and follicle-stimulating hormone (FSH) response to a challenge with LH-releasing hormone (LHRH) (mean peak response and maximum increment) and on the maximal unstimulated concentration of plasma estradiol in the girls and of plasma testosterone in the boys. Note the relatively rapid change from pubertal values to prepubertal values. For conversion to SI units, see the legends of Figures 24–17 and 24–18. (From Styne DM, Harris DA, Egli CA, et al. Treatment of true precocious puberty with a potent luteinizing hormone releasing factor agonist: effect on growth, sexual maturation, pelvic sonography, and the hypothalamic pituitary gonadal axis. J Clin Endocrinol Metab 1985; 61:142–181. © by The Endocrine Society.)

therapy starting before 6 years of age than after 8 years of age[1794, 1795]; the age that is optimal for discontinuation of therapy is still open to question as the post-treatment growth spurt is important in determining adult height.[1796, 1797] The remaining challenge is the rapid diagnosis of central precocious puberty and early initiation of GnRH therapy if final height is to be preserved.

Children with true precocious puberty have higher mean concentrations of circulating IGF-I for chronologic age, consistent with the increased secretion of gonadal steroids and comparable to the typical elevated IGF-I levels of normal puberty. The IGF-I concentration correlates best with the stage of puberty and the plasma concentration of testosterone or estradiol.[209] Treatment with LHRH agonists reduces the level of IGF-I to the normal range for bone age but not for chronologic age.[209] This indicates that gonadal steroids increase plasma IGF-I concentrations in true precocious puberty as well as in normal puberty. Secretion of GH is increased in true precocious puberty to a level comparable to that in normal puberty.[192, 193] Treatment with LHRH agonists usually results in a decrease in GH secretion, most strikingly during sleep, and in a decrease in GH response to provocative stimuli. It is suggested that the serum concentration of GH and GH-BP activity better reflect the suppression of growth velocity with LHRH agonist than serum IGF-I and IGF-BP-3.[1798, 1799] The reason for the fall in GH secretion is unclear, but it may involve both a decrease in plasma gonadal steroid levels and an increase in BMI.

The serum concentrations of the propeptide of type III procollagen in normal puberty and in true precocious puberty parallel the normal pubertal growth curve. Serum levels of the propeptide of type III procollagen also parallel the changes in growth rate in children treated with LHRH agonists.

When used chronically, LHRH agonists induce a pharmacologic gonadectomy with reversion to a prepubertal level of gonadal steroid output. The use of depot formulations of LHRH agonists provides continuous exposure to the agonist with a single intramuscular injection every 4 weeks and minimizes the problem of compliance.[1229, 1511, 1649, 1800, 1801] However, irregular or inadequate treatment or poor compliance results in persistent or intermittent increases in the concentrations of plasma gonadal steroids. Regular assessment is essential, initially at intervals of 1 to 3 months. Such assessment involves periodic determinations of plasma testosterone levels in boys and estradiol levels in girls; the change in basal concentrations of LH and FSH in third-generation assays or the LH and FSH response to exogenous LHRH; measurement of growth, bone age, and secondary sexual characteristics; and in girls serial evaluations of ovarian morphology and uterine size by pelvic sonography. Although the urinary excretion of LH correlates with the stage of pubertal development in normal individuals, urinary gonadotropin determinations are not sufficiently sensitive to be used for monitoring purposes.[1385] A

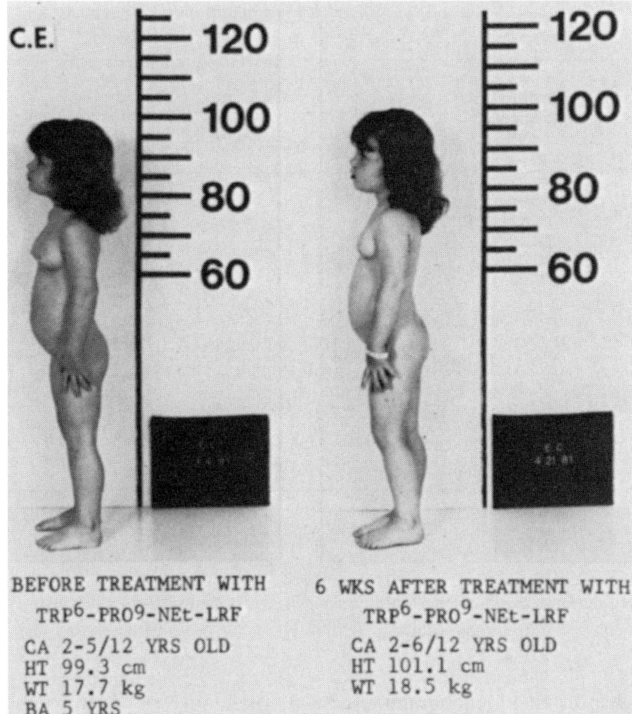

Figure 24–67. A 2 5/12-year-old girl with true precocious puberty after 6 weeks of deslorelin therapy (4 μg/day subcutaneously). Note the regression in the size of the breasts; however, the rapid rate of growth had not decreased. At the end of 1 year of therapy, growth rate was suppressed to 4 cm/year, and bone age advanced only 1 year. CA, chronologic age; HT, height; WT, weight; BA, bone age. (From Styne DM, Grumbach MM. Puberty in the male and female: its physiology and disorders. In Yen SCC, Jaffe RB [eds]. Reproductive Endocrinology, 2nd ed. Philadelphia, WB Saunders, 1986, pp 313–384.)

decrease in the size of ovaries and uterus on pelvic sonography occurs with successful treatment with LHRH agonist.[1718, 1802] Regularly scheduled visits also provide the opportunity for continued counseling.

Increasing numbers of patients are now completing treatment after years of therapy, and the return of gonadal function has been assessed. In 46 girls treated for at least 2 years who completed therapy at a mean age of 11 years, menarche occurred at a mean age of 12.1 years, which represents an average of 1.2 years after discontinuing therapy. Ovulation occurred in 50% of girls 1 year after menarche and in 90% of those studied 2 or more years after menarche.[1803] Spontaneous menses occurred at a mean of 18 months in another follow-up study after LHRH agonist therapy ceased with a range of 0 to 60 months.[1804] This pattern is quite similar to that of normal pubertal maturation. There is no delay in the development of the hypothalamic-pituitary axis in girls with true precocious puberty treated with LHRH agonist therapy.[1805] Reports on boys with true precocious puberty after LHRH therapy was discontinued confirm the reversible nature of the therapy. Gonadotropins in the basal or LHRH-stimulated state return to normal pubertal values by 1 year after cessation of therapy.[1719] However, testicular size may take longer to reach normal values.

The criteria for treatment of patients with true precocious puberty are listed in Table 24–42. Therapy is not indicated if a pubertal pattern of pulsatile LH secretion during sleep is not present or if the LH response to exogenous LHRH is prepubertal. Before beginning treatment, it is essential to establish the rapidly progressive nature of the sexual precocity.[1669, 1792] Girls without a reduced height potential do not require LHRH agonist therapy to ensure an appropriate final height outcome; these girls tend to have lower serum IGF-I and estradiol concentrations and may have fewer signs of estrogenization.[1806, 1807] The most severely affected girls are the ones who respond best to LHRH agonist therapy.[1792, 1808] In a subset of girls, the tempo is relatively slow and the sexual precocity may not be sustained.[871, 1774, 1809] The growth rate slows to normal for age, skeletal maturation progresses in accordance with chronologic age, and there is little to no risk of impairment of final height. In some girls, we have observed within a 1- to 2-month period the return of a pubertal pattern of LH pulsatility during sleep, of a pubertal LH response to LHRH,

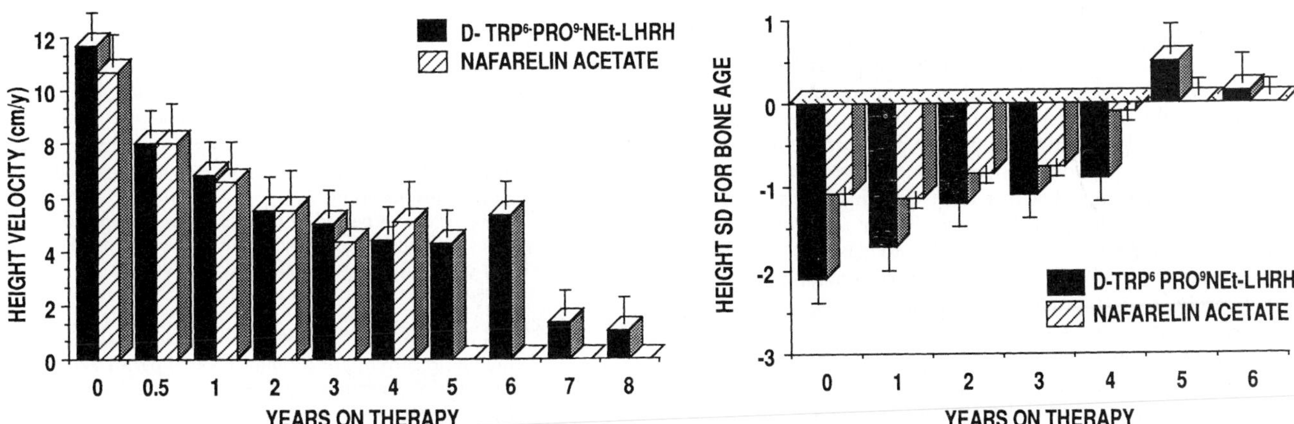

Figure 24–68. Effect of luteinizing hormone–releasing hormone (LHRH) agonist therapy in true precocious puberty on growth. *Left,* Changes in mean height velocity (cm/year ± 1 SE) after the initiation of LHRH agonist therapy with DTrp^{6}Pro^{9}Net (LHRH) (deslorelin) *(filled bars)* or with nafarelin *(hatched bars).* A sharp decrease in height velocity occurred within 1 year. *Right,* Mean (±1 SE) height for bone age before and during LHRH agonist treatment. The discrepancy between height and the more advanced bone age decreases (reverts to normal) with chronic LHRH agonist treatment. (From Kaplan SL, Grumbach MM. True precocious puberty: treatment with GnRH agonists. In Delemarre-Van de Waal H, Plant TM, van Rees GP, et al [eds]. Control of the Onset of Puberty III. Amsterdam, Elsevier, 1989, pp 357–373.)

Table 24–41. Comparison of Current Height (Final or Near Final) and Height Gain of Luteinizing Hormone–Releasing Hormone Agonist–Treated Patients

	No. of Patients	Mean Current Ht (cm)		Mean Ht Gain (cm)[a]
		Female	Male	
Untreated[b]				
Total	116	152.7 ± 8.6	155.6 ± 7.7	
<5 yr	41	150.2 ± 7.6	153.3 ± 7.1	
>5 yr	75	153.4 ± 8.4	161.3 ± 6.0	
LHRH-treated[d]				
UCSF	26	160.5 ± 6.6	166.3 ± 12.2	
<5 yr[c]	11	164.3 ± 7.7	172.1	10.0 (female); 11.1 (male)
>5 yr[c]	15	157.6 ± 6.6	163.3 ± 13.0	4.0 (female); 6.0 (male)
Ref.				
Oerter[2138]	40	157.8 ± 5.9	168.8 ± 8.3	5.2 (female), 6.7 (male)
Kaull[1790]	8	151.2 ± 5.9		5.8 (female)
Boepple[2139]	26	154.4		4.1 (female)

[a]Final predicted height − initial predicted height (Bayley-Pinneau method).
[b]Final height.
[c]CA at start of therapy.
[d]Final or nearly final height.
From Paul D, Conte FA, Grumbach MM, Kaplan SL. Long-term effect of gonadotropin-releasing hormone agonist therapy on final and near-final height in 26 children with true precocious puberty treated at a median age of less than 5 years. J Clin Endocrinol Metab 1995; 80:546–551.

and of the concentration of plasma estradiol to a pubertal state; unlike the typical patients, such girls do not exhibit the initial hyperresponse of plasma estradiol and LH to the LHRH agonist. Many girls in this subset have clinical and hormonal features that fall between those of premature thelarche and true precocious puberty and are typical of neither condition,[1810] so-called exaggerated thelarche.

About 10% of girls with apparently classical premature thelarche progress to definite true precocious puberty with no signs at the time of first presentation to differentiate them from girls who continued with the pattern of premature thelarche; in the majority in this situation, the onset of breast development is noted after 2 years of age.[1811] Psychosocial factors and parental anxiety that adversely affect the well-being of the child need to be assessed in the decision to initiate LHRH agonist treatment.

Adverse Effects

Untoward reactions to LHRH agonists in the treatment of true precocious puberty have so far been minimal but include local and systemic allergic reactions in a few patients, including asthmatic episodes when the agent is given intranasally. However, the prevalence of a sterile abscess at the site of intramuscular injection of long-acting repository preparations, including leuprorelin and triptorelin, is clearly increased (5% to 10%), unpredictable, and intermittent and in most instances is related to the polylactic and polyglycotic polymer and not to the LHRH agonist itself.[1781, 1812] Switching to daily subcutaneous injections or to intranasal administration of nondepot preparations is rarely associated with a recurrence.

When treatment is discontinued, even after 8 years, the gonadal suppression is reversed within a few weeks to months with a rise in the concentration of plasma gonadal steroids, progression of sexual maturation, and return of menses.[1789, 1804, 1813] A small increase in serum prolactin above normal limits, but not galactorrhea, has been described in girls following treatment with LHRH agonist.[1814] Areal BMD, but not volumetric bone, is increased in children with central precocious puberty.[1815] Although a decrease in bone density has been reported in LHRH agonist–treated patients,[311] later studies indicated that volumetric BMD and peak bone mass are normal during and after discontinuation of LHRH therapy.[310, 1789, 1815] Despite these encouraging results, one must be alert to the possible emergence of unforeseen long-term side effects. Four patients developed slipped capital femoral epiphyses during or just after treatment of central precocious puberty with LHRH agonist.[1816]

LHRH agonists are effective in both boys and girls with idiopathic true precocious puberty, the androgen-induced form of secondary true precocious puberty after therapy for virilizing congenital adrenal hyperplasia with glucocorticoids, and organic or neurogenic forms of true precocious puberty associated with hamartomas of the tuber cinereum, hypothalamic neoplasms, and other CNS lesions.[1718, 1770, 1818] Although there are reports in the literature of surgical removal of hamartomas of the tuber cinereum,[888, 1705, 1716, 1819–1822] the ease of medical treatment of the sexual precocity associated with this congenital malformation, the finding that the mass does not enlarge on MRI or CT brain scans, and the risks of an adverse outcome of surgical intervention in this region of the CNS[888]

Table 24–42. Indications for Therapy with Luteinizing Hormone–Releasing Hormone Agonists in True or Central Precocious Puberty

In children with clinical and unequivocal endocrine features of idiopathic true precocious puberty:
- Rapid advancement over a period of 6 mo to 1 yr of secondary sex characteristics, height, height velocity, and bone age (increased >2.5 SD for chronologic age) in affected boys and girls
- A plasma testosterone concentration sustained >2.5 nmol/L (>75 ng/dL) in boys younger than 8 yr of age determined by sensitive, specific immunoassay
- A plasma estradiol, recurrently ≥36 pmol/L (≥10 pg/mL) determined by a sensitive, specific assay capable of quantifying low concentrations of estradiol
- Onset of menarche (and recurrent menses) in girls younger than 9 yr of age
- Psychosocial factors and parental anxiety, including evidence that the child's psychosocial well-being is adversely affected
- In children with neurogenic or organic true precocious puberty, especially those with associated GH deficiency, the course is almost invariably progressive and LHRH treatment should not be delayed

Table 24–43. Potential Use of Aromatase Inhibitors or Estrogen Receptor Antagonists to Restrain Skeletal Maturation in Disorders of Growth and Sexual Maturation

Growth disorders or variants of normal growth (to restrain epiphyseal maturation)
Isolated growth hormone deficiency
Genetic short stature/constitutional delay in growth
Sexual precocity
Congenital virilizing adrenal hyperplasia in male and female
To reduce dose of glucocorticoid
To inhibit conversion of C19 steroids to estrogens (or estrogen action)
With/without use of C17/20 lyase inhibitor or anti-androgen
Testotoxicosis
To inhibit conversion of C19 steroids to estrogens
McCune-Albright syndrome
To inhibit conversion of C19 steroids to estrogens (or estrogen action)
Adolescent gynecomastia
To inhibit estrogen synthesis (or estrogen action)

From Grumbach MM. Estrogen, bone, growth, and sex: a sea change in conventional wisdom. J Pediatr Endocrinol Metab 2000; 13(suppl 6):1439–1455.

support the choice of LHRH agonists over surgical intervention.

The LHRH agonists are useful in conjunction with GH in the management of organic or neurogenic true precocious puberty, especially when associated with GH deficiency (usually as a result of radiation of the brain). Such a regimen allows a longer period of GH treatment before epiphyseal fusion.[1606] As the course of neurogenic true precocious puberty is almost invariably progressive, after appropriate evaluation of the tempo of puberty, it is advisable to initiate LHRH agonist treatment. A few, usually short-term, studies utilized GH and LHRH agonist in short normal children or those with intrauterine growth retardation in an attempt to increase final height. Some, but not all, studies suggest that an increase in predicted final height is possible. This regimen is experimental; its cost-effectiveness needs to be considered (see the earlier section considering the hormonal control of the pubertal growth spurt).[1023, 1024, 1572, 1823–1827] On the other hand, the combination of LHRH agonist and GH is useful for increasing final height in GH-deficient patients of pubertal age.[1828]

An aromatase inhibitor, such as letrozole, decreases or eliminates the effect of estrogen on bone age advancement. This effect may be useful to improve height prognosis in sexual precocity in boys.[172, 173] Controlled studies are necessary to establish safety and efficacy (Table 24–43).

Psychosocial Aspects

Psychological management is a critical aspect of the care of children with true precocious puberty.[875, 1585, 1722, 1817] With the advanced physical maturation for chronologic age, they tend to seek friends closer to their size, strength, and physical development. Difficulties may arise because they lack the social skills of older children. Sex education of the child and the family is essential and must be given in a skillful, sensitive, and explicit manner; the risks of sexual abuse in both sexes and of pregnancy in girls need to be discussed. The parents need to be informed about the management of menses. The onset of sexual activity may be earlier than average but generally remains within the normal range.[1671]

It is imperative to provide support in handling the increased height, advanced sexual maturation, and effects of gonadal steroids on behavior, activity, and emotional stability. The unrealistic demands and expectations that arise from the discrepancy between the physique and the chronologic, mental, and psychosexual age require wise counseling, as do the reaction to ridicule by peers and the concern about being different from age mates. Some of these problems have been mitigated by school acceleration, advancing the child one or two grades, if this is consistent with the mental and emotional development. These comments are applicable to children with all forms of sexual precocity. The effectiveness of LHRH agonists has reduced but not eliminated many of these issues in true precocious puberty.[1722]

Incomplete Form of Isosexual Precocity: Luteinizing Hormone–Releasing Hormone–Independent Sexual Precocity

In this group of disorders, the secretion of testosterone in boys and of estrogen in girls is independent of the hypothalamic LHRH pulse generator (see Table 24–32). Affected individuals do not exhibit a pubertal-type LH response to administration of LHRH or a pubertal pattern of pulsatile LH secretion, nor do they respond to chronic administration of an LHRH agonist with suppression of gonadal steroid output. Incomplete isosexual precocity or precocious pseudopuberty is a consequence of gonadal or adrenal steroid secretion independent of LHRH, of iatrogenic exposure to gonadal steroids, or, in boys, of rare hCG- or LH-secreting tumors.

Boys

Chorionic Gonadotropin-Secreting Tumors

Several types of germ cell tumors can secrete a glycoprotein hormone that has the bioactivity of LH or hCG and can cross-react in some polyclonal LH radioimmunoassay systems. Studies using highly specific antisera to the β subunit of hCG, however, confirm that the gonadotropin is hCG. Boys with these hCG-secreting neoplasms may have slightly enlarged testes (although not usually to a size consonant with the size of the phallus and other male secondary sex characteristics) and may be difficult to differentiate from boys with true precocious puberty on the basis of physical examination alone.[871, 1829, 1830] However, plasma hCG levels are elevated without an increase in the concentration of FSH or LH.[1829] Hepatomas and hepatoblastomas are among the most serious of these tumors and cause firm, irregular nodular or smooth hepatic enlargement (Fig. 24–69). The hCG has been localized to the multinucleated tumor giant cells; in one case, α-fetoprotein was found in the embryonal-type tumor cells spread throughout the hepatoblastoma.[1831] The average survival is only 10.7 months after diagnosis; the mean age at onset is 2 years, 8 months.[1830–1833]

Some teratomas, chorioepitheliomas, or mixed germ cell tumors in the hypothalamic region (or in the mediastinum, the lungs, the gonads, or the retroperitoneum) and certain hypothalamic pineal tumors (usually a germ cell tumor or mixed germ cell tumor,[1829, 1834, 1835] less commonly a chorioepithelioma or its variants) cause sexual precocity in boys by secreting hCG rather than by activating the hypothalamic LHRH pulse generator and the pituitary gonadotropin–gonadal axis.[1829] The prevalence of hCG-secreting embryonal neoplasms, especially of the mediastinum, is increased in boys with 47,XXY or mosaic Klinefelter's syndrome. About 20% of mediastinal germ cell tumors occur in boys with Klinefelter's syndrome, a prevalence 30 to 50 times that in unaffected boys.[1359, 1836, 1837] Plasma α-fetoprotein is a useful additional marker for yolk sac (endodermal sinus) or mixed germ cell tumors[1838]; the cells in the tumor that secrete α-fetoprotein appear to differ from those that secrete hCG. Intracranial germ cell tumors are 2.6 times more common in males than females[1839]; in females, germ cell tumors do not cause gonadotropin-induced isosexual precocity because of the paucity of

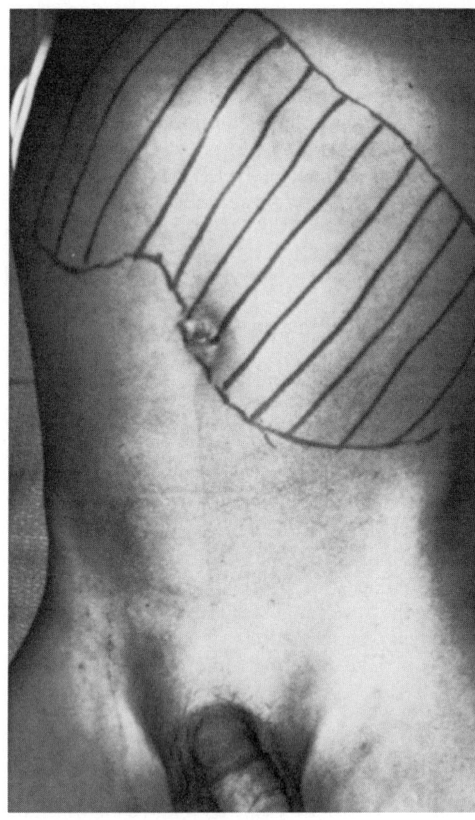

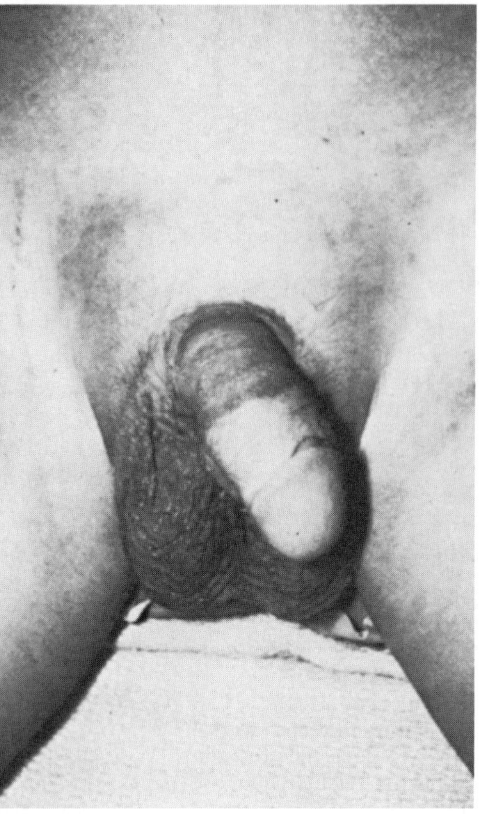

Figure 24–69. A 1 5/12-year-old boy with a human chorionic gonadotropin (hCG)–secreting hepatoblastoma. Note the outline of the large liver *(left)* and the penile enlargement *(right)*. The testes were 2 × 1 cm, and pubic hair was stage 2. The plasma hCG level was 50 mIU/mL; plasma testosterone 168 ng/dL; and plasma α-fetoprotein 160,000 ng/mL. Metastatic lesions in both lungs were seen on the radiograph of the chest. To convert testosterone values to SI units, see the legend of Figure 24–17. To convert hCG values to international units per liter, multiply by 1.0. To convert α-fetoprotein values to micrograms per liter, multiply by 1.0. (From Kaplan SL, Grumbach MM. Pathogenesis of sexual precocity. In Grumbach MM, Sizonenko PC, Aubert ML [eds]. Control of the Onset of Puberty. Baltimore, Williams & Wilkins, 1990, pp 620–660. © 1990, the Williams & Wilkins Co., Baltimore.)

effects of hCG in prepubertal females. However, they can cause true precocious puberty through disinhibition of the hypothalamic LHRH pulse generator by local effects; rarely, the germ cells contain sufficient aromatase activity to convert circulating C_{19} precursors (of adrenal origin after adrenarche) to estradiol, which in some instances is sufficient to induce breast development.[1050, 1840–1842]

"True" pure CNS germ cell tumors (germinomas) secrete insufficient hCG to be readily detectable in the circulation, but in some patients hCG can be detected in the cerebrospinal fluid.[1048] In mixed germ cell tumors, on the other hand, hCG is commonly present in the blood as well as in cerebrospinal fluid.

In children, germ cell tumors in the suprasellar-hypothalamic region do not exhibit a sex predominance and are generally associated with pituitary hormone deficiencies including diabetes insipidus.[1048] Germ cell tumors that secrete hCG are rarely located in the thalamus and basal ganglia. Intracranial germ cell tumors account for 3% to 11% of malignant CNS tumors in children and adolescents, with a predominance in the Far East.[1843, 1844] Germ cell tumors of the hypothalamus or pineal region constitute less than 1% of primary CNS tumors in Western countries but account for 4.5% of such tumors in Japan.[1845] Mixed germ cell tumors and especially pure germinomas are radiosensitive, and regression of sexual precocity may occur if the bone age is less than 11 years, only to progress later into normal puberty.[1829] Long-term survival was reported to be 88% after appropriate therapy.[1846] Calcification of the pineal is found in 8% to 11% of 8- to 11-year-old children and by itself is not indicative of a tumor. Gonadotropin-secreting pituitary adenomas are exceedingly rare in children. An LH- and prolactin-secreting pituitary adenoma caused sexual precocity in two boys.[1845, 1847] The concentration of serum LH was strikingly elevated (900 IU/L) and did not rise further after the administration of LHRH. The elevated serum testosterone (7 nmol/L, 200 ng/dL) and prolactin (215 μg/L) levels and the high concentration of LH fell to prepubertal values after removal of a "chromophobe" adenoma with suprasellar extension.

Precocious Androgen Secretion Caused by Congenital Adrenal Hyperplasia, Virilizing Adrenal Tumor, or Leydig Cell Tumor

Virilizing congenital adrenal hyperplasia caused by a defect in 21-hydroxylation (CYP21, cytochrome $P450_{c21}$ deficiency) leads to elevated androgen concentrations and masculinization and is a common cause of LHRH-independent sexual precocity in boys[1330] (see Chapter 22).[1848] Approximately 75% of patients with $P450_{c21}$ deficiency have salt loss resulting from impaired aldosterone secretion and have low serum sodium and high serum potassium concentrations. Increased plasma concentrations of 17-hydroxyprogesterone, increased levels of urinary 17-ketosteroids and pregnanetriol, and advanced bone age and rapid growth are characteristic. Treatment with glucocorticoids suppresses the abnormal androgen secretion and arrests virilization; treatment with mineralocorticoids, when necessary, corrects the electrolyte imbalance. A rarer form of virilizing adrenal hyperplasia is usually accompanied by hypertension and is caused by 11β-hydroxylase deficiency; the progressive virilization ceases and the blood pressure falls to normal with glucocorticoid therapy.

All forms of congenital adrenal hyperplasia are inherited as autosomal recessive traits.[1330] Virilizing congenital adrenal hyperplasia, if untreated, can cause anovulatory amenorrhea in females and oligospermia in males; with treatment, the infertility is usually corrected (see Chapter 22). Treatment of virilizing congenital adrenal hyperplasia may unmask LHRH-dependent sexual precocity (secondary true precocious puberty) as a consequence of the advanced somatic and presumably hypothalamic maturation because of exposure to androgen before glucocorticoid therapy is initiated.

Virilizing adrenal carcinomas or adenomas secrete large amounts of DHEA and DHEAS and on occasion testosterone. Glucocorticoids do not suppress the increased secretion of adrenal androgens or the urinary excretion of 17-ketosteroids to the normal range for age in carcinoma, but they readily decrease plasma 17-hydroxyprogesterone or 11-deoxycortisol levels and 17-ketosteroid excretion in congenital adrenal hyperplasia. Cushing's syndrome resulting from adrenal carcinoma may cause isosexual precocity and growth failure in boys. Rarely, an adrenal adenoma may produce both testosterone and aldosterone, leading to sexual precocity and hypertension with hypokalemia.[1849]

Adrenal rests, or heterotopic adrenal tissue in the testes, may enlarge with endogenous ACTH stimulation in boys with untreated or inadequately treated virilizing congenital adrenal hyperplasia and may mimic bilateral or unilateral interstitial cell tumors. Rarely, the adrenal rests may lead to massive enlargement of the testes (see Chapter 22). MRI sonography including Doppler flow studies of the testes is useful in defining the extent and nature of the testicular masses. In boys in whom the testicular tumors are unresponsive to glucocorticoid therapy or improved compliance, surgical management including enucleation of the tumor has been useful in preventing further damage to the testes and improving the potential for fertility.[1850] LH receptors have been detected on adrenal or cortical cells.[1851–1854] Although some of the testicular masses may become autonomous, it seems possible that LH stimulation is a factor in some patients.

Infrequently, a Leydig cell tumor in boys is the cause of sexual precocity; unilateral enlargement (often nodular) of the testis usually occurs in this neoplasm (although 5% to 10% are bilateral), in contrast to the usually normal size of both testes for chronologic age in boys with congenital adrenal hyperplasia or a virilizing adrenal tumor.[675, 1855] Of interest, an LH receptor–activating mutation was detected in three boys with a sporadic Leydig cell adenoma (see later).[1856]

Women with a previous history of congenital adrenal hyperplasia or a virilizing tumor may exhibit ovarian hyperandrogenism associated with persistent elevation of LH in spite of successful treatment of their initial virilizing condition in childhood: this is not usually the case in women who have late-onset congenital adrenal hyperplasia.[1857]

Familial or Sporadic Testotoxicosis (Familial Male-Limited Gonadotropin-Independent Sexual Precocity with Premature Leydig Cell and Germ Cell Maturation)

A unique form of sexual precocity in males is pituitary gonadotropin–independent familial premature Leydig cell and germ cell maturation, or testotoxicosis.[1845, 1858–1864] Although it has been recognized as an LHRH-independent form of male isosexual precocity only since 1981, this disorder was described more than 50 years ago. Indeed, Andrew Shenker brought to our attention a report by Stone in 1852.[1865] Affected boys have secondary sexual development with penile enlargement, which may be present at birth,[1859] and bilateral enlargement of testes to the early or midpubertal range, although the testes are often smaller than expected in relation to penile growth and pubertal maturation (Fig. 24–70). The testes show premature Leydig and Sertoli cell maturation and spermatogenesis; in some instances, Leydig cell hyperplasia is present.[1858, 1859, 1861] The rate of linear growth is rapid, skeletal maturation is advanced, and muscular development is prominent. Serum hormone determinations reveal prepubertal basal and LHRH-stimulated gonadotropin concentrations and lack of a pubertal pattern of LH pulsatility, whether measured by immunologic or bioassay techniques[1859] (Table 24–44). In affected boys, plasma testosterone values are in the normal pubertal or adult range with normal clearance of testosterone. The onset of adrenarche and its biochemical marker, serum DHEAS, correlates with bone age rather than chronologic age.

Treatment with an LHRH agonist does not suppress the testicular function or maturation.[1859, 1863] When most untreated affected individuals reach late childhood or early adolescence, fertility is achieved and an adult pattern of LH secretion and response to LHRH is demonstrable[1860]; secondary LHRH-dependent true precocious puberty is superimposed on the substrate of testotoxicosis.[1860, 1861, 1866] In some adults, impaired spermatogenic function is associated with elevated concentrations of plasma FSH.[1860] This disorder, although it occurs sporadically, quite likely as a consequence of a germ line mutation or even a postzygotic one, is inherited as a sex-limited autosomal dominant trait[1860] and probably accounts for the earlier descriptions of "true" precocious puberty in families in which only males were affected. A kindred with nine generations of affected males has been reported[1860]; obligatory female carriers of the trait were unaffected as constitutional activation of the LH receptor on the ovary causes no ill effects.[1860, 1866]

In 1993, Shenker[1867] and Kremer[1868] and their colleagues independently described heterozygous activating mutations of the heterotrimeric Gs protein–coupled LH/CG receptor that in concert transduce the LH/CG signal to the main effector, adenyl cyclase (Fig. 24–71). The receptors for pituitary and placental gonadotropins and TSH belong to a subfamily of the seven-transmembrane-spanning, G protein–coupled receptors. The LH receptor, first cloned from the rat[1869] and pig[1870] and later the human,[1871, 1872] is a glycoprotein of 80 to 90 kd. It is encoded by a gene localized to chromosome 2p21 (the same as the FSH receptor) that spans at least 70 kb and contains 11 exons separated by 10 introns. The large glycosylated amino-terminal extracellular hormone-binding domain of the 701-amino-acid LH/hCG receptor[1872] is encoded by exons 1 to 10. A single exon, the large exon 11, encodes the entire G-linked transmembrane domain with its 7α-helical segments connected by alternating extracellular and intracellular loops, the intracellular domain, and the 3′ untranslated region—almost two thirds of the receptor[1384, 1873–1875] (see Fig. 24–71).

Thirteen constitutively activating heterozygous missense mutations (in over 60 reported patients) all residing within exon 11 have been reported (see Fig. 24–71); six involve the transmembrane helix VI, two involve the flanking third cytoplasmic loop, there is one each in helix V and helix II, and less commonly there are mutations in the first transmembrane helix.[1867, 1868, 1876–1880] Thus, nine mutations are between amino acid residues 542 and 581, suggesting a hot spot. There appears to be a limited repertoire of mutations in American boys, consistent with a founder effect; European pedigrees are more diverse.[1881, 1882] A model of the transmembrane domain of the receptor provides novel suggestions concerning the structural and functional effects of these activating mutations.[1883] Transfected cultured cells with these mutations exhibited increased basal cAMP production in the absence of agonist, observations consistent with a constitutive activating mutation.[1881] The conformational changes in the LH receptor that lead to its constitutive activation have yet to be established, but various possibilities have been considered.[1884] LHRH-dependent puberty usually ensues in adolescence. Infertility related to testicular damage can occur in adult men.[1562, 1860] Inactivating mutations of the LH/CG receptor and their clinical consequences are discussed in Chapter 22.

In one Polish family, the disorder, a mutation of *M298T* in the second transmembrane domain of the LH receptor, led to sexual precocity in one boy but not in the mother, who carried

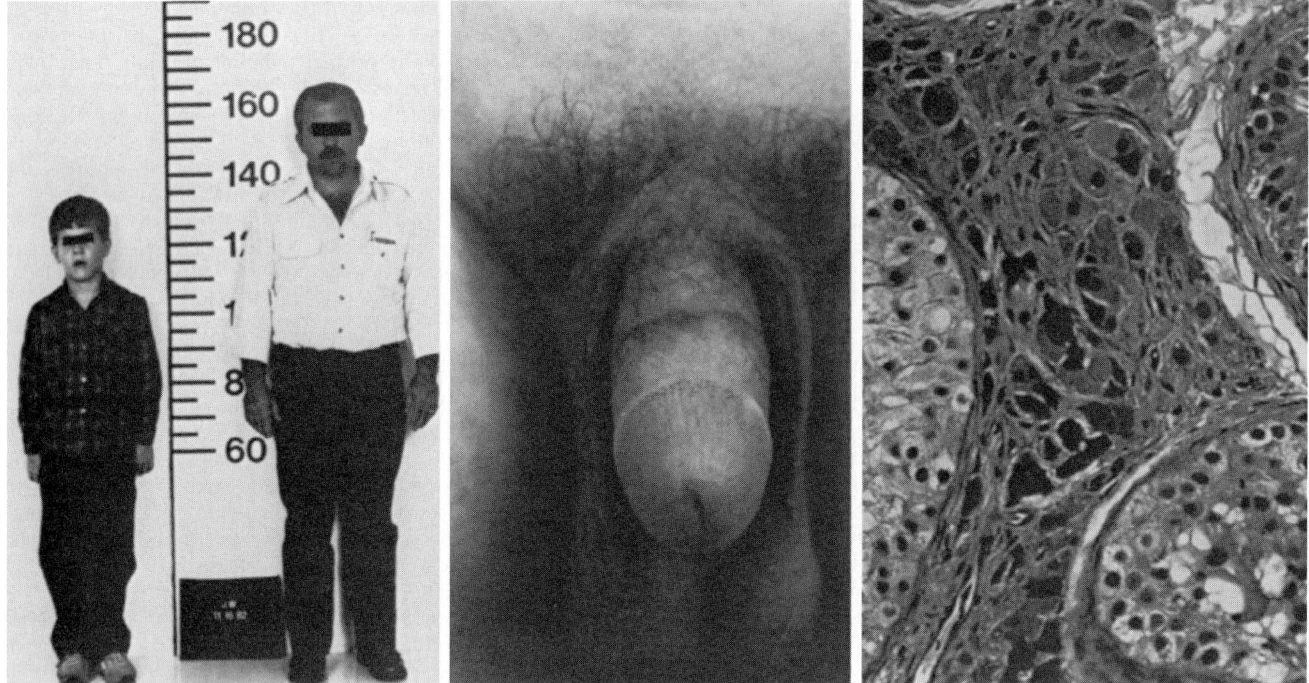

Figure 24–70. Familial testotoxicosis. *Left,* A 5½-year-old boy and his 28-year-old father with the disorder. The boy exhibited signs of sexual precocity by 3 years of age. Height was 130.6 cm (+4.8 SD); bone age 12½ years. The plasma testosterone level was 267 ng/dL; dihydrotestosterone 46 ng/dL; dehydroepiandrosterone sulfate (DHEAS) 23 μg/dL. The plasma luteinizing hormone (LH) and follicle-stimulating hormone (FSH) levels were low, and neither rose after treatment. Pulsatile LH secretion was not demonstrable. Treatment with deslorelin, an LHRH agonist, was without effect. The father had begun sexual maturation by 3 years of age and had reached a final height of 162.6 cm in his early teens. The plasma testosterone level was 294 ng/dL; LH 0.5 ng/mL (LER-960); and FSH 0.5 ng/mL (LER-869). The father had an adult-type LH and FSH response to LHRH; the LH level increased to 7.5 ng/mL, and the FSH level to 2 ng/mL. At least 28 male family members over nine generations are affected. To convert dihydrotestosterone values to nanomoles per liter, multiply by 0.03467. For other conversions to SI units, see the legends of Figures 24–17 and 24–18. *Center,* External genitalia of the 5½-year-old boy. The penis measured 12 × 2.8 cm; the right testis was 4 × 2 cm, and the left testis 3.5 × 2.5 cm. *Right,* Testis of the boy showed Leydig cell maturation without Reinke crystalloids and spermatogenesis (Mallory trichome).

the same mutation, or in her father or his son, the maternal uncle, suggesting the involvement of epigenetic factors.[1885] Three boys with sexual precocity related to a sporadic Leydig cell adenoma had an Asp 578 His mutation in the tumor[710, 1856] (Fig. 24–72).

The remarkable association of testotoxicosis and pseudohypoparathyroidism type Ia due to a mutation in the subunit of Gs is considered in the following. Boys with LHRH-independent, pituitary gonadotropin–independent maturation of the testes do not respond to chronic administration of an LHRH agonist with suppression of testosterone secretion, in contrast to the characteristic response in patients with true precocious puberty.[1859] However, testosterone secretion, height velocity and rate of bone maturation, and aggressive and hyperactive behavior have been decreased by treatment with oral medroxyprogesterone acetate.[875, 1859]

Two other therapies have been used (Table 24–45). Ketoconazole, an orally active substituted imidazole derivative, suppresses gonadal and adrenal biosynthesis at several steps.[1886] At the dosage used in testotoxicosis (200 mg every 8 to 12 hours orally),[1862, 1887] ketoconazole mainly inhibits the enzyme cytochrome $P450_{c17}$, which regulates both 17-hydroxylation and the scission (17,20-lyase) of α-hydroxypregnenolone to dehydroepiandrosterone (see adrenarche in this chapter). However, even at the recommended dose, the agent produces a mild transient decrease in cortisol secretion and interferes with binding of testosterone to TeBG. Secondary true precocious puberty often occurs when the bone age advances to or has already reached the pubertal range (usually > 11.5 years), at which time addition of an LHRH agonist is appropriate.[1862] Ketoconazole can cause hepatic injury, which is usually mild and reversible, but hepatotoxicity is rarely severe.[1886] Further, reversible renal injury, rash, and interstitial pneumonia have been reported in a patient who tolerated lower doses, suggesting a dose-response effect.[1888]

Another therapeutic approach has been the use of the antiandrogen (and antimineralocorticoid) spironolactone combined with testolactone, an inhibitor of cytochrome P450 aro-

Table 24–44. Testotoxicosis: Clinical and Laboratory Characteristics

Sex-limited autosomal dominant inheritance; activating mutation in the gene encoding the LH receptor
Early onset of sexual precocity in boys with bilateral testicular enlargement
Prepubertal immunologic and biologic LH response to LHRH, prepubertal LH pulse secretory pattern
Concentration of plasma testosterone in pubertal range
Premature Leydig cell and seminiferous tubule maturation
No CNS, adrenal, or testicular abnormalities demonstrable by radiologic or hormonal studies
Lack of suppression of plasma testosterone or physical signs of puberty by LHRH agonist

CNS, central nervous system; LH, luteinizing hormone; LHRH, LH-releasing hormone.

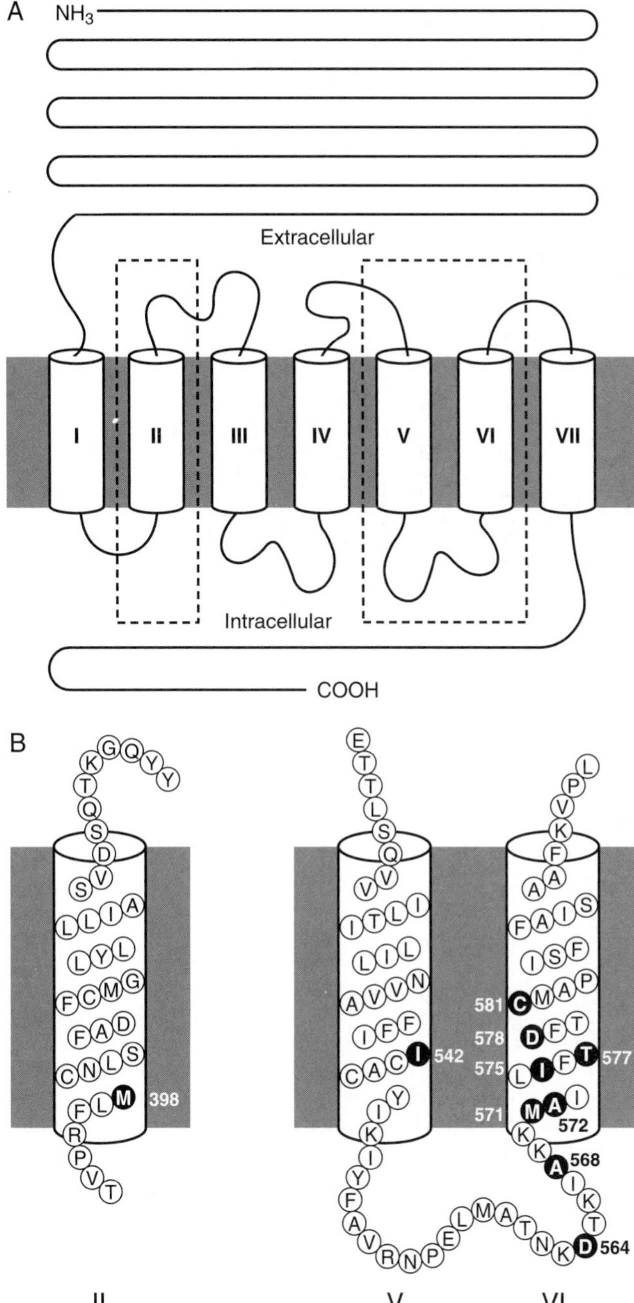

Figure 24–71. *A,* The serpentine seven transmembrane G_s protein coupled hLH/hCG receptor with its large extracellular domain and the intracellular domain. The seven helical transmembrane domains are indicated by Roman numerals. *B,* The two-dimensional seven-transmembrane topology of the hLH/hCG receptor with positions of constitutively activating mutations causing testotoxicosis (male-limited autosomal dominant sexual precocity). The mutations are indicated by solid circles and the residue number. Note the cluster of mutations in the VI transmembrane helix and third cytoplasmic loop. The aspartine 578–glycine mutation is the most common. (Redrawn from Yano K, Kohn LD, Saji M, et al. A case of male limited precocious puberty caused by a point mutation in the second transmembrane domain of the luteinizing hormone choriogonadotropin receptor gene. Biochem Biophys Res Commun 1996; 220:1036–1042.)

matase (CYP19), the key enzyme in the conversion of androgens to estrogens.[1889] Because these boys often experience secondary central precocious puberty after control with spironolactone and testolactone, the addition of an LHRH agonist is a useful step to suppress pituitary gonadotropin secretion.[1890] More potent and specific nonsteroidal antiandrogens such as flutamide and nilutamide[1891] and aromatase inhibitors, such as letrozole[1892, 1893] to inhibit the rate of skeletal maturation and linear growth by suppressing estradiol synthesis, are now available and have potentially greater therapeutic efficacy.[172, 173] Table 24–45 lists the various agents used in the treatment of testotoxicosis; which of these agents or combination of agents will be effective for long-term treatment and safe remains to be determined.

Girls

Incomplete isosexual precocity in girls (see Table 24–32) is caused by conditions in which estrogen is secreted autonomously by an ovarian cyst or tumor, by an adrenal neoplasm, or because of inadvertent exposure to estrogen. In a pure hCG-secreting tumor in girls, signs of isosexual precocity are absent. Girls harboring a teratoma or teratocarcinoma (or a CNS germ cell tumor) that secretes hCG have had sexual precocity caused by concurrent estrogen secretion by the tumor; these girls may also have galactorrhea, especially if chorionic somatomammotropin (human chorionic somatomammotropin, human placental lactogen) is also secreted.

Autonomous Ovarian Follicular Cysts

The most common estrogen-secreting ovarian mass and ovarian cause of sexual precocity is the follicular cyst.[1894] Antral follicles up to about 8 mm in diameter are common in the ovaries of normal prepubertal girls[122, 1895–1897] and may be seen in third-trimester fetuses and newborn infants.[1898–1902] They may appear and regress spontaneously. Large follicular cysts may be discovered because of the presence of an abdominal mass or abdominal pain, especially after torsion or as an unexpected finding on pelvic sonography performed for other reasons. Occasionally, the antral follicles secrete estrogen and may enlarge to form large masses, or the follicular cysts may recur and cause recurrent signs of sexual precocity and acyclic vaginal bleeding.

Enlarged antral follicles or cysts occur in premature thelarche, true precocious puberty, and transient or incomplete sexual precocity.[871, 1689, 1903–1905] With some ovarian follicular cysts, the transient or recurrent sexual precocity is LHRH-independent (Fig. 24–73). The concentration of estradiol fluctuates, usually correlating with changes in the size of the follicular cyst when monitored by pelvic sonography,[1906] and may increase to levels found in a granulosa cell tumor.[492, 871, 1905] The concentration of LH is suppressed, a pubertal pattern of pulsatile LH secretion is absent, and the LH rise induced by LHRH is prepubertal.[871, 1689, 1904, 1905]

It is curious that a constitutive activating mutation of the FSH receptor is undescribed in a female, especially because a heterozygous mutation, Asp 567 Gly, has been detected in the third intracellular loop of the FSH receptor in a hypophysectomized man who, despite the gonadotropin deficiency, was fertile and had normal-sized testes.[1907] This is a site of activating mutations in the LH receptor. Accordingly, the possibility that some girls with recurrent ovarian cysts harbor an activating mutation of the FSH receptor seems worthy of study. The McCune-Albright syndrome needs to be considered in any girl with recurrent ovarian cysts, even with apparent initial absence of other features of this disorder, because of somatic activating mutations in the gene encoding the α subunit of the heterotrimeric Gs protein (see below).

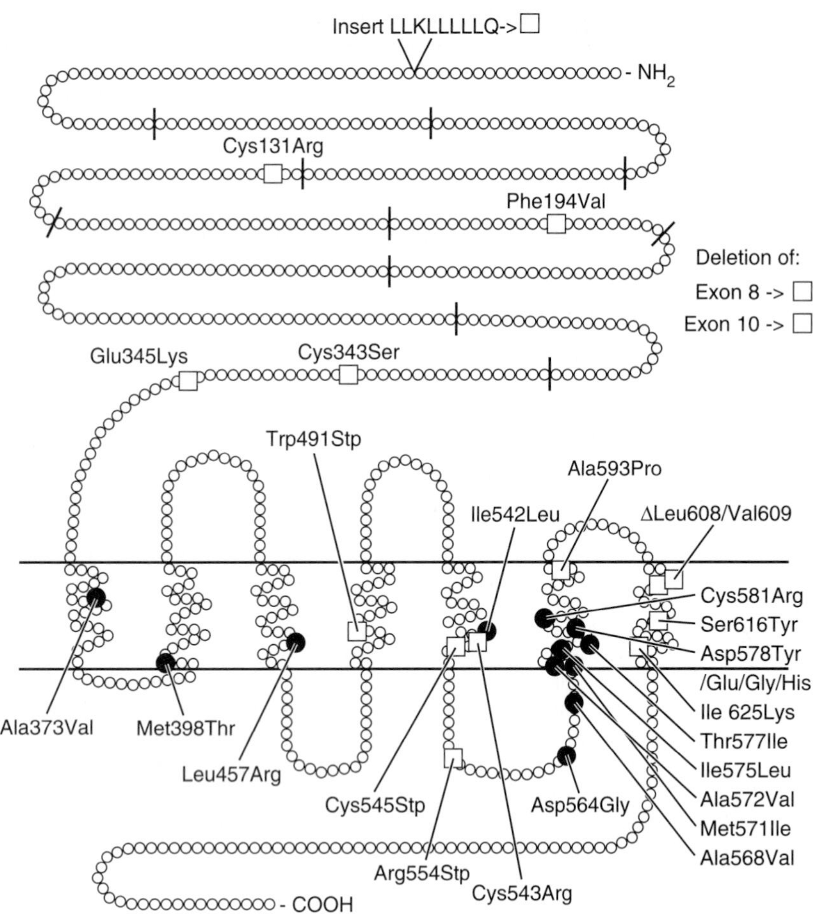

Figure 24–72. Mutations in the luteinizing hormone (LH) receptor protein. Schematic structure of the LH receptor protein and localization of the inactivating (*open squares*) and activating (*filled circles*) mutations currently known in the human LH receptor. The *short lines* across the amino acid chain separate the 11 exons. (From Themmen APN, Huhtaniemi IT. Mutations of gonadotropins and gonadotropin receptors. Endocr Rev 2000;21(5):551–583.)

An unusual syndrome of estradiol-secreting ovarian cysts in preterm infants born before 30 weeks of gestation is associated with edema of the labia majora and, in some instances, of the lower abdominal wall.[1900] In four preterm neonates the syndrome appeared weeks after birth and 1 to 4 weeks before the putative date of a full-term gestation. The follicular cysts, which may be unilateral or bilateral, were detected by abdominal and pelvic sonography. The LH and FSH response to LHRH suggested that the cysts were LHRH-dependent. Treatment with medroxyprogesterone acetate was associated with regression of the cysts. LHRH agonists are useful in the treatment of ovarian follicular cysts associated with true precocious puberty (LHRH-dependent) but not so-called autonomous cysts. However, girls with autonomously functioning

Table 24–45. Pharmacologic Therapy for Sexual Precocity

Disorder	Treatment	Action and Rationale
LHRH dependent		
True or central precocious puberty	LHRH agonists	Desensitization of gonadotropes; blocks action of endogenous LHRH
LHRH independent		
Incomplete sexual precocity		
Girls		
Autonomous ovarian cysts	Medroxyprogesterone acetate	Inhibition of ovarian steroidogenesis; regression of cyst (inhibition of FSH release)
McCune-Albright syndrome	Medroxyprogesterone acetate*	Inhibition of ovarian steroidogenesis; regression of cyst (inhibition of FSH release)
	Third-generation aromatase inhibitor, e.g., letrozole	Inhibition of P-450 aromatase; blocks estrogen synthesis
Boys		
Familial testotoxicosis	Ketoconazole*	Inhibition of P-450-c17 (CYP17) (mainly 17,20-lyase activity)
	Spironolactone* or flutamide and letrozole	Antiandrogen Inhibition of aromatase; blocks estrogen synthesis
	Medroxyprogesterone acetate*	Inhibition of testicular steroidogenesis

*If true precocious puberty develops, an LHRH agonist can be added.
LHRH, luteinizing hormone–releasing hormone.
Modified from Grumbach MM, Kaplan SL. Recent advances in the diagnosis and management of sexual precocity. Acta Paediatr Jpn 1988; 30(suppl):155–175.

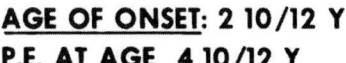

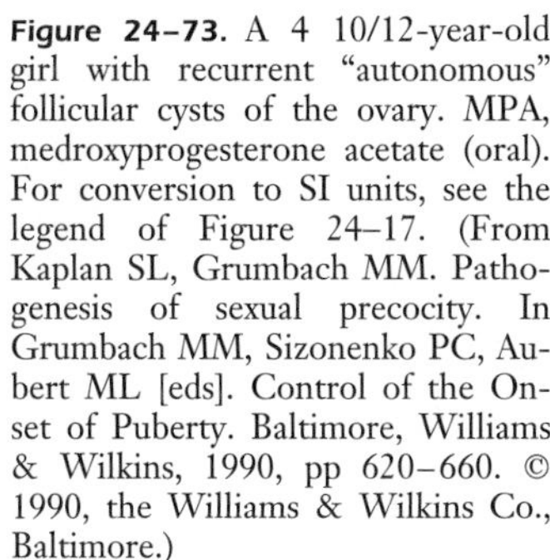

Figure 24–73. A 4 10/12-year-old girl with recurrent "autonomous" follicular cysts of the ovary. MPA, medroxyprogesterone acetate (oral). For conversion to SI units, see the legend of Figure 24–17. (From Kaplan SL, Grumbach MM. Pathogenesis of sexual precocity. In Grumbach MM, Sizonenko PC, Aubert ML [eds]. Control of the Onset of Puberty. Baltimore, Williams & Wilkins, 1990, pp 620–660. © 1990, the Williams & Wilkins Co., Baltimore.)

ovarian follicular cysts, whether recurrent or an isolated episode, often respond to treatment with oral medroxyprogesterone acetate but not to LHRH agonists. Medroxyprogesterone acetate also seems to prevent recurrence and accelerate involution of the follicular cysts[871, 1905] and reduce the risk of torsion. The use of one of the new, potent aromatase inhibitors such as letrozole to reduce estradiol secretion is another potential approach to treatment.[1908] Surgical intervention is rarely indicated; a large or persistent cyst can be reduced by puncture at laparoscopy. The size of the cyst can be monitored readily by pelvic sonography.

Plasma estradiol concentrations in girls with recurrent cysts (>7 cm) may increase to high levels indistinguishable from those in granulosa cell tumors of the ovary,[871, 1905] but they do not have increased plasma granulosa cell tumor markers such as AMH and inhibin. Alternatively, the levels of estrogen in blood and urine may be in the early pubertal range. A characteristic feature in girls with recurrent cysts is waxing and waning of estrogen levels that correlate with changes in the appearance of the ovary on pelvic sonography. Pelvic sonography is useful for visualization of ovarian cysts and estimation of functional activity.[1906, 1909] In occasional patients, exploratory laparotomy or laparoscopy may be necessary to differentiate these cysts from ovarian neoplasms or to rupture the cyst; the latter, if indicated, can also be performed by percutaneous aspiration guided by sonography. The luteinization of follicular cysts may be related to subtle elevations and increased pulses of plasma FSH. A cyst that secretes estrogen autonomously differs from the follicular cysts that may occur in girls as a result of true precocious puberty. In the latter case, removal or reduction of the cyst does not correct the sexual precocity.[1905, 1910] Furthermore, the autonomously secreting cysts are not associated with augmented pulsatile LH secretion or with a pubertal LH response to LHRH administration. Ovarian cysts and sexual precocity have been associated with the fragile X syndrome in girls.[1911]

Granulosa Cell Tumor of the Ovary

This tumor is rare in childhood, and theca cell tumors are even less common.[1910, 1912] Juvenile granulosa cell tumors have distinctive features that differentiate them from the tumors in adults. Characteristic histologic features include nodular architecture, follicle formation, abundant interstitial and intrafollicular acid mucopolysaccharide–rich fluid, irregular microcysts, individual cell necrosis, and high mitotic activity (mean activity, 11 mitotic figures per 10 high-power fields). Size can vary from 2.5 to 25 cm with a mean diameter of 12 cm. The interstitial mucinous fluid consists predominantly of hyaluronic acid.[1913] The prognosis is good as only about 3% of patients die of the disease. Approximately 80% of granulosa cell tumors can be palpated on bimanual examination. Less than 5% are bilateral or clinically malignant. The concentration of plasma estradiol may increase to high levels[492]; FSH and LH concentrations are usually suppressed. The tumor secretes AMH and inhibin, which are sensitive tumor markers.[1914–1918] Sonograms of the ovary facilitate diagnosis. After surgical removal, measurements of plasma estradiol and AMH levels are a useful screen for metastases; if the patient is younger than 9 years an elevated estradiol and at any age an abnormal rise in concentration of plasma AMH or inhibin suggests recurrence or metastasis.

Occasionally, gonadoblastomas in streak gonads, rare lipoid tumors, cystadenomas, and ovarian carcinomas secrete estrogens, androgens, or both hormones. Even with successful resection of a gonadal sex steroid–secreting neoplasm, the child is at risk for secondary central precocious puberty developing in the future. Gonadal tumors composed of a mixture of germ cells and sex cord stromal cells that are distinct from gonadoblastoma are usually benign when discovered in female infants or children with 46,XX karyotypes,[1919, 1920] although neoplastic transformation is a risk.[1921, 1922] Two cases of metastasizing malignant mixed germ cell–sex cord–stromal tumors have been described in prepubertal girls with isosexual precocity.[1922] Some of these neoplasms secrete α-fetoprotein and other tumor markers. Ovarian tumors are rare in the prepubertal period, accounting for about 1% of all tumors in girls younger than 17 years, and most are benign.[1923–1925] The majority of ovarian tumors arise from germ cells or sex cord stromal cells in childhood and less than 20% are of epithelial origin, whereas in adults the majority of tumors are of epithelial origin.[1926, 1927] Early diagnosis of most childhood tumors of the ovary, unlike ovarian cancer in women, allows successful cure.[1928]

Peutz-Jeghers Syndrome

This autosomal dominant syndrome of mucocutaneous pigmentation of the lips, buccal mucosa, fingers, and toes; gastrointestinal hamartomatous polyposis; and a predisposition to malignancy is associated with a rare, distinctive sex cord tumor with annular tubules in both boys and girls.[1929–1931] Estrogen secretion by the tumor may lead to feminization and incomplete sexual precocity in boys as well as girls. Less frequently, an epithelial tumor of the ovary, dysgerminoma, or a feminizing Sertoli-Leydig cell tumor has been found in patients with Peutz-Jeghers syndrome.[1932, 1933] Children with this disorder should be examined at regular intervals for the presence of gonadal tumors by pelvic sonography. The syndrome is due to mutations in the gene on 9p13.3 encoding a serine/threonine protein kinase STK11 leading to haploinsufficiency of this novel tumor-suppressing gene.[1934–1937]

Sex cord–stromal tumors derive from the coelomic epithelium or mesenchymal cells of the embryonic gonads and are composed of granulose, theca, Leydig, and Sertoli cells. Estrogen secretion from these tumors can cause pseudoprecocious puberty, and androgen secretion can cause virilization. Both inhibin A and B activin are produced as well as antimüllerian factor; all serve as useful tumor markers.[1916, 1938, 1939] Sex cord–stromal tumors not associated with Peutz-Jeghers syndrome are malignant in 25% of patients; these tumors may grow quite large, whereas those associated with Peutz-Jeghers syndrome are often small and multiple, and contain calcifications.[1940]

Adrenal Adenomas

Adrenocortical tumors are rare in childhood (reported to be 0.6% of all childhood tumors and 0.3% of all malignant childhood tumors), but most produce steroid hormones in childhood whereas those in adults usually do not. The median age of diagnosis is 4 years, with various studies stating mean ages of 2, 4.3, and 5 years. Forty-one percent appear before 2 years and 71% before 5 years of age. Most cause virilization or Cushing's syndrome, but adrenal tumors may produce estrogen as well as androgens and cause sexual precocity in a girl or gynecomastia in a boy. One adrenal adenoma found in a 7-year-old girl expressed the gene for aromatase, demonstrating that the tumor could directly produce estrogen.[1941] There was substantial production of estrogen leading to a serum estradiol concentration of 145 pg/mL, a value in the range that is found in adrenal carcinomas as well as adenomas.

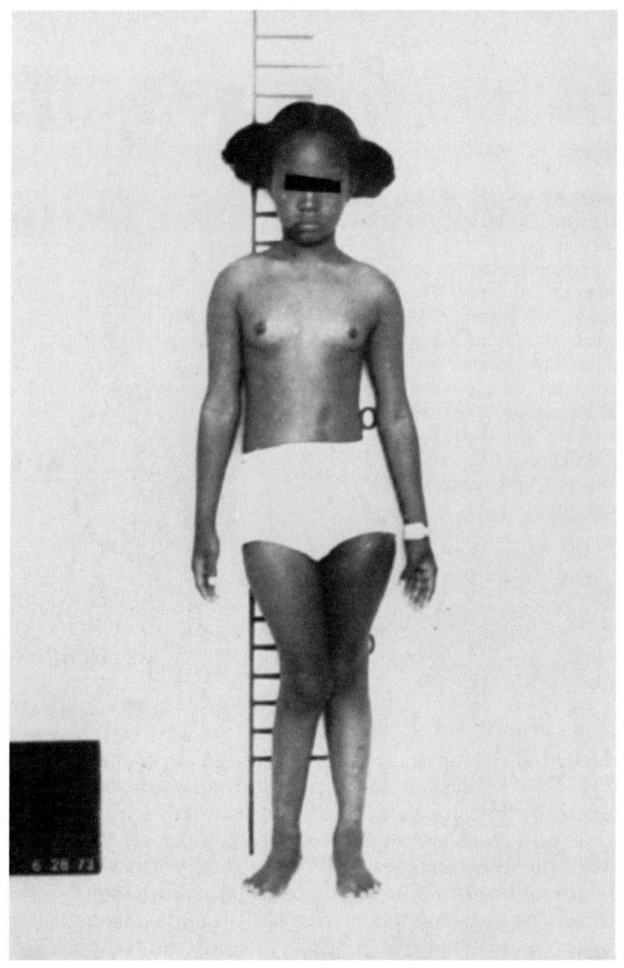

Figure 24–74. A 7 4/12-year-old girl with luteinizing hormone–releasing hormone (LHRH)–independent sexual precocity associated with McCune-Albright syndrome. She had breast development since infancy, and it increased noticeably at about 3 years of age; 6 months later episodes of recurrent vaginal bleeding began. Growth of pubic hair was noted at about 4 to 5 years of age. At age 5 1/12 years the bone age was 6 11/12 years; height was +1 SD above the mean value for age. By 6½ years of age, when she was seen at the University of California, San Francisco, the bone age had advanced to 9 years, and height was at +1 SD. Breasts were at Tanner stage 4; pubic hair at stage 3. Extensive irregular café-au-lait macules cover the right side of the face, left lower abdomen and thigh, and both buttocks. A bone survey showed widespread involvement of the long bones with typical polyostotic fibrous dysplasia, and the floor of the anterior fossa of the skull was sclerotic and the diploetic space widened. She has had two pathologic fractures through bone cysts in the right upper femur. Note the osseous deformities. Plasma estradiol concentrations were consistently in the pubertal range; LH response to LHRH was prepubertal. Results of thyroid function studies were normal, including the thyrotropin response to thyrotropin-releasing hormone administration and antithyroid antibodies were not detected. Treatment with oral medroxyprogesterone acetate suppressed menses and arrested pubertal development but did not slow skeletal maturation. Her final height is 142 cm (−2.5 SD). Menstrual cycles are regular.

Incomplete Sexual Precocity: Boys and Girls

McCune-Albright Syndrome

This sporadic syndrome,[1942, 1943] which occurs about twice as often in girls as in boys, is due to somatic activating mutations in the gene (*GNAS1*) encoding the α subunit of the trimeric guanosine triphosphate (GTP)-binding protein ($G_{s\alpha}$) that stimulates adenyl cyclase. It is characterized by the triad of irregularly edged hyperpigmented macules (café-au-lait spots); a slowly progressive bone disorder, polyostotic fibrous dysplasia, that can involve any bone and is frequently associated with facial asymmetry and hyperostosis of the base of the skull; and, more commonly in girls, LHRH-independent sexual precocity[1662, 1944, 1945] (Fig. 24–74 and Table 24–46). Autonomous hyperfunction most commonly involves the ovary, but other endocrine involvement includes thyroid (nodular hyperplasia with thyrotoxicosis or, remarkably, with euthyroid status),[1365] adrenal (multiple hyperplastic nodules with Cushing's syndrome),[1945] pituitary (adenoma or mammosomatotroph hyperplasia with gigantism and acromegaly and hyperprolactinemia),[1946] and parathyroids (adenoma or hyperplasia with hyperparathyroidism).[1662] In addition, hypophosphatemic vitamin D–resistant rickets or osteomalacia can occur in this syndrome because of either overproduction of a phosphaturic factor, phosphatonin,[1947] secreted by the bone lesions or an

Table 24–46. Clinical Manifestations of McCune-Albright Syndrome in 158 Reported Patients*

Manifestation	Patients (%) (n = 158)	Male (n = 53)	Female (n = 105)	Age at Diagnosis (yr)	(range)	Comments
Fibrous dysplasia	97	51	103	7.7	(0–52)	Polyostotic more common than monostotic
Café-au-lait lesion	85	49	86	7.7	(0–52)	Variable size and number of lesions, irregular border ("coast of Maine")
Sexual precocity	52	8	74	4.9	(0.3–9)	Common initial manifestation
Acromegaly/gigantism	27	20	22	14.8	(0.2–42)	17/26 with adenoma on MRI/CT
Hyperprolactinemia	15	9	14	16.0	(0.2–42)	23/42 of acromegalic with ↑ PRL
Hyperthyroidism	19	7	23	14.4	(0.5–37)	Euthyroid goiter is common
Hypercortisolism	5	4	5	4.4	(0.2–17)	All primary adrenal
Myxomas	5	3	5	34	(17–50)	Extremity myxomas
Osteosarcoma	2	1	2	36	(34–37)	At site of fibrous dysplasia, not related to prior radiation therapy
Rickets/osteomalacia	3	1	3	27.3	(8–52)	Responsive to phosphorus plus calcitriol
Cardiac abnormalities	11	8	9		(0.1–66)	Arrhythmias and CHF reported
Hepatic abnormalities	10	6	10	1.9	(0.3–4)	Neonatal icterus is most common

*Evaluations include clinical and biochemical data; other rarely described manifestations include metabolic acidosis, nephrocalcinosis, developmental delay, thymic and splenic hyperplasia, and colonic polyps.

MRI, magnetic resonance imaging; CT, computed tomography; PRL, prolactin; CHF, congestive heart failure.

Modified from Ringel MD, Schwindinger WF, Levine MA. Clinical implication of genetic defects in G proteins: the molecular basis of McCune-Albright syndrome and Albright hereditary osteodystrophy. Medicine (Baltimore) 1996; 75:171–184.

intrinsic renal abnormality leading to excess generation of nephrogenous cAMP in the proximal tubule and, as a result, decreased reabsorption of phosphate.[1948] At least two of the features must be present to consider the diagnosis. Hepatocellular dysfunction may be due to expression of the mutant-activating gene in liver cells.[1949] This is a sporadic condition that can be concordant or discordant in monozygotic twins.[1950]

The skin manifestations may not be conspicuous in infancy, although the majority of patients have pigmented skin lesions in infancy that usually increase in size along with body growth.[1951] The irregular-bordered café-au-lait macules usually do not cross the midline, are often located on the same side as the main bone lesions, and have a segmented distribution.[1942]

The skeletal lesions in the cortex are dysplastic and are filled with spindle cells with poorly organized collagen support; they take the form of scattered cystic areas of rarefaction on radiography and often result in pathologic fractures and progressive deformities[1952] (Fig. 24–75). Technetium bone scintigraphy has been the most sensitive approach to the detection of bone lesions before they are visible radiographically. If the skull is involved, there may be entrapment and compression of optic or auditory nerve foramina, which can lead to blindness, deafness, facial asymmetry, and ptosis. Fifty percent of affected children in one series manifested bone abnormalities by 8 years of age.[1951] Increased serum GH levels have an adverse effect on the skull deformities.

The sexual precocity, the onset of which is often in the first 2 years of life and is frequently heralded by menstrual bleeding, is due to an autonomously functioning luteinized follicular cyst of the ovary (see Table 24–47).[871, 1662] The ovaries contain multiple follicular cysts but not corpora lutea and commonly exhibit asymmetrical enlargement as a result of a large solitary cyst that characteristically enlarges and spontaneously regresses only to recur (Fig. 24–76).[871, 1662, 1863, 1945, 1953, 1954] Serum estradiol is elevated (at times to extraordinarily high levels); in contrast, the LH response to LHRH is prepubertal and the pubertal pattern of nighttime LH pulses is absent at the onset and during the initial years.[871, 1955, 1956] Later in the course of the sexual precocity, when the bone age approaches 12 years, the LHRH pulse generator becomes operative and ovulatory cycles ensue. Thus, an affected girl may progress from LHRH-independent puberty to LHRH-dependent puberty[871, 1955, 1957] (see Table 24–45). LHRH agonists are not effective for treatment in the LHRH-independent stage. Testolactone (40 mg/kg per day orally),[1958] a relatively weak aromatase inhibitor, has been of equivocal usefulness[1959] and some patients become resistant to the drug.[1960] The new, highly potent, specific, third-generation aromatase inhibitors, for example, letrozole, should be more effective.[172, 173] Antiestrogens offer another method of control of the estrogenic effects of the disorder. A single case report of treatment with tamoxifen showed decreases in bone age advancement, growth rate, menses, and pubertal development.[1961] Multicenter trials of antiestrogen and antiaromatase therapy in this disorder are in progress.

Sexual precocity is rare in boys with McCune-Albright syndrome.[1662, 1944, 1962, 1963] Affected boys may have asymmetrical enlargement of the testes in addition to signs of sexual precocity. The histologic changes are reminiscent of those in testotoxicosis; the seminiferous tubules are enlarged and exhibit spermatogenesis, and Leydig cells may be hyperplastic.[1962] The LH response to LHRH was prepubertal in two cases. The hormonal data (although scant) and the testicular findings appear similar to those in boys with familial testotoxicosis.[1662] A 3.8-year-old boy with McCune-Albright syndrome (Arg 201 His mutation detected in bone and testis tissue) had the unusual feature of macro-orchidism (right testis 9 mL, left testis 7 mL) and absence of sexual precocity. He had several café-au-lait lesions on the back and a radiograph of the skeleton showed polyostotic fibrous dysplasia. Gonadotropins, the LHRH stimulation test, and sex steroid levels were prepubertal but serum inhibin B and AMH concentrations were strikingly elevated. The testes on histology showed that most seminiferous tubules were "slightly" increased in diameter and filled with Sertoli cells but lacked a lumen. The tubules stained intensively for inhibin B_B subunit; mature Leydig cells were absent.[1964]

The pathogenesis of the sporadic McCune-Albright syndrome was uncertain since its first description. It may occur concordantly or discordantly in monozygotic twins; familial cases have not been described. In 1986, Happle[1965] posited that the disorder is caused by an autosomal dominant lethal gene that results in loss of the zygote in utero and that cells bearing

Table 24–47. A Patient with McCune-Albright Syndrome and Recurrent Ovarian Cysts

Chronologic Age (yr)	Bone Age (yr)	Height (cm)	Physical Signs*	Basal and Post-LHRH‡	Plasma Estradiol, pmol/L (pg/mL)	Radiograph, Long Bones
1 4/12	1 3/12	81.1	Café au lait pigmentation, B2, PH1 Vaginal bleeding (× 2 mo)	LH 0.6–1.3† (LER-960) FSH 1.9–3.2† (LER-869) (DHEAS <0.14 μmol/L [<50 ng/mL])	40 (11)	Normal
1 8/12			B1, PH1			
2 6/12	2 6/12	92.4	B2, PH2 Vaginal bleeding	LH 0.6–1.1 FSH 1.9–3.2 (DHEAS <0.14 μmol/L [<50 ng/mL])	55–66 (15–18)	Normal
3 3/12		98.3	B1, PH1			
3 10/12	3 10/12		B2, PH1	LH 1.1–2.0 FSH 1–1.7	51–95 (14–26)	Normal
4 3/12			B1, PH1		7.3–7.3 (20–20)	Polyostotic fibrous dysplasia of femurs
5 11/12	6	123.4	B3, PH2 Vaginal bleeding (× 2 mo)	LH 1.1–4.3 FSH 1.0–2.0		
6 6/12	7 10/12	128.5	B3, PH2 Oral medroxyprogesterone acetate, 10 mg bid started		<5	
7 10/12	8 10/12	136.8				
8 7/12		142.2				

*B2, breast stage 2; PH1, pubic hair stage 1.
†ng/mL To convert ng/mL to IU/L, multiply LH value by 3.8 and FSH value by 8.4.
‡Note the prepubertal LH response to LHRH consistent with LHRH-independent sexual precocity until age 5 11/12 y, and the pubertal LH response at 5 11/12 yr consistent with the development of secondary true precocious puberty (LHRH-dependent). Note discrepancy between gonadarche and adrenarche as evidenced by preadrenarchal concentration of DHEAS.

nine 201 residue is critical for α subunit GTPase activity, and each of the two mutations decreases the GTPase activity of the $G_{s\alpha}$ subunit and leads to constitutive activation. These activating mutations have been found in all tissues affected in the syndrome,[1979, 1980] including bone lesions.

Manifestations of the McCune-Albright syndrome in infancy include Cushing's syndrome related to macronodular adrenal cortical hyperplasia, hyperthyroidism caused by thyroid adenomas, jaundice associated with hepatobiliary disease, and pancreatitis.[1949] Another nonendocrine manifestation is cardiac disease that carries the risk of cardiac arrhythmia and sudden death.

Gonadotropin-Independent Sexual Precocity and Pseudohypoparathyroidism Type Ia Caused by a $G_{s\alpha}$ Mutation

Mutations in $G_{s\alpha}$ can either constitutively activate or inactivate adenyl cyclase.[1967] Two boys who presented in infancy with classical pseudohypoparathyroidism type Ia, a disorder characterized by resistance to hormones whose action is mediated by cAMP, developed signs of sexual precocity with the hormonal characteristics of testotoxicosis (gonadotropin-independent sexual precocity) at about 24 months of age.[1981] They both had a unique alanine 366 to serine mutation[1981] in one allele of the $G_{s\alpha}$ gene; the alanine residue is absolutely conserved in all heterotrimeric G proteins. Pseudohypoparathyroidism type Ia is due to a wide variety of inactivating mutations in $G_{s\alpha}$ that lead to about a 50% reduction in $G_{s\alpha}$ activity in functional assays.[1944]

The paradox of a $G_{s\alpha}$ mutation causing both inactivation and pseudohypoparathyroidism and constitutive activation and testotoxicosis was resolved by in vitro studies.[1982] In cultured cells, the $G_{s\alpha}$ Ala 366 Ser mutant protein was rapidly degraded at 37°C but constitutively activated adenyl cyclase at 33°C.[1982] Unlike other activating mutations of $G_{s\alpha}$, which involve mutations inhibiting its intrinsic GTPase activity and decreasing the rate of hydrolysis of GTP to GDP, the mutation in the two boys caused accelerated dissociation of GDP at 33°C in transfected Leydig cells but rapid degradation at 37°C in a lymphoma cell line[1982] and in skin fibroblasts at both 33 and 37°C[1981] transfected with the mutation. These observations explain the clinical consequences of increased $G_{s\alpha}$ activity in the testes, which are 3 to 5°C cooler than the body, and the tissue specificity and temperature dependence of the mutation.[1982] The mother of one patient appeared to be a mosaic for the $G_{s\alpha}$ mutation, whereas a germ line mutation is likely in the other boy.[1981]

Juvenile Hypothyroidism

Long-standing untreated primary hypothyroidism, usually a consequence of Hashimoto's thyroiditis, is an uncommon cause of incomplete isosexual precocity[225, 1983, 1984] in both girls and boys and occurs in association with impaired growth and delayed skeletal maturation. If the concentration of plasma prolactin is elevated, galactorrhea may be demonstrable, more commonly in affected girls than boys (Fig. 24–78). The signs of sexual maturation are not accompanied by a pubertal growth spurt; instead, growth is impaired[225] (Fig. 24–79). Girls have breast development, enlarged labia minora, and estrogenic changes in the vaginal smear, usually without the appearance of pubic hair[225, 1985–1987]; some girls have irregular vaginal bleeding,[225, 1988] and solitary or multiple ovarian cysts may be demonstrable by pelvic sonography or by physical examination.[225] In about 80% of boys with juvenile hypothyroidism, the testes are enlarged because of an increase in the size of the

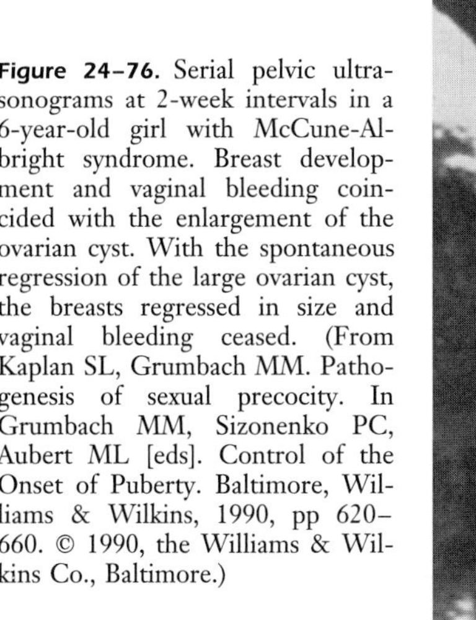
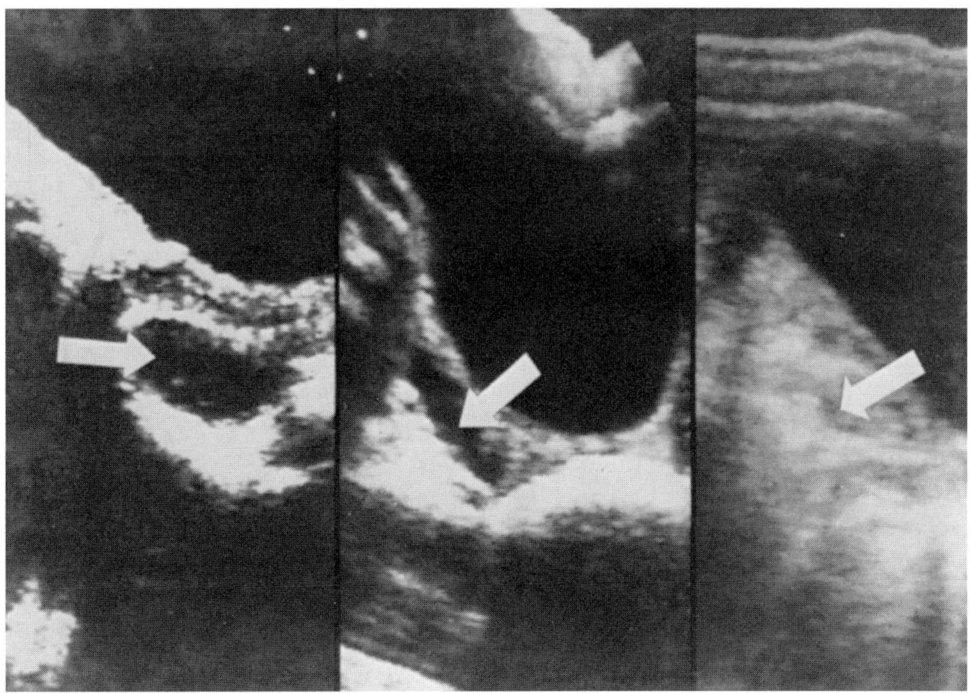

Figure 24–76. Serial pelvic ultrasonograms at 2-week intervals in a 6-year-old girl with McCune-Albright syndrome. Breast development and vaginal bleeding coincided with the enlargement of the ovarian cyst. With the spontaneous regression of the large ovarian cyst, the breasts regressed in size and vaginal bleeding ceased. (From Kaplan SL, Grumbach MM. Pathogenesis of sexual precocity. In Grumbach MM, Sizonenko PC, Aubert ML [eds]. Control of the Onset of Puberty. Baltimore, Williams & Wilkins, 1990, pp 620–660. © 1990, the Williams & Wilkins Co., Baltimore.)

seminiferous tubules, but signs of virilization and Leydig cell maturation are absent[1989, 1990] and the plasma concentration of testosterone is prepubertal. Enlargement of the sella turcica and the pituitary gland (see Fig. 24–79) has led to the misdiagnosis of a pituitary neoplasm. The hypothyroidism, incomplete sexual maturation, galactorrhea, and pituitary enlargement are reversed or corrected by levothyroxine therapy within a few months.[225]

In 1960, Van Wyk and Grumbach[225] suggested that the syndrome resulted from hormonal "overlap" in negative feedback regulation with increased secretion of gonadotropins, prolactin, and TSH as a consequence of the chronic hypothyroidism. With the advent of radioimmunoassays for pituitary hormones, increased prolactin secretion was documented in children[1984] and adults with primary hypothyroidism and in affected girls with the syndrome.[1985]

Hyperprolactinemia correlated with the increased production of TSH. GH release is usually decreased as in uncomplicated primary hypothyroidism.[1991, 1992] Hypothalamic TRH stimulates the release of both prolactin and TSH, and the increased TRH concentration in children with primary hypothyroidism seems to account for the rise in serum prolactin and TSH levels.

However, the explanation for the sexual maturation remains uncertain. Pubertal development in primary hypothyroidism is usually delayed and is only rarely advanced for chronologic age. By using radioimmunoassays for FSH and LH in which the cross-reaction with TSH is negligible, an increased (pubertal) concentration of plasma immunoreactive and bioactive FSH but not LH has been detected.[1991–1993] Bioactive LH activity is also low. In addition, increased FSH pulsatility, mainly at night, but not LH release was demonstrated in patients with the syndrome and in some children with primary hypothyroidism who did not exhibit premature sexual maturation.[1991–1993] The increased FSH release and the high FSH/LH ratio (in contrast to that in normal puberty) seem to account for the increased ovarian estrogen secretion in girls and for the enlarged testes without signs of virilization in affected boys; the suggestion here is that FSH-induced Sertoli cell proliferation is an important determinant of mature testis size.[139, 1994, 1995] An LHRH-independent mechanism is quite likely as LHRH agonist did not suppress the pubertal LH levels.[1993] Pulsatile TSH release is increased at night, and administration of TRH appears to increase FSH release in normal children (but not adults). Moreover, the FSH response to TRH, but not LHRH, is augmented in primary hypothyroidism[1992] and this FSH response to TRH can occur in gonadotropin-secreting pituitary adenomas.

If the latter observations are confirmed, it is likely that the incomplete sexual precocity and the increased prolactin secretion and galactorrhea are a consequence of the increased release of TRH, the increased sensitivity of the mammotrophs and gonadotrophs to TRH, or both. This mechanism,[225] which has gained support,[1993] would explain the relatively rapid and complete reversal of the syndrome by levothyroxine treatment. Human recombinant TSH at a dose about 1000-fold greater than hFSH evoked a dose-dependent cAMP response in COS-7 cells transfected with the human FSH receptor, which suggests another possible but less likely mechanism for the FSH-dependent (or FSH-like–dependent) but LHRH-independent sexual precocity.[1996] A direct effect of severe hypothyroidism on the prepubertal testis that leads to overproliferation of Sertoli cells has also been advanced to explain the macro-orchidism.[1990]

Diagnosis of Sexual Precocity

See Table 24–48 and Figures 24–80 to 24–82. The separation of patients with self-limited benign disorders, such as premature adrenarche or premature thelarche or normal but early puberty, from those with serious or even potentially fatal disorders is the first step in evaluation. The history may reveal symptoms suggesting perinatal abnormalities or injuries, previous infections, adventitious ingestion of or exposure to gonadal steroids, or the presence of similar conditions in family members. In addition, previous measurements should be plotted on a growth chart to determine height velocity and the age of onset of any increase in the rate of growth.

Important aspects of the physical examination include description of the secondary sexual development according to

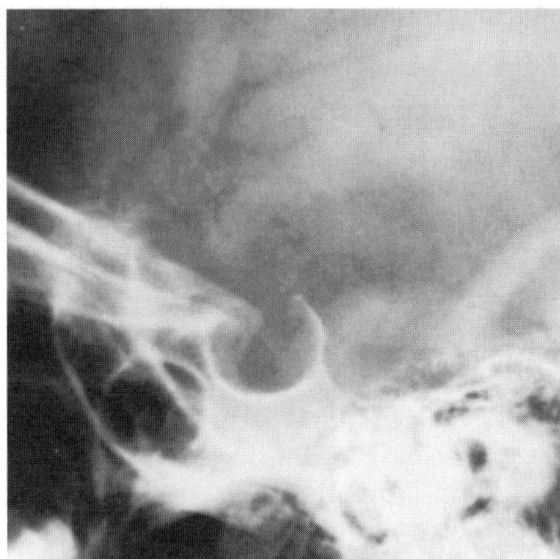

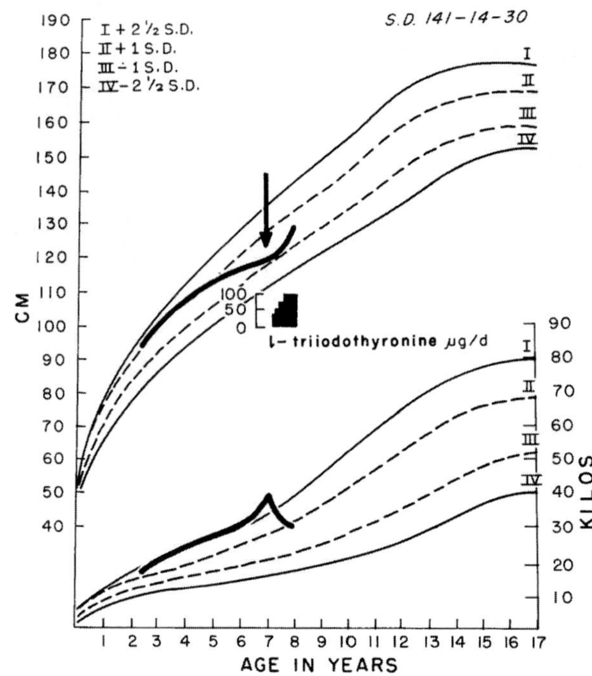

Figure 24–79. *Left,* Radiograph of the skull of a patient with hypothyroidism illustrating an enlarged pituitary fossa in the lateral view. The dorsum sellae was thin and demineralized, and the floor had a double contour line. The area of the sella turcica was 150 mm^2. Pneumoencephalography showed a suprasellar mass impinging on the cisterna chiasmatica. After thyroid hormone treatment for 8 months, the area of the sella had decreased 30% in volume to 100 mm^2, the dorsum sellae had remineralized, and the double floor was no longer evident. *Right,* Growth curve illustrating the decrease in growth rate despite the sexual precocity and the catch-up growth induced by thyroid hormone therapy. (From Van Wyk JJ, Grumbach MM. Syndrome of precocious menstruation and galactorrhea in juvenile hypothyroidism: an example of hormonal overlap in pituitary feedback. J Pediatr 1960; 57:416–435.)

elevated plasma concentrations of cortisol and urinary free cortisol and 17-hydroxycorticosteroid values confirm the latter diagnosis. The appearance in a girl of pubic hair and other signs of virilization, such as clitoral enlargement, acne, deepening voice, muscular development, or growth spurt, is caused by congenital virilizing adrenal hyperplasia, virilizing adrenal tumor, or virilizing ovarian tumor; Cushing's syndrome caused by an adrenocortical carcinoma can cause virilization associated with growth failure. Virilizing ovarian tumors can be detected by pelvic ultrasonography.

The appearance of pubic hair without other signs of puberty in boys or girls is usually a result of premature adrenarche but may be the first sign of sexual precocity or of adrenal virilism of other causes.

In a girl, breast development associated with dulling and thickening of the vaginal mucosa and enlargement of the labia minora indicates significant estrogen secretion or iatrogenic exposure to estrogen. The differential diagnosis includes true precocious puberty, an estrogen-secreting neoplasm, and a cyst of the ovary. If the plasma concentrations of gonadotropins are in the pubertal range, if LH pulses of pubertal amplitude are detected, or if a pubertal LH response to LHRH is elicited, true precocious puberty is present. Estrogen concentrations in girls early in normal or true precocious puberty are in the prepubertal range much of the day, and a single determination may be inadequate to reflect ovarian function[173, 871] (see Fig. 24–60). A CNS tumor is less likely in girls than in boys to be the cause of this premature reactivation of the hypothalamic LHRH pulse generator–pituitary gonadal system. However, studies using MRI or CT brain scans indicate that the hypothalamic hamartoma is more prevalent in both boys and girls with so-called idiopathic true precocious puberty than was previously suspected.

If the concentration of plasma estradiol is elevated but gonadotropin levels are low, an estrogen-secreting cyst or neoplasm is present. Ovarian tumors of moderate size can be palpated by bimanual examination. Advances in pelvic sonography allow the delineation of ovarian cysts or tumors and the determination of uterine size, and this procedure has become an essential component of the diagnostic evaluation.[127] An estrogen-secreting neoplasm of the ovary is usually accompanied by high estradiol concentrations. However, some ovarian cysts are associated with concentrations of estradiol as high as those in granulosa cell tumors; the differential diagnosis between these cysts and ovarian neoplasms rarely requires exploratory laparotomy or laparoscopy and can usually be made by pelvic sonography and by the use of tumor markers. Breast development in the absence of other estrogen effects is almost always a result of premature thelarche.

Iatrogenic Sexual Precocity

Prepubertal children are remarkably sensitive to exogenous gonadal steroids and may show signs of sexual maturation resulting from overlooked sources of androgens or estrogens, such as ingested or absorbed tonics, lotions, or creams that contain or are inadvertently contaminated with an estrogen.[2009–2011] Interest in the effects of environmental estrogens or disruptors on reproductive development in girls and boys is mounting.[2012, 2013]

Estrogen exposure may come from cosmetics. Hair creams and straighteners may contain estrogenic substances; this source of exogenous estrogens is more frequently encountered in a black population.[2014] The amount of estrogen available from these sources is unclear, but it is estimated that a dermal exposure to estrogen might add up to more than 300 µg, far in excess of a therapeutic dose[2015] and possibly greater in infants and children exposed to estrogen dermal gel. Children

Table 24–48. Differential Diagnosis of Sexual Precocity

	Plasma Gonadotropins	LH Response to LHRH	Serum Sex Steroid Concentration	Gonadal Size	Miscellaneous
True Precocious Puberty (premature reactivation of LHRH pulse generator)	Prominent LH pulses, initially during sleep	Pubertal LH response	Pubertal values of testosterone or estradiol	Normal pubertal testicular enlargement or ovarian and uterine enlargement (by ultrasonography)	MRI of brain to rule out CNS tumor or other abnormality; skeletal survey for McCune-Albright syndrome
Incomplete Sexual Precocity (pituitary gonadotropin-independent)					
Males					
Chorionic gonadotropin-secreting tumor in males	High hCG, low LH	Prepubertal LH response	Pubertal value of testosterone	Slight to moderate uniform enlargement of testes	Hepatomegaly suggests hepatoblastoma; CT scan of brain if chorionic gonadotropin-secreting CNS tumor suspected
Leydig cell tumor in males	Suppressed	No LH response	Very high testosterone	Irregular asymmetrical enlargement of testes	
Familial testotoxicosis	Suppressed	No LH response	Pubertal values of testosterone	Testes symmetrical and larger than 2.5 cm but smaller than expected for pubertal development; spermatogenesis occurs	Familial; probably sex-limited, autosomal dominant trait
Virilizing congenital adrenal hyperplasia	Prepubertal	Prepubertal LH response	Elevated 17-OHP in CYP21 deficiency or elevated 11-deoxycortisol in CYP11B1 deficiency	Testes prepubertal	Autosomal recessive, may be congenital or late-onset form, may have salt loss in CYP21 deficiency or hypertension in CYP11B1 deficiency
Virilizing adrenal tumor	Prepubertal	Prepubertal LH response	High DHEAS and androstenedione values	Testes prepubertal	CT, MRI, or ultrasonography of abdomen
Premature adrenarche	Prepubertal	Prepubertal LH response	Prepubertal testosterone, DHEAS, or urinary 17-ketosteroid values appropriate for pubic hair stage 2	Testes prepubertal	Onset usually after 6 years of age; more frequent in CNS-injured children
Females					
Granulosa cell tumor (follicular cysts may present similarly)	Suppressed	Prepubertal LH response	Very high estradiol	Ovarian enlargement on physical examination, CT, or ultrasonography	Tumor often palpable on abdominal examination
Follicular cyst	Suppressed	Prepubertal LH response	Prepubertal to very high estradiol	Ovarian enlargement on physical examination, CT, or ultrasonography	Single or recurrent episodes of menses and/or breast development; exclude McCune-Albright syndrome
Feminizing adrenal tumor	Suppressed	Prepubertal LH response	High estradiol and DHEAS values	Ovaries prepubertal	Unilateral adrenal mass
Premature thelarche	Prepubertal	Prepubertal LH, pubertal estradiol response	Prepubertal or early	Ovaries prepubertal	Onset usually before 3 years of age
Premature adrenarche	Prepubertal	Prepubertal LH response	Prepubertal estradiol; DHEAS or urinary 17-ketosteroid values appropriate for pubic hair stage 2	Ovaries prepubertal	Onset usually after 6 years of age; more frequent in brain-injured children
Late-onset virilizing congenital adrenal hyperplasia	Prepubertal	Prepubertal LH response	Elevated 17-OHP in basal or corticotropin-stimulated state	Ovaries prepubertal	Autosomal recessive

Table continued on following page

Table 24–48. Differential Diagnosis of Sexual Precocity *Continued*

	Plasma Gonadotropins	LH Response to LHRH	Serum Sex Steroid Concentration	Gonadal Size	Miscellaneous
In Both Sexes					
McCune-Albright syndrome	Suppressed	Suppressed	Sex steroids pubertal or higher	Ovarian (on ultrasound); slight testicular enlargement	Skeletal survey for polyostotic fibrous dysplasia and skin examination for café au lait spots
Primary hypothyroidism	LH prepubertal; FSH may be slightly elevated	Prepubertal FSH may be increased	Estradiol may be pubertal	Testicular enlargement; ovaries cystic	TSH and prolactin elevated; T_4 low

CNS, central nervous system; CT, computed tomography; DHEAS, dehydroepiandrosterone sulfate; hCG, human chorionic gonadotropin; LH, luteinizing hormone; MRI, magnetic resonance imaging; 17-OHP, 17-hydroxyprogesterone; T_4, thyroxine; TSH, thyrotropin.

who inhaled estrogen dust have developed sexual precocity. A short course of application of estrogen cream is used to treat labial adhesions, but long courses may lead to breast development or even withdrawal bleeding. In addition to breast development, pigmentation of the areolae and the linea alba and the appearance of pubic hair may be seen in children exposed to estrogen.

Food is another potential source of estrogen.[2016] Epidemics of gynecomastia in boys and thelarche in girls have occurred in schoolchildren in Italy[2017, 2018]; meat contaminated by estrogens was suspected in some cases.[2019] However, no etiology was uncovered in Milan and environs, where 21.1% of 1- to 2-year-old girls and 36.6% of 1- to 2-year-old boys were reported with premature thelarche or gynecomastia.[2020] During a 10-year period more than 600 cases of gynecomastia in boys and premature thelarche or incomplete sexual precocity in girls

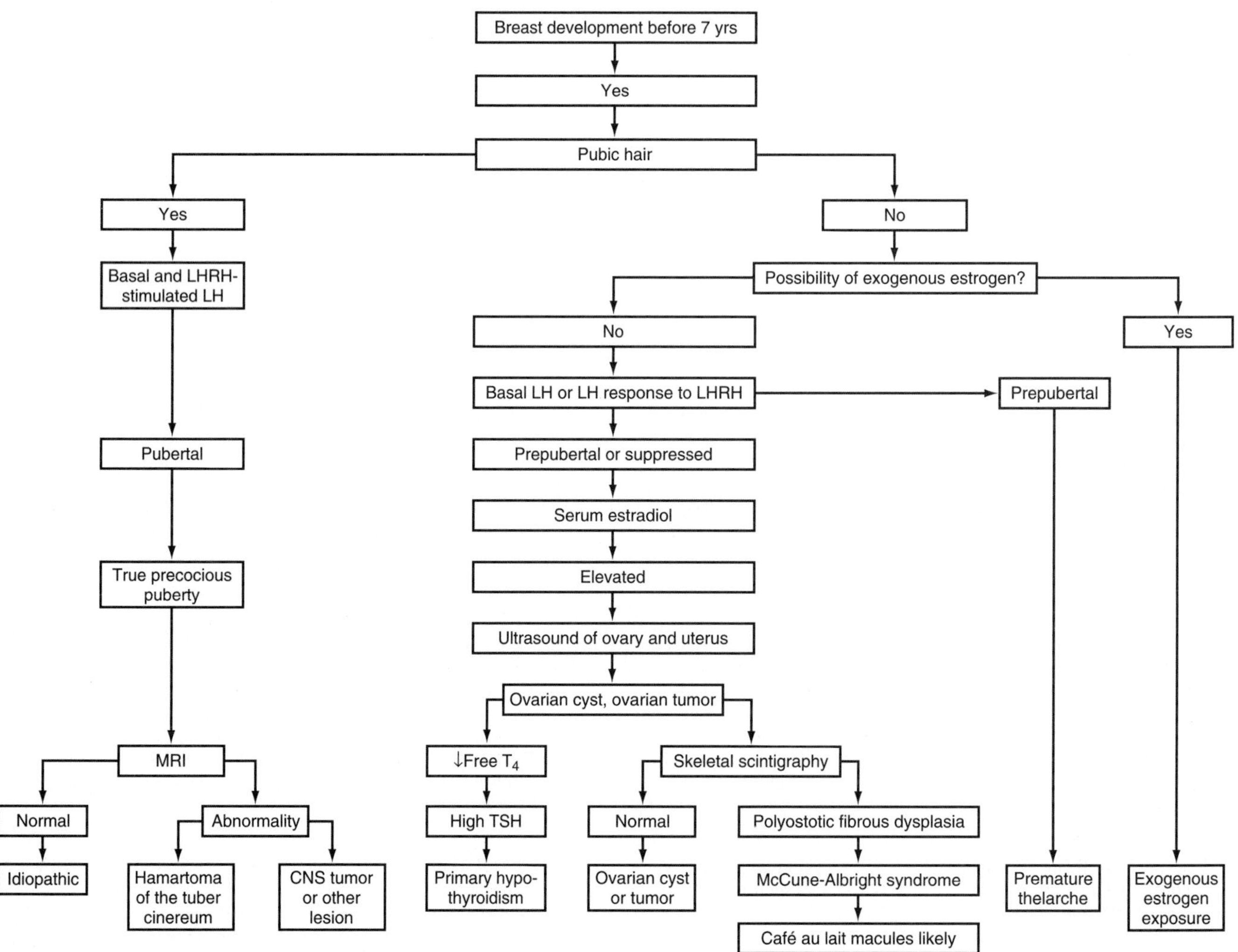

Figure 24–80. The diagnosis of sexual precocity in girls.

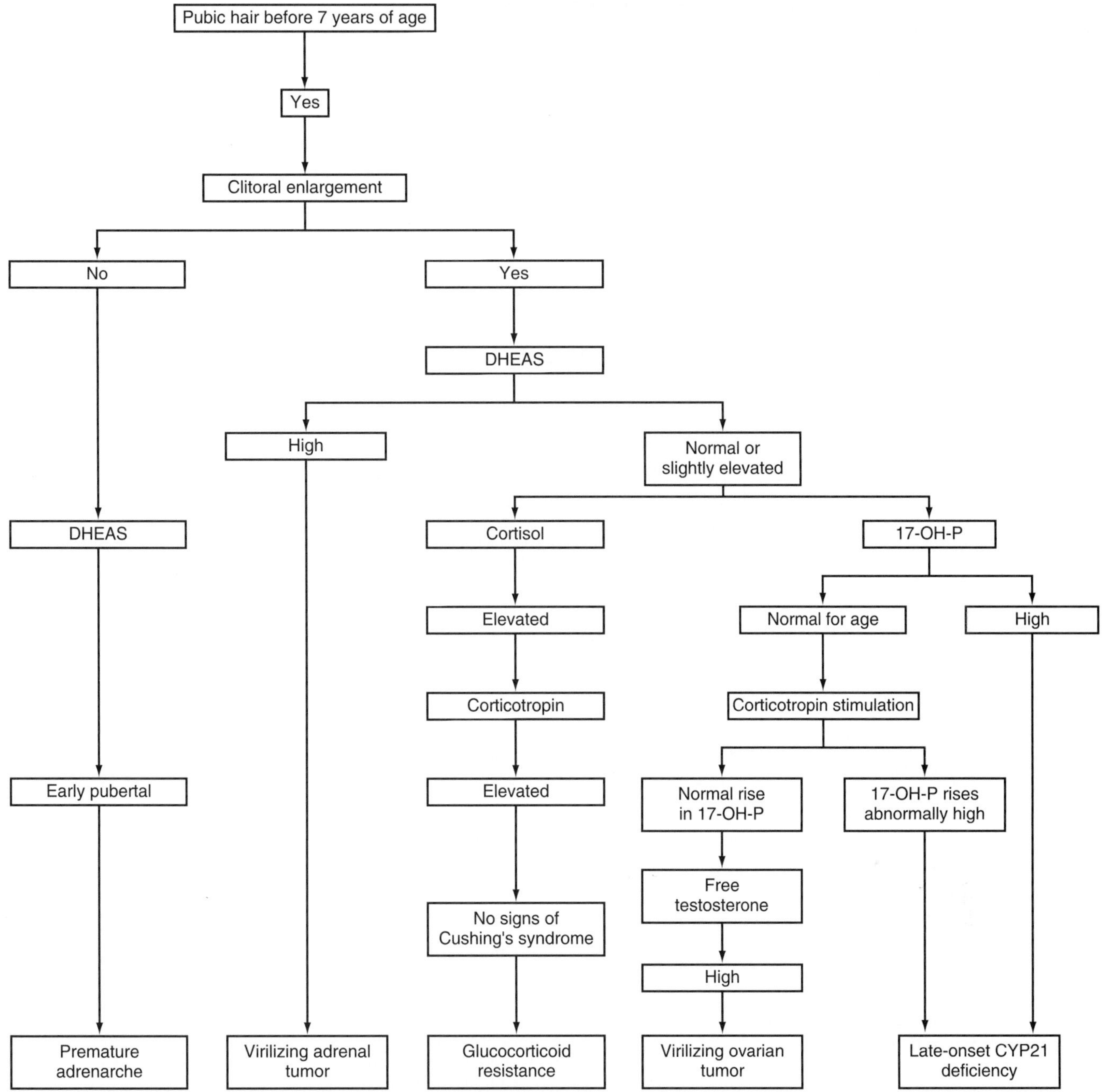

Figure 24–81. The evaluation of pubic hair in normal phenotypic girls before 7 years.

were discovered in Puerto Rico, the highest prevalence noted in the world, about 10 to 15 times higher than the prevalence in a survey in Olmsted, Minnesota.[2021–2023] Maternal ovarian cysts were demonstrated in two thirds of affected Puerto Rican girls.[2021, 2024]

The wide publicity given these observations and the questions raised about contamination of the food supply by the clandestine use of estrogens as growth-promoting agents for meat production caused anxiety among parents, cattle raisers, and farmers. It was suggested that the use of estrogen preparations in animals to stimulate weight gain led to ingestion of estrogen-contaminated meat. Although this idea has not been confirmed by selected analyses of meat, poultry, and milk in Puerto Rico by the U.S. Department of Agriculture, it has not been excluded.[2024] Guidelines from the FDA define a limit of not more than 1% of normal daily estrogen production of prepubertal children as a safe intake of estrogen,[2025] which translates into 0.43 ng/day for boys and 3.24 ng/day for girls using the latest data from extremely sensitive estrogen assays.[2011] A possible association has been advanced between plasticizers with documented estrogenic and antiandrogenic activity and premature thelarche in Puerto Rico. Significantly elevated concentrations of phthalates and their major metabolites were found in 28 girls (68%) of a cohort with premature breast development.[2026]

Girls breast-fed following an accidental exposure of their mothers to polybrominated biphenyls experienced early menarche (by about 1 year) and early appearance of pubic hair but not breast development compared with girls who were not exposed and girls who were not breast-fed.[2027]

The administration of hCG to boys with undescended testes may induce secretion of testosterone sufficient to cause incom-

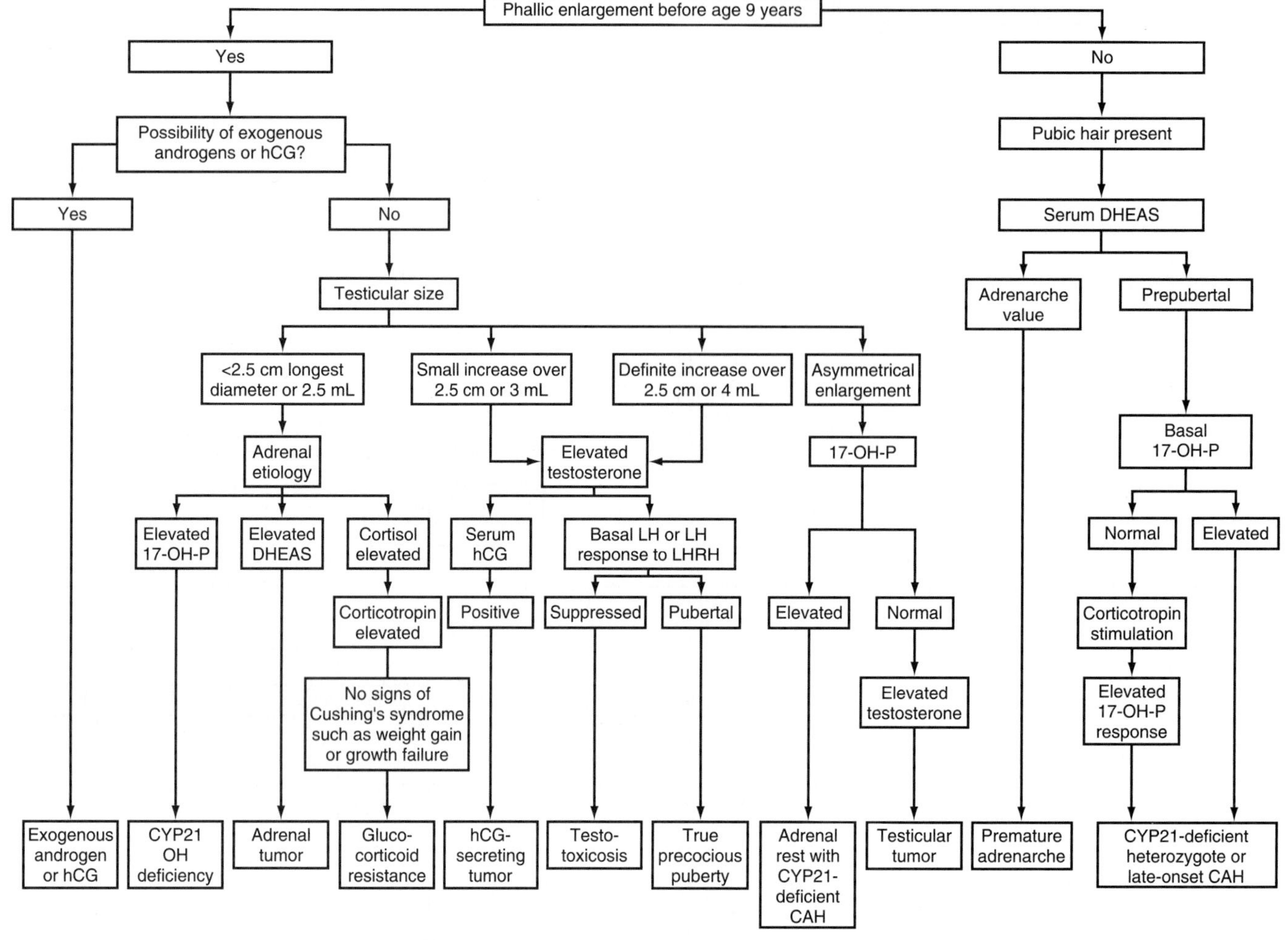

Figure 24–82. The diagnosis of sexual precocity in a phenotypic male.

plete sexual precocity. From these examples it is clear that careful investigation of sources of possible exposure to exogenous hormones is mandatory in every case of sexual precocity.

Feminization in Boys and Virilization in Girls (Contrasexual Precocity)

Boys

Feminization in a boy before the age of puberty is rare. Rarely, an estrogen-secreting adrenal adenoma[2028] or a chorionepithelioma may cause gynecomastia. Gynecomastia has been reported in a 1-year-old boy with 11-hydroxylase deficiency[2029] and in boys with late-onset congenital adrenal hyperplasia.

Aromatase Excess Syndrome

Gynecomastia in prepubertal boys can also be caused by increased extraglandular aromatization of C_{19}-steroids of adrenal origin such as androstenedione and hence increased extraglandular estrogen production in sporadic or familial cases.[2030–2032] This autosomal dominant disorder leading to excess estrogen synthesis from C_{19} precursors because of aromatase overexpression, especially in fat and skin, is a consequence of novel gain-of-function mutations of *CYP19*, the gene encoding aromatase, related to a chromosome arrangement that give rise to a cryptic promoter.[2033]

Feminizing Testicular Tumors

Feminizing testicular tumors may cause gynecomastia in boys younger than age 6 with the Peutz-Jeghers syndrome.[1929–1931] Both testes may be enlarged, and the histology indicates sex cord or Sertoli cell tumors that form annular tubules and often have areas of calcification; increased estradiol secretion is noted in the basal state, and a further rise occurs after hCG administration. Otherwise, feminizing Sertoli cell tumors are rare in boys.[1933] Sonography or MRI scans of the testes may be useful in the diagnosis.[1933, 2034]

Girls

Virilization in a girl indicates organic disease except for premature adrenarche. Congenital adrenal hyperplasia resulting from 21-hydroxylase or 11β-hydroxylase deficiency and androgen-producing tumors of the adrenal can cause virilization, and these were discussed earlier as occurring in males. 3β-Hydroxydehydrogenase/$\Delta^{4,5}$-isomerase deficiency is a rare type of congenital adrenal hyperplasia characterized by elevated 5,17-hydroxypregnenolone, DHEA, and DHEAS levels and, in the severe form, decreased secretion of aldosterone and cortisol. Severely affected patients have mineralocorticoid and glucocorticoid deficiency and may die in infancy. Excess adrenal androgens lead to virilization in utero and to ambiguous external genitalia, including clitoral enlargement in females with continued virilization after birth[1330] (see Chapter 22). Milder forms of this disorder can cause hirsutism in women. 46,XY phenotypic women with incomplete forms of androgen resistance syndrome or with 17β-hydroxysteroid dehydrogenase (17β-HSD) type 3 deficiency may have virilization as well as breast development at the time of expected puberty. Mutations in the *CYP19* gene that encodes aromatase are associated not only with intrauterine masculinization of the external genitalia in affected XX individuals but also with progressive virilization, lack of female secondary sex characteristics, multicystic ovaries at the age of puberty, tall stature, and osteopenia[180, 182] (see Chapter 22).

Cushing's syndrome resulting from adrenal carcinoma is usually manifest as growth failure with or without virilization, obesity, and moon facies; striae may not appear until months to years later.

The syndrome of glucocorticoid resistance is manifest in various degrees. Some patients demonstrate hyperandrogenic signs such as acne, hirsutism, male-type baldness, menstrual irregularities, and oligoanovulation and infertility.[2035] Dexamethasone decreased the excessive adrenal androgen secretion, virilization, and advancing bone age found in a prepubertal boy with general glucocorticoid resistance.[2036]

Arrhenoblastoma, the most common virilizing ovarian tumor, is rare in children. Lipoid cell tumor of the ovary and gonadoblastoma are even more unusual sources of androgens.[2037, 2038]

Variations of Pubertal Development

Premature Thelarche

Unilateral or bilateral breast enlargement without other signs of sexual maturation (e.g., sexual hair and growth of the labia minora and the uterus) is not uncommon in infancy and childhood and has been referred to as premature thelarche. The disorder usually occurs by age 2 (in over 80%) and rarely after age 4.[2039, 2040] In a retrospective study in Minnesota, premature thelarche occurred with an incidence of 21.2 per 100,000 patient-years, 60% of cases were noted between 6 months and 2 years of age, and most regressed in 6 months to 6 years after diagnosis, although a few persisted until puberty. A 10- to 35-year follow-up was available in 25 cases, and no untoward effects on later health, growth, or fertility were evident.[2041] The breast enlargement usually regresses after a few months[2040, 2042] but occasionally persists for years or lasts until the onset of normal puberty; in about half of affected girls the breast development, which is characteristically cyclic, lasts 3 to 5 years. Usually, significant nipple and areolae development is absent and estrogen-induced thickening and dulling of the vaginal mucosa are uncommon. Enlargement of the uterus on ultrasonography (>1.8 mL volume and length > 36 mm) is rare. Measurement of the ellipsoid volume of the uterus (V = longitudinal diameter $\times$ anteroposterior diameter $\times$ transverse diameter $\times$ 0.523) is the most sensitive and specific discriminator between premature thelarche and early true precocious puberty[128] and provides better early discrimination than the LH response to LHRH. Growth in stature is normal.[675, 2039, 2043–2045]

Premature thelarche is a benign, self-limited disorder compatible with normal pubertal development at an appropriate age; only reassurance and follow-up are usually necessary. The appearance of premature thelarche can, however, be the harbinger of further sexual maturation in a minority of cases as discussed earlier.[675, 2040, 2043, 2046, 2047] Because the development may be unilateral, it is important to consider the condition in girls with unilateral breast development so that needless worry about a breast neoplasm is not stimulated in the parents and no unnecessary surgical procedure is carried out. Indeed, the removal of tissue in premature thelarche may leave the child with no possibility of future breast development.[1564] In selected instances, sonography of the breast is useful in distinguishing unilateral premature thelarche from less benign conditions.[2048]

The most common cause of breast mass in the pubertal girl is fibroadenoma; although metastatic disease may locate in the pubertal breast, breast carcinoma is exceedingly rare.[2048]

Plasma estradiol levels are slightly high for age in premature thelarche when determined by a highly sensitive estrogen assay.[2049] However, there is usually no increase in plasma levels of TeBG or in thyroxine-binding globulin, indicators of estrogen action on circulating plasma proteins,[2050] although a modest increase of TeBG for age has been reported.[1596] The urocytogram often reveals an estrogen effect on squamous epithelial cells in the urine.[492, 2051]

The concentration of serum FSH may be in the pubertal range, nocturnal FSH pulsatility has been detected, and the rise in FSH elicited by the administration of LHRH may be augmented for chronologic age, with an FSH/LH ratio higher in precocious thelarche than in normal individuals or girls with true precocious puberty.[945, 1690, 2039, 2052] However, these results overlap those in normal prepubertal girls.

Sonograms of the ovary often show one or several cysts larger than 0.5 cm that disappear and reappear, usually correlating with changes in the size of the breasts,[1909, 2052] but the volume of the ovary and uterus is prepubertal.[128, 2053]

As noted, there is evidence for intermittent secretion of small amounts of estrogen from the ovary. Thus, as postulated for some recurrent ovarian cysts, premature thelarche appears to result from the ovarian response to transient increases in FSH levels and possible variations in ovarian sensitivity to FSH.[945, 2051] The LH response to LHRH is prepubertal in all cases.[945, 2054] Plasma inhibin and activin concentrations have not been reported; the possible role of a paracrine-acting pituitary factor in stimulating FSH independently of LHRH is not known.

"Exaggerated" thelarche is described as premature thelarche with the added findings of advanced bone age and increased growth rate, estrogen effects in addition to thelarche. The endocrine measurements in the basal state are in the normal prepubertal range, whereas after LHRH agonist stimulation, the FSH but not LH rose higher than in control subjects or those with true precocious puberty.[2055]

Premature Isolated Menarche

Rarely, girls begin periodic vaginal bleeding at age 1 to 9 without any other signs of secondary sexual development.[2056, 2057] The bleeding can recur for 1 to 6 years and then cease. At the normal age of puberty (3 to 11 years later), secondary sexual development and menses ensue and follow a normal pattern, as does stature. Fertility was later demonstrated after a normal onset of puberty in women with this variant of pubertal development. The etiology is uncertain, but it may be a counterpart of premature thelarche.

Isolated menarche may appear before other manifestations of sexual precocity in the McCune-Albright syndrome and in the premature sexual maturation that can occur in juvenile hypothyroidism.

Before the diagnosis of premature menarche is accepted, all other causes of vaginal bleeding and precocious estrogen secretion and of exposure to exogenous estrogens should be excluded, including neoplasms, granulomas, infection of the vagina or cervix, or a foreign body.[2058] In a series of 50 girls who had vaginal bleeding before age 10, a local lesion was found in about 50%; half of the latter had a malignant neoplasm (usually a rhabdomyosarcoma) and the other half had no discernible cause.[2059] In another report, a foreign body was responsible for 25% of vaginal bleeding in prepubertal girls.[2060] A careful examination for trauma, such as that caused by sexual abuse, is indicated. Urethral prolapse may be misdiagnosed as vaginal bleeding.

Premature Adrenarche (Pubarche)

Premature adrenarche[2061–2063] is the precocious appearance of pubic hair or axillary hair, or both, and less commonly an apocrine odor, comedones, and acne without other signs of puberty or virilization; it is characterized by premature and mild adrenal hyperandrogenism.[671] In the past, this designation was assigned to the appearance of these clinical features before age 8 in girls or age 9 in boys. Although in boys the age of 9 still seems appropriate, the age of 8 can no longer be used for American girls. In a well carried out cross-sectional study involving 17,077 girls with physical examination by practitioners, striking ethnic differences were detected in pubic hair (and breast) development between black and white girls. At 6 years of age, 9.5% (range 5.7% to 16.4%) and at 8 years of age, 34.3% of black girls had Tanner stage 2 or greater pubic hair whereas 1.4% (range 0.9% to 2.2%) and 7.7% of white girls at these ages, respectively, had pubic hair[27] (mean ages are shown in Table 24–3). Accordingly, we recommend that the diagnosis of premature pubarche be limited to black girls younger than 5 years of age and white American girls younger than 7 years, which should affect the age at which laboratory studies are initiated unless there are other signs of virilization such as clitoromegaly or rapid growth.

Premature adrenarche is about 10 times more common in girls than boys. The prevalence is increased in children with CNS abnormalities without a clear sex difference; the electroencephalogram may be abnormal[699, 1664] in the absence of other neurologic findings. Familial transmission is uncommon.[2064] Premature adrenarche is commonly slowly progressive and does not have an untoward effect on either the onset or normal progression of gonadarche or final adult height.[224] Nonetheless, there is a relationship between reduced fetal growth leading to intrauterine growth retardation, the increased prevalence of premature adrenarche, and hyperinsulinism and ovarian hyperandrogenism in life[2065] (see later).

Plasma concentrations of DHEA, DHEAS, androstenedione, testosterone, 17-hydroxyprogesterone, and 17-hydroxypregnenolone are comparable to values normally found in pubic hair stage 2.[971, 2061, 2066–2068] ACTH stimulation increases serum DHEA and DHEAS concentrations and the excretion of urinary 17-ketosteroids, but the concentrations of plasma 17-hydroxyprogesterone and 17-hydroxypregnenolone do not increase to the levels found in individuals with virilizing forms of congenital adrenal hyperplasia.[2067, 2069, 2070] As in congenital adrenal hyperplasia, dexamethasone suppresses adrenal androgen and androgen precursor secretion.[2067, 2068] Serum gonadotropin levels in the basal state and after LHRH are in the prepubertal range in premature adrenarche.[945, 2071] Premature adrenarche occurs independently of gonadarche and is due to some factor other than increased secretion of LHRH or ACTH[969] (see the discussion of adrenarche). Bone age and height are slightly advanced for chronologic age but normal adult height is commonly achieved,[2072, 2073] with the rare exception of some individuals with unusually high values of adrenal androgens, hirsutism, acne, and a bone age more than 2.5 SD above the mean value for chronologic age. In a follow-up study of 20 girls, the functional adrenal hyperandrogenism in premature adrenarche was limited to childhood.[2073]

In our view, premature adrenarche is a developmentally regulated, normal variation in the differentiation, growth, and function of the zona reticularis of the adrenal cortex, marked biochemically by the precocious increase in the concentration of plasma DHEAS to ≥40 μg/dL.[224] The latter is quite likely related to the independent increase of 17,20-lyase activity in the developing zona reticularis mediated by the increased phosphorylation of serine and threonine residues on the $P450_{c17}$ enzyme, and the increased abundance of cytochrome b_5 and of electron-donating redox partners such as cytochrome P450 oxidoreductase and cytochrome b_5, essential for the 17,20-lyase activity of this functional microsomal enzyme (see Fig. 24–43).[2069] Nonetheless, the factor stimulating the development and function of the zona reticularis, independent of ACTH, remains elusive (see adrenarche). In the past, failure to recognize the earlier onset of adrenarche, particularly the striking ethnic differences in black, Hispanic, and Latin populations, has contributed to the overdiagnosis of premature adrenarche[2072, 2074, 2075] and, in some instances, needless laboratory studies.

The concept of exaggerated adrenarche[2076] was first advanced[2077] in relation to a postulated childhood antecedent of PCOS, the hallmarks of which are hyperandrogenism, hirsutism, anovulation, amenorrhea or oligomenorrhea, and insulin resistance and compensatory hyperinsulinemia with its attendant risk of major metabolic sequelae including type 2 diabetes mellitus, dyslipidemia, an increased propensity for coronary heart disease, and in about 50% of affected women obesity.[2074, 2078–2082] It has been extended to include rare instances of premature adrenarche associated with excessive responses of 17-hydroxypregnenolone, DHEAS, and androstenedione to ACTH found in women with functional adrenal hyperandrogenism.

Although premature adrenarche is usually considered a benign condition with no substantial long-term risk, accumulating observations indicate that girls with premature adrenarche are at increased risk of developing functional ovarian hyperandrogenism and the polycystic ovarian syndrome, hyperinsulinism, acanthosis nigricans, and dyslipidemia in adolescence and adult life, especially if fetal growth was reduced and the birth weight was low.[671] Premature adrenarche is a risk factor for the later development of PCOS and functional ovarian hyperandrogenism in adolescent and adult women; the magnitude of this risk is unknown, but it appears to be rare with the exception of girls with a history of decreased fetal growth.[671, 2065, 2073, 2076, 2083, 2084] Plasma plasminogen activator inhibitor-1, a marker of risk for cardiovascular disease including women with PCOS, was increased in girls with premature adrenarche, especially those with low birth weights, and may be useful in the identification of those with a greater risk of developing PCOS.[2085] Girls with reduced fetal growth are at risk for a reduced number of ovarian primordial follicles at birth, small ovaries and uterus at puberty, and an increased serum FSH level and decreased estradiol concentrations, suggesting relative ovarian resistance to FSH. Girls from certain ethnic groups, especially black and Hispanic girls, have a higher risk of the association of premature adrenarche with syndrome X (obesity, hyperinsulinism, dyslipidemia, and later coronary heart disease) and the development of PCOS in late adolescence and early adulthood,[671, 2086–2088] especially if decreased insulin sensitivity and acanthosis nigricans accompany the premature adrenarche.[2087] Of interest, the adrenal steroid pattern in the black and Hispanic patients in the latter study[2088] did not differ from that in children with uncomplicated premature adrenarche.

As discussed previously, hyperinsulinism is associated with many metabolic and endocrine conditions and functional ovarian hyperandrogenism that in some cases is heralded by premature adrenarche.[2089] When the role of insulin resistance and hyperinsulinism was recognized in the pathogenesis of PCOS, therapeutic approaches to reduce insulin resistance were introduced, especially the use of insulin sensitizers. Among the latter, the most widely used drug is metformin because of its low prevalence of adverse effects and therapeutic efficacy. In early studies, this at present experimental agent in the treatment of PCOS decreased insulin resistance, ovarian hyperandrogenism, and hirsutism in both obese and nonobese patients.[1553, 2090–2092] The safety and efficacy of metformin in 82 children and adolescents with type 2 diabetes mellitus (10 to 16 years of age) were supported by a short-term randomized control trial,[2093] providing useful preliminary data to support its use in adolescents with insulin resistance and functional ovarian hyperandrogenism. Troglitazone is another potent insulin sensitizer that improved hirsutism and ovulation in PCOS in a well-controlled study.[2094] In an in vitro study, troglitazone but not metformin directly inhibited the steroidogenic enzymes $P450_{c17}$ and 3β-HSD.[2095] These are promising approaches to a still poorly understood syndrome that often becomes manifest during adolescence. Many aspects need to be addressed in the management of this heterogeneous disorder and include, apart from pharmacologic agents, concern about nutrition and physical activity.

Premature pubarche can be associated with nonclassical congenital adrenal hyperplasia caused by homozygous or compound heterozygous missense mutations in the *CYP21* gene encoding cytochrome $P450_{c21}$[2096] and can readily be detected by a plasma 17-hydroxyprogesterone response to ACTH that is at least 6 SD above the mean value. The prevalence of nonclassical 21-hydroxylase deficiency in children with premature adrenarche is low[2073, 2076, 2097] except in some ethnic groups[2098–2100] (e.g., Hispanics, Italians, and Ashkenazi Jews; see Chapter 22), in whom the prevalence may be as high as 20% to 30%.[2099, 2100] 21-Hydroxylase deficiency can be excluded by determining the plasma 17-hydroxyprogesterone response to ACTH. Premature adrenarche is also associated with the rare nonclassical 11β-hydroxylase deficiency.

There has been controversy about the prevalence and significance of 3β-HSD2 deficiency and the pervasive belief that a mutation in the gene encoding this enzyme was a common cause of premature adrenarche and nonclassical 3β-HSD deficiency.[2099] The possibility of a mutation in the open receding frame of 3β-HSD of the type 2 or type 1 gene has been excluded as all but an uncommon cause of this condition.[2101–2103] Mutations in the 3β-HSD type 2 gene have been associated with a 17-hydroxypregnenolone response to ACTH that exceeds or equals the mean normal value by 6 SD. Of 26 families studied, only one family with a mutation, alanine 82 threonine, had affected females who exhibited premature pubarche; in this family the affected male was a male pseudohermaphrodite.[2104] Thus, a mutation in the 3β-HSD type 2 or type 1 gene is an uncommon cause of premature pubarche, exaggerated adrenarche, and hirsutism in adolescent girls and women. The cause of the "mild deficiency" in 3β-HSD activity is unknown, but it may be multifactorial and lead to a wide range in the secretory capacity of the zona reticularis. A family constellation was described with a dominant pattern of inheritance[2064] of elevated adrenal androgens and androgen precursors that occurred as premature pubarche; later affected individuals developed hirsutism and anovulation.[2143] Thus there is controversy as to the limits of differential diagnosis between 3β-HSD deficiency and premature pubarche. Recent analyses of boys and girls with either congenital adrenal and/or gonadal 3β-HSD deficiency and apparent premature pubarche and girls with pubertal hirsutism led to recommendations to improve the accuracy of the diagnosis of inherited 3β-HSD deficiency. According to this study, ACTH-stimulated 17-hydroxypregnenolone (Δ5-17P) levels in children with premature pubarche at or greater than 294 nmol/L equivalent to or greater than 54 SD above Tanner II pubic hair stage matched control mean level [17 ± 5 (SD) nmol/L] or ACTH-stimulated ratio of Δ5-17P to F (cortisol) in children with premature pubarche at or greater than 363 equivalent to or greater than 38 SD above the control mean ratio [20 ± 9 (SD)], support the diagnosis of 3β-HSD deficiency. However, ACTH-stimulated Δ5-17P levels in children with premature pubarche up to 72 nmol/L equivalent to up to 11 SD above the control mean level, and ACTH-stimulated Δ5-17P to F ratio in children with premature pubarche up to 67, equivalent to up to 5 SD above the control mean ratio, are not consistent with 3β-HSD deficiency congenital adrenal hyperplasia. These criteria are stricter than those utilized in the past.[2143]

DHEA is a stimulus to sebaceous gland activity[2105] and prepubertal acne or comedones may appear in association with elevated serum DHEAS concentrations in some children without the appearance of pubic hair, suggesting a variant of premature adrenarche may be manifest in this manner.[2106–2108] Androgen effects such as clitoral or penile enlargement, rapid growth, hirsutism, and deepening of the voice, for example, exclude premature adrenarche and indicate a more severe form of hyperandrogenism.

Adolescent Gynecomastia

Normal pubertal boys, usually in the early stages of puberty, may have either unilateral breast enlargement (approximately 25% of boys)[2109] or bilateral breast enlargement (approximately 50% to 65% of boys)[2110] of varying degrees, commonly between chronologic ages 14 to 14½ years or pubic hair stages 3 and 4. In these boys the plasma concentrations of testosterone and estrogen are normal for the stage of puberty. Pubertal gynecomastia is usually associated with an elevated ratio of the concentration of serum estradiol to testosterone.[2111–2114]

In a prospective study, adolescent boys with gynecomastia had a lower mean free testosterone concentration, lower weight, higher plasma TeBG levels, and a tendency toward earlier onset of puberty and more rapid progression through puberty.[2109] In one study a significant decrease in the concentration ratio of plasma androstenedione to estrone and estradiol and a similarly low ratio of DHEAS to estrone and estradiol were described in boys with pubertal gynecomastia who had normal ratios of plasma testosterone to estrone and estradiol. It was postulated that either decreased adrenal production of androgens or more likely increased peripheral conversion of adrenal androgens to estrogens was a factor in the development of pubertal gynecomastia.[2115] An elevated ratio of testosterone to dihydrotestosterone, presumably related to a decrease in 5α-reductase activity, was suggested in the etiology of gynecomastia as well.[2116] Immunoreactive estrogen, androgen, and progesterone receptors localized to the nucleus of ductal cells was detected in all of 30 patients with gynecomastia, but aromatase immunoreactivity, limited to stromal cells, was detected in only 37% of cases.[2117]

Pubertal gynecomastia usually resolves spontaneously within 1 to 2 years of onset, and reassurance and continued observation are often adequate treatment. Nevertheless, some boys have conspicuous gynecomastia and sufficient psychological distress to warrant a reduction mammoplasty.[2118] Liposuction is an alternative approach, but its efficacy in adolescent gynecomastia remains to be established. Rarely, untreated gynecomastia persists into adulthood, as illustrated by a patient who had persistent unilateral gynecomastia that began during puberty and contralateral Poland's syndrome of hypoplasia of the chest, breast tissue, and nipple.[2119]

Gynecomastia is a component of Klinefelter's syndrome, anorchia, primary and secondary hypogonadism, biosynthetic defects in testosterone synthesis, increased aromatase activity in adipose and other tissues (aromatase excess syndrome), Sertoli cell tumors, adventitious exposure to estrogens in meat or cosmetics, and variants of the androgen resistance syndromes, including Rosewater's syndrome (familial hypogonadism and gynecomastia) and Reifenstein's syndrome (hypospadias, hypogonadism, and gynecomastia). These disorders usually have characteristic findings that allow ready differentiation from the normal gynecomastia of puberty[1330] (see Chapter 22). Gynecomastia has been described in association with the administration of drugs such as cimetidine, spironolactone, digitalis, and phenothiazines as well as with GH therapy[2120] and the use of marijuana.

Macro-Orchidism

Fragile X syndrome is the most common inherited cause of mental retardation.[2121] This condition is due to multiple repeats of a CCC expansion that leads to hypermethylation of the *FMR1* gene (Xq,27fra) that prevents transcription and translation of the FMRP protein. Affected individuals have mental retardation in association with multiple physical anomalies including large testes.[2122] Eighty percent to 95% of adolescents or adults with fragile X syndrome have testicular volume greater than 30 mL with an average of 45 mL, although the 95th percentile for the syndrome is 70 mL.[2123, 2124] In most cases the enlargement begins at 8 to 9 years of age, prior to the appearance of pubic hair, although some prepubertal children already have a testicular volume greater than 4 mL.[2125]

The enlarged testes are due to increased interstitial volume and excessive connective tissue, including increased peritubular collagen fibers,[2126] rather than to increase in the seminiferous tubules. Testicular biopsy has demonstrated normal Leydig and Sertoli cells, normal to slightly decreased spermatogenic cells, and an increase in testicular interstitial fluid. Although there may be subtle elevation of serum gonadotropins that might be part of the etiology of macro-orchidism, affected males are fertile, although most are not sexually active. Other associated anomalies include increased birth weight, high forehead, large ears, prognathism, pale irises, and an increased head circumference.

Macro-orchidism without androgenization is a rare manifestation of the McCune-Albright syndrome.[1964] Macro-orchidism is an occasional finding in prepubertal boys with long-standing primary hypothyroidism. This form of testicular enlargement appears to result from increased FSH secretion independent of a pubertal increase in LH secretion or a pubertal LH response to LHRH (see above). Testicular adrenal rests in congenital adrenal hyperplasia (see Chapter 22) and a lymphoma can cause bilateral macro-orchidism. It was a feature of severe aromatase deficiency in a young male adult[182] and in men with an FSH-secreting pituitary macroadenoma. Bilateral megalotestis (testicular volume 26 mL) in adults can occur as a normal variant.[2127] One may speculate that some instances of bilateral macro-orchidism are due to a heterozygous constitutive activating mutation of the FSH receptor.

Disorders of Sexual Differentiation with Both Virilization and Feminization at Puberty

Virilization as well as feminization at puberty may occur in a phenotypic female who has a 46,XY karyotype in certain types of male pseudohermaphrodism (see Chapter 22). 17β-HSD type 3 deficiency (a testosterone biosynthetic defect) and incomplete forms of androgen resistance (resulting from defects in the androgen receptor) may occur in this manner; however, ambiguous genitalia are usually noted early in life in these conditions. True hermaphrodites with ovarian and testicular tissue may undergo both virilization and feminization at puberty.[1330]

References

1. Grumbach MM. Onset of puberty. In Berenberg SR (ed). Puberty, Biologic and Social Components. Leiden, HE Stenfert Kroese, 1975, pp 1–21.
2. Bogin B. Growth and development: recent evolutionary and biocultural research. In Boaz NT, Wolfe DL (eds). Biological Anthropology: The State of the Science. Bend, Ore, International Institute for Human Evolutionary Research, 1995, pp 49–70.
3. Dean C, Leakey MG, Reid D, et al. Growth processes in teeth distinguish modern humans from *Homo erectus* and earlier hominids. Nature 2001; 414:628–631.
4. Moggi-Cecchi J. Questions of growth. Nature 2001; 414:595–597.
5. Bogin B. Adolescence in evolutionary perspective. Acta Paediatr Suppl 1994; 406:29–35; discussion 36.
6. Conroy GC, Kuykendall K. Paleopediatrics: or when did human infants really become human? Am J Phys Anthropol 1995; 98: 121–131.
7. Tattersall I. Out of Africa again . . . and again? Sci Am 1997; 276(4):60–67.
8. Mayr E. The objects of selection. Proc Natl Acad Sci USA 1997; 94:2091–2094.
9. Tanner JM. Aristotle: De generatione animalium. In Tanner JM (ed). A History of the Study of Human Growth. Cambridge, Cambridge University Press, 1981, p 7.
10. Marshall WA, Tanner JM. Puberty. In Falkner F, Tanner JM (eds). Human Growth. New York, Plenum, 1986, pp 171–209.
11. Tanner JM. A History of the Study of Human Growth. Cambridge, Cambridge University Press, 1981, pp 286–298.
12. Tanner JM. Growth at Adolescence. Springfield, Ill, Charles C Thomas, 1962.
13. Wyshak G, Frisch RE. Evidence for a secular trend in age of menarche. N Engl J Med 1982; 306:1033–1035.
14. Okasha M, McCarron P, McEwen J, Smith GD. Age at menarche: secular trends and association with adult anthropometric measures. Ann Hum Biol 2001; 28:68–78.
15. Zacharias L, Wurtman RJ, Schatzoff M. Sexual maturation in contemporary American girls. Am J Obstet Gynecol 1970; 108: 833–846.
16. Nicholson AB, Hanley C. Indices of physiological maturity: derivation and interrelationships. Child Dev 1953; 24:3–38.
17. Damon A. Larger body size and earlier menarche: the end may be in sight. Soc Biol 1974; 21:8–11.
18. Gerver WJ, De Bruin R, Drayer NM. A persisting secular trend for body measurements in Dutch children. The Oosterwolde II Study. Acta Paediatr 1994; 83:812–814.
19. Whincup PH, Gilg JA, Odoki K, et al. Age of menarche in contemporary British teenagers: survey of girls born between 1982 and 1986. BMJ 2001; 322:1095–1096.
20. Loesch DZ, Stokes K, Huggins RM. Secular trend in body height and weight of Australian children and adolescents. Am J Phys Anthropol 2000; 111:545–556.
21. Olesen AW, Jeune B, Boldsen JL. A continuous decline in menarcheal age in Denmark. Ann Hum Biol 2000; 27:377–386.
22. Marrodan MD, Mesa MS, Arechiga J, Perez-Magdaleno A. Trend in menarcheal age in Spain: rural and urban comparison during a recent period. Ann Hum Biol 2000; 27:313–319.
23. Kac G, Auxiliadora de Santa Cruz Coel, Velasquez-Melendez G. Secular trend in age at menarche for women born between 1920 and 1979 in Rio de Janeiro, Brazil. Ann Hum Biol 2000; 27: 423–428.
24. Kill V. Stature and growth of Norwegian men during past 200 years. Skr Nor Vidensk Akad 1939; 2(6):1–175.
25. Zacharias L, Rand M, Wurtman R. A prospective study of sexual development in American girls: the statistics of menarche. Obstet Gynecol Surv 1976; 31:325–337.
26. MacMahon B. Age at menarche. In National Health Survey. DHEW Publication No (HRA) 74–1615, Series 11, No 133. Washington, DC, Government Printing Office, 1973.
27. Herman-Giddens ME, Slora EJ, Wasserman RC, et al. Secondary sexual characteristics and menses in young girls seen in office practice: a study from the Pediatric Research in Office Settings network. Pediatrics 1997; 99:505–512.
28. Harlan WR, Harlan EA, Grillo GP. Secondary sex characteristics of girls 12 to 17 years of age: the U.S. Health Examination Survey. J Pediatr 1980; 96:1074–1078.
29. Matsuo N, Anzo M, Sato S, et al. Testicular volume in Japanese boys up to the age of 15 years. Eur J Pediatr 2000; 159:843–845.
30. Veronesi FM, Gueresi P. Trend in menarcheal age and socioeconomic influence in Bologna (northern Italy). Ann Hum Biol 1994; 21:187–196.

31. Cole TJ. Secular trends in growth. Proc Nutr Soc 2000; 59: 317–324.
32. Artaria MD, Henneberg M. Why did they lie? Socio-economic bias in reporting menarcheal age. Ann Hum Biol 2000; 27:561–569.
33. Koo MM, Rohan TE. Accuracy of short-term recall of age at menarche. Ann Hum Biol 1997; 24:61–64.
34. Williams RL, Cheyne KL, Houtkooper LK, Lohman TG. Adolescent self-assessment of sexual maturation: effects of fatness classification and actual sexual maturation stage. J Adolesc Health Care 1988; 9:480–482.
35. Tryggvadottir L, Tulinius H, Larusdottir M. A decline and a halt in mean age at menarche in Iceland. Ann Hum Biol 1994; 21:179–186.
36. Morabia A, Costanza MC. Reproductive factors and incidence of breast cancer: an international ecological study. Soz Praventivmed 2000; 45:247–257.
37. Gao YT, Shu XO, Dai Q, et al. Association of menstrual and reproductive factors with breast cancer risk: results from the Shanghai Breast Cancer Study. Int J Cancer 2000; 87:295–300.
38. Stoll BA, Vatten LJ, Kvinnsland S. Does early physical maturity influence breast cancer risk? Acta Oncol 1994; 33:171–176.
39. MacMahon B, Trichopoulos D, Brown J, et al. Age at menarche, urine estrogens and breast cancer risk. Int J Cancer 1982; 30:427–431.
40. Apter D, Vihko R. Early menarche, a risk factor for breast cancer, indicates early onset of ovulatory cycles. J Clin Endocrinol Metab 1983; 57:82–86.
41. Persson I. Estrogens in the causation of breast, endometrial and ovarian cancers: evidence and hypotheses from epidemiological findings. J Steroid Biochem Mol Biol 2000; 74:357–364.
42. Mucci LA, Kuper HE, Tamimi R, et al. Age at menarche and age at menopause in relation to hepatocellular carcinoma in women. BJOG 2001; 108:291–294.
43. Berkey CS, Gardner JD, Frazier AL, Colditz GA. Relation of childhood diet and body size to menarche and adolescent growth in girls. Am J Epidemiol 2000; 152:446–452.
44. Morrison JA, Barton B, Biro FM, et al. Sexual maturation and obesity in 9- and 10-year-old black and white girls: the National Heart, Lung, and Blood Institute Growth and Health Study. J Pediatr 1994; 124:889–895.
45. Adair LS, Gordon-Larsen P. Maturational timing and overweight prevalence in US adolescent girls. Am J Public Health 2001; 91:642–644.
46. Garn SM, LaVelle M, Rosenberg KR, Hawthorne VM. Maturational timing as a factor in female fatness and obesity. Am J Clin Nutr 1986; 43:879–883.
47. Hartz AJ, Barboriak PN, Wong A, et al The association of obesity with infertility and related menstrual abnormalities in women. Int J Obes 1979; 3:57–73.
48. Harlan WR, Harlan EA, Grillo GP. Secondary sex characteristics of girls 12 to 17 years of age: the U.S. Health Examination Survey. J Pediatr 1980; 96:1074–1078.
49. Buffon H. Histoire naturelle. In Tanner JM (ed). A History of the Study of Human Growth. Cambridge, Cambridge University Press, 1981, p 83.
50. Daw SF. Age of boys' puberty in Leipzig, 1727–49, as indicated by voice breaking in J.S. Bach's choir members. Hum Biol 1970; 42:87–89.
51. Sasco AJ. Epidemiology of breast cancer: An environmental disease? APMIS 2001; 109(5):321–332.
52. Delemarre-Van de Waal HA. Environmental factors influencing growth and pubertal development. Environ Health Perspect 1993; 101(suppl 2):39–44.
53. Morabia A, Costanza MC. International variability in ages at menarche, first livebirth, and menopause. World Health Organization Collaborative Study of Neoplasia and Steroid Contraceptives. Am J Epidemiol 1998; 148:1195–1205.
54. Worthman C. Bio-cultural interactions in human development. In Pereira M, Fairbanks L (eds). Juvenile Primates: Life History, Development and Behavior. Oxford, Oxford University Press, 1993, pp 339–358.
55. Smecuol E, Maurino E, Vazquez H, et al. Gynaecological and obstetric disorders in coeliac disease: Frequent clinical onset during pregnancy or the puerperium. Eur J Gastroenterol Hepatol 1996; 8:63–89.
56. Panter-Brick C, Worthman CM. Hormones, health, and behavior: A socioecological and lifespan perspective. New York: Cambridge University Press, 1999.
57. Rosenstock SJ, Jorgensen T, Andersen LP, Bonnevie O. Association of *Helicobacter pylori* infection with lifestyle, chronic disease, body-indices, and age at menarche in Danish adults. Scand J Public Health 2000; 28:32–40.
58. Patel P, Mendall MA, Khulusi S, et al. *Helicobacter pylori* infection in childhood: risk factors and effect on growth. BMJ 1994; 309:1119–1123.
59. Zacharias L, Wurtman RJ. Blindness: its relation to age of menarche. Science 1964; 144:1154–1155.
60. Freyre EA, Ortiz MV. The effect of altitude on adolescent growth and development. J Adolesc Health Care 1988; 9:144–149.
61. Warren MP. The effects of exercise on pubertal progression and reproductive function in girls. J Clin Endocrinol Metab 1980; 51:1150–1157.
62. Osler DC, Crawford JD. Examination of the hypothesis of a critical weight at menarche in ambulatory and bedridden mentally retarded girls. Pediatrics 1973; 51:674–679.
63. McClintock MK. Menstrual synchrony and suppression. Nature 1971; 229:244–245.
64. Wilson HC. A critical review of menstrual synchrony research. Psychoneuroendocrinology 1992; 17:565–591.
65. Casper RC. Women's Health: Hormones, Emotions, and Behavior. Cambridge, Cambridge University Press, 1998.
66. Persky H. Psychoendocrinology of Human Sexual Behavior. New York, Praeger, 1987.
67. Zacharias L, Wurtman RJ. Age at menarche. N Engl J Med 1969; 280:868–875.
68. Meyer JM, Eaves LJ, Heath AC, Martin NG. Estimating genetic influences on the age-at-menarche: a survival analysis approach. Am J Med Genet 1991; 39:148–154.
69. Loesch DZ, Huggins R, Rogucka E, et al. Genetic correlates of menarcheal age: a multivariate twin study. Ann Hum Biol 1995; 22:470–490.
70. Loesch DZ, Hopper JL, Rogucka E, Huggins RM. Timing and genetic rapport between growth in skeletal maturity and height around puberty: similarities and differences between girls and boys. Am J Hum Genet 1995; 56:753–759.
71. Fischbein S. Onset of puberty in MX and DZ twins. Acta Genet Med Gemellol (Roma) 1977; 26:151–158.
72. Fischbein S. Intra-pair similarity in physical growth of opposite-sex twin pairs during puberty. Ann Hum Biol 1983; 10:135–145.
73. Graber JA, Brooks-Gunn J, Warren MP. The antecedents of menarcheal age: heredity, family environment, and stressful life events. Child Dev 1995; 66:346–359.
74. Hayward C, Killen JD, Wilson DM, et al. Psychiatric risk associated with early puberty in adolescent girls. J Am Acad Child Adolesc Psychiatry 1997; 36:255–262.
75. Moffitt TE, Caspi A, Belsky J, Silva PA. Childhood experience and the onset of menarche: a test of a sociobiological model. Child Dev 1992; 63:47–58. [Published erratum appears in Child Dev 1993;64(4): following table of contents].
76. Campbell BC, Udry JR. Stress and age at menarche of mothers and daughters. J Biosoc Sci 1995; 27:127–134.
77. Duke PM, Litt IF, Gross RT. Adolescents' self-assessment of sexual maturation. Pediatrics 1980; 66:918–920.
78. Dorn LD, Susman EJ, Nottelmann ED, et al. Perceptions of puberty: adolescent, parent, and health care personnel. Dev Psychol 1990; 26:322–329.
79. Schlossberger NM, Turner RA, Irwin CEJ. Validity of self-report of pubertal maturation in early adolescents. J Adolesc Health 1992; 13:109–113.
80. Taylor SJ, Whincup PH, Hindmarsh PC, et al. Performance of a new pubertal self-assessment questionnaire: a preliminary study. Paediatr Perinat Epidemiol 2001; 15:88–94.
81. Finkelstein JW, D'Arcangelo MR, Susman EJ, et al. Self-assessment of physical sexual maturation in boys and girls with delayed puberty. J Adolesc Health 1999; 25:379–381.
82. Wu Y, Schreiber GB, Klementowicz V, et al. Racial differences in accuracy of self-assessment of sexual maturation among young black and white girls. J Adolesc Health 2001; 28:197–203.
83. Rillema JA. Development of the mammary gland and lactation. Trends Endocrinol Metab 1994; 5:149–154.

84. Drife JO. Breast development in puberty. Ann NY Acad Sci 1986; 464:58–65.
85. Stratz CH. Der Korper des Kindes und Seine Pflege. Stuttgart, Ferdinand Enke, 1909, p 245.
86. Reynolds EL, Wines JV. Individualized differences in physical changes associated with adolescence in girls. Am J Dis Child 1948; 75:329–350.
87. O'Hare PM, Frieden IJ. Virginal breast hypertrophy. Pediatr Dermatol 2000; 17:277–281.
88. Rohn RD. Papilla (nipple) development during female puberty. J Adolesc Health Care 1982; 2:217–220.
89. Paavonen J. Physiology and ecology of the vagina. Scand J Infect Dis Suppl 1983; 40:31–35.
90. McCann J. Color Atlas of Child Sexual Abuse. Chicago, Year Book Medical, 1989.
91. Zachmann M, Prader A, Kind HP, et al. Testicular volume during adolescence: cross-sectional and longitudinal studies. Helv Paediatr Acta 1974; 29:61–72.
92. Taskinen S, Taavitsainen M, Wikstrom S. Measurement of testicular volume: comparison of 3 different methods. J Urol 1996; 155:930–933.
93. Biro FM, Lucky AW, Huster GA, Morrison JA. Pubertal staging in boys. J Pediatr 1995; 127:40–46.
94. Sutherland RS, Kogan BA, Baskin LS, et al. The effect of prepubertal androgen exposure on adult penile length. J Urol 1996; 156:783–787.
95. Rohn RD. Papilla (nipple) development in puberty: the adolescent male. J Adolesc Health Care 1985; 6:429–432.
96. Harlan WR, Grillo GP, Cornoni-Huntley J, Leaverton PE. Secondary sex characteristics of boys 12 to 17 years of age: the U.S. Health Examination Survey. J Pediatr 1979; 95:293–297.
97. Roche AF, Wellens R, Attie KM, Siervogel RM. The timing of sexual maturation in a group of U.S. white youths. J Pediatr Endocrinol 1995; 8:11–18.
98. Herman-Giddens ME, Wang L, Koch G. Secondary sexual characteristics in boys. Arch Pediatr Adolesc Med 2001; 155: 1022–1028.
99. Reiter EO, Lee PA. Have the onset and tempo of puberty changed? Arch Pediatr Adolesc Med 2001; 155:988–989.
100. Kaplowitz PB, Oberfield SE. Reexamination of the age limit for defining when puberty is precocious in girls in the United States: implications for evaluation and treatment. Drug and Therapeutics and Executive Committees of the Lawson Wilkins Pediatric Endocrine Society. Pediatrics 1999; 104:936–941.
101. Marti-Henneberg C, Vizmanos B. The duration of puberty in girls is related to the timing of its onset. J Pediatr 1997; 131: 618–621.
102. Lee PA, Guo SS, Kulin HE. Age of puberty: data from the United States of America. APMIS 2001; 109:81–88.
103. Troiano RP, Flegal KM, Kuczmarski RJ, et al. Overweight prevalence and trends for children and adolescents. The National Health and Nutrition Examination Surveys, 1963 to 1991. Arch Pediatr Adolesc Med 1995; 149:1085–1091.
104. Styne DM. Childhood and adolescent obesity: prevalence and significance. Pediatr Clin North Am 2001; 48:823–854.
105. Kaplowitz PB, Slora EJ, Wasserman RC, et al. Earlier onset of puberty in girls: relation to increased body mass index and race. Pediatrics 2001; 108:347–353.
106. He Q, Karlberg J. BMI in childhood and its association with height gain, timing of puberty, and final height. Pediatr Res 2001; 49:244–251.
107. Berkey CS, Dockery DW, Wang X, et al. Longitudinal height velocity standards for U.S. adolescents. Stat Med 1993; 12:403–414.
108. Peschel ER, Peschel RE. Medical insights into the castrati in opera. Am Sci 1987; 75:578–583.
109. Harries M, Hawkins S, Hacking J, Hughes I. Changes in the male voice at puberty: vocal fold length and its relationship to the fundamental frequency of the voice. J Laryngol Otol 1998; 112:451–454.
110. Harries ML, Walker JM, Williams DM, et al. Changes in the male voice at puberty. Arch Dis Child 1997; 77:445–447.
111. Karlberg P, Taranger J. The somatic development of children in a Swedish urban community. Acta Paediatr Scand Suppl 1976; 258:1–148.
112. Amy de la Breteque B, Sanchez S. [A comparative acoustic study of the speaking and singing voice during the adolescent's break of the voice]. Rev Laryngol Otol Rhinol (Bord) 2000; 121:325–328.
113. Lucky AW, Biro FM, Simbartl LA, et al. Predictors of severity of acne vulgaris in young adolescent girls: results of a five-year longitudinal study. J Pediatr 1997; 130:30–39.
114. Traupe H, Von Muhlendahl KE, Bramswig J, Happle R. Acne of the fulminans type following testosterone therapy in three excessively tall boys. Arch Dermatol 1988; 124:414–417.
115. Addy M, Hunter ML, Kingdon A, et al. An 8-year study of changes in oral hygiene and periodontal health during adolescence. Int J Paediatr Dent 1994; 4:75–80.
116. Nakagawa S, Fujii H, Machida Y, Okuda K. A longitudinal study from prepuberty to puberty of gingivitis: correlation between the occurrence of Prevotella intermedia and sex hormones. J Clin Periodontol 1994; 21:658–665.
117. Gusberti FA, Mombelli A, Lang NP, Minder CE. Changes in subgingival microbiota during puberty: a 4-year longitudinal study. J Clin Periodontol 1990; 17:685–692.
118. Grumbach MM, Gluckman PD. The human fetal hypothalamus and pituitary gland; the maturation of neuroendocrine mechanisms controlling the secretion of fetal pituitary growth hormone, prolactin, gonadotropin, and adrenocorticotropin-related peptides and thyrotropin. In Tulchinsky D, Little AB (eds). Maternal-Fetal Endocrinology. Philadelphia, WB Saunders, 1994, pp 193–261.
119. Rabinovici J, Jaffe RB. Development and regulation of growth and differentiated function in human and subhuman primate fetal gonads. Endocr Rev 1990; 11:532–551.
120. Ross GT. Follicular development: the life cycle of the follicle and puberty. In Grumbach MM, Sizonenko PC, Aubert MI (eds). Control of the Onset of Puberty. Baltimore, Williams & Wilkins, 1990, pp 376–386.
121. Gougeon A. Regulation of ovarian follicular development in primates: facts and hypotheses. Endocr Rev 1996; 17:121–155.
122. Peters H, Byskov AG, Grinsted J. Follicular growth in fetal and prepubertal ovaries of humans and other primates. Clin Endocrinol Metab 1978; 7:469–485.
123. Hillier SG. Gonadotropic control of ovarian follicular growth and development. Mol Cell Endocrinol 2001; 179:39–46.
124. Richards JS. Perspective: the ovarian follicle—a perspective in 2001. Endocrinology 2001; 142:2184–2193.
125. Shikone T, Yamoto M, Kokawa K, et al. Apoptosis of human corpora lutea during cyclic luteal regression and early pregnancy. J Clin Endocrinol Metab 1996; 81:2376–2380.
126. Hsueh AJ, Eisenhauer K, Chun SY, et al. Gonadal cell apoptosis. Recent Prog Horm Res 1996; 51:433–455; discussion 455–456.
127. Fleischer AC, Shawker TH. The role of sonography in pediatric gynecology. Clin Obstet Gynecol 1987; 30:735–746.
128. Haber HP, Wollmann HA, Ranke MB. Pelvic ultrasonography: early differentiation between isolated premature thelarche and central precocious puberty. Eur J Pediatr 1995; 154:182–186.
129. Salardi S, Orsini LF, Cacciari E, et al. Pelvic ultrasonography in premenarcheal girls: relation to puberty and sex hormone concentrations. Arch Dis Child 1985; 60:120–125.
130. Bridges NA, Cooke A, Healy MJ, et al. Standards for ovarian volume in childhood and puberty. Fertil Steril 1993; 60:456–460.
131. Onat J, Ertem B. Age at menarche: relationship to socioeconomic status, growth rate in stature and weight, and skeletal and sexual maturation. Am J Hum Biol 1995; 7:741–750.
132. Mitan LA, Slap GB. Adolescent menstrual disorders: update. Med Clin North Am 2000; 84:851–868.
133. Apter D, Vihko R. Serum pregnenolone, progesterone, 17-hydroxyprogesterone, testosterone and 5 alpha-dihydrotestosterone during female puberty. J Clin Endocrinol Metab 1977; 45:1039–1048.
134. Pakarinen A, Hammond GL, Vihko R. Serum pregnenolone, progesterone, 17alpha-hydroxyprogesterone, androstenedione, testosterone, 5alpha-dihydrotestosterone and androsterone during puberty in boys. Clin Endocrinol (Oxf) 1979; 11:465–474.
135. Metcalf MG, MacKenzie JA. Incidence of ovulation in young women. J Biosoc Sci 1980; 12:345–352.
136. Lemarchand-Beraud T, Zufferey MM, Reymond M. Maturation of the hypothalamo-pituitary ovarian axis in adolescent girls. J Clin Endocrinol Metab 1982; 54:241–246.

137. Births: final data for 2000. National Vital Statistics Reports. CDC, 2002, p 50.
138. Chemes HE. Infancy is not a quiescent period of testicular development. Int J Androl 2001; 24:2–7.
139. Cortes D, Muller J, Skakkebaek NE. Proliferation of Sertoli cells during development of the human testis assessed by stereological methods. Int J Androl 1987; 10:589–596.
140. Gondos B, Kogan SJ. Testicular development during puberty. In Grumbach MM, Sizonenko PC, Aubert ML, et al (eds). Control of the Onset of Puberty. Baltimore, Williams & Wilkins, 1990, pp 387–402.
141. Saez JM. Leydig cells: endocrine, paracrine, and autocrine regulation. Endocr Rev 1994; 15:574–626.
142. Prince FP. The triphasic nature of Leydig cell development in humans, and comments on nomenclature. J Endocrinol 2001; 168:213–216.
143. Aumuller G, Riva A. Morphology and functions of the human seminal vesicle. Andrologia 1992; 24:183–196.
144. Paltiel HJ, Rupich RC, Babcock DS. Maturational changes in arterial impedance of the normal testis in boys: Doppler sonographic study. AJR 1994; 163:1189–1193.
145. Pedersen JL, Nysom K, Jorgensen M, et al. Spermaturia and puberty. Arch Dis Child 1993; 69:384–387.
146. Nielsen CT, Skakkebaek NE, Darling JA, et al. Longitudinal study of testosterone and luteinizing hormone (LH) in relation to spermarche, pubic hair, height and sitting height in normal boys. Acta Endocrinol Suppl (Copenh) 1986; 279:98–106.
147. Richardson DW, Short RV. Time of onset of sperm production in boys. J Biosoc Sci Suppl 1978; (5):15–25.
148. Weissenberg R, Hirsch M, Shemesh J, et al. Evaluation of the morphology of sperm in urine of adolescent boys. Int J Androl 1984; 7:348–351.
149. Janczewski Z, Bablok L. Semen characteristics in pubertal boys. II. Semen quality in relation to bone age. Arch Androl 1985; 15: 207–211.
150. Janczewski Z, Bablok L. Semen characteristics in pubertal boys. III. Semen quality and somatosexual development. Arch Androl 1985; 15:213–218.
151. Nysom K, Pedersen JL, Jorgensen M, et al. Spermaturia in two normal boys without other signs of puberty. Acta Paediatr 1994; 83:520–521.
152. Laron Z, Arad J, Gurewitz R, et al. Age at first conscious ejaculation: a milestone in male puberty. Helv Paediatr Acta 1980; 35:13–20.
153. Marshall WA, Tanner JM. Variations in pattern of pubertal changes in girls. Arch Dis Child 1969; 44:291–303.
154. Largo RH, Prader A. Pubertal development in Swiss girls. Helv Paediatr Acta 1983; 38:229–243.
155. Tanner JM, Whitehouse RH, Marubini E, Resele LF. The adolescent growth spurt of boys and girls of the Harpenden growth study. Ann Hum Biol 1976; 3:109–126.
156. Largo RH, Gasser TH, Prader A. Analysis of the adolescent growth spurt using smoothing spline functions. Ann Hum Biol 1978; 5:421–434.
157. Karlberg J, Fryer JG, Engstrom I, Karlberg P. Analysis of linear growth using a mathematical model. II. From 3 to 21 years of age. Acta Paediatr Scand Suppl 1987; 337:12–29.
158. Limony Y, Zadik Z, Pic AK, Leiberman E. Improved method for predicting adult height of pubertal boys using a mathematical model. Horm Res 1993; 40:117–122.
159. Tanner JM, Davies PSW. Clinical longitudinal standards for height and height velocity for North American children. J Pediatr 1985; 107:317–329.
160. Vanden Eynde B, Vienne D, Vuylsteke-Wauters M, et al. Aerobic power and pubertal peak height velocity in Belgian boys. Eur J Appl Physiol 1988; 57:430–434.
161. Calvo MS, Eyre DR, Gundberg CM. Molecular basis and clinical application of biologic markers of bone turnover. Endocr Rev 1996; 17:333–368.
162. Johansen JS, Giwercman A, Hartwell D, et al. Serum bone Gla-protein as a marker of bone growth in children and adolescents: correlation with age, height, serum insulin-like growth factor I, and serum testosterone. J Clin Endocrinol Metab 1988; 67:273–278.
163. Crofton PM, Stirling HF, Schonau E, Kelnar CJ. Bone alkaline phosphatase and collagen markers as early predictors of height velocity response to growth-promoting treatments in short normal children. Clin Endocrinol (Oxf) 1996; 44:385–394.
164. Fujimoto S, Kubo T, Tanaka H, et al. Urinary pyridinoline and deoxypyridinoline in healthy children and in children with growth hormone deficiency. J Clin Endocrinol Metab 1995; 80: 1922–1928.
165. Rauch F, Schnabel D, Seibel MJ, et al. Urinary excretion of galactosyl-hydroxylysine is a marker of growth in children. J Clin Endocrinol Metab 1995; 80:1295–1300.
166. Sen AT, Derman O, Kinik E. The relationship between osteocalcin levels and sexual stages of puberty in male children. Turk J Pediatr 2000; 42:281–285.
167. Garbagnati E. Urate changes in lean and obese boys during pubertal development. Metabolism 1996; 45:203–205.
168. Bourguignon JP. Linear growth as a function of age at onset of puberty and sex steroid dosage: therapeutic implications. Endocr Rev 1988; 9:467–488.
169. Hägg U, Juranger J. Height and height velocity in early, average and late maturers followed to the age of 25: a prospective longitudinal study of Swedish urban children from birth to adulthood. Ann Hum Biol 1991; 18:47–56.
170. McKusick VA. Heritable Disorders of Connective Tissue. St. Louis, CV Mosby, 1972, pp 73–74.
171. Tanner JM, Whitehouse RH, Hughes PCR, et al. Relative importance of growth hormone and sex steroids for the growth at puberty of trunk length, limb length, and muscle width in growth hormone–deficient children. J Pediatr 1976; 89:1000–1008.
172. Grumbach MM, Auchus RJ. Estrogen: consequences and implication of human mutations in synthesis and action. J Clin Endocrinol Metab 1999; 84:4677–4694.
173. Grumbach MM. Estrogen, bone, growth, and sex: a sea change in conventional wisdom. J Pediatr Endocrinol Metab 2000; 13(suppl 6):1439–1455.
174. Rochira V, Balestrieri A, Faustini-Fustini M, Carani C. Role of estrogen on bone in the human male: insights from the natural models of congenital estrogen deficiency. Mol Cell Endocrinol 2001; 178:215–220.
175. Elster AD, Chen MY, Williams DW 3rd, Key LL. Pituitary gland: MR imaging of physiologic hypertrophy in adolescence. Radiology 1990; 174:681–685.
176. Attie KM, Ramirez NR, Conte FA, et al. The pubertal growth spurt in eight patients with true precocious puberty and growth hormone deficiency: evidence for a direct role of sex steroids. J Clin Endocrinol Metab 1990; 71:975–983.
177. Van Wyk JJ, Smith EP. Insulin-like growth factors and skeletal growth: possibilities for therapeutic interventions. J Clin Endocrinol Metab 1999; 84:4349–4354.
178. Rogol AD. Growth at puberty: interaction of androgens and growth hormone. Med Sci Sports Exerc 1994; 26:767–770.
179. Riggs BL, Khosla S, Melton LJ. Sex steroids and conservation of the adult skeleton. Endocr Rev 2002; 23:279–302.
180. Conte FA, Grumbach MM, Ito Y, et al. A syndrome of female pseudohermaphrodism, hypergonadotropic hypogonadism and multicystic ovaries associated with missense mutations in the gene encoding aromatase (P450 arom). J Clin Endocrinol Metab 1994; 78:1287–1292.
181. Smith EP, Boyd J, Frank GR, et al. Estrogen resistance caused by a mutation in the estrogen-receptor gene in a man. N Engl J Med 1994; 331:1056–1061.
182. Morishima A, Grumbach MM, Simpson ER, et al. Aromatase deficiency in male and female siblings caused by a novel mutation and the physiological role of estrogens. J Clin Endocrinol Metab 1995; 80:3689–3698.
183. Bilezikian JP, Morishima A, Bell J, Grumbach MM. Increased bone mass as a result of estrogen therapy in a man with aromatase deficiency. N Engl J Med 1998; 339:599–603.
184. Carani C, Qin K, Simoni M, et al. Effect of testosterone and estradiol in a man with aromatase deficiency. N Engl J Med 1997; 337:91–95.
185. Rochira V, Faustini-Fustini M, Balestrieri A, Carani C. Estrogen replacement therapy in a man with congenital aromatase deficiency: effects of different doses of transdermal estradiol on bone mineral density and hormonal parameters. J Clin Endocrinol Metab 2000; 85:1841–1845.
186. Stratakis CA, Vottero A, Brodie A, et al. The aromatase excess

syndrome is associated with feminization of both sexes and autosomal dominant transmission of aberrant P450 aromatase gene transcription. J Clin Endocrinol Metab 1998; 83:1348–1357.
187. Weise M, De Levi S, Barnes KM, et al. Effects of estrogen on growth plate senescence and epiphyseal fusion. Proc Natl Acad Sci USA 2001; 98:6871–6876.
188. Manolagas SC. Birth and death of bone cells: basic regulatory mechanisms and implications for the pathogenesis and treatment of osteoporosis. Endocr Rev 2000; 21:115–137.
189. Schoenau E, Neu CM, Rauch F, Manz F. The development of bone strength at the proximal radius during childhood and adolescence. J Clin Endocrinol Metab 2001; 86:613–618.
190. Marcus R, Leary D, Schneider DL, et al. The contribution of testosterone to skeletal development and maintenance: lessons from the androgen insensitivity syndrome. J Clin Endocrinol Metab 2000; 85:1032–1037.
191. Miller JD, Tannenbaum GS, Colle E, et al. Daytime pulsatile growth hormone secretion during childhood and adolescence. J Clin Endocrinol Metab 1982; 55:989–994.
192. Ross JL, Pescovitz OH, Barnes K, et al. Growth hormone secretory dynamics in children with precocious puberty. Ann Hum Biol 1989; 16:397–406.
193. Costin G, Kaufman FR. Growth hormone secretory patterns in children with short stature. J Pediatr 1987; 110:362–368.
194. Costin G, Kaufman FR, Brasel JA. Growth hormone secretory dynamics in subjects with normal stature. J Pediatr 1989; 115: 537–544.
195. Garnier P, Raynaud F, Job JC. Growth hormone secretion during sleep. I. Comparison with GH responses to conventional pharmacologic stimuli in pubertal and early pubertal short subjects. Effects of treatment with human GH in patients with discrepant measurements of GH secretion. Horm Res 1988; 29: 133–139.
196. Link K, Blizzard RM, Evans WS, et al. The effect of androgens on the pulsatile release and the twenty-four-hour mean concentration of growth hormone in peripubertal males. J Clin Endocrinol Metab 1986; 62:159–164.
197. Martha PM Jr, Rogol AD, Veldhuis JD. Alterations in the pulsatile properties of circulating growth hormone concentrations during puberty in boys. J Clin Endocrinol Metab 1989; 69:563–570.
198. Mauras N, Blizzard RM, Link K, et al. Augmentation of growth hormone secretion during puberty: evidence for a pulse amplitude-modulated phenomenon. J Clin Endocrinol Metab 1987; 64:596–601.
199. Wennink JM, Delemarre-van de Waal HA, Schoemaker R, et al. Growth hormone secretion patterns in relation to LH and estradiol secretion throughout normal female puberty. Acta Endocrinol (Copenh) 1991; 124:129–135.
200. Martha PMJ, Gorman KM, Blizzard RM, et al. Endogenous growth hormone secretion and clearance rates in normal boys, as determined by deconvolution analysis: relationship to age, pubertal status, and body mass. J Clin Endocrinol Metab 1992; 74:336–344.
201. Veldhuis JD, Roemmich JN, Rogol AD. Gender and sexual maturation–dependent contrasts in the neuroregulation of growth hormone secretion in prepubertal and late adolescent males and females: a general clinical research center–based study. J Clin Endocrinol Metab 2000; 85:2385–2394.
202. Marin G, Domene HM, Barnes KM, et al. The effects of estrogen priming and puberty on the growth hormone response to standardized treadmill exercise and arginine-insulin in normal girls and boys. J Clin Endocrinol Metab 1994; 79:537–541.
203. Bouix O, Brun JF, Fedou C, et al. Plasma beta-endorphin, corticotrophin and growth hormone responses to exercise in pubertal and prepubertal children. Horm Metab Res 1994; 26:195–199.
204. Loche S, Cambiaso P, Carta D, et al. The growth hormone–releasing activity of hexarelin, a new synthetic hexapeptide, in short normal and obese children and in hypopituitary subjects. J Clin Endocrinol Metab 1995; 80:674–678.
205. Bellone J, Aimaretti G, Bartolotta E, et al. Growth hormone-releasing activity of hexarelin, a new synthetic hexapeptide, before and during puberty. J Clin Endocrinol Metab 1995; 80: 1090–1094.
206. Metzger DL, Kerrigan JR. Estrogen receptor blockade with tamoxifen diminishes growth hormone secretion in boys: evidence for a stimulatory role of endogenous estrogens during male adolescence. J Clin Endocrinol Metab 1994; 79:513–518.
207. Kerrigan JR, Veldhuis JD, Rogol AD. Androgen-receptor blockade enhances pulsatile luteinizing hormone production in late pubertal males: evidence for a hypothalamic site of physiologic androgen feedback action. Pediatr Res 1994; 35:102–106.
208. Keenan BS, Richards GE, Ponder SW, et al. Androgen-stimulated pubertal growth: the effects of testosterone and dihydrotestosterone on growth hormone and insulin-like growth factor-I in the treatment of short stature and delayed puberty. J Clin Endocrinol Metab 1993; 76:996–1001.
209. Harris DA, Van Vliet G, Egli CA, et al. Somatomedin-C in normal puberty and in true precocious puberty before and after treatment with a potent luteinizing hormone–releasing hormone agonist. J Clin Endocrinol Metab 1985; 61:152–159.
210. Mansfield MJ, Rudlin CR, Crigler JF Jr, et al. Changes in growth and serum growth hormone and plasma somatomedin-C levels during suppression of gonadal sex steroid secretion in girls with central precocious puberty. J Clin Endocrinol Metab 1988; 66:3–9.
211. Rimoin DL, Merimee TJ, Rabinowitz D, McKusick VA. Genetic aspects of clinical endocrinology. Recent Prog Horm Res 1968; 24:365–437.
212. Phillips JA III. Inherited defects in growth hormone synthesis and action. In Scriver CR, Beaudet AI, Sly WS, et al (eds). The Metabolic and Molecular Bases of Inherited Disease. New York, McGraw-Hill/Medical Publishing Division, 2001, Vol 3, pp 4159–4180.
213. de Boer JA, Schoemaker J, van der Veen EA. Impaired reproductive function in women treated for growth hormone deficiency during childhood. Clin Endocrinol (Oxf) 1997; 46:681–689.
214. Aynsley-Green A, Zachmann M, Prader A. Interrelation of the therapeutic effects of growth hormone and testosterone on growth in hypopituitarism. J Pediatr 1976; 89:992–999.
215. Bala RM, Lopatka J, Leung A. Serum immunoreactive somatomedin levels in normal adults, pregnant women at term, children at various ages, and children with constitutionally delayed growth. J Clin Endocrinol Metab 1981; 52:508–512.
216. Lofqvist C, Andersson E, Gelander L, et al. Reference values for IGF-I throughout childhood and adolescence: a model that accounts simultaneously for the effect of gender, age, and puberty. J Clin Endocrinol Metab 2001; 86:5870–5876.
217. Juul A, Bang P, Hertel NT, et al. Serum insulin-like growth factor-I in 1030 healthy children, adolescents, and adults: relation to age, sex, stage of puberty, testicular size, and body mass index. J Clin Endocrinol Metab 1994; 78:744–752.
218. Sjogren K, Liu JL, Blad K, et al. Liver-derived insulin-like growth factor I (IGF-I) is the principal source of IGF-I in blood but is not required for postnatal body growth in mice. Proc Natl Acad Sci USA 1999; 96:7088–7092.
219. Yakar S, Liu JL, Stannard B, et al. Normal growth and development in the absence of hepatic insulin-like growth factor I. Proc Natl Acad Sci USA 1999; 96:7324–7329.
220. Zachman M, Prader A, Sobel E, et al. Pubertal growth in patients with androgen insensitivity: indirect evidence for the importance of estrogens in pubertal growth of girls. J Pediatr 1986; 108:694–697.
221. Klein KO, Baron J, Colli MJ, et al. Estrogen levels in childhood determined by an ultrasensitive recombinant cell bioassay. J Clin Invest 1994; 94:2475–2480.
222. Ikegami S, Moriwake T, Tanaka H, et al. An ultrasensitive assay revealed age-related changes in serum oestradiol at low concentrations in both sexes from infancy to puberty. Clin Endocrinol 2001; 55:789–795.
223. Klein KO, Martha PMJ, Blizzard RM, et al. A longitudinal assessment of hormonal and physical alterations during normal puberty in boys. II. Estrogen levels as determined by an ultrasensitive bioassay. J Clin Endocrinol Metab 1996; 81:3203–3207.
224. Grumbach MM, Richards GE, Conte FA, et al. Clinical disorders of adrenal function and puberty: an assessment of the role of the adrenal cortex in normal and abnormal puberty in man and evidence for an ACTH-like pituitary adrenal androgen stimulating hormone. In James VHT, Serio M, Giusti G, et al (eds). The Endocrine Function of the Human Adrenal Cortex,

Serono Symposium. New York, Academic Press, 1977, pp 583–612.

225. Van Wyk JJ, Grumbach MM. Syndrome of precocious menstruation and galactorrhea in juvenile hypothyroidism: an example of hormonal overlap in pituitary feedback. J Pediatr 1960; 57: 416–435.
226. Greulich WS, Pyle SI. Radiographic Atlas of Skeletal Development of the Hand and Wrist. Stanford, CA, Stanford University Press, 1959.
227. Tanner JM, Whitehouse RH, Marshall WA, et al. Assessment of Skeletal Maturity and Prediction of Adult Height: TW 2 Method. New York, Academic Press, 1975.
228. Aicardi G, Vignolo M, Milani S, et al. Assessment of skeletal maturity of the hand-wrist and knee: a comparison among methods. Am J Hum Biol 2000; 12:610–615.
229. Marshall WA. Inter-relationships of skeletal maturation, sexual development and somatic growth in man. Ann Hum Biol 1974; 1:29–40.
230. Loesch DZ, Hopper JL, Rogucka E, Huggins RM. Timing and genetic rapport between growth in skeletal maturity and height around puberty: similarities and differences between girls and boys. Am J Hum Genet 1995; 56:753–759.
231. Hauspie R, Bielicki T, Koniarek J. Skeletal maturity at onset of the adolescent growth spurt and at peak height velocity for growth in height: a threshold effect? Ann Hum Biol 1995; 18: 23–29.
232. Bayley N, Pinneau SR. Tables for predicting adult height from skeletal age: revised for use with the Greulich-Pyle standards. J Pediatr 1952; 40:441.
233. Roche AF, Wainer H, Thissen D. The RWT method for the prediction of adult stature. Pediatrics 1975; 56:1026–1033.
234. Walker RN. Standards for somatotyping children. I. Prediction of young adult height from children's growth data. Ann Hum Biol 1974; 1:149–158.
235. Roche AF. Skeletal maturity of children 6–11 years: racial, geographic area of residence, socioeconomic differentials. In National Health Survey. DHEW Vital and Health Statistics Series 11, No 149. Washington, DC, Government Printing Office, 1975.
236. Tanner JM, Gibbons RD. Automatic bone age measurement using computerized image analysis. J Pediatr Endocrinol 1994; 7:141–145.
237. Gross GW, Boone JM, Bishop DM. Pediatric skeletal age: determination with neural networks. Radiology 1995; 195:689–695.
238. Van Teunenbroek A, De Waal W, Roks A, et al. Computer-aided skeletal age scores in healthy children, girls with Turner syndrome, and in children with constitutionally tall stature. Pediatr Res 1996; 39:360–367.
239. Roberts CD, Vogtle L, Stevenson RD. Effect of hemiplegia on skeletal maturation. J Pediatr 1994; 125:824–828.
240. Seeman E. From density to structure: growing up and growing old on the surfaces of bone. J Bone Miner Res 1997; 12:509–521.
241. Seeman E. Clinical review 137: sexual dimorphism in skeletal size, density, and strength. J Clin Endocrinol Metab 2001; 86: 4576–4584.
242. Lu PW, Cowell CT, Lloyd-Jones SA, et al. Volumetric bone mineral density in normal subjects, aged 5–27 years. J Clin Endocrinol Metab 1996; 81:1586–1590.
243. Bass S, Delmas PD, Pearce G, et al. The differing tempo of growth in bone size, mass, and density in girls is region-specific. J Clin Invest 1999; 104:795–804.
244. Weaver CM, Peacock M, Martin BR, et al. Calcium retention estimated from indicators of skeletal status in adolescent girls and young women. Am J Clin Nutr 1996; 64:67–70.
245. Carrie Fassler AL, Bonjour JP. Osteoporosis as a pediatric problem. Pediatr Clin North Am 1995; 42:811–824.
246. Matkovic V, Jelic T, Wardlaw GM, et al. Timing of peak bone mass in Caucasian females and its implication for the prevention of osteoporosis: inference from a cross-sectional model. J Clin Invest 1994; 93:799–808.
247. del Rio L, Carrascosa A, Pons F, et al. Bone mineral density of the lumbar spine in white Mediterranean Spanish children and adolescents: changes related to age, sex, and puberty. Pediatr Res 1994; 35:362–366.
248. Proesmans W, Goos G, Emma F, et al. Total body mineral mass measured with dual photon absorptiometry in healthy children. Eur J Pediatr 1994; 153:807–812.
249. Kroger H, Kotaniemi A, Kroger L, Alhava E. Development of bone mass and bone density of the spine and femoral neck: a prospective study of 65 children and adolescents. Bone Miner 1993; 23:171–182.
250. Bachrach LK. Bone mineralization in childhood and adolescence. Curr Opin Pediatr 1993; 5:467–473.
251. Bachrach LK, Hastie T, Wang MC, et al. Bone mineral acquisition in healthy Asian, Hispanic, black, and Caucasian youth: a longitudinal study. J Clin Endocrinol Metab 1999; 84:4702–4712.
252. Grimston SK, Morrison K, Harder JA, Hanley DA. Bone mineral density during puberty in western Canadian children. Bone Miner 1992; 19:85–96.
253. Theintz G, Buchs B, Rizzoli R, et al. Longitudinal monitoring of bone mass accumulation in healthy adolescents: evidence for a marked reduction after 16 years of age at the levels of lumbar spine and femoral neck in female subjects. J Clin Endocrinol Metab 1992; 75:1060–1065.
254. Bonjour JP, Theintz G, Buchs B, et al. Critical years and stages of puberty for spinal and femoral bone mass accumulation during adolescence. J Clin Endocrinol Metab 1991; 73:555–563.
255. Loro ML, Sayre J, Roe TF, et al. Early identification of children predisposed to low peak bone mass and osteoporosis later in life. J Clin Endocrinol Metab 2000; 85:3908–3918.
256. Bailey DA, Martin AD, McKay HA, et al. Calcium accretion in girls and boys during puberty: a longitudinal analysis. J Bone Miner Res 2000; 15:2245–2250.
257. Nguyen TV, Maynard LM, Towne B, et al. Sex differences in bone mass acquisition during growth: The Fels Longitudinal Study. J Clin Densitom 2001; 4(2):147–157.
258. Bonjour JP, Theintz G, Law F, et al. Peak bone mass. Osteoporos Int 1994; 4(suppl 1):7–13.
259. Bradney M, Karlsson MK, Duan Y, et al. Heterogeneity in the growth of the axial and appendicular skeleton in boys: implications for the pathogenesis of bone fragility in men. J Bone Miner Res 2000; 15:1871–1878.
260. Mora S, Goodman WG, Loro ML, et al. Age-related changes in cortical and cancellous vertebral bone density in girls: assessment with quantitative CT. AJR 1994; 162:405–409.
261. Lloyd T, Rollings N, Andon MB, et al. Determinants of bone density in young women. I. Relationships among pubertal development, total body bone mass, and total body bone density in premenarchal females. J Clin Endocrinol Metab 1992; 75:383–387.
262. Moreira-Andres MN, Papapietro K, Canizo FJ, et al. Correlations between bone mineral density, insulin-like growth factor I and auxological variables. Eur J Endocrinol 1995; 132:573–579.
263. Rico H, Revilla M, Villa LF, et al. Determinants of total-body and regional bone mineral content and density in postpubertal normal women. Metabolism 1994; 43:263–266.
264. van der Meulen MC, Ashford MWJ, Kiratli BJ, et al. Determinants of femoral geometry and structure during adolescent growth. J Orthop Res 1996; 14:22–29.
265. Lehtonen-Veromaa M, Mottonen T, Irjala K, et al. A 1-year prospective study on the relationship between physical activity, markers of bone metabolism, and bone acquisition in peripubertal girls. J Clin Endocrinol Metab 2000; 85:3726–3732.
266. Lehtonen-Veromaa M, Mottonen T, Nuotio I, et al. Influence of physical activity on ultrasound and dual-energy x-ray absorptiometry bone measurements in peripubertal girls: a cross-sectional study. Calcif Tissue Int 2000; 66:248–254.
267. Lehtonen-Veromaa M, Mottonen T, Svedstrom E, et al. Physical activity and bone mineral acquisition in peripubertal girls. Scand J Med Sci Sports 2000; 10:236–243.
268. Genanat HK, Engelke K, Fuerst T, et al. Noninvasive assessment of bone mineral and structure: state of the art. J Bone Miner Res 1992; 7:137–145.
269. Lu PW, Briody JN, Ogle GD, et al. Bone mineral density of total body, spine, and femoral neck in children and young adults: a cross-sectional and longitudinal study. J Bone Miner Res 1994; 9:1451–1458.
270. Schoenau E, Neu CM, Rauch F, Manz F. The development of bone strength at the proximal radius during childhood and adolescence. J Clin Endocrinol Metab 2001; 86:613–618.

271. Lappe JM, Stegman M, Davies KM, et al. A prospective study of quantitative ultrasound in children and adolescents. J Clin Densitom 2000; 3:167–175.
272. Lum CK, Wang MC, Moore E, et al. A comparison of calcaneus ultrasound and dual x-ray absorptiometry in healthy North American youths and young adults. J Clin Densitom 1999; 2: 403–411.
273. Kardinaal AF, Hoorneman G, Vaananen K, et al. Determinants of bone mass and bone geometry in adolescent and young adult women. Calcif Tissue Int 2000; 66:81–89.
274. Bachrach LK. Acquisition of optimal bone mass in childhood and adolescence. Trends Endocrinol Metab 2001; 12:22–28.
275. Weaver CM, Peacock M, Johnston CC Jr. Adolescent nutrition in the prevention of postmenopausal osteoporosis. J Clin Endocrinol Metab 1999; 84:1839–1843.
276. Rubin K, Schirduan V, Gendreau P, et al. Predictors of axial and peripheral bone mineral density in healthy children and adolescents, with special attention to the role of puberty. J Pediatr 1993; 123:863–870.
277. Sentipal JM, Wardlaw GM, Mahan J, Matkovic V. Influence of calcium intake and growth indexes on vertebral bone mineral density in young females. Am J Clin Nutr 1991; 54:425–428.
278. Dibba B, Prentice A, Ceesay M, et al. Effect of calcium supplementation on bone mineral accretion in Gambian children accustomed to a low-calcium diet. Am J Clin Nutr 2000; 71:544–549.
279. Abrams SA, Stuff JE. Calcium metabolism in girls: current dietary intakes lead to low rates of calcium absorption and retention during puberty. Am J Clin Nutr 1994; 60:739–743.
280. Anderson JJ, Pollitzer WS. Ethnic and genetic differences in susceptibility to osteoporotic fractures. Adv Nutr Res 1994; 9: 129–149.
281. Gilsanz V, Roe TF, Mora S, et al. Changes in vertebral bone density in black girls and white girls during childhood and puberty. Am J Med Genet 1991; 41:313–318.
282. Chan GM, Hoffman K, McMurry M. Effects of dairy products on bone and body composition in pubertal girls. J Pediatr 1995; 126:551–556.
283. Anderson JJ, Metz JA. Contributions of dietary calcium and physical activity to primary prevention of osteoporosis in females. J Am Coll Nutr 1993; 12:378–383.
284. Johnston CCJ, Miller JZ, Slemenda CW, et al. Calcium supplementation and increases in bone mineral density in children. N Engl J Med 1992; 327:82–87.
285. Matkovic V. Calcium and peak bone mass. J Intern Med 1992; 231:151–160.
286. Lee WT, Leung SS, Leung DM, Cheng JC. A follow-up study on the effects of calcium-supplement withdrawal and puberty on bone acquisition of children. Am J Clin Nutr 1996; 64:71–77.
287. Bonjour JP, Chevalley T, Ammann P, et al. Gain in bone mineral mass in prepubertal girls 3.5 years after discontinuation of calcium supplementation: a follow-up study. Lancet 2001; 358: 1208–1212.
288. Abrams SA, Copeland KC, Gunn SK, et al. Calcium absorption, bone mass accumulation, and kinetics increase during early pubertal development in girls. J Clin Endocrinol Metab 2000; 85: 1805–1809.
289. Teegarden D, Lyle RM, Proulx WR, et al. Previous milk consumption is associated with greater bone density in young women. Am J Clin Nutr 1999; 69:1014–1017.
290. Abrams SA. Calcium turnover and nutrition through the life cycle. Proc Nutr Soc 2001; 60(2):283–289.
291. Nickols-Richardson SM, Modlesky CM, O'Connor PJ, Lewis RD. Premenarcheal gymnasts possess higher bone mineral density than controls. Med Sci Sports Exerc 2000; 32:63–69.
292. Lloyd T, Chinchilli VM, Johnson-Rollings N, et al. Adult female hip bone density reflects teenage sports-exercise patterns but not teenage calcium intake. Pediatrics 2000; 106:40–44.
293. Mauras N, Haymond MW, Darmaun D, et al. Calcium and protein kinetics in prepubertal boys. Positive effects of testosterone. J Clin Invest 1994; 93:1014–1019.
294. Zamberlan N, Radetti G, Paganini C, et al. Evaluation of cortical thickness and bone density by roentgen microdensitometry in growing males and females. Eur J Pediatr 1996; 155:377–382.
295. Finkelstein JS, Neer RM, Biller BM, et al. Osteopenia in men with a history of delayed puberty. N Engl J Med 1992; 326: 600–604.
296. Finkelstein JS, Klibanski A, Neer RM. A longitudinal evaluation of bone mineral density in adult men with histories of delayed puberty. J Clin Endocrinol Metab 1996; 81:1152–1155.
297. Finkelstein JS, Klibanski A, Neer RM. Evaluation of lumbar spine bone mineral density (BMD) using dual energy x-ray absorptiometry (DXA) in 21 young men with histories of constitutionally-delayed puberty. J Clin Endocrinol Metab 1999; 84: 3400–3401.
298. Behre HM, Simoni M, Nieschlag E. Strong association between serum levels of leptin and testosterone in men. Clin Endocrinol (Oxf) 1997; 47:237–240.
299. Bertelloni S, Baroncelli GI, Battini R, et al. Short-term effect of testosterone treatment on reduced bone density in boys with constitutional delay of puberty. J Bone Miner Res 1995; 10: 1488–1495.
300. Bertelloni S, Baroncelli GI, Ferdeghini M, et al. Normal volumetric bone mineral density and bone turnover in young men with histories of constitutional delay of puberty. J Clin Endocrinol Metab 1998; 83:4280–4283.
301. Bertelloni S, Baroncelli GI, Saggese G. Normal volumetric bone mineral density in young men with histories of constitutional delay of puberty: author's response. J Clin Endocrinol Metab 1999; 84:3403.
302. Arisaka O, Arisaka M, Nakayama Y, et al. Effect of testosterone on bone density and bone metabolism in adolescent male hypogonadism. Metabolism 1995; 44:419–423.
303. Kubler A, Schulz G, Cordes U, et al. The influence of testosterone substitution on bone mineral density in patients with Klinefelter's syndrome. Exp Clin Endocrinol 1992; 100:129–132.
304. Hergenroeder AC. Bone mineralization, hypothalamic amenorrhea, and sex steroid therapy in female adolescents and young adults. J Pediatr 1995; 126:683–689.
305. Fabbri G, Petraglia F, Segre A, et al. Reduced spinal bone density in young women with amenorrhoea. Eur J Obstet Gynecol Reprod Biol 1991; 41:117–122.
306. Grinspoon S, Thomas E, Pitts S, et al. Prevalence and predictive factors for regional osteopenia in women with anorexia nervosa. Ann Intern Med 2000; 133:790–794.
307. Saggese G, Bertelloni S, Baroncelli GI, et al. Reduction of bone density: an effect of gonadotropin releasing hormone analogue treatment in central precocious puberty. Eur J Pediatr 1993; 152:717–720.
308. Saggese G, Bertelloni S, Baroncelli GI, et al. Bone loss during gonadotropin-releasing hormone agonist treatment in girls with true precocious puberty is not due to an impairment of calcitonin secretion. J Endocrinol Invest 1991; 14:231–236.
309. Verrotti A, Chiarelli F, Montanaro AF, Morgese G. Bone mineral content in girls with precocious puberty treated with gonadotropin-releasing hormone analog. Gynecol Endocrinol 1995; 9:277–281.
310. Neely EK, Bachrach LK, Hintz RL, et al. Bone mineral density during treatment of central precocious puberty. J Pediatr 1995; 127:819–822.
311. Antoniazzi F, Bertoldo F, Zamboni G, et al. Bone mineral metabolism in girls with precocious puberty during gonadotrophin-releasing hormone agonist treatment. Eur J Endocrinol 1995; 133:412–417.
312. Simberg N, Titinen A, Silfvast A, et al. High bone density in hyperandrogenic women: effect of gonadotropin-releasing hormone agonist alone or in conjunction with estrogen-progestin replacement. J Clin Endocrinol Metab 1995; 80:646–651.
313. Buchanan JR, Hospodar C, Myers C, et al. Effect of excess androgens on bone density in young women. J Clin Endocrinol Metab 1988; 67:937–943.
314. Orwel ES. Androgens as anabolic agents for bone. Trends Endocrinol Metab 1996; 7:77–84.
315. Lonzer MD, Imrie R, Rogers D, et al. Effects of heredity, age, weight, puberty, activity, and calcium intake on bone mineral density in children. Clin Pediatr (Phila) 1996; 35:185–189.
316. McKay HA, Bailey DA, Wilkinson AA, Houston CS. Familial comparison of bone mineral density at the proximal femur and lumbar spine. Bone Miner 1994; 24:95–107.
317. Blumsohn A, Hannon RA, Wrate R, et al. Biochemical markers of bone turnover in girls during puberty. Clin Endocrinol (Oxf) 1994; 40:663–670.

318. Molina RM, Bouchard C. Growth, Maturation and Physical Activity. Champaign, Ill, Human Kinetics, 1991.
319. Holliday MA. Body composition and energy needs during growth. In Falkner F, Tanner JM (eds). Human Growth, Postnatal Growth. New York, Plenum, 1986, pp 101–117.
320. Rico H, Revilla M, Villa LF, et al. Body composition in children and Tanner's stages: a study with dual-energy x-ray absorptiometry. Metabolism 1993; 42:967–970.
321. Cheek DB. Body composition, hormones, nutrition and adolescent growth. In Grumbach MM, Grave GD, Mayer FE (eds). Control of the Onset of Puberty. New York, John Wiley & Sons, 1974, pp 424–447.
322. Forbes GB. Puberty: body composition. In Berenberg SR (ed). Puberty, Biologic and Social Components. Leiden, HE Stenfert Kroese, 1975, pp 132–145.
323. Forbes GB. Body composition in adolescence. In Falkner F, Tanner JM (eds). Human Growth, Postnatal Growth. New York, Plenum, 1986, pp 119–145.
324. Frisancho AR, Flegel PN. Advanced maturation with centripetal fat pattern. Hum Biol 1982; 54:717–727.
325. Garn SM. Fat weight and fat placement in the female. Science 1957; 125:1091–1092.
326. Kissebah AH, Krakower GR. Regional adiposity and morbidity. Physiol Rev 1994; 74:761–811.
327. Rolland-Cachera MF. Body composition during adolescence: methods, limitations and determinants. Horm Res 1993; 39(suppl 3):25–40.
328. Rosenthal M, Bain SH, Bush A, Warner JO. Weight/height as a screening test for obesity or thinness in schoolage children. Eur J Pediatr 1994; 153:876–883.
329. Ellis KJ, Shypailo RJ, Pratt JA, et al. Accuracy of dual-energy x-ray absorptiometry for body-composition measurements in children. Am J Clin Nutr 1994; 60:660–665.
330. de Ridder CM, de Boer RW, Seidell JC, et al. Body fat distribution in pubertal girls quantified by magnetic resonance imaging. Int J Obes Relat Metab Disord 1992; 16:443–449.
331. Goran MI. Measurement issues related to studies of childhood obesity: assessment of body composition, body fat distribution, physical activity and food intake. Pediatrics 1998; 101:505–518.
332. Fox KR, Peters DM, Sharpe P, Bell M. Assessment of abdominal fat development in young adolescents using magnetic resonance imaging. Int J Obes Relat Metab Disord 2000; 24:1653–1659.
333. Goran MI, Gower BA, Treuth M, Nagy TR. Prediction of intra-abdominal and subcutaneous abdominal adipose tissue in healthy pre-pubertal children. Int J Obes Relat Metab Disord 1998; 22:549–558.
334. Roemmich JN, Rogol AD. Hormonal changes during puberty and their relationship to fat distribution. Am J Hum Biol 1999; 11:209–224.
335. Gidding SS. Preventive pediatric cardiology: tobacco, cholesterol, obesity, and physical activity. Pediatr Clin North Am 1999; 46:253–262.
336. Goran MI. Energy expenditure, body composition, and disease risk in children and adolescents. Proc Nutr Soc 1997; 56:195–209.
337. Goran MI, Kaskoun M, Shuman WP. Intra-abdominal adipose tissue in young children. Int J Obes Relat Metab Disord 1995; 19:279–283.
338. Hammer LD, Wilson DM, Litt IF, et al. Impact of pubertal development on body fat distribution among white, Hispanic, and Asian female adolescents. J Pediatr 1991; 118:975–980.
339. de Ridder CM, Bruning PF, Zonderland ML, et al. Body fat mass, body fat distribution, and plasma hormones in early puberty in females. J Clin Endocrinol Metab 1990; 70:888–893.
340. Caserta F, Tchkonia T, Civelek VN, et al. Fat depot origin affects fatty acid handling in cultured rat and human preadipocytes. Am J Physiol 2001; 280:E238–E247.
341. Frisch RE, Revelle R. Height and weight at menarche and a hypothesis of critical body weights and adolescent events. Science 1970; 169:397–399.
342. Obesity and cardiovascular disease risk factors in black and white girls: the NHLBI Growth and Health Study. Am J Public Health 1992; 82:1613–1620.
343. Morrison JA, Barton B, Biro FM, et al. Sexual maturation and obesity in 9- and 10-year-old black and white girls: the National Heart, Lung, and Blood Institute Growth and Health Study. J Pediatr 1994; 124:889–895.
344. Wong WW, Butte NF, Ellis KJ, et al. Pubertal African-American girls expend less energy at rest and during physical activity than Caucasian girls. J Clin Endocrinol Metab 1999; 84:906–911.
345. Kaplan AS, Zemel BS, Stallings VA. Differences in resting energy expenditure in prepubertal black children and white children. J Pediatr 1996; 129:643–647.
346. Morrison JA, Alfaro MP, Khoury P, et al. Determinants of resting energy expenditure in young black girls and young white girls. J Pediatr 1996; 129:637–642.
347. Sun M, Gower BA, Bartolucci AA, et al. A longitudinal study of resting energy expenditure relative to body composition during puberty in African American and white children. Am J Clin Nutr 2001; 73:308–315.
348. Gunn VL, Nechyloa C. Harriet Lane Handbook, 16th ed. St. Louis, Mosby, 2002.
349. Schur EA, Sanders M, Steiner H. Body dissatisfaction and dieting in young children. Int J Eat Disord 2000; 27:74–82.
350. Javier Nieto F, Szklo M, Comstock GW. Childhood weight and growth rate as predictors of adult mortality. Am J Epidemiol 1992; 136:201–213.
351. Neumark-Sztainer D, Hannan PJ. Weight-related behaviors among adolescent girls and boys: results from a national survey. Arch Pediatr Adolesc Med 2000; 154:569–577.
352. Schreiber GB, Robins M, Striegel-Moore R, et al. Weight modification efforts reported by black and white preadolescent girls: National Heart, Lung, and Blood Institute Growth and Health Study. Pediatrics 1996; 98:63–70.
353. Neumark-Sztainer D, Rock CL, Thornquist MD, et al. Weight-control behaviors among adults and adolescents: associations with dietary intake. Prev Med 2000; 30:381–391.
354. Knishkowy B, Palti H, Tun N, et al. Cardiovascular risk factors by ethnic group and menstrual status among 13- and 14-year-old Israeli schoolchildren. Public Health Rev 1994; 22:55–73.
355. Gunnell DJ, Frankel SJ, Nanchahal K, et al. Childhood obesity and adult cardiovascular mortality: a 57-y follow-up study based on the Boyd Orr cohort. Am J Clin Nutr 1998; 67:1111–1118.
356. Must A, Jacques PF, Dallal GE, et al. Long-term morbidity and mortality of overweight adolescents: a follow-up of the Harvard Growth Study of 1922 to 1935. N Engl J Med 1992; 327:1350–1355.
357. Nieto FJ, Szklo M, Comstock GW. Childhood weight and growth rate as predictors of adult mortality. Am J Epidemiol 1992; 136:201–213.
358. Mossberg HO. 40-year follow-up of overweight children. Lancet 1989; 2:491–493.
359. Hoffmans MD, Kromhout D, Coulander CD. Body mass index at the age of 18 and its effects on 32-year-mortality from coronary heart disease and cancer: a nested case-control study among the entire 1932 Dutch male birth cohort. J Clin Epidemiol 1989; 42:513–520.
360. Hoffmans MD, Kromhout D, de Lezenne CC. The impact of body mass index of 78,612 18-year old Dutch men on 32-year mortality from all causes. J Clin Epidemiol 1988; 41:749–756.
361. Freedman DS, Dietz WH, Srinivasan SR, Berenson GS. The relation of overweight to cardiovascular risk factors among children and adolescents: the Bogalusa Heart Study. Pediatrics 1999; 103:1175–1182.
362. Csabi G, Torok K, Jeges S, Molnar D. Presence of metabolic cardiovascular syndrome in obese children. Eur J Pediatr 2000; 159:91–94.
363. Akerblom HK, Viikari J, Raitakari OT, Uhari M. Cardiovascular Risk in Young Finns Study: general outline and recent developments. Ann Med 1999; 31:45–54.
364. Ronnemaa T, Knip M, Lautala P, et al. Serum insulin and other cardiovascular risk indicators in children, adolescents and young adults. Ann Med 1991; 23:67–72.
365. Gallistl S, Sudi KM, Borkenstein MH, et al. Determinants of haemostatic risk factors for coronary heart disease in obese children and adolescents. Int J Obes Relat Metab Disord 2000; 24:1459–1464.
366. McGill HJ, McMahan CA, Zieske AW, et al. Association of coronary heart disease risk factors with microscopic qualities of coronary atherosclerosis in youth. Circulation 2000; 102:374–379.

367. Lauer RM, Lee J, Clarke WR. Factors affecting the relationship between childhood and adult cholesterol levels: the Muscatine Study. Pediatrics 1988; 82:309–318.
368. Lauer RM, Lee J, Clarke WR. Predicting adult cholesterol levels from measurements in childhood and adolescence: the Muscatine Study. Bull NY Acad Med 1989; 65:1127–1142.
369. Bao W, Srinivasan SR, Berenson GS. Persistent elevation of plasma insulin levels is associated with increased cardiovascular risk in children and young adults: the Bogalusa Heart Study. Circulation 1996; 93:54–59.
370. Chen W, Bao W, Begum S, et al. Age-related patterns of the clustering of cardiovascular risk variables of syndrome X from childhood to young adulthood in a population made up of black and white subjects: the Bogalusa Heart Study. Diabetes 2000; 49:1042–1048.
371. Hulman S, Kushner H, Katz S, Falkner B. Can cardiovascular risk be predicted by newborn, childhood, and adolescent body size? An examination of longitudinal data in urban African Americans. J Pediatr 1998; 132:90–97.
372. Leccia G, Marotta T, Masella MR, et al. Sex-related influence of body size and sexual maturation on blood pressure in adolescents. Eur J Clin Nutr 1999; 53:333–337.
373. Voors AW, Webber LS, Frerichs RR, et al. Body height and body mass as determinants of basal blood pressure in children: the Bogalusa Heart Study. Am J Epidemiol 1977; 106:101–108.
374. Adrogue HE, Sinaiko AR. Prevalence of hypertension in junior high school–aged children: effect of new recommendations in the 1996 Updated Task Force Report. Am J Hypertens 2001; 14:412–414.
375. Bao W, Dalferes ER, Srinivasan SR, et al. Normative distribution of complete blood count from early childhood through adolescence: the Bogalusa Heart Study. Prev Med 1993; 22: 825–837.
376. Berkey CS, Gardner J, Colditz GA. Blood pressure in adolescence and early adulthood related to obesity and birth size. Obes Res 1998; 6:187–195.
377. Deckelbaum RJ, Williams CL. Childhood obesity: the health issue. Obes Res 2001; 9(suppl 4):239S–243S.
378. Falkner B. Hypertension in childhood and adolescence. Clin Exp Hypertens 1993; 15:1315–1326.
379. Feld LG, Springate JE, Waz WR. Special topics in pediatric hypertension. Semin Nephrol 1998; 18:295–303.
380. Flynn JT. What's new in pediatric hypertension? Curr Hypertens Rep 2001; 3:503–510.
381. He Q, Ding ZY, Fong DY, Karlberg J. Blood pressure is associated with body mass index in both normal and obese children. Hypertension 2000; 36:165–170.
382. Modesti PA, Pela I, Cecioni I, et al. Changes in blood pressure reactivity and 24-hour blood pressure profile occurring at puberty. Angiology 1994; 45:443–450.
383. Nelson MJ, Ragland DR, Syme SL. Longitudinal prediction of adult blood pressure from juvenile blood pressure levels. Am J Epidemiol 1992; 136:633–645.
384. Resnicow K, Futterman R, Vaughan RD. Body mass index as a predictor of systolic blood pressure in a multiracial sample of US schoolchildren. Ethn Dis 1993; 3:351–361.
385. Rocchini AP, Katch V, Anderson J, et al. Blood pressure in obese adolescents: effect of weight loss. Pediatrics 1988; 82:16–23.
386. Rosner B, Prineas R, Daniels SR, Loggie J. Blood pressure differences between blacks and whites in relation to body size among US children and adolescents. Am J Epidemiol 2000; 151: 1007–1019.
387. Liker HR, Barnes KM, Comite F, et al. Blood pressure and body size in precocious puberty. Acta Paediatr Scand 1988; 77: 294–298.
388. Lurbe E, Alvarez V, Liao Y, et al. The impact of obesity and body fat distribution on ambulatory blood pressure in children and adolescents. Am J Hypertens 1998; 11:418–424.
389. Dietz WH. Health consequences of obesity in youth: childhood predictors of adult disease. Pediatrics 1998; 101:518–525.
390. Bartosh SM, Aronson AJ. Childhood hypertension: an update on etiology, diagnosis, and treatment. Pediatr Clin North Am 1999; 46:235–252.
391. Voors AW, Harsha DW, Webber LS, et al. Relation of blood pressure to stature in healthy young adults. Am J Epidemiol 1982; 115:833–840.
392. Watanabe T, Nagashima M, Hojo Y. Circadian rhythm of blood pressure in children with reference to normal and diseased children. Acta Paediatr Jpn 1994; 36:683–689.
393. Bao W, Threefoot SA, Srinivasan SR, Berenson GS. Essential hypertension predicted by tracking of elevated blood pressure from childhood to adulthood: the Bogalusa Heart Study. Am J Hypertens 1995; 8:657–665.
394. Janz KF, Dawson JD, Mahoney LT. Predicting heart growth during puberty: the Muscatine Study. Pediatrics 2000; 105:E63.
395. Huttenlocher PR. Synaptic density in human frontal cortex: developmental changes and effects of aging. Brain Res 1979; 163: 195–205.
396. Feinberg I, Carlson VR. Sleep variables as a function of age in man. Arch Gen Psychiatry 1968; 18:18239–18250.
397. Feinberg I, Thode HC Jr, Chugani HT, March JD. Gamma distribution model describes maturational curves for delta wave amplitude, cortical metabolic rate and synaptic density. J Theor Biol 1990; 142:149–161.
398. Anokhin AP, Birbaumer N, Lutzenberger W, et al. Age increases brain complexity. Electroencephalogr Clin Neurophysiol 1996; 99:63–68.
399. Feinberg I. Changes in sleep cycle patterns with age. J Psychiatr Res 1974; 10:283–306.
400. Wolf P. Epilepsy and puberty. In Bourguignon JP, Plant TM (eds). The Onset of Puberty in Perspective. Amsterdam, Elsevier, 2000, pp 157–164.
401. Wu FC. Neurosignaling and the onset of puberty-integration. In Bourguignon JP, Plant TM (eds). The Onset of Puberty in Perspective. Amsterdam, Elsevier, 2001, pp 179–183.
402. Gordon CT, Frazier JA, McKenna K, et al. Childhood-onset schizophrenia: an NIMH study in progress. Schizophr Bull 1994; 20:697–712.
403. Lewis DA. Schizophrenia and peripubertal refinements in prefrontal cortical circuitry. In Bourguignon JP, Plant TM (eds). The Onset of Puberty in Perspective. Amsterdam, Elsevier, 2000, pp 165–183.
404. Hamburg BA. Psychosocial Development. In Freidman SB, Fisher M, Schoenberg SK, Alderman EA (eds). Comprehensive Adolescent Health Care. St. Louis, Mosby, 1998, pp 38–48.
405. Michael RP, Zumpke D. Behavioral changes associated with puberty in higher primates and the human. In Grumbach MM, Sizonenko PC, Aubert ML (eds). Control of the Onset of Puberty. Baltimore, Williams & Wilkins, 1990, pp 574–587.
406. Remschmidt H. Psychosocial milestones in normal puberty and adolescence. Horm Res 1994; 41(suppl 2):19–29.
407. Slap GB, Khalid N, Paikoff RL, et al. Evolving self-image, pubertal manifestations, and pubertal hormones: preliminary findings in young adolescent girls. J Adolesc Health 1994; 15: 327–335.
408. Weiner IB, del Gaudio AC. Psychopathology in adolescence: an epidemiological study. In Chess S, Thomas A (eds). Annual Progress in Child Psychiatry and Child Development. New York, Brunner/Mazel, 1977, pp 471–488.
409. Susman EJ, Nottelmann ED, Inoff-Germain G, et al. Hormonal influences on aspects of psychological development during adolescence. J Adolesc Health Care 1987; 8:492–504.
410. Klerman LV. The influence of economic factors on health-related behaviors in adolescents. In Millstein SG, Petersen AC, Nightingale EO (eds). Promoting the Health of Adolescents: New Directions for the Twenty-First Century. New York, Oxford University Press, 1993, pp 38–57.
411. Petersen AC. Presidential address: Creating adolescents: the role of context and process in developmental trajectories. J Res Adolesc 1993;3:1–18.
412. Brooks-Gunn J, Graber JA. Puberty as a biological and social event: implications for research on pharmacology. J Adolesc Health 1994; 15:663–671.
413. Steinberg L, Morris AS. Adolescent development. Annu Rev Psychol 2001; 52:83–110.
414. Hall GS. Adolescence: Its Psychology and Its Relations to Physiology, Anthropology, Sociology, Sex, Crime, Religion and Education. New York, Appleton, 1904.
415. Offer D. The Psychological World of the Teenager: A Study of Normal Adolescent Boys. New York, Basic Books, 1969.
416. Masterson JFJ. The psychiatric significance of adolescent turmoil. Am J Psychiatry 1968; 124:1549–1554.

417. Udry RR, Billy JOG, Morris NM, et al. Serum androgenic hormones motivate sexual behavior in boys. Fertil Steril 1985; 43:90–94.
418. Casper RC. Women's Health: Hormones, Emotions, and Behavior. Cambridge, Cambridge University Press, 1998.
419. Offer D, Schonert-Reichl KA. Debunking the myths of adolescence: findings from recent research. J Am Acad Child Adolesc Psychiatry 1992; 31:1003–1014.
420. Warren MP, Brooks-Gunn J. Mood and behavior at adolescence: evidence for hormonal factors. J Clin Endocrinol Metab 1989; 69:77–83.
421. Murphy DG, DeCarli C, Daly E, et al. X-chromosome effects on female brain: a magnetic resonance imaging study of Turner's syndrome. Lancet 1993; 342:1197–1200.
422. Rao U, Weissman MM, Martin JA, Hammond RW. Childhood depression and risk of suicide: a preliminary report of a longitudinal study. J Am Acad Child Adolesc Psychiatry 1993; 32:21–27.
423. Angold A, Costello EJ, Worthman CM. Puberty and depression: the roles of age, pubertal status and pubertal timing. Psychol Med 1998; 28:51–61.
424. Angold A, Worthman CW. Puberty onset of gender differences in rates of depression: a developmental, epidemiologic and neuroendocrine perspective. J Affect Disord 1993; 29:145–158.
425. Angold A, Costello EJ, Erkanli A, Worthman CM. Pubertal changes in hormone levels and depression in girls. Psychol Med 1999; 29:1043–1053.
426. Ryan ND. Psychoneuroendocrinology of children and adolescents. Psychiatr Clin North Am 1998; 21:435–441.
427. Dorn LD, Chrousos GP. The neurobiology of stress: understanding regulation of affect during female biological transitions. Semin Reprod Endocrinol 1997; 15:19–35.
428. Swedo SE, Pleeter JD, Richter DM, et al. Rates of seasonal affective disorder in children and adolescents. Am J Psychiatry 1995; 152:1016–1019.
429. Birmaher B, Dahl RE, Williamson DE, et al. Growth hormone secretion in children and adolescents at high risk for major depressive disorder. Arch Gen Psychiatry 2000; 57:867–872.
430. Hafner H, an der Heiden W, Behrens S, et al. Causes and consequences of the gender difference in age at onset of schizophrenia. Schizophr Bull 1998; 24:99–113.
431. Hayward C, Killen JD, Hammer LD, et al. Pubertal stage and panic attack history in sixth- and seventh-grade girls. Am J Psychiatry 1992; 149:1239–1243.
432. Solomon S. Migraine diagnosis and clinical symptomatology. Headache 1994; 34:S8–S12.
433. Orr DP, Ingersoll GM. The contribution of level of cognitive complexity and pubertal timing to behavioral risk in young adolescents. Pediatrics 1995; 95:528–533.
434. Wilson DM, Killen JD, Hayward C, et al. Timing and rate of sexual maturation and the onset of cigarette and alcohol use among teenage girls. Arch Pediatr Adolesc Med 1994; 148:789–795.
435. Tschann JM, Adler NE, Irwin CEJ, et al. Initiation of substance use in early adolescence: the roles of pubertal timing and emotional distress. Health Psychol 1994; 13:326–333.
436. Andrade MM, Benedito-Silva AA, Domenice S, et al. Sleep characteristics of adolescents: a longitudinal study. J Adolesc Health 1993; 14:401–406.
437. Strickland AL. Long-term results of treatment with low-dose fluoxymesterone in constitutional delay of growth and puberty and in genetic short stature. Pediatrics 1993; 91:716–720.
438. Carskadon MA, Acebo C, Richardson GS, et al. An approach to studying circadian rhythms of adolescent humans. J Biol Rhythms 1997; 12:278–289.
439. Rodgers JL. Development of sexual behavior. In Freidman SB, Fisher M, Schonberg SK (eds). Comprehensive Adolescent Health Care. St. Louis, Quality Medical Publishing, 1998, pp 49–54.
440. Brindis CD, Irwin CE Jr, Millstein SG. United States profile. In McAnarney ER, Kreipe RE, Irr DP, Comerci GD (eds). Textbook of Adolescent Medicine. Philadelphia, WB Saunders, 1992, p 12.
441. National Research Council (U.S.). Panel on adolescent pregnancy and childbearing Cobassae. Risking the future: Adolescent sexuality, pregnancy and childbearing. Washington, DC, National Academy Press, 1987.
442. Halpern CT, Udry JR, Campbell B, Suchindran C. Testosterone and pubertal development as predictors of sexual activity: a panel analysis of adolescent males. Psychosom Med 1993; 55: 436–447.
443. Udry JR, Billy JO, Morris NM, et al. Serum androgenic hormones motivate sexual behavior in adolescent boys. Fertil Steril 1985; 43:90–94.
444. Halpern CT, Udry JR, Campbell B, Suchindran C. Testosterone and pubertal development as predictors of sexual activity: a panel analysis of adolescent males. Psychosom Med 1993; 55: 436–447.
445. Halpern CT, Udry JR, Suchindran C. Monthly measures of salivary testosterone predict sexual activity in adolescent males. Arch Sex Behav 1998; 27:445–465.
446. Hutchinson KA. Androgens and sexuality. Am J Med 1995; 98: 111S–115S.
447. Money J. Sexual revolution and counter-revolution. Horm Res 1994; 41(suppl 2):44–48.
448. Friedman HL. Changing patterns of adolescent sexual behavior: consequences for health and development. J Adolesc Health 1992; 13:345–350.
449. Halpern CT, Udry JR, Campbell B, et al. Testosterone and religiosity as predictors of sexual attitudes and activity among adolescent males: a biosocial model. J Biosoc Sci 1994; 26:217–234.
450. Udry JR, Talbert LM, Morris NM. Biosocial foundations for adolescent female sexuality. Demography 1986; 23:217–230.
451. Halpern CT, Udry JR, Suchindran C. Testosterone predicts initiation of coitus in adolescent females. Psychosom Med 1997; 59:161–171.
452. Finkelstein JW, Susman EJ, Chinchilli VM, et al. Effects of estrogen or testosterone on self-reported sexual responses and behaviors in hypogonadal adolescents. J Clin Endocrinol Metab 1998; 83:2281–2285.
453. Halpern CT, Joyner K, Udry JR, Suchindran C. Smart teens don't have sex (or kiss much either). J Adolescent Health 2000; 26:213–225.
454. Graber JA, Lewinsohn PM, Seeley JR, Brooks-Gunn J. Is psychopathology associated with the timing of pubertal development? J Am Acad Child Adolesc Psychiatry 1997; 36:1768–1776.
455. Blyth DA, Simmons RG, Blucroft R, et al. The effects of physical development on self-image and satisfaction with body-image for early adolescent males. In Simmon RG (ed). Research in Community and Mental Health. Norwalk, Conn, JAI Press, 1981, pp 43–73.
456. Apter A, Galatzer A, Weizman A, et al. Psychological aspects of developmental endocrinopathies in adolescence. Isr J Psychiatry Relat Sci 1994; 31:246–253.
457. Lewis VG, Money J, Bobrow NA. Idiopathic pubertal delay beyond age fifteen: psychologic study of twelve boys. Adolescence 1977; 12:1–11.
458. Hayward C, Killen JD, Wilson DM, et al. Psychiatric risk associated with early puberty in adolescent girls. J Am Acad Child Adolesc Psychiatry 1997; 36:255–262.
459. Newcombe N, Dubas JS. Individual differences in cognitive ability: are they related to timing of puberty? In Lerner RM, Foch TT (eds). Biological-Psychosocial Interactions in Early Adolescence. Hillsdale, NJ, Lawrence Erlbaum Associates, 1987, pp 249–302.
460. Brooks-Gunn J, Warren MP. Mother-daughter differences in menarcheal age in adolescent girls attending national dance company schools and non-dancers. Ann Hum Biol 1988; 15:35–43.
461. Brooks-Gunn J. Pubertal processes and girls' psychological adaptation. In Lerner RM, Foch TT (eds). Biological-Psychosocial Interactions in Early Adolescence. Hillsdale, NJ, Lawrence Erlbaum Associates, 1987, pp 123–153.
462. Grumbach MM, Roth JC, Kaplan SL, et al. Hypothalamic-pituitary regulation of puberty in man: evidence and concepts derived from clinical research. In Grumbach MM, Grave GD, Mayer FE (eds). Control of the Onset of Puberty. New York, John Wiley & Sons, 1974, pp 115–166.
463. Grumbach MM, Kaplan SL. The neuroendocrinology of human puberty: an ontogenetic perspective. In Grumbach MM, Sizonenko PC, Aubert ML (eds). Control of the Onset of Puberty. Baltimore, Williams & Wilkins, 1990, pp 1–68.

464. Kaplan SL, Grumbach MM, Aubert ML. The ontogenesis of pituitary hormones and hypothalamic factors in the human fetus: maturation of central nervous system regulation of anterior pituitary function. Recent Prog Horm Res 1976; 32:161–243.
465. Dunkel L, Alfthan H, Stenman U, et al. Pulsatile secretion of LH and FSH in prepubertal and early pubertal boys revealed by ultrasensitive time-resolved immunofluorometric assays. Pediatr Res 1990; 27:215–219.
466. Dunkel L, Alfthan H, Stenman U, et al. Gonadal control of pulsatile secretion of luteinizing hormone and follicle-stimulating hormone in prepubertal boys evaluated by ultrasensitive time-resolved immunofluorometric assays. J Clin Endocrinol Metab 1990; 70:107–114.
467. Albertsson-Wikland K, Rosberg S, Lannering B, et al. Twenty-four-hour profiles of luteinizing hormone, follicle-stimulating hormone, testosterone, and estradiol levels: a semilongitudinal study throughout puberty in healthy boys. J Clin Endocrinol Metab 1997; 82:541–549.
468. Wu FC, Butler GE, Kelnar CJ, et al. Ontogeny of pulsatile gonadotropin releasing hormone secretion from midchildhood, through puberty, to adulthood in the human male: a study using deconvolution analysis and an ultrasensitive immunofluorometric assay. J Clin Endocrinol Metab 1996; 81:1798–1805.
469. Apter D, Butzow TL, Laughlin GA, Yen SS. Gonadotropin-releasing hormone pulse generator activity during pubertal transition in girls: pulsatile and diurnal patterns of circulating gonadotropins. J Clin Endocrinol Metab 1993; 76:940–949.
470. Mitamura R, Yano K, Suzuki N, et al. Diurnal rhythms of luteinizing hormone, follicle-stimulating hormone, and testosterone secretion before the onset of male puberty. J Clin Endocrinol Metab 1999; 84:29–37.
471. Mitamura R, Yano K, Suzuki N, et al. Diurnal rhythms of luteinizing hormone, follicle-stimulating hormone, testosterone, and estradiol secretion before the onset of female puberty in short children. J Clin Endocrinol Metab 2000; 85:1074–1080.
472. Corley KP, Valk TW, Kelch RP, et al. Estimation of GnRH pulse amplitude during pubertal development. Pediatr Res 1981; 15:157–162.
473. Jakacki RI, Kelch RP, Sauder SE, et al. Pulsatile secretion of luteinizing hormone in children. J Clin Endocrinol Metab 1982; 55:453–458.
474. Kelch RP, Clemens LE, Markovs M, et al. Metabolism and effects of synthetic gonadotropin-releasing hormone (GnRH) in children and adults. J Clin Endocrinol Metab 1975; 40:53–61.
475. Hassing JM, Padmanabhan V, Kelch RP, et al. Differential regulation of serum immunoreactive luteinizing hormone and bioactive follicle-stimulating hormone by testosterone in early pubertal boys. J Clin Endocrinol Metab 1990; 70:1082–1089.
476. Clark PA, Iranmanesh A, Veldhuis JD, Rogol AD. Comparison of pulsatile luteinizing hormone secretion between prepubertal children and young adults: evidence for a mass/amplitude-dependent difference without gender or day/night contrasts. J Clin Endocrinol Metab 1997; 82:2950–2955.
477. Styne DM, Grumbach MM. Puberty in boys and girls. In Pfaff DW (ed). Hormone, Brain and Behavior. Philadelphia, Elsevier, 2002, pp 661–716.
478. Plant TM. Neurobiological bases underlying the control of the onset of puberty in the rhesus monkey: a representative higher primate. Front Neuroendocrinol 2001; 22:107–139.
479. Yen SS, Apter D, Butzow T, Laughlin GA. Gonadotrophin releasing hormone pulse generator activity before and during sexual maturation in girls: new insights. Hum Reprod 1993; 8(suppl 2):66–71.
480. Boyar RM, Finkelstein J, Roffwarg H, et al. Synchronization of augmented luteinizing hormone secretion with sleep during puberty. N Engl J Med 1972; 287:582–586.
481. Wennink JM, Delemarre-Van de Waal HA, van Kessel H, et al. Luteinizing hormone secretion patterns in boys at the onset of puberty measured using a highly sensitive immunoradiometric assay. J Clin Endocrinol Metab 1988; 67:924–928.
482. Roth JC, Kelch RP, Kaplan SL, Grumbach MM. FSH and LH response to luteinizing hormone–releasing factor in prepubertal and pubertal children, adult males and patients with hypogonadotropic and hypertropic hypogonadism. J Clin Endocrinol Metab 1972; 35:926–930.
483. Roth JC, Grumbach MM, Kaplan SL. Effect of synthetic luteinizing hormone–releasing factor on serum testosterone and gonadotropins in prepubertal, pubertal, and adult males. J Clin Endocrinol Metab 1973; 37:680–686.
484. Job JC, Garnier PE, Chaussain JL, Milhaud G. Elevation of serum gonadotropins (LH and FSH) after releasing hormone (LH-RH) injection in normal children and in patients with disorders of puberty. J Clin Endocrinol Metab 1972; 35:473–476.
485. Boyar RM, Rosenfeld RS, Kapen S, et al. Simultaneous augmented secretion of luteinizing hormone and testosterone during sleep. J Clin Invest 1974; 54:609–618.
486. Kapen S, Boyar RM, Hellman L, Weitzman ED. Twenty-four-hour patterns of luteinizing hormone secretion in humans: ontogenetic and sexual considerations. Prog Brain Res 1975; 42:103–113.
487. Hale PM, Khoury S, Foster CM, et al. Increased luteinizing hormone pulse frequency during sleep in early to midpubertal boys: effects of testosterone infusion. J Clin Endocrinol Metab 1988; 66:785–791.
488. Apter D, Cacciatore B, Alfthan H, et al. Serum luteinizing hormone concentrations increase 100-fold in females from 7 years to adulthood, as measured by time-resolved immunofluorometric assay. J Clin Endocrinol Metab 1989; 68:53–57.
489. Burr IM, Sizonenko PC, Kaplan SL, et al. Hormonal changes in puberty. I. Correlation of serum luteinizing hormone and follicle stimulating hormone with stages of puberty, testicular size, and bone age in normal boys. Pediatr Res 1970; 4:25–35.
490. Sizonenko PC, Burr IM, Kaplan SL, et al. Hormonal changes in puberty. II. Correlation of serum luteinizing hormone and follicle stimulating hormone with stages of puberty and bone age in normal girls. Pediatr Res 1970; 4:36–45.
491. August GP, Grumbach MM, Kaplan SL. Hormonal changes in puberty. 3. Correlation of plasma testosterone, LH, FSH, testicular size, and bone age with male pubertal development. J Clin Endocrinol Metab 1972; 34:319–326.
492. Jenner MR, Kelch RP, Kaplan SL, Grumbach MM. Hormonal changes in puberty. IV. Plasma estradiol, LH, and FSH in prepubertal children, pubertal females, and in precocious puberty, premature thelarche, hypogonadism, and in a child with a feminizing ovarian tumor. J Clin Endocrinol Metab 1972; 34:521–530.
493. Belgorosky A, Chahin S, Chaler E, et al. Serum concentrations of follicle stimulating hormone and luteinizing hormone in normal girls and boys during prepuberty and at early puberty. J Endocrinol Invest 1996; 19:88–91.
494. Faiman C, Winter JSD. Gonadotropins and sex hormone patterns in puberty: clinical data. In Grumbach MM, Grave GD, Mayer FE (eds). Control of the Onset of Puberty. New York, John Wiley & Sons, 1974, pp 32–61.
495. Garibaldi LR, Picco P, Magier S, et al. Serum luteinizing hormone concentrations, as measured by a sensitive immunoradiometric assay, in children with normal, precocious or delayed pubertal development. J Clin Endocrinol Metab 1991; 72:888–898.
496. Spratt DI, Crowley WFJ. Pituitary and gonadal responsiveness is enhanced during GnRH-induced puberty. Am J Physiol 1988; 254:E652–E657.
497. Beitins IZ, Padmanabhan V. Bioactivity of gonadotropins. Endocrinol Metab Clin North Am 1991; 20:85–120.
498. Demir A, Voutilainen R, Juul A, et al. Increase in first morning voided urinary luteinizing hormone levels precedes the physical onset of puberty. J Clin Endocrinol Metab 1996; 81:2963–2967.
499. Cavallo A, Zhou XH. LHRH test in the assessment of puberty in normal children. Horm Res 1994; 41:10–15.
500. Ghai K, Rosenfield RL. Maturation of the normal pituitary-testicular axis, as assessed by gonadotropin-releasing hormone agonist challenge. J Clin Endocrinol Metab 1994; 78:1336–1340.
501. Ghai K, Cara JF, Rosenfield RL. Gonadotropin releasing hormone agonist (nafarelin) test to differentiate gonadotropin deficiency from constitutionally delayed puberty in teen-age boys: a clinical research center study. J Clin Endocrinol Metab 1995; 80:2980–2986.
502. Veldhuis JD, Pincus SM, Mitamura R, et al. Developmentally delimited emergence of more orderly luteinizing hormone and testosterone secretion during late prepuberty in boys. J Clin Endocrinol Metab 2001; 86:80–89.

503. Wang C, Zhong CQ, Leung A, Low LC. Serum bioactive follicle-stimulating hormone levels in girls with precocious sexual development. J Clin Endocrinol Metab 1990; 70:615–619.
504. Reiter EO, Beitins IZ, Ostrea T, Gutai JP. Bioassayable luteinizing hormone during childhood and adolescence and in patients with delayed pubertal development. J Clin Endocrinol Metab 1982; 54:155–161.
505. Reiter EO, Biggs DE, Veldhuis JD, Beitins IZ. Pulsatile release of bioactive luteinizing hormone in prepubertal girls: discordance with immunoreactive luteinizing hormone pulses. Pediatr Res 1987; 21:409–413.
506. Lucky AW, Rich BH, Rosenfield RL, et al. LH bioactivity increases more than immunoreactivity during puberty. J Pediatr 1980; 97:205–213.
507. Dunger DB, Villa AK, Matthews DR, et al. Pattern of secretion of bioactive and immunoreactive gonadotrophins in normal pubertal children. Clin Endocrinol (Oxf) 1991; 35:267–275.
508. Schroor EJ, van Weissenbruch MM, Engelbregt M, et al. Bioactivity of luteinizing hormone during normal puberty in girls and boys. Horm Res 1999; 51:230–237.
509. Huhtaniemi IT, Haavisto AM, Anttila R, et al. Sensitive immunoassay and in vitro bioassay demonstrate constant bioactive/immunoreactive ratio of luteinizing hormone in healthy boys during the pubertal maturation. Pediatr Res 1996; 39:180–184.
510. Baenziger JU. Glycosylation: to what end for the glycoprotein hormones (editorial)? Endocrinology 1996; 137:1520–1522.
511. Ulloa-Aguirre A, Midgley AR Jr, Beitins IZ, Padmanabhan V. Follicle-stimulating isohormones: characterization and physiological relevance. Endocr Rev 1995; 16:765–787.
512. Wide L, Albertsson-Wikland K, Phillips DJ. More basic isoforms of serum gonadotropins during gonadotropin-releasing hormone agonist therapy in pubertal children. J Clin Endocrinol Metab 1996; 81:216–221.
513. Kasa-Vubu JZ, Padmanabhan V, Kletter GB, et al. Serum bioactive luteinizing and follicle-stimulating hormone concentrations in girls increase during puberty. Pediatr Res 1993; 34:829–833.
514. Kletter GB, Padmanabhan V, Brown MB, et al. Serum bioactive gonadotropins during male puberty: a longitudinal study. J Clin Endocrinol Metab 1993; 76:432–438.
515. Phillips DJ, Wide L. Serum gonadotropin isoforms become more basic after an exogenous challenge of gonadotropin-releasing hormone in children undergoing pubertal development. J Clin Endocrinol Metab 1994; 79:814–819.
516. Weinstein RL, Kelch RP, Jenner MR, et al. Secretion of unconjugated androgens and estrogens by the normal and abnormal human testis before and after hCG. J Clin Invest 1974; 53:1–6.
517. Peterson RE, Imperato-McGinley J, Gautier T, Sturla E. Male pseudohermaphroditism due to steroid 5-alpha-reductase deficiency. Am J Med 1977; 62:170–191.
518. Knoor D, Bidlingmaier F, Butenandt O, et al. Plasma testosterone in male puberty. I. Physiology of plasma testosterone. Acta Endocrinol (Copenh) 1974; 75:181–194.
519. Corbier P, Edwards DA, Roffi J. The neonatal testosterone surge: a comparative study. Arch Int Physiol Biochim Biophys 1992; 100:127–131.
520. Forest MG, Sizonenko PC, Cathiard AM, Bertrand J. Hypophyso-gonadal function in humans during the first year of life. 1. Evidence for testicular activity in early infancy. J Clin Invest 1974; 53:819–828.
521. Gendrel D, Chaussain JL, Roger M, Job JC. Simultaneous postnatal rise of plasma LH and testosterone in male infants. J Pediatr 1980; 97:600–602.
522. Judd HL, Parker DC, Yen SS. Sleep-wake patterns of LH and testosterone release in prepubertal boys. J Clin Endocrinol Metab 1977; 44:865–869.
523. Goji K, Tanikaze S. Spontaneous gonadotropin and testosterone concentration profiles in prepubertal and pubertal boys: temporal relationship between luteinizing hormone and testosterone. Pediatr Res 1993; 34:229–236.
524. Dehennin L, Delgado A, Peres G. Urinary profile of androgen metabolites at different stages of pubertal development in a population of sporting male subjects. Eur J Endocrinol 1994; 130:53–59.
525. Kratzsch J, Keller E, Hoepffner W, et al. The DSL analog free testosterone assay: serum levels are not related to sex hormone-binding globulin in normative data throughout childhood and adolescence. Clin Lab 2001; 47:73–77.
526. Raivio T, Palvimo JJ, Dunkel L, et al. Novel assay for determination of androgen bioactivity in human serum. J Clin Endocrinol Metab 2001; 86:1539–1544.
527. Boas SR, Cleary DA, Lee PA, Orenstein DM. Salivary testosterone levels in male adolescents with cystic fibrosis. Pediatrics 1996; 97:361–363.
528. Ohzeki T, Manella B, Gubelin-De Campo C, Zachmann M. Salivary testosterone concentrations in prepubertal and pubertal males: comparison with total and free plasma testosterone. Horm Res 1991; 36:235–237.
529. Inkster S, Yue W, Brodie A. Human testicular aromatase: immunocytochemical and biochemical studies. J Clin Endocrinol Metab 1995; 80:1941–1947.
530. Brodie A, Inkster S. Aromatase in the human testis. J Steroid Biochem Mol Biol 1993; 44:549–555.
531. Norjavaara E, Ankarberg C, Albertsson-Wikland K. Diurnal rhythm of 17 beta-estradiol secretion throughout pubertal development in healthy girls: evaluation by a sensitive radioimmunoassay. J Clin Endocrinol Metab 1996; 81:4095–4102.
532. Goji K. Twenty-four-hour concentration profiles of gonadotropin and estradiol (E2) in prepubertal and early pubertal girls: the diurnal rise of E2 is opposite the nocturnal rise of gonadotropin. J Clin Endocrinol Metab 1993; 77:1629–1635.
533. Angsusingha K, Kenny FM, Nankin HR, Taylor FH. Unconjugated estrone, estradiol and FSH and LH in prepubertal and pubertal males and females. J Clin Endocrinol Metab 1974· 39: 63–68.
534. Lindstedt G, Lundberg P, Hammond GL, et al. Sex hormone binding globulin: still many questions. Scand J Clin Lab Invest 1985; 45:1–6.
535. Apter D, Bolton NJ, Hammond GL, Vihko R. Serum sex hormone–binding globulin during puberty in girls and in different types of adolescent menstrual cycles. Acta Endocrinol (Copenh) 1984; 107:413–419.
536. Lee IR, Lawder LE, Townend DC, et al. Plasma sex hormone binding globulin concentration and binding capacity in children before and during puberty. Acta Endocrinol (Copenh) 1985; 109:276–280.
537. Pugeat M, Cousin P, Baret C, et al. Sex hormone–binding globulin during puberty in normal and hyperandrogenic girls. J Pediatr Endocrinol Metab 2000; 13(suppl 5):1277–1279.
538. Maruyama Y, Aoki N, Suzuki Y, et al. Sex-steroid-binding plasma protein (SBP), testosterone, oestradiol and dehydroepiandrosterone (DHEA) in prepuberty and puberty. Acta Endocrinol (Copenh) 1987; 114:60–67.
539. August GP, Tkachuk M, Grumbach MM. Plasma testosterone-binding affinity and testosterone in umbilical cord plasma, late pregnancy, prepubertal children and adults. J Clin Endocrinol Metab 1969; 29:891–899.
540. Anderson DC. Sex hormone–binding globulin. Clin Endocrinol (Oxf) 1974; 3:69–95.
541. Horst HJ, Bartsch W, Dirksen-Thiedens I. Plasma testosterone, sex hormone binding globulin binding capacity and per cent binding of testosterone and 5alpha-dihydrotestosterone in prepubertal, pubertal and adult males. J Clin Endocrinol Metab 1977; 45:522–527.
542. Bartsch W, Horst HJ, Derwahl DM. Interrelationships between sex hormone-binding globulin and 17 beta-estradiol, testosterone, 5 alpha-dihydrotestosterone, thyroxine, and triiodothyronine in prepubertal and pubertal girls. J Clin Endocrinol Metab 1980; 50:1053–1056.
543. Cunningham SK, McKenna TJ. Evaluation of an immunoassay for plasma sex hormone–binding globulin: comparison with steroid-binding assay under physiological and pathological conditions. Ann Clin Biochem 1988; 25:360–366.
544. Cunningham SK, Loughlin T, Culliton M, McKenna TJ. Plasma sex hormone–binding globulin levels decrease during the second decade of life irrespective of pubertal status. J Clin Endocrinol Metab 1984; 58:915–918.
545. Rudd BT, Rayner PH, Thomas PH. Observations on the role of GH/IGF-1 and sex hormone binding globulin (SHBG) in the pubertal development of growth hormone deficient (GHD) children. Acta Endocrinol Suppl (Copenh) 1986; 279:164–169.
546. Holly JM, Dunger DB, al-Othman SA, et al. Sex hormone

binding globulin levels in adolescent subjects with diabetes mellitus. Diabet Med 1992; 9:371–374.
547. Aubert ML, Sizonenko PC, Kaplan SL, et al. The ontogenesis of human prolactin from fetal life to puberty. In Crosignani PG, Robyn C (eds). Prolactin and Human Reproduction. New York, Academic Press, 1977, pp 9–20.
548. Vale W, Bilezikjian LM, Rivier C. Reproductive and other roles of inhibins and activins. In Knobil E, Neil JD (eds). Physiology of Reproduction. New York, Raven Press, 1994, pp 1861–1878.
549. Mather JP. Follistatins and α_2-macroglobulin are soluble binding proteins for inhibin and activin. Horm Res 1996; 45:207–210.
550. Groome NP, Evans LW. Does measurement of inhibin have a clinical role? Ann Clin Biochem 2000; 37:419–431.
551. Hayes FJ, Pitteloud N, DeCruz S, et al. Importance of inhibin B in the regulation of FSH secretion in the human male. J Clin Endocrinol Metab 2001; 86:5541–5546.
552. Welt CK, Smith ZA, Pauler DK, Hall JE. Differential regulation of inhibin A and inhibin B by luteinizing hormone, follicle-stimulating hormone, and stage of follicle development. J Clin Endocrinol Metab 2001; 86:2531–2537.
553. McLachlan RI, Robertson DM, Burger HG, et al. The radioimmunoassay of bovine and human follicular fluid and serum inhibin. Mol Cell Endocrinol 1986; 46:175–185.
554. Groome NP, Illingworth PJ, O'Brien M, et al. Measurement of dimeric inhibin B throughout the human menstrual cycle. J Clin Endocrinol Metab 1996; 81:1401–1405.
555. Robertson DM, Cahir N, Findlay JK, et al. The biological and immunological characterization of inhibin A and B forms in human follicular fluid and plasma. J Clin Endocrinol Metab 1997; 82:889–896.
556. Meachem SJ, Nieschlag E, Simoni M. Inhibin B in male reproduction: pathophysiology and clinical relevance. Eur J Endocrinol 2001; 145:561–571.
557. Wallace E, Riley SM, Crossley JA, et al. Dimeric inhibins in amniotic fluid, maternal serum, and fetal serum in human pregnancy. J Clin Endocrinol Metab 1997; 82:218–222.
558. Fowler PA, Evans LW, Groome NP, et al. A longitudinal study of maternal serum inhibin-A, inhibin-B, activin-A, activin-AB, pro-alphaC and follistatin during pregnancy. Hum Reprod 1998; 13:3530–3536.
559. Majdic G, McNeilly AS, Sharpe RM, et al. Testicular expression of inhibin and activin subunits and follistatin in the rat and human fetus and neonate and during postnatal development in the rat. Endocrinology 1997; 138:2136–2147.
560. Debieve F, Beerlandt S, Hubinont C, Thomas K. Gonadotropins, prolactin, inhibin A, inhibin B, and activin A in human fetal serum from midpregnancy and term pregnancy. J Clin Endocrinol Metab 2000; 85:270–274.
561. Burger HG, McLachlan RI, Bangah M, et al. Serum inhibin concentrations rise throughout normal male and female puberty. J Clin Endocrinol Metab 1988; 67:689–694.
562. Manasco PK, Umbach DM, Muly SM, et al. Ontogeny of gonadotropin, testosterone, and inhibin secretion in normal boys through puberty based on overnight serial sampling. J Clin Endocrinol Metab 1995; 80:2046–2052.
563. Bergada I, Rojas G, Ropelato G, et al. Sexual dimorphism in circulating monomeric and dimeric inhibins in normal boys and girls from birth to puberty. Clin Endocrinol 1999; 51:455–560.
564. Andersson A-M, Juul A, Petersen JH, et al. Serum inhibin B in healthy pubertal and adolescent boys: relation to age, stage of puberty and FSH, LH, testosterone, and estradiol levels. J Clin Endocrinol Metab 1997; 82:3976–3981.
565. Byrd W, Bennett MJ, Carr BR, et al. Regulation of biologically active dimeric inhibin A and B from infancy to adulthood in the male. J Clin Endocrinol Metab 1998; 83:2849–2854.
566. Groome NP, Tsigou A, Cranfield M, et al. Enzyme immunoassays for inhibins, activins and follistatins. Mol Cell Endocrinol 2001; 180:73–77.
567. Anawalt BD, Bebb RA, Matsumoto AM, et al. Serum inhibin B levels reflect Sertoli cell function in normal men and in men with testicular dysfunction. J Clin Endocrinol Metab 1996; 81: 3341–3345.
568. Andersson A, Skakkebaek NE. Serum inhibin B levels during male childhood and puberty. Mol Cell Endocrinol 2001; 180: 103–107.
569. Raivio T, Perheentupa A, McNeilly AS, et al. Biphasic increase in serum inhibin B during puberty: a longitudinal study of healthy Finnish boys. Pediatr Res 1998; 44:552–556.
570. Crofton PM, Evans AE, Groome NP, et al. Inhibin B in boys from birth to adulthood: relationship with age, pubertal stage, FSH and testosterone. Clin Endocrinol (Oxf) 2002; 56:215–221.
571. Crofton PM, Evans AE, Groome NP, et al. Dimeric inhibins in girls from birth to adulthood: relationship with age, pubertal stage, FSH and oestradiol. Clin Endocrinol (Oxf) 2002; 56:223–230.
572. Foster CM, Phillips DJ, Wyman T, et al. Changes in serum inhibin, activin and follistatin concentrations during puberty in girls. Hum Reprod 2000; 15:1052–1057.
573. Mitchell R, Schaefer F, Morris ID, et al. Elevated serum immunoreactive inhibin levels in peripubertal boys with chronic renal failure. Cooperative Study Group on Pubertal Development in Chronic Renal Failure (CSPCRF). Clin Endocrinol (Oxf) 1993; 39:27–33.
574. Lee PA, Coughlin MT, Bellinger MF. No relationship of testicular size at orchiopexy with fertility in men who previously had unilateral cryptorchidism. J Urol 2001; 166:236–239.
575. Dunkel L, Siimes MA, Bremner WJ. Reduced inhibin and elevated gonadotropin levels in early pubertal boys with testicular defects. Pediatr Res 1993; 33:514–518.
576. Andersson AM, Muller J, Skakkebaek NE. Different roles of prepubertal and postpubertal germ cells and Sertoli cells in the regulation of serum inhibin B levels. J Clin Endocrinol Metab 1998; 83:4451–4458.
577. Kubini K, Zachmann M, Albers N, et al. Basal inhibin B and the testosterone response to human chorionic gonadotropin correlate in prepubertal boys. J Clin Endocrinol Metab 2000; 85: 134–138.
578. Hudson PL, Dougas I, Donahoe PK, et al. An immunoassay to detect human mullerian inhibiting substance in males and females during normal development. J Clin Endocrinol Metab 1990; 70:16–22.
579. Josso N, Legeai L, Forest MG, et al. An enzyme linked immunoassay for anti-mullerian hormone: a new tool for the evaluation of testicular function in infants and children. J Clin Endocrinol Metab 1990; 70:23–27.
580. Donahoe PK. Mullerian inhibiting substance in reproduction and cancer. Mol Reprod Dev 1992; 32:168–172.
581. Lee MM, Donahoe PK, Hasegawa T, et al. Müllerian inhibiting substance in humans: normal levels from infancy to adulthood. J Clin Endocrinol Metab 1996; 81:571–576.
582. Rey R, Mebarki F, Forest MG, et al. Anti-müllerian hormone in children with androgen insensitivity. J Clin Endocrinol Metab 1994; 79:960–964.
583. Baker ML, Hutson JM. Serum levels of müllerian inhibiting substance in boys throughout puberty and in the first two years of life. J Clin Endocrinol Metab 1993; 76:245–247.
584. Josso N. Paediatric applications of anti-müllerian hormone research. Horm Res 1995; 43:243–248.
585. Lee MM, Donahoe PK, Silverman BL, et al. Measurements of serum Müllerian inhibiting substance in the evaluation of children with nonpalpable gonads. N Engl J Med 1997; 336:1480–1486.
586. Randell EW, Diamandis EP, Ellis G. Serum prostate-specific antigen measured in children from birth to age 18 years. Clin Chem 1996; 42:420–423.
587. Vieira JG, Nishida SK, Pereira AB, et al. Serum levels of prostate-specific antigen in normal boys throughout puberty. J Clin Endocrinol Metab 1994; 78:1185–1187.
588. Juul A, Holm K, Kastrup KW, et al. Free insulin-like growth factor I serum levels in 1430 healthy children and adults, and its diagnostic value in patients suspected of growth hormone deficiency. J Clin Endocrinol Metab 1997; 82:2497–2502.
589. Martha PM Jr, Rogol AD, Veldhuis JD, et al. Alterations in the pulsatile properties of circulating growth hormone concentrations during puberty in boys. J Clin Endocrinol Metab 1989; 69: 563–570.
590. Albertsson-Wikland K, Rosberg S, Karlberg J, Groth T. Analysis of 24-hour growth hormone profiles in healthy boys and girls of normal stature: relation to puberty. J Clin Endocrinol Metab 1994; 78:1195–1201.
591. Eakman GD, Dallas JS, Ponder SW, Keenan BS. The effects of

testosterone and dihydrotestosterone on hypothalamic regulation of growth hormone secretion. J Clin Endocrinol Metab 1996; 81:1217–1223.
592. Mericq V, Cassorla F, Garcia H, et al. Growth hormone (GH) responses to GH-releasing peptide and to GH-releasing hormone in GH-deficient children. J Clin Endocrinol Metab 1995; 80:1681–1684.
593. Laron Z, Bowers CY, Hirsch D, et al. Growth hormone–releasing activity of growth hormone–releasing peptide-1 (a synthetic heptapeptide) in children and adolescents. Acta Endocrinol (Copenh) 1993; 129:424–426.
594. Skinner AM, Price DA, Addison GM, et al. The influence of age, size, pubertal status and renal factors on urinary growth hormone excretion in normal children and adolescents. Growth Regul 1992; 2:156–160.
595. Crowne EC, Wallace WH, Shalet SM, et al. Relationship between urinary and serum growth hormone and pubertal status. Arch Dis Child 1992; 67:91–95.
596. Main KM, Jarden M, Angelo L, et al. The impact of gender and puberty on reference values for urinary growth hormone excretion: a study of 3 morning urine samples in 517 healthy children and adults. J Clin Endocrinol Metab 1994; 79:865–871.
597. Patel L, Skinner AM, Price DA, Clayton PE. The influence of body mass index on growth hormone secretion in normal and short statured children. Growth Regul 1994; 4:29–34.
598. Martha PMJ, Rogol AD, Blizzard RM, et al. Growth hormone–binding protein activity is inversely related to 24-hour growth hormone release in normal boys. J Clin Endocrinol Metab 1991; 73:175–181.
599. Argente J, Barrios V, Pozo J, et al. Normative data for insulin-like growth factors (IGFs), IGF-binding proteins, and growth hormone–binding protein in a healthy Spanish pediatric population: age- and sex-related changes. J Clin Endocrinol Metab 1993; 77:1522–1528.
600. Merimee TJ, Russell B, Quinn S. Growth hormone–binding proteins of human serum: developmental patterns in normal man. J Clin Endocrinol Metab 1992; 75:852–854.
601. Massa G, Bouillon R, Vanderschueren-Lodeweyckx M. Serum levels of growth hormone–binding protein and insulin-like growth factor-I during puberty. Clin Endocrinol (Oxf) 1992; 37: 175–180.
602. Martha PMJ, Rogol AD, Carlsson LM, et al. A longitudinal assessment of hormonal and physical alterations during normal puberty in boys. I. Serum growth hormone–binding protein. J Clin Endocrinol Metab 1993; 77:452–457.
603. Juul A, Fisker S, Scheike T, et al. Serum levels of growth hormone binding protein in children with normal and precocious puberty: relation to age, gender, body composition and gonadal steroids. Clin Endocrinol (Oxf) 2000; 52:165–172.
604. Hasegawa Y, Hasegawa T, Takada M, Tsuchiya Y. Plasma free insulin-like growth factor I concentrations in growth hormone deficiency in children and adolescents. Eur J Endocrinol 1996; 134:184–189.
605. Rosenfield RL, Furlanetto R, Bock D. Relationship of somatomedin-C concentrations to pubertal changes. J Pediatr 1983; 103:723–728.
606. Luna AM, Wilson DM, Wibbelsman CJ, et al. Somatomedins in adolescence: a cross-sectional study of the effect of puberty on plasma insulin-like growth factor I and II levels. J Clin Endocrinol Metab 1983; 57:268–271.
607. Hesse V, Jahreis G, Schambach H, et al. Insulin-like growth factor I correlations to changes of the hormonal status in puberty and age. Exp Clin Endocrinol 1994; 102:289–298.
608. Juul A, Dalgaard P, Blum WF, et al. Serum levels of insulin-like growth factor (IGF)–binding protein-3 (IGFBP-3) in healthy infants, children, and adolescents: the relation to IGF-I, IGF-II, IGFBP-1, IGFBP-2, age, sex, body mass index, and pubertal maturation. J Clin Endocrinol Metab 1995; 80:2534–2542.
609. Juul A, Bang P, Hertel NT, et al. Serum insulin-like growth factor-I in 1030 healthy children, adolescents, and adults: relation to age, sex, stage of puberty, testicular size, and body mass index. J Clin Endocrinol Metab 1994; 78:744–752.
610. Juul A, Flyvbjerg A, Frystyk J, et al. Serum concentrations of free and total insulin-like growth factor-I, IGF binding proteins-1 and -3 and IGFBP-3 protease activity in boys with normal or precocious puberty. Clin Endocrinol (Oxf) 1996; 44:515–523.
611. Wilson DM, Stene MA, Killen JD, et al. Insulin-like growth factor binding protein-3 in normal pubertal girls. Acta Endocrinol (Copenh) 1992; 126:381–386.
612. Amiel SA, Caprio S, Sherwin RS, et al. Insulin resistance of puberty: a defect restricted to peripheral glucose metabolism. J Clin Endocrinol Metab 1991; 72:277–282.
613. Bloch CA, Clemons P, Sperling MA. Puberty decreases insulin sensitivity. J Pediatr 1987; 110:481–487.
614. Amiel SA, Sherwin RS, Simonson DC, et al. Impaired insulin action in puberty: a contributing factor to poor glycemic control in adolescents with diabetes. N Engl J Med 1986; 315:215–219.
615. Hindmarsh PC, Matthews DR, Di Silvio L, et al. Relation between height velocity and fasting insulin concentrations. Arch Dis Child 1988; 63:665–666.
616. Rosenbloom AL, Wheeler L, Bianchi R, et al. Age-adjusted analysis of insulin responses during normal and abnormal glucose tolerance tests in children and adolescents. Diabetes 1975; 4:820–828.
617. Hindmarsh P, Di Silvio L, Pringle PJ, et al. Changes in serum insulin concentration during puberty and their relationship to growth hormone. Clin Endocrinol (Oxf) 1988; 28:381–388.
618. Godsland IF. The influence of female sex steroids on glucose metabolism and insulin action. J Intern Med Suppl 1996; 738:1–60.
619. Goran MI, Gower BA. Longitudinal study on pubertal insulin resistance. Diabetes 2001; 50:2444–2450.
620. Arslanian SA. Type 2 diabetes mellitus in children: pathophysiology and risk factors. J Pediatr Endocrinol Metab 2000; 13(suppl 6):1385–1394.
621. Caprio S, Cline G, Boulware S, et al. Effects of puberty and diabetes on metabolism of insulin-sensitive fuels. Am J Physiol 1994; 266:E885–E891.
622. Hoffman RP, Vicini P, Sivitz WI, Cobelli C. Pubertal adolescent male-female differences in insulin sensitivity and glucose effectiveness determined by the one compartment minimal model. Pediatr Res 2000; 48(3):384–388.
623. McFarlane SI, Banerji M, Sowers JR. Insulin resistance and cardiovascular disease. J Clin Endocrinol Metab 2001; 86:713–718.
624. Ibanez L, Potau N, Zampolli M, et al. Hyperinsulinemia in postpubertal girls with a history of premature pubarche and functional ovarian hyperandrogenism. J Clin Endocrinol Metab 1996; 81:1237–1243.
625. Ibanez L, Potau N, Marcos MV, de Zegher F. Adrenal hyperandrogenism in adolescent girls with a history of low birthweight and precocious pubarche. Clin Endocrinol (Oxf) 2000; 53:523–527.
626. Ibanez L, Potau N, de Zegher F. Endocrinology and metabolism after premature pubarche in girls. Acta Paediatr Suppl 1999; 88:73–77.
627. Ibanez L, de Zegher F, Potau N. Premature pubarche, ovarian hyperandrogenism, hyperinsulinism and the polycystic ovary syndrome: from a complex constellation to a simple sequence of prenatal onset. J Endocrinol Invest 1998; 21:558–566.
628. Maffeis C, Moghetti P, Grezzani A, et al. Insulin resistance and the persistence of obesity from childhood into adulthood. J Clin Endocrinol Metab 2002; 87:71–76.
629. Svec F, Nastasi K, Hilton C, et al. Black-white contrasts in insulin levels during pubertal development. The Bogalusa Heart Study. Diabetes 1992; 41:313–317.
630. Arslanian SA, Kalhan SC. Correlations between fatty acid and glucose metabolism: potential explanation of insulin resistance of puberty. Diabetes 1994; 43:908–914.
631. Travers SH, Jeffers BW, Bloch CA, et al. Gender and Tanner stage differences in body composition and insulin sensitivity in early pubertal children. J Clin Endocrinol Metab 1995; 80:172–178.
632. Caprio S, Amiel SA, Merkel P, Tamborlane WV. Insulin-resistant syndromes in children. Horm Res 1993; 39(suppl 3):112–114.
633. Holl RW, Heinze E, Seifert M, et al. Longitudinal analysis of somatic development in paediatric patients with IDDM: genetic influences on height and weight. Diabetologia 1994; 37:925–929.
634. Brown M, Ahmed ML, Clayton KL, Dunger DB. Growth during childhood and final height in type 1 diabetes. Diabet Med 1994; 11:182–187.

635. Normann EK, Evald U, Dahl-Jorgensen K, et al. Decreased serum insulin-like growth factor I during puberty in children with insulin dependent diabetes mellitus (IDDM). Ups J Med Sci 1994; 99:147–154.
636. Pal BR, Matthews DR, Edge JA, et al. The frequency and amplitude of growth hormone secretory episodes as determined by deconvolution analysis are increased in adolescents with insulin dependent diabetes mellitus and are unaffected by short-term euglycaemia. Clin Endocrinol (Oxf) 1993; 38:93–100.
637. Menon RK, Arslanian S, May B, et al. Diminished growth hormone–binding protein in children with insulin-dependent diabetes mellitus. J Clin Endocrinol Metab 1992; 74:934–938.
638. Stoll BA. Obesity and breast cancer. Int J Obes Relat Metab Disord 1996; 20:389–392.
639. Stoll BA. Timing of weight gain in relation to breast cancer risk. Ann Oncol 1995; 6:245–248.
640. Stoll BA, Secreto G. New hormone-related markers of high risk to breast cancer. Ann Oncol 1992; 3:435–438.
641. Stoll BA. Breast cancer risk in Japanese women with special reference to the growth hormone–insulin-like growth factor axis. Jpn J Clin Oncol 1992; 22:1–5.
642. Islam AH, Yamashita S, Kotani K, et al. Fasting plasma insulin level is an important risk factor for the development of complications in Japanese obese children: results from a cross-sectional and a longitudinal study. Metabolism 1995; 44:478–485.
643. Kokkonen J, Laatikainen L, van Dickhoff K, et al. Ocular complications in young adults with insulin-dependent diabetes mellitus since childhood. Acta Paediatr 1994; 83:273–278.
644. Algvere P. Prepubertal diabetes duration increases the risk of retinopathy. Acta Paediatr 1994; 83:341.
645. Flack A, Kaar ML, Laatikainen L. A prospective, longitudinal study examining the development of retinopathy in children with diabetes. Acta Paediatr 1996; 85:313–319.
646. Fairchild JM, Hing SJ, Donaghue KC, et al. Prevalence and risk factors for retinopathy in adolescents with type 1 diabetes. Med J Aust 1994; 160:757–762.
647. Flack AA, Kaar ML, Laatikainen LT. Prevalence and risk factors of retinopathy in children with diabetes: a population-based study on Finnish children. Acta Ophthalmol (Copenh) 1993; 71: 801–809.
648. McNally PG, Raymond NT, Swift PG, et al. Does the prepubertal duration of diabetes influence the onset of microvascular complications? Diabet Med 1993; 10:906–908.
649. Goldstein DE, Blinder KJ, Ide CH, et al. Glycemic control and development of retinopathy in youth-onset insulin-dependent diabetes mellitus: results of a 12-year longitudinal study. Ophthalmology 1993; 100:1125–1131; discussion 1131–1132.
650. de Abreu JR, Silva R, Cunha-Vaz JG. The blood-retinal barrier in diabetes during puberty. Arch Ophthalmol 1994; 112:1334–1338.
651. Janner M, Knill SE, Diem P, et al. Persistent microalbuminuria in adolescents with type I (insulin- dependent) diabetes mellitus is associated to early rather than late puberty: results of a prospective longitudinal study. Eur J Pediatr 1994; 153:403–408.
652. Type 2 diabetes in children and adolescents. American Diabetes Association. Diabetes Care 2000; 23:381–389.
653. Glaser NS. Non–insulin-dependent diabetes mellitus in childhood and adolescence. Pediatr Clin North Am 1997; 44:307–337.
654. Glaser N, Jones KL. Non–insulin-dependent diabetes mellitus in children and adolescents. Adv Pediatr 1996; 43:359–396.
655. Todd JA. Transcribing diabetes. Nature 1996; 384:407–408.
656. Kirkland RT, Keenan BS, Probstfield JL, et al. Decrease in plasma high-density lipoprotein cholesterol levels at puberty in boys with delayed adolescence: correlation with plasma testosterone levels. JAMA 1987; 257:502–507.
657. LaRosa JC. Lipids and cardiovascular disease: do the findings and therapy apply equally to men and women? Womens Health Issues 1992; 2:102–111; discussion 111–113.
658. Sorva R, Kuusi T, Dunkel L, et al. Effects of endogenous sex steroids on serum lipoproteins and postheparin plasma lipolytic enzymes. J Clin Endocrinol Metab 1988; 66:408–413.
659. Cobbaert C, Deprost L, Mulder P, et al. Pubertal serum lipoprotein (a) and its correlates in Belgian schoolchildren. Int J Epidemiol 1995; 24:78–87.
660. Haffner SM, Frangos M, Williamson J, et al. Lp(a) concentrations and phenotypes in children with insulin-dependent diabetes mellitus. Chem Phys Lipids 1994; 67–68:223–231.
661. Srinivasan SR, Wattigney W, Webber LS, Berenson GS. Race and gender differences in serum lipoproteins of children, adolescents, and young adults—emergence of an adverse lipoprotein pattern in white males: the Bogalusa Heart Study. Prev Med 1991; 20:671–684.
662. Wilcken DE, Lynch JF, Marshall MD, et al. Relevance of body weight to apolipoprotein levels in Australian children. Med J Aust 1996; 164:22–25.
663. Flodmark CE, Sveger T, Nilsson-Ehle P. Waist measurement correlates to a potentially atherogenic lipoprotein profile in obese 12–14-year-old children. Acta Paediatr 1994; 83:941–945.
664. Cameron JL. Metabolic cues for the onset of puberty. Horm Res 1991; 36:97–103.
665. Brambilla P, Manzoni P, Sironi S, et al. Peripheral and abdominal adiposity in childhood obesity. Int J Obes Relat Metab Disord 1994; 18:795–800.
666. DiPietro L, Mossberg HO, Stunkard AJ. A 40-year history of overweight children in Stockholm: life-time overweight, morbidity, and mortality. Int J Obes Relat Metab Disord 1994; 18:585–590.
667. Kiess W, Meidert A, Dressendorfer RA, et al. Salivary cortisol levels throughout childhood and adolescence: relation with age, pubertal stage, and weight. Pediatr Res 1995; 37:502–506.
668. Grumbach MM. The neuroendocrinology of puberty. In Krieger DT, Hughes JC, et al (eds). Neuroendocrinology. Sunderland, Mass, Sinauer Associates, 1980, pp 249–258.
669. Grumbach MM, Kaplan SL. Fetal pituitary hormones and the maturation of central nervous system regulation of anterior pituitary function. In Gluck L (ed). Modern Perinatal Medicine. Chicago, Year Book Medical, 1974, pp 247–271.
670. Reiter EO, Grumbach MM. Neuroendocrine control mechanisms and the onset of puberty. Annu Rev Physiol 1982; 44: 595–613.
671. Ibanez L, DiMartino-Nardi J, Potau N, Saenger P. Premature adrenarche: normal variant or forerunner of adult disease? Endocr Rev 2000; 21:671–696.
672. Kaplan SL, Grumbach MM. Pituitary and placental gonadotropins and sex steroids in the human and sub-human primate fetus. Clin Endocrinol Metab 1978; 7:487–511.
673. Donovan BT, van der Werff JJ. Physiology of Puberty. Baltimore, Williams & Wilkins, 1965.
674. Critchlow V, Bar-Sela ME. Control of the onset of puberty. In Martini L, Ganong WF (eds). Neuroendocrinology. New York, Academic Press, 1967, pp 101–162.
675. Wilkins L. The Diagnosis and Treatment of Endocrine Disorders in Childhood and Adolescence. Springfield, Ill, Charles C Thomas, 1965.
676. King JC, Anthony ELP, Fitzgerald DM, et al. Luteinizing hormone–releasing hormone neurons in human preoptic/hypothalamus: differential intraneuronal localization of immunoreactive forms. J Clin Endocrinol Metab 1985; 60:88–97.
677. Knobil E. The neuroendocrine control of the menstrual cycle. Recent Prog Horm Res 1980; 36:53–88.
678. Karlsson M, Bass S, Seeman E. The evidence that exercise during growth or adulthood reduces the risk of fragility fractures is weak. Best Pract Res Clin Rheumatol 2001; 15:429–450.
679. Mellon PL, Windle JJ, Goldsmith PC, et al. Immortalization of hypothalamic GnRH neurons by genetically targeted tumorigenesis. Neuron 1990; 5:1–10.
680. Knobil E. The GnRH pulse generator. Am J Obstet Gynecol 1990; 163:1721–1727.
681. Martinez de la Escalera G, Choi ALH, Weiner RI. Generation and synchronization of gonadotropin-releasing hormone (GnRH) pulses: intrinsic properties of the GT1-1 gonadotropin-releasing hormone (GnRH) neuronal cell line. Proc Natl Acad Sci USA 1992; 89:1852–1855.
682. Adelman JP, Mason AJ, Hayflick JS, et al. Isolation of the gene and hypothalamic cDNA for the common precursor of gonadotropin-releasing hormone and prolactin release–inhibiting factor in human and rat. Proc Natl Acad Sci USA 1986; 83:179–183.
683. Wetsel W, ValenHa MM, Merchenthaler I. Intrinsic pulsatile secretory activity of immortalized luteinizing hormone–releasing hormone–secreting neurons. Proc Natl Acad Sci USA 1992; 89: 4149–4153.

684. Kusano K, Frushko S, Gainer H, Wray S. Electrical and synaptic properties of embryonic luteinizing hormone–releasing hormone neurons in explant cultures. Proc Natl Acad Sci USA 1995; 92:3918–3922.
685. Grumbach MM. The neuroendocrinology of human puberty revisited. Hormone Res 2002; 57(Suppl 2):2–14.
686. Marshall PE, Goldsmith PC. Neuroregulatory and neuroendocrine GnRH pathways in the hypothalamus and forebrain of the baboon. Brain Res 1980; 193:353–372.
687. Witkin JW, Silverman AJ. Synaptology of LHRH neurons in rat preoptic area. Peptides 1985; 6:263–271.
688. Tabensky A, Duan Y, Edmonds J, Seeman E. The contribution of reduced peak accrual of bone and age-related bone loss to osteoporosis at the spine and hip: insights from the daughters of women with vertebral or hip fractures. J Bone Miner Res 2001; 16:1101–1107.
689. Seeman E. Raloxifene. J Bone Miner Metab 2001; 19:65–75.
690. Karlsson MK, Duan Y, Ahlborg H, et al. Age, gender, and fragility fractures are associated with differences in quantitative ultrasound independent of bone mineral density. Bone 2001; 28: 118–122.
691. Adachi JD, Saag KG, Delmas PD, et al. Two-year effects of alendronate on bone mineral density and vertebral fracture in patients receiving glucocorticoids: a randomized, double-blind, placebo-controlled extension trial. Arthritis Rheum 2001; 44: 202–211.
692. Seeman E. Hip fractures and osteoporosis in men. Med J Aust 1997; 167:404–405.
693. Duan Y, Tabensky A, DeLuca V, Seeman E. The benefit of hormone replacement therapy on bone mass is greater at the vertebral body than posterior processes or proximal femur. Bone 1997; 21:447–451.
694. Pitts GR, Nunemaker CS, Moenter SM. Cycles of transcription and translation do not comprise the gonadotropin-releasing hormone pulse generator in GT1 cells. Endocrinology 2001; 142: 1858–1864.
695. Mahachoklertwattana P, Black SM, Kaplan SL, et al. Nitric oxide synthesized by gonadotropin-releasing hormone neurons is a mediator of *N*-methyl-D-aspartate (NMDA)–induced GnRH secretion. Endocrinology 1994; 135:1709–1712.
696. Morreto M, Lopez FJ, Negro-Villar A. Nitric oxide regulates luteinizing hormone–releasing hormone secretion. Endocrinology 1993; 133:2399–2402.
697. Gorski RA. Extrahypothalamic influences on gonadotropin secretion. In Grumbach MM, Grave GD, Mayer FE (eds). Control of the Onset of Puberty. New York, John Wiley & Sons, 1974, p 182.
698. Gorski RA. Maturation of neural mechanisms and the pubertal process. In Grumbach MM, Sizonenko PC, Aubert ML (eds). Control of the Onset of Puberty. Baltimore, Williams & Wilkins, 1990, pp 259–281.
699. Reichlin S. Neuroendocrinology. In Wilson JD, Foster DW (eds). Williams Textbook of Endocrinology. Philadelphia, WB Saunders, 1992, pp 135–219.
700. Gallo RV. Neuroendocrine regulation of pulsatile luteinizing hormone in the rat. Neuroendocrinology 1980; 20:122–131.
701. Ojeda SR, Andrews WW, Advis JP. Recent advances in the endocrinology of puberty. Endocr Rev 1980; 1:228–257.
702. Thind KK, Goldsmith PC. Infundibular gonadotropin-releasing hormone neurons are inhibited by direct opioid and autoregulatory synapses in juvenile monkeys. Neuroendocrinology 1988; 47:203–216.
703. Goldsmith PC, Thind KK, Perera AD, Plant TM. Glutamate-immunoreactive neurons and their gonadotropin-releasing hormone–neuronal interactions in the monkey hypothalamus. Endocrinology 1994; 134:858–868.
704. De Jong FH. Inhibin. Physiol Rev 1988; 68:555–607.
705. Ying S-Y. Inhibins, activins, and follistatins: gonadal proteins modulating the secretion of follicle-stimulating hormone. Endocr Rev 1988; 9:267–293.
706. Wetsel WC. Immortalized hypothalamic luteinizing hormone–releasing hormone (LHRH) neurons: a new tool for dissecting the molecular and cellular basis of LHRH physiology. Cell Mol Neurobiol 1995; 15:43–78.
707. Martinez de la Escalera G, Choi ALH, Weiner RI. Signaling pathways involved in GnRH secretion in GT1 cells. Neuroendocrinology 1995; 61:310–317.
708. Krsmanovic LZ, Stojilkovic SS, Catt KJ. Pulsatile gonadotropin-releasing hormone release and its regulation. Trends Endocrinol Metab 1996; 7:56–59.
709. Shacham S, Harris D, Ben-Shlomo H, et al. Mechanism of GnRH receptor signaling on gonadotropin release and gene expression in pituitary gonadotrophs. Vitam Horm 2001; 63:63–90.
710. Themmen APN, Huhtaniemi IT. Mutations of gonadotropins and gonadotropin receptors: elucidating the physiology and pathophysiology of pituitary-gonadal function. Endocr Rev 2000; 21:551–583.
711. Huckle W, Conn PM. Molecular mechanisms of gonadotropin releasing hormone action. II. The effector system. Endocr Rev 1988; 9:387–395.
712. Hazum E, Conn PM. Molecular mechanism of gonadotropin releasing hormone (GnRH) action. I. The GnRH receptor. Endocr Rev 1988; 9:379–386.
713. Sealfon SC, Weinstein H, Millar RP. Molecular mechanisms of ligand interaction with the gonadotropin-releasing hormone receptor. Endocr Rev 1997; 18:180–205.
714. Short RV. The evolution of human reproduction. Proc R Soc Med 1976; 195:3–24.
715. Bronson FH, Rissman EF. The biology of puberty. Biol Rev 1986; 61:157–195.
716. Terasawa E, Fernandez DL. Neurobiological mechanisms of the onset of puberty in primates. Endocr Rev 2001; 22:111–151.
717. Germak JA, Knobil E. Control of puberty in the rhesus monkey. In Grumbach MM, Sizonenko PC, Aubert ML (eds). Control of the Onset of Puberty. Baltimore, Williams & Wilkins, 1990, pp 69–81.
718. Plant TM. Puberty in primates. In Knobil E, Neill JD (eds). The Physiology of Reproduction. New York, Raven Press, 1994, pp 1763–1788.
719. Mitsushima D, Hei DL, Terasawa E. Gamma-Aminobutyric acid is an inhibitory neurotransmitter restricting the release of luteinizing hormone–releasing hormone before the onset of puberty. Proc Natl Acad Sci USA 1994; 91:395–399.
720. Mitsushima D, Marzban F, Luchansky LL, et al. Role of glutamic acid decarboxylase in the prepubertal inhibition of the luteinizing hormone releasing hormone release in female rhesus monkeys. J Neurosci 1996; 16:2563–2573.
721. Spratt DI, O'Dea LS, Schoenfeld D. Neuroendocrine-gonadal axis in men: frequent sampling of LH, FSH, and testosterone. Am J Physiol 1988; 254:E658–E666.
722. Crowley WF, Filicori M, Spratt DI. The physiology of gonadotropin releasing hormone (GnRH) secretion in men and women. Recent Prog Horm Res 1985; 41:473–526.
723. Wildt L, Hausler A, Marshall G, et al. Frequency and amplitude of gonadotropin-releasing hormone stimulation and gonadotropin secretion in the rhesus monkey. Endocrinology 1981; 109:376–385.
724. Gross KM, Matsumoto AM, Brenner WJ. Differential control of luteinizing hormone and follicle-stimulating hormone secretion by luteinizing hormone–releasing hormone pulse frequency in man. J Clin Endocrinol Metab 1987; 64:675–680.
725. Finkelstein JS, Budger TM, O'Dea LS, et al. Effects of decreasing the frequency of gonadotropin-releasing hormone stimulation on gonadotropin secretion in gonadotropin-releasing hormone–deficient men and perfused rat pituitary cells. J Clin Invest 1988; 81:1725–1733.
726. Belchetz PE, Plant TM, Nakai Y, et al. Hypophyseal responses to continuous and intermittent delivery of hypothalamic gonadotropin-releasing hormone. Science 1978; 202:631–633.
727. Nett TM, Crowder ME, Moss GE, et al. GnRH-receptor interaction. V. Down-regulation of pituitary receptors for GnRH in ovariectomized ewes by infusion of homologous hormone. Biol Reprod 1981; 24:1145–1155.
728. Schwanzel-Fukuda M, Pfaff DW. Origin of luteinizing hormone–releasing hormone neurons. Nature 1989; 338:161–164.
729. Wray S, Grant P, Gainer H. Evidence that cells expressing luteinizing hormone–releasing hormone mRNA in the mouse are derived from progenitor cells in the olfactory placode. Proc Natl Acad Sci USA 1989; 86:8132–8136.
730. Wray S, Nieburgs A, Elkabes S. Spatiotemporal cell expression for luteinizing hormone–releasing hormone in the prenatal mouse: evidence for an embryonic origin in the olfactory placode. Dev Brain Res 1989; 46:309–318.

731. Henry MJ, Pasco JA, Seeman E, et al. Assessment of fracture risk: value of random population-based samples—the Geelong Osteoporosis Study. J Clin Densitom 2001; 4:283–289.
732. Ronnekleiv OK, Resko JA. Ontogeny of gonadotropin-releasing hormone–containing neurons in early fetal development of rhesus macaques. Endocrinology 1990; 126:498–511.
733. Magnusson HI, Westlin NE, Nyqvist F, et al. Abnormally decreased regional bone density in athletes with medial tibial stress syndrome. Am J Sports Med 2001; 29:712–715.
734. Schwanzel-Fukuda M, Bick D, Pfaff DW. Luteinizing hormone–releasing hormone (LHRH)–expressing cells do not migrate normally in an inherited hypogonadal (Kallmann) syndrome. Mol Brain Res 1989; 6:311–326.
735. Schwanzel-Fukuda M, Crossin KL, Pfaff DW, et al. Migration of luteinizing hormone–releasing hormone (LHRH) neurons in early human embryos. J Comp Neurol 1996; 366:547–557.
736. Parhar I, Pfaff D, Schwanzel-Fukuda M. Genes and behavior as studied through gonadotropin-releasing hormone (GnRH) neurons: comparative and functional aspects. Cell Mol Neurobiol 1995; 15:107–116.
737. Gluckman PD, Grumbach MM, Kaplan SL. The neuroendocrine regulation and function of growth hormone and prolactin in the mammalian fetus. Endocr Rev 1981; 2:363–395.
738. Thliveris JA, Currie RW. Observations on the hypothalamo-hypophyseal portal vasculature in the developing human fetus. Am J Anat 1980; 157:441–444.
739. Clark SJ, Ellis N, Styne DM, et al. Hormone ontogeny in the ovine fetus. XVII. Demonstration of pulsatile luteinizing hormone secretion by the fetal pituitary gland. Endocrinology 1984; 115:1774–1779.
740. Clark SJ, Hauffa BP, Rodens KP, et al. Hormone ontogeny in the ovine fetus. XIX. The effect of a potent luteinizing hormone–releasing factor agonist on gonadotropin and testosterone release in the fetus and neonate. Pediatr Res 1989; 25:347–352.
741. Huhtaniemi I, Lautala P. Stimulation of steroidogenesis in human fetal testes by the placenta during perfusion. J Steroid Biochem 1979; 10:109–113.
742. Molsberry RL, Carr BR, Mendelson CR, et al. Human chorionic gonadotropin binding to human fetal testes as a function of gestational age. J Clin Endocrinol Metab 1982; 55:791–794.
743. Huhtaniemi IT, Yamamoto M, Ranta T, et al. Follicle-stimulating hormone receptors appear earlier in the primate fetal testis than in the ovary. J Clin Endocrinol Metab 1987; 65:1210–1214.
744. Huhtaniemi I, Pelliniemi J. Fetal Leydig cells: cellular origin, morphology, life span and special functional feature. Proc Soc Exp Biol Med 1992; 201:125–140.
745. Huhtaniemi I. Ontogeny of luteinizing hormone action in the male. In Payne AH, Jardy MP, Russel LD (eds). The Leydig Cell. Vienna, Ill, Cache River Press, 1996, pp 366–382.
746. Saez JM. Leydig cells: endocrine, paracrine and autocrine regulation. Endocr Rev 1994; 15:574–626.
747. Seeman E. During aging, men lose less bone than women because they gain more periosteal bone, not because they resorb less endosteal bone. Calcif Tissue Int 2001; 69:205–208.
748. Baker RG, Scrimgeour JB. Development of the gonad in normal and anencephalic human fetuses. J Reprod Fertil 1980; 68:193–199.
749. Beck-Peccoz P, Padmanabhan V, Baggiani AM, et al. Maturation of hypothalamic-pituitary-gonadal function in normal human fetuses: circulating levels of gonadotropins, their common alpha subunit and free testosterone, and discrepancy between immunological and biological activities of circulating follicle-stimulating hormone. J Clin Endocrinol Metab 1991; 73:525–532.
750. Massa G, de Zegher F, Vanderschueren-Lodeweyckx M. Serum levels of immunoreactive inhibin, FSH and LH in human infants at preterm and term birth. Biol Neonate 1992; 61:150–155.
751. Gluckman PD, Marti Henneberg C, Kaplan SL, et al. Hormone ontogeny in the ovine fetus. XIV. The effect of 17β-estradiol infusion on fetal plasma gonadotropins and prolactin and the maturation of sex steroid–dependent negative feedback. Endocrinology 1983; 112:1618–1623.
752. Groom GV, Boyns AR. Effect of hypothalamic releasing factor and steroids on release of gonadotrophins by organ culture of human fetal pituitary glands. J Endocrinol 1973; 59:511–522.
753. Jaffe AB, Mulcahey JJ, DiBabio AM, et al. Peptide regulation of pituitary and target tissue function and growth in the primate fetus. Recent Prog Horm Res 1988; 44:431–544.
754. Takagi ST, Yoshida T, Tsubata K, et al. Sex differences in fetal gonadotropins and androgens. J Steroid Biochem 1977; 8:609–620.
755. Davies JL, Naftolin F, Ryan KJ, et al. A specific high affinity limited capacity estrogen binding component in the cytosol of human fetal pituitary and brain tissues. J Clin Endocrinol Metab 1975; 40:909–912.
756. Cuttler L, Egli CA, Styne DM, et al. Hormone ontogeny in the ovine fetus. XVIII. The effect of an opioid antagonist on luteinizing hormone secretion. Endocrinology 1985; 116:1997–2002.
757. Mesiano S, Hart CS, Heyer BW, et al. Hormone ontogeny in the ovine fetus. XXVI. A sex difference in the effect of castration on the hypothalamic-pituitary gonadotropin unit in the ovine fetus. Endocrinology 1991; 129:3073–3079.
758. Van den Pol AN, Wuarin JP, Dudek FE. Glutamate, the dominant excitatory transmitter in neuroendocrine regulation. Science 1990; 250:1276–1278.
759. Bettendorf M, de Zegher F, Albers N, et al. Acute *N*-methyl-D,L-aspartate administration stimulates the luteinizing hormone releasing hormone pulse generator in the ovine fetus. Horm Res 1999; 51:25–30.
760. Dhandapani KM, Brann DW. The role of glutamate and nitric oxide in the reproductive neuroendocrine system. Biochem Cell Biol 2000; 78:165–179.
761. Albers N, Bettendorf M, Hart CS, et al. Hormone ontogeny in the ovine fetus. XXIII. Pulsatile administration of follicle-stimulating hormone stimulates inhibin production and decreases testosterone synthesis in the ovine fetal gonad. Endocrinology 1989; 124:3089–3094.
762. Albers N, Hart CS, Kaplan SL, et al. Hormone ontogeny in the ovine fetus. XXIV. Porcine follicular fluid "inhibins" selectively suppress plasma follicle-stimulating hormone in the ovine fetus. Endocrinology 1989; 125:675–678.
763. Corbier P, Dehenin L, Castanier M, et al. Sex differences in serum luteinizing hormone and testosterone in the human neonate during the first few hours after birth. J Clin Endocrinol Metab 1990; 71:1347–1348.
764. Lustig RH, Conte FA, Kogan BA, et al. Ontogeny of gonadotropin secretion in congenital anorchism: sexual dimorphism versus syndrome of gonadal dysgenesis and diagnostic considerations. J Urol 1987; 138:587–591.
765. Plant TM. The effects of neonatal orchidectomy on the developmental pattern of gonadotropin secretion in the male rhesus monkey (*Macaca mulatta*). Endocrinology 1980; 106:1451–1454.
766. Terasawa E, Fernandez DL. Neurobiological mechanisms of the onset of puberty in primates. Endocr Rev 2001; 22:111–151.
767. Muller J, Skakkebaek NE. Fluctuations in the number of germ cells during the late foetal and early postnatal periods in boys. Acta Endocrinol (Copenh) 1984; 105:271–274.
768. Winter JSD, Faiman C, Hobson WC, et al. Pituitary-gonadal regulations in infancy. I. Patterns of serum gonadotropin concentrations from birth to four years of age in man and chimpanzee. J Clin Endocrinol Metab 1975; 40:545–551.
769. Forest MG. Pituitary gonadotropin and sex steroid secretion during the first two years of life. In Grumbach MM, Sizonenko PC, Aubert AU (eds). Control of the Onset of Puberty. Baltimore, Williams & Wilkins, 1990, pp 451–478.
770. Grumbach MM. The central nervous system and the onset of puberty. In Falkner F, Tanner JM (eds). Human Growth. New York, Plenum, 1978, pp 215–238.
771. Gennari C, Seeman E. The First International Conference on Osteoporosis in Men. Siena, Italy, February 23–25, 2001. Calcif Tissue Int 2001; 69:177–178.
772. Perola M, Ohman M, Hiekkalinna T, et al. Quantitative-trait-locus analysis of body-mass index and of stature, by combined analysis of genome scans of five Finnish study groups. Am J Hum Genet 2001; 69:117–123.
773. Lander ES, Schork NJ. Genetic dissection of complex traits. Science 1994; 265:2037–2048.
774. Frankel WN, Schork N. Who's afraid of epistasis? Nat Genet 1996; 14:371–373.
775. Paterson AH. Molecular dissection of quantitative traits: progress and prospects. Genome Res 1995; 5:321–333.

776. Risch N, Merikangas K. The future of genetic studies of complex human diseases. Science 1996; 273:1516–1517.
777. Mackay TF. The genetic architecture of quantitative traits. Annu Rev Genet 2001; 35:303–339.
778. Brookes AJ. Rethinking genetic strategies to study complex diseases. Trends Mol Med 2001; 7:512–516.
779. Frisch RE. Fatness of girls from menarche to age 18 with a nomogram. Hum Biol 1976; 48:353–359.
780. Frisch RE, McArthur JW. Menstrual cycles: fatness as a determinant of minimum weight for height necessary for their maintenance or onset. Science 1974; 185:949–951.
781. Frisch RE. Pubertal adipose tissue: is it necessary for normal sexual maturation? Evidence from the rat and human female. Fed Proc 1980; 39:2395–2400.
782. Garn SM, LaVelle M. Reproductive histories of low weight girls and women. Am J Clin Nutr 1983; 37:862–866.
783. Garn SM, LaVelle M, Pilkington JJ. Comparison of fatness in premenarchial and postmenarchial girls of the same age. J Pediatr 1983; 103:328–331.
784. Forbes GB. Body size and composition of perimenarchial girls. Am J Dis Child 1992; 146:63–66.
785. Bronson FH, Manning JM. Minireview: the energetic regulation of ovulation; a realistic role of body fat. Biol Reprod 1991; 44: 945–950.
786. Malina RM. Menarche in athletes: a synthesis and hypothesis. Ann Hum Biol 1983; 10:1–24.
787. Wellens R, Malina RM, Roche AF, et al. Body size and fatness in young adults in relation to age of menarche. Am J Hum Biol 1992; 4:783–787.
788. Frisch RE. Body fat, puberty and fertility. Biol Rev Camb Philos Soc 1984; 59:161–188.
789. Hartz AJ, Barboriak PN, Wong A. The association of obesity with infertility and related menstrual abnormalities in women. Int J Obes 1979; 3:57–73.
790. Boyar RM, Katz J, Finkelstein JW, et al. Anorexia nervosa: immaturity of the 24-hour luteinizing hormone secretory pattern. N Engl J Med 1974; 291:861–865.
791. Frisch RE, Wyshak G, Vincent L. Delayed menarche and amenorrhea in ballet dancers. N Engl J Med 1980; 303:17–19.
792. de Souza MJ, Metzger DA. Reproductive dysfunction in amenorrheic athletes and anorexic patients: a review. Med Sci Sports Exerc 1991; 23:995–1007.
793. Frisch RE, Gotz-Welbergen AV, McArthur JW, et al. Delayed menarche and amenorrhea of college athletes in relation to age of onset of training. JAMA 1981; 246:1559–1564.
794. McArthur JW, Bullen BA, Beitins IZ, et al. Hypothalamic amenorrhea in runners of normal body composition. Endocr Res Commun 1980; 7:13–25.
795. Cameron N, Mitchell J, Meyer D, et al. Secondary sexual development of 'Cape Coloured' girls following kwashiorkor. Ann Hum Biol 1988; 15:65–75.
796. Johnston FE, Roche AF, Schell LM, et al. Critical weight at menarche. Am J Dis Child 1975; 129:19–23.
797. Cameron N. Weight and skinfold variation at menarche and the critical body weight hypothesis. Ann Hum Biol 1976; 3:279–282.
798. Billewicz WS, Fellowes HM, Hytten CA. Comments on the critical metabolic mass and the age of menarche. Ann Hum Biol 1976; 3:51–59.
799. Penny R, Goldstein IP, Frasier SD. Gonadotropin excretion and body composition. Pediatrics 1978; 61:294–300.
800. Vizmanos B, Marti-Henneberg C. Puberty begins with a characteristic subcutaneous body fat mass in each sex. Eur J Clin Nutr 2000; 54:203–208.
801. de Ridder CM, Thijssen JH, Bruning PF, et al. Body fat mass, body fat distribution, and pubertal development: a longitudinal study of physical and hormonal sexual maturation of girls. J Clin Endocrinol Metab 1992; 75:442–446.
802. Legro RS, Lin HM, Demers LM, Lloyd T. Rapid maturation of the reproductive axis during perimenarche independent of body composition. J Clin Endocrinol Metab 2000; 85:1021–1025.
803. Kennedy GC, Mitra J. Body weight and food intake as initiating factors for puberty in the rat. J Physiol (Lond) 1963; 166:408–418.
804. Zhang Y, Proenca R, Maffel M, et al. Positional cloning of the mouse obese gene and its human analogue. Nature 1994; 372: 425–432.
805. Campfield LA, Smith FJ, Guisez Y, et al. Recombinant mouse OB protein: evidence for a peripheral signal linking adiposity and central neural networks. Science 1995; 269:546–549.
806. Halaas JL, Gajiwala KS, Maffei M, et al. Weight-reducing effects of the plasma protein encoded by the obese gene. Science 1995; 269:543–549.
807. Spiegelman BM, Flier JS. Adipogenesis and obesity: rounding out the big picture. Cell 1996; 87:377–389.
808. Pelleymounter MA, Cullen MJ, Baker MB, et al. Effects of the obese gene product on body weight regulation in *ob/ob* mice. Science 1995; 269:540–543.
809. Caro JF, Sinha MK, Kolacznski JW, et al. Leptin: the tale of an obesity gene. Diabetes 1996; 45:1455–1462.
810. Tartaglia LA, Dembski M, Weng X, et al. Identification and expression cloning of a leptin receptor, OB-R. Cell 1995; 83: 1263–1271.
811. Sinha MK, Opentanova I, Ohannesian JP, et al. Evidence of free and bound leptin in human circulation. Studies in lean and obese subjects and during short-term fasting. J Clin Invest 1996; 98:1277–1282.
812. Licinio J, Mantzoros C, Negraao AB, et al. Human leptin levels are pulsatile and inversely related to pituitary-adrenal function. Nat Med 1997; 3:575–579.
813. Ahima RS, Saper CB, Flier JS, Elmquist JK. Leptin regulation of neuroendocrine systems. Front Neuroendocrinol 2000; 21: 263–307.
814. Wauters M, Considine RV, Van Gaal LF. Human leptin: from an adipocyte hormone to an endocrine mediator. Eur J Endocrinol 2000; 143:293–311.
815. Klein KO, Larmore KA, de Lancey E, et al. Effect of obesity on estradiol level, and its relationship to leptin, bone maturation, and bone mineral density in children. J Clin Endocrinol Metab 1998; 83:3469–3475.
816. Quinton ND, Smith RF, Clayton PE, et al. Leptin binding activity changes with age: the link between leptin and puberty. J Clin Endocrinol Metab 1999; 84:2336–2341.
817. Caprio M, Fabbrini E, Isidori AM, et al. Leptin in reproduction. Trends Endocrinol Metab 2001; 12:65–72.
818. Lee GH, Proenca R, Montez JM, et al. Abnormal splicing of the leptin receptor in diabetic mice. Nature 1996; 379:632–635.
819. Coleman DL. Obese and diabetes: two mutant genes causing diabetes-obesity syndromes in mice. Diabetologia 1978; 14:141–148.
820. Chehab FF, Lim ME, Lu R. Correction of the sterility defect in homozygous obese female mice by treatment with the human recombinant leptin. Nat Genet 1996; 12:318–320.
821. Chehab FF. A broader role for leptin. Nat Med 1996; 2:723–724.
822. Chehab FF. Leptin as a regulator of adipose mass and reproduction. Trends Pharmacol Sci 2000; 21:309–314.
823. Mounzih K, Lu R, Chehab FF. Leptin treatment rescues the sterility of genetically obese *ob/ob* males. Endocrinology 1997; 138:1190–1193.
824. Ahima RS, Dushay J, Flier SN, et al. Leptin accelerates the onset of puberty in normal female mice. J Clin Invest 1997; 99: 391–395.
825. Chehab FF, Mounzih K, Lu R, Lim ME. Early onset of reproductive function in normal female mice treated with leptin. Science 1997; 275:88–90.
826. Bronson FH. Puberty in female mice is not associated with increases in either body fat or leptin. Endocrinology 2001; 142: 4758–4761.
827. Gruaz NM, Lalaoui M, Pierroz DD, et al. Chronic administration of leptin into the lateral ventricle induces sexual maturation in severely food-restricted female rats. J Neuroendocrinol 1998; 10:627–633.
828. Cheung CC, Clifton DK, Steiner RA. Perspectives on leptin's role as a metabolic signal for the onset of puberty. Front Horm Res 2000; 26:87–105.
829. Magni P, Vettor R, Pagano C, et al. Expression of a leptin receptor in immortalized gonadotropin-releasing hormone-secreting neurons. Endocrinology 1999; 140:1581–1585.
830. Zamorano PL, Mahesh VB, De Sevilla L, Brann DW. Excitatory amino acid receptors and puberty. Steroids 1998; 63:268–270.
831. Woller M, Tessmer S, Neff D, et al. Leptin stimulates gonado-

tropin releasing hormone release from cultured intact hemihypothalami and enzymatically dispersed neurons. Exp Biol Med (Maywood) 2001; 226:591–596.
832. Yu WH, Kimura M, Walczewska A, et al. Role of leptin in hypothalamic-pituitary function. Proc Natl Acad Sci USA 1997; 94:1023–1028.
833. Parent AS, Lebrethon MC, Gerard A, et al. Leptin effects on pulsatile gonadotropin releasing hormone secretion from the adult rat hypothalamus and interaction with cocaine and amphetamine regulated transcript peptide and neuropeptide Y. Regul Pept 2000; 92:17–24.
834. Plant TM, Durrant AR. Circulating leptin does not appear to provide a signal for triggering the initiation of puberty in the male rhesus monkey (*Macaca mulatta*). Endocrinology 1997; 138: 4505–4508.
835. Urbanski HF, Pau KY. A biphasic developmental pattern of circulating leptin in the male rhesus macaque *Macaca mulatta*. Endocrinology 1998; 139:2284–2286.
836. Finn PD, Cunningham MJ, Pau KY, et al. The stimulatory effect of leptin on the neuroendocrine reproductive axis of the monkey. Endocrinology 1998; 139:4652–4662.
837. Cheung CC, Thornton JE, Nurani SD, et al. A reassessment of leptin's role in triggering the onset of puberty in the rat and mouse. Neuroendocrinology 2001; 74:12–21.
838. Mantzoros CS, Flier JS, Rogol AD. A longitudinal assessment of hormonal and physical alterations during normal puberty in boys. V. Rising leptin levels may signal the onset of puberty. J Clin Endocrinol Metab 1997; 82:1066–1070.
839. Clayton PE, Gill MS, Hall CM, et al. Serum leptin through childhood and adolescence. Clin Endocrinol (Oxf) 1997; 46: 727–733.
840. Blum WF, Englaro P, Hanitsch S, et al. Plasma leptin levels in healthy children and adolescents: dependence on body mass index, body fat mass, gender, pubertal stage, and testosterone. J Clin Endocrinol Metab 1997; 82:2904–2910.
841. Ahmed ML, Ong KK, Morrell DJ, et al. Longitudinal study of leptin concentrations during puberty: sex differences and relationship to changes in body composition. J Clin Endocrinol Metab 1999; 84:899–905.
842. Horlick MB, Rosenbaum M, Nicolson M, et al. Effect of puberty on the relationship between circulating leptin and body composition. J Clin Endocrinol Metab 2000; 85:2509–2518.
843. Palmert MR, Radovick S, Boepple PA. The impact of reversible gonadal sex steroid suppression on serum leptin concentrations in children with central precocious puberty. J Clin Endocrinol Metab 1998; 83:1091–1096.
844. Andreelli F, Hanaire-Broutin H, Laville M, et al. Normal reproductive function in leptin-deficient patients with lipoatropic diabetes. J Clin Endocrinol Metab 2000; 85:715–719.
845. Clayton PE, Trueman JA. Leptin and puberty. Arch Dis Child 2000; 83:1–4.
846. Ozata M, Ozdemir IC, Licinio J. Human leptin deficiency caused by a missense mutation: multiple endocrine defects, decreased sympathetic tone, and immune system dysfunction indicate new targets for leptin action, greater central than peripheral resistance to the effects of leptin, and spontaneous correction of leptin-mediated defects. J Clin Endocrinol Metab 1999; 84:3686–3695.
847. Clement K, Vaisse C, Lahlou N, et al. A mutation in the human leptin receptor gene causes obesity and pituitary dysfunction. Nature 1998; 392:398–401.
848. Farooqi IS, Jebb SA, Langmack G, et al. Effects of recombinant leptin therapy in a child with congenital leptin deficiency. N Engl J Med 1999; 341:879–884.
849. Comuzzie AG, Hixson JE, Almasy L, et al. A major quantitative trait locus determining serum leptin levels and fat mass is located on human chromosome 2. Nat Genet 1997; 15:273–276.
850. Brown DC, Kelnar CJ, Wu FC. Energy metabolism during male human puberty. I. Changes in energy expenditure during the onset of puberty in boys. Ann Hum Biol 1996; 23:273–279.
851. Brown DC, Kelnar CJ, Wu FC. Energy metabolism during male human puberty. II. Use of testicular size in predictive equations for basal metabolic rate. Ann Hum Biol 1996; 23: 281–284.
852. Odell WD, Swerdloff RS. Etiologies of sexual maturation: a model system based on the sexually maturing rat. Recent Prog Horm Res 1976; 32:245–288.
853. Davidson JM. Hypothalamic-pituitary regulation of puberty: evidence from animal experimentation. In Grumbach MM, Grave GD, Mayer FE (eds). Control of the Onset of Puberty. New York, John Wiley & Sons, 1974, pp 79–103.
854. Ramirez VD. Endocrinology of puberty. Female reproductive system. Part 1. In Greep RO, Astwood EB (eds). Handbook of Physiology. Sect 7: Endocrinology. Washington, DC, American Physiological Society, 1973, pp 1–28.
855. Lenko HL, Lang U, Aubert ML, et al. Hormonal changes in puberty. VII. Lack of variation of daytime plasma melatonin. J Clin Endocrinol Metab 1982; 54:1056–1058.
856. Cohen HN, Hay ID, Annesley TM, et al. Serum immunoreactive melatonin in boys with delayed puberty. Clin Endocrinol (Oxf) 1982; 17:517–521.
857. Reppert SM, Weaver DR. Melatonin madness. Cell 1995; 83: 1059–1062.
858. Luboshitzky R, Lavi S, Thuma I, Lavie P. Increased nocturnal melatonin secretion in male patients with hypogonadotropic hypogonadism and delayed puberty. J Clin Endocrinol Metab 1995; 80:2144-2148.
859. Cavallo A. Melatonin and human puberty: current perspectives. J Pineal Res 1993; 15:115–121.
860. Cavallo A. Melatonin secretion during adrenarche in normal human puberty and in pubertal disorders. J Pineal Res 1992; 12: 71–78.
861. Cavallo A. Plasma melatonin rhythm in normal puberty: interactions of age and pubertal stages. Neuroendocrinology 1992; 55: 372–379.
862. Cavallo A, Ritschel WA. Pharmacokinetics of melatonin in human sexual maturation. J Clin Endocrinol Metab 1996; 81: 1882–1886.
863. Luboshitzky R, Lavi S, Thuma I, Lavie P. Testosterone treatment alters melatonin concentrations in male patients with gonadotropin-releasing hormone deficiency. J Clin Endocrinol Metab 1996; 81:770–774.
864. Okatani Y, Sagara Y. Amplification of nocturnal melatonin secretion in women with functional secondary amenorrhoea: relation to endogenous oestrogen concentration. Clin Endocrinol (Oxf) 1994; 41:763–770.
865. Salti R, Galluzzi F, Bindi G, et al. Nocturnal melatonin patterns in children. J Clin Endocrinol Metab 2000; 85:2137–2144.
866. Foster DL, Ryan KD. Puberty in the lamb: sexual maturation of a seasonal breeder in a changing environment. In Grumbach MM, Sizonenko PC, Aubert ML (eds). Control of the Onset of Puberty. Baltimore, Williams & Wilkins, 1990, pp 143–155.
867. Ojeda SR, Smith-White S, Advis JP, et al. First preovulatory gonadotropin surge in the rodent. In Grumbach MM, Sizonenko PC, Aubert ML (eds). Control of the Onset of Puberty. Baltimore, Williams & Wilkins, 1990, pp 156–182.
868. Donovan BT. Puberty in the guinea pig and rabbit. In Grumbach MM, Sizonenko PC, Aubert ML (eds). Control of the Onset of Puberty. Baltimore, Williams & Wilkins, 1990, pp 143–144.
869. Vandenbergh JG. Pheromones and mammalian reproduction. In Knobil E, Neill JD (eds). The Physiology of Reproduction. New York, Raven Press, 1994, pp 1679–1696.
870. Grumbach MM, Styne DM. Puberty, ontogeny, neuroendocrinology, physiology, and disorders. In Wilson JD, Foster DW, Kronenberg MD, Larsen PR (eds). Williams Textbook of Endocrinology. Philadelphia, WB Saunders, 1998, pp 1509–1625.
871. Kaplan SL, Grumbach MM. Pathogenesis of sexual precocity. In Grumbach MM, Sizonenko PC, Aubert ML (eds). Control of the Onset of Puberty. Baltimore, Williams & Wilkins, 1990, pp 620–660.
872. Conte FA, Grumbach MM, Kaplan SL, Reiter EO. Correlation of luteinizing hormone–releasing factor–induced luteinizing hormone and follicle-stimulating hormone release from infancy to 19 years with the changing pattern of gonadotropin secretion in agonadal patients: relation to the restraint of puberty. J Clin Endocrinol Metab 1980; 50:163–168.
873. Conte FA, Grumbach MM, Kaplan SL. A diphasic pattern of gonadotropin secretion in patients with the syndrome of gonadal dysgenesis. J Clin Endocrinol Metab 1975; 40:670–674.
874. Kelch RP, Kaplan SL, Grumbach MM. Suppression of urinary and plasma follicle-stimulating hormone by exogenous estrogens in prepubertal and pubertal children. J Clin Invest 1973; 52: 1122–1128.

875. Grumbach MM, Kaplan SL. Recent advances in the diagnosis and management of sexual precocity. Acta Paediatr Jpn 1988; 30(suppl):155–175.
876. Voigt P, Ma YJ, Gonzalez D, et al. Neural and glial mediated effects of growth factors acting via tyrosine kinase receptors on luteinizing hormone–releasing hormone neurons. Endocrinology 1997; 137:2593–2605.
877. Wetsel WC, Hill DF, Ojeda SR. Basic fibroblast growth factor regulates the conversion of pro-luteinizing hormone releasing hormone (pro-LHRH) to LHRH in immortalized hypothalamic neurons. Endocrinology 1997; 137:2606–2616.
878. Junier MP, Ma YJ, Costa ME, et al. Transforming growth factor alpha contributes to the mechanism by which hypothalamic injury induces precocious puberty. Proc Natl Acad Sci USA 1991; 88:9743–9747.
879. Olson BR, Scott DC, Wetsel WC, et al. Effects of insulin-like growth factors I and II and insulin on the immortalized hypothalamic GTI-7 cell line. Neuroendocrinology 1995; 62:155–165.
880. Ojeda SR, Dissen GA, Junier M-P. Neutrophilic factors and female sexual development. Front Neuroendocrinol 1992; 13: 120–162.
881. Hiney JK, Srivastava V, Nyberg CL, et al. Insulin-like growth factor I of peripheral origin acts centrally to accelerate the initiation of female puberty. Endocrinology 1996; 137:3717–3728.
882. Gallo F, Morale MC, Avola R, Marchetti B. Cross-talk between luteinizing hormone–releasing hormone (LHRH) neurons and astroglia cells: developing glia release factors that accelerate neuronal differentiation and stimulate LHRH release from GT neuronal cell line and LHRH neurons induce astroglia proliferation. Endocrine 1995; 3:863–874.
883. Watanabe G, Terasawa E. In vivo luteinizing hormone releasing hormone increases with puberty in the female rhesus monkey. Endocrinology 1989; 125:92–99.
884. Terasawa E, Noonan JJ, Nass TE, Loose MD. Posterior hypothalamic lesions advance the onset of puberty in the female rhesus monkey. Endocrinology 1984; 115:2241–2250.
885. Schultz NJ, Terasawa E. Posterior hypothalamic lesions advance the time of the pubertal changes in luteinizing hormone release in ovariectomized female rhesus monkeys. Endocrinology 1988; 123:445–455.
886. Pohl CR, deRidder CM, Plant TM. Gonadal and nongonadal mechanisms contribute to the prepubertal hiatus in gonadotropin secretion in the female rhesus monkey (*Macaca mulatta*). J Clin Endocrinol Metab 1995; 80:2094–2101.
887. Hochman HI, Judge DM, Reichlin S. Precocious puberty and hypothalamic hamartoma. Pediatrics 1981; 67:236–244.
888. Judge DM, Kulin HE, Santen R, et al. Hypothalamic hamartoma: a source of luteinizing-hormone–releasing factor in precocious puberty. N Engl J Med 1977; 296:7–10.
889. Mahachoklertwattana P, Kaplan SL, Grumbach MM. The luteinizing hormone–releasing hormone–secreting hypothalamic hamartoma is a congenital malformation: natural history. J Clin Endocrinol Metab 1993; 77:118–124.
890. Krieger DT, Perlow MJ, Gibson MJ, et al. Brain grafts reverse hypogonadism of gonadotropin-releasing hormone deficiency. Nature 1982; 298:468–472.
891. Silverman AJ, Gibson M. Hypothalamic transplantation. Repair of defects in hypogonadal mice. Trends Endocrinol Metab 1990; 1:403–408.
892. Arslan M, Pohl CR, Plant TM. DL-2-Amino-5-phosphonopentanoic acid, a specific *N*-methyl-D-aspartic acid receptor antagonist, suppresses pulsatile LH release in the rat. Neuroendocrinology 1988; 47:465–468.
893. Bettendorf M, Albers N, de Zegher F, et al. A neuroexcitatory amino acid analogue, *N*-methyl-D,L-aspartate (NMDA), elicits LH and FSH release in the ovine fetus by a central mechanism. Endocr Soc Abstr 1988; 288.
894. Gambacciani M, Yen SS, Rasmussen D. GnRH release from the mediobasal hypothalamus: in vitro inhibition by corticotropin releasing factor. Neuroendocrinology 1986; 43:533–536.
895. Kuljis RO, Advis JP. Immunocytochemical and physiological evidence of a synapse between dopamine- and luteinizing hormone releasing hormone–containing neurons in the ewe median eminence. Endocrinology 1989; 124:1579–1581.
896. MacLusky NJ, Naftolin F, Leranth C. Immunocytochemical evidence for direct synaptic connections between corticotrophin-releasing factor (CRF) and gonadotrophin-releasing hormone (GnRH)–containing neurons in the preoptic area of the rat. Brain Res 1988; 439:391–395.
897. Plant TM, Gay VL, Marshall GR, et al. Puberty in monkeys is triggered by chemical stimulation of the hypothalamus. Proc Natl Acad Sci USA 1989; 86:2506–2510.
898. Wilson RC, Kesner JS, Kaufman JM, et al. Central electrophysiologic correlates of pulsatile luteinizing hormone secretion in the rhesus monkey. Neuroendocrinology 1984; 39:256–260.
899. Ozata M, Bulur M, Bingol N, et al. Daytime plasma melatonin levels in male hypogonadism. J Clin Endocrinol Metab 1996; 81:1877–1881.
900. Kelch RP, Foster CM, Kletter GB. Neuroendocrine regulation of puberty in boys. In Sizonenko PC, Aubert ML (eds). Developmental Endocrinology. New York, Raven Press, 1990, pp 103–115.
901. Fraioli F, Cappa M, Fabbri A, et al. Lack of endogenous opioid inhibitory tone on LH secretion in early puberty. Clin Endocrinol (Oxf) 1984; 20:299–305.
902. Petraglia F, Bernasconi S, Iughetti L, et al. Naloxone-induced luteinizing hormone secretion in normal, precocious, and delayed puberty. J Clin Endocrinol Metab 1986; 63:1112–1116.
903. Mauras N, Veldhuis JD, Rogol AD. Role of endogenous opiates in pubertal maturation: opposing actions of naltrexone in prepubertal and late pubertal boys. J Clin Endocrinol Metab 1986; 62:1256–1263.
904. Saunder SE, Case GD, Hopwood NJ, et al. the effects of opiate antagonism on gonadotropin secretion in children and in women with hypothalamic amenorrhea. Pediatr Res 1984; 18: 322–328.
905. Mitsushima D, Marzban F, Luchansky LL, et al. Role of glutamic acid decarboxylase in the prepubertal inhibition of the luteinizing hormone releasing hormone release in female rhesus monkeys. J Neuroscience 1996; 16:2563–2573.
906. Terasawa E. Control of luteinizing hormone–releasing hormone pulse generation in nonhuman primates. Cell Mol Neurobiol 1995; 15:141–164.
907. Kasuya E, Nyberg CL, Mogi K, Terasawa E. A role of gamma-amino butyric acid (GABA) and glutamate in control of puberty in female rhesus monkeys: effect of an antisense oligodeoxynucleotide for GAD67 messenger ribonucleic acid and MK801 on luteinizing hormone–releasing hormone release. Endocrinology 1999; 140:705–712.
908. Keen KL, Burich AJ, Mitsushima D, et al. Effects of pulsatile infusion of the GABA(A) receptor blocker bicuculline on the onset of puberty in female rhesus monkeys. Endocrinology 1999; 140:5257–5266.
909. Terasawa E, Luchansky LL, Kasuya E, Nyberg CL. An increase in glutamate release follows a decrease in gamma aminobutyric acid and the pubertal increase in luteinizing hormone releasing hormone release in the female rhesus monkeys. J Neuroendocrinol 1999; 11:275–282.
910. Martinez de la Escalera G, Choi ALH, Weinter RI. Biphasic gabaergic regulation of GnRH secretion in GT1 cell lines. Neuroendocrinology 1994; 59:420–425.
911. Hales TG, Sanderson MJ, Charles AC. GABA has excitatory actions on GnRH-secreting immortalized hypothalamic (GT1-7) neurons. Neuroendocrinology 1994; 59:297–308.
912. El Etr M, Akwa Y, Fiddes RJ, et al. A progesterone metabolite stimulates the release of gonadotropin-releasing hormone from GT1-1 hypothalamic neurons via the gamma- aminobutyric acid type A receptor. Proc Natl Acad Sci USA 1995; 92:3769–3773.
913. Cherubini E, Gaiarsa JL, Ben Ari Y. GABA: an excitatory transmitter in early postnatal life. Trends Neurosci 1991; 14:515–519.
914. Ganguly K, Schinder AF, Wong ST, Poo M. GABA itself promotes the developmental switch of neuronal GABAergic responses from excitation to inhibition. Cell 2001; 105:521–532.
915. El Majdoubi M, Sahu A, Ramaswamy S, Plant TM. Neuropeptide Y: a hypothalamic brake restraining the onset of puberty in primates. Proc Natl Acad Sci USA 2000; 97:6179–6184.
916. Ma YJ, Costa ME, Ojeda SR. Developmental expression of the genes encoding transforming growth factor alpha and its receptor in the hypothalamus of female rhesus macaques. Neuroendocrinology 1994; 60:346–359.

917. Plant TM. Neurobiological bases underlying the control of the onset of puberty in the rhesus monkey: a representative higher primate. Front Neuroendocrinol 2001; 22:107–139.
918. Cheung CC, Clifton DK, Steiner RA. Galanin: an unassuming neuropeptide moves to center stage in reproduction. Trends Endocrinol Metab 1996; 7:301–306.
919. Urbanski HF, Ojeda SR. Activation of luteinizing hormone–releasing hormone release advances the onset of female puberty. Neuroendocrinology 1987; 46:273–276.
920. Price MT, Olney JW, Cicero TJ. Acute elevations of serum luteinizing hormone induced by kainic acid, *N*-methyl aspartic acid or homocystic acid. Neuroendocrinology 1978; 26:352–358.
921. Gay VL, Plant TM. *N*-Methyl-D,L-aspartate elicits hypothalamic gonadotropin-releasing hormone release in prepubertal male rhesus monkeys (*Macaca mulatta*). Endocrinology 1987; 120:2289–2296.
922. Wilson RC, Knobil E. Acute effects of *N*-methyl-DL-aspartate on the release of pituitary gonadotropins and prolactin in the adult female rhesus monkey. Brain Res 1982; 248:177–179.
923. Bourguignon JP, Gerard A, Mathieu J, et al. Pulsatile release of gonadotropin-releasing hormone from hypothalamic explants is restrained by blockade of *N*-methyl-D,L-aspartate receptors. Endocrinology 1989; 125:1090–1096.
924. Hardelin JP, Levilliers J, Young J, et al. Xp22.3 deletions in isolated familial Kallmann's syndrome. J Clin Endocrinol Metab 1993; 76:827–831.
925. Terasawa E, Luchansky LL, Kasuya E, Nyberg CL. An increase in glutamate release follows a decrease in gamma aminobutyric acid and the pubertal increase in luteinizing hormone releasing hormone release in the female rhesus monkeys. J Neuroendocrinol 1999; 11:275–282.
926. Van den Pol AN, Trombley PQ. Glutamate neurons in hypothalamus regulate excitatory transmission. J Neurosci 1993; 13: 2829–2836.
927. Terasawa E. Hypothalamic control of the onset of puberty. Curr Opin Endocrinol Diabet 1999; 6:44–49.
928. Claypool LE, Kasuya E, Saitoh Y, et al. *N*-Methyl D,L-aspartate induces the release of luteinizing hormone–releasing hormone in the prepubertal and pubertal female rhesus monkey as measured by in vivo push-pull perfusion in the stalk-median eminence. Endocrinology 2000; 141:219–228.
929. Mahachoklertwattana P, Sanchez J, Kaplan SL, et al. *N*-Methyl-D-aspartate (NMDA) receptors mediate the release of hormone (GnRH) by NMDA in a hypothalamic neuronal cell line (GT1-1). Endocrinology 1994; 134:1023–1030.
930. Ojeda SR, Ma YJ. Glial-neuronal interactions in the neuroendocrine control of mammalian puberty: facilitatory effects of gonadal steroids. J Neurobiol 1999; 40:528–540.
931. Ma YJ, Hill DF, Creswick KE, et al. Neuregulins signaling via a glial erbB-2-erbB-4 receptor complex contribute to the neuroendocrine control of mammalian sexual development. J Neurosci 1999; 19:9913–9927.
932. Ojeda SR, Ma YJ, Lee BJ, Prevot V. Glia-to-neuron signaling and the neuroendocrine control of female puberty. Recent Prog Horm Res 2000; 55:197–223.
933. Jung H, Carmel P, Schwartz MS, et al. Some hypothalamic hamartomas contain transforming growth factor α, a puberty-inducing growth factor, not luteinizing hormone releasing hormone neurons. J Clin Endocrinol Metab 1999; 84:4695–4701.
934. Rebar RW, Yen SSC. Endocrine rhythms in gonadotropins and ovarian steroids with reference to reproductive processes. In Krieger DT (ed). Endocrine Rhythms. New York, Raven Press, 1979, pp 259–298.
935. Kelch RP, Marshall JC. Pulsatile gonadotropin-releasing hormone and the induction of puberty in human beings. In Grumbach MM, Sizonenko PC, Aubert ML (eds). Control of the Onset of Puberty. Baltimore, Williams & Wilkins, 1990, pp 82–107.
936. Boyar RM, Finkelstein JW, Roffwarg H, et al. Twenty-four patterns of luteinizing hormone and follicle-stimulating hormone secretory patterns in gonadal dysgenesis. J Clin Endocrinol Metab 1973; 37:521–525.
937. Kulin HE, Moore RGJ, Santner SJ. Circadian rhythms in gonadotropin excretion in prepubertal and pubertal children. J Clin Endocrinol Metab 1976; 42:770–773.
938. Waldhauser F, Weissenbacher G, Frisch H, Pollak A. Pulsatile secretion of gonadotropins in early infancy. Eur J Pediatr 1981; 137:71–74.
939. Penny R, Olambiwonnu NO, Frasier SD. Episodic fluctuations of serum gonadotropins in pre- and post-pubertal girls and boys. J Clin Endocrinol Metab 1977; 45:307–311.
940. Boyar R, Finkelstein JW, David R, et al. Twenty-four hour patterns of plasma luteinizing hormone and follicle-stimulating hormone in sexual precocity. N Engl J Med 1973; 289:282–286.
941. Kletter GB, Foster CM, Brown MB, et al. Nocturnal naloxone fails to reverse the suppressive effects of testosterone infusion on luteinizing hormone secretion in pubertal boys. J Clin Endocrinol Metab 1994; 79:1147–1151.
942. Watanabe G, Terasawa E. In vivo release of luteinizing hormone releasing hormone increases with puberty in the female rhesus monkey. Endocrinology 1989; 125:92–99.
943. Yen SSC, Lasley BL, Wang FC, et al. The operating characteristics of the hypothalamic-pituitary system during the menstrual cycle and observations of biological action of somatostatin. Recent Prog Horm Res 1975; 31:321–363.
944. Keye WR, Jaffe RB. Strength-duration characteristics of estrogen effects on gonadotropin response to gonadotropin-releasing hormone in women. I. Effects of varying duration of estradiol administration. J Clin Endocrinol Metab 1975; 41:1003–1008.
945. Reiter EO, Kaplan SL, Conte FA, Grumbach MM. Responsivity of pituitary gonadotropes to luteinizing hormone–releasing factor in idiopathic precocious puberty, precocious thelarche, precocious adrenarche, and in patients treated with medroxyprogesterone acetate. Pediatr Res 1975; 9:111–116.
946. Crowley WF Jr, McArthur JW. Stimulation of the normal menstrual cycle in Kallmann's syndrome by pulsatile administration of luteinizing hormone-releasing hormone (LHRH). J Clin Endocrinol Metab 1980; 51:173–175.
947. Yoshimoto Y, Moridera K, Imura H. Restoration of normal pituitary gonadotropin reserve by administration of luteinizing hormone releasing hormone in patients with hypogonadotropic hypogonadism. N Engl J Med 1975; 292:242–245.
948. Jacobson RI, Seyler LE, Tamborlane WV, et al. Pulsatile subcutaneous nocturnal administration of Gn-RH by portable infusion pump in hypogonadotropic hypogonadism: initiation of gonadotropin responsiveness. J Clin Endocrinol Metab 1979; 49: 652–654.
949. Marshall JC, Kelch RP. Low dose pulsatile gonadotropin-releasing hormone in anorexia nervosa: a model of human pubertal development. J Clin Endocrinol Metab 1979; 49:712–718.
950. Valk TW, Corley KP, Kelch RP, et al. Hypogonadotropic hypogonadism: hormonal responses to low dose pulsatile administration of gonadotropin-releasing hormone. J Clin Endocrinol Metab 1980; 51:730–737.
951. Pohl GR, Knobil E. The role of the central nervous system in the control of ovarian function in higher primates. Annu Rev Physiol 1982; 44:583–593.
952. Knobil E, Plant TM. The neuroendocrine control of gonadotropin secretion in the female rhesus monkey. Front Neuroendocrinol 1978; 4:249–264.
953. Wildt L, Marshall G, Knobil E. Experimental induction of puberty in the infantile female rhesus monkey. Science 1980; 207: 1373–1375.
954. Boyar RM, Finkelstein JW, Witkin M, et al. Studies of endocrine function in "isolated" gonadotropin deficiency. J Clin Endocrinol Metab 1973; 36:64–72.
955. Winter JS, Taraska S, Faiman C. The hormonal response to HCG stimulation in male children and adolescents. J Clin Endocrinol Metab 1972; 34:348–353.
956. Sizonenko PC, Cuendet A, Paunier L. FSH. 1. Evidence for its mediating role on testosterone secretion in cryptorchidism. J Clin Endocrinol Metab 1973; 37:68–73.
957. Ross GT, Cargille CM, Lipsett MB, et al. Pituitary and gonadal hormones in women during spontaneous and induced ovulatory cycles. Recent Prog Horm Res 1970;26:1–62.
958. Reiter EO, Kulin HE, Hamwood SM. The absence of positive feedback between estrogen and luteinizing hormone in sexually immature girls. Pediatr Res 1974; 8:740–745.
959. Presl J, Horejsi J, Strouflova A, et al. Sexual maturation in girls and the development of estrogen-induced gonadotropic hormone release. Ann Biol Anim Biochim Biophys 1976; 16:377–383.

960. Hayes FJ, Seminara SB, DeCruz S, et al. Aromatase inhibition in the human male reveals a hypothalamic site of estrogen feedback. J Clin Endocrinol Metab 2000; 85:3027–3035.
961. Knobil E, Plant TM, Wildt L, et al. Control of the rhesus monkey menstrual cycle: permissive role of the hypothalamic gonadotropin-releasing hormone. Science 1980; 207:1371–1373.
962. Doring GK. Uber die relativ Sterilitat in den Jahren nach der Menarche. Geburtsh Frauenheilkd 1963; 23:30–36.
963. Hansen JW, Hoffman HJ, Ross GT. Monthly gonadotropin cycles in premenarcheal girls. Science 1975; 190:161–163.
964. Winter JSD, Faiman C. Pituitary-gonadal relations in female children and adolescents. Pediatr Res 1973; 7:948–953.
965. van Hooff MH, Voorhorst FJ, Kaptein MB, et al. Insulin, androgen, and gonadotropin concentrations, body mass index, and waist to hip ratio in the first years after menarche in girls with regular menstrual cycles, irregular menstrual cycles, or oligomenorrhea. J Clin Endocrinol Metab 2000; 85:1394–1400.
966. Warren MP, Shantha S. The female athlete. Baillieres Best Pract Res Clin Endocrinol Metab 2000; 14:37–53.
967. Warren MP, Voussoughian F, Geer EB, et al. Functional hypothalamic amenorrhea: hypoleptinemia and disordered eating. J Clin Endocrinol Metab 1999; 84:873–877.
968. Cutler GBJ, Loriaux DL. Adrenarche and its relationship to the onset of puberty. Fed Proc 1980; 39:2384–2390.
969. Sklar CA, Kaplan SL, Grumbach MM. Evidence for dissociation between adrenarche and gonadarche: studies in patients with idiopathic precocious puberty, gonadal dysgenesis, isolated gonadotropin deficiency, and constitutionally delayed growth and adolescence. J Clin Endocrinol Metab 1980; 51:548–556.
970. Hopper BR, Yen SSC. Circulating concentrations of dehydroepiandrosterone and dehydroepiandrosterone sulfate during puberty. J Clin Endocrinol Metab 1975; 40:458–461.
971. Sizonenko PC, Paunier LC. Correlation of plasma dehydroepiandrosterone, testosterone, FSH, and LH with stages of puberty and bone age in normal boys and girls and in patients with Addison's disease or hypogonadism or with premature or late adrenarche. J Clin Endocrinol Metab 1975; 41:894–904.
972. Reiter EO, Fuldauer VG, Root AW. Secretion of the adrenal androgen, dehydroepiandrosterone sulfate, during normal infancy, childhood, and adolescence, in sick infants, and in children with endocrinologic abnormalities. J Pediatr 1977; 90:766–770.
973. Apter D, Pakarinen A, Hammond GL, Vihko R. Adrenocortical function in puberty: serum ACTH, cortisol and dehydroepiandrosterone in girls and boys. Acta Paediatr Scand 1979; 68:599–604.
974. Dhom G. The prepuberal and puberal growth of the adrenal (adrenarche). Beitr Pathol 1973; 150:357–377.
975. Endoh A, Kristiansen SB, Casson PR, et al. The zona reticularis is the site of biosynthesis of dehydroepiandrosterone and dehydroepiandrosterone sulfate in the adult human adrenal cortex resulting from its low expression of 3β-hydroxysteroid dehydrogenase. J Clin Endocrinol Metab 1996; 81:3558–3565.
976. Kennerson AR, McDonald DA, Adams JB. Dehydroepiandrosterone sulfotransferase localization in human adrenal glands: a light and electron microscope study. J Clin Endocrinol Metab 1983; 56:786–790.
977. Gell JS, Carr BR, Sasano H, et al. Adrenarche results from development of a 3beta-hydroxysteroid dehydrogenase–deficient adrenal reticularis. J Clin Endocrinol Metab 1998; 83:3695–3701.
978. Dupont E, Luu-The V, Lubrie F, et al. Ontogeny of the 3β-hydroxysteroid dehydrogenase/Δ5-Δ4 isomerase (3β-HSD) in human adrenal gland performed by immunochemistry. Mol Cell Endocrinol 1990; 74:R7–R10.
979. Parker CR Jr, Stankovic AK, Falany CN, et al. Immunocytochemical analyses of dehydroepiandrosterone sulfotransferase in cultured human fetal adrenal cells. J Clin Endocrinol Metab 1995; 80:1027–1031.
980. Khoury EL, Greenspan JS, Greenspan FS. Adrenocortical cells of the zona reticularis normally express HLA-DR antigenic determinants. Am J Pathol 1987; 127:580–591.
981. Marx C, Bornstein SR, Wolkersdorfer GW. Relevance of MHC class II expression as a hallmark for the cellular differentiation in the human adrenal cortex. J Clin Endocrinol Metab 1997; 82:3136–3140.
982. Kitamura M, Bucko E, Dufau ML. Dissociation of hydroxylase and lyase activities by site directed mutagenesis of the rat P450c17. Steroids 1991; 5:1373–1380.
983. Miller WL, Auchus RJ, Geller DH. The regulation of 17,20 lyase activity. Steroids 1997; 62:133–142.
984. Geller DH, Auchus RJ, Mendonca BB, Miller WL. The genetic and functional basis of isolated 17,20-lyase deficiency. Nat Genet 1997; 17:201–205.
985. Zhang L, Rodriguez H, Ohno S, Miller WL. Serine phosphorylation of human P450c17 increases 17,20 lyase activity: implications for adrenarche and for the polycystic ovary syndrome. Proc Natl Acad Sci USA 1995; 92:10619–10623.
986. Auchus RJ, Miller WL. Molecular modeling of human P450c17 (17alpha-hydroxylase/17,20-lyase): insights into reaction mechanisms and effects of mutations. Mol Endocrinol 1999; 13:1169–1182.
987. Miller WL. The molecular basis of premature adrenarche: an hypothesis. Acta Paediatr Suppl 1999; 88:60–66.
988. Ibanez L, Potau N, Marcos MV, de Zegher F. Corticotropin-releasing hormone as adrenal androgen secretagogue. Pediatr Res 1999; 46:351–353.
989. Ibanez L, Potau N, Marcos MV, de Zegher F. Corticotropin-releasing hormone: a potent androgen secretagogue in girls with hyperandrogenism after precocious pubarche. J Clin Endocrinol Metab 1999; 84:4602–4606.
990. Smith R, Mesiano S, Chan EC, et al. Corticotropin-releasing hormone directly and preferentially stimulates dehydroepiandrosterone sulfate secretion by human fetal adrenal cortical cells. J Clin Endocrinol Metab 1998; 83:2916–2920.
991. Karteris E, Randeva HS, Grammatopoulos DK, et al. Expression and coupling characteristics of the CRH and orexin type 2 receptors in human fetal adrenals. J Clin Endocrinol Metab 2001; 86:4512–4519.
992. Remer T, Manz F. Role of nutritional status in the regulation of adrenarche. J Clin Endocrinol Metab 1999; 84:3936–3944.
993. Reiter EO, Grumbach MM, Kaplan SL, et al. The response of pituitary gonadotropes to synthetic LRF in children with glucocorticoid-treated congenital adrenal hyperplasia: lack of effect of intrauterine and neonatal androgen excess. J Clin Endocrinol Metab 1975; 40:318–325.
994. Butler GE, McKie M, Ratcliffe SG. The cyclical nature of prepubertal growth. Ann Hum Biol 1990; 17:177-198.
995. Remer T, Manz F. The midgrowth spurt in healthy children is not caused by adrenarche. J Clin Endocrinol Metab 2001; 86:4183–4186.
996. Prader A. Delayed adolescence. Clin Endocrinol Metab 1975; 4:143–155.
997. Counts DR, Pescovitz OH, Barnes KM, et al. Dissociation of adrenarche and gonadarche in precocious puberty and in isolated hypogonadotropic hypogonadism. J Clin Endocrinol Metab 1987; 64:1174–1178.
998. Du Caju MV, Op De Beeck L, Sys SU, et al. Progressive deceleration in growth as an early sign of delayed puberty in boys. Horm Res 2000; 54:126–130.
999. Rikken B, Wit JM. Prepubertal height velocity references over a wide age range. Arch Dis Child 1992; 67:1277–1280.
1000. Gourmelen M, Pham-Huu-Trung MT, Girard F. Transient partial hGH deficiency in prepubertal children with delay of growth. Pediatr Res 1979; 13:221–224.
1001. Bierich JR. Serum growth hormone levels in provocation tests and during nocturnal spontaneous secretion: a comparative study. Acta Paediatr Scand Suppl 1987; 337:48–59.
1002. Saggese G, Cesaretti G, Giannessi N, et al. Stimulated growth hormone (GH) secretion in children with delays in pubertal development before and after the onset of puberty: relationship with peripheral plasma GH-releasing hormone and somatostatin levels. J Clin Endocrinol Metab 1992; 74:272–278.
1003. Stanhope R, Hindmarsh P, Pringle PJ, et al. Oxandrolone induces a sustained rise in physiological growth hormone secretion in boys with constitutional delay of growth and puberty. Pediatrician 1987; 14:183–188.
1004. Loche S, Corda R, Lampis A, et al. The effect of oxandrolone on the growth hormone response to growth hormone releasing hormone in children with constitutional growth delay. Clin Endocrinol 1986; 25:195–200.
1005. Clayton PE, Shalet SM, Price DA, Addison GM. Growth and

growth hormone responses to oxandrolone in boys with constitutional delay of growth and puberty (CDGP). Clin Endocrinol (Oxf) 1988; 29:123–130.
1006. Stolecke H, Gilessen G. Oxandrolone and spontaneous hGH secretion (abstract). Pediatr Res 1984; 18:1216.
1007. Cara JF, Rosenfield RL. Insulin-like growth factor I and insulin potentiate luteinizing hormone–induced androgen synthesis by rat ovarian theca-interstitial cells. Endocrinology 1988; 123:733–739.
1008. Apter D. Self-image in adolescents with delayed puberty and growth retardation. J Youth Adolesc 1981; 10:501–505.
1009. Mussen PH, Jones MC. Self conceptions, motivations and interpersonal attitudes of late and early maturing boys. Child Dev 1957; 28:243–256.
1010. Gordon M, Crouthamel C, Post EM. Psychosocial aspects of constitutional short stature: social competence, behavior problems, self esteem and family functioning. J Pediatr 1982; 101: 477–480.
1011. Crowne EC, Shalet SM, Wallace WH, et al. Final height in boys with untreated constitutional delay in growth and puberty. Arch Dis Child 1990; 65:1109–1112.
1012. Blethen SL, Gaines S, Weldon V. Comparison of predicted and adult heights in short boys: effect of androgen therapy. Pediatr Res 1984; 18:467–469.
1013. Crowne EC, Shalet SM, Wallace WH, et al. Final height in girls with untreated constitutional delay in growth and puberty. Eur J Pediatr 1991; 150:708–712.
1014. LaFranchi S, Hanna CE, Mandel SH. Constitutional delay of growth: expected versus final adult height. Pediatrics 1991; 87: 82–87.
1015. Albanese A, Stanhope R. Predictive factors in the determination of final height in boys with constitutional delay of growth and puberty. J Pediatr 1995; 126:545–550.
1016. Albanese A, Stanhope R. Does constitutional delayed puberty cause segmental disproportion and short stature? Eur J Pediatr 1993; 152:293–296.
1017. Rensonnet C, Kanen F, Coremans C, et al. Pubertal growth as a determinant of adult height in boys with constitutional delay of growth and puberty. Horm Res 1999; 51:223–229.
1018. Adan L, Souberbielle JC, Brauner R. Management of the short stature due to pubertal delay in boys. J Clin Endocrinol Metab 1994; 78:478–482.
1019. Bierich JR, Nolte K, Drews K, Brugmann G. Constitutional delay of growth and adolescence. Results of short-term and long-term treatment with GH. Acta Endocrinol (Copenh) 1992; 127:392–396.
1020. Volta C, Bernasconi S, Tondi P, et al. Combined treatment with growth hormone and luteinizing hormone releasing hormone-analogue (LHRHa) of pubertal children with familial short stature. J Endocrinol Invest 1993; 16:763–767.
1021. Municchi G, Rose SR, Pescovitz OH, et al. Effect of deslorelin-induced pubertal delay on the growth of adolescents with short stature and normally timed puberty: preliminary results. J Clin Endocrinol Metab 1993; 77:1334–1339.
1022. Saggese G, Cesaretti G, Andreani G, Carlotti C. Combined treatment with growth hormone and gonadotropin-releasing hormone analogues in children with isolated growth hormone deficiency. Acta Endocrinol (Copenh) 1992; 127:307–312.
1023. Carel JC, Hay F, Coutant R, et al. Gonadotropin-releasing hormone agonist treatment of girls with constitutional short stature and normal pubertal development. J Clin Endocrinol Metab 1996; 81:3318–3322.
1024. Yanovski JA, Rose SR, Filmer KM. Deslorelin-induced delay of puberty increases adult height of adolescents with short stature: results of randomized, placebo-controlled trial (abstract). Pediatr Res 1996; 39:101A.
1025. Saggese G, Federico G, Barsanti S, Cerri S. Is there a place for combined therapy with GnRH agonist plus growth hormone in improving final height in short statured children? J Pediatr Endocrinol Metab 2000; 13(suppl 1):821–826.
1026. Kamp GA, Mul D, Waelkens JJ, et al. A randomized controlled trial of three years growth hormone and gonadotropin-releasing hormone agonist treatment in children with idiopathic short stature and intrauterine growth retardation. J Clin Endocrinol Metab 2001; 86:2969–2975.
1027. Kaplowitz PB. If gonadotropin-releasing hormone plus growth hormone (GH) really improves growth outcomes in short non–GH-deficient children, then what? J Clin Endocrinol Metab 2001; 86:2965–2968.
1028. Wickman S, Sipila I, Ankarberg-Lindgren C, et al. A specific aromatase inhibitor and potential increase in adult height in boys with delayed puberty: a randomised controlled trial. Lancet 2001; 357:1743–1748.
1029. Spratt DI, Carr DH, Merriam GR, et al. The spectrum of abnormal patterns of gonadotropin-releasing hormone secretion in men with idiopathic hypogonadotropic hypogonadism: clinical and laboratory correlations. J Clin Endocrinol 1987; 64:283–291.
1030. Byrne MN, Sessions DG. Nasopharyngeal craniopharyngioma: case report and literature review. Ann Otol Rhinol Laryngol 1990; 99:633–639.
1031. Fukushima T, Hirakawa K, Kimura M. Intraventricular craniopharyngioma: its characteristics in magnetic resonance imaging and successful total removal. Surg Neurol 1990; 33:22–27.
1032. Banna M. Craniopharyngioma: based on 160 cases. Br J Radiol 1976; 49:206–223.
1033. Banna M, Hoare RD, Stanley P. Craniopharyngioma in children. J Pediatr 1973; 83:781–785.
1034. Thomsett MJ, Conte FA, Kaplan SL, et al. Endocrine and neurologic outcome in childhood craniopharyngioma: review of effect of treatment in 42 patients. J Pediatr 1980; 97:728–735.
1035. Baumgartner JE, Wilson CB, Edwards MSB, et al. Management of craniopharyngioma in children. Part 1. The effect of surgery and radiation therapy on outcome magnetic resonance imaging of pituitary and parasellar abnormalities. J Neurosurg 1989; 27: 265–281.
1036. Chakeres DW, Curtin A, Ford G. Magnetic resonance imaging of pituitary and parasellar abnormalities. Radiol Clin North Am 1989; 27:265–281.
1037. Fahlbusch R, Honegger J, Paulus W, et al. Surgical treatment of craniopharyngiomas: experience with 168 patients. J Neurosurg 1999; 90:237–250.
1038. Curtis J, Daneman D, Hoffman HJ, Ehrlich RM. The endocrine outcome after surgical removal of craniopharyngiomas. Pediatr Neurosurg 1994; 21(suppl 1):24–27.
1039. Weiss M, Sutton L, Marcial V. The role of radiation therapy in the management of childhood craniopharyngioma. Int J Radiat Oncol Biol Phys 1989; 17:1313–1321.
1040. Fischer EG, Welch K, Shillito J Jr. Craniopharyngiomas in children: long term effects of conservative surgical procedures combined with radiation therapy. J Neurosurg 1990; 73:534–540.
1041. Warnick RE, Edwards MSB. Pediatric brain tumors. Curr Probl Pediatr 1991; 21:129–173.
1042. Paja M, Lucas T, Garcia-Uria J. Hypothalamic-pituitary dysfunction in patients with craniopharyngioma. Clin Endocrinol 1995; 42:467–473.
1043. De Vile CJ, Grant DB, Hayward RD. Obesity in childhood craniopharyngioma: relation to post-operative hypothalamic damage shown by magnetic resonance imaging. J Clin Endocrinol Metab 1996; 81:2734–2737.
1044. Bray GA. Genetic, hypothalamic, and endocrine features of clinical and experimental obesity. Prog Brain Res 1992; 93:333–341.
1045. Palm L, Nordin V, Elmqvist D, et al. Sleep and wakefulness after treatment for craniopharyngioma in childhood; influence on the quality and maturation of sleep. Neuropediatrics 1992; 23:39–45.
1046. Mukherjee S, Louie SG, Campbell M, et al. Ductal growth is impeded in mammary glands of C-neu transgenic mice. Oncogene 2000; 19:5982–5987.
1047. Dayan AD, Marshall AHE, Miller AA. Atypical teratomas of the pineal and hypothalamus. J Pathol Bacteriol 1966; 92:1–28.
1048. Mootha SL, Barkovich AJ, Grumbach MM, et al. Idiopathic hypothalamic diabetes insipidus, pituitary stalk thickening and the occult intracranial germinoma in children and adolescents. J Clin Endocrinol Metab 1997; 82:1362–1367.
1049. Sklar CA, Grumbach MM, Kaplan SL, et al. Hormonal and metabolic abnormalities associated with central nervous system germinoma in children and adolescents and the effect of therapy: report of 10 patients. J Clin Endocrinol Metab 1981; 52:9–16.

1050. Kitanaka C, Matsutani M, Sora S, et al. Precocious puberty in a girl with an hCG-secreting suprasellar immature teratoma: case report. J Neurosurg 1994; 81:601–604.
1051. Spiegel AM, Giovanni DC, Gordon P. Diagnosis of radiosensitive hypothalamic tumors without craniotomy. Ann Intern Med 1976; 85:290–293.
1052. Kilgore DP, Strother CM, Starshak RJ, et al. Pineal germinoma: MR imaging. Radiology 1986; 158:435–438.
1053. Schmidt F, Penka B, Trauner M, et al. Lack of pineal growth during childhood. J Clin Endocrinol Metab 1995; 80:1221–1225.
1054. Wara WM, Fellows FC, Sheline GE. Radiation therapy for pineal tumors and suprasellar germinomas. Radiology 1977; 124: 221–223.
1055. Saxena KM. Endocrine manifestations of neurofibromatosis in children. Am J Dis Child 1970; 120:265–272.
1056. Fienman NL, Yakovac WC. Neurofibromatosis in childhood. J Pediatr 1970; 76:339–346.
1057. Kibirige MS, Birch JM, Campbell RH. A review of astrocytoma in childhood. Pediatr Hematol Oncol 1989; 6:319–329.
1058. De Menis E, Visentin A, Billeci D, et al. Pituitary adenomas in childhood and adolescence. Clinical analysis of 10 cases. J Endocrinol Invest 2001; 24:92–97.
1059. Job JC, Chaussain JL, Toublanc JE. Delayed puberty. In Grumbach MM, Sizonenko PC, Aubert ML (eds). Control of the Onset of Puberty. Baltimore, Williams & Wilkins, 1990, pp 588–619.
1060. Cheyne KL, Lightner ES, Comerci GD. Bromocriptine-unresponsive prolactin macroadenoma in a prepubertal female. J Adolesc Health Care 1988; 9:331–334.
1061. Patton ML, Woolf PD. Hyperprolactinemia and delayed puberty: a report of three cases and their response to therapy. Pediatrics 1983; 71:572–575.
1062. Mahachoklertwattana P, Conte FA, Grumbach MM, et al. Prolactinomas in children and adolescents: Effect on pubertal onset and long term outcome following selective transsphenoidal adenomectomy. In preparation 2002.
1063. Koenig MP, Zuppinger K, Liechti B. Hyperprolactinemia as a cause of delayed puberty: successful treatment with bromocriptine. J Clin Endocrinol Metab 1977; 45:825–828.
1064. Willman CL, Busque L, Griffith BB. Langerhans'-cell histiocytosis (histiocytosis X): a clonal proliferative disease. N Engl J Med 1994; 331:154–160.
1065. Herzog KM, Tubbs RR. Langerhans cell histiocytosis. Adv Anat Pathol 1998; 5:347–358.
1066. Vogel JM, Vogel P. Idiopathic histiocytosis: a discussion of eosinophilic granuloma, the Hand-Schüller-Christian syndrome, and the Letterer-Siwe syndrome. Semin Hematol 1972; 9:349–364.
1067. Sims DG. Histiocytosis X: follow-up of 43 cases. Arch Dis Child 1977; 52:433–440.
1068. Egeler RM, Nesbit ME. Langerhans cell histiocytosis and other disorders of monocyte-histiocyte lineage. Crit Rev Oncol Hematol 1995; 18:9–35.
1069. Maghnie M, Cosi G, Genovese E, et al. Central diabetes insipidus in children and young adults. N Engl J Med 2000; 343: 998–1007.
1070. Nanduri VR, Bareille P, Pritchard J, Stanhope R. Growth and endocrine disorders in multisystem Langerhans' cell histiocytosis. Clin Endocrinol (Oxf) 2000; 53:509–515.
1071. Kaltsas GA, Powles TB, Evanson J, et al. Hypothalamo-pituitary abnormalities in adult patients with Langerhans cell histiocytosis: clinical, endocrinological, and radiological features and response to treatment. J Clin Endocrinol Metab 2000; 85:1370–1376.
1072. Willis B, Ablin A, Weinberg V, et al. Disease course and late sequelae of Langerhans' cell histiocytosis: 25-year experience at the University of California, San Francisco. J Clin Oncol 1996; 14:2073–2082.
1073. Broadbent V, Dunger DB, Yeomans E, Kendall B. Anterior pituitary function and computed tomography/magnetic resonance imaging in patients with Langerhans cell histiocytosis and diabetes insipidus. Med Pediatr Oncol 1993; 21:649–654.
1074. Gadner H, Grois N, Arico M, et al. A randomized trial of treatment for multisystem Langerhans' cell histiocytosis. J Pediatr 2001; 138:728–734.
1075. Lavin PT, Osband ME. Evaluating the role of therapy in histiocytosis X: clinical studies, staging, and scoring. Hematol Oncol Clin North Am 1987; 1:35–47.
1076. Egeler RM, D'Angio GJ. Langerhans cell histiocytosis. J Pediatr 1995; 127:1–11.
1077. Asherson RA, Jackson WPU, Lewis B. Abnormalities of development associated with hypothalamic calcification after tuberculous meningitis. Br Med J 1965; 2:839–843.
1078. Fiedler R, Krieger DT. Endocrine disturbances in patients with congenital aqueductal stenosis. Acta Endocrinol (Copenh) 1975; 80:1–13.
1079. Cholley F, Trivin C, Sainte-Rose C, et al. Disorders of growth and puberty in children with non-tumoral hydrocephalus. J Pediatr Endocrinol Metab 2001; 14:319–327.
1080. Richards GE, Wara WM, Grumbach MM, et al. Delayed onset of hypopituitarism: sequelae of therapeutic irradiation of central nervous system, eye, and middle ear tumors. J Pediatr 1976; 89: 553–559.
1081. Schmiegelow M, Lassen S, Poulsen HS, et al. Gonadal status in male survivors following childhood brain tumors. J Clin Endocrinol Metab 2001; 86:2446–2452.
1082. Shalet SM, Crowne EC, Didi MA, et al. Irradiation-induced growth failure. Baillieres Clin Endocrinol Metab 1992; 6:513–526.
1083. Oberfield SE, Soranno D, Nirenberg A, et al. Age at onset of puberty following high-dose central nervous system radiation therapy. Arch Pediatr Adolesc Med 1996; 150:589–592.
1084. Stubberfield TG, Byrne GC, Jones TW. Growth and growth hormone secretion after treatment for acute lymphoblastic leukemia in childhood: 18-Gy versus 24-Gy cranial irradiation. J Pediatr Hematol Oncol 1995; 17:167–171.
1085. Bath LE, Anderson RA, Critchley HO, et al. Hypothalamic-pituitary-ovarian dysfunction after prepubertal chemotherapy and cranial irradiation for acute leukaemia. Hum Reprod 2001; 16:1838–1844.
1086. Hokken-Koelega AC, van Doorn JW, Hahlen KST, et al. Long-term effects of treatment for acute lymphoblastic leukemia with and without cranial irradiation on growth and puberty: a comparative study. Pediatr Res 1993; 33:577–582.
1087. Hanna CE, Mandel SH, LaFranchi SH. Puberty in the syndrome of septo-optic dysplasia. Am J Dis Child 1989; 143:186–189.
1088. Kaplan SL, Grumbach MM, Hoyt WF. A syndrome of hypopituitary dwarfism, hypoplasia of optic nerves, and malformation of prosencephalon: report of 6 patients (abstract). Pediatr Res 1970; 4:480–481.
1089. Badawy SZ, Pisarska MD, Wasenko JJ, Buran JJ. Congenital hypopituitarism as part of suprasellar dysplasia: a case report. J Reprod Med 1994; 39:643–648.
1090. Dattani MT, Martinez-Barbera JP, Thomas PQ, et al. Mutations in the homeobox gene *HESX1/Hesx1* associated with septo-optic dysplasia in human and mouse. Nat Genet 1998; 19: 125–133.
1091. Parks JS, Brown MR, Hurley DL, et al. Hereditable disorders of pituitary development. J Clin Endocrinol Metab 1999; 84: 4362–4370.
1092. Netchine I, Sobrier ML, Krude H, et al. Mutations in *LHX3* result in a new syndrome revealed by combined pituitary hormone deficiency. Nat Genet 2000; 25:182–186.
1093. Wu W, Cogan JD, Pfeaffle RW, et al. Mutations in *PROP1* cause familial combined pituitary hormone deficiency. Nat Genet 1998; 18:147–149.
1094. Fluck C, Deladoey J, Rutishauser K, et al. Phenotypic variability in familial combined pituitary hormone deficiency caused by a *PROP1* gene mutation resulting in the substitution of ArgCys at codon 120 (R120C). J Clin Endocrinol Metab 1998; 83:3727–3734.
1095. Deladoey J, Fluck C, Buyukgebiz A, et al. "Hot spot" in the *PROP1* gene responsible for combined pituitary hormone deficiency. J Clin Endocrinol Metab 1999; 84:1645–1650.
1096. Asteria C, Oliveira JH, Abucham J, Beck-Peccoz P. Central hypocortisolism as part of combined pituitary hormone deficiency due to mutations of *PROP-1* gene. Eur J Endocrinol 2000; 143:347–352.
1097. Kollias SS, Ball WS, Prenger EC. Review of the embryologic development of the pituitary gland and report of a case of

hypophyseal duplication detected by MRI. Neuroradiology 1995; 37:3–12.

1098. Perrone L, Del Gaizo D, D'Angelo E, et al. Endocrine studies in children with myelomeningocele. J Pediatr Endocrinol 1994; 7:219–223.

1099. Elias ER, Sadeghi-Nejad A. Precocious puberty in girls with myelodysplasia. Pediatrics 1994; 93:521–522.

1100. Seminara SB, Hayes FJ, Crowley WFJ. Gonadotropin-releasing hormone deficiency in the human (idiopathic hypogonadotropic hypogonadism and Kallmann's syndrome): pathophysiological and genetic considerations. Endocr Rev 1999; 19:521–539.

1101. Layman LC. Mutations in human gonadotropin genes and their physiologic significance in puberty and reproduction. Fertil Steril 1999; 71:201–218.

1102. Seminara SB, Oliveira LM, Beranova M, et al. Genetics of hypogonadotropic hypogonadism. J Endocrinol Invest 2000; 23: 560–565.

1103. Weinstein RL, Reitz RE. Pituitary-testicular responsiveness in male hypogonadotropic hypogonadism. J Clin Invest 1974; 53: 408–415.

1104. Van Dop C, Burstein S, Conte FA, et al. Isolated gonadotropin deficiency in boys: clinical characteristics and growth. J Pediatr 1987; 111:684–692.

1105. Pitteloud N, Hayes FJ, Boepple PA, et al. The role of prior pubertal development, biochemical markers of testicular maturation, and genetics in elucidating the phenotypic heterogeneity of idiopathic hypogonadotropic hypogonadism. J Clin Endocrinol Metab 2002; 87:152–160.

1106. Layman LC. Genetics of human hypogonadotropic hypogonadism. Am J Med Genet 1999; 89:240–248.

1107. Achermann JC, Weiss J, Lee EJ, Jameson JL. Inherited disorders of the gonadotropin hormones. Mol Cell Endocrinol 2001; 179:89–96.

1108. de Roux N, Milgrom E. Inherited disorders of GnRH and gonadotropin receptors. Mol Cell Endocrinol 2001; 179:83–87.

1109. Uriarte MM, Baron J, Garcia HB, et al. The effect of pubertal delay on adult height in men with isolated hypogonadotropic hypogonadism [published erratum appears in J Clin Endocrinol Metab 1992;75:1009]. J Clin Endocrinol Metab 1992; 74:436–440.

1110. Seeburg PH, Mason AJ, Steward TA, et al. The mammalian GnRH gene and its pivotal role in reproduction. Recent Prog Horm Res 1987; 43:69–107.

1111. Kallmann F, Schonfeld WA, Barrera SW. Genetic aspects of primary eunuchoidism. Am J Ment Defic 1944; 48:203–236.

1112. Seminara SB, Hayes FJ, Crowley WJ. Gonadotropin-releasing hormone deficiency in the human (idiopathic hypogonadotropic hypogonadism and Kallmann's syndrome): pathophysiological and genetic considerations. Endocr Rev 1998; 19:521–539.

1113. Wortsman J, Hughes LF. Case report: olfactory function in a fertile eunuch with Kallmann syndrome. Am J Med Sci 1996; 311:135–138.

1114. Bauman A. Markedly delayed puberty or Kallmann's syndrome variant. J Androl 1986; 7:224–227.

1115. Quinton R, Cheow HK, Tymms DJ, et al. Kallmann's syndrome: is it always for life? Clin Endocrinol 1999; 50:481–485.

1116. Doty RL, Shaman P, Dann M. The development of the University of Pennsylvania smell identification test: a standardized microencapsulated test of olfactory function. Physiol Behav 1984; 32:501–507.

1117. Santen RJ, Paulsen CA. Hypogonadotropic eunuchoidism. I. Clinical study of the mode of inheritance. J Clin Endocrinol Metab 1973; 36:47–54.

1118. Prager D, Braunstein GD. X-chromosome-linked Kallmann's syndrome: pathology at the molecular level (editorial). J Clin Endocrinol Metab 1993; 76:824–826.

1119. Kirk JMW, Grant DB, Besser GM, et al. Unilateral renal aplasia in X-linked Kallmann's syndrome. Clin Genet 1994; 46:260–262.

1120. Dunek A, Heye B, Schroedter R. Cortically evoked motor responses in patients with Xp22.3-linked Kallmann's syndrome and in female gene carriers. Am J Neuroradiol 1992; 31:299–304.

1121. Duke VM, Winyard PJ, Thorogood P, et al. *KAL*, a gene mutated in Kallmann's syndrome, is expressed in the first trimester of human development. Mol Cell Endocrinol 1995; 110: 73–79.

1122. Klingmuller D, Dewes W, Krahe T, et al. Magnetic resonance imaging of the brain in patients with anosmia and hypothalamic hypogonadism (Kallmann's syndrome). J Clin Endocrinol Metab 1987; 65:581–584.

1123. Truwit CL, Barkovich AJ, Grumbach MM, et al. Magnetic resonance imaging of Kallmann syndrome, a genetic disorder of neuronal migration affecting the olfactory and genital systems. AJNR 1993; 14:827–838.

1124. Quinton R, Duke VM, de Zoysa PA, et al. The neuroradiology of Kallmann's syndrome: a genotypic and phenotypic analysis. J Clin Endocrinol Metab 1996; 81:3010–3017.

1125. Wu FC, Butler GE, Kelnar CJ, et al. Patterns of pulsatile luteinizing hormone and follicle-stimulating hormone secretion in prepubertal (midchildhood) boys and girls and patients with idiopathic hypogonadotropic hypogonadism (Kallmann's syndrome): a study using an ultrasensitive time-resolved immunofluorometric assay. J Clin Endocrinol Metab 1991; 72:1229–1237.

1126. Oliveira LM, Seminara SB, Beranova M, et al. The importance of autosomal genes in Kallmann syndrome: genotype-phenotype correlations and neuroendocrine characteristics. J Clin Endocrinol Metab 2001; 86:1532–1538.

1127. Hardelin JP, Julliard AK, Moniot B, et al. Anosmin-1 is a regionally restricted component of basement membranes and interstitial matrices during organogenesis: implications for the developmental anomalies of X chromosome–linked Kallmann syndrome. Dev Dyn 1999; 215:26–44.

1128. Hardelin JP. Kallmann syndrome: towards molecular pathogenesis. Mol Cell Endocrinol 2001; 179:75–81.

1129. Ballabio A, Bardoni B, Carrozzo R, et al. Contiguous gene syndromes due to deletions in the distal short arm of the human X chromosome. Proc Natl Acad Sci USA 1989; 86:10001–10005.

1130. Legouis R, Hardelin J-P, Levilliers J, et al. The candidate gene for the X-linked Kallmann syndrome encodes a protein related to adhesion molecules. Cell 1991; 67:423–435.

1131. Cohen-Salmon M, Tronche F, del Castillo I, Petit C. Characterization of the promoter of the human *KAL* gene responsible for the X-chromosome–linked Kallmann syndrome. Gene 1995; 164:235–242.

1132. Santen RJ, Paulsen CA. Hypogonadotropic eunuchoidism. II. Gonadal responsiveness to exogenous gonadotropins. J Clin Endocrinol Metab 1973; 36:55–63.

1133. Merriam GR, Beitins IZ, Bode HH. Father to son transmission of hypogonadism with anosmia. Am J Dis Child 1977; 131: 1216–1219.

1134. White BJ, Rogol AD, Brown KS, et al. The syndrome of anosmia with hypogonadotropic hypogonadism: a genetic study of 18 new families and a review. Am J Med Genet 1983; 15:417–435.

1135. Hipkin LJ, Casson IF, Davis JC. Identical twins discordant for Kallmann's syndrome. J Med Genet 1990; 27:198–199.

1136. Quinton R, Duke VM, de Zoysa PA, et al. The neuroradiology of Kallmann's syndrome: a genotypic and phenotypic analysis. J Clin Endocrinol Metab 1996; 81:3010–3017. [Published erratum appears in J Clin Endocrinol Metab 1996;81:3614].

1137. de Roux N, Young J, Misrahi M, et al. A family with hypogonadotropic hypogonadism and mutations in the gonadotropin-releasing hormone receptor. N Engl J Med 1997; 337:1597–1602.

1138. de Roux N, Young J, Misrahi M, et al. Loss of function mutations of the GnRH receptor: a new cause of hypogonadotropic hypogonadism. J Pediatr Endocrinol Metab 1999; 12(suppl 1): 267–275.

1139. de Roux N, Young J, Brailly-Tabard S, et al. The same molecular defects of the gonadotropin-releasing hormone receptor determine a variable degree of hypogonadism in affected kindred. J Clin Endocrinol Metab 1999; 84:567–572.

1140. Beranova M, Oliveira LM, Bedecarrats GY, et al. Prevalence, phenotypic spectrum, and modes of inheritance of gonadotropin-releasing hormone receptor mutations in idiopathic hypogonadotropic hypogonadism. J Clin Endocrinol Metab 2001; 86: 1580–1588.

1141. Kottler ML, Chauvin S, Lahlou N, et al. A new compound heterozygous mutation of the gonadotropin-releasing hormone receptor (L314X, Q106R) in a woman with complete hypogonadotropic hypogonadism: chronic estrogen administration amplifies the gonadotropin defect. J Clin Endocrinol Metab 2000; 85:3002–3008.

1142. Pralong FP, Gomez F, Castillo E, et al. Complete hypogonadotropic hypogonadism associated with a novel inactivating mutation of the gonadotropin-releasing hormone receptor. J Clin Endocrinol Metab 1999; 84:3811–3816.

1143. Pitteloud N, Boepple PA, DeCruz S, et al. The fertile eunuch variant of idiopathic hypogonadotropic hypogonadism: spontaneous reversal associated with a homozygous mutation in the gonadotropin-releasing hormone receptor. J Clin Endocrinol Metab 2001; 86:2470–2475.

1144. Seminara SB, Beranova M, Oliveira LM, et al. Successful use of pulsatile gonadotropin-releasing hormone (GnRH) for ovulation induction and pregnancy in a patient with GnRH receptor mutations. J Clin Endocrinol Metab 2000; 85:556–562.

1145. Bin-Abbas B, Conte FA, Grumbach MM, Kaplan SL. Congenital hypogonadotropic hypogonadism and micropenis: effect of testosterone treatment on adult penile size why sex reversal is not indicated. J Pediatr 1999; 134:579–583.

1146. Burstein S, Grumbach MM, Kaplan SL. Early determination of androgen-responsiveness is important in the management of microphallus. Lancet 1979; 2:983–986.

1147. Zanarla E, Muscatelli F, Bardoni B, et al. An unusual member of the nuclear hormone receptor superfamily responsible for X-linked adrenal hypoplasia congenita. Nature 1994; 372:635–641.

1148. Muscatelli F, Strom TM, Walker AP, et al. Mutations in the *DAX-1* gene give rise to both X-linked adrenal hypoplasia congenita and hypogonadotropic hypogonadism. Nature 1994; 372: 672–676.

1149. Guo W, Burris TP, Zhang Y-H, et al. Genomic sequence of the *DAX1* gene: an orphan nuclear receptor responsible for X-linked adrenal hypoplasia congenita and hypogonadotropic hypogonadism. J Clin Endocrinol Metab 1996; 81:2481–2486.

1150. Burris TP, Guo W, McCabe ERB. The gene responsible for adrenal hypoplasia congenita, *DAX-1*, encodes a nuclear hormone receptor that defines a new class within the superfamily. Recent Prog Horm Res 1996; 51:241–260.

1151. McCabe ERB. Adrenal hypoplasias and aplasias. In Scriver CR, Beaudet AL, Sly WS, et al (eds). The Metabolic and Molecular Basis of Inherited Diseases. New York, McGraw Hill, 2001, pp 4263–4274.

1152. Ito M, Yu R, Jameson JL. DAX-1 inhibits SF-1–mediated transactivation via a carboxy-terminal domain that is deleted in adrenal hypoplasia congenita. Mol Cell Biol 1997; 17:1476–1483.

1153. Lalli E, Bardoni B, Zazopoulos E, et al. A transcriptional silencing domain in DAX-1 whose mutation causes adrenal hypoplasia congenita. Mol Endocrinol 1997; 11:1950–1960.

1154. Burris TP, Guo W, Le T, McCabe ER. Identification of a putative steroidogenic factor-1 response element in the DAX-1 promoter. Biochem Biophys Res Commun 1995; 214:576–581.

1155. Vilain E, Guo W, Zhang YH, McCabe ER. *DAX1* gene expression upregulated by steroidogenic factor 1 in an adrenocortical carcinoma cell line. Biochem Mol Med 1997; 61:1–8.

1156. Ingraham HA, Lala DS, Ikeda Y, et al. The nuclear receptor steroidogenic factor 1 acts at multiple levels of the reproductive axis. Genes Dev 1994; 8:2302–2312.

1157. Prader A, Zachmann M, Illig KR. Luteinizing hormone deficiency in hereditary congenital adrenal hypoplasia. J Pediatr 1975; 86:421–422.

1158. Kruse K, Sippell WG, Schnakenburg KV. Hypogonadism in congenital adrenal hypoplasia: evidence for a hypothalamic origin. J Clin Endocrinol Metab 1984; 58:12–17.

1159. Hay ID, Smail PJ, Forsyth CC. Familial cytomegalic adrenocortical hypoplasia: an X-linked syndrome of pubertal failure. Arch Dis Child 1981; 56:715–721.

1160. Kikuchi K, Kaji M, Momoi T, et al. Failure to induce puberty in a man with X-linked congenital adrenal hypoplasia and hypogonadotropic hypogonadism by pulsatile administration of low-dose gonadotropin-releasing hormone. Acta Endocrinol (Copenh) 1987; 114:153–160.

1161. Kletter GB, Gorski JL, Kelch RP. Congenital adrenal hypoplasia and isolated gonadotropin deficiency. Trends Endocrinol Metab 1991; 2:123–128.

1162. Uttley WS. Familial congenital adrenal hypoplasia. Arch Dis Child 1968; 43:724–730.

1163. Seltzer WK, Firminger H, Klein L, et al. Adrenal dysfunction in glycerol kinase deficiency. Biochem Med 1985; 33:189–199.

1164. Mantovani G, Ozisik G, Achermann JC, et al. Hypogonadotropic hypogonadism as a presenting feature of late-onset X-linked adrenal hypoplasia congenita. J Clin Endocrinol Metab 2002; 87:44–48.

1165. Reutens AT, Achermann JC, Ito M, et al. Clinical and functional effects of mutations in the *DAX-1* gene in patients with adrenal hypoplasia congenita. J Clin Endocrinol Metab 1999; 84:504–511.

1166. Peter M, Viemann M, Partsch CJ, Sippell WG. Congenital adrenal hypoplasia: clinical spectrum, experience with hormonal diagnosis, and report on new point mutations of the DAX-1 gene. J Clin Endocrinol Metab 1998; 83:2666–2674.

1167. Tabarin A, Achermann JC, Recan D, et al. A novel mutation in *DAX1* causes delayed-onset adrenal insufficiency and incomplete hypogonadotropic hypogonadism. J Clin Invest 2000; 105:321–328.

1168. Merke DP, Tajima T, Baron J, Cutler GJ. Hypogonadotropic hypogonadism in a female caused by an X-linked recessive mutation in the *DAX1* gene. N Engl J Med 1999; 340:1248–1252.

1169. McCabe ER. Vulnerability within a robust complex system—*DAX-1* mutations and steroidogenic axis development (editorial). J Clin Endocrinol Metab 2002; 87:41–43.

1170. Achermann JC, Wen-xia G, Kotlar J, et al. Mutational analysis of *DAX1* in patients with hypogonadotropic hypogonadism or pubertal delay. J Clin Endocrinol Metab 1999; 84:4497–4500.

1171. Guo W, Mason JS, Stone CG Jr, et al. Diagnosis of X-linked adrenal hypoplasia congenita by mutation analysis of the *DAX1* gene. JAMA 1995; 274:324–330.

1172. Yanase T, Takayanagi R, Oba K, et al. New mutations of DAX-1 genes in two Japanese patients with X-linked congenital adrenal hypoplasia and hypogonadotropic hypogonadism. J Clin Endocrinol Metab 1996; 81:530–535.

1173. Guo W, Burris TP, McCabe ERB. Expression of *DAX-1*, the gene responsible for X-linked adrenal hypoplasia congenita and hypogonadotropic hypogonadism, in the hypothalamic-pituitary-adrenal/gonadal axis. Biochem Mol Med 1995; 56:8–13.

1174. Habiby RL, Boepple P, Nachtigall L, et al. Adrenal hypoplasia congenita with hypogonadotropic hypogonadism: evidence that *DAX-1* mutations lead to combined hypothalamic and pituitary defects in gonadotropin production. J Clin Invest 1996; 98: 1055–1062.

1175. Takahashi T, Shoji Y, Shoji Y, et al. Active hypothalamic-pituitary-gonadal axis in an infant with X-linked adrenal hypoplasia congenita. J Pediatr 1997; 130:485–488.

1176. Kaiserman KB, Nakamoto JM, Geffner ME, McCabe ER. Minipuberty of infancy and adolescent pubertal function in adrenal hypoplasia congenita. J Pediatr 1998; 133:300–302.

1177. Takahashi I, Takahashi T, Shoji Y, Takada G. Prolonged activation of the hypothalamus-pituitary-gonadal axis in a child with X-linked adrenal hypoplasia congenita. Clin Endocrinol (Oxf) 2000; 53:127–129.

1178. Domenice S, Latronico AC, Brito VN, et al. Adrenocorticotropin-dependent precocious puberty of testicular origin in a boy with X-linked adrenal hypoplasia congenita due to a novel mutation in the *DAX1* gene. J Clin Endocrinol Metab 2001; 86: 4068–4071.

1179. Seminara SB, Achermann JC, Genel M, et al. X-linked adrenal hypoplasia congenita: a mutation in *DAX1* expands the phenotypic spectrum in males and females. J Clin Endocrinol Metab 1999; 84:4501–4509.

1180. Phelan JK, McCabe ER. Mutations in *NR0B1* (*DAX1*) and *NR5A1* (*SF1*) responsible for adrenal hypoplasia congenita. Hum Mutat 2001; 18:472–487.

1181. Worley KC, Ellison KA, Zhang Y-H et al. Yeast artificial chromosome cloning in the glycerol kinase and adrenal hypoplasia congenita region of Xp21. Genomics 1993; 16:407–416.

1182. Smals AGH, Kloppenborg PWC, Van Haelst UJG, et al. Fertile eunuch syndrome versus classic hypogonadotrophic hypogonadism. Acta Endocrinol (Copenh) 1978; 87:389–399.

1183. Weiss J, Axelrod L, Whitcomb RW, et al. Hypogonadism caused by a single amino acid substitution in the beta subunit of luteinizing hormone. N Engl J Med 1992; 326:179–183.

1184. Lovinger RD, Kaplan SL, Grumbach MM. Congenital hypopituitarism associated with neonatal hypoglycemia and microphal-

lus: four cases secondary to hypothalamic hormone deficiencies. J Pediatr 1975; 87:1171–1181.
1185. Layman LC, Lee EJ, Peak DB, et al. Delayed puberty and hypogonadism caused by mutations in the follicle-stimulating hormone beta-subunit gene. N Engl J Med 1997; 337:607–611.
1186. Matthews C, Chatterjee VK. Isolated deficiency of follicle-stimulating hormone re-revisited. N Engl J Med 1997; 337:642.
1187. Matthews CH, Borgato S, Beck-Peccoz P, et al. Primary amenorrhoea and infertility due to a mutation in the beta-subunit of follicle-stimulating hormone. Nat Genet 1993; 5:83–86.
1188. Rabin D, Spitz I, Bercovici B, et al. Isolated deficiency of follicle-stimulating hormone: clinical and laboratory features. N Engl J Med 1972; 287:1313–1317.
1189. Lindstedt G, Nystrom E, Matthews C, et al. Follitropin (FSH) deficiency in an infertile male due to FSHbeta gene mutation: a syndrome of normal puberty and virilization but underdeveloped testicles with azoospermia, low FSH but high lutropin and normal serum testosterone concentrations. Clin Chem Lab Med 1998; 36:663–665.
1190. Phillip M, Arbelle JE, Segev Y, Parvari R. Male hypogonadism due to a mutation in the gene for the beta-subunit of follicle-stimulating hormone. N Engl J Med 1998; 338:1729–1732.
1191. Jackson RS, Creemers JW, Ohagi S, et al. Obesity and impaired prohormone processing associated with mutations in the human prohormone convertase 1 gene. Nat Genet 1997; 16:303–306.
1192. Goodman HG, Grumbach MM, Kaplan SL. Growth and growth hormone. II. A comparison of isolated growth-hormone deficiency and multiple pituitary-hormone deficiencies in 35 patients with idiopathic hypopituitary dwarfism. N Engl J Med 1968; 278:57–68.
1193. Tanner JM, Whitehouse RH. A note on the bone age at which patients with true isolated growth hormone deficiency enter puberty. J Clin Endocrinol Metab 1975; 41:788–790.
1194. Phillips JA III. Inherited defects in growth hormone synthesis and action. In Scriver CR, Beaudet AI, Sly WS, et al (eds). The Metabolic Basis of Inherited Disease, 6th ed. New York, McGraw-Hill, 1989, pp 1965–1983.
1195. Rosenbloom AL, Almonte AS, Brown MR, et al. Clinical and biochemical phenotype of familial anterior hypopituitarism from mutation of the *PROP1* gene. J Clin Endocrinol Metab 1999; 84:50–57.
1196. Pernasetti F, Toledo SP, Vasilyev VV, et al. Impaired adrenocorticotropin-adrenal axis in combined pituitary hormone deficiency caused by a two-base pair deletion (301-302delAG) in the prophet of Pit-1 gene. J Clin Endocrinol Metab 2000; 85:390–397.
1197. Arrigo T, Crisafulli G, Salamone A, et al. Adult height exceeding target height in a patient with congenital panhypopituitarism diagnosed after the age of 25 years. J Pediatr Endocrinol 1994; 7:269–272.
1198. Saggese G, Federico G, Barsanti S, Fiore L. The effect of administering gonadotropin-releasing hormone agonist with recombinant-human growth hormone (GH) on the final height of girls with isolated GH deficiency: results from a controlled study. J Clin Endocrinol Metab 2001; 86:1900–1904.
1199. Albanese A, Stanhope R. Treatment of growth delay in boys with isolated growth hormone deficiency. Eur J Endocrinol 1994; 130:65–69.
1200. Bray GA, Dahms WT, Swerdloff RS, et al. The Prader-Willi syndrome: a study of 40 patients and a review of the literature. Medicine (Baltimore) 1983; 62:59–80.
1201. Prader A, Labhart A, Willi H. Ein syndrom von Adipositas, Kleinwuchs, Kryptorchidismus und Oligophrenie nach Myatonieartigem Zustad im Neugeborenalter. Schweiz Med Wochenschr 1956; 86:1260–1261.
1202. Tolis G, Lewis W, Verdy M, et al. Anterior pituitary function in the Prader-Labhart-Willi (PLW) syndrome. J Clin Endocrinol Metab 1974; 39:1061–1066.
1203. Linde R, McNeil L, Rabin D. Induction of menarche by clomiphene citrate in a fifteen-year-old girl with the Prader-Labhart-Willi syndrome. Fertil Steril 1982; 37:118–120.
1204. Holm VA, Cassidy SB, Butler MG, et al. Prader-Willi syndrome: consensus diagnostic criteria. Pediatrics 1993; 91:398–402.
1205. Cassidy SB, Schwartz S. Prader-Willi and Angelman syndromes: disorders of genomic imprinting. Medicine (Baltimore) 1998; 77:140–151.
1206. Eiholzer U, Bachmann S, l'Allemand D. Is there growth hormone deficiency in Prader-Willi syndrome? Six arguments to support the presence of hypothalamic growth hormone deficiency in Prader-Willi syndrome. Horm Res 2000; 53(suppl 3): 44–52.
1207. Lindgren AC, Ritzen EM. Five years of growth hormone treatment in children with Prader-Willi syndrome. Swedish National Growth Hormone Advisory Group. Acta Paediatr Suppl 1999; 88:109–111.
1208. Lindgren AC, Hagenas L, Muller J, et al. Growth hormone treatment of children with Prader-Willi syndrome affects linear growth and body composition favourably. Acta Paediatr 1998; 87:28–31.
1209. Carrel AL, Myers SE, Whitman BY, Allen DB. Sustained benefits of growth hormone on body composition, fat utilization, physical strength and agility, and growth in Prader-Willi syndrome are dose-dependent. J Pediatr Endocrinol Metab 2001; 14:1097–1105.
1210. Cassidy SB, Ledbetter DH. Prader-Willi syndrome. Neurol Clin 1989; 7:37–54.
1211. Knoll JHM, Nicholls RD, Magenis RE, et al. Angleman and Prader-Willi share a common chromosome 15 deletion but differ in parental origin of the deletion. Am J Med Genet 1989; 32:285–290.
1212. Nicholls RD. Imprinting mechanisms and genes involved in Prader-Willi and Angelman syndromes. Dev Biol 1994; 5:311–322.
1213. Saitoh S, Buiting K, Rogan PK, et al. Minimal definition of the imprinting region center and fixation of a chromosome 15q11-q13 epigenotype by imprinting mutations. Proc Natl Acad Sci USA 1996; 93:7811–7815.
1214. Nicholls RD, Knoll JHM, Butler MG, et al. Genetic imprinting suggested by maternal hetero-disomy in non-deletion Prader-Willi syndrome. Nature 1989; 342:281–285.
1215. Meguro M, Mitsuya K, Sui H, et al. Evidence for uniparental, paternal expression of the human GABAA receptor subunit genes, using microcell-mediated chromosome transfer. Hum Mol Genet 1997; 6:2127–2133.
1216. OzHelik R, Leff S, Robinson W, et al. Small nuclear ribonucleoprotein polypeptide N (SNRPN), an expressed gene in the Prader-Willi syndrome critical region. Nat Genet 1992; 2:259–269.
1217. Lalande M. In and around SNRPN. Nat Genet 1994; 8:5–6.
1218. Swaab DF, Purba JS, Hoffman MA. Alterations in the paraventricular nucleus and its oxytocin neurons (putative satiety cells) in Prader-Willi syndrome: a study of five cases. J Clin Endocrinol Metab 1995; 80:573–579.
1219. Laurence JZ, Moon RC. Four cases of "retinitis pigmentosa," occurring in the same family, and accompanied by general imperfections of development. Ophthalmic Rev 1866; 2:32–41.
1220. Stiggelbout T. The (Laurence Moon) Bardet Biedl syndrome. The Netherlands, Van Gorcum, 1969.
1221. Kulin HE, Bwibo N, Mutie D, et al. The effect of chronic childhood malnutrition on pubertal growth and development. Am J Clin Nutr 1982; 36:527–536.
1222. Katsanis N, Ansley SJ, Badano JL, et al. Triallelic inheritance in Bardet-Biedl syndrome, a mendelian recessive disorder. Science 2001; 293:2256–2259.
1223. Nishimura DY, Searby CC, Carmi R, et al. Positional cloning of a novel gene on chromosome 16q causing Bardet-Biedl syndrome (BBS2). Hum Mol Genet 2001; 10:865–874.
1224. Burghes AH, Vaessin HE, de La Chapelle A. Genetics: the land between mendelian and multifactorial inheritance. Science 2001; 293:2213–2214.
1225. Kulin HE, Bwibo N, Mutie D, Santner SJ. Gonadotropin excretion during puberty in malnourished children. J Pediatr 1984; 105:325–328.
1226. Maki M, Kallonen K, Lahdeaho ML, et al. Changing pattern of childhood coeliac disease in Finland. Acta Paediatr Scand 1988; 77:408–412.
1227. Vigersky R, Anderson AE, Thompson RH, et al. Hypothalamic dysfunction in secondary amenorrhea associated with simple weight loss. N Engl J Med 1977; 297:1141–1145.
1228. Landon C, Rosenfeld RG. Short stature and pubertal delay in male adolescents with cystic fibrosis: androgen treatment. Am J Dis Child 1984; 138:388–391.

1229. Johannesson M, Gottlieb C, Hjelte L. Delayed puberty in girls with cystic fibrosis despite good clinical status. Pediatrics 1997; 99:29–34.
1230. Reiter EO, Stern RC, Root AW. The reproductive endocrine system in cystic fibrosis. I. Basal gonadotropin and sex steroid levels. Am J Dis Child 1981; 135:422–426.
1231. Stern RC, Boat TF, Doershuk CF, et al. Course of cystic fibrosis in 95 patients. J Pediatr 1976; 89:406–411.
1232. Taussig LM, Lobeck CC, di Sant'Agnese PA, et al. Fertility in males with cystic fibrosis. N Engl J Med 1972; 287:586–589.
1233. Tizzano EF, Silver MM, Chitayat D, et al. Differential cellular expression of cystic fibrosis transmembrane regulator in human reproductive tissues: clues for the infertility in patients with cystic fibrosis. Am J Pathol 1994; 144:906–914.
1234. Vazquez-Levin MH, Kupchik GS, Torres Y, et al. Cystic fibrosis and congenital agenesis of the vas deferens, antisperm antibodies and CF-genotype. J Reprod Immunol 1994; 27:199–212.
1235. Serjeant GR, Singhal A, Hambleton IR. Sickle cell disease and age at menarche in Jamaican girls: Observations from a cohort study. Arch Dis Child 2001; 85(5):375–378.
1236. Zago MA, Kerbauy J, Souza HM, et al. Growth and sexual maturation of Brazilian patients with sickle cell diseases. Trop Geogr Med 1992; 44:317–321.
1237. Olatunji Olambiwonnu N, Penny R, Frasier SD. Sexual maturation in subjects with sickle cell anemia: studies of serum gonadotropin concentration, height, weight, and skeletal age. J Pediatr 1975; 87:459–464.
1238. Kwan EY, Lee AC, Li AM, et al. A cross-sectional study of growth, puberty and endocrine function in patients with thalassaemia major in Hong Kong. J Paediatr Child Health 1995; 31: 83–87.
1239. Grundy RG, Woods KA, Savage MO, Evans JP. Relationship of endocrinopathy to iron chelation status in young patients with thalassaemia major. Arch Dis Child 1994; 71:128–132.
1240. De Sanctis V, Galimberti M, Lucarelli G, et al. Pubertal development in thalassaemic patients after allogenic bone marrow transplantation [published erratum appears in Eur J Pediatr 1994;153:470]. Eur J Pediatr 1993; 152:993–997.
1241. Yesilipek MA, Bircan I, Oygur N, et al. Growth and sexual maturation in children with thalassemia major. Haematologica 1993; 78:30–33.
1242. Chatterjee R, Katz M. Reversible hypogonadotrophic hypogonadism in sexually infantile male thalassaemic patients with transfusional iron overload. Clin Endocrinol (Oxf) 2000; 53:33–42.
1243. Borgna Pignatti C, De Stefano P, Zonta L, et al. Growth and sexual maturation in thalassemia major. J Pediatr 1985; 106: 150–155.
1244. Italian Working Group on Endocrine Complications in Nonendocrine Diseases. Multicentre study on prevalence of endocrine complications in thalassemia major. Clin Endocrinol (Oxf) 1995; 42:581–586.
1245. Wang C, Tso SC, Todd D. Hypogonadotropic hypogonadism in severe beta-thalassemia: effect of chelation and pulsatile gonadotropin-releasing hormone therapy. J Clin Endocrinol Metab 1989; 68:511–516.
1246. Balducci R, Toscano V, Finocchi G, et al. Effect of hCG or hCG+ treatments in young thalassemic patients with hypogonadotropic hypogonadism. J Endocrinol Invest 1990; 13:1–7.
1247. De Sanctis V, Vullo C, Katz M, et al. Gonadal function in patients with beta thalassaemia major. J Clin Pathol 1988; 41: 133–137.
1248. Sklar CA, Lew LQ, Yoon DJ, et al. Adrenal function in thalassemia major following long-term treatment with multiple transfusions and chelation therapy: evidence for dissociation of cortisol and adrenal androgen secretion. Am J Dis Child 1987; 141: 327–330.
1249. Soliman AT, elZalabany MM, Ragab M, et al. Spontaneous and GnRH-provoked gonadotropin secretion and testosterone response to human chorionic gonadotropin in adolescent boys with thalassaemia major and delayed puberty. J Trop Pediatr 2000; 46:79–85.
1250. Gertner JM, Kaufman FR, Donfield SM, et al. Delayed somatic growth and pubertal development in human immunodeficiency virus-infected hemophiliac boys: Hemophilia Growth and Development Study. J Pediatr 1994; 124:896–902.
1251. Brain CE, Savage MO. Growth and puberty in chronic inflammatory bowel disease. Baillieres Clin Gastroenterol 1994; 8:83–100.
1252. Cacciari E, Corazza GR, Salardi S, et al. What will be the adult height of coeliac patients? Eur J Pediatr 1991; 150:407–409.
1253. Ferraris J, Saenger P, Levine L, et al. Delayed puberty in males with chronic renal failure. Kidney Int 1980; 18:344–350.
1254. Schaefer F, Stanhope R, Scheil H, et al. Pulsatile gonadotropin secretion in pubertal children with chronic renal failure. Acta Endocrinol (Copenh) 1989; 120:14–19.
1255. Kulin H, Demers L, Chinchilli V, et al. Usefulness of sequential urinary follicle-stimulating hormone and luteinizing hormone measurements in the diagnosis of adolescent hypogonadotropism in males. J Clin Endocrinol Metab 1994; 78:1208–1211.
1256. Rees L, Greene SA, Adlard P, et al. Growth and endocrine function in steroid sensitive nephrotic syndrome. Arch Dis Child 1988; 63:484–490.
1257. Polito C, Di Toro R. Delayed pubertal growth spurt in glomerulopathic boys receiving alternate-day prednisone. Child Nephrol Urol 1992; 12:202–207.
1258. van Diemen-Steenvoorde R, Donckerwolcke RA, Brackel H, et al. Growth and sexual maturation in children after kidney transplantation. J Pediatr 1987; 110:351–356.
1259. Martin LW, McEnery PT, Rosenkrantz JG, et al. Renal homotransplantation in children. J Pediatr Surg 1979; 14:571–576.
1260. Ferraris JR, Domene HM, Escobar ME, et al. Hormonal problems in pubertal females with chronic renal failure: before and under hemodialysis and after renal transplantation. Acta Endocrinol (Copenh) 1987; 115:289–296.
1261. van Diemen-Steevoorde MD, Donckerwolcke RA, Brakel H, et al. Growth and sexual maturation in children after kidney transplantation. J Pediatr 1987; 110:351–356.
1262. Belgorosky A, Ferraris JR, Ramirez JA, et al. Serum sex hormone–binding globulin and serum nonsex hormone–binding globulin–bound testosterone fractions in prepubertal boys with chronic renal failure. J Clin Endocrinol Metab 1991; 73:107–110.
1263. Hokken-Koelega AC, Stijnen T, De Muinck Keizer-Schrama SM, et al. Levels of growth hormone, insulin-like growth factor-I (IGF-I) and -II, IGF-binding protein-1 and -3, and cortisol in prednisone-treated children with growth retardation after renal transplantation. J Clin Endocrinol Metab 1993; 77:932–938.
1264. Siris ES, Leventhal BG, Vaitukaitis JL. Effects of childhood leukemia and chemotherapy on puberty and reproductive function in girls. N Engl J Med 1976; 294:1143–1146.
1265. Vilska S, Lahteenmaki P, Kaihola HL, Salmi TT. Endocrine status and growth after malignancy treated in childhood or adolescence. Int J Fertil 1988; 33:283–290.
1266. Lannering B, Rosberg S, Marky I, et al. Reduced growth hormone secretion with maintained periodicity following cranial irradiation in children with acute lymphoblastic leukaemia. Clin Endocrinol (Oxf) 1995; 42:153–159.
1267. Cicognani A, Cacciari E, Rosito P, et al. Longitudinal growth and final height in long-term survivors of childhood leukaemia. Eur J Pediatr 1994; 153:726–730.
1268. Ochs J, Mulhern R. Long-term sequelae of therapy for childhood acute lymphoblastic leukaemia. Baillieres Clin Haematol 1994; 7:365–376.
1269. Davies HA, Didcock E, Didi M, et al. Disproportionate short stature after cranial irradiation and combination chemotherapy for leukaemia. Arch Dis Child 1994; 70:472–475.
1270. Holm K, Nysom K, Hertz H, Muller J. Normal final height after treatment for acute lymphoblastic leukemia without irradiation. Acta Paediatr 1994; 83:1287–1290.
1271. Chou RH, Wong GB, Kramer JH, et al. Toxicities of total-body irradiation for pediatric bone marrow transplantation. Int J Radiat Oncol Biol Phys 1996; 34:843–851.
1272. Didi M, Didcock E, Davies HA, et al. High incidence of obesity in young adults after treatment of acute lymphoblastic leukemia in childhood. J Pediatr 1995; 127:(1):63–67.
1273. Pantsiouou S, Stanhope R, Uruena M, et al. Growth prognosis and growth after menarche in primary hypothyroidism. Arch Dis Child 1991; 66:838–840.
1274. Mauriac P. Hépatomalie de l'enfance avec troubles de la croissance et du métabolisme des glucides. Paris (Med) 1987; 2:206–208.

1275. Arreola F, Junco E, Partida-Hernandez G, et al. HbA1, height velocity and weight gain as indicators of metabolic control in type I diabetic children: a 5 year survey. Arch Invest Med (Mex) 1991; 22:303–307.
1276. Wise JE, Kolb EL, Sauder SE. Effect of glycemic control on growth velocity in children with IDDM. Diabetes Care 1992; 15:826–830.
1277. Travis LB. Diabetes Mellitus in Children and Adolescents. Philadelphia, WB Saunders, 1987, p 206.
1278. Dills DG, Allen C, Palta M, et al. Insulin-like growth factor-I is related to glycemic control in children and adolescents with newly diagnosed insulin-dependent diabetes. J Clin Endocrinol Metab 1995; 80:2139–2143.
1279. Styne DM, Grumbach MM, Kaplan SL, et al. Treatment of Cushing's disease in childhood and adolescence by transsphenoidal microadenomectomy. N Engl J Med 1984; 310:889–893.
1280. Devoe DJ, Miller WL, Conte FA, et al. Long-term outcome in children and adolescents after transsphenoidal surgery for Cushing's disease. J Clin Endocrinol Metab 1997; 82:3196–3202.
1281. Mindermann T, Wilson CB. Pediatric pituitary adenomas. Neurosurgery 1995; 36:259–268.
1282. Diagnostic and Statistical Manual of Mental Disorders: DSM-IV. Washington, DC, American Psychiatric Association, 1994.
1283. Crisp AH. The dyslipophobias: a view of the psychopathologies involved and the hazards of construing anorexia nervosa and bulimia nervosa as 'eating disorders'. Proc Nutr Soc 1996; 54: 701–709.
1284. Graber JA, Brooks-Gunn J, Warren MP. The vulnerable transition: puberty and the development of eating pathology and negative mood. Womens Health Issues 1999; 9:107–114.
1285. Schwabe AD, Lippe BM, Chang RJ, et al. Anorexia nervosa. Ann Intern Med 1981; 94:371–381.
1286. Silverman JA. Anorexia nervosa: clinical and metabolic observations in a successful treatment plan. In Vigersky RA (ed). Anorexia Nervosa. New York, Raven Press, 1977, pp 331–339.
1287. Warren MP, Vande Wile RL. Clinical and metabolic features of anorexia nervosa. Am J Obstet Gynecol 1973; 117:435–449.
1288. Polivy J, Herman CP. Causes of eating disorders. Annu Rev Psychol 2002; 53:187–213.
1289. Kaye WH, Klump KL, Frank GK, Strober M. Anorexia and bulimia nervosa. Annu Rev Med 2000; 51:299–313.
1290. Danziger Y, Mukamel M, Zeharia A, et al. Stunting of growth in anorexia nervosa during the prepubertal and pubertal period. Isr J Med Sci 1994; 30:581–584.
1291. De Lange WE, Sluiter WJ, Van Zanten AK, Doorenbos H. The effect of injection and infusion of LH-RH on serum LH and FSH in normal males and in boys with delayed puberty. Neth J Med 1974; 17:196–201.
1292. van Binsbergen CJM, Coelingh Bennink HJT, Odink J, et al. A comparative and longitudinal study on endocrine changes related to ovarian function in patients with anorexia nervosa. J Clin Endocrinol Metab 1990; 71:705–711.
1293. Beaumont PJV, George GCW, Pimstone BL, et al. Body weight and the pituitary response to hypothalamic releasing hormones in patients with anorexia nervosa. J Clin Endocrinol Metab 1976; 43:487–496.
1294. Grinspoon S, Gulick T, Askari H, et al. Serum leptin levels in women with anorexia nervosa. J Clin Endocrinol Metab 1996; 81:3861–3863.
1295. Ferron F, Considine RV, Peino R, et al. Serum leptin concentrations in patients with anorexia nervosa, bulimia nervosa and non-specific eating disorders correlate with the body mass index but are independent of the respective disease. Clin Endocrinol 1997; 46:289–293.
1296. Casanueva FF, Dieguez C, Popovic V, et al. Serum immunoreactive leptin concentrations in patients with anorexia nervosa before and after partial weight recovery. Biochem Mol Med 1997; 60:116–120.
1297. Waldhauser F, Toifl K, Spona J, et al. Diminished prolactin response to thyrotropin and insulin in anorexia nervosa. J Clin Endocrinol Metab 1984; 59:538–544.
1298. Stoving RK, Hangaard J, Hagen C. Update on endocrine disturbances in anorexia nervosa. J Pediatr Endocrinol Metab 2001; 14:459–480.
1299. Warren MP. Metabolic factors and the onset of puberty. In Grumbach MM, Sizonenko PC, Aubert ML (eds). Control of the Onset of Puberty. Baltimore, Williams & Wilkins, 1990, pp 553–573.
1300. Yen SSC, Rebar R, VandenBerg G, Judd H. Hypothalamic amenorrhea and hypogonadotropinism: responses to synthetic LRF. J Clin Endocrinol Metab 1973; 36:811–816.
1301. Couzinet B, Young J, Brailly S, et al. Functional hypothalamic amenorrhoea: a partial and reversible gonadotrophin deficiency of nutritional origin. Clin Endocrinol (Oxf) 1999; 50:229–235.
1302. Warren MP, Voussoughian F, Geer EB, et al. Functional hypothalamic amenorrhea: Hypoleptinemia and disordered eating. Submitted for publication, 1997.
1303. Russell GFM. Bulimia nervosa: an ominous variant of anorexia nervosa. Psychol Med 1979; 9:429–448.
1304. Eisenstein TD, Gerson MJ. Psychosocial growth retardation in adolescence: a reversible condition secondary to severe stress. J Adolesc Health Care 1988; 9:436–440.
1305. Constantini NW, Warren MP. Special problems of the female athlete. Baillieres Clin Rheumatol 1994; 8:199–219.
1306. Carpenter SE. Psychosocial menstrual disorders: stress, exercise and diet's effect on the menstrual cycle. Curr Opin Obstet Gynecol 1994; 6:536–539.
1307. Warren MP, Perlroth NE. The effects of intense exercise on the female reproductive system. J Endocrinol 2001; 170:3–11.
1308. Sundgot-Borgen J. Risk and trigger factors for the development of eating disorders in female elite athletes. Med Sci Sports Exerc 1994; 26:414–419.
1309. Loucks AV, Horvath SB. Athletic amenorrhea: a review. Med Sci Sports Exerc 1985; 17:56–72.
1310. Claessens AL, Malina RM, Lefevre J, et al. Growth and menarcheal status of elite female gymnasts. Med Sci Sports Exerc 1992; 24:755–763.
1311. Georgopoulos N, Markou K, Theodoropoulou A, et al. Growth and pubertal development in elite female rhythmic gymnasts. J Clin Endocrinol Metab 1999; 84:4525–4530.
1312. Warren MP. The effects of exercise on pubertal progression and reproductive function in girls. J Clin Endocrinol Metab 1980; 51:1150–1157.
1313. Constantini NW, Warren MP. Menstrual dysfunction in swimmers: a distinct entity. J Clin Endocrinol Metab 1995; 80:2740–2744.
1314. Theintz GE, Howald H, Weiss U, Sizonenko PC. Evidence for a reduction of growth potential in adolescent female gymnasts. J Pediatr 1993; 122:306–313.
1315. Lindholm C, Hagenfeldt K, Ringertz BM. Pubertal development in elite juvenile gymnasts: effects of physical training. Acta Obstet Gynecol Scand 1994; 73:269–273.
1316. Baxter-Jones AD, Helms P, Baines-Preece J, Preece M. Menarche in intensively trained gymnasts, swimmers and tennis players. Ann Hum Biol 1994; 21:407–415.
1317. Damsgaard R, Bencke J, Matthiesen G, et al. Is prepubertal growth adversely affected by sport? Med Sci Sports Exerc 2000; 32:1698–1703.
1318. Damsgaard R, Bencke J, Matthiesen G, et al. Body proportions, body composition and pubertal development of children in competitive sports. Scand J Med Sci Sports 2001; 11:54–60.
1319. Baxter-Jones A, Maffulli N, Helms P. Low injury rates in elite athletes. Arch Dis Child 1993; 68:130–132.
1320. Goldberg CJ, Dowling FE, Fogarty EE. Adolescent idiopathic scoliosis: early menarche, normal growth. Spine 1993; 18:529–535.
1321. Hagglund G, Karlberg J, Willner S. Growth in girls with adolescent idiopathic scoliosis. Spine 1992; 17:108–111.
1322. Carr AJ, Jefferson RJ, Turner-Smith AR. Family stature in idiopathic scoliosis. Spine 1993; 18:20–23.
1323. Brisson GR, Volle MA, Desharnais M, et al. Exercise induced dissociation of the blood prolactin response in young women according to their sports habits. Horm Metab Res 1980; 21: 201–205.
1324. Harmon J, Aliapoulios MA. Gynecomastia in marihuana user. N Engl J Med 1972; 287:936–1080.
1325. Copeland KC, Underwood LE, Van Wyk JJ. Marihuana smoking and pubertal arrest. J Pediatr 1980; 96:1079–1080.
1326. Granovsky-Grisaru S, Aboulafia Y, Diamant YZ, et al. Gynecologic and obstetric aspects of Gaucher's disease: a survey of 53 patients. Am J Obstet Gynecol 1995; 172:1284–1290.
1327. Maayan C, Sela O, Axelrod F, et al. Gynecological aspects of female familial dysautonomia. Isr Med Assoc J 2000; 2:679–683.

1328. Rosenfeld RG, Northcraft GB, Hintz RL. A prospective, randomized study of testosterone treatment of constitutional delay of growth and development in male adolescents. Pediatrics 1982; 69:681–687.
1329. Susman EJ, Finkelstein JW, Chinchilli VM, et al. The effect of sex hormone replacement therapy on behavior problems and moods in adolescents with delayed puberty. J Pediatr 1998; 133: 521–525.
1330. Grumbach MM, Conte FA. Disorders of sexual differentiation. In Wilson JD, Foster DW, Kroneberg HM, Larsen PR (eds). Williams Textbook of Endocrinology. Philadelphia, WB Saunders, 1998, pp 1509–1626.
1331. Klinefelter HF Jr, Reifenstein EC Jr, Albright F. Syndrome characterized by gynecomastia, aspermatogenesis without A-leydigism, and increased excretion of follicle-stimulating hormone. J Clin Endocrinol 1942; 2:615–627.
1332. Wittenberg DF, Padayachi T, Norman RJ. Hypogonadotrophic variant of Klinefelter's syndrome: a case report S Afr Med J 1988; 74:181–183.
1333. Caldwell PD, Smith DW. The XXY (Klinefelter's) syndrome in childhood: detection and treatment. J Pediatr 1972; 80:250–258.
1334. Sagawa I, Kazama T, Terada T, et al. Hormonal profiles in Klinefelter's syndrome with and without testicular epidermoid cyst. Arch Androl 1988; 21:205–209.
1335. Salbenblatt JA, Bender BG, Puck MH, et al. Pituitary-gonadal function in Klinefelter syndrome before and during puberty. Pediatr Res 1985; 19:82–86.
1336. Plymate SR, Leonard JM, Paulsen CA. Sex hormone–binding globulin changes with androgen replacement. J Clin Endocrinol Metab 1983; 57:645–648.
1337. Wieland RG, Zorn EM, Johnson MW. Elevated testosterone-binding globulin in Klinefelter's syndrome. J Clin Endocrinol Metab 1980; 51:1199–1200.
1338. Eberle AJ, Sparrow JT, Keenan BS. Treatment of persistent pubertal gynecomastia with dihydrotestosterone heptanoate. J Pediatr 1986; 109:144–149.
1339. Rovet J, Netley C, Keenan M, et al. The psychoeducational profile of boys with Klinefelter syndrome. J Learn Disabil 1996; 29:180–196.
1340. Boone KB, Swerdloff RS, Miller BL, et al. Neuropsychological profiles of adults with Klinefelter syndrome. J Int Neuropsychol Soc 2001; 7:446–456.
1341. Rovet J, Netley C, Bailey J, et al. Intelligence and achievement in children with extra X aneuploidy: a longitudinal perspective. Am J Med Genet 1995; 60:356–363.
1342. Netley C, Rovet J. Hemispheric lateralization in 47,XXY Klinefelter's syndrome boys. Brain Cogn 1984; 3:10–18.
1343. Netley C, Rovet J. Relations between a dermatoglyphic measure, hemispheric specialization, and intellectual abilities in 47,XXY males. Brain Cogn 1987; 6:153–160.
1344. Stewart DA, Bailey JD, Netley CT, et al. Growth and development of children with X and Y chromosome aneuploidy from infancy to pubertal age: the Toronto study. Birth Defects Orig Artic Ser 1982; 18:99–154.
1345. Collaer ML, Hines M. Human behavioral sex differences: a role for gonadal hormones during early development? Psychol Bull 1995; 118:55–107.
1346. Geschwind N, Galaburda AM. Cerebral lateralization. Biological mechanisms, associations, and pathology: I. A hypothesis and a program for research. Arch Neurol 1985; 42:428–459.
1347. Geschwind DH, Boone KB, Miller BL, Swerdloff RS. Neurobehavioral phenotype of Klinefelter syndrome. Ment Retard Dev Disabil Res Rev 2000; 6:107–116.
1348. Nielsen J, Pelsen B, Sorensen K. Follow-up of 30 Klinefelter males treated with testosterone. Clin Genet 1988; 33:262–269.
1349. Kleczkowska A, Fryns JP, Van den Berghe H. X-chromosome polysomy in the male: the Leuven experience 1966–1987. Hum Genet 1988; 80:16–22.
1350. Nielsen J, Pelsen B. Follow-up 20 years later of 34 Klinefelter males with karyotype 47,XXY and 16 hypogonadal males with karyotype 46,XY. Hum Genet 1987; 77:188–192.
1351. Sorenson K, Porter ME, Gardner HA, DeFeudis P. Verbal deficits in Klinefelter (XXY) adults living in the community. Clin Genet 1988; 33:246–253.
1352. Price WH, Clayton JF, Wilson J. Causes of death in X chromatin positive males (Klinefelter's syndrome). J Epidemiol Community Health 1985; 39:330–336.
1353. Scheike O, Visfeldt J, Peterson B. Male breast cancer: III. Breast carcinoma in association with the Klinefelter syndrome. Acta Pathol Microbiol Scand Suppl 1973; 81:352–358.
1354. Bizzarro A, Valentini G, DiMartino G. Influence of testosterone therapy on clinical and immunological features of autoimmune diseases associated with Klinefelter's syndrome. J Clin Endocrinol Metab 1987; 64:32–36.
1355. Fialkow PJ. Genetic aspects of autoimmunity. Prog Med Genet 1969; 6:117–167.
1356. Foresta C, Busnardo B, Zanatta G. Lower calcitonin levels in young hypogonadic men with osteoporosis. Horm Metab Res 1983; 15:206–207.
1357. Dexeus FH, Logothetis CJ, Chong C, et al. Genetic abnormalities in men with germ cell tumors. J Urol 1988; 140:80–84.
1358. Billmire D, Vinocur C, Rescorla F, et al. Malignant mediastinal germ cell tumors: an intergroup study. J Pediatr Surg 2001; 36: 18–24.
1359. Derenoncourt AN, Castro-Magana M, Jones KL. Mediastinal teratoma and precocious puberty in a boy with mosaic Klinefelter syndrome. Am J Med Genet 1995; 55:38–42.
1360. Von Muhlendahl KE, Heinrich U. Sexual precocity in Klinefelter syndrome: report on two new cases with idiopathic central precocious puberty. Eur J Pediatr 1994; 153:322–324.
1361. Hasle H, Jacobsen BB, Asschenfeldt P, Andersen K. Mediastinal germ cell tumour associated with Klinefelter syndrome: a report of case and review of the literature. Eur J Pediatr 1992; 151: 735–739.
1362. Bramswig JH, Heimes U, Heiermann E, et al. The effects of different cumulative doses of chemotherapy on testicular function: results in 75 patients treated for Hodgkin's disease during childhood or adolescence. Cancer 1990; 65:1298–1302.
1363. Afify Z, Shaw PJ, Clavano-Harding A, Cowell CT. Growth and endocrine function in children with acute myeloid leukaemia after bone marrow transplantation using busulfan/cyclophosphamide. Bone Marrow Transplant 2000; 25:1087–1092.
1364. Kenney LB, Laufer MR, Grant FD, et al. High risk of infertility and long term gonadal damage in males treated with high dose cyclophosphamide for sarcoma during childhood. Cancer 2001; 91:613–621.
1365. Watson AR, Rance CP, Bain J. Long term effects of cyclophosphamide on testicular function. Br Med J (Clin Res Ed) 1985; 291:1457–1460.
1366. Penso J, Lippe B, Ehrlich R, Smith FGJ. Testicular function in prepubertal and pubertal male patients treated with cyclophosphamide for nephrotic syndrome. J Pediatr 1974; 84:831–836.
1367. Callis L, Nieto J, Vila A, et al. Chlorambucil treatment in minimal lesion nephrotic syndrome: a reappraisal of its gonadal toxicity. J Pediatr 1980; 97:653–656.
1368. Hoorweg-Nijman JJ, Delemarre-van de Waal HA, de Waal FC, Behrendt H. Cyclophosphamide-induced disturbance of gonadotropin secretion manifesting testicular damage. Acta Endocrinol (Copenh) 1992; 126:143–148.
1369. Dhabhar BN, Malhotra H, Joseph R, et al. Gonadal function in prepubertal boys following treatment for Hodgkin's disease. Am J Pediatr Hematol Oncol 1993; 15:306–310.
1370. Mustieles C, Munoz A, Alonso M, et al. Male gonadal function after chemotherapy in survivors of childhood malignancy. Med Pediatr Oncol 1995; 24:347–351.
1371. Bramswig JH, Heimes U, Heiermann E, et al. The effects of different cumulative doses of chemotherapy on testicular function. Cancer 1990; 65:1298–1302.
1372. Ben Arush MW, Solt I, Lightman A, et al. Male gonadal function in survivors of childhood Hodgkin and non-Hodgkin lymphoma. Pediatr Hematol Oncol 2000; 17:239–245.
1373. Barrett A, Nicholls J, Gibson B. Late effects of total body irradiation. Radiother Oncol 1987; 9:131–135.
1374. Ogilvy-Stuart AL, Shalet SM. Effect of radiation on the human reproductive system. Environ Health Perspect 1993; 101(suppl 2):109–116.
1375. Aslam I, Fishel S, Moore H, et al. Fertility preservation of boys undergoing anti-cancer therapy: a review of the existing situation and prospects for the future. Hum Reprod 2000; 15:2154–2159.
1376. Muller J, Sonksen J, Sommer P, et al. Cryopreservation of semen from pubertal boys with cancer. Med Pediatr Oncol 2000; 34:191–194.

1377. Schover LR, Agarwal A, Thomas AJ Jr. Cryopreservation of gametes in young patients with cancer. J Pediatr Hematol Oncol 1998; 20:426–428.
1378. Tesarik J, Bahceci M, Ozcan C, et al. Restoration of fertility by in-vitro spermatogenesis. Lancet 1999; 353:555–556.
1379. Antinori S, Versaci C, Dani G, et al. Successful fertilization and pregnancy after injection of frozen-thawed round spermatids into human oocytes. Hum Reprod 1997; 12:554–556.
1380. Bosson D, Wolter R, Toppet M, et al. Partial 17,20-desmolase and 17 alpha-hydroxylase deficiencies in a 16-year-old boy. J Endocrinol Invest 1988; 11:527–533.
1381. Bose HS, Sugawara T, Strauss JF 3rd, Miller WL. The pathophysiology and genetics of congenital lipoid adrenal hyperplasia. International Congenital Lipoid Adrenal Hyperplasia Consortium. N Engl J Med 1996; 335:1870–1878.
1382. Bose HS, Pescovitz OH, Miller WL. Spontaneous feminization in a 46,XX female patient with congenital lipoid adrenal hyperplasia due to a homozygous frameshift mutation in the steroidogenic acute regulatory protein. J Clin Endocrinol Metab 1997; 82:1511–1515.
1383. Fujieda K, Tajima T, Nakae J, et al. Spontaneous puberty in 46,XX subjects with congenital lipoid adrenal hyperplasia: ovarian steroidogenesis is spared to some extent despite inactivating mutations in the steroidogenic acute regulatory protein (StAR) gene. J Clin Invest 1997; 99:1265–1271.
1384. Dufau ML. The luteinizing hormone receptor. Annu Rev Physiol 1998; 60:461–496.
1385. David R, Yoon DJ, Landin L, et al. A syndrome of gonadotropin resistance possibly due to a luteinizing hormone receptor defect. J Clin Endocrinol Metab 1984; 59:156–160.
1386. Gromoll J, Eiholzer U, Nieschlag E, Simoni M. Male hypogonadism caused by homozygous deletion of exon 10 of the luteinizing hormone (LH) receptor: differential action of human chorionic gonadotropin and LH. J Clin Endocrinol Metab 2000; 85:2281–2286.
1387. Latronico AC, Anasti J, Arnhold IJ, et al. Brief report: testicular and ovarian resistance to luteinizing hormone caused by inactivating mutations of the luteinizing hormone–receptor gene. N Engl J Med 1996; 334:507–512.
1388. Martens JW, Verhoef-Post M, Abelin N, et al. A homozygous mutation in the luteinizing hormone receptor causes partial Leydig cell hypoplasia: correlation between receptor activity and phenotype. Mol Endocrinol 1998; 12:775–784.
1389. Winkler L, Offner G, Krull F, Brodehl J. Growth and pubertal development in nephropathic cystinosis. Eur J Pediatr 1993; 152:244–249.
1390. Lee P. Fertility in cryptorchidism: does treatment make a difference? Endocrinol Metab Clin North Am 1993; 22:479–490.
1391. Hutson JM, Hasthorpe S, Heyns CF. Anatomical and functional aspects of testicular descent and cryptorchidism. Endocr Rev 1997; 18:259–280.
1392. Lee PA, Coughlin MT. Fertility after bilateral cryptorchidism: evaluation by paternity, hormone, and semen data. Horm Res 2001; 55:28–32.
1393. Saez J, Forest MG. Kinetics of human chorionic gonadotropin–induced steroidogenic response of the human testis. I. Plasma testosterone: implications for human chorionic gonadotropin stimulation test. J Clin Endocrinol Metab 1979; 49:278–283.
1394. Hurwitz RS, Kaptein JS. How well does contralateral testis hypertrophy predict the absence of the nonpalpable testis? J Urol 2001; 165:588–592.
1395. Laron Z, Dickerman Z, Ritterman I, Kaufman H. Follow-up of boys with unilateral compensatory testicular hypertrophy. Fertil Steril 1980; 33:297–301.
1396. Pyorala S, Huttunen N-P, Uhari M. A review and meta analysis of hormonal treatment of cryptorchidism. J Clin Endocrinol Metab 1995; 80:2795–2799.
1397. Huff DS, Fenig DM, Canning DA, et al. Abnormal germ cell development in cryptorchidism. Horm Res 2001; 55:11–17.
1398. Grasso M, Buonaguidi A, Lania C, et al. Postpubertal cryptorchidism: review and evaluation of the fertility. Eur Urol 1991; 20:126–128.
1399. Docimo SG. The results of surgical therapy for cryptorchidism: a literature review and analysis. J Urol 1995; 154:1148–1152.
1400. Cortes D, Thorup JM, Visfeldt J. Cryptorchidism: aspects of fertility and neoplasms. A study including data of 1,335 consecutive boys who underwent testicular biopsy simultaneously with surgery for cryptorchidism. Horm Res 2001; 55:21–27.
1401. Nistal M, Riestra ML, Paniagua R. Correlation between testicular biopsies (prepubertal and postpubertal) and spermiogram in cryptorchid men. Hum Pathol 2000; 31(9):1022–1030.
1402. Mininberg DT, Rodger JC, Bedford JM. Ultrastructural evidence of the onset of testicular pathological conditions in the cryptorchid human testis within the first year of life. J Urol 1982; 128:782–784.
1403. Cendron M, Keating MA, Huff DS, et al. Cryptorchidism, orchiopexy and infertility: a critical long-term retrospective analysis. J Urol 1989; 142:559–562.
1404. Huff DS, Hadziselimovic F, Snyder HM III, et al. Postnatal testicular maldevelopment in unilateral cryptorchidism. J Urol 1989; 142:546–548.
1405. Lin YM, Hsu CC, Lin JS. Successful testicular sperm extraction and fertilization in an azoospermic man with postpubertal mumps orchitis. BJU Int 1999; 83:526–527.
1406. Heaton ND, Davenport M, Pryor JP. Fertility after correction of bilateral undescended testes at the age of 23 years. Br J Urol 1993; 71:490–491.
1407. Shin D, Lemack GE, Goldstein M. Induction of spermatogenesis and pregnancy after adult orchiopexy. J Urol 1997; 158:2242.
1408. Giwercman A, Hansen LL, Skakkebaek NE. Initiation of sperm production after bilateral orchiopexy: clinical and biological implications. J Urol 2000; 163:1255–1256.
1409. Lee PA, Jaffe RB, Midgley ARJ. Serum gonadotropin, testosterone and prolactin concentrations throughout puberty in boys: a longitudinal study. J Clin Endocrinol Metab 1974; 39:664–672.
1410. Moller H, Jorgensen N, Forman D. Trends in incidence of testicular cancer in boys and adolescent men. Int J Cancer 1995; 61:761–764.
1411. Skakkebaek NE, Rajpert-De Meyts E, Main KM. Testicular dysgenesis syndrome: an increasingly common developmental disorder with environmental aspects. Hum Reprod 2001; 16: 972–978.
1412. United Kingdom Testicular Cancer Study Group. Aetiology of testicular cancer: association with congenital abnormalities, age at puberty, infertility, and exercise. BMJ 1994; 308:1393–1399.
1413. Parkinson MC, Swerdlow AJ, Pike MC. Carcinoma in situ in boys with cryptorchidism: when can it be detected? Br J Urol 1994; 73:431–435.
1414. Giwercman A, von der Maase H, Skakkebaek NE. Epidemiological and clinical aspects of carcinoma in situ of the testis. Eur Urol 1993; 23:104–110; discussion 111–114.
1415. Thomas DB, Jimenez LM, McTiernan A, et al. Breast cancer in men: risk factors with hormonal implications. Am J Epidemiol 1992; 135:734–748.
1416. Rosenfeld RG, Grumbach MM. Turner Syndrome. New York, Marcel Decker, 1990, pp 1–512.
1417. Ranke MB, Rosenfeld RG (eds). Turner Syndrome: Growth Promoting Therapies. Amsterdam, Excerpta Medica, 1991.
1418. Hibi I, Takano K (eds). Basic and Clinical Approach to Turner Syndrome. Amsterdam, Excerpta Medica, 1993.
1419. Albertsson Wikland K, Ranke MB (eds). Turner Syndrome in a Life Span Perspective: Research and Clinical Aspects. Amsterdam, Elsevier Science, 1995.
1420. Elsheikh M, Dunger DB, Conway GS, Wass JA. Turner's syndrome in adulthood. Endocr Rev 2002; 23:120–140.
1421. Ranke MB, Saenger P. Turner's syndrome. Lancet 2001; 358: 309–314.
1422. Hook EB, Warburton D. The distribution of chromosomal genotypes associated with Turner's syndrome: livebirth prevalence rates and evidence for diminished fetal mortality and severity in genotypes associated with structural X abnormalities or mosaicism. Hum Genet 1983; 64:24–27.
1423. Turner HH. A syndrome of infantilism, congenital webbed neck and cubitus valgus. Endocrinology 1938; 23:566–574.
1424. Carr DH, Gedeon M. Population cytogenetics in human abortuses. In Hook EB, Porter IH (eds). Population Cytogenetics. New York, Academic Press, 1977, pp 1–9.
1425. Warburton D, Kline J, Stein I. Monosomy X: a chromosomal anomaly associated with young maternal age. Lancet 1980; 1: 167–169.
1426. Saenger P, Wikland KA, Conway GS, et al. Recommendations for the diagnosis and management of Turner syndrome. J Clin Endocrinol Metab 2001; 86:3061–3069.

1427. Roa E, Weiss B, Fukami M, et al. Pseudoautosomal deletions encompassing a novel homeobox gene cause growth failure in idiopathic short stature and Turner syndrome. Nat Genet 1997; 16:54–62.
1428. Ellison JW, Wardak Z, Young MF, et al. PHOG, a candidate gene for involvement in the short stature of Turner syndrome. Hum Molec Genet 1997; 6(8):1341–1347.
1429. Belin V, Cusin V, Viot G, et al. *SHOX* mutations in dyschondrosteosis (Leri-Weill syndrome). Nat Genet 1998; 19:67–69.
1430. Kosho T, Muroya K, Nagai T, et al. Skeletal features and growth patterns in 14 patients with haploinsufficiency of SHOX: implications for the development of Turner syndrome. J Clin Endocrinol Metab 1999; 84:4613–4621.
1431. Blaschke RJ, Rappold GA. SHOX: growth, Leri-Weill and Turner syndromes. Trends Endocrinol Metab 2000; 11:227–230.
1432. Ogata T, Muroya K, Matsuo N, et al. Turner syndrome and Xp deletions: clinical and molecular studies in 47 patients. J Clin Endocrinol Metab 2001; 86:5498–5508.
1433. Ogata T, Matsuo N, Nishimura G. SHOX haploinsufficiency and overdosage: impact of gonadal function status. J Med Genet 2001; 38:1–6.
1434. Clement-Jones M, Schiller S, Rao E, et al. The short stature homeobox gene SHOX is involved in skeletal abnormalities in Turner syndrome. Hum Mol Genet 2000; 9:695–702.
1435. Ogata T, Kosho T, Wakui K, et al. Short stature homeobox-containing gene duplication on the der(X) chromosome in a female with 45,X/46,X, der(X), gonadal dysgenesis, and tall stature. J Clin Endocrinol Metab 2000; 85:2927–2930.
1436. Szpunar J. Middle ear disease in Turner's syndrome. Arch Otolaryngol Head Neck Surg 1968; 87:34–40.
1437. Barreñas M, Landin-Wilhelmsen K, Hanson C. Ear and hearing in relation to genotype and growth in Turner syndrome. Hear Res 2000; 144:21–28.
1438. Palmer CG, Reichman A. Chromosomal and clinical findings in 110 females with Turner syndrome. Hum Genet 1976; 35:35–49.
1439. Lin AE, Lippe BM, Geffner ME, et al. Aortic dilation, dissection, and rupture in patients with Turner syndrome. J Pediatr 1986; 109:820–826.
1440. Lippe BM, Geffner ME, Dietrich RB, et al. Renal malformations in patients with Turner syndrome: imaging in 141 patients. Pediatrics 1988; 82:852–856.
1441. Arulanantham K, Kramer MS, Gryboski JD. The association of inflammatory bowel disease and X-chromosomal abnormality. Pediatrics 1980; 66:63–67.
1442. Knudtzon J, Svane S, Price WH. Turner's syndrome associated with chronic inflammatory bowel disease: a case report and review of the literature. Acta Med Scand 1979; 16:263–266.
1443. Price WH. A high incidence of chronic inflammatory bowel disease in patients with Turner syndrome. J Med Genet 1979; 16:263–266.
1444. Gravholt CH, Juul S, Naeraa RW, Hansen J. Morbidity in Turner syndrome. J Clin Epidemiol 1998; 51:147–158.
1445. Elsheikh M, Wass JA, Conway GS. Autoimmune thyroid syndrome in women with Turner's syndrome: the association with karyotype. Clin Endocrinol (Oxf) 2001; 55:223–226.
1446. Nielsen J, Johansen K, Yde H. The frequency of diabetes mellitus in patients with Turner's syndrome and pure gonadal dysgenesis. Acta Endocrinol (Copenh) 1969; 62:251–269.
1447. Silbert A, Wolffe PH, Lilienthal J. Spatial and temporal processing in patients with Turner's syndrome. Behav Genet 1977; 7:11–21.
1448. Swillen A, Fryns JP, Kleczkowska A, et al. Intelligence, behaviour and psychosocial development in Turner syndrome: a cross-sectional study of 50 pre-adolescent and adolescent girls (4–20 years). Genet Couns 1993; 4:7–18.
1449. Garron DC. Intelligence among persons with Turner's syndrome. Behav Genet 1977; 7:105–127.
1450. Ross JL, Roeltgen D, Kushner H, et al. The Turner syndrome–associated neurocognitive phenotype maps to distal Xp. Am J Hum Genet 2000; 67:672–681.
1451. Cummings DE, Clement K, Purnell JQ, et al. Elevated plasma ghrelin levels in Prader Willi syndrome. Nat Med 2002; 8:643–644.
1452. Skuse DH, James RS, Bishop DVM, et al. Evidence from Turner's syndrome of an imprinted X-linked locus affecting cognitive function. Nature 1997; 387:705–708.
1453. McGuffin P, Scourfield J. A father's imprint on his daughter's thinking. Nature 1997; 387:652–653.
1454. Rovet J, Ireland L. Behavioral phenotype in children with Turner syndrome. J Pediatr Psychol 1994; 19:779–790.
1455. Migeon BR, Luo S, Jani M, Jeppesen P. The severe phenotype of females with tiny ring X chromosomes is associated with inability of these chromosomes to undergo X inactivation. Am J Hum Genet 1994; 55:497–504.
1456. Even L, Cohen A, Marbach N, et al. Longitudinal analysis of growth over the first 3 years of life in Turner's syndrome. J Pediatr 2000; 137:460–464.
1457. Brook CGD, Murset G, Zachmann M, et al. Growth in children with 45,XO Turner's syndrome. Arch Dis Child 1974; 73: 789–795.
1458. Lyon AJ, Preece MA, Grant DB. Growth curve for girls with Turner syndrome. Arch Dis Child 1985; 60:932–935.
1459. Ranke MB, Stubbe P, Majewski F, et al. Spontaneous growth in Turner's syndrome. Acta Paediatr Scand Suppl 1988; 343:22–30.
1460. Ranke MB, Grauer ML. Adult height in Turner syndrome: results of a multinational survey 1993. Horm Res 1994; 42:90–94.
1461. Massa G, Vanderschueren-Lodeweyckx M, Malvaux P. Linear growth in patients with Turner syndrome: influence of spontaneous puberty and parental height. Eur J Pediatr 1990; 149: 246–250.
1462. Sas TC, de Muinck Keizer-Schrama S, Stijnen T, et al. Normalization of height in girls with Turner syndrome after long-term growth hormone treatment: results of a randomized dose-response trial. J Clin Endocrinol Metab 1999; 84:4607–4612.
1463. Carel JC, Mathivon L, Gendrel C, et al. Near normalization of final height with adapted doses of growth hormone in Turner's syndrome. J Clin Endocrinol Metab 1998; 83:1462–1466.
1464. Cacciari E, Mazzanti L. Final height of patients with Turner's syndrome treated with growth hormone (GH): indications for GH therapy alone at high doses and late estrogen therapy. Italian Study Group for Turner Syndrome. J Clin Endocrinol Metab 1999; 84:4510–4515.
1465. Rosenfeld RG, Attie KM, Frane J, et al. Growth hormone therapy of Turner's syndrome: beneficial effect on adult height. J Pediatr 1998; 132:319–324.
1466. Ranke MB, Lindberg A, Chatelain P, et al. Prediction of long-term response to recombinant human growth hormone in Turner syndrome: development and validation of mathematical models. KIGS International Board. Kabi International Growth Study. J Clin Endocrinol Metab 2000; 85:4212–4218.
1467. Betts PR, Butler GE, Donaldson MD, et al. A decade of growth hormone treatment in girls with Turner syndrome in the UK. UK KIGS Executive Group. Arch Dis Child 1999; 80:221–225.
1468. Takano K, Ogawa M, Tanaka T, et al. Clinical trials of GH treatment in patients with Turner's syndrome in Japan: a consideration of final height. The Committee for the Treatment of Turner's Syndrome. Eur J Endocrinol 1997; 137:138–145.
1469. Sas TC, Gerver WJ, De Bruin R, et al. Body proportions during long-term growth hormone treatment in girls with Turner syndrome participating in a randomized dose-response trial. J Clin Endocrinol Metab 1999; 84:4622–4628.
1470. Chernausek SD, Attie KM, Cara JF, et al. Growth hormone therapy of Turner syndrome: the impact of age of estrogen replacement on final height. Genentech, Inc., Collaborative Study Group. J Clin Endocrinol Metab 2000; 85:2439–2445.
1471. Savendahl L, Davenport ML. Delayed diagnoses of Turner's syndrome: proposed guidelines for change. J Pediatr 2000; 137: 455–459.
1472. Sas TC, de Muinck Keizer-Schrama S, Stijnen T, et al. Carbohydrate metabolism during long-term growth hormone (GH) treatment and after discontinuation of GH treatment in girls with Turner syndrome participating in a randomized dose-response study. Dutch Advisory Group on Growth Hormone. J Clin Endocrinol Metab 2000; 85:769–775.
1473. Cicognani A, Mazzanti L, Tassinari D, et al. Differences in carbohydrate tolerance in Turner syndrome depending on age and karyotype. Eur J Pediatr 1988; 148:64–68.
1474. Ross JL, Feuillan P, Long LM, et al. Lipid abnormalities in Turner syndrome. J Pediatr 1995; 126:242–245.

1475. Sklar CA, Kaplan SL, Grumbach MM. Lack of effect of oestrogens on adrenal androgen secretion in children and adolescents with a comment on oestrogens and pubic hair growth. Clin Endocrinol (Oxf) 1981; 14:311–320.
1476. Sas TC, de Muinck Keizer-Schrama SM, Stijnen T, et al. Bone mineral density assessed by phalangeal radiographic absorptiometry before and during long-term growth hormone treatment in girls with Turner's syndrome participating in a randomized dose-response study. Pediatr Res 2001; 50:417–422.
1477. Bechtold S, Rauch F, Noelle V, et al. Musculoskeletal analyses of the forearm in young women with Turner syndrome: a study using peripheral quantitative computed tomography. J Clin Endocrinol Metab 2001; 86:5819–5823.
1478. Bertelloni S, Cinquanta L, Baroncelli GI, et al. Volumetric bone mineral density in young women with Turner's syndrome treated with estrogens or estrogens plus growth hormone. Horm Res 2000; 53:72–76.
1479. Ross JL, Stefanatos G, Roeltgen D, et al. Ullrich-Turner syndrome: neurodevelopmental changes from childhood through adolescence. Am J Med Genet 1995; 58:74–82.
1480. Ross JL, Kushner H, Roeltgen DP. Developmental changes in motor function in girls with Turner syndrome. Pediatr Neurol 1996; 15:317–322.
1481. Temple CM, Carney R. Reading skills in children with Turner's syndrome: an analysis of hyperplexia. Cortex 1996; 32:335–345.
1482. Robinson A, Bender BG, Linden MG. Prognosis of prenatally diagnosed children with sex chromosome aneuploidy. Am J Med Genet 1992; 44:365–368.
1483. Reiss AL, Mazzocco MM, Greenlaw R, et al. Neurodevelopmental effects of X monosomy: a volumetric imaging study. Ann Neurol 1995; 38:731–738.
1484. Murphy DG, Mentis MJ, Pietrini P, et al. A PET study of Turner's syndrome: effects of sex steroids and the X chromosome on brain. Biol Psychiatry 1997; 41:285–298.
1485. Voeller KK. Right-hemisphere deficit syndrome in children. Am J Psychiatry 1986; 143:1004–1009.
1486. Mazzocco MM. A process approach to describing mathematics difficulties in girls with Turner syndrome. Pediatrics 1998; 102: 492–496.
1487. Van Dyke DL, Wiktor A, Palmer CG, et al. Ullrich-Turner syndrome with a small ring X chromosome and presence of mental retardation. Am J Med Genet 1992; 43:996–1005.
1488. Downey J, Elkin EJ, Ehrhardt AA, et al. Cognitive ability and everyday functioning in women with Turner syndrome. J Learn Disabil 1991; 24:32–39.
1489. Swillen A, Fryns JP, Kleczkowska A, et al. Intelligence, behaviour and psychosocial development in Turner syndrome. A cross-sectional study of 50 pre-adolescent and adolescent girls (4–20 years). Genet Couns 1993; 4:7–18.
1490. Nyborg H. Hormones, Sex and Society. Westport, Conn, Praeger, 1994, pp 1–207.
1491. Romans SM, Stefanatos G, Roeltgen DP, et al. Transition to young adulthood in Ullrich-Turner syndrome: neurodevelopmental changes. Am J Med Genet 1998; 79:140–147.
1492. Ross JL, Roeltgen D, Feuillan P, et al. Effects of estrogen on nonverbal processing speed and motor function in girls with Turner's syndrome. J Clin Endocrinol Metab 1998; 83:3198–3204.
1493. Johnson R Jr, Rohrbaugh JW, Ross JL. Altered brain development in Turner's syndrome: an event-related potential study. Neurology 1993; 43:801–808.
1494. Rovet J, Holland J. Psychological aspects of the Canadian randomized controlled trial of human growth hormone and low-dose ethinyl oestradiol in children with Turner syndrome. The Canadian Growth Hormone Advisory Group. Horm Res 1993; 39(suppl 2):60–64.
1495. Lagrou K, Xhrouet-Heinrichs D, Heinrichs C, et al. Age-related perception of stature, acceptance of therapy, and psychosocial functioning in human growth hormone-treated girls with Turner's syndrome. J Clin Endocrinol Metab 1998; 83:1494–1501.
1496. Ross JL, Feuillan P, Kushner H, et al. Absence of growth hormone effects on cognitive function in girls with Turner syndrome. J Clin Endocrinol Metab 1997; 82:1814–1817.
1497. Siegel PT, Clopper R, Stabler B. The psychological consequences of Turner syndrome and review of the National Cooperative Growth Study psychological substudy. Pediatrics 1998; 102:488–491.
1498. Ross JL, Roeltgen D, Feuillan P, et al. Use of estrogen in young girls with Turner syndrome: effects on memory. Neurology 2000; 54:164–170.
1499. Phillips SM, Sherwin BB. Variations in memory function and sex steroid hormones across the menstrual cycle. Psychoneuroendocrinology 1992; 17:497–506.
1500. Phillips SM, Sherwin BB. Effects of estrogen on memory function in surgically menopausal women. Psychoneuroendocrinology 1992; 17:485–495.
1501. Rickert VI, Hassed SJ, Hendon AE, Cunniff C. The effects of peer ridicule on depression and self-image among adolescent females with Turner syndrome. J Adolesc Health 1996; 19:34–38.
1502. McCauley E, Kay T, Ito J, Treder R. The Turner syndrome: cognitive deficits, affective discrimination, and behavior problems. Child Dev 1987; 58:464–473.
1503. Mazzocco MM, Baumgardner T, Freund LS, Reiss AL. Social functioning among girls with fragile X or Turner syndrome and their sisters. J Autism Dev Disord 1998; 28:509–517.
1504. Gnanapavan S, Kola B, Bustin SA, et al. The tissue distribution of the mRNA of ghrelin and subtypes of its receptor, GHS-R, in humans. J Clin Endocrinol Metab 2002; 87:2988–2991.
1505. Skuse DH. Genomic imprinting of the X chromosome: a novel mechanism for the evolution of sexual dimorphism. J Lab Clin Med 1999; 133:23–32.
1506. Bishop DV, Canning E, Elgar K, et al. Distinctive patterns of memory function in subgroups of females with Turner syndrome: evidence for imprinted loci on the X-chromosome affecting neurodevelopment. Neuropsychologia 2000; 38:712–721.
1507. Mazzanti L, Nizzoli G, Tassinari D, et al. Spontaneous growth and pubertal development in Turner's syndrome with different karyotypes. Acta Paediatr 1994; 83:299–304.
1508. Cuseen LJ, MacMahan RA. Germ cells and ova in dysgenetic gonads of a 46-XY female dizygotic twin. Am J Dis Child 1979; 133:373–375.
1509. Scully RE. Gonadoblastoma: a review of 74 cases. Cancer 1970; 25:1340–1356.
1510. Khodr GS, Cadena GD, Ong TC. Y-autosome translocation, gonadal dysgenesis, and gonadoblastoma. Am J Dis Child 1979; 133:277–282.
1511. Tartaglia M, Kalides K, Shaw A, et al. PTPN 11 Mutations in Noonans syndrome: Molecular spectrum, genotype-phenotype correlations and phenotypic heterogeneity. Am J Hum Genet 2002; 70:1555–1563.
1512. Umehara F, Tate G, Itoh K, et al. A novel mutation of desert hedgehog in a patient with 46,XY partial gonadal dysgenesis accompanied by minifascicular neuropathy. Am J Hum Genet 2000; 67:1302–1305.
1513. Thibaud E, Ramirez M, Brauner R, et al. Preservation of ovarian function by ovarian transposition performed before pelvic irradiation during childhood. J Pediatr 1992; 121:880–884.
1514. Quigley C, Cowell C, Jimenez M, et al. Normal or early development of puberty despite gonadal damage in children treated for acute lymphoblastic leukemia. N Engl J Med 1989; 321: 143–151.
1515. Lahteenmaki PM, Toppari J, Ruokonen A, et al. Low serum inhibin B concentrations in male survivors of childhood malignancy. Eur J Cancer 1999; 35:612–619.
1516. Ahmed SR, Shalet SM, Campbell RH, et al. Primary gonadal damage following treatment of brain tumors in childhood. J Pediatr 1983; 103:562–565.
1517. Perrone L, Sinisi AA, Sicuranza R, et al. Prepubertal endocrine follow-up in subjects with Wilms' tumor. Med Pediatr Oncol 1988; 16:255–258.
1518. Nicosia SV, Matus Ridley M, Meadows AT. Gonadal effects of cancer therapy in girls. Cancer 1985; 55:2364–2372.
1519. Matus Ridley M, Nicosia SV, Meadows AT. Gonadal effects of cancer therapy in boys. Cancer 1985; 55:2353–2363.
1520. Paulino AC, Wen BC, Brown CK, et al. Late effects in children treated with radiation therapy for Wilms' tumor. Int J Radiat Oncol Biol Phys 2000; 46:1239–1246.
1521. Byrne J, Fears TR, Gail MH, et al. Early menopause in long-term survivors of cancer during adolescence. Am J Obstet Gynecol 1992; 166:788–793.

1522. Longhi A, Porcu E, Petracchi S, et al. Reproductive functions in female patients treated with adjuvant and neoadjuvant chemotherapy for localized osteosarcoma of the extremity. Cancer 2000; 89:1961–1965.
1523. Hoek A, Schoemaker J, Drexhage HA. Premature ovarian failure and ovarian autoimmunity. Endocr Rev 1997; 18:107–134.
1524. Irvine WJ. Autoimmunity in endocrine disease. Recent Prog Horm Res 1980; 36:509–556.
1525. Ahonen P, Myllarniemi S, Sipila I, et al. Clinical variation of autoimmune polyendocrinopathy–candidiasis–ectodermal dystrophy (APECED) in a series of 68 patients. N Engl J Med 1990; 322:1829–1836.
1526. Lucky AW, Rebar RW, Blizzard RM, Goren EM. Pubertal progression in the presence of elevated serum gonadotropins in girls with multiple endocrine deficiencies. J Clin Endocrinol Metab 1977; 45:673–678.
1527. Betterle C, Rossi A, Dalla Pria S, et al. Premature ovarian failure: autoimmunity and natural history. Clin Endocrinol (Oxf) 1993; 39:35–43.
1528. Chen S, Sawicka J, Betterle C, et al. Autoantibodies to steroidogenic enzymes in autoimmune polyglandular syndrome, Addison's disease, and premature ovarian failure. J Clin Endocrinol Metab 1996; 81:1871–1876.
1529. Scott HS, Heino M, Peterson P, et al. Common mutations in autoimmune polyendocrinopathy–candidiasis–ectodermal dystrophy patients of different origins. Mol Endocrinol 1998; 12: 1112–1119.
1530. Flora S, Bottazzo GF, Doniach D. Immunofluorescence studies on antibodies to steroid producing cells, and to germ line cells in endocrine disease and infertility. Clin Exp Immunol 1980; 39: 97–111.
1531. Arif S, Underhil JA, Donaldson P, et al. J Clin Endocrinol Metab 1999; 84:1056–1060.
1532. Dewhurst CJ, Dekoos EB, Ferreira HP. The resistant ovary syndrome. Br J Obstet Gynaecol 1975; 82:341–345.
1533. Evers JLH, Rolland RT. The gonadotropin resistant ovary syndrome: a curable disease? Clin Endocrinol (Oxf) 1981; 14:99–103.
1534. Davis CJ, Davison RM, Payne NN, et al. Female sex preponderance for idiopathic familial premature ovarian failure suggests an X chromosome defect: opinion. Hum Reprod 2000; 15: 2418–2422.
1535. Gibson JB. Gonadal function in galactosemics and in galactose-intoxicated animals. Eur J Pediatr 1995; 154(suppl 2):S14–S20.
1536. Schweitzer S, Shin Y, Jakobs C, Brodehl J. Long-term outcome in 134 patients with galactosaemia. Eur J Pediatr 1993; 152:36–43.
1537. Kaufman FR, Kogut MD, Donnell GN, et al. Hypergonadotropic hypogonadism in female patients with galactosemia. N Engl J Med 1981; 304:994–998.
1538. Crisponi L, Deiana M, Loi A, et al. The putative forkhead transcription factor FOXL2 is mutated in blepharophimosis/ptosis/epicanthus inversus syndrome. Nat Genet 2001; 27:159–166.
1539. Nicolino M, Bost M, David M, Chaussain JL. Familial blepharophimosis: an uncommon marker of ovarian dysgenesis. J Pediatr Endocrinol Metab 1995; 8:127–133.
1540. Jaeken J, Matthijs G. Congenital disorders of glycosylation. Annu Rev Genomics Hum Genet 2001; 2:129–151.
1541. Kristiansson B, Stibler H, Wide L. Gonadal function and glycoprotein hormones in the carbohydrate-deficient glycoprotein (CDG) syndrome. Acta Paediatr 1995; 84:655–660.
1542. de Zegher F, Jaeken J. Endocrinology of the carbohydrate-deficient glycoprotein syndrome type 1 from birth through adolescence. Pediatr Res 1995; 37:395–401.
1543. Sprengel R, Braun T, Nikolics K, et al. The testicular receptor for follicle-stimulating hormone: structure and functional expression of cloned with DNA. Mol Endocrinol 1990; 4:525–530.
1544. Simoni M, Gromoll J, Nieschlag E. The follicle-stimulating hormone receptor: biochemistry, molecular biology, physiology, and pathophysiology. Endocr Rev 1997; 18:739–773.
1545. Conway GS. Clinical manifestations of genetic defects affecting gonadotrophins and their receptors. Clin Endocrinol 1996; 45(6):657–663.
1546. Aittomaki K, Herva R, Stenman U-H, et al. Clinical features of primary ovarian failure caused by a point mutation in the follicle-stimulating hormone receptor gene. J Clin Endocrinol Metab 1996; 81:3722–3726.
1547. Kumar TR, Wang Y, Lu N, Matzuk MM. Follicle stimulating hormone is required for ovarian follicle maturation but not male fertility. Nat Genet 1997; 15:201–204.
1548. Aittomaki K, Dieguez Lucena JL, Pakarinen P, et al. Mutation in the follicle-stimulating hormone receptor gene causes hereditary hypergonadotropic ovarian failure. Cell 1995; 82:959–968.
1549. Tapanainen JS, Aittomaki K, Min J, et al. Men homozygous for an inactivating mutation of the follicle-stimulating hormone (FSH) receptor gene present variable suppression of spermatogenesis and fertility. Nat Genet 1997; 15:205–206.
1550. Latronico AC, Anasti J, Arnhold IJP, et al. Testicular and ovarian resistance to luteinizing hormone caused by inactivating mutations of the luteinizing hormone receptor gene. N Engl J Med 1996; 344:507–512.
1551. Stanhope R, Adams J, Brook CG. Evolution of polycystic ovaries in a girl with delayed menarche: a case report. J Reprod Med 1988; 33:482–484.
1552. Porcu E, Venturoli S, Magrini O, et al. Circadian variation of luteinizing hormone can have two different profiles in adolescent anovulation. J Clin Endocrinol Metab 1987; 65:488–493.
1553. Dunaif A, Thomas A. Current concepts in the polycystic ovary syndrome. Annu Rev Med 2001; 52:401–419.
1554. Elsawi MM, Pryor JP, Klufio G, et al. Genital tract function in men with Noonan syndrome. J Med Genet 1994; 31:468–470.
1555. Witt DR, Keena BA, Hall JG, Allanson JE. Growth curves for height in Noonan syndrome. Clin Genet 1986; 30:150–153.
1556. Kelnar CJ. Growth hormone therapy in Noonan syndrome. Horm Res 2000; 53(suppl 1):77–81.
1557. MacFarlane CE, Brown DC, Johnston LB, et al. Growth hormone therapy and growth in children with Noonan's syndrome: results of 3 years' follow-up. J Clin Endocrinol Metab 2001; 86: 1953–1956.
1558. Takagi M, Miyashita Y, Koga M, et al. Estrogen deficiency is a potential cause for osteopenia in adult male patients with Noonan's syndrome. Calcif Tissue Int 2000; 66:200–203.
1559. Carrascosa A, Gussinye M, Terradas P, et al. Spontaneous, but not induced, puberty permits adequate bone mass acquisition in adolescent Turner syndrome patients. J Bone Miner Res 2000; 15:2005–2010.
1560. King LR, Siegel MJ, Solomon AL. Usefulness of ovarian volume and cysts in female isosexual precocious puberty. J Ultrasound Med 1993; 12:577–581.
1561. Bailey WA, Zwingman TA, Reznik VM, et al. End-stage renal disease and primary hypogonadism associated with a 46,XX karyotype. Am J Dis Child 1992; 146:1218–1223.
1562. John H, Schmid C. Kallmann's syndrome: clues to clinical diagnosis. Int J Impot Res 2000; 12:269–271.
1563. Gilger JW, Geary DC, Eisele LM. Reliability and validity of retrospective self-reports of the age of pubertal onset using twin, sibling, and college student data. Adolescence 1991; 26: 41–53.
1564. Carskadon MA, Acebo C. A self-administered rating scale for pubertal development. J Adolesc Health 1993; 14:190–195.
1565. Bonneville JF, Cattin F. The role of magnetic resonance imaging in the diagnosis of endocrine tumours of the sellar region in children. Horm Res 1995; 43:151–153.
1566. Massarano AA, Adams J, Preece MA, et al. Ovarian ultrasound appearances in the Turner syndrome. J Pediatr 1989; 114:568–573.
1567. Spitz IM, Hirsch HJ, Trestian S. The prolactin response to thyrotropin-releasing hormone differentiates isolated gonadotropin deficiency from delayed puberty. N Engl J Med 1983; 308: 575–579.
1568. Buyukgebiz A, Oktay S. The role of TRH-stimulated prolactin responses in distinguishing gonadotropin deficiency from constitutional delayed puberty. J Pediatr Endocrinol 1994; 7:325–330.
1569. Winters SJ, Johnsonbaugh RE, Sherins RJ. The response of prolactin to chlorpromazine stimulation in men with hypogonadotrophic hypogonadism and early pubertal boys: relationship to sex steroid exposure. Clin Endocrinol (Oxf) 1982; 16:321–330.
1570. Cristiano AM, Munabi A, el Sabbagh H, et al. Prolactin response to metoclopramide does not distinguish patients with hypogonadotrophic hypogonadism from delayed puberty. Clin Endocrinol (Oxf) 1988; 28:75–82.

2028. Howard CP, Takahashi H, Hayles AB. Feminizing adrenal adenoma in a boy. Mayo Clin Proc 1977; 52:354–357.
2029. MacLaren NL, Migeon CH, Raiti S. Gynecomastia with congenital virilizing adrenal hyperplasia (11-β-hydroxylase deficiency). J Pediatr 1975; 86:579–581.
2030. Hemsell DL, Edman CD, Marks JF, et al. Massive extraglandular aromatization of plasma androstenedione resulting in feminization of a prepubertal boy. J Clin Invest 1977; 60:455–464.
2031. Berkovitz GD, Guerami A, Brown TR, et al. Familial gynecomastia with increased extraglandular aromatization of plasma carbon19-steroids. J Clin Invest 1985; 75:1763–1769.
2032. Stratakis CA, Vottero A, Brodie A, et al. The aromatase excess syndrome is associated with feminization of both sexes and autosomal dominant transmission of aberrant P450 aromatase gene transcription. J Clin Endocrinol Metab 1998; 83:1348–1357.
2033. Shozu M, Sebastian S, Takayama K, et al. Prepubertal gynecomastia due to estrogen excess associated with novel gain-of-function mutations affecting the aromatase gene. N Engl J Med. In press.
2034. Wilson DM, Pitts WC, Hintz RL, et al. Testicular tumors with Peutz-Jeghers syndrome. Cancer 1986; 57:2238–2240.
2035. Arai K, Chrousos GP. Syndromes of glucocorticoid and mineralocorticoid resistance. Steroids 1995; 60:173–179.
2036. Malchoff CD, Reardon G, Javier EC, et al. Dexamethasone therapy for isosexual precocious pseudopuberty caused by generalized glucocorticoid resistance. J Clin Endocrinol Metab 1994; 79:1632–1636.
2037. Young RH, Scully RE. Ovarian Sertoli cell tumors: a report of 10 cases. Int J Gynecol Pathol 1984; 2:349–363.
2038. Tavassoli FA, Norris HJ. Sertoli tumors of the ovary: a clinicopathologic study of 28 cases with ultrastructural observations. Cancer 1980; 46:2282–2297.
2039. Ilicki A, Lewin P, Kauli LR, et al. Premature thelarche: natural history and sex hormone secretion in 68 girls. Acta Paediatr Scand 1984; 73:756–762.
2040. Volta C, Bernasconi S, Cisternino M, et al. Isolated premature thelarche and thelarche variant: clinical and auxological follow-up of 119 girls. J Endocrinol Invest 1998; 21:180–183.
2041. Van Winter JT, Noller KL, Zimmerman D, Melton LJ 3rd. Natural history of premature thelarche in Olmsted County, Minnesota, 1940 to 1984. J Pediatr 1990; 116:278–280.
2042. Date Y, Kojima M, Hosoda H, et al. Ghrelin, a novel growth hormone-releasing acylated peptide, is synthesized in a distinct endocrine cell type in the gastrointestinal tracts of rats and humans. Endocrinology 2000; 141:4255–4261.
2043. Lutfallah C, Wang W, Mason JI, et al. Newly proposed hormonal criteria via genotypic proof for type II 3beta-hydroxysteroid dehydrogenase deficiency. Submitted for publication, 1997.
2044. Caparo VJ, Bayonet-Rivera NP, Thomas A, et al. Premature thelarche. Obstet Gynecol Surg 1971; 26:2–7.
2045. Ferrier P, Shepard TH, Smith FK. Growth disturbances and values for hormone excretion in various forms of precocious sexual development. Pediatrics 1961; 28:258–275.
2046. Rosenfield RL. Normal and almost normal precocious variations in pubertal development premature pubarche and premature thelarche revisited. Horm Res 1994; 41(suppl 2):7–13.
2047. Salardi S, Cacciari E, Mainetti B, et al. Outcome of premature thelarche: relation to puberty and final height. Arch Dis Child 1998; 79:173–174.
2048. Simmons PS. Diagnostic considerations in breast disorders of children and adolescents. Obstet Gynecol Clin North Am 1992; 19:91–102.
2049. Klein KO, Mericq V, Brown-Dawson JM, et al. Estrogen levels in girls with premature thelarche compared with normal prepubertal girls as determined by an ultrasensitive recombinant cell bioassay. J Pediatr 1999; 134:190–192.
2050. Wenick GB, Chasalow FI, Blethen SL. Sex hormone–binding globulin and thyroxine-binding globulin levels in premature thelarche. Steroids 1988; 52:543–550.
2051. Collett-Solberg PR, Grumbach MM. A simplified procedure for evaluating estrogenic effects and the sex chromatin pattern in exfoliated cells in urine: studies in premature thelarche and gynecomastia of adolescence. J Pediatr 1965; 66:883–890.
2052. Stanhope R, Abdulwahid NA, Adams J, et al. Studies of gonadotrophin pulsatility and pelvic ultrasound examinations distinguish between isolated premature thelarche and central precocious puberty. Eur J Pediatr 1986; 145:190–194.
2053. Verrotti A, Ferrari M, Morgese G, Chiarelli F. Premature thelarche: a long-term follow-up. Gynecol Endocrinol 1996; 10: 241–247.
2054. Caufriez H, Wolter R, Gouaerts M, et al. Gonadotropins and prolactin pituitary reserve in premature thelarche. J Pediatr 1977; 91:751–753.
2055. Garibaldi LR, Aceto TJ, Weber C. The pattern of gonadotropin and estradiol secretion in exaggerated thelarche. Acta Endocrinol (Copenh) 1993; 128:345–350.
2056. Murram D, Dewhurst J, Grant DB. Premature menarche: a follow-up study. Arch Dis Child 1983; 58:142–143.
2057. Blanco-Garcia M, Eva-Brion D, Roger M, et al. Isolated menses in prepubertal girls. Pediatrics 1985; 76:43–47.
2058. Fishman A, Paldi E. Vaginal bleeding in premenarchal girls: a review. Obstet Gynecol Surv 1991; 46:457–460.
2059. Hill NCW, Oppenheimer LW, Morton KE. The aetiology of vaginal bleeding in children: a 20-year review. Br J Obstet Gynaecol 1989; 96:467–470.
2060. David L, Betand B, Berlier P, et al. Les hémorragie génitales de la fille avant la puberté. Ann Pediatr (Paris) 1984; 31:55–61.
2061. Silverman SH, Migeon CJ, Rosenberg E, et al. Precocious growth of sexual hair without other secondary sexual development; "premature pubarche," a constitutional variation of adolescence. Pediatrics 1952; 10:426–431.
2062. Thamdrup E. Premature pubarche, a hypothalamic disorder? Acta Endocrinol (Copenh) 1955; 18:564–567.
2063. Rappaport R. Plasma androgens and LH in scoliotic patients with premature pubarche. J Clin Endocrinol Metab 1974; 38: 401–406.
2064. Lee PA, Migeon CJ, Bias WB, et al. Familial hypersecretion of adrenal androgens transmitted as a dominant, non-HLA linked trait. Obstet Gynecol 1987;259–264.
2065. Ibanez L, Potau N, de Zegher F. Recognition of a new association: reduced fetal growth, precocious pubarche, hyperinsulinism and ovarian dysfunction. Ann Endocrinol (Paris) 2000; 61:141–142.
2066. Ferrier P, Shepard TH, Smith FK. Growth disturbances and values for hormone excretion in various forms of precocious sexual development. Pediatrics 1961; 28:258–275.
2067. Korth-Schutz S, Levine LS, New MI. Serum androgens in normal prepubertal and pubertal children and in children with precocious adrenarche. J Clin Endocrinol Metab 1976; 42:117–124.
2068. Rosenfield RL. Plasma 17-ketosteroids and 17-beta-hydroxysteroid in girls with premature development of sexual hair. J Pediatr 1971; 79:260–266.
2069. Miller WL, Auchus RJ, Geller DH. The regulation of 17,20 lyase activity. Steroids 1997; 62:133–142.
2070. Apter D, Bhtzow T, Laughlin GA, Yen SSC. Metabolic features of polycystic ovary syndrome are found in adolescent girls with hyperandrogenism. J Clin Endocrinol Metab 1995; 80:2966–2973.
2071. Lee PA, Gareis FJ. Gonadotropin and sex steroid response to luteinizing hormone–releasing hormone in patients with premature adrenarche. J Clin Endocrinol Metab 1976; 43:195–197.
2072. Ibanez L, Virdio R, Potau N, et al. Natural history of premature pubarche: an auxological study. J Clin Endocrinol Metab 1992; 74:254–257.
2073. Pere A, Perheentupa J, Peter M, Voutilainen R. Follow up of growth and steroids in premature adrenarche. Eur J Pediatr 1995; 154:346–352.
2074. Diamanti-Kandarakis E, Dunaif A. New perspectives in polycystic ovary syndrome. Trends Endocrinol Metab 1996; 7:267–271.
2075. Oberfield SE, Mayes DM, Levine LS. Adrenal steroidogenic function in a black and Hispanic population with precocious pubarche. J Clin Endocrinol Metab 1990; 70:76–82.
2076. Likitmaskul S, Cowell CT, Donaghue K, et al. 'Exaggerated adrenarche' in children presenting with premature adrenarche. Clin Endocrinol (Oxf) 1995; 42:265–272.
2077. Yen SCC. The polycystic ovary syndrome. Clin Endocrinol (Oxf) 1980; 12:177–207.
2078. Franks S. Polycystic ovary syndrome. N Engl J Med 1995; 333: 853–861.

2079. Ehrman DA, Barnes RB, Rosenfield RL. Polycystic ovary syndrome as a form of functional ovarian hyperandrogenism due to dysregulation of androgen secretion. Endocr Rev 1995; 16:322–353.
2080. Morales AJ, Laughlin GA, Bhtzow T, et al. Insulin somatotropic and luteinizing hormone axes in lean and obese women with polycystic ovary syndrome: common and distinct features. J Clin Endocrinol Metab 1996; 81:2854–2864.
2081. Dunaif A, Segal KR, Shelley DR, et al. Evidence for distinctive and intrinsic defects in insulin action in polycystic ovary syndrome. Diabetes 1992; 41:1257–1266.
2082. Dunaif A, Xia J, Book CB, et al. Excessive insulin receptor serine phosphorylation in cultured fibroblasts and in skeletal muscle: a potential mechanism for insulin resistance in the polycystic ovary syndrome. J Clin Invest 1995; 96:801–810.
2083. Ibanez L, Potau N, Francois I, de Zegher F. Precocious pubarche, hyperinsulinism, and ovarian hyperandrogenism in girls: relation to reduced fetal growth. J Clin Endocrinol Metab 1998; 83:3558–3562.
2084. Ibanez L, de Zegher F, Potau N. Anovulation after precocious pubarche: early markers and time course in adolescence. J Clin Endocrinol Metab 1999; 84:2691–2695.
2085. Ibanez L, Aulesa C, Potau N, et al. Plasminogen activator inhibitor-1 in girls with precocious pubarche: a premenarcheal marker for polycystic ovary syndrome? Pediatr Res 2002; 51: 244–248.
2086. Ibaenez L, Potau N, Zampolli M, et al. Source localization of androgen excess in adolescent girls. J Clin Endocrinol Metab 1994; 79:1778–1784.
2087. Oppenheimer E, Linder B, DiMartino-Nardi J. Decreased insulin sensitivity in prepubertal girls with premature adrenarche and acanthosis nigricans. J Clin Endocrinol Metab 1995; 80: 614–618.
2088. Ibaenez L, Potau N, Zampolli M, et al. Hyperinsulinemia in postpubertal girls with a history of premature pubarche and functional ovarian hyperandrogenism. J Clin Endocrinol Metab 1996; 81:1237–1243.
2089. Ibanez L, Potau N, de Zegher F. Ovarian hyporesponsiveness to follicle stimulating hormone in adolescent girls born small for gestational age. J Clin Endocrinol Metab 2000; 85:2624–2626.
2090. Oberfield SE. Metabolic lessons from the study of young adolescents with polycystic ovary syndrome: is insulin, indeed, the culprit? J Clin Endocrinol Metab 2000; 85:3520–3525.
2091. Ibanez L, Valls C, Potau N, et al. Sensitization to insulin in adolescent girls to normalize hirsutism, hyperandrogenism, oligomenorrhea, dyslipidemia, and hyperinsulinism after precocious pubarche. J Clin Endocrinol Metab 2000; 85:3526–3530.
2092. Arslanian S, Lewy V, Danadian K, et al. Metformin therapy in adolescents with PCOS: lowering of adrenal cytochrome P450c17á activity and attenuation of hyperandrogenemia with reduction of an insulinemia (abstract). Pediatr Res 2001; 49: 109A.
2093. Jones KL, Arslanian S, Peterokova VA, et al. Effect of metformin in pediatric patients with type 2 diabetes: a randomized controlled trial. Diabetes Care 2002; 25:89–94.
2094. Azziz R, Ehrmann D, Legro RS, et al. Troglitazone improves ovulation and hirsutism in the polycystic ovary syndrome: a multicenter, double blind, placebo-controlled trial. J Clin Endocrinol Metab 2001; 86:1626–1632.
2095. Arlt W, Auchus RJ, Miller WL. Thiazolidinediones but not metformin directly inhibit the steroidogenic enzymes P450c17 and 3beta-hydroxysteroid dehydrogenase. J Biol Chem 2001; 276:16767-16771.
2096. Wilson R, Mercado A, Cheng K, et al. Steroid 21-hydroxylase deficiency: genotype may not predict phenotype. J Clin Endocrinol Metab 1995; 80:2322–2329.
2097. Morris AH, Reiter EO, Geffner ME, et al. Absence of nonclassical congenital adrenal hyperplasia in patients with precocious adrenarche. J Clin Endocrinol Metab 1989; 69:709–715.
2098. Speiser PW, Dupont B, Rubenstein P, et al. High frequency of nonclassical steroid 21-hydroxylase deficiency. Am J Hum Genet 1985; 35:650–667.
2099. Temeck JW, Pang S, Nelson C, et al. Genetic defects of steroidogenesis in premature pubarche. J Clin Endocrinol Metab 1987; 64:609–617.
2100. Balducci R, Boscherini B, Mangiantini A, et al. Isolated precocious pubarche: an approach. J Clin Endocrinol Metab 1994; 79: 582–589.
2101. Zerah M, Rheaume E, Mani P, et al. No evidence of mutations in the genes for type I and type II 3β- hydroxysteroid dehydrogenase (3β-HSD) in nonclassical 3β-HSD deficiency. J Clin Endocrinol Metab 1994; 79:1811–1817.
2102. Chang YT, Zhang L, Alkaddour HS, et al. Absence of molecular defect in type II 3β-hydroxysteroid dehydrogenase (3β-HSD) gene in premature pubarche children and hirsute female patients with moderately decreased adrenal 3β-HSD activity. Pediatr Res 1995; 37:820–824.
2103. Morel Y, Mebarki F, Rheaume E, et al. Structure-function relationships of 3β-hydroxysteroid dehydrogenase: contribution made by the molecular genetics of 3β- hydroxysteroid dehydrogenase deficiency. Steroids 1997; 62:176–184.
2104. Mendonca BB, Russell AJ, Vasconcelos-Leite M, et al. Mutation in 3 beta-hydroxysteroid dehydrogenase type II associated with pseudohermaphroditism in males and premature pubarche or cryptic expression in females. J Mol Endocrinol 1994; 12:119–122.
2105. Deplewski D, Rosenfield RL. Role of hormones in pilosebaceous unit development. Endocr Rev 2000; 21:363–392.
2106. Lucky AW, Biro FM, Huster GA, et al. Acne vulgaris in premenarchal girls: an early sign of puberty associated with rising levels of dehydroepiandrosterone. Arch Dermatol 1994; 130: 308–314.
2107. Yamamoto A, Ito M. Sebaceous gland activity and urinary androgen levels in children. J Dermatol Sci 1992; 4:98–104.
2108. Stewart ME, Downing DT, Cook JS, et al. Sebaceous gland activity and serum dehydroepiandrosterone sulfate levels in boys and girls. Arch Dermatol 1992; 128:1345–1348.
2109. Biro FM, Lucky AW, Huster GA, Morrison JA. Hormonal studies and physical maturation in adolescent gynecomastia. J Pediatr 1990; 116:450–455.
2110. Nydick M, Bustos J, Dale JH, et al. Gynecomastia in adolescent boys. JAMA 1961; 178:449–454.
2111. Large DM, Anderson DC. Twenty-four hour profiles of circulating androgens and oestrogens in male puberty with and without gynaecomastia. Clin Endocrinol (Oxf) 1979; 11:505–521.
2112. Carlson SE. Gynecomastia. N Engl J Med 1980; 404:795–799.
2113. LaFranchi SH, Parlow AF, Lippe BM, et al. Pubertal gynecomastia and transient elevation of serum estradiol level. Am J Dis Child 1975; 129:927–931.
2114. Siiteri PK, MacDonald PC. The role of extraglandular estrogen in human endocrinology. In Greep RO, Astwood EB (eds). Handbook of Physiology. Sect 7: Endocrinology. Vol II. Part 1. Female Reproductive System. Washington, DC, American Physiological Society, 1973, pp 615–629.
2115. Moore DC, Schlaepfer LV, Punier L, et al. Hormonal changes during puberty. V. Transient pubertal gynecomastia: abnormal androgen-estrogen ratios. J Clin Endocrinol Metab 1997; 58: 492–499.
2116. Villalpando S, Mondragon L, Barron C, et al. Role of testosterone and dihydrotestosterone in spontaneous gynecomastia of adolescents. Arch Androl 1992; 28:171–176.
2117. Sasano H, Kimura M, Shizawa S, et al. Aromatase and steroid receptors in gynecomastia and male breast carcinoma: an immunohistochemical study. J Clin Endocrinol Metab 1996; 81:3063–3067.
2118. McGrath MH, Mukerji S. Plastic surgery and the teenage patient. J Pediatr Adolesc Gynecol 2000; 13:105–118.
2119. Mohoney J, Hynes B. Concurrent Poland's syndrome and gynecomastia: a case report. Can J Surg 1990; 33:58–60.
2120. Glass AR. Gynecomastia. Endocrinol Metab Clin North Am 1994; 23:825–837.
2121. Hagerman RJ. Neurodevelopmental Disorders. New York, Oxford University Press, 1999.
2122. Merenstein SA, Sobesky WE, Taylor AK, et al. Molecular-clinical correlations in males with an expanded *FMR1* mutation. Am J Med Genet 1996; 64:388–394.
2123. Butler MG, Brunschwig A, Miller LK, Hagerman RJ. Standards for selected anthropometric measurements in males with the fragile X syndrome. Pediatrics 1992; 89:1059–1062.
2124. Hagerman RJ. Physical and behavioral phenotype. In Hagerman

RJ, Cronister A (eds). Fragile X Syndrome: Diagnosis, Treatment and Research. Baltimore, Johns Hopkins University Press, 1996, pp 3–87.

2125. Lachiewicz AM, Dawson DV. Do young boys with fragile X syndrome have macroorchidism? Pediatrics 1994; 93:992–995.
2126. Chudley AE, Hagerman RJ. Fragile X syndrome. J Pediatr 1987; 110:821–830.
2127. Meschede D, Behre HM, Nieschlag E. Endocrine and spermatologic characteristics of 135 patients with bilateral megalotestis. Andrologia 1995; 207–212.
2128. Marshall WA, Tanner JM. Variations in the pattern of pubertal changes in boys. Arch Dis Child 1970; 45:13–23.
2129. Dupertuis CW, Atkinson WB, Elftman H. Sex differences in pubic hair distribution. Hum Biol 2002; 16:137–142.
2130. Billewicz WZ, Fellowes HM, Thomson AM. Pubertal changes in boys and girls in Newcastle upon Tyne. Ann Hum Biol 1981; 8:211–219.
2131. Roy MP, Sempe M, Orssaud E, Pedron G. [Clinical course of puberty in girls (somatic longitudinal study of 80 adolescents)] Evolution clinique de la puberte de la fille (etude longitudinale somatique de 80 adolescentes. Arch Fr Pediatr 1972; 29:155–168.
2132. Van Wieringen JD, Wafelbakker F, Verbrugge HP. Growth Diagrams 1965 Netherlands: Second National Survey on 0–24 Year Olds. Netherlands Institute for Preventative Medicine TNO. Groningen, Wolters-Noordhoof Publishing, 1971.
2133. Neyzi O, Alp H, Yalcindag A, Yakacikli S, Orr DP. Sexual Maturation in Turkish boys. Ann Hum Biol 1975; 2(3):251–259.
2134. Villarreal SF, Martorell R, Mendoza F. Sexual maturation of Mexican-American adolescents. Am J Hum Biol 1989; 1:87–95.
2135. Taranger J, Engstrom I, Lichtenstein H, Svennberg RI. VI. Somatic pubertal development. Acta Paediatr Scand [Suppl] 1976; 121–135.
2136. Waaler PE, Thorsen T, Stoba C, et al. Studies in normal male puberty. Acta Paediatr Scand [Suppl] 1974; 1–36.
2137. Bachrach LK, Hastie T, Wang M, et al. Bone mineral acquisition in healthy Asian, Hispanic, black and Caucasian youth: A longitudinal study. J Clin Endocrinol Metab 1999; 84:4702–4712.
2138. Oerter KE, Manasco P, Barnes KM, Jones J, Hill S, Cutler GBJ. Adult height in precocious puberty after long-term treatment with deslorelin. J Clin Endocrinol Metab 1991; 73:1235–1240.
2139. Boepple PA, Crowley WFJ. Gonadotrophin-releasing hormone analogues as therapeutic probes in human growth and development: Evidence from children with central precocious puberty. Acta Paediatr Scand [Suppl] 1991; 372:33–38.
2140. Rappaport R, Fontoura M, Brauner R. Treatment of central precocious puberty with an LHRH agonist (Buserelin): Effect on growth and bone maturation after three years of treatment. Horm Res 1987; 28:149–154.
2141. Suwa S, Hibi I, Kato K, Nakazima H. LH-RH agonistic analog (buserelin) treatment of precocious puberty: Collaborative study in Japan. Acta Paediatr Jpn 1988; 30(Supp):176–184.
2142. Luder AS, Holland FJ, Costigan DC, Jenner MR, Wielgosz G, Fazekas AT. Intranasal and subcutaneous treatment of central precocious puberty in both sexes with a long-acting analog of luteinizing hormone-releasing hormone. J Clin Endocrinol Metab 1984; 58:966–972.
2142a. Oostdijk W, Hummelink R, Odink RJ, Partsch CJ, Drop SL, Lorenzen F, et al. Treatment of children with central precocious puberty by a slow-release gonadotropin-releasing hormone agonist. Eur J Pediatr 1990; 149:308–313.
2143. Donaldson MD, Stanhope R, Lee TJ, Price DA, Brook CG, Savage DC. Gonadotrophin responses to GnRH in precocious puberty treated with GnRH analogue. Clin Endocrinol (Oxf) 1984; 21:499–503.
2144. Bourguignon JP, Van Vliet G, Vandeweghe M, et al. Treatment of central precocious puberty with an intranasal analogue of GnRH (buserelin). Eur J Pediatr 1987; 146:555–560.
2145. Rime JL, Zumsteg U, Blumberg A, Hadziselimovic F, Girard J, Zurbrugg RP. Long-term treatment of central precocious puberty with an intranasal LHRH analogue: Control of pituitary function by urinary gonadotropins. Eur J Pediatr 1988; 147: 263–269.
2146. Kauli R, Pertzelan A, Ben-Zeev Z, Lewin RP, Kaufman H, Schally AM, et al. Treatment of precocious puberty with LHRH analogue in combination with cyproterone acetate-further experience. Clin Endocrinol (Oxf) 1984; 20:377–387.
2147. Stanhope R, Pringle PJ, Brook CG. Growth, growth hormone and sex steroid secretion in girls with central precocious puberty treated with a gonadotrophin releasing hormone (GnRH) analogue. Acta Paediatr Scand 1988; 77:525–530.

25 Endocrinology and Aging

Steven W. J. Lamberts

The average length of human life is currently 75 to 78 years and may increase to 85 years during the coming ten years,[1] but it is not clear whether these additional years will be satisfactory. Most data indicate a modest gain in the number of healthy years lived but a far greater increase in years of compromised physical, mental, and social function.[2] The number of days with restricted activity and admissions to hospitals and nursing homes increases sharply after 70 years of age.[3] The U.S. National Health Interview Survey indicated that more than 25 million aging people suffer from physical impairment and the number of persons requiring assistance with the activities of daily living increases from 14% at ages 65 to 75 years to 45% in people older than age 85 years.[4, 5]

AGING AND PHYSICAL FRAILTY

Throughout adult life, all physiologic functions start to decline gradually.[6] There is a diminished capacity for cellular protein synthesis, a decline in immune function, an increase in fat mass, a loss of muscle mass and strength, and a decrease in bone mineral density.[6] Most older adults die of atherosclerosis, cancer, or dementia, but in an increasing number of the "healthy" oldest old, loss of muscle strength is the limiting factor that determines their chances of an independent life until death.

Age-related disability is characterized by generalized weakness, impaired mobility and balance, and poor endurance. In the oldest old, this state is termed *physical frailty*, defined as "a state of reduced physiological reserves associated with increased susceptibility to disability."[7] Clinical correlates of physical frailty include falls, fractures, impairment in activities of daily living, and loss of independence. Falls contribute to 40% of admissions to nursing homes.[8]

Loss of muscle strength is an important factor in the development of frailty. Muscle weakness can be caused by aging of muscle fibers and their innervation, osteoarthritis, and chronic debilitating diseases.[9] A sedentary lifestyle, decreased physical activity, and disuse, however, are also important determinants of the decline in muscle strength.

In a study of 100 frail nursing home residents (average age, 87 years), lower extremity muscle mass and strength were closely related.[10] Supervised resistance exercise training (45 minutes three times a week for 10 weeks) doubled muscle strength and significantly increased gait velocity and stair-climbing power. This finding demonstrates that frailty in the elderly population is not an irreversible effect of aging and disease but can be influenced and perhaps even prevented.[10] Further, in nondisabled elderly persons living in the community, objective measures of lower extremity function are highly predictive of subsequent disability.[11] Prevention of frailty can be achieved only by working (training). However, exercise is difficult to implement in the daily routine of the aging population, and the number of dropouts from exercise programs is very high.

Part of the aging process involving body composition (i.e., loss of muscle [strength] and bone, increase in fat mass) might also be related to changes in the endocrine system.[6] Current knowledge has shed light on the effects of long-term hormonal replacement therapy on body composition as well as on atherosclerosis, cancer formation, and cognitive function.

THE ENDOCRINOLOGY OF AGING

The two most important clinical changes in endocrine activity during aging involve the pancreas and the thyroid gland.

Approximately 40% of individuals aged 65 to 74 years and 50% of those older than 80 years have impaired glucose tolerance or diabetes mellitus, and in nearly 50% of elderly adults with diabetes the disease is undiagnosed.[12] These adults are at risk for development of secondary, mainly macrovascular, complications at an accelerated rate. Pancreatic, insulin receptor, and postreceptor changes associated with aging are critical components of the endocrinology of aging. Apart from decreased (relative) insulin secretion by the beta cells, peripheral insulin resistance related to poor diet, physical inactivity, in-

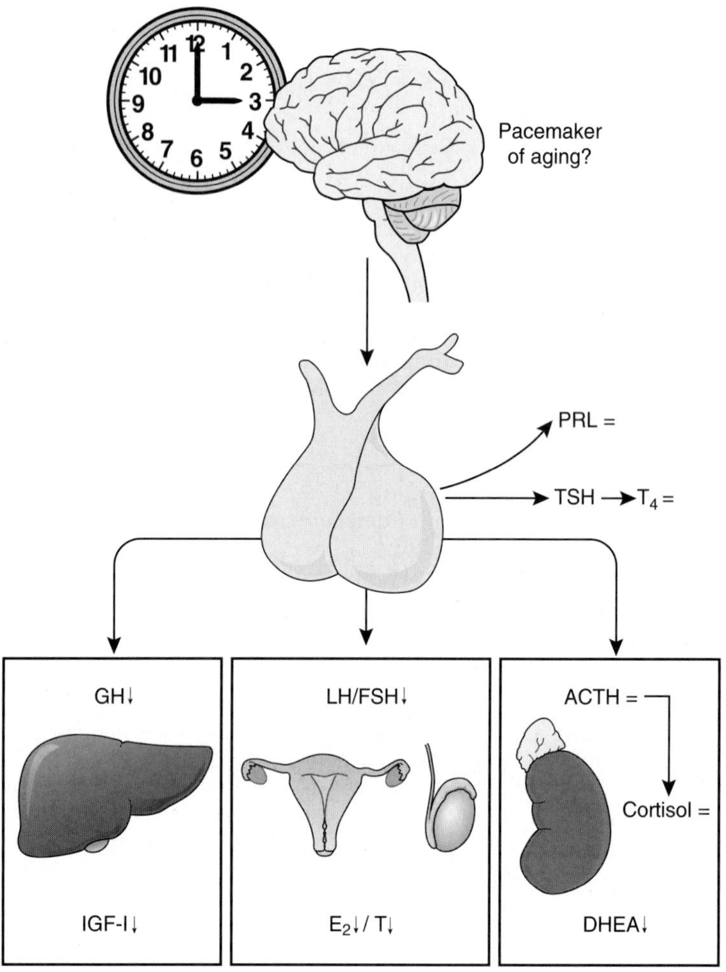

Figure 25–1. During aging, declines in the activities of a number of hormonal systems occur. PRL, prolactin; T_4, thyroxine; TSH, thyrotropin.

Left, A decrease in growth hormone (GH) release by the pituitary gland causes a decrease in the production of insulin-like growth factor I (IGF-I) by the liver and other organs (somatopause).

Middle, A decrease in release of gonadotropin luteinizing hormone (LH) and follicle-stimulating hormone (FSH) and decreased secretion at the gonadal level (from the ovaries, decreased estradiol [E_2] from the testicle, decreased testosterone [T]) cause menopause and andropause, respectively. (Immediately after the initiation of menopause, serum LH and FSH levels increase sharply.)

Right, The adrenocortical cells responsible for the production of dehydroepiandrosterone (DHEA) decrease in activity (adrenopause) without clinically evident changes in corticotropin (adrenocorticotropic hormone, ACTH) and cortisol secretion. A central pacemaker in the hypothalamus or higher brain areas (or both) is hypothesized, which together with changes in the peripheral organs (the ovaries, testicles, and adrenal cortex) regulates the aging process of these endocrine axes.

creased abdominal fat mass, and decreased lean body mass contributes to the deterioration of glucose metabolism.[12] Dietary management, exercise, oral hypoglycemic agents, and insulin are the four components of treatment for these patients, whose medical care is costly and intensive (see Chapter 27).

Age-related thyroid dysfunction is also common.[13] Lowered plasma thyroxine (T_4) and increased thyrotropin concentrations occur in 5% to 10% of elderly women.[13] These abnormalities are mainly caused by autoimmunity and are thus an expression of age-associated disease rather than a consequence of the aging process. Normal aging is accompanied by a slight decrease in pituitary thyrotropin release but especially by decreased peripheral degradation of T_4, which results in a gradual age-dependent decline in serum triiodothyronine (T_3) concentrations without changes in T_4 levels.[13] This slight decrease in plasma T_3 concentrations occurs largely within the broad normal range of the healthy elderly population and has not been convincingly related to functional changes during the aging process. At present, the question of whether healthy aging subjects might benefit from T_3 replacement therapy remains unresolved.

Changes in insulin sensitivity and thyroid function that occur in the aging population are frequently of clinical importance and recognized and treated as diseases. Three other hormonal systems exhibit lowered circulating hormone concentrations during normal aging, and these changes have thus far been considered mainly physiologic (Figs. 25–1 and 25–2). Hormone replacement strategies have been developed, but many aspects remain controversial, and replenishing hormone blood levels to those found in 30- to 50-year-old patients has not yet uniformly proved beneficial and safe.

The most dramatic and rapidly occurring change in women around age 50 years is *menopause*.[14] Cycling estradiol production during the reproductive years is replaced by very low, constant estradiol levels. For many years, the prevailing view was that menopause resulted from exhaustion of ovarian follicles. An alternative perspective is that age-related changes in the central nervous system and the hypothalamic-pituitary unit initiate the menopausal transition. The evidence that both the ovary and the brain are key pacemakers in menopause is compelling.[14]

Changes in the activity of the hypothalamic-pituitary-gonadal axis in men are slower and more subtle. During aging, a gradual decline in serum total and free testosterone levels occurs.[15] *Andropause* is characterized by a decrease in testicular Leydig cell numbers and their secretory capacity as well as by

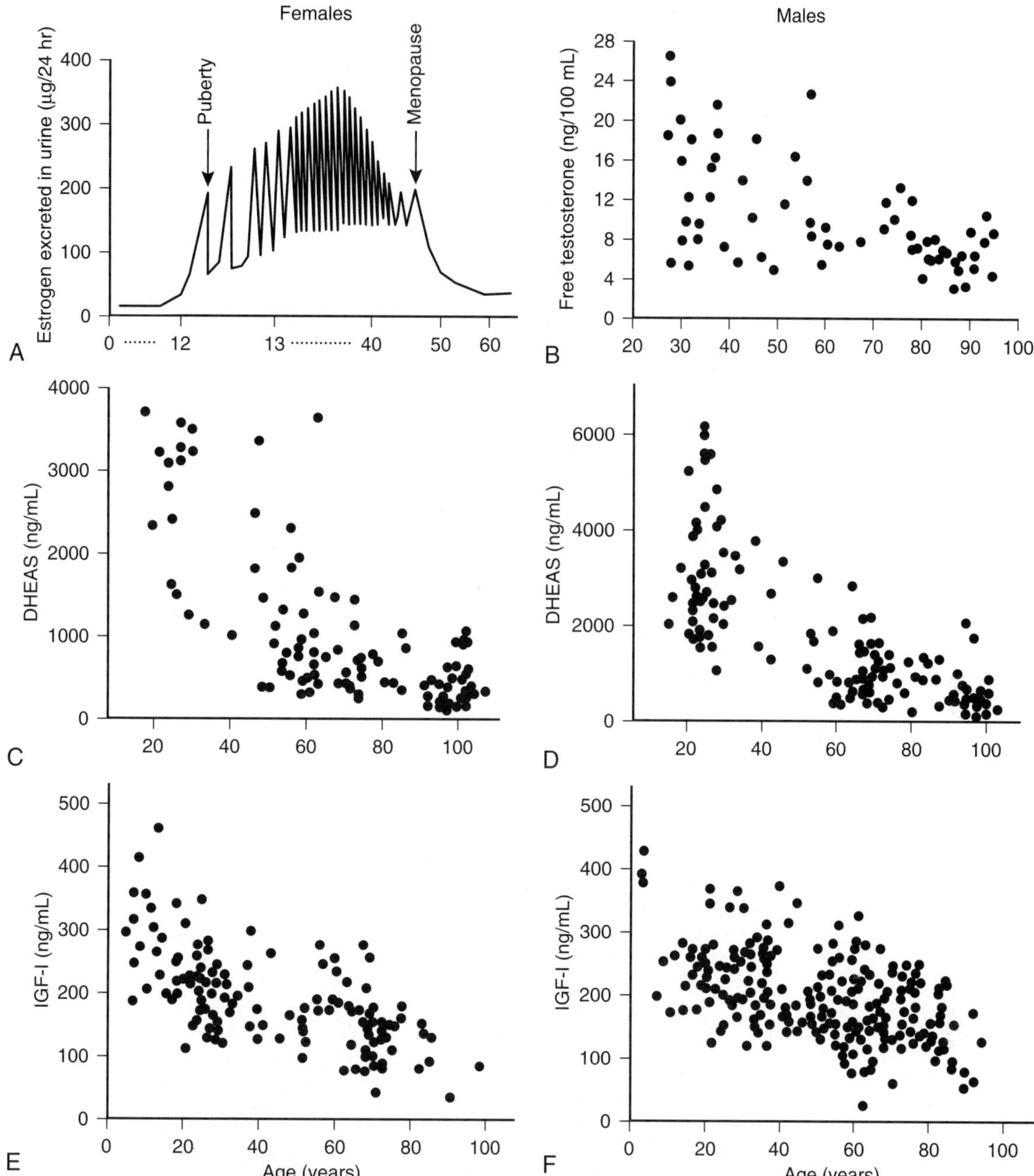

Figure 25–2. Changes in the hormone levels of normal women (*left*) and men (*right*) during the aging process.
A and *B*, Estrogen secretion throughout an individual normal woman's life (expressed as urinary estrogen excretion) (*A*) and mean free testosterone (T) index (the ratio of serum total T to sex hormone–binding globulin levels) during the life span of healthy men (*B*). (From Guyton AC. In Guyton AC [ed]. Textbook of Medical Physiology, 8th ed. Philadelphia, WB Saunders, 1991, pp 899–914.[22])
C and *D*, Serum dehydroepiandrosterone sulfate (DHEAS) concentrations in 114 healthy women (*C*) and 163 healthy men (*D*). (Adapted from Ravaglia G, et al. J Clin Endocrinol Metab 1996; 81:1173–1178.[19])
E and *F*, The course of serum insulin-like growth factor I (IGF-I) concentrations in 131 healthy women (*E*) and 223 healthy men (*F*) during aging. Note the difference in the distribution of ages in the different panels. (Adapted from Corpas E, et al. Endocr Rev 1993; 14:20–39.[21])

an age-related decrease in episodic and stimulated gonadotropin secretion.[16, 17]

The second hormonal system demonstrating age-related changes is *adrenopause*, a term that describes the gradual decline in circulating levels of dehydroepiandrosterone (DHEA) and its sulfate (DHEAS).[18, 19] Adrenal secretion of DHEA gradually decreases over time, while corticotropin secretion, which is physiologically linked to plasma cortisol levels, remains largely unchanged. The decline in DHEA and DHEAS levels in both sexes, therefore, contrasts with the maintenance of plasma cortisol levels and seems to be caused by a selective decrease in the number of functional zona reticularis cells in the adrenal cortex instead of being regulated by a central (hypothalamic) pacemaker of aging.[20]

The third endocrine system that gradually declines in activity during aging is the growth hormone (GH)–insulin-like

Table 25–1. Lifetime Disease Probability for a 50-Year-Old White Woman with or without Treatment with Long-Term Hormone Replacement

Disease	Lifetime Probability* (%) No Treatment	E_2 + P	Relative Risk
Coronary heart disease	46.1	30.4†	0.66
Stroke	19.8	19.3	0.96
Fractures	30–40	15–28	0.50–0.70
Dementia	16.3	11.5†	0.71
Breast cancer	10.2	13.5–18.4	1.35–1.80
Endometrial cancer	2.6	2.6	1.00
Life expectancy (years)	82.8	83.8	

*The estimated lifetime probabilities of developing the conditions mentioned have been derived from mortality and incidence data from the 1987 Vital Statistics of the United States. The relative risks are the best estimates of the relative risk for developing each condition in long-term hormone users compared with nonusers. These estimates were derived from a model of the risks and benefits of hormone therapy developed by Grady et al.[26]

A number of limitations and assumptions must be considered when interpreting this table: The duration of the use and dose regimens of E_2 + P varied considerably between studies included in the meta-analysis (duration, 2–10 years). It was assumed that the addition of progestagen to the estrogen regimen would increase the risk for breast cancer from 1.35 to 1.80.[31]

†Data from Barrett-Connor. BMJ 1998; 317:457–461.[27]

E_2 + P, estrogen plus progestagen.

From a meta-analysis by Grady D, Rubin SM, Petitti DB, et al. Hormone therapy to prevent disease and prolong life in postmenopausal women. Ann Intern Med 1992; 117:1016–1037.

growth factor I (IGF-I) axis (see Fig. 25–2).[6, 21] Mean pulse amplitude and duration and fraction of GH secreted, but not pulse frequency, gradually decrease during aging. In parallel, a progressive drop in circulating IGF-I levels occurs in both sexes.[21, 23] There is no evidence for a peripheral factor in this process of *somatopause*, and its triggering pacemaker seems mainly localized in the hypothalamus because pituitary somatotropes, even of the oldest old, can be restored to their youthful secretory capacity by treatment with GH-releasing peptides (see later).

It is unclear whether changes in gonadal function (menopause, andropause) are interrelated with the processes of adrenopause and somatopause, which occur in both men and women. Also, functional correlates (muscle size and function, fat and bone mass, progression of atherosclerosis, and changes in cognitive function) have not been related to these changes in endocrine activity. However, a number of effects of normal aging closely resemble features of (isolated) hormonal deficiency (hypogonadism, GH deficiency), which in subjects in middle adulthood are successfully reversed by replacement of the appropriate hormone.[24, 25] Although aging does not simply result from a variety of hormone deficiency states, medical intervention in the processes of menopause, andropause, adrenopause, or somatopause might prevent or delay some aspects of the aging process.

MENOPAUSE

Menopause is the permanent cessation of menstruation resulting from the loss of ovarian follicular function and is diagnosed retrospectively after 12 months of amenorrhea.

In most women, vasomotor reactions, depressed mood, and urogenital complaints accompany this period of estrogen decline. In the subsequent years, the loss of estrogens is followed by a high incidence of cardiovascular disease, loss of bone mass, and cognitive impairment. The average age of menopause (51.4 years) has not changed over time and seems to be largely determined by genetic factors.

The use of *hormone replacement therapy* (HRT), consisting of estrogen or estrogen plus progestagen, can alleviate the symptoms of menopause (*perimenopausal* use), but long-term use of HRT (5 to 10 years or more) may also be advantageous in preventing cardiovascular disease, bone loss, and cognitive impairment.[26–29]

Perimenopausal Use of Hormone Replacement Therapy

Typical symptoms that result from the sudden decrease in estrogen production around menopause are menstrual cycle disorders, vasomotor changes (hot flushes, night sweats), and urogenital complications (atrophic vaginal irritation and dryness, dyspareunia, atrophic urethral epithelium leading to micturition disorders). Additional symptoms are irritability, mood swings, joint pain, and sleep disturbances. Frequency, severity, onset, and duration of symptoms vary widely between individuals and between ethnic groups. About 75% of women in Western societies experience so few troublesome symptoms during the menopausal transition that HRT is not needed or requested.[27]

HRT rapidly alleviates the symptoms of menopause. Hot flushes and vasomotor instability as well as symptoms of urogenital atrophy rapidly disappear upon the start of HRT.

Long-Term Hormone Replacement Therapy

Because life expectancy is increasing, the time a woman spends after menopause constitutes more than one third of her life. Long-term use of HRT (5 to 10 years) seems to have advantages with regard to the prevention of the three chronic disorders most common in the elderly: (1) cardiovascular diseases, (2) osteoporosis, and (3) dementia. There are, however, also important adverse effects of long-term estrogen-progestagen replacement therapy after menopause. The most compelling problem is the increased incidence of breast cancer.[26, 28, 30, 31]

Lifetime probabilities of disease occurrence for a 50-year-old white woman entering menopause without or with subsequent HRT are presented in Table 25–1.[26]

Coronary Heart Disease and Stroke

Nearly every observational study has demonstrated a decreased risk of heart disease in women who ever used estrogen. Meta-analyses of 25 published studies of women who used estrogen and 7 studies that separately assessed estrogen plus progestagen treatment found summary relative risks of 0.70 and 0.66, respectively, for coronary heart disease among women.[27] The apparent benefit is largely limited to current or recent estrogen use. HRT does not play a role in *secondary* prevention; progression of coronary atherosclerosis in women with established disease was not influenced.[32] HRT was not consistently associated with a reduced risk of stroke.[26]

The mechanism of cardioprotection remains uncertain but probably involves multiple actions. Estrogen is an antioxidant and calcium blocker and induces beneficial effects on concentrations of serum low-density lipoprotein (LDL) cholesterol (lowering) and high-density lipoprotein (HDL) cholesterol (increasing). Added progestagen attenuates these estradiol-mediated effects experimentally, but epidemiologically there is no convincing evidence for a decreased effect of combined therapy in comparison with estrogen alone in the primary prevention of coronary disease.[27]

Bone Loss

Osteoporosis is characterized by low bone mass and microarchitectural deterioration of bone tissue, leading to increased bone fragility and, therefore, to fracture susceptibility. The lifetime risk of fractures in 50-year-old white women is 30% to 40% (see Table 25–1).

The efficacy of HRT on the main sites of osteoporotic fractures has been documented in case-control and cohort studies but only in a few prospective controlled trials.[26, 33] Current use of HRT, especially long-term use, is associated with a reduction in the risk of hip fractures by about 30% and of spine fractures by about 50%. Most osteoporotic fractures occur after age 65. Long-term use is necessary to decrease the incidence of fractures substantially. After HRT is stopped, bone loss resumes within a year and bone turnover increases to the levels observed in untreated women within 3 to 6 months, which probably accounts for the lack of fracture protection in past users.[34]

Estrogen reduces bone turnover and increases bone density in postmenopausal women in part because it improves calcium homeostasis. The addition of calcium potentiates the effect of estrogen on bone mass. The further addition of androgens (low-dose testosterone) or an antiresorptive drug (bisphosphonates) may further increase bone formation in women most at risk for fractures.

Dementia

A number of experimental studies indicate that estrogens may directly influence the brain by a number of mechanisms, including activation of the cholinergic system, inhibition of oxidative stress and neuronal apoptosis, and an increase in synaptic plasticity. Estrogen may also, through its effects on the cardiovascular system, reduce the risk of vascular dementia.[35]

Several studies have suggested that HRT improves cognition, prevents development of dementia, and decreases the severity of dementia, but other studies have not shown this benefit of estrogen use.[36, 37]

It is now well recognized that cognition improves in perimenopausal women using HRT. However, most studies suggest that this improvement occurs because menopausal symptoms are alleviated and that there is no clear beneficial effect of HRT on cognition in asymptomatic women.[37]

Ten observational studies have measured the effect of postmenopausal estrogen use on the risk of development of dementia. A meta-analysis of these studies suggested a 29% decreased risk of dementia among estrogen users.[37] However, results of eight small uncontrolled trials of estrogen use in women with dementia or Alzheimer's disease did not demonstrate a clear benefit for cognition.[38]

Given the limited data, no definite conclusions can be reached about the effect of HRT in reducing cognitive decline and dementia in older women. Although the data available are promising, HRT is not currently recommended for the prevention or treatment of dementia.[39]

Other Benefits

HRT is associated with slightly longer overall survival. Apart from the clear, rapidly occurring effect on menopausal symptoms, no improvement in quality of life was observed in asymptomatic older women receiving HRT.

Breast and Endometrial Cancer

Late menopause has long been known to be associated with an increased risk, and early menopause with a reduced risk, of breast cancer. This observation is consistent with the idea that prolonged exposure to endogenous estrogen is an adverse risk factor. For every 1-year increase in age at menopause, there is about a 3% increase in the risk of breast cancer.[30]

Most studies have found no increased risk of breast cancer in women who had ever used estrogen, usually for less than 2 years in the perimenopausal period. The relative risk increase for breast cancer in HRT users seems largely confined to current or recent use.

A meta-analysis of more than 50 studies clearly demonstrated that the risk of breast cancer increases with long-term estrogen use.[40] Among women who used estrogen for 5 years or longer (median use, 11 years), the summary relative risk for breast cancer was 1.35. Among 1000 women who used HRT continuously for 10 years starting at age 50 years, it was estimated that there would be an additional six breast cancers, raising the incidence from a background of 45 cases to 51 cases. However, these data mainly refer to the use of estrogens only. In the Breast Cancer Detection Demonstration Project, in which 46,000 women participated, the estrogen-progestagen regimens were associated with greater increases in breast cancer risk compared with estrogen alone.[31] The excess risk increased by 8% for each year of combined hormone use and by 1% for each year of estrogen-only use. Thus, risk of breast cancer would be predicted to increase by approximately 80% after 10 years of estrogen-progestagen use.[41]

An association between endometrial cancer and estrogen use was observed many years ago. Ten years of unopposed estrogen use increases the risk for endometrial cancer 10-fold.[26] For this reason, the HRT regimens were supplemented with progestagens, which almost completely prevented this excess risk for endometrial cancer.

Other Risks

HRT doubles a woman's risk of needing gallbladder surgery. It also doubles the risk of deep vein thrombosis and pulmonary embolism; however, the absolute risk is low, about 3 cases per 10,000 treated women per year.

Hormone Replacement Regimens

As described by Barrett-Connor,[27] presently advised doses of estrogen were designed to prevent bone loss, and progestagen regimens were proposed to prevent endometrial cancer. The advice, however, has not been based on studies of a wide range of doses. Several estrogen and progestagen preparations are available for HRT (Table 25–2). Components of available preparations vary in their effects on different target tissues. Commercial preparations differ in their clinical effects by design, and individual women differ in their responses. HRT can be administered orally, transdermally, topically, intranasally, or as subcutaneous implants.

Estrogen has distinct route-dependent effects on somatotropic action. Oral estrogens probably lower serum IGF-I concentrations through impairment of hepatic IGF-I production. This effect does not occur after transdermal estrogen administration.[43] Increasing evidence suggests that transdermally administered estrogen thus has more beneficial effects on protein metabolism and body composition.

Prevention of endometrial hyperplasia and cancer induction by estrogen depends on both dose and duration of progestagen use. Uterine protection requires 12 days of cyclic progestagens or combined continuous regimens. The former causes sched-

Table 25–2. Hormone Replacement Regimens

Bone-Conserving Estrogen Doses*	
Conjugated equine estrogens	0.625 mg/day
Estrogen sulfate	1.5 mg/day
Estradiol 17β	
Oral	1–2 mg/day
Transdermal	0.05 mg/day
Implant	50 mg 6 monthly
***Oral Progesterone Doses for Endometrial Protection*†**	
Norgestrel	0.15 mg
Noresthisterone	1 mg
Medroxyprogesterone acetate‡	10 mg
Dydrogesterone	10 mg
Micronized progesterone	200 mg

*These are average doses for a postmenopausal woman in her sixth decade. Younger women may require higher doses; older women may require less.

†These minimum doses are protective when given for 12 days per calendar month.

‡Equally protective as 2.5 mg daily continually throughout calendar month.

Data from Barrett-Connor E. BMJ 1998; 317:457–461[27]; Clinical Synthesis Panel on HRT. Lancet 1999; 354:152–155[28]; and Stevenson JC. Menopause 1996; 243–245.[42]

uled bleeding and the latter causes unpredictable spotting or bleeding, which usually resolves within 9 months.[28, 42]

Initially after the start of HRT, side effects, including mastalgia, bloating, bleeding, premenstrual tension, and depression, can occur. To prevent these side effects but also to increase compliance, it is generally recommended that the patient start with half the estrogen dose.

Data indicate a close relationship between endogenous circulating estrogen levels and bone loss, bone mineral density, and fractures.[44] Women with detectable serum estradiol concentrations (8 to 92 pmol/L; 5 to 25 pg/mL) had higher bone mineral density, significantly less bone loss, and a lower risk for subsequent hip fractures than women with undetectable estradiol levels. These findings suggest that much lower estrogen doses might be sufficient to maintain bone than those indicated in Table 25–2.

Indications for Hormone Replacement Therapy

Perimenopausal or menopausal HRT is strongly indicated for women having premature menopause, women with clinically important symptoms of the menopausal transition, and women entering menopause with osteoporosis.

The concept that long-term HRT after menopause is an effective risk reduction strategy for coronary heart disease, fractures, and cognitive decline has to be balanced against the increased risk of breast cancer. The decision to start long-term HRT should be based on an individual's risk factors, attitude toward hormonal treatment, and knowledge of its risks and benefits. Individualization of the treatment decision is mandatory. Both knowledge and education influence the decision to start HRT; in a Swedish study, only 24% of women 54 years of age but 72% of female general practitioners and 88% of female gynecologists were receiving estrogen-progestagen replacement therapy.[45]

Selective Estrogen Receptor Modulators

A new development in the search for optimal hormone replacement therapy during menopause came from observations that tamoxifen has variable antiestrogenic and estrogenic actions in different tissues.[46, 47] Tamoxifen suppresses the growth of estrogen receptor–positive breast cancer cells. Long-term treatment of menopausal patients with breast cancer with tamoxifen also lowered the incidence of new (contralateral) breast cancer by 40%. In addition, the number of cardiovascular incidents decreased by 70%, and the age-related decrease in bone mineral density was partially prevented.[48–50]

These initially puzzling observations were explained by the fact that tamoxifen and other compounds such as raloxifene have selective estrogen receptor–modulating effects, exerting antiestrogenic actions on normal and cancerous breast tissue but agonistic actions on bone, lipids, and the blood vessel walls.[51–53] These effects of tamoxifen and raloxifene may be explained by differential stabilization of the conformation of the estrogen receptor but might also be related to the activation of different estrogen receptor forms, in which the α form is the classical estrogen receptor, whereas a β form mediates the vascular and bone effects of estrogens.[54, 55]

Raloxifene is the second selective estrogen receptor modulator (SERM) available for clinical use in menopausal women. It demonstrates estrogen agonist activity on bone and lipid metabolism and has estrogen antagonist activity in uterine and breast tissue. The 60-mg dose is currently approved for the prevention and treatment of postmenopausal osteoporosis.

The efficacy and safety of raloxifene for the prevention of osteoporosis in postmenopausal women were proved in a study that demonstrated a 2.5% increase in bone mineral density in the lumbar spine and hip in a group of postmenopausal nonosteoporotic women treated with raloxifene for 2 years.[56] A significant reduction of vertebral fracture risk by raloxifene was subsequently demonstrated.[57] A total of 7705 postmenopausal women with existing osteoporosis were studied. After 36 months, bone mineral density at the hip and spine increased in the women treated with 60 mg of raloxifene by 2.1% and 2.6%, respectively, compared with those receiving placebo. At 36 months, 7.4% of women had at least one new vertebral fracture, including 10.1% of women receiving placebo and 6.6% of those receiving raloxifene at 60 mg/day. Compared with the placebo group, those receiving 60 mg of raloxifene had a relative risk for fracture of 0.7 ($P < .001$). Forty-six subjects needed raloxifene at 60 mg for 3 years to prevent one vertebral fracture in menopausal women without an existing fracture; for those with an existing fracture, 16 subjects required treatment.

Raloxifene has effects on lipids similar to those of estrogen, except for a relatively small effect on high-density lipoprotein cholesterol and no significant effect on triglycerides.[56, 58] Data on cardiovascular event rates and on cognitive function are not yet available.

Raloxifene, in contrast to tamoxifen and estrogen, does not stimulate endometrial thickness or vaginal bleeding.[56, 59] With regard to side effects, raloxifene causes an increased incidence of leg cramps and hot flashes.[60]

A most promising effect of raloxifene is its chemoprotective action against breast cancer. Cummings and colleagues[61] reported the effects in 7705 postmenopausal women (mean age, 66.5 years) with osteoporosis who were treated for a median of 40 months with placebo or raloxifene at 60 or 120 mg/day. Thirteen cases of breast cancer were confirmed among the women assigned to raloxifene compared with 27 among the women assigned to placebo (relative risk 0.24; $P < .001$). To prevent one case of breast cancer, 126 women would need to be treated. Raloxifene decreased the risk of estrogen receptor–positive breast cancer by 90% but did not affect the risk of estrogen receptor–negative invasive breast cancer. This important study demonstrated that among postmenopausal women with osteoporosis, the risk of invasive breast cancer was decreased by 76% during 3 years of treatment with raloxifene (Fig. 25–3).

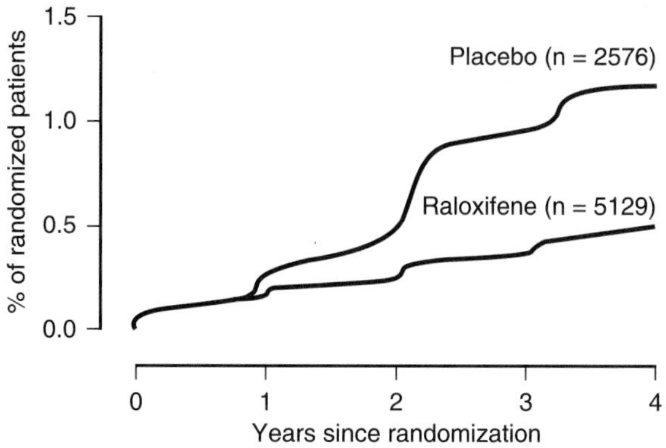

Figure 25–3. Effect of raloxifene administration (60 to 120 mg/day) on the cumulative incidence of breast cancer in 7705 postmenopausal women (mean age, 66.5 years) with osteoporosis. Statistical significance of the difference between the groups was $P < .001$. (From Cummings SR, Eckert S, Krueger KA, et al. The effect of raloxifene on risk of breast cancer in postmenopausal women: results from the MORE randomized trial. Multiple Outcomes of Raloxifene Evaluation. JAMA 1999; 281:2189–2197.)

Hormone Replacement Therapy, Selective Estrogen Receptor Modulators, or No Treatment?

The issue of hormonal intervention for postmenopausal women is controversial, and many aspects remain unresolved. The idea that HRT is a global risk reduction strategy is being reevaluated.[27, 29] Although the general clinical benefits of HRT in the short term during and after the menopausal transition are clear, the balance of the beneficial effects of long-term HRT after menopause versus negative effects, especially on breast cancer incidence, remains worrisome.

Currently, a vast armamentarium of pharmacologic treatments to reduce cardiovascular and bone risks is available; these include cholesterol-lowering statins, β-blockers, SERMs, and bisphosphonates. An optimal choice of these different lifestyle drugs for menopausal women requires individualization of the treatment decision. Coronary artery disease, for example, is a complex disorder, resulting from an interaction of genetic predisposition and environmental factors. Risk factor modification (diet, smoking, physical activity) should be advised. Primary prevention of coronary artery disease with HRT seems effective; more effective for existing atherosclerosis are lipid-lowering drugs, aspirin, nitrates, and β-blockers.[62]

For women with existing osteoporosis, HRT is very effective. However, SERMs and bisphosphonates come close in their fracture-reducing effects. Recognition of an increased risk for breast cancer in menopausal women is an important consideration in the choice of SERMs. If the impressive preventive effect of raloxifene on breast cancer is confirmed to last much longer than 3 years, chemoprevention of breast cancer will probably become a major consideration in the pharmacologic choice for risk reduction in the long-term preventive treatment of postmenopausal women.

ANDROPAUSE

Role of Testosterone during Aging

Age-associated hypogonadism does not develop as clearly in men at andropause as in women at menopause. The key difference is the gradual, often subtle change in androgen levels in men versus the precipitate fall of estrogen production in women. It is generally agreed that as men age, there is a decline in serum total testosterone concentration that begins after the age of 40 years. In cross-sectional studies, the annual decline in total and free testosterone is 0.4% and 1.2%, respectively. The higher decline in free testosterone levels is related to the increase in sex hormone–binding globulin (SHBG) levels with age.[15, 63]

It remains unclear whether the well-known biologic changes occurring during aging in men (e.g., reduced sexual activity, muscle mass and strength, and skeletal mineralization) are causally related to these changes in testosterone bioactivity (andropause).

In a group of more than 400 independently living elderly men (mean age, 78 years; range, 73 to 94 years), Beld and colleagues[64] observed a positive association between total and free serum testosterone concentrations and muscle strength as well as an inverse relationship with fat mass. Low bioavailable testosterone was associated with a depressed mood[65] in a population-based study of 856 men aged 50 to 89 years.

Testosterone Replacement Therapy

Many persuasive reports in the literature demonstrate that testosterone replacement in men of all ages (young, adult, and old) with clear clinical and biochemical hypogonadism instantly reverses vasomotor activity (flushes and sweats); improves libido, sexual activity, and mood; increases muscle mass, strength, and bone mineralization; prevents fractures; decreases fat mass; and decreases fatigue and poor concentration.[24, 63, 66] Also, the treatment of normal adult men with supraphysiologic doses of testosterone, especially when combined with resistance exercise training, increased fat-free mass and muscle size and strength.[67]

Most studies reporting the results of androgen therapy in older men were small, short-term, noncontrolled, and without uniform end points. The results of a large randomized study in healthy elderly men have now been published and seem representative for effects expected of androgen therapy.[68, 69] Ninety-six men (mean age 73 years) wore a testosterone patch on their scrotum (6 mg of testosterone per 24 hours) or a placebo patch for 36 months. Mean serum testosterone concentrations in the men treated with testosterone increased from 12.7 ± 2.9 nmol/L (367 ± 7.9 ng/dL) before treatment to 21.7 ± 8.6 nmol/L (625 ± 249 ng/dL; $P < .001$) at 6 months of treatment and remained at that level for the duration of the study. The decrease in fat mass (−3.0 ± 0.5 kg) in the testosterone-treated men during the 36 months of treatment was significantly different from the decrease (−0.7 ± 0.5 kg) in the placebo-treated men ($P < .001$) (Fig. 25–4). The increase in lean mass (1.9 ± 0.3 kg) in the testosterone-treated men was significantly different from that in the placebo-treated men (0.2 ± 0.2 kg; $P < .001$).

Changes in knee extension and flexion strength, hand grip, walking speed, and other parameters of muscle strength and function were not significantly different in the two groups. Bone mineral density in the lumbar spine increased in both the testosterone-treated (4.2% ± 0.8%) and placebo-treated (2.5% ± 0.6%) groups, but mean changes did not differ between groups (see Fig. 25–4). However, the lower the pretreatment serum testosterone concentration, the greater the effects of testosterone treatment on lumbar spine bone density after 36 months ($P = .02$). A minimal effect (0.9 ± 1.0%) of testosterone treatment on bone mineral density was observed in men with a pretreatment serum testosterone concentration of 13.9 nmol/L (400 ng/dL), but an increase of 5.9% ± 2.2% was found in men with a pretreatment testosterone concentration of 6.9 nmol/L (200 ng/dL).

The subjective perception of physical function decreased significantly during the 36 months of treatment in the placebo-

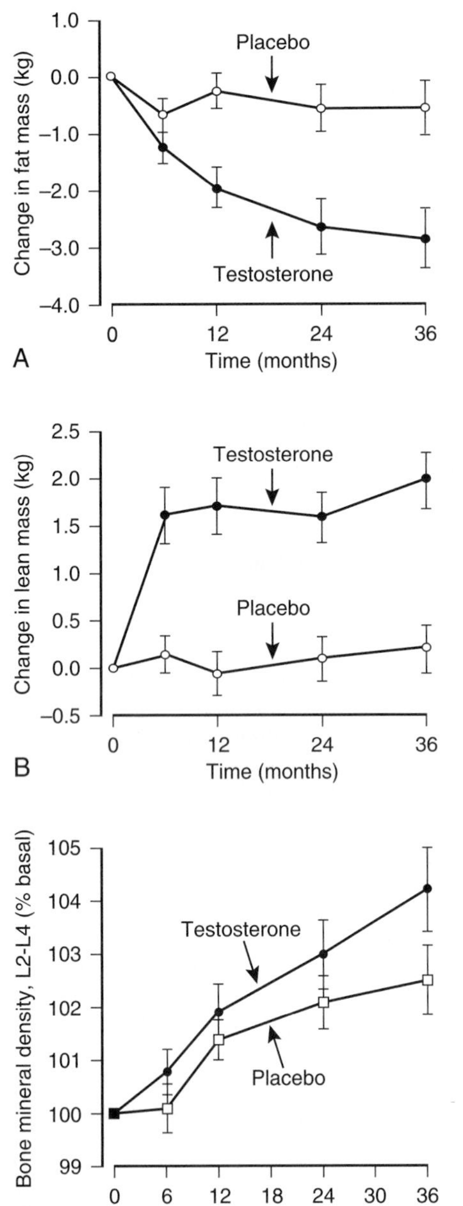

Figure 25–4. *A–C,* Mean (± standard error) change from baseline in fat mass, lean mass, and bone mineral density of the lumbar spine (L2 to L4) as determined by dual-energy x-ray absorptiometry in 108 men older than 65 years who were treated with either testosterone or placebo (54 men each). The decrease in fat mass ($P < .005$) and the increase in lean mass ($P < .01$) in the testosterone-treated subjects were significantly different from those in placebo-treated subjects at 36 months. Bone mineral density increased significantly in both groups. (*A* and *B*, from Snyder PJ, et al. J Clin Endocrinol Metab 1999; 84: 1966–1972[68]; *C*, from Snyder PJ, et al. J Clin Endocrinol Metab 1999; 84:2647–2653.[69])

treated ($P < .001$) but not in the testosterone-treated group. Interestingly, the effect of testosterone treatment on the perception of physical functioning varied inversely with the pretreatment serum testosterone concentration ($P < .01$). There was no significant difference between the two treatment groups with regard to the subjective perception of energy or sexual functions.

With regard to the potential adverse effects of testosterone treatment in healthy elderly men, again the study by Snyder and colleagues[68] seems representative. The mean serum prostate-specific antigen (PSA) concentration did not change during the 36 months of treatment in the placebo-treated group but increased by a relatively small but statistically significant ($P < .001$) amount by 6 months of treatment in the testosterone-treated group and remained relatively stable for the remainder of the study. The urine flow rate, volume of urine in the bladder after voiding, and number of clinically significant prostate events during the 3 years of the study were similar in the two groups. Hemoglobin and hematocrit did not change in the placebo-treated group during treatment, but both increased significantly ($P < .001$) in the testosterone-treated group within 6 months and remained relatively stable for the remainder of the study. Three men treated with testosterone developed persistent erythrocytosis (hemoglobin > 17.5 g/dL; hematocrit > 52%) during treatment.

Other androgen replacement studies in older men have demonstrated that lipid profiles are not adversely affected by this therapy, but the incidence of cardiovascular events in healthy elderly men who receive androgens for extended periods has not been studied.[63, 70, 71]

Numerous studies of large populations of healthy men have shown a marked rise in the incidence of impotence to over 50% in men 60 to 70 years old.[72] Although this increased rate occurs in the same age group who show a clear decline in serum (free) testosterone levels, no causal relationships have been demonstrated. In most instances, testosterone replacement therapy in elderly men is not effective for the treatment of loss of libido or impotence in individuals with serum testosterone concentrations within the normal range in age-matched subjects. Other factors, such as atherosclerosis, alcohol consumption, smoking, and the quality of personal relationships, seem to be more important.[73, 74] Only in the case of clear hypogonadism is the decrease in libido and testosterone restored by potency therapy.[24, 66] This result suggests that there is a threshold level of testosterone in the low normal range below which libido and sexual function are impaired and above which there is no further enhancement of response.[75]

Summarizing the available literature, the indiscriminate (preventive) treatment of healthy elderly men with testosterone at a dose that increases serum testosterone concentrations to those observed in 20- to 30-year-olds has limited anabolic effects on body composition (a slight decrease in fat mass and a slight increase in muscle mass). No beneficial effects on muscle strength or physical performance are observed.

Detailed analyses of a number of studies of elderly men selected on the basis of low pretreatment serum testosterone concentrations indicated a beneficial effect of testosterone replacement therapy on muscle strength, bone mineral density, mood, and (subjective) aspects of the quality of life.[70, 73, 76] This introduces the question of how to select elderly men who might benefit from testosterone treatment.

There is great interindividual variation in serum testosterone concentrations among healthy men. In adulthood, the biochemical definition of male hypogonadism is generally accepted if serum total testosterone is below 10.4 to 12.1 nmol/L (300 to 500 ng/dL), depending on the population studied[63] (Fig. 25–5). Of healthy men between the ages of 60 to 80 years, 20% demonstrated a serum testosterone concentration below 10.4 nmol/L (300 ng/dL). In the same study, non-SHBG testosterone levels were below the lower limit for young men (<1.6 nmol/L) in over 60% of these men.[63]

An important question is how to define true hypogonadism in elderly men. Because many signs and symptoms of hypogonadism coincide with those observed during the normal aging process, no good single measure of clinically significant hypogonadism is available.[63] In a discussion of testosterone replacement in older men,[71, 73] it was suggested that the biochemical diagnosis of hypogonadism seems certain if the serum total testosterone concentration is less than 7.0 nmol/L (200

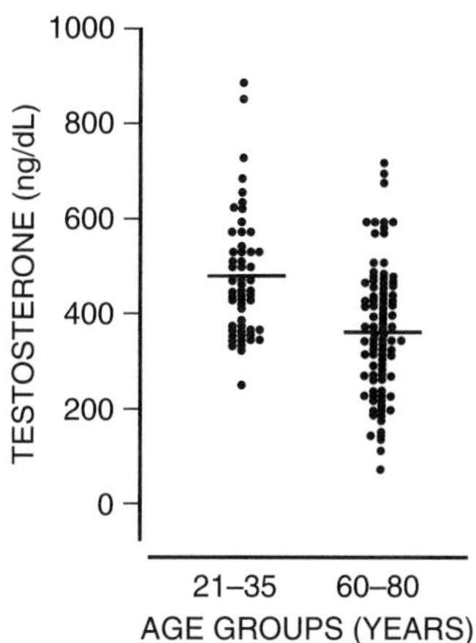

Figure 25–5. Serum total testosterone levels in a group of healthy young (*n* = 58; aged 21 to 35 years) and older (*n* = 96; aged 60 to 80 years) men. Mean ± standard deviation. Serum total testosterone is 18.2 ± 4.2 nmol/L (525 ± 122 ng/dL) for the young men and 14.5 ± 4.5 nmol/L (420 ± 12.9 ng/dL) for the older men. (From Tenover JS. Androgen administration to aging men. Endocrinol Metab Clin North Am 1994; 23:877–892.)

ng/dL). This cutoff remains arbitrary and does not answer the question of whether healthy elderly men with testosterone levels between 7.0 and 10.4 nmol/L are hypogonadal or whether such men would benefit from replacement therapy with testosterone. Also, it has been demonstrated that intercurrent diseases frequently result in a transient, sharp drop in serum testosterone concentrations,[77] whereas frail, elderly men in general tend to have testosterone levels 10% to 15% lower than those of healthy, age-matched control subjects.[78]

When a serum testosterone concentration is found to be below 7.0 nmol/L (200 ng/dL), an additional evaluation with measurements of serum gonadotropins and prolactin is mandatory in order to exclude pituitary pathology.

Conclusions

Testosterone at supraphysiologic doses, when administered to eugonadal men, increases muscle mass and strength. Replacement therapy directed at restoring serum testosterone in healthy elderly men to levels observed between the ages of 30 and 50 years lowers fat mass and increases lean mass to a limited extent without a beneficial effect on muscle strength and physical performance. It remains uncertain whether testosterone replacement produces clinically meaningful improvements in muscle function without significant adverse effects in frail older men or in elderly men with serum testosterone concentrations between 7.0 and 11.4 nmol/L.

If one decides to start testosterone replacement, the major goal of therapy is to return testosterone levels to values as close to "physiologic" levels in age-matched controls as possible. The dose should thus be titrated according to serum levels. Considerations concerning the choice of testosterone preparation as well as the route of administration (oral, injectable, implantable, or transdermal) are discussed in Chapter 8.

At present, the duration of testosterone administration is uncertain. Control of prostate size, PSA levels, and hematocrit is mandatory. The identification of elderly men who might benefit most from testosterone treatment remains uncertain, and the risks to the prostate and possible effects on the process of atherosclerosis require further study. The development of androgenic compounds with variable biologic action in different organs (selective androgen receptor modulation) is currently being pursued.[79]

ADRENOPAUSE

Role of Dehydroepiandrosterone during Aging

Humans are unique among primates and rodents because the human adrenal cortex secretes large amounts of the steroid precursor DHEA and its sulfate derivative DHEAS.[80] Serum DHEAS concentrations in adult men and women are 100 to 500 times higher than those of testosterone and 1000 to 10,000 times higher than those of estradiol. In normal subjects, serum concentrations of DHEA and its sulfate are highest in the third decade of life, after which the concentrations of both gradually decrease, so that by the age of 70 to 80 years, the values are about 20% of peak values in men and 30% of peak values in women[19] (see Fig. 25–2).

DHEA and DHEAS seem to be inactive precursors that are transformed within human tissues by a complicated network of enzymes into androgens or estrogens, or both (Fig. 25–6). The key enzymes are aromatase, steroid sulfatase, 3β-hydroxysteroid dehydrogenases (3β-HSD-1, -2), and at least seven organ-specific 17β-hydroxysteroid dehydrogenases (17β-HSD-1 to -7). Labrie and colleagues[80] introduced the term *intracrinology* to describe this synthesis of active steroids in peripheral target tissues in which the action is exerted in the same cells in which synthesis takes place, without release into the extracellular space and general circulation.

In postmenopausal women, nearly 100% of sex steroids are synthesized in peripheral tissues from precursors of adrenal origin except for a small contribution from ovarian or adrenal testosterone and androstenedione. Thus, in postmenopausal women, virtually all active sex steroids are made in target tissues by an intracrine mechanism. In elderly men, the intracrine production of androgens is also important; less than 50% of the androgen supply is derived from testicular production.

The high secretion rate of adrenal precursor sex steroids in men and women differs from that in laboratory animal models, in which the secretion of sex steroids occurs exclusively in the gonads. In rats and mice, long-term administration of DHEA prevented obesity, diabetes mellitus, cancer, and heart disease and enhanced immune function.[18, 20, 81]

These experimental animal data have been used to argue that DHEA administration in adult or elderly individuals prolongs life span and might be an "elixir of youth." Supportive data in humans are few, however, and highly controversial. Epidemiologic studies indeed point to a mild cardioprotective effect of higher DHEAS levels in both men and women.[82] Functional parameters of activities of daily living in men older than 90 years were lowest in those with the lowest serum DHEAS concentrations,[19] and in healthy elderly individuals there was an association between the ratio of cortisol to DHEAS levels and cognitive impairment.[83]

Dehydroepiandrosterone Replacement Therapy

Several randomized placebo-controlled studies demonstrated that oral administration of DHEA was beneficial.[84–86] Three months of daily treatment with 50 mg of DHEA in 20 healthy adults, most of whom were not elderly, increased serum DHEA and DHEAS concentrations to young adult levels, increased androgen and IGF-I concentrations, and induced a remarkable increase in perceived physical and psychological well-being in both sexes without an effect on libido (Fig. 25–7).[85] In a subsequent study, treatment with 100 mg of DHEA for 6 months in eight adult men and eight adult women increased lean body mass in both sexes but increased muscle strength only in the men (Fig. 25–8).[86] A number of shorter,

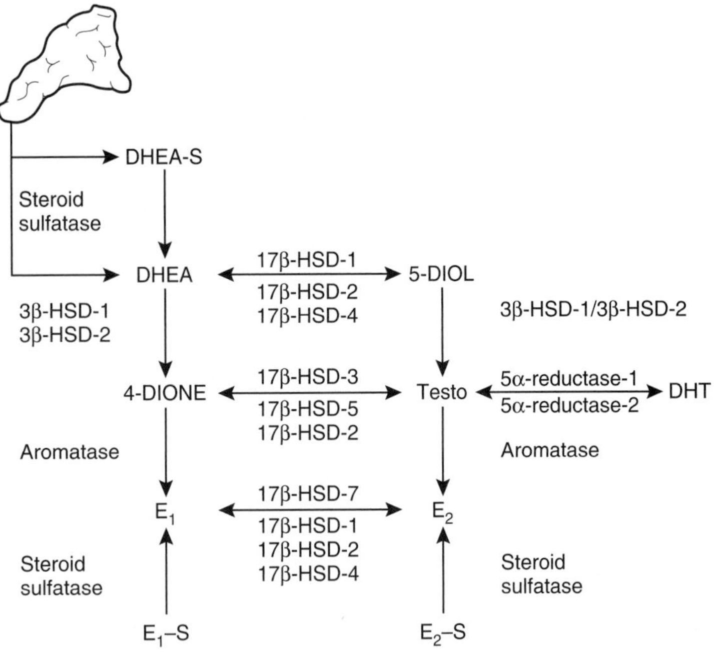

Figure 25–6. Human steroidogenic enzymes in peripheral intracrine tissues. DHEA, dehydroepiandrosterone; DHEAS, DHEA sulfate; DHT, dihydrotestosterone; 5-DIOL, androstene-5-ene-3β,17β-diol; 4-Dione, androstenedione; E_1, estrone; E_2, estradiol; 3β-HSD, 3β-hydroxysteroid dehydrogenase; 17β-HSD, 17β-hydroxysteroid dehydrogenase; Testo, testosterone. (Modified and adapted from Labrie F, Luu-The V, Lin SX, et al. Intracrinology: role of the family of 17 beta-hydroxysteroid dehydrogenases in human physiology and disease. J Mol Endocrinol 2000; 25:1–16.)

well-controlled trials with DHEA subsequently did not demonstrate a clinically significant effect on the parameters just mentioned.[87]

After 280 healthy elderly women and men, aged 60 to 79 years, were given DHEA at 50 mg or placebo orally daily for 1 year in a randomized trial, no adverse effects were noted. A significant increase in most parameters related to libido was observed in older women. Improved skin status, including hydration, epidermal thickness, serum production, and pigmentation, was also noted, particularly in women. In women older than 70 years, bone turnover slightly improved as a result of a decrease in osteoclast activity.[88]

A physiologic functional role of DHEA in women has been ascertained in a careful double-blind study. In women with adrenal insufficiency,[89] DHEA administration (50 mg/day) normalized serum concentrations of DHEA, DHEAS, androstenedione, and testosterone. DHEA significantly improved overall well-being as well as scores for depression and anxiety, the frequency of sexual thoughts, sexual interest, and satisfaction with both mental and physical aspects of sexuality.

Conclusions

No prospective long-term randomized studies of DHEA administration have been carried out in frail elderly people or in the elderly individuals with the lowest serum DHEA and DHEAS concentrations. DHEAS is a universal precursor for the peripheral local production and action of estrogens and androgens in elderly people. The data suggest that serum estradiol concentrations (which might be a surrogate marker for tissue concentrations) and serum luteinizing hormone concentrations (which reflect serum androgen and estrogen activity) demonstrate important positive relations with bone mineral density, quality of life, cognitive decline, and degree of atherosclerosis.[63, 90–92]

The addition of DHEA (50 mg) to the existing large pool of DHEA and DHEAS in unselected elderly individuals has limited clinical effects, especially in elderly women. It is not known whether the increase in sex steroid levels induced by long-term DHEA administration is safe with regard to development of ovarian, prostate, or other types of steroid-depen-

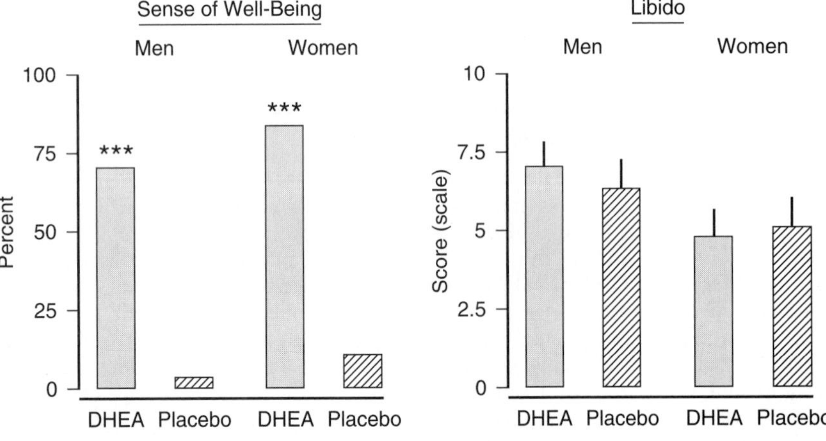

Figure 25–7. Percentage of healthy adult men and women who reported an improved sense of well-being after 12 weeks of oral administration of 50 mg of DHEA nightly in comparison with placebo: $^{***}P < .005$ compared with placebo values. Scored values of libido on a Visual Analogue Scale in men and women did not change during DHEA administration. (From Morales AJ, Nolan JJ, Nelson JC, et al. Effects of replacement dose of dehydroepiandrosterone in men and women of advancing age. J Clin Endocrinol Metab 1994; 78: 1360–1367.)

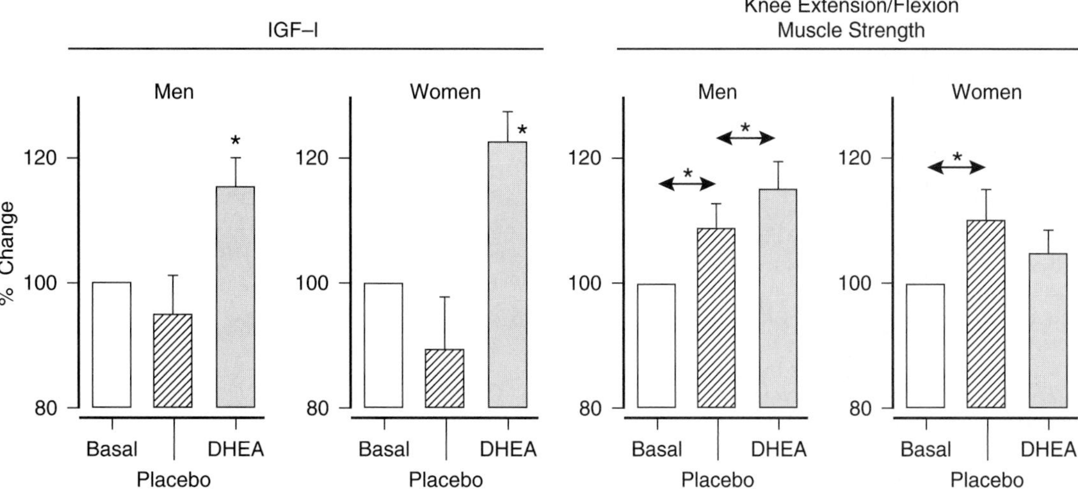

Figure 25–8. Knee extension-flexion muscle strength at baseline (100%) and percentage change in response to placebo and DHEA (100 mg/day) in aging men (n = 8) and women (n = 8), expressed as number of feet. *$P < .05$, placebo versus baseline; *$P < .05$, DHEA versus placebo. (From Yen SS, Morales AJ, Khorram O. Replacement of DHEA in aging men and women. Potential remedial effects. Ann NY Acad Sci 1995; 774:128–142.)

dent cancers. DHEA is currently widely used in the United States as an unapproved treatment against aging. With the scientific verdict still out, without further confirmation of the reported beneficial actions of DHEA in humans, and without a better understanding of its potential risks, it is premature to recommend the routine use of DHEA for delaying or preventing the physiologic consequences of aging.[93, 94]

SOMATOPAUSE

Role of Growth Hormone and Insulin-like Growth Factor I during Aging

Elderly men and women secrete GH less frequently and at lower amplitude than do young people.[21] In fact, GH secretion declines approximately 14% per decade in normal individuals.[95, 96] In parallel, serum levels of IGF-I (see Fig. 25–2) are 20% to 80% lower in healthy elderly individuals than in healthy young adults.[97] The concept that this decline in GH and IGF-I secretion contributes to the decline of functional capacity in elderly people (somatopause) is mainly derived from studies in which GH replacement therapy in GH-deficient adults was shown to increase muscle mass, muscle strength, bone mass, and the quality of life. A beneficial effect on the lipid profile and an important decrease in fat mass were also observed in these patients.[25, 98, 99] As in hypogonadal individuals, adult GH deficiency can thus be considered a model of normal aging because a number of catabolic processes that are central in the biology of aging can be reversed by GH replacement.

Several studies of the relationship between body composition and functional capacity and serum IGF-I concentrations demonstrated contradictory results. In a study of healthy individuals of a broad age range, an association was observed between the maximum aerobic capacity and circulating IGF-I levels.[100] However, no relationship with IGF-I was demonstrated in a group of highly active older people when grip strength, physical performance, and cognitive state were measured.[101, 102]

Growth Hormone Replacement Therapy

Rudman and colleagues,[103] after a ground-breaking randomized controlled trial in healthy men 61 to 81 years old with serum IGF-I concentrations in the lower third for their age, reported in 1990 that GH treatment (30 μg/kg thee times weekly for 6 months) restored the men's IGF-I levels to "normal." In the treatment group, lean body mass rose by 8.8% and lumbar vertebral density increased by 1.6%. The magnitudes of these initial changes were equivalent to a reversal of the age-related changes by 10 to 20 years. However, during continuation of this study to 12 months, the significant positive effect on bone mineral density at any site was lost.[104]

In the subsequent years, it became clear that GH administration in healthy elderly individuals frequently caused acute adverse effects such as carpal tunnel syndrome, gynecomastia, fluid retention, and hyperglycemia, which were severe enough for an appreciable number of individuals to drop out of these studies. The most disappointing aspect, however, was that no positive effects of GH administration were observed on muscle strength, maximal oxygen consumption, or functional capacity. (In contrast, when GH was administered in combination with resistance exercise training, a significant positive effect on muscle mass and muscle strength was recorded that did not differ from that seen with placebo treatment, which suggests that GH does not add to the beneficial effects of exercise.[106, 107]) A representative example of a well-controlled study[105] of GH administration in unselected elderly men is given in Table 25–3.

Earlier studies demonstrated that pharmacologic doses of GH prevent the *autocannibalistic* effects of acute diseases on muscle mass.[108] This finding prompted us to carry out a randomized, placebo-controlled trial of 6 weeks of GH administration in elderly individuals with an acute hip fracture. Our preliminary results indicate that in patients older than 75 years, GH administration causes an earlier return to independent living after the fracture.[109] Comparable studies are being done in several countries, and confirmation is needed before GH can gain a place in the treatment of acute catabolic states in frail elderly people.

Other components in the regulation of the GH–IGF-I axis

are effective in activating GH and IGF-I secretion. Long-acting derivatives of the hypothalamic peptide growth hormone–releasing hormone (GHRH), given twice daily subcutaneously for 14 days to healthy 70-year-old men, increased GH and IGF-I levels to those encountered in 35-year-olds.[110] These studies suggest that somatopause is driven primarily by the hypothalamus and that pituitary somatotropes retain their capacity to synthesize and secrete high levels of GH.

GH-releasing peptides (GHRPs) are oligopeptides with even more powerful GH-releasing effects.[111] They were originally developed by design. Their effects on GH secretion are mediated through endogenous specific receptors.[112, 113] Nonpeptide analogues (e.g., MK-677 and L-692,429) have powerful GH-releasing effects, restoring IGF-I secretion in older adults to levels typical of young adults.[114, 115] Long-term oral administration of MK-677 to healthy elderly individuals increased lean body mass but not muscle strength. If proven to be GH-specific, these orally active GHRP derivatives might be important alternatives to subcutaneously administered GH for studies of the reversal of somatopause, prevention of frailty, and reversal of acute catabolism.[116]

The long-term safety of activating GH and IGF-I levels in older people has become a concern because of reports of an association between serum IGF-I concentrations and cancer risk. Individuals with high IGF-I levels (or low IGF-binding protein 3 levels) within the broad normal range have an increased risk of prostate, colon, and breast cancer.[117–119] These epidemiologic studies, together with experimental data, suggest that the IGF-I system is involved in tumor development and progression. However, no causal relationship between IGF-I levels and cancer risk has yet been established, and possible medical intervention directed at increasing IGF-I bioactivity in elderly people will in most instances be given toward the end of life, presumably not allowing enough time to affect tumor development or progression.

Table 25–3. Effects of Growth Hormone Administration (30 μg/kg three times a week) for 6 Months in 52 Healthy Men (69 years) with Well-Preserved Functional Ability but Low Levels of Insulin-like Growth Factor I

	Mean Change in Variable		
	GH (n = 26)	Placebo (n = 26)	P Value
IGF-I (ng/mL)	119.2	7.6	< .0001
Body Weight and Composition			
Weight, kg	0.5	1.0	> .2
Lean mass, %	4.3	− 0.1	< .001
Fat mass, %	− 13.1	− 0.3	< .001
Bone mineral content, %	0.9	− 0.1	.05
Skin thickness, %	13.4	1.1	.09
***Muscle Strength*, %**			
Knee extension	3.8	1.3	> .2
Knee flexion	10.0	8.2	> .2
Hand grip	− 1.5	3.8	.11
Maximum oxygen consumption, %	2.5	− 2.0	> .2

GH, growth hormone; IGF-I, insulin-like growth factor I.

From Papadakis MA, Grady D, Black D, et al. Growth hormone replacement in healthy older men improves body composition but not functional ability. Ann Intern Med 1996; 124:708–716.

Conclusions

During the aging process, GH–IGF-I axis activity declines. It is unclear whether changes in body composition and functional capacity are directly related. GH administration in older adults causes an increase in lean body mass and an appreciable loss of fat mass. However, the very limited ability of GH treatment to improve muscle strength and functional capacity in elderly people, despite restoration of circulating IGF-I concentrations to young adult levels, limits its application. Furthermore, most dose regimens of GH cause appreciable adverse effects, and long-term safety with regard to tumor development and progression remains uncertain. GHRP and its orally active analogues are capable of restoring GH and IGF-I levels in the elderly population.

In the near future, clinical trials with such orally active molecules in frail elderly people or in elderly individuals with clearly lowered IGF-I levels, or both, should be able to delineate the precise role of the GH–IGF-I axis in the aging process. In such trials, much emphasis must be given to safety aspects. At present, there is insufficient evidence to recommend medical intervention in the GH–IGF-I axis to rejuvenate healthy elderly people.[116, 120, 121] Only elderly patients with GH deficiency caused by organic diseases, such as pituitary adenomas, clearly benefit from GH replacement therapy.[122]

THE CONCEPT OF SUCCESSFUL AGING

There is considerable variation in the effects of aging on healthy individuals, with some people exhibiting greater and others evidencing few or no age-related alterations in physiologic functions. It has been suggested that it might be useful to distinguish between usual and successful patterns of aging.[123] Genetic factors, lifestyle, and societal investments in a safe and healthful environment are important aspects of successful aging.[124] Traditionally, the aging process, including the development of physical frailty toward the end of life, has been considered physiologic and unavoidable.

It has recently become evident, however, that it might not be necessary to accept the grim stereotype of aging as an unalterable process of decline and loss.[123] As life expectancy rises further in the coming decades, the overarching goal should be "an increase in years of healthy life with a full range of functional capacity at each stage of life."[125] Such a compression of morbidity can be achieved by adapting lifestyle measures, but a number of aspects of the aging process of the endocrine system invite the development of routine medical intervention programs offering long-term replacement therapy with one or more hormones in order to delay the aging process and to allow humans to live for a longer period in a relatively intact state.[126]

References

1. Fries JF. Aging, natural death, and the compression of morbidity. N Engl J Med 1980; 303:130–135.
2. Campion EW. The oldest old. N Engl J Med 1994; 330:1819–1820.
3. Kosorok MR, Omenn GS, Diehr P, et al. Restricted activity days among older adults. Am J Public Health 1992; 82:1263–1267.
4. Moss AJ, Parsons VL. Current estimates from the National Health Interview Survey. United States, 1985. Vital Health Stat 10 1986; (160):i–iv, 1–182.
5. Brody JA. Prospects for an ageing population. Nature 1985; 315: 463–466.
6. Rudman D, Rao MP. Serum insulin-like growth factor I in healthy older men in relation to physical activity. In Morley JE, Korenman SG (eds). Endocrinology and Metabolism in the Elderly. Oxford, Blackwell Scientific, 1992, pp 50–68.

7. Buchner DM, Wagner EH. Preventing frail health. Clin Geriatr Med 1992; 8:1–17.
8. Tinetti ME, Speechley M, Ginter SF. Risk factors for falls among elderly persons living in the community. N Engl J Med 1988; 319:1701–1707.
9. Kallman DA, Plato CC, Tobin JD. The role of muscle loss in the age-related decline of grip strength: cross-sectional and longitudinal perspectives. J Gerontol 1990; 45:M82–M88.
10. Fiatarone MA, O'Neill EF, Ryan ND, et al. Exercise training and nutritional supplementation for physical frailty in very elderly people. N Engl J Med 1994; 330:1769–1775.
11. Guralnik JM, Ferrucci L, Simonsick EM, et al. Lower-extremity function in persons over the age of 70 years as a predictor of subsequent disability. N Engl J Med 1995; 332:556–561.
12. Peters AL, Davidson MB. Aging and diabetes. In Alberti KGMM, Zimmet P, Defrozo RA (eds). International Textbook of Diabetes Mellitus. Chichester, UK, John Wiley & Sons, 1997, pp 1151–1176.
13. Mariotti S, Franceschi C, Cossarizza A, et al. The aging thyroid. Endocr Rev 1995; 16:686–715.
14. Wise PM, Krajnak KM, Kashon ML. Menopause: the aging of multiple pacemakers. Science 1996; 273:67–70.
15. Vermeulen A. Clinical review 24: androgens in the aging male. J Clin Endocrinol Metab 1991; 73:221–224.
16. Harman SM, Tsitouras PD. Reproductive hormones in aging men. I. Measurement of sex steroids, basal luteinizing hormone, and Leydig cell response to human chorionic gonadotropin. J Clin Endocrinol Metab 1980; 51:35–40.
17. Harman SM, Tsitouras PD, Costa PT, et al. Reproductive hormones in aging men. II. Basal pituitary gonadotropins and gonadotropin responses to luteinizing hormone–releasing hormone. J Clin Endocrinol Metab 1982; 54:547–51.
18. Herbert J. The age of dehydroepiandrosterone. Lancet 1995; 345:1193–1194.
19. Ravaglia G, Forti P, Maioli F, et al. The relationship of dehydroepiandrosterone sulfate (DHEAS) to endocrine-metabolic parameters and functional status in the oldest-old. Results from an Italian study on healthy free-living over-ninety-year-olds. J Clin Endocrinol Metab 1996; 81:1173–1178.
20. Hornsby PJ. Biosynthesis of DHEAS by the human adrenal cortex and its age-related decline. Ann NY Acad Sci 1995; 774:29–46.
21. Corpas E, Harman SM, Blackman MR. Human growth hormone and human aging. Endocr Rev 1993; 14:20–39.
22. Guyton AC (ed). Textbook of Medical Physiology, 8th ed. Philadelphia, WB Saunders, 1991, pp 899–914.
23. Blackman MR. Pituitary hormones and aging. Endocrinol Metab Clin North Am 1987; 16:981–994.
24. Wang C, Swedloff RS, Iranmanesh A, et al. Transdermal testosterone gel improves sexual function, mood, muscle strength, and body composition parameters in hypogonadal men. Testosterone Gel Study Group. J Clin Endocrinol Metab 2000; 85:2839–2853.
25. Attanasio AF, Lamberts SW, Matranga AM, et al. Adult growth hormone (GH)–deficient patients demonstrate heterogeneity between childhood onset and adult onset before and during human GH treatment. Adult Growth Hormone Deficiency Study Group. J Clin Endocrinol Metab 1997; 82:82–88.
26. Grady D, Rubin SM, Petitti DB, et al. Hormone therapy to prevent disease and prolong life in postmenopausal women. Ann Intern Med 1992; 117:1016–1037.
27. Barrett-Connor E. Hormone replacement therapy. BMJ 1998; 317:457–461.
28. Clinical Synthesis Panel on HRT. Hormone replacement therapy. Lancet 1999; 354:152–155.
29. Santoro NF, Col NF, Eckman MH, et al. Therapeutic controversy: hormone replacement therapy—where are we going? J Clin Endocrinol Metab 1999; 84:1798–1812.
30. Jacobs HS. Hormone replacement therapy and breast cancer. Endocr Relat Cancer 2000; 7:53–61.
31. Schairer C, Lubin J, Troisi R, et al. Menopausal estrogen and estrogen-progestin replacement therapy and breast cancer risk. JAMA 2000; 283:485–491.
32. Herrington DM, Reboussin DM, Brosnihan KB, et al. Effects of estrogen replacement on the progression of coronary-artery atherosclerosis. N Engl J Med 2000; 343:522–529.
33. Lufkin EG, Wahner HW, O'Fallon WM, et al. Treatment of postmenopausal osteoporosis with transdermal estrogen. Ann Intern Med 1992; 117:1–9.
34. Kanis JA. Estrogens, the menopause, and osteoporosis. Bone 1996; 19(Suppl):185S–190S.
35. Burns A, Murphy D. Protection against Alzheimer's disease? Lancet 1996; 348:420–421.
36. Tang MX, Jacobs D, Stern Y, et al. Effect of oestrogen during menopause on risk and age at onset of Alzheimer's disease. Lancet 1996; 348:429–432.
37. Yaffe K, Sawaya G, Lieberburg I, et al. Estrogen therapy in postmenopausal women: effects on cognitive function and dementia. JAMA 1998; 279:688–695.
38. Mulnard RA, Cotman CW, Kawas C, et al. Estrogen replacement therapy for treatment of mild to moderate Alzheimer disease: a randomized controlled trial. Alzheimer's Disease Cooperative Study. JAMA 2000; 283:1007–1015.
39. Shaywitz BA, Shaywitz SE. Estrogen and Alzheimer disease: plausible theory, negative clinical trial. JAMA 2000; 283:1055–1056.
40. Collaborative Group on Hormonal Factors in Breast Cancer. Breast cancer and hormone replacement therapy: collaborative reanalysis of data from 51 epidemiological studies of 52,705 women with breast cancer and 108,411 women without breast cancer. Lancet 1997; 350:1047–1059.
41. Willett WC, Colditz G, Stampfer M. Postmenopausal estrogens—opposed, unopposed, or none of the above. JAMA 2000; 283:534–535.
42. Stevenson JC. Do we need different galenic forms of estrogens and progestogens? Menopause 1996; 3:243–245.
43. O'Sullivan AJ, Crampton LJ, Freund J, Ho KK. The route of estrogen replacement therapy confers divergent effects on substrate oxidation and body composition in postmenopausal women. J Clin Invest 1998; 102:1035–1040.
44. Cummings SR, Browner WS, Bauer D, et al. Endogenous hormones and the risk of hip and vertebral fractures among older women. Study of Osteoporotic Fractures Research Group. N Engl J Med 1998; 339:733–738.
45. Andersson K, Mattsson LA, Milsom I. Use of hormone replacement therapy. Lancet 1996; 348:1521.
46. Santen RJ. Long-term tamoxifen therapy: can an antagonist become an agonist? J Clin Endocrinol Metab 1996; 81:2027–2029.
47. Grainger DJ, Metcalfe JC. Tamoxifen: teaching an old drug new tricks? Nat Med 1996; 2:381–385.
48. Love RR, Mazess RB, Barden HS, et al. Effects of tamoxifen on bone mineral density in postmenopausal women with breast cancer. N Engl J Med 1992; 326:852–856.
49. Grey AB, Stapleton JP, Evans MC, et al. The effect of the antiestrogen tamoxifen on bone mineral density in normal late postmenopausal women. Am J Med 1995; 99:636–641.
50. Rutqvist LE, Mattsson A. Cardiac and thromboembolic morbidity among post-menopausal women with early-stage breast cancer in a randomized trial of adjuvant tamoxifen. The Stockholm Breast Cancer Study Group. J Natl Cancer Inst 1993; 85:1398–1406.
51. Black LJ, Sato M, Rowley ER, et al. Raloxifene (LY139481 HCI) prevents bone loss and reduces serum cholesterol without causing uterine hypertrophy in ovariectomized rats. J Clin Invest 1994; 93:63–69.
52. Draper MW, Flowers DE, Huster WJ, et al. A controlled trial of raloxifene (LY139481) HCl: impact on bone turnover and serum lipid profile in healthy postmenopausal women. J Bone Miner Res 1996; 11:835–842.
53. Yang NN, Bryant HU, Hardikar S, et al. Estrogen and raloxifene stimulate transforming growth factor-beta 3 gene expression in rat bone: a potential mechanism for estrogen- or raloxifene-mediated bone maintenance. Endocrinology 1996; 137:2075–2084.
54. McDonnell DP, Clemm DL, Hermann T, et al. Analysis of estrogen receptor function in vitro reveals three distinct classes of antiestrogens. Mol Endocrinol 1995; 9:659–669.
55. Korach KS, Couse JF, Curtis SW, et al. Estrogen receptor gene disruption: molecular characterization and experimental and clinical phenotypes. Recent Prog Horm Res 1996; 51:159–186.
56. Delmas PD, Bjarnason NH, Mitlak BH, et al. Effects of raloxifene on bone mineral density, serum cholesterol concentrations, and uterine endometrium in postmenopausal women. N Engl J Med 1997; 337:1641–1647.
57. Ettinger B, Black DM, Mitlak BH, et al. Reduction of vertebral fracture risk in postmenopausal women with osteoporosis treated

with raloxifene: results from a 3-year randomized clinical trial. Multiple Outcomes of Raloxifene Evaluation (MORE) Investigators. JAMA 1999; 282:637–645.
58. Walsh BW, Kuller LH, Wild RA, et al. Effects of raloxifene on serum lipids and coagulation factors in healthy postmenopausal women. JAMA 1998; 279:1445–1451.
59. Goldstein SR, Scheele WH, Rajagopalan SK, et al. A 12-month comparative study of raloxifene, estrogen, and placebo on the postmenopausal endometrium. Obstet Gynecol 2000; 95:95–103.
60. Davies GC, Huster WJ, Lu Y, et al. Adverse events reported by postmenopausal women in controlled trials with raloxifene. Obstet Gynecol 1999; 93:558–565.
61. Cummings SR, Eckert S, Krueger KA, et al. The effect of raloxifene on risk of breast cancer in postmenopausal women: results from the MORE randomized trial. Multiple Outcomes of Raloxifene Evaluation. JAMA 1999; 281:2189–2197.
62. Nabel EG. Coronary heart disease in women—an ounce of prevention. N Engl J Med 2000; 343:572–574.
63. Tenover JS. Androgen administration to aging men. Endocrinol Metab Clin North Am 1994; 23:877–892.
64. Beld AW van den, de Jong FH, Grobbee DE, et al. Measures of bioavailable serum testosterone and estradiol and their relationships with muscle strength, bone density, and body composition in elderly men. J Clin Endocrinol Metab 2000; 85:3276–3282.
65. Barrett-Connor E, Von Muhlen DG, Kritz-Silverstein D. Bioavailable testosterone and depressed mood in older men: the Rancho Bernardo Study. J Clin Endocrinol Metab 1999; 84:573–577.
66. Wang C, Eyre DR, Clark R, et al. Sublingual testosterone replacement improves muscle mass and strength, decreases bone resorption, and increases bone formation markers in hypogonadal men—a clinical research center study. J Clin Endocrinol Metab 1996; 81:3654–3662.
67. Bhasin S, Storer TW, Berman N, et al. The effects of supraphysiologic doses of testosterone on muscle size and strength in normal men. N Engl J Med 1996; 335:1–7.
68. Snyder PJ, Peachey H, Hannoush P, et al. Effect of testosterone treatment on bone mineral density in men over 65 years of age. J Clin Endocrinol Metab 1999; 84:1966–1972.
69. Snyder PJ, Peachey H, Hannoush P, et al. Effect of testosterone treatment on body composition and muscle strength in men over 65 years of age. J Clin Endocrinol Metab 1999; 84:2647–2653.
70. Tenover JL. Testosterone and the aging male. J Androl 1997; 18: 103–106.
71. Bhasin S, Bagatell CJ, Bremner WJ, et al. Issues in testosterone replacement in older men. J Clin Endocrinol Metab 1998; 83: 3435–3448.
72. Pearlman CK, Kobashi LI. Frequency of intercourse in men. J Urol 1972; 107:298–301.
73. Bhasin S, Bremner WJ. Clinical review 85: emerging issues in androgen replacement therapy. J Clin Endocrinol Metab 1997; 82:3–8.
74. Bagatell CJ, Bremner WJ. Androgens in men—uses and abuses. N Engl J Med 1996; 334:707–714.
75. Hayes FJ. Testosterone—fountain of youth or drug of abuse? J Clin Endocrinol Metab 2000; 85:3020–3023.
76. Sih R, Morley JE, Kaiser FE, et al. Testosterone replacement in older hypogonadal men: a 12-month randomized controlled trial. J Clin Endocrinol Metab 1997; 82:1661–1667.
77. Morley JE, Melmed S. Gonadal dysfunction in systemic disorders. Metabolism 1979; 28:1051–1073.
78. Gray A, Feldman HA, McKinlay JB, et al. Age, disease, and changing sex hormone levels in middle-aged men: results of the Massachusetts Male Aging Study. J Clin Endocrinol Metab 1991; 73:1016–1025.
79. Negro-Vilar A. Selective androgen receptor modulators (SARMs): a novel approach to androgen therapy for the new millennium. J Clin Endocrinol Metab 1999; 84:3459–3462.
80. Labrie F, Luu-The V, Lin SX, et al. Intracrinology: role of the family of 17 beta-hydroxysteroid dehydrogenases in human physiology and disease. J Mol Endocrinol 2000; 25:1–16.
81. Labrie F, Belanger A, Simard J, et al. DHEA and peripheral androgen and estrogen formation: intracrinology. Ann NY Acad Sci 1995; 774:16–28.
82. Barrett-Connor E, Goodman-Gruen D. The epidemiology of DHEAS and cardiovascular disease. Ann NY Acad Sci 1995; 774: 259–270.
83. Kalmijn S, Launer LJ, Stolk RP, et al. A prospective study on cortisol, dehydroepiandrosterone sulfate, and cognitive function in the elderly. J Clin Endocrinol Metab 1998; 83:3487–3492.
84. Baulieu EE. Studies on dehydroepiandrosterone (DHEA) and its sulphate during aging. C R Acad Sci III 1995; 318:7–11.
85. Morales AJ, Nolan JJ, Nelson JC, et al. Effects of replacement dose of dehydroepiandrosterone in men and women of advancing age. J Clin Endocrinol Metab 1994; 78:1360–1367.
86. Yen SS, Morales AJ, Khorram O. Replacement of DHEA in aging men and women. Potential remedial effects. Ann NY Acad Sci 1995; 774:128–142.
87. Flynn MA, Weaver-Osterholtz D, Sharpe-Timms KL, et al. Dehydroepiandrosterone replacement in aging humans. J Clin Endocrinol Metab 1999; 84:1527–1533.
88. Baulieu EE, Thomas G, Legrain S, et al. Dehydroepiandrosterone (DHEA), DHEA sulfate, and aging: contribution of the DHEAge Study to a sociobiomedical issue. Proc Natl Acad Sci USA 2000; 97:4279–4284.
89. Arlt W, Callies F, van Vlijmen JC, et al. Dehydroepiandrosterone replacement in women with adrenal insufficiency. N Engl J Med 1999; 341:1013–1020.
90. Barrett-Connor E, Mueller JE, von Muhlen DG, et al. Low levels of estradiol are associated with vertebral fractures in older men, but not women: the Rancho Bernardo Study. J Clin Endocrinol Metab 2000; 85:219–223.
91. van den Beld A, Huhtaniemi IT, Pettersson KS, et al. Luteinizing hormone and different genetic variants, as indicators of frailty in healthy elderly men. J Clin Endocrinol Metab 1999; 84:1334–1339.
92. Yaffe K, Lui LY, Grady D, et al. Cognitive decline in women in relation to non-protein-bound oestradiol concentrations. Lancet 2000; 356:708–712.
93. Nestler JE. Regulation of human dehydroepiandrosterone metabolism by insulin. Ann NY Acad Sci 1995; 774:73–81.
94. Skolnick AA. Scientific verdict still out on DHEA. JAMA 1996; 276:1365–1367.
95. Toogood AA, O'Neill PA, Shalet SM. Beyond the somatopause: growth hormone deficiency in adults over the age of 60 years. J Clin Endocrinol Metab 1996; 81:460–465.
96. Toogood A, Jones J, O'Neill P, et al. The diagnosis of severe growth hormone deficiency in elderly patients with hypothalamic pituitary disease. Clin Endocrinol 1998; 48:569–576.
97. Borst SE, Millard WJ, Lowenthal DT, et al. Growth hormone, exercise, and aging: the future of therapy for the frail elderly. J Am Geriatr Soc 1994; 42:528–535.
98. Nass R, Huber RM, Klauss V, et al. Effect of growth hormone (hGH) replacement therapy on physical work capacity and cardiac and pulmonary function in patients with hGH deficiency acquired in adulthood. J Clin Endocrinol Metab 1995; 80:552–557.
99. Salomon F, Cuneo RC, Hesp R, et al. The effects of treatment with recombinant human growth hormone on body composition and metabolism in adults with growth hormone deficiency. N Engl J Med 1989; 321:1797–1803.
100. Poehlman ET, Copeland KC. Influence of physical activity on insulin-like growth factor-I in healthy younger and older men. J Clin Endocrinol Metab 1990; 71:1468–1473.
101. Papadakis MA, Grady D, Tierney MJ, et al. Insulin-like growth factor 1 and functional status in healthy older men. J Am Geriatr Soc 1995; 43:1350–1355.
102. Rudman D. Growth hormone, body composition, and aging. J Am Geriatr Soc 1985; 33:800–807.
103. Rudman D, Feller AG, Nagraj HS, et al. Effects of human growth hormone in men over 60 years old. N Engl J Med 1990; 323:1–6.
104. Rudman D, Feller AG, Cohn L. Effects of GH on body composition in elderly men. Horm Res 1991; 36:73–81.
105. Papadakis MA, Grady D, Black D, et al. Growth hormone replacement in healthy older men improves body composition but not functional ability. Ann Intern Med 1996; 124:708–716.
106. Taaffe DR, Pruitt L, Reim J, et al. Effect of recombinant human growth hormone on the muscle strength response to resistance exercise in elderly men. J Clin Endocrinol Metab 1994; 79:1361–1366.
107. Yarasheski KE, Zachwieja JJ, Campbell JA, et al. Effect of growth hormone and resistance exercise on muscle growth and strength in older men. Am J Physiol 1995; 268:E268–E276.

108. Herndon DN, Barrow RE, Kunkel KR, et al. Effects of recombinant human growth hormone on donor-site healing in severely burned children. Ann Surg 1990; 212:424–429.
109. van der Lely AJ, Lamberts SWJ, Jauch KW, et al. Use of human GH in elderly patients with accidental hip fracture. Eur J Endocrinol 2000; 143:585–592.
110. Corpas E, Harman SM, Pineyro MA, et al. Growth hormone (GH)–releasing hormone-(1–29) twice daily reverses the decreased GH and insulin-like growth factor-I levels in old men. J Clin Endocrinol Metab 1992; 75:530–535.
111. Bowers CY, Momany FA, Reynolds GA, et al. On the in vitro and in vivo activity of a new synthetic hexapeptide that acts on the pituitary to specifically release growth hormone. Endocrinology 1984; 114:1537–1545.
112. Howard AD, Feighner SD, Cully DF, et al. A receptor in pituitary and hypothalamus that functions in growth hormone release. Science 1996; 273:974–977.
113. Pong SS, Chaung LY, Dean DC, et al. Identification of a new G-protein–linked receptor for growth hormone secretagogues. Mol Endocrinol 1996; 10:57–61.
114. Chapman IM, Hartman ML, Pezzoli SS, et al. Enhancement of pulsatile growth hormone secretion by continuous infusion of a growth hormone–releasing peptide mimetic, L-692,429, in older adults—a clinical research center study. J Clin Endocrinol Metab 1996; 81:2874–2880.
115. Chapman IM, Bach MA, Van Cauter E, et al. Stimulation of the growth hormone (GH)–insulin-like growth factor I axis by daily oral administration of a GH secretogogue (MK-677) in healthy elderly subjects. J Clin Endocrinol Metab 1996; 81:4249–4257.
116. Chapman IM. Hypothalamic growth hormone–IGF-I axis. In Morley JE, van den Berg L (eds). Endocrinology of Aging. Totowa, NJ, Humana Press, 2000, pp 23–40.
117. Chan JM, Stampfer MJ, Giovannucci E, et al. Plasma insulin-like growth factor-I and prostate cancer risk: a prospective study. Science 1998; 279:563–566.
118. Hankinson SE, Willett WC, Colditz GA, et al. Circulating concentrations of insulin-like growth factor-I and risk of breast cancer. Lancet 1998; 351:1393–1396.
119. Ma J, Pollak MN, Giovannucci E, et al. Prospective study of colorectal cancer risk in men and plasma levels of insulin-like growth factor (IGF)-I and IGF-binding protein-3. J Natl Cancer Inst 1999; 91:620–625.
120. Martin F. Frailty and the somatopause. Growth Horm IGF Res 1999; 9:3–10.
121. Rosen CJ. Growth hormone and aging. Endocrine 2000; 12:197–201.
122. Shalet SM. GH deficiency in the elderly: the case for GH replacement. Clin Endocrinol 2000; 53:279–280.
123. Rowe JW, Kahn RL. Human aging: usual and successful. Science 1987; 237:143–149.
124. Hazzard WR. Weight control and exercise. Cardinal features of successful preventive gerontology. JAMA 1995; 274:1964–1965.
125. Healthy People 2000: National and Health Promotion and Disease Prevention Objectives. Washington, DC, Government Printing Office, 1991.
126. Lamberts SW, van den Beld AW, van der Lely AJ. The endocrinology of aging. Science 1997; 278:419–424.

	Calcium ions	Phosphate ions
Extracellular		
Concentration		
total, in serum	2.5×10^{-3} M	1.00×10^{-3} M
free	1.2×10^{-3} M	0.85×10^{-3} M
Functions	bone mineral blood coagulation membrane excitability	bone mineral
Intracellular		
Concentration	10^{-7} M	$1–2 \times 10^{-3}$ M
Functions	signal for: • neuronal activation • hormone secretion • muscle contraction	• structural role • high-energy bonds • regulation of proteins by phosphorylation

Figure 26–1. Distribution and function of calcium and phosphate. Note the dramatic differences between intracellular and extracellular concentrations of calcium ion and the dramatically different functions of calcium and phosphate inside cells.

becoming better understood with the identification of specific receptors for calciotropic signaling molecules such as the inositol triphosphate (IP_3) receptor and ryanodine receptors.

Phosphate is more widely distributed to nonosseous tissues than is calcium. Eighty-five percent of body phosphate is in the mineral phase of bone, and the remainder is located in inorganic or organic form throughout the extracellular and intracellular compartments. In human serum, inorganic phosphate (P_i) is present at a concentration of approximately 1 mM and exists almost entirely in ionized form as either $H_2PO_4^-$ or HPO_4^{2-}. Only 12% of serum phosphate is protein-bound, and an additional small fraction is loosely complexed with calcium, magnesium, and other cations. Intracellular free phosphate concentrations are generally comparable to those in the extracellular fluid (i.e., 1 to 2 mM), although the inside-negative electrical potential of the cell creates a significant energy requirement for translocation of phosphate into cells. This process generally is accomplished through sodium-phosphate cotransport driven by the transmembrane sodium gradient. A number of sodium-phosphate cotransporters have been cloned; various cells and tissues employ different species of such transporters with distinctive regulatory characteristics.

Organic phosphate is a key component of virtually all classes of structural, informational, and effector molecules that are essential for normal genetic, developmental, and physiologic processes. Phosphate is an integral constituent of nucleic acids; phospholipids; complex carbohydrates; glycolytic intermediates; structural, signaling, and enzymatic phosphoproteins; and nucleotide cofactors for enzymes and G proteins. Of particular importance are the high-energy phosphate ester bonds present in molecules such as adenosine triphosphate (ATP), diphosphoglycerate, and creatine phosphate that store chemical energy. Phosphate plays a particularly prominent role as the key substrate or recognition site in numerous kinase and phosphatase regulatory cascades. Cytosolic phosphate per se also directly regulates a number of crucial intracellular reactions, including those involved in glucose transport, lactate production, and synthesis of ATP. In light of these diverse roles, it is not surprising that disorders of phosphate homeostasis associated with severe depletion of intracellular phosphate lead to profound and global impairment of organ function.

Magnesium is the fourth most abundant cation in the body. Roughly half is found in bone and half in muscle and other soft tissues. As much as half of the magnesium in bone is not sequestered in the mineral phase but is freely exchangeable with ions in the extracellular fluid and therefore may serve as a buffer against changes in extracellular magnesium concentration. Less than 1% of all magnesium in the body is present in the extracellular fluid, where the magnesium concentration is approximately 0.5 mM.[1] The concentration of magnesium in serum normally is 0.7 to 1.0 mM, of which roughly a third is protein bound, 15% is loosely complexed with phosphate or other anions, and 55% is present as the free ion.[1] Over 95% of intracellular magnesium is bound to other molecules, most notably ATP, the concentration of which is approximately 5 mM. The intracellular cytosolic free magnesium concentration is approximately 0.5 mM—that is, 1000-fold higher than that of calcium—and is maintained by an active sodium-magnesium antiporter. The mechanism whereby magnesium enters cells, presumably down a favorable electrochemical gradient, is unknown, although some evidence for regulated channels has been obtained.

Intracellular magnesium, like phosphate, is necessary for a wide range of cellular functions. It is an essential cofactor in enzymatic reactions, including most of the same glycolytic, kinase, and phosphatase pathways that also involve phosphate. Magnesium serves to directly stabilize the structures of a variety of macromolecules and complexes, including deoxyribonucleic acid (DNA), ribonucleic acid (RNA), and ribosomes; is a key activator of the many ATPase-coupled ion transporters; and plays a direct role in mitochondrial oxidative metabolism. As a result, magnesium is critical for energy metabolism and the maintenance of a normal intracellular environment. Extracellular magnesium is crucial for normal neuromuscular excitability and nerve conduction, and many of the clinical consequences of magnesium deficiency or excess reflect abnormalities in this sphere.

The importance of the mineral ions for normal cellular physiology as well as skeletal integrity is reflected in the powerful endocrine control mechanisms that have evolved to maintain their extracellular concentrations within relatively narrow limits. The following topics describe the structures, secretory controls, actions, and interactions of parathyroid hormone, calcitonin, and 1,25-dihydroxyvitamin D ($1{,}25(OH)_2D_3$ or calcitriol)—the major hormones involved in mineral ion homeostasis. Subsequent topics cover the wide variety of clinical disorders that accompany abnormalities in this hormonal network.

PARATHYROID HORMONE

Parathyroid hormone (PTH) is the peptide hormone that controls the minute-to-minute level of ionized calcium in the blood and extracellular fluids. PTH binds to cell surface receptors in bone and kidney, thereby triggering responses that increase blood calcium (Fig. 26–2). PTH also increases renal synthesis of $1{,}25(OH)_2D_3$, the hormonally active form of vitamin D, which then acts on the intestine to augment absorption of dietary calcium, in addition to promoting calcium fluxes into blood from bone and kidney. The resulting increase in blood calcium (and in $1{,}25(OH)_2D_3$) feeds back on the parathyroid glands to decrease the secretion of PTH. The parathyroid glands, bones, kidney, and gut are thus the crucial organs that participate in PTH-mediated calcium homeostasis.

Parathyroid Gland Biology

Parathyroid chief cells have three properties vital to their homeostatic function:

1. They rapidly secrete stored hormone in response to changes in blood calcium.

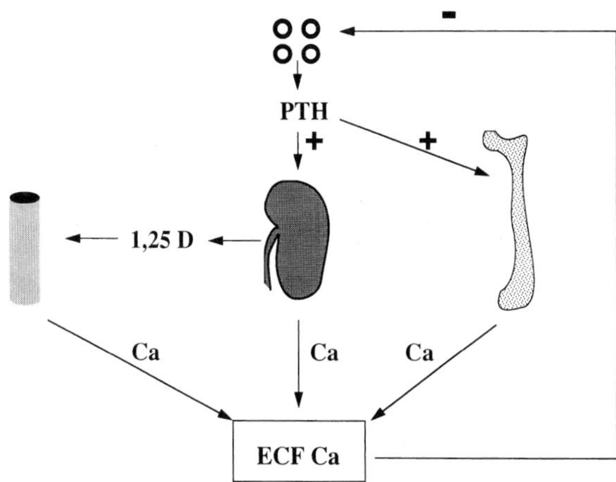

Figure 26–2. Parathyroid hormone (PTH)-calcium feedback loop that controls calcium homeostasis. Four organs—the parathyroid glands, intestine, kidney, and bone—together determine the parameters of calcium homeostasis. +, positive effect; −, negative effect.

2. They can synthesize, process, and store large amounts of PTH in a regulated manner.
3. They replicate when chronically stimulated.

These functional attributes allow for short-term, intermediate-term, and long-term adaptation, respectively, to changes in calcium availability.

```
                          PRE                ↓ PRO ↓      PTH
          -31                                -6      +1       +10
human     MIPAKDMAKVMIVMLAICFLTKSDG  KSVKKR  SVSEIQLMHN
bovine    MMSAKDMVKVMIVMLAICFLARSDG  KSVKKR  AVSEIQFMHN
porcine   MMSAKDTVKVMVVMLAICFLARSDG  KPIKKR  SVSEIQLMHN
rat       MMSASTMAKVMILMLAVCLLTQADG  KPVKKR  AVSEIQLMHN
canine    MMSAKDMVKVMIVMFAICFLAKSDG  KPVKKR  SVSEIQFMHN
chicken   MTSTKNLAKAIVILYAICFFTNSDG  RPMMKR  SVSEMQLMHN

                   +20       +30       +40        +50
human     LGKHLNSMERVEWLRKKLQDVHNFVALGAPLAPRDAGSQRPRK
bovine    LGKHLSSMERVEWLRKKLQDVHNFVALGASIAYRDGSSQRPRK
porcine   LGKHLSSLERVEWLRKKLQDVHNFVALGASIVHRDGGSQRPRK
rat       LGKHLASVERMQWLRKKLQDVHNFVSLGVQMAAREGSYQRPTK
canine    LGKHLSSMERVEWLRKKLQDVHNFVALGAPIAHRDGSSQRPLK
chicken   LGEHRHTVERQDWLQMKLQDVH..SALE.....DARTQRPRN

                +60           +70                 +80
human     KEDNVLVE...SHEKSLGEA.........DKADVNVLTKAKSQ
bovine    KEDNVLVE...SHQKSLGEA.........DKADVDVLIKAKPQ
porcine   KEDNVLVE...SHQKSLGEA.........DKAAVDVLIKAKPQ
rat       KEENVLVD...GNSKSLGEG.........DKADVDVLVKAKSQ
canine    KEDNVLVE...SYQKSLGEA.........DKADVDVLTKAKSQ
chicken   KEDIVLGEIRNRRLLPEHLRAAVQKKSIDLDKAYMNVLFKTKP.
```

Figure 26–3. Sequences of pre-proparathyroid hormone from six species. Completely conserved residues are in boldface. Arrows indicate the sites of signal sequence ("pre") and "pro" sequence cleavage. Numbers start at residue +1 of mature parathyroid hormone (PTH); because of gaps, the numbers correspond only to the mammalian and not to the chicken sequence. Amino acids are indicated by the single letter code: A, Ala; R, Arg; N, Asn; D, Asp; C, Cys; Q, Gln; E, Glu; G, Gly; H, His; I, Ile, L, Leu; K, Lys; M, Met; F, Phe; P, Pro; S, Ser; T, Thr; W, Trp; Y, Tyr; V, Val.

Parathyroid Hormone Biosynthesis

PTH, a protein of 84 amino acids, is synthesized as a larger precursor, pre-proparathyroid hormone (pre-pro-PTH). Figure 26–3 illustrates the reported pre-pro-PTH sequences. These pre-pro-PTH sequences share a 25-residue "pre" or signal sequence and a 6-residue "pro" sequence. The signal sequence, along with the short pro sequence, functions to direct the protein into the secretory pathway (Fig. 26–4). During transit across the membrane of the endoplasmic reticulum, the signal sequence is cleaved off and rapidly degraded. The importance of the signal sequence for normal secretion of PTH is illustrated by the hypoparathyroidism inherited in families carrying mutations in the signal sequence of pre-pro-PTH.[2–4]

The role of the short pro sequence is not completely understood; it may help the signal sequence work efficiently and ensure accurate cleavage of the precursor.[5] After cleavage of the pro sequence, the mature PTH(1–84) is concentrated in secretory vesicles and granules. One morphologically distinct subtype of granule contains both PTH and the proteases cathepsin B and cathepsin H.[6] This co-localization of proteases and PTH in secretory granules probably explains the observation that a portion of the PTH secreted from parathyroid glands consists of carboxy-terminal PTH fragments.[7] No amino-terminal fragments of PTH are secreted. Although the possible functions of carboxy-terminal fragments of PTH are still poorly characterized, these fragments do not activate the PTH/PTHrP receptor (see later). Thus, the intracellular fragmentation of PTH probably represents an inactivating pathway. The intracellular degradation of newly synthesized PTH provides an important regulatory mechanism. Under conditions of hypercalcemia, the secretion of PTH is substantially decreased, and most of what is secreted consists of carboxy-terminal fragments.[8–11]

Parathyroid Hormone Secretion

Although catecholamines, magnesium, and other stimuli can affect PTH secretion,[12] the major regulator of PTH secretion is the concentration of ionized calcium in blood. Increased serum ionized calcium leads to a decrease in PTH secretion (Fig. 26–5*A*). The shape of the dose-response curve is sigmoid.[13] Properties of the parathyroid cell determine the conformation of the sigmoid curve but do not alone determine the point on the curve that represents a physiologic steady state for an individual. This point, usually between the mid-point and the bottom of the curve, is determined by how vigorously target organs respond to PTH.[14] Figure 26–5*C* (*solid line*) shows how an individual's calcium level rises in response to increases in PTH; the parathyroid gland's sigmoid curve is the *dotted line*. In the steady state, an individual's blood levels of PTH and calcium represent the intersection of the two lines.

The sigmoid curve reveals several important physiologic properties of the parathyroid gland. The minimal secretory

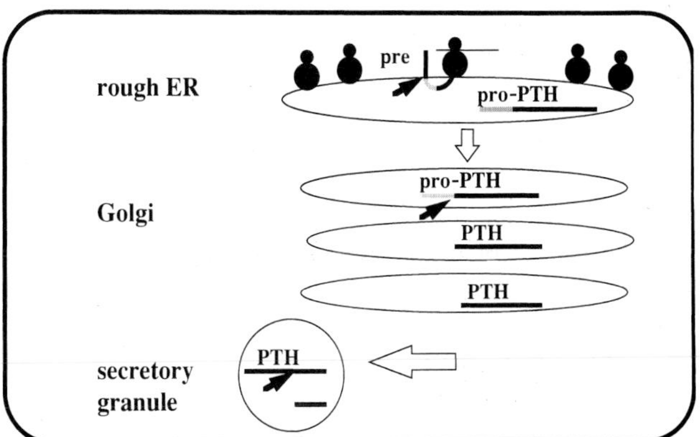

Figure 26–4. Intracellular processing of pre-proparathyroid hormone (pre-pro-PTH). Diagonal arrows indicate sites of cleavage by enzymes that generate pro-PTH in the rough endoplasmic reticulum (ER), PTH in the Golgi, and carboxy-terminal fragments of PTH in the secretory granule.

studies show that acute hypocalcemia in rats leads, within an hour, to an increase in PTH messenger RNA (mRNA).[35, 36] In contrast, hypercalcemia leads to little[36] or no[35] change in PTH mRNA. Thus, under normal conditions, the inhibition by calcium of PTH biosynthesis already is nearly maximal, just as it is for PTH secretion. The parathyroid gland is poised to respond to a fall in calcium much more readily than to a rise. The mechanism for the increase in PTH mRNA in response to hypocalcemia is uncertain; differing experimental paradigms suggest regulation at the levels of gene transcription,[37] mRNA stability,[38] and mRNA translation.[39]

For decades it has been known that phosphate elevation stimulates PTH secretion,[40] largely by lowering blood calcium and $1,25(OH)_2D_3$ levels. More recently, a series of studies in vitro[41, 42] and in vivo[43, 44] have demonstrated that phosphate can increase PTH secretion directly, independent of effects on blood calcium and $1,25(OH)_2D_3$. Phosphate increases PTH secretion acutely only after a delay and probably works largely through regulation of PTH mRNA levels. The direct effects of phosphate may be important only at very high and very low levels, although these effects may be important in the setting of renal failure.

The regulation of the PTH gene has particular clinical relevance in patients with renal failure. Hypocalcemia, low levels of $1,25(OH)_2D_3$, hyperphosphatemia, and, possibly, uremic toxins disrupt normal calcium homeostasis in this setting. Therapy with $1,25(OH)_2D_3$ and calcium increases calcium absorption and also inhibits PTH synthesis by direct effects on the parathyroid gland. Prevention of hyperphosphatemia avoids the direct and indirect actions of phosphate to stimulate PTH secretion.

Regulation of Parathyroid Cell Number

Parathyroid cells divide during the growth of young animals but replicate little in adulthood.[45] Parathyroid cell number can dramatically increase, however, in the setting of hypocalcemia, low levels of $1,25(OH)_2D_3$, hyperphosphatemia, or uremia and during neoplastic growth.

Calcium, acting through the parathyroid calcium-sensing receptor, restrains parathyroid proliferation. This effect has been demonstrated clinically in patients who lack both copies of the calcium-sensing receptor gene. These neonates exhibit severe primary hyperparathyroidism with large, diffusely hyperplastic glands that presumably have developed because of insufficient activation of the parathyroid calcium-sensing receptor by extracellular calcium. Furthermore, administration of the calcimimetic compound NPS R-568, which activates the calcium-sensing receptor directly, prevents parathyroid cell proliferation in experimental uremia.[46]

The role of $1,25(OH)_2D_3$, independent of blood calcium, in regulating parathyroid cell proliferation is less well established than that of calcium. That $1,25(OH)_2D_3$ can dramatically affect parathyroid cell number has been shown in vivo in many settings,[47, 48] but such studies cannot rigorously eliminate effects of transient changes in blood calcium. The suppression of proliferation of cultured parathyroid cells by $1,25(OH)_2D_3$[49, 50] certainly suggests that $1,25(OH)_2D_3$ can directly inhibit parathyroid cell replication. Nevertheless, modest changes in $1,25(OH)_2D_3$ have no effect on parathyroid cell proliferation in vivo,[51] and calcium alone can prevent parathyroid cell hyperplasia in mice engineered to lack vitamin D receptors.[52] Thus, the importance of regulation of parathyroid cell number by $1,25(OH)_2D_3$ in vivo has not been established.

Although the ability to increase parathyroid cell number in response to physiologic challenge represents an important defense against hypocalcemia, it is a slow response that is not easily reversible. When the need for an increased number of parathyroid cells disappears (e.g., after renal transplantation for uremia), persistent hyperparathyroidism can cause vexing clinical problems for months and years thereafter. The mechanisms for decreasing parathyroid cell number, if they exist, are poorly understood. Apoptosis of normal parathyroid cells in response to experimental manipulation has not been demonstrated.[51]

Parathyroid Gland Development

Genes involved in making parathyroid cells during development may also regulate PTH synthesis and parathyroid cell number throughout life; thus, an understanding of parathyroid cell development may have broad clinical implications. Although the genetic mechanisms used to generate parathyroid chief cells during development are largely unknown, the importance of four specific genes has become clear. Studies of gene knockout mice have shown that the hoxa3[53] and pax 9[54] transcription factors are needed to form parathyroid glands as well as many other pharyngeal pouch derivatives, such as the thymus. People with mutations in the gene encoding the transcription factor GATA3 exhibit a syndrome of hypoparathyroidism, sensorineural deafness, and renal anomalies when only one copy of the gene is mutated.[55] Furthermore, mice[56] or humans[57] missing the *gcm2* and *GCMB* genes, respectively, have no parathyroid glands. In both species, the deletion of *gcm2* or *GCMB* (the human equivalent) is very specific for controlling parathyroid development because no abnormalities in other tissues have been noted. Mice, which have only two parathyroid glands normally, still make PTH in a small number of cells in the thymus after *gcm2* gene ablation and secrete this PTH into the circulation. A human patient without *GCMB* had no detectable circulating PTH at birth and low levels of PTH several years later.

Peripheral Metabolism of Parathyroid Hormone

The earliest radioimmunoassays for PTH demonstrated that the molecular forms of PTH in the circulation differ from those in the parathyroid gland.[58] Characterization of the metabolism of PTH and its fragments has clarified the origins and significance of immunoreactive PTH molecules in the blood stream. As noted previously, both PTH(1–84) and carboxy-terminal fragments of PTH are secreted from the parathyroid gland[7]; the ratio of inactive PTH to active PTH secretion increases with increasing blood calcium. Secreted intact PTH(1–84) is extensively metabolized by liver (70%) and kidney (20%) and disappears from the circulation with a half-life of 2 minutes. This rapid peripheral metabolism of PTH is unaffected by widely varying levels of blood calcium or $1,25(OH)_2D_3$.[59] Less than 1% of the secreted hormone finds its way to PTH receptors on physiologic target organs.[60] These features of PTH metabolism ensure that the blood level of PTH is determined principally by the activity of the parathyroid glands and that the PTH level can respond rapidly to small changes in the rate of secretion of the hormone.

In the liver, a small amount of PTH binds to physiologically relevant PTH receptors but most of the intact PTH is cleaved, initially after residues 33 and 36, probably by cathepsins.[61] In the kidney, a small amount of intact PTH binds to physiologic PTH receptors, but most of the intact PTH is filtered at the glomerulus and subsequently bound by a large, membrane-bound luminal protein, megalin[62]; this binding leads to internalization and degradation of PTH by the tubules.[63] Carboxy-terminal fragments are also cleared efficiently by glomerular filtration. In fact, the kidney is the only known site of clearance of carboxy-terminal PTH fragments; these fragments thus accumulate dramatically when the glomerular filtration rate (GFR) falls. Even in the presence of normal renal function, the half-life of carboxy-terminal fragments of PTH exceeds that of

PTH(1–84) by several-fold. Consequently, the concentration of carboxy-terminal fragments in the circulation exceeds that of intact PTH, even though intact PTH usually is the major form of PTH secreted from the parathyroid gland.

Careful analysis of PTH fragments using high-performance liquid chromatography (HPLC) and immunologic methods have revealed almost full-length PTH fragments missing the first several amino acids of the hormone, but containing most or all of the remaining hormone sequence.[64] These still incompletely characterized fragments are both secreted from the parathyroid gland and generated by peripheral metabolism of the hormone. Because they are missing the amino-terminal portion of PTH, they cannot stimulate cyclic adenosine monophosphate (cAMP) production by the PTH/parathyroid hormone–related protein (PTHrP) receptor, and except in renal failure, they circulate in small amounts.[65] Nevertheless, the possible biologic activity of these and other PTH fragments, possibly through novel receptors, remains an unsettled issue. Experiments with PTH(7–84) suggest that such extended carboxyl fragments may exert potent effects in vivo, antagonistic to those of intact PTH.[66]

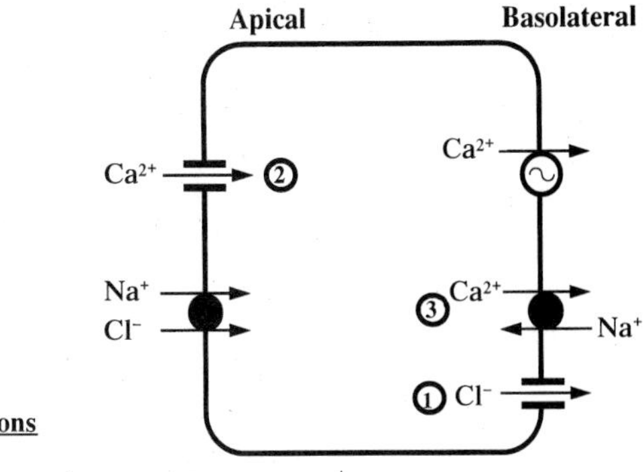

Figure 26–7. Effects of parathyroid hormone (PTH) on distal tubular calcium transport. PTH acts to increase chloride efflux through channels in the basolateral membrane. As indicated, this increase leads to calcium influx through apical calcium channels. PTH also increases basolateral Ca^{2+}-Na^+ exchange. The apical Na^+-Cl^- cotransporter allows chloride to enter the cell and is the target of thiazide diuretics. Cl_i^-, intracellular chloride. (Adapted from Friedman PA, Gesek FA. Calcium transport in renal epithelial cells. Am J Physiol 1993; 264: F181–F198.)

Actions of Parathyroid Hormone

Actions on the Kidney

Stimulation of Calcium Reabsorption

Almost all of the calcium in the initial glomerular filtrate is reabsorbed by the renal tubules. Sixty-five percent is reabsorbed by the proximal convoluted and straight tubules via a passive, paracellular route.[67, 68] Changes in the transepithelial voltage gradient, determined largely by the rate of sodium reabsorption, control the rate of calcium transport in the proximal tubule; PTH does little to affect calcium flux in this region. The remaining calcium is largely reabsorbed more distally—20% of the initial filtrate in the cortical thick ascending limb (cTAL) of Henle's loop and 10% in the distal convoluted and connecting tubules. In the cTAL, calcium reabsorption also is mainly passive and paracellular, although some transcellular, active calcium transport may occur as well.[69]

Efficient paracellular calcium and magnesium movement requires expression of a unique tight junction protein, paracellin-1; mutant paracellin-1 genes underlie a rare renal calcium- and magnesium-wasting disorder.[70] Because paracellular cation transport in the cTAL is driven by the lumen-positive transepithelial voltage gradient that is established by active Na-K-Cl_2 reabsorption, calcium reabsorption there is strongly inhibited by loop diuretics such as furosemide. The calcium-sensing receptor, initially characterized in the parathyroid, also is expressed in the cTAL.[71] When activated by high blood calcium or magnesium, this receptor inhibits Na-K-Cl_2 reabsorption in the cTAL. Consequently, renal concentrating capacity and calcium reabsorption are inhibited as well. This inhibition provides a parathyroid-independent mechanism for controlling renal calcium handling in direct response to changes in blood calcium concentration.

Although PTH modestly stimulates paracellular calcium reabsorption in the cTAL, the primary site for hormonal regulation of renal calcium reabsorption is the distal nephron, which normally reabsorbs nearly all of the remaining 10% of filtered calcium by a unique transcellular active transport mechanism. As depicted in Figure 26–1, the intracellular level of calcium is extremely low, about 150 nM, compared with the millimolar levels in the glomerular filtrate and the blood. Calcium enters the distal tubular cell from the tubular lumen through voltage-sensitive calcium channels, one subtype of which (ECaC in the rabbit, CaT2 in the rat) has been cloned.[72, 73] This conductance is passive but is regulated directly by the electrochemical gradient across the apical membrane. PTH increases this conductance (② in Fig. 26–7) by increasing the transmembrane voltage gradient (i.e., by hyperpolarizing the cell),[74, 75] probably by increasing chloride exit through basolateral chloride channels (① in Fig. 26–7).

A similar hyperpolarizing effect is exerted by thiazide-type diuretics, which reduce intracellular chloride (by inhibiting apical sodium chloride [NaCl] transporters) and thereby also open apical calcium channels, increasing calcium entry. To protect the low physiologic level of cytosolic free calcium from the relatively large amounts of incoming calcium, these cells express the calcium-binding protein calbindin-D28K, which avidly binds entering calcium at the apical membrane and transports it to the basolateral membrane, where it is then ejected via active processes involving sodium-calcium exchange and an ATP-driven calcium pump. Expression of calbindin-D28K is increased by PTH directly and also indirectly, via increased synthesis of $1,25(OH)_2D_3$.[76, 77] Sodium-calcium exchange also is increased by PTH (③ in Fig. 26–7).[78]

The amount of calcium in the final urine reflects all of the tubular reabsorption processes just enumerated but also depends crucially on the initial filtered load of calcium. All of PTH's actions serve to raise the blood calcium level, so that the filtered load of calcium is high in states of PTH excess. In that setting, even though the rate of distal tubular calcium reabsorption is increased by PTH, the total amount of calcium in the final urine is likely to be high, because of the high initial filtered load.

Inhibition of Phosphate Transport

Phosphate reabsorption occurs mainly in the proximal renal tubules, which reclaim roughly 80% of the filtered load. Some additional phosphate (8% to 10%) is reabsorbed in the distal tubule (but not in Henle's loop), leaving about 10% to 12% for excretion in the urine. The normal overall fractional tubular reabsorption of phosphate (TRP), therefore, is about 88%, although a more reliable measure of renal phosphate handling is the *phosphate threshold* (TmP/GFR), which can be derived from the TRP through the use of a nomogram (Fig. 26–8) based on studies of experimental phosphate infusions in

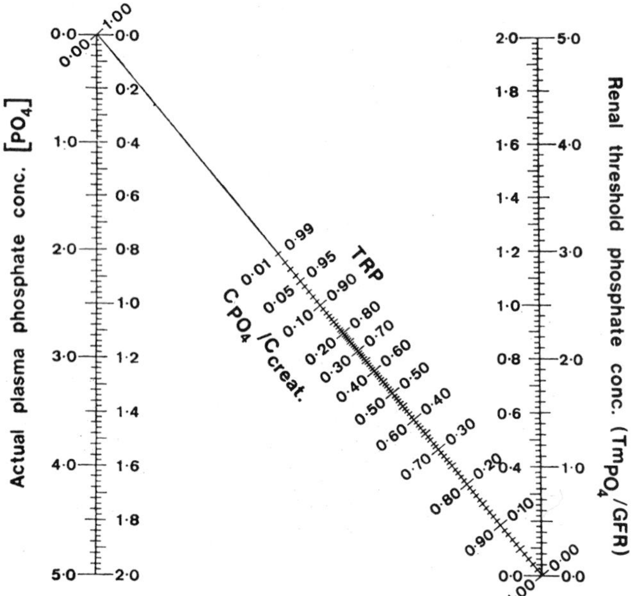

Figure 26–8. Nomogram for determining renal threshold phosphate concentration (Tm_{PO_4}/GFR) from the plasma phosphate concentration and the fractional reabsorption of filtered phosphate (TRP) or fractional excretion of filtered phosphate (1−TRP, or $C_{PO_4}C_{creat}$). Because the blood level of phosphate influences the renal handling of phosphate, the renal threshold phosphate concentration best separates normal from abnormal renal phosphate handling. C, clearance; creat, creatinine; GFR, glomerular filtration rate; TRP, tubular resorption of phosphate. (From Walton RJ, Bijvoet OLM. Nomogram of derivation of renal threshold phosphate concentration. Lancet 1975; 2:309–310.)

healthy persons and in patients with a variety of diseases that affect phosphate excretion.[79]

Phosphate reabsorption in both proximal and distal tubules is strongly inhibited by PTH, although the proximal effect is quantitatively the more important. Phosphate is reabsorbed by a transepithelial route. Transport from the glomerular filtrate into the cell is mediated by specific sodium–(inorganic) phosphate (NaP_i) cotransporters.[80, 81] The low level of sodium within the cell drives the cotransport of sodium and phosphate, even though the phosphate travels up an electrochemical gradient. In response to PTH, the V_{max} for sodium-phosphate cotransport decreases because NaP_i cotransporters are rapidly (by 15 minutes) sequestered within subapical endocytic vesicles, after which they are delivered to lysosomes and undergo proteolysis.[82] Conversely, in hypoparathyroidism expression of NaP_i protein and mRNA is strongly up-regulated.[83]

Dietary intake of phosphate also reciprocally regulates the expression and activity of NaP_i cotransporters and thus the proximal tubular absorption of phosphate by a mechanism that is independent of PTH. Dietary deprivation of phosphate, for example, leads to a stimulation of phosphate reabsorption that can override the effects of PTH on the proximal tubule. Although not yet demonstrated experimentally, a likely candidate to mediate this effect of dietary phosphate is the putative hormone "phosphatonin," excessive action of which is implicated in the humoral hypophosphatemic syndromes X-linked hypophosphatemic rickets and oncogenous osteomalacia (see "Disorders of Phosphate Metabolism," later).

Other Renal Effects of Parathyroid Hormone

PTH stimulates the synthesis of $1,25(OH)_2D_3$ in the proximal tubule by rapidly inducing transcription of the 25-hydroxyvitamin D [25(OH)D] 1α-hydroxylase gene, an effect that can be overridden by hypercalcemia or by the action of $1,25(OH)_2D_3$.[84, 85] PTH inhibits proximal tubular transcription of the 25(OH)D 24-hydroxylase gene and antagonizes the up-regulation of 24-hydroxylase activity by $1,25(OH)_2D_3$[86, 87] (see "Vitamin D Metabolism"). PTH inhibits proximal tubular sodium, water, and bicarbonate reabsorption,[88] mainly via inhibition of the apical amiloride-sensitive Na^+-H^+ exchanger (NHE3) and the basolateral Na^+-K^+-ATPase.[89, 90] PTH also stimulates proximal tubular gluconeogenesis[91] and acts directly on glomerular podocytes to decrease both single-nephron and whole-kidney GFR.[92]

Actions of Parathyroid Hormone on Bone

The actions of PTH on bone are complicated because PTH acts on a number of cell types both directly and indirectly. PTH increases both bone formation and bone resorption. With regard to calcium homeostasis, the effect of PTH on bone resorption is dominant; continuous administration of PTH leads to a net release of calcium from bone. But this straightforward net effect of PTH on calcium homeostasis belies the highly variable effects of the hormone on bone, which depend on the type of bone (trabecular or cortical), the particular target cell type, and the pattern of PTH administration.

Figure 26–9 illustrates the cells of the osteoblast lineage (see also Chapter 27). Osteoblasts are derived from multipotent mesenchymal stem cells that can differentiate into chondrocytes, adipocytes, osteoblasts, and probably other cell types.[93] Within the osteoblast lineage, committed osteoprogenitor cells divide, become preosteoblastic stromal cells (which can divide further), and then become osteoblasts. Osteoblasts no longer divide and are cuboidal cells found on the bone surface actively laying down new bone. When these cells become surrounded by bone, they become stellate osteocytes. If, instead, osteoblasts stop synthesizing matrix and remain on the bone surface, they flatten out as bone lining cells. Not all preosteoblasts and osteoblasts mature; a variable number die by apoptotic, programmed cell death.[94]

Receptors for PTH are found on preosteoblasts, osteoblasts, lining cells, and osteocytes. PTH changes the osteoblast lineage cell population by stimulating cell proliferation[95]; by decreasing apoptosis of preosteoblasts and osteoblasts, thereby increasing the number of osteocytes; and perhaps by converting inactive lining cells to osteoblasts.[96] When added to cells in culture, PTH stops preosteoblastic cells from becoming mature osteoblasts.[97] Furthermore, PTH changes the activity of mature osteoblasts by a variety of mechanisms. When PTH is added to isolated osteoblasts in vitro, the osteoblasts decrease their synthesis of collagen I and other matrix proteins, at least in part by steering the essential transcription factor core-binding factor-α1 (CBFA1) toward proteosomal destruction.[98] In vivo, however, the most obvious effects of PTH are to increase bone formation, probably by indirect actions such as stimulation of synthesis of insulin-like growth factor I (IGFI) and other growth factors by osteoblast lineage cells. This action of PTH can be mimicked in vitro by intermittent administration of PTH to osteoblasts in organ culture[95] or as dispersed cells.[99]

Surprisingly, osteoclasts, the bone-resorbing cells derived from hematopoietic precursors, have no PTH receptors. Instead, preosteoblasts and osteoblasts signal to osteoclast precursors to cause them to fuse and form mature osteoclasts and signal to those osteoclasts to allow them to resorb bone and to avoid apoptosis (Fig. 26–10). Two osteoblast surface proteins, macrophage colony-stimulating factor (M-CSF) and RANK ligand (RANKL), are essential for stimulation of osteoclastogenesis,[100, 101] and RANKL is essential for the activation of mature osteoclasts. The growth factor M-CSF (or CSF1), is expressed both as a secreted protein and as a cell surface protein; the production of both forms is stimulated by PTH.[102]

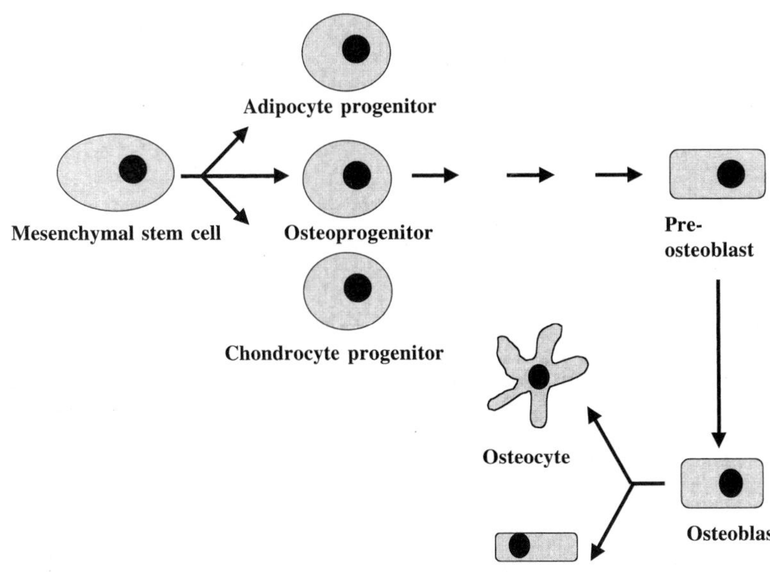

Figure 26–9. Osteoblast lineage. All precursors of osteoblasts can proliferate; osteoblasts are transformed to osteocytes and lining cells without further proliferation. Some data suggest that lining cells may revert to osteoblast function after parathyroid hormone stimulation. At each stage in the lineage, apoptotic cell death is probably an alternative fate.

RANKL—also named osteoprotegerin ligand (OPGL), osteoclast-differentiating factor (ODF), and TRANCE—is a membrane-bound member of the tumor necrosis factor (TNF) family; its synthesis is also increased by PTH. RANKL binds to its receptor, RANK, a member of the TNF receptor family. RANK is found both on osteoclast precursors and on mature osteoclasts. The binding of RANKL to RANK can be blocked by osteoprotegerin (OPG), another member of the TNF receptor family. OPG (also called OCIF and TR1) circulates and is also secreted by cells of the osteoblastic lineage. PTH decreases the synthesis and secretion of OPG from these cells.[103] Thus, PTH, by increasing RANK and decreasing OPG locally in bone, serves to increase bone resorption.

Because PTH can both increase bone formation and increase resorption, the net effect of PTH on bone mass varies from one part of bone to another and also varies dramatically according to whether PTH is administered continuously or intermittently. Intermittent administration of low doses of PTH causes dramatic net increase in trabecular bone mass with little effect on cortical bone in humans. Continuous administration of PTH, in contrast, leads to a decrease in cortical bone mass; the net effect of PTH on trabecular bone depends on the dose. In mild hyperparathyroidism, there is little net effect of PTH on trabecular bone and a decrease in cortical bone. In all of these settings, the rate of bone formation is increased; the varying rate of osteoclastic resorption determines the net effect of PTH on bone mass.

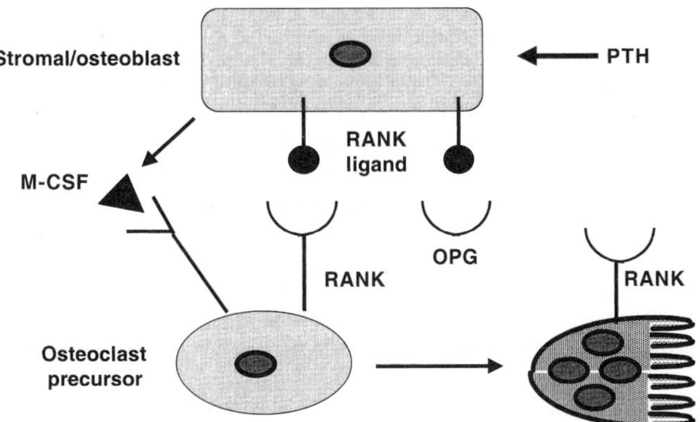

Figure 26–10. Stromal cell control of osteoclastogenesis and osteoclast activity. Parathyroid hormone (PTH) acts on PTH/PTH-related protein (PTHrP) receptors on precursors of osteoblasts to increase the production of macrophage colony–stimulating factor (M-CSF) and RANK ligand and to decrease the production of osteoprotegerin (OPG). M-CSF and RANK ligand stimulate the production of osteoclasts and increase the activity of mature osteoclasts by binding to the receptor RANK. OPG blocks the interaction of RANK ligand and RANK.

Molecular Basis of Parathyroid Hormone Action

Ever since the discovery that PTH stimulates the secretion of cAMP into the urine,[104] PTH has been thought to act by triggering a cascade of intracellular second messengers. This guiding hypothesis, in its current form, postulates that all of the actions of PTH result from the binding of the hormone to a receptor on the plasma membrane of target tissues. This receptor is a member of a large family of G protein–linked receptors that span the plasma membrane seven times (Fig. 26–11). The binding of hormone on the outside of the membrane causes conformational changes in the receptor molecule that activate the receptor's ability to release guanosine diphosphate (GDP) from the α subunit of a G protein bound to the receptor. The G protein then binds guanosine triphosphate (GTP) in place of GDP. The GTP-binding α subunit of the G protein then separates from the $\beta\gamma$ subunits, and the separate subunits of the G protein then modulate the activity of enzymes and channels. The activity of these enzymes and channels then affects proteins further downstream, eventually leading to the physiologic responses of bone and kidney cells.

Parathyroid Hormone and Parathyroid Hormone–Related Receptors

DNA encoding a PTH/PTHrP receptor has been isolated from rat, opossum, human, pig, *Xenopus* (toad), and zebrafish cells and tissues.[105–107] The receptor mediates actions of both PTH and PTHrP. The predicted amino acid sequence of the receptor and direct mapping of inserted epitopes suggest that the receptor spans the plasma membrane seven times, but the sequence does not closely resemble the sequences of most known G protein–linked receptors. Instead, it is a member of a distinct subfamily of closely related receptors. Most of these

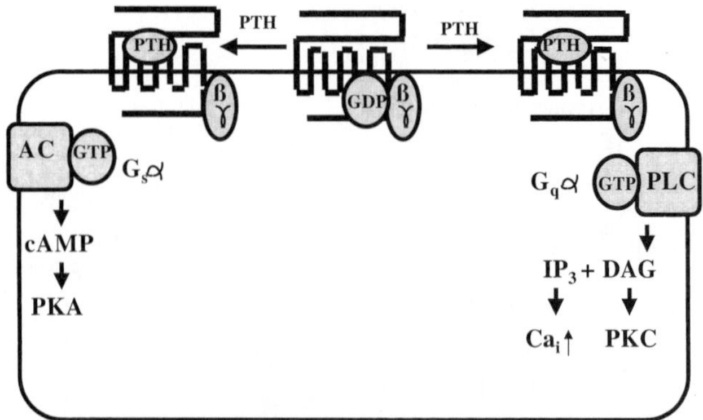

Figure 26–11. Parathyroid hormone (PTH)/PTH-related protein (PTHrP) receptors act as nucleotide exchangers. PTH binding to the receptor leads to exchange of guanosine triphosphate (GTP) for guanosine diphosphate (GDP) bound to $G\alpha$ subunits. $G\alpha$ subunits bound to GTP are released from the receptor and from the $\beta\gamma$ subunits and then activate effectors. $G_s\alpha$ activates adenylate cyclase, leading to the formation of cyclic AMP (cAMP), which then activates protein kinase A (PKA). $G_q\alpha$ and related α subunits activate phospholipase C (PLC). PLC hydrolyzes phosphotidyl inositol (1,4,5)tris-phosphate to generate diacyl glycerol (DAG) and inositol (1,4,5)tris-phosphate (IP_3). The DAG then activates protein kinase C (PKC), and the IP_3 activates a receptor on microsomal vesicles that directs the movement of calcium from microsomal vesicles into the cytosol.

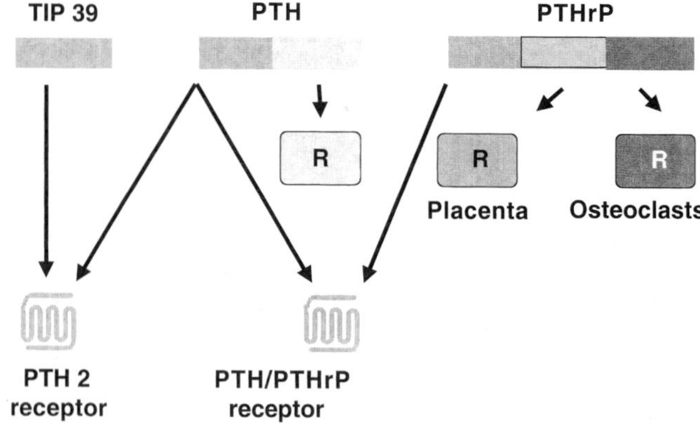

Figure 26–12. Network of parathyroid hormone (PTH) ligands and receptors (R). PTH and PTH-related protein (PTHrP) closely resemble each other at the amino-terminal region; TIP39 is more distantly related. Although only the PTH/PTHrP receptor and the PTH2 receptors have been cloned, biologic actions suggest receptors specific for the carboxy-terminal portion of PTH, as well as distinct receptors for the mid-region of PTHrP and for a more distal region of PTHrP. Not shown are possible nuclear sites of action of PTHrP.

receptors bind peptides of 30 to 40 amino acids in length. Known members include receptors for the secretin family of peptides (secretin, vasoactive intestinal peptide (VIP), glucagon, glucagon-like peptide, growth hormone–releasing hormone, pituitary adenylate cyclase–activating peptide, gastric inhibitory peptide), corticotropin-releasing hormone, calcitonin, and insect diuretic hormones related to corticotropin-releasing hormone. The PTH/PTHrP receptor most closely resembles receptors of the secretin group. The gene encoding the PTH/PTHrP receptor has a complicated structure, with 13 introns interrupting the coding sequence.[108, 109]

In the mouse, an upstream promoter is used primarily in kidney and to some extent in liver; a downstream promoter is used in all tissues that express the gene, including bone.[109, 110] The human promoter uses the same start sites, but the kidney-specific promoter is much less active in humans, and a third, distinct start site is used in many tissues.[111]

The cloned PTH/PTHrP receptor binds amino-terminal fragments of PTH and PTHrP with equal affinity. The receptor is expressed at high levels in kidney and in osteoblasts of bone but is also expressed in a wide variety of tissues, such as smooth muscle, brain, and a variety of fetal tissues, which are thought to be target tissues more for PTHrP than for PTH.[112] In response to binding of PTH or PTHrP, the receptor activates several G proteins, including $G_s\alpha$, $G_q\alpha$ and its close relatives, $G_i\alpha$, and perhaps other G proteins.[113–115]

The PTH/PTHrP receptor probably mediates many of the actions of both PTH and PTHrP. The ligand-binding and signaling properties of the receptor, the pattern of expression of the receptor, and the consequences of mutation of the receptor sequence (see later) are persuasive evidence in this regard. Nevertheless, the scheme of PTH action illustrated in Figure 26–11 should be considered a simplified outline. It is unlikely that all of the actions of PTH can be explained by interactions with the cloned PTH/PTHrP receptor: Fragments of PTH that seem not to bind the receptor may be biologically active[116–118]; some cells respond to PTH in ways not mimicked by the cloned receptor.[119–122] Furthermore, the carboxyl-terminal portion of PTH(1–84) binds a cell surface protein distinct from the PTH/PTHrP receptor.[123]

A second PTH receptor, which can be activated by PTH but not by PTHrP, called the PTH2 receptor (PTH2R), has been cloned.[124] This receptor is expressed in multiple tissues, including brain, vascular endothelium and smooth muscle, endocrine cells of the gastrointestinal tract, and sperm.[125] Expression is not seen in osteoblasts or renal tubules, however. Although PTH activates human PTH2R well, PTH only poorly activates the rat PTH2R.[126] Furthermore, a novel ligand called TIP39 has been characterized and shown to be a potent activator of PTH2R.[127] TIP39 bears only a weak resemblance to PTH or PTHrP and is likely to be a physiologically relevant activator of that receptor. The functional role of the PTH2R is unknown; this receptor may well not mediate actions of PTH in vivo. The two cloned PTHRs, as well as distinct receptors for fragments of PTHrP (see later), probably are part of a complex network of ligands and receptors (Fig. 26–12).

Functional Implications of Parathyroid Hormone Structure

Amino-terminal fragments of PTH as short as PTH(1–34) have potency at least as great as that of the full-length PTH(1–84).[128] Several discrete portions of the PTH(1–34) peptide interact with the receptor.[129] The first several residues of PTH are particularly important for triggering the conformational change in the receptor that results in activation of G_s and adenylate cyclase. Sequences responsible for transmembrane activation of G_s make up most of the first 13 residues of PTH[130]; it is these residues that are highly conserved between PTH and PTHrP. At high concentrations, PTH(1–14) by itself can activate the PTH/PTHrP receptor.[131] This activation domain interacts with the receptor's transmembrane domains and extracellular loops.[132–134] When the first nine residues of PTH are covalently linked to the receptor's transmembrane domains and extracellular loops, they can activate the receptor.[135] An analogue of PTH(1–14) can trigger G_q activation, thus activating phospholipase C.[136] These data, plus the observation that a PTH analogue modified at position 1 selectively loses its ability to activate phospholipase C,[137] demonstrate that the amino-terminal portion of PTH is essential for activation of both G_s and G_q. More distal regions of PTH(1–34) can activate protein kinase C and can raise intracellular calcium levels by mechanisms that have not been fully clarified.

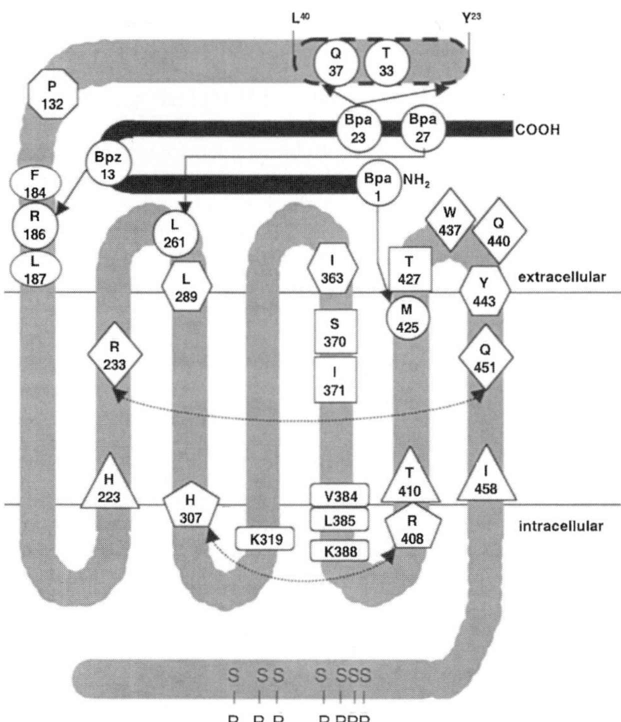

Figure 26–13. Interactions between parathyroid hormone (PTH) and the PTH/PTH-related protein (PTHrP) receptor. Key residues involved in PTH–PTH receptor function are indicated (amino acid residues and position numbers correspond to the human PTH/PTHrP receptor sequence): circles, residues identified in crosslinking studies; octagon, a site involved in Blomstrand's chondrodysplasia; ovals, hydrophobic residues important for PTH(1–34) and PTH(1–14) binding; triangles, residues mutated in patients with Jansen's chondrodysplasia; hexagons, sites at which the corresponding residues in the PTH2 receptor play a role in discriminating between PTH and PTHrP; squares, residues that determine agonist versus antagonist action of Arg2-PTH(1–34); diamonds, sites at which mutations impair PTH(1–34) binding but not PTH(3–34) binding; rectangles, residues that when mutated alter G protein coupling; and dashed curves with arrows, interdomain interactions as determined by paired mutations affecting PTH(1–34) interaction (R233 and Q451) or by zinc chelation studies (H307 and R408). (From DeGroot LJ (ed). Endocrinology, 4th ed. Philadelphia, WB Saunders, 2001, p 986.)

The more carboxy-terminal portions of PTH(1–34) contribute importantly to the specificity and tight binding of PTH to the PTH/PTHrP receptor, at least partly through interactions with the receptor's amino-terminal extracellular domain.[138] A variety of studies of genetically altered receptors and biochemical studies using photoactivated crosslinks between PTH and the receptor have reinforced each other and show that the carboxy-terminal portion of PTH makes multiple contacts with the amino-terminal extension of the receptor and with its extracellular loops[139, 140] (Fig. 26–13).

Studies of the structure of PTH by nuclear magnetic resonance spectroscopy[141, 142] suggest that the activation domain and the carboxy-terminal domain are discrete entities dominated by α-helices separated by a flexible loop of variable size, depending on the hydrophobicity of the solvent. In the crystal structure of human PTH(1–34), the flexible loop is entirely replaced with helical structure.[143] Taken together, these studies suggest that the carboxy-terminal portion of PTH makes multiple contacts with the receptor that allow high-affinity binding and position the amino-terminal portion of PTH to activate the receptor through contacts with transmembrane domains and associated loops.

Activation of Second Messengers

Precisely how binding of PTH to the extracellular domains of the PTH/PTHrP receptor leads to activation of G proteins is not understood. The crystal structure of rhodopsin,[144] another member of the seven-transmembrane receptor family, as well as the behavior of certain mutant PTH/PTHrP receptors,[134, 145] suggest that the seven transmembrane domains of the PTH/PTHrP receptors form a ring, with the seventh transmembrane domain adjacent to the first and second domains. Presumably, binding of PTH to several different regions of the receptor changes the relationships of the transmembrane domains such that the receptor's three intracellular loops and carboxy-terminal tail interact with G proteins in an altered way.

Receptors with certain point mutations in the second,[146] sixth,[147] and seventh[148] transmembrane domains can activate G_s even without stimulation by hormone. These mutant receptors were discovered by analyzing the PTH/PTHrP receptors in patients with Jansen's metaphyseal chondrodystrophy.[149, 150] Patients with this disorder have signs of parathyroid overactivity (hypercalcemia, hypophosphatemia, high levels of $1,25(OH)_2D_3$, and urinary cAMP) but low PTH and PTHrP levels. The mutations must change the conformation of the intracellular face of the receptor in a way that resembles the effect of binding of PTH to the normal receptor. The observation that inappropriate activation of the PTH/PTHrP receptor in Jansen's chondrodystrophy leads to all of the metabolic abnormalities found in primary hyperparathyroidism is one of the most persuasive pieces of evidence that the cloned PTH/PTHrP receptor does, in fact, mediate the actions of PTH in bone and kidney in vivo.

Second Messengers and Distal Effects of Parathyroid Hormone

The activation of multiple G proteins by PTH[114, 115, 151] raises questions about the individual roles of each second messenger and their possible interactions. The importance of cAMP as a mediator of the physiologic actions of PTH has been demonstrated by studies in vivo[104, 152–154] and in vitro.[155–158] Furthermore, patients with pseudohypoparathyroidism type I, who cannot increase urinary cAMP levels in response to PTH, show clear renal resistance to PTH (see later).

Phospholipase C, with concomitant activation of protein kinase C and synthesis of IP_3, may mediate physiologic actions of PTH as well,[159] such as inhibition of sodium-phosphate cotransport[160] and stimulation of the renal 25(OH)D 1α-hydroxylase.[161] Some actions of PTH may require activation of both adenylate cyclase and phospholipase C for optimal activity.

Target Cell Responsiveness to Parathyroid Hormone

Physiologic responses to PTH depend not only on the concentration of PTH in blood but also on the responsiveness of target cells to PTH. This responsiveness can be modified by previous exposure to PTH or by exposure to a variety of other hormones and paracrine factors. Responsiveness can be changed by alterations at virtually every step in the cellular response to PTH.

Major regulators of PTH/PTHrP receptor gene expression include, not surprisingly, PTH and $1,25(OH)_2D_3$, both of which can decrease PTH/PTHrP receptor mRNA in certain target cells.[162–166] In some settings, PTH decreases the amount of immunoreactive and functional receptor on the cell surface without changing the levels of PTH/PTHrP mRNA.[167, 168] This decrease reflects ligand-induced internalization and degradation of receptors. Internalization of receptor is stimulated by PTH binding[169] and is modulated by sequences found in the membrane-proximal portion of the receptor's cytoplasmic tail.[170] The precise mechanism of PTH-induced internalization of the PTH/PTHrP receptor is not fully understood and may vary in different cellular contexts.[171–173] Even without change in receptor number, previous exposure to PTH leads to inefficient triggering of G proteins (desensitization).[168]

PARATHYROID HORMONE–RELATED PROTEIN

Parathyroid hormone–related protein (PTHrP) was discovered because the secretion of PTHrP by a wide variety of tumors contributes to the humoral hypercalcemia of malignancy. For this reason, the initial studies of PTHrP in humans and animals stressed the PTH-like structure and properties of the molecule. Subsequent studies soon showed, however, that PTHrP, unlike PTH, is made by a wide variety of tissues, in which it acts locally in ways that may have little relevance to the control of blood calcium.

Gene and Protein Structure

PTHrP sequences from human, rat, mouse, dog, bovine species, chicken, fugufish, and sea bream have been cloned[174–176] (Fig. 26–14). In humans, alternative RNA splicing yields transcripts that encode three distinct proteins of 139, 141, and 173 residues that differ only after residue 139.

Inspection of these sequences suggests that PTHrP has several functionally distinct domains. Eight or nine of the first 13 residues of PTHrP are identical to those in known mammalian PTH sequences. These sequences encompass the known "activation" domain of PTH (see earlier) and are instrumental in the ability of PTHrP to activate PTH/PTHrP receptors. The conserved histidine at position 5 of all PTHrP molecules, which differs from the hydrophobic residue found at the corresponding position of all PTHs, allows PTHrP to activate the PTH/PTHrP receptor but not the PTH2 receptor.[177, 178]

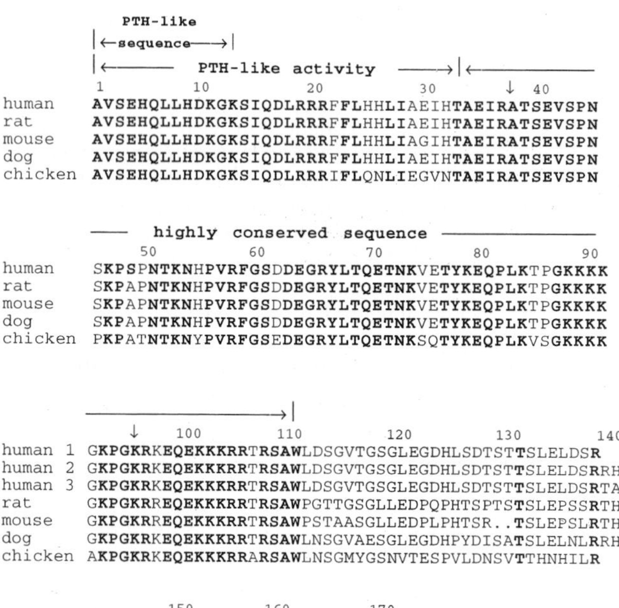

Figure 26–14. Sequences of parathyroid hormone–related protein (PTHrP) from five species. Completely conserved residues are in **boldface**; note the high level of conservation through residue 111. *Arrows* indicate sites of internal cleavage after residues 37 and 95, which lead to generation of PTHrP(38–94) amide and PTHrP(38–95). Another site of cleavage, generating PTHrP(38–101) and, perhaps, PTHrP(107–139) is not shown.[165] The three human sequences represent proteins synthesized from alternatively spliced mRNAs and differ only after residue 139. Amino acids are indicated by the single letter code; see legend to Figure 26–3 for code.

The sequences in PTHrP(14–34) are also highly conserved. Although these sequences little resemble the corresponding region of PTH, they can displace PTH from the PTH/PTHrP receptor. Studies of the secondary and tertiary structures of PTHrP(1–34) and PTH(1–37) suggest that they have similar structures dominated by α-helices connected by a flexible hinge.[179–181]

The remaining portion of the PTHrP molecule bears no resemblance to corresponding sequences in PTH. Nevertheless, residues 35 to 111 of PTHrP are strikingly well conserved, with only nine residues differing between mammalian and chicken PTHrP sequences. This sequence conservation is considerably greater than that found in the carboxyl-terminal portion of PTH, suggesting that this region of PTHrP has unique and important functions. After residue 111, the PTHrP sequences vary considerably from species to species.

Interspersed within the PTHrP sequences are multiple sites containing one or several basic residues that might serve as post-translational cleavage sites (see Fig. 26–14). Extensive analysis of PTHrP fragments in tumors, cell lines, and transfected cells has shown that several of these sites are, in fact, functional cleavage signals.[182] PTHrP is cleaved after the arginine at residue 37[183]; this cleavage, followed by carboxypeptidase cleavage, generates a PTH-like PTHrP(1–36) fragment as well as the fragments PTHrP(38–94)amide, PTHrP(38–95), and PTHrP(38–101).[184] More carboxy-terminal fragments of PTHrP have been detected in cells as well.

In the blood of patients with humoral hypercalcemia of malignancy, multiple immunoreactive species of PTHrP have been found that may well correspond to the fragments of PTHrP in cells and tissue culture media, although precise characterization of these various immunoreactive species is incomplete (see later).[185–188] Full-length PTHrP may well not circulate, since an amino-terminal–specific immunoaffinity column was unable to extract carboxy-terminal immunoreactivity from the serum of patients with malignant hypercalcemia.[187]

Functions of Parathyroid Hormone–Related Protein

The first actions of PTHrP to be defined were the PTH-like actions associated with the humoral hypercalcemia of malignancy. In this pathologic entity, PTHrP acts as a hormone; it is secreted from the tumor into the blood stream and then acts on bone and kidney to raise calcium levels[189–191] (see "Hypercalcemia of Malignancy" later). Whether or not PTHrP circulates at high enough levels in normal adults to contribute to normal calcium homeostasis is an unanswered question. With metastases of breast cancer to bone, locally produced PTHrP can raise serum calcium without necessarily raising blood levels of PTHrP.[192]

Growing evidence suggests that PTHrP acts as a calciotropic hormone during fetal life and in lactation. PTHrP secreted from the fetal parathyroid gland stimulates transport of calcium across the placenta in sheep.[193, 194] PTH, in contrast, has no effect on placental calcium transport. Furthermore, fetal mice missing the PTHrP gene transport ^{45}Ca across the placenta inefficiently.[195] This action of PTHrP requires only the mid-region of PTHrP and probably involves a receptor distinct from the PTH/PTHrP receptor.

The second possible setting for humoral actions of PTHrP is lactation. Secretion of PTHrP from the breast into the blood stream may influence the movement of calcium from maternal bone into breast milk.[196–201] PTHrP, therefore, probably contributes to the dramatic but largely reversible bone loss during lactation, which is only minimally affected by calcium supplementation.[202] An exaggeration of this lactational role of PTHrP may explain the rare presentation of hypercalcemia and high PTHrP levels in pregnant and lactating women.[203–205] Large amounts of PTHrP are also secreted into breast milk, although the role of PTHrP in milk is unknown.

Most of the actions of PTHrP are likely to be paracrine or autocrine.[206, 207] PTHrP is synthesized at one time or another during fetal life in virtually every tissue. Its role in the development of fetal bone has been demonstrated through the striking abnormalities found in genetically engineered mice missing the PTHrP gene.[208] These abnormalities suggest that PTHrP normally keeps chondrocytes proliferating in orderly columns, thereby delaying chondrocyte differentiation. The role of PTHrP in many other fetal tissues may analogously involve regulation of proliferation and differentiation. The widespread expression of the PTHrP in fetal life probably underlies the expression of PTHrP in a wide variety of malignancies. As is often the case in malignancy, the expression of PTHrP represents the reinitiation of a fetal pattern of gene expression.

PTHrP is synthesized by many adult tissues.[206] In tissues such as skin, hair, and breast, it is likely that PTHrP regulates cell proliferation and differentiation.[209] PTHrP is also synthesized in response to stretch in the smooth muscle of blood vessels and of the gastrointestinal tract, uterus, and bladder and acts in an autocrine fashion to relax the smooth muscle.[210] PTHrP is also widely expressed in neurons of the central nervous system; its function in the brain is unknown, but it may protect neurons from excitotoxicity by decreasing flux through voltage-gated calcium channels[211]; an analogous mechanism may explain the role of PTHrP in smooth muscle relaxation.

Many of the actions of PTHrP are mediated by the PTH/PTHrP receptor. Others, such as the activation of placental calcium transport, are probably mediated by a distinct receptor, and other actions on bone cells probably involve yet another receptor responsive to more distal portions of PTHrP.[212, 213] Increasing evidence suggests, furthermore, that some actions of PTHrP involve direct nuclear actions of PTHrP.[214–216] Thus, both PTH and PTHrP are likely to use multiple mechanisms to stimulate cells (see Fig. 26–12).

CALCITONIN

Calcitonin has an important role in regulating blood calcium in fish and a demonstrable role in rodents; however, the importance of calcitonin in human calcium homeostasis remains uncertain.

The existence of a second calcium-regulating hormone, in addition to PTH, was first demonstrated during perfusion studies of the thyroid and parathyroid glands of dogs.[217] High-level calcium perfusion resulted in a rapid decrease in plasma calcium, even more rapid than after parathyroidectomy. This effect suggested that calcium had stimulated the secretion of a hormone that lowered blood calcium. It was subsequently demonstrated that this missing hormone, named *calcitonin* for its role in regulating the "tone" or level of calcium, was elaborated by the thyroid gland, not the parathyroids. Calcitonin is found in the nonfollicular cells of the thyroid, called *C cells*, which originate from the neural crest.[218] In fish, the location of the C cells in discrete organs led to the rapid isolation of calcitonin from these ultimobranchial bodies in dogfish, salmon, and several other species. The identification of the glandular origin of calcitonin enabled the isolation of sufficient quantities of calcitonin for sequence analysis[219, 220] and studies of its structure and biologic function.

Synthesis and Secretion

Calcitonin consists of a 32-amino-acid polypeptide with an intrachain disulfide bond provided by the cysteines at positions 1 and 7 (Fig. 26–15). These two cysteine residues, along with the carboxy-terminal proline-amide and six additional residues are the only amino acids conserved among the calcitonins isolated from various species. The disulfide linkage and proline-amide residues are important for the function of the molecule, although biologically active analogues lacking disulfide bonds have been developed.

Of interest, fish calcitonin is more potent in mammals than is the mammalian hormone. The mature peptide is derived from the middle of a 136-amino-acid precursor.[221] The human calcitonin gene, located on the short arm of chromosome 11, contains six exons that are alternatively spliced in a tissue-specific manner to yield the mRNAs encoding calcitonin or calcitonin gene–related peptide (CGRP) (Fig. 26–16). The mRNA encoding calcitonin is derived by splicing together the first four exons[222] and represents over 95% of mature transcripts in the thyroid C cells. The splicing of the first three exons to exons 5 and 6 results in an mRNA that encodes the 37-amino-acid α-CGRP. The mRNA encoding α-CGRP is expressed in multiple tissues and is the only mature transcript of the calcitonin gene detected in neural tissue. A second CGRP gene encodes the closely related β-CGRP. In humans, the predicted sequence of the mature peptide differs from that of α-CGRP by only three amino acids (see Fig. 26–15). The β-CGRP gene is also found on chromosome 11[223]; its tissue distribution is the same as that of α-CGRP.

The synthesis and secretion of calcitonin are tightly regu-

Peptide	Species	Sequence
Calcitonin	Human	**C**GNLST**C**MLGTYTQDFNKFHTFPQTAIGVGAP -NH$_2$
	Salmon-1	**C**S----**C**V--KLS-ELH-LQTY-R-NT-SGT- -NH$_2$
	Salmon-2	**C**S----**C**V--KLS-DLH-LQTF-R-NT-AGV- -NH$_2$
	Salmon-3	**C**S----**C**M--KLS-DLH-LQTF-R-NT-AGV- -NH$_2$
CGRP	Human-α	A**C**DTAT**C**VTHRLAGLLSRSGGVVKNNFVPTNVGSKAF -NH$_2$
	Human-β	-**C**N---**C**------GL-S-----VKS------------ -NH$_2$
	Salmon	-**C**N---**C**------DF-N-----GNS------------ -NH$_2$
Amylin	Human	A**C**DTAT**C**VTHRLAGLLSRSGGVVKNNFVPTNVGSKAF -NH$_2$
ADM	Human	YRQSMNNFQGLRSFG**C**RFGT**C**TVQKLAHQIYQFTDKDKDNVAPRSKISPQGY -NH$_2$

Figure 26–15. The amino acid sequences of calcitonin, calcitonin gene–related peptide (CGRP), and amylin and adrenomedullin (ADM) from selected species. The bold **C**s represent the cysteine residues that form the disulfide linkages critical for the secondary structure of these peptides. The other residues conserved among species are indicated by a dashed line. See the legend to Figure 26–3 for the single-letter amino acid codes.

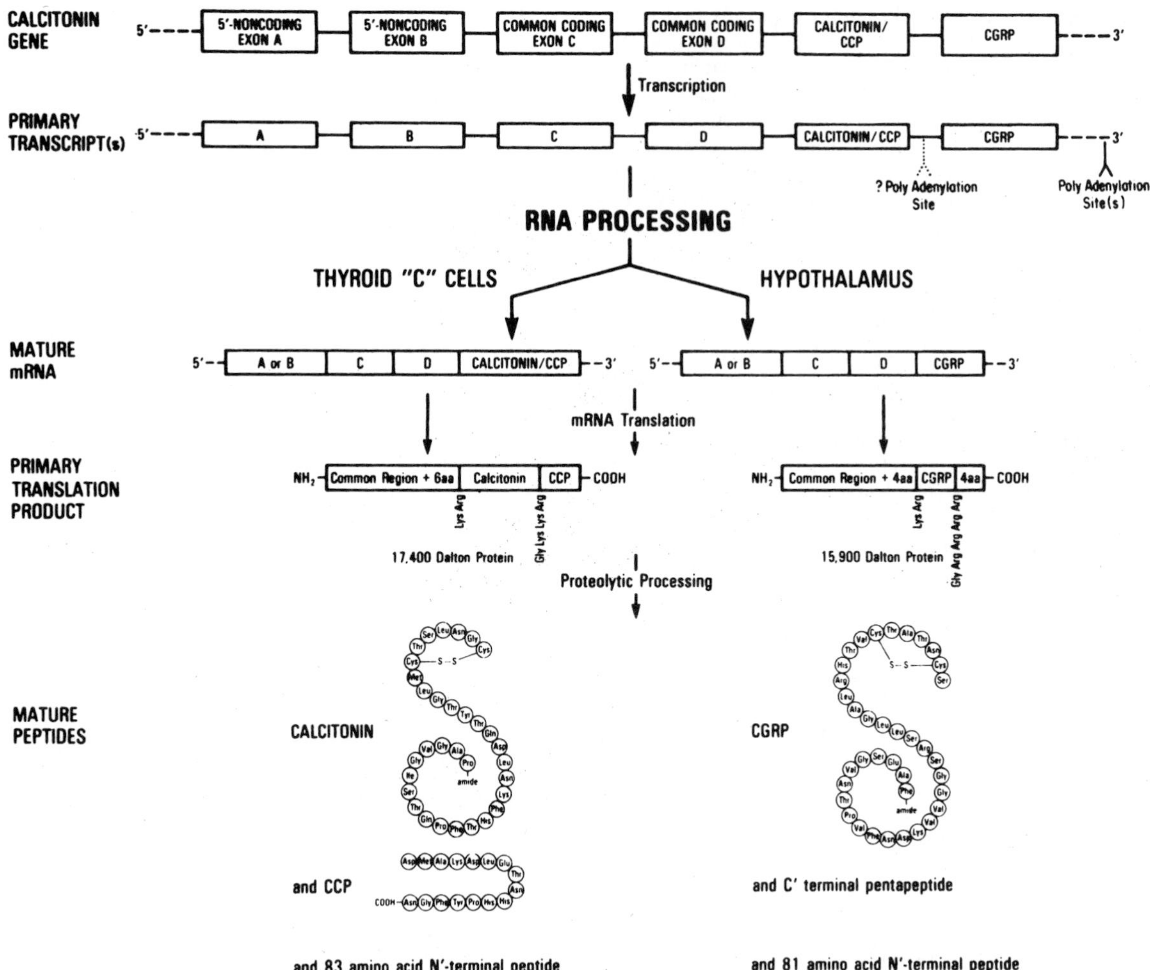

Figure 26–16. Tissue-specific expression of the calcitonin gene. Splicing of alternative exons leads to two different messenger RNAs (mRNAs). The mRNA encoding calcitonin is found predominantly in the thyroid C cell; the mRNA encoding calcitonin gene related-peptide (CGRP) is found predominantly in the hypothalamus and other nervous tissue. (From Amara SG, Jonas V, Rosenfeld MG, et al. Alternative RNA processing in calcitonin gene expression generates mRNAs encoding different polypeptide products. Nature 1982; 298:240–244.)

lated. Studies in a porcine model reveal a linear relationship between the secretion of calcitonin and ambient calcium levels.[224] Cell culture studies using calcium ionophores and calcium channel blockers demonstrate that the calcium ion concentration within the C cell determines this secretion rate.[225] The calcium-sensing receptor cloned from parathyroid cells is also expressed in C cells[226] and contributes to the regulation of calcitonin secretion.[227] Other calcitonin secretagogues include glucocorticoids, CGRP, glucagon, enteroglucagon, gastrin, pentagastrin, pancreozymin, and β-adrenergic agents.[228, 229]

The physiologic role of the gastrointestinal hormones in regulating calcitonin remains unclear; however, they have been postulated to play a role in the regulation of postprandial hypercalcemia. The secretion of calcitonin is inhibited by somatostatin, which is also secreted by the thyroidal C cells. In vivo[230] and in vitro[231, 232] studies have demonstrated that $1,25(OH)_2D_3$ decreases calcitonin mRNA levels by a transcriptional mechanism.

Calcitonin, when administered acutely, decreases tubular resorption of calcium[233] and impairs osteoclast-mediated bone resorption by a direct action on osteoclasts.[234] In rodents, calcitonin is known to play a role in the regulation of postprandial hypercalcemia.[235] Studies in calcitonin knockout mice reveal a doubling of bone formation rate in the absence of hormone, accompanied by resistance to ovariectomy-induced bone loss.[236] The physiologic role of calcitonin in humans, however, remains elusive. The effect of calcitonin on bone density was examined in patients with long-term hypercalcitoninemia secondary to medullary carcinoma of the thyroid gland (MCT) and in patients with subtotal thyroidectomy resulting in lack of calcitonin secretory reserve.[237] Bone density at the lumbar spine and distal radius were not influenced by the abnormal calcitonin levels. Furthermore, no physiologic abnormalities have been reported with long-term, high-dose administration of exogenous calcitonin.[238]

Many of the effects of calcitonin are mediated by a G protein–coupled cell surface receptor in the PTH/secretin receptor family.[239] The mRNA encoding this receptor has been found in multiple tissues, including kidney, brain, and osteoclasts. The coupling of this receptor to different G proteins results in the activation of either adenylate cyclase or phospholipase C; in some settings, this effect is cell cycle–dependent.[240] Glycosylation of the receptor is important for both binding and signal transduction.[241] Several isoforms of the calcitonin receptor have been described,[242–246] but the functional significance of these various isoforms is not known.

Calcitonin Family: Calcitonin Gene–Related Peptide, Amylin, and Adrenomedullin

CGRP, amylin, and adrenomedullin all have been shown to have high-affinity binding sites, and displacement studies suggest that several receptor subtypes are present. However, cloning of specific receptors for these ligands proved difficult because the functional receptors consist of heterodimers between G protein–coupled receptors and single transmembrane proteins of the RAMP (receptor activity–modifying protein) family.[247] Interaction of the calcitonin receptor–like receptor, a relative of the calcitonin receptor, with RAMP1 results in a CGRP receptor, whereas RAMP2 and RAMP3 interactions with the same calcitonin receptor–like receptor generate adrenomedullin receptors. Interaction of RAMP1 with the calcitonin receptor creates an amylin receptor.[248]

CGRP is thought to act as a neurotransmitter and vasodilator rather than as a hormone. In support of this hypothesis, mice lacking α-CGRP have an increase in mean arterial pressure.[249] Immunohistochemical studies of CGRP in the brain and peripheral nervous system suggest that this neuropeptide also plays an important role in sensory and integrative motor functions.

Amylin is highly homologous to CGRP and calcitonin (see Fig. 26–15). The striking presence of amylin in the pancreas of patients with type 2 diabetes mellitus suggests an etiologic role for this peptide in this disorder.[250, 251]

Adrenomedullin (see Fig. 26–15) has vasodilatory effects similar to those of CGRP. In addition to activating CGRP receptors, adrenomedullin binds to specific receptors in the vascular system.[252] The physiologic roles of amylin and adrenomedullin and the functional correlates of their receptor interactions have not yet been clarified.[253]

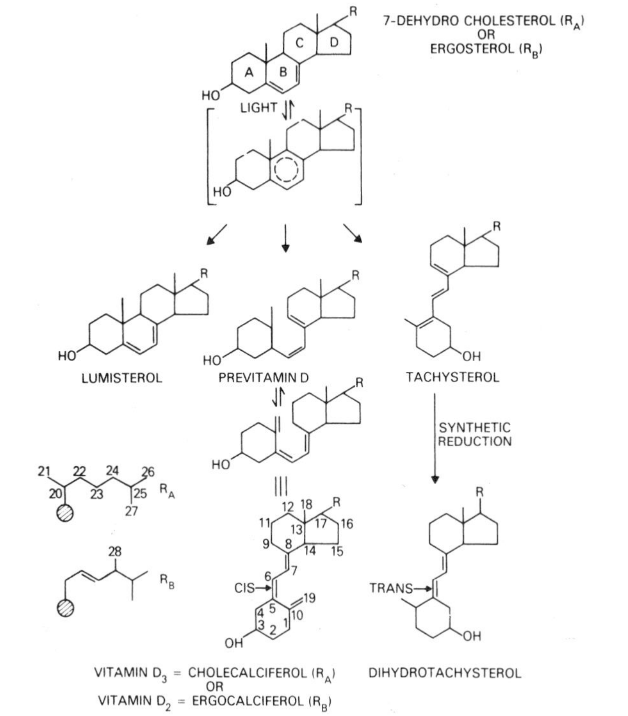

Figure 26–17. Vitamin D precursors and alternative reaction products. The numbering system for vitamin D carbons and the distinct structures of vitamin D_2 (ergocalciferol) and D_3 (cholecalciferol) are noted, as is the structure of dihydrotachysterol, a synthetic product not produced in vivo. Note that the 3-hydroxyl group of dihydrotachysterol is in a pseudo–1-hydroxyl configuration. This may explain the relatively high potency of dihydrotachysterol in conditions associated with low 1-hydroxylase activity.

Calcitonin in Human Disease

Calcitonin is secreted by several endocrine malignancies and can therefore serve as a tumor marker. Basal and pentagastrin-stimulated calcitonin levels have been used to identify and follow persons at risk for, or affected by, medullary carcinoma of the thyroid gland (see Chapter 13), although abnormal basal and stimulated levels may be observed in patients on chronic hemodialysis.[254] Calcitonin may also be ectopically secreted by other tumors, including insulinomas, VIPomas, and lung cancers. Severely ill patients, including those with burn inhalation injury,[255] toxic shock syndrome,[256] and pancreatitis,[257] also may have elevated calcitonin levels.

Therapeutic Uses

The observation that calcitonin inhibits osteoclastic bone resorption has led to its therapeutic use for the treatment of several disorders associated with excess bone resorption, including osteoporosis and Paget's disease (see Chapter 27). Calcitonin has also been shown to have an analgesic effect in the treatment of vertebral crush fractures, osteolytic metastases, and phantom limb.[258, 259]

VITAMIN D

Metabolism of Vitamin D

Vitamin D is not a true vitamin, since nutritional supplementation is not required in humans who have adequate sun exposure. When the skin is exposed to ultraviolet radiation, the cutaneous precursor of vitamin D, 7-dehydrocholesterol, undergoes photochemical cleavage of the carbon bond between carbons 9 and 10 of the steroid ring (Fig. 26–17). The resultant product, pre–vitamin D, is thermally labile and over a period of 48 hours undergoes a temperature-dependent molecular rearrangement that results in the production of vitamin D.[260] Alternatively, this thermally labile product can isomerize to two biologically inert products, luminosterol and tachysterol. This alternative photoisomerization prevents production of excessive amounts of vitamin D with prolonged sun exposure. The degree of skin pigmentation, which increases in response to solar exposure, also regulates the conversion of 7-dehydrocholesterol to vitamin D by blocking the penetration of ultraviolet rays.

The alternative source of vitamin D is dietary. The elderly, the institutionalized, and those living in northern climates probably obtain most of their vitamin D from dietary sources. However, with increasing avoidance of sun exposure by the general population, ensuring adequate dietary intake of vitamin D has become important for the population at large. Vitamin D deficiency is prevalent[261] and has been shown to contribute significantly to osteopenia and fracture risk. The major dietary sources of vitamin D are fortified dairy products, although the lack of monitoring of this supplementation results in marked variation in the amount of vitamin D provided.[262] Other dietary sources include egg yolks, fish oils, and fortified cereal products. Vitamin D provided by plant sources is in the form of vitamin D_2, whereas that provided by animal sources is in the form of vitamin D_3 (see Fig. 26–17). These two forms have equivalent biologic potencies and are activated equally efficiently by the hydroxylases in humans.

Vitamin D is absorbed into the lymphatics and enters the

and may play a role in this process, as may the $1,25(OH)_2D_3$-inducible calcium binding protein calbindin 9K.[314]

Transcellular Transport

The best-studied effect of vitamin D on the enterocyte is the induction of synthesis of the intestinal calcium-binding protein calbindin 9K. This protein has an EF hand structure that permits the binding of two calcium ions per molecule. The affinity of calbindin for calcium is approximately four times that of the brush border calcium-binding components; thus, calcium is preferentially transferred to calbindin. Calbindin serves to buffer the intracellular free calcium concentration during calcium absorption. It associates with microtubules and may play a role in the transport of calcium across the enterocyte. Organelles such as the mitochondria, Golgi, and endoplasmic reticulum also serve as repositories for intracellular calcium.

Exit from the Enterocyte

The transport of calcium across the antiluminal surface of the enterocyte, the final process involved in intestinal calcium absorption, is dependent on $1,25(OH)_2D_3$. The main mechanism of calcium extrusion is the $1,25(OH)_2D_3$-inducible[315] ATP-dependent Ca^{2+} pump. The affinity of the pump for calcium is approximately 2.5 times that of calbindin.[316] With high calcium intake, a $1,25(OH)_2D_3$-independent Na^{+}-Ca^{2+} exchanger may play a role in the transfer of calcium across the basolateral membrane as well.

Actions on the Parathyroid Gland

1,25-Dihydroxyvitamin D_3 has been shown to regulate gene transcription and cell proliferation in the parathyroid glands. The hormone also inhibits the proliferation of dispersed parathyroid cells in culture, although the relative contribution of calcium and $1,25(OH)_2D_3$ in the regulation of parathyroid cell proliferation in vivo has not been established. Normocalcemic mice lacking functional vitamin D receptors have normal serum PTH levels and normal-size parathyroid glands, demonstrating that the genomic actions of $1,25(OH)_2D_3$ are not essential for parathyroid cellular homeostasis.[52] 1,25-Dihydroxyvitamin D_3, however, decreases the transcription of the PTH gene both in vivo and in vitro.[26–28] This action has been exploited in the use of $1,25(OH)_2D_3$ in the treatment of the secondary hyperparathyroidism associated with chronic renal failure (see "Parathyroid Hormone Biosynthesis" earlier and "Vitamin D Deficiency" later).

Actions on Bone

The effects of $1,25(OH)_2D_3$ on bone are numerous. 1,25-Dihydroxyvitamin D_3 is a major transcriptional regulator of the two most abundant bone matrix proteins: it represses the synthesis of type I collagen[317] and induces the synthesis of osteocalcin.[318] 1,25-Dihydroxyvitamin D_3 promotes the differentiation of osteoclasts from monocyte-macrophage stem cell precursors in vitro, and it also increases osteoclastic bone resorption in high doses in vivo, by stimulating production of osteoclast-differentiating factor (ODF—i.e., RANK ligand) by osteoblasts.[319] Despite the multiple effects of $1,25(OH)_2D_3$ on the biology of bone in vitro, results of in vivo studies in $1,25(OH)_2D_3$-deficient rats[320, 321] and in mice lacking functional vitamin D receptors[52, 305] suggest that the major osseous consequences of hormone and receptor deficiency can be reversed when mineral ion homeostasis is normalized. In addition, parenteral calcium infusions have been shown to heal the osteomalacic lesions in children with mutant vitamin D receptors.[303] These observations suggest that the major role of $1,25(OH)_2D_3$ in bone is to provide the proper microenvironment for bone mineralization through stimulation of the intestinal absorption of calcium and phosphate.

Other Actions of Vitamin D

The effects of $1,25(OH)_2D_3$ on phosphate transport are less well studied than those on calcium transport; however, vitamin D promotes the already efficient intestinal phosphate absorption.

One of the striking clinical features of profound vitamin D deficiency that remains unexplained is the severe proximal myopathy.[322] Muscle cells express vitamin D receptors, and $1,25(OH)_2D_3$ has nongenomic effects on muscle.[323] Furthermore, $1,25(OH)_2D_3$ increases amino acid uptake and alters phospholipid metabolism in vitro in muscle cells.[322] Vitamin D administration has been shown to increase the concentration of troponin C, a calcium-binding protein that plays a role in excitation coupling and increases the rate of uptake of calcium by the sarcoplasmic reticulum.[324] However, little is known regarding the direct role of vitamin D in normal muscle physiology. The myopathy that accompanies vitamin D deficiency is characterized by normal creatine kinase levels, a myopathic electromyogram, and biopsy findings of loss of myofibrils, fatty infiltration, and interstitial fibrosis. The myopathy resolves within days to weeks of vitamin D replacement and is not related to normalization of mineral ion homeostasis.

Vitamin D Analogues

The recognition that $1,25(OH)_2D_3$ promotes cellular differentiation and inhibits cellular proliferation has led to efforts directed at producing new analogues that retain these effects but do not cause hypercalcemia. Several analogues have been shown to have antiproliferative effects on normal cells as well as on malignant cells in vitro and in xenografts in immunosuppressed mice.[325–328] In addition, analogues of vitamin D have been shown to synergize with cyclosporine in preventing rejection of transplanted pancreatic islet cells in a murine model.[329] One analogue, 22-oxacalcitriol, suppresses PTH synthesis and secretion in rats,[330] at doses that stimulate intestinal calcium absorption less than that caused by $1,25(OH)_2D_3$. This finding suggests that such analogues may be useful in preventing and treating hyperparathyroidism. The antiproliferative effects of vitamin D have been exploited clinically in the treatment of psoriasis.[331] Although analogues with reduced calcemic activity are predominantly used, hypercalcemic crisis after excessive topical use of such compounds can occur.[332]

The physiologic processes underlying the differential biologic effects of these analogues are not completely understood. Altered affinity for the vitamin D–binding protein, metabolism by target tissues,[333] and effects on recruitment of coactivators by the vitamin D receptor may contribute to the unique properties of vitamin D analogues.[334–337]

CALCIUM AND PHOSPHATE HOMEOSTASIS

The cytosolic concentrations of intracellular calcium, phosphorus, and magnesium differ markedly, as reviewed previously, and their physiologic roles within cells are diverse and largely unrelated (see Fig. 26–1). In contrast, the concentrations of these mineral ions in extracellular fluid are quite comparable (i.e., 1 to 2 mM), and it is here that they exert important interactions, both with cells and with one another, that are critical for bone mineralization, neuromuscular function, and normal mineral ion homeostasis. Extracellular calcium and phosphate, in particular, exist so close to the limits of their mutual solubility that stringent regulation of their concentrations is required to avoid diffuse precipitation of calcium phosphate crystals in tissues.

Serum concentrations and total body balances of the mineral ions are maintained within narrow limits by powerful, interactive homeostatic mechanisms. PTH and $1,25(OH)_2D_3$ regulate mineral ion levels, mineral ion levels regulate PTH and $1,25(OH)_2D_3$ secretion, and both hormones regulate the production of each other. Calcium-sensing receptors in the parathyroid glands control PTH secretion by monitoring the blood concentration of ionized calcium, whereas those in the kidney act to adjust tubular calcium reabsorption, independent of PTH or $1,25(OH)_2D_3$. The operation of these homeostatic mechanisms can easily be appreciated by considering specific examples of how the organism adapts to changes in calcium loads (Fig. 26–20).

Dietary calcium restriction, for example, is followed by an increase in the efficiency of intestinal calcium absorption. This increased efficiency results from a sequence of homeostatic responses in which lowered blood ionized calcium activates secretion of PTH, PTH augments synthesis of $1,25(OH)_2D_3$ by the proximal tubules of the kidney, and $1,25(OH)_2D_3$ then acts directly upon enterocytes to increase active transcellular transport of calcium. Enhanced intestinal calcium absorption is quantitatively the most important response to calcium deprivation, but a series of other homeostatic events also occur that limit the impact of this stress. Renal tubular calcium reabsorption is increased by PTH, an effect that is enhanced by increased $1,25(OH)_2D_3$-stimulated expression of calbindin-D28K in the distal tubules. Calcium reabsorption is also enhanced directly by any tendency to hypocalcemia, which is detected by calcium-sensing receptors in Henle's loop (and possibly also in the distal nephron) that control transepithelial calcium movements independent of PTH or $1,25(OH)_2D_3$.

The impact of dietary calcium deprivation is reduced by approximately 15% through release of calcium from bone in response to PTH and $1,25(OH)_2D_3$. The concomitant increase in net bone resorption causes release of phosphate as well as calcium into the extracellular fluid. Intestinal phosphate absorption also is increased by $1,25(OH)_2D_3$. These phosphate loads are problematic, in that phosphate directly lowers ionized calcium in extracellular fluid, suppresses renal synthesis of $1,25(OH)_2D_3$, and directly inhibits bone resorption. These potentially negative effects of phosphate are obviated by the powerful phosphaturic action of PTH.

Finally, the possibility of unrestrained secretion of PTH, leading to excessive bone resorption and severe hypophosphatemia, is prevented by the effects of calcium on PTH secretion and by the direct suppressive effect of $1,25(OH)_2D_3$ on the synthesis of PTH and of PTH receptors. As a result of these homeostatic responses, calcium-deprived people maintain near-normal serum calcium and phosphate concentrations but display increased intestinal calcium absorption, increased bone resorption and progressive osteopenia, increased renal tubular calcium reabsorption, decreased renal tubular phosphate reabsorption, low urinary calcium excretion, elevated urinary phosphate excretion, and high serum concentrations of PTH and $1,25(OH)_2D_3$.

Calcium loads induce an opposite series of adaptations: parathyroid suppression, inhibition of renal $1,25(OH)_2D_3$ synthesis, decreased intestinal active transport of calcium, increased renal excretion of calcium and decreased renal excretion of phosphate (secondary to functional hypoparathyroidism), and a decrease in bone resorption sufficient to allow positive skeletal calcium balance. The decline in intestinal calcium absorption is the major safeguard against calcium overload, although this mechanism may be overridden with extraordinarily high intakes of calcium because of the persistence of the passive, non–vitamin D–dependent mode of calcium absorption. Moreover, nonenteral sources of calcium, such as intravenous calcium infusion or excessive net bone resorption (as from immobilization or malignancy), may readily overwhelm the limited homeostatic adaptations that remain once suppressed intestinal calcium absorption is bypassed. In such situations, the kidney rather than the intestine becomes the principal defense against hypercalcemia, and calcium homeostasis becomes critically de-

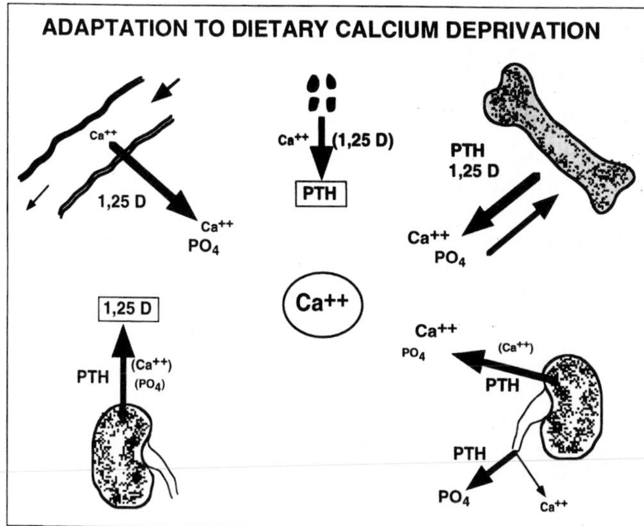

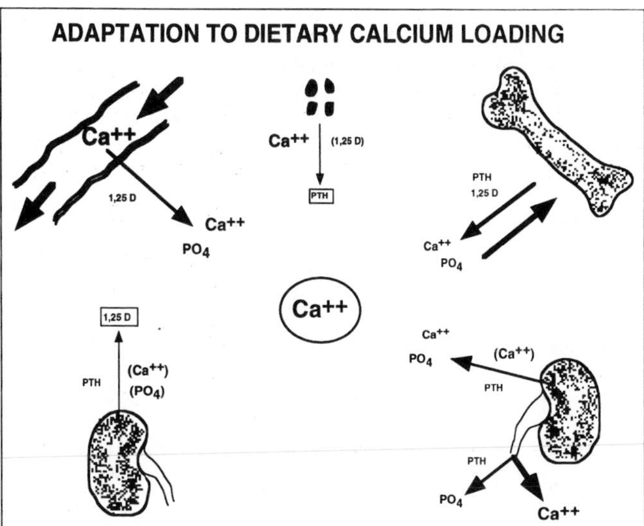

Figure 26–20. Homeostatic responses to variations in dietary calcium content. Major homeostatic responses to dietary calcium deprivation or loading are depicted. Arrow thickness indicates relative activity of transport or secretory mechanisms, whereas amounts of hormones or transported ions are related to the size of their notations. Parentheses indicate an inhibitory regulation. Note that the extracellular calcium concentration is well maintained, although different underlying mechanisms are involved in the two circumstances (see text for details).

pendent on adequate renal function. If renal function is impaired in these settings, as frequently occurs clinically, severe hypercalcemia and pathologic calcium deposition in extraskeletal sites may ensue.

LABORATORY ASSESSMENT OF MINERAL METABOLISM

Parathyroid Hormone

The major challenges in the measurement of blood PTH have been the low levels of circulating PTH and the presence of inactive PTH fragments in far greater abundance than for the intact, biologically active PTH molecule. The measurement of inactive fragments would not be a concern if the ratio of inactive to active PTH molecules remained constant. However, this ratio does change in response to changes in GFR and in parathyroid gland secretory activity (see "Parathyroid Hormone Secretion" and "Peripheral Metabolism of Parathyroid Hormone" earlier). Consequently, radioimmunoassays of PTH have suffered from lack of sensitivity and from the inability to measure the biologically active hormone directly.

For these reasons, two-site assays that require the presence of amino-terminal and carboxy-terminal sequences of full-length PTH(1–84) on the same molecule have generally replaced older radioimmunoassays.[338] It is reassuring that for all assays of this type, the normal ranges for blood PTH are very similar. The assays are sensitive enough to detect PTH in all normal persons. The assays have demonstrated modest circadian variation in PTH levels and some pulsatility in PTH secretion, but these variations have not interfered with the diagnostic usefulness of randomly drawn PTH measurements. Some studies have reported modest increases of PTH levels with age, although others have not. Unlike older radioimmunoassays, the two-site assays demonstrate virtually no overlap in PTH levels between patients with primary hyperparathyroidism and those with nonparathyroid hypercalcemia (Fig. 26–21). Because this distinction represents the most important challenge in the clinical setting, the use of the two-site assay has dramatically facilitated the clinician's task.

This straightforward picture has been complicated by the realization that many two-site assays do detect small amounts of PTH fragments that are large but do not extend to the hormone's amino-terminus.[64] These fragments accumulate in significant amounts in patients with renal failure.[65] The clinical importance of the detection of large fragments of PTH by most two-site assays is unknown.

Parathyroid Hormone–Related Protein

The measurement of PTHrP in serum presents a series of challenges that have made the development of clinically useful assays for PTHrP more difficult than for PTH assays. The concentration of PTHrP in the blood stream, even in some patients with PTHrP-mediated malignant hypercalcemia, is not high, and the molecular definition of circulating, biologically active fragments is incomplete. Despite these problems, several groups of investigators have developed assays for PTHrP that can be helpful in the evaluation of a subset of hypercalcemic patients.[339] Radioimmunoassays for amino-terminal portions of PTHrP[340, 341] and two-site assays for amino-terminal and mid-region PTHrP[186, 187, 342] separate healthy persons and patients with nonmalignant hypercalcemia from most patients with the humoral hypercalcemia of malignancy (Fig. 26–22). When measured with the most recently developed assays, PTHrP levels are elevated in almost all patients with malignant hypercalcemia without bone metastases and in most patients with hypercalcemia and bone metastases.

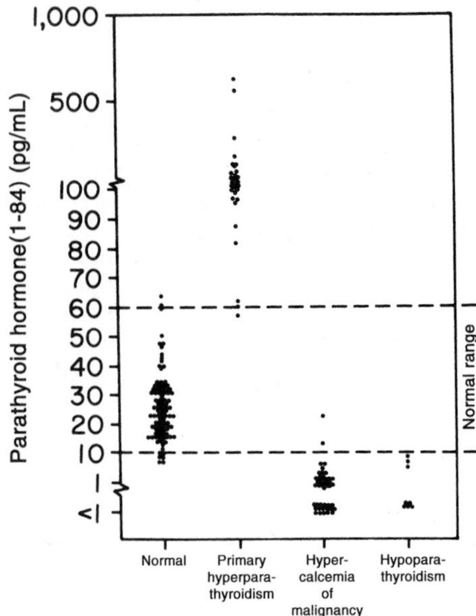

Figure 26–21. Intact immunoreactive parathyroid hormone (PTH) determined using a two-site immunoradiometric assay in normal and three different patient groups. Note some overlap between normal people and patients with primary hyperparathyroidism, but no overlap between hypercalcemic patients with primary hyperparathyroidism and those with hypercalcemia of malignancy. (From Segre GV. Advances in techniques for measurement of parathyroid hormone: current applications in clinical medicine and directions for future research. Trends Endocrinol Metab 1990; 1:243–247.)

In occasional patients, the PTHrP assay has helped distinguish an occult malignancy from other causes of non–PTH-dependent hypercalcemia.[198] Nevertheless, because the diagnosis of malignancy as the cause of hypercalcemia is usually clinically obvious, and the PTH assay can be used to diagnose primary hyperparathyroidism, the role of PTHrP assays in clinical practice is likely to be limited. Further improvement in assay sensitivity and further understanding of the normal functions of circulating PTHrP fragments may lead to changes in this assessment.

Calcitonin

Several assays for measuring serum calcitonin are commercially available. The measurements are based on single-antibody or double-antibody radioimmunoassays or enzyme immunoassays, several of which are sufficiently sensitive to detect calcitonin deficiency.[343, 344] The calcitonin monomer is thought to be the biologically active molecule; therefore, some investigators believe that extraction of the multimeric forms before radioimmunoassay[345] provides a more sensitive and specific measurement of serum calcitonin levels. However, the double-antibody radioimmunoassay is thought by others to provide the same information with less sample manipulation.[346] The only clinical use of the calcitonin assay is as a tumor marker, primarily in medullary carcinoma of the thyroid.

Vitamin D Metabolites

The currently used radioligand assays for determining the levels of vitamin D metabolites require fractionation and extraction of the hormone from serum proteins by HPLC or silica cartridges.[347] These assays are sufficiently sensitive to

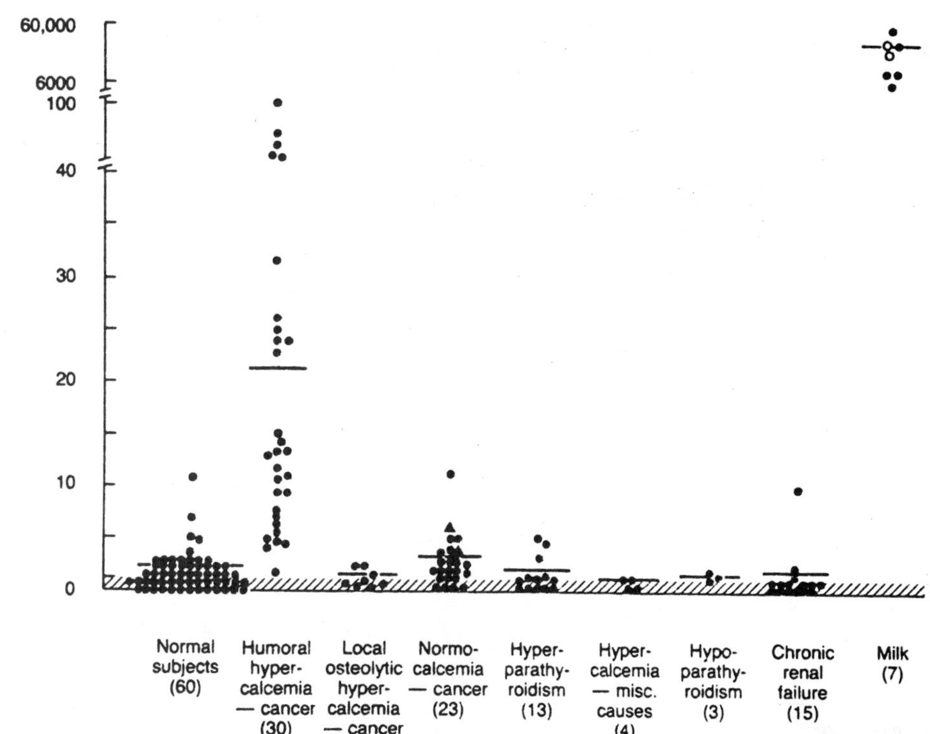

Figure 26–22. Plasma PTHrP(1–74) determined by two-site immunoradiometric assay in selected patient groups and normals. Also shown are concentrations of PTHrP in human milk (*filled circles*) and in bovine milk (*open circles*). Two normocalcemic patients with cancer (*filled triangles*) subsequently became hypercalcemic. *Hatched area* denotes levels too low to detect with this assay. PTHrP, parathyroid hormone–related protein. (Adapted from Burtis WJ, Brady TG, Orloff JJ, et al. Immunochemical characterization of circulating parathyroid hormone–related protein in patients with humoral hypercalcemia of cancer. N Engl J Med 1990; 322:1106–1112.)

detect subnormal values. Because the assays measure both protein-bound and unbound vitamin D metabolites, results may not always reflect the levels of biologically relevant ("free") metabolites. This limitation may lead to misleading results in patients with nephrotic syndrome and vitamin D intoxication.

The levels of 25(OH)D correlate better with the clinical signs and symptoms of vitamin D deficiency than do the levels of $1,25(OH)_2D_3$. Because the 25-hydroxylation of vitamin D is not tightly regulated, measurements of 25(OH)D more accurately reflect body stores of vitamin D. Measurement of this metabolite should therefore be performed when vitamin D deficiency is suspected.

Measurements of $1,25(OH)_2D_3$ should be reserved for cases when excessive or impaired 1α-hydroxylation is suspected. High $1,25(OH)_2D_3$ levels can be seen in sarcoidosis, lymphomas, Williams' syndrome, and intoxication with 1α-hydroxylated metabolites (see "Hypercalcemic Disorders"). Impaired 1α-hydroxylation can contribute to the hypocalcemia occurring in patients with renal dysfunction, oncogenic osteomalacia, and hereditary defects of vitamin D metabolism (see "Hypocalcemic Disorders").

CLINICAL DISORDERS

HYPERCALCEMIC DISORDERS

Parathyroid-Dependent Hypercalcemia

It is useful to delineate two categories of hypercalcemia: (1) that associated with dysfunction of the parathyroid cell and (2) that in which hypercalcemia occurs despite appropriate parathyroid suppression. This distinction is particularly useful clinically, because it emphasizes the centrality of the PTH assay in the diagnostic approach to the hypercalcemic patient. Abnormal parathyroid glands are associated with hypercalcemia in three settings: (1) primary hyperparathyroidism, (2) familial hypocalciuric hypercalcemia (FHH), and (3) lithium-induced hypercalcemia.

Primary Hyperparathyroidism

In primary hyperparathyroidism, a primary abnormality of parathyroid tissue leads to inappropriate secretion of PTH. (In contrast, increased secretion of PTH that is an appropriate response to hypocalcemia is called secondary hyperparathyroidism.) The inappropriately high serum concentration of PTH in primary hyperparathyroidism, in turn, sustains excessive renal calcium reabsorption, phosphaturia, and $1,25(OH)_2D_3$ synthesis as well as increased bone resorption. These actions of PTH produce the characteristic biochemical phenotypic features of hypercalcemia and hypophosphatemia, loss of cortical bone, hypercalciuria, and the various clinical sequelae of chronic hypercalcemia. Primary hyperparathyroidism results most often—in 75% to 80% of the cases—from the occurrence of one or more adenomas in previously normal parathyroid glands, although in 20% of the cases, diffuse hyperplasia of all parathyroid glands may be present or, rarely, parathyroid carcinoma may be found (less than 1% to 2%).[348–351]

Classical Primary Hyperparathyroidism

The bone disease *osteitis fibrosa cystica* was first described by von Recklinghausen in 1891, but the etiologic link between this disease and parathyroid neoplasms was not established until 1925, when Mandl observed clinical improvement following removal of a parathyroid adenoma from a young man with severe bone disease. In early clinical descriptions of primary hyperparathyroidism,[352, 353] the disease emerged as a distinctly uncommon disorder with significant morbidity and mortality, in which nearly all affected patients had radiographically significant or symptomatic skeletal or renal involvement, or both.

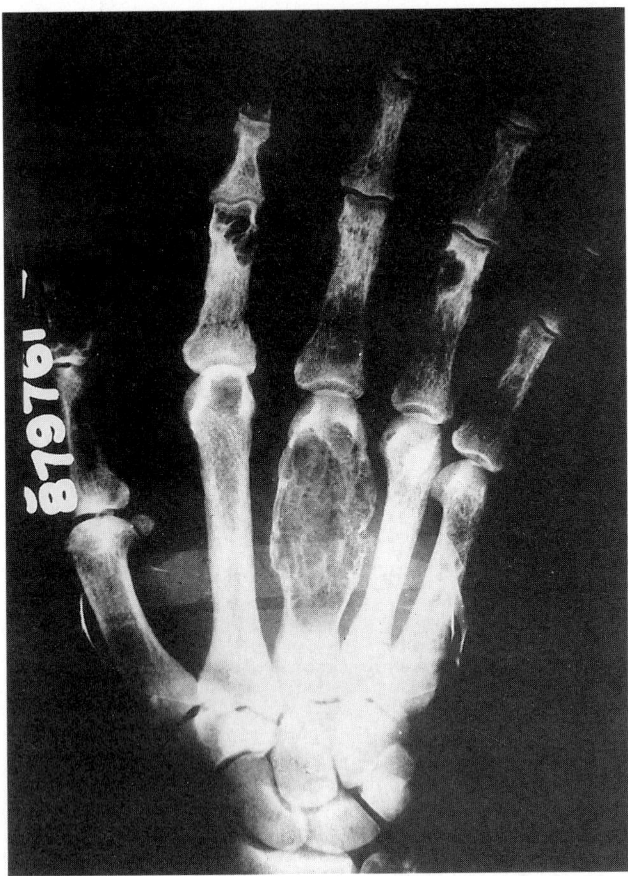

Figure 26–23. Radiograph of hand from a patient with severe primary hyperparathyroidism. Note the dramatic remodeling associated with the intense region of high bone turnover in the third metacarpal in addition to widespread evidence of subperiosteal, endosteal, and trabecular resorption. (Courtesy of Fuller Albright Collection, Massachusetts General Hospital.)

The skeletal involvement in "classical" primary hyperparathyroidism reflects a striking and generalized increase in osteoclastic bone resorption, which is accompanied by fibrovascular marrow replacement and increased osteoblastic activity. The radiographic appearance (Fig. 26–23) features *generalized demineralization* of bone, with coarsening of the trabecular pattern (due to osteoclastic resorption of the smaller trabeculae); characteristic *subperiosteal resorption*, often most evident in the phalanges of the hands, which gives an irregular, serrated appearance to the outer, subperiosteal cortex and may progress to extensive cortical resorption; *bone cysts*, usually multiple, which contain a brownish serous or mucoid fluid, tend to occur in the central medullary portions of the shafts of the metacarpals, ribs, or pelvis, and may expand into and disrupt the overlying cortex; *osteoclastomas*, or "*brown tumors*," composed of numerous multinucleated osteoclasts ("giant cells") admixed with stromal cells and matrix, which are found most often in trabecular portions of the jaw, long bones, and ribs; and pathologic *fractures*.

The skull may exhibit a finely mottled, "salt-and-pepper" radiographic appearance, with loss of definition of the inner and outer cortices. Dental radiographs typically show erosion or disappearance of the lamina dura due to subperiosteal resorption, often with extension into the adjacent mandibular bone. The erosion and demineralization of cortical bone may lead to radiographic disappearance of some bones, most notably the tufts of the distal phalanges of the hands, the inferolateral cortex of the distal third of the clavicles, the distal ulna, the inferior margin of the femoral neck and pubis, and the medial aspect of the proximal tibia. The clinical correlates of these changes may include aching bone pain and tenderness, "bowing" of the shoulders, kyphosis and loss of height, and collapse of lateral ribs and pelvis with "pigeon breast" and triradiate deformities, respectively.

The renal manifestations of classical severe primary hyperparathyroidism include recurrent calcium nephrolithiasis, nephrocalcinosis, and renal functional abnormalities that range from impaired concentrating ability to end-stage renal failure. Associated signs and symptoms include recurrent flank pain, polyuria, and polydypsia. No unique features of the stone disease in primary hyperparathyroidism serve to distinguish it from that associated with other, more common causes of calcium kidney stones. The stone disease more often may be recurrent and severe, and in some patients, the stones may be composed entirely of calcium phosphate, instead of the pure oxalate or mixtures of oxalate and phosphate more commonly encountered in other disorders. In patients diagnosed before 1965, the frequency with which nephrolithiasis complicated primary hyperparathyroidism was as high as 60% to 80% (the frequency is currently less than 25%), yet in studies of unselected patients conducted throughout the past 50 years, primary hyperparathyroidism has accounted for fewer than 5% of all calcium kidney stones.

Nephrocalcinosis refers to the presence of bilateral, extensive but minute calcifications that are evident on plain abdominal radiographs, usually in the renal pyramids and medullary regions, and that correlate with the presence of deposits of calcium in the epithelium of the renal tubules. In classical severe primary hyperparathyroidism, nephrocalcinosis was observed with roughly one-third the frequency of symptomatic stone disease, although it may occur in the absence of stones.

Other clinical features that have been reported in association with classical severe primary hyperparathyroidism are conjunctival calcifications, band keratopathy, hypertension (50%), gastrointestinal signs and symptoms (anorexia, nausea, vomiting, constipation, or abdominal pain), peptic ulcer disease, and acute or chronic pancreatitis. The issue of whether primary hyperparathyroidism increases the risk for peptic ulcer disease and pancreatitis remains controversial. Although hyperparathyroidism is associated with a higher risk of hypertension, successful parathyroidectomy has not been shown to correct the hypertension.

Signs and symptoms in primary hyperparathyroidism may result from the involvement of bone (fracture, bone pain) or kidneys (renal colic, renal failure), peptic ulcer disease, pancreatitis, or hypercalcemia per se (weakness, apathy, depression, polyuria, constipation, coma). The presence and severity of neuropsychiatric symptoms, in particular, correlate poorly with the serum calcium concentration, although few patients with severe hypercalcemia are entirely asymptomatic. Elderly persons are most likely to exhibit such symptoms. A peculiar neuromuscular syndrome, first described in 1949 but rarely encountered now, includes symmetrical proximal weakness and gait disturbance, with muscle atrophy, characteristic electromyographic abnormalities, generalized hyperreflexia, and tongue fasciculations.[354]

Modern Primary Hyperparathyroidism

The clinical spectrum of primary hyperparathyroidism was changed dramatically in the early 1970s by the introduction of routine multichannel serum chemistry screening, which unearthed a large population of patients with previously unsuspected asymptomatic disease. In Rochester, Minnesota, for example, the annual incidence of the disease increased abruptly from 0.15 to 1.12 per 1000 persons between the prescreening era (1965–1974) and 1975, the year after routine screening was introduced.[355] The peak incidence occurs in the sixth decade of life, and the disease rarely is encountered in patients younger than 15 years of age. It is two to three times more common in women, who are slightly older than men at diagnosis.

Annual incidence rates, widely reported to be 0.1 to 0.3 per 1000 persons in the wake of this surge of ascertainment in Europe and the United States, appear to have declined substantially in the past decade to levels as low as 0.04 per 1000.[355] This decrease may represent a true decline in disease incidence or may simply be the residual effect of "sweeping" the population of prevalent subclinical disease over the past three decades.

Ascertainment of mild or asymptomatic disease may decline even further in the future because of prevalent economic disincentives to routine serum chemistry screening in the primary care setting. On the other hand, insistence upon overt hypercalcemia as a diagnostic criterion may underestimate the true incidence of the disease. For example, when serum calcium and immunoreactive PTH (iPTH) were measured in a large population of Swedish women undergoing routine mammographic screening, the prevalence of unsuspected primary hyperparathyroidism, defined by criteria that included the combination of high-normal serum calcium plus elevated or high-normal iPTH, was 2.1%.[356] Two thirds of these women (72 of 109) were normocalcemic (10.0 to 10.4 mg/dL), yet bone density was reduced in the group as a whole, and the disease was confirmed histologically in 98% of the 61 who underwent surgery.

It is not surprising, given that primary hyperparathyroidism now usually is diagnosed incidentally, that few patients are found to have overt signs or symptoms of the classical disease and thus are considered to be "asymptomatic." For example, only 2% of patients with primary hyperparathyroidism residing in Olmsted County, Minnesota, and only 17% of 121 patients studied at an academic referral center in New York City had classical disease symptoms.[355, 357] In most of these, the relevant symptom was urolithiasis. Many clinicians argue, however, that most patients regarded as having "asymptomatic" primary hyperparathyroidism and only minimally elevated serum calcium actually suffer from various neuropsychiatric or other symptoms that may abate following curative surgery.[358–360] However, these symptoms, which include fatigability, weakness, forgetfulness, depression, somatization, polydipsia, polyuria, and bone and joint pain, are common in otherwise normal persons.

The difficulties in designing appropriately controlled studies to determine whether these symptoms can be confidently ascribed to the parathyroid disorder are well described.[361] Although as yet unresolved, this is a critical issue, as the advent of less invasive operative approaches and concerns regarding fracture, cancer, and mortality risk have lowered the threshold for consideration of surgery in many patients with the disease (see later on). Throughout this chapter, "asymptomatic primary hyperparathyroidism" refers to patients who lack signs or symptoms of the classical disease, whether or not they experience any of the subtle symptoms mentioned previously.

The natural history of untreated asymptomatic primary hyperparathyroidism, as currently detected, remains incompletely understood. Few patients seem to experience progression of disease, as measured by extreme elevations of serum or urinary calcium, appearance of renal dysfunction or nephrocalcinosis, or worsening osteopenia, over many years of observation.[357, 362] On the other hand, an excess risk of mortality, mainly from cardiovascular disease, has been noted during extended follow-up of large cohorts of patients with chronic hypercalcemia (and presumed primary hyperparathyroidism) identified by population health screening in Sweden,[363] and similar observations have been made during extended follow-up of postsurgical patients with hyperparathyroidism.[360, 364] Associations of hypertension, hyperuricemia, and glucose intolerance with primary hyperparathyroidism have been implicated, together with hypercalcemia per se, as contributors to this elevated risk.[365, 366] Abnormal cardiac calcification and left ventricular hypertrophy (reversible after successful parathyroidectomy) have been reported in primary hyperparathyroidism as well.[367] Increased cardiovascular mortality may be a feature only of severe hyperparathyroidism, as it was restricted to patients with serum calcium values in the highest quartile in the Olmsted County study, which otherwise showed an overall decreased risk of death.[368] A 40% excess risk of malignancy also was reported among 4163 Swedish patients who had undergone surgery more than a year earlier for (presumably symptomatic) primary hyperparathyroidism.[369] It has been argued that these increased risks for mortality and malignancy, even if confirmed, may apply only to persons with primary hyperparathyroidism that is more severe than the "asymptomatic" version typically encountered today.[366]

Abnormalities of bone in modern, mild primary hyperparathyroidism are far subtler than those associated with the classical disease. Histologically, the rate at which new bone remodeling cycles are activated is increased. Because the phase of restorative bone formation at each remodeling site is much longer than the initial resorptive phase, such an increase in remodeling rate inevitably increases the effective volume of the *remodeling space* and thus the porosity of bone. Depending on the rate and extent of the accompanying increase in osteoblastic activity and the resulting local balance between net bone formation and resorption, mineralized bone volume may decrease further, remain stable, or even increase (despite an increased remodeling space). For reasons not yet understood, the balance achieved between increased resorption and formation of bone in primary hyperparathyroidism depends not only on the severity of the hyperparathyroidism but also on skeletal location. Thus, net resorption of endosteal bone may predominate in cortical bone sites, whereas net apposition of mineral may occur in trabecular bone[370, 371] (Fig. 26–24).

In mild primary hyperparathyroidism, osteopenia generally is not evident radiographically, although bone mineral density may be reduced, particularly at sites of predominantly cortical bone such as the mid-radius, by as much as 10% to 20%.[372, 373] The mass of trabecular or cancellous bone, as represented in the vertebral bodies, is preferentially preserved and often is normal.[374] A curious finding is that the reduced cortical bone density at the forearm is not improved by successful parathyroidectomy, whereas density at trabecular bone–rich sites such as the hip and spine may increase by 10% to 15% over several years postoperatively.[357]

The critical issue of whether fracture risk is increased in patients with primary hyperparathyroidism was addressed by a retrospective analysis of fracture incidence within a cohort of 407 residents of Rochester, Minnesota, who were diagnosed with the disease between 1965 and 1992.[375] Compared with the expected age-adjusted and sex-adjusted rates of incident fractures in that community, the relative risk among persons with hyperparathyroidism was significantly elevated for fractures of the vertebrae (3.2-fold), distal forearm (2.2-fold), and ribs (2.7-fold), although not for fractures of the hip (1.4-fold). Overall risk of fracture at any site was significantly increased as well (1.3-fold) and was as high in persons in whom primary hyperparathyroidism was diagnosed incidentally (following the institution of automated chemistry screening in 1974) as in those in whom the disorder was diagnosed before that time. These results are consistent with those of several previous studies involving smaller cohorts of patients and, absent data from an appropriately controlled prospective study, strongly support the conclusion that patients with primary hyperparathyroidism should be considered to be at increased risk for fracture. This presumably is true of those with both sympto-

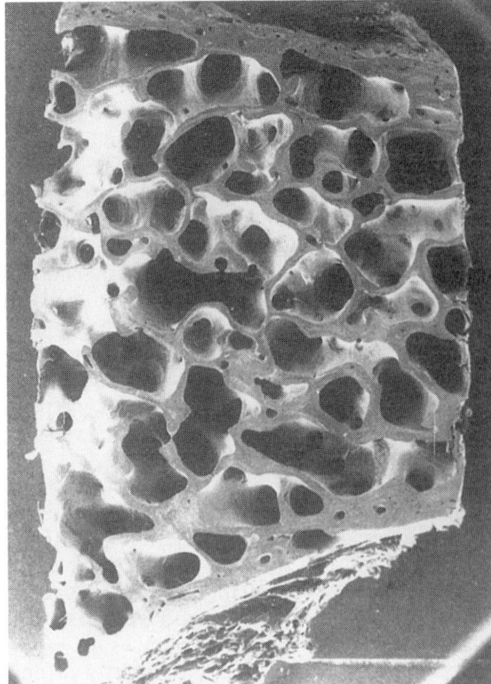
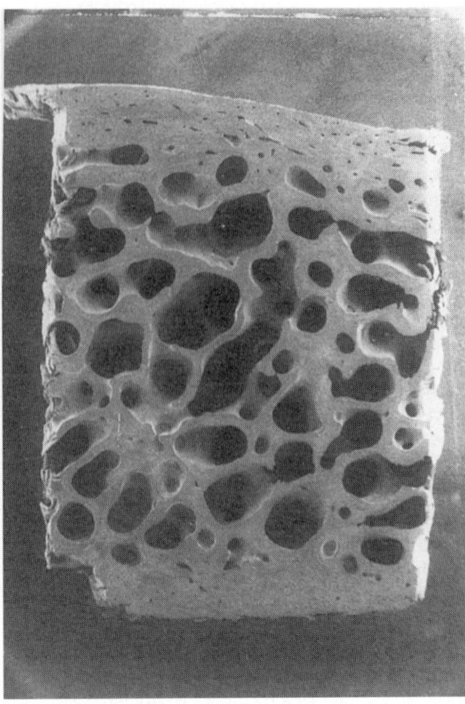

Figure 26–24. Iliac crest biopsy specimens from a patient with primary hyperparathyroidism (*left*) and a normal control (*right*), viewed by scanning electron microscopy. Note the thin cortices and contrasting maintenance of trabecular bone in the patient. (From Parisien M, Silverberg SJ, Shane E, et al. The histomorphometry of bone in primary hyperparathyroidism: preservation of cancellous bone structure. J Clin Endocrinol Metab 1990; 70:930–938.)

matic and asymptomatic disease, as less than 10% of the post-screening Rochester cohort had symptoms or complications of primary hyperparathyroidism.[355] What is not yet known is whether fracture risk is reduced by successful parathyroidectomy.

Kidney stones now are reported in only 10% to 25% of patients with primary hyperparathyroidism, although some degree of renal dysfunction, either a significant reduction in creatinine clearance or impaired concentrating or acidifying ability, may be found in up to a third of those with asymptomatic disease.[376] As with the reduction in cortical bone mineral density, these renal abnormalities are not progressive in a majority of affected patients.[357, 377] The association of kidney stones with primary hyperparathyroidism generally is viewed as an indication for parathyroidectomy, however, because successful surgery usually prevents further symptomatic stone disease.[357, 360] Yet it is not possible at present to confidently predict, from biochemical measurements in blood or urine, which asymptomatic patients with hyperparathyroidism will go on to develop new stone disease. Stone formers are more likely to be hypercalciuric than not, but less than one third of hypercalciuric patients with hyperparathyroidism actually develop stones.[378] As noted later on, however, marked hypercalciuria (calcium levels of >400 mg/day) generally is viewed as an indication for surgery in otherwise asymptomatic patients.[379]

Etiology and Pathogenesis

Parathyroid adenomas are caused by mutations in the DNA of parathyroid cells; these mutations confer a proliferative or survival advantage for affected cells over their normal neighbors.[380, 381] As a consequence of this advantage, the descendants of one particular parathyroid cell, a clone of cells, undergo clonal expansion to produce an adenoma.

Multiple chromosomal regions are missing in the parathyroid cells of individual parathyroid adenomas. These genetic deletions probably reflect the deletion of tumor suppressor genes. These chromosomal loci include portions of chromosome 1p–pter (in 40% of adenomas),[382] 6q (in 32% of adenomas),[383] 15q (in 30% of adenomas),[383] and 11q (in 25% to 30% of adenomas).[384, 385] Many of the 11q deletions are associated, in the undeleted chromosome 11, with mutations in the gene encoding the transcription factor menin, the gene mutated in multiple endocrine neoplasia type 1 (MEN 1).[386] Thus, this gene is also involved commonly in somatic mutations in patients with sporadic parathyroid adenomas. The widespread presence of somatic mutations in sporadic parathyroid adenomas, which are detectable only because large numbers of cells in any one tumor contain the same deletion, constitutes the strongest evidence that parathyroid adenomas are clonal expansions of mutant cells.

One parathyroid proto-oncogene, the PRAD 1 or cyclin D1 gene, has been identified.[387] This gene was discovered at the breakpoint of an inversion on chromosome 11 in a parathyroid adenoma. This inversion led to the juxtaposition of the PTH gene's regulatory region and the DNA encoding cyclin D1. As a consequence, the cyclin D1 gene was overexpressed. Cyclin D1 is an important regulator of the transition from the G_1 phase of the cell cycle (which follows mitosis) to the S phase (associated with DNA synthesis) and is mutated or amplified in a wide variety of malignancies.[381] Cyclin D1 is overexpressed in about 20% of parathyroid adenomas,[388] though cyclin D1 gene rearrangements have been documented in only 5% of adenomas. Portions of chromosomes 16p and 19p are amplified in a subset of parathyroid adenomas; presumably, the amplified regions contain uncharacterized proto-oncogenes.[389]

As expected for a disease caused by mutations in DNA, parathyroid adenomas occur more frequently in patients who underwent neck irradiation decades earlier, with greater radiation exposure leading to higher risk.[390] Most patients have no definite history of exposure to specific mutagens, however. An intriguing clue that abnormalities of vitamin D physiology may predispose to primary hyperparathyroidism has come from the observation that patients with parathyroid adenomas are more likely than others to inherit a particular allele of the vitamin D receptor gene.[391] These patients have tumors with particularly low levels of mRNA encoding the vitamin D receptor.[392]

The cause of sporadic primary parathyroid hyperplasia is unknown. The known stimulus for parathyroid cell proliferation—low levels of blood calcium or $1,25(OH)_2D_3$—is not present in this disease. Presumably, some other stimulus outside the parathyroid glands or a genetic abnormality present in all four parathyroid glands leads to inappropriate cell proliferation. Such abnormalities have been found in several inherited forms of parathyroid hyperplasia (see later), but most cases of parathyroid hyperplasia are not found in familial clusters.

The theoretical distinction between adenoma as a clonal proliferation and hyperplasia as a polyclonal growth is clear-cut. In some settings, however, clonal expansion can occur in the context of preexisting nonclonal proliferation. The clearest example of this complication has been found in the large glands associated with severe renal failure. In many such glands removed surgically because of hypercalcemia or severe parathyroid-dependent bone disease, evidence for clonal proliferation complicating secondary hyperplasia has been found.[393, 394] Analogous mechanisms may be operative in a number of settings associated with stimuli to parathyroid cell proliferation, such as X-linked hypophosphatemia[395] and long-term lithium therapy.[396, 397] Furthermore, just as clonal tumors can arise in the setting of *secondary* parathyroid hyperplasia, they can also arise in the setting of sporadic *primary* parathyroid hyperplasia[396] and in MEN 1.[384, 398]

The distinction between adenoma and hyperplasia is clinically important, because removal of the one abnormal gland can be expected to cure a parathyroid adenoma, whereas removal of multiple glands is required to cure parathyroid hyperplasia. Unfortunately, differentiating adenoma from hyperplasia from normal parathyroid tissue at pathologic examination is not straightforward. Pathologists distinguish normal from abnormal parathyroid glands by the increase in size and the paucity of fat in abnormal glands. Attempts have been made to distinguish an adenoma from an individual hyperplastic gland on the basis of morphologic features, but no criteria have proved completely reliable.[349] The formation of clonal neoplasms in originally hyperplastic tumors may explain some of the difficulty in pathologic diagnosis.

An increase in cell number is not the only abnormality in primary hyperparathyroidism. The ability of the normal parathyroid cell to suppress PTH secretion in response to hypercalcemia might be expected to protect the individual from sustained hypercalcemia, even if the number of parathyroid cells increased moderately. Unfortunately, parathyroid cells in parathyroid adenomas usually demonstrate abnormalities in their responsiveness to calcium, with a shift in set-point to the right[399] (Fig. 26–25). This set-point shift, combined with the nonsuppressible component of PTH secretion, leads to a new steady state in which both the PTH level and the blood calcium level are higher than normal. The molecular underpinning of the abnormal parathyroid cell responsiveness is beginning to be understood. Parathyroid cells from adenomas respond to changes in extracellular calcium with smaller than normal increases in intracellular calcium,[400] and the amount of calcium-sensing receptor protein on the cell surface is reduced.[401, 402]

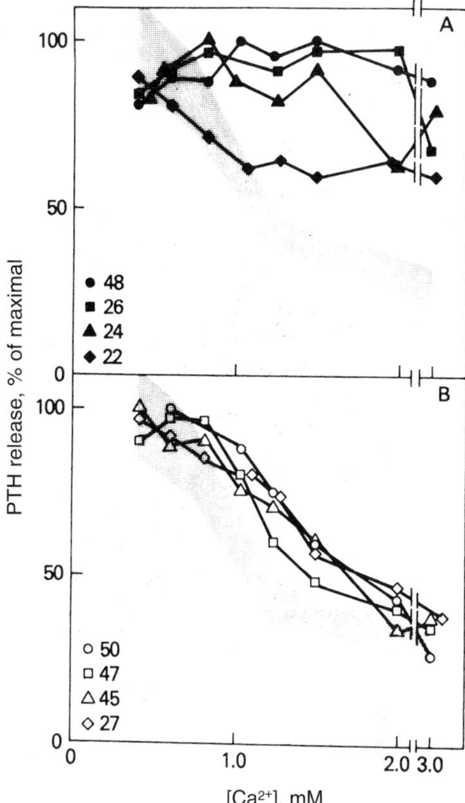

Figure 26–25. Abnormal patterns of parathyroid hormone (PTH) secretion from cells prepared from adenomatous glands and stimulated with varying levels of calcium in tissue culture. The *shaded area* shows the pattern of PTH release (±1 SD) from normal human parathyroid cells. Panel A illustrates the pattern from four patients with little suppression of PTH secretion by calcium. Panel B illustrates the pattern from four patients with relatively intact mechanism of suppression of PTH secretion by calcium. Even in this group the set-point for calcium suppression is shifted to the right. (From Brown, EM. Calcium-regulated parathyroid hormone release in primary hyperparathyroidism, studies in vitro with dispersed parathyroid cells. Am J Med 1979; 66:923–931.)

Inherited Primary Hyperparathyroidism

Although uncommon, inherited forms of primary hyperparathyroidism are clinically important for several reasons. The management of the parathyroid tumors found in familial parathyroid syndromes often differs from that of sporadic primary hyperparathyroidism. Furthermore, extra-parathyroidal manifestations of inherited syndromes may need treatment, and awareness of familial clustering should prompt systematic family screening.

Multiple Endocrine Neoplasia Type 1

MEN 1 is caused by inactivating mutations in the tumor suppressor gene encoding menin[386] Menin is a ubiquitously expressed transcription factor. Although MEN 1 includes tumors of the parathyroid, anterior pituitary, and pancreatic islets, the parathyroid tumors are far more prevalent than the others; 95% of affected patients eventually develop hyperparathyroidism. Most of the parathyroid tumors harbor mutations in both copies of the menin gene; one mutation is inherited and the second occurs in the parathyroid cell whose progeny form the tumor.

The onset of hypercalcemia occurs in the second and third decades of life, though occasional patients present in the first decade. Hypercalcemia never presents at birth or in infancy. The disease involves all four parathyroid glands, although the involvement can be asymmetrical and apparently asynchronous. Apart from the earlier age at diagnosis, the presenting clinical picture generally resembles that of sporadic primary hyperparathyroidism. One common complicating feature is that hypercalcemia can dramatically increase the gastrin levels and symptomatology of patients who also have gastrinomas.

Treatment of the parathyroid disease in this setting can greatly simplify the management of the gastric hyperacidity. After parathyroid surgery, hypoparathyroidism and recurrent hyperparathyroidism are more common than in other forms of hyperparathyroidism.[403, 404] The timing and type of surgery are therefore more complicated issues than in sporadic primary hyperparathyroidism. Most authorities agree that parathyroid disease recurs eventually, if fewer than three glands are removed. Some surgeons prefer subtotal parathyroidectomy, whereas others prefer total parathyroidectomy with forearm implantation of a small amount of parathyroid tissue.

Multiple Endocrine Neoplasia Type 2a

Parathyroid disease is a usually late and infrequent (5% to 20%) occurrence in MEN 2a, a disease defined by the clustering of medullary carcinoma of the thyroid, pheochromocytoma, and hyperparathyroidism. In some families, hyperparathyroidism is more common; however, these families have the same mutations in the *RET* gene that are found in families without frequent hyperparathyroidism.[405] Both parathyroid hyperplasia and adenoma have been noted at surgery. Because asymptomatic parathyroid hyperplasia has been noted at the time of thyroid surgery, a progression from hyperplasia to adenoma in MEN 2a has been suggested. The approach to diagnosis and treatment of hyperparathyroidism is similar to that in sporadic primary hyperparathyroidism, but hyperplasia is more frequently the underlying disorder. The pathogenesis of the hyperparathyroidism is uncertain, but the *RET* gene, mutated in virtually all cases of MEN 2a,[406, 407] is expressed in parathyroid cells,[408] so abnormal ret expression in parathyroid cells may directly cause parathyroid tumorigenesis. Hyperparathyroidism does not occur in MEN 2b, the variant associated with mucosal neuromas.

Other Inherited Syndromes

Several other distinct autosomal dominant syndromes of primary hyperparathyroidism have been characterized. Patients with hereditary isolated primary hyperparathyroidism[409] present with parathyroid tumors that can be multiple and occasionally are malignant. No other endocrine glands are abnormal in affected families, and the disease maps to neither the MEN 1 nor MEN 2a locus. Patients with hereditary hyperparathyroidism–jaw tumor syndrome[410, 411] present with parathyroid adenomas that are usually cystic and with fibrous jaw tumors that are unrelated to the hyperparathyroidism. Parathyroid cancer, Wilms' tumor, and polycystic renal disease also have occurred in affected families. This syndrome maps to chromosome 1q21–q31. Occasional families with apparently isolated familial hyperparathyroidism have inherited mutations in the MEN 1 gene, but most such families do not.

Management of Primary Hyperparathyroidism

The strategy for management of primary hyperparathyroidism has evolved in parallel with the changing presentation of the disease. The only opportunity for permanent cure is surgical removal of the abnormal gland(s), an approach that clearly was appropriate for virtually all patients in whom the classical, severe form of the disease was diagnosed four to five decades ago and which still is the treatment of choice for those patients who do present with recurrent kidney stones, nephrocalcinosis, clinically overt bone disease, or severe hypercalcemia.

In contrast, the choice of surgical versus medical management for patients with asymptomatic primary hyperparathyroidism remains an open and hotly debated question. Investigators who favor surgery point to the expected improvement in bone mineral density (at the hip and spine) and reversibility of left ventricular hypertrophy following successful surgical intervention; evidence of increased risk for fracture, cardiovascular mortality, malignancy, and neuropsychiatric symptoms associated with primary hyperparathyroidism; and the recent successful development of effective minimally invasive surgical procedures (see later on).

Investigators who favor an observational approach emphasize the evidence for lack of disease progression in most asymptomatic patients; the small but finite risk of surgical failure and postoperative complications; the probability that excess mortality and cancer risks documented in patients with relatively severe disease may not apply to those with mild, asymptomatic primary hyperparathyroidism; the difficulty in assigning vague neuropsychiatric symptoms to the parathyroid disorder; the lack of evidence (or negative evidence) that patients with hypertension or possibly increased risk of cancer, fracture, or cardiovascular mortality, or who already have such disease, are benefited by successful parathyroidectomy; and the availability of sensitive techniques for monitoring disease status in nonoperated patients.[366]

Unfortunately, no prospective studies have compared outcomes in patients with asymptomatic primary hyperparathyroidism randomly assigned to surgery with those in patients assigned to medical management. Furthermore, no large trials of differing strategies in medical management of the disease have been conducted. Surgical series generally reflect outcomes in patients preselected to receive interventional treatment; thus, results may not be readily extrapolated to those with mild, asymptomatic disease. Evidence that the true incidence of the disease may be declining, and that economic forces may increasingly limit detection to more symptomatic cases of the disease, may indicate that yet another change in the clinical character of the disease is in the offing. For all of these reasons, opinion in this area is rapidly evolving, and all recommendations thus should be considered provisional.

One set of such provisional recommendations was issued by a National Institutes of Health (NIH)-sponsored Consensus Development Conference held in 1990.[379] The major conclusion of the Conference group was that although surgery always should be considered an appropriate option, many patients with asymptomatic primary hyperparathyroidism can be safely monitored without surgery. These patients were defined as those who lacked "significant bone, renal, gastrointestinal, or neuromuscular symptoms typical of primary hyperparathyroidism" and who also did not meet the other criteria listed in Table 26–1. Such patients account for at least 50% of persons who currently present with primary hyperparathyroidism.

In other Consensus Conference recommendations, surgery may be preferable if the patient desires surgery even when asymptomatic, if the probability of consistent monitoring seems low, if concomitant illness seems likely to complicate management or obscure significant disease progression, or if the patient is relatively young (under 50 years of age). These recommendations reflect the absence of reliable information about the natural history of the disease over many decades of follow-up, as well as the cumulative cost of medical monitoring, which begins to exceed that of surgery by 5 to 10 years. Conversely, age alone is not a contraindication to parathyroidectomy, as the procedure has been accomplished with excellent results, with a perioperative mortality of 1% to 3%, in large numbers of appropriately selected patients older than 75 years of age.[412, 413] Because hypertension is not thought to be a feature of mild primary hyperparathyroidism,[362, 376, 414] and because hypertension generally is not corrected by parathyroidectomy, hypertension is not viewed as an indication for surgery.

Table 26–1. Indications for Surgery in Primary Hyperparathyroidism

1. Overt clinical manifestations of primary hyperparathyroidism
   a. Radiographic nephrolithiasis or otherwise documented kidney stone(s)
   b. Reduced creatinine clearance (not otherwise explained)
   c. Radiographically evident hyperparathyroid bone disease
   d. Classical hyperparathyroid neuromuscular disease
   e. Symptoms attributable to hypercalcemia per se
   f. Previous episode of life-threatening hypercalcemia
2. Serum calcium concentration greater than 12 mg/dL (2.99 mM)
3. Urinary calcium excretion greater than 400 mg/day (9.98 mmol/day)
4. Low or declining bone mineral density
   a. Less than 2 SDs below age/sex-matched controls (any site) *or*
   b. Vertebral osteopenia* *or*
   c. Declining vertebral bone density*
5. Age younger than 50 years
6. Uncertain prospect for successful medical monitoring
   a. Patient requests surgery
   b. Consistent follow-up seems unlikely
   c. Coexistent illness that may contribute to, or confound detection of, disease progression

*Not among original recommendations of NIH Consensus Conference.
SD, standard deviation.

Although the Consensus Conference recommendations provide a useful framework for decision making, supporting data from large clinical trials are lacking. In a series of 52 asymptomatic patients selected for nonoperative management mainly on the basis of the Consensus Conference criteria and whose course was followed for 10 years, approximately 25% developed one or more new indications for surgery[357] (Table 26–1). Patients who do not meet the Consensus Conference criteria for surgery may nevertheless experience the same postsurgical increase in bone density as occurs in those who do.[415] Some investigators have emphasized that evidence of baseline vertebral osteopenia, an unusual finding in primary hyperparathyroidism, should be added to the original Consensus Conference criteria for surgery (see Table 26–1)[374] and that surgery also should be considered for menopausal women who exhibit vertebral bone loss in the setting of primary hyperparathyroidism.[357, 366]

A common dilemma is the inability to ascertain whether vague but troublesome symptoms such as fatigue, lethargy, weakness (without objective muscle weakness), or depression are due to hyperparathyroidism and thus qualify as "significant" in the context of the decision regarding surgery. Most clinicians do not routinely recommend parathyroidectomy on the basis of such symptoms alone, although dramatic responses to surgery are occasionally seen. With the availability of improved, minimally invasive surgical approaches, the threshold for considering surgery for patients who are significantly disabled by such symptoms clearly is lower now than in the past. Some authorities have advocated, in selected cases, a limited trial of medical therapy to reduce serum calcium (i.e., strict dietary calcium restriction, estrogen, oral phosphate, or bisphosphonate; see later), thereby attempting to predict the symptomatic response to surgical cure.[379] The severity of such symptoms generally cannot be shown to correlate with serum calcium concentration, however, and may be related to other factors, such as blood PTH concentration.

Medical Monitoring of Primary Hyperparathyroidism

The NIH Consensus Conference recommended that patients be followed carefully, at least semiannually initially and at longer intervals if stable, for appearance of symptoms; appearance of adverse effects on blood pressure and serum or urinary calcium or creatinine; review of annual abdominal radiographs; and serial determination of bone mineral density at 1- or 2-year intervals. The most appropriate bone densitometric site was considered to be one that reflects mainly changes in cortical bone (i.e., distal forearm or total body), although the importance of monitoring vertebral bone density, as well, has been emphasized more recently.[357, 374]

Patients undergoing nonoperative medical management must be cautioned to maintain adequate hydration, to avoid diuretics and prolonged immobilization, and to seek prompt medical attention in the event of illnesses accompanied by significant vomiting or diarrhea. Dietary calcium probably should not exceed the recommended daily allowance (RDA) of 800 mg/day, even though short-term studies in highly selected patients with elevated serum $1,25(OH)_2D_3$ levels have demonstrated that a high-calcium diet may reduce serum $1,25(OH)_2D_3$ and PTH, albeit at the expense of a mild increase in serum and urinary calcium.[416]

Estrogen therapy may be a consideration in postmenopausal women with mild primary hyperparathyroidism or in those who are symptomatic but yet refuse or cannot safely undergo surgery. Estrogens may reduce serum calcium and phosphorus, and urinary calcium and hydroxyproline, and histologic evidence of bone resorption in women with primary hyperparathyroidism, although serum PTH remains elevated and serum $1,25(OH)_2D_3$ increases, owing mainly to increased concentrations of the vitamin D binding protein.[417–419] Progestins may exert similar effects on serum calcium and may slow bone loss in elderly women with primary hyperparathyroidism, but concern over their adverse effects on blood lipids have limited use of these agents in this population.[418, 419] Selective estrogen receptor modulators such as tamoxifen or raloxifene may prove useful in postmenopausal women with osteopenia due to primary hyperparathyroidism, but a beneficial effect has not yet been shown.

Oral phosphate therapy has been advocated for use in occasional patients with primary hyperparathyroidism who have failed or refused surgery and who may have recurrent calcium kidney stones or other serious symptoms. Phosphate in this setting may act by inhibiting both renal synthesis of $1,25(OH)_2D_3$ and osteoclastic bone resorption, by promoting precipitation of calcium into bone and soft tissues, and, in the gut, by binding intraluminal calcium and impairing its absorption. Oral phosphate does reduce serum and urinary calcium as well as serum $1,25(OH)_2D_3$, but it increases serum PTH, and the long-term effect on bone is unknown.[420]

Bisphosphonates have been employed successfully in the urgent therapy of hypercalcemia due to primary hyperparathyroidism, but their use in chronic management of mild primary hyperparathyroidism has been limited by several adverse effects, including stimulation of PTH secretion and a lowering of the renal phosphate threshold, which aggravates hypophosphatemia and may augment renal $1,25(OH)_2D_3$ synthesis.[421] Although not yet available for routine clinical use, calcimimetic drugs capable of binding to and activating the parathyroid calcium-sensing receptor are in development and may offer a new avenue for control of hyperparathyroidism.[422]

Surgical Treatment of Primary Hyperparathyroidism

Parathyroidectomy is a safe and highly effective approach to definitive treatment of primary hyperparathyroidism. The most serious potential complications of parathyroid surgery—vocal cord paralysis and permanent hypoparathyroidism—occur after less than 1% and 4%, respectively, of procedures performed by highly skilled surgeons, although the rates for these complications can be much higher with less experienced operators.[348]

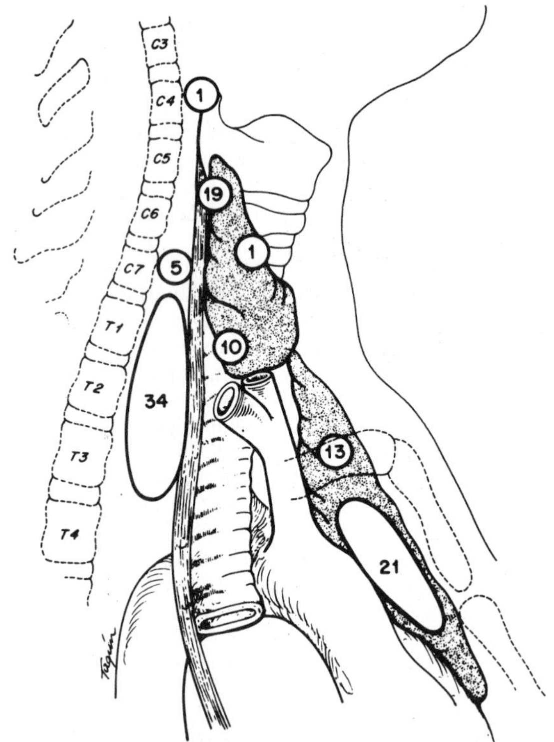

Figure 26–26. Sites of ectopic location of 104 parathyroid glands found at reoperation for primary hyperparathyroidism. (From Wang C-A. A clinical and pathological study of 112 cases. Ann Surg 1977; 186:140–145.)

Such complications occur most often in patients who require subtotal parathyroid resection for hyperplasia or resection of carcinoma. The surgical cure rate for primary hyperparathyroidism in the best hands is at least 95%.[348, 423, 424] Apart from operator inexperience, the usual cause of initial surgical failure—"persistent disease"—is the presence of either unrecognized (often very asymmetrical) parathyroid hyperplasia or ectopic parathyroid tissue (i.e., intrathyroidal, undescended, retroesophageal, or mediastinal glands)[424, 425] (Fig. 26–26). Up to one in five parathyroid glands may be located ectopically—especially supernumerary glands.[348, 426, 427] The incidence of recurrent disease, defined as that occurring after an interval of at least 6 to 12 months of normocalcemia, ranges from 2% to 16%. Recurrent hyperparathyroidism usually arises in unresected hyperplastic glands, but rarely it may be due to parathyroid carcinoma, to a second adenoma, or to a multicentric or miliary "parathyromatosis" engendered by inadvertent local seeding of parathyroid tissue into the neck during previous parathyroid surgery.[348, 428]

Until recently, there was broad agreement that the best approach is a bilateral neck exploration in which all four parathyroids are identified and all enlarged glands removed.[426, 429–431] With this procedure, preoperative parathyroid localization studies before initial cervical exploration are superfluous, as the positive predictive value of even the best technique (technetium Tc 99m sestamibi scanning) falls well short of the success rate of experienced surgeons unaided by previous imaging.[348, 423, 424, 432–434] Some surgeons prefer to biopsy all identified glands, even though this approach risks a 20% to 40% incidence of transient postoperative hypocalcemia, whereas others report excellent results without routine biopsy of nonenlarged glands.[349, 426] In the event that one gland is not identified after extensive exploration, ipsilateral thyroid lobectomy commonly is performed, as the frequency of intrathyroidal parathyroid glands is approximately 5%.

With the advent of preoperative technetium Tc 99m sestamibi scanning, which can accurately localize 80% to 90% of the single adenomas that account for 75% to 85% of cases, there has been renewed interest in performance of directed unilateral explorations, which reduce operative and recovery room time, minimize the number of frozen sections required, are associated with significantly fewer postoperative complications, and can more readily be performed using minimally invasive techniques (including local anesthesia and intravenous sedation) that enable same-day discharge.[435, 436] Sestamibi scanning also can identify the occasional mediastinal adenoma and thereby direct the surgeon away from neck exploration. On the other hand, because the sensitivity of sestamibi scanning ranges from 75% to 90% and the technique is least reliable in the presence of multiglandular disease (hyperplasia or double adenomas), the test may falsely localize an adenoma or miss the presence of bilateral disease in 10% to 20% of patients.[436–439] To reduce this failure rate, which is unacceptably high in comparison with that of bilateral exploration, supplemental preoperative ultrasonic imaging (with or without needle biopsy) has been employed, and rapid intraoperative PTH assays have been developed to verify successful excision.[440–442]

Because the half-life of intact PTH in blood is very short (<2 minutes), a decline of 50% or more from baseline within 10 minutes or so can signal successful removal of all hyperfunctioning parathyroid tissue. This approach has worked well in patients with single adenomas but can be misleading in those with multiglandular disease unless more stringent criteria for cure are applied (i.e., >70% decline in, or even normalization of, iPTH levels at 20 minutes).[440] No surgical series has analyzed a sufficient number of patients with hyperplasia to permit rigorous definition of the role of intraoperative PTH measurements.

Another adjunct to minimally invasive parathyroidectomy has been the use of a hand-held gamma probe intraoperatively, both to map the location of abnormal glands and to verify their removal, following immediate preoperative imaging technetium Tc 99m using sestamibi.[443] The challenging logistics of arranging the sequence of injection, imaging, and surgery necessary for success with this technique have limited its use to a few specialized centers, however.

At present, preoperative imaging enables consideration of a minimally invasive unilateral parathyroidectomy in approximately 70% of those patients thought preoperatively to have sporadic primary hyperparathyroidism due to a solitary adenoma. The ultimate dominance of this approach will depend on the balance between advantages (reduced operative and recovery time, fewer ancillary procedures, and lower hospital charge) and disadvantages (the added costs of the imaging and intraoperative PTH assays and the possibly greater demands for surgical skill and experience). Alternatively, successful application of minimally invasive techniques to bilateral explorations has begun. In one center, for example, 97% of patients with primary hyperparathyroidism currently undergo bilateral exploration under local anesthesia, with completion of the procedure in less than 1 hour and discharge to home within 6 hours.[444]

In patients found or suspected to have multiglandular hyperplasia, several different approaches have been recommended, including removal of all but approximately 30 to 50 mg of parathyroid tissue ("3½-gland parathyroidectomy"), removal of all enlarged glands (but at least two) with biopsy of the remaining normal-sized glands, and total resection of all parathyroid tissue from the neck followed by autotransplantation of gland fragments to the forearm, with cryopreservation of remaining tissue.[348, 426, 427, 445] A concerted effort is made to search for a possible fifth gland, and any unresected (or transplanted) parathyroid tissue is marked with clips or sutures to facilitate identification in the event that reoperation becomes necessary. Great care must be taken by both the surgeon and the pathologist to describe the origin of, and label, all resected putative parathyroid tissue, particularly in parathyroid hyperplasia, as one of the most common handicaps facing the surgeon, should a subsequent operation become necessary, is inadequate knowledge of the original surgical findings and pathology. In contrast to initial cervical exploration, preoperative localization should be attempted routinely in those few patients who require reoperation for failed surgery, and intraoperative PTH determinations may be helpful in guiding the surgeon during these often difficult procedures.[440, 446]

The incidence of parathyroid carcinoma in primary hyperparathyroidism is less than 1%,[348, 350, 427] but this possibility should be strongly considered in patients with unusually severe hyperparathyroidism, a palpable neck mass, hoarseness, evidence of local invasion at surgery, or recurrent hypercalcemia (see later on). Even so, parathyroid carcinoma rarely is suspected preoperatively and often eludes diagnosis at the time of initial surgery. When the disease is recognized, vigorous attempts should be made to remove the tumor en bloc. The incidence of local recurrence approaches 50%, however, and distant metastases, particularly to lung, may be heralded by recurrent, severe hyperparathyroidism.[348, 426, 427]

The immediate postoperative management of parathyroidectomy focuses on establishing the success of the surgery and monitoring the patient closely for symptomatic hypocalcemia and for uncommon but potentially serious acute complications such as bleeding, vocal cord paralysis, or laryngospasm. After successful resection of a parathyroid adenoma, serum intact PTH levels decline rapidly, often to undetectable concentrations, with a disappearance half-time of about 2 minutes, whereas serum calcium typically reaches a nadir between 24 and 36 hours. Serum PTH returns to the normal range within 30 hours, although measurements of the parathyroid secretory response to hypocalcemia suggest that it does not fully normalize for at least several weeks.[447, 448]

In the past, patients generally were maintained on a low-calcium diet until normalization of serum calcium was clearly documented, ampules of injectable calcium and other seizure precautions were maintained at the bedside, serum calcium was measured at least every 12 hours until the patient was stable, and symptomatic hypocalcemia was promptly treated with calcium, either intravenously (90-mg bolus, 50 to 100 mg/hour) or orally (1.5 to 3.0 g/day). This approach is no longer appropriate for most patients, who are discharged less than 24 hours after surgery. Instead, oral calcium supplements routinely are provided as soon as oral intake is re-established, and moderate doses of $1,25(OH)_2D_3$ (0.5 to 1.0 μg daily) are added in those with large adenomas and severe hyperparathyroidism or in whom alkaline phosphatase had been elevated preoperatively—that is, patients in whom an impressive calcium requirement can be anticipated, often for many weeks postoperatively, as they remineralize their skeletons. This *hungry bone syndrome* is associated with hypocalcemia, hypophosphatemia, and low urinary calcium excretion.

Serum calcium should be checked at intervals of several days initially to guide adjustment of calcium and vitamin D therapy as needed to achieve a stable result. In patients in whom hypocalcemia persists for more than several days, serum PTH should be measured to exclude the possibility of postoperative hypoparathyroidism. In view of evidence that bone mineral density continues to increase for at least a year after successful parathyroidectomy,[357] it is prudent to continue calcium supplementation for at least that long.

The approach to patients with persistent or recurrent hyperparathyroidism is informed by the recognition that parathyroid hyperplasia or carcinoma, ectopic or supernumerary parathyroid tissue, and postoperative hypoparathyroidism and other complications of further surgery all are more common in this population.[348, 424, 434] The first issue to address is whether surgery is indicated. When a presumed adenoma is not identified initially, the original indications for surgery generally still exist, although some patients may not be suitable candidates for more extensive surgery, such as a median sternotomy, because of concurrent medical illness. Patients with parathyroid hyperplasia have experienced significant clinical improvement even after incomplete parathyroidectomy, although those with MEN 1 are likely to experience further progression of their disease.[403]

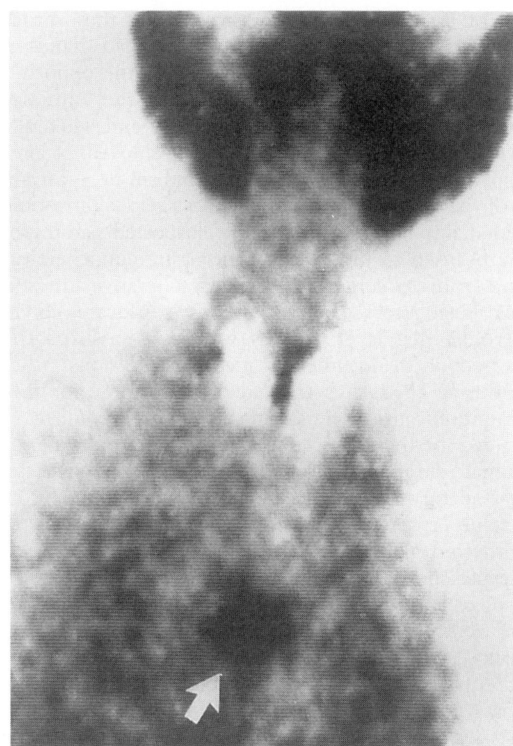

Figure 26–27. Technetium Tc 99m sestamibi ^{123}I subtraction scanning of a patient with persistent hyperparathyroidism after two previous unsuccessful operations. *Arrow* points to parathyroid adenoma, shown as increased tracer uptake in the aortopulmonary window. (From Thule P, Thakore K, Vansant J, et al. Preoperative localization of parathyroid tissue with technetium-99m sestamibi ^{123}I subtraction scanning. J Clin Endocrinol Metab 1994; 78:77–82.)

As noted previously, preoperative localization studies, although unnecessary for initial neck exploration, are justified for patients in whom a first operation failed to effect a cure or in whom the disease has recurred. Scanning with technetium Tc 99m sestamibi offers the highest sensitivity and accuracy, although other studies—ultrasonography, computed tomography (CT), or magnetic resonance imaging (MRI)—may provide additional or confirmatory information. Sestamibi does localize to thyroid nodules, which may accompany parathyroid disease in 20% to 40% of patients,[449] although it tends to wash out of thyroid tissue much more rapidly than from parathyroids. Technetium Tc 99m sestamibi can be combined with ^{123}I scanning to improve distinction of parathyroids from thyroid nodules or with single photon emission CT (SPECT) imaging to achieve accuracy in localization not possible with planar imaging[434, 450–452] (Fig. 26–27). On the other hand, sestamibi scanning may fail to reveal small glands or to demonstrate multiple abnormal glands in cases of parathyroid hyperplasia, the most common cause of persistent postoperative hyperparathyroidism.

More invasive techniques have been employed as well, including angiography and selective venous sampling for measurement of PTH, although the sensitivity of these procedures for detection of residual abnormal parathyroid glands is only 50% to 65%.[434, 453] Angiography does offer the opportunity to attempt angioablation of any identified tissue, although this procedure is not routinely successful,[453, 454] and when all other parathyroid tissue has been previously removed, it precludes the opportunity to avoid hypoparathyroidism by autotransplantation of parathyroid fragments at surgery. Ultrasound- or CT-guided fine-needle aspiration of suspected parathyroid tissue may be used to obtain cytologic or immunochemical confirmation prior to surgery,[455] and intraoperative ultrasonography has been useful in some cases to locate cervical or intrathyroidal glands.[434] Success with video-assisted thoracoscopic resection of documented mediastinal lesions[456, 457] offers a less invasive alternative to median sternotomy for this relatively common cause of persistent hyperparathyroidism.

The need for these procedures depends on the experience of the original surgeon and the surgeon's confidence that the neck was adequately explored initially. For example, at reoperation at one center, more than half of the "missed" hyperplastic parathyroid glands in those cases previously explored by a highly experienced parathyroid surgeon were found in the mediastinum or another ectopic location, whereas more than 90% of those referred by less experienced surgeons were discovered in a normal anatomic location in the neck.[348]

After successful surgery for primary hyperparathyroidism, bone mass generally improves by as much as 5% to 10% in the first year at sites rich in trabecular bone (spine, femoral neck) but does not improve at cortical bone sites (distal radius).[357] Bone density increases at trabecular bone sites may continue for several years, to as much as 12% to 15% after 10 years, although normal bone mineral density may not be achieved.[357, 372, 373, 458] This improvement, which is most apparent in patients with the greatest preoperative reductions in bone mass, may be related in part to rapid remineralization of the previously enlarged portion of bone undergoing remodeling,[372, 373, 415, 459] but the continued improvement over years suggests a more sustained increase in net bone formation and total bone volume, as well.[357]

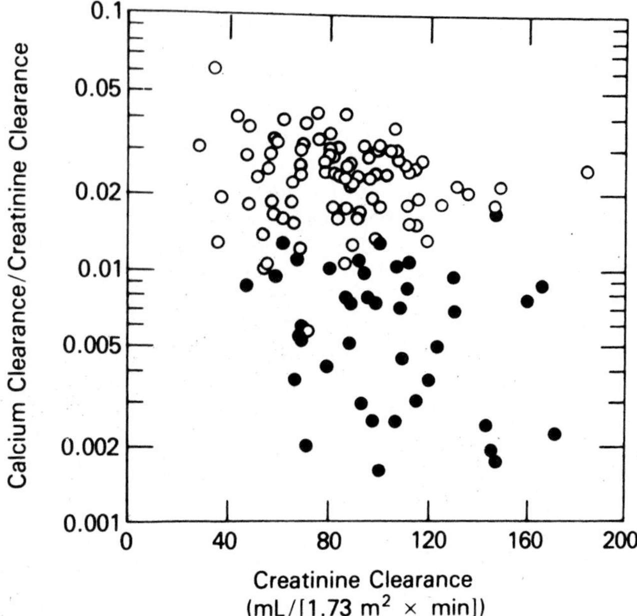

Figure 26–28. Index of urinary excretion rate for calcium as a function of creatinine clearance. Each point represents the mean of multiple determinations for a hypercalcemic patient with familial hypocalciuric hypercalcemia (*filled circles*) or with typical primary hyperparathyroidism (*open circles*). The data are based on average 24-hour urinary excretion values and average fasting serum samples. (From Marx SJ, Attie MF, Levine M, et al. The hypocalciuric or benign variant of familial hypercalcemia: clinical and biochemical features in fifteen kindreds. Medicine 1981; 60:397–412.)

Familial Hypocalciuric Hypercalcemia

Familial hypocalciuric hypercalcemia (FHH), also appropriately called *familial benign hypercalcemia*, is, in most families, a disorder of autosomal dominant inheritance caused by mutations of the calcium-sensing receptor gene found in parathyroid glands, kidney, and other organs[20] (see earlier discussion of calcium sensing). The mutations, which cause complete or partial loss of function of the calcium-sensing receptor, lead to a shift in the parathyroid cell's set-point for calcium.[460] As a consequence, higher than normal levels of blood calcium are needed to suppress PTH secretion. Furthermore, abnormal function of the calcium-sensing receptor in the renal thick ascending limb leads to increased, PTH-independent calcium reabsorption and consequent hypocalciuria.

The presence of one normal sensing receptor gene with the abnormal one usually leads to a very mild clinical disorder, although the receptor functions as a dimer, and certain mutations can worsen the function of the normal allele.[461, 462] Rare patients who inherit mutant calcium-sensing receptor genes from both parents present at birth with severe, life-threatening, primary hyperparathyroidism and almost always require immediate parathyroid surgery. In another genetic variation, a familial form of calcium-sensing receptor–dependent hypercalcemia has been described in association with other autoimmune disorders such as Hashimoto's hypothyroidism and celiac sprue, in which autoantibodies directed against the sensor apparently antagonize calcium recognition by the parathyroids and renal tubules.[463]

FHH is manifested at birth by hypercalcemia. Although some controversy exists, most observers note that the condition is asymptomatic and that apparent symptoms represent ascertainment bias.[23] Possible exceptions include the occurrence of chondrocalcinosis and perhaps pancreatitis. The blood calcium level is usually less than 12 mg/dL but can be higher. Phosphate measurements are low, as in primary hyperparathyroidism. Blood magnesium levels are high normal or slightly elevated. PTH levels are inappropriately normal for the degree of hypercalcemia and are occasionally modestly elevated. Urine calcium is usually low, though one novel mutation in the receptor's intracellular tail has been associated with hypercalciuria, possibly because of only mild dysfunction in the kidney.[464]

When patients present as adults, the distinction from mild primary hyperparathyroidism can be difficult. The distinction between FHH and primary hyperparathyroidism is a crucial one, however. Young patients with primary hyperparathyroidism are usually treated surgically and cured. In contrast, hypercalcemia always recurs after surgery for FHH, unless the patient is rendered hypoparathyroid by the removal of all parathyroid tissue. Therefore, surgery is contraindicated as therapy for FHH, except in the very rare patient with severe, symptomatic hypercalcemia. No blood or urine measurements are completely reliable for distinguishing between the two conditions, though the ratio of calcium clearance to creatinine clearance distinguishes most patients with FHH from those with primary hyperparathyroidism[465] (Fig. 26–28). The most helpful diagnostic information is the presence of hypercalcemia in an infant relative; such early hypercalcemia does not occur in MEN 1. Furthermore, a past history of clearly normal blood calcium, considerably lower than current measurements, makes FHH unlikely, if no other reason for a change in blood calcium exists.

Lithium Toxicity

Treatment of bipolar affective disorders with lithium commonly leads to mild, persistent increases in blood calcium[396, 466] occasionally out of the normal range, in affected persons. After several years of therapy, clear elevations of PTH levels and modest increases in parathyroid gland size, detected by ultrasonography, often occur.[396] Usually, when lithium therapy is stopped, the blood calcium and PTH normalize within several months. Uncommonly, substantial hypercalcemia and clear hyperparathyroidism ensue. At surgery, parathyroid hyperplasia and, occasionally, parathyroid adenomas have been found.

The management of patients with mild, lithium-induced hypercalcemia is somewhat complicated. Like patients with mild primary hyperparathyroidism, patients taking lithium usually tolerate mild hypercalcemia without obvious symptoms. These patients can be monitored with protocols similar to those for patients with asymptomatic primary hyperparathyroidism. Close attention must be paid to urine concentrating ability in these patients, however, because the nephrogenic diabetes insipidus associated with lithium therapy can lead to dehydration and sudden worsening of hypercalcemia. Substantial hypercalcemia should lead to withdrawal of lithium therapy, if possible, with substitution of newer psychopharmacologic agents. If hypercalcemia persists after withdrawal of lithium, decisions about surgery follow the same guidelines as those for patients with primary hyperparathyroidism.

Lithium increases the set-point for PTH secretion when it is added to isolated parathyroid cells in vitro.[467] The set-point for PTH secretion in vivo is shifted to the right in patients who have received lithium for several years as well.[468] A corresponding shift in the concentration of extracellular calcium needed to raise intracellular calcium levels[469] suggests that lithium interferes with the action of the parathyroid calcium-sensing receptor, perhaps by interfering with inositol phosphate metabolism.

Parathyroid-Independent Hypercalcemia

In parathyroid-independent hypercalcemia, PTH secretion is appropriately suppressed. PTH levels, measured using two-site assays, are invariably lower than 25 pg/mL and are usually lower than normal or undetectable. Most affected patients have malignant hypercalcemia, although parathyroid-independent hypercalcemia occurs in a number of other settings as well.

Hypercalcemia of Malignancy

The diagnosis of malignant hypercalcemia is seldom a subtle one. Most malignancies produce hypercalcemia only when they are far advanced; the diagnosis becomes evident after routine studies, guided by the history and physical examination. Patients with malignant hypercalcemia usually die a month or two after hypercalcemia is discovered.[470] Patients present with the classic signs and symptoms of hypercalcemia: confusion, polydypsia, polyuria, constipation, nausea, and vomiting. Perhaps because of the acuteness of the hypercalcemia and the elderly patient population involved, dramatic changes in mental status, culminating in coma, are relatively common. The diagnosis can be missed because the manifestations often overlap those of the underlying malignancy and because low blood albumin may lead to an apparently normal total blood calcium, despite an elevated blood ionized calcium. Even though the overall prognosis is grim, the diagnosis of malignant hypercalcemia is important to make.

Treatment is usually simple and effective in the short term; such treatment can importantly reverse the patient's symptoms for several weeks, and even provide time for a fundamental attack on the underlying tumor, if it is treatable. Only effective treatment of the underlying neoplasm can significantly influence the long-term prognosis for patients with malignant hypercalcemia.

Although mechanisms in a given patient may be multiple, it is still useful to distinguish hypercalcemia associated with local involvement of bone from that caused by humoral mechanisms. In all cases, resorption of bone plays a pivotal role in the pathogenesis.

Local Osteolytic Hypercalcemia

Hypercalcemia resulting from tumors invading bone occurs most clearly in multiple myeloma and some patients with breast cancer. There is little evidence that the tumor cells themselves resorb bone. Instead, active osteoclasts found near the tumor cells are thought to be the proximate mediators of bone resorption.[471] Myeloma cells and marrow cells associated with myeloma cells secrete numerous cytokines capable of stimulating bone resorption, including lymphotoxin (tumor necrosis factor-β) and interleukins 1β and 6 (IL-1β and IL-6).[472, 473] RANKL is also found on the surface of myeloma cells and therefore may stimulate the production and activity of osteoclasts, just as RANKL on the surface of osteoblast-like cells can. In patients with myeloma, treatment with intermittent intravenous pamidronate (a bisphosphonate) inhibits this resorption and reduces the incidence of bone pain, fracture, and hypercalcemia.[474]

The pathogenesis of hypercalcemia in breast cancer is not completely understood. Extensive metastases to bone are detected in most patients with hypercalcemia and breast cancer; this finding suggests that factors produced in bone by the metastatic tumor cells may be important. Breast cancer cells make a host of cytokines capable of resorbing bone.[471] The role of tumor-produced PTHrP may be particularly important.[192] A majority of breast cancer patients with hypercalcemia have elevated blood levels of PTHrP.[340, 342, 475] This circulating PTHrP, as well as PTHrP produced in bone by metastatic tumor cells, may generate the hypercalcemia. Primary breast tumors that stain for PTHrP are more likely to result in bone metastases than are those that do not stain for PTHrP[475]; this PTHrP may be instrumental in the establishment of lytic metastases.[476] Animal models indicate that transforming growth factor-β (TGF-β), released from bone matrix by PTHrP-stimulated osteoclastic resorption, may further augment PTHrP secretion by the tumor cells.[477] The latter may be further promoted by estrogen, which may explain the occasional occurrence of hypercalcemia following institution of estrogen or tamoxifen therapy in this disease.[478]

Humoral Hypercalcemia of Malignancy

Albright, in 1941, was the first to propose that a PTH-like humoral factor caused the hypercalcemia in patients with malignancy but few or no bone metastases.[479] Four decades later biochemical analysis demonstrated that such patients have high blood calcium levels, low blood phosphate levels, and high urinary cAMP levels like those found in primary hyperparathyroidism, but no elevation in iPTH levels.[480] The stimulation of cAMP production was used as an assay to eventually purify PTHrP from human tumors associated with the humoral hypercalcemia of malignancy.[174, 481–483]

The evidence that PTHrP mediates the humoral hypercalcemia of malignancy in most patients is substantial. As noted previously, PTHrP binds to the PTH/PTHrP receptor and mimics all of the actions of amino-terminal fragments of PTH.[189–191] Blood levels of PTHrP are elevated in most patients with solid tumors and hypercalcemia.[187, 198, 342] In animal models of the humoral hypercalcemia of malignancy, antibodies against PTHrP can reverse the hypercalcemia.[341, 484]

The acute actions of PTHrP cannot explain all of the findings in patients with the hypercalcemia of malignancy, however. Acutely administered PTHrP, like PTH, increases blood levels of $1,25(OH)_2D_3$ by stimulating the renal 1α-hydroxylase. Nevertheless, patients with the humoral hypercalcemia of malignancy usually have low levels of $1,25(OH)_2D_3$.[480] This finding is particularly puzzling, because human tumors associated with low $1,25(OH)_2D_3$ levels stimulate $1,25(OH)_2D_3$ synthesis after they are transplanted into nude mice.[485] Possible explanations for the low $1,25(OH)_2D_3$ levels in patients include inhibition of the 1α-hydroxylase by hypercalcemia[486] or by tumor products.[487]

A second disparity between the acute actions of PTHrP and the findings in patients with malignant hypercalcemia involves the rate of bone formation. Acutely, PTHrP, like PTH, leads to increased bone formation. Nevertheless, in patients with malignant hypercalcemia, bone formation is markedly lower than normal. The explanation for this effect may well lie in the action of other cytokines, immobilization, or particular fragments of PTHrP with novel properties.

The tumors most commonly associated with humoral hypercalcemia include squamous cell cancers of the lung, head and neck, esophagus, cervix, vulva, and skin; breast cancer; renal cell cancer; and bladder cancer. Benign or malignant pheochromocytomas, islet cell tumors, and carcinoids can also overproduce PTHrP, causing hypercalcemia. The aggressive T-cell lymphoma associated with human T-cell lymphotropic virus-1 (HTLV-1) infection is the only hematologic malignancy commonly associated with PTHrP overproduction and hypercalcemia.

It is unlikely that PTHrP is the sole cause of the humoral hypercalcemia of malignancy. As noted previously, many cytokines produced by tumors can stimulate bone resorption. The actions of these cytokines have been shown to synergize with those of PTHrP in a number of experimental models.[488] The hypercalcemia observed in rare patients with VIP-secreting pancreatic islet cell tumors may reflect tumor cell secretion of PTHrP as well as direct bone-resorbing actions of VIP and of the systemic acidosis that results from VIP-induced diarrhea. Furthermore, in hypercalcemic patients with non-Hodgkin's lymphoma, blood levels of $1,25(OH)_2D_3$ were found to be higher than otherwise expected.[489] In these patients, the relative importance of $1,25(OH)_2D_3$ cytokines, like those implicated in multiple myeloma, PTHrP, and immobilization, needs to be clarified.

In a few reported cases, malignant tumors secrete PTH and not PTHrP.[490–494] Although this phenomenon has now been well documented, it should be stressed that in almost all patients with cancer and high PTH levels, concurrent primary hyperparathyroidism, not ectopic PTH production, is the cause of the hyperparathyroidism.

Vitamin D Intoxication

Because the synthesis of $1,25(OH)_2D_3$ is so tightly regulated, extremely large doses of vitamin D, on the order of 100,000 units per day, are required to cause hypercalcemia. Such doses are available in the United States only by prescription; therefore, most cases of vitamin D intoxication are iatrogenic. Occasionally, inadvertent ingestion occurs.[284] Patients present with nausea, vomiting, weakness, and altered level of consciousness. Hypercalcemia can be severe and prolonged, because of the storage of vitamin D in fat. As expected, PTH levels are suppressed, and levels of 25(OH)D, which are poorly regulated and reflect levels of ingested vitamin D, are dramatically elevated. In contrast, the levels of $1,25(OH)_2D_3$ are only modestly elevated or can be normal or even low. The modest changes in $1,25(OH)_2D_3$ levels result from the down-regulation of the renal 1α-hydroxylase by low levels of PTH and high levels of phosphate, calcium, and $1,25(OH)_2D_3$ itself. The cause of the hypercalcemia, when it occurs in the face of normal levels of $1,25(OH)_2D_3$, is uncertain but may reflect the direct action of 25(OH)D and possibly other vitamin D metabolites, which are capable of binding the $1,25(OH)_2D_3$ receptor weakly. Also, the weaker vitamin D metabolites may displace $1,25(OH)_2D_3$ from the circulating D-binding protein and increase the concentration of active, free $1,25(OH)_2D_3$.[284]

The hypercalcemia of vitamin D intoxication results both from increased intestinal absorption of calcium and from the direct effect of $1,25(OH)_2D_3$ to increase resorption of bone. In severe cases, therefore, glucocorticoid therapy, which counters the action of $1,25(OH)_2D_3$ on both bone and intestine, should be added to the therapeutic regimen of hydration and omission of dietary calcium.[495]

Sarcoidosis and Other Granulomatous Diseases

Sarcoidosis may be associated with hypercalcemia and, even more commonly, hypercalciuria.[496] Hypercalcemic patients have high levels of $1,25(OH)_2D_3$[497]; the high level of $1,25(OH)_2D_3$ probably causes the hypercalcemia, although overproduction of bone-resorbing cytokines and PTHrP may contribute in some patients.[498] As expected in $1,25(OH)_2D_3$-dependent hypercalcemia, intestinal absorption of calcium is increased and PTH levels are suppressed. Furthermore, the hypercalcemia and high levels of $1,25(OH)_2D_3$ fall upon treatment with glucocorticoids. The unregulated synthesis of $1,25(OH)_2D_3$, found even in an anephric patient,[274] occurs not in the kidney but rather in the sarcoid granulomas. Removal of a large amount of granulomatous tissue can reverse hypercalcemia.[499] Furthermore, isolated sarcoid macrophages can synthesize $1,25(OH)_2D_3$ from 25(OH)D, as can normal macrophages stimulated with interferon γ.[500, 501] Such macrophages express the gene encoding the identical 25(OH)D 1α-hydroxylase found in the kidney.[502]

The unregulated synthesis of $1,25(OH)_2D_3$ by activated macrophages explains many of the findings in sarcoid patients. These patients have unusual sensitivity to vitamin D and can become hypercalcemic in response to ultraviolet radiation or oral vitamin D intake.[497] Abnormalities in calcium metabolism are usually found only in patients with active disease and large, clinically obvious total-body burdens of granulomas. Nevertheless, hypercalcemia can present in patients without obvious pulmonary disease. Furthermore, subtle abnormalities of vitamin D metabolism can be demonstrated even in patients with mildly active sarcoidosis. For example, patients without elevated levels of angiotensin-converting enzyme in their blood have normal levels of $1,25(OH)_2D_3$, but these levels do not fall normally in response to an oral calcium challenge.[503]

Hypercalcemia is also associated with other granulomatous diseases, such as tuberculosis, fungal infections,[504] and berylliosis and has been reported in Wegener's granulomatosis,[505] in acquired immunodeficiency syndrome (AIDS)-related *Pneumocystis carinii* infection,[506] and even in association with extensive granulomatous foreign body reactions.

Hyperthyroidism

Mild hypercalcemia can result from thyrotoxicosis.[507] Blood calcium levels seldom exceed 11mg/dL, but mild elevations are found in a quarter of patients.[508] Patients have low PTH levels, low $1,25(OH)_2D_3$ levels, and hypercalciuria. The hypercalcemia is caused by a direct action of thyroid hormone to stimulate bone resorption.[509] Beta-adrenergic blocking agents can reverse the hypercalcemia.[510]

Vitamin A Intoxication

Excess ingestion of vitamin A (retinol) results in a syndrome of dry skin, pruritus, headache from pseudotumor cerebri, bone pain, and, occasionally, hypercalcemia. Hypercalcemia occurs only with the ingestion of 10 times the RDA (5000 IU/day). The identical syndrome can result from ingestion of the vitamin A derivatives isotretinoin (13-*cis*-retinoic acid [Accutane]) and tretinoin (all-*trans*-retinoic acid [Retin-A]), used to treat acne.[511] Bones can show characteristic periosteal calcification on radiographs.[512] The hypercalcemia is probably caused by the action of retinoids to directly stimulate bone resorption. The diagnosis is made by the association of a history of excess ingestion of retinoids with the characteristic syndrome and abnormal results of liver function tests; elevated vitamin A levels confirm the diagnosis. Treatment involves hydration and, if necessary, glucocorticoids.

Adrenal Insufficiency

Hypercalcemia occurs in the setting of adrenal insufficiency. Blood calcium is elevated partly as a result of hemoconcentration and increased albumin levels,[513] but the level of ionized calcium can be increased as well.[514] The hypercalcemia in one well-studied case[514] resulted from a combination of influx of calcium into the vascular space, probably from bone, combined with low renal clearance.

Thiazide Diuretics

Thiazide diuretics do not cause hypercalcemia by themselves, but can exacerbate the hypercalcemia of primary hyperparathyroidism. The mechanism of the hypercalcemia may involve the action of thiazide diuretics to increase distal tubular calcium reabsorption.[67] Thiazides block sodium chloride cotransport into these cells (see Fig. 26–7). The fall in intracellular chloride hyperpolarizes the cell, thereby increasing calcium influx through voltage-sensitive channels.[233] Decreased renal clearance of calcium alone would be expected to raise blood calcium in the normal human only transiently because the transient hypercalcemia would be expected to suppress PTH secretion and lead to return of the blood calcium to normal.

As predicted by this model, thiazide administration leads to chronic hypercalcemia only in patients with abnormal parathyroid physiology.[515] In primary hyperparathyroidism, thiazide administration exacerbates the hypercalcemia, and in hypoparathyroidism, thiazide administration facilitates the maintenance of normocalcemia when given in conjunction with $1,25(OH)_2D_3$ and calcium.[516]

Milk-Alkali Syndrome

The triad of hypercalcemia, metabolic alkalosis, and renal failure can be the consequence of massive ingestion of calcium and absorbable alkali.[517] This syndrome was first described when milk and sodium bicarbonate were used in large amounts to treat peptic ulcer disease. With the change in ulcer treatment to nonabsorbable antacids and suppression of acid secretion, milk-alkali syndrome became rare. In the last several years, however, the increased use of calcium carbonate to treat dyspepsia and osteoporosis has led to the reappearance of milk-alkali syndrome.[518, 519] In most cases, a history of ingestion of several grams per day of calcium in the form of calcium carbonate can be elicited. The pathogenesis of the syndrome is not understood in detail but may well involve a vicious circle in which alkalosis decreases renal calcium clearance and hypercalcemia helps maintain alkalosis. Nephrocalcinosis, nephrogenic diabetes insipidus, decrease in GFR associated with hypercalcemia, and hypovolemia from vomiting all lead to renal failure, which can be severe. PTH levels, measured with currently available two-site assays, are invariably low in hypercalcemic patients[518, 519] as are levels of $1,25(OH)_2D_3$. After clearance of the calcium by hydration or dialysis, if necessary, renal function generally returns to normal, unless the disorder has been severe and long-standing.

Immobilization

Immobilization can lead to bone resorption sufficient to cause hypercalcemia. The immobilization is usually caused by spinal cord injury or extensive casting after fractures. Hypercalcemia of immobilization occurs predominantly in the young or in patients with other reasons for a high rate of bone turnover, such as Paget's disease or extensive fractures. Hypercalciuria and substantial bone loss are more common than hypercalcemia is. After spinal cord injury, the hypercalciuria is maximal at 4 months and can persist for more than a year.[520] PTH and $1,25(OH)_2D_3$ levels are suppressed[521]; bone biopsies show increased resorption and decreased formation of bone.[522] The combination of calcitonin and bisphosphonates[523] or simply bisphosphonates alone[524] have been used to reverse the hypercalcemia and hypercalciuria of spinal cord injury.

Renal Failure

Following rhabdomyolysis, during the oliguric phase of acute renal failure, severe hypocalcemia can result from acute hyperphosphatemia and calcium deposition in muscle.[525, 526] PTH levels are high. In the diuretic phase that follows, hypercalcemia can occur. The hypercalcemia results from the high $1,25(OH)_2D_3$ levels observed in some patients and from mobilization of the calcium deposits.[527]

In chronic renal failure, hypercalcemia can result from tertiary hyperparathyroidism or may appear during therapy of aplastic bone disease associated with low PTH levels and sometimes with aluminum toxicity.[528]

Williams' Syndrome

Williams' syndrome is a developmental disorder in which supravalvular aortic stenosis is associated with elfin facies and mental retardation.[529, 530] Hypercalcemia can occur transiently in the first four years of life. Affected hypercalcemic infants have been found to have increased intestinal absorption of calcium and associated elevations of $1,25(OH)_2D_3$ that fall to normal as the blood calcium normalizes.[531] Levels of 25(OH)D are normal. The hypercalcemia can generally be controlled by dietary manipulation.

Molecular analysis has clarified the origin of the connective tissue component of Williams' syndrome.[532, 533] Isolated supravalvular aortic stenosis is associated with deletion or translocation of the distal portion of the elastin gene. Williams' syndrome, with more protean connective tissue abnormalities and mental retardation, is associated with large deletions that include the elastin gene and a gene encoding the protein kinase LIM-kinase 1.[534] It is possible that the subgroup of patients with infantile hypercalcemia have deletion of another gene near the elastin locus. This possible genetic heterogeneity may explain the conflicting literature, which has found no consistent abnormality of calcium metabolism in normocalcemic patients with Williams' syndrome.[535]

Jansen's Metaphyseal Chondrodysplasia

Jansen's metaphyseal chondrodysplasia is a rare disease in which affected persons present in childhood with short stature

Table 26–5. Types of Pseudohypoparathyroidism

Disorder	Urinary cAMP Response to PTH	Urinary PO_4 Response to PTH	Other Hormonal Resistance	AHO	Pathophysiology
Pseudohypoparathyroidism Ia	Decreased	Decreased	Yes	Yes	$G_s\alpha$ mutation
Pseudo-pseudohypoparathyroidism	Normal	Normal	No	Yes	$G_s\alpha$ mutation
Pseudohypoparathyroidism Ib	Decreased	Decreased	No	No	20q13.3 defect (*GNAS1* locus)
Pseudohypoparathyroidism Ic	Decreased	Decreased	Yes	Yes	$G_s\alpha$ function normal
Pseudohypoparathyroidism II	Normal	Decreased	No	No	Vitamin D deficiency or myotonic dystrophy in some cases

AHO, Albright's hereditary osteodystrophy; cAMP, cyclic adenosine monophosphate; PO_4, phosphate.

the mutant gene is inherited from the mother but have normal expression in the cortex when the mutant gene is inherited from the father. No such imprinting pattern is seen in the inner medulla; this finding correlates with demonstration of PTH but not vasopressin resistance in the mice (and patients).[593]

Patients with PHP type Ib present with hypocalcemia and high PTH levels, and PTH infusions fail to increase urinary cAMP production. However, this disorder is not accompanied by any of the clinical features of AHO, nor is it associated with abnormal $G_s\alpha$ levels in fibroblasts. Renal resistance to PTH is the only consistent feature of type Ib; therefore, several investigators had postulated that this syndrome is due to an isolated abnormality of the PTH receptor. However, a search for mutations in the coding exons of the receptor gene failed to reveal a functional receptor abnormality.[595] The target organ manifestations of PHP Ib are variable, with some affected persons demonstrating PTH overactivity in bone and PTH resistance in kidney. Cultured osteoblast-like cells from a patient with this disorder demonstrated normal cAMP responsiveness to PTH, despite the lack of renal responsiveness.[596]

The locus responsible for PHP Ib has been found to reside on chromosome 20q13.3,[597] the same region that contains the *GNAS1* gene, encoding $G_s\alpha$. The disease is inherited with the imprinting characteristic of PHP Ia, but mapping studies suggest that the disease mutations are close to but distinct from the $G_s\alpha$-coding region; furthermore, some kindreds have no abnormalities in $G_s\alpha$ exonic sequences.[598] In contrast, in one family, a 3-base-pair deletion in the $G_s\alpha$ gene was found in three brothers with the syndrome of PHP Ib and in their unaffected mother.[599] In vitro studies demonstrated that this mutation prevented coupling of $G_s\alpha$ to the PTH/PTHrP receptor, but not to the TSH or LH receptors. The mutations in a large majority of patients, which do not involve the $G_s\alpha$-coding region, remain to be defined.

Several patients with AHO and PTH resistance have been found to have normal $G_s\alpha$ activity; the disorder in this subgroup has been designated PHP Ic. Biochemical characterization in one case[600] revealed a significant decrease in the manganese-stimulated adenylate cyclase activity in fibroblast membranes of the affected person, raising the possibility that a second defect in the cAMP pathway may lead to the phenotype of PHP Ic. In a more recently analyzed patient with PHP Ic, a small deletion in the $G_s\alpha$ gene blocked activation by receptors but did not change $G_s\alpha$ activity in the usual in vitro assays.[600a]

A second bone disorder distinct from AHO has been associated with $G_s\alpha$ gene mutations that are paternally inherited. These patients have progressive osseous heteroplasia, a disabling disorder associated with ossification of skin, muscle, and other connective tissue.[600b]

In PHP II, PTH infusions increase urinary cAMP normally; however, PTH does not elicit a phosphaturic response.[601] In this syndrome, as in PHP Ib, signs of AHO or resistance to other hormones are lacking, but unlike in PHP Ib, the disorder is not familial in origin. The age at onset of this disorder is variable, ranging from infancy to senescence, suggesting that it is an acquired defect or that the biochemical phenotype may be unmasked by intercurrent abnormalities. A subset of patients with myotonic dystrophy display the biochemical features of PHP II, the degree of PTH resistance correlating with the degree of expansion of the pathogenetic CTG repeats in the myotonin protein kinase gene.[602] A similar biochemical phenotype can also be observed in vitamin D deficiency, and some authors have suggested that PHP II is a manifestation of vitamin D deficiency rather than a distinct clinical entity.[603]

Minagawa and colleagues reported on cases of three neonates with no signs of rickets and with normal levels of vitamin D who presented with transient PHP II that resolved at about 6 months of age.[604] These workers postulated that PTH responsiveness is subject to maturation during fetal and neonatal development. PHP II, therefore, seems to reflect a heterogeneous clinical disorder associated with defects in PTH responsiveness distal to cAMP generation or involving a separate signal transduction pathway.[605]

The resistance to PTH in PHP has not been documented in bone cells; rather, several patients with PHP Ib have been reported to have skeletal changes consistent with hyperparathyroidism.[606–609] Patients with PHP have lower bone density than that in normal persons and hypoparathyroid patients. Basal urinary hydroxyproline excretion in patients with PHP is twice that in hypoparathyroid patients, and they have similar increases in response to parathyroid extract.[610] Because the markers of bone turnover in patients with PHP are not as high as those in hyperparathyroid patients with similar or lower PTH levels, it has been postulated by some authors that the PTH resistance in bone is relative.[608] However, normal cAMP response has been documented in osteoblasts isolated from patients with PHP Ia[611] and PHP Ib.[596] This finding suggests that the hypocalcemia in PHP is not secondary to skeletal resistance but is a consequence of the renal resistance to PTH that results in both increased urinary calcium losses and impaired 25(OH)D 1α-hydroxylation. The lack of activation of vitamin D results in diminished intestinal calcium absorption and osteomalacia, both of which further exacerbate the hypocalcemia. Deficiency of $1,25(OH)_2D_3$ and the resultant hypocalcemia can, in turn, impair the phosphaturic responses to PTH but not the urinary cAMP responses to PTH[612]; therefore, it is imperative that studies to confirm the diagnosis of PHP II be performed in normocalcemic patients who have normal vitamin D status.

Vitamin D–Related Disorders

Hypocalcemia secondary to vitamin D deficiency or resistance to the biologic effects of $1,25(OH)_2D_3$ is easily differentiated from the hypocalcemia of hypoparathyroidism by routine clinical and laboratory evaluation. The primary cause of hypocalcemia in vitamin D deficiency is decreased intestinal absorption of calcium. In the setting of normal renal function, the hypocalcemia of vitamin D deficiency, unlike that of hypoparathyroidism, is accompanied by hypophosphatemia and increased renal phosphate clearance. This increase in phosphate clearance is a direct result of compensatory (secondary) hyperparathyroidism. The hyperparathyroidism is a consequence of the hypocalcemic stimulus to PTH secretion and the stimulation of PTH gene expression and parathyroid cell proliferation caused by hypocalcemia (see "Parathyroid Hormone Biosynthesis" earlier). Therefore, measurement of serum phosphate and PTH are very useful in distinguishing these disorders from hypoparathyroidism. The secondary hyperparathyroidism results in increased calcium mobilization from the skeleton, increased renal reabsorption of calcium, and increased renal 1α-hydroxylation of 25(OH)D. In severe vitamin D deficiency, the increased levels of PTH no longer lead to increased bone resorption, perhaps because osteoclasts appear not to resorb unmineralized osteoid.

In profound vitamin D deficiency, the level of $1,25(OH)_2D_3$ is usually low; in moderate vitamin D deficiency, the stimulation of the renal 1α-hydroxylase by PTH can result in a normal or even elevated $1,25(OH)_2D_3$ level. These high levels of $1,25(OH)_2D_3$ reflect the action of PTH on the renal 1α-hydroxylase. The ineffectiveness of the high levels of total $1,25(OH)_2D_3$ to normalize serum calcium may be explained by increased binding of this metabolite to vitamin D–binding protein when the levels of 25(OH)D are very low.

Vitamin D Deficiency

Because the two sources of vitamin D are the diet and cutaneous synthesis after ultraviolet radiation, lack of solar radiation and decreased intake or impaired absorption of vitamin D can lead to vitamin D deficiency. As the population has become increasingly educated about the risks of skin cancer from solar radiation, the avoidance of long periods of intense sun exposure, coupled with the use of high-SPF (sun protection factor) sun blocks, has resulted in increased reliance on dietary sources of vitamin D. The RDA for vitamin D is 200 IU; however, in the absence of solar exposure, this recommendation is two to three times lower than that required to prevent vitamin D deficiency.[261, 613, 614]

Vitamin D is present in many food sources, both vegetable and animal. In addition, many prepared foods, especially cereals, are fortified with vitamin D. Although dairy products have been fortified with vitamin D as well, the actual amount of vitamin D provided does not correlate well with the purported content.[262] The vitamin D derived from vegetable sources is vitamin D_2, and that from animal sources is vitamin D_3. These two forms of vitamin D are metabolized identically and have equivalent biologic potency in humans. Both forms have been used to fortify foods.

Early vitamin D deficiency can be detected when the serum level of 25(OH)D falls below 15 ng/dL, because this level has been shown to be associated with the development of secondary hyperparathyroidism. Although elderly, homebound individuals are at high risk, several studies have demonstrated that vitamin D deficiency is prevalent in the general population (reviewed in reference 261). The clinical relevance of this vitamin D deficiency has been confirmed by a study demonstrating that vitamin D administration (800 IU/day) to an ambulatory elderly population decreases serum PTH levels as well as the incidence of hip fracture.[615]

Malabsorption also remains an important cause of vitamin D deficiency in all age groups. Because vitamin D is a fat-soluble vitamin, its absorption is dependent on emulsification by bile acids. Any cause of fat malabsorption or short bowel syndrome can result in vitamin D deficiency; therefore, malabsorption should be ruled out in patients with low 25(OH)D levels (<8 ng/dL).

Accelerated Loss of Vitamin D

25-Hydroxyvitamin D and $1,25(OH)_2D_3$ are secreted with bile salts and undergo enterohepatic circulation[616]; therefore, intestinal disease may also result in vitamin D deficiency owing to excessive losses. Increased metabolism of vitamin D, leading to low blood levels of 25(OH)D, is seen in individuals given anticonvulsant medications and antituberculous therapy. Phenobarbital, primidone, phenytoin,[617] rifampin, and glutethimide[618] all have been reported to accelerate the hepatic inactivation of vitamin D.

Impaired 25-Hydroxylation of Vitamin D

The vitamin D that is absorbed undergoes 25-hydroxylation in the liver; therefore, severe hepatic parenchymal damage can result in 25(OH)D deficiency. Clinically, severe vitamin D deficiency secondary to liver disease is rare, because the degree of hepatic destruction necessary to impair 25-hydroxylation is incompatible with long-term survival. However, isoniazid has been shown to decrease the 25-hydroxylation of vitamin D.[619] Two kindreds have been described in whom the clinical and biochemical presentations and therapeutic responses suggest an inherited 25-hydroxylation defect.[620]

Impaired 1α-Hydroxylation of 25-Hydroxyvitamin D

The final step in the activation of vitamin D is the hydroxylation of 25(OH)D by the renal 1α-hydroxylase to yield $1,25(OH)_2D_3$. Renal parenchymal damage, therefore, can result in deficiency of the active metabolite of vitamin D. Impaired 1α-hydroxylation is observed once creatinine clearance decreases to approximately 30 to 40 mL/minute. Unlike the situation of liver failure, with renal failure, dialysis permits long-term survival; therefore, deficiency of $1,25(OH)_2D_3$ secondary to impaired renal 1α-hydroxylation is a common and important clinical entity.

The metabolic consequences of chronic renal failure on the parathyroid glands and the skeleton are complex (see Chapter 27). Impaired renal 1α-hydroxylation leads to decreased intestinal absorption of calcium, resulting in hypocalcemia. The diminished phosphate clearance associated with renal failure leads to elevated levels of blood phosphate; this change, in turn, further lowers levels of calcium and $1,25(OH)_2D_3$. The resultant secondary hyperparathyroidism increases release of calcium and phosphate from bone; however, because of the renal insufficiency, PTH does not have a phosphaturic effect. As a result, the increased serum phosphate rises further.

Oral phosphate binders are used to lower blood phosphate. Calcium-containing antacids are now used as oral phosphate binders, in preference to the more toxic aluminum-containing antacids (see Chapter 27). Calcium administration also attenuates the hypocalcemic stimulus to parathyroid secretion. 1,25-Dihydroxyvitamin D_3 therapy is crucial for the absorption of this calcium and should be instituted early in the course of renal failure (when the creatinine clearance falls below 30 to 40 mL/min) to avoid the development of secondary hyperparathyroidism, with careful monitoring to avoid hypercalcemia. Once secondary hyperparathyroidism has developed, pharmacologic doses of $1,25(OH)_2D_3$, delivered intravenously[621] or orally,[622–625] may be required to suppress PTH gene transcription and parathyroid cellular proliferation.

Table 26–8. Causes of Hypophosphatemia

Reduced Renal Tubular Phosphate Reabsorption
- PTH/PTHrP-Dependent
  - Primary hyperparathyroidism
  - PTHrP-dependent hypercalcemia of malignancy
  - Secondary hyperparathyroidism
    - Vitamin D deficiency/resistance
    - Calcium starvation or malabsorption
    - Rapid, selective correction of severe hypomagnesemia
- PTH-Independent
  - Familial hypophosphatemic rickets (X-linked hypophosphatemic rickets)
  - Fanconi syndrome(s), other renal tubular disorders
    - Cystinosis
    - Amyloidosis
    - Hemolytic uremic syndrome
    - Following renal transplantation
    - Rewarming or hyperthermia
    - Wilson's disease
    - Multiple myeloma
    - Heavy metal toxicity
    - Magnesium deficiency
  - Oncogenous osteomalacia syndrome
  - Idiopathic hypercalciuria
  - Poorly controlled diabetes, alcoholism
  - Hyperaldosteronism
  - Drugs or toxins
    - Ethanol
    - Acetazolamide, other diuretics
    - High-dose glucocorticoids
    - Bicarbonate
    - Toluene
    - Heavy metals (lead, cadmium)
    - Calcitonin
    - High-dose estrogens
    - Ifosfamide
    - Cisplatin
    - Suramin
    - Foscarnet
    - *N*-methyl formamide
    - Pamidronate

Impaired Intestinal Phosphate Absorption
- Aluminum-containing antacids

Shifts of Extracellular Phosphate into Cells or Bone
- Acute intracellular shifts
  - Intravenous glucose, fructose, glycerol
  - Insulin therapy for hyperglycemia, diabetic ketoacidosis
  - Catecholamines (epinephrine, albuterol, terbutaline, dopamine)
  - Acute respiratory alkalosis, salicylate intoxication, acute gout
  - Gram-negative sepsis, toxic shock syndrome
  - Recovery from acidosis, starvation
  - Rapid cellular proliferation
    - Leukemic blast crisis
    - Intensive erythropoetin, G-CSF therapy

Accelerated Net Bone Formation
- Following parathyroidectomy
- Osteoblastic metastases
- Treatment of vitamin D deficiency
- Calcitonin therapy

G-CSF, granulocyte colony-stimulating factor; PTH, parathyroid hormone; PTHrP, PTH-related protein.

phosphatemia as hypocalcemia persists and PTH secretion increases.

Renal phosphate clearance may be increased in a variety of conditions that do not involve increases in PTH or PTHrP. These conditions include the proximal tubular dysfunction associated with Fanconi's syndrome, severe hypokalemia or hypomagnesemia, acute metabolic alkalosis induced by bicarbonate infusion, and exposure to certain drugs or toxins (see Table 26–7). Excessive phosphaturia also may occur in some patients with idiopathic hypercalciuria or primary hyperaldosteronism, with severe glycosuria in poorly controlled diabetes, following renal transplantation, and in Reye's syndrome.

Two syndromes—familial X-linked hypophosphatemic rickets (XLH)[697, 698] and oncogenic osteomalacia[699, 700]—result from renal tubular phosphate wasting that appears to be driven by humoral mechanisms. Involvement of a humoral mediator is clear-cut in oncogenic osteomalacia, as the syndrome resolves following extirpation of the responsible neoplasm, but is still inferential in XLH, where it is suggested by studies in a related animal model. Both syndromes include renal tubular phosphate wasting, impaired renal synthesis of $1,25(OH)_2D_3$, borderline hypocalcemia, hypocalciuria, and rickets or osteomalacia. Serum PTH generally is normal or only slightly elevated, and $1,25(OH)_2D_3$ is inappropriately normal. The bone disease dominates the clinical picture (see Chapter 27).

Rapid egress of extracellular phosphate into cells is the cause of hypophosphatemia that develops acutely during administration of intravenous glucose, insulin therapy for hyperglycemia, or administration of catecholamines (pressors or bronchodilators) or in profound respiratory alkalosis or leukemic blast crisis. Hypophosphatemia in these situations is most pronounced when there is underlying phosphate depletion, as in hyperparathyroidism or vitamin D deficiency, or following prolonged malnutrition or with alcoholism or glycosuria. Accelerated uptake of phosphate into cells, principally into muscle and bone, is particularly likely in postsurgical or trauma patients, in whom it may be promoted by high levels of circulating catecholamines and exacerbated by concurrent respiratory alkalosis, fever, volume expansion, sepsis, and hypokalemia. Similar mechanisms may pertain in nonsurgical illnesses such as acute myocardial infarction. Hypophosphatemia complicating administration of hematopoietic growth factors such as erythropoietin or G-CSF is due to the high demand for new intracellular phosphate imposed by rapid cellular proliferation in the bone marrow.

Clinical Features

The clinical significance of hypophosphatemia has been the subject of some controversy and probably depends on the presence and severity of underlying phosphate depletion. Unfortunately, the status of the total-body phosphorus pool is reflected only indirectly by the concentration of phosphate in the extracellular fluid, which contains less than 5% of body phosphorus. Thus, although serum phosphate concentrations generally are used to characterize hypophosphatemia as severe (<1–1.5 mg/dL, or <0.3–0.5 mM), moderate (1.5–2.2 mg/dL, or 0.5–0.7 mM), or mild (2.2–3.0 mg/dL, or 0.75–1.0 mM), the serum phosphate level may be normal or even high (depending on renal function) in the presence of profound intracellular phosphate deficiency. Conversely, it may be low when intracellular phosphate is relatively normal, as following a sudden movement of extracellular phosphate into cells.

The prevalence of severe hypophosphatemia among hospitalized patients is less than 1%, whereas mild or moderate hypophosphatemia may be detected in 2% to 5%.[701–703] Hypophosphatemia is recognized most often in critically ill patients, alcoholics or other malnourished individuals, decompensated diabetics, and those with acute infectious or pulmonary disorders.[701–704]

The clinical manifestations of severe hypophosphatemia are protean. Among the most common are various neuromuscular symptoms, ranging from progressive lethargy, muscle weakness, and paresthesias to paralysis, coma, and even death, depending on the severity of the phosphate depletion. Confusion, profound weakness, paralysis, seizures, and other major sequelae generally are limited to patients with serum phosphate concentrations below 0.8 to 1.0 mg/dL.[694, 705–708]

Biochemical evidence of muscle injury is observed within 1 or 2 days in over a third of patients whose serum phosphate concentrations fall to less than 2 mg/dL.[709] Overt rhabdomyolysis also may occur, especially in the setting of chronic alcoholism with underlying malnutrition and phosphate depletion.[710, 711] However, by the time this problem is recognized, the serum phosphate often has been raised by the large amounts of cellular phosphate released from damaged muscle.

Reversible respiratory failure due to respiratory muscle

weakness may preclude successful weaning from ventilatory support.[712–714] Left ventricular dysfunction, heart failure, and ventricular arrhythmias may result from profound hypophosphatemia but may not be significant if serum phosphate is greater than 1.5 mg/dL.[689, 715–718] In one study, correction of moderate hypophosphatemia (phosphate level of <2 mg/dL) in patients with septic shock led to a significant increase in blood pressure as well as improvement of left ventricular function and arterial pH.[716] Hematologic sequelae of severe hypophosphatemia include hemolysis, platelet dysfunction with bleeding, and impaired leukocyte function (phagocytosis and killing).[719–721] Erythrocytes demonstrate increased fragility; altered membrane composition, rigidity, and microspherocytosis; and reduced levels of ATP and 2,3-diphosphoglycerate (2,3-DPG).[719] The reduction in erythrocyte 2,3-DPG impairs oxyhemoglobin dissociation, thereby potentially reducing oxygen delivery to tissues. This problem, together with accelerated hemolysis, may provoke a substantial increase in cardiac output. The blockade in cellular glycolysis becomes demonstrable at levels of serum phosphate between 1 and 2mg/dL.[722] Glucose intolerance and insulin resistance also have been demonstrable in affected patients.[723]

Treatment

Hypophosphatemia appears most often in acutely or critically ill persons. Accordingly, it often is difficult to discern whether hypophosphatemia is responsible for features of the multiple organ dysfunction commonly encountered in this population. For example, although depression of intracellular high-energy organophosphates has been demonstrated during treatment of diabetic ketoacidosis, and phosphate repletion leads to more rapid recovery of erythrocyte 2,3-DPG concentrations, opinion is divided as to whether phosphate therapy in this setting hastens recovery, prevents complications, or reduces mortality.[724–726] Nevertheless, because severe hypophosphatemia has been associated, in a variety of clinical settings, with serious neuromuscular, cardiovascular, and hematologic dysfunction that is at least partially reversible with phosphate repletion, most authorities now agree that a relatively low threshold for treatment should be adopted.[689, 713, 716]

The decision to correct hypophosphatemia urgently should be guided by the estimated severity of the cellular phosphate deficit, the presence of signs or symptoms suggestive of phosphate depletion, and the overall clinical status of the patient. The presence of renal insufficiency (a risk for iatrogenic hyperphosphatemia), concomitant administration of intravenous glucose (alone or as a component of hyperalimentation solutions), and the potential for aggravating coexistent hypocalcemia also should be considered.

Limited data are available from clinical trials to predict the appropriate dose and rate of phosphate administration. In patients without severe renal insufficiency or hypocalcemia, administration of intravenous phosphate at rates of 2 to 8 mmol/hour of elemental phosphorus over 4 to 8 hours frequently corrects hypophosphatemia without provoking hyperphosphatemia or hypocalcemia.[702, 727–729] Suggested guidelines based on serum phosphate concentration are shown in Table 26–9. It is essential that serum calcium and phosphate be monitored every 6 to 12 hours during and after phosphate therapy, both to detect untoward consequences and because many patients require additional infusions for recurrent hypophosphatemia within 24 to 48 hours of apparently successful repletion. Less acute or severe hypophosphatemia should be managed with oral (or enteral) phosphate supplements if possible, generally given as a total of 1.0 to 2.0 g/day (as elemental phosphate) of neutral sodium or potassium phosphate in divided doses three to four times a day (see Table 26–6). In many patients, however, oral phosphate therapy is limited by gastrointestinal symptoms such as nausea or diarrhea.

Table 26–9. Urgent Therapy of Hypophosphatemia

Consider
- Severity of hypophosphatemia
- Likelihood of underlying phosphate depletion
- Clinical condition of the patient
- Renal function
- Serum calcium
- Concurrent parenteral therapy (glucose, hyperalimentation)

Guidelines

Serum Phosphate (mg/dL)	Rate of Infusion* (mmol/hr)	Duration (hr)	Total Phosphate (mmol)
<2.5	2.0	6	12
<1.5	4.0	6	24
<1.0	8.0	6	48

*Rates shown are normalized for a 70-kg person. Most formulations available in the United States provide 3 mMol/mL of sodium or potassium phosphate.

DISORDERS OF MAGNESIUM METABOLISM

The fourth most abundant extracellular cation, magnesium, like calcium, plays a critical physiologic role, particularly in neuromuscular function.[730] The importance of intracellular magnesium in energy metabolism, as a cofactor for ATP and a wide variety of enzymes and transporters, is reflected in the fairly global clinical effects that accompany disorders of magnesium homeostasis. Hypomagnesemia and hypermagnesemia are among the most common electrolyte disturbances; one or the other of these abnormalities is observed in as many as 20% of hospitalized patients and even more frequently (i.e., in 30% to 40%) among those admitted to intensive care units.[731, 732]

Hypermagnesemia

Magnesium homeostasis is achieved mainly through highly efficient regulation of tubular magnesium reabsorption in the loop of Henle.[733] As normal kidneys can readily excrete even large amounts of magnesium (i.e., 500 mEq/day), high filtered loads of magnesium rarely cause hypermagnesemia except in patients with severe acute or chronic renal failure.[734, 735] Increased magnesium loads in such cases may arise from ingestion of large amounts of oral magnesium salts, typically given as cathartics or antacids, or from extensive soft tissue ischemia or necrosis in patients with trauma, sepsis, cardiopulmonary arrest, burns, or shock[734] (Table 26–10). Hypermagnesemia may result from parenteral administration of magnesium salts, as when magnesium is used to treat preeclampsia.[736, 737] The infants of such hypermagnesemic mothers may manifest transient hypermagnesemia as well, along with parathyroid suppression and neurobehavioral symptoms.[738, 739] The use of oral magnesium preparations as laxatives may lead to hypermagnesemia if absorption is increased by intestinal ileus, obstruction, or perforation.[740, 741]

The most prominent clinical manifestations of hypermagnesemia are vasodilatation and neuromuscular blockade, which may involve both pre- and postsynaptic inhibition of neuromuscular transmission.[742–744] Signs and symptoms generally do not appear unless the serum magnesium concentration exceeds

Table 26–10. Causes of Hypermagnesemia

Excessive Magnesium Intake
Cathartics, antacids, enemas
Dead Sea drowning
Parenteral magnesium administration
Magnesium-rich urologic irrigants
Intestinal obstruction or perforation following magnesium ingestion
Rapid Mobilization from Soft Tissues
Trauma
Shock, sepsis
Cardiac arrest
Burns
Impaired Magnesium Excretion
Renal failure
Familial hypocalciuric hypercalcemia
Other
Adrenal insufficiency
Hypothyroidism
Hypothermia

4 mEq/L.[730, 734] Hypotension, often refractory to pressors and volume expansion, may be one of the earliest signs of progressive hypermagnesemia.[743–745] Lethargy, nausea, and weakness, accompanied by reduction in or loss of deep tendon reflexes, may progress to stupor or coma with respiratory insufficiency or quadriparesis at serum concentrations in excess of 8 to 10 mEq/L. Gastrointestinal hypomotility or ileus is common. Facial flushing and pupillary dilatation may be observed. Hypotension may be complicated by a paradoxical relative bradycardia, and other cardiac effects may be evident, including prolongation of the PR, QRS, and QT_c intervals and appearance of heart block and, ultimately, asystole as serum concentrations approach 20 mEq/L.

Hypermagnesemia also causes hypocalcemia and increased urinary calcium excretion, the result of both a direct suppression of PTH secretion and a PTH-independent inhibition of renal tubular calcium reabsorption.[736, 746–748] Severe hypocalcemia opposes the effect of hypermagnesemia on PTH secretion, so that serum PTH typically remains within the normal range but is still inappropriate for the serum calcium level.[749, 750]

Successful treatment of hypermagnesemia requires identification and interruption of the source of magnesium, together with measures to increase clearance of magnesium from the extracellular fluid. Use of magnesium-free cathartics or enemas to accelerate clearance of ingested magnesium from the gastrointestinal tract, together with vigorous intravenous hydration, generally has been successful in reversing hypermagnesemia. Refractory cases, especially those in patients with advanced renal insufficiency, may require hemodialysis.[735] Intravenous calcium (100 to 200 mg) infusions have been advocated as an effective antidote to hypermagnesemia, and there are examples in which this approach has apparently been successful, at least temporarily.[734, 744, 751]

Hypomagnesemia

Hypomagnesemia may occur because of impaired intestinal absorption of magnesium or defective renal tubular reabsorption of magnesium, or a combination of these (Table 26–11).[752] Because only 1% of the body's magnesium content is present in extracellular fluid, measurements of serum magnesium concentration typically do not adequately reflect total-body magnesium or the magnesium status of the intracellular compartment in critical tissues such as muscle.[1, 753] Thus, patients with deficiency of tissue magnesium may fail to manifest overt hypomagnesemia[754] but will exhibit abnormal retention (i.e., >50% in 24 hours) of infused magnesium, a maneuver that may be employed to assess magnesium status.[755, 756]

Etiology

Intestinal Causes of Hypomagnesemia

Selective dietary magnesium deficiency does not occur, and it is remarkably difficult, in fact, to induce magnesium depletion experimentally by feeding magnesium-deficient diets, probably because renal magnesium conservation is so efficient. Large amounts of magnesium may be lost in chronic diarrheal states (this fluid may contain more than 10 mEq of magnesium per liter), or via intestinal fistulae or prolonged gastrointestinal drainage.[757] More commonly, magnesium becomes trapped within fatty acid "soaps" in disorders associated with chronic malabsorption.[758–761] In a rare but informative genetic syn-

Table 26–11. Causes of Hypomagnesemia

Impaired Intestinal Magnesium Absorption
Primary infantile hypomagnesemia
Malabsorption syndromes
Increased Intestinal Magnesium Losses
Protracted vomiting or diarrhea
Intestinal drainage
Intestinal fistulas
Impaired Renal Tubular Magnesium Reabsorption
Congenital magnesium-wasting syndromes
Bartter's syndrome
Gitelman's syndrome
Magnesuria with nephrocalcinosis
Acquired renal disease
Tubulointerstitial disease
Postobstruction, acute tubular necrosis (diuretic phase)
Renal transplantation
Drugs and toxins
Ethanol
Diuretics (loop, thiazide, osmotic)
Cisplatin
Pentamidine
Cyclosporine
Aminoglycosides
Foscarnet
Amphotericin B
Endocrine and metabolic abnormalities
Extracellular fluid volume expansion
Hyperaldosteronism (primary, secondary)
Inappropriate antidiuretic hormone secretion
Diabetes mellitus
Hypercalcemia
Phosphate depletion
Metabolic acidosis
Hyperthyroidism
Rapid Shifts of Magnesium out of Extracellular Fluid
Intracellular redistribution
Recovery from diabetic ketoacidosis
Refeeding syndrome
Correction of respiratory acidosis
Catecholamines
Accelerated net bone formation
Following parathyroidectomy
Osteoblastic metastases
Treatment of vitamin D deficiency
Calcitonin therapy
Other losses
Pancreatitis
Blood transfusions
Extensive burns
Excessive sweating
Pregnancy (third trimester) and lactation

drome termed *primary hypomagnesemia*, a defect in the saturable component of intestinal magnesium absorption causes hypomagnesemia that can be partially overcome by administering large amounts of oral magnesium.[762, 763]

Renal Causes of Hypomagnesemia

Renal magnesium wasting may result from a primary tubular transport defect, as occurs in Bartter's syndrome and a number of other rare inherited magnesium-wasting renal tubular disorders[764–768] (see Table 26–11). Most often, however, it is attributable to an acquired abnormality in tubular magnesium reabsorption. In normal persons, magnesium reabsorption is virtually complete within several days of instituting experimental dietary magnesium deficiency, even before serum magnesium has declined substantially.[769] Thus, the finding of more than 1 mEq/day of urinary magnesium in a frankly hypomagnesemic patient indicates a defect in renal tubular magnesium reabsorption. Acquired primary renal tubular magnesium wasting occurs in various tubulointerstitial disorders, recovery from acute tubular necrosis or obstruction, renal transplantation, various endocrinopathies, alcoholism, and exposure to certain drugs (see Table 26–11).

Hypomagnesemia or magnesium depletion due to subnormal renal reabsorption may complicate a variety of endocrinopathies, including hyperaldosteronism, hyperthyroidism, and disorders associated with hypercalcemia, hypercalciuria, or phosphate depletion.[756] In primary hyperparathyroidism, PTH stimulates increased tubular magnesium reabsorption, but this increase is opposed by a direct tubular effect of hypercalcemia. As a result, the serum magnesium level in primary hyperparathyroidism generally is normal or only slightly reduced.[770] In hypoparathyroidism, serum and urinary magnesium levels are low. The magnesium depletion in hypoparathyroidism is consistent with loss of both the magnesium-retaining renal action of PTH and the stimulatory effect of $1,25(OH)_2D_3$ on intestinal magnesium absorption.[771]

Diabetes is among the most common medical disorders associated with hypomagnesemia.[772, 773] The severity of the hypomagnesemia in diabetics correlates with indices of glycosuria and poor glycemic control,[774] which suggests that urinary losses of magnesium on the basis of glycosuria may partly explain the magnesium depletion. Rapid correction of hyperglycemia with insulin therapy causes magnesium to enter cells and may further lower the extracellular magnesium concentration during treatment.

Alcoholism is another very common clinical setting in which hypomagnesemia occurs.[775] Magnesium depletion in alcoholism may result in part from nutritional deficiency of magnesium, overall caloric starvation and ketosis, and gastrointestinal losses due to vomiting or diarrhea,[730, 774, 776] but an acute magnesuric effect of alcohol ingestion probably plays the major role.[775, 777–779] This effect of alcohol is most evident when blood alcohol levels are rising and may be related to transient suppression of PTH secretion.[777, 779] Other factors that may contribute to hypomagnesemia in alcoholism include pancreatitis, malabsorption, secondary hyperaldosteronism, respiratory alkalosis, and elevation in plasma catecholamines, which increase intracellular sequestration of magnesium.[756]

Numerous drugs have been identified as causes of defective renal tubular magnesium reabsorption and hypomagnesemia.[756] These agents include diuretics of all classes (especially loop diuretics), cisplatin, pentamidine, cyclosporine, aminoglycosides, foscarnet, and amphotericin. Most often, drug-induced hypomagnesemia is mild and reversible, particularly that associated with diuretic therapy. In over half of patients undergoing cisplatin therapy, hypomagnesemia is noted within days or weeks and roughly half of those who develop the abnormality exhibit persistent hypomagnesemia many months or even years later. The median duration of hypomagnesemia in cisplatin-treated patients is about 2 months, but recovery has been observed up to 2 years after treatment.[780] Cisplatin may induce a more generalized nephropathy and azotemic renal failure, but the magnesium wasting appears to be an isolated functional abnormality. There is some evidence that the renal magnesium-wasting syndrome can be prevented by intravenous magnesium administration (24 to 40 mEq) before or during cisplatin infusion.[781] Such findings suggest that cisplatin may selectively impair magnesium reabsorption by binding competitively to sites or cells involved in binding and transport of magnesium.

A syndrome very similar to that seen with cisplatin therapy is observed frequently in transplant recipients who receive cyclosporin A.[782–784] The frequency of this complication has approached 100% in some series.[783] It is possible that concomitant use of other agents, especially aminoglycosides or amphotericin B, has colored the presentation in these patients.

Other Causes of Hypomagnesemia

Magnesium, like phosphate, is a major intracellular ion, and significant shifts of magnesium from the extracellular compartment may therefore occur during recovery from chronic respiratory acidosis or acute ketoacidosis, with refeeding, during administration of hyperalimentation solutions, and in response to elevation of circulating catecholamines.[756] Other rapid losses of extracellular magnesium may occur during periods of greatly accelerated net bone formation (as after parathyroidectomy, during recovery from vitamin D deficiency, or with osteoblastic metastases)[775] or with large losses due to pancreatitis,[785] cardiopulmonary bypass surgery,[786] massive transfusion,[787] extensive burns,[788] excessive sweating,[789] or pregnancy or lactation.[790]

Consequences of Hypomagnesemia

Most of the signs and symptoms of hypomagnesemia reflect alterations in neuromuscular function: tetany, hyperreflexia, Chvostek's and Trousseau's signs, tremors, fasciculations, seizures, ataxia, nystagmus, vertigo, choreoathetosis, muscle weakness, apathy, depression, irritability delirium, and psychosis.[730, 756, 769] Patients usually are not symptomatic unless serum magnesium concentration falls below 1 mEq/L, although occurrence of symptoms, as with levels of intracellular magnesium, may not correlate well with serum magnesium concentration. Atrial or ventricular arrhythmias may occur, as may various electrocardiographic abnormalities—prolonged PR or QT intervals, T wave flattening or inversion, or ST segment straightening.[756, 791] Hypomagnesemia also increases myocardial sensitivity to digitalis toxicity.[792, 793]

Hypomagnesemia evokes important alterations in mineral ion and potassium homeostasis that frequently aggravate the clinical syndrome. Magnesium-deprived humans or animals develop hypocalcemia, hypocalciuria, hypokalemia (owing to impaired tubular reabsorption of potassium), and positive calcium and sodium balance.[769, 794] Sustained correction of hypocalcemia or hypokalemia cannot be achieved by administration of calcium or potassium alone, respectively, whereas both abnormalities respond to administration of magnesium.[761, 795]

The etiology of hypocalcemia in the setting of hypomagnesemia may be multifactorial. Inappropriately normal or low serum PTH, despite hypocalcemia, is common and indicates a defect in PTH secretion.[575, 796, 797] Other evidence indicates that hypomagnesemia also may impair PTH action on target cells in bone and kidney, although some investigators have observed normal responsiveness, and the issue remains controversial.[574–576, 795–798]

Vitamin D resistance also is a feature of hypomagnesemic

states.[760, 799] This abnormality appears to be due mainly to impaired renal 1α-hydroxylation of 25(OH)D, although tissue resistance to $1,25(OH)_2D_3$ also may play a role.[771, 800] The serum $1,25(OH)_2D_3$ concentration usually is low during hypomagnesemia, which may result from magnesium depletion per se, parathyroid insufficiency, or coexistent vitamin D deficiency.[801–803] Deficiency of $1,25(OH)_2D_3$ is probably not the main cause of hypocalcemia in these patients, however, because hypocalcemia can be rapidly corrected (within hours to days) by magnesium therapy alone, well in advance of any increase in the serum $1,25(OH)_2D_3$ concentration.[801, 802]

Therapy of Hypomagnesemia

Mild, asymptomatic hypomagnesemia may be treated with oral magnesium salts—$MgCl_2$, MgO, or $Mg(OH)_2$—usually given in divided doses totaling 40 to 60 mEq (480 to 720 mg) per day (see Table 26–6). Diarrhea sometimes occurs with larger doses but generally is not a problem. The gluconate form (supplying 58 mg of magnesium per gram) is said to cause less diarrhea.[756] Patients with malabsorption or ongoing urinary magnesium losses may require chronic oral therapy to avoid recurrent magnesium depletion. Although intestinal magnesium absorption is severely impaired in renal failure,[804] oral magnesium must be administered with great caution in this setting, especially in patients receiving concomitant therapy with $1,25(OH)_2D_3$.

Symptomatic or severe hypomagnesemia (magnesium concentration of <1 mEq/L), especially if complicated by hypocalcemia, usually signifies magnesium deficits of at least 1 to 2 mEq/kg and is best treated promptly with parenteral magnesium salts. The use of intramuscular magnesium sulfate ($MgSO_4$) is to be discouraged, as the injections are painful and provide relatively little magnesium (2 mL of 50% $MgSO_4$ supplies only 8 mEq of magnesium, as compared with typical magnesium deficits in excess of 100 mEq). Moreover, because unretained sulfate ions also may increase urinary calcium excretion, administration of intravenous magnesium chloride or gluconate probably is the most logical approach to initial parenteral therapy for patients who also may be hypocalcemic.

In adult hypomagnesemic patients with normal renal function, rates of infusion of 2 to 4 mEq/hour (i.e., 50 to 100 mEq/day) generally are needed to maintain serum magnesium concentrations in the range of 2 to 3 mEq/L.[761, 801, 805] Up to 100 mEq/day for 2 days can be safely administered without elevating serum magnesium concentration above 4 mEq/L, whereas doses of 200 mEq/day may increase serum magnesium to 4.5 to 5.5 mEq/L and thus are excessive.[805] In patients with active seizures or other urgent indications, the infusion may be preceded by a slowly administered bolus of 10 to 20 mEq, followed by a higher rate of infusion (i.e., 10 to 15 mEq/hour) for the first 1 or 2 hours only. Patients with normal renal function can readily excrete over 400 mEq/day of magnesium in the urine without becoming hypermagnesemic, but even mild renal failure may greatly limit magnesium excretion. Therefore, doses of magnesium supplements should be reduced two- to threefold and careful serial monitoring of serum magnesium performed in patients with compromised renal function.

It is important to appreciate that a large fraction of parenterally administered magnesium may be excreted in the urine, even in patients with profound magnesium deficiency. Many such patients excrete as much as 50% to 75% of infused magnesium; in normal subjects, this fraction approaches 100%.[761] Moreover, because equilibration of the intracellular and extracellular magnesium pools is relatively slow, it is generally necessary to continue magnesium therapy for 3 to 5 days to achieve adequate repletion of the typical deficit of 1 to 2 mEq/kg. Because serum magnesium may become normal well before tissue stores are repleted, monitoring of urinary magnesium excretion is a more reliable measure of the approach to full repletion, especially after patients are switched to oral therapy.

The need for calcium, potassium, and phosphate supplementation should be considered in the usual clinical setting of hypomagnesemia. Vitamin D deficiency also frequently coexists and should be treated with oral or parenteral vitamin D or 25(OH)D. Use of $1,25(OH)_2D_3$ is not necessary, does not hasten recovery, and may actually worsen hypomagnesemia by suppressing PTH secretion and thereby promoting renal magnesium excretion.[806] Initial parenteral magnesium therapy in hypocalcemic patients may produce dramatic hypophosphatemia via the rapid stimulation of PTH secretion. This effect is most likely to be problematic in patients with underlying phosphate depletion (as in malabsorption, alcoholism, or diabetes), in whom it may provoke acute neuromuscular dysfunction, and may be avoided by concomitant intravenous calcium therapy.

References

1. Elin RJ, Armstrong WD, Singer L. Body fluid electrolyte composition of chronically magnesium-deficient and control rats. Am J Physiol 1971; 220:543–548.
2. Arnold A, Horst SA, Gardella RJ, et al. Mutation of the signal peptide–encoding region of the preproparathyroid hormone gene in familial isolated hypoparathyroidism. J Clin Invest 1990; 86: 1084–1087.
3. Karaplis AC, Lim S-K, Baba H, et al. Inefficient membrane targeting, translocation, and proteolytic processing by signal peptidase of a mutant preproparathyroid hormone protein. J Biol Chem 1995; 270:1629–1635.
4. Sunthornthepvarakul T, Churesigaew S, Ngowngarmratana S. A novel mutation of the signal peptide of the preproparathyroid hormone gene associated with autosomal recessive familial isolated hypoparathyroidism. Clin Endocrinol Metab 1999; 84:3792–3796.
5. Wiren KM, Potts JT Jr, Kronenberg HM. Importance of the propeptide sequence of human preproparthyroid hormone for signal sequence function. J Biol Chem 1988; 263:19771–19777.
6. Hashizume Y, Waguri S, Watanabe T, et al. Cysteine proteinases in rat parathyroid cells with special reference to their correlation with parathyroid hormone (PTH) in storage granules. J Histochem Cytochem 1993; 41:273–282.
7. Flueck JA, DiBella FP, Edis AJ, et al. Immunoheterogeneity of parathyroid hormone in venous effluent serum of hyperfunctioning parathyroid glands. J Clin Invest 1977; 69:1367–1375.
8. Mayer GP, Keaton JA, Hurst JG, et al. Effects of plasma calcium concentration on the relative proportion of hormone and carboxyl fragments in parathyroid venous blood. Endocrinology 1979; 104:1778–1784.
9. D'Amour P, Palardy J, Bahsali G, et al. The modulation of circulating parathyroid hormone immunoheterogeneity in man by ionized calcium concentration. J Clin Endocrinol Metab 1992; 74:525–532.
10. Habener JF, Kemper B, Potts JT Jr. Calcium-dependent intracellular degradation of parathyroid hormone: a possible mechanism for the regulation of hormone stores. Endocrinology 1975; 97: 431–441.
11. Chu LLH, MacGregor RR, Anast CS, et al. Studies on the biosynthesis of rat parathyroid hormone and proparathyroid hormone: adaptation of the parathyroid gland to dietary restriction of calcium. Endocrinology 1973; 93:915–924.
12. Brown EM. PTH secretion in vivo and in vitro. Miner Electrolyte Metab 1982; 8:130–150.
13. Brown EM. Four-parameter model of the sigmoidal relationship between parathyroid hormone release and extracellular calcium concentration in normal and abnormal parathyroid tissue. J Clin Endocrinol Metab 1983; 56:572–581.
14. Parfitt AM. Calcium homeostasis. In Mundy GR, Martin TJ (eds). Physiology and Pharmacology of Bone. Berlin, Springer-Verlag, 1993, pp 1–65.
15. Grant FD, Conlin PR, Brown EM. Rate and concentration dependence of parathyroid hormone dynamics during stepwise

changes in serum ionized calcium in normal humans. J Clin Endocrinol Metab 1990; 71:370–378.
16. Brown EM, Gamba G, Riccardi D, et al. Cloning and characterization of an extracellular Ca^{2+}-sensing receptor from bovine parathyroid. Nature 1993; 366:575–580.
17. Garrett JE, Capuano IV, Hammerland LG, et al. Molecular cloning and functional expression of human parathyroid calcium receptor cDNAs. J Biol Chem 1995; 270:12919–12925.
18. Chattopadhyay N, Mithal A, Brown EM. The calcium-sensing receptor: a window into the physiology and pathophysiology of mineral ion metabolism. Endocr Rev 1996; 17:289–307.
19. Rogers KV, Dunn CK, Hebert SC, et al. Pharmarcological comparison of bovine parathyroid, human parathyroid, and rat kidney calcium receptors expressed in HEK 293 cells. Bone Miner Res 1995; 10(Suppl 1):S483.
20. Pollak MR, Brown EM, Chou YHW, et al. Mutations in the human Ca^{2+}-sensing receptor gene cause familial hypocalciuric hypercalcemia and neonatal severe hyperparathyroidism. Cell 1993; 75:1297–1303.
21. Pearce SHS, Williamson C, Kifor O, et al. A familial syndrome of hypocalcemia with hypercalciuria due to mutations in the calcium-sensing receptor. N Engl J Med 1996; 335:1115–1122.
22. Ho C, Conner DA, Pollack MR, et al. A mouse model of human familial hypocalciuric hypercalcemia and neonatal severe hyperparathyroidism. Nat Genet 1995; 11:389–394.
23. Heath H III, Sanguinetti EL, Oglesby S, et al. Inhibition of human parathyroid hormone secretion in vivo by NPS R-568, a calcimimetic drug that targets the parathyroid cell-surface calcium receptor. Bone 1995; 16:85S.
24. Silverberg SJ, Bone HG, Marriott TB, et al. Short-term inhibition of parathyroid hormone secretion by a calcium-receptor agonist in patients with primary hyperparathyroidism. N Engl J Med 1997; 337:1506–1510.
25. Conigrave AD, Quinn SJ, Brown EM. L-Amino acid sensing by the extracellular Ca^{2+}-sensing receptor. Proc Natl Acad Sci USA 2000; 97:4814–4819.
26. Silver J, Russell J, Sherwood LM. Regulation by vitamin D metabolites of messenger ribonucleic acid for preproparathyroid hormone in isolated bovine parathyroid cells. Proc Natl Acad Sci USA 1985; 82:4270–4273.
27. Russell J, Lettieri D, Sherwood LM. Suppression by $1,25(OH)_2D_3$ of transcription of the pre-proparathyroid hormone gene. Endocrinology 1986; 119:2864–2866.
28. Silver J, Naveh-Many T, Mayer H, et al. Regulation by vitamin D metabolites of parathyroid hormone gene transcription in vivo in the rat. J Clin Invest 1986; 78:1296–1301.
29. Hawa NS, O'Riordan JLH, Farrow SM. Binding of 1,25-dihydroxyvitamin D_3 receptors to the 5′-flanking region of the bovine parathyroid hormone gene. Endocrinology 1994; 142:53–60.
30. Demay MB, Kiernan MS, DeLuca HF, et al. Sequences in the human parathyroid hormone gene that bind the 1,25-dihydroxyvitamin D_3 receptor and mediate transcriptional repression in response to 1,25-dihydroxyvitamin D_3. Proc Natl Acad Sci USA 1992; 89:8097–8101.
31. Russell J, Ashok S, Koszewski N. Vitamin D receptor interactions with the rat parathyroid hormone gene: synergistic effects between two negative vitamin D response elements. J Bone Miner Res 1999; 14:1828–1837.
32. Brown AJ, Zhong M, Finch J, et al. The roles of calcium and 1,25-dihydroxyvitamin D_3 in the regulation of vitamin D receptor expression by rat parathyroid glands. Endocrinology 1995; 136: 1419–1425.
33. Russell J, Bar A, Sherwood LM, et al. Interaction between calcium and 1,25-dihydroxyvitamin D_3 in the regulation of preproparathyroid hormone and vitamin D receptor mRNA in avian parathyroids. Endocrinology 1993; 132:2639–2643.
34. Sela-Brown A, Russell J, Koszewski NJ, et al. Calreticulin inhibits vitamin D's action on the PTH gene in vitro and may prevent vitamin D's effect in vivo in hypocalcemic rats. Mol Endocrinol 1998; 12:1193–1200.
35. Naveh-Many T, Friedlaender MM, Mayer H, et al. Calcium regulates parathyroid hormone messenger ribonucleic acid (mRNA), but not calcitonin mRNA in vivo in the rat. Dominant role of 1,25-dihydroxyvitamin D. Endocrinology 1989; 125:275–280.
36. Yamamoto M, Igarashi T, Muramatsu M, et al. Hypocalcemia increases and hypercalcemia decreases the steady state level of parathyroid hormone messenger ribonucleic acid in the rat. J Clin Invest 1989; 83:1053–1058.
37. Russell J, Sherwood LM. The effects of $1,25(OH)_2D_3$ and high calcium on transcription of the pre-proparathyroid hormone gene are direct. Trans Assoc Am Physicians 1987; 100:256–262.
38. Sela-Brown A, Silver J, Brewer G, et al. Identification of AUF1 as a parathyroid hormone mRNA 3′-untranslated region–binding protein that determines parathyroid hormone mRNA stability. J Biol Chem 2000; 275:7424–7429.
39. Hawa NS, O'Riordan JLH, Farrow SM. Post-transcriptional regulation of bovine parathyroid hormone synthesis. Mol Endocrinol 1993; 10:43–49.
40. Sherwood LM, Mayer GP, Ramberg CF Jr, et al. Regulation of parathyroid hormone secretion: proportional control by calcium, lack of effect of phosphate. Endocrinology 1968; 83:1043–1051.
41. Almaden Y, Canalejo A, Hernandez A, et al. Direct effect of phosphorus on PTH secretion from whole rat parathyroid glands in vitro. J Bone Miner Res 1996; 11:970–976.
42. Slatopolsky E, Finch J, Denda M, et al. Phosphorus restriction prevents parathyroid gland growth. J Clin Invest 1996; 97:2534–2540.
43. Kilav R, Silver J, Naveh-Many T. Parathyroid hormone gene expression in hypophosphatemic rats. J Clin Invest 1995; 96:327–333.
44. Estepa JC, Aguilera-Tejero E, Lopez I, et al. Effect of phosphate on parathyroid hormoe secretion in vivo. J Bone Miner Res 1999; 14:1848–1854.
45. Parfitt AM. Parathyroid growth: normal and abnormal. In Bilezikian JP (ed). The Parathyroids. New York, Raven Press, 1994, pp 373–405.
46. Wada M, Nagano N, Furuya Y, et al. Calcimimetic NPS R-568 prevents parathyroid hyperplasia in rats with severe secondary hyperparathyroidism. Kidney Int 2000; 57:50–58.
47. Szabo A, Merke J, Beier E, et al. $1,25(OH)_2$ vitamin D_3 inhibits parathyroid cell proliferation in experimental uremia. Kidney Int 1989; 35:1049–1056.
48. Henry HL, Taylor AN, Norman AW. Response of chick parathyroid glands to the vitamin D metabolites, 1,25-dihydroxycholecalciferol and 24,25-dihydroxycholecalciferol. J Nutrit 1977; 107:1918–1926.
49. Kremer R, Bolivar I, Goltzman D, et al. Influence of calcium and 1,25-dihydroxycholecalciferol on proliferation and proto-oncogene expression in primary cultures of bovine parathyroid cells. Endocrinology 1989; 125:935–941.
50. Nygren P, Larsson R, Johansson H, et al. $1,25(OH)_2D_3$ inhibits hormone secretion and proliferation but not functional dedifferentiation of cultured bovine parathyroid cells. Calcif Tissue Int 1988; 43:213–218.
51. Naveh-Many T, Rahamimov R, Livni N, et al. Parathyroid cell proliferation in normal and chronic renal failure rats: the effects of calcium, phosphate and vitamin D. J Clin Invest 1995; 96: 1786–1793.
52. Li YC, Amling M, Pirro AE, et al. Normalization of mineral ion homeostasis by dietary means prevents hyperparathyroidism, rickets, and osteomalacia but not alopecia in vitamin D receptor–ablated mice. Endocrinology 1998; 139:4391–4396.
53. Manley NR, Capecchi MR. Hox group 3 paralogs regulate the development and migration of the thymus, thyroid, and parathyroid glands. Dev Biol 1998; 195:1–15.
54. Peters H, Neubüser A, Kratochwil K, et al. *Pax9*-deficient mice lack pharyngeal pouch derivatives and teeth and exhbit craniofacial and limb abnormalities. Genes Dev 1998; 12:2735–2747.
55. Van Esch H, Groenen P, Nesbit MA, et al. GATA3 haploinsufficiency causes human HDR syndrome. Nature 2000; 406: 419–422.
56. Günther T, Chen Z-F, Kim J, et al. Genetic ablation of parathyroid glands reveals another source of parathyroid hormone. Nature 2000; 406:199–203.
57. Ding C, Buckingham B, Levine MA. Familial isolated hypoparathyroidism caused by a mutation in the gene for the transcription factor GCMB. J Clin Invest 2001; 108:1215–1220.
58. Berson SA, Yallow RS. Immunochemical heterogeneity of parathyroid hormone in plasma. J Clin Endocrinol Metab 1968; 28: 1037–1047.
59. Bringhurst FR, Stern AM, Yotts M, et al. Peripheral metabolism

of [35S]parathyroid hormone in vivo: influence of alterations in calcium availability and parathyroid status. J Endocrinol 1989; 122:237–245.
60. Rouleau MF, Warshawsky H, Goltzman D. Parathyroid hormone binding in vivo to renal, hepatic, and skeletal tissues of the rat using a radioautographic approach. Endocrinology 1986; 118: 919–931.
61. Segre GV, D'Amour P, Potts JT Jr. Metabolism of radioiodinated bovine parathyroid hormone in the rat. Endocrinology 1976; 99:1645–1652.
62. Hilpert J, Nykjaer A, Jacobsen C, et al. Megalin antagonizes activation of the parathyroid hormone receptor. J Biol Chem 1999; 274:5620–5625.
63. Martin KJ, Hruska KA, Freitag JJ, et al. The peripheral metabolism of parathyroid hormone. N Engl J Med 1979; 302:1092–1098.
64. Lepage R, Roy L, Brossard JH, et al. A non-(1-84) circulating parathyroid hormone (PTH) fragment interferes significantly with intact PTH commercial assay measurements in uremic samples. Clin Chem 1998; 44:805–809.
65. John MR, Goodman WG, Gao P, et al. A novel immunoradiometric assay detects full-length human PTH but not amino-terminally truncated fragments: implications for PTH measurements in renal failure. J Clin Endocrinol Metab 1999; 84:4287–4290.
66. Slatopolsky E, Finch J, Clay P, et al. A novel mechanism for skeletal resistance in uremia. Kidney Int 2000; 58:753–761.
67. Friedman PA, Gesek FA. Calcium transport in renal epithelial cells. Am J Physiol 1993; 264:F181–F198.
68. Bourdeau JE. Mechanisms and regulation of calcium transport in the nephron. Semin Nephrol 1993; 13:191–201.
69. Friedman PA, Gesek FA. Cellular calcium transport in renal epithelia: measurement, mechanisms and regulation. Physiol Rev 1995; 75:429–471.
70. Simon DB, Lu Y, Choate KA, et al. Paracellin-1, a renal tight junction protein required for paracellar Mg^{2+} resorption. Science 1999; 285:103–106.
71. Brown EM, Pollak M, Hebert SC. The extracellular calcium-sensing receptor: its role in health and disease. Ann Rev Med 1998; 49:15–29.
72. Hoenderop JG, van der Kemp AW, Hartog A, et al. The epithelial calcium channel, ECaC, is activated by hyperpolarization and regulated by cytosolic calcium. Biochem Biophys Res Commun 1999; 261:488–492.
73. Peng J-B, Chen X-Z, Berger UV, et al. A rat kidney–specific calcium transporter in the distal nephron. J Biol Chem 2000; 275:28186–28194.
74. Gesek FA, Friedman PA. On the mechanisms of parathyroid hormone stimulation of calcium uptake by mouse distal convoluted tubule cells. J Clin Invest 1992; 90:749–758.
75. Shimizu T, Yoshitomi K, Nakamura M, et al. Effect of parathyroid hormone on the connecting tubule from the rabbit kidney: biphasic response of transmural voltage. Pfleugers Arch Eur J Physiol 1990; 416:254–261.
76. Rhoten WB, Bruns ME, Christakos S. Presence and localization of two vitamin D–dependent calcium binding proteins in kidneys of higher vertebrates. Endocrinology 1985; 117:674–683.
77. Hemmingsen C, Staun M, Lewin E, et al. Effect of parathyroid hormone on renal calbindin-D28k. J Bone Miner Res 1996; 11: 1086–1093.
78. Bouhtiauy I, LaJeunesse D, Brunette MG. The mechanism of parathyroid hormone action on calcium reabsorption by the distal tubule. Endocrinology 1991; 128:251–258.
79. Bijvoet OLM. Relation of plasma phosphate concentration to renal tubular reabsorption of phosphate. Clin Sci 1969; 37:23–36.
80. Tenenhouse HS. Cellular and molecular mechanisms of renal phosphate transport. J Bone Miner Res 1997; 12:159–164.
81. Murer H, Lotscher M, Kaissling B, et al. Renal brush border membrane Na/P_i-cotransport: molecular aspects in PTH-dependent and dietary regulation. Kidney Int 1996; 49:1769–1773.
82. Lotscher M, Scarpetta Y, Levi M, et al. Rapid downregulation of rat renal Na/P(i) cotransporter in response to parathyroid hormone involves microtubule rearrangement. J Clin Invest 1999; 104:483–494.
83. Kilav R, Silver J, Biber J, et al. Coordinate regulation of rat renal parathyroid hormone receptor mRNA and Na-P_i cotransporter mRNA and protein. Am J Physiol 1995; 268:F1017–F1022.
84. Murayama A, Takeyama K, Kitanaka S, et al. Positive and negative regulations of the renal 25-hydroxyvitamin D_3 1α-hydroxylase gene by parathyroid hormone, calcitonin, and $1\alpha,25(OH)_2D_3$ in intact animals. Endocrinology 1999; 140:2224–2231.
85. Weisinger JR, Favus MJ, Langman CB, et al. Regulation of 1,25-dihydroxyvitamin D_3 by calcium in the parathyroidectomized, parathyroid hormone–replete rat. J Bone Miner Res 1989; 4: 929–935.
86. Reinhardt TA, Horst RL. Parathyroid hormone down-regulates 1,25-dihydroxyvitamin D receptors (VDR) and VDR messenger ribonucleic acid in vitro and blocks homologous up-regulation of VDR in vivo. Endocrinology 1990; 127:942–948.
87. Yang W, Friedman PA, Kumar R, et al. Expression of $25(OH)D_3$ 24-hydroxylase in distal nephron: coordinate regulation by $1,25(OH)_2D_3$ and cAMP or PTH. Am J Physiol 1999; 276:E793–E805.
88. Alpern RJ. Cell mechanisms of proximal tubule acidification. Physiol Rev 1990; 70:79–114.
89. Hensley CB, Bradley ME, Mircheff AK. Parathyroid hormone–induced translocation of Na-H antiporters in rat proximal tubules. Am J Physiol 1989; 257:C637–C645.
90. Derrickson BH, Mandel LJ. Parathyroid hormone inhibits Na(+)-K(+)-ATPase through Gq/G11 and the calcium-independent phospholipase A_2. Am J Physiol 1997; 272:F781–F788.
91. Wang MS, Kurokawa K. Renal gluconeogenesis: axial and internephron heterogeneity and the effect of parathyroid hormone. Am J Physiol 1984; 246:F59–F66.
92. Humes HD, Ichikawa I, Troy JL, et al. Evidence for a parathyroid hormone–dependent influence of calcium on the glomerular ultrafiltration coefficient. J Clin Invest 1978; 61:32–40.
93. Aubin J. Bone stem cells. J Cell Biochem Suppl 1998; 30/31:73–82.
94. Manolagas SC. Birth and death of bone cells: basic regulatory mechanisms and implications for the pathogenesis and treatment of osteoporosis. Endocr Rev 2000; 21:115–137.
95. Canalis E, Centrella M, Burch W, et al. Insulin-like growth factor 1 mediates selective anabolic effects of parathyroid hormone in bone cultures. J Clin Invest 1989; 83:60–65.
96. Dobnig H, Turner RT. Evidence that intermittent treatment with parathyroid hormone increases bone formation in adult rats by activation of bone lining cells. Endocrinology 1995; 136:3632–3638.
97. Bellows CG, Ishida H, Aubin JE, et al. Parathyroid hormone reversibly suppresses the differentiation of osteoprogenitor cells into functional osteoblasts. Endocrinology 1990; 127:3111–3116.
98. Tintut Y, Farhad P, Le V, et al. Inhibition of osteoblast-specific transcription factor Cbfa1 by the cAMP pathway in osteoblastic cells. J Biol Chem 1999; 274:28875–28879.
99. Ishizuya T, Yokose S, Hori M, et al. Parathyroid hormone exerts disparate effects on osteoblast differentiation depending on exposure time in rat osteoblastic cells. J Clin Invest 1997; 99:2961–2970.
100. Suda T, Takahashi N, Udagawa N, et al. Modulation of osteoclast differentiation and function by the new members of the tumor necrosis factor receptor and ligand families. Endocr Rev 1999; 20:345–357.
101. Hofbauer LC, Heufelder AE. The role of receptor activator of nuclear factor-κB ligand and osteoprotegerin in the pathogenesis and treatment of metabolic bone diseases. J Clin Endocr Metab 2000; 85:2355–2363.
102. Yao G-Q, Sun B, Hammond EE, et al. The cell-surface form of colony-stimulating factor-1 is regulated by osteotropic agents and supports formation of multinucleated osteoclast-like cells. J Biol Chem 1998; 273:4119–4128.
103. Horwood NJ, Elliott J, Martin TJ, et al. Osteotropic agents regulate the expression of osteoclast differentiation factor and osteoprotegerin in osteoblastic stromal cells. Endocrinology 1998; 139:4743–4746.
104. Chase LR, Aurbach GD. Parathyroid function and the renal secretion of 3′,5′-adenylic acid. Proc Natl Acad Sci USA 1967; 58: 518–525.
105. Jüppner H, Abou-Samra A-B, Freeman M, et al. A G protein–linked receptor for parathyroid hormone and parathyroid hormone–related peptide. Science 1991; 254:1024–1026.
106. Abou-Samra AB, Jüppner H, Force T, et al. Expression cloning of a common receptor for parathyroid hormone and parathyroid

hormone–related peptide from rat osteoblast-like cells: a single receptor stimulates intracellular accumulation of both cAMP and inositol triphosphates and increases intracellular free calcium. Proc Natl Acad Sci USA 1992; 89:2732–2736.
107. Rubin DA, Juppner H. Zebrafish express the common parathyroid hormone/parathyroid hormone–related peptide receptor (PTH1R) and a novel receptor (PTH3R) that is preferentially activated by mammalian and fugufish parathyroid hormone–related peptide. J Biol Chem 1999; 274:28185–28190.
108. Kong XF, Schipani E, Lanske B, et al. The rat, mouse and human genes encoding the receptor for parathyroid hormone and parathyroid hormone–related peptide are highly homologous. Biochem Biophys Res Commun 1994; 200:1290–1299.
109. McCuaig KA, Lee HS, Clarke JC, et al. Parathyroid hormone/parathyroid hormone–related peptide receptor gene transcripts are expressed from tissue-specific and ubiquitous promoters. Nucleic Acids Res 1995; 23:1948–1955.
110. Joun H, Lanske B, Abou-Samra AB. Tissue-specific transcription start sites and 5′-alternative splicing of the PTH/PTHrP receptor gene. J Bone Miner Res 1995; 10(Suppl 1):S468.
111. Bettoun JD, Minagawa M, Hendy GN, et al. Developmental upregulation of human parathyroid hormone (PTH)/PTH-related peptide receptor gene expression from conserved and human-specific promoters. J Clin Invest 1998; 102:958–967.
112. Lee K, Deeds JD, Segre GV. Expression of parathyroid hormone–related peptide and its receptor messenger ribonucleic acids during fetal development of rats. Endocrinology 1995; 136: 453–463.
113. Schwindinger WF, Fredericks J, Watkins L, et al. Coupling of the PTH/PTHrP receptor to multiple G-proteins. Endocrine 1998; 8:201–209.
114. Offermanns S, Iida-Klein A, Segre GV, et al. Gαq family members couple PTH/PTHrP and calcitonin receptors to phospholipase C in COS-7 cells. Mol Endocrinol 1996; 10:566–574.
115. Mitchell J, Mayeenuddin L, Sargeant J. Dual, G protein–mediated regulation of phospholipase C activity in osteosarcoma cells. J Bone Miner Res 1995; 10(Suppl 1):S321.
116. Murray TM, Rao LG, Muzaffar SA, et al. Human parathyroid hormone carboxyterminal peptide(53–84) stimulates alkaline phosphatase activity in dexamethasone-treated rat osteosarcoma cells in vitro. Endocrinology 1989; 124:1097–1099.
117. Kaji H, Sugimoto T, Kanatani M, et al. Carboxyl-terminal parathyroid hormone fragments stimulate osteoclast-like cell formation and osteoclastic-like cell formation and osteoclastic activity. Endocrinology 1994; 134:1897–1904.
118. Schlüter K-D, Hellstern H, Wingender E, et al. The central part of parathyroid hormone stimulates thymidine incorporation of chondrocytes. J Biol Chem 1989; 264:11087–11092.
119. Orloff JJ, Ganz MB, Ribaudo AE, et al. Analysis of PTHrP binding and signal transduction mechanisms in benign and malignant squamous cells. Am J Physiol 1992; 262:E599–E607.
120. Whitfield JF, Chakravarthy BR, Durkin JP, et al. Parathyroid hormone stimulates protein kinase C but not adenylate cyclase in mouse epidermal keratinocytes. J Cell Physiol 1992; 150:299–303.
121. Gaich G, Orloff JJ, Atillasoy EJ, et al. Amino-terminal parathyroid hormone–related protein: specific binding and cytosolic calcium responses in rat insulinoma cells. Endocrinology 1993; 132: 1402–1409.
122. Orloff JJ, Kats Y, Urena P, et al. Further evidence for a novel receptor for amino-terminal parathyroid hormone–related protein on keratinocytes and squamous carcinoma cell lines. Endocrinology 1995; 136:3016–3023.
123. Inomata N, Akiyama M, Kubota N, et al. Characterization of a novel parathyroid hormone (PTH) receptor with specificity for the carboxyl-terminal region of PTH-(1-84). Endocrinology 1995; 136:4732–4740.
124. Usdin TB, Gruber C, Bonner TI. Identification and functional expression of a receptor selectively recognizing parathyroid hormone, the PTH2 receptor. J Biol Chem 1995; 270:15455–15458.
125. Usdin TB, Hilton J, Vertesi T, et al. Distribution of the parathyroid hormone 2 receptor in rat: immunolocalization reveals expression by several endocrine cells. Endocrinology 1999; 140: 3363–3371.
126. Hoare SRJ, Bonner TI, Usdin TB. Comparison of rat and human parathyroid hormone 2 (PTH2) receptor activation: PTH is a low potency partial agonist at the rat PTH2 receptor. Endocrinology 1999; 140:4419–4425.
127. Usdin TB, Hoare SRJ, Wang T, et al. TIP39: a new neuropeptide and PTH2-receptor agonist from hypothalamus. Nat Neurosci 1999; 2:941–943.
128. Chorev M, Rosenblatt M. Structure-function analysis of parathyroid hormone and parathyroid hormone-related protein. In Bilezikian JP (ed). The Parathyroids. New York, Raven Press, 1994, pp 139–156.
129. Nussbaum SR, Rosenblatt M, Potts JT Jr. Parathyroid hormone/renal receptor interactions: demonstration of two receptor-binding domains. J Biol Chem 1980; 255:10183–10187.
130. Nutt RF, Caulfield MP, Levy JJ, et al. Removal of partial agonism from parathyroid hormone (PTH)–related protein-(7-34) NH_2 by substitution of PTH amino acids at positions 10 and 11. Endocrinology 1990; 127:491–493.
131. Luck MD, Carter PC, Gardella TJ. The (1–14) fragment of parathyroid hormone (PTH) activates intact and amino-terminally truncated PTH-1 receptors. Mol Endocrinol 1999; 13:670–680.
132. Gardella TJ, Jüppner H, Wilson AK, et al. Determinants of [Arg2]PTH-(1–34) binding and signaling in the transmembrane region of the parathyroid hormone receptor. Endocrinology 1994; 135:1186–1194.
133. Lee CW, Luck MD, Jüppner H, et al. Homolog scanning mutagenesis of the parathyroid hormone (PTH) receptor reveals PTH(1–34) binding determinants in the third extracellular loop. Mol Endocrinol 1995; 9:1269–1278.
134. Gardella TJ, Luck MD, Fan MH, et al. Mutations in the transmembrane domains of the PTH receptor impair binding of PTH-(1–34) but not PTH-(3–34). J Biol Chem 1996; 271: 12820–12825.
135. Shimizu M, Carter PH, Gardella TJ. Autoactivation of type-1 parathyroid hormone receptors containing a tethered ligand. J Biol Chem 2000; 275:19456–19460.
136. Shimizu M, Potts JT Jr, Gardella TJ. Minimization of parathyroid hormone. J Biol Chem 2000; 275:21836–21843.
137. Takasu H, Gardella T, Luck MD, et al. Amino-terminal modifications of human parathyroid hormone (PTH) selectively alter phospholipase C signaling via the type 1 PTH receptor: implications for design of signal-specific PTH ligands. Biochemistry 1999; 38:13453–13460.
138. Bergwitz C, Gardella TJ, Flannery MR, et al. Full activation of chimeric receptors by hybrids between parathyroid hormone and calcitonin. J Biol Chem 1996; 271:26469–26472.
139. Mannstadt M, Jüppner H, Gardella TJ. Receptors for PTH and PTHrP: their biological importance and functional properties. Am J Physiol 1999; 277:F665–F675.
140. Adams AE, Bisello A, Chorev M, et al. Arginine 186 in the extracellular N-terminal region of the human parathyroid hormone 1 receptor is essential for contact with position 13 of the hormone. Mol Endocrinol 1998; 12:1673–1683.
141. Pellegrini M, Royo M, Rosenblatt M, et al. Addressing the tertiary structure of human parathyroid hormone-(1–34). J Biol Chem 1998; 273:10420–10427.
142. Marx UC, Adermann K, Bayer P, et al. Solution structures of human parathyroid hormone fragments hPTH(1–34) and hPTH(1–39) and bovine parathyroid hormone fragment bPTH(1–37). Biochem Biophys Res Commun 2000; 267:213–220.
143. Jin L, Briggs SL, Chandrasekhar S, et al. Crystal structure of human parathyroid hormone 1–34 at 0.9-Å resolution. J Biol Chem 2000; 275:27238–27244.
144. Palczewski K, Kumasaka T, Hori T, et al. Crystal structure of rhodopsin: a G protein–coupled receptor. Science 2000; 289: 739–745.
145. Sheikh SP, Vilardarga JP, Baranski T, et al. Similar structures and shared switch mechanisms of the $beta_2$-adrenoceptor and the parathyroid hormone receptor. Zn(II) bridges between helices III and VI block activation. J Biol Chem 1999; 274:17033–17041.
146. Schipani E, Kruse K, Jüppner H. A constitutively active mutant PTH-PTHrP receptor in Jansen-type metaphyseal chondrodysplasia. Science 1995; 268:98–100.
147. Schipani E, Langman CB, Parfitt AM, et al. Constitutively activated receptors for PTH and PTHrP in Jansens metaphyseal chondrodysplasia. N Engl J Med 1996; 335:708–714.

148. Schipani E, Langman C, Hunzelman J, et al. A novel parathyroid hormone (PTH)/PTH-related peptide receptor mutation in Jansen's metaphyseal chondrodysplasia. J Clin Endocrinol Metab 1999; 84:3052–3057.
149. DeHaas WHD, DeBoer W, Griffioen F. Metaphysial dysostosis. J Bone Joint Surg Br 1969; 51:290–299.
150. Kruse K, Schütz C. Calcium metabolism in the Jansen type of metaphyseal dysplasia. Eur J Pediatr 1993; 152:912–915.
151. Schwindinger WF, Watkins L, Pines M, et al. Direct demonstration that the PTH/PTHrP receptor activates G-proteins G_s and $G_{Q/11}$ (abstract OR41-6). Paper presented at the 77th Annual Meeting of the Endocrine Society, June 14–17, 1995, Washington, DC.
152. Wells H, Lloyd W. Hypercalcemic and hypophosphatemic effects of dibutyryl cyclic AMP in rats after parathyroidectomy. Endocrinology 1969; 84:861–867.
153. Agus ZS, Puschett JB, Senesky D, et al. Mode of action of parathyroid hormone and adenosine 3′,5′-cyclic monophosphate on renal tubular phosphate reabsorption in the dog. J Clin Invest 1971; 50:617–626.
154. Sugimoto T, Fukase M, Tsutsumi M, et al. Additive effects of parathyroid hormone and calcitonin on adenosine 3′,5′-monophosphate release in newly established perfusion system of rat femur. Endocrinology 1985; 117:1901–1905.
155. Caverzasio J, Rizzoli R, Bonjour JV. Sodium-dependent phosphate transport inhibited by parathyroid hormone and cyclic AMP stimulation in an opossum kidney cell line. J Biol Chem 1986; 261:3233–3237.
156. Civitelli R, Hruska KA, Jeffrey JJ, et al. Second messenger signaling in the regulation of collagenase production by osteogenic osteosarcoma cells. Endocrinology 1989; 124:2928–2934.
157. Bringhurst FR, Zajac JD, Daggett AS, et al. Inhibition of parathyroid hormone responsiveness in clonal osteoblastic cells expressing a mutant form of 3′,5′-cyclic adenosine monophosphate–dependent protein kinase. Mol Endocrinol 1989; 3:60–67.
158. Segal JH, Pollock AS. Transfection-mediated expression of a dominant cAMP-resistant phenotype in the opossum-kidney (OK) cell line prevents parathyroid hormone–induced inhibition of Na-phosphate cotransport. J Clin Invest 1990; 86:1442–1450.
159. Dunlay R, Hruska K. PTH receptor coupling to phospholipase C is an alternate pathway of signal transduction in bone and kidney. Am J Physiol 1990; 258:F223–F231.
160. Malstrom K, Stange G, Murer H. Intracellular cascades in the parathyroid-hormone dependent regulation of Na_+ phosphate cotransport in OK cells. Biochem J 1988; 251:207–213.
161. Janulis M, Tembe V, Favus MJ. Role of protein kinase C in parathyroid hormone stimulation of renal 1,25-dihydroxyvitamin D_3 secretion. J Clin Invest 1992; 90:2278–2283.
162. Fukayama S, Tashjian AH Jr, Davis JN, et al. Signaling by N- and C-terminal sequences of parathyroid hormone–related protein in hippocampal neurons. Proc Natl Acad Sci USA 1995; 92: 10182–10186.
163. Gonzalez EA, Zhong M, Brown AJ, et al. Effects of dietary calcium and calcitriol administration of the levels of parathyroid hormone, serum calcium and PTH receptor mRNA in vitamin D deficient rats. J Bone Miner Res 1995; 10(Suppl 1):S483.
164. Turner G, Coureau C, Rabin MR, et al. Parathyroid hormone (PTH)/PTH-related protein receptor messenger ribonucleic acid expression and PTH response in a rat model of secondary hyperparathyroidism associated with vitamin D deficiency. Endocrinology 1995; 136:3751–3758.
165. Xie LY, Leung A, Segre GV, et al. Dramatic downregulation of the PTH/PTHrP receptor protein and transcript by $1,25(OH)_2$ vitamin D_3 in the osteoblast-like ROS 17/2.8 cells. Am J Physiol 1996; 270:E654–E660.
166. Amizuka N, Kwan MY, Goltzman D, et al. Vitamin D_3 differentially regulates parathyroid hormone/parathyroid hormone–related peptide receptor expression in bone and cartilage. J Clin Invest 1999; 103:373–381.
167. Urena P, Iida-Klein A, Kong XF, et al. Regulation of parathyroid hormone (PTH)/PTH-related peptide receptor messenger ribonucleic acid by glucocorticoids and PTH in ROS 17/2.8 and OK cells. Endocrinology 1994; 134:451–456.
168. Abou-Samra AB, Goldsmith PK, Xie LY, et al. Down-regulation of parathyroid (PTH)/PTH-related peptide receptor immunoreactivity and PTH binding in opossum kidney cells by PTH and dexamethasone. Endocrinology 1994; 135:2588–2594.
169. Huang Z, Bambino T, Chen Y, et al. Biochemical and confocal microscopic studies of constitutive and agonist-stimulated endocytosis of the PTH-PTHrP receptor. J Bone Miner Res 1995; 10(Suppl 1):S94.
170. Huang Z, Chen Y, Nissenson RA. The cytoplasmic tail of the G-protein–coupled receptor for parathyroid hormone and parathyroid hormone–related protein contains positive and negative signals for endocytosis. J Biol Chem 1995; 270:151–156.
171. Ferrari SL, Behar V, Chorev M, et al. Endocytosis of ligand–human parathyroid hormone receptor 1 complexes is protein kinase C–dependent and involves β-arrestin$_2$. J Biol Chem 1999; 274:29968–29975.
172. Huang Z, Bambino T, Chen Y, et al. Role of signal transduction in internalization of the G protein–coupled receptor for parathyroid hormone (PTH) and PTH-related protein. Endocrinology 1999; 140:1294–1300.
173. Qian F, Tawfeek H, Abou-Samra A. The role of phosphorylation of PTH/PTHrP receptor internalization. J Bone Miner Res 1999; 14(Suppl 1):S543.
174. Suva LJ, Winslow GA, Wettenhall RE, et al. A parathyroid hormone–related protein implicated in malignant hypercalcemia: cloning and expression. Science 1987; 237:893–896.
175. Wojcik SF, Schanbacher FL, McCauley LK, et al. Cloning of bovine parathyroid hormone–related protein (PTHrP) cDNA and expression of PTHrP mRNA in the bovine mammary gland. J Mol Endocrinol 1998; 20:271–280.
176. Power D, Ingleton P, Flanagan J, et al. Genomic structure and expression of parathyroid hormone–related protein gene (PTHrP) in a teleost, *Fugu rubripes*. Gene 2000; 250:67–76.
177. Gardella TJ, Luck MD, Jensen GS, et al. Converting parathyroid hormone–related peptide (PTHrP) into a potent PTH-2 receptor agonist. J Biol Chem 1996; 271:19888–19893.
178. Behar V, Nakamoto C, Greenberg Z, et al. Histidine at position 5 is the specificity "switch" between two parathyroid hormone receptor subtypes. Endocrinology 1996; 137:4217–4224.
179. Barden JA, Kemp BE. NMR study of a 34-residue N-terminal fragment of the parathyroid-hormone–related protein secreted during humoral hypercalcemia of malignancy. Eur J Biochem 1989; 184:379–394.
180. Weidler M, Marx UC, Seidel G, et al. The structure of human parathyroid hormone–related protein(1–34) in near-physiological solution. FEBS Lett 1999; 444:239–244.
181. Peggion E, Mammi S, Schievano E, et al. Conformational studies of parathyroid hormone (PTH)/PTH-related protein (PTHrP) point-mutated hybrids. Biopolymers 1999; 50:525–535.
182. Orloff JJ, Reddy D, DePapp AE, et al. Parathyroid hormone–related protein as a prohormone: posttranslational processing and receptor interactions. Endocr Rev 1994; 15:40–59.
183. Soifer NE, Dee KE, Insogna KL, et al. Parathyroid hormone–related protein. J Biol Chem 1992; 267:18236–18243.
184. Wu TL, Vasavada RC, Yang KH, et al. Structural and physiologic characterization of the mid-region secretory species of parathyroid hormone–related protein. J Biol Chem 1996; 271:24371–24381.
185. Henderson JE, Shustik C, Kremer R, et al. Circulating concentrations of parathyroid hormone-like peptide in malignancy and in hyperparathyroidism. J Bone Miner Res 1990; 5:105–113.
186. Ratcliffe WA, Norbury S, Stott RA, et al. Immunoreactivity of plasma parathyrin-related peptide: three region-specific radioimmunoassays and a two-site immunoradiometric assay compared. Clin Chem 1991; 37:1781–1787.
187. Burtis WJ, Brady TG, Orloff JJ, et al. Immunochemical characterization of circulating parathyroid hormone–related protein in patients with humoral hypercalcemia of cancer. N Engl J Med 1990; 322:1106–1112.
188. Burtis WJ, Dann P, Gaich GA, et al. A high abundance midregion species of parathyroid hormone–related protein: immunological and chromatographic characterization in plasma. J Clin Endocrinol Metab 1994; 78:317–322.
189. Martin TJ. Parathyroid hormone–related protein: molecular biology, chemistry, and actions. In Mundy GR, Martin TJ (eds). Physiology and Pharmacology of Bone. Berlin, Springer-Verlag, 1993, pp 617–639.
190. Orloff JJ, Wu TL, Stewart AF. PTH-like protein, biochemical responses, and receptor interactions. Endocr Rev 1989; 10:476–495.

191. Strewler GJ, Nissenson RA. Peptide mediators of hypercalcemia in malignancy. Annu Rev Med 1990; 41:35–44.
192. Guise TA, Yin JJ, Taylor SD, et al. Evidence for a causal role of parathyroid hormone–related protein in the pathogenesis of human breast cancer–mediated osteolysis. J Clin Invest 1996; 98: 1544–1549.
193. Rodda CP, Kubota M, Heath JA, et al. Evidence for a novel parathyroid hormone–related protein in fetal lamb parathryoid glands and sheep placenta: comparisons with a similar protein implicated in humoral hypercalcaemia of malignancy. J Endocrinol 1988; 117:261–271.
194. Abbas SK, Pickard DW, Rodda CP, et al. Stimulation of ovine placental calcium transport by purified natural and recombinant parathyroid hormone–related protein (PTHrP) preparations. Q J Exp Physiol 1989; 74:549–552.
195. Kovacs CS, Lanske B, Karaplis A, et al. PTHrP knockout mice have reduced ionized calcium, fetal-maternal calcium gradient and 45-calcium transport in utero. J Bone Miner Res 1995; 10(Suppl 1):S157.
196. Halloran BP, DeLuca HF. Skeletal changes during pregnancy and lactation: the role of vitamin D. Endocrinology 1980; 107: 1923–1929.
197. Hodnett DW, DeLuca HF, Jorgensen NA. Bone mineral loss during lactation occurs in absence of parathyroid tissue. Am J Physiol 1992; 262:E230–E233.
198. Ratcliffe WA, Hutchesson ACJ, Bundred NJ, et al. Role of assays for parathyroid-hormone–related protein in investigation of hypercalcaemia. Lancet 1992; 339:164–167.
199. Yamamoto M, Duong LT, Fisher JE, et al. Suckling-mediated increases in urinary phosphate and 3′,5′-cyclic adenosine monophosphate excretion in lactating rats: possible systemic effect of parathyroid hormone–related protein. Endocrinology 1991; 129: 2614–2622.
200. Grill V, Hillary J, Ho PMW, et al. Parathyroid hormone–related protein: a possible endocrine function in lactation. Clin Endocrinol 1992; 37:405–410.
201. Bucht E, Rong H, Bremme K, et al. Midmolecular parathyroid hormone–related peptide in serum during pregnancy, lactation and in umbilical cord blood. Eur J Endocrinol 1995; 132:438–443.
202. Kalkwarf HJ, Specker BL, Bianchi DC, et al. The effect of calcium supplementation on bone density during lactation and after weaning. N Engl J Med 1997; 337:523–528.
203. Khosla S, van Heerden JA, Gharib H, et al. Parathyroid hormone–related protein and hypercalcemia secondary to massive mammary hyperplasia. N Engl J Med 1990; 322:1157.
204. Lepre F, Grill V, Ho PWM, et al. Hypercalcemia in pregnancy and lactation associated with parathyroid hormone–related protein. N Engl J Med 1993; 328:666–667.
205. Sato K, Taira M, Yoshiwara I, et al. A case of humoral hypercalcemia of pregnancy: hypercalcemic crisis at the postpartum period due to markedly elevated plasma PTHrP levels without malignancy. J Bone Miner Res 1995; 10(Suppl 1):S401.
206. Philbrick WM, Wysolmerski JJ, Galbraith S, et al. Defining the roles of parathyroid hormone–related protein in normal physiology. Physiol Rev 1996; 76:127–173.
207. Strewler GJ. The physiology of parathyroid hormone–related protein. N Engl J Med 2000; 342:177–185.
208. Karaplis AC, Luz A, Glowacki J, et al. Lethal skeletal dysplasia from targeted disruption of the parathyroid hormone–related peptide gene. Genes Dev 1994; 8:277–289.
209. Wysolmerski JJ, Philbrick WM, Dunbar ME, et al. Rescue of the parathyroid hormone–related protein knockout mouse demonstrates that parathyroid hormone–related protein is essential for mammary gland development. Development 1998; 125:1285–1294.
210. Maeda S, Sutliff RL, Qian J, et al. Targeted overexpression of parathyroid hormone–related protein (PTHrP) to vascular smooth muscle in transgenic mice lowers blood pressure and alters vascular contractility. Endocrinology 1999; 140:1815–1825.
211. Brines ML, Ling Z, Broadus A. Parathyroid hormone–related protein protects against kainic acid excitotoxicity in rat cerebellar granule cells by regulating L-type channel calcium flux. Neurosci Lett 1999; 274:13–16.
212. Fenton AJ, Kemp BE, Kent GN, et al. A carboxyl-terminal peptide from the parathyroid hormone–related protein inhibits bone resorption by osteoclasts. Endocrinology 1991; 129:1762–1768.
213. Cornish J, Callon KE, Nicholson GC, et al. Parathyroid hormone–related protein-(107–139) inhibits bone resorption in vivo. Endocrinology 1997; 138:1299–1304.
214. Henderson JE, Amizuka N, Warshawsky H, et al. Nucleolar localization of parathyroid hormone–related peptide enhances survival of chondrocytes under conditions that promote apoptotic cell death. Mol Cell Biol 1995; 15:4064–4075.
215. Nguyen MTA, Karaplis AC. The nucleus: a target site for parathyroid hormone–related peptide (PTHrP) action. J Cell Biochem 1998; 70:193–199.
216. Lam MHC, Briggs LJ, Hu W, et al. Importin β recognizes parathyroid hormone–related protein with high affinity and mediates its nuclear import in the absence of importin α. J Biol Chem 1999; 274:7391–7398.
217. Copp DH, Cameron EC, Cheney B, et al. Evidence for calcitonin—a new hormone from the parathyroid that lowers blood calcium. Endocrinology 1962; 70:638–649.
218. Pearse AGE. The cytochemistry of the thyroid C cells and their relationship to calcitonin. Proc R Soc London 1966; 170:71–80.
219. Neher R, Riniker B, Rittel W, et al. Menschliches calcitonin III. Struktur von calcitonin M und D. Helv Chim Acta 1968; 51: 1900–1905.
220. Potts JT, Niall HD, Keutmann HT, et al. The amino acid sequence of porcine thyrocalcitonin. Proc Natl Acad Sci USA 1968; 59:1321–1328.
221. Jacobs JW, Goodman RH, Chin WW, et al. Calcitonin messenger RNA encodes multiple polypeptides in a single precursor. Science 1981; 213:457–459.
222. Amara SG, Jones V, Rosenfeld MG, et al. Alternative RNA processing in calcitonin gene expression generates mRNAs encoding different polypeptide products. Nature 1982; 298:240–244.
223. Hoppener JWM, Steenbergh PH, Zandberg J, et al. The second human calcitonin/CGRP gene is located on chromosome 11. Hum Genet 1985; 70:259–263.
224. Care AD, Cooper CW, Duncan T, et al. A study of thyrocalcitonin secretion by direct measurement of in vivo secretion rates in pigs. Endocrinology 1968; 83:161–169.
225. Cooper CW, Borosky SA, Farrell PE, et al. Effects of the calcium channel activator BAY-K-8644 on in vitro secretion of calcitonin and parathyroid hormone. Endocrinology 1986; 118:545–549.
226. Garrett JE, Tamir H, Kifor O, et al. Calcitonin-secreting cells of the thyroid express an extracellular calcium receptor gene. Endocrinology 1995; 136:5202–5211.
227. Fox J, Lowe SH, Conklin RL, et al. Calcimimetic compound NPS R-568 stimulates calcitonin secretion but selectively targets parathyroid gland Ca(2+) receptor in rats. J Pharmacol Exp Ther 1999; 290:480–486.
228. Care AD. The regulation of the secretion of calcitonin. Bone Miner 1992; 16:182–185.
229. Cote GJ, Gagel RF. Dexamethasone differentially affects the levels of calcitonin and calcitonin gene–related peptide mRNAs expressed in a human medullary thyroid carcinoma cell line. J Biol Chem 1986; 261:15524–15528.
230. Naveh-Many T, Raue F, Grauer A, et al. Regulation of calcitonin gene expression by hypocalcemia, hypercalcemia, and vitamin D in the rat. J Bone Miner Res 1992; 7:1233–1237.
231. Peleg S, Abruzzese RV, Cooper CW, et al. Down-regulation of calcitonin gene transcription by vitamin D requires two widely separated enhancer sequences. Mol Endocrinol 1993; 7:999–1008.
232. Cote GJ, Rodgers DG, Huang ESC, et al. The effect of 1,25-dihydroxyvitamin D_3 treatment on calcitonin and calcitonin gene–related peptide mRNA levels in cultured human thyroid C-cells. Biochem Biophys Res Commun 1987; 149:239–243.
233. Friedman PA, Gesek FA. Cellular calcium transport in renal epithelial: measurement, mechanisms and regulation. Physiol Rev 1995; 75:429–471.
234. Chambers TJ, McSheehy PM, Thomson BM, et al. The effect of calcium-regulating hormones and prostaglandins on bone resorption by osteoclasts disaggregated from neonatal rabbit bones. Endocrinology 1985; 116:234–239.
235. Talmage RV, Vanderwiel CJ, Decker SA, et al. Changes produced in postprandial urinary calcium excretion by thyroidectomy and calcitonin administration in rats on different calcium regimes. Endocrinology 1979; 105:459–464.

236. Catala-Lehnen P, Hoff AO, Thomas PM, et al. Calcitonin/CGRP deficiency results in high bone mass in mice and protects against osteopenia caused by gonadal failure. J Bone Miner Res 2000; 15(Suppl 1):A1054.
237. Hurley DL, Tiegs RD, Wahner HW, et al. Axial and appendicular bone mineral density in patients with long-term deficiency or excess of calcitonin. N Engl J Med 1987; 317:537–541.
238. Wimalawansa SJ. Long- and short-term side effects and safety of calcitonin in man: a prospective study. Calcif Tissue Int 1993; 52: 90–93.
239. Lin HY, Harris TL, Flannery MS, et al. Expression cloning of an adenylate cyclase–coupled calcitonin receptor. Science 1991; 254:1022–1024.
240. Chakraborty M, Chatterjee D, Kellokumpu S, et al. Cell cycle–dependent coupling of the calcitonin receptor to different G proteins. Science 1991; 251:1078–1082.
241. Ho H, Gilbert M, Nussenzveig D, et al. Glycosylation is important for binding to human calcitronin receptors. Biochemistry 1999; 38:1866–1872.
242. Houssami S, Findley DM, Brady CL, et al. Isoforms of the rat calcitonin receptor: consequences for ligand binding and signal transduction. Endocrinology 1994; 135:183–190.
243. Ikegame M, Rakopoulos M, Zhou H, et al. Calcitonin receptor isoforms in mouse and rat osteoclasts. J Bone Miner Res 1995; 10:59–65.
244. Nakamura M, Hashimoto T, Nakajima T, et al. A new type of human calcitonin receptor isoform generated by alternative splicing. Biochem Biophys Res Commun 1995; 209:744–751.
245. Nussenzveig DR, Mathew S, Gershengorn MC. Alternative splicing of a 48-nucleotide exon generates two isoforms of the human calcitonin receptor. Endocrinology 1995; 136:2047–2051.
246. Yamin M, Gorn AH, Flannery MR, et al. Cloning and characterization of a mouse brain calcitonin receptor complementary deoxyribonucleic acid and mapping of the calcitonin receptor gene. Endocrinology 1994; 135:2635–2643.
247. McLatchie L, Fraser N, Main M, et al. RAMPs regulate the transport and ligand specificity of the calcitonin-receptor–like receptor. Nature 1998; 393:333–339.
248. Zumpe E, Tilakaratne N, Fraser N, et al. Multiple ramp domains are required for generation of amylin receptor phenotype from the calcitonin receptor gene product. Biochem Biophys Res Commun 2000; 267:368–372.
249. Gangula P, Zhao H, Supowit S, et al. Increased blood presure in alpha-calcitonin gene–related peptide/calcitonin gene knockout mice. Hypertension 2000; 35:470–475.
250. Wilding JPH, Khandan-Nia N, Bennet WM, et al. Lack of acute effect of amylin (islet associated polypeptide) on insulin sensitivity during hyperinsulinaemic euglycaemic clamp in humans. Diabetologia 1994; 37:166–169.
251. Lorenzo A, Razzaboni B, Weir GC, et al. Pancreatic islet cell toxicity of amylin associated with type-2 diabetes mellitus. Nature 1994; 368:756–757.
252. Hinson JP, Kapas S, Smith DM. Adrenomedullin, a multifunctional regulatory peptide. Endocr Rev 2000; 21:138–167.
253. Poyner D. Pharmacology of receptors for calcitonin gene–related peptide and amylin. Trends Pharmacol Sci 1995; 16:424–428.
254. Niccoli P, Brunet P, Roubicek C, et al. Abnormal calcitonin basal levels and pentagastrin response in patients with chronic renal failure on maintenance hemodialysis. Eur J Endocrinol 1995; 132: 75–81.
255. O'Neill WJ, Jordan MH, Lewis MS, et al. Serum calcitonin may be a marker for inhalation injury in burns. J Burn Care Rehabil 1992; 13:605–616.
256. Sperber SJ, Blevins DD, Francis JB. Hypercalcitoninemia, hypocalcemia, and toxic shock syndrome. Rev Infect Dis 1990; 12: 736–739.
257. Canale DD, Donabedian RK. Hypercalcitoninemia in acute pancreatitis. J Clin Endocrinol Metab 1975; 40:738–741.
258. Szanto J, Ady N, Jozsef S. Pain killing with calcitonin nasal spray in patients with malignant tumors. Oncology 1992; 49:180–182.
259. Jaeger H, Maier C. Calcitonin in phantom limb pain: a double-blind study. Pain 1992; 48:21–27.
260. Holick MF, MacLaughlin JA, Clark MB, et al. Photosynthesis of previtamin D_3 in human skin and the physiologic consequences. Science 1980; 210:203–205.
261. Thomas M, Demay M. Vitamin D deficiency and disorders of vitamin D metabolism. Endocrinol Metab Clin North Am 2000; 29:611–627.
262. Holick MF, Shao Q, Liu WW, et al. The vitamin D content of fortified milk and infant formula. N Engl J Med 1992; 326:1178–1181.
263. Bikle DD, Gee E, Halloran B, et al. Assessment of the free fraction of 25-hydroxyvitamin D in serum and its regulation by albumin and the vitamin D–binding protein. J Clin Endocrinol Metab 1986; 63:954–959.
264. Bikle DD, Siiteri PK, Ryzen E, et al. Serum protein binding of 1,25-dihydroxyvitamin D: a reevaluation by direct measurement of free metabolite levels. J Clin Endocrinol Metab 1985; 61:969–975.
265. Safadi F, Thornton P, Magiera H, et al. Osteopathy and resistance to vitamin D toxicity in mice null for vitamin D binding protein. J Clin Invest 1999; 103:239–251.
266. Nykjaer A, Dragun D, Walther D, et al. An endocytic pathway essential for renal uptake and activation of the steroid 25-(OH) vitamin D_3. Cell 1999; 96:507–515.
267. Takeyama K, Kitanaka S, Sato T, et al. 25-Hydroxyvitamin D_3 1α-hydroxylase and vitamin D synthesis. Science 1997; 277:1827–1830.
268. St-Arnaud R, Messerlian S, Moir J, et al. The 25-hydroxyvitamin D 1α-hydroxylase gene maps to the pseudovitamin D–deficiency rickets (PDDR) disease locus. J Bone Miner Res 1997; 12:1552–1559.
269. Fu G, Lin D, Zang M, et al. Cloning of human 25-hydroxyvitamin D_1-α-hydroxylase and mutations causing vitamin D–dependent rickets type 1. Mol Endocrinol 1997; 11:1961–1970.
270. Tanaka Y, DeLuca HF. The control of 25-hydroxyvitamin D metabolism by inorganic phosphorus. Arch Biochem Biophys 1973; 154:566–574.
271. Glass AR, Eil C. Ketoconazole-induced reduction in serum 1,25-dihydroxyvitamin D and total serum calcium in hypercalcemic patients. J Clin Endocrinol Metab 1988; 66:934–938.
272. Tanaka Y, Halloran B, Schnoes HK, et al. In vitro production of 1,25-dihydroxyvitamin D_3 by rat placental tissue. Proc Natl Acad Sci USA 1979; 76:5033–5035.
273. Breslau NA, McGuire JL, Zerwekh JE, et al. Hypercalcemia associated with increased serum calcitriol levels in three patients with lymphoma. Ann Intern Med 1984; 100:1–7.
274. Barbour GL, Coburn JW, Slatopolsky E, et al. Hypercalcemia in an anephric patient with sarcoidosis: evidence for extrarenal generation of 1,25-dihydroxyvitamin D. N Engl J Med 1981; 305: 440–443.
275. Overbergh L, Decallonne B, Valckx D, et al. Identification and immune regulation of 25-hydroxyvitamin D_{-1}-alpha-hydroxylase in murine macrophages. Clin Exp Immunol 2000; 120:139–146.
276. Adams JS, Sharma OP, Diz MM, et al. Ketoconazole decreases the serum 1,25-dihydroxyvitamin D and calcium concentration in sarcoidosis-associated hypercalcemia. J Clin Endocrinol Metab 1990; 70:1090–1095.
277. Adams JS, Diz MM, Sharma OP. Effective reduction in the serum 1,25-dihydroxyvitamin D and calcium concentration in sarcoidosis-associated hypercalcemia with short-course chloroquine therapy. Ann Intern Med 1989; 111:437–438.
278. Ohyama Y, Noshiro M, Okuda K. Cloning and expression of cDNA encoding 25-hydroxyvitamin D_3 24-hydroxylase. FEBS Lett 1991; 278:195–198.
279. DeLuca HF. The vitamin D story: a collaborative effort of basic science and clinical medicine. FASEB J 1988; 2:224–236.
280. St-Arnaud R, Arabian A, Travers R, et al. Deficient mineralization of intramembranous bone in vitamin D-24-hydroxylase–ablated mice is due to elevated 1,25-dihydroxyvitamin D and not to the absence of 24,25-dihydroxyvitamin D. Endocrinology 2000; 141:2658–2666.
281. Canterbury JM, Gavellas G, Bourgoignie JJ, et al. Metabolic consequences of oral administration of 24,25-dihydroxycholecalciferol to uremic dogs. J Clin Invest 1980; 65:571–576.
282. Schwartz Z, Brooks B, Swain L, et al. Production of 1,25-dihydroxyvitamin D_3 and 24,25-dihydroxyvitamin D_3 by growth zone and resting zone chondrocytes is dependent on cell maturation and is regulated by hormones and growth factors. Endocrinology 1992; 130:2495–2504.
283. Baker AR, McDonnell DP, Hughes M, et al. Cloning and expression of full-length cDNA encoding human vitamin D receptor. Proc Natl Acad Sci USA 1988; 85:3294–3298.

284. Pettifor JM, Bikle DD, Cavaleros M, et al. Serum levels of free 1,25-dihydroxyvitamin D in vitamin D toxicity. Ann Intern Med 1995; 122:511–513.
285. Rachez C, Freedman LP. Mechanisms of gene regulation by vitamin D_3 receptor—a network of coactivator interactions. Gene 2000; 246:9–21.
286. Demay MB, Kiernan MS, DeLuca HF, et al. Characterization of 1,25-dihydroxyvitamin D_3 receptor interactions with target sequences in the rat osteocalcin gene. Mol Endocrinol 1992; 6: 557–562.
287. Noda M, Vogel RL, Craig AM, et al. Identification of a DNA sequence responsible for binding of the 1,25-dihydroxyvitamin D_3 receptor and 1,25-dihydroxyvitamin D_3 enhancement of mouse secreted phosphoprotein 1 (Spp-1 or osteopontin) gene expression. Proc Natl Acad Sci USA 1990; 87:9995–9999.
288. Gill RK, Christakos S. Identification of sequence elements in mouse calbindin-D_{28k} gene that confer 1,25-dihydroxyvitamin D_3- and butyrate-inducible responses. Proc Natl Acad Sci USA 1993; 90:2984–2988.
289. Cao X, Ross FP, Zhang L, et al. Cloning of the promoter for the avian integrin β_3 subunit gene and its regulation by 1,25-dihydroxyvitamin D_3. J Biol Chem 1993; 268:27371–27380.
290. Chen K-S, DeLuca HF. Cloning of the human 1-alpha,25-dihydroxyvitamin D_3 24-hydroxylase gene promoter and identification of two vitamin D–responsive elements. Biochim Biophys Acta 1995; 1263:1–9.
291. Inoue T, Kamiyama J, Sakai T. Sp1 and NF-Y synergistically mediate the effect of vitamin D_3 in the $p27^{Kip1}$ gene promotor that lacks vitamin D response elements. J Biol Chem 1999; 274: 32309–32317.
292. Murayama A, Takeyama K, Asahina T, et al. Cloning of a novel transcription factor mediating the negative vitamin D responsiveness through the human 25-hydroxyvitamin D 1-alpha-hydroxylase nVDRE. J Bone Miner Res 2000; 15(Suppl 1):A1244.
293. Nishishita T, Okazaki T, Ishikawa T, et al. A negative vitamin D response DNA element in the human parathyroid hormone–related peptide gene binds to vitamin D receptor along with Ku antigen to mediate negative gene regulation by vitamin D. J Biol Chem 1998; 273:10901–10907.
294. Godschalk M, Levy JR, Downs RW Jr. Glucocorticoids decrease vitamin D receptor number and gene expression in human osteosarcoma cells. J Bone Miner Res 1992; 7:21–27.
295. Iida K, Shinki T, Yamaguchi A, et al. A possible role of vitamin D receptors in regulating vitamin D activation in the kidney. Proc Natl Acad Sci USA 1995; 92:6112–6116.
296. Caffrey JM, Farach-Carson MC. Vitamin D_3 metabolites modulate dihydropyridine-sensitive calcium currents in clonal rat osteosarcoma cells. J Biol Chem 1989; 264:20265–20274.
297. Nemere I, Dormanen MC, Hammond MW, et al. Identification of a specific binding protein for 1α,25-dihydroxyvitamin D_3 in basal-lateral membranes of chick intestinal epithelium and relationship to transcaltachia. J Biol Chem 1994; 269:23750–23756.
298. Norman AW, Okamura WH, Farach-Carson MC, et al. Structure-function studies of 1,25-dihydroxyvitamin D_3 and the vitamin D endocrine system. J Biol Chem 1993; 268:13811–13819.
299. Barsony J, Marx SJ. Rapid accumulation of cyclic GMP near activated vitamin D receptors. Proc Natl Acad Sci USA 1991; 88: 1436–1440.
300. Hughes MR, Malloy PJ, Kieback DG, et al. Point mutations in the human vitamin D receptor gene associated with hypocalcemic rickets. Science 1988; 242:1702–1705.
301. Li YC, Pirro AE, Amling M, et al. Targeted ablation of the vitamin D receptor: an animal model of vitamin D–dependent rickets type II with alopecia. Proc Nat Acad Sci USA 1997; 94: 9831–9835.
302. Yoshizawa T, Handa Y, Uematsu Y, et al. Mice lacking the vitamin D receptor exhibit impaired bone formation, uterine hypoplasia and growth retardation after weaning. Nat Genet 1997; 16:391–396.
303. Balsan S, Garabedian M, Larchet M, et al. Long-term nocturnal calcium infusions can cure rickets and promote normal mineralization in hereditary resistance to 1,25-dihydroxyvitamin D. J Clin Invest 1986; 77:1661–1667.
304. Li YC, Amling M, Pirro AE, et al. Normalization of mineral ion homeostasis by dietary means prevents hyperparathyroidism, rickets, and osteomalacia, but not alopecia in vitamin D receptor–ablated mice. Endocrinology 1998; 139:4391–4396.
305. Amling M, Priemel M, Holzmann T, et al. Rescue of the skeletal phenotype of vitamin D receptor–ablated mice in the setting of normal mineral ion homeostasis: formal histomorphometric and biomechanical analyses. Endocrinology 1999; 140:4982–4987.
306. van Os CH. Transcellular calcium transport in intestinal and renal epithelial cells. Biochim Biophys Acta 1987; 906:195–222.
307. Wasserman RH, Fullmer CS. Calcium transport proteins, calcium absorption, and vitamin D. Annu Rev Physiol 1983; 45: 375–390.
308. Karbach U. Paracellular calcium transport across the small intestine. J Nutr 1992; 122:672–677.
309. de Boland AR, Nemere I, Norman AW. Ca^{2+}-channel agonist BAY K8644 mimics $1,25(OH)_2$-vitamin D_3 rapid enhancement of Ca^{2+} transport in chick perfused duodenum. Biochem Biophys Res Commun 1990; 166:217–222.
310. Nemere I, Norman AW. 1,25-Dihydroxyvitamin D_3-mediated vesicular transport of calcium in intestine: time-course studies. Endocrinology 1988; 122:2962–2969.
311. Fullmer CS. Intestinal calcium absorption: calcium entry. J Nutr 1992; 122:644–650.
312. Peng J, Chen X, Berger UV, et al. Molecular cloning and characterization of a channel-like transporter mediating intestinal calcium absorption. J Biol Chem 1999; 274:22739–22746.
313. Hoenderop JG, van der Kemp AWCM, Hartog A, et al. Molecular indentification of the Apical Ca^{2+} channel in 1,25-dihydroxyvitamin D_3–responsive epithelia. J Biol Chem 1999; 274:8375–8378.
314. Kaune R, Munson S, Bikle DD. Regulation of calmodulin binding to the ATP extractable 110 kDa protein (myosin I) from chicken duodenal brush border by $1,25(OH)_2D_3$. Biochim Biophys Acta 1994; 1190:329–336.
315. Cai Q, Chandler JS, Wasserman RH, et al. Vitamin D and adaptation to dietary calcium and phosphate deficiencies increase intestinal plasma membrane calcium pump gene expression. Proc Natl Acad Sci USA 1993; 90:1345–1349.
316. Wasserman RH, Chandler JS, Meyer SA, et al. Intestinal calcium transport and calcium extrusion processes at the basolateral membrane. J Nutr 1992; 122:662–671.
317. Harrison JR, Petersen DN, Lichtler AC, et al. 1,25-Dihydroxyvitamin D_3 inhibits transcription of type I collagen genes in the rat osteosarcoma line ROS 17/2.8. Endocrinology 1989; 125:327–333.
318. Price PA. Vitamin K–dependent bone proteins. In Cohn DV, Martin TJ, Meunier PJ (eds) Calcium Regulation and Bone Metabolism: Basic and Clinical Aspects. Amsterdam, Exerpta Medica, 1987, pp 419–426.
319. Yasuda H, Shima N, Nakagawa N, et al. Osteoclast differentiation factor is a ligand for osteoprotegerin/osteoclastogenesis-inhibitory factor and is identical to TRANCE/RANKL. Proc Natl Acad Sci USA 1998; 95:3597–3602.
320. Underwood JL, DeLuca HF. Vitamin D is not directly necessary for bone growth and mineralization. Am J Physiol 1984; 246: E493–E498.
321. Weinstein RS, Underwood JL, Hutson MS, et al. Bone histomorphometry in vitamin D–deficient rats infused with calcium and phosphorus. Am J Physiol 1984; 246:E499–E506.
322. Kumar R. Vitamin D and calcium transport. Kidney Int 1991; 40:1177–1189.
323. Massheimer V, Fernandez LM, Boland R, et al. Regulation of Ca^{2+} uptake in skeletal muscle by 1,25-dihydroxyvitamin D_3; role of phosphorylation and calmodulin. Mol Cell Endocrinol 1992; 84:15–22.
324. Pointon JJ, Francis MJO, Smith R. Effect of vitamin D deficiency on sarcoplasmic reticulum function and troponin C concentration of rabbit skeletal muscle. Clin Sci 1979; 57:257–263.
325. Zhou JY, Norman AW, Chen DL, et al. 1,25-Dihydroxy-16-ene-23-yne-vitamin D_3 prolongs survival time of leukemic mice. Proc Natl Acad Sci USA 1990; 87:3929–3932.
326. Shabahang M, Buras RR, Davoodi F, et al. Growth inhibition of HT-29 human colon cancer cells by analogues of 1,25-dihydroxyvitamin D_3. Cancer Res 1994; 54:4057–4064.
327. Halline AG, Davidson NO, Skarosi SF, et al. Effects of 1,25-dihydroxyvitamin D_3 on proliferation and differentiation of Caco-2 cells. Endocrinology 1994; 134:1710–1717.
328. Colston KW, Mackay AG, James SY, et al. EB 1089: a new vitamin D analogue that inhibits the growth of breast cancer cells in vivo and in vitro. Biochem Pharmacol 1992; 44:2273–2280.

329. Mathieu C, Laureys J, Waer M, et al. Prevention of autoimmune destruction of transplanted islets in spontaneously diabetic NOD mice by KH1060, a 20-epi analog of vitamin D: synergy with cyclosporine. Transplant Proc 1994; 26:3128–3129.
330. Brown AJ, Ritter CR, Finch JL, et al. The noncalcemic analogue of vitamin D, 22-oxacalcitriol, suppresses parathyroid hormone synthesis and secretion. J Clin Invest 1989; 84:728–732.
331. Holick MF, Smith E, Pincus S. Skin as the site of vitamin D synthesis and target tissue for 1,25-dihydroxyvitamin D_3. Use of calcitriol (1,25-dihydroxyvitamin D_3) for treatment of psoriasis. Arch Dermatol 1987; 123:1677–1683.
332. Hoeck HC, Laurberg G, Laurberg P. Hypercalcemia crisis after excessive topical use of a vitamin D derivative. J Intern Med 1994; 235:281–282.
333. Kamimura S, Gallieni M, Kubodera N, et al. Differential catabolism of 22-oxacalcitriol and 1,25-dihydroxyvitamin D_3 by normal human peripheral monocytes. Endocrinology 1993; 133:2719–2722.
334. Gill HS, Londowski JM, Corradino RA, et al. The synthesis and biological activity of 25-hydroxy-26,27-dimethylvitamin D_3 and 1,25-dihydroxy-26,27-dimethylvitamin D_3; highly potent novel analogs of vitamin D_3. J Steroid Biochem 1988; 31:147–160.
335. Peleg S, Sastry M, Collins ED, et al. Distinct conformational changes induced by 20-epi analogues of 1α,25-dihydroxyvitamin D_3 are associated with enhanced activation of the vitamin D receptor. J Biol Chem 1995; 270:10551–10558.
336. Norman AW, Sergeev IN, Bishop JE, et al. Selective biological response by target organs (intestine, kidney, and bone) to 1,25-dihydroxyvitamin D_3 and two analogues. Cancer Res 1993; 53: 3935–3942.
337. Liu Y, Collins E, Norman AW, et al. Differential interaction of 1α25-dihydroxyvitamin D_3 analogues and their 20-epi homologues with the vitamin D receptor. J Biol Chem 1997; 272: 3336–3345.
338. Nussbaum SR, Zahradnik RJ, Lavigne JR, et al. Highly sensitive two-site immunoradiometric assay of parathyrin and its clinical utility in evaluating patients with hypercalcemia. Clin Chem 1987; 33:1364–1367.
339. Bilezikian JP. Clinical utility of assays for parathyroid hormone–related protein. Clin Chem 1992; 38:179–181.
340. Grill V, Ho P, Body JJ, et al. Parathyroid hormone–related protein: elevated levels in both humoral hypercalcemia of malignancy and hypercalcemia complicating metastatic breast cancer. J Clin Endocrinol Metab 1991; 73:1309–1315.
341. Henderson J, Bernier S, D'Amour P, et al. Effects of passive immunization against PTH-like peptide in hypercalcemic tumor-bearing rats and normocalcemic controls. Endocrinology 1990; 127:1310–1316.
342. Pandian MR, Morgan CH, Carlton E, et al. Modified immunoradiometric assay of parathyroid hormone–related protein: clinical application in the differential diagnosis of hypercalcemia. Clin Chem 1992; 38:282–288.
343. Weissel M, Kainz H, Tyl E, et al. Clinical evaluation of new assays for determination of serum calcitonin concentrations. Acta Endocrinologica 1991; 124:540–544.
344. Isomura M, Honda N, Kawada A, et al. Development of a highly sensitive enzyme immunoasay for human calcitonin using solid phase coupled with multiple antibodies. Ann Clin Biochem 1999; 36:629–635.
345. Kao PC, Gharib H. Clinical performance of an extraction calcitonin radioimmunoassay. Mayo Clin Proc 1993; 68:1165–1170.
346. Wimalawansa SJ, Bailey F. Validation, role in perioperative assessment, and clinical applications of an immunoradiometric assay for human calcitonin. Peptides 1995; 16:307–312.
347. Hollis B. Quantitation of 25-hydroxyvitamin D and 1,25-dihydroxyvitamin D by radioimmunoaay using radioiodinated tracers. Methods Enzymol 1997; 282:174–186.
348. Weber CJ, Sewell CW, McGarity WC. Persistent and recurrent sporadic primary hyperparathyroidism: histopathology, complications, and results of reoperation. Surgery 1994; 116:991–998.
349. LiVolsi VA. Embryology, anatomy, and pathology of the parathyroids. In Bilezikian JP (ed). The Parathyroids. New York, Raven Press, 1994, pp 1–14.
350. Rosen IB, Young JEM, Archibald SD, et al. Parathyroid cancer: clinical variations and relationships to autotransplantation. Can J Cancer 1994; 37:465–469.
351. Shane E, Bilezikian JP. Parathyroid carcinoma: a review of 62 patients. Endocr Rev 1982; 3:218–226.
352. Albright F, Aub J, Bauer W. Hyperparathyroidism. A common and polymorphic condition as illustrated by seventeen proved cases from one clinic. JAMA 1934; 102:1276–1287.
353. Cope O. The study of hyperparathyroidism at the Massachusetts General Hospital. N Engl J Med 1966; 274:1174–1182.
354. Patten BM, Bilezikian JP, Mallette LE, et al. Neuromuscular disease in hyperparathyroidism. Ann Intern Med 1974; 80:182–193.
355. Wermers RA, Khosla S, Atkinson EJ, et al. The rise and fall of primary hyperparathyroidism: a population-based study in Rochester, Minnesota, 1965–1992. Ann Intern Med 1997; 126:433–440.
356. Lundgren E, Rastad J, Thrufjell E, et al. Population-based screening for primary hyperparathyroidism with serum calcium and parathyroid hormone values in menopausal women. Surgery 1997; 121:287–294.
357. Silverberg SJ, Shane E, Jacobs TP, et al. A 10-year prospective study of primary hyperparathyroidism with or without parathyroid surgery. N Engl J Med 1999; 341:1249–1255.
358. Clark OH. Presidential address: "Asymptomatic" primary hyperparathyroidism: is parathyroidectomy indicated? Surgery 1994; 116:947–953.
359. Pasieka JL, Parsons LL. Prospective surgical outcome study of relief of symptoms following surgery in patients with primary hyperparathyroidism. World J Surg 1998; 22:513–518.
360. Walgenbach S, Hommel G, Junginger T. Outcome after surgery for primary hyperparathyroidism: ten-year prospective follow-up study. World J Surg 2000; 24:564–569.
361. Kleerekoper M, Bilezkian JP. A cure in search of a disease: parathyroidectomy for nontraditional features of primary hyperparathyroidism. (editorial). Am J Med 1994; 96:99–100.
362. Rao DS, Wilson RJ, Kleerekoper M, et al. Lack of biochemical progression or continuation of accelerated bone loss in mild asymptomatic primary hyperparathyroidism: evidence for biphasic disease course. J Clin Endocrinol Metab 1988; 67:1294–1298.
363. Palmer M, Adami HO, Bergstrom R, et al. Mortality after surgery for primary hyperparathyroidism: a follow-up of 441 patients operated on from 1956 to 1979. Surgery 1987; 102:1–7.
364. Hedback G, Tisell LE, Bengtsson BA, et al. Premature death in patients operated on for primary hyperparathyroidism. World J Surgery 1990; 14:829–836.
365. Leifsson BG, Ahren B. Serum calcium and survival in a large health screening program. J Clin Endocrinol Metab 1996; 81: 2149–2153.
366. Silverberg SJ, Bilezikian JP, Bone HG, et al. Therapeutic controversies in primary hyperparathyroidism. J Clin Endocrinol Metab 1999; 84:2275–2285.
367. Stefenelli T, Abela C, Frank H, et al. Cardiac abnormalities in patients with primary hyperparathyroidism: implications for follow-up. J Clin Endocrinol Metab 1997; 82:106–112.
368. Wermers RA, Khosla S, Atkinson EJ, et al. Survival after the diagnosis of hyperparathyroidism: a population-based study. Am J Med 1998; 104:115–122.
369. Palmer M, Adami HO, Krusemo UB, et al. Increased risk of malignant diseases after surgery for primary hyperparathyroidism. A nationwide cohort study. Am J Epidemiol 1988; 127:1031–1040.
370. Parisien M, Silverberg SJ, Shane E, et al. The histomorphometry of bone in primary hyperparathyroidism: preservation of cancellous bone structure. J Clin Endocrinol Metab 1990; 70:930–938.
371. Silverberg S, Shane E, de la Cruz L, et al. Skeletal disease in primary hyperparathyroidism. J Bone Miner Res 1989; 4:283–291.
372. Martin P. Long-term irreversibility of bone loss after surgery. Arch Intern Med 1990; 150:1495–1497.
373. Silverberg SJ, Gartenberg F, Jacobs TP, et al. Longitudinal measurements of bone density and biochemical indices in untreated primary hyperparathyroidism. J Clin Endocrinol Metab 1995; 80: 723–728.
374. Silverberg SJ, Locker FG, Bilezikian JP. Verterbral osteopenia: a new indication for surgery in primary hyperparathyroidism. J Clin Endocrinol Metab 1996; 81:4007–4012.
375. Khosla S, Melton LJI, Wermers RA, et al. Primary hyperparathyroidism and the risk of fracture: a population-based study. J Bone Miner Res 1999; 14:1700–1707.

376. Mitlak B, Daly M, Potts JJ, et al. Asymptomatic primary hyperparathyroidism. J Bone Miner Res 1991; 6(Suppl):S103–S110.
377. Parfitt AM, Rao DS, Kleerekoper M. Asymptomatic primary hyperparathyroidism discovered by multichannel biochemical screening: clinical course and considerations bearing on the need for surgical intervention. J Bone Miner Res 1991; 6(Suppl):S97–S101.
378. Silverberg SJ, Shane E, Jacobs TP, et al. Nephrolithiasis and bone involvement in primary hyperparathyroidism. Am J Med 1990; 89:327–334.
379. Potts JT Jr (ed). Proceedings of the NIH Consensus Development Conference on Diagnosis and Management of Asymptomatic Primary Hyperparathyroidism. J Bone Miner Res 1991; 6(Suppl):S9–S13.
380. Arnold A, Staunton CE, Kim HG, et al. Monoclonality and abnormal parathyroid hormone genes in parathyroid adenomas. N Engl J Med 1988; 318:658–662.
381. Arnold A. Molecular basis of hyperparathyroidism. In Bilezikian JP (ed). The Parathyroids. Second edition. New York, Raven Press, 2nd ed 2001, pp 331–347.
382. Cryns VL, Yi SM, Tahara H, et al. Frequent loss of chromosome arm 1p DNA in parathyroid adenomas. Genes Chromosomes Cancer 1995; 13:9–17.
383. Tahara H, Smith AP, Gas RD, et al. Genomic localization of novel candidate tumor suppressor gene loci in human parathyroid adenomas. Cancer Res 1996; 56:599–605.
384. Friedman E, Sakaguchi K, Bale AE, et al. Clonality of parathyroid tumors in familial multiple endocrine neoplasia type I. N Engl J Med 1989; 321:213–218.
385. Bystrom C, Larsson C, Blomberg C, et al. Localization of the MEN 1 gene to a small region within chromosome 11q13 by deletion mapping in tumors. Proc Natl Acad Sci USA 1990; 87: 1968–1972.
386. Marx SJ, Agarwal SK, Kester MB, et al. Multiple endocrine neoplasia type 1: clinical and genetic features of the hereditary endocrine neoplasias. Recent Prog Horm Res 1999; 54:397–439.
387. Motokura T, Bloom T, Kim HG, et al. A BCL1-linked candidate oncogene which is rearranged in parathyroid tumors encodes a novel cyclin. Nature 1991; 350:512–515.
388. Hsi E, Zukerberg LR, Yang WI, et al. Cyclin D1/PRAD1 expression in parathyroid adenomas: an immunohistochemical study. J Clin Endocrinol Metab 1996; 81:1736–1739.
389. Palanisamy N, Imanishi Y, Rao PH, et al. Novel chromosomal abnormalities identified by comparative genomic hybridizatin in parathyroid adenomas. J Clin Endocrinol Metab 1998; 83:1766–1770.
390. Schneider AB, Gierlowski TC, Shore-Freedman E, et al. Dose-response relationships for radiation-induced hyperparathyroidism. J Clin Endocrinol Metab 1995; 80:254–257.
391. Carling T, Kindmark A, Hellman P, et al. Vitamin D receptor genotypes in primary hyperparathyroidism. Nat Med 1995; 1: 1309–1311.
392. Carling T, Rastad J, Åkerström G, et al. Vitamin D receptor (VDR) and parathyroid hormone messenger ribonucleic acid levels correspond to polymorphic VDR alleles in human parathyroid tumors. J Clin Endocrinol Metab 1998; 83:2255–2259.
393. Falchetti A, Bale AE, Amorosi A, et al. Progression of uremic hyperparathyroidism involves allelic loss on chromosome 11. J Clin Endocrinol Metab 1993; 76:139–144.
394. Arnold A, Brown MF, Urena P, et al. Monoclonality of parathyroid tumors in chronic renal failure and in primary parathyroid hyperplasia. J Clin Invest 1995; 95:2047–2053.
395. Davies M. Hyperparathyroidism in X-linked hypophosphataemic osteomalacia. Clin Endocrinol 1995; 42:205–206.
396. Mallette LE, Khouri K, Zengotita H, et al. Lithium treatment increases intact and midregion parathyroid hormone and parathyroid volume. J Clin Endocrinol Metab 1989; 68:654–660.
397. Stancer HC, Forbath N. Hyperparathyroidism, hypothyroidism and impaired renal function after 10 to 20 years of lithium treatment. Arch Intern Med 1989; 149:1042–1045.
398. Thakker RV, Bouloux P, Wooding C, et al. Association of parathyroid tumors in multiple endocrine neoplasia type 1 with loss of alleles on chromosome 11. N Engl J Med 1989; 321:218–224.
399. Brown EM, Gardner DG, Brennan MF, et al. Calcium-regulated parathyroid hormone release in primary hyperparathyroidism. Am J Med 1979; 66:923–931.
400. LeBoff MS, Shoback D, Brown EM, et al. Regulation of parathyroid hormone release and cytosolic calcium by extracellular calcium in dispersed and cultured bovine and pathological human parathyroid cells. J Clin Invest 1985; 75:49–57.
401. Kifor O, Moore FD, Wang P, et al. Reduced immunostaining for the extracellular Ca^{2+}-sensing receptor in primary and uremic secondary hyperparathyroidism. J Clin Endocrinol Metab 1996; 81:1598–1606.
402. Corbetta S, Mantovani G, Lania A, et al. Calcium-sensing receptor expression and signalling in human parathyroid adenomas and primary hyperplasia. Clin Endocrinol (Oxf) 2000; 52:339–348.
403. Rizzoli R, Green J, Marx SJ. Primary hyperparathyroidism in familial multiple endocrine neoplasia type 1. Am J Med 1985; 78: 467–474.
404. Hellman P, Skogseid B, Juhlin C, et al. Findings and long-term results of parathyroid surgery in multiple endocrine neoplasia type 1. World J Surg 1992; 16:718–723.
405. Schuffenecker I, Virally-Monod M, Brohet R, et al. Risk and penetrance of primary hyperparathyroidism in multiple endocrine neoplasia type 2A families with mutations at codon 634 of the *RET* proto-oncogene. J Clin Endocrinol Metab 1998; 83:487–491.
406. Hofstra RMW, Landsvater RM, Ceccherini I, et al. A mutation in the *RET* proto-oncogene associated with multiple endocrine neoplasia type 2B and sporadic medullary thyroid carcinoma. Nature 1994; 367:375–383.
407. Santoro M, Carlomagno F, Romano A, et al. Activation of *RET* as a dominant transforming gene by germline mutations of MEN2A and MEN2B. Science 1995; 267:381–383.
408. Pausova Z, Soliman E, Amizuka N, et al. Expression of the *ret* proto-oncogene in hyperparathyroid tissues: implications for the pathogenesis of the parathyroid disease in men 2A. J Bone Miner Res 1995; 10(Suppl 1):S191.
409. Wassif WS, Moniz CF, Friedman E, et al. Familial isolated hyperparathyroidism: a distinct genetic entity with an increased risk of parathyroid cancer. J Clin Endocrinol Metab 1993; 77:1485–1489.
410. Szabo J, Heath B, Hill VM, et al. Heredity hyperparathyroidism–jaw tumor syndrome: the endocrine tumor gene *HRPT2* maps to chromosome 1q21–q31. Am J Hum Genet 1995; 56:944–950.
411. Haven CJ, Wong FK, van Dam EWM, et al. A genotypic and histopathological study of a large Dutch kindred with hyperparathyroidism–jaw tumor syndrome. J Clin Endocrinol Metab 2000; 85:1449–1454.
412. Ohrvall U, Akerstrom G, Ljunghall S, et al. Surgery for sporadic primary hyperparathyroidism in the elderly. World J Surg 1994; 18:612–618.
413. Chigot JP, Menegaux F, Achrafi H. Should primary hyperparathyroidism be treated surgically in elderly patients older than 75 years? Surgery 1995; 117:397–401.
414. Scholz DA, Purnell DC. Asymptomatic primary hyperparathyroidism. 10-year prospective study. Mayo Clin Proc 1981; 56: 473–478.
415. Nakaoka D, Sugimoto T, Kobayashi T, et al. Prediction of bone mass change after parathyroidectomy in patients with primary hyperparathyroidism. J Clin Endocrinol Metab 2000; 85:1901–1907.
416. Insogna KL, Mitnick ME, Stewart AF, et al. Sensitivity of the parathyroid hormone–1,25-dihydroxyvitamin D axis to variations in calcium intake in patients with primary hyperparathyroidism. N Engl J Med 1985; 313:1126–1130.
417. Gallagher JC, Wilkinson R. The effect of ethinyloestradiol on calcium and phosphorus metabolism of post-menopausal women with primary hyperparathyroidism. Clin Sci Mol Med 1973; 45: 782–785.
418. Marcus R. Estrogens and progestins in the management of primary hyperparathyroidism. J Bone Miner Res 1991; 6(Suppl): S125–S129.
419. Selby PL, Peacock M. Ethinyl estradiol and norethindrone in the treatment of primary hyperparathyroidism in postmenopausal women. N Engl J Med 1986; 314:1481–1485.
420. Broadus AE, Magee JS. A detailed evaluation of oral phosphate therapy in selected patients with primary hyperparathyroidism. J Clin Endocrinol Metab 1983; 56:953–961.
421. Reasner CA, Stone MD, Hosking DJ, et al. Acute changes in calcium homeostasis during treatment of primary hyperparathy-

514. Muls E, Bouillon R, Boelaert J, et al. Etiology of hypercalcemia in a patient with Addison's disease. Calcif Tissue Int 1982; 34: 523–526.
515. Christensson T, Hellstrom K, Wengle B. Hypercalcemia and primary hyperparathyroidism: prevalence in patients receiving thiazides as detected in a health screen. Arch Intern Med 1977; 137:1138–1142.
516. Porter RH, Cox BG, Heaney P, et al. Treatment of hypoparathyroid patients with chlorthalidone. N Engl J Med 1978; 298: 577–581.
517. McMillan DE, Freeman RB. The milk alkali syndrome: a study of the acute disorder with comments on the development of the chronic condition. Medicine 1965; 44:485–501.
518. Abreo K, Adlakha A, Kilpatrick S, et al. The milk-alkali syndrome. Arch Intern Med 1993; 153:1005–1010.
519. Beall DP, Scofield RH. Milk-alkali syndrome associated with calcium carbonate consumption. Medicine 1995; 74:89–96.
520. Naftchi NE, Viaa AT, Sell GH, et al. Mineral metabolism in spinal cord injury. Arch Phys Med Rehabil 1980; 61:139–142.
521. Stewart AF, Alder M, Byers CM. Calcium homeostasis in immobilization: an example of resorptive hypercalciuria. N Engl J Med 1982; 306:1136–1140.
522. Minaire P, Meunier P, Edouard C, et al. Quantitative histological data on disuse osteoporosis—comparison with biological data. Calcif Tissue Res 1974; 17:57–73.
523. Meythaler JM, Tuel SM, Cross LL. Successful treatment of immobilization hypercalcemia using calcitonin and etidronate. Arch Phys Med Rehabil 1993; 74:316–319.
524. Massagli TL, Cardenas DD. Immobilization hypercalcemia treatment with pamidronate disodium after spinal cord injury. Arch Phys Med Rehabil 1999; 80:998–1000.
525. Llach F, Felsenfeld AJ, Haussler MR. The pathophysiology of altered calcium metabolism in rhabdomyolysis-induced acute renal failure. N Engl J Med 1981; 305:117–123.
526. Akmal M, Bishop JE, Telfer N, et al. Hypocalcemia and hypercalcemia in patients with rhabdomyolysis with and without acute renal failure. J Clin Endocrinol Metab 1986; 63:137–142.
527. Hadjis T, Grieff M, Lockhart D, et al. Calcium metabolism in acute renal failure due to rhabdomyolysis. Clin Nephrol 1993; 39:22–27.
528. Coburn JW, Salusky IB. Hyperparathyroidism in renal failure. In Bilezikian JP (ed). The Parathyroids. New York, Raven Press, 1994, pp 721–745.
529. Williams JCP, Barratt-Boyes BG, Lowe JB. Supravalvular aortic stenosis. Circulation 1961; 24:1311–1318.
530. Jones KL. Williams syndrome: an historical perspective of its evolution, natural history, and etiology. Am J Med Genet 1990; 6:89–96.
531. Garabedian M, Jacqz E, Guillozo H, et al. Elevated plasma 1,25-dihydroxyvitamin D concentrations in infants with hypercalcemia and an elfin facies. N Engl J Med 1985; 312:948–952.
532. Ewart AK, Morris CA, Atkinson D, et al. Hemizygosity at the elastin locus in a developmental disorder, Williams syndrome. Nature 1993; 5:11–16.
533. Ewart AK, Jin W, Atkinson D, et al. Supravalvular aortic stenosis associated with a deletion disrupting the elastin gene. J Clin Invest 1994; 93:1071–1077.
534. Frangiskakis JM, Ewart AK, Morris CA, et al. LIM-kinase 1 hemizygosity implicated in impaired visuospacial constructive cognition. Cell 1996; 86:59–69.
535. Kruse K, Pankau R, Gosch A, et al. Calcium metabolism in Williams-Beuren syndrome. J Pediatr 1992; 121:902–907.
536. Parfitt AM, Schipani E, Rao DS, et al. Hypercalcemia due to constitutive activity of the parathyroid hormone (PTH)/PTH-related peptide receptor: comparison with primary hyperparathyroidism. J Clin Endocrinol Metab 1996; 81:3584–3588.
537. Weir E, Philbrick W, Neff L, et al. Targeted overexpression of parathyroid hormone–related peptide in chondrocytes causes skeletal dysplasia and delayed osteogenesis. J Bone Miner Res 1995; 10(Suppl 1):S11.
538. Schipani E, Lanske B, Hunzelman J, et al. Targeted expression of constitutively active receptors for parathyroid hormone and parathyroid hormone–related peptide delays endochondral bone formation and rescues mice that lack parathyroid hormone–related peptide. Proc Natl Acad Sci USA 1997; 94:13689–13694.
539. Bilezikian JP. Management of acute hypercalcemia. N Engl J Med 1992; 326:1196.
540. Suki WN, Yiumm JJ, vonMinden M, et al. Acute treatment of hypercalcemia with furosemide. N Engl J Med 1970; 283:836–840.
541. Wimalawansa SJ. Optimal frequency of administration of pamidronate in patients with hypercalcemia of malignancy. Clin Endocrinol 1994; 41:591–595.
542. Hosking DJ, Gilson D. Comparison of the renal and skeletal actions of calcitonin in the treatment of severe hypercalcemia of malignancy. Q J Med 1984; 53:359–368.
543. Ralston SH, Alzaid AA, Gardner MD, et al. Treatment of cancer-associated hypercalcaemia with combined aminohydroxypropylidene disphonate and calcitonin. Br Med J 1986; 292:1549–1550.
544. Warrell RP, Israel R, Frisone M, et al. Gallium nitrate for acute treatment of cancer-related hypercalcemia: a randomized, double-blind comparison to calcitonin. Ann Intern Med 1988; 108:669–674.
545. Shackney S, Hasson J. Precipitous fall in serum calcium, hypotension, and acute renal failure after intravenous phosphate therapy for hypercalcemia: report of two cases. Ann Intern Med 1967; 66:906–916.
546. Doroghazi RM, Childers R. Time-related changes in the Q-T interval in acute myocardial infarction: possible relation to local hypocalcemia. Am J Cardiol 1978; 41:684–688.
547. Reddy CVR, Gould L, Gomprecht RF. Unusual electrocardiographic manifestations of hypocalcemia. Angiology 1974; 25:764–768.
548. Connor TB, Rosen BL, Blaustein MP, et al. Hypocalcemia precipitating congestive heart failure. N Engl J Med 1982; 307:869–872.
549. Tambyah PA, Ong BKC, Lee KO. Reversible parkinsonism and asymptomatic hypocalcemia with basal ganglia calcification from hypoparathyroidism 26 years after thyroid surgery. Am J Med 1993; 94:444.
550. Zaloga GP, Willey S, Tomasic P, et al. Free fatty acids alter calcium binding: a cause for misinterpretation of serum calcium values and hypocalcemia in critical illness. J Clin Endocrinol Metab 1987; 64:1010–1014.
551. Ding C, Buckingham B, Levine MA. Neonatal hypoparathyroidism attributable to homozygous partial deletion of the human glial cell missing gene-B (abstract 1690). Paper presented at the 82nd Annual Meeting of the Endocrine Society, 2000.
552. Thakker RV, Davies KE, Whyte MP, et al. Mapping the gene causing X-linked recessive idiopathic hypoparathyroidism to Xq26–Xq27 by linkage studies. J Clin Invest 1990; 86:40–45.
553. Garabedian M. Hypocalcemia and chromosome 22q11 microdeletion. Genet Couns 1999; 10:389–394.
554. Karayiorgou M, Morris MA, Morrow B, et al. Schizophrenia susceptibility associated with interstitial deletions of chromosome 22q11. Proc Natl Acad Sci USA 1995; 92:7612–7616.
555. Budarf ML, Collins J, Gong W, et al. Cloning a balanced translocation associated with DiGeorge syndrome and identification of a disrupted candidate gene. Nat Genet 1995; 10:269–278.
556. Scire G, Dallapiccola B, Iannetti P, et al. Hypoparathyroidism as the major manifestation in two patients with 22q11 deletions. Am J Med Genet 1994; 52:478–482.
557. Daw SC, Taylor C, Kraman M, et al. A common region of 10p deleted in DiGeorge and velocardiofacial syndromes. Nat Genet 1996; 13:458–460.
558. Van Esch H, Groenen P, Nesbit MA, et al. GATA3 haplo-insufficiency causes human HDR syndrome. Nature 2000; 406: 419–422.
559. Bockman DE, Kriby ML. Dependence of thymus development on derivatives of the neural crest. Science 1984; 223:498–500.
560. Chisaka O, Capecchi MR. Regionally restricted developmental defects resulting from targeted disruption of the mouse homeobox gene hox-1.5. Nature 1991; 350:473–479.
561. Dionisi-Vici C, Garavaglia B, Burlina A, et al. Hypoparathyroidism in mitochondrial trifunctional protein deficiency. J Pediatr 1996; 129:159–162.
562. Papadimitriou A, Hadjigeorgiou G, Divari R, et al. The influence of coenzyme Q10 on total serum calcium concentration in two patients with Kearns-Sayre syndrome and hypoparathyroidism. Neuromuscul Disord 1996; 6:49–53.
563. Ahn TG, Antonarakis SE, Kronenberg HM, et al. Familial isolated hypoparathyroidism: a molecular genetic analysis of 8 families with 23 affected persons. Medicine 1986; 65:73–81.

564. Baldellou A, Bone J, Tamparillas M, et al. Congenital hypoparathyroidism, ocular colobomata, unilateral renal agenesis and dysmorphic features. Genet Couns 1991; 2:245–247.
565. Dahlberg PJ, Borer WZ, Newcomer KL, et al. Autosomal or X-linked recessive syndrome of congenital lymphedema, hypoparathyroidism, nephropathy, prolapsing mitral valve, and brachytelephalangy. Am J Med Genet 1983; 16:99–104.
566. Bilous RW, Murty G, Parkinson DB, et al. Brief report: autosomal dominant familial hypoparathyroidism, sensorineural deafness, and renal dysplasia. N Engl J Med 1992; 327:1069–1074.
567. Sunthornthepvarakul T, Churesigaew S, Ngowngarmratana S. A novel mutation of the signal peptide of the preproparathyroid hormone gene associated with autosomal recessive familial isolated hypoparathyroidism. J Clin Endocrinol Metab 1999; 84: 3792–3796.
568. Parkinson DB, Thakker RV. A donor splice site mutation in the parathyroid hormone gene is associated with autosomal recessive hypoparathyroidism. Nat Genet 1992; 2:149–152.
569. Northcutt RC, Levinson JD, Earnest JB. Hypocalcemia resulting from infarction of a parathyroid adenoma. Ann Intern Med 1969; 70:353–356.
570. Hammes M, DeMory A, Sprague SM. Hypocalcemia in end-stage renal disease: a consequence of spontaneous parathyroid gland infarction. Am J Kidney Dis 1994; 24:519–522.
571. Burch WM, Posillico JT. Hypoparathyroidism after I-131 therapy with subsequent return of parathyroid function. J Clin Endocrinol Metab 1983; 57:398–401.
572. Gertner JM, Broadus AE, Anast CS, et al. Impaired parathyroid response to induced hypocalcemia in thalassemia major. J Pediatr 1979; 95:210–213.
573. Carpenter TO, Carnes DL, Anast CS. Hypoparathyroidism in Wilson's disease. N Engl J Med 1983; 309:873–877.
574. Suh SM, Tashjian AH, Matsuo N, et al. Pathogenesis of hypocalcemia in primary hypomagnesemia: normal end-organ responsiveness to parathyroid hormone, impaired parathyroid gland function. J Clin Invest 1973; 52:153–160.
575. Rude RK, Oldham SB, Singer FR. Functional hypoparathyroidism and parathyroid hormone end-organ resistance in human magnesium deficiency. Clin Endocrinol 1976; 5:209–224.
576. Estep H, Shaw WA, Watlington C, et al. Hypocalcemia due to hypomagnesemia and reversible parathyroid hormone unresponsiveness. J Clin Endocrinol Metab 1969; 29:842–848.
577. Krapf R, Jaeger P, Hulter HN, et al. Chronic respiratory alkalosis induces renal PTH-resistance, hyperphosphatemia and hypocalcemia in humans. Kidney Int 1992; 42:727–734.
578. Pearce S, Williams C, Kifor O, et al. A familial syndrome of hypocalcemia with hypercalciuria due to mutations in the calcium-sensing receptor. N Engl J Med 1996; 335:1115–1122.
579. Leinhardt A, Garabédian M, Bai M, et al. A large homozygous or heterozygous in-frame deletion within the calcium-sensing receptor's carboxylterminal cytoplasmic tail that causes autosomal dominant hypocalcemia. J Clin Endocrinol Metab 2000; 85: 1695–1702.
580. Albright F, Burnett CH, Smith PH, et al. Pseudo-hypoparathyroidism—an example of "Seabright-Bantam syndrome." Endocrinology 1942; 30:922–932.
581. Chase LR, Melson GL, Aurbach GD. Pseudohypoparathyroidism: defective excretion of 3′,5′-AMP in response to parathyroid hormone. J Clin Invest 1969; 48:1832–1844.
582. Farfel Z, Brickman AS, Kaslow HR, et al. Defect of receptor-cyclase coupling protein in pseudohypoparathyroidism. N Engl J Med 1980; 303:237–242.
583. Mallette LE, Kirkland JL, Gagel RF, et al. Synthetic human parathyroid hormone-(1–34) for the study of pseudohypoparathyroidism. J Clin Endocrinol Metab 1988; 67:964–972.
584. Carter A, Bardin C, Collins R, et al. Reduced expression of multiple forms of the α subunit of the stimulatory GTP-binding protein in pseudohypoparathyroidism type 1a. Proc Natl Acad Sci USA 1987; 84:7266–7269.
585. Levine MA, Ahn TG, Klupt SF, et al. Genetic deficiency of the α subunit of the guanine nucleotide–binding protein G_s as the molecular basis for Albright hereditary osteodystrophy. Proc Natl Acad Sci USA 1988; 85:617–621.
586. Patten JL, Johns DR, Valle D, et al. Mutation in the gene encoding the stimulatory G protein of adenylate cyclase in Albright's hereditary osteodystrophy. N Engl J Med 1990; 322: 1412–1419.
587. Weinstein LS, Gejman PV, de Mazancourt P, et al. A heterozygous 4-bp deletion mutation in the $G_s\alpha$ gene (GNAS1) in a patient with Albright hereditary osteodystrophy. Genomics 1992; 13:1319–1321.
588. Farfel Z, Friedman E. Mental deficiency in pseudohypoparathyroidism type I is associated with Ns-protein deficiency. Ann Intern Med 1986; 105:197–199.
589. Iiri T, Herzmark P, Nakamoto JM, et al. Rapid GDP release from $Gs\alpha$ in patients with gain and loss of endocrine function. Nature 1994; 371:164–168.
590. Levine MA, Jap TS, Mauseth RS, et al. Activity of the stimulatory guanine nucleotide–binding protein is reduced in erythrocytes from patients with pseudohypoparathyroidism and pseudopseudohypoparathyroidism: biochemical, endocrine and genetic analysis of Albright's hereditary osteodystrophy in six kindreds. J Clin Endocrinol Metab 1986; 62:497–502.
591. Davies SJ, Hughes HE. Imprinting in Albright's hereditary osteodystrophy. J Med Genet 1993; 30:101–103.
592. Wilson LC, Oude Luttikhuis ME, Clayton PT, et al. Parental origin of G_s alpha gene mutations in Albright's hereditary osteodystrophy. J Med Genet 1994; 31:835–839.
593. Yu S, Yu D, Lee E, et al. Variable and tissue-specific hormone resistance in heterotrimeric G_s protein α-subunit ($G_s\alpha$) knockout mice is due to tissue-specific imprinting of the $G_s\alpha$ gene. Proc Natl Acad Sci USA 1998; 95:8715–8720.
594. Farfel Z, Bourne H, Iiri T. The expanding spectrum of G protein diseases. N Engl J Med 1999; 340:1012–1020.
595. Schipani E, Weinstein LS, Bergwitz C, et al. Pseudohypoparathyroidism Type Ib is not caused by mutations in the coding exons of the human parathyroid hormone (PTH)/PTH-related peptide receptor gene. J Clin Endocrinol Metab 1995; 80:1611–1621.
596. Murray TM, Rao LG, Wong MM, et al. Pseudohypoparathyroidism with osteitis fibrosa cystica: direct demonstration of skeletal responsiveness to parathyroid hormone in cells cultured from bone. J Bone Miner Res 1993; 8:83–91.
597. Jüppner H, Schipani E, Bastepe M, et al. The gene responsible for pseudohypoparathyroidism type Ib is paternally imprinted and maps in four unrelated kindreds to chromosome 20q13.3. Proc Natl Acad Sci USA 1998; 95:11798–11803.
598. Bastepe M, Pincus JE, Sugimoto T, et al. Positional dissociation between the genetic mutation responsible for pseudohypoparathyroidism type Ib and the associated methylation defect at exon A/B: evidence for a long-range regulatory element within the imprinted GNAS1 locus. Human Molec Gen 2001; 10:1231–1241.
599. Wu WI, Schwindinger WF, Aparicio LF, et al. Selective resistance to parathyroid hormone caused by a novel uncoupling mutation in the carboxyl terminus of G alpha(s): a cause of pseudohypoparathyroidism type Ib. J Biol Chem 2000; Oct 11.
600. Barrett D, Breslau NA, Wax MB, et al. New form of pseudohypoparathyroidism with abnormal catalytic adenylate cyclase. Am J Physiol 1989; 257:E277–E283.
600a. Linglart A, Carel JC, Garabedian M, et al. GNAS1 lesions in pseudohypoparathyroidism Ia and Ic: genotype phenotype relationship and evidence of the maternal transmission of the hormonal resistance. J Clin Endoc Metab 2002; 87:189–197.
600b. Shore EM, Ahn J, de Beur SJ, et al. Paternally inherited inactivating mutations of the GNAS1 gene in progressive osseous heteroplasia. N Engl J Med 2002; 346:99–106.
601. Drezner M, Neelon FA, Lebovitz HE. Pseudohypoparathyroidism Type II: a possible defect in the reception of the cyclic AMP signal. N Engl J Med 1973; 289:1056–1060.
602. Kinoshita M, Komori T, Ohtake T, et al. Abnormal calcium metabolism in myotonic dystrophy as shown by the Ellsworth-Howard test and its relation to CTG triplet repeat length. J Neurol 1997; 244:613–622.
603. Rao DS, Parfitt AM, Kleerekoper M, et al. Dissociation between the effects of endogenous parathyroid hormone on adenosine 3′,5′-monophosphate generation and phosphate reabsorption in hypocalcemia due to vitamin D depletion: an acquired disorder resembling pseudohypoparathyroidism type II. J Clin Endocrinol Metab 1985; 61:285–290.
604. Minagawa M, Yasuda T, Kobayashi Y, et al. Transient pseudohypoparathyroidism of the neonate. Eur J Endocrinol 1995; 133: 151–155.
605. Silve C. Pseudohypoparathyroidism syndromes: the many faces of

parathyroid hormone resistance. Eur J Endocrinol 1995; 133: 145–146.
606. Kidd GS, Schaaf M, Adler RA, et al. Skeletal responsiveness in pseudohypoparathyroidism. Am J Med 1980; 68:772–781.
607. Kolb FO, Steinbach HL. Pseudohypoparathyroidism with secondary hyperparathyroidism and osteitis fibrosa. J Clin Endocrinol Metab 1962; 22:59–70.
608. Kruse K, Kracht U, Wohlfart K, et al. Biochemical markers of bone turnover, intact serum parathyroid hormone and renal calcium excretion in patients with pseudohypoparathyroidism and hypoparathyroidism before and during vitamin D treatment. Eur J Pediatr 1989; 148:535–539.
609. Frame B, Hanson CA, Frost HM, et al. Renal resistance to parathyroid hormone with osteitis fibrosa. Am J Med 1972; 52: 311–321.
610. Breslau NA, Moses AM, Pak CYC. Evidence for bone remodeling but lack of calcium mobilization response to parathyroid hormone in pseudohypoparathyroidism. J Clin Endocrinol Metab 1983; 57:638–644.
611. Ish-Shalom S, Rao LG, Levine MA, et al. Normal parathyroid hormone responsiveness of bone-derived cells from a patient with pseudohypoparathyroidism. J Bone Miner Res 1996; 11:8–14.
612. Rao DS, Parfitt AM, Kleerekoper M, et al. Dissociation between the effects of endogenous parathyroid hormone on adenosine 3′,5′-monophosphate generation and phosphate reabsorption in hypocalcemia due to vitamin D depletion: an acquired disorder resembling pseudohypoparathyroidism Type II. J Clin Endocrinol Metab 1985; 61:285–290.
613. Holick MF. The use and interpretation of assays for vitamin D and its metabolites. J Nutr 1990; 120:1464–1469.
614. Thomas M, Lloyd-Jones DM. Thadhani R, et al. Hypovitaminosis D in medical patients. N Engl J Med 1998; 338:777–783.
615. Chapuy MC, Arlot ME, Duboeuf F, et al. Vitamin D_3 and calcium to prevent hip fractures in elderly women. N Engl J Med 1992; 327:1637–1642.
616. Arnaud C, Maijer R, Reade T, et al. Vitamin D dependency: an inherited postnatal syndrome with secondary hyperparathyroidism. Pediatrics 1970; 46:871–880.
617. Hahn TJ, Hendin BA, Scharp CR, et al. Effect of chronic anticonvulsant therapy on serum 25-hydroxycalciferol levels in adults. N Engl J Med 1972, 287:900–904.
618. Greenwood RH, Pruntz FTG, Silver J. Osteomalacia after prolonged glutethimide administration. Br Med J 1973; 1:643–645.
619. Brodie MJ, Boobis AR, Hillyard CJ, et al. Effect of rifampicin and isoniazid on vitamin D metabolism. Clin Pharmacol Ther 1982; 32:525–530.
620. Casella SJ, Reiner BJ, Chen TC, et al. A possible genetic defect in 25-hydroxylation as a cause of rickets. J Pediatr 1994; 124: 929–932.
621. Andress DL, Norris KC, Coburn JW, et al. Intravenous calcitriol in the treatment of refractory osteitis fibrosa of chronic renal failure. N Engl J Med 1989; 321:274–279.
622. Mazzaferro S, Pasquali M, Ballanti P, et al. Intravenous versus oral calcitriol therapy in renal osteodystrophy: results of a prospective, pulsed and dose-comparable study. Miner Electrolyte Metab 1994; 20:122–129.
623. Martin KJ, Ballal HS, Domoto DT, et al. Pulse oral calcitriol for the treatment of hyperparathyroidism in patients on continuous ambulatory peritoneal dialysis: preliminary observations. Am J Kidney Dis 1992; 19:540–545.
624. Liou HH, Chiang SS, Huang TP, et al. Comparative effect of oral or intravenous calcitriol on secondary hyperparathyroidism in chronic hemodialysis patients. Miner Electrolyte Metab 1994; 20:97–102.
625. Shigematsu T, Kawaguchi Y, Unemura S, et al. Suppression of secondary hyperparathyroidism in chronic dialysis patients by single oral weekly dose of 1,25-dihydroxycholecalciferol. Intern Med 1993; 32:695–701.
626. Drezner MK, Feinglos MN. Osteomalacia due to 1α,25-dihydroxycholecalciferol deficiency. J Clin Invest 1977; 60:1046–1053.
627. Delvin EE, Glorieux FH, Marie PJ, et al. Vitamin D dependency: replacement therapy with calcitriol. Pediatrics 1981; 99: 26–34.
628. Scriver CR, Reade TM, DeLuca HF, et al. Serum 1,25-dihydroxyvitamin D levels in normal subjects and in patients with hereditary rickets or bone disease. N Engl J Med 1978; 299:976–979.
629. Fraser D, Kooh SW, Kind HP, et al. Pathogenesis of hereditary vitamin-D-dependent rickets: an inborn error of vitamin D metabolism involving defective conversion of 25-hydroxyvitamin D to 1α,25-dihydroxyvitamin D. N Engl J Med 1973; 289:817–822.
630. Kitnaka S, Takeyama K-I, Muryama A, et al. Inactivating mutations in the 25-hydroxyvitamin D, 1α-hydroxylase gene in patients with pseudovitamin D-deficiency rickets. N Engl J Med 1998; 338:653–661.
631. Wang J, Lin C-J, Burridge S, et al. Genetics of vitamin D 1α-hydroxylase deficiency in 17 families. Am J Hum Genet 1998; 63: 1694–1702.
632. Glorieux FH. Calcitriol treatment in vitamin D-dependent and vitamin D-resistant rickets. Metabolism 1990; 39:10–12.
633. Reade TM, Scriver CR, Glorieux FH, et al. Response to crystalline 1α-hydroxyvitamin D_3 in vitamin D dependency. Pediatr Res 1975; 9:593–599.
634. Hughes M, Malloy P, Kieback D, et al. Human vitamin D receptor mutations: identification of molecular defects in hypocalcemic vitamin D resistant rickets. Adv Exp Med Biol 1989; 255:491–503.
635. Hughes MR, Malloy PJ, O'Malley BW, et al. Genetic defects of the 1,25-dihydroxyvitamin D_3 receptor. J Recept Res 1991; 11: 699–716.
636. Saijo T, Ito M, Takeda E, et al. A unique metation in the vitamin D receptor gene in three Japanese patients with vitamin D-dependent rickets type II: utility of single-strand conformation polymorphism analysis for heterozygous carrier detection. Am J Hum Genet 1991; 49:668–673.
637. Sone T, Scott RA, Hughes MR, et al. Mutant vitamin D receptors which confer hereditary resistance to 1,25-dihydroxyvitamin D_3 in humans are transcriptionally inactive in vitro. J Biol Chem 1989; 264:20230–20234.
638. Sone T, Marx SJ, Liberman UA, et al. A unique point mutation in the human vitamin D receptor chromosomal gene confers hereditary resistance to 1,25-dihydroxyvitamin D_3. Mol Endocrinol 1990; 4:623–631.
639. Yagi H, Ozono K, Miyake H, et al. A new point mutation in the deoxyribonucleic acid-binding domain of the vitamin D receptor in a kindred with hereditary 1,25-dihydroxyvitamin D-resistant rickets. J Clin Endocrinol Metab 1993; 76:509–512.
640. Ritchie HH, Hughes MR, Thompson ET, et al. An ochre mutation in the vitamin D receptor gene causes hereditary 1,25-dihydroxyvitamin D_3-resistant rickets in three families. Proc Natl Acad Sci USA 1989; 86:9783–9787.
641. Brooks MH, Bell NH, Love L, et al. Vitamin D-dependent rickets Type II: resistance of target organs to 1,25-dihydroxyvitamin D. N Engl J Med 1978; 298:996–999.
642. Fraher LJ, Karmali R, Hinde FRJ, et al. Vitamin D-dependent rickets type II: extreme end organ resistance to 1,25-dihydroxy vitamin D_3 in a patient without alopecia. Eur J Pediatr 1986; 145:389–395.
643. Liberman UA, Halabe A, Samuel R, et al. End-organ resistance to 1,25-dihydroxycholecalciferol. Lancet 1980; 1:504–506.
644. Bell NH. Vitamin D-dependent rickets type II. Calcif Tissue Int 1980; 31:89–91.
645. Li YC, Pirro AE, Demay MB. Analysis of vitamin D-dependent calcium-binding protein messenger ribonucleic acid expression in mice lacking the vitamin D receptor. Endocrinology 1998; 139: 847–851.
646. Chen TL, Hirst MA, Cone CM, et al. 1,25-Dihydroxyvitamin D resistance, rickets, and alopecia: analysis of receptors and bioresponse in cultured fibroblasts from patients and parents. J Clin Endocrinol Metab 1984; 59:383–388.
647. Eil C, Liberman UA, Marx SJ. The molecular basis for resistance to 1,25-dihydroxyvitamin D: studies in cells cultured from patients with hereditary hypocalcemic $1,25(OH)_2D_3$-resistant rickets. Adv Exp Med Biol 1986; 196:407–422.
648. Takeda E, Yokota I, Kawakami I, et al. Two siblings with vitamin-D-dependent rickets type II: no recurrence of rickets for 14 years after cessation of therapy. Eur J Pediatr 1989; 149:54–57.
649. Marx SJ, Liberman UA, Eil C, et al. Hereditary resistance to 1,25-dihydroxyvitamin D. Recent Prog Horm Res 1984; 40:589–615.
650. Harrison HC, Harrison HE. Inhibition of vitamin D-stimulated active transport of calcium of rat intestine by diphenylhydantoin-phenobarbital treatment. Proc Soc Exp Biol Med 1976; 153:220–224.

651. Kido Y, Okamura T, Tomikawa M, et al. Hypocalcemia associated with 5-fluorouracil and low dose leucovorin in patients with advanced colorectal or gastric carcinomas. Cancer 1996; 78:1794–1797.
652. Relkin R. Hypocalcemia resulting from calcium accretion by a chondrosarcoma. Cancer 1974; 34:1834–1837.
653. Dembinski TC, Yatscoff RW, Blandford DE. Thyrotoxicosis and hungry bone syndrome—a cause of posttreatment hypocalcemia. Clin Biochem 1994; 27:69–74.
654. Jacobson MA, Gambertoglio JG, Aweeka FT, et al. Foscarnet-induced hypocalcemia and effects of foscarnet on calcium metabolism. J Clin Endocrinol Metab 1991; 72:1130–1135.
655. Aggeler PM, Perkins HA, Watkins HB. Hypocalcemia and defective hemostasis after massive blood transfusion. Report of a case. Transfusion 1967; 7:35–39.
656. Greco RJ, Hartford CE, Haith LR, et al. Hydrofluoric acid–induced hypocalcemia. J Trauma 1988; 28:1593–1596.
657. Kao W, Dart R, Kuffner E, et al. Ingestion of low-concentration hyrofluoric acid: an insidious and potentially fatal poisoning. Ann Emerg Med 1999; 34:35–41.
658. Tsang RC, Kleinman LI, Sutherland JM, et al. Hypocalcemia in infants of diabetic mothers. J Pediatr 1972; 80:384–395.
659. Tsang RC, Light IJ, Sutherland JM, et al. Possible pathogenetic factors in neonatal hypocalcemia of prematurity. J Pediatr 1973; 82:423–429.
660. Kaplan EL, Burrington JD, Klementschitsch P, et al. Primary hyperparathyroidism, pregnancy and neonatal hypocalcemia. Surgery 1984; 96:717–722.
661. Kuehn EW, Anders HJ, Bogner JR, et al. Hypocalcaemia in HIV infection and AIDS. J Intern Med 1999; 245:69–73.
662. Lind L, Carlstedt F, Rastad J, et al. Hypocalcemia and parathyroid hormone secretion in critically ill patients. Critical Care Med 2000; 28:93–99.
663. Stewart AF, Longo W, Kreutter D, et al. Hypocalcemia associated with calcium-soap formation in a patient with a pancreatic fistula. N Engl J Med 1986; 315:496–498.
664. Dettelbach MA, Deftos LJ, Stewart AF. Intraperitoneal free fatty acids induce severe hypocalcemia in rats: a model for the hypocalcemia of pancreatitis. J Bone Miner Res 1990; 5:1249–1255.
665. Norberg HP, DeRoos J, Kaplan EL. Increased parathyroid hormone secretion and hypocalcemia in experimental pancreatitis: necessity for an intact thyroid gland. Surgery 1975; 77:773–779.
666. Weir GC, Lesser PB, Drop LJ, et al. The hypocalcemia of acute pancreatitis. Ann Intern Med 1975; 83:185–189.
667. Desai TK, Carlson RW, Geheb MA. Prevalence and clinical implications of hypocalcemia in acutely ill patients in a medical intensive care setting. Am J Med 1988; 84:209–214.
668. Winer KK, Yanovski JA, Sarani B, et al. A randomized, cross-over trial of once-daily versus twice-daily parathyroid hormone 1-34 in treatment of hypoparathyroidism. J Clin Endocrinol Metab 1998; 83:3480–3486.
669. Slatopolsky E, Robson AM, Elkan I, et al. Control of phosphate excretion in uremic man. J Clin Invest 1968; 47:1865–1874.
670. Okano K, Furukawa Y, Hirotoshi M, et al. Comparative efficacy of various vitamin D metabolites in the treatment of various types of hypoparathyroidism. J Clin Endocrinol Metab 1982; 55: 238–242.
671. Howard JE, Hopkins TR, Connor TB. On certain physiologic responses to intravenous injection of calcium salts into normal, hyperparathyroid and hypoparathyroid persons. J Clin Endocrinol 1953; 13:1–19.
672. Corvilain J, Abramow M. Growth and renal control of plasma phosphate. J Clin Endocrinol Metab 1972; 34:452–459.
673. Hammerman MR, Karl IE, Hruska KA. Regulation of canine renal vesicle P_i transport by growth hormone and parathyroid hormone. Biochim Biophys Acta 1980; 603:322–335.
674. Schwartz E, Wiedman E, Simon S, et al. Estrogenic antagonism of metabolic effects of administered growth hormone. J Clin Endocrinol Metab 1969; 29:1176.
675. Recker RR, Hassing GS, Lau JR, et al. The hyperphosphatemic effect of disodium ethane-1-hydroxy-1,1-diphosphonate (EHDP): renal handling of phosphorus and the renal response to parathyroid hormone. J Lab Clin Med 1973; 81:258–260.
676. Lyles KW, Halsey DL, Friedman NE, et al. Correlations of serum concentrations of 1,25-dihydroxyvitamin D, phosphorus, and parathyroid hormone in tumoral calcinosis. J Clin Endocrinol Metab 1988; 67:88–92.
677. Lufkin EG, Kumar R, Heath H III. Hyperphosphatemic tumoral calcinosis: effects of phosphate depletion on vitamin D metabolism, and of acute hypocalcemia on parathyroid hormone secretion and action. J Clin Endocrinol Metab 1983; 56:1319–1322.
678. Prince MG, Schaefer PC, Goldsmith RS, et al. Hyperphosphatemic tumoral calcinosis: association with elevation of serum 1,25-dihydroxycholecalciferol concentration. Ann Intern Med 1982; 96:586–591.
679. Chernow B, Rainey TG, Georges LP, et al. Iatrogenic hyperphosphatemia: a metabolic consideration in critical care medicine. Crit Care Med 1981; 9:772–774.
680. McConnell TH. Fatal hypocalcemia from phosphate absorption from laxative preparation. JAMA 1971; 216:147–148.
681. Chesney RW, Houghton PB. Tetany following phosphate enemas in chronic renal disease. Am J Dis Child 1974; 127:584–586.
682. Biberstein M, Parker BA. Enema induced hyperphosphatemia. Am J Med 1985; 79:645–646.
683. Jimenez RAH, Larson EB. Tumoral calcinosis: an unusual complication of the laxative abuse syndrome. Am J Med Sci 1981; 282:141–147.
684. Oxnard SA, O'Bell J, Grupe WE. Severe tetany in an azotemic child related to a sodium phosphate enema. Pediatrics 1974; 53: 105–106.
685. Tsokos GL, Balow JE, Spiegel RJ, et al. Renal and metabolic complication of undifferentiated and lymphoblastic lymphomas. Medicine 1981; 60:218–229.
686. Zusman J, Brown DM, Nesbit ME. Hyperphosphatemia, hyperphosphaturia and hypocalcemia in acute lymphoblastic leukemia. N Engl J Med 1973; 289:1335–1340.
687. Brereton HD, Anderson T, Johnston RE, et al. Hyperphosphatemia and hypocalcemia in Burkitt lymphoma. Arch Intern Med 1975; 135:307–309.
688. Armata J, Depowska T. Hyperphosphatemia and hypocalcemia in neoplastic disorders. N Engl J Med 1974; 290:858.
689. O'Connor LR, Klein KL, Bethune JE. Hyperphosphatemia in lactic acidosis. N Engl J Med 1977; 297:707–709.
690. Miller PD, Heinig RE, Waterhouse C. Treatment of alcoholic ketoacidosis. Arch Intern Med 1978; 138:57–72.
691. Oster JR, Perez GO, Vaamode CA. Relationship between blood pH and potassium and phosphorus during acute metabolic acidosis. Am J Physiol 1978; 235:345–351.
692. Tranquada RE, Grant WJ, Peterson CR. Lactic acidosis. Arch Intern Med 1982; 117:192–202.
693. Spencer H, Lewin I, Samachson J, et al. Changes in metabolism in obese persons during starvation. Am J Med 1966; 40:27–37.
694. Silvis SE, Paragas PU Jr. Paresthesias, weakness, seizures and hypophosphatemia in patients receiving hyperalimentation. Gastroenterology 1972; 62:513–520.
695. Eisenberg E. Effects of serum calcium level and parathyroid extracts on phosphate and calcium excretion in hypoparathyroid patients. J Clin Invest 1965; 44:942–946.
696. Amiel C, Kuntziger H, Couette S, et al. Evidence for a parathyroid hormone–independent calcium modulation of phosphate transport along the nephron. J Clin Invest 1976; 57:256–263.
697. Reid IR, Hardy DC, Murphy WA, et al. X-linked hypophosphatemia: a clinical, biochemical and histopathologic assessment of morbidity in adults. Medicine 1989; 68:336–352.
698. Hruska KA, Rifas L, Cheng SL, et al. X-linked hyposphosphatemic rickets and the murine Hyp homologue. Am J Phys 1995; 268:F357–F362.
699. Ryan EA, Reiss E. Oncogenous osteomalacia. A review of the world literature of 42 cases and report of two new cases. Am J Med 1984; 77:501–512.
700. Cai Q, Hodgson SF, Kao PC, et al. Inhibition of renal phosphate transport by a tumor product in a patient with oncogenic osteomalacia. N Engl J Med 1994; 330:1645–1649.
701. Larsson L, Rebel K, Sorbo B. Severe hypophosphatemia. A hospital survey. Acta Med Scand 1983; 214:221–223.
702. Daily WH, Tonnesen AS, Allen SJ. Hypophosphatemia. Incidence, etiology and prevention in the trauma patient. Crit Care Med 1990; 18:1210–1214.
703. Betro MG, Pain RW. Hypophosphatemia and hyperphosphatemia in a hospital population. Br Med J 1972; 1:273–276.
704. Fiaccadori E, Coffrini E, Ronda N, et al. Hypophosphatemia in course of chronic obstructive pulmonary disease. Prevalence, mechanisms, and relationships with skeletal muscle phosphorus content. Chest 1990; 97:857–868.

705. Vanneste J, Hage J. Acute severe hypophosphatemia mimicking Wernicke's encephalopathy. Lancet 1986; 1:44.
706. Weintraub MI, Chakravorty HP. Nutrient deficiencies after intensive parenteral alimentation. N Engl J Med 1974; 291:799.
707. Silvis SE, DiBartolomeo AG, Aaker HM. Hypophosphatemia and neurological changes secondary to oral caloric intake. Am J Gastroenterol 1980; 73:215–222.
708. Furlan AJ, Hanson M, Cooperman A, et al. Acute areflexic paralysis. Association with hyperalimentation and hypophosphatemia. Arch Neurol 1975; 32:706–707.
709. Singhal PC, Kumar A, Desroches L, et al. Prevalence and predictors of rhabdomyolysis in patients with hypophosphatemia. Am J Med 1992; 92:458–464.
710. Gabow PA, Kaehny WD, Kelleher SP. The spectrum of rhabdomyolysis. Medicine 1982; 61:141–152.
711. Knochel JR, Bilbrey GL, Fuller TJ, et al. The muscle cell in chronic alcoholism: the possible role of phosphate depletion in alcoholic myopathy. Ann NY Acad Sci 1975; 252:274–286.
712. Agusti AG, Torres A, Estopa R, et al. Hypophosphatemia as a cause of failed weaning: the importance of metabolic factors. Crit Care Med 1984; 12:142–143.
713. Aubier M, Murciano D, Lecocguic Y, et al. Effect of hypophosphatemia on diaphragmatic contractility in patients with acute respiratory failure. N Engl J Med 1985; 3131:420–424.
714. Newman JH, Neff TA, Ziporin P. Acute respiratory failure associated with hypophosphatemia. N Engl J Med 1977; 296:1101–1103.
715. Davis SV, Olichwier KK, Chakko SC. Reversible depression of myocardial performance in hypophosphatemia. Am J Med Sci 1988; 295:183–187.
716. Bollaert PE, Levy B, Nace L, et al. Hemodynamic and metabolic effects of rapid correction of hypophosphatemia in patients with septic shock. Chest 1995; 107:1698–1701.
717. Rasmussen A, Buus S, Hessov I. Postoperative myocardial performance during glucose-induced hypophosphatemia. Acta Chir Scand 1985; 151:13–15.
718. Vered Z, Battler A, Motro M, et al. Left ventricular function in patients with chronic hypophosphatemia. Am Heart J 1984; 107: 796–798.
719. Lichtman MA, Miller DR, Cohen J, et al. Reduced red cell glycolysis, 2,3-diphosphoglycerate and adenosine triphosphate concentration and increased hemoglobin oxygen affinity caused by hypophosphatemia. Ann Intern Med 1971; 74:562–568.
720. Craddock PR, Yawata Y, VanSanten L, et al. Acquired phagocyte dysfunction. A complication of the hypophosphatemia of parenteral hyperalimentation. N Engl J Med 1974; 290:1403–1407.
721. Yawata Y, Hebbel RP, Silvis S, et al. Blood cell abnormalities complicating the hypophosphatemia of hyperalimentation: erythrocyte and platelet ATP deficiency associated with hemolytic anemia and bleeding in hyperalimented dogs. J Lab Clin Med 1974; 84:643–653.
722. Travis SF, Sugerman HJ. Alterations in red-cell glycolytic intermediates and oxygen transport as a consequence of hypophosphatemia in patients receiving intravenous hyperalimentation. N Engl J Med 1971; 285:763–768.
723. DeFronzo RA, Lang R. Hypophosphatemia and glucose interolerance: evidence for tissue insensitivity to insulin. N Engl J Med 1980; 202:1259-1263.
724. Franks M, Berris RF, Kaplan NO, et al. Metabolic studies in diabetic acidosis. II. The effect of the administration of sodium phosphate. Arch Intern Med 1948; 81:42–55.
725. Wilson HK, Keuer SP, Lea AS, et al. Phosphate therapy in diabetic ketoacidosis. Arch Intern Med 1982; 142:517–520.
726. Keller U, Berger W. Prevention of hypophosphatemia by phosphate infusion during treatment of diabetic ketoacidosis and hyperosmolar coma. Diabetes 1980; 29:87–95.
727. Rosen GH, Boullata JI, O'Rangers EA, et al. Intravenous phosphate repletion regimen for critically ill patients with moderate hypophosphatemia. Crit Care Med 1995; 23(7):1204–1210.
728. Clark CL, Sacks GS, Dickerson RN, et al. Treatment of hypophosphatemia in patients receiving specialized nutrition support using a graduated dosing scheme: results from a prospective clinical trial. Crit Care Med 1995; 23:1504–1511.
729. Kingston M, Al Siba'I MB. Treatment of severe hypophosphatemia. Crit Care Med 1985; 13:16–18.
730. Wacker WEC, Parisi AF. Magnesium metabolism. N Engl J Med 1968; 278:712–717.
731. Reinhart RA, Desbiens NA. Hypomagnesemia in patients entering the ICU. Crit Care Med 1985; 13:506–507.
732. Broner CW, Stidham GL, Westenkirchner DF, et al. Hypermagnesemia and hypocalcemia as predictors of high mortality in critically ill pediatric patients. Crit Care Med 1990; 18:921–928.
733. de Rouffignac C, Quamme G. Renal magnesium handling and its hormonal control. Physiol Rev 1994; 74:305–322.
734. Mordes JP, Wacker WE. Excess magnesium. Pharmacol Rev 1978; 29:273–300.
735. Alfrey AC, Terman DS, Brettschneider L, et al. Hypermagnesemia after renal homotransplantation. Ann Intern Med 1970; 73: 367–371.
736. Cruikshank DP, Pitkin RM, Reynolds WA, et al. Effects of magnesium sulfate treatment on perinatal calcium metabolism. I. Maternal and fetal responses. Am J Obstet Gynecol 1979; 134:243–249.
737. Green KW, Key TC, Coen R, et al. The effects of maternally administered magnesium sulfate on the neonate. Am J Obstet Gynecol 1983; 146:29–33.
738. Rasch DK, Huber PA, Richardson CJ, et al. Neurobehavioral effects of neonatal hypermagnesemia. J Pediatr 1982; 100:272–276.
739. Donovan EF, Tsang RC, Steichen JJ, et al. Neonatal hypermagnesemia: effect on parathyroid hormone and calcium homeostasis. J Pediatr 1980; 96:305–310.
740. Brand JM, Greer FR. Hypermagnesemia and intestinal perforation following antacid administration in a premature infant. Pediatrics 1990; 85:121–124.
741. Zwanger ML. Hypermagnesemia and perforated viscus. Ann Emerg Med 1986; 15:1219–1220.
742. Engbaek L. The pharmacological actions of magnesium ions with particular reference to the neuromuscular and the cardiovascular system. Pharmacol Rev 1952; 4:396–414.
743. Randall RE, Cohen MD, Spray CC, et al. Hypermagnesemia and renal failure: etiology and toxic manifestations. Ann Intern Med 1964; 61:73–88.
744. Mordes JP, Swartz R, Arky RA. Extreme hypermagnesemia as a cause of refractory hypotension. Ann Intern Med 1975; 83:657–658.
745. Ferdinandus J, Pederson JA, Whang R. Hypermagnesemia as a cause of refractory hypotension, respiratory depression, and coma. Arch Intern Med 1981; 141:669–670.
746. Suzuki K, Nonaka K, Kono N, et al. Effects of the intravenous administration of magnesium sulfate on corrected serum calcium level and nephrogenous cyclic AMP excretion in normal human subjects. Calcif Tissue Int 1986; 39:304–309.
747. Cholst IN, Steinberg SF, Tropper PJ, et al. The influence of hypermagnesemia on serum calcium and parathyroid hormone levels in human subjects. N Engl J Med 1984; 310:1221–1225.
748. Carney SL, Wong NLM, Quamme GA, et al. Effect of magnesium deficiency on renal magnesium and calcium transport in the rat. J Clin Invest 1980; 65:180–188.
749. Cruikshank DP, Pitkin RM, Donnelly E, et al. Urinary magnesium, calcium, and phosphate excretion during the magnesium sulfate infusion. Obstet Gynecol 1981; 58:430–443.
750. Buckle RM, Care AD, Cooper CW, et al. The influence of plasma magnesium concentration on parathyroid hormone secretion. J Endocrinol 1968; 42:529–534.
751. Fassler CA, Rodriguez RM, Badesch DB, et al. Magnesium toxicity as a cause of hypotension and hypoventilation. Occurrence in patients with normal renal function. Arch Intern Med 1985; 145: 1604–1606.
752. Rude RK. Magnesium deficiency: a cause of heterogeneous disease in humans. J Bone Miner Res 1998; 13:749–758.
753. Alfrey AC, Miller NL, Butkus D. Evaluation of body magnesium stores. J Lab Clin Med 1974; 84:153–162.
754. Lim P, Jacob E. Magnesium status of alcoholic patients. Metabolism 1972; 21:1045–1051.
755. Ryzen E, Elbaum N, Singer FR, et al. Parenteral magnesium tolerance testing in the evaluation of magnesium deficiency. Magnesium 1985; 4:137–147.
756. Al-Ghamdi SMG, Cameron EC, Sutton RAL. Magnesium deficiency: pathophysiologic and clinical overview. Am J Kid Dis 1994; 24:737–752.
757. Barnes BA. Magnesium conservation: a study of surgical patients. Ann NY Acad Sci 1969; 162:786–801.

758. Goldman AS, Van Fossan DD, Baird EE. Magnesium deficiency in celiac disease. Pediatrics 1962; 29:948–952.
759. Booth CC, Hanna S, Babouris N, et al. Incidence of hypomagnesaemia in intestinal malabsorption. Br Med J 1963; 2:141–144.
760. Heaton FW, Fourman P. Magnesium deficiency and hypocalcaemia in intestinal malabsorption. Lancet 1965; 2:50–52.
761. Rude RK, Singer FR. Magnesium deficiency and excess. Annu Rev Med 1981; 32:245–259.
762. Milla PJ, Aggett PJ, Wolff OH, et al. Studies in primary hypomagnesemia: evidence for defective carrier-mediated small intestinal transport of magnesium. Gut 1979; 20:1028–1033.
763. Pronicka E, Gruszczynska B. Familial hypomagnesemia with secondary hypocalcemia—autosomal or X-linked inheritance? J Inherit Metab Dis 1991; 14:397–399.
764. Bettinelli A, Bianchetti MG, Borella P, et al. Genetic heterogeneity in tubular hypomagnesemia-hypokalemia with hypocalcuria (Gitelman's syndrome). Kidney Int 1995; 47:547–551.
765. Evans RA, Carter JN, George CRP, et al. The congenital "magnesium-losing kidney." Q J Med 1981; 197:39–52.
766. Manz F, Scharer K, Janka P, et al. Renal magnesium wasting, incomplete tubular acidosis, hypercalciuria and nephrocalcinosis in siblings. Eur J Pediatr 1978; 128:67–79.
767. Smilde TJ, Haverman JF, Schipper P, et al. Familial hypokalemia/hypomagnesemia and chondrocalcinosis. J Rheumatol 1994; 21:1515–1519.
768. Tsukamoto T, Kobayashi T, Kawamoto K, et al. Possible discrimination of Gitelman's syndrome from Bartter's syndrome by renal clearance study: report of two cases. Am J Kidney Dis 1995; 25:637–641.
769. Shils ME. Experimental human magnesium depletion. Medicine 1969; 48:61–85.
770. King RG, Stanbury SW. Magnesium metabolism in primary hyperparathyroidism. Clin Sci 1970; 39:281–303.
771. Jones KH, Fourman P. Effects of infusions of magnesium and of calcium in parathyroid insufficiency. Clin Sci 1966; 30:139–150.
772. Jackson CE, Meier DW. Routine serum magnesium analysis. Ann Intern Med 1968; 69:743–748.
773. Mather HM, Nisbet JA, Burton GH, et al. Hypomagnesemia in diabetes. Clin Chim Acta 1979; 95:235–242.
774. Martin HE. Clinical magnesium deficiency. Ann NY Acad Sci 1969; 162:891–900.
775. Heaton FW, Pyrah LN, Beresford CC, et al. Hypomagnesaemia in chronic alcoholism. Lancet 1962; 2:802–805.
776. Drenick EJ, Hunt IF, Swendseid ME. Magnesium depletion during prolonged fasting of obese males. J Clin Endocrinol Metab 1969; 29:1341–1348.
777. Laitinen K, Lamberg-Allardt C, Tunninen R, et al. Transient hypoparathyroidism during acute alcohol intoxication. N Engl J Med 1991; 324:721–727.
778. McCollister RJ, Flink EB, Lewis MD. Urinary excretion of magnesium in man following the ingestion of ethanol. Am J Clin Nutr 1963; 12:415–420.
779. Mendelson JH, Ogata M, Mello NK. Effects of alcohol ingestion and withdrawal on magnesium states of alcoholics: clinical and experimental findings. Ann NY Acad Sci 1969; 169:918–933.
780. Schilsky RI, Anderson T. Hypomagnesemia and renal magnesium wasting in patients receiving cisplatin. Ann Intern Med 1979; 90: 929–931.
781. Martin M, Diaz RE, Casado A, et al. Intravenous and oral magnesium supplementations in the prophylaxis of cisplatin-induced hypomagnesemia. Results of a controlled trial. Am J Clin Oncol 1992; 15:348–351.
782. Barton CH, Vaziri ND, Martin DC, et al. Hypomagnesemia and renal magnesium wasting in renal transplant recipients receiving cyclosporine. Am J Med 1987; 83:693–699.
783. Millane TA, Jennison SH, Mann JM, et al. Myocardial magnesium depletion associated with prolonged hypomagnesemia: a longitudinal study in heart transplant patients. J Am Coll Cardiol 1992; 20:806–812.
784. Thompson CB, June CH, Sullivan KM, et al. Association between cyclosporin neurotoxicity and hypomagnesaemia. Lancet 1984; 2:1116–1120.
785. Edmundson HA, Berne CJ, Homann RE Jr, et al. Calcium, potassium, magnesium and amylase disturbances in acute pancreatitis. Am J Med 1952; 12:34–42.
786. England MR, Gordon G, Salem M, et al. Magnesium administration and dysrhythmias after cardiac surgery. A placebo-controlled, double-blind, randomized trial. JAMA 1992; 268:2395–2402.
787. McLellan BA, Reid SR, Lane PL. Massive blood transfusion causing hypomagnesemia. Crit Care Med 1984; 12:146–147.
788. Broughton A, Anderson IRM, Bowden CH. Magnesium-deficiency syndrome in burns. Lancet 1968; 2:1156–1158.
789. Consolazio CF, Matoush LO, Nelson RA, et al. Excretion of sodium, potassium, magnesium amd iron in human sweat and the relation of each to balance and requirements. J Nutr 1963; 79: 407–415.
790. Greenwald JH, Dubin A, Cardon L. Hypomagnesemic tetany due to excessive lactation. Am J Med 1963; 35:854–860.
791. Iseri LT, Freed J, Bures AR. Magnesium deficiency and cardiac disorders. Am J Med 1975; 58:837–846.
792. Seller RH, Cangiano J, Kim KE, et al. Digitalis toxicity and hypomagnesemia. Am Heart J 1970; 79:57–68.
793. Beller GA, Hood DB, Smith TW, et al. Correlation of serum magnesium levels and cardiac digitalis intoxication. Am J Cardiol 1974; 33:225–229.
794. Whang R, Morosi HJ, Rodgers D, et al. The influence of sustained magnesium deficiency on muscle potassium repletion. J Lab Clin Med 1967; 70:895–902.
795. Muldowney FP, McKenna TJ, Kyle LH, et al. Parathormone-like effect of magnesium replenishment in steatorrhea. N Engl J Med 1970; 281:61–68.
796. Allgrove J, Adami S, Fraher L, et al. Hypomagnesemia: studies of parathyroid hormone secretion and function. Clin Endocrinol 1984; 21:435–449.
797. Anast CS, Winnacker JL, Forte LR, et al. Impaired release of parathyroid hormone in magnesium deficiency. J Clin Endocrinol Metab 1976; 42:707–717.
798. Johannesson AJ, Raisz LG. Effects of low medium magnesium concentration on bone resorption in response to parathyroid hormone and 1,25-dihydroxyvitamin D in organ culture. Endocrinology 1983; 113:2294–2298.
799. Medalle R, Waterhouse C, Hahn TJ. Vitamin D resistance in magnesium deficiency. Am J Clin Nutr 1976; 29:854–858.
800. Rosler A, Rabinowitz D. Magnesium induced reversal of vitamin D resistance in hypoparathyroidism. Lancet 1973; 1:803–805.
801. Rude RK, Adams JS, Ryzen E, et al. Low serum concentrations of 1,25-dihydroxyvitamin D in human magnesium deficiency. J Clin Endocrinol Metab 1985; 61:933–940.
802. Fuss M, Cogan E, Gillet C, et al. Magnesium administration reverses the hypocalcemia secondary to hypomagnesemia despite low circulating levels of 25-dihydroxyvitamin D and 1,25-dihydroxyvitamin D. Clin Endocrinol 1985; 22:807–815.
803. Fuss M, Bergmann P, Bergans A, et al. Correction of low circulating levels of 1,25-dihydroxyvitamin D by 25-hydroxyvitamin D during reversal of hypomagnesaemia. Clin Endocrinol 1989; 31: 31–38.
804. Brannan PG, Vergne-Marini P, Pak CYC, et al. Magnesium absorption in the human small intestine. J Clin Invest 1976; 57: 1412–1418.
805. Flink EB. Therapy of magnesium deficiency. Ann NY Acad Sci 1969; 162:901–905.
806. Sutton RAL, Walker VR, Halabe A, et al. Chronic hypomagnesemia caused by cisplatin: effect of calcitriol. J Lab Clin Med 1991; 117:40–43.

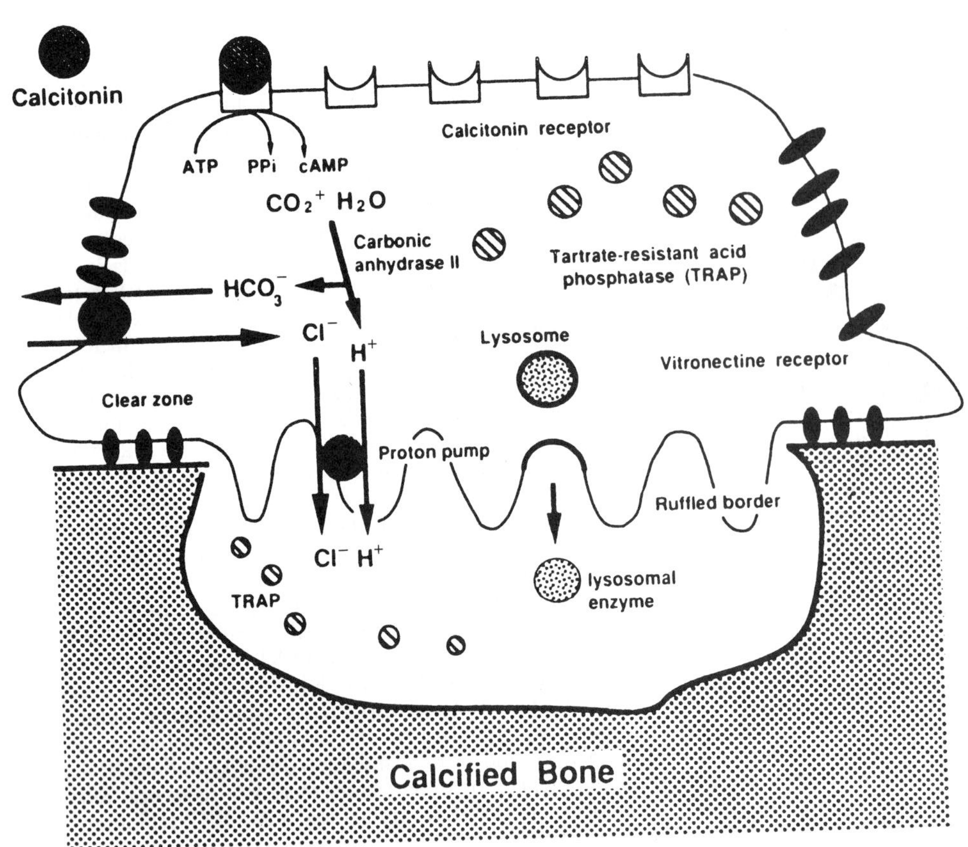

Figure 27–7. Functional elements of the fully differentiated osteoclast. (From Suda T, Takahashi N, Martin TJ. Modulation of osteoclast differentiation. Endocr Rev 1992; 13:66–80. Copyright © 1992, by The Endocrine Society.)

clast is limited. As osteoclasts become inactive, they die by apoptosis. Hormones that enhance bone resorption may delay apoptosis, and inhibitors of resorption can accelerate it. The mechanisms that limit the extent of osteoclastic resorption are incompletely understood and may involve inhibition by calcium ions, which accumulate under the osteoclast resorbing surface, or by local inhibitory factors, such as transforming growth factor β (TGF-β), which are released and activated during resorption.

The mature osteoclast is a unique and highly specialized cell (Fig. 27–7). It usually contains 10 to 20 nuclei, but giant osteoclasts with up to 100 nuclei can be seen in Paget's disease or giant cell tumors of bone. The large size of osteoclasts is probably essential for their resorptive function, which depends on their ability to isolate a region of the bone surface from the extracellular fluid and produce a local environment that can dissolve bone mineral and degrade matrix. The resorbing apparatus consists of a central ruffled border area, which secretes hydrogen ions and proteolytic enzymes, surrounded by a clear or sealing zone that anchors the cell to the bone surface by a ring of contractile proteins linked to integrin receptors. The osteoclast may secrete adhesion proteins, such as osteopontin and bone sialoprotein, that anchor the cell to bone by binding both to mineral and to cell-surface integrins.

Acidification of the ruffled border area requires that osteoclasts have proton pumps. These pumps are similar to the vacuolar proton pumps that acidify intracellular organelles, but in the osteoclast they are exteriorized to increase the extracellular hydrogen ion concentration.[17] The hydrogen ions dissociate from carbonic acid, which is synthesized by carbonic anhydrase; the bicarbonate generated by this dissociation is removed from the cell by chloride-bicarbonate exchange. Ion pumps can transport the dissolved calcium from the bone surface through the cell to the extracellular fluid.

However, calcium can also reach the extracellular fluid directly if the sealing zone is disrupted. The proteolytic enzymes produced by the osteoclast include lysosomal enzymes and metalloproteinases. Lysosomal proteases can degrade collagen at the low pH present in the ruffled border area. Cathepsin K is probably the most important of these.[18] Metalloproteinases, which are active at neutral pH, have also been detected at the resorption site.[19] In trabecular bone, osteoclasts characteristically resorb to a limited depth and then move laterally to produce irregular, plate-like resorption areas that are termed Howship's lacunae. In cortical remodeling, the path of directed resorption is longer, possibly because of renewal of osteoclasts from hematopoietic cells brought to the site through the haversian canal.

BONE REMODELING AND ITS REGULATION

After peak bone mass has been achieved, the cellular activity in the skeleton is largely devoted to an orderly sequence of bone resorption and formation, termed *remodeling*.[20, 21] This process produces plate-like structures on trabecular surfaces and cylindrical structures (osteons) in cortical bone called *basic multicellular* or *basic structural units*. The remodeling cycle can be divided into four steps: (1) activation, (2) resorption, (3) reversal, and (4) formation (Figs. 27–8 and 27–9).

Similar sequences are seen in trabecular and cortical remodeling. In young adults, this cycle is tightly coupled and the amount of new bone formed by osteoblasts is equal to the amount that is resorbed by osteoclasts. Postmenopausal and age-related bone loss begins when resorption increases and formation no longer keeps pace. The activation of new remodeling sites may also increase with age.

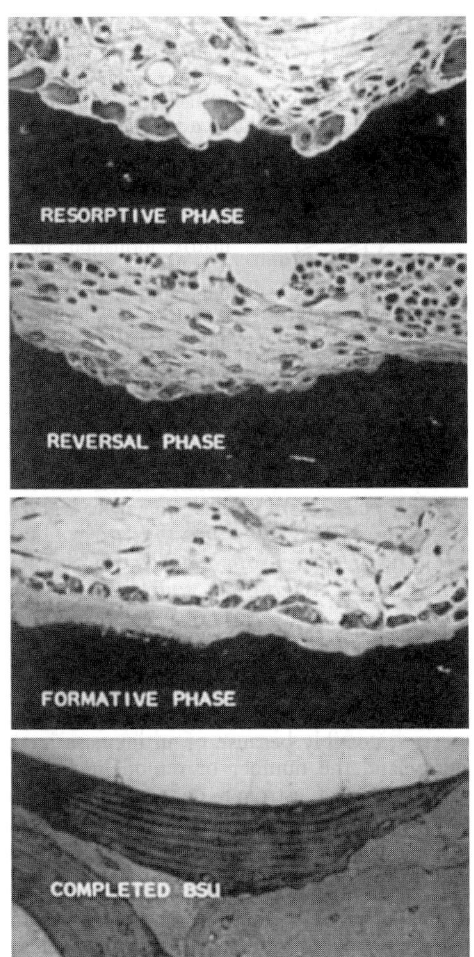

Figure 27–8. Stages of bone remodeling. The resorptive, reversal, and formative phases of bone remodeling and a completed bone structural unit (BSU) on a trabecular surface are illustrated. The morphologic features of the activation step have not been defined. (Courtesy of Dr. Robert E. Schenk, University of Berne, Switzerland.)

Although 80% of skeletal mass is cortical bone, the surface area of cortical bone is only about one fifth that of cancellous bone. Moreover, more osteoclast precursor cells are available in cancellous bone and on the endosteal surfaces of cortical bone. Consequently, turnover is greater on these surfaces than on those of periosteal bone, which normally undergoes little remodeling. However, subperiosteal resorption can be activated in hyperparathyroidism, and the periosteal surface contains preosteoblasts that may become active late in life and cause an age-related increase in the periosteal diameter of long bones. This periosteal expansion may maintain bone strength and compensate for losses at the endosteal surfaces and in cancellous bone.

Remodeling can be activated by both systemic and local factors and probably serves several physiologic functions. Changes in mechanical force can activate remodeling to improve the skeletal strength. Remodeling may serve to repair microdamage, particularly in cortical bone, and this may explain the fact that remodeling is sustained in the aging skeleton.[22] However, loss of osteocytes with age may impair this response.[23] Systemic hormones influence bone remodeling to regulate the movement of mineral from bone to extracellular fluid and as part of their overall effects on growth. Local factors mediate the response to mechanical forces and may also modulate the effects of systemic hormones.

Calcium-Regulating Hormones

Parathyroid Hormone

PTH acts on bone to stimulate resorption but does not act on osteoclasts in the absence of cells of the osteoblastic lineage; moreover, PTH receptors are abundant on osteoblasts but not on osteoclasts. PTH acts on osteoblasts to cause cell contraction; to induce immediate-early response genes, including c-*fos* and the inducible form of prostaglandin G/H synthase (cyclooxygenase); and to increase the synthesis of local mediators, including insulin-like growth factor I (IGF-I) and IL-6.[24] High concentrations of PTH in vitro inhibit expression of type I collagen, but intermittent administration of PTH in vivo or in vitro can stimulate bone formation. PTH induces production of RANKL by cells of the osteoblast lineage and thereby increases osteoclastogenesis and the activity of osteoclasts. In some settings, PTH increases proliferation of cells of the osteoblast lineage and decreases their death by apoptosis.[25]

Vitamin D

The hormonal form of vitamin D—$1,25(OH)_2D$—is necessary for intestinal calcium and phosphorus absorption and, therefore, for mineralization. This form of vitamin D also has effects on the skeleton,[26] but its physiologic role in bone remodeling is not clear. By increasing RANKL production by osteoblasts, it is a potent stimulator of osteoclast formation in cell culture, and high concentrations increase osteocalcin synthesis by osteoblasts and inhibit collagen synthesis. Lower concentrations may increase bone formation but not to the extent seen with intermittent administration of PTH.

Calcitonin

Calcitonin inhibits bone resorption by acting directly on the osteoclast but appears to play a small role in the regulation of bone turnover in adults. Bone mass is not greatly altered in patients with medullary thyroid carcinoma, who have an excess of calcitonin production, or in athyreotic patients receiving adequate thyroid hormone replacement, who have low calcitonin levels.[27] In fact, bone turnover is increased in patients with medullary thyroid carcinoma.[28] Nevertheless, subtle alterations in calcitonin production or response may play a role in metabolic bone disease.

Other Systemic Hormones

Growth Hormone

Deficiency and excess of growth hormone have marked effects on skeletal growth.[29] Growth hormone increases both circulating and local levels of IGF-I, which mediates the skeletal effects of growth hormone. Both exogenous growth hormone and IGF-I increase bone remodeling. Growth hormone also stimulates cartilage growth, probably through an increase in local IGF production and direct stimulation of cartilage cell proliferation. Whether systemic IGF plays a role in skeletal growth is not known, but low levels of growth hormone receptors are present in bone cells and administration of IGF-I together with its major binding protein, IGFBP-3, can increase skeletal growth.

Glucocorticoids

Glucocorticoids exert biphasic effects on bone formation and resorption.[30] In vivo, glucocorticoids may increase bone resorption indirectly by diminishing calcium absorption and producing secondary hyperparathyroidism. Low levels of glucocorticoids increase osteoclastic activity in organ culture, whereas

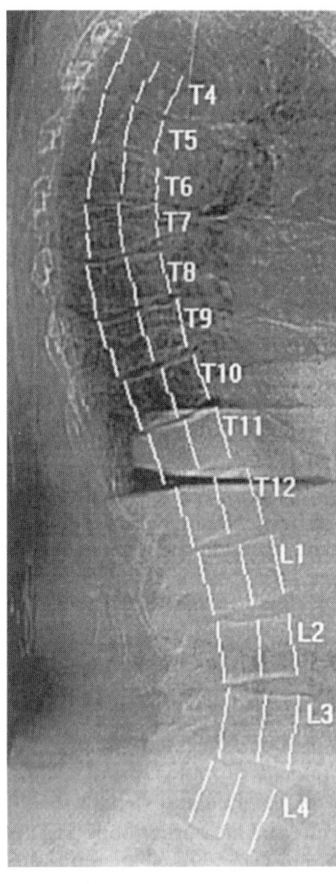

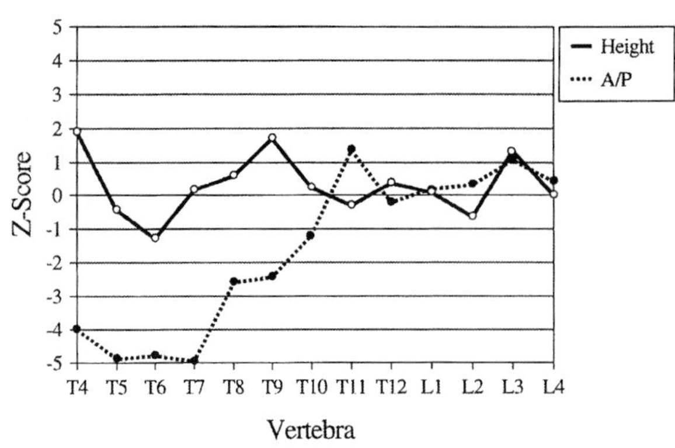

Region	HEIGHT (mm)	Z	A/P Ratio	Z
T4 >	18.6	+1.9	0.74	-4.0
T5 >	16.2	-0.5	0.69	-4.9
T6 >	15.6	-1.4	0.66	-4.8
T7 >	17.6	+0.2	0.64	-5.0
T8	18.7	+0.7	0.77	-2.6
T9	20.7	+1.8	0.81	-2.5
T10	20.0	+0.2	0.88	-1.2
T11	20.5	-0.3	1.00	+1.4
T12	23.5	+0.4	0.93	-0.2
L1	24.4	+0.1	0.96	+0.2
L2	23.9	-0.7	1.01	+0.4
L3	28.3	+1.5	1.07	+1.1
L4	25.7	+0.1	1.07	+0.5

Figure 27–10. Use of dual-energy x-ray absorptiometry for vertebral body morphometry. Posterior vertebral body heights and the ratio of anterior to posterior (A/P) height are presented in terms of standard deviation scores. Note that minor anterior wedging alone may not indicate an osteoporotic fracture. (Courtesy of Dr. Richard B. Mazess.)

older patients are subject to errors caused by aortic calcification and osteoarthritic changes.[72]

The last disadvantage can be overcome by performing lateral densitometry of the lumbar spine, but this measurement is less precise. Newer DXA systems may also have sufficient resolution to measure changes in vertebral body height in thoracic as well as the lumbar vertebrae. Detection of the new vertebral compressions by this method may be particularly useful in follow-up for patients with vertebral fractures (Fig. 27–10).[73, 74]

Quantitative Computed Tomography

QCT, which employs instruments available in most radiology departments, can be used to assess true bone density (g/cm^3) and to separate cancellous and cortical bone in the vertebral body. QCT has also been used to measure cortical and trabecular bone density in the appendicular skeleton. The radiation exposure (100 to 300 mrem) is larger than for DXA, and the precision and accuracy are lower but within the acceptable range. A major disadvantage may be cost, but this varies widely.

Peripheral Densitometry

A number of methods to measure bone mass and density in the appendicular skeleton have been developed that are less expensive, faster, and more portable than DXA or QCT.[75] Measurement of cortical bone in the shaft of the radius and ulna and trabecular bone in the distal radius by radiography, photon absorptiometry, or CT scanning is precise and can be used to predict fracture risk in populations, but it cannot predict BMD of the spine and hip in individual patients. The advantages of ultrasonography, particularly of the calcaneus, are that (1) it does not use x-rays, (2) it is rapid and portable, and (3) it has the capability of predicting fracture risk. These measurements may be particularly useful for large-scale screening programs.

Biochemical Measurements

One of the most important advances in metabolic bone disease has been the development of more accurate biochemical measurements that can assess rates of bone formation and resorption. In population studies, these methods have been used to show that increased turnover (i.e., high rates of both resorption and formation) correlates inversely with bone mass and may predict a high rate of bone loss and an increased risk of fracture.[76, 77] However, markers currently available are characterized by a wide normal range and considerable variability, which limit their use in individual patients.[78] The most common current clinical use of these assays in care of patients is to obtain a more rapid assessment of the response to antiresorptive agents, which can be detected at 3 to 6 months, before changes in BMD.[79, 80]

Markers of Bone Formation

Alkaline Phosphatase

Total serum alkaline phosphatase is measured to assess osteoblastic activity in Paget's disease, primary hyperparathyroidism, osteomalacia, and rickets. An immunoassay that selectively measures the bone isoenzyme may increase the usefulness of this test in osteoporosis, in which changes in osteoblastic activity are smaller. High bone-specific alkaline phosphatase values have been shown to predict bone loss and fractures.[81]

Osteocalcin

Osteocalcin, a bone carboxyglutamic acid–containing protein, is one of the few proteins that are relatively specific for skeletal tissue. A fraction of the osteocalcin synthesized by osteoblasts is released into the circulation. Carboxyl-terminal cleavage of the molecule may occur after release, but both the intact and amino-terminal portions can be measured by specific immunoassays. Serum osteocalcin correlates with skeletal growth rates in childhood and puberty and is increased when bone turnover is accelerated (e.g., in hyperparathyroidism, hyperthyroidism). In Paget's disease, osteocalcin is elevated to a lesser degree than alkaline phosphatase.

Because osteocalcin production is increased by $1,25(OH)_2D$, the levels may be low in osteomalacia and rickets even when alkaline phosphatase is elevated. Conversely, osteocalcin levels may be selectively reduced in patients given glucocorticoids to a greater degree than other formation markers. Undercarboxylated osteocalcin is present in vitamin K and vitamin D deficiency, increases with age, and is associated with increased fracture risk.

Procollagen Peptides

The amino-terminal and carboxyl-terminal extension peptides of procollagen (see Fig. 27–2), which are removed during processing of collagen, are released into the circulation. The N-terminal propeptide assay may be more sensitive and reliable than the C-terminal assay.[82] Their measurement is an index of total-body synthesis of collagen, the bulk of which is derived from bone. Procollagen peptide levels correlate with histologic measures of bone formation. Levels of procollagen peptides are high in infants and may provide a clinically useful index of growth.

Markers of Bone Resorption

Calcium

Measurement of fasting urinary calcium excretion is convenient but shows wide variation, reflecting the net result of intestinal absorption, bone resorption, and mineralization as well as renal tubular handling of calcium. Markedly increased urinary calcium occurs with a marked increase in osteoclastic activity with little change in formation, for example, in some patients with osteolytic bone metastases.

Hydroxyproline

Collagen degradation releases hydroxyproline into the circulation in both free and peptide-bound forms. Because bone resorption is by far the largest contributor to collagen breakdown, urinary hydroxyproline excretion has been used as a measure of bone resorption. However, 80% to 90% of the released hydroxyproline is metabolized, and hydroxyproline from collagen or gelatin in the diet is excreted in urine. Therefore, the sample should be obtained after a 12-hour fast or while the patient is receiving a gelatin-free diet. The hydroxyproline assay has been most useful in conditions in which resorption is markedly increased, such as Paget's disease, hyperparathyroidism, and malignancy. Because cross-link excretion can also be used in these conditions, hydroxyproline assays are used less frequently in clinical assessment.

Collagen Cross-Links

Unlike hydroxyproline, the pyridinoline and deoxypyridinoline cross-links that stabilize collagen in the extracellular matrix (Fig. 27–11) are not metabolized but are excreted in the urine in either a free or peptide-bound form. The deoxypyridinoline cross-link is almost entirely derived from skeletal tissue and therefore is a more sensitive indicator of bone resorption than pyridinoline, which is also found in skin and other connective tissues.

Measurement of total urinary pyridinoline and particularly deoxypyridinoline by high-performance liquid chromatography (HPLC) probably provides the best measure of bone resorption but is expensive and time-consuming. Immunoassays have been developed for free pyridinoline and deoxypyridinoline as well as for peptides that include these cross-links and are released during resorption. These assays can now be carried out in serum as well as urine.[77, 80, 83, 84] Measurements correlate with bone turnover and change in response to agents that affect resorption. Hence, they are useful in assessing changes in resorption in the course of disease or in response to therapy. They may also be valuable in identifying patients with high bone turnover, who not only have low bone mass but also lose bone rapidly and are more likely to develop osteoporosis.

All of these assays have shown diurnal variation and may also be affected by meals. For urine assays, a fasting, second-voided morning urine sample is probably the most reliable.

Other Assays

Tartrate-resistant acid phosphatase is secreted by osteoclasts into serum and may be useful as a measure of bone resorption. Other collagen breakdown products, such as glycosylated hydroxylysines, may be used to assess resorption. Bone sialoprotein is a product of osteoblasts but apparently is not released during bone formation; it correlates best with other measures of bone resorption.[85]

Bone Biopsy

Transiliac bone biopsy can provide direct information about cancellous bone volume, the density of connections between trabecular plates (connectivity), and the function of bone cells.[86] The rate of bone formation and mineralization can be measured by this technique with the use of dynamic histomorphometry after tetracycline labeling (Fig. 27–12), but bone resorption is more difficult to assess by bone biopsy. Bone biopsy necessitates the use of a large needle with a 7- to 9-mm internal bore and the technical skill to obtain a sample that is not crushed or distorted. The sample must be processed without decalcification and stained appropriately. Unstained sections are needed in order for one to see fluorescent tetracycline labels. Special stains may be used to identify mast cells in mastocytosis or aluminum in renal osteodystrophy.

Bone biopsies are rarely indicated in the clinical care of patients with osteoporosis but may be indicated for patients with unusual skeletal lesions or for young men or women who have osteoporotic fractures with no evident secondary cause. However, therapeutic decisions can generally be made without biopsies. Biopsies may be indicated more frequently in renal osteodystrophy because the different forms of this disorder are managed differently.[87, 88]

Radiographs and Bone Scans

The use of radiographs and bone scans in diagnosis is covered under the discussions of specific disorders. Radiographs are very important in detecting fractures.[89] High-resolution radiographs and CT images have also been used to assess cortical porosity.

Bone scans using technetium 99m linked to a bisphosphonate are useful in localization of bone lesions.[90] Uptake is a

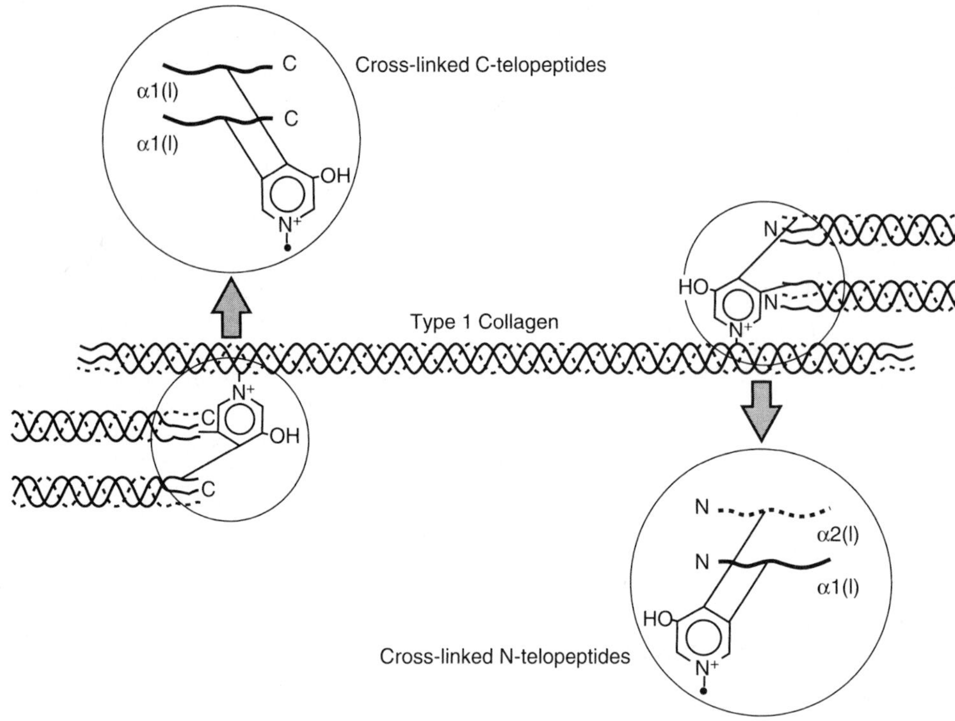

Figure 27–11. Collagen cross-links. Cross-links are formed between the COOH-terminal and NH_2-terminal nonhelical portions of collagen and adjacent helical molecules. Immunoassays are available for the pyridinoline and deoxypyridinoline molecules themselves and for the adjacent nonhelical peptides. (Redrawn from Eyre DR. The specificity of collagen cross-links as markers of bone and connective tissue degradation. Acta Orthop Scand 1995; 266:166–170.)

function of blood flow to the region and the amount of mineralizing bone. The test does not give information about the nature of the lesion but may serve as a guide for further studies. The current systems for MRI may be used to assess bone structure. Moreover, the type of tissue in the marrow or surrounding the bone can be identified. MRI is particularly useful in the detection of small soft tissue masses or vascular lesions in bone.

OSTEOPOROSIS

Primary Osteoporosis

Definition

Osteoporosis is by far the most common metabolic bone disease. One in two white and Asian postmenopausal women and at least one in eight older men and women of other racial backgrounds are likely to have an osteoporotic fracture at some time during their lifetime (Fig. 27–13). Osteoporosis has been better defined by the Consensus Development Conference[91] as "a disease characterized by low bone mass and microarchitectural deterioration of bone tissue, leading to enhanced bone fragility and a consequent increase in fracture risk."

Currently, diagnostic categories for postmenopausal women are based on measurements of BMD (Table 27–2).[92] These categories are clearly arbitrary but do give some indication of fracture risk. However, the risk of fracture at any given BMD increases markedly with age and can be affected by a number of other factors.[93]

A more rational approach to diagnosis and management might be to obtain an estimate of fracture risk based on all factors in individual patients. The use of T-scores to categorize BMD measurements as indicating the presence or absence of osteoporosis is complicated by the fact that the estimation of fracture risk is both site and method specific.[94] Despite great advances, there are still many unresolved questions in defining and diagnosing osteoporosis.[95]

Epidemiology

Osteoporosis has been considered a disorder of postmenopausal women of Northern European descent because they have high rates of fractures.[96, 97] However, the frequency of osteoporotic fractures is also high in other populations and is likely to increase further as life expectancy increases. Moreover, the age-adjusted incidence of hip fractures around the world is rising, possibly related to increasing industrialization and decreasing physical activity. Most of the epidemiologic data are for hip fractures, but vertebral fractures are equally common. In one study, the lifetime risk of osteoporotic fractures of the hip, spine, or wrist after age 50 years was about 40% in women and 13% in men (Table 27–3). The temporal pattern of the increase in fracture incidence differs for the hip, spine, and wrist (Fig. 27–14).

The incidence of osteoporotic fractures varies among populations, possibly because of variations in skeletal architecture and turnover and in bone mass. For example, in South Africa the incidence of hip fracture in Bantus is only a fraction of that in whites, although the Bantus have lower bone densities.[98]

Pathogenesis

Understanding of the pathogenesis of primary osteoporosis remains largely descriptive.[99] Decreased bone mass and increased fragility can occur because of (1) failure to achieve optimal peak bone mass, (2) bone loss caused by increased bone resorption, or (3) inadequate replacement of lost bone as a result of decreased bone formation. Moreover, an analysis of the pathogenesis of osteoporosis must take into account the heterogeneity of clinical expression.

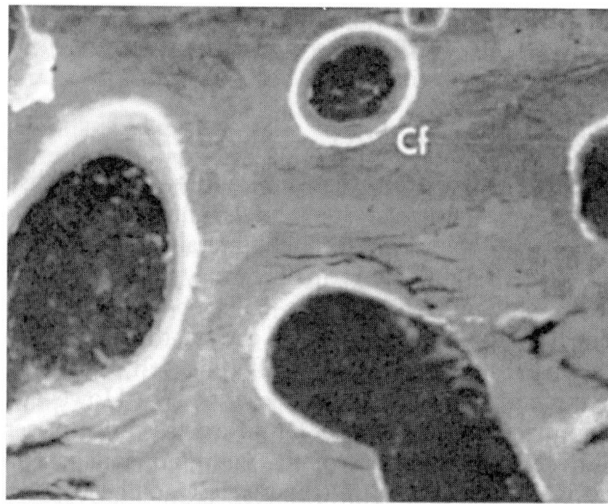

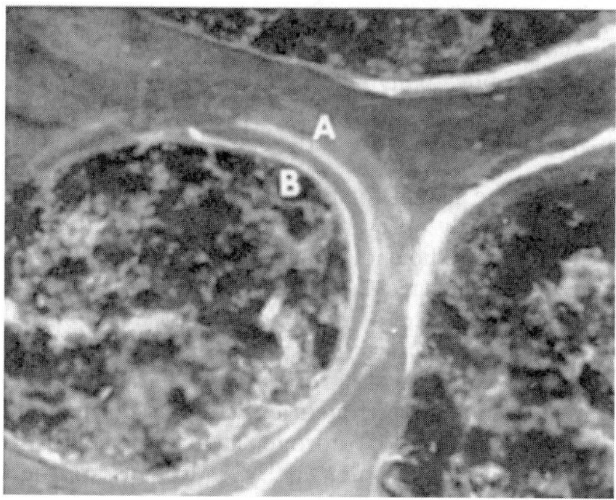

Figure 27–12. Tetracycline labels sites of active mineralization and is deposited at the calcification front (Cf) *(top)*. A double-label technique can be used to measure the rate of mineralization; label A was administered about 10 days before label B *(bottom)*. Undecalcified iliac crest, ultraviolet light, ×113. (From Aaron J. Histology and microanatomy of bone. In Nordin BEC [ed]. Calcium, Phosphate and Magnesium Metabolism. Edinburgh, Churchill Livingstone, 1976, pp 298–356.)

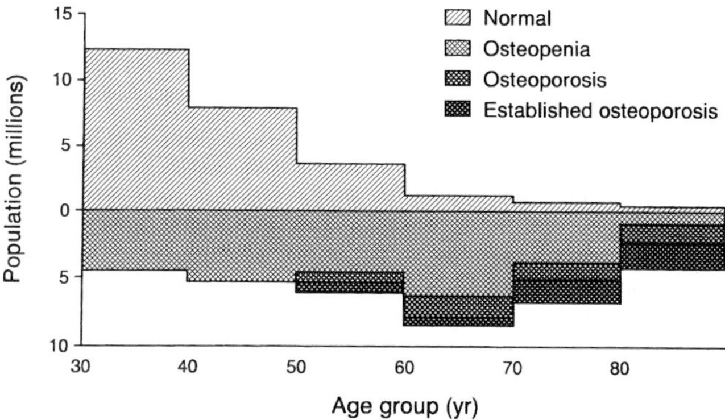

Figure 27–13. Estimation of the current prevalence of osteoporosis in the United States. On the basis of World Health Organization criteria, more than 9 million women in the United States have osteoporosis; more than half of these women have established osteoporosis with fractures. In addition, 17 million postmenopausal women have osteopenia (low bone mass) and are at risk for development of osteoporosis. (From Melton LJ. How many women have osteoporosis now? J Bone Miner Res 1995; 10:175–177.)

Table 27–2. Diagnostic Categories for Osteoporosis Based on Measurements of Bone Mineral Density and Bone Mineral Content

Category	Definition
Normal	A value for BMD or BMC ± 1 SD of the young adult reference mean
Low bone mass (osteopenia)	A value for BMD or BMC > 1 SD and < 2.5 SD lower than the young adult mean
Osteoporosis	A value for BMD or BMC > 2.5 SD lower than the young adult mean
Severe osteoporosis (established osteoporosis)	A value for BMD or BMC > 2.5 SD lower than the young adult mean in the presence of one or more fragility fractures

BMC, bone mineral content; BMD, bone mineral density; SD, standard deviation.

Inadequate Peak Bone Mass

Studies of twins suggest that genetic determinants are responsible for up to 85% of the variation in peak bone mass.[100, 101] However, genetic factors may be less important in determining fracture incidence in elderly people.[102] Polymorphisms of candidate genes, including vitamin D and estrogen receptors, collagen, cytokines, apolipoprotein E, and growth factors, have been analyzed to assess their possible roles in determining peak bone mass, remodeling, and fracture risk.[103–105] The results generally show small effects or are inconsistent. This problem may reflect the fact that it is difficult to determine the appropriate control population or that these polymorphisms may reflect effects of linked genes. Moreover, gene effects may be influenced by environmental factors.

A broader search for quantitative trait loci associated with differences in bone mass has identified a number of chromosomes that may be involved.[106] This approach is likely to lead to the identification of a number of genes that influence the skeleton and are determinants not only of peak bone mass but also of microarchitecture and turnover. Furthermore, microarchitectural features of the skeleton, such as the length of the femoral neck, are genetically determined and can influence fracture incidence.[107] High levels of physical activity and good calcium intake during childhood and puberty can help achieve maximal peak bone mass.[108]

Skeletal development involves a number of systemic hormones, including glucocorticoids, growth hormone, thyroid hormones, and particularly gonadal steroids. Gonadal hormones are responsible for the initiation of the pubertal growth

Table 27–3. Estimated Lifetime Fracture Risk in Women and Men from Rochester, Minnesota, at Age 50 Years

Fracture Site	Women (% [95% Confidence Interval])	Men (% [95% Confidence Interval])
Proximal femur	17.5 (16.8–18.2)	6.0 (5.6–6.5)
Vertebra*	15.6 (14.8–16.3)	5.0 (4.6–5.4)
Distal forearm	16.0 (15.7–16.7)	2.5 (2.2–3.1)
Any of the above	39.7 (38.7–40.6)	13.1 (12.4–13.7)

*Clinically diagnosed fractures.

From Melton LJ III, Chrischilles EA, Cooper C, et al. How many women have osteoporosis? J Bone Miner Res 1992; 7:1005–1010.

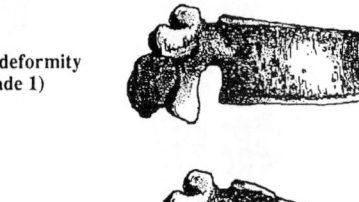

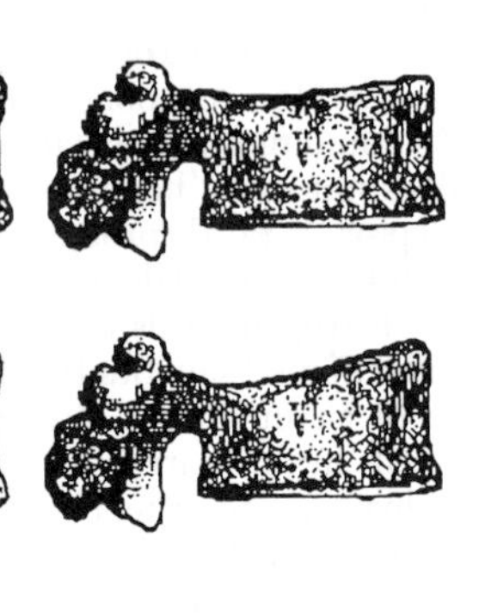

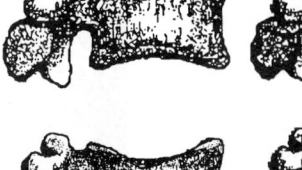

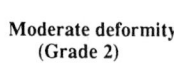

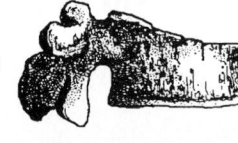

Figure 27–16. Types of vertebral compression fractures. Changes in vertebral height can be quantitated by measuring percent change or standard deviations from expected normal heights. (From Genant HK, Wu CY, van Kuijk C, Nevitt MC. Vertebral fracture assessment using a semiquantitative technique. J Bone Miner Res 1993; 8:1137–1148.)

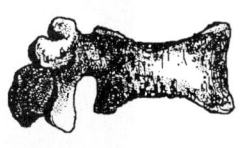

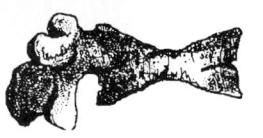

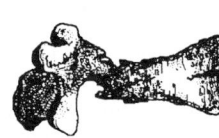

arthritis, particularly in the spinal facets. Osteoporosis itself rarely compresses nerve roots or the spinal cord. Although patients with severe osteoarthritis are somewhat less likely to have osteoporosis, these two common disorders commonly occur in the same patient.[153]

Hip Fracture

Fractures of the proximal femur are a major cause of morbidity and mortality in older people. Most fractures are in the femoral neck or at the base of the greater trochanter and are associated with trauma, although the trauma may be minimal. The risk is influenced by factors that increase the risk of falling and by the type of fall as well as the structure of the skeleton and surrounding soft tissue.[154] The increased incidence of hip fractures with age is caused both by increased falls and by continued bone loss. Vitamin D deficiency may play a role.[125]

Hip fracture is usually treated surgically, and the costs are substantial. In addition, perioperative and postoperative complications are associated with a 5% to 20% mortality rate. Many elderly patients cannot return to their previous level of activity after hip fracture and require long-term nursing home care. It is important to perform a diagnostic evaluation and to develop a prevention plan for these patients because a second hip fracture or a fragility fracture at another site is likely to occur. Unfortunately, most patients with hip fractures do not undergo evaluation or treatment to prevent progression of osteoporosis and additional fractures.[155]

Colles' Fracture

Colles' fractures of the distal radius, which is composed largely of trabecular bone, are caused by falling on the outstretched hand. The incidence in women begins to increase after age 40 years and may be associated with premenopausal and perimenopausal bone loss[156] and with genetic factors.[157] Unlike that of vertebral and hip fractures, the incidence of Colles' fractures in men does not increase with age. Colles' fractures usually heal well and only occasionally result in long-term morbidity. Women with a Colles' fracture should be assessed for osteoporosis so that an appropriate treatment plan can be provided.

Other Fractures

Fractures at any site, with the possible exception of the face and skull, can be associated with osteoporosis. Measurements of bone mass and further diagnostic work-up are indicated for all fractures that occur with minimal trauma.

Osteoporosis in Men

The incidence of hip and spine fractures in men increases with age and is about one third that in women.[158] Men often have vertebral deformities associated with trauma earlier in life. In men, the increase in hip fractures tends to occur later in life, and a higher proportion of men have definable secondary causes.[159] Bone histomorphometry shows increased resorption in most patients.[160]

Osteoporosis in men is associated with low estrogen and high SHBG levels.[161] Abnormalities of the IGF system are also implicated.[162, 163] A diagnostic work-up and therapeutic plan should be provided for men with fragility fractures, but this is rarely carried out in practice. Screening for osteoporosis in older men who do not have fractures has not yet been evaluated but may be justified now that preventive therapy is available.

Juvenile Osteoporosis

Juvenile osteoporosis[164] is a rare, self-limiting disease that can begin between the ages of 8 and 14 years with back pain and vertebral compression. If bone turnover is high, antiresorptive or anti-inflammatory agents may be beneficial.[165] However, deficient bone formation may be the critical defect leading to fractures in these children.[166] A mutation in type I collagen has been reported in one family with this disorder.[167] Spontaneous remission usually occurs, and the disorder usually does not lead to permanent deformity.

Idiopathic Osteoporosis

Osteoporosis with no obvious secondary cause in premenopausal women or younger men is called *idiopathic osteoporosis.* The term is not used consistently, and patients so defined include individuals with both high and low bone turnover.[168] Some patients have a transient, self-limited condition, whereas others have a progressive and disabling disease. Idiopathic osteoporosis can be associated with nonspecific inflammatory changes, and these cases may be caused by abnormal cytokine activity. A careful evaluation, including consideration of bone biopsy, should be made to search for secondary causes.

Osteoporosis in Pregnancy

Osteoporosis in pregnancy is rare and may represent bone disease that has been present before pregnancy. Ordinarily, maternal bone loss is modest,[169] presumably because the high levels of estrogen protect the skeleton and high levels of $1,25(OH)_2D$ stimulate calcium absorption. Bone loss can occur, however, particularly in adolescents.[170] Lactation is associated with transient bone loss but is not a risk factor for osteoporosis.[171]

Localized Osteoporosis

Immobilization is the most common cause of localized osteoporosis (see later). Transient osteoporosis of the hip has been reported in middle-aged men and in pregnancy.[172] Regional migratory osteoporosis can occur without immobilization, particularly in the lower extremities.[173] This phenomenon may be associated with local inflammation or autonomic dysfunction with vasomotor changes and hyperesthesia, a syndrome called *reflex sympathetic dystrophy.*[174]

Secondary Osteoporosis

The division of osteoporosis into primary and secondary forms is somewhat arbitrary.[175] For example, patients with diseases that lead to hypogonadism early in life are considered to have *secondary* osteoporosis, whereas osteoporosis in women with natural menopause and older men with low sex hormone levels is termed *primary.* Moreover, many patients have a combination of primary and secondary causes. Although most postmenopausal women and older men do not have a definable secondary cause, the few who do can be treated more effectively. Therefore, this possibility should be considered in every patient. There are many causes of secondary osteoporosis (Table 27–4), only a few of which are discussed here.

Table 27–4. Causes of Secondary Osteoporosis

Endocrine Disorders
Hyperparathyroidism
Cushing's syndrome
Hypogonadism
Hyperthyroidism
Prolactinoma
Diabetes mellitus
Acromegaly
Pregnancy and lactation
Hematopoietic Disorders
Plasma cell dyscrasias: multiple myeloma and macroglobulinemia
Systemic mastocytosis
Leukemias and lymphomas
Sickle cell disease and thalassemia minor
Lipidoses: Gaucher's disease
Myeloproliferative disorders: polycythemia
Connective Tissue Disorders
Osteogenesis imperfecta
Ehlers-Danlos syndrome
Marfan's syndrome
Homocystinuria and lysinuria
Menkes' syndrome
Scurvy
Drug-Induced Disorders
Glucocorticoids
Heparin
Anticonvulsants
Methotrexate, cyclosporine
Luteinizing hormone–releasing hormone (LHRH) agonist or antagonist therapy
Aluminum-containing antacids
Immobilization
Renal Disease
Chronic renal failure
Renal tubular acidosis
Nutritional and Gastrointestinal Disorders
Malabsorption
Total parenteral nutrition
Gastrectomy
Hepatobiliary disease
Chronic hypophosphatemia
Miscellaneous
Familial dysautonomia (Riley-Day syndrome)
Reflex sympathetic dystrophy

Glucocorticoid-Induced Osteoporosis

The most common form of secondary osteoporosis is that induced by exogenous glucocorticoids.[176] Cushing's syndrome, caused by an excess of endogenous glucocorticoids, is less common but may also involve osteoporosis at presentation. Patients with rheumatoid arthritis, chronic pulmonary disease, or gastrointestinal disease who receive exogenous glucocorticoids are at additional risk because disease-associated inflammation, poor nutrition, and immobilization can worsen bone loss. Glucocorticoid-induced osteoporosis is particularly common in postmenopausal women, presumably because they also have primary osteoporosis. However, fragility fractures can occur in any patient receiving moderate to high doses of glucocorticoids. The increased fracture risk appears within a few months of initiating therapy and rapidly declines after cessation of treatment.[177]

Glucocorticoid-induced osteoporosis is a result of both increased bone resorption and decreased bone formation. Increased resorption may be caused by decreased calcium absorption and the resulting secondary hyperparathyroidism. Decreased bone formation is probably caused by direct inhibition of osteoblasts, which are highly sensitive to glucocorticoids. For example, as little as 2.5 mg of prednisone given at bedtime can block the normal nocturnal rise in osteocalcin.[178] Glucocorticoids decrease osteoblast formation[179] and increase osteoblast and osteocyte apoptosis.[179, 180] Glucocorticoids also increase urinary calcium and phosphate and can inhibit gonadal hormone production by blocking gonadotropin release. Levels of testosterone are low in men receiving prednisone, 20 mg/day or more.[181] Exogenous glucocorticoids decrease secretion of corticotropin, thereby decreasing the production of adrenal androgens, which are the major precursors for estrogen formation in postmenopausal women.

Clinically, glucocorticoid-induced osteoporosis is similar to primary osteoporosis. Initial bone loss is predominantly trabecular and is best assessed in the spine or distal radius. However, rib fractures and aseptic necrosis of the femoral or humeral heads or the vertebrae are common in glucocorticoid-induced osteoporosis, although they are rare in primary osteoporosis. Glucocorticoid-induced osteoporosis can be reversible, particularly in young patients who are cured of Cushing's syndrome.[182] In patients who cannot discontinue glucocorticoid therapy, early preventive therapy may be effective. Bisphosphonates and PTH prevent bone loss in patients with glucocorticoid-induced osteoporosis.[183–185] Bisphosphonates also decrease fracture risk[186]; they may act in part by suppressing osteoblast and osteocyte apoptosis.[187]

Hypogonadism

Hypogonadism can occur in either men or women and has multiple causes. Patients with primary hypogonadism related to ovarian or testicular failure or secondary hypogonadism related to hypothalamic or pituitary disease lose bone rapidly and often have fragility fractures. The hypogonadotropic group includes patients with anorexia nervosa, athletic amenorrhea, prolactinoma, or lesions of the pituitary gland or hypothalamus, including tumors.[188] Undernutrition and hypercortisolism may also contribute to bone loss in anorexia nervosa and athletic amenorrhea. Loss of growth hormone may play a role in the osteoporosis of pituitary tumors. Patients with prolactinomas can secrete parathyroid hormone–related protein (PTHrP), which may cause bone loss.[189]

Drug-induced hypogonadism is increasing in frequency. The drugs implicated include long-acting progestins used for contraception in young women[190, 191] and gonadotropin-releasing hormone (GnRH) analogues used to block hormone production in women with endometriosis and men with prostate cancer.[192]

Other Endocrine Causes

Hyperthyroidism can produce bone loss[193]; however, the increase in formation in young persons is usually adequate, and, if the disease is treated early, changes in bone mass are small. Although there is no general increase in fracture risk in hyperthyroid patients, long-term thyroid hormone excess may lead to bone loss and increased risk of fractures.[31, 129] In individuals at risk for osteoporosis, primary hyperthyroidism may be missed or excessive amounts of exogenous thyroid hormone may be administered for many years. Osteoporosis has been seen in patients with growth hormone deficiency,[194] acromegaly, and prolactinoma and may be caused by gonadotropin deficiency and the loss of gonadal hormones with any large pituitary tumor.[195, 196]

Patients with insulin-dependent diabetes mellitus, especially men,[197, 198] often have low bone mass and diminished bone formation, but osteoporotic fractures are not a major problem. The role of non–insulin-dependent diabetes mellitus in the pathogenesis of osteoporosis is unclear. Bone loss may occur, particularly in patients who are not obese, but the data on fracture incidence are inconsistent.[199, 200]

Malignancy

Multiple myeloma and other lymphoproliferative malignancies can produce a clinical picture that resembles primary osteoporosis.[201, 202] It is particularly important to exclude myeloma in patients with rapidly progressive vertebral crush fracture syndrome. Metastases to the spine may also cause vertebral compression and should be considered in the differential diagnosis, particularly for patients with normal bone density. These lesions can usually be detected by MRI.[203]

Other Diseases

The incidence and severity of osteoporosis are increased in patients with chronic hepatic and intestinal disorders, probably for nutritional reasons and because these patients often receive glucocorticoids or other drugs that affect the skeleton.[204] Abnormal cytokine production may be a factor in inflammatory bowel disease.[205] Although it was initially thought that impairment of vitamin D function in hepatic and intestinal disease would cause osteomalacia, the most common lesion in such patients is osteoporosis. Unfortunately, these patients often do not respond to vitamin D supplementation. People with severe alcoholism can also have osteoporosis; however, low intakes of ethanol may be associated with increased bone mass and a decreased fracture risk.[206]

Mastocytosis causes both osteoporosis and osteosclerosis, and the number of mast cells may be increased in the marrow of patients with primary osteoporosis.[207–209] The functional significance of the mast cells is not known, although mast cells produce heparin, which can cause bone loss. Hyperplastic anemias, such as thalassemia, can also cause bone loss,[210] partly because of bone erosion by the marrow and partly because of hypogonadism associated with transfusion-induced hemochromatosis.[211] Osteoporosis after organ transplantation is common and results both from the underlying disease and from the drugs used to prevent graft rejection.[212]

Drugs

A number of drugs can produce osteoporosis.[213] Heparin stimulates bone resorption and inhibits bone formation and can cause osteoporosis. Patients receiving anticonvulsants, including phenytoin, barbiturates, and carbamazepine, often have low bone mass. Impairment of vitamin D metabolism has been described, but most patients have osteoporosis with normal mineralization. Immunosuppressive agents, such as cyclosporine and FK506, are associated with bone loss. GnRH analogues, which decrease production of gonadal hormones, can lead to osteoporosis.[214] Some agents used in cancer chemotherapy probably act both by inhibiting osteoblasts and by suppressing gonadal hormones.

Diagnosis

As indicated by the World Health Organization, osteoporosis can be diagnosed before fracture occurs by measuring bone density. The frequency of diagnosis, therefore, depends on the frequency, site, and timing of bone density measurements.[94] There is no general agreement about who should be screened or when screening should be done. A suggested approach is illustrated in Figure 27–17.

Screening at menopause is recommended for women who have multiple risk factors, such as low body weight or a personal or family history of fragility fractures (appendicular or axial fractures after a fall from standing height or less).[128, 215, 216] Universal screening of postmenopausal women after age 65 years has been recommended as cost-effective.[93] Bone density should also be measured in men and premenopausal women with fragility fractures. BMD measurements may also be useful in early postmenopausal women under consideration for hormone replacement therapy. Bone density measurements not only establish the severity of bone loss but also provide a baseline for monitoring the patient's therapeutic response. The test may also enhance health-related behavior.[217] The subsequent work-up should be the same whether osteoporosis is diagnosed on the basis of screening or after the finding of a fragility fracture.

The history should include a detailed analysis of calcium intake and nutrition, changes in height or weight, physical activity and lifestyle, smoking history, menstrual and reproductive history, and personal or family history of fragility fractures or other metabolic or endocrine disorders that may affect the

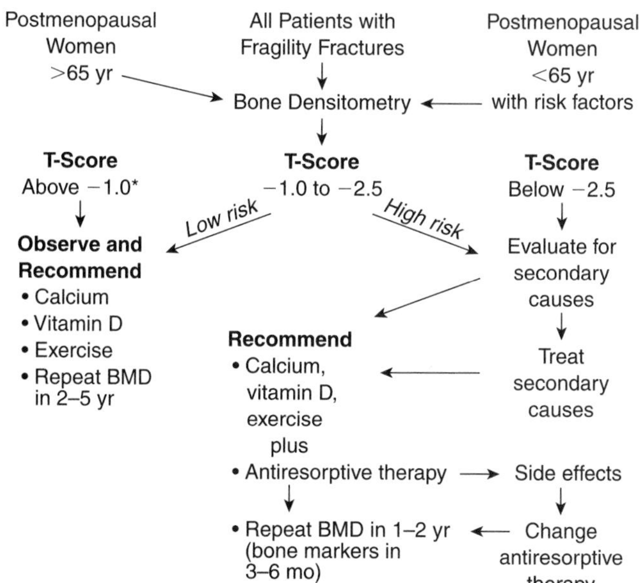

Figure 27–17. Diagnosis and management of osteoporosis. The diagram outlines an approach based largely on evidence from studies of postmenopausal white women, with dual-energy x-ray absorptiometry used to measure bone mineral density (BMD). Its application to other populations, including patients with secondary osteoporosis and other methods of assessing BMD, is not established.

skeleton. Physical examination should include a careful height measurement, assessment of the spine, and evaluation for thyroid or adrenal disease.

Radiologic assessment of fractures may be possible using DXA[218] as well as ordinary radiographs. In addition, MRI or CT may be indicated if there are neurologic changes or if fractures are associated with normal bone density, raising the possibility of malignancy.

A minimal laboratory screen should include measurement of serum calcium, preferably as ionized calcium or with albumin to permit correction for protein-bound calcium and fasting calcium excretion (most easily measured as the calcium/creatinine ratio in the second-voided morning specimen). Appropriate tests to exclude secondary causes of osteoporosis should be based on the history and physical findings. Serum phosphorus and alkaline phosphatase are useful in ruling out hyperparathyroidism and osteomalacia. Measurements of vitamin D metabolites, urine phosphorus, and PTH are indicated if the screening test results are abnormal. Serum electrophoresis, blood count, and erythrocyte sedimentation rate can help to rule out myeloma, and thyroid function should be assessed. Laboratory studies for Cushing's syndrome are indicated in patients with suggestive clinical features. Measurements of gonadal and pituitary hormones are indicated for younger patients with osteoporosis. Gluten-sensitive enteropathy should be ruled out in patients with weight loss or frequent bowel movements.

Despite the inverse correlation between markers of bone resorption and formation and bone mass, these measurements have wide variations and cannot substitute for measurements of BMD in the diagnosis of osteoporosis. Because elevated values of both resorption and formation markers do indicate increased risk for bone loss and fractures, these measurements may become useful in determining the need for therapy, particularly if they can be made more accurate and less expensive.

Prevention and Therapy

Although it is important to relieve pain and to limit the impact of deformities in established osteoporosis, the primary goal of treatment is to prevent fractures. Therefore, prevention and therapy are considered together.

Nutrition and Calcium Supplementation

The calcium intakes recommended for prevention and treatment of osteoporosis range from 1 to 2 g/day.[219] In children and adolescents, intakes of 1000 to 1200 mg/day are recommended.[108] Most studies indicate that calcium supplementation slows bone loss,[220] and there is limited evidence that calcium supplementation alone can decrease fracture risk.[221] Moreover, low calcium intakes in the presence of low calcium absorption increase the risk of hip fractures.[222] High calcium intakes are generally safe, although it may be worthwhile to check urinary calcium levels.

There is no clear advantage for any particular calcium formulation. *Calcium carbonate* is inexpensive and, when taken with meals, is usually well absorbed, even in patients with achlorhydria.[223] *Calcium citrate* and other salts may be absorbed better than calcium carbonate in the fasting state.

It is also worthwhile to include foods high in calcium in the diet. Patients should be informed about the calcium content of the major food sources, such as dairy products.

Vitamin D intake should be at least 400 U/day, and up to 2000 U/day is probably safe; higher levels may produce hypercalciuria or hypercalcemia. Calcium and vitamin D increase bone mass, decrease seasonal bone loss,[224] and decrease the incidence of fractures, particularly in populations likely to have deficient intakes or limited sun exposure.[221, 225] Other forms of vitamin D have been used, including calcidiol (25[OH]D), calcitriol ($1,25[OH]_2D$), and $1\alpha(OH)D$, but there is no direct evidence that these are superior to ordinary vitamin D, which is less expensive.[226] Dietary intakes of other minerals and of vitamins C and K, which are important for bone matrix synthesis, as well as protein should be adequate.

Exercise, Lifestyle, and Prevention of Falls

The role of exercise in treatment of osteoporosis has not been defined. On the basis of limited data, ½ hour of weight-bearing exercise per day is recommended for patients who can tolerate it. Epidemiologic data suggest that lifetime leisure exercise is associated with higher BMD at the hip but may have no effect on fracture incidence.[227–229] Patients are often better able to develop and maintain a suitable exercise program under the supervision of a physical therapist. Patients should also be instructed in body mechanics and posture in order to minimize musculoskeletal damage and the likelihood of falls. They should stop smoking and limit their intake of alcohol.

Medicines that cause prolonged sedation[230] or postural hypertension should be avoided in elderly people. Older patients at high risk may be able to avoid hip fractures by wearing a hip protector.[231] Help should be provided for coping with osteoporosis and for designing a lifestyle that maintains function and minimizes fracture risk.[232] Excessive sodium intake should be avoided because it can increase urinary calcium excretion.

Management of Fractures

Fractures of the hip as well as other appendicular fractures are generally treated surgically. Vertebral fractures may require transient bed rest. A careful but intensive program of rehabilitation is critical in patients with fractures of the hip and spine.

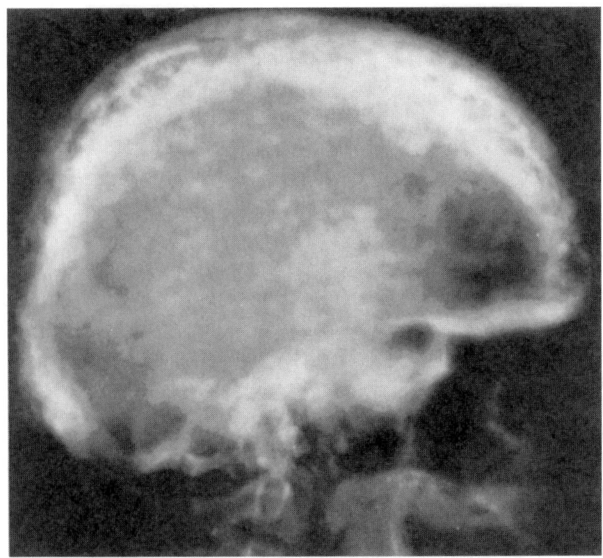

Figure 27–22. Radiograph of the skull of a patient with advanced Paget's disease showing thickening, disordered new bone formation (cotton-wool patches), and basilar impression. (From Singer FR. Paget's Disease of Bone. New York, Plenum, 1977.)

centration or after a routine radiograph. In older persons with deformities or bone pain, the diagnosis should be considered and a careful family history and review of the musculoskeletal system by both history and physical examination should be obtained. A bone scan should be carried out to localize possible pagetic sites. Positive scans do not necessarily indicate Paget's disease, and radiographs should be obtained to confirm that Paget's disease is the cause of the increased uptake. Rarely, pagetic sites in bone are not evident on bone scan because there is a minimal formation response in the lesion. Such pagetic lesions in the skull are termed *osteoporosis circumscripta*.

An audiogram should be obtained in patients with involvement of the petrous bone or in those with complaints of hearing loss. Because of the possible increased incidence of hyperparathyroidism, ionized calcium levels should be measured in the initial work-up. Monostotic Paget's disease, particularly in the vertebrae, may be difficult to distinguish from metastatic disease. In addition, some patients with vertebral disease may have impingement on the spinal canal. In these individuals, the area should be examined by CT or MRI. Bone biopsies can be useful in atypical cases. An ordinary aspiration biopsy sometimes yields the giant osteoclasts that are pathognomonic of Paget's disease. Samples of bone that show the irregular *marble bone pattern* can also be diagnostic.

After the initial evaluation has been completed, the patient can usually be monitored biochemically by serial measurements of total or bone-specific alkaline phosphatase and a marker of bone resorption.[319] Urinary hydroxyproline measurements may be used, as may serum or urinary levels of type I collagen breakdown products such as C-telopeptide or N-telopeptide or measurements of pyridinoline or deoxypyridinoline in the urine. Although 24-hour urine measurements of hydroxyproline are often recommended, a morning fasting measurement avoids the dual problems of collecting a 24-hour sample and maintaining a diet free of gelatin products.

Therapy

In the past, patients with Paget's disease were often simply observed until symptoms were clear-cut or until there was evidence of progression in critical areas of the skeleton. With the newer bisphosphonates, treatment is instituted earlier. Pamidronate is available for IV use. The recommended dose for Paget's disease is 30 mg infused over 4 hours on 3 consecutive days for a total of 90 mg. Patients with more extensive disease may require retreatment and should be evaluated by measuring levels of bone turnover markers at regular intervals. IV pamidronate is generally safe, although transient fever and a transient increase in bone pain may occur. Rare idiosyncratic reactions include uveitis.

Other bisphosphonates are given orally. Alendronate (40 mg/day for 6 months), risedronate (30 mg/day for 2 months), and tiludronate (400 mg/day for 3 months) are approved in the United States. As with pamidronate, patients may require repeated therapy with oral bisphosphonates after a drug-free period that varies with each agent (6 months for alendronate, 2 months for risedronate, and 3 months for tiludronate). Oral bisphosphonates need to be taken in a manner that minimizes the development of esophagitis or interactions with food and other therapeutics in the stomach. These treatments have largely replaced therapy with calcitonin, etidronate, or plicamycin. All of these agents act by inhibiting osteoclastic activity, and the earliest indication of therapeutic response is a drop in resorption markers followed by a decrease in formation markers.

The indications for treatment are pain that can be attributed to Paget's disease and deformities that might produce neurologic changes or are likely to lead to fracture, such as the osteolytic *flame lesion* or *blade of grass lesion* in weight-bearing bones (see Fig. 27–20). Hearing loss may be an indication for therapy, although most patients do not show major improvement after treatment.

Patients with heart disease and extensive Paget's disease should be treated in the hope that decreased pagetic activity will improve management. With the advent of safe and effective therapy, patients with mild to moderate disease, particularly those with the potential for complications (i.e., those with lesions in weight-bearing bone, the vertebral bodies, or the base of the skull), are being treated before symptoms develop. Early treatment is logical in young patients with Paget's disease because it is hoped that therapy may prevent progression. However, proof of this hypothesis is not conclusive.

Many patients with Paget's disease have pain associated with joint damage that does not respond to antipagetic therapy. These patients may respond to anti-inflammatory drugs. If osteoarthritis is advanced, knee and hip replacement may be appropriate but biochemical remission should be obtained before surgery.

A high calcium intake may be useful in Paget's disease. Bisphosphonate therapy can lower the serum calcium level and cause secondary hyperparathyroidism, which is probably not advantageous; increased calcium intake may prevent this development. Moreover, calcium loading can produce an increase in endogenous calcitonin secretion that may have beneficial effects. It is also important to monitor serum 25(OH)D levels periodically in patients with Paget's disease who are to be treated with bisphosphonates, as osteomalacia is not uncommon in the elderly population who are at risk for this condition and low serum vitamin D levels may exacerbate the potential of bisphosphonates to cause hypocalcemia. Urinary calcium should be checked before calcium or vitamin D supplementation is given because an increase in the incidence of renal stones has been reported in pagetic patients.

Hereditary Hyperphosphatasia

Although hereditary hyperphosphatasia has been termed *juvenile Paget's disease*, it involves all of the skeleton and develops in infants.[320] The serum alkaline phosphatase levels are very high. There are severe bone deformities, and the histologic appearance resembles that of Paget's disease with high bone turnover, although the osteoclasts are not enlarged. Treatment with bisphosphonates or calcitonin may be effective in reducing bone turnover and improving bone lesions. A new familial form with expansile long bone lesions has been described.[321, 322]

OSTEOGENESIS IMPERFECTA

Osteogenesis imperfecta, or *brittle bone disease*, is a heterogeneous, congenital disorder in which increased bone fragility leads to fractures and deformity.[323] It ranges in severity from a lethal perinatal form to a mild disorder that results only in increased fractures.

Pathogenesis

Most patients with osteogenesis imperfecta have defects in the genes for *type I* collagen. Bones, ligaments, skin, sclerae, and teeth are affected. The incidence of osteogenesis imperfecta is estimated to be 1 in 200,000 to 500,000. The heterogeneity of the features is caused by the variety of genetic defects, although phenotypic variation occurs even with the same genetic abnormality (see Table 27–5). The more severe forms, *type II* and *type III*, involve mutations in the helical portion of the collagen molecule that prevent normal assembly and produce unstable triple helices. Point mutations in this portion of the collagen gene can be associated with mild disease *(type IV)*.

Type I osteogenesis imperfecta differs from the other forms in that there is usually a deletion of one allele of the $\alpha1$(I) procollagen gene, resulting in decreased collagen production but a normal molecular structure.[324] This disorder is of particular interest because familial osteoporosis may also exhibit such defects.[325] Bone biopsies show decreased cortical width and trabecular bone volume, increased turnover, and decreased bone formation in patients with type I disease.[326] The disorder in a subgroup of patients with low turnover and ligamentous calcifications has been designated type V osteoporosis imperfecta.[327]

Classification and Clinical Features

The classification devised by Sillence and modified by Byers[323] is summarized in Table 27–5. In addition to the bone involvement, there may be ligament laxity, joint hypermobility, and easy bruising. Dentin formation is often abnormal, and the teeth are fragile and discolored. Blue sclerae are a variable manifestation and do not correlate with severity. Because of the thoracic deformities, patients with severe manifestations are predisposed to pulmonary infections and usually have a shortened life span. Intelligence is not affected, and individuals with marked deformities can be highly productive if appropriate conditions are provided.

Diagnosis

In patients with moderate to severe disease, the clinical features make the diagnosis relatively straightforward; in patients with the milder forms, however, the diagnosis may be missed. In children without deformities, multiple fractures are usually attributed to trauma; in infants, the presence of such fractures may lead to an accusation of parental abuse. In the absence of typical clinical features, the diagnosis can be made only biochemically. Culture of fibroblasts from skin biopsies and analysis of the collagen by gel electrophoresis can point to a defect, and the techniques of molecular biology can identify the mutation more specifically. This analysis is useful for families because specific deoxyribonucleic acid (DNA) polymorphisms may allow prenatal diagnosis if the mutation has already been identified in other affected family members.

In children and adolescents with multiple fractures but no deformity, measurements of bone density and turnover may point toward the diagnosis. In the type I disorder, both bone density and serum type I procollagen peptide levels are likely to be decreased.[328] However, because excretion of collagen cross-links is increased in most types of osteogenesis imper-

Table 27–5. Classification of Osteogenesis Imperfecta

Type	Clinical Features	Inheritance	Common Biochemical Abnormality
I	Normal stature, little or no deformity, blue sclerae, hearing loss in 50% of families Dentinogenesis imperfecta may distingush a subset.	AD	Nonfunctional allele of the $\alpha1$(I) procollagen gene (*COL1A1*)
II	Lethal in the perinatal period; minimal calvarial mineralization, beaded ribs, compressed femurs, marked long bone deformity, platyspondyly	AD (new mutations) AR (rare)	Substitution of glycine in triple helix of *COL1A1* or *COL1A2*
III	Progressively deforming bones, usually with moderate deformity at birth Scleral hue varies, often lightening with age Dentinogenesis imperfecta common, hearing loss common Stature very short	AD AR (uncommon)	Substitution of glycine in triple helix of *COL1A1* or *COL1A2*
IV	Normal sclerae, mild to moderate bone deformity, and variable short stature; dentinogenesis imperfecta is common and hearing loss occurs in some families	AD	Substitution of glycine in triple helix of *COL1A1* or *COL1A2*; exon skipping in *COL1A2*

AD, autosomal dominant; AR autosomal recessive.

Classification from Sillence et al, as modified from Byers PH. Osteogenesis imperfecta. In Royce PM, Steinman B (eds). Connective Tissue and Its Heritable Disorders: Molecular, Genetic and Medical Aspects. New York, Wiley-Liss, 1993, pp 317–350. Reprinted by permission of Wiley-Liss, Inc., a subsidiary of John Wiley & Sons, Inc.

357. Lala R, Matarazzo P, Bertelloni S, et al. Pamidronate treatment of bone fibrous dysplasia in nine children with McCune-Albright syndrome. Acta Paediatr 2000; 89:188–193.
358. Zacharin M, O'Sullivan M. Intravenous pamidronate treatment of polyostotic fibrous dysplasia associated with the McCune-Albright syndrome. J Pediatr 2000; 137:403–409.
359. Hou WS, Bromme D, Zhao Y, et al. Characterization of novel cathepsin K mutations in the pro and mature polypeptide regions causing pyknodysostosis. J Clin Invest 1999; 103:731–738.
360. Fujita Y, Nakata K, Yasui N, et al. Novel mutations of the cathepsin K gene in patients with pyknodysostosis and their characterization. J Clin Endocrinol Metab 2000; 85:425–431.
361. Haagerup A, Hertz JM, Christensen MF. Cathepsin K gene mutations and 1q21 haplotypes in patients with pyknodysostosis in an outbred population. Eur J Hum Genet 2000; 8:431–436.
362. Hernandez MV, Peris P, Guanabens N, et al. Biochemical markers of bone turnover in Camurati-Engelmann disease: a report on four cases in one family. Calcif Tissue Int 1997; 61:48–51.
363. Janssens K, Gershoni-Baruch R, Van Hul E. Localisation of the gene causing diaphyseal dysplasia (Camurati-Engelmann disease) to chromosome 19q13. J Med Genet 2000; 37:245–249.
364. Janssens K, Gershoni-Baruch R, Guanabens N, et al. Mutations in the gene encoding the latency-associated peptide of TGF-beta 1 cause Camurati-Engelmann disease. Nat Genet 2000; 26:273–275.
365. Balemans W, Van Den Ende J, Freire Paes-Alves F, et al. Localization of the gene for sclerosteosis to the van Buchem disease-gene region on chromosome 17q12-q21. Am J Hum Genet 1999; 64:1661–1669.
366. Van Hul W, Balemans W, Van Hul E, et al. Van Buchem disease (hyperostosis corticalis generalisata) maps to chromosome 17q12-q21. Am J Hum Genet 1998; 62:391–399.
367. Lazar CM, Braunstein EM, Econs MJ. Clinical vignette: osteopathia striata with cranial sclerosis. J Bone Miner Res 1999; 14: 152–153.
368. Kim JE, Kim EH, Han EH, et al. A TGF-β–inducible cell adhesion molecule, βig-h3, is downregulated in melorheostosis and involved in osteogenesis. J Cell Biochem 2000; 77:169–178.
369. Greenspan A, Azouz EM. Bone dysplasia series. Melorheostosis: review and update. Can Assoc Radiol J 1999; 50:324–330.
370. Nevin NC, Thomas PS, Davis RI, Cowie GH. Melorheostosis in a family with autosomal dominant osteopoikilosis. Am J Med Genet 1999; 19:409–414.
371. Deniaux-Domenech B, Bonjour JP, Rizzoli R. Axial osteomalacia: report of a new case with selective increase in axial bone mineral density. Bone 1996; 18:633–637.
372. Sissons HA. Fibrogenesis imperfecta ossium (Baker's disease): a case studied at autopsy. Bone 2000; 27:865–873.
373. Sinha GP, Curtis P, Haigh D, et al. Pachydermoperiostosis in childhood. Br J Rheumatol 1997; 36:1224–1227.
374. Gardiner JS, Zauk AM, Donchey SS, et al. Prostaglandin-induced cortical hyperostosis: case report and review of the literature. J Bone Joint Surg Am 1995; 77:932–936.
375. Thometz JG, DiRaimondo CA. A case of recurrent Caffey's disease treated with naproxen. Clin Orthop 1996; 323:304–309.
376. Freebourn TM, Barber DB, Able AC. The treatment of immature heterotopic ossification in spinal cord injury with combination surgery, radiation therapy and NSAID. Spinal Cord 1999; 37:50–53.
377. Kluger G, Kochs A, Holthausen H. Heterotopic ossification in childhood and adolescence. J Child Neurol 2000; 15:406–413.
378. Savaci N, Avundduk MC, Tosun Z. Hyperphosphatemic tumoral calcinosis. Plast Reconstr Surg 2000; 205:162–165.
379. Yamaguchi T, Sugimoto T, Imai Y, et al. Successful treatment of hyperphosphatemic tumoral calcinosis with long-term acetazolamide. Bone 1995; 16:S247–S250.
380. Thakur A, Hines OJ, Thakur V, et al. Tumoral calcinosis regression after subtotal parathyroidectomy: a case presentation and review of the literature. Surgery 1999; 126:95–98.
381. Cohen RB, Hahn GV, Tabas JA, et al. The natural history of heterotopic ossification in patients who have fibrodysplasia ossificans progressiva: a study of forty-four patients. J Bone Joint Surg Am 1993; 75:215–219.
382. Feldman G, Li M, Martin S, et al. Fibrodysplasia ossificans progressiva, a heritable disorder of severe heterotopic ossification, maps to human chromosome 4q27-31. Am J Hum Genet 2000; 66:128–135.
383. Gannon FH, Kaplan FS, Olmsted E, et al. Bone morphogenetic protein 2/4 in early fibromatous lesions of fibrodysplasia ossificans progressiva. Hum Pathol 1997; 28:339–343.
384. Kaplan FS, Shore EM. Progressive osseous heteroplasia. J Bone Miner Res 2000; 15:2084–2094.
385. Gong Y, Slee RB, Fukai N, et al. LDL receptor-related protein 5 (LRP5) affects bone accrual and eye development. Cell 2001; 107:513–523.
386. Little RD, Carulli JP, DelMastro RG, et al: A mutation in the LDL receptor-related protein 5 gene results in the autosomal dominant high-bone-mass trait. Am J Hum Genet 2002; 70:11–19.

28 Kidney Stones

Rebeca D. Monk and David A. Bushinsky

Nephrolithiasis is a common disorder with an incidence greater than one case per 1000 patients per year. The incidence peaks in the third and fourth decades. The prevalence in industrialized nations is close to 10% and increases with age until approximately age 70 years.[1–4] In general, stones may be composed of calcium oxalate, calcium phosphate, uric acid, magnesium ammonium phosphate (struvite), or cystine, or a combination thereof. A variety of pathogenetic mechanisms determine the type of stone formed.

Stones tend to localize in the renal tubules and collecting system but are also commonly found within the ureters and bladder. Nephrolithiasis rarely results in renal insufficiency or life-threatening illness but is responsible for substantial morbidity. The severe pain of renal colic can lead to frequent hospitalization, shock wave lithotripsy, or invasive surgical procedures. Insight into the mechanisms involved in stone formation can help direct appropriate therapy, which is known to decrease the incidence of stone disease and its associated morbidity.

EPIDEMIOLOGY OF STONE FORMATION

Numerous factors determine the prevalence of stones, including sex, age, race, and geographic distribution. Nephrolithiasis is more common in men than women at a ratio of 2:1 to 4:1.[1–4] In the United States, blacks, Hispanic Americans, and Asian Americans are much less likely to have stones than whites. Geography also appears to influence stone formation in the United States, with a decreasing prevalence from south to north and, to some degree, from east to west.

The greater exposure to sunlight in the southeastern United States may be responsible for the increased rates of nephrolithiasis in that area. Sun exposure can lead to more concentrated urine by increasing insensible fluid losses due to sweating; in addition, it may result in intestinal calcium absorption and urinary calcium excretion by stimulating vitamin D production.[5]

Geographic location can also influence the type of stone formed. Uric acid stones, for example, predominate in Mediterranean and Middle Eastern countries, where they constitute up to 75% of all the stones formed. In the United States, however, fewer than 10% are pure uric acid stones, and more than 70% of stones formed are composed of calcium and an associated anion. Less common are magnesium ammonium phosphate (struvite or infection) stones, which account for about 10% to 15% of stones formed, and cystine stones, which are due to an autosomal recessive disorder and constitute only about 1% of all stones formed (Table 28–1).[2, 6, 7]

PATHOGENESIS OF STONE FORMATION

Kidney stones form when urine becomes oversaturated with respect to the specific components of the stone. Saturation is dependent on chemical free ion activities of the stone constituents. Factors that affect chemical free ion activity include urinary ion concentration, pH, and complexing with other substances. For example, an increase in the quantity of urinary calcium or a decrease in urine volume increases the free ion activity of calcium ions in the urine. Urinary pH can also modify chemical free ion activity. A low urinary pH increases the free ion activity of uric acid ions but decreases the activity of calcium and phosphate ions. Citrate combines with calcium ions to form soluble complexes and can thereby decrease their free ion activity. When the chemical free ion activities are increased, the urine becomes oversaturated and new stones may form or established stones grow. In the setting of decreased free ion activity, urine becomes undersaturated and stones do not grow and may even dissolve. The equilibrium solubility product is the degree of chemical free ion activity of stone components in a solution in which the stone neither grows nor dissolves.

Formation of stones occurs through either *homogeneous* or *heterogeneous* nucleation:

1. Homogeneous. Progressive oversaturation can eventually result in formation of small clusters of ions; these clusters grow in size to form a permanent solid phase.

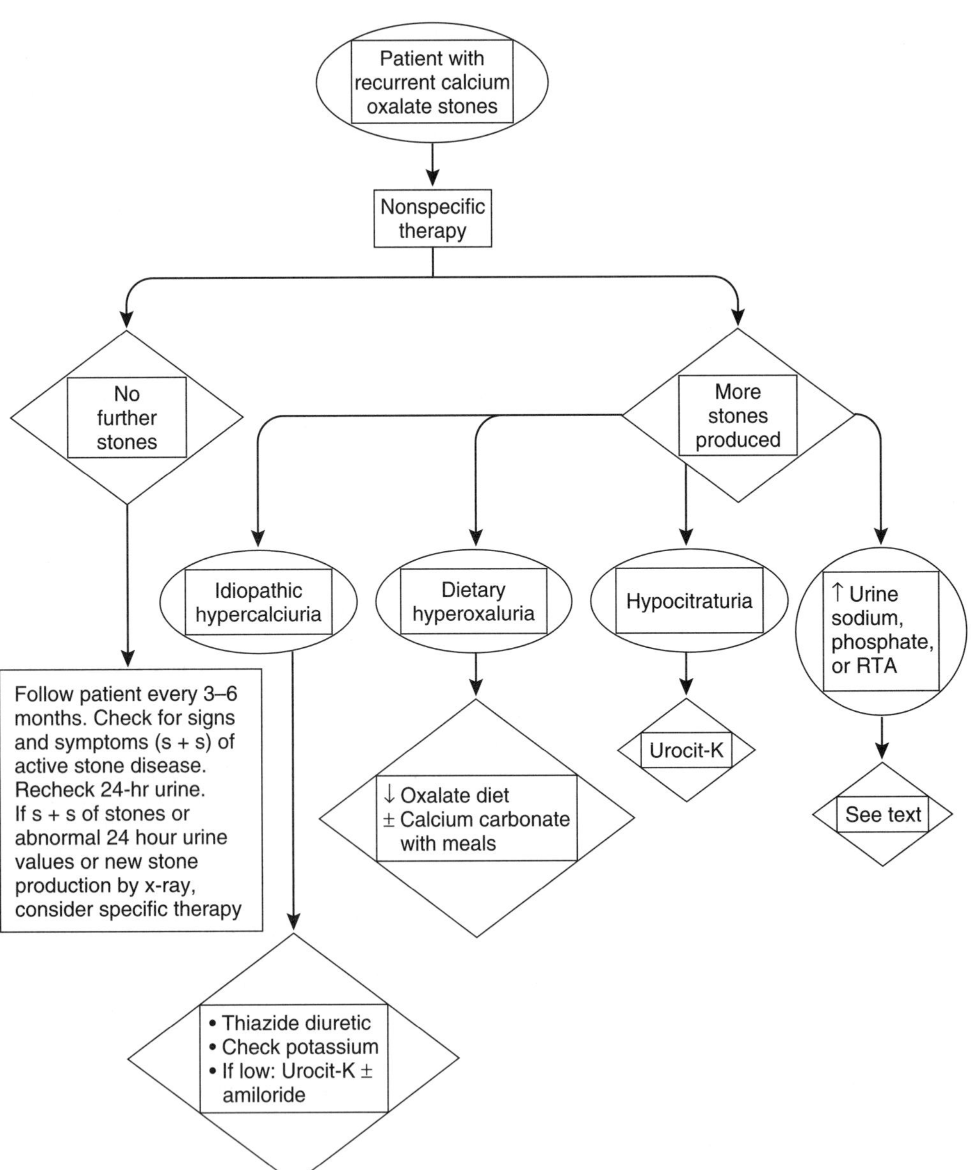

Figure 28–3. Treatment of the patient with recurrent calcium oxalate stones. phos, phosphorus; RTA, renal tubular acidosis.

gens, and acetazolamide. Men tend to have lower urinary citrate concentrations than women, which may be responsible for the higher incidence of stone formation in men. Furthermore, women with nephrolithiasis have lower urinary citrate concentrations than non–stone-forming women.[98, 99]

Along with therapy for the underlying condition, such as moderating dietary protein intake, potassium citrate is prescribed. This salt is preferable to sodium citrate because sodium excretion promotes calcium excretion. Again, potassium citrate in the wax matrix formulation is preferred to the liquid preparation because of increased palatability. Large amounts may be required (30 to 75 mEq/day) in divided doses in order to raise the urinary citrate concentration to more than 320 mg/day. Potassium and bicarbonate levels should be closely monitored, especially in patients with renal insufficiency. If metabolic alkalosis ensues, partial supplementation with potassium chloride may be necessary.[1, 85, 100]

Renal Tubular Acidosis

Distal (type 1) RTA is a disorder in which distal tubular hydrogen ion excretion is impaired, resulting in a non–anion gap metabolic acidosis and a persistently alkaline urine. The acidosis leads to calcium and phosphate release from bone as well as enhanced proximal tubular reabsorption of citrate. The net result is an increased filtered load of calcium and phosphate, severe hypocitraturia, and an elevated urinary pH, all of which promote calcium phosphate precipitation. Nephrocalcinosis, or renal parenchymal calcification, is frequently seen in this setting.

Twenty-four-hour urinary citrate levels are commonly below 100 mg in patients with distal RTA. Therapy consists of potassium citrate or potassium bicarbonate supplementation in order to treat both the metabolic acidosis and hypocitraturia. Large doses of these medications are often required—1 to 2 mEq/kg per day in two or three divided doses.[11, 12, 99, 101]

Nephrocalcinosis

Nephrocalcinosis is a process in which calcium is deposited in the renal parenchyma. There are two forms:

1. *Dystrophic calcification*. Calcium deposition arises from tissue necrosis secondary to neoplasm, infarction, or infection. It

may be seen in the setting of renal transplant rejection, renal cortical necrosis, chronic glomerulonephritis, ethylene glycol toxicity, acquired immunodeficiency syndrome (AIDS)–related infections, and Alport's syndrome. In general, serum calcium and phosphorus levels are normal and calcium-phosphate deposition occurs predominantly in the renal cortex.

2. *Metastatic calcification.* Patients may have elevated serum calcium and phosphate levels or an elevated urinary pH. Calcification in this setting occurs more commonly in the renal medulla. Common causes include RTA, primary hyperparathyroidism (or any disorder resulting in elevated serum calcium levels), medullary sponge kidney, papillary necrosis, acetazolamide, amphotericin B, triamterene, and primary hyperoxaluria. Primary hyperoxaluria can result in both medullary and cortical calcifications.

Both medullary and cortical parenchymal calcifications are easily noted with ultrasonography and CT scanning, even before they can be detected on plain radiographs. Therapy consists of treating the underlying disorder whenever possible. Otherwise, measures aimed at reducing hypercalcemia, oxalosis, and hyperphosphatemia should be attempted.[46]

Uric Acid Stones (see Table 28–4)

Although uric acid stones make up only about 5% to 10% of all calculi formed in the United States, the prevalence of uric acid lithiasis is much greater in Mediterranean countries. These stones tend to be round, smooth, and yellow-orange. Because they are radiolucent, they are not visible on plain films but can be detected by ultrasonography or CT or as filling defects on IVP. Uric acid is a purine metabolite and is also found in large quantities within cells. The three main causes of uric acid stone formation are (1) low urine volume, (2) low urinary pH, and (3) elevated urinary uric acid levels.

Urine Volume and pH

Any disorder that results in low urine volume (e.g., diarrheal disorders, diaphoresis, reduced fluid intake) can contribute to uric acid lithiasis. Diarrhea and diets high in animal protein can also contribute to an acidic urinary pH. Uric acid is increasingly soluble at an alkaline urinary pH such that urine with a pH of 6.5 can contain more than five times more uric acid than urine at pH 5.3 without inducing precipitation and may actually dissolve existing stones.[51, 97]

Hyperuricosuria

Hyperuricosuria may be evident in patients who ingest large quantities of dietary purine or animal protein. Foods high in purine include organ meats, shellfish, certain fish, meat extracts, yeast, gravies, and stocks (Table 28–8). Hyperuricemic disorders such as gout, myeloproliferative disorders, tumor lysis syndrome, and certain inborn errors of metabolism (e.g., glucose-6-phosphatase deficiency, Lesch-Nyhan syndrome) may also contribute to an increased urinary filtered load of uric acid. Certain medications such as salicylates and probenecid can be hyperuricosuric as well.[4, 99]

Therapy for patients with uric acid stones begins with nonspecific measures such as increasing fluid intake to maintain urine volume at about 3 L/day. Patients are prescribed a low-purine diet to decrease uric acid production. Despite dietary intervention, hyperuricemia often persists, especially in patients with disorders of cellular catabolism. In this setting, allopurinol should be prescribed at a starting dose of 100 mg/day, increasing to 300 mg/day as needed.[88, 102, 103]

A diet low in animal protein is also beneficial because the decreased endogenous acid production raises urinary pH. Ideally, the urinary pH should be elevated to approximately 6.5 to 7.0, a level that can dissolve existing crystals and stones. A urinary pH higher than 7.0 should be avoided, however, as calcium phosphate deposition may result. Potassium citrate at doses of 30 mEq by mouth twice a day or greater may be required to raise the urinary pH sufficiently. (See "Hypercalciuria" and "Hypocitruria" on available potassium citrate preparations.) Prescription of Nitrazine paper allows patients to monitor the urinary pH at various times of day and adjust their potassium citrate intake accordingly.

Although sodium bicarbonate may effectively alkalinize the urine, it should be avoided because the additional sodium excretion encourages sodium urate formation. Sodium urate in the setting of alkaline urine can serve as a nidus for calcium oxalate precipitation. If the urinary pH cannot be raised adequately despite high doses of potassium citrate or if the dose prescribed results in hyperkalemia, the carbonic anhydrase inhibitor acetazolamide may be initiated. This medication results in an alkaline urine and mild systemic metabolic acidosis, a pattern similar to that in type 1 RTA. Again, the urinary pH should be maintained at less than 7.0 in order to avoid calcium phosphate precipitation.[11, 51, 88]

Table 28–8. Foods High in Purine

Organ meats
Brain, heart, kidney, liver, sweetbreads
Meat extracts
Bouillon, consomme, stock, gravies
Meat
Beef, chicken, goose, lamb, pork
Shellfish
Clams, mussels, scallops, shrimp, oysters
Fish
Anchovies, fish roe, herring, mackerel, sardines, others
Certain vegetables
Asparagus, cauliflower, kidney beans, lentils, lima beans, mushrooms, peas, spinach

Adapted from Monk RD, Bushinsky DA. Nephrolithiasis and nephrocalcinosis. In Johnson R, Frehally J (eds). Comprehensive Clinical Nephrology. London, Mosby, 2000, pp 973–989[4]; and Wainer L, Resnik BA, Resnik MI. Nutritional Aspects of Stone Disease. Boston, Martinus Nijhoff, 1987.[88]

Struvite Stones (see Table 28–4)

Struvite stones have also been termed *triple phosphate stones*, *magnesium ammonium phosphate stones*, and *infection stones*. Although they make up only about 10% to 15% of all stones formed, most staghorn calculi (i.e., large stones that extend beyond a single renal calix) are composed of struvite. The propensity of these stones to grow rapidly to a large size, to recur despite therapy, and to result in significant morbidity (and potential mortality) has also led to the appellation *stone cancer*. Infection with urease-producing bacteria must be present for these stones to form, and therefore severe renal infections as well as sepsis and loss of renal function may develop.

In contrast to other stone types, struvite stones occur with a higher incidence in women than in men, largely because of women's increased susceptibility to urinary tract infections. Other groups at risk for development of struvite stones because of urinary stasis or infection include elderly people and patients with neurogenic bladders, indwelling urinary catheters, spinal cord lesions, or genitourinary abnormalities. Even in the absence of stone analysis, struvite stones should be suspected in patients with large stones, an alkaline urinary pH (>7), and

47. Sakhaee K. Pathogenesis and medical management of cystinuria. Semin Nephrol 1996; 16:435–447.
48. Danpure CJ, Smith LH. The Primary Hyperoxalurias. In Coe FL, Favus MJ, Pak CYC, et al (eds). Kidney Stones: Medical and Surgical Management. Philadelphia, Lippincott-Raven, 1996, pp 859–881.
49. Asplin J, Chandhoke PS. The stone-forming patient. In Coe FL, Parks JH, Pak CYC, et al (eds). Kidney Stones: Medical and Surgical Management. Philadelphia, Lippincott-Raven, 1996, pp 337–352.
50. Preminger GM, Harvey JA. Diagnostic Considerations. Boston, Martinus Nijhoff, 1987.
51. Bleyer A, Agus ZS. Approach to nephrolithiasis. Kidney 1992; 25: 2, 1–10.
52. Kopp JB, Miller KD, Mican JM, et al. Crystalluria and urinary tract abnormalities associated with indinavir. Ann Intern Med 1997; 127:119–125.
53. Curhan GC, Willett WC, Rimm EB, Stampfer MJ. A prospective study of dietary calcium and other nutrients and the risk of symptomatic kidney stones. N Engl J Med 1993; 328:833–838.
54. Lemann J, Pleuss JA, Worcester EM, et al. Urinary oxalate excretion increases with body size and decreases with increasing dietary calcium intake among healthy adults. Kidney Int 1996; 49:200–208.
55. Rodman JS. Struvite stones. In Pak CYC (ed). Renal Stone Disease: Pathogenesis, Prevention, and Treatment. Boston, Martinus Nijhoff, 1987, pp 225–251.
56. Brand E, Harris MM, Billion S. Cystinuria: excretion of a cystine complex which decomposes in the urine with the liberation of free cystine. J Biol Chem 1930; 86:315–331.
57. Worchester EM. Stones Due to Bowel Disease. In Coe FL, Favus MJ, Pak CYC, et al (eds). Kidney Stones: Medical and Surgical Management. Philadelphia, Lippincott-Raven, 1996, pp 883–903.
58. Denton ER, Mackenzie A, Greenwell T, et al. Unenhanced helical CT for renal colic—is the radiation dose justifiable? Clin Radiol 1999; 54:444–447.
59. Smith RC, Coll DM. Helical computed tomography in the diagnosis of ureteric colic. BJU Int 2000; 86:33–41.
60. Nakada SY, Hoff DG, Attai S, et al. Determination of stone composition by noncontrast spiral computed tomography in the clinical setting. Urology 2000; 55:816–819.
61. Chen MY, Zagoria RJ. Can noncontrast helical computed tomography replace intravenous urography for evaluation of patients with acute urinary tract colic? J Emerg Med 1999; 17:299–303.
62. Smith RC, Verga M, McCarthy S, Rosenfield AT. Diagnosis of acute flank pain: value of unenhanced helical CT. AJR 1996; 166: 97–101.
63. Smith RC, Rosenfield AT, Choe KA, et al. Acute flank pain: comparison of non-contrast-enhanced CT and intravenous urography. Radiology 1995; 159:735–740.
64. Dalrymple NC, Verga M, Anderson KR, et al. The value of unenhanced helical computerized tomography in the management of acute flank pain. J Urol 1998; 159:735–740.
65. Uribarri J, Oh MS, Carroll HJ. The first kidney stone. Ann Intern Med 1989; 111:1006–1009.
66. Pak CYC. Prevention of recurrent nephrolithiasis. In Pak CYC (ed). Renal Stone Disease: Pathogenesis, Prevention, and Treatment. Boston, Martinus Nijhoff, 1987, pp 165–199.
67. Hosking DH, Erickson SB, Van Den Berg CJ, et al. The stone clinic effect in patients with idiopathic calcium urolithiasis. J Urol 1983; 130:1115–1118.
68. Muldowney FP, Freaney R, Moloney MF. Importance of dietary sodium in the hypercalciuria syndrome. Kidney Int 1972; 22:292–296.
69. Breslau NA, McGuire JL, Zerwekh JE, Pak CYC. The role of dietary sodium on renal excretion and intestinal absorption of calcium and on vitamin D metabolism. J Clin Endocrinol Metab 1982; 55:369–373.
70. Lemann JJ, Worcester EA, Gray RW. Hypercalciuria and stones. Am J Kidney Dis 1991; 17:386–391.
71. Chen Y, Cann MJ, Litvin TN, et al. Soluble adenylyl cyclase as an evolutionarily conserved bicarbonate sensor. Science 2000; 289:625–628.
72. Lemann J Jr, Litzow JR, Lennon EJ. The effects of chronic acid loads in normal man: further evidence for the participation of bone mineral in the defense against chronic metabolic acidosis. J Clin Invest 1966; 45:1608–1614.
73. Lemann J Jr, Litzow JR, Lennon EJ. Studies of the mechanism by which chronic metabolic acidosis augments urinary calcium excretion in man. J Clin Invest 1967; 46:1318–1328.
74. Allen LH, Oddoye EA, Margen S. Protein induced hypercalciuria: a longer term study. Am J Clin Nutr 1979; 32:741–749.
75. Licata A, Bou E, Bartter FC, Cox J. Effects of dietary protein on urinary calcium in normal subjects and in patients with nephrolithiasis. Metabolism 1979; 28:895–900.
76. Lemann J. Idiopathic hypercalciuria, in nephrolithiasis. In Coe FL, Brenner BM, Stein JH (eds). Contemporary Issues in Nephrology. New York, Churchill Livingstone, 1980, pp 86–135.
77. Allen LH, Bartlett RS, Block GD. Reduction of renal calcium reabsorption in man by consumption of dietary protein. J Nutr 1979; 109:1345–1350.
78. Hamm LL. Renal handling of citrate. Kidney Int 1990; 38:728–735.
79. Velentzas C, Oreopoulos DG, Meema S, et al. Dietary calcium restriction may be good for patients' stones—but not for their bones. In Smith LH, Robertson WG, Finlayson B (eds). Urolithiasis, Clinical and Basic Research. New York, Plenum, 1981, pp 847–854.
80. Jaeger P, Lippuner K, Casez JP, et al. Low bone mass in idiopathic renal stone formers: magnitude and significance. J Bone Miner Res 1994; 9:1525–1532.
81. Stauffer JQ. Hyperoxaluria and intestinal disease: the role of steatorrhea and dietary calcium in regulating intestinal oxalate absorption. Dig Dis 1977; 22:921–928.
82. Saunders DR, Sillery J, McDonald GB. Regional differences in oxalate absorption by rat intestine: evidence for excessive absorption by the colon in steatorrhea. Gut 1975; 16:543–554.
83. Mandel GS, Mandel N. Analysis of Stones. In Coe FL, Favus MJ, Pak CYC, et al (eds). Kidney Stones: Medical and Surgical Management. Philadelphia, Lippincott-Raven, 1996, pp 323–335.
84. Coe FL, Parks JH, Bushinsky DA, et al. Chlorthalidone promotes mineral retention in patients with idiopathic hypercalciuria. Kidney Int 1988; 33:1140–1146.
85. Pak CYC, Fuller C, Sakhaee K, et al. Long-term treatment of calcium oxalate nephrolithiasis with potassium citrate. J Urol 1985; 134:11–19.
86. Smith LH. Hyperoxaluric states. In Coe FL, Favus MJ (eds). Disorders of Bone and Mineral Metabolism. New York, Raven Press, 2000, pp 707–727.
87. Smith LH. Diet and hyperoxaluria in the syndrome of idiopathic calcium oxalate urolithiasis. Am J Kidney Dis 1991; 17:370–375.
88. Wainer L, Resnik BA, Resnick MI. Nutritional Aspects of Stone Disease. Boston, Martinus Nijhoff, 1987.
89. Nordenvall B, Backman L, Larsson L, Tiselius HG. Effects of calcium, aluminum, magnesium and cholestyramine on hyperoxaluria in patients with jejunoileal bypass. Acta Chir Scand 1983; 149:93–98.
90. Clarke AM, McKenzie RG. Ileostomy and the risk of urinary uric acid stones. Lancet 1969; 2:395–397.
91. Gigax JH, Leach JR. Uric acid calculi associated with ileostomy for ulcerative colitis. J Urol 1971; 105:797–799.
92. Rudman D, Dedonis JL, Fountain MT, et al. Hypocitruria in patients with gastrointestinal malabsorption. N Engl J Med 1980; 303:657–661.
93. Rumsby G. Biochemical and genetic diagnosis of the primary hyperoxalurias: a review. Mol Urol 2000; 4:349–354.
94. Milliner DS, Wilson DM, Smith LH. Phenotypic expression of primary hyperoxaluria: comparative features of types I and II. Kidney Int 2001; 59:31–36.
95. Petrarulo M, Vitale C, Facchini P, Marangella M. Biochemical approach to diagnosis and differentiation of primary hyperoxalurias: an update. J Nephrol 2001; 11:23–28.
96. Watts RWE, Danpure CJ, de Pauw L, et al. Combined liver-kidney and isolated liver transplantations for primary hyperoxaluria type 1. The European experience. Nephrol Dial Transplant 1991; 6:502–511.
97. Millman S, Strauss AL, Parks JH, et al. Pathogenesis and clinical course of mixed calcium oxalate and uric acid nephrolithiasis. Kidney Int 1982; 366–370.
98. Parks JH, Coe FL. A urinary calcium-citrate index for the evaluation of nephrolithiasis. Kidney Int 1986; 30:85–90.

99. Breslau NA, Sakhaee K. Pathophysiology of Nonhypercalciuric Causes of Stones. Boston, Martinus Nijhoff, 1987.
100. Pak CYC, Fuller C. Idiopathic hypocitraturic calcium oxalate nephrolithiasis successfully treated with potassium citrate. Ann Intern Med 1986; 104:33–37.
101. Bushinsky DA. Net calcium efflux from live bone during chronic metabolic, but not respiratory, acidosis. Am J Physiol 1989; 256: F836–F842.
102. Coe FL, Raisen L. Allopurinol treatment of uric-acid disorders in calcium-stone formers. Lancet 1973; 1:129–131.
103. Ettinger B, Tang A, Citron JT, et al. Randomized trial of allopurinol in the prevention of calcium oxalate calculi. N Engl J Med 1986; 315:1386–1389.
104. Griffith DP. Struvite stones. Kidney Int 1978; 13:372–383.
105. Wong HY, Riedl CR, Griffith DP. Medical management and prevention of struvite stones. In Coe FL, Favus MJ, Pak CYC, et al (eds). Kidney Stones: Medical and Surgical Management. Philadelphia, Lippincott-Raven, 1996, pp 941–950.
106. Michaels EK. Surgical management of struvite stones. In Coe FL, Favus MJ, Pak CYC, et al (eds). Kidney Stones: Medical and Surgical Management. Philadelphia, Lippincott-Raven, 1996, pp 951–970.
107. Sant GR, Blaivas JG, Meares EM Jr. Hemiacidrin irrigation in the management of struvite calculi: long-term results. J Urol 1983; 130:1048–1050.
108. Kolb FO, Earll JM, Harper HA. “Disappearance” of cystinuria in a patient treated with prolonged low methionine diet. Metabolism 1967; 16:378–381.
109. Pak CYC. Cystine lithiasis. In Resnick MI, Pak CYC (eds). Urolithiasis: A Medical and Surgical Reference. Philadelphia, WB Saunders, 1990, pp 133–143.
110. Bushinsky DA, Monk RD. Calcium. Lancet 1998; 352:306–311.

DISORDERS OF CARBOHYDRATE AND LIPID METABOLISM

29 Type 2 Diabetes Mellitus

John B. Buse, Kenneth S. Polonsky, and Charles F. Burant

EPIDEMIOLOGY

Type 2 diabetes is the predominant form of diabetes worldwide, accounting for 90% of cases globally.[1, 2] An epidemic of type 2 diabetes is under way in both developed and developing countries, although the brunt of the disorder is felt disproportionately in non-European populations as evidenced by studies in Hispanic populations, Native American and Canadian communities, Pacific and Indian Ocean island populations, and in India and Australian Aboriginal communities.[3–5] In the Pacific island of Nauru, diabetes was virtually unknown 50 years ago and is now present in approximately 40% of adults. Globally, the number of people with diabetes is expected to rise from the current estimate of 150 million to 220 million in 2010 and 300 million in 2025. Alarming increases in the prevalence of diabetes have occurred in various Chinese populations. Type 2 diabetes has become one of the world's most important public health problems.

Considerable information is available on the factors that are responsible for the development of type 2 diabetes, and these are summarized in Table 29–1.

Type 2 diabetes is currently thought to occur in genetically predisposed individuals who are exposed to a series of environmental influences that precipitate the onset of clinical disease. The genetic basis of type 2 diabetes is discussed in detail later in this chapter, but the syndrome consists of monogenic and polygenic forms that can be differentiated both on clinical grounds and in terms of the genes that are involved in the pathogenesis of these disorders.

Sex, age, and ethnic background are important factors in determining risk for the development of type 2 diabetes.[6–8] The disorder is more common in females, and the increased prevalence in certain racial and ethnic minority groups has already been alluded to. Age is also a critical factor. Type 2 diabetes has been viewed in the past as a disorder of aging with an increasing prevalence with age. This remains true today. However, a disturbing trend has become apparent in which the prevalence of obesity and type 2 diabetes in children is rising dramatically. In the past, it was believed that the overwhelming majority of children with diabetes had type 1 diabetes, with only 1% to 2% of children considered to have type 2 or other rare forms of diabetes.[9] Later reports suggest that as many as 8% to 45% of children with newly diagnosed diabetes have non–immune-mediated diabetes. The majority of these children have type 2 diabetes, but other types are being increasingly identified. An idiopathic non–immune-mediated form of diabetes has been reported particularly in the black population.

Table 29–1. Epidemiologic Determinants and Risk Factors of Type 2 Diabetes

Genetic factors
Genetic markers, family history, "thrifty gene(s)"
Demographic characteristics
Sex, age, ethnicity
Behavioral and lifestyle-related risk factors
Obesity (including distribution of obesity and duration)
Physical inactivity
Diet
Stress
Westernization, urbanization, modernization
Metabolic determinants and intermediate risk categories of type 2 diabetes
Impaired glucose tolerance
Insulin resistance
Pregnancy-related determinants (parity, gestational diabetes, diabetes in offspring of women with diabetes during pregnancy, intrauterine malnutrition or overnutrition)

From Zimmet P, Alberti KG, Shaw J. Global and societal implications of the diabetes epidemic. Nature 2001; 414:782–787.

DIAGNOSTIC CRITERIA FOR DIABETES MELLITUS

The diagnosis of diabetes rests on the measurement of plasma glucose levels. The diagnostic criteria for diabetes were changed in 1997[10] with the most significant changes being the level of fasting plasma glucose (FPG) that is recognized as diagnostic for diabetes, which was decreased from 140 to 126 mg/dL, and the introduction of a category of impaired fasting glucose (IFG). Current criteria for the diagnosis of diabetes, impaired fasting glucose and impaired glucose tolerance (IGT), are shown in Table 29–2.

Because plasma glucose concentrations range as a continuum, the criteria are based on estimates of the threshold for the complications of diabetes. The primary end point used to evaluate the relationship between glucose levels and complications is retinopathy. The prevalence of retinopathy in comparison with FPG and 2-hour plasma glucose has been evaluated in two relatively large studies.[11, 12] Both diagnostic criteria were able to predict the presence of retinopathy and, by inference, glucose levels that are diagnostic of diabetes (Fig. 29–1). There is also an association between FPG and 2-hour plasma glucose and risk of macrovascular and cardiovascular disease.[13–15] For instance, the Paris Prospective Study showed that the incidence of fatal coronary heart disease was related to both FPG and 2-hour plasma glucose that were determined at a baseline examination.[16] Rates of disease were markedly increased at FPG greater than 125 mg/dL (6.9 mmol/L) or 2-hour plasma glucose greater than 140 mg/dL (7.8 mmol/L).

Reproducibility of the plasma glucose concentration is an important issue in the interpretation of the results of diagnostic tests for diabetes. There is significant variation in the results of repeated tests in adults after a 2- to 6-week interval. The intraindividual coefficient of variation in one study was 6.4% for the FPG and 16.7% for the 2-hour plasma glucose value. Thus, it is essential that abnormal results be confirmed by a repeated test. Although the oral glucose tolerance test (OGTT) is an invaluable tool in research, it is not recommended for routine use in the diagnosis of diabetes. It is

Table 29–2. Criteria for the Diagnosis of Diabetes

Normoglycemia	Impaired Fasting Glucose or Impaired Glucose Tolerance	Diabetes*
FPG <110 mg/dL	FPG ≥110 and <126 mg/dL (IFG)	FPG ≥126 mg/dL
2-hr PG <140 mg/dL	2-hr PG ≥140 and <200 mg/dL (IGT)	2-hr PG ≥200 mg/dL
		Symptoms of diabetes and casual plasma glucose concentration ≥200 mg/dL

*A diagnosis of diabetes must be confirmed, on a subsequent day, by measurement of FPG, 2-hour PG, or random plasma glucose (if symptoms are present). The FPG test is greatly preferred because of ease of administration, convenience, acceptability to patients, and lower cost. Fasting is defined as no caloric intake for at least 8 hours.

FPG, fasting plasma glucose; IFG, impaired fasting glucose; IGT, impaired glucose tolerance; PG, plasma glucose.

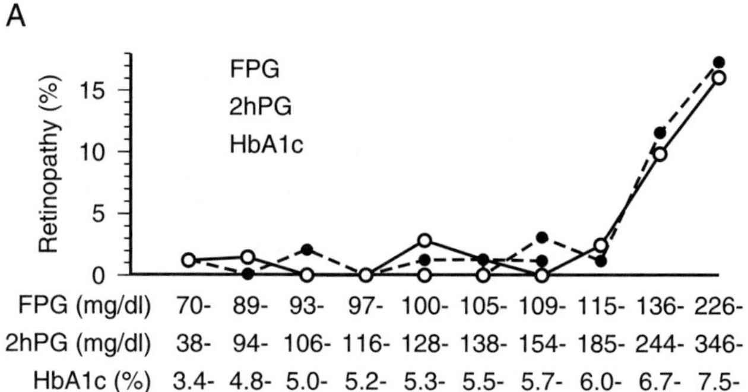

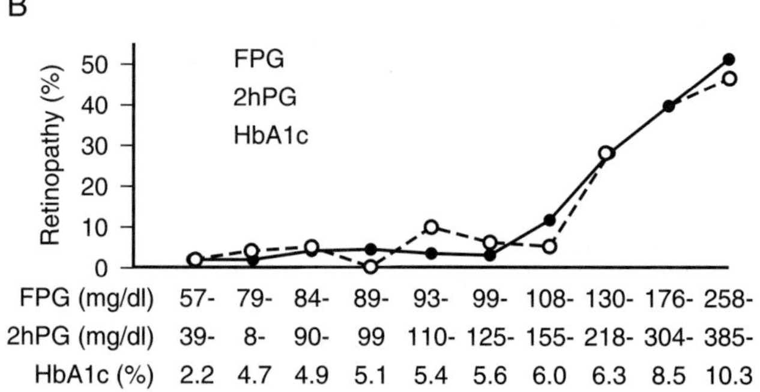

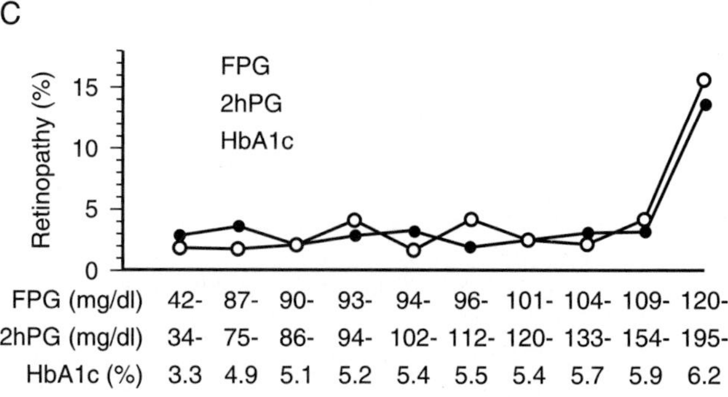

Figure 29–1. American Diabetes Association consensus.

inconvenient for patients, and in the vast majority of cases the diagnosis can be made on the basis of either an elevated fasting glucose concentration or an elevated random glucose determination in the presence of hyperglycemic symptoms.

Levels of hemoglobin A_{1c} (HbA_{1c}) are not currently recommended for the diagnosis of diabetes. The major reasons are the lack of standardization of the assays for HbA_{1c} and the imperfect correlation between HbA_{1c} and FPG and 2-hour plasma glucose. However, HbA_{1c} remains the most effective method for monitoring the effectiveness of diabetes treatment.

SCREENING FOR TYPE 2 DIABETES

Undiagnosed type 2 diabetes is common, with an estimated lag of 5 to 7 years between the onset of diabetes and diagnosis.[17–19] It is estimated that in up to 50% of affected people the disease is undiagnosed.[20] Subjects with IGT and undiagnosed type 2 diabetes are at significantly increased risk for coronary heart disease, stroke, and peripheral vascular disease. Thus, this delay in the diagnosis of type 2 diabetes causes an increase in microvascular and macrovascular disease. In addition, affected individuals have a greater likelihood of having dyslipidemia, hypertension, and obesity. Therefore, it is important for the clinician to screen for diabetes in a cost-effective manner in subjects who demonstrate major risk factors for diabetes as summarized in Table 29–3. Recommendations for screening are summarized in Table 29–4.

Table 29–4. Summary of Major Recommendations for Screening

Recommendations
Evaluation for type 2 diabetes should be performed within the health care setting. Patients should be screened at 3-year intervals beginning at age 45; testing should be considered at an earlier age or be carried out more frequently if diabetes risk factors are present.
Diabetes risk factors include a family history of diabetes; overweight, defined as BMI ≥25 kg/m²; habitual physical inactivity; belonging to a high-risk ethnic or racial group; previously identified IFG or IGT; hypertension; dyslipidemia; history of GDM or delivery of a baby weighing >9 lb; and polycystic ovary syndrome.
The FPG is the recommended screening test. The OGTT may be necessary for the diagnosis of diabetes when the FPG is normal. The FPG is preferred for screenings because it is faster and easier to perform, more convenient, acceptable to patients, and less expensive.
Diagnostic testing should be performed in any clinical situation in which such testing is warranted; health care providers should not consider whether a person meets screening criteria in such cases.
Screening outside of health care settings, or community screening, has not been shown to be beneficial and may result in some harm; this type of screening is not recommended.

BMI, body mass index; FPG, fasting plasma glucose; GDM, gestational diabetes mellitus; IFG, impaired fasting glucose; IGT, impaired glucose tolerance; OGTT, oral glucose tolerance test.

From Screening for diabetes. Diabetes Care 2002; 25:21–24.

PATHOGENESIS OF TYPE 2 DIABETES

The pathogenesis of type 2 diabetes is complex and involves the interaction of genetic and environmental factors. A number of environmental factors have been shown to play a critical role in the development of the disease, particularly excessive caloric intake leading to obesity and a sedentary lifestyle. The clinical presentation is also heterogeneous with a wide range in age of onset, severity of associated hyperglycemia, and degree of obesity. From a pathophysiologic standpoint, persons with type 2 diabetes consistently demonstrate three cardinal abnormalities: (1) resistance to the action of insulin in peripheral tissues, particularly muscle and fat but also liver; (2) defective insulin secretion, particularly in response to a glucose stimulus; and (3) increased glucose production by the liver.

Table 29–3. Major Risk Factors for Type 2 Diabetes

Risk factor
Family history of diabetes (i.e., parents or siblings with diabetes)
Overweight (BMI ≥25 kg/m²)
Habitual physical inactivity
Race/ethnicity (e.g., African Americans, Hispanic Americans, Native Americans, Asian Americans and Pacific Islanders)
Previously identified IFG or IGT
Hypertension (≥140/90 mm Hg in adults)
HDL cholesterol ≤35 mg/dL (0.90 mmol/L) and/or a triglyceride level ≥250 mg/dL (2.82 mmol/L)
History of GDM or delivery of a baby weighing >9 lb
Polycystic ovary syndrome

BMI, body mass index; GDM, gestational diabetes mellitus; HDL, high-density lipoprotein; IFG, impaired fasting glucose; IGT, impaired glucose tolerance.

From Screening for diabetes. Diabetes Care 2002; 25:21–24.

Although the precise manner in which these genetic, environmental, and pathophysiologic factors interact to lead to the clinical onset of type 2 diabetes is not known, our understanding of these processes has increased substantially. With the exception of specific monogenic forms of the disease that may result from defects largely confined to the pathways that regulate insulin action in muscle, liver, and fat or defects in insulin secretory function in the pancreatic beta cell, there is an emerging consensus that the common forms of type 2 diabetes are polygenic in nature and are due to a combination of abnormal insulin secretion and insulin resistance. From a pathophysiologic standpoint, it is the inability of the pancreatic beta cell to adapt to the reductions in insulin sensitivity that occur over the lifetime of human subjects in response to puberty or pregnancy, a sedentary lifestyle, or overeating leading to weight gain that precipitates the onset of type 2 diabetes. An underlying genetic predisposition appears to be a critical factor in determining the frequency with which this occurs.

Genetic Factors in the Development of Type 2 Diabetes

Genetically, type 2 diabetes consists of monogenic and polygenic forms.[21, 22] The monogenic forms, although relatively uncommon, are nevertheless important and a number of the genes involved have been identified and characterized. The genes involved in the common polygenic form or forms of the disorder have been far more difficult to identify and characterize.

Monogenic Forms of Diabetes

In the monogenic forms of diabetes, the gene involved is both necessary and sufficient to cause disease. In other words, environmental factors play little or no role in determining whether or not a genetically predisposed individual develops clinical diabetes. The monogenic forms of diabetes generally occur in young individuals, often in the first two to three decades of life, although if only mild asymptomatic elevations in blood glucose occur the diagnosis may be missed until later in life.

Table 29–5. Monogenic Forms of Diabetes

Associated with insulin resistance
- Mutations in the insulin receptor gene
  - Type A insulin resistance
  - Leprechaunism
  - Rabson-Mendenhall syndrome
- Lipoatrophic diabetes
- Mutations in the PPAR-γ gene

Associated with defective insulin secretion
- Mutations in the insulin or proinsulin genes
- Mitochondrial gene mutations
- Maturity-onset diabetes of the young (MODY)
  - Mutations in the genes for
    - HNF-4α (MODY 1)
    - Glucokinase (MODY 2)
    - HNF-1α (MODY 3)
    - IPF-1 (MODY 4)
    - HNF-1β (MODY 5)
    - NeuroD1/Beta2 (MODY 6)

HNF, hepatocyte nuclear factor; IPF, insulin promoter factor; MODY, maturity-onset diabetes of the young; NeuroD1/Beta2, neurogenic differentiation 1/ beta cell E-box *trans*-activator 2; PPAR, peroxisome proliferator-activated receptor.

The monogenic forms of diabetes are summarized in Table 29–5 and can be divided into those in which the mechanism is a defect in insulin secretion and those that involve defective responses to insulin or insulin resistance.

Monogenic Forms of Diabetes Associated with Insulin Resistance

Mutations in the Insulin Receptor

More than 70 mutations have been identified in the insulin receptor gene in various insulin-resistant patients.[23] There are at least three clinical syndromes caused by mutations in the insulin receptor gene. Type A insulin resistance is defined by the presence of insulin resistance, acanthosis nigricans, and hyperandrogenism.[24] Patients with leprechaunism have multiple abnormalities, including intrauterine growth retardation, fasting hypoglycemia, and death within the first 1 to 2 years of life.[25–27] The Rabson-Mendenhall syndrome is associated with short stature, protuberant abdomen, and abnormalities of teeth and nails; pineal hyperplasia was a characteristic in the original description of this syndrome.[28]

These mutations may impair receptor function by a number of different mechanisms, including decreasing the number of receptors expressed on the cell surface (e.g., by decreasing the rate of receptor biosynthesis [class 1], accelerating the rate of receptor degradation [class 5], or inhibiting the transport of receptors to the plasma membrane [class 2]). The intrinsic function of the receptor may be abnormal if the affinity of insulin binding is reduced (class 3) or receptor tyrosine kinase is inactivated (class 4). The insulin resistance that is associated with insulin receptor mutations may be severe and present in the neonatal period, as with leprechaunism and the Rabson-Mendenhall syndrome, or occur in a milder form in adulthood leading to insulin-resistant diabetes with marked hyperinsulinemia, acanthosis nigricans, and hyperandrogenism.

Lipoatrophic Diabetes

In another monogenic form of diabetes, so-called lipoatrophic diabetes, severe insulin resistance is associated with lipoatrophy and lipodystrophy. This form of diabetes is characterized by a paucity of fat, insulin resistance, and hypertriglyceridemia.[29] The disease has several genetic forms, including face-sparing partial lipoatrophy (the Dunnigan syndrome or the Koberling-Dunnigan syndrome), an autosomal dominant form caused by mutations in the lamin A/C gene,[30] and congenital generalized lipoatrophy (the Seip-Berardinelli syndrome), an autosomal recessive form.[31]

Mutations in Peroxisome Proliferator–Activated Receptor γ

It has been demonstrated that mutations in the transcription factor peroxisome proliferator–activated receptor γ (PPARγ) can cause type 2 diabetes of early onset.[32] Two different heterozygous mutations were identified in the ligand-binding domain of PPARγ in three subjects with severe insulin resistance. In the PPARγ crystal structure, the mutations destabilize helix 12, which mediates *trans*-activation. Both receptor mutants showed markedly decreased transcriptional activation and inhibited the action of coexpressed wild-type PPARγ in a dominant negative manner. A common amino acid polymorphism (Pro12Ala) in PPARγ has been associated with type 2 diabetes. People homozygous for the Pro12 allele are more insulin resistant than those having one Ala12 allele and have a 1.25-fold increased risk of diabetes. There is also evidence for interaction between this polymorphism and fatty acids, linking this locus with diet.

Monogenic Forms of Diabetes Associated with Defects in Insulin Secretion

Mutant Insulin Syndromes

The first syndrome associated with diabetes to be characterized in terms of the clinical picture, genetic mechanisms, and clinical pathophysiology was that associated with mutant insulin or proinsulin.[33] Persons with this disorder present clinically with a mild non–insulin-dependent form of diabetes. Affected individuals characteristically have marked hyperinsulinemia on routine insulin assays. Increases in the concentration of insulin in association with diabetes are usually indicative of insulin resistance, but in this syndrome insulin resistance can be easily excluded because the patients respond normally to administration of exogenous insulin. Characterization of the insulin by high-performance liquid chromatography reveals that the hyperinsulinemia is due to the presence of the abnormal insulin or proinsulin and related breakdown products. The increased concentrations of insulin appear to be related to the presence of mutations in regions of the insulin molecule that are important for receptor binding, particularly the COOH terminus of the insulin B chain.

Because the liver is the major site of insulin clearance and the first-step hepatic insulin uptake and degradation are mediated by the insulin receptor, mutant forms of insulin with diminished insulin receptor binding ability are cleared more slowly from the circulation, and this reduction in insulin clearance leads to hyperinsulinemia. Alternatively, mutations in proinsulin may reduce the conversion of proinsulin to insulin, leading to accumulation of proinsulin.[34, 35] Because proinsulin is cleared more slowly from the circulation than insulin, proinsulin levels increase. Proinsulin cross-reacts in most commercially available assays, and this insulin-like immunoreactivity can be characterized as related to the presence of proinsulin rather than insulin only by high-performance liquid chromatography or by the use of assays that are specific for insulin and proinsulin.

A patient with a mutation in prohormone convertase 1, one of the enzymes responsible for the conversion of proinsulin to insulin, has been described.[36]

Mitochondrial Diabetes

An A-to-G transition in the mitochondrial tRNALeu(UUR) gene at base pair 3243 has been shown to be associated with maternally transmitted diabetes and sensorineural hearing loss.[37] In other subjects, this mutation is associated with diabetes and the syndrome of mitochondrial myopathy, encephalopathy, lactic acidosis, and stroke-like episodes (MELAS syndrome). The mitochondrion plays a key role in the regulation of insulin secretion, particularly in response to glucose. We have documented abnormal insulin secretion on at least one of a battery of tests in subjects with this mitochondrial mutation, even in subjects with normal or impaired glucose tolerance who have not developed overt diabetes.[38]

MODY

Maturity-onset diabetes of the young (MODY) is a genetically and clinically heterogeneous group of disorders characterized by nonketotic diabetes mellitus, an autosomal dominant mode of inheritance, onset usually before 25 years of age and frequently in childhood or adolescence, and a primary defect in pancreatic beta cell function. A detailed review of MODY has been published,[39] and the information contained in that review is summarized.

MODY can result from mutations in any one of at least six different genes. One of these genes encodes the glycolytic enzyme glucokinase (*MODY2*)[40] and the other five encode transcription factors, hepatocyte nuclear factor (HNF)-4α (*MODY1*),[41] HNF-1α (*MODY3*),[42] insulin promoter factor-1 (IPF-1) (*MODY4*),[43] HNF-1β (*MODY5*),[44] and neurogenic differentiation 1/beta cell E-box *trans*-activator 2 (NeuroD1/BETA2) (*MODY6*).[45] All of these genes are expressed in the insulin-producing pancreatic beta cell, and heterozygous mutations cause diabetes related to beta cell dysfunction. Abnormalities in liver and kidney function may occur in some forms of MODY, reflecting expression of the transcription factors in these tissues. Nongenetic factors that affect insulin sensitivity (infection, puberty, pregnancy, and rarely obesity) may trigger diabetes onset and affect the severity of hyperglycemia in MODY but do not play a significant role in the development of MODY.

The most common clinical presentation of MODY is a mild asymptomatic increase in blood glucose in a child, adolescent, or young adult with a prominent family history of diabetes often in successive generations, suggesting an autosomal dominant mode of inheritance. Some patients may have mild hyperglycemia for many years, whereas others have varying degrees of glucose intolerance for several years before the onset of persistent hyperglycemia.[39] The diagnosis may be made only in adulthood even though the elevation in plasma glucose has been present for many years. Prospective testing indicates that in most patients the disease onset occurs in childhood or adolescence. In some patients, there may be a rapid progression to overt asymptomatic or symptomatic hyperglycemia necessitating therapy with an oral hypoglycemic drug or insulin. The presence of persistently normal plasma glucose levels in subjects with mutations in any of the known MODY genes is unusual, and the majority eventually experience diabetes (with the exception of many patients with glucokinase mutations; see later).

Although the exact prevalence of MODY is not known, current estimates suggest that MODY may account for 1% to 5% of all cases of diabetes in the United States and other industrialized countries.[39] Several clinical characteristics distinguish patients with MODY from those with type 2 diabetes, including a prominent family history of diabetes in three or more generations, young age at presentation, and absence of obesity.

Functional Effects of MODY Genes

The identification of several genes associated with diabetes has provided a unique opportunity to characterize the pathophysiologic mechanisms by which genetic mutations can lead to an increase in the plasma glucose concentration. All the susceptibility genes identified to date cause impaired insulin secretory responses to glucose, although the mechanisms differ.

Glucokinase

Glucokinase is expressed at its highest levels in the pancreatic beta cell and the liver. It catalyzes the transfer of phosphate from adenosine triphosphate (ATP) to glucose to generate glucose-6-phosphate (Fig. 29–2).

This reaction is the first rate-limiting step in glucose metabolism. Glucokinase functions as the glucose sensor in the beta cell by controlling the rate of entry of glucose into the glycolytic pathway (glucose phosphorylation) and its subsequent metabolism. In the liver glucokinase plays a key role in the ability to store glucose as glycogen, particularly in the postprandial state. Heterozygous mutations leading to partial deficiency of glucokinase are associated with MODY, and homozygous mutations resulting in complete deficiency of this enzyme lead to permanent neonatal diabetes mellitus.[46] As predicted by the physiologic functions of glucokinase, the increase in plasma glucose concentrations seen in patients with this form of diabetes is due to a combination of reduced glucose-induced insulin secretion from the pancreatic beta cell and reduced glycogen storage in the liver after glucose ingestion.

Liver-Enriched Transcription Factors: Hepatocyte Nuclear Factor-1α, Hepatocyte Nuclear Factor-1β, and Hepatocyte Nuclear Factor-4α

The transcription factors HNF-1α, HNF-1β, and HNF-4α play a key role in the tissue-specific regulation of gene expression in the liver[47] and are also expressed in other tissues including pancreatic islets, kidney, and genital tissues. HNF-1α and HNF-1β are members of the homeodomain-containing family of transcription factors, and HNF-4α is an orphan nuclear receptor.[47, 48] HNF-1α, HNF-1β, and HNF-4α make up part of an interacting network of transcription factors that function together to control gene expression during embryonic development and in adult tissues in which they are coexpressed. In the pancreatic beta cell, these transcription factors regulate the expression of the insulin gene as well as proteins involved in glucose transport and metabolism and mitochondrial metabolism, all linked to insulin secretion, and lipoprotein metabolism.[49] The expression of HNF-1α is regulated at least in part by HNF-4α. Persons with diabetes related to mutations in these genes have defects in insulin secretory responses to a variety of secretagogues, particularly glucose, that are present before the onset of hyperglycemia, suggesting that they represent the primary functional defect in the syndrome. Reduced glucagon responses to arginine have also been observed, suggesting that the pancreatic alpha cell is also involved in a broader pancreatic developmental abnormality.

Insulin Promoter Factor-1

IPF-1 is a homeodomain-containing transcription factor that was originally isolated as a transcriptional regulator of the insulin and somatostatin genes. It also plays a central role in the development of the pancreas as well as the regulation of expression of a variety of pancreatic islet genes including, besides insulin, glucokinase, islet amyloid polypeptide, and glucose transporter 2 genes. IPF-1 also appears to mediate glucose-induced stimulation of insulin gene transcription.[50]

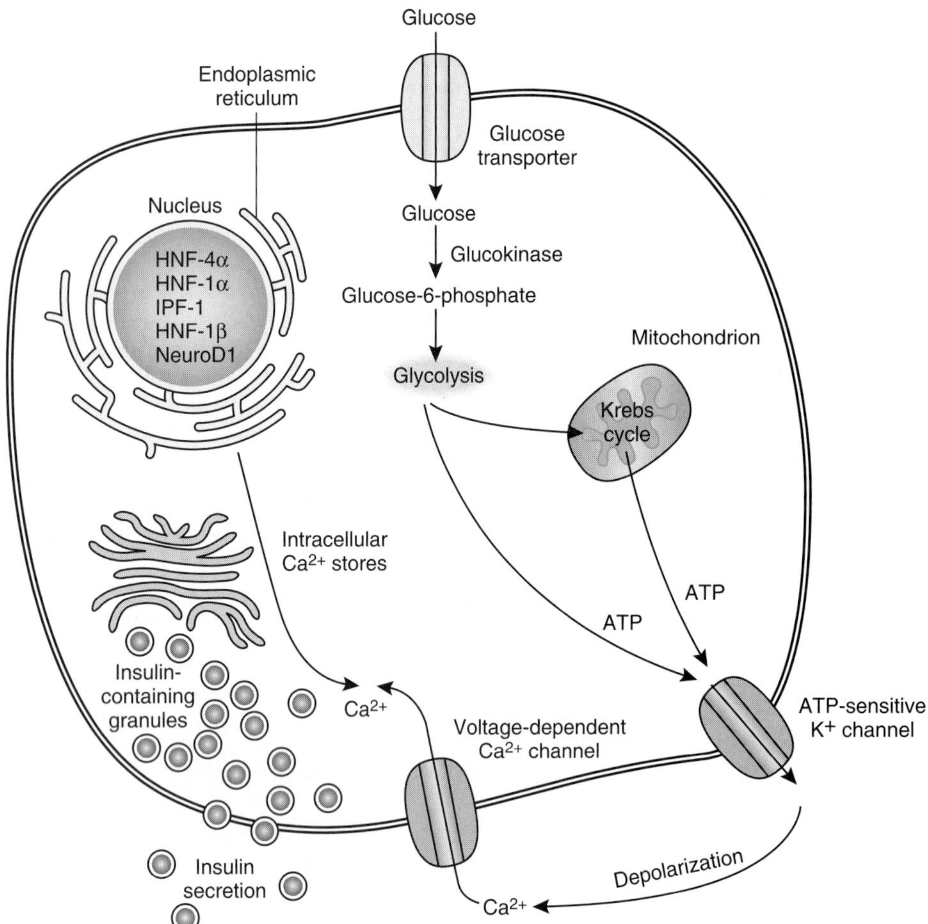

Figure 29–2. Model of a pancreatic beta cell and the proteins implicated in maturity-onset diabetes of the young. From Fajans SS, Bell GI, Polonsky KS. Molecular mechanisms and clinical pathophysiology of maturity-onset diabetes of the young. N Engl J Med 2001; 345:973.

A child born with pancreatic agenesis was shown to have a mutation in IPF-1 that lacked the homeodomain required for deoxyribonucleic acid (DNA) binding and nuclear localization. Heterozygous carriers of an IPF-1 mutation from the same kindred developed an early-onset autosomal dominant form of diabetes (i.e., MODY) caused by dominant negative inhibition of transcription of the insulin gene and other beta cell-specific genes regulated by the mutant IPF-1.[51] Additional IPF-1 mutations have been discovered in pedigrees with late-onset type 2 diabetes.[52] Thus, mutations in IPF-1 may cause a range of phenotype manifestations, depending on whether the subjects have homozygous or heterozygous mutations and the severity of the functional effects.

Neurogenic Differentiation-1 (NeuroD1/BETA2)

The basic helix-loop-helix transcription factor NeuroD1/BETA2 was isolated on the basis of its ability to activate transcription of the insulin gene and is required for normal pancreatic islet development. Two patients with heterozygous mutations in NeuroD1 and diabetes have been described,[45] and a third has been identified in an Icelandic population.[53] Studies in other populations have failed to detect mutations in NeuroD1 even in subjects with a MODY phenotype. It therefore appears that mutations in NeuroD1 are a rare cause of MODY.

Genetics of the Polygenic Forms of Type 2 Diabetes

As alluded to earlier, the common polygenic form of type 2 diabetes has complex pathophysiology with genetic and environmental factors both playing a major role. The phenotypic manifestations of the disease are also complex, and subjects with established type 2 diabetes demonstrate abnormalities in a number of tissues that play a key role in the regulation of glucose metabolism. These include resistance to the action of insulin in muscle, fat, and liver; defects in insulin secretory responses from the pancreatic beta cell; and increases in hepatic glucose production. However, the primary defect or defects responsible for the development of the syndrome remain elusive and are likely not to be defined until more is known about the genes responsible for diabetes and the nature of the gene-environment interactions that are ultimately responsible for the development of the disorder in predisposed individuals.

Insulin resistance is present in individuals predisposed to type 2 diabetes before the onset of hyperglycemia, and this finding has been interpreted by some to indicate that insulin resistance is the primary abnormality that is responsible for the development of type 2 diabetes. However, defective beta cell function is also present before the onset of type 2 diabetes when IGT is present and in first-degree relatives of persons with type 2 diabetes who have completely normal plasma glucose concentrations. Thus, although there is still controversy about whether insulin resistance or abnormal insulin secretion represents the primary defect in type 2 diabetes, there is general consensus that both defects are present in essentially all subjects with the disorder, frequently from an early preclinical stage.

It is therefore evident that the identification and characterization of the genes responsible for type 2 diabetes will add an essential level to our understanding of the pathophysiology of the disorder. Unfortunately, progress in identifying these genes has been slow for reasons that are discussed in greater detail in the following.

The candidate gene approach has not been successful in identifying genes responsible for the common polygenic forms of type 2 diabetes. This approach involves identifying and then cloning genes known to be involved in pathways that regulate glucose metabolism, screening for variants in these genes, and assessing the frequency of the variants in cases and controls.

Because the candidate gene approach has not been productive in identifying the genes for the common forms of type 2 diabetes, linkage analysis has been applied.[54] This approach involves defining regions of chromosomal DNA shared to excess by affected family members. Parents are genotyped at a particular marker, and the offspring are scored for sharing of zero, one, or two alleles inherited from their parents. Markers are genotyped in family members in the regions of polymorphic repeats called microsatellites or simple tandem repeats. Because in the case of type 2 diabetes (as well as other common polygenic human diseases), there is no prior knowledge of the gene defect, microsatellites at defined chromosomal locations are typed either in family members or in affected sibling pairs. In order to screen the whole genome, 300 to 400 microsatellites are genotyped in the study subjects at roughly 10-centimorgan intervals. This is generally adequate to define chromosomal regions sharing single gene defects. The evidence for linkage usually extends over a broad region, which may be 10 to 20 cM, and positional cloning strategies are then utilized to find the gene within this broad region.

This approach has demonstrated that genetic variation in the gene that encodes a ubiquitously expressed member of the calpain-like cysteine protease family, calpain-10 (*CAPN10*), is associated with increased risk for type 2 diabetes.[55]

Until the observation was made on the grounds of genetic studies that calpains may be involved in the pathophysiology of diabetes, this possibility had not been considered. It is now critical that the role of calpains in regulating the metabolic pathways responsible for the maintenance of insulin secretion and insulin action be defined. Data available from the initial studies that have addressed these questions have begun to provide clues to the mechanisms that may be involved.

It appears that the effects of the at-risk polymorphisms are mediated by decreasing calpain-10 expression in relevant tissues. Thus, Baier and colleagues[56] demonstrated that the polymorphism in calpain-10 that is responsible for the linkage to type 2 diabetes is associated with reduced muscle messenger ribonucleic acid (mRNA) and insulin resistance in Pima Indians, a population at extremely high risk for the development of type 2 diabetes. In order to simulate the physiologic effects of reduced calpain activity or expression, we have exposed rodent pancreatic islets or muscle strips to various calpain inhibitors for either 4 to 6 or 48 hours.[57] The effects on pancreatic islets were dependent on the duration of the exposure. After 4 to 6 hours, inhibition of calpain activity was associated with enhanced glucose-induced insulin secretion that appeared to be mediated by effects on the secretion process itself. Exposure of mouse islets to calpain inhibitors of different structure and mechanism of action for 48 hours reversibly suppressed glucose-induced insulin secretion by 40% to 80%. Exposure of islets to other protease inhibitors (cathepsin B and proteasome) did not result in similar effects. The 48-hour incubation with calpain inhibitors also attenuated insulin secretory responses to the mitochondrial fuel α-ketoisocaproate and the Ca^{2+}-independent exocytosis trigger mastoparan. Glucose metabolism and intracellular calcium $(Ca^{2+})_i$, responses to glucose or α-ketoisocaproate were also reduced, as was the exocytosis of insulin granules (measured by cell capacitance) in single beta cells. Thus, inhibition of calpain activity in islets attenuates insulin secretion, possibly by limiting the rate of glucose metabolism and exocytosis of insulin.

Exposure of rodent muscle strips to calpain inhibitors was shown to induce insulin resistance by impairing insulin-induced glucose transport and glycogen synthesis. Thus, these preliminary investigations suggest that calpain-sensitive pathways are present in pancreatic islet and muscle. Clearly, more detailed studies are needed to identify the specific calpain targets involved and to define their role in the normal control of insulin secretion and action and in the abnormalities in these processes that are responsible for the development of type 2 diabetes.

Why has it been so difficult to identify the genes responsible for the polygenic forms of type 2 diabetes, and what are the prospects for future progress? A perspective on the subject published by Cox[58] emphasized that the experience to date gained from studies on *CAPN10* is likely to provide a preview of the challenges that need to be overcome in the future.

The first important issue is that the *CAPN10* variation implicated in susceptibility to type 2 diabetes was located in a noncoding rather than a coding sequence and leads to a significant reduction in skeletal muscle calpain-10 mRNA levels as well as insulin resistance. The latter functional result could not have been predicted from the genetic analyses and knowledge of the biology of calpains and could be obtained only from studies of the functional effects of *CAPN10* variation in nondiabetic Pima Indians.

The second critical issue is that the mechanism for *CAPN10* effects is complex and combinations of variants are more strongly associated with disease than individual polymorphisms. In the case of *CAPN10*, individuals heterozygous for the two different haplotypes that form the high-risk haplotype combination have approximately threefold increased risk compared with all other combinations of haplotypes and approximately eightfold increased risk compared with the lowest risk haplotype combination. Individuals homozygous for either of the haplotypes in the high-risk combination were not at increased risk of developing type 2 diabetes.

The third issue is that the physiologic mechanism or mechanisms by which genetic susceptibility loci cause disease may not be clear and may be difficult to determine. This is certainly the case with *CAPN10* and with calpains in general, for which the primary physiologic function is unclear.

The fourth issue is that because multiple genetic mechanisms as well as environmental factors are involved in disease pathogenesis, replication may be difficult as the importance of specific genetic variations may differ in different populations.

In summary, therefore, as we move from studies of the monogenic forms of diabetes to studies that aim to understand the genetic, molecular, and physiologic basis of the polygenic forms of this condition, additional serious challenges must be met. However, in light of the complex nature of these disorders, understanding the genetic basis of these conditions is still the most likely pathway to solving the nature of these disorders.

INSULIN RESISTANCE AND THE RISK OF TYPE 2 DIABETES

Insulin Resistance

A substantial amount of data indicates that insulin resistance plays a major role in the development of glucose intolerance and diabetes. Insulin resistance is a consistent finding in patients with type 2 diabetes, and resistance is present years before the onset of diabetes.[59–64] Prospective studies show that insulin resistance predicts the onset of diabetes.[60, 61]

The term *insulin resistance* indicates the presence of an impaired biologic response to either exogenously administered or endogenously secreted insulin. Insulin resistance is manifested by decreased insulin-stimulated glucose transport and metabolism in adipocytes and skeletal muscle and by impaired suppression of hepatic glucose output. Insulin sensitivity is influenced by a number of factors including age,[65] weight, ethnicity, body fat (especially abdominal), physical activity, and medications. Insulin resistance is associated with the progression to IGT and type 2 diabetes,[66] although diabetes is rarely seen in insulin-resistant persons without some degree of beta cell dysfunction.[64] First-degree relatives of type 2 diabetics have insulin resistance even at a time when they are nonobese, implying a strong genetic component in the development of insulin resistance.[60, 66, 67] There is also a strong influence of environmental factors on the genetic predisposition to insulin resistance and therefore to diabetes.[68, 69]

Obesity and Type 2 Diabetes

The association of obesity with type 2 diabetes has been recognized for decades. A close association between obesity and insulin resistance is seen in all ethnic groups and is found across the full range of body weights, across all ages, and in both sexes[70–72] (Fig. 29–3). A number of large epidemiologic studies showed that the risk for diabetes, and presumably insulin resistance, rises as body fat content increases from the very

DIABETES BY AGE

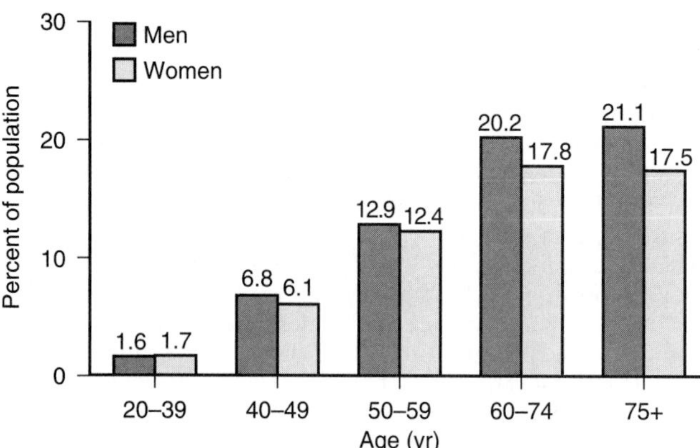

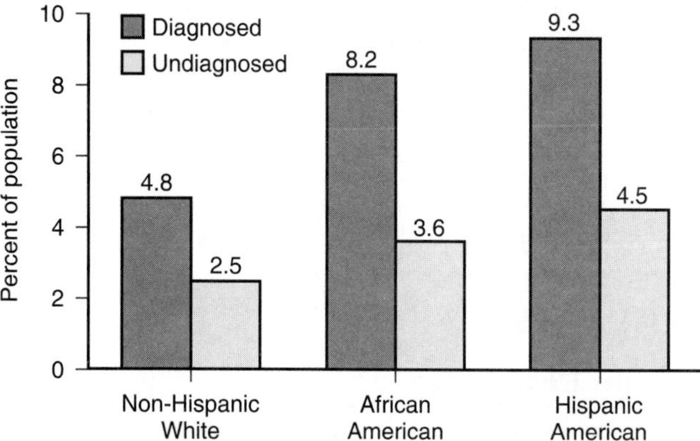

Figure 29–3. Prevalence of diabetes by age *(A)* and by ethnicity *(B)*. (From Harris MI, Flegal KM, Cowie CC, et al. Prevalence of diabetes, impaired fasting glucose, and impaired glucose tolerance in U.S. adults. The Third National Health and Nutrition Examination Survey, 1988–1994. Diabetes Care 1998; 21:518–524.)

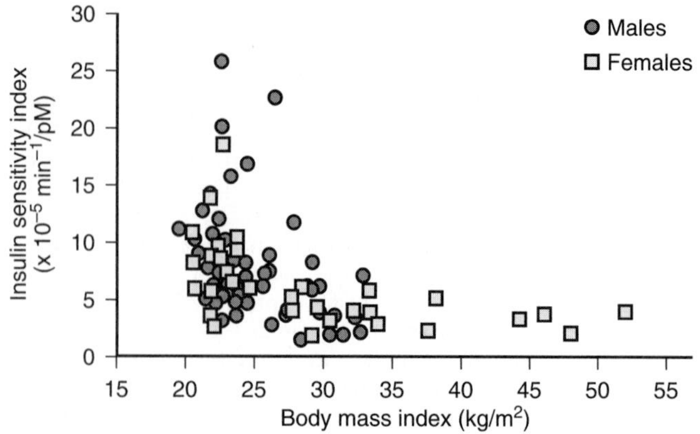

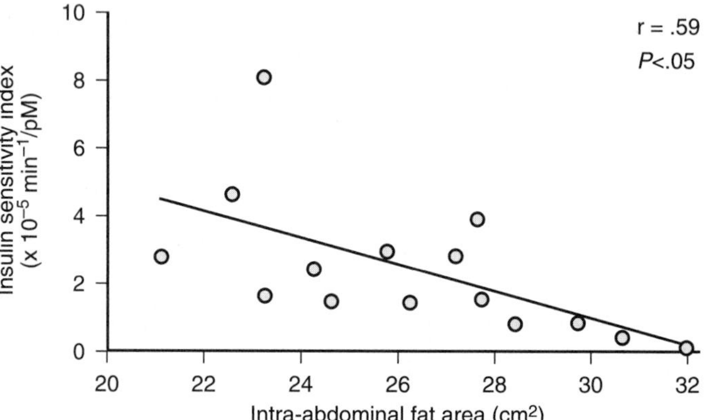

Figure 29–4. Relationship between body mass index *(A)* or intra-abdominal fat *(B)* and insulin sensitivity. (*A*, From Fujimoto WY, Bergstrom RW, Boyko EJ, et al. Obesity Res 1995; Suppl 2:1795–1863; *B*, from Kahn SE, Prigeon RL, McCulloch DK, et al. Quantification of the relationship between insulin sensitivity and beta-cell function in human subjects: evidence for a hyperbolic function. Diabetes 1993; 42: 1663–1672.)

lean to the very obese, implying that the absolute amount of body fat has an effect on insulin sensitivity across a broad range[73–75] (Fig. 29–4*A*). However, central (intra-abdominal) adiposity is more strongly linked to insulin resistance (Fig. 29–4*B*) and a number of important metabolic variables, including plasma glucose, insulin, total plasma cholesterol and triglyceride concentrations, and decreased plasma high-density lipoprotein (HDL) cholesterol concentration, than is total adiposity.[76–82] In addition, the effect of accumulation of abdominal fat on glucose tolerance is independent of total adiposity.[83, 84]

The reason for the relationship to intra-abdominal fat with abnormal metabolism is not clearly defined, but a number of hypotheses, which are not mutually exclusive, have been proposed. First, abdominal fat is more lipolytically active than subcutaneous fat, perhaps because of its greater complement of adrenergic receptors.[85, 86] In addition, the abdominal adipose store is resistant to the antilipolytic effects of insulin[87] including alterations in lipoprotein lipase activity, which leads to increased lipase activity and a greater flux of fatty acids into the circulation with the portal circulation receiving the greatest fatty acid load. The role of the liver in insulin resistance and hyperglycemia is discussed subsequently.

Skeletal Muscle Insulin Resistance

The primary site of glucose disposal after a meal is skeletal muscle, and the primary mechanism of glucose storage is

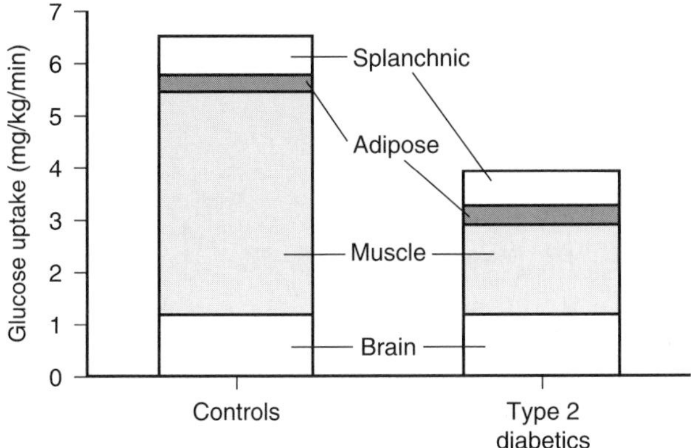

Figure 29–5. Tissue uptake of glucose in nondiabetic and insulin-resistant diabetic subjects during a hyperinsulinemic-euglycemic clamp. (From DeFronzo RA. Lilly lecture 1987. The triumvirate: beta-cell, muscle, liver. A collusion responsible for NIDDM. Diabetes 1988; 37: 667–687.)

through its conversion to glycogen. Studies using the hyperinsulinemic-euglycemic clamp technique have demonstrated that in insulin-resistant people with and without type 2 diabetes, there is a deficiency in the nonoxidative disposal of glucose related primarily to a defect in glycogen synthesis[88, 89] (Fig. 29–5).

Free Fatty Acids and Insulin Resistance

Elevated free fatty acids (FFAs) predict the progression from IGT to diabetes.[90, 91] In the periphery, FFAs may not be markedly elevated because of efficient extraction by the liver and skeletal muscle. Thus, normal or minimally elevated FFA levels may not reflect the true exposure of fatty acids to peripheral tissues. Increases in fatty acid flux to skeletal muscle related to the increased visceral lipolysis have been implicated in the inhibition of muscle glucose uptake.

The Randle hypothesis, or the glucose-fatty acid cycle, was originally proposed to account for the ability of FFAs to inhibit muscle glucose utilization. Randle and colleagues[92] demonstrated that fatty acids compete with glucose for substrate oxidation in isolated muscle. The increase in fatty acid metabolism leads to an increase in the intramitochondrial acetyl coenzyme A (CoA)/CoA and reduced nicotinamide adenine dinucleotide (NADH)/NAD^+ ratios with subsequent inhibition of pyruvate dehydrogenase. The resulting increased intracellular mitochondrial (and cytosolic) citrate concentrations result in allosteric inhibition of phosphofructokinase, the key rate-controlling enzyme in glycolysis. Subsequent accumulation of glucose-6-phosphate would inhibit hexokinase II activity, resulting in an increase in intracellular glucose concentrations and decreased glucose uptake.

However, later studies have suggested that the primary effect of fatty acids, at least in the presence of raised insulin levels, is a decrease in glucose transport as measured by a reduction in the rate of accumulation of intracellular glucose and glycogen using ^{13}C and ^{31}P nuclear magnetic resonance spectroscopy. In normal subjects, elevated fatty acids, achieved by infusion of triglyceride emulsions and heparin (to activate lipoprotein lipase), resulted in a fall in intracellular glucose and glucose-6-phosphate concentrations that preceded the fall in glycogen accumulation.[93, 94] These results challenge the Randle hypothesis (which predicts a rise in intracellular glucose-6-phosphate concentrations) as the basis of the reduction in insulin sensitivity seen with elevated fatty acids. Similar decreases in glucose transport have been seen in patients with type 2 diabetes[95] and lean, normoglycemic insulin-resistant offspring of type 2 diabetic individuals.[96, 97] These studies also found a decrease in the activity of phosphatidylinositol 3-phosphate kinase (PI 3-kinase) and increased protein kinase C-θ activity that may, in part, mediate the effect of high FFAs.[98, 99]

Intramuscular Triglyceride and Insulin Resistance

It has been found that insulin-stimulated glucose uptake is inversely related to the amount of intramuscular triglycerides. A strong correlation between intramuscular triglyceride concentration and insulin resistance has been demonstrated by evaluating intramuscular triglyceride with biopsy,[100] computed tomographic scanning,[101] and magnetic resonance imaging measurements.[102] The latter method has been a valuable addition because the magnetic resonance signal can distinguish intramyocellular from extramyocellular fat and demonstrates the increased triglyceride accumulation within the myofiber itself.[103] First-degree relatives of type 2 diabetics have an increase in intramyocellular fat, and in this group there is also a correlation with insulin resistance.[102]

The mechanism for accumulation of triglyceride in the skeletal muscle of obese and insulin-resistant individuals is probably related to the mismatching of FFA uptake and oxidation. During resting postabsorptive conditions, about 30% of fatty acid flux in the plasma pool is accounted for by oxidation, with the remaining 70% of flux recycled into triglyceride, indicating a physiologic reserve that exceeds immediate tissue needs for oxidative substrates. The equilibrium between oxidation and reesterification within muscle is paramount in determining fatty acid storage within tissue. The uptake, transport, and metabolism of fatty acids are highly regulated processes (Fig. 29–6), and alteration of the balance between uptake and oxidation in skeletal muscle leads to increased intramyocellular triglyceride. The increased lipolysis associated with obesity provides an increased amount of FFA presented to muscle.

Increased muscle triglyceride content is not invariably linked to insulin resistance because exercise training is associated with increased muscle triglyceride content,[104] and chronic exercise increases insulin sensitivity as well as the capacity for fatty acid oxidation.[105–109]

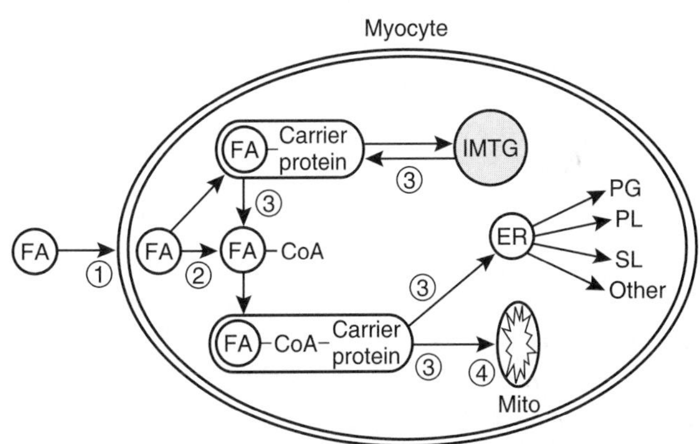

Figure 29–6. Simplified schematic diagram demonstrating fatty acid (FA) uptake, activation (formation of FA–coenzyme A [CoA]), and intracellular transport to different organelles within a muscle cell. IMTG, intramuscular triglyceride; PG, prostaglandin; PL, phospholipid; SL, sphingolipid.

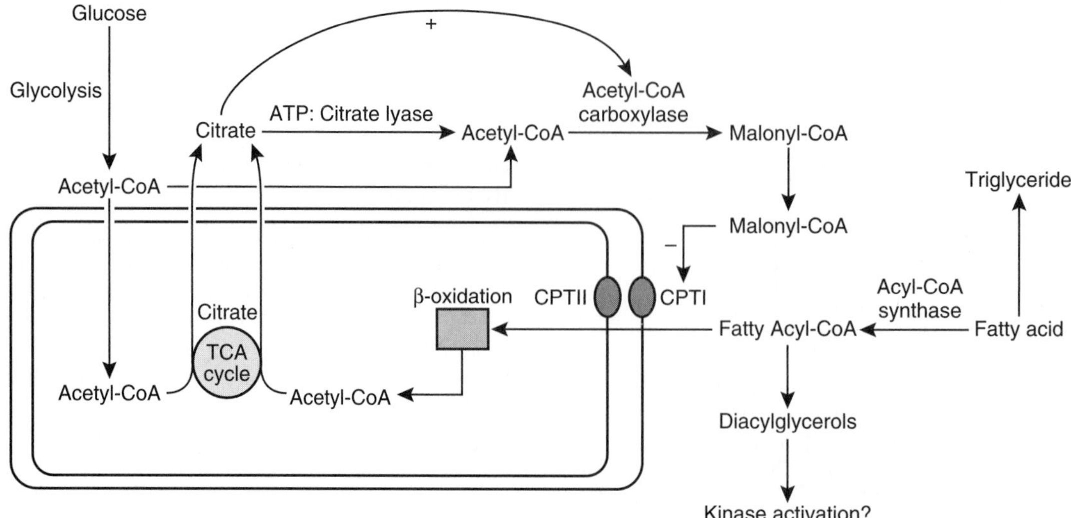

Figure 29–7. Glucose effect on triglyceride metabolism. Increased uptake of glucose results in an increase in the production of acetyl coenzyme A (CoA) as a product of glycolysis. The increased tricarboxylic acid (TCA) cycle activity associated with oxidation of both triglycerides and glucose increases the production of citrate, which is shuttled to the cytoplasm, activates the enzyme acetyl-CoA carboxylase (ACC) by allosteric mechanisms, and increases the susceptibility of ACC to phosphatases. This leads to increased ACC activity converting acetyl CoA to malonyl CoA. Malonyl CoA is a potent inhibitor of carnitine palmitoyltransferase I (CPT-I) on the outer mitochondrial membrane, which leads to accumulation of fatty acyl CoAs in the cytoplasm. This can result in the production of signaling molecules that can increase the activity of kinases and other enzymes and lead to insulin resistance.

Fatty Acid Metabolism in Skeletal Muscle, Relationship to Insulin Sensitivity

The uptake of fatty acid from the serum, where it is mostly bound to albumen, is mediated by at least three families of proteins: fatty acid translocase, plasma membrane fatty acid binding protein (FABP-pm), and fatty acid transport protein.[110–112] The levels of the putative transport proteins are regulated by exercise,[113] are correlated with body weight at least in women, and can be modulated by insulin infusion.[114]

FABPs are capable of binding multiple hydrophobic ligands, including fatty acids, eicosanoids, and retinoids with high affinity.[115] FABPs are thought to facilitate uptake of fatty acids and promote subsequent intracellular transport to subcellular organelles.[116] There is a direct correlation between heart-type FABP content and oxidative capacity observed during development and among different muscle types.[117, 118] In mice with a disruption of the heart[119] or adipocyte[120] isoform of FABP, plasma fatty acid concentrations were significantly elevated while plasma glucose was decreased, suggesting a key role in normal regulation in fatty acid oxidation. Some,[121] but not all[122] studies have shown a decrease in heart-type FABP in insulin-resistant humans.

Carnitine palmitoyltransferase I (CPT-I) has been the subject of intense scrutiny for many years because of its central role in the balance between mitochondrial glucose and fatty acid metabolism, primarily because of inhibition of mitochondrial fatty acid uptake by malonyl CoA.[123, 124] A specific isoform contributes 97% of the CPT-I in muscle and has 100-fold lower sensitivity to inhibition by malonyl CoA.[125] This lower sensitivity to malonyl CoA inhibition suggests that the levels of CPT-I itself may be important in the balance of uptake and oxidation of fatty acids. Evidence for this in skeletal muscle stems from the finding that, as with other fatty acid-oxidizing enzymes, muscle CPT-I mRNA is regulated by PPARα activators, fat feeding, and exercise in rodents and is inversely correlated with obesity in humans.[126–129]

Long-chain fatty acids, after passing through the inner mitochondrial membrane as acylcarnitines, are metabolized at the surface of the inner mitochondrial membrane by CPT-II and the long chain–specific oxidation system consisting of very-long-chain acyl CoA dehydrogenase (VLCAD) and the trifunctional protein (TFP) oxidation complex (Fig. 29–7). Transfer of the acyl chain from carnitine to CoA catalyzed by CPT-II is followed by one cycle of oxidation catalyzed by VLCAD and TFP to yield a chain-shortened acyl CoA that can recycle through the same oxidation system.[130] In actuality, four different acyl CoA dehydrogenase enzymes catalyze the initial dehydrogenation of straight-chain fatty acids in mitochondria. Three of them—short-chain acyl CoA dehydrogenase (SCAD), medium-chain acyl CoA dehydrogenase (MCAD), and long-chain acyl CoA dehydrogenase (LCAD)—are soluble enzymes located in the mitochondrial matrix as homotetramers. A fourth, VLCAD, is attached to the inner membrane as a homodimer. Their names derive from the length of the fatty acids that they process. VLCAD and LCAD shorten the long-chain fatty acids into medium-chain fatty acids that can then be processed by MCAD and SCAD.[131] The SCAD, MCAD, and LCAD monomers share a high degree of homology between them but not with VLCAD. At least some of these enzymes can be regulated in humans during exercise training.[132]

Uncoupling protein-1 (UCP1) is clearly related to the uncoupling of oxidative phosphorylation in brown adipose tissue.[95] UCP2 and UCP3 have structural similarities to UCP1, but it is not clear that they are actually uncouplers of oxidative phosphorylation.[133] Newer members of the family, brain mitochondrial carrier protein 1 (BMCP1) and UCP4, have an even more distant sequence relationship.[134] BMCP1 and UCP4 are predominantly expressed in neural tissues, namely the brain. UCP3 mRNA is found primarily in skeletal muscle and in brown adipose tissue. UCP2 has a ubiquitous tissue distribution. UCP2 and UCP3 mRNA levels have been correlated with different physiologic states, and numerous studies indicate that expression of UCP2 and UCP3 is stimulated by thyroid hormones and in the presence of high levels of fatty acids.[135] In humans, the levels of UCP2 and UCP3 mRNAs were up-regulated by a high-fat diet and the up-regulation was more pronounced in humans with high proportions of type IIA fibers.[136] In a small study, exercise training in humans increased mitochondrial oxidative capacity but did not change UCP2 or UCP3 levels.[137] Obesity itself was shown to be positively correlated with a splice isoform of UCP3.[138] A unique polymorphism in the promoter region of UCP3 correlated with the expression of UCP3 in skeletal muscle.[139]

Glucose Influence on Fatty Acid Metabolism

An emerging concept that could couple the increased fatty acid flux into skeletal muscle with impaired insulin action is the central role of malonyl CoA in regulating fatty acid and glucose oxidation[140] (see Fig. 29–7). Malonyl CoA is an allosteric inhibitor of CPT-I, the enzyme that controls the transfer of long-chain fatty acyl CoAs into the mitochondria.[123, 141, 142] Even in insulin-resistant skeletal muscle, glucose uptake into the skeletal muscle is higher, especially at the elevated levels of glucose found in type 2 diabetes.[143, 144] The glucose is shunted toward the glycolytic pathway, generating acetyl CoA that can be converted to malonyl CoA in the cytoplasm by the action of the highly regulated enzyme acetyl CoA carboxylase (ACC).

In humans an infusion of insulin and glucose at a high rate leads to increases in the concentration of malonyl CoA in skeletal muscle and to decreases in whole-body and, presumably, muscle fatty acid oxidation.[145] In the presence of elevated glucose and insulin levels, the tricarboxylic acid (TCA) cycle is activated, resulting in an increase in citrate in the cytoplasm through increased malate cycling in the mitochondria. The increased citrate is converted to acetyl CoA through citrate lyase and thus provides an indirect substrate for ACC. Citrate also allosterically activates ACC and makes ACC a better substrate for phosphatases that activate the enzyme.[146, 147] ACC is also regulated by a phosphorylation-dephosphorylation cycle, with adenosine monophosphate (AMP)–dependent protein kinase an important kinase, which inhibits both ACC basal activity and activation by citrate.[148] ACC then generates malonyl CoA that in turn allosterically inhibits CPT-I residing on the outer mitochondrial membrane, inhibiting uptake of acyl CoA. The resulting buildup of long-chain acyl CoAs and diacylglycerols is proposed to activate one or more protein kinase C isoforms or other lipid-activated proteins, resulting in insulin resistance.[140] Support for this hypothesis is the finding that exercise, which activates AMP-dependent kinase, inactivates ACC, lowers intracellular long-chain acyl CoA levels, and has an acute insulin-sensitizing effect.[149]

Hyperinsulinemia and Insulin Resistance

Hyperinsulinemia per se has been proposed to cause insulin resistance. Elevated concentrations of insulin can cause insulin resistance by down-regulating insulin receptors and desensitizing postreceptor pathways.[150] Del Prato and associates showed that 24 and 72 hours of sustained physiologic hyperinsulinemia in normal individuals specifically inhibited the ability of insulin to increase nonoxidative glucose disposal in association with an impaired ability of insulin to stimulate glycogen synthase activity.[151] Suppression of insulin secretion in obese, insulin-resistant people results in increased insulin sensitivity.[152, 153]

Insulin Signaling Abnormalities in Insulin Resistance

The pathways that are critical for insulin regulation of glucose and lipid metabolism are being clarified. However, the complete cascade of events remains to be determined. Besides intermediary metabolism of glucose and lipid, signaling by insulin affects other cellular processes such as amino acid transport and metabolism, protein synthesis, cell growth, differentiation, and apoptosis.

Insulin Signaling

Insulin signaling is initiated through the binding to and activation of its cell-surface receptor and initiates a cascade of phosphorylation and dephosphorylation events, second messenger generation, and protein-protein interactions that result in the diverse metabolic events in nearly every tissue (Fig. 29–8). The insulin receptor consists of two insulin-binding α subunits and two catalytically active β subunits that are disulfide linked into an $\alpha 2\beta 2$ heterotetrameric complex. Insulin binds to the extracellular α subunits, activating the intracellular tyrosine kinase domain of the β subunit.[154] One receptor β subunit phosphorylates its partner on specific tyrosine residues that may have distinct functions such as stimulation of intermolecular association of signaling molecules such as Shc and Grb, members of the insulin receptor substrate family (IRS1, 2, 3, 4), Shc adapter protein isoforms, and SIRP (signal regulatory protein) family members, Gab-1, Cbl, CAP, and APS[155, 156]; stimulation of mitogenesis[157]; and receptor internalization.[158]

Insulin receptor β subunit has also been shown to undergo serine-threonine phosphorylation, which may decrease the ability of the receptor to autophosphorylate. The activities of a number of protein kinase C isoforms that catalyze the serine or threonine phosphorylation of the insulin receptor are elevated in animal models of insulin resistance and in insulin-resistant humans.[159, 160] Interventions that decrease serine phosphorylation of the insulin receptor result in increased insulin signaling.[161] Termination of the insulin signaling event occurs by internalization and dephosphorylation of the receptor by protein tyrosine phosphatases. Increased activity of protein tyrosine phosphatase can attenuate insulin signaling. Two protein tyrosine phosphatases that have been shown to negatively regulate insulin signaling, PTP1B and LAR (leukocyte antigen related), have been reported to be elevated in insulin-resistant patients.[162, 163] Conversely, disruption of PTB1B in mice resulted in a marked increase in insulin sensitivity and resistance to diet-induced obesity.[164]

Mutations in the insulin receptor are associated with rare forms of insulin resistance. These mutations affect insulin receptor number, splicing, trafficking, binding, and phosphorylation. The affected patients demonstrate severe insulin resistance, manifest as clinically diverse syndromes including the type A syndrome, leprechaunism, Rabson-Mendenhall syndrome, and lipoatrophic diabetes.[165, 166]

Downstream Events Following Insulin Receptor Phosphorylation

IRSs act as multifunctional docking proteins activated by tyrosine phosphorylation.[167] The IRS proteins have multiple functional domains, including Pleckstrin homology (PH) and phosphotyrosine binding (PTB) and SH domains that interact with other proteins to mediate the insulin signaling events. Disruption of IRS1 in mice resulted in mild insulin resistance and growth retardation, whereas disruption of IRS2 resulted in beta cell failure and secondary insulin resistance.[168]

PI 3-kinase, which is regulated by interaction with IRS proteins, is necessary but not sufficient for the stimulation of the glucose transporter GLUT4-mediated increase in glucose transport in insulin-sensitive tissues.[169] In addition, inhibition of PI 3-kinase activity with the fungal inhibitor wortmannin inhibited insulin-stimulated glucose uptake, glycogen synthesis, triglyceride accumulation, protein synthesis, and modulation of gene expression.[170] PI 3-kinase generates 3,4,5-phosphoinositol, which activates several PIP3 (phosphatidylinositol-3,4,5 tri-

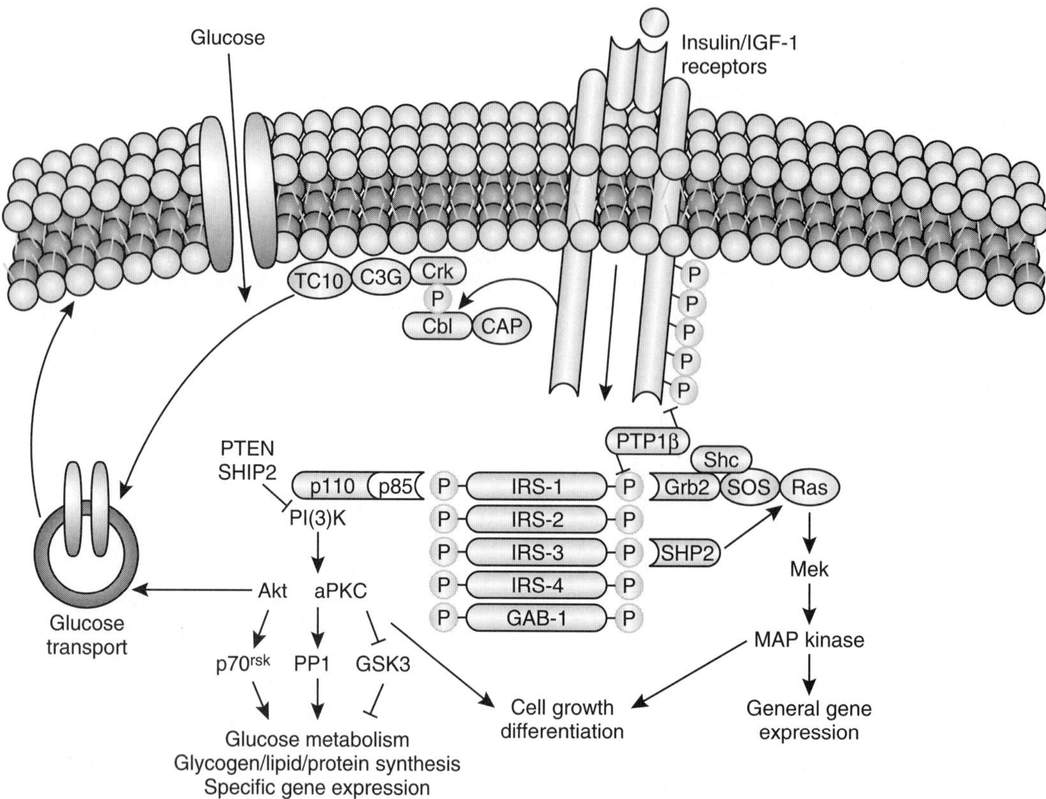

Figure 29–8. Insulin signaling. The insulin receptor is autophosphorylated on multiple tyrosine residues, allowing the docking and activation of multiple signaling molecules, which mediates the increases in glucose uptake and metabolism as well as changes in protein and lipid metabolism. (From Saltiel AR, Kahn CR. Insulin signalling and the regulation of glucose and lipid metabolism. Nature 2001; 414:799–806.)

phosphate)-dependent serine-threonine kinases, such as PI-dependent protein kinases 1 and 2, which in turn activates Akt, salt- and glucocorticoid-induced kinases,[113] protein kinase C, wortmannin-sensitive and insulin-stimulated serine kinase, and others.

Akt kinase (also known as protein kinase B) exists as three distinct isoforms that are activated by phosphorylation on specific threonine and serine residues.[171] Activated Akt has the ability to phosphorylate proteins that regulate lipid synthesis, glycogen synthesis, protein synthesis, and apoptosis. Disruption of Akt2 resulted in insulin resistance and diabetes in mice.[172] Several investigators have examined the role of PI 3-kinase and Akt in individuals with insulin resistance. Studies have shown a decrease in IRS-associated PI 3-kinase[173] and Akt[174] activity in insulin-resistant skeletal muscle; however, in some patients with reduced PI 3-kinase activity there was normal activation of Akt.[175]

A primary effect of insulin is to stimulate translocation of the glucose transporter GLUT4 from an intracellular pool to the surface of cells, primarily in skeletal muscle and adipose tissue and heart.[176] The mechanism by which the signaling pathways converge on the intracellular GLUT4-containing vesicles to cause GLUT4 translocation is not well understood. It appears that the number of glucose transporters in skeletal muscle of insulin-resistant persons is not changed but the ability of insulin to effect this translocation is disrupted.[177–179]

Glucocorticoid-Induced Insulin Resistance

Cushing's syndrome and exogenous glucocorticoid treatment have long been known to induce significant insulin resistance in humans. The exact mechanism is unknown, but it is associated with redistribution of fat from the periphery to the central compartment. Elevations in triglyceride and FFA levels also occur. At a molecular level, dexamethasone has differential effects on the proteins involved in the early steps in insulin action in liver and muscle. In both tissues, dexamethasone treatment results in a reduction in insulin-stimulated IRS1-associated PI 3-kinase, which may play a role in the pathogenesis of insulin resistance at the cellular level in these animals.

Tumor Necrosis Factor α

Studies in humans and animal models of obesity have identified changes in the expression and activity of key molecules involved in the insulin signaling pathway. Decreases in the number and the kinase activity of insulin receptors[180] and impairment in the activation of IRS1,[181] PI 3-kinase,[182–183] and protein kinase B[184] have been observed. Although the basis for the changes is, in general, unknown, a tumor necrosis factor α (TNF-α)–mediated mechanism for the decreased activity in the initial steps of the insulin signaling cascade has been proposed. TNF-α, made and secreted by adipocytes, is elevated in a variety of experimental models of obesity.[185] The kinase activity of the insulin receptor in rats[186] or in 3T3-L1 adipocytes[185] treated with TNF-α was reduced, possibly by increased serine phosphorylation.[187] Fat-fed mice with genetic ablation of TNF-α production had increased kinase activity of the insulin receptor compared with control mice and demonstrated increased insulin sensitivity.[188] In addition, rats treated with neutralizing antisera or soluble TNF receptors demonstrated an amelioration of their insulin resistance. As described later, other interventions to decrease TNF-α action result in increased insulin sensitivity.

Glucotoxicity, Glucosamine

Hyperglycemia is a primary factor in the development of the complications of diabetes, and decreases in average blood glucose have a profound effect to prevent complications in both type 1[189] and type 2 diabetes.[190] Hyperglycemia itself can cause insulin resistance. In Pima Indians, the level of fasting glycemia is the primary determinant of insulin sensitivity.[191] The defect is primarily in skeletal muscle[192] and is related to the degree of hyperglycemia.

Entry of glucose into the cell results in its phosphorylation to glucose-6-phosphate, which has multiple metabolic fates. The enzyme glutamine:fructose-6-phosphate amidotransferase (GFAT) carries out the rate-limiting step of the hexosamine pathway.[193] Evidence suggests that the hexosamine pathway underlies the defect in glucose utilization associated with hyperglycemia. Hexosamines, such as glucosamine, when incubated with adipose tissue, induce insulin resistance in fat cells[194] and in skeletal muscle.[195] Infusion of glucosamine into rats resulted in a dose-dependent increase in insulin resistance of skeletal muscle.[195] Finally, transgenic mice that overexpress GFAT specifically in skeletal muscle acquired severe insulin resistance.[196] By a pathway that is unclear, glucosamine overproduction resulted in a disruption of the ability of insulin to cause translocation of GLUT4 to the cell surface.[197] Through its anti-insulin action, the hexosamine pathway has been hypothesized to be a glucose sensor that allows the cell to sense and adapt to the prevailing level of glucose.[192]

Insulin Resistance and Lipodystrophy Associated with Human Immunodeficiency Virus Infection

A syndrome with many of the clinical and metabolic features of insulin resistance is increasingly being recognized in patients with human immunodeficiency virus (HIV) infection.[198] An unusual form of lipodystrophy is observed in certain of these patients in whom there is significant fat redistribution from the extremities and face to the torso with accumulation of intra-abdominal and intrascapular fat. This form of lipodystrophy is associated with significant insulin resistance and type 2 diabetes, dyslipidemia with elevated total and low-density lipoprotein (LDL) cholesterol and suppressed HDL cholesterol concentrations, and a susceptibility to lactic acidemia.[199]

Epidemiologic studies have associated this syndrome with previous or current treatment with antiretroviral protease inhibitors or nucleoside reverse transcriptase inhibitors. There is also an association with increased age.[198] Other possible contributing factors are male sex, diagnosis of the acquired immunodeficiency syndrome, responsiveness to antiretroviral treatment, and increases in CD4 T-cell counts. An increased emphasis has been placed on the role of protease inhibitors in the pathogenesis of the syndrome. Administration of these drugs or ritonavir to normal subjects caused increases in plasma triglyceride and very-low-density lipoprotein (VLDL) cholesterol and decreased plasma HDL cholesterol levels.[200] Indinavir administration for 4 weeks resulted in small increases in serum glucose and insulin levels and decreased insulin-mediated glucose disposal as assessed with a hyperinsulinemic, euglycemic clamp. In this study there were no changes in lipoprotein, triglycerides, or FFA levels.[201]

The molecular basis of the metabolic syndrome is not clear. A number of protease inhibitors can inhibit glucose transport in vitro and in vivo, and there is evidence for a direct interaction with the GLUT4 glucose transporter[202] that could inhibit glucose uptake specifically in insulin-responsive tissue. Mitochondrial abnormalities have been described in subcutaneous adipose tissue biopsy specimens of HIV-infected patients with lipodystrophy compared with those without the syndrome.[203] A direct effect of protease inhibitors on differentiation of adipocytes has also been described.[204–206] At present, the precise mechanism for the lipodystrophy associated with HIV infection is not known.

Mechanisms of Reducing Insulin Resistance

The most effective measures to improve insulin sensitivity are weight loss and exercise. Both modalities are effective and can be additive in their ability to improve insulin action. Later in this chapter, the role of these interventions in the treatment of patients with type 2 diabetes is discussed. The scientific basis and molecular mechanisms responsible for the improvements in insulin sensitivity seen with these interventions are now summarized.

Mechanisms for Improved Insulin Sensitivity with Weight Loss

Weight loss can be a highly effective treatment for overweight patients with type 2 diabetes and other cardiovascular risk factors, and indeed it is advocated as the first line of therapy. Weight loss may also play a role in the prevention of type 2 diabetes.[73, 207] In overweight patients with type 2 diabetes, weight loss can reduce hepatic glucose production, insulin resistance, and fasting hyperinsulinemia and can improve glycemic control. Weight loss in type 2 diabetes is also associated with a reduction in blood pressure and an improvement in the lipid profile. These benefits can occur with as little as 5% to 10% weight loss.[208–210] Moreover, preventing obesity in primates with long-term caloric restriction attenuates the development of insulin resistance.

One possible mechanism for improvements in insulin sensitivity through weight loss may be effects on the pattern of muscle fatty acid metabolism and the accumulation of lipid within muscle. In this context, it would be important to know whether alterations in the pathways of fatty acid utilization in skeletal muscle represent primary defects in obese individuals or arise secondarily, after an individual has become obese. This question cannot be answered by cross-sectional comparisons of lean and obese subjects. One prospective clinical study indicated that lower rates of lipid oxidation were a predisposing factor for greater weight gain,[139] and collateral studies implicated altered skeletal muscle enzyme activities in impaired lipid oxidation.[140, 141] A reduced reliance on lipid oxidation has also been identified as a risk factor for weight regain after weight loss.[142] These data raise the possibility that a potential impairment in the capacity for lipid oxidation may be a primary defect in obesity. Weight loss can markedly improve insulin-resistant glucose metabolism in skeletal muscle. When the patient's response indicates a substantial acquired or secondary component of obesity-related insulin-resistant glucose metabolism, it is important to determine whether weight loss can modulate patterns of skeletal muscle metabolism of fatty acids, including the content of fat within muscle.

Mechanisms for Improved Insulin Sensitivity with Exercise

Exercise is clearly effective in increasing insulin sensitivity in animals and in humans. There appear to be two separable but related effects of exercise on insulin action. A single bout of exercise can result in an acute increase in insulin-independent glucose transport measurable during and for a relatively short period after exercise.[211–215] Like insulin, exercise and muscle contractions increase glucose transport by translocation of intracellular GLUT4 glucose transporters to the cell surface.[216–218]

Acute Exercise

The signaling pathway leading to the exercise-induced increase in glucose transporter translocation and glucose transport is unknown, although there is ample evidence that the pathway is independent of the insulin-stimulated, receptor-mediated pathway. The effect of exercise and contractions on translocation and transport is additive to the maximal effect of insulin.[211, 218–221] Insulin-stimulated glucose transport in muscle is inhibited by specific inhibitors of PI 3-kinase, such as wortmannin, whereas transport or translocation stimulated by muscle contractions is insensitive to these inhibitors.[218, 222, 223] Stimulation of muscle contractions in situ and exercise do not increase insulin receptor phosphorylation or tyrosine kinase activity, IRS phosphorylation, or PI 3-kinase activity.[217, 224] In addition, in many insulin-resistant states the acute exercise-stimulated (but not insulin-stimulated) glucose transport and GLUT4 translocation is normal. This has been demonstrated in the obese, insulin-resistant Zucker rat[225] and in type 2 diabetic patients.[179] Finally, hypoxia, a stimulus for glucose transport that is also independent of the insulin receptor–mediated pathway, is effective in increasing glucose transport in muscle strips from obese, insulin-resistant individuals and in patients with type 2 diabetes.[226]

The acute effect of exercise and hypoxia may be mediated by AMP-dependent protein kinase (AMPK). AMPK is thought to be a sensor of intracellular energy stores and is activated by increases in intracellular AMP. A stable AMP analogue, 5-amino-4-imidazole carboxamide ribotide (ZMP), can be generated intracellularly from 5-aminoimidazole-4-carboxamide ribonucleoside (AICAR) and can activate AMPK in cells, leading to increased phosphorylation of known substrates for AMPK including 3-hydroxy-3-methylglutaryl CoA reductase, acyl-CoA carboxylase, and creatine kinase.[227] Treatment of incubated skeletal muscle with AICAR resulted in increased glucose uptake and glucose transporter translocation.[228] Similarly, the inclusion of 2 mM AICAR in the perfusate of the rat hindlimb resulted in inactivation of ACC, decreases in malonyl CoA levels and a twofold increase in glucose uptake.[229, 230] The euglycemic clamp technique has been used in conscious rats to demonstrate that infusion of AICAR resulted in a more than twofold increase in glucose utilization. Uptake of the glucose analogue 2-deoxyglucose was also increased twofold in vivo in soleus and gastrocnemius muscles. As with previous studies, this uptake was not associated with PI 3-kinase activation, again indicating a separate pathway from that of insulin.

A second effect of exercise, which becomes evident as the acute effect on glucose transport reverses, is a large increase in the sensitivity of glucose transport to stimulation by insulin.[231–234] This effect is due to translocation of more GLUT4 glucose transporters to the cell surface for any given dose of insulin.[235, 236] As with the acute stimulation of transport by exercise, the cellular mechanisms leading to enhanced translocation in response to submaximally effective stimuli are unknown. However, several studies have shown that steps in the insulin signaling cascade leading to activation of PI 3-kinase are not enhanced after a bout of exercise. There is no change in insulin binding to its receptor,[224, 237] insulin stimulation of receptor tyrosine kinase activity,[224, 238] increase in insulin-stimulated tyrosine phosphorylation of IRS1,[235] or PI 3-kinase activity associated with IRS1.[217, 238]

Exercise Training

Exercise training also results in increases in insulin sensitivity[239, 240] and can delay or prevent the onset of type 2 diabetes in those at high risk.[241] Using the hyperinsulinemic-euglycemic clamp, Perseghin and co-workers[242] compared exercise training for 45 minutes on a stair-climbing machine 4 days per week for 6 weeks in normal insulin-sensitive subjects and a group of high-risk, insulin-resistant relatives of type 2 diabetics. A 100% increase in insulin sensitivity was seen in both groups without a significant change in body weight. Interestingly, the higher basal and glucose-stimulated insulin release seen in the insulin-resistant subjects was not altered after exercise training. The effect of exercise training on insulin sensitivity has been proposed to be due to up-regulation of glucose transporter number, changes in capillary density, and increases in the number of red, glycolytic (type IIa) fibers.[243, 244]

Mechanisms That Link Cardiovascular Disease and Insulin Resistance: Syndrome X

Myocardial infarction, stroke, and nonischemic cardiovascular disease are the cause of death in up to 80% of individuals with type 2 diabetes. Independent of other risk factors, type 2 diabetes increases the risk for cardiovascular morbidity and mortality but also provides a synergistic interaction with other risk factors such as smoking, hypertension, and dyslipidemia.[245] In a Finnish population, diabetes increased the risk for myocardial infarction fivefold,[246] and insulin resistance as measured by elevated fasting insulin levels increased the risk of death from heart disease.[247] Women are particularly vulnerable to the cardiovascular effects of type 2 diabetes as they appear to lose the protective effects of estrogen in the premenopausal period.[248, 249]

A constellation of metabolic derangements that are frequently seen in patients with insulin resistance and type 2 diabetes are individually associated with an increased risk of cardiovascular disease. These patients have been variously designated as having syndrome X; the dysmetabolic syndrome; hypertension, obesity, non–insulin-dependent diabetes mellitus (NIDDM), dyslipidemia, and atherosclerotic cardiovascular disease (HONDA); or the "deadly quartet."[250, 251] The syndrome has also been associated with easily oxidized, small LDL particles; heightened blood-clotting activity (e.g., increased plasminogen activator inhibitor 1); and elevated serum uric acid concentration. The central abnormality associated with syndrome X has been proposed to be insulin resistance. Some of the abnormalities have also been proposed to contribute *to* insulin resistance.

Perhaps the overriding risk factor for coronary artery disease in insulin resistance and type 2 diabetes is the associated dyslipidemia. The profile includes hypertriglyceridemia, low plasma HDL, and small, dense LDL particle concentrations. The percentage of men with type 2 diabetes with abnormal cholesterol levels is not different from that of nondiabetic men. However, diabetic women have nearly double the rate of hypercholesterolemia[252] and greater changes in other lipid parameters that increase the risk for cardiovascular disease (Fig. 29–9). The physiologic basis for this abnormal lipid profile appears to be overproduction of apolipoprotein B-containing VLDL particles. The apolipoprotein B production by the liver is primarily post-translational[253] and augmented by insulin and by the increased availability of FFAs in the portal circulation,[254–258] probably as a result of increased lipolysis in the visceral adipose tissue.[259–261] Part of the post-translational regulation may be due to insulin and fatty acid-mediated increases in microsomal triglyceride transfer protein levels that catalyze the transfer of lipids to apolipoprotein B and decrease the ubiquination-dependent degradation of apolipoprotein B.[262–264]

The overproduction of VLDL triglyceride results in increased transfer of VLDL triglyceride to HDL particles in exchange for HDL cholesterol esters mediated by the cholesterol ester transfer protein.[265] The triglyceride-rich HDL is hydrolyzed by hepatic lipase, which results in the generation of

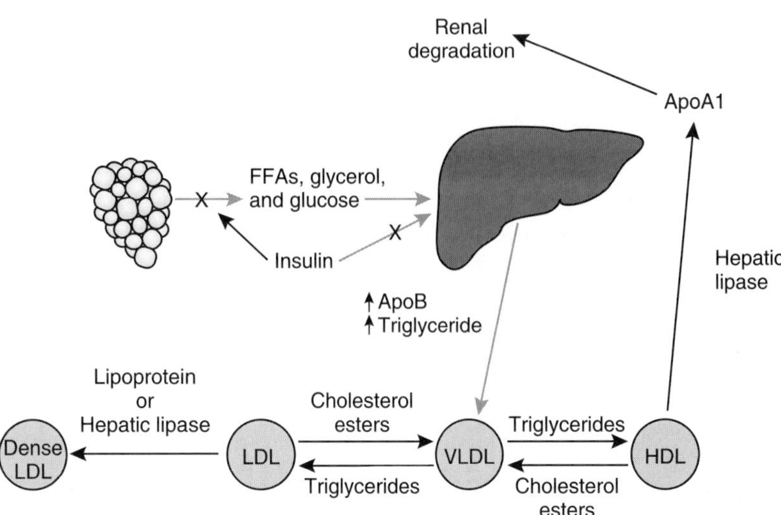

Figure 29–9. Insulin resistance and dyslipidemia. The suppression of lipoprotein lipase and very-low-density lipoprotein (VLDL) production by insulin is defective in insulin resistance, leading to increased free fatty acid (FFA) flux to the liver, and increased VLDL production, which results in increased circulating triglyceride concentrations. The triglycerides are transferred to low-density lipoprotein (LDL) and high-density lipoprotein (HDL) and the VLDL particle gains cholesterol esters by the action of the cholesterol ester transfer protein (CETP). This leads to increased catabolism of HDL particles by the liver and loss of apolipoprotein A (ApoA), resulting in low HDL concentrations. The triglyceride-rich LDL particle is stripped of the triglycerides, resulting in the accumulation of atherogenic small, dense LDL particles.

small HDL, which is degraded more readily by the kidney, resulting in low HDL levels in serum. Cholesterol ester transfer protein–mediated exchange of VLDL triglyceride for LDL cholesterol esters and subsequent triglyceride hydrolysis by hepatic lipase probably result in the generation of the small, dense LDL particles found in insulin-resistant subjects.[266–269]

The increased risk of heart disease in patients with diabetes has prompted the recommendation that individuals with diabetes be treated for their dyslipidemia as aggressively as individuals who have had a previous myocardial infarction. In addition, individuals with the metabolic syndrome of insulin resistance and obesity are considered to be in a higher risk category and should also be aggressively treated in order to lower lipids.[270]

Hypertension and overt diabetes double the risk of cardiovascular disease. Defects in vasodilatation and alterations in blood flow may provide a link to hypertension in insulin-resistant subjects. The normal vasodilatory response of insulin is disrupted in obese, insulin-resistant, and diabetic individuals,[271] perhaps through inability of insulin to increase the production of the potent vasodilator nitric oxide by endothelial cells.[272, 273] The defect may be magnified by increases in plasma FFAs.[274] Other proposed mechanisms for insulin resistance leading to hypertension are the activation of the sympathetic nervous system by insulin[275–277] and the intrinsic ability of insulin to cause salt and water readsorption in the kidney resulting in expanded plasma volume.[278–280]

Hypertension itself, independent of other risk factors, has been associated with the propensity to become diabetic.[281] A prospective cohort study found that type 2 diabetes was nearly 2.5 times more likely to develop in subjects with hypertension than in subjects with normal blood pressure.[282] A possible mechanism is that an intrinsic defect in vasodilatation may contribute to insulin resistance by decreasing the surface area of the vasculature perfusing skeletal muscle, decreasing the efficiency of glucose uptake.[274] Conversely, vasodilatory agents may improve glucose uptake and may even prevent the onset of diabetes, as has been observed with angiotensin-converting enzyme inhibitor therapy.[283]

Several factors involved in clotting and fibrinolysis, including fibrinogen, factor VII, and plasminogen activator inhibitor 1 (PAI-1), have been shown to be increased in individuals with insulin resistance.[284–289] PAI-1 has been extensively studied, and there is a clear relationship between elevated PAI-1 levels and risk for coronary artery disease.[290] Insulin increased PAI-1 expression in hepatocytes, endothelial cells, and abdominal adipose tissue,[291–293] and insulin-sensitizing thiazolidinediones decreased PAI-1 activity.[294]

Upper body rather than lower body obesity (the apple rather than the pear shape) is highly correlated with insulin resistance and risk for type 2 diabetes. Thus, the anatomic distribution of fat, rather than the overall degree of obesity, appears to determine risk for the metabolic syndrome. The reported association between increased abdominal (upper body) fat and an increased risk of coronary heart disease is related to visceral fat, for which the waist-to-hip ratio is a convenient index. A waist-to-hip ratio greater than 1.0 in men and 0.8 in women indicates abdominal obesity.[295] Recently the National Cholesterol Education Program (NCEP) has suggested that a waist circumference >40 inches in men and >35 inches in women is a marker for the metabolic syndrome.[295a]

The Role of Increased Hepatic Glucose Production in the Hyperglycemia of Type 2 Diabetes and Impaired Glucose Tolerance

The disposal of glucose after meals depends on the ability of insulin to increase peripheral glucose uptake and simultaneously decrease endogenous glucose production. Although studies have suggested that the kidney can contribute up to 25% of endogenous glucose production,[296, 297] the defect in type 2 diabetes is primarily in defective regulation of glucose production from the liver (hepatic glucose output [HGO]). Two routes of glucose production by the liver are glycogenolysis of stored glycogen and gluconeogenesis from two- and three-carbon substrates derived primarily from skeletal muscle.[298–299] Under different conditions and at different times postprandially, the contribution of each of these to maintenance of glucose levels may vary. Using ^{13}C nuclear magnetic resonance spectroscopy combined with measurement of whole-body glucose production in normal human subjects at different intervals after fasting, it was found that gluconeogenesis accounted for 50% to 96% of glucose production with the proportion increasing with increasing duration of fasting.[300, 301]

The production of glucose by the liver is regulated primarily by the relative actions of glucagon and insulin to activate or suppress glucose production, respectively, although the nervous system[302] and glucose autoregulation of hepatic glucose production probably play less important roles.[303] The ability of insulin to reduce HGO is an important mechanism for maintaining normal glucose tolerance.[304, 305] Under normal circumstances, insulin suppresses up to 85% of glucose production in normal individuals by directly inhibiting glycogenolysis, espe-

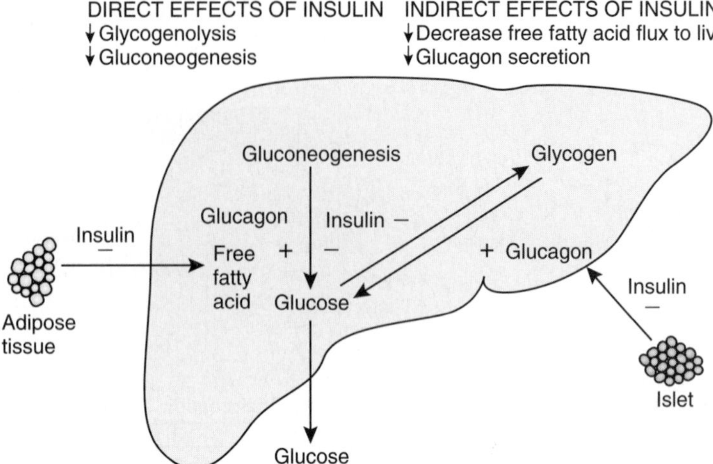

Figure 29–10. Insulin suppresses hepatic glucose production by direct and indirect mechanisms. In insulin resistance, insulin's ability to suppress lipolysis in adipose tissue and glucagon secretion by alpha cells in the islet results in increased gluconeogenesis. In addition, insulin inhibition of glycogenolysis is impaired. Thus, both hepatic and peripheral insulin resistance results in abnormal glucose production by the liver.

cially at lower insulin concentrations.[306] Under circumstances in which glycogenolysis is enhanced by glucagon, the effects of insulin to suppress hepatic glucose production may be even greater.[307] Glucagon increases glycogenolysis by activation of the classical protein kinase cascade involving cyclic AMP (cAMP)–dependent protein kinase and phosphorylase and also increases gluconeogenesis in part by increasing the transcription of phosphoenolpyruvate carboxykinase through the cAMP response element binding protein.[305, 308, 309]

Insulin produces decreases in endogenous glucose production by both direct and indirect mechanisms[310] (Fig. 29–10). In its direct action, portal insulin suppresses glucose production by inhibiting glycogenolysis through an increase in phosphodiesterase activity[311, 312] or changes in the assembly of protein phosphatase complexes.[313, 314] Insulin can also directly suppress gluconeogenesis by inhibiting the activation of phosphoenolpyruvate carboxykinase transcription through the insulin-dependent phosphorylation of the forkhead transcription factor, sequestering it in the cytoplasm.[315–317]

The indirect or peripheral effect of insulin in controlling glucose production by the liver is twofold. First, insulin has a profound effect on decreasing glucagon secretion by the alpha cell of the pancreas through systemic and paracrine effects.[318, 319] The decrease in glucagon secretion decreases the activation of glycogenolysis and gluconeogenesis. The second important peripheral action of insulin is decreasing FFA levels by suppressing lipolysis. FFAs increase hepatic glucose production by stimulating gluconeogenesis.[320] When the reduction in plasma FFAs during a hyperinsulinemic clamp was prevented by infusion of triglyceride emulsions with heparin (which results in increased FFA levels by activation of lipoprotein lipase), insulin-mediated suppression of HGO was reduced.[298, 321] The suppression of glucagon secretion and decrease in FFA delivery to the liver are additive in reducing liver glucose production.[322]

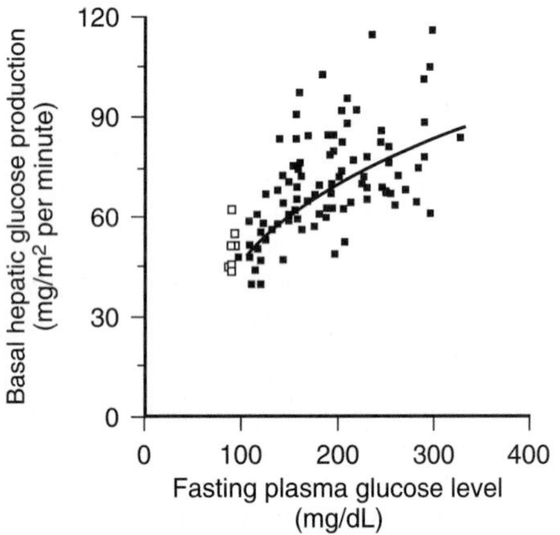

Figure 29–11. Relationship between fasting hepatic glucose output and fasting plasma glucose levels. *Open squares* represent nondiabetic control subjects; *closed squares* represent diabetic subjects. (From Maggs DG, Buchanan TA, Burant CF, et al. Metabolic effects of troglitazone monotherapy in type 2 diabetes mellitus: a randomized, double-blind, placebo-controlled trial. Ann Intern Med 1998; 128:176–185.)

Hepatic insulin resistance plays an important role in the hyperglycemia of type 2 diabetes,[323–326] and the impairment in suppression of HGO appears to be quantitatively similar to or even larger than the defect in the stimulation of peripheral glucose disposal.[324, 327] There is a direct relationship between increases in HGO and fasting hyperglycemia[328] (Fig. 29–11). Insulin-mediated suppression of HGO is impaired at both low and high plasma insulin levels in type 2 diabetic patients,[327, 329–331] and hepatic glucose production is elevated early in the course of the disease[323] but may be normal in lean, relatively insulin-sensitive type 2 diabetics.[332] Treatment of patients with metformin, which suppress hepatic glucose production, results in improvements in glucose tolerance.[333]

Alterations in both the direct and indirect effects of insulin in type 2 diabetics appear to play a role in the elevation in hepatic glucose production. Defects in the direct effect of insulin to suppress hepatic glucose production that have been demonstrated in humans[334] appear to be due to a large rightward shift in the steep dose-response curve for insulin's inhibition of glycogenolysis.[335] However, peripheral insulin resistance may play the bigger role in elevated hepatic glucose production in type 2 diabetes. The resistance of adipose tissue, especially visceral fat, to suppression of lipolysis by insulin is responsible for part of the inability of insulin to suppress hepatic glucose production by the indirect route, resulting in enhanced gluconeogenesis.[336, 337] In addition, the suppression of glucagon levels in humans with insulin resistance may be impaired, again leading to an increase in endogenous glucose production.[338]

INSULIN SECRETION AND TYPE 2 DIABETES

Normal insulin secretory function is essential for the maintenance of normal glucose tolerance, and abnormal insulin secretion is invariably present in patients with type 2 diabetes. In

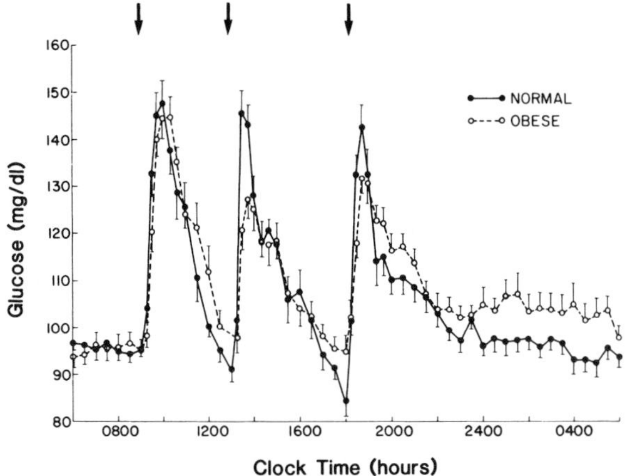

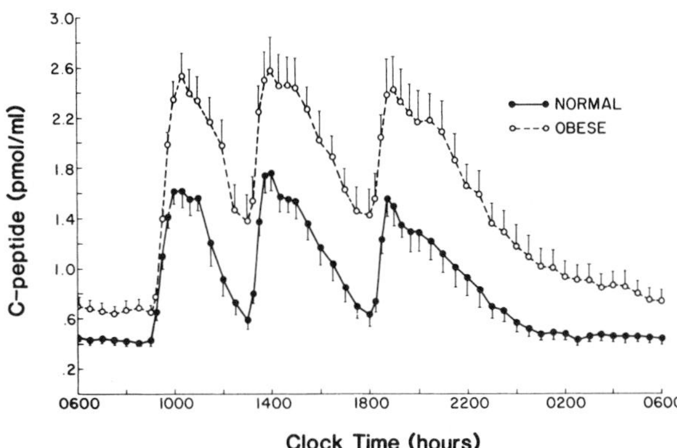

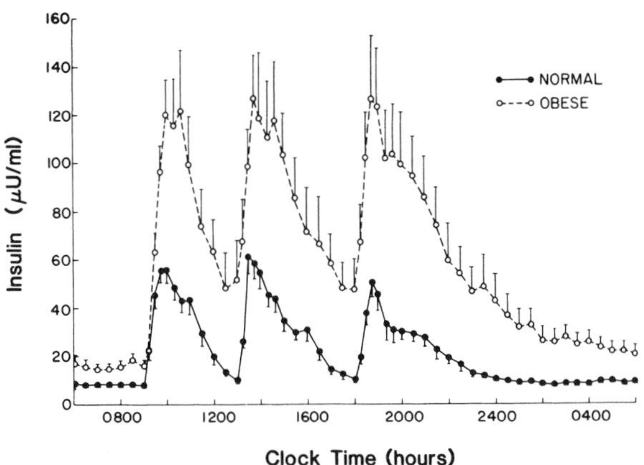

Figure 29–12. Mean 24-hour profiles of plasma concentrations of glucose, C peptide, and insulin in normal and obese subjects. (From Polonsky KS, Given BD, van Cauter E. Twenty-four-hour profiles and pulsatile patterns of insulin secretion in normal and obese subjects. J Clin Invest 1988; 81:442–448.)

this section, the physiology of normal insulin and the alterations that are present in persons with type 2 diabetes are reviewed.

Quantitation of Beta Cell Function

The measurement of peripheral insulin concentrations by radioimmunoassay is still the most widely used method for quantifying beta cell functions in vivo.[339] Although this approach provides valuable information, it is limited by the fact that 50% to 60% of the insulin produced by the pancreas is extracted by the liver without ever reaching the systemic circulation.[340, 341] The standard radioimmunoassay for the measurement of insulin concentrations is also unable to distinguish between endogenous and exogenous insulin, making it ineffective as a measure of endogenous beta cell reserve in the insulin-treated diabetic patient. Anti-insulin antibodies that may be present in patients treated with insulin interfere with the insulin radioimmunoassay, making insulin measurements in insulin-treated patients inaccurate. Conventional insulin radioimmunoassays are also unable to distinguish between levels of circulating proinsulin and true levels of circulating insulin.

Insulin is derived from a single-chain precursor, proinsulin.[342] Within the Golgi apparatus of the pancreatic beta cell, proinsulin is cleaved by convertases to form insulin, C peptide, and two pairs of basic amino acids. Insulin is subsequently released into the circulation at concentrations equimolar with those of C peptide.[343, 344] In addition, small amounts of intact proinsulin and proinsulin conversion intermediates are released. Proinsulin and its related conversion intermediates can be detected in the circulation, where they constitute 20% of the total circulating insulin-like immunoreactivity.[345] In vivo, proinsulin has a biologic potency that is only about 10% of that of insulin[346, 347] and the potency of split proinsulin intermediates is between those of proinsulin and insulin.[348, 349] C peptide has no known conclusive effects on carbohydrate metabolism,[350, 351] although certain physiologic effects of C peptide have been proposed.[352] Unlike insulin, C peptide is not extracted by the liver[341, 353, 354] and is excreted almost exclusively by the kidneys. Its plasma half-life of approximately 30 minutes[355] contrasts sharply with that of insulin, which is approximately 4 minutes.

Because C peptide is secreted in equimolar concentrations with insulin and is not extracted by the liver, many investigators have used levels of C peptide as a marker of beta cell function. The use of plasma C-peptide levels as an index of beta cell function is dependent on the critical assumption that the mean clearance rates of C peptide are constant over the range of C-peptide levels observed under normal physiologic conditions. This assumption has been shown to be valid for both dogs and humans,[341, 356] and this approach can be used to derive rates of insulin secretion from plasma concentrations of C peptide under steady-state conditions.[356] However, because of the long plasma half-life of C peptide, under non–steady-state conditions (e.g., after a glucose infusion) peripheral plasma levels of C peptide do not change in proportion to the changing insulin secretory rate.[356, 357] Thus, under these conditions, insulin secretion rates are best calculated with use of the two-compartment model initially proposed by Eaton and coworkers.[358] Modifications to the C-peptide model of insulin secretion have been introduced. This approach combines the minimal model of insulin action with the two-compartment model of C-peptide kinetics and allows insulin secretion and insulin sensitivity to be derived after either intravenous or oral administration of glucose.[359–362]

Signaling Pathways in the Beta Cell and Insulin Secretion

Figure 29–12 depicts the signaling pathways in the pancreatic beta cell that are involved in the stimulus-secretion coupling of insulin release. These pathways provide the mechanism whereby insulin secretion rates respond to changes in blood glucose concentrations. Glucose enters the pancreatic beta cell by a process of facilitated diffusion mediated by the glucose transporter GLUT2. Although levels of GLUT2 on the beta cell membrane are reduced in diabetic states for various reasons, it is not currently believed that this is a rate-limiting step in the regulation of insulin secretion.

The first rate-limiting step in this process is the phosphorylation of glucose to glucose-6-phosphate. This reaction is mediated by the enzyme glucokinase.[363, 364] There is considerable evidence that glucokinase, by determining the rate of glycolysis, functions as the glucose sensor of the beta cell and that this is the primary mechanism whereby the rate of insulin secretion adapts to changes in blood glucose. According to this view, as blood glucose levels increase more glucose enters the beta cell, the rate of glycolysis increases, and the rate of insulin secretion increases. A fall in blood glucose levels results in a fall in the rate of glycolysis and a reduction in the rate of insulin secretion.

Glucose metabolism produces an increase in cytosolic ATP, the key signal that initiates insulin secretion by causing blockade of the ATP-dependent K^+ channel (K_{ATP}) on the beta cell membrane. Blockade of this channel induces membrane depolarization, which leads to an increase in cytosolic Ca^{2+} and insulin secretion. The biochemical events that link the increase in glycolysis to an increase in ATP are complex. Dukes and co-workers[365] proposed the glycolytic production of NADH during the oxidation of glyceraldehyde-3-phosphate as the key process because NADH is subsequently processed into ATP by mitochondria through the operation of specific shuttle systems.

The rate of pyruvate generation has also been proposed as an explanation for the link between glucose metabolism and the increase in insulin secretion.[366] According to this view, pyruvate generated by the glycolytic pathway enters the mitochondria and is metabolized further in the TCA cycle. Electron transfer from the TCA cycle to the respiratory chain by NADH and reduced flavin adenine dinucleotide ($FADH_2$) promotes the generation of ATP, which is exported into the cytosol. The increase in ATP closes ATP-sensitive K^+ channels, which depolarizes the beta cell membrane and opens the voltage-dependent Ca^{2+} channels, leading to an increase in intracellular Ca^{2+}. The increase in cytosolic Ca^{2+} is the main trigger for exocytosis, the process by which insulin-containing secretory granules fuse with the plasma membrane, leading to the release of insulin into the circulation. The increase in ATP not only closes K_{ATP} channels but also serves as a major permissive factor for movement of insulin granules and for priming of exocytosis.

Cyclic AMP also plays an important role in beta cell signal transduction pathways. This second messenger is generated at the plasma membrane from ATP and potentiates glucose-stimulated insulin secretion, particularly in response to glucagon, glucagon-like peptide 1 (GLP-1), and gastric inhibitory polypeptide. The cAMP-dependent pathways appear to be particularly important in the exocytotic machinery.

K_{ATP} channels play an essential role in beta cell stimulus-secretion coupling. The reader is directed to an excellent review for more complete information.[367] K_{ATP} channels comprise sulfonylurea receptors (SURs) and potassium inward rectifiers, KIR6.1 and KIR6.2, that assemble to form a large octameric channel with a (SUR/KIR6.x) stoichiometry. In the pancreatic beta cell the SUR1/KIR6.2 pairs constitute the K_{ATP} channel. K_{ATP} channels control the flux of potassium ions driven by an electrochemical potential. Opening these channels can set the resting membrane potential of beta cells below the threshold for activation of voltage-gated Ca^{2+} channels when plasma glucose levels are low, thus reducing insulin secretion. Changes in the cytosolic concentrations of ATP and adenosine diphosphate (ADP) as summarized earlier lead to closure of the channels and depolarization of the beta cell membrane. Mutations in both components of the beta cell K_{ATP}, SUR1, and KIR6.2 have been shown to lead to hypersecretion of insulin resulting clinically in either a recessive form of familial hyperinsulinemia or persistent hyperinsulinemic hypoglycemia of infancy.

Physiologic Factors Regulating Insulin Secretion

Carbohydrate Nutrients

The most important physiologic substance involved in the regulation of insulin release is glucose.[368–370] The effect of glucose on the beta cell is dose-related. Dose-dependent increases in concentrations of insulin and C peptide and in rates of insulin secretion have been observed after oral and intravenous glucose loads, with 1.4 units of insulin, on average, being secreted in response to an oral glucose load as small as 12 g.[371–374] The insulin secretory response is greater after oral than after intravenous glucose administration.[374–377] Known as the incretin effect,[373, 378] this enhanced response to oral glucose has been interpreted as an indication that absorption of glucose by way of the gastrointestinal tract stimulates the release of hormones and other mechanisms that ultimately enhance the sensitivity of the beta cell to glucose (see following discussion of hormonal factors). In a study involving nine normal volunteers in whom glucose was infused at a rate designed to achieve levels previously attained after an oral glucose load, the amount of insulin secreted in response to the intravenous load was 26% less than that secreted in response to the oral load.[377]

Insulin secretion does not respond as a linear function of glucose concentration. The relationship of glucose concentration to the rate of insulin release follows a sigmoidal curve, with a threshold corresponding to the glucose levels normally seen under fasting conditions and with the steep portion of the dose-response curve corresponding to the range of glucose levels normally achieved postprandially.[379–381] The sigmoidal nature of the dose-response curve has been attributed to a gaussian distribution of thresholds for stimulation among the individual beta cells.[381–383]

When glucose is infused intravenously at a constant rate, an initial biphasic secretory response is observed that consists of a rapid, early insulin peak followed by a second, more slowly rising peak.[368, 384, 385] The significance of the first-phase insulin release is unclear, but it may reflect the existence of a compartment of readily releasable insulin within the beta cell or a transient rise and fall of a metabolic signal for insulin secretion.[386] Despite early suggestions to the contrary,[387, 388] a subsequent study demonstrated that the first-phase response to intravenous glucose is highly reproducible within subjects.[389] After the acute response, a second phase of insulin release occurs that is directly related to the level of glucose elevation. In vitro studies of isolated islet cells and the perfused pancreas have identified a third phase of insulin secretion commencing 1.5 to 3.0 hours after exposure to glucose and characterized by a spontaneous decline in secretion to 15% to 25% of the amount released during peak secretion—a level subsequently maintained for more than 48 hours.[390–393]

In addition to its acute secretagogue effects on insulin secretion, glucose has intermediate and longer term effects that are physiologically and clinically relevant. In the intermediate term, exposure of the pancreatic beta cell to a high concentration of glucose primes its response to a subsequent glucose stimulus leading to a shift to the left in the dose-response curve relating glucose and insulin secretion.[394, 395] However, when pancreatic islets are exposed to high concentrations for prolonged periods, a reduction of insulin secretion is seen. Although all the precise mechanisms responsible for these adverse effects that have been termed *glucotoxicity* are not known, there is evidence that long-term exposure to high glucose reduces expression of a number of genes that are critical to normal beta cell function, including the insulin gene.[396, 397]

Noncarbohydrate Nutrients

Amino acids have been shown to stimulate insulin release in the absence of glucose, the most potent secretagogues being the essential amino acids leucine, arginine, and lysine.[398, 399] The effects of arginine and lysine on the beta cell appear to be more potent than that of leucine. The effects of amino acids on insulin secretion are potentiated by glucose.[399–401]

In contrast to amino acids, various lipids and their metabolites appear to have only minor effects on insulin release in vivo. Although carbohydrate-rich fat meals stimulate insulin secretion, carbohydrate-free fat meals have minimal effects on beta cell function.[402] Ketone bodies and short- and long-chain fatty acids have been shown to stimulate insulin secretion acutely both in islet cells and in humans.[403–407] The effects of elevated FFAs in the insulin secretory responses to glucose are related to the duration of the exposure. Zhou and Grill[408] first suggested that long-term exposure of pancreatic islets to FFAs inhibited glucose-induced insulin secretion and biosynthesis. This observation has been confirmed in rats.[409] In humans, it was demonstrated that the insulin resistance induced by an acute (90-minute) elevation in FFAs was compensated for by an appropriate increase in insulin secretion.[410] After chronic elevation of FFAs (48 hours), the beta cell compensatory response for insulin resistance was not adequate. Additional studies have demonstrated that the adverse effects of prolonged FFAs on glucose-induced insulin secretion are not seen in individuals with type 2 diabetes. From these results, it appears that elevated FFAs may contribute to the failure of beta cell compensation for insulin resistance.

Hormonal Factors

The release of insulin from the beta cell after a meal is facilitated by a number of gastrointestinal peptide hormones, including glucose-dependent insulinotropic peptide (GIP), cholecystokinin, and GLP-1.[378, 411–418] These hormones are released from small intestinal endocrine cells postprandially and travel in the blood stream to reach the beta cells, where they act through second messengers to increase the sensitivity of these islet cells to glucose. In general, these hormones are not of themselves secretagogues, and their effects are evident only in the presence of hyperglycemia.[411–413] The release of these peptides may explain why the modest postprandial glucose levels achieved in normal subjects in vivo have such a dramatic effect on insulin production, whereas similar glucose concentrations in vitro elicit a much smaller response.[418] Similarly, this incretin effect could account for the greater beta cell response observed after oral as opposed to intravenous glucose administration.

Whether impaired postprandial secretion of incretin hormones plays a role in the inadequate insulin secretory response to oral glucose and to meals in IGT or diabetes is controversial,[419–426] but pharmacologic doses of these peptides may have future therapeutic benefit. Subcutaneous administration of GLP-1, the most potent of the incretin peptides, lowers glucose in type 2 diabetic patients by stimulating endogenous insulin secretion and perhaps by inhibiting glucagon secretion and gastric empyting.[427, 428] Because of its short half-life, however, its longer acting analogue, exendin-4, has greater therapeutic promise.[429] Treatment with supraphysiologic doses of GIP during hyperglycemia has been shown to augment insulin secretion in normal[430, 431] but not in diabetic humans.[422, 431] Although cholecystokinin has the ability to augment insulin secretion in humans, whether it is an incretin at physiologic levels is not firmly established.[432–435] Its effects are also seen largely at pharmacologic doses.[436]

The postprandial insulin secretory response may also be influenced by other intestinal peptide hormones, including vasoactive intestinal polypeptide,[437] secretin,[438–441] and gastrin,[438, 442] but the precise role of these hormones remains to be elucidated.

The hormones produced by pancreatic alpha and beta cells also modulate insulin release. Whereas glucagon has a stimulatory effect on the beta cell,[443] somatostatin suppresses insulin release.[444] It is currently unclear whether these hormones reach the beta cell by traveling through the islet cell interstitium (thus exerting a paracrine effect) or through islet cell capillaries. Indeed, the importance of these two hormones in regulating basal and postprandial insulin levels under normal physiologic circumstances is in doubt. Paradoxically, the low insulin levels observed during prolonged periods of starvation have been attributed to the elevated glucagon concentrations seen in this setting.[402, 445–448] Other hormones that exert a stimulatory effect on insulin secretion include growth hormone,[449] glucocorticoids,[450] prolactin,[451–453] placental lactogen,[454] and the sex steroids.[455]

Whereas all of the preceding hormones may stimulate insulin secretion indirectly by inducing a state of insulin resistance, some may also act directly on the beta cell, possibly to augment its sensitivity to glucose. Thus, hyperinsulinemia is associated with conditions in which these hormones are present in excess, such as acromegaly, Cushing's syndrome, and the second half of pregnancy. Furthermore, treatments with placental lactogen,[456] hydrocortisone,[457] and growth hormone[457, 458] are all effective in reversing the reduction in insulin response to glucose that is observed in vitro after hypophysectomy. Although hyperinsulinemia after an oral glucose load has been observed in patients with hyperthyroidism,[459, 460] the increased concentration of immunoreactive insulin in this setting may reflect elevations in serum proinsulin rather than a true increase in serum insulin.[461]

Neural Factors

The islets are innervated by both the cholinergic and adrenergic limbs of the autonomic nervous system. Although both sympathetic stimulation and parasympathetic stimulation enhance secretion of glucagon,[462, 463] the secretion of insulin is stimulated by vagal nerve fibers and inhibited by sympathetic nerve fibers.[462–467] Adrenergic inhibition of the beta cell appears to be mediated by the α-adrenoceptor because its effect is attenuated by the α-antagonist phentolamine[463] and reproduced by the α_2-agonist clonidine.[468] There is also considerable evidence that many indirect effects of sympathetic nerve stimulation play a role in regulation of beta cell function through stimulation or inhibition of somatostatin, β_2-adrenoceptors, and neuropeptides galanin and neuropeptide Y.[469]

Parasympathetic stimulation of islets results in stimulation of insulin, glucagon, and pancreatic polypeptide directly and through the neuropeptides vasoactive intestinal polypeptide, gastrin-releasing polypeptide, and pituitary adenylate cyclase–activating polypeptide.[469] In addition, sensory innervation of islets may play a role in tonic inhibition of insulin secretion through the neuropeptides calcitonin gene–related peptide[470–472] and, less clearly, substance P.[473, 474]

The importance of the autonomic nervous system in regulating insulin secretion in vivo is unclear. The neural effects on beta cell function cannot be entirely dissociated from the hormonal effects because some of the neurotransmitters of the autonomic nervous system are, in fact, hormones. Furthermore, the secretion of insulinotropic hormones such as GIP and GLP-1 postprandially has been shown to be under vagal[475, 476] and adrenergic[477, 478] control.

Temporal Pattern of Insulin Secretion

It has been estimated that, in any 24-hour period, 50% of the total insulin secreted by the pancreas is secreted under basal conditions and the remainder is secreted in response to meals.[479, 480] The estimated basal insulin secretion rates range from 18 to 32 units per 24 hours (0.7 to 1.3 mg).[356, 358, 371, 479] After meal ingestion, the insulin secretory response is rapid and insulin secretion increases approximately fivefold over baseline to reach a peak within 60 minutes (Fig. 29–13; see Fig. 29–12). In these studies subjects consumed 20% of calories with breakfast and 40% with lunch and dinner, respectively. However, the amount of insulin secreted after each meal did not differ significantly. The rapidity of the insulin secretory response to breakfast is underscored by the fact that 71.6% ± 1.6% of the insulin secreted in the 4 hours after the meal was produced in the first 2 hours and the remainder in the next 2 hours. Insulin secretion did not decrease as rapidly after lunch and dinner and 62.8% ± 1.6% and 59.6% ± 1.4% of the total meal response were secreted in the first 2 hours after these meals.

The normal insulin secretory profile is characterized by a series of insulin secretory pulses. After breakfast, 1.8 ± 0.2 secretory pulses were identified in normal volunteers and the peaks of these pulses occurred 42.8 ± 3.4 minutes after the meal. Multiple insulin secretory pulses were also identified after lunch and dinner. After these meals, up to four pulses of insulin secretion were identified in both groups of subjects. Thus, in the 5-hour time interval between lunch and dinner, an average of 2.5 ± 0.3 secretory pulses were identified, and 2.6 ± 0.2 were identified in the same period after dinner.

Pulses of insulin secretion that did not appear to be meal-related were also identified. Between 11:00 PM and 6:00 AM and in the 3 hours before breakfast, on average 3.9 ± 0.3 secretory pulses were present in normal subjects. Thus, over the 24-hour period of observation, a total of 11.1 ± 0.5 pulses were identified in normal subjects. Close to 90% (87% ± 3%) of postmeal pulses in insulin secretion but only 47% ± 8% of non–meal-related pulses were concomitant with a pulse in glucose.

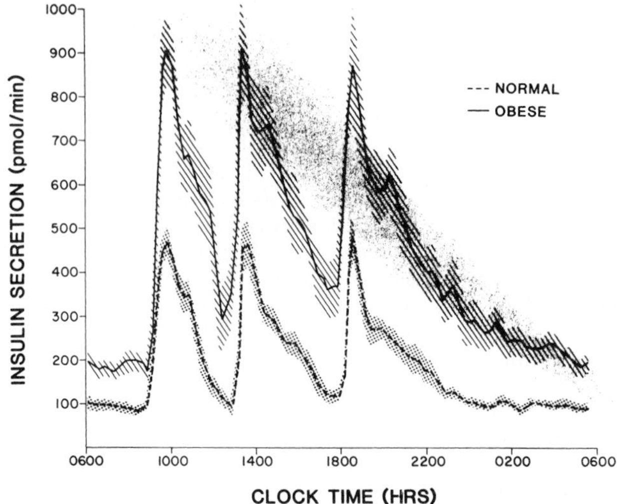

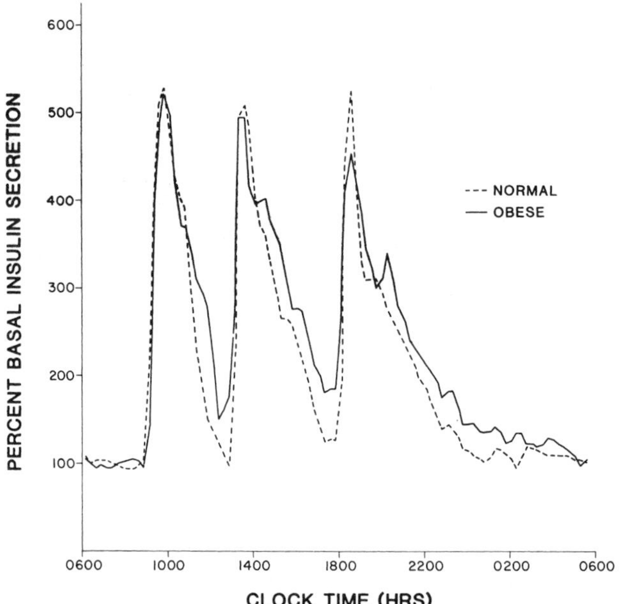

Figure 29–13. Mean 24-hour profiles of insulin secretion rates in normal and obese subjects *(top)*. The *hatched areas* represent ± 1 standard error of the mean. The curves in the lower panel were derived by dividing the insulin secretion rate measured in each subject by the basal secretion rate derived in the same subject. Mean data for the normal *(dashed line)* and obese *(solid line)* subjects are shown. (From Polonsky KS, Given BD, van Cauter E. Twenty-four-hour profiles and pulsatile patterns of insulin secretion in normal and obese subjects. J Clin Invest 1988; 81:442–448.)

Oscillatory Insulin Secretion

In vivo studies of beta cell secretory function have demonstrated that insulin is released in a pulsatile manner. This behavior is characterized by rapid oscillations occurring every 8 to 15 minutes that are superimposed on slower (ultradian) oscillations occurring at a periodicity of 80 to 150 minutes.[481] The rapid oscillations persist in vitro and are therefore likely to be the result of metabolic pathways in the pancreatic beta cell that involved negative feedback loops with time lags.

The rapid oscillations of insulin are of small amplitude in the systemic circulation, averaging between 0.4 and 3.2 μU/mL in several published human studies.[482–484] Because these values are close to the limits of sensitivity of most standard insulin radioimmunoassays, the characterization of these oscillations is subject to considerable pitfalls,[485] not the least of which is the need to differentiate between true oscillations of small amplitude and random assay noise. The latter problem has been overcome by the development of extremely sensitive enzyme-linked immunosorbent assays that allow the detection of extremely small changes in peripheral insulin concentrations. The application of these assays in studies involving frequent sampling from the peripheral circulation has led to a series of studies of the role of these oscillations in the overall regulation of insulin secretion.[486–490]

These studies have suggested that increases in overall insulin secretion seen in response to a variety of secretagogues in various physiologic and pathophysiologic states are due to an increase in the amplitude of the bursts of insulin secretion. The studies have proposed that 75% of insulin secretion is accounted for by secretory bursts and the responses to GLP-1, sulfonylureas, and oral glucose are all mediated by an increase in the amplitude of insulin secretory pulses. Furthermore, consistent with observations made by O'Rahilly and colleagues[491] a number of years ago, relatives of patients with type 2 diabetes demonstrate a disorderly profile of the insulin secretory oscillations. A number of mathematical programs have been developed that allow these insulin secretory oscillations to be evaluated and studied.[492] The latest addition to the list is the development of ApEn and cross ApEn, which are statistics that measure temporal regularity of the oscillations in the insulin secretory profile.[493]

The low amplitude of the rapid oscillations in the systemic circulation contrasts sharply with observations in the portal vein, where pulse amplitudes of 20 to 40 μU/mL have been recorded in dogs.[494] Although the physiologic importance of these low-amplitude rapid pulses in the periphery is unclear, they are likely to be of physiologic importance in the portal

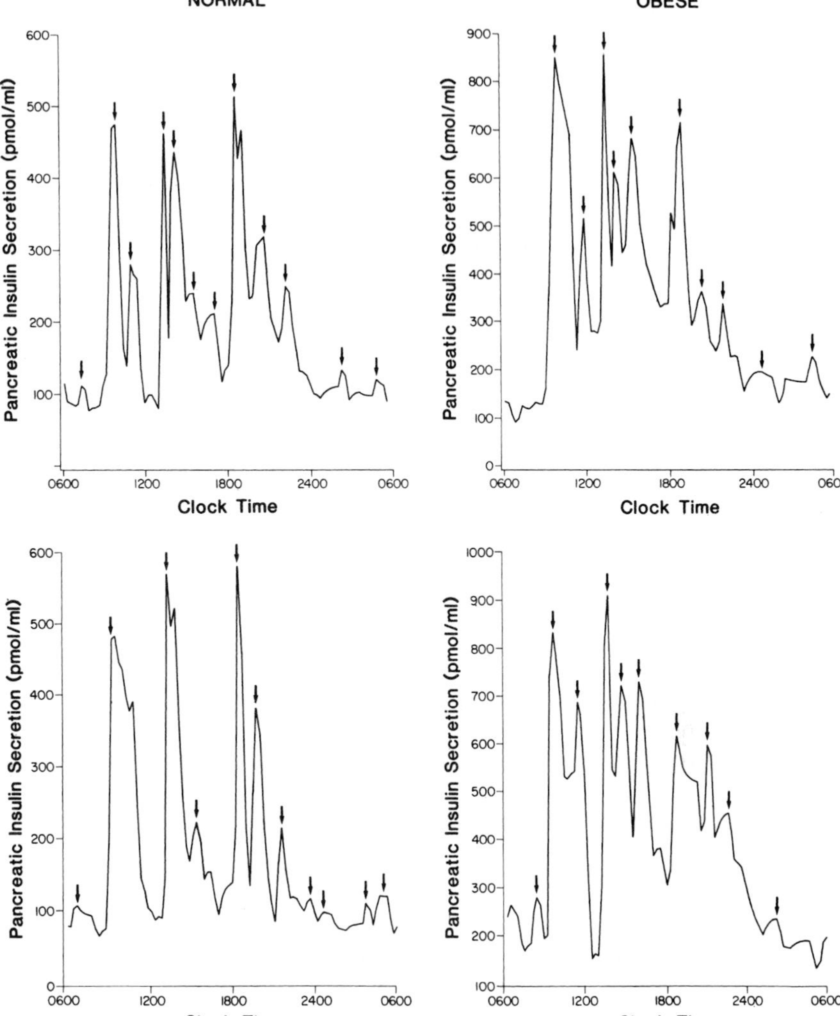

Figure 29–14. Patterns of insulin secretion in normal and obese subjects. Four representative 24-hour profiles from two normal-weight subjects *(left)* and two obese subjects *(right)*. Meals were consumed at 0900, 1300, and 1800 hours. Statistically significant pulses of secretion are shown by the *arrows*. (From Polonsky KS, Given BD, van Cauter E. Twenty-four-hour profiles and pulsatile patterns of insulin secretion in normal and obese subjects. J Clin Invest 1988; 81:442–448.)

vein. It is possible that the liver responds more readily to insulin delivered in a pulsatile fashion than to insulin delivered at a constant rate.[495–497]

In contrast to the rapid oscillations, the slower (ultradian) oscillations are of much larger amplitude in the peripheral circulation. They are present under basal conditions but are amplified postprandially (Fig. 29–14) and have been observed in subjects receiving intravenous glucose, suggesting that they are not generated by intermittent absorption of nutrients from the gut. Furthermore, they do not appear to be related to fluctuations in glucagon or cortisol levels[388] and are not regulated by neural factors because these oscillations are also present in recipients of successful pancreas transplants.[498, 499] Many of these ultradian insulin and C-peptide pulses are synchronous with pulses of similar oscillatory period in glucose, raising the possibility that these oscillations are a product of the insulin-glucose feedback mechanism. Ultradian oscillations are self-sustained during constant glucose infusion at various rates, they are increased in amplitude after stimulation of insulin secretion without change in frequency, and there is a slight temporal advance of the glucose versus the insulin oscillation.

These findings suggest that the ultradian oscillations may be entirely accounted for by the major dynamic characteristics of the insulin-glucose feedback system, with no need to postulate the existence of an intrapancreatic pacemaker.[500] In support of this hypothesis, Sturis and colleagues[501] demonstrated that when glucose is administered in an oscillatory pattern, ultradian oscillations in plasma glucose and insulin secretion are generated that are 100% concordant with the oscillatory period of the exogenous glucose infusion. This close relationship between the ultradian oscillations in insulin secretion and similar oscillations in plasma glucose was further exemplified in a series of dose-response studies in which the largest amplitude oscillations in insulin secretion were observed in the subjects exhibiting the largest amplitude glucose oscillations, which in turn were directly related to the infusion dose of glucose. It has been shown that in normal humans, insulin is more effective in reducing plasma glucose levels when administered intravenously as a 120-minute oscillation than when delivered at a constant rate. These results indicate that the ultradian oscillations have functional significance.

Circadian variations in the secretion of insulin have also been reported. When insulin secretory responses were measured during a 24-hour period during which subjects received three standard meals, the maximal postprandial responses were observed after breakfast.[480, 502, 503] These findings are mirrored by the results of studies in which subjects were tested for oral glucose tolerance at different times of the day and were found to exhibit maximal insulin secretory responses in the morning and lower responses in the afternoon and evening.[504–506] These diurnal differences are also noted in tests for intravenous glucose tolerance. Furthermore, although ultradian glucose and insulin oscillations are closely correlated during a constant 24-hour glucose infusion, the nocturnal rise in mean glucose lev-

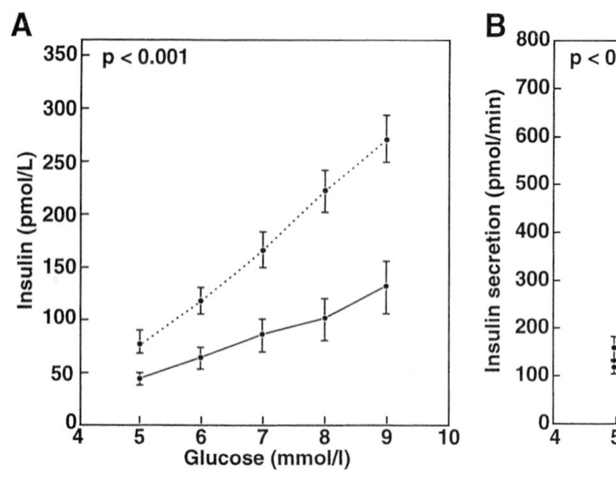

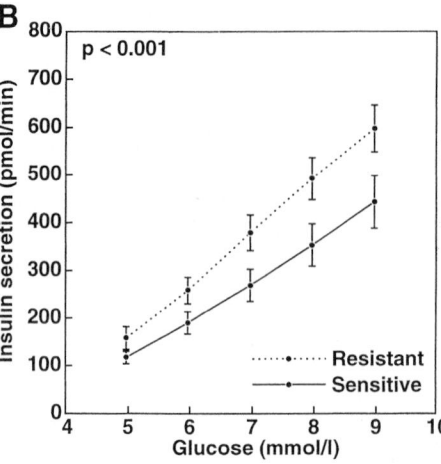

Figure 29–15. Plasma insulin concentrations *(A)* and insulin secretion rates *(B)* in response to molar increments in the plasma glucose concentration during the graded glucose infusion in the insulin-resistant *(dotted line)* and insulin-sensitive *(solid line)* groups. (From Jones CNO, Pei D, Staris P, et al. Alterations in the glucose-stimulated insulin secretory dose-response curve and in insulin clearance in nondiabetic insulin-resistant individuals. J Clin Endocrinol Metab 1997; 82:1834–1838.)

els is not accompanied by a similar increase in the insulin secretory rate.[507] It has been postulated that these diurnal differences may reflect diminished responsiveness of the beta cell to glucose in the afternoon and evening.[506]

Insulin Secretion in Obesity and Insulin Resistance

Obesity and other insulin-resistant states are associated with a substantially greater risk for the development of type 2 diabetes. The ability of the pancreatic beta cell to compensate for insulin resistance determines whether blood glucose levels remain normal in insulin-resistant subjects or whether the subjects develop glucose intolerance or diabetes.

The nature of the beta cell compensation for insulin resistance involves hypersecretion of insulin even in the presence of normal glucose concentrations. This can occur only if beta cell sensitivity to glucose is increased. The increase in beta cell sensitivity to glucose seen in obesity appears to be mediated by two factors. First, increased beta cell mass is observed in obesity and other insulin-resistant states.[508] Second, insulin resistance appears to be associated with increased expression of hexokinase in the beta cell relative to the expression of glucokinase.[509] Because hexokinase has a significantly lower Michaelis constant (Km) for glucose than glucokinase, the functional effect of increased hexokinase expression is to shift the glucose–insulin secretion dose-response curve to the left, leading to increased insulin secretion across a wide range of glucose concentrations.

Assessment of the adequacy of the beta cell compensation for insulin resistance is important because this is the major determinant of the development of diabetes. In insulin-resistant states it is important to evaluate beta cell function in relation to the degree of insulin resistance. Kahn and coworkers[510] studied the relationship between insulin sensitivity and beta cell function in 93 relatively young, apparently healthy human subjects of varying degrees of obesity. The sensitivity index SI was calculated using the minimal model of Bergman as a measure of insulin sensitivity and was then compared with various measures of insulin secretion.[361, 511] The relationship between the SI and the beta cell measures was curvilinear and reciprocal for fasting insulin ($P < .0001$), first-phase insulin response (AIR (acute insulin response) glucose; $P < .0001$), glucose potentiation slope ($n = 56$; $P < .005$), and beta cell secretory capacity (AIRmax; $n = 43$; $P < .0001$). The curvilinear relationship between SI and the beta cell measures could not be distinguished from a hyperbola, that is, SI × beta cell function = constant. The nature of this relationship is consistent with a regulated feedback loop control system such that for any difference in SI, a proportionate reciprocal difference occurs in insulin levels and responses in subjects with similar carbohydrate tolerance. Thus, in human subjects with normal glucose tolerance and varying degrees of obesity, beta cell function varies quantitatively with differences in insulin sensitivity. The increase in insulin secretion that is observed with a fall in SI should be viewed as the beta cell compensation that allows normal glucose tolerance to be maintained in the presence of insulin resistance.

The insulin resistance of obesity is characterized by hyperinsulinemia. Hyperinsulinemia in this setting reflects a combination of increased insulin production and decreased insulin clearance, but most evidence suggests that increased insulin secretion is the predominant factor.[512, 513] Both basal and 24-hour insulin secretory rates are three to four times higher in obese subjects and are strongly correlated with body mass index. Insulin secretory responses to intravenous glucose have been studied in otherwise healthy insulin-resistant subjects in comparison with insulin-sensitive subjects by means of a graded glucose infusion.

Figure 29–15 depicts insulin concentrations and insulin secretion rates at each level of plasma glucose achieved, thereby constructing a glucose-insulin or glucose–insulin secretion rate dose-response relationship. Both insulin concentrations and insulin secretion rates are increased in insulin-resistant subjects, resulting from a combination of increased insulin secretion and decreased insulin clearance. For each level of glucose, insulin secretion rates are higher in the insulin-resistant subjects, reflecting an adaptive response of the beta cell to peripheral insulin resistance. Similar compensatory hyperinsulinemia has been demonstrated using other clinical techniques such as the frequently sampled intravenous glucose tolerance test in obesity and other insulin-resistant states such as late pregnancy.[510, 514]

The temporal pattern of insulin secretion is unaltered in obese subjects compared with normal subjects. Basal insulin secretion in obese subjects accounts for 50% of the total daily production of insulin, and secretory pulses of insulin occur every 1.5 to 2 hours.[503, 512] However, the amplitude of these pulses postprandially is greater in obese subjects. Nevertheless, when these postprandial secretory responses are expressed as a percentage of the basal secretory rate, the postprandial responses in obese and normal subjects are identical.

Insulin Secretion in Subjects with Impaired Glucose Tolerance

It has been suggested that insulin secretion may be normal in subjects with IGT. However, substantial defects in insulin

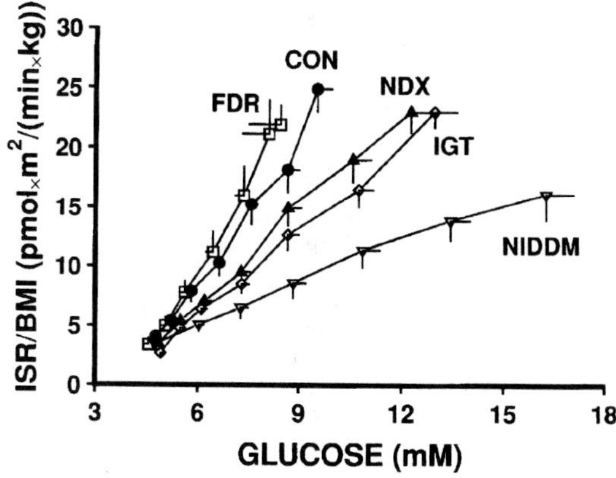

Figure 29–16. Dose-response relationship between glucose and insulin secretory rate (ISR) after an overnight fast in control subjects (CON), normoglycemic subjects with a family history of non–insulin dependent diabetes mellitus (FDR), subjects with a nondiagnostic OGTT (NDX), subjects with impaired glucose tolerance (IGT), and subjects with non–insulin-dependent diabetes mellitus (NIDDM). BME, body mass index. (From Byrne MM, Sturis J, Sobel RJ, Polonsky KS. Elevated plasma glucose 2 h postchallenge predicts defects in beta-cell function. Am J Physiol 1996; 270:E572–E579. The American Physiological Society, copyright 1996.)

secretion have been demonstrated in people with normal fasting glucose and glycosylated hemoglobin concentrations with glucose values greater than 140 mg/dL or 7.8 mmol/L 2 hours after ingestion of 75 g of glucose orally. Thus, defects in insulin secretion can be detected before the onset of overt hyperglycemia.

Detailed study of insulin secretion in patients with IGT has demonstrated that consistent quantitative and qualitative defects are seen in this group. During oral glucose tolerance testing, there is a delay in the peak insulin response.[515–517] The glucose–insulin secretion dose-response relationship is flattened and shifted to the right (Fig. 29–16), and first-phase insulin responses to an intravenous glucose bolus are consistently decreased in relation to ambient insulin sensitivity.[518, 519] Further, abnormalities in first-phase insulin secretion were observed in first-degree relatives of patients with type 2 diabetes who exhibited only mild intolerance to glucose,[520] and an attenuated insulin response to oral glucose was observed in normoglycemic co-twins of patients with type 2 diabetes.[521] This pattern of insulin secretion during the so-called prediabetic phase was also seen in subjects with IGT who later developed type 2 diabetes[401, 522, 523] and in normoglycemic obese subjects with a recent history of gestational diabetes,[524] another group at high risk for type 2 diabetes.[525] Beta cell abnormalities may therefore precede the development of overt type 2 diabetes by many years.

The temporal pattern of insulin secretory responses is altered in IGT and is similar to but not as pronounced as that seen in diabetic subjects (see later). There is a loss of coordinated insulin secretory responses during oscillatory glucose infusion, indicating that the ability of the beta cell to sense and respond appropriately to parallel changes in the plasma glucose level is impaired (Fig. 29–17). Abnormalities in rapid oscillations of insulin secretion have also been observed in first-degree relatives of patients with type 2 diabetes who have only mild glucose intolerance,[491] further suggesting that abnormalities in the temporal pattern of beta cell function may be an early manifestation of beta cell dysfunction preceding the development of type 2 diabetes. Because an elevation in serum proinsulin is seen in subjects with diabetes, the contribution of proinsulin to the hyperinsulinemia of IGT has been questioned. The hyperinsulinemia of IGT has not been accounted

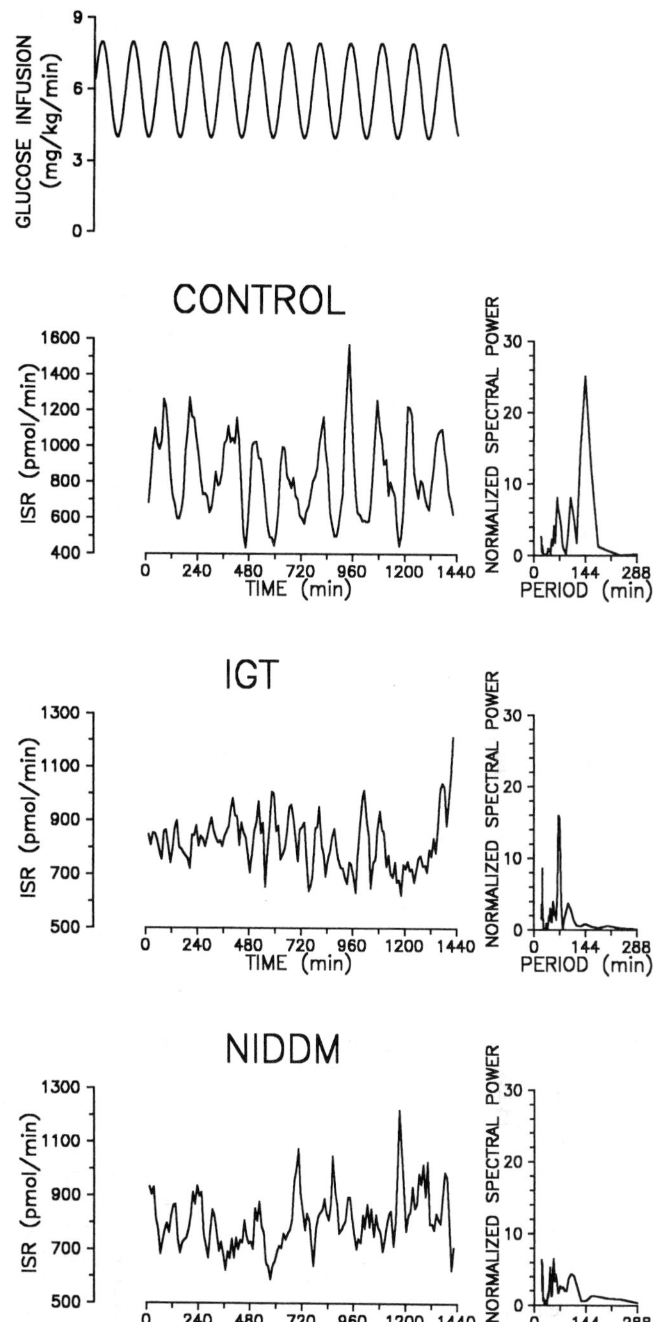

Figure 29–17. Oscillatory glucose infusions were administered with a periodicity of 144 minutes in representative subjects with type 2 diabetes, impaired glucose tolerance (IGT), and normal glucose tolerance. In the control subject, the insulin secretion rate (ISR) adjusts and responds to the 144-minute oscillations in glucose, resulting in sharp spectral peak at 144 minutes. In the subjects with IGT and type 2 diabetes, the ISR does not respond to the oscillatory glucose stimulus and although oscillations in insulin secretion are evident, they are irregular, resulting in markedly reduced spectral peaks at 144 minutes and small-amplitude high-frequency spectral peaks. (Adapted from O'Meara NM, Sturis J, Van Cauter E, Polonsky KS. Lack of control by glucose of ultradian insulin secretory oscillations in impaired glucose tolerance and in non–insulin-dependent diabetes mellitus. J Clin Invest 1993; 92:262–271.)

for by an increase in proinsulin, although elevations in fasting and stimulated proinsulin or proinsulin/insulin ratios have been found by many, although not all, investigators.[526–531] Correlation of elevated proinsulin levels in IGT as a predictor of future conversion to diabetes has also been observed.[532–534]

Insulin Secretion in Type 2 Diabetes Mellitus

Because of the presence of concomitant insulin resistance, patients with type 2 diabetes are often hyperinsulinemic, but the degree of hyperinsulinemia is inappropriately low for the prevailing glucose concentrations. Nevertheless, many of these patients have sufficient beta cell reserve to maintain a euglycemic state by dietary restriction with or without an oral agent. The beta cell defect in patients with type 2 diabetes mellitus is characterized by an absent first-phase insulin and C-peptide response to an intravenous glucose load and a reduced second-phase response.[535] Although hyperglycemia may play a role in mediating these changes, the abnormal first-phase response to intravenous glucose persists in patients whose diabetic control has been greatly improved,[536, 537] consistent with the idea that patients with type 2 diabetes have an intrinsic defect in the beta cell. Furthermore, abnormalities in first-phase insulin secretion have also been observed in first-degree relatives of patients with type 2 diabetes who have only mild glucose intolerance, and an attenuated insulin response to oral glucose has been observed in normoglycemic co-twins of patients with type 2 diabetes—a group at high risk for type 2 diabetes and who can legitimately be classified as prediabetic.[538] This pattern of insulin secretion during the so-called prediabetic phase is also seen in subjects with IGT who later develop type 2 diabetes and in normoglycemic obese subjects with a recent history of gestational diabetes, who are also at high risk for type 2 diabetes. Beta cell abnormalities may therefore precede the development of overt type 2 diabetes by many years.

Type 2 diabetes also affects proinsulin levels in serum. Increased levels of proinsulin are consistently seen in association with increases in the proinsulin/insulin molar ratio.[535] The amount of proinsulin produced in this setting appears to be related to the degree of glycemic control rather than to the duration of the diabetic state, and in one series proinsulin levels contributed almost 50% of the total insulin immunoreactivity in type 2 diabetes patients who had marked hyperglycemia. In addition to intact proinsulin, the beta cell secretes one or more of the four major proinsulin conversion products (split 32,33-, split 65,66-, des-31,32-, and des-64,65-proinsulin) into the circulation. These conversion products are produced within the secretory granules of the islet as a result of the activity of specific conversion enzymes at the two cleavage sites in proinsulin linking the C peptide to the A and B chains.

The composition of the elevated proinsulin-like immunodeficiency (PLI) in patients with type 2 diabetes compared with control subjects has not been fully characterized. Hales and colleagues[539] have developed immunoradiometric assays for this purpose. Using these assays, split 32,33-proinsulin was reported to be the predominant proinsulin conversion product in the circulation, although des-31,32-proinsulin levels may also be elevated. Insulin, proinsulin, and conversion product concentrations were also measured with these assays 30 minutes after oral glucose in patients with type 2 diabetes. Insulin was reduced in all patients, with no overlap between patients and controls, and concentrations of proinsulin and conversion products were elevated in the diabetic patients. These data highlight the importance of the potentially confounding effects of proinsulin and proinsulin conversion products in the interpretation of circulating immunoreactive insulin in patients with type 2 diabetes and emphasize the need to measure the concentrations of the individual peptides.

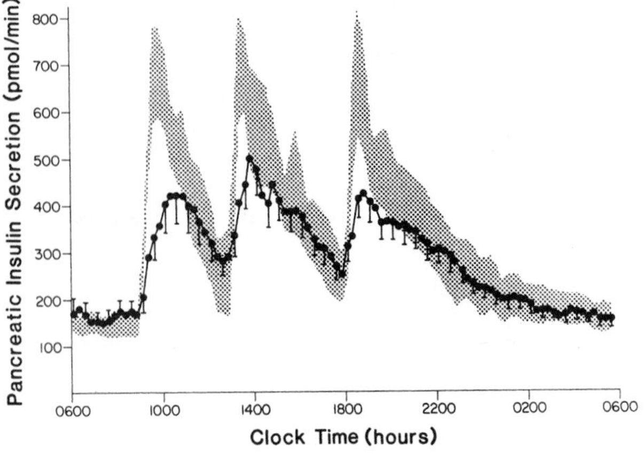

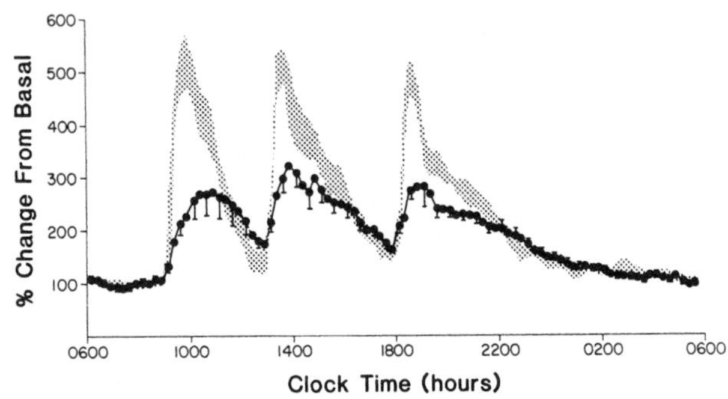

Figure 29–18. Mean (± standard error of the mean [SEM]) rates of insulin secretion in type 2 diabetic patients compared with control subjects. The *shaded area* corresponds to 1 SEM above and below the mean in control subjects. The curves in the lower panel were derived by dividing, for each subject, the insulin secretion rate at each sampling time by the average fasting secretion rate measured between 6 AM and 9 AM in the same subject.

Abnormalities in the temporal pattern of insulin secretion have also been demonstrated in patients with type 2 diabetes. In contrast to normal subjects, in whom equal amounts of insulin are secreted basally and postprandially in a given 24-hour period, patients with type 2 diabetes secrete a greater proportion of their daily insulin under basal conditions[540] (Fig. 29–18). This reduction in the proportion of insulin secreted postprandially appears to be related in part to a reduction in the amplitude of the secretory pulses of insulin occurring after meals rather than to a reduction in the number of pulses. In contrast to normal subjects, patients with type 2 diabetes have ultradian oscillations in insulin secretion that are less tightly coupled with oscillations in plasma glucose (Fig. 29–19). Similar findings were observed in patients with IGT studied under the same experimental conditions and in a further group of type 2 diabetic patients studied under fasting conditions. The rapid insulin pulses are also abnormal in type 2 diabetes because the persistent regular rapid oscillations present in normal subjects are not observed. Instead, the cycles are of shorter duration and are irregular in nature. Similar findings were observed in a group of first-degree relatives of patients with type 2 diabetes who had only mild glucose intolerance, suggesting that abnormalities in oscillatory activity may be an early manifestation of beta cell dysfunction.[518]

The effects of therapy on beta cell function in patients with type 2 diabetes have also been investigated. Although interpre-

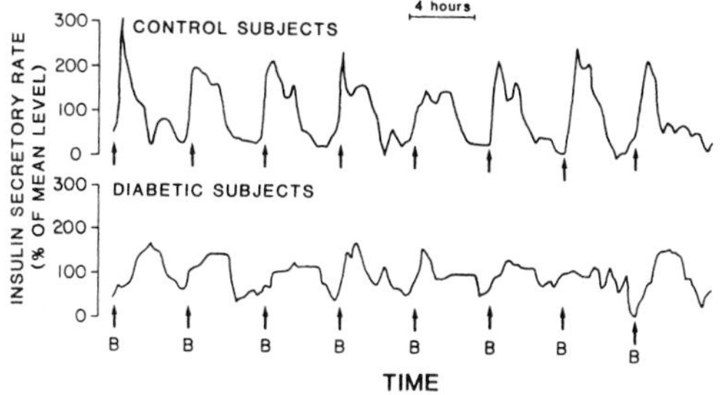

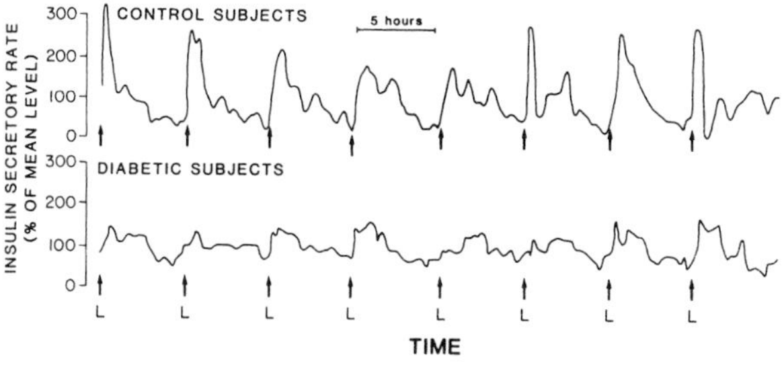

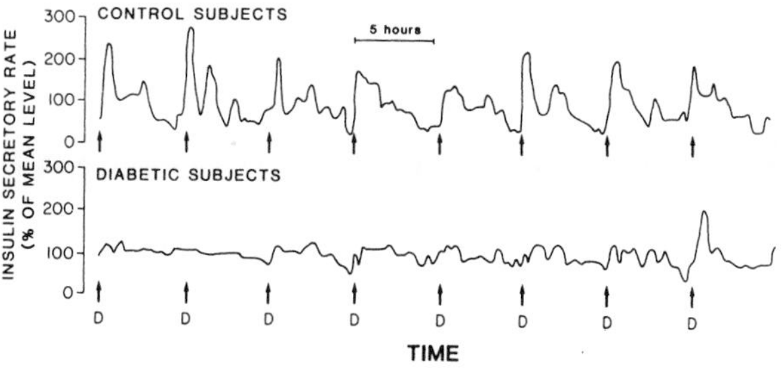

Figure 29–19. Temporal variations in postbreakfast, postlunch, and postdinner rates of insulin secretion in control and diabetic subjects. In each subject, the secretion rates during the 30 minutes before the meal and the 4 hours after breakfast or the 5 hours after lunch or dinner were expressed as a percentage of the mean rate of insulin secretion during that interval. The curves were obtained by concatenating the resulting postmeal profiles in eight representative subjects. The times at which the meals were served to successive subjects in the series are indicated by *arrows*. (From Polonsky KS, Given BD, Hirsch LJ, et al. Abnormal patterns of insulin secretion in non–insulin-dependent diabetes mellitus. N Engl J Med 1988; 318:1231–1239.)

tation of the results in many instances is limited by the fact that beta cell function was not always studied at comparable levels of glucose before and during therapy, the majority of the studies indicated that improvements in diabetic control are associated with an enhancement of beta cell secretory activity. This increased endogenous production of insulin appears to be independent of the mode of treatment and is in particular associated with increases in the amount of insulin secreted postprandially.[537, 541] The enhanced beta cell secretory activity after meals reflects an increase in the amplitude of existing secretory pulses rather than an increased number of pulses. Despite improvements in glycemic control, beta cell function is not normalized after therapy, suggesting that the intrinsic defect in the beta cell persists.

Treatment with the sulfonylurea glyburide increases the amount of insulin secreted in response to meals but does not correct the underlying abnormalities in the pattern of insulin secretion. In particular, the abnormalities in the pulsatile pattern of ultradian insulin secretory oscillations persist on treatment with glyburide despite the increase in the amount of insulin secreted.

We have also investigated the effects on insulin secretion of improving insulin resistance in subjects with IGT by using the insulin-sensitizing agent troglitazone, a thiazolidinedione. Troglitazone therapy improved insulin sensitivity, and this was associated with enhanced ability of the pancreatic beta cell to respond to a glucose stimulus as judged by improvements in the dose-response relationships between glucose and insulin secretion as well as enhanced ability of the pancreatic beta cell to detect and respond to small oscillations in the plasma glucose concentration.[542]

RODENT MODELS OF TYPE 2 DIABETES

A number of spontaneous and genetically selected animal models of type 2 diabetes have been identified. Most of the models combine the two main features of type 2 diabetes, obesity-associated insulin resistance and beta cell dysfunction with or without diminished beta cell mass. As with diabetes in humans, the different rodent models of type 2 diabetes have similarities but a number of overt and subtle differences make them useful surrogates for intensive study of the syndromes associated with type 2 diabetes.

An interesting observation is the striking sexual dimorphism in most rodent models of type 2 diabetes, with the male most often being affected exclusively, earlier, or more severely in most instances. In this regard, it is not like the human situation. The advent of transgenic and knockout technology in mice has produced a wide range of models of insulin resistance and beta cell dysfunction that results in hyperglycemia. It is beyond the scope of this chapter to review each of these, and the reader is referred to the primary literature for review of these animals. We limit our discussion to the well-documented spontaneous or derived models of the disease in rodents.

Mouse Models of Type 2 Diabetes

Leptin (*Lep^{ob}*) and the Leptin Receptor (*db*)

The *ob* mutation, now designated *Lep^{ob}*, was first described in 1950,[543] but the gene mutation responsible for the syndrome was not described until the *ob* mutation was found to be in the gene for leptin.[544] Mice homozygous for the *ob* mutation do not produce the satiety factor leptin and become markedly hyperphagic, obese, insulin-resistant, and hyperinsulinemic. They have a multitude of other hypothalamic dysfunctions that render them hypometabolic, contribute to the obesity, and also result in infertility.[545, 546] Leptin treatment of these mice results in decreased food intake and reverses many of their other metabolic defects.[547–551] The *ob* mice develop obesity at weaning that becomes progressive because of hyperphagia. Insulin resistance is seen in muscle, adipose tissue, and liver, with a variety of signaling defects that are also reversible with insulin administration.[552] The *ob* mouse becomes hyperglycemic and has a profound hyperinsulinemia associated with beta cell hyperplasia with up to a 10-fold increase in islet mass.[553, 554]

Parabiotic experiments between the *ob* and *db* mice suggested that the *db* mutation would be in the receptor for ob. This was confirmed with the identification of multiple mutations in the leptin receptor in *db*.[555, 556] Like *ob* mice, *db* mice are hyperphagic and begin to surpass their littermates in weight at weaning. They are progressively hyperinsulinemic, become hyperglycemic at 6 to 8 weeks, and because of a decline in beta cell function[557–560] become markedly hyperglycemic at 4 to 6 months. The reason for the more severe diabetes in the *db* mouse is not clear, but it may be due to background strain differences as similar defects in insulin signaling are seen in this animal model as well.[561–563] Treatment of both *ob* and *db* mice with insulin-sensitizing agents such as thiazolidinediones reversed the insulin resistance and ameliorated or prevented the onset of diabetes.[564, 565]

Agouti Mouse

Dominant "yellow" mutations in the *agouti* gene produce obesity and hyperglycemia. Depending on the background strain, the *agouti* mutation has a variable phenotype. In susceptible strains, the onset of hyperinsulinemia begins at 6 weeks of age and insulin levels continue to increase with age with beta cell hyperplasia and hypertrophy.[566, 567] The *agouti* mutation results in systemic production of a protein normally expressed in the skin, most frequently because of a retrotransposon insertion into the promoter region of the gene.[568] Interestingly, a number of genes, including the fatty acid synthase gene, have both insulin and agouti response elements, which result in a marked increase in expression leading to increased hepatic fatty acid synthesis and enhanced fat deposition in adipocytes.[556, 569, 570] The hyperglycemia is postprandial, and the fasting glucose levels are usually normal. The exact function of the *agouti* gene is unknown, but the animals are hyperphagic and show enhanced growth.

KK Mouse

These mice were originally bred for enhanced size but are not as obese as most other obese mice (usually less than 60 g). Breeding the KK into various background strains has produced variable insulin resistance, hyperinsulinemia, and hyperglycemia. The most studied stain is the KKA^y produced in Japan.[571] This mouse has markedly increased insulin levels (>1000 μU/mL) when fed a high-fat diet.[572, 573] As the male mouse ages, glucose levels fall toward the normal range. The mutation responsible for the KK phenotype is unknown.

NZO Mouse

New Zealand obese (NZO) mice were derived by inbreeding of abdominally obese outbred mice.[554, 574–576] NZO neonates have high birth weights, and mice of both sexes are large and at weaning exhibit an elevated carcass fat content.[574] Approximately 40% to 50% of group-caged NZO males, but not females, develop type II diabetes between 12 and 20 weeks of age when maintained with a chow diet containing 4.5% fat.[577] Obesity in NZO mice is characterized by widespread accumulation of subcutaneous as well as visceral fat. The obesity in these mice is accompanied by glucose intolerance in males associated with increased hepatic and peripheral insulin resistance. In contrast to those in *ob* and *db* mice, genes encoding certain gluconeogenic and glycolytic enzymes in the liver retain normal responsiveness to insulin, although there is evidence for an inappropriately active fructose-1,6-biphosphatase.[578–580] Defective beta cell insulin secretion from NZO islets in vitro and in vivo has been described.[574] There appears be a defect in the glycolytic pathway in beta cells leading to defective glucose-stimulated insulin release.[581]

The genetics of NZO mice show a polygenic disorder, and none of the allelic variants have been discovered. Complicating the analysis of the model is the susceptibility of the mice to autoimmune disorders including a lupus-like syndrome[582, 583] and the insulin receptor.[584] There is also a maternal influence in the peripartum period in the development of the disorder, which may reflect substances in the maternal milk.[585]

Gold Thioglucose-Induced Diabetes

Gold thioglucose induces specific lesions in the ventromedial hypothalamus and induces an initial chronic hyperinsulinemia that leads to hypoglycemia, hyperphagia, obesity, and the development of insulin resistance and hyperglycemia.[586] This model has been used as an example of pancreatic dysfunction preceding the induction of insulin resistance as opposed to pancreatic compensation for insulin resistance.

Diabetes Induced by Fat Ablation

Three models of insulin-resistant diabetes have been created in which adipose tissue has been genetically eliminated by overproduction of foreign genes using the fat-specific promoter aP2. Expression of an attenuated diphtheria toxin in adipose tissue resulted in an age-dependent loss of fat, progressive insulin resistance, hyperinsulinemia, and significant diabetes.[587, 588] Adipose-specific expression of a constitutively active form of the sterol regulatory element-binding protein SREBP-1c also resulted in fat ablation.[589] Lipoatrophy has also been induced by fat-specific overexpression of a dominant-negative form of the transcription factor A-ZIP/F.[590, 591] The A-ZIP/F protein heterodimerizes with and inactivates basic zipper (B-ZIP) transcription factors, including activating protein-1 (AP-1) and CCAAT/enhancer binding protein (C/EBP) isoforms, probably disrupting normal fat development. The lack of fat in the various models leads to hepatomegaly, insulin resistance with hyperinsulinemia, hypoleptinemia and significant glucose intolerance, and diabetes. These mice represent a model of the human condition lipodystrophic diabetes and demonstrate the importance of fat in normal glucose homeostasis. It has been suggested that the lack of fat depots results in elevated fatty acid delivery to liver and muscle and the development of insulin resistance. The diabetes in these animals can be variously treated by thiazolidinediones,[587] leptin administration,[592] and fat transplantation.[591] Interestingly, human lipodystrophy also responds to thiazolidinedione treatment,[593] suggesting that some of the effects of these compounds are not wholly dependent upon adipose tissue.

C57BL/6J Mice Fed a High-Fat Diet

Male C57BL/6J (also know as B6) mice fed a high-fat, high-carbohydrate diet (58% fat by kilocalories) or a "Western" diet developed hyperglycemia, hyperinsulinemia, hyperlipidemia, and increased adiposity.[594, 595] Glucose-stimulated insulin secretion was blunted, and there was significant insulin resistance.[596, 597] Despite obesity, plasma leptin levels in the Western diet-fed B6 mice were significantly lower than in control mice in the absence of hyperphagia.[594, 598] The weight gain is due primarily to an increase in mesenteric adiposity, which makes this a good model for adult-onset type 2 diabetes.

Nagoya-Shibata-Yasuda (NSY) Mice

The NSY mouse shows male-specific, mild IGT with only a minority of the females becoming diabetic.[599] An impairment in beta cell function and obesity are present. These mice do not show the typical islet hyperplasia associated with insulin resistance.

TallyHo Mice

The TallyHo mouse also has a male-only development of diabetes associated with beta cell hyperplasia. Both male and female TallyHo mice are obese, hyperinsulinemic, and hyperlipidemic, with the males having glucose levels greater than 500 mg/dL.[600]

Rat Models of NIDDM

Zucker Diabetic Fatty (ZDF) Rat

The orthologue of the *db* mouse, the obese Zucker rat (*fa/fa*), has a mutation in the leptin receptor that results in significant hyperphagia.[601] The *fa* mutation is distinct from the mutations in *db* in that it does not disrupt leptin receptor gene expression and does not affect ligand binding.[601, 602] This mutation results in a constitutive intracellular signaling domain, which may induce a desensitization of the leptin signaling pathways.[603]

The selection of the inbred ZDF strain utilized Zucker (*fa/fa*) rats that had progressed to a diabetic phenotype. Brother-sister mating resulted in nearly 100% diabetes in the male rats receiving a 5% fat diet.[604] Hyperglycemia begins to develop in males at 7 weeks of age, with serum glucose levels rising to 500 mg/dL by 12 weeks of age. The hyperinsulinemia precedes hyperglycemia with marked islet hyperplasia with dysmorphogenesis,[605] but by 19 weeks of age insulin levels drop concomitantly with islet atrophy, in part because of an imbalance of hyperplasia and apoptosis.[606] The islets of prediabetic ZDF rats secrete significantly more insulin in response to glucose with elevated basal levels of insulin secretion and a leftward shift but a blunted glucose dose-response curve.[607, 608] Islets of prediabetic male ZDF rats also have defects in the normal oscillatory pattern of insulin secretion.[607]

In contrast to the male ZDF rat, the female rat has significant insulin resistance but does not become diabetic unless given a proprietary high-fat diet (GMI 13004).[609] The high-fat diet appears to have a direct effect on the beta cell as there is no change in peripheral insulin sensitivity (P. Hansen and C. F. Burant, unpublished). Interestingly, there is a decrease in peripheral triglyceride and FFA levels in the female rat after the institution of the high-fat diet.

The underlying genetic defect that results in beta cell failure in the ZDF rat is unknown. The beta cell number and insulin content are not different from those in homozygous normal animals, but insulin promoter activity is doubled in the ZDF rat.[610] Insulin promoter mapping studies suggest that a critical region in the promoter of the insulin gene is affected. A number of other gene expression differences have been described in ZDF islets, including decreases in the expression of GLUT2[611, 612]; increases in glucokinase and hexokinase activity[608]; decreases in mitochondrial metabolism[608]; accumulation of intraislet lipid and long-chain fatty acyl CoA, which is associated with abnormal beta cell secretion[613–615]; and increases in nitric oxide and ceramide accumulation,[616, 617] which is associated with apoptosis. Other gene expression changes are also found in the prediabetic rat islet.[618] Which of these defects are important for the development of the diabetes is not clear. Despite the fixed genetic defect in the male animal that leads to diabetes, this defect interacts with the insulin resistance because treatment with insulin-sensitizing agents can prevent the onset of diabetes in the male and female.[615, 619] These agents are not effective in the male after establishment of diabetes; however, the female rat can respond to thiazolidinediones, even after significant hyperglycemia.

Goto-Kakizaki (GK) Rats

The GK inbred rat strain was derived from outbred Wistar rats by selection for IGT.[620] Early in the development of diabetes, there are mild elevations of both glucose and insulin levels in the GK rat, but as the animals age, reduced beta cell mass is evident with markedly diminished insulin stores and abnormal secretory responses to glucose.[621, 622] A number of biochemical defects have been described in the islets of these animals, including decreased energy production,[623–625] expression of proteins involved in insulin granule movement,[626] and decreased adenylate cyclase activity.[627] Defects in peripheral signaling include decreased maximal and submaximal insulin-stimulated IRS1 tyrosine phosphorylation, IRS1-associated PI 3-kinase activity, and Akt activation in muscle[628] and defective regulation of protein phosphatase-1 (PP-1), PP-2A, and mitogen-activated protein kinase activation by upstream insulin signaling components in adipocytes.[629] Some of these defects may be due to hyperglycemia because they can be reversed by phlorizin-induced normalization of serum glucose.[628]

Bureau of Home Economics (BHE/Cdb) Rats

The BHE/Cdb rat is a subline of the parent BHE obtained by selection for hyperglycemia and dyslipidemia without obesity.[630] Glucose-stimulated insulin secretion is markedly diminished in these rats, a trait that is maternally inherited.[631] A significant defect appears to be in the liver, where increased gluconeogenesis and lipogenesis precede the hyperglycemia, which may be due to defects in mitochondrial respiration associated with mitochondrial DNA mutations.[632, 633]

Psammomys obesus (Sand Rat)

This is a nutritionally induced obesity model of type 2 diabetes. Genetically, the Sand Rat is in reality a gerbil and the animal usually lives on a low-calorie vegetable diet.[634] When given a high-carbohydrate diet, the Sand Rat rapidly becomes hyperglycemic secondary to weight gain associated with significant insulin resistance[635] and enhanced hepatic glucose production.[636] When a relatively hypocaloric diet is restored, the metabolic syndrome reverts to normoglycemia. A subpopulation of the Sand Rat develops frank beta cell failure and becomes ketotic.

Otsuka Long-Evans Tokushima Fatty (OLETF) Rats

The OLETF rat strain was derived from the Long-Evans rat with polyuria, polydipsia, and mild obesity.[637] About 90% of the male animals become diabetic by 1 year of age. Statistical tests have determined that the locus containing the cholecystokinin A receptor is responsible for about 50% of the NIDDM in the OLETF rats.[638] The receptor is disrupted in the OLETF rat because of a 165-bp deletion in exon 1.[639, 640] Genetic segregation analysis has also shown interaction with a second locus, *Obd2*, which acts in a synergistic fashion to result in NIDDM, and both of these loci are required in homozygous OLETF rats to cause elevated plasma glucose.[641]

The role of sex hormones is pronounced in this strain as orchiectomy markedly reduces the incidence of diabetes whereas ovariectomy increases hyperglycemia to 30% in the female. Further, treatment of castrated males with testosterone restores the incidence to 89%. The islets undergo a progressive inflammatory reaction with progressive fibrosis. This reaction is associated with the impairment of beta cell function.[642] Obesity and insulin resistance appear to precede the development of beta cell failure.[643] Studies have also shown that obesity is necessary for the development of NIDDM in OLETF males and that insulin resistance may be closely related to fat deposition in the abdominal cavity.[644] Troglitazone and metformin have been used successfully to treat the diabetes in the OLETF rat, with troglitazone completely preventing the beta cell morphologic and functional deterioration.[645]

Neonatal Streptozotocin

Two models have been described in which a single dose of the beta cell toxin streptozotocin is given to 2-day-old female Wistar[646, 647] or male Sprague-Dawley rats.[648, 649] These animals have a transient hyperglycemia but develop IGT at 4 to 6 weeks of age. There is an initial reduction of beta cell mass with regeneration resulting in an approximately 50% reduction in adulthood.

MANAGEMENT OF TYPE 2 DIABETES

Over the last 10 years, a conceptual transformation in the principles of management of type 2 diabetes has occurred. Fundamentally, there has been a change in the level of concern about diabetes as a public health issue as well as in attitudes toward its treatment. Dramatic advances in the spectrum of pharmacologic agents and monitoring technology available for the treatment of diabetes have made it possible to lower glucose safely to the near-normal range in the majority of patients. Great strides have been made in establishing an evidence base for guidelines regarding glycemic control and efforts to reduce the risk of complications. Both corporate and government health insurance providers have greatly improved the extent to which diabetes equipment and supplies are covered.

A comprehensive review of all the subtleties of diabetes management in the 21st century is beyond the scope of this chapter. In the following pages, we deal with the salient features of the epidemiology of the complications of type 2 diabetes, diagnostic strategies, treatment guidelines, lifestyle interventions, and pharmacotherapy before turning briefly to a discussion of preventive measures for type 2 diabetes and its complications. An excellent source of information on these issues that is updated annually is the American Diabetes Association's *Clinical Practice Recommendations*. It is published as the first supplement to the journal *Diabetes Care* each January and is available on line at *www.diabetes.org* by clicking "For Health Care Professionals"; near the end of that document is a listing of technical reviews, which are generally recent, fairly exhaustive treatments of most areas of interest in diabetes care.

Scope of the Problem

Type 2 diabetes is estimated to affect some 17 million to 20 million people in the United States. There is an epidemic of diabetes nationwide with a 6% annual growth rate in the prevalence of the disease. Worldwide, the prevalence of diabetes is increasing even faster. This increase is driven by population aging; population growth, particularly among ethnic groups with greater susceptibility to the disease; and dramatic increases in rates of obesity as a consequence of increasingly sedentary lifestyles and greater consumption of simple sugars and high-caloric-density foods. At least in the United States, opportunistic screening for diabetes in high-risk populations is recommended by professional societies and many insurers, resulting in an increase in the proportion of affected individuals diagnosed in this country from approximately one half a decade ago to about two thirds.[650–653]

The morbidity, mortality, and expense associated with diabetes are staggering. In Western society, people with diabetes are three times more likely to be hospitalized than nondiabetic individuals. In the United States, diabetes is the leading cause of blindness and accounts for over 40% of the new cases of end-stage renal disease. The risk of heart disease and stroke is 2 to 4 times higher and the risk of lower extremity amputation is approximately 20 times higher for people with diabetes than for those without. Life expectancy is reduced by approximately 10 years in people with diabetes, and although diabetes is the seventh leading cause of death in the United States, this is clearly an underestimate. Despite the fact that some 70% of people with diabetes die of heart disease and stroke, only approximately 10% have diabetes listed as a contributing cause on death certificates.

Tragically, this enormous burden of death and disability has not been reduced by huge health care expenditures. In fact, the epidemic of diabetes is one of the drivers of increasing health care costs, with annual disbursements for people with diabetes approximately three to five times higher per capita than those for individuals without diabetes. In the United States, at least 15% of health care expenditures are related to the treatment of people with diabetes. Nevertheless, whereas rates of coronary artery disease are declining in the United States in general, this is not the case for people with diabetes. However, there is evidence that increased effort to control diabetes and its comorbidities can even reduce costs associated with diabetes and that a public health approach to diabetes can reduce the burden of complications of diabetes.[654–660]

Screening and Diagnosis

The role of screening to make the diagnosis of diabetes in asymptomatic individuals is an area of substantial controversy. No prospective randomized trials have examined the benefit of such a screening program. On the other hand, it seems self-evident that early diagnosis and intervention have at least the potential to reduce complications in a disease in which 20% to 50% of patients have a complication at the time of diagnosis. The cost-effectiveness of universal approaches to diabetes screening has been called into question. The American Diabetes Association (ADA) recommendations[661] for screening are based on a review that concludes, "Periodic, targeted, and opportunistic screening within the existing health care system seems to offer the greatest yield and likelihood of appropriate follow-up and treatment."[662] The ADA suggests that patients (i.e., screening should be performed only in the context of a routine health care setting) should be screened at 3-year intervals beginning at age 45 and that testing should be considered at an earlier age or be carried out more frequently if diabetes risk factors are present. Those risk factors are listed in Table 29–3.

Most groups recommend FPG as the most practical screening test, although it is recognized that its sensitivity is substantially lower than that of the OGTT. More recent data suggest that alternative screening strategies may have advantages. In a study employing glucose meters to measure random capillary blood glucose, values of 120 mg/dL or higher obtained at random without regard to meals were 75% to 84% sensitive and 86% to 90% specific for detecting diabetes as defined by either FPG or oral glucose tolerance testing.[663] In the future, it is possible that well-validated models will allow us to predict diabetes risk from standard biologic measures such as body mass index, blood pressure, and lipids with greater precision than today.[664]

Classically, diabetes has been diagnosed on the basis of prospective epidemiologic data associating circulating glucose levels with the future development of diabetic retinopathy. In 1997, recommendations were made by an expert committee to change the diagnostic criteria for diabetes to improve the sensitivity of FPG for the diagnosis of diabetes.[665] They determined, from a review of several large data sets, that FPG greater than or equal to 126 mg/dL (7.0 mM) identified a population of people with a risk of retinopathy similar to that of those with a 2-hour value in an OGTT of 200 mg/dL or higher. In an effort to simplify the OGTT, only the 2-hour plasma glucose after a 75-g oral glucose load needs to be measured for diagnostic purposes. Furthermore, patients with classical symptoms of diabetes in association with a random glucose level of 200 mg/dL or higher also meet diagnostic criteria for diabetes. To avoid misclassification, it is further suggested that patients should meet one of the three diagnostic criteria on at least two separate days before making the diagnosis of diabetes.

Because macrovascular disease accounts for the majority of the morbidity and almost all the mortality associated with diabetes and the diagnosis of diabetes is associated with more stringent guidelines for the treatment of comorbidities such as dyslipidemia and hypertension, it seems likely that the diagnostic criteria for diabetes will be lowered again to make the fasting glucose cut points more sensitive. This seems appropriate, as it is clear that glucose levels above normal but below the current thresholds for diabetes are associated with increased cardiovascular risk. A debate unlikely to be answered in the next decade is whether it is acceptable to measure only fasting glucose as an index of glucose intolerance or whether it is cost-effective to use an oral challenge to ascertain fully glucose-related risks.[666–669]

Glucose Treatment Guidelines

Prospective randomized clinical trials have documented improved rates of microvascular complications in patients with type 2 diabetes treated to lower glycemic targets. In the UK Prospective Diabetes Study (UKPDS),[670] patients with new-onset diabetes were treated with diet and exercise for 3 months with an average reduction in glycosylated hemoglobin or HbA_{1c} from approximately 9% to 7% (upper limit of normal 6%). Those with FPG greater than 108 mg/dL (6 mM) were randomly assigned to two treatment policies. In the standard intervention, subjects continued the lifestyle intervention. Pharmacologic therapy was initiated only if the FPG reached 15 mM (270 mg/dL) or the patient became symptomatic. In the more intensive treatment program, all patients were randomly assigned and treated with either sulfonylurea, metformin, or insulin as initial therapy, with the dose increased to try to achieve an FPG less than 108 mg/dL. Combinations of agents were used only if the patients became symptomatic or FPG became greater than 270 mg/dL (15 mM). As a consequence of the design, although the HbA_{1c} fell initially to about 6%, over the average 10 years of follow-up it rose to approximately 8%. The average HbA_{1c} in the standard treatment group was approximately 1% higher. The risk of severe hypoglycemia was small—on the order of 1% to 5% per year in the insulin-treated group—and weight gain was modest; both were higher in patients randomly assigned to insulin and lower in those receiving metformin.[671] Associated with this improvement in glycemic control, there was a reduction in the risk of microvascular complications (retinopathy, nephropathy, and neuropathy) in the intensive group. Although there was a trend toward reduced rates of macrovascular events in the more intensively treated group, it did not reach statistical significance.[670]

Similar reductions in microvascular events were observed in another trial of entirely different design and much smaller size. In the Kumamoto study, Japanese patients of normal weight with type 2 diabetes treated with insulin were randomly assigned to standard treatment or an intensive program of insulin therapy designed to achieve normal glycemia. The control group maintained HbA_{1c} values at approximately 9%, whereas the HbA_{1c} in the intensive group was reduced to approximately 7% and the separation maintained for 6 years. Again, there was a modest increased risk of hypoglycemia and weight gain, a reduction in microvascular complications, and a non-statistically significant trend toward reduced rates of vascular end points.[672]

Table 29–6. Glycemic Targets

Parameter	Normal	ADA	ACE
Premeal plasma glucose (mg/dL)	<110 (mean ~90)	90–130	<110
Postprandial plasma glucose (mg/dL)	<140		<140
HbA_{1c}	4%–6%	<7%	<6.5%

ACE, American College of Endocrinologists; ADA, American Diabetes Association; HbA_{1c}, hemoglobin A_{1c}.

From American Diabetes Association. Standards of medical care for patients with diabetes mellitus. Diabetes Care 2002; 25(suppl 1):S33–S49; American College of Endocrinologists. American College of Endocrinology consensus statement on guidelines for glycemic control. Endocr Pract 2002; Jan/Feb. 8(suppl 1): 5–11.

Although no interventional studies have documented a reduced risk of vascular end points associated with an improvement in glycemic control, multiple epidemiologic studies have suggested that there is an association between cardiovascular risk and HbA_{1c}, FPG, and the 2-hour level in the OGTT.[669, 673, 674] In the UKPDS epidemiologic analysis, there was a 16% reduction in cardiovascular disease rates per 1% reduction in HbA_{1c} without evidence of a threshold or lower limit of benefit all the way into the normal range.[674]

In Table 29–6, guidelines from the ADA and the American College of Endocrinology (ACE) are presented. The ADA suggests that the goal of treatment in the management of diabetes should be an HbA_{1c} value less than 7%.[675] Although initially developed on an ad hoc basis, this goal is supported by the clinical trial data as this level of glycemia was associated with improved outcomes in patients with type 2 diabetes in the preceding studies. The ACE, on the basis of the fact that in the same outcome studies normal glucose levels were targeted and achieved in at least some subjects and that epidemiologic analyses suggest no threshold to the benefit of glucose lowering, has recommended an HbA_{1c} goal of less than 6.5%.[676] Because the average HbA_{1c} in the United States is estimated to be in the 7.5% to 9.5% range, the argument about whether the HbA_{1c} target should be 6.5% or 7% is of limited practical significance.

However, it should be recognized that there are potential adverse events related to pursuit of more aggressive targets—hypoglycemia, long-term exposure to poorly studied combinations of medications, expense, life disruption caused by greater attention and effort to achieve lower glycemic targets, and the potential that great efforts expended in achieving extremely stringent glycemic goals will result in less attention to other health risks by patient or provider. No cohort of patients of substantial size has ever been reported in which an average HbA_{1c} level less than 7% has been achieved over a time frame that exceeds more than a few months. Several adequately powered, randomized controlled clinical trials are under way or being planned to explore the effects of seeking more intensive glycemic targets ($HbA_{1c} < 6\%$). Although it is clear that many patients can achieve lower glucose levels with currently available drugs and lifestyle interventions, it remains theoretically possible that the risks would exceed the benefits of seeking glucose targets less than 7%.

With respect to fasting, premeal, or postprandial targets, there is little support for any particular level of glycemic control in the management of type 2 diabetes as no large-scale outcome study has targeted particular levels of glucose with home glucose monitoring. The ADA target of fasting and premeal plasma glucose levels of 90 to 130 mg/dL is based on an estimate of the range of average glucose values that would be associated with a low risk of hypoglycemia and HbA_{1c} less than 7%.[675] The ACE target of less than 110 mg/dL is an effort to achieve normal levels of glycemia.[676] However, it should be recognized that consistent fasting and premeal glucose levels less than 110 mg/dL would be expected to be associated with an HbA_{1c} of approximately 5.5%.[677]

The ADA has not set any treatment goals for postprandial glucose levels because there are no published studies in which even safety, much less outcome, is documented for targeting a particular level of postprandial glucose.[675] However, the ADA statement on postprandial glucose recognizes that there are effective HbA_{1c}-lowering agents that primarily target postprandial glucose levels and suggests that monitoring postprandial glucose levels may allow dose adjustment of these agents.[678] Furthermore, they recognize that there are patients with diabetes who have average fasting glucose levels within targets but whose HbA_{1c} is elevated and that monitoring and specifically treating postprandial elevations in these patients may provide improvements in HbA_{1c}, perhaps with a lower risk of hypoglycemia and weight gain than further lowering fasting and premeal glucose levels. The ACE recommends targeting a 2-hour postprandial glucose less than 140 mg/dL (7.8 mM) in an effort to achieve near-normal glycemia.[676] Consistent postprandial glucose values less than 140 mg/dL would be associated with average HbA_{1c} levels of approximately 5%.[677]

Lifestyle Intervention

The components of lifestyle intervention include medical nutrition counseling, exercise recommendations, and comprehensive diabetes education with the purpose of changing the paradigm of care in diabetes from provider-focused to patient-focused. Arguably, over the last 5 years, nothing has changed more fundamentally than the emphasis on lifestyle intervention. For decades, physicians and patients have paid lip service to the notion that lifestyle intervention is important. Now we have significant clinical trial evidence that each component of lifestyle intervention, when appropriately administered, can contribute to improved outcomes. Furthermore, since the Balanced Budget Act of 1997 and the passage of complementary legislation in most state governments, lifestyle intervention has been a covered benefit for most people. Although full implementation of these regulations is still in progress, they have dramatically expanded the proportion of the population with diabetes with insurance coverage for these essential services.

Education of Patients

Diabetes is a lifelong disease, and health care providers have almost no control over the extent to which patients adhere to the day-to-day treatment regimen. The appropriate role of the health care provider is to serve as a coach to the patient, who has primary responsibility for the delivery of daily care.

As a result, health care providers must carefully engage patients as partners in the therapeutic process. It is critical for the health care professional to understand the context in which patients are taking care of their disease. Using a prescriptive approach in which patients are told what to do can work in some situations but fails more often than not because of unrecognized barriers to the execution of a particular plan. For long-term success, diabetes self-management education is critical.

As defined by the ADA,[679] diabetes self-management education is the process of providing the person with diabetes with the knowledge and skills needed to perform self-care, manage crises, and make lifestyle changes. As a result of this process, the patient must become a knowledgeable and active participant in the management of his or her disease. To achieve this task, patients and providers work together in a long-term, ongoing process. Minimal diabetes education should be universally provided and individualized with emphasis on the issues highlighted in Table 29–7. There are many more specialized topics relevant to almost all patients, such as how to adjust therapy when eating out or during travel as well as review of available local health care resources such as support groups and insurance issues. Although there are only limited studies, they do provide support for the concept that diabetes education can be cost-effective and can improve outcomes.[680, 681]

Table 29–7. Curricular Areas That Should Be Addressed in Diabetes Self-Management Education

Pathophysiology of the patient's diabetes and its relationship to treatment options
Incorporating appropriate nutritional management
Incorporating physical activity into lifestyle
Utilizing medications (if applicable) for therapeutic effectiveness
Monitoring blood glucose, urine ketones (when appropriate), and using the results to improve control
Preventing, detecting, and treating acute complications including "sick day rules" and hypoglycemia
Preventing, detecting, and treating chronic complications
Goal setting to promote health, and problem solving for daily living
Integrating psychosocial adjustment to daily life
Promoting preconception care, management during pregnancy, and gestational diabetes management (if applicable)

Adapted from American Diabetes Association. National standards for diabetes self-management education. Diabetes Care 2002; 25(suppl 1):140–147.

A team of providers is generally required to implement fully the process of diabetes self-management education as the amount of information that needs to be exchanged is large and the range of expertise broad. It is generally not possible to cover the recommended content fully in the context of several or even many brief encounters with a physician in an office setting. Potential providers in a team care approach could include nurses, dietitians, exercise specialists, behavioral therapists, pharmacists, and other medical specialists including diabetologists or endocrinologists, podiatrists, medical subspecialists, obstetrician-gynecologists, psychiatrists, and surgeons. The potential role of the community in which the patient lives and works in the diabetes self-care process is enormous, including family, friends, employers, and health care insurance providers. Each potential member of the team has a role to play in the process, which must be reviewed and assessed frequently (Table 29–8). The primary role of the providers in this process is to provide guidance in goal setting to manage the risk of complications, suggest strategies to achieve goals and techniques to overcome barriers, provide training in skills, and help screen for complications. For this process to be a success, the patient must commit to the principles of self-care, participate fully in the development of a treatment plan, make ongoing decisions regarding self-care from day to day, and communicate honestly and with sufficient frequency with the team.

Fortunately, barriers to providing team care are becoming less daunting. Diabetes education programs are being established at a rapid rate. The American Association of Diabetes Educators (800-TEAM-UP4) and the ADA (800-DIABETEs) can provide information regarding diabetes educators and education programs in your area.

For team care to be most effective, communication, trust, and mutual respect are critical. Unfortunately, in many communities, the full benefit of the consultation and ongoing care with diabetes educators, nurses, dietitians, pharmacists, or others is not achieved because of overly hierarchic approaches to care. Nonphysicians, including patients, ought to provide suggestions regarding medication and lifestyle adjustments and

Table 29–8. Team Care: Roles of the Players

Primary care provider
- To be a source of accurate information and to refer to and coordinate with other sources of information as necessary
- To provide guidance in developing goals of treatment
- To screen for complications and evaluate progress in meeting treatment goals
- To help develop strategies to achieve treatment goals and avoid complications

Other providers
- To be a source of accurate information and to communicate with the primary care provider as well as coordinate with other sources of information as necessary
- To provide guidance in developing goals of treatment and to help the primary care provider develop strategies to achieve treatment goals and avoid complications

Patient
- To commit to diabetes self-management (as defined above)
- To be an active participant in the process
- To communicate with other team members when goals are not achieved or barriers or problems are encountered

Community
- To provide support to encourage ongoing diabetes self-care

help in the process of identifying barriers to effective management such as lack of knowledge, lack of time, and lack of resources and strategies to overcome those barriers.

Perhaps some of the most overlooked contributors to ineffective care in the setting of type 2 diabetes are the relatively common barriers created by psychiatric, neurocognitive function, and adjustment disorders, which are largely responsive to psychosocial therapies.[682]

Nutrition

With respect to self-management education, a technical review documents the effect of medical nutrition therapy and specific advice on diabetes-related outcomes such as HbA_{1c}, weight, and proteinuria.[683] These are summarized in Table 29–9. A comprehensive, individually negotiated nutrition program in which each patient's circumstances, preferences, and cultural background as well as the overall treatment program are considered is most likely to result in optimal outcomes. Because of the complexity of both the medical and nutritional issues for most patients, it is recommended that a registered dietitian, with specific skill and experience in implementing nutrition therapy in diabetes management, work collaboratively with the patient and other health care team members in providing medical nutrition therapy.

Analogously, physicians and other members of the health care team need to understand the major issues in diabetes and nutrition and support the nutritional plan developed collaboratively. Individualized dietary advice can be developed by a physician from a brief diet history obtained by asking: "What do you eat for breakfast? . . . lunch? . . . supper? Do you have snacks between breakfast and lunch? . . . lunch and supper? . . . supper and bedtime? What do you drink during the day?" Ideally, this information should be obtained at each visit, with specific suggestions for change that both patient and provider agree are important and achievable.

Easy issues to address include caloric beverages, which tend to elevate glucose levels dramatically and can generally be replaced quite painlessly by artificially sweetened alternatives. Juices are generally perceived as healthy but can significantly affect glycemic control and total calorie intake. Substituting low-fat products for higher fat alternatives is useful but needs to be done with the recognition that they are generally higher in carbohydrates. "Fat-free" and "sugar-free" foods need to be recognized as food that is not "free." Portion control and recipe modification are excellent dietary techniques, particularly for meats and fried foods.

Adequate spacing between meals is usually good advice for patients with type 2 diabetes because postprandial glucose levels generally peak 2 hours after a meal, when a snack would normally be taken. Eating approximately every 4 hours while awake is the most practical dietary plan for most overweight people. Frequent small meals have been shown to be of benefit when used in a controlled inpatient setting, but in general when overweight patients are encouraged to eat more frequently they often overeat more frequently. At a minimum, avoiding high-calorie snacks is reasonable advice for most people with diabetes. A repeated diet history and additional modest changes negotiated every few weeks to months by all health care providers (doctor, nurse, or dietitian) allow assessment of whether previously agreed to changes were enacted, reinforcement of the importance of dietary efforts, and slow enticement of patients into more healthful dietary choices.

In general, the critical nutrient for glycemic consistency is carbohydrate. Essentially every molecule of carbohydrate consumed is converted to glucose in the gut and requires the action of insulin to be cleared from the circulation. A dietary technique called carbohydrate counting can be used in patients with type 2 diabetes to facilitate consistent carbohydrate intake or to allow insulin dose adjustment in response to changes in carbohydrates consumed.[684] Whereas the beta cell in type 2 diabetes has generally lost its responsiveness to glucose, the second phase of insulin secretion is largely spared in type 2 diabetes and is in part driven by amino acids and fatty acids. Therefore, including some protein and fat in each meal and snack is useful.

Dietary fat is the nutrient most closely associated in epidemiologic studies with the risk of developing type 2 diabetes. Although dietary fats clearly have an impact on total caloric intake related to their caloric density and on circulating lipids, they have a minimal impact on glycemia acutely. Fat intake is a contributor to obesity and the critical nutrient for cardiovascular risk management. It is generally recommended that people with diabetes (and all people in general) consume a diet that is modestly restricted in calories (if they are overweight) containing less than 10% of total calories as saturated fat and less than 10% as polyunsaturated fat. Some would advocate substituting foods high in monounsaturated fatty acids—seeds, nuts, avocado, olives, olive oil, and canola oil—for carbohydrate, but most patients do not find adequate variety in the monounsaturated fatty acid category and often overeat these high-caloric-density foods. Higher carbohydrate diets may raise postprandial glucose and triglycerides but are much less calorically dense and have a higher thermic effect, both of which tend to promote weight loss.

Dietary protein similarly has a minimal impact on glucose levels, although amino acids do promote insulin secretion, which may be advantageous in the setting of type 2 diabetes. Metabolism of protein results in the formation of acids and nitrogenous waste, which may result in bone demineralization and glomerular hyperfiltration. At least 0.8 g of high-quality protein per kilogram is generally recommended; otherwise, restriction of protein intake to 10% to 20% of total calories minimizes potential adverse long-term effects of high protein intake.

The role of vitamins, trace minerals, and nutritional supplements in the treatment of diabetes is poorly understood. There are some who are absolutely convinced of the utility of soluble fiber, magnesium, chromium, zinc, folic acid, pyridoxine, cyanocobalamin, vitamin A, vitamin C, vitamin E, vanadium, selenium, garlic, and others. Clinical trial data to support their safety and efficacy are inconclusive. Many patients are convinced that nutritional supplementation is healthful, and it is

Table 29–9. Major Nutrition Recommendations for Diabetes

Carbohydrate

- Foods containing carbohydrate from whole grains, fruits, vegetables, and low-fat milk are important components, and should be included, in a healthy diet.
- With regard to the glycemic effects of carbohydrates, the total amount of carbohydrate in meals or snacks is more important than the source or type.
- Individuals receiving intensive insulin therapy should adjust their premeal insulin doses based on the carbohydrate content of meals.
- As sucrose does not increase glycemia to a greater extent than isocaloric amounts of starch, sucrose and sucrose-containing foods do not need to be restricted by people with diabetes; however, they should be substituted for other carbohydrate sources or, if added, covered with insulin or other glucose-lowering medication.
- Nonnutritive sweeteners are safe when consumed within the acceptable daily intake levels established by the Food and Drug Administration.
- Individuals receiving fixed daily insulin doses should try to be consistent in day-to-day carbohydrate intake.
- Although the use of low-glycemic-index foods may reduce postprandial hyperglycemia, there is not sufficient evidence of long-term benefit to recommend use of low-glycemic-index diets as a primary strategy in food or meal planning.
- As with the general public, consumption of dietary fiber is to be encouraged; however, there is no reason to recommend that people with diabetes consume a greater amount of fiber than other Americans.
- Carbohydrate and monounsaturated fat should together provide 60%–70% of energy intake. However, the metabolic profile and need for weight loss should be considered when determining the monounsaturated fat content of the diet.
- Sucrose and sucrose-containing foods should be eaten in the context of a healthy diet.

Protein

- In persons with controlled type 2 diabetes, ingested protein does not increase plasma glucose concentrations, although protein is just as potent a stimulant of insulin secretion as carbohydrate.
- For persons with diabetes, especially those not in optimal glucose control, the protein requirement may be greater than the recommended dietary allowance (RDA) but not greater than usual intake.
- For persons with diabetes, there is no evidence to suggest that usual protein intake (15%–20% of total daily energy) should be modified if renal function is normal.
- The long-term effects of diets high in protein and low in carbohydrate are unknown. Although such diets may produce short-term weight loss and improved glycemia, it has not been established that weight loss is maintained long-term. The long-term effect of such diets on low-density lipoprotein (LDL) cholesterol is also a concern.

Fat

- Less than 10% of energy intake should be derived from saturated fats. Some individuals (i.e., persons with LDL cholesterol ≥100 mg/dL) may benefit from lowering saturated fat intake to less than 7% of energy intake.
- To lower LDL cholesterol, energy derived from saturated fat can be reduced if weight loss is desirable or replaced with either carbohydrate or monounsaturated fat if weight loss is not a goal.
- Dietary cholesterol intake should be less than 300 mg/day. Some individuals (i.e., persons with LDL cholesterol ≥100 mg/dL) may benefit from lowering dietary cholesterol to less than 200 mg per day.
- Intake of *trans*-unsaturated fatty acids should be minimized.
- Polyunsaturated fat intake should be approximately 10% of energy intake.
- Reduced-fat diets, when maintained long-term, contribute to modest loss of weight and improvement in dyslipidemia.

Energy balance and obesity

- In insulin-resistant individuals, reduced energy intake and modest weight loss improve insulin resistance and glycemia in the short term.
- Structured programs which emphasize lifestyle changes including education, reduced fat (<30% of daily energy) and energy intake, regular physical activity, and regular participant contact can produce long-term weight loss on the order of 5% to 7% of starting weight.
- Exercise and behavior modification are most useful as adjuncts to other weight loss strategies. Exercise is helpful in maintenance of weight loss.
- Standard weight reduction diets, when used alone, are unlikely to produce long-term weight loss. Structured, intensive lifestyle programs are necessary.

Micronutrients

- There is no clear evidence of benefit from vitamin or mineral supplementation in people with diabetes who do not have underlying deficiencies.
- Routine supplementation of the diet with antioxidants is not advised because of uncertainties related to long-term efficacy and safety.

Alcohol

- If individuals choose to drink alcohol, daily intake should be limited to one drink for adult women and two drinks for adult men. One drink is defined as 12 oz of beer, 5 oz of wine, or 1.5 oz of ~80 proof spirits.
- To reduce risk of hypoglycemia, alcohol should be consumed with food.

Children and adolescents with diabetes

- Individualized food or meal plans and intensive insulin regimens can provide flexibility for children and adolescents with diabetes to accommodate irregular mealtimes and schedules, varying appetite, and varying activity levels.
- Nutrient requirements for children and adolescents with type 1 or type 2 diabetes appear to be similar to those of other same-age children and adolescents.

Older adults

- Energy requirements for older adults are less than for younger adults.
- Physical activity should be encouraged.
- In the elderly, undernutrition is more likely than overnutrition and therefore caution should be exercised when prescribing weight loss diets.

Acute complications

- Glucose is the preferred treatment for hypoglycemia, although any form of carbohydrate that contains glucose may be used.
- Ingestion of 15 to 20 g of glucose is an effective treatment for hypoglycemia but blood glucose may be corrected only temporarily.
- Blood glucose should be evaluated in approximately 60 minutes, as additional treatment may be necessary.
- During acute illnesses, testing blood glucose and blood or urine for ketones, drinking adequate amounts of fluids, and ingesting carbohydrates are important.

Hypertension

- In both normotensive and hypertensive individuals, a reduction in sodium intake lowers blood pressure. The goal should be to reduce sodium intake to 2400 mg (100 mmol) or 6000 mg sodium chloride (salt) per day.
- A modest amount of weight loss beneficially affects blood pressure.

Table 29–9. Major Nutrition Recommendations for Diabetes *Continued*

Dyslipidemia
- For persons with elevated LDL cholesterol, saturated fatty acids and *trans*-saturated fatty acids should be limited to less than 10% and perhaps to less than 7% of energy.
- Energy derived from saturated fat can be reduced if weight loss is desirable or replaced with either carbohydrates or monounsaturated fats if weight loss is not a goal.
- For persons with elevated plasma triglycerides, reduced high-density lipoprotein (HDL) cholesterol, and small dense LDL cholesterol (the metabolic syndrome), improved glycemic control, modest weight loss, dietary saturated fat restriction, increased physical activity, and incorporation of monounsaturated fats may be beneficial.

Nephropathy
- In individuals with microalbuminuria, reduction of protein to 0.8 to 1.0 g/kg body weight per day and in individuals with overt nephropathy, reduction to 0.8 g/kg body weight per day may slow the progression of nephropathy.

Catabolic illness
- The energy needs of most hospitalized patients can be met by providing 25–35 kcal/kg body weight.
- Protein needs are between 1.0 to 1.5 g/kg body weight; the higher end of the range being for more stressed patients.

Prevention of diabetes
- Structured programs which emphasize lifestyle changes including education, reduced fat and energy intake, regular physical activity and regular participant contact can produce long-term weight loss of 5%–7% of starting weight and reduce the risk for developing diabetes.
- All individuals, especially family members of persons with type 2 diabetes, should be encouraged to engage in regular physical activity to decrease risk of developing type 2 diabetes.

Adapted from American Diabetes Association. Evidence-based nutrition principles and recommendations for the treatment and prevention of diabetes and related complications. Diabetes Care 2002; 25:202–212.

often counterproductive to engage in scholarly discussion of the nature of the evidence base for their decision. At a minimum, discussion should include the documented efficacy of more classical lifestyle and pharmacologic intervention and the idea that these efforts should not be left by the wayside when budgetary constraints affect potentially more effective interventions.[685, 686] A multivitamin containing at least 400 μg of folic acid is probably a reasonable nutritional supplement for most patients with type 2 diabetes, and supplementation with folic acid (1 mg), vitamin B_{12} (400 μg), and pyridoxine (10 mg) has been shown to reduce the rate of restenosis after coronary angioplasty, presumably by reducing homocysteine levels.[687]

Although there are proponents of a wide range of dietary composition, there are few data to support these recommendations from long-term outcome studies of prescribed diets. Mixed meals containing 10% to 20% of calories from protein, no more than 10% of calories from saturated fat, and the remainder largely from monounsaturated fats (seeds, nuts, avocados, olives, olive oil, canola oil) and carbohydrates, particularly whole grains, fruit, vegetables, and low-fat milk, are probably most reasonable. There is evidence to suggest that a diet rich in complex carbohydrates and low in fat and animal protein is a beneficial component of comprehensive lifestyle management in the setting of cardiovascular disease.[688]

Weight loss is a goal of many patients with and without diabetes and certainly is associated with improvements in glycemic control, insulin resistance, circulating lipids, and blood pressure. Numerous clinical studies document that intensive lifestyle programs involving frequent contact with patients, individualized counseling, and education aimed at reducing dietary fat and calorie intake coupled with regular physical activity and efforts to understand and control behaviors that result in overeating can produce modest weight loss that can be largely maintained with sustained effort.[689–692]

Exercise

There is a substantial body of literature supporting exercise as a modality of treatment in type 2 diabetes.[689–694] Exercise is perhaps the single most important lifestyle intervention in diabetes as it is associated with improved glycemic control, insulin sensitivity, cardiovascular fitness, and remodeling. Aerobic exercise and resistance (strength) training both have a positive impact on glucose control. Improvements in glycemic control are generally apparent immediately, become maximal after a few weeks of consistent exercise, but may persist for only 3 to 6 days after the cessation of training, hence the rationale for negotiating a minimum of three exercise sessions a week to maintain the benefit of the intervention.

The key concept is to promote an increase in activity using an approach similar to the one discussed for diet. Goals, methods, intensity, and frequency have to be negotiated with patients with great sensitivity to recognizing barriers and helping patients discover solutions. The role of educators, exercise specialists, physical therapists, and social supports in this process is critical. The major role for the physician is to screen for complications (neuropathy, nephropathy, retinopathy, vascular disease) and discover ways for patients to be able to exercise safely. Exercise in the presence of uncontrolled diabetes, hypertension, retinopathy, nephropathy, neuropathy, and cardiovascular disease can create devastating problems. These can all be addressed creatively and should never provide an insurmountable barrier to increasing physical activity.

Some authorities recommend that all patients older than 35 years have stress tests before exercise. Their utility is potentially limited by their poor sensitivity and specificity.[654, 695] If the exercise program contemplated does not involve more strenuous (intensity and duration) activity than the patient has engaged in recently but merely involves more frequent activity, screening cardiovascular stress testing is unlikely to be useful. However, when sedentary patients plan to embark on a program of strenuous exercise, stress testing is prudent to evaluate for subclinical coronary disease. Even when stress testing is employed and negative results are obtained, encouraging patients not to overexert and to recognize exertional chest, jaw, or arm discomfort as well as palpitations and dyspnea as symptoms of cardiac dysfunction is reasonable. Over time, improved exercise tolerance should be viewed as a measure of improving cardiorespiratory function.

For aerobic exercise to be most useful in improving insulin resistance, it should be performed at 60% to 80% of maximal aerobic capacity (tachypnea that is not severe enough to prevent one from carrying on a conversation) for at least 20 minutes (recognizing that 30 minutes is about twice as beneficial as 20 minutes) at least every 48 hours. For the average patient with type 2 diabetes starting an exercise program, this equates to quite low level activity initially, such as walking at a pace of 2 miles an hour. Initially, it may even be advantageous to negotiate once-weekly walks or shorter duration exercise sessions, or both, and proceed from there. Over time, patients are encouraged to pick up the pace as tolerated and increase the duration and frequency of exercise sessions slowly to avoid overuse injuries. It is not unreasonable to suggest to patients that if they are going to incorporate exercise in their diabetes management program, they must think of exercise as a treatment that takes the place of a pill and thus requires adherence to produce benefit.

Self-Monitoring of Blood Glucose

Self-monitoring of blood glucose (SMBG) has not been demonstrated in clinical trials to change outcomes in type 2 diabetes when evaluated in isolation.[696] However, many diabetes self-management programs have been demonstrated to help reduce complications. In all of these, SMBG is an integral part of the process, suggesting that SMBG is at least a component of effective therapy. The frequency and type of monitoring in diabetes therapy should be determined in consultation with the patient, taking into account the nature of the diabetes, the overall treatment plan and goals, and the patient's abilities. SMBG is particularly recommended for all patients with type 2 diabetes taking insulin or sulfonylureas as it allows the identification of minimal or asymptomatic episodes of hypoglycemia. Although severe hypoglycemia is relatively rare in type 2 diabetes, it can have devastating consequences such as trauma or self-injury or change in the perceived ability of a patient to continue to live independently as a result of confusion or loss of consciousness. Also, it is essential to have patients critically assess the nature of any hypoglycemic symptoms that may occur. Many patients are fearful or overconcerned about hypoglycemia and routinely consume extra calories in response to a variety of life's circumstances such as when they are hungry, sweaty, nervous, or upset. Monitoring studies generally document that most symptoms in patients with type 2 diabetes are not related to hypoglycemia and should not be treated with excessive caloric consumption.

Timing of SMBG varies depending on the diabetes therapy. It is important to advise patients to vary the time of the day at which blood glucose levels are checked. For some patients, the highest blood glucose of the day is the morning glucose, whereas for others the highest is before bed. Particularly in early diabetes, gestational diabetes, and well-controlled diabetes, monitoring 1 to 2 hours after meals allows patients to assess the effect of their lifestyle and pharmacologic efforts in controlling postprandial glucose levels, which are usually the only glycemic abnormality present. Monitoring and thus targeting therapy at just one time of day can leave the patient with a less than ideal overall response to therapy.

When glucose control is poor, having patients concentrate on premeal glucose levels is adequate. Once the premeal glucose levels reach the middle to low 100s, many advocate that patients switch to checking 1- to 2-hour postprandial glucose levels because it amplifies the observed effect of diet on glycemic control and enables patients to see that moderate changes in meal plan, activity, and medications have a significant impact on glycemic control. Even after substantial inappropriate changes in food intake, activity, or timing or dose of medication, blood sugar values often return to near-normal levels overnight or by the time of the next meal.

The frequency of glucose monitoring needs to be matched to individual patients' needs and treatment. Many clinicians ask patients to monitor at least once a day, varying among before breakfast, lunch, supper, bedtime, and midsleep as well as with hypoglycemic symptoms. Others ask intensively insulin-treated patients to monitor with intensity similar to that described for patients with type 1 diabetes (four times per day before meals with weekly checks at least once after breakfast, lunch, supper, and at midsleep as well as with symptoms). Some ask for sets of glycemic readings more infrequently (e.g., fasting and 1 hour after the biggest meal). In the subset of patients who achieve stable blood glucose levels without significant hypoglycemia, it is generally appropriate to decrease the frequency of SMBG to a few times a week. It is critical that SMBG be frequent enough that both patient and provider have a good understanding of both the adequacy of the treatment regimen and the stability of glycemic control.

It has been widely assumed that the benefits of SMBG stem from the effect of putting patients in a situation in which they can be in control of their own therapy. If patients are aware of the glycemic targets associated with the outcomes they seek to achieve, SMBG enables them to evaluate critically their response to therapy and assure themselves that they are reaching their goals. It is generally useful for patients to keep a daily diary of their SMBG results, not only so that they can assess their results periodically but also so that they can share them with the health care team. Unfortunately, many patients faithfully perform daily or more frequent SMBG, record the results as instructed, and discuss them with their health care team only at quarterly or semiannual visits despite the fact that their control is inadequate. Unless SMBG results are entirely within agreed to targets, they should be communicated and reviewed at least monthly with a member of the health care team by telephone, fax, mail, or e-mail or at an interim visit to trigger changes in therapy as the need arises. Unfortunately, such services are generally unreimbursed and may become an unsustainable burden on health care teams.

Finally, one of the most difficult areas in which to keep current is the area of available equipment and supplies, particularly for glucose monitoring. A useful resource in this regard is the annual *Resource Guide*, which comes out as the January issue of *Diabetes Forecast*, a magazine for lay people with diabetes and their families. It is available on line at the ADA Web site (*www.diabetes.org*) by clicking on "Community and Resources" on the left and then "Diabetes Forecast" below and finally on "Back Issues" to find the most recent January issue.

Pharmacotherapy of Type 2 Diabetes

The revolution in the treatment of type 2 diabetes since 1995 in the United States has been driven by the release of multiple new classes of drugs that independently address different pathophysiologic mechanisms that contribute to the development of diabetes. The available oral antidiabetic agents can be divided by mechanism of action into insulin sensitizers with primary action in the liver, insulin sensitizers with primary action in peripheral tissues, insulin secretagogues, and agents that slow the absorption of carbohydrates. Insulin therapy in the setting of type 2 diabetes effectively is a supplement to endogenous insulin secretion. The relative benefits of lifestyle intervention and the six classes of drugs available for the management of type 2 diabetes are found in Table 29–10. This area has been the subject of extensive reviews.[697–700] Because of limitations of space, in the following discussion the principles outlined in these reviews are summarized and limited additional references provided.

Insulin Sensitizers with Predominant Action in the Liver: Biguanides

Metformin is the only biguanide available in the United States. Phenformin was removed from the United States market in the 1970s because of deaths associated with lactic acidosis. Phenformin and buformin remain available in some countries around the world. Although metformin has been available

Table 29–10. Comparisons of Therapies for Type 2 Diabetes

Property	Lifestyle	Insulins	Sulfonylureas	Metformin	α-Glucosidase Inhibitors	"Glitazones" Pioglitazone (P) Rosiglitazone (R)	"Glinides" Repaglinide (R) Nateglinide (N)
Target tissue	Muscle or fat	Beta cell supplement	Beta cell	Liver	Gut	Muscle	Beta cell
Δ HbA_{1c} (monotherapy)	Variable	1%–>2%	1%–2%	1%–2%	0.5%–1%	0.5%–2%	R:1%–2% N:0.5%–1%
Fasting effect	Good	Excellent	Good	Good	Poor	Good	R: Moderate N: Poor
Postprandial effect	Good	Excellent	Good	Good	Excellent	Good	R: Good N: Excellent
Severe hypoglycemia	No	Yes	Yes	No	No	No	R:Yes N:No
Dosing interval	Continuous	qd to continuous	qd to tid	bid or tid	bid to qid	P:qd R:qd or bid	tid to qid with meals
Δ Weight (lb/yr)	+1	+3	+1–3	0 to −6	0 to −10	+1 to 13	+1–3
Δ Insulin	Variable	Increase	Increase	Modest decrease	Modest decrease	Decrease	Increase
Δ LDL	Minimal decrease	Minimal decrease	None	Decrease	Minimal decrease	P: None R: Increase	None
ΔHDL	Minimal increase	None	None	Increase	None	Increase	None
Δ TG	Minimal decrease	Decrease	None	Decrease	Minimal decrease	P: Decrease R: None	None
Common problem	Recidivism, injury	Hypoglycemia, weight gain	Hypoglycemia, weight gain	Transient GI	Flatulence	Weight gain, edema, anemia	Hypoglycemia
Rare problem				Lactic acidosis		Hepatotoxicity?	
Contraindications	None	None	Allergy	Renal failure Liver failure CHF >80 yr old	Intestinal disease	Hepatocellular disease CHF	
Cost ($ per month)	0–200	15–100+	5–25	20–90	25–60	70–150	50–90
Maximum effective dose		1–2 U/kg/day	1/2 maximum or double starting	1000 mg bid	50 tid	P: 45 mg qd R: 4 mg bid	R: 2 mg tid N: 120 mg tid

CHF, Congestive heart failure; GI, gastrointestinal; HbA_{1c}, hemoglobin A_{1c}; HDL, high-density lipoprotein; LDL, low-density lipoprotein; TG, triglyceride.

in Europe for almost 40 years, it has been marketed in the United States only since 1995. The precise mechanism of action of metformin is unknown. Its major activity is to reduce hepatic insulin resistance and thereby gluconeogenesis and glucose production. It has more inconsistently demonstrated effects to improve insulin sensitivity in peripheral tissues. Because of its limited duration of action, it is generally taken at least twice daily, although a sustained-release formulation is now available.

As biguanides do not increase insulin levels, they are not associated with a significant risk of hypoglycemia. The most common adverse events are gastrointestinal—nausea, diarrhea, crampy abdominal pain, and dysgeusia. About one third of patients have some gastrointestinal distress, particularly early in their course of treatment. This distress can be minimized by starting with a low dose once daily with meals and titrating upward slowly (over weeks) to effective doses. Sustained-release metformin is associated with less frequent and severe upper gastrointestinal symptoms, the more common of the adverse effects of metformin, but can increase the frequency of diarrhea, a much less common adverse effect overall. The vast majority of patients note no adverse effects with metformin therapy, and at least 90% tolerate it adequately with long-term use. Perhaps as a result of clinical or subclinical gastrointestinal effects, metformin is associated with less weight gain than other antidiabetic agents and in some studies modest mean weight loss.

The other side effect of concern with metformin is lactic acidosis, which is quite rare and occurs almost exclusively in patients who are at high risk of developing lactic acidosis apart from metformin therapy. As a result, it is recommended that high-risk patients avoid use of metformin.[701] The package insert suggests that metformin is absolutely contraindicated in patients with renal insufficiency as the drug is cleared renally; it states that the drug should not be used in males with a serum creatinine greater than or equal to 1.5 mg/dL and in females at 1.4 mg/dL.

Obviously, there is a complex relationship between serum creatinine and renal function. Thus, reasonable practice would generally involve avoiding the use of metformin entirely in patients with an estimated creatinine clearance from the Cockcroft-Gault equation of less than 50 mL/min and avoiding greater than half-maximal doses of metformin in patients with an estimated creatinine clearance between 50 and 70 mL/min. As a reminder, according to the Cockcroft-Gault equation, creatinine clearance equals [(140 − age)*(weight in kg)]/(72 ×

serum creatinine in mg/dL) in males, and this is multiplied by 0.85 in females. Therefore, a 30-year-old, 250-pound construction worker with a creatinine of 1.6 has a normal creatinine clearance of 103 mL/min, whereas an 80-year-old, 110-pound woman with a creatinine of 0.8 has a low creatinine clearance of 44 mL/min. Metformin is also contraindicated in patients with congestive heart failure requiring treatment, in those with hepatic insufficiency, and in the setting of alcohol abuse. Caution is required in elderly people, patients with acute illness or poorly controlled chronic illness, and in the setting of simultaneous treatment with nephrotoxic drugs (e.g., contrast dye).

The glucose-lowering efficacy and the prevalence of adverse gastrointestinal effects increase proportionately in the dose range 500 to 2000 mg/day. The maximal dose of 2550 mg does not generally provide additional benefit beyond that seen at 2000 mg daily. A new formulation of metformin combined with glyburide has been developed to maximize glucose-lowering effectiveness through the synergy of using an insulin secretagogue and thereby minimize gastrointestinal effects and is available in tablets with metformin/glyburide ratios of 250/1.25, 500/2.5, and 500/5. The formulations containing proportionally lower glyburide doses (250/1.25 and 500/2.5) seem to perform similarly to the higher dose combinations and thus are preferred.

Arguably, metformin has the best record of accomplishment among oral antidiabetic agents in outcome studies. In the UKPDS, among overweight subjects, those randomly assigned to metformin not only had improvements in microvascular complications similar to those of subjects randomly assigned to insulin and sulfonylurea but also demonstrated a reduction in diabetes-related deaths and myocardial infarction.[671] The validity of this observation has been challenged because of unusual responses in a subsequent subrandomization. The beneficial effect of metformin on macrovascular complications through mechanisms independent of glycemic control is certainly plausible and supported by such observations as metformin-associated modest reductions in LDL, triglycerides, blood pressure, and procoagulant factors.

Insulin Sensitizers with Predominant Action in Peripheral Insulin-Sensitive Tissues: Thiazolidinediones

The thiazolidinedione class of drugs, often termed TZDs or glitazones, has engendered great enthusiasm and controversy since the first agent, troglitazone, was approved in 1997.[702] Troglitazone was withdrawn from the United States market in the year 2000, largely because the remaining agents (pioglitazone and rosiglitazone) were thought to be safer than troglitazone, with which rare fatal hepatotoxicity was associated. These agents are believed to work through binding and modulation of the activity of a family of nuclear transcription factors termed peroxisome proliferator-activated receptors (PPARs). They are associated with slow improvement in glycemic control over weeks to months in parallel with an improvement in insulin sensitivity and reduction of FFA levels.

Each of these agents varies in important ways with regard to potency, pharmacokinetics, metabolism, binding characteristics, and demonstrated lipid effects. At the same time, all are effective glucose-lowering agents that are remarkably well tolerated with weight gain and fluid retention (and associated edema formation and hemodilution) as the only significant adverse effects. There is no substantial evidence that these newer agents are associated with hepatotoxicity, but this record of safety has been established in the setting of careful liver function test monitoring. Therefore, it is important to continue to recommended that the glitazones not be used in patients with active hepatocellular disease or in patients with unexplained serum alanine aminotransferase (ALT) levels greater than 2.5 times the upper limit of normal as well as to recommend serum ALT monitoring before initiating therapy, every 2 months for the first year and intermittently thereafter.

Whether there are clinically important differences between the two currently available agents is hotly debated,[703] but definitive answers await adequately powered head-to-head studies that are under way. The promise of the glitazone class to reverse or prevent the negative cardiovascular associations of insulin resistance in parallel with its demonstrated effect of improving insulin sensitivity is exciting but unproven and under formal study in a series of randomized prospective clinical trials. Almost all of the available data with regard to vascular effects of this class come from studies with troglitazone and include the following tantalizing clinical associations: reduced carotid intimal medial thickness, normalization of vascular endothelial function, improvements in dyslipidemia, lower blood pressure, and improved fibrinolytic and coagulation parameters. A second attribute of the glitazones that has generated great enthusiasm is an effect to improve insulin secretory dynamics in subjects with diabetes and IGT. These observations provide hope that glitazone therapy may be useful in preventing diabetes or in halting the progression of established diabetes, thereby reducing the need for additional drug therapy over time. It is critical to recognize that the proven effects of pioglitazone and rosiglitazone to date are limited to improvements in glycemic control and changes in lipid parameters.

The adverse effect that has engendered the greatest concern regarding this class of drugs is weight gain. Careful study indicates that the weight gain is a result of subcutaneous and not visceral fat accumulation and that there is, in fact, a reduction in visceral fat, hepatic fat, and intramyocellular fat. Thus, the weight gain observed with glitazones, while having obvious negative consequences from the cosmetic standpoint, is perhaps less likely to cause significant adverse cardiovascular effects. Both weight gain and fluid retention are more common and severe in patients with the greatest glycemic responses, making expectant management of these adverse effects mandatory. All patients prescribed glitazones should be counseled to redouble lifestyle efforts to minimize weight gain.

With regard to edema, with appropriate caution almost no one should need to withdraw from therapy as a result of fluid retention. The patients most likely to experience edema are those treated with insulin and those with preexisting edema. Thus, women, overweight patients, and those with diastolic dysfunction or renal insufficiency are at greatest risk. It is prudent to teach patients with preexisting edema how to assess pitting pretibial edema at home and suggest that they make a habit of checking nightly. If they note a pattern of increasing edema at home, patients can be instructed to restrict sodium intake, to start a diuretic, or to increase their diuretic by some specified quantity on their own as needed.

In the edematous patient, people treated with insulin, and those at higher risk of fluid retention, it is prudent to initiate therapy with the lowest marketed dose of glitazone. When patients return for their 2-month ALT check, if the glycemic response has been inadequate and significant edema has not developed, increasing the dose of glitazone further with continued expectant management of edema can be accomplished. Most patients with mild edema respond to a low-dose thiazide diuretic (e.g., hydrochlorothiazide [HCTZ] at 25 mg). In patients with more extensive edema, a combination of low-dose thiazide diuretic with moderate-dose loop diuretic is sometimes required. Anecdotal reports suggest that avoidance of nonsteroidal anti-inflammatory agents and dihydropyridine calcium channel blockers can reduce the frequency of edema as an adverse event. It should be noted that fluid retention to the point of congestive heart failure and anasarca has been reported and that in some patients edema is refractory to diuretic therapy.

Insulin Secretagogues

Currently available insulin secretagogues all bind to the sulfonylurea receptor (SUR1), a subunit of the ATP-sensitive potassium channel (K_{ATP}) on plasma membrane of pancreatic beta cells. The SUR1 subunit regulates the activity of the channel and also binds ATP and ADP, effectively functioning as a glucose sensor and trigger for insulin secretion. Sulfonylurea binding as well as increases in intracellular ATP and decreases in ADP as a result of fuel metabolism lead to closing of the channel. The membrane depolarization that ensues causes the opening of voltage-dependent L-type calcium channels. Subsequent calcium influx results in an increase in intracellular calcium, which leads to insulin secretion. Differences in pharmacokinetic and binding properties of the various insulin secretagogues result in the specific responses that each agent produces. The major difference between them seems to be related to duration of action and to fairly subtle variations in their hypoglycemic potential.

Sulfonylureas

The sulfonylureas have been available since the 1950s. They have a relatively slow onset of action and variable duration of action. There are numerous choices available (Table 29–11), which can be divided into first- and second-generation agents. In general, the second-generation agents are more potent and as a result have fewer adverse effects and drug-drug interactions. Glipizide-GITS (gastrointestinal therapeutic system) and glimepiride are preferred agents as they can be given as a once-daily dose (without additional effect with twice-daily dosing) in the vast majority of patients and involve a relatively low risk of hypoglycemia and weight gain. Glyburide is one of the most commonly prescribed insulin secretagogues despite the fact that essentially all marketed oral secretagogues have been shown to have a significantly lower hypoglycemic potential.

An unusual characteristic of sulfonylureas is that the maximum marketed dose is generally two to four times higher than the maximally effective dose. There has been concern over the years that sulfonylureas may result in increased arrhythmic cardiovascular events in patients with diabetes as a result of their activity on vascular and cardiac SUR2 receptors with an effect of blunting ischemic preconditioning, a protective autoregulatory mechanism in the heart. There is some evidence to suggest that this may be less likely to occur with glimepiride than with glyburide, but it is also a rationale to avoid high-dose sulfonylurea therapy.[704] Sulfonylureas are arguably the most cost-effective glucose-lowering agents and therefore are clearly worthy of their widespread use. In general, limiting the dose to one-fourth maximal, unless higher doses are clearly demonstrated to provide significant benefits in glycemic control, minimizes both costs and adverse events. Small doses of sulfonylurea (e.g., 0.5 to 1 mg of glimepiride or 2.5 mg of glipizide-GITS) are remarkably effective, particularly in patients on concomitant insulin- sensitizing therapy, and are almost uniformly well tolerated.

Repaglinide

Repaglinide is a member of the meglitinide family of insulin secretagogues, distinct from the sulfonylureas. It has a short half-life and a distinct SUR1 binding site. As a result of more rapid absorption, it produces a generally faster and briefer stimulus to insulin secretion. As a result, it is generally taken with each meal and provides better postprandial control and generally less hypoglycemia and weight gain than glyburide. Repaglinide does seem to have a long residence time on the sulfonylurea receptor and a prolonged effect on fasting glucose despite the fact that its pharmacologic half-life is quite short. Repaglinide is available in 0.5, 1, and 2 mg tablets. The maximal dose is 4 mg with each meal. As is the case with the sulfonylureas, there is a modest glucose-lowering advantage of high doses versus moderate doses of repaglinide.

Nateglinide

Nateglinide is a derivative of phenylalanine, structurally distinct from both sulfonylureas and the meglitinides. It has a quicker onset and shorter duration of action than repaglinide. Its interaction with SUR1 is fleeting. As a result, its effect in lowering postprandial glucose is quite specific and it has little effect in lowering fasting glucose. This provides advantages (less hypoglycemia) and disadvantages (less overall glucose-lowering effectiveness). Therefore, nateglinide is most appropriately used when fasting glucose levels are modestly elevated in the setting of early diabetes or in combination with insulin sensitizers or long-acting evening insulin. Nateglinide is available as 120-mg tablets and is taken with each meal. A 60-mg tablet is available but is not generally used except in patients with minimal hyperglycemia.

The rationale for stimulating insulin secretion in a way that minimizes fasting hyperinsulinemia and maximizes postprandial control is compelling. Furthermore, these newer agents demonstrate little binding to the vascular smooth muscle and cardiac SUR2 receptors. However, the use in the United States of these newer glinide agents has been modest, in part because of the need for multiple daily doses, greater expense than with sulfonylureas, and lack of head-to-head comparative studies that demonstrate superiority over newer sulfonylureas already perceived as having low potential for producing hypoglycemia and weight gain.

Carbohydrate Absorption Inhibitors: α-Glucosidase Inhibitors

α-Glucosidase inhibitors (AGIs) work to inhibit the terminal step of carbohydrate digestion at the brush border of the intestinal epithelium. As a result, carbohydrate absorption is shifted more distally in the intestine and is therefore delayed, allowing the sluggish insulin secretory dynamics characteristic of type 2 diabetes to catch up with carbohydrate absorption. There are two currently available agents, acarbose and miglitol. Their use in the United States has been limited by a number of factors, including the need to administer the medication at the beginning of each meal, flatulence as a common side effect, and only modest reductions in blood glucose. These factors should be balanced against the AGI's ability to lower postprandial glucose, thereby improving glycemia without increasing weight or hypoglycemic risk. Even though they may potentially lower glucose in everyone, the extent of the lowering is generally modest, calling into question their utility in the presence of substantial expense and side effects. To maximize the potential for these agents to be well tolerated, start with a low dose such as one fourth of the maximum dose just once daily and increase over a period of weeks to months to one-fourth to one-half maximal dose with each meal.

Insulins

Insulin has been commercially available since the early 1920s and is arguably still the mainstay of therapy for the majority of people with type 2 diabetes worldwide. Subcutaneous injection

Table 29–11. Characteristics of Sulfonylureas

Generic Name	Initial Daily Dose	Maximum Daily Dose	Equivalent Doses (mg)	Duration of Action	Comments
Acetohexamide	250 mg	1500 mg, divided bid	500	Intermediate 12–18 hr	Metabolized by liver to active metabolite (twice as potent as parent compound). Has diuretic activity. Has uricosuric activity.
Chlorpropamide	100 mg	750 mg qd (500 mg in older patients)	250	Very long 60 hr	70% metabolized by liver to less active metabolites; 30% excreted intact by kidneys. Can potentiate ADH. Disulfiram (Antabuse) like reaction with alcohol occurs in nearly a third of patients.
Tolazamide	100 mg	1000 mg, divided bid	250	Intermediate 12–24 hr	Metabolized by liver to less active and inactive products. Has diuretic activity.
Tolbutamide	250–500 mg	3000 mg, divided bid or tid	1000	Short 6–12 hr	Metabolized by liver to inactive product.
Glipizide	5 mg	40 mg, divided bid	5	Intermediate 12–24 hr	Metabolized by liver to inactive products that are excreted in the urine and, to a lesser extent, in the bile. Mild diuretic activity.
Glipizide-GITS	5 mg	20 mg qd		Long >24 hr	
Glyburide	2.5 mg	20 mg, divided bid	5	Intermediate 16–24 hr	Metabolized by liver to weakly active and inactive products, excreted in urine and bile. Mild diuretic activity. Highest risk of hypoglycemia.
Micronized glyburide	3 mg	6 mg bid	3	Shorter	
Glimepiride	1 mg	8 mg qd	2	Long >24 hr	Metabolized to inactive metabolities by liver, excreted in urine and bile.

GITS, gastrointestinal therapeutic system.
Adapted from Facts and Comparisons, drug information monthly update service. St. Louis, JB Lippincott.

of insulin in type 2 diabetes is designed to supplement endogenous production of insulin both in the basal state to modulate hepatic glucose production and in the postprandial state, in which a surge in insulin release normally facilitates glucose clearance into muscle and fat for storage to allow intraprandial metabolism. Currently, the vast majority of insulin used worldwide is of recombinant human origin. The available formulations largely differ in their pharmacokinetics as reviewed in Table 29–12.

Insulin lispro and insulin aspart are rapid-acting insulin analogues that have an onset of action in 5 to 15 minutes, peak activity in approximately 1 hour, and a duration of activity of approximately 4 hours. Regular insulin is approximately half as fast as the rapid-acting analogue with onset in 30 minutes, a peak at 2 to 4 hours, and a duration of action of 6 to 8 or more hours. Intermediate-acting insulin—neutral protamine Hagedorn (NPH) and Lente—is approximately twice as slow as regular insulin with an onset of action in 1 to 2 hours, a peak at 4 to 8 hours, and a duration of action of 12 to 16 hours. Ultralente insulin is purportedly long acting, but the pharmacokinetics of human Ultralente are not dramatically different from those of NPH or Lente. Insulin glargine is a novel long-acting insulin analogue with distinctive properties. It provides a flat, peakless profile of activity with a duration of action of more than 24 hours in most patients. Premixed insulin formulations provide greater convenience and accuracy of mixing than those mixed by patients. Premixed formulations available in the United States are 70/30 and 50/50 mixtures of NPH and regular insulin, a 75/25 mixture of lispro insulin in its NPH-like formulation with insulin lispro, and a 70/30 mixture of insulin aspart with its NPH-like congener. Premixed insulin provides a profile of activity as expected from the addition of the activities of its components.

Adverse events associated with insulin are well known and include weight gain and hypoglycemia. It is interesting that both fast-acting and long-acting insulin analogues have been shown to provide a modest reduction in hypoglycemia. Insulin allergies are rare, as are chronic skin reactions—lipodystrophy and lipohypertrophy. It should be noted that the absolute risk of severe hypoglycemia in patients with type 2 diabetes is relatively small, approximately one third to one tenth as high as in similarly treated patients with type 1 diabetes. This risk can be further minimized with appropriate education of patients and expectant home glucose monitoring at times when

Table 29–12. Pharmacology of Insulin

Insulin	Onset (hr)	Peak (hr)	Duration (hr)	IM or IV Dosing	Forms and Modifiers	Variability in Absorption
Lispro, Aspart	0.10–0.25	0.75–2.0	3.0–4.0	No	Insulin analogue, monomeric	Minimal
Regular	0.5–1.0	1.0–4.0	4.0–10	$t_{1/2}$ IM 20 min $t_{1/2}$ IV 10 min	None	Moderate
NPH	1.0–3.0	5.0–7.0	13–18	No	Protamine	High
Lente	1.5–4.0	4.0–8.0	13–20	No	Zinc	High
Ultralente	2.0–6.0	8.0–12	18–30	No	Zinc	Very High
Glargine	~2	No discrete peak	~24	No	Insulin analogue, precipitates at neutral pH	Moderate

IM, intramuscular; IV, intravenous; NPH, neutral protamine Hagedorn.

unrecognized hypoglycemia is most likely to occur—midsleep or during unplanned or strenuous activity. There are rare examples of patients who develop irritation at injection sites (more common but rarely dose limiting with insulin glargine) or allergies.

Newer insulin needles cause less discomfort than those previously available because of a finer gauge, shorter length, sharper points, and smoother surfaces. Insulin pen technology makes teaching a patient to take insulin much easier and provides greater convenience and accuracy of dosing. Insulin pump therapy has been used in patients with type 2 diabetes but is not widely accepted as cost-effective in routine use. Even though the vast majority of patients now find insulin therapy much easier and more effective than they had anticipated, there is still substantial resistance to initiating insulin therapy on the part of patients and providers.

Practical Aspects of Initiating and Progressively Managing Type 2 Diabetes

A significant challenge in clinical decision making in diabetes is that the increased availability of therapeutic options for antidiabetic therapy is ahead of adequate prospective outcome studies. Currently available clinical trial data have not identified the preferred agents in type 2 diabetes, either as initial therapy or in subsequent care. Each class of drugs and even agents within each class have advantages and limitations, and individual issues may significantly affect the appropriate choice of therapy in particular patients. Table 29–10 highlights some of the relative advantages and disadvantages of various agents and classes.

A general approach in the absence of any patient-specific factors is suggested in the algorithm presented in Figure 29–20. A growing body of experience indicates that the use of metformin as initial therapy in combination with diet and exercise can provide impressive lowering of glucose with essentially no risk of hypoglycemia. Because this agent is available as a generic preparation, relative cost is low, and if the response is judged to be inadequate a thiazolidinedione, sulfonylurea, or glinide can be added. It has been proposed that the use of metformin alone or in combination with a thiazolidinedione may lead to a greater reduction in cardiovascular risk than similarly effective (with respect to glycemia) approaches that increase insulin levels. At present, the data are not definitive on this point.

Patients with higher levels of glucose (generally FPG > 200 mg/dL) almost always require agents to increase insulin levels. Because insulin, sulfonylureas, and glinides provide much faster improvements in overall control that metformin, glitazones, or AGIs, they are preferred in patients with higher levels of glucose either as monotherapy or as part of initial combined therapy. Starting a patient with a low dose of a glimepiride, glipizide-GITS, or insulin combined with either metformin, glitazone, or AGI is a reasonable initial approach to the poorly controlled condition.

In patients who have reasonable control of fasting and preprandial plasma glucose levels (more than 50% of values less than 130 mg/dL) whose overall control as assessed by HbA_{1c} is still higher than desired, monitoring may be either inaccurate or ineffective or postprandial plasma glucose (PPG) levels may be elevated. As it can be more difficult to have patients monitor in the postprandial state, it is important to remember that without specific therapy, almost all patients with type 2 diabetes have elevated PPG. Thus, in such patients, targeting presumed PPG elevations with the use of AGIs, glinides, or rapid-acting insulin analogues can theoretically lower average glucose with a lower risk of weight gain and hypoglycemia than with sulfonylureas or long-acting insulin.

The most critical issue in long-term glycemic management is that of continuously reassessing with patients the adequacy of their control, examining glucose monitoring logs and HbA_{1c} values, and refining treatment regimens to achieve optimal control with the lowest dose of the least number of medications. Most patients in specialty care require two or more drugs to achieve recommended targets. Many patients require three or more (particularly if you consider long-acting and short-acting insulin as two agents). Fortunately, almost all the possible two-drug combinations and many of the three-drug combinations have been examined in modest-sized studies and have been shown to be safe and effective. Generally, it is preferred to add agents if there was an improvement in control with the first agent selected and to continue to add agents as

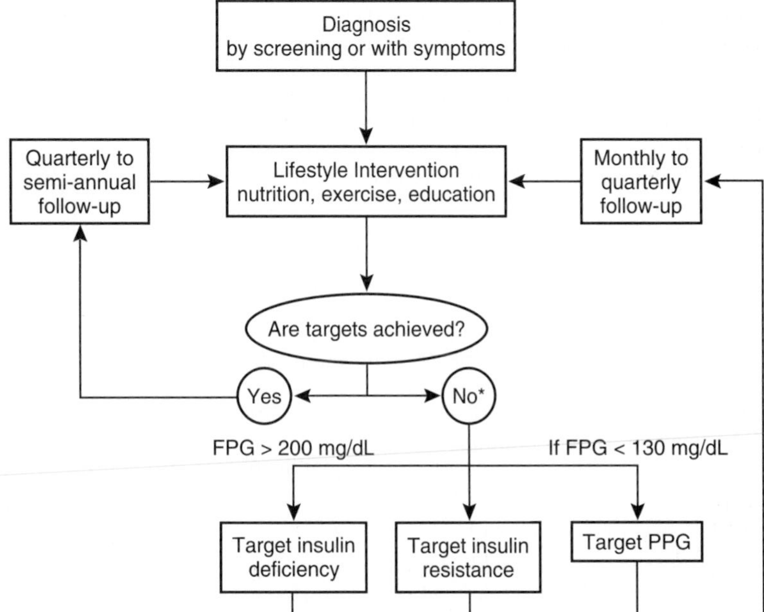

Figure 29–20. Treatment algorithm for type 2 diabetes. FPG, fasting plasma glucose; PPG, postprandial plasma glucose.

needed to achieve goals. Subsequent back-titration to optimize treatment is often possible when glycemic goals are achieved. The selection of initial therapy should be based on mutually (patient and provider) recognized priorities. Increasingly, practitioners are using submaximal doses of agents in combination to increase the ratio of efficacy to adverse effects and in recognition of the potential synergy of sensitizers and secretagogues as well as the value of treatment of postprandial glucose and fasting glucose in combination therapy.

When adding insulin in the management of inadequately controlled type 2 diabetes, some practitioners prefer to stop the oral antidiabetic agents and switch to insulin. Most generally continue the oral agents and add an evening dose of insulin. Classically, bedtime NPH insulin and more lately bedtime insulin glargine have been preferred for initiating insulin therapy. In more overweight patients (>120% of ideal body weight), the use of mixed insulin (or premixed insulin) at supper can help clear glucose elevations after the evening meal, generally the largest meal of the day. This works quite well in most patients, although some experience nocturnal hypoglycemia, which is less common with mixtures employing rapid-acting insulin analogues. There are data suggesting that glargine given at bedtime can similarly provide for lower morning glucose values with less nocturnal hypoglycemia than NPH insulin, particularly in more overweight patients. Many patients eventually require more complex regimens—twice-daily injections, split-mix insulin, multiple injection regimens, and rarely insulin pump therapy. It should be noted that a minority of patients with type 2 diabetes have a better response to insulin administered in the morning than in the evening.

It is important that both patient and health care provider agree on how to reach the goals of therapy. Therefore, biases and concerns of the patient should be addressed when trying to determine which agent should be prescribed. These biases can be elucidated in interviews with patients through discussions of various strategies.

Strategies

Minimal Cost Strategy

For a large proportion of patients, particularly those who are elderly, drug costs are an overwhelming issue. Diet and exercise can be extremely effective and almost free. The least expensive drugs for the treatment of diabetes are the sulfonylureas; metformin has become available in generic formulations. Thus, a minimum cost strategy could start with a sulfonylurea and progress to the addition of generic metformin or bedtime or presupper insulin and finally two or more insulin injections per day if necessary. In the Veterans Administration Cooperative Study, excellent control was achieved in the context of a comprehensive program of diabetes education using a combination of daytime sulfonylurea and evening insulin. Although insulin is relatively inexpensive, in high doses (1 U/kg or more) the costs begin to rise, creating a rationale for adding metformin or a thiazolidinedione. It should be noted that most pharmaceutical companies have programs to provide no-cost or low-cost medication to the poor. Many of these are listed with links at *www.needymeds.com*. Furthermore, for increasing numbers of patients, the major driving force in their drug expenses is the number of prescriptions as each is associated with a copayment, providing a rationale for using combination agents.

Minimum Weight Gain Strategy

Weight gain associated with the treatment of diabetes is of concern to most clinicians and is often an overriding issue with patients. A strategy to minimize weight gain would emphasize diet and exercise and would almost certainly employ metformin or an AGI as initial therapy with the addition of the other agent if one was inadequate. As sulfonylureas and repaglinide seem to have a modest weight-sparing effect in combination therapy with insulin, one or the other could be added before insulin administration in such a strategy. As discussed earlier, the weight gain associated with thiazolidinediones, although certainly a cosmetic issue, may not be associated with increased cardiovascular risk.

Minimal Injection Strategy

Too many patients are determined to avoid insulin injections at any cost. The minimal injection strategy involves sulfonylureas, metformin, AGIs, and thiazolidinediones, which can be added in any order. Insulin, probably as a bedtime or presupper dose to minimize the inconvenience, would be added only if absolutely necessary. The strategy of using thiazolidinediones early in the course of diabetes in the hope that this may reduce the rate of progressive beta cell dysfunction remains unproved. It is important to try to dispel notions that insulin therapy is difficult, ominous, or fraught with peril by highlighting its efficacy and the great strides that have been made in insulin formulations and delivery devices. Most patients require insulin at some point in their lifetime.

Minimal Insulin Resistance Strategy

The possible atherogenic effects of insulin have been widely touted in the lay press and by marketing programs within the pharmaceutical industry. The relationship between circulating insulin levels and cardiovascular risk in nondiabetic populations is incontrovertible but probably related to the presence of insulin resistance rather than the insulin concentrations per se. Furthermore, in essentially all studies of intensive management with insulin, improved outcomes were observed with insulin treatment. There are no clinical data to suggest that exogenous insulin is associated with adverse side effects or long-term complications beyond its hypoglycemic effects and the associated weight gain. In any case, this strategy is analogous to the minimal injection strategy except that the order of introduction of agents is perhaps important. The thiazolidinediones have the greatest efficacy in reducing insulin resistance, metformin is second, and AGIs are third, with nateglinide associated with more specific stimulation of insulin levels after meals than the other insulin secretagogues, which all increase peripheral insulin levels less than injected insulin.

Minimal Effort Strategy

Many patients are capable of making only a minimal effort with regard to their diabetes. Questioning patients about their pill-taking history and their realistic ability to comply with a prescribed frequency of therapy is important. Taking a once-a-day sulfonylurea or thiazolidinedione requires the least effort by the patient. Taking bedtime insulin is actually relatively well accepted by patients to whom this consideration is important. Developing strategies to improve adherence and increase motivation is certainly a long-term goal in this population.

Hypoglycemia Avoidance Strategy

This is another important consideration for many patients. The AGIs have been reported in small studies to reduce "reactive" hypoglycemia. Other oral agents could be added in any order with the exception that insulin secretagogues would be added last, their dose minimized, and glyburide avoided. Nateglinide in particular among the secretagogues is associated with an exceptionally low risk of significant hypoglycemia. The insulin analogues are associated with a lower risk of hypoglycemia than human insulin.

Postprandial Targeting Strategy

Achieving postprandial glucose targets is generally associated with better control than just meeting premeal targets.[705] On the basis of epidemiologic studies, it has been suggested that PPG is more highly correlated with cardiovascular disease risk than fasting glucose levels. Correction for confounding variables such as components of the multiple metabolic syndrome has not been performed, however. Furthermore, there are no outcome studies that have demonstrated the superiority of these approaches in the setting of type 2 diabetes. Control of postprandial glycemia can be achieved only with specific lifestyle efforts and pharmacologic agents, which target postprandial glucose. Postprandial glucose monitoring is helpful in this regard as it reinforces the goals and is the most effective measure to assess the effectiveness of treatment. Techniques that can improve postprandial control include lowering the carbohydrate content of meals, adding fiber, substituting monounsaturated fats for carbohydrates, encouraging physical activity after meals, adding AGIs with meals, and using rapid-acting insulin analogues. Nateglinide and repaglinide provide a theoretical advantage in this situation compared with other secretagogues, although formal head-to-head studies have not been completed comparing the glinides with glimepiride and glipizide-GITS.

Prevention of Type 2 Diabetes

The possibility that type 2 diabetes can be prevented in high-risk individuals has been formally tested in a series of large-scale clinical trials. The Da Qing study randomly assigned clinics in an industrial city in China to a dietary intervention, exercise intervention, combined diet and exercise, or no intervention at all. Among the clinics, 577 subjects with IGT were studied. In this study, the interventions were quite modest and conducted largely in group settings. All three interventions led to reductions in the risk of conversion to diabetes of 31% to 46% compared with the control groups.[691] In a Finnish study, a similar number of middle-aged obese subjects with IGT were randomly assigned to a control group that received minimal lifestyle advice or to intensive, individualized instruction on food intake, increased physical activity, and weight reduction. The intensive lifestyle therapy group demonstrated a 58% relative risk reduction compared with the control group in the incidence of diabetes.[692] In the United States, the Diabetes Prevention Program enrolled over 3000 middle-aged, overweight subjects with IGT including substantial representation from high-risk minority groups. The intensive lifestyle group in this study also demonstrated a 58% relative risk reduction in the progression to diabetes.[690] In the Diabetes Prevention Program, there was another arm of the study that evaluated the ability of metformin at 500 mg twice a day to prevent the development of diabetes. It was moderately successful, with a 31% relative reduction in the progression of diabetes, although the benefit seemed to be greater in younger, more overweight, and more hyperglycemic subjects. In other studies not yet fully published, other oral antidiabetic agents—troglitazone in the Troglitazone in the Prevention of Diabetes (TRIPOD) study[690a] and acarbose in the STOP-NIDDM study[690b]—have been reported to reduce the risk of developing diabetes. Patients and families as well as health care professionals are excited about the possibilities of preventing the disease.

The success of the lifestyle interventions is impressive, demonstrating conclusively that with a variety of techniques it is possible for patients to achieve physiologically relevant changes in body weight. Medications overall had less positive impact than lifestyle intervention, although troglitazone did perform remarkably well in diabetes prevention. The questions that arise from these results are how to screen for people at risk and what intervention should be initiated in those with an interest in prevention.

It seems reasonable to screen on the basis of current recommendations as outlined earlier primarily for case finding but also recognizing that patients with abnormal glucose values (fasting greater than 110 mg/dL or IGT with an OGTT) would be ideal candidates for preventive strategies. Certainly, high-risk individuals should be counseled on nutritional approaches to achieve weight loss, instructed to increase physical activity, and observed prospectively to determine whether progression of hyperglycemia has occurred. Treatment for other cardiovascular risk factors should also be considered if they are present. In the absence of outcome studies, it is difficult to recommend drug therapy to prevent diabetes because significant complications are unlikely to develop in the short window of time during which glucose levels increase from a fasting glucose of 110 to 126 mg/dL. An extension phase of the Diabetes Prevention Program that is under way should provide evidence concerning whether prevention or delay in the development of diabetes will prevent death or disability.

Future Directions

The present-day management of type 2 diabetes is significantly more effective and easier for patients than the situation that prevailed even 10 years ago. A better understanding of the barriers to effective diabetes management and how to overcome them would be of great benefit. The epidemic in diabetes and obesity that is under way coupled with the predicted early death and disability that follow threatens to overwhelm our health care system. Practical, cost-effective public health approaches to stem this tide are desperately needed.[706]

Novel pharmaceutical agents including glucagon receptor antagonists, inhibitors of gluconeogenic and glycogenolytic pathways, activators of the insulin signaling pathways, modifiers of lipid metabolism, and antiobesity agents are areas of early pharmaceutical development.[707]

There is tremendous interest in developing novel PPAR modulators that preserve the glucose-lowering effectiveness of the glitazones, enhance the lipid benefits, and mitigate the effects on fluid retention and weight gain. As these PPAR-active agents are thought to exert their action in the nucleus, there is reason to believe that such a goal is achievable. There are dozens of compounds in early stages of development and several already in phase III trials. The major barrier to success in this arena is the lack of well-validated animal models to predict human responses.[708] Novel methods of insulin delivery similarly have generated a great deal of enthusiasm among patients, particularly techniques to deliver insulin orally or by inhalation.[709] There is considerable controversy in the endocrine community in this regard. On the one hand, it seems unlikely that oral insulin delivery would be efficient enough to treat insulin resistance effectively; on the other hand, any delivery into the portal system could be more effective and perhaps have an improved safety profile because of preferential inhibition of hepatic glucose production.

The area of gut hormones offers promise for advances in treatment of type 2 diabetes. Amylin, the second beta cell hormone, is known to act centrally to suppress postprandial glucagon secretion, slow gastric emptying, and increase satiety. Synthetic amylin is in late-phase trials, and although only modestly effective as a glucose-lowering agent, it does seem to be well tolerated and is associated with weight reduction.[710]

GLP-1 is a gut hormone secreted from intestinal cells that has an overlapping but generally more robust profile of action than amylin with the additional effect of preserving functioning beta cell mass. GLP-1 is rapidly degraded in the circulation, and thus inhibitors of the degrading enzyme (dipeptidylpeptidase IV [DP-IV]) as well as DP-IV–resistant analogues are being investigated in clinical trials.[711] Additional studies will determine whether glucagon-like peptides provide the next major class of antidiabetic agents.

References

1. Zimmet P, Alberti KG, Shaw J. Global and societal implications of the diabetes epidemic. Nature 2001; 414:782–787.
2. King H, Aubert RE, Herman WH. Global burden of diabetes, 1995–2025: prevalence, numerical estimates, and projections. Diabetes Care 1998; 21:1414–1431.
3. Boyko EJ, de Cowten M, Zimmer PZ, et al. Features of the metabolic syndrome predict higher risk of diabetes and impaired glucose tolerance: A prospective study in Mauritius. Diabetes Care 2000; 23:1242–1248.
4. Ramachandran A, Snehalatha C, Latha E, et al. Rising prevalence of NIDDM in an urban population in India. Diabetologia 1997; 40:232–237.
5. O'Dea K. Westernisation, insulin resistance and diabetes in Australian aborigines. Med J Aust 1991; 155:258–264.
6. Harris MI, Flegal KM, Cowie CC, et al. Prevalence of diabetes, impaired fasting glucose, and impaired glucose tolerance in U.S. adults. The Third National Health and Nutrition Examination Survey, 1988–1994. Diabetes Care 1998; 21:518–524.
7. Harris MI, Eastman RC, Cowie CC, et al. Comparison of diabetes diagnostic categories in the U.S. population according to the 1997 American Diabetes Association and 1980–1985 World Health Organization diagnostic criteria. Diabetes Care 1997; 20: 1859–1862.
8. Mokdad AH, Bowman BA, Ford ES, et al. The continuing epidemics of obesity and diabetes in the United States. JAMA 2001; 286:1195–1200.
9. Type 2 diabetes in children and adolescents. American Diabetes Association. Diabetes Care 2000; 23:381–389.
10. Report of the Expert Committee on the Diagnosis and Classification of Diabetes Mellitus. Diabetes Care 1997; 20:1183–1197.
11. McCance DR, Hanson RL, Charles MA, et al. Comparison of tests for glycated haemoglobin and fasting and two hour plasma glucose concentrations as diagnostic methods for diabetes. BMJ 1994; 308:1323–1328.
12. Engelgau MM, Thompson TJ, Herman WH, et al. Comparison of fasting and 2-hour glucose and HbA1c levels for diagnosing diabetes: diagnostic criteria and performance revisited. Diabetes Care 1997; 20:785–791.
13. Jackson CA, Yudkin JS, Forrest RD. A comparison of the relationships of the glucose tolerance test and the glycated haemoglobin assay with diabetic vascular disease in the community. The Islington Diabetes Survey. Diabetes Res Clin Pract 1992; 17: 111–123.
14. Beks PH, Mackaay AJ, de Vries H, et al. Carotid artery stenosis is related to blood glucose level in an elderly Caucasian population: the Hoorn Study. Diabetologia 1997; 40:290–298.
15. Fuller JH, Shipley MJ, Rose G, et al. Coronary-heart-disease risk and impaired glucose tolerance: the Whitehall study. Lancet 1980; 1:1373–1376.
16. Charles MA, Shipley MJ, Rose G, et al. Risk factors for NIDDM in white population: Paris prospective study. Diabetes 1991; 40: 796–799.
17. Harris MI, Klein R, Welbom JA, Knuiman MW. Onset of NIDDM occurs at least 4–7 yr before clinical diagnosis. Diabetes Care 1992; 15:815–819.
18. Harris MI. Undiagnosed NIDDM: clinical and public health issues. Diabetes Care 1993; 16:642–652.
19. Harris MI, Eastman RC. Early detection of undiagnosed diabetes mellitus: a US perspective. Diabetes Metab Res Rev 2000; 16: 230–236.
20. Harris MI, Hadden WC, Knowler WC, Bennett PH. Prevalence of diabetes and impaired glucose tolerance and plasma glucose levels in U.S. population aged 20–74 yr. Diabetes 1987; 36:523–534.
21. Almind K, Doria A, Kahn CR. Putting the genes for type II diabetes on the map. Nat Med 2001; 7:277–279.
22. Bell GI, Polonsky KS. Diabetes mellitus and genetically programmed defects in beta-cell function. Nature 2001; 414:788–791.
23. Taylor SI, Arioglu E. Genetically defined forms of diabetes in children. J Clin Endocrinol Metab 1999; 84:4390–4396.
24. Kahn CR, Flier JS, Bar RS, et al. The syndromes of insulin resistance and acanthosis nigricans: insulin-receptor disorders in man. N Engl J Med 1976; 294:739–745.
25. Donohue W. Leprechaunism: a euphemism for a rare familial disorder. J Pediatr 1954; 45:505–519.
26. Elders MJ, Schedewie HK, Olefsky J, et al. Endocrine-metabolic relationships in patients with leprechaunism. J Natl Med Assoc 1982; 74:1195–1210.
27. Rosenberg AM, Haworth JC, Degroot GW, et al. A case of leprechaunism with severe hyperinsulinemia. Am J Dis Child 1980; 134:170–175.
28. Rabson S, Mendenhall E. Familial hypertrophy of pineal body, hyperplasia of adrenal cortex and diabetes mellitus. Am J Clin Pathol 1956; 26:283–290.
29. Garg A. Lipodystrophies. Am J Med 2000; 108:143–152.
30. Vigouroux C, Magre J, Vantyghem MC, et al. Lamin A/C gene: sex-determined expression of mutations in Dunnigan-type familial partial lipodystrophy and absence of coding mutations in congenital and acquired generalized lipoatrophy. Diabetes 2000; 49: 1958–1962.
31. Magre J, Delepine M, Khallouf E, et al. Identification of the gene altered in Berardinelli-Seip congenital lipodystrophy on chromosome 11q13. Nat Genet 2001; 28:365–370.
32. Barroso I, Gurnell M, Crowley VE, et al. Dominant negative mutations in human PPARgamma associated with severe insulin resistance, diabetes mellitus and hypertension. Nature 1999; 402: 880–883.
33. Haneda M, Polonsky KS, Bergenstal RM, et al. Familial hyperinsulinemia due to a structurally abnormal insulin: definition of an emerging new clinical syndrome. N Engl J Med 1984; 310:1288–1294.
34. Gruppuso PA, Gorden P, Kahn CR, et al. Familial hyperproinsulinemia due to a proposed defect in conversion of proinsulin to insulin. N Engl J Med 1984; 311:629–634.
35. Shibasaki Y, Kawakami T, Kanazawa Y, et al. Posttranslational cleavage of proinsulin is blocked by a point mutation in familial hyperproinsulinemia. J Clin Invest 1985; 76:378–380.
36. O'Rahilly S, Gray H, Humphreys PJ, et al. Brief report: impaired processing of prohormones associated with abnormalities of glucose homeostasis and adrenal function. N Engl J Med 1995; 333: 1386–1390.
37. Ballinger SW, Shoffner JM, Hedaya EV, et al. Maternally transmitted diabetes and deafness associated with a 10.4 kb mitochondrial DNA deletion. Nat Genet 1992; 1:11–15.
38. Velho G, Byrne MM, Clement K, et al. Clinical phenotypes, insulin secretion, and insulin sensitivity in kindreds with maternally inherited diabetes and deafness due to mitochondrial tRNALeu(UUR) gene mutation. Diabetes 1996; 45:478–487.
39. Fajans SS, Bell GI, Polonsky KS. Molecular mechanisms and clinical pathophysiology of maturity-onset diabetes of the young. N Engl J Med 2001; 345:971–980.
40. Froguel P, Zouali H, Vionnet N, et al. Familial hyperglycemia due to mutations in glucokinase: definition of a subtype of diabetes mellitus. N Engl J Med 1993; 328:697–702.
41. Yamagata K, Furuta H, Oda N, et al. Mutations in the hepatocyte nuclear factor-4alpha gene in maturity-onset diabetes of the young (MODY1). Nature 1996; 384:458–460.
42. Yamagata K, Oda N, Kaisaki PJ, et al. Mutations in the hepatocyte nuclear factor-1alpha gene in maturity-onset diabetes of the young (MODY3). Nature 1996; 384:455–458.
43. Stoffers DA, Ferrer J, Clarke WL, Habener N. Early-onset type-II diabetes mellitus (MODY4) linked to IPF1. Nat Genet 1997; 17:138–139.
44. Horikawa Y, Iwasaki N, Hara N, et al. Mutation in hepatocyte nuclear factor-1 beta gene (TCF2) associated with MODY. Nat Genet 1997; 17:384–385.
45. Malecki MT, Jhala US, Antonellis A, et al. Mutations in *NEUROD1* are associated with the development of type 2 diabetes mellitus. Nat Genet 1999; 23:323–328.

46. Njolstad PR, Sovik O, Cuesta-Munoz A, et al. Neonatal diabetes mellitus due to complete glucokinase deficiency. N Engl J Med 2001; 344:1588–1592.
47. Cereghini S. Liver-enriched transcription factors and hepatocyte differentiation. FASEB J 1996; 10:267–282.
48. Duncan SA, Navas MA, Dufort D, et al. Regulation of a transcription factor network required for differentiation and metabolism. Science 1998; 281:692–695.
49. Stoffel M, Duncan SA. The maturity-onset diabetes of the young (MODY1) transcription factor HNF4alpha regulates expression of genes required for glucose transport and metabolism. Proc Natl Acad Sci USA 1997; 94:13209–13214.
50. Edlund H. Factors controlling pancreatic cell differentiation and function. Diabetologia 2001; 44:1071–1079.
51. Stoffers DA, Stanojevic V, Habener JF. Insulin promoter factor-1 gene mutation linked to early-onset type 2 diabetes mellitus directs expression of a dominant negative isoprotein. J Clin Invest 1998; 102:232–241.
52. Hani EH, Stoffers DA, Chevre JC, et al. Defective mutations in the insulin promoter factor-1 (IPF-1) gene in late-onset type 2 diabetes mellitus. J Clin Invest 1999; 104:R41–R48.
53. Kristinsson SY, Thorolfsdottir ET, Talseth B, et al. MODY in Iceland is associated with mutations in HNF-1alpha and a novel mutation in NeuroD1. Diabetologia 2001; 44:2098–2103.
54. Permutt MA, Hattersley AT. Searching for type 2 diabetes genes in the post-genome era. Trends Endocrinol Metab 2000; 11:383–393.
55. Horikawa Y, Oda N, Cox NJ, et al. Genetic variation in the gene encoding calpain-10 is associated with type 2 diabetes mellitus. Nat Genet 2000; 26:163–175.
56. Baier LJ, Permana PA, Yang X, et al. A calpain-10 gene polymorphism is associated with reduced muscle mRNA levels and insulin resistance. J Clin Invest 2000; 106:R69–R73.
57. Sreenan SK, Zhou YP, Otani K, et al. Calpains play a role in insulin secretion and action. Diabetes 2001; 50:2013–2020.
58. Cox NJ. Challenges in identifying genetic variation affecting susceptibility to type 2 diabetes: examples from studies of the calpain-10 gene. Hum Mol Genet 2001; 10:2301–2305.
59. Himsworth H, Kerr RB. Insulin-sensitive and insulin-insensitive types of diabetes mellitus. Clin Sci 1939; 4:119–152.
60. Warram JH, Martin BC, Krowelski AS, et al. Slow glucose removal rate and hyperinsulinemia precede the development of type II diabetes in the offspring of diabetic parents. Ann Intern Med 1990; 113:909–915.
61. Lillioija S, Mott DM, Howard BV, et al. Impaired glucose tolerance as a disorder of insulin action: longitudinal and cross-sectional studies in Pima Indians. N Engl J Med 1988; 318:1217–1225.
62. Haffner SM, Stern MP, Dunn J, et al. Diminished insulin sensitivity and increased insulin response in nonobese, nondiabetic Mexican Americans. Metabolism 1990; 39:842–847.
63. Reaven GM, Bernstein R, Davis B, Olefsky JM. Nonketotic diabetes mellitus: insulin deficiency or insulin resistance? Am J Med 1976; 60:80–88.
64. DeFronzo RA. Lilly lecture 1987. The triumvirate: beta-cell, muscle, liver. A collusion responsible for NIDDM. Diabetes 1988; 37:667–687.
65. Paolisso G, Tagliamonte MR, Rizzo MR, Giugliano D. Advancing age and insulin resistance: new facts about an ancient history. Eur J Clin Invest 1999; 29:758–769.
66. Groop L. Genetics of the metabolic syndrome. Br J Nutr 2000; 83(suppl 1):S39–S48.
67. Lehtovirta M, Kaprio J, Forsblom C, et al. Insulin sensitivity and insulin secretion in monozygotic and dizygotic twins. Diabetologia 2000; 43:285–293.
68. Mayer EJ, Newman B, Austin MA, et al. Genetic and environmental influences on insulin levels and the insulin resistance syndrome: an analysis of women twins. Am J Epidemiol 1996; 143: 323–332.
69. Hong Y, Pedersen NL, Brismar K, de Faire U. Genetic and environmental architecture of the features of the insulin-resistance syndrome. Am J Hum Genet 1997; 60:143–152.
70. Fujioka S, Matsuzawa Y, Tokunaga K, Tarui S. Contribution of intra-abdominal fat accumulation to the impairment of glucose and lipid metabolism in human obesity. Metabolism 1987; 36:54–59.
71. Brambilla P, Manzoni P, Sironi S, et al. Peripheral and abdominal adiposity in childhood obesity. Int J Obes Relat Metab Disord 1994; 18:795–800.
72. Berman DM, Rodriguez LM, Nicklas BJ, et al. Racial disparities in metabolism, central obesity, and sex hormone–binding globulin in postmenopausal women. J Clin Endocrinol Metab 2001; 86:97–103.
73. Hu FB, Manson JE, Stampfer MJ, et al. Diet, lifestyle, and the risk of type 2 diabetes mellitus in women. N Engl J Med 2001; 345:790–797.
74. Tuomilehto J, Lindstrom J, Eriksson G, et al. Prevention of type 2 diabetes mellitus by changes in lifestyle among subjects with impaired glucose tolerance. N Engl J Med 2001; 344:1343–1350.
75. Must A, Spadano J, Coakley EH, et al. The disease burden associated with overweight and obesity. JAMA 1999; 282:1523–1529.
76. Cefalu WT, Werbel S, Bell-Farrow AD, et al. Insulin resistance and fat patterning with aging: relationship to metabolic risk factors for cardiovascular disease. Metabolism 1998; 47:401–408.
77. Larsson B, Svardsudd K, Welin L, et al. Abdominal adipose tissue distribution, obesity, and risk of cardiovascular disease and death: 13 year follow up of participants in the study of men born in 1913. Br Med J (Clin Res Ed) 1984; 288:1401–1404.
78. Despres JP, Tremblay A, Perusse L, et al. Abdominal adipose tissue and serum HDL-cholesterol: association independent from obesity and serum triglyceride concentration. Int J Obes 1988; 12:1–13.
79. Landin K, Krotkiewski M, Smith U. Importance of obesity for the metabolic abnormalities associated with an abdominal fat distribution. Metabolism 1989; 38:572–576.
80. Heitmann BL. The variation in blood lipid levels described by various measures of overall and abdominal obesity in Danish men and women aged 35–65 years. Eur J Clin Nutr 1992; 46:597–605.
81. Reeder BA, Senthilselvan A, Despres JP, et al. The association of cardiovascular disease risk factors with abdominal obesity in Canada. Canadian Heart Health Surveys Research Group. Can Med Assoc J 1997; 157(suppl 1):S39–S45.
82. Lamarche B. Abdominal obesity and its metabolic complications: implications for the risk of ischaemic heart disease. Coron Artery Dis 1998; 9:473–481.
83. Evans DJ, Hoffmann RG, Kalkhoff RK, Kissebah AH. Relationship of body fat topography to insulin sensitivity and metabolic profiles in premenopausal women. Metabolism 1984; 33:68–75.
84. Peiris AN, Mueller RA, Smith GA, et al. Splanchnic insulin metabolism in obesity. Influence of body fat distribution. J Clin Invest 1986; 78:1648–1657.
85. Arner P, Hellstrom L, Wahrenberg H, Bronnegard M. Beta-adrenoceptor expression in human fat cells from different regions. J Clin Invest 1990; 86:1595–1600.
86. Nicklas BJ, Rogus EM, Colman EG, Goldberg AP. Visceral adiposity, increased adipocyte lipolysis, and metabolic dysfunction in obese postmenopausal women. Am J Physiol 1996; 270:E72–E78.
87. Mittelman SD, Van Citters GW, Kim SP, et al. Longitudinal compensation for fat-induced insulin resistance includes reduced insulin clearance and enhanced beta-cell response. Diabetes 2000; 49:2116–2125.
88. Del Prato S, Bonadonna RC, Bonora E, et al. Characterization of cellular defects of insulin action in type 2 (non–insulin-dependent) diabetes mellitus. J Clin Invest 1993; 91:484–494.
89. Freymond D, Bogardus C, Okubo M, et al. Impaired insulin-stimulated muscle glycogen synthase activation in vivo in man is related to low fasting glycogen synthase phosphatase activity. J Clin Invest 1988; 82:1503–1509.
90. Charles MA, Eschwege E, Thibult N, et al. The role of non-esterified fatty acids in the deterioration of glucose tolerance in Caucasian subjects: results of the Paris Prospective Study. Diabetologia 1997; 40:1101–1106.
91. Paolisso G, Tataranni PA, Foley JE, et al. A high concentration of fasting plasma non-esterified fatty acids is a risk factor for the development of NIDDM. Diabetologia 1995; 38:1213–1217.
92. Garland PB, Newsholme EA, Randle PJ. Regulation of glucose uptake by muscle. 9. Effects of fatty acids and ketone bodies, and of alloxan-diabetes and starvation, on pyruvate metabolism and on lactate-pyruvate and L-glycerol 3-phosphate-dihydroxyacetone phosphate concentration ratios in rat heart and rat diaphragm muscles. Biochem J 1964; 93:665–678.

93. Roden M, Price TB, Perseghin G, et al. Mechanism of free fatty acid-induced insulin resistance in humans. J Clin Invest 1996; 97: 2859–2865.
94. Jucker BM, Rennings AJ, Cline GW, Shulman GI. ^{13}C and ^{31}P NMR studies on the effects of increased plasma free fatty acids on intramuscular glucose metabolism in the awake rat. J Biol Chem 1997; 272:10464–10473.
95. Adams SH. Uncoupling protein homologs: emerging views of physiological function. J Nutr 2000; 130:711–714.
96. Rothman DL, Magnusson I, Cline G, et al. Decreased muscle glucose transport/phosphorylation is an early defect in the pathogenesis of non–insulin-dependent diabetes mellitus. Proc Natl Acad Sci USA 1995; 92:983–987.
97. Price TB, Parseghin G, Duleba A, et al. NMR studies of muscle glycogen synthesis in insulin-resistant offspring of parents with non–insulin-dependent diabetes mellitus immediately after glycogen-depleting exercise. Proc Natl Acad Sci USA 1996; 93:5329–5334.
98. Itani SI, Pories WJ, Macdonald KG, Dohm GL. Increased protein kinase C theta in skeletal muscle of diabetic patients. Metabolism 2001; 50:553–557.
99. Griffin ME, Marcucci MJ, Cline GW, et al. Free fatty acid-induced insulin resistance is associated with activation of protein kinase C theta and alterations in the insulin signaling cascade. Diabetes 1999; 48:1270–1274.
100. Pan DA, Lillioja S, Kriketos AD, et al. Skeletal muscle triglyceride levels are inversely related to insulin action. Diabetes 1997; 46:983–988.
101. Goodpaster BH, Thaete FL, Simoneau JA, Kelley DE. Subcutaneous abdominal fat and thigh muscle composition predict insulin sensitivity independently of visceral fat. Diabetes 1997; 46:1579–1585.
102. Perseghin G, Scifo P, De Cobelli F, et al. Intramyocellular triglyceride content is a determinant of in vivo insulin resistance in humans: a ^{1}H-^{13}C nuclear magnetic resonance spectroscopy assessment in offspring of type 2 diabetic parents. Diabetes 1999; 48:1600–1606.
103. Boesch C, Slotboom J, Hoppeler H, Kreis R. In vivo determination of intra-myocellular lipids in human muscle by means of localized ^{1}H-MR-spectroscopy. Magn Reson Med 1997; 37:484–493.
104. Carlson LA, Ekelund LG, Froberg SO. Concentration of triglycerides, phospholipids and glycogen in skeletal muscle and of free fatty acids and beta-hydroxybutyric acid in blood in man in response to exercise. Eur J Clin Invest 1971; 1:248–254.
105. Laws A, Reaven GM. Effect of physical activity on age-related glucose intolerance. Clin Geriatr Med 1990; 6:849–863.
106. Gollnick PD, Saltin B. Significance of skeletal muscle oxidative enzyme enhancement with endurance training. Clin Physiol 1982; 2:1–12.
107. Turcotte LP, Richter EA, Kiens B. Increased plasma FFA uptake and oxidation during prolonged exercise in trained vs. untrained humans. Am J Physiol 1992; 262:E791–E799.
108. Romijn JA, Klein S, Coyle EF, et al. Strenuous endurance training increases lipolysis and triglyceride-fatty acid cycling at rest. J Appl Physiol 1993; 75:108–113.
109. Phillips SM, Green HJ, Tamopolsky MA, et al. Effects of training duration on substrate turnover and oxidation during exercise. J Appl Physiol 1996; 81:2182–2191.
110. Stremmel W, Strohmeyer G, Borchard F, et al. Isolation and partial characterization of a fatty acid binding protein in rat liver plasma membranes. Proc Natl Acad Sci USA 1985; 82:4–8.
111. Abumrad NA, el-Maghrabi MR, Amri EZ, et al. Cloning of a rat adipocyte membrane protein implicated in binding or transport of long-chain fatty acids that is induced during preadipocyte differentiation: homology with human CD36. J Biol Chem 1993; 268:17665–17668.
112. Stahl A, Gimeno RE, Tartaglia LA, Lodish HF. Fatty acid transport proteins: a current view of a growing family. Trends Endocrinol Metab 2001; 12:266–273.
113. Luiken JJ, Glatz JF, Bonen A. Fatty acid transport proteins facilitate fatty acid uptake in skeletal muscle. Can J Appl Physiol 2000; 25:333–352.
114. Binnert C, Koistinen HA, Martin G, et al. Fatty acid transport protein-1 mRNA expression in skeletal muscle and in adipose tissue in humans. Am J Physiol 2000; 279:E1072–E1079.
115. Veerkamp JH. Fatty acid transport and fatty acid-binding proteins. Proc Nutr Soc 1995; 54:23–37.
116. Schaap FG, van der Vusse GJ, Glatz JF. Fatty acid-binding proteins in the heart. Mol Cell Biochem 1998; 180:43–51.
117. Van Nieuwenhoven FA, Verstijnen CP, Abumrad NA, et al. Putative membrane fatty acid translocase and cytoplasmic fatty acid-binding protein are co-expressed in rat heart and skeletal muscles. Biochem Biophys Res Commun 1995; 207:747–752.
118. Linssen MC, Vork MM, de Jong YF, et al. Fatty acid oxidation capacity and fatty acid-binding protein content of different cell types isolated from rat heart. Mol Cell Biochem 1990; 98:19-25.
119. Binas B, Danneberg H, McWhir J, et al. Requirement for the heart-type fatty acid binding protein in cardiac fatty acid utilization. FASEB J 1999; 13:805–812.
120. Hotamisligil GS, Johnson RS, Distel RJ, et al. Uncoupling of obesity from insulin resistance through a targeted mutation in aP2, the adipocyte fatty acid binding protein. Science 1996; 274: 1377–1379.
121. Blaak EE, Wagenmakers AJ, Glatz JF, et al. Plasma FFA utilization and fatty acid-binding protein content are diminished in type 2 diabetic muscle. Am J Physiol 2000; 279:E146–E154.
122. Simoneau JA, Veerkamp JH, Turcotte LP, Kelley DE. Markers of capacity to utilize fatty acids in human skeletal muscle: relation to insulin resistance and obesity and effects of weight loss. FASEB J 1999; 13:2051–2060.
123. McGarry JD. Glucose–fatty acid interactions in health and disease. Am J Clin Nutr 1998; 67(3 suppl):500S–504S.
124. McGarry JD. Malonyl-CoA and satiety? Food for thought. Trends Endocrinol Metab 2000; 11:399–400.
125. Zammit VA, Price NT, Fraser F, Jackson VN. Structure-function relationships of the liver and muscle isoforms of carnitine palmitoyltransferase I. Biochem Soc Trans 2001; 29:287–292.
126. Minnich A, Tian N, Byan L, Bilder G. A potent PPARalpha agonist stimulates mitochondrial fatty acid beta-oxidation in liver and skeletal muscle. Am J Physiol 2001; 280:E270–E279.
127. Power GW, Newsholme EA. Dietary fatty acids influence the activity and metabolic control of mitochondrial carnitine palmitoyltransferase I in rat heart and skeletal muscle. J Nutr 1997; 127:2142–2150.
128. Hildebrandt AL, Neufer PD. Exercise attenuates the fasting-induced transcriptional activation of metabolic genes in skeletal muscle. Am J Physiol 2000; 278:E1078–E1086.
129. Kim JY, Hickner RC, Cartright RL, et al. Lipid oxidation is reduced in obese human skeletal muscle. Am J Physiol 2000; 279: E1039–E1044.
130. Eaton S, Bartlett K, Pourfarzam M. Mammalian mitochondrial beta-oxidation. Biochem J 1996; 320:345–357.
131. Nada MA, Rhead WJ, Sprecher H, et al. Evidence for intermediate channeling in mitochondrial beta-oxidation. J Biol Chem 1995; 270:530–535.
132. Horowitz JF, Leone TC, Feng W, et al. Effect of endurance training on lipid metabolism in women: a potential role for PPARalpha in the metabolic response to training. Am J Physiol 2000; 279:E348–E355.
133. Porter RK. Mitochondrial proton leak: a role for uncoupling proteins 2 and 3? Biochim Biophys Acta 2001; 1504:120–127.
134. Bouillaud F, Couplan E, Pecqueur C, Rigquier D. Homologues of the uncoupling protein from brown adipose tissue (UCP1): UCP2, UCP3, BMCP1 and UCP4. Biochim Biophys Acta 2001; 1504:107–119.
135. Boss O, Muzzin P, Giacobino JP. The uncoupling proteins, a review. Eur J Endocrinol 1998; 139:1–9.
136. Schrauwen P, Hoppeler H, Billeter R, et al. Fiber type dependent upregulation of human skeletal muscle UCP2 and UCP3 mRNA expression by high-fat diet. Int J Obes Relat Metab Disord 2001; 25:449–456.
137. Tonkonogi M, Krook A, Walsh B, Sahlin K. Endurance training increases stimulation of uncoupling of skeletal muscle mitochondria in humans by non-esterified fatty acids: an uncoupling-protein-mediated effect? Biochem J 2000; 351:805–810.
138. Bao S, Kennedy A, Wojciechowski B, et al. Expression of mRNAs encoding uncoupling proteins in human skeletal muscle: effects of obesity and diabetes. Diabetes 1998; 47:1935–1940.
139. Schrauwen P, Xia J, Wakler K, et al., A novel polymorphism in the proximal UCP3 promoter region: effect on skeletal muscle UCP3 mRNA expression and obesity in male non-diabetic Pima Indians. Int J Obes Relat Metab Disord 1999; 23:1242–1245.

140. Ruderman NB, Saha AK, Vavvas D, Witters LA. Malonyl-CoA, fuel sensing, and insulin resistance. Am J Physiol 1999; 276:E1–E18.
141. McGarry JD. Malonyl-CoA and carnitine palmitoyltransferase I: an expanding partnership. Biochem Soc Trans 1995; 23:481–485.
142. Swanson ST, Foster DW, McGarry JD, Brown NF. Roles of the N- and C-terminal domains of carnitine palmitoyltransferase I isoforms in malonyl-CoA sensitivity of the enzymes: insights from expression of chimaeric proteins and mutation of conserved histidine residues. Biochem J 1998; 335:513–519.
143. Kelley DE, Simoneau JA. Impaired free fatty acid utilization by skeletal muscle in non–insulin-dependent diabetes mellitus. J Clin Invest 1994; 94:2349–2356.
144. Kelley DE, Mandarino LJ. Hyperglycemia normalizes insulin-stimulated skeletal muscle glucose oxidation and storage in non-insulin-dependent diabetes mellitus. J Clin Invest 1990; 86:1999–2007.
145. Bavenholm PN, Pigon J, Saha AK, et al. Fatty acid oxidation and the regulation of malonyl-CoA in human muscle. Diabetes 2000; 49:1078–1083.
146. Jamil H, Madsen NB. Phosphorylation state of acetyl-coenzyme A carboxylase. I. Linear inverse relationship to activity ratios at different citrate concentrations. J Biol Chem 1987; 262:630–637.
147. Jamil H, Madsen NB. Phosphorylation state of acetyl-coenzyme A carboxylase. II. Variation with nutritional condition. J Biol Chem 1987; 262:638–642.
148. Winder WW, Wilson HA, Hardie DG, et al. Phosphorylation of rat muscle acetyl-CoA carboxylase by AMP-activated protein kinase and protein kinase A. J Appl Physiol 1997; 82:219–225.
149. Dean D, Daugaard JR, Young ME, et al. Exercise diminishes the activity of acetyl-CoA carboxylase in human muscle. Diabetes 2000; 49:1295–1300.
150. Olefsky JM, Revers RR, Prince M, et al. Insulin resistance in non–insulin dependent (type II) and insulin dependent (type I) diabetes mellitus. Adv Exp Med Biol 1985; 189:176–205.
151. Del Prato S, Leonetti F, Simonson DC, et al. Effect of sustained physiologic hyperinsulinaemia and hyperglycaemia on insulin secretion and insulin sensitivity in man. Diabetologia 1994; 37: 1025–1035.
152. Ratzmann KP, Ruhnke R, Kohnert KD. Effect of pharmacological suppression of insulin secretion on tissue sensitivity to insulin in subjects with moderate obesity. Int J Obes 1983; 7:453–458.
153. Alemzadeh R, Langley G, Upchurch L, et al. Beneficial effect of diazoxide in obese hyperinsulinemic adults. J Clin Endocrinol Metab 1998; 83:1911–1915.
154. White MF, Kahn CR. The insulin signaling system. J Biol Chem 1994; 269:1–4.
155. Ward CW, Gough KH, Rashke M, et al. Systematic mapping of potential binding sites for Shc and Grb2 SH2 domains on insulin receptor substrate-1 and the receptors for insulin, epidermal growth factor, platelet-derived growth factor, and fibroblast growth factor. J Biol Chem 1996; 271:5603–5609.
156. Pessin JE, Saltiel AR. Signaling pathways in insulin action: molecular targets of insulin resistance. J Clin Invest 2000; 106:165–169.
157. McClain DA, Maegawa H, Thies RS, Olefsky JM. Dissection of the growth versus metabolic effects of insulin and insulin-like growth factor-I in transfected cells expressing kinase-defective human insulin receptors. J Biol Chem 1990; 265:1678–1682.
158. McClain DA. Mechanism and role of insulin receptor endocytosis. Am J Med Sci 1992; 304:192–201.
159. Formisano P, Beguinot F. The role of protein kinase C isoforms in insulin action. J Endocrinol Invest 2001; 24:460–467.
160. Itani SI, Zhou Q, Pories WJ, et al. Involvement of protein kinase C in human skeletal muscle insulin resistance and obesity. Diabetes 2000; 49:1353–1358.
161. Peraldi P, Xu M, Spiegelman BM. Thiazolidinediones block tumor necrosis factor-alpha–induced inhibition of insulin signaling. J Clin Invest 1997; 100:1863–1869.
162. Goldstein BJ, Ahmad F, Ding W, et al. Regulation of the insulin signalling pathway by cellular protein-tyrosine phosphatases. Mol Cell Biochem 1998; 182:91–99.
163. Drake PG, Bevan AP, Burgess JW, et al. A role for tyrosine phosphorylation in both activation and inhibition of the insulin receptor tyrosine kinase in vivo. Endocrinology 1996; 137:4960–4968.
164. Elchebly M, Payette P, Michaliszyn E, et al. Increased insulin sensitivity and obesity resistance in mice lacking the protein tyrosine phosphatase-1B gene. Science 1999; 283:1544–1548.
165. Krook A, O'Rahilly S. Mutant insulin receptors in syndromes of insulin resistance. Baillieres Clin Endocrinol Metab 1996; 10:97–122.
166. Taylor SI, Arioglu E. Syndromes associated with insulin resistance and acanthosis nigricans. J Basic Clin Physiol Pharmacol 1998; 9:419–439.
167. White MF. The IRS-signaling system: a network of docking proteins that mediate insulin and cytokine action. Recent Prog Horm Res 1998; 53:119–138.
168. Previs SF, Withers DJ, Ren JM, et al. Contrasting effects of IRS-1 versus IRS-2 gene disruption on carbohydrate and lipid metabolism in vivo. J Biol Chem 2000; 275:38990–38994.
169. Czech MP, Corvera S. Signaling mechanisms that regulate glucose transport. J Biol Chem 1999; 274:1865–1868.
170. Kido Y, Nakae J, Accili D. Clinical review 125: the insulin receptor and its cellular targets. J Clin Endocrinol Metab 2001; 86: 972-979.
171. Kohn AD, Barthel A, Kovacina KS, et al. Construction and characterization of a conditionally active version of the serine/threonine kinase Akt. J Biol Chem, 1998; 273:11937–11943.
172. Cho H, Mu J, Kim JK, et al. Insulin resistance and a diabetes mellitus-like syndrome in mice lacking the protein kinase Akt2 (PKB beta). Science 2001; 292:1728–1731.
173. Zierath JR, Krook A, Wallberg-Henriksson H. Insulin action in skeletal muscle from patients with NIDDM. Mol Cell Biochem 1998; 182:153–160.
174. Krook A, Roth RA, Jiang XJ, et al. Insulin-stimulated Akt kinase activity is reduced in skeletal muscle from NIDDM subjects. Diabetes 1998; 47:1281–1286.
175. Kim YB, Nikoulina SE, Ciaraldi TP, et al. Normal insulin-dependent activation of Akt/protein kinase B, with diminished activation of phosphoinositide 3-kinase, in muscle in type 2 diabetes. J Clin Invest 1999; 104:733–741.
176. Zorzano A, Sevilla L, Tomas E, et al. Trafficking pathway of GLUT4 glucose transporters in muscle. Int J Mol Med 1998; 2: 263–271.
177. Davidson MB. Role of glucose transport and GLUT4 transporter protein in type 2 diabetes mellitus. J Clin Endocrinol Metab 1993; 77:25–26.
178. Garvey WT, Maianu L, Zhu JH, et al. Multiple defects in the adipocyte glucose transport system cause cellular insulin resistance in gestational diabetes: heterogeneity in the number and a novel abnormality in subcellular localization of GLUT4 glucose transporters. Diabetes 1993; 42:1773–1785.
179. Kennedy JW, Hirshman MF, Gervino EV, et al. Acute exercise induces GLUT4 translocation in skeletal muscle of normal human subjects and subjects with type 2 diabetes. Diabetes 1999; 48:1192–1197.
180. Gumbiner B, Mucha JF, Lindstrom JE, et al. Differential effects of acute hypertriglyceridemia on insulin action and insulin receptor autophosphorylation. Am J Physiol 1996; 270:E424–E429.
181. Saad MJ, Araki E, Miralpeix M, et al. Regulation of insulin receptor substrate-1 in liver and muscle of animal models of insulin resistance. J Clin Invest 1992; 90:1839–1849.
182. Zierath JR, Houseknecht KL, Gnudi L, Kahn BB. High-fat feeding impairs insulin-stimulated GLUT4 recruitment via an early insulin-signaling defect. Diabetes 1997; 46:215–223.
183. Anai M, Funaki M, Ogihara T, et al. Altered expression levels and impaired steps in the pathway to phosphatidylinositol 3-kinase activation via insulin receptor substrates 1 and 2 in Zucker fatty rats. Diabetes 1998; 47:13–23.
184. Krook A, Kawano Y, Song XM, et al. Improved glucose tolerance restores insulin-stimulated Akt kinase activity and glucose transport in skeletal muscle from diabetic Goto-Kakizaki rats. Diabetes 1997; 46:2110–2114.
185. Hotamisligil GS, Spiegelman BM. Tumor necrosis factor alpha: a key component of the obesity-diabetes link. Diabetes 1994; 43: 1271–1278.
186. Miles PD, Romeo OM, Higo K, et al. TNF-alpha–induced insulin resistance in vivo and its prevention by troglitazone. Diabetes 1997; 46:1678–1683.
187. Hotamisligil GS, Peraldi P, Budavari A, et al. IRS-1–mediated inhibition of insulin receptor tyrosine kinase activity in TNF-

alpha– and obesity-induced insulin resistance. Science 1996; 271: 665–668.
188. Uysal KT, Wiesbrock SM, Marino MW, Hotamisligil GS. Protection from obesity-induced insulin resistance in mice lacking TNF-alpha function. Nature 1997; 389:610–614.
189. The effect of intensive treatment of diabetes on the development and progression of long-term complications in insulin-dependent diabetes mellitus. The Diabetes Control and Complications Trial Research Group. N Engl J Med 1993; 329:977–986.
190. Turner RC. The U.K. Prospective Diabetes Study. A review. Diabetes Care 1998; 21(suppl 3):C35–C38.
191. Sakul H, Pratley R, Cardon L, et al. Familiality of physical and metabolic characteristics that predict the development of non-insulin-dependent diabetes mellitus in Pima Indians. Am J Hum Genet 1997; 60:651–656.
192. Yki-Jarvinen H, Sahlin K, Ren JM, Koivisto VA. Localization of rate-limiting defect for glucose disposal in skeletal muscle of insulin-resistant type I diabetic patients. Diabetes 1990; 39:157–167.
193. Kornfeld R. Studies on L-glutamine D-fructose 6-phosphate amidotransferase. I. Feedback inhibition by uridine diphosphate-*N*-acetylglucosamine. J Biol Chem 1967; 242:3135–3141.
194. Marshall S, Bacote V, Traxinger RR. Discovery of a metabolic pathway mediating glucose-induced desensitization of the glucose transport system: role of hexosamine biosynthesis in the induction of insulin resistance. J Biol Chem 1991; 266:4706–4712.
195. Robinson KA, Weinstein ML, Lindenmayer GE, Buse MG. Effects of diabetes and hyperglycemia on the hexosamine synthesis pathway in rat muscle and liver. Diabetes 1995; 44:1438–1446.
196. Hebert LF Jr, Daniels MC, Zhou J, et al. Overexpression of glutamine: fructose-6-phosphate amidotransferase in transgenic mice leads to insulin resistance. J Clin Invest 1996; 98:930–936.
197. Baron AD, Zhu JS, Zhu JH, et al. Glucosamine induces insulin resistance in vivo by affecting GLUT 4 translocation in skeletal muscle: implications for glucose toxicity. J Clin Invest 1995; 96: 2792–2801.
198. Mallon PW, Cooper DA, Carr A. HIV-associated lipodystrophy. HIV Med 2001; 2:166–173.
199. Shevitz A, Wanke CA, Falutz J, Kotler DP. Clinical perspectives on HIV-associated lipodystrophy syndrome: an update. AIDS 2001; 15:1917–1930.
200. Purnell JQ, Zambon A, Knopp RH, et al. Effect of ritonavir on lipids and post-heparin lipase activities in normal subjects. AIDS 2000; 14:51–57.
201. Noor MA, Lo JC, Mulligan K, et al. Metabolic effects of indinavir in healthy HIV-seronegative men. AIDS 2001; 15:F11–F18.
202. Murata H, Hruz PW, Mueckler M. The mechanism of insulin resistance caused by HIV protease inhibitor therapy. J Biol Chem 2000; 275:20251–20254.
203. Shikuma CM, Hu N, Milne C, et al. Mitochondrial DNA decrease in subcutaneous adipose tissue of HIV-infected individuals with peripheral lipoatrophy. AIDS 2001; 15:1801–1809.
204. Caron M, Auclair M, Vigouroux C, et al. The HIV protease inhibitor indinavir impairs sterol regulatory element–binding protein-1 intranuclear localization, inhibits preadipocyte differentiation, and induces insulin resistance. Diabetes 2001; 50:1378–1388.
205. Dowell P, Flexner C, Kwiterovich PO, Lane MD. Suppression of preadipocyte differentiation and promotion of adipocyte death by HIV protease inhibitors. J Biol Chem 2000; 275:41325–41332.
206. Carr A, Samaras K, Chisholm DJ, Cooper DA. Pathogenesis of HIV-1-protease inhibitor–associated peripheral lipodystrophy, hyperlipidaemia, and insulin resistance. Lancet 1998; 351:1881–1883.
207. Knowler WC, Barrett-Connor E, Fowler SE, et al. Reduction in the incidence of type 2 diabetes with lifestyle intervention or metformin. N Engl J Med 2002; 346:393–403.
208. Kelley DE, Mandarino LJ. Fuel selection in human skeletal muscle in insulin resistance: a reexamination. Diabetes 2000; 49:677–683.
209. Long SD, O'Brien K, MacDonald KG Jr, et al. Weight loss in severely obese subjects prevents the progression of impaired glucose tolerance to type II diabetes: a longitudinal interventional study. Diabetes Care 1994; 17:372–375.
210. Wing RR, Venditti E, Jakicic JM, et al. Lifestyle intervention in overweight individuals with a family history of diabetes. Diabetes Care 1998; 21:350–359.
211. Nesher R, Karl IE, Kipnis DM. Dissociation of effects of insulin and contraction on glucose transport in rat epitrochlearis muscle. Am J Physiol 1985; 249:C226–C232.
212. Wallberg-Henriksson H, Holloszy JO. Activation of glucose transport in diabetic muscle: responses to contraction and insulin. Am J Physiol 1985; 249:C233–C237.
213. Wallberg-Henriksson H, Constable SH, Young DA, Holloszy JO. Glucose transport into rat skeletal muscle: interaction between exercise and insulin. J Appl Physiol 1988; 65:909–913.
214. Young DA, Wallberg-Henriksson H, Sleeper MD, Holloszy JO. Reversal of the exercise-induced increase in muscle permeability to glucose. Am J Physiol 1987; 253:E331–E335.
215. Douen AG, Ramlal T, Rastogi S, et al. Exercise induces recruitment of the "insulin-responsive glucose transporter." Evidence for distinct intracellular insulin- and exercise-recruitable transporter pools in skeletal muscle. J Biol Chem 1990; 265:13427–13430.
216. Goodyear LJ, Hirshman MF, King PA, et al. Skeletal muscle plasma membrane glucose transport and glucose transporters after exercise. J Appl Physiol 1990; 68:193–198.
217. Goodyear LJ, Giorgino F, Balon TW, et al. Effects of contractile activity on tyrosine phosphoproteins and PI 3-kinase activity in rat skeletal muscle. Am J Physiol 1995; 268:E987–E995.
218. Lund S, Holman GD, Schmitz O, Pedersen O. Contraction stimulates translocation of glucose transporter GLUT4 in skeletal muscle through a mechanism distinct from that of insulin. Proc Natl Acad Sci USA 1995; 92:5817–5821.
219. Zorzano A, Balon TW, Goodman MN, Ruderman NB. Additive effects of prior exercise and insulin on glucose and AIB uptake by rat muscle. Am J Physiol 1986; 251:E21–E26.
220. Henriksen EJ, Bourey RE, Rodnick KJ, et al. Glucose transporter protein content and glucose transport capacity in rat skeletal muscles. Am J Physiol 1990; 259:E593–E598.
221. Gao J, Ren J, Gulve EA, Holloszy JO. Additive effect of contractions and insulin on GLUT-4 translocation into the sarcolemma. J Appl Physiol 1994; 77:1597–1601.
222. Lee AD, Hansen PA, Holloszy JO. Wortmannin inhibits insulin-stimulated but not contraction-stimulated glucose transport activity in skeletal muscle. FEBS Lett 1995; 361:51–54.
223. Yeh JI, Gulve EA, Rameh L, Birnbaum MJ. The effects of wortmannin on rat skeletal muscle: dissociation of signaling pathways for insulin- and contraction-activated hexose transport. J Biol Chem 1995; 270:2107–2111.
224. Treadway JL, James DE, Burcel E, Ruderman B. Effect of exercise on insulin receptor binding and kinase activity in skeletal muscle. Am J Physiol 1989; 256:E138–E144.
225. Brozinick JT Jr, Etgen GJ Jr, Yaspelkis BB 3rd, Ivy JL. Contraction-activated glucose uptake is normal in insulin-resistant muscle of the obese Zucker rat. J Appl Physiol 1992; 73:382–387.
226. Azevedo JL Jr, Carey JO, Pories WJ, et al. Hypoxia stimulates glucose transport in insulin-resistant human skeletal muscle. Diabetes 1995; 44:695–698.
227. Winder WW, Hardie DG. AMP-activated protein kinase, a metabolic master switch: possible roles in type 2 diabetes. Am J Physiol 1999; 277:E1–E10.
228. Hayashi T, Hirshman MF, Kurth EJ, et al. Evidence for 5′ AMP-activated protein kinase mediation of the effect of muscle contraction on glucose transport. Diabetes 1998; 47:1369–1373.
229. Merrill GF, Kurth EJ, Hardie DG, Winder WW. AICA riboside increases AMP-activated protein kinase, fatty acid oxidation, and glucose uptake in rat muscle. Am J Physiol 1997; 273:E1107–E1112.
230. Bergeron R, Russell RR 3rd, Young LH, et al. Effect of AMPK activation on muscle glucose metabolism in conscious rats. Am J Physiol 1999; 276:E938–E944.
231. Richter EA, Garetto LP, Goodman MN, Ruderman NB. Muscle glucose metabolism following exercise in the rat: increased sensitivity to insulin. J Clin Invest 1982; 69:785–793.
232. Garetto LP, Richter EA, Goodman MN, Ruderman NB. Enhanced muscle glucose metabolism after exercise in the rat: the two phases. Am J Physiol 1984; 246:E471–E475.
233. Cartee GD, Young DA, Sleeper MD, et al. Prolonged increase in insulin-stimulated glucose transport in muscle after exercise. Am J Physiol 1989; 256:E494–E499.
234. Richter EA, Young DA, Sleeper MD, et al. Effect of exercise on insulin action in human skeletal muscle. J Appl Physiol 1989; 66: 876–885.

235. Hansen PA, Nolte LA, Chen MM, Holloszy JO. Increased GLUT-4 translocation mediates enhanced insulin sensitivity of muscle glucose transport after exercise. J Appl Physiol 1998; 85: 1218–1222.
236. Thorell A, Hirshman MF, Nygren J, et al. Exercise and insulin cause GLUT-4 translocation in human skeletal muscle. Am J Physiol 1999; 277:E733–E741.
237. Zorzano A, Balon TW, Garetto LP, et al. Muscle alpha-aminoisobutyric acid transport after exercise: enhanced stimulation by insulin. Am J Physiol 1985; 248:E546–E552.
238. Wojtaszewski JF, Hansen BF, Kiens B, Richter EA. Insulin signaling in human skeletal muscle: time course and effect of exercise. Diabetes 1997; 46:1775–1781.
239. Oshida Y, Yamanouchi K, Hayamizu S, Sato Y. Long-term mild jogging increases insulin action despite no influence on body mass index or VO_2 max. J Appl Physiol 1989; 66:2206–2210.
240. DeFronzo RA, Sherwin RS, Kraemer N. Effect of physical training on insulin action in obesity. Diabetes 1987; 36:1379–1385.
241. Helmrich SP, Rayland DR, Leung RW, Paffenbarger RS Jr. Physical activity and reduced occurrence of non–insulin-dependent diabetes mellitus. N Engl J Med 1991; 325:147–152.
242. Perseghin G, Price TB, Petersen KF, et al. Increased glucose transport-phosphorylation and muscle glycogen synthesis after exercise training in insulin-resistant subjects. N Engl J Med 1996; 335:1357–1362.
243. Ebeling P, Bourey R, Koranyi L, et al. Mechanism of enhanced insulin sensitivity in athletes. Increased blood flow, muscle glucose transport protein (GLUT-4) concentration, and glycogen synthase activity. J Clin Invest 1993; 92:1623–1631.
244. Houmard JA, Egan PC, Neufer PD, et al. Elevated skeletal muscle glucose transporter levels in exercise-trained middle-aged men. Am J Physiol 1991; 261:E437–E443.
245. Stamler J, Vaccaro O, Neaton JD, Wentworth D. Diabetes, other risk factors, and 12-yr cardiovascular mortality for men screened in the Multiple Risk Factor Intervention Trial. Diabetes Care 1993; 16:434–444.
246. Haffner SM, Lehto S, Ronnemaa T, et al. Mortality from coronary heart disease in subjects with type 2 diabetes and in nondiabetic subjects with and without prior myocardial infarction. N Engl J Med 1998; 339:229–234.
247. Fontbonne AM, Eschwege EM. Insulin and cardiovascular disease. Paris Prospective Study. Diabetes Care 1991; 14:461–469.
248. Willeit J, Kiechl S, Egger G, et al. The role of insulin in age-related sex differences of cardiovascular risk profile and morbidity. Atherosclerosis 1997; 130:183–189.
249. Hu FB, Stampfer MJ, Soloman CG, et al. The impact of diabetes mellitus on mortality from all causes and coronary heart disease in women: 20 years of follow-up. Arch Intern Med 2001; 161: 1717–1723.
250. Reaven GM. Banting Lecture 1988. Role of insulin resistance in human disease. Nutrition 1997; 13:65; discussion 64, 66.
251. Reaven GM. Role of insulin resistance in human disease (syndrome X): an expanded definition. Annu Rev Med 1993; 44:121–131.
252. Siegel RD, Cupples A, Schaefer EJ, Wilson PW. Lipoproteins, apolipoproteins, and low-density lipoprotein size among diabetics in the Framingham offspring study. Metabolism 1996; 45:1267–1272.
253. Davidson NO, Shelness GS. Apolipoprotein B: mRNA editing, lipoprotein assembly, and presecretory degradation. Annu Rev Nutr 2000; 20:169–193.
254. Lewis GF, Steiner G. Acute effects of insulin in the control of VLDL production in humans: implications for the insulin-resistant state. Diabetes Care 1996; 19:390–393.
255. Riches FM, Watts GF, Naoumova RP, et al. Hepatic secretion of very-low-density lipoprotein apolipoprotein B-100 studied with a stable isotope technique in men with visceral obesity. Int J Obes Relat Metab Disord 1998; 22:414–423.
256. Wang SL, Du EZ, Martin TD, Davis RA. Coordinate regulation of lipogenesis, the assembly and secretion of apolipoprotein B–containing lipoproteins by sterol response element binding protein 1. J Biol Chem 1997; 272:19351–19358.
257. Moberly JB, Cole TG, Alpers DH, Schonfeld G. Oleic acid stimulation of apolipoprotein B secretion from HepG2 and Caco-2 cells occurs post-transcriptionally. Biochim Biophys Acta 1990; 1042:70–80.
258. Ellsworth JL, Erickson SK, Cooper AD. Very low and low density lipoprotein synthesis and secretion by the human hepatoma cell line Hep-G2: effects of free fatty acid. J Lipid Res 1986; 27: 858–874.
259. Kobatake T, Matsuzawa Y, Tokunaga K, et al. Metabolic improvements associated with a reduction of abdominal visceral fat caused by a new alpha-glucosidase inhibitor, AO-128, in Zucker fatty rats. Int J Obes 1989; 13:147–154.
260. Matsuzawa Y, Shimomura I, Nakamura T, et al. Pathophysiology and pathogenesis of visceral fat obesity. Diabetes Res Clin Pract 1994; 24(suppl):S111–S116.
261. Nguyen TT, Mijares AH, Johnson CM, Jensen MD. Postprandial leg and splanchnic fatty acid metabolism in nonobese men and women. Am J Physiol 1996; 271:E965–E972.
262. Gordon DA, Jamil H, Sharp D, et al. Secretion of apolipoprotein B–containing lipoproteins from HeLa cells is dependent on expression of the microsomal triglyceride transfer protein and is regulated by lipid availability. Proc Natl Acad Sci USA 1994; 91: 7628–7632.
263. Gordon DA, Jamil H. Progress towards understanding the role of microsomal triglyceride transfer protein in apolipoprotein-B lipoprotein assembly. Biochim Biophys Acta 2000; 1486:72–83.
264. Liao W, Kobayashi K, Chan L. Adenovirus-mediated overexpression of microsomal triglyceride transfer protein (MTP): mechanistic studies on the role of MTP in apolipoprotein B-100 biogenesis. Biochemistry 1999; 38:7532–7544.
265. Horowitz BS, Goldberg IJ, Merab J, et al. Increased plasma and renal clearance of an exchangeable pool of apolipoprotein A-I in subjects with low levels of high density lipoprotein cholesterol. J Clin Invest 1993; 91:1743–1752.
266. Lemieux I, Couillard C, Pascot A, et al. The small, dense LDL phenotype as a correlate of postprandial lipemia in men. Atherosclerosis 2000; 153:423–432.
267. Tan KC, Cooper MB, Ling KL, et al. Fasting and postprandial determinants for the occurrence of small dense LDL species in non–insulin-dependent diabetic patients with and without hypertriglyceridaemia: the involvement of insulin, insulin precursor species and insulin resistance. Atherosclerosis 1995; 113:273–287.
268. Austin MA, Selby JV. LDL subclass phenotypes and the risk factors of the insulin resistance syndrome. Int J Obes Relat Metab Disord 1995; 19(suppl 1):S22–S26.
269. Stewart MW, Laker MF, Dyer RG, et al. Lipoprotein compositional abnormalities and insulin resistance in type II diabetic patients with mild hyperlipidemia. Arterioscler Thromb 1993; 13: 1046–1052.
270. Alexander JK. Obesity and coronary heart disease. Am J Med Sci 2001; 321:215–224.
271. Laakso M, Edelman SV, Brechtel G, Baron AD. Impaired insulin-mediated skeletal muscle blood flow in patients with NIDDM. Diabetes 1992; 41:1076–1083.
272. Steinberg HO, Brechtel G, Johnson A, et al. Insulin-mediated skeletal muscle vasodilation is nitric oxide dependent. A novel action of insulin to increase nitric oxide release. J Clin Invest 1994; 94:1172–1179.
273. Baron AD, Zhu JS, Marshall S, et al. Insulin resistance after hypertension induced by the nitric oxide synthesis inhibitor L-NMMA in rats. Am J Physiol 1995; 269:E709–E715.
274. Steinberg HO, Paradisi G, Hook G, et al. Free fatty acid elevation impairs insulin-mediated vasodilation and nitric oxide production. Diabetes 2000; 49:1231–1238.
275. Landsberg L. Insulin resistance, energy balance and sympathetic nervous system activity. Clin Exp Hypertens A 1990; 12:817–830.
276. Weidmann P, de Courten M, Bohlen L. Insulin resistance, hyperinsulinemia and hypertension. J Hypertens Suppl 1993; 11(suppl 5):S27–S38.
277. Masuo K, Mikami H, Itoh M, et al. Sympathetic activity and body mass index contribute to blood pressure levels. Hypertens Res 2000; 23:303–310.
278. DeFronzo RA. Insulin and renal sodium handling: clinical implications. Int J Obes 1981; 5(suppl 1):93–104.
279. DeFronzo RA, Goldberg M, Agus ZS. The effects of glucose and insulin on renal electrolyte transport. J Clin Invest 1976; 58:83–90.
280. DeFronzo RA, Cooke CR, Andres R, et al. The effect of insulin on renal handling of sodium, potassium, calcium, and phosphate in man. J Clin Invest 1975; 55:845–855.

281. Welborn TA, Breckenridge A, Rubinstein AH, et al. Serum-insulin in essential hypertension and in peripheral vascular disease. Lancet 1966; 1:1336–1337.
282. Gress TW, Nieto FJ, Shahar E, et al. Hypertension and antihypertensive therapy as risk factors for type 2 diabetes mellitus. Atherosclerosis Risk in Communities Study. N Engl J Med 2000; 342:905–912.
283. Yusuf S, Sleight P, Pogue J, et al. Effects of an angiotensin-converting-enzyme inhibitor, ramipril, on cardiovascular events in high-risk patients. The Heart Outcomes Prevention Evaluation Study Investigators. N Engl J Med 2000; 342:145–153.
284. Sebestjen M, Zegura B, Guzic-Salobir B, Keber I. Fibrinolytic parameters and insulin resistance in young survivors of myocardial infarction with heterozygous familial hypercholesterolemia. Wien Klin Wochenschr 2001; 113:113–118.
285. Juhan-Vague I, Alessi MC, Morange PE. Hypofibrinolysis and increased PAI-1 are linked to atherothrombosis via insulin resistance and obesity. Ann Med 2000; 32(suppl 1):78–84.
286. Fujii S, Goto D, Zaman T, et al. Diminished fibrinolysis and thrombosis: clinical implications for accelerated atherosclerosis. J Atheroscler Thromb 1998; 5:76–81.
287. Sobel BE. The potential influence of insulin and plasminogen activator inhibitor type 1 on the formation of vulnerable atherosclerotic plaques associated with type 2 diabetes. Proc Assoc Am Physicians 1999; 111:313–318.
288. Festa A, D'Agostino R Jr, Mykkanan L, et al. Relative contribution of insulin and its precursors to fibrinogen and PAI-1 in a large population with different states of glucose tolerance. The Insulin Resistance Atherosclerosis Study (IRAS). Arterioscler Thromb Vasc Biol 1999; 19:562–568.
289. Lormeau B, Aurousseau MH, Valensi P, et al. Hyperinsulinemia and hypofibrinolysis: effects of short-term optimized glycemic control with continuous insulin infusion in type II diabetic patients. Metabolism 1997; 46:1074–1079.
290. Hamsten A, Eriksson P, Karpe F, Silveira A. Relationships of thrombosis and fibrinolysis to atherosclerosis. Curr Opin Lipidol 1994; 5:382–389.
291. Grenett HE, Benza RL, Li XN, et al. Expression of plasminogen activator inhibitor type I in genotyped human endothelial cell cultures: genotype-specific regulation by insulin. Thromb Haemost 1999; 82:1504–1509.
292. Chomiki N, Henry M, Alessi MC, et al. Plasminogen activator inhibitor-1 expression in human liver and healthy or atherosclerotic vessel walls. Thromb Haemost 1994; 72:44–53.
293. Koistinen HA, Dusserre E, Ebeling P, et al. Subcutaneous adipose tissue expression of plasminogen activator inhibitor-1 (PAI-1) in nondiabetic and type 2 diabetic subjects. Diabetes Metab Res Rev 2000; 16:364–369.
294. Kruszynska YT, Yu JG, Olefsky JM, Sobel BE. Effects of troglitazone on blood concentrations of plasminogen activator inhibitor 1 in patients with type 2 diabetes and in lean and obese normal subjects. Diabetes 2000; 49:633–639.
295. Stunkard AJ. Current views on obesity. Am J Med 1996; 100: 230–236.
295a. Expert Panel on Detection, Evaluation and Treatment of High Blood Cholesterol in Adults. Executive Summary of the Third Report of the National Cholesterol Education Program (NCEP) Expert Panel on Detection, Evaluation and Treatment of High Blood Cholesterol in Adults (Adult Treatment Panel III). JAMA 285:2486–2497.
296. Gerich JE, Meyer C, Woerle HJ, Stumvoll M. Renal gluconeogenesis: its importance in human glucose homeostasis. Diabetes Care 2001; 24:382–391.
297. Meyer C, Stumvoll M, Nadkami V, et al. Abnormal renal and hepatic glucose metabolism in type 2 diabetes mellitus. J Clin Invest 1998; 102:619–624.
298. Rebrin K, Steil GM, Mittelman SD, Bergman RN. Causal linkage between insulin suppression of lipolysis and suppression of liver glucose output in dogs. J Clin Invest 1996; 98:741–749.
299. Mittelman SD, Fu YY, Rebrin K, et al. Indirect effect of insulin to suppress endogenous glucose production is dominant, even with hyperglucagonemia. J Clin Invest 1997; 100:3121–3130.
300. Rothman DL, Magnusson I, Katz LD, et al. Quantitation of hepatic glycogenolysis and gluconeogenesis in fasting humans with ^{13}C NMR. Science 1991; 254:573–576.
301. Petersen KF, Price T, Cline GW, et al. Contribution of net hepatic glycogenolysis to glucose production during the early postprandial period. Am J Physiol 1996; 270:E186–E191.
302. Nonogaki K. New insights into sympathetic regulation of glucose and fat metabolism. Diabetologia 2000; 43:533–549.
303. Moore MC, Connolly CC, Cherrington AD. Autoregulation of hepatic glucose production. Eur J Endocrinol 1998; 138:240–248.
304. Bavenholm PN, Pigon J, Ostenson CG, Efendic S. Insulin sensitivity of suppression of endogenous glucose production is the single most important determinant of glucose tolerance. Diabetes 2001; 50:1449–1454.
305. Mitrakou A, Kelley D, Mokan M, et al. Role of reduced suppression of glucose production and diminished early insulin release in impaired glucose tolerance. N Engl J Med 1992; 326:22–29.
306. McCall RH, Wiesenthal SR, Shi ZQ, et al. Insulin acutely suppresses glucose production by both peripheral and hepatic effects in normal dogs. Am J Physiol 1998; 274:E346–E356.
307. Lewis GF, Vranic M, Giacca A. Glucagon enhances the direct suppressive effect of insulin on hepatic glucose production in humans. Am J Physiol 1997; 272:E371–E378.
308. Herzig S, Long F, Jhala US, et al. CREB regulates hepatic gluconeogenesis through the coactivator PGC-1. Nature 2001; 413:179–183.
309. Yoon JC, Puigserver P, Chen G, et al. Control of hepatic gluconeogenesis through the transcriptional coactivator PGC-1. Nature 2001; 413:131–138.
310. Cherrington AD, Edgerton D, Sindelar DK. The direct and indirect effects of insulin on hepatic glucose production in vivo. Diabetologia 1998; 41:987–996.
311. Chiasson JL, Liljenquist JE, Finger FE, Lacy WW. Differential sensitivity of glycogenolysis and gluconeogenesis to insulin infusions in dogs. Diabetes 1976; 25:283–291.
312. Rossetti L, Giaccari A, Barzilai N, et al. Mechanism by which hyperglycemia inhibits hepatic glucose production in conscious rats: implications for the pathophysiology of fasting hyperglycemia in diabetes. J Clin Invest 1993; 92:1126–1134.
313. Gasa R, Jansen PB, Berman HK, et al. Distinctive regulatory and metabolic properties of glycogen-targeting subunits of protein phosphatase-1 (PTG, GL, GM/RGl) expressed in hepatocytes. J Biol Chem 2000; 275:26396–26403.
314. Newgard CB, Brady MJ, O'Doherty RM, Saltiel AR. Organizing glucose disposal: emerging roles of the glycogen targeting subunits of protein phosphatase-1. Diabetes 2000; 49:1967–1977.
315. Yeagley D, Guo S, Unterman T, Quinn PG. Gene- and activation-specific mechanisms for insulin inhibition of basal and glucocorticoid-induced insulin-like growth factor binding protein-1 and phosphoenolpyruvate carboxykinase transcription: roles of forkhead and insulin response sequences. J Biol Chem 2001; 276: 33705–33710.
316. Jackson JG, Kreisberg JI, Koterba AP, et al. Phosphorylation and nuclear exclusion of the forkhead transcription factor FKHR after epidermal growth factor treatment in human breast cancer cells. Oncogene 2000; 19:4574–4581.
317. Hall RK, Yamasaki T, Kucera T, et al. Regulation of phosphoenolpyruvate carboxykinase and insulin-like growth factor-binding protein-1 gene expression by insulin: the role of winged helix/forkhead proteins. J Biol Chem 2000; 275:30169–30175.
318. Asplin CM, Paquette TL, Palmer JP. In vivo inhibition of glucagon secretion by paracrine beta cell activity in man. J Clin Invest 1981; 68:314–318.
319. Shi ZQ, Wasserman D, Vranic M. Metabolic implications of exercise and physical fitness in physiology and diabetes. In Porte D, Sherwin R (eds). Ellenberg and Rifkin Diabetes Mellitus. Norwalk, Conn, Appleton & Lange, 1997, pp 653–687.
320. Chen X, Iqbal N, Boden G. The effects of free fatty acids on gluconeogenesis and glycogenolysis in normal subjects. J Clin Invest 1999; 103:365–372.
321. Boden G. Fatty acids and insulin resistance. Diabetes Care 1996; 19:394–395.
322. Lewis GF, Vranic M, Giacca A. Role of free fatty acids and glucagon in the peripheral effect of insulin on glucose production in humans. Am J Physiol 1998; 275:E177–E186.
323. Perriello G, Pampanelli S, Del Sindaco P, et al. Evidence of increased systemic glucose production and gluconeogenesis in an early stage of NIDDM. Diabetes 1997; 46:1010–1016.
324. DeFronzo RA, Bonadonna RC, Ferrannini E. Pathogenesis of NIDDM: a balanced overview. Diabetes Care 1992; 15:318–368.

325. DeFronzo RA, Simonson D, Ferrannini E. Hepatic and peripheral insulin resistance: a common feature of type 2 (non–insulin-dependent) and type 1 (insulin-dependent) diabetes mellitus. Diabetologia 1982; 23:313–319.
326. Bogardus C, Lillioja S, Howard BV, et al. Relationships between insulin secretion, insulin action, and fasting plasma glucose concentration in nondiabetic and noninsulin-dependent diabetic subjects. J Clin Invest 1984; 74:1238–1246.
327. Hother-Nielsen O, Beck-Nielsen H. Insulin resistance, but normal basal rates of glucose production in patients with newly diagnosed mild diabetes mellitus. Acta Endocrinol (Copenh) 1991; 124:637–645.
328. DeFronzo RA. Lilly lecture 1987. The triumvirate: beta-cell, muscle, liver. A collusion responsible for NIDDM. Diabetes 1988; 37:667–687.
329. Hother-Nielsen O, Beck-Nielsen H. On the determination of basal glucose production rate in patients with type 2 (non–insulin-dependent) diabetes mellitus using primed-continuous 3-^{3}H-glucose infusion. Diabetologia 1990; 33:603–610.
330. Firth R, Bell P, Rizza R. Insulin action in non–insulin-dependent diabetes mellitus: the relationship between hepatic and extrahepatic insulin resistance and obesity. Metabolism 1987; 36:1091–1095.
331. Groop LC, Bonadonna RC, Shank M, et al. Role of free fatty acids and insulin in determining free fatty acid and lipid oxidation in man. J Clin Invest 1991; 87:83–89.
332. Pigon J, Giacca A, Ostenson CG, et al. Normal hepatic insulin sensitivity in lean, mild noninsulin-dependent diabetic patients. J Clin Endocrinol Metab 1996; 81:3702–3708.
333. Stumvoll M, Nurjhan N, Perriello G, et al. Metabolic effects of metformin in non-insulin-dependent diabetes mellitus. N Engl J Med 1995; 333:550–554.
334. Lewis GF, Carpentier A, Vranic N, Giacca A. Resistance to insulin's acute direct hepatic effect in suppressing steady-state glucose production in individuals with type 2 diabetes. Diabetes 1999; 48:570–576.
335. Staehr P, Hother-Nielsen O, Levin K, et al. Assessment of hepatic insulin action in obese type 2 diabetic patients. Diabetes 2001; 50:1363–1370.
336. Magnusson I, Rothman DL, Gerard DP, et al. Contribution of hepatic glycogenolysis to glucose production in humans in response to a physiological increase in plasma glucagon concentration. Diabetes 1995; 44:185–189.
337. Magnusson I, Rothman DL, Katz LD, et al. Increased rate of gluconeogenesis in type II diabetes mellitus: a ^{13}C nuclear magnetic resonance study. J Clin Invest 1992; 90:1323–1327.
338. Baron AD, Schaeffer L, Shragg P, Kolterman OG. Role of hyperglucagonemia in maintenance of increased rates of hepatic glucose output in type II diabetics. Diabetes 1987; 36:274–283.
339. Yalow R, Berson S. Immunoassay of endogenous plasma insulin in man. J Clin Invest 1960; 39:1157–1175.
340. Polonsky K, Jaspan J, Emmanouel D, et al. Differences in the hepatic and renal extraction of insulin and glucagon in the dog: evidence for saturability of insulin metabolism. Acta Endocrinol (Copenh) 1983; 102:420–427.
341. Polonsky K, Jaspan J, Pugh W, et al. Metabolism of C-peptide in the dog: in vivo demonstration of the absence of hepatic extraction. J Clin Invest 1983; 72:1114–1123.
342. Steiner DF, James DE. Cellular and molecular biology of the beta cell. Diabetologia 1992; 35(suppl 2):S41–S48.
343. Melani F, Ryan WG, Rubenstein AH, Steirer DF. Proinsulin secretion by a pancreatic beta-cell adenoma. Proinsulin and C-peptide secretion. N Engl J Med 1970; 283:713–719.
344. Horwitz D, Starr JI, Mako ME, et al. Proinsulin, insulin, and C-peptide concentrations in human portal and peripheral blood. J Clin Invest 1975; 55:1278–1283.
345. Melani F, Rubenstein A, Steiner D. Human serum proinsulin. J Clin Invest 1970; 49:497–507.
346. Bergenstal R, Cohen RM, Lever E, et al. The metabolic effects of biosynthetic human proinsulin in individuals with Type I diabetes. J Clin Endocrinol Metab 1984; 58:973–979.
347. Revers R, Henry R, Schmeiser L, et al. The effects of biosynthetic human proinsulin on carbohydrate metabolism. Diabetes 1984; 33:762–770.
348. Peavy D, Brunner MR, Duckworth W, et al. Receptor binding and biological potency of several split forms (conversion intermediates) of human proinsulin: studies in cultured IM-9 lymphocytes and in vivo and in vitro in rats. J Biol Chem 1985; 260:13989–13994.
349. Gruppuso P, Frank B, Schwartz R. Binding of proinsulin and proinsulin conversion intermediates to human placental insulin-like growth factor 1 receptors. J Clin Endocrinol Metab 1988; 67:197.
350. Polonsky K, Rubenstein A. C-peptide as a measure of the secretion and hepatic extraction of insulin: pitfalls and limitations. Diabetes 1984; 33:486–494.
351. Wojcikowski C, Blackman J, Ostrega D, et al. Lack of effect of high-dose biosynthetic human C-peptide on pancreatic hormone release in normal subjects. Metabolism 1990; 39:827–832.
352. Wahren J, Ekberg K, Johansson J, et al. Role of C-peptide in human physiology. Am J Physiol 2000; 278:E759–E768.
353. Polonsky K, Pugh W, Jaspan JB, et al. C-peptide and insulin secretion: relationship between peripheral concentrations of C-peptide and insulin and their secretion rates in the dog. J Clin Invest 1984; 74:1821–1829.
354. Bratusch-Marrain P, Waldhausl WK, Gasic S, Hofer A. Hepatic disposal of biosynthetic human insulin and porcine C-peptide in humans. Metabolism 1984; 33:151–157.
355. Faber O, Hagen C, Binder C, et al. Kinetics of human connecting peptide in normal and diabetic subjects. J Clin Invest 1978; 62:197–203.
356. Polonsky K, Licinio-Paixas J, Given BD, et al. Use of biosynthetic human C-peptide in the measurement of insulin secretion rates in normal volunteers and type I diabetic patients. J Clin Invest 1986; 77:98–105.
357. Shapiro E, Tillil H, Rubenstein H, Polonsky KS. Peripheral insulin parallels changes in insulin secretion more closely than C-peptide after bolus intravenous glucose administration. J Clin Endocrinol Metab 1988; 67:1094–1099.
358. Eaton R, Allen RC, Schade DS, et al. Prehepatic insulin production in man: kinetic analysis using peripheral connecting peptide behavior. J Clin Endocrinol Metab 1980; 51:520–528.
359. Welch S, Gebhart SS, Bergman RN, Phillips LS. Minimal model analysis of intravenous glucose tolerance test-derived insulin sensitivity in diabetic subjects. J Clin Endocrinol Metab 1990; 71:1508–1518.
360. Breda E, Cavaghan MK, Toffolo G, et al. Oral glucose tolerance test minimal model indexes of beta-cell function and insulin sensitivity. Diabetes 2001; 50:150–158.
361. Bergman R, Phillips L, Cobelli C. Physiologic evaluation of factors controlling glucose tolerance in man: measurement of insulin sensitivity and beta-cell glucose sensitivity from the response to intravenous glucose. J Clin Invest 1981; 68:1456–1467.
362. Caumo A, Bergman R, Cobelli C. Insulin sensitivity from meal tolerance tests in normal subjects: a minimal model index. J Clin Endocrinol Metab 2000; 85:4396–4402.
363. Davis EA, Cuesta-Munoz A, Raoul M, et al. Mutants of glucokinase cause hypoglycaemia and hyperglycaemia syndromes and their analysis illuminates fundamental quantitative concepts of glucose homeostasis. Diabetologia 1999; 42:1175–1186.
364. Matschinsky FM, Glaser B, Magnuson MA. Pancreatic beta-cell glucokinase: closing the gap between theoretical concepts and experimental realities. Diabetes 1998; 47:307–315.
365. Dukes ID, McIntyre MS, Mertz RJ, et al. Dependence on NADH produced during glycolysis for beta-cell glucose signaling. J Biol Chem 1994; 269:10979–10982.
366. Maechler P, Wollheim CB. Mitochondrial function in normal and diabetic beta-cells. Nature 2001; 414:807–812.
367. Aguilar-Bryan L, Bryan J, Nakazaki M. Of mice and men: K(ATP) channels and insulin secretion. Recent Prog Horm Res 2001; 56:47–68.
368. Porte DJ, Pupo A. Insulin responses to glucose: evidence for a two-pooled system in man. J Clin Invest 1969; 48:2309–2319.
369. Chen M, Porte DJ. The effect of rate and dose of glucose infusion on the acute insulin response in man. J Clin Endocrinol Metab 1976; 42:1168–1175.
370. Ward W, Beard JC, Halter JB, et al. Pathophysiology of insulin secretion in non-insulin-dependent diabetes mellitus. Diabetes Care 1984; 7:491–502.
371. Waldhäus W, Bratusch-Marrain P, Gasic S, et al. Insulin production rate following glucose ingestion estimated by splanchnic C-peptide output in normal man. Diabetologia 1979; 17:221–227.

372. Eaton R, Allen R, Schade D. Hepatic removal of insulin in normal man: dose response to endogenous insulin secretion. J Clin Endocrinol Metab 1983; 56:1294–1300.
373. Nauck M, Homberger E, Siegel EG, et al. Incretin effects of increasing glucose loads in man calculated from venous insulin and C-peptide responses. J Clin Endocrinol Metab 1986; 63:492–498.
374. Tillil H, Shapiro ET, Miller MA, et al. Dose-dependent effects of oral and intravenous glucose on insulin secretion and clearance in normal humans. Am J Physiol 1988; 254:E349–E357.
375. Faber O, Madsbad S, Kehlet H, Binder C. Pancreatic beta cell secretion during oral and intravenous glucose administration. Acta Med Scand Suppl 1979; 624:61–64.
376. Madsbad S, Kehlet H, Hilsted J, Tronier B. Discrepancy between plasma C-peptide and insulin response to oral and intravenous glucose. Diabetes 1983; 32:436–438.
377. Shapiro E, Tillil H, Miller MA, et al. Insulin secretion and clearance: comparison after oral and intravenous glucose. Diabetes 1987; 93:1120–1130.
378. Creutzfeldt W, Ebert R. New developments in the incretin concept. Diabetologia 1985; 28:565–576.
379. Pagliara A, Stillings SN, Hover B, et al. Glucose modulation of amino acid-induced glucagon and insulin release in the isolated perfused rat pancreas. J Clin Invest 1974; 54:819–832.
380. Gerich J, Charles M, Grodsky G. Characterization of the effects of arginine and glucose on glucagon and insulin release from the perfused rat pancreas. J Clin Invest 1974; 54:833–847.
381. Grodsky G. The kinetics of insulin release. In Hasselblatt A, Bruchhausen F. Handbook of Experimental Pharmacology, vol 32. Berlin, Springer-Verlag, 1975, pp 1–19.
382. Salomon D, Meda P. Heterogeneity and contact-dependent regulation of hormone secretion by individual β cells. Exp Cell Res 1986; 162:507–520.
383. Schmitz O, Porksen N, Nyholm B, et al. Disorderly and nonstationary insulin secretion in relatives of patients with NIDDM. Am J Physiol 1997; 272:E218–E226.
384. Cerasi E, Luft R. The plasma insulin response to glucose infusion in healthy subjects and in diabetes mellitus. Acta Endocrinol (Copenh) 1967; 55:278–304.
385. Bennett L, Grodsky G. Multiphasic aspects of insulin release after glucose and glucagon. Diabetes. Proceedings of the Sixth Congress of the International Diabetes Federation. Amsterdam, Excerpta Medica, 1967.
386. Grodsky G. A threshold distribution hypothesis for packet storage of insulin and its mathematical modeling. J Clin Invest 1972; 51:2047–2059.
387. Smith C, Tam AC, Thomas JM, et al. Between and within subject variation of the first phase insulin response to intravenous glucose. Diabetologia 1988; 31:123–125.
388. Bardet S, Pasqual C, Maugendre D, et al. Inter and intra individual variability of acute insulin response during intravenous glucose tolerance tests. Diabetes Metab 1989; 15:224–232.
389. Rayman G, Clark P, Schneider AE, Hales CN. The first phase insulin response to intravenous glucose is highly reproducible. Diabetologia 1990; 33:631–634.
390. Bolaffi J, Haldt A, Lewis LD, Grodsky GM. The third phase of in vitro insulin secretion: evidence for glucose insensitivity. Diabetes 1986; 35:370–373.
391. Curry D. Insulin content and insulinogenesis by the perfused rat pancreas: effects of long term glucose stimulation. Endocrinology 1986; 118:170–175.
392. Hoenig M, MacGregor L, Matschinsky F. In vitro exhaustion of pancreatic β-cells. Am J Physiol 1986; 250:E502–E511.
393. Grodsky G. A new phase of insulin secretion: how will it contribute to our understanding of β-cell function? Diabetes 1989; 38: 673–678.
394. Cerasi E. Potentiation of insulin release by glucose in man. Acta Endocrinol (Copenh) 1975; 79:511–534.
395. Grill V. Time and dose dependencies for priming effect of glucose on insulin secretion. Am J Physiol 1981; 240:E24–E31.
396. Poitout V, Robertson RP. Minireview: secondary beta-cell failure in type 2 diabetes—a convergence of glucotoxicity and lipotoxicity. Endocrinology 2002; 143:339–342.
397. Leahy JL. Natural history of beta-cell dysfunction in NIDDM. Diabetes Care 1990; 13:992–1010.
398. Levin S, Karam JH, Hane S, et al. Enhancement of arginine-induced insulin secretion in man by prior administration of glucose. Diabetes 1971; 20:171–176.
399. Fajans S, Floyd J. Stimulation of islet cell secretion by nutrients and by gastrointestinal hormones released during digestion. In Steiner D, Freinkel N (eds). Handbook of Physiology. Section 7. Endocrinology. Washington, DC, American Physiological Society, 1972, pp 473–493.
400. Ward W, Bolgiano DC, McKnight B, et al. Diminished β-cell secretory capacity in patients with non–insulin dependent diabetes mellitus. J Clin Invest 1984; 74:1318–1328.
401. Kadowaki T, Miyake Y, Hagura R, et al. Risk factors for worsening to diabetes in subjects with impaired glucose tolerance. Diabetologia 1984; 26:44–49.
402. Muller W, Faloona G, Unger R. The influence of the antecedent diet upon glucagon and insulin secretion. N Engl J Med 1971; 285:1450–1454.
403. Goberna R, Tamarit J Jr, Osorio J, et al. Action of β-hydroxybutyrate, acetoacetate and palmitate on the insulin release from the perfused isolated rat pancreas. Horm Metab Res 1974; 6:256–260.
404. Crespin S, Greenough D, Steinberg D. Stimulation of insulin secretion by long-chain free fatty acids. J Clin Invest 1973; 52: 1979–1984.
405. Crespin S, Greenough W, Steinberg D. Stimulation of insulin secretion by infusion of fatty acids. J Clin Invest 1969; 48:1934–1943.
406. Paolisso G, Gambardella M, Amato L, et al. Opposite effects of short- and long-term fatty acid infusion on insulin secretion in healthy subjects. Diabetologia 1995; 38:1295–1299.
407. Boden G, Chen X. Effects of fatty acids and ketone bodies on basal insulin secretion in type 2 diabetes. Diabetes 1999; 48:577–583.
408. Zhou Y-P, Grill V. Long term exposure of rat pancreatic islets to fatty acids inhibits glucose-induced insulin secretion and biosynthesis through a glucose fatty acid cycle. J Clin Invest 1994; 93: 870–876.
409. Mason T, Goh T, Tchipashvili V, et al. Prolonged elevation of plasma free fatty acids desensitizes the insulin secretory response to glucose in vivo in rats. Diabetes 1999; 48:524–530.
410. Carpentier A, Mittelman SD, Lamarche B, et al. Acute enhancement of insulin secretion by FFA in humans is lost with prolonged FFA elevation. Am J Physiol 1999; 276:E1055–E1066.
411. Dupre J, Ross SA Watson D, Brown JC. Stimulation of insulin secretion by gastric inhibitory polypeptide in man. J Clin Endocrinol Metab 1973; 37:826–828.
412. Andersen D, Elahi D, Brown JC, et al. Oral glucose augmentation of insulin secretion: interactions of gastric inhibitory polypeptide with ambient glucose and insulin levels. J Clin Invest 1978; 62:152–161.
413. Schmidt W, Siegel E, Creutzfeldt W. Glucagon-like peptide-2 stimulates insulin release from isolated rate pancreatic islets. Diabetologia 1985; 28:704–707.
414. Kreymann B, Williams G, Ghatei MA, Bloom SR. Glucagon-like peptide-1 7–36: a physiological incretin in man. Lancet 1987; 2: 1300–1304.
415. Zawalich W, Diaz V. Prior cholecystokinin exposure sensitizes islets of Langerhans to glucose stimulation. Diabetes 1987; 36: 118–227.
416. Zawalich W. Synergistic impact of cholecystokinin and gastric inhibitory polypeptide on the regulation of insulin secretion. Metabolism 1988; 37:778–781.
417. Weir G, Mojsovs S, Hendrick GK, Habener JF. Glucagon-like peptide 1(7–37) actions on endocrine pancreas. Diabetes 1989; 38:338–342.
418. Rasmussen H, Zawalich KC, Ganesan S, et al. Physiology and pathophysiology of insulin secretion. Diabetes Care 1990; 13: 655–666.
419. Fukase N, Manaka H, Sugiyama K, et al. Response of truncated glucagon-like peptide-1 and gastric inhibitory polypeptide to glucose ingestion in non–insulin dependent diabetes mellitus. Effect of sulfonylurea therapy. Acta Diabetol 1995; 32:165–169.
420. Groop P. The influence of body weight, age and glucose tolerance on the relationship between GIP secretion and beta-cell function in man. Scand J Clin Lab Invest 1989; 49:367–379.
421. Creutzfeldt W, Ebert R, Nauck M, Stockmann F. Disturbances of the entero-insulin axis. Scand J Gastroenterol 1983; 83(suppl): 111–119.

422. Nauck M, Heimesaat MM, Orskov C, et al. Preserved incretin activity of glucagon-like peptide 1 (7–36 amide) but not of synthetic human gastric inhibitory polypeptide in patients with type 2 diabetes mellitus. J Clin Invest 1993; 91:301–307.
423. Ahrén B, Larsson H, Holst J. Reduced gastric inhibitory polypeptide but normal glucagon-like peptide 1 response to oral glucose in postmenopausal women with impaired glucose tolerance. Eur J Endocrinol 1997; 137:127–131.
424. Rushakoff R, Goldfine ID, Beccaria LJ, et al. Reduced postprandial cholecystokinin (CCK) secretion in patients with noninsulin-dependent diabetes mellitus: evidence for a role for CCK in regulating postprandial hyperglycemia. J Clin Endocrinol Metab 1993; 76:489–493.
425. Meguro T, Shimosegawa T, Satoh A, et al. Gallbladder emptying and cholecystokinin and pancreatic polypeptide responses to a liquid meal in patients with diabetes mellitus. J Gastroenterol 1997; 32:628–634.
426. Hasegawa H, Shirohara H, Okabayashi Y, et al. Oral glucose ingestion stimulates cholecystokinin release in normal subjects and patients with non-insulin-dependent diabetes mellitus. Metabolism 1996; 45:196–202.
427. Nauck M, Wollschlager D, Werner J, et al. Effects of subcutaneous glucagon-like peptide 1 (GLP-1 (7-36 amide)) in patients with NIDDM. Diabetologia 1996; 39:1546–1553.
428. Creutzfeldt W, Kleine N, Willms B, et al. Glucagonostatic actions and reduction of fasting hyperglycemia by exogenous glucagon-like peptide I(7-36) amide in type I diabetic patients. Diabetes Care 1996; 19:580–586.
429. Young A, Gedulin BR, Bhavsar S, et al. Glucose-lowering and insulin-sensitizing actions of exendin-4: studies in obese diabetic (*ob/ob*, *db/db*) mice, diabetic fatty Zucker rats, and diabetic rhesus monkeys (*Macaca mulatta*). Diabetes 1999; 48:1026–1034.
430. Nauck M, Bartels E, Orskov C, et al. Additive insulinotropic effects of exogenous synthetic human gastric inhibitory polypeptide and glucagon-like peptide-1-(7-36) amide infused at near-physiological insulinotropic hormone and glucose concentrations. J Clin Endocrinol Metab, 1993; 76:912–917.
431. Elahi D, McAloon-Dyke M, Fukagawa NK, et al. The insulinotropic actions of glucose-dependent insulinotropic polypeptide (GIP) and glucagon-like peptide-1 (7-37) in normal and diabetic subjects. Regul Pept 1994; 51:63–74.
432. Niederau C, Schwarzendrube J, Luthen R, et al. Effects of cholecystokinin receptor blockade in circulating concentrations of glucose, insulin, C-peptide, and pancreatic polypeptide after various meals in healthy human volunteers. Pancreas 1992; 7:1–10.
433. Fieseler P, Bridenbaugh S, Nustede R, et al. Physiological augmentation of amino acid–induced insulin secretion by GIP and GLP-I but not by CCK-8. Am J Physiol 1995; 268:E949–E955.
434. Reimers J, Nauck M, Creutzfeldt W, et al. Lack of insulinotropic effect of endogenous and exogenous cholecystokinin in man. Diabetologia 1988; 31:271–280.
435. Rushakoff R, Goldfine ID, Carter JD, Liddle RA. Physiological concentrations of cholecystokinin stimulate amino acid-induced insulin release in humans. J Clin Endocrinol Metab 1987; 65: 395–401.
436. Ahrén B, Holst J, Efendic S. Antidiabetogenic action of cholecystokinin-8 in type 2 diabetes. J Clin Endocrinol Metab 2000; 85: 1043–1048.
437. Schebalin M, Said S, Makhlouf G. Stimulation of insulin and glucagon secretion by vasoactive intestinal peptide. Am J Physiol 1977; 232:E197–E200.
438. Dupre J, Curtis JD, Unger RH, et al. Effects of secretin, pancreozymin, or gastrin on the response of the endocrine pancreas to administration of glucose or arginine in man. J Clin Invest 1969; 48:745–757.
439. Halter J, Porte DJ. Mechanisms of impaired acute insulin release in adult onset diabetes: studies with isoproterenol and secretin. J Clin Endocrinol Metab 1978; 46:952–960.
440. Glaser B, Shapiro B, Glowniak J, et al. Effects of secretin on the normal and pathological beta-cell. J Clin Endocrinol Metab 1988; 66:1138–1143.
441. Bertrand G, Puech R, Maisonnasse Y, et al. Comparative effects of PACAP and VIP on pancreatic endocrine secretions and vascular resistance in rat. Br J Pharmacol 1996; 117:764–770.
442. Rehfeld J, Stadil F. The effect of gastrin on basal- and glucose-stimulated insulin secretion in man. J Clin Invest 1973; 52:1415–1426.
443. Samols E, Marri G, Marks V. Promotion of insulin secretion by glucagon. Lancet 1965; 2:15–16.
444. Alberti K, Christensen NJ, Christensen SE, et al. Inhibition of insulin secretion by somatostatin. Lancet 1973; 2:1299–1301.
445. Aguilar-Parada E, Eisentraut A, Unger R. Effects of starvation on plasma pancreatic glucagon in normal man. Diabetes 1969; 18: 717–723.
446. Marliss E, Aoki TT, Unger RH, et al. Glucagon levels and metabolic effects in fasting man. J Clin Invest 1970; 49:2256–2270.
447. Malaisse W, Malaisse L, Wright P. Effect of fasting upon insulin secretion in the rat. Am J Physiol 1967; 213:843–848.
448. Zawalich W, Dye ES, Pagliara AS, et al. Starvation diabetes in the rat: onset, recovery and specificity of reduced responsiveness of pancreatic β-cells. Endocrinology 1979; 104:1344–1351.
449. Felig P, Marliss E, Cahill JG. Metabolic response to human growth hormone during prolonged starvation. J Clin Invest 1971; 50:411–421.
450. Kalhan S, Adam P. Inhibitory effect of prednisone on insulin secretion in man: model for duplication of blood glucose concentration. J Clin Endocrinol Metab 1975; 41:600–610.
451. Landgraf R, Landgraf-Luers MM, Weissmann A, et al. Prolactin: a diabetogenic hormone. Diabetologia 1977; 13:99–104.
452. Gustafson A, Banasiak MF, Kalkhoff RK, et al. Correlation of hyperprolactinemia with altered plasma insulin and glucagon: similarity to effects of late human pregnancy. J Clin Endocrinol Metab 1980; 51:242–246.
453. Brelje T, Sorenson R. Nutrient and hormonal regulation of the threshold of glucose-stimulated insulin secretion in isolated rat pancreases. Endocrinology 1988; 123:1582–1590.
454. Beck P, Daughaday W. Human placental lactogen: studies of its acute metabolic effects and disposition in normal man. J Clin Invest 1967; 46:103–110.
455. Ensinck J, Williams R. Hormonal and nonhormonal factors modifying man's response to insulin. In Steiner D, Freinkel N (eds). Handbook of Physiology. Section 7. Endocrinology. Washington, DC, American Physiological Society, 1972, pp 665–669.
456. Martin J, Friesen H. Effect of human placental lactogen on the isolated islets of Langerhans in vitro. Endocrinology 1969; 84: 619–621.
457. Curry D, Bennett L. Dynamics of insulin release by perfused rat pancreases: effects of hypophysectomy, growth hormone, adrenocorticotropic hormone and hydrocortisone. Endocrinology 1973; 93:602–609.
458. Malaisse W, Malaisse-Lagae F, King S, Wright PH. Effect of growth hormone on insulin secretion. Am J Physiol 1968; 215: 423–428.
459. Randin J, Scazziga B, Jequier E, Felber JP. Study of glucose and lipid metabolism by continuous indirect calorimetry in Graves' disease: effect of an oral glucose load. J Clin Endocrinol Metab 1985; 61:1165–1171.
460. Foss M, Paccola GM, Saad MJ, et al. Peripheral glucose metabolism in human hyperthyroidism. J Clin Endocrinol Metab 1990; 70:1167–1172.
461. Sestoft L, Heding L. Hypersecretion of proinsulin in thyrotoxicosis. Diabetologia 1981; 21:103–107.
462. Nishi S, Seino Y, Ishida H, et al. Vagal regulation of insulin, glucagon, and somatostatin secretion in vitro in the rat. J Clin Invest 1987; 79:1191–1196.
463. Kurose T, Seino Y, Nishi S, et al. Mechanism of sympathetic neural regulation of insulin, somatostatin, and glucagon secretion. Am J Physiol 1990; 251:E220–E227.
464. Woods S, Porte DJ. Neural control of the endocrine pancreas. Physiol Rev 1974; 54:596–619.
465. Bloom SR, Edwards A. Certain pharmacological characteristics of the release of pancreatic glucagon in response to stimulation of the splanchnic nerves. J Physiol (Lond) 1978; 280:25–35.
466. Porte D Jr, Girardier L, Seydoux J, et al. Neural regulation of insulin secretion in the dog. J Clin Invest 1973; 52:210–214.
467. Roy M, Lee KC, Jones MS, Miller RE. Neural control of pancreatic insulin and somatostatin secretion. Endocrinology 1984; 115:770–775.
468. Skoglund G, Lundquist I, Ahren B. Selective alpha 2-adrenoceptor activation by clonidine: effects on $^{45}Ca^{2+}$ efflux and insulin secretion from isolated rat islets. Acta Physiol Scand 1988; 132: 289–296.

469. Ahrén B. Autonomic regulation of islet hormone secretion: implications for health and disease. Diabetologia 2000; 43:393–410.
470. Pettersson M, Ahrén B. Calcitonin gene-related peptide inhibits insulin secretion: studies on ion fluxes and cyclic AMP in isolated rat islets. Diabetes Res Clin Pract 1990; 15:9–14.
471. Pettersson M, Ahrén B, Bottcher G, Sundler F. Calcitonin gene-related peptide: occurrence in pancreatic islets in the mouse and the rat and inhibition of insulin secretion in the mouse. Diabetologia 1986; 119:865–869.
472. Ahrén B, Mårtensson H, Nobin A. Effects of calcitonin gene-related peptide (CGRP) on islet hormone secretion in the pig. Diabetologia 1987; 30:354–359.
473. Lundquist I, Sundler F, Ahrén B, et al. Somatostatin, pancreatic polypeptide, substance P, and neurotensin: cellular distribution and effects on stimulated insulin secretion in the mouse. Endocrinology 1979; 104:832–838.
474. Hermansen K. Effects of substance P and other peptides on the release of somatostatin, insulin and glucagon in vitro. Endocrinology 1980; 107:256–261.
475. Larrimer J, Mazzaferri EL, Cataland S, Mekhjian HS. Effect of atropine on glucose-stimulated gastric inhibitory polypeptide. Diabetes 1978; 27:638–642.
476. Rocca A, Brubaker P. Role of the vagus nerve in mediating proximal nutrient-induced glucagon-like peptide-1 secretion. Endocrinology 1999; 140:1687–1694.
477. Flaten O, Sand T, Myren J. Beta-adrenergic stimulation and blockade of the release of gastric inhibitory polypeptide and insulin in man. Scand J Gastroenterol 1982; 17:283–288.
478. Claustre J, Brechet S, Plaisancie P, et al. Stimulatory effect of beta-adrenergic agonists on ileal L cell secretion and modulation by alpha-adrenergic activation. J Endocrinol 1999; 162:271–278.
479. Kruszynska Y, Home PD, Hanning I, Alberti KG. Basal and 24-h C-peptide and insulin secretion rate in normal man. Diabetologia 1987; 30:16–21.
480. Polonsky KS, Given BD, Van Cauter E. Twenty-four-hour profiles and pulsatile patterns of insulin secretion in normal and obese subjects. J Clin Invest 1988; 81:442–448.
481. Polonsky KS. Lilly Lecture 1994. The beta-cell in diabetes: from molecular genetics to clinical research. Diabetes 1995; 44:705–717.
482. Lang DA, Matthews DR, Peto J, Turner RC. Cyclic oscillations of basal plasma glucose and insulin concentrations in human beings. N Engl J Med 1979; 301:1023–1027.
483. Hansen BC, Jen KC, Belbez Pek S, Wolfe RA. Rapid oscillations in plasma insulin, glucagon, and glucose in obese and normal weight humans. J Clin Endocrinol Metab 1982; 54:785–792.
484. Matthews DR, Lang DA, Burnett MA, Turner RC. Control of pulsatile insulin secretion in man. Diabetologia 1983; 24:231–237.
485. O'Meara NM, Sturis J, Van Cauter E, Polonsky KS. Lack of control by glucose of ultradian insulin secretory oscillations in impaired glucose tolerance and in non-insulin-dependent diabetes mellitus. J Clin Invest 1993; 92:262–271.
486. Porksen N, Grafte B, Nyholm B, et al. Glucagon-like peptide 1 increases mass but not frequency or orderliness of pulsatile insulin secretion. Diabetes 1998; 47:45–49.
487. Porksen N, Nyholm B, Veldhuis JD, et al. In humans at least 75% of insulin secretion arises from punctuated insulin secretory bursts. Am J Physiol 1997; 273:E908–E914.
488. Porksen N, Hussain MA, Bianda TL, et al. IGF-I inhibits burst mass of pulsatile insulin secretion at supraphysiological and low IGF-I infusion rates. Am J Physiol 1997; 272:E352–E358.
489. Porksen NK, Munn SR, Steers JL, et al. Mechanisms of sulfonylurea's stimulation of insulin secretion in vivo: selective amplification of insulin secretory burst mass. Diabetes 1996; 45:1792–1797.
490. Porksen N, Munn S, Steers J, et al. Effects of glucose ingestion versus infusion on pulsatile insulin secretion. The incretin effect is achieved by amplification of insulin secretory burst mass. Diabetes 1996; 45:1317–1323.
491. O'Rahilly S, Turner RC, Matthews DR. Impaired pulsatile secretion of insulin in relatives of patients with non-insulin-dependent diabetes. N Engl J Med 1988; 318:1225–1230.
492. Van Cauter E. Estimating false-positive and false-negative errors in analyses of hormonal pulsatility. Am J Physiol 1988; 254: E786–E794.
493. Pincus SM. Quantification of evolution from order to randomness in practical time series analysis. Methods Enzymol 1994; 240:68–89.
494. Jaspan JB, Lever E, Polonsky KS, Van Cauter E. In vivo pulsatility of pancreatic islet peptides. Am J Physiol 1986; 251:E215–E226.
495. Matthews DR, Naylor BA, Jones RG, et al. Pulsatile insulin has greater hypoglycemic effect than continuous delivery. Diabetes 1983; 32:617–621.
496. Bratusch-Marrain PR, Komjati M, Waldhausl WK. Efficacy of pulsatile versus continuous insulin administration on hepatic glucose production and glucose utilization in type I diabetic humans. Diabetes 1986; 35:922–926.
497. Ward GM, Walters JM, Aitken PM, et al. Effects of prolonged pulsatile hyperinsulinemia in humans. Enhancement of insulin sensitivity. Diabetes 1990; 39:501–507.
498. Sonnenberg GE, Hoffmann RG, Johnson CP, Kissebah AH. Low- and high-frequency insulin secretion pulses in normal subjects and pancreas transplant recipients: role of extrinsic innervation. J Clin Invest 1992; 90:545–553.
499. Blackman JD, Polonsky KS, Jaspan JB, et al. Insulin secretory profiles and C-peptide clearance kinetics at 6 months and 2 years after kidney-pancreas transplantation. Diabetes 1992; 41:1346–1354.
500. Sturis J, Polonsky KS, Mosekilde E, Van Cauter E. Computer model for mechanisms underlying ultradian oscillations of insulin and glucose. Am J Physiol 1991; 260:E801–E809.
501. Sturis J, Van Cauter E, Blackman JD, Polonsky KS. Entrainment of pulsatile insulin secretion by oscillatory glucose infusion. J Clin Invest 1991; 87:439–445.
502. Malherbe C, De Gasparo M, De Hertogh R, Hoet JJ. Circadian variations of blood sugar and plasma insulin levels in man. Diabetologia 1969; 5:397–404.
503. Polonsky K, Given B, Van Cauter E. Twenty-four-hour profiles and pulsatile patterns of insulin secretion in normal and obese subjects. J Clin Invest 1988; 81:442–448.
504. Jarrett RJ, Baker IA, Keen H, Oakley NW. Diurnal variation in oral glucose tolerance: blood sugar and plasma insulin levels morning, afternoon, and evening. Br Med J 1972; 1:199–201.
505. Carroll KF, Nestel PJ. Diurnal variation in glucose tolerance and in insulin secretion in man. Diabetes 1973; 22:333–348.
506. Aparicio NJ, Puchulu FE, Gagliardino JJ, et al. Circadian variation of the blood glucose, plasma insulin and human growth hormone levels in response to an oral glucose load in normal subjects. Diabetes 1974; 23:132–137.
507. Van Cauter E, Desir D, Decoster C, et al. Nocturnal decrease in glucose tolerance during constant glucose infusion. J Clin Endocrinol Metab 1989; 69:604–611.
508. Pick A, Clark J, Kubstrup P, et al. Role of apoptosis in failure of beta-cell mass compensation for insulin resistance and beta-cell defects in the male Zucker diabetic fatty rat. Diabetes 1998; 47: 358–364.
509. Cockburn BN, Ostrega DM, Sturis J, et al. Changes in pancreatic islet glucokinase and hexokinase activities with increasing age, obesity, and the onset of diabetes. Diabetes 1997; 46:1434–1439.
510. Kahn SE, Prigeon RL, McCulloch DK, et al. Quantification of the relationship between insulin sensitivity and beta-cell function in human subjects: evidence for a hyperbolic function. Diabetes 1993; 42:1663–1672.
511. Toffolo G, Bergman RN, Finegood DT, et al. Quantitative estimation of beta cell sensitivity to glucose in the intact organism: a minimal model of insulin kinetics in the dog. Diabetes 1980; 29: 979–990.
512. Polonsky KS, Given BD, Hirsch L, et al. Quantitative study of insulin secretion and clearance in normal and obese subjects. J Clin Invest 1988; 81:435–441.
513. Jones CN, Pei D, Staris P, et al. Alterations in the glucose-stimulated insulin secretory dose-response curve and in insulin clearance in nondiabetic insulin-resistant individuals. J Clin Endocrinol Metab 1997; 82:1834–1838.
514. Buchanan TA, Metzger BE, Freinkel N, Bergman RN. Insulin sensitivity and B-cell responsiveness to glucose during late pregnancy in lean and moderately obese women with normal glucose tolerance or mild gestational diabetes. Am J Obstet Gynecol 1990; 162:1008–1014.

515. Reaven GM, Bernstein R, Davis B, Olefsky JM. Nonketotic diabetes mellitus: insulin deficiency or insulin resistance? Am J Med 1976; 60:80–88.
516. Bergstrom RW, Wahl PW, Leonetti DL, Fujimoto WY. Association of fasting glucose levels with a delayed secretion of insulin after oral glucose in subjects with glucose intolerance. J Clin Endocrinol Metab 1990; 71:1447–1453.
517. Phillips DI, Clark PM, Hales CN, Osmond C. Understanding oral glucose tolerance: comparison of glucose or insulin measurements during the oral glucose tolerance test with specific measurements of insulin resistance and insulin secretion. Diabet Med 1994; 11:286–292.
518. Byrne MM, Sturis J, Sobel RJ, Polonsky KS. Elevated plasma glucose 2 h postchallenge predicts defects in beta-cell function. Am J Physiol 1996; 270:E572–E579.
519. Ahrén B, Pacini G. Impaired adaptation of first-phase insulin secretion in postmenopausal women with glucose intolerance. Am J Physiol 1997; 273:E701–E707.
520. O'Rahilly SP, Nugent Z, Rudenski AS, et al. Beta-cell dysfunction, rather than insulin insensitivity, is the primary defect in familial type 2 diabetes. Lancet 1986; 2:360–364.
521. Barnett AH, Spiliopoulos AJ, Pyke DA, et al. Metabolic studies in unaffected co-twins of non–insulin-dependent diabetics. Br Med J (Clin Res Ed) 1981; 282:1656–1658.
522. Kosaka K, Hagura R, Kuzuya T. Insulin responses in equivocal and definite diabetes, with special reference to subjects who had mild glucose intolerance but later developed definite diabetes. Diabetes 1977; 26:944–952.
523. Efendic S, Luft R, Wajngot A. Aspects of the pathogenesis of type 2 diabetes. Endocr Rev 1984; 5:395–410.
524. Ward WK, Johnston CL, Beard JC, et al. Insulin resistance and impaired insulin secretion in subjects with histories of gestational diabetes mellitus. Diabetes 1985; 34:861–869.
525. O'Sullivan JB. Body weight and subsequent diabetes mellitus. JAMA 1982; 248:949–952.
526. Yoshioka N, Kuzuya T, Matsuda A, et al. Serum proinsulin levels at fasting and after oral glucose load in patients with type 2 (non–insulin-dependent) diabetes mellitus. Diabetologia 1988; 31: 355–360.
527. Saad MF, Kahn SE, Nelson RG, et al. Disproportionately elevated proinsulin in Pima Indians with noninsulin-dependent diabetes mellitus. J Clin Endocrinol Metab 1990; 70:1247–1253.
528. Reaven GM, Chen YD, Hollenbeck CB, et al. Plasma insulin, C-peptide, and proinsulin concentrations in obese and nonobese individuals with varying degrees of glucose tolerance. J Clin Endocrinol Metab 1993; 76:44–48.
529. Larsson H, Ahren B. Relative hyperproinsulinemia as a sign of islet dysfunction in women with impaired glucose tolerance. J Clin Endocrinol Metab 1999; 84:2068–2074.
530. Snehalatha C, Ramachandran A, Satyavani K, et al. Specific insulin and proinsulin concentrations in nondiabetic South Indians. Metabolism 1998; 47:230–233.
531. Birkeland KI, Torjesen PA, Eriksson J, et al. Hyperproinsulinemia of type II diabetes is not present before the development of hyperglycemia. Diabetes Care 1994; 17:1307–1310.
532. Inoue I, Takahashi K, Katayama S, et al. A higher proinsulin response to glucose loading predicts deteriorating fasting plasma glucose and worsening to diabetes in subjects with impaired glucose tolerance. Diabet Med 1996; 13:330–336.
533. Kahn SE, Leonetti DL, Prigeon RL, et al. Proinsulin levels predict the development of non–insulin-dependent diabetes mellitus (NIDDM) in Japanese-American men. Diabet Med 1996; 13(9 suppl 6):S63–S66.
534. Heine RJ, Nijpels G, Mooy JM. New data on the rate of progression of impaired glucose tolerance to NIDDM and predicting factors. Diabet Med 1996; 13(3 suppl 2):S12–S14.
535. Porte D Jr. Clinical importance of insulin secretion and its interaction with insulin resistance in the treatment of type 2 diabetes mellitus and its complications. Diabetes Metab Res Rev 2001; 17: 181–188.
536. Ferner RE, Ashworth L, Tronier B, Alberti KG. Effects of short-term hyperglycemia on insulin secretion in normal humans. Am J Physiol 1986; 250:E655–E661.
537. O'Meara NM, Shapiro ET, Van Cauter E, Polonsky KS. Effect of glyburide on beta cell responsiveness to glucose in non–insulin-dependent diabetes mellitus. Am J Med 1990; 89:11S–16S; discussion 51S-53S.
538. Gerich JE. The genetic basis of type 2 diabetes mellitus: impaired insulin secretion versus impaired insulin sensitivity. Endocr Rev 1998; 19:491–503.
539. Clark PM, Levy JL, Cox L, et al. Immunoradiometric assay of insulin, intact proinsulin and 32-33 split proinsulin and radioimmunoassay of insulin in diet-treated type 2 (non–insulin-dependent) diabetic subjects. Diabetologia 1992; 35:469–474.
540. Polonsky KS, Given BD, Hirsch LJ, et al. Abnormal patterns of insulin secretion in non–insulin-dependent diabetes mellitus. N Engl J Med 1988; 318:1231–1239.
541. Block MB, Rosenfield RL, Mako ME, et al. Sequential changes in beta-cell function in insulin-treated diabetic patients assessed by C-peptide immunoreactivity. N Engl J Med 1973; 288:1144–1148.
542. Cavaghan MK, Ehrmann DA, Byrne MM, Polonsky KS. Treatment with the oral antidiabetic agent troglitazone improves beta cell responses to glucose in subjects with impaired glucose tolerance. J Clin Invest 1997; 100:530–537.
543. Ingalls AM, Dickie MM, Snell GD. Obese, a new mutation in the house mouse. Obes Res 1996; 4:101.
544. Zhang Y, Proenca R, Maffei M, et al. Positional cloning of the mouse obese gene and its human homologue. Nature 1994; 372: 425–432.
545. Pelleymounter MA, Cullen MJ, Baker MB, et al. Effects of the obese gene product on body weight regulation in *ob/ob* mice. Science 1995; 269:540–543.
546. Halaas JL, Gajiwala KS, Maffei M, et al. Weight-reducing effects of the plasma protein encoded by the obese gene. Science 1995; 269:543–546.
547. Friedman JM, Halaas JL. Leptin and the regulation of body weight in mammals. Nature 1998; 395:763–770.
548. Friedman JM. Leptin and the regulation of body weight. Harvey Lect 1999; 95:107–136.
549. Halaas JL, Boozer C, Blair-West J, et al. Physiological response to long-term peripheral and central leptin infusion in lean and obese mice. Proc Natl Acad Sci USA 1997; 94:8878–8883.
550. Friedman JM. The alphabet of weight control. Nature 1997; 385: 119–120.
551. Friedman JM. Leptin, leptin receptors and the control of body weight. Eur J Med Res 1997; 2:7–13.
552. Kerouz NJ, Horsch D, Pons S, Kahn CR. Differential regulation of insulin receptor substrates-1 and -2 (IRS-1 and IRS-2) and phosphatidylinositol 3-kinase isoforms in liver and muscle of the obese diabetic (*ob/ob*) mouse. J Clin Invest 1997; 100:3164–3172.
553. Genuth SM, Przybylski RJ, Rosenberg DM. Insulin resistance in genetically obese, hyperglycemic mice. Endocrinology 1971; 88: 1230–1238.
554. Herberg L, Coleman DL. Laboratory animals exhibiting obesity and diabetes syndromes. Metabolism 1977; 26:59–99.
555. Lee GH, Proenca R, Montez JM, et al. Abnormal splicing of the leptin receptor in diabetic mice. Nature 1996; 379:632–635.
556. Chen H, Charlat O, Tartaglia LA, et al. Evidence that the diabetes gene encodes the leptin receptor: identification of a mutation in the leptin receptor gene in *db/db* mice. Cell 1996; 84:491–495.
557. Coleman DL, Hummel KP. Hyperinsulinemia in pre-weaning diabetes (*db*) mice. Diabetologia 1974; 10(suppl):607–610.
558. Like AA, Chick WL. Studies in the diabetic mutant mouse. I. Light microscopy and radioautography of pancreatic islets. Diabetologia 1970; 6:207–215.
559. Lavine RL, Chick WL, Like AA, Makdisi TW. Glucose tolerance and insulin secretion in neonatal and adult mice. Diabetes 1971; 20:134–139.
560. Like AA, Chick WL. Studies in the diabetic mutant mouse. II. Electron microscopy of pancreatic islets. Diabetologia 1970; 6: 216–242.
561. Shargill NS, Tatoyan A, el-Rafai MF, et al. Impaired insulin receptor phosphorylation in skeletal muscle membranes of *db/db* mice: the use of a novel skeletal muscle plasma membrane preparation to compare insulin binding and stimulation of receptor phosphorylation. Biochem Biophys Res Commun 1986; 137:286–294.
562. Hummel KP, Coleman DL, Lane PW. The influence of genetic background on expression of mutations at the diabetes locus in the mouse. I. C57BL-KsJ and C57BL-6J strains. Biochem Genet 1972; 7:1–13.
563. Coleman DL, Hummel KP. The influence of genetic background

on the expression of the obese (*Ob*) gene in the mouse. Diabetologia 1973; 9:287–293.
564. Cantello BC, Cawthorne MA, Cottam GP, et al. ((omega-(Heterocyclylamino)alkoxy)benzyl)-2,4-thiazolidinediones as potent antihyperglycemic agents. J Med Chem 1994; 37:3977–3985.
565. Lohray BB, Bhushan V, Rao BP, et al. Novel euglycemic and hypolipidemic agents. 1. J Med Chem 1998; 41:1619–1630.
566. Frigeri LG, Wolff GL, Robel G. Impairment of glucose tolerance in yellow (Avy/A) (BALB/c X VY) F-1 hybrid mice by hyperglycemic peptide(s) from human pituitary glands. Endocrinology 1983; 113:2097–2105.
567. Warbritton A, Gill AM, Yen TT, et al. Pancreatic islet cells in preobese yellow Avy/- mice: relation to adult hyperinsulinemia and obesity. Proc Soc Exp Biol Med 1994; 206:145–151.
568. Michaud EJ, Bultman SJ, Klebig ML, et al. A molecular model for the genetic and phenotypic characteristics of the mouse lethal yellow (*Ay*) mutation. Proc Natl Acad Sci USA 1994; 91:2562–2566.
569. Claycombe KJ, Wang Y, Jones BH, et al. Transcriptional regulation of the adipocyte fatty acid synthase gene by agouti: interaction with insulin. Physiol Genomics 2000; 3:157–162.
570. Claycombe KJ, Wang Y, Jones BH, et al. Regulation of leptin by agouti. Physiol Genomics 2000; 2:101–105.
571. Kondo ZK, Nozawa K, Tomito T, Ezaki K. Inbred strains resulting from Japanese mice. Bull Exp Anim 1957; 5:107–116.
572. Iwatsuka H, Shino A, Suzuoki Z. General survey of diabetic features of yellow KK mice. Endocrinol Jpn 1970; 17:23–35.
573. Matsuo T, Shino A, Iwatsuka H, Suzuoki Z. Induction of overt diabetes in KK mice by dietary means. Endocrinol Jpn 1970; 17: 477–488.
574. Veroni MC, Proietto J, Larkins RG. Evolution of insulin resistance in New Zealand obese mice. Diabetes 1991; 40:1480–1487.
575. Cameron DP, Opat F, Insch S. Studies of immunoreactive insulin secretion in NZO mice in vivo. Diabetologia 1974; 10(suppl): 649–654.
576. Bielschowsky M, Bielschowsky F. A new strain of mice with hereditary obesity. Proc Univ Otago Med Sch 1953; 31:29–31.
577. Leiter EH, Reifsnyder PC, Flurkey K, et al. NIDDM genes in mice: deleterious synergism by both parental genomes contributes to diabetogenic thresholds. Diabetes 1998; 47:1287–1295.
578. Thorburn A, Andrikopoulos S, Proietto J. Defects in liver and muscle glycogen metabolism in neonatal and adult New Zealand obese mice. Metabolism 1995; 44:1298–1302.
579. Andrikopoulos S, Proietto J. The biochemical basis of increased hepatic glucose production in a mouse model of type 2 (non–insulin-dependent) diabetes mellitus. Diabetologia 1995; 38:1389–1396.
580. Andrikopoulos S, Rosella G, Kacmarczyk SJ, et al. Impaired regulation of hepatic fructose-1,6-biphosphatase in the New Zealand obese mouse: an acquired defect. Metabolism 1996; 45:622–626.
581. Larkins RG, Simeonova L, Veroni MC. Glucose utilization in relation to insulin secretion in NZO and C57Bl mouse islets. Endocrinology 1980; 107:1634–1638.
582. Melez KA, Harrison LC, Gilliam JN, Steinberg AD. Diabetes is associated with autoimmunity in the New Zealand obese (NZO) mouse. Diabetes 1980; 29:835–840.
583. Melez KA, Reeves JP, Steinberg AD. Regulation of the expression of autoimmunity in NZB × NZW F1 mice by sex hormones. J Immunopharmacol 1978; 1:27–42.
584. Harrison LC, Itin A. A possible mechanism for insulin resistance and hyperglycaemia in NZO mice. Nature 1979; 279:334–336.
585. Reifsnyder PC, Churchill G, Leiter EH. Maternal environment and genotype interact to establish diabesity in mice. Genome Res 2000; 10:1568–1578.
586. Blair SC, Caterson ID, Cooney GJ. Glucose and lipid metabolism in the gold-thioglucose injected mouse model of diabesity. In Shafir E (ed). Lessons from Animal Diabetes VI. Boston, Birkhauser, 1996, pp 239–267.
587. Burant CF, Sreenan S, Hirano K, et al. Troglitazone action is independent of adipose tissue. J Clin Invest 1997; 100:2900-2908.
588. Ross SR, Graves RA, Choy L, et al. Transgenic mouse models of disease: altering adipose tissue function in vivo. Ann NY Acad Sci 1995; 758:297–313.
589. Shimomura I, Hammer RE, Richardson JA, et al. Insulin resistance and diabetes mellitus in transgenic mice expressing nuclear SREBP-1c in adipose tissue: model for congenital generalized lipodystrophy. Genes Dev 1998; 12:3182–3194.
590. Reitman ML, Gavrilova O. A-ZIP/F-1 mice lacking white fat: a model for understanding lipoatrophic diabetes. Int J Obes Relat Metab Disord 2000; 24(suppl 4):S11–S14.
591. Gavrilova O, Marcus-Samuels B, Graham D, et al. Surgical implantation of adipose tissue reverses diabetes in lipoatrophic mice. J Clin Invest 2000; 105:271–278.
592. Shimomura I, Hammer RE, Ikemoto S, et al. Leptin reverses insulin resistance and diabetes mellitus in mice with congenital lipodystrophy. Nature 1999; 401:73–76.
593. Arioglu E, Duncan-Marin J, Sebring N, et al. Efficacy and safety of troglitazone in the treatment of lipodystrophy syndromes. Ann Intern Med 2000; 133:263–274.
594. Surwit RS, Feinglos MN, Rodin J, et al. Differential effects of fat and sucrose on the development of obesity and diabetes in C57BL/6J and A/J mice. Metabolism 1995; 44:645–651.
595. Rebuffe-Scrive M, Surwit R, Feinglos M, et al. Regional fat distribution and metabolism in a new mouse model (C57BL/6J) of non–insulin-dependent diabetes mellitus. Metabolism 1993; 42:1405–1409.
596. Wencel HE, Smothers C, Opara ED, et al. Impaired second phase insulin response of diabetes-prone C57BL/6J mouse islets. Physiol Behav 1995; 57:1215–1220.
597. Lee SK, Opara EC, Surwit RS, et al. Defective glucose-stimulated insulin release from perifused islets of C57BL/6J mice. Pancreas 1995; 11:206–211.
598. Parekh PI, Petro AE, Tiller JM, et al. Reversal of diet-induced obesity and diabetes in C57BL/6J mice. Metabolism 1998; 47: 1089–1096.
599. Shibata M, Yasuda B. (Spontaneously occurring diabetes in NSY mice). Jikken Dobutsu 1979; 28:584–590.
600. Kim JH, Sen S, Avery CS, et al. Genetic analysis of a new mouse model for non–insulin-dependent diabetes. Genomics 2001; 74: 273–286.
601. Phillips MS, Liu Q, Hammond HA, et al. Leptin receptor missense mutation in the fatty Zucker rat. Nat Genet 1996; 13:18–19.
602. Chua SC Jr, White DW, Wu-Peng XS, et al. Phenotype of fatty due to Gln269Pro mutation in the leptin receptor (Lepr). Diabetes 1996; 45:1141–1143.
603. White DW, Wang DW, Chua SC Jr, et al. Constitutive and impaired signaling of leptin receptors containing the Gln → Pro extracellular domain fatty mutation. Proc Natl Acad Sci USA 1997; 94:10657–10662.
604. Peterson RG, et al. Zucker diabetic fatty rat as a model for non-insulin-dependent diabetes mellitus. ILAR News 1990; 32:16–19.
605. Janssen SW, Hermus AR, Lange WP, et al. Progressive histopathological changes in pancreatic islets of Zucker diabetic fatty rats. Exp Clin Endocrinol Diabetes 2001; 109:273–282.
606. Pick A, Clark J, Kubstrup C, et al. Role of apoptosis in failure of beta-cell mass compensation for insulin resistance and beta-cell defects in the male Zucker diabetic fatty rat. Diabetes 1998; 47: 358–364.
607. Cockburn BN, Ostrega DM, Sturis J, et al. Changes in pancreatic islet glucokinase and hexokinase activities with increasing age, obesity, and the onset of diabetes. Diabetes 1997; 46:1434–1439.
608. Zhou YP, Cockburn BN, Pugh W, Polonsky KS. Basal insulin hypersecretion in insulin-resistant Zucker diabetic and Zucker fatty rats: role of enhanced fuel metabolism. Metabolism 1999; 48:857–864.
609. Corsetti JP, Sparks JD, Peterson RG, et al. Effect of dietary fat on the development of non–insulin dependent diabetes mellitus in obese Zucker diabetic fatty male and female rats. Atherosclerosis 2000; 148:231–241.
610. Griffen SC, Wang J, German MS. A genetic defect in beta-cell gene expression segregates independently from the fa locus in the ZDF rat. Diabetes 2001; 50:63–68.
611. Johnson JH, Ogawa A, Chen L, et al. Underexpression of beta cell high K_m glucose transporters in noninsulin-dependent diabetes. Science 1990; 250:546–549.
612. Orci L, Ravazzola M, Baetens D, et al. Evidence that down-regulation of beta-cell glucose transporters in non–insulin-dependent diabetes may be the cause of diabetic hyperglycemia. Proc Natl Acad Sci USA 1990; 87:9953–9957.
613. Unger RH. Lipotoxicity in the pathogenesis of obesity-dependent NIDDM: genetic and clinical implications. Diabetes 1995; 44: 863–870.

614. Lee Y, Hirose H, Zhou YT, et al. Increased lipogenic capacity of the islets of obese rats: a role in the pathogenesis of NIDDM. Diabetes 1997; 46:408–413.

615. Sreenan S, Keck S, Fuller T, et al. Effects of troglitazone on substrate storage and utilization in insulin-resistant rats. Am J Physiol 1999; 276:E1119–E1129.

616. Shimabukuro M, Ohneda M, Lee Y, Unger RH. Role of nitric oxide in obesity-induced beta cell disease. J Clin Invest 1997; 100:290–295.

617. Shimabukuro M, Higa M, Zhou YT, et al. Lipoapoptosis in beta-cells of obese prediabetic fa/fa rats: role of serine palmitoyltransferase overexpression. J Biol Chem 1998; 273:32487–32490.

618. Tokuyama Y, Sturis J, DePaoli AM, et al. Evolution of beta-cell dysfunction in the male Zucker diabetic fatty rat. Diabetes 1995; 44:1447–1457.

619. Sreenan S, Sturis J, Pugh W, et al. Prevention of hyperglycemia in the Zucker diabetic fatty rat by treatment with metformin or troglitazone. Am J Physiol 1996; 271:E742–E747.

620. Goto Y, Kakizaki M, Masaki N. Spontaneous diabetes produced by selective breeding of normal Wistar rats. Proc Jpn Acad 1975; 51:80–85.

621. Movassat J, Saulnier C, Serradas P, Portha B. Impaired development of pancreatic beta-cell mass is a primary event during the progression to diabetes in the GK rat. Diabetologia 1997; 40: 916–925.

622. Movassat J, Saulnier C, Portha B. Beta-cell mass depletion precedes the onset of hyperglycaemia in the GK rat, a genetic model of non-insulin-dependent diabetes mellitus. Diabet Metab 1995; 21:365–370.

623. Ostenson CG, Khan A, Abdel-Halim SM, et al. Abnormal insulin secretion and glucose metabolism in pancreatic islets from the spontaneously diabetic GK rat. Diabetologia 1993; 36:3–8.

624. Ostenson CG, Abdel-Halim SM, Rasschaert J, et al. Deficient activity of FAD-linked glycerophosphate dehydrogenase in islets of GK rats. Diabetologia 1993; 36:722–726.

625. Abdel-Halim SM, Guenifi A, Efendic S, Ostenson CG. Both somatostatin and insulin responses to glucose are impaired in the perfused pancreas of the spontaneously noninsulin-dependent diabetic GK (Goto-Kakizaki) rats. Acta Physiol Scand 1993; 148: 219–226.

626. Nagamatsu S, Nakamichi Y, Yamamura C, et al. Decreased expression of t-SNARE, syntaxin 1, and SNAP-25 in pancreatic beta-cells is involved in impaired insulin secretion from diabetic GK rat islets: restoration of decreased t-SNARE proteins improves impaired insulin secretion. Diabetes 1999; 48:2367–2373.

627. Guenifi A, Portela-Gomes GM, Grimelius L, et al. Adenylyl cyclase isoform expression in non-diabetic and diabetic Goto-Kakizaki (GK) rat pancreas: evidence for distinct overexpression of type-8 adenylyl cyclase in diabetic GK rat islets. Histochem Cell Biol 2000; 113:81–89.

628. Song XM, Kawano Y, Krook A, et al. Muscle fiber type–specific defects in insulin signal transduction to glucose transport in diabetic GK rats. Diabetes 1999; 48:664–670.

629. Begum N, Ragolia L. Altered regulation of insulin signaling components in adipocytes of insulin-resistant type II diabetic Goto-Kakizaki rats. Metabolism 1998; 47:54–62.

630. Berdanier CD. The BHE strain to rat: an example of the role of inheritance in determining metabolic controls. Fed Proc 1976; 35:2295–2299.

631. Berdanier CD, Tobin RB, DeVore V. Effects of age, strain, and dietary carbohydrate on the hepatic metabolism of male rats. J Nutr 1979; 109:261–271.

632. Mathews CE, McGraw RA, Dean R, Berdanier CD. Inheritance of a mitochondrial DNA defect and impaired glucose tolerance in BHE/Cdb rats. Diabetologia 1999; 42:35–40.

633. McCusker RH, Deaver OE Jr, Berdanier CD. Effect of sucrose or starch feeding on the hepatic mitochondrial activity of BHE and Wistar rats. J Nutr 1983; 113:1327–1334.

634. Borenshtein D, Ofri R, Werman M, et al. Cataract development in diabetic sand rats treated with alpha-lipoic acid and its gamma-linolenic acid conjugate. Diabetes Metab Res Rev 2001; 17:44–50.

635. Ikeda Y, Olsen GS, Ziv E, et al. Cellular mechanism of nutritionally induced insulin resistance in *Psammomys obesus*: overexpression of protein kinase Cepsilon in skeletal muscle precedes the onset of hyperinsulinemia and hyperglycemia. Diabetes 2001; 50:584–592.

636. Kanety H, Moshe S, Shafrir E, et al. Hyperinsulinemia induces a reversible impairment in insulin receptor function leading to diabetes in the sand rat model of non-insulin- dependent diabetes mellitus. Proc Natl Acad Sci USA 1994; 91:1853–1857.

637. Kawano K, Hirashima T, Mori S, et al. Spontaneous long-term hyperglycemic rat with diabetic complications: Otsuka Long-Evans Tokushima Fatty (OLETF) strain. Diabetes 1992; 41: 1422–1428.

638. Moralejo DH, Ogino T, Zhu M, et al. A major quantitative trait locus co-localizing with cholecystokinin type A receptor gene influences poor pancreatic proliferation in a spontaneously diabetogenic rat. Mamm Genome 1998; 9:794–798.

639. Takiguchi S, Takata Y, Takahashi N, et al. A disrupted cholecystokinin A receptor gene induces diabetes in obese rats synergistically with *ODB1* gene. Am J Physiol 1998; 274:E265–E270.

640. Takiguchi S, Takata Y, Funakoshi A, et al. Disrupted cholecystokinin type-A receptor (*CCKAR*) gene in OLETF rats. Gene 1997; 197:169–175.

641. Hirashima T, Kawano K, Mori S, Natori T. A diabetogenic gene, *ODB2*, identified on chromosome 14 of the OLETF rat and its synergistic action with *ODB1*. Biochem Biophys Res Commun 1996; 224:420–425.

642. Shi K, Mizuno A, Sano T, et al. Sexual difference in the incidence of diabetes mellitus in Otsuka-Long-Evans-Tokushima-Fatty rats: effects of castration and sex hormone replacement on its incidence. Metabolism 1994; 43:1214–1220.

643. Ishida K, Mizuno A, Murakami T, Shima K. Obesity is necessary but not sufficient for the development of diabetes mellitus. Metabolism 1996; 45:1288–1295.

644. Okauchi N, Mizuno A, Zhu M, et al. Effects of obesity and inheritance on the development of non–insulin-dependent diabetes mellitus in Otsuka-Long-Evans-Tokushima fatty rats. Diabetes Res Clin Pract 1995; 29:1–10.

645. Kosegawa I, Chen S, Awata T, et al. Troglitazone and metformin, but not glibenclamide, decrease blood pressure in Otsuka Long Evans Tokushima fatty rats. Clin Exp Hypertens 1999; 21: 199–211.

646. Triadou N, Portha B, Picon L, Rosselin G. Experimental chemical diabetes and pregnancy in the rat: evolution of glucose tolerance and insulin response. Diabetes 1982; 31:75–79.

647. Portha B, Picon L, Rosselin G. Chemical diabetes in the adult rat as the spontaneous evolution of neonatal diabetes. Diabetologia 1979; 17:371–377.

648. Kodama T, Iwase M, Nunoi K, et al. A new diabetes model induced by neonatal alloxan treatment in rats. Diabetes Res Clin Pract 1993; 20:183–189.

649. Iwase M, Nunoi K, Wakisaka M, et al. Spontaneous recovery from non-insulin-dependent diabetes mellitus induced by neonatal streptozotocin treatment in spontaneously hypertensive rats. Metabolism 1991; 40:10–14.

650. Bjork S. The cost of diabetes and diabetes care. Diabetes Res Clin Pract 2001; 54(suppl 1):S13–S18.

651. Boyle JP, Honeycutt AA, Narayan KM, et al. Projection of diabetes burden through 2050: impact of changing demography and disease prevalence in the U.S. Diabetes Care 2001; 24:1936–1940.

652. Harris MI, Eastman RC, Cowie CC, et al. Comparison of diabetes diagnostic categories in the U.S. population according to the 1997 American Diabetes Association and 1980–1985 World Health Organization diagnostic criteria. Diabetes Care 1997; 20: 1859–1862.

653. Mokdad AH, Bowman BA, Ford ES, et al. The continuing epidemics of obesity and diabetes in the United States. JAMA 2001; 286:1195–1200.

654. Consensus development conference on the diagnosis of coronary heart disease in people with diabetes: 10–11 February 1998, Miami, Florida. American Diabetes Association. Diabetes Care 1998; 21:1551–1559.

655. Bojestig M, Arnqvist HJ, Hermansson G, et al. Declining incidence of nephropathy in insulin-dependent diabetes mellitus. N Engl J Med 1994; 330:15–18.

656. Gu K, Cowie CC, Harris MI. Mortality in adults with and without diabetes in a national cohort of the U.S. population, 1971–1993. Diabetes Care 1998; 21:1138–1145.

657. Gu K, Cowie CC, Harris MI. Diabetes and decline in heart disease mortality in US adults. JAMA 1999; 281:1291–1297.

658. Rubin RJ, Altman WM, Mendelson DN. Health care expenditures for people with diabetes mellitus, 1992. J Clin Endocrinol Metab 1994; 78:809A–809F.
659. Wagner EH, Sandhu N, Newton KM, et al. Effect of improved glycemic control on health care costs and utilization. JAMA 2001; 285:182–189.
660. Zimmet P, Alberti KG, Shaw J. Global and societal implications of the diabetes epidemic. Nature 2001; 414:782–787.
661. Screening for diabetes. American Diabetes Association. Diabetes Care 2002; 25(suppl 1):S21–S24.
662. Engelgau MM, Narayan KM, Herman WH. Screening for type 2 diabetes. Diabetes Care 2000; 23:1563–1580.
663. Rolka DB, Narayan KM, Thompson TJ, et al. Performance of recommended screening tests for undiagnosed diabetes and dysglycemia. Diabetes Care 2001; 24:1899–1903.
664. Stern M, Williams K, Haffner S. Identification of individuals at high risk of type 2 diabetes: do we need the oral glucose tolerance test? Ann Intern Med 2002; 136:575–581.
665. Expert committee on the diagnosis and classification of diabetes mellitus. Report on the Diagnosis and Classification of Diabetes Mellitus. American Diabetes Association. Diabetes Care 2002; 25(suppl 1):S5–S20.
666. Bjornholt JV, Erikssen G, Aaser E, et al. Fasting blood glucose: an underestimated risk factor for cardiovascular death. Results from a 22-year follow-up of healthy nondiabetic men. Diabetes Care 1999; 22:45–49.
667. Khaw KT, Wareham N, Luben R, et al. Glycated haemoglobin, diabetes, and mortality in men in Norfolk cohort of European prospective investigation of cancer and nutrition (EPIC-Norfolk). BMJ 2001; 322:15–18.
668. Saydah SH, Miret M, Sung J, et al. Postchallenge hyperglycemia and mortality in a national sample of U.S. adults. Diabetes Care 2001; 24:1397–1402.
669. Glucose tolerance and cardiovascular mortality: comparison of fasting and 2-hour diagnostic criteria. Arch Intern Med 2001; 161:397–405.
670. Intensive blood-glucose control with sulphonylureas or insulin compared with conventional treatment and risk of complications in patients with type 2 diabetes (UKPDS 33). UK Prospective Diabetes Study (UKPDS) Group. Lancet 1998; 352:837–853.
671. Effect of intensive blood-glucose control with metformin on complications in overweight patients with type 2 diabetes (UKPDS 34). UK Prospective Diabetes Study (UKPDS) Group. Lancet 1998; 352:854–865.
672. Ohkubo Y, Kishikawa H, Araki E, et al. Intensive insulin therapy prevents the progression of diabetic microvascular complications in Japanese patients with non–insulin-dependent diabetes mellitus: a randomized prospective 6-year study. Diabetes Res Clin Pract 1995; 28:103–117.
673. Smith NL, Barzilay JI, Shaffer D, et al. Fasting and 2-hour postchallenge serum glucose measures and risk of incident cardiovascular events in the elderly: the Cardiovascular Health Study. Arch Intern Med 2002; 162:209–216.
674. Stratton IM, Adler AI, Neil HA, et al. Association of glycaemia with macrovascular and microvascular complications of type 2 diabetes (UKPDS 35): prospective observational study. BMJ 2000; 321:405–412.
675. Standards of medical care for patients with diabetes mellitus. American Diabetes Association. Diabetes Care 2002; 25(suppl 1): S33–S49.
676. American College of Endocrinology consensus statement on guidelines for glycemic control. American College of Endocrinologists. Endocr Pract 2002; 8(suppl 1):5–11.
677. Rohlfing CL, Wiedmeyer HM, Little RR, et al. Defining the relationship between plasma glucose and HbA_{1c}: analysis of glucose profiles and HbA_{1c} in the Diabetes Control and Complications Trial. Diabetes Care 2002; 25:275–278.
678. Postprandial blood glucose. American Diabetes Association. Diabetes Care 2001; 24:775–778.
679. National standards for diabetes self-management education. American Diabetes Association. Diabetes Care 2002; 25(suppl 1): S140–S147.
680. Klonoff DC, Schwartz DM. An economic analysis of interventions for diabetes. Diabetes Care 2000; 23:390–404.
681. Norris SL, Engelgau MM, Narayan KM. Effectiveness of self-management training in type 2 diabetes: a systematic review of randomized controlled trials. Diabetes Care 2001; 24:561–587.
682. Delamater AM, Jacobson AM, Anderson B, et al. Psychosocial therapies in diabetes: report of the Psychosocial Therapies Working Group. Diabetes Care 2001; 24:1286–1292.
683. Evidence-based nutrition principles and recommendations for the treatment and prevention of diabetes and related complications. Diabetes Care 2002; 25:202–212.
684. Gillespie SJ, Kulkarni KD, Daly AE. Using carbohydrate counting in diabetes clinical practice. J Am Diet Assoc 1998; 98:897–905.
685. Egede LE, Ye K, Zhang D, Silverstein MD. The prevalence and pattern of complementary and alternative medicine use in individuals with diabetes. Diabetes Care 2002; 25:324–329.
686. Ernst E. Complementary medicine: its hidden risks. Diabetes Care 2001; 24:1486–1488.
687. Schnyder G, Roffi M, Pin R, et al. Decreased rate of coronary restenosis after lowering of plasma homocysteine levels. N Engl J Med 2001; 345:1593–1600.
688. Connor WE, Connor SL. Should a low-fat, high-carbohydrate diet be recommended for everyone? The case for a low-fat, high-carbohydrate diet. N Engl J Med 1997; 337:562-563; discussion, 566-567.
689. Kanaley J, Weinstock R. Nonpharmacologic therapy in the treatment of insulin resistance. Curr Opin Endocrinol Diabetes 2001; 8:219–225.
690. Knowler WC, Barrett-Connor E, Fowler SE, et al. Reduction in the incidence of type 2 diabetes with lifestyle intervention or metformin. N Engl J Med 2002; 346:393–403.
690a. Buchanan. Diabetes 2002, in press.
690b. Chiasson JL, Josse RG, Gomis R, et al. Acarbose for prevention of type 2 diabetes mellitus: The STOP-NIDDM randomised trial. Lancet 2002; 359(9323):2072–2077.
691. Pan XR, Li GW, Hu YH, et al. Effects of diet and exercise in preventing NIDDM in people with impaired glucose tolerance. The Da Qing IGT and Diabetes Study. Diabetes Care 1997; 20: 537–544.
692. Tuomilehto J, Lindstrom J, Eriksson JG, et al. Prevention of type 2 diabetes mellitus by changes in lifestyle among subjects with impaired glucose tolerance. N Engl J Med 2001; 344:1343–1350.
693. Diabetes mellitus and exercise. American Diabetes Association. Diabetes Care 2002; 25(suppl 1):S64–S68.
694. Boule NG, Haddad E, Kenny GP, et al. Effects of exercise on glycemic control and body mass in type 2 diabetes mellitus: a meta-analysis of controlled clinical trials. JAMA 2001; 286:1218–1227.
695. Inzucchi SE. Noninvasive assessment of the diabetic patient for coronary artery disease. Diabetes Care 2001; 24:1519–1521.
696. Faas A, Schellevis FG, Van Eijk JT. The efficacy of self-monitoring of blood glucose in NIDDM subjects: a criteria-based literature review. Diabetes Care 1997; 20:1482–1486.
697. Buse JB. Overview of current therapeutic options in type 2 diabetes: rationale for combining oral agents with insulin therapy. Diabetes Care 1999; 22(suppl 3):C65–C70.
698. DeFronzo RA. Pharmacologic therapy for type 2 diabetes mellitus. Ann Intern Med 2000; 133:73–74.
699. Inzucchi SE. Oral antihyperglycemic therapy for type 2 diabetes: scientific review. JAMA 2002; 287:360–372.
700. Lebovitz HE. Oral therapies for diabetic hyperglycemia. Endocrinol Metab Clin North Am 2001; 30:909–933.
701. Chan NN, Brain HP, Feher MD. Metformin-associated lactic acidosis: a rare or very rare clinical entity? Diabet Med 1999; 16: 273–281.
702. Parulkar AA, Pendergrass ML, Granda-Ayala R, et al. Nonhypoglycemic effects of thiazolidinediones. Ann Intern Med 2001; 134:61–71.
703. King AB. A comparison in a clinical setting of the efficacy and side effects of three thiazolidinediones. Diabetes Care 2000; 23: 557.
704. Klepzig H, Kober G, Matter C, et al. Sulfonylureas and ischaemic preconditioning; a double-blind, placebo-controlled evaluation of glimepiride and glibenclamide. Eur Heart J 1999; 20: 439–446.
705. Buse JB, Hroscikoski M. The case for a role for postprandial glucose monitoring in diabetes management. J Fam Pract 1998; 47(5 suppl):S29–S36.
706. Narayan KM, Gregg EW, Engelgau MM, et al. Translation re-

search for chronic disease: the case of diabetes. Diabetes Care 2000; 23:1794–1798.

707. Moller DE. New drug targets for type 2 diabetes and the metabolic syndrome. Nature 2001; 414:821–827.
708. Olefsky JM, Saltiel AR. PPAR gamma and the treatment of insulin resistance. Trends Endocrinol Metab 2000; 11:362–368.
709. Cefalu WT. Novel routes of insulin delivery for patients with type 1 or type 2 diabetes. Ann Med 2001; 33:579–586.
710. Weyer C, Maggs DG, Young AA, Kolterman OG. Amylin replacement with pramlintide as an adjunct to insulin therapy in type 1 and type 2 diabetes mellitus: a physiological approach toward improved metabolic control. Curr Pharm Des 2001; 7:1353–1373.
711. Drucker DJ. Development of glucagon-like peptide-1–based pharmaceuticals as therapeutic agents for the treatment of diabetes. Curr Pharm Des 2001; 7:1399–1412.

30 Type 1 Diabetes Mellitus

George S. Eisenbarth, Kenneth S. Polonsky, and
John B. Buse

In 1984, Sutherland and co-workers[1] transplanted the tail of the pancreas from nondiabetic identical twins to their twin mates with type 1 diabetes. In contrast to the transplantation of organs such as kidneys, in which the transplants are accepted between identical twins, pancreatic islets but not acinar pancreas were rapidly destroyed.[1] The diabetes of the twin transplant recipients was cured for only a matter of weeks. In retrospect, the results of these transplants were predictable, given the autoimmune nature of type 1A diabetes and similar results in animal models of the disorder.[2] Following this clinical study, type 1 diabetes became one of the most intensively studied autoimmune disorders, and the National Institutes of Health has designated type 1A diabetes a Priority One target for the development of a preventive immunologic vaccine. Knowledge of the immunogenetics and immunopathogenesis of type 1A diabetes is beginning to influence clinical care,[3] greatly influences current clinical research, and will, we hope, lead to disease prevention.[4]

DIFFERENTIAL DIAGNOSIS OF TYPE 1 DIABETES

An expert committee of the American Diabetes Association, with its etiologic diagnostic criteria (Table 30–1), has recommended dividing type 1 diabetes into type 1A (immune-mediated) and type 1B (other forms of diabetes with severe insulin deficiency).[5] At the onset of diabetes, distinguishing type 1A diabetes from type 2 diabetes, let alone type 1B diabetes, is not always a simple task. The best current criterion for diagnosis of type 1A diabetes is the presence of anti-islet autoantibodies measured with highly specific (and reasonably sensitive) autoantibody radioassays.[6]

The presence of autoantibodies with assays defined as positive in less than 1 of 100 control subjects (specificity $\geq$ 99%) is reasonably diagnostic of type 1A diabetes. Non-Hispanic white children presenting with diabetes usually have type 1A diabetes, whereas adults older than 40 years usually have type 2 diabetes.[7] More than 90% of such children presenting with diabetes express one of three commonly measured autoantibodies (see later). In contrast, among black or Hispanic American children, almost one half lack any autoantibody.[8–10] Most of these children appear to have an early age of onset of type 2 diabetes mellitus, and many have attendant risk factors such as obesity and lack human leukocyte antigen (HLA) alleles associated with type 1A diabetes (see later). Imagawa and co-workers[11] described an unusual form of diabetes. The patients had normal hemoglobin A_{1c} (HbA_{1c}) despite severe hyperglycemia, suggesting that the diabetes had been present for only a short time. Histologic examination of pancreatic sections demonstrated pancreatitis but no insulitis, and anti-islet autoantibodies were not detected. It is likely that this represents one of the first examples of type 1B diabetes although a fulminant type 1A is possible.

susceptibility are similar in diverse countries, with specific alleles of those genes differing in their frequency.[72] Several monogenic forms of type 1A diabetes can now be identified. It is not clear whether these genetically characterized forms of diabetes should now be included in the group of "Other Defined Causes of Diabetes."[5] For the great majority of patients with type 1A diabetes, most of the genes causing diabetes susceptibility remain to be identified.

Monogenic Forms of Type 1A Diabetes

Autoimmune Polyendocrine Syndrome Type I (*AIRE* Gene)

The autoimmune polyendocrine syndrome type I (APS-I) is rare, with an increased incidence in Finland, Sardinia, and among Iranian Jews, but has a worldwide occurrence. The disorders of the syndrome such as type 1 diabetes, mucocutaneous candidiasis, hypoparathyroidism, Addison's disease, and hepatitis (see Chapter 37 for more detailed discussion) identify a unique syndrome, and patients with this group of disorders almost always have mutations of the *AIRE* (autoimmune regulator) gene on chromosome 21. This gene apparently encodes a deoxyribonucleic acid (DNA) binding protein. The function of the gene is unknown, but its expression in lymphoid tissue and the clinical syndrome suggests an essential role in maintaining self-tolerance. There is considerable variability in the diseases expressed even for siblings with the same mutation. Some of this variability is likely to be influenced by genetic loci other than the *AIRE* gene. One example is the observation that although 18% of patients with APS-I develop type 1 diabetes, those with the common diabetes-protective HLA allele DQB1*0602 appear to have some protection from diabetes although not from Addison's disease.

X-Linked Polyendocrinopathy, Immune Dysfunction, and Diarrhea (*Scurfy* Gene)

The syndrome of X-linked polyendocrinopathy, immune dysfunction, and diarrhea (XPID) is associated with overwhelming neonatal autoimmunity, with most children dying in the first few days of life or as infants.[73–76] In this syndrome lymphocytes invade multiple organs. It is associated with insulitis and beta cell destruction as well as lymphocytic intestinal inflammation with flattened villi and severe malabsorption. It is inherited as an X-linked recessive disease affecting only males, with a frequent clinical history of lack of male births. The disease apparently results from mutations of the *scurfy* gene, whose function is currently unknown but which, like the *AIRE* gene of APS-I, is a transcription factor.[73, 77]

Idiopathic Type 1A Diabetes

Descriptive Genetics

In the United States, the risk of childhood diabetes is approximately 1 in 300.[78] This is 15-fold less than the diabetes risk for a first-degree relative of a patient with type 1 diabetes (Table 30–2). It is 150-fold less than the risk for a monozygotic twin of a patient with type 1 diabetes.[79, 80] Although the population risk of type 1 diabetes in Japan is 15-fold less than in the United States, the risk for an identical twin in Japan is similar to that for an identical twin in the United States.[81, 82] This suggests that when genetic susceptibility is present, either in Japan or in the United States, the diabetes risk is extremely high. Although the risk of diabetes is much greater for relatives of patients with type 1A diabetes, it is important to realize that most (>85%) individuals in whom type 1A diabetes develops do not have a first-degree relative with the disease. The frequency of sporadic cases results in part from the fact that almost 40% of individuals in the general population carry high-risk HLA alleles for type 1A diabetes (see "The Major Histocompatibility Complex").

The highest known incidence of type 1A diabetes is found in Finland and Sardinia. Finland now has an annual incidence approaching 50 per 100,000 children. Over the past four decades the incidence has increased almost threefold, suggesting a dramatic environmental change (either an increase of causative factors or a decrease of protective factors).

Twin Studies

Twin studies of diabetes have an impressive pedigree. The study of monozygotic twins of patients with diabetes by Pyke and co-workers[83] contributed to the recognition of distinct forms of diabetes, initially termed adult-onset and juvenile-onset, subsequently termed insulin-dependent and non–insulin-dependent, and now termed type 1 and type 2 diabetes.[5] The concordance rate for monozygotic and dizygotic twins

Table 30–2. Risk of Type 1A Diabetes

Proband with Diabetes	% Childhood Diabetes Mellitus (incidence/yr)	Islet Autoantibody	Comment
General population (United States)	0.3% (15–25/100,000)	3% single Ab	Japanese incidence 1/100,000
		0.3% multiple Abs	Incidence increasing in United States as in many European countries (e.g., in Colorado now 25/1,000,000)
Offspring	1%	4.1%	
Sibling	3.2%, 6% lifetime	7.4%	
Dizygotic twin	6%	10%	
Mother	2%	5%	Lower risk than offspring of father with diabetes mellitus
Father	4.6%	6.5%	
Father and mother	10% ?	?	
Monozygotic twin	50% Incidence varies with age of index twin	50%	MZT in Japan, 40% risk of diabetes

Ab, antibody; MZT, monozygotic twin.

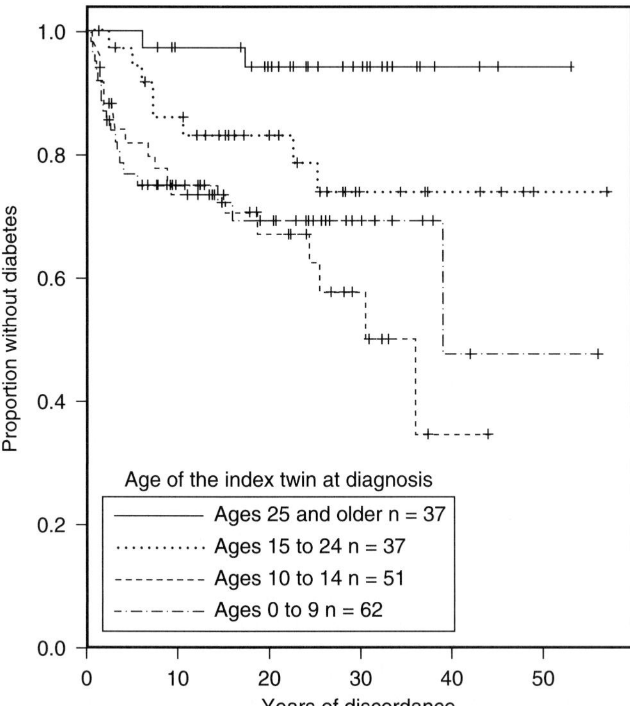

Figure 30–1. Progression to diabetes of initially discordant monozygotic twins of patients with type 1 diabetes subdivided by the age of diabetes onset of the first twin to develop diabetes (proband). Late progression to diabetes is evident, with some twins becoming diabetic more than 20 years after their twin mate. For discordant twins whose twin mate developed diabetes after age 25, the risk of diabetes is less than 10%. (From Redondo MJ, Yu L, Hawa M, et al. Heterogeneity of type 1 diabetes: analysis of monozygotic twins in Great Britain and the United States. Diabetologia 2001; 44:354–362.)

provides important information regarding genetic factors contributing to a disease because monozygotic twins share all germ line–inherited polymorphisms or mutations whereas dizygotic twins are similar to siblings of patients with a disease and have only one half of genes in common. For a locus that contributes to disease in a recessive manner, only one fourth of dizygotic twins would be homozygous to a sibling with diabetes at that locus but all monozygotic twins would be homozygous for all recessive loci of their diabetic twin mate. Although overall concordance rates of monozygotic twins for type 1 diabetes are calculated, it is likely that type 1 diabetes is heterogeneous and that groups of monozygotic twins may have different genetic etiologies. With such genetic heterogeneity, one would expect different concordance rates for different genetic diseases.

Redondo and co-workers[84] have analyzed prospective follow-up data from a large series of initially discordant monozygotic twins from Great Britain combined with a series from the United States. Progression to diabetes was identical for both series of twins. Of note, there was no length of time of discordance beyond which a monozygotic twin mate did not have a risk of type 1 diabetes. Nevertheless, the hazard rate for development of diabetes decreased as the period of discordance increased. There was also a marked variation in the risk of diabetes relative to the age at which diabetes developed in the index twin. The overall rate of concordance for monozygotic twins was 50%. However, if type 1 diabetes developed in the index twin after age 25, the concordance rate by life table analysis was less than 10% (Fig. 30–1). If diabetes developed in the index twin prior to age 5, the concordance rate was 70% by 40 years of follow-up. This analysis of monozygotic twins suggests genetic heterogeneity but also confirms that a significant subset of monozygotic twins do not progress to diabetes. This suggests that either environmental factors, random factors, or non–germ line–inherited variations (e.g., imprinting, T-cell receptor polymorphisms, somatic mutations) contribute to diabetes risk.

An important unanswered question (given the limited number and size of studies) is whether dizygotic twins of patients with type 1A diabetes have a diabetes risk greater than that of siblings. If the risk is identical, it suggests that environmental factors whose presence is time-dependent (e.g., uncommon infections) may have little influence on the development of diabetes. Dizygotic twins differ from siblings in terms of a greater commonality of environment over time (e.g., common pregnancy). Studies of dizygotic twins suggest that their risk of diabetes may not differ from that of siblings or at most is increased by a factor of 2 compared with the 10-fold increase for monozygotic twins.

Genetic factors influence not only the development of diabetes but also the expression of anti-islet autoantibodies. For identical twins the expression of anti-islet autoantibodies is tightly linked to the eventual progression to overt diabetes, and monozygotic twins have a high prevalence of expression of autoantibodies. Dizygotic twins much less often express anti-islet autoantibodies, and the prevalence is similar to that of siblings.[85]

Associated Autoimmune Disorders

Because type 1A diabetes is an immune-mediated illness that develops in a genetically susceptible individual, it is not surprising that most patients with type 1A have one or more additional autoimmune diseases. The most common associated disorders are thyroid autoimmunity (Graves' disease or Hashimoto's thyroiditis) and celiac disease (Table 30–3).

The Major Histocompatibility Complex

The most important loci determining the risk of type 1 diabetes are within the MHC on chromosome 6p21 (Fig. 30–2), in particular HLA class II molecules (DR, DQ, and DP).[19, 89–91] In addition, standard class I loci (HLA A, B, and C) influence disease, and it is likely that additional loci within the MHC that influence immune function contribute to diabetes risk.[92] Figure 30–2 illustrates the MHC. The nomenclature for alleles of this region is somewhat daunting, but with definitions of several terms and a description of the basis for classification it is comprehensible.

HLA molecules function to present peptides to T lymphocytes. Each molecule is made up of two chains, with each chain encoded by a separate gene. These molecules are extremely polymorphic in amino acid sequence. Each polymorphic variant of each chain is designated with a gene locus name (e.g., DRB1) followed by an asterisk (*), followed by two

Table 30–3. Associated Autoimmune Diseases

Disease	Autoantibody	Disease Prevalence (%)
Thyroiditis or Graves' disease	25% (peroxidase or thyroglobulin)	4
Celiac disease	12% (transglutaminase)[86]	6
Addison's disease	1.5% (21-hydroxylase)[87]	0.5
Pernicious anemia	21% (parietal cell)[88]	2.6[88]

Other viruses are being evaluated for association with the triggering of autoimmunity. One study from Australia found an association with rotavirus infection.[125] Rotavirus infection is common in young children. The Australian study did not find an increase in rotavirus infection compared with that in control subjects but reported an association of rotavirus infection with increases of anti-islet autoantibodies. Studies from Denver did not indicate an increase in rotavirus infection in infants developing autoantibodies.

Vaccination

It has been claimed that the timing of routine childhood vaccinations influences the development of type 1A diabetes.[126] This is an important health concern if parents alter their family's childhood vaccination because of concern about development of diabetes. A series of studies have been carried out[127–129] and do not provide evidence that childhood vaccinations influence the development of diabetes.

Diet

A disease such as celiac disease is critically dependent on the ingestion of a specific food, namely the wheat protein gliadin.[130] In addition, a number of dietary modifications altered the development of diabetes in NOD mice and BB rats.[131] Investigators have championed the hypothesis that early introduction of bovine milk increases the development of diabetes. This hypothesis is primarily based on retrospective studies associating early or increased bovine milk ingestion (or less breast-feeding) with an increased risk of type 1A diabetes.[132] Several prospective studies in which infants are observed until the development of anti-islet autoantibodies have failed to find an association or have found a weak association with either breast-feeding or bovine milk ingestion.[133–136] Pilot studies of an infant formula lacking bovine milk proteins have been initiated in Finland. Preliminary data suggest that such a restricted diet may produce a small decrease of cytoplasmic islet cell autoantibodies but not of GAD65 autoantibodies.

NATURAL HISTORY OF TYPE 1A DIABETES

We typically divide the development of type 1A diabetes into a series of stages beginning with genetic susceptibility and ending with essentially complete beta cell destruction (Fig. 30–3). It is, however, likely that both genes and environmental factors influence the course of development of type 1A diabetes during the complete prediabetic period. For instance, injection of immunostimulants such as Freund's adjuvant can prevent progression to diabetes in animals with insulitis. Mathis and co-workers[136a] have proposed the existence of "checkpoints" in the development of diabetes, and such checkpoints may have a strong genetic component. As discussed subsequently, type 1A diabetes is quite predictable given specific immunologic, genetic, and metabolic characteristics, and it is such characteristics that set the stage for preventive trials.

Genetic and Immunologic Heterogeneity by Age of Onset

Type 1A diabetes can develop at any age, from the neonatal period to the sixth decade of life. In that identical twins can become concordant 30 years after their twin mate, not all age heterogeneity can be ascribed to different genetic syndromes.[85] Nevertheless, there is an overall correlation between the age at which diabetes develops in one twin or sibling and the age of development of diabetes in his or her relative. As discussed earlier, children in whom type 1A diabetes develops at an early age more often are DR3/4, DQ8/2 heterozygotes. In addition, there is evidence that class I HLA alleles (or other non–class II genes with the HLA region) may influence the age of diabetes onset (e.g., the A24 allele).[137] At the other end of the age spectrum, there is evidence that the protective HLA allele DQA1*0102, DQB1*0602 is not as protective for young adults as it is for children.[138]

The most characteristic difference related to the age of diabetes onset is the presence of higher levels of insulin autoantibodies in children who develop the disease at an early age (e.g., younger than 5 years).[139, 140] The high levels and frequent

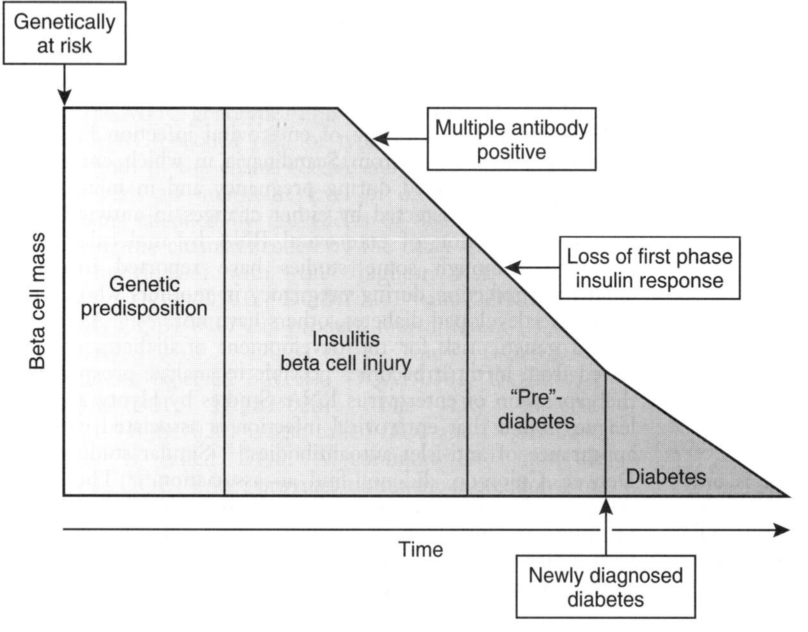

Figure 30–3. Hypothetical stages in the development of type 1A diabetes beginning with genetic susceptibility and ending with complete beta cell destruction. (Modified from Eisenbarth GS. Type 1 diabetes mellitus: A chronic autoimmune disorder. N Engl J Med 1986, with modifications by Jay Skyler, University of Miami.)

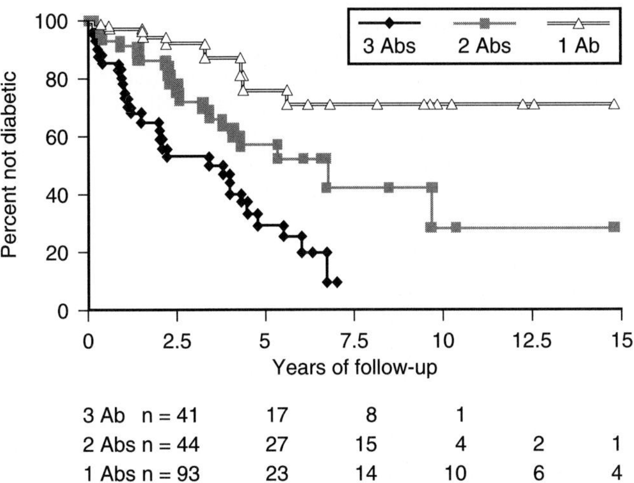

Figure 30–4. Progression to type 1 diabetes of first-degree relatives of patients with diabetes subdivided by the number of anti-islet autoantibodies of insulin, GAD65 (glutamic acid decarboxylase), and ICA512 (IA-2) expressed. (From Verge CF, Gianani R, Kawasaki E, et al. Prediction of type 1 diabetes in first-degree relatives using a combination of insulin, GAD, and ICA512 bdc/IA-2 autoantibodies. Diabetes 45:926–933, 1996.)

positivity of insulin autoantibodies make measurement of IAA (insulin autoantibodies) the best single marker for diabetes development in young children. For children in whom autoantibodies arise in the first 3 years of life, insulin autoantibodies often appear first. In contrast, GAD65 autoantibodies are more often positive in adults developing type 1A diabetes. The correlation of levels of insulin autoantibodies and age of diabetes onset may be related to children with higher levels progressing more rapidly to diabetes.[141] Such rapid progression, however, occurs only if insulin autoantibodies are present with another islet autoantibody (see "Combinatorial Autoantibody Prediction") (Fig. 30–4).

Combinatorial Autoantibody Prediction

The most specific anti-islet autoantibody assays are usually set with cutoffs above the 99th percentile of control populations. Thus, with three major autoantibody assays (GAD65, ICA512 [islet cell antibody], and insulin) one would predict that approximately 3 of 100 normal individuals would express one or more of the three autoantibodies. Because approximately 3 of 1000 children develop type 1A diabetes, this suggests that in the great majority of antibody-positive individuals, diabetes never develops or may develop late in life.

A relatively low positive predictive value for single antibodies may be due to methodologic limitations or the presence of autoantibodies identical to those of prediabetics but found in some individuals who do not progress to diabetes. It is likely that both occur. For example, a low positive (but > 99th percentile) autoantibody result of a control subject is often not confirmed on repeated testing. Autoantibodies of prediabetic individuals usually react with multiple epitopes of the ICA512 molecule, whereas false-positive autoantibodies frequently react with only one or no clearly defined epitope of the molecule, suggesting that false-positive and diabetes-associated anti-ICA512 autoantibodies differ. There are, however, individuals, usually adult relatives of patients with type 1A diabetes (often with DQB1*0602), with extremely high levels of GAD65 autoantibodies that react with multiple GAD epitopes with no evidence of progression to diabetes.[142]

Assessment of the significance of an autoantibody result (as for any diagnostic test) is improved by taking into account the prior probability of disease. A patient with overt diabetes and expression of a single anti-islet autoantibody has a high probability of type 1A diabetes. An individual from the general population or even a relative expressing a single autoantibody (and remaining with a single autoantibody) has a much lower risk of progressing to type 1A diabetes.

Usually, in attempting to improve the specificity of a test, one sacrifices sensitivity. For prediction of type 1A diabetes, because three biochemical autoantibodies are measurable, one can combine the tests with the observation that the presence of two or more autoantibodies is associated with a very high risk of diabetes.[143, 144] Approximately 1 of 350 individuals from the general population express two or more of the GAD65, ICA512, or insulin autoantibodies, which approaches population estimates of type 1A diabetes. Among first-degree relatives of patients with type 1A diabetes, two or more autoantibodies indicate a risk over 10 years of more than 90%, whereas a single autoantibody is associated with a risk of less than 20% over 10 years.[143]

Metabolic Progression before Hyperglycemia

The intravenous glucose tolerance test aids in evaluating the time to onset of diabetes among individuals expressing anti-islet autoantibodies.[145] Most commonly, glucose is given at 0.5 g/kg over 5 minutes (maximum 35 g, 25 g/dL) and insulin levels are measured before and 1 and 3 minutes after the glucose infusion.[146, 147] Most individuals within a year of overt diabetes have no first-phase insulin secretion after intravenous glucose. The diagnosis of type 1A diabetes usually relies upon the presence of fasting hyperglycemia, but with prospective evaluation many individuals have diabetes by the 120-minute criteria on oral glucose tolerance with nondiagnostic fasting glucose.

C-Peptide Loss after Hyperglycemia

Following the diagnosis of diabetes, levels of C peptide can be utilized to assess remaining beta cell function. C-peptide levels are usually measured in the fasting state or after intravenous glucagon or with a standard meal (e.g., Sustacal). Such measurements are primarily of importance for trials of therapies to alleviate loss of insulin secretion after diagnosis. Determination of C peptide provides the best current measure for assessing the impact of new therapies. As shown in the Diabetes Control and Complications Trial (DCCT), a small amount of remaining C peptide is associated with impressive metabolic benefit.[148]

Type 1A Diabetes with Pregnancy

Approximately 5% of women with gestational diabetes (diabetes diagnosed during pregnancy) have an early form of type 1A diabetes that is discovered during pregnancy.[149] These women express anti-islet autoantibodies and progress to overt diabetes more rapidly after pregnancy.

Latent Autoimmune Diabetes of Adults

Type 1A diabetes can occur at any age. Depending on the population, between 5% and 15% of individuals with what appears to be type 2 diabetes express anti-islet autoantibodies.[150, 151] Multiple studies have demonstrated that such individuals progress relatively rapidly (within 3 years) to insulin-requiring diabetes. The HLA alleles of such individuals reflect that of type 1A diabetes.[152]

Transient Hyperglycemia

A significant number of children are evaluated by endocrinologists for transient hyperglycemia. The usual history is of severe stress associated with hyperglycemia that resolves within days to a month. Such children may be in the "honeymoon" phase of type 1A diabetes or may truly have a transient episode of hyperglycemia. Rarely, diabetes in children is misdiagnosed (e.g., the authors have seen a child with normal HbA_{1c} values for several years who stopped insulin and was subsequently found to have renal glucosuria and not diabetes). Children without severe stress with transient hyperglycemia or with a relative with type 1A diabetes are more likely to have early type 1A diabetes. Absence of anti-islet autoantibodies and a normal intravenous glucose tolerance test are strongly indicative of transient hyperglycemia and not type 1A diabetes.[153] It is not known whether children with transient hyperglycemia are at increased risk for type 2 diabetes later in life.

IMMUNOTHERAPY OF TYPE 1A DIABETES

At the onset of type 1A diabetes, a major clinical research goal is the prevention of further beta cell destruction. At present there is no proven safe and effective therapy to prevent such further destruction or to prevent the development of type 1A diabetes in those at risk (e.g., genetically at risk individuals with anti-islet autoantibodies). A number of clinical trials have been completed and a large number of trials are under way or about to be initiated.

Immunosuppression

The earliest studies of therapies to prevent beta cell destruction utilized immunosuppressive agents. Large trials of cyclosporine indicated that while administered it prevented further loss of C-peptide secretion and improved metabolic function.[154–157] It did not, however, maintain a nondiabetic state when therapy was instituted after the onset of diabetes, and with discontinuation of the drug individuals rapidly lost C-peptide reserve. The combination of inability to "cure" diabetes and toxicities associated with cyclosporine (in particular nephrotoxicity and concern about increased risk of malignancy) has ruled out its use. Other immunosuppressive agents such as prednisone or azathioprine had relatively little effect.[158–160] A small study suggested that methotrexate, another common immunotherapeutic agent, is ineffective.[161] Thus, at present, although type 1A diabetes is an immune-mediated disorder, it is not treated with common immunotherapeutic agents. A pilot study of a specific antibody to CD3 has been reported and further essential trials are underway.[160a]

Immunologic Vaccination

In animal models (especially the NOD mouse) it is relatively easy to prevent type 1 diabetes.[14] Potentially the most exciting modalities utilize forms of immunologic vaccination. Much of the excitement derives from the specificity of the therapy and relatively low risk compared with immunosuppression and not from demonstrated efficacy in humans. The basic concept behind the bulk of such therapies is the induction of lymphocytes that target a given islet antigen and upon encountering their target antigen (e.g., insulin) produce cytokines that suppress autoimmunity and tissue destruction.[38, 162]

A general class of T lymphocytes termed TH2 T cells produce the cytokine interleukin-4 rather than interferon γ and interleukin-2 (TH1 T cells) and decrease cell-mediated immune destruction. Induction of a protective immune response may depend upon the route of administration of the given antigen (e.g., oral tolerance) or the utilization of an altered antigen (e.g., altered peptide ligands). For example, insulin given either orally or by subcutaneous injection prevented diabetes in NOD mice.[163, 164] Intact insulin is not necessary because insulin B chain and an immunodominant B:9-23 peptide of insulin were also effective.[40] The latter molecules have no insulin-like metabolic effect but are able to activate T lymphocytes that target insulin.

The Diabetes Prevention Trial Type 1 is studying both oral insulin and parenteral injections of low doses of insulin. The results of the parenteral trial did not demonstrate a reduction in the risk of developing diabetes. The oral trial will continue for several more years (relatives of patients with type 1A diabetes can be screened for this trial by calling 1-800-HALT-DM1). A peptide of a heat shock protein (p277) is being studied,[165] and trials of the GAD65 molecule are about to be initiated.

Other Therapies

A review by Atkinson and Leiter[14] pointed out that more than 100 different interventions prevent diabetes in NOD mice. The relative ease of diabetes prevention in this animal model provides the basis for a number of trials initiated in humans. The largest such European trial (ENDIT, European Nicotinamide Trial) utilizes nicotinamide in gram doses. Nicotinamide is able to prevent diabetes induced by the drug streptozotocin and probably acts by preserving nicotinamide adenine dinucleotide levels in islet cells or blocking cytokine-induced destruction. There have been a number of studies of nicotinamide, including a randomized placebo-controlled trial in children and a small trial in at-risk relatives, that found no effect of nicotinamide.[166] Other trials suggest some preservation in adult patients presenting with type 1A diabetes.[167] The ENDIT trial should provide definitive information concerning the potential effect (or lack of effect) of nicotinamide.

IMMUNOLOGY OF ISLET-PANCREATIC TRANSPLANTATION

Pancreatic transplantation for patients requiring a kidney transplant is an accepted clinical procedure.[168] Patients with a kidney transplant receive immunosuppressive drugs, and results for pancreatic transplantation in this setting have progressively improved. With a successful pancreas transplant, hyperglycemia is "immediately" reversed and there is some evidence of improved long-term outcomes.[168, 169] Nevertheless, the surgery is extensive and there are multiple potential complications associated with the transplant. Diabetes can recur because of either recurrent autoimmunity or more often allograft rejection.[170] It is difficult to monitor specific islet destruction, and with the development of hyperglycemia it is usually not possible to restore euglycemia.

Up until studies from Edmonton the results of islet transplantation have been poor, with less than 10% of patients with type 1A diabetes becoming insulin independent at 1 year.[171] In contrast, with autotransplants of patients with pancreatitis most patients become insulin independent and remain so. The Edmonton group has utilized meticulous islet isolation techniques, transplantation of islets from two pancreases, and an immunosuppressive regimen utilizing the new drug rapamycin.[171] With this regimen more than a dozen patients have had successful transplants, and the longest duration after transplantation has been 18 months. With the Edmonton regimen, insulin antibodies decreased and there was no new development or increase of either GAD65 or ICA512 autoantibodies. With other regimens, marked increases of such autoantibodies appeared to herald loss of islet function.

The Edmonton protocol is now being tested in a series of specialized centers throughout North America and Europe, and the applicability of the technique should be rapidly evaluated. Even if the Edmonton results are reproduced at multiple centers, the number of islets available from cadaveric donors for transplantation is limited. Further research to allow xenogeneic transplantation or production of islets from stem cells is essential.

INSULIN AUTOIMMUNE SYNDROME

The insulin autoimmune syndrome, also termed Hirata syndrome, is rare and typically associated with hypoglycemia.[172] These patients have extremely high concentrations of autoantibodies reacting with human insulin. It is thought that inappropriate (nonregulated) release of autoantibody-bound insulin produces the hypoglycemia. The disease occurs most commonly in Asian individuals. Among 50 Japanese patients with the syndrome and the typical polyclonal anti-insulin autoantibodies, 96% had a DRB1, DR4 allele and 84% (42 of 50) the DRB1*0406 allele.[173] In contrast, patients with monoclonal anti-insulin autoantibodies do not have such a remarkable HLA association. Most patients develop the disease in association with treatment with sulfhydryl-containing medications, in particular methimazole. Treatment usually consists of stopping these medications, and for more than 75% the disease remits.[173]

INSULIN ALLERGY

Mild forms of immune reactivity to insulin are not uncommon. Essentially all patients treated with human insulin produce anti-insulin autoantibodies measurable with sensitive fluid phase radioassays. The levels of these autoantibodies are relatively low and they do not appear to interfere with insulin therapy, although there are reports correlating insulin antibodies with macrosomia.[174] With the introduction of recombinant human insulin replacing animal insulins, symptomatic immune responses to insulin such as immediate hypersensitivity, delayed hypersensitivity, lipoatrophy, and lipohypertrophy have decreased.[175] Allergic reactions can occur with insulin analogues, although this is uncommon. More common perhaps are allergies to protamine used to complex insulin in neutral protamine Hagedorn (NPH) formulations as well as to the lubricants, preservatives, and plastics in bottles, stoppers, syringes, and needles. The usual therapy consists of switching the type or formulation of insulin followed by oral antihistamines for immunoglobulin E–mediated local reactions, followed by insulin desensitization or addition of small amounts of glucocorticoids to the insulin injected for local delayed hypersensitivity reactions.

ANTI–INSULIN RECEPTOR AUTOANTIBODIES

Anti–insulin receptor autoantibodies (type B insulin resistance) are associated with both hypoglycemia and insulin resistance.[176] It appears that anti–insulin receptor autoantibodies can act as either an antagonist or agonist. This syndrome is rare and is often associated with non–organ specific autoimmunity.[177]

CLINICAL PRESENTATION

The peak age of presentation of type 1 diabetes in children is around the age of puberty. The symptoms and signs are related to the presence of hyperglycemia and the resulting effects on fluid and electrolyte balance. They generally include polyuria, polydipsia, polyphagia, weight loss, and blurred vision. Because infection may have precipitated the initial presentation, symptoms of infection may also be present such as fever, sore throat, cough, or dysuria. In children in particular the onset of symptoms may occur over a brief period and families may be able to date their onset with considerable accuracy. Onset of symptoms may also be insidious, particularly in older persons with type 1 diabetes, and may occur over a time frame of weeks or even months.

If onset of type 1 diabetes is associated with ketoacidosis, which is not uncommon, additional symptoms related to this acute metabolic complication of diabetes are also present. These symptoms can include abdominal pain, nausea, and vomiting. Variable effects on mental status may be seen, ranging from slight drowsiness to profound lethargy and even coma if the condition has been untreated for a significant period of time.

Laboratory Findings

Plasma glucose concentrations at presentation are elevated, usually in the range 300 to 500 mg/dL. If the presentation is uncomplicated, the remainder of the fluid and electrolyte measurements may be completely normal. On the other hand, if diabetic ketoacidosis is present, the measurements reflect the presence of an acidosis as well as more severe dehydration. Thus, in diabetic ketoacidosis, the serum sodium value is frequently at the lower limit of normal or even mildly reduced, reflecting the osmotic effect of hyperglycemia and on occasion the presence of vomiting with continued water intake. A sodium value less than 120 mmol/L is usually associated with severe hypertriglyceridemia that can lead to spurious hyponatremia. Despite significant losses of potassium in the urine and total-body potassium deficits, the presence of acidosis usually leads to an elevated serum potassium concentration at the time of the initial presentation. Serum bicarbonate concentrations are usually less than 10 mg/dL, and elevations in serum concentrations of triglyceride and free fatty acids are found. Levels of ketone bodies are also elevated. Because dehydration is invariably present, this leads to increases in the concentrations of blood urea nitrogen and creatinine. In conjunction with the increase in serum glucose, the increases in blood urea nitrogen invariably increase the serum osmolality, often to greater than 300 mmol/kg.

TREATMENT OF TYPE 1 DIABETES

Importance of Tight Glucose Control

The overriding principle in the treatment of the majority of patients with type 1 diabetes is that a health care team that includes a physician, diabetes nurse educator, nutritionist, and other health care professionals as appropriate should work closely with the patient to achieve blood glucose concentrations as close to normal as possible because these are associated with a reduced risk of diabetic complications. Although studies in animal models[178–180] and epidemiologic studies[181–183] suggested that tighter glucose control was associated with better long-term outcomes for the diabetic patient in terms of a reduced risk of complications, the most definitive study in this regard has been the Diabetes Control and Complications Trial (DCCT) that was completed in 1993.[184] This landmark study was performed in a total of 1441 patients with type 1 diabetes—726 with no retinopathy at baseline (the primary prevention cohort) and 715 with mild retinopathy (the secondary intervention cohort) who were randomly assigned to intensive therapy or conventional therapy.

Intensive therapy consisted of insulin administration by an external pump or by three or more daily insulin injections. The dosage was adjusted according to the results of self-monitoring of the blood glucose performed at least four times per day as well as in response to dietary intake and anticipated exercise. The goals of intensive therapy were to achieve blood glucose concentrations between 70 and 120 mg/dL before meals, values less than 180 mg/dL after meals, a weekly 3 AM measurement greater than 65 mg/dL, and an HbA_{1c} value within the normal range (6.05% or less). Patients in the intensive treatment group visited their centers each month and had more frequent contacts with a member of the health care team, generally weekly, to review and adjust their regimens.

Conventional therapy consisted of one or two daily injections of insulin, including mixed intermediate and rapid-acting insulins, daily self-monitoring of urine or blood glucose, and education about diet and exercise. The goals of conventional therapy included absence of symptoms of hyperglycemia; absence of ketonuria; maintenance of normal growth, development, and ideal body weight; and freedom from frequent severe hypoglycemia.

The entire cohort of patients was observed for a mean of 6.5 years and 99% of the patients completed the study. Although only 5% of the subjects in the intensive treatment group were able to sustain the goal of a normal HbA_{1c} over time, they nevertheless did have significantly lower average values (approximately 7%) over time than the subjects in the conventional treatment group (approximately 9%). Average capillary blood glucose profiles in the intensive treatment group were 155 ± 30 mg/dL compared with 231 ± 55 mg/dL in the conventional therapy group ($P < .0001$). These differences in glucose control formed the basis of analyses to determine the effects of lower levels of glycemia on diabetic complications.

When both the primary prevention and secondary intervention cohorts were considered, intensive therapy reduced the risk of proliferative or severe nonproliferative retinopathy by 47% and the need for treatment by photocoagulation by 56%. Intensive therapy reduced the mean adjusted risk of microalbuminuria (defined as urinary albumin excretion of > 40 mg per 24 hours) by 34% in the primary prevention cohort and by 43% in the secondary intervention cohort. The risk of albuminuria was reduced by 56% in the secondary intervention cohort. Intensive therapy reduced the appearance of neuropathy by 69% in the primary prevention cohort and by 57% in the secondary intervention cohort.

There has been considerable controversy regarding potential adverse effects of aggressive insulin therapy in exacerbating the predisposition to macrovascular disease. In this study intensive insulin therapy reduced the development of hypercholesterolemia, defined as a serum concentration of low-density lipoprotein cholesterol greater than 160 mg/dL, by 34% and the risk of macrovascular disease by 41%, although the latter differences were not statistically significant.[185]

Was there an increase in adverse events associated with the intensive treatment regimen? Overall mortality did not differ in the two treatment groups and was actually less than expected on the basis of population-based mortality studies. However, the incidence of severe hypoglycemia was approximately three times higher in the intensive therapy group than in the conventional therapy group ($P < .001$). Some of the episodes of hypoglycemia were quite severe, resulting in motor vehicle accidents or the need for hospitalization. Severe hypoglycemia occurred more often during sleep,[186] and of episodes that occurred while the patients were awake, a significant proportion (approximately one third) were not associated with warning symptoms. In intensively treated subjects predictors of hypoglycemia included a history of severe hypoglycemia, longer duration of diabetes, higher baseline HbA_{1c}, and a lower recent HbA_{1c}.

Weight gain also occurred more frequently in the intensively treated patients. Intensive therapy was associated with a 33% increase in risk of becoming overweight, defined as a body weight more than 120% above the ideal. Five years into the trial, patients being treated intensively had gained a mean of 4.6 kg more than patients receiving conventional therapy. Among subjects in the top quartile of weight gain, changes in plasma lipids, blood pressure, and body fat distribution were observed that were similar to those seen with insulin resistance.[187]

Goals of Treatment

On the basis of these results, the authors of the study recommended that most patients with type 1 diabetes be treated with an intensive treatment regimen under the close supervision of a health care team consisting of a physician, nurses, nutritionist, and behavioral and exercise specialists as needed. However, for certain groups of patients this recommendation may need to be modified because the risk-benefit ratio may not be as favorable as it was in the cohorts with mild or no diabetic complications that were studied in the DCCT. Patients for whom it may be appropriate to be more cautious about instituting intensive treatment regimens include children younger than 13 years, elderly people, and patients with advanced complications such as end-stage renal disease or significant cardiovascular or cerebrovascular disease. It has also been reported[188–190] that instituting aggressive insulin therapy in subjects with proliferative or severe nonproliferative retinopathy may lead to accelerated progression of retinopathy after the start of intensive therapy. Treatment of the eye disease should be considered before instituting an aggressive insulin regimen. In addition, patients who do not experience warning adrenergic symptoms of hypoglycemia (hypoglycemia unawareness) are at significantly greater risk for severe recurrent hypoglycemia, and this may prevent the safe institution of tight glucose control.[191]

Table 30–5. Glycemic Control for Nonpregnant Individuals with Diabetes*

Values	Normal	Goal	Additional Action Suggested†
Plasma values‡			
Average preprandial glucose (mg/dL)	<110	90–130	<90/>150
Average bedtime glucose (mg/dL)	<120	110–150	<110/>180
Whole blood values§			
Average preprandial glucose (mg/dL)	<100	80–120	<80/>140
Average bedtime glucose (mg/dL)	<110	100–140	<100/>160
A_{1c} (%)	<6	<7	>8

*The values shown in this table are by necessity generalized to the entire population of individuals with diabetes. Patients with comorbid diseases, the very young and older adults, and others with unusual conditions or circumstances may warrant different treatment goals. These values are for nonpregnant adults.

†Values above or below these levels are not goals, nor are they acceptable in most patients. They are an indication for a significant change in the treatment plan. Additional action suggested depends on individual patients' circumstances. Such actions may include enhanced diabetes self-management education, comanagement with a diabetes team, referral to an endocrinologist, change in pharmacologic therapy, initiation of or increase in self-monitored blood glucose, or more frequent contact with the patient. A_{1c} is referenced to a nondiabetic range of 4.0–6.0% (mean 5.0%, standard deviation 0.5%).

‡Values calibrated to plasma glucose.

§Measurement of capillary blood glucose.

From Diabetes Care 2002; 25:S33–S49, Table 6.

The American Diabetes Association revises and publishes treatment guidelines annually as the first supplement to *Diabetes Care*. The recommendations for 2002 are listed in Table 30–5. The goal of therapy is to achieve average preprandial plasma glucose concentrations in the range of 90 to 130 mg/dL, average bedtime plasma glucose values between 110 and 150 mg/dL, and A_{1c} values less than 7%.[192]

It is recognized that in order to achieve glucose control at this level patients need to monitor glucose levels at least three or four times per day and receive nutritional counseling and training in self-management of the insulin doses and problem solving to allow them to deal with the problems that they encounter in their daily lives. Hospitalization may be necessary for the initiation of therapy.

Team Approach to Treatment

As alluded to previously, because of the complex nature of modern intensive diabetes treatment regimens and the need for regular feedback and modification of the parameters of treatment, it has now become generally accepted that intensive insulin regimens can be instituted more effectively by a health care team rather than a physician alone. Members of the team can include diabetes nurse educators, nutritionists, psychologists, or medical social workers, and others such as exercise physiologists may also be included depending on the needs of a particular patient. A critical aspect of intensive diabetes treatment is the need to monitor continuously the effectiveness of specific components of the regimen and to make adjustments in response to changing life circumstances of the patient.

Pharmacokinetics of Available Insulin Preparations

In the past, insulin for human use was obtained from animal sources—beef and pig. With advances in recombinant DNA technology, it is now possible to produce large quantities of insulin with an amino acid structure identical to that of human insulin using laboratory strains of *Escherichia coli* bacteria or yeast that have been genetically altered by the addition of the gene for human insulin production. All forms of insulin have identical physiologic effects. They differ in the rapidity of the onset of action, the time from injection to peak action, and the duration of action depending on the chemical nature of the particular insulin preparation. These data are summarized in Table 30–6. The available insulins can be divided into three broad categories on a pharmacokinetic basis.

Rapid-Acting Insulins

These insulins have an onset of action within an hour or less and are used to reduce the peak of glycemia that occurs after meal ingestion.

1. *Regular insulin.* This form of insulin consists of zinc-insulin crystals dissolved in a clear fluid. The pharmacokinetic profile of regular insulin is related to the fact that after subcutaneous injection it tends to self-associate, first into dimers and then into hexamers, which result from the self-association of three dimers. Only the monomeric and dimeric forms can be absorbed to any appreciable degree.[193] The resulting relative delay in the onset and duration of action of regular insulin limits its effectiveness in controlling postprandial glucose.

2. *Insulin lispro* of recombinant DNA origin is a human insulin analogue created when amino acids at positions 28 and 29 on the human insulin B chain are reversed. Insulin lispro was the first insulin analogue to receive approval by the United States Food and Drug Administration. It is chemically Lys(B28), Pro(B29) insulin and is created in a special nonpathogenic laboratory strain of *E. coli* bacteria that has been genetically altered by the addition of the gene for insulin lispro. The effect of this amino acid rearrangement is to reduce the capacity of the insulin to self-aggregate in subcutaneous tissues, resulting in behavior similar to that of monomeric insulin. This leads to more rapid absorption and shorter duration of action of lispro compared with regular insulin when given by subcutaneous injection. However, lispro is not intrinsically more active and on a molar basis is equipotent to human insulin. When they are given by intravenous injection, the pharmacokinetic profiles of lispro and human regular insulin are similar. Because of its rapid onset of action within 5 to 15 minutes of administration and peak action within 1 to 2 hours, lispro is the first insulin that mimics the time course of the increase in plasma glucose seen after ingestion of a carbohydrate-rich meal.

3. *Insulin aspart* differs from human insulin by substitution

Table 30–6. Pharmacokinetic Properties of Insulin Preparation

Preparation	Onset	Peak	Duration
Rapid acting			
Regular	½–1 hr	2–4 hr	6–8 hr
Lispro	15 min	1 hr	3–4 hr
Aspart	15 min	1 hr	3–4 hr
Intermediate acting			
NPH	1–3 hr	6–8 hr	12–16 hr
Lente	1–4 hr	6–10 hr	14–18 hr
Long acting			
Ultralente	2–4 hr	8–10 hr	16–24 hr
Glargine	6 hr	Broad peak of activity lasting ~24 hr	

NPH, neutral protamine Hagedorn.

of aspartic acid for proline in position 28 on the chain, and this also leads to a more rapid onset and duration of action analogous to those of insulin lispro.

Whether there are substantial differences between the two available rapid-acting insulin analogues is controversial. Although little difference is observed in most cases by either patients or providers, there certainly may be differences at least in subsets of patients that could be exploited to improve glycemic control.

In general, treatment with monomeric insulin analogues (lispro and aspart) is associated with a lower risk of hypoglycemia, particularly in sleep, than treatment with regular insulin. It is quite easy to document improved glycemic control in the postprandial state. Finally, patients may inject these insulin analogues immediately before or after meals instead of 30 to 60 minutes before meals as is classically recommended with regular insulin, providing greater convenience. These features have been exploited in clinical trials to produce modest improvements in overall control with monomeric insulin analogues versus regular insulin.

Intermediate-Acting Insulins

These forms of insulin have a significantly longer delay in their onset and duration of action. In the setting of type 1 diabetes they are generally used in combination with a rapidly acting form of insulin although they may be given before bedtime to limit hyperglycemia overnight and in the early hours of the morning.

1. *NPH insulin.* This is a crystalline suspension of insulin with protamine and zinc providing an intermediate-acting insulin with onset of action in 1 to 3 hours, duration of action up to 24 hours, and peak action from 6 to 8 hours.
2. *Lente insulin.* This is an amorphous and crystalline suspension of insulin with zinc resulting in an intermediate pharmacokinetic profile. It generally has a slightly longer onset, peak, and duration of action than NPH insulin.

Long-Acting Insulins

Even after an overnight fast, the normal pancreas continues to secrete insulin. Investigators have long attempted to develop forms of insulin with pharmacokinetic properties that simulate the basal production of insulin.

1. *Ultralente insulin.* Ultralente insulin is also a preparation of insulin consisting of zinc insulin crystals. It has an onset of action in 2 to 4 hours and a prolonged duration that may be as long as 24 hours. The peak of action is broad and spans 8 to 16 hours. This formulation of insulin is arguably the most variably absorbed and can be associated in some patients with substantial variability in glycemic control.
2. *Insulin glargine.* Insulin glargine is a recombinant human insulin analogue that is long acting. It differs from human insulin in that the amino acid asparagine at position A21 is replaced by glycine and two arginines are added to the C-terminus of the B chain. In the injection solution at pH 4, insulin glargine is completely soluble. However, it has low aqueous solubility at neutral pH. After injection into the subcutaneous tissue, the acidic solution is neutralized, leading to the formation of microprecipitates from which small amounts of insulin glargine are slowly released, resulting in a broad increase in concentration over a 24-hour period with no pronounced peak. It thus simulates the basal production of insulin. In other respects the mechanism of action of glargine insulin is similar to that of human insulin, and on a molar basis its glucose-lowering effects are similar to those of human insulin when given intravenously. Because this insulin is provided in an acid vehicle, it cannot be mixed with other forms of insulin or intravenous fluids and some patients have greater discomfort with injection at least some of the time. In general, glargine is less variably absorbed than Ultralente, NPH, and Lente insulin and in clinical trials in patients with type 1 diabetes has been associated with a reduced risk of hypoglycemia, particularly nocturnal hypoglycemia. In about 10% of patients, insulin glargine must be taken twice daily to provide 24-hour coverage of basal insulin needs. In a smaller proportion of patients, there may be a modest peak in effect approximately 2 hours after injection.

Approach to the Treatment of Type 1 Diabetes

Levels of glucose control equivalent to those achieved in the intensive treatment group in the DCCT are not possible in the majority of patients unless the insulin regimen utilizes more than two injections of insulin with the patient adjusting the insulin dose depending on the results of self-monitoring of glucose as well as on the basis of dietary intake and physical activity. The reason for this is relatively simple. In patients with little or no endogenous insulin production, the exogenous insulin regimen needs to simulate the multiphasic profile of insulin secretory responses to meals and snacks present in normal subjects if levels of glycemia approaching normal are to be achieved.

A number of regimens have been used to achieve these ends. Three basic approaches are reviewed, although it is clear that other possible approaches may be effective in individual patients. Achieving the glycemic goals of therapy is far more important than the details of the insulin regimen. Nevertheless, one of the following three general approaches to therapy is most likely to lead to the desired outcome.

Combination of Rapid-Acting and Intermediate-Acting Insulin with Breakfast and Dinner and Intermediate-Acting Insulin at Bedtime

The rationale for these regimens is that the rapid-acting insulin (regular, lispro, or aspart) limits the postprandial glycemia after breakfast and dinner, the intermediate-acting insulin (NPH or Lente) administered before breakfast limits glycemia in the afternoon, and the intermediate-acting insulin before dinner limits glycemia in the early hours of the morning. Although such a regimen may be sufficient to achieve glucose targets in some patients, in many individuals the intermediate-acting insulin given before dinner is insufficient to control elevations in blood glucose commonly seen in the early morning (dawn phenomenon). Attempts to increase the dose of intermediate-acting insulin at dinner expose the patient to a greater risk of hypoglycemia in the middle of the night, hence the need for a smaller dose at bedtime to provide sufficient insulin to restrain the dawn phenomenon the following morning while moderating the risk of nocturnal hypoglycemia. This three-injection regimen was the mainstay of therapy in the DCCT but is rapidly being supplanted by regimens that take greater advantage of the availability of insulin analogues.

Combination of Rapid-Acting Insulin Given with Meals and Long-Acting Insulin at Bedtime

This combination of insulins can also simulate the pattern of insulin production that occurs normally. Use of monomeric insulin analogues provides excellent meal coverage. Use of insulin glargine provides excellent control of the fasting plasma glucose. This combination of rapid-acting monomeric insulin analogues with insulin glargine is rapidly supplanting human insulin–based treatment regimens as it seems to be associated with less variability in glycemic control associated with lower risks of hypoglycemia. Human Ultralente can be used as the basal insulin in such a regimen but would generally need to be administered twice daily.

Insulin Administration by an External Insulin Pump

An alternative method of delivering insulin is by an external mechanical pump. This approach involves the administration of a rapidly acting insulin preparation delivered by continuous subcutaneous infusion through a catheter usually inserted into the subcutaneous tissues of the anterior abdominal wall. The pumps deliver insulin as a preprogrammed basal infusion as well as patient-directed boluses given before meals or snacks or in response to elevations in the blood glucose concentration outside the desired range. With currently available pumps, the basal insulin infusion rate (usually approximately 1 U/hour) can be programmed either to continue at a constant rate over the 24-hour period or more commonly to increase and decrease at predetermined times of the day to prevent anticipated excursions in the blood glucose concentration, for example, morning rises in glucose. Newer pumps provide the ability to use multiple basal profiles to deal with recurrent patterns (e.g., menstruation, weekends, activity). Protocols for insulin administration by the pump usually require approximately half the insulin to be administered as a basal infusion and the remainder as premeal boluses.

Insulin administration by an external pump has some advantages over regimens that utilize multiple insulin injections. Only rapidly acting insulin is used in the insulin pump. Consequently, adjustments to the basal insulin infusion rate or changes in the size and timing of the insulin boluses result in more rapid changes in the blood glucose concentration than are possible when adjustments are made to the dose of intermediate-acting or long-acting insulin. This leads to greater flexibility for the patient. It has been suggested that use of lispro insulin may lead to a lower risk of hypoglycemia.[194, 195]

However, there are also disadvantages of insulin pump therapy. There is a significant initial cost of the pump itself. Furthermore, the tubing, which needs to be changed every 24 to 72 hours, and other supplies are expensive. The risk of infection at the site of insulin administration is significant. Infections occur on average once annually per patient even in the best of practices, and although these can usually be treated by changing the site of infusion and giving a short course of oral antibiotics, if an abscess develops surgical drainage may be necessary. In addition, because only rapidly acting insulin is used, pump failure as a result of mechanical malfunction or catheter-related problems can quickly result in severe hyperglycemia and even ketoacidosis. Patients treated with insulin pump therapy must monitor glucose frequently and always be alert to the possibility of failure of the infusion system.

Controlled clinical trials have indicated that on average intensive insulin regimens that use multiple insulin injections lead to levels of glucose control similar to those achieved with the insulin pump. On the other hand, there are some patients who never achieve adequate control with multiple daily injections but experience dramatic improvements with pump therapy. According to the Clinical Practice Recommendations of the American Diabetes Association,[196] the insulin pump should be used only by candidates strongly motivated to improve glucose control and willing to work with their health care provider in assuming substantial responsibility for their day-to-day care. They must also understand and demonstrate use of the insulin pump and self-monitoring of blood glucose and be able to use the data obtained in an appropriate fashion.

Algorithms of Insulin Administration

An essential component of intensive regimens of insulin replacement is the need to make regular adjustments to the insulin dose depending on the prevailing blood glucose concentration. Algorithms have been developed to guide these adjustments that aim to simulate the normal feedback control of insulin secretion whereby hyperglycemia stimulates and hypoglycemia inhibits insulin secretion. They all involve frequent monitoring of the blood glucose concentration, generally three or four times per day or more, with increases in the insulin dose if glucose levels are above the target upper level that is judged to be acceptable and reductions in the insulin dose if glucose levels are below the acceptable lower level. Many algorithms are in use; one example is shown in Table 30–7.

Table 30–7. Sample Algorithm for Premeal Insulin Lispro Supplements*

Premeal Blood Glucose				
mmol/L	**mg/dL**	**Insulin Dose**	**Lag Time†**	**Comments**
<2.8	<50	Decrease by 2 U	Inject during meal	Include at least 10 g of simple carbohydrate in the meal
2.8–4.4	50–80	Decrease by 1 U	0	
4.4–7.2	80–130	No change	0	
7.2–8.3	130–150	Increase by 1 U	0	
8.3–11.1	150–200	Increase by 2 U	10 min	
11.1–13.9	200–250	Increase by 3 U	15 min	
13.9–16.7	250–300	Increase by 4 U	20 min	Urinary ketones, especially with CSII
16.7–19.4	300–350	Increase by 5 U	25 min	Urinary ketones, especially with CSII; if moderate or large, increase fluid intake, consider additional insulin

(From Hirsch IB. Intensive treatment of type 1 diabetes. Med Clin North Am 1998; 82:689–719.)

*Assumes preprandial target of 4.4 to 7.2 mmol/L (60 to 130 mg/dL). Initial supplements may be based on previous experience or *1500 rule* (1500/total insulin dose = the effect of 1 U insulin on blood glucose decrease in mg/dL). Plans should be individualized for each patient. This example would likely be treated with ~50 units per day of insulin.

†Refers to the amount of time between injecting the insulin and eating.

CSII, continuous subcutaneous insulin infusion.

Complications of Insulin Therapy

Hypoglycemia

The most serious complication of intensive regimens of insulin replacement is hypoglycemia, and this is generally the factor that limits patients' ability to achieve tight glucose control. In the DCCT, patients in the intensive treatment group had an approximately threefold greater risk of hypoglycemia than those in the conventional treatment group. Hypoglycemia may be life-threatening, leading to motor vehicle accidents, serious falls with fractures, and seizures. Patients with type 1 diabetes have serious defects in mechanisms responsible for glucose counterregulation, and this is a major underlying reason for the predisposition to hypoglycemia. Glucose counterregulation is reviewed in detail in Chapter 32.

The risk of hypoglycemia can be reduced if all patients treated with intensive regimens of insulin replacement are carefully educated about recognition of hypoglycemic symptoms and measures that should be taken to avoid more serious hypoglycemia after symptoms are initially experienced. Certain patients, particularly those with long-standing diabetes and autonomic neuropathy, may not subjectively sense symptoms of hypoglycemia even in the presence of low glucose concentrations. Glycemic targets of therapy should be adjusted upward in these subjects because they are at particularly high risk of hypoglycemia. Similarly, patients with advanced end-stage microvascular or macrovascular diabetic complications in whom the benefit of intensive glucose control is likely to be less should not be exposed to the increased risk of hypoglycemia that is inherent in extremely intensive insulin treatment regimens.

In addition to the availability of glucose tablets, hard candy or other sources of a readily absorbable form of carbohydrate, all patients with type 1 diabetes should have emergency glucagon kits at home and at work, assuming that there are people in those settings who can be trained in their use. The administration of 0.5 to 1 mg of glucagon intramuscularly to a severely symptomatic person with hypoglycemia rapidly raises the plasma glucose concentration to an acceptable range and avoids the difficulties and dangers associated with attempting to get a stuporous or disoriented individual to ingest glucose by mouth. Nevertheless, because of occasional failures of glucagon to reverse hypoglycemia fully, friends and family members should always be instructed to call for medical assistance as soon as the injection is provided.

Weight Gain

Improvement in glucose control with a reduction in glycosuria is invariably associated with weight gain as the leakage of calories into the urine is reduced or eliminated. In addition, increased food intake to treat or prevent hypoglycemia can contribute to weight gain. Insulin itself may stimulate appetite. As a result of the combination of all these effects, weight gain is common, particularly with intensive regimens of insulin replacement.

Worsening of Retinopathy

Institution of regimens of tight glucose control has been reported to exacerbate the underlying retinopathy. Thus, if a patient with serious background or proliferative retinopathy presents in poor glucose control, consideration should be given to ophthalmologic treatment of the retinopathy before instituting tight glucose control.

Insulin Allergy

Insulin allergy has become much less common with the use of human insulin. Most manifestations of allergic reactions to insulin consist of local wheal-and-flare reactions at the site of injection. The allergic reaction can be to the insulin itself or to other components of the insulin preparation such as the protamine in NPH insulin. Occasionally, more generalized allergic reactions occur, and even more rarely anaphylactic reactions take place. In general, mild local allergic reactions to insulin can be treated with antihistamines. More severe reactions require desensitization. Admission to the hospital is necessary, and under close supervision of a physician with access to equipment for emergency resuscitation a protocol is followed in which the patient is exposed to gradually increasing amounts of insulin administered according to a set schedule.[197]

ACUTE DIABETIC EMERGENCIES: DIABETIC KETOACIDOSIS

Diabetic ketoacidosis (DKA) is a life-threatening condition in which severe insulin deficiency leads to hyperglycemia, excessive lipolysis, and unrestrained fatty acid oxidation producing the ketone bodies acetone, β-hydroxybutyrate, and acetoacetate. This results in metabolic acidosis, dehydration, and deficits in fluid and electrolytes. Excess secretion of primarily glucagon as well as catecholamines, glucocorticoids, and growth hormone in combination with insulin deficiency produces hyperglycemia by stimulating glycogenolysis and gluconeogenesis and impairing glucose disposal. DKA is a far more characteristic feature of type 1 than of type 2 diabetes but may be seen in persons with type 2 diabetes under conditions of stress such as occurs with serious infections, trauma, and cardiovascular or other emergencies.

Clinical Presentation

Patients with uncontrolled diabetes present with nonspecific complaints. If the disease follows an indolent course over months to years, patients can manifest profound wasting, cachexia, and prostration similar in degree to those of patients with long-standing malignancy or chronic infection. With significant physical or emotional stress, sudden metabolic decompensation can occur. The cases of DKA that are misdiagnosed usually occur in patients with new-onset diabetes. Polyuria (or at least nocturia) and weight loss are almost always present, although often not reported by the patient. Any patient with severe illness (acute or chronic) or neurologic changes should have glucose and electrolytes measured.

In DKA, metabolic decompensation usually develops over a period of hours to a few days. Patients with DKA classically present with lethargy and a characteristic hyperventilation pattern with deep slow breaths (Kussmaul's respirations) associated with the fruity odor of acetone. They often complain of nausea and vomiting, with abdominal pain being somewhat less frequent. The abdominal pain can be quite severe and may be associated with distention, ileus, and tenderness without rebound but usually resolves relatively quickly with therapy unless there is underlying abdominal pathology. Most patients are normotensive, tachycardic, and tachypneic with signs of mild to moderate volume depletion. Hypothermia has been described in DKA, and patients with underlying infection may not manifest fever. Cerebral edema does occur, generally during therapy. Patients with DKA can be stuporous with obvious profound dehydration and often demonstrate focal neurologic deficits such as Babinski's reflexes, asymmetric reflexes, cranial nerve findings, paresis, fasciculations, and aphasia.

Laboratory Test Results and Differential Diagnosis

Laboratory tests that would be routinely monitored in the setting of DKA include the following:

1. Hemoglobin, white blood cell and differential count.
2. Glucose, electrolytes, blood urea nitrogen (BUN), creatinine.
3. Changes in Na, K, Cl, P, BUN, creatinine.

The sine qua non of DKA is acidosis, and the serum HCO_3 concentration is usually less than 10 mEq/L. The acidosis is due to production and accumulation of ketones in the serum. Three ketones are produced in DKA—two ketoacids, β-hydroxybutyrate and acetoacetate, as well as the neutral ketone acetone. Ketones can be detected in serum and urine using the nitroprusside reaction on diagnostic strips for use at the patient's bedside or in the clinical laboratory. This test detects acetoacetate more effectively than acetone and does not detect an increased concentration of β-hydroxybutyrate. Particularly in severe DKA, β-hydroxybutyrate is the predominant ketone, and it is possible although unusual to have a negative serum nitroprusside reaction in the presence of severe ketosis. However, under these circumstances the serum HCO_3 is still markedly reduced and the anion gap is increased, indicative of the presence of metabolic acidosis. The urinary β-hydroxybutyrate can be measured at many centers and commercially but is not usually readily available. The anion gap is a readily available index for unmeasured anions in the blood (normal < 14 mEq/L):

$$\text{Anion gap} = \text{sodium} - (\text{chloride} + \text{bicarbonate})$$

Most patients with DKA present with an anion gap greater than 20 mEq/L and some with a gap greater than 40 mEq/L. However, occasional patients have a hyperchloremic metabolic acidosis without a significant anion gap.[198] Patients with DKA almost invariably have large amounts of ketones in their urine. The serum glucose in DKA is usually in the 500 mg/dL range. However, an entity known as euglycemic DKA has been described, particularly in the presence of decreased oral intake or in pregnancy, in which the serum glucose is normal or near normal but the patient requires insulin therapy for the clearance of ketoacidosis.[199] The arterial pH is commonly less than 7.3 and can be as low as 6.5. There is partial respiratory compensation with hypocarbia. Patients are often mildly hyperosmolar, although osmolalities greater than 330 mOsm/kg are unusual without mental status changes.

Not all patients with hyperglycemia and an anion gap metabolic acidosis have DKA and other causes of metabolic acidosis must be considered in these patients, particularly if the serum or urine ketone measurements are not elevated. The following causes of metabolic acidosis need to be considered in the differential diagnosis of DKA.

1. *Lactic acidosis* is the most common cause of metabolic acidosis in hospitalized patients and can be seen in patients with uncomplicated diabetes as well as those with DKA. Lactic acidosis usually occurs in the setting of decreased tissue oxygen delivery resulting in the nonoxidative metabolism of glucose to lactic acid. Lactic acidosis complicates other primary metabolic acidoses as a consequence of dehydration or shock, and assessing its relative contribution can be difficult. The presentation is identical to that of DKA. In pure lactic acidosis, the serum glucose and ketones should be normal and the serum lactate concentration should be greater than 5 mM. The therapy of lactic acidosis is directed at the underlying cause and optimizing tissue perfusion.[200]

2. *Starvation ketosis* results from inadequate carbohydrate availability resulting in physiologically appropriate lipolysis and ketone production to provide fuel substrates for muscle. The blood glucose is usually normal. Although the urine can have large amounts of ketones, the blood rarely does. Arterial pH is normal, and the anion gap is at most mildly elevated.

3. *Alcoholic ketoacidosis* is a more severe form of starvation ketosis wherein the appropriate ketogenic response to poor carbohydrate intake is increased through as yet poorly defined effects of alcohol on the liver. Classically, these patients are long-standing alcoholics for whom ethanol has been the main caloric source for days to weeks. The ketoacidosis occurs when for some reason alcohol and caloric intake decreases. In isolated alcoholic ketoacidosis, the metabolic acidosis is usually mild to moderate in severity. The anion gap is elevated. Serum and urine ketones are always present. However, alcoholic ketoacidosis produces an even higher ratio of β-hydroxybutyrate to acetoacetate than DKA, and negative or weakly positive nitroprusside reactions are common. Respiratory alkalosis associated with delirium tremens, agitation, or pulmonary processes often normalizes the pH but should be evident with careful analysis of acid-base status. Usually, the patient is normoglycemic or hypoglycemic, although mild hyperglycemia is occasionally present. Patients who are significantly hyperglycemic should be treated as if they have DKA. The therapy of alcoholic ketoacidosis consists of thiamine, carbohydrates, fluids, and electrolytes with special attention to the more severe consequences of alcohol toxicity, alcohol withdrawal, and chronic malnutrition. In more severely ill patients in whom alcoholic ketoacidosis is considered a possibility, there is usually another underlying illness such as pancreatitis, gastrointestinal bleeding, hepatic encephalopathy, delirium tremens, or infection complicated by concomitant lactic acidosis.[201, 202]

4. *Uremic acidosis* is characterized by extremely large elevations in the BUN (often > 200) and creatinine (>10) with normoglycemia. The pH and anion gap are usually only mildly abnormal. The treatment is supportive with careful attention to fluid and electrolytes until dialysis can be performed. Rhabdomyolysis is a cause of renal failure in which the anion gap can be significantly elevated and acidosis can be severe. There should be marked elevation of creatine phosphokinase and myoglobin. It should be noted that mild rhabdomyolysis is not uncommon in DKA, but the presence of hyperglycemia and ketonemia leaves no doubt about the primary etiology of the acidosis.[203]

5. *Toxic ingestions* can be differentiated from DKA by history and laboratory investigation. Salicylate intoxication produces an anion gap metabolic acidosis usually with a respiratory alkalosis. The plasma glucose is normal or low, the osmolality normal, ketones negative, and salicylates can be detected in the urine or blood. It should be noted that salicylates can cause a false-positive glucose determination when using the cupric sulfate method and a false-negative result when using the glucose oxidase reaction. Methanol and ethylene glycol also produce an anion gap metabolic acidosis without hyperglycemia or ketones but need to be kept in mind primarily because they produce an increase in the measured serum osmolality but not in the calculated serum osmolality—an osmolar gap. Their serum levels can also be measured. Isopropyl alcohol does not cause a metabolic acidosis but should be remembered because it is metabolized to acetone, which can produce a positive result in the nitroprusside reaction commonly used for the detection of ketoacids. These intoxications must be appropriately treated.[204–206] Rare cases of anion gap acidoses have been reported with other ingestions including toluene, iron, hydrogen sulfide, nalidixic acid, papaverine, paraldehyde, strychnine, isoniazid, and outdated tetracycline.

When DKA is considered, the diagnosis can be made quickly with routine laboratory tests. Blood and urine glucose and ketones can be obtained in minutes with glucose oxidase–impregnated strips and the nitroprusside reaction, respectively.

Osmolarity

The increase in osmolarity that occurs in DKA must be differentiated from the increase in osmolarity seen in hyperosmolar-hyperglycemic nonketotic (diabetic) coma (HHNC). The osmolarity can be measured by freezing point depression or estimated using the following formula:

$$\text{Osmolarity (mOsm/L)} = 2 \times \text{sodium} + \text{glucose}/18 + \text{BUN}/2.8 + \text{ethanol}/4.6$$

Patients with DKA not uncommonly present with hyperosmolarity and coma. In HHNC, the osmolarity is generally greater than 350 mOsm/L and can exceed 400 mOsm/L. The serum sodium and potassium can be high, normal, or low and do not reflect total-body levels, which are uniformly depleted. The glucose is usually greater than 600 mg/dL, and levels over 1000 mg/dL are quite common. In pure HHNC, there is not a significant metabolic acidosis or anion gap.

It should be remembered that patients often present with combinations of the preceding findings. HHNC can involve mild to moderate ketonemia and acidosis. Alcoholic ketoacidosis can contribute to either DKA or HHNC. Lactic acidosis is common in severe DKA and HHNC. Any patient with hyperglycemia greater than 250 mg/dL and an anion gap metabolic acidosis should be treated by the general principles outlined in the following with special consideration of other possible contributing metabolic acidoses.

Therapy

The optimal management of DKA has been the source of considerable controversy over the past half-century. Only recently have prospective studies of various therapeutic approaches been performed. The guidelines we propose rely heavily on prospective studies of DKA by Kitabchi[207] and coworkers. The general approach is to (1) provide necessary fluids to restore the circulation, (2) treat insulin deficiency with continuous insulin, (3) treat electrolyte disturbances, (4) observe the patient closely and carefully, and (5) search for underlying causes of metabolic decompensation.

Fluids

Volume contraction is one of the hallmarks of DKA. It can contribute to acidosis through lactic acid production as well as decreased renal clearance of organic and inorganic acids. It contributes to hyperglycemia by decreasing renal clearance of glucose. If decreased tissue perfusion is significant, it causes insulin resistance by decreasing insulin delivery to the sites of insulin-mediated glucose disposal, namely muscle and adipose tissue, as well as through stimulation of catecholamine and glucocorticoid secretion. Fluid deficits on the order of 5 to 10 L are common in DKA. It should be remembered that the urine produced during the osmotic diuresis of hyperglycemia is approximately half-normal with respect to sodium. Therefore, water deficits are in excess of sodium deficits. Historically, large quantities of isotonic intravenous fluids have been administered rapidly to patients in DKA. For patients with a history of congestive heart failure, chronic or acute renal failure, severe hypotension, or significant pulmonary disease, early invasive hemodynamic monitoring should be considered.

When there is physical evidence of dehydration—that is, hypotension, decreased skin turgor, or dry mucous membranes—generally administer 1 L of normal saline over the first hour and 200 to 500 mL/hour in subsequent hours until hypotension resolves and adequate circulation is maintained. If hypotension is severe with clinical evidence of hypoperfusion and does not respond to crystalloid, therapy with colloid is considered, often in combination with invasive hemodynamic monitoring. If there is no hypotension and no concern about renal failure, administer 1 L of half-normal saline over the first hour.

During that first hour, the laboratory data usually return and can be quite helpful in planning further therapy. Despite the excess of water losses over sodium, the measured sodium is usually low because of osmotic effects of glucose. These osmotic effects can be corrected using a simple formula:

$$\text{Corrected sodium concentration} = \text{measured sodium} + 0.016(\text{glucose} - 100)$$

Severe hypertriglyceridemia, which is common in severe diabetes, can cause a false decrease in the serum sodium concentration by approximately 1.0 mEq/L at a serum lipid concentration of 460 mg/dL.[197] An estimated water deficit can be calculated using the corrected sodium:

$$\text{Water deficit in liters} = 0.6\ (\text{weight in kg})\ [(\text{sodium}/140) - 1]$$

Using these formulas, a 70-kg patient with a measured sodium level of 140 mEq/L and a glucose concentration of 1000 mg/dL would have a calculated water deficit of 4.3 L. If the patient is normotensive after the first liter of fluids, it would be reasonable to aim to replace urinary losses with one-half normal saline and also provide approximately one half the water deficit as 5% dextrose over the first 12 to 24 hours (using the preceding example, 2 L) and the remainder over the subsequent 24 hours. The plan for fluid therapy should be continuously reevaluated in light of the clinical and laboratory response of the patient. When the serum glucose reaches 250 to 300 mg/dL, all fluids should contain 5% dextrose and therapy should be aimed at maintaining the serum glucose in that range for 24 hours to allow slow equilibration of osmotically active substances across cell membranes.

The primary goal of fluid therapy is to maintain an adequate circulation and secondly to maintain a brisk diuresis. Beyond that, pulmonary edema, hyperchloremic metabolic acidosis, and a rapid fall in the serum osmolality should be avoided by frequent monitoring of the patient, glucose, and electrolytes. It has been demonstrated that fluid administration and subsequent continued osmotic diuresis are responsible for a large portion of the initial decline in glucose during therapy.

Insulin

Insulin is the mainstay of therapy of DKA because it is essentially an insulin-deficient state. In the past, high doses of insulin (upward of 50 U/hour) were favored. In later studies, low-dose insulin therapy (0.1 U/kg per hour) has been shown to be as effective as higher doses in producing a decrease in serum glucose and clearance of ketones. Furthermore, low-dose therapy results in a reduction in the major morbidity of intensive insulin therapy, namely hypoglycemia and hypokalemia.

Studies have also shown that intravenous insulin is significantly more effective than intramuscular or subcutaneous insulin in lowering the ketone body concentration over the first 2 hours of therapy. The subcutaneous route is inappropriate for the critically ill patient because of the possibility of tissue hypoperfusion and slower kinetics of absorption. There are numerous studies that attest to the efficacy of intramuscular therapy in severe DKA. In cases in which there is insufficient nursing monitoring or intravenous access to allow safe intravenous administration, intramuscular therapy would be the route of choice.

Lastly, it has been shown that a 10-U intravenous insulin priming dose when insulin therapy is started significantly improves the glycemic response to the first hour of therapy. The rationale is to saturate insulin receptors fully before beginning continuous therapy and to avoid the lag time necessary to achieve steady-state insulin levels. When mixing insulin in normal saline, it does not seem to be necessary to add albumin to prevent insulin adsorption to the infusion set. However, the intravenous tubing should be flushed with the insulin infusate before use.

In the rare instances in which the glucose does not decrease at least 10% or 50 mg/dL in an hour, the insulin infusion rate should be increased by 50% to 100% and a second bolus of intravenous insulin administered. As the glucose level decreases, it is usually necessary to decrease the rate of infusion. After the glucose reaches approximately 250 mg/dL, it is prudent to decrease the insulin infusion rate and administer dextrose. It usually takes an additional 12 to 24 hours to clear ketones from the circulation after hyperglycemia is controlled. With resolution of ketosis, the rate of infusion approaches the physiologic range of 0.3 to 0.5 U/kg per day.

When the decision is made to feed the patient, the patient should be switched from intravenous or intramuscular therapy to subcutaneous therapy. Subcutaneous insulin should be administered before a meal and the insulin drip discontinued approximately 30 minutes later. The glucose should be checked in 2 hours and at least every 4 hours subsequently until a relatively stable insulin regimen is determined.

Potassium

Potassium losses during the development of DKA are usually quite high (3 to 10 mEq/kg) and are mediated by shifts to the extracellular space secondary to acidosis and protein catabolism compounded by hyperaldosteronism and osmotic diuresis. Although most patients with DKA or HHNC have normal or even high serum potassium at presentation, the initial therapy with fluids and insulin causes it to fall.

Our approach has been to monitor the electrocardiogram (ECG) for signs of hyperkalemia (peaked T wave, QRS widening) initially and to administer potassium if these are absent and the serum potassium is less than 5.5 mEq/L. If the patient is oliguric, we do not administer potassium unless the serum concentration is less than 4 mEq/L or there are ECG signs of hypokalemia (U wave), and even then it is done with extreme caution. With therapy of DKA, the potassium level always falls, usually reaching a nadir after several hours. We usually replace potassium at 10 to 20 mEq/hour, one half as potassium chloride and one half as potassium phosphate, and monitor serum levels at least every 2 hours initially as well as follow ECG morphology. Occasionally, patients with DKA who have had protracted courses with vomiting present with hypokalemia and acidosis and may require 40 to 60 mEq/hour by central line to avoid further decreases in the serum potassium.

Phosphate

Like potassium, phosphate is depleted in patients with DKA. Although patients usually present with elevated serum phosphate, the serum level declines with therapy. No well-documented clinical significance of these findings has been determined and no benefit of phosphate administration has been demonstrated, but most authorities recommend phosphate therapy as before and monitoring for its possible complications—hypocalcemia and hypomagnesemia.

Bicarbonate

Serum bicarbonate is always low in DKA, but a true deficit is not present because the ketoacid and lactate anions are metabolized to bicarbonate during therapy. The use of bicarbonate in the therapy of DKA is highly controversial. No benefit of bicarbonate therapy has been demonstrated in clinical trials. In fact, in two trials, hypokalemia was more common in bicarbonate-treated patients. There are theoretical considerations against the use of bicarbonate. Cellular levels of 2,3-diphosphoglycerate are depleted in DKA, causing a shift in the oxyhemoglobin dissociation curve to the left and thus impairing tissue oxygen delivery. Acidemia has the opposite effect, and therefore reversing acidosis acutely could decrease tissue oxygen delivery. In addition, there are in vitro data suggesting that pH is a regulator of cellular lactate metabolism and correction of acidosis could increase lactate production. These observations are of questionable clinical relevance, however.

We reserve bicarbonate therapy for use (1) in patients with severe acidosis (pH < 6.9), (2) in the presence of hemodynamic instability if the pH is less than 7.1, or (3) in cases of hyperkalemia with ECG findings. When bicarbonate is used, it should be used sparingly and considered a temporizing measure while definitive therapy with insulin and fluids is under way. Approximately 1 mEq/kg of bicarbonate is administered as a rapid infusion over 10 to 15 minutes with further therapy based on repeated arterial blood gases every 30 to 120 minutes. Potassium therapy should be considered before treatment with bicarbonate as transient hypokalemia is not an uncommon complication of the administration of alkali.

Monitoring

It is possible to manage many cases of mild DKA without admission to the intensive care unit, depending on staff availability. We routinely admit patients with DKA to the intensive care unit if they have a pH less than 7.3. If mental status is compromised, prophylactic intubation is considered and nasogastric suctioning is always performed because of frequent ileus and danger of aspiration. If the patient cannot void at will, bladder catheterization is necessary to follow urine output adequately. ECG monitoring is continuous with hourly documentation of QRS intervals as well as T-wave morphology. Initially, serum glucose, electrolytes, BUN, creatinine, calcium, magnesium, phosphate, ketones, lactate, creatine phosphokinase, and liver function tests as well as urinalysis, ECG, upright chest radiograph, complete blood count, and arterial blood gases are obtained. If there is any concern about possible toxic ingestions, toxicology screening is also performed. Subsequently, glucose and electrolytes are measured at least hourly; calcium, magnesium, and phosphate every 2 hours; and BUN, creatinine, and ketones every 6 to 24 hours.

It is often not necessary to monitor arterial blood gases routinely because bicarbonate and anion gap are relatively good indices of the response to therapy. Monitoring venous pH has also been shown to reflect acidemia and response to therapy adequately. Usually, frequent blood work is necessary only for the first 12 hours or so. In the severely ill patient with obvious underlying disease, the course is often more protracted and, particularly when venous access is a problem, early consideration should be given to placement of an arterial line. A flow sheet tabulating these findings as well as mental status, vital signs, insulin dose, fluid and electrolytes administered, and urine output allows easy analysis of response to therapy. When the acidosis begins to resolve and the response to therapy becomes predictable, it is reasonable to curtail laboratory use. If cardiovascular status is unclear or troublesome, invasive hemodynamic monitoring is an appropriate guide for fluid therapy. The goals should be to achieve hemodynamic stability rapidly and to correct DKA fully in 12 to 36 hours.

Search for Underlying Causes

After stabilizing the patient, a careful history and physical examination and a diagnostic strategy should be aimed at determining the precipitating event. In most inner-city practices, the most common cause of DKA is noncompliance with insulin therapy and is usually easily treated. The second most common cause is infection, with viral syndromes, urinary tract infection, pelvic inflammatory disease, and pneumonia predominating. It is often difficult to determine initially whether the patient is infected. Fever can be absent in a significant proportion of patients with diabetic emergencies. The white blood cell count is not uncommonly elevated in the range of 20,000 or higher even in the absence of infection.[208] As a result, cultures should be performed for most patients, and if there is significant concern about infection, empirical broad antibiotic coverage should be considered pending microbiologic findings.

Special consideration should be given to ruling out meningitis in the patient with altered mental status. In this regard, most would perform lumbar punctures in all patients with meningismus and in patients with disproportionate mental status changes. If the index of suspicion is lower, gear the antibiotic therapy to cover bacterial meningitis and perform a lumbar puncture if the mental status does not improve quickly with therapy. The cerebrospinal fluid glucose is not particularly useful in determining whether the fluid is infected, and a cerebrospinal fluid glucose level less than 100 mg/dL is unusual when the serum glucose is greater than 250 mg/dL.[209] The relative frequency of sinus infection (particularly *Mucor*), foot infection, bacterial arthritis, cholecystitis, cellulitis, and necrotizing fascitis should also be considered.

Pneumonia can be difficult to diagnose in patients with dehydration because the alveolar edema fluid that shows up as an infiltrate on chest radiographs is often not present but develops along with progressive hypoxia during hydration. To avoid this occurrence, we administer intravenous fluid judiciously to patients we suspect have pneumonia. Pancreatitis and pregnancy are common precipitants and should be especially considered when assessing the abdominal pain that is almost ubiquitous at presentation. Abdominal guarding and tenderness associated with vomiting are common, and rebound is occasionally present. These symptoms and findings usually resolve quickly with therapy in the absence of intra-abdominal pathology. The serum amylase is often elevated without pathologic significance, although lipase is usually more specific.[210] Acute myocardial infarction and stroke as well as thromboembolic phenomena are frequent precipitants and complications of DKA.

The more insulin resistant the patient seems to be, the more likely one is to find a precipitating cause. If a precipitating cause is found, treatment is essential if adequate metabolic control is to be achieved.

Complications and Prognosis

It should now be possible to treat almost all cases of DKA successfully. The most troublesome complication is cerebral edema. It is common particularly in children and can be fatal. In most series, specific causes could not be assigned, although aggressive hydration, particularly with hypotonic fluids, may contribute.[211] In 50% of patients who subsequently had a respiratory arrest, there were premonitory symptoms, and despite early intervention only half of them avoided severe or fatal brain damage. Other complications of life-threatening severity that have been reported include the acute respiratory distress syndrome and bronchial mucous plugging.[212–214] Arterial and venous thromboembolic events are quite common. Standard prophylactic low-dose heparin is certainly reasonable in patients with DKA, but currently no indication exists for full anticoagulation.

References

1. Sutherland DE, Sibley R, Xu XA, et al. Twin-to-twin pancreas transplantation: reversal and reenactment of the pathogenesis of type I diabetes. Trans Assoc Am Physicians 1984; 97:80–87.
2. Wang YO, Ponteselli RG, Gill RG, et al. The role of CD4 and CD8 T cells in the destruction of islet grafts by diabetic NOD mice. Proc Natl Acad Sci USA 1991; 88:527–531.
3. Gottlieb PA, Eisenbarth GS. Human autoimmune diabetes (type 1A diabetes). Unpublished work, 1999.
4. Bach JF. Etiology and pathogenesis of human insulin-dependent diabetes mellitus. In Volpe R (ed). Contemporary Endocrinology: Autoimmune Endocrinopathies. Totowa, NJ, Humana Press, 1999, pp 293–307.
5. American Diabetes Association. Report of the Expert Committee on the Diagnosis and Classification of Diabetes Mellitus. Diabetes Care 1997; 20:1183–1197.
6. Leslie RD, Atkinson MA, Notkins AL. Autoantigens IA-2 and GAD in type I (insulin-dependent) diabetes. Diabetologia 1999; 42:3–14.
7. Rewers M, Norris JM. Epidemiology of type I diabetes. In Eisenbarth GS, Lafferty KJ (eds). Type I Diabetes: Molecular, Cellular, and Clinical Immunology, 1st ed. New York, Oxford University Press, 1996, pp 172–208.
8. Pinhas-Hamiel O, Dolan LM, Daniels SR, et al. Increased incidence of non–insulin dependent diabetes mellitus among adolescents. J Pediatr 1996; 128:608–615.
9. Pinhas-Haniel O, Dolan LM, Zeitlers PS. Diabetic ketoacidosis among obese African-American adolescents with NIDDM. Diabetes Care 1997; 20:484–486.
10. Rosenbloom AL, House DV, Winter WE. Non–insulin dependent diabetes mellitus (NIDDM) in minority youth: research priorities and needs. Clin Pediatr (Phila) 1998; 37:143–152.
11. Imagawa A, Hanafusa T, Miyagawa J. A novel subtype of type 1 diabetes mellitus characterized by a rapid onset and an absence of diabetes-related antibodies. N Engl J Med 2000; 342:301–307.
12. Ziegler A-G, Hummel M, Schenker M, Bonifacio E. Autoantibody appearance and risk for development of childhood diabetes in offspring of parents with type 1 diabetes: the 2-year analysis of the German BABYDIAB study. Diabetes 1999; 48:460–468.
13. Mordes JP, Bortell R, Doukas J, et al. The BB/Wor rat and the balance hypothesis of autoimmunity. Diabetes Metab Rev 1996; 12:103–109.
14. Atkinson MA, Leiter EH. The NOD mouse model of type 1 diabetes: as good as it gets? Nat Med 1999; 5:601–604.
15. Thomas HE, Kay TW. Beta cell destruction in the development of autoimmune diabetes in the non-obese diabetic (NOD) mouse. Diabetes Metab Res Rev 2000; 16:251–261.
16. Wong FS, Janeway CAJ. Insulin-dependent diabetes mellitus and its animal models. Curr Opin Immunol 1999; 11:643–647.
17. Leiter EH. Lessons from the animal models: the NOD mouse. In Palmer JP (ed). Prediction, Prevention, and Genetic Counseling in IDDM. Chichester, England, Wiley, 1996, pp 201–227.
18. Hattori M, Buse JB, Jackson RA, et al. The NOD mouse: recessive diabetogenic gene within the major histocompatibility complex. Science 1986; 231:733–735.
19. Noble JA, Valdes AM, Cook M, et al. The role of HLA class II genes in insulin-dependent diabetes mellitus: molecular analysis of 180 Caucasian, multiplex families. Am J Hum Genet 1996; 59: 1134–1148.
20. Todd JA, Bell JI, McDevitt HO. *HLA-DQB* gene contributes to susceptibility and resistance to insulin-dependent diabetes mellitus. Nature 1987; 329:599–604.
21. Nishimoto H, Kikutani H, Yamamura K, Kishimoto T. Prevention of autoimmune insulitis by expression of I-E molecules in NOD mice. Nature 1987; 328:432–434.
22. Singer SM, Tisch R, Yang XD, et al. Prevention of diabetes in NOD mice by a mutated I-Ab transgene. Diabetes 1998; 47: 1570–1577.
23. Lyons PA, Hancock WW, Denny P, et al. The NOD Idd9

genetic interval influences the pathogenicity of insulitis and contains molecular variants of Cd30, Tnfr2, and Cd137. Immunity 2000; 13:107–115.
24. Mathews CE, Graser RT, Serreze DV, Leiter EH. Reevaluation of the major histocompatibility complex genes of the NOD-progenitor CTS/Shi strain. Diabetes 2000; 49:131–134.
25. Yui MA, Muralidharan K, Moreno-Altamirano B, et al. Production of congenic mouse strains carrying NOD-derived diabetogenic genetic intervals: an approach for the genetic dissection of complex traits. Mamm Genome 1996; 7:331–334.
26. Wicker LS, Miller BJ, Coker LZ, et al. Genetic control of diabetes and insulitis in the nonobese diabetic (NOD) mouse. J Exp Med 1987; 165:1639–1654.
27. Yu L, Robles DT, Abiru N, et al. Early expression of anti-insulin autoantibodies of man and the NOD mouse: evidence for early determination of subsequent diabetes. Proc Natl Acad Sci USA 2000; 97:1701–1706.
28. Sreenan S, Pick AJ, Levisetti M, et al. Increased β-cell proliferation and reduced mass before diabetes onset in the nonobese diabetic mouse. Diabetes 1999; 48:989–996.
29. Dilts SM, Lafferty KJ. Autoimmune diabetes: the involvement of benign and malignant autoimmunity. J Autoimmun 1999; 12: 229–232.
30. Shimada A, Charlton B, Taylor-Edwards C, Fathman CG. β-cell destruction may be a late consequence of the autoimmune process in nonobese diabetic mice. Diabetes 1996; 45:1063–1067.
31. Chatenoud L, Primo J, Bach JF. CD3 antibody–induced dominant self tolerance in overtly diabetic NOD mice. J Immunol 1997; 158:2947–2954.
32. Wegmann DR, Eisenbarth GS. It's Insulin. J Autoimmun 2000; 15:286–291.
33. Nagata M, Santamaria P, Kawamura T, et al. Evidence for the role of CD8$^+$ cytotoxic T cells in the destruction of pancreatic β-cells in nonobese diabetic mice. J Immunol 1994; 152:2042–2050.
34. Schmidt D, Amrani A, Verdaguer J, et al. Autoantigen-independent deletion of diabetogenic CD4$^+$ thymocytes by protective MHC class II molecules. J Immunol 1999; 162:4627–4636.
35. Haskins K. T cell receptor gene usage in autoimmune diabetes. Int Rev Immunol 1999; 18:61–81.
36. Wegmann DR, Norbury-Glaser M, Daniel D. Insulin-specific T cells are a predominant component of islet infiltrates in prediabetic NOD mice. Eur J Immunol 1994; 24:1853–1857.
37. Tian J, Atkinson M, Clare-Salzer M, et al. Nasal administration of glutamate decarboxylase (GAD65) peptides induces Th2 responses and prevents murine insulin dependent diabetes. J Exp Med 1996; 183:1561–1567.
38. Muir A, Peck A, Clare-Salzler M, et al. Insulin immunization of nonobese diabetic mice induces a protective insulitis characterized by diminished intraislet interferon-gamma transcription. J Clin Invest 1995; 95:628–634.
39. Cetkovic-Cvrlje M, Gerling IC, Muir A, et al. Retardation or acceleration of diabetes in NOD/Lt mice mediated by intrathymic administration of candidate β-cell antigens. Diabetes 1997; 46:1975–1982.
40. Daniel D, Wegmann DR. Protection of nonobese diabetic mice from diabetes by intranasal or subcutaneous administration of insulin peptide B-(9-23). Proc Natl Acad Sci USA 1996; 93:956–960.
41. Awata T, Guberski DL, Like AA. Genetics of the BB rat: association of autoimmune disorders (diabetes, insulitis, and thyroiditis) with lymphopenia and major histocompatibility complex class II. Endocrinology 1995; 136:5731–5735.
42. Eisenbarth GS. Isotypes of anti-islet autoantibodies. Diabetes Care 2000; 23:151–152.
43. Jacob HJ, Pettersson A, Wilson D, et al. Genetic dissection of autoimmune type I diabetes in the BB rat. Nat Genet 1992; 2: 56–60.
44. Gottlieb PA, Handler ES, Appel MC, et al. Insulin treatment prevents diabetes mellitus but not thyroiditis in RT 6–depleted diabetes resistant BB/Wor rats. Diabetologia 1991; 34:296–300.
45. Song HY, Abad MM, Mahoney CP, McEvoy RC. Human insulin B chain but not A chain decreases the rate of diabetes in BB rats. Diabetes Res Clin Pract 1999; 46:109–114.
46. Kawano K, Hirashima T, Moris S, et al. New inbred strain of Long-Evans Tokushima lean rats with IDDM without lymphopenia. Diabetes 1991; 40:1375–1381.
47. Yokoi N, Kanazawa M, Kitada K, et al. A non-MHC locus essential for autoimmune type I diabetes in the Komeda diabetes-prone rat. J Clin Invest 1997; 100:2015–2021.
48. Uchigata Y, Yamamoto H, Nagai H, Okamoto H. Effect of poly(ADP-ribose) synthetase inhibitor administration to rats before and after injection of alloxan and streptozotocin on islet proinsulin synthesis. Diabetes 1983; 32:316–318.
49. Tanaka SI, Nakajima AS, Inoue S, et al. Genetic control by I-A subregion in H-2 complex of incidence of streptozotocin-induced autoimmune diabetes in mice. Diabetes 1990; 39:1298–1304.
50. Ellerman KE, Like AA. Susceptibility to diabetes is widely distributed in normal class IIu haplotype rats. Diabetologia 2000; 43:890–898.
51. Birk OS, Elias D, Weiss AS, et al. NOD mouse diabetes: the ubiquitous mouse hsp60 is a beta-cell target antigen of autoimmune T cells. J Autoimmun 1996; 9:159–166.
52. Ablamunits V, Elias D, Reshef T, Cohen IR. Islet T cells secreting IFN-gamma in NOD mouse diabetes: arrest by p277 peptide treatment. J Autoimmun 1998; 11:73–81.
53. Pipeleers D, Ling Z. Pancreatic beta cells in insulin-dependent diabetes. Diabetes Metab Rev 1992; 8:209–227.
54. Foulis AK, Clark A. Pathology of the pancreas in diabetes mellitus. In Kahn CR, Weir GC (eds). Joslin's Diabetes Mellitus, 13th ed. Philadelphia, Lea & Febiger, 1994, pp 265–281.
55. Doniach D, Morgan AG. Islets of Langerhans in juvenile diabetes mellitus. Clin Endocrinol (Oxf) 1973; 2:233–248.
56. Gepts W, LeCompte PM. The pancreatic islets in diabetes. Am J Med 1981; 70:105–115.
57. Foulis AK, Liddle CN, Farquharson MA, et al. The histopathology of the pancreas in type I diabetes (insulin dependent) mellitus: a 25-year review of deaths in patients under 20 years of age in the United Kingdom. Diabetologia 1986; 29:267–274.
58. Foulis AK, Farquharson MA, Hardman R. Aberrant expression of class II major histocompatibility complex molecules by β cells and hyperexpression of class I major histocompatibility complex molecules by insulin containing islets in type 1 (insulin dependent) diabetes mellitus. Diabetologia 1987; 30:333–343.
59. Huang X, Yuan J, Goddard A, et al. Interferon expression in the pancreases of patients with type I diabetes. Diabetes 1995; 44: 658–664.
60. Suri A, Katz JD. Dissecting the role of CD4$^+$ T cells in autoimmune diabetes through the use of TCR transgenic mice. Immunol Rev 1999; 169:55–65.
61. Amrani A, Verdaguer J, Thiessen S, et al. IL-1alpha, IL-1beta, and IFN-gamma mark beta cells for fas-dependent destruction by diabetogenic CD4$^+$ T lymphocytes. J Clin Invest 2000; 105:459–468.
62. Itoh N, Imagawa A, Hanafusa T, et al. Requirement of Fas for the development of autoimmune diabetes in nonobese diabetic mice. J Exp Med 1997; 186:613–618.
63. Chervonsky AV, Wang Y, Wong FS, et al. The role of Fas in autoimmune diabetes. Cell 1997; 89:17–24.
64. Thomas HE, Kay TW. Beta cell destruction in the development of autoimmune diabetes in the non-obese diabetic (NOD) mouse. Diabetes Metab Res Rev 2000; 16:251–261.
65. Sarvetnick N. Etiology of autoimmunity. Immunol Res 2000; 21: 357–362.
66. Lo D. Immune regulation: susceptibility and resistance to autoimmunity. Immunol Res 2000; 21:239–246.
67. Wong FS, Janeway CAJ. The role of CD4 vs. CD8 T cells in IDDM. J Autoimmun 1999; 13:290–295.
68. Dilts SM, Solvason N, Lafferty KJ. The role of CD4 and CD8 T cells in the development of autoimmune diabetes. J Autoimmun 1999; 13:285–290.
69. Wong FS, Dittel BN, Janeway CAJ. Transgenes and knockout mutations in animal models of type 1 diabetes and multiple sclerosis. Immunol Rev 1999; 169:93–104.
70. Foulis AK, McGill M, Farquharson MA, Hilton DA. A search for evidence of viral infection in pancreases of newly diagnosed patients with IDDM. Diabetologia 1997; 40:53–61.
71. Thorsby E. Invited anniversary review: HLA associated diseases. Hum Immunol 1997; 53:1–11.
72. Park Y, Eisenbarth GS. Genetic susceptibility factors of type 1 diabetes in Asians and their functional evaluation. Diabetes Metab Res Rev 2001; 17:2–11.
73. Clark LB, Appleby MW, Brunkow ME, et al. Cellular and mo-

lecular characterization of the scurfy mouse mutant. J Immunol 1999; 162:2546–2554.
74. Powell BR, Buist NR, Stenzel P. An X-linked syndrome of diarrhea, polyendocrinopathy, and fatal infection in infancy. J Pediatr 1982; 100:731–737.
75. Roberts J, Searle J. Neonatal diabetes mellitus associated with severe diarrhea, hyperimmunoglobulin E syndrome, and absence of islets of Langerhans. Pediatr Pathol Lab Med 1995; 15:477–483.
76. Cilio CM, Bosco A, Moretti C, et al. Congenital autoimmune diabetes mellitus (letter). N Engl J Med 2000; 342:1529–1531.
77. Kanangat S, Blair P, Reddy R, et al. Disease in the scurfy (sf) mouse is associated with overexpression of cytokine genes. Eur J Immunol 1996; 26:161–165.
78. Eisenbarth GS. Genetic basis of autoimmune diabetes. In Williams G, Habener JF (eds). Metabolic Basis of Common Inherited Diseases. Philadelphia, Harcourt Health Sciences/WB Saunders, 2000.
79. Redondo MJ, Yu L, Hawa M, et al. Late progression to type 1 diabetes of discordant twins of patients with type 1 diabetes: combined analysis of two twin series (United States and United Kingdom) (abstract). Diabetes 1999; 48:780.
80. Kyvik KO, Green A, Beck-Nielsen H. Concordance rates of insulin dependent diabetes mellitus: a population based study of young Danish twins. BMJ 1995; 311:913–917.
81. Anonymous. Diabetes mellitus in twins: a cooperative study in Japan. Committee on Diabetic Twins, Japan Diabetes Society. Diabetes Res Clin Pract 1988; 5:271–280.
82. Ikegami H, Ogihara T. Genetics of insulin-dependent diabetes mellitus. Endocr J 1996; 43:605–613.
83. Barnett AH, Eff C, Leslie RD, Pyke DA. Diabetes in identical twins: a study of 200 pairs. Diabetologia 1981; 20:87–93.
84. Redondo MJ, Yu L, Hawa M, et al. Heterogeneity of type 1 diabetes: analysis of monozygotic twins in Great Britain and the United States. Diabetologia 2001; 44:354–362.
85. Redondo MJ, Rewers M, Yu L, et al. Genetic determination of islet cell autoimmunity in monozygotic twin, dizygotic twin, and non-twin siblings of patients with type 1 diabetes: prospective twin study. BMJ 1999; 318:698–702.
86. Bao F, Yu L, Babu S, et al. One third of HLA DQ2 homozygous patients with type 1 diabetes express celiac disease associated transglutaminase autoantibodies. J Autoimmun 1999; 13:143–148.
87. Yu L, Brewer KW, Gates S, et al. DRB1*04 and DQ alleles: expression of 21-hydroxylase autoantibodies and risk of progression to Addison's disease. J Clin Endocrinol Metab 1999; 84:328–335.
88. De Block CE, De Leeuw IH, Van Gaal LF. High prevalence of manifestations of gastric autoimmunity in parietal cell antibody–positive type 1 (insulin-dependent) diabetic patients. The Belgian Diabetes Registry. J Clin Endocrinol Metab 1999; 84:4062–4067.
89. Nepom GT, Kwok WW. Perspectives in diabetes: molecular basis for HLA-DQ associations with IDDM. Diabetes 1998; 47:1177–1184.
90. McDevitt HO. The role of MHC class II molecules in susceptibility and resistance to autoimmunity. Curr Opin Immunol 1998; 10:677–681.
91. Eisenbarth GS. Genetic counseling for type 1 diabetes. In Lebovitz HE (ed). Therapy for Diabetes Mellitus and Related Disorders, 3rd ed. Alexandria, VA, American Diabetes Association, 1998, pp 8–19.
92. Nakanishi K, Kobayashi T, Murase T, et al. Human leukocyte antigen-A24 and -DQA1*0301 in Japanese insulin-dependent diabetes mellitus: independent contributions to susceptibility to the disease and additive contributions to acceleration of beta-cell destruction. J Clin Endocrinol Metab 1999; 84:3721–3725.
93. Rewers M, Bugawan TL, Norris JM, et al. Newborn screening for HLA markers associated with IDDM: diabetes autoimmunity study in the young (DAISY). Diabetologia 1996; 39:807–812.
94. Kulmala P, Savola K, Reijonen H, et al. Genetic markers, humoral autoimmunity, and prediction of type 1 diabetes in siblings of affected children. Childhood Diabetes in Finland Study Group. Diabetes 2000; 49:48–58.
95. Redondo MJ, Kawasaki E, Mulgrew CL, et al. DR and DQ associated protection from type 1 diabetes: comparison of DRB1*1401 and DQA1*0102-DQB1*0602. J Clin Endocrinol Metab 2000; 85:3793–3797.
96. Kawasaki E, Noble J, Erlich H, et al. Transmission of DQ haplotypes to patients with type 1 diabetes. Diabetes 1998; 47:1971–1973.
97. Morel PA, Dorman JS, Todd JA, et al. Aspartic acid at position 57 of the HLA-DQ beta chain protects against type I diabetes: a family study. Proc Natl Acad Sci USA 1988; 85:8111–8115.
98. Bell GI, Horita S, Karam JH. A polymorphic locus near the human insulin gene is associated with insulin-dependent diabetes mellitus. Diabetes 1984; 33:176–183.
99. Bennett ST, Lucassen AM, Gough SCL, et al. Susceptibility to human type I diabetes at IDDM2 is determined by tandem repeat variation at the insulin gene minisatellite locus. Nat Genet 1995; 9:284–292.
100. Pugliese A, Zeller M, Fernandez A, et al. The insulin gene is transcribed in the human thymus and transcription levels correlate with allelic variation at the INS VNTR-IDDM2 susceptibility locus for type I diabetes. Nat Genet 1997; 15:293–297.
101. Vafiadis P, Bennett ST, Todd JA, et al. Insulin expression in human thymus is modulated by INS VNTR alleles at the IDDM2 locus. Nat Genet 1997; 15:289–292.
102. Hanahan D. Peripheral-antigen-expressing cells in thymic medulla: factors in self-tolerance and autoimmunity. Curr Opin Immunol 1998; 10:656–662.
103. Todd JA, Farrall M. Panning for gold: genome-wide scanning for linkage in type I diabetes. Hum Mol Genet 1996; 5:1443–1448.
104. Concannon P, Gogolin-Ewens KJ, Hinds DA, et al. A second-generation screen of the human genome for susceptibility to insulin-dependent diabetes mellitus. Nat Genet 1998; 19:292–296.
105. Lernmark Å, Ott J. Sometimes it's hot, sometimes it's not. Nat Genet 1998; 19:213–214.
106. Larsen ZM, Kristiansen OP, Mato E, et al. IDDM12 (CTLA4) on 2q33 and IDDM13 on 2q34 in genetic susceptibility to type 1 diabetes (insulin-dependent). Autoimmunity 1999; 31:35–42.
107. Delepine M, Pociot F, Habita C, et al. Evidence of a non-MHC susceptibility locus in type I diabetes linked to HLA on chromosome 6. Am J Hum Genet 1997; 60:174–187.
108. Verge CF, Vardi P, Babu S, et al. Evidence for oligogenic inheritance of type 1A diabetes in a large Bedouin Arab family. J Clin Invest 1998; 102:1569–1575.
109. Eisenbarth GS, Elsey C, Yu L, Rewers M. Infantile anti-islet autoimmunity: DAISY study (abstract). Diabetes 1998; 47:A210.
110. Schenker M, Hummel M, Ferber K, et al. Early expression and high prevalence of islet autoantibodies for DR3/4 heterozygous and DR4/4 homozygous offspring of parents with type I diabetes: the German BABYDIAB study. Diabetologia 1999; 42:671–677.
111. Robles DT, Eisenbarth GS. Type 1A diabetes induced by infection and immunization. J Autoimmun 2001; 16:355–362.
112. Ellerman KE, Richards CA, Guberski DL, et al. Kilham rat virus triggers T-cell-dependent autoimmune diabetes in multiple strains of rat. Diabetes 1996; 45:557–562.
113. Gardner SG, Bingley PJ, Sawtell PA, et al. Rising incidence of insulin dependent diabetes in children aged under 5 years in the Oxford region: time trend analysis. BMJ 1997; 315:713–717.
114. Tuomilehto J, Karvonen M, Pitkaniemi J, et al. Record-high incidence of type I (insulin-dependent) diabetes mellitus in Finnish children. The Finnish Childhood Type I Diabetes Registry Group. Diabetologia 1999; 42:655–660.
115. Feltbower RG, McKinney PA, Bodansky HJ. Rising incidence of childhood diabetes is seen at all ages and in urban and rural settings in Yorkshire, United Kingdom (letter). Diabetologia 2000; 43:682–684.
116. Shaver KA, Boughman JA, Nance WE. Congenital rubella syndrome and diabetes: a review of epidemiologic, genetic, and immunologic factors. Am Ann Deaf 1985; 130:526–532.
117. Rubenstein P. The HLA system in congenital rubella patients with and without diabetes. Diabetes 1982; 31:1088–1091.
118. Clarke WL, Shaver KA, Bright GM, et al. Autoimmunity in congenital rubella syndrome. J Pediatr 1984; 104:370–373.
119. Ou D, Jonsen LA, Metzger DL, Tingle AJ. $CD4^+$ and $CD8^+$ T-cell clones from congenital rubella syndrome patients with IDDM recognize overlapping GAD65 protein epitopes: implications for HLA class I and II allelic linkage to disease susceptibility. Hum Immunol 1999; 60:652–664.
120. Rabinowe SL, George KL, Loughlin R, et al. Congenital rubella: monoclonal antibody–defined T cell abnormalities in young adults. Am J Med 1986; 81:779–782.

121. Yoon JW, Austin M, Onodera T, Notkins A. Isolation of a virus from the pancreas of a child with diabetic ketoacidosis. N Engl J Med 1979; 300:1173–1179.
122. Nigro G, Pacella ME, Patane E, Midulla M. Multi-system coxsackie virus B-6 infection with findings suggestive of diabetes mellitus. Eur J Pediatr 1986; 145:557–559.
123. Lonnrot M, Korpela K, Knip M, et al. Enterovirus infection as a risk factor for beta-cell autoimmunity in a prospectively observed birth cohort: the Finnish Diabetes Prediction and Prevention Study. Diabetes 2000; 49:1314–1318.
124. Graves PM, Rewers M. The role of enteroviral infections in the development of IDDM: limitations of current approaches. Diabetes 1997; 46:161–168.
125. Honeyman MC, Coulson BS, Stone NL, et al. Association between rotavirus infection and pancreatic islet autoimmunity in children at risk of developing type 1 diabetes. Diabetes 2000; 49: 1319–1324.
126. Classen DC, Classen JB. The timing of pediatric immunization and the risk of insulin-dependent diabetes mellitus. Infect Dis Clin Pract 1997; 6:449–454.
127. Karvonen M, Cepaitis Z, Tuomilehto J. Association between type 1 diabetes and *Haemophilus influenzae* type b vaccination: birth cohort study. BMJ 1999; 318:1169–1172.
128. Lindberg B, Ahlfors K, Carlsson A, et al. Previous exposure to measles, mumps, and rubella—but not vaccination during adolescence—correlates to the prevalence of pancreatic and thyroid autoantibodies. Pediatrics 1999; 104:e12.
129. Graves PM, Barriga KJ, Norris JM, et al. Lack of association between early childhood immunizations and beta-cell autoimmunity. Diabetes Care 1999; 22:1694–1697.
130. Bao F, Rewers M, Scott F, Eisenbarth GS. Celiac disease. In Eisenbarth GS (ed). Endocrine and Organ Specific Autoimmunity. Austin, Tex, RG Landes, 1999, pp 85–96.
131. Scott FW, Cloutier HE, Kleemann R, et al. Potential mechanisms by which certain foods promote or inhibit the development of spontaneous diabetes in BB rats. Diabetes 1997; 46:589–598.
132. Akerblom HK, Savilahti E, Saukkonen TT, et al. The case for elimination of cow's milk in early infancy in the prevention of type 1 diabetes: the Finnish experience. Diabetes Metab Rev 1993; 9:269–278.
133. Virtanen SM, Laara E, Hypponen E, et al. Cow's milk consumption, HLA-DQB1 genotype, and type 1 diabetes: a nested case-control study of siblings of children with diabetes. Childhood Diabetes in Finland Study Group. Diabetes 2000; 49:912–917.
134. Virtanen SM, Rasanen L, Aro A, et al. Infant feeding in Finnish children less than 7 yr of age with newly diagnosed IDDM. Childhood Diabetes in Finland Study Group. Diabetes Care 1991; 14:415–417.
135. Couper JJ, Steele C, Beresford S, et al. Lack of association between duration of breast-feeding or introduction of cow's milk and development of islet autoimmunity. Diabetes 1999; 48:2145–2149.
136. Norris JM, Beaty B, Klingensmith G, et al. Lack of association between early exposure to cow's milk protein and β-cell autoimmunity: Diabetes Autoimmunity Study in the Young (DAISY). JAMA 1996; 276:609–614.
136a. Andre I, Gonzalez A, Wong B, et al. Checkpoints in the progression of autoimmune disease: Lessons from diabetes models. Proc Natl Acad Sci U S A 1996; 93:2260–2263.
137. Fennessy M, Metcalfe K, Hitman GA, et al. A gene in the HLA class I region contributes to susceptibility to IDDM in the Finnish population. Childhood Diabetes in Finland (DiMe) Study Group. Diabetologia 1994; 37:937–944.
138. Kockum I, Sanjeevi CB, Eastman S, et al. Population analysis of protection by HLA-DR and DQ genes from insulin-dependent diabetes mellitus in Swedish children with insulin-dependent diabetes and controls. Eur J Immunogenet 1995; 22:443–465.
139. Vardi P, Ziegler AG, Matthews JH, et al. Concentration of insulin autoantibodies at onset of type I diabetes: inverse log-linear correlation with age. Diabetes Care 1988; 11:736–739.
140. Arslanian SL, Becker DJ, Rabin B, et al. Correlates of insulin antibodies in newly diagnosed children with insulin-dependent diabetes before insulin therapy. Diabetes 1985; 34:926–930.
141. Eisenbarth GS, Gianani R, Yu L, et al. Dual parameter model for prediction of type 1 diabetes mellitus. Proc Assoc Am Physicians 1998; 110:126–135.
142. Pugliese A, Kawasaki E, Zeller M, et al. Sequence analysis of the diabetes-protective human leukocyte antigen-DQB1*0602 allele in unaffected, islet cell antibody–positive first degree relatives and in rare patients with type 1 diabetes. J Clin Endocrinol Metab 1999; 84:1722–1728.
143. Verge CF, Gianani R, Kawasaki E, et al. Prediction of type I diabetes in first-degree relatives using a combination of insulin, GAD, and ICA512bdc/IA-2 autoantibodies. Diabetes 1996; 45: 926–933.
144. Bingley PJ, Bonifacio E, Williams AJK, et al. Prediction of IDDM in the general population: strategies based on combinations of autoantibody markers. Diabetes 1997; 46:1701–1710.
145. Chase HP, Cuthbertson DD, Dolan LM, et al. First phase insulin release during the intravenous glucose tolerance test as a risk factor for type 1 diabetes. J Pediatr 2001; 138:244–249.
146. Bingley PJ, Colman P, Eisenbarth GS, et al. Standardization of IVGTT to predict IDDM. Diabetes Care 1992; 15:1313–1316.
147. Bingley PJ. Interactions of age, islet cell antibodies, insulin autoantibodies, and first-phase insulin response in predicting risk of progression to IDDM in ICA+ relatives: the ICARUS data set. Diabetes 1996; 45:1720–1728.
148. Anonymous. Epidemiology of severe hypoglycemia in the diabetes control and complications trial. The DCCT Research Group. Am J Med 1991; 90:450–459.
149. Füchtenbusch M, Ferber K, Standl E, et al. Prediction of type I diabetes postpartum in patients with gestational diabetes mellitus by combined islet cell autoantibody screening: a prospective multicenter study. Diabetes 1997; 46:1459–1467.
150. Zimmet PZ, Tuomi T, Mackay IR, et al. Latent autoimmune diabetes mellitus in adults (LADA): the role of antibodies to glutamic acid decarboxylase in diagnosis and prediction of insulin dependency. Diabet Med 1994; 11:299–303.
151. Turner R, Stratton I, Horton V, et al. UKPDS 25: autoantibodies to islet-cell cytoplasm and glutamic acid decarboxylase for prediction of insulin requirement in type 2 diabetes. UK Prospective Diabetes Study Group. Lancet 1997; 350:1288–1293.
152. Horton V, Stratton I, Bottazzo GF, et al. Genetic heterogeneity of autoimmune diabetes: age of presentation in adults is influenced by HLA DRB1 and DQB1 genotypes (UKPDS 43). UK Prospective Diabetes Study (UKPDS) Group. Diabetologia 1999; 42:608–616.
153. Ricker AT, Herskowitz R, Wolfsdorf JI, et al. Prognostic factors in children and young adults presenting with transient hyperglycemia or impaired glucose tolerance (abstract). Diabetes 1986; 35(suppl 1):93A.
154. Assan R, Feutren G, Debray-Sachs M, et al. Metabolic and immunological effects of cyclosporine in recently diagnosed type I diabetes mellitus. Lancet 1985; 1:67–71.
155. Chase HP, Butler-Simon N, Garg SK, et al. Cyclosporine A for the treatment of new-onset insulin-dependent diabetes mellitus. Pediatrics 1990; 85:241–245.
156. Stiller CR, Dupre J, Gent M, et al. Effects of cyclosporine immunosuppression in insulin-dependent diabetes mellitus of recent onset. Science 1984; 223:1362–1367.
157. Carel J-C, Boitard C, Eisenbarth G, et al. Cyclosporine delays but does not prevent clinical onset in glucose intolerant pre–type 1 diabetic children. J Autoimmun 1996; 9:739–745.
158. Cook JJ, Hudson I, Harrison LC, et al. Double-blind controlled trial of azathioprine in children with newly diagnosed type I diabetes. Diabetes 1989; 38:779–783.
159. Silverstein J, Maclaren N, Riley W, et al. Immunosuppression with azathioprine and prednisone in recent-onset insulin-dependent diabetes mellitus. N Engl J Med 1988; 319:599–604.
160. Eisenbarth GS, Srikanta S, Jackson R, et al. Anti-thymocyte globulin and prednisone immunotherapy of recent onset type I diabetes mellitus. Diabetes Res 1985; 2:271–276.
160a. Herold KC, Hagopian W, Auger JA, et al. Anti-CD3 monoclonal antibody in new-onset type 1 diabetes mellitus. N Engl J Med 2002; 346:1692–1698.
161. Buckingham BA, Sandborg CI. A randomized trial of methotrexate in newly diagnosed patients with type 1 diabetes mellitus. Clin Immunol 2000; 96:86–90.
162. Weiner HL, Miller A, Khoury SJ, et al. Suppression of organ-specific autoimmune diseases by oral administration of autoantigens. Proceedings of the 8th International Congress on Immunology, 1992, pp 627–634.

163. Zhang ZJ, Davidson L, Eisenbarth G, Weiner HL. Suppression of diabetes in nonobese diabetic mice by oral administration of porcine insulin. Proc Natl Acad Sci USA 1991; 88:10252–10256.
164. Atkinson MA, Maclaren NK, Luchetta R. Insulitis and diabetes in NOD mice reduced by prophylactic insulin therapy. Diabetes 1990; 39:933–937.
165. Elias D, Meilin A, Ablamunits V, et al. Hsp60 peptide therapy of NOD mouse diabetes induces a Th2 cytokine burst and downregulates autoimmunity to various β-cell antigens. Diabetes 1997; 46:758–764.
166. Lampeter EF, Klinghammer A, Scherbaum WA, et al. The Deutsche Nicotinamide Intervention Study: an attempt to prevent type 1 diabetes. DENIS Group. Diabetes 1998; 47:980–984.
167. Pozzilli P, Visalli N, Signore A, et al. Double blind trial of nicotinamide in recent-onset IDDM (the IMDIAB III study). Diabetologia 1995; 38:848–852.
168. Robertson RP, Sutherland DER, Kendall DM, et al. Metabolic characterization of long-term successful pancreas transplants in type I diabetes. J Investig Med 1996; 44:549–555.
169. Robertson RP, Kendall D, Teuscher A, Sutherland DER. Long-term metabolic control with pancreatic transplantation. Transplant Proc 1994; 26:386–387.
170. Nakhleh RE, Gruessner RWG, Swanson PE, et al. Pancreas transplant pathology: a morphologic, immunohistochemical, and electron microscopic comparison of allogeneic grafts with rejection, syngeneic grafts, and chronic pancreatitis. Am J Surg Pathol 1991; 15:246–256.
171. Shapiro AM, Lakey JR, Ryan EA, et al. Islet transplantation in seven patients with type 1 diabetes mellitus using a glucocorticoid-free immunosuppressive regimen. N Engl J Med 2000; 343: 230–238.
172. Uchigata Y, Kuwata S, Tsushima T, et al. Patients with Graves' disease who developed insulin autoimmune syndrome (Hirata disease) possess HLA-Bw62/Cw4/DR4 carrying DRB1*0406. J Clin Endocrinol Metab 1993; 77:249–254.
173. Uchigata Y, Hirata Y. Insulin autoimmune syndrome (IAS, Hirata disease). In Eisenbarth G (ed). Molecular Mechanisms of Endocrine and Organ Specific Autoimmunity. Austin, Tex, RG Landes, 1999, pp 133–148.
174. Menon RK, Cohen RM, Sperling MA, et al. Transplacental passage of insulin in pregnant women with insulin-dependent diabetes mellitus: its role in fetal macrosomia. N Engl J Med 1990; 323:309–315.
175. Schernthaner G. Immunogenicity and allergenic potential of animal and human insulins. Diabetes Care 1993; 16:155–165.
176. Taylor SI, Grunberger G, Marcus-Samuels B, et al. Hypoglycemia associated with antibodies to the insulin receptor. N Engl J Med 1982; 307:1422–1426.
177. Dons RF, Havlik R, Taylor SI, et al. Clinical disorders associated with autoantibodies to the insulin receptor: simulation by passive transfer of immunoglobulins to rats. J Clin Invest 1983; 72:1072–1080.
178. Engerman R, Bloodworth JM Jr, Nelson S. Relationship of microvascular disease in diabetes to metabolic control. Diabetes 1977; 26:760–769.
179. Engerman RL, Kern TS. Progression of incipient diabetic retinopathy during good glycemic control. Diabetes 1987; 36:808–812.
180. Cohen AJ, McGill PD, Rossetti RG, et al. Glomerulopathy in spontaneously diabetic rat: impact of glycemic control. Diabetes 1987; 36:944–951.
181. Klein R, Klein BE, Moss SE, et al. The Wisconsin epidemiologic study of diabetic retinopathy. II. Prevalence and risk of diabetic retinopathy when age at diagnosis is less than 30 years. Arch Ophthalmol 1984; 102:520–526.
182. Klein R, Klein BE, Moss SE, et al. Glycosylated hemoglobin predicts the incidence and progression of diabetic retinopathy. JAMA 1988; 260:2864–2871.
183. Chase HP, Jackson WE, Hoops SL, et al. Glucose control and the renal and retinal complications of insulin-dependent diabetes. JAMA 1989; 261:1155–1160.
184. The effect of intensive treatment of diabetes on the development and progression of long-term complications in insulin-dependent diabetes mellitus. The Diabetes Control and Complications Trial Research Group. N Engl J Med 1993; 329:977–986.
185. Effect of intensive diabetes management on macrovascular events and risk factors in the Diabetes Control and Complications Trial. Am J Cardiol 1995; 75:894–903.
186. Sherwin R, Felig P. Hypoglycemia. In Felig P (ed). Endocrinology and Metabolism, 2nd ed. New York, McGraw-Hill, 1987, pp 1043–1178.
187. Purnell JQ, Hokanson JE, Marcovina SM, et al. Effect of excessive weight gain with intensive therapy of type 1 diabetes on lipid levels and blood pressure: results from the DCCT. Diabetes Control and Complications Trial. JAMA 1998; 280:140–146.
188. Blood glucose control and the evolution of diabetic retinopathy and albuminuria: a preliminary multicenter trial. The Kroc Collaborative Study Group. N Engl J Med 1984; 311:365–372.
189. Lauritzen T, Frost-Larsen K, Larsen HW, Deckert T. Effect of 1 year of near-normal blood glucose levels on retinopathy in insulin-dependent diabetics. Lancet 1983; 1:200–204.
190. Dahl-Jorgensen K, Brinchmann-Hansen O, Hansen KF, et al. Rapid tightening of blood glucose control leads to transient deterioration of retinopathy in insulin dependent diabetes mellitus: the Oslo study. Br Med J (Clin Res Ed) 1985; 290:811–815.
191. Cryer PE. Hypoglycemia-associated autonomic failure in diabetes. Am J Physiol 2001; 281:E1115–E1121.
192. Standards of medical care for patients with diabetes mellitus. American Diabetes Association. Diabetes Care 2002; 25(suppl 1): 33–49.
193. Hirsch IB. Intensive treatment of type 1 diabetes. Med Clin North Am 1998; 82:689–719.
194. Lougheed WD, Zinman B, Strack TR, et al. Stability of insulin lispro in insulin infusion systems. Diabetes Care 1997; 20:1061–1065.
195. Bode BW, Steed RD, Davidson PC. Reduction in severe hypoglycemia with long-term continuous subcutaneous insulin infusion in type I diabetes. Diabetes Care 1996; 19:324–327.
196. Continuous subcutaneous insulin infusion. American Diabetes Association. Diabetes Care 2002; 25(suppl 1):116.
197. Weisberg LS. Pseudohyponatremia: A reappraisal. Am J Med 1989; 86:315–318.
198. Adrogue HJ, Wilson H, Boyd AE 3rd, et al. Plasma acid-base patterns in diabetic ketoacidosis. N Engl J Med 1982; 307:1603–1610.
199. Munro JF, Campbell IW, McCuish AC, Duncan LJ. Euglycaemic diabetic ketoacidosis. Br Med J 1973; 2:578–580.
200. Madias NE. Lactic acidosis. Kidney Int 1986; 29:752–774.
201. Fulop M. Alcoholism, ketoacidosis, and lactic acidosis. Diabetes Metab Rev 1989; 5:365–378.
202. Duffens K, Marx JA. Alcoholic ketoacidosis: a review. J Emerg Med 1987; 5:399–406.
203. Moller-Petersen J, Andersen PT, Hjorne N, Ditzel J. Nontraumatic rhabdomyolysis during diabetic ketoacidosis. Diabetologia 1986; 29:229–234.
204. Brenner BE, Simon RR. Management of salicylate intoxication. Drugs 1982; 24:335–340.
205. Turk J, Morrell L. Ethylene glycol intoxication. Arch Intern Med 1986; 146:1601–1603.
206. Rich J, Scheife RT, Katz N, Caplan LR. Isopropyl alcohol intoxication. Arch Neurol 1990; 47:322–324.
207. Kitabchi AE. Low-dose insulin therapy in diabetic ketoacidosis: fact or fiction? Diabetes Metab Rev 1989; 5:337–363.
208. Burris AS. Leukemoid reaction associated with severe diabetic ketoacidosis. South Med J 1986; 79:647–648.
209. Powers WJ. Cerebrospinal fluid to serum glucose ratios in diabetes mellitus and bacterial meningitis. Am J Med 1981; 71:217–220.
210. Campbell IW, Duncan LJ, Innes JA, et al. Abdominal pain in diabetic metabolic decompensation: clinical significance. JAMA 1975; 233:166–168.
211. Rosenbloom AL. Intracerebral crises during treatment of diabetic ketoacidosis. Diabetes Care 1990; 13:22–33.
212. Brun-Buisson CJ, Bonnet F, Bergeret S, et al. Recurrent high-permeability pulmonary edema associated with diabetic ketoacidosis. Crit Care Med 1985; 13:55–56.
213. Brandstetter RD, Tamarin FM, Washington D, et al. Occult mucous airway obstruction in diabetic ketoacidosis. Chest 1987; 91:575–578.
214. Hansen LA, Prakash UB, Colby TV. Pulmonary complications in diabetes mellitus. Mayo Clin Proc 1989; 64:791–799.

31 Complications of Diabetes Mellitus

Michael Brownlee, Lloyd P. Aiello, Eli Friedman,
Aaron I. Vinik, Richard W. Nesto, and
Andrew J. M. Boulton

BIOCHEMISTRY AND MOLECULAR CELL BIOLOGY

All forms of diabetes, both inherited and acquired, are characterized by hyperglycemia, a relative or absolute lack of insulin, and the development of diabetes-specific microvascular pathology in the retina, renal glomerulus, and peripheral nerve. Diabetes is also associated with accelerated atherosclerotic macrovascular disease affecting arteries that supply the heart, brain, and lower extremities. Pathologically, this condition resembles macrovascular disease in nondiabetic patients but is more extensive and progresses more rapidly. As a consequence of its microvascular pathology, diabetes mellitus is now the leading cause of new blindness in people 20 to 74 years of age and the leading cause of end-stage renal disease (ESRD).

People with diabetes mellitus are the fastest growing group of renal dialysis and transplant recipients. The life expectancy of patients with diabetic end-stage renal failure is only 3 or 4 years. More than 60% of diabetic patients are affected by neuropathy, which includes *distal symmetrical polyneuropathy* (DSPN), mononeuropathies, and a variety of autonomic neuropathies causing erectile dysfunction, urinary incontinence, gastroparesis, and nocturnal diarrhea. Accelerated lower extremity arterial disease in conjunction with neuropathy makes diabetes mellitus account for 50% of all nontraumatic amputations in the United States. The risk of cardiovascular complications is increased by twofold to sixfold in subjects with diabetes. Overall, life expectancy is about 7 to 10 years shorter than for people without diabetes mellitus because of increased mortality from diabetic complications.[1]

Large, prospective clinical studies show a strong relationship between glycemia and diabetic microvascular complications in both type 1 and type 2 diabetes mellitus.[2, 3] There is a continuous, though not linear, relationship between level of glycemia and the risk of development and progression of these complications (Fig. 31–1).[4, 5] Hyperglycemia and the dyslipidemia induced by insulin resistance both appear to play important roles in the pathogenesis of macrovascular complications.[6–10]

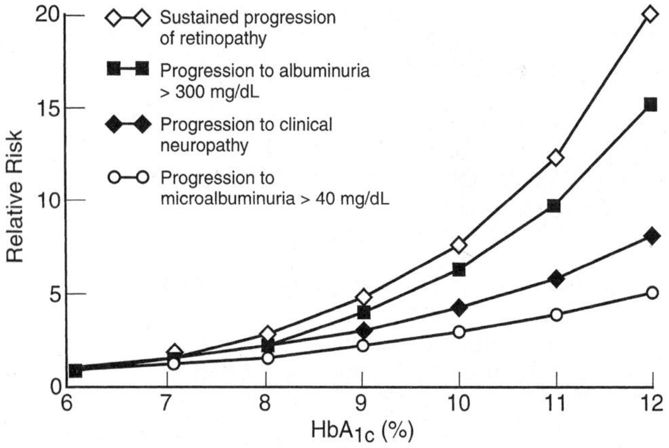

Figure 31–1. Relative risks for the development of diabetic complications at different levels of mean hemoglobin A_{1c} (HbA_{1c}, glycated hemoglobin), obtained from the Diabetes Control and Complications Trial. (Adapted from Skyler J: Diabetic complications: the importance of glucose control. Endocrinol Metab Clin North Am 1996; 25:243–254.)

SHARED PATHOPHYSIOLOGIC FEATURES OF MICROVASCULAR COMPLICATIONS

In the retina, glomerulus, and vasa nervorum, diabetes-specific microvascular disease is characterized by similar pathophysiologic features.

Requirement for Intracellular Hyperglycemia

Clinical and animal model data indicate that chronic hyperglycemia is the central initiating factor for all types of diabetic microvascular disease. Duration and magnitude of hyperglycemia are both strongly correlated with the extent and rate of progression of diabetic microvascular disease. In the Diabetes Control and Complications Trial (DCCT), for example, type 1 diabetic patients whose intensive insulin therapy resulted in hemoglobin A_{1c} (Hb A_{1c}) levels 2% lower than those receiving conventional insulin therapy had a 76% lower incidence of retinopathy, a 54% lower incidence of nephropathy, and a 60% reduction in neuropathy.[2, 3]

Although all diabetic cells are exposed to elevated levels of plasma glucose, hyperglycemic damage is limited to those cell types (e.g., endothelial cells) that develop intracellular hyperglycemia. Endothelial cells develop intracellular hyperglycemia because, unlike many other cells, they cannot down-regulate glucose transport when exposed to extracellular hyperglycemia. As illustrated in Figure 31–2, vascular smooth muscle cells, which are not damaged by hyperglycemia, show an inverse relationship between extracellular glucose concentration and subsequent rate of glucose transport measured as 2-deoxyglucose uptake (Fig. 31–2*A*). In contrast, vascular endothelial cells show no significant change in subsequent rate of glucose transport after exposure to elevated glucose concentrations (Fig. 31–2*B*).[11] That intracellular hyperglycemia is necessary and sufficient for the development of diabetic pathology is further demonstrated by the fact that overexpression of the GLUT1 glucose transporter in mesangial cells cultured in a normal glucose milieu mimics the diabetic phenotype, inducing the same increases in collagen type IV, collagen type I, and fibronectin gene expression as diabetic hyperglycemia (Fig. 31–3).[12]

Abnormal Endothelial Cell Function

Early in the course of diabetes mellitus, before structural changes are evident, hyperglycemia causes abnormalities in blood flow and vascular permeability in the retina, glomerulus, and peripheral nerve vasa nervorum.[13, 14] The increase in blood flow and intracapillary pressure is thought to reflect hyperglycemia-induced decreased nitric oxide (NO) production on the efferent side of capillary beds, and possibly an increased sensitivity to angiotensin II. As a consequence of increased intracapillary pressure and endothelial cell dysfunction, retinal capillaries exhibit increased leakage of fluorescein and glomerular capillaries have an elevated albumin excretion rate (AER). Comparable changes occur in the vasa vasorum of peripheral nerve. Early in the course of diabetes, increased permeability is reversible; as time progresses, however, it becomes irreversible.

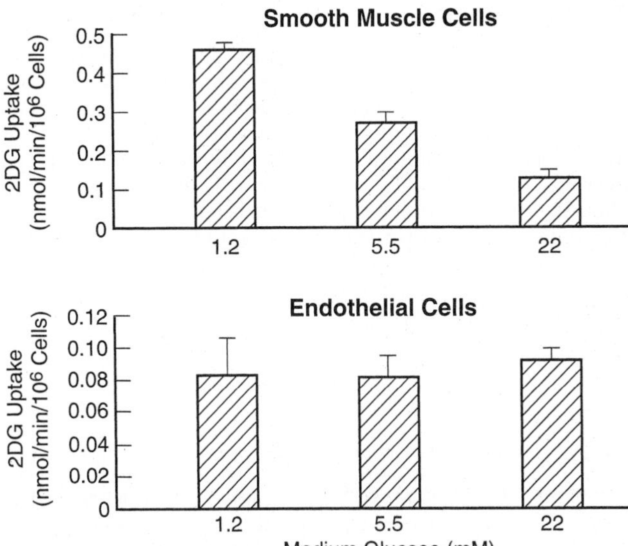

Figure 31–2. Lack of down-regulation of glucose transport in cells affected by diabetic complications. *Upper*, 2-deoxyglucose (2DG) uptake in vascular smooth muscle cells preexposed to either 1.2, 5.5, or 22 mM glucose. *Lower*, 2DG uptake in bovine endothelial cells preexposed to either 1.2, 5.5, or 22 mM glucose. (From Kaiser N, Feener EP, Boukobza-Vardi N, et al. Differential regulation of glucose transport and transporters by glucose in vascular endothelial and smooth muscle cells. Diabetes 1993; 42:80–89.)

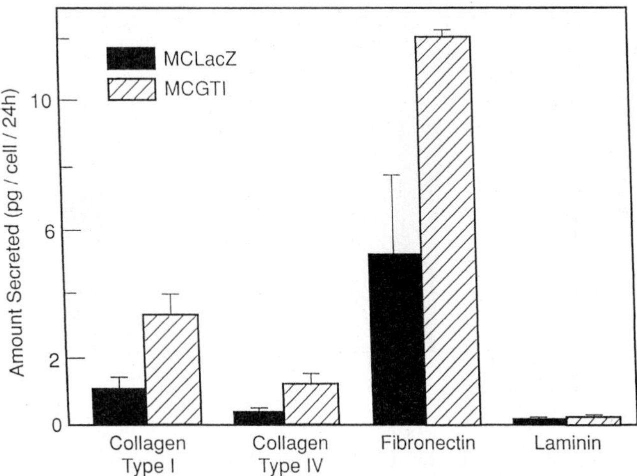

Figure 31–3. Overexpression of *GLUT1* in mesangial cells cultured in normal glucose mimics the diabetic phenotype. Mesangial cells transfected with either *LacZ* (MCLacZ)- or *GLUT1* (MCGT1)-expressing constructs were cultured in 5-mM glucose, and the amount of the indicated matrix components secreted was determined. (From Heilig CW, Concepcion LA, Riser BL, et al. Overexpression of glucose transporters in rat mesangial cells cultured in a normal glucose milieu mimics the diabetic phenotype. J Clin Invest 1995; 96:1802–1814.)

Increased Vessel Wall Protein Accumulation

The common pathophysiologic feature of diabetic microvascular disease is progressive narrowing and eventual occlusion of vascular lumina, which results in inadequate perfusion and function of the affected tissues. Early hyperglycemia-induced microvascular hypertension and increased vascular permeability contribute to irreversible microvessel occlusion by three processes:

The first is an abnormal leakage of periodic acid–Schiff (PAS)-positive, carbohydrate-containing plasma proteins, which are deposited in the capillary wall and which may stimulate perivascular cells such as pericytes and mesangial cells to elaborate growth factors and extracellular matrix.

The second is extravasation of growth factors, such as transforming growth factor β_1 (TGF-β_1), which directly stimulates overproduction of extracellular matrix components,[15] and may induce apoptosis in certain complication-relevant cell types.

The third is hypertension-induced stimulation of pathologic gene expression by endothelial cells and supporting cells, which include glut-1 glucose transporters, growth factors, growth factor receptors, extracellular matrix components, and adhesion molecules that can activate circulating leukocytes.[16] The observation that unilateral reduction in the severity of diabetic microvascular disease occurs on the side with ophthalmic or renal artery stenosis is consistent with this concept.[17, 18]

Microvascular Cell Loss and Vessel Occlusion

The progressive narrowing and occlusion of diabetic microvascular lumina are also accompanied by microvascular cell loss. In the retina, diabetes mellitus induces programmed cell death of Müller cells and ganglion cells,[19] pericytes, and endothelial cells.[20] In the glomerulus, declining renal function is associated with widespread capillary occlusion and podocyte loss, but the mechanisms underlying glomerular cell loss are not yet known. In the vasa nervorum, endothelial cell and pericyte degeneration occur,[21] and these microvascular changes

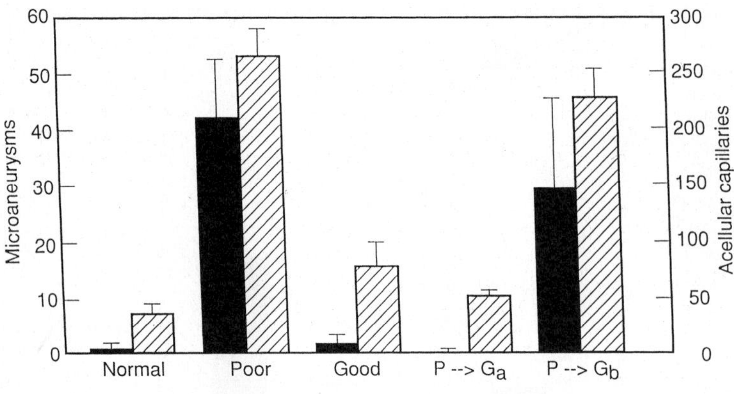

Figure 31–4. Development of retinopathy during posthyperglycemic normoglycemia ("hyperglycemic memory"). Quantitation of retinal microaneurysms and acellular capillaries in normal dogs, dogs with poor glycemic control for 5 years, dogs with good glycemic control for 5 years, dogs with poor glycemic control for 2.5 years (P → G_a), and the same dogs after a subsequent 2.5 years of good glycemic control (P → G_b). (Adapted from Engerman RL, Kern TS. Progression of incipient diabetic retinopathy during good glycemic control. Diabetes 1987; 36:808–812.)

appear to precede the development of diabetic peripheral neuropathy.[22] The multifocal distribution of axonal degeneration in diabetes supports a causal role for microvascular occlusion, but hyperglycemia-induced decreases in neurotrophins may contribute by preventing normal axonal repair and regeneration.[23]

Development of Microvascular Complications During Posthyperglycemic Euglycemia ("Hyperglycemic Memory")

Another common feature of diabetic microvascular disease has been termed *hyperglycemic memory*, or the persistence or progression of hyperglycemia-induced microvascular alterations during subsequent periods of normal glucose homeostasis. The most striking example of this phenomenon is the development of severe retinopathy in histologically normal eyes of diabetic dogs that occurred entirely during a 2.5-year period of normalized blood glucose that followed 2.5 years of hyperglycemia (Fig. 31–4).[24] Normal dogs were compared to diabetic dogs with either poor control for 5 years, good control for 5 years, or poor control for 2.5 years (P → G_a) followed by good control for the next 2.5 years (P → G_b). Hb A_1 values for both the good control group and the P → G_b group were identical to the normal group. Hyperglycemia-induced increases in selected matrix gene transcription also persist for weeks after restoration of normoglycemia in vivo, and a less pronounced, but qualitatively similar, prolongation of hyperglycemia-induced increase in selected matrix gene transcription occurs in cultured endothelial cells.[25]

Data from the DCCT study suggest that hyperglycemic memory occurs in patients. In the secondary-intervention cohort, there was no difference in the incidence of sustained progression of retinopathy for the first 3 years, no difference in development of clinical albuminuria for 4 years, and no difference in the rate of change in creatinine clearance during the entire study. For neuropathy, the sural nerve sensory conduction velocity did not differ between the groups for 4 years, and intensive therapy did not slow the rate of decline of autonomic function at all.[2, 26–28] Even more strikingly, the effects of former intensive and conventional therapy on the occurrence and severity of retinopathy and nephropathy were shown to persist for 4 years after the DCCT, despite nearly identical glycosylated hemoglobin values during the 4-year follow-up (8.2% versus 7.9%, respectively) (Fig. 31–5).[29] Together, these observations from animal and clinical studies imply that hyperglycemia induces prolonged and sometimes irreversible changes in long-lived intracellular molecules that persist and cause continued pathologic function in the absence of continued hyperglycemia.

Genetic Determinants of Susceptibility to Microvascular Complications

Clinicians have long observed that different patients with similar duration and degree of hyperglycemia differed markedly in their susceptibility to microvascular complications. Such observations suggested that genetic differences existed that affected the pathways by which hyperglycemia damaged microvascular cells. The leveling of risk of overt proteinuria after 30 years' duration of type 1 diabetes at 27% is evidence that only a subset of patients are susceptible to development of diabetic nephropathy.[30]

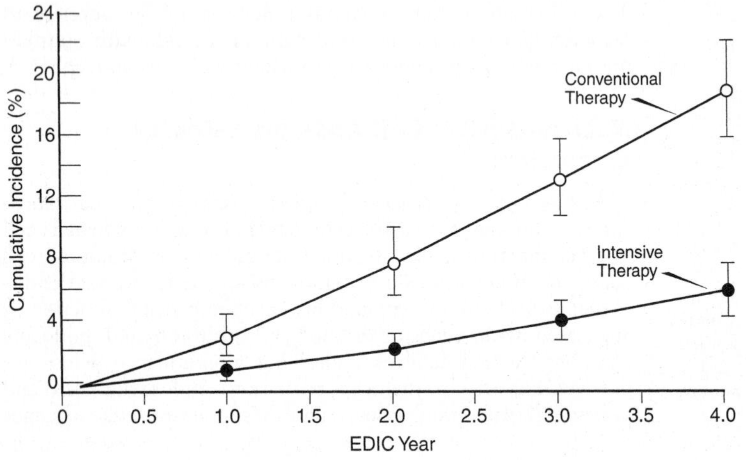

Figure 31–5. Cumulative incidence of further progression of retinopathy 4 years after the end of the Diabetes Control and Complications Trial. Median glycosylated hemoglobin was 8.2% for the conventional therapy group and 7.9% for the intensive therapy group. EDIC, Epidemiology of Diabetes Interventions and Complications [Research Group]. (From Retinopathy and nephropathy in patients with type 1 diabetes four years after a trial of intensive therapy. The Diabetes Control and Complications Trial/Epidemiology of Diabetes Interventions and Complications Research Group. N Engl J Med 2000; 342:381–389.)

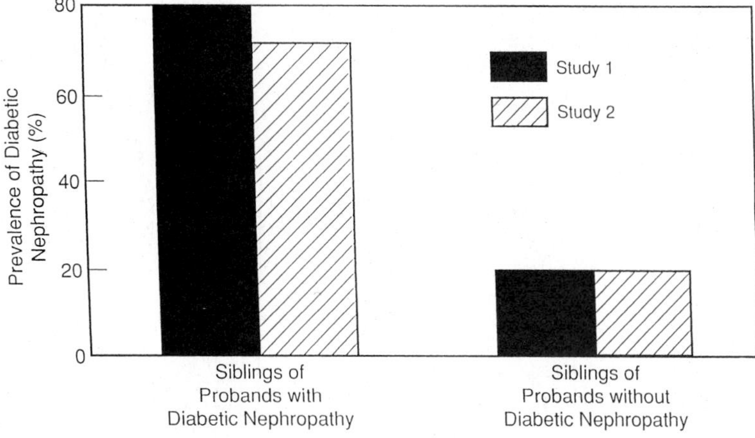

Figure 31–6. Familial clustering of diabetic nephropathy. Prevalence of diabetic nephropathy in two studies of diabetic siblings of probands with or without diabetic nephropathy. (Adapted from Seaquist ER, Goetz FC, Rich S, Barbosa J. Familial clustering of diabetic kidney disease: evidence for genetic susceptibility to diabetic nephropathy. N Engl J Med 1989; 320:1161–1165; and Quinn M, Angelico MC, Warram JH, Krolewski AS. Familial factors determine the development of diabetic nephropathy in patients with IDDM. Diabetologia 1996; 39:940–945.)

A role for genetic determinant of susceptibility to diabetic nephropathy is most strongly supported by the demonstration of familial clustering of diabetic nephropathy. In two studies of families with two or more siblings having type 1 diabetes, if one diabetic sibling had advanced diabetic nephropathy, the other diabetic sibling had a nephropathy risk of 83% or 72%; in contrast, the risk was only 17% or 22% if the index patient did not have diabetic nephropathy (Fig. 31–6).[31, 32] For retinopathy, the DCCT reported familial clustering as well, with an odds ratio of 5.4 for the risk of severe retinopathy in diabetic relatives of positive versus negative subjects from the conventional treatment group.[33]

Numerous associations have been made between various genetic polymorphisms and the risk of various diabetic complications. Examples include the 5′ insulin gene polymorphism,[34] the G2m^{23+} immunoglobulin allotype,[35] angiotensin-converting enzyme (ACE) insertion/deletion polymorphisms,[36, 37] HLA-DQB1*0201/0302 alleles,[38] polymorphisms of the aldose reductase gene,[39] and a polymorphic CCTTT (n) repeat of NO synthetase (NOS) 2A.[40] In all of these studies, there is no indication that the polymorphic gene actually plays a functional role rather than simply being in linkage disequilibrium with the locus encoding the unidentified relevant genes.

PATHOPHYSIOLOGIC FEATURES OF MACROVASCULAR COMPLICATIONS

Unlike microvascular disease, which occurs only in patients with diabetes mellitus, macrovascular disease resembles that in subjects without diabetes. However, subjects with diabetes have more rapidly progressive and extensive cardiovascular disease (CVD), with a greater incidence of multivessel disease and a greater number of diseased vessel segments than nondiabetic persons.[41] Although dyslipidemia and hypertension occur with great frequency in type 2 diabetic populations, there is still excess risk in diabetic subjects after adjusting for these other risk factors.[42, 43] Diabetes itself may confer 75% to 90% of the excess risk of coronary disease in these diabetic subjects, and it enhances the deleterious effects of the other major cardiovascular risk factors (Fig. 31–7).[44, 45]

In subjects with or without diabetes, atherosclerosis begins with endothelial dysfunction or injury.[46] These endothelial changes or injury induce the secretion of chemokines such as monocyte chemoattractant protein 1 (MCP-1), increase the expression of endothelial adhesion molecules for leucocytes and platelets, and enhance permeability to lipoproteins and other plasma constituents. As detailed in Chapter 34, this leads to recruitment of monocyte-macrophages to the subendothelial space and to the infiltration of plasma LDL, which binds to arterial proteoglycan. The retained LDL then undergoes oxidation and is taken up by macrophages.

Activated macrophages and other leukocytes, as well as adherent aggregated platelets, stimulate smooth muscle cell proliferation and elaboration of extracellular matrix, culminating in the formation of a complex lesion filled with prothrombotic material contained by a fibrin cap. Rupture of this fibrin cap by matrix metalloproteinases causes thrombus formation and arterial occlusion.[47–49] Because macrovascular disease also occurs in nondiabetic subjects, diabetes is thought to accelerate the process by increasing endothelial cell dysfunction and by exacerbating dyslipidemia.

The pathogenesis of endothelial cell dysfunction in diabetic arteries appears to involve both insulin resistance and hyperglycemia. In vitro studies suggest that insulin has both antiatherogenic and proatherogenic effects (Fig. 31–8).[50, 51] One major antiatherogenic effect is the stimulation of endothelial NO production. NO released from endothelial cells is a potent inhibitor of platelet aggregation and adhesion to the vascular wall. Endothelial NO also controls the expression of genes involved in atherogenesis. It decreases expression of the chemoattractant protein MCP-1, and of surface adhesion molecules such as CD11/CD18, P-selectin, vascular cell adhesion molecule-1 (VCAM-1), and intercellular adhesion molecule-1 (ICAM-1). Endothelial cell NO also reduces vascular permeability and decreases the rate of oxidation of low-density lipoprotein (LDL) to its proatherogenic form.

Finally, endothelial cell NO inhibits proliferation of vascular smooth muscle cells.[52] Two major proatherogenic effects of insulin are the potentiation of platelet-derived growth factor (PDGF)–induced vascular smooth muscle cell (VSMC) proliferation and the stimulation of VSMC plasminogen activator inhibitor 1 (PAI-1) production.[53, 54] Since insulin-induced NO production is mediated by the insulin receptor substrate →PI3 kinase signal transduction pathway, while the effects on smooth muscle cells are mediated by the ras →raf →mekk →map kinase signal transduction pathway,[50, 51] it has been proposed that pathway-selective insulin resistance in arterial cells may contribute to diabetic atherosclerosis. Recently, evidence of such selective vascular resistance to insulin has been demonstrated in the obese zucker rat.[55]

Hyperglycemia also inhibits arterial endothelial NO production, both in vivo and in vitro.[56–59] Similarly, hyperglycemia potentiates PDGF-induced VSMC proliferation and stimulates endothelial cell PAI-1 production.[60, 58] In addition, hyperglycemia has a variety of other proatherogenic effects on endothelial

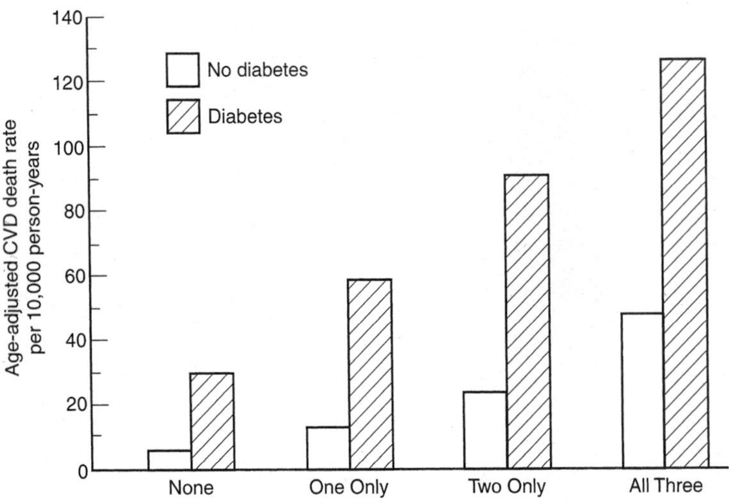

Figure 31–7. Adjusted death rates by number of cardiovascular disease (CVD) risk factors for diabetic and nondiabetic men. Subjects are participants from the Multiple Risk Factor Intervention Trial (MRFIT) study; risk factors are hypercholesterolemia, hypertension, and cigarette smoking. (From Stamler J, Vaccaro O, Neaton JD, Wentworth D. Diabetes, other risk factors, and 12-year cardiovascular mortality for men screened in the Multiple Risk Factor Intervention Trial. Diabetes Care 1993; 2:434–444.)

cells, platelets, and monocyte/macrophages. These include increased expression of MCP-1,[61] up-regulation of adhesion molecules such as ICAM-1 and VCAM-1,[62–64] potentiation of collagen-induced platelet activation,[65] and increased secretion of collagen type IV and fibronectin.[66, 67]

Both insulin resistance and hyperglycemia have been implicated in the pathogenesis of diabetic dyslipidemia as well. Insulin resistance is associated with a characteristic lipoprotein profile that includes a high very-low-density lipoprotein (VLDL), a low high-density lipoprotein (HDL), and small, dense LDL. Both low HDL and small, dense LDL are each independent risk factors for macrovascular disease. This profile arises as a direct result of increased net free fatty acid (FFA) release by insulin resistant adipocytes (Fig. 31–9).[68] Increased FFA flux into hepatocytes stimulates VLDL secretion. In the presence of cholesteryl ester transfer protein, excess VLDL transfers significant amounts of triglyceride to both HDL and LDL while depleting HDL and LDL of cholesteryl ester. The resultant triglyceride-enriched HDL carries less cholesteryl ester for reverse cholesterol transport to the liver, and loss of Apo1A-1, from these particles reduces the total concentration of HDL available for reverse cholesterol transport. The triglyceride-enriched, cholesteryl ester–depleted LDL is smaller and denser than normal LDL, allowing it to penetrate the vessel wall and be oxidized more easily.

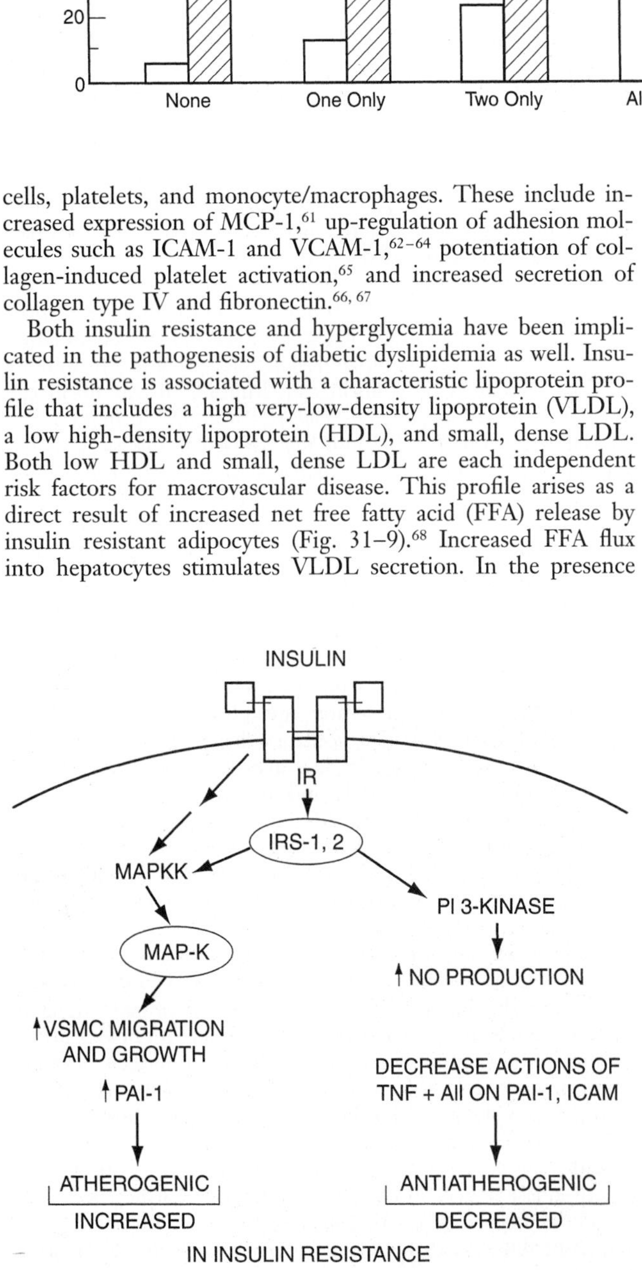

Hyperglycemia appears to contribute to diabetic dyslipidemia by causing delayed clearance of postprandial lipoproteins, resulting in elevated levels of atherogenic cholesterol-enriched remnant particles.[9] This remnant clearance defect is caused by a hyperglycemia-induced reduction in expression of the heparan sulfate proteoglycan perlecan on hepatocytes. Perlecan interaction with apoB-48–containing lipoprotein remnant particles is necessary for efficient uptake by the LDL receptor-related protein.

The importance of hyperlipidemia in the pathogenesis of diabetic macrovascular disease in patients with type 2 diabetes is underscored by recent studies validating that effective treatment of hyperlipidemia in such patients substantially reduces their risk of CVD.[7, 8] The importance of hyperglycemia in the pathogenesis of diabetic macrovascular disease is suggested by the observation that carotid wall thickness is increased in persons with established diabetes but not in persons with impaired glucose tolerance.[6]

The United Kingdom Prospective Diabetes Study (UKPDS) identified hyperglycemia as an important risk factor for macrovascular disease in type 2 diabetes, and numerous correlational studies show that hyperglycemia is a continuous risk factor for macrovascular disease.[69–73] Similarly, glycohemoglobin A_1 is an independent risk factor for CVD[74] in type 1 diabetes. The relative importance of hyperglycemia in type 1 patients is suggested by the 41% reduction in macrovascular disease (P = .06) observed in the intensive therapy group of the DCCT.[2]

INSULIN
IR
IRS-1, 2
MAPKK
MAP-K
↑VSMC MIGRATION AND GROWTH
↑PAI-1
PI 3-KINASE
↑NO PRODUCTION
DECREASE ACTIONS OF TNF + AII ON PAI-1, ICAM
ATHEROGENIC
INCREASED
ANTIATHEROGENIC
DECREASED
IN INSULIN RESISTANCE

Figure 31–8. Schematic summary of proatherosclerotic and antiatherosclerotic actions of insulin on vascular cells. See text for abbreviations. (Adapted from King G, Brownlee M. The cellular and molecular mechanisms of diabetic complications. Endocrinol Metab Clin North Am 1996; 2:255–270; and Hsueh WA, Law RE. Cardiovascular risk continuum: implications of insulin resistance and diabetes. Am J Med 1998; 105:4S-14S.)

MECHANISMS OF HYPERGLYCEMIA-INDUCED DAMAGE

Four major hypotheses about how hyperglycemia causes diabetic complications have generated a large amount of data as

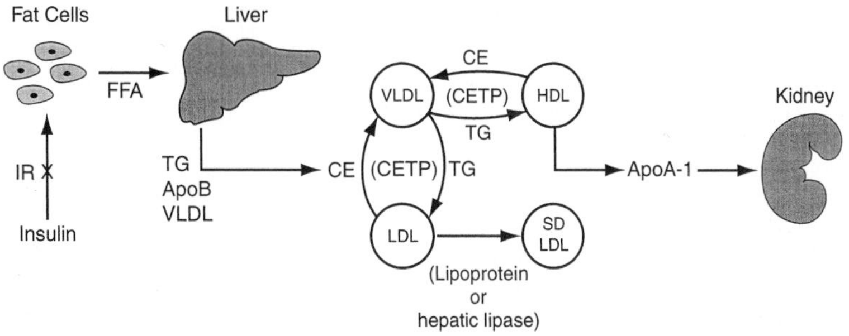

Figure 31–9. Schematic summary relating insulin resistance (IR) to the characteristic dyslipidemia of type 2 diabetes mellitus. IR at the adipocyte results in increased free fatty acid (FFA) release. Increased FFA flux stimulates very-low-density lipoprotein (VLDL) secretion, causing hypertriglyceridemia (TG). VLDL stimulates a reciprocal exchange of TG to cholesteryl ester (CE) from both high-density lipoprotein (HDL) and low-density lipoprotein (LDL), catalyzed by CE transfer protein (CETP). TG-enriched HDL dissociates from ApoA-1, leaving less HDL for reverse cholesterol transport. TG-enriched LDL serves as a substrate for lipases that convert it to atherogenic small, dense LDL particles (SD LDL). (From Ginsberg HN. Insulin resistance and cardiovascular disease. J Clin Invest 2000; 106:453–458.)

well as several clinical trials based on specific inhibitors of these mechanisms. Until recently, there was no unifying hypothesis linking these four mechanisms together, nor was there an obvious connection between any of these mechanisms, each of which responds quickly to normalization of hyperglycemia, and the phenomenon of hyperglycemic memory (see earlier).

Increased Polyol Pathway Flux

Aldose Reductase Function

Aldose reductase (alditol:NAD(P)$^+$ 1-oxidoreductase, EC 1.1.1.21) is a cytosolic, monomeric oxidoreductase that catalyzes the NADPH-dependent reduction of a wide variety of carbonyl compounds including glucose. Triphosphopyridine nucleotide, reduced form of NADP (NADPH) is the cofactor in both this reaction and in the regeneration of glutathione by glutathione reductase. Aldose reductase has a low affinity (high Michaelis constant [K_m]) for glucose, and at the normal glucose concentrations found in nondiabetic patients, metabolism of glucose by this pathway constitutes a small percentage of total glucose utilization. In a hyperglycemic environment, however, increased intracellular glucose results in increased enzymatic conversion to the polyalcohol sorbitol, with concomitant decreases in NADPH. In the polyol pathway, sorbitol is oxidized to fructose by the enzyme sorbitol dehydrogenase, with NAD$^+$ reduced to NADH (Fig. 31–10).

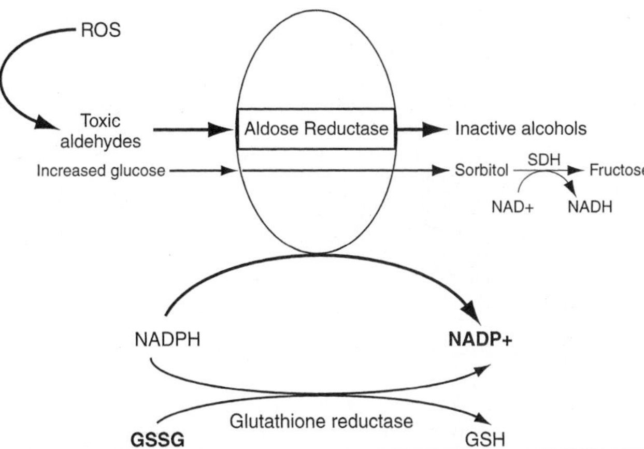

Figure 31–10. Aldose reductase and the polyol pathway. Aldose reductase reduces reactive oxygen species (ROS)-generated toxic aldehydes to inactive alcohols, and glucose to sorbitol, using triphosphopyridine nucleotide, reduced form of NADP (NADPH) as a cofactor. In cells where aldose reductase activity is sufficient to deplete reduced glutathione (GSH), oxidative stress would be augmented. Sorbitol dehydrogenase (SDH) oxidizes sorbitol to fructose using nicotinamide-adenine dinucleotide (NAD$^+$) as a cofactor. GSSG, oxidized glutathione.

Biochemical Consequences of Increased Polyol Pathway Flux

A number of mechanisms have been proposed to explain the potential detrimental effects of hyperglycemia-induced increases in polyol pathway flux. These include sorbitol-induced osmotic stress, decreased Na^+/K^+ ATPase activity, increased cytosolic NADH/NAD$^+$, and decreased cytosolic NADPH. Sorbitol does not diffuse easily across cell membranes, and it was originally suggested that this resulted in osmotic damage to microvascular cells. However, sorbitol concentrations measured in diabetic vessels and nerves are far too low to cause osmotic damage.

Another early suggestion was that increased flux through the polyol pathway decreased Na^+/K^+ ATPase activity. Although this was originally thought to be mediated by polyol-pathway–linked decreases in phosphatidylinositol synthesis, it has been shown to result from activation of protein kinase C (PKC) (see later). Hyperglycemia-induced activation of PKC increases cytosolic phospholipase A_2 activity, which increases the production of two inhibitors of Na^+/K^+ ATPase, arachidonate and prostaglandin E_2 (PGE_2).[75]

More recently, it has been proposed that oxidation of sorbitol by NAD$^+$ increases the cytosolic ratio of NADH/NAD$^+$, thereby inhibiting activity of the enzyme glyceraldehyde-3-phosphate dehydrogenase and increasing concentrations of triose phosphate.[76] Elevated triose phosphate concentrations could increase formation of both methylglyoxal, a precursor of advanced glycation end products (AGEs), and diacylglycerol (DAG) (via α-glycerol-3-phosphate), thus activating PKC (discussed in subsequent sections). Although increased NADH production is supported by the observation that hyperglycemia increases both lactate concentration and the lactate/pyruvate ratio, there is no direct evidence that the concentrations of NADH and NAD$^+$, as opposed to NADH and NAD$^+$ flux, are altered. In endothelial cells, where aldose reductase activity is low, increased NADH production may also reflect hyperglycemia-induced increased flux through glycolysis[77] and through the glucuronic acid pathway.[78]

Other evidence presented in support of this hypothesis includes the observation that administration of pyruvate can prevent diabetes-related endothelial dysfunction in some systems. However, the observed effects of pyruvate on microvascular function may reflect its potent antioxidant properties rather than effects on the NADH/NAD$^+$ ratio, because reactive oxygen species (ROS) also partially inhibit glyceraldehyde-3-phosphate dehydrogenase and increase glyceraldehyde-3-phosphate levels.[79, 80] The source of hyperglycemia-induced ROS is discussed later in this section.

It has also been proposed that reduction of glucose to sorbitol by NADPH consumes the cofactor NADPH. Because NADPH is required for regenerating reduced glutathione (GSH), this could induce or exacerbate intracellular oxidative stress. Less reduced glutathione has in fact been found in the lens of transgenic mice that overexpress aldose reductase, and this is the most likely mechanism by which increased flux through the polyol pathway has deleterious consequences.[81] Hyperglycemia-induced inhibition of glucose-6-phosphate dehydrogenase, the major source of NADPH regeneration, may further reduce NADPH concentration in some vascular cells or neuronal cells.[82]

Increased Intracellular Advanced Glycation End-Product Formation

Advanced Glycation End Products Are Formed from Intracellular Dicarbonyl Precursors

AGEs are found in increased amounts in extracellular structures of diabetic retinal vessels[83–85] and renal glomeruli,[86–88] where they can cause damage by mechanisms described later in this section. These AGEs were originally thought to arise from nonenzymatic reactions between extracellular proteins and glucose. However, the rate of AGE formation from glucose is orders of magnitude slower than the rate of AGE formation from glucose-derived dicarbonyl precursors generated intracellularly, and it now seems likely that intracellular hyperglycemia is the primary initiating event in the formation of both intracellular and extracellular AGEs.[89] AGEs can arise from intracellular auto-oxidation of glucose to glyoxal,[90] decomposition of the Amadori product to 3-deoxyglucosone (perhaps accelerated by an Amadoriase), and fragmentation of glyceraldehyde-3-phosphate to methylglyoxal[91] (Fig. 31–11). These reactive intracellular dicarbonyls react with amino groups of intracellular and extracellular proteins to form AGEs. Methylglyoxal and glyoxal are detoxified by the glyoxalase system.[91] All three AGE precursors are also substrates for other reductases.[92, 93]

Intracellular production of AGE precursors damages target cells by three general mechanisms (Fig. 31–12):

1. Intracellular proteins modified by AGEs have altered function.
2. Extracellular matrix components modified by AGE precursors interact abnormally with other matrix components and with matrix-receptors (integrins) on cells.
3. Plasma proteins modified by AGE precursors bind to AGE receptors on cells such as macrophages, inducing receptor-mediated ROS production. This AGE receptor ligation activates the pleiotrophic transcription factor NFκB, causing pathologic changes in gene expression.[94]

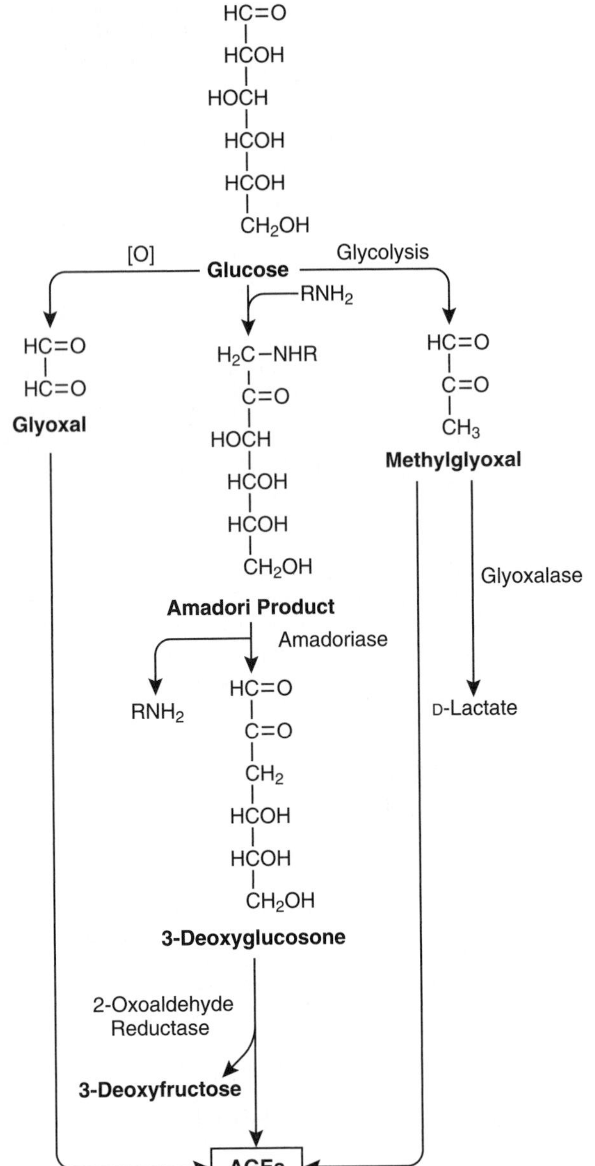

Figure 31–11. Potential pathways leading to the formation of advanced glycation end product (AGE) from intracellular dicarbonyl precursors. Glyoxal arises from the auto-oxidation of glucose, 3-deoxyglucosone arises from decomposition of the Amadori product, and methylglyoxal arises from fragmentation of glyceraldehyde 3-phosphate. These reactive dicarbonyls react with amino groups of proteins to form AGEs. Methylglyoxal and glyoxal are detoxified by the glyoxalase system. (Adapted from Shinohara M, Thornalley PJ, Giardino I, et al. Overexpression of glyoxalase-I in bovine endothelial cells inhibits intracellular advanced glycation end-product formation and prevents hyperglycemia-induced increases in macromolecular endocytosis. J Clin Invest 1998; 101:1142.)

Advanced Glycation End Products Alter Intracellular Protein Function

In endothelial cells, intracellular AGE formation occurs quickly. Within 1 week, AGE content increases 13.8-fold in endothelial cells cultured in media containing high levels of glucose.[95] Basic fibroblast growth factor (bFGF) is one of the major AGE-modified proteins in endothelial cells.[95] Endothelial cell cytosol mitogenic activity is reduced 70% by AGE formation when cytosolic AGE-bFGF is increased 6.1-fold. Proteins involved in macromolecular endocytosis are also modified by AGEs, because the 2.2-fold increase in endocytosis induced by hyperglycemia is prevented by overexpression of the methylglyoxal-detoxifying glyoxalase I.[96] Glyoxalase I overexpression also completely prevents the fourfold hyperglycemia-induced increase in Müller cell expression of angiopoietin

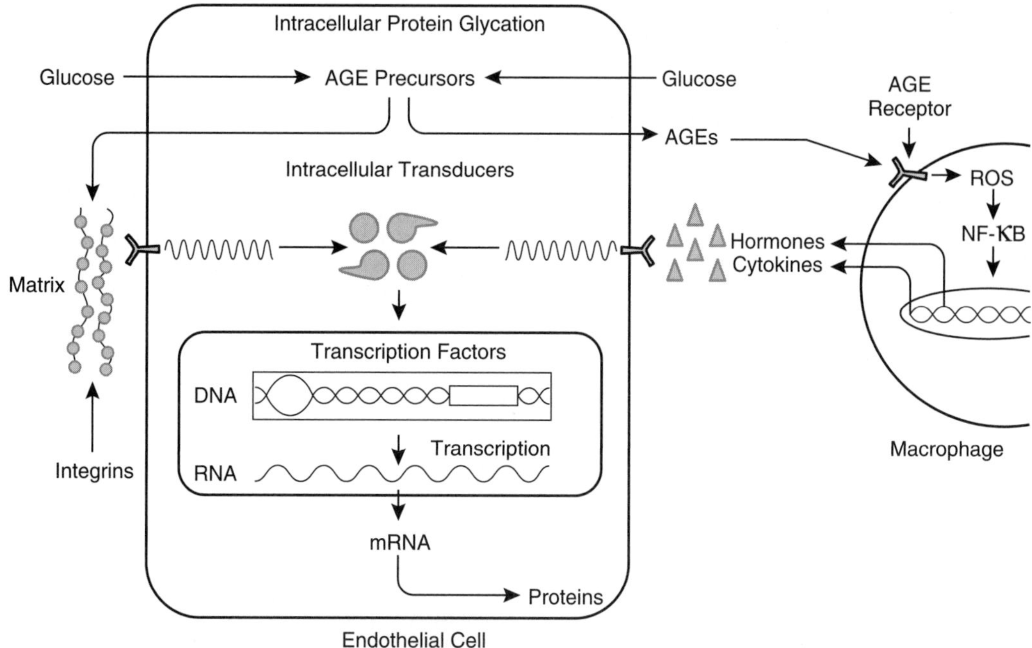

Figure 31–12. Potential mechanisms by which intracellular production of advanced glycation end-product (AGE) precursors damages vascular cells. First, intracellular protein modification alters protein function. Second, extracellular matrix modified by AGE precursors has abnormal functional properties. Third, plasma proteins modified by AGE precursors bind to AGE receptors on adjacent cells such as macrophages, thereby inducing receptor-mediated production of deleterious gene products such as cytokines. mRNA, messenger RNA; NFκB, neurotropic factor-κB; ROS, reactive oxygen species. (Adapted from Brownlee M. Lilly Lecture 1993: Glycation and Diabetic Complications. Diabetes 1994; 43:836–841.)

2 (Matsumura and associates, unpublished), a factor that has been implicated in both pericyte loss and capillary regression.[97–99] This observation suggests that the α-oxoaldehyde AGE precursors methylglyoxal and glyoxal modify transcriptional complex proteins and thereby activate gene expression.

Advanced Glycation End Products Interfere with Normal Matrix-Matrix and Matrix-Cell Interactions

AGE formation alters the functional properties of several important matrix molecules. Collagen was the first matrix protein used to demonstrate that glucose-derived AGEs form covalent, intermolecular bonds. This process is partly mediated by H_2O_2 production.[100, 101] On type I collagen, this cross-linking induces an expansion of the molecular packing.[102] These AGE-induced cross-links alter the function of intact vessels. For example, AGEs decrease elasticity in large vessels from diabetic rats, even after vascular tone is abolished, and increase fluid filtration across the carotid artery.[103] AGE formation on type IV collagen from basement membrane inhibits lateral association of these molecules into a normal network-like structure by interfering with binding of the noncollagenous NC1 domain to the helix-rich domain.[104] AGE formation on laminin causes decreased polymer self-assembly, decreased binding to type IV collagen, and decreased binding of heparan sulfate proteoglycan.[105] In vitro AGE formation on intact glomerular basement membrane increases its permeability to albumin in a manner that resembles the abnormal permeability of diabetic nephropathy.[106, 107]

AGE formation on extracellular matrix interferes not only with matrix-matrix interactions but also with matrix-cell interactions. For example, AGE modification of type IV collagen's cell-binding domains decreases endothelial cell adhesion,[108] and AGE modification of a 6–amino acid growth-promoting sequence in the A chain of the laminin molecule markedly reduces neurite outgrowth.[109] AGE modification of vitronectin reduces cell attachment–promoting activity.[110]

Advanced Glycation End-Product Receptors Mediate Pathologic Changes in Gene Expression

Specific receptors for AGEs were first identified on monocytes and macrophages. Two AGE-binding proteins isolated from rat liver are both present on monocyte/macrophages. Antisera to either the 60-kd or 90-kd protein, recently identified as OST-48 and 80K-H, respectively,[111] block AGE binding.[112] AGE protein binding to this receptor stimulates macrophage production of interleukin 1, insulin-like growth factor (IGF)-I, tumor necrosis factor α, TGF-β, macrophage colony-stimulating factor, and granulocyte/macrophage colony-stimulating factor at levels that have been shown to increase glomerular synthesis of type IV collagen and to stimulate proliferation and chemotaxis of both arterial smooth muscle cells and macrophages.[113–121] The macrophage scavenger receptor type 2 and galectin 3 have also been shown to recognize AGEs.[122–125]

AGE receptors have also been identified on glomerular mesangial cells. *In vitro*, AGE protein binding to its receptor on mesangial cells stimulates PDGF secretion, which, in turn, mediates production of type IV collagen, laminin, and heparan sulfate proteoglycan.[126, 127]

Vascular endothelial cells also express AGE-specific receptors (RAGE). A 35-kd and a 46-kd AGE-binding protein have been purified to homogeneity from endothelial cells.[128–130] The N-terminal sequence of the 35-kd protein was identical to lactoferrin, whereas the 46-kd protein was novel. A full-length, 1.5-kb complementary DNA (cDNA) for the 46-kd protein was cloned and sequenced. This novel AGE-binding protein appears to be a member of the immunoglobulin superfamily,

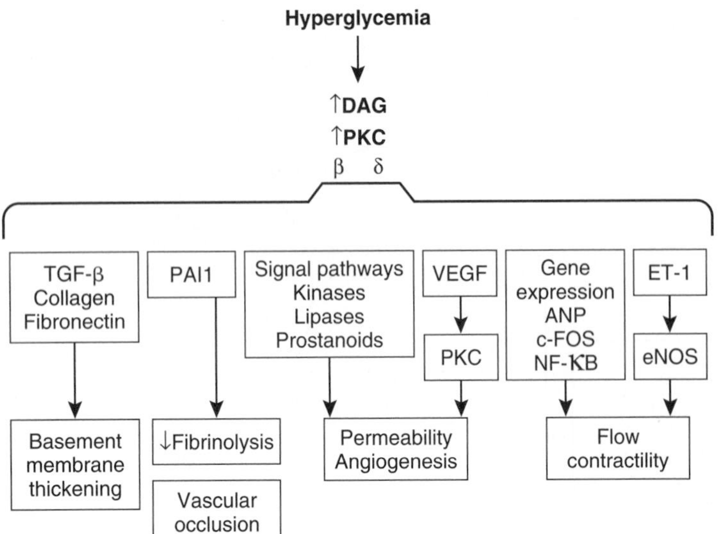

Figure 31–13. Potential consequences of hyperglycemia-induced protein kinase C (PKC) activation. Hyperglycemia increases diacylglycerol (DAG) content, which activates PKC, primarily the β and δ isoforms. Activated PKC has a number of pathogenic consequences. See text for additional abbreviations. (Adapted from Koya D, Jirousek MR, Lin YW, et al. Characterization of protein kinase C beta isoform activation on the gene expression of transforming growth factor-beta, extracellular matrix components, and prostanoids in the glomeruli of diabetic rats. J Clin Invest 1997; 100:115–126.).

with three disulfide-bonded immunoglobulin homology units. RAGE has been shown to mediate signal transduction via generation of ROS, activation of NFκB, and p21 ras.[131–133] AGE signaling is blocked in cells by expression of RAGE antisense cDNA[134] or anti-RAGE ribozyme.[135]

In endothelial cells, AGE binding to its receptor induces changes in gene expression that include alterations in thrombomodulin, tissue factor, and VCAM-1.[136–139] These changes induce procoagulatory changes in the endothelial surface and increase the adhesion of inflammatory cells to the vessel wall. In addition, endothelial RAGE binding appears to mediate in part the hyperpermeability induced by diabetes, probably through the induction of vascular endothelial growth factor (VEGF).[140–142] The potential importance of AGEs in the pathogenesis of diabetic macrovascular disease is highlighted by the observation that infusion of the soluble extracellular domain of RAGE suppressed macrovascular disease in an atherosclerosis-prone type 1 diabetic mouse model in a glucose- and lipid-independent fashion.[143]

Activation of Protein Kinase C

Mechanism of Hyperglycemia-Induced Protein Kinase C Activation

PKCs are a family of at least 11 isoforms, 9 of which are activated by the lipid second-messenger DAG. Intracellular hyperglycemia increases DAG content in cultured microvascular cells and in the retina and renal glomeruli of diabetic animals.[144–146] Intracellular hyperglycemia appears to increase DAG content primarily by increasing its de novo synthesis from the glycolytic intermediate glyceraldehyde-3-phosphate via reduction to glycerol-3-phosphate and stepwise acylation.[145, 147] Increased de novo synthesis of DAG activates PKC both in cultured vascular cells[146, 148–150] and in retina and glomeruli of diabetic animals.[145, 146, 148] Increased DAG primarily activates the β and δ isoforms of PKC, but increases in other isoforms have also been found, such as PKC-α and PKC-ϵ isoforms in the retina[151] and PKC-α and PKC-δ in the glomerulus[152, 153] of diabetic rats.

Consequences of Hyperglycemia-Induced Protein Kinase C Activation

In early experimental diabetes, activation of PKC-β isoforms has been shown to mediate retinal and renal blood flow abnormalities,[154] perhaps by depressing NO production and increasing endothelin-1 activity (Fig. 31–13). Abnormal activation of PKC has been implicated in the decreased glomerular production of NO induced by experimental diabetes[155] and in the decreased smooth muscle cell NO production induced by hyperglycemia.[156] PKC activation also inhibits insulin-stimulated expression of endothelial nitric oxide synthase (eNOS) messenger RNA (mRNA) in cultured endothelial cells.[157] Hyperglycemia increases endothelin 1–stimulated mitogen-activated protein kinase activity in glomerular mesangial cells by activating PKC isoforms.[158] The increased endothelial cell permeability induced by high glucose in cultured cells is mediated by activation of PKC-α, however.[159] Activation of PKC by elevated glucose levels also induces expression of the permeability-enhancing factor VEGF in smooth muscle cells.[160]

In addition to affecting hyperglycemia-induced abnormalities of blood flow and permeability, activation of PKC contributes to increased microvascular matrix protein accumulation by inducing the expression of TGF-β_1, fibronectin, and α1 (IV) collagen in both cultured mesangial cells[161, 162] and in the glomeruli of diabetic rats.[163] This effect appears to be mediated through PKC's inhibition of NO production.[164] Hyperglycemia-induced expression of laminin C1 in cultured mesangial cells is independent of PKC activation, however.[165] Hyperglycemia-induced activation of PKC has also been implicated in the overexpression of the fibrinolytic inhibitor PAI-1[166] and in the activation of the pleiotrophic transcription factor NF-κB in cultured endothelial cells and vascular smooth muscle cells.[167, 168]

Increased Hexosamine Pathway Flux

A fourth hypothesis about how hyperglycemia causes diabetic complications has recently been formulated,[169–172] in which glucose is shunted into the hexosamine pathway (Fig. 31–14). In this pathway, fructose-6-phosphate is diverted from glycolysis to provide substrates for reactions that require UDP-*N*-acetylglucosamine, such as proteoglycan synthesis and the formation of *O*-linked glycoproteins. Inhibition of the rate-limiting enzyme in the conversion of glucose to glucosamine, glutamine:fructose-6-phosphate amidotransferase, blocks hyperglycemia-induced increases in the transcription of both TGF-α[169] and TGF-β_1.[170] This pathway has previously been shown to play an important role in hyperglycemia-induced and fat-induced insulin resistance.[173–175]

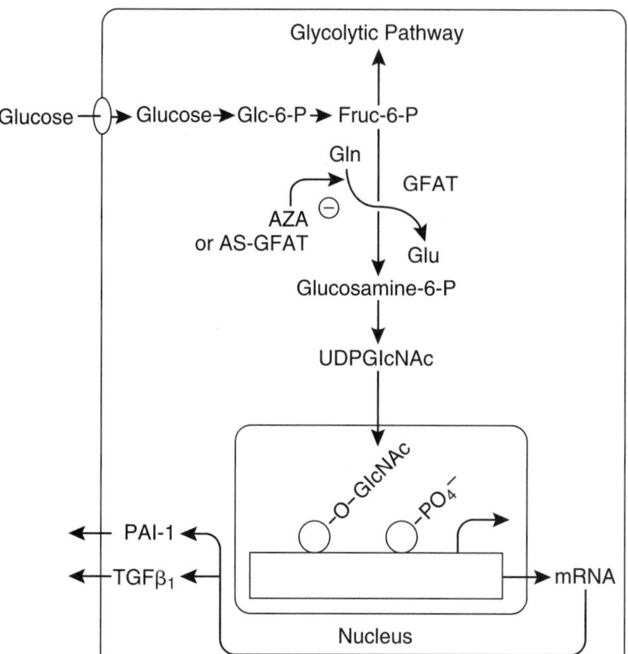

Figure 31–14. Schematic representation of the hexosamine pathway. The glycolytic intermediate fructose-6-phosphate (Fruc-6-P) is converted to glucosamine-6-phosphate (Glc-6-P) by the enzyme glutamine:fructose 6-phosphate amidotransferase (GFAT). Increased donation of N-Acetylglucosamine moieties to serine and threonine residues of transcription factors such as Sp1 increases production of such complication-promoting factors as PAI-1 and TGF-β_1. See text for additional abbreviations. (Adapted from Du XL, Edelstein D, Rossetti L, et al. Hyperglycemia-induced mitochondrial superoxide overproduction activates the hexosamine pathway and induces plasminogen activator inhibitor-1 expression by increasing Sp1 glycosylation. Proc Natl Acad Sci USA 2000; 97:12222–12226.)

The mechanism by which increased flux through the hexosamine pathway mediates hyperglycemia-induced increases in gene transcription has not been clear, but the observation that Sp1 sites regulate hyperglycemia-induced activation of the PAI-1 promoter in vascular smooth muscle cells[176] suggests that covalent modification of Sp1 by *N*-acetylglucosamine may explain the link between hexosamine pathway activation and hyperglycemia-induced changes in gene transcription. Virtually every RNA polymerase II transcription factor examined has been found to be *0*-Glc*N*acylated,[177] and the glycosylated form of Sp1 appears to be more transcriptionally active than the deglycosylated form of the protein.[178] A four-fold increase in Sp1 *0*-GlcNacylation caused by inhibition of the enzyme *0*-GlcNac-β-N-acetylglucosaminidase resulted in a reciprocal 30% decrease in its level of serine/threonine phosphorylation, supporting the concept that *0*-GlcNacylation and phosphorylation compete to modify the same sites on this protein.[179]

GlcNac modification of Sp1 may regulate other glucose-responsive genes in addition to TGF-β_1 and PAI-1. Glucose-responsive transcription is regulated by Sp1 sites in the acetyl-CoA carboxylase gene, the rate-limiting enzyme for fatty acid synthesis, for example, and it appears that post-translational modification of Sp1 is responsible for this effect.[180, 181] Because virtually every RNA polymerase II transcription factor examined has been found to be *O*-GlcNacylated,[177] it is possible that reciprocal modification by *O*-GlcNacylation and phosphorylation of transcription factors other than Sp1 may function as a more generalized mechanism for regulating glucose-responsive gene transcription.

In addition to transcription factors, many other nuclear and cytoplasmic proteins are dynamically modified by *O*-GlcNAc moieties and may exhibit reciprocal modification by phosphorylation in a manner analogous to Sp1.[177] Thus, activation of the hexosamine pathway by hyperglycemia may result in many changes in both gene expression and in protein function that together contribute to the pathogenesis of diabetic complications.

DIFFERENT PATHOGENIC MECHANISMS REFLECT A SINGLE HYPERGLYCEMIA-INDUCED PROCESS

Although specific inhibitors of aldose reductase activity, AGE formation, and PKC activation each ameliorate various diabetes-induced abnormalities in animal models, there has been no apparent common element linking the four mechanisms of hyperglycemia-induced damage discussed in the preceding section.[154, 182–185] It has also been conceptually difficult to explain the phenomenon of hyperglycemic memory (discussed in an earlier section) as a consequence of four processes that quickly normalize when euglycemia is restored. These issues have now been resolved by the recent discovery that each of the four different pathogenic mechanisms reflects a single hyperglycemia-induced process: overproduction of superoxide by the mitochondrial electron transport chain.[77, 186]

Hyperglycemia increases ROS production inside cultured bovine aortic endothelial cells.[187] To understand how this occurs, a brief overview of glucose metabolism is helpful. Intracellular glucose oxidation begins with glycolysis in the cytoplasm, which generates NADH and pyruvate. Cytoplasmic NADH can donate reducing equivalents to the mitochondrial electron transport chain via two shuttle systems, or it can reduce pyruvate to lactate, which exits the cell to provide substrate for hepatic gluconeogenesis. Pyruvate can also be transported into the mitochondria, where it is oxidized by the tricarboxylic acid (TCA) cycle to produce carbon dioxide (CO_2), water (H_2O), four molecules of NADH, and one molecule of $FADH_2$. Mitochondrial NADH and $FADH_2$ provide energy for adenosine triphosphate (ATP) production via oxidative phosphorylation by the electron transport chain.

Electron flow through the mitochondrial electron transport chain is carried out by four inner membrane–associated enzyme complexes, plus cytochrome-*c* and the mobile carrier ubiquinone.[188] NADH derived from both cytosolic glucose oxidation and mitochondrial TCA cycle activity donates electrons to NADH:ubiquinone oxidoreductase *(Complex I)*. Complex I ultimately transfers its electrons to ubiquinone. Ubiquinone can also be reduced by electrons donated from several $FADH_2$-containing dehydrogenases, including succinate:ubiquinone oxidoreductase *(Complex II)* and glycerol-3-phosphate dehydrogenase. Electrons from reduced ubiquinone are then transferred to ubiquinol:cytochrome c oxidoreductase *(Complex III)* by the ubisemiquinone radical-generating Q cycle.[189] Electron transport then proceeds through cytochrome-*c*, cytochrome-*c* oxidase *(Complex IV)*, and finally, molecular oxygen.

Electron transfer through Complexes I, III, and IV generates a proton gradient that drives ATP synthase *(Complex V)*. When the electrochemical potential difference generated by this proton gradient is high, the life of superoxide-generating electron transport intermediates such as ubisemiquinone is prolonged. There appears to be a threshold value above which superoxide production is markedly increased (Fig. 31–15).[190]

Using inhibitors of both the shuttle that transfers cytosolic

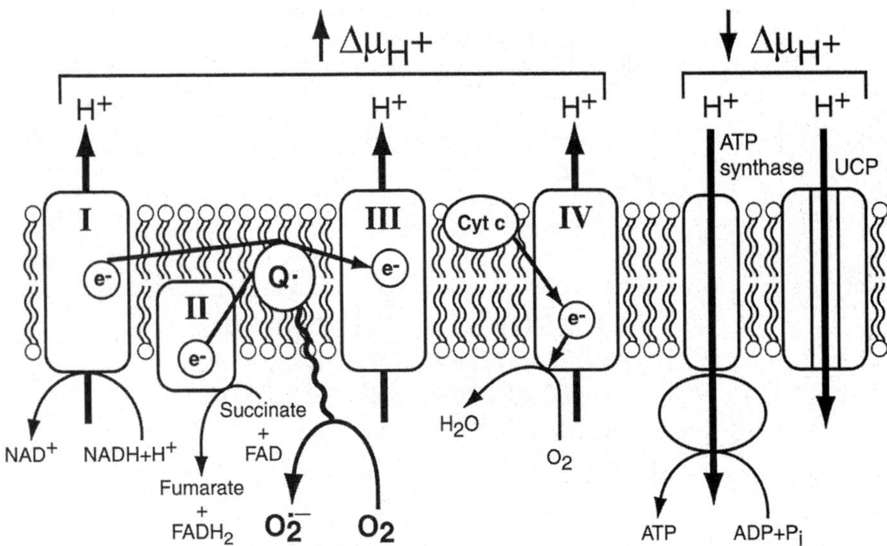

Figure 31–15. Production of superoxide by the mitochondrial electron transport chain. Increased hyperglycemia-derived electron donors from the tricarboxylic acid cycle (NADH and $FADH_2$) generate a high mitochondrial membrane potential ($\Delta\mu H^+$) by pumping protons across the mitochondrial inner membrane. This inhibits electron transport at complex III and increases the half-life of free radical intermediates of coenzyme Q, which reduce O_2 to superoxide. See text for abbreviations. (From Boss O, Hagen T, Lowell BB. Uncoupling proteins 2 and 3: potential regulators of mitochondrial energy metabolism. Diabetes 2000; 49:143–156.)

NADH into mitochondria, and the transporter that transfers cytosolic pyruvate into the mitochondria, the TCA cycle was shown to be the source of hyperglycemia-induced ROS in endothelial cells. Overexpression of uncoupling protein 1 (UCP-1), a specific protein uncoupler of oxidative phosphorylation capable of collapsing the proton electrochemical gradient,[191] also prevented the effect of hyperglycemia. These results demonstrate that hyperglycemia-induced intracellular ROS are produced by the proton electrochemical gradient generated by the mitochondrial electron transport chain. Overexpression of manganese superoxide dismutase, the mitochondrial form of this antioxidant enzyme,[192] also prevented the effect of hyperglycemia. This result demonstrates that superoxide is the reactive oxygen radical produced by this mechanism.

The effect of hyperglycemia-induced mitochondrial superoxide overproduction on polyol pathway flux was evaluated after first determining that sorbitol in these cells was exclusively derived from aldose reductase activity. Sorbitol levels were 2.6-fold higher than baseline (5-mM glucose) when endothelial cells were incubated in 30-mM glucose (Fig. 31–16). Hyperglycemia-induced sorbitol accumulation was completely prevented by UCP-1 and superoxide dismutase (Mn-SOD) (see Fig. 31–16), indicating that mitochondrial superoxide overproduction stimulates aldose reductase activity. This effect appears to reflect the well-described reversible inhibition of glyceraldehyde-3-phosphate dehydrogenase by ROS,[80, 186] which increases glyceraldehyde-3-phosphate levels and the levels of proximal glycolytic metabolites, including glucose (Fig. 31–17).

Next, the effect of hyperglycemia-induced mitochondrial superoxide overproduction on intracellular AGE formation was determined. In bovine aortic endothelial cells, hyperglycemia increases intracellular AGEs primarily, if not exclusively, by increasing the formation of AGE-forming methylglyoxal.[96] Therefore, the effect of UCP-1 and Mn-SOD on hyperglycemia-induced formation of intracellular methylglyoxal-derived AGEs was examined (see Fig. 31–16). Each of these agents completely prevented hyperglycemia-induced formation of intracellular AGEs (see Fig. 31–16), indicating that mitochondrial superoxide initiates intracellular AGE formation. Because methylglyoxal is formed by fragmentation of glyceraldehyde-3-phosphate, this dependency on increased mitochondrial superoxide production also likely reflects increased glyceraldehyde-3-phosphate levels due to inhibition of glyceraldehyde-3-phosphate dehydrogenase by ROS (see Fig. 31–17).

The effect of UCP-1 and Mn-SOD on hyperglycemia-induced activation of PKC was also evaluated (see Fig. 31–16). Each of these agents completely inhibited PKC activation, suggesting that mitochondrial superoxide overproduction initiates the hyperglycemia-induced de novo synthesis of DAG that activates PKC.[151] Most likely this too reflects increased glyceraldehyde-3-phosphate levels due to inhibition of glyceraldehyde-3-phosphate dehydrogenase by ROS (see Fig. 31–17).

Finally, the effect of hyperglycemia-induced mitochondrial superoxide overproduction on the hexosamine pathway was determined.[186] Hyperglycemia induced an increase in hexosamine pathway activity that was completely prevented by UCP-1, Mn-SOD, and azaserine, an inhibitor of the rate-limiting enzyme in the hexosamine pathway.

Hyperglycemia-induced activation of the redox-sensitive pleiotropic transcription factor NF-κB was also prevented by inhibition of mitochondrial superoxide overproduction.[77]

A POSSIBLE MOLECULAR BASIS FOR HYPERGLYCEMIC MEMORY

In contrast to the four known hyperglycemia-inducible abnormalities of intracellular metabolism, hyperglycemia-induced mitochondrial superoxide production may provide an explanation for the development of complications during posthyperglycemic normoglycemia *(hyperglycemic memory)*. Hyperglycemia-induced increases in superoxide would not only increase aldose reductase activity, AGE formation, PKC activity, and hexosamine pathway activity but may also induce mutations in mitochondrial DNA (mtDNA).[193] Mitochondria are more vulnerable to mutation because mtDNA contains virtually no introns, lacks protective histones, and has no effective DNA repair mechanism.[194–196] mtDNA has a 10- to 20-fold higher mutation rate than nuclear DNA.[197, 198] Defective electron transport complex subunits encoded by mutated mtDNA would eventually cause increased superoxide production at physiologic concentrations of glucose, with resultant continued activation of the four pathways despite the absence of hyperglycemia.

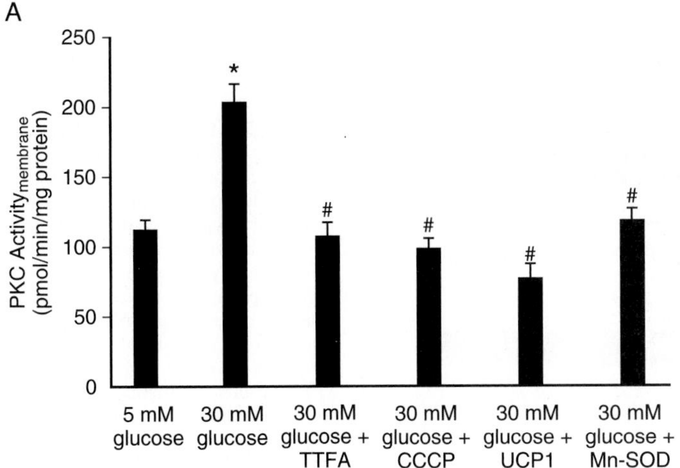

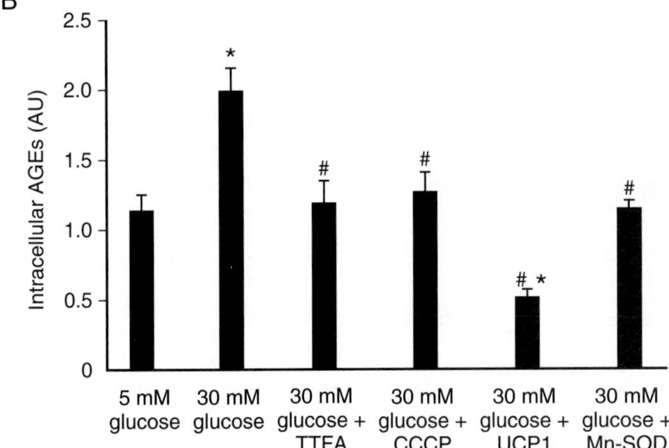

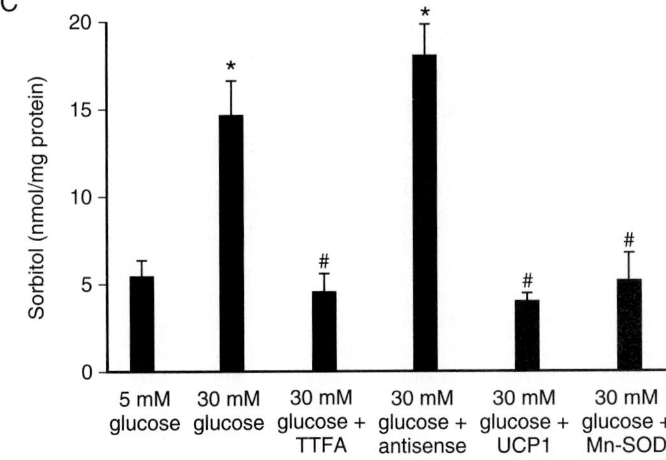

Figure 31–16. Effect of agents that alter mitochondrial electron transport chain function on the three main pathways of hyperglycemic damage. *A*, Hyperglycemia-induced protein kinase C (PKC) activation. *B*, Intracellular advanced glycation end-product (AGE) formation. *C*, Sorbitol accumulation. Cells were incubated in 5-mM glucose, 30-mM glucose alone, and 30-mM glucose plus either agents that uncouple oxidative phosphorylation and reduce the high mitochondrial membrane potential (TTFA, CCCP, UCP-1), or dismutate superoxide (Mn-SOD). See text for additional abbreviations. (From Nishikawa T, Edelstein D, Du XL, et al. Normalizing mitochondrial superoxide production blocks three pathways of hyperglycaemic damage. Nature 2000; 404:787–790.)

PROSPECTS FOR PHARMACOLOGIC INTERVENTION

Aldose Reductase Inhibitors

In vivo studies of polyol pathway inhibition have yielded promising results with neuropathy but disappointing results in other target tissues of diabetic complications. During the course of a 5-year study, nerve conduction velocity (NCV) progressively decreased in untreated diabetic dogs, whereas this decrease was prevented by treatment with an aldose reductase inhibitor (ARI).[182] Positive effects of ARIs on human diabetic neuropathy have been reported.[199, 200] In contrast, aldose reductase inhibition failed to prevent retinopathy in the 5-year study in dogs, nor did it prevent capillary basement membrane thickening in the retina, kidney, or muscles.[201] A 3-year human trial also failed to show any effect on diabetic retinopathy.[202]

Advanced Glycation End-Product Inhibitors

The hydrazine compound aminoguanidine was the first AGE inhibitor discovered,[101] and its effect on diabetic pathology has been investigated in the retina, kidney, nerve, and artery. In the rat retina, diabetes causes a 19-fold increase in the number of acellular capillaries. Aminoguanidine treatment of diabetics prevented excess AGE accumulation and reduced the number of acellular capillaries by 80%. Diabetes-induced pericyte dropout also was markedly reduced by aminoguanidine treatments.[83]

Similar results have been obtained in animal models of diabetic kidney disease.[203–205] Diabetes increased AGEs in the renal glomerulus, and aminoguanidine treatment prevented this diabetes-induced increase. Untreated diabetic animals developed albuminuria that averaged 30 mg every 24 hours for 32 weeks. This was more than a 10-fold increase above control levels. In aminoguanidine-treated diabetic rats, the level of AER was reduced nearly 90%.[75] Untreated diabetic animals also developed the characteristic structural feature of human diabetic nephropathy (i.e., increased fractional mesangial volume). When diabetic animals were treated with aminoguanidine, the increase was completely prevented. A structurally unrelated AGE inhibitor, OPB-9195, also prevented the development and progression of experimental diabetic nephropathy by blocking type IV collagen overproduction and normalizing the expression of TGF-β.[206, 207]

In the peripheral nerve of diabetic rats, both motor nerve and sensory NCVs are decreased after 8 weeks of diabetes.[208] Nerve action potential amplitude is decreased by 37% and peripheral nerve blood flow is decreased by 57% after 24 weeks of diabetes.[209] Aminoguanidine treatment prevented each of these abnormalities of diabetic peripheral nerve function.[208, 209]

In a large randomized, double-blind, placebo-controlled, multicenter trial of aminoguanidine in type 1 diabetic patients with overt nephropathy, aminoguanidine lowered total urinary protein and slowed progression of nephropathy, over and above the effects of existing optimal care. In addition, aminoguanidine reduced the progression of diabetic retinopathy (defined as an increase by three or more steps in the Early Treatment Diabetic Retinopathy Study [ETDRS] scale).[210, 211]

Protein Kinase C Inhibitors

The recent development of a β isoform–specific PKC inhibitor has allowed in vivo studies to go forward, because the

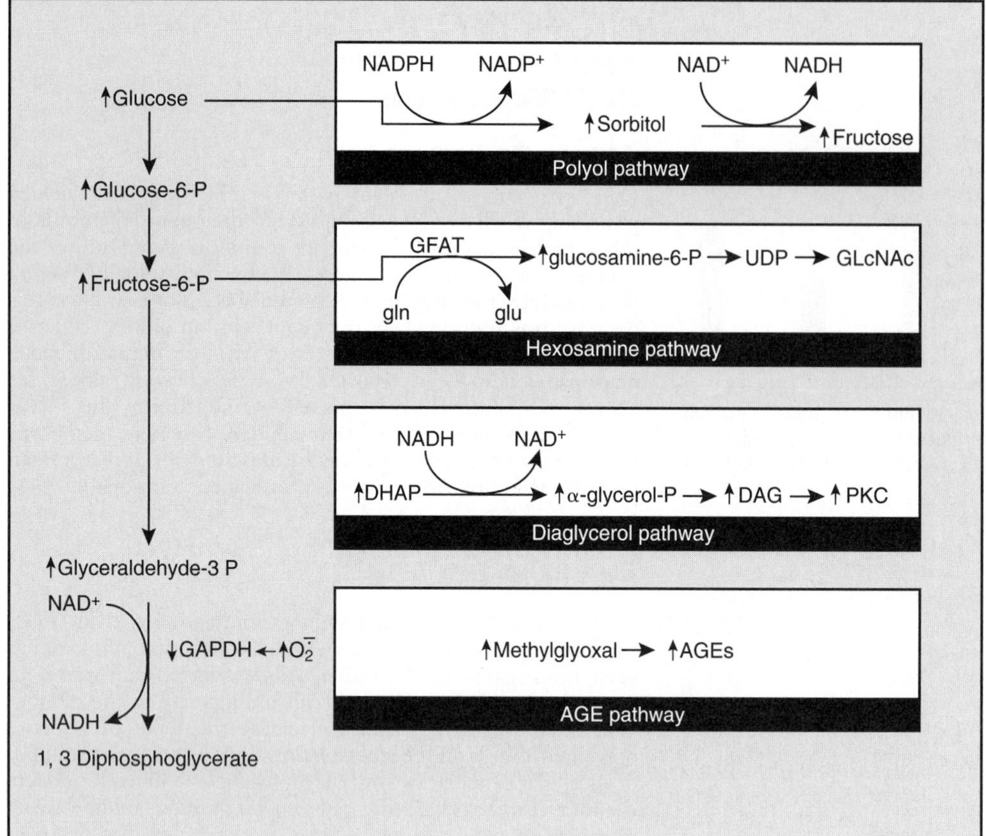

Figure 31–17. Potential mechanism by which hyperglycemia-induced mitochondrial superoxide overproduction activates four pathways of hyperglycemic damage. Excess superoxide partially inhibits the glycolytic enzyme glyceraldehyde-3-phosphate dehydrogenase, thereby diverting upstream metabolites from glycolysis into pathways of glucose overutilization. This results in increased flux of triose phosphate to diacylglycerol (DAG), an activator of protein kinase C (PKC), and to methylglyoxal, the major intracellular advanced glycation end-product (AGE) precursor. Increased flux of fructose-6-phosphate to UDP-*N*-acetylglucosamine increases modification of proteins by hexosamine, and increased glucose flux through the polyol pathway consumes NADPH and depletes GSH. See text for additional abbreviations.

toxicity of non-selective PKC inhibitors precludes their use. LY333531 inhibits PKC-β_1 and PKC-β_2 with a half-maximal inhibitory constant (IC_{50}) that is at least 50-fold less than for other PKC isoforms.[154] Treatment with LY333531 significantly reduced PKC activity in the retina and renal glomeruli of diabetic animals. Concomitantly, LY333531 treatment significantly reduced diabetes-induced increases in retinal mean circulation time, normalized diabetes-induced increases in glomerular filtration rate (GFR), and partially corrected urinary AER. Treatment of db/db mice with LY333531 for a longer period also ameliorated accelerated glomerular mesangial expansion.[212] Clinical trials of LY333531 in human diabetic patients are currently in progress.

Future Drug Targets

The recent discovery that each of the four different pathogenic mechanisms discussed in this section reflect a single hyperglycemia-induced process[77, 186] suggests that interrupting the overproduction of superoxide by the mitochondrial electron transport chain would normalize polyol pathway flux, AGE formation, PKC activation, hexosamine pathway flux, and NF-κB activation. Novel compounds that act as superoxide dismutase/catalase mimetics already exist,[213–215] and these compounds have been shown to normalize hyperglycemia-induced mitochondrial superoxide overproduction.[186] These and the other agents described in this section may have unique clinical efficacy in preventing the development and progression of diabetic complications.

RETINOPATHY, MACULAR EDEMA, AND OTHER OCULAR COMPLICATIONS*

Diabetic retinopathy is a well-characterized, sight-threatening, chronic microvascular complication that eventually afflicts virtually all patients with diabetes mellitus.[218] Diabetic retinopathy is characterized by gradually progressive alterations in the retinal microvasculature, leading to areas of retinal nonperfusion, increased vasopermeability, and pathologic intraocular proliferation of retinal vessels. The complications associated with the increased vasopermeability, termed *macular edema*, and uncontrolled neovascularization, termed *proliferative diabetic retinopathy* (PDR), can result in severe and permanent visual loss. Despite decades of research, there is presently no known means of preventing diabetic retinopathy and, despite effective therapies, diabetic retinopathy remains the leading cause of new-onset blindness in working-aged Americans.[218] With ap-

*Portions of this section draw on, among others, (1) *Principles and Practices of Ophthalmology: The Harvard System* (Aiello LP, et al. *Ocular Complications of Diabetes*, 2nd ed., WB Saunders, 2000); (2) *Diabetic Retinopathy: Technical Review* (Aiello LP, et al. American Diabetes Association. Diabetes Care 1998; 21:143–156); and (3) *Diabetic Retinopathy* (Aiello LP, Cavellerano J. Diabetic retinopathy. In Johnstone MT, Veves A [eds]. Contemporary Cardiology. Diabetes and Cardiovascular Disease. Humana Press, 2001, pp 385–398).

propriate medical and ophthalmologic care, however, more than 90% of visual loss resulting from diabetic retinopathy can be prevented.[219]

Thus, until a cure for diabetes is discovered, the primary clinical care emphasis for the prevention of vision loss is appropriately directed at the early identification, accurate classification, and timely treatment of retinopathy. Emphasis must also be placed on ensuring compliant life-long routine ophthalmologic follow-up of the diabetic patient and optimization of associated systemic disorders.

EPIDEMIOLOGY AND IMPACT

Sixteen million Americans have diabetes mellitus, but only half are aware that they have the disease.[218, 220] Diabetic retinopathy is the leading cause of new cases of legal blindness among Americans between the ages of 20 and 74 years.[221] There is a higher risk of more frequent and severe ocular complications in type 1 diabetes.[222] Approximately 25% of patients with type 1 diabetes have retinopathy after 5 years, with this figure increasing to 60% and 80% after 10 and 15 years, respectively. However, because there are more adult-onset cases than juvenile-onset cases, type 2 disease accounts for a higher proportion of patients with visual loss. The most threatening form of retinopathy (PDR) is present in approximately 25% of type 1 patients with diabetes of 15 years' duration.[223]

An estimated 700,000 persons have PDR, 130,000 with high-risk PDR, 500,000 with macular edema, and 325,000 with *clinically significant macular edema* (CSME) in the United States.[224–228] An estimated 63,000 cases of PDR, 29,000 high-risk PDR, 80,000 macular edema, 56,000 CSME, and 5000 new cases of legal blindness occur each year as a result of diabetic retinopathy.[224, 225] Blindness has been estimated to be 25 times more common in persons with diabetes than in those without the disease.[229, 230]

Estimates of the medical and economic impact of retinopathy-associated morbidity have been performed using computer simulations that incorporate clinical trial and cost reimbursement data to model effects of applying accepted evaluation and treatment techniques to patients with type 1 and type 2 diabetic retinopathy.[226, 228, 231–239] The models predict that in the absence of good glycemic control, 72% of patients with type 1 diabetes will develop PDR requiring panretinal photocoagulation (PRP) over their lifetime and that 42% will develop macular edema.[231] If patients with type 1 diabetes receive currently suggested treatment, there is a predicted cost of $966 per person-year of vision saved from PDR and $1120 per person-year of central acuity saved from macular edema as of 1990. Indeed, current estimates are that only 60% of patients in need of retinopathy treatment are receiving appropriate ophthalmic care.[240] If all patients with both type 1 and type 2 diabetes were to receive care according to currently suggested guidelines, annual savings of $624 million and 173,540 person-years of sight would be realized.[226, 232]

The DCCT showed that both the rate of development of any retinopathy as well as the rate of retinopathy progression once it was present were significantly reduced after 3 years of intensive insulin therapy,[241] an effect maintained even 4 years after conclusion of the study.[26, 29, 242] Applying DCCT intensive insulin therapy to all persons in the United States with insulin-dependent diabetes mellitus would result in a gain of 920,000 person-years of sight,[243] although the costs of intensive therapy are three times that of conventional therapy.[244]

PATHOPHYSIOLOGY

A detailed discussion of the pathophysiologic mechanisms underlying diabetic retinopathy and other diabetes-related complications has been presented earlier in this chapter. The earliest histologic effects of diabetes mellitus in the eye include loss of retinal vascular pericytes (supporting cells for retinal endothelial cells), thickening of vascular endothelium basement membrane, and alterations in retinal blood flow (Fig. 31–18).[24, 245–250] With increasing loss of retinal pericytes, the retinal vessel wall develops outpouchings *(microaneurysms)* and becomes fragile.

Clinically, microaneurysms and small retinal hemorrhages may not always be readily distinguishable and are evaluated together as "hemorrhages and microaneurysms" (Fig. 31–19*A*) (see also Color Plate). Rheologic changes occur in diabetic retinopathy resulting from increased platelet aggregation, integrin-mediated leukocyte adhesion, and endothelial damage.[251–253] Disruption of the blood retinal barrier may ensue, characterized by increased vascular permeability.[254, 255] The subsequent leakage of blood and serum from the retinal vessels results in retinal hemorrhages, retinal edema, and hard exudates (Fig. 31–19*A* and *C*). Moderate visual loss follows if the fovea is affected by the leakage.[239]

With time, increasing sclerosis and endothelial cell loss lead to narrowing of the retinal vessels, which decreases vascular perfusion and may ultimately lead to obliteration of the capillaries and small vessels (Fig. 31–19*B*). The resulting retinal ischemia is a potent inducer of angiogenic growth factors. Several angiogenic growth factors have been isolated from eyes with diabetic retinopathy, including IGFs, bFGF, hepatocyte growth factor (HGF), and VEGF.[256–259] These factors promote the development of new vessel growth and retinal vascular permeability.[260–264] Indeed, inhibition of molecules such as VEGF and their signaling pathways can suppress the development of retinal neovascularization and retinal vascular permeability.[261, 265–269]

New vessels tend to grow in regions of strong vitreous adhesion to the retina, such as at the optic disc and major vascular arcades (Fig. 31–19*D* and *E*). The posterior vitreous face also serves as a scaffold for pathologic neovascularization, and the new vessels commonly arise at the junctions between perfused and nonperfused retina. When the retina is severely ischemic, the concentration of angiogenic growth factors may reach sufficient concentration in the anterior chamber to cause abnormal new vessel proliferation on the iris and the anterior chamber angle.[258, 270] Uncontrolled anterior segment neovascularization may result in rubeotic glaucoma because the fibrovascular proliferation in the angle of the eye causes blockage of aqueous outflow through the trabecular meshwork.[271]

Proliferating new vessels in diabetic retinopathy have a tendency to bleed, which results in preretinal and vitreous hemorrhages (VHs) (Fig. 31–19*E* and *F*). Although the presence of a large amount of blood in the preretinal space or vitreous cavity per se is not damaging to the retina, these intraocular hemorrhages often cause prolonged visual loss by blocking the visual axis. Membranes on the retinal surface can be induced by blood and result in wrinkling and traction on the retina. Although all retinal neovascularization eventually becomes quiescent, as with most scarring processes there is progressive fibrosis of the new vessel complexes that is associated with contraction. However, in the eye, such forces may exert traction on the retina, leading to tractional retinal detachment and retinal tears that may result in severe and permanent visual loss if left untreated (Fig. 31–19*G* and *H*).

In short, causes of visual loss from complications of diabetes mellitus include retinal ischemia involving the fovea, macular

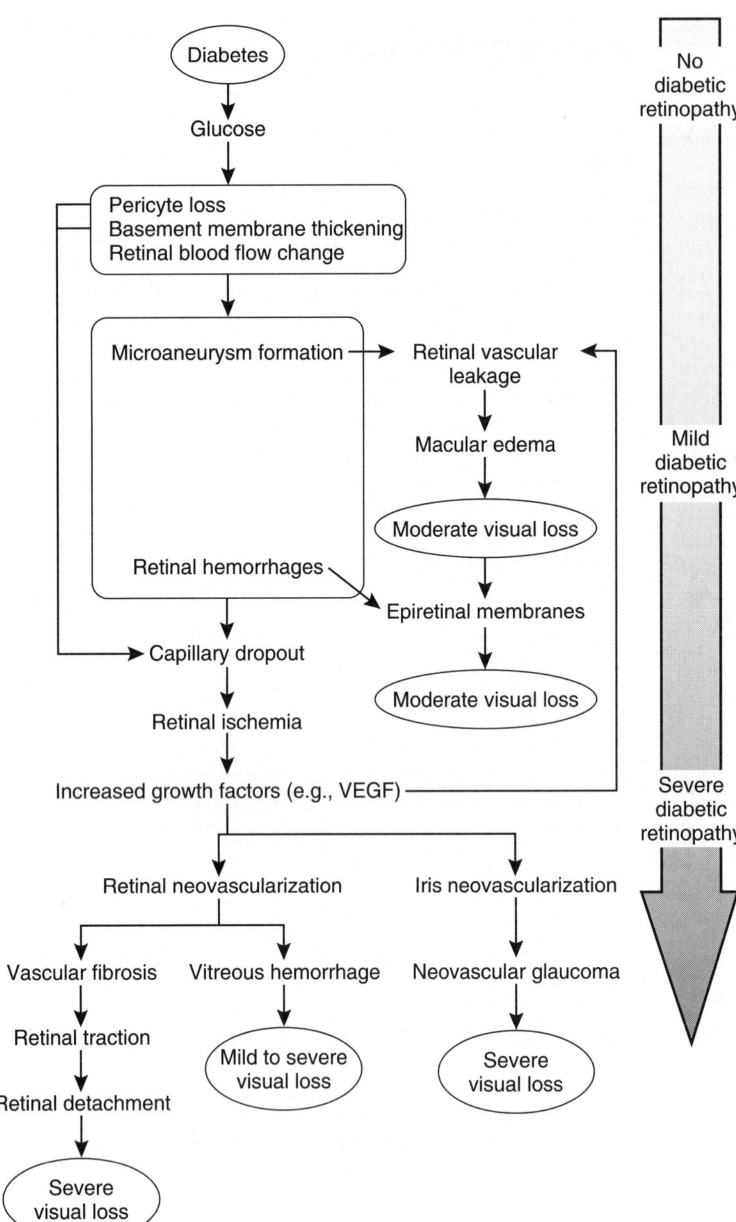

Figure 31–18. Diabetic retinopathy pathogenesis flow chart. The schematic flow chart represents the major preclinical and clinical findings associated with the full spectrum of diabetic retinopathy and macular edema. VEGF, vascular endothelial growth factor.

edema at or near the fovea, preretinal or vitreous hemorrhages, retinal detachment, and neovascular glaucoma. Visual loss may also result from more indirect effects of disease progression in diabetic patients, such as retinal vessel occlusion, accelerated atherosclerotic disease, and embolic phenomena.

CLINICAL FEATURES

Risk Factors

Duration of diabetes is closely associated with the onset and severity of diabetic retinopathy. Diabetic retinopathy is rare in prepubescent patients with type 1 diabetes, but nearly all patients with type 1 diabetes and more than 60% of patients with type 2 diabetes develop some degree of retinopathy after 20 years.[218, 223, 272] In patients with type 2 diabetes, approximately 20% have retinopathy at the time of diabetes diagnosis and most have some degree of retinopathy over subsequent decades.

Diabetic retinopathy is the most frequent cause of new-onset blindness among American adults aged 20 to 74 years. In the Wisconsin Epidemiologic Study of Diabetic Retinopathy, approximately 4% of patients younger than 30 years of age at diagnosis and nearly 2% of patients older than 30 years of age at diagnosis were legally blind. In the younger-onset group, 86% of blindness was attributable to diabetic retinopathy. In the older-onset group, where other eye diseases were also common, 33% of the cases of legal blindness were due to diabetic retinopathy.[223, 272]

Lack of glycemic control is another significant risk factor for the onset and progression of diabetic retinopathy. The DCCT demonstrated a clear relationship between hyperglycemia and diabetic microvascular complications, including retinopathy in 1441 patients with type 1 diabetes.[26, 27, 273–275] In patients monitored 4 to 9 years, the DCCT showed that intensive insulin therapy reduced or prevented the development of retinopathy

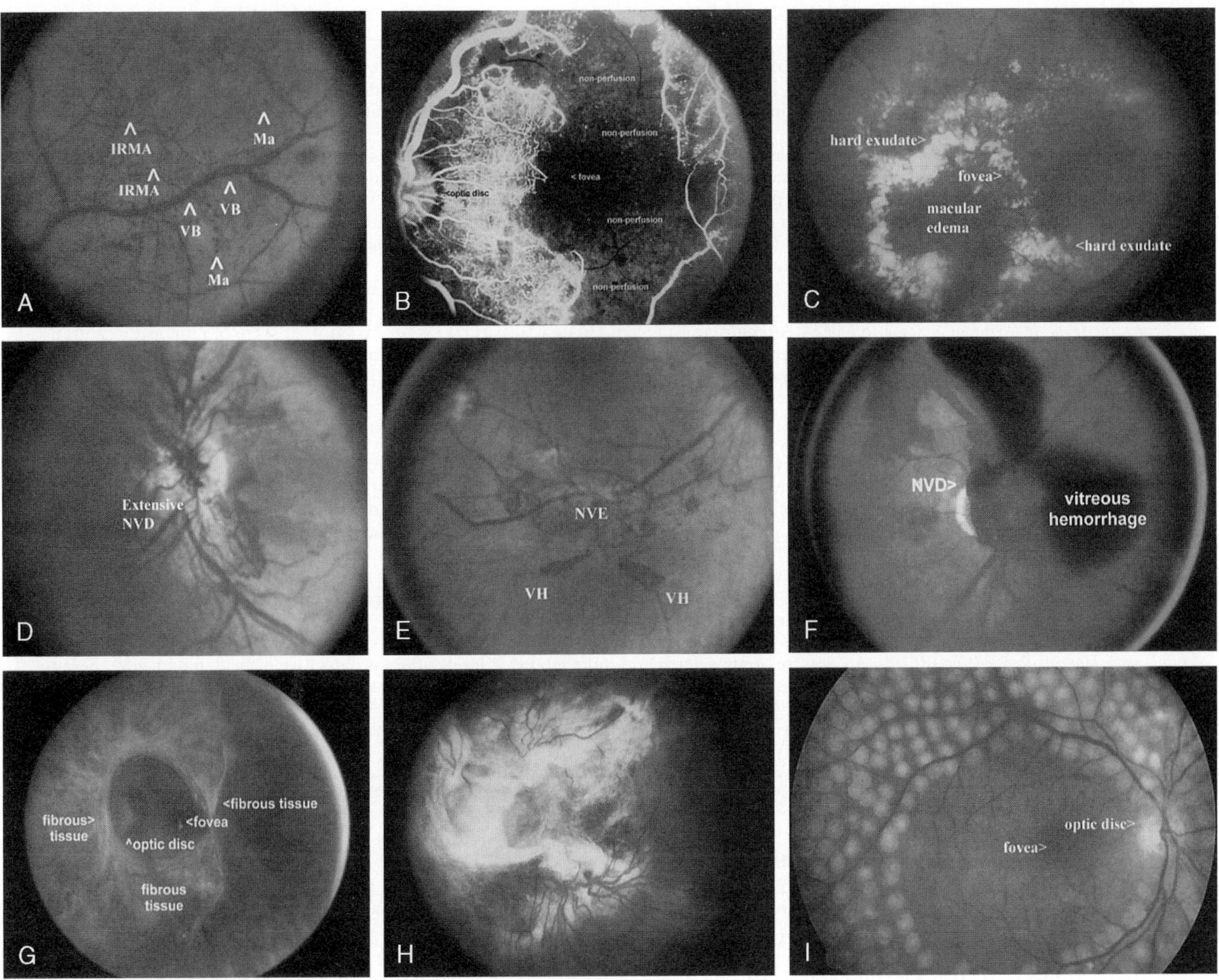

Figure 31–19. Clinical features of diabetic retinopathy: some typical findings in human diabetic retinopathy. *A*, Findings in severe nonproliferative diabetic retinopathy, including microaneurysms (Ma), venous beading (VB), and intraretinal microvascular abnormalities (IRMA). *B*, Fluorescein angiogram showing marked capillary nonperfusion. *C*, Clinically significant macular edema with retinal thickening and hard exudates involving the fovea. *D*, Extensive neovascularization of the optic disc (NVD). This is high-risk proliferative diabetic retinopathy. *E*, Neovascularization elsewhere (NVE) and two small vitreous hemorrhages (VH). *F*, Extensive vitreous hemorrhage arising from severe neovascularization of the disc (NVD). *G*, Severe fibrovascular proliferation surrounding the fovea. *H*, Traction retinal detachment from extensive fibrovascular proliferation. *I*, Panretinal (scatter) laser photocoagulation. The macula and fovea and optic disc are not treated to preserve central vision. Laser burns are evident as white retinal lesions. (*A* to *I*, Adapted from Aiello LP. Eye complications of diabetes. In Korenman SG, Kahn CR [eds]. Atlas of Clinical Endocrinology. Vol 2: Diabetes. Philadelphia, Blackwell Scientific, 1999.) (See also Color Plate.)

by 27% as compared with conventional therapy. Additionally, intensive insulin therapy reduced the progression of diabetic retinopathy by 34% to 76% and had a substantial beneficial effect over the entire range of retinopathy severity. This improvement was achieved with an average 10% reduction in Hb A_{1c} from 8% to 7.2%. These results underscore that although intensive therapy does not prevent retinopathy completely, it reduces the risk of retinopathy onset and progression.

Renal disease, as manifested by microalbuminuria and proteinuria, is yet another significant risk factor for onset and progression of diabetic retinopathy.[276, 277] Hypertension is associated with PDR and is an established risk factor for the development of macular edema.[278] Additionally, elevated serum lipid levels are associated with extravasated lipid in the retina (hard exudates) and visual loss.[279]

Clinical Findings

Clinical findings associated with early and progressing diabetic retinopathy include hemorrhages or microaneurysms (H/Ma), cotton-wool spots (CWSs), hard exudates, intraretinal microvascular abnormalities (IRMAs), and venous caliber abnormalities (VCABs), such as venous loops, venous tortuosity, and venous beading (see Fig. 31–19*A* and C). Microaneurysms are saccular outpouchings of the capillary walls that can leak fluid and result in intraretinal hemorrhages. The intraretinal

Table 31–1. Glossary & Abbreviations Pertinent to Diabetic Eye Disease

Background Diabetic Retinopathy (BDR): An outdated term referring to some stages of nonproliferative diabetic retinopathy. Because this terminology is not closely associated with disease progression, it has been replaced by the various levels of nonproliferative diabetic retinopathy.
Clinically Significant Macular Edema (CSME): Thickening of the retina in the macular region of sufficient extent and location to threaten central visual function.
Cotton Wool Spot: A gray or white area lesion in the nerve fiber layer of the retina resulting from stasis of axoplasmic flow as a result of infarction.
Diabetes Control & Complications Trial (DCCT): A multicenter randomization, clinical trial designed to address whether intensive insulin therapy could prevent or slow the progression of systemic complications of diabetes mellitus.
Diabetic Retinopathy (DR): Retinal pathology related to the underlying systemic disease of diabetes mellitus.
Diabetic Retinopathy Study (DRS): The first multicenter randomized clinical trial to demonstrate the value of laser scatter (panretinal) photocoagulation in reducing the risk of visual loss among patients with all levels of diabetic retinopathy.
Diabetic Retinopathy Vitrectomy Study (DRVS): A multicenter clinical trial demonstrating the value of early vitrectomy for patients with very advanced diabetic retinopathy.
Early Treatment Diabetic Retinopathy Study (ETDRS): A multicenter randomized clinical trial that addressed at what stage of retinopathy scatter (panretinal) photocoagulation was indicated, whether focal photocoagulation was effective for preventing moderate visual loss from clinically significant macular edema, and whether aspirin therapy altered the risks for outcome or treatment of diabetic retinopathy.
Focal or Grid Laser Photocoagulation: A type of laser treatment used for patients with clinically significant macular edema whose main goal is to reduce vascular leakage either by focal treatment of leaking retinal microaneurysms or by application of therapy in a grid-like pattern.
Hard Exudate: Lipid accumulation within the retina as a result of increased vasopermeability.
High-Risk-Characteristic Proliferative Diabetic Retinopathy (HRC-PDR): Proliferative diabetic retinopathy of a defined extent, location, and/or clinical findings that is particularly associated with severe visual loss.
Microaneurysm (Ma): An early vascular abnormality consisting of an outpouching of the retinal microvasculature.
Neovascular Glaucoma (NVG): Elevation of intraocular pressure caused by the development of neovascularization in the anterior segment of the eye.
Neovascularization at the Disc (NVD): Retina neovascularization occurring at or within 1500 μm of the optic disc.
Neovascularization Elsewhere (NVE): Retinal neovascularization that is located more than 1500 μm away from the optic disc.
Neovascularization of the Iris (NVI): Neovascularization occurring on the iris (rubeosis iris), usually as a result of extensive retinal ischemia.
No Light Perception (NLP): The inability to perceive light.
Nonproliferative Diabetic Retinopathy (NPDR): Severities of diabetic retinopathy that precede the development of proliferative diabetic retinopathy.
Preproliferative Diabetic Retinopathy (PPDR): An outdated term referring to more advanced levels of nonproliferative diabetic retinopathy. Because this terminology is not closely associated with disease progression, it has been replaced by the various levels of nonproliferative diabetic retinopathy.
Proliferative Diabetic Retinopathy (PDR): an advanced level of diabetic retinopathy, where proliferation of new vessels occurs on or within the retina.
Rubeosis Iridis: see Neovascularization of the Iris (NVI).

hemorrhages can be "flame-shaped" or "dot/blot"–like in appearance, reflecting the architecture of the layer of the retina in which they occur. IRMAs are either new vessel growth within the retinal tissue itself or shunt vessels through areas of poor vascular perfusion. It is common for IRMAs to be adjacent to CWSs, which are caused by microinfarcts in the nerve fiber layer. VCABs are a sign of severe retinal hypoxia. In some cases of extensive vascular loss, however, the retina may actually appear free of nonproliferative lesions. Such areas are termed "featureless retina" and are a sign of severe retinal hypoxia.

Vision loss from diabetic retinopathy generally results from persistent, nonclearing vitreous hemorrhage, traction retinal detachment, or *diabetic macular edema* (DME) (see Figs. 31–18 and 31–19). Neovascularization with fibrous tissue contraction can distort the retina and lead to traction retinal detachment. The new vessels may bleed, causing preretinal or vitreous hemorrhage. The most common cause of vision loss from diabetes, however, is macular disease and macular edema. Macular edema is more likely to occur in patients with type 2 diabetes, which represents 90% of the diabetic population. In diabetic macular disease, macular edema involving the fovea or nonperfusion of the capillaries in the central macula is responsible for the loss of vision.

Classification of Diabetic Retinopathy

Diabetic retinopathy is broadly classified into *non-PDR* (NPDR) and *PDR* categories.[280, 281] Macular edema may coexist with either group and is not used in the classification of level of retinopathy. The historical terms *background retinopathy* and *preproliferative diabetic retinopathy* have been replaced to reflect the specific characteristics and risk stratification of the prognostically important subgroups in NPDR (Table 31–1).

Generally, diabetic retinopathy progresses from no retinopathy, through mild, moderate, severe, and very severe nonproliferative disease and eventually on to PDR. Level of NPDR is determined by the extent and location of clinical manifestations of retinopathy. Mild NPDR is characterized by limited microvascular abnormalities such as H/Ma, CWS, and increased vascular permeability. Moderate and severe NPDR are characterized by increasing severity of H/Ma, VCABs, IRMA, and vascular closure.

PDR is characterized by vasoproliferation of the retina and its complications, including new vessels on the optic disc (NVD), new vessels elsewhere on the retina (NVE), preretinal hemorrhage (PRH), vitreous hemorrhage, and fibrous tissue proliferation (FP). On the basis of the extent and location of these lesions, PDR is classified as *early PDR* or *high-risk PDR*. Larger areas of these complications as well as new vessels that are near the optic disc are associated with greater risks of visual loss. The level of NPDR establishes the risk of progression to sight-threatening retinopathy and dictates appropriate clinical management and follow-up.

Classification of Diabetic Macular Edema

Diabetic macular edema can be present with any level of diabetic retinopathy. When it involves or threatens the center of the macula, it is called *CSME* (defined earlier). CSME exists if there is retinal thickening at or within 500 μm of the fovea, hard exudates with adjacent retinal thickening at or within 500 μm of the fovea, or an area of retinal thickening 1500 μm or more in diameter, any part of which is within 1500 μm of the fovea.[280, 282, 283] CSME is a clinical diagnosis that is not dependent on visual acuity or results of ancillary testing such as fluorescein angiography.

Other Ocular Manifestations of Diabetes

All structures of the eye are susceptible to complications of diabetes. The consequence of these changes can range from being unnoticed by both patient and physician, to symptomatic but not sight-threatening, to requiring evaluation to rule out potentially life-threatening underlying causes other than diabetes.

Mononeuropathies of the third, fourth, or sixth cranial nerves may arise in association with diabetes, with the fourth cranial nerve being least likely diabetes-associated.[284–286] Nerve palsies present a significant diagnostic challenge because misdiagnosis may result in a life-threatening lesion remaining untreated. In one review of cranial nerve palsies treated in a diabetic patient population in 1967, 42% of mononeuropathies were not diabetic in origin.[285] This finding underscores the danger of routinely attributing mononeuropathies to the diabetic condition itself without carefully ruling out other potential causes. The percentage of all extraocular muscle palsies attributable to diabetes mellitus is estimated at 4.5% to 6%.[286] Mononeuropathies may be the initial presenting sign of new-onset diabetes, and diabetes should therefore be considered in the differential diagnosis of any mononeuropathy affecting the extraocular muscles, even in patients who do not claim a history of diabetes. Diabetes-induced third-, fourth-, and sixth-nerve palsies are usually self-limited and should resolve spontaneously in 2 to 6 months. Palsies may recur or subsequently develop in the contralateral eye.

The optic disc can be affected by diabetes in a variety of ways other than NVD or NVE. Diabetic papillopathy must be distinguished from other causes of disc swelling such as true papilledema from increased intracranial pressure, pseudopapilledema such as optic nerve head drusen, toxic optic neuropathies, neoplasms of the optic nerve, and hypertension.[287] Optic disc pallor can occur following spontaneous remission of proliferative retinopathy or remission following scatter (panretinal) laser photocoagulation (see Fig. 31–19*I*). Because diabetes poses an increased risk for the development of open-angle glaucoma, the disc pallor following remission of retinopathy or PRP must be considered when evaluating the optic nerve head for glaucoma.

A potentially serious diabetic ocular complication is neovascularization of the iris (NVI). Usually the new iris vessels are first observed at the pupillary border, followed by a fine network of vessels over the iris tissue progressing into the filtration angle of the eye. Closure of the angle by the fibrovascular network results in neovascular glaucoma.[288] Neovascular glaucoma is difficult to manage and requires aggressive treatment. Diabetes is the second leading cause of neovascular glaucoma, accounting for 32% of cases.[289] NVI occurs in 4% to 7% of diabetic eyes and may be present in up to 40% to 60% of eyes with proliferative retinopathy.[290, 291] When possible, scatter (panretinal) laser photocoagulation is the principal therapy for NVI, although other approaches such as goniophotocoagulation, topical/systemic antiglaucoma medications, and antiglaucomatous filtration surgery are available when needed.[292–294]

The cornea of the diabetic person is more susceptible to injury and slower to heal after injury than is the nondiabetic cornea.[295, 296] The diabetic cornea is also more prone to infectious corneal ulcers, which can lead to rapid loss of vision, need for corneal transplant, or loss of the eye if not treated aggressively. Consequently, diabetic patients using contact lenses should exercise caution and maintain careful monitoring.

Open-angle glaucoma is 1.4 times more common in the diabetic population than in the nondiabetic population.[297] The prevalence of glaucoma increases with age and duration of diabetes, but medical therapy for open-angle glaucoma is generally effective.

Diabetes effects on the crystalline lens can result in transitory refractive changes, alterations in accommodative ability,[298] and cataracts. Refractive change can be significant and is related to fluctuation of blood glucose levels with osmotic lens swelling.[289] Cataracts occur earlier in life and progress more rapidly in the presence of diabetes.[299, 300] Cataracts are 1.6 times more common in people with diabetes than in those without diabetes.[300, 301] In patients with earlier-onset diabetes, duration of diabetes, retinopathy status, diuretic use, and glycosylated hemoglobin are risk factors.[302] In patients with later-onset diabetes, age of the patient, lower intraocular pressure, smoking, and lower diastolic blood pressure (BP) may be additional risk factors.[303, 304] Diabetic patients undergoing simultaneous kidney or pancreas transplantation are at an increased risk of developing all types of cataract, independent of the use of corticosteroids after transplantation.[305] Both phacoemulsification and extracapsular cataract extraction with intraocular lens implantation are appropriate surgical therapies. The principal determinant of postoperative vision and progression of retinopathy is related to the preoperative presence of diabetic macular edema and level of NPDR.[306, 307]

Other findings with higher frequency among patients with diabetes include xanthelasma,[284] microaneurysms of the bulbar conjunctiva,[308] posterior vitreous detachment,[309] and the rare but frequently fatal orbital fungal infection Mucorales (phycomycosis).[290, 291] Prompt diagnosis and treatment of *Mucor* is crucial, although the survival rate still remains at only 57%.[291, 310]

MONITORING AND TREATMENT OF DIABETIC RETINOPATHY

Appropriate clinical management of diabetic retinopathy has been defined by results of four major, randomized, multicentered clinical trials (Fig. 31–20): the Diabetic Retinopathy Study (DRS),[311] the ETDRS,[312] the Diabetic Retinopathy Vitrectomy Study (DRVS),[313] and the DCCT.[314] These studies have elucidated the progression rates of each level of diabetic retinopathy; defined follow-up intervals; and elucidated the proper delivery, timing, and resulting effectiveness of glycemic control and laser photocoagulation surgery (Figs. 31–21 to 31–24). They have also established guidelines for vitrectomy surgery.

Comprehensive Eye Examination

An accurate ocular examination detailing the extent and location of retinopathy-associated findings is critical for making monitoring and treatment decisions in patients with diabetic retinopathy. As detailed later, most of the blindness associated with advanced stages of retinopathy can be averted with appropriate and timely diagnosis and therapy. Unfortunately, many diabetic patients do not receive adequate eye care at an appropriate stage in their disease.[240, 315] In one study, 55% of patients with high-risk PDR and CSME had never had laser photocoagulation.[240] In fact, 11% of type 1 and 7% of type 2 patients with high-risk PDR necessitating prompt treatment had not been examined by an ophthalmologist within the past 2 years.[315]

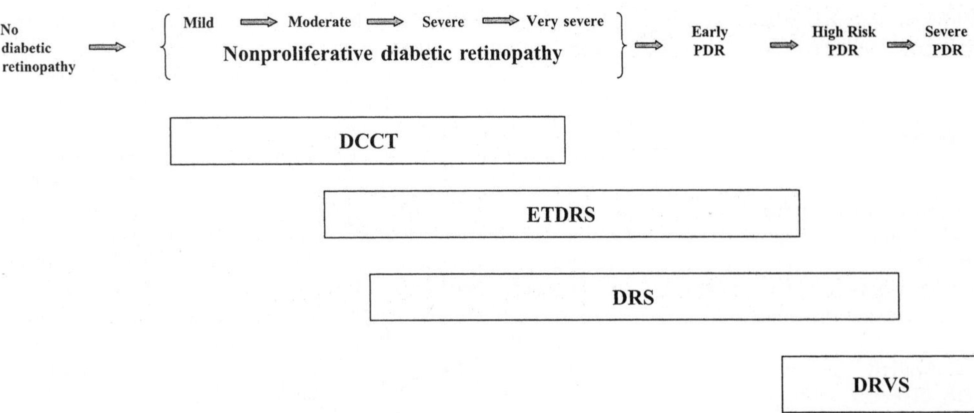

Figure 31–20. Major multicenter clinical trials of diabetic retinopathy. Schematic representation of the major multicenter clinical trials of diabetic retinopathy and the levels of diabetic retinopathy that they primarily addressed. DCCT, Diabetes Control and Complications Trial; DRS, Diabetic Retinopathy Study; DRVS, Diabetic Retinopathy Vitrectomy Study; ETDRS, Early Treatment Diabetic Retinopathy Study; PDR, proliferative diabetic retinopathy.

The comprehensive eye examination is the mainstay of such evaluation and is necessary on a repetitive, life-long basis for patients with diabetes.[280, 316] Such an evaluation has four major components: history, examination, diagnosis, and treatment. The fundamentals of a comprehensive eye examination for the nondiabetic patient have been detailed by the American Academy of Ophthalmology[316] and the American Optometric Association.[317] The examination of the patient with diabetes should be similar, with additional emphasis on portions of the examination that relate to problems particularly relevant to diabetes.

Dilated ophthalmic examination is superior to nondilated evaluation because only 50% of eyes are correctly classified as to presence and severity of retinopathy through undilated pupils.[318, 319] Appropriate ophthalmic evaluation entails pupillary dilation, slit lamp biomicroscopy, examination of the retinal periphery with indirect ophthalmoscopy or mirrored contact lens, and sometimes gonioscopy.[316, 317] Because of the complexities of the diagnosis and treatment of PDR and CSME, ophthalmologists with specialized knowledge and experience in the management of diabetic retinopathy are required to determine

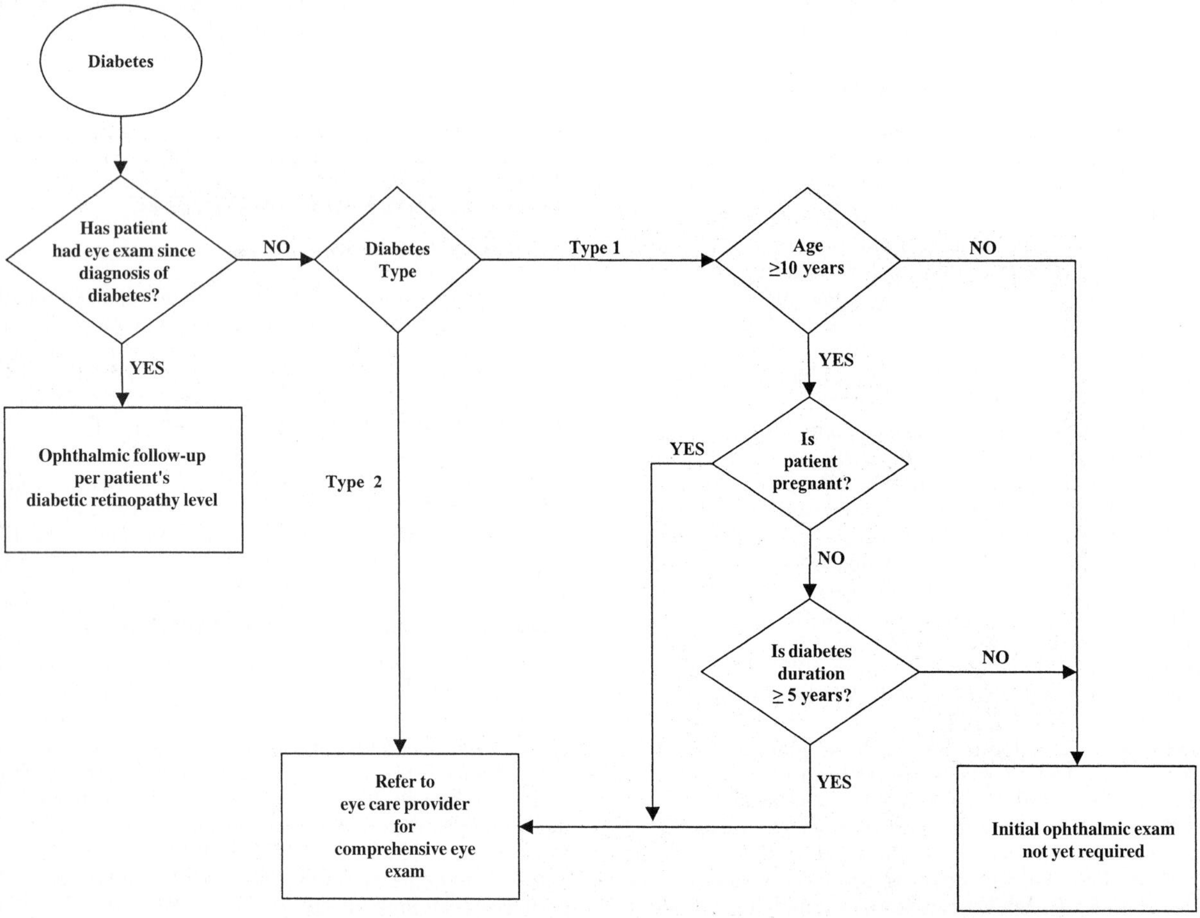

Figure 31–21. Initial ophthalmic examination flow chart. Schematic flow chart of major principles involved in determining the timing of initial ophthalmic examination following diagnosis of diabetes mellitus. These are maximal recommended guidelines. Ocular symptoms, complaints, or other associated medical issues may necessitate earlier evaluation.

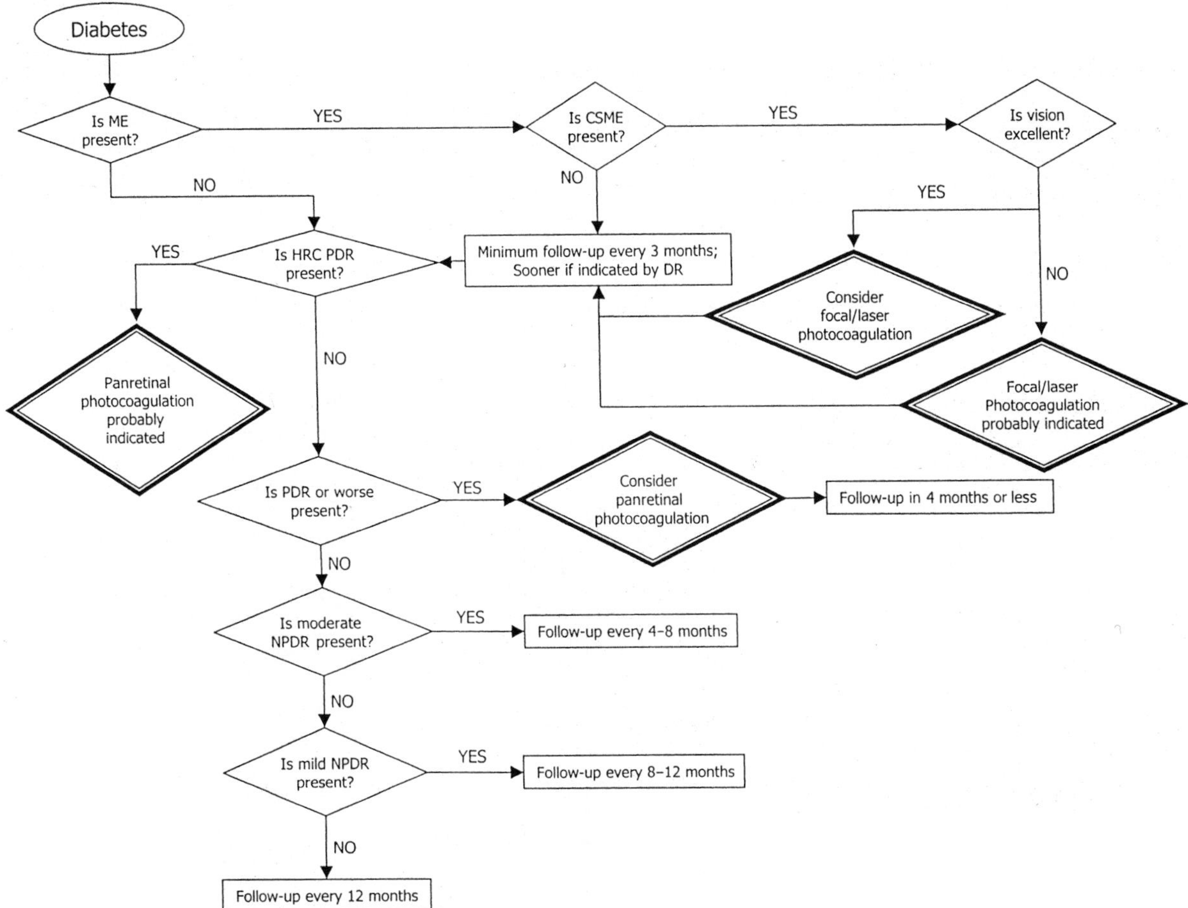

Figure 31–22. Diabetic retinopathy and macular edema examination and treatment flow chart: nonpregnant patients. The schematic flow chart is of major principles involved in determining routine ophthalmic follow-up and indications for treatment in nonpregnant patients with diabetes. These are only general, maximal recommended guidelines. Ocular symptoms, complaints, or other associated ophthalmic or medical issues may necessitate earlier evaluation and/or an altered approach. CSME, clinically significant macular edema; DR, diabetic retinopathy; HRC PDR, high-risk character proliferative diabetic retinopathy; ME, macular edema; NPDR, nonproliferative diabetic retinopathy; PDR, proliferative diabetic retinopathy.

and provide appropriate surgical intervention.[320] Thus, it is recommended that all patients with diabetes should have dilated ocular examinations by an experienced eye care provider (ophthalmologist or optometrist) and should be under the direct or consulting care of an ophthalmologist experienced in the management of diabetic retinopathy at least by the time severe diabetic retinopathy or diabetic macular edema is present.[280]

Initial Ophthalmic Evaluation

The recommendation for initial ocular examination in persons with diabetes is based on prevalence rates of retinopathy (see Fig. 31–21). Approximately 80% of type 1 patients have retinopathy after 15 years of disease, but only about 25% have any retinopathy after 5 years.[223] The prevalence of PDR is less than 2% at 5 years and 25% by 15 years. For type 2 diabetes, the onset date of diabetes is frequently unknown, and more severe disease can be observed at diagnosis. Up to 3% of patients first diagnosed after age 30 (type 2) can have CSME or high-risk PDR at the time of initial diagnosis of diabetes.[321] Thus, in patients older than 10 years of age, initial ophthalmic examination is recommended beginning 5 years after the diagnosis of type 1 diabetes mellitus and on diagnosis of type 2 diabetes mellitus (see Fig. 31–21).[280, 322, 323]

Puberty and pregnancy can accelerate retinopathy progression. The onset of vision-threatening retinopathy is rare in children prior to puberty, regardless of the duration of diabetes.[223, 323–326] However, if diabetes is diagnosed between the ages of 10 and 30, significant retinopathy may arise within 6 years of disease.[327] Diabetic retinopathy can become particularly aggressive during pregnancy in patients with diabetes.[328, 329] In the past, the prognosis for pregnancy in the diabetic patient with microvascular complications was so poor that pregnant diabetic patients were frequently advised to avoid or terminate pregnancies.[330] With recognition of the importance of glycemic control, many diabetic patients in the child-bearing age now experience a safe and satisfying pregnancy and childbirth with minimal risk to both the mother and the baby. There are excellent recent reviews on this subject.[331]

Ideally, patients with diabetes who are planning pregnancy should have a comprehensive eye examination within 1 year prior to conception (see Fig. 31–23). Patients who become pregnant should have a comprehensive eye examination in the first trimester of pregnancy. Close follow-up throughout pregnancy is indicated, with subsequent examinations determined by the findings present at the first-trimester examination.[280, 322] This guideline does not apply to women who develop gestational diabetes, because such individuals are not at increased risk of developing diabetic retinopathy.

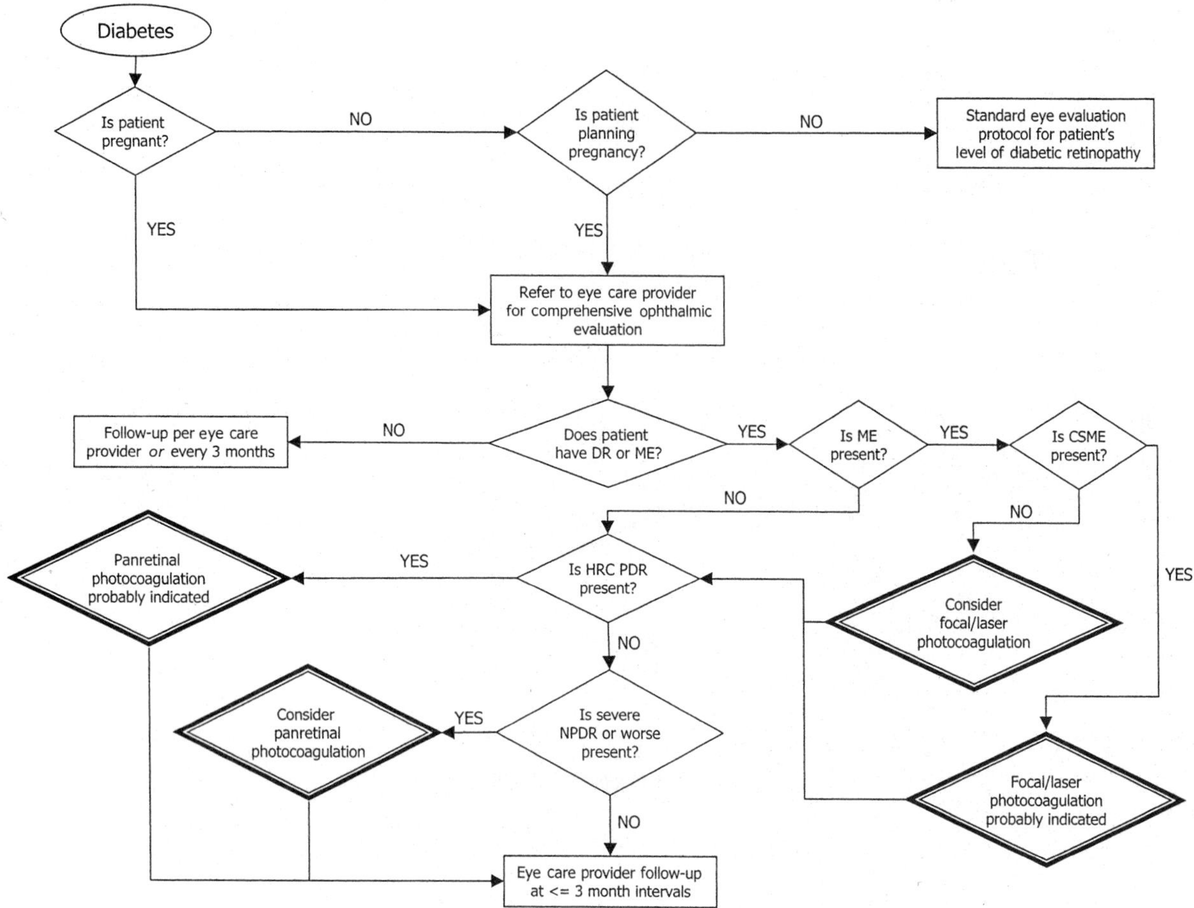

Figure 31–23. Diabetic retinopathy and macular edema examination and treatment flow chart: pregnant patients. The schematic flow chart is of major principles involved in determining routine ophthalmic follow-up and indications for treatment in pregnant patients with diabetes. These are only general, maximal recommended guidelines. Ocular symptoms, complaints, or other associated ophthalmic or medical issues may necessitate earlier evaluation and/or an altered approach. Because retinopathy may progress rapidly in patients with diabetes, careful and more frequent evaluation is often indicated. CSME, clinically significant macular edema; DR, diabetic retinopathy; HRC PDR, high-risk character proliferative diabetic retinopathy; ME, macular edema; NPDR, nonproliferative diabetic retinopathy.

Follow-up Ophthalmic Examination

Follow-up ocular examination is determined from the risk of disease progression at any particular retinopathy level (see Fig. 31–22). As described earlier, NPDR is categorized into four levels of severity based on clinical findings compared to stereo fundus photographic standards: mild, moderate, severe, and very severe.[332] Progression of nonproliferative retinopathy to the visually threatening level of high-risk PDR is closely correlated with NPDR level (Table 31–2). Progression rates from each individual NPDR level to any other retinopathy level are also known. These are used to define standard minimal follow-up intervals as detailed in Figure 31–22 and Table 31–3. Patients with no clinically evident diabetic retinopathy and no known ocular problems require annual comprehensive ophthalmic examinations even if totally asymptomatic.

Diabetic Retinopathy

As detailed earlier, the extent and location of neovascularization determine the level of PDR.[333, 334] PDR is best evaluated by dilated examination using slit lamp biomicroscopy, combined with indirect ophthalmoscopy, and/or stereo fundus photography. Without photocoagulation, eyes with high-risk PDR have a 28% risk of severe visual loss within 2 years. This compares with a 7% risk of severe visual loss after 2 years for eyes with PDR but without high-risk characteristics.[333] Severe visual loss is defined as best-corrected acuity of 5/200 or worse on two consecutive visits 4 months apart. The DRS demonstrated that scatter (panretinal) laser photocoagulation was effective in reducing the risk of severe vision loss from PDR by 50% or more. The ETDRS demonstrated that PRP applied when an eye approaches or just reaches high-risk PDR reduces the risk of severe vision loss to less than 4%. Prompt PRP is indicated for all patients with high-risk PDR, often indicated for patients with PDR less than high risk and, on occasion, advisable for patients with severe or very severe NPDR, especially in the setting of type 2 diabetes (see Fig. 31–22).[239, 333–336] Recent progression of the eye disease, status of the fellow eye, compliance with follow-up, concurrent health concerns such as hypertension or kidney disease, and other factors must be considered in determining if laser surgery should be performed in these patients. In particular, patients with type 2 diabetes should be considered for PRP prior to the development of high-risk PDR because the risk of severe visual loss and the need for pars plana vitrectomy (PPV) can be reduced by 50% in these patients, especially when macular edema is present.[336]

In scatter PRP, 1200 to 1800 laser burns are applied to the peripheral retinal tissue, actually focally destroying the outer photoreceptor and retinal pigment epithelium of the retina (see Fig. 31–19*I*). Large vessels are avoided, as are areas of

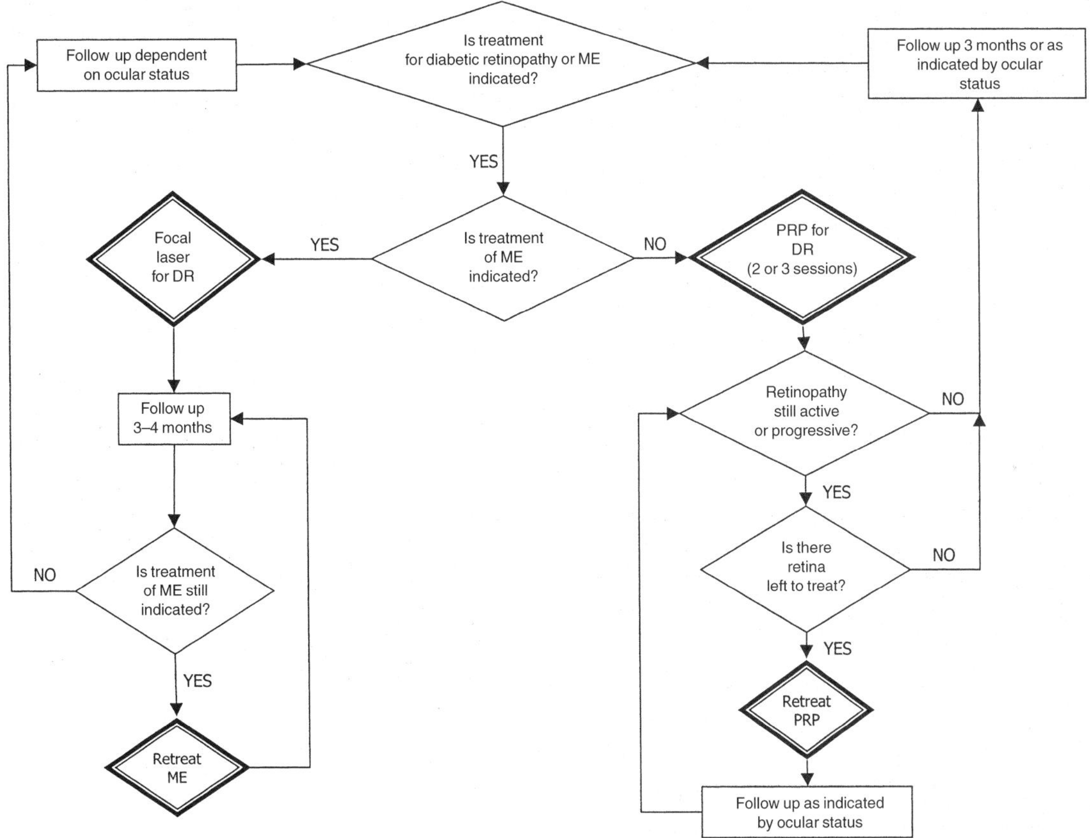

Figure 31–24. Photocoagulation flow chart. The schematic flow chart details general photocoagulation treatment approaches in patients with diabetic retinopathy and/or diabetic macular edema. These are only general guidelines, and actual treatment choices can be affected by numerous other factors, including findings in the same eye, contralateral eye, systemically, and others. DR, diabetic retinopathy; ME, macular edema; PRP, panretinal (scatter) photocoagulation.

preretinal hemorrhage. The treatment is thought to exert its effect by increasing oxygen delivery to the inner retina and decreasing viable hypoxic growth factor–producing cells. The total treatment is usually applied over two or three sessions, spaced 1 to 2 weeks apart. Follow-up evaluation usually occurs at 3 months.

The response to PRP varies. The most desirable effect is to see a regression of the new vessels, although stabilization of the neovascularization with no further growth may result. This later situation requires careful clinical monitoring. In some cases, new vessels continue to proliferate, requiring additional PRP (see Fig. 31–24).

Table 31–2. Progression to PDR by NPDR Level

Retinopathy Level	Chance (%) of high-risk PDR: 1 Year	5 Years
Mild NPDR	1	16
Moderate NPDR	3–8	27–39
Severe NPDR	15	56
Very severe NPDR	45	71
PDR with < high-risk characteristics	22–46	64–75

NPDR, nonproliferative diabetic retinopathy; PDR, proliferative diabetic retinopathy. From Aiello LP, Gardner TW, King GL, et al. Diabetic retinopathy: technical review. Diabetes Care 1998; 21: 143–156.

The DRVS, completed in 1989, demonstrated that early PPV in persons with severe fibrovascular proliferation was more likely to result in better vision and less likely to result in poor vision, particularly in patients with type 1 diabetes.[313] PPV is surgery within the eye aimed primarily at removing abnormal fibrovascular tissue, alleviating retinal traction, and removing vitreous opacities such as vitreous hemorrhage. The actual outcome data from this study may not be totally applicable due to the dramatic advances in surgical techniques and the advent of laser endophotocoagulation that have occurred in the intervening years.

Macular Edema

Untreated CSME is associated with an approximately 25% chance of moderate visual loss after 3 years (defined as at least doubling the visual angle, e.g., 20/40 to 20/80).[239] Macular edema is best evaluated by dilated examination using slit lamp biomicroscopy or stereo fundus photography. Focal laser photocoagulation is generally indicated for patients with CSME (see Figs. 31–19*C* and 31–22). The ETDRS demonstrated that focal laser photocoagulation for CSME reduced the 5-year risk of moderate vision loss from nearly 30% to less than 15%.[337] In focal laser photocoagulation, lesions from 300 to 3000 μm from the center of the macula that are contributing to thickening of the macular area are directly photocoagulated. These lesions are generally identified by fluorescein angiography and consist primarily of leaking microaneurysms. When leakage is diffuse, or microaneurysms innumerable, photocoag-

tions. However, the exact threshold for hemorrhage from the abnormal new vessels in PDR is unknown, with up to 84% of vitreous hemorrhages associated with exercise no more strenuous than walking in some studies.[389] In general, people with PDR should avoid anaerobic exercise and exercise that involves straining, jarring, near-maximal isometric contractions, or Valsalva-type maneuvers such as high-impact aerobics, jogging, or heavy weight training. Beneficial low-risk exercises include stationary cycling, low-intensity machine rowing, swimming, and walking. Because of the beneficial effects, all patients with diabetes should be encouraged to participate in regular physical exercise programs specifically tailored to their individual ocular status.

As conclusively demonstrated by the ETDRS, the use of aspirin in diabetic patients is not associated with an increased risk of hemorrhage and has no demonstrated impact on the progression of retinopathy or macular edema.[390, 391] There is one case report of vitreous hemorrhage associated with retinopathy after thrombolysis.[392] However, approximately 90,000 patients have been involved in clinical trials of thrombolytic agents in myocardial infarction, of which 10% had diabetes mellitus without any reports of ocular complications.[393–396]

Smoking is a certain risk factor for CVD, progression of albuminuria to proteinuria, and nephropathy in both type 1 and 2 diabetic patients. However, the effects of smoking on diabetic retinopathy are unclear, because some studies have suggested an association[397, 398] whereas others have not.[345, 399–401] Because smoking has detrimental effects on the cardiovascular system and the development of nephropathy, smoking in patients with diabetes mellitus should be discouraged in the strongest possible terms.

Low hematocrit was an independent risk factor in the ETDRS analysis of baseline risk factors for development of high-risk PDR and of severe visual loss.[402] A cross-sectional study involving 1691 patients revealed a twofold increased risk of any retinopathy in patients with a hemoglobin level of less than 12 g/dL as compared to those with a higher hemoglobin concentration using multivariate analyses controlling for serum creatinine, proteinuria, and other factors.[403] In patients with retinopathy, those with low hemoglobin levels have a fivefold increased risk of severe retinopathy compared with those with higher hemoglobin levels. There have been limited reports of resolution of macular edema and hard exudate with improvement or stabilization of visual acuity in erythropoietin-treated patients after an increase in mean hematocrit.[404] In view of the potential association of low hematocrit and diabetic retinopathy, it is important to ensure that patients with diabetic retinopathy and anemia are receiving appropriate management.

In summary, diabetes is clearly a multisystem disease requiring a medical team approach. Even with regard to ocular health, this necessitates the involvement of multiple health care specialists for optimal patient care.

Investigational Approaches

Our understanding of the basic molecular mechanisms underlying the development, progression, and damage from diabetic retinopathy has markedly expanded in recent years. There is considerable evidence to suggest that significant beneficial effects may be achieved using pharmacologic interventions to prevent or delay the development of nonproliferative retinopathy, suppress retinal vascular leakage, and inhibit intraocular neovascularization. Such efforts hold promise for the prevention of visual loss without the retinal damage inherent with current photocoagulation therapies. Indeed, numerous pharmacologic agents are in or approaching clinical trial for indications involving diabetic retinopathy, macular edema, and other ocular disorders. Results from these trials should become available within the next few years and may herald a new era in our therapeutic approach to diabetic ocular complications.

DIABETIC NEPHROPATHY

Diabetic nephropathy is clinically defined by persistent proteinuria greater than 500 mg/24 hours in a person with diabetic retinopathy without other renal disease.[405] Listed as the chief cause of end-stage renal disease (ESRD) in North America, Japan, Korea, and most industrialized European nations, diabetic nephropathy in 1998 accounted for 44.5% of incident ESRD patients funded by Medicare (Fig. 31–26).[406] Typically, diabetic ESRD patients have serious co-morbid conditions, especially heart, eye, and peripheral vascular diseases. It is not surprising, therefore, that caring for afflicted individuals imposes a major financial burden on family members and governments. In 1998, Medicare spent more than $4 billion for the care of diabetic ESRD patients.[406]

Both type 1 and type 2 diabetes cause renal disease. Compared to type 1, a slightly smaller and imperfectly defined proportion of type 2 patients progress to ESRD, but they represent more than 90% of those receiving renal replacement therapy with the diagnosis of diabetes.[407, 408] The distribution of renal disease due to type 2 diabetes is uneven among racial groups. American Indians, African Americans, and Mexican Americans have a greater incidence than non-Hispanic whites.[407, 409–411] Genetic predisposition, environmental factors, delayed diagnosis of type 2 diabetes, and subadequate medical care in minority groups contribute in undefined amounts to such disparity.[409, 412–414]

PATHOLOGY

Kidney injury in diabetes is indistinguishable by diabetes type and affects glomeruli, arterioles, tubules, and interstitium.[415–417] Glomerular lesions include diffuse and nodular forms of intracapillary glomerulosclerosis (Fig. 31–27*A* to *C*) (see also Color Plate). The diffuse type is characterized by mesangial expansion with increased PAS-positive matrix material, thickening of capillary wall and basement membrane. In

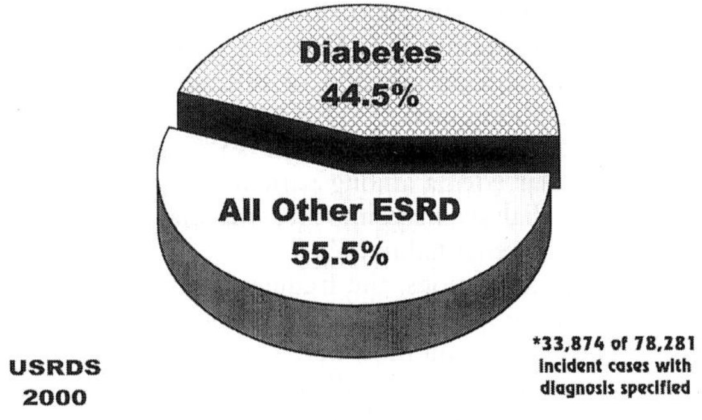

Figure 31–26. End-stage renal disease (ESRD) among Medicare patients in 1998 with diagnosis specified. USRDS, United States Renal Data System. (From The absence of a glycemic threshold for the development of long-term complications: the perspective of the Diabetes Control and Complications Trial. Diabetes 1996; 45:1289–1298.)

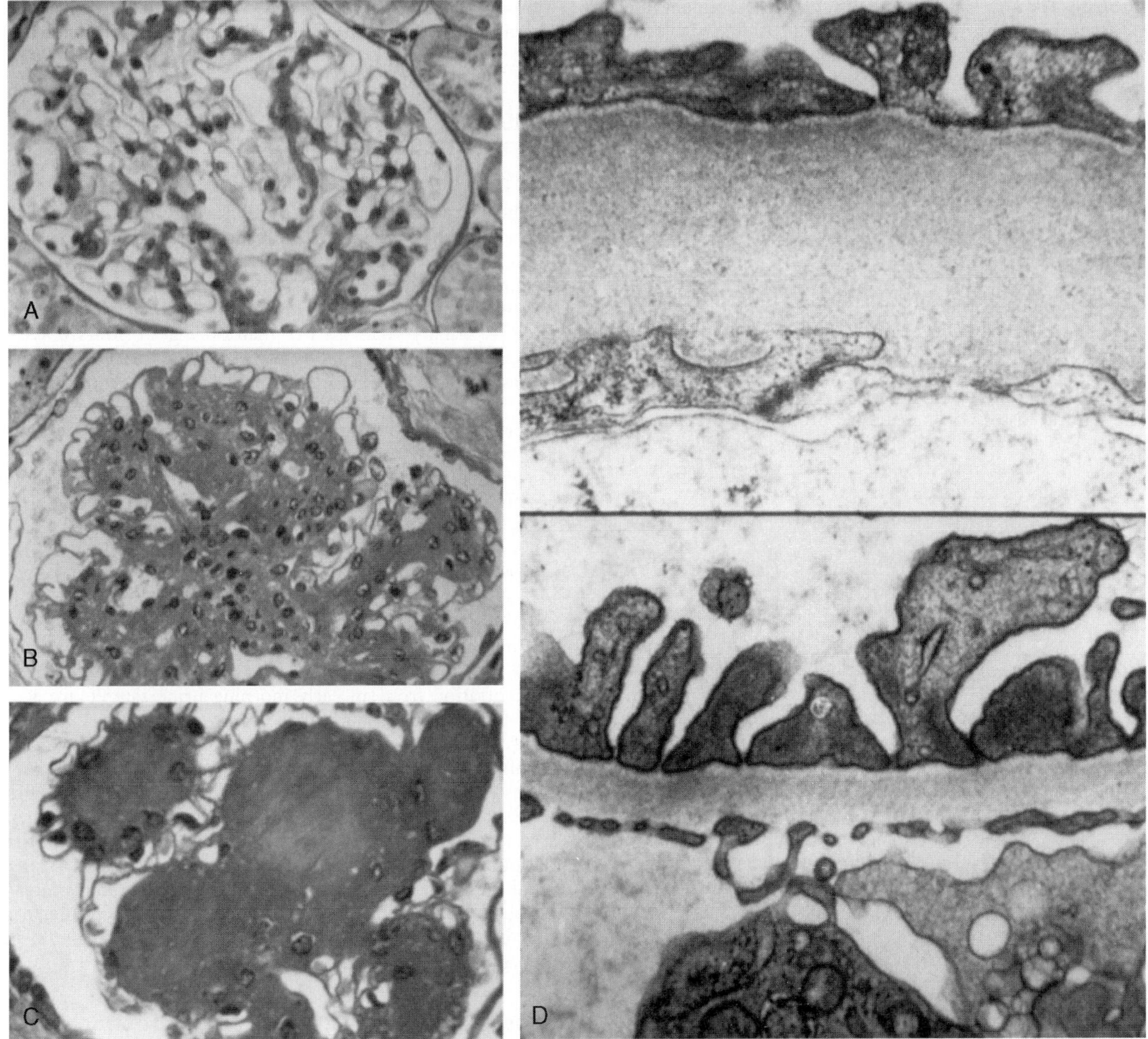

Figure 31–27. *A*, Periodic acid–Schiff (PAS) stain of a normal glomerulus sectioned through the vascular pole. The mesangial cellularity and matrix are normal. *B*, Glomerulus showing marked diffuse diabetic glomerulosclerosis. There is extreme expansion of the mesangium with both matrix and cellular material (PAS). *C*, Example of nodular diabetic glomerulosclerosis (Kimmelstiel-Wilson lesions). Note the reduction of glomerular capillary luminal space (PAS). *D*, Electron photomicrograph showing a normal glomerular basement membrane width *(bottom panel)* and diffuse thickening of the glomerular basement membrane secondary to diabetes *(upper panel)*.

type 1 diabetes, an early structural abnormality of diabetic nephropathy is glomerular basement membrane thickening (Fig. 31–27*D*).[418] Also noted in early and sequential biopsies is an increase in mesangial fractional volume (mesangial volume per glomerulus).[418, 419] With progression, capillary wall thickening and mesangial widening lead to capillary narrowing and reduced glomerular capillary filtration surface area. In diabetic patients, there is good correlation between the degree of mesangial expansion and the severity of clinical diabetic nephropathy.[420, 421]

Although nodular lesions were first thought to be pathognomonic for diabetic glomerulopathy, they may also be noted by light microscopy in amyloidosis, dysproteinemias (multiple myeloma and heavy chain disease), and glomerulonephritis (mesangial proliferative and membranoproliferative).[422–424] Typical nodules are well-demarcated, PAS-positive globular structures exaggerating the diffuse lesions, and they occur at the periphery of the glomeruli.

Additionally, hyaline deposits (so-called exudative or insudative lesions), consisting of plasma proteins and lipids, are present in arterioles (hyaline arteriosclerosis), capillary walls (fibrin caps), and Bowman's capsules (capsular drops).[422] Hyaline arteriosclerosis or arteriolar hyalinosis, prominent in diabetic nephropathy, affects afferent as well as efferent arterioles.[422] Initially, collections of hyaline material (hyaline drops) aggregate in the wall of juxtaglomerular arterioles. Gradually, these drops increase in size and replace the entire wall structure. Progression of glomerular and arteriolar changes ends in complete sclerosis. Østerby and associates demonstrated that a high rate of glomerular occlusion in type 1 patients correlated significantly with decreased GFR.[425]

Although diabetes is primarily a vascular disease, diabetic

nephropathy is also associated with tubular basement membrane thickening and interstitial space expansion.[426] Several reports note that thickening of the basement membrane of proximal tubules and interstitial expansion are present early in diabetic nephropathy.[426–428] Expansion of the interstitial space correlates with loss of renal function.[429] Deterioration of renal function in diabetic nephropathy is thus a product of several forces acting in concert, including glomerular capillary narrowing, hyaline arteriosclerosis, glomerular sclerosis or occlusion, and interstitial fibrosis.[430]

NEPHROPATHY IN TYPE 1 DIABETES

The natural history of diabetic nephropathy has been extensively studied in type 1 diabetes because it is usually possible to specify the exact time of onset. As first described by Mogensen, there are five distinct stages.[405] The course of diabetic nephropathy can be followed by two main variables: proteinuria and GFR (Fig. 31–28).

Stage 1: Glomerular Hyperfiltration and Renal Enlargement

Glomerular hyperfiltration and kidney enlargement typify the first stage. In 1934, Cambier noted that inulin clearances were greater than normal in type 1 diabetes.[431] Subsequent studies, using creatinine clearance or radionuclide techniques, validated this finding.[432–434] At onset of type 1 diabetes, approximately one third of individuals have an elevated GFR that is 20% to 40% higher than that of age-matched normal subjects.[435] No single pathophysiologic mechanism totally explains both kidney enlargement and glomerular hyperfiltration. Hyperglycemia, hormonal and vasoactive factors, enhanced renal plasma flow, and elevated transglomerular hydrostatic pressure gradient have been proposed as determinants of diabetic hyperfiltration.[435–438] With intensive insulin therapy, hyperglycemia decreases and GFR starts to decline within 3 to 8 days and drops further over the next few months.[435, 439] Thus, hyperfiltration may be an early indicator of individual susceptibility to hyperglycemia-induced renal changes. Hyperfiltration is a predictor of clinical nephropathy in some individuals. Mogensen's initial findings[440] that an elevated GFR predicts subsequent glomerulopathy in type 1 patients, previously contested, were confirmed by two different reports.[441, 442] In an 8-year prospective study of diabetic adolescents, Rudberg and colleagues showed that an increase of the initial GFR significantly predicted nephropathy.[443] Recently, Chiarelli and associates, in a 10-year longitudinal study, indicated glomerular hyperfiltration increased the risk of developing microalbuminuria in diabetic children.[444] Short-term or long-term intensive insulin treatments did not reduce kidney size in type 1 diabetic individuals.[455–457]

Stage 2: Early Glomerular Lesions or Silent Stage with Normal Albumin Excretion

Early glomerular lesions, consisting of glomerular basement membrane thickening and mesangial matrix expansion,[418, 419] characterize the second stage. Those structural changes appear 18 to 36 months after onset of type 1 diabetes[448] and may become prominent after 3.5 to 5 years.[449] During this stage of morphologic changes, microalbuminuria, seen only after exercise or during episodes of very poor metabolic control, may be the only clinically detectable evidence of renal involvement.[405] Otherwise, nephropathy is silent with normal AER (<25 mg/day).

Stage 3: Incipient Diabetic Nephropathy or Microalbuminuric Stage

The third stage, also called *incipient diabetic nephropathy*, is characterized by persistent and usually increasing microalbuminuria.[405] Hypertension may also be a feature of the microalbuminuric stage.[450–452] Hyperfiltration and renal enlargement persist, though to a lesser degree.[453, 454] *Microalbuminuria*, defined as urinary AER greater than 30 mg/24 hours or 20 μg/minute and less than 300 mg/24 hours or 200 μg/minute, represents the first laboratory evidence of diabetic renal disease.[455] Total daily AER varies greatly and is increased by hypertension, strenuous exercise, fever, poor glycemic control, and congestive heart failure (CHF).[456, 457] Therefore, a diagnosis of incipient diabetic nephropathy is made only when microalbuminuria is detected in at least two of three urine specimens over several months.

Hemodynamic abnormalities and variable glomerular charge-selective properties due to loss of negatively charged proteoglycans contribute to variability of microalbuminuria.[458] Measurements of urinary AER can be carried out by 24-hour, overnight, or short-term urine collections.[459, 460] Determinations of albumin:creatinine ratio (30:300 mg/g) or albumin concentration from an early morning urine sample are acceptable for screening, but timed urine collection is more accurate.[460] The prevalence of microalbuminuria varies from 25% to 40% in individuals with type 1 diabetes for 5 to 15 years.[461, 462] Persistent microalbuminuria rarely occurs during the first 5 years of type 1 diabetes or before puberty.[463, 464] Consequently, screening in type 1 subjects should start after 3 years of diabetes duration or with puberty. Microalbuminuria is a sign of renal damage in both types of diabetes that predicts later nephropathy and, ultimately, ESRD.[405, 465–468] Therefore, detection of microalbuminuria represents a vital step in the early management of diabetic renal disease.

Stage 4: Clinical or Overt Diabetic Nephropathy: Proteinuria and Falling Glomerular Filtration Rate

Albuminuria greater than 300 mg/24 hours, relentless decline of renal function, and hypertension define the fourth stage of diabetic nephropathy.[405, 469] This stage, though variable, usually occurs 15 to 20 years after the onset of type 1 diabetes and after 5 or more years of diagnosed type 2 diabetes. The amount of urinary protein can be as little as 500 mg, but it can reach massive proportions, such as 20 to 40 g/24 hours. Continuing urinary protein loss of this magnitude is associated with increased glomerular pore size. There is a high mortality rate associated with proteinuria. Median survival is 10 years from the onset of proteinuria.

Diagnoses other than diabetic nephropathy should be pursued whenever a nephrotic syndrome develops in a patient with short-term type 1 diabetes or in the absence of retinopathy. Similarly, a diagnosis of diabetic nephropathy is prudently doubted when progressive renal insufficiency in a diabetic patient is not accompanied by macroalbuminuria (AER > 300 mg/24 hours). Percutaneous renal biopsy to clarify the renal disorder is indicated in such instances. In the follow-up of more than 90 patients with insulin-dependent diabetes and diabetic nephropathy, Viberti and co-workers have not encountered a single case of progressive renal failure without macroalbuminuria.[470]

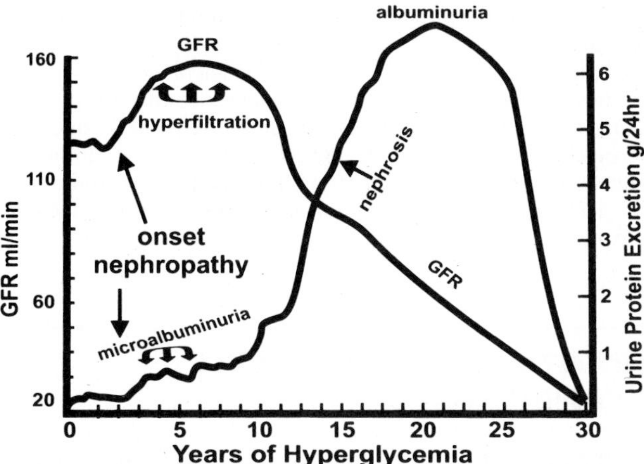

Figure 31–28. Schematic representation of the progression of diabetic nephropathy. Glomerular hyperfiltration and microalbuminuria are the earliest manifestations of glomerulopathy. Subsequently, urinary protein increases to nephrotic range (>3.5 g/day) and glomerular filtration rate (GFR) declines relentlessly.

In subjects with type 1 diabetes, the prevalence of arterial hypertension ranges from 65% to 79% when macroalbuminuria is present.[468, 471] Hypertension intensifies the rate of progression of established diabetic renal disease.[472–474] When structural kidney changes are advanced, GFR will invariably decrease. Without treatment, GFR usually declines in a linear fashion at a rate ranging from 7.5 to 28 mL/minute per year.[469, 475, 476]

Stage 5: End-Stage Renal Disease

After 20 to 30 years of type 1 diabetes, about 30% to 40% of patients progress to ESRD. Recently, the interval between the onset of persistent proteinuria and the final stage of diabetic nephropathy has been lengthened by early and intensive treatment of hypertension and enhanced metabolic control of hyperglycemia.

NEPHROPATHY IN TYPE 2 DIABETES

Although renal structural changes and severity of target organ damage are similar in both types of diabetes,[417] delayed diagnosis has complicated the construction of the natural history of diabetic renal disease in type 2 diabetes. The results of studies about renal hemodynamics and hypertrophy in newly diagnosed and established patients have been inconsistent. For example, Vora and associates reported that 45% of their 110 patients with type 2 diabetes had a GFR higher than 120 mL/minute per 1.73 m^2 and 16% had frank hyperfiltration (GFR > 140 mL/minute per 1.73 m^2).[477] By contrast, Schmitz and colleagues did not observe hyperfiltration in their newly diagnosed patients with type 2 diabetes (GFR 106 ± 14 mL/minute per 1.73 m^2).[478]

Fourteen percent to 24% of newly diagnosed patients with type 2 diabetes have microalbuminuria, which is associated with hyperglycemia, elevated BP, smoking, and hyperlipidemia.[479–481] Microalbuminuria in type 2 diabetes is partially reversed by reduction of hyperglycemia and high BP.[480] In a systematic review of the literature linking microalbuminuria to cardiovascular mortality in individuals with type 2 diabetes, Dinneen and Gerstein[482] found that the prevalence of microalbuminuria ranged from 20% to 36% in diabetic patients. There was also a significant association between microalbuminuria and total or cardiovascular mortality. Microalbuminuria raised the overall odds ratio for death to 2.4 and cardiovascular mortality to 2.0 over those without microalbuminuria.[482] For older people, other causes of microalbuminuria should be considered before attributing this abnormality to type 2 diabetes.[483] In a population-based study in southern Wisconsin, the prevalence of overt proteinuria in a 10-year interval was 33%.[484] GFR of diabetic Arizona Pima Indians with macroalbuminuria declined by 35% over a 4-year period.[485] Hypertension is highly characteristic of renal disease in type 2 diabetes, whether the individuals are normoalbuminuric, microalbuminuric, or macroalbuminuric.

PATHOGENESIS OF DIABETIC NEPHROPATHY

The pathogenesis of diabetic nephropathy is a multistage process starting with a genetic predisposition to injury by an elevated glucose concentration. The biochemical mechanisms by which hyperglycemia may induce diabetic renal damage are discussed in the chapter part entitled "Biochemistry and Molecular Cell Biology." Because a significant number of type 1 patients do not develop diabetic nephropathy, however, hyperglycemia appears to be necessary but not sufficient for the development of diabetic nephropathy. Genetically determined differences in the renal response to hyperglycemia may affect glucose transporter function, ROS formation, the polyol pathway, PKC activation, AGE formation, or the hexosamine pathway. These differences in renal response to hyperglycemia may also affect more distal mediators of diabetic renal pathology, such as TGF-β and other growth factors causing increased matrix deposition. In addition to growth factors, gene products causing altered glomerular hemodynamics may also be differentially affected.

In humans with type 1 diabetes, several investigators have demonstrated that hyperfiltration is a predictor of clinical nephropathy.[440, 443, 444] Glomerular hyperfiltration characterizes the early stages of diabetes in experimental animals and in humans. In moderately hyperglycemic rats, single-nephron GFR increases by 40% as compared to normal rats.[486] Hyperfiltration results from increased glomerular capillary plasma flow rate (hyperperfusion) and increased hydraulic pressure (hypertension), which are subsequently associated with morphologic changes and progressive albuminuria.[486–489] The rise in glomerular pressure is due to less resistance in the afferent than in the efferent arterioles. These changes in arteriolar resistance facilitate transmission of normal or elevated systemic pressures to glomeruli.

Relaxation factors affecting afferent arteriolar tone such as atrial natriuretic peptide (ANP), NO, and vasodilator prostaglandins or constriction factors affecting efferent arteriolar tone such as angiotensin II, endothelin, and vasoconstrictor prostanoids could both play a significant role in the pathogenesis of diabetic hyperfiltration by creating glomerular capillary hypertension.[490] Neutralization of elevated plasma ANP levels with an antibody or a specific receptor antagonist decreases hyperfiltration in diabetic rats.[491, 492] Nonspecific inhibitors of NO synthases block NO synthesis and decrease GFR in diabetic rats with glomerular hyperfiltration.[493, 494] Prevention of glomerular capillary hypertension in diabetic rats with an ACE inhibitor protects against subsequent development of glomerular structural injury and proteinuria.[488]

Increased blood flow, acting through shear stress, can alter glomerular cell gene expression. Expansion of glomerular capillaries and stretching of the mesangium in response to glomerular hypertension may promote increased mesangial matrix and glomerular basement membrane thickening.[495] In addition to its vasoconstrictive effect on the efferent arteriole, angiotensin II enlarges glomerular membrane pore size.[496] Increased protein filtration through enlarged membrane pores causes further damage and leads to additional nephron loss.

As discussed earlier, extension of these findings to renal hemodynamics in type 2 diabetes is inconsistent.[477, 478] This lack of consistency is explained, in part, by the difficulty in determining the exact time of onset in type 2 diabetes and its association with nondiabetic renal diseases.[495]

OTHER DIABETES-ASSOCIATED RENAL DISEASES

Three other renal conditions are associated with diabetes: (1) urinary tract infection, (2) papillary necrosis, and (3) radiocontrast-induced renal failure. In long-standing type 1 diabetes, diabetic women, but not diabetic men, have an increased frequency of urinary tract infection.[497] Diabetic patients are also at risk for emphysematous pyelonephritis, a rare, life-threatening complication of upper urinary tract infections, characterized by gas in the renal parenchyma or perirenal space.[498] Renal ultrasonography or computed tomographic (CT) scanning is necessary to detect upper urinary tract complications early for appropriate treatment.[499] Parenteral antimicrobial therapy and close metabolic control of diabetes with insulin therapy are mandatory, but nephrectomy or drainage is often necessary to preserve life.

Renal papillary necrosis, a severe destruction of renal parenchyma due to impaired blood flow to the inner medulla and papilla of the kidney, although observed in urinary infections, analgesic abuse, and sickle cell disease, is most common in diabetes. Clinical manifestations comprise flank pain, hematuria, chills, fever, and septicemia. Red and white blood cells, bacteria, and fragments of renal papillae can be seen in strained urine. Ureteral obstruction due to papilla fragments should be relieved promptly.[500, 501]

Radiocontrast-induced renal failure occurs more frequently in type 1 and 2 diabetic patients than in nondiabetic patients when the serum creatinine level is higher than 2 mg/dL.[502, 503] The use of radiographic contrast medium in a diabetic patient with renal insufficiency should be limited whenever possible. When angiography is unavoidable, patients should be aware of the risk of acute renal failure. Hydration before and after contrast injection may reduce the risk of nephropathy. A highly encouraging report indicates that pretreatment with acetylcysteine may protect against radiographic contrast media nephropathy.[504]

HYPORENINEMIC HYPOALDOSTERONISM

Hyporeninemic hypoaldosteronism is prevalent in patients with renal insufficiency due to diabetic nephropathy. The syndrome of hyporeninemic hypoaldosteronism is characterized by normal cortisol levels, hyperkalemia, and low plasma renin, angiotensin II, and aldosterone levels. Most patients with the syndrome manifest a coexistent hyperchloremic metabolic acidosis.[505] In diabetes mellitus, low plasma renin activity is due to defective conversion of prorenin to active renin.[506] Increased extracellular volume due to diabetic nephropathy may, in part, diminish renin release. In this case, hyporeninemia is corrected by diuresis.[507]

Clark and co-workers suggest that an increase in ANP contributes to hypoaldosteronism and hyperkalemia in the syndrome of acquired hypoaldosteronism.[508] ACE inhibitors, nonsteroidal anti-inflammatory drugs (NSAIDs), cyclosporine, potassium-sparing diuretics, trimethoprim, and pentamidine all can accentuate the hyperkalemia of hyporeninemic hypoaldosteronism.[509–512]

TREATMENT OF DIABETIC NEPHROPATHY

Experience of the past two decades convincingly demonstrates that intensive control of hyperglycemia and adequate lowering of hypertensive BP are the key components of diabetic nephropathy management. Control of both hyperglycemia and hypertension has modified the natural course of diabetic nephropathy by reversing functional changes and by stabilizing progression of structural abnormalities (Fig. 31–29).[513, 514]

Glycemic Control

Large-scale, prospective trials provide compelling evidence that intensive glycemic control prevents diabetic nephropathy.[2, 3] The DCCT, which strived for near-normoglycemia in patients with type 1 diabetes, showed a 39% reduction in the risk of developing microalbuminuria and a 54% reduction in the occurrence of albuminuria. The UKPDS, comparing intensive blood glucose with conventional therapy in type 2 diabetes, found a 25% risk reduction (7% to 40%; $P = .0099$) in microvascular complications, including progressive nephropathy. Degradation of insulin is compromised in renal failure. Consequently, progressive reductions in oral agent and insulin doses are necessary to minimize hypoglycemia.[515] Metformin, a powerful hypoglycemic drug, is contraindicated in renal insufficiency (serum creatinine $>$ 2.0 mg/dL) because of the risk of fatal lactic acidosis.

Blood Pressure Control

Early diagnosis and intensive treatment of arterial hypertension, whether with ACE inhibitors or other antihypertensive drugs in combination with low-dose diuretics, are essential for diabetic patients with diabetic renal disease. Effective BP control reduces albuminuria, delays progression of nephropathy, postpones renal insufficiency, and improves survival in type 1 and type 2 diabetic patients with diabetic nephropathy. Moreover, risk of fatal or nonfatal cardiovascular events is decreased in diabetic patients when systolic hypertension is treated.

The National Kidney Foundation Hypertension and Diabetes Executive Committees Working Group has lowered the previously recommended BP level of 130/85 to 130/80 mm Hg to optimally preserve renal function and reduce cardiovascular events in diabetic nephropathy. Two or more antihypertensive drugs are usually required to achieve this new target.[516] Additionally, BP levels lower than 125/75 mm Hg are recommended for people who have proteinuria higher than 1 g/day and renal insufficiency regardless of etiology.[517] Hypoproteinemic diabetic patients with renal insufficiency are susceptible to striking fluid retention, making BP control refractory to usual antihypertensive therapy. Dietary salt restriction and a combination of loop diuretics plus metolazone, a quinazoline diuretic, are necessary. A regimen of furosemide, 80 mg twice a day, and metolazone (Zaroxolyn), 10 mg twice a day, usually

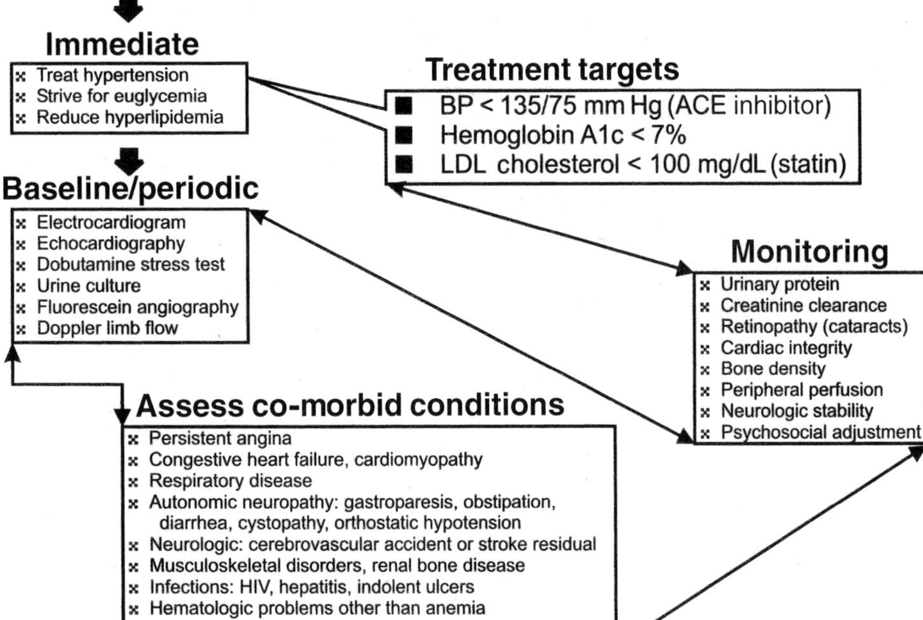

Figure 31–29. Flow chart illustrating the management of patients with diabetic nephropathy before the onset of renal failure. ACE, angiotensin-converting enzyme; HIV, human immunodeficiency virus; LDL, low-density lipoprotein.

is effective as long as the creatinine clearance is higher than 10 mL/minute.

ACE inhibitors are efficient in both types of diabetes. Apart from reducing arterial BP, they are renoprotective due to their ability to decrease intraglomerular pressure.

Several randomized, controlled trials in normotensive type 1 and type 2 diabetic subjects with incipient nephropathy demonstrate that ACE inhibitors reduce microalbuminuria and may even preempt progression to overt nephropathy.[518, 519] Bakris and associates suggest that combining a calcium antagonist with an ACE inhibitor results in a greater decrease in urinary protein excretion and slower GFR decline. In addition, this combination permits equivalent BP reduction by lower doses of both drugs.[520] ACE inhibitors can worsen hyperkalemia in diabetic patients with hyporeninemic hypoaldosteronism and induce temporary renal failure in those with bilateral renal artery stenosis or single-kidney and renal stenosis. Approximately one in five diabetic patients treated with ACE inhibitors discontinued the drug because of persistent nonproductive cough.

A related class of antihypertensive drugs, the angiotensin receptor blockers, block angiotensin II at the receptor level. Whether angiotensin receptor blockers will match the ACE inhibitors in improving the natural history of renal diseases is the subject of two large prospective, randomized trials in type 2 diabetic patients.

Dietary Protein and Lipid Restriction

Rodent studies show that a low-protein diet reduces glomerular hypertension and prevents glomerular injury and albuminuria.[521] In type 1 diabetic subjects with microalbuminuria and glomerular hyperfiltration, short-term dietary protein restriction (0.6 to 0.8 g/kg per day) decreases urinary AER and hyperfiltration.[522] Long-term studies of protein restriction have been criticized for using creatinine clearance or the reciprocal of the serum creatinine instead of inulin clearance or radionuclide techniques to assess renal function. From a meta-analysis of five studies, Pedrini and colleagues[523] concluded that dietary protein restriction delayed progression of diabetic nephropathy in subjects with type 1 diabetes, a finding disputed by Parving.[524] In type 2 diabetes, trials of protein restriction are few and positive results have not been attained.[525]

Abnormal lipid metabolism is highly prevalent in diabetic individuals with nephropathy, especially in those with a nephrotic syndrome. Although rodent studies imply that hyperlipidemia is important in the pathogenesis of glomerular injury, only suggestive data in humans have been reported.[526, 527] Nevertheless, treatment of dyslipidemia is paramount in the overall management of diabetes because it decreases the risk of CVDs.

Uremia Therapy

While renal function relentlessly deteriorates, patients with diabetic renal disorder should be instructed as to the available options in uremia therapy, including home or facility hemodialysis, continuous ambulatory peritoneal dialysis, continuous cyclic peritoneal dialysis, living related or cadaveric kidney transplant, and combined pancreas and kidney transplant (Table 31–4). A small number of uremic diabetic patients, severely debilitated by extensive co-morbid conditions, may choose death instead of renal replacement therapy. As reported by the U.S. Renal Data System (USRDS) in 2000,[406] for 102,942 diabetic patients receiving uremia therapy in 1998, about 74% were treated with facility hemodialysis, but only 7.5% elected peritoneal dialysis. A few (0.7%) adopted home hemodialysis, although this therapy, by consensus, is superior to facility dialysis. Approximately 17% of diabetic ESRD patients had a functioning kidney transplant in the United States in 1998. Kidney transplantation, the best option in uremia therapy for diabetic patients, provides patient survival and rehabilitation that is greater than the best dialytic therapy.[528]

Although combined pancreas plus kidney transplantation, when successful, offers exquisite glycemic control and better quality of life, the prospective recipient risks a serious surgical complication rate.[529]

type 2 diabetes mellitus and additionally in various forms of acquired diabetes.[541]

The major morbidity associated with somatic neuropathy is foot ulceration, the precursor of gangrene and limb loss. DSPN increases the risk of amputation 1.7-fold: 12-fold if there is deformity (itself a consequence of neuropathy) and 36-fold if there is a history of previous ulceration.[542] About 85,000 amputations are performed in the United States each year—one every 2 minutes—and neuropathy is considered to be the major contributor in 87% of cases. It is also the most life-spoiling of the diabetic complications and has tremendous ramifications for the quality of life of the person with diabetes. Once autonomic neuropathy sets in, life can become quite dismal, and the mortality rate approximates 25% to 50% within 5 to 10 years.[543, 544]

NATURAL HISTORY

The natural history of diabetic neuropathy separates patients into two very distinctive entities: (1) those who progress gradually with increasing duration of diabetes mellitus and (2) those who have a relatively explosive onset and experience remission almost completely. Sensory and autonomic neuropathies generally progress, whereas mononeuropathies, radiculopathies, and acute painful neuropathies, although symptoms are severe, are short-lived and tend to recover.[545]

Progression of DSPN is related to glycemic control in both type 1 and type 2 diabetes mellitus.[2, 546] The most rapid deterioration of nerve function occurs soon after the onset of type 1 diabetes mellitus, and within 2 to 3 years there is a slowing of the progress with a shallower slope to the curve of dysfunction. In contrast, slowing of NCVs in type 2 diabetes mellitus may be one of the earliest neuropathic abnormalities and is often present at diagnosis.[547] After diagnosis, slowing of NCV generally progresses at a steady rate of approximately 1 m/second each year, and the level of impairment is positively correlated with duration of diabetes mellitus. Although most studies have documented that symptomatic patients are more likely to have slower NCVs than patients without symptoms, these do not relate to the severity of symptoms.

In a long-term follow-up study of patients with type 2 diabetes mellitus,[548] electrophysiologic abnormalities in the lower limb increased from 8% at baseline to 42% after 10 years, and a decrease in sensory and motor amplitudes, indicating axonal destruction, was more pronounced than the slowing of the NCVs. An increase of about 2 points in an 80-point clinical symptom and sign scale (*neurologic symptom score* [NSS] and *neurologic impairment score* [NIS] can be expected per year. These scales contain information on motor, sensory, and autonomic signs and symptoms. Using objective measures of sensory function such as the VPT test, the rate of decline in function has been reported as 1 or 2 vibration units per year.

In a 6-year cohort study,[549] elevated VPT (>6.5 vibrations) was found in 62.5% of patients. The risk factors were male sex, age, and increased AER. However, there now appears to be a decline in this rate of evolution. For example, in the *nerve growth factor* (NGF) study, the VPT at the beginning of the study in the placebo group was identical to that at the end of 1 year.[550, 551] This is particularly important in planning studies on the treatment of DSPN, which have always relied on differences between drug treatment and placebo and have been successful because of the decline in nerve function in the placebo-treated patients.[552] According to the earlier data on rates of change, clinically meaningful loss of VPT and NCV has been estimated to take at least 3 years, dictating a future need to carry out studies over a longer period when considering only large-fiber dysfunction.

We must recognize that DSPN is a disorder in which the prevailing abnormality is loss of axons that electrophysiologically translates to a reduction in amplitudes and not conduction velocities, and changes in NCV may not be an appropriate means of monitoring progress or deterioration of nerve function. It has always been advocated that diabetes mellitus affects the longest fibers first, hence, the increased predisposition in taller individuals.[553] Now it seems that small-fiber involvement may herald the onset of neuropathy and even diabetes mellitus itself. Small-fiber function is not detectable using standard electrodiagnostic methods and requires measurement of sensory, neurovascular, and autonomic thresholds and cutaneous nerve fiber density.[554–556]

There are few data on the longitudinal trends in small-fiber dysfunction[548] and the mutual concurrence and development of peripheral somatic and autonomic neuropathies.[557] Toyry and associates[558] reported that the development of autonomic and peripheral somatic neuropathies was divergent in patients with type 2 diabetes mellitus, suggesting different pathophysiologic processes for these neuropathies. Much remains to be learned of the natural history of diabetic autonomic neuropathy.[558]

Karamitsos and colleagues[559] reported that the progression of diabetic autonomic neuropathy is significant during the 2 years subsequent to its discovery. The mortality for diabetic patients with autonomic neuropathy has been estimated to be 44% within 2.5 years of diagnosing symptomatic autonomic neuropathy.[543] A meta-analysis[560] of 14 longitudinal studies revealed that the mortality rate after 5.8 years of diabetes with asymptomatic autonomic neuropathy was 27%.

CLASSIFICATION

Diabetic neuropathy is not a single entity but a number of different syndromes, ranging from subclinical to clinical manifestations depending on the classes of nerve fibers involved. According to the San Antonio Convention,[561] the main groups of neurologic disturbance in diabetes mellitus include the following:

1. *Subclinical neuropathy*, determined by abnormalities in electrodiagnostic and quantitative sensory testing without concomitant clinical sign and symptoms.
2. *Diffuse clinical neuropathy*, which may be proximal or distal and have large symmetrical sensorimotor or small-fiber and autonomic dysfunction.
3. *Focal neuropathies*, which include mononeuropathies and entrapment syndromes.

The onset of neuropathy may be acute, with pain or, insidious, with chronic pain as well as clinical features of a mixed sensorimotor dysfunction.

PATHOGENESIS

Focal Neuropathies

Mononeuropathies are caused by microscopic vasculitis and subsequent ischemia or infarction of nerve.[562–564] Focal ischemia results in segmental demyelination followed by remyelination. In diabetic patients, remyelination is defective and delays the repair of focal deficits. Delayed remyelination may be a consequence of diabetes-induced Schwann cell dysfunction.[565] However, in most cases, recovery does occur because adjacent fascicles take over the function of the damaged ones.

It is not clear why diabetic nerves are more susceptible to

entrapment syndromes. Upton and McComas[566] suggested that serial constrictions impairing axoplasmic flow may combine to cause nerve dysfunction and that diabetic patients who have severely impaired axoplasmic flow are more frequent. It was thought that mechanical rather than microvascular factors account for pathologic features of compressed nerves.[567] However, the increased prevalence may be related to repeated undetected trauma, susceptibility of diabetic nerves to injury, accumulation of AGEs, or accumulation of fluid or edema within the confined space of the carpal tunnel.[568]

Distal Symmetrical Polyneuropathy

For a detailed discussion of the different theories on pathogenesis of DSPN, the reader is referred to several excellent recent reviews.[569–571] However, we do review the principal theories on pathogenesis. DSPN is a heterogeneous disease with widely varying pathology, suggesting differences in pathogenic mechanisms for the different clinical syndromes. Recognition of the clinical homologue of these pathologic processes is the first step in achieving the appropriate form of intervention. Figure 31–32 summarizes our current view of the pathogenesis of DSPN. This figure depicts multiple causes, including metabolic, vascular, autoimmune, oxidative stress, and neurohormonal growth factor deficiency.

Metabolic Hypothesis of Nerve Damage

Although there is increasing evidence that the pathogenesis of DSPN consists of several mechanisms, the prevailing theory is that persistent hyperglycemia is the primary factor.[18] Persistent hyperglycemia (or glucose toxicity) or insulin deficiency may precipitate metabolic or vascular events.[572, 573] Metabolic defects include alteration of the polyol or sorbitol pathway,[18, 574] abnormalities in lipid metabolism, deficiencies of dihomo-γ-linolenic acid (GLA) and *N*-acetyl-L-carnitine (which are significant in diabetics)[574] glycation or AGE formation,[575, 576] increased oxidative stress,[577–579] and diabetes mellitus–induced growth factor defects.[580] The results of the DCCT[546] endorse the importance of glycemic control in preventing neuropathy. However, it seems unlikely that metabolic factors can account for all patients with neuropathy or for the heterogeneity of the clinical syndromes.

Immune Hypothesis of Nerve Damage

Data from several large epidemiologic studies show that neurologic signs precede the diagnosis of diabetes in up to 11% of diabetes patients.[541] The neuropathogenic process in some patients with diabetes mellitus may be independent of hyperglycemia. A number of autoantigens have been described in these patients that might induce immune system responses, including antiphospholipid antibodies (PLAs), a family of closely related immunoglobulins that interact with one or more negatively charged phospholipids (constituents of nervous tissues), and sera with high titers of IgG-PLA that inhibit cell growth and differentiation in a neuroblastoma cell line.[581] Anti-PLAs have been found in 88% of a diabetic population with neuropathy compared with 32% in diabetes mellitus patients without apparent neurologic complications and 2% in the general population.[581] Because PLAs are associated with a tendency to vascular thrombosis, their presence may provide a link between the immune and vascular theories of causation of neuropathy.

Autoantibodies to the gangliosides, sialo- and asialo-GM1, have been described in diabetes mellitus patients with neuropathy[568] characterized by a slight emphasis on a motor deficit with electrophysiologic signs of demyelination. It is argued that anti-GM1 antibodies are not pathogenic but passively reflect cellular destruction.[582] A number of observations, however, suggest that they have pathogenic potential.[583–585] Indeed, there may be differences in responsiveness based on the distribution of these antibodies among the immunoglobulin classes. As yet, there is no known autoimmune mechanism in the pathogenesis of the disease, but our understanding of autoimmune neuropathies is constantly being fueled by new evidence. This area of research in diabetes promises to be exciting and fruitful.[586]

Microvascular Hypothesis

The peripheral and autonomic nervous system has an important role in the control and regulation of microvascular function. As a corollary, microvascular perfusion is essential for the integrity of nerves. Microvascular insufficiency due to impaired vasoconstriction and vasodilation to various stimuli has been proposed as a possible cause of DSPN by a number of investigators.[587–589] The interest in microvascular derangements in DSPN arises from studies suggesting that absolute or relative ischemia may exist in the nerves of diabetes mellitus subjects due to altered function of the endoneural and epineurial blood vessels.[590] Histopathologic studies show the presence of different degrees of endoneurial and epineurial microvasculopathy,[591] mainly vessel basement membrane thickening and obstruction of vasa nervorum.[592, 593]

A number of functional disturbances are found in the microvasculature of the nerves of patients with diabetes mellitus. These include decreased neural blood flow,[594] increased vascular resistance, decreased neural PO_2,[594, 595] and altered vascular permeability characteristics, such as loss of the anionic charge barrier and decreased charge selectivity. Decreased neural blood flow and increased vascular resistance in diabetes mellitus may result from alterations in microvascular reactivity, such as impaired dilator responses to substance P, calcitonin gene-related peptide (CGRP), and reactive hyperemia. Vasomotion, the rhythmic contraction exhibited by arterioles and small arteries, is disordered in diabetes mellitus patients,[596] and the warm thermal sensory threshold correlated significantly with the mean amplitude of vasomotion. This indicates an interaction between C-fiber function and vasomotion, but it is not clear whether the neurologic deficit precedes or follows the loss of normal vascular motility.

It also has been shown that abnormalities of cutaneous blood flow correlated with indices of small fiber neuropathy.[597, 598] Metabolic dysfunction of both central and reflex vasoconstrictor sympathetic nerves, together with abnormal vascular smooth muscle metabolism, may alter vascular tone and increase arteriolar and shunt blood flow, both of which would increase capillary pressure. This might be similar to the mechanism of disordered kidney function in diabetes. In contrast, disordered endothelial and smooth muscle metabolism, resulting in impaired NO generation, or resistance to the vasodilatory actions of NO[599, 600] would lead to reduced microvascular responses to both flow-mediated vasodilation following ischemia and hyperemia following injury. These defects have now been reported prior to the onset of diabetes mellitus,[597, 601, 602] in family members,[597, 602] and co-segregate with other components of the metabolic syndrome, including hypertension, dyslipidemia with elevated triglyceride levels, and insulin resistance.

Thus, it is possible that ischemia precedes neuropathy or that both conditions are the result of separate processes caused by the same etiologic factors and each accelerates the other's progress; that is, vascular insufficiency causes nerve damage and nerve dysfunction impairs blood flow. Whatever the case, the loss of the neurovascular function reduces the required nutritional delivery to skin and subcutaneous tissue and, coupled with impaired perception, predisposes the limb to injury, ulceration, and infection that may culminate in gangrene.

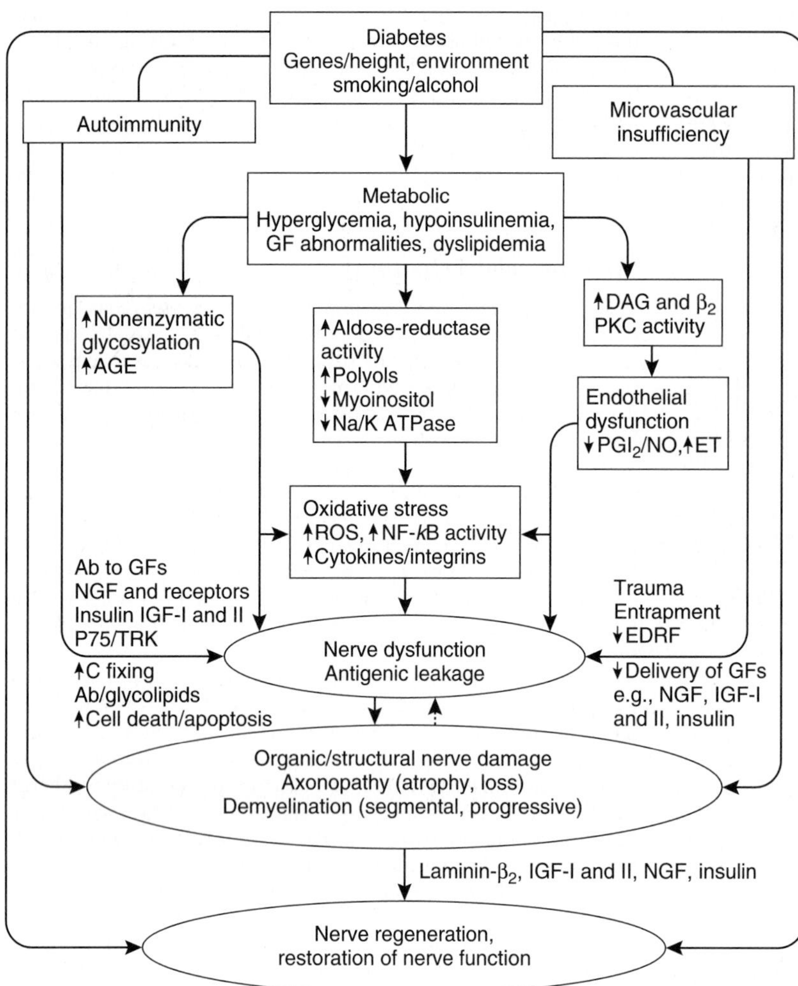

Figure 31–32. A theoretical framework for the development of diabetic neuropathy. Ab, antibody; AGE, advanced glycation end product; C', complement; DAG, diacylglycerol; EDRF, endothelium-derived relaxing factor; ET, endothelin; GF, growth factor; IGF, insulin-like growth factor; NGF, nerve growth factor; NO, nitric oxide; PKC, protein kinase C; ROS, reactive oxygen species. (Adapted from Vinik AI, Newlon P, Lauterio TJ, et al. Diabetes Rev 1995; 3:139–157.)

Neurotrophic Hypothesis

The basic neurotrophic factor concept is defined by the hypothesis that trophic proteins are synthesized in target tissues and delivered to the neuronal soma via retrograde transport, where they exert a trophic and survival effect.[603, 604] The abnormalities in the synthesis and availability of these neurotrophic factors have been implicated in the pathogenesis of DSPN.[605, 606] These factors (see Fig. 31–32) include neurotrophins such as NGF, brain-derived neurotrophic factor, neurotrophin 3, and neurotrophin 4/5; IGFs[607]; and cytokine-like growth factors (ciliary neurotrophic factor and glial-derived neurotrophic factor).[608]

Adult dorsal root ganglia and sympathetic neurons, both of which are affected in DSPN, are dependent on NGF for their maintenance or survival.[609] NGF has been implicated in diverse and widespread activities, including vasodilatation, gut motility, and nociception.[609] Numerous data suggest that a decline in NGF synthesis in diabetes mellitus plays a role in the pathogenesis of DSPN by causing a functional deficit in small fibers. These fibers have a role in pain and thermal sensation. The effect of NGF depletion may be mediated through the down-regulation of neurofilament gene expression[610, 611] or mRNAs that encode the precursor molecules of substance P,[606] both shown to be NGF-dependent. Another member of the neurotrophin family, neurotrophin 3, may be important for the survival and function of the large nerve fibers subserving position, vibration, and possibly motor functions.

IGF-I and IGF-II, which are implicated in the growth and differentiation of neurons and IGF receptors, are present in nerve tissues (i.e., neurons, Schwann cells, ganglia) involved in DSPN.[612] IGFs and their binding proteins are regulated by insulin and the glycemic state.[613] One consequence of insulin insufficiency in diabetes mellitus is a reduction in circulating IGF-I concentration.[614] It seems reasonable to hypothesize that abnormal IGF-I and IGF-II metabolism plays a role in some aspect of DSPN. Little is known, however, about the other effects of diabetes mellitus on local expression, synthesis, and transport of these growth factors in nerve tissue.

Laminin, a large heterotrimeric protein present in the basal lamina of nerves, appears to be important in nerve regeneration and its expression.[615] Laminin also exerts antiapoptotic properties against the neurotoxicity of sera of patients with diabetes mellitus.[616]

Oxidative Stress Hypothesis

Reactive oxygen species (ROS) can regulate multiple signaling mediators linked with important processes that may involve various components of the nerve, dorsal root ganglia, and the vasa nervorum. These processes include metabolism, immune response, cell-cell adhesion, inflammation, cell proliferation, aging, and cell death.[619] Hyperglycemia generates free radicals primarily through increasing flux through the mitochondrial electron transport chain. Formation of AGEs and interaction with the AGE receptor may also lead to the generation of ROS in some cell types.

A prominent role of these reactive molecules as mediators of cellular processes that lead to endothelial cell dysfunction in diabetes mellitus has been suggested.[620–623] One of the most extensively investigated redox-sensitive molecular paths is that involving a nuclear factor, NF-κB. It is a classic member of the Rel family of transcription factors and is known to regulate a diverse set of cellular functions, such as cell growth, immune response, cell survival and development. There are five members of the family, and they tend to form homodimers as well as heterodimers with other members of the family. High glucose and AGE-mediated activation of NF-κB is regarded as a key event in the transformation of the vasculature and accelerated vascular disease as well as smooth muscle dysfunction in diabetes mellitus. It is also potentially reversible with the powerful antioxidant, α-lipoic acid.[624, 625]

In summary, DSPN is a heterogeneous disease with widely varying pathology, suggesting differences in pathogenic mechanisms for the different clinical syndromes. Recognition of the clinical homologue of these pathologic processes is the first step in achieving the appropriate form of intervention.

CLINICAL PRESENTATION AND TREATMENT OPTIONS

The spectrum of clinical neuropathic syndromes described in patients with diabetes mellitus includes dysfunction of almost every segment of the somatic peripheral and autonomic nervous system[568] (Fig. 31–33). Each syndrome can be distinguished by its pathophysiologic, therapeutic, and prognostic features.

Focal Neuropathies

Mononeuropathies

Mononeuropathies occur primarily in the older population, their onset is generally acute and associated with pain, and their course is self-limiting, resolving within 6 to 8 weeks. These are due to vascular obstruction after which adjacent neuronal fascicles take over the function of those infarcted by the clot.[563]

Treatment

Treatment is predominantly symptomatic for pain. If there is weakness such as of the facial muscles, physical therapy and electrical stimulation may be necessary to prevent the weakness from becoming permanent.

Entrapment Syndromes

Entrapment syndromes that start slowly, progress, and persist without intervention must be distinguished from mononeuropathies. Common entrapment sites in diabetes mellitus patients involve median, ulnar, radial, femoral, and lateral cutaneous nerves of the thigh, peroneal nerves, and medial and lateral plantar nerves. Entrapment syndromes are found in one third of patients with diabetes. For example, carpal tunnel syndrome occurs twice as frequently in people with diabetes mellitus compared with a normal healthy population. It is important, therefore, to elicit a detailed history of the distribution of pain and weakness and to perform the equivalent of Tinel's test at various levels of entrapment. If recognized, the diagnosis can be confirmed by electrophysiologic studies.

Treatment

The mainstays of nonsurgical treatment are resting the joint traversed by the nerve, aided by the placement of splints in a neutral position for day and night use; diuretics to reduce edema; addition of nonsteroidal anti-inflammatory drugs (NSAIDs), and steroids and local anesthetic injections. Surgical treatment consists of sectioning the constrictive tendon sheath. The decision to proceed with surgery is based on many considerations, including severity of symptoms, appearance of motor weakness, and failure of nonsurgical treatment.

Diffuse Neuropathies

Proximal Motor Neuropathies

For many years, proximal motor neuropathy has been considered to be a component of diabetic neuropathy. Its patho-

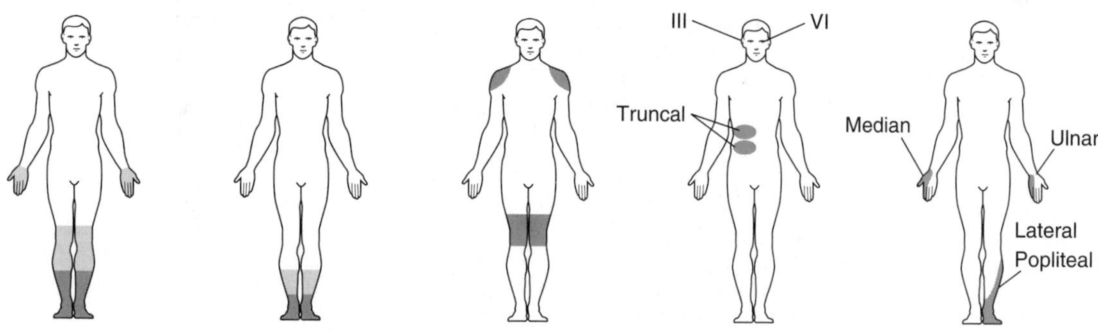

Large-fiber Neuropathy	Small-fiber Neuropathy	Proximal motor neuropathy	Acute mononeuropathies	Pressure palsies
Sensory loss: 0→+++ (Touch, vibration) Pain: +→++± Tendon reflex: N→↓↓↓ Motor deficit 0→+++	Sensory loss: 0→± (thermal, allodynia) Pain: +→++± Tendon reflex: N→↓ Motor deficit: 0	Sensory loss: 0→± Pain: +→++± Tendon reflex: ↓↓ Proximal motor deficit: +→++±	Sensory loss: 0→± Pain: +→++± Tendon reflex: N Motor deficit: +→+++	Sensory loss in Nerve distribution: +→++± Pain: +→± Tendon reflex: N Motor deficit: +→++±

Figure 31–33. Different clinical presentations of diabetic neuropathies. (Modified from Pickup J, Williams G [eds]. Textbook of Diabetes, Vol 1. Oxford, England, Blackwell Scientific, 1997.)

genesis was not understood,[629] and its treatment was neglected with the anticipation that the patient would eventually recover, albeit over a period of some 1 to 2 years, suffering considerable pain, weakness, and disability. The condition is known by a number of synonyms: proximal neuropathy, femoral neuropathy, diabetic amyotrophy, and diabetic neuropathic cachexia. Proximal motor neuropathy can be clinically identified based on recognition of the following common features:

1. Primarily affects the elderly.
2. Gradual or abrupt onset.
3. Begins with pain in the thighs and hips or buttocks, followed by significant weakness of the proximal muscles of the lower limbs with inability to rise from the sitting position (positive Gower's maneuver).
4. Begins unilaterally and spreads bilaterally.
5. Coexists with DSPN.
6. Is characterized by spontaneous or percussion-provoked muscle fasciculation.

Proximal motor neuropathy is now recognized as being secondary to a variety of causes unrelated to diabetes mellitus but that occur more frequently in patients with diabetes mellitus than in the general population. The condition includes patients with chronic inflammatory demyelinating polyneuropathy (CIDP), monoclonal gammopathy, circulating GM1 antibodies and antibodies to neuronal cells, and inflammatory vasculitis.[630, 631] It was formerly thought to resolve spontaneously in 1.5 to 2 years, but now, if found to be immune-mediated, it can resolve within days of initiation of immunotherapy. The condition is readily recognizable clinically with prevailing weakness of the iliopsoas, obturator, and adductor muscles, together with relative preservation of the gluteus maximus and minimus and hamstrings.[632]

Affected patients have great difficulty rising out of chairs unaided and often use their arms to assist themselves. Heel or toe standing is surprisingly good. In the classic form of diabetic amyotrophy, axonal loss is the predominant process and the proximal motor neuropathy coexists with DSPN.[562]

Electrophysiologic evaluation reveals lumbosacral plexopathy.[632] In contrast, if demyelination predominates and the motor deficit affects proximal and distal muscle groups, the diagnosis of CIDP, monoclonal gammopathy of unknown significance, and vasculitis should be considered.[633, 634] Biopsy of the obturator nerve reveals deposition of immunoglobulin, demyelination, and inflammatory cell infiltrate of the vasa nervorum.[635] Cerebrospinal fluid protein content is high, and the lymphocyte count is elevated.

Treatment

Treatment options include intravenous immunoglobulin for CIDP, plasma exchange for monoclonal gammopathy of unknown significance, steroids and azathioprine for vasculitis, and withdrawal from drugs or other agents that may have caused a vasculitis. It is important to divide proximal syndromes into these two subcategories, because the CIDP variant responds dramatically to intervention,[633, 636] whereas amyotrophy runs its own course over months to years. Until more evidence is available, they should be considered separate syndromes.

Distal Symmetrical Polyneuropathy

Distal symmetrical polyneuropathy (DSPN) is the most common and widely recognized form of diabetic neuropathy. The onset is usually insidious but occasionally is acute, following stress or initiation of therapy for diabetes mellitus. DSPN may be either sensory or motor and involve small nerve fibers, large nerve fibers, or both.[637] Small-fiber dysfunction usually occurs early and often is present without objective signs or electrophysiologic evidence of nerve damage.[638] It is manifested by early lower limb symptoms of pain and hyperalgesia in the lower limbs, followed by a loss of thermal sensitivity and reduced light touch and pinprick sensation.[568] DSPN may be accompanied by loss of cutaneous nerve fibers that stain positive for the neuronal antigen protein gene product (PGP) 9.5 (Fig. 31–34)[639] as well as impaired neurovascular blood flow (Fig. 31–35).[597] Small-fiber neuropathies, however, can present in a variety of ways.

Small-Fiber Neuropathy

Acute Painful Neuropathy

In some patients, a predominantly *small-fiber neuropathy* develops, manifested by pain and paresthesias early in the course of diabetes mellitus (Table 31–5). It may be associated with the onset of insulin therapy and has been termed *insulin neuritis*.[640] By definition, it has been present for less than 6 months. Symptoms often are exacerbated at night and are manifested in the feet more than the hands. Spontaneous episodes of pain can be severely disabling. The pain varies in intensity and character. In some patients, the pain has been variably described as burning, lancinating, stabbing, or sharp. Paresthesias or episodes of distorted sensation, such as pins and needles, tingling, coldness, numbness, or burning, often accompany the pain.[637] The lower legs may be exquisitely tender to touch, with any disturbance of the hair follicles resulting in excruciating pain. Because pain can be exacerbated by repeated contact of the lower limbs with foreign objects, even basic daily activities, such as sitting at a desk, may be disrupted. Pain often occurs at the onset of the disease and is often worsened by initiation of therapy with insulin or sulfonylureas.[640]

It may be associated with profound weight loss and severe depression, termed *diabetic neuropathic cachexia*.[641] This syndrome occurs predominantly in male patients and may occur at any time in the course of both type 1 and type 2 diabetes mellitus. It is self-limiting and invariably responds to simple symptomatic treatment. Conditions such as Fabry's disease, amyloid, human immunodeficiency viral infection, heavy metal poisoning (e.g., as with arsenic), and excess alcohol consumption should be excluded. It does overlap with the idiopathic variety of acute, painful small-fiber neuropathy that is also a diagnosis by exclusion.[642]

Treatment

The treatment of the acute neuropathic pain syndrome is purely symptomatic because most cases resolve spontaneously and there is no need for other forms of intervention. However, there may be a significant component of depression and weight loss, and antidepressive agents are useful for their combined effects of relieving pain and mood elevation. The condition may appear soon after initiation of therapy.[640] A striking amelioration of symptoms with the intravenous administration of insulin can be achieved[643] in the absence of change in blood glucose control.

Chronic Painful Neuropathy

Another variety of painful polyneuropathy is characterized by an onset occurring later (often years) in the course of diabetes mellitus, in which the pain persists for longer than 6 months and becomes debilitating. This condition may result in tolerance to narcotics and analgesics and, finally, to addiction. It is extremely resistant to all forms of intervention and is most frustrating to both patient and physician.

The mechanism of pain in DSPN is not well understood. Interacting pathophysiologic mechanisms at the peripheral and

A

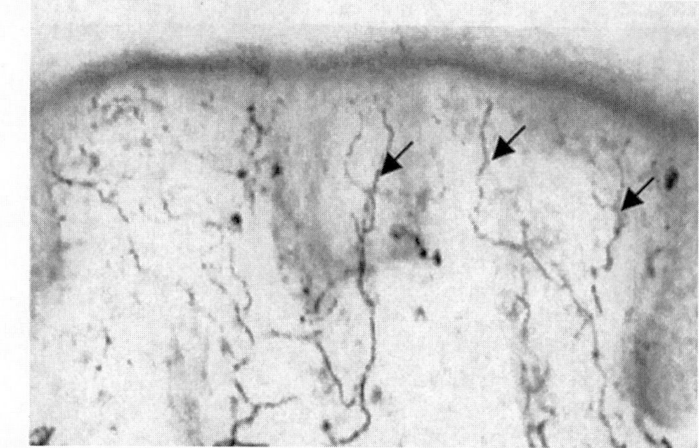

B

C

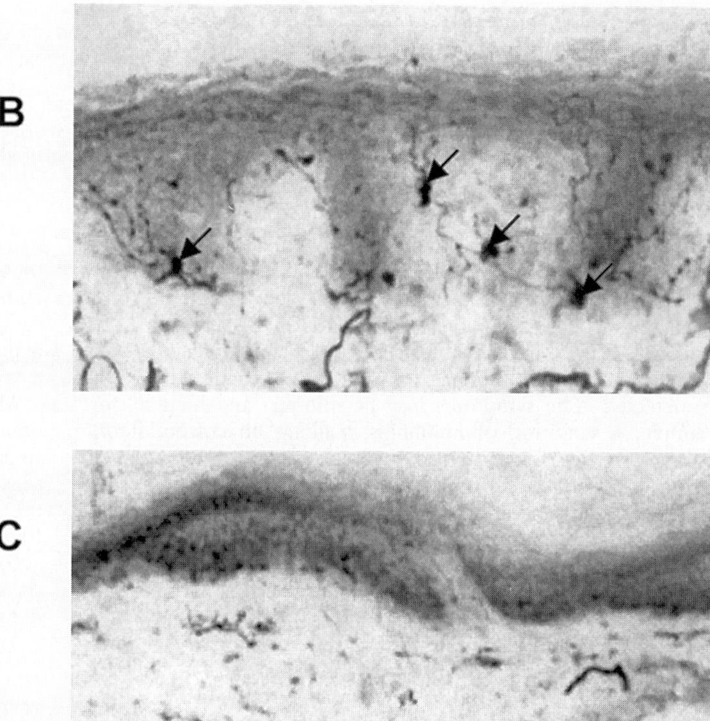

Figure 31–34. Loss of cutaneous nerve fibers that stain positive for the neuronal antigen protein gene product 9.5 in sensory neuropathy. *A*, Normal epidermal fibers in back. *B*, Slightly reduced density and swelling in proximal thigh. *C*, Complete clearance in calf. (From McArthur JC, Stocks EA, Hauer P. Epidermal nerve fiber density: normative reference range and diagnostic efficiency. Arch Neurol 1998; 55:1513–1520.)

central nervous system may be responsible for initiation and maintenance of chronic neuropathic pain (Fig. 31–36). Hyperglycemia may be a factor in lowering the pain threshold. There is a sequence in DSPN, beginning when nerve function is good and there is no pain, hyperalgesia, hyperesthesia, or allodynia. Progression of the condition results in nerve dysfunction and pain, increased sensitivity to painful stimuli, and allodynia.

Chronic Small-Fiber Neuropathy

Disappearance of these symptoms may not necessarily reflect nerve recovery but rather nerve death. When patients volunteer the "apparent improvement," progression of the neuropathy must be excluded by careful examination. Pain, however, may persist *even with dead nerves*. The objective physical features include loss of warm thermal perception, decreased heat pain, cold pain, loss of touch pressure perception, and impairment of blood flow. A foot with these findings is at risk for repeated minor trauma, foot ulceration, infection, and gangrene. Small-fiber neuropathies have profound effects on quality of life and mortality.[644]

Large-Fiber Neuropathies

Large-fiber neuropathies may involve sensory nerves, motor nerves, or both (Table 31–6). These tend to be the neuropathies of signs rather than symptoms. Large fibers subserve motor function, vibration perception, position sense, and cold thermal perception. Unlike the small nerve fibers, these are

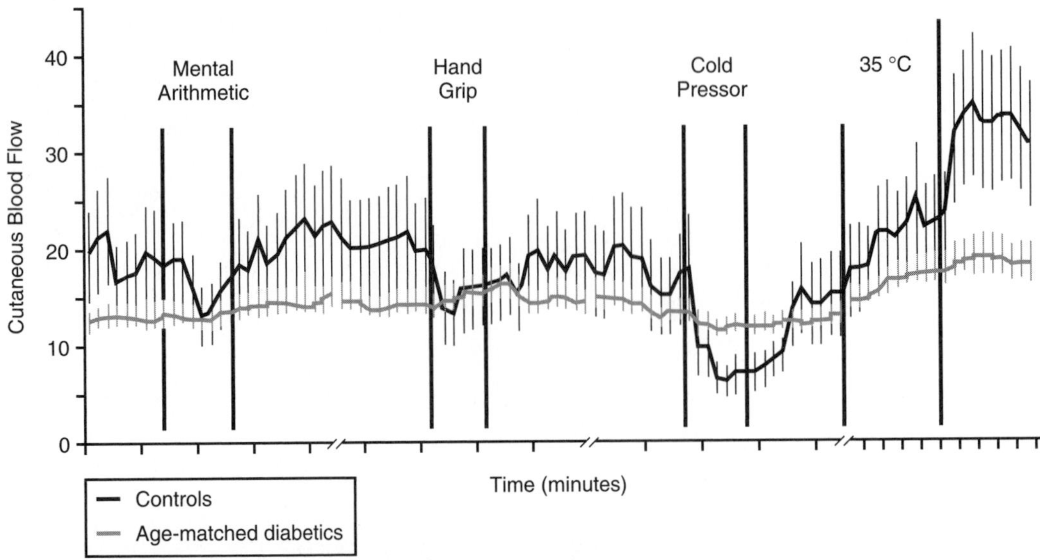

Figure 31–35. Impaired neurovascular blood flow. (From Stansberry KB, Hill MA, Shapiro SA et al. Impairment of peripheral blood flow responses in diabetes resembles an enhanced aging effect. Diabetes Care 1997; 20:1711–1716.)

the myelinated, rapidly conducting fibers that begin in the toes and have their first synapse in the medulla oblongata. They tend to be affected first because of their length and the tendency in diabetes for nerves to "die back." Because they are myelinated, they are the fibers represented in the electromyogram, and subclinical abnormalities in nerve function are readily detected. The symptoms may be minimal and include, for example, a sensation of numbness, walking on cotton, floors feeling "strange," inability to turn the pages of a book, or inability to discriminate among coins.

Characteristic features are wasting of the interosseous muscles of the hands and feet, giving rise to the hammertoe deformities and pes equinus, and the loss of hand grip strength and the ability to tie knots and do buttons. There is a significant impact on activities of daily living.[644]

Objective findings include loss of reflexes, decreased vibration perception, ataxic gait, and inability to perform a tandem stand or one-legged stand for longer than 30 seconds.[645] There is no impairment of blood flow, the feet are often hot, and there is a susceptibility to osteopenia of the feet and a risk of Charcot's neuroarthropathy. The concurrence of equinus leads to repeated midfoot trauma, widening of Lisfranc's joint, and foot deformity that can be relieved by Achilles tendon lengthening. The ataxia and loss of strength increase the susceptibility to falling and fractures. The tendency is increased in aging diabetic patients[645, 646] and requires preventive measures and exercise and strength training.

Most patients with DSPN, however, have a "mixed" variety of neuropathy, with both large-fiber and small-fiber damages. In the case of DSPN, a "glove-and-stocking" distribution of sensory loss is almost universal.[568, 647, 648] Early in the course of the neuropathic process, multifocal sensory loss also might be found. In some patients, severe distal muscle weakness can accompany the sensory loss, resulting in an inability to stand on the toes or heels. Some grading systems use this as a definition of severity.

Table 31–5. Clinical Manifestations of Small-Fiber Neuropathies

1. Symptoms prominent. Pain is of the C-fiber type. It is burning and superficial and associated with allodynia, i.e., interpretation of all stimuli as painful (e.g., touch).
2. Late in the condition, hypoalgesia.
3. Defective warm thermal sensation.
4. Defective autonomic function with decreased sweating, dry skin, impaired vasomotion and blood flow, and a cold foot.
5. Remarkable intactness of reflexes, motor strength.
6. Electrophysiologically silent.
7. Loss of cutaneous nerve fibers using PGP 9.5 staining.
8. Diagnosed clinically by reduced sensitivity to 1.0-g Semmes Weinstein monofilament and pricking sensation using the Waardenberg wheel or similar instrument.
9. Abnormalities in thresholds for warm thermal perception, neurovascular function, pain, quantitative sudorimetry, and quantitative autonomic function tests.
10. Risks are foot ulceration and subsequent gangrene.

DIAGNOSIS AND DIFFERENTIAL DIAGNOSIS OF DISTAL SYMMETRICAL POLYNEUROPATHY

The 1988 San Antonio conference on DSPN[561] and the 1992 conference of the American Academy of Neurology recommended that at least one parameter from each of the following five categories be measured to classify DSPN:

- Symptom profiles
- Neurologic examination
- Quantitative sensory test (QST)
- Nerve conduction velocity (NCV) study
- Quantitative autonomic function test (QAFT)

The diagnosis of DSPN rests heavily on a careful history for which a number of questionnaires for the neurologic symptom score and the neurologic impairment score have been developed by Boulton,[538] Dyck,[649] Vinik,[650] and others.[651, 652] The initial neurologic evaluation should be directed toward the detection of the specific part of the nervous system affected by

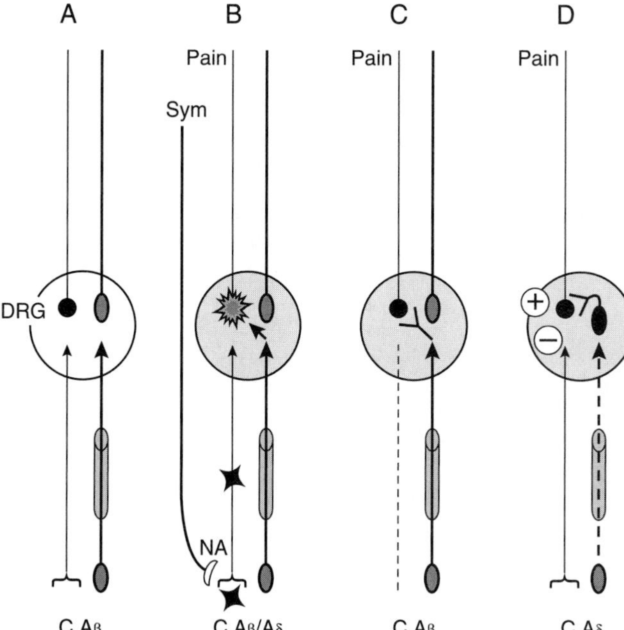

Figure 31–36. Mechanisms of neuropathic pain. *A*, Normal. *B*, C-fiber sensitization. Peripheral nociceptive fibers can be abnormally sensitized and then central nociceptive second-order neurons in the spinal cord dorsal horn can also be sensitized. Then they are hyperexcitable and start responding to non-noxious stimuli. *C*, C-fiber loss or degeneration may trigger anatomic sprouting of low-threshold mechanosensitive terminals to central nociceptive neurons and may subsequently induce synaptic reorganization in the dorsal horn. *D*, Central disinhibition and cold hyperalgesia. A selective damage of cold-sensitive A delta (Aδ) fibers leads to a loss of central inhibition mediated by interneurons (disinhibition), resulting in cold hyperalgesia. DRG, dorsal root ganglion.

Table 31–6. Clinical Presentation of Large-Fiber Neuropathies

1. Impaired vibration perception (often the first objective evidence) and position sense.
2. Depressed tendon reflexes.
3. A delta type deep-seated gnawing, dull, like a toothache in the bones of the feet, or even crushing or cramp-like pain.
4. Sensory ataxia (waddling like a duck).
5. Wasting of small muscles of feet with hammertoes (intrinsic minus feet and hands) with weakness of hands and feet.
6. Shortening of the Achilles tendon with pes equinus.
7. Increased blood flow (hot foot).
8. Risk is Charcot's neuroarthropathy.

diabetes mellitus (Fig. 31–37). Bedside neurologic examination is quick and easy but provides nominal or ordinal measures and contains substantial interindividual and intraindividual variation. The least reliable measure is the neurologic symptom score.[546]

For example, it is useless to measure VPT with a tuning fork other than one that has a frequency of 128 Hz. Similarly, using a 10-g monofilament is good for predicting foot ulceration, as is the Achilles reflex, but both are insensitive to the early detection of neuropathy, and a 1.0-g monofilament increases the sensitivity from 60% to 90%.[653] Sensory function must be evaluated on both sides of the feet and hands if one wants to be sure not to miss entrapment syndromes. Tinel's sign not only is useful for carpal tunnel problems but also can be applied to the ulnar notch, the head of the fibula, and below the medial tibial epicondyle for ulnar, peroneal and medial plantar entrapments, respectively. The QST and QAFT are objective indices of neurologic functional status. Combined, these tests cover vibratory, proprioceptive, light touch, pain, thermal, and autonomic function. Developments of a number of relatively inexpensive devices allow suitable assessment of somatosensory function, including vibration, thermal, light touch, and pain perception.[654] These types of instruments allow for cutaneous sensory functions to be assessed noninvasively, and their measurements are correlated with specific neural fiber function.

QAFT consists of a series of simple, noninvasive tests for detecting cardiovascular autonomic neuropathy.[638, 655] These tests are based on detection of heart rate and BP response to a series of maneuvers. Specific tests are used in evaluating disordered regulation of gastrointestinal, genitourinary, and pseudomotor function and peripheral skin blood flow induced by autonomic neuropathy.[653] Subclinical neuropathy is diagnosed on the basis of the following:

1. Abnormal electrodiagnostic tests with decreased NCV or decreased amplitudes;
2. Abnormal QST for vibration perception, light touch, thermal warming, and cooling thresholds;
3. QAFT revealing diminished heart rate variation with deep breathing, Valsalva maneuver, and postural testing.

Biopsy of nerve tissue may be helpful for excluding other causes of neuropathy and in the determination of predominant pathologic changes in patients with complex clinical findings as a means of dictating choice of treatment.[562, 656] Skin biopsy has some clinical advantages in diagnosis of small-fiber neuropathies by quantification of PGP 9.5, when all other measures, including electromyography, are negative and there are no objective physical signs.[554, 657] Diabetes mellitus as the cause of neuropathy is diagnosed by exclusion of various other causes of neuropathy (see Fig. 31–37).[568, 658]

MANAGEMENT OF DISTAL SYMMETRICAL POLYNEUROPATHY

Once DSPN is diagnosed, therapy can then be instituted with the goal of both ameliorating symptoms and preventing the progression of neuropathy. Successful management of these syndromes may eventually be geared to the individual pathogenic processes. At present, however, control of hyperglycemia and meticulous foot care (Table 31–7) are the mainstays of therapy.

Management Aimed at Pathogenetic Mechanisms

Control of Hyperglycemia

Retrospective and prospective studies have suggested a relationship between hyperglycemia and the development and severity of DSPN.[546] Pirart[659] followed 4400 diabetic patients over 25 years and showed an increase in prevalence of clinically detectable DSPN from 12% of patients at the time of diagnosis of diabetes mellitus to almost 50% after 25 years. The highest prevalence occurred in those people with poorest diabetes control.

The DCCT research group[2, 546] reported significant effects of intensive insulin therapy on progression of neuropathy. In type 1 diabetes, the prevalence rates for clinical or electrophysiologic evidence of neuropathy were reduced by 64% in those treated by intensive insulin therapy after 5 years of follow-up

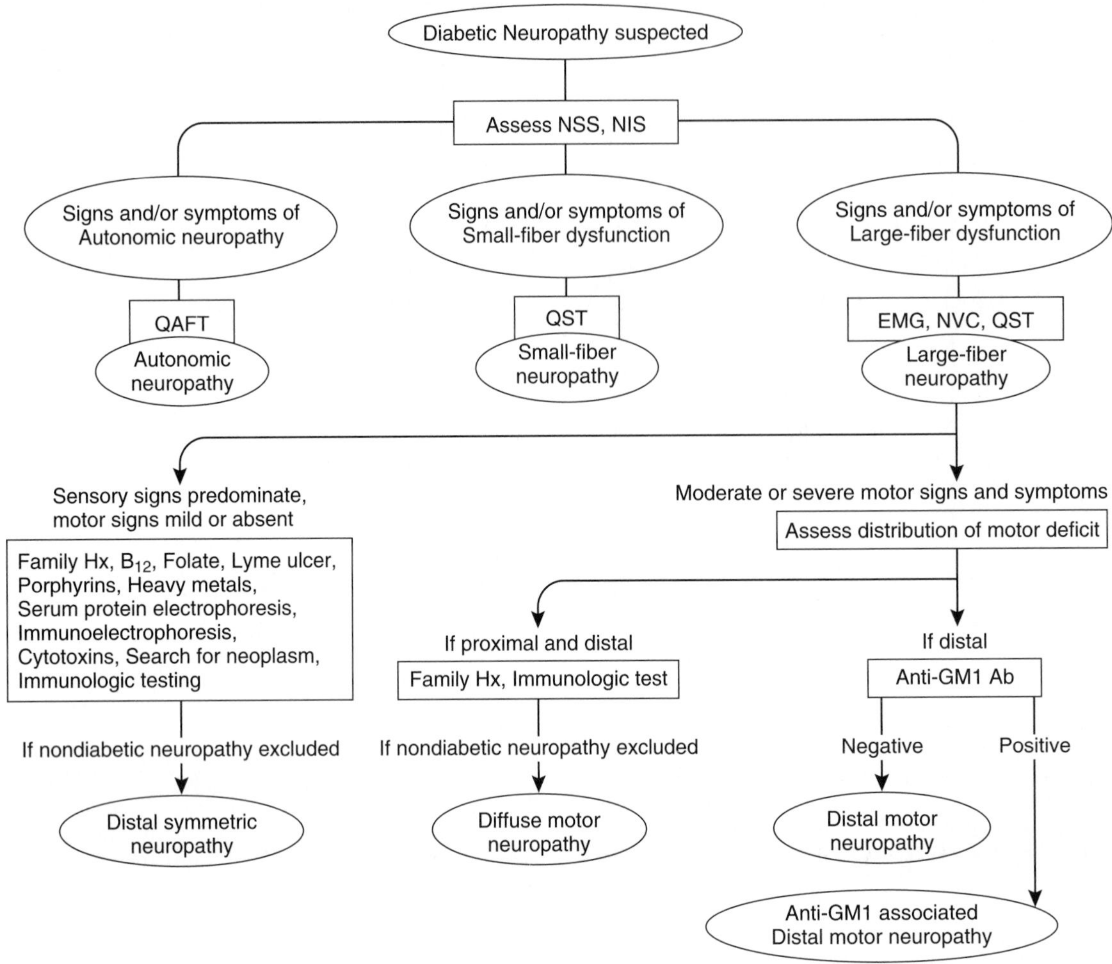

Figure 31-37. Diagnostic algorithm for assessment of neurologic deficit and classification of neuropathic syndrome. Ab, antibody; EMG, electromyography; Hx, history; NCV, nerve conduction velocity; NIS, neurologic impairment score; NSS, neurologic symptom score; QAFT, quantitative autonomic function test; QST, quantitative sensory test.

in combined cohort (5% of the intensive therapy group compared with 13% of the conventional therapy group).[546] In the secondary intervention cohort, intensive insulin therapy significantly reduced the prevalence of clinical neuropathy by 61% (7% in intensive insulin therapy group versus 17% in conventional therapy group). The results of the DCCT study support the necessity for strict glycemic control, but the effect of insulin as a growth factor and immunomodulator, aside from its metabolic effects, must also be investigated.

In the UKPDS, control of blood glucose was associated with improvement in VPT.[3, 660, 661] In the Steno trial,[662] a reduction of the odds ratio for the development of autonomic neuropathy to 0.32 was reported. This stepwise, progressive study involved treatment of type 2 diabetes mellitus patients with hypotensive drugs, including ACE inhibitors, and calcium channel antagonists, hypoglycemic agents, aspirin, hypolipidemic agents, and antioxidants. These findings argue strongly for the multifactorial nature of neuropathy and for the need to address the multiple metabolic abnormalities with potentially efficacious mechanism-targeted therapies in the future.

Table 31-7. Managing Small-Fiber Neuropathies

1. Patients must be instructed on foot care with daily foot inspection.
2. Patients must have a mirror in the bathroom for inspection of the soles of the feet.
3. Providing patients with a monofilament for self-testing reduces ulcers.
4. All diabetic patients should wear padded socks.
5. Shoes must fit well with adequate support and must be inspected for the presence of foreign bodies (e.g., nails, pins, teeth) before donning. Examine the feet and the shoes daily.
6. Patients must exercise care with exposure to heat (no falling asleep in front of fires).
7. Emollient creams should be used for the skin drying and cracking.
8. After bathing, feet should be thoroughly dried and powdered between the toes.
9. Nails should be cut transversely, preferably by a podiatrist.

Aldose Reductase Inhibitors

ARIs reduce the flux of glucose through the polyol pathway, inhibiting tissue accumulation of sorbitol and fructose and preventing reduction of redox potentials.

In a placebo-controlled, double-blind study of tolrestat, 219 diabetes mellitus patients with symmetrical polyneuropathy, as defined by at least one pathologic cardiovascular reflex, were treated for 1 year.[663] Patients who received tolrestat showed significant improvement in autonomic function tests as well as in vibration perception, whereas placebo-treated patients showed deterioration in most of the parameters measured.[664]

In a 12-month study of zenarestat,[665] there was a dose-dependent improvement in nerve fiber density, particularly of small unmyelinated nerve fibers. This was accompanied by an increase in NCV, although the changes in NCV occurred at a dose of the drug that did not change the nerve fiber density.[665] Impaired cardiac ejection fractions can be improved with zopolrestat.[666] It is also becoming clear that aldose reductase inhibition may be insufficient in its own right to achieve the desirable degree of metabolic enhancement in patients with a multitude of biochemical abnormalities. Combinations of therapy with ARIs and antioxidants may become critical if we are to abate the relentless progress of DSPN.

Alpha-Lipoic Acid

Lipoic acid (1,2-dithiolane-3-pentanoic acid), a derivative of octanoic acid, is present in food and is also synthesized by the liver. It is a natural cofactor in the pyruvate dehydrogenase complex where it binds acyl groups and transfers them from one part of the complex to another α-lipoic acid. It is effective in ameliorating both the somatic and autonomic neuropathies in diabetes mellitus.[667–669] Lipoic acid is currently undergoing extensive trials in the United States as an antidiabetic agent and as a therapy for DSPN.

Gamma-Linolenic Acid

Linoleic acid, an essential fatty acid, is metabolized to GLA, which serves as an important constituent of neuronal membrane phospholipids and also as a substrate for prostaglandin formation, seemingly important for preservation of nerve blood flow. In diabetes mellitus, conversion of linoleic acid to γ-linolenic acid and subsequent metabolites is impaired, possibly contributing to the pathogenesis of DSPN.[670] A multicenter double-blind, placebo-controlled trial using GLA for 1 year demonstrated significant improvements in both clinical measures and electrophysiologic tests.[671]

Aminoguanidine

Animal studies using aminoguanidine, an inhibitor of the formation of AGEs and a free radical scavenger, show improvement in NCV in streptozotocin-induced DSPN in rats.[623, 672, 673] Controlled clinical trials to determine its efficacy in humans have been discontinued because of toxicity. However, successors to aminoguanidine and other drugs hold promise for this approach.[674, 675]

Human Intravenous Immunoglobulin

Immune intervention with human intravenous immunoglobulin (IVIg) has become appropriate in some patients with forms of peripheral DSPN that are associated with signs of antineuronal autoimmunity.[633, 636] Treatment with immunoglobulin is well tolerated and is considered safe, especially with respect to viral transmission.[676] The major toxicity of IVIg has been an anaphylactic reaction, but the frequency of these reactions is now low and confined mainly to patients with immunoglobulin (usually immunoglobulin A) deficiency. Patients may experience severe headache due to aseptic meningitis, which resolves spontaneously. In some instances, it may be necessary to combine treatment with prednisone and/or azathioprine. Relapses may occur requiring repeated courses of therapy.

Neurotrophic Therapy

In animal models of diabetes mellitus, the evidence now suggests that decreased expression of NGF and its receptor trk A reduces retrograde axonal transport of NGF and diminishes support of small unmyelinated neurons and their neuropeptides, such as substance P and CGRP—both potent vasodilators.[677–679] Furthermore, recombinant human NGF (rhNGF) administration restores these neuropeptide levels toward normal and prevents the manifestations of sensory neuropathy in animals.[680]

In a 15-center, double-blind, placebo-controlled study of the safety and efficacy of rhNGF in 250 subjects with symptomatic small-fiber neuropathy,[550] rhNGF improved the neurologic impairment score of the lower limbs as well as small nerve fiber function cooling threshold (A delta fibers) and the ability to perceive heat pain (C-fiber) compared with placebo. These results were consistent with the postulated actions of NGF on trk A receptors present on small-fiber neurons. This finding led to two large multicenter studies conducted in the United States[551, 681] and the rest of the world. Regrettably, rhNGF was not found to have beneficial effects over and above placebo. The reason for this dichotomy has not been resolved, but this has somewhat dampened the enthusiasm for growth factor therapy of DSPN. Nonetheless, several new agents are able to bring about nerve growth, proliferation, and differentiation in vitro and have neurotrophic potential; these agents are now being evaluated in early phase II studies.

Management Aimed at Symptoms

Pain Control

Control of pain constitutes one of the most difficult management issues in DSPN. In essence, simple measures are tried first (Fig. 31–38). If no distinction is made for pain syndromes, the numbers needed to treat (NNT) in DSPN to reduce pain by 50% is 1.4 for optimal-dose tricyclic antidepressants, 1.9 for dextromethorphan, 3.3 for carbamazepine, 3.4 for tramadol, 3.7 for gabapentin, 5.9 for capsaicin, 6.7 for

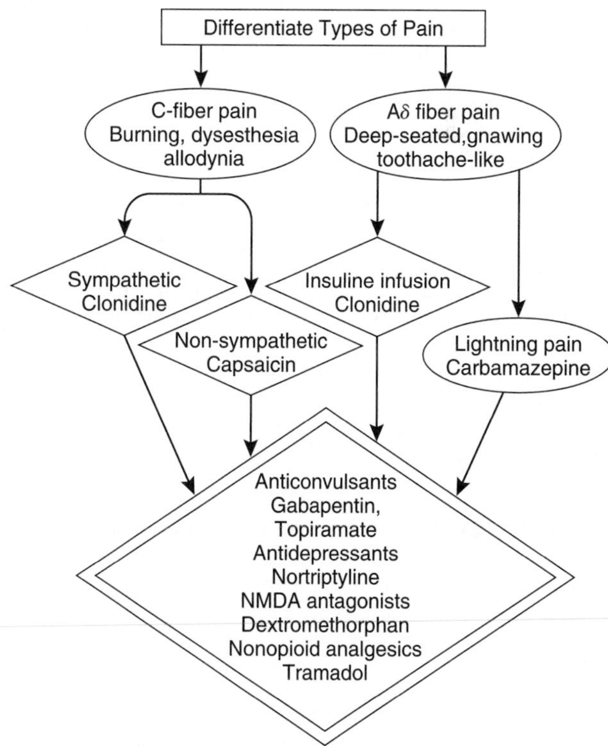

Figure 31–38. Management of painful diabetic neuropathy. (Modified from Vinik AI, Holland MT, LeBeau JM, et al. Diabetic neuropathies. Diabetes Care 1992; 15:1926–1975.)

selective serotonin reuptake inhibitors, and 10.0 for mexiletine.[682] If pain is divided according to its derivation from different nerve fiber type (A delta versus C-fiber), however, different types of pain respond to different therapies (see Fig. 31–38), as described next.

C-Fiber Pain

Initially, when there is ongoing damage to the nerves, the patient experiences the pain of the burning, lancinating, dysesthetic type often accompanied by hyperalgesia and allodynia. Because the peripheral sympathetic nerve fibers are also small unmyelinated C-fibers, sympathetic blocking agents (clonidine) may improve the pain. Loss of sympathetic regulation of sweat glands and arteriovenous shunt vessels in the foot creates a favorable environment for bacteria to penetrate, multiply, and wreak havoc with the foot. These fibers use the neuropeptide substance P as their neurotransmitter, and depletion of axonal substance P (capsaicin) often leads to amelioration of the pain. However, when the destructive forces persist, the individual becomes pain free and develops impaired warm temperature and pain thresholds. Disappearance of pain in these circumstances should be hailed as a warning that the neuropathy is progressing.

Capsaicin

Capsaicin is extracted from chili peppers. A simple, cheap mixture is formed by adding 1 to 3 teaspoons of cayenne pepper to a jar of cold cream and applying to the area of pain. The capsaicinoid receptor, or vanilloid receptor (VR1), is present on C and A delta fibers.[683] When it is activated, it produces desensitization or degeneration of the sensory afferents.

VR1 is essential for selective modalities of pain sensation and for tissue injury–induced thermal hyperalgesia.[684] Prolonged application of capsaicin depletes stores of substance P and, possibly, other neurotransmitters from sensory nerve endings. This reduces or abolishes the transmission of painful stimuli from the peripheral nerve fibers to the higher centers.[685] Care must be taken to avoid eyes and genitals, and gloves must be worn. Because of capsaicin's volatility, it is safer to cover the affected areas with plastic wrap. There is an initial exacerbation of symptoms that is followed by relief in 2 to 3 weeks.

Clonidine

There is an element of sympathetic-mediated C-fiber–type pain that can be overcome with clonidine (α_2-adrenergic agonist) or phentolamine. Clonidine can be applied topically,[686] but the dose titration may be more difficult. Unresponsive patients are treated as outlined in Figure 31–38.

A Delta Fiber pain

A delta fiber pain is a more deep-seated, dull, and gnawing ache, which often does not respond to the previously described measures. A number of different agents have been used for the pain associated with these fibers with varying success.

Insulin

Continuous intravenous insulin infusion without resort to blood glucose lowering may be useful in some patients. A response with reduction of pain usually occurs within 48 hours,[643] and the insulin infusion can be discontinued. If this measure fails, several medications are available that may abolish the pain.

Tramadol and Dextromethorphan

There are two possible targeted therapies. Tramadol is a nonopioid centrally acting analgesic for use in treating moderate to severe pain. It has recently been reported to provide pain relief in DSPN.[687] Another spinal cord target for pain relief is the excitatory glutaminergic *N*-methyl-D-aspartate (NMDA) receptor. Blockade of NMDA receptors is believed to be one mechanism by which dextromethorphan exerts analgesic efficacy.[688] An accomplished pharmacist can procure a sugar-free solution of dextromethorphan.

Antidepressants

Clinical trials have focused on interrupting pain transmission using antidepressant drugs that inhibit the reuptake of norepinephrine or serotonin. This central action accentuates the effects of these neurotransmitters in activation of endogenous pain-inhibitory systems in the brain that modulate pain transmission cells in the spinal cord.[689] Side effects, including dysautonomia and dry mouth, can be troublesome. Switching to nortriptyline may lessen some of the anticholinergic effects of amitriptyline.

Carbamazepine

Several double-blind, placebo-controlled studies have demonstrated carbamazepine to be effective in the management of pain in DSPN.[568] Toxic side effects may limit its use in some patients. However, it is useful for those patients with lightning or shooting pain.

Gabapentin

Gabapentin, which is structurally related to the neurotransmitter γ-aminobutyric acid, is an effective anticonvulsant whose mechanism is not well understood yet holds additional promise as an analgesic agent in painful neuropathy.[690] In a multicenter study in the United States,[691] gabapentin monotherapy appeared to be efficacious for the treatment of pain and sleep interference associated with DSPN. It also exhibited positive effects on mood and quality of life.[692]

Transcutaneous Electrical Nerve Stimulation (TENS)

TENS occasionally may be helpful and certainly represents one of the more benign therapies for painful neuropathy.[693] Care should be taken to move the electrodes around to identify sensitive areas and obtain maximal relief.

Analgesics

Analgesics are rarely of much benefit in the treatment of painful neuropathy, although they may be of some use on a short-term basis for some of the self-limited syndromes, such as painful diabetic third nerve palsy. Use of narcotics in the setting of chronic pain generally is avoided because of the risk of addiction.

MANAGEMENT OF LARGE-FIBER NEUROPATHIES

Patients with large-fiber neuropathies are uncoordinated and ataxic. As a result, they are more likely to fall than are non-neuropathic age-matched people.[694] It has been demonstrated that high-intensity strength training in older people increases

Table 31-8. Management of Large-Fiber Neuropathies

1. Gait and strength training.
2. Pain management as detailed in text.
3. Orthotics should be fitted with proper shoes for the deformities.
4. Tendon lengthening for Achilles tendon shortening.
5. Bisphosphonates may be given for osteopenia.
6. Surgical reconstruction and full-length casting as necessary.

muscle strength in a variety of muscles. More important, the strength training results in improved coordination and balance quantifiable with backward tandem walking (Table 31–8).[695] Thus, it is vital to embark on a program of strength training and improvement of balance.

AUTONOMIC NEUROPATHIES

Diabetic autonomic neuropathy may involve any system in the body. Involvement of the autonomic nervous system can occur as early as the first year after diagnosis, and major manifestations are cardiovascular, gastrointestinal, and genitourinary system dysfunction (Table 31–9).[568, 696] Reduced exercise tolerance, edema, paradoxic supine or nocturnal hypertension, and intolerance to heat due to defective thermoregulation are a consequence of autonomic neuropathy.

Common peripheral autonomic function tests are the quantitative sudomotor axon reflex test and the sympathetic skin response,[697] which in most hands are not reliable and sufficiently variable to be of no use clinically. Defective blood flow in the small capillary circulation is found with decreased responsiveness to mental arithmetic, cold pressor, hand grip, and heating.[597] The defect is associated with a reduction in the amplitude of vasomotion[596] and resembles premature aging.[597] There are differences in the glabrous and hairy skin circulations. In hairy skin, a functional defect is found prior to the development of neuropathy[556] and is correctable with antioxidants.[698] The clinical counterpart is a dry, cold skin; loss of sweating; and development of fissures and cracks that are portals of entry for organisms leading to infectious ulcers and gangrene. Silent myocardial infarction, respiratory failure, amputations, and sudden death are hazards for diabetic patients with cardiac autonomic neuropathy.[560, 699] Therefore, it is vitally important to make this diagnosis early so that appropriate intervention can be instituted.[700–703]

Table 31-9. Clinical Features of Autonomic Neuropathies

Cardiovascular
- Resting tachycardia
- Orthostatic hypotension
- Silent myocardial infarction, congestive heart failure, and sudden death

Gastrointestinal
- Gastroparesis
- Diarrhea, constipation

Genitourinary
- Bladder dysfunction
- Erectile dysfunction

Peripheral
- Gustatory sweating
- Pupillary abnormalities
- Disturbed neurovascular flow
- Edema

Metabolic
- Hypoglycemia unawareness, hypoglycemia unresponsiveness

Management of Autonomic Neuropathy

Prevention and Reversibility of Autonomic Neuropathy

It has now become clear that strict glycemic control[546]; a stepwise, progressive management of hyperglycemia, lipid levels, and BP; and the use of antioxidants[668] and ACE inhibitors[704] reduce the odds ratio for autonomic neuropathy to 0.32 (Fig. 31–39).[662] It has also been shown that mortality is a function of loss of beat-to-beat variability with myocardial infarction. This mortality can be reduced by 33% with acute administration of insulin.[705]

Kendall and coworkers[706] reported that successful pancreas transplantation improves epinephrine response and normalizes hypoglycemia symptom recognition in patients with longstanding diabetes mellitus and established autonomic neuropathy. Burger and associates[707] showed that a reversible metabolic component of cardiac autonomic neuropathy exists in patients in the early stages of the neuropathy.

Postural Hypotension

The syndrome of postural hypotension is posture-related dizziness and syncope. Patients who have type 2 diabetes mellitus and orthostatic hypotension are hypovolemic and have sympathoadrenal insufficiency; both factors contribute to the pathogenesis of orthostatic hypotension.[708] Postural hypotension in the patient with diabetic autonomic neuropathy can present a difficult management problem. Elevating the BP in the standing position must be balanced against preventing hypertension in the supine position.

Supportive Garments

Whenever possible, attempts should be made to increase venous return from the periphery by means of total body stockings. However, leg compression alone is less effective, presumably reflecting the large capacity of the abdomen relative to the legs.[709] Patients should be instructed to put the stockings on while lying down and to avoid removing them until returning to the supine position.

Drug Therapy

Some patients with postural hypotension may benefit from treatment with 9-fluorohydrocortisone. Unfortunately, symptoms do not improve until edema occurs, and there is a significant risk for development of CHF and hypertension. If fluorohydrocortisone does not work satisfactorily, various adrenergic agonists and antagonists may be used. If the adrenergic receptor status is known, therapy can be guided to the appropriate agent. Metoclopramide may be helpful in patients with dopamine excess or increased sensitivity to dopaminergic stimulation. Patients with α_2-adrenergic receptor excess may respond to the α_2-antagonist yohimbine. Those few patients in whom β receptors are increased may be helped with propranolol.

α_2-Adrenergic receptor deficiency can be treated with the α_2-agonist, clonidine, which in this setting may paradoxically increase BP. One should start with small doses and gradually

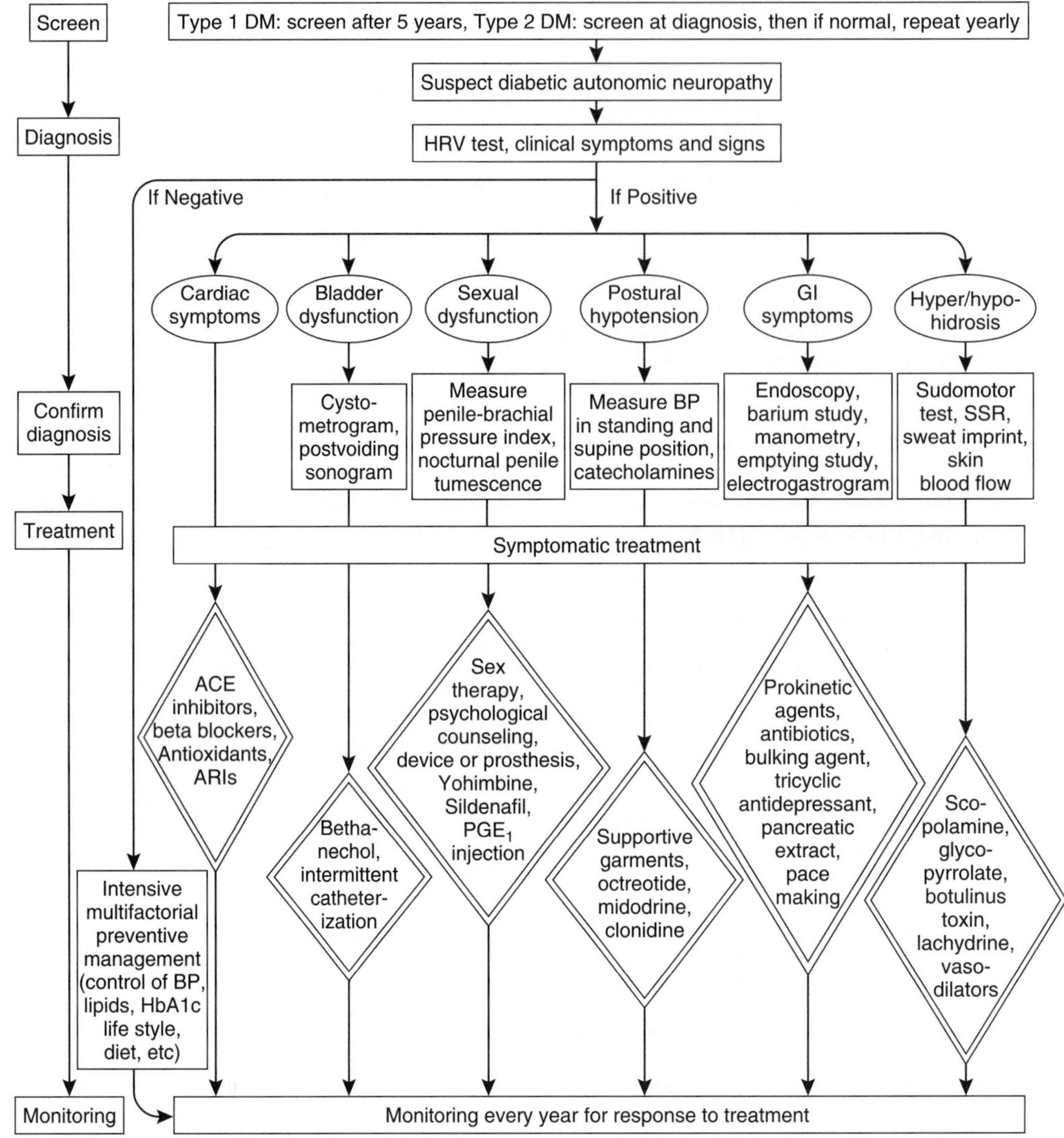

Figure 31–39. Diagnosis and treatment algorithm of diabetic autonomic neuropathy. ACE, angiotensin-converting enzyme; ARI, aldose reductase inhibitor; BP, blood pressure; DM, diabetes mellitus; GI, gastrointestinal; HRV, heart rate variability; PGE_1, prostaglandin E_1; SSR, sympathetic skin response.

increase the dose. If the preceding measures fail, midodrine, an α_1-adrenergic agonist, or dihydroergotamine in combination with caffeine may help. A particularly refractory form of postural hypotension occurs in some patients postprandially and may respond to therapy with octreotide given subcutaneously in the mornings.

Gastropathy

Gastrointestinal motor disorders are common and widespread in patients with type 2 diabetes mellitus, regardless of symptoms,[710] and there is a poor correlation between symptoms and objective evidence of functional or organic defects. The first step in management of diabetic gastroparesis consists of multiple, small feedings. The amount of fat should be decreased because it tends to delay gastric emptying. Maintenance of glycemic control is important.[711, 712] Metoclopramide may be used; when gastroparesis is severe, it is important to administer it intravenously, in liquid form, or as a suppository. When emptying becomes normal, the oral form may be resumed. Tachyphylaxis is common, and withdrawal from the drug periodically restores responsiveness.

Domperidone has been effective in some patients,[713, 714] although probably no more so than metoclopramide. Erythromycin, given as either a liquid or a suppository, may also be helpful. Erythromycin acts on the motilin receptor, "the sweeper of the gut," and shortens gastric emptying time.[715] If medications are unsuccessful and severe gastroparesis persists, jejunostomy placement into normally functioning bowel may be needed.

Enteropathy

Enteropathy involving the small bowel and colon can produce both chronic constipation and explosive diabetic diarrhea, making treatment of this particular complication difficult.

Diet

Patients with poor digestion may benefit from a gluten-free diet. The physician should be aware that certain fibers in the neuropathic patient can lead to bezoar formation because of bowel stasis in the gastroparetic or constipated state.

Antibiotics

Stasis of bowel contents with bacterial overgrowth may contribute to the diarrhea. Treatment with broad-spectrum antibiotics is the mainstay of therapy, including tetracycline or trimethoprim and sulfamethoxazole. Metronidazole appears to be the most effective and should be continued for at least 3 weeks.

Cholestyramine

Retention of bile may occur and can be highly irritating to the gut. Chelation of bile salts with cholestyramine 4 g three times daily mixed with fluid may offer relief of symptoms.

Diphenoxylate plus Atropine

Diphenoxylate plus atropine may help control diarrhea; toxic megacolon can occur, however, and extreme care should be used.

Somatostatin

In refractory cases, small doses of octreotide can be helpful in controlling diarrhea.

Cystopathy

Patients with neurogenic bladder should be instructed to palpate the bladder, and if they cannot initiate micturition when the bladder is full, they should be advised to use Credé's maneuver to start the flow of urine. Parasympathomimetics such as bethanechol are sometimes helpful, although often they do not help fully empty the bladder. Extended sphincter relaxation can be achieved with an α_1-adrenergic blocker, such as doxazosin.[568] Self-catheterization can be particularly useful in this setting, with the risk of infection generally being low.

Sexual Dysfunction

Erectile dysfunction (ED) occurs in 50% to 75% of diabetic men and tends to occur at an earlier age than in the general population. The incidence of ED in diabetic men aged 20 to 29 years is 9% and increases to 95% by age 70. It may be the presenting symptom of diabetes. More than 50% notice the onset of ED within 10 years of the diagnosis, but it may precede the other complications of diabetes.

The cause of ED in diabetes is multifactorial. Neuropathy, vascular disease, diabetes control, nutrition, endocrine disorders, and psychogenic factors as well as drugs used in the treatment of diabetes mellitus and its complications play a role.[716, 717] The diagnosis of the cause of ED is made by a logical, stepwise progression[716, 717] in all instances.

Sildenafil (Viagra), an orally active selective inhibitor of phosphodiesterase type 5, can be used in diabetic ED.[717] Most diabetic patients require 50 or 100 mg, and treatment should never be started without an evaluation of cardiac function. Patients with diabetic neuropathy are notorious for silent myocardial ischemia and poor ejection fractions,[696] and cardiovascular function must be evaluated before the prescription is written. The concomitant use with nitrites or nitrates is contraindicated because of the profound hypotension that may occur.[718]

Gustatory Sweating

Gustatory sweating is more common than previously believed, and topically applied glycopyrrolate, an antimuscarinic compound, is effective treatment in reducing both the severity and frequency of sweating of the head and neck region while eating food that triggers this reflex.[719, 720]

DIABETIC HEART DISEASE

IMPACT OF CARDIOVASCULAR DISEASE IN PATIENTS WITH DIABETES MELLITUS

It is widely underappreciated that CVD is the leading cause of mortality in patients with diabetes mellitus. Approximately 75% of the cardiovascular deaths attributed to diabetes are directly related to coronary artery disease. The economic burden of CVD in patients with diabetes far exceeds that of ESRD.[721] Despite the well-recognized benefits of tight glycemic control in reducing the risk of microvascular complications of diabetes, as evidenced from the results of large randomized clinical trials, a similar corollary for macrovascular complications has not been firmly established.

As the treatment of diabetic microvascular disease improves, an even greater increase in the incidence and prevalence of diabetic macrovascular disease can be expected. The steady increase in both the prevalence of overt diabetes and impaired glucose tolerance in the United States further highlights the need for a comprehensive and aggressive approach to cardiovascular risk factor management in these patients.[722] The "graying" of populations in most Westernized countries will also likely lead to a substantially larger social and economic burden from the cardiovascular complications of diabetes.

CORONARY HEART DISEASE MORBIDITY AND MORTALITY IN TYPE 1 AND TYPE 2 DIABETES

The last decades have been witness to substantial declines in coronary heart disease (CHD) mortality in the general population in the United States. However, significantly less improvement in CHD mortality has been seen in diabetic men and women during this same period.[723] More than 90% of all patients with diabetes have type 2 diabetes, and it is this population (most middle-aged and elderly) that has been evaluated in the majority of studies of CHD risk. In these studies, the excess morbidity and mortality associated with diabetes and elevated glucose remained even after adjustment for traditional CHD risk factors.

Data from the Framingham Study showed a twofold to threefold elevation in the risk of clinically evident atherosclerotic disease in patients with type 2 diabetes compared to those without diabetes.[724] Diabetic men in the Multiple Risk Factor Intervention Trial (MRFIT) study had an absolute risk of CHD death more than three times higher than that in the

23. Tomlinson DR, Fernybough P, Diemel LT. Role of neurotrophins in diabetic neuropathy and treatment with nerve growth factors. Diabetes 1997; 46(Suppl 2):S43–S49.
24. Engerman RL, Kern TS. Progression of incipient diabetic retinopathy during good glycemic control. Diabetes 1987; 36:808–812.
25. Roy S, Sala R, Cagliero E, Lorenzi M. Overexpression of fibronectin induced by diabetes or high-glucose phenomenon with a memory. Proc Natl Acad Sci USA 1990; 87:404–408.
26. The effect of intensive treatment of diabetes on the development and progression of long-term complications in insulin-dependent diabetes mellitus. The Diabetes Control and Complications Trial Research Group. N Engl J Med 1993; 329:977–986.
27. Effect of intensive therapy on the development and progression of diabetic nephropathy in the Diabetes Control and Complications Trial. The Diabetes Control and Complications (DCCT) Research Group. Kidney Int 1995; 47:1703–1712.
28. The effect of intensive diabetes therapy on the development and progression of neuropathy. The Diabetes Control and Complications Trial Research Group. Ann Intern Med 1995; 122:561–568.
29. Retinopathy and nephropathy in patients with type 1 diabetes four years after a trial of intensive therapy. The Diabetes Control and Complications Trial/Epidemiology of Diabetes Interventions and Complications Research Group. N Engl J Med 2000; 342: 381–389.
30. Krolewski AS, Warren JH, Freire MB. Epidemiology of late diabetic complications: a basis for the development and evaluation of preventive programs. Endocrinol Metab Clin North Am 1996; 25:217–242.
31. Seaquist ER, Goetz FC, Rich S, Barbosa J. Familial clustering of diabetic kidney disease: evidence for genetic susceptibility to diabetic nephropathy. N Engl J Med 1989; 320:1161–1165.
32. Quinn M, Angelico MC, Warram JH, Krolewski AS. Familial factors determine the development of diabetic nephropathy in patients with IDDM. Diabetologia 1996; 39:940–945.
33. Clustering of long-term complications in families with diabetes in the diabetes control and complications trial. The Diabetes Control and Complications Trial Research Group. Diabetes 1997; 46: 1829–1839.
34. Raffel LJ, Vadheim CM, Roth MP, et al. The 5′ insulin gene polymorphism and the genetics of vascular complications in type 1 (insulin-dependent) diabetes mellitus. Diabetologia 1991; 34: 680–683.
35. Stewart LL, Field LL, Ross S, McArthur RG. Genetic risk factors in diabetic retinopathy. Diabetologia 1993; 36:1293–1298.
36. Marre M, Bernadet P, Gallois Y, et al. Relationships between angiotensin I–converting enzyme gene polymorphism, plasma levels, and diabetic retinal and renal complications. Diabetes 1994; 43:384–388.
37. Marre M, Jeunemaitre X, Gallois Y, et al. Contribution of genetic polymorphism in the renin-angiotensin system to the development of renal complications in insulin-dependent diabetes: Genetique de la Nephropathie Diabetique (GENEDIAB) study group. J Clin Invest 1997; 99:1585–1595.
38. Agardh D, Gaur LK, Agardh E, et al. LADQB1*0201/0302 is associated with severe retinopathy in patients with IDDM. Diabetologia 1996; 39:1313–1317.
39. Oates PJ, Mylari BL. Aldose reductase inhibitors: therapeutic implications for diabetic complications. Exp Opin Invest Drugs 1999; 8:1–25.
40. Warpeha KM, Xu W, Liu L, et al. Genotyping and functional analysis of a polymorphic (CCTTTn) repeat of NOS2A in diabetic retinopathy. FASEB J 1999; 13:1825–1832.
41. Granger CB, Califf RM, Young S. Outcome of patients with diabetes mellitus and acute myocardial infarction treated with thrombolytic agents. The Thrombolysis and Angioplasty in Myocardial Infarction (TAMI) Study Group. J Am Coll Cardiol 1993; 21:920–925.
42. Stamler J, Vaccaro O, Neaton JD, Wentworth D. Diabetes, other risk factors, and 12-year cardiovascular mortality for men screened in the Multiple Risk Factor Intervention Trial. Diabetes Care 1993; 2:434–444.
43. Fitzgerald AP, Jarrett RJ. Are conventional risk factors for mortality relevant in type 2 diabetes? Diabet Med 1991; 8:475–480.
44. Fuller JH, Shipley MJ, Rose G, et al. Coronary heart disease risk and impaired glucose tolerance. The Whitehall Study. Lancet 1980; 1:1373–1376.
45. Rosengren A, Welin L, Tsipogianni A, et al. Impact of cardiovascular risk factors on coronary heart disease and mortality among middle-aged diabetic men: a general population study. BMJ 1989; 299:1127–1131.
46. Ross R. Atherosclerosis: an inflammatory disease. N Engl J Med 1999; 340:115–126.
47. Ross R. The pathogenesis of atherogenesis: a perspective for the 1990s. Nature 1993; 362:801–809.
48. Falk E, Shan PK, Fuster V. Pathogenesis of plaque disruption. In Fuster V, Ross R, Topol EJ (eds). Atherosclerosis and Coronary Artery Disease, Vol 2. Philadelphia, Lippincott-Raven, 1996, pp 492–510.
49. Davies MJ. A macro and micro view of coronary vascular insult in ischemic heart disease. Circulation 1990; 82(Suppl II): II-38–II-46.
50. King G, Brownlee M. The cellular and molecular mechanisms of diabetic complications. Endocrinol Metab Clin North Am 1996; 25:255–270.
51. Hsueh WA, Law RE. Cardiovascular risk continuum: implications of insulin resistance and diabetes. Am J Med 1998; 105:4S-14S.
52. Li H, Forstermann U. Nitric oxide in the pathogenesis of vascular disease. J Pathol 2000; 190:244–254.
53. Banskota NK, Taub R, Zellner K, King GL. Insulin, insulin-like growth factor I, and platelet-derived growth factor interact additively in the induction of the protooncogene *c-myc* and cellular proliferation in cultured bovine aortic smooth muscle cells. Mol Endocrinol 1989; 8:1183–1190.
54. Stolar MW. Atherosclerosis in diabetes: the role of hyperinsulinemia. Metabolism 1988; 7(Suppl 1):1–9.
55. Jiang ZY, Lin YW, Clemont A, et al. Characterization of selective resistance to insulin signaling in the vasculature of obese Zucker (fa/fa) rats. J Clin Invest 1999; 104:447–457.
56. Akbari CM, Saouaf R, Barnhill DF, et al. Endothelium-dependent vasodilatation is impaired in both microcirculation and macrocirculation during acute hyperglycemia. J Vasc Surg 1998; 28: 687–694.
57. Williams SB, Goldfine AB, Timimi FK, et al. Acute hyperglycemia attenuates endothelium-dependent vasodilation in humans in vivo. Circulation 1998; 97:1695–1701.
58. Du XL, Edelstein D, Rossetti L, et al. Hyperglycemia-induced mitochondrial superoxide overproduction activates the hexosamine pathway and induces plasminogen activator inhibitor-1 expression by increasing Sp1 glycosylation. Proc Natl Acad Sci USA 2000; 97:12222–12226.
59. Du XL, Edelstein D, Dimmler S, et al. Hyperglycemia inhibits endothelial nitric oxide synthase activity by altering its post-translational modification at the Akt site. J Clin Invest 2001; 108: 1341–1348.
60. Yamagishi S, Edelstein D, Du XD, Brownlee M. Hyperglycemia potentiates platelet-derived growth factor induced proliferation of smooth muscle cells through mitochondrial superoxide overproduction. Am J Pathol, submitted 2002.
61. Sassy-Prigent C, Heudes D, Mandet C, et al. Early glomerular macrophage recruitment in streptozotocin-induced diabetic rats Diabetes 2000; 49:466–475.
62. Gilcrease MZ, Hoover RL. Examination of monocyte adherence to endothelium under hyperglycemic conditions. Am J Pathol 1991; 139:1089–1097.
63. Ceriello A, Falleti E, Motz E. Hyperglycemia-induced circulating ICAM-1 increased in diabetes mellitus: the possible role of oxidative stress. Horm Metab Res 1998; 30:146–149.
64. Kim JA, Berliner JA, Natarajan RD, Nadler JL. Evidence that glucose increases monocyte binding to human aortic endothelial cells. Diabetes 1994; 43:1103–1107.
65. Yamagishi Y, Edelstein D, Du XD, Brownlee M. Hyperglycemia potentiates collagen-induced platelet activation through mitochondrial superoxide overproduction. Diabetes 2001; 50:1491–1494.
66. Cagliero E, Maiello M, Boeri D, et al. Increased expression of basement membrane components in human endothelial cells cultured in high glucose. J Clin Invest 1988; 82:735–738.
67. Cagliero E, Roth T, Roy S, et al. Expression of genes related to the extracellular matrix in human endothelial cells: differential

modulation by elevated glucose concentrations, phorbol esters, and cAMP. J Biol Chem 1991; 266:14244–14250.
68. Ginsberg HN. Insulin resistance and cardiovascular disease. J Clin Invest 2000; 106:453–458.
69. Gerstein HC. Is glucose a continuous risk factor for cardiovascular mortality? Diabetes Care 1999; 22:659–660.
70. Gall MA, Borch-Johnsen K, Hougaard P, et al. Albuminuria and poor glycemic control predict mortality in NIDDM. Diabetes 1995; 44:1303–1309.
71. Kuusisto J, Mykkanen L, Pyorala K, Laakso M. NIDDM and its metabolic control predict coronary heart disease in elderly subjects. Diabetes 1994; 43:960–967.
72. Salomaa V, Riley W, Kark JD, et al. Non–insulin-dependent diabetes mellitus and fasting glucose and insulin concentrations are associated with arterial stiffness indexes. The Atherosclerosis Risk in Communities (ARIC) Study. Circulation 1995; 91:1432–1443.
73. Laakso M, Kuusisto J. Epidemiological evidence for the association of hyperglycaemia and atherosclerotic vascular disease in non–insulin-dependent diabetes mellitus. Ann Med 1996; 28: 415–418.
74. Lehto S, Ronnemma T, Pyorala K, Laakso M. Poor glycemic control predicts coronary heart disease events in patients with type I diabetes without nephropathy. Arterioscler Thromb Vasc Biol 1999; 19:1014–1019.
75. Xia P, Kramer RM, King GL: Identification of the mechanism for the inhibition of Na,K-adenosine triphosphatase bv hyperglycemia involving activation of protein kinase C and cytosolic phospholipase A2. J Clin Invest 1995; 96:733.
76. Williamson JR, Chang K, Frangos M, et al. Hyperglycemic pseudohypoxia and diabetic complications. Diabetes 1993; 42:801–813.
77. Nishikawa T, Edelstein D, Du XL, et al. Normalizing mitochondrial superoxide production blocks three pathways of hyperglycaemic damage. Nature 2000; 404:787–790.
78. Marano CW, Szwergold BS, Kappler F, et al. Human retinal pigment epithelial cells cultured in hyperglycemic media accumulate increased amounts of glycosaminoglycan precursors. Invest Ophthalmol Vis Sci 1992; 33:2619–2625.
79. Beyer-Mears A, Diecke FP, Mistry K, et al. Effect of pyruvate lens myo-inositol transport and polyol formation in diabetic cataract. Pharmacology 1997; 55:78–86.
80. Knight RJ, Koefoed KF, Schelbert HR, Buxton DB. Inhibition of glyceraldehyde-3-phosphate dehydrogenase in post-ischaemic myocardium. Cardiovasc Res 1996; 32:1016–1023.
81. Lee AY, Chung SS. Contributions of polyol pathway to oxidative stress in diabetic cataract. FASEB J 1999; 13:23–30.
82. Zhang Z, Apse K, Pang J, Stanton RC. High glucose decreases glucose-6-phosphate dehydrogenase (G6PD) activity and impairs G6PD response to oxidative stress, thus predisposing cells to cell death in cultured bovine aortic endothelial cells. Diabetes 1999; 48(Suppl 1):A127.
83. Hammes H-P, Martin S, Federlin K, et al. Amino-guanidine treatment inhibits the development of experimental diabetic retinopathy. Proc Natl Acad Sci USA 1991; 88:11555–11559.
84. Stitt AW, Moore JE, Sharkey JA, et al. Advanced glycation end products in vitreous: structural and functional implications for diabetic vitreopathy. Invest Ophthalmol Vis Sci 1998; 39:2517–2521.
85. Stitt AW, Li YM, Gardiner TA, et al. Advanced glycation end products (AGEs) co-localize with AGE receptors in the retinal vasculature of diabetic and of AGE-infused rats. Am J Pathol 1997; 150:523–528.
86. Nishino T, Horri Y, Shikki H, et al. Immunohistochemical detection of advanced glycosylation end products within the vascular lesions and glomeruli in diabetic nephropathy. Hum Pathol 1995; 26:308–312.
87. Horie K, Miyata T, Maeda K, et al. Immunohistochemical colocalization of glycoxidation products and lipid peroxidation products in diabetic renal glomerular lesions: implication for glycoxidative stress in the pathogenesis of diabetic nephropathy. J Clin Invest 1997; 100:2995–2999.
88. Niwa T, Katsuzaki T, Miyazaki S, et al. Immunohistochemical detection of imidazolone, a novel advanced glycation end product, in kidneys and aortas of diabetic patients. J Clin Invest 1997; 99:1272–1276.
89. Degenhardt TP, Thorpe SR, Baynes JW. Chemical modification of proteins by methylglyoxal. Cell Mol Biol 1998; 44:1139–1145.
90. Wells-Knecht KJ, Zyzak DV, Litchfield JE, et al. Mechanism of autoxidative glycosylation: identification of glyoxal and arabinose as intermediates in the autoxidative modification of proteins by glucose. Biochemistry 1995; 34:3702.
91. Thornalley PJ. The glyoxalase system: new developments towards functional characterization of a metabolic pathway fundamental to biological life. Biochem J 1990; 269:1.
92. Takahashi M, Fujii J, Teshima T, et al. Identity of a major 3-deoxyglucosone reducing enzyme with aldehyde reductase in rat liver established by amino acid sequencing and cDNA expression. Gene 1993; 127:249.
93. Suzuki K, Koh YH, Mizuno H, et al. Overexpression of aldehyde reductase protects PC12 cells from the cytotoxicity of methylglyoxal or 3-deoxyglucosone. J Biochem 1998; 123:353.
94. Chang EY, Szallasi Z, Acs P, et al. Functional effects of overexpression of protein kinase C-alpha, -beta, -delta, -epsilon, and -eta in the mast cell line RBL-2H3. J Immunol 1997; 1159: 2624–2632.
95. Giardino I, Edelstein D, Brownlee M. Nonenzymatic glycosylation in vitro and in bovine endothelial cells alters basic fibroblast growth factor activity: a model for intracellular glycosylation in diabetes. J Clin Invest 1994; 94:110.
96. Shinohara M, Thornalley PJ, Giardino I, et al. Overexpression of glyoxalase-I in bovine endothelial cells inhibits intracellular advanced glycation end-product formation and prevents hyperglycemia-induced increases in macromolecular endocytosis. J Clin Invest 1998; 101:1142.
97. Maisonpierre PC, Suri C, Jones PF, et al. Angiopoietin-2, a natural antagonist for Tie2 that disrupts in vivo angiogenesis. Science 1997; 277:55–60.
98. Papapetropoulos A, Garcia-Cardena G, Dengler TJ, et al. Direct actions of angiopoietin-1 on human endothelium: evidence for network stabilization, cell survival, and interaction with other angiogenic growth factors. Lab Invest 1999; 79:213–223.
99. Hanahan D. Signaling vascular morphogenesis and maintenance. Science 1997; 277:48–50.
100. Elgawish A, Glomb M, Friedlander M, Monnier VM. Involvement of hydrogen peroxide in collagen cross-linking by high glucose in vitro and in vivo. J Biol Chem 1996; 271:129–164.
101. Brownlee M, Vlassara H, Kooney T, et al. Aminoguanidine prevents diabetes-induced arterial wall protein cross-linking. Science 1986; 232:1629.
102. Tanaka S, Avigad G, Brodsky B, Eikenberry EF. Glycation induces expansion of the molecular packing of collagen. J Mol Biol 1988; 203:495.
103. Huijberts MSP, Wolffenbuttel BRH, Struijker Boudier HAJ, et al. Aminoguanidine treatment increases elasticity and decreases fluid filtration of large arteries from diabetic rats. J Clin Invest 1993; 92:1407.
104. Tsilbary EC, Charonis AS, Reger LA, et al. The effect of nonenzymatic glucosylation the binding of the main noncollagenous NC1 domain to type IV collagen. J Biol Chem 1990; 263:4302.
105. Charonis AS, Reger LA, Dege JE, et al. Laminin alterations after in vitro nonenzymatic glucosylation. Diabetes 1988; 39:807.
106. Cochrane SM, Robinson GB. In vitro glycation of a glomerular basement membrane alters its permeability: a possible mechanism in diabetic complications. FEBS Lett 1995; 375:41.
107. Boyd-White J, Williams JC Jr. Effect of cross-linking on matrix permeability: a model for AGE-modified basement membranes. Diabetes 1996; 45:348.
108. Haitoglou CS, Tsilibary EC, Brownlee M, Charonis AS. Altered cellular interactions between endothelial cells and nonenzymatically glucosylated laminin/type IV collagen. J Biol Chem 1992; 267:12404.
109. Federoff HJ, Lawrence D, Brownlee M. Nonenzymatic glycosylation of laminin and the laminin peptide CIKVAVS inhibits neurite outgrowth. Diabetes 1993; 42:509.
110. Hammes HP, Weiss A, Hess S, et al. Modification of vitronectin by advanced glycation alters functional properties in vitro and in the diabetic retina. Lab Invest 1996; 75:325–338.
111. Li YM, Mitsuhashi T, Wojciechowicz D, et al. Molecular identity and cellular distribution of advanced glycation end-product receptors: relationship of p60 to OST-48 and p90 to 80K-H membrane proteins. Proc Natl Acad Sci USA 1996; 93:11047.

290. Schwartz JN, Donnelly EH, Klintworth GK. Ocular and orbital phycomycosis. Surv Ophthalmol 1977; 22:3–28.
291. Blitzer A, Lawson W, Meyers BR, Biller HF. Patient survival factors in paranasal sinus mucormycosis. Laryngoscope 1980; 90: 635–648.
292. Wand M, Dueker DK, Aiello LM, Grant WM. Effects of panretinal photocoagulation on rubeosis iridis, angle neovascularization, and neovascular glaucoma. Am J Ophthalmol 1978; 86:332–339.
293. Aiello LM, Wand M, Liang G. Neovascular glaucoma and vitreous hemorrhage following cataract surgery in patients with diabetes mellitus. Ophthalmology 1983; 90:814–820.
294. Simmons RJ, Dueker DK, Kimbrough RL, Aiello LM. Goniophotocoagulation for neovascular glaucoma. Trans Am Acad Ophthalmol Otolaryngol 1977; 83:80–89.
295. Hyndiuk RA, Kazarian EL, Schultz RO, Seideman S. Neurotrophic corneal ulcers in diabetes mellitus. Arch Ophthalmol 1977; 95:2193–2196.
296. Khodadoust AA, Silverstein AM, Kenyon DR, Dowling JE. Adhesion of regenerating corneal epithelium: the role of basement membrane. Am J Ophthalmol 1968; 65:339–348.
297. Klein BE, Klein R, Moss SE. Intraocular pressure in diabetic persons. Ophthalmology 1984; 91:1356–1360.
298. Marmor MF. Transient accommodative paralysis and hyperopia in diabetes. Arch Ophthalmol 1973; 89:419–421.
299. Klein BE, Klein R, Moss SE. Prevalence of cataracts in a population-based study of persons with diabetes mellitus. Ophthalmology 1985; 92:1191–1196.
300. Ederer F, Hiller R, Taylor HR. Senile lens changes and diabetes in two population studies. Am J Ophthalmol 1981; 91:381–395.
301. Klein BE, Klein R, Moss SE. Prevalence of cataracts in a population-based study of persons with diabetes mellitus. Ophthalmology 1985; 92:1191–1196.
302. Bursell SE, Baker RS, Weiss JN, et al. Clinical photon correlation spectroscopy evaluation of human diabetic lenses. Exp Eye Res 1989; 49:241–258.
303. Klein BE, Klein R, Moss SE. Incidence of cataract surgery in the Wisconsin Epidemiologic Study of Diabetic Retinopathy. Am J Ophthalmol 1995; 119:295–300.
304. Klein BE, Klein R, Wang Q, Moss SE. Older-onset diabetes and lens opacities: the Beaver Dam Eye Study. Ophthalmic Epidemiol 1995; 2:49–55.
305. Pai RP, Mitchell P, Chow VC, et al. Posttransplant cataract: lessons from kidney-pancreas transplantation (see comments). Transplantation 2000; 69:1108–1114.
306. Dowler JG, Hykin PG, Hamilton AM. Phacoemulsification versus extracapsular cataract extraction in patients with diabetes. Ophthalmology 2000; 107:457–462.
307. Borrillo JL, Mittra RA, Dev S, et al. Retinopathy progression and visual outcomes after phacoemulsification in patients with diabetes mellitus. Trans Am Ophthalmol Soc 1999; 97:435–445. Article in Am J Ophthalmol 2000 June; 129:832.
308. Funahashi T, Fink AI. The pathology of the bulbar conjunctiva in diabetes mellitus: I. Microaneurysms. Am J Ophthalmol 1963; 55:504–511.
309. Tagawa H, McMeel JW, Trempe CL. Role of the vitreous in diabetic retinopathy: II. Active and inactive vitreous changes. Ophthalmology 1986; 93:1188–1192.
310. Fleckner RA, Goldstein JH. Mucormycosis. Br J Ophthalmol 1969; 53:542–548.
311. The Diabetic Retinopathy Study Research Group. Photocoagulation treatment of proliferative diabetic retinopathy: clinical application of Diabetic Retinopathy Study (DRS) findings, DRS Report No. 8. Ophthalmology 1981; 88:583–600.
312. The Early Treatment Diabetic Retinopathy Study Research Group. Early photocoagulation for diabetic retinopathy. ETDRS Report No. 9. Ophthalmology 1991; 98(5 Suppl):766–785.
313. Diabetic Retinopathy Vitrectomy Study Group. Two-year course of visual acuity in severe proliferative diabetic retinopathy with conventional management. Diabetic Retinopathy Vitrectomy Study (DRVS) Report No. 1. Ophthalmology 1985; 92:492–502.
314. The Diabetes Control and Complications Trial Research Group. The effect of intensive diabetes treatment on the progression of diabetic retinopathy in insulin-dependent diabetes mellitus: the Diabetes Control and Complications Trial. Arch Ophthalmol 1995; 113:36–51.
315. Witkin SR, Klein R. Ophthalmologic care for persons with diabetes. JAMA 1984; 251:2534–2537.
316. Comprehensive Adult Eye Evaluation: Preferred Practice Pattern, 1989. San Francisco, American Academay of Ophthalmology, 1989.
317. Comprehensive Adult Eye and Vision Examination: Optometric Clinical Practice Guideline, 1994. American Optometric Association, St. Louis, Missouri.
318. Klein R, Klein BE, Neider MW, et al. Diabetic retinopathy as detected using ophthalmoscopy, a nonmydriatic camera, and a standard fundus camera. Ophthalmology 1985; 92:485–491.
319. Moss SE, Klein R, Kessler SD, Richie KA. Comparison between ophthalmoscopy and fundus photography in determining severity of diabetic retinopathy. Ophthalmology 1985; 92:62–67.
320. Sussman EJ, Tsiaras WG, Soper KA. Diagnosis of diabetic eye disease. JAMA 1982; 247:3231–3234.
321. Klein R, Moss SE, Klein BE. New management concepts for timely diagnosis of diabetic retinopathy treatable by photocoagulation. Diabetes Care 1987; 10:633–638.
322. Aiello LP, Gardner TW, King GL, et al. Diabetic retinopathy. Diabetes Care 1998; 21:143–156.
323. Klein R, Klein BE, Moss SE, et al. Retinopathy in young-onset diabetic patients. Diabetes Care 1985; 8:311–315.
324. Krolewski AS, Warram JH, Rand LI, et al. Risk of proliferative diabetic retinopathy in juvenile-onset type I diabetes: a 40-year follow-up study. Diabetes Care 1986; 9:443–452.
325. Klein BE, Moss SE, Klein R. Is menarche associated with diabetic retinopathy? Diabetes Care 1990; 13:1034–1038.
326. Kostraba JN, Klein R, Dorman JS, et al. The epidemiology of diabetes complications study: IV. Correlates of diabetic background and proliferative retinopathy. Am J Epidemiol 1991; 133: 381–391.
327. Klein R, Klein BE, Moss SE, Cruickshanks KJ. The Wisconsin Epidemiologic Study of Diabetic Retinopathy: XV. The long-term incidence of macular edema. Ophthalmology 1995; 102:7–16.
328. Sunness JS. The pregnant woman's eye. Surv Ophthalmol 1988; 32:219–238.
329. Klein BE, Moss SE, Klein R. Effect of pregnancy on progression of diabetic retinopathy. Diabetes Care 1990; 13:34–40.
330. White P. Diabetes mellitus in pregnancy. Clin Perinatol 1974; 1: 331–347.
331. Best RM, Chakravarthy U. Diabetic retinopathy in pregnancy. Br J Ophthalmol 1997; 81:249–251.
332. The Early Treatment Diabetic Retinopathy Study Research Group. Grading diabetic retinopathy from stereoscopic color fundus photographs—an extension of the modified Airlie House classification: ETDRS Report No. 10. Ophthalmology 1991; 98(5 Suppl):786–806.
333. The Diabetic Retinopathy Study Research Group. Indications for photocoagulation treatment of diabetic retinopathy: Diabetic Retinopathy Study Report No. 14. Int Ophthalmol Clin 1987; 27: 239–253.
334. The Diabetic Retinopathy Study Research Group. Photocoagulation treatment of proliferative diabetic retinopathy: the second report of diabetic retinopathy study findings. Ophthalmology 1978; 85:82–106.
335. The Early Treatment Diabetic Retinopathy Study Research Group. Photocoagulation for diabetic macular edema. Early Treatment Diabetic Retinopathy Study Report No. 1. Arch Ophthalmol 1985; 103:1796–1806.
336. Ferris F. Early photocoagulation in patients with either type 1 or type 2 diabetes. Trans Am Ophthalmol Soc 1996; 94:505–537.
337. The Early Treatment Diabetic Retinopathy Study Research Group. Photocoagulation for diabetic macular edema: Early Treatment Diabetic Retinopathy Study Report No. 4. Int Ophthalmol Clin 1987; 27:265–272.
338. LaPiana FG, Penner R. Anaphylactoid reaction to intravenously administered fluorescein. Arch Ophthalmol 1968; 79:161–162.
339. Butner RW, McPherson AR. Adverse reactions in intravenous fluorescein angiography. Ann Ophthalmol 1983; 15:1084–1086.
340. Wittpenn JR, Rapoza P, Sternberg P, et al. Respiratory arrest following retrobulbar anesthesia. Ophthalmology 1986; 93:867–870.
341. Klein R, Klein BE, Lee KE, et al. The incidence of hypertension in insulin-dependent diabetes. Arch Intern Med 1996; 156:622–627.
342. Vascular complications in non–insulin-dependent diabetics in

Thailand. Thai Multicenter Research Group on Diabetes Mellitus. Diabetes Res Clin Pract 1994; 25:61–69.

343. Klein R, Klein BE, Moss SE, DeMets DL. Blood pressure and hypertension in diabetes. Am J Epidemiol 1985; 122:75–89.
344. Fujimoto WY, Leonetti DL, Kinyoun JL, et al. Prevalence of complications among second-generation Japanese-American men with diabetes, impaired glucose tolerance, or normal glucose tolerance. Diabetes 1987; 36:730–739.
345. Klein R, Klein BE, Moss SE, Cruickshanks KJ. The Wisconsin Epidemiologic Study of Diabetic Retinopathy: XVII. The 14-year incidence and progression of diabetic retinopathy and associated risk factors in type 1 diabetes (see comments). Ophthalmology 1998; 105:1801–1815.
346. Zander E, Heinke P, Herfurth S, et al. Relations between diabetic retinopathy and cardiovascular neuropathy: a cross-sectional study in IDDM and NIDDM patients. Exp Clin Endocrinol Diabetes 1997; 105:319–326.
347. Diabetes Drafting Group. Prevalence of small vessel and large vessel disease in diabetic patients from 14 centres: the World Health Organization Multinational Study of Vascular Disease in Diabetes. Diabetologia 1985; 28:615–640.
348. Agardh CD, Agardh E, Torffvit O. The association between retinopathy, nephropathy, cardiovascular disease, and long-term metabolic control in type 1 diabetes mellitus: a 5-year follow-up study of 442 adult patients in routine care. Diabetes Res Clin Pract 1997; 35:113–121.
349. Lopes de Faria JM, Jalkh AE, Trempe CL, McMeel JW. Diabetic macular edema: risk factors and concomitants. Acta Ophthalmol Scand 1999; 77:170–175.
350. Marshall G, Garg SK, Jackson WE, et al. Factors influencing the onset and progression of diabetic retinopathy in subjects with insulin-dependent diabetes mellitus. Ophthalmology 1993; 100: 1133–1139.
351. Tight blood pressure control and risk of macrovascular and microvascular complications in type 2 diabetes: UKPDS 38. UK Prospective Diabetes Study Group (see comments) (published erratum appears in BMJ 1999; 318:29). BMJ 1998; 317:703–713.
352. Schrier RW, Estacio RO, Jeffers B. Appropriate Blood Pressure Control in NIDDM (ABCD) Trial. Diabetologia 1996; 39:1646–1654.
353. Klein R, Klein BE, Moss SE, et al. The Wisconsin Epidemiology Study of Diabetic Retinopathy: V. Proteinuria and retinopathy in a population of diabetic persons diagnosed prior to 30 years of age. In Friedman EA, L'Esperance FA Jr (eds). Diabetic Renal-Retinal Syndrome, 3rd ed. Orlando, Grune & Stratton, 1986, pp 245–264.
354. Kullberg CE, Arnqvist HJ. Elevated long-term glycated haemoglobin precedes proliferative retinopathy and nephropathy in type 1 (insulin-dependent) diabetic patients. Diabetologia 1993; 36: 961–965.
355. Klein R, Moss SE, Klein BE. Is gross proteinuria a risk factor for the incidence of proliferative diabetic retinopathy? Ophthalmology 1993; 100:1140–1146.
356. Mathiesen ER, Ronn B, Storm B, et al. The natural course of microalbuminuria in insulin-dependent diabetes: a 10-year prospective study. Diabet Med 1995; 12:482–487.
357. Park JY, Kim HK, Chung YE, et al. Incidence and determinants of microalbuminuria in Koreans with type 2 diabetes. Diabetes Care 1998; 21:530–534.
358. Hasslacher C, Bostedt-Kiesel A, Kempe HP, Wahl P. Effect of metabolic factors and blood pressure on kidney function in proteinuric type 2 (non–insulin-dependent) diabetic patients. Diabetologia 1993; 36:1051–1056.
359. Collins VR, Dowse GK, Plehwe WE, et al. High prevalence of diabetic retinopathy and nephropathy in Polynesians of Western Samoa. Diabetes Care 1995; 18:1140–1149.
360. Lee ET, Lee VS, Kingsley RM, et al. Diabetic retinopathy in Oklahoma Indians with NIDDM: incidence and risk factors. Diabetes Care 1992; 15:1620–1627.
361. Esmatjes E, Castell C, Gonzalez T, et al. Epidemiology of renal involvement in type II diabetics (NIDDM) in Catalonia. The Catalan Diabetic Nephropathy Study Group. Diabetes Res Clin Pract 1996; 32:157–163.
362. Savage S, Estacio RO, Jeffers B, Schrier RW. Urinary albumin excretion as a predictor of diabetic retinopathy, neuropathy, and cardiovascular disease in NIDDM. Diabetes Care 1996; 19:1243–1248.
363. Fujisawa T, Ikegami H, Yamato E, et al. Association of plasma fibrinogen level and blood pressure with diabetic retinopathy, and renal complications associated with proliferative diabetic retinopathy, in type 2 diabetes mellitus. Diabet Med 1999; 16:522–526.
364. Cruickshanks KJ, Ritter LL, Klein R, Moss SE. The association of microalbuminuria with diabetic retinopathy. The Wisconsin Epidemiologic Study of Diabetic Retinopathy. Ophthalmology 1993; 100:862–867.
365. Roy MS. Diabetic retinopathy in African Americans with type 1 diabetes—the New Jersey 725: II. Risk factors. Arch Ophthalmol 2000; 118:105–115.
366. Klein R, Klein BE, Moss SE, Cruickshanks KJ. Ten-year incidence of gross proteinuria in people with diabetes. Diabetes 1995; 44:916–923.
367. Mogensen CE, Chachati A, Christensen CK, et al. Microalbuminuria: an early marker of renal involvement in diabetes. Uremia Invest 1985; 9:85–95.
368. Villarosa IP, Bakris GL. The Appropriate Blood Pressure Control in Diabetes (ABCD) Trial. J Hum Hypertens 1998; 12:653–655.
369. Nelson RG, Knowler WC, Pettitt DJ, et al. Incidence and determinants of elevated urinary albumin excretion in Pima Indians with NIDDM. Diabetes Care 1995; 18:182–187.
370. Gomes MB, Lucchetti MR, Gazzola H, et al. Microalbuminuria and associated clinical features among Brazilians with insulin-dependent diabetes mellitus. Diabetes Res Clin Pract 1997; 35: 143–147.
371. Predictors of the development of microalbuminuria in patients with type 1 diabetes mellitus: a seven-year prospective study. The Microalbuminuria Collaborative Study Group (see comments). Diabet Med 1999; 16:918–925.
372. Ravid M, Brosh D, Ravid-Safran D, et al. Main risk factors for nephropathy in type 2 diabetes mellitus are plasma cholesterol levels, mean blood pressure, and hyperglycemia. Arch Intern Med 1998; 158:998–1004.
373. Gall MA, Hougaard P, Borch-Johnsen K, Parving HH. Risk factors for development of incipient and overt diabetic nephropathy in patients with non–insulin-dependent diabetes mellitus: prospective, observational study (see comments). BMJ 1997; 314: 783–788.
374. Kordonouri O, Danne T, Hopfenmuller W, et al. Lipid profiles and blood pressure: are they risk factors for the development of early background retinopathy and incipient nephropathy in children with insulin-dependent diabetes mellitus? Acta Paediatr 1996; 85:43–48.
375. Larsson LI, Alm A, Lithner F, et al. The association of hyperlipidemia with retinopathy in diabetic patients aged 15–50 years in the county of Umea. Acta Ophthalmol Scand 1999; 77:585–591.
376. Sjolie AK, Stephenson J, Aldington S, et al. Retinopathy and vision loss in insulin-dependent diabetes in Europe. The EURODIAB IDDM Complications Study. Ophthalmology 1997; 104:252–260.
377. Verrotti A, Lobefalo L, Chiarelli F, et al. Lipids and lipoproteins in diabetic adolescents and young adults with retinopathy. Eye 1997; 11:876–881.
378. Klein BE, Moss SE, Klein R, Surawicz TS. The Wisconsin Epidemiologic Study of Diabetic Retinopathy: XIII. Relationship of serum cholesterol to retinopathy and hard exudate. Ophthalmology 1991; 98:1261–1265.
379. El-Asrar AM, Al-Rubeaan KA, Al-Amro SA, et al. Risk factors for diabetic retinopathy among Saudi diabetics. Int Ophthalmol 1998; 22:155–161.
380. Ferris FL, Chew EY, Hoogwerf BJ. Serum lipids and diabetic retinopathy. Early Treatment Diabetic Retinopathy Study Research Group. Diabetes Care 1996; 19:1291–1293.
381. Chew EY, Klein ML, Ferris FL, et al. Association of elevated serum lipid levels with retinal hard exudate in diabetic retinopathy. Early Treatment Diabetic Retinopathy Study (ETDRS) Report No. 22. Arch Ophthalmol 1996; 114:1079–1084.
382. National Cholesterol Education Program. Report of the NECP expert panel on detection, evaluation, and treatment of high blood cholesterol in adults. Arch Intern Med 1988; 148:36–39.
383. Rasmidatta S, Khunsuk-Mengrai K, Warunyuwong C. Risk factors of diabetic retinopathy in non–insulin-dependent diabetes mellitus. J Med Assoc Thai 1998; 81:169–174.
384. Cruickshanks KJ, Moss SE, Klein R, Klein BE. Physical activity

and proliferative retinopathy in people diagnosed with diabetes before age 30 years. Diabetes Care 1992; 15:1267–1272.
385. LaPorte RE, Dorman JS, Tajima N, et al. Pittsburgh Insulin-Dependent Diabetes Mellitus and Mortality Study: physical activity and diabetic complications. Pediatrics 1986; 78:1027–1033.
386. Kriska AM, LaPorte RE, Patrick SL, et al. The association of physical activity and diabetic complications in individuals with insulin-dependent diabetes mellitus: The Epidemiology of Diabetic Complications Study VII. J Clin Epidemiol 1991; 44:1207–1214.
387. Orchard TJ, Dorman JS, Maser RE, et al. Factors associated with avoidance of severe complications after 25 years of IDDM. Pittsburgh Epidemiology of Diabetes Complications Study I. Diabetes Care 1990; 13:741–747.
388. Cruickshanks KJ, Moss SE, Klein R, Klein BE. Physical activity and the risk of progression of retinopathy or the development of proliferative retinopathy. Ophthalmology 1995; 102:1177–1182.
389. Anderson B Jr. Activity and diabetic vitreous hemorrhages. Ophthalmology 1980; 87:173–175.
390. Early Treatment Diabetic Retinopathy Study Research Group. Effects of aspirin treatment on diabetic retinopathy. ETDRS Report No. 8. Ophthalmology 1991; 98(Suppl):757–765.
391. Chew EY, Klein ML, Murphy RP, et al. Effects of aspirin on vitreous/preretinal hemorrhage in patients with diabetes mellitus. Early Treatment Diabetic Retinopathy Study Report No. 20. Arch Ophthalmol 1995; 113:52–55.
392. Caramelli B, Tranchesi B Jr, Gebara OC, et al. Retinal haemorrhage after thrombolytic therapy (letter). Lancet 1991; 337:1356–1357.
393. Barbash GI, White HD, Modan M, Van de WF. Significance of diabetes mellitus in patients with acute myocardial infarction receiving thrombolytic therapy. Investigators of the International Tissue Plasminogen Activator/Streptokinase Mortality Trial. J Am Coll Cardiol 1993; 22:707–713.
394. Randomised trial of intravenous streptokinase, oral aspirin, both, or neither among 17,187 cases of suspected acute myocardial infarction: ISIS-2. ISIS-2 (Second International Study of Infarct Survival) Collaborative Group (see comments). Lancet 1988; 2: 349–360.
395. ISIS-3: a randomised comparison of streptokinase versus tissue plasminogen activator versus anistreplase and of aspirin plus heparin versus aspirin alone among 41,299 cases of suspected acute myocardial infarction. ISIS-3 (Third International Study of Infarct Survival) Collaborative Group (see comments). Lancet 1992; 339:753–770.
396. GISSI-2: a factorial randomised trial of alteplase versus streptokinase and heparin versus no heparin among 12,490 patients with acute myocardial infarction. Gruppo Italiano per lo Studio della Sopravvivenza nell'Infarto Miocardico (see comments). Lancet 1990; 336:65–71.
397. Muhlhauser I, Sawicki P, Berger M. Cigarette smoking as a risk factor for macroproteinuria and proliferative retinopathy in type 1 (insulin-dependent) diabetes. Diabetologia 1986; 29:500–502.
398. Muhlhauser I, Bender R, Bott U, et al. Cigarette smoking and progression of retinopathy and nephropathy in type 1 diabetes. Diabet Med 1996; 13:536–543.
399. West KM, Erdreich LS, Stober JA. Absence of a relationship between smoking and diabetic microangiopathy. Diabetes Care 1980; 3:250–252.
400. Chen MS, Kao CS, Chang CJ, et al. Prevalence and risk factors of diabetic retinopathy among non–insulin-dependent diabetic subjects. Am J Ophthalmol 1992; 114:723–730.
401. Muhlhauser I. Cigarette smoking and diabetes: an update. Diabet Med 1994; 11:336–343.
402. Davis MD, Fisher MR, Gangnon RE, et al. Risk factors for high-risk proliferative diabetic retinopathy and severe visual loss: Early Treatment Diabetic Retinopathy Study Report No. 18. Invest Ophthalmol Vis Sci 1998; 39:233–252.
403. Qiao Q, Keinanen-Kiukaanniemi S, Laara E. The relationship between hemoglobin levels and diabetic retinopathy. J Clin Epidemiol 1997; 50:153–158.
404. Friedman EA, Brown CD, Berman DH. Erythropoietin in diabetic macular edema and renal insufficiency. Am J Kidney Dis 1995; 26:202–208.
405. Mogensen CE: Definition of diabetic renal disease in insulin-dependent diabetes mellitus based on renal function tests. In Mogensen CE (ed). The Kidney and Hypertension in Diabetes Mellitus, 5th ed. Boston, Kluwer, 2000, pp 13–28.
406. U.S. Renal Data System (USRDS) 2000 Annual Data Report, National Institutes of Health, National Institute of Diabetes and Digestive and Kidney Diseases, Bethesda, MD, June 2000.
407. Pugh JA, Medina RA, Cornell JC, et al: NIDDM is the major cause of diabetic end-stage renal disease: more evidence of a tri-ethnic community. Diabetes 1995; 44:1375–1380.
408. Lippert J, Ritz E, Schwarzbeck A, et al: The rising of end-stage renal failure from diabetic nephropathy type II: an epidemiologic analysis. Nephrol Dial Transplant 1995; 10:462–467.
409. Brancati FL, Whittle JC, Whelton PK, et al: The excess incidence of diabetic end-stage renal disease among blacks: a population-based study of potential explanatory factors. JAMA 1992; 268:3079–3079.
410. Smith SR, Svetkey LP, Dennis VW: Racial differences in the incidence and progression of renal diseases. Kidney Int 1991; 40: 815–822.
411. Nelson RG, Knowler WC, Pettitt DJ, et al: Diabetic kidney disease in Pima Indians. Diabetes Care 1993; 16:335–341.
412. Imperatore G, Knowler WC, Pettitt DJ, et al: Segregation analysis of diabetic nephropathy in Pima Indians. Diabetes 2000; 49: 1049–1056.
413. National Diabetes Fact Sheet, 1998. National Estimates and General Information on Diabetes in the Unites States, rev ed. Atlanta, U.S. Department of Health and Human Services, Centers for Disease Control and Prevention, 1998.
414. Krop JS, Soresh J, Chambless LE: A community-based study of explanatory factors for the excess for early renal function decline in blacks versus whites with diabetes: the Atherosclerotic Risk in Communities study. Arch Intern Med 1999; 159:1777–1783.
415. Østerby R, Gall M-A, Schmitz A, et al: Glomerular structure and function in proteinuric type 2 (non–insulin-dependent) diabetic patients. Diabetologia 1993; 36:1064–1070.
416. Hayashi H, Karasawa R, Inn H, et al: An electron microscopic study of glomeruli in Japanese patients with non–insulin-dependent diabetes mellitus. Kidney Int 1992; 41:749–757.
417. White KE, Bilous RW: Type 2 diabetic patients with nephropathy show structural-functional relationships that are similar to type 1 disease. J Am Soc Nephrol 2000; 11:1667–1673.
418. Østerby R: Glomerular structural changes in type 1 (insulin-dependent) diabetes mellitus: causes, consequences, and prevention. Diabetologia 1992; 35:803–812.
419. Fioretto P, Steffes MW, Sutherland DE, et al: Sequential renal biopsies in insulin-dependent diabetic patients: structural factors associated with clinical progression. Kidney Int 1995; 48:1929–1935.
420. Mauer SM, Steffes MW, Ellis EN, et al: Structural-functional relationships in diabetic nephropathy. J Clin Invest 1984; 74: 1143–1155.
421. Steffes MW, Bilous RW, Sutherland DER, et al: Cell and matrix components of the glomerular mesangium in type I diabetes. Diabetes 1992; 41:679–684.
422. Olsen S: Light microscopy of diabetic glomerulopathy: the classic lesions. In Mogensen CE (ed): The Kidney and Hypertension in Diabetes Mellitus, 2nd ed. Boston, Kluwer Academic, 2000, pp 201–210.
423. Da Silva EC, Saldanha LB, Pestolazzi MS, et al: Nodular diabetic glomerulosclerosis without diabetes mellitus. Nephron 1992; 62:289–291.
424. Gallo GR, Feiner HD, Katz LA, et al: Nodular glomerulopathy associated with nonamyloidotic kappa light chain deposits and excess immunoglobulin light synthesis. Am J Pathol 1980; 99: 621–644.
425. Østerby R, Schmitz A, Nyberg G: Renal structural changes in insulin-dependent diabetic patients with albuminuria: comparison of cases with onset of albuminuria after short or long duration. APMIS 1998; 106:361–370.
426. Brito PL, Fioretto P, Drummond K, et al: Proximal tubular basement width in insulin-dependent diabetes mellitus. Kidney Int 1998; 53:754–761.
427. Dalla Vestra M, Saller A, Bortoloso E, et al: Structural involvement in type 1 and type 2 diabetic nephropathy. Diabetes Metab 2000; 26(Suppl 4):8–14.
428. Bangstad HJ, Østerby R, Dahl-Jorgensen K, et al: Early glomerulopathy is present in young, type 1 (insulin-dependent) diabetic patients with microalbuminuria. Diabetologia 1993; 36:523–529.

429. Bader R, Bader H, Grund KE, et al: Structure and function of the kidney in diabetic glomerulosclerosis: correlations between morphological and functional parameters. Pathol Res Pract 1980; 167:204–216.
430. Lane PH, Steffes MW, Fioretto P, et al: Renal expansion in insulin-dependent diabetes mellitus. Kidney Int 1993; 43:661–667.
431. Cambier P: [Application de la théorie de Rehberg a l-étude clinique des affections rénales and du diabète.] Annu Med 1934; 35: 273–299.
432. Ditzel J, Schwartz M: Abnormally increased glomerular filtration rate in short-term insulin-treated diabetic subjects. Diabetes 1967; 16:264–267.
433. Mogensen CE: Kidney function and glomerular permeability to macromolecules in early juvenile diabetes. Scand J Clin Lab Invest 1971; 28:79–90.
434. Mogensen CE, Christensen CK: Predicting diabetic nephropathy in insulin-dependent patients. N Engl J Med 1984; 311:89–93.
435. Christiansen JS, Frandsen M, Parving HH: The effect of intravenous insulin infusion on kidney function in insulin-dependent diabetes mellitus. Diabetologia 1981; 20:199–204.
436. Christiansen JS, Gammelgaard J, Frandsen M, et al: Increased kidney size, glomerular filtration rate, and renal plasma flow in short-term insulin-dependent diabetics. Diabelogia 1981; 20:451–456.
437. Christiansen JS: On the pathogenesis of the increased glomerular filtration rate in short-term insulin-dependent diabetes. Dan Med Bull 1984; 31:349–361.
438. Bank N: Mechanisms of diabetic hyperfiltration. Kidney Int 1991; 40:792–807.
439. Christensen CK, Christiansen JS, Schmitz A, et al: Effect of continuous subcutaneous insulin infusion on kidney function and size in IDDM patients: a 2-year controlled study. J Diabetic Complications 1987; 1:91–95.
440. Mogensen CE: Early glomerular hyperfiltration in insulin-dependent diabetics and late nephropathy. Scand J Clin Lab Invest 1986; 46:201–206.
441. Lervang HH, Jensen S, Brøchner-Mortensen J, et al: Early glomerular hyperfiltration and the development of late nephropathy in type I insulin-dependent diabetes mellitus. Diabetologia 1988; 31:723–723.
442. Jones SL, Wiseman MJ, Viberti GC: Glomerular hyperfiltration as a risk factor for diabetic nephropathy: five-year report of a prospective study. Diabetologia 1991; 34:59–60.
443. Rudberg S, Persson B, Dahlquist G: Increased glomerular filtration rate as a predictor of diabetic nephropathy: an 8-year prospective study. Kidney Int 1992; 41:822–828.
444. Chiarelli F, Verrotti A, Morgese G: Glomerular hyperfiltration increases the risk of developing microalbuminuria in diabetic children. Pediatr Nephrol 1995; 9:154–158.
445. Christiansen JS, Gammelgaard J, Tronier B, et al: Kidney function and size in diabetics before and during initial treatment. Kidney Int 1982; 21:683–688.
446. Wiseman MJ, Saunders AJ, Keen H, et al: Effect of glucose control on increased glomerular filtration rate and kidney size in insulin-dependent diabetes. N Engl J Med 1985; 12:617–621.
447. Christensen CK, Christiansen JS, Schmitz A, et al: Effect of continuous subcutaneous insulin infusion on kidney function and size in IDDM patients: a 2-year controlled study. HNO 1987; 1: 91–95.
448. Østerby R: Early phases in the development of diabetic glomerulopathy: quantitative electron microscopic study. Acta Med Scand 1974; S574(Suppl):3–82.
449. Østerby R, Gundersen HJG: Glomerular size and structure in diabetes mellitus: I. Early abnormalities. Diabetologia 1975; 11: 225–229.
450. NØrgaard K, Feldt-Rasmussen B, Borch-Johnsen K, et al: Prevalence of hypertension in type 1 (insulin-dependent) diabetes mellitus. Diabetologia 1990; 33:407–410.
451. Molitch ME, Steffes MW, Cleary PA, et al: Baseline analysis of renal function in the diabetes control and complications trial. Kidney Int 1993; 43:668–674.
452. Mogensen CE: Diabetic renal disease: the quest for normotension and beyond. Diabetic Med 1995; 12:756–769.
453. Feldt-Rasmussen B, Hegedus L, Mthiesen ER, et al: Kidney volume in type 1 (insulin-dependent) diabetic patients with normal or increased urinary albumin excretion: effect of long-term improvement of metabolic control. Scand J Clin Lab Invest 1991; 51:31–36.
454. Ellis EN, Steffes MW, Goetz FC, et al: Relationship of renal size to nephropathy in type 1 (insulin-dependent) diabetes. Diabetologia 1985; 28:12–15.
455. Mortensen HB: Microalbuminuria in young patients with type 1 diabetes. In Mogensen CE (ed). The Kidney and Hypertension in Diabetes Mellitus, 5th ed. Boston, Kluwer, 2000, pp 363–379.
456. Gibb DM, Shah V, Preece M, et al: Variability of urine albumin excretion in normal and diabetic children. Pediatr Nephrol 1989; 3:414–419.
457. Mogensen CE, Vestbo E, Poulsen PL, et al: Microalbuminuria and potential confounders: a review and some observations on variability of urinary albumin excretion. Diabetes Care 1995; 15: 572–581.
458. Brenner BM, Hostetter TH, Humes HD: Molecular basis of proteinuria of glomerular origin. N Engl J Med 1978; 298:826–833.
459. Schwab SJ, Dunn FL, Feinglos MN: Screening for microalbuminuria: a comparison of single sample of collection and techniques of albumin analysis. Diabetes Care 1992; 15:1581–1584.
460. Eshøj O, Feldt-Rasmussen B, Larsen ML, et al: Comparison of overnight, morning, and 24-hour urine collection in the assessment of diabetic microalbuminuria. Diabet Med 1987; 4:531–533.
461. Viberti GC, Keen H: The pattern of proteinuria in diabetes mellitus: relevance to pathogenesis and prevention of diabetic nephropathy. Diabetes 1984; 33:686–692.
462. Mogensen CE: Microalbuminuria as a predictor of clinical diabetic nephropathy. Kidney Int 1987; 31:673–689.
463. Mathiesen ER, Saurbrey N, Hommel E, et al: Prevalence of microalbuminuria in children with type 1 (insulin-dependent) diabetes mellitus. Diabetologia 1986; 29:640–643.
464. Dahlquist G, Rudberg S: The prevalence of microalbuminuria in diabetic children and adolescents and its relation to puberty. Acta Paediatr Scand 1987; 76:795–800.
465. Mathiesen ER, Øxenboll B, Johansen K, et al: Incipient nephropathy in type 1 insulin-dependent diabetes. Diabetologia 1984; 26: 406–410.
466. Viberti GC, Hill RD, Jarrett RJ, et al: Microalbuminuria as a predictor of clinical nephropathy in insulin-dependent diabetes mellitus. Lancet 1982; 1:1430–1432.
467. Bangstad HJ, Østerby R, Dahl-Jorgensen K: Early glomerulopathy is present in young, type 1 (insulin-dependent) diabetic patients with microalbuminuria. Diabetologia 1993; 36:523–529.
468. Parving HH, Hommel E, Mathiesen E, et al: Prevalence of microalbuminuria, arterial hypertension, retinopathy, and neuropathy in patients with insulin-dependent diabetes. BMJ 1988; 296: 156–160.
469. Parving HH, Smidt UM, Friisberg B, et al: A prospective study of glomerular filtration rate and arterial blood pressure in insulin-dependent diabetics with diabetic nephropathy. Diabetologia 1981; 20:457–461.
470. Viberti GC, Wiseman MJ, Pinto JR, et al: Diabetic nephropathy. In Kahn CR, Weir GC (eds). Joslin's Diabetes Mellitus, 13th ed. Philadelphia, Lea & Febiger, 1994, pp 691–737.
471. Tarnow L, Rossing P, Gall MA, et al: Prevalence of arterial hypertension in diabetic patients before and after the JNC-V. Diabetes Care 1994; 17:1247–1251.
472. Hasslacher C, Stech W, Wahl P, et al: Blood pressure and metabolic control as risk factors for nephropathy in type 1 (insulin-dependent) diabetes. Diabetologia 1985; 28:6–11.
473. Taft JL, Nolan CJ, Yeung SP,et al: Clinical and histological correlations of decline in renal function in diabetic patients with proteinuria. Diabetes 1994; 43:1046–1051.
474. Breyer JA, Bain RP, Evans JK, et al: Predictors of the progression of renal insufficiency in patients with insulin-dependent diabetes and overt diabetic nephropathy. The Collaborative Study Group. Kidney Int 1996; 50:1651–1658.
475. Mogensen CE: Progression of nephropathy in long-term diabetics with proteinuria and effect of initial antihypertensive treatment. Scan J Clin Lab Invest 1976; 36:383–388.
476. Viberti GC, Bilous RW, Mackintosh C: Monitoring glomerular function in diabetic nephropathy: a prospective study. Am J Med 1983; 74:256–264.

477. Vora JP, Dolben J, Dean JD, et al: Renal hemodynamics in newly presenting non–insulin-dependent diabetes mellitus. Kidney Int 1992; 41:829–835.
478. Schmitz A, Hansen HH, Christensen T: Kidney function in newly diagnosed type 2 (non–insulin-dependent) diabetic patients, before and during treatment. Diabetologia 1989; 32:434–439.
479. Olivarius NF, Andreasen AH, Keiding N, et al: Epidemiology of renal involvement in newly diagnosed middle-aged and elderly diabetic patients: cross-sectional from the population-based study "Diabetes Care in General Practice," Denmark. Diabetologia 1993; 36:1007–1016.
480. UK Prospective Diabetes Study (UKPDS): X. Urinary albumin excretion over 3 years in diet-treated type 2, (non–insulin-dependent) diabetic patients, and association with hypertension, hyperglycaemia, and hypertriglyceridaemia. Diabetologia 1993; 36:1021–1029.
481. Standl E, Stiegler H: Microalbuminuria in a random cohort of recently diagnosed type 2 (non–insulin-dependent) diabetic patients living in the greater Munich area. Diabetologia 1993; 36:1017–1023.
482. Dinneen SF, Gerstein HC: The association of microalbuminuria and mortality in non–insulin-dependent diabetes mellitus: a systematic overview of the literature. Arch Intern Med 1997; 157:1413–1418.
483. Parving H-H, Gall M-A, Skøtt P, et al: Prevalence and causes of albuminuria in non–insulin-dependent diabetic (NIDDM) patients (abstract). Kidney Int 1990; 37:243.
484. Klein R, Klein BE, Moss SE, et al: Ten-year incidence of gross proteinuria in people with diabetes. Diabetes 1995; 44:916–923.
485. Nelson RG, Bennett PH, Beck GJ, et al: Development and progression of renal disease in Pima Indians with non–insulin-dependent diabetes mellitus. Diabetic Renal Disease Study Group. N Engl J Med 1996; 335:1636–1642.
486. Hostetter TH, Troy JL, Brenner BM: Glomerular hemodynamics in experimental diabetes diabetes mellitus. Kidney Int 1981; 19:410–415.
487. Zatz R, Meyer TW, Renneke HG, et al: Predominance of hemodynamic rather than metabolic factors in the pathogenesis of diabetic glomerulopathy. Proc Natl Acad Sci USA 1985; 82:5963–5967.
488. Zatz R, Dunn BR, Meyer TW, et al: Prevention of diabetic glomerulopathy by pharmacological amelioration of glomerular capillary hypertension. J Clin Invest 1986; 77:1925–1930.
489. Anderson S, Brenner BM: Pathogenesis of diabetic glomerulopathy: hemodynamic considerations. Diabetes Metab Rev 1988; 4:163–177.
490. Anderson S, Komers R: Pathogenesis of diabetic glomerulopathy: the role of glomerular hemodynamic factors. In Mogensen CE (ed). The Kidney and Hypertension in Diabetes Mellitus, 5th ed. Boston, Kluwer, 2000, pp 281–294.
491. Ortola FV, Ballerman BJ, Anderson S, et al: Elevated plasma atrial natriuretic peptide levels in diabetic rats. J Clin Invest 1987; 80:670–674.
492. Zhang PL, Mackenzie HS, Troy JL: Effects of an atrial natriuretic peptide receptor antagonist on glomerular hyperfiltration in diabetic rats. J Am Soc Nephrol 1994; 4:1564–1570.
493. Bank N, Aynedjian HS: Role of EDRF (nitric oxide) in diabetic renal hyperfiltration. Kidney Int 1993; 43:1306–1312.
494. Tolins JP, Shultz PJ, Raij L, et al: Abnormal renal hemodynamic response to reduced renal perfusion pressure in diabetic rats: role of NO. Am J Physiol 1993; 265:F886–F895.
495. O'Bryan GT, Hostetter TH: The renal hemodynamic basis of diabetic nephropathy. Semin Nephrol 1997; 17:93–100.
496. Remuzzi G, Bertani T: Pathophysiology of progressive nephropathies. N Engl J Med 1998; 339:1448–1456.
497. Inberg CM, Palmer M, Schvarcz E, et al: Prevalence of urinary tract symptoms in long-standing type 1 diabetes mellitus. Diabetes Metab 1998; 24:351–354.
498. Pagnoux C, Cazaala JG, Mejean A, et al: Emphysematous pyelonephritis in diabetics. Rev Med Interne 1997; 18:888–892.
499. Patterson JE, Andriole VT: Bacterial urinary tract infections in diabetes. Infect Dis Clin North Am 1997; 11:735–750.
500. Eknoyan G, Qunibi WY, Grisson RT, et al: Renal papillary necrosis: an update. Medicine (Baltimore) 1982; 61:55–73.
501. Griffin MD, Bergtralhn EJ, Larson TS: Renal papillary necrosis: a sixteen-year clinical experience. J Am Soc Nephrol 1995; 6:248–256.
502. Parfrey PS, Griffiths SM, Barrett BJ, et al: Contrast material–induced renal failure in patients with diabetes mellitus, renal insufficiency, or both: a prospective, controlled study. N Engl J Med 1989; 320:143–149.
503. Taliercio CP, Vlietstra RE, Fisher LD: Risks of renal dysfunction with cardiac angiography. Ann Intern Med 1986; 104:501–504.
504. Tepel M, van der Giet M, Scnwarzfeld C, et al: Prevention of radiographic contrast agent–induced reductions in renal function by α-acetylcystein. N Engl J Med 2000; 343:180–184.
505. DeFronzo RA: Hyperkalemia in hyporeninemic hypoaldosteronism. Kidney Int 1980; 17:118–134.
506. Lush DJ, King JA, Fray JC: Pathophysiology of low renin syndromes: sites of renal secretory impairment and prorenin overexpression. Kidney Int 1993; 43:983–999.
507. Oh MS, Carroll HJ, Clemmons JE, et al: A mechanism for hyporeninemic hypoaldosteronism in chronic renal disease. Metabolism 1974; 23:1157–1166.
508. Clark BA, Brown RS, Epstein FH: Effect of atrial natriuretic peptide on potassium-stimulated aldosterone secretion: potential relevance to hypoaldosteronism. J Clin Endocrinol Metab 1992; 75:399–403.
509. Zimran A, Kramer M, Plaskin M, et al: Incidence of hyperkalemia induced by indomethacin in a hospital population. BMJ 1985; 291:107–108.
510. Oates JA, Fitzgerald GA, Branch RA, et al: Clinical implications of prostaglandin and thromboxane A_2 formation. N Engl J Med 1988; 319:761–767.
511. Textor SC, Bravo EL, Fouad FM, et al: Hyperkalemia in azotemic patients during angiotensin-converting enzyme inhibition and aldosterone reduction with captopril. Am J Med 1982; 73:7119–7125.
512. Bantle JP, Nath KA, Sutherland DE, et al: Effect of cyclosporine on the renin-angiotensin system and potassium excretion in renal transplant recipients. Arch Intern Med 1985; 145:505–508.
513. Bangstad HJ, Østerby R, Dahl-Jorgensen K, et al: Improvement of blood glucose control retards the progression of morphological changes in early diabetic nephropathy. Diabetologia 1994; 37:483–490.
514. Rudberg S, Østerby R, Bangstad HJ, et al: Effect of angiotensin-converting enzyme inhibitor or beta blocker on glomerular structural changes in young microalbuminuric patients with type 1 (insulin-dependent) diabetes mellitus. Diabetologia 1999; 42:589–595.
515. Weinrauch LA, Healy RW, Leland OS, et al: Decreased insulin requirement in acute failure in diabetic nephropathy. Arch Intern Med 1978; 138:399–402.
516. Bakris GL, Williams M, Dworkin L, et al: Preserving renal function in adults with hypertension and diabetes: a consensus approach. Am J Kidney Dis 2000; 36:646–661.
517. Lazarus JM, Bourgoignie JJ, Buckalew VM, et al: Achievement and safety of a low BP goal in chronic renal disease. The Modification of Diet in Renal Disease Study Group. Hypertension 1997; 29:641–650.
518. The Microalbuminuria Captopril Study Group: Captopril reduces the risk of nephropathy in IDDM patients with microalbuminuria. Diabetologia 1996; 39:587–593.
519. Ahmad J, Siddiqui MA, Ahmad H: Effective postponement of diabetic nephropathy with enalapril in normotensive type 2 diabetic patients with microalbuminuria. Diabetes Care 1997; 20:1576–1581.
520. Bakris GL, Barnhill BW, Sadler R: Treatment of arterial hypertension in diabetic humans: importance of therapeutic selection. Kidney Int 1992; 41:912–919.
521. Zatz R, Brenner BM: Pathogenesis of diabetic microangiopathy: the hemodynamic view. Am J Med 1986; 80:443–453.
522. Cohen D, Dodds RA, Viberti GC: Effect of protein restriction in insulin-dependent diabetics at risk of nephropathy. BMJ 1987; 294:795–798.
523. Pedrini MT, Levey AS, Lau J, et al: The effect of dietary protein restriction on the progression of diabetic and nondiabetic renal diseases: meta-analysis. Ann Intern Med 1996; 124:627–632.
524. Parving HH: Effects of dietary protein on renal disease. Ann Intern Med 1997; 126:330–331.
525. Jameel N, Pugh JA, Mitchell BD, et al: Dietary protein intake is

not correlated with clinical proteinuria in NIDDM. Diabetes Care 1992; 15:178–183.

526. Joles JA, Kunter U, Janssen U, et al: Early mechanisms of renal injury in hypercholesterolemic or hypertriglyceridemic rats. J Am Soc Nephol 2000; 11:669–683.
527. Oda H, Keane WF: Recent advances in statins and the kidney. Kidney Int 1999; 71(Suppl):S2-S5.
528. Pirson Y: The diabetic patient with ESRD: how to select the modality of renal replacement. Nephrol Dial Transplant 1996; 11:1511–1513.
529. Gruessner RW, Sutherland DE, Troppmann C, et al: The surgical risk of pancreas transplantation in the cyclosporine era: an overview. J Am Coll Surg 1997; 185:128–144.
530. Churchill DN, Thorpe KE, Vonesh EF, et al: Lower probability of survival with continuous peritoneal dialysis in United States compared with Canada. Canada-USA (CANUSA) Peritoneal Dialysis Study Group. J Am Soc Nephol 1997; 8:965–971.
531. Jungers P, Zingraff J, Albouze P: Late referral to maintenance dialysis: detrimental consequences. Nephrol Dial Transplant 1993; 8:1089–1093.
532. Woods JD, Port FK: The impact of vascular access for haemodialysis on patient survival. Nephrol Dial Transplant 1997; 12:657–659.
533. Lameire N, Van Biesen W, Dombros N, et al: The referral pattern of patients with ESRD is a determinant in the choice of dialysis modality. Perit Dial Int 1997; 17(Suppl 2):S161-S166.
534. Weiner P, Parente ST, Garnick DW, et al: Variations in office-based quality: a claims-based profile of care provided to Medicare patients with diabetes. JAMA 1995; 273:1503–1508.
535. Vinik AI, Mitchell BD, Leichter SB, et al. Epidemiology of the complications of diabetes. In Leslie RDG, Robbins DC (eds). Diabetes: Clinical Science in Practice. Cambridge, England, Cambridge University Press, 1995, pp 221–287.
536. Holzer SE, Camerota A, Martens L, et al. Costs and duration of care for lower extremity ulcers in patients with diabetes. Clin Ther 1998; 20:169–181.
537. Caputo GM, Cavanagh PR, Ulbrecht JS, et al. Assessment and management of foot disease in patients with diabetes. N Engl J Med 1994; 331:854–860.
538. Young MJ, Boulton AJM, MacLeod AF, et al. A multicentre study of the prevalence of diabetic peripheral neuropathy in the United Kingdom hospital clinic population. Diabetologia 1993; 36:1–5.
539. Shaw J, Zimmet PZ. The epidemiology of diabetic neuropathy. Diabetes Rev 1999; 7:245–252.
540. Vinik A. Diabetic neuropathy: pathogenesis and therapy. Am J Med 1999; 107:17S-26S.
541. Dyck PJ, Kratz KM, Karnes JL, et al. The prevalence by staged severity of various types of diabetic neuropathy, retinopathy, and nephropathy in a population-based cohort: the Rochester Diabetic Neuropathy Study. Neurology 1993; 43:817–824.
542. Armstrong DG, Lavery LA, Harkless LB. Validation of a diabetic wound classification system: the contribution of depth, infection, and ischemia to risk of amputation. Diabetes Care 1998; 21:855–859.
543. Levitt NS, Stansberry KB, Wychanck S, et al. Natural progression of autonomic neuropathy and autonomic function tests in a cohort of IDDM. Diabetes Care 1996; 19:751–754.
544. Rathmann W, Ziegler D, Jahnke M, et al. Mortality in diabetic patients with cardiovascular autonomic neuropathy. Diabet Med 1993; 10:820–824.
545. Watkins PJ. Progression of diabetic autonomic neuropathy. Diabet Med 1993; 10(Suppl 2):77S–78S.
546. DCCT Research Group. The effect of intensive diabetes therapy on the development and progression of neuropathy. Ann Intern Med 1995; 122:561–568.
547. Ziegler D, Cicmir I, Mayer P, et al. Somatic and autonomic nerve function during the first year after diagnosis of type 1 (insulin-dependent) diabetes. Diabetes Res 1988; 7:123–127.
548. Partanen J, Niskanen L, Lehtinen J, et al. Natural history of peripheral neuropathy in patients with non–insulin-dependent diabetes mellitus. N Engl J Med 1995; 333:89–94.
549. Olsen BS, Sjolie A, Hougaard P, et al. A 6-year nationwide cohort study of glycaemic control in young people with type 1 diabetes: risk markers for the development of retinopathy, nephropathy, and neuropathy. J Diabetes Complications 2000; 14: 295–300.
550. Apfel SC, Kessler JA, Adornato BT, et al. Recombinant human nerve growth factor in the treatment of diabetic polyneuropathy. Neurology 1998; 51:695–702.
551. Vinik AI. Treatment of diabetic polyneuropathy (DPN) with recombinant human nerve growth factor (rhNGF). Diabetes 1999; 48(Suppl 1):A54–A55.
552. Dyck PJ, Kratz KM, Lehman KA, et al. The Rochester Diabetic Neuropathy Study: design, criteria for types of neuropathy, selection bias, and reproducibility of neuropathic tests. Neurology 1991; 41:799–807.
553. Oh SJ. Clinical electromyelography: nerve conduction studies. In Oh SJ (ed). Nerve Conduction in Polyneuropathies. Baltimore, Williams & Wilkins, 1993, pp 579–591.
554. Kennedy WR, Wendelschafer-Crabb G, Johnson T. Quantitation of epidermal nerves in diabetic neuropathy. Neurology 1996; 47: 1042–1048.
555. Herrmann DN, Griffin JW, Hauer P, et al. Epidermal nerve fiber density and sural nerve morphometry in peripheral neuropathies. Neurology 1999; 53:1634–1640.
556. Stansberry KB, Peppard HR, Babyak LM, et al. Primary nociceptive afferents mediate the blood flow dysfunction in non-glabrous (hairy) skin of type 2 diabetes. Diabetes Care 1999; 22:1549–1554.
557. Toyry JP, Partanen JV, Niskanen LK, et al. Divergent development of autonomic and peripheral somatic neuropathies in NIDDM. Diabetologia 1997; 40:953–958.
558. Toyry JP, Niskanen LK, Mantysaari MJ, et al. Occurrence, predictors, and clinical significance of autonomic neuropathy in NIDDM: ten-year follow-up from the diagnosis. Diabetes 1996; 45:308–315.
559. Karamitsos DT, Didangelos TP, Athyros VG, et al. The natural history of recently diagnosed autonomic neuropathy over a period of 2 years. Diabetes Res Clin Pract 1998; 42:55–63.
560. Ziegler D. Diabetic cardiovascular autonomic neuropathy: prognosis, diagnosis, and treatment. Diabetes Metab Rev 1994; 10: 339–383.
561. Consensus Statement. Report and recommendations of the San Antonio conference on diabetic neuropathy. American Diabetes Association American Academy of Neurology. Diabetes Care 1988; 11:592–597.
562. Said G, Goulon-Goreau C, Lacroix C, et al. Nerve biopsy findings in different patterns of proximal diabetic neuropathy. Ann Neurol 1994; 35:559–569.
563. Vinik AI, Suwanwalaikorn S. Autonomic neuropathy. In DeFronzo RA (ed). Current Therapy of Diabetes Mellitus. St Louis, Mosby–Year Book, 1997, pp 165–176.
564. Dyck PJ, Norell JE, Dyck PJ. Microvasculitis and ischemia in diabetic lumbosacral radiculoplexus neuropathy. Neurology 1999; 53:2113–2121.
565. Jaffey PB, Gelman BB. Increased vulnerability to demyelination in streptozotocin diabetic rats. J Comp Neurol 1996; 373:55–61.
566. Upton AR, McComas AJ. The double crush in nerve entrapment syndromes. Lancet 1973; 7825:359–362.
567. Dyck PJ, Lais AC, Giannini C, et al. Structural alterations of nerve during cuff compression. Proc Natl Acad Sci USA 1990; 87:9828–9832.
568. Vinik AI, Holland MT, LeBeau JM, et al. Diabetic neuropathies. Diabetes Care 1992; 15:1926–1975.
569. Sima AAF, Sugimoto K. Experimental diabetic neuropathy: an update. Diabetologia 1999; 42:773–788.
570. Zochodne DW. Diabetic neuropathies: features and mechanisms. Brain Pathol 1999; 9:369–391.
571. Greene DA, Stevens MJ, Obrosova I, et al. Glucose-induced oxidative stress and programmed cell death in diabetic neuropathy. Eur J Pharmacol 1999; 375:217–223.
572. Cameron NE, Cotter MA, Ferguson K, et al. Effects of chronic α–adrenergic receptor blockade on peripheral nerve conduction, hypoxic resistance, polyols, Na^+,K^+-ATPase activity and vascular supply in STZ-D rats. Diabetes 1991; 40:1652–1658.
573. Cameron NE, Cotter MA, Low PA. Nerve blood flow in early experimental diabetes in rats: relation to conduction deficits. Am J Physiol 1991; 261:E1–E8.
574. Greene DA, Lattimer SA, Sima AA. Sorbitol, phosphoinositides, and sodium-potassium-ATPase in the pathogenesis of diabetic complications. N Engl J Med 1987; 316:599–606.
575. Schmidt AM, Hasu M, Zhang JH, et al. Receptor for advanced

glycation end products (AGEs) has central role in vessel wall interactions and gene activation in response to circulating AGE proteins. Proc Natl Acad Sci USA 1994; 91:881–887.

576. Varma SD, Devamanoharan PS, Ali AH. Formation of advanced glycation end (AGE) products in diabetes: prevention by pyruvate and alpha-ketoglutarate. Mol Cell Biochem 1997; 171:23–28.
577. Cameron NE, Cotter MA. Neurovascular dysfunction in diabetic rats: potential contribution of auto-oxidation and free radicals examined using transition metal-chelating agents. J Clin Invest 1995; 96:1159–1163.
578. Van Dam PS, Van Asbeck BS, Erkelens DW, et al. The role of oxidative stress in neuropathy and other diabetic complications. Diabetes Metab Rev 1995; 11:181–192.
579. Low PA, Nickander KK, Tritschler HJ. The roles of oxidative stress and antioxidant treatment in experimental diabetic neuropathy. Diabetes 1997; 46(Suppl 2):S38-S42.
580. Hellweg R, Hartung HD. Endogenous levels of nerve growth factor (NGF) are altered in experimental diabetes mellitus: a possible role for NGF in the pathiogenesis of diabetic neuropathy. J Neurosci Res 1990; 26:258–267.
581. Vinik AI, Pittenger GL, Stansberry KB, et al. Phospholipid and glutamic acid decarboxylase autoantibodies in diabetic neuropathy. Diabetes Care 1995; 18:1225–1232.
582. Bansal AS, Abdul-Karim B, Malik RA, et al. IgM ganglioside GM1 antibodies in patients with autoimmune disease or neuropathy, and controls. J Clin Pathol 1994; 47:300–302.
583. Ohsawa T, Miyatake T, Yuki N. Anti–B series ganglioside-recognizing autoantibodies in an acute sensory neuropathy patient cause cell death of rat dorsal root ganglion neurons. Neurosci Lett 1993; 157:167–170.
584. Ogino M, Orazio N, Latov N. IgG anti-GM1 antibodies from patients with acute motor neuropathy are predominantly of the IgG1 and IgG3 subclasses. J Neuroimmunol 1995; 58:77–80.
585. Guijo CG, Garcia-Merino A, Rubio G. Presence and isotype of anti-ganglioside antibodies in healthy persons, motor neuron disease, peripheral neuropathy, and other disease of the nervous system. J Neuroimmunol 1995; 56:27–33.
586. Vinik AI, Pittenger GL, Milicevic Z et al. Autoimmune Mechanisms in the Pathogenesis of Diabetic Neuropathy. In Eisenbarth RG (ed). Molecular Mechanisms of Endocrine and Organ Specific Autoimmunity. Georgetown, Landes, 1998, pp 217–251.
587. Tesfaye S, Malik RA, Ward JD. Vascular factors in diabetic neuropathy. Diabetologia 1994; 37:847–854.
588. Younger DS, Rosoklija G, Hays AP. Diabetic peripheral neuropathy. Semin Neurol 1998; 18:95–104.
589. Young MJ, Bennett JL, Liderth SA, et al. Rheological and microvascular parameters in diabetic peripheral neuropathy. Clin Sci 1996; 90:183–187.
590. McKenzie D, Nukada H, van Rij AM, et al. Endoneurial microvascular abnormalities of sural nerve in non-diabetic chronic atherosclerotic occlusive disease. J Neurol Sci 1999; 162:84–88.
591. Malik RA, Tesfaye S, Thompson SD, et al. Transperineurial capillary abnormalities in the sural nerve of patients with diabetic neuropathy. Microvasc Res 1994; 48:236–245.
592. Britland ST, Young RJ, Sharma AK, et al. Relationship of endoneurial capillary abnormalities to type and severity of diabetic polyneuropathy. Diabetes 1990; 39:909–913.
593. Malik RA, Veves A, Masson EA, et al. Endoneurial capillary abnormalities in human diabetic neuropathy. J Neurol Neurosurg Psychiatry 1992; 55:557–561.
594. Tesfaye S, Harris N, Jakubowski J, et al. Impaired blood flow and arteriovenous shunting in human diabetic neuropathy: a novel technique of nerve photography and fluorescein angiography. Diabetologia 1993; 36:1266–1274.
595. Young MJ, Veves A, Walker MG, et al. Correlations between nerve function and tissue oxygenation in diabetic patients: further clues to the aetiology of diabetic neuropathy? Diabetologia 1992; 35:1146–1150.
596. Stansberry KB, Shapiro SA, Hill MA, et al. Impaired peripheral vasomotion in diabetes. Diabetes Care 1996; 19:715–721.
597. Stansberry KB, Hill MA, Shapiro SA, et al. Impairment of peripheral blood flow responses in diabetes resembles an enhanced aging effect. Diabetes Care 1997; 20:1711–1716.
598. Benbow SJ, Pryce DW, Noblett K, et al. Flow motion in peripheral diabetic neuropathy. Clin Sci 1995; 88:191–196.
599. Veves A, Quist W, Caballero E, et al. Expression of endothelial nitric oxide synthase (eNOS) in the skin microvasculature. Diabetes 2000; 49:A150.
600. Stansberry KB, Scanelli JA, McNitt PM, et al. Nitric oxide production mediates neurogenic vasodilation in human skin but is not impaired in type 2 diabetes. Diabetes 2000; 49(Suppl 1):A33.
601. Tooke J, Goh K. Vascular function in type 2 diabetes mellitus and pre-diabetes: the case for intrinsic endotheliopathy. Diabet Med 1999; 16:710–715.
602. Caballero AE, Arora S, Saouaf R, et al. Microvascular and macrovascular reactivity is reduced in subjects at risk for type 2 diabetes. Diabetes 1999; 48:1856–1862.
603. Liu GZ, Ishihara H, Osada R, et al. Nitric oxide mediates the change of proteoglycan synthesis in the human lumbar intervertebral disc in response to hydrostatic pressure. Spine 2001; 26:134–141.
604. Apfel SC. Neurotrophic factors in peripheral neuropathies: therapeutic implications. Brain Pathol 1999; 9:393–413.
605. Ishii DN. Implications of insulin-like growth factors in the pathogenesis of diabetic neuropathy. Brain Res Rev 1995; 20:47–67.
606. Tomlinson DR, Fernygough P. Neurotrophism in diabetic neuropathy. In Sima AAF (ed). Frontiers in Animal Diabetes Research: Chronic Complications in Diabetes. Amsterdam, Harwood, 1999, pp 167–182.
607. Schmidt RE, Dorsey DA, Beaudet LN, et al. Insulin-like growth factor I reverses experimental diabetic autonomic neuropathy. Am J Pathol 1999; 155:1651–1660.
608. Apfel SC. Neurotrophic factors in the therapy of diabetic neuropathy. Am J Med 1999; 107(Suppl 2):34S-42S.
609. Rask CA. Biological actions of nerve growth factor in the peripheral nervous system. Eur Neurol 1999; 41(Suppl 1):14–19.
610. Verge VM, Tetzlaff W, Bisby MA, et al. Influence of nerve growth factor on neurofilament gene expression in mature primary sensory neurons. J Neurosci 1990; 10:2018–2025.
611. Gold BG, Mizisin A, Matheson SF. Regulation of axonal caliber, neurofilament content, and nuclear localization in mature sensory neurons by nerve growth factor. J Neurosci 1991; 11:943–955.
612. Ishii DN. Insulin and related neurotrophic factors in diabetic neuropathy. Diabetic Med 1993; 10(Suppl 2):14S-15S.
613. Russell JW, Feldman EL. Insulin-like growth factor-I prevents apoptosis in sympathetic neurons exposed to high glucose. Horm Metab Res 1999; 31:90–96.
614. Cortizo AM, Lee PD, Cedola NV, et al. Relationship between non-enzymatic glycosylation and changes in serum insulin-like growth factor-1 (IGF-1) and IGF-binding protein-3 levels in patients with type 2 diabetes mellitus. Acta Diabetol 1998; 35:85–90.
615. Rivas RJ, Burneister DWA, Goldberg DJ. Rapid effects of laminin on the growth cone. Neuron 1992; 8:107–115.
616. Pittenger G, Erbas T, Burcus N, et al. Serum from patients with diabetic neuropathy impairs laminin neuroprotection by altering laminin receptor integrin expression. Diabetes 2000; 49(Suppl 1): A34.
617. Gold BG. Neuroimmunophilin ligands: evaluation of their therapeutic potential for the treatment of neurological disorders. Expert Opin Investig Drug 2000; 9:2331–2342.
618. Coyle JT. The Nagging Question of the function of *N*-acetylaspartylglutamate. Neurobiol Dis 1997; 4:231–238.
619. Sen CK. Redox signaling and the emerging therapeutic potential of thiol antioxidants. Biochem Pharmacol 1998; 55:1747–1758.
620. Kashiwagi A, Asahina T, Nishio Y, et al. Glycation, oxidative stress, and scavenger activity: glucose metabolism and radical scavenger dysfunction in endothelial cells. Diabetes 1996; 45:S84-S86.
621. Giugliano D, Ceriello A, Paolisso G. Oxidative stress and diabetic vascular complications. Diabetes Care 1996; 19:257–267.
622. Pieper GM, Langenstroer P, Siebeneich W. Diabetic-induced endothelial dysfunction in rat aorta: role of hydroxyl radicals. Cardiovasc Res 1997; 34:145–156.
623. Brownlee M. Negative consequences of glycation. Metabolism 2000; 49:9–13.
624. Bierhaus A, Chevion S, Chevion M, et al. Advanced glycation end product–induced activation of NF-kappa B is suppressed by alpha-lipoic acid in cultured endothelial cells. Diabetes 1997; 46: 1481–1490.
625. Collins T, Read MA, Neish AS, et al. Transcriptional regulation

of endothelial cell adhesion molecules: NF-kappa B and cytokine-inducible enhancers. FASEB J 1995; 9:899–909.
626. Chang MH, Lee SS, Ger LP, et al. Oral drug of choice in carpal tunnel syndrome. Neurology 1998; 51:390–393.
627. O'Gradaigh D, Merry P. Corticosteroid injection for the treatment of carpal tunnel syndrome. Ann Rheum Dis 2000; 59:918–919.
628. Arle JE, Zager EL. Surgical treatment of common entrapment neuropathies in the upper limbs. Muscle Nerve 2000; 23:1160–1174.
629. Llewelyn JG, Thomas PK, King RH. Epineurial microvasculitis in proximal diabetic neuropathy. J Neurol 1998; 245:159–165.
630. Vinik AI, Pittenger GL, Milicevic Z, et al. Autoimmune mechanisms in the pathogenesis of diabetic neuropathy. In Eisenbarth RG (ed). Molecular Mechanisms of Endocrine and Organ-Specific Autoimmunity. Georgetown, Landes, 1999, pp 217–251.
631. Steck AJ, Kappos L. Gangliosides and autoimmune neuropathies: classification and clinical aspects of autoimmune neuropathies. J Neurol Neurosurg Psychiatry 1994; 57(Suppl):26–28.
632. Sander HW, Chokroverty S. Diabetic amyotrophy: current concepts. Semin Neurol 1996; 16:173–178.
633. Krendel DA, Costigan DA, Hopkins LC. Successful treatment of neuropathies in patients with diabetes mellitus. Arch Neurol 1995; 52:1053–1061.
634. Britland ST, Young RJ, Sharma AK, et al. Acute and remitting painful diabetic polyneuropathy: a comparison of peripheral nerve fibre pathology. Pain 1992; 48:361–370.
635. Milicevic Z, Newlon PG, Pittenger GL, et al. Antiganglioside GM1 antibody and distal symmetrical "diabetic polyneuropathy" with dominant motor features. Diabetologia 1997; 40:1364–1365.
636. Barada A, Reljanovic M, Milicevic Z, et al. Proximal diabetic neuropathy: response to immunotherapy. Diabetes 1999; 48(Suppl 1):A148.
637. Bird SJ, Brown MJ. The clinical spectrum of diabetic neuropathy. Semin Neurol 1996; 16:115–122.
638. Hanson PH, Schumaker P, Debugne TH, et al. Evaluation of somatic and autonomic small-fiber neuropathy in diabetes. Am J Phys Med Rehabil 1992; 71:44–47.
639. McArthur JC, Stocks EA, Hauer P. Epidermal nerve fiber density: normative reference range and diagnostic efficiency. Arch Neurol 1998; 55:1513–1520.
640. Tesfaye S, Malik R, Harris N, et al. Arterio-venous shunting and proliferating new vessels in acute painful neuropathy of rapid glycaemic control (insulin neuritis). Diabetologia 1996; 39:329–335.
641. Van Heel DA, Levitt NS, Winter TA. Diabetic neuropathic cachexia: the importance of positive recognition and early nutritional support. Int J Clin Pract 1998; 52:591–592.
642. Holland NR, Crawford TO, Hauer P. Small-fiber sensory neuropathies: clinical course and neuropathology of idiopathic cases. Ann Neurol 1998; 44:47–59.
643. Said G, Bigo A, Ameri A, et al. Uncommon early-onset neuropathy in diabetic patients. J Neurol 1998; 245:61–68.
644. Vinik EJ, Stansberry KB, Zarrabi L, et al. Development of a sensitive, specific quality of life inventory for peripheral neuropathy. Diabetes 2000; 49(Suppl 1):A819.
645. Resnick H, Vinik A, Schwartz A, et al. Independent effects of peripheral nerve dysfunction on lower extremity physical function in old age. Diabetes Care 2000; 23:1642–1647.
646. Vinik A. Diagnosis and management of diabetic neuropathy. Clin Geriatr Med 1999; 15:293–319.
647. Vinik AI, Park TS, Stansberry KB, et al. Diabetic neuropathies. Diabetologia 2000; 48:957–973.
648. Vinik AI. Diagnosis and management of diabetic neuropathy. Can J Diabetes Care 2000; 24:56–76.
649. Dyck PJ. Detection, characterization, and staging of polyneuropathy: assessed in diabetes. Muscle Nerve 1988; 11:21–32.
650. Vinik AI, Mitchell B. Clinical aspects of diabetic neuropathies. Diabetes Metab Rev 1988; 4:223–253.
651. Ziegler D, Hanefeld M, Ruhnau KJ, et al. Treatment of symptomatic diabetic peripheral neuropathy with the antioxidant alpha-lipoic acid: a 3-week multicentre randomized controlled trial (ALADIN Study). Diabetologia 1995; 38:1425–1433.
652. Feldman EL, Stevens MJ, Thomas PK, et al. A practical two-step quantitative clinical and electrophysiological assessment for the diagnosis and staging of diabetic neuropathy. Diabetes Care 1994; 17:1281–1289.
653. Vinik AI, Newlon P, Milicevic Z, et al. Diabetic neuropathies: an overview of clinical aspects. In LeRoith D, Taylor SI, Olefsky JM (eds). Diabetes Mellitus: A Fundamental and Clinical Text. Philadelphia, Lippincott-Raven, 1996, pp 737–751.
654. Vinik AI, Suwanwalaikorn S, Stansberry KB, et al. Quantitative measurement of cutaneous perception in diabetic neuropathy. Muscle Nerve 1995; 18:574–584.
655. Ducher M, Thivolet C, Cerutti C, et al. Noninvasive exploration of cardiac autonomic neuropathy. Diabetes Care 1999; 22:388–393.
656. Jaradeh SS, Prieto TE, Lobeck LJ. Progressive polyradiculoneuropathy in diabetes: correlation of variables and clinical outcome after immunotherapy. J Neurol Neurosurg Psychiatry 1999; 67: 607–612.
657. Periquet MI, Novak V, Collins MP, et al. Painful sensory neuropathy: prospective evaluation using skin biopsy. Neurology 1999; 53:1641–1647.
658. Krendel DA, Zacharias A, Younger DS. Autoimmune diabetic neuropathy. Neurol Clin 1997; 15:959–971.
659. Pirart J. (Diabetes mellitus and its degenerative complications: a prospective study of 4,400 patients observed between 1947 and 1973 (3rd and last part) (author's transl)). Diabetes Metab 1977; 3:245–256.
660. UK Prospective Diabetes Study (UKPDS) Group. Effect of intensive blood-glucose control with metformin on complications in overweight patients with type 2 diabetes (UKPDS 34). Lancet 1998; 352:854–865.
661. UK Prospective Diabetes Study Group. Tight blood pressure control and risk of macrovascular and microvascular complications in type 2 diabetes: UKPDS 38. BMJ 1998; 317:703–713.
662. Gaede P, Vedel P, Parving HH, et al. Intensified multifactorial intervention in patients with type 2 diabetes mellitus and microalbuminuria: the Steno type 2 randomised study. Lancet 1999; 353:617–622.
663. Boulton AJM, Levin S, Comstock J. A multicentre trial of the aldose reductase inhibitor, tolrestat, in patients with symptomatic diabetic neuropathy. Diabetologia 1990; 33:431–437.
664. Didangelos TP, Karamitsos DT, Athyros VG, et al. Effect of aldose reductase inhibition on cardiovascular reflex tests in patients with definite diabetic autonomic neuropathy. J Diabetes Complications 1998; 12:201–207.
665. Greene DA, Arezzo JC, Brown MB. Effect of aldose reductase inhibition on nerve conduction and morphometry in diabetic neuropathy. Zenarestat Study Group. Neurology 1999; 53:580–591.
666. Johnson BF, Law G, Nesto R, et al. Aldose reductase inhibitor zopolrestat improves systolic function in diabetics. Diabetes 1999; 48(Suppl 1):A133.
667. Ziegler D, Schatz H, Conrad F, et al. Effects of treatment with the antioxidant alpha-lipoic acid on cardiac autonomic neuropathy in NIDDM patients: a 4-month randomized controlled multicenter trial (DEKAN Study). Deutsche Kardiale Autonome Neuropathie. Diabetes Care 1997; 20:369–373.
668. Ziegler D, Gries FA. Alpha-lipoic acid in the treatment of diabetic peripheral and cardiac autonomic neuropathy. Diabetes 1997; 46(Suppl 2):S62-S66.
669. Ziegler D, Hanefeld M, Ruhnau KJ, et al. Treatment of symptomatic diabetic polyneuropathy with the antioxidant alpha-lipoic acid: a 7-month multicenter randomized controlled trial (ALADIN III Study). ALADIN III Study Group. Alpha-Lipoic Acid in Diabetic Neuropathy. Diabetes Care 1999; 22:1296–1301.
670. Jamal GA. The use of gamma linolenic acid in the prevention and treatment of diabetic neuropathy. Diabet Med 1994; 11:145–149.
671. Keen H, Payan J, Allawi J, et al. Treatment of diabetic neuropathy with γ-linolenic acid. Diabetes Care 1993; 16:8–15.
672. Miyauchi Y, Shikama H, Takasu T, et al. Slowing of peripheral motor nerve conduction was ameliorated by aminoguanidine in streptozocin-induced diabetic rats. Eur J Endocrinol 1996; 134: 467–473.
673. Schmidt RE, Dorsey DA, Beaudet LN, et al. Effect of aminoguanidine on the frequency of neuroaxonal dystrophy in the superior mesenteric sympathetic autonomic ganglia of rats with streptozotocin-induced diabetes. Diabetes 1996; 45:284–290.
674. Rahbar S, Kumar Yernini K, Scott S, et al. Novel inhibitors of

advanced glycation end products. Biochem Biophys Res Commun 1999; 262:651–656.

675. Nargi SE, Colen LB, Liuzzi F, et al. PTB treatment restores joint mobility in a new model of diabetic cheirothropathy. Diabetes 1999; 48(Suppl 1):A17.
676. Suez D. Intravenous immunoglobulin therapy: indication, potential side effects, and treatment guidelines. J Intraven Nurs 1995; 18:178–190.
677. Diemel LT, Stevens JC, Willars GB, et al. Depletion of substance P and calcitonin gene-related peptide in sciatic nerve of rats with experimental diabetes: effects of insulin and aldose reductase inhibition. Neurosci Lett 1992; 137:253–256.
678. Hellweg R, Wohrle M, Hartung HD. Diabetes mellitus associated decrease in nerve growth factor levels is reversed by allogenetic pancreatic islet transplantation. Neurosci Lett 1991; 125:1–4.
679. Tomlinson DR, Fernyhough P, Diemel LT. Neurotrophins and peripheral neuropathy. Philos Trans R Soc Lond B Biol Sci 1996; 351:455–462.
680. Apfel SC, Kessler JA. Neurotropic factors in the therapy of peripheral neuropathy. Bailliere Clin Neuropath 1995; 4:593–606.
681. Apfel SC, Schwartz S, Adornato BT, et al. Efficacy and safety of recombinant human nerve growth factor in patients with diabetic polyneuropathy: a randomized, controlled trial. JAMA 2000; 284: 2215–2221.
682. Sindrup SH, Jensen TS. Efficacy of pharmacological treatments of neuropathic pain: an update and effect related to mechanism of drug action. Pain 1999; 83:389–400.
683. Szallasi A, Di Marzo V. New perspectives on enigmatic vanilloid receptors. Trends Neurosci 2000; 23:491–497.
684. Caterina MJ, Leffler A, Malmberg AB, et al. Impaired nociception and pain sensation in mice lacking the capsaicin receptor. Science 2000; 288:306–313.
685. Rains C, Bryson HM. Topical capsaicin: a review of its pharmacological properties and therapeutic potential in post-herpetic neuralgia, diabetic neuropathy, and osteoarthritis. Drugs Aging 1995; 7:317–328.
686. Bays-Smith MG, Max MB, Muir J, et al. Transdermal clonidine compared to placebo in painful diabetic neuropathy using a two-stage "enriched enrollment" design. Pain 1995; 60:267–274.
687. Harati Y, Gooch C, Swenson M, et al. Double-blind randomized trial of tramadol for the treatment of the pain of diabetic neuropathy. Neurology 1998; 50:1842–1846.
688. Nelson KA, Park KM, Robinovitz E, et al. High-dose oral dextromethorphan versus placebo in painful diabetic neuropathy and postherpetic neuralgia. Neurology 1997; 48:1212–1218.
689. Max M, Lynch S, Muir J. Effects of desipramine, amitryptylline, and fluoxetine on pain in diabetic neuropathy. N Engl J Med 1992; 326:1250–1256.
690. Gorson KC, Schott C, Herman R, et al. Gabapentin in the treatment of painful diabetic neuropathy: a placebo-controlled, double-blind, crossover trial. J Neurol Neurosurg Psychiatry 1999; 66:251–252.
691. Backonja M, Beydoun A, Edwards KR, et al. Gabapentin for the symptomatic treatment of painful neuropathy in patients with diabetes mellitus. JAMA 1998; 280:1831–1836.
692. Vinik A, Fonseca V, LaMoreaux L, et al. Neurontin (gabapentin, GBP) improves quality of life (QOL) in patients with painful diabetic peripheral neuropathy. Diabetes 1998; 47(Suppl 1):A374.
693. Somers DL, Somers MF. Treatment of neuropathic pain in a patient with diabetic neuropathy using transcutaneous electrical nerve stimulation applied to the skin of the lumbar region. Phys Ther 1999; 79:767–775.
694. Cavanagh PR, Derr JA, Ulbrecht JS, et al. Problems with gait and posture in neuropathic patients with insulin-dependent diabetes mellitus. Diabet Med 1992; 9:469–474.
695. Nelson ME, Fiatarone MA, Morganti CM, et al. Effects of high-intensity strength training on multiple risk factors for osteoporotic fractures: a randomized, controlled trial. JAMA 1994; 272: 1909–1914.
696. Zola BE, Vinik AI. Effects of autonomic neuropathy associated with diabetes mellitus on cardiovascular function. Coron Artery Dis 1992; 3:33–41.
697. Hilz MJ, Hecht MJ, Berghoff M, et al. Abnormal vasoreaction to arousal stimuli: an early sign of diabetic sympathetic neuropathy demonstrated by laser Doppler flowmetry. J Clin Neurophysiol 2000; 17:419–425.
698. Haak ES, Usadel KH, Kohleisen M, et al. The effect of alpha-lipoic acid on the neurovascular reflex arc in patients with diabetic neuropathy assessed by capillary microscopy. Microvasc Res 1999; 58:28–34.
699. Valensi P. Diabetic autonomic neuropathy: what are the risks? Diabetes Metab 1998; 24:66–72.
700. Vinik AI, Suwanwalaikorn S. Autonomic neuropathy. In DeFronzo RA (ed). Current Therapy of Diabetes Mellitus. St. Louis, Mosby, 1997, pp 165–176.
701. Vinik A, Erbas T, Stansberry KB. Gastrointestinal, genitourinary, and neurovascular disturbances in diabetes. Diabetes Rev 1999; 7: 358–378.
702. Vinik A, Glass L. Diabetic autonomic neuropathy. Clin Diabetes Mellitus 2000; 3:637–647.
703. Mancia G, Paleari F, Parati G. Early diagnosis of diabetic autonomic neuropathy: present and future approaches. Diabetologia 1997; 40:482–484.
704. Athyros VG, Didangelos TP, Karamitsos DT, et al. Long-term effect of converting enzyme inhibition on circadian sympathetic and parasympathetic modulation in patients with diabetic autonomic neuropathy. Acta Cardiol 1998; 53:201–209.
705. Malmberg K, Norhammar A, Wedel H, et al. Glycometabolic state at admission. Important risk marker of mortality in conventionally treated patients with diabetes mellitus and acute myocardial infarction: long-term results from the Diabetes and Insulin-Glucose Infusion in Acute Myocardial Infarction (DIGAMI) study. Circulation 1999; 99:2626–2632.
706. Kendall DM, Rooney DP, Smets YF, et al. Pancreas transplantation restores epinephrine response and symptom recognition during hypoglycemia in patients with long-standing type I diabetes and autonomic neuropathy. Diabetes 1997; 46:249–257.
707. Burger AJ, Weinrauch LA, D'Elia JA, et al. Effects of glycemic control on heart rate variability in type I diabetic patients with cardiac autonomic neuropathy. Am J Cardiol 1999; 84:687–691.
708. Laederach-Hofmann K, Weidmann P, Ferrari P. Hypovolemia contributes to the pathogenesis of orthostatic hypotension in patients with diabetes mellitus. Am J Med 1999; 106:50–58.
709. Denq JC, Opfer-Gehrking TL, Giuliani M, et al. Efficacy of compression of different capacitance beds in the amelioration of orthostatic hypotension. Clin Auton Res 1997; 7:321–326.
710. Annese V, Bassotti G, Caruso N, et al. Gastrointestinal motor dysfunction, symptoms, and neuropathy in non–insulin-dependent (type 2) diabetes mellitus. J Clin Gastroenterol 1999; 29: 171–177.
711. Melga P, Mansi C, Ciuchi E, et al. Chronic administration of levosulpiride and glycemic control in IDDM patients with gastroparesis. Diabetes Care 1997; 20:55–58.
712. Stacher G, Schernthaner G, Francesconi M, et al. Cisapride versus placebo for 8 weeks on glycemic control and gastric emptying in insulin-dependent diabetes: a double-blind cross-over trial. J Clin Endocrinol Metab 1999; 84:2357–2362.
713. Barone JA. Domperidone: a peripherally acting dopamine$_2$-receptor antagonist. Ann Pharmacother 1999; 33:429–440.
714. Silvers D, Kipnes M, Broadstone V, et al. Domperidone in the management of symptoms of diabetic gastroparesis: efficacy, tolerability, and quality-of-life outcomes in a multicenter controlled trial. DOM-USA-5 Study Group. Clin Ther 1998; 20:438–453.
715. Erbas T, Varoglu E, Erbas B, et al. Comparison of metoclopramide and erythromycin in the treatment of diabetic gastroparesis. Diabetes Care 1993; 16:1511–1514.
716. Vinik AI, Richardson D. Erectile dysfunction in diabetes. Diabetes Rev 1998; 6:16–33.
717. Vinik AI, Richardson D. Erectile dysfunction in diabetes: pills for penile failure. Clin Diabetes 1998; 16:108–119.
718. Cheitlin MD, Hutter AM, Brindis RG, et al. Use of sildenafil (Viagra) in patients with cardiovascular disease. Technology and Practice Executive Committee. Circulation 1999; 99:168–177.
719. Shaw JE, Parker R, Hollis S, et al. Gustatory sweating in diabetes mellitus. Diabet Med 1996; 13:1033–1037.
720. Shaw JE, Abbott CA, Tindle K, et al. A randomised, controlled trial of topical glycopyrrolate, the first specific treatment for diabetic gustatory sweating. Diabetologia 1997; 40:299–301.
721. Selby JV, Ray GT, Zhang D, et al. Excess costs of medical care for patients with diabetes in a managed care population. Diabetes Care 1997; 20:1396–1402.
722. Harris MI. Diabetes in America: epidemiology and scope of the problem. Diabetes Care 1998; 21(Suppl 3):C11–C14.

723. Gu K, Cowie CC, Harris MI. Diabetes and decline in heart disease mortality in US adults. JAMA 1999; 281:1291–1297.
724. Kannel WB, McGee DL. Diabetes and cardiovascular disease. The Framingham study. JAMA 1979; 241:2035–2038.
725. Stamler J, Vaccaro O, Neaton JD, et al. Diabetes, other risk factors, and 12-year cardiovascular mortality for men screened in the Multiple Risk Factor Intervention Trial. Diabetes Care 1993; 16:434–444.
726. Haffner SM, Lehto S, Ronnemaa T, et al. Mortality from coronary heart disease in subjects with type 2 diabetes and in nondiabetic subjects with and without prior myocardial infarction. N Engl J Med 1998; 339:229–234.
727. Krolewski AS, Warram JH, Rand LI, et al. Epidemiologic approach to the etiology of type I diabetes mellitus and its complications. N Engl J Med 1987; 317:1390–1398.
728. Wilson PW, Kannel WB, Silbershatz H, et al. Clustering of metabolic factors and coronary heart disease. Arch Intern Med 1999; 159:1104–1109.
729. Turner RC. The UK Prospective Diabetes Study: a review. Diabetes Care 1998; 21(Suppl 3):C35–C38.
730. Andersson DK, Svardsudd K. Long-term glycemic control relates to mortality in type II diabetes. Diabetes Care 1995; 18:1534–1543.
731. Wei M, Gaskill SP, Haffner SM, et al. Effects of diabetes and level of glycemia on all-cause and cardiovascular mortality. The San Antonio Heart Study. Diabetes Care 1998; 21:1167–1172.
732. Klein R, Klein BE, Moss SE. The Wisconsin Epidemiologic Study of Diabetic Retinopathy: XVI. The relationship of C-peptide to the incidence and progression of diabetic retinopathy. Diabetes 1995; 44:796–801.
733. Wingard DL, Barrett-Connor EL, Scheidt-Nave C, et al. Prevalence of cardiovascular and renal complications in older adults with normal or impaired glucose tolerance or NIDDM: a population-based study. Diabetes Care 1993; 16:1022–1025.
734. Folsom AR, Eckfeldt JH, Weitzman S, et al. Relation of carotid artery wall thickness to diabetes mellitus, fasting glucose and insulin, body size, and physical activity. Atherosclerosis Risk in Communities (ARIC) Study Investigators. Stroke 1994; 25:66–73.
735. Temelkova-Kurktschiev TS, Koehler C, Leonhardt W, et al. Increased intimal-medial thickness in newly detected type 2 diabetes: risk factors. Diabetes Care 1999; 22:333–338.
736. Wagenknecht LE, D'Agostino RB Jr, Haffner SM, et al. Impaired glucose tolerance, type 2 diabetes, and carotid wall thickness. The Insulin Resistance Atherosclerosis Study. Diabetes Care 1998; 21:1812–1818.
737. Hanefeld M, Koehler C, Schaper F, et al. Postprandial plasma glucose is an independent risk factor for increased carotid intima-media thickness in non-diabetic individuals. Atherosclerosis 1999; 144:229–235.
738. Bonora E, Kiechl S, Willeit J, et al. Prevalence of insulin resistance in metabolic disorders. The Bruneck Study. Diabetes 1998; 47:1643–1649.
739. Deedwania PC. The deadly quartet revisited. Am J Med 1998; 105:1S-3S.
740. Howard G, O'Leary DH, Zaccaro D, et al. Insulin sensitivity and atherosclerosis. The Insulin Resistance Atherosclerosis Study (IRAS) Investigators. Circulation 1996; 93:1809–1817.
741. Despres JP, Lamarche B, Mauriege P, et al. Hyperinsulinemia as an independent risk factor for ischemic heart disease. N Engl J Med 1996; 334:952–957.
742. Abraira C, Colwell J, Nuttall F, et al. Cardiovascular events and correlates in the Veterans Affairs Diabetes Feasibility Trial. Veterans Affairs Cooperative Study on Glycemic Control and Complications in Type II Diabetes. Arch Intern Med 1997; 157:181–188.
743. Gowri MS, Van der Westhuyzen DR, Bridges SR, et al. Decreased protection by HDL from poorly controlled type 2 diabetic subjects against LDL oxidation may be due to the abnormal composition of HDL. Arterioscler Thromb Vasc Biol 1999; 19: 2226–2233.
744. The Long-Term Intervention with Pravastatin in Ischemic Disease (LIPID) Study Group. Prevention of cardiovascular events and death in pravastatin I patients with coronary heart disease and a broad range of initial cholesterol levels. N Engl J Med 1998; 339:1349–1357.
745. Haffner SM, Alexander CM, Cook TJ, et al. Reduced coronary events in simvastatin-treated patients with coronary heart disease and diabetes or impaired glucose levels. Arch Intern Med 1999; 159:2661–2667.
746. Rubins HB, Robins SJ, Collins D, et al. Gemfibrozil for the secondary prevention of coronary heart disease in men with low levels of high-density lipoprotein cholesterol. Veterans Affairs High-Density Lipoprotein Cholesterol Intervention Trial Study Group. N Engl J Med 1999; 341:410–418.
747. Expert Panel on Detection, Evaluation, and Treatment of High Blood Cholesterol in Adults. Executive Summary of the Third Report of the National Cholesterol Education Program (NCEP) Expert Panel on Detection, Evaluation, and Treatment of High Blood Cholesterol in Adults (Adult Treatment Panel III). JAMA 2001; 285:2486–2497.
748. Joint National Committee on Prevention, Detection, Evaluation, and Treatment of High Blood Pressure. The Sixth Report of the Joint National Committee on Prevention, Detection, Evaluation, and Treatment of High Blood Pressure (JNC VI). Arch Intern Med 1997; 157:2413–2446.
749. Curb JD, Pressel SL, Cutler JA, et al. Effect of diuretic based antihypertensive treatment on cardiovascular disease risk in older diabetic patients with isolated systolic hypertension. JAMA 1996; 276:1886–1892.
750. Tuomilehto J, Rastenyte D, Birkenhager WH, et al. Effects of calcium-channel blockade in older patients with diabetes and systolic hypertension. Systolic Hypertension in Europe Trial Investigators. N Engl J Med 1999; 340:677–684.
751. The Heart Outcomes Prevention Evaluation Study Investigators. Effects of an angiotensin-converting enzyme inhibitor, ramipril, on cardiovascular events in high-risk patients. N Engl J Med 2000; 342:145–153.
752. Efficacy of atenolol and captopril in reducing risk of macrovascular and microvascular complications in type 2 diabetes: UKPDS 39. UK Prospective Diabetes Study Group. BMJ 1998; 317:713–720.
753. Hansson L, Zanchetti A, Carruthers SG, et al. Effects of intensive blood pressure lowering and low-dose aspirin in patients with hypertension: principal results of the Hypertension Optimal Treatment (HOT) randomised trial. HOT Study Group. Lancet 1998; 351:1755–1762.
754. Nesto RW, Zarich S: Acute myocardial infarction in diabetes mellitus: lessons learned from ACE inhibition. Circulation 1998; 97:12–15.
755. Jacoby RM, Nesto RW. Acute myocardial infarction in the diabetic patient: pathophysiology, clinical course and prognosis. J Am Coll Cardiol 1992; 20:736–744.
756. Iwasaka T, Takahashi N, Nakamura S, et al. Residual left ventricular pump function after acute myocardial infarction in NIDDM patients. Diabetes Care 1992; 15:1522–1526.
757. Bernardi L, Ricordi L, Lazzari P, et al. Impaired circadian modulation of sympathovagal activity in diabetes: a possible explanation for altered temporal onset of cardiovascular disease. Circulation 1992; 86:1443–1452.
758. Zarich S, Waxman S, Freeman RT, et al. Effect of autonomic nervous system dysfunction on the circadian pattern of myocardial ischemia in diabetes mellitus. J Am Coll Cardiol 1994; 24: 956–962.
759. Muller JE, Tofler GH, Stone PH. Circadian variation and triggers of onset of acute cardiovascular disease. Circulation 1989; 79:733–743.
760. Imperatore G, Riccardi G, Iovine C, et al. Plasma fibrinogen—a new factor of the metabolic syndrome: a population-based study. Diabetes Care 1998; 21:649–654.
761. Sobel BE, Woodcock-Mitchell J, Schneider DJ, et al. Increased plasminogen activator inhibitor type 1 in coronary artery atherectomy specimens from type 2 diabetic compared with nondiabetic patients: a potential factor predisposing to thrombosis and its persistence. Circulation 1998; 97:2213–2221.
762. Meigs JB, Mittleman MA, Nathan DM, et al. Hyperinsulinemia, hyperglycemia, and impaired hemostasis. The Framingham Offspring Study. JAMA 2000; 283:221–228.
763. Woodfield SL, Lundergan CF, Reiner JS, et al. Angiographic findings and outcome in diabetic patients treated with thrombolytic therapy for acute myocardial infarction: the GUSTO-I experience. J Am Coll Cardiol 1996; 28:1661–1669.

764. Mak KH, Moliterno DJ, Granger CB, et al. Influence of diabetes mellitus on clinical outcome in the thrombolytic era of acute myocardial infarction. GUSTO-I Investigators. Global Utilization of Streptokinase and Tissue Plasminogen Activator for Occluded Coronary Arteries. J Am Coll Cardiol 1997; 30:171–179.
765. Sun D, Nguyen N, DeGrado T, et al. Ischemia-induced translocation of the insulin-responsive glucose transporter GLUT4 in the plasma membrane of cardiac myocytes. Circulation 1994; 89: 793–798.
766. Oliver M, Opie H. Effects of glucose and fatty acids on myocardial ischaemia and arrhythmias. Lancet 1994; 343:155–158.
767. Zola B, Vinik A. Effects of autonomic neuropathy associated with diabetes mellitus on cardiovascular function. Coron Artery Dis 1992; 3:33–41.
768. Bellodi G, Manicardi V, Malavasi V, et al. Hyperglycemia and prognosis of acute myocardial infarction in patients without diabetes mellitus. Am J Cardiol 1989; 64:885–888.
769. Oswald GA, Smith CC, Betteridge DJ, et al. Determinants and importance of stress hyperglycaemia in non-diabetic patients with myocardial infarction. BMJ 1986; 293:917–922.
770. Fava S, Aquilina O, Azzopardi J, et al: The prognostic value of blood glucose in diabetic patients with acute myocardial infarction. Diabetes Med 1996; 13:80–83.
771. Capes SE, Hunt D, Malmberg K, et al. Stress hyperglycemia and increased risk of death after myocardial infarction in patients with and without diabetes: a systematic overview. Lancet 2000; 355: 773–778.
772. Malmberg K, Ryden L, Efendic S, et al. Randomized trial of insulin-glucose infusion followed by subcutaneous insulin treatment in diabetic patients with acute myocardial infarction (DIGAMI study): effects on mortality at 1 year. J Am Coll Cardiol 1995; 26:57–65.
773. Garratt KN, Brady PA, Hassinger NL, et al. Sulfonylurea drugs increase early mortality in patients with diabetes mellitus after direct angioplasty for acute myocardial infarction. J Am Coll Cardiol 1999; 33:119–124.
774. Cleveland JC Jr, Meldrum DR, Cain BS, et al. Oral sulfonylurea hypoglycemic agents prevent ischemic preconditioning in human myocardium: two paradoxes revisited. Circulation 1997; 96:29–32.
775. Katsuda Y, Egashira K, Ueno H, et al. Glibenclamide, a selective inhibitor of ATP-sensitive K^+ channels, attenuates metabolic coronary vasodilatation induced by pacing tachycardia in dogs. Circulation 1995; 92:511–517.
776. Davis CA III, Sherman AJ, Yaroshenko Y, et al. Coronary vascular responsiveness to adenosine is impaired additively by blockade of nitric oxide synthesis and a sulfonylurea. Am J Cardiol 1998; 31:816–822.
777. O'Driscoll G, Green D, Maiorana A, et al. Improvement in endothelial function by angiotensin-converting enzyme inhibition in non–insulin-dependent diabetes mellitus. J Am Coll Cardiol 1999; 33:1506–1511.
778. Vaughan DE, Rouleau JL, Ridker PM, et al. Effects of ramipril on plasma fibrinolytic balance in patients with acute anterior myocardial infarction. HEART Study Investigators. Circulation 1997; 96:442–447.
779. Torlone E, Britta M, Rambotti AM, et al. Improved insulin action and glycemic control after long-term angiotensin-converting enzyme inhibition in subjects with arterial hypertension and type II diabetes. Diabetes Care 1993; 16:1347–1355.
780. Zuanetti G, Latini R, Maggioni A, et al. Effect of the ACE-inhibitor lisinopril on mortality in diabetic patients with acute myocardial infarction: the data from the GISSI-3 study. Circulation 1997; 96:4239–4245.
781. Gustafsson I, Torp-Pedersen C, Kober L, et al. Effect of the angiotensin-converting enzyme inhibitor trandolapril on mortality and morbidity in diabetic patients with left ventricular dysfunction after acute myocardial infarction. Trace Study Group. J Am Coll Cardiol 1999; 34:83–89.
782. Lakshman MR, Reda DJ, Materson BJ, et al. Diuretics and beta-blockers do not have adverse effects at 1 year on plasma lipid and lipoprotein profiles in men with hypertension. Department of Veterans Affairs Cooperative Study Group on Antihypertensive Agents. Arch Intern Med 1999; 159:551–558.
783. Shorr RI, Ray WA, Daugherty JR, et al. Antihypertensives and the risk of serious hypoglycemia in older persons using insulin or sulfonylureas. JAMA 1997; 278:40–43.
784. Chen J, Marciniak TA, Radford MJ, et al. Beta-blocker therapy for secondary prevention of myocardial infarction in elderly diabetic patients. Results from the National Cooperative Cardiovascular Project. J Am Coll Cardiol 1999; 34:1388–1394.
785. Giugliano D, Acampora R, Marfella R. Metabolic and cardiovascular effects of carvedilol and atenolol in non–insulin-dependent diabetes mellitus and hypertension. Ann Intern Med 1997; 126: 955–959.
786. Aspirin effects on mortality and morbidity in patients with diabetes mellitus. Early Treatment Diabetic Retinopathy Study report 14. ETDRS Investigators. JAMA 1992; 268:1292–1300.
787. Aspirin therapy in diabetes. American Diabetes Association. Diabetes Care 1997; 20:772–1773.
788. Davi G, Catalano I, Averna M, et al. Thromboxane biosynthesis and platelet function in type II diabetes mellitus. N Engl J Med 1990; 322:1769–1774.
789. Inhibition of the platelet glycoprotein IIb/IIIa receptor with tirofiban in unstable angina and non–Q-wave myocardial infarction. Platelet Receptor Inhibition in Ischemic Syndrome Management in Patients Limited by Unstable Signs and Symptoms (PRISM-PLUS) Study Investigators. N Engl J Med 1998; 338:1488–1497.
790. Platelet glycoprotein IIb/IIIa receptor blockade and low-dose heparin during percutaneous coronary revascularization. The EPILOG Investigators. N Engl J Med 1997; 336:1689–1696.
791. Lincoff AM, Califf RM, Moliterno DJ, et al. Complementary clinical benefits of coronary artery stenting and blockade of platelet glycoprotein IIb/IIIa receptors: Evaluation of Platelet IIb/IIIa Inhibition in Stenting Investigators. N Engl J Med 1999; 341: 319–327.
792. Comparison of coronary bypass surgery with angioplasty in patients with multivessel disease. The Bypass Angioplasty Revascularization Investigation (BARI) Investigators. N Engl J Med 1996; 335:217–225.
793. Kannel WB, Hjortland M, Castelli WP. Role of diabetes in congestive heart failure. The Framingham study. Am J Cardiol 1974; 34:29–34.
794. Jacoby R, Nesto R. Acute myocardial infarction in the diabetic patient: pathophysiology, clinical course, and prognosis. J Am Coll Cardiol 1992; 20:736–744.
795. Aronson D, Rayfield E, Cheseboro J. Mechanisms determining course and outcome of diabetic patients who have had acute myocardial infarction. Ann Intern Med 1997; 126:296–306.
796. Cabin H, Roberts W. Quantitative comparison of extent of coronary narrowing and size of healed myocardial infarct in 33 necropsy patients with clinically recognized and in 28 with clinically unrecognized ("silent") previous acute myocardial infarction. Am J Cardiol 1982; 50:677–681.
797. van Hoeven KH, Factor SM. A comparison of the pathological spectrum of hypertensive, diabetic, and hypertensive-diabetic heart disease. Circulation 1990; 82:848–855.
798. Kawaguchi M, Techigawara M, Ishihata T, et al. A comparison of ultrastructural changes on endomyocardial biopsy specimens obtained from patients with diabetes mellitus with and without hypertension. Heart Vessels 1997; 12:267–274.
799. Nahser P, Brown R, Oskarsson H, et al. Maximal coronary flow reserve and metabolic coronary vasodilation in patients with diabetes mellitus. Circulation 1995; 91:635–640.
800. Depre C, Vanoverschelde JL, Taegtmeyer H. Glucose for the heart. Circulation 1999; 99:578–588.
801. Azzarelli A, Dini F, Cristofani R, et al. NIDDM as unfavorable factor to the postinfarction ventricular function in the elderly: echocardiography study. Coron Artery Dis 1995; 6:629–634.
802. Iwasaka T, Takahashi N, Nakamura S, et al. Residual left ventricular pump function after acute myocardial infarction in NIDDM patients. Diabetes Care 1992; 15:1522–1526.
803. Korup E, Dalsgaard D, Nyvad O, et al. Comparison of degrees of left ventricular dilation within three hours and up to six days after onset of first acute myocardial infarction. Am J Cardiol 1997; 80:449–453.
804. Mayfield JA, Reiber GE, Maynard C, et al: Trends in lower limb amputation in the Veterans Health Administration, 1989–1998. J Rehabil Res Dev 2000; 37:23–30.
805. Vileikyte L. Psychological and behavioural issues in diabetic neu-

ropathic foot ulceration. In Boulton AJM, Connor H, Cavanagh PR (eds). The Foot in Diabetes, 3rd ed. Chichester, United Kingdom, John Wiley, 2000, pp 121–130.
806. Bowker JH, Pfeifer MA (eds). Levin & O'Neal's The Diabetic Foot, 6th ed. St Louis, CV Mosby, 2000.
807. Boulton AJM, Connor H, Cavanagh PR (eds). The Foot in Diabetes, 3rd ed. Chichester, United Kingdom, John Wiley, 2000.
808. Schaper NC, Bakker K, Rauwerda JA (eds). The Diabetic Foot: Proceedings of the Third International Symposium on the Diabetic Foot. Diabet Metab Res Rev 2000; 16(Suppl 1):S1–S92.
809. Jude EB, Boulton AJM. End-stage complications of diabetic neuropathy. Diabet Rev 1999; 7:395–410.
810. Boulton AJM, Vileikyte L. The diabetic foot: the scope of the problem. J Fam Pract 2000; 49(Suppl):S3–S8.
811. Ramsey DS, Newton K, Blough D, et al: Incidence, outcomes, and cost of foot ulcers in patients with diabetes. Diabetes Care 1999; 22:382–387.
812. Abbott CA, Vileikyte L, Williamson S, et al: Multicentre study of the incidence of and predictive risk factors for diabetic neuropathic foot ulceration. Diabetes Care 1998; 21:1071–1074.
813. Pomposelli FB Jr, Maracaccio E, Gobbons GW, et al. Dorsalis pedis arterial bypass: durable limb salvage for foot ischemia in patients with diabetes mellitus. J Vasc Surg 1995; 21:375–384.
814. Reiber GE, Vileikyte L, Boyko EJ, et al. Causal pathways for incident lower extremity ulcers in patients with diabetes from two settings. Diabetes Care 1999; 22:157–162.
815. Booth J, Young MJ: Differences in the performance of commercially available 10 g monofilaments. Diabetes Care 2000; 23:984–988.
816. Edmonds ME, Blundell MP, Morris ME, et al. Improved survival of the diabetic foot: the role of a specialized foot clinic. Q J Med 1986; 60:763.
817. Boulton AJM. Why bother educating the multidisciplinary team and the patient? The example of prevention of lower extremity amputation in diabetes. Patient Educ Counsel 1995; 26:183–188.
818. Armstrong DG, Lavery LA, Harkless LB. Validation of a diabetic wound classification system. Diabet Med 1998; 14:855–859.
819. Oyibo S, Jude EB, Tarawneh I, et al. A comparision of two diabetic foot ulcer classification systems: the Wagner and the University of Texas wound classification systems. Diabetes Care 2001; 24:84–88.
820. Steed DL, Donohoe D, Webster MW, et al: Effect of extensive débridement and treatment on the healing of diabetic foot ulcers. J Am Coll Surg 1996; 183:61–64.
821. Consensus statement on diabetic foot wound care. Diabetes Care 1999; 22:1354–1360.
822. Armstrong DG, Nguyen HC, Lavery LA, et al: Off-loading the diabetic foot wound: a randomized, controlled trial. Diabetes Care 2001; 24:1019–1022.
823. Smiell J, Wieman TJ, Steed DL, et al: Efficacy and safety of becaplermin in patients with non-healing lower extremity diabetic ulcers: a combined analysis of four randomised, controlled studies. Wound Rep Regen 1999; 7:335–346.

32 Glucose Homeostasis and Hypoglycemia

Philip E. Cryer

Glucose is an obligate metabolic fuel for the brain under physiologic conditions. In contrast, other organs oxidize fatty acids as well as glucose. Because of this unique dependence on glucose and because it cannot synthesize glucose or store more than a few minutes' supply as glycogen, the brain requires a continuous supply of glucose from the circulation. Facilitated diffusion of glucose from the blood to the brain is a direct function of the arterial plasma glucose concentration. At normal plasma glucose concentrations, the rate of blood-to-brain glucose transport exceeds the rate of brain glucose metabolism. However, as the plasma glucose concentration falls below the physiologic range, blood-to-brain glucose transport becomes limiting to brain energy metabolism and, thus, to survival. Given the immediate survival value of maintenance of the plasma glucose concentration, it is not surprising that physiologic mechanisms that prevent or rapidly correct hypoglycemia have evolved. Indeed, these mechanisms are so effective that hypoglycemia is an uncommon clinical event except in people who use drugs that lower glucose levels (e.g., insulin, sulfonylureas, or alcohol).

Insight into the physiology of glucose counterregulation—the mechanisms that normally prevent or rapidly correct hypoglycemia—and its pathophysiology in the context of clinical hypoglycemia, which has been reviewed in detail,[1-3] has improved the management of hypoglycemia. Nonetheless, major gaps in understanding remain. Both are discussed here.

The author's work cited has been supported by National Institutes of Health grants R37 DK27085, M01 RR00036, P01 NS06833, P60 DK20579, and T32 DK07120; grants and a fellowship award from the American Diabetes Association; and grants from the Juvenile Diabetes Foundation International.

PHYSIOLOGY OF SYSTEMIC GLUCOREGULATION

Cellular and molecular glucoregulation is discussed in Chapter 29. Glucose metabolism and systemic glucose balance and their regulation are summarized here, with emphasis on the aspects relevant to glucose counterregulation and the prevention of hypoglycemia.

Glucose Metabolism

Origins and Fates of Glucose

Glucose is derived from three sources: intestinal *absorption* that follows digestion of dietary carbohydrates; *glycogenolysis*, the breakdown of glycogen, which is the polymerized storage form of glucose; and *gluconeogenesis*, the formation of glucose from precursors including lactate (and pyruvate), amino acids (especially alanine and glutamine), and, to a lesser extent, glycerol (Fig. 32–1).

Although most tissues express the enzyme systems required to synthesize (glycogen synthase) and hydrolyze (phosphorylase) glycogen, only the liver and kidneys express glucose-6-phosphatase, the enzyme necessary for the release of glucose into the circulation, at levels sufficient to permit these organs to contribute to the systemic glucose pool. The liver and kidneys also express the enzymes necessary for gluconeogenesis (including the critical gluconeogenic enzymes pyruvate carboxylase, phosphoenolpyruvate carboxykinase, and fructose-1,6-bisphosphatase).

There are multiple potential metabolic fates for glucose that is transported into cells (external losses are normally negligible) (see Fig. 32–1). It may be stored as glycogen, or may

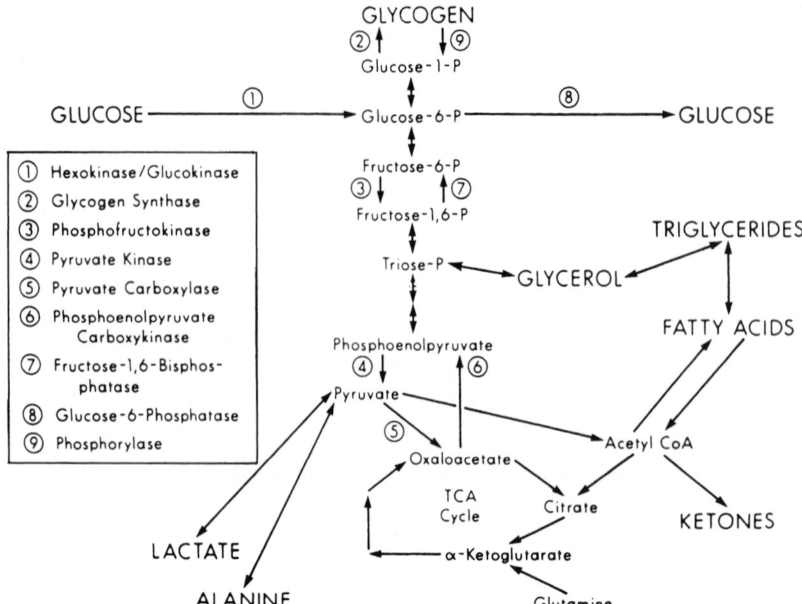

Figure 32–1. Schematic representation of glucose metabolism. TCA, tricarboxylic acid.

undergo glycolysis to pyruvate, which can be reduced to lactate, transaminated to form alanine, or converted to acetyl coenzyme A (CoA), which in turn can be oxidized to carbon dioxide and water through the tricarboxylic acid cycle, converted to fatty acids (and stored as triglycerides), or utilized for ketone body (acetoacetate, β-hydroxybutyrate) or cholesterol synthesis. Finally, glucose may be released into the circulation. As summarized in the following paragraphs, these outcomes differ in different organs.

Hepatic (and Renal) Glucose Metabolism

The liver is remarkably flexible in its role in glucose homeostasis and is the major source of net endogenous glucose production (through glycogenolysis and gluconeogenesis). Under conditions of high glucose output (e.g., fasting), the energy needs of the liver are largely provided by the beta oxidation of fatty acids. Conversely, the liver can also be an organ of net glucose uptake, with glucose stored as glycogen, oxidized for energy, or converted to fat, which can either remain in the liver or be transported to other tissues as very-low-density lipoproteins. The kidneys also produce (through gluconeogenesis) and utilize glucose.[4, 5]

Glucose Utilization

Muscle can store glucose as glycogen or metabolize glucose through glycolysis to pyruvate, which either is reduced to lactate or transaminated to form alanine or is oxidized. Lactate (and pyruvate) released from muscle is transported to the liver, where it serves as a gluconeogenic precursor (the Cori or glucose-lactate cycle). However, to the extent that lactate and pyruvate carbons are derived from glucose, they cannot result in net new glucose formation. Alanine, glutamine, and other amino acids may also flow from muscle to liver, where they too serve as gluconeogenic precursors. Circulating alanine is also largely derived from glucose (glucose-alanine cycle). Glutamine is also a major precursor for new glucose formation, although it too is partially derived from glucose (glucose-glutamine cycle).[6] During a fast, muscle can reduce its glucose uptake virtually to zero, oxidize fatty acids for its energy needs, and, through proteolysis, mobilize amino acids for transport to the liver to serve as gluconeogenic precursors for net glucose formation.

Although quantitatively less important than muscle, adipose tissue can also use glucose for fatty acid synthesis or formation of glycerol-3-phosphate, which can then esterify fatty acids (derived largely from circulating very-low-density lipoproteins) to form triglycerides. During a fast, adipocytes decrease their glucose utilization and satisfy energy needs from the beta oxidation of fatty acids. Other tissues, such as the formed elements of the blood and the renal medullae, do not have the capacity to decrease glucose utilization during fasting and therefore produce lactate at relatively fixed rates.

As mentioned earlier, glucose is the predominant metabolic fuel used by the brain under most conditions. Glucose undergoes terminal oxidation to carbon dioxide and water in the brain. The brain respiratory quotient is approximately 1.0. Although the adult brain constitutes only about 2.5% of body weight its oxidative metabolism accounts for approximately 25% of the basal metabolic rate under physiologic conditions. However, when ketones are plentiful in the circulation, as during prolonged fasting, they can support the majority of the energy needs of the brain and thus reduce its glucose utilization.

Systemic Glucose Balance

Normally, rates of endogenous glucose influx into the circulation and those of glucose efflux out of the circulation into tissues other than the brain are coordinately regulated—largely by the plasma glucose–lowering (regulatory) hormone insulin and the plasma glucose–raising (counterregulatory) hormones glucagon and epinephrine—such that systemic glucose balance is maintained, hypoglycemia (as well as hyperglycemia) is prevented, and a continuous supply of glucose to the brain is assured. This is accomplished despite wide variations in exogenous glucose influx (e.g., after feeding versus during fasting) and in glucose efflux (e.g., during exercise versus during rest). Hypoglycemia occurs when rates of glucose appearance in the circulation (the sum of endogenous glucose production, from the liver through both glycogenolysis and gluconeogenesis) (see Fig. 32–1) and, to a lesser extent, from the kidneys through gluconeogenesis, and of exogenous glucose delivery from ingested carbohydrates) fail to keep pace with rates of glucose disappearance from the circulation (the sum of ongoing brain glucose metabolism and of variable glucose utilization by tissues such as muscle and fat as well as the liver and kidneys, among others).

Fasting

The postabsorptive state is the interdigestive period that begins approximately 5 to 6 hours after a meal. However, the term is most commonly used to refer to data obtained after a 10- to 14-hour overnight fast. In healthy adults, the physiologic postabsorptive (fasting) plasma glucose concentration is approximately 4.0 to 6.0 mmol/L (72 to 108 mg/dL) with a mean of approximately 5.0 mmol/L (90 mg/dL). In the postabsorptive steady state, rates of glucose production and utilization are equal. They average 12 μmol/kg/minute (2.2 mg/kg/minute) and range from about 10 to 14 μmol/kg/minute (1.8 to 2.6 mg/kg/minute) in healthy adults after an overnight fast.[7] (These rates are as much as threefold higher in infants, at least in part because of their greater brain mass relative to their body weight.)

Approximately 60% of basal glucose utilization is accounted for by the brain. The remainder is used by glycolyzing tissues, such as the formed elements of the blood and the renal medullae and to some extent muscle and fat. Hepatic glucose production results from both glycogenolysis and gluconeogenesis even after an overnight fast.[8]

The liver is the predominant source of net endogenous glucose production after an overnight fast. The kidneys, which both use and produce glucose, contribute little to net glucose production.[4, 5] However, renal, like hepatic, glucose production is regulated.[9] It is suppressed by insulin and stimulated by epinephrine (but not by glucagon). Thus, the common practice of equating endogenous glucose production with hepatic glucose production is not precise.

The importance of gluconeogenesis in providing new glucose and supporting hepatic glycogen stores after an overnight fast becomes apparent when one considers the limited availability of preformed glucose. The glucose pool, namely free glucose in the extracellular fluid and in the cells of certain tissues (primarily in the liver but also small amounts in the kidneys, intestinal mucosa, pancreatic islet cells, brain, and blood cells), is about 83 to 111 mmol (15 to 20 g) in the normal adult. Glycogen that can be mobilized to provide circulating glucose (e.g., hepatic glycogen) contains approximately 390 mmol glucose (70 g), with a range of about 135 to 722 mmol (25 to 130 g). Thus, in an adult of average size, preformed glucose can provide as little as a 3-hour supply of glucose and less than an 8-hour supply on average, even at the diminished rate of glucose utilization that occurs in the postabsorptive state. Clearly, therefore, gluconeogenesis is important for maintenance of the plasma glucose concentration even during an overnight fast.

If fasting is prolonged to 24 to 48 hours, the plasma glucose level declines and then stabilizes, hepatic glycogen content falls to less than 55 mmol (10 g), and gluconeogenesis becomes the sole source of glucose production.[8] Because amino acids are the main gluconeogenic precursors that result in net glucose formation, muscle protein is degraded. Glucose utilization by muscle and fat virtually ceases. As lipolysis and ketogenesis accelerate and circulating ketone levels rise, ketones become a major source of fuel for the brain. Thus, glucose utilization by the brain declines by about half, resulting in a decrease in the rate of gluconeogenesis required to maintain the plasma glucose concentration and hence in diminished protein wasting. After prolonged fasting (40 days), ketones provide an estimated 80% to 90% of the energy used by the brain and renal gluconeogenesis provides up to half of the endogenous glucose production.[10]

Feeding

After a meal, glucose absorption into the circulation is more than twice the rate of postabsorptive endogenous glucose production, depending on the carbohydrate content of the meal and the rate of its digestion and absorption. As glucose is absorbed, endogenous glucose production is suppressed and glucose utilization by liver, muscle, and fat accelerates. Thus, exogenous glucose is assimilated and the plasma glucose concentration returns to the postabsorptive level.

Exercise

Exercise increases glucose utilization (by muscle) to rates that can be severalfold greater than those of the postabsorptive state. Endogenous glucose production normally accelerates to match the utilization so that the plasma glucose concentration is maintained.

From these examples, it is clear that the plasma glucose concentration is normally maintained within a narrow range despite wide variations in glucose flux, a homeostatic feat accomplished by hormonal, neural, and substrate glucoregulatory factors.[1, 2] From a mechanistic perspective, hypoglycemia could result from decreased glucose production, increased glucose utilization, or both.

Glucoregulatory Factors

Hormonal Glucoregulatory Factors

Hormones are the most important glucoregulatory factors, and the regulation of their secretion is complex. Glucose, specifically the plasma glucose concentration, is the most important determinant of the secretion of glucoregulatory hormones, including insulin, glucagon, epinephrine, growth hormone, and cortisol.

Insulin, the dominant glucose-lowering hormone, suppresses endogenous glucose production and stimulates glucose utilization by insulin-sensitive tissues, thereby lowering the plasma glucose concentration. Insulin is secreted from beta cells of the pancreatic islets into the hepatic portal circulation and acts on the liver and peripheral tissues. It inhibits hepatic glycogenolysis and gluconeogenesis and, in concert with other factors (including hyperglycemia and hypoglucagonemia), converts the liver into an organ of net glucose uptake and fuel storage (glycogen and triglycerides). It also suppresses renal glucose production and stimulates glucose uptake, storage, and utilization by tissues such as muscle and fat. In the postabsorptive state, insulin regulates the plasma glucose concentration primarily by restraining hepatic glucose production.[11] Higher levels, such as those that occur after meals, are required to stimulate glucose utilization.[11]

Conversely, decreased insulin secretion causes increased hepatic (and renal) glucose production and decreased glucose utilization by insulin-sensitive tissues such as muscle and thus tends to raise the plasma glucose concentration. Insulin is therefore both a glucose-lowering (regulatory) and a glucose-raising (counterregulatory) hormone. The rate of insulin secretion is regulated by a number of factors, the most important of which is glucose. A fall in the plasma glucose concentration has an immediate inhibitory effect on insulin secretion, thereby limiting a further fall in the plasma glucose level. Insulin is a potent and critical hormone. Either profound insulin deficiency or marked insulin excess can be lethal. But it is not the only glucoregulatory hormone.

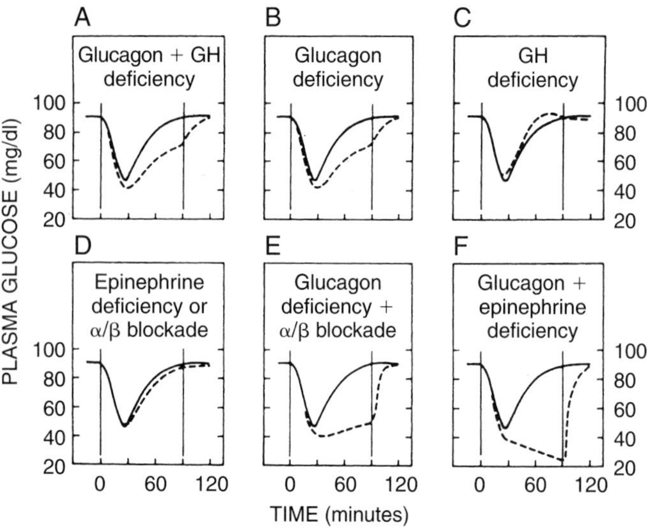

Figure 32–4. Summary of studies of the mechanisms of glucose recovery from short-term hypoglycemia in healthy humans. Insulin was injected intravenously at time 0 minutes. Interventions were started at time 0 minutes and stopped at time 90 minutes (i.e., between the vertical lines in each panel). Plasma glucose curves during control studies (*solid curves*, same in all six panels) and as modified (*dashed curves*) by the following. *A*, Somatostatin infusion (glucagon plus growth hormone [GH] deficiency. *B*, somatostatin infusion plus growth hormone replacement (glucagon deficiency). *C*, Somatostatin infusion plus glucagon replacement (GH deficiency). *D*, Phentolamine and propranolol infusion (combined α-adrenergic and β-adrenergic blockade) or studies performed in bilaterally adrenalectomized individuals (epinephrine deficiency). *E*, Somatostatin, phentolamine, and propranolol infusion (glucagon deficiency + α-adrenergic and β-adrenergic blockade). *F*, Somatostatin infusion in bilaterally adrenalectomized individuals (glucagon + epinephrine deficiency). (*Curves* derived from data in Clarke WL et al. Am J Physiol 1979; 236:E147–E152[49]; Gerich JE et al. Am J Physiol 1979; 236:E370–E385[50]; and Rizza RA et al. J Clin Invest 1979; 64:62–71.[51] From Cryer PE. Glucose counterregulation in man. Diabetes 1981; 30:261–264. Copyright 1981, American Diabetes Association, Alexandria, Va.)

people with poorly controlled diabetes (who often have symptoms of hypoglycemia at higher than normal glucose levels) and to lower plasma glucose concentrations in people who suffer recurrent hypoglycemia, such as those with well-controlled diabetes or with an insulinoma (who often tolerate subnormal glucose levels without symptoms).

Glucose Counterregulation

The physiology of glucose counterregulation—the mechanisms that normally prevent or rapidly correct hypoglycemia[7, 49–66]—has been reviewed in detail.[1, 2] Early studies of the mechanisms of the correction of short-term insulin-induced hypoglycemia[49–51] and of more prolonged insulin-induced hypoglycemia[59, 60, 64, 65] are summarized in Figures 32–4 and 32–5, respectively. These and studies of the prevention of hypoglycemia are detailed elsewhere.[2]

The principles of glucose counterregulation are three.[1, 2] First, the prevention and the correction of hypoglycemia involve both waning of insulin and activation of glucose counterregulatory factors. These are not due solely to waning of insulin. Second, although insulin is the dominant plasma glucose–lowering factor, there are redundant glucose counterregulatory factors including a decrease in insulin and increases in glucagon and epinephrine. Thus, there is a fail-safe system that prevents failure of the counterregulatory process even when one, or perhaps more, of the components of the system fails. Third, there is a hierarchy among the counterregulatory factors. Some are more important than others.

The physiology of glucose counterregulation is also summarized in Table 32–1. The first defense against falling plasma glucose concentrations is decreased insulin secretion. Among the counterregulatory factors, increased glucagon secretion plays a primary role. Glucose recovery from hypoglycemia is impaired and postabsorptive plasma glucose concentrations decline but then level off when glucagon secretion is deficient. Glucagon is the second defense against falling plasma glucose concentrations. Albeit demonstrably involved, increased epinephrine secretion is not normally critical. It becomes critical when glucagon is deficient. Epinephrine is the third defense against falling plasma glucose concentrations. Hypoglycemia develops or progresses when both glucagon and epinephrine are deficient and insulin is present despite the actions of the other glucose counterregulatory factors. Thus, insulin, glucagon, and epinephrine stand high in the hierarchy of redundant glucose counterregulatory factors.

Growth hormone and cortisol, both of which tend to increase plasma glucose concentrations after several hours, are involved in defense against prolonged hypoglycemia.[59, 60] However, neither is critical to recovery from even prolonged hypoglycemia or, at least in adults, to prevention of hypoglycemia after an overnight fast.[61]

There is some evidence that glucose autoregulation is involved although only during severe hypoglycemia.[62, 63] Other hormones, neurotransmitters, and substrates other than glucose (and fatty acids that may mediate part of the effect of epinephrine) may also be involved. If so, they play relatively minor roles.

PATHOPHYSIOLOGY OF HYPOGLYCEMIA

Clinical Manifestations of Hypoglycemia

Whipple's triad—symptoms consistent with hypoglycemia, a low plasma glucose concentration, and relief of those symptoms when the plasma glucose concentration is raised—provides compelling evidence of hypoglycemia.

Symptoms of hypoglycemia can be divided into two categories, *neuroglycopenic* and *neurogenic* (autonomic) symptoms.[1, 35] Neuroglycopenic symptoms are the direct result of CNS neuronal glucose deprivation. They include behavioral changes, confusion, fatigue or weakness, warmth, visual changes, seizure, loss of consciousness, and, if hypoglycemia is severe and prolonged, death. Neurogenic symptoms are the result of the perception of physiologic changes caused by the autonomic nervous system discharge triggered by hypoglycemia. They include adrenergic symptoms such as palpitations, tremor, and anxiety and cholinergic symptoms such as sweating, hunger, and paresthesias.[35] Adrenergic symptoms are mediated by norepinephrine released from sympathetic postganglionic neurons, the adrenal medullae, or both and epinephrine released from the adrenal medullae. The relative contributions of these are not known, but palpitations have been attributed to circulating epinephrine and tremor to sympathetic neural norepinephrine. Cholinergic symptoms, at least sweating, are thought to be mediated by acetylcholine released from sympathetic postganglionic neurons.

Representative neurogenic and neuroglycopenic symptoms of hypoglycemia are listed in Figure 32–6, which also illustrates that awareness of hypoglycemia—the extent to which individuals perceive that their blood sugar is low—is largely the result

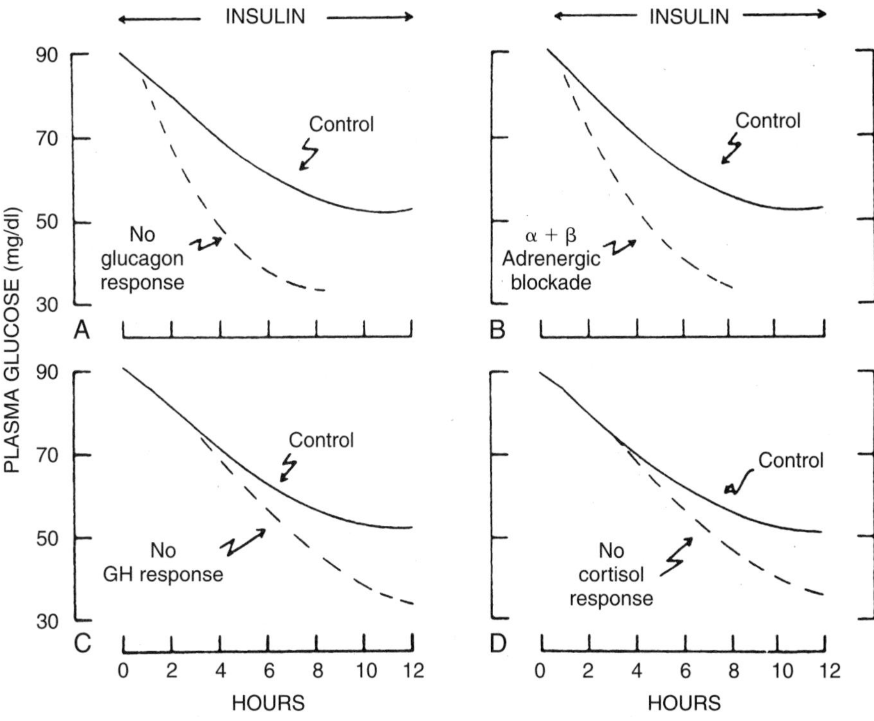

Figure 32–5. Summary of studies of the mechanisms of defense against prolonged hypoglycemia in healthy humans. Plasma glucose curves during control studies (*solid curves*, same in all panels) and as modified (*dashed curves*) by the following. *A*, Somatostatin infusion and metyrapone administration with cortisol and growth hormone (GH) replacement and endogenous epinephrine secretion (no glucagon response). *B*, Somatostatin infusion and metyrapone administration with glucagon, cortisol, and growth hormone replacement and endogenous epinephrine secretion and phentolamine and propranolol infusion (α-adrenergic + β-adrenergic blockade). *C*, Somatostatin infusion and metyrapone administration with glucagon and cortisol replacement and endogenous epinephrine secretion (no growth hormone response). *D*, Somatostatin infusion and metyrapone administration with glucagon and growth hormone replacement (no cortisol response). (Data from DeFeo P, et al. Am J Physiol 1989: 256:E835–E843[59]; DeFeo P, et al. Am J Physiol 1989; 257: E35–E42[60]; DeFeo P et al. Am J Physiol 1991; 260:E203–E212[64]; and DeFeo P et al. Am J Physiol 1991; 261:E725–E736.[65] From Gerich JE. Glucose counterregulation and its impact on diabetes mellitus. Diabetes 1988; 37:1608–1617. Copyright 1988, American Diabetes Association, Alexandria, Va.)

of the perception of neurogenic symptoms. The autonomic, including the sympathochromaffin, response to hypoglycemia is initiated by glucose-sensitive neurons, including those in the ventromedial hypothalamus, that increase firing as extracellular glucose levels fall. Thus, although both neurogenic and neuroglycopenic symptoms could be viewed as fundamentally neuroglycopenic in origin, their mechanisms are different. Some prefer the term autonomic rather than neurogenic symptoms because they may be mediated by a circulating hormone (epinephrine) as well as by a neurotransmitter. Nonetheless, the autonomic response is CNS-mediated and, therefore, the resulting symptoms are fundamentally neurogenic.

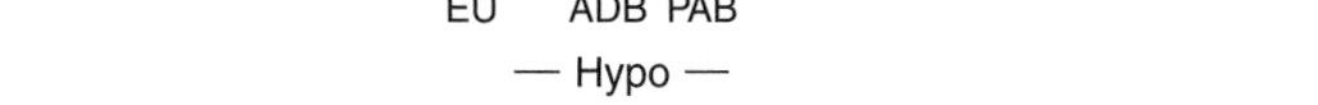

NEUROGENIC
Sweaty
Hungry
Tingling
Shaky/tremulous
Heart pounding
Nervous/anxious

Blood sugar low
($P < .001$)
3 Δ
2 *
1 †
0
EU ADB PAB
— Hypo —

NEUROGLYCOPENIC
Warm
Weak
Difficulty Thinking/confused
Tired/drowsy
Faint
Dizzy
Difficulty speaking
Blurred vision

Figure 32–6. Neurogenic (autonomic) and neuroglycopenic symptoms of hypoglycemia in normal humans. Among the neurogenic symptoms, "sweaty," "hungry," and "tingling" are cholinergic and "shaky/tremulous," "heart pounding," and "nervous/anxious" are adrenergic. See text for discussion. Mean (±SE) subject scores for awareness of hypoglycemia (blood sugar low) during clamped euglycemia (EU) and during hypoglycemia (Hypo) alone (*closed column*), with combined α-adrenergic and β-adrenergic blockade with infused phentolamine and propranolol (ADB, *crosshatched column*), and with combined α-adrenergic and β-adrenergic blockade plus muscarinic cholinergic blockade with atropine, panautonomic blockade (PAB, *open column*), are also shown. Data from Towler DA et al. Diabetes 1993; 42:1791–1798.[35] (From Cryer PE. Hypoglycemia: the limiting factor in the management of IDDM. Diabetes 1994; 43:1378–1389. Copyright, 1994, American Diabetes Association, Alexandria, Va.)

Common signs of hypoglycemia include pallor and diaphoresis. Heart rate and systolic blood pressure are typically increased, but these findings may not be prominent. To the extent that they are observable, the neuroglycopenic manifestations are often valuable, albeit nonspecific, signs. Transient neurologic defects occur occasionally. Permanent neurologic damage is rare.

The magnitude of the responses to hypoglycemia is an inverse function of the nadir plasma glucose concentration rather than the rate of decrease in plasma glucose.[67–69] It was once thought that neurogenic symptoms are less prominent when hypoglycemia develops gradually. However, the relative paucity of symptoms at a given low plasma glucose concentration in individuals with recurrent hypoglycemia, such as those with tightly controlled diabetes[70] or with an insulinoma,[71] is attributable to a shift in glycemic thresholds for responses to lower plasma glucose concentrations. Conversely, the threshold shifts to higher plasma glucose concentrations in patients with chronic hyperglycemia result in symptoms of hypoglycemia at relatively high glucose levels.[72] The mechanism of these shifts in thresholds is unknown. Potential mechanisms are discussed later in this chapter.

Diagnosis of Hypoglycemia

The manifestations of hypoglycemia are nonspecific, vary among individuals, and may change from time to time in the same individual. They are also typically episodic. Thus, although the history is of fundamental importance in suggesting the possibility of hypoglycemia, the diagnosis cannot be made solely on the basis of symptoms and signs.

The diagnosis of hypoglycemia should also not be made solely on the basis of plasma glucose measurements unless they are unequivocally subnormal. It is not possible to define a plasma glucose concentration below which neuroglycopenia invariably occurs and above which neuroglycopenia never occurs. Although symptoms commonly occur with plasma glucose levels less than 3.0 mmol/L (54 mg/dL),[46–48] they can occur at higher plasma glucose levels in poorly controlled diabetes[70, 72] and only at lower glucose levels in well-controlled diabetes[70] or in other conditions that result in recurrent hypoglycemia such as insulinoma.[71] In addition, venous plasma glucose concentrations substantially less than 3.0 mmol/L (54 mg/dL) may occur in normal individuals late after glucose ingestion (arterial glucose levels are higher) and in some women and children during fasting without producing recognizable symptoms. This is not to say that distinctly low plasma glucose measurements should be ignored. Some patients with endogenous hyperinsulinism[71] or intensively treated diabetes[70] tolerate glucose levels that are unequivocally subnormal, as mentioned earlier. Because these patients can have hypoglycemic symptoms at other times (presumably when glucose levels are even lower), it would be inappropriate to deny that they have hypoglycemia.

In general, venous plasma glucose concentrations greater than 3.9 mmol/L (70 mg/dL) after an overnight fast are normal, those between 2.8 and 3.9 mmol/L (50 and 70 mg/dL) are suggestive of hypoglycemia, and those less than 2.8 mmol/L (50 mg/dL) indicate postabsorptive hypoglycemia. Because substantial glucose extraction occurs across the forearm under hyperinsulinemic conditions, arterial glucose concentrations (those relevant to brain function) are as much as 30% higher than venous glucose concentrations after an oral glucose load. Artifactually low measured glucose levels can result from glycolysis in vitro (pseudohypoglycemia), particularly in the presence of leukocytosis or polycythemia, or both, or if separation of plasma from the formed elements of the blood is delayed. The diagnosis of hypoglycemia is most convincingly established when it is based on Whipple's triad: symptoms consistent with hypoglycemia, a low plasma glucose concentration, and relief of those symptoms when the plasma glucose concentration is increased to normal levels.

Postabsorptive versus Postprandial Hypoglycemia

Reproducible hypoglycemia in the postabsorptive state implies the presence of disease and requires diagnostic explanation and therapy. This condition is commonly referred to as postabsorptive, or fasting, hypoglycemia. However, it need not be apparent initially or exclusively during prolonged fasting or after an overnight fast; it may become symptomatic during the latter portion of any interdigestive period especially with exercise. In contrast, postprandial (reactive, stimulative) hypoglycemia usually does not imply a serious underlying disorder. Thus, the distinction between postabsorptive and postprandial hypoglycemia is useful.

Mechanisms of Hypoglycemia

Hypoglycemia indicates that the rate of glucose efflux from the circulation exceeds that of glucose influx into the circulation. It can result from excessive glucose efflux (excessive utilization, external losses) or deficient glucose influx (deficient endogenous production in the absence of exogenous glucose delivery), or both. Conditions in which glucose utilization is increased include exercise, pregnancy, and sepsis; renal losses can occur at physiologic plasma glucose concentrations (e.g., renal glycosuria, pregnancy). However, because of the capacity of the normal liver (and kidneys) to increase glucose production severalfold, as discussed earlier, clinical hypoglycemia rarely results solely from excessive glucose efflux. Rather it is commonly the result of inappropriately low glucose production relative to the rate of glucose utilization.

Hypoglycemia can be caused by regulatory, enzymatic, or substrate defects. Glucoregulatory defects include excessive secretion of insulin or deficient secretion of glucose counterregulatory hormones. Enzymatic defects in glucose production may be primary or may result from hepatic disease. Substrate defects include failure to mobilize or utilize gluconeogenic substrates.

Clinical Classification of Hypoglycemia

Hypoglycemia can be classified on the basis of glucose kinetic patterns, pathogenic mechanisms, or disease groups. The last approach is used in this chapter (Table 32–2). Postabsorptive, or fasting, hypoglycemia can be the result of drugs, critical illnesses including hepatic or renal failure, hormonal deficiencies, non–beta cell tumors, endogenous hyperinsulinism (including that caused by pancreatic beta cell tumors), or metabolic disorders of infancy and childhood. Postprandial, or reactive, hypoglycemia is rarely caused by congenital enzyme defects but can follow gastric surgery and perhaps occurs rarely as an idiopathic disorder.

Most episodes of hypoglycemia result from drugs, particularly insulin, sulfonylureas, or alcohol. In one series of patients treated in an emergency room for hypoglycemia, two thirds had diabetes mellitus and two thirds had been drinking alcohol.[73] Clearly, the combination of drug-treated diabetes and alcohol ingestion can be devastating. Nearly one fourth of the patients were septic, but diabetes or alcohol ingestion was common even in those patients. Drugs are also a common cause of hypoglycemia in inpatients.[74] In this case, however, critical illnesses such as renal or hepatic failure, sepsis, and inanition are common. Hypoglycemia resulting from hormonal

Table 32–2. Clinical Classification of Hypoglycemia

Postabsorptive (Fasting) Hypoglycemia

- Drugs
  - Especially insulin, sulfonylureas, alcohol
  - Also pentamidine, quinine
  - Rarely, salicylates, sulfonamides
  - Others
- Critical illnesses
  - Hepatic failure
  - Cardiac failure
  - Renal failure
  - Sepsis
  - Inanition
- Hormonal deficiencies
  - Cortisol or growth hormone, or both
  - Glucagon and epinephrine
- Non–beta cell tumors
- Endogenous hyperinsulinism
  - Pancreatic beta cell disorders
    - Tumor (insulinoma)
    - Nontumor
  - Beta cell secretagogue (e.g., sulfonylureas)
  - Autoimmune hypoglycemia
    - Insulin antibodies
    - Insulin receptor antibodies
    - ? Beta cell antibodies
  - ? Ectopic insulin secretion
- Hypoglycemias of infancy and childhood

Postprandial (Reactive) Hypoglycemia

- Congenital deficiencies of enzymes of carbohydrate metabolism
  - Hereditary fructose intolerance
  - Galactosemia
- Alimentary hypoglycemia
- Idiopathic (functional) postprandial hypoglycemia

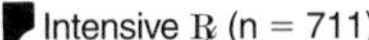

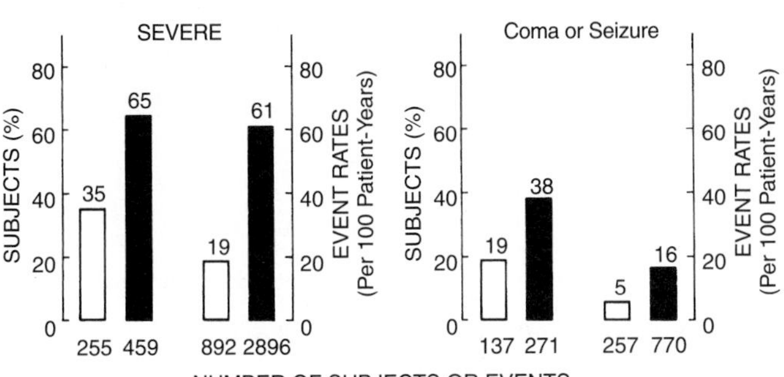

Figure 32–7. Proportion of patients affected and event rates for severe hypoglycemia (*left*) and severe hypoglycemia with coma or seizure (*right*) in the Diabetes Control and Complications Trial. (Data from The Diabetes Control and Complications Trial Research Group. Diabetes 1997; 46:271–286.[80] From Cryer PE. Hypoglycemia: the limiting factor in the management of IDDM. Diabetes 1994; 43:1378–1389. Copyright 1994, American Diabetes Association, Alexandria, Va.)

Table 32–3. Severe Hypoglycemia during Aggressive Glycemic Therapy of Diabetes

	Episodes Per 100 Patient-Years
Type 1 Diabetes	
Edinburgh (Diabet Med 1993; 10:238)	170
Utrecht (Diabetes Care 2000; 23:1467)	150
Stockholm Diabetes Intervention Study (Diabetes 1994; 43:313)	110
Diabetes Control and Complications Trial (N Engl J Med 1993; 329:977)	62
Type 2 Diabetes	
Edinburgh (Diabet Med 1993; 10:238)	73
Veterans Affairs Pump Study* (JAMA 1996; 276:1322)	10
Veterans Affairs Cooperative Study (Diabetes Care 1993; 8:1113)	3

*Multiple daily insulin injection subset.

deficiencies is uncommon but often treatable by hormone replacement. Hypoglycemia caused by non–beta cell tumors or by endogenous hyperinsulinism is rare.

HYPOGLYCEMIA IN DIABETES MELLITUS

Clinical Context

It is now well established that comprehensive care makes a difference for people with diabetes. A fundamentally important component of comprehensive care of diabetes is glycemic control because it prevents or delays the long-term specific complications of diabetes (retinopathy, nephropathy, and neuropathy) and may reduce its macrovascular complications.[75–77] However, iatrogenic hypoglycemia is the limiting factor[1, 78] in the glycemic management of both *type 1 diabetes mellitus* (T1DM)[75, 76, 79–81] and *type 2 diabetes mellitus* (T2DM)[77, 82] both conceptually and in practice.

Conceptually, were it not for the potentially devastating effects of hypoglycemia on the brain, hyperglycemia would be rather easy to treat. Administration of enough insulin (or any effective medication) to lower plasma glucose levels to or below the normal range would eliminate symptoms of hyperglycemia; prevent diabetic ketoacidosis and hyperosmolar coma; almost assuredly prevent diabetic retinopathy, nephropathy, and neuropathy; and probably reduce atherosclerotic risk. The devastating effects of hypoglycemia are real, however, and the glycemic management of diabetes is therefore complex.

In practice, euglycemia, even near euglycemia, cannot be achieved and maintained safely in most patients with T1DM[75, 76] and many patients with T2DM[77] because of the barrier of iatrogenic hypoglycemia. Because of that barrier, retinopathy, nephropathy, and neuropathy develop or progress in some patients with T1DM[75, 76] or T2DM[77] despite aggressive attempts to achieve glycemic control, albeit at lower rates than during less aggressive therapy. Indeed, the inability to maintain euglycemia over time, because of the barrier of hypoglycemia, may explain the limited impact of aggressive glycemic therapy on the atherosclerotic complications of diabetes.[75–77]

In T1DM, aggressive attempts to achieve glycemic control increase the risk of severe, at least temporarily disabling, iatrogenic hypoglycemia (i.e., that requiring the assistance of another individual) more than threefold (Fig. 32–7). Documented in both of the controlled clinical trials with sample sizes large enough to demonstrate beneficial effects of intensive therapy on the long-term complications of diabetes, the Diabetes Control and Complications Trial (DCCT)[75, 79, 80] and the Stockholm Diabetes Intervention Study,[76, 81] that fact was confirmed in a meta-analysis that also included 12 smaller controlled clinical trials of intensive therapy.[83] However, it is possible to reduce the risk of hypoglycemia during aggressive therapy of T1DM. For example, the sixfold increased risk of severe hypoglycemia during intensive therapy in the feasibility phase of the DCCT[6] was reduced by half in the full-scale trial.[75, 80]

Because of the interplay of therapeutic insulin excess and compromised physiologic and behavioral defenses against falling plasma glucose concentrations, as discussed later in this chapter, people with T1DM are at ongoing risk for episodes of hypoglycemia.[1] Those attempting to achieve glycemic control suffer untold numbers of episodes of asymptomatic hypoglycemia—plasma glucose levels may be lower than 2.8 mmol/L (50 mg/dL) as much as 10% of the time—and an average of two episodes of symptomatic hypoglycemia per week. They suffer an episode of severe, at least temporarily disabling hypoglycemia, often with seizure or coma, every year or two on average (Table 32–3). Although seemingly complete recovery from even severe hypoglycemia is the rule, permanent neurologic deficits can result. It has been estimated that 2% to 4% of deaths of people with T1DM are caused by hypoglycemia.[1, 84] In addition, hypoglycemia can cause recurrent or even persistent psychosocial morbidity. The reality of hypoglycemia, the rational fear of hypoglycemia, or both can be a barrier to glycemic control.

Iatrogenic hypoglycemia is generally less frequent in T2DM.[3, 77, 82] However, it occurs during treatment with sulfonylureas or other insulin secretagogues (and has been reported in patients treated with metformin) or with insulin (Table 32–4; see Table 32–3). The frequency of hypoglycemia approaches that in T1DM in those who reach the insulin-deficient end of the spectrum of T2DM.[82] Indeed, in one series, the frequency of severe hypoglycemia was similar in patients with T2DM and T1DM matched for duration of insulin therapy.[85] The United Kingdom Prospective Diabetes

Table 32–4. Cumulative Incidence of Hypoglycemia (Any, Major) in Type 2 Diabetes over 6 Years in the United Kingdom Prospective Diabetes Study

Therapy*	N	Hemoglobin A_{1c} HbA_{1c} (%)	Percent with Hypoglycemia Any	Major†
Diet	379	8.0	3.0	0.2
Sulfonylurea	922	7.1	45.0	3.3
Insulin	689	7.1	76.0	11.2‡
Diet	297	8.2	2.8	0.4
Metformin	251	7.4	17.6	2.4

*Taking assigned medication.
†Requiring medical assistance or admission to hospital.
‡Compared with severe hypoglycemia (that requiring the assistance of another individual) in 65% of intensively treated patients over 6.5 years in the Diabetes Control and Complications Trial.
From The United Kingdom Prospective Diabetes Study Research Group. Overview of 6 years of therapy of type II diabetes: a progressive disease. Diabetes 1995; 44:1249–1258.

Table 32–5. Comprehensive Risk Factors for Hypoglycemia in Diabetes

Premise: Iatrogenic hypoglycemia in type 1 diabetes is the result of the interplay of therapeutic insulin excess and compromised glucose counterregulation.
1. Absolute or relative therapeutic insulin excess (the conventional risk factors)
   a. Insulin doses excessive, ill-timed, wrong type
   b. Decreased food intake
   c. Increased glucose utilization (e.g., exercise)
   d. Decreased glucose production (e.g., alcohol)
   e. Increased sensitivity to insulin (e.g., after exercise, during the night, glycemic control, weight loss)
   f. Decreased insulin clearance (e.g., renal failure)
2. Compromised glucose counterregulation
   a. Absolute insulin deficiency (C-peptide negativity)
      β-Cell destruction: No ↓ in insulin in response to ↓ glucose
      Unknown: No ↑ in glucagon in response to ↓ glucose
   b. History of severe hypoglycemia or aggressive therapy per se (lower glucose goals, lower hemoglobin A_{1c})
      Episodes of hypoglycemia: Attenuated autonomic (including ↑ epinephrine) activation and symptoms in response to ↓ glucose (defective glucose counterregulation and hypoglycemia unawareness)

Study investigators concluded that over time hypoglycemia becomes limiting in the treatment of T2DM just as it is in the treatment of T1DM.[82]

Given the now well-established long-term benefits of glycemic control and the short-term potentially devastating effects of iatrogenic hypoglycemia, it is clear that the goals of both reducing mean glycemia and minimizing hypoglycemia are important for people with diabetes. Minimizing the risk of hypoglycemia in T1DM involves both application of the principles of aggressive therapy—education and empowerment of patients, frequent self-monitoring of blood glucose, flexible insulin regimens, individualized glycemic goals, and ongoing professional guidance and support—and implementation of hypoglycemia risk reduction. As discussed later in this chapter, hypoglycemia risk reduction requires consideration of the roles of both therapeutic insulin excess and compromised physiologic and behavioral defenses against developing hypoglycemia.

Risk Factors

Insulin Excess

The conventional risk factors for iatrogenic hypoglycemia in T1DM[1] (Table 32–5) are based on the premise that relative or absolute therapeutic insulin excess, which must occur from time to time because of the gross pharmacokinetic imperfections of all current insulin replacement regimens, is the sole determinant of risk.

Relative or absolute therapeutic insulin excess occurs when:

1. Insulin doses are excessive, ill-timed, or of the wrong type.
2. The influx of exogenous glucose is decreased (as during the overnight fast or after missed meals or snacks).
3. Insulin-independent glucose utilization is increased (as during exercise).
4. Endogenous glucose production is decreased (as after alcohol ingestion or administration or other drugs and with loss of renal parenchyma).
5. Sensitivity to insulin is increased (as after exercise; in the middle of the night; with glycemic control; with increased fitness, weight loss, or both; or with administration of certain drugs).
6. Insulin clearance is decreased (as in renal failure).

These are the issues with which people with diabetes and their health care providers deal routinely as they attempt to minimize iatrogenic hypoglycemia. However, it became clear early in the DCCT that these conventional risk factors explain only a minority of episodes of severe iatrogenic hypoglycemia.[79] Indeed, in a multivariate model none was found to be statistically significant. Clearly, we must look beyond these risk factors if we are to understand the majority of episodes of severe hypoglycemia in T1DM.

Interplay of Insulin Excess and Compromised Glucose Counterregulation

Iatrogenic hypoglycemia in T1DM is more appropriately viewed as the result of the interplay of relative or absolute therapeutic insulin excess (the conventional risk factors) and compromised glucose counterregulation (see Table 32–5). Three clinically well-documented risk factors for iatrogenic hypoglycemia in T1DM are (1) absolute insulin deficiency (i.e., C-peptide negativity),[80, 86, 87] (2) a history of severe hypoglycemia,[80, 87] and (3) aggressive glycemic therapy per se as evidenced by lower glycemic goals or lower hemoglobin A_{1c} levels.[80, 87] (Obviously, iatrogenic hypoglycemia occurs in people with diabetes who are not C peptide–negative, have no history of severe hypoglycemia, and are not practicing aggressive glycemic therapy. Nonetheless, these are associated with a substantially increased risk of hypoglycemia.[80, 86, 87]) These three risk factors are clinical surrogates of compromised physiologic and behavioral defenses against falling plasma glucose concentrations—the clinical syndromes of defective glucose counterregulation and of hypoglycemia unawareness and the pathophysiologic concept of hypoglycemia-associated autonomic failure.

Pathophysiology of Glucose Counterregulation in Diabetes

As the person with T1DM becomes absolutely insulin-deficient over the first few months or years of clinical T1DM, circulating insulin levels—then simply the passive result of

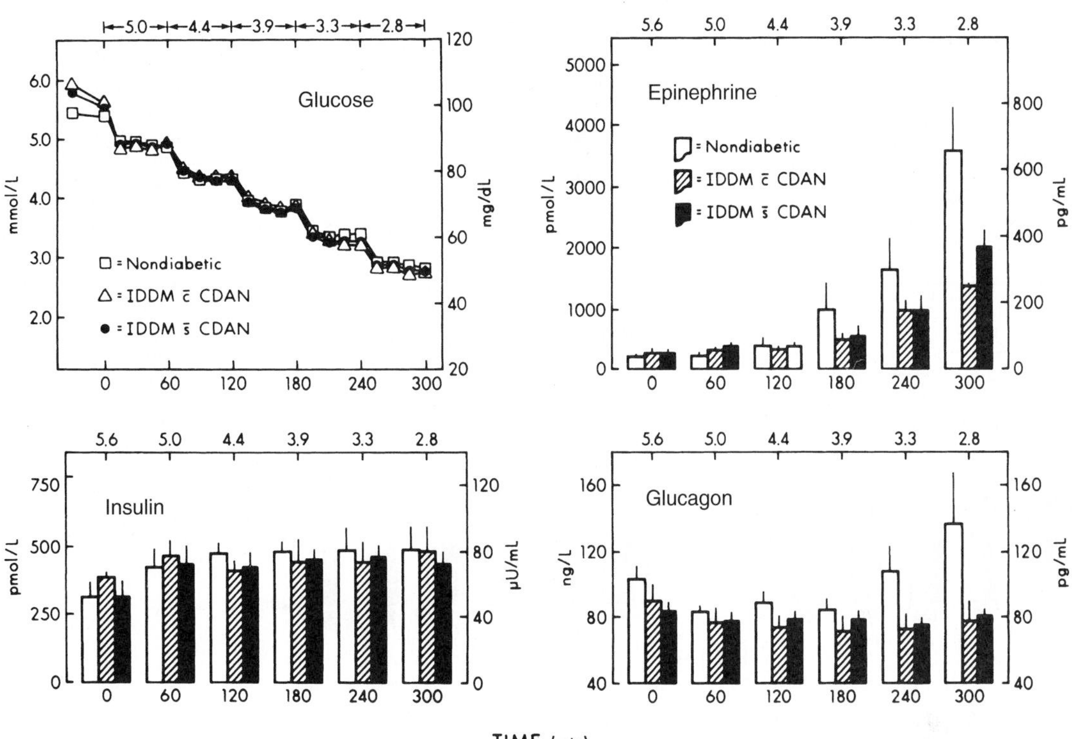

Figure 32–8. Mean (±SE) plasma glucose, insulin, epinephrine, and glucagon concentrations during hyperinsulinemic stepped hypoglycemic glucose clamps in nondiabetic subjects (*open squares* and *columns*), people with type 1 diabetes mellitus (IDDM, insulin-dependent diabetes mellitus) with classic diabetic autonomic neuropathy (CDAN, *open triangles* and *crosshatched columns*), and people with type 1 diabetes mellitus without CDAN (*closed circles* and *columns*). (From Dagogo-Jack SE, Craft S, Cryer PE. Hypoglycemia-associated autonomic failure in insulin dependent diabetes mellitus. J Clin Invest 1993; 91:819–828. Copyright, 1994, American Society for Clinical Investigation, New York.)

absorption of exogenous insulin—do not fall as plasma glucose levels decline. The first defense against hypoglycemia is lost.

Over the same time frame, the glucagon response to hypoglycemia is lost in T1DM.[88, 89] This is a selective defect; the glucagon responses to other stimuli are largely, if not entirely, intact. The mechanism of the defect is unknown, but it is tightly linked to absolute insulin deficiency.[86] Given that and the finding that a decrease in intraislet secretion is normally a potent stimulus to the glucagon secretory response to hypoglycemia,[40] the absent glucagon response may be a direct result of absent insulin secretion. Thus, the clinical hypoglycemia risk factor of C-peptide negativity[80, 86, 87] indicates that the first defense against hypoglycemia (decreased insulin secretion) is lost and predicts accurately that the second defense against hypoglycemia (increased glucagon secretion) is lost. Therefore, patients with established (i.e., C peptide–negative) T1DM are largely dependent on the third defense against hypoglycemia, increased epinephrine secretion.

The epinephrine response to hypoglycemia is attenuated in many patients with T1DM[1, 70, 89–92] (Fig. 32–8), particularly those with the other clinical risk factors for hypoglycemia such as a history of severe hypoglycemia or aggressive glycemic therapy per se as evidenced by lower glycemic goals, lower hemoglobin A_{1c} levels, or both. The former indicates and the latter implies recurrent episodes of prior hypoglycemia. In contrast to the absent glucagon response, the attenuated epinephrine response represents a threshold shift; an epinephrine response can be elicited, but lower plasma glucose concentrations are required[70, 92] (see Fig. 32–8). This threshold shift to lower plasma glucose concentrations is largely the result of recent antecedent iatrogenic hypoglycemia.

Recent antecedent hypoglycemia reduces autonomic (including adrenomedullary epinephrine) and symptomatic, among other, responses to a given level of subsequent hypoglycemia in nondiabetic individuals[93–97] and in patients with T1DM[92, 98, 99] (Figs. 32–9 and 32–10). It shifts the glycemic thresholds for these responses to lower plasma glucose concentrations. As a result, it also impairs glycemic defense against hyperinsulinemia and developing hypoglycemia in T1DM[92] (Fig. 32–11). In addition to this functional threshold shift, there may be an anatomic component—loss of adrenomedullary chromaffin cells—of the reduced epinephrine response in patients with classical diabetic autonomic neuropathy.[100, 101] Nonetheless, the epinephrine response is typically reduced in patients with no clinical evidence of classical diabetic autonomic neuropathy[92, 100, 101] (see Fig. 32–8).

The development of an attenuated epinephrine response to falling glucose levels—loss of the third defense against hypoglycemia—is a critical pathophysiologic event. Patients with T1DM who have combined deficiencies of glucagon and epinephrine responses have been shown in prospective studies to suffer severe hypoglycemia at rates 25-fold[102] or more[103] higher than those of patients with absent glucagon but intact epinephrine responses during aggressive glycemic therapy. They have the clinical syndrome of *defective glucose counterregulation*. The mechanisms of altered and defective glucose counterregulation are illustrated in Figure 32–12.

By reducing the autonomic, specifically the sympathochromaffin, responses to subsequent hypoglycemia, recent antecedent iatrogenic hypoglycemia also causes loss of the warning, largely if not exclusively neurogenic, symptoms of developing hypoglycemia[92, 98, 99] that previously allowed the patient to rec-

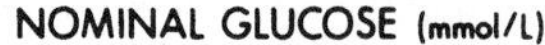

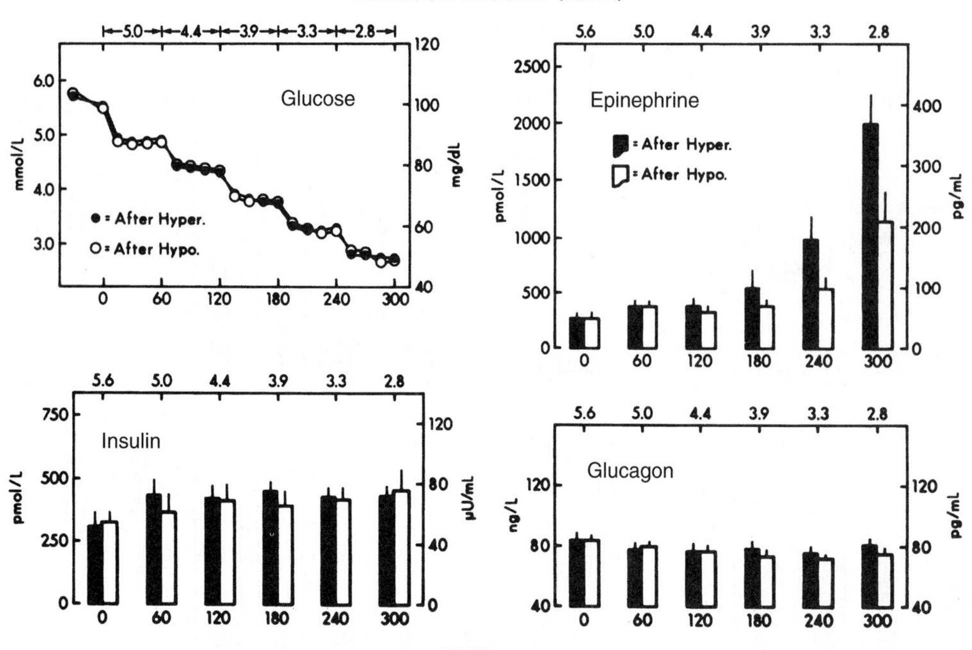

Figure 32–9. Mean (±SE) plasma glucose, insulin, epinephrine, and glucagon concentrations during hyperinsulinemic stepped hypoglycemic glucose clamps in patients with type 1 diabetes mellitus (IDDM, insulin-dependent diabetes mellitus) without classical diabetic autonomic neuropathy on mornings following afternoon hyperglycemia (Hyper., *closed circles* and *columns*) and on mornings following afternoon hypoglycemia (Hypo., *open circles* and *columns*). (From Dagogo-Jack SE, Craft S, Cryer PE. Hypoglycemia-associated autonomic failure in insulin dependent diabetes mellitus. J Clin Invest 1993; 91:819–828. Copyright, 1993, American Society for Clinical Investigation, New York.)

ognize that glucose levels were falling and prompted the appropriate behavioral response (e.g., ingestion of food) to abort the episode. Thus, the first clinical manifestation of a hypoglycemic episode is neuroglycopenia, and it is often too late for the patient to recognize and self-treat the episode. This is the clinical syndrome of *hypoglycemia unawareness*. It, too, has been shown in a prospective study to be associated with a high frequency of severe iatrogenic hypoglycemia.[104]

The concept of *hypoglycemia-associated autonomic failure* in T1DM, a functional disorder distinct from the fixed autonomic failure of classical diabetic autonomic neuropathy, was formulated[105] and then verified experimentally[92, 106–109] to unify the pathogenesis of the clinical syndromes of defective glucose counterregulation and hypoglycemia unawareness.

The concept of hypoglycemia-associated autonomic failure in T1DM (Fig. 32–13) posits that:

1. Periods of relative or absolute therapeutic insulin excess in the setting of absent glucagon responses lead to episodes of hypoglycemia.
2. These episodes, in turn, cause reduced autonomic (including adrenomedullary epinephrine) responses to falling glucose concentrations on subsequent occasions.
3. These reduced autonomic responses result in reduced symptoms of, and therefore behavioral responses to, developing hypoglycemia (i.e., hypoglycemia unawareness) and—because epinephrine responses are reduced in the setting of absent glucagon response—impaired physiologic defenses against developing hypoglycemia (i.e., defective glucose counterregulation).

Thus, a vicious circle of recurrent hypoglycemia is created and perpetuated.

Perhaps the most compelling support for the concept of hypoglycemia-associated autonomic failure in T1DM is the finding, in three independent laboratories,[109–111] that hypoglycemia unawareness (Fig. 32–14) and, at least in part, the reduced epinephrine component of defective glucose counterregulation are reversible after as little as 2 weeks of scrupulous avoidance of iatrogenic hypoglycemia in most affected patients. This involves a shift of glycemic thresholds for autonomic and symptomatic responses back toward higher plasma glucose concentrations.

The basic mechanism of hypoglycemia-associated autonomic failure remains to be determined. There is evidence that it is mediated by the cortisol response to previous hypoglycemia,[112, 113] although that remains to be confirmed independently. Evidence, obtained with the Kety-Schmidt technique, that it involves increased brain glucose uptake during hypoglycemia has been reported.[114, 115] However, evidence that recent antecedent hypoglycemia does not increase blood-to-brain glucose transport or cerebral glucose metabolism, measured with [$1-{}^{11}C$]glucose and positron emission tomography, or cerebral blood flow, measured with [${}^{15}O$] water, has been presented.[116] The latter data do not exclude regional increments in blood-to-brain glucose transport. Alternatively, the alteration may lie beyond the blood-brain barrier.

Consistent with the concept of hypoglycemia-associated autonomic failure in T1DM, recent antecedent hypoglycemia also shifts glycemic thresholds for hypoglycemic cognitive dysfunction to lower plasma glucose concentrations[106–108] and impairs detection of hypoglycemia in the clinical setting in patients with T1DM.[107] In addition to shifting the thresholds for the adrenomedullary (plasma epinephrine) and parasympathetic (plasma pancreatic polypeptide) response to lower plasma glucose concentrations, recent antecedent hypoglycemia has been reported to reduce the sympathetic neural response to subsequent hypoglycemia,[97, 112, 113] although the latter has been questioned.[117]

There is also evidence that reduced sensitivity to catecholamines, measured as a reduced heart rate response to the β-adrenergic agonist isoproterenol, contributes to the pathogenesis of hypoglycemia unawareness in T1DM.[118–121] Hypoglycemia has been reported to reduce β-adrenergic sensitivity, tested about 10 hours later, in T1DM (but not in nondiabetic individuals).[120] Thus, it is conceivable that both reduced activation of the sympathochromaffin system and reduced sensitivity to released catecholamines might play a role in the pathogenesis of hypoglycemia unawareness and defective glucose counterregulation induced by recent antecedent iatrogenic hypoglycemia.

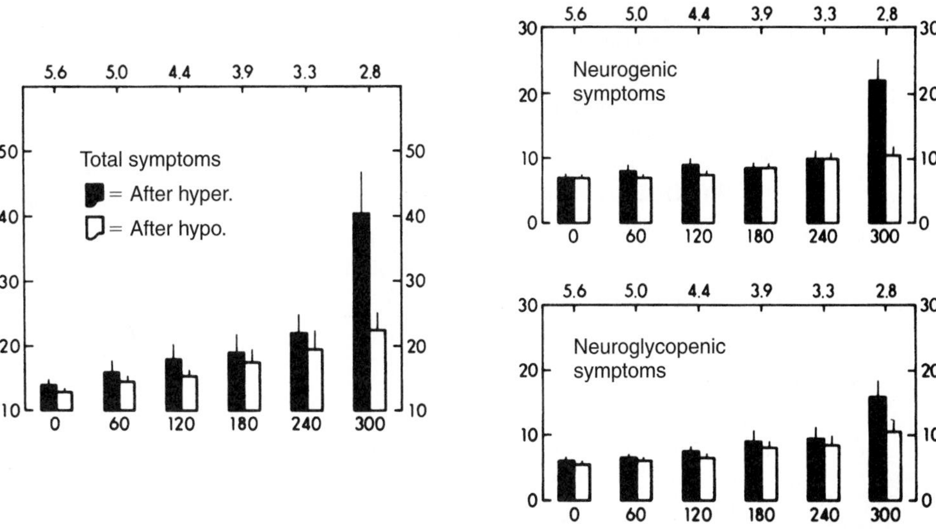

Figure 32-10. Mean (±SE) total, neurogenic, and neuroglycopenic symptom scores during hyperinsulinemic, stepped hypoglycemic glucose clamps in patients with type 1 diabetes mellitus (IDDM, insulin-dependent diabetes mellitus) without classic diabetic autonomic neuropathy on mornings following afternoon hyperglycemia (hyper., *closed columns*) and on mornings following afternoon hypoglycemia (hypo., *open columns*). (From Dagogo-Jack SE, Craft S, Cryer PE. Hypoglycemia-associated autonomic failure in insulin dependent diabetes mellitus. J Clin Invest 1993; 91: 819–828. Copyright, 1993, American Society for Clinical Investigation, New York.)

The extent to which these pathophysiologic concepts, developed in T1DM, apply to patients with T2DM remains to be assessed in detail. They may well apply to those approaching the insulin-deficient end of the spectrum of T2DM because hypoglycemia becomes limiting to glycemic control in such patients.[82] Indeed, in one series the frequency of severe hypoglycemia was found to be similar in patients with T2DM and T1DM matched for duration of insulin therapy.[85] This issue is complicated by the fact that some patients with apparent T2DM may actually have late-onset T1DM.[122] Nonetheless, patients with advanced T2DM have been reported to have reduced glucagon responses to hypoglycemia[123] (Table 32–6), a key feature of defective glucose counterregulation in T1DM. Furthermore, patients with T2DM have reduced epinephrine and neurogenic symptom responses to hypoglycemia after episodes of hypoglycemia, key features of defective glucose counterregulation, hypoglycemia unawareness, and hypoglycemia-associated autonomic failure in T1DM.[123]

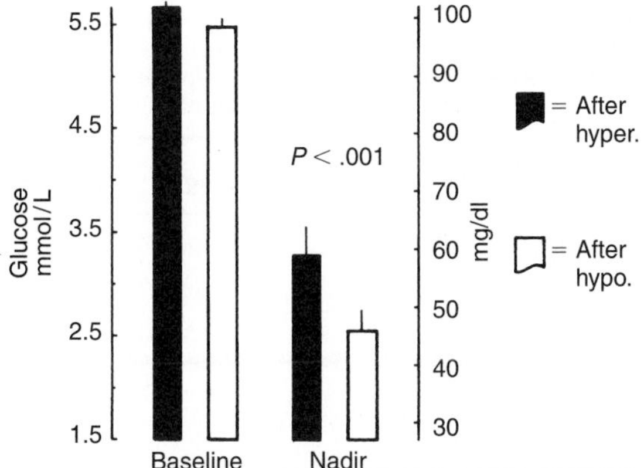

Figure 32-11. Mean (±SE) baseline and nadir plasma glucose concentrations during morning insulin infusion tests following afternoon hyperglycemia (hyper., *closed columns*) and following afternoon hypoglycemia (hypo., *open columns*) in people with type 1 diabetes without classic diabetic autonomic neuropathy. (Data from Dagogo-Jack SE, Craft S, Cryer PE. Hypoglycemia-associated autonomic failure in insulin dependent diabetes mellitus. J Clin Invest 1993; 91:819–828. Copyright, 1993, American Society for Clinical Investigation, New York.)

The concept of hypoglycemia-associated autonomic failure in T1DM is illustrated in Figure 32–13, and the comprehensive risk factors for iatrogenic hypoglycemia in T1DM, viewed in the context of the interplay of therapeutic insulin excess and compromised glucose counterregulation, are outlined in the Table 32–5.

Hypoglycemia Risk Reduction in Diabetes

Clearly, every effort must be made to minimize the risk of iatrogenic hypoglycemia and eliminate the risk of severe hypoglycemia while pursuing the greatest degree of glycemic control that can be achieved safely in an individual person with diabetes. Hypoglycemia risk reduction involves (1) addressing the issue of hypoglycemia in every contact with the patient, (2) applying the principles of aggressive glycemic therapy, and (3) considering each of the comprehensive risk factors for hypoglycemia.

In addition to questioning the patient about episodes of symptomatic and biochemical hypoglycemia and looking for

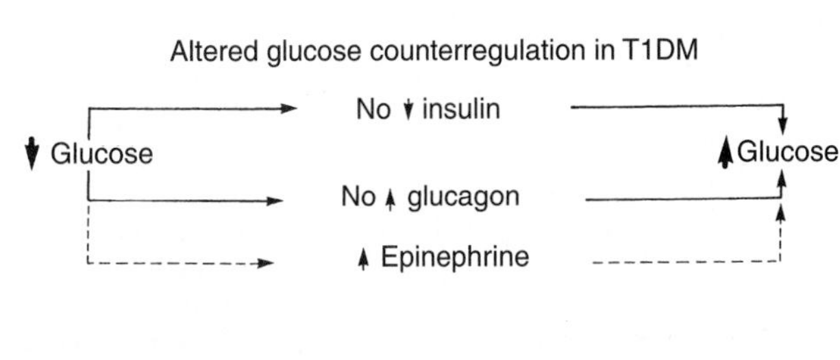

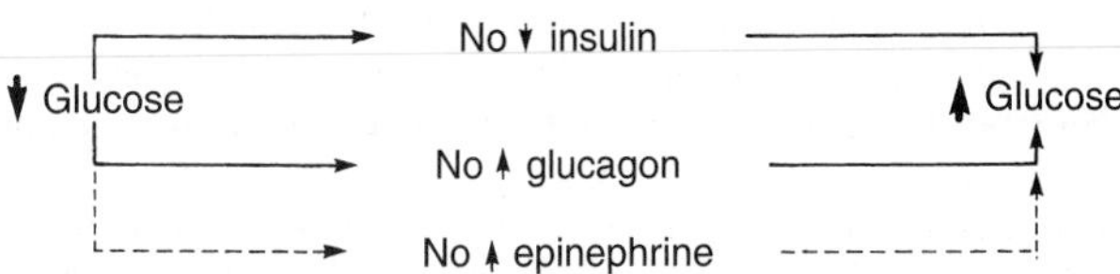

Figure 32-12. Schematic representation of the pathophysiology of glucose counterregulation in people with type 1 diabetes mellitus (T1DM). See text for discussion.

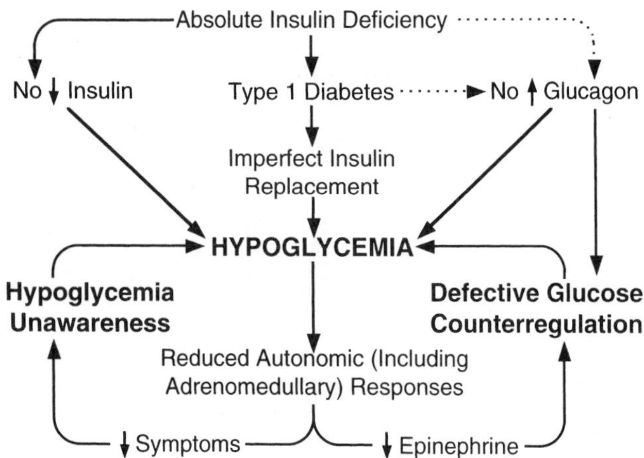

Figure 32–13. Schematic representation of the concept of hypoglycemia-associated autonomic failure in type 1 diabetes. See text for discussion. (Modified from Cryer PE. Iatrogenic hypoglycemia as a cause of hypoglycemia-associated autonomic failure in IDDM: a vicious cycle. Diabetes 1992; 41:255–260. Copyright 1992, American Diabetes Association, Alexandria, Va.)

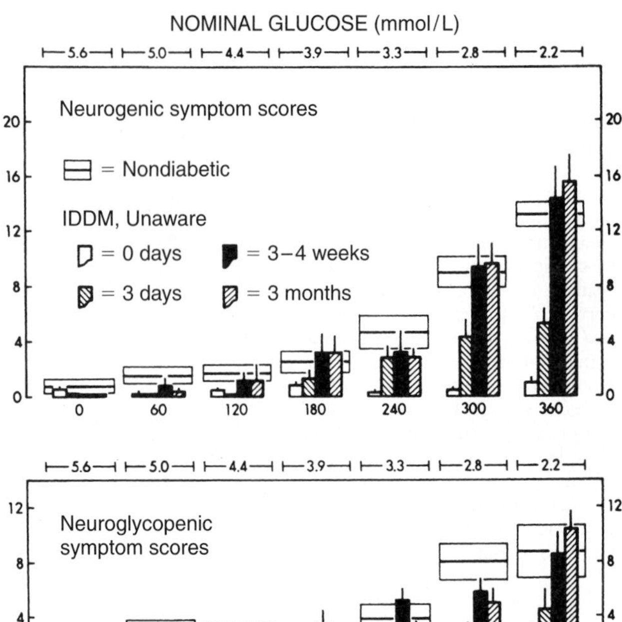

Figure 32–14. Mean (±SE) neurogenic (autonomic) and neuroglycopenic symptom scores during hyperinsulinemic stepped hypoglycemic glucose clamps in nondiabetic subjects (*rectangles*) and people with type 1 diabetes (IDDM, insulin-dependent diabetes mellitus) selected for hypoglycemia unawareness studied at baseline before (0 days, *open columns*), and after 3 days (*first set of cross-hatched columns*), 3 to 4 weeks (*closed columns*), and 3 months (*second set of crosshatched columns*) of scrupulous avoidance of iatrogenic hypoglycemia. (From Dagogo-Jack S, Rattarasarn C, Cryer PE. Reversal of hypoglycemia unawareness, but not defective glucose counterregulation, in IDDM. Diabetes 1994; 43:1426–1434.[109] Copyright, 1994, American Diabetes Association, Alexandria, Va.)

low values in the self-monitoring of the blood glucose (SMBG) log, it is important to assess the patient's awareness of hypoglycemia. A history of hypoglycemia unawareness identifies that clinical syndrome (and also implies defective glucose counterregulation). It is also important to determine the extent to which the patient is concerned about the reality or the possibility of hypoglycemia. Fear of hypoglycemia can be a barrier to glycemic control. If episodes of hypoglycemia are identified, their frequency, severity, timing, and clinical contexts need to be determined.

Once the problem of iatrogenic hypoglycemia is recognized, it is appropriate to review the treatment plan with respect to the principles of aggressive glycemic therapy. These include (1) education and empowerment of the patient; (2) frequent SMBG; (3) flexible insulin (or other drug) regimens; (4) rational, individualized glycemic goals; and (5) ongoing professional guidance and support. Particularly in T1DM, but also in advanced T2DM, glycemic control is achieved safely by a well-informed, thoughtful person with diabetes who must make judgments about the management of his or her diabetes several times each day. The patient must be given the resources to make those judgments.

In the context of these therapeutic principles, hypoglycemia risk reduction requires consideration of both the conventional risk factors that lead to episodes of absolute or relative insulin excess—insulin (or other drug) dose, timing, and type; patterns of food ingestion and of exercise; interactions with alcohol or other drugs; and altered sensitivity to or clearance of insulin—and the risk factors for compromised glucose counterregulation that impair physiologic and behavioral defenses against developing hypoglycemia (see Table 32–5). The underlying principle is that iatrogenic hypoglycemia is the result of the interplay of insulin excess and compromised glucose counterregulation rather than insulin excess alone.

As discussed earlier, the clinical surrogates of risk attributable to compromised glucose counterregulation include absolute insulin deficiency—which may be apparent from a history of ketosis-prone diabetes requiring insulin therapy from diagnosis, although it is now recognized that absolute insulin deficiency can sometimes develop more gradually in late-onset T1DM[122] or advanced T2DM[77, 82]—and a history of recurrent hypoglycemia or, absent that, aggressive glycemic therapy per se as evidenced by lower glycemic goals, lower hemoglobin A_{1c} levels, or both.[80, 86, 87] It is possible to test for defective glucose counterregulation with an insulin infusion test,[102, 103] but that is generally neither practical nor useful given the now recognized dynamic nature of hypoglycemia unawareness and the reduced epinephrine component of defective glucose counterregulation discussed earlier. On the other hand, a diagnosis of partial or

Table 32–6. Glucagon and Epinephrine Responses to Hypoglycemia in Type 2 Diabetes

Reference	Glucagon	Epinephrine
Boden et al (Diabetes 1983; 32: 1055)	Normal	Normal
Bolli et al (J Clin Invest 1984; 73: 1532)	↓	Normal
Heller et al (Diabetologia 1987; 30: 924)	Normal	Normal
Meneilly et al (Diabetes 1994; 43: 403)	↓	↑
Shamoon et al (J Clin Invest 1994; 93:2562)	↓	↑
Peacey et al (Diabetes Care 2000; 23:1023)	Normal	Normal
Segel et al (Diabetes 2000; 49: A131)	↓*	Normal*

*In advanced type 2 diabetes, as evidenced by the requirement for therapy with insulin for an average of 5 years and reduced plasma C-peptide levels.

complete hypoglycemia unawareness can be made from the history.

Clinical hypoglycemia unawareness (which also suggests defective glucose counterregulation) implies recurrent antecedent iatrogenic hypoglycemia whether that has or has not been documented. If such hypoglycemia is not apparent to the patient or to his or her family or in the SMBG log, it is probably occurring during the night. Indeed, hypoglycemia—including severe hypoglycemia—occurs most commonly during the night in people with T1DM.[75, 79, 80] That is typically the longest interdigestive period and time between SMBG and the time of maximal sensitivity to insulin.[124] In addition, sleep limits the recognition of warning symptoms of developing hypoglycemia, and thus the appropriate behavioral response, and has been found to further reduce the epinephrine response to hypoglycemia[125] and thus to further compromise the physiologic defense against developing hypoglycemia.

In addition to regimen adjustments, approaches to the problem of nocturnal hypoglycemia include use of newer insulin analogues and bedtime treatments. Substitution of a preprandial rapid-acting insulin analogue (e.g., lispro or aspart) for short-acting (regular) insulin during the day reduces the frequency of nocturnal hypoglycemia.[126] Substitution of a long-acting insulin analogue (e.g., glargine) for neutral protamine Hagedorn (NPH) or Ultralente insulin at bedtime may also reduce the frequency of nocturnal hypoglycemia.[127] Bedtime treatments intended to reduce nocturnal hypoglycemia include bedtime snacks, although their efficacy is largely limited to the first half of the night.[128] Experimental approaches include bedtime administration of uncooked cornstarch,[129, 130] of the glucagon-releasing amino acid alanine[128, 131] or of the epinephrine-simulating β_2-adrenergic agonist terbutaline.[128, 131] The efficacy of uncooked cornstarch in the 5.0-g dose recommended remains to be established. Although bedtime alanine and bedtime terbutaline have been shown to prevent nocturnal hypoglycemia more effectively than a conventional bedtime snack, alanine is probably impractical and terbutaline has not been studied further in a large clinical trial.

Obviously, with a history of recurrent hypoglycemia, one should determine when it occurs and adjust the treatment regimen appropriately. With a basal-bolus insulin regimen, morning fasting hypoglycemia implicates the long-acting or immediate-acting basal insulin, daytime hypoglycemia implicates the rapid-acting or short-acting insulin, and nighttime hypoglycemia may implicate either, all in the context of the other risk factors for insulin excess. A history of severe iatrogenic hypoglycemia—that requiring the assistance of another individual—is a clinical red flag. Unless it was the result of an easily remediable factor, such as a missed meal after insulin administration or vigorous exercise without the appropriate regimen adjustment, a substantive change in the regimen must be made. If it is not, the risk of recurrent severe hypoglycemia is unacceptably high.[80, 87]

In a patient with hypoglycemia unawareness, a 2- to 3-week period of scrupulous avoidance of iatrogenic hypoglycemia is advisable and can be assessed by return of awareness of hypoglycemia. This return of awareness has been accomplished without[110, 111] or with minimal[109] compromise of glycemic control, but that required substantial involvement of health professionals. In practice, it can involve acceptance of somewhat higher glucose levels over the short term. However, with the return of symptoms of developing hypoglycemia, empirical approaches to better glycemic control can be tried.

Hypoglycemia is a fact of life for people with T1DM (and some with T2DM) who attempt to achieve near-euglycemia.[1, 75–77, 79–83, 87] Because of the pharmacokinetic imperfections of all current insulin replacement regimens, it is not practical to maintain euglycemia while eliminating episodes of asymptomatic and even symptomatic hypoglycemia in T1DM. That awaits the ultimate goal of the prevention and cure of diabetes or, in the shorter term, development of clinical strategies for perfect insulin replacement (e.g., transplantation of insulin-secreting cells or development of a closed-loop insulin replacement system) or for near-perfect insulin replacement coupled with measures that prevent, correct, or compensate for compromised glucose counterregulation.

Treatment of Hypoglycemia in Diabetes

Most episodes of asymptomatic hypoglycemia (detected by SMBG) and mild to moderate symptomatic hypoglycemia are effectively self-treated by ingestion of glucose tablets or carbohydrate in the form of juices, soft drinks, milk, crackers, candy, or a meal.[131–133] A commonly recommended dose of glucose is 20 g (0.3 g/kg in children). However, the glycemic response to oral glucose is transient, usually less than 2 hours in insulin-induced hypoglycemia in T1DM[131] (Fig. 32–15). Thus, ingestion of a more substantial mixed snack or meal shortly after the plasma glucose level is raised is generally advisable.

Parenteral treatment is necessary when a hypoglycemic patient is unable or unwilling (because of neuroglycopenia) to take carbohydrate orally. Glucagon is commonly injected subcutaneously or intramuscularly by a spouse or family member.[131, 132, 134–136] The standard dose, 1 mg (15 μg/kg in children), can cause substantial but transient hyperglycemia[131] (see Fig. 32–15). Intranasal administration of glucagon causes a glycemic response similar to that to injected glucagon.[137–139] Although glucagon can be administered intravenously by medical personnel,[134] intravenous glucose, 25 g initially, is the standard intravenous therapy. Because the glycemic response is transient, a subsequent glucose infusion is often needed and food should be provided orally as soon as the patient is able to take it safely.

HYPOGLYCEMIC DISORDERS

Hypoglycemia is most often caused by drugs, including those used to treat diabetes, just discussed, and alcohol.[73, 74,] Other causes of hypoglycemia (see Table 32–2) include several critical illnesses (hepatic, cardiac, and renal failure; sepsis; and inanition), endocrine deficiencies (cortisol, growth hormone, or both), non–beta cell tumors (non–islet cell tumor hypoglycemia), and endogenous as well as exogenous hyperinsulinemia (insulinoma among others). Some hypoglycemic disorders are unique to, or typically have their onset in, infancy and childhood. Clinical hypoglycemia in general[1] and that not resulting from the treatment of diabetes[140] have been reviewed in detail.

The Fasting (Postabsorptive) Hypoglycemias

Drugs

Drugs are the most common cause of hypoglycemia.[73, 74, 140, 141] Among these, insulin, sulfonylureas, and perhaps metformin, used to treat diabetes, are the common offenders as discussed earlier in this chapter. Insulin and particularly sulfonylureas are possible causative agents even when there is no history of diabetes because these are sometimes taken surreptitiously, administered with criminal intent, or taken as the result of a pharmacy or other error.[142] Established and putative hypoglycemia-causing drugs are listed in Table 32–7.

Ethanol inhibits gluconeogenesis,[143] possibly because its metabolism to acetaldehyde and then acetate (by alcohol dehydro-

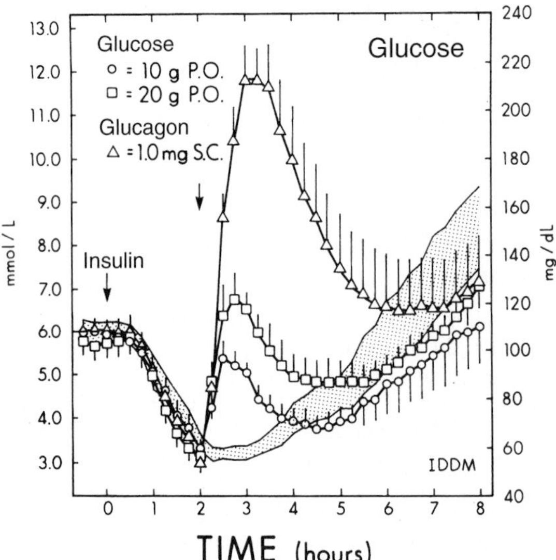

Figure 32–15. Mean (±SE) plasma glucose concentrations during hypoglycemia produced by subcutaneous insulin injection in people with type 1 diabetes in response to 10 g (*circles*) and 20 g (*squares*) of oral (p.o.) glucose and 1.0 mg of subcutaneous (S.C.) glucagon (*triangles*) compared with placebo (*shaded area*). (From Wiethop BV, Cryer PE. Alanine and terbutaline in the treatment of hypoglycemia in IDDM. Diabetes Care 1993; 16:1131–1136. Copyright, 1993, American Diabetes Association, Alexandria, Va.)

genase and aldehyde dehydrogenase, respectively) depletes nicotinamide adenine dinucleotide, a cofactor critical to the entry of most precursors into the gluconeogenic pathway. It does not inhibit glycogenolysis. Ethanol also inhibits cortisol and growth hormone[143] responses and may delay the epinephrine[143] and glucagon[143, 144] responses to hypoglycemia. In healthy humans ethanol administration does not cause postabsorptive hypoglycemia[145] or impair recovery from short-term hypoglycemia,[144] presumably because of intact glucagon and epinephrine secretion and responsive hepatic glycogenolysis coupled with decreased sensitivity to insulin.[144, 146, 147] However, because gluconeogenesis becomes the dominant route of glucose production during prolonged hypoglycemia,[143] ethanol can contribute to the progression of hypoglycemia in patients with drug-treated diabetes. It can also cause postabsorptive hypoglycemia in states of glycogen depletion.[142]

Clinical alcohol-induced hypoglycemia typically follows (by 6 to 36 hours) a binge of moderate to heavy alcohol consumption during which the person eats little food (i.e., in the setting of glycogen depletion).[141] Hypoglycemia can be profound, and alcohol-induced hypoglycemia can be fatal. However, with restoration of normal glucose levels and supportive care, complete recovery is the rule. Ethanol is typically measurable in blood at the time of presentation, but its levels correlate poorly with glucose levels. On the other hand, hypoglycemia may be a late feature of alcoholic ketoacidosis and ethanol may not be measurable in the blood at the time of presentation.[141]

Salicylates in relatively large doses (4 to 6 g/day) can lower plasma glucose concentrations[148] and produce hypoglycemia in children and, rarely, in adults.[149, 150] Sulfonamides also rarely produce hypoglycemia.[151] The mechanisms of salicylate- and sulfonamide-induced hypoglycemia are unknown but, at least for the latter, may involve stimulation of insulin secretion.

Pentamidine is a beta cell toxin. Initially, it can cause hypoglycemia by causing insulin release. Ultimately, it can cause diabetes mellitus. In one series of immunocompromised patients with *Pneumocystis* pneumonia treated with pentamidine,

Table 32–7. Established and Putative Hypoglycemia-Causing Drugs

Disorder Treated	Drug
	Established
Diabetes mellitus	Insulin, sulfonylureas and other insulin secretagogues, metformin
	Alcohol
Infections	Pentamidine, quinine, sulfonamides
Arrhythmias	Quinidine, disopyramide, cibenzoline
Pain	Acetylsalicylic acid
	Putative
Infection	Ciprofloxacin, chloramphenicol, ketoconazole, oxytetracycline, ethionamide, isoniazid, *p*-aminosalicylic acid, *p*-aminobenzoate
Pain	Acetaminophen, indomethacin, propoxyphene, phenylbutazone
Hypertension, heart disease	β-Adrenergic antagonists (nonselective > β_1-selective), angiotensin-converting enzyme inhibitors
Edema	Furosemide, acetazolamide
Depression	Monoamine oxidase inhibitors, fluoxetine, imipramine
Psychoses	Haloperidol, chlorpromazine, perhexiline
Hyperlipidemia	Clofibrate, bezafibrate
Allergies	Orphenadrine, diphenhydramine
Gastric hyperacidity	Cimetidine, ranitidine
Gout	Colchicine, sulfinpyrazone
Seizures	Phenytoin
(Anesthetics)	Enflurane, halothane
(Chelation)	Penicillamine
Miscellaneous	Hypoglycins (in Jamaican akee fruit), thalidomide, selegiline, others

7% experienced hypoglycemia, 14% experienced hypoglycemia followed by diabetes, and 18% experienced diabetes without detected hypoglycemia.[152] Risk factors for pentamidine-induced hypoglycemia include therapy of longer duration and increased doses, previous pentamidine therapy, and renal insufficiency.[152, 153]

Hypoglycemia occurs commonly in severe malaria. Although associated with relative hyperinsulinemia attributed to quinine-induced insulin release in some patients,[154] hypoglycemia can occur in the absence of quinine therapy[155] and in the absence of hyperinsulinemia in quinine-treated patients.[156] Nonetheless, quinine has been reported to cause hypoglycemia in persons not afflicted by malaria,[157] and treatment of malaria with quinine, compared with the artemisinin-derivative artesunate, has been associated with higher plasma insulin/glucose ratios and lower glucose turnover rates and reported to produce higher rates of postadmission hypoglycemia.[158] Among antiarrhythmic drugs, quinidine, disopyramide,[159] and cibenzoline[160] have been reported to cause hypoglycemia.

Hypoglycemia has been attributed to many other drugs (see Table 32–7). In many of the cases, other potential causes of hypoglycemia have been present. For example, although hypoglycemia attributed to propranolol has been reported in healthy children,[161, 162] most of the reported incidents occurred in insulin-treated diabetes. Although nonselective β-adrenergic antagonists such as propranolol would be expected to reduce symptoms of developing hypoglycemia and impair epinephrine-mediated glucose counterregulation,[163] compelling evidence that these drugs increase the frequency of clinical hypoglycemia in insulin-treated diabetes has not been forthcoming. Nonetheless, it would be reasonable to use a relatively selective

β_1-adrenergic receptor antagonist (e.g., metoprolol or atenolol) in such patients.

Critical Illnesses

Among hospitalized patients, drugs, particularly insulin, are still the most common cause of hypoglycemia.[74] However, serious diseases—particularly renal failure but also hepatic or cardiac failure, sepsis, or inanition—are second only to drugs.

In addition to appropriate glucoregulatory signals and a sufficient supply of gluconeogenic precursors, maintenance of the postabsorptive plasma glucose concentration requires a structurally and functionally intact liver. Renal glucose production notwithstanding, total hepatectomy results in profound hypoglycemia.[164] Extensive liver disease is required to produce hypoglycemia. Hepatogenous hypoglycemia occurs most commonly when destruction of the liver is rapid and massive (e.g., toxic hepatitis). It has been reported in fulminant viral hepatitis,[165] in fatty liver attributed to alcohol ingestion, and in cholangitis and bilary obstruction. It is unusual in common forms of cirrhosis and hepatitis, although glucose metabolism is altered demonstrably (with lower postabsorptive plasma glucose concentrations, diminished glycemic responses to glucagon, and reduced hepatic glycogen contents) in uncomplicated viral hepatitis.[166] It is also unusual in metastatic liver disease despite extensive hepatic replacement.[167] Hypoglycemia can be caused by primary malignant tumors but is the result of a glucoregulatory abnormality, insulin-like growth factor II overproduction (see "Non–Beta Cell Tumors").

The pathogenesis of hypoglycemia in occasional patients with severe cardiac failure is unknown. Possibilities include hepatic congestion and hypoxia, inanition, and gluconeogenic precursor limitation. The finding of elevated blood lactate levels associated with hypoglycemia[168] raises the possibility of inhibited gluconeogenesis.

Postabsorptive hypoglycemia occurs in some patients with renal failure,[169–173] and the finding of a high frequency of renal insufficiency among patients with low plasma glucose levels[74] suggests that compromised glucose counterregulation may be a feature of renal failure. However, the pathogenesis of hypoglycemia in such patients is not known; it may involve multiple mechanisms. Most patients with hypoglycemia attributed to renal failure are cachectic. One such patient had reduced glucose turnover, diminished gluconeogenesis from alanine, and reduced alanine turnover.[171] During fasting, plasma glucose levels fell, blood lactate levels did not increase, and blood alanine levels fell. Hypoglycemia was attributed to substrate limitation of gluconeogenesis. However, at least one patient did not respond to substrate (glycerol, alanine) administration.[172] Glycemic responses to glucagon have been found to be reduced, suggesting impaired glycogenolysis, in some[173, 174] but not all[175] studies.

Some patients with hypoglycemia attributed to renal failure have had diabetes,[169, 171] but hypoglycemia persisted or recurred after insulin or oral hypoglycemic agents were withdrawn. The kidneys are a major site of insulin clearance, and decreasing insulin requirements parallel decreasing renal function in patients with insulin-treated diabetes. In the absence of insulin or insulin secretagogue therapy, however, endogenous insulin secretion should decrease as glucose levels decline and hypoglycemia would, therefore, not be expected. The extent to which reduced renal glucose production contributes to hypoglycemia in end-stage renal disease is unknown. However, given the capacity of the normal liver to produce substantial amounts of glucose, loss of glucose-producing renal parenchyma would not be expected to produce hypoglycemia. Indeed, renal transplantation does not correct postabsorptive hypoglycemia in patients with glucose-6-phosphatase deficiency.[176] Thus, one functioning kidney is not sufficient to provide normal endogenous glucose production in the virtual absence of hepatic glucose production.

Sepsis is a relatively common cause of hypoglycemia.[73, 74, 177] Increased glucose utilization (by skeletal muscle[178] and by macrophage-rich tissues such as liver, spleen, and ileum[179]) and, at least initially, glucose production characterize experimental sepsis.[180, 181] Hypoglycemia develops when hepatic glucose production decreases.[181, 182] The factors responsible for the increased glucose turnover and the ultimate failure of glucose production to keep pace in sepsis are not entirely clear. Cytokines such as tumor necrosis factor α (TNF-α) and interleukin-6, among others, are thought to increase glucose utilization.[182–186] The initial increase in glucose production is at least in part mediated by increased glucagon[187] and catecholamine[185, 188, 189] release, appropriate physiologic responses to accelerated glucose utilization. These may also be stimulated by cytokines.[186, 190] For example, TNF-α infusion increases glucose production, an effect attributable to TNF-α–stimulated glucagon secretion, in dogs.[186] The later decline in glucose production, which results in hypoglycemia, is not the result of glucose counterregulatory failure. Rather, it appears to be the result of decreased hepatic responsiveness to appropriate glucoregulatory stimuli, that is, low insulin and high glucagon and epinephrine levels.[191] Hepatic hypoperfusion is a plausible mechanism. It has been suggested that inactivation (oxidation) of catecholamines by superoxide anions plays a role in the pathogenesis of septic shock.[192]

Hypoglycemia caused by inanition[193] is thought to be rare in developed countries but has been reported in the United States.[194] Because hypoglycemia can persist despite high rates of glucose infusion, such patients must have high rates of glucose utilization. Beyond this, the pathogenesis of hypoglycemia is unknown. An entirely speculative suggestion is that glucose becomes the sole oxidative fuel in the setting of total body fat depletion and that high rates of glucose utilization exceed the capacity to produce glucose because of limitation of substrate (e.g., amino acids). Postabsorptive hypoglycemia (with low blood alanine levels) has been reported in some patients with profound muscle atrophy.[195]

Hormonal Deficiencies

With the notable exception of defective glucose counterregulation in patients with established T1DM and advanced T2DM, discussed earlier in this chapter, hormonal glucoregulatory abnormalities resulting in hypoglycemia are not common. These abnormalities include hyperinsulinism, discussed later, and deficiencies of glucose counterregulatory hormones.

Most adults with deficient secretion of cortisol, growth hormone, or both do not experience hypoglycemia. Indeed, plasma glucose concentrations (and endogenous glucose production) after an overnight fast are not distinguishable from normal in glucocorticoid-withdrawn patients with panhypopituitarism never treated with growth hormone.[61] Nonetheless, postabsorptive hypoglycemia can occur in patients with chronic deficiencies of these hormones, particularly in the neonatal period and in children younger than 5 years of age.[196, 197, 198] Indeed, severely glucocorticoid-deficient (corticotropin-releasing hormone knockout) newborn male mice became more hypoglycemic than wild mice during fasting.[199]

Hypoglycemia in children with deficient secretion of cortisol, growth hormone, or both is generally preceded by a period of caloric deprivation. That is consistent with the observation that hypoglycemia can sometimes be provoked by 24 to 30 hours of fasting in children with hypopituitarism who do not exhibit hypoglycemia after an overnight fast.[200, 201] This intolerance of fasting is largely corrected by glucocorticoid

Table 32–8. Biochemical Patterns in Patients with Various Causes of Hyperinsulinemic Hypoglycemia

Insulin	C Peptide	Proinsulin	Sulfonylurea	Insulin Antibody	Diagnosis
↑	↓	↓	−	−	Exogenous insulin
↑	↑	↑*	−	−	Insulinoma, CHI†
↑	↑	↑	+	−	Sulfonylurea
↑	↑‡	↑‡	−	+	Insulin autoimmune
±↑	↓	↓	−	−	Insulin receptor autoimmune§

*> 20% of insulin value.
†Congenital hyperinsulinism.
‡Free C peptide and proinsulin ↓.
§Insulin receptor antibody +.

replacement, whereas growth hormone replacement has a lesser effect.[200, 201] These findings suggest that a defect in gluconeogenesis causes hypoglycemia when hepatic glycogen stores are depleted.

Cortisol supports gluconeogenesis both by increasing gluconeogenic enzyme activities and by mobilizing gluconeogenic precursors to the liver (and the kidneys).[200, 202, 203] Postabsorptive hypoglycemia in hypopituitarism is associated with low levels of circulating gluconeogenic precursors.[200, 204] However, oral alanine administration only partially reverses hypoglycemia.[204] Finally, because cortisol deficiency causes reduced epinephrine secretion[205]—presumably because of reduced induction of adrenomedullary phenylethanolamine *N*-methyltransferase by adrenocortical cortisol—epinephrine deficiency might contribute to the pathogenesis of hypoglycemia in this setting. Glucagon secretion is not reduced in such patients. Thus, given the key role of glucagon in glucose counterregulation, it is not surprising that glucose recovery, at least from short-term hypoglycemia, is generally normal in children with deficient secretion of cortisol, growth hormone, or both.[206] Adults with hypopituitarism occasionally suffer postabsorptive hypoglycemia, particularly when glucose utilization or loss is increased, as during exercise or in pregnancy, respectively,[207] or when gluconeogenesis is impaired, as after alcohol ingestion.[208] Again, these observations suggest that impaired gluconeogenesis becomes limiting to glucose production in the setting of glycogen depletion resulting from caloric deprivation.

As discussed earlier (see "Glucose Counterregulation"), hypoglycemia develops or progresses when both glucagon and epinephrine are deficient and insulin is present[1, 2] (see Table 32–1). This combination occurs in patients with established T1DM. They must be treated with insulin, have no glucagon response to hypoglycemia, and typically have a reduced epinephrine response to hypoglycemia and are, as a result, at high risk for iatrogenic hypoglycemia[1, 2] as discussed earlier (see "Hypoglycemia in Diabetes Mellitus"). However, systematic studies of an unusual patient[209] suggest that clinical postabsorptive hypoglycemia may not develop when both glucagon and epinephrine are deficient but insulin secretion decreases normally as plasma glucose levels decline. That patient, with hypopituitarism attributed to sarcoidosis involving the hypothalamus, was shown to have no glucagon or epinephrine response to insulin-induced hypoglycemia; glucose recovery from that short-term experimental hypoglycemia was impaired markedly, as expected. Plasma glucose concentrations were relatively low after overnight fasts (3.2 ± 0.5 mmol/L, 58 ± 8 mg/dL). However, during a 72-hour fast plasma insulin levels declined to about 30 pmol/L (5 μU/mL); glucose levels declined to only 2.8 mmol/L (50 mg/dL), a value indistinguishable from that of similarly fasted healthy subjects; and symptoms of hypoglycemia did not occur.

Table 32–9. Plasma Glucose, Insulin, C-Peptide, and Proinsulin Concentrations used by Service (1999)[140] and by Marks and Teale (1996)[243] to Diagnose Fasting Hypoglycemia Caused by Endogenous Hyperinsulinism (e.g., in a Patient with an Insulinoma)

	Service	Marks and Teale
Glucose		
mmol/L	≤2.5	<3.0
mg/dL	≤45	<54
Insulin		
pmol/L	≥36	>30
μU/mL	≥6	>5
C peptide		
nmol/L	≥0.2	>0.3
ng/mL	≥0.6	>0.9
Proinsulin		
pmol/L	≥5	>20

Hypoglycemia is not a feature of the epinephrine-deficient state that results from bilateral adrenalectomy if glucocorticoid replacement is appropriate,[51, 56, 210] and hypoglycemia does not occur during pharmacologic blockade of catecholamine actions when other glucose counterregulatory systems are intact.[18, 51, 53, 56, 58, 211] Hypoglycemia has been attributed to epinephrine deficiency. For example, urinary[212, 213] and plasma[214] epinephrine responses to hypoglycemia are reduced in ketotic hypoglycemia of childhood, and therapeutic responses to ephedrine, a catecholamine-releasing drug, have been reported in uncontrolled studies of such patients.[215, 216] Also, some patients have been reported to have diminished glycemic responses to glucagon during fasting.[215–217]

Postabsorptive hypoglycemia has also been attributed to epinephrine deficiency in one member of each of three sets of twins.[218, 219] Compared with their unaffected twins, the hypoglycemic children had reduced, but not absent, urinary epinephrine responses to infused 2-deoxyglucose and to hypoglycemia induced by fasting. However, the glucagon secretory responses were not evaluated, and the affected infants had inappropriately high insulin levels while they were hypoglycemic.[218] Finally, reduced epinephrine excretion in infants of diabetic mothers has been associated with the occurrence of neonatal hypoglycemia.[220]

Isolated glucagon deficiency would be expected to result in lowered postabsorptive plasma glucose concentrations but not frank hypoglycemia if insulin secretion was suppressed appropriately and epinephrine secretion were intact.[1, 53] A seemingly convincing example of hypoglycemia attributable to isolated glucagon deficiency has been described in an abstract[221] but the case was never published. Postabsorptive hypoglycemia has been reported in another glucagon-deficient adult, but cortisol secretion and growth hormone secretion were also deficient.[222] Neonatal hypoglycemia has also been attributed to glucagon deficiency.[223, 224] However, plasma insulin levels were inappropriately high during hypoglycemia.

Elevated plasma levels of glucose counterregulatory hormones during hypoglycemia exclude deficiencies of these. Levels that are not elevated during a spontaneous episode of hypoglycemia provide a diagnostic clue that requires definitive testing. In a patient with postabsorptive hypoglycemia that is not readily explained, it is my practice to seek clinical clues of hypopituitarism or primary adrenocortical insufficiency—and often assess the plasma cortisol response to cosyntropin (synthetic ACTH)—and to pursue such clues with definitive testing (e.g., the responses to insulin-induced hypoglycemia). Given the evidence, just summarized, that isolated glucagon deficiency or isolated epinephrine deficiency rarely if ever causes postabsorptive hypoglycemia, these theoretical possibilities are generally not pursued.

Non–Beta Cell Tumors

Postabsorptive hypoglycemia is occasionally caused by non–beta cell tumors (non–islet cell tumor hypoglycemia).[1] The majority are large retroperitoneal, intra-abdominal or intrathoracic tumors that are typically slow-growing albeit malignant. Epithelial tumors that can cause hypoglycemia include hepatomas,[225] adrenocortical carcinomas, and carcinoid tumors. More common carcinomas and hematologic or lymphoid malignancies rarely cause hypoglycemia. Affected patients often have relatively high rates of glucose utilization,[226–228] a pattern resembling that of hyperinsulinism. Reports of a few patients with hypoglycemia attributed to ectopic insulin secretion have been published,[229–235] but plasma insulin and C-peptide levels are suppressed appropriately during hypoglycemia in the vast majority of patients with non–beta cell tumor hypoglycemia.

Similarly, insulin-like growth factor I (IGF-I) levels are typically suppressed. Overproduction of insulin-like growth factor II (IGF-II), specifically an incompletely processed form ("big IGF-II") that does not complex normally with circulating binding proteins and thus more readily gains access to target tissues, is the cause of hypoglycemia in most patients.[236–242] The diagnosis is usually not difficult. The tumors are often apparent clinically and plasma insulin, C-peptide, and proinsulin levels are low during hypoglycemia. Free IGF-II levels (and levels of pro–IGF-II [E1–21]) are elevated.[240–242] It should be noted, however, that both of these are often elevated in patients with renal failure. Presumably because of negative feedback mediated by IGF-II, growth hormone secretion is suppressed. Thus, serum IGF-I levels are low and the ratio of IGF-II to IGF-I is distinctly elevated.

Endogenous Hyperinsulinemia

Hypoglycemia related to excessive endogenous insulin secretion[1, 141, 243] can be caused by:

1. A primary pancreatic islet beta cell disorder, typically a beta cell tumor (insulinoma), sometimes multiple insulinomas, or, especially in infants or young children, a functional beta cell disorder with beta cell hyperplasia or without an anatomic correlate.
2. A beta cell secretagogue, often a sulfonylurea, theoretically a beta cell–stimulating autoantibody.
3. An antibody to insulin.

None of these is common. Endogenous hyperinsulinism is more likely in an overtly well individual with postabsorptive hypoglycemia, that is, a person with no relevant drug history or critical illness and no clinical clues to hormone deficiencies or a non–beta cell tumor. In such an individual, accidental, surreptitious, or even malicious administration of a sulfonylurea, another insulin-releasing drug, or insulin should also be considered.

The critical pathophysiologic feature of endogenous hyperinsulinism is failure of insulin secretion, assessed by plasma insulin and C-peptide levels, to fall to very low rates during hypoglycemia.[1, 141, 243] The plasma insulin, C-peptide, proinsulin, sulfonylurea, and insulin antibody patterns in the various diagnostic categories (including exogenous as well as endogenous hyperinsulinism) are shown in Table 32–8.

The plasma glucose, insulin, C-peptide, and proinsulin levels advocated by Service[140] and by Marks and Teale[243] for the diagnosis of endogenous hyperinsulinism are summarized in Table 32–9. Insulin and C-peptide levels need not be high in the absolute (i.e., relative to euglycemic postabsorptive norms) but only inappropriately high during postabsorptive hypoglycemia. The diagnostic concept of relative hyperinsulinemia is fundamentally important. Measurements of insulin and C-peptide levels when the patient is not hypoglycemic are not useful diagnostically. Insulin, C-peptide, and proinsulin (and sulfonylurea) levels need to be determined when the patient is clearly hypoglycemic—plasma glucose at least less than 2.8 mmol/L (50 mg/dL), preferably with symptoms—in the postabsorptive state. This determination accomplishes two diagnostic goals:

1. It generally establishes that the patient does, in fact, have postabsorptive hypoglycemia. Even during a prolonged (e.g., 48 to 72 hours) fast, plasma glucose levels rarely fall to less than 2.8 mmol/L in healthy adult men although lower levels sometimes occur in healthy adult women and children.[244, 245] However, healthy subjects should not have symptoms of hypoglycemia and their insulin, C-peptide, and proinsulin levels should be low.
2. It determines whether the patient has hyperinsulinemic or hypoinsulinemic hypoglycemia, the latter excluding hyperinsulinism as a diagnostic consideration.

Plasma C-peptide levels are low in exogenous hyperinsulinism, whether that is therapeutic, surreptitious, or malicious.[246] Plasma proinsulin concentrations, like insulin and C-peptide levels, are disproportionately high in patients with insulinomas and related disorders.[247–249] Sulfonylureas produce glucose, insulin, and C-peptide patterns indistinguishable from those produced by a primary beta cell disorder,[248] but a sulfonylurea is measurable. (This potential diagnostic problem could be confounded by the availability of new nonsulfonylurea insulin-releasing drugs such as repaglinide and nateglinide.) Antibodies to insulin[250–258] produce hypoglycemia during the transition from the postprandial to the postabsorptive state as insulin—secreted in response to the earlier meal and bound to the antibodies—slowly dissociates from the antibodies and causes relative hyperinsulinism. Total and free plasma insulin concentrations are inappropriately high. Insulin secretion is suppressed appropriately and free plasma C-peptide (and proinsulin) levels are low, but total C-peptide (and proinsulin) levels are high because of cross-reactivity with antibody-bound proinsulin including its C-peptide sequence.[253]

Hypoglycemia can also be caused, rarely, by insulin receptor–stimulating autoantibodies.[259–264] Plasma glucose and C-peptide levels are low but insulin levels tend to be high, presumably because receptor-bound antibodies impair the clearance of insulin.[262] Antibodies that stimulate beta-cell insulin secretion in vitro have been described in sera from patients with hypoglycemia,[265–267] but a corresponding clinical syndrome has not been defined. Finally, as noted earlier, ectopic insulin secretion has been described.[229–235] Nonetheless, insulin arteriovenous differences across such tumors remain to be documented.

In summary, the diagnostic strategy is to measure plasma

mone levels), structural and enzymatic integrity of the liver (and kidneys), and availability of sufficient gluconeogenic precursors are essential. In the setting of relatively low plasma glucose concentrations, the combination of hypoinsulinemia and activated glucose counterregulatory systems also favors lipolysis. High nonesterified fatty acid levels provide an alternative fuel for tissues other than the brain and limit glucose utilization by muscle and fat. They also drive ketogenesis, thus providing an alternative fuel for the brain during neonatal life. These glucoregulatory signals also favor mobilization of gluconeogenic precursors. Impairment of any of these adaptations to extrauterine life can cause transient neonatal hypoglycemia. Persistent defects cause recurrent or persistent hypoglycemia.

Transient intolerance of fasting occurs in preterm or small-for-gestational age infants; in hypopituitarism, adrenal hypoplasia, or congenital adrenal hyperplasia; or, later, in ketotic hypoglycemia of childhood. At least in the absence of seizure or coma, neonatal hypoglycemia (that developing in the first 72 hours after birth) is usually transient.[293] It is particularly common in preterm or small-for-gestational age infants and is thought to result from incomplete development of gluconeogenic mechanisms,[299] although glucose counterregulatory signals may be impaired.[300] Deficiencies of cortisol, growth hormone, or both can be congenital and cause hypoglycemia through mechanisms discussed earlier.

In general, children tolerate fasting less well than adults. Indeed, hypoglycemia is the rule after 24 to 48 hours of fasting in normal children.[245] The syndrome of ketotic hypoglycemia of childhood, which typically has its onset between ages 2 and 5 years and remits spontaneously before age 10 years, may account for the fraction of children who are least tolerant of fasting.[301] Hypoglycemia occurs when feeding is interrupted, typically during an intercurrent illness. The syndrome appears to involve diminished mobilization of gluconeogenic precursors including alanine.[302, 303] Blood alanine levels are low during hypoglycemia, and alanine infusion increases plasma glucose levels. Glycogenolytic and gluconeogenic mechanisms appear to be intact and, aside from low epinephrine levels,[212–217] glucoregulatory signals are appropriate. Deficient epinephrine secretion might impair alanine mobilization because epinephrine stimulates alanine turnover in humans.[304] Nonetheless, epinephrine deficiency per se does not cause hypoglycemia, as discussed earlier.

The most common cause of hyperinsulinemic neonatal hypoglycemia is maternal diabetes.[293] Infants of diabetic mothers are hyperglycemic (in proportion to the mother's hyperglycemia) and correspondingly hyperinsulinemic. Presumably reflecting chronic stimulation of fetal insulin secretion in utero and its failure to become suppressed normally as glucose levels fall shortly after birth, transient neonatal hypoglycemia occurs. Transient hyperinsulinemia also underlies neonatal hypoglycemia in infants with Rh factor incompatibility or with the Beckwith-Wiedemann syndrome (macroglossia, omphalocele, and visceromegaly). Hypoglycemia, resulting from hyperinsulinemia stimulated by glucose infusion during the procedure, can also follow exchange transfusion. Neonatal hypoglycemia can be caused by drugs given to the mother, including agents that stimulate fetal insulin secretion (e.g., a sulfonylurea) or that produce maternal and fetal hyperglycemia and thus fetal hyperinsulinemia (e.g., a β_2-adrenergic agonist used to delay labor). Accidental or malicious administration of a sulfonylurea or insulin is a rare cause of hyperinsulinemic hypoglycemia in children.

In contrast to these causes of transient neonatal hyperinsulinemic hypoglycemia, congenital hyperinsulinism (or persistent hyperinsulinemic hypoglycemia of infancy) may persist from the neonatal period or become apparent clinically in the first year of life.[293–295, 305] (Patients in that age range rarely have a discrete insulinoma, although insulinomas are found in children who develop hyperinsulinemic hypoglycemia after the first year.) Although partial pancreatectomy may become necessary, patients with congenital hyperinsulinism are treated medically initially—with glucose administration for stabilization; frequent feedings; and diazoxide (often with a thiazide), octreotide, and glucagon, often tried in that sequence—in the anticipation of amelioration of hypoglycemia over time because there is a high frequency of diabetes late after partial pancreatectomy.[294, 295, 305]

Congenital hyperinsulinism is the most common cause of nontransient neonatal hypoglycemia. It is often inherited as an autosomal recessive trait and the result of mutations of the genes that encode adenosine triphosphate–sensitive potassium (KATP) channels, specifically the sulfonylurea receptor (SUR1) or the channel itself (Kir6.2).[305–310] Homozygous mutations result in diffuse beta-cell hypersecretion; focal beta-cell hypersecretion has been attributed to loss of maternal heterozygosity and expression of the paternal KATP mutation.[309, 310] In general, patients with KATP channel mutations suffer from severe neonatal hypoglycemia that is unresponsive to diazoxide. Successful treatment with the calcium channel antagonist nifedipine has been reported.[311, 312] Other causes of congenital hyperinsulinism[305]—which typically cause less marked hypoglycemia and are more likely to be responsive to diazoxide—include autosomal dominant activating mutations of the glutamate dehydrogenase gene (the hyperinsulinism-hyperammonemia syndrome)[313, 314] and of the glucokinase gene.[315–317] Hyperinsulinemic hypoglycemia has also been reported in an infant with phosphomannose isomerase deficiency and was found to be responsive to mannose administration.[318]

Hypoglycemia that develops in infancy or childhood and persists into adulthood with effective therapy[319] can also be caused by enzymatic defects in carbohydrate metabolism (e.g., glycogen storage disease types I, III, and IV; glycogen synthase deficiency; fructose-1,6-bisphosphatase, phosphoenolpyruvate carboxykinase, or pyruvate kinase deficiency; fructose-1-phosphate aldolase deficiency; galactose-1-phosphate uridyltransferase deficiency; or glucose transporter defects),[319–339] in protein metabolism (e.g., branched-chain α-keto acid dehydrogenase complex deficiency),[340–343] or in fat metabolism (e.g., various defects in fatty acid oxidation).[294, 344–352] All of these disorders cause postabsorptive hypoglycemia except for hereditary fructose intolerance caused by fructose-1-phosphate aldolase deficiency and galactosemia caused by galactose uridyltransferase deficiency, which cause postprandial hypoglycemia. Although clinical features and biochemical patterns suggest a subset of diagnostic possibilities and in some instances provide a specific diagnosis, definitive diagnosis often requires either documentation of deficient enzyme activity in affected tissues or, increasingly, identification of a mutation in the relevant gene.

As first documented by Cori and Cori[320] in 1952, deficient glucose-6-phosphatase activity causes glycogen storage disease type I (von Gierke's disease).[294, 321–323] Type I glycogen storage disease is the prototype glycogen storage disease. Because hydrolysis of glucose-6-phosphate to glucose is the common pathway for systemic glucose production from both hepatic glycogenolysis and gluconeogenesis (and renal gluconeogenesis), glucose-6-phosphatase deficiency causes (1) profound postabsorptive hypoglycemia with hypoinsulinemia; (2) activated glucose counterregulatory systems with elevated lactate, alanine, nonesterified fatty acid, ketone body, and triglyceride levels; and (3) metabolic acidosis with hyperuricemia. Hepatomegaly (caused by hepatocyte accumulation of fat as well as glycogen) is a universal finding. With the exception of hepatomegaly, the abnormalities can be reversed by the prevention of hypoglycemia with frequent feedings during waking hours and continuous intragastric glucose infusion during sleep[324] or with bedtime administration of large doses of uncooked cornstarch.[325] Liver transplantation corrects hypoglycemia and the associated metabolic abnormalities.[326] Adults with (presumably inadequately treated) type I glycogen storage disease have a high incidence of hepatic adenomas and renal disease.[319, 327] Interestingly, renal transplantation does not correct hypoglycemia.[321] The mechanism by which these patients maintain some level of endogenous glucose production is unclear.[338]

The glucose-6-phosphatase system is complex. Most patients with type I glycogen storage disease have mutations of the gene encoding the catalytic subunit (type Ia). Others do not have such mutations; the defect has been attributed to mutations in the glucose-6-phosphate translocase gene (type Ib-Ic or non–type Ia).[294, 322, 323] Hypoglycemia is less prominent in type III (amylo-1,6-glucosidase deficiency)[319] and type IV (branching enzyme deficiency) and rare in type VI and IX (phosphorylase complex deficiency) glycogen storage diseases. Hypoglycemia can also be caused by glycogen synthase deficiency,[330, 331] which, unlike the glycogen storage diseases, does not cause hepatomegaly. Because it blocks gluconeogenesis, fructose-1,6-bisphosphatase deficiency causes profound postabsorptive hypoglycemia with lactic acidosis, ketosis, and elevated alanine levels.[332, 333] Hyperlipidemia, hyperuricemia, and hepatomegaly (related to fat accumulation) occur as in type I glycogen storage disease. Hypoglycemia has also been attributed to phosphoenolpyruvate carboxykinase and pyruvate carboxylase deficiencies.[333]

Finally, with respect to postabsorptive hypoglycemia and defects in glucose metabolism, CNS glucopenia occurs in patients with mutations of the GLUT-1 glucose transporter gene.[294, 334–336] Plasma glucose levels are normal but cerebrospinal glucose levels are low because of reduced GLUT-1–mediated glucose transport across the blood-brain barrier. Treatment includes a ketogenic (low-carbohydrate) diet designed to raise ketone levels and thus provide an alternative fuel to the brain. Hypoglycemia has also been attributed to GLUT-2 deficiency in the Fanconi-Bickel syndrome.[336]

Postprandial, rather than postabsorptive, hypoglycemia can be a feature of hereditary fructose intolerance[337] and, rarely, galactosemia.[338] Fructose-1-phosphate aldolase deficiency, the enzymatic defect in hereditary fructose intolerance, causes vomiting and severe hypoglycemia after fructose ingestion. Fructose-1-phosphate accumulates and inhibits glycogenolysis (at the phosphorylase level) and gluconeogenesis (at the mutant aldolase level). The patients are well when fructose is omitted from the diet. Galactose uridyltransferase deficiency, one of the causes of galactosemia, can also cause postprandial hypoglycemia, which has been attributed to inhibition of glycogenolysis.[338, 339]

Deficiencies of enzymes involved in protein metabolism that can cause postabsorptive hypoglycemia include that of the branched-chain keto acid dehydrogenase complex, the basis of branched-chain ketoaciduria (maple syrup urine disease).[340] The levels of leucine, isoleucine, and valine—particularly leucine—in plasma and urine are elevated. The pathogenesis of hypoglycemia is not entirely clear, although it results from defective gluconeogenesis.[341, 342] Hypoglycemia related to impaired gluconeogenesis also occurs in methylmalonic aciduria.[343]

Several defects that ultimately impair fatty acid oxidation result in postabsorptive hypoglycemia with *hypo*ketonemia.[294, 344–352] Normally,[353] low-insulin, high-glucagon (and catecholamine) states such as fasting favor the mobilization of fatty acids from fat (lipolysis) and their transport to other tissues including the liver and skeletal and cardiac muscle. These regulatory conditions also favor fatty acid oxidation (with ATP formation) and ketogenesis over triglyceride, phospholipid, and cholesterol ester synthesis and peroxisomal oxidation. Mitochondrial fatty acid oxidation and ketogenesis require transport of fatty acids across the plasma membrane, formation of fatty acyl-CoA derivatives, and transport of the derivatives into mitochondria. Because the inner mitochondrial membranes are not permeable to long-chain (as opposed to medium-chain and short-chain) fatty acyl-CoA esters, the long-chain fatty acyl-CoA esters are transesterified to fatty acylcarnitines at the outer surface of the membranes (by carnitine palmitoyltransferase I, CPT-I), transported across the membranes (by a translocase), and reconverted to the fatty acyl-CoA esters (by carnitine palmitoyltransferase II, CPT-II) at the inner surface of the membranes. Then they can be oxidized or converted to ketones.

Insulin decreases fat oxidation and ketogenesis by decreasing lipolysis and by increasing lipogenesis and the formation of malonyl-CoA, which inhibits CPT-I. Conversely, low insulin levels favor fatty acid oxidation and ketogenesis. High glucagon levels do so by decreasing malonyl-CoA. Catecholamines do so largely by stimulating lipolysis. Any defect in this sequence—defects in the carnitine cycle (carnitine transport defect, CPT-I deficiency, carnitine-acylcarnitine translocase deficiency, CPT-II deficiency), defects in the beta oxidation spiral (long-chain acyl-CoA dehydrogenase [LCAD] deficiency, long-chain L-3-hydroxylacyl-CoA dehydrogenase [LCHAD] deficiency, short-chain L-3-hydroxyacyl-CoA dehydrogenase [SCHAD] deficiency, 2,4-dienoyl-CoA reductase deficiency, medium-chain acyl-CoA dehydrogenase [MCAD] deficiency, short-chain acyl-CoA dehydrogenase [SCAD] deficiency), several defects of electron transfer or defects in ketogenesis (hydroxymethylglutaryl [HMG]-CoA lyase deficiency, HMG-CoA synthetase deficiency)—decreases fatty acid oxidation (and ketogenesis) and reciprocally increases glucose oxidation, resulting in hypoketonemic postabsorptive hypoglycemia. Reduced plasma carnitine levels (20% to 50% of normal) are the rule in these disorders, but extremely low carnitine levels characterize the carnitine transport defect, a true carnitine deficiency state that is responsive to carnitine supplementation.[344, 350] CPT-I deficiency, a rare disorder, is treatable by administration of medium-chain triglycerides, which do not require the CPT system for oxidation, or by a high-carbohydrate, low-fat diet.[354] CPT-II deficiency, which is typically seen with episodes of muscle pain and myoglobinuria but can also cause hypoglycemia, is more common.[355, 356]

The child affected with a disorder of fatty acid oxidation typically presents with hypoketonemic hypoglycemia; intravenous glucose causes prompt improvement. Some have presented with Reye's syndrome. All are at risk for sudden death, presumably from cardiac causes. Treatment includes provision of an adequate caloric intake, avoidance of fasting, and support of the plasma glucose concentration during intercurrent illnesses. The diagnosis of specific fatty acid oxidation defects is typically accomplished by blood acylcarnitine profiling,[357, 358] although molecular diagnosis is increasingly possible. Interestingly, the presence of a defect in fatty acid oxidation in a fetus may have implications for the mother. While carrying a fetus with a specific mutation (Glu474Gln) causing long-chain 3-hydroxyacyl-CoA dehydrogenase deficiency, 15 (79%) of 19 mothers suffered fatty liver of pregnancy or the HELLP (hemolysis, elevated liver enzyme levels, and low platelet count) syndrome.[359]

Given the array of causes of hypoglycemia in infancy and childhood just summarized, it is reasonable to suggest an extensive biochemical assessment during a hypoglycemic episode when the hypoglycemic mechanism is obscure.[294, 295] In addition to the concurrent plasma glucose concentration, this might include (1) plasma insulin, C peptide, sulfonylureas, growth hormone, and cortisol; (2) plasma or blood lactate, amino acids (including alanine), nonesterified fatty acids, and β-hydroxybutyrate; (3) serum liver enzymes; (4) plasma acylcarnitine profile; and (5) urine ketones and organic acid profile.

The Postprandial (Reactive) Hypoglycemias

Postprandial (reactive, stimulative) hypoglycemia occurs exclusively after meals, typically within 4 hours after food ingestion. All disorders that cause postabsorptive hypoglycemia can also result in hypoglycemia detected after a meal. However, the diagnostic and therapeutic approach is that of postabsorptive hypoglycemia in such a patient.

Congenital deficiencies of enzymes of carbohydrate metabolism, such as those that cause hereditary fructose intolerance[337] and galactosemia,[338] discussed earlier, are rare causes of postprandial hypoglycemia that becomes apparent early in life. Postprandial hypoglycemia can occur in individuals who have undergone gastric surgery that results in rapid movement of ingested food into the small intestine.[360] Termed *alimentary hypoglycemia*, this is thought to be the result of marked early hyperinsulinemia caused by rapid increments in plasma glucose, enhanced secretion of incretins (gut factors that enhance glucose-stimulated insulin secretion),[361] or both. Hypoglycemia occurs 1.5 to 3.0 hours after food ingestion. Symptoms of hypoglycemia must be distinguished from those of the dumping syndrome—abdominal fullness, nausea, and weakness—which occur less than an hour after ingestion. Administration of an α-glucosidase inhibitor (e.g., acarbose or miglitol) is a conceptually attractive treatment for alimentary hypoglycemia, although controlled trials indicating its efficacy are lacking.

The frequency, and even the existence, of clinically relevant idiopathic (functional) postprandial hypoglycemia is a matter of debate.[362, 363] Idiopathic postprandial hypoglycemia is often erroneously diagnosed by patients and by physicians. For example, only 16 of 118 patients suspected of having postprandial hypoglycemia in one series had both a plasma glucose concentration lower than the 10th percentile of asymptomatic control subjects and typical symptoms after an oral glucose load; only 5 of those 16 patients had similar symptoms after their regular meals.[364] Furthermore, most patients thought to have hypoglycemic symptoms and low glucose levels after glucose ingestion have normal glucose levels after a mixed meal.[365–367] In one series in which blood glucose was measured during symptomatic episodes, only 5% of 132 episodes were associated with blood glucose levels of 2.8 mmol/L (50 mg/dL) or less.[367]

Service and colleagues[368] reported on five adults judged to have hyperinsulinemic ("pancreatogenous") postprandial hypoglycemia. The patients were assessed thoroughly, and insulinomas were not found. Insulin levels were judged to be inappropriately high during hypoglycemia (but norms from prolonged fasts were used); antibodies to insulin were not reported. Mutations of the Kir6.2 and SUR1 genes were not found. An alternative theoretical possibility would be an attenuated resumption of glucagon secretion during the transition from the postprandial to the postabsorptive state. That would plausibly explain the pathogenesis of the postprandial syndrome including compensatory enhancement of epinephrine secretion, the production of symptoms attributable to the enhanced sympathochromaffin response, and the prevention of severe hypoglycemia and restoration of euglycemia.

Lower plasma glucagon levels in persons with plasma glucose nadirs less than 2.8 mmol/L (50 mg/dL) than in those with higher nadir glucose levels after an oral glucose load have been reported.[369] However, glucagon levels were also lower at baseline and were not discernibly lower after glucose ingestion in the two individuals with the lowest plasma glucose nadirs (1.5 mmol/L [27 mg/dL] and 1.3 mmol/L [2.3 mg/dL]). On the other hand, in another report, similarly selected individuals (nadir glucose less than 2.8 mmol/L [50 mg/dL]) had normal pancreatic glucagon levels after glucose ingestion.[370] Nonetheless, enhanced, presumably compensatory, plasma epinephrine responses have been reported in individuals with sweating, tremor, and greater heart rates temporally related to the glucose nadir late after glucose ingestion.[371] In such individuals, the postprandial syndrome may be the result of an appropriately enhanced sympathochromaffin response to falling plasma glucose concentrations rather than hypoglycemia per se.

A diagnosis of postprandial hypoglycemia should not be made on the basis of seemingly low plasma glucose concentrations during an oral glucose tolerance test. The lower limits of normal for venous plasma glucose concentrations late after glucose ingestion can be defined statistically. For example, in 650 individuals who remained asymptomatic after ingestion of 100 g of glucose, nadir glucose concentrations were lower 5th percentile, 2.4 mmol/L (43 mg/dL); lower 10th percentile, 2.6 mmol/L (47 mg/dL); and lower 25th percentile, 3.0 mmol/L (54 mg/dL).[365] (The absence of symptoms in response to such seemingly low plasma glucose concentrations is most plausibly explained by venous sampling. Although glucose arteriovenous differences are negligible in the postabsorptive state, there is substantial glucose extraction across the forearm under hyperinsulinemic conditions. Thus, arterial glucose levels—those relevant to glucose delivery to the brain—were undoubtedly considerably higher than the reported venous glucose levels.) Because the lowest glucose levels in these individuals cause no recognizable symptoms, have no known long-term ill effects, are self-limited, and do not imply the presence of disease, there is no reason to classify 2.5% or 5% of the population arbitrarily as abnormal. The diagnosis requires documentation of appropriate symptoms temporally related to a low plasma glucose concentration after a mixed meal and relief of those symptoms as the plasma glucose concentration rises (Whipple's triad). The diagnosis cannot be made on the basis of an oral glucose tolerance test.

Diets low in carbohydrate and high in protein are commonly recommended to patients thought to have postprandial hypoglycemia. Their efficacy has not been established by controlled clinical trials. Frequent feedings and avoidance of simple sugars are also advised. Anticholinergic drugs have been reported to be beneficial in uncontrolled studies of patients with the postprandial syndrome hypoglycemia but may cause undesirable side effects.[372] The β-adrenergic antagonist propranolol reduces symptoms (except diaphoresis) in patients with postgastrectomy postprandial hypoglycemia, and administration of pectin is said to decrease symptoms in such patients.[373] As mentioned earlier, to the extent that an excessive initial increase in plasma glucose plays a role in the pathogenesis of alimentary hypoglycemia, administration of an α-glucosidase inhibitor to delay carbohydrate digestion is a conceptually attractive treatment. Finally, such patients have been treated surgically with reversal of a segment of proximal jejunum.[374]

TREATMENT OF POSTABSORPTIVE HYPOGLYCEMIA

In view of the vulnerability of the brain to prolonged hypoglycemia, the plasma glucose concentration must be raised at least to normal levels as rapidly as possible and recurrence of hypoglycemia must be prevented. Because it is self-limited, postprandial hypoglycemia rarely requires urgent treatment. In contrast, postabsorptive hypoglycemias are typically persistent or progressive and require short-term and long-term therapy.

The urgent treatment of iatrogenic hypoglycemia in individuals with diabetes—with oral carbohydrate or glucose per se or with parenteral glucagon or glucose—was discussed earlier under "Hypoglycemia in Diabetes Mellitus." Clinical improvement should occur within about 15 to 20 minutes after the plasma glucose level is increased and maintained provided that brain damage has not occurred. Whenever possible, the presence of hypoglycemia should be documented before therapy and the response to therapy should be followed by frequent measurements of the plasma glucose level. If these are not available and there is no clinical response within 15 minutes, the initial therapy should be repeated and access to plasma glucose monitoring and intravenous glucose infusion should be obtained as soon as possible. Even if there is a response to initial therapy, glucose monitoring is essential to ensure maintenance of the plasma glucose concentration.

Although CNS function usually recovers promptly after restoration of the plasma glucose level, recovery may be delayed, perhaps because of cerebral edema. Unconsciousness lasting more than 30 minutes after the plasma glucose concentration has been raised to normal and maintained is referred to as posthypoglycemic coma.[375] It has been treated with intravenous mannitol (40 g as a 20% solution over 20 minutes) or glucocorticoids (e.g., dexamethasone, 10 mg), or both,[375–377] along with maintenance of normal plasma glucose levels.

Definitive treatment of the postabsorptive hypoglycemias requires correction of the underlying defect whenever possible. When that is not possible, attempts must be made to increase exogenous delivery or endogenous glucose production and to limit glucose utilization by tissues other than the brain. Although the judicious use of snacks is a useful component of therapy for individuals with diabetes, frequent feedings are less than ideal for the long-term treatment of chronic hypoglycemia. One problem is weight gain. However, frequent feedings, even overnight gastric infusions, are sometimes necessary when other measures are inadequate.

Hypoglycemia caused by drugs is limited to the duration of action of the offending drug. The management is straightforward: discontinuation of the drug (at least temporarily), maintenance of the plasma glucose level while drug action continues, and adjustment of subsequent drug regimens to avoid recurrent hypoglycemia if the causative drug is known. Therapy is more difficult if the drug is used surreptitiously or given accidentally or maliciously.

As discussed earlier, postabsorptive hypoglycemia related to endogenous hyperinsulinism is often curable by the surgical removal of an insulinoma. If this is not possible because of multiple or metastatic tumors or the absence of a definable lesion, diazoxide is sometimes effective.[284–287] Diazoxide (100 to 800 mg/day in adults and 5 to 30 mg/kg/day in infants) raises the plasma glucose concentration by suppressing insulin secretion.[378] Diazoxide is bound tightly to albumin and has a plasma half-time of 20 to 30 hours.[379] When given by rapid intravenous injection, it is a potent hypotensive drug, but when given orally or by slow intravenous infusion, it has little hypotensive action; indeed, hypertensive responses may occur. Although chemically related to the thiazide diuretics, diazoxide causes sodium retention. Coadministration of a thiazide diuretic both limits sodium retention and potentiates the hyperglycemic action of diazoxide.[286, 287] Both edema formation and gastrointestinal side effects (anorexia, nausea, sometimes vomiting) are dose-related. Generalized growth of lanugo hair (hypertrichosis lanuginosa) may occur during prolonged therapy. Allergic reactions, including skin rashes and agranulocytosis, are rare. Other treatments include octreotide[295] and calcium channel antagonists.[311, 312]

The treatment of hypoglycemia associated with non–beta cell tumors involves short-term measures pending effective medical, surgical, or radiotherapeutic treatment of the tumor. Administration of a glucocorticoid or growth hormone sometimes alleviates hypoglycemia. The former, but not the latter, has been reported to reduce IGF-II levels.[380, 381] Hypoglycemia resulting from glucocorticoid deficiency is corrected by replacement therapy. Hypoglycemia is rarely an indication for growth hormone replacement. Remissions of autoimmune hypoglycemias have been associated with immunosuppressive therapy, including glucocorticoids, but controlled trials are lacking. The treatment of hypoglycemia related to inanition, hepatic or renal disease, cardiac failure, or sepsis includes short-term measures and, when possible, treatment or management of the underlying disease process. The treatment of the hypoglycemias of infancy and childhood and that of postprandial hypoglycemia were discussed earlier.

APPROACH TO THE PATIENT WITH HYPOGLYCEMIA

In addition to recognition and documentation of hypoglycemia and often urgent treatment, management of hypoglycemia requires diagnosis of the hypoglycemic mechanism leading to treatment that prevents, or at least minimizes, recurrent hypoglycemia. The differential diagnosis of hypoglycemia, discussed earlier, is summarized in Table 32–2. A diagnostic algorithm is shown in Figure 32–16. The thought process is summarized in Table 32–12.

Recognition and Documentation of Hypoglycemia

Hypoglycemia is sometimes detected serendipitously. However, a report of a distinctly low plasma glucose measurement in a person who does not have a history of corresponding symptoms raises the possibility of pseudohypoglycemia—a measured low glucose level resulting from ongoing metabolism

Table 32–12. Diagnostic Approach to an Adult with Documented Fasting Hypoglycemia

1. Think of drugs, critical illness, endocrine deficiency, non–beta cell tumor, and hyperinsulinism while supporting the plasma glucose concentration if necessary.
2. Search the history, physical examination, and available laboratory data for clinical clues to the hypoglycemic mechanism and pursue the plausible mechanism or mechanisms:

a. Insulin-treated or sulfonylurea-treated diabetes	a. Adjust the therapeutic regimen
b. Use of other drugs known or suspected to cause hypoglycemia	b. Discontinue the drug (substitute an alternative if necessary)
c. Hepatic, renal, or cardiac failure; sepsis; or inanition	c. Treat the underlying disorder
d. Anorexia, weight loss, change in skin pigmentation, known pituitary or adrenocortical disease, hypotension, hypoatremia, hyperkalemia	d. Evaluate for adrenocortical insufficiency
e. Known non–beta cell tumor, mass on examination or imaging studies	e. Check for high IGF-II/IGF-I ratio

3. In the absence of clinical clues, consider medication error, endogenous hyperinsulinism, and surreptitious or malicious sulfonylurea or insulin administration.
4. A metabolic enzyme deficiency is rarely first detected in an adult.

IGF, insulin-like growth factor.

of glucose by the formed elements of the blood after the sample is drawn. Pseudohypoglycemia is particularly common when leukocyte, thrombocyte, or erythrocyte counts are abnormally high, but it can occur in the absence of these if separation of the plasma or serum from the formed elements is delayed. Nonetheless, a report of a distinctly low plasma glucose concentration measured in a reliable laboratory cannot be ignored.

Hypoglycemia is often sought because of a history of suggestive symptoms. But the symptoms are not specific for hypoglycemia, and a normal plasma glucose concentration measured when the patient is free of those symptoms does not exclude the possibility of hypoglycemia at the time of those earlier symptoms.

Convincing documentation of hypoglycemia requires demonstration of Whipple's triad—symptoms consistent with hypoglycemia, a low plasma glucose concentration, and relief of those symptoms after the plasma glucose concentration is raised. This can be accomplished easily, by measuring the plasma glucose concentration and then administering glucose, if the patient is seen while symptomatic. When the patient is not symptomatic when seen but has a history of a previous low measured plasma glucose concentration, of previous symptoms suggestive of hypoglycemia, or both, the initial diagnostic strategy is to obtain samples from the patient under conditions in which Whipple's triad would be expected to be demonstrable if a hypoglycemic disorder exists. In most instances, that condition would be the postabsorptive state, initially after an overnight fast but after a longer fast if necessary. If the history suggests only postprandial hypoglycemia, that condition would be after a mixed meal.

Urgent Treatment

If the patient is hypoglycemic when seen, urgent treatment is often necessary. When possible, a sample for documentation of the plasma glucose concentration by a quantitative analytical method (not a blood glucose monitor) should be obtained prior to treatment. Obviously, glucose administration—based on clinical suspicion of hypoglycemia, a low monitor-measured glucose level, or both—need not be delayed until the result for the initial sample is reported. The potential detrimental effects of delayed treatment of hypoglycemia far outweigh any ill effect of unnecessary treatment. In addition, if the hypoglycemic mechanism is obscure, plasma samples for insulin, C peptide, sulfonylureas, and ethanol, at a minimum, should be obtained before glucose administration.

Oral treatment, with glucose tablets or glucose-containing fluids, candy, or food, is appropriate if the patient is able and willing to take these. A reasonable initial dose is 20 g of glucose (see Fig. 32–15).[131] If the patient is unable or unwilling (because of neuroglycopenia) to take oral feedings, parenteral therapy is necessary. Intravenous glucose, 25 g initially, is preferable. If intravenous therapy is not practical, subcutaneous, intramuscular, or even intranasal glucagon can be used.

All of these urgent treatments raise plasma glucose concentrations only transiently (see Fig. 32–15). The plasma glucose concentration, as well as the patient's clinical status, should be monitored after treatment. Intravenous glucose infusion is often necessary, and the patient should eat as soon as that is practicable.

Diagnosis of the Hypoglycemic Mechanism

In a patient with documented hypoglycemia, a plausible hypoglycemic mechanism (see Table 32–2) is usually apparent clinically from the history, physical examination, and available laboratory data. Iatrogenic hypoglycemia is reasonably assumed in the vast majority of instances in a patient treated with insulin, a sulfonylurea, or another insulin secretagogue or metformin for diabetes. In an adult who does not have diabetes, the use of a relevant drug, including alcohol; the presence of a relevant critical illness (hepatic, renal, or cardiac failure, sepsis, or inanition); clues to deficient secretion of cortisol, growth hormone, or both; or evidence of a non–beta cell tumor leads to a presumptive mechanistic diagnosis and guides further diagnostic evaluation. Absent such clues, one must consider medication error, endogenous hyperinsulinism, or surreptitious or malicious sulfonylurea or insulin administration (see Fig. 32–16). Congenital metabolic defects are occasionally first recognized in an adult. The same differential diagnosis should be considered for children and even infants, although the hypoglycemic disorders unique to infancy and childhood, discussed earlier, must also be considered.

Prevention of Recurrent Hypoglycemia

Prevention of recurrent hypoglycemia in the long term requires treatment that corrects or circumvents the hypoglycemic mechanism. Offending drugs can be discontinued or their doses reduced. Underlying critical illnesses can often be treated. Cortisol (and growth hormone) can be replaced. Surgical, radiotherapeutic, or chemotherapeutic reduction of a non–beta cell tumor can alleviate hypoglycemia even if the tumor cannot be cured; glucocorticoid (or growth hormone) administration may alleviate hypoglycemia in such patients. Surgical resection of an insulinoma is often curative; medical therapy with diazoxide, octreotide, or both can be used if that is not possible and in patients with a nontumor primary beta-cell disorder. The treatment of autoimmune hypoglycemia (e.g., with a glucocorticoid) is more problematic, but the disorder is typically self-limited. Failing these treatments, provision of exogenous glucose with frequent feedings, large doses of uncooked cornstarch at bedtime, or even overnight intragastric glucose infusion may be necessary.

Acknowledgments

The author acknowledges the substantive contributions of several colleagues and collaborators that shaped the views expressed in this chapter; the assistance of the nursing, dietary, laboratory, informatics, and biostatistical staffs of the Washington University General Clinical Research Center and the laboratory staff of the Washington University Diabetes Research and Training Center in the performance of the original work cited; and the help of Ms. Karen Muehlhauser in the preparation of the manuscript.

References

1. Cryer PE. Hypoglycemia: Pathophysiology, Diagnosis and Treatment. New York, Oxford University Press, 1997.
2. Cryer PE. The prevention and correction of hypoglycemia. In Jefferson LS, Cherrington AD (eds). The Endocrine Pancreas and Regulation of Metabolism, vol II, The Endocrine System. Handbook of Physiology. New York, Oxford University Press, 2001, pp 1057–1092.
3. Cryer PE. Hypoglycaemia: The limiting factor in the glycaemic management of type I and type II diabetes. Diabetologia 2002; 45:937–948.
4. Gerich JE, Meyer C, Woerle HJ, Stumvoll M. Renal gluconeogenesis. Diabetes Care 2001; 24:382–391.
5. Ekberg K, Landau BR, Wajngot A, et al. Contributions by kidney and liver to glucose production in the postabsorptive state and after 60 h of fasting. Diabetes 1999; 48:292–298.
6. Perriello G, Jorde R, Nurjhan N, et al. Estimation of glucose-alanine-lactate-glutamine cycles in postabsorptive humans: role of skeletal muscle. Am J Physiol 1995; 269:E443–E450.

7. Garber AJ, Cryer PE, Santiago JV, et al. The role of adrenergic mechanisms in the substrate and hormonal response to insulin induced hypoglycemia in man. J Clin Invest 1976; 58:7–15.
8. Rothman DL, Magnusson I, Katz LD, et al. Quantitation of hepatic glycogenolysis and gluconeogenesis in fasting humans with ^{13}C NMR. Science 1991; 254:573–576.
9. Stumvoll M, Chintalapudi U, Perriello G, et al. Uptake and release of glucose by the human kidney. J Clin Invest 1995; 96: 2528–2533.
10. Owen OE, Felig P, Morgan AP, et al. Liver and kidney metabolism during prolonged starvation. J Clin Invest 1969; 48:574–583.
11. Rizza RA, Mandarino L, Gerich JE. Dose-response characteristics for the effects of insulin on production and utilization of glucose in man. Am J Physiol 1981; 240:630–639.
12. Rizza RA, Gerich JE. Persistent effect of sustained hyperglucagonemia on glucose production in man. J Clin Endocrinol Metab 1979; 48:352–353.
13. Cryer PE. Catecholamines, pheochromocytoma and diabetes. Diabetes Rev 1993; 1:309–317.
14. Rizza RA, Cryer PE, Haymond MW, et al. Adrenergic mechanisms for the effect of epinephrine on glucose production and clearance in man. J Clin Invest 1980; 65:682–689.
15. Berk MA, Clutter WE, Skor D, et al. Enhanced glycemic responsiveness to epinephrine in insulin dependent diabetes mellitus is the result of the inability to secrete insulin. J Clin Invest 1985; 75:1842–1851.
16. Gerich JE, Lorenzi M, Tsalikian E, et al. Studies on the mechanisms of epinephrine induced hyperglycemia in man. Diabetes 1976; 25:65–71.
17. Rosen SG, Clutter WE, Shah SD, et al. Direct α-adrenergic stimulation of hepatic glucose production in postabsorptive man. Am J Physiol 1983; 245:E616–E626.
18. Laurent D, Petersen KF, Russell RR, et al. Effect of epinephrine on muscle glycogenolysis and insulin-stimulated muscle glycogen synthesis in humans. Am J Physiol 1998; 274:E130–E138.
19. MacGorman LR, Rizza RA, Gerich JE. Physiological concentrations of growth hormone exert insulin-like and insulin antagonist effects on both hepatic and extrahepatic tissues in man. J Clin Endocrinol Metab 1981; 53:556–559.
20. Shamoon H, Hendler R, Sherwin RS. Synergistic interactions among anti-insulin hormones in the pathogenesis of stress hyperglycemia in humans. J Clin Endocrinol Metab 1981; 52:1235–1241.
21. Lautt WW. Hepatic nerves: a review of their functions and effects. Can J Physiol Pharmacol 1980; 58:105–123.
22. Nobin ABF, Ingemansson S, Jarhult J, et al. Organization and function of the sympathetic innervation of the human liver. Acta Physiol Scand 1977; 452(Suppl):103–106.
23. Boyle PJ, Liggett SB, Shah SD, et al. Direct muscarinic cholinergic inhibition of hepatic glucose production in humans. J Clin Invest 1988; 82:445–449.
24. Liljenquist JE, Mueller GL, Cherrington AD, et al. Hyperglycemia per se (insulin and glucagon withdrawn) can inhibit hepatic glucose production in man. J Clin Endocrinol Metab 1979; 48: 171–174.
25. Sacca L, Sherwin R, Hendler R, et al. Influence of continuous physiologic hyperinsulinemia on glucose kinetics and counterregulatory hormones in normal and diabetic humans. J Clin Invest 1979; 63:849–857.
26. Ahrén B. Autonomic regulation of islet hormone secretion: implications for health and disease. Diabetologia 2000; 43:393–410.
27. Frizell RT, Jones EM, Davis SN, et al. Counterregulation during hypoglycemia is directed by widespread brain regions. Diabetes 1993; 42:1253–1261.
28. Taborsky GJ Jr, Ahrén B, Havel PJ. Autonomic mediation of glucagon secretion during hypoglycemia. Diabetes 1998; 47:995–1005.
29. Ensinck JW, Walter RM, Palmer JP, et al. Glucagon responses to hypoglycemia in adrenalectomized man. Metabolism 1976; 25: 227–232.
30. Brodows RG, Ensinck JW, Campbell RG. Mechanism of cyclic AMP response to hypoglycemia in man. Metabolism 1976; 25: 659–663.
31. Palmer JP, Henry DP, Benson JW, et al. Glucagon response to hypoglycemia in sympathectomized man. J Clin Invest 1976; 57: 522–525.
32. Frier BM, Corrall RJM, Ratcliffe JG, et al. Autonomic neural control mechanisms of substrate and hormonal responses to acute hypoglycemia in man. Clin Endocrinol 1991; 14:425–433.
33. Palmer JP, Werner PL, Hollander P, et al. Evaluation of the control of glucagon secretion by the parasympathetic nervous system in man. Metabolism 1979; 28:549–552.
34. Hilsted J, Frandsen H, Holst JJ, et al. Plasma glucagon and glucose recovery after hypoglycemia: the effect of total autonomic blockade. Acta Endocrinol 1991; 125:466–469.
35. Towler DA, Havlin CE, Craft S, et al. Mechanisms of awareness of hypoglycemia: perception of neurogenic (predominantly cholinergic) rather than neuroglycopenic symptoms. Diabetes 1993; 42:1791–1798.
36. Coiro VM, Passeri M, Volpi R, et al. Effect of muscarinic and nicotinic cholinergic blockade on the glucagon response to insulin-induced hypoglycemia in normal man. Horm Metab Res 1989; 21:102–103.
37. Havel P, Ahrén B. Activation of autonomic nerves and the adrenal medulla contributes to increased glucagon secretion during moderate insulin-induced hypoglycemia in women. Diabetes 1997; 46:801–807.
38. Pipeleers DG, Schuitt FC, van Schravendijk CFH, et al. Interplay of nutrients and hormones in the regulation of glucagon release. Endocrinology 1985; 117:817–823.
39. Samols E, Stagner JI, Ewart RBL, et al. The order of islet microvascular cellular perfusion is B → A → D in the perfused rat pancreas. J Clin Invest 1988; 82:350–353.
40. Banarer S, McGregor VP, Cryer PE. Intraislet hyperinsulinemia prevents the glucagon response to hypoglycemia despite an intact autonomic response. Diabetes 2002; 51:958–965.
41. Mathias CJ, Christensen NJ, Corbett JL, et al. Plasma catecholamines during paroxysmal neurogenic hypertension in quadriplegic man. Circ Res 1976; 39:204–208.
42. Brodows RG, Pi-Sunyer FX, Campbell RG. Neural control of counterregulatory events during glucopenia in man. J Clin Invest 1973; 52:1841–1844.
43. Borg, WP, Sherwin RS, During MJ, et al. Local ventromedial hypothalamus glucopenia triggers counterregulatory hormone release. Diabetes 1995; 44:180–184.
44. Lynch RM, Tompkins LS, Brooks HL, et al. Localization of glucokinase gene expression in the rat brain. Diabetes 2000; 49: 693–700.
45. Heavener AL, Bergman RN, Donovan CM. Portal vein afferents are critical for the sympathoadrenal response to hypoglycemia. Diabetes 2000; 49:8–12.
46. Schwartz NS, Shah SD, Clutter WE, et al. Glycemic thresholds for activation of glucose counterregulatory systems are higher than the threshold for symptoms. J Clin Invest 1987; 79:777–781.
47. Mitrakou A, Ryan C, Veneman T, et al. Hierarchy of glycemic thresholds for counterregulatory hormone secretion, symptoms and cerebral dysfunction. Am J Physiol 1991; 260:E67–E74.
48. Fanelli C, Pampanelli S, Epifano L, et al. Relative roles of insulin and hypoglycaemia on induction of neuroendocrine responses to, symptoms of and deterioration of cognitive function in hypoglycemia in male and female humans. Diabetologia 1994; 37:797–807.
49. Clarke WL, Santiago JV, Thomas L, et al. Adrenergic mechanisms in recovery from hypoglycemia in man: adrenergic blockade. Am J Physiol 1979; 236:E147–E152.
50. Gerich JE, Davis J, Lorenzi M, et al. Hormonal mechanisms of recovery from insulin-induced hypoglycemia in man. Am J Physiol 1979; 236:E380–E385.
51. Rizza RA, Cryer PE, Gerich JE. Role of glucagon, epinephrine and growth hormone in human glucose counterregulation: effects of somatostatin and adrenergic blockade on plasma glucose recovery and glucose flux rates following insulin induced hypoglycemia. J Clin Invest 1979; 64:62–71.
52. Popp DA, Shah SD, Cryer PE. The role of epinephrine mediated adrenergic mechanisms in hypoglycemic glucose counterregulation and posthypoglycemic hyperglycemia in insulin-dependent diabetes mellitus. J Clin Invest 1982; 69:315–326.
53. Rosen SG, Clutter WE, Berk MA, et al. Epinephrine supports the postabsorptive plasma glucose concentration, and prevents hypoglycemia, when glucagon secretion is deficient in man. J Clin Invest 1984; 73:405–411.

54. Rosen SG, Clutter WE, Berk MA, et al. Insulin, glucagon and catecholamines in the prevention of hypoglycemia during fasting in humans. Am J Physiol 1989; 256:E651–E661.
55. Tse TF, Clutter WE, Shah SD, et al. Neuroendocrine response to glucose ingestion in man: specificity, temporal relationships and quantitative aspects. J Clin Invest 1983; 721:270–277.
56. Tse TF, Clutter WE, Shah SD, et al. Mechanisms of postprandial glucose counterregulation in man: physiologic roles of glucagon and epinephrine vis-à-vis insulin in the prevention of hypoglycemia late after glucose ingestion. J Clin Invest 1983; 72: 278–286.
57. Hirsch IB, Marker JC, Smith L, et al. Insulin and glucagon in the prevention of hypoglycemia during exercise in humans. Am J Physiol 1991; 260:E695–E704.
58. Marker JC, Hirsch IB, Smith L, et al. Catecholamines in the prevention of hypoglycemia during exercise in humans. Am J Physiol 1991; 260:E705–E712.
59. DeFeo P, Periello G, Torlone E, et al. Demonstration of a role for growth hormone in glucose counterregulation. Am J Physiol 1989; 256:E835–E843.
60. DeFeo P, Periello G, Torlone E, et al. Contribution of cortisol to glucose counterregulation. Am J Physiol 1989; 257:E35–E42.
61. Boyle PJ, Cryer PE. Growth hormone, cortisol, or both are involved in defense against, but are not critical to recovery from, prolonged hypoglycemia in humans. Am J Physiol 1991; 260: E395–E402.
62. Bolli G, DeFeo P, Periello G, et al. Role of hepatic autoregulation in defense against hypoglycemia in humans. J Clin Invest 1985; 75:1623–1631.
63. Hansen I, Firth R, Haymond M, et al. The role of autoregulation of hepatic glucose production in man. Diabetes 1986; 35: 186–191.
64. DeFeo P, Perriello G, Torlone E, et al. Evidence against important catecholamine compensation for absent glucagon counterregulation. Am J Physiol 1991; 260:E203–E212.
65. DeFeo P, Perriello G, Torlone E, et al. Contribution of adrenergic mechanisms to glucose counterregulation in humans. Am J Physiol 1991; 261:E725–E736.
66. Heller SR, Cryer PE. Hypoinsulinemia is not critical to glucose recovery from hypoglycemia in humans. Am J Physiol 1991; 261: E41–E48.
67. Santiago JV, Clarke WL, Shah SD, et al. Epinephrine, norepinephrine, glucagon and growth hormone release in association with physiological decrements in the plasma glucose concentration in normal and diabetic man. J Clin Endocrinol Metab 1980; 51:877–883.
68. Amiel SA, Simonson DC, Tamborlane WV, et al. Rate of glucose fall does not affect counterregulatory hormone responses to hypoglycemia in normal and diabetic humans. Diabetes 1987; 36: 518–522.
69. Mitrakou A, Mokan M, Ryan C, et al. Influence of plasma glucose rate of decrease on hierarchy of responses to hypoglycemia. J Clin Endocrinol Metab 1993; 76:462–465.
70. Amiel SA, Sherwin RS, Simonson DC, et al. Effect of intensive insulin therapy on glycemic thresholds for counterregulatory hormone release. Diabetes 1988; 37:901–907.
71. Mitrakou A, Fanelli C, Veneman T, et al. Reversibility of hypoglycemia unawareness. N Engl J Med 1993; 329:834–839.
72. Boyle PJ, Schwartz NS, Shah SD, et al. Plasma glucose concentrations at the onset of hypoglycemic symptoms in patients with poorly controlled diabetes and nondiabetics. N Engl J Med 1988; 318:1487–1492.
73. Malouf R, Brust JCM. Hypoglycemia: causes, neurological manifestations, and outcome. Ann Neurol 1985; 17:421–430.
74. Fischer KF, Lees JA, Newman JH. Hypoglycemia in hospitalized patients: causes and outcomes. N Engl J Med 1986; 315:1245–1250.
75. The Diabetes Control and Complications Trial Research Group. The effect of intensive treatment of diabetes on the development and progression of long-term complications in insulin-dependent diabetes mellitus. N Engl J Med 1993; 329:977–986.
76. Reichard P, Nilsson B-Y, Rosenqvist U. The effect of long-term intensified insulin treatment on the development of microvascular complications of diabetes mellitus. N Engl J Med 1993; 329:304–309.
77. The United Kingdom Prospective Diabetes Study Group. Intensive blood-glucose control with sulfonylureas or insulin compared with conventional treatment and risk of complications in patients with type 2 diabetes. Lancet 1998; 352:837–853.
78. Cryer PE. Hypoglycemia *is* the limiting factor in the management of diabetes. Diabetes Metab Res Rev 1999; 15:42–46.
79. The Diabetes Control and Complications Trial Research Group. Epidemiology of severe hypoglycemia in the Diabetes Control and Complications Trial. Am J Med 1991; 90:450–459.
80. The Diabetes Control and Complications Trial Research Group. Hypoglycemia in the Diabetes Control and Complications Trial. Diabetes 1997; 46:271–286.
81. Reichard P, Berglund B, Britz A, et al. Intensified conventional insulin treatment retards the microvascular complications of insulin-dependent diabetes mellitus: the Stockholm Diabetes Intervention Study after 5 years. J Intern Med 1990; 230:101–108.
82. The United Kingdom Prospective Diabetes Study Group. A 6-year, randomized, controlled trial comparing sulfonylurea, insulin and metformin therapy in patients with newly diagnosed type 2 diabetes that could not be controlled with diet therapy. Ann Intern Med 1998; 128:165–175.
83. Egger M, Davey Smith G, Stettler C, et al. Risk of adverse effects of intensified treatment in insulin-dependent diabetes mellitus: a meta-analysis. Diabet Med 1997; 14:919–928.
84. Laing SP, Swerdlow AJ, Slater SD, et al. The British Diabetic Association Cohort Study. II. Cause-specific mortality in patients with insulin-treated diabetes mellitus. Diabet Med 1999; 16:466–471.
85. Hepburn DA, MacLeod KM, Pell ACH, et al. Frequency and symptoms of hypoglycemia experienced by patients with type 2 diabetes treated with insulin. Diabet Med 1993; 10:231–237.
86. Fukuda M, Tanaka A, Tahara Y, et al. Correlation between minimal secretory capacity of pancreatic β-cells and stability of diabetic control. Diabetes 1988; 37:81–88.
87. Mühlhauser I, Overmann H, Bender R, et al. Risk factors for severe hypoglycaemia in adult patients with type 1 diabetes: a prospective population based study. Diabetologia 1997; 41:1274–1282.
88. Gerich JE, Langlois M, Noacco C, et al. Lack of glucagon response to hypoglycemia in diabetes: evidence for an intrinsic pancreatic alpha cell defect. Science 1973; 182:171–173.
89. Bolli G, De Feo P, Compagnucci P, et al. Abnormal glucose counterregulation after subcutaneous insulin in insulin dependent diabetes mellitus: interaction of anti-insulin antibodies and impaired glucagon and epinephrine secretion. Diabetes 1983; 32: 134–141.
90. Boden G, Reichard GA Jr, Hoeldtke RD, et al. Severe insulin-induced hypoglycemia associated with deficiencies in the release of counterregulatory hormones. N Engl J Med 1981; 305:1200–1205.
91. Hirsch BR, Shamoon H. Defective epinephrine and growth hormone responses in type 1 diabetes are stimulus specific. Diabetes 1987; 36:20–26.
92. Dagogo-Jack SE, Craft S, Cryer PE. Hypoglycemia-associated autonomic failure in insulin dependent diabetes mellitus. J Clin Invest 1993; 91:819–828.
93. Heller SR, Cryer PE. Reduced neuroendocrine and symptomatic responses to subsequent hypoglycemia after one episode of hypoglycemia in nondiabetic humans. Diabetes 1991; 40:223–226.
94. Davis MR, Shamoon H. Counterregulatory adaptation to recurrent hypoglycemia in normal humans. J Clin Endocrinol Metab 1991; 73:995–1001.
95. Widom B, Simonson DC. Intermittent hypoglycemia impairs glucose counterregulation. Diabetes 1992; 41:1597–1602.
96. Veneman T, Mitrakou A, Mokan M, et al. Induction of hypoglycemia unawareness by asymptomatic nocturnal hypoglycemia. Diabetes 1993; 42:1233–1237.
97. Davis SN, Shavers C, Mosqueda-Garcia R, Costa F. Effects of differing antecedent hypoglycemia on subsequent counterregulation in normal humans. Diabetes 1997; 46:1328–1335.
98. Davis MR, Mellman M, Shamoon H. Further defects in counterregulatory responses induced by recurrent hypoglycemia in IDDM. Diabetes 1992; 41:1335–1340.
99. Lingenfelser T, Renn W, Sommerwerck U, et al. Compromised hormonal counterregulation, symptom awareness, and neurophysiological function after recurrent short-term episodes of insulin-induced hypoglycemia in IDDM patients. Diabetes 1993; 42:610–618.

100. Bottini P, Boschetti E, Pampanelli S, et al. Contribution of autonomic neuropathy to reduced plasma adrenaline responses to hypoglycemia in IDDM: evidence for a nonselective defect. Diabetes 1997; 46:814–823.
101. Meyer C, Grobmann R, Mitrakou A, et al. Effects of autonomic neuropathy on counterregulation and awareness of hypoglycemia in type 1 diabetic patients. Diabetes Care 1998; 21:1960–1966.
102. White NH, Skor D, Cryer PE, et al. Identification of type 1 diabetic patients at increased risk for hypoglycemia during intensive therapy. N Engl J Med 1983; 308:485–491.
103. Bolli GG, De Feo P, De Cosmo S, et al. A reliable and reproducible test for adequate glucose counterregulation in type 1 diabetes. Diabetes 1984; 33:732–737.
104. Gold AE, MacLeod KM, Frier BM. Frequency of severe hypoglycemia in patients with type 1 diabetes with impaired awareness of hypoglycemia. Diabetes Care 1994; 17:697–703.
105. Cryer PE. Iatrogenic hypoglycemia as a cause of hypoglycemia-associated autonomic failure in IDDM: a vicious cycle. Diabetes 1992; 41:255–260.
106. Hvidberg A, Fanelli CG, Hershey TG, et al. Impact of recent antecedent hypoglycemia on hypoglycemic cognitive dysfunction in nondiabetic humans. Diabetes 1996; 45:1030–1036.
107. Ovalle F, Fanelli CG, Paramore DS, et al. Brief twice weekly episodes of hypoglycemia reduce detection of clinical hypoglycemia in type 1 diabetes mellitus. Diabetes 1998; 47:1472–1479.
108. Fanelli CG, Paramore DS, Hershey T, et al. Impact of nocturnal hypoglycemia on hypoglycemia cognitive dysfunction in type 1 diabetes mellitus. Diabetes 1998; 47:1920–1927.
109. Dagogo-Jack S, Rattarasarn C, Cryer PE. Reversal of hypoglycemia unawareness, but not defective glucose counterregulation, in IDDM. Diabetes 1994; 43:1426–1434.
110. Fanelli CG, Pampanelli S, Epifano L, et al. Long-term recovery from unawareness, deficient counterregulation and lack of cognitive dysfunction during hypoglycemia following institution of rational intensive therapy in IDDM. Diabetologia 1994; 37:1265–1276.
111. Cranston I, Lomas J, Maran A, et al. Restoration of hypoglycemia unawareness in patients with long duration insulin-dependent diabetes mellitus. Lancet 1994; 344:283–287.
112. Davis SN, Shavers C, Costa F, Mosqueda-Garcia R. Role of cortisol in the pathogenesis of deficient counterregulation after antecedent hypoglycemia in normal humans. J Clin Invest 1996; 98:680–691.
113. Davis SN, Shavers C, Davis B, Costa F. Prevention of an increase in plasma cortisol during hypoglycemia preserves subsequent counterregulatory responses. J Clin Invest 1997; 100:429–438.
114. Boyle PJ, Nagy RJ, O'Connor AM, et al. Adaptation in brain glucose uptake following recurrent hypoglycemia. Proc Natl Acad Sci USA 1994; 91:9352–9356.
115. Boyle PJ, Kempers SF, O'Connor AM, Nagy RJ. Brain glucose uptake and unawareness of hypoglycemia in patients with insulin dependent diabetes mellitus. N Engl J Med 1995; 333:1726–1731.
116. Segel S, Fanelli C, Dence C, et al. Blood-to-brain glucose transport, cerebral glucose metabolism and cerebral blood flow are not increased following hypoglycemia. Diabetes 2001; 50:911–917.
117. Paramore DS, Fanelli CG, Shah SD, Cryer PE. Hypoglycemia per se stimulates sympathetic neural as well as adrenomedullary activity but, unlike the adrenomedullary response, the forearm sympathetic neural response is not reduced following recent hypoglycemia. Diabetes 1999; 48:1429–1436.
118. Berlin I, Grimaldi A, Payan C, et al. Hypoglycemic symptoms and decreased β-adrenergic sensitivity in insulin dependent diabetic patients. Diabetes Care 1987; 10:742–747.
119. Korytkowski M, Mokan M, Veneman T, et al. Reduced β-adrenergic sensitivity in insulin dependent diabetic patients. Diabetes Care 1998; 21:1939–1943.
120. Fritsche A, Stumvoll M, Grüb M, et al. Effect of hypoglycemia on β-adrenergic sensitivity in normal and type 1 diabetic subjects. Diabetes Care 1998; 21:1505–1510.
121. Fritsche A, Stumvoll M, Häring H-U, Gerich JE. Reversal of hypoglycemia unawareness in a long-term type 1 diabetic patient by improvement of β-adrenergic sensitivity after prevention of hypoglycemia. J Clin Endocrinol Metab 2000; 85:523–525.
122. Turner R, Stratton I, Horton V, et al. Autoantibodies to islet cell cytoplasm and glutamic acid decarboxylase for prediction of insulin requirement in type 2 diabetes. Lancet 1997; 350:1288–1293.
123. Segel SA, Paramore DS, Cryer PE. Hypoglycemia-associated autonomic failure in advanced type 2 diabetes. Diabetes 2002; 51: 724–733.
124. Perriello G, De Feo P, Torlone E, et al. The dawn phenomenon in type 1 (insulin dependent) diabetes mellitus: magnitude, frequency, variability, and dependence on glucose counterregulation and insulin sensitivity. Diabetes 1991; 34:21–28.
125. Jones TW, Porter P, Sherwin RS, et al. Decreased epinephrine responses to hypoglycemia during sleep. N Engl J Med 1998; 338:1657–1662.
126. Heller SR, Amiel SA, Mansell P, et al. Effect of the fast acting insulin analog lispro on the risk of nocturnal hypoglycemia during intensified insulin therapy. Diabetes Care 1999; 22:1607–1611.
127. Ratner RE, Hirsch IB, Neifing JL, et al. Less hypoglycemia with insulin glargine in intensive insulin therapy for type 1 diabetes. Diabetes Care 2000; 23:639–643.
128. Saleh TY, Cryer PE. Alanine and terbutaline in the prevention of nocturnal hypoglycemia in IDDM. Diabetes Care 1997; 20:1231–1236.
129. Ververs MTC, Rouwé C, Smit GPA. Complex carbohydrates in the prevention of nocturnal hypoglycaemia in diabetic children. Eur J Clin Nutr 1993; 47:268–273.
130. Kaufman FR, Devgan S. Use of uncooked cornstarch to avert nocturnal hypoglycemia in children and adolescents with type 1 diabetes. J Diabetes Complications 1996; 10:84–87.
131. Wiethop BV, Cryer PE. Alanine and terbutaline in the treatment of hypoglycemia in IDDM. Diabetes Care 1993; 16:1131–1136.
132. MacCuish AC. Treatment of hypoglycemia. In Frier BM, Fisher BM (eds). Diabetes and Hypoglycaemia. London, Edward Arnold, 1993, pp 212–221.
133. Brodows RG, Williams C, Amatruda JM. Treatment of insulin reactions in diabetics. JAMA 1984; 252:3378–3381.
134. Collier A, Steedman DJ, Patrick AW, et al. Comparison of intravenous glucagon and dextrose in treatment of severe hypoglycemia in an accident and emergency department. Diabetes Care 1987; 10:712–715.
135. Namba M, Hanafusa T, Kono N, et al. Clinical evaluation of biosynthetic glucagon treatment for recovery from hypoglycemia developed in diabetic patients. Diabetes Res Clin Pract 1993; 19: 133–138.
136. Hvidberg AM, Jørgensen S, Hilsted J. The effect of genetically engineered glucagon on glucose recovery after hypoglycaemia in man. Br J Clin Pharmacol 1992; 34:547–550.
137. Pontiroli AE, Pozza G. Intranasal administration of peptide hormones: factors affecting transmucosal absorption. Diabet Med 1990; 7:770–774.
138. Slama G, Alamowitch C, Desplanque N, et al. A new noninvasive method for treating insulin-reaction: intranasal lyophilized glucagon. Diabetologia 1990; 33:671–674.
139. Rosenfalck AM, Bendtson I, Jørgensen S, et al. Nasal glucagon in the treatment of hypoglycaemia in type I (insulin-dependent) diabetic patients. Diabetes Res Clin Pract 1992; 17:43–50.
140. Service FJ. Hypoglycemic disorders. Endocrinol Metab Clin North Am 1999; 28:467–661.
141. Marks V, Teale JD. Drug-induced hypoglycemia. Endocrinol Metab Clin North Am 1999; 28:555–578.
142. Marks V, Teale JD. Hypoglycemia: factitious and felonious. Endocrinol Metab Clin North Am 1999; 28:579–601.
143. Lecavalier L, Bolli G, Cryer P, et al. Contributions of gluconeogenesis and glycogenolysis during glucose counterregulation in normal humans. Am J Physiol 1989; 256:E844–E851.
144. Kolaczynski JW, Ylikahri R, Hrkonen M, et al. The acute effect of ethanol on counterregulatory response and recovery from insulin induced hypoglycemia. J Clin Endocrinol Metab 1988; 67: 384–388.
145. Yki-Järvinen H, Koivisto VA, Ylikahri R, et al. Acute effects of ethanol and acetate on glucose kinetics in normal subjects. Am J Physiol 1988; 254:E175–E180.
146. Shelmet JJ, Reichard GA, Skutches CL, et al. Ethanol causes acute inhibition of carbohydrate, fat and protein oxidation and insulin resistance. J Clin Invest 1988; 81:1137–1145.
147. Avogaro A, Valerio A, Miola M, et al. Ethanol impairs insulin-mediated glucose uptake by an indirect mechanism. J Clin Endocrinol Metab 1996; 81:2285–2290.

148. Fang V, Foyle WO, Robinson SM, et al. Hypoglycemic activity and chemical structure of salicylates. J Pharm Sci 1968; 57:2111–2116.
149. Arena FP, Dugowson C, Saudek CD. Salicylate-induced hypoglycemia and ketoacidosis in a nondiabetic adult. Arch Intern Med 1978; 138:1153–1156.
150. Raschke R, Arnold-Capell PA, Richeson R, et al. Refractory hypoglycemia secondary to topical salicylate intoxication. Arch Intern Med 1991; 151:591–593.
151. Poretsky L, Moses AC. Hypoglycemia associated with trimethoprim/sulfamethoxazole therapy. Diabetes Care 1984; 7:508–509.
152. Assan R, Perronne C, Assan D, et al. Pentamidine-induced derangements of glucose metabolism. Diabetes Care 1995; 18:47–55.
153. Waskin H, Stehr-Green JK, Helmick CG, et al. Risk factors for hypoglycemia associated with pentamidine therapy for *Pneumocystis* pneumonia. JAMA 1988; 260:345–347.
154. White NJ, Warrell DA, Chanthavanich P, et al. Severe hypoglycemia and hyperinsulinemia in falciparum malaria. N Engl J Med 1983; 309:61–66.
155. White NJ, Miller KD, Marsh K, et al. Hypoglycaemia in African children with severe malaria. Lancet 1987; 1:708–711.
156. Taylor TE, Molyneux ME, Wirima JJ, et al. Blood glucose levels in Malawian children before and during the administration of intravenous quinine for severe falciparum malaria. N Engl J Med 1988; 319:1040–1047.
157. Limburg PJ, Katz H, Grant CS, et al. Quinine-induced hypoglycemia. Ann Intern Med 1993; 119:218–219.
158. Agbenyega T, Angus BJ, Bedu-Addo G, et al. Glucose and lactate kinetics in children with severe malaria. J Clin Endocrinol Metab 2000; 85:1569–1576.
159. Cacoub P, Deray G, Baumelou A, et al. Disopyramide-induced hypoglycemia: case report and review of the literature. Fundam Clin Pharmacol 1989; 3:527–535.
160. Moore N, Kreft-Jais C, Haramburu F, et al. Report of hypoglycaemia associated with use of ACE inhibitors and other drugs: a case/non-case study in French pharmacovigilance system database. Br J Pharmacol 1997; 44:513–518.
161. Hesse B, Pedersen JT. Hypoglycemia after propranolol in children. Acta Med Scand 1973; 193:551–552.
162. McBride JT, McBride MC, Vites PH. Hypoglycemia associated with propranolol. Pediatrics 1973; 51:1085–1087.
163. Hirsch IB, Boyle PJ, Craft S, et al. Higher glycemic thresholds for symptoms during β-adrenergic blockade in IDDM. Diabetes 1991; 40:1177–1186.
164. Mann FC, Magath TB. Studies on the physiology of the liver. II: The effect of the removal of the liver on the blood sugar level. Arch Intern Med 1922; 30:73–84.
165. Samson RL, Trey C, Timme AH, et al. Fulminant hepatitis with recurrent hypoglycemia and hemorrhage. Gastroenterology 1967; 53:291–300.
166. Felig P, Brown WV, Levine RA, et al. Glucose homeostasis in viral hepatitis. N Engl J Med 1970; 283:1436–1440.
167. Younus S, Soterakis J, Sosi AJ, et al. Hypoglycemia secondary to metastases to the liver. Gastroenterology 1977; 72:334–337.
168. Medalle R, Webb R, Waterhouse C. Lactic acidosis and hypoglycemia. Arch Intern Med 1971; 128:273–278.
169. Block MB, Rubenstein AH. Spontaneous hypoglycemia in diabetic patients with renal insufficiency. JAMA 1970; 213:1863–1866.
170. Frizell M, Larsen PR, Field JB. Spontaneous hypoglycemia associated with chronic renal failure. Diabetes 1973; 22:493–498.
171. Garber AJ, Bier DM, Cryer PE, et al. Hypoglycemia in compensated chronic renal insufficiency. Diabetes 1974; 23:982–986.
172. Rutsky EA, McDaniel HG, Tarpe DL, et al. Spontaneous hypoglycemia in chronic renal failure. Arch Intern Med 1978; 138: 1364–1368.
173. Arem R. Hypoglycemia associated with renal failure. Endocrinol Metab Clin North Am 1989; 18:103–121.
174. Schmitz O. Peripheral and hepatic resistance to insulin and hepatic resistance to glucagon in uraemic patients. Acta Endocrinol 1988; 118:125–134.
175. Baylor P, Shilo S, Zonszein J, et al. Adrenergic contribution to glucagon-induced glucose production and insulin secretion in uremia. Am J Physiol 1986; 251:E322–E327.
176. Chen YT, Burchell A. Glycogen storage diseases. In Scriver CR, Beaudetal AL, Sly WS, Valle D (eds). The Metabolic and Molecular Bases of Inherited Disease, 7th ed. New York, McGraw Hill, 1995, pp 935–965.
177. Miller SI, Wallace RJ Jr, Musher DM, et al. Hypoglycemia as a manifestation of sepsis. Am J Med 1980; 68:649–653.
178. Meszaros K, Bagby GJ, Lang CH, et al. Increased uptake and phosphorylation of 2-deoxyglucose by skeletal muscles in endotoxin-treated rats. Am J Physiol 1987; 253:E33–E39.
179. Lang CH, Dobrescu C. Sepsis-induced increases in glucose uptake by macrophage-rich tissues persist during hypoglycemia. Metabolism 1991; 40:585–593.
180. Hargrove DM, Bagby GJ, Lang CH, et al. Adrenergic blockade prevents endotoxin-induced increases in glucose metabolism. Am J Physiol 1988; 255:E629–E635.
181. Naylor JM, Kronfeld DS. In vivo studies of hypoglycemia and lactic acidosis in endotoxic shock. Am J Physiol 1985; 248:E309–E316.
182. Lang CH, Spolarics Z, Ohlakan A, et al. Effect of high dose endotoxin on glucose production and utilization. Metabolism 1993; 42:1351–1358.
183. Lee MD, Zentella A, Pekala PH, et al. Effect of endotoxin-induced monokines on glucose metabolism in the muscle cell line L6. Proc Natl Acad Sci USA 1987; 84:2590–2594.
184. Wolfe RR, Elahi D, Spitzer JJ. Glucose and lactate kinetics after endotoxin administration in dogs. Am J Physiol 1977; 232:E180–E185.
185. Mathison JC, Wolfson E, Ulevitch RJ. Participation of tumor necrosis factor in the mediation of gram negative bacterial lipopolysaccharide–induced injury in rabbits. J Clin Invest 1988; 81: 1925–1937.
186. Sakurai Y, Zhang X-J, Wolfe RR. TNF directly stimulates glucose uptake and leucine oxidation and inhibits FFA flux in conscious dogs. Am J Physiol 1996; 270:E864–E872.
187. Lang CH, Bagby GJ, Blakesley HL, et al. Importance of hyperglucagonemia in eliciting the sepsis-induced increase in glucose production. Circ Shock 1989; 29:181–191.
188. McKechnie K, Dean HG, Furman BL, et al. Plasma catecholamines during endotoxin infusion in conscious unrestrained rats: effects of adrenal demedullation and/or guanethidine treatment. Circ Shock 1985; 17:85–94.
189. Bagby GJ, Lang CH, Skrepnik N, et al. Attenuation of glucose metabolic changes resulting from TNF administration by adrenergic blockade. Am J Physiol 1992; 262:R628–R635.
190. Stouthard JML, Romijn JA, van der Poll T, et al. Endocrinologic and metabolic effects of interleukin-6 in humans. Am J Physiol 1995; 268:E813–E819.
191. Hargrove DM, Lang CH, Bagby GJ, et al. Epinephrine-induced increase in glucose turnover is diminished during sepsis. Metabolism 1989; 38:1070–1076.
192. Macarthur H, Westfall TC, Riley DP, et al. Inactivation of catecholamines by superoxide gives new insight on the pathogenesis of septic shock. Proc Natl Acad Sci USA 2000; 97:9753–9758.
193. Wharton B. Hypoglycemia in children with kwashiorkor. Lancet 1970; 1:171–173.
194. Elias AN, Gwinup G. Glucose-resistant hypoglycemia in inanition. Arch Intern Med 1982; 142:743–746.
195. Bruce AK, Jacobsen E, Dossing H, et al. Hypoglycaemia in spinal muscular atrophy. Lancet 1995; 346:609–610.
196. Maleribi D, Liberman B, Guirno-Filho A, et al. Glucocorticoids and glucose metabolism: hepatic glucose production in untreated addisonian patients and on two different levels of glucocorticoid administration. Clin Endocrinol (OXF) 1988; 28:415–422.
197. Artavia-Loria E, Chaussian JL, Bougneres PF, Job JC. Frequency of hypoglycemia in children with adrenal insufficiency. Acta Endocrinol Suppl (Copenh) 1986; 279:275–277.
198. Goodman HG, Grumbach MM, Kaplan SL. Growth and growth hormone. II: A comparison of isolated growth hormone deficiency and multiple pituitary hormone deficiencies in 35 patients with idiopathic hypopituitary dwarfism. N Engl J Med 1968; 278: 57–68.
199. Muglia L, Jacobsen L, Dikkies P, et al. Corticotropin-releasing hormone deficiency reveals major fetal but not adult glucocorticoid need. Nature 1995; 373:427–432.
200. Haymond MW, Karl I, Weldon VV, et al. The role of growth hormone and cortisone in glucose and gluconeogenic substrate regulation in fasted hypopituitary children. J Clin Endocrinol Metab 1976; 42:846–856.

302. Pagliara AS, Karl IE, DeVivo DC, et al. Hypoal concomitant of ketotic hypoglycemia. J Clin Inves 1440–1449.
303. Haymond MW, Karl IE, Pagliara AS. Ketotic hypo amino acid substrate limited disorder. J Clin Endoc 1974; 38:521–530.
304. Miles JM, Nissen S, Gerich J, et al. Effects of epine sion on leucine and alanine kinetics in humans. A 1984; 247:E166–E172.
305. Glaser B, Thornton P, Otonkoski T, et al. Genetics hyperinsulinism. Arch Dis Child Fetal Neonatal E F79–F86.
306. Thomas PM, Cote GJ, Wohllk N, et al. Mutations nylurea receptor gene in familial hyperinsulinemic h of infancy. Science 1995; 268:426–429.
307. Thomas P, Ye Y, Lightner E. Mutation of the pa inward rectifier Kir6.2 also leads to familial persiste linemic hypoglycemia of infancy. Hum Mol Genet 1 1812.
308. Nestorowicz A, Inagaki N, Gonol T et al. A nonse in the inward rectifier potassium channel gene, Kir ated with familial hyperinsulinism. Diabetes 1997; 46
309. Ryan FD, Devaney D, Joyce C, et al. Hyperinsulin lecular aetiology of focal disease. Arch Dis Child 1 447.
310. Verkarre V, Fournet JC, de Lonlay P, et al. Paterna the sulfonylurea receptor SUR1 gene and maternal imprinted genes lead to persistent hyperinsulinism nomatous hyperplasia. J Clin Invest 1998; 102:1286–
311. Eichmann D, Hufnagel M, Quick P, et al. Treatme sulinaemic hypoglycaemia with nifedipine. Eur J 158:204–206.
312. Bas F, Darendeliler F, Demirkol D, et al. Successful calcium channel blocker (nifedipine) in persistent ne insulinemic hypoglycemia of infancy. J Pediatr End 1999; 12:873–878.
313. Stanley CA, Lieu YK, Hsu BYL, et al. Hyperin hyperammonemia in infants with regulatory mutatio tamate dehydrogenase gene. N Engl J Med 199 1357.
314. Stanley CA, Fang J, Kutyna K, et al. Molecular basi terization of the hyperinsulinism/hyperammonem predominance of mutations in exons 11 and 12 of t dehydrogenase gene. Diabetes 2000; 49:667–673.
315. Glaser B, Kesavan P, Heyman M, et al. Familial h caused by an activating glucokinase mutation. N 1998; 338:226–230.
316. Davis EA, Cuesta-Muñoz A, Raoul M, et al. Muta nase cause hypoglycaemia and hyperglycaemia s their analysis illuminates fundamental quantitativ glucose homeostasis. Diabetologia 1999; 42:1175–1
317. Mahalingam B, Cuesta-Muñoz A, Davis EA, et model of human glucokinase in complex with gluc Diabetes 1999; 48:1698–1705.
318. De Lonlay P, Cuer M, Vuillaumier-Barrot S, et al. emic hypoglycemia as a presenting sign in ph isomerase deficiency: a new manifestation of carb cient glycoprotein syndrome treatable with mann 1999; 135:379–383.
319. Talente GM, Coleman RA, Alter C, et al. Gly disease in adults. Ann Intern Med 1994; 120:218–2
320. Cori GT, Cori CF. Glucose-6-phosphatase of the gen storage disease. J Biol Chem 1952; 199:661–66
321. Chen YT, Burchell A. Glycogen storage diseases. Beaudet AL, Sly WS, Valle D (eds). The Metaboli lar Bases of Inherited Disease, 7th ed. New York, 1995, pp 935–965.
322. Chou JY, Mansfield BC. Molecular genetics of ty storage diseases. Trends Endocrinol Metab 1999;
323. Van de Werve G, Lange A, Newgard C, et al. the regulation of glucose metabolism taught by phosphatase system. Eur J Biochem 2000; 267:1533
324. Greene HL, Slonim AE, Burr IM, et al. Type 1 g disease: five years of management with noctur feeding. J Pediatr 1989; 96:590–595.
325. Wolfsdorf JI, Ehrlich S, Landy HS, et al. Optimal

201. Wolfsdorf JI, Sadeghi-Nejad A, Senior B. Hypoketonemia and age-related fasting hypoglycemia in growth hormone deficiency. Metabolism 1983; 32:457–462.
202. Frizell RT, Campbell PJ, Cherrington AD. Gluconeogenesis and hypoglycemia. Diabetes Metab Rev 1988; 4:51–70.
203. Rizza RA, Mandarino L, Gerich JE. Cortisol induced insulin resistance in man: impaired suppression of glucose production and stimulation of glucose utilization due to a postreceptor defect of insulin action. J Clin Endocrinol Metab 1981; 54:131–138.
204. Aynsley-Green A, Moncrieff MW, Ratter S, et al. Isolated ACTH deficiency. Arch Dis Child 1978; 53:499–502.
205. Rudman D, Moffitt SD, Fernhoff PM, et al. Epinephrine deficiency in hypocorticotropic hypopituitary children. J Clin Endocrinol Metab 1981; 53:722–729.
206. Voorhees ML, Jakubowski AF, MacGillivray MH. The adrenomedullary and glucagon responses of hypopituitary children to insulin induced hypoglycemia. Pediatr Res 1981; 15:912–915.
207. Smallridge RC, Corrigan DF, Thomason AM, et al. Hypoglycemia in pregnancy: occurrence due to adrenocorticotropic hormone and growth hormone deficiency. Arch Intern Med 1980; 140:564–565.
208. Steer P, Marnell R, Werk EE Jr. Clinical alcohol hypoglycemia and isolated adrenocorticotropic hormone deficiency. Ann Intern Med 1969; 71:343–348.
209. Fery F, Plat L, Van de Borne P, et al. Impaired counterregulation of glucose in a patient with hypothalamic sarcoidosis. N Engl J Med 1999; 340:852–856.
210. Shah SD, Tse TF, Clutter WE, et al. The human sympathochromaffin system. Am J Physiol 1984; 247:E380–E384.
211. Clarke WL, Santiago JV, Thomas L, et al. Adrenergic mechanisms in recovery from hypoglycemia in man: adrenergic blockade. Am J Physiol 1979; 236:E147–E152.
212. Broberger O, Jungner I, Zetterstrom R. Studies in spontaneous hypoglycemia in childhood failure to increase epinephrine secretion in insulin-induced hypoglycemia. J Pediatr 1959; 55:713–719.
213. Tietze HU, Zurbrug RP, Zuppinger KA, et al. Occurrence of impaired cortisol regulation in children with hypoglycemia associated with adrenal medullary hyporesponsiveness. J Clin Endocrinol Metab 1972; 34:948–958.
214. Christensen NJ. Hypoadrenalinemia during insulin hypoglycemia in children with ketotic hypoglycemia. J Clin Endocrinol Metab 1974; 38:107–112.
215. Rosenbloom AL, Tiwary CM. Ketotic (idiopathic glucagon unresponsive) hypoglycemia: catecholamine excretion and effects of ephedrine therapy. Arch Dis Child 1972; 47:924–926.
216. Court JM, Dunlop ME, Boulton TJC. Effect of ephedrine in ketotic hypoglycemia. Arch Dis Child 1974; 49:63–65.
217. Sizonenko PC, Paunier L, Vallotton MB, et al. Response to 2-deoxy-glucose and to glucagon in "ketotic hypoglycemia" of childhood: evidence for epinephrine deficiency and altered alanine availability. Pediatr Res 1973; 7:983–993.
218. Kerr DS, Brooke OG, Robinson HM. Fasting energy utilization in the smaller of twins with epinephrine-deficient hypoglycemia. Metabolism 1981; 30:6–17.
219. Kerr DS, Picou DIM. Fasting glucose production in the smaller of twins with epinephrine-deficient hypoglycemia. Metabolism 1981; 30:18–26.
220. Light IJ, Sutherland JM, Loggie JM, et al. Impaired epinephrine release in hypoglycemic infants of diabetic mothers. N Engl J Med 1967; 277:394–398.
221. Bleicher SJ, Levy LJ, Zarowitz H, et al. Glucagon deficiency hypoglycemia: a new syndrome? (abstract) Clin Res 1970; 19:355.
222. Starke AAR, Valverde I, Botazzo GF, et al. Glucagon deficiency associated with hypoglycaemia and the absence of islet cell antibodies in the polyglandular failure syndrome before the onset of insulin-dependent diabetes mellitus: a case report. Diabetologia 1983; 25:336–339.
223. Vidnes J, Oyaseater S. Glucagon deficiency causing severe neonatal hypoglycemia in a patient with normal insulin secretion. Pediatr Res 1977; 11:943–949.
224. Kollee LA, Monnens LA, Cejka V, et al. Persistent neonatal hypoglycemia due to glucagon deficiency. Arch Dis Child 1978; 53:422–424.
225. McFadzean AJS, Yeung RTT. Further observations of hypoglycaemia in hepato-cellular carcinoma. Am J Med 1969; 47:220–235.
226. Benn JJ, Firth RGR, Sönksen PH. Metabolic effects of an insulin-like factor causing hypoglycaemia in a patient with a hemangiopericytoma. Clin Endocrinol (OxF) 1990; 32:769–780.
227. Møller N, Blum WF, Mengel A, et al. Basal and insulin stimulated substrate metabolism in tumor induced hypoglycaemia: evidence for increased muscle glucose uptake. Diabetologia 1991; 34:17–20.
228. Eastman RC, Carson RE, Orloff DG, et al. Glucose utilization in a patient with hepatoma and hypoglycemia. J Clin Invest 1992; 89:1958–1963.
229. Olefsky S, Bailey L, Samols E, et al. A fibrosarcoma with hypoglycemia and high serum insulin levels. Lancet 1962; 2:378–380.
230. Lyall SS, Marieb MJ, Wise JK, et al. Hyperinsulinemic hypoglycemia associated with a neurofibrosarcoma. Arch Intern Med 1975; 135:865–867.
231. Kiang DT, Bauer GE, Kennedy BJ. Immunoassayable insulin in carcinoma of the cervix associated with hypoglycemia. Cancer 1973; 31:801–805.
232. Shames JM, Dhurandhar NE, Blackard WG. Insulin-secreting bronchial carcinoid tumor with widespread metastases. Am J Med 1968; 44:632–636.
233. Appleyard TN, Losowsky MD. A pancreatic tumor with carcinoid syndrome and hypoglycemia. Postgrad Med J 1970; 46:159–171.
234. Marks V, Samols E. Hypoglycemia of nonendocrine origin. Proc R Soc Med 1966; 59:338–340.
235. Seckl MJ, Mulholland PJ, Bishop AE, et al. Hypoglycemia due to an insulin-secreting small cell carcinoma of the cervix. N Engl J Med 1999; 341:733–736.
236. Daughaday WH, Emanuelle MA, Brooks MH, et al. Synthesis and secretion of insulin-like growth factor II by a leiomyosarcoma with associated hypoglycemia. N Engl J Med 1988; 319:1434–1440.
237. Lowe WL, Roberts CT, LeRoith D, et al. Insulin-like growth factor-II in nonislet cell tumors associated with hypoglycemia: increased levels of messenger ribonucleic acid. J Clin Endocrinol Metab 1989; 69:1153–1159.
238. Wu J-C, Daughaday WH, Lee S-D, et al. Radioimmunoassay of serum IGF-I and IGF-II in patients with chronic liver diseases and hepatocellular carcinoma with or without hypoglycemia. J Lab Clin Med 1988; 112:589–594.
239. Zapf J, Futo E, Peter M, et al. Can "big" insulin-like growth factor II in serum of tumor patients account for the development of extrapancreatic tumor hypoglycemia? J Clin Invest 1992; 90:2574–2584.
240. Daughaday WH, Trivedi B, Baxter RC. Serum "big insulin-like growth factor II" from patients with tumor hypoglycemia lacks normal E-domain O-linked glycosylation, a possible determinant of normal propeptide processing. Proc Natl Acad Sci USA 1993; 90:5823–5827.
241. Fukuda I, Hizuka N, Takano K, et al. Circulating forms of insulin-like growth factor II (IGF-II) in patients with non–islet cell tumor hypoglycemia. Endocrinol Metab 1994; 1:89–95.
242. Daughaday WH. The pathophysiology of IGF-II hypersecretion in non-islet tumor hypoglycemia. Diabetes Rev 1995; 3:62–72.
243. Marks V, Teale JD. Investigation of hypoglycaemia. Clin Endocrinol (OxF) 1996; 44:133–136.
244. Merrimee TJ, Fineberg SE. Homeostasis during fasting. II. Hormone substrate differences between men and women. J Clin Endocrinol Metab 1973; 37:698–702.
245. Haymond MW, Karl IE, Clark WL, et al. Differences in circulating gluconeogenic substrate during short-term fasting in men, women and children. Metabolism 1982; 31:33–42.
246. Grunberger G, Weiner JL, Silverman R, et al. Factitious hypoglycemia due to surreptitious administration of insulin. Ann Intern Med 1988; 108:252–257.
247. Cohen RM, Given BD, Licinio-Paixo J, et al. Proinsulin radioimmunoassay in the evaluation of insulinomas and familial hyperproinsulinemia. Metabolism 1986; 36:1137–1146.
248. Hamptom SM, Beyzavi K, Teale D, et al. A direct assay for proinsulin in plasma and its application in hypoglycaemia. Clin Endocrinol (OxF) 1988; 29:9–16.
249. Kao PC, Taylor RL, Service FJ. Proinsulin by immunochemiluminometric assay for the diagnosis of insulinoma. J Clin Endocrinol Metab 1994; 78:1048–1051.
250. Hirata Y, Tominaga M, Ito JI, et al. Spontaneous hypoglycemia

with insulin autoimmunity in Graves' disease. /
1974; 81:214–218.
251. Ichihara K, Shima K, Saito Y, et al. Mechanism
observed in a patient with autoimmune syndrome
26:500–506.
252. Anderson JH, Blackard WG, Goldman J, et a
hypoglycemia due to insulin antibodies. Am J Me
872.
253. Goldman J, Baldwin D, Rubenstein AH, et al.
of circulating insulin and proinsulin binding antil
mune hypoglycemia. J Clin Invest 1979; 63:1050
254. Redmon B, Pyzdrowski KL, Elson MK, et al. Br
glycemia due to a monoclonal insulin-binding ai
ple myeloma. N Engl J Med 1992; 326:994–998.
255. Burch HB, Clement S, Sokol MS, et al. Reacti
coma due to insulin autoimmune syndrome: case
ature review. Am J Med 1992; 92:681–685.
256. Uchigata Y, Tokunaga K, Nepom G, et al. Diffi
genetic determinants of polyclonal insulin autoir
(Hirata's disease) and monoclonal insulin autoin
Diabetes 1995; 44:1227–1232.
257. Arnqvist HJ, Halban PA, Mathiesen UL, et al
caused by atypical insulin antibodies in a pat
monoclonal gammopathy. J Intern Med 1993; 2
258. Redmon JB, Nuttall FQ. Autoimmune hypoglyc
Metab Clin North 1999; 28:603–618.
259. Taylor SI, Barbetti F, Accili D, et al. Syndrom
ity and hypoglycemia. Endocrinol Metab Clin
18:123–143.
260. Moller DE, Ratner RE, Borenstein DG, et al.
the insulin receptor as a cause of autoimmune
systemic lupus erythematosus. Am J Med 1988;
261. Rocket N, Blanche S, Carel JC, et al. Hypogly
antibodies to insulin receptor following a bone r
tation in an immuno-deficient child. Diabetolo
172.
262. Kiyokawa H, Kono N, Hamaguchi T, et al.
due to impaired insulin clearance associated wit
cemia and postprandial hyperglycemia: an an
with antiinsulin antibodies. J Clin Endocrinol
616–621.
263. De Pirro R, Borboni P, Marini MA, et al. Anti
the insulin receptor: clinical aspects and applic
of insulin action. J Endocrinol Invest 1990; 13:
264. Di Paolo S, Giogrino R. Insulin resistance and
patient with systemic lupus erythematosus: des
sulin receptor antibodies that enhance insulin b
insulin actions. J Clin Endocrinol Metab 1991;
265. Wilkin TJ, Hammonds P, Mirza JH, et al. Gr
β-cell: glucose dysregulation due to islet-cell st
ies. Lancet 1988; 2:1155–1158.
266. Wilkin TJ. Receptor autoimmunity in endo
Engl J Med 1990; 323:1318–1324.
267. Foggensteiner L, Bone AJ, Webster KA, et
proinsulin mRNA in pancreatic islets incubat
stimulating antibodies from serums of type I
Diabetes 1990; 39:1165–1169.
268. McMahon MM, O'Brien PC, Service FJ. Dia
tion of the intravenous tolbutamide test for
Clin Proc 1989; 64:1481–1488.
269. Service FJ, O'Brien PC, Kao PC, et al. C-p
test: effects of gender, age and body mass ind
for diagnosis of insulinoma. J Clin Endocrin
204–210.
270. Service FJ, McMahon MM, O'Brien PC, et al
linoma: incidence, recurrence, and long-term
Mayo Clin Proc 1991; 66:711–719.
271. Perry RR, Vinik AI. Diagnosis and managem
islet cell tumors. J Clin Endocrinol Metab 199
272. Philippe J, Powers AC, Mojsov S, et al. Ex
hormone genes in human islet cell tumors.
647–651.
273. D'Arcangues CM, Awoke S, Lawrence GD
noma with long survival and glucagonoma syn
Med 1984; 100:233–235.
274. Rizza RA, Haymond MW, Verdonk CA, et

349. Glasgow AM, Engel AG, Bier DM, et al. Hypoglycemia, hepatic dysfunction, muscle weakness, cardiomyopathy, free carnitine deficiency and long chain acylcarnitine excess responsive to medium chain triglyceride diet. Pediatr Res 1983; 17:319–326.
350. Nezu J, Tamai I, Oku A, et al. Primary systemic carnitine deficiency is caused by mutations in a gene encoding sodium ion-dependent carnitine transporter. Nat Genet 1999; 21:91–94.
351. Jist LI, Mandel H, Oostheim W, et al. Molecular basis of hepatic carnitine palmitoyltransferase I deficiency. J Clin Invest 1998; 102:527–531.
352. Infante JP, Huszagh VA. Secondary carnitine deficiency and impaired decoxahexaenoic (22:6n-3) acid synthesis: a common denominator in the pathophysiology of diseases of oxidative phosphorylation and β-oxidation. FEBS Lett 2000; 468:1–5.
353. McGarry JD, Brown NF. The mitochondrial carnitine palmitoyltransferase system. Eur J Biochem 1997; 244:1–14.
354. Bougnieres PF, Saudubray JM, Marsac C, et al. Fasting hypoglycemia resulting from hepatic carnitine palmitoyltransferase deficiency. J Pediatr 1981; 98:742–746.
355. Taroni F, Verderio E, Fiorucci S, et al. Molecular characterization of inherited carnitine palmitoyltransferase II deficiency. Proc Natl Acad Sci USA 1992; 89:8429–8433.
356. Yamamoto S, Abe H, Kohgo T, et al. Two novel gene mutations (Glu174→Lys, Phe 383→Tyr) causing the "hepatic" form of carnitine palmitoyltransferase II deficiency. Hum Genet 1996; 98: 116–118.
357. Vianey-Saban C, Guffan N, Delolne F, et al. Diagnosis of inborn errors of metabolism by acylcarnitine profiling in blood using tandem mass spectrometry. J Inherit Metab Dis 1997; 20:411–414.
358. Vreben P, van Lint AE, Bootsma AH, et al. Rapid diagnosis of organic acidemias and fatty acid oxidation defects by quantitative electrospray tandem-MS acyl-carnitine analysis in plasma. Adv Exp Med Biol 1999; 466:327–337.
359. Ibdah JA, Bennett MJ, Rinaldo P, et al. A fetal fatty-acid oxidation disorder as a cause of liver disease in pregnant women. N Engl J Med 1999; 340:1723–1731.
360. Shultz KT, Neelon FA, Nilsen LB, et al. Mechanism of postgastrectomy hypoglycemia. Arch Intern Med 1971; 128:240–246.
361. Toft-Nilsen M, Madsbad S, Holst JJ. Exaggerated secretion of glucagon-like peptide-1 (GLP-1) can explain reactive hypoglycemia (abstract). Diabetes 1996; 45:223A.
362. Lefebvre PJ, Andreani D, Marks V, et al. Statement on "postprandial" or "reactive" hypoglycemia. In Andreani D, Marks V, Lefebvre PJ (eds). Hypoglycemia. New York, Raven Press, 1987, p 79.
363. Service FJ. Hypoglycemic disorders. N Engl J Med 1995; 332: 1144–1152.
364. Charles MA, Hofeldt F, Shackelford A, et al. Comparison of oral glucose tolerance tests and mixed meals in patients with apparent idiopathic postabsorptive hypoglycemia. Diabetes 1981; 30:465–470.
365. Lev-Ran A, Anderson RW. The diagnosis of postprandial hypoglycemia. Diabetes 1981; 30:996–999.
366. Betteridge DJ. Reactive hypoglycemia. Br Med J 1987; 295:286–287.
367. Palardy J, Havrankova J, Lepage R, et al. Blood glucose measurements during symptomatic episodes in patients with suspected postprandial hypoglycemia. N Engl J Med 1989; 321:1421–1425.
368. Service FJ, Natt N, Thompson GB, et al. Noninsulinoma pancreatogenous hypoglycemia: a novel syndrome of hyperinsulinemic hypoglycemia in adults independent of mutations in Kir6.2 and SUR1 genes. J Clin Endocrinol Metab 1999; 84:1582–1589.
369. Foa PP, Dunbar JC, Klein SP, et al. Reactive hypoglycemia and A-cell ("pancreatic") glucagon deficiency in the adult. JAMA 1980; 244:2281–2285.
370. Shima K, Tabata M, Tanaka A, et al. Exaggerated response of plasma glucagon-like immunoreactivity to oral glucose in patients with reactive hypoglycemia. Endocrinol Jpn 1981; 28:249–256.
371. Chalew SA, McLaughlin JV, Mersey J, et al. The use of the plasma epinephrine response in the diagnosis of idiopathic postprandial syndrome. JAMA 1984; 251:612–615.
372. Permutt MA, Keller D, Santiago JV. Cholinergic blockade in reactive hypoglycemia. Diabetes 1977; 26:121–127.
373. Jenkins DJA, Bloom SR, Albuquerque RH, et al. Pectin and complications after gastric surgery: normalization of postprandial glucose and endocrine responses. Gut 1980; 21:574–579.
374. Fink WJ, Hucke ST, Gray TW, et al. Treatment of postoperative reactive hypoglycemia by a reversed intestinal segment. Am J Surg 1976; 131:19–22.
375. Kay WW. The treatment of prolonged insulin coma. J Ment Sci 1961; 107:194–238.
376. MacCuish AC, Munro JF, Duncan LJP. Treatment of hypoglycaemic coma with glucagon, intravenous dextrose, and mannitol infusion in a hundred diabetics. Lancet 1970; 2:946–949.
377. Hoffbrand BI, Sevitt LH. Use of mannitol in prolonged coma due to insulin overdosage. Lancet 1966; 1:402.
378. Anderson JH, Byrd GW, Blackard WG. Hyperresponsiveness to tolbutamide of dogs pretreated with diazoxide. Metabolism 1971; 20:1023–1030.
379. Koch-Weser J. Diazoxide. N Engl J Med 1976; 294:1271–1273.
380. Baxter RC, Holman SR, Corbould A, et al. Regulation of the insulin-like growth factors and their binding proteins by glucocorticoid and growth hormone in nonislet cell tumor hypoglycemia. J Clin Endocrinol Metab 1995; 80:2700–2708.
381. Baxter RC. The role of insulin-like growth factors and their binding proteins in tumor hypoglycemia. Horm Res 1996; 46: 195–201.

33 Obesity

Samuel Klein and Johannes A. Romijn

Obesity is a chronic disease that is causally related to serious medical illnesses. In the United States alone, the consequences of obesity account for an estimated 300,000 deaths per year.[1] The medical expenses and cost of lost productivity related to obesity are greater than $100 billion per year.[2] This chapter addresses the important clinical and pathophysiologic issues in obesity.

DEFINITION

Body Mass Index

Body mass index (BMI) is calculated by dividing weight (in kilograms) by height (in meters squared) or by dividing weight (in pounds) multiplied by 704 by height (in inches squared). There is a strong curvilinear relation between BMI and relative body fat mass.[3] However, the current practical definition of obesity is based on the relationship between BMI and health outcome rather than BMI and body composition.

Table 33–1 summarizes the guidelines for classifying weight status by BMI, proposed by the major national and international health organizations.[4–7] Large epidemiologic studies have established that there is a strong inverse relationship between BMI and mortality.[8, 9] Men and women with a BMI of 25.0 to 29.9 kg/m^2 are considered overweight, and those with a BMI 30 kg/m^2 or greater are considered obese. Obese persons have higher risk for adverse health consequences than those who are overweight (Fig. 33–1). These criteria for overweight and obesity represent imposed cutoff values along a continuum between mortality rate and BMI. The prevalence of obesity-related diseases, such as diabetes, begins to increase at BMI values below 25 kg/m^2 (Fig. 33–2).

Factors Affecting Body Mass Index–Related Risk

As shown in Table 33–1, several factors influence BMI-related health risk. For example, obese persons with excess abdominal fat are at higher risk for diabetes, hypertension, dyslipidemia, and ischemic heart disease than obese persons whose fat is located predominantly in the lower body.[10] Waist circumference is highly correlated with abdominal fat mass and is therefore often used as a surrogate marker for abdominal (upper body) obesity. Waist circumference values denoting increased risk for metabolic diseases have been proposed on the basis of epidemiologic data. For men, a waist circumference greater than 102 cm (40 inches) and, for women, a waist circumference greater than 88 cm (35 inches) have been proposed as cutoff values for increased risk.[5] However, this proposal imposes arbitrary cutoff values on the continuous relationship between waist circumference and metabolic disease risk.

Another factor that modifies the risk of obesity-related complications is weight gain during adulthood. In both men and women, weight gain of 5 kg or more since age 18 to 20 years is associated with an increased risk of diabetes, hypertension, and coronary heart disease, and the risk of disease increases with the amount of weight gained.[11–16]

Risks of developing obesity-associated diabetes or cardiovascular disease can also be modified by aerobic fitness. Blair and colleagues monitored more than 8000 men for an average of 6 years. Across a range of body adiposity, incidences of diabetes[17] and cardiovascular mortality[18] were lower in those who were fit, as defined by maximal ability to consume oxygen during exercise, than in those who were unfit.

BMI-associated health risk is also influenced by ethnicity.[19] For example, when the subjects are matched on BMI, the risk

Table 33–3. Adipocyte-Secreted Proteins

Category	Protein
Potential hormone	Leptin, resistin, angiotensinogen, Adiponectin/ACRP 30, estrogens
Cytokine	Interleukin-6, tumor necrosis factor α
Extracellular matrix protein	Type I, III, IV, and VI collagen, fibronectin, osteonectin, laminin, entactin, matrix metalloproteinases 2 and 9
Complement factor	Adipsin, complement C3, factor B
Enzyme	Cholester ester transfer protein, lipoprotein lipase
Acute phase response proteins	α_1-Acid glycoprotein, haptoglobin
Other	Fatty acids Plasminogen activator inhibitor-1 Prostacyclin

tween excess body fat and pathologic states, such as insulin resistance and type 2 diabetes mellitus.[61, 62]

Leptin

Adipocytes produce leptin and secrete it into the blood stream. Leptin has pleiotropic effects on food intake, hypothalamic neuroendocrine regulation, reproductive function, and energy expenditure.[63, 64] There is a direct relationship between plasma leptin concentrations and BMI or percent body fat.[65] However, there can be considerable variability in leptin concentrations among persons with the same BMI, suggesting that leptin production is also regulated by factors other than adipose tissue mass per se.

Leptin levels decrease rapidly within 12 hours after the start of starvation; conversely, they increase in response to overfeeding.[66] Therefore, plasma leptin concentrations reflect adipose tissue mass and are influenced by energy balance. In this perspective, leptin is a bidirectional signal that switches physiologic regulation between fed and starved states. Plasma leptin concentrations increase with increasing fat mass and decrease rapidly during early fasting. At present, the relative importance of the central versus peripheral effects of leptin remains to be elucidated.[67]

Resistin

Resistin is another signaling polypeptide secreted by adipocytes.[68] Resistin levels are increased in mice with diet-induced and genetic forms of obesity and insulin resistance. Administration of recombinant resistin to normal mice impaired glucose tolerance and insulin action. Neutralization of resistin reduced hyperglycemia in obese, insulin-resistant mice, in part by improving insulin sensitivity. It has therefore been proposed that resistin is a hormone that links obesity to diabetes by inducing insulin resistance.

Estrogens

Adipose tissue has aromatase activity. This enzyme is important for transforming androstenedione into estrone. Estrone is the second major circulating estrogen in premenopausal women and the most important estrogen in postmenopausal women.[62] The rate of conversion of androstenedione to estrone increases with age and obesity and is higher in lower body than in upper body obesity. In addition to a role in endocrine regulation, the effects of P450 aromatase on estrogen metabolism may have a role in autocrine or paracrine action because estrogen receptors are present in adipose tissue.

Tumor Necrosis Factor α

Adipocytes secrete TNF-α, and TNF-α expression is increased in the enlarged adipocytes of obese subjects.[69] However, plasma TNF-α levels are generally at or below the detection limit of available assays, which suggests that the TNF-α produced within adipose tissue has paracrine rather than endocrine functions. The multiple effects of TNF-α on adipocytes include impairment of insulin signaling. Therefore, it has been proposed that TNF-α may partially contribute to insulin resistance in obesity.[61]

ADIPOCYTE BIOLOGY

Obesity is associated with an increased number of adipocytes. A lean adult has about 35 billion adipocytes, each containing about 0.4 to 0.6 μg of triglyceride; an extremely obese adult can have four times as many adipocytes (125 billion), each containing twice as much lipid (0.8 to 1.2 μg of triglyceride).[70]

Our understanding of adipocyte differentiation is largely derived from studies of preadipocytes in culture. The current concept is that adipocytes are derived from fibroblast precursor cells after the concerted actions of extracellular signals and intrinsic transcription factors and coactivators. Many extranuclear factors and intracellular transduction pathways influence the adipogenic potential of cells in vitro and in vivo (Fig. 33–3).[71] Although in the future it may be possible to regulate adipogenesis in vivo, decreasing adipogenesis without altering energy balance may result in the deposition of triglycerides in other tissues. Excessive triglycerides in nonadipose tissues can have deleterious effects, as suggested by the liver steatosis,

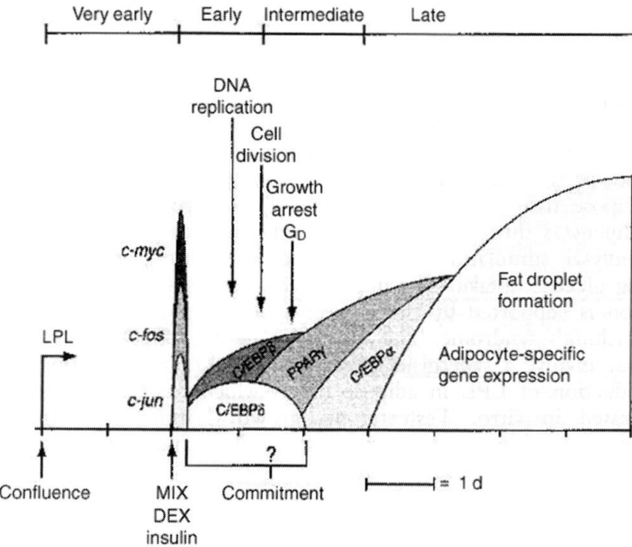

Figure 33–3. Progression of 3T3-L1 preadipocyte differentiation with subsequent changes in cellular characteristics. The distinct stages of differentiation (very early, early, intermediate, and late) are shown. C/EBP, CCAAT/enhancer binding protein; DEX, dexamethasone; LPL, lipoprotein lipase; MIX, methylisobutylxanthine; PPAR, peroxisome proliferator–activated receptor. (Modified from Ntambi JM, Kim Y-C. Adipocyte differentiation and gene expression. J Nutr 2000; 130: 3122S–3126S.)

dyslipidemia, and diabetes observed when adipogenesis was prevented in mice.[72]

The cornerstone of obesity therapy is to increase the utilization of endogenous fat stores as fuel by reducing energy intake below energy expenditure. With dieting, weight loss is composed of approximately 75% to 85% fat and 15% to 25% *fat-free mass* (FFM).[73] An energy deficit of approximately 3500 kcal is required to oxidize 1 pound of adipose tissue. However, because of the oxidation of lean tissue and associated water losses, a 3500-kcal energy deficit reduces body weight by more than 1 pound. The distribution of fat loss is characterized by regional heterogeneity.[74, 75] Particularly in men and women with initially increased intra-abdominal fat, there are greater relative losses of intra-abdominal fat than of total body fat mass. A decrease in the size (triglyceride content) of existing adipocytes accounts for most, if not all, of the fat loss.[76] In humans, there is also evidence that the number of adipocytes is reduced with large, long-term fat loss.[77] However, it is possible that this perception of decreased fat cell number is false because standard cell-counting techniques may fail to detect adipocytes that have undergone marked shrinkage.

There are two possible mechanisms through which weight loss can eliminate fat cells: (1) *dedifferentiation*, the morphologic and biochemical reversion of mature adipocytes to preadipocytes, and (2) *apoptosis*. Adipocyte dedifferentiation has been observed in vitro, but there is no evidence that it occurs in vivo.[78] Adipocyte apoptosis has been induced in vitro[79] and has been shown to occur in vivo in some patients with cancer.[80] To date, it is not known whether diet-mediated weight loss induces adipocyte apoptosis.

PREVALENCE OF OBESITY

The worldwide prevalence of obesity has increased dramatically over the last several decades. In the United States alone, an estimated 61% (110 million) of adults 20 to 74 years of age are now considered overweight or obese.[81] According to national population surveys conducted since 1960, the prevalence of overweight in the United State increased only slightly from 30.5% to 34.0% but the prevalence of obesity (BMI >30 kg/m^2) more than doubled, from 12.8% to 27%.[81, 82] In the United States, the prevalence of obesity increases progressively from 20 to 50 years of age but then declines after 60 to 70 years of age.

The prevalence of obesity has also risen in children and adolescents. As defined by a BMI greater than the 95th percentile for age and gender from the revised National Center for Health Statistics growth charts, 10% to 15% of 6- to 17-year-old children and adolescents in the United States are overweight.[83] These data indicate that overweight prevalence rates for children and adolescents, reported by earlier surveys, have doubled. Diseases commonly associated with obesity in adults, such as type 2 diabetes mellitus, hypertension, hyperlipidemia, gallbladder disease, nonalcoholic steatohepatitis, sleep apnea, and orthopedic complications, are now increasingly observed in children.[84]

CLINICAL FEATURES AND COMPLICATIONS OF OBESITY

Obesity is strongly associated with many serious medical complications that impair quality of life and lead to increased morbidity and premature death (Fig. 33–4). The complications

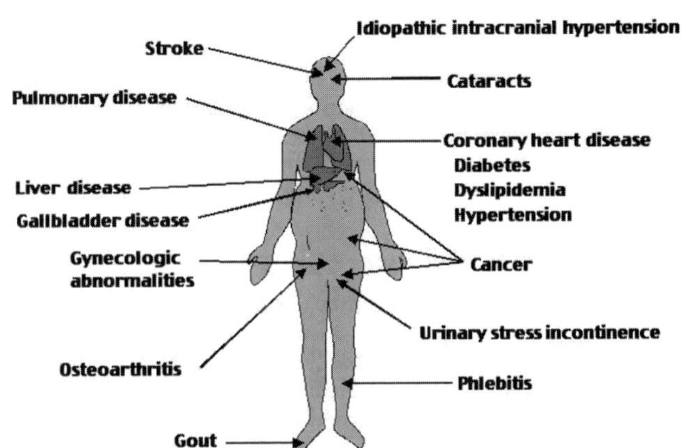

Figure 33–4. Medical complications associated with obesity.

associated with obesity have been reviewed in detail previously.[5]

Endocrine and Metabolic Disease

The Metabolic or Insulin Resistance Syndrome

In the metabolic or insulin resistance syndrome, also known as *syndrome X*, the specific phenotype of upper body or abdominal obesity is associated with a cluster of metabolic risk factors for coronary heart disease (CHD). Features of this syndrome include:

1. Insulin resistance, including hyperinsulinemia, impaired glucose tolerance, impaired insulin-mediated glucose disposal, and type 2 diabetes mellitus.
2. Dyslipidemia, characterized by hypertriglyceridemia and low serum high-density lipoprotein (HDL) cholesterol levels.
3. Hypertension.

Abdominal obesity has also been associated with the metabolic risk factors of (1) increased serum levels of apolipoprotein B; (2) small, dense low-density lipoprotein (LDL) particles; and (3) plasminogen activator inhibitor 1 with impaired fibrinolysis.[85, 86] The metabolic syndrome does not affect only those with frank obesity; it has also been reported in persons of normal weight, who presumably have an increased amount of abdominal fat.[87]

The metabolic syndrome was originally identified and defined on the basis of epidemiologic associations. The underlying pathogenesis and the interrelationships between the individual features have not been completely elucidated. Insulin resistance has been hypothesized to be the common underlying pathogenic mechanism.[88] However, according to a factor analysis of data from nondiabetic subjects in the Framingham Offspring Study, insulin resistance may not be the only precedent condition and more than one independent physiologic process may be involved.[89] Abdominal obesity is clearly associated with insulin resistance. It is not clear whether the visceral (omental and mesenteric) or subcutaneous depots of abdominal fat are more closely related to insulin resistance because data from different studies are contradictory. In addition, it is difficult to define the relationship between each abdominal adipose tissue depot and insulin resistance because the size of the depots is closely correlated. Furthermore, it is not known whether visceral fat and abdominal fat actually participate in the pathogenesis of the metabolic syndrome or merely serve as markers of increased risk for the metabolic complications of obesity.[90]

There is increasing evidence that the ectopic distribution of triglycerides in nonadipose tissue may be involved in the com-

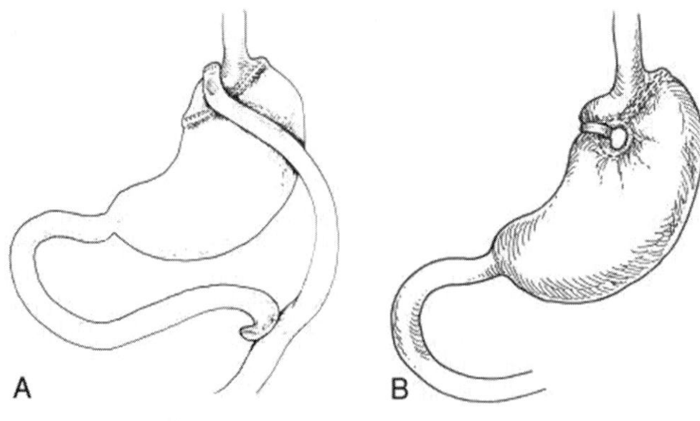

Figure 33–6. Schematic diagram of the gastric bypass procedure *(A)* and vertical banded gastroplasty *(B)*. (From Klein S, Wadden TA, Sugerman H. American Gastroenterological Association technical review: clinical issues in obesity. Gastroenterology [in press].)

cedure include marginal ulcers, stomal stenosis, dilatation of the bypassed stomach, staple line disruption, internal hernias, malabsorption of specific nutrients, and dumping syndrome.

Gastroplasty

Vertical banded and Silastic ring gastroplasties, also known as *gastric stapling,* involve creating a small pouch from the gastroesophageal junction along the lesser curvature of the stomach, which has a stoma that is restricted by a 1-cm polypropylene or Silastic ring and empties into the rest of the stomach (Fig. 33–6*B*).[265, 266] Specific complications associated with gastroplasty include staple line disruption, stomal stenosis, and gastroesophageal reflux.

Gastric Bypass versus Gastroplasty

Data from four prospective, randomized trials showed that weight loss several years after surgery was consistently greater with the gastric bypass procedure (loss of ~65% of excess weight) than with gastroplasty (loss of ~40% of excess weight)[267–270] (Fig. 33–7). In addition, independent evaluations of each procedure suggest better long-term (10 to 14 years) results with the gastric bypass procedure than gastroplasty.[168, 271] As a result of these findings, most centers now consider gastric bypass the "gold standard" for obesity surgery.

Gastric Banding

In the *laparoscopically inserted adjustable silicone gastric band* (LASGB) procedure, a silicone band is placed around the upper stomach, just below the gastroesophageal junction. The band's circumference can be adjusted by inflating or deflating a balloon connected to a subcutaneously implanted port with percutaneous access.

This operation is currently the most popular bariatric surgical procedure performed in Europe and has been approved for use in the United States. The degree of weight loss achieved with this procedure has been similar to that achieved with vertical banded gastroplasty[272] but on average has been much less than that achieved with the gastric bypass procedure.[273]

Associated complications include esophageal dilatation, erosion of the band into the stomach, band slippage, band or port infections, and balloon or system leaks that lead to inadequate weight loss.[274, 275] Esophageal dilatation and dysphagia can result from the placement of the band at the gastroesophageal junction.[274] Although loosening the band usually relieves the dilatation, removal of the band is sometimes necessary.[275] In some patients, the band erodes into the stomach and must be surgically removed. When the posterior stomach wall herniates through the band, band slippage occurs. Band slippage can cause gastric obstruction and necessitates surgical revision.

Partial Biliopancreatic Bypass Procedures

The partial biliopancreatic bypass and the partial biliopancreatic bypass with duodenal switch result in both gastric restriction and maldigestion or malabsorption. Both procedures involve a partial gastrectomy and bypassing a considerable amount of small intestine from biliary and pancreatic secretions.[276, 277] Partial biliopancreatic bypass induces malabsorption of protein, fat, fat-soluble vitamins, iron, calcium, and vitamin B_{12} and thus promotes more nutritional deficits than gastric restrictive procedures.[276, 278] The incidence of protein deficiency is probably less common and gastrointestinal side effects are not as severe after partial biliopancreatic bypass with duodenal switch than after partial biliopancreatic bypass with distal gastric resection. Presumably, these procedures cause greater weight loss (~75% of excess weight) than a standard gastric bypass, but they have never been compared directly in a prospective randomized trial.

Jejunoileal Bypass

Jejunoileal bypass was first described in 1969. This procedure was designed to bypass the major portion of the small intestine and thereby promote weight loss by inducing the malabsorption of ingested nutrients.[279, 280] The procedure is no longer performed because of an unacceptable incidence of serious side effects. The serious side effects of jejunoileal bypass result from protein-calorie malnutrition, bacterial overgrowth and translocation, and excess oxalate absorption (e.g., cirrhosis, interstitial nephritis, migratory arthritis, bypass enteritis, erythema nodosum, oxalate urolithiasis, hypocalcemia, and electrolyte imbalances).[281–285] Oral metronidazole is effective in treating the complications of jejunoileal bypass related to bacterial overgrowth (e.g., migratory arthritis, elevated liver enzymes, bleeding from inflammation in the bypassed intestine).[284, 285]

Inadequate Weight Loss After Surgery

About 15% of patients fail to lose more than 40% of their excess weight (10% to 15% of total weight) after a gastric

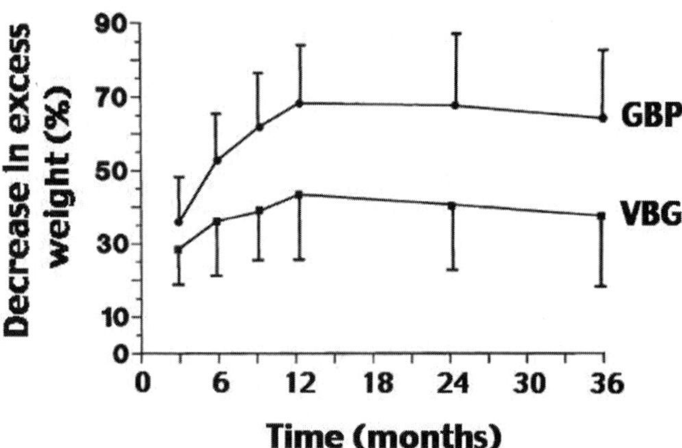

Figure 33–7. Percentage of excess weight (mean ± standard deviation) lost over 36 months after the gastric bypass procedure (GBP) and vertical banded gastroplasty (VBGP). (Adapted from Sugerman HJ, Starkey JV, Birkenhauer R. A randomized prospective trial of gastric bypass versus vertical banded gastroplasty for morbid obesity and their effects on sweets versus non-sweets eaters. Ann Surg 1987; 205:613–624.)

Table 33–6. Suggested Weight Loss Treatment Options Based on Body Mass Index and Risk Factors

Treatment	BMI Category (kg/m²)				
	25.0–26.9	27.0–29.9	30.0–34.9	35.0–39.9	≥40.0
Diet, physical activity, and behavior therapy	With CHD risk factor or obesity-related disease	With CHD risk factor or obesity-related disease	Yes	Yes	Yes
Pharmacotherapy*		With obesity-related disease	Yes	Yes	Yes
Surgery†				With obesity-related disease	Yes

*Pharmacotherapy should be considered only in patients who are not able to achieve adequate weight loss with available conventional therapy (diet, physical activity, and behavior therapy) and who do not have any absolute contraindications for drug therapy.

†Bariatric surgery should be considered only in patients who are unable to lose weight with available conventional therapy and do not have any absolute contraindications for surgery.

BMI, body mass index; CHD, coronary heart disease.

bypass procedure.[168, 286] The percentage of patients who cannot lose this amount of weight after a gastroplasty procedure is even greater.[271] The major cause of inadequate weight loss after gastric bypass is the frequent ingestion of high-calorie soft foods and liquids (e.g., ice cream, cookies, milk shakes, and sodas) and high-fat snacks and fried foods (e.g., potato chips and fried potatoes). In patients who have undergone either a stapled gastroplasty or gastric bypass, increased food intake may be related to staple line disruption, particularly if the patient is able to eat much larger quantities of food at a time.

Perioperative Mortality

The perioperative mortality rate after open surgical procedures for obesity reported in studies involving large numbers of patients was usually less than 1.5%.[168, 267] Approximately 75% of the deaths were due to anastomotic leaks and peritonitis, and 25% were due to pulmonary embolism.

TREATMENT GUIDELINES

A practical guide to the management of overweight and obesity was developed by the North American Association for the Study of Obesity in conjunction with the NIH.[245] An overview of these guidelines is shown in Table 33–6. According to these guidelines, all overweight or obese patients who have type 2 diabetes should attempt to modify diet and physical activity behaviors. Certain behaviors are common among patients who have achieved successful long-term weight loss without bariatric surgery.[287] Therefore, these four behaviors should be a goal for all patients:

1. Consume a diet that is low in calories (1300 to 1400 kcal/day) and fat (~25% kcal as fat).
2. Engage in high levels of regular physical activity (expending about 2800 kcal/week equivalent to walking about 4 miles/day).
3. Monitor food intake and physical activity.
4. Check weight regularly.

Weight management is a key component in the treatment of overweight or obese patients with type 2 diabetes. Even a modest weight loss of 5% of initial body weight improves glycemic control and reduces the need for hypoglycemic medication. Moreover, modest weight loss improves other diabetes-related risk factors for CHD.

Unfortunately, successful weight management is more difficult to achieve in obese patients with type 2 diabetes than in those without diabetes.[175, 176] In fact, treatment of diabetes itself is usually associated with an increase in body weight.[177] Therefore, the first principle of weight management in patients with diabetes is to use hypoglycemic therapy that is associated with the least amount of weight gain. Metformin is the preferred oral hypoglycemic agent because it produces minimal weight gain or slight weight loss.[288, 289] In addition, providing long-acting insulin at night is associated with less weight gain than more frequent dosing.[290, 291]

References

1. Allison DB, Fontaine KR, Manson JE, et al. Annual deaths attributable to obesity in the United States. JAMA 1999; 282:1530–1538.
2. Wolf AM, Colditz GA. Current estimates of the economic cost of obesity in the United States. Obes Res 1998; 6:97–106.
3. Gallagher D, Heymsfield SB, Heo M, et al. Health percentage body fat ranges: an approach for developing guidelines based on body mass index. Am J Clin Nutr 2000; 72:694–701.
4. World Health Organization. Obesity: Preventing and Managing the Global Epidemic. Report of a WHO Consultation on Obesity. Geneva: World Health Organization, 1998.
5. National Institutes of Health, National Heart, Lung, and Blood Institute. Clinical guidelines on the identification, evaluation, and treatment of overweight and obesity in adults: the evidence report. Obes Res 1998; 6(Suppl 2):51S–209S.
6. US Department of Health and Human Services. Nutrition and overweight. In: Healthy People 2010. Washington, DC: Government Printing Office, 2000.
7. US Department of Agriculture and US Department of Health and Human Services. Nutrition and Your Health: Dietary Guidelines for Americans, 5th ed (Home and Garden Bulletin No 232). Washington, DC: Government Printing Office, 2000.
8. Troiano RP, Frongillo EA Jr, Sobal J, Levitsky DA. The relationship between body weight and mortality: a quantitative analysis of combined information from existing studies. Int J Obes 1996; 20:63–75.
9. Calle EE, Thun MJ, Petrelli JM, et al. Body-mass index and mortality in a prospective cohort of U.S. adults. N Engl J Med 1999; 341:1097–1105.
10. Kissebah AH, Videlingum N, Murray R, et al. Relation of body fat distribution to metabolic complications of obesity. J Clin Endocrinol Metab 1982; 54:254–260.
11. Willett WC, Manson JE, Stampfer MJ, et al. Weight, weight change, and coronary heart disease in women: risk within the 'normal' weight range. JAMA 1995; 273:461–465.
12. Rimm EB, Stampfer MJ, Giovannucci E, et al. Body size and fat distribution as predictors of coronary heart disease among middle-aged and older US men. Am J Epidemiol 1995; 141:1117–1127.

13. Colditz GA, Willett WC, Rotnitzky A, Manson JE. Weight gain as a risk factor for clinical diabetes mellitus in women. Ann Intern Med 1995; 122:481–486.
14. Chan JM, Rimm EB, Colditz GA, et al. Obesity, fat distribution, and weight gain as risk factors for clinical diabetes in men. Diabetes Care 1994; 17:961–969.
15. Huang Z, Willett WC, Manson JE, et al. Body weight, weight change, and risk for hypertension in women. Ann Intern Med 1998; 128:81–88.
16. Maclure KM, Hayes KC, Colditz GA, et al. Weight, diet, and risk of symptomatic gallstones in middle-aged women. N Engl J Med 1989; 321:563–569.
17. Wei M, Gibbons L, Mitchell T, et al. The association between cardiorespiratory fitness and impaired fasting glucose and type 2 diabetes mellitus in men. Ann Intern Med 1999; 130:89–96.
18. Lee CD, Blair SN, Jackson AS. Cardiorespiratory fitness, body composition, and all-cause and cardiovascular disease mortality in men. Am J Clin Nutr 1999; 69:373–380.
19. McKeigue P, Shah B, Marmont MG. Relation of central obesity and insulin resistance with high diabetes prevalence and cardiovascular risk in South Asians. Lancet 1991; 337:382–386.
20. Rosenbaum M, Leibel RL, Hirsch J. Obesity. N Engl J Med 1997; 337:396–408.
21. Bouchard C, Perusse L. Genetics of obesity. Annu Rev Nutr 1993; 3:337–354.
22. Pratley RE. Gene-environment interactions in the pathogenesis of type 2 diabetes mellitus: lessons learned from the Pima Indians. Proc Nutr Soc 1998; 57:175–181.
23. O'Dea K, White N, Sinclair A. An investigation of nutrition-related risk factors in an isolated Aboriginal community in northern Australia: advantages of a traditionally-orientated life style. Med J Aust 1988; 148:177–180.
24. O'Dea K. Marked improvement in carbohydrate and lipid metabolism in diabetic Australian Aborigines after temporary reversion to traditional lifestyle. Diabetes 1983; 33:596-603.
25. Whitaker RC, Wright JA, Pepe MS, et al. Predicting obesity in young adulthood from childhood and parental obesity. N Engl J Med 1997; 337:869–873.
26. Montague CT, Farooqi IS, Whitehead JP, et al. Congenital leptin deficiency is associated with severe early-onset obesity in humans. Nature 1997; 387:903–908.
27. Strobel A, Issad T, Camoin L, et al. A leptin missense mutation associated with hypogonadism and morbid obesity. Nat Genet 1998; 18:213–215.
28. Farooqi IS, Jebb SA, Langmack G, et al. Effects of recombinant leptin therapy in a child with congenital leptin deficiency. N Engl J Med 1999; 341:879–884.
29. Consadine RV, Sinha MK, Heiman ML, et al. Serum immunoreactive-leptin concentrations in normal-weight and obese humans. N Engl J Med 1996; 334:292-295.
30. Clement K, Vaisse C, Lahlou N, et al. A mutation in the human leptin receptor gene causes obesity and pituitary dysfunction. Nature 1998; 392:398–401.
31. Jackson RS, Creemers JW, Ohagi S, et al. Obesity and impaired prohormone processing associated with mutation of the human prohormone convertase 1 gene. Nat Genet 1997; 16:218–220.
32. Krude H, Biebermann H, Luck W, et al. Severe early-onset obesity, adrenal insufficiency and red hair pigmentation caused by *POMC* mutations in humans. Nat Genet 1998; 19:155–157.
33. Farooqi IS, Yeo GS, Keogh JM, et al. Dominant and recessive inheritance of morbid obesity associated with melanocortin 4 receptor deficiency. J Clin Invest 2000; 106:271–279.
34. Holder JL Jr, Butte NF, Zinn AR. Profound obesity associated with a balanced translocation that disrupts the *SIM1* gene. Hum Mol Genet 2000; 9:101-108.
35. Pérusse L, Chagnon YC, Weisnagel J, et al. The human obesity gene map: the 2000 update. Obes Res 2001; 9:135-169.
36. Ravussin E, Burnand B, Schutz Y, Jequier E. Twenty-four-hour energy expenditure and resting metabolic rate in obese, moderately obese, and control subjects. Am J Clin Nutr 1982; 35:566–573.
37. Skov AR, Toubro S, Buemann B, Astrup A. Normal levels of energy expenditure in patients with reported 'low metabolism.' Clin Physiol 1997; 17:279–285.
38. Lichtman SW, Pisarka K, Berman ER, et al. Discrepancy between self-reported and actual caloric intake and exercise in obese subjects. N Engl J Med 1992; 327:1893–1898.
39. Segal KR, Presta E, Gutin B. Thermic effect of food during graded exercise in normal weight and obese men. Am J Clin Nutr 1984; 40:95–100.
40. de Jonge L, Bray GA. The thermic effect of food and obesity: a critical review. Obes Res 1997; 5:622–631.
41. Roberts SB, Savage J, Coward WA, et al. Energy expenditure and intake from infants born to lean and overweight mothers. N Engl J Med 1988; 318:461–466.
42. Stunkard AJ, Berkowitz RI, Stallings VA, Schoeller DA. Energy intake, not energy output, is a determinant of body size in infants. Am J Clin Nutr 1999; 69:524–530.
43. Ravussin E, Stephen Lillioja MB, Knowler WC, et al. Reduced rate of energy expenditure as a risk factor for body-weight gain. N Engl J Med 1988; 318:467–472.
44. Seidell JC, Muller DC, Sorkin JD, Andres R. Fasting respiratory exchange ratio and resting metabolic rate as predictors of weight gain: the Baltimore Longitudinal Study on Aging. Int J Obes Relat Metab Disord 1992; 16:667–674.
45. Bouchard C, Tremblay A, Despres JP, et al. The response to long-term overfeeding in identical twins. N Engl J Med 1990; 322:1477–1482.
46. Levine JA, Eberhardt NL, Jensen MD. Role of nonexercise activity thermogenesis in resistance to fat gain in humans. Science 1999; 282:212–214.
47. Wadden TA, Foster GD, Letizia KA, Mullen JL. Long-term effects of dieting on resting metabolic rate in obese outpatients. JAMA 1990; 264:707–711.
48. Amatruda JM, Statt MC, Welle SL. Total resting energy expenditure in obese women reduced to ideal body weight. J Clin Invest 1993; 92:1236–1242.
49. Weinsier RL, Nagy TR, Hunter GR, et al. Do adaptive changes in metabolic rate favor weight regain in weight-reduced individuals? An examination of the set-point theory. Am J Clin Nutr 2000; 72:1088–1094.
50. Astrup A, Gotzsche PC, van de Werken K, et al. Meta-analysis of resting metabolic rate in formerly obese subjects. Am J Clin Nutr 1999; 69:1117–1122.
51. Leiter LA, Marliss EB. Survival during fasting may depend on fat as well as protein stores. JAMA 1982; 248:2306–2307.
52. Stewart WK, Fleming LW. Features of a successful therapeutic fast of 382 days duration. Postgrad Med J 1973; 49:203–209.
53. Angel A, Bray GA. Synthesis of fatty acids and cholesterol by the liver, adipose tissue and intestinal mucosa from obese and control patients. Eur J Clin Invest 1979; 9:355–362.
54. Ramsay TG. Fat cells. Endocrinol Metab Clin North Am 1996; 25:847–870.
55. Simsolo RB, Ong JM, Saffari B, Kern PA. Effect of improved diabetes control on the expression of lipoprotein lipase in human adipose tissue. J Lipid Res 1992; 33;89–95.
56. Heiling VJ, Miles JM, Jensen MD. How valid are isotopic measurements of fatty acid oxidation? Am J Physiol 1991; 261:E572-E577.
57. Leweis GF. Fatty acid regulation of very low density lipoprotein production. Curr Opin Lipidol 1997; 8:146–153.
58. Jensen MD. Diet effects on fatty acid metabolism in lean and obese subjects. Am J Clin Nutr 1998; 67:531S–534S.
59. Jensen MD, Haymond MW, Rizza RA, et al. Influence of body fat distribution on free fatty acid metabolism in obesity. J Clin Invest 1989; 83:12168–12173.
60. Martin ML, Jensen MD. Effects of body fat distribution on regional lipolysis in obesity. J Clin Invest 1991; 88:609–613.
61. Kahn BB, Flier JS. Obesity and insulin resistance. J Clin Invest 2000; 106:473–481.
62. Wajchenberg BL. Subcutaneous and visceral adipose tissue: their relation to the metabolic syndrome. Endocr Rev 2000; 21:697–738.
63. Friedman JM. Obesity in the new millennium. Nature 2000; 404: 632–634.
64. Lee Y, Wang MY, Wang ZW, et al. Liporegulation in diet-induced obesity: the antisteatotic role of hyperleptinemia. J Biol Chem 2001; 276:5629–5635.
65. Considine RV, Sinha MK, Heiman ML, et al. Serum immunoreactive leptin concentrations in normal weight and obese humans. N Engl J Med 1996; 334:292–295.
66. Kolaczynsky JW, Ohammesian JP, Considine RV, et al. Response of leptin to short-term and prolonged overfeeding in humans. J Clin Endocrinol Metab 1996; 81:4162–4165.

67. Flier JS. Clinical review 94: what's in a name? In search of leptin's physiologic role. J Clin Endocrinol Metab 1998; 83: 1407–1413.
68. Steppan CM, Bailey ST, Bhat S, et al. The hormone resistin links obesity to diabetes. Nature 2001; 409:307–312.
69. Peraldi P, Spiegelman B. TNF alpha and insulin resistance: summary and future prospects. Mol Cell Biochem 1998; 182:169-171.
70. Hirsch J, Knittle JL. Cellularity of obese and non-obese human adipose tissue. Fed Proc 1970; 29:1516–1521.
71. Ntambi JM, Kim Y-C. Adipocyte differentiation and gene expression. J Nutr 2000; 130:3122S–3126S.
72. Shimomura I, Hammer RE, Richardson JA, et al. Insulin resistance and diabetes mellitus in transgenic mice expressing nuclear SREBP-1c in adipose tissue: model for congenital generalized lipodystrophy. Genes Dev 1998; 12:3182–3194.
73. Ballor DL, Poehlman ET. Exercise-training enhances fat-free mass preservation during diet-induced weight loss: a meta-analytical finding. Int J Obes Relat Metab Disord 1994; 18:35–40.
74. Ross R, Rissanen J, Pedwell H, et al. Influence of diet and exercise on skeletal muscle and visceral adipose tissue in men. J Appl Physiol 1996; 81:2445–2455.
75. Smith SR, Zachwieja JJ. Visceral adipose tissue: a critical review of intervention strategies. Int J Obes Relat Metab Disord 1999; 23:329–335.
76. Knittle JL, Ginsberg-Fellner F. Effect of weight reduction on in vitro adipose tissue lipolysis and cellularity in obese adolescents and adults. Diabetes 1972; 21:754–761.
77. Naslund I, Hallgren P, Sjostrom L. Fat cell weight and number before and after gastric surgery for morbid obesity in women. Int J Obes 1988; 12:191–197.
78. Prins JB, O'Rahilly S. Regulation of adipose cell number in man. Clin Sci 1997; 92:3–11.
79. Prins JB, Walker NL, Winterford CM, Cameron DP. Apoptosis of human adipocyte in vitro. Biochem Biophys Res Commun 1994; 201:500–507.
80. Prins JB, Walker NL, Winterford CM, Cameron DP. Human adipocyte apoptosis occurs in malignancy. Biochem Biophys Res Commun 1994; 205:625–630.
81. National Center for health Statistics, Centers for Disease Control and Prevention. Available at www.cdc.gov.nchs/products/pubs/pubd/hestats/obese/obse99.htm (accessed December 14, 2000).
82. Flegal KM, Carroll MD, Kuczmarski RJ, Johnson CL. Overweight and obesity in the United States: prevalence and trends, 1960–1994. Int J Obes Relat Metab Disord 1998; 22:39–47.
83. Flegal KM, Troiano RP. Changes in the distribution of body mass index of adults and children in the US population. Int J Obes Relat Metab Disord 2000; 24:807–818.
84. Barlow SE, Dietz WH. Obesity evaluation and treatment: Expert Committee recommendations. The Maternal and Child Health Bureau, Health Resources and Services Administration and the Department of Health and Human Services. Pediatrics 1998; 102: E29.
85. Landin K, Stigendal L, Eriksson E, et al. Abdominal obesity is associated with an impaired fibrinolytic activity and elevated plasminogen activator inhibitor-1. Metabolism 1990; 39:1044–1048.
86. Lemieux I, Pascot A, Couillard C, et al. Hypertriglyceridemic waist: a marker of the atherogenic metabolic triad (hyperinsulinemia; hyperapolipoprotein B; small, dense LDL) in men? Circulation 2000; 102:179–184.
87. Ruderman N, Chisholm D, Pi-Sunyer X, Schneider S. The metabolically obese, normal-weight individual revisited. Diabetes 1998; 47:699–713.
88. Reaven GM. Role of insulin resistance in human disease. Diabetes 1988; 37:1595–1607.
89. Meigs JB, D'Agostino RB, Wilson WF, et al. Risk variable clustering in the insulin resistance syndrome. Diabetes 1997; 46: 1594–1600.
90. Frayn KN. Visceral fat and insulin resistance: causative or correlative? Br J Nutr 2000; 83(Suppl 1):S71–S77.
91. Krssak M, Petersen KF, Dresner A, et al. Intramyocellular lipid concentrations are correlated with insulin sensitivity in humans: a ^{1}H NMR spectroscopy study. Diabetologia 1999; 42:113–116.
92. Dobbins RL, Szczepaniak LS, Bentley B, et al. Prolonged inhibition of muscle carnitine palmitoyltransferase I promotes intramyocellular lipid accumulation and insulin resistance in rats. Diabetes 2001; 50:123–130.
93. Harris MI, Flegal KM, Cowie CC, et al. Prevalence of diabetes, impaired fasting glucose, and impaired glucose tolerance in U.S. adults. The Third National Health and Nutrition Examination Survey, 1988–1994. Diabetes Care 1998; 21:518–524.
94. Colditz GA, Willett WC, Stampfer MJ, et al. Weight as a risk factor for clinical diabetes in women. Am J Epidemiol 1990; 132: 501–513.
95. Ohlson LO, Larsson B, Svardsudd K, et al. The influence of body fat distribution on the incidence of diabetes mellitus. Diabetes 1985; 34:1055–1058.
96. Lundgren H, Bengtsson C, Blohme G, et al. Adiposity and adipose tissue distribution in relation to incidence of diabetes in women: results from a prospective population study in Gothenburg, Sweden. Int J Obes 1989; 13:413–423.
97. Kaye SA, Folsom AR, Sprafka JM, et al. Increased incidence of diabetes mellitus in relation to abdominal adiposity in older women. J Clin Epidemiol 1991; 44:329–334.
98. Reaven GM, Chen YDI, Jeppesen J, et al. Insulin resistance and hyperinsulinemia in individuals with small, dense, low density lipoprotein particles. J Clin Invest 1993; 92:141–146.
99. Terry RB, Wood PD, Haskell WL, et al. Regional adiposity pattern in relation to lipids, lipoprotein cholesterol, and lipoprotein subfraction mass in men. J Clin Endocrinol Metab 1989; 68: 191–199.
100. Brown CD, Higgins M, Donato KA, et al. Body mass index and the prevalence of hypertension and dyslipidemia. Obes Res 2000; 8:605–619.
101. Assmann G, Schulte H. Relation of high-density lipoprotein cholesterol and triglycerides to incidence of atherosclerotic coronary artery disease (the PROCAM experience). Am J Cardiol 1992; 70:733–737.
102. Lamarche B, Lemieux I, Despres JP. The small, dense LDL phenotype and the risk of coronary heart disease: epidemiology, patho-physiology and therapeutic aspects. Diabetes Metab 1999; 25:199–211.
103. Hubert HB, Feinleib M, McNamara PM, Castelli WP. Obesity as an independent risk factor for cardiovascular disease: a 26-year follow-up of participants in the Framingham Heart Study. Circulation 1983; 67:968–977.
104. Stamler R, Stamler J, Riedlinger WF, et al. Weight and blood pressure: findings in hypertension screening of 1 million Americans. JAMA 1978; 240:1607–1609.
105. Kannel W, Brand N, Skinner J, et al. The relation of adiposity to blood pressure and development of hypertension. The Framingham Study. Ann Intern Med 1967; 67:48–59.
106. Stamler J, Wentworth D, Neaton JD. Is relationship between serum cholesterol and risk of premature death from coronary disease continuous or graded? Findings in 356,222 primary screenees of the Multiple Risk Factor Intervention Trial (MRFIT). JAMA 1986; 256:2823–2828.
107. Rexrode KM, Carey VJ, Hennekens CH, et al. Abdominal adiposity and coronary heart disease in women. JAMA 1998; 280: 1843–1848.
108. Manson JE, Willett WC, Stampfer MJ, et al. Body weight and mortality among women. N Engl J Med 1995; 333:677–685.
109. Eckel RH, Krauss RM. American Heart Association call to action: obesity as a major risk factor for coronary heart disease. Circulation 1998; 97:2099–2100.
110. Krause RM, Eckel RH, Howard B, et al. AHA Dietary guidelines revision 2000: a statement for healthcare professionals from the nutrition committee of the American Heart Association. Circulation 2000; 102:2296–2311.
111. Walker SP, Rimm EB, Ascherio A, et al. Body size and fat distribution as predictors of stroke among US men. Am J Epidemiol 1996; 144:1143–1150.
112. Rexrode KM, Hennekens CH, Willett WC, et al. A prospective study of body mass index, weight change, and risk of stroke in women. JAMA 1997; 277:1539–1545.
113. Hansson PO, Eriksson H, Welin L, et al. Smoking and abdominal obesity: risk factors for venous thromboembolism among middle-aged men: "the study of men born in 1913." Arch Intern Med 1999; 159:1886–1890.
114. Sugerman HJ, Windsor ACJ, Bessos MK, Wolfe L. Abdominal pressure, sagittal abdominal diameter and obesity co-morbidity. J Intern Med 1997; 241:71–79.
115. Visser M, Bouter LM, McQuillan GM, et al. Elevated C-reactive

protein levels in overweight and obese adults. JAMA 1999; 282: 2131–2135.
116. Strohl KP, Strobel RJ, Parisi RA. Obesity and pulmonary function. In: Bray GA, Bouchard C, James WPT, eds. Handbook of Obesity. New York, Marcel Dekker, 1998, pp 725–739.
117. Vgontzas AN, Tan TL, Bixler EO, et al. Sleep apnea and sleep disruption in obese patients. Arch Intern Med 1994; 154:1705–1711.
118. Davies RJ, Stradling JR. The relationship between neck circumference, radiographic pharyngeal anatomy, and the obstructive sleep apnoea syndrome. Eur Respir J 1990; 3:509–514.
119. Katz I, Stradling J, Slutsky AS, et al. Do patients with obstructive sleep apnea have thick necks? Am Rev Respir Dis 1990; 141: 1228–1231.
120. Roubenoff R, Klag MJ, Mead LA, et al. Incidence and risk factors for gout in white men. JAMA 1991; 266:3004–3007.
121. Cigolini M, Targher G, Tonoli M, et al. Hyperuricaemia: relationships to body fat distribution and other components of the insulin resistance syndrome in 38-year-old healthy men and women. Int J Obes Relat Metab Disord 1995; 19:92–96.
122. Felson DT, Anderson JJ, Naimark A, et al. Obesity and knee osteoarthritis. The Framingham Study. Ann Intern Med 1988; 109:18–24.
123. Cicuttini FM, Baker JR, Spector TD. The association of obesity with osteoarthritis of the hand and knee in women: a twin study. J Rheumatol 1996; 23:1221–1226.
124. Lew EA, Garfinkel L. Variations in mortality by weight among 750,000 men and women. J Chronic Dis 1979; 32:563–576.
125. Giovannucci E, Ascherio A, Rimm EB, et al. Physical activity, obesity, and risk for colon cancer and adenoma in men. Ann Intern Med 1995; 122:327–334.
126. Potter JD, Slattery ML, Bostick RM, Gapstur SM. Colon cancer: a review of the epidemiology. Epidemiol Rev 1993; 15:499–545.
127. Huang Z, Hankinson SE, Colditz GA, et al. Dual effects of weight and weight gain on breast cancer risk. JAMA 1997; 278: 1407–1411.
128. Willett WC, Browne ML, Bain C, et al. Relative weight and risk of breast cancer among premenopausal women. Am J Epidemiol 1985; 122:731–740.
129. Grodstein F, Goldman MB, Cramer DW. Body mass index and ovulatory infertility. Epidemiology 1994; 5:247–250.
130. Johnson SR, Kolberg BH, Varner MW, Railsback LD. Maternal obesity and pregnancy. Surg Gynecol Obstet 1987; 164:431–437.
131. Garbaciak JA Jr, Richter M, Miller S, Barton JJ. Maternal weight and pregnancy complications. Am J Obstet Gynecol 1985; 152: 238–245.
132. Prentice A, Goldberg G. Maternal obesity increases congenital malformations. Nutr Rev 1996; 54:146–152.
133. Dwyer PL, Lee ETC, Hay DM. Obesity and urinary incontinence in women. Br J Obstet Gynaecol 1988; 95:91–96.
134. Bump RC, Sugerman HJ, Fantl JA, McClish DK. Obesity and lower urinary tract function in women: effect of surgically induced weight loss. Am J Obstet Gynecol 1992; 167:392–399.
135. Durcan FJ, Corbett JJ, Wall M. The incidence of pseudotumor cerebri: population studies in Iowa and Louisiana. Arch Neurol 1988; 45:875–877.
136. Giuseffi V, Wall M, Siegel PZ, Rojas PB. Symptoms and disease associations in idiopathic intracranial hypertension (pseudotumor cerebri): a case-control study. Neurology 1991; 41:239–244.
137. Sugerman HJ, Felton WL, Sismanis A, et al. Effects of surgically induced weight loss on pseudotumor cerebri in morbid obesity. Neurology 1995; 45:1655–1659.
138. Sugerman HJ, Felton WL III, Sismanis A, et al. Gastric surgery for pseudotumor cerebri associated with severe obesity. Ann Surg 1999; 229:634–642.
139. Glynn RJ, Christen WG, Manson JE, et al. Body mass index: an independent predictor of cataract. Arch Ophthalmol 1995; 113: 1131–1137.
140. Romero Y, Cameron AJ, Locke GR III, et al. Familial aggregation of gastroesophageal reflux in patients with Barrett's esophagus and esophageal adenocarcinoma. Gastroenterology 1997; 113: 1449–1456.
141. Locke GR, Talley NJ, Fett SL, et al. Risk factors associated with symptoms of gastroesophageal reflux. Am J Med 1999; 106:642–649.
142. Lagergren JM, Bergeström R, Nyrén O. No relation between body mass and gastro-oesophageal reflux symptoms in a Swedish population-based study. Gut 2000; 47:26–29.
143. Fisher BL, Pennathur A, Mutnick JLM, Little AG. Obesity correlates with gastroesophageal reflux. Dig Dis Sci 1999; 44:2290–2294.
144. Lundell L, Ruth M, Sandberg N, Bove-Nielsen M. Does massive obesity promote abnormal gastroesophageal reflux? Dig Dis Sci 1995; 40:1632–1635.
145. Stampfer MJ, Maclure KM, Colditz GA, et al. Risk of symptomatic gallstones in women. Am J Clin Nutr 1992; 55:652–658.
146. Hay DW, Carey MC. Pathophysiology and pathogenesis of cholesterol gallstone formation. Semin Liver Dis 1990; 10:159–170.
147. Weinsier RL, Wilson LJ, Lee J. Medically safe rate of weight loss for the treatment of obesity: a guideline based on risk of gallstone formation. Am J Med 1995; 98:115-117.
148. Broomfield PH, Chopra R, Sheinbaum RC, et al. Effects of ursodeoxycholic acid and aspirin on the formation of lithogenic bile gallstones during loss of weight. N Engl J Med 1988: 319: 1567–1572.
149. Shiffman ML, Kaplan GD, Brinkman-Kaplan V, Vickers FF. Prophylaxis against gallstone formation with ursodeoxycholic acid in patients participating in a very-low-calorie diet program. Ann Intern Med 1995; 122:899–905.
150. Wattchow DA, Hall JC, Whiting MJ, et al. Prevalence and treatment of gall stones after gastric bypass surgery for morbid obesity. Br Med J (Clin Res Ed) 1983; 286:763.
151. Stone BG, Ansel HJ, Peterson FJ, Gebhard RL. Gallbladder emptying stimuli in obese and normal weight subjects. Hepatology 1990; 12:795–798.
152. Festi D, Colecchia A, Orsini M, et al. Gallbladder motility and gallstone formation in obese patients following very low calorie diets: use it (fat) to lose it (well). Int J Obes 1998; 22:592–600.
153. Shoheiber O, Biskupiak JE, Nash DB. Estimation of the cost savings resulting from the use of ursodiol for the prevention of gallstones in obese patients undergoing rapid weight reduction Int J Obes Relat Metab Disord 1997; 21:1038–1045.
154. Funnell IC, Bornman PC, Weakley SP. Obesity: an important prognostic factor in acute pancreatitis. Br J Surg 1993; 80:484–486.
155. Matteoni C, Younossi ZM, McCullough A. Nonalcoholic fatty liver disease: a spectrum of clinical pathological severity. Gastroenterology 1999; 116:1413–1419.
156. Wanless IR, Lentz JS. Fatty liver hepatitis (steatohepatitis) and obesity: an autopsy study with analysis of risk factors. Hepatology 1990; 12:1106–1110.
157. Luyckx FH, Desaive C, Thiry A, et al. Liver abnormalities in severely obese subjects: effect of a drastic weight loss after gastroplasty. Int J Obes Relat Metab Disord 1998; 22:222–226.
158. Bellentani S, Saccocio G, Masutti F, et al. Prevalence of and risk factors for hepatic steatosis in Northern Italy. Ann Intern Med 2000; 132:112–117.
159. Marchesini G, Brizi M, Morselli-Labate M, et al. Association of nonalcoholic fatty liver disease with insulin resistance. Am J Med 1999; 107:450–455.
160. Cigolini M, Targher G, Agostino G, et al. Liver steatosis and its relation to plasma haemostatic factors in apparently healthy men: role of the metabolic syndrome. Thromb Haemost 1996; 76:69–73.
161. Day CO, James OFW. Steatohepatitis: a tale of two 'hits.' Gastroenterology 1998; 114:842–845.
162. Tilg H, Diehl AM. Cytokines in alcoholic and nonalcoholic steatohepatitis. N Engl J Med 2000; 343:1467–1476.
163. Palmer M, Schaffner F. Effect of weight reduction on hepatic abnormalities in overweight patients. Gastroenterology 1990; 99: 1408–1413.
164. Andersen T, Gluud C, Franzmann MB, Christoffersen P. Hepatic effects of dietary weight loss in morbidly obese subjects. J Hepatol 1991; 12:224–226.
165. Sjostrom CD, Lissner L, Wedel H, Sjostrom L. Reduction in incidence of diabetes, hypertension and lipid disturbances after intentional weight loss induced by bariatric surgery: the SOS Intervention Study. Obes Res 1999; 7:477–484.
166. Moore LL, Visioni AJ, Wilson PW, et al. Can sustained weight loss in overweight individuals reduce the risk of diabetes mellitus? Epidemiology 2000; 11:269–273.
167. Wing RR, Koeske R, Epstein LH, et al. Long-term effects of

modest weight loss in type II diabetic patients. Arch Intern Med 1987; 147:1749–1753.
168. Pories WJ, Swanson MS, MacDonald KG, et al. Who would have thought it? An operation proves to be the most effective therapy for adult-onset diabetes mellitus. Ann Surg 1995; 222: 339-350.
169. Karason K, Wikstrand J, Sjostrom L, Wendelhag I. Weight loss and progression of early atherosclerosis in the carotid artery: a four-year controlled study of obese subjects. Int J Obes Relat Metab Disord 1999; 23:948–956.
170. Hughes TA, Gwynne JT, Switzer BR, et al. Effects of caloric restriction and weight loss on glycemic control, insulin release and resistance, and atherosclerotic risk in obese subjects with type II diabetes mellitus. JAMA 1984; 77:7–17.
171. Markovic TP, Jenkins AB, Campbell LV, et al. The determinants of glycemic responses to diet restriction and weight loss in obesity and NIDDM. Diabetes Care 1998; 21:687–694.
172. Pan XR, Li GW, Hu YH, et al. Effects of diet and exercise in preventing NIDDM in people with impaired glucose tolerance: the Da Qing IGT and Diabetes Study. Diabetes Care 1997; 20: 537–544.
173. Sjostrom CD, Peltonen M, Wedel H, Sjostrom L. Differentiated long-term effects of intentional weight loss on diabetes and hypertension. Hypertension 2000; 36:20–25.
174. Tuomilehto J, Lindstrom J, Eriksson JG, et al. Prevention of type 2 diabetes mellitus by changes in lifestyle among subjects with impaired glucose tolerance. N Engl J Med 2001; 344:1343-1350.
175. Wing RR, Marcus MD, Epstein LH, Salata R. Type II diabetic subjects lose less weight than their overweight nondiabetic spouses. Diabetes Care 1987; 10:563–566.
176. Khan MA, St Peter JV, Breen GA, et al. Diabetes disease stage predicts weight loss outcomes with long-term appetite suppressants. Obes Res 2000; 8:43–48.
177. UK Prospective Diabetes Study (UKPDS) Group. Intensive blood-glucose control with sulphonylureas or insulin compared with conventional treatment and risk of complications in patients with type 2 diabetes (UKPDS 33). Lancet 1998; 352:837–853.
178. Dattilo AM, Kris-Etherton PM. Effects of weight reduction on blood lipids and lipoproteins: a meta-analysis. Am J Clin Nutr 1992; 56:320–328.
179. Wadden TA, Anderson DA, Foster GD. Two-year changes in lipids and lipoproteins associated with the maintenance of a 5% to 10% reduction in initial weight: some findings and some questions. Obes Res 1999; 7:170–178.
180. Stefanick ML, Mackey S, Sheehan M, et al. Effects of diet and exercise in men and postmenopausal women with low levels of HDL cholesterol and high levels of LDL cholesterol. N Engl J Med 1998; 339:12–20.
181. Effects of weight loss and sodium reduction intervention on blood pressure and hypertension incidence in overweight people with high-normal blood pressure. The Trials of Hypertension Prevention, phase II. The Trials of Hypertension Prevention Collaborative Research Group. Arch Intern Med 1997; 157:657–667.
182. Stevens VJ, Obarzanek E, Cook NR, et al. Long-term weight loss and changes in blood pressure: results of the Trials of Hypertension Prevention, phase II. Ann Intern Med 2001; 134:1–11.
183. Carson JL, Ruddy ME, Duff AE, et al. The effect of gastric bypass surgery on hypertension in morbidly obese patients. Arch Intern Med 1994; 154:193–200.
184. Sjöström CD, Peltonen M, Wedel H, Sjöström L. Differentiated long-term effects of intentional weight loss on diabetes and hypertension. Hypertension 2000; 36:20–25.
185. Huang Z, Willett WC, Manson JE, et al. Body weight, weight change, and risk for hypertension in women. Ann Intern Med 1998; 128:81–88.
186. Wilson PW, Kannel WB, Silbershatz H, D'Agostino RB. Clustering of metabolic factors and coronary heart disease. Arch Intern Med 1999; 159:1104–1109.
187. MacMahon SW, Wilcken D, MacDonald GJ. The effect of weight reduction on left ventricular mass. N Engl J Med 1986; 314:334–339.
188. Karason K, Lindroos AK, Stenlof K, Sjostrom L. Relief of cardiorespiratory symptoms and increased physical activity after surgically induced weight loss: results from the Swedish Obese Subjects Study. Arch Intern Med 2000; 160:1797–1802.
189. Sugerman HJ, Fairman RP, Sood RK, et al. Long-term effects of gastric surgery for treating respiratory insufficiency of obesity. Am J Clin Nutr 1992; 55:597S–601S.
190. Smith PL, Gold AR, Meyers DA, et al. Weight loss in mildly to moderately obese patients with obstructive sleep apnea. Ann Intern Med 1985; 103:850–855.
191. Sugerman HJ, Baron PL, Fairman RP, et al. Hemodynamic dysfunction in obesity hypoventilation syndrome and the effects of treatment with surgically induced weight loss. Ann Surg 1988; 207:604–613.
192. Andres R, Muller DC, Sorkin JD. Long-term effects of change in body weight on all-cause mortality: a review. Ann Intern Med 1993; 119:737–743.
193. Williamson DF, Pamuk E, Thun M, et al. Prospective study of intentional weight loss and mortality in never-smoking overweight U.S. white women aged 40–64 years. Am J Epidemiol 1995; 141:1128–1141.
194. Williamson DF, Pamuk E, Thun M, et al. Prospective study of intentional weight loss and mortality in overweight weight white women aged 40–64 years. Am J Epidemiol 1999; 149:491–503.
195. Williamson DF, Thompson TJ, Thun M, et al. Intentional weight loss and mortality among overweight individuals with diabetes. Diabetes Care 2000; 23:1499–1504.
196. Atkinson RL, Dietz WH, Foreyt JP, et al. Weight cycling. National Task Force on the Prevention and Treatment of Obesity. JAMA 1994; 272:1196–1202.
197. Lissner L, Odell PM, D'Agostino RB, et al. Variability of body weight and health outcomes in the Framingham population. N Engl J Med 1991; 324:1839–1844.
198. Harris JA, Benedict FG. Standard basal metabolism constants for physiologists and clinicians. In: A Biometric Study of Basal Metabolism in Man (Publication 279, The Carnegie Institute of Washington). Philadelphia, JB Lippincott, 1919.
199. World Health Organization. WHO/FAO/UNO Report: Energy and Protein Requirements (WHO Technical Report Series, No 724). Geneva: World Health Organization, 1985.
200. Wing RR, Marcus MD, Salata R, et al. Effects of a very-low-calorie diet on long-term glycemic control in obese type 2 diabetic subjects. Arch Intern Med 1991; 151:1334–1340.
201. Torgerson JS, Lissner L, Lindross AK, et al. VLCD plus dietary and behavioral support versus support alone in the treatment of severe obesity: a randomised two-year clinical trial. Int J Obes Relat Metab Disord 1997; 21:987–994.
202. Wadden TA, Foster GD, Letizia KA. One-year behavioral treatment of obesity: comparison of moderate and severe caloric restriction and the effects of weight maintenance therapy. J Consult Clin Psychol 1994; 62:165–171.
203. Wadden TA, Stunkard AJ. A controlled trial of very-low-calorie diet, behavior therapy, and their combination in the treatment of obesity. J Consult Clin Psychol 1986; 4:482–488.
204. Miura J, Arai K, Ohno M, Ikeda Y. The long term effectiveness of combined therapy by behavior modification and very low calorie diet: 2 year follow-up. Int J Obes 1989; 13:73–77.
205. Torgerson JS, Lissner L, Lindross AK, et al. VLCD plus dietary and behavioral support versus support alone in the treatment of severe obesity: a randomised two-year clinical trial. Int J Obes Relat Metab Disord 1997; 21:987–994.
206. Ryttig KR, Flaten H, Rossner S. Long-term effects of a very low calorie diet (Nutrilett) in obesity treatment: a prospective, randomized comparison between VLCD and a hypocaloric diet + behavior modification and their combination. Int J Obes Relat Metab Disord 1997; 21:574–579.
207. Foster GD, Wadden TA, Peterson FJ, et al. A controlled comparison of three very-low-calorie diets: effects on weight, body composition, and symptoms. Am J Clin Nutr 1992; 55:811–817.
208. Bray GA, Popkin BM. Dietary fat intake does affect obesity! Am J Clin Nutr 1998; 68:1157–1173.
209. Yu-Poth S, Zhao G, Etherton T, et al. Effects of the National Cholesterol Education Program's Step I and Step II dietary intervention programs on cardiovascular disease risk factors: a meta-analysis. Am J Clin Nutr 1999; 69:632–646.
210. Astrup A, Grunwald GK, Melanson EL, et al. The role of low-fat diets in body weight control: a meta-analysis of ad libitum dietary intervention studies. Int J Obes Relat Metab Disord 2000; 24:1545–1552.

211. Rolls BJ, Bell EA. Dietary approaches to the treatment of obesity. Med Clin North Am 2000; 84:401–418.
212. Duncan KH, Bacon JA, Weinsier RL. The effects of high and low energy density diets on satiety, energy intake, and eating time of obese and nonobese subjects. Am J Clin Nutr 1983; 37: 763–767.
213. Stubbs RJ, Harbron CG, Murgafroyd PR, et al. Covert manipulation of dietary fat and energy density: effect on substrate flux and food intake in men eating ad libitum. Am J Clin Nutr 1995; 62:316–329.
214. Bell EA, Castellanos VH, Pelkman CL, et al. Energy density of foods affects energy intake in normal-weight women. Am J Clin Nutr 1998; 67:412–420.
215. Yang M-U, Van Itallie TB. Composition of weight lost during short-term weight reduction. J Clin Invest 1976; 58:722–730.
216. Atkins RC. Dr. Atkins' New Diet Revolution. New York, Avon Books, 1992.
217. Council on Foods and Nutrition. A critique of low-carbohydrate ketogenic weight reduction regimens. JAMA 1973; 224:1415–1419.
218. Westman EC, Yancy WS, Edman JS, et al. Effects of a very-low-carbohydrate diet program on body weight: a pilot study (abstract). Obes Res 2000; 8(Suppl 1):73S.
219. Ballor DL, Poehlman ET. A meta-analysis of the effects of exercise and/or dietary restriction on resting metabolic rate. Eur J Appl Physiol Occup Physiol 1995; 71:535–542.
220. Ballor DL, Poehlman ET. Exercise-training enhances fat-free mass preservation during diet-induced weight loss: a meta-analytical finding. Int J Obes Relat Metab Disord 1994; 18:35–40.
221. Garrow JS, Summerbell CD. Meta-analysis: effect of exercise, with or without dieting, on the body composition of overweight subjects. Eur J Clin Nutr 1995; 49:1–10.
222. Warwick PM, Garrow JS. The effect of addition of exercise to a regime of dietary restriction on weight loss, nitrogen balance, resting metabolic rate and spontaneous physical activity in three obese women in a metabolic ward. Int J Obes Relat Metab Disord 1981; 5:25–32.
223. Holloszy JO, Schultz J, Kusnierkiewicz J, et al. Effects of exercise on glucose tolerance and insulin resistance. Acta Med Scand 1986; 711:55–65.
224. Helmrich SP, Ragland DR, Leung RW, Paffenbarger RS Jr. Physical activity and reduced occurrence of non–insulin-dependent diabetes mellitus. N Engl J Med 1991; 325:147–152.
225. Wei M, Gibbons L, Mitchell T, et al. The association between cardiorespiratory fitness and impaired fasting glucose and type 2 diabetes mellitus in men. Ann Intern Med 1999; 130:89–96.
226. Lee CD, Blair SN, Jackson AS. Cardiorespiratory fitness, body composition, and all-cause and cardiovascular disease mortality in men. Am J Clin Nutr 1999; 69:373–380.
227. Wood PD, Stefanick ML, Dreon DM, et al. Changes in plasma lipids and lipoproteins in overweight men during weight loss through dieting as compared with exercise. N Engl J Med 1988; 319:1173–1179.
228. Klem ML, Wing RR, McGuire MT, et al. A descriptive study of individuals successful at long-term maintenance of substantial weight loss. Am J Clin Nutr 1997; 66:239–246.
229. Kayman S, Bruvold W, Stern JS. Maintenance and relapse after weight loss in women: behavioral aspects. Am J Clin Nutr 1990; 52:800–807.
230. Hill JO, Schlundt DG, Sbrocco T, et al. Evaluation of an alternating-calorie diet with and without exercise in the treatment of obesity. Am J Clin Nutr 1989; 50:284–254.
231. Wing RR. Physical activity in the treatment of the adulthood overweight and obesity: current evidence and research issues. Med Sci Sports Exerc 1999; 31(Suppl 11):S547–S551.
232. Schoeller DA, Shay K, Kushner RF. How much physical activity is needed to minimize weight gain in previously obese women? Am J Clin Nutr 1997; 66:551–556.
233. Jakicic JM, Wing RR, Winters D. Effects of intermittent exercise and use of home exercise equipment on adherence, weight loss, and fitness in overweight women. JAMA 1999; 282:1554–1560.
234. Wadden TA, Sarwer DB, Berkowitz RI. Behavioural treatment of the overweight patient. Baillieres Clin Endocrinol Metab 1999; 13:93–107.
235. Wadden TA, Foster GD. Behavioral treatment of obesity. Med Clin North Am 2000; 84:441–461.
236. Perri MG, Nezu AM, Viegener BJ. Improving the Long-Term Management of Obesity: Theory, Research and Clinical Guidelines. New York, John Wiley & Sons, 1992.
237. Sjostrom L, Rissanen A, Andersen T, et al. Randomised placebo-controlled trial of orlistat for weight loss and prevention of weight regain in obese patients. Lancet 1998; 352:167–172.
238. Weintraub M, Sundaresan PR, Schuster B, et al. Long-term weight control study. V (weeks 190 to 210). Follow-up of participants after cessation of medication. Clin Pharmacol Ther 1992; 51:615–618.
239. Lean ME. Sibutramine: a review of clinical efficacy. Int J Obes Relat Metab Disord 1997; 21(Suppl 1):S30–S36.
240. Wadden TA, Berkowitz RI, Sarwer DB, et al. Benefits of life style modification in the pharmacologic treatment of obesity. Arch Intern Med 2001; 161:218–227.
241. Khan MA, Herzog CA, St Peter JV, et al. The prevalence of cardiac valvular insufficiency assessed by transthoracic echocardiography in obese patients treated with appetite-suppressant drugs. N Engl J Med 1998; 339:713–718.
242. Kernan WN, Viscoli CM, Brass LM, et al. Phenylpropanolamine and the risk of hemorrhagic stroke. N Engl J Med 2000; 343: 1826–1832.
243. Bray GA, Greenway FL. Current and potential drugs for treatment of obesity. Endocr Rev 1999; 20:805-875.
244. Hansen DL, Toubro S, Stock MJ, et al. Thermogenic effects of sibutramine in humans. Am J Clin Nutr 1998; 68:1180–1186.
245. National Institutes of Health, National Heart, Lung, and Blood Institute and North American Association for the Study of Obesity. Practical Guide to the Identification, Evaluation, and Treatment of Overweight and Obesity in Adults (NIH Publication No. 00-4084). October 2000.
246. Bray GA, Blackburn GL, Ferguson JM, et al. Sibutramine produces dose-related weight loss. Obes Res 1999; 7:189–198.
247. Smith IG, Goulder MA. Randomized placebo-controlled trial of long-term treatment with sibutramine in mild to moderate obesity. J Fam Prac 2001; 50:505–512.
248. McMahon FG, Fujioka K, Singh BN, et al. Efficacy and safety of sibutramine in obese white and African American patients with hypertension: a 1-year, double-blind, placebo-controlled, multicenter trial. Arch Intern Med 2000; 160:2185–2191.
249. Apfelbaum M, Vague P, Ziegler O, et al. Long-term maintenance of weight loss after a very-low-calorie diet: a randomized blinded trial of the efficacy and tolerability of sibutramine. Am J Med 1999; 106:179–184.
250. James WPT, Astrup A, Finer N, et al. Effect of sibutramine on weight maintenance after weight loss: a randomized trial. Lancet 2000; 356:2119–2125.
251. Hadvary P, Lengsfield H, Wolfer H. Inhibition of pancreatic lipase in vitro by the covalent inhibitor tetrahydrolipstatin. Biochem J 1998; 256:357-361.
252. Zhi J, Melia AT, Guerciolini R, et al. Retrospective population-based analysis of the dose-response (fecal fat excretion) relationship of orlistat in normal and obese volunteers. Clin Pharmacol Ther 1994; 56:82–86.
253. Zhi J, Melia AT, Funk C, et al. Metabolic profiles of minimally absorbed orlistat in obese/overweight volunteers. J Clin Pharmacol 1996; 36:1006–1011.
254. Sjöström L, Rissanen A, Andersen T, et al. Randomised placebo-controlled trial of orlistat for weight loss and prevention of weight regain in obese patients. Lancet 1998; 352:167–172.
255. Davidson MH, Hauptman J, DiGirolamo M, et al. Weight control and risk factor reduction in obese subjects treated for 2 years with orlistat. JAMA 1999; 281:235–242.
256. Rössner S, Sjöström L, Noack R, et al. Weight loss, weight maintenance, and improved cardiovascular risk factors after 2 years treatment with orlistat for obesity. Obes Res 2000; 8:49–61.
257. Finer N, James WP, Kopelman PG, et al. One-year treatment of obesity: a randomized, double-blind, placebo-controlled, multicentre study of orlistat, a gastrointestinal lipase inhibitor. Int J Obes Relat Metab Disord 2000; 24:306–313.
258. Hauptman J, Lucas C, Boldrin MN, et al. Orlistat in the long-term treatment of obesity in primary care settings. Arch Fam Med 2000; 9:160–167.
259. Hollander PA, Elbein SC, Hirsch IB, et al. Role of orlistat in the treatment of obese patients with type 2 diabetes. Diabetes Care 1998; 21:1288–1294.

260. Lindgarde F. The effect of orlistat on body weight and coronary heart disease risk profile in obese patients: the Swedish Multimorbidity Study. J Intern Med 2000; 248:245–254.
261. Mittendorfer B, Ostlund R, Patterson BW, Klein S. Orlistat inhibits dietary cholesterol absorption. Obes Res 2000; 8(Suppl 1): 43S.
262. Colman E, Fossler M. Reduction in blood cyclosporin concentrations by orlistat. N Engl J Med 2000; 342:1141–1142.
263. NIH Conference: Gastrointestinal surgery for severe obesity: Consensus Development Conference Panel. Ann Intern Med 1991; 115:956–961.
264. Brolin RE, Kenler HA, Gorman JH, Cody RP. Long-limb gastric bypass in the superobese: a prospective randomized study. Ann Surg 1992; 215:387–395.
265. Mason EE. Vertical banded gastroplasty for obesity. Arch Surg 1982; 117:701–706.
266. Eckhout GV, Willibanks OL, Moore JT. Vertical ring gastroplasty for morbid obesity: five year experience with 1,463 patients. Am J Surg 1986; 152:713–716.
267. MacLean LD, Rhode BM, Sampalis J, Forse RA. Results of the surgical treatment of obesity. Am J Surg 1993; 165:155–162.
268. Sugerman HJ, Starkey JV, Birkenhauer RA. A randomized prospective trial of gastric bypass versus vertical banded gastroplasty and their effects on sweets versus non sweets eaters. Ann Surg 1987; 205:613–624.
269. Hall JC, Watts JM, O'Brien PE, et al. Gastric surgery for morbid obesity. The Adelaide Study. Ann Surg 1990; 211:419–427.
270. Howard L, Malone M, Michalek A, et al. Gastric bypass and vertical banded gastroplasty: a prospective randomized comparison and 5-year follow-up. Obes Surg 1995; 5:55–60.
271. Balsiger BM, Kelly KA, Poggio JL, et al. Long term prospective follow-up (>10 years) after vertical banded gastroplasty (VBG). Gastroenterology 2000; 118:A1060.
272. Belachew M, Legrand M, Vincent V, et al. Laparoscopic adjustable gastric banding. World J Surg 1998; 22:955–963.
273. DeMaria EJ, Sugerman HJ, Kellum JM, et al. High failure rate following laparoscopic adjustable silicone gastric banding for treatment of morbid obesity. Ann Surg 2001; 233:809–818.
274. Hauri P, Steffen R, Ricklin T, et al. Treatment of morbid obesity with the Swedish adjustable gastric band (SAGB): complication rate during a 12-month follow-up period. Surgery 2000; 127: 484–488.
275. Gustavsson S. Laparoscopic adjustable gastric banding: a caution. Surgery 2000; 127:489–490.
276. Scopinaro N, Adami GF, Marinari GM, et al. Biliopancreatic diversion. World J Surg 1998; 22:936-946.
277. Marceau P, Hould FS, Simard S, et al. Biliopancreatic diversion with duodenal switch. World J Surg 1998; 22:947-954.
278. Clare MW. Reversals on 504 biliopancreatic surgeries over 12 years. Obes Surg 1993; 3:169-173.
279. Payne JH, DeWind LT. Surgical treatment of obesity. Am J Surg 1969; 118:141–147.
280. Scott HW Jr, Dean RH, Shull HJ, Gluck F. Results of jejunoileal bypass in two hundred patients with morbid obesity. Surg Gynecol Obstet 1977; 145:661–673.
281. Hocking MP, Duerson MC, O'Leary JP, Woodward ER. Jejunoileal bypass for morbid obesity: late follow-up in 100 cases. N Engl J Med 1983; 308:995–999.
282. Drenick EJ, Bassett LW, Stanley TM. Rheumatoid arthritis associated with jejunoileal bypass. Arthritis Rheum 1984; 27:1300–1305.
283. Drenick EJ, Stanley TM, Wills CE. Renal damage after intestinal bypass. Int J Obes Relat Metab Disord 1981; 5:501–508.
284. Drenick EJ, Fisler J, Johnson D. Hepatic steatosis after intestinal bypass: prevention and reversal with metronidazole, irrespective of protein-calorie malnutrition. Gastroenterology 1982; 82:535–548.
285. Drenick EJ, Ament ME, Finegold SM, Passaro E Jr. Bypass enteropathy: an inflammatory process in the excluded segment with systemic complications. Am J Clin Nutr 1977; 30:76–89.
286. Sugerman HJ, Kellum JM, Engle KM, et al. Gastric bypass for treating severe obesity. Am J Clin Nutr 1992; 55:560S–566S.
287. Klem ML, Wing RR, McGuire MT, et al. A descriptive study of individuals successful at long-term maintenance of substantial weight loss. Am J Clin Nutr 1997; 66:239–246.
288. De Fronzo RA, Goodman AM. Efficacy of metformin in patients with non–insulin-dependent diabetes mellitus. N Engl J Med 1995; 333:541–549.
289. Johansen K. Efficacy of metformin in the treatment of NIDDM: a meta-analysis. Diabetes Care 1999; 22:33–37.
290. Yki-Jarvinen H, Kauppila M, Kujansuu E, et al. Comparison of insulin regimens in patients with non–insulin-dependent diabetes mellitus. N Engl J Med 1992; 327:1426–1433.
291. Landstedt-Hallin L, Adamson U, Arner P, et al. Comparison of bedtime NPH or preprandial regular insulin combined with glibenclamide in secondary sulfonylurea failure. Diabetes Care 1995; 18:1183–1186.

34 Disorders of Lipid Metabolism

Robert W. Mahley, Karl H. Weisgraber, and
Robert V. Farese, Jr.

LIPID BIOCHEMISTRY AND CHOLESTEROL METABOLISM

Lipids are hydrophobic molecules that are insoluble or minimally soluble in water. They are found in cell membranes, which maintain cellular integrity and allow the cytoplasm to be compartmentalized into specific organelles. Lipids function as a major form of stored nutrients (triglycerides), as precursors of adrenal and gonadal steroids and bile acids (cholesterol), and as extracellular and intracellular messengers (e.g., prostaglandins, phosphatidylinositol). Lipoproteins provide a vehicle for transporting the complex lipids in the blood as water-soluble complexes and deliver lipids to cells throughout the body.

Classes of Lipids: Structure and Function

Fatty Acids

Fatty acids vary in length and in the number and position of double bonds (Fig. 34–1). Saturated fatty acids lack double bonds (all carbon atoms have a full complement of hydrogen), and unsaturated fatty acids have one or more double bonds. Monounsaturated fatty acids have one double bond, and polyunsaturated fatty acids have two or more. The major fatty acids and their sources in foods are listed in Table 34–1.

Fatty acids are a readily available source of energy. In tissues, they can be esterified to other organic molecules to form complex lipids (e.g., triglycerides). In the blood, they may be transported on lipoproteins as complex lipids, or they may be

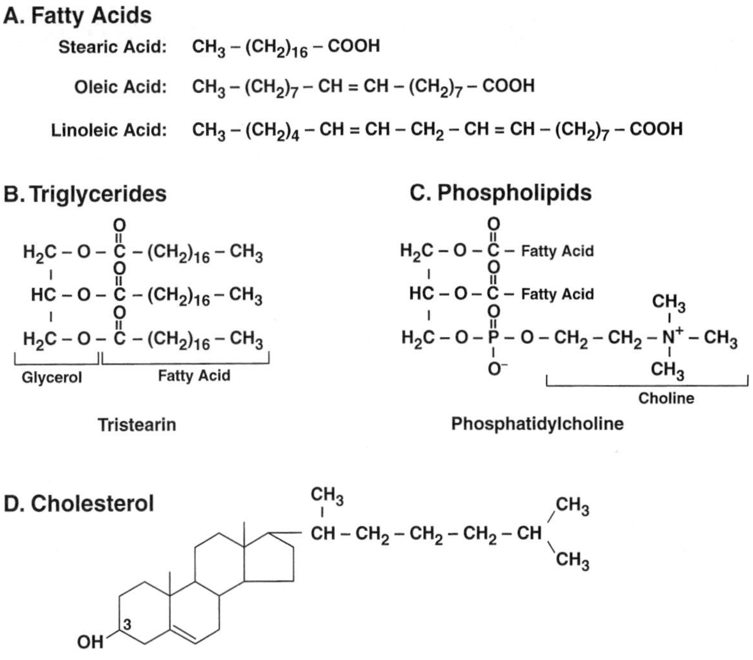

A. Fatty Acids

Stearic Acid: $CH_3-(CH_2)_{16}-COOH$

Oleic Acid: $CH_3-(CH_2)_7-CH=CH-(CH_2)_7-COOH$

Linoleic Acid: $CH_3-(CH_2)_4-CH=CH-CH_2-CH=CH-(CH_2)_7-COOH$

B. Triglycerides

Glycerol | Fatty Acid

Tristearin

C. Phospholipids

Fatty Acid

Fatty Acid

Choline

Phosphatidylcholine

D. Cholesterol

Figure 34–1. Structures of the common lipids.

transported in the nonesterified state as free fatty acids bound to albumin.

Table 34–1. Major Fatty Acids

Chemical Designation*	Common Name	Common Food Sources
Saturated fatty acids (no double bonds)		
C12:0	Lauric	Coconut oil
C14:0	Myristic	Coconut oil, butter fat
C16:0	Palmitic	Butter, cheese, meat
C18:0	Stearic	Beef, chocolate
Monounsaturated fatty acids (one double bond)		
C18:1Δ^9	Oleic	Olive oil, canola oil
Polyunsaturated fatty acids (two or more double bonds)		
Omega-6 fatty acids		
C18:2ω6Δ^9, Δ^{12}	Linoleic	Sunflower, corn, soybean, and safflower oils
C20:4ω6Δ^5, Δ^8, Δ^{11}, Δ^{14}	Arachidonic	
Omega-3 fatty acids		
C20:5ω3	Eicosapentaenoic (EPA)	Salmon, cod, mackerel, tuna
C22:6ω3	Docosahexaenoic (DHA)	Salmon, cod, mackerel, tuna

*The numeral after the C indicates the number of carbon atoms; the numeral after the colon indicates the number of double bonds. Carbon number 1 is the carboxylic acid carbon, and the ω carbon atom is the carbon most distant from the carboxyl group. The placement of the double bonds is shown by the Δ designations (e.g., Δ^9 indicates a double bond between carbons 9 and 10). In omega-6 fatty acids the first double bond occurs after the sixth carbon atom from the ω carbon atom (indicated by ω6), and in omega-3 fatty acids it occurs after the third carbon atom from the ω carbon atom (ω3).

Cholesterol

Cholesterol is a four-ring hydrocarbon with an eight-carbon side chain (see Fig. 34–1). It plays a critical role as a major component of cell membranes and as a precursor of steroid hormones (adrenal and gonadal hormones). Cholesterol is also a precursor of bile acids, which are formed in the liver, stored in the gallbladder, and secreted in the intestine to participate in the absorption of fat. In the blood, about two thirds of the cholesterol is esterified (i.e., has a fatty acid esterified to the hydroxyl group at position 3).

Complex Lipids

Triglycerides (Triacylglycerol)

Triglycerides consist of three fatty acid molecules esterified to a glycerol molecule (see Fig. 34–1). Diglycerides (diacylglycerols) contain two fatty acids, and monoglycerides have only one fatty acid per glycerol molecule. Triglycerides serve to store fatty acids and form large lipid droplets in adipose tissue. They are also transported as a component of certain lipoproteins. When triglycerides are hydrolyzed in adipocytes or on lipoprotein particles, free fatty acid molecules are released to be used as a source of energy.

Phospholipids

Phospholipids have fatty acids esterified at two of the three hydroxyl groups of glycerol (see Fig. 34–1). The third hydroxyl group is esterified to phosphate (this complex lipid is referred to as phosphatidic acid). Typically, in mammalian tissue, the phosphatidic acid is esterified to the hydroxyl group of a hydrophilic molecule, such as choline, serine, or ethanolamine, to form phosphatidylcholine (commonly called lecithin), phosphatidylserine, or phosphatidylethanolamine, respectively. Lysolecithin is phosphatidylcholine from which one of the fatty acids has been removed. The combination of hydrophobic and hydrophilic regions in phospholipids enables them to be miscible at the water-lipid interface and makes them ideal components of membranes and of surface coats of lipoproteins. They are the most hydrophilic of the complex lipids.

Cholesterol Biosynthesis and the Low-Density Lipoprotein Receptor Pathway

Cholesterol is either absorbed from the diet or synthesized by cells in the body. All dietary cholesterol is of animal origin (i.e., from meats, dairy products, and eggs). Plants do not produce cholesterol; plant membranes contain sitosterol, which, except in a rare genetic disease, is not absorbed. Cholesterol is produced in many tissues (e.g., liver, skin, adrenals, gonads, brain, intestine). In most mammals, including humans, about 10% to 20% of the total synthesis of cholesterol occurs in the liver.[1–8]

Cholesterol Biosynthesis

Cholesterol synthesis, illustrated schematically in Figure 34–2*A*, begins with acetate. Three molecules of acetate are condensed to form 3-hydroxy-3-methylglutaryl coenzyme A (HMG-CoA), which is then converted to mevalonic acid by the enzyme HMG-CoA reductase. Through a series of steps, mevalonic acid is converted to cholesterol. The key (rate-limiting) step regulating cholesterol biosynthesis involves HMG-CoA reductase. Competitive inhibitors of this enzyme (the statins) reduce cholesterol biosynthesis and lower plasma cholesterol levels. Increased cholesterol content of cells feeds back on the HMG-CoA reductase and decreases its activity, thereby decreasing cholesterol biosynthesis. Conversely, a deficiency of intracellular cholesterol increases reductase activity and increases cholesterol biosynthesis[1–8] (see later discussion).

Cholesterol cannot be eliminated by catabolism to carbon dioxide and water; it must be either excreted as free cholesterol in the bile or converted to bile acids and secreted into the intestine.[9] About 50% of the cholesterol entering the intestine is reabsorbed and recirculates to the liver; the remainder is eliminated in the feces. Almost all of the secreted bile acids (97%) are reabsorbed from the intestine and transported back to the liver. This recirculation of cholesterol and bile acids from the intestine to the liver is called the *enterohepatic circulation* (Fig. 34–2*B*). The reabsorbed cholesterol and bile acids regulate de novo cholesterol and bile acid synthesis in the liver. For example, if the amount of bile acids returning to the liver is decreased (as occurs in the intestine during treatment with bile acid–binding resins), bile acid synthesis is increased, enhancing the amount of cholesterol being converted to bile acids.

A. Cholesterol Biosynthesis

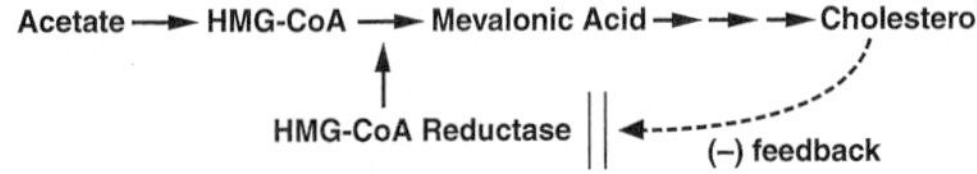

B. Enterohepatic Circulation

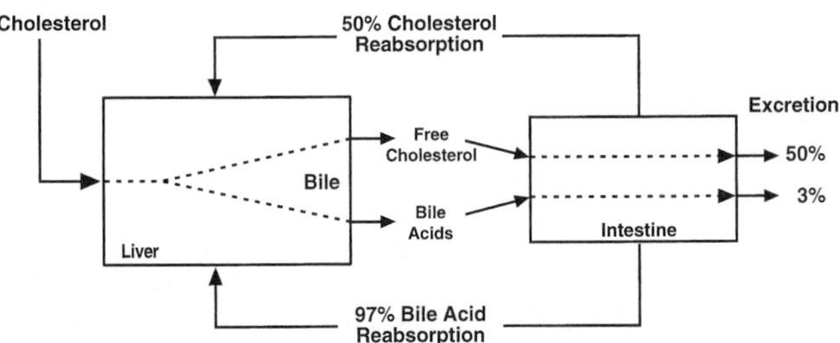

Figure 34–2. *A*, Cholesterol biosynthesis. 3-Hydroxy-3-methylglutaryl coenzyme A (HMG-CoA) reductase is a rate-limiting enzyme regulating cholesterol biosynthesis. The enzyme is down-regulated by excess cholesterol in the cell. *B*, Enterohepatic circulation of cholesterol and bile acids. About 50% of cholesterol and 97% of bile acids are reabsorbed from the intestine and recirculated to the liver. (*A*, modified from Brown MS, Goldstein JL. A receptor-mediated pathway for cholesterol homeostasis. Science 1986; 232:34–47.)

Cholesterol 7α-Hydroxylase

This enzyme of about 57 kDa (503 amino acids), known as CYP7A (formerly $P450_{7\alpha}$), converts free cholesterol to 7α-hydroxycholesterol. This is the rate-limiting step in bile acid synthesis, and it is under feedback regulation by recirculated bile acids. The interruption of bile acid recirculation increases cholesterol 7α-hydroxylase activity. This enzyme and HMG-CoA reductase are closely coupled, and their activities usually change in parallel (for a review see references 3, 5, and 10 to 13). In this way, the intracellular cholesterol level for bile acid production remains rather constant.

Low-Density Lipoprotein Receptor

Cholesterol levels in the blood are controlled primarily through the low-density lipoprotein (LDL) receptor pathway.[4, 14] This receptor is present on the surface of all cells throughout the body, including hepatocytes, and mediates the uptake of cholesterol-rich lipoproteins (e.g., LDL) from the blood. Specific proteins on the surface of certain lipoproteins (apolipoprotein [apo] B100 and apo-E) interact with the LDL receptor and facilitate lipoprotein internalization by cells. By this mechanism, cells that require cholesterol can obtain the preformed sterol. The LDL receptor also allows the liver (the principal site for LDL catabolism) to take up LDL and eliminate cholesterol from the body (discussed in "Lipoprotein Receptors Controlling Lipoprotein Metabolism").

The number of LDL receptors on the cell surface is tightly regulated.[4, 14] If the cholesterol content of a cell is elevated, fewer receptors are synthesized (i.e., receptor expression is down-regulated). On the other hand, if a cell requires cholesterol, expression of LDL receptors is up-regulated and synthesis increases. This system keeps the intracellular cholesterol concentration relatively constant and prevents excessive and possibly toxic accumulation. Within the cell, cholesterol can be esterified by the enzyme acyl-CoA:cholesterol acyltransferase (ACAT).

Acyl-Coenzyme A:Cholesterol Acyltransferase

ACAT is an enzyme of the endoplasmic reticulum (ER) (about 45 to 50 kDa, 550 amino acids) that catalyzes the formation of cholesteryl esters from long-chain fatty acyl-CoA (e.g., oleoyl-CoA) and free cholesterol substrates.[15–19] When lipoproteins enter the cell by receptor-mediated endocytosis and are degraded within the lysosomes, the free cholesterol released can be transported to the ER, where it is esterified by ACAT. There are two ACAT enzymes. ACAT1 is present in macrophages, steroidogenic tissues, and sebaceous glands,[20] and its action in macrophages has been implicated in foam cell formation and atherogenesis.[21, 22] ACAT2 is found in liver and intestine,[23–25] where it plays a role in providing cholesteryl esters for assembly of apo-B–containing lipoproteins. In the intestine, ACAT2 acts to promote the absorption of dietary cholesterol.[26] Agents that inhibit intestinal ACAT activity may provide a means to limit cholesterol absorption by the intestine.[19, 26]

Cholesteryl ester hydrolysis by cholesterol ester hydrolase generates free cholesterol, either for efflux from the cells or to serve as a biosynthetic substrate (e.g., for steroid hormones and cell membranes) within the cells. The pool of intracellular cholesterol and cholesteryl esters is dynamic.

Metabolism of Dietary Lipids

The digestion of dietary fats begins in the stomach and continues in the proximal small intestine.[27–31] Triglycerides are hydrolyzed to free fatty acids and small amounts of monoglycerides and diglycerides, cholesteryl esters are hydrolyzed to free cholesterol, and phospholipids are converted primarily to lysolecithin. Bile salt micelles disperse and partially solubilize water-insoluble lipids; this facilitates the intestinal transport and delivery of lipids to the unstirred water layer of intestinal epithelial cells, where they can be taken up by the cells. Bile acids also activate pancreatic lipase, which participates in the hydrolysis of triglycerides. Long-chain fatty acids are taken up primarily by the enterocytes of the duodenum and proximal jejunum, reesterified into triglycerides, and used in the biosynthesis of intestinal lipoproteins (chylomicrons), which are delivered to the mesenteric lymph and enter the general circulation with the thoracic duct lymph. Medium-chain fatty acids ($\leq$10 carbons) are absorbed into the portal blood without being esterified and are cleared directly from the blood by the liver. Bile acids are reabsorbed primarily from the ileum, enter the portal blood, and are taken up by the liver.

Triglyceride and Free Fatty Acid Metabolism

Storage and Use

Free fatty acids are released from triglycerides of chylomicrons and very-low-density lipoproteins (VLDLs) through the action of lipoprotein lipase (LPL). LPL is bound to the capillary endothelial cells adjacent to adipose, muscle, and breast tissue, where it liberates free fatty acids from lipoprotein triglyceride. The level of LPL in tissues differs under different physiologic circumstances[32] so that free fatty acids are directed to tissues requiring them as substrates or energy sources. During fasting, for example, LPL activity decreases in adipose tissue and increases in heart muscle. In the breast, LPL levels are low until parturition, when they increase 10-fold to promote milk formation.

In adipose tissue, high levels of glucose and insulin promote the conversion of free fatty acids to triglyceride for storage. Insulin stimulates LPL activity and fatty acid esterification through the formation of glycerol phosphate and decreases free fatty acid release through the inhibition of hormone-sensitive lipase.[33] Insulin deficiency, as in diabetes mellitus, is associated with decreased LPL activity. Insulin and glucose also stimulate the biosynthesis of free fatty acids in the liver and, to a lesser degree, in adipocytes when dietary fat is replaced by carbohydrates. As a result, hepatic free fatty acids are converted to triglyceride and packaged into VLDL particles (discussed in the section on plasma lipoproteins).

Acyl-Coenzyme A:Diacylglycerol Acyltransferase

Triglyceride (triacylglycerol) synthesis is catalyzed by the enzyme acyl-CoA:diacylglycerol acyltransferase (DGAT)[34–36] (Fig. 34–3). A DGAT gene, which is expressed in all tissues, has been identified.[37] Interestingly, the inactivation of this gene in mice has revealed that multiple pathways exist for triglyceride synthesis.[38] These alternative mechanisms might include a second DGAT or fatty acyl-CoA–independent mechanisms.[39] The gene inactivation study also revealed that DGAT plays an important role in energy metabolism.[38, 40]

Fatty Acid Release from Adipose Tissue

The net release of free fatty acids and glycerol from adipose triglyceride stores occurs during various physiologic conditions, including stress, exercise, fasting, and uncontrolled diabetes mellitus. This release occurs in response to hormones (Table 34–2), most of which act by means of cyclic adenosine monophosphate to activate a hormone receptor-coupled protein kinase that in turn activates a hormone-sensitive lipase (Fig. 34–4).[33] In contrast to numerous hormones, insulin inhibits rather than stimulates hormone-sensitive lipase in adipose tissue. Growth hormone liberates free fatty acids by a different mechanism, which requires enhanced synthesis of hormone-sensitive lipase.

After triglyceride hydrolysis in adipose tissue, the released free fatty acids bind to albumin and circulate in the plasma. Released glycerol is taken up by the liver and kidney for triglyceride synthesis or for gluconeogenesis. The fate of the free fatty acid–albumin complexes is determined in part by

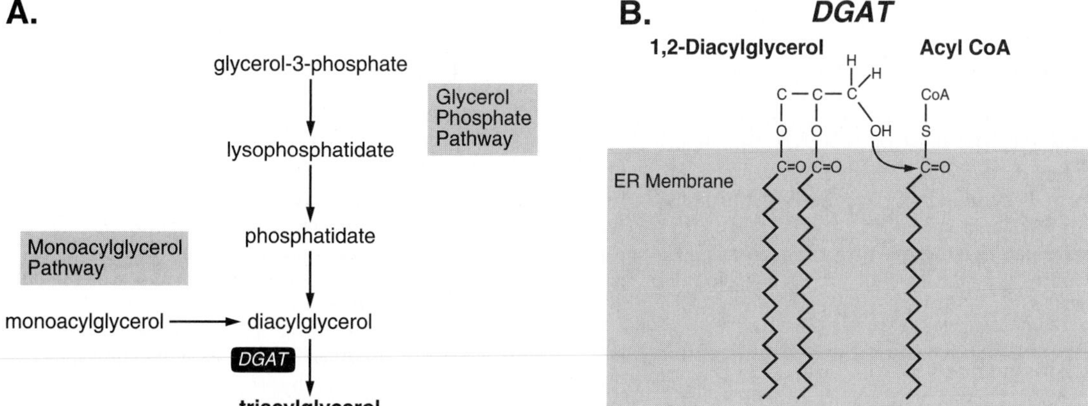

Figure 34–3. Triglyceride synthesis and the *DGAT* reaction. *A*, Two major pathways of triglyceride synthesis have been described: the glycerol-phosphate pathway and the monoacylglycerol pathway, which is prominent in the small intestine. *B*, *DGAT* catalyzes a reaction in which 1,2-diacylglycerol and fatty acyl CoA react to form triacylglycerol at the surface of the endoplasmic reticulum. (From Farese RV Jr, Cases S, Smith SJ. Triglyceride synthesis: insights from the cloning of diacylglycerol acyltransferase. Curr Opin Lipidol 2000; 11:229–234.)

Table 34–2. Hormones That Affect Lipolysis in Vitro

Rapid Stimulation	Slow Stimulation
Catecholamines (β-1 agonists)	Glucocorticoids
Corticotropin	Growth hormone
Glucagon	**Suppression**
Placental lactogen	Insulin
Prolactin	Gastric inhibitory polypeptide
Secretion	Oxytocin
Thyrotropin	Prostaglandin
Vasoactive intestinal peptide	Somatomedins
Vasopressin	

Modified from Bierman EL, Glomset JA. Disorders of lipid metabolism. In Wilson JD, Foster DW (eds). Williams' Textbook of Endocrinology, 8th ed. Philadelphia, WB Saunders, 1992, pp. 1367–1395.

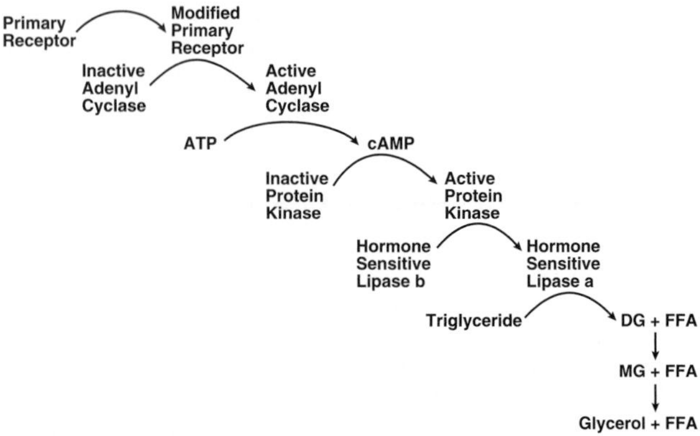

Figure 34–4. Cascade of reactions involved in activation of hormone-sensitive lipase. ATP, adenosine triphosphate; cAMP, cyclic adenosine monophosphate; DG, diglyceride; FFA, free fatty acid; MG, monoglyceride. (From Steinberg D, Huttunen JK. The role of cyclic AMP in activation of hormone-sensitive lipase of adipose tissue. Adv Cyclic Nucleotide Res 1972; 1:47–62.)

blood flow. With intense exercise and diminished blood flow to the splanchnic bed, free fatty acids are targeted to muscle. Depending on the metabolic state, free fatty acids taken up by the liver are reused for triglyceride or phospholipid synthesis (exported on VLDL), oxidized to carbon dioxide, or converted to ketone bodies.

Fatty Acid Oxidation and Ketogenesis

Both oxidation and ketogenesis of fatty acids take place in the mitochondria, except for very-long-chain fatty acids (C-24 and C-26), which are oxidized in peroxisomes. Because free fatty acids and their CoA derivatives can penetrate only the outer leaflet of the mitochondrial membrane, they are converted to carnitine derivatives within the mitochondrial membrane to allow transport across the inner membrane. Once inside the mitochondria, they are reconverted to CoA derivatives and undergo beta oxidation, which produces acetyl-CoA and the reduced forms of nicotinamide-adenine dinucleotide (NADH) and flavin-adenine dinucleotide (FADH).

With a normal flux of free fatty acids, the NADH and FADH enter the electron transport system, resulting in the formation of adenosine triphosphate and water. The condensation of acetyl-CoA with oxaloacetic acid yields citrate, which can enter the citric acid cycle, where it is oxidized to carbon dioxide or is transported out of the mitochondria and converted again to free fatty acids. If free fatty acid flux to the liver is massively increased, as in insulin-deficient states such as prolonged fasting or uncontrolled diabetes mellitus, the production of VLDL triglyceride from free fatty acids is limited. As a result, NADH, FADH, and acetyl-CoA accumulate in the mitochondria and give rise to the products of ketogenesis: acetoacetate, β-hydroxybutyrate, and acetone.

Ketogenesis occurs in several steps. Initially, acetyl-CoA condenses in two steps to form acetoacetyl-CoA and then HMG-CoA. The latter is cleaved to acetoacetate and acetyl-CoA, which leads to the liberation of CoA and its use in beta oxidation of free fatty acids. Acetoacetate can be reduced by NADH to form β-hydroxybutyrate; the NAD produced can be used for continued beta oxidation of fatty acids. Alternatively, the acetoacetate can decompose to form acetone. The ketones are released into the plasma and, if they accumulate, cause ketoacidosis.

Fatty Acid Biosynthesis

Under normal conditions, the diet supplies sufficient fatty acids through the ingestion of fat. However, increases in the ratio of carbohydrate to fat in the diet stimulate fatty acid synthesis by the liver and adipose tissue. Fatty acids are synthesized from two carbon units of acetyl-CoA. Because acetyl-CoA is produced in the mitochondria, it must first be converted to citrate by condensation with oxaloacetate and then transported into the cytosol, where it is reconverted to acetyl-CoA and oxaloacetate. Eight acetyl-CoA units are condensed to form palmitic acid (16 carbon atoms) in a series of reactions involving the enzymes fatty acid synthase and acetyl-CoA carboxylase. Longer fatty acids, such as stearic acid (18 carbon atoms) or oleic acid (18 carbon atoms with a single double bond), are synthesized from palmitic acid by chain extension. In this way, fatty acid synthesis can meet most of the body's requirements.

Certain essential polyunsaturated fatty acids cannot be synthesized in humans and must be supplied in the diet. These include linoleic acid (18 carbon atoms with two double bonds) and linolenic acid (18 carbon atoms with three double bonds). Essential fatty acids are required for a number of special functions, including prostaglandin synthesis.[41–43]

PLASMA LIPOPROTEINS: APOLIPOPROTEINS, RECEPTORS, AND ENZYMES

General Structure and Major Classes of Lipoproteins

Lipoproteins function as vehicles to transport lipids in the blood in the form of soluble complexes of lipids and proteins. The lipids include triglycerides, cholesteryl esters, free cholesterol, and phospholipids. About 10 different protein moieties, called apolipoproteins, are associated with various lipoproteins and are given letter designations (Table 34–3).[44–47] Lipoproteins also transport fat-soluble vitamins (A, D, and E), drugs (e.g., probucol, cyclosporine), some viruses, and certain antioxidant enzymes (e.g., paraoxonase[48] and platelet-derived activating factor hydrolase[49]).

Lipoproteins are spherical particles with a core of mostly hydrophobic lipids (triglycerides and cholesteryl esters) and a surface layer of more hydrophilic constituents, namely protein, free cholesterol, and phospholipids (Fig. 34–5). Six major classes of lipoproteins play different roles in lipid transport (Table 34–4), and the specific apolipoproteins on the surface determine the fate of the lipoproteins. To understand lipoprotein metabolism and the diseases associated with lipid abnormalities, it is necessary to consider the roles of the in-

Table 34–3. Characteristics and Major Functions of Human Apolipoproteins

Apolipoprotein	Average Plasma Concentration (mg/dL)	Chromosome	Gene (bases)	Molecular Weight (× 1000)	Mature Protein (amino acids)	Major Sites of Synthesis	Major Functions
AI	130	11	1863	~29	243	Liver, intestine	Structural protein/HDL. Cofactor for LCAT. Ligand for putative HDL receptor.
AII	40	1	1330	~17 (dimer)	77	Liver	Inhibits apo-E binding to receptors (through the E–AII complex).
AIV	40	11	2600	~45	376	Intestine	May facilitate cholesterol efflux from cells. Activator of LCAT. Possible role in triglyceride metabolism.
B100	85	2	43,000	~513	4536	Liver	Structural protein/VLDL and LDL. Ligand for LDL receptor.
B48	Variable			~241	2152	Intestine	Structural protein/chylomicrons.
CI	6	19	4653	~6.6	57	Liver	Modulates remnant binding to receptors. Activates LCAT.
CII	3	19	3320	8.9	79	Liver	Cofactor for LPL.
CIII	12	11	3133	8.8	79	Liver	Modulates remnant binding to receptors.
E	5	19	3597	~34	299	Liver, brain, skin, testes, spleen	Ligand for LDL and remnant receptors. Local lipid redistribution. Reverse cholesterol transport (HDL with apo-E).
Apo(a)	Variable	6	Variable	~400–800	4000–6000	Liver	Modulates thrombosis/fibrinolysis.
D	10	3	12,000	~20	169	Liver, intestine	Activator of LCAT (?)

Apo-E, apolipoprotein E; HDL, high-density lipoprotein; LCAT, lecithin:cholesterol acyltransferase; LDL, low-density lipoprotein; LPL, lipoprotein lipase; VLDL, very-low-density lipoprotein.

dividual apolipoproteins in regulating lipid metabolism. Some of their properties are summarized in Table 34–4 and Figure 34–6.[8, 45, 46]

Major Apolipoproteins Regulating Lipoprotein Metabolism

Apolipoprotein B

In human plasma, apo-B occurs in two forms, apo-B100 and apo-B48, which are derived from a single gene[50–54] on the short arm of chromosome 2. The human apo-B gene comprises 29 exons and 28 introns and is approximately 45 kilobases in length. A unique ribonucleic acid (RNA)–editing mechanism is responsible for the synthesis of apo-B100 and apo-B48 from the apo-B messenger RNA (mRNA) (Fig. 34–7) (for a review see references 52 and 55 to 57). An editing protein (or proteins) interacts with the apo-B mRNA in the human intestine to change a single nucleotide, resulting in the synthesis of a truncated form of apo-B (apo-B48). In humans, this modification of the apo-B mRNA occurs only in the intestine and not in the liver; therefore, the liver produces the full-length apo-B100. Apo-B100 (but not apo-B48) is also expressed in the yolk sac of mammals.

The editing of apo-B mRNA results in the change of cytosine-6666 in the apo-B100 mRNA to a uracil.[58–60] This cytosine is part of the codon CAA, which encodes a glutamine at amino acid residue 2153 in apo-B100, whereas the codon UAA is a stop codon and terminates translation of the protein chain (see Fig. 34–7). Therefore, apo-B48 possesses only 2152 amino acids, compared with the 4536 in apo-B100. Apo-B100, a 513-kd protein, is synthesized in the liver; it serves as a structural protein of VLDL and of intermediate-density lipoproteins (IDLs) and is the exclusive protein constituent of LDL. Each VLDL, IDL, and LDL particle contains one molecule of apo-B100. The primary structure of apo-B contains many hydrophobic and amphipathic sequences, forming alpha helices and beta strands, that occur throughout the molecule and appear to function as lipid-binding domains. In addition to its structural role, apo-B100 functions as a ligand for the LDL receptor.

Apo-B48, a 241-kd protein, is a structural constituent of chylomicrons.[50–52] Each chylomicron appears to possess one or

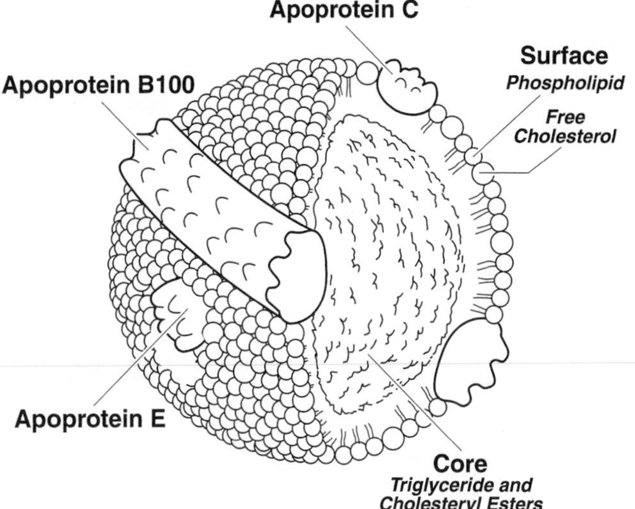

Figure 34–5. General structure of lipoproteins (a schematic representation of very-low-density lipoprotein, VLDL).

Table 34–4. Major Classes of Plasma Lipoproteins

Type	Density (g/mL)	Electrophoretic Mobility	Site of Origin	Major Lipids	Major Apolipoproteins
Chylomicrons	<0.95	Origin	Intestine	85% Triglyceride	B48, AI, AIV (E, CI, CII, CIII—by transfer from HDL)
Chylomicron remnants	<1.006	Origin	Intestine	60% Triglyceride, 20% cholesterol	B48, E
VLDL*	<1.006	Pre-β	Liver	55% Triglyceride, 20% cholesterol	B100, E, CI, CII, CIII
IDL*	1.006–1.019	β	Derived from VLDL	35% Cholesterol, 25% triglyceride	B100, E
LDL	1.019–1.063	β	Derived from IDL	60% Cholesterol, 5% triglyceride	B100
HDL	1.063–1.21	α	Liver, intestine, plasma	25% Phospholipid, 20% cholesterol, 5% triglyceride (50% protein)	AI, AII, CI, CII, CIII, E
HDL_2	1.063–1.125	α			
HDL_3	1.125–1.21	α			

*Small, partially lipolyzed VLDL and IDL are often called VLDL remnants.
HDL, high-density lipoprotein; IDL, intermediate-density lipoprotein; LDL, low-density lipoprotein; VLDL, very-low-density lipoprotein.

possibly two molecules of apo-B48. Because it lacks the carboxyl-terminal domain of apo-B100, apo-B48 cannot bind to the LDL receptor. The carboxyl-terminal domain of apo-B100 in the region of amino acids 3000 to 3700 is critical for the binding of apo-B100 to the LDL receptor (Fig. 34–8).[61, 62] Selective chemical modification of the apo-B100 of LDL demonstrated that the positively charged (basic) amino acids arginine and lysine are important in the interaction of LDL with its receptor. When apo-B100 was sequenced, several regions enriched in arginines and lysines became candidates for receptor binding.[61–63] It is now apparent that the basic residues in the region of amino acids 3359 to 3369 are critical for receptor binding. However, it is also clear that the carboxyl-terminal region of apo-B100 in the vicinity of amino acid 3500 can modulate receptor-binding activity.[64] Patients expressing apo-B defective in binding have hypercholesterolemia and high LDL levels. This genetic disorder, familial defective apo-B100 (see later discussion), is caused by the substitution of glutamine for arginine at amino acid 3500 of apo-B100.[65]

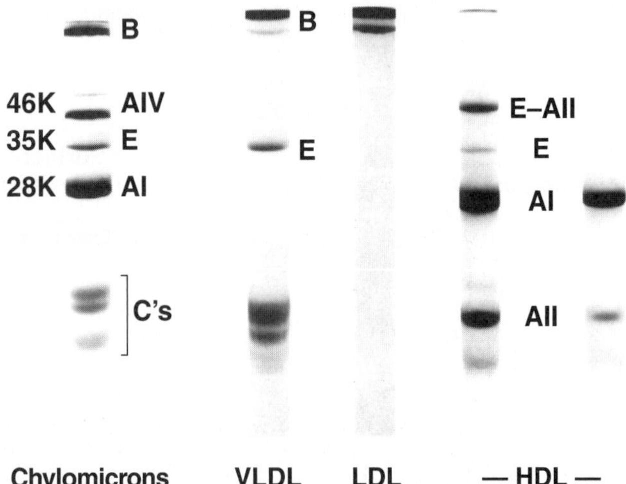

Figure 34–6. Polyacrylamide gel showing the various apolipoproteins characteristic of each type of plasma lipoprotein particle. HDL, high-density lipoprotein; LDL, low-density lipoprotein; VLDL, very-low-density lipoprotein. (Modified from Mahley RW, Innerarity TL. Lipoprotein receptors and cholesterol homeostasis. Biochim Biophys Acta 1983; 737:197–222. With permission from Elsevier Science-NL, Sara Burgerhartstraat 25, 1055 KV Amsterdam, The Netherlands.)

Role of Apolipoprotein B in Lipid Metabolism

Apo-B100 and apo-B48 play critical roles in the biosynthesis of apo-B–containing lipoproteins (for a review, see references 8, 45 to 47, 50, 51, 63, and 66 to 68). In addition, the apo-B100 in LDL interacts with the LDL receptor. Although it is also a constituent of VLDL and IDL, apo-B100 does not play a major role in the binding of these lipoproteins to LDL receptors. Apo-E is responsible for most of the receptor-mediated clearance of VLDL and IDL; presumably, the lipid or apolipoprotein content of the VLDL and IDL masks or alters the conformation of the receptor-binding domain of the apo-B100 on these particles. Apo-B100 is, however, the major (or exclusive) protein moiety of LDL and is responsible for directing the clearance of these lipoproteins through the LDL receptor pathway.

Overexpression of apo-B in transgenic mice increases the levels of LDL and other apo-B–containing lipoproteins,[69–74] resulting in increased susceptibility to diet-induced atheroscle-

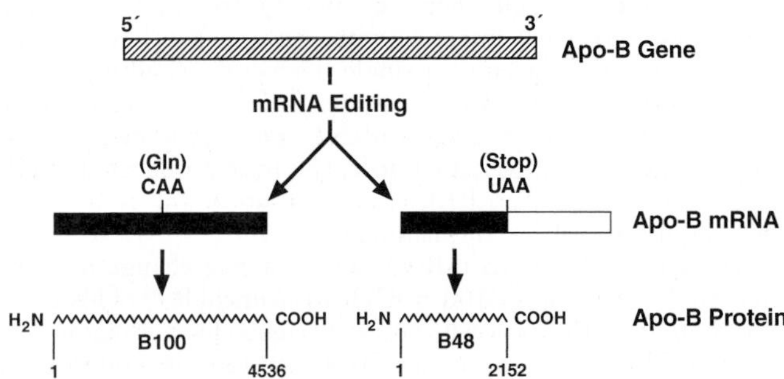

Figure 34–7. Synthesis of apolipoprotein B100 (apo-B100) and apo-B48 by a unique messenger ribonucleic acid (mRNA)–editing mechanism. In the human intestine, a specific cytosine (C) is changed to a uracil (U) in the apo-B mRNA. This change results in a stop codon and the formation of apo-B48, which contains only the first 2152 amino acids of the full-length apo-B100 (4536 amino acids).

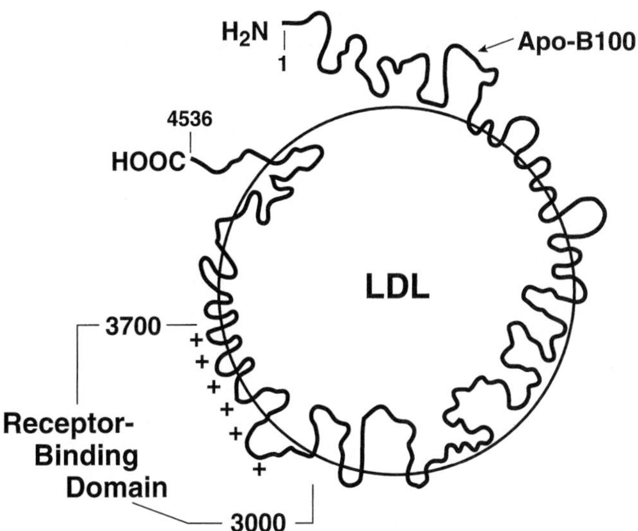

Figure 34–8. Schematic representation of apolipoprotein B100 (apo-B100) on the surface of a low-density lipoprotein (LDL) particle. The receptor-binding domain may form a cluster of positively charged arginine and lysine residues (a basic patch) capable of interacting with critical negatively charged glutamic and aspartic acid residues in the ligand-binding domain of the LDL receptor. (Adapted from Yang C-Y, Gu Z-W, Weng S-A, et al. Structure of apolipoprotein B-100 of human low density lipoproteins. Arteriosclerosis 1989; 9:96–108.)

rosis.[73] Knockout of the apo-B gene in mice is embryonically lethal.[74, 75] Production of apo-B in the yolk sac appears to play an essential role in the delivery of lipids to the developing mouse embryo; delivery of α-tocopherol may be particularly important to embryonic tissues.[76]

Apolipoprotein E

Apo-E[77–79] mediates the interaction of apo-E–containing lipoproteins with the LDL receptor and with the chylomicron remnant (apo-E) receptor, presumably the LDL receptor–related protein (LRP). As a consequence, apo-E plays a critical role in determining the metabolic fate of several classes of lipoproteins and is of central importance in cholesterol metabolism. In addition, apo-E appears to participate in cholesterol transport to cells undergoing proliferation and repair and may modulate lymphocyte response and smooth muscle cell proliferation (for a review, see references 77, 78, and 80).

Apo-E, a 34-kDa protein composed of 299 amino acids,[77] circulates in the plasma both as a constituent of chylomicrons, chylomicron remnants, VLDL, and IDL and as a component of a minor subclass of high-density lipoproteins (HDLs), referred to as HDL with apo-E or HDL_1 (see Fig. 34–6). Normal plasma apo-E levels range from 30 to 70 μg/mL, approximately half of which is associated with HDL and serves as a reservoir of apo-E for redistribution to chylomicrons and VLDLs as they enter the plasma. In lymph and interstitial fluid, apo-E is associated with lipid complexes (phospholipid–apo-E discs) or with HDL.

Approximately 75% of plasma apo-E is synthesized by hepatocytes, and the remainder is synthesized in a variety of tissues. Macrophages can synthesize and secrete the protein, especially when they are loaded with cholesterol, and are responsible for a portion of the apo-E found in interstitial fluid. Smooth muscle cells of arteries and keratinocytes in the skin also synthesize apo-E (see Table 34–3). The tissue with the second highest level of apo-E mRNA (after the liver) is the brain, where apo-E is synthesized primarily by astrocytes. Cerebrospinal fluid contains apo-E derived from the brain (approximately 0.3 mg/dL, or 5% to 10% of plasma apo-E levels). Apo-E appears to play a key role in cholesterol transport in both the central and peripheral nervous systems and may be involved in the pathogenesis of Alzheimer's disease (for a review, see references 77 and 80 to 84).

The apo-E gene is located on chromosome 19 and is part of a gene cluster that includes the genes for apo-CI and apo-CII. The apo-E gene locus has multiple alleles that give rise to a common genetic protein polymorphism.[77–80, 83, 85, 86] The three major forms of apo-E—apo-E2, apo-E3, and apo-E4—arise from three alleles, referred to as ε2, ε3, and ε4, that occur in several populations with a frequency of about 8%, 77%, and 15%, respectively (Fig. 34–9). There are three homozygous (E2/2, E3/3, and E4/4) and three heterozygous (E3/2, E4/2, and E4/3) phenotypes. About 60% of individuals are homozygous for apo-E3.

These genetic polymorphisms are caused by amino acid differences at two sites in the protein (see Fig. 34–9).[46, 63, 77, 78, 83, 86, 87] Apo-E3 has cysteine at position 112 and arginine at position 158, whereas apo-E2 has cysteine at both positions and apo-E4 has arginine. In addition, apo-E displays a second type of polymorphism, post-translational glycosylation. Carbohydrate attachment at threonine-194 and the presence of multiple sialic acid residues give rise to minor acidic isoforms.

Apo-E functions in both receptor binding and lipid binding, and the different isoforms have different activities. Apo-E3 and apo-E4 are equally capable of interacting with LDL receptors, but the binding of apo-E2 to LDL receptors is impaired and is associated with the development of type III hyperlipoproteinemia under certain conditions.[86, 88] Apo-E isoforms also interact

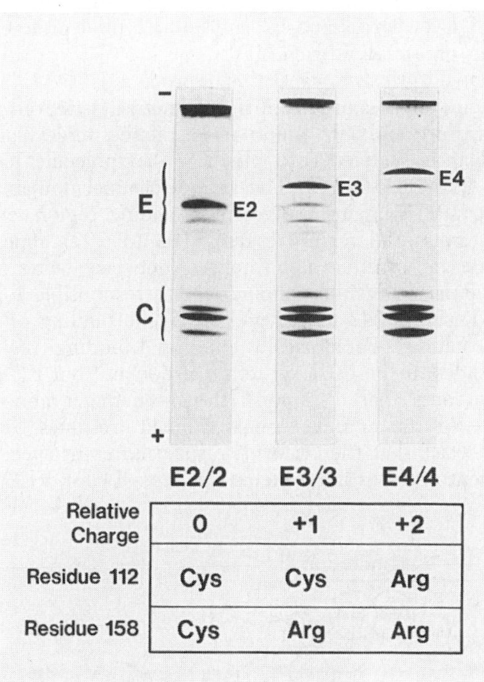

	E2/2	E3/3	E4/4
Relative Charge	0	+1	+2
Residue 112	Cys	Cys	Arg
Residue 158	Cys	Arg	Arg

Figure 34–9. Isoelectric focusing gels of very-low-density lipoprotein (VLDL) apolipoproteins from three individuals homozygous for the common apo-E phenotypes. The relative charge differences among the different apo-E isoforms are accounted for by the specific amino acid substitutions that are responsible for the three isoforms. The minor, more acidic apo-E isoforms represent sialylated forms of the protein. (From Mahley RW, Rall SC Jr. Type III hyperlipoproteinemia (dysbetalipoproteinemia): the role of apolipoprotein E in normal and abnormal lipoprotein metabolism. In Scriver CR, Beaudet AL, Sly WS, et al [eds]. The Metabolic and Molecular Bases of Inherited Disease, 7th ed. New York, McGraw-Hill, 1995, pp 1953–1980.)

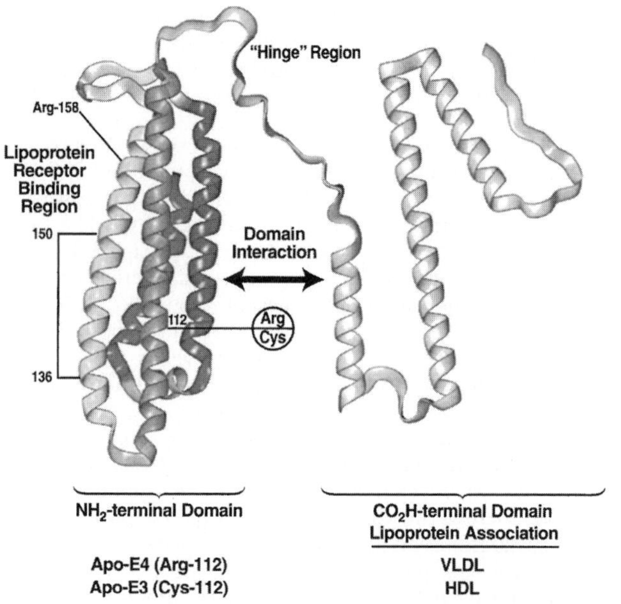

Figure 34–10. Predicted secondary structure of apolipoprotein E (apo-E). The majority of the structure is composed of alpha helices, beta-sheet structures, and beta turns. A region of random structure encompassing residues 165 to 200 appears to form a boundary or hinge region between the two functional domains. HDL, high-density lipoprotein; VLDL, very-low-density lipoprotein.

differently with specific types of lipids and lipoproteins.[78] Apo-E4 binds preferentially to large, triglyceride-rich lipoproteins (e.g., VLDL), whereas apo-E3 and apo-E2 bind preferentially to smaller, phospholipid-rich HDL.

The apo-E primary translational product is a 317-amino-acid protein; an 18-amino-acid signal peptide is cleaved before the mature protein (299 amino acids, relative molecular mass ≅ 34 kDa) is secreted into plasma. The molecule has two domains (Fig. 34–10).[77, 78] The amino-terminal domain (residues 1 to 191) contains the receptor-binding region, and the carboxyl-terminal domain (residues 192 to 299) appears to have three amphipathic alpha helices (one face being hydrophilic and the other hydrophobic) and is responsible for lipid binding. Residues 242 to 272 are key in the binding of apo-E to lipoproteins.[89] Paradoxically, the lipid-binding region of apo-E resides in the carboxyl-terminal domain, but the amino acid differences that distinguish the three major apo-E isoforms are in the amino-terminal domain (residues 112 and 158). The fact that the isoforms display different specificities for different types of lipoproteins (i.e., apo-E4 for VLDL and apo-E3 and apo-E2 for HDL) suggests that the amino-terminal and carboxyl-terminal domains interact so that specific residues in the amino terminus alter the conformation and specificity of the lipid-binding domain in the carboxyl terminus for certain types of lipoproteins (for a more complete discussion, see references 78, 83, and 89).

The amino acids of apo-E that mediate its binding to the LDL receptor are in the vicinity of residues 134 to 160 (Fig. 34–11).[77, 78, 86, 87] Positively charged arginines and lysines between amino acids 136 and 150 may interact with the negatively charged glutamic and aspartic acids in the ligand-binding region of the LDL receptor. As shown by x-ray crystallography, the amino-terminal domain of apo-E (residues 1 to 191) forms a four-helix bundle (Fig. 34–12).[89–91] The fourth helix encompasses residues 130 to 165, the area envisioned to contain the receptor-binding region. The basic residues in the vicinity of amino acids 134 to 150 are oriented away from the surface of the molecule and are probably involved in the direct interaction of apo-E with the LDL receptor.[90, 91]

The identification of naturally occurring mutants of apo-E that are defective in receptor binding has provided key insights into the specific residues involved (see Fig. 34–11). The most common variant that is defective in binding is apo-E2 (Arg-158 → Cys). This substitution appears to impair receptor binding secondarily by altering the conformation of residues in the 136 to 150 region of apo-E.[91, 92] Other variants that are defective in binding involve single amino acid substitutions: Arg-136 → Ser, Arg-142 → Cys, Arg-145 → Cys, and Lys-146 → Gln or Glu. Site-directed mutagenesis showed that Arg-150 also plays a key role in receptor binding. A rare apo-E mutation, apo-E Leiden, involves a duplication of seven amino acids (residues 121 to 127) inserted in tandem at the junction between helices 3 and 4. This insertion probably disrupts receptor binding by altering the conformation of the 136 to 150 receptor-binding region.

Apo-E also binds to heparin and to heparan sulfate proteoglycans (HSPGs).[83, 93] As discussed later, binding of apo-E to HSPG is important in the clearance of remnant lipoproteins by the LRP pathway. Residues in the 136 to 150 region of apo-E are responsible for the ionic interaction with the sulfate groups of heparin-like molecules and for binding to the LRP.

Roles of Apolipoprotein E in Lipid Metabolism

Apo-E functions in two aspects of lipid and cholesterol transport.[77, 80, 84] The first, involving chylomicron and VLDL metabolism, provides a global transport role for apo-E. The knockout of apo-E by gene targeting in mice results in marked hyperlipidemia and the development of severe atherosclerosis, confirming the importance of this protein in cholesterol homeostasis and lipid transport.[94, 95] The second aspect involves

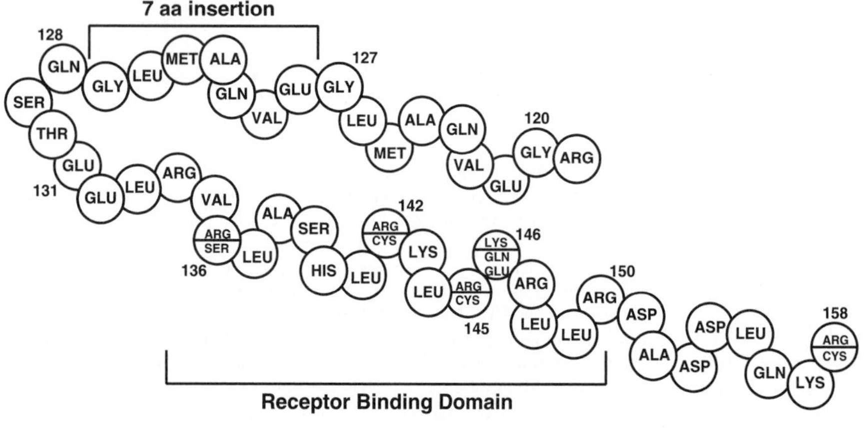

Figure 34–11. Schematic representation of the receptor-binding domain of apolipoprotein E, indicating the location and identity of naturally occurring amino acid substitutions that lead to type III hyperlipoproteinemia. In each substitution, the bottom amino acid represents the mutant.

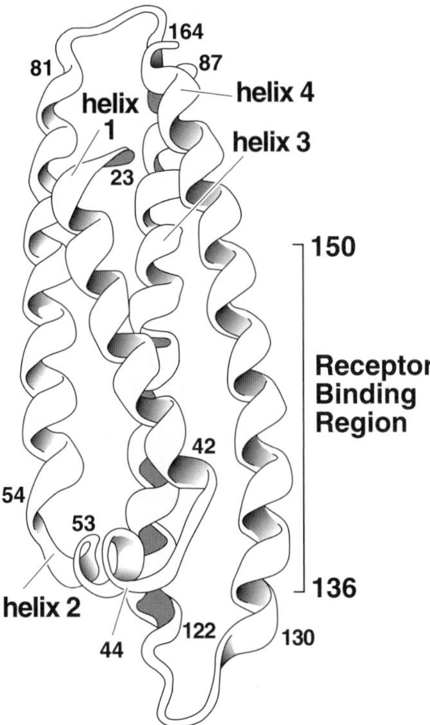

Figure 34–12. Three-dimensional structure of the amino-terminal region (residues 1 to 191) of apolipoprotein E, which forms a four-helix bundle. The receptor-binding domain resides in helix 4. (Modified from Wilson C, Wardell MR, Weisgraber KH, et al. Three-dimensional structure of the LDL receptor-binding domain of human apolipoprotein E. Science 1991; 252:1817–1822.)

the redistribution of lipids (including cholesterol) among cells within a tissue or organ. This local transport role redistributes lipids from cells with excess cholesterol to those requiring cholesterol, phospholipids, and other lipids for repair, proliferation, or other purposes. This pathway may involve lipid-laden HDL and apo-E that can acquire tissue lipids or apo-E–lipid complexes formed in the interstitial fluid. As stated previously, apo-E is synthesized and secreted by a variety of cells and is available in interstitial fluid to transport lipids. Cells requiring cholesterol up-regulate their LDL receptors, and apo-E targets the apo-E–containing HDL or lipid complexes to cells deficient in necessary lipids. For example, the local transport pathway for apo-E is involved in lipid redistribution within a nerve after injury and during regeneration.[77, 81, 83]

Apolipoprotein AI

Apo-AI is a 29-kDa protein encoded by a gene on the long arm of chromosome 11, part of a cluster that includes genes for apo-CIII and apo-AIV.[45, 96–99] The apo-AI gene is 1863 base pairs in length, and its mRNA encodes a 267-amino-acid protein that includes an 18-amino-acid prepeptide and a 6-amino-acid propeptide. The propeptide is cleaved extracellularly to yield the mature circulating protein of 243 amino acids (see Table 34–3).

Apo-AI is synthesized by the human intestine and liver and is a constituent of chylomicrons and HDL. It binds to lipids of these lipoproteins, mainly through a series of 22-amino-acid amphipathic alpha helices separated by helix-breaking proline residues.[99] The polar face of the amphipathic helix is exposed to the aqueous environment, whereas the nonpolar face binds to the lipid (primarily phospholipid) on the surface of the particle. There are eight complete 22-amino-acid amphipathic helices and two 11-amino-acid repeats in apo-AI.

In addition to its role as a structural protein in HDL, apo-AI activates lecithin:cholesterol acyltransferase (LCAT), which esterifies free cholesterol on HDL particles. It may facilitate the interaction of LCAT with phosphatidylcholine, the substrate of LCAT, and activate the enzyme. The specific regions of apo-AI involved in LCAT activation have been identified, including the amino acid residues responsible for enhanced catalytic activity.[100] Other apolipoproteins, such as apo-AIV and apo-CI, which have similar lipid-binding properties, can also activate LCAT (discussed in detail in a later section).

Apo-AI–associated particles, either HDL or its phospholipid-rich precursor, pre-β HDL, serve as acceptors for cholesterol released from cells.[47, 96, 99] The efflux of cholesterol to HDL represents part of the so-called reverse cholesterol transport pathway (discussed in "Metabolic Pathways Involving High-Density Lipoproteins").[101–103] Apo-AI may also serve as the recognition protein for the binding of HDL to a putative HDL receptor that mediates cholesterol uptake by cells.[104, 105]

Mutations that give rise to apo-AI deficiency are characterized by absent or low levels of HDL (discussed in "Primary Disorders of High-Density Lipoprotein Metabolism").[98, 99] Apo-AI synthesis is required for HDL production. Apo-AI deficiency causes a variety of manifestations: planar xanthomas, corneal clouding, and sometimes premature coronary heart disease (CHD). Apo-AI is often described as an antiatherogenic apolipoprotein. Although apo-E–deficient mice typically develop extensive atherosclerosis,[94, 95] overexpression of human apo-AI in these mice causes an increase in HDL and a significant decrease in atherosclerosis.[106, 107]

Apolipoprotein AII

The apo-AII gene is on the long arm of chromosome 1.[45, 96, 97, 99] The mRNA encodes a 100-amino-acid protein, but the mature circulating form of apo-AII is 77 amino acids in length. In the plasma, human apo-AII exists primarily as a homodimer. A cysteine at residue 6 of apo-AII forms a disulfide bond with a second apo-AII molecule. Heterodimers of apo-AII and apo-E occur only in persons with apo-E2 and apo-E3, which possess free cysteine residues. Heterodimer formation interferes with the ability of apo-E to bind to the LDL receptor.

Apo-AII is synthesized primarily in the liver.[45, 97, 99] It is found together with apo-AI on a subfraction of HDL referred to as LpAI/AII particles. Apo-AII may play a role in the activation of hepatic lipase and the inhibition of LCAT. The genetic absence of apo-AII in two sisters did not produce any obvious phenotypic effects and did not cause low HDL levels.[108]

Overexpression of apo-AII in mice leads to an increased susceptibility to atherosclerosis,[109] possibly because apo-AII displaces apo-AI from HDL. This could interfere with the normal ability of apo-AI–containing HDL to transport cellular cholesterol to the liver for excretion. Therefore, apo-AII is considered a proatherogenic apolipoprotein.

C Apolipoproteins

The genes for apo-CI and apo-CII reside on chromosome 19 near the gene that encodes apo-E, whereas the apo-CIII gene is part of the apo-AI and apo-AIV gene cluster on chromosome 11 (for a review, see references 8 and 45 to 47). The C apolipoproteins (see Table 34–3 and Fig. 34–6) readily exchange among various lipoproteins and are synthesized primarily by the liver. (Apo-CI is also produced by macrophages and, in small amounts, by the intestine.) HDLs appear to serve as a reservoir for the C apolipoproteins, which can then be transferred to triglyceride-rich lipoproteins. The C apolipoproteins appear to regulate triglyceride metabolism and to influence the inverse relation between triglyceride levels and HDL cholesterol (HDL-C). Apo-CI (6.6 kDa) modulates the uptake of triglyceride-rich lipoprotein (chylomicron remnants, VLDL, and IDL) by interfering with the ability of apo-E to mediate binding to lipoprotein receptor pathways. Similarly, apo-CIII (8.8 kDa) may prevent the normal interaction of triglyceride-rich, apo-E–containing lipoproteins with receptors and cell-surface HSPG. Apo-CI and apo-CIII may displace apo-E from the particles. Apo-CII (8.9 kDa) is a cofactor for LPL, and mutations in the apo-CII gene result in a marked hypertriglyceridemia (discussed later).

Overexpression of apo-CI, apo-CII, or apo-CIII in transgenic mice results in hypertriglyceridemia (for a review, see references 45 and 110). In the case of apo-CI and apo-CIII, the resulting hyperlipidemia appears to be caused by displacement of apo-E from triglyceride-rich particles, which results in impaired receptor-mediated uptake, displacement of apo-CII, and impaired lipolytic processing. A polymorphism of the apo-CIII gene promoter region in mice is also associated with increased levels of apo-CIII and hypertriglyceridemia.[111]

The hypertriglyceridemia that follows the overexpression of apo-CII was initially puzzling[45] because apo-CII is a cofactor that activates LPL-mediated hydrolysis of triglycerides. However, the triglyceride-rich lipoproteins that accumulate in the plasma are poor in apo-E and do not interact well enough with cell-surface HSPG to allow lipase activity to occur or with receptors in the proteoglycan-rich matrices of the cell surface to allow uptake. Therefore, either overproduction or underproduction of apo-CII can cause hypertriglyceridemia.

Lipoprotein Receptors Controlling Lipoprotein Metabolism

Low-Density Lipoprotein Receptor Gene Family

Mammalian members of this gene family, in addition to the LDL receptor itself, include the LRP, the glycoprotein 330 (gp330)/megalin receptor, the VLDL receptor, and the apo-E receptor 2.[112–115] Nonmammalian members include the chicken vitellogenin receptor, a *Caenorhabditis elegans* receptor, and the Y1 protein in the fruit fly *Drosophila melanogaster*.[114] These receptors share common structural motifs, including a single transmembrane domain, a short cytoplasmic tail, and an extracellular ligand-binding domain that contains various numbers of cysteine-rich repeats of approximately 40 amino acids each. It has become apparent that the functions of this gene family extend far beyond mediating lipid uptake by cells and include serving as transducers of extracellular signals involved in normal brain development.[116]

Low-Density Lipoprotein Receptor

The LDL receptor, a glycoprotein with an apparent molecular weight of 160,000, is expressed on the surface of most cells and especially in liver. It functions in the uptake of apo-B– and apo-E–containing lipoproteins, including LDL, chylomicron remnants, VLDL, VLDL remnants, IDL, and HDL_1.[46, 63, 77] Most HDL particles lack apo-E and do not interact with the LDL receptor. Cells can acquire cholesterol from the plasma by taking up these lipoproteins through the LDL receptor. The LDL receptor was first identified in 1973, and its gene was characterized in 1985 in the laboratory of Nobel laureates Joseph L. Goldstein and Michael S. Brown.[14, 117–119] Two proteins on the lipoprotein surface, apo-B100 and apo-E, bind to the LDL receptor, which for this reason is sometimes referred to as the apo-B100/apo-E receptor.

After the lipoprotein binds to the LDL receptor, the resulting complex becomes localized to a specialized area of the cell membrane called a coated pit. The "coat" contains a protein complex called clathrin, which clusters the receptors in a region of the cell membrane that can invaginate and form an intracellular vesicle to contain the lipoprotein. As these internalized vesicles, or endosomes, move into the cytoplasm, the internal environment becomes progressively more acidic, causing the receptor and the lipoprotein to dissociate. The lipoproteins are degraded in the lysosomes, and the unoccupied receptors recycle to the cell surface (Fig. 34–13).

The LDL receptor is synthesized in the ER as a protein of 839 amino acids[117, 119] with an apparent molecular weight of 120,000. Glycosylation of the protein in the ER and in the Golgi apparatus increases its weight to about 160,000. The LDL receptor has five distinct structural and functional domains[119] (Fig. 34–14). Mutations within these domains disrupt the normal function of the receptor in lipoprotein metabolism and cause the genetic disorder familial hypercholesterolemia (FH)[119] (discussed later).

Ligand-Binding Domain

The ligand-binding domain of the LDL receptor consists of the 292 amino acids at the amino terminus (see Fig. 34–14). This region of the molecule is rich in cysteines and contains glutamic and aspartic acids that mediate the binding to apo-B and apo-E. It is composed of seven repeats of approximately 40 amino acids each. Each repeat contains six cysteines that form three intrarepeat disulfide bonds, resulting in a very stable structure. In addition, each repeat contains a Ser-Asp-Glu triplet that mediates the interaction of apo-B– and apo-E–containing lipoproteins with the LDL receptor. The ligand-receptor binding is an ionic interaction between positively charged arginines and lysines in apo-B100 and apo-E and negatively charged aspartic and glutamic acids in the ligand-binding domain of the LDL receptor.

Site-directed mutagenesis and analysis of naturally occurring mutants of the LDL receptor associated with FH have pro-

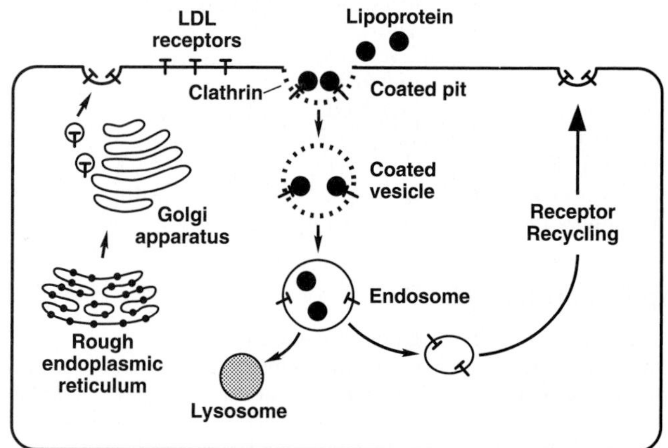

Figure 34–13. Low-density lipoprotein (LDL) receptor pathway. The LDLs interact with their receptors on the cell surface. The complex enters the coated pit and is internalized. The coated vesicle loses its clathrin coat and becomes an endosome, the site of lipoprotein and receptor dissociation. The receptors recycle to the cell surface, and the lipoproteins are degraded. Alternatively, new receptors are synthesized in the rough endoplasmic reticulum and transported to the cell surface. (Modified from Brown MS, Goldstein JL. A receptor-mediated pathway for cholesterol homeostasis. Science 1986; 232:34–47; and Myant NB. Cholesterol Metabolism, LDL, and the LDL Receptor. San Diego, Academic Press, 1990.)

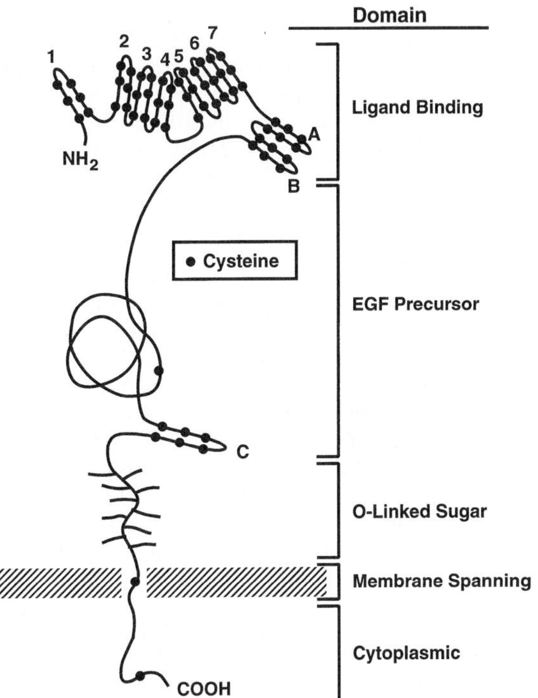

Figure 34–14. Functional domains of the low-density lipoprotein receptor. See text for complete description. EGF, epidermal growth factor.

vided insights into the roles of specific repeats and residues in ligand binding.[119] Ligand-binding domain repeat 1 does not play a major role in the binding of either apo-B–containing (LDL) or apo-E–containing (β-VLDL) lipoproteins. The deletion of repeats 2 through 7, however, markedly impairs the binding of LDL. The binding of β-VLDL is mediated by apo-E and is impaired only if repeat 5 is deleted. Therefore, the requirements for the binding of LDL are more stringent than those for the binding of β-VLDL.

Single amino acid substitutions of critical residues in the ligand-binding repeats also impair binding activity. For example, in patients with FH Puerto Rico, in which the serine of the ligand-binding triplet (Ser-Asp-Glu) in repeat 4 is changed to a leucine, the LDL fails to bind, although apo-E–containing β-VLDL binds with near-normal affinity. In FH Mexico, in which lysine is substituted for the glutamic acid of the ligand-binding triplet of repeat 5, neither LDL nor β-VLDL binds normally.

The defect in the Watanabe heritable hyperlipidemic (WHHL) rabbit with hypercholesterolemia and accelerated atherosclerosis involves a deletion of four amino acids in repeat 4. Although this defect is associated with a reduced number of receptors reaching the cell surface, those that do reach the surface retain the ability to bind β-VLDL (apo-E) but not LDL (apo-B).[119]

As demonstrated in the WHHL rabbit, mutations in the ligand-binding domain can also disrupt the normal transport of the LDL receptor to the cell surface. The decreased transport of the mutant receptor from the ER to the Golgi apparatus and to the cell surface is undoubtedly caused by improper folding of the molecule and increased intracellular degradation. For example, FH Afrikaner, which is caused by the presence of a glutamic acid rather than aspartic acid in the triplet of repeat 5, results in defective transport and lack of normal expression of the receptor on the cell surface.

Epidermal Growth Factor Precursor Homology Domain

This region is composed of 400 amino acids and is about 33% identical to the sequence of the human EGF precursor.[117–119] It contains three cysteine-rich repeats (A, B, and C), each approximately 40 amino acids in length. The repeats are not homologous to the 40-amino-acid repeats of the ligand-binding domain but are related to the EGF. Repeat A is involved in the binding of LDL, and its deletion markedly inhibits LDL binding (β-VLDL binding is retained). The EGF precursor domain also plays a role in allowing the LDL receptor or receptors to dissociate from the lipoproteins and recycle to the cell surface. Deletion of the EGF precursor homology domain allows normal binding and internalization of β-VLDL but prevents dissociation of the ligand and receptor. As a result, receptors do not recycle to the cell surface. The role of the EGF precursor domain was established by site-directed mutagenesis studies, and FH Osaka was subsequently found to have the same deletion.

O-Linked Sugar Domain

This domain is composed of 58 amino acids,[117–119] primarily serines and threonines, many of which are sites for the attachment of O-linked carbohydrate chains. No functional role for this domain has been described, and its deletion has no functional consequences.

Membrane-Spanning Domain

The 22 amino acids in this domain are hydrophobic and serve to anchor the receptor within the plasma membrane (see Fig. 34–14).[117–119] Truncation mutations that exclude this region are characterized by secretion of the receptor from the cell so that lipoproteins are not internalized.

Cytoplasmic Domain

The carboxyl-terminal region of the LDL receptor is composed of 50 amino acids[117–119] and contains the sequence NPXY (N, asparagine; P, proline; X, any amino acid; Y, tyrosine), which is responsible for clustering the receptors in coated pits and mediating internalization of the receptors by the cells. One of the early mutations associated with FH (J.D. allele, FH Bari) provided insights into the role of a critical residue for directing internalization. In the mutant form of the receptor, tyrosine-807 is changed to a cysteine. Site-directed mutagenesis demonstrated that this position must be occupied by an aromatic amino acid (tyrosine, phenylalanine, or tryptophan) for normal internalization. The tetrameric sequence Asn-Pro-Val-Tyr, in which tyrosine-807 occurs, is the signal directing the receptors to the coated pit.

Regulation of the Low-Density Lipoprotein Receptor Gene

The LDL receptor gene is 45 kilobases in length and is located on the distal portion of the short arm of chromosome 19. Synthesis of the LDL receptor is regulated by deoxyribonucleic acid (DNA) sequences in the 5′-flanking region of the LDL receptor gene (Fig. 34–15).[120–123] A sequence of approximately 10 bases in this region, called the sterol regulatory element (SRE), and two other repeats that bind the transcription factor Sp1 are necessary for the regulation of the LDL receptor mRNA levels. If intracellular sterol levels are high, LDL receptor mRNA is not transcribed. When the sterol content of the cells decreases, the expression of LDL receptors on the cell surface increases, causing increased uptake of apo-

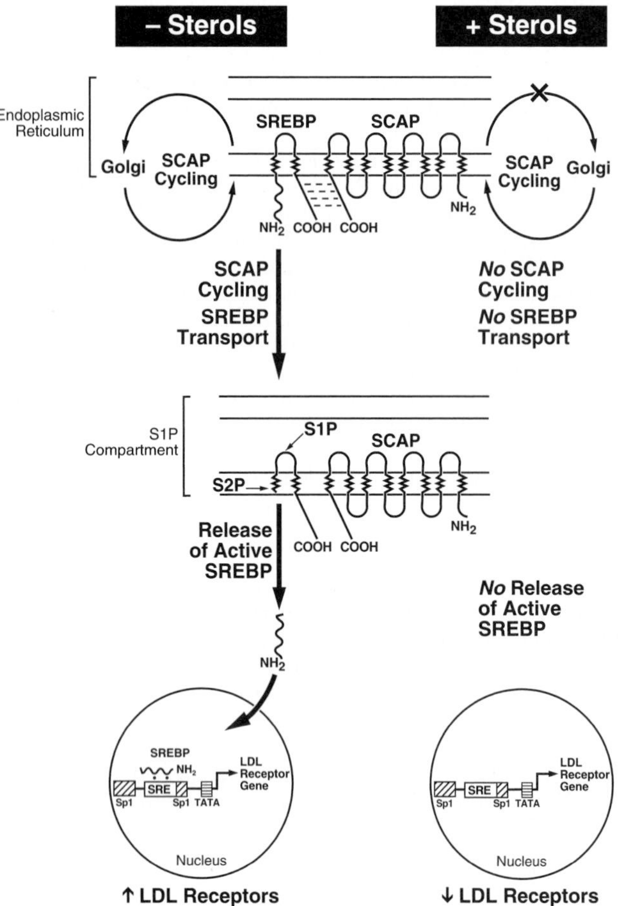

Figure 34–15. Low-density lipoprotein (LDL) receptor gene regulation. SREBP, sterol regulatory element–binding protein.

B– and apo-E–containing lipoproteins and increased delivery of cholesterol to the cells. The LDL receptor gene "senses" the sterol level of the cell and appropriately controls receptor mRNA production and protein biosynthesis to meet the needs of the cell.

The control mechanism of LDL receptor expression has been elucidated in considerable detail.[120–122, 124, 125] Currently, there are three structurally related transcription factors, SRE-binding proteins (SREBPs) 1a, 1c, and 2, which regulate the level of LDL receptors and other genes encoding enzymes involved in the biosynthesis of cholesterol, unsaturated fatty acids, and triglycerides. SREBP-1a and SREBP-1c arise from the same gene but use different promoters and have different first introns; SREBP-2 arises from a separate gene. The intact 125-kDa SREBPs are three-domain integral membrane proteins containing two membrane-spanning regions (see Fig. 34–15). The amino-terminal domain of SREBPs represents transcription factors of the loop-helix leucine zipper family and contains sequences that recognize the SREs on the genes that they control.

To become active transcription factors, the intact SREBPs must be cleaved in the correct order by two proteases in a post-ER compartment and then translocated to the nucleus to interact with the SREs. The first protease, designated site-1 protease (S1P), cleaves the loop connecting the amino-terminal and carboxyl-terminal domains, both of which remain membrane bound after cleavage. The second protease, site-2 protease (S2P), further cleaves the amino-terminal domain just within the first membrane-spanning region, releasing the transcription factor to enter the nucleus and interact with the SREs (see Fig. 34–15).

Sterol control is exerted through a two-domain regulatory protein, SREBP cleavage activating protein (SCAP), that is required for S1P cleavage of the SREBP. SCAP is membrane associated (eight transmembrane regions) and is tightly complexed to the SREBPs through its carboxyl-terminal domain. Five of the eight membrane-spanning segments serve as a sterol-sensing domain. It is not clear whether the sensing domain interacts directly or indirectly with sterols. What is known is that sterols regulate the ability of SCAP to transport SREBPs to the post-ER compartment where S1P is located.[126] SCAP cycles between the ER and Golgi apparatus, and whether SCAP transports the SREBPs to the S1P compartment is dependent on the processing of its N-linked carbohydrates by the Golgi apparatus. In sterol-depleted cells, SCAP cycles to the Golgi apparatus and its N-linked carbohydrates are modified; the modified SCAP returns to the ER to transport the SREBPs. Sterols block the movement of SCAP from the ER to the Golgi apparatus, preventing carbohydrate modification and the ability of SCAP to transport the SREBPs for S1P cleavage.

Low-Density Lipoprotein Receptor–Related Protein

The LRP is an integral membrane receptor composed of two components: a 515-kDa amino-terminal extracellular domain and an 85-kDa cytoplasmic and membrane-spanning domain (the precursor protein, composed of 4525 amino acids, is cleaved after synthesis).[127, 128] This large protein is equivalent structurally to approximately four LDL receptors and possesses 31 ligand-binding domains. The LRP contains the four structural motifs characteristic of other members of the LDL receptor gene family: multiple ligand-binding repeats, EGF repeats and EGF precursor homology domains, a single membrane-spanning region, and two NPXY internalization signals. The LRP is expressed primarily in liver (parenchymal cells), brain (neurons), and placenta (syncytiotrophoblast cells).[112, 113, 129]

The LRP interacts with approximately 18 ligands and has several functions. With respect to lipoprotein metabolism, the LRP binds with high affinity to apo-E–enriched chylomicron remnants and VLDL remnants and internalizes them. Interaction of these lipoproteins with the LRP requires the addition of multiple apo-E molecules per particle, which serve as ligands. Initial binding of the lipoprotein to cell-surface HSPG is necessary to facilitate the interaction or transfer of the apo-E–enriched remnants to the LRP[93] (discussed further in "Chylomicron Remnant Receptors in Remnant Catabolism"). The LRP does not bind LDL.

The LRP can also interact with LPL[130] and hepatic lipase.[131] This interaction could mediate the hepatic binding and uptake of remnant lipoproteins possessing these enzymes on their surface. Other ligands for the LRP that are not directly related to lipid metabolism include α_2-macroglobulin, plasminogen activators and inhibitors, and bacterial toxins.[112, 113] Knockout of the LRP in mice is lethal, demonstrating its critical importance,[132] but the reason for the lethality remains to be elucidated.

A receptor-associated protein (RAP) of 39 kDa can be isolated along with purified LRP and effectively competes with all the ligands for the LRP binding. This protein also binds to the gp330 and VLDL receptors (described later) and blocks ligand binding to these receptors as well. However, RAP does not appear to be secreted from the cells, and it may serve as an intracellular chaperone that occupies the ligand-binding sites for transport of the LRP to the cell surface. The knockout of RAP by gene targeting in mice markedly reduces the expression of LRP in both liver and brain, further suggesting an intracellular transport role for this protein.[133] Alternatively, it may participate in the intracellular recycling of the receptors. Regardless of its physiologic role, RAP inhibits the interaction of LRP and its ligands both in cultured cells and in intact animals.

Glycoprotein 330

The gp330/megalin receptor, also referred to as the major Heymann nephritis antigen, is a large protein (about 600 kDa) that possesses many of the structural motifs of the LDL receptor.[112, 113] It is expressed in the proximal tubules of the kidney and the ependymal cells in the brain and is not present in liver. Although gp330 binds apo-E–containing lipoproteins and LDL, its role in lipoprotein metabolism is unknown. The knockout of gp330 by gene targeting does not have an obvious effect on lipoprotein metabolism, but it causes developmental abnormalities of the central nervous system (holoprosencephaly).[134]

Very-Low-Density Lipoprotein Receptor

The VLDL receptor closely resembles the LDL receptor except that it has an eighth ligand-binding repeat.[135] The VLDL receptor (about 130 kDa) binds apo-E–containing lipoproteins and is present primarily in muscle, fat, and brain. In the nervous system, it is present in the choroid plexus and in some neurons. It is absent from liver, and its role in lipoprotein metabolism remains to be determined. It has been suggested, because the receptor is present in tissues that metabolize VLDL-derived fatty acids, that it may function to deliver triglyceride-rich lipoproteins to target tissues.[114]

Apolipoprotein E Receptor 2

The apo-E receptor 2 (~106 kDa) is the newest member of the LDL receptor family to be described; it is expressed primarily in the brain and to a lesser extent in the placenta and can be expressed as various splice variants.[136] Although this receptor, like the LDL receptor, contains seven cysteine-rich repeats in the ligand-binding domain, the repeats are more closely related structurally to the VLDL receptor. Because the receptor is primarily expressed in the brain, it is likely to play a role in lipoprotein metabolism in the central nervous system. In addition to their roles in lipoprotein metabolism, the apo-E receptor 2 and the VLDL receptor have been implicated in normal brain development by transducing extracellular signals.[116]

Scavenger Receptors

Originally, it was thought that a single scavenger receptor existed on macrophages.[137] Also known as the acetyl-LDL receptor,[138] this receptor was characterized by its ability to interact with chemically modified LDL but not with native LDL. LDL particles that had been modified by acetylation, acetoacetylation, or malondialdehyde were taken up by high-affinity cell-surface receptors on macrophages, resulting in marked cholesterol accumulation. As a result of cloning efforts, it became apparent that the scavenger receptor actually represented a large family of receptors with specificities for a broad range of unrelated ligands and involvement in a spectrum of physiologic processes, including atherosclerosis, host defense, and central nervous system disorders.[139, 140]

Currently, there are five subclasses (A to E) of the scavenger receptor family. Class A receptors include types I, II, and III and MARCO. The type I and type II receptors are generated by alternative splicing of the mRNA encoded by a gene on chromosome 8.[112] The predicted structure is that of a trimer (~220 kDa) composed of three identical subunits (each about 77 kDa). The type I receptor contains six domains: a cytoplasmic, amino-terminal domain (50 amino acids); a transmembrane domain (26 amino acids); a spacer (74 amino acids); an alpha-helical coiled-coil domain (121 amino acids); a collagen-like domain (72 amino acids with a Gly-X-Tyr repeat); and a cysteine-rich domain (110 amino acids). The type II scavenger receptor is identical to the type I receptor except that it lacks the carboxyl-terminal cysteine-rich domain; its collagen-like domain is responsible for ligand binding. Clusters of positively charged residues (lysines) appear to mediate the interaction with the chemically modified lipoproteins (see section on the LDL paradox and oxidized lipids for a discussion of the role of the scavenger receptor in atherogenesis). In addition to binding acetyl-LDL, class A scavenger receptors bind anionic proteins, polynucleotides, and bacterial endotoxins (lipopolysaccharides).[141] Their main function appears to involve the clearance of microbial pathogens, senescent cells, and altered lipoproteins.

Class B scavenger receptors include CD36 and murine SR-BI (human homologue CLA-1). These receptors possess two membrane-spanning regions and bind both oxidized and native lipoproteins. CD36 is expressed on the surface of platelets, capillary endothelial cells, adipose cells, circulating monocytes, and other cell types. The role of the SR-BI as a receptor for HDL and its involvement in reverse cholesterol transport are discussed in the section "Transport Facilitated by a Cell-Surface Binding Protein." CD36 is also implicated in platelet adhesion and aggregation, phagocytosis of apoptotic cells, and clearance of *Plasmodium falciparum*–infected cells (for a review, see reference 139).

Class C is represented by a single member, SR-C from *D. melanogaster*. It contains domains that are homologous to the vertebrate complement control protein and a mucin-like domain. Class D and E scavenger receptors are also represented by single members, Lox-1 and endothelial scavenger receptor, respectively. Lox-1 is characterized by a C-type lectin structure and the endothelial scavenger receptor by multiple EGF repeats.[140] Regardless of the class, all scavenger receptors share the common property of binding oxidized or modified LDLs, or both.

Enzymes and Transfer Proteins Involved in Lipid and Lipoprotein Metabolism

Lipoprotein Lipase

Human LPL is a protein composed of 448 amino acids (approximately 50 kDa). It is synthesized by adipocytes, by myocytes in skeletal and cardiac muscle, and by macrophages but is not produced by hepatocytes. After secretion from adipocytes and myocytes, LPL is transported to the surface of capillary endothelial cells of these tissues, where it attaches to HSPG and interacts with chylomicrons and VLDL in the circulation and mediates the hydrolysis of their triglycerides to release free fatty acids for use by the tissues. The fatty acids are stored as triglyceride in adipocytes and used as a source of energy in muscle and for triglyceride synthesis in the formation of hepatic VLDL.[142–146]

The active form of LPL is a dimer. Although its crystal structure is not known, LPL has a high degree of homology with another serine esterase, pancreatic lipase, whose structure is known. Based on similarities between LPL and pancreatic lipase, a model for LPL function has been suggested (Fig. 34–16), and five functional domains have been identified in LPL on the basis of structural and mutational studies.[142, 146]

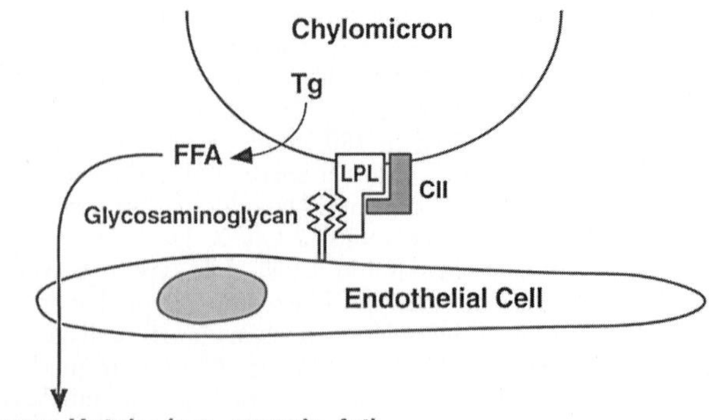

Figure 34–16. Lipoprotein lipase (LPL), attached by interaction with glycosaminoglycans on the endothelial cells, interacts with chylomicrons to catalyze the hydrolysis of the chylomicron triglycerides (Tg) to form free fatty acids (FFA). Apolipoprotein CII on the lipoprotein serves as a cofactor for LPL.

Heparin-Binding Site

The heparin-binding site mediates the interaction of LPL with HSPG on endothelial cells. Clusters of positively charged arginines and lysines on one face of LPL, particularly those in the carboxyl terminus, appear to mediate this interaction.

Lipid-Binding Site

The domain of the protein that allows the enzyme to interact with the surface of the chylomicron lies in the carboxyl terminus, particularly around residues 245 to 253.

Apolipoprotein CII–Binding Site

Apo-CII, an essential cofactor for LPL, binds to the carboxyl terminus at a site that has not been identified precisely.

Catalytic Site

This site mediates the hydrolysis of triglycerides, primarily to fatty acids and monoglyceride, and is postulated to involve serine-132, aspartic acid–156, and histidine-241, which are at the bottom of a hydrophobic channel that is covered by a flap or catalytic lid. The lid may mediate the interaction with the lipid substrate by assuming an open or closed conformation. LPL is a serine esterase with triglyceride hydrolase activity and, to a lesser extent, phospholipase activity.

LRP-Binding Site

The LRP-binding site is distinct from the heparin-binding site and involves the carboxyl-terminal domain. Through its interaction with the LRP, LPL can facilitate the binding and uptake of lipoproteins associated with the enzyme.

Hepatic Lipase

Hepatic lipase (about 53 kDa, 477 amino acids) is primarily a phospholipase but also possesses triglyceride hydrolase activity.[45, 47, 93, 144, 145, 147] It is synthesized by hepatocytes and is present primarily on liver endothelial cells and on HSPG in the space of Disse. Hepatic lipase is transported from the liver to the capillary endothelium of the adrenals, ovaries, and testes, where it functions in the release of lipids from lipoproteins for use in these organs. Its activity is increased by androgens and reduced by estrogens. Little is known about the structural domains of hepatic lipase except by analogy to similar domains within LPL, but the catalytic triad includes serine-145, aspartic acid–171, and histidine-256.

Hepatic lipase has several roles in lipoprotein metabolism.[93, 144, 147–149] First, it hydrolyzes triglycerides and possibly excess surface phospholipids in the final processing of chylomicron remnants. As suggested, this enzyme may be active in the space of Disse. It binds heparan sulfate and facilitates the interaction of remnant lipoproteins with the LRP, thereby delivering these lipoproteins to the receptor for internalization by hepatocytes. Second, it completes the processing of IDL to LDL (discussed in the section on IDL). Third, it participates in the conversion of HDL_2 to HDL_3 by the removal of triglyceride and phospholipid from HDL_2 (discussed in "Metabolic Pathways Involving High-Density Lipoproteins"). High levels of hepatic lipase activity decrease total HDL levels.

Contrasting Lipoprotein Lipase and Hepatic Lipase

LPL requires apo-CII as a cofactor to stimulate its catalytic activity, but apo-CII is not a cofactor for hepatic lipase. In contrast, apo-E may facilitate both triglyceride and phospholipid hydrolysis by hepatic lipase and may be a cofactor for its enzymatic activity.[150] In other respects, the enzymes are similar. After intravenous injection of heparin, both enzymes are released from endothelial cells of the liver and peripheral tissues and are referred to as postheparin lipase. Therefore, measurements of total plasma lipolytic activity after heparin injection reflect the activities of both enzymes.

Mutations that impair or inactivate LPL cause hypertriglyceridemia[145, 146] (discussed later). Likewise, deficiency of apo-CII prevents normal activation of LPL and also causes hypertriglyceridemia. Hepatic lipase deficiencies result in a variable and diverse pattern of lipoprotein changes, including the accumulation of remnant lipoproteins, IDL, and HDL_2. These changes are predictable on the basis of the functional roles of hepatic lipase. Knockout of the LPL gene in mice causes a particularly severe hypertriglyceridemia that becomes evident as soon as the newborns begin to suckle and causes death within the first 24 hours.[45] On the other hand, knockout of the hepatic lipase gene causes less severe manifestations, including changes in HDL and increased plasma phospholipid levels.[151] In the mouse, LPL may take on some of the functions subserved by hepatic lipase in other species. Overexpression of human hepatic lipase in transgenic mice[152] and rabbits[153] markedly decreases HDL and IDL.

Lecithin:Cholesterol Acyltransferase

LCAT circulates in association with HDL in the plasma and functions to esterify free cholesterol.[154] In humans, most of the cholesteryl esters in plasma lipoproteins are formed by the action of LCAT. The major substrate for LCAT is the small HDL particle; to a lesser extent, LDL is also a substrate. The enzyme catalyzes the transfer of long-chain fatty acids from phosphatidylcholine (linoleic acid at position 2 of lecithin preferred) to the hydroxyl group at position 3 on cholesterol. The structure and function of LCAT are discussed more thoroughly in the context of HDL metabolism.

Cholesteryl Ester Transfer Protein

The cholesteryl ester transfer protein (CETP) transfers cholesteryl esters from the larger HDL to VLDL, IDL, and remnant lipoproteins.[155, 156] In return, triglyceride from these lipoproteins is transferred to HDL. LCAT and CETP function in concert in HDL metabolism, and the structure and function of CETP are discussed further in the section on HDL.

PLASMA LIPOPROTEINS: STRUCTURE, FUNCTION, AND METABOLISM

Chylomicrons

Characteristics

Chylomicrons (density [*d*] < 0.95 g/mL) are the largest of the plasma lipoproteins (>1000 Å in diameter) and readily float after ultracentrifugation of plasma. They are composed of 98% to 99% lipid (85% to 90% triglyceride) and 1% to 2% protein (see Table 34–4). Chylomicrons are present in postprandial plasma (but absent after an overnight fast) and contain several apolipoproteins, including apo-B48, apo-AI, apo-AIV, apo-E, and the C apolipoproteins (see Fig. 34–6). The distinctive apolipoprotein is apo-B48, a form of apo-B that has an apparent molecular mass 48% that of apo-B100. Because it is the only form of apo-B synthesized by the intestine, apo-B48 is a marker for human lipoproteins produced by the intestinal epithelium.[8, 50–52]

Origin

Chylomicrons are produced by the epithelial cells of the small intestine (duodenum and proximal jejunum) when dietary fat and cholesterol are presented to the brush border of the epithelial cell membranes as bile acid micelles. Free fatty acids and monoglycerides taken up by the intestinal epithelial cells are synthesized into triglycerides in the ER in the apical region of the intestinal cells. Triglycerides, phospholipids, and cholesterol (absorbed or synthesized by the intestinal cells) are used for chylomicron formation in the Golgi apparatus, where some of the apolipoproteins undergo final carbohydrate processing, and the chylomicrons are secreted into the space along the lateral borders of the intestinal cells. From there, they enter the mesenteric lymph and proceed through the thoracic duct lymph to the general circulation. Newly synthesized chylomicrons possess apo-B48, apo-AI, and apo-AIV (intestinally synthesized apolipoproteins); they acquire apo-E and C apolipoproteins in the lymph and blood, primarily from HDL.

Metabolic Fate

In the circulation, LPL catalyzes the release of free fatty acids from chylomicron triglycerides and converts them into triglyceride-poor, cholesterol-enriched chylomicron remnants (Fig. 34–17). The free fatty acids are taken up by various tissues to be stored as triglyceride, oxidized as an energy source, or reutilized in hepatic lipoprotein–triglyceride synthesis. Hepatic lipase, acting primarily as a phospholipase and secondarily as a glyceride hydrolase, also plays a role in the final preparation of chylomicron remnants for uptake by hepatocytes. Chylomicron remnants are cleared rapidly from the plasma by the liver.[86, 93, 112, 113, 129] The metabolic pathways involved in their catabolism are discussed later in the chapter.

The pathways responsible for chylomicron remnant clearance are understood (Figs. 34–18 and 34–19). The remnants rapidly appear in the liver in the space of Disse, which is bounded by endothelial cells lining the liver blood sinusoids and by liver cells covered with microvilli. Apo-E on the surface of chylomicron remnants and newly secreted by hepatocytes is critical for initiating plasma clearance of these lipoproteins, but both the plasma clearance and the catabolism of these particles are complex.[77, 86, 93, 129]

Sequestration of chylomicron remnants within the space of Disse (see Fig. 34–18) appears to involve binding of the remnant lipoproteins to HSPG mediated by apo-E (or possibly LPL or hepatic lipase). The microvilli-covered surface of hepatocytes is coated with HSPG, which is abundant in the space of Disse. HSPGs bind apo-E by an ionic interaction between negatively charged sulfate groups of HSPG and basic amino acids within the 136 to 150 region of apo-E. The absence of proteoglycans on the cell surface impairs uptake of the particles.[93] Apo-E secreted by the hepatocytes appears to be bound to the cell-surface HSPG and further enhances the apo-E–mediated binding of remnant lipoproteins.

Chylomicron remnants may be *further processed* by lipases or other enzymes in the space of Disse. LPL is carried into the space of Disse on chylomicron remnants, and hepatic lipase produced by the liver may be localized there. These lipases facilitate the binding and uptake of remnants by interacting with the LRP.

The actual uptake of the particles by hepatocytes may involve two or more receptors (see Fig. 34–18), the *LDL recep-*

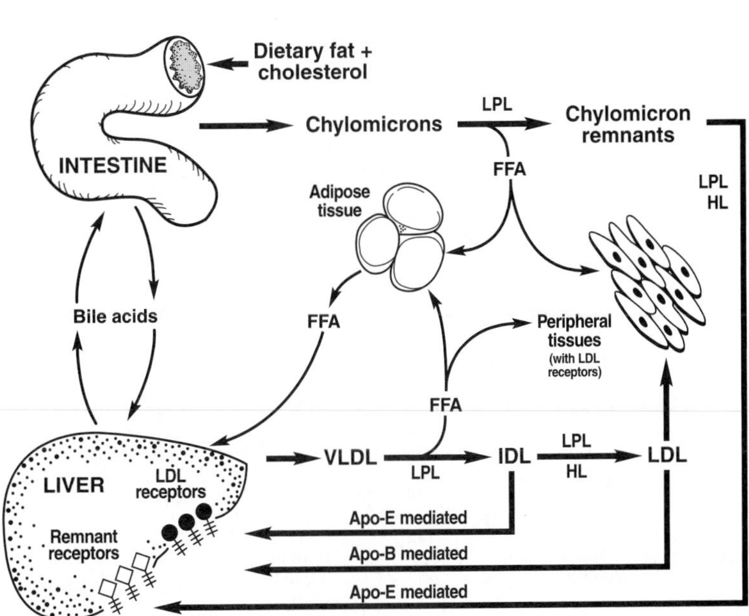

Figure 34–17. General scheme summarizing the major pathways involved in the metabolism of chylomicrons synthesized by the intestine and very-low-density lipoprotein (VLDL) synthesized by the liver. Apo-E, apolipoprotein E; FFA, free fatty acid; HL, hepatic lipase; IDL, intermediate-density lipoprotein. (Modified from Mahley RW. Biochemistry and physiology of lipid and lipoprotein metabolism. In Becker KL [ed]. Principles and Practice of Endocrinology and Metabolism, 2nd ed. Philadelphia, JB Lippincott, 1995, pp 1369–1378.)

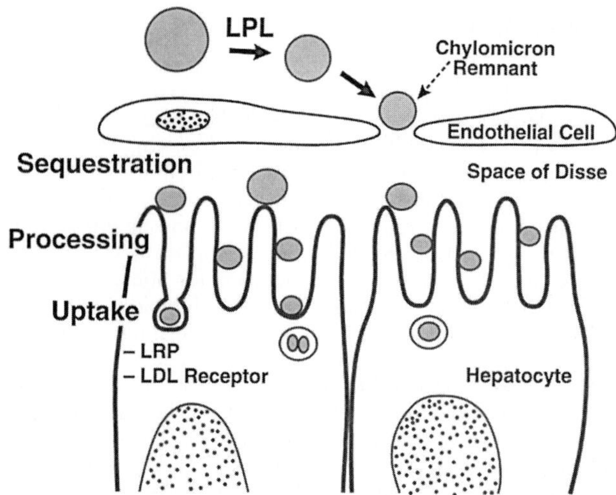

Figure 34–18. Pathways involved in chylomicron remnant metabolism. In *sequestration*, chylomicron remnants are trapped in the space of Disse, possibly through apolipoprotein E–mediated proteoglycan binding. In *processing*, enzymes, including lipases, may continue processing the remnants to smaller particles. In *uptake*, receptors involved in the uptake of the remnants appear to include the low-density lipoprotein (LDL) receptor and the LDL receptor–related protein (LRP).

tor, which interacts with lipoproteins containing apo-B100 and apo-E,[157] and possibly a unique apo-E or chylomicron remnant receptor, now known to be the LRP.[112, 113, 129, 158]

Whereas remnant particles with LPL or hepatic lipase on their surfaces may interact by means of these molecules with the HSPG in the space of Disse and facilitate binding and uptake by the LRP,[130, 131] apo-E–mediated interactions with HSPG and the LRP or the LDL receptor are critical in remnant metabolism. Patients with apo-E mutations that prevent interaction with HSPG or lipoprotein receptors develop hyperlipidemia characterized by remnant lipoprotein accumulation despite having normal lipase activity.[86, 93] In addition, knockout of apo-E by gene targeting in mice causes a massive accumulation of remnant lipoproteins.[95, 99]

Role of the Low-Density Lipoprotein Receptor in Remnant Catabolism

The LDL receptor plays a key role in chylomicron remnant uptake by the liver.[113, 157] The lack of accumulation of chylomicrons or chylomicron remnants in patients with absent or defective LDL receptors could reflect the fact that remnant clearance requires several steps, as described. For example, sequestration of the particles in the space of Disse (HSPG binding) is normal in patients with defective LDL receptors and could prevent the accumulation of remnants in plasma. Furthermore, the HSPG/LRP pathway can compensate for deficiency of LDL receptors. Both receptors probably function in the uptake of the remnants, and in the absence of one the other continues to function.

Chylomicron Remnant Receptors in Remnant Catabolism

Evidence suggests that the LRP is the chylomicron remnant (apo-E) receptor, which belongs to the LDL receptor gene family (discussed previously).[112, 113] As noted earlier, the LRP binds with high affinity to apo-E–enriched lipoproteins but does not bind LDL to a significant extent. Apo-E must be added to remnant lipoproteins before they bind to the LRP with high affinity. Apo-E exists in the space of Disse in high concentration, probably because it is secreted by hepatocytes and binds to HSPG in the space of Disse. The HSPG may serve as a reservoir for apo-E, allowing enrichment of the remnants with this apolipoprotein (see Fig. 34–19).[86, 93, 113, 129]

These and other observations have led to the hypothesis that apo-E functions in a process called *secretion-capture*.[93, 158–160] It is envisioned that apo-E combines with lipids or lipoproteins and directs them to cells expressing LDL receptors or the LRP. In the liver, the LRP and apo-E could interact in this way to capture chylomicron remnants (see Fig. 34–19). The LRP is also present in other tissues, including brain, and may function locally in the uptake of lipids. The secretion-capture role of apo-E functions in peripheral nerve injury and repair and in the normal maintenance of neurons.[77, 81–83]

As already stated, LRP-mediated uptake of remnants requires the initial interaction of apo-E–containing lipoproteins with cell-surface HSPG (see Fig. 34–19).[93] If HSPGs are hydrolyzed by treating cells with heparinase in vitro or by infusing heparinase into the portal vein of mice, apo-E–enriched remnants do not bind to the cell surface and do not interact with the LRP even though the receptor is present. After the lipoproteins interact with HSPG, the remnants may be transferred to the LRP for internalization by the cells, or the HSPG/LRP complex may be internalized. This two-step process involving cell-surface proteoglycans and receptors is referred to as the HSPG/LRP pathway; a similar two-step proc-

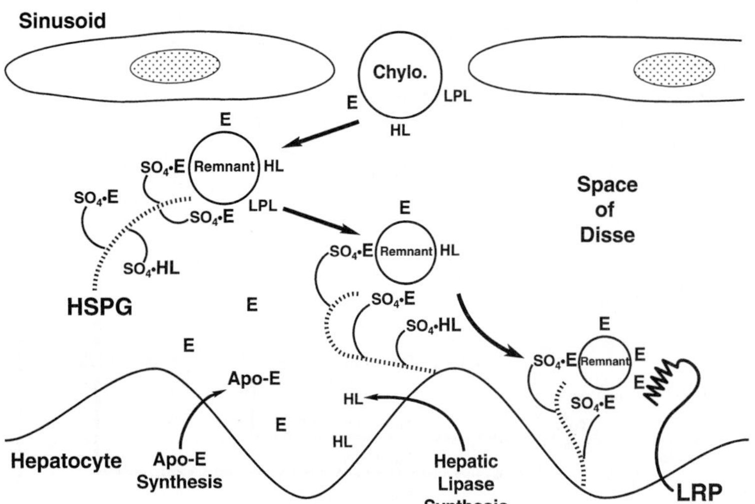

Figure 34–19. Heparan sulfate proteoglycan (HSPG)/low-density lipoprotein (LDL) receptor–related protein (LRP) pathway. Apo-E, apolipoprotein E; HL, hepatic lipase; LPL, lipoprotein lipase.

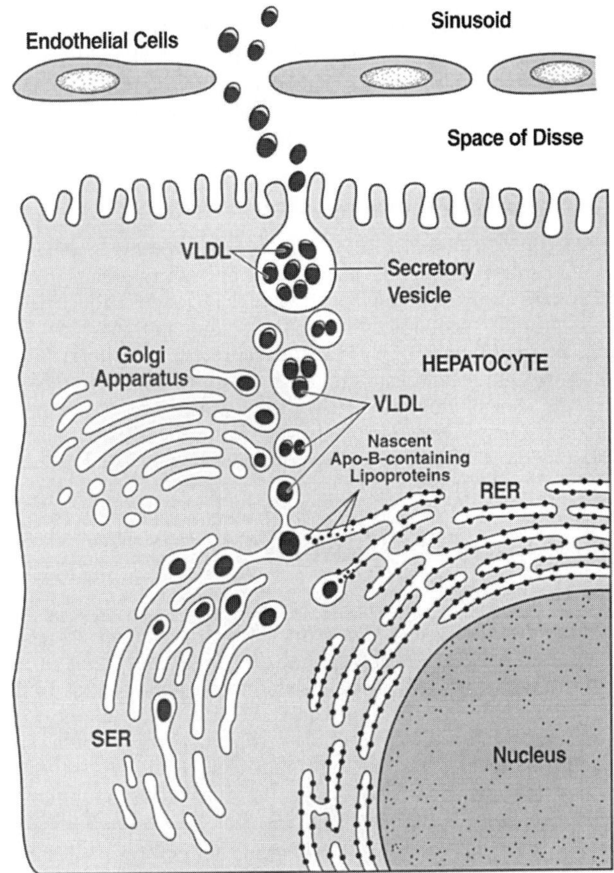

Figure 34–20. Very-low-density lipoprotein (VLDL) biosynthesis by hepatocytes. The nascent apolipoprotein B (apo-B)–containing apolipoproteins synthesized by the rough endoplasmic reticulum (RER) apparently combine with the lipids in the smooth endoplasmic reticulum (SER). The VLDLs are processed in the Golgi apparatus and accumulate in large secretory vesicles. They are then released into the space of Disse, from which they enter the plasma. (Modified from Alexander CA, Hamilton RL, Havel RJ. Subcellular localization of B apoprotein of plasma lipoproteins in rat liver. J Cell Biol 1976; 69: 241–263; by copyright permission of The Rockefeller University Press)

ess has also been described for growth factors.[83, 93, 160–162] It is also possible that HSPG alone can mediate remnant uptake directly without the LRP.

The LRP interacts not only with apo-E–containing lipoproteins but also with an unrelated protein, α_2-macroglobulin, a broad-spectrum endopeptidase inhibitor that is involved in clearing of proteases from the plasma by the liver. The binding of protease activates α_2-macroglobulin, which then binds to the LRP. Activated α_2-macroglobulin competes with remnants for binding to the LRP.[129] Radiolabeled chylomicron remnants are rapidly cleared from the plasma of mice, but the injection of α_2-macroglobulin along with the chylomicron remnants impairs remnant clearance. This finding indicates that α_2-macroglobulin and the remnants are binding to the same receptor, the LRP.

Herz and colleagues demonstrated that the LRP is the chylomicron remnant (apo-E) receptor and documented its importance in remnant catabolism.[112–114] These studies used RAP, which blocks the interaction of all ligands with the LRP, to demonstrate the role of the LRP in remnant clearance in mice. Knockout of RAP in mice results in a loss of LRP expression in the liver. Double-knockout mice, in which both RAP and the LDL receptor are missing, develop hyperlipidemia characterized by the accumulation of remnant lipoproteins in the plasma.[133]

In summary, the catabolism of chylomicron remnants involves several steps and several components: sequestration, further lipolytic processing, and receptor-mediated endocytosis utilizing both the LDL receptor pathway and the HSPG/LRP pathway.

Very-Low-Density Lipoproteins

Characteristics

VLDLs are particles 300 to 700 Å in diameter that float on ultracentrifugation at a density of less than 1.006 g/mL (see Table 34–4). They are composed of 85% to 90% lipid (about 55% triglyceride, 20% cholesterol, and 15% phospholipid) and 10% to 15% protein. The distinctive apolipoprotein is apo-B100, the hepatic form of apo-B. VLDLs also contain apo-E and C apolipoproteins (see Fig. 34–6). VLDLs have pre-β or α_2-electrophoretic mobility and were previously called pre-β lipoproteins.[4, 8, 46, 47]

Origin

VLDLs are synthesized by the liver, and their production is stimulated by increased delivery of free fatty acids to the hepatocytes, either from a high intake of dietary fat or from the mobilization of fatty acids from adipose tissue with fasting or uncontrolled diabetes mellitus. Triglycerides and phospholipids to be used in the formation of VLDL are synthesized in the liver, whereas VLDL cholesterol can be synthesized de novo or reutilized from LDL cholesterol (LDL-C). The VLDL particles are first visible at the junction of the rough ER and the smooth ER (transitional elements) before they enter the Golgi apparatus.[163] Several of the apolipoproteins undergo carbohydrate processing within the Golgi apparatus. Large Golgi secretory vesicles migrate to the brush border surface of the hepatocytes, fuse with the plasma membrane, and release the VLDL particles into the space of Disse, where they enter the plasma (Fig. 34–20). The major protein constituents of the newly synthesized VLDLs are apo-B100, apo-E, and small amounts of the C apolipoproteins. In plasma, VLDLs acquire additional C apolipoproteins and apo-E, primarily from HDL.

Control of Very-Low-Density Lipoprotein Secretion Rate

The quantity of VLDL secreted from the liver is not controlled by changes in apo-B100 mRNA levels. Apo-B100 is constitutively expressed and is not highly variable.[164–167] Newly synthesized apo-B100 is subject to two fates: (1) it can be combined with lipid to form VLDL particles, or (2) it can be degraded, in which case a VLDL particle is not secreted.[168] If there is a stimulus for VLDL production, such as the delivery of free fatty acids to the liver, the balance is shifted away from apo-B100 degradation to the formation and secretion of apo-B100–containing VLDL.

Biosynthesis of Very-Low-Density Lipoproteins

Newly synthesized apo-B100 is translocated across the rough ER membrane. If not sufficiently lipidated as it is translocated, apo-B100 is destined to be degraded. If sufficient lipid is available, the apo-B100 binds the lipid as it enters the ER and forms triglyceride-rich particles. These particles can increase in size, enter the secretory pathway, and exit from the cell as mature VLDLs (see Fig. 34–20).[67, 68, 167, 169]

The newly synthesized apo-B100 could associate with the

inner leaflet of the ER and serve as a lipid nucleation site capable of accepting triglycerides to form a central core for the VLDL particles. Triglycerides and possibly cholesteryl esters and phospholipids are transferred into the particle by the microsomal triglyceride transfer protein (MTP),[170, 171] and additional triglyceride, cholesterol, and phospholipid may be added as the VLDL precursor passes through the lumen of the rough ER. At the junction of the rough and smooth ER, lipid-rich particles lacking apo-B have been identified in rat liver, and these particles may fuse with the apo-B–containing VLDL precursors to form the mature particle.[163, 172] However, because rat liver synthesizes both apo-B100– and apo-B48–containing VLDLs, the fusion step may apply only to apo-B48 VLDL and may be more relevant to apo-B48–containing chylomicron synthesis by the intestine.

Microsomal Triglyceride Transfer Protein

MTP is produced in the liver at sites where apo-B100–containing VLDLs are synthesized and in the intestine at sites where apo-B48–containing chylomicrons are synthesized. MTP (97 kDa) occurs as a heterodimer complex with the 58-kDa protein disulfide isomerase, an association required for MTP activity. Protein disulfide isomerase reshuffles disulfide bonds of cysteine residues and therefore may play a role in altering the conformation of apo-B for lipidation. In addition to transferring triglycerides to these lipoprotein particles, MTP transfers cholesteryl esters and phospholipids.[170, 171]

More than a dozen mutations of MTP interfere with its activity. Defective MTP is responsible for the lipid disorder abetalipoproteinemia, a condition in which patients essentially lack apo-B–containing lipoproteins in plasma.[171] Therefore, MTP is critical for the biosynthesis of both apo-B100 VLDLs in the liver and apo-B48 chylomicrons in the intestine.

The luminal surfaces of the hepatocytes express LDL receptors and the LRP, and VLDLs possess both apo-B100 and apo-E that can react with these receptors. How then do VLDLs traverse the space of Disse and enter the blood? First, lipids such as phosphatidylethanolamine on the surface of the newly secreted VLDLs may alter the reactivity of the lipoproteins with the receptors. Newly secreted VLDLs are rich in phosphatidylethanolamine, but VLDLs in the circulation are poor in phosphatidylethanolamine. This phospholipid may prevent the particle from interacting with the receptors (i.e., specific lipids may mask the receptor-binding domains of apo-B100 and apo-E).

Second, other apolipoproteins may mask the receptor-binding domains of the VLDL apo-B100 and apo-E. Although they are present in small amounts on newly secreted VLDLs, the C apolipoproteins may alter the conformation or availability of apolipoproteins that interact with lipoprotein receptors. Specifically, when VLDLs are formed in the liver and acquire apo-E, the C apolipoproteins may be positioned so as to mask the apo-E and thereby block its ability to react with the receptor or with proteoglycans in the space of Disse. Alternatively, apo-E associated with the particles intracellularly may not be available to bind to the receptors; only newly acquired apo-E obtained from HDL may have the appropriate conformation for receptor binding.

Metabolic Fate

VLDL triglycerides are hydrolyzed by the actions of LPL and hepatic lipase. They are converted to smaller and smaller particles that become increasingly rich in cholesterol (see Fig. 34–17). The products of VLDL catabolism are IDLs (d = 1.006 to 1.019 g/mL). IDLs retain apo-B100 and apo-E but have lost most of the C apolipoproteins. IDLs are processed to LDLs (d = 1.019 to 1.063 g/mL) by LPL with final processing by hepatic lipase. Approximately half of VLDLs are converted to LDLs, and the remainder are cleared directly by the liver as VLDL remnants (small VLDL) and IDLs (see Fig. 34–17). The uptake of VLDL remnants and IDLs by liver parenchymal cells is mediated by apo-E, and the uptake of LDL by the LDL receptor is mediated by apo-B100.[4, 14, 47, 77]

Intermediate-Density Lipoproteins

IDLs (d = 1.006 to 1.019 g/mL) are normally present in low concentrations in the plasma and are intermediate in size and composition between VLDL and LDL (see Table 34–4). Their primary proteins are apo-B100 and apo-E.[4, 8, 47] The IDLs are precursors of LDLs and represent metabolic products of VLDL catabolism in the plasma by the action of lipases. As shown in Figure 34–17, IDLs may be further processed by hepatic lipase or removed from the plasma by the LDL receptor. IDLs are often considered to be VLDL remnants and to be atherogenic.

Low-Density Lipoproteins

Characteristics

LDLs (d = 1.019 to 1.063 g/mL), which are about 200 Å in diameter, are the major cholesterol-carrying lipoproteins in the plasma; about 70% of total plasma cholesterol is in LDL. LDLs are composed of approximately 75% lipid (about 35% cholesteryl ester, 10% free cholesterol, 10% triglyceride, and 20% phospholipid) and 25% protein (see Table 34–4). Apo-B100 is the principal protein in these particles, along with trace amounts of apo-E (see Fig. 34–6). LDLs have β-electrophoretic mobility and were previously referred to as β lipoproteins.[1, 4, 8, 47]

Origin

LDLs are the end products of lipase-mediated hydrolysis of VLDLs (see Fig. 34–17). Moreover, as the triglyceride-rich core of the larger VLDL particles is removed, the surface lipids and proteins are remodeled and excess surface constituents are transferred to HDL, resulting in the formation of a small, cholesterol-rich LDL devoid of almost all apolipoproteins except apo-B100.

Metabolic Fate

About 75% of LDL is taken up by hepatocytes. Other tissues take up smaller amounts of LDL. Approximately two thirds of the uptake is mediated by the LDL receptor, and the remainder is mediated by a poorly defined process that does not involve receptors. LDLs are considered to be atherogenic.

Apolipoproteins B and E Determine Rate of Plasma Lipoprotein Clearance

The rate of clearance of lipoproteins from the plasma is determined by the apolipoprotein that mediates the interaction with the receptor and by the number of receptors expressed on the cell surface (primarily in the liver). VLDL and IDL are rapidly cleared from the plasma (their half-lives are measured in minutes to a few hours). Apo-E mediates their binding to the LDL receptors. Multiple apo-E molecules per lipoprotein can interact with more than one receptor or with multiple sites on a receptor. Multiple interactions enhance binding affinity and increase the clearance of these particles from the plasma. The clearance of LDL is mediated by apo-B100. The affinity of apo-B100 for the LDL receptor is lower than that of apo-E, and clearance of LDL is much slower (with a half-life of 2 to

3 days). Compared with apo-B100–containing LDLs, apo-E–containing lipoproteins have 20-fold greater affinity for the LDL receptor.[8, 46, 63, 77]

This difference in affinity may affect the circulating levels of lipoproteins containing apo-B100 and apo-E. In the presence of high levels of apo-E associated with remnants, VLDL, and IDL, these lipoproteins compete effectively with LDL for binding to the LDL receptor, and LDL levels can rise. Conversely, in the presence of low levels of apo-E or apo-E that is defective in receptor-binding activity (apo-E2 associated with type III hyperlipoproteinemia), these lipoproteins do not compete effectively with LDL for the LDL receptor; as a result, the LDL concentrations are lower. Thus, the difference in the affinities of apo-B100 and apo-E plays a role in plasma cholesterol homeostasis.

Role for Lipoprotein Cholesterol in Cellular Metabolism

All cells can synthesize cholesterol de novo.[1, 2, 4–6] However, LDL serves as a source of cholesterol for many cells. Cholesterol taken up by the liver has several fates: membrane biosynthesis, VLDL biosynthesis, excretion as cholesterol in the bile, and conversion to bile acids. Cholesterol is used as a precursor for steroid hormone production in the adrenals, ovaries, and testes. In other peripheral tissues, cholesterol is used in membrane biosynthesis for cell repair and proliferation.

Factors Affecting Low-Density Lipoprotein Levels in the Blood

Plasma LDL levels can be increased through two primary mechanisms: (1) increased VLDL biosynthesis and secretion caused by increased flux of free fatty acids to the liver from dietary fats or from mobilization from adipose tissue and (2) decreased LDL catabolism. Decreased catabolism can result from (1) decreased LDL receptor levels in hepatic and extrahepatic tissues (LDL receptor expression is down-regulated when cells have enough cholesterol for their metabolic needs or when diets are high in saturated fat and cholesterol), (2) increased numbers of high-affinity apo-E–containing lipoproteins that compete with LDL for receptor interaction (as discussed previously), (3) defective LDL receptors incapable of normal interaction with apo-B100, and (4) defective apo-B100 incapable of normal interaction with LDL receptors.

High-Density Lipoproteins

Characteristics

HDLs are small particles (70 to 120 Å in diameter) that float at densities of 1.063 to 1.21 g/mL. They are somewhat arbitrarily divided into two major subclasses: HDL_2 (d = 1.063 to 1.125 g/mL) and HDL_3 (d = 1.125 to 1.21 g/mL). HDLs contain about 50% lipid (25% phospholipid, 15% cholesteryl ester, 5% free cholesterol, and 5% triglyceride) and 50% protein (see Table 34–4). Their major apolipoproteins are apo-AI (65%), apo-AII (25%), and smaller amounts of the C apolipoproteins and apo-E (see Fig. 34–6). Apo-E is a minor component of a subclass of HDL referred to as HDL_1, but about 50% of total plasma apo-E is in this HDL fraction. The major classes of HDLs lack apo-E and therefore do not interact with the LDL receptor. HDLs serve as a reservoir for apo-E and the C apolipoproteins to be distributed to other lipoproteins when they enter the plasma (e.g., chylomicrons, VLDLs). Subclasses of HDL may contain only apo-AI (called LpAI) or apo-AI and apo-AII (called LpAI/AII). Although LpAI and LpAI/AII do not correspond directly to the ultracentrifugal fractions, LpAI corresponds primarily to HDL_2 and LpAI/AII to HDL_3. The HDLs as a class have α-electrophoretic mobility and previously were referred to as α lipoproteins.[8, 45, 47, 96, 97, 99]

Origin

HDLs originate from three major sources (Fig. 34–21). First, the liver secretes an apo-AI–phospholipid disc called nascent or precursor HDL. Second, the intestine directly synthesizes a small apo-AI–containing HDL particle. Third, HDLs are derived from surface material (primarily apo-AI and phospholipid) that comes from chylomicrons and VLDLs during lipolysis. As chylomicrons and VLDLs are acted on by LPL and the triglyceride-rich core is hydrolyzed, excess material is shed from the surface of the particle in combination with apo-AI to form small HDL discs. The phospholipid transfer protein facilitates the shedding of the surface material during lipolytic processing of triglyceride-rich lipoproteins to generate the HDL precursors.[173]

Maturation of High-Density Lipoproteins

The nascent or precursor HDL particles exist as apo-AI–phospholipid discs. Designated pre-β_1, pre-β_2, and pre-β_3,[47, 99, 174] these discs are excellent acceptors of free cholesterol from cell membranes with excess cholesterol or from other lipoproteins. The pre-β phospholipid discs can accommodate only a limited amount of free cholesterol. However, esterification of the cholesterol with a long-chain fatty acid increases its hydrophobicity, and the newly formed cholesteryl ester moves away from the surface of the disc, beginning the process of forming a cholesteryl ester–rich core and converting the disc to a sphere. The enzyme in plasma that converts free cholesterol to cholesteryl ester is LCAT.

The small, spherical, mature HDL particles (HDL_3) also serve as acceptors for free cholesterol; as more free cholesterol is acquired and esterified, the particles increase in size, forming HDL_2. These HDL subclasses can include LpAI, or they can be converted to LpAI/AII particles by the addition of apo-AII.

In some animals and to a lesser extent in humans, HDL_2 can be further enriched in cholesteryl ester and at the same time acquire apo-E (Fig. 34–22). These apo-E–containing HDL_1 are a minor but metabolically active subclass of HDL.[8, 46, 63] The presence of apo-E targets the HDL_1 to cells expressing the LDL receptor. Typical HDLs lack apo-E and do not interact with the LDL receptor. The HDL_1 represent a major HDL class in many lower species and in humans with abetalipoproteinemia or CETP deficiency.

HDL_1 can also arise from a precursor particle that displays γ-electrophoretic mobility and is called γLp-E.[175] This particle is approximately 80% protein and 20% lipid (primarily sphin-

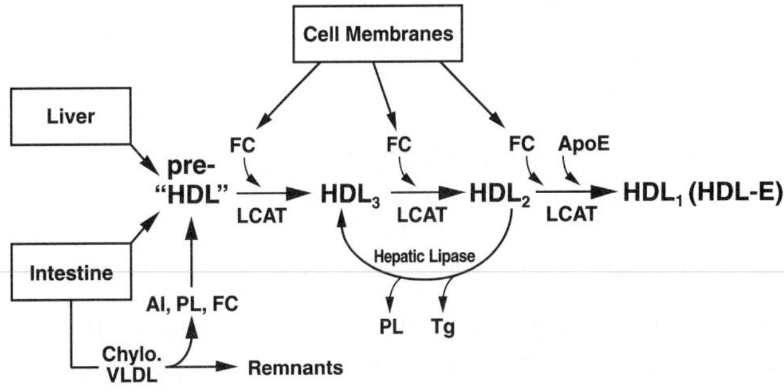

Figure 34–21. Origin of high-density lipoprotein (HDL) from liver, intestine, and surface material from chylomicrons and very-low-density lipoprotein (VLDL). AI, apo-AI; FC, free cholesterol; HDL-E, HDL with apo-E; LCAT, lecithin:cholesterol acyltransferase; PL, phospholipid; Tg, triglyceride.

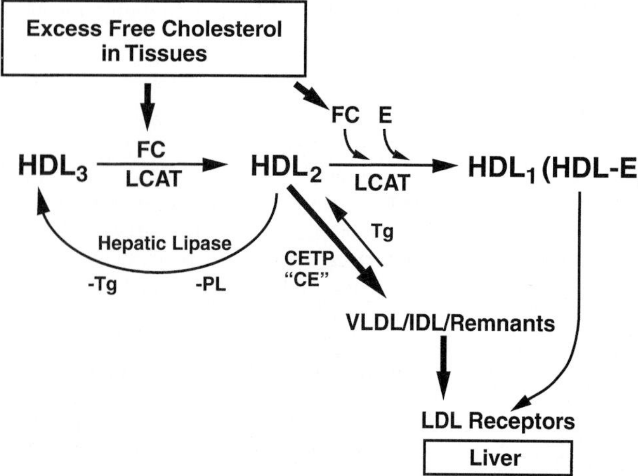

Figure 34–22. Role of high-density lipoprotein (HDL) in the redistribution of lipids from cells with excess cholesterol to cells requiring cholesterol or to the liver for excretion. The reverse cholesterol transport pathway is indicated by bold arrows (net transfer of cholesterol from cells → HDL → LDL → liver). CETP, cholesteryl ester transfer protein; FC, free cholesterol; HDL-E, HDL-with apolipoprotein E; IDL, intermediate-density lipoprotein; LCAT, lecithin:cholesterol acyltransferase; LDL, low-density lipoprotein; PL, phospholipid; Tg, triglyceride; VLDL, very-low-density lipoprotein.

gomyelin and phosphatidylcholine, with some free cholesterol). The γLp-E is a good acceptor of free cholesterol from cells and appears to be converted to the larger HDL_1 by the action of LCAT. HDL_1 also contains apo-AI and sometimes apo-AII. It is difficult to fractionate these various subclasses of HDL.

Acquisition of Cholesterol by High-Density Lipoproteins

HDL, especially HDL_3, precursors of mature HDL, and lipid-poor apo-AI, can acquire cholesterol from cells by two mechanisms: aqueous transfer from cells and transport facilitated by a cell-surface binding protein.[176]

Aqueous Transfer from Cells

The HDLs come in close contact with cells having excess cholesterol and acquire free cholesterol (not cholesteryl ester) from the cell surface. Free cholesterol follows a physicochemical concentration gradient from the cell to the HDL particle, from a high concentration of free cholesterol in the membranes of cells with excess cholesterol to a low concentration at the surface of the HDL. This process is referred to as passive desorption.[177]

Transport Facilitated by a Cell-Surface Binding Protein

At least two cell-surface proteins facilitate the efflux of free cholesterol from cells possessing excess cholesterol. The class B, type I scavenger receptor (SR-BI) binds HDL particles to the cell surface. This receptor may alter the organization of the cell membrane lipids facilitating the efflux of free cholesterol from the membrane to the lipoprotein. The HDLs are not internalized by the cell and are released into the circulation when the particle is enriched in cholesterol.[178–180] The second receptor that participates in the efflux of cholesterol from cells is the ATP binding cassette transporter A1 (ABCA1). It appears to bind apo-AI or a pre-β HDL disc to the cell membrane and facilitate the transfer of free cholesterol and phospholipid from the cell to enrich the HDL precursors in these lipids.[181, 182] Mutations in ABCA1 prevent the efflux of cholesterol from cells, resulting in absence of mature HDL and rapid catabolism of apo-AI and causing the lipid disorder called Tangier disease.[183, 184]

Enzyme Involved in High-Density Lipoprotein Metabolism: Lecithin:Cholesterol Acyltransferase

LCAT (47 kDa, 416 amino acids) is synthesized as a glycoprotein (25% of total mass is carbohydrate) primarily by the liver and to a lesser extent in the brain and testes.[148, 154, 185–187] In the plasma, it is associated primarily with LpAI or pre-β_3 and small mature HDL and to a lesser extent with LDL. Activated by apo-AI (and by apo-CI and apo-AIV), LCAT is responsible for the production of most cholesteryl esters in plasma lipoproteins in humans. Although HDLs are the preferred substrate for LCAT, a small proportion of free cholesterol is esterified on LDLs; LCAT has both α-LCAT activity (acting on HDL) and β-LCAT activity (acting on LDL). In the human disorder called fish-eye disease, a single amino acid substitution of threonine for isoleucine-123 blocks the ability of LCAT to esterify cholesterol in HDL, but the mutated protein still catalyzes the esterification of cholesterol on LDL. Therefore, this form of LCAT deficiency is less severe than complete LCAT deficiency.

LCAT has two different enzymatic activities. First, *lecithin cleavage (phospholipase activity)* involves the ester bond of the fatty acid in position 2 of lecithin, which is usually linoleic acid (C18:2), yielding lysolecithin and the fatty acid. The fatty acid becomes covalently linked to serine-181 in the LCAT molecule. Second, *transesterification (transacylase activity)* involves the transfer of the fatty acid attached to LCAT to the 3β-hydroxyl position of cholesterol, forming a cholesteryl ester. The mechanism for the transfer of the fatty acid to cholesterol has not been well defined.

Much has been learned about the normal function of LCAT in lipoprotein metabolism by studying patients who have low or undetectable activity of this enzyme in plasma. LCAT deficiency can be caused by mutations that affect the structure of LCAT or of apo-AI. The disorder is manifested by low levels of cholesteryl esters, low levels of HDL, and clinical features ranging from mild symptoms such as corneal clouding (caused by accumulation of free cholesterol in the cornea) to severe disorders such as renal failure (see "Lecithin:Cholesterol Acyltransferase Deficiency").

Metabolic Pathways Involving High-Density Lipoproteins

HDLs function in the redistribution of lipids among lipoproteins and cells by a process called *reverse cholesterol transport*.[188] HDLs acquire cholesterol from cells and transport it to the liver for excretion or to other cells that require cholesterol. The scheme is shown in Figure 34–22.[8, 99, 154]

HDL_3 particles are converted to HDL_2 and then to HDL_1, as described earlier. Apo-E, which is associated with HDL_1, targets this minor HDL subclass to cells expressing LDL receptors.[46, 63] In this way, cholesterol can be redistributed from cells with excess cholesterol to cells that require cholesterol. This apo-E–mediated pathway may also deliver cholesterol to the liver for excretion. HDL_1 is a major transport pathway for cholesteryl ester delivery to the liver in some species (mice, rats, and dogs) but not in humans.

A second pathway of cholesterol redistribution involves CETP (see Fig. 34–22).[101–103, 150, 156, 189] CETP transfers cholesteryl ester from HDL_2 to VLDL, IDL, LDL, and remnants.

The cholesterol is thus delivered indirectly to the liver through VLDL and chylomicron remnant pathways. In exchange for transfer of the cholesteryl ester, CETP transfers triglyceride from VLDL, IDL, LDL, and remnants to HDL_2, which becomes enriched with triglycerides. The CETP pathway is the major route for the transport and delivery of cholesteryl esters from HDL to the liver in humans, nonhuman primates, and rabbits.

HDL_2 Is Reconverted to HDL_3 to Regenerate These Cholesterol Acceptors

As stated previously, HDL_2 particles are partially depleted of cholesteryl esters and enriched in triglycerides by the action of CETP. Hepatic lipase can then act on the large, triglyceride-enriched HDL_2 to hydrolyze the triglycerides (and possibly excess phospholipids), converting HDL_2 to HDL_3.[149, 190] HDL_3 serves as an acceptor of free cholesterol, thus perpetuating the HDL_2-HDL_3 cycle (see Fig. 34–22).[8, 47, 99, 174]

The catabolism of HDL is not entirely understood. Specific lipid moieties of HDL can be taken up by cells without removal of the intact particle from the plasma compartment. For example, cholesteryl esters are removed from the particle by selective uptake and preferentially delivered to the liver, adrenal glands, and gonads.[179, 191] The SR-BI can facilitate the transfer of cholesteryl esters from HDL to cells without the lipoprotein particle entering the cell or being degraded. The SR-BI appears to function by transferring cholesteryl ester through a hydrophilic channel formed in the cell membrane.[179] Hepatic lipase may be involved in the selective uptake of cholesterol from the HDL by hydrolyzing the phospholipids on the particles and creating a chemical gradient that promotes the transfer of cholesterol from the particle to the cell. Recall that hepatic lipase is localized in the space of Disse of the liver and in the adrenal glands and ovaries. In the kidneys, apo-AI is removed in preference to cholesterol; this apo-AI may be dissociated from the HDL particle, filtered, and degraded. Ultimately, intact HDL can be taken up by hepatocytes and degraded. Although HDL_1 represents a small fraction of total HDL, it is taken up directly by LDL receptors and degraded in the liver through the LDL pathway.

Selective Uptake of Cholesterol by Steroidogenic Cells

HDL is more efficient than LDL in delivering cholesterol to steroidogenic cells of the adrenal, ovary, and testis. In these organs, the lipoproteins concentrate on the surface of cells in microvillar channels.[179, 192] The channels appear to represent flaps of cell-surface membrane that form a 150- to 250-Å–wide cleft in which the lipoproteins are trapped at least transiently. Within these channels, cholesteryl ester and free cholesterol can be extracted from the HDLs without the particles' being endocytosed or degraded. Hepatic lipase is selectively localized to the same organs and is believed to modify HDL so as to facilitate the selective uptake of cholesterol. Presumably, the particles are released to reenter the circulation after some cholesterol is extracted.

The importance of HDL and specifically apo-AI–containing HDL for delivery of cholesterol to steroidogenic cells has been shown in apo-AI knockout mice.[179] In the adrenal glands, the reticularis and fasciculata cells are usually loaded with lipid droplets. In knockout mice, however, there is no lipid in these cells, lipoproteins are absent from the microvillar channels, and luteal cells of the ovary and Leydig's cells of the testis have markedly reduced levels of lipid. However, lipid and cell-surface lipoprotein particles are present in the adrenal gland, ovary, or testis of knockout mice lacking apo-AII or apo-E. Therefore, apo-AI appears to play an important role, possibly by targeting the particles to the channels or by providing particles with the proper composition to allow their entry into the channels for selective delivery of cholesterol to the cells. The importance of the apo-AI–HDL pathway in delivering cholesterol to the adrenal is further shown by the blunted synthesis and secretion of glucocorticoids in apo-AI knockout mice that are acutely stressed.

Cholesteryl Ester Transfer Protein

CETP facilitates the transfer of cholesteryl esters from HDL to the lower density, triglyceride-rich lipoproteins (primarily VLDL, IDL, and remnants).[155] CETP plays a pivotal role in lipid metabolism and may affect susceptibility or resistance to the development of atherosclerosis.[193, 194] For example, humans, nonhuman primates, and rabbits have significant amounts of CETP activity in their plasma. As a consequence, they form only small amounts of HDL_1; they dispose of most of their HDL cholesteryl esters by delivering them to lower density lipoproteins (see Fig. 34–22). Ultimately, most of the cholesteryl esters leave the plasma by the LDL pathway. These species are susceptible to atherosclerosis and tend to have higher levels of LDL. On the other hand, rats, mice, and dogs have no CETP activity, readily form HDL_1, and can deliver the cholesterol directly to the liver by the apo-E–mediated pathway. These animals have very low levels of LDL and are resistant to the development of atherosclerosis. These observations suggest that high levels of CETP activity accelerate atherogenesis and that inhibition of CETP may be beneficial in treating certain types of hyperlipidemia.

However, this concept has been brought into question by the observation that Japanese Americans with a deficiency of CETP have increased HDL but nevertheless develop CHD.[155, 195] The HDL in these subjects tends to be the large HDL_1, and levels of the smaller HDL_3 are decreased. If these data concerning the atherogenicity of low CETP activity are confirmed, it may mean that low levels of HDL_3, which serves as the most potent acceptor of cellular cholesterol, are a major risk factor for CHD in these subjects; alternatively, high levels of the large apo-E–containing HDL_1 may be atherogenic.

Data obtained through overexpression of CETP in transgenic mice do not clarify whether high levels are protective or detrimental.[45, 97, 155, 194] In one study, overexpression of CETP led to accelerated atherogenesis,[196] but in a study in which CETP was overexpressed in hypertriglyceridemic mice expressing high levels of apo-CIII, there was less atherosclerosis even though the mice were hyperlipidemic and had low HDL levels.[155] The potential therapeutic value of lowering CETP to retard atherogenesis must be questioned until these inconsistencies are sorted out.

High-Density Lipoproteins as Antiatherogenic Lipoproteins

Numerous studies have demonstrated that high levels of HDL-C are associated with a lower incidence of CHD. Conversely, low levels of HDL-C are associated with a higher incidence of CHD.[197] The protective mechanism involving HDL may be related to its role in reverse cholesterol transport, which results in redistribution of cholesterol away from the artery wall. Although low HDL-C is a major CHD risk factor, it must be kept in mind that the HDLs are a heterogeneous group of molecules having different metabolic roles. Some may be protective (e.g., LpAI, HDL_2), and others may not be (e.g., LpAI/AII). As the complex nature of HDL is unraveled, it may be possible to define an antiatherogenic spectrum of HDL particles and determine the metabolic and therapeutic measures needed to alter these HDLs selectively.

LIPIDS AND ATHEROSCLEROSIS

Atherosclerosis causes a reduction of blood flow and insufficient delivery of oxygen and nutrients to affected organs. Insufficient oxygen results in ischemia or infarction, leading to angina or myocardial infarction in the case of restricted blood flow to the heart muscle, to stroke with reduced blood flow to the brain, or to intermittent claudication with restricted blood flow to the lower extremities. CHD is the leading cause of death in the United States and in western Europe.

The restricted arterial blood flow in atherosclerosis is caused by changes in the vessel wall characterized by lipid deposition and cell proliferation. Narrowing of the vessel lumen may lead to obstruction and, more important, to unstable plaques susceptible to ulceration or fissure formation causing thrombosis.[198] The deposited lipids are derived from plasma lipoproteins, and elevated plasma cholesterol represents a major risk factor. Other important risk factors include low HDL levels, cigarette smoking, hypertension, male sex, diabetes mellitus, obesity, stress, and lack of exercise.[9, 199] The discussion here focuses on plasma lipoproteins and the cholesterol-diet-heart hypothesis.

Cholesterol-Diet-Heart Hypothesis

For the last 40 years, evidence linking high plasma cholesterol concentrations with an increased risk for CHD has been accumulating,[9, 28–30, 200, 201] and the evidence is now overwhelming and indisputable. The cholesterol-diet-heart hypothesis states (1) that increased plasma cholesterol concentrations increase the risk of CHD, (2) that diets high in fat (especially saturated fat) and cholesterol result in increased levels of plasma cholesterol, and (3) that lowering plasma cholesterol levels results in a decreased risk of CHD.

Animal Models

Numerous animal models have demonstrated that diets enriched in cholesterol and saturated fat elevate plasma cholesterol levels and lead to atherosclerosis with many features of the human disease.[202–205] Studies in monkeys are particularly relevant.[204, 205] Feeding monkeys a diet that approximates the typical Western diet (500 mg cholesterol per day and 20% of calories as saturated fat) resulted in elevation of plasma LDL concentrations and atherosclerotic lesions almost identical to those seen in humans.[204] Eliminating the saturated fat and cholesterol from the diet reduced LDL levels and caused lesions to regress. In addition to elevations in LDL concentrations, cholesterol-fat feeding in animals caused accumulation of β-VLDL. These cholesterol-enriched remnant lipoproteins are derived from lipoproteins secreted by the intestine and liver and also accumulate in type III hyperlipoproteinemia (discussed later).[46, 86, 202, 203]

Single-gene mutations in animals have also demonstrated the link between hypercholesterolemia and atherosclerosis. The WHHL rabbit is a model of FH in which the LDL receptors are defective; elevated LDL concentrations result from retarded clearance rates.[206] Another model of FH is the LDL receptor–deficient mouse, in which functional receptors have been eliminated by gene targeting.[207] As discussed previously, apo-E–deficient mice represent another model of defective remnant lipoprotein clearance.[94, 95] As a result of high levels of remnant accumulation, these animals develop severe spontaneous atherosclerosis, even when fed a low-fat diet.

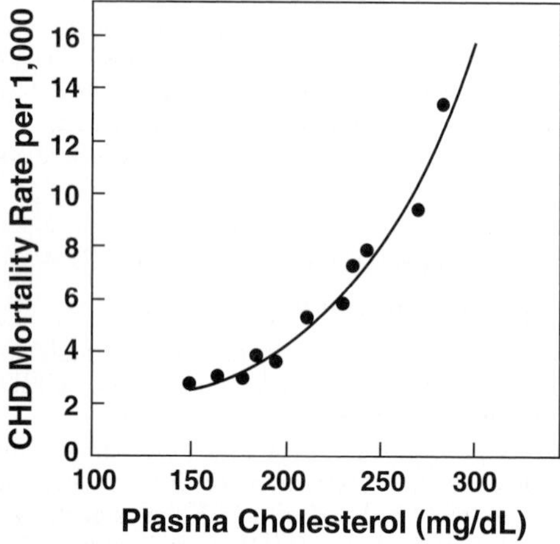

Figure 34–23. Relation between plasma cholesterol levels and coronary heart disease (CHD) mortality in the Multiple Risk Factor Intervention Trial. (Modified from Stamler J, Wentworth D, Neaton JD. Is relationship between serum cholesterol and risk of premature death from coronary heart disease continuous and graded? Findings in 356,222 primary screenees of the Multiple Risk Factor Intervention Trial (MRFIT). JAMA 1986; 256:2823–2828; Copyright © 1986, by the American Medical Association.)

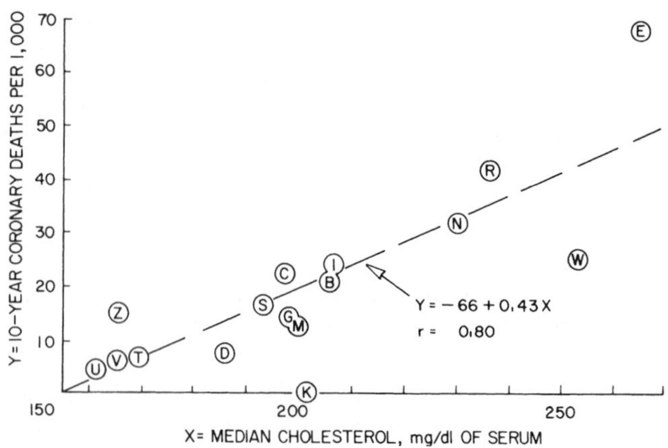

Figure 34–24. Coronary heart disease mortality (10-year death rates) versus median serum cholesterol (mg/dL). All men were free of heart disease at the beginning of the study. B = Belgrade, Serbia; C = Crevalcore, Italy; D = Dalmatia, Croatia; E = East Finland; G = Corfu, Greece; I = Italian railroad workers (Rome division); K = Crete, Greece; M = Montegiorgio, Italy; N = Zutphen, The Netherlands; R = American railroad workers (Green Bay, WI; San Francisco, CA; Seattle, WA); S = Slavonia, Croatia; T = Tanushimaru, Japan; U = Ushibuka, Japan; W = West Finland; Z = Zrenjanin, Serbia. (From Keys A. Seven Countries: A Multivariate Analysis of Death and Coronary Heart Disease. Cambridge, Mass, Harvard University Press, 1980.)

Epidemiologic Evidence

Several epidemiologic studies have demonstrated a relation between the plasma cholesterol level and the risk of CHD. For example, the Multiple Risk Factor Intervention Trial (Fig. 34–23) showed that there is increased risk at levels above 5.2 mmol/L (200 mg/dL).[208] The Seven Countries Study also demonstrated a relation between an increased incidence of CHD and high plasma cholesterol levels (Fig. 34–24).[30, 201]

The causal relationship between elevated plasma cholesterol levels and accelerated atherosclerosis is established. Epidemiologic studies have linked the intake of high levels of dietary fat, especially saturated fats, with increased plasma cholesterol levels.[9, 27–30] Likewise, diets high in cholesterol also tend to increase plasma cholesterol levels.[27–29] Therefore, restriction of saturated fat and cholesterol is the cornerstone of dietary therapy to reduce elevated blood cholesterol levels.

Familial Hypercholesterolemia

Some of the most compelling evidence for the deleterious effects of elevated plasma cholesterol has come from studies of FH.[14, 119] This genetic disorder results from a series of mutations in the LDL receptor that cause LDL to accumulate in the plasma as a result of defective clearance of LDL by the receptors. These studies conclusively demonstrate that increased plasma concentrations of LDL cause atherosclerosis.

Experimental Evidence in Humans

Final compelling evidence supporting the cholesterol-diet-heart hypothesis came from several human clinical trials examining the efficacy of several lipid-lowering drugs in reducing CHD (reviewed in the section on treatment of lipid disorders, clinical trials). In all groups examined, including patients with and without preexisting CHD over a range of initial plasma cholesterol levels, the results unequivocally demonstrated that lowering plasma cholesterol levels reduces the risk of CHD.

In summary, the current evidence overwhelmingly supports the cholesterol-diet-heart hypothesis and upholds the conclusion of the Cholesterol Consensus Conference on Lowering Blood Cholesterol to Prevent Coronary Heart Disease organized by the National Heart, Lung, and Blood Institute that the cause-and-effect relation between cholesterol and CHD is clearly established.[209]

Atherogenic Lipoproteins

In addition to LDL, almost all classes of lipoproteins that contain apo-B (VLDL, β-VLDL, IDL, Lp(a), and oxidized LDL) are considered to be atherogenic. A common feature of these atherogenic lipoproteins is that they contain various amounts of cholesteryl esters and either apo-B100 or apo-B48. In addition, Lp(a) contains apo(a), a protein that is disulfide-linked to apo-B and is homologous to plasminogen; apo(a) may contribute to atherogenesis by mechanisms related to thrombosis.[210, 211] Finally, the atherogenic potential of LDL differs among the various LDL size and density subclasses, with the small, dense LDL subclass being the most atherogenic.[212]

Apo-B–containing remnant lipoproteins appear to be especially atherogenic[202, 203, 213] because β-VLDLs, which accumulate in the plasma of cholesterol-fed animals and in patients with type III hyperlipoproteinemia, are associated with accelerated formation of atherosclerotic lesions. These particles, representing chylomicron remnants and VLDL remnants (IDL), are taken up by macrophages, including, presumably, macrophages in the artery wall, in a nonsaturable manner. This uptake results in massive intracellular accumulation of cholesteryl esters in the form of lipid droplets. The lipid-engorged macrophages resemble the foam cells of the early fatty streak (discussed subsequently).

Another related class of potentially atherogenic apo-B–containing lipoproteins is triglyceride-rich lipoproteins, which are associated with postprandial lipemia after ingestion of a fatty meal.[214] Whereas chylomicrons and large, triglyceride-rich VLDLs are not believed to be atherogenic, remnants derived from these particles are.

The Low-Density Lipoprotein Paradox and Oxidized Lipids

Because LDL-C levels are a strong predictor of CHD and atherosclerosis, it was expected that LDL would be taken up avidly by macrophages, leading to the formation of foam cells. However, in vitro experiments showed that only low levels of normal plasma LDL are taken up by macrophages. This low uptake presumably occurred because of the highly regulated LDL receptor pathway; the delivery of LDL-C to macrophages down-regulates LDL receptor expression, thereby protecting the cells from overaccumulation of LDL-C. These results led to the so-called LDL paradox: How do LDLs contribute to atherosclerosis if only limited quantities are taken up by macrophages?[137] The explanation turned out to be that LDLs that have been modified are taken up by macrophages in an unregulated manner through receptors unrelated to the LDL receptor.[138] These receptors for modified LDL were originally referred to as acetyl-LDL receptors[138] but are now commonly referred to as scavenger receptors (discussed in "Scavenger Receptors").[137]

In vitro experiments have demonstrated that a number of chemical modifications, including acetylation, acetoacetylation, and reaction with malondialdehyde,[215] circumvent the LDL receptor pathway and cause massive amounts of modified LDL to enter macrophages by means of scavenger receptors.[138] Furthermore, macrophages can alter LDL so that these particles can be taken up by macrophages in an unregulated manner.[216] Other cells, including smooth muscle cells, can also modify LDL.[137, 217, 218]

The physiologically important LDL modification probably involves oxidation and results in lipid peroxidation. The oxidized-LDL hypothesis proposes that unsaturated lipids on the particle undergo oxidative modification, which subsequently leads to oxidation of apo-B, which alters the protein's affinity for cell-surface receptors. As a corollary, antioxidant vitamins (such as A, C, and E), drugs (such a probucol), and enzymes (such as paraoxonase) may limit these oxidative processes. It appears that production of reactive oxygen species (i.e., free radicals) is an integral part of the modification and may be related to the general aging process, in which lipid peroxidation may be a component.[219, 220] Two products of lipid peroxidation, 4-hydroxynonenal and malondialdehyde, modify amino acids of apo-B100, resulting in its fragmentation. Modification is inhibited by antioxidants. Phospholipase and lipoxygenases have also been implicated in LDL modification.[217, 218] In addition to macrophage uptake, oxidized LDLs may participate directly in atherogenesis because they are cytotoxic,[221] may serve as chemoattractants for circulating monocyte-macrophages,[222] and are immunogenic.[223]

The role of oxidized LDL as a major contributor to atherosclerosis remains to be proved in vivo.[224] However, what appear to be oxidatively modified forms of LDL have been identified in atherosclerotic lesions and inflammatory fluid.[223, 225] Also, epitopes of malondialdehyde- and 4-hydroxynonenal–modified apo-B100 have been observed in lesions.[223] Therefore, the formation of oxidized LDL, which may contribute to atherogenesis in a number of ways, is an attractive solution to the LDL paradox.

The most probable mechanism by which oxidized or modified LDLs are taken up by macrophages is by one or more of the scavenger receptors (see "Scavenger Receptors"). The roles of the various scavenger receptors and their relative importance in atherogenesis are still being clarified (for a review, see reference 139). However, the receptor whose primary function is to take up oxidized or modified LDL within the artery wall and to contribute to the development and progression of atherosclerosis may well remain to be identified.

Overview of Atherogenesis

Until the last several years, two theories of atherogenesis prevailed. The first, referred to initially as the lipid infiltration hypothesis, proposed that excess blood lipids in the form of lipoproteins infiltrate into the arterial wall. This theory was supported by epidemiologic evidence and the identification of atherogenic lipoproteins. The second theory was the endothelial injury hypothesis, which proposed that injury to the endothelial surface is required and results in removal of these cells, exposing a thrombogenic surface to which platelets adhere. Platelet adherence was suggested to result in the release of platelet-derived growth factor, which would stimulate the smooth muscle cell proliferation and migration that are characteristic of early lesion formation. Endothelial denudation would also remove the endothelial barrier, allowing lipoproteins to enter the vessel wall more readily. The current view of atherosclerosis development combines features of both hypotheses.[226–232] However, loss of endothelial cells is not required for an atherosclerotic lesion to develop, and atherogenic lipoproteins can and do penetrate intact endothelium to enter the artery wall.

A unifying modification of this general view of atherogenesis is the response-to-retention hypothesis. According to this view, one key early event in atherosclerosis is the retention of atherogenic, cholesterol-rich lipoproteins bound to arterial proteoglycans in the arterial subendothelium.[233] Oxidation and other modifications of the retained lipoproteins could initiate a series of responses that lead to the transformation of healthy, normal arteries into diseased, lesioned arteries. An important component of the artery wall involved in the retention is chondroitin 6-sulfate proteoglycans, which are known to bind LDL. Although oxidation may be a major fate of the retained lipoproteins, it is not the only possibility. Nonpancreatic secretory phospholipase A_2 has been proposed to generate proinflammatory modified lipid components from aggregated but nonoxidized lipoproteins.[234] Also, induction of cell-adhesion molecules such as vascular cell adhesion molecule 1, leading to recruitment of inflammatory cells, appears to be triggered by nonoxidized, retained lipoproteins.[235]

Consistent with a prominent role for inflammation, atherosclerotic lesions share many features with wound healing or inflammation: (1) proliferation of smooth muscle cells and accumulation of macrophages; (2) formation, by smooth muscle cells, of a connective tissue matrix composed of elastic fibers, collagen, and proteoglycans; and (3) deposition of lipid, primarily cholesterol, both intracellularly and extracellularly.[229, 230] The pattern of lesion formation does not occur randomly within the arterial tree but is focal in nature. Susceptible regions are more permeable to plasma components, and endothelial cell turnover is greater, although the endothelial surface appears to be intact. The focal nature of atherosclerosis suggests that local hemodynamic factors are involved.

Normally, the endothelium forms a relatively impermeable barrier. The endothelial cells and the relatively narrow region beneath them (subendothelial space), which contains an occasional smooth muscle cell, constitute the intima of the artery wall (Fig. 34–25*A*). Beneath the intima is a layer of many smooth muscle cells, the media, which constitutes the bulk of the artery wall. The adventitia is the outermost layer of the artery wall and is composed of loose connective tissue.

A current model of atherogenesis is depicted in Figure 34–25*B* through *E*. The major cell types involved include endothelial cells, smooth muscle cells, and inflammatory mononuclear cells, such as macrophages and possibly lymphocytes. One of the initial events is the focal attachment of circulating monocytes to the endothelial surface (see Fig. 34–25*B*). It is not entirely clear which factors are responsible for the adherence of monocytes, although oxidized or modified LDLs or other atherogenic lipoproteins retained in the subendothelium are probably a major initiating factor; areas of microinjury may contribute as well. The monocytes modify the endothelial surface and induce the expression of leukocyte adhesion molecules such as vascular cell adhesion molecule 1.[236] Once adhered, the monocytes migrate between endothelial cells, enter the subendothelial space, and differentiate into macrophages (see Fig. 34–25*B*). In addition, LDLs and other atherogenic lipoproteins can enter this space. Within the wall, LDLs may become entrapped in the matrix and undergo oxidation or further

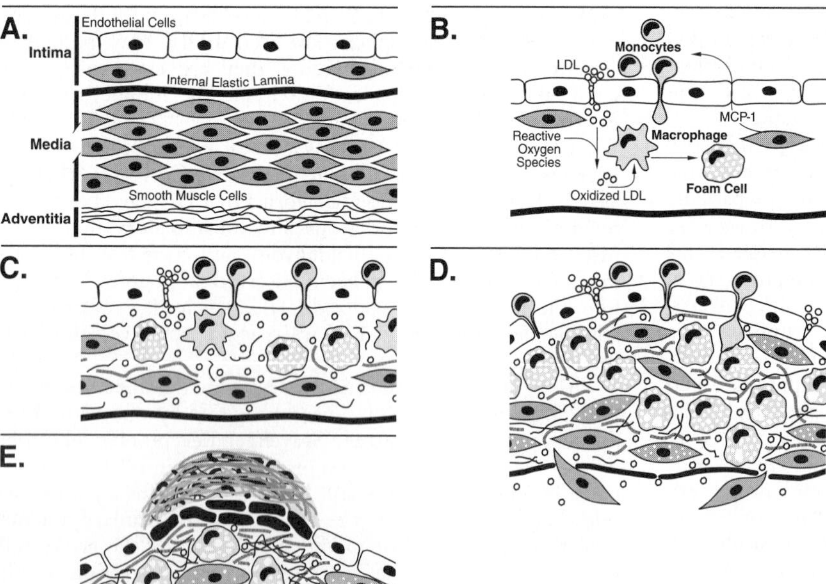

Figure 34–25. Schematic representation of the progression of atherogenesis. *A*, Normal artery wall showing the three major regions of the vessel wall: intima, media, and adventitia. The thickness of the intima beneath the endothelial cell layer is exaggerated relative to the media to allow illustration of the changes that occur within the subendothelial intima. *B*, Initial events in lesion formation include recruitment of monocyte-macrophages to the subendothelial space and the infiltration of plasma low-density lipoproteins (LDLs) *(small circles)*, which are oxidized by unknown mechanisms that may include reactive oxygen species. Oxidized LDLs are taken up by macrophages, leading to the formation of foam cells. MCP-1, monocyte chemoattractant protein 1. *C*, Fatty streak lesion. Further recruitment of monocyte-macrophages from the plasma takes place along with smooth muscle cell proliferation and collagen synthesis *(rows of vertical lines)*. Elastin fibers *(thin curved lines)* begin to accumulate. *D*, Proliferative or fibrous lesion. Atherogenesis continues as the lesion begins to extend into the vessel lumen. Necrosis of foam cells begins, and smooth muscle cells start to migrate from the media through the disrupted internal elastic lamina. Some smooth muscle cells accumulate lipid droplets. *E*, Complicated lesion. The endothelial cell layer covering the lesion is lost. As a result, the surface of the lesion becomes thrombogenic, inducing thrombus formation. Cellular debris increases. Calcification and appearance of cholesterol crystals can occur.

chemical modifications. The macrophages take up the oxidized or modified LDLs and begin to take on the appearance of foam cells as lipid accumulates. These initial steps set in motion a chain of events that includes the expression of growth factors (mediators of cell proliferation and chemotaxis) and cytokines (mediators involved in inflammation and immunity).

Monocyte chemoattractant protein 1 (MCP-1), produced by endothelial and smooth muscle cells, plays a role in further monocyte recruitment into lesions and may be induced by the presence of oxidized LDL. The role of MCP-1 in macrophage recruitment in the early stages of lesion development was established in MCP-1–deficient mice.[237–239] When the MCP-1–deficient mice were crossed with apo-E–deficient mice, a common mouse model of atherosclerosis, and fed a high-fat Western-type diet for 5 weeks, fewer macrophages were present in the aortas of the doubly transgenic mice than in the apo-E–deficient control mice. After 5 to 26 weeks of the diet, the doubly transgenic mice displayed significantly smaller lesions. These results establish a role for MCP-1 in the recruitment of macrophages into the artery wall at an early stage of lesion formation and establish MCP-1 as an important factor for atherogenesis.

Other growth factors that have been implicated in atherosclerosis include platelet-derived growth factor, basic fibroblast growth factor, insulin-like growth factors, interleukin-1, tumor necrosis factor, and transforming growth factor β.[226, 227] These mitogenic factors, which can stimulate smooth muscle cell proliferation, are not expressed in the normal artery wall but are present in developing lesions. Several of these mitogens are also chemoattractants with the potential to attract smooth muscle cells or monocytes-macrophages into a developing lesion. Inflammatory response cytokines include interleukin-1, interferon γ, tissue necrosis factor α, interleukin-2, and the colony-stimulating factors. It is unlikely that the various factors act in isolation from each other, but they probably act through a network of cellular interactions operating in a paracrine or autocrine manner.[226]

The first grossly visible atherosclerotic lesion is referred to as a fatty streak (see Fig. 34–25*C*). Macrophages accumulate in abundance in the subendothelial space and are converted to foam cells, presumably through the uptake of oxidized LDLs or remnant lipoproteins. The recruitment of monocytes continues, and smooth muscle cells begin to migrate into the intima. Fatty streaks probably come and go, depending on the local stimuli present in the artery wall.

As the cycle of interactions continues, the fatty streak matures into a proliferative or fibrous plaque, which is raised and begins to extend into the lumen of the vessel (see Fig. 34–25*D*). The foam cells begin to necrose, probably because of the cytotoxicity of the accumulated lipid; as the lesion progresses, cholesterol crystals develop. The death of foam cells leads to extracellular lipid deposition, accompanied by collagen synthesis and smooth muscle cell migration and proliferation. In the continued presence of factors that promote atherogenesis (e.g., high plasma concentrations of atherogenic lipoproteins), the plaque progresses to the complicated lesion stage (see Fig. 34–25*E*).

The surfaces of complicated lesions may become thrombogenic as endothelial cells are lost and the subendothelial space is exposed. Platelets can adhere to this exposed surface, promoting thrombus formation. Alternatively, a fissure forms in the unstable plaques and blood actually dissects into the artery wall, leading to the formation of a large thrombus. At late stages in complicated lesions, T lymphocytes infiltrate the lesion and there is evidence of an autoimmune response characterized by lymphocyte infiltration of the adventitia. Calcification is also a feature of late lesions. Advanced lesions can weaken the elasticity and integrity of the artery wall, with the potential to lead to an aneurysm of the vessel. As experiments in humans have shown, removal or reduction of the atherogenic stimulus can result in plaque regression, leaving a remnant devoid of lipid that resembles a wound scar.

HYPERLIPIDEMIA: DEFINITIONS AND OVERVIEW

Plasma lipid levels vary among individuals of different populations owing to genetic and dietary factors. For example, the mean plasma cholesterol concentration for Western men is 5.4 mmol/L (210 mg/dL),[240] whereas for Japanese men it is 4.3 mmol/L (165 mg/dL).[241] Historically, *hyperlipidemia* has been arbitrarily defined from population distributions as the upper 5% to 10% of values (i.e., the 90th to 95th percentile). For Western adults, cholesterol concentrations higher than 6.2 mmol/L (240 mg/dL) or triglyceride concentrations higher than 2.3 mmol/L (200 mg/dL) constitute significant hyperlipidemia.

In agreement with these definitions, guidelines from the 2001 National Cholesterol Education Program (NCEP) suggest that plasma cholesterol levels less than 5.2 mmol/L (200 mg/dL) are desirable, that those between 5.2 and 6.2 mmol/L (200 to 240 mg/dL) are borderline elevated, and that levels greater than 6.2 mmol/L (240 mg/dL) are high.[242] Because plasma lipid levels increase with age,[243] cutoff values for hyperlipidemia in children are lower (5.2 mmol/L [200 mg/dL] and 1.6 mmol/L [140 mg/dL], respectively, for cholesterol and triglycerides). Conversely, *hypolipidemia* can be defined as plasma cholesterol concentrations less than 3.4 mmol/L (130 mg/dL). Although these boundaries are arbitrary, the designation of plasma cholesterol concentrations higher than 6.2 mmol/L (240 mg/dL) as hyperlipidemic has support from clinical observations indicating that the risk for atherosclerotic CHD increases markedly when the cholesterol concentration reaches or exceeds this level[244] (see Fig. 34–23).

Hyperlipidemia is caused by increased concentrations of plasma lipoproteins. One or more classes of lipoproteins may accumulate in the blood stream because of increased production or secretion into the circulation or because of decreased clearance or removal from the circulation; in some cases, both processes coexist. Alterations in metabolic processes are often related to alterations in the proteins involved in lipoprotein metabolism (see "Plasma Lipoproteins: Apolipoproteins, Receptors, and Enzymes"). Alterations resulting from genetic defects are classified as *primary* disorders of lipid metabolism. Alternatively, other factors that alter lipoprotein metabolism, such as diabetes mellitus or hypothyroidism, lead to increased plasma lipoprotein concentrations; these are classified as *secondary* disorders of lipid metabolism. Often, hyperlipidemia results from mixed primary and secondary causes, such as when diabetes mellitus occurs in a subject who has an inherited defect in one of the proteins involved in lipoprotein metabolism. In cases in which no known cause of hyperlipidemia can be identified, the disorder is classified as sporadic or possibly polygenic in origin.

When considering the causes of hyperlipidemia, it is useful to classify the various possibilities by the pattern of plasma lipoprotein elevation (or the lipoprotein phenotype). This was once commonly done by performing plasma electrophoresis to separate and determine the relative concentrations of the plasma lipoproteins[245] (Table 34–5). Although such a classification is still useful in some instances, it has generally lost utility[246] because it has been recognized that certain disorders can manifest different phenotypes at different times in the same person and that different phenotypes may occur in different family members with the same disorder. Furthermore, classifi-

Table 34–5. Lipoprotein Pattern Types Based on Plasma Electrophoresis

Type	Predominant Elevated Plasma Lipoprotein	Predominant Elevated Plasma Lipid	Plasma Appearance After Refrigeration	Example
I	Chylomicrons	Triglycerides	Cream layer	LPL deficiency
IIa	LDL	Cholesterol	Clear	Familial hypercholesterolemia
IIb	VLDL + LDL	Triglycerides and cholesterol	Usually clear	Familial combined hyperlipidemia
III	Remnants (β-VLDL)	Triglycerides and cholesterol	Turbid	Type III hyperlipoproteinemia
IV	VLDL	Triglycerides	Turbid	Familial hypertriglyceridemia
V	Chylomicrons + VLDL	Triglycerides and cholesterol	Cream layer, turbid below	Apo-CII deficiency

Apo-CII, apolipoprotein CII; LDL, low-density lipoproteins; LPL, lipoprotein lipase; VLDL, very-low-density lipoproteins.

cation based on electrophoresis is not necessary to determine a therapeutic plan. Nevertheless, many of the terms still used to describe lipoprotein disorders (e.g., *hypoalphalipoproteinemia, hypobetalipoproteinemia, abetalipoproteinemia, type III hyperlipoproteinemia, dysbetalipoproteinemia*) are derived from the patterns observed on plasma electrophoresis gels.

It is also possible to create a differential diagnosis on the basis of whether the concentration of plasma cholesterol, triglycerides, or both is elevated. Table 34–6 illustrates such a diagnostic strategy. More extensive lists of primary and secondary disorders are given in Table 34–7 and Table 34–8. Although it is often not essential to diagnose a genetic disorder in a hyperlipidemic subject for treatment purposes, the understanding of genetic causes may have important implications for family members. The recognition of secondary disorders is of great importance because therapy should be directed, at least in part, toward correcting the underlying disorder.

PRIMARY DISORDERS OF HYPERLIPIDEMIA

Familial Hypercholesterolemia

FH is a relatively common disorder caused by mutations in the LDL receptor gene that result in LDL receptor malfunction or absence in cells of the liver and peripheral tissues, leading to elevation of plasma LDL and total cholesterol concentrations.[117–119] Heterozygous subjects typically have plasma cholesterol concentrations that are twofold to threefold above average, and homozygous subjects have cholesterol concentrations that are elevated threefold to sixfold.

Clinical Features

Heterozygosity for FH occurs with a frequency of about 1 in 500 in the population and is found in many ethnic groups.[266] Typically, the plasma cholesterol concentration is higher than 7.8 mmol/L (300 mg/dL), and the LDL-C concentration is higher than 6.5 mmol/L (250 mg/dL). Plasma triglycerides are not elevated. The hyperlipidemia is present at birth, and the diagnosis can be suspected from elevated cholesterol concentrations in umbilical cord blood. Plasma electrophoresis exhibits a type IIa pattern, reflecting increased concentrations of β-migrating LDLs.

The characteristic physical finding in approximately 75% of affected subjects is the presence of tendon xanthomas (Fig. 34–26*C* and *D*), usually located on the Achilles tendons or extensor tendons of the hands. Xanthomas of the Achilles tendon can cause recurrent episodes of Achilles tendinitis.[267] These xanthomas may be subtle and apparent only as a thickening of the tendon (see Fig. 34–26*C*). Other common physical findings include xanthelasma (see Fig. 34–26*A;* see color section) and premature arcus corneae (i.e., in persons younger than 40 years).[268] A minority of affected subjects have no physical findings. Premature coronary artery disease is common; the average age of onset of coronary disease is 45 years in men and 55 years in women.[269]

Homozygosity for FH is rare, occurring at a frequency of about 1 in 10^6 in the population (i.e., ~250 persons in the United States population). These subjects come to clinical attention early in life because of marked hypercholesterolemia or premature CHD. Typical plasma cholesterol concentrations range from 15.5 mmol/L (600 mg/dL) to 25.9 mmol/L (1000 mg/dL), and LDL-C concentrations range from 14.2 mmol/L (550 mg/dL) to 24.6 mmol/L (950 mg/dL). In addition to the xanthelasma and tendon xanthomas found in heterozygotes,

Table 34–6. Differential Diagnosis of Hyperlipidemia Including Common Secondary Disorders

	Major Plasma Lipid Abnormality		
Type of Disorder	**Increased Cholesterol**	**Increased Cholesterol and Triglyceride**	**Increased Triglyceride**
Primary	Familial hypercholesterolemia Familial defective apo-B100 Polygenic hypercholesterolemia	Familial combined hyperlipidemia Type III hyperlipoproteinemia (dysbetalipoproteinemia)	Familial hypertriglyceridemia LPL deficiency Apo-CII deficiency Sporadic hypertriglyceridemia
Secondary	Hypothyroidism Nephrotic syndrome	Hypothyroidism Nephrotic syndrome Diabetes mellitus	Diabetes mellitus Alcoholic hyperlipidemia Estrogen therapy

Apo-B100, apolipoprotein B100; LPL, lipoprotein lipase.

Table 34–7. Major Genetic Hyperlipoproteinemias Resulting from Single-Gene Mutations

Disorder	Mutant Gene	Inheritance	Estimated Population Frequency	Lipoprotein Pattern	Typical Clinical Manifestations: Xanthomas	Pancreatitis	Premature Vascular Disease
Familial LPL deficiency	LPL	Autosomal recessive	$1/10^6$	I, V	Eruptive	+	—
Familial apo-CII deficiency	Apo-CII	Autosomal recessive	$1/10^6$	I, V	Eruptive (rarely)	+	—
Familial hypercholesterolemia	LDL receptor	Autosomal dominant	1/500 (heterozygous); $1/10^6$ (homozygous)	IIa (rarely IIb)	Tendon; xanthelasma	—	+
Familial defective apo-B100	Apo-B	Autosomal dominant	1/1000	IIa	Tendon	—	+
Familial type III hyperlipoproteinemia	Apo-E	Autosomal recessive (rarely dominant)	1/10000	III	Palmar; tuberous	—	+
Familial combined hyperlipidemia	Unknown	Autosomal dominant	1/100	IIa, IIb, IV (rarely V)	—	—	+
Familial hypertriglyceridemia	Unknown	Autosomal dominant	Uncertain	IV (rarely V)	—	—	+(?)

Apo, apolipoprotein; LDL, low-density lipoproteins; LPL, lipoprotein lipase.

Table 34–8. Clinical Disorders Associated with Secondary Hyperlipidemia

Disorder	Lipoprotein Type	Elevated Plasma Lipoprotein	Proposed Mechanism	References*
Endocrine-Metabolic				
Diabetes mellitus	IV, V	VLDL, chylomicrons	Increased VLDL production; decreased VLDL catabolism	See text
Hypothyroidism	IIa (rarely III)	LDL (rarely β-VLDL)	Decreased LDL clearance	See text
Estrogen therapy	IV (rarely V)	VLDL	Increased VLDL production (especially in genetically predisposed)	See text
Glucocorticoid therapy	IIa or IIb	VLDL, LDL	Increased VLDL production with conversion to LDL	247–249
Hypopituitarism (ateliotic dwarfism)	IIb	VLDL, LDL	Increased VLDL production with conversion to LDL	250
Acromegaly	IV	VLDL	Increased VLDL production	251
Anorexia nervosa	IIa	LDL	Decreased biliary excretion of cholesterol and bile acids	252, 253
Lipodystrophy (congenital or acquired)	IV	VLDL	Increased VLDL production	254
Werner's syndrome	IIa	LDL	Unknown	255
Acute intermittent porphyria	IIa	LDL	Unknown	256
Glycogen storage disease	IV (rarely V)	VLDL	Increased VLDL production; decreased VLDL catabolism	257, 258
Nonendocrine				
Alcohol	IV (rarely V)	VLDL (rarely chylomicrons)	Increased VLDL production (especially in genetically predisposed)	See text
Nephrotic syndrome	IIa or IIb	VLDL, LDL	Increased VLDL production	See text
Uremia	IV	VLDL	Decreased VLDL clearance	259
Biliary obstruction or cholestasis	—	LP-X	Diversion of biliary cholesterol and phospholipid into circulation	260
Hepatitis	IV	VLDL	Decreased LCAT	261, 262
Systemic lupus erythematosus	I	Chylomicrons	Antibodies bind heparin and thereby decrease LPL activity	263
Monoclonal gammopathy	IIa, III, IV	VLDL, IDL, LDL	Antibodies bind lipoproteins and interfere with catabolism	264, 265

*References are given for disorders not discussed in the text. For a thorough review of the metabolism associated with many of the secondary hyperlipidemic disorders, see Havel RJ, Goldstein JL, Brown MS. Lipoproteins and lipid transport. In Bondy PK, Rosenberg LE (eds). Metabolic Control and Disease, 8th ed. Philadelphia, WB Saunders, 1980, pp 393–494.

LCAT, lecithin:cholesterol acyltransferase; LDL, low-density lipoproteins; LPL, lipoprotein lipase; VLDL, very-low-density lipoproteins.

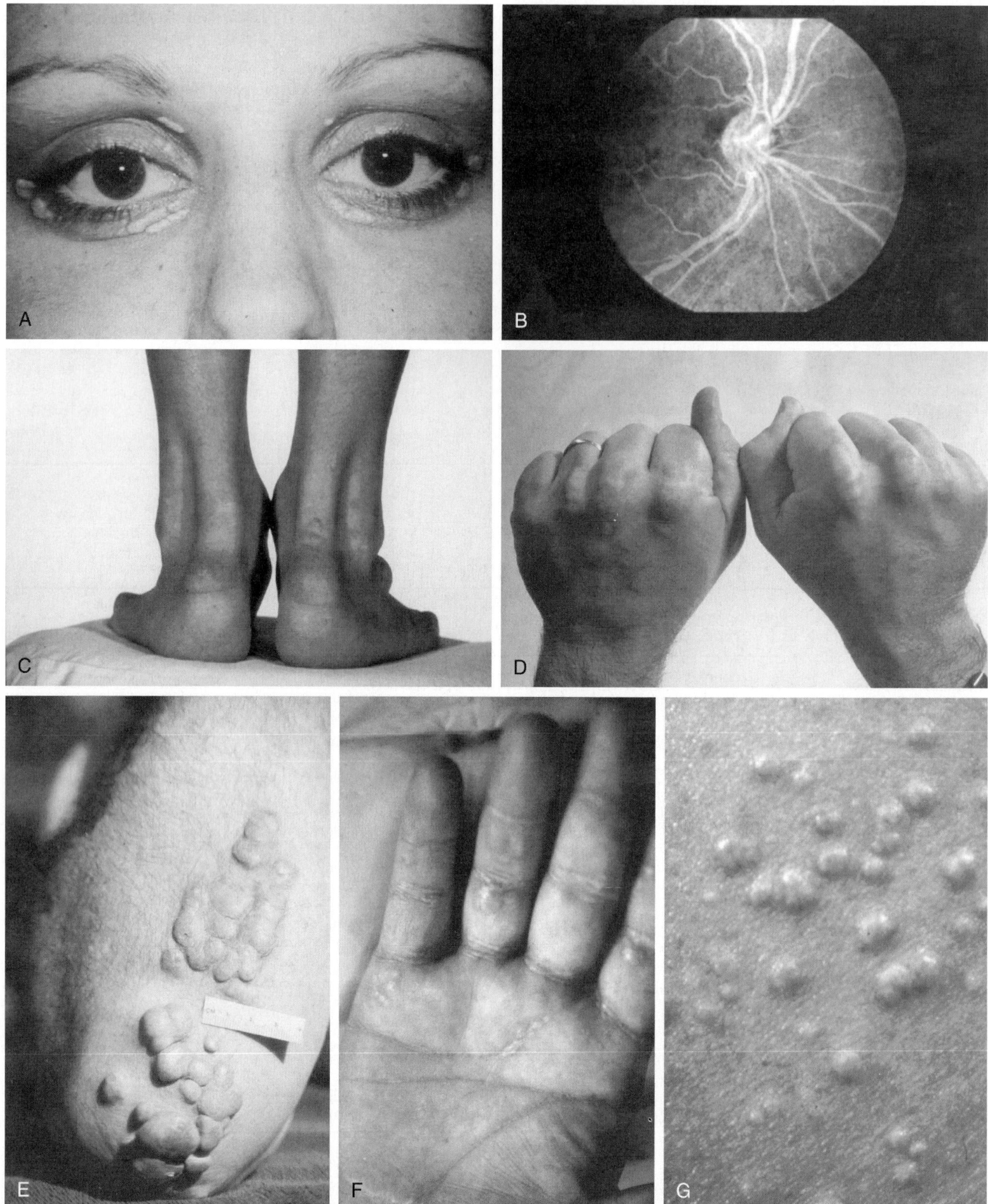

Figure 34–26. Physical examination findings associated with hyperlipidemia (see also Color Plate). *A*, Xanthelasma. *B*, Lipemia retinalis. *C*, Achilles tendon xanthomas. Note the marked thickening of the tendons. *D*, Tendon xanthomas. *E*, Tuberous xanthomas. *F*, Palmar xanthomas. *G*, Eruptive xanthomas. (*A* and *B*, Courtesy of Dr. Mark Dresner and Hospital Practice [May 1990, p 15]. *C*, *D*, *E*, and *F*, Courtesy of Dr. Tom Bersot. *G*, Courtesy of Dr. Alan Chait.)

homozygous individuals frequently have planar xanthomas, which are almost unique to this disorder and almost always noticed by age 6. These xanthomas are raised plaques of cholesterol deposits that occur in the skin at areas of trauma, such as the elbows and knees. Symptoms of CHD may occur before age 10,[270] and, if not treated, these homozygous individuals usually die from myocardial infarction by age 20. Myocardial infarction has been reported as early as age 18 months.[271] Homozygotes are also susceptible to both valvular and supravalvular aortic stenosis.[272]

Origin and Pathogenesis

FH is an autosomal dominant disorder caused by mutations in the LDL receptor gene.[14, 119, 273] Many different types of mutations have been described, including null mutations or nonsense mutations that affect the production of a functional protein, mutations that affect the ability of the receptor to bind to its ligands on lipoproteins, and mutations in which receptors bind LDL normally but are unable to internalize the lipoprotein.[117, 118] A milder phenotype occurs when the ability to bind LDL is impaired but not absent. Different LDL receptor mutations occur in different ethnic groups; for example, there is an increased prevalence (about 60%) of a large deletion mutation in French Canadians with heterozygous FH.[274]

The lack of LDL receptors impairs the clearance of lipoproteins that rely on the LDL receptor for this purpose; these include LDLs, in which apo-B100 is the ligand, and remnant lipoproteins (IDLs) that are cleared by apo-E. This results in a twofold to threefold increase in the plasma cholesterol concentration in heterozygotes and in a threefold to sixfold increase in homozygotes. The high levels of LDL in the plasma are taken up by scavenger receptors on macrophages in a nonsaturable manner, possibly after the LDL undergoes oxidative modification.[217, 275, 276] As a consequence, cholesterol accumulates in tissue macrophages in the arterial wall, tendons, and skin and causes the pathologic processes observed in these tissues.

Diagnosis

The diagnosis of heterozygous FH is suggested by the presence of high plasma levels of total cholesterol and LDL-C, normal plasma triglycerides, tendon xanthomas, and a family history of premature CHD. Up to 25% of subjects do not have xanthomas. Heterozygous FH should be suspected in any person with premature heart disease. In one study, heterozygous FH accounted for 4% of men who survived myocardial infarction before age 60.[277] The differential diagnosis includes familial defective apo-B100,[278] which has many of the same phenotypic characteristics, including tendon xanthomas. The pattern of isolated high LDL-C also occurs in the more common disorder of polygenic hypercholesterolemia, but tendon xanthomas are not usually a feature of the latter.

The diagnosis of FH is primarily a clinical diagnosis because tests to detect one of the many LDL receptor gene mutations or to demonstrate diminished LDL receptor function are performed only in specialized research laboratories. The diagnosis can be confirmed in the laboratory by culturing skin fibroblasts and demonstrating a reduced ability of LDL to bind to receptors on the cells.[279] The diagnosis of FH is important not only for proper treatment of the affected subject but also for identification of other family members who may be at high risk of developing CHD.

The diagnosis of homozygous FH should be suspected in any child with extremely high plasma cholesterol (typically > 12.9 mmol/L [500 mg/dL]) or xanthomas. Both parents are obligate heterozygotes and should manifest the phenotype of heterozygous FH.

Treatment

Treatment of heterozygous FH[280] consists of a diet low in total and saturated fat (approximately 20% and 6% of calories, respectively) and low in cholesterol (<2.6 mmol/day [100 mg/day])[281] and drug therapy. Dietary modifications usually result in only minor decreases in the plasma cholesterol levels (5% to 15%). With the development of more potent HMG-CoA reductase inhibitors, adequate cholesterol lowering in these patients can sometimes be achieved by a single therapeutic drug.[282] However, combinations of two or three drugs are often needed to reduce plasma cholesterol to desired levels.[283] Effective drug combinations usually include low doses of bile acid sequestrants together with HMG-CoA reductase inhibitors[284] or niacin[285, 286] or all three agents combined.[287] Bile acid sequestrants and HMG-CoA reductase inhibitors both work by depleting cholesterol from hepatic cells (see later discussion), thereby causing increased expression of functional LDL receptors (from the normal allele) on cells, which in turn lowers the plasma cholesterol.[288]

Because high Lp(a) concentrations appear to be an adverse risk factor for patients with heterozygous FH,[289] the plasma Lp(a) level should be determined; if it is elevated, niacin should be considered in the drug regimen because this agent can lower plasma Lp(a) levels.[290] On the basis of studies in animal models of FH,[291, 292] antioxidant agents may be of therapeutic benefit for preventing CHD, but this has not been demonstrated directly in humans. Probucol treatment has resulted in xanthoma regression.[293] Ileal bypass surgery,[294] which, like bile acid sequestrants, causes decreased reabsorption of bile acids from the gut, may be considered in patients who cannot tolerate lipid-lowering drugs.

The age at which treatment should begin in heterozygous FH is somewhat controversial. On the one hand, development of atherosclerosis in these subjects is a long process that begins early in life, and one could argue that treatment should begin during the early stages of lesion development. On the other hand, CHD is usually not symptomatic until the third or fourth decade of life in men and 10 years later in women. Because established CHD is reversible,[295, 296] one could argue that medicines can be withheld until after age 25 in men or age 35 in women. A rational approach may be to use diet therapy and bile acid sequestrants, which do not have systemic toxicity, in the early years and to add more potent drug combinations later. The presence of additional risk factors (e.g., high plasma Lp(a) levels, low plasma HDL-C levels, smoking) in an affected subject is an indication for more aggressive treatment at a young age.

Unless the causative mutation is such that there is some residual LDL binding, drug therapy for FH homozygotes is usually ineffective for lowering plasma cholesterol, except with high doses of atorvastatin and simvastatin.[297, 298] However, the most effective means of therapy in these patients is selective removal of LDL from the plasma by extracorporeal pheresis combined with LDL immunoadsorption[299, 300] performed every 1 to 3 weeks. Experimental therapies include liver transplantation,[301, 302] which provides functional LDL receptors, portacaval shunting,[303, 304] and gene therapy.[305, 306]

Familial Defective Apolipoprotein B100

Familial defective apo-B100 is a relatively common disorder caused by a mutation in apo-B100, the ligand for the LDL receptor, that results in high plasma LDL and total cholesterol levels and increased susceptibility to CHD. It is phenotypically similar to FH.

Clinical Features

This disorder occurs with a frequency of 1 in 500 to 1 in 750 in white persons with hypercholesterolemia.[65, 307, 308] The prevalence of familial defective apo-B100 was 0.08% in an ethnically diverse, unselected population.[309] Familial defective apo-B100 had not been described in nonwhite populations until 1993, when it was detected in an individual of Chinese ancestry.[310] The clinical features of heterozygous familial defective apo-B100 overlap extensively with those of heterozygous FH and include isolated elevations of plasma LDL-C (type IIa pattern), tendon xanthomas, xanthelasmas, and premature CHD.[278, 307, 311, 312]

Although there is extensive overlap, familial defective apo-B100 is usually milder in its manifestations than FH.[65, 312] Subjects who are homozygous for the familial defective apo-B100 mutation also appear to have a milder clinical phenotype than FH homozygotes.[313–315] In one report, a 66-year-old man and his 69-year-old sister with homozygous familial defective apo-B100 had total plasma cholesterol levels of 9.6 mmol/L (370 mg/dL) and 11.9 mmol/L (460 mg/dL), respectively, and only the man had evidence of CHD.[314] Presumably, the less severe phenotype is related to the fact that the binding of apo-B to LDL receptors is defective but not totally absent in familial defective apo-B100, whereas the apo-E–mediated clearance of remnant particles, which is impaired in FH, is normal in persons with familial defective apo-B100.

Origin and Pathogenesis

Familial defective apo-B100 is caused by a mutation in apo-B100 that impairs its ability to bind to the LDL receptor.[316–318] To date, a single mutation, the substitution of glutamine for arginine at amino acid 3500, accounts for almost all cases of familial defective apo-B100.[65] Apo-B allele haplotype analysis of DNA from affected subjects has indicated that almost all cases can be traced back to an original founder.[309] Only after extensive screening was this mutation detected in persons with a different apo-B haplotype for the allele carrying the mutation, one of whom was of Chinese ancestry[310] and one in a kindred from Germany.[319]

The mutation located at apo-B amino acid 3500 disrupts the conformation of the protein in the receptor-binding domain[320] and reduces receptor binding of LDL from heterozygotes to levels that are about one third of normal in tissue culture assays.[316] Isolation of the binding-defective LDL from affected subjects demonstrated that it binds with 4% to 9% of normal activity to LDL receptors.[321] Decreased affinity of the defective apo-B100 for its receptor delays the clearance of LDL from the plasma (by about 50%)[318] and leads to elevation of plasma LDL-C levels. Defective LDL particles accumulate in the plasma in increased proportions relative to normal LDL. A second mutation at amino acid 3500 (tryptophan for arginine) has been reported.[322]

Another mutation located near the receptor-binding region of the apo-B molecule (a substitution of cysteine for arginine at amino acid 3531) also impairs binding of apo-B to the LDL receptor.[323] This mutation decreases LDL binding to LDL receptors by 35% to 40% in tissue culture assays and is associated with moderate elevations in plasma LDL-C levels.

Diagnosis

As in heterozygous FH, the diagnosis of familial defective apo-B100 is suggested by the presence of increased plasma LDL-C and normal triglyceride levels, especially in the presence of tendon xanthomas and a family history of premature CHD. Without specialized testing, however, familial defective apo-B100 is clinically indistinguishable from FH. Because familial defective apo-B100 is caused primarily by one mutation, in contrast to the many mutations that cause FH,[117] it is possible to screen easily for the familial defective apo-B100 mutation using a polymerase chain reaction–based assay of genomic DNA isolated from blood.[324] This test is available only in specialized laboratories.

Treatment

Treatment of familial defective apo-B100 is similar to that of heterozygous FH and consists of a low-fat, low-cholesterol diet and a combination drug regimen.[278] Drugs that either decrease LDL production (e.g., niacin[325]) or increase the expression of LDL receptors to facilitate clearance of the normal apo-B100–containing particles effectively lower the plasma LDL-C level.[278, 326] In two patients with homozygous familial defective apo-B100 whose LDL had receptor-binding affinities 10% to 20% of normal, treatment with HMG-CoA reductase inhibitors markedly reduced plasma cholesterol levels.[314] Family members at risk should also be screened for the dominant mutation.

Familial Combined Hyperlipidemia

Originally described in 1973,[277, 327, 328] familial combined hyperlipidemia is a common disorder of unknown genetic cause associated with elevations of plasma cholesterol and triglyceride levels and increased susceptibility to CHD. It is inherited as an autosomal dominant trait. The phenotype of familial combined hyperlipidemia overlaps with and may be the same as that in familial hyperapobetalipoproteinemia[329], in subjects with plasma elevations of small, dense LDL particles[330], and in subjects with *syndrome X* or the *metabolic syndrome*, a disorder that includes insulin resistance, increased plasma levels of small, dense LDL, elevated plasma triglycerides, and low plasma HDL levels.[331]

Clinical Features

The features of familial combined hyperlipidemia include moderate elevations of plasma cholesterol, triglycerides, or both within subjects of an affected kindred, corresponding to lipoprotein pattern type IIa, IIb, or IV on plasma electrophoresis. The predominant lipid abnormality may vary in a single person over time or among affected family members[277]; the variable phenotype in this disorder led in part to the decreased utility of pattern typing of hyperlipoproteinemia by plasma electrophoresis in the clinical evaluation.[246] Levels of HDL-C are often moderately decreased,[332] especially in the setting of increased plasma triglycerides.

Although it was originally thought that lipid abnormalities usually develop after puberty, it is now known that the phenotype can be detected in children.[277, 333] Neither xanthomas nor xanthelasma is a feature of familial combined hyperlipidemia. Associated metabolic disturbances may include glucose intolerance, obesity, and hyperuricemia. Premature CHD is a common feature; in one study of male survivors of myocardial infarction, familial combined hyperlipidemia was found in 11.3% of those younger than 60 years of age.[277] CHD is often present in men by age 50.

Origin and Pathogenesis

Although familial combined hyperlipidemia is a common disorder (estimated prevalence, 0.5% to 2.0%),[277, 334] neither its genetic cause nor its metabolic pathogenesis is clear. Given the dominant pattern of inheritance, it was initially presumed that familial combined hyperlipidemia is caused by a single gene defect.[277] Now it is believed that multiple genes may be involved, with one or two genes playing a large role and other genes acting as modifiers.[335] A candidate gene locus was identified in syntenic chromosomal regions in mice and humans,[336, 337] suggesting that an important contributing gene may reside at this locus. The phenotype of this disorder has also been mapped to loci on chromosomes 11[338] and 19,[339] and several different loci may underlie the expression of the phenotype.[335, 340, 341] Heterozygous LPL deficiency may constitute a subset of familial combined hyperlipidemia.[342]

A significant problem with mapping this disorder is the difficult task of assigning phenotypes to individuals because of the fluctuating and indistinct clinical features. Familial hyperapobetalipoproteinemia, a disorder characterized by high plasma levels of apo-B and normal plasma cholesterol levels,[329] overlaps with the phenotype of familial combined hyperlipidemia,[334] as do both the familial syndrome characterized by small, dense LDL[330] and syndrome X characterized by insulin resistance and other metabolic abnormalities.[331] The metabolic defect that leads to the hypercholesterolemia or hypertriglyceridemia, or both, is also unclear, but overproduction of apo-B may be a contributing factor[343, 344]; apo-B overproduction can result in elevations in plasma VLDL, LDL, or both.[345] Similarly, the pathogenesis of the low HDL in this disorder remains unclear. Low HDL-C is commonly associated with hypertriglyceridemia. This finding could be related either to decreased substrate for HDL formation because of impaired catabolism of the apo-B–containing lipoproteins or to enhanced CETP-mediated cholesteryl ester transfer from HDL to the apo-B–containing lipoproteins.

Diagnosis

Familial combined hyperlipidemia should be suspected in subjects with moderate hypertriglyceridemia or moderate hypercholesterolemia (lipoprotein type IIa, IIb, or IV), or both, especially in the setting of a family history of premature CHD. Xanthomas are not a feature of this disorder. Low plasma HDL-C, obesity, insulin resistance, and hyperuricemia are often present. The diagnosis is a clinical one; it requires demonstration of the clinical phenotype in the affected subject and family members and exclusion of other primary or secondary disorders. Secondary disorders that produce a similar phenotype include diabetes mellitus, nephrotic syndrome, and occasionally hypothyroidism. Many patients with diabetes mellitus and combined hyperlipidemia may have a genetic susceptibility related to inheritance of familial combined hyperlipidemia.

Treatment

Weight reduction and dietary treatment can help correct metabolic abnormalities, such as obesity and insulin resistance, that contribute to the hyperlipidemia. Drug therapy should be directed at the predominant lipid abnormality. For example, plasma elevations of total cholesterol and LDL-C can be treated with HMG-CoA reductase inhibitors, niacin, or bile acid sequestrants.[282] Of these, HMG-CoA reductase inhibitors may be preferable because niacin can cause or worsen glucose intolerance and hyperuricemia and bile acid sequestrants can cause hypertriglyceridemia.[346] Gemfibrozil can lower triglyceride and raise HDL-C levels, and it reduced the incidence of coronary events in the Helsinki Heart Study.[347] Low HDL-C levels can be treated with niacin, gemfibrozil, or HMG-CoA reductase inhibitors.[348] Because familial combined hyperlipidemia is associated with premature CHD, affected family members should be identified.

Type III Hyperlipoproteinemia (Familial Dysbetalipoproteinemia)

Type III hyperlipoproteinemia, or familial dysbetalipoproteinemia, is an uncommon disorder of lipoprotein metabolism characterized by moderate to severe hypertriglyceridemia and hypercholesterolemia caused by the accumulation of cholesterol-rich remnant particles in the plasma.[86, 88] Premature peripheral vascular disease and coronary artery disease are common. The cause is mutations in apo-E that result in defective binding to lipoprotein receptors. The disorder is associated with the apo-E2 isoform (described previously) and in most instances is inherited as an autosomal recessive trait that requires a secondary exacerbating metabolic factor (either genetic or environmental) for expression of the phenotype. Several rare apo-E mutations result in the dominant expression of the disorder.

Clinical Features

Type III hyperlipoproteinemia is usually diagnosed in adulthood and is rarely detected in persons younger than 20 years, with the exception of those with the rare autosomal dominant apo-E mutations.[86] The disorder is more common in men and is usually not manifested in women until after menopause. It is characterized by moderately severe elevations in plasma triglyceride and cholesterol levels; typically, these values range from 3.4 to 4.5 mmol/L (300 to 400 mg/dL) and 7.8 to 10.3 mmol/L (300 to 400 mg/dL), respectively. Concentrations of HDL-C are normal, and LDL-C is almost always reduced.

Xanthomas are present in more than half of affected subjects.[86, 88] The presence of palmar xanthomas, which are planar xanthomas in the palmar creases (see Fig. 34–26*F*), is virtually pathognomonic for this disorder. Tuberous or tuberoeruptive xanthomas (see Fig. 34–26*E*; see color section) are also common but are less specific for this disorder. Tendon xanthomas and xanthelasma occur in some patients. Premature vascular disease is common, and peripheral vascular disease occurs in addition to premature CHD.[86] Type III hyperlipoproteinemia accounts for 0.2% to 1.0% of lipid disorders associated with myocardial infarction in persons younger than 60 years. Coexisting metabolic conditions that exacerbate the phenotype of type III hyperlipoproteinemia, such as obesity, alcohol consumption, diabetes mellitus, and hypothyroidism, are often present.

Origin and Pathogenesis

Type III hyperlipoproteinemia is caused by the plasma accumulation of cholesterol-rich remnants of VLDL, IDL, and chylomicron particles.[86, 88] The clearance defect is caused by mutant apo-E that binds defectively to remnant receptors, including LDL receptors (discussed in "Roles of Apolipoprotein E in Lipid Metabolism"). The remnants that accumulate have lost much of their triglyceride through LPL-mediated triglyceride hydrolysis and therefore are cholesterol rich. The predominant remnant particles are termed β-VLDL and can be isolated in the VLDL ultracentrifugation density range (<1.006 g/mL). In contrast to normal VLDLs, which migrate as pre-β particles, these remnants are characterized by β-migration on agarose gel electrophoresis.

Homozygosity for the apo-E2 isoform occurs at a frequency of about 1 in 100 in the general population. Despite this high frequency, the type III hyperlipoproteinemia phenotype is relatively rare; the dyslipidemia develops in about 1 in 10 to 1 in 100 apo-E2 homozygotes (overall prevalence of 1 in 10,000). Manifestation of the dyslipidemia appears to require the presence of a secondary factor, such as a metabolic condition that contributes to the phenotype of impaired remnant clearance.

Clinical Features

Subjects with familial hypertriglyceridemia typically have plasma triglyceride levels in the range of 2.3 to 5.6 mmol/L (200 to 500 mg/dL) and normal LDL-C levels. As the level of LDL-C considered to be normal has declined, the prevalence of individuals with isolated elevations of plasma triglycerides has also diminished. The hypertriglyceridemia is often associated with low plasma HDL-C levels.[376] The elevated triglyceride levels are usually not evident until adulthood[277] and may be exacerbated by secondary factors, including hypothyroidism, estrogen therapy, or alcohol ingestion. Such exacerbations can be associated with severe elevations of triglycerides (>11.3 mmol/L [1000 mg/dL]), placing subjects at risk for eruptive xanthomas and pancreatitis. However, xanthomas are usually not present. Obesity and insulin resistance are common. Although familial hypertriglyceridemia was originally thought to be associated with increased risk for CHD,[277] this relation has been questioned.[377] The association of decreased HDL-C levels with hypertriglyceridemia may contribute to increased CHD risk.[376]

Origin and Pathogenesis

Familial hypertriglyceridemia appears to be caused by overproduction of VLDL triglycerides in the presence of near-normal apo-B production,[343, 344, 378] which leads to the secretion of large, triglyceride-rich VLDL. Secondary disorders (e.g., insulin resistance) that lead to VLDL overproduction can exacerbate the syndrome. The low plasma HDL levels commonly found in hypertriglyceridemia are associated with enhanced fractional catabolism of apo-AI.[379, 380] The genetic defect in familial hypertriglyceridemia is unknown. It is likely that the genetic loci involved in causing hypertriglyceridemia in familial combined hyperlipidemia are also involved in causing isolated hypertriglyceridemia. Whether the large, triglyceride-rich VLDLs are atherogenic is unclear; an enhanced risk for premature CHD may be related to whether concomitant decreases in HDL-C occur.

Diagnosis

Familial hypertriglyceridemia should be suspected in individuals with increased plasma triglyceride levels and normal plasma cholesterol. The disorder can be diagnosed only if hypertriglyceridemia is found in half of the first-degree relatives at risk, and it can be difficult to distinguish from familial combined hyperlipidemia, which may also occur as isolated hypertriglyceridemia related to increased plasma VLDL (type IV pattern). Measurement of plasma lipid levels in children does not help to distinguish these disorders because lipid abnormalities are usually not present until after puberty in either disorder. The elevated VLDL levels can be observed as a cloudy appearance of the plasma after overnight refrigeration.

Treatment

In addition to dietary fat restriction, secondary disorders such as diabetes mellitus, estrogen administration, or alcohol intake should be screened for and treated. Drugs that lower triglyceride levels (e.g., niacin, gemfibrozil) may be useful. Because niacin can impair glucose tolerance, it should be used cautiously in patients with underlying insulin resistance.

Elevated Plasma Lp(a)

This disorder consists of elevations of modified LDL particles in the plasma, in which the apo-B protein of LDL is covalently bonded to apo(a).[381–384] Apo(a) is a protein of unknown function that shares high sequence homology with plasminogen but is not catalytically active.[385] Some[332, 386–388] but not all[389–393] studies suggest that elevated plasma Lp(a) concentrations are associated with an increased risk for CHD.

Clinical Features

There are no characteristic physical findings or lipoprotein patterns to suggest elevated plasma Lp(a) levels. Elevated Lp(a) (>30 mg/dL) may be suspected, however, in patients with premature CHD. Plasma Lp(a) concentrations are influenced by heredity[394–396] and vary among different ethnic populations.[397] For example, African populations have higher levels.[382] Some data suggest that elevations of plasma Lp(a) may be atherogenic only in the presence of high concentrations of LDL.[398] In support of this, elevated Lp(a) concentrations are a risk factor for development of CHD in subjects with FH.[289] Thus, high Lp(a) levels may be viewed as a potent risk factor for CHD in predisposed individuals.[399]

Origin and Pathogenesis

Apo(a) is found only in humans, nonhuman primates, and hedgehogs.[382] Its function from an evolutionary perspective is unclear. Nevertheless, the presence of high plasma levels of apo(a) appears to have been selected for in certain populations.[397] Apo(a) is attached by disulfide bonds to the apo-B protein of LDL.[400] Plasma Lp(a) levels are in large part determined by heredity and appear to be related to the number of repeats of a so-called kringle motif in the protein.[394] The larger isoforms that contain more kringle repeats are found in lower concentrations in the plasma,[401] possibly related to impaired processing of these large forms for secretion by hepatocytes. The factors that control the production and clearance of Lp(a) are largely unknown. An increased susceptibility to atherosclerosis associated with high plasma levels of Lp(a) could be related to impaired fibrinolysis caused by competition for plasminogen receptors,[402, 403] to effects on smooth muscle proliferation,[404] or to unknown factors.

Diagnosis

The diagnosis of high plasma Lp(a) levels is made by specific assays of plasma for apo(a) or intact Lp(a) particles; care should be taken to ensure that samples are collected and stored appropriately and that the assay does not detect plasminogen. Lp(a) levels greater than 30 mg/dL are considered high.

Treatment

Of the hypolipidemic drugs currently available, only niacin appears to lower plasma Lp(a) levels.[290] Treatment with niacin (4 g/day) lowers Lp(a) levels by 35% to 40%. In postmenopausal women, estrogen therapy lowers Lp(a) levels by about 20%.[405, 406]

Polygenic Hypercholesterolemia

Hypercholesterolemia is defined as a cholesterol value that exceeds the 95th percentile for the population. A study by Goldstein and co-workers[277] suggested that about 10% of patients with hypercholesterolemia have familial combined hyperlipidemia and about 5% have FH. In a large proportion of the remaining 85%, the cause of the hypercholesterolemia is unknown but probably largely involves combinations of genetic and environmental factors. Other genetic factors that contribute to hypercholesterolemia may involve physiologic processes that influence cholesterol absorption, bile acid metabolism, or intracellular cholesterol metabolism. Polygenic hypercholesterolemia is diagnosed by excluding other primary genetic causes, by the absence of tendon xanthomas, and by demonstrating that hypercholesterolemia is present in no more than 10% of first-degree relatives.[277] The hypercholesterolemia is treated according to NCEP guidelines (described later).

Sporadic Hypertriglyceridemia

As with high plasma cholesterol, unknown genetic and environmental factors can result in elevated plasma triglyceride levels.[277] This so-called sporadic hypertriglyceridemia can be distinguished from familial syndromes by the absence of hypertriglyceridemia in relatives. The condition is treated with dietary fat restriction, treatment of secondary conditions that exacerbate hypertriglyceridemia, and drugs that lower triglyceride levels, such as niacin or gemfibrozil.

PRIMARY DISORDERS OF HIGH-DENSITY LIPOPROTEIN METABOLISM

Several genetic disorders can result in decreased or increased plasma levels of HDL-C (Table 34–9).

Familial Hypoalphalipoproteinemia

The autosomal dominant disorder familial hypoalphalipoproteinemia is manifested by low plasma HDL-C levels and an increased risk for premature CHD.[332, 407, 408] The diagnosis is suggested by HDL-C levels that are less than the 10th percentile (<0.8 mmol/L [30 mg/dL] in men or 1.0 mmol/L [40 mg/dL] in premenopausal women). There are no characteristic physical findings, but there is often a family history of low HDL-C levels and premature CHD. The genetic and metabolic defects that lead to low plasma HDL levels are unknown, but it appears that up to 50% of low HDL-C levels can be linked to the hepatic lipase or apo-AI/apo-CIII/apo-AIV gene locus.[409] The lack of HDL in the plasma accelerates the development of atherosclerosis, presumably because reverse cholesterol transport or other protective effects of HDL are impaired.[410, 411]

Drug therapy should be aimed at raising the plasma HDL concentration or lowering the plasma LDL concentration, or both.[348, 412] Treatments to raise HDL levels include estrogen therapy for postmenopausal women,[413–415] aerobic exercise,[416] and the drug niacin or gemfibrozil.[347, 348] Because increasing HDL-C is difficult with current therapies, lowering the LDL-C concentration may be the most effective approach, with the premise that the lowering of atherogenic LDL particles can overcome some, if not all, of the effects of low HDL.[348]

Low HDL levels have been found in specific ethnic groups. For example, Southeast Asians, specifically people from the Indian subcontinent, have very low HDL levels in the context of insulin resistance.[416a, 416b] In Turks, however, low HDL levels are associated with elevated hepatic lipase activity without insulin resistance.[417, 418]

Apolipoprotein AI Mutations

Mutations in the apo-AI gene[98, 99, 419, 420] can decrease HDL formation and result in low plasma HDL-C levels. Apo-AI deficiency can be caused by point mutations in the apo-AI gene or by deletions or gene rearrangements at the apo-AI/apo-CIII/apo-AIV gene locus.[419] Apo-AI deficiency typically results in plasma HDL-C levels less than 0.3 mmol/L (10 mg/dL).[420] Manifestations include a predisposition to premature CHD, xanthomas, and corneal opacities.[420] The molecular diagnosis can be made only by specialized analysis, including electrophoresis of the plasma apolipoproteins and DNA analysis to identify the mutation. Inasmuch as it is difficult to raise the plasma apo-AI or HDL-C levels in these disorders, the treatment should be directed toward lowering the levels of plasma non–HDL-C.

Other rare variants of apo-AI exist,[419] including apo-AI_{Milano},[421] which is caused by a substitution of cysteine for arginine at amino acid 173 and results in lower plasma HDL-C levels. This mutation is inherited as an autosomal dominant trait and has not been associated with premature CHD. Whether the mutation protects against the development of atherosclerosis or

Table 34–9. Genetic Disorders of High-Density Lipoprotein Metabolism

Disorder	Mutant Gene	Mode of Inheritance	Population Frequency	Typical Plasma HDL-C (mmol/L [mg/dL])	Typical Clinical Manifestations: Corneal Opacifications	Typical Clinical Manifestations: Premature Vascular Disease
Familial hypoalphalipoproteinemia	Unknown	Autosomal dominant	~1/400	0.5–0.8 (20–30)	–	+
Familial apo-AI and apo-CIII deficiency	Apo-AI or apo-AI/apo-CIII	Autosomal recessive	Rare	<0.1 (5)	+	+
Apo-AI_{Milano}	Apo-AI	Autosomal dominant	Rare	~0.3 (10)	–	–
LCAT deficiency	LCAT	Autosomal recessive	Rare	<0.3 (10)	+	+
Fish-eye disease	LCAT	Autosomal recessive	Rare	<0.3 (10)	+	–
Tangier disease*	ABCA1	Autosomal recessive	Rare	<0.1 (5)	+	+
CETP deficiency	CETP	Autosomal recessive	Rare	>2.6 (100)	–	–

*Clinical manifestations also include orange tonsils.

ABCA1, adenosine triphosphate binding cassette transporter A1; apo-AI, apolipoprotein AI; CETP, cholesteryl ester transfer protein; LCAT, lecithin:cholesterol acyltransferase.

whether this kindred has mitigating genetic or environmental factors is not known. Other apo-AI variants are associated with amyloidosis.[422–424]

Cholesteryl Ester Transfer Protein Deficiency

CETP deficiency is a hereditary syndrome in which plasma HDL-C levels are increased because of diminished activity of plasma CETP.[156, 425, 426] Once thought to be rare, the disorder is not uncommon in the Japanese population.[195] Its features include marked elevations of plasma HDL-C in homozygotes (usually >2.6 mmol/L [100 mg/dL]) and possible protection against development of CHD.[425] Heterozygotes have moderately elevated HDL-C levels. The diminished activity of CETP results in diminished transport of cholesteryl esters from HDL to the apo-B–containing lipoproteins. As a result, more cholesteryl esters are found in HDL, and the ratio of total cholesterol to HDL-C is markedly reduced. Presumably, the combination of reduced amounts of atherogenic LDL and increased antiatherogenic HDL decreases susceptibility to atherosclerosis.

Studies in transgenic mice have confirmed this relation between CETP and atherosclerosis. Although mice normally do not have significant plasma CETP activity and have high plasma HDL-C levels, transgenic mice that express CETP have increased plasma LDL-C, decreased HDL-C, and increased susceptibility to atherosclerosis.[196, 427, 428] Nevertheless, as discussed previously, subjects who are heterozygous for CETP deficiency experience CHD despite high plasma HDL,[195] and it remains to be determined whether lowering CETP activity in humans would have therapeutic value. The molecular diagnosis of CETP deficiency requires the measurement of plasma CETP activity in vitro or identification of the DNA mutation. At present, there is no specific treatment.

Lecithin:Cholesterol Acyltransferase Deficiency

LCAT deficiency is a rare autosomal recessive disorder that causes corneal opacities,[268] normochromic anemia, and renal failure in young adults.[429, 430] About 30 kindreds of LCAT deficiency and a number of mutations have been described.[430, 431] LCAT deficiency results in decreased esterification of cholesterol to cholesteryl esters on HDL particles.[432] As a result, free cholesterol accumulates on lipoprotein particles and in peripheral tissues such as the cornea, red blood cell membranes, and renal glomeruli, presumably because reverse cholesterol transport is impaired. Plasma cholesterol levels in LCAT deficiency are variable, HDL-C levels are reduced, and the ratio of free cholesterol to esterified cholesterol in the plasma is increased.[431] Normally, free cholesterol accounts for about one third of the total cholesterol in the plasma; in LCAT deficiency, free cholesterol accounts for most of the plasma cholesterol. The accumulation of free cholesterol in vascular tissues can lead to premature CHD. At present, there is no means to increase the plasma activity of LCAT; therefore, the treatment is preventive (by dietary fat restriction) and symptomatic (e.g., renal transplantation).

A variant of LCAT deficiency is called fish-eye disease.[430, 433] Although this disorder is also caused by mutations of the LCAT gene,[434–436] the phenotype is less severe than that seen in complete LCAT deficiency. Fish-eye disease is characterized by low plasma HDL-C levels and corneal opacities; anemia, renal disease, and premature atherosclerosis are not present.[185] The phenotypic differences between LCAT deficiency and fish-eye disease have been attributed to whether LCAT activity is absent from both HDL and apo-B–containing lipoproteins (LCAT deficiency) or from HDL only (fish-eye disease)[437]; however, one subject with phenotypic fish-eye disease had normal HDL-associated LCAT activity.[438]

Tangier Disease

Tangier disease is a rare autosomal recessive disorder associated with hypolipidemia, including decreases in both plasma HDL and LDL-C levels, and the presence of orange tonsils.[98, 439] Other features include corneal opacities,[268] hepatosplenomegaly, peripheral neuropathy, and premature CHD.[440] Metabolic studies have demonstrated that the disorder is associated with enhanced catabolism of plasma HDL.[441] Mutations in *ABCA1* have been causally linked to Tangier disease.[442–444] ABCA1 appears to promote cholesterol efflux from cells such as macrophages; the loss of this function apparently accounts for the impaired efflux of cholesterol from Tangier cells.[184, 445–447] As a result, massive amounts of cholesteryl esters accumulate in macrophages of the reticuloendothelial system. The orange tonsils observed in this disorder are caused by cholesterol deposits. There is currently no specific treatment. The degree to which heterozygosity for *ABCA1* mutations contributes to inherited low-HDL syndromes remains to be determined.

PRIMARY GENETIC HYPOLIPIDEMIAS

Familial Hypobetalipoproteinemia

Familial hypobetalipoproteinemia, an autosomal dominant disorder of apo-B metabolism, is associated with plasma cholesterol and LDL-C levels that are less than one half of normal in heterozygotes and with marked hypocholesterolemia (<1.3 mmol/L [50 mg/dL]) in homozygotes.[50, 448]

Clinical Features

Heterozygous subjects, about 1 in 500 persons, are usually asymptomatic but come to attention because of the detection of low plasma cholesterol levels. Typically, the total plasma cholesterol level is less than the fifth percentile, and it may be less than 2.6 mmol/L (100 mg/dL). Plasma LDL-C levels are also reduced by one half or more, and HDL-C levels are normal or slightly increased.[449] Plasma triglyceride levels are reduced in some kindreds. Although heterozygotes are usually asymptomatic, fat malabsorption has been reported.[450, 451] The syndrome is associated with longevity,[452] probably the result of a low risk for CHD.

Subjects who are homozygotes or compound heterozygotes for these apo-B mutations are rare, about 1 in 10^6 persons. Homozygotes may be detected at a young age because of fat malabsorption and decreased plasma cholesterol levels. Fat malabsorption is caused by inability to form chylomicrons in the intestine and subsequent failure to absorb fats and fat-soluble vitamins. Fat malabsorption may be accompanied by retinitis pigmentosa, acanthocytosis, and a progressive neurologic degenerative disease resulting from vitamin E deficiency. The acanthocytosis is caused by alterations in red blood cell membrane lipids. Despite the low plasma cholesterol levels, steroidogenesis appears to be normal except when demands are quite high.[453, 454] Homozygous subjects who produce enough of a truncated isoform of apo-B to facilitate some fat absorption may have a milder phenotype.

Origin and Pathogenesis

Most cases of known origin result from mutations in the apo-B gene.[448] More than 30 mutations have been described;

most are either nonsense or frameshift mutations that lead to the formation of truncated apo-B proteins.[455] Metabolic turnover studies indicate that these apo-B gene mutations impair the synthesis of apo-B–containing lipoproteins in some cases[456] and enhance the clearance of apo-B–containing lipoproteins from the plasma in others.[457] The decreased levels of apo-B–containing lipoproteins in the plasma cause low plasma cholesterol and triglyceride levels. Although most known cases of hypobetalipoproteinemia involve apo-B mutations, additional undefined genetic factors can result in low cholesterol levels.[458–460]

In homozygous subjects, the absence of apo-B leads to impaired intestinal chylomicron formation, which in turn leads to impaired absorption of fats and fat-soluble vitamins. Cholesterol absorption is probably also impaired, as demonstrated in transgenic mice lacking intestinal apo-B expression and chylomicron formation.[461] As noted, vitamin E malabsorption results in low tissue stores of tocopherol and a degenerative neurologic disease. Retinal degeneration may also be related to deficiencies of fat-soluble vitamins.[462]

Diagnosis

The diagnosis of familial hypolipoproteinemia is suggested by low plasma total and LDL cholesterol levels inherited as an autosomal dominant trait. The homozygous condition is suggested by extremely low plasma cholesterol and triglyceride levels in an infant or child with fat malabsorption. The differential diagnosis of the homozygous state includes abetalipoproteinemia (see later discussion) and Anderson's disease (chylomicron retention disease).[408, 463, 464] The molecular diagnosis of hypobetalipoproteinemia can be performed only in specialized laboratories by gel electrophoresis of plasma apo-B or by DNA analysis to identify specific mutations.

Treatment and Prognosis

Because heterozygous subjects are almost always asymptomatic, no specific treatment is indicated, but dietary supplementation of fat-soluble vitamins (especially vitamin E) is reasonable. Heterozygotes should be informed that if their spouse also has a very low plasma cholesterol level, their children could have homozygous or compound heterozygous hypobetalipoproteinemia; in this scenario, subjects should be referred to a lipid clinic for genetic counseling.

Subjects with homozygous hypobetalipoproteinemia (phenotypic abetalipoproteinemia) should be treated with large doses of vitamin E orally (100 to 300 mg/kg/day), which can raise the tissue vitamin E concentrations and prevent the neurologic complications.[374, 465] It is imperative to make the diagnosis and begin treatment at an early age to prevent nutritional deficiencies. Fat should be provided in the diet up to a level that symptoms allow (usually 15% to 20% of calories). Supplementation with medium-chain triglycerides is probably contraindicated because of reports of liver toxicity.[375]

Abetalipoproteinemia

Abetalipoproteinemia is a rare autosomal recessive disorder caused by a deficiency in MTP, which results in a virtual absence of apo-B–containing lipoproteins in the plasma.[170, 466–468]

Clinical Features

Abetalipoproteinemia occurs in fewer than 1 in 10^6 persons and has the same phenotype as homozygous hypobetalipoproteinemia (described previously), including malabsorption of fat and fat-soluble vitamins from the intestine, which can lead to neurologic disease related to vitamin E deficiency. The disorder is frequently detected in infancy because of fat malabsorption associated with marked decreases in plasma cholesterol and triglyceride levels.

Origin and Pathogenesis

Abetalipoproteinemia is caused by a deficiency of MTP,[466] a protein that transfers triglycerides or phospholipids onto nascent apo-B–containing lipoproteins during their formation in the ER. Insufficient lipidation of nascent particles impairs the synthesis and secretion of these particles by the intestine and the liver, and little if any apo-B is found in the plasma. Several mutations in the MTP gene have been described.[170, 468] The lack of MTP in the intestine leads to impaired chylomicron formation and malabsorption of fats and fat-soluble vitamins.

Diagnosis

The diagnosis is suggested by fat malabsorption associated with extremely low levels of plasma cholesterol (usually <1.3 mmol/L [50 mg/dL]) and triglyceride in an infant or young child.[467] Cholesterol levels in the parents, who are obligate heterozygotes, are normal. The demonstration of the molecular defect requires a specialized laboratory for detection of low or absent MTP in intestinal biopsy specimens or DNA analysis to identify specific mutations. The differential diagnosis of abetalipoproteinemia includes homozygous hypobetalipoproteinemia, in which the obligate heterozygote parents have low plasma lipid levels, and Anderson's disease.[408, 463, 464] Also called chylomicron retention syndrome, the latter disorder is a rare condition that is phenotypically similar to abetalipoproteinemia. Subjects with Anderson's disease cannot secrete chylomicrons from the intestine owing to an as yet undefined recessive mutation.

Treatment

Abetalipoproteinemia is treated in the same way as homozygous hypobetalipoproteinemia. Large doses of vitamin E are given by mouth to prevent the neurologic sequelae of vitamin E deficiency.

OTHER RARE PRIMARY LIPID DISORDERS

Hepatic Lipase Deficiency

Hepatic lipase deficiency is a disorder associated with lack of hepatic lipase activity in the plasma.[469–474] Its features include combined hyperlipidemia, with elevated levels of plasma cholesterol (6.5 to 38.8 mmol/L [250 to 1500 mg/dL]) and triglyceride (4.5 to 92.6 mmol/L [395 to 8200 mg/dL]); palmar and tuboeruptive xanthomas; and premature arcus corneae. β-VLDL levels are increased (however, the VLDL cholesterol/triglyceride ratio is <0.3, in contrast to type III hyperlipoproteinemia), and there is a threefold to fivefold enrichment of triglyceride in the LDL and HDL fractions. HDL-C levels are normal or slightly increased. Susceptibility to atherosclerosis is thought to be increased. The demonstration of hepatic lipase deficiency requires specialized in vitro assays of hepatic lipase activity in plasma or DNA analysis to identify mutations. Dietary restriction of fat and cholesterol can lower the plasma lipid levels.

Sitosterolemia

In this rare disorder, dietary sitosterol and other plant sterols, which are not normally absorbed in significant quantities in the intestine, are absorbed in large amounts, resulting in their accumulation in the plasma and in peripheral tissues.[475] Premature atherosclerosis can occur.[476] The molecular defect was mapped to chromosome 2p21[477] and was identified as mutations in the genes encoding ABCG8 and ABCG5.[478, 479] Clinically, affected children have tendon xanthomas and normal to high plasma levels of LDL-C; the differential diagnosis includes FH and cerebrotendinous xanthomatosis. The diagnosis can be confirmed by gas-liquid chromatography of plasma lipids to demonstrate the abnormal sterols. Treatment consists of restriction of plant sterols in the diet.

Cerebrotendinous Xanthomatosis

Cerebrotendinous xanthomatosis[475, 480] is a rare disorder of sterol metabolism associated with neurologic disease, tendon xanthomas, and cataracts in young adults. Neurologic manifestations include cerebellar ataxia, dementia, spinal cord paresis, and subnormal intelligence. Premature atherosclerosis is common.[481] Osteoporosis has been reported and is presumably caused by alterations in vitamin D metabolism.[482] The disorder results from mutations that cause deficiencies of 27-hydroxylase, a key enzyme in cholesterol oxidation and bile acid synthesis.[483] As a result, high levels of cholesterol and cholestanol, a 5α-dihydro derivative of cholesterol, accumulate in the plasma, tendons, and tissues of the nervous system. Treatment is with chenodeoxycholic acid,[484] often in combination with an HMG-CoA reductase inhibitor.[485, 486]

Acid Cholesteryl Ester Hydrolase Deficiency

Acid cholesteryl ester hydrolase deficiency is an autosomal recessive disorder caused by deficiency of a lysosomal esterase, which results in massive accumulation of cholesteryl esters and triglycerides in lysosomes.[487–489] In the variant called Wolman's disease, which is usually fatal in the first year of life, there is a complete deficiency of the lysosomal esterase. Cholesteryl ester storage disease is a milder variant in which there may be some residual esterase activity; affected subjects can survive past childhood but may develop premature CHD.

Familial Isolated Vitamin E Deficiency

Familial isolated vitamin E deficiency is a rare disorder characterized by low plasma levels of vitamin E in association with progressive neurologic degenerative disease.[490, 491] It is caused by lack of hepatic α-tocopherol transfer protein,[492] which is thought to facilitate the incorporation of α-tocopherol onto nascent VLDLs during their formation in the liver. In the absence of the protein, there is a lack of vitamin E on VLDL, which is a major transport mechanism for delivery of vitamin E to peripheral tissues. Treatment consists of daily supplementation with high doses of oral vitamin E.

SECONDARY DISORDERS OF LIPID METABOLISM

A number of metabolic diseases and drug therapies influence plasma lipids.[254, 493, 494] The secondary disorders of hyperlipidemia are listed in Table 34–8. Factors that affect HDL levels are listed in Table 34–10.

Table 34–10. Factors Affecting Plasma High-Density Lipoprotein Levels

Factors That Increase HDL
Estrogens
Exercise
Alcohol
Drugs: nicotinic acid, fibrates, HMG-CoA reductase inhibitors
Factors That Decrease HDL
Androgens
Progestins
Cigarette smoking
Obesity
Low-fat diet
Drugs: probucol, β-blockers

HDL, high-density lipoproteins; HMG-CoA, 3-hydroxy-3-methylglutaryl coenzyme A.

Diabetes Mellitus

Of the common diseases, diabetes mellitus exerts some of the most profound effects on plasma lipid metabolism.[495–498] Hypertriglyceridemia is found in up to one third of all diabetic patients and is related to the critical role of insulin in the production and clearance of triglyceride-rich lipoproteins from the plasma.[495] In addition, diabetic patients frequently have high plasma levels of atherogenic lipoproteins and low plasma HDL, predisposing them to premature CHD, a leading cause of death in diabetes.

In type 1 diabetes, insulin deficiency and poor glycemic control are associated with increases in the plasma levels of triglycerides and of apo-B–containing lipoproteins because of effects on plasma lipid metabolism in peripheral tissues and the liver. In peripheral tissues, insulin deficiency results in impaired LPL activity and diminished clearance of triglyceride-rich particles.[499] Insulin deficiency also causes enhanced lipolysis, which results in increased free fatty acid flux to the liver. In the liver, increased free fatty acid flux drives triglyceride synthesis and VLDL triglyceride synthesis and secretion. Plasma LDL-C levels may also be increased, possibly because insulin stimulates LDL receptor–mediated degradation of LDL[500] and this is diminished in type 1 diabetes.

In its most severe form, insulin deficiency can cause a chylomicronemia syndrome known as *diabetic lipemia*.[499, 501] In this disorder, massive increases in plasma triglyceride levels (>22.6 mmol/L [2000 mg/dL]) can result in lipemia retinalis, eruptive xanthomas, fatty liver, and pancreatitis. This disorder arises from an acquired LPL deficiency[499] and is relatively rare in the modern era of insulin therapy. The acquired lack of LPL activity results in accumulation of chylomicrons in the plasma (type I pattern), similar to that seen in primary genetic LPL deficiency. The disorder may result from the occurrence of diabetes mellitus in combination with some underlying disorder of triglyceride metabolism.[502] The hyperlipidemia related to insulin deficiency and type 1 diabetes is reversible with intensive insulin therapy. Persistent lipid abnormalities in patients with type 1 diabetes with excellent glycemic control suggest that another disorder of lipid metabolism is present.

In type 2 diabetes, which accounts for more than 90% of cases, the metabolic defect is related to insulin resistance and relative insulin deficiency. The insulin resistance appears to be caused by both genetic and acquired factors; metabolic abnormalities that accompany the insulin resistance include obesity, hyperglycemia, hypertension, plasma lipid abnormalities, and hyperuricemia, which are referred to as syndrome X or the metabolic syndrome.[331] One of the most common lipid abnormalities in type 2 diabetes is a moderate hyperlipidemia characterized by an increase in VLDL (type IV pattern), which can be accompanied by various degrees of chylomicronemia (type V pattern), depending on the dietary fat intake.[331] This disorder is characterized by the accumulation of apo-B–containing lipoproteins, which are likely to be proatherogenic, in the plasma. The plasma triglyceride and cholesterol levels are often moderately elevated, the HDL-C concentration may be low,[503, 504] and IDLs, or remnants, which are probably atherogenic, are also often increased.[505] Plasma levels of LDL are increased in some but not all subjects. However, the hyperlipidemia in type 2 diabetes is often characterized by an increase in the small, dense LDLs (LDL subclass pattern B),[506] which are particularly atherogenic; this increase occurs even in the absence of hyperlipidemia.[506] In addition, a portion of the plasma LDL undergoes glycosylation, which may increase susceptibility to oxidation.[507] Xanthomas are usually absent in this disorder.

Factors that contribute to the lipoprotein abnormalities in type 2 diabetes include decreased LPL activity in muscle and adipose tissue and increased free fatty acid flux to the liver from peripheral adipose tissue stores.[496] Combined with hepatic overproduction of apo-B, which occurs in insulin resistance,[508] the free fatty acid flux drives triglyceride synthesis and VLDL production in the liver.[509] The lipid abnormalities associated with VLDL overproduction may be exacerbated by a primary genetic disorder of lipid metabolism.[502, 510]

The mainstay of therapy for patients with type 2 diabetes with hyperlipidemia is glycemic control through diet, oral hypoglycemic agents, or insulin therapy. Periodic monitoring of the glycosylated hemoglobin is helpful in assessing the glycemic control. However, in contrast to the situation in type 1 diabetes, the hyperlipidemia in type 2 diabetes may be difficult to eradicate even with excellent glycemic control because these subjects have accompanying genetic and acquired metabolic abnormalities that are not resolved by returning blood sugar levels to normal. Decreasing insulin resistance through weight loss can, however, have dramatic effects on both the hyperglycemia and the hyperlipidemia. Metformin, a hypoglycemic agent, may lower plasma glucose levels and produce a modest lowering of plasma lipid levels.[511] In addition to glycemic control, drugs for diabetic hyperlipidemia include gemfibrozil and HMG-CoA reductase inhibitors. Niacin should be used with caution as it can impair or worsen glucose tolerance. Treatment with insulin can lower plasma LDL-C levels in both type 1[512] and type 2[513] diabetes mellitus.

Hypothyroidism

Alterations in thyroid function can have profound effects on plasma lipids,[493, 514, 515] and all patients with significant hyperlipidemia should be screened for hypothyroidism. The classical manifestation of hypothyroidism is an elevation of the plasma LDL-C level (6.5 to 15.5 mmol/L [250 to 600 mg/dL]), but this disorder can also be associated with high plasma triglyceride levels.[514, 516] Levels of HDL-C are usually unchanged or slightly lower in hypothyroidism and may be reduced in hyperthyroidism[517, 518]; the latter effect may be related to alterations in hepatic lipase activity.[517, 519] The elevations of plasma LDL-C in hypothyroidism are associated with impaired clearance of LDL,[520–522] probably reflecting decreased LDL receptor expression.[523] The high LDL-C levels in hypothyroidism are associated with an increased risk for atherosclerosis,[524] but risk for myocardial infarction is not necessarily increased,[524, 525] perhaps because hypothyroidism decreases myocardial oxygen demand. Subclinical hypothyroidism, in which metabolic abnormalities are present without symptoms, can also cause hypercholesterolemia that responds to treatment with thyroid hormone.[526] Hypothyroidism is also associated with low LPL activity,[514, 527] predisposing to increased plasma triglyceride levels. Hyperlipidemia with hypothyroidism may be more marked in those with an underlying genetic susceptibility,[354, 516] but it responds dramatically to thyroid hormone replacement. In elderly patients with CHD or significant risk factors, thyroid hormone should be replaced cautiously because rapid replacement can exacerbate underlying ischemic heart disease.

Estrogen Therapy

Estrogen therapy increases plasma triglyceride levels[240, 528] and can occasionally cause marked hypertriglyceridemia, especially in predisposed individuals.[529] The hypertriglyceridemia appears to be dose-related.[413] Although most women taking either oral contraceptives or postmenopausal estrogens maintain triglyceride levels in the normal range, massive hypertriglyceridemia can on occasion cause pancreatitis.[529] For this reason, triglyceride levels should be measured in women before estrogen therapy is initiated. Estrogens appear to cause hypertriglyceridemia through increased production of VLDL.[530] LPL activity in adipose tissue is not altered.

Estrogen therapy also enhances the clearance of LDL from the circulation[528] and lowers plasma LDL-C. Enhanced LDL clearance probably results from increased hepatic LDL receptor expression.[531] Treatment of postmenopausal women with estrogen can lower LDL-C by 15%.[415, 528] Estrogens can also reduce the hyperlipidemia of type III hyperlipoproteinemia.[355]

Estrogens have significant effects on HDL metabolism, increasing HDL-C in postmenopausal women by more than 15%,[415, 528] primarily by increasing the HDL_2 subfraction. Women have higher HDL-C levels than men at all ages after puberty. This is presumably a result of the effects of androgens because HDL-C levels decrease at puberty in men but remain constant in women.[243] The mechanism by which gonadal hormones alter the HDL-C levels is uncertain but may involve differences in hepatic lipase activity. The effects of estrogen, which raises HDL and lowers LDL-C levels, can be offset if estrogens are combined with progestational agents, which lower HDL and raise LDL cholesterol levels.[532] Because estrogens tend to lower LDL and raise HDL-C, estrogen therapy in postmenopausal women appears to decrease CHD risk significantly.[533, 534] However, more recent studies have brought this into question.[535, 536]

Alcohol Consumption

The regular consumption of large amounts of alcohol can significantly affect plasma triglyceride metabolism.[537] Alcohol metabolism results in increased NADH levels, which inhibit fatty acid oxidation in the liver. This inhibition leads to increased triglyceride synthesis, fatty liver, and enhanced VLDL production.[538] The enhanced VLDL production raises plasma triglycerides and occasionally causes massive hypertriglyceridemia and pancreatitis, especially in persons with an underlying genetic susceptibility.[363] Plasma electrophoresis reveals an accumulation of VLDL in the plasma (type IV pattern) and occasionally a superimposed chylomicronemia (type V pattern) as these particles compete for saturable clearance mechanisms.[539] Subjects with type III hyperlipoproteinemia are particularly sensitive to the effects of alcohol consumption because the alcohol-induced overproduction of VLDL and associated remnant particles occurs in the setting of impaired remnant clearance. Hypertriglyceridemia can be an important contributor to pancreatitis associated with alcohol consumption.

Alcohol consumption is also associated with higher plasma levels of HDL-C,[540] which in turn may explain why moderate alcohol consumption may protect against CHD.[538, 541, 542] Indeed, moderate consumption of alcohol in the form of wine may be inversely correlated with CHD mortality.[543]

Nephrotic Syndrome

Hyperlipidemia, which almost always accompanies the nephrotic syndrome, is caused predominantly by elevation of LDL (type IIa pattern) but can also be caused by high VLDL levels (type IV pattern). Total cholesterol, VLDL, LDL-C, total triglycerides, and plasma apo-B are all elevated.[544] The ratio of total cholesterol to HDL-C is increased, consistent with an atherogenic phenotype. Plasma Lp(a) levels can also be elevated.[545] The pathogenesis of the hyperlipidemia appears to be related to increased rates of production of LDL or VLDL or both.[544, 546, 547] The cause of VLDL overproduction is unclear, but it may be related to a generalized hypersecretion phenomenon in the liver. Because myocardial infarction ranks second only to renal failure as the cause of death in subjects with nephrotic syndrome, the hyperlipidemia should be treated vigorously. HMG-CoA reductase inhibitors appear to be particularly effective.[548]

Protease Inhibitor Use in Human Immunodeficiency Virus Infection

Combination therapy with protease inhibitors for human immunodeficiency virus infection has been associated with metabolic changes, including hyperlipidemia, lipodystrophy, and insulin resistance, in many patients.[549–552] The cause of this syndrome is currently unknown. With the improved life expectancy in patients receiving protease inhibitor regimens, there is increased concern about the risk of CHD related to the metabolic side effects. Although data concerning CHD risk and treatment guidelines are lacking, many affected subjects are currently treated with regimens similar to those used in patients with insulin resistance or diabetes not associated with human immunodeficiency virus infection.

Other Drugs

In addition to estrogens, other therapeutic agents can cause hyperlipidemia.[519] These agents include glucocorticoids[247–249] and antihypertensive agents such as thiazide diuretics and β-adrenergic blockers.[519, 553–555] Exogenous androgens can reduce HDL-C levels.[556, 557]

TREATMENT OF LIPID DISORDERS

Clinical Trials Providing Rationale for Treating Hyperlipidemia

In addition to proving the cholesterol-diet-heart hypothesis, clinical trials in humans demonstrated that lowering plasma lipid levels reduces the incidence of symptomatic CHD in patients at risk. The Lipid Research Clinics Coronary Primary Prevention Trial was the first of the trials and followed approximately 3800 men (ages 35 to 59) with plasma cholesterol concentrations higher than 6.7 mmol/L (260 mg/dL) and with no prior evidence of CHD.[558] The men were divided into two groups. The control group was given a placebo and minimal dietary advice, while the experimental group was given the lipid-lowering drug cholestyramine and dietary management. Over the 7-year study, reductions of 19%, 19%, and about 25% were seen in total and LDL cholesterol concentrations, in the incidence of fatal and nonfatal myocardial infarction, and in the incidence of angina, respectively. At high doses of cholestyramine, the results were even more dramatic, with 35% and 50% reductions in LDL-C levels and in the incidence of symptomatic CHD, respectively.

The Familial Atherosclerosis Treatment Study took the cholesterol-diet-heart hypothesis a step further.[295] In this study, 120 high-risk men were treated aggressively with lipid-lowering protocols for 2.5 years. All subjects had plasma cholesterol and LDL concentrations higher than 7.0 mmol/L (270 mg/dL) and 4.7 mmol/L (180 mg/dL), respectively, and all had angiographically documented CHD. Digitized quantitative coronary arteriography was used for documentation. Men receiving either drug treatment (lovastatin and colestipol or niacin and colestipol) displayed dramatic reductions in plasma LDL concentrations and in the progression of coronary atherosclerosis. More important, established atherosclerotic lesions actually regressed.

Despite the impressive results of these intervention trials, critics continued to question recommendations for diet and drug therapy to reduce the risk of CHD[559, 560] on the basis of the fact that the trials, although they clearly demonstrated a marked reduction in CHD-related events, did not conclusively prove that lowering cholesterol prolonged life. Concern was expressed that an increased risk of death from other causes could result from the treatment. Two important prospective studies have addressed these concerns: the Scandinavian Simvastatin Survival Study (4S), conducted in high-risk patients with preexisting coronary disease (a so-called secondary prevention study),[561] and the West of Scotland Coronary Prevention Study (WOSCOPS), conducted in men without preexisting coronary disease (a so-called primary prevention study).[562]

The 4S trial included 4444 patients, of whom 19% were women, with angina pectoris or a previously documented myocardial infarction and with elevated plasma cholesterol concentrations (5.5 to 8.0 mmol/L [214 to 311 mg/dL]). The subjects, who previously received a lipid-lowering diet, were randomly divided into placebo and treatment groups; the drug tested was simvastatin, an HMG-CoA reductase inhibitor. The groups were observed for an average of 5.4 years (the time interval at which 10% of the study participants died). The mean changes in total plasma cholesterol, LDL-C, and HDL-C in the drug group compared with the placebo group were −25%, −35%, and 8%, respectively. The placebo group had 256 (12%) deaths, and the simvastatin group had 182 (8%), for a relative risk of death of 0.70. Deaths from CHD-related events were 189 in the placebo group and 111 in the simvastatin group, for a relative risk of death of 0.58 in the drug group. There were no differences in noncardiovascular deaths between the two groups (49 versus 46, respectively). In addition, the relative risk for one or more coronary events was 0.66 for the drug group, and there was a 37% reduction in the need for myocardial procedures.[561] In this study, cholesterol lowering prolonged life in persons with established CHD.

The results from the WOSCOPS trial were equally impressive.[562] This trial was designed to test the effect of another HMG-CoA reductase inhibitor (pravastatin) in men (6595 subjects, 45 to 65 years old) with elevated plasma cholesterol concentrations (average 7.0 ± 0.6 mmol/L [272 ± 23 mg/dL]) but with no prior history of cardiac disease. The dosage of pravastatin was 40 mg/day, and the subjects were followed for an average of 4.9 years. Drug treatment lowered plasma cholesterol and LDL-C concentrations by 20% and 26%, respectively, whereas the placebo group had no changes in these levels. The placebo group had 248 documented coronary events (either nonfatal myocardial infarction or death from CHD) compared with 174 for the drug group, representing a 31% reduction in risk with treatment. The drug group had a 32% reduction in death from all cardiovascular causes and a 22% reduction in the risk of death from any cause. Furthermore, reduction in clinical cardiac events was evident within 6 to 12 months. Again, cholesterol lowering in men at high risk for CHD reduced death from cardiovascular events without increasing the risk of noncardiovascular death.

The efficacy and safety of treatment with statins were further demonstrated in subsequent trials. In the Cholesterol and Recurrent Events (CARE) trial and the Long-term Intervention with Pravastatin in Ischemic Disease (LIPID) study, subjects with established CHD at baseline were studied for 5 years.[563] In CARE the average baseline plasma cholesterol was 209 mg/dL (139 and 39 mg/dL for LDL-C and HDL-C, respectively), and in LIPID it was 218 mg/dL (150 and 36 mg/dL for LDL-C and HDL-C, respectively). Treatment with pravastatin (40 mg/day) reduced LDL-C by 25% in CARE and by 28% in LIPID. These decreases were associated with a 24% reduction in CHD in LIPID and 29% and 28% reductions in nonfatal myocardial infarctions in LIPID and CARE, respectively.

The CARE and LIPID studies along with 4S demonstrate that patients with CHD and LDL-C levels above 130 mg/dL benefit from lipid-lowering therapy. Although patients in these studies with LDL-C levels between 100 and 130 mg/dL did not display a consistent benefit from treatment, the Veterans Affairs High Density Lipoprotein Intervention Trial demonstrated that CHD patients with LDL-C of 104 mg/dL did benefit from gemfibrozil therapy.[564] Thus, the results from these four trials clearly suggest that treatment of CHD patients with LDL-C higher than 100 mg/dL with hypolipidemic drugs is of benefit and that the target of treatment of CHD patients should be to reduce LDL-C to less than 100 mg/dL.

Like the WOSCOPS trial, the Air Force/Texas Coronary Atherosclerosis Prevention Study (AFCAPS/TexCAPS) targeted men and women without CHD but with moderately elevated LDL-C (average, 156 mg/dL) who were also at risk because of age (men older than 45 years; women older than 55 years) coupled with low HDL-C levels (average, 37 mg/dL).[565] In this trial, lovastatin reduced LDL-C by 26% and primary end-point events, including fatal and nonfatal myocardial infarction and unstable angina pectoris, by 37%.

In addition to proving the diet-cholesterol-heart disease hypothesis, the clinical trials confirm and extend the recommended guidelines for treatment of dyslipidemic patients established by the NCEP, which are discussed in a later section.[199]

Approach to the Hyperlipidemic Patient

Individuals come to attention for evaluation for a lipid disorder because of the presence of atherosclerotic vascular disease, pancreatitis, xanthomas, or xanthelasma or because of detection of a high plasma cholesterol or triglyceride level. The initial evaluation of these patients includes a history and physical examination, including assessment of CHD risk factors, and measurement of plasma lipids.

Risk Factors

The initial examination should include an assessment of risk factors for atherosclerotic CHD. Table 34–11 lists the risk factors, as specified by the NCEP in 2001.[242] Diabetes mellitus is considered to be a disorder equivalent to established CHD with regard to risk.[566, 567] In addition, data indicate that obesity is an independent risk factor for CHD.[568] Particular emphasis should be placed on obtaining a detailed history of all first-degree relatives to identify cholesterol disorders or premature CHD.

Table 34–11. Major Risk Factors for Coronary Heart Disease

Positive
1. Age (men ≥45 yr; women ≥55 yr)
2. Family history of premature CHD (male parent or sibling <55 yr, female parent or sibling <65 yr)
3. Current cigarette smoking
4. Hypertension (blood pressure ≥140/90 mm Hg or receiving antihypertensive medication)
5. Low HDL-C (<1.0 mmol/L [<40 mg/dL])
6. Diabetes mellitus*

Negative
1. High HDL-C (≥1.6 mmol/L [≥60 mg/dL])

*Diabetes is regarded as a CHD equivalent, that is, >20% risk of a CHD event within 10 years.

Adapted from National Cholesterol Education Program Expert Panel. Executive summary of the third report of the National Cholesterol Education Program (NCEP) Expert Panel on Detection, Evaluation, and Treatment of High Blood Cholesterol in Adults (Adult Treatment Panel III). JAMA 2001; 285:2486–2497.

CHD, coronary heart disease; HDL-C, high-density lipoprotein cholesterol.

Physical Examination

A thorough physical examination should be performed with emphasis on the cardiovascular system and the manifestations of hyperlipidemia. Elevated plasma lipids (cholesterol or triglycerides) can accumulate in macrophage reticuloendothelial cells in certain tissues, particularly skin, tendons, eye, liver, and spleen. Deposits in the skin or tendons are manifest as xanthomas or xanthelasmas. In almost all cases, these tissue lipid deposits are reversible with lipid-lowering therapy. Several of the clinical findings are illustrated in Figure 34–26.

Xanthelasmas (see Fig. 34–26*A*) are small, raised, yellowish macules that typically appear on or near the eyelids above and around the medial canthus. They are seen in FH, familial defective apo-B100, and type III hyperlipoproteinemia. Xanthelasmas occasionally occur in patients with normal plasma cholesterol levels, possibly as the result of enhanced uptake of oxidized or modified lipoproteins by tissue macrophages. Xanthelasmas typically regress with cholesterol lowering and can often be treated effectively in the setting of normal cholesterol levels with low doses of probucol, an antioxidant drug. *Lipemia retinalis* (see Fig. 34–26*B*), a condition in which lipemic plasma can be visualized by routine ophthalmologic examination of the fundi, is typically seen only when the triglyceride levels are 22.6 mmol/L (2000 mg/dL) or higher.

Tendon xanthomas (see Fig. 34–26*C* and *D*) are nodular deposits of cholesterol that accumulate in tissue macrophages in the Achilles and other tendons, including the extensor tendons in the hands, knees, and elbows. Tendon xanthomas are often present in FH (approximately 75% of subjects), in familial defective apo-B100, and sometimes in type III hyperlipoproteinemia. Small tendon xanthomas can be overlooked if not specifically sought. The examination of the Achilles tendon should include an assessment for thickness and for irregularities of contour (see Fig. 34–26*C*). Achilles tendon xanthomas can also be detected by xeroradiography.

Tuberous or *tuboeruptive xanthomas* (see Fig. 34–26*E*) are subcutaneous nodules that develop in the skin over areas susceptible to trauma such as the elbows and knees. They may be singular or multiple and may range from pea-sized to lemon-sized. Tuberous xanthomas are most often seen in type III hyperlipoproteinemia and also occur in FH. *Palmar xanthomas* (see Fig. 34–26*F*) are cutaneous deposits in the palmar and digital creases of the hands. This type of xanthoma is almost pathognomonic for high plasma levels of β-VLDL and type III hyperlipoproteinemia.

Eruptive xanthomas (see Fig. 34–26*G*) are cutaneous xanthomas that appear as small, yellowish, round papules that contain a pale center and an erythematous base. They can be mistaken for acne. The distribution of eruptive xanthomas includes the abdominal wall, the back, the buttocks, and other pressure contact areas. They are caused by accumulation of triglyceride in dermal histiocytes and generally occur when the plasma triglyceride level is 11.3 to 22.6 mmol/L (1000 to 2000 mg/dL) or more. They can disappear rapidly with lowering of the plasma triglyceride level.

Screening for Secondary Disorders

The history and physical examination should be directed toward uncovering secondary disorders of lipid metabolism (e.g., diabetes mellitus, hypothyroidism, or the nephrotic syndrome) and toward identifying agents that could cause hyperlipidemia (e.g., estrogens, alcohol, or β-adrenergic blockers). In addition, laboratory studies should be performed to measure fasting blood sugar or glycosylated hemoglobin or both and to assess renal and hepatic function and urinary protein. To screen for hypothyroidism, the plasma thyroid-stimulating hormone (thyrotropin) level should be assessed because the prevalence of hypothyroidism is increased in dyslipidemic subjects.[569]

Measurement of Plasma Lipids

Ideally, plasma lipids should be measured at least twice under fasting steady-state conditions before therapeutic decisions are made. Although plasma lipids are usually measured after a 12-hour fast, the plasma lipid response in the postabsorptive state, which may include significant elevations in atherogenic remnant lipoproteins, may be important in atherogenesis. Because cholesterol is a minor component of chylomicrons, plasma cholesterol can be measured in either the fasting or nonfasting state. Of note, plasma lipids can be decreased in the setting of acute myocardial infarction,[570] and follow-up measurements are essential in these patients.

Most clinical laboratories measure plasma levels of total triglycerides, total cholesterol, and HDL-C; the last analysis is performed after apo-B–containing lipoproteins are precipitated from the plasma with an agent such as heparin. The plasma LDL-C concentration is then calculated from these measurements by the Friedewald formula[571]:

$$\text{LDL cholesterol} = \text{total cholesterol} - \text{HDL-C} - \text{VLDL cholesterol (triglycerides} \div 5)$$

This formula relies on an estimate of the VLDL cholesterol that is about 20% of the plasma triglyceride level and is reliable for triglyceride levels of 4.5 mmol/L (400 mg/dL) or less. Plasma LDL concentrations calculated by this formula may be inaccurate in the setting of severe hypertriglyceridemia. Specialized lipid laboratories separate the plasma into different density fractions (e.g., VLDL, LDL, and HDL) by sequential ultracentrifugation of the plasma and then measure the lipid concentrations in each fraction. The main advantage of the latter technique is that VLDL cholesterol, which can reflect atherogenic remnant lipoproteins, is measured directly.

Because the plasma lipids can be divided roughly into the *proatherogenic* apo-B–containing lipoproteins and the *antiatherogenic* HDL, assessment of the relative proportions of cholesterol in these two fractions can be valuable in the individual lipid profile. One method is to assess absolute levels of HDL and non-HDL cholesterol.[572] Another method is to determine the ratio of total cholesterol to HDL-C[573–575]; it is desirable for the ratio to be about 4.5 or lower (i.e., to have at least 25% of the plasma cholesterol in the HDL fraction). Both methods allow incorporation of the potentially atherogenic apo-B–containing lipoproteins in the assessment of cardiovascular risk from hyperlipidemia by including VLDL cholesterol levels in the assessment.

Several caveats for interpretation of the plasma triglyceride level deserve mention. First, a triglyceride level higher than 11.3 mmol/L (1000 mg/dL) usually signifies the presence of two or more abnormalities of lipid metabolism (e.g., estrogen therapy in the presence of underlying familial hypertriglyceridemia).[576] Second, elevated plasma triglyceride levels can fluctuate markedly in a single person over short periods. The fluctuation occurs because the LPL-mediated clearance mechanisms for triglyceride-rich particles become saturated at plasma triglyceride concentrations of approximately 5.6 mmol/L (500 mg/dL), and above this level plasma triglyceride levels largely reflect dietary influences. In this range, the plasma triglyceride levels may rise precipitously with high dietary fat intake and fall rapidly with dietary fat restriction.[363]

In some instances, visual inspection of plasma after it has been refrigerated overnight can be helpful in understanding a disorder of lipoprotein metabolism. To accomplish this, plasma should be collected in a tube containing ethylenediaminetetraacetic acid (EDTA) and refrigerated overnight. A cream-like layer on the top signifies the presence of chylomicrons (type I hyperlipoproteinemia), which are less dense than plasma and float to the surface. A turbid plasma infranatant signifies high levels of VLDL (type IV hyperlipoproteinemia). The combination of a cream-like top layer and turbid plasma indicates the presence of both chylomicrons and VLDL (type V hyperlipoproteinemia). Plasma can also be analyzed by electrophoresis on paper or agarose gels and stained for neutral lipids to analyze the amount of lipids in the various lipoprotein classes.[245] This type of analysis is now rarely used because it has little utility in the classification or treatment of lipid disorders.[246] Nevertheless, much of the terminology used to describe lipoprotein disorders is derived from the originally described patterns (see Table 34–5).

Specialized tests used to assess plasma lipid disorders include measurements of plasma Lp(a) levels and plasma apolipoproteins and screening of genomic DNA for mutations. Plasma Lp(a) levels can be determined by enzyme-linked immunoabsorbent assays, if warranted. The Lp(a) assay must distinguish the apo(a) protein from plasminogen, which is highly homologous. Plasma Lp(a) measurement may be helpful in assessing CHD risk, and high levels of Lp(a) may suggest the use of niacin as a therapeutic agent.[290] Plasma apo-B and apo-AI levels may be of great value in predicting CHD risk[577]; however, because the assays for these apolipoproteins are difficult to perform and add minimal information to that obtained from plasma cholesterol measurements, they are not routinely used. Specialized tests such as in vitro assays for enzyme activities (e.g., LPL, CETP) or DNA screening for mutations (e.g., the familial defective apo-B100 mutation) are currently performed in specialized laboratories.

Selection of Patients for Plasma Lipid Measurements

Guidelines published by the NCEP in 2001 recommend that a complete plasma lipid profile (total cholesterol, LDL-C, HDL-C, and triglycerides) be measured in all adults 20 years of age and older at least once every 5 years.[242] The classification of plasma lipid levels is shown in Table 34–12. An analysis of large, long-term cohort studies has provided evidence that young men with hypercholesterolemia are at substantially

Table 34–12. Classification of Plasma Lipid Levels

Level	Classification
Total Cholesterol	
<200 mg/dL	Desirable
200–239 mg/dL	Borderline high
≥240 mg/dL	High
HDL-C	
<40 mg/dL	Low (consider < 50 mg/dL as low for women)
>60 mg/dL	High
LDL-C	
<100 mg/dL	Optimal
100–129 mg/dL	Near optimal
130–159 mg/dL	Borderline high
160–189 mg/dL	High
≥190 mg/dL	Very high
Triglycerides	
<150 mg/dL	Normal
150–199 mg/dL	Borderline high
200–499 mg/dL	High
≥500 mg/dL	Very high

HDL-C, high-density lipoprotein cholesterol, LDL-C, low-density lipoprotein cholesterol.

Adapted from National Cholesterol Education Program Expert Panel. Executive summary of the third report of the National Cholesterol Education Program (NCEP) Expert Panel on Detection, Evaluation, and Treatment of High Blood Cholesterol in Adults (Adult Treatment Panel III). JAMA 2001; 285:2486–2497.

increased risk for morbidity and mortality from CHD.[578] Others have suggested that cost-benefit analyses of the impact of such screening programs on health care and the potential reversibility of atherosclerosis make it questionable whether to screen young, healthy people without significant risk factors for development of premature coronary artery disease[579]; these researchers recommend delaying plasma lipid screening until an older age.[580]

Plasma triglycerides should be measured in all patients with pancreatitis. The lipemic plasma seen in hypertriglyceridemia can interfere with some assays for serum amylase.[581] In these instances, serum lipase or urinary amylase measurements can be helpful.

Selection of Patients for Treatment

The 2001 NCEP treatment guidelines are based on measurements of plasma cholesterol levels and risk factor assessment.[242] The first step in risk assessment is to determine whether CHD or a CHD equivalent (e.g., diabetes mellitus) is present, as these disorders confer more than 20% risk of a CHD event within 10 years. Framingham risk scores (Table 34–13)[242] are used to identify additional subjects with multiple risk factors conferring a 10-year risk of more than 20%. Treatment options, based on risk stratification, are discussed below. Other criteria for assessing risk in primary prevention have been proposed, including an assessment that places more emphasis on age.[582] Guidelines for managing dyslipidemia based on risk assessment were also published by the European Atherosclerosis Society in 1998.[583]

Treatment decisions can be divided into two major categories: treatment of hyperlipidemia in patients with *established* CHD and treatment of patients for the *primary prevention* of CHD. Subjects with hyperlipidemia and established CHD should be aggressively treated to lower plasma cholesterol to NCEP treatment guideline levels. The rationale for this recommendation is that lowering of plasma cholesterol in patients with established CHD decreases subsequent risk for cardiac events[294, 295, 584–587] and decreases mortality from cardiac events.[588] One study demonstrated a reduction in CHD-related and overall mortality in treated patients[561]; this benefit extended to elderly patients as well. In subjects with established CHD, lipid-lowering therapy causes atherosclerotic lesions to stabilize or regress.[294–296, 589–591] However, despite the overwhelming evidence demonstrating the benefits of lipid-lowering treatment, many people with hypercholesterolemia and CHD remain untreated.

The use of lipid-lowering therapies in subjects with hypercholesterolemia and no known CHD (i.e., therapy for primary prevention) has been more controversial.[592] This issue arises in part because there is no easy noninvasive test for assessing the degree of atherosclerosis in human coronary arteries. Therefore, treatment recommendations for asymptomatic persons have been based largely on studies of hypercholesterolemic populations. Primary prevention trials showed that lipid lowering in such patients decreased cardiac events and CHD-related mortality[347, 558] but not overall mortality.[593, 594] However, the WOSCOPS trial (discussed previously) showed that lipid-lowering treatment for 5 years decreased both CHD-related mortality and overall mortality in middle-aged hypercholesterolemic men.[562] This study also established that lipid-lowering therapy improves survival in asymptomatic hypercholesterolemic men. Because the costs of such treatment are high, a noninvasive test to evaluate the coronary arteries and identify which hypercholesterolemic subjects are at the highest risk would be useful.

The treatment of hypercholesterolemia in persons older than 65 years is controversial, and few prospective studies have addressed the benefits of treatment in this population. Nevertheless, CHD accounts for a high proportion of deaths in this age group, and the 4S trial demonstrated the survival benefits of treatment in elderly individuals who have established CHD.[561]

Patients with type 2 diabetes mellitus have at least a twofold increase in the risk for CHD,[566] and diabetics without diagnosed CHD have the same risk as nondiabetics with established CHD.[567] In post hoc analyses, clinical trials with HMG-CoA reductase inhibitors (e.g., 4S, CARE, AFCAPS/TexCAPS, and LIPID) demonstrated 20% to 55% reductions in CHD events. For these reasons, the American Heart Association and American Diabetes Association have recommended that guidelines for treatment of hyperlipidemia in diabetics be the same as for patients with CHD.[566] Accordingly, the latest NCEP guidelines[242] recommend considering diabetes mellitus as a CHD equivalent, with identical treatment goals. HMG-CoA reductase inhibitors have been recommended as a first-line treatment.

Severe hypertriglyceridemia (>11.3 mmol/L [1000 mg/dL]) should be treated aggressively because it is associated with a high risk for pancreatitis, a potentially fatal disease.[363]

Treatment Goals

The treatment goals of the 2001 NCEP guidelines, based on LDL-C and risk assessment, are summarized in Table 34–14. For patients with clinical CHD, the treatment goal for LDL-C should be a level less than 2.6 mmol/L (100 mg/dL). A useful rule is to lower total cholesterol to roughly 4.1 mmol/L (160 mg/dL) and LDL-C to 2.6 mmol/L (100 mg/dL). These values are similar to the average cholesterol levels in the Japanese population, in which CHD is much less prevalent. In general, LDL-C levels should be lowered to less than 4.1 mmol/L (160 mg/dL) for patients with minimal risk (10-year risk <10%) and to less than 3.4 mmol/L (130 mg/dL) in those with moderate risk (10-year risk 10–20%). It is also useful to monitor the ratio of total cholesterol to HDL-C, which should be 4.5 or less.

Table 34-13. Framingham Risk Scoring Tables

Estimate of 10-Year Risk for Men

Age (yr)	Points
20–34	−9
35–39	−4
40–44	0
45–49	3
50–54	6
55–59	8
60–64	10
65–69	11
70–74	12
75–79	13

Total Cholesterol (mg/dL)	Points: Age 20–39 yr	Age 40–49 yr	Age 50–59 yr	Age 60–69 yr	Age 70–79 yr
<160	0	0	0	0	0
160–199	4	3	2	1	0
200–239	7	5	3	1	0
240–279	9	6	4	2	1
≥280	11	8	5	3	1

	Points: Age 20–39 yr	Age 40–49 yr	Age 50–59 yr	Age 60–69 yr	Age 70–79 yr
Nonsmoker	0	0	0	0	0
Smoker	8	5	3	1	1

HDL (mg/dL)	Points
≥60	−1
50–59	0
40–49	1
<40	2

Systolic BP (mm Hg)	If Untreated	If Treated
<120	0	0
120–129	0	1
130–139	1	2
140–159	1	2
≥160	2	3

Point Total	10-yr Risk (%)
<0	<1
0	1
1	1
2	1
3	1
4	1
5	2
6	2
7	3
8	4
9	5
10	6
11	8
12	10
13	12
14	16
15	20
16	25
≥17	≥30

Estimate of 10-Year Risk for Women

Age (yr)	Points
20–34	−7
35–39	−3
40–44	0
45–49	3
50–54	6
55–59	8
60–64	10
65–69	12
70–74	14
75–79	16

Total Cholesterol (mg/dL)	Points: Age 20–39 yr	Age 40–49 yr	Age 50–59 yr	Age 60–69 yr	Age 70–79 yr
<160	0	0	0	0	0
160–199	4	3	2	1	1
200–239	8	6	4	2	1
240–279	11	8	5	3	2
≥280	13	10	7	4	2

	Points: Age 20–39 yr	Age 40–49 yr	Age 50–59 yr	Age 60–69 yr	Age 70–79 yr
Nonsmoker	0	0	0	0	0
Smoker	9	7	4	2	1

HDL (mg/dL)	Points
≥60	−1
50–59	0
40–49	1
<40	2

Systolic BP (mm Hg)	If Untreated	If Treated
<120	0	0
120–129	1	3
130–139	2	4
140–159	3	5
≥160	4	6

Point Total	10-yr Risk (%)
<9	<1
9	1
10	1
11	1
12	1
13	2
14	2
15	3
16	4
17	5
18	6
19	8
20	11
21	14
22	17
23	22
24	27
≥25	≥30

Adapted from National Cholesterol Education Program Expert Panel. Executive summary of the third report of the National Cholesterol Education Program (NCEP) Expert Panel on Detection, Evaluation, and Treatment of High Blood Cholesterol in Adults (Adult Treatment Panel III). JAMA 2001; 285:2486–2497.

HDL, high-density lipoproteins; BP, blood pressure.

Table 34–14. National Cholesterol Education Program: Treatment Recommendations Based on Risk Assessment*

Risk Category	LDL-C Goal, mmol/L (mg/dL)	LDL-C Level at Which to Initiate Therapeutic Lifestyle Changes† mmol/L (mg/dL)	LDL-C Level at Which to Consider Drug Therapy, mmol/L (mg/dL)
CHD or CHD risk equivalent (10-yr risk >20%)	<2.6 (100)	≥2.6 (100)	≥3.4 (130) [2.6–3.3 (100–129): drug optional]
2+ Risk factors (10-yr risk <20%)	<3.4 (130)	≥3.4 (130)	10-yr risk 10%–20%: ≥3.4 (130) 10-yr risk <10%: ≥4.1 (160)
0–1 Risk factor	<4.1 (160)	≥4.1 (160)	≥4.9 (190) [4.1–4.8 (160–189): drug optional]

*Risk assessment is based on major risk factors (Table 34–11) and Framingham risk scores (Table 34–12).

†Therapeutic lifestyle changes are shown in Table 34–13.

Adapted from National Cholesterol Education Program Expert Panel. Executive summary of the third report of the National Cholesterol Education Program (NCEP) Expert Panel on Detection, Evaluation, and Treatment of High Blood Cholesterol in Adults (Adult Treatment Panel III). JAMA 2001; 285:2486–2497.

CHD, coronary heart disease; LDL-C, low-density lipoprotein cholesterol.

If severe hypertriglyceridemia is present, the goals for triglyceride lowering are to lower the plasma triglyceride level to less than 4.5 mmol/L (400 mg/dL), which markedly reduces the risk for development of pancreatitis. The 2001 NCEP guidelines[242] reflect the fact that even moderate hypertriglyceridemia (>1.7 mmol/L, or 150 mg/dL) is associated with increased CHD risk. If plasma triglycerides remain above 2.3 mmol/L (200 mg/dL) after the LDL-C goal is reached, further reduction may be achieved by increasing the drug therapy.

Treatment of Hyperlipidemia

The treatment of hyperlipidemia is directed primarily at lowering plasma cholesterol levels to prevent morbidity and mortality from CHD. The rationale and the use of diet or drugs for this purpose have been reviewed.[572, 595, 596] Treatment modalities recommended by the NCEP include therapeutic lifestyle changes, which include diet, weight management, and physical activity recommendations, and drug therapy.[242] A major goal in the treatment of hypertriglyceridemia is to prevent pancreatitis. Patients with CHD or CHD equivalent should immediately start appropriate lipid-lowering therapy. Patients without CHD or CHD equivalent should receive lifestyle advice for 3 to 6 months before starting drug therapy.

Table 34–15. Clinical Identification of the Metabolic Syndrome

Risk Factor	Defining Level
Abdominal obesity*	Waist circumference†
Men	>102 cm (>40 in)
Women	>88 cm (>35 in)
Triglycerides	≥150 mg/dL
HDL-C	
Men	<40 mg/dL
Women	<50 mg/dL
Blood pressure	≥130/≥85 mm Hg
Fasting glucose	≥110 mg/dL

*Overweight and obesity are associated with insulin resistance and the metabolic syndrome. However, the presence of abdominal obesity is more highly correlated with the metabolic risk factors than is an elevated body mass index. Therefore, the simple measurement of waist circumference is recommended to identify the body weight component of the metabolic syndrome.

†Some male patients can develop multiple metabolic risk factors when the waist circumference is only marginally increased, for example, 94–102 cm (37–39 in). Such patients may have a strong genetic contribution to insulin resistance and, like men with categorical increases in waist circumference, they should benefit from changes in life habits.

Adapted from National Cholesterol Education Program Expert Panel. Executive summary of the third report of the National Cholesterol Education Program (NCEP) Expert Panel on Detection, Evaluation, and Treatment of High Blood Cholesterol in Adults (Adult Treatment Panel III). JAMA 2001; 285:2486–2497.

HDL-C, high-density lipoprotein cholesterol.

The 2001 NCEP guidelines recognize the increased CHD risk associated with the metabolic syndrome, which is characterized by the presence of at least three of five CHD risk factors (Table 34–15). In addition to treating increased LDL-C levels, treatment for these patients should focus on weight loss and increased physical activity, as obesity appears to exacerbate these metabolic abnormalities.

Dietary Treatment

All patients should receive instruction about restriction of dietary saturated fat and cholesterol. On average, the Western diet contains 35% to 40% of calories as fat (about 15% to 20% saturated fat, 10% polyunsaturated fat, and 10% monounsaturated fat) and approximately 380 mg of cholesterol per day. In contrast, the average diet in many underdeveloped countries is closer to 10% of calories as fat. The American Heart Association has recommended a single diet, termed Step 1 Dietary Therapy by the NCEP, for all persons older than 2 years.[597] The diet consists of 50% of calories in the form of carbohydrate (complex carbohydrate preferred), 20% as protein, and no more than 30% as fat. Saturated fat should constitute less than 10% of total calories, monounsaturated fat 10% to 15% of calories, and polyunsaturated fat up to 10% of total calories. Cholesterol intake should be limited to 250 mg/day or less. A more stringent restriction of saturated fat (<7% of calories) and cholesterol (≤200 mg/day) intake (Step 2 diet) is recommended for patients with established coronary artery disease.[595] This diet is similar to the therapeutic lifestyle changes diet proposed by the NCEP (Table 34–16). In patients with established CHD, drug therapy should be instituted concomitantly with dietary therapy.

Changing from a typical Western diet to a Step 1 diet lowers plasma cholesterol levels by only 5% to 10%.[598, 599] The adoption of a Step 2 diet (25% of calories as fat) has produced mixed results in two noteworthy studies. In one study, restricting fat intake to 25% of calories lowered cholesterol levels by only 5%; however, in this outpatient study, it was not clear that the diets were strictly adhered to, as evidenced by comparison of the expected and the actual weight loss in participants.[600] In an inpatient (metabolic ward) study, reducing fat intake from 43% to 25% of calories lowered total cholesterol levels by 17% and LDL-C levels by 23%.[601] Even more stringent limitation of fat intake (e.g., 10% of calories) can further lower plasma lipids. In conjunction with modifications of other lifestyle factors, this diet achieved a reduction of about 25% in total plasma cholesterol levels, an average weight loss of 10 kg, and angiographic regression of coronary artery disease.[590] The

Table 34–16. National Cholesterol Education Program: Therapeutic Lifestyle Changes for Reducing Coronary Heart Disease Risk

1. Diet:
   Saturated fat (and *trans*-esterified fatty acids) less than 7% of total calories
   Polyunsaturated fat up to 10% of total calories
   Monounsaturated fat up to 20% of total calories
   Total fat 25%–35% of total calories
   Carbohydrates (predominantly complex) 50%–60% of total calories
   Fiber 20–30 g/d*
   Protein ~15% of total calories
   Cholesterol <5.2 mmol/L (200 mg/dL)
   Consider plant stanols/sterols (2 g/d) to enhance LDL-C lowering
2. Weight reduction
3. Increased physical activity

*Adapted from National Cholesterol Education Program Expert Panel. Executive summary of the third report of the National Cholesterol Education Program (NCEP) Expert Panel on Detection, Evaluation, and Treatment of High Blood Cholesterol in Adults (Adult Treatment Panel III). JAMA 2001; 285:2486–2497.
LDL-C, low-density lipoprotein cholesterol.

latter studies suggest that dietary restriction of fat intake can lower plasma cholesterol levels provided the diet is followed. The typical saturated fat and cholesterol contents of common foods are indicated in Table 34–17.

The effects of various types of fat in the diet have been studied extensively.[597, 602] Current recommendations are that dietary fat intake be lowered, primarily by restricting saturated fat intake because saturated fats appear to have the greatest propensity to elevate plasma cholesterol levels.[29] The mechanism of this effect appears to involve decreased receptor-mediated clearance of LDL from the plasma.[603] Similarly, high levels of cholesterol intake raise plasma cholesterol by reducing receptor-mediated catabolism of LDL and by increasing LDL synthesis.[604]

Polyunsaturated fats, such as linoleic acid, which are chiefly found in vegetable oils, have less deleterious effects on plasma cholesterol levels than saturated fats.[29, 605] However, because the long-term effects of consumption of large amounts of polyunsaturated fats are unknown, current recommendations are that polyunsaturated fat constitute no more than 10% of total calories.[597] Polyunsaturated fats that have been hardened by hydrogenation (e.g., in margarines) result in the conversion of some double bonds in the fatty acid from the *cis* to the *trans* configuration; these *trans* fatty acids appear to exert effects on plasma cholesterol that are comparable to those of saturated fatty acids.[606]

Fish oils are rich in a particular subset of long-chain polyunsaturated fats containing double bonds at the n-3 or omega (ω)-3 position, such as eicosapentaenoic acid (C-20) or docosahexaenoic acid (C-22). Because the incidence of CHD is decreased in populations that consume relatively large amounts of fish oils,[607] these polyunsaturated fatty acids have been evaluated for the treatment of hyperlipidemia and the prevention of CHD.[608] Although they lower VLDL levels and are effective for treating hypertriglyceridemia, fish oils appear to have little effect on total cholesterol levels and increase LDL levels in many patients with hypertriglyceridemia.[608, 609] Fish oils may have beneficial effects on cardiovascular disease by means other than their effects on lipoproteins, such as inhibition of platelet aggregation,[610] but a prospective study of male health professionals found no protective effects of increased intake of dietary fish oil on the development of CHD.[611] In addition, fish oil supplementation can worsen glycemic control in persons with type 2 diabetes.[612]

Of all the types of fatty acids, monounsaturated fats may have the least deleterious effects on plasma lipoprotein metabolism.[29, 597, 613] Monounsaturated fats, such as oleic acid, are found in high quantities in olive oil and canola oil. When substituted for saturated fats, monounsaturated fats lowered total plasma cholesterol levels without lowering plasma HDL-C levels.[613]

Other dietary components may influence plasma lipid levels. For example, soluble fibers such as psyllium or oat bran, which may bind bile acids in the gut and promote net cholesterol excretion, can result in modest (<10%) decreases in LDL-C levels.[614–616] Margarine containing sitostanol, a nonabsorbed plant sterol that inhibits cholesterol absorption, reduces serum cholesterol by about 10%.[617] Garlic[618] and walnuts[619] are reported to result in modest decreases in plasma cholesterol levels.

Drug Treatment

Categories of drugs for treatment of lipid abnormalities[282, 572, 620] are listed in Table 34–18. These include drugs that interfere with bile acid absorption from the gut, such as bile acid sequestrants, or with cholesterol biosynthesis in cells, such as HMG-CoA reductase inhibitors. These agents reduce cholesterol levels and increase LDL receptor expression in cells, thereby lowering plasma LDL concentrations. Other agents, including niacin and gemfibrozil, either inhibit VLDL synthesis and secretion or enhance the clearance of triglyceride-rich particles by enhancing VLDL-mediated catabolism. Finally, drugs that work primarily as antioxidants are being tested. The choice of drug for treatment of hyperlipidemia depends primarily on the type of disorder (Table 34–19) and on the side effects of each drug. In cases of severe hypercholesterolemia (e.g., FH), combinations of agents may act to reduce plasma cholesterol concentrations with great efficacy.

HMG-CoA Reductase Inhibitors

Several potent inhibitors of HMG-CoA reductase, the enzyme that catalyzes the rate-limiting step in cholesterol biosynthesis, are available (Table 34–20).[282, 620] Inhibition of cholesterol biosynthesis up-regulates cellular LDL receptors and enhances clearance of LDL from the plasma into cells.[288] The inhibitors differ in their side chains, which can affect their relative hydrophobicity.[621] For example, lovastatin and simvastatin are relatively hydrophobic and lipophilic compared with

Table 34–17. Cholesterol and Saturated Fat Content in Some Common Foods

Food	Cholesterol (mg/100 g)	Saturated Fat (g/100 g)
Eggs	500	3
Organ meats (liver, kidney)	>300	2
Butter	230	50
Shrimp, crab, lobster	110	1
Cheese	110	21
Meat (beef, pork, lamb)	90–100	5–13
Poultry (no skin)	90	1
Fish	70	1
Ice cream (10% fat)	40	7
Sherbet; frozen yogurt	4	<1
Milk, whole (3.5%)	14	2
Milk, skim	2	0
Cottage cheese	6	<1
Margarine, soft	0	16
Vegetable oil	0	13
Coconut oil, cocoa butter	0	75

Adapted from Connor WE, Connor SL. The dietary treatment of hyperlipidemia: rationale, technique and efficacy. Med Clin North Am 1982; 66:485–518.

Table 34–18. Drugs Commonly Used for Treating Hyperlipidemia

Class	Drugs Available	Dosage	Major Lipoprotein Decreased	Mechanism	Side Effects
Bile acid sequestrants	Cholestyramine Colestipol	4–12 g bid 5–15 g bid	LDL	Increase sterol excretion; increase LDL receptor–mediated removal of LDL	Gastrointestinal symptoms; can increase triglycerides; binds other drugs
Nicotinic acid	Niacin	1–2 g tid	VLDL (LDL)	Decrease VLDL production	Flushing; hyperglycemia; hepatic dysfunction; gout
Fibric acid derivatives	Gemfibrozil Clofibrate Fenofibrate	600 mg bid 1 g bid 67–201 mg qd	VLDL (LDL)	Decrease VLDL production; enhance LPL action	Gallstones; myopathy
HMG-CoA reductase inhibitors	Lovastatin Pravastatin Simvastatin Fluvastatin Atorvastatin	10–80 mg qd 10–40 mg qd 5–80 mg qd 20–80 mg qd 10–80 mg qd	LDL	Decrease cholesterol synthesis; increase LDL receptor–mediated removal of LDL	Hepatic dysfunction; myopathy

HMG-CoA, 3-hydroxy-3-methylglutaryl coenzyme A; LDL, low-density lipoprotein; VLDL, very-low-density lipoprotein.

pravastatin, which is more hydrophilic; these properties appear to have little effect on the ability to lower LDL levels. Therapeutic doses of these agents reduce total cholesterol and LDL-C levels by 20% to 55% (see Table 34–20).[622, 623] Plasma triglyceride levels greater than 250 mg/dL are reduced by amounts that are comparable to the reductions in LDL-C.[624] High doses of the most potent statins reduce triglyceride levels by 35% to 40%. In patients with triglyceride levels less than 250 mg/dL, statins reduce triglyceride levels by less than 25%.[624] Statins increase plasma HDL-C levels by 5% to 10%. In addition to lipid-lowering effects, a multitude of potentially cardioprotective effects are being ascribed to statins, including improved endothelial function, increased plaque stability, decreased inflammation, decreased lipoprotein oxidation, and improved circulation.[282, 625]

The reductase inhibitors are well tolerated and cause few side effects. The most serious potential side effect is myopathy, which occurs in less than 1% of persons taking lovastatin[622] and can cause myoglobinuria and renal failure.[626] Patients taking HMG-CoA reductase inhibitors in whom myalgias develop should have serum creatine phosphokinase measurements, and the drug should be stopped immediately if evidence of myositis is found. The risk of myopathy is increased if an HMG-CoA reductase inhibitor is used in combination with niacin[627] or gemfibrozil,[626] which can cause myopathy by themselves, or with drugs that are metabolized by the 3A4 isoform of cytochrome P450 (CYP3A4), such as erythromycin, cyclosporine, nefazodone, or protease inhibitors.[282, 628–630] Of the available statins, only pravastatin and fluvastatin are not extensively metabolized by CYP3A4. Although these drugs may be less likely to cause myopathy when used with other CYP3A4-metabolized drugs, myopathy has been reported with their use.

Table 34–19. Drug Selection Based on Major Lipid Abnormality

Major Elevated Plasma Lipid(s)	Drugs
Cholesterol	HMG-CoA reductase inhibitor Niacin Bile acid sequestrants
Cholesterol and triglyceride	Niacin Fibric acid derivative HMG-CoA reductase inhibitor
Triglyceride	Niacin Fibric acid derivative Fish oils
Lp(a)	Niacin

HMG-CoA, 3-hydroxy-3-methylglutaryl coenzyme A.

To minimize the risk of myopathy, drug combinations should be avoided. However, statins may be used with a predisposing drug without increasing myopathy risk if the statin is administered at no more than 25% of its maximal dose.[630] The plasma creatine kinase level should probably be monitored if the combinations are used. Serum transaminase elevations (greater than three times normal) occur in 2% to 3% of patients.[622] The long-term side effects of HMG-CoA reductase inhibitor therapy are not known, but no significant long-term toxicities have been observed with lovastatin, which has now been in use for more than 15 years.

Bile Acid Sequestrants

Bile acid sequestrants are anion-exchange resins that exchange chloride for negatively charged bile acids.[282] The bound bile acids are then excreted in the feces.[631] The increased excretion of bile acids causes increased oxidation of cholesterol to form bile acids in hepatocytes, and the resultant up-regulation of hepatic LDL receptors in turn lowers plasma LDL concentrations.[632] Because bile acid sequestrants act in the intestine, the side effects are limited to local effects in the gastrointestinal system (e.g., bloating, gas, constipation). At therapeutic doses, these agents can lower plasma cholesterol levels by 15% to 25%. However, they can increase plasma triglyceride levels[633] and must be used with caution in patients predisposed to hypertriglyceridemia. In addition, because they bind negatively charged molecules in the intestine, these agents can interfere with the absorption of other medications, including levothyroxine, digoxin, warfarin, and thiazide diuretics. Therefore, resins are given at least 4 hours before or 1 hour after other medications.

Niacin

The most inexpensive drug for treating hyperlipidemia is the B vitamin niacin. Therapeutic doses of niacin (typically 2.0 to 4.5 g/day) lower both total and LDL cholesterol by 15% to 30%, lower triglyceride levels by 30% to 40%, and raise HDL-C levels by 15% to 25%.[282, 634] Maximal HDL increases usually occur with therapeutic doses of 1.5 to 2.0 g/day. Niacin

Table 34–20. Doses (mg) of Statins Required to Achieve Various Reductions in Low-Density Lipoprotein Cholesterol from Baseline

Drug	20%–25%	26%–30%	31%–35%	36%–40%	41%–50%	51%–55%
Atorvastatin	—	—	10	20	40	80
Fluvastatin	20	40	80			
Lovastatin	10	20	40	80		
Pravastatin	10	20	40			
Simvastatin	—	10	20	40	80	

also lowers plasma Lp(a) concentrations by up to 40%.[290, 635] The preparation must be niacin and not niacinamide, which has no efficacy. The mechanism whereby niacin affects plasma lipids is unclear but seems to be associated with decreased hepatic VLDL production.

The most troublesome side effect of niacin therapy is a flushing syndrome that occurs shortly after taking the medicine. Flushing can be minimized by initiating therapy with small doses (e.g., 100 mg) and gradually increasing the dosage to the therapeutic range over weeks to months. Repeated dosing is associated with a gradual tolerance to the flushing syndrome. In addition, taking an aspirin about 1 hour before the niacin can diminish the flushing, possibly by inhibiting prostaglandin-mediated side effects.

The most serious complication of niacin therapy is hepatotoxicity, and therapy should be accompanied by monitoring of serum liver function tests. Mild increases in serum transaminases are common when doses are increased rapidly; however, therapy should be discontinued if transaminases reach highly elevated levels (e.g., >10 times normal). Because hepatotoxicity appears to be more common with sustained-release preparations of niacin,[636] the immediate-release crystalline form is preferred. Other side effects of niacin therapy include impairment or worsening of glucose tolerance and hyperuricemia. Data suggest that niacin can be used safely in patients with glucose intolerance or diabetes mellitus,[637] but the drug should be used with great caution in patients with a history of gout and is contraindicated in patients with active peptic ulcer disease.

Fibric Acid Derivatives

The fibric acid derivatives, clofibrate and gemfibrozil, lower plasma triglycerides by about 40% and increase HDL-C levels by about 10%[347] but have only minor effects on LDL-C.[282] These agents act by activating the peroxisome proliferator–activated receptor α, a nuclear hormone receptor that is expressed in the liver and other tissues.[638] This results in increased fatty acid oxidation, increased LPL synthesis, and reduced expression of apo-CIII, all of which contribute to lowering plasma triglycerides.[638] The physiologic results are a decrease in VLDL triglyceride production and an increase in LPL-mediated catabolism of triglyceride-rich lipoproteins.[639] This receptor also stimulates the expression of apo-AI and apo-AII, leading to increased HDL levels. These agents are given twice a day and are well tolerated. Side effects include gastrointestinal discomfort and possibly an increased incidence of cholesterol gallstones. Fibric acid derivatives should be used with great caution in the setting of renal insufficiency because patients with this condition have an increased risk of myopathy.[640]

Clofibrate received adverse publicity because of a large clinical trial in which slightly more cancer deaths were noted in the clofibrate-treated group.[641] However, a later analysis did not substantiate this finding,[642] and there is no firm evidence that the drug is carcinogenic in humans. In two subsequent trials, the Helsinki Heart Study (primary prevention) and the Veterans Affairs High Density Lipoprotein Intervention Trial (secondary prevention), gemfibrozil treatment reduced fatal and nonfatal CHD events without changes in mortality rates.[347, 564]

Combination Therapy

For patients with severe elevations of plasma cholesterol (e.g., >7.8 mmol/L [300 mg/dL]), in whom treatment goals are to reduce the plasma and LDL cholesterol levels by 50% or more, combination drug therapy is usually required.[282, 620] Often this can be achieved with combinations that employ lower doses than needed when these agents are used as single agents. For example, combined therapy with an HMG-CoA reductase inhibitor and either niacin[285, 286] or a bile acid sequestrant[284] can lower plasma cholesterol levels by more than 50%. Occasionally, in patients with severe hypercholesterolemia, combinations that include an HMG-CoA reductase inhibitor, niacin, and a bile acid sequestrant can achieve the desired lipid-lowering effect.[287] Patients with diabetes mellitus who have high plasma levels of triglyceride and VLDL cholesterol may benefit from combination therapy with a low dose of an HMG-CoA reductase inhibitor and gemfibrozil. Because the use of HMG-CoA reductase inhibitors with niacin or gemfibrozil is associated with a higher risk of myopathy, such combinations must be used with caution. Monitoring of the serum creatine kinase level may be helpful, and only low doses of the reductase inhibitors (20 mg/day of lovastatin or the equivalent) should be used in most patients.

Drugs on the Horizon

A number of strategies to improve the treatment of dyslipidemia are under development.[282] For example, more potent statins capable of lowering LDL-C levels by more than 65% are being developed.[643] Inhibitors of MTP represent another strategy.[644] These agents have the potential to lower both plasma triglycerides and cholesterol levels by inhibiting hepatic VLDL production. Agents that impair cholesterol absorption, such as ezetimibe[645] or an ACAT2 inhibitor,[26] may offer alternative strategies for lowering plasma cholesterol levels. Inhibitors of CETP have the potential to raise HDL levels and inhibit atherosclerosis.[646]

There has been intense interest in the use of antioxidants to treat or prevent atherosclerosis. Probucol, a potent antioxidant transported on lipoproteins, protected against the development of atherosclerotic lesions in animals.[291, 292] However, in a trial in humans,[647] probucol failed to benefit patients with established peripheral vascular disease. A number of new antioxidants are under development. The antioxidant vitamins (the fat-soluble vitamins E and A and the water-soluble vitamin C) may also be antiatherogenic.[224] Evidence to support this comes from population studies in which high intake of antioxidants was associated with decreased coronary events.[648] However, a prospective trial examining β-carotene supplementation failed to show a benefit.[649] In a prospective trial of vitamin E supplementation, 400 IU/day reduced the risk of nonfatal infarction in patients with established CHD.[650] More prospective data demonstrating that supplemental antioxidant vitamin therapy can prevent atherosclerosis or CHD events in humans are needed before a recommendation can be made.

Estrogen Replacement Therapy and Coronary Heart Disease

Because estrogen replacement therapy in postmenopausal women reduces LDL-C and Lp(a) levels and raises HDL-C levels and because CHD risk increases substantially in postmenopausal women, there has been intense interest in using estrogens to prevent CHD.[651] However, two clinical trials have shown no benefit of estrogen replacement therapy in women with established CHD.[535, 536] It remains to be determined whether estrogen replacement will be effective in the primary prevention of CHD. Estrogen replacement has been shown to have multiple noncardiovascular benefits.[651]

Surgical Treatment

Partial ileal bypass surgery has been used to reduce lipid levels in patients with severe hypercholesterolemia who cannot tolerate lipid-lowering drugs. This surgical therapy can reduce total cholesterol levels by 20% to 25% and cause regression of angiographically measured atherosclerotic lesions.[294] In addition, liver transplantation[301, 302] and portacaval shunting[303, 304] have been used as experimental therapies for homozygous FH (see previous discussion).

Treatment to Raise High-Density Lipoprotein Cholesterol

Patients with familial hypoalphalipoproteinemia may have normal or modestly increased plasma cholesterol levels but have very low HDL-C levels, resulting in a predisposition to CHD. Such patients may have high ratios of total cholesterol to HDL-C (e.g., >10) despite having a normal plasma cholesterol level. At present, there are no highly effective therapies to raise HDL-C levels.[412] Estrogens can be given to postmenopausal women,[413–415] and exercise in sustained amounts may modestly increase HDL-C levels.[416] HDL-C levels increased by approximately 2 mg/dL for every 10 miles run per week in one study of recreational runners.[652] Alcohol, when consumed in modest quantities, can also increase HDL-C levels.[540] Of the available drug therapies, niacin results in the largest increase in HDL-C levels (about 15% to 25%)[634]; gemfibrozil and HMG-CoA reductase inhibitors increase HDL-C by about 10%. However, the potent ability of HMG-CoA reductase inhibitors to lower total cholesterol can improve the ratio of total cholesterol to HDL-C.[348]

Treatment of the Chylomicronemia Syndrome

Patients with the chylomicronemia syndrome often present with acute pancreatitis and severe hypertriglyceridemia (triglycerides >22.6 mmol/L [2000 mg/dL]).[363] These patients should be treated with total fat restriction until the triglyceride level falls to a safe range (e.g., <11.3 mmol/L [1000 mg/dL]), at which time a fat-restricted diet (e.g., <10% of calories) can be instituted and the plasma triglyceride level further monitored. The goal is to maintain the triglyceride level at less than 11.3 mmol/L (1000 mg/dL) and preferably less than 4.5 mmol/L (400 mg/dL). Often this can be accomplished by modifying the diet and eliminating or modifying secondary causes of hyperlipidemia such as drugs, glucose intolerance, or alcohol consumption. However, such patients often require a triglyceride-lowering drug, such as gemfibrozil or niacin, to maintain the plasma triglyceride level in a range that should prevent subsequent episodes of pancreatitis. Recommendations for the management of the hypertriglyceridemia associated with pregnancy have been described.[653]

References

1. Myant NB. Cholesterol Metabolism, LDL, and the LDL Receptor. San Diego, Academic Press, 1990.
2. Rudney H, Panini SR. Cholesterol biosynthesis. Curr Opin Lipidol 1993; 4:230–237.
3. Edwards PA, Fogelman AM. Cellular enzymes of cholesterol metabolism. Curr Opin Lipidol 1990; 1:136–139.
4. Brown MS, Goldstein JL. The hyperlipoproteinemias and other disorders of lipid metabolism. In Isselbacher KJ, Braunwald E, Wilson JD, et al (eds). Harrison's Principles of Internal Medicine, 13th ed. New York, McGraw-Hill, 1994, pp 2058–2069.
5. Angelin B. Studies on the regulation of hepatic cholesterol metabolism in humans. Eur J Clin Invest 1995; 25:215–224.
6. Dietschy JM, Turley SD, Spady DK. Role of liver in the maintenance of cholesterol and low density lipoprotein homeostasis in different animal species, including humans. J Lipid Res 1993; 34:1637–1659.
7. Goldstein JL, Brown MS. Regulation of the mevalonate pathway. Nature 1990; 343:425–430.
8. Mahley RW. Biochemistry and physiology of lipid and lipoprotein metabolism. In Becker KL (ed). Principles and Practice of Endocrinology and Metabolism, 2nd ed. Philadelphia, JB Lippincott, 1995, pp 1369–1378.
9. Grundy SM. Cholesterol and Atherosclerosis. Diagnosis and Treatment. Philadelphia, JB Lippincott, 1990.
10. Jelinek DF, Andersson S, Slaughter CA, Russell DW. Cloning and regulation of cholesterol 7α-hydroxylase, the rate-limiting enzyme in bile acid biosynthesis. J Biol Chem 1990; 265:8190–8197.
11. Li YC, Wang DP, Chiang JYL. Regulation of cholesterol 7α-hydroxylase in the liver: cloning, sequencing, and regulation of cholesterol 7α-hydroxylase mRNA. J Biol Chem 1990; 265:12012–12019.
12. Russell DW, Setchell KDR. Bile acid biosynthesis. Biochemistry 1992; 31:4737–4749.
13. Björkhem I, Eggertsen G. Genes involved in initial steps of bile acid synthesis. Curr Opin Lipidol 2001; 12:97–103.
14. Brown MS, Goldstein JL. A receptor-mediated pathway for cholesterol homeostasis. Science 1986; 232:34–47.
15. Chang CCY, Huh HY, Cadigan KM, Chang TY. Molecular cloning and functional expression of human acyl-coenzyme A: cholesterol acyltransferase cDNA in mutant Chinese hamster ovary cells. J Biol Chem 1993; 268:20747–20755.
16. Chang T-Y, Doolittle GM. Acyl coenzyme A:cholesterol *O*-acyltransferase. In Boyer PD (ed). The Enzymes, vol 16. New York, Academic Press, 1983, pp 523–539.
17. Suckling KE, Stange EF. Role of acyl-CoA:cholesterol acyltransferase in cellular cholesterol metabolism. J Lipid Res 1985; 26:647–671.
18. Pape ME, Schultz PA, Rea TJ, et al. Tissue specific changes in acyl-CoA:cholesterol acyltransferase (ACAT) mRNA levels in rabbits. J Lipid Res 1995; 36:823–838.
19. Sliskovic DR, White AD. Therapeutic potential of ACAT inhibitors as lipid lowering and anti-atherosclerotic agents. Trends Pharmacol Sci 1991; 12:194–199.
20. Meiner V, Tam C, Gunn MD, et al. Tissue expression studies of mouse acyl CoA:cholesterol acyltransferase gene (*Acact*): findings supporting the existence of multiple cholesterol esterification enzymes in mice. J Lipid Res 1997; 38:1928–1933.
21. Bocan TMA, Mueller SB, Uhlendorf PD, et al. Comparison of CI-976, an ACAT inhibitor, and selected lipid-lowering agents for antiatherosclerotic activity in iliac-femoral and thoracic aortic lesions: a biochemical, morphological, and morphometric evaluation. Arterioscler Thromb 1991; 11:1830–1843.
22. Accad M, Smith SJ, Newland DL, et al. Massive xanthomatosis

and altered composition of atherosclerotic lesions in hyperlipidemic mice lacking acyl CoA:cholesterol acyltransferase 1. J Clin Invest 2000; 105:711–719.

23. Cases S, Novak S, Zheng Y-W, et al. ACAT-2, a second mammalian acyl-CoA:cholesterol acyltransferase: its cloning, expression, and characterization. J Biol Chem 1998; 273:26755–26764.
24. Anderson RA, Joyce C, Davis M, et al. Identification of a form of acyl-CoA:cholesterol acyltransferase specific to liver and intestine in nonhuman primates. J Biol Chem 1998; 273:26747-26754.
25. Oelkers P, Behari A, Cromley D, et al. Characterization of two human genes encoding acyl coenzyme A:cholesterol acyltransferase–related enzymes. J Biol Chem 1998; 273:26765–26771.
26. Buhman KK, Accad M, Novak S, et al. Resistance to diet-induced hypercholesterolemia and gallstone formation in ACAT2-deficient mice. Nat Med 2000; 6:1341–1347.
27. Connor WE, Connor SL. The key role of nutritional factors in the prevention of coronary heart disease. Prev Med 1972; 1:49–83.
28. Gotto AM. Cholesterol intake and serum cholesterol level. N Engl J Med 1991; 324:912–913.
29. Grundy SM, Denke MA. Dietary influences on serum lipids and lipoproteins. J Lipid Res 1990; 31:1149–1172.
30. Keys A, Menotti A, Karvonen MJ, et al. The diet and 15-year death rate in the Seven Countries Study. Am J Epidemiol 1986; 124:903–915.
31. Carey MC, Small DM, Bliss CM. Lipid digestion and absorption. Annu Rev Physiol 1983; 45:651–677.
32. Kuwajima M, Foster DW, McGarry JD. Regulation of lipoprotein lipase in different rat tissues. Metabolism 1988; 37:597–601.
33. Stråfors P, Olsson H, Belfrage P. Hormone-sensitive lipase. In Boyer PD, Krebs EG (eds). The Enzymes, vol 18, 3rd ed. Orlando, Fla, Academic Press, 1987, pp 147–177.
34. Bell RM, Coleman RA. Enzymes of glycerolipid synthesis in eukaryotes. Annu Rev Biochem 1980; 49:459–487.
35. Brindley DN. Metabolism of triacylglycerols. In Vance DE, Vance JE (eds). Biochemistry of Lipids, Lipoproteins and Membranes. Amsterdam, Elsevier, 1991, pp 171–203.
36. Lehner R, Kuksis A. Biosynthesis of triacylglycerols. Prog Lipid Res 1996; 35:169–201.
37. Cases S, Smith SJ, Zheng Y-W, et al. Identification of a gene encoding an acyl CoA:diacylglycerol acyltransferase, a key enzyme in triacylglycerol synthesis. Proc Natl Acad Sci USA 1998; 95:13018–13023.
38. Smith SJ, Cases S, Jensen DR, et al. Obesity resistance and multiple mechanisms of triglyceride synthesis in mice lacking DGAT. Nat Genet 2000; 25:87–90.
39. Farese RV Jr, Cases S, Smith SJ. Triglyceride synthesis: insights from the cloning of diacylglycerol acyltransferase. Curr Opin Lipidol 2000; 11:229–234.
40. Chen HC, Farese RV Jr. DGAT and triglyceride synthesis: a new target for obesity treatment? Trends Cardiovasc Med 2000; 10:188–192.
41. Needleman P, Turk J, Jakschik BA, et al. Arachidonic acid metabolism. Annu Rev Biochem 1986; 55:69–102.
42. Neuringer M, Anderson GJ, Connor WE. The essentiality of n-3 fatty acids for the development and function of the retina and brain. Annu Rev Nutr 1988; 8:517–541.
43. Crawford MA, Hassam AG, Stevens PA. Essential fatty acid requirements in pregnancy and lactation with special reference to brain development. Prog Lipid Res 1982; 20:31–40.
44. Assmann G. Lipid Metabolism and Atherosclerosis. Stuttgart, FK Schattauer Verlag, 1982.
45. Breslow JL. Insights into lipoprotein metabolism from studies in transgenic mice. Annu Rev Physiol 1994; 56:797–810.
46. Mahley RW, Innerarity TL, Rall SC Jr, Weisgraber KH. Plasma lipoproteins: apolipoprotein structure and function. J Lipid Res 1984; 25:1277–1294.
47. Havel RJ, Kane JP. Introduction: structure and metabolism of plasma lipoproteins. In Scriver CR, Beaudet AL, Sly WS, et al (eds). The Metabolic and Molecular Bases of Inherited Disease, vol 2, 8th ed. New York, McGraw-Hill, 2001, pp 2705–2716.
48. Mackness MI, Durrington PN. HDL, its enzymes and its potential to influence lipid peroxidation. Atherosclerosis 1995; 115: 243–253.
49. Tjoelker LW, Wilder C, Eberhardt C, et al. Anti-inflammatory properties of a platelet-activating factor acetylhydrolase. Nature 1995; 374:549–553.
50. Mahley RW, Young SG. Hyperlipidemia: molecular defects of apolipoproteins B and E responsible for elevated blood lipids. In Mockrin SC (ed). Molecular Genetics and Gene Therapy of Cardiovascular Disease. New York, Marcel Dekker, 1996, pp 173–207.
51. Young SG. Recent progress in understanding apolipoprotein B. Circulation 1990; 82:1574–1594.
52. Innerarity TL, Borén J, Yamanaka S, Olofsson S-O. Biosynthesis of apolipoprotein B48–containing lipoproteins: regulation by novel post-transcriptional mechanisms. J Biol Chem 1996; 271: 2353–2356.
53. Schumaker VN, Phillips ML, Chatterton JE. Apolipoprotein B and low-density lipoprotein structure: implications for biosynthesis of triglyceride-rich lipoproteins. Adv Protein Chem 1994; 45: 205–248.
54. Chan L. Apolipoprotein B, the major protein component of triglyceride-rich and low density lipoproteins. J Biol Chem 1992; 267:25621–25624.
55. Hodges P, Scott J. Apolipoprotein B mRNA editing: a new tier for the control of gene expression. Trends Biochem Sci 1992; 17: 77–81.
56. Davidson NO, Anant S, MacGinnitie AJ. Apolipoprotein B messenger RNA editing: insights into the molecular regulation of post-transcriptional cytidine deamination. Curr Opin Lipidol 1995; 6:70–74.
57. Anant S, Davidson NO. Molecular mechanisms of apolipoprotein B mRNA editing. Curr Opin Lipidol 2001; 12:159–165.
58. Powell LM, Wallis SC, Pease RJ, et al. A novel form of tissue-specific RNA processing produces apolipoprotein-B48 in intestine. Cell 1987; 50:831–840.
59. Driscoll DM, Casanova E. Characterization of the apolipoprotein B mRNA editing activity in enterocyte extracts. J Biol Chem 1990; 265:21401–21403.
60. Boström K, Garcia Z, Poksay KS, et al. Apolipoprotein B mRNA editing: direct determination of the edited base and occurrence in non–apolipoprotein B-producing cell lines. J Biol Chem 1990; 265:22446–22452.
61. Knott TJ, Pease RJ, Powell LM, et al. Complete protein sequence and identification of structural domains of human apolipoprotein B. Nature 1986; 323:734–738.
62. Yang C-Y, Gu Z-W, Weng S-A, et al. Structure of apolipoprotein B-100 of human low density lipoproteins. Arteriosclerosis 1989; 9:96–108.
63. Mahley RW, Innerarity TL. Lipoprotein receptors and cholesterol homeostasis. Biochim Biophys Acta 1983; 737:197–222.
64. Borén J, Lee I, Zhu W, et al. Identification of the low density lipoprotein receptor-binding site in apolipoprotein B100 and the modulation of its binding activity by the carboxyl terminus in familial defective apo-B100. J Clin Invest 1998; 101:1084–1093.
65. Innerarity TL, Mahley RW, Weisgraber KH, et al. Familial defective apolipoprotein B100: a mutation of apolipoprotein B that causes hypercholesterolemia. J Lipid Res 1990; 31:1337–1349.
66. Hamilton RL. Apolipoprotein-B–containing plasma lipoproteins in health and in disease. Trends Cardiovasc Med 1994; 4:131–139.
67. Kang S, Davis RA. Cholesterol and hepatic lipoprotein assembly and secretion. Biochim Biophys Acta 2000; 1529:223–230.
68. Shelness GS, Sellers JA. Very-low-density lipoprotein assembly and secretion. Curr Opin Lipidol 2001; 12:151–157.
69. Chiesa G, Johnson DF, Yao Z, et al. Expression of human apolipoprotein B100 in transgenic mice: editing of human apolipoprotein B100 mRNA. J Biol Chem 1993; 268:23747–23750.
70. Linton MF, Farese RV Jr, Chiesa G, et al. Transgenic mice expressing high plasma concentrations of human apolipoprotein B100 and lipoprotein(a). J Clin Invest 1993; 92:3029–3037.
71. Young SG, Farese RV Jr, Pierotti VR, et al. Transgenic mice expressing human $apoB_{100}$ and $apoB_{48}$. Curr Opin Lipidol 1994; 5:94–101.
72. Callow MJ, Stoltzfus LJ, Lawn RM, Rubin EM. Expression of human apolipoprotein B and assembly of lipoprotein(a) in transgenic mice. Proc Natl Acad Sci USA 1994; 91:2130–2134.
73. Purcell-Huynh DA, Farese RV Jr, Johnson DF, et al. Transgenic mice expressing high levels of human apolipoprotein B develop severe atherosclerotic lesions in response to a high-fat diet. J Clin Invest 1995; 95:2246–2257.
74. Farese RV Jr, Ruland SL, Flynn LM, et al. Knockout of the

mouse apolipoprotein B gene results in embryonic lethality in homozygotes and protection against diet-induced hypercholesterolemia in heterozygotes. Proc Natl Acad Sci USA 1995; 92: 1774–1778.

75. Huang L-S, Voyiaziakis E, Markenson DF, et al. Apo B gene knockout in mice results in embryonic lethality in homozygotes and neural tube defects, male infertility, and reduced HDL cholesterol ester and apo A-I transport rates in heterozygotes. J Clin Invest 1995; 96:2152–2161.
76. Farese RV Jr, Cases S, Ruland SL, et al. A novel function for apolipoprotein B: lipoprotein synthesis in the yolk sac is critical for maternal-fetal lipid transport in mice. J Lipid Res 1996; 37: 347–360.
77. Mahley RW. Apolipoprotein E: cholesterol transport protein with expanding role in cell biology. Science 1988; 240:622–630.
78. Weisgraber KH. Apolipoprotein E: structure-function relationships. Adv Protein Chem 1994; 45:249–302.
79. Davignon J, Gregg RE, Sing CF. Apolipoprotein E polymorphism and atherosclerosis. Arteriosclerosis 1988; 8:1–21.
80. Mahley RW, Rall SC Jr. Apolipoprotein E: far more than a lipid transport protein. Annu Rev Genomics Hum Genet 2000; 1:507–537.
81. Mahley RW, Nathan BP, Bellosta S, Pitas RE. Apolipoprotein E: impact of cytoskeletal stability in neurons and the relationship to Alzheimer's disease. Curr Opin Lipidol 1995; 6:86–91.
82. Weisgraber KH, Mahley RW. Human apolipoprotein E: the Alzheimer's disease connection. FASEB J 1996; 10:1485–1494.
83. Mahley RW. Apolipoprotein E: structure and function in lipid metabolism and neurobiology. In Rosenberg RN, Prusiner SB, DiMauro S, Barchi RL (eds). The Molecular and Genetic Basis of Neurological Disease, 2nd ed. Boston, Butterworth-Heinemann, 1997, pp 1037–1049.
84. Mahley RW, Huang Y. Apolipoprotein E: from atherosclerosis to Alzheimer's disease and beyond. Curr Opin Lipidol 1999; 10: 207–217.
85. Utermann G, Kindermann I, Kaffarnik H, Steinmetz A. Apolipoprotein E phenotypes and hyperlipidemia. Hum Genet 1984; 65: 232–236.
86. Mahley RW, Rall SC Jr. Type III hyperlipoproteinemia (dysbetalipoproteinemia): the role of apolipoprotein E in normal and abnormal lipoprotein metabolism. In Scriver CR, Beaudet AL, Sly WS, et al (eds). The Metabolic and Molecular Bases of Inherited Disease, vol 2, 8th ed. New York, McGraw-Hill, 2001, pp 2835–2862.
87. Mahley RW, Innerarity TL, Rall SC Jr, et al. Apolipoprotein E: genetic variants provide insights into its structure and function. Curr Opin Lipidol 1990; 1:87–95.
88. Mahley RW, Huang Y, Rall SC Jr. Pathogenesis of type III hyperlipoproteinemia (dysbetalipoproteinemia): questions, quandaries, and paradoxes. J Lipid Res 1999; 40:1933–1949.
89. Dong L-M, Wilson C, Wardell MR, et al. Human apolipoprotein E: role of arginine 61 in mediating the lipoprotein preferences of the E3 and E4 isoforms. J Biol Chem 1994; 269:22358–22365.
90. Wilson C, Wardell MR, Weisgraber KH, et al. Three-dimensional structure of the LDL receptor-binding domain of human apolipoprotein E. Science 1991; 252:1817–1822.
91. Wilson C, Mau T, Weisgraber KH, et al. Salt bridge relay triggers defective LDL receptor binding by a mutant apolipoprotein. Structure 1994; 2:713–718.
92. Dong L-M, Parkin S, Trakhanov SD, et al. Novel mechanism for defective receptor binding of apolipoprotein E2 in type III hyperlipoproteinemia. Nat Struct Biol 1996; 3:718–722.
93. Mahley RW, Ji Z-S. Remnant lipoprotein metabolism: key pathways involving cell-surface heparan sulfate proteoglycans and apolipoprotein E. J Lipid Res 1999; 40:1–16.
94. Zhang SH, Reddick RL, Piedrahita JA, Maeda N. Spontaneous hypercholesterolemia and arterial lesions in mice lacking apolipoprotein E. Science 1992; 258:468–471.
95. Plump AS, Smith JD, Hayek T, et al. Severe hypercholesterolemia and atherosclerosis in apolipoprotein E–deficient mice created by homologous recombination in ES cells. Cell 1992; 71: 343–353.
96. Tall AR, Breslow JL. Plasma high-density lipoproteins and atherogenesis. In Fuster V, Ross R, Topol EJ (eds). Atherosclerosis and Coronary Artery Disease, vol 1. Philadelphia, Lippincott-Raven, 1996, pp 105–128.
97. Schultz JR, Rubin EM. The properties of HDL in genetically engineered mice. Curr Opin Lipidol 1994; 5:126–137.
98. Assmann G, von Eckardstein A, Brewer HB Jr. Familial analphalipoproteinemia: Tangier disease. In Scriver CR, Beaudet AL, Sly WS, et al (eds). The Metabolic and Molecular Bases of Inherited Disease, vol 2, 8th ed. New York, McGraw-Hill, 2001, pp 2937–2960.
99. Tall AR, Breslow JL, Rubin EM. Genetic disorders affecting plasma high-density lipoproteins. In Scriver CR, Beaudet AL, Sly WS, et al (eds). The Metabolic and Molecular Bases of Inherited Disease, vol 2, 8th ed. New York, McGraw-Hill, 2001, pp 2915–2936.
100. Cho K-H, Durbin DM, Jonas A. Role of individual amino acids of apolipoprotein A-I in the activation of lecithin:cholesterol acyltransferase and in HDL rearrangements. J Lipid Res 2001; 42: 379–389.
101. Fielding CJ. Reverse cholesterol transport. Curr Opin Lipidol 1991; 2:376–378.
102. Swenson TL. Transfer proteins in reverse cholesterol transport. Curr Opin Lipidol 1992; 3:67–74.
103. Brown ML, Hesler C, Tall AR. Plasma enzymes and transfer proteins in cholesterol metabolism. Curr Opin Lipidol 1990; 1: 122–127.
104. Acton S, Rigotti A, Landschulz KT, et al. Identification of scavenger receptor SR-BI as a high density lipoprotein receptor. Science 1996; 271:518–520.
105. Liadaki KN, Liu T, Xu S, et al. Binding of high density lipoprotein (HDL) and discoidal reconstituted HDL to the HDL receptor scavenger receptor class B type I: effect of lipid association and apoA-I mutations on receptor binding. J Biol Chem 2000; 275:21262–21271.
106. Plump AS, Scott CJ, Breslow JL. Human apolipoprotein A-I gene expression increases high density lipoprotein and suppresses atherosclerosis in the apolipoprotein E–deficient mouse. Proc Natl Acad Sci USA 1994; 91:9607–9611.
107. Pászty C, Maeda N, Verstuyft J, Rubin EM. Apolipoprotein AI transgene corrects apolipoprotein E deficiency–induced atherosclerosis in mice. J Clin Invest 1994; 94:899–903.
108. Deeb SS, Takata K, Peng R, et al. A splice-junction mutation responsible for familial apolipoprotein A-II deficiency. Am J Hum Genet 1990; 46:822–827.
109. Warden CH, Hedrick CC, Qiao J-H, et al. Atherosclerosis in transgenic mice overexpressing apolipoprotein A-II. Science 1993; 261:469–472.
110. Taylor JM, Simonet WS, Bucay N, et al. Expression of the human apolipoprotein E/apolipoprotein C-I gene locus in transgenic mice. Curr Opin Lipidol 1991; 2:73–80.
111. Dammerman M, Sandkuijl LA, Halaas JL, et al. An apolipoprotein CIII haplotype protective against hypertriglyceridemia is specified by promoter and 3′ untranslated region polymorphisms. Proc Natl Acad Sci USA 1993; 90:4562–4566.
112. Krieger M, Herz J. Structures and functions of multiligand lipoprotein receptors: macrophage scavenger receptors and LDL receptor–related protein (LRP). Annu Rev Biochem 1994; 63:601–637.
113. Herz J, Willnow TE. Lipoprotein and receptor interactions in vivo. Curr Opin Lipidol 1995; 6:97–103.
114. Willnow TE. The low-density lipoprotein receptor gene family: multiple roles in lipid metabolism. J Mol Med 1999; 77:306–315.
115. Nimpf J, Schneider WJ. From cholesterol transport to signal transduction: low density lipoprotein receptor, very low density lipoprotein receptor, and apolipoprotein E receptor-2. Biochim Biophys Acta 2000; 1529:287–298.
116. Willnow TE, Nykjaer A, Herz J. Lipoprotein receptors: new roles for ancient proteins. Nat Cell Biol 1999; 1:E157–E162.
117. Hobbs HH, Russell DW, Brown MS, Goldstein JL. The LDL receptor locus in familial hypercholesterolemia: mutational analysis of a membrane protein. Annu Rev Genet 1990; 24:133–170.
118. Hobbs HH, Brown MS, Goldstein JL. Molecular genetics of the LDL receptor gene in familial hypercholesterolemia. Hum Mutat 1992; 1:445–466.
119. Goldstein JL, Hobbs HH, Brown MS. Familial hypercholesterolemia. In Scriver CR, Beaudet AL, Sly WS, et al (eds). The Metabolic and Molecular Bases of Inherited Disease, vol 2, 8th ed. New York, McGraw-Hill, 2001, pp 2863–2913.
120. Sato R, Yang J, Wang X, et al. Assignment of the membrane

attachment, DNA binding, and transcriptional activation domains of sterol regulatory element-binding protein-1 (SREBP-1). J Biol Chem 1994; 269:17267–17273.

121. Wang X, Pai J-T, Wiedenfeld EA, et al. Purification of an interleukin-1β converting enzyme–related cysteine protease that cleaves sterol regulatory element–binding proteins between the leucine zipper and transmembrane domains. J Biol Chem 1995; 270:18044–18050.
122. Hua X, Sakai J, Ho YK, et al. Hairpin orientation of sterol regulatory element–binding protein-2 in cell membranes as determined by protease protection. J Biol Chem 1995; 270:29422–29427.
123. Brown MS, Goldstein JL. Sterol regulatory element binding proteins (SREBPs): controllers of lipid synthesis and cellular uptake. Nutr Rev 1998; 56:S1–S3.
124. Brown MS, Goldstein JL. A proteolytic pathway that controls the cholesterol content of membranes, cells, and blood. Proc Natl Acad Sci USA 1999; 96:11041–11048.
125. Edwards PA, Tabor D, Kast HR, Venkateswaran A. Regulation of gene expression by SREBP and SCAP. Biochim Biophys Acta 2000; 1529:103–113.
126. Nohturfft A, DeBose-Boyd RA, Scheek S, et al. Sterols regulate cycling of SREBP cleavage–activating protein (SCAP) between endoplasmic reticulum and Golgi. Proc Natl Acad Sci USA 1999; 96:11235–11240.
127. Herz J, Hamann U, Rogne S, et al. Surface location and high affinity for calcium of a 500-kd liver membrane protein closely related to the LDL-receptor suggest a physiological role as lipoprotein receptor. EMBO J 1988; 7:4119–4127.
128. Strickland DK, Ashcom JD, Williams S, et al. Sequence identity between the α_2-macroglobulin receptor and low density lipoprotein receptor–related protein suggests that this molecule is a multifunctional receptor. J Biol Chem 1990; 265:17401–17404.
129. Mahley RW, Hussain MM. Chylomicron and chylomicron remnant catabolism. Curr Opin Lipidol 1991; 2:170–176.
130. Beisiegel U, Weber W, Bengtsson-Olivecrona G. Lipoprotein lipase enhances the binding of chylomicrons to low density lipoprotein receptor–related protein. Proc Natl Acad Sci USA 1991; 88:8342–8346.
131. Ji Z-S, Lauer SJ, Fazio S, et al. Enhanced binding and uptake of remnant lipoproteins by hepatic lipase–secreting hepatoma cells in culture. J Biol Chem 1994; 269:13429–13436.
132. Herz J, Clouthier DE, Hammer RE. LDL receptor–related protein internalizes and degrades uPA–PAI-1 complexes and is essential for embryo implantation. Cell 1992; 71:411–421.
133. Willnow TE, Armstrong SA, Hammer RE, Herz J. Functional expression of low density lipoprotein receptor–related protein is controlled by receptor-associated protein in vivo. Proc Natl Acad Sci USA 1995; 92:4537–4541.
134. Willnow TE, Hilpert J, Armstrong SA, et al. Defective forebrain development in mice lacking gp330/megalin. Proc Natl Acad Sci USA 1996; 93:8460–8464.
135. Jingami H, Yamamoto T. The VLDL receptor: wayward brother of the LDL receptor. Curr Opin Lipidol 1995; 6:104–108.
136. Kim D-H, Iijima H, Goto K, et al. Human apolipoprotein E receptor 2: a novel lipoprotein receptor of the low density lipoprotein receptor family predominantly expressed in brain. J Biol Chem 1996; 271:8373–8380.
137. Steinberg D. Lipoproteins and the pathogenesis of atherosclerosis. Circulation 1987; 76:508–514.
138. Brown MS, Goldstein JL. Lipoprotein metabolism in the macrophage: implications for cholesterol deposition in atherosclerosis. Annu Rev Biochem 1983; 52:223–261.
139. Yamada Y, Doi T, Hamakubo T, Kodama T. Scavenger receptor family proteins: roles for atherosclerosis, host defence and disorders of the central nervous system. Cell Mol Life Sci 1998; 54: 628–640.
140. Platt N, Gordon S. Scavenger receptors: diverse activities and promiscuous binding of polyanionic ligands. Chem Biol 1998; 5: R193–R203.
141. Dhaliwal BS, Steinbrecher UP. Scavenger receptors and oxidized low density lipoproteins. Clin Chim Acta 1999; 286:191–205.
142. Olivecrona T, Bengtsson-Olivecrona G. Lipases involved in lipoprotein metabolism. Curr Opin Lipidol 1990; 1:116–121.
143. Lalouel J-M, Wilson DE, Iverius P-H. Lipoprotein lipase and hepatic triglyceride lipase: molecular and genetic aspects. Curr Opin Lipidol 1992; 3:86–95.
144. Hayden MR, Ma Y, Brunzell J, Henderson HE. Genetic variants affecting human lipoprotein and hepatic lipases. Curr Opin Lipidol 1991; 2:104–109.
145. Brunzell JD, Deeb SS. Familial lipoprotein lipase deficiency, apo C-II deficiency, and hepatic lipase deficiency. In Scriver CR, Beaudet AL, Sly WS, et al (eds). The Metabolic and Molecular Bases of Inherited Disease, vol 2, 8th ed. New York, McGraw-Hill, 2001, pp 2789–2816.
146. Santamarina-Fojo S, Dugi KA. Structure, function and role of lipoprotein lipase in lipoprotein metabolism. Curr Opin Lipidol 1994; 5:117–125.
147. Kern PA. Lipoprotein lipase and hepatic lipase. Curr Opin Lipidol 1991; 2:162–169.
148. Applebaum-Bowden D. Lipases and lecithin:cholesterol acyltransferase in the control of lipoprotein metabolism. Curr Opin Lipidol 1995; 6:130–135.
149. Cohen JC, Vega GL, Grundy SM. Hepatic lipase: new insights from genetic and metabolic studies. Curr Opin Lipidol 1999; 10: 259–267.
150. Thuren T, Weisgraber KH, Sisson P, Waite M. Role of apolipoprotein E in hepatic lipase catalyzed hydrolysis of phospholipid in high-density lipoproteins. Biochemistry 1992; 31:2332–2338.
151. Homanics GE, de Silva HV, Osada J, et al. Mild dyslipidemia in mice following targeted inactivation of the hepatic lipase gene. J Biol Chem 1995; 270:2974–2980.
152. Busch SJ, Barnhart RL, Martin GA, et al. Human hepatic triglyceride lipase expression reduces high density lipoprotein and aortic cholesterol in cholesterol-fed transgenic mice. J Biol Chem 1994; 269:16376–16382.
153. Fan J, Wang J, Bensadoun A, et al. Overexpression of hepatic lipase in transgenic rabbits leads to a marked reduction of plasma high density lipoproteins and intermediate density lipoproteins. Proc Natl Acad Sci USA 1994; 91:8724–8728.
154. Glomset JA, Assmann G, Gjone E, Norum KR. Lecithin:cholesterol acyltransferase deficiency and fish eye disease. In Scriver CR, Beaudet AL, Sly WS, Valle D (eds). The Metabolic and Molecular Bases of Inherited Disease, vol 2, 7th ed. New York, McGraw-Hill, 1995, pp 1933–1951.
155. Tall A. Plasma lipid transfer proteins. Annu Rev Biochem 1995; 64:235–257.
156. Tall AR. Plasma cholesteryl ester transfer protein. J Lipid Res 1993; 34:1255–1274.
157. Choi SY, Fong LG, Kirven MJ, Cooper AD. Use of an anti–low density lipoprotein receptor antibody to quantify the role of the LDL receptor in the removal of chylomicron remnants in the mouse in vivo. J Clin Invest 1991; 88:1173–1181.
158. Brown MS, Herz J, Kowal RC, Goldstein JL. The low-density lipoprotein receptor–related protein: double agent or decoy? Curr Opin Lipidol 1991; 2:65–72.
159. Ji Z-S, Fazio S, Lee Y-L, Mahley RW. Secretion-capture role for apolipoprotein E in remnant lipoprotein metabolism involving cell surface heparan sulfate proteoglycans. J Biol Chem 1994; 269:2764–2772.
160. Shimano H, Namba Y, Ohsuga J, et al. Secretion-recapture process of apolipoprotein E in hepatic uptake of chylomicron remnants in transgenic mice. J Clin Invest 1994; 93:2215–2223.
161. Ji Z-S, Brecht WJ, Miranda RD, et al. Role of heparan sulfate proteoglycans in the binding and uptake of apolipoprotein E–enriched remnant lipoproteins by cultured cells. J Biol Chem 1993; 268:10160–10167.
162. Ji Z-S, Brecht WJ, Miranda RD, et al. Intravenous heparinase hydrolysis of hepatic heparan sulfate proteoglycans inhibits remnant lipoprotein clearance in vivo (abstract). Circulation 1994; 90: I-290.
163. Alexander CA, Hamilton RL, Havel RJ. Subcellular localization of B apoprotein of plasma lipoproteins in rat liver. J Cell Biol 1976; 69:241–263.
164. Pullinger CR, North JD, Teng B-B, et al. The apolipoprotein B gene is constitutively expressed in HepG2 cells: regulation of secretion by oleic acid, albumin, and insulin, and measurement of the mRNA half-life. J Lipid Res 1989; 30:1065–1077.
165. Sorci-Thomas M, Wilson MD, Johnson FL, et al. Studies on the expression of genes encoding apolipoproteins B100 and B48 and the low density lipoprotein receptor in nonhuman primates: comparison of dietary fat and cholesterol. J Biol Chem 1989; 264: 9039–9045.

166. Boström K, Borén J, Wettesten M, et al. Studies on the assembly of apo B-100–containing lipoproteins in HepG2 cells. J Biol Chem 1988; 263:4434–4442.
167. Borén J, Rustaeus S, Wettesten M, et al. Influence of triacylglycerol biosynthesis rate on the assembly of apoB-100–containing lipoproteins in Hep G2 cells. Arterioscler Thromb 1993; 13: 1743–1754.
168. Ginsberg HN. Synthesis and secretion of apolipoprotein B from cultured liver cells. Curr Opin Lipidol 1995; 6:275–280.
169. Olofsson S-O, Asp L, Borén J. The assembly and secretion of apolipoprotein B–containing lipoproteins. Curr Opin Lipidol 1999; 10:341–346.
170. Sharp D, Blinderman L, Combs KA, et al. Cloning and gene defects in microsomal triglyceride transfer protein associated with abetalipoproteinaemia. Nature 1993; 365:65–69.
171. Gregg RE, Wetterau JR. The molecular basis of abetalipoproteinemia. Curr Opin Lipidol 1994; 5:81–86.
172. Raabe M, Véniant MM, Sullivan MA, et al. Analysis of the role of microsomal triglyceride transfer protein in the liver of tissue-specific knockout mice. J Clin Invest 1999; 103:1287–1298.
173. Jiang X-C, Bruce C, Mar J, et al. Targeted mutation of plasma phospholipid transfer protein gene markedly reduces high-density lipoprotein levels. J Clin Invest 1999; 103:907–914.
174. Tall AR, Jiang X-C, Luo Y, Silver D. 1999 George Lyman Duff Memorial Lecture. Lipid transfer proteins, HDL metabolism, and atherogenesis. Arterioscler Thromb Vasc Biol 2000; 20: 1185–1188.
175. Huang Y, von Eckardstein A, Wu S, et al. A plasma lipoprotein containing only apolipoprotein E and with γ mobility on electrophoresis releases cholesterol from cells. Proc Natl Acad Sci USA 1994; 91:1834–1838.
176. Yokoyama S. Release of cellular cholesterol: molecular mechanism for cholesterol homeostasis in cells and in the body. Biochim Biophys Acta 2000; 1529:231–244.
177. Johnson WJ, Mahlberg FH, Rothblat GH, Phillips MC. Cholesterol transport between cells and high-density lipoproteins. Biochim Biophys Acta 1991; 1085:273–298.
178. Krieger M. Charting the fate of the "good cholesterol": identification and characterization of the high-density lipoprotein receptor SR-BI. Annu Rev Biochem 1999; 68:523–558.
179. Williams DL, Connelly MA, Temel RE, et al. Scavenger receptor BI and cholesterol trafficking. Curr Opin Lipidol 1999; 10: 329–339.
180. Trigatti BL, Rigotti A, Braun A. Cellular and physiological roles of SR-BI, a lipoprotein receptor which mediates selective lipid uptake. Biochim Biophys Acta 2000; 1529:276–286.
181. Oram JF, Vaughan AM. ABCA1-mediated transport of cellular cholesterol and phospholipids to HDL apolipoproteins. Curr Opin Lipidol 2000; 11:253–260.
182. Schmitz G, Langmann T. Structure, function and regulation of the ABC1 gene product. Curr Opin Lipidol 2001; 12:129–140.
183. Schmitz G, Kaminski WE, Orsó E. ABC transporters in cellular lipid trafficking. Curr Opin Lipidol 2000; 11:493–501.
184. Oram JF. Tangier disease and ABCA1. Biochim Biophys Acta 2000; 1529:321–330.
185. Assmann G, von Eckardstein A, Funke H. Lecithin:cholesterol acyltransferase deficiency and fish-eye disease. Curr Opin Lipidol 1991; 2:110–117.
186. Yang C-Y, Manoogian D, Pao Q, et al. Lecithin:cholesterol acyltransferase: functional regions and a structural model of the enzyme. J Biol Chem 1987; 262:3086–3091.
187. Jonas A. Lecithin cholesterol acyltransferase. Biochim Biophys Acta 2000; 1529:245–256.
188. Tall AR. An overview of reverse cholesterol transport. Eur Heart J 1998; 19(suppl A):A31–A35.
189. Yamashita S, Hirano K-I, Sakai N, Matsuzawa Y. Molecular biology and pathophysiological aspects of plasma cholesteryl ester transfer protein. Biochim Biophys Acta 2000; 1529:257–275.
190. Rye K-A, Clay MA, Barter PJ. Remodelling of high density lipoproteins by plasma factors. Atherosclerosis 1999; 145:227–238.
191. Glass C, Pittman RC, Weinstein DB, Steinberg D. Dissociation of tissue uptake of cholesterol ester from that of apoprotein A-I of rat plasma high density lipoprotein: selective delivery of cholesterol ester to liver, adrenal, and gonad. Proc Natl Acad Sci USA 1983; 80:5435–5439.
192. Reaven E, Tsai L, Azhar S. Cholesterol uptake by the 'selective' pathway of ovarian granulosa cells: early intracellular events. J Lipid Res 1995; 36:1602–1617.
193. Ha YC, Barter PJ. Differences in plasma cholesteryl ester transfer activity in sixteen vertebrate species. Comp Biochem Physiol B 1982; 71:265–269.
194. Morton RE. Cholesteryl ester transfer protein and its plasma regulator: lipid transfer inhibitor protein. Curr Opin Lipidol 1999; 10:321–327.
195. Inazu A, Jiang X-C, Haraki T, et al. Genetic cholesteryl ester transfer protein deficiency caused by two prevalent mutations as a major determinant of increased levels of high density lipoprotein cholesterol. J Clin Invest 1994; 94:1872–1882.
196. Marotti KR, Castle CK, Boyle TP, et al. Severe atherosclerosis in transgenic mice expressing simian cholesteryl ester transfer protein. Nature 1993; 364:73–75.
197. Genest JJ, McNamara JR, Salem DN, Schaefer EJ. Prevalence of risk factors in men with premature coronary artery disease. Am J Cardiol 1991; 67:1185–1189.
198. Stary HC. The sequence of cell and matrix changes in atherosclerotic lesions of coronary arteries in the first forty years of life. Eur Heart J 1990; 11(suppl E):3–19.
199. National Cholesterol Education Program. Second report of the Expert Panel on Detection, Evaluation, and Treatment of High Blood Cholesterol in Adults (Adult Treatment Panel II). Circulation 1994; 89:1333–1445.
200. Keys A. Coronary heart disease: the global picture. Atherosclerosis 1975; 22:149–192.
201. Keys A. Seven Countries. A Multivariate Analysis of Death and Coronary Heart Disease. Cambridge, Mass, Harvard University Press, 1980.
202. Mahley RW. Development of accelerated atherosclerosis: concepts derived from cell biology and animal model studies. Arch Pathol Lab Med 1983; 107:393–399.
203. Mahley RW. Atherogenic lipoproteins and coronary artery disease: concepts derived from recent advances in cellular and molecular biology. Circulation 1985; 72:943–948.
204. Vesselinovitch D. Animal models and the study of atherosclerosis. Arch Pathol Lab Med 1988; 112:1011–1017.
205. Faggiotto A, Ross R, Harker L. Studies of hypercholesterolemia in the nonhuman primate. I. Changes that lead to fatty streak formation. Arteriosclerosis 1984; 4:323–340.
206. Buja LM, Clubb FJ Jr, Bilheimer DW, Willerson JT. Pathobiology of human familial hypercholesterolaemia and a related animal model, the Watanabe heritable hyperlipidaemic rabbit. Eur Heart J 1990; 11(suppl E):41–52.
207. Ishibashi S, Goldstein JL, Brown MS, et al. Massive xanthomatosis and atherosclerosis in cholesterol-fed low density lipoprotein receptor-negative mice. J Clin Invest 1994; 93:1885–1893.
208. The Multiple Risk Factor Intervention Trial Research Group. Mortality rates after 10.5 years for participants in the Multiple Risk Factor Intervention Trial: findings related to a priori hypotheses of the trial. JAMA 1990; 263:1795–1801.
209. Consensus Conference. Lowering blood cholesterol to prevent heart disease. JAMA 1985; 253:2080–2086.
210. Scanu AM. Lipoprotein(a): a genetic risk factor for premature coronary heart disease. JAMA 1992; 267:3326–3329.
211. Berg K. Lp(a) lipoprotein: an overview. Chem Phys Lipids 1994; 67/68:9–16.
212. Krauss RM. Low-density lipoprotein subclasses and risk of coronary artery disease. Curr Opin Lipidol 1991; 2:248–252.
213. Mahley RW, Weisgraber KH, Innerarity TL, Rall SC Jr. Genetic defects in lipoprotein metabolism: elevation of atherogenic lipoproteins caused by impaired catabolism. JAMA 1991; 265:78–83.
214. Havel R. McCollum Award Lecture, 1993: triglyceride-rich lipoproteins and atherosclerosis—new perspectives. Am J Clin Nutr 1994; 59:795–799.
215. Haberland ME, Fless GM, Scanu AM, Fogelman AM. Malondialdehyde modification of lipoprotein(a) produces avid uptake by human monocyte-macrophages. J Biol Chem 1992; 267:4143–4151.
216. Henriksen T, Mahoney EM, Steinberg D. Enhanced macrophage degradation of low density lipoprotein previously incubated with cultured endothelial cells: recognition by receptors for acetylated low density lipoproteins. Proc Natl Acad Sci USA 1981; 78: 6499–6503.

217. Steinberg D, Parthasarathy S, Carew TE, et al. Beyond cholesterol: modifications of low-density lipoprotein that increase its atherogenicity. N Engl J Med 1989; 320:915–924.
218. Witztum JL. The oxidation hypothesis of atherosclerosis. Lancet 1994; 344:793–795.
219. Stadtman ER. Protein oxidation and aging. Science 1992; 257: 1220–1224.
220. Harman D. Free radical theory of aging: role of free radicals in the origination and evolution of life, aging, and disease processes. In Johnson JE Jr, Walford R, Harman D, Miquel J (eds). Free Radicals, Aging, and Degenerative Diseases. New York, Alan R Liss, 1986, pp 3–49.
221. Chisolm GM. Cytotoxicity of oxidized lipoproteins. Curr Opin Lipidol 1991; 2:311–316.
222. Quinn MT, Parthasarathy S, Fong LG, Steinberg D. Oxidatively modified low density lipoproteins: a potential role in recruitment and retention of monocyte/macrophages during atherogenesis. Proc Natl Acad Sci USA 1987; 84:2995–2998.
223. Palinski W, Ylä-Herttuala S, Rosenfeld ME, et al. Antisera and monoclonal antibodies specific for epitopes generated during oxidative modification of low density lipoprotein. Arteriosclerosis 1990; 10:325–335.
224. Steinberg D. Is there a potential therapeutic role for vitamin E or other antioxidants in atherosclerosis? Curr Opin Lipidol 2000; 11:603–607.
225. Haberland ME, Fong D, Cheng L. Malondialdehyde-altered protein occurs in atheroma of Watanabe heritable hyperlipidemic rabbits. Science 1988; 241:215–218.
226. Ross R. The pathogenesis of atherosclerosis: a perspective for the 1990s. Nature 1993; 362:801–809.
227. Schwartz CJ, Valente AJ, Sprague EA. A modern view of atherogenesis. Am J Cardiol 1993; 71:9B–14B.
228. Gimbrone MA Jr. Vascular endothelium: nature's blood container. In Gimbrone MA Jr (ed). Vascular Endothelium in Hemostasis and Thrombosis. Edinburgh, Churchill Livingstone, 1986, pp 1–13.
229. Ross R. Atherosclerosis: an inflammatory disease. N Engl J Med 1999; 340:115–126.
230. Libby P. Changing concepts of atherogenesis. J Intern Med 2000; 247:349–358.
231. Lusis AJ. Atherosclerosis. Nature 2000; 407:233–241.
232. Glass CK, Witztum JL. Atherosclerosis: the road ahead. Cell 2001; 104:503–516.
233. Williams KJ, Tabas I. The response-to-retention hypothesis of early atherogenesis. Arterioscler Thromb Vasc Biol 1995; 15: 551–561.
234. Romano M, Romano E, Björkerud S, Hurt-Camejo E. Ultrastructural localization of secretory type II phospholipase A_2 in atherosclerotic and nonatherosclerotic regions of human arteries. Arterioscler Thromb Vasc Biol 1998; 18:519–525.
235. Allen S, Khan S, Al-Mohanna F, et al. Native low density lipoprotein–induced calcium transients trigger VCAM-1 and E-selectin expression in cultured human vascular endothelial cells. J Clin Invest 1998; 101:1064–1075.
236. Cybulsky MI, Gimbrone MA Jr. Endothelial expression of a mononuclear leukocyte adhesion molecule during atherogenesis. Science 1991; 251:788–791.
237. Boring L, Gosling J, Chensue SW, et al. Impaired monocyte migration and reduced type 1 (Th1) cytokine responses in C-C chemokine receptor 2 knockout mice. J Clin Invest 1997; 100: 2552–2561.
238. Boring L, Gosling J, Cleary M, Charo IF. Decreased lesion formation in $CCR2^{-/-}$ mice reveals a role for chemokines in the initiation of atherosclerosis. Nature 1998; 394:894–897.
239. Peters W, Charo IF. Involvement of chemokine receptor 2 and its ligand, monocyte chemoattractant protein-1, in the development of atherosclerosis: lessons from knockout mice. Curr Opin Lipidol 2001; 12:175–180.
240. Wallace RB, Hoover J, Sandler D, et al. Altered plasma-lipids associated with oral contraceptive or œstrogen consumption. The Lipid Research Clinic program. Lancet 1977; 2:11–14.
241. Verschuren WMM, Jacobs DR, Bloemberg BPM, et al. Serum total cholesterol and long-term coronary heart disease mortality in different cultures: twenty-five-year follow-up of the Seven Countries Study. JAMA 1995; 274:131–136.
242. National Cholesterol Education Program Expert Panel. Executive summary of the third report of the National Cholesterol Education Program (NCEP) Expert Panel on Detection, Evaluation, and Treatment of High Blood Cholesterol in Adults (Adult Treatment Panel III). JAMA 2001; 285:2486–2497.
243. Heiss G, Tamir I, Davis CE, et al. Lipoprotein-cholesterol distributions in selected North American populations: the Lipid Research Clinics Program Prevalence Study. Circulation 1980; 61: 302–315.
244. Martin MJ, Hulley SB, Browner WS, et al. Serum cholesterol, blood pressure, and mortality: implications from a cohort of 361 662 men. Lancet 1986; 2:933–936.
245. Beaumont JL, Carlson LA, Cooper GR, et al. Classification of hyperlipidaemias and hyperlipoproteinaemias. Bull World Health Organ 1970; 43:891–907.
246. Fredrickson DS. It's time to be practical. Circulation 1975; 51: 209–211.
247. Bagdade JD, Porte D Jr, Bierman EL. Steroid-induced lipemia: a complication of high-dosage corticosteroid therapy. Arch Intern Med 1970; 125:129–134.
248. Taskinen M-R, Nikkilä EA, Pelkonen R, Sane T. Plasma lipoproteins, lipolytic enzymes, and very low density lipoprotein triglyceride turnover in Cushing's syndrome. J Clin Endocrinol Metab 1983; 57:619–626.
249. Ettinger WH Jr, Hazzard WR. Prednisone increases very low density lipoprotein and high density lipoprotein in healthy men. Metabolism 1988; 37:1055–1058.
250. Merimee TJ, Hollander W, Fineberg SE. Studies of hyperlipidemia in the HGH-deficient state. Metabolism 1972; 21:1053–1061.
251. Nikkilä EA, Pelkonen R. Serum lipids in acromegaly. Metabolism 1975; 24:829–838.
252. Klinefelter HF. Hypercholesterolemia in anorexia nervosa. J Clin Endocrinol Metab 1965; 25:1520–1521.
253. Crisp AH, Blendis LM, Pawan GLS. Aspects of fat metabolism in anorexia nervosa. Metabolism 1968; 17:1109–1118.
254. Havel RJ, Goldstein JL, Brown MS. Lipoproteins and lipid transport. In Bondy PK, Rosenberg LE (eds). Metabolic Control and Disease, 8th ed. Philadelphia, WB Saunders, 1980, pp 393–494.
255. Epstein CJ, Martin GM, Schultz AL, Motulsky AG. Werner's syndrome: a review of its symptomatology, natural history, pathologic features, genetics and relationship to the natural aging process. Medicine (Baltimore) 1966; 45:177–221.
256. Lees RS, Song CS, Levere RD, Kappas A. Hyperbeta-lipoproteinemia in acute intermittent porphyria. N Engl J Med 1970; 282:432–433.
257. Hülsmann WC, Eijkenboom WHM, Koster JF, Fernandes J. Glucose-6-phosphatase deficiency and hyperlipaemia. Clin Chim Acta 1970; 30:775–778.
258. Jakovcic S, Khachadurian AK, Hsia DY-Y. The hyperlipidemia in glycogen storage disease. J Lab Clin Med 1966; 68:769–779.
259. Goldberg A, Sherrard DJ, Brunzell JD. Adipose tissue lipoprotein lipase in chronic hemodialysis: role in plasma triglyceride metabolism. J Clin Endocrinol Metab 1978; 47:1173–1182.
260. McIntyre N, Harry DS, Pearson AJG. The hypercholesterolaemia of obstructive jaundice. Gut 1975; 16:379–391.
261. Simon JB. Lecithin:cholesterol acyltransferase in human liver disease. Scand J Clin Lab Invest 1974; 33(suppl 137):107–113.
262. Sabesin SM, Hawkins HL, Kuiken L, Ragland JB. Abnormal plasma lipoproteins and lecithin-cholesterol acyltransferase deficiency in alcoholic liver disease. Gastroenterology 1977; 72:510–518.
263. Glueck CJ, Kaplan AP, Levy RI, et al. A new mechanism of exogenous hyperglyceridemia. Ann Intern Med 1969; 71:1051–1062.
264. Taylor JS, Lewis LA, Battle JD Jr, et al. Plane xanthoma and multiple myeloma with lipoprotein-paraprotein complexing. Arch Dermatol 1978; 114:425–431.
265. Kihara S, Matsuzawa Y, Kubo M, et al. Autoimmune hyperchylomicronemia. N Engl J Med 1989; 320:1255–1259.
266. Goldstein JL, Brown MS. The LDL receptor locus and the genetics of familial hypercholesterolemia. Annu Rev Genet 1979; 13:259–289.
267. Shapiro JR, Fallat RW, Tsang RC, Glueck CJ. Achilles tendinitis and tenosynovitis: a diagnostic manifestation of familial type II hyperlipoproteinemia in children. Am J Dis Child 1974; 128: 486–490.

268. Barchiesi BJ, Eckel RH, Ellis PP. The cornea and disorders of lipid metabolism. Surv Ophthalmol 1991; 36:1–22.
269. Stone NJ, Levy RI, Fredrickson DS, Verter J. Coronary artery disease in 116 kindred with familial type II hyperlipoproteinemia. Circulation 1974; 49:476–488.
270. Sprecher DL, Schaefer EJ, Kent KM, et al. Cardiovascular features of homozygous familial hypercholesterolemia: analysis of 16 patients. Am J Cardiol 1984; 54:20–30.
271. Coetzee GA, van der Westhuyzen DR, Berger GMB, et al. Low density lipoprotein metabolism in cultured fibroblasts from a new group of patients presenting clinically with homozygous familial hypercholesterolemia. Arteriosclerosis 1982; 2:303–311.
272. Allen JM, Thompson GR, Myant NB, et al. Cardiovascular complications of homozygous familial hypercholesterolaemia. Br Heart J 1980; 44:361–368.
273. Lehrman MA, Goldstein JL, Brown MS, et al. Internalization-defective LDL receptors produced by genes with nonsense and frameshift mutations that truncate the cytoplasmic domain. Cell 1985; 41:735–743.
274. Hobbs HH, Brown MS, Russell DW, et al. Deletion in the gene for the low-density-lipoprotein receptor in a majority of French Canadians with familial hypercholesterolemia. N Engl J Med 1987; 317:734–737.
275. Goldstein JL, Ho YK, Basu SK, Brown MS. Binding site on macrophages that mediates uptake and degradation of acetylated low density lipoprotein, producing massive cholesterol deposition. Proc Natl Acad Sci USA 1979; 76:333–337.
276. Brown MS, Deuel TF, Basu SK, Goldstein JL. Inhibition of the binding of low-density lipoprotein to its cell surface receptor in human fibroblasts by positively charged proteins. J Supramol Struct 1978; 8:223–234.
277. Goldstein JL, Schrott HG, Hazzard WR, et al. Hyperlipidemia in coronary heart disease. II. Genetic analysis of lipid levels in 176 families and delineation of a new inherited disorder, combined hyperlipidemia. J Clin Invest 1973; 52:1544–1568.
278. Myant NB. Familial defective apolipoprotein B-100: a review, including some comparisons with familial hypercholesterolaemia. Atherosclerosis 1993; 104:1–18.
279. Brown MS, Goldstein JL. Familial hypercholesterolemia: defective binding of lipoproteins to cultured fibroblasts associated with impaired regulation of 3-hydroxy-3-methylglutaryl coenzyme A reductase activity. Proc Natl Acad Sci USA 1974; 71:788–792.
280. Packard CJ, Shepherd J. Current concepts in the treatment of familial hypercholesterolaemia. Curr Opin Lipidol 1995; 6:57–61.
281. Connor WE, Connor SL. Importance of diet in the treatment of familial hypercholesterolemia. Am J Cardiol 1993; 72:42D–53D.
282. Mahley RW, Bersot TP. Drug therapy for hypercholesterolemia and dyslipidemia. In Hardman JG, Limbird LE, Gilman AG (eds). Goodman & Gilman's The Pharmacological Basis of Therapeutics, 10th ed. New York, McGraw-Hill, 2002, pp 971–1002.
283. Illingworth DR. How effective is drug therapy in heterozygous familial hypercholesterolemia? Am J Cardiol 1993; 72:54D–58D.
284. Mabuchi H, Sakai T, Sakai Y, et al. Reduction of serum cholesterol in heterozygous patients with familial hypercholesterolemia: additive effects of compactin and cholestyramine. N Engl J Med 1983; 308:609–613.
285. Kane JP, Malloy MJ, Tun P, et al. Normalization of low-density-lipoprotein levels in heterozygous familial hypercholesterolemia with a combined drug regimen. N Engl J Med 1981; 304:251–258.
286. Illingworth DR, Phillipson BE, Rapp JH, Connor WE. Colestipol plus nicotinic acid in treatment of heterozygous familial hypercholesterolaemia. Lancet 1981; 1:296–298.
287. Malloy MJ, Kane JP, Kunitake ST, Tun P. Complementarity of colestipol, niacin, and lovastatin in treatment of severe familial hypercholesterolemia. Ann Intern Med 1987; 107:616–623.
288. Bilheimer DW, Grundy SM, Brown MS, Goldstein JL. Mevinolin and colestipol stimulate receptor-mediated clearance of low density lipoprotein from plasma in familial hypercholesterolemia heterozygotes. Proc Natl Acad Sci USA 1983; 80:4124–4128.
289. Seed M, Hoppichler F, Reaveley D, et al. Relation of serum lipoprotein(a) concentration and apolipoprotein(a) phenotype to coronary heart disease in patients with familial hypercholesterolemia. N Engl J Med 1990; 322:1494–1499.
290. Carlson LA, Hamsten A, Asplund A. Pronounced lowering of serum levels of lipoprotein Lp(a) in hyperlipidaemic subjects treated with nicotinic acid. J Intern Med 1989; 226:271–276.
291. Carew TE, Schwenke DC, Steinberg D. Antiatherogenic effect of probucol unrelated to its hypocholesterolemic effect: evidence that antioxidants in vivo can selectively inhibit low density lipoprotein degradation in macrophage-rich fatty streaks and slow the progression of atherosclerosis in the Watanabe heritable hyperlipidemic rabbit. Proc Natl Acad Sci USA 1987; 84:7725–7729.
292. Kita T, Nagano Y, Yokode M, et al. Probucol prevents the progression of atherosclerosis in Watanabe heritable hyperlipidemic rabbit, an animal model for familial hypercholesterolemia. Proc Natl Acad Sci USA 1987; 84:5928–5931.
293. Yamamoto A, Matsuzawa Y, Yokoyama S, et al. Effects of probucol on xanthomata regression in familial hypercholesterolemia. Am J Cardiol 1986; 57:29H–35H.
294. Buchwald H, Varco RL, Matts JP, et al. Effect of partial ileal bypass surgery on mortality and morbidity from coronary heart disease in patients with hypercholesterolemia: report of the Program on the Surgical Control of the Hyperlipidemias (POSCH). N Engl J Med 1990; 323:946–955.
295. Brown G, Albers JJ, Fisher LD, et al. Regression of coronary artery disease as a result of intensive lipid-lowering therapy in men with high levels of apolipoprotein B. N Engl J Med 1990; 323:1289–1298.
296. Kane JP, Malloy MJ, Ports TA, et al. Regression of coronary atherosclerosis during treatment of familial hypercholesterolemia with combined drug regimens. JAMA 1990; 264:3007–3012.
297. Raal FJ, Pappu AS, Illingworth DR, et al. Inhibition of cholesterol synthesis by atorvastatin in homozygous familial hypercholesterolemia. Atherosclerosis 2000; 150:421–428.
298. Raal FJ, Pilcher GJ, Illingworth DR, et al. Expanded-dose simvastatin is effective in homozygous familial hypercholesterolaemia. Atherosclerosis 1997; 135:249–256.
299. Stoffel W, Borberg H, Greve V. Application of specific extracorporeal removal of low density lipoprotein in familial hypercholesterolaemia. Lancet 1981; 2:1005–1007.
300. Gordon BR, Saal SD. Advances in LDL-apheresis for the treatment of severe hypercholesterolemia. Curr Opin Lipidol 1994; 5:69–73.
301. Bilheimer DW, Goldstein JL, Grundy SM, et al. Liver transplantation to provide low-density-lipoprotein receptors and lower plasma cholesterol in a child with homozygous familial hypercholesterolemia. N Engl J Med 1984; 311:1658–1664.
302. Valdivielso P, Escolar JL, Cuervas-Mons V, et al. Lipids and lipoprotein changes after heart and liver transplantation in a patient with homozygous familial hypercholesterolemia. Ann Intern Med 1988; 108:204–206.
303. Forman MB, Baker SG, Mieny CJ, et al. Treatment of homozygous familial hypercholesterolaemia with portacaval shunt. Atherosclerosis 1982; 41:349–361.
304. McNamara DJ, Ahrens EH Jr, Kolb R, et al. Treatment of familial hypercholesterolemia by portacaval anastomosis: effect on cholesterol metabolism and pool sizes. Proc Natl Acad Sci USA 1983; 80:564–568.
305. Brown MS, Goldstein JL, Havel RJ, Steinberg D. Gene therapy for cholesterol. Nat Genet 1994; 7:349–350.
306. Grossman M, Raper SE, Kozarsky K, et al. Successful ex vivo gene therapy directed to liver in a patient with familial hypercholesterolaemia. Nat Genet 1994; 6:335–341.
307. Schuster H, Rauh G, Kormann B, et al. Familial defective apolipoprotein B-100: comparison with familial hypercholesterolemia in 18 cases detected in Munich. Arteriosclerosis 1990; 10:577–581.
308. Tybjærg-Hansen A, Gallagher J, Vincent J, et al. Familial defective apolipoprotein B-100: detection in the United Kingdom and Scandinavia, and clinical characteristics of ten cases. Atherosclerosis 1990; 80:235–242.
309. Ludwig EH, McCarthy BJ. Haplotype analysis of the human apolipoprotein B mutation associated with familial defective apolipoprotein B100. Am J Hum Genet 1990; 47:712–720.
310. Bersot TP, Russell SJ, Thatcher SR, et al. A unique haplotype of the apolipoprotein B-100 allele associated with familial defective apolipoprotein B-100 in a Chinese man discovered during a study of the prevalence of this disorder. J Lipid Res 1993; 34:1149–1154.
311. Rauh G, Keller C, Kormann B, et al. Familial defective apolipo-

protein B_{100}: clinical characteristics of 54 cases. Atherosclerosis 1992; 92:233–241.

312. Miserez AR, Keller U. Differences in the phenotypic characteristics of subjects with familial defective apolipoprotein B-100 and familial hypercholesterolemia. Arterioscler Thromb Vasc Biol 1995; 15:1719–1729.
313. März W, Baumstark MW, Scharnagl H, et al. Accumulation of "small dense" low density lipoproteins (LDL) in a homozygous patient with familial defective apolipoprotein B-100 results from heterogenous interaction of LDL subfractions with the LDL receptor. J Clin Invest 1993; 92:2922–2933.
314. Gallagher JJ, Myant NB. The affinity of low-density lipoproteins and of very-low-density lipoprotein remnants for the low-density lipoprotein receptor in homozygous familial defective apolipoprotein B-100. Atherosclerosis 1995; 115:263–272.
315. Funke H, Rust S, Seedorf U, et al. Homozygosity for familial defective apolipoprotein B-100 (FDB) is associated with lower plasma cholesterol concentrations than homozygosity for familial hypercholesterolemia (FH) (abstract). Circulation 1992; 86:I-691.
316. Innerarity TL, Weisgraber KH, Arnold KS, et al. Familial defective apolipoprotein B-100: low density lipoproteins with abnormal receptor binding. Proc Natl Acad Sci USA 1987; 84:6919–6923.
317. Soria LF, Ludwig EH, Clarke HRG, et al. Association between a specific apolipoprotein B mutation and familial defective apolipoprotein B-100. Proc Natl Acad Sci USA 1989; 86:587–591.
318. Vega GL, Grundy SM. In vivo evidence for reduced binding of low density lipoproteins to receptors as a cause of primary moderate hypercholesterolemia. J Clin Invest 1986; 78:1410–1414.
319. Rauh G, Schuster H, Schewe CK, et al. Independent mutation of $arginine_{(3500)} \rightarrow glutamine$ associated with familial defective apolipoprotein B-100. J Lipid Res 1993; 34:799–805.
320. Lund-Katz S, Innerarity TL, Arnold KS, et al. ^{13}C NMR evidence that substitution of glutamine for arginine 3500 in familial defective apolipoprotein B-100 disrupts the conformation of the receptor-binding domain. J Biol Chem 1991; 266:2701–2704.
321. Arnold KS, Balestra ME, Krauss RM, et al. Isolation of allele-specific, receptor-binding–defective low density lipoproteins from familial defective apolipoprotein B-100 subjects. J Lipid Res 1994; 35:1469–1476.
322. Gaffney D, Reid JM, Cameron IM, et al. Independent mutations at codon 3500 of the apolipoprotein B gene are associated with hyperlipidemia. Arterioscler Thromb Vasc Biol 1995; 15:1025–1029.
323. Pullinger CR, Hennessy LK, Chatterton JE, et al. Familial ligand-defective apolipoprotein B: identification of a new mutation that decreases LDL receptor binding affinity. J Clin Invest 1995; 95:1225–1234.
324. Hansen PS, Rüdiger N, Tybjaerg-Hansen A, et al. Detection of the apoB-3500 mutation (glutamine for arginine) by gene amplification and cleavage with MspI. J Lipid Res 1991; 32:1229–1233.
325. Schmidt EB, Illingworth DR, Bacon S, et al. Hypolipidemic effects of nicotinic acid in patients with familial defective apolipoprotein B-100. Metabolism 1993; 42:137–139.
326. Schmidt EB, Illingworth DR, Bacon S, et al. Hypocholesterolemic effects of cholestyramine and colestipol in patients with familial defective apolipoprotein B-100. Atherosclerosis 1993; 98: 213–217.
327. Rose HG, Kranz P, Weinstock M, et al. Inheritance of combined hyperlipoproteinemia: evidence for a new lipoprotein phenotype. Am J Med 1973; 54:148–160.
328. Nikkilä EA, Aro A. Family study of serum lipids and lipoproteins in coronary heart-disease. Lancet 1973; 1:954–959.
329. Sniderman A, Shapiro S, Marpole D, et al. Association of coronary atherosclerosis with hyper*apo*betalipoproteinemia [increased protein but normal cholesterol levels in human plasma low density (β) lipoproteins]. Proc Natl Acad Sci USA 1980; 77:604–608.
330. Krauss RM. Dense low density lipoproteins and coronary artery disease. Am J Cardiol 1995; 75:53B–57B.
331. Reaven GM. Pathophysiology of insulin resistance in human disease. Physiol Rev 1995; 75:473–486.
332. Genest JJ Jr, Martin-Munley SS, McNamara JR, et al. Familial lipoprotein disorders in patients with premature coronary artery disease. Circulation 1992; 85:2025–2033.
333. Cortner JA, Coates PM, Gallagher PR. Prevalence and expression of familial combined hyperlipidemia in childhood. J Pediatr 1990; 116:514–519.
334. Grundy SM, Chait A, Brunzell JD. Familial combined hyperlipidemia workshop. Arteriosclerosis 1987; 7:203–207.
335. Pajukanta P, Terwilliger JD, Perola M, et al. Genomewide scan for familial combined hyperlipidemia genes in Finnish families, suggesting multiple susceptibility loci influencing triglyceride, cholesterol, and apolipoprotein B levels. Am J Hum Genet 1999; 64:1453–1463.
336. Castellani LW, Weinreb A, Bodnar J, et al. Mapping a gene for combined hyperlipidaemia in a mutant mouse strain. Nat Genet 1998; 18:374–377.
337. Pajukanta P, Nuotio I, Terwilliger JD, et al. Linkage of familial combined hyperlipidaemia to chromosome 1q21-q23. Nat Genet 1998; 18:369–373.
338. Wojciechowski AP, Farrall M, Cullen P, et al. Familial combined hyperlipidaemia linked to the apolipoprotein AI-CIII-AIV gene cluster on chromosome 11q23-q24. Nature 1991; 349:161–164.
339. Nishina PM, Johnson JP, Naggert JK, Krauss RM. Linkage of atherogenic lipoprotein phenotype to the low density lipoprotein receptor locus on the short arm of chromosome 19. Proc Natl Acad Sci USA 1992; 89:708–712.
340. Rotter JI, Bu X, Cantor R, et al. Multilocus genetic determination of LDL particle size in coronary artery disease families (abstract). Clin Res 1994; 42:16A.
341. Aouizerat BE, Allayee H, Bodnar J, et al. Novel genes for familial combined hyperlipidemia. Curr Opin Lipidol 1999; 10:113–122.
342. Babirak SP, Iverius P-H, Fujimoto WY, Brunzell JD. Detection and characterization of the heterozygote state for lipoprotein lipase deficiency. Arteriosclerosis 1989; 9:326–334.
343. Chait A, Albers JJ, Brunzell JD. Very low density lipoprotein overproduction in genetic forms of hypertriglyceridaemia. Eur J Clin Invest 1980; 10:17–22.
344. Janus ED, Nicoll AM, Turner PR, et al. Kinetic bases of the primary hyperlipidaemias: studies of apolipoprotein B turnover in genetically defined subjects. Eur J Clin Invest 1980; 10:161–172.
345. Brunzell JD, Albers JJ, Chait A, et al. Plasma lipoproteins in familial combined hyperlipidemia and monogenic familial hypertriglyceridemia. J Lipid Res 1983; 24:147–155.
346. Crouse JR III. Hypertriglyceridemia: a contraindication to the use of bile acid binding resins. Am J Med 1987; 83:243–248.
347. Frick MH, Elo O, Haapa K, et al. Helsinki Heart Study: primary-prevention trial with gemfibrozil in middle-aged men with dyslipidemia. Safety of treatment, changes in risk factors, and incidence of coronary heart disease. N Engl J Med 1987; 317: 1237–1245.
348. Vega GL, Grundy SM. Lipoprotein responses to treatment with lovastatin, gemfibrozil, and nicotinic acid in normolipidemic patients with hypoalphalipoproteinemia. Arch Intern Med 1994; 154:73–82.
349. Havel RJ, Kotite L, Kane JP, et al. Atypical familial dysbetalipoproteinemia associated with apolipoprotein phenotype E3/3. J Clin Invest 1983; 72:379–387.
350. Rall SC Jr, Newhouse YM, Clarke HRG, et al. Type III hyperlipoproteinemia associated with apolipoprotein E phenotype E3/3: structure and genetics of an apolipoprotein E3 variant. J Clin Invest 1989; 83:1095–1101.
351. Koo C, Wernette-Hammond ME, Innerarity TL. Uptake of canine β-very low density lipoproteins by mouse peritoneal macrophages is mediated by a low density lipoprotein receptor. J Biol Chem 1986; 261:11194–11201.
352. Morganroth J, Levy RI, Fredrickson DS. The biochemical, clinical, and genetic features of type III hyperlipoproteinemia. Ann Intern Med 1975; 82:158–174.
353. Hixson JE, Vernier DT. Restriction isotyping of human apolipoprotein E by gene amplification and cleavage with *Hha*I. J Lipid Res 1990; 31:545–548.
354. Hazzard WR, Bierman EL. Aggravation of broad-β disease (type 3 hyperlipoproteinemia) by hypothyroidism. Arch Intern Med 1972; 130:822–828.
355. Kushwaha RS, Hazzard WR, Gagne C, et al. Type III hyperlipoproteinemia: paradoxical hypolipidemic response to estrogen. Ann Intern Med 1977; 87:517–525.
356. Hoogwerf BJ, Bantle JP, Kuba K, et al. Treatment of type III hyperlipoproteinemia with four different treatment regimens. Atherosclerosis 1984; 51:251–259.
357. Schaefer EJ (discussant). Type III hyperlipoproteinemia: diagno-

sis, molecular defects, pathology, and treatment. Dietary and drug treatment. Ann Intern Med 1983; 98:633–640.

358. Hoogwerf BJ, Peters JR, Frantz ID Jr, Hunninghake DB. Effect of clofibrate and colestipol singly and in combination on plasma lipids and lipoproteins in type III hyperlipoproteinemia. Metabolism 1985; 34:978–981.
359. Illingworth DR, O'Malley JP. The hypolipidemic effects of lovastatin and clofibrate alone and in combination in patients with type III hyperlipoproteinemia. Metabolism 1990; 39:403–409.
360. Stuyt PMJ, Mol MJTM, Stalenhoef AFH. Long-term effects of simvastatin in familial dysbetalipoproteinaemia. J Intern Med 1991; 230:151–155.
361. Feussner G, Eichinger M, Ziegler R. The influence of simvastatin alone or in combination with gemfibrozil on plasma lipids and lipoproteins in patients with type III hyperlipoproteinemia. Clin Investig 1992; 70:1027–1035.
362. Wiklund O, Angelin B, Bergman M, et al. Pravastatin and gemfibrozil alone and in combination for the treatment of hypercholesterolemia. Am J Med 1993; 94:13–20.
363. Chait A, Brunzell JD. Chylomicronemia syndrome. Adv Intern Med 1991; 37:249–273.
364. Santamarina-Fojo S, Brewer HB Jr. The familial hyperchylomicronemia syndrome: new insights into underlying genetic defects. JAMA 1991; 265:904–908.
365. Brunzell JD, Bierman EL. Chylomicronemia syndrome: interaction of genetic and acquired hypertriglyceridemia. Med Clin North Am 1982; 66:455–468.
366. Chait A, Robertson HT, Brunzell JD. Chylomicronemia syndrome in diabetes mellitus. Diabetes Care 1981; 4:343–348.
367. Heilman KM, Fisher WR. Hyperlipidemic dementia. Arch Neurol 1974; 31:67–68.
368. Mathew NT, Meyer JS, Achari AN, Dodson RF. Hyperlipidemic neuropathy and dementia. Eur Neurol 1976; 14:370–382.
369. Steffes MW, Freier EF. A simple and precise method of determining true sodium, potassium, and chloride concentrations in hyperlipemia. J Lab Clin Med 1976; 88:683–688.
370. Wilson DE, Emi M, Iverius P-H, et al. Phenotypic expression of heterozygous lipoprotein lipase deficiency in the extended pedigree of a proband homozygous for a missense mutation. J Clin Invest 1990; 86:735–750.
371. Fojo SS, Brewer HB. Hypertriglyceridaemia due to genetic defects in lipoprotein lipase and apolipoprotein C-II. J Intern Med 1992; 231:669–677.
372. Gagné C, Brun L-D, Julien P, et al. Primary lipoprotein-lipase-activity deficiency: clinical investigation of a French Canadian population. Can Med Assoc J 1989; 140:405–411.
373. Eckel RH. Lipoprotein lipase: a multifunctional enzyme relevant to common metabolic diseases. N Engl J Med 1989; 320:1060–1068.
374. Illingworth DR, Connor WE, Miller RG. Abetalipoproteinemia: report of two cases and review of therapy. Arch Neurol 1980; 37: 659–662.
375. Partin JS, Partin JC, Schubert WK, McAdams AJ. Liver ultrastructure in abetalipoproteinemia: evolution of micronodular cirrhosis. Gastroenterology 1974; 67:107–118.
376. Schaefer EJ. Familial lipoprotein disorders and premature coronary artery disease. Med Clin North Am 1994; 78:21–39.
377. Brunzell JD, Schrott HG, Motulsky AG, Bierman EL. Myocardial infarction in the familial forms of hypertriglyceridemia. Metabolism 1976; 25:313–320.
378. Chuntharapai A, Lee J, Burnier J, et al. Neutralizing monoclonal antibodies to human IL-8 receptor A map to the NH_2-terminal region of the receptor. J Immunol 1994; 152:1783–1789.
379. Schaefer EJ, Zech LA, Jenkins LL, et al. Human apolipoprotein A-I and A-II metabolism. J Lipid Res 1982; 23:850–862.
380. Brinton EA, Eisenberg S, Breslow JL. Increased apo A-I and apo A-II fractional catabolic rate in patients with low high density lipoprotein-cholesterol levels with or without hypertriglyceridemia. J Clin Invest 1991; 87:536–544.
381. Berg K. A new serum type system in man: the Lp system. Acta Pathol Microbiol Scand 1963; 59:369–382.
382. Utermann G. The mysteries of lipoprotein(a). Science 1989; 246: 904–910.
383. Scanu AM, Fless GM. Lipoprotein (a): heterogeneity and biological relevance. J Clin Invest 1990; 85:1709–1715.
384. Gaw A, Hobbs HH. Molecular genetics of lipoprotein (a): new pieces to the puzzle. Curr Opin Lipidol 1994; 5:149–155.
385. McLean JW, Tomlinson JE, Kuang W-J, et al. cDNA sequence of human apolipoprotein(a) is homologous to plasminogen. Nature 1987; 330:132–137.
386. Dahlen GH, Guyton JR, Attar M, et al. Association of levels of lipoprotein Lp(a), plasma lipids, and other lipoproteins with coronary artery disease documented by angiography. Circulation 1986; 74:758–765.
387. Sandkamp M, Funke H, Schulte H, et al. Lipoprotein(a) is an independent risk factor for myocardial infarction at a young age. Clin Chem 1990; 36:20–23.
388. Genest J Jr, Jenner JL, McNamara JR, et al. Prevalence of lipoprotein (a) [Lp(a)] excess in coronary artery disease. Am J Cardiol 1991; 67:1039–1045.
389. Gurewich V, Mittleman M. Lipoprotein(a) in coronary heart disease: is it a risk factor after all? JAMA 1994; 271:1025–1026.
390. Ridker PM, Hennekens CH, Stampfer MJ. A prospective study of lipoprotein(a) and the risk of myocardial infarction. JAMA 1993; 270:2195–2199.
391. Jauhiainen M, Koskinen P, Ehnholm C, et al. Lipoprotein (a) and coronary heart disease risk: a nested case-control study of the Helsinki Heart Study participants. Atherosclerosis 1991; 89:59–67.
392. Schaefer EJ, Lamon-Fava S, Jenner JL, et al. Lipoprotein(a) levels and risk of coronary heart disease in men. The Lipid Research Clinics Coronary Primary Prevention Trial. JAMA 1994; 271:999–1003.
393. Rosengren A, Wilhelmsen L, Eriksson E, et al. Lipoprotein (a) and coronary heart disease: a prospective case-control study in a general population sample of middle aged men. Br Med J 1990; 301:1248–1251.
394. Boerwinkle E, Leffert CC, Lin J, et al. Apolipoprotein(a) gene accounts for greater than 90% of the variation in plasma lipoprotein(a) concentrations. J Clin Invest 1992; 90:52–60.
395. Lamon-Fava S, Jimenez D, Christian JC, et al. The NHLBI Twin Study: heritability of apolipoprotein A-I, B, and low density lipoprotein subclasses and concordance for lipoprotein(a). Atherosclerosis 1991; 91:97–106.
396. Berg K. Twin research in coronary heart disease. Prog Clin Biol Res 1981; 69C:117–130.
397. Sandholzer C, Hallman DM, Saha N, et al. Effects of the apolipoprotein(a) size polymorphism on the lipoprotein(a) concentration in 7 ethnic groups. Hum Genet 1991; 86:607–614.
398. Maher VMG, Brown BG, Marcovina SM, et al. Effects of lowering elevated LDL cholesterol on the cardiovascular risk of lipoprotein(a). JAMA 1995; 274:1771–1774.
399. Stein JH, Rosenson RS. Lipoprotein Lp(a) excess and coronary heart disease. Arch Intern Med 1997; 157:1170–1176.
400. McCormick SPA, Ng JK, Taylor S, et al. Mutagenesis of the human apolipoprotein B gene in a yeast artificial chromosome reveals the site of attachment for apolipoprotein(a). Proc Natl Acad Sci USA 1995; 92:10147–10151.
401. Gavish D, Azrolan N, Breslow JL. Plasma Lp(a) concentration is inversely correlated with the ratio of Kringle IV/Kringle V encoding domains in the apo(a) gene. J Clin Invest 1989; 84:2021–2027.
402. Hajjar KA, Gavish D, Breslow JL, Nachman RL. Lipoprotein(*a*) modulation of endothelial cell surface fibrinolysis and its potential role in atherosclerosis. Nature 1989; 339:303–305.
403. Miles LA, Fless GM, Levin EG, et al. A potential basis for the thrombotic risks associated with lipoprotein(*a*). Nature 1989; 339: 301–303.
404. Grainger DJ, Kirschenlohr HL, Metcalfe JC, et al. Proliferation of human smooth muscle cells promoted by lipoprotein(a). Science 1993; 260:1655–1658.
405. Espeland MA, Marcovina SM, Miller V, et al. Effect of postmenopausal hormone therapy on lipoprotein(a) concentration. Circulation 1998; 97:979–986.
406. Shlipak MG, Simon JA, Vittinghoff E, et al. Estrogen and progestin, lipoprotein(a), and the risk of recurrent coronary heart disease events after menopause. JAMA 2000; 283:1845–1852.
407. Third JLHC, Montag J, Flynn M, et al. Primary and familial hypoalphalipoproteinemia. Metabolism 1984; 33:136–146.
408. Vergani C, Bettale G. Familial hypo-alpha-lipoproteinemia. Clin Chim Acta 1981; 114:45–52.
409. Cohen JC, Wang Z, Grundy SM, et al. Variation at the hepatic lipase and apolipoprotein AI/CIII/AIV loci is a major cause of

500. Chait A, Bierman EL, Albers JJ. Low-density lipoprotein receptor activity in cultured human skin fibroblasts: mechanism of insulin-induced stimulation. J Clin Invest 1979; 64:1309–1319.
501. Bagdade JD, Porte D Jr, Bierman EL. Diabetic lipemia: a form of acquired fat-induced lipemia. N Engl J Med 1967; 276:427–433.
502. Brunzell JD, Hazzard WR, Motulsky AG, Bierman EL. Evidence for diabetes mellitus and genetic forms of hypertriglyceridemia as independent entities. Metabolism 1975; 24:1115–1121.
503. Laakso M, Pyörälä K, Sarlund H, Voutilainen E. Lipid and lipoprotein abnormalities associated with coronary heart disease in patients with insulin-dependent diabetes mellitus. Arteriosclerosis 1986; 6:679–684.
504. Manzato E, Crepaldi G. Dyslipoproteinaemia in manifest diabetes. J Intern Med 1994; 236(suppl 736):27–31.
505. Joven J, Vilella E, Costa B, et al. Concentrations of lipids and apolipoproteins in patients with clinically well-controlled insulin-dependent and non–insulin-dependent diabetes. Clin Chem 1989; 35:813–816.
506. Feingold KR, Grunfeld C, Pang M, et al. LDL subclass phenotypes and triglyceride metabolism in non–insulin-dependent diabetes. Arterioscler Thromb 1992; 12:1496–1502.
507. Bowie A, Owens D, Collins P, et al. Glycosylated low density lipoprotein is more sensitive to oxidation: implications for the diabetic patient? Atherosclerosis 1993; 102:63–67.
508. Sparks JD, Sparks CE. Insulin modulation of hepatic synthesis and secretion of apolipoprotein B by rat hepatocytes. J Biol Chem 1990; 265:8854–8862.
509. Tobey TA, Greenfield M, Kraemer F, Reaven GM. Relationship between insulin resistance, insulin secretion, very low density lipoprotein kinetics, and plasma triglyceride levels in normotriglyceridemic man. Metabolism 1981; 30:165–171.
510. Eto M, Watanabe K, Sato T, Makino I. Apolipoprotein-E2 and hyperlipoproteinemia in noninsulin-dependent diabetes mellitus. J Clin Endocrinol Metab 1989; 69:1207–1212.
511. DeFronzo RA, Goodman AM, the Multicenter Metformin Study Group. Efficacy of metformin in patients with non–insulin-dependent diabetes mellitus. N Engl J Med 1995; 333:541–549.
512. Rosenstock J, Vega GL, Raskin P. Effect of intensive diabetes treatment on low-density lipoprotein apolipoprotein B kinetics in type I diabetes. Diabetes 1988; 37:393–397.
513. Taskinen M-R, Kuusi T, Helve E, et al. Insulin therapy induces antiatherogenic changes of serum lipoproteins in noninsulin-dependent diabetes. Arteriosclerosis 1988; 8:168–177.
514. Valdemarsson S, Hansson P, Hedner P, Nilsson-Ehle P. Relations between thyroid function, hepatic and lipoprotein lipase activities, and plasma lipoprotein concentrations. Acta Endocrinol (Copenh) 1983; 104:50–56.
515. Kinlaw WB III. Atherosclerosis and the thyroid. Thyroid Today 1991; 14:1–8.
516. Abrams JJ, Grundy SM, Ginsberg H. Metabolism of plasma triglycerides in hypothyroidism and hyperthyroidism in man. J Lipid Res 1981; 22:307–322.
517. Hansson P, Valdemarsson S, Nilsson-Ehle P. Experimental hyperthyroidism in man: effects on plasma lipoproteins, lipoprotein lipase and hepatic lipase. Horm Metab Res 1983; 15:449–452.
518. Agdeppa D, Macaron C, Mallik T, Schnuda ND. Plasma high density lipoprotein cholesterol in thyroid disease. J Clin Endocrinol Metab 1979; 49:726–729.
519. Henkin Y, Como JA, Oberman A. Secondary dyslipidemia. Inadvertent effects of drugs in clinical practice. JAMA 1992; 267:961–968.
520. Thompson GR, Soutar AK, Spengel FA, et al. Defects of receptor-mediated low density lipoprotein catabolism in homozygous familial hypercholesterolemia and hypothyroidism in vivo. Proc Natl Acad Sci USA 1981; 78:2591–2595.
521. Scarabottolo L, Trezzi E, Roma P, Catapano AL. Experimental hypothyroidism modulates the expression of the low density lipoprotein receptor by the liver. Atherosclerosis 1986; 59:329–333.
522. Sykes M, Cnoop-Koopmans WM, Julien P, Angel A. The effects of hypothyroidism, age, and nutrition on LDL catabolism in the rat. Metabolism 1981; 30:733–738.
523. Chait A, Bierman EL, Albers JJ. Regulatory role of triiodothyronine in the degradation of low density lipoprotein by cultured human skin fibroblasts. J Clin Endocrinol Metab 1979; 48:887–889.
524. Vanhaelst L, Neve P, Chailly P, Bastenie PA. Coronary-artery disease in hypothyroidism: observations in clinical myxœdema. Lancet 1967; 2:800–802.
525. Steinberg AD. Myxedema and coronary artery disease: a comparative autopsy study. Ann Intern Med 1968; 68:338–344.
526. Arem R, Patsch W. Lipoprotein and apolipoprotein levels in subclinical hypothyroidism: effect of levothyroxine therapy. Arch Intern Med 1990; 150:2097–2100.
527. Pykälistö O, Goldberg AP, Brunzell JD. Reversal of decreased human adipose tissue lipoprotein lipase and hypertriglyceridemia after treatment of hypothyroidism. J Clin Endocrinol Metab 1976; 43:591–600.
528. Walsh BW, Schiff I, Rosner B, et al. Effects of postmenopausal estrogen replacement on the concentrations and metabolism of plasma lipoproteins. N Engl J Med 1991; 325:1196–1204.
529. Davidoff F, Tishler S, Rosoff C. Marked hyperlipidemia and pancreatitis associated with oral contraceptive therapy. N Engl J Med 1973; 289:552–555.
530. Glueck CJ, Fallat RW, Scheel D. Effects of estrogenic compounds on triglyceride kinetics. Metabolism 1975; 24:537–545.
531. Windler EET, Kovanen PT, Chao Y-S, et al. The estradiol-stimulated lipoprotein receptor of rat liver: a binding site that mediates the uptake of rat lipoproteins containing apoproteins B and E. J Biol Chem 1980; 255:10464–10471.
532. Wahl P, Walden C, Knopp R, et al. Effect of estrogen/progestin potency on lipid/lipoprotein cholesterol. N Engl J Med 1983; 308:862–867.
533. Psaty BM, Heckbert SR, Atkins D, et al. A review of the association of estrogens and progestins with cardiovascular disease in postmenopausal women. Arch Intern Med 1993; 153:1421–1427.
534. Stampfer MJ, Colditz GA, Willett WC, et al. Postmenopausal estrogen therapy and cardiovascular disease: ten-year follow-up from the Nurses' Health Study. N Engl J Med 1991; 325:756–762.
535. Hulley S, Grady D, Bush T, et al. Randomized trial of estrogen plus progestin for secondary prevention of coronary heart disease in postmenopausal women. JAMA 1998; 280:605–613.
536. Herrington DM, Reboussin DM, Brosnihan KB, et al. Effects of estrogen replacement on the progression of coronary-artery atherosclerosis. N Engl J Med 2000; 343:522–529.
537. Janus ED, Lewis B. Alcohol and abnormalities of lipid metabolism. Clin Endocrinol Metab 1978; 7:321–332.
538. Steinberg D, Pearson TA, Kuller LH. Alcohol and atherosclerosis. Ann Intern Med 1991; 114:967–976.
539. Brunzell JD, Hazzard WR, Porte D Jr, Bierman EL. Evidence for a common, saturable, triglyceride removal mechanism for chylomicrons and very low density lipoproteins in man. J Clin Invest 1973; 52:1578–1585.
540. Hulley SB, Gordon S. Alcohol and high-density lipoprotein cholesterol: causal inference from diverse study designs. Circulation 1981; 64:III-57–III-63.
541. Gaziano JM, Buring JE, Breslow JL, et al. Moderate alcohol intake, increased levels of high-density lipoprotein and its subfractions, and decreased risk of myocardial infarction. N Engl J Med 1993; 329:1829–1834.
542. Suh I, Shaten BJ, Cutler JA, Kuller LH. Alcohol use and mortality from coronary heart disease: the role of high-density lipoprotein cholesterol. Ann Intern Med 1992; 116:881–887.
543. Criqui MH, Ringel BL. Does diet or alcohol explain the French paradox? Lancet 1994; 344:1719–1723.
544. Joven J, Villabona C, Vilella E, et al. Abnormalities of lipoprotein metabolism in patients with the nephrotic syndrome. N Engl J Med 1990; 323:579–584.
545. Wanner C, Rader D, Bartens W, et al. Elevated plasma lipoprotein(a) in patients with the nephrotic syndrome. Ann Intern Med 1993; 119:263–269.
546. Kekki M, Nikkilä EA. Plasma triglyceride metabolism in the adult nephrotic syndrome. Eur J Clin Invest 1971; 1:345–351.
547. Warwick GL, Caslake MJ, Boulton-Jones JM, et al. Low-density lipoprotein metabolism in the nephrotic syndrome. Metabolism 1990; 39:187–192.
548. Grundy SM. Management of hyperlipidemia of kidney disease. Kidney Int 1990; 37:847–853.
549. Carr A, Samaras K, Thorisdottir A, et al. Diagnosis, prediction, and natural course of HIV-1 protease-inhibitor–associated lipodystrophy, hyperlipidaemia, and diabetes mellitus: a cohort study. Lancet 1999; 353:2093–2099.

550. Mulligan K, Grunfeld C, Tai VW, et al. Hyperlipidemia and insulin resistance are induced by protease inhibitors independent of changes in body composition in patients with HIV infection. J Acquir Immune Defic Syndr 2000; 23:35–43.
551. Tsiodras S, Mantzoros C, Hammer S, Samore M. Effects of protease inhibitors on hyperglycemia, hyperlipidemia, and lipodystrophy: a 5-year cohort study. Arch Intern Med 2000; 160: 2050–2056.
552. Vigouroux C, Gharakhanian S, Salhi Y, et al. Adverse metabolic disorders during highly active antiretroviral treatments (HAART) of HIV disease. Diabetes Metab 1999; 25:383–392.
553. Lardinois CK, Neuman SL. The effects of antihypertensive agents on serum lipids and lipoproteins. Arch Intern Med 1988; 148:1280–1288.
554. Pollare T, Lithell H, Berne C. A comparison of the effects of hydrochlorothiazide and captopril on glucose and lipid metabolism in patients with hypertension. N Engl J Med 1989; 321: 868–873.
555. Rohlfing JJ, Brunzell JD. The effects of diuretics and adrenergic-blocking agents on plasma lipids. West J Med 1986; 145:210–218.
556. Haffner SM, Kushwaha RS, Foster DM, et al. Studies on the metabolic mechanism of reduced high density lipoproteins during anabolic steroid therapy. Metabolism 1983; 32:413–420.
557. Webb OL, Laskarzewski PM, Glueck CJ. Severe depression of high-density lipoprotein cholesterol levels in weight lifters and body builders by self-administered exogenous testosterone and anabolic-androgenic steroids. Metabolism 1984; 33:971–975.
558. Lipid Research Clinics Program. The Lipid Research Clinics Coronary Primary Prevention Trial results. II. The relationship of reduction in incidence of coronary heart disease to cholesterol lowering. JAMA 1984; 251:365–374.
559. Oliver MF. Doubts about preventing coronary heart disease: multiple interventions in middle aged men may do more harm than good. Br Med J 1992; 304:393–394.
560. Smith GD, Pekkanen J. Should there be a moratorium on the use of cholesterol lowering drugs? Br Med J 1992; 304:431–434.
561. Scandinavian Simvastatin Survival Study Group. Randomised trial of cholesterol lowering in 4444 patients with coronary heart disease: the Scandinavian Simvastatin Survival Study (4S). Lancet 1994; 344:1383–1389.
562. Shepherd J, Cobbe SM, Ford I, et al. Prevention of coronary heart disease with pravastatin in men with hypercholesterolemia. N Engl J Med 1995; 333:1301–1307.
563. Sacks FM, Pfeffer MA, Moye LA, et al. The effect of pravastatin on coronary events after myocardial infarction in patients with average cholesterol levels. N Engl J Med 1996; 335:1001–1009.
564. Rubins HB, Robins SJ, Collins D, et al. Gemfibrozil for the secondary prevention of coronary heart disease in men with low levels of high-density lipoprotein cholesterol. N Engl J Med 1999; 341:410–418.
565. Downs JR, Clearfield M, Weis S, et al. Primary prevention of acute coronary events with lovastatin in men and women with average cholesterol levels: results of AFCAPS/TexCAPS. JAMA 1998; 279:1615–1622.
566. Grundy SM, Benjamin IJ, Burke GL, et al. Diabetes and cardiovascular disease: a statement for healthcare professionals from the American Heart Association. Circulation 1999; 100:1134–1146.
567. Haffner SM, Lehto S, Rönnemaa T, et al. Mortality from coronary heart disease in subjects with type 2 diabetes and in nondiabetic subjects with and without prior myocardial infarction. N Engl J Med 1998; 339:229–234.
568. Pi-Sunyer FX, Becker DM, Bouchard C, et al. Clinical Guidelines on the Identification, Evaluation, and Treatment of Overweight and Obesity in Adults. The Evidence Report (NIH Publication No 98-4083). Bethesda, Md, US Department of Health and Human Services, Public Health Service, National Institutes of Health, 1998, pp 58–59.
569. Diekman T, Lansberg PJ, Kastelein JJP, Wiersinga WM. Prevalence and correction of hypothyroidism in a large cohort of patients referred for dyslipidemia. Arch Intern Med 1995; 155: 1490–1495.
570. Watson WC, Buchanan KD, Dickson C. Serum cholesterol levels after myocardial infarction. Br Med J 1963; 2:709–712.
571. Friedewald WT, Levy RI, Fredrickson DS. Estimation of the concentration of low-density lipoprotein cholesterol in plasma, without use of the preparative ultracentrifuge. Clin Chem 1972; 18:499–502.
572. Havel RJ, Rapaport E. Management of primary hyperlipidemia. N Engl J Med 1995; 332:1491–1498.
573. Castelli WP, Garrison RJ, Wilson PWF, et al. Incidence of coronary heart disease and lipoprotein cholesterol levels. The Framingham Study. JAMA 1986; 256:2835–2838.
574. Castelli WP, Abbott RD, McNamara PM. Summary estimates of cholesterol used to predict coronary heart disease. Circulation 1983; 67:730–734.
575. Arntzenius AC, Kromhout D, Barth JD, et al. Diet, lipoproteins, and the progression of coronary atherosclerosis. The Leiden Intervention Trial. N Engl J Med 1985; 312:805–811.
576. Chait A, Brunzell JD. Severe hypertriglyceridemia: role of familial and acquired disorders. Metabolism 1983; 32:209–214.
577. Stampfer MJ, Sacks FM, Salvini S, et al. A prospective study of cholesterol, apolipoproteins, and the risk of myocardial infarction. N Engl J Med 1991; 325:373–381.
578. Stamler J, Daviglus ML, Garside DB, et al. Relationship of baseline serum cholesterol levels in 3 large cohorts of younger men to long-term coronary, cardiovascular, and all-cause mortality and to longevity. JAMA 2000; 284:311–318.
579. Hulley SB, Newman TB, Grady D, et al. Should we be measuring blood cholesterol levels in young adults? JAMA 1993; 269: 1416–1419.
580. American College of Physicians. Guidelines for using serum cholesterol, high-density lipoprotein cholesterol, and triglyceride levels as screening tests for preventing coronary heart disease in adults. Ann Intern Med 1996; 124:515–517.
581. Salt WB II, Schenker S. Amylase—its clinical significance: a review of the literature. Medicine (Baltimore) 1976; 55:269–289.
582. Avins AL, Browner WS. Improving the prediction of coronary heart disease to aid in the management of high cholesterol levels. JAMA 1998; 279:445–449.
583. Wood D, De Backer G, Faergeman O, et al. Prevention of coronary heart disease in clinical practice: recommendations of the Second Joint Task Force of European and other Societies on Coronary Prevention. Summary of recommendations. Eur Heart J 1998; 19:1434–1503.
584. Carlson LA, Rosenhamer G. Reduction of mortality in the Stockholm Ischaemic Heart Disease Secondary Prevention Study by combined treatment with clofibrate and nicotinic acid. Acta Med Scand 1988; 223:405–418.
585. Canner PL, Berge KG, Wenger NK, et al. Fifteen year mortality in Coronary Drug Project patients: long-term benefit with niacin. J Am Coll Cardiol 1986; 8:1245–1255.
586. Trial of clofibrate in the treatment of ischaemic heart disease: five-year study by a group of physicians of the Newcastle upon Tyne region. Br Med J 1971; 4:767–775.
587. Leren P. The effect of plasma cholesterol lowering diet in male survivors of myocardial infarction: a controlled clinical trial. Acta Med Scand Suppl 1966; 466:1–92.
588. Rossouw JE, Lewis B, Rifkind BM. The value of lowering cholesterol after myocardial infarction. N Engl J Med 1990; 323: 1112–1119.
589. Blankenhorn DH, Nessim SA, Johnson RL, et al. Beneficial effects of combined colestipol-niacin therapy on coronary atherosclerosis and coronary venous bypass grafts. JAMA 1987; 257: 3233–3240.
590. Ornish D, Brown SE, Scherwitz LW, et al. Can lifestyle changes reverse coronary heart disease? The Lifestyle Heart Trial. Lancet 1990; 336:129–133.
591. Brown BG, Zhao X-Q, Sacco DE, Albers JJ. Lipid lowering and plaque regression: new insights into prevention of plaque disruption and clinical events in coronary disease. Circulation 1993; 87: 1781–1791.
592. Criqui MH. Cholesterol, primary and secondary prevention, and all-cause mortality. Ann Intern Med 1991; 115:973–976.
593. Muldoon MF, Manuck SB, Matthews KA. Lowering cholesterol concentrations and mortality: a quantitative review of primary prevention trials. Br Med J 1990; 301:309–314.
594. MacMahon S. Lowering cholesterol: effects on trauma death, cancer death and total mortality. Aust NZ J Med 1992; 22:580–582.
595. The Expert Panel. Summary of the second report of the National Cholesterol Education Program (NCEP) Expert Panel on Detec-

tion, Evaluation, and Treatment of High Blood Cholesterol in Adults (Adult Treatment Panel II). JAMA 1993; 269:3015–3023.
596. Connor WE, Connor SL. The dietary treatment of hyperlipidemia: rationale, technique and efficacy. Med Clin North Am 1982; 66:485–518.
597. Dietary guidelines for healthy American adults: a statement for physicians and health professionals by the Nutrition Committee, American Heart Association. Circulation 1988; 77:721A–724A.
598. Denke MA, Grundy SM. Individual responses to a cholesterol-lowering diet in 50 men with moderate hypercholesterolemia. Arch Intern Med 1994; 154:317–325.
599. Ginsberg HN, Barr SL, Gilbert A, et al. Reduction of plasma cholesterol levels in normal men on an American Heart Association Step 1 diet or a Step 1 diet with added monounsaturated fat. N Engl J Med 1990; 322:574–579.
600. Hunninghake DB, Stein EA, Dujovne CA, et al. The efficacy of intensive dietary therapy alone or combined with lovastatin in outpatients with hypercholesterolemia. N Engl J Med 1993; 328: 1213–1219.
601. Cobb MM, Teitelbaum HS, Breslow JL. Lovastatin efficacy in reducing low-density lipoprotein cholesterol levels on high- vs low-fat diets. JAMA 1991; 265:997–1001.
602. Willett WC. Diet and health: what should we eat? Science 1994; 264:532–537.
603. Spady DK, Dietschy JM. Dietary saturated triacylglycerols suppress hepatic low density lipoprotein receptor activity in the hamster. Proc Natl Acad Sci USA 1985; 82:4526–4530.
604. Packard CJ, McKinney L, Carr K, Shepherd J. Cholesterol feeding increases low density lipoprotein synthesis. J Clin Invest 1983; 72:45–51.
605. Mensink RP, Katan MB. Effect of a diet enriched with monounsaturated or polyunsaturated fatty acids on levels of low-density and high-density lipoprotein cholesterol in healthy women and men. N Engl J Med 1989; 321:436–441.
606. Mensink RP, Katan MB. Effect of dietary trans fatty acids on high-density and low-density lipoprotein cholesterol levels in healthy subjects. N Engl J Med 1990; 323:439–445.
607. Kromhout D, Bosschieter EB, de Lezenne Coulander C. The inverse relation between fish consumption and 20-year mortality from coronary heart disease. N Engl J Med 1985; 312:1205–1209.
608. Harris WS. Fish oils and plasma lipid and lipoprotein metabolism in humans: a critical review. J Lipid Res 1989; 30:785–807.
609. Sullivan DR, Sanders TAB, Trayner IM, Thompson GR. Paradoxical elevation of LDL apoprotein B levels in hypertriglyceridaemic patients and normal subjects ingesting fish oil. Atherosclerosis 1986; 61:129–134.
610. Leaf A, Weber PC. Cardiovascular effects of n-3 fatty acids. N Engl J Med 1988; 318:549–556.
611. Ascherio A, Rimm EB, Stampfer MJ, et al. Dietary intake of marine n-3 fatty acids, fish intake, and the risk of coronary disease among men. N Engl J Med 1995; 332:977–982.
612. Friday KE, Childs MT, Tsunehara CH, et al. Elevated plasma glucose and lowered triglyceride levels from omega-3 fatty acid supplementation in type II diabetes. Diabetes Care 1989; 12:276–281.
613. Grundy SM. Comparison of monounsaturated fatty acids and carbohydrates for lowering plasma cholesterol. N Engl J Med 1986; 314:745–748.
614. Connor WE. Dietary fiber: nostrum or critical nutrient? N Engl J Med 1990; 322:193–195.
615. Jenkins DJA, Wolever TMS, Rao AV, et al. Effect on blood lipids of very high intakes of fiber in diets low in saturated fat and cholesterol. N Engl J Med 1993; 329:21–26.
616. Sprecher DL, Harris BV, Goldberg AC, et al. Efficacy of psyllium in reducing serum cholesterol levels in hypercholesterolemic patients on high- or low-fat diets. Ann Intern Med 1993; 119: 545–554.
617. Miettinen TA, Puska P, Gylling H, et al. Reduction of serum cholesterol with sitostanol-ester margarine in a mildly hypercholesterolemic population. N Engl J Med 1995; 333:1308–1312.
618. Warshafsky S, Kamer RS, Sivak SL. Effect of garlic on total serum cholesterol: a meta-analysis. Ann Intern Med 1993; 119: 599–605.
619. Sabaté J, Fraser GE, Burke K, et al. Effects of walnuts on serum lipid levels and blood pressure in normal men. N Engl J Med 1993; 328:603–607.
620. Ginsberg HN. Update on the treatment of hypercholesterolemia, with a focus on HMG-CoA reductase inhibitors and combination regimens. Clin Cardiol 1995; 18:307–315.
621. Grundy SM. HMG-CoA reductase inhibitors for treatment of hypercholesterolemia. N Engl J Med 1988; 319:24–33.
622. Bradford RH, Shear CL, Chremos AN, et al. Expanded Clinical Evaluation of Lovastatin (EXCEL) Study results. I. Efficacy in modifying plasma lipoproteins and adverse event profile in 8245 patients with moderate hypercholesterolemia. Arch Intern Med 1991; 151:43–49.
623. Vega GL, Grundy SM. Treatment of primary moderate hypercholesterolemia with lovastatin (mevinolin) and colestipol. JAMA 1987; 257:33–38.
624. Stein EA, Lane M, Laskarzewski P. Comparison of statins in hypertriglyceridemia. Am J Cardiol 1998; 81:66B–69B.
625. Davignon J, Laaksonen R. Low-density lipoprotein–independent effects of statins. Curr Opin Lipidol 1999; 10:543–559.
626. Marais GE, Larson KK. Rhabdomyolysis and acute renal failure induced by combination lovastatin and gemfibrozil therapy. Ann Intern Med 1990; 112:228–230.
627. Reaven P, Witztum JL. Lovastatin, nicotinic acid, and rhabdomyolysis. Ann Intern Med 1988; 109:597–598.
628. East C, Alivizatos PA, Grundy SM, et al. Rhabdomyolysis in patients receiving lovastatin after cardiac transplantation. N Engl J Med 1988; 318:47–48.
629. Christians U, Jacobsen W, Floren LC. Metabolism and drug interactions of 3-hydroxy-3-methylglutaryl coenzyme A reductase inhibitors in transplant patients: are the statins mechanistically similar? Pharmacol Ther 1998; 80:1–34.
630. Fichtenbaum C, Gerber J, Rosenkranz S, et al. Pharmacokinetic interactions between protease inhibitors and selected HMG-CoA reductase inhibitors (abstract). Seventh Conference on Retroviruses and Opportunistic Infections, San Francisco, 2000, p 236.
631. Ast M, Frishman WH. Bile acid sequestrants. J Clin Pharmacol 1990; 30:99–106.
632. Shepherd J, Packard CJ, Bicker S, et al. Cholestyramine promotes receptor-mediated low-density-lipoprotein catabolism. N Engl J Med 1980; 302:1219–1222.
633. Beil U, Crouse JR, Einarsson K, Grundy SM. Effects of interruption of the enterohepatic circulation of bile acids on the transport of very low density-lipoprotein triglycerides. Metabolism 1982; 31:438–444.
634. Packard CJ, Stewart JM, Third JLHC, et al. Effects of nicotinic acid therapy on high-density lipoprotein metabolism in type II and type IV hyperlipoproteinaemia. Biochim Biophys Acta 1980; 618:53–62.
635. Gurakar A, Hoeg JM, Kostner G, et al. Levels of lipoprotein Lp(a) decline with neomycin and niacin treatment. Atherosclerosis 1985; 57:293–301.
636. McKenney JM, Proctor JD, Harris S, Chinchili VM. A comparison of the efficacy and toxic effects of sustained- vs immediate-release niacin in hypercholesterolemic patients. JAMA 1994; 271: 672–677.
637. Elam MB, Hunninghake DB, Davis KB, et al. Effect of niacin on lipid and lipoprotein levels and glycemic control in patients with diabetes and peripheral arterial disease. The ADMIT study: a randomized trial. JAMA 2000; 284:1263–1270.
638. Kersten S, Desvergne B, Wahli W. Roles of PPARs in health and disease. Nature 2000; 405:421–424.
639. Kissebah AH, Adams PW, Harrigan P, Wynn V. The mechanism of action of clofibrate and tetranicotinoylfructose (bradilan) on the kinetics of plasma free fatty acid and triglyceride transport in type IV and type V hypertriglyceridaemia. Eur J Clin Invest 1974; 4:163–174.
640. Pierides AM, Alvarez-Ude F, Kerr DNS, Skillen AW. Clofibrate-induced muscle damage in patients with chronic renal failure. Lancet 1975; 2:1279–1282.
641. Committee of Principal Investigators. A co-operative trial in the primary prevention of ischaemic heart disease using clofibrate: report from the Committee of Principal Investigators. Br Heart J 1978; 40:1069–1118.
642. Heady JA, Morris JN, Oliver MF. WHO clofibrate/cholesterol trial: clarifications. Lancet 1992; 340:1405–1406.
643. Olsson AG, Pears JS, McKellar J, et al. Pharmacodynamics of new HMG-CoA reductase inhibitor ZD4522 in patients with primary hypercholesterolaemia (abstract). Atherosclerosis 2000; 151:39.

644. Wetterau JR, Gregg RE, Harrity TW, et al. An MTP inhibitor that normalizes atherogenic lipoprotein levels in WHHL rabbits. Science 1998; 282:751–754.
645. van Heek M, Farley C, Compton DS, et al. Comparison of the activity and disposition of the novel cholesterol absorption inhibitor, SCH58235, and its glucuronide, SCH60663. Br J Pharmacol 2000; 129:1748–1754.
646. Okamoto H, Yonemori F, Wakitani K, et al. A cholesteryl ester transfer protein inhibitor attenuates atherosclerosis in rabbits. Nature 2000; 406:203–207.
647. Walldius G, Erikson U, Olsson AG, et al. The effect of probucol on femoral atherosclerosis: the Probucol Quantitative Regression Swedish Trial (PQRST). Am J Cardiol 1994; 74:875–883.
648. Jha P, Flather M, Lonn E, et al. The antioxidant vitamins and cardiovascular disease: a critical review of epidemiologic and clinical trial data. Ann Intern Med 1995; 123:860–872.
649. Hennekens CH, Buring JE, Manson JE, et al. Lack of effect of long-term supplementation with beta carotene on the incidence of malignant neoplasms and cardiovascular disease. N Engl J Med 1996; 334:1145–1149.
650. Stephens NG, Parsons A, Schofield PM, et al. Randomised controlled trial of vitamin E in patients with coronary disease: Cambridge Heart Antioxidant Study (CHAOS). Lancet 1996; 347:781–786.
651. Mosca L. The role of hormone replacement therapy in the prevention of postmenopausal heart disease. Arch Intern Med 2000; 160:2263–2272.
652. Williams PT. High-density lipoprotein cholesterol and other risk factors for coronary heart disease in female runners. N Engl J Med 1996; 334:1298–1303.
653. Sanderson SL, Iverius P-H, Wilson DE. Successful hyperlipemic pregnancy. JAMA 1991; 265:1858–1860.

sues do so only because of their effects on cell proliferation and accumulation. Such genes need not influence hormonal function. Furthermore, a mutant gene that alters hormonal function but confers no selective growth advantage is not tumorigenic. Nevertheless, the frequent coexistence of growth deregulation and hormonal hyperfunction in endocrine tumors does indicate that the tumor-causing genes may directly or indirectly alter hormone control pathways.

In certain instances, such as a mutation affecting the α subunit of stimulatory G protein ($G_{\alpha s}$) in growth hormone–producing and thyroid adenomas, a single mutant gene can directly contribute to both cell proliferation and hormonal hyperfunction. In general, however, the relationship between hypercellularity caused by clonally selected mutant genes and hormonal hyperfunction is poorly understood.

Hyperplasia versus Neoplasia

Not all hypercellular expansions are monoclonal. For instance, the generalized proliferative response of all cells of a tissue to an extrinsic stimulus yields a polyclonal expansion, examples of which include the hyperthyroidism of Graves' disease and the early, reversible secondary hyperparathyroidism in states of chronic hypocalcemia. Such polyclonal expansions represent biologic hyperplasia, whereas any monoclonal growth (benign or malignant) is a true neoplasm. Analyses of tumor clonality have been used to distinguish between these types of tumorigenic mechanisms. Nevertheless, the genesis of some tumors may involve both types of processes. For example, a generalized stimulus to polyclonal hyperplasia can, by increasing the chances of mitosis-related DNA damage in one cell, foster the emergence of a monoclonal population capable of eventually overwhelming or replacing its hyperplastic neighbors.

The clinical and histopathologic use of the term *hyperplasia* does not necessarily correspond to the biologic meaning described earlier, a situation that has engendered much confusion. For example, the usual tumors responsible for primary hyperparathyroidism have been clinicopathologically classified as adenomas when a single gland is abnormal and as hyperplasia when the individual patient has multiple hypercellular glands. No histopathologic criteria can reliably predict whether a single or multiple glands are involved on the basis of analysis of only one such gland. Not only are clinical adenomas monoclonal neoplasms,[1] but many parathyroid glands from patients with multigland "hyperplasia" are also monoclonal.[2] It is therefore important to ensure that the terms used in the description of endocrine tumorigenesis are clearly defined.

Insights into Tumor Pathogenesis

The clonal status of a cellular proliferation is of fundamental importance in deciphering its pathogenesis; thus, endocrine tumors have been studied to determine whether the expansion is monoclonal or polyclonal. One way of determining that a tumor is monoclonal is to identify a DNA or chromosomal lesion that, because of its tumor specificity and presence in all or most of the neoplastic cells, directly defines the expansion as monoclonal. Examples of cytogenetically defined clonal abnormalities are chromosome translocations such as the t(9;22) Philadelphia chromosome in chronic myelogenous leukemia and the t(14;18) translocation in follicular lymphoma.

The use of classical cytogenetics is technically more difficult in solid tumors than in hematopoietic tumors because hematopoietic cells divide in culture much more readily and yield excellent metaphase chromosomal spreads. Specimens of endocrine tumors are difficult to obtain for culture and to analyze cytogenetically. Fortunately, improved methods for the cytogenetic and molecular cytogenetic study of tumors, including fluorescence in situ hybridization, comparative genomic hybridization, and chromosome painting, promise to open up new avenues for the detection of clonal chromosomal lesions in endocrine tumors.[3–5]

Examples of monoclonal abnormalities defined by molecular methods in endocrine neoplasia include (1) $G_{\alpha s}$ gene mutations in growth hormone–producing pituitary tumors,[6] (2) thyrotropin (TSH) receptor gene mutations in thyroid tumors,[7] and (3) cyclin D1 or *PRAD1* gene rearrangements in parathyroid adenomas.[8] Identification of tumor-specific changes, such as deletions of DNA markers in particular regions of the tumor genome, also serves as evidence of monoclonality, even though the specific genes affected by such deletions may not be known.[9–14]

Indirect methods can determine the clonal status of tumors without the necessity of identifying the specific genes or chromosomal regions that are clonally mutated and involved in tumorigenesis. These methods have generally exploited the phenomenon of random X chromosome inactivation (the *Lyon phenomenon*) in women.[15] Random X chromosome inactivation occurs early in female embryonic development in all somatic cells. In any cell, the choice of which X chromosome is inactivated is random; once that choice is made, however, the decision is faithfully transmitted to all progeny of that cell (Fig. 35–1*A*). Usually, therefore, the maternally derived X chromosome is inactive in about 50% of the cells in a normal tissue, and the paternally derived X chromosome is inactive in about 50%.

Polyclonal growth, representing a generalized expansion of many or all original cells within a tissue, maintains the relatively even mix of active maternal and paternal X chromosomes characteristic of the normal tissues. In contrast, the neoplastic cells within a monoclonal tumor are derived from a single progenitor and all should reflect an identical X chromosome pattern, with either the maternal or the paternal X chromosome uniformly inactivated (see Fig. 35–1*A*).

A unifying feature of methods based on the analysis of X chromosome inactivation to determine the clonal status of a tumor is the use of a normally occurring variant, or *polymorphism*, at the genetic or protein level to distinguish between a woman's two X chromosomes. The other step involves assaying some property that reflects the state of X chromosome inactivation imposed on the tumor cell chromosomes at the polymorphic site. Assays to reflect X chromosome inactivation status include assessment of gene expression (RNA or protein levels) or regional DNA methylation.

A polymorphism in glucose-6-phosphate dehydrogenase (G6PD) was the first to be used in X chromosome inactivational analyses of tumor clonality.[16] A disadvantage of the G6PD system is that only a small minority of women are heterozygous for electrophoretically distinguishable isoforms of this X chromosome–encoded enzyme. Thus, most tumors have been unsuitable for clonal analysis. Furthermore, the method fails to detect the monoclonality of certain tumors,[1, 17, 18] perhaps because of differences in the level of G6PD expression in tumor cells compared with "contaminating" admixed normal cells within the analyzed samples.

DNA polymorphisms are now preferred for clonal analyses to distinguish between the two X chromosomes. High rates of heterozygosity make it possible to analyze most tumors. Some multiallelic polymorphisms, based on differences in the number of highly repeated sequence units in a genomic location, are heterozygous in more than 90% of women, and a large number of DNA polymorphisms have been described on the X chromosome (and on all chromosomes). Most, however, cannot be used in clonality studies because they have not been characterized for detectable changes that correlate with the

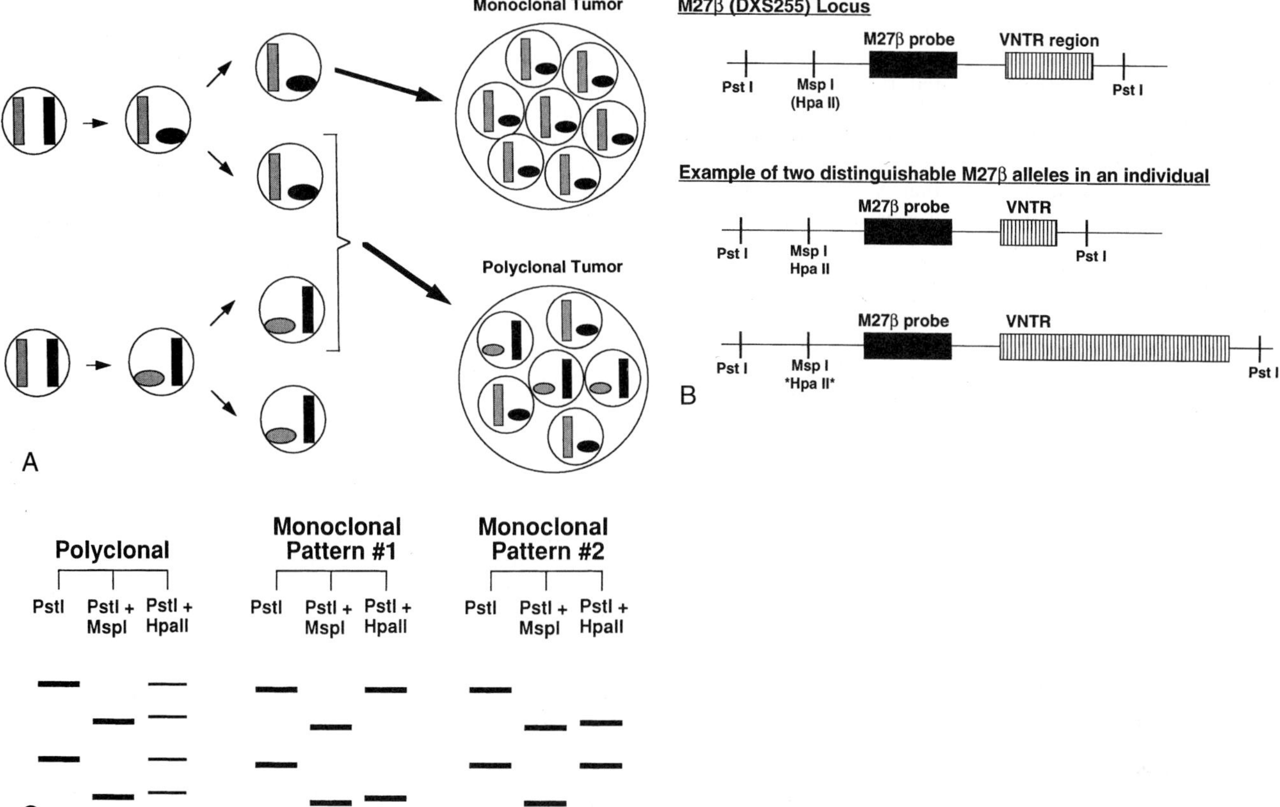

Figure 35–1. X chromosome inactivation analysis of tumor clonality with the use of the M27β polymorphism.

A, Diagrammatic illustration of general principles. *Left*, Lightly shaded and dark rectangles represent the maternally and paternally inherited copies of the two X chromosomes of somatic cells early in the development of a female embryo. As embryogenesis proceeds, one of the X chromosomes in each somatic cell is randomly chosen for inactivation (lyonization); the inactivated chromosome is represented as a small oval with shading corresponding to its origin. Subsequently, daughter cells *(third column)* faithfully maintain the same selection of inactivated X chromosome as found in their parent cells. Accordingly, an adult tissue typically contains a mixture of approximately 50% cells with the maternally inherited X chromosome inactive and 50% with the paternally inherited X chromosome inactive. *Lower right*, A polyclonal tumor arising from a large number of cells in a tissue, maintains this relatively even mixture of cells with different X inactivation patterns. *Upper right*, A monoclonal tumor, derived from a single somatic cell, has a uniform pattern of X chromosome inactivation in all cells.

B, Partial restriction endonuclease map of the M27β locus (DXS255) and an example of two distinguishable M27β alleles.The variable number of tandem repeat (VNTR, minisatellite) region, which is highly variable in its length from person to person, is shown in stripes. A 2.5-kb DNA fragment used as the hybridization probe is shown as a solid rectangle. Cleavage sites for restriction enzyme *Pst*I flank the locus. The enzyme *Msp*I cleaves the sequence CCGG whether or not the internal cytosine is methylated. In contrast, the enzyme *Hpa*II cleaves this sequence only if the internal cytosine is unmethylated. The diagrammed *Msp*I-*Hpa*II site actually represents a 270-base-pair region containing three such sites, two of which vary in their methylation status in accord with location on the active versus the inactive X chromosome.[20] In the example of two distinguishable alleles, variation in size of the minisatellite repeat region (VNTR) causes a difference in the size of the *Pst*I restriction fragment detectable by hybridization to the labeled M27β probe. If an individual with these two alleles had a monoclonal tumor, in which the larger allele was uniformly associated with the active X chromosome, the *Msp*I-*Hpa*II site of this allele would be consistently methylated and, therefore, resistant to cleavage by *Hpa*II *(asterisks)*. The resulting Southern blot pattern would correspond to monoclonal pattern 1 in *C*.

C, Schematic diagram of prototypical Southern blot hybridization patterns for X inactivation analysis using M27β. A monoclonal tumor can exhibit only one of the two monoclonal patterns shown. The *Pst*I + *Msp*I control digestion is useful for marking the sizes of fully cleaved alleles.

(*A* to *C*, From Arnold A, Brown MF, Urena P, et al. Monoclonality of parathyroid tumors in chronic renal failure and in primary parathyroid hyperplasia. J Clin Invest 1995; 95:2047–2053. Copyright, The American Society for Clinical Investigation.)

state of activity of the X chromosome on which an allele resides. Some of the X-linked polymorphisms that have been valuable in clonal analyses of human tumors include restriction fragment length polymorphisms in the *HPRT* and *PGK* gene regions,[19] a minisatellite repeat (>10 nucleotide core repeated unit) region called M27β or DXS255,[2, 20] and a microsatellite repeat (<10 nucleotide core repeated unit) locus within the androgen receptor gene.[21, 22]

Changes in DNA methylation in the vicinity of certain polymorphic sites on the X chromosome correlate with the activity of that X chromosome and are useful in clonal analyses. Methylation of specific cytosine nucleotides is an epigenetic process functioning adrenocortical nodules, growth hormone–secreting pituitary tumors, and male precocious puberty caused by hormonally active testicular tumors.[45]

Cyclin D1 (*PRAD1*) in Hyperparathyroidism and General Oncology

Another illustrative example is that of the cyclin D1, or *PRAD1*, oncogene. Unlike many endocrine tumor–associated oncogenes, cyclin D1 is also commonly involved in nonendocrine tumors. Interestingly, this gene, now appreciated to be of central importance to molecular oncology and to normal cellular physiology, was discovered in the molecular dissection of an endocrine tumor.

Many human oncogenes were discovered because they are adjacent to nonrandom chromosome breakpoints in tumors. Chromosome breaks and rearrangements probably occur often in normal cells but are recognized only when they result in deregulation of the expression of a growth-related gene and confer a selective advantage on the cell. Cyclin D1 or *PRAD1* was identified as the putative oncogene adjacent to one such breakpoint on chromosome 11 in a subset of parathyroid adenomas (Fig. 35–2).[8, 46–48] On the 11q13 side of the inversion breakpoint, the promoter and coding exons of the cyclin D1 gene remain in contiguity with each other. Across the breakpoint are regulatory sequences from the upstream region of the parathyroid hormone *(PTH)* gene on 11p15 that normally function to enhance *PTH* gene transcription in the presence of parathyroid tissue–specific signals (likely to be DNA binding proteins found in the nucleus). Such transcriptional enhancer sequences can act over distances of many kilobases to enhance transcription, and cyclin D1 transcription is increased in these tumors.[49] Although the variability in potential breakpoint sites makes it difficult to determine the true incidence of such rearrangements, cyclin D1 protein levels are elevated in 20% to 40% of parathyroid adenomas.[50–52]

In a broader context, the tissue-specific enhancer-driven expression of cyclin D1 in parathyroid tumors is analogous to the activation of oncogenes such as *BCL2* or *MYC* in B-cell lymphomas.[48] In these tumors, chromosomal rearrangements lead to a juxtaposition of immunoglobulin gene enhancer elements and the oncogene, which is thereby inappropriately activated.

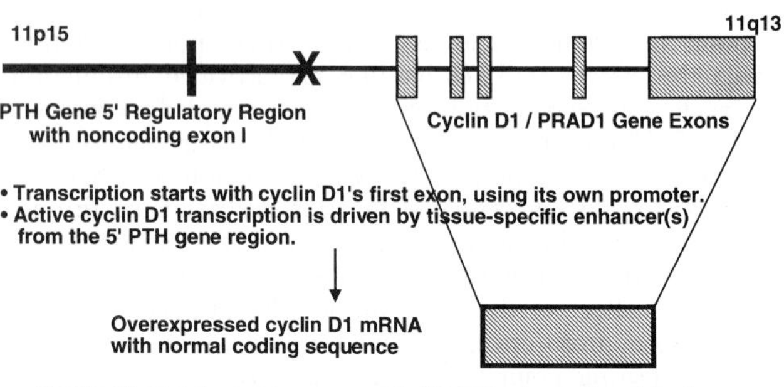

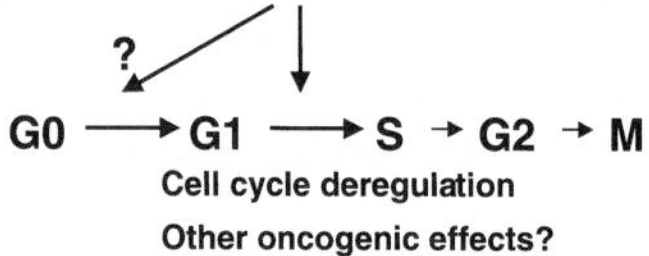

Figure 35–2. Diagram of the molecular structure of the parathyroid hormone–cyclin D1 DNA rearrangement in a subset of parathyroid adenomas and its functional consequences. The dark X represents the chromosome breakpoint between the *PTH* gene regulatory region, plus *PTH* noncoding exon 1 *(solid light vertical bar)* and part of its first intron, from 11p15 *(left)*, and the intact promoter and five exons of the cyclin D1 gene from 11q13. Cyclin D1 gene transcription proceeds in a left-to-right direction, as drawn. (Modified from Arnold A. Genetic basis of endocrine disease: 5. Molecular genetics of parathyroid gland neoplasia. J Clin Endocrinol Metab 1993; 77:1108–1112. Copyright 1993, The Endocrine Society.)

The PRAD1 gene product was initially recognized as a cyclin by virtue of its structural relationship to the cyclin family of proteins, known to be involved in controlling the cell cycle. However, before discovery of *PRAD1* (cyclin D1), no mammalian cyclins were known to participate in the control of the critical transition from G_1 to S phase; this checkpoint would be an appropriate site for attack by an oncogenic protein because movement into S phase commits a cell to the remainder of the cycle and another mitosis.[53–55] It is now widely accepted that cyclin D1 is a G_1 cyclin that functions to push the cell toward or through this key juncture.[54]

One cautionary note: This functional assignment for cyclin D1 is overwhelmingly derived from cultured cell systems, which might not fully reflect the true in vivo roles of this key oncoprotein. Thus, the detailed mechanism of action of cyclin D1, both normally and when dysregulated in tumorigenesis, should be further explored.

Cyclins are regulatory subunits of holoenzymes whose catalytic subunits are cyclin-dependent kinases (CDKs). The major kinase partner for cyclin D1 appears to be CDK4 or, in some cell types, CDK6. The protein product of the retinoblastoma tumor suppressor gene, pRB, has been recognized as one substrate for phosphorylation by cyclin D–cdk complexes. Whether all such relevant phosphorylations occur in G_1 phase progression or might in part push quiescent G_0 cells into an active G_1 cycling mode, for example, requires further study.

Natural inhibitors of CDK function also exist, and $p16^{INK4a}$ is recognized as a key inhibitor of cyclin D–CDK4/6 complexes. Thus, inactivation of p16 might be expected to be as oncogenic as cyclin D1 overexpression, and p16 is, indeed, a tumor suppressor gene in familial melanoma and several types of sporadic human tumors.[55] Interestingly, inactivating mutations of p16 are uncommon, if they occur at all, in parathyroid adenomas.[56] Hence, the cellular consequences of p16 loss and cyclin D1 activation may not precisely overlap. Interestingly, some early evidence exists for possible non–cdk-dependent actions of cyclin D1.[57]

The significance of cyclin D1 in human neoplasia extends far beyond its involvement in endocrine tumors. It is the long-sought *BCL1* oncogene that is deregulated by the characteristic t(11;14) translocation in mantle cell or centrocytic B-cell lymphomas.[48] Thus, assessment of cyclin D1 gene rearrangement or expression is clinically useful in the molecular diagnosis of B-cell neoplasia. In addition, cyclin D1 is a key oncogene in breast cancer, squamous cell cancer of the head and neck, esophageal cancer, and a variety of other tumors.[48] Cyclin D1 and other members of its oncogenic pathway or pathways may serve as targets for development of antineoplastic therapies.

RET Gene Rearrangements in Papillary Thyroid Cancer

Activating mutations of the *RET* proto-oncogene are responsible for multiple endocrine neoplasia type 2 (see Chapter 36), but this gene is also involved in human disease through another mechanism: Clonal somatic rearrangements of this gene are found in about 25% of papillary thyroid cancers but not in other types of thyroid (or nonthyroidal) cancer.[58–60]

RET encodes a member of the receptor tyrosine kinase superfamily, and one endogenous ligand that binds to and activates RET is the glial cell line–derived neurotrophic factor (GDNF).[61, 62] Normally, *RET* acts mainly during embryogene-

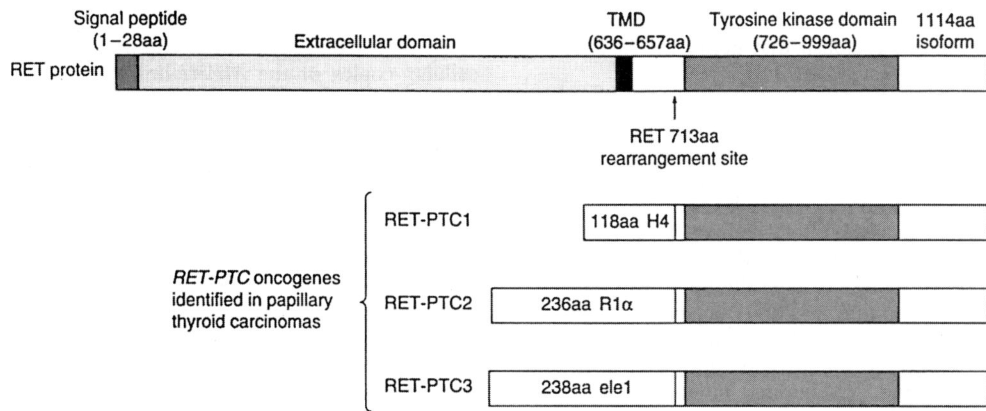

Figure 35–3. Schematic representation of the normal RET protein *(upper)* and the oncoproteins created by selected *RET-PTC* oncogenes in papillary thyroid cancer *(lower)*. For each indicated rearranged oncoprotein, the number of N-terminal amino acids contributed by the specified partner gene is shown, fused to the tyrosine kinase domain and C-terminus of *RET*. aa, amino acid; TMD, transmembrane domain. (From Pasini B, Ceccherini I, Romeo G. RET mutations in human disease. Trends Genet 1996; 12:138–144. Copyright 1996, Elsevier Science.)

sis, with expression in cells derived from the neural crest and in the developing central and peripheral nervous systems and kidney.[60, 63] Inactivating germ line mutations of *RET* are a cause of Hirschsprung's disease, in which parasympathetic ganglia fail to migrate properly in the gastrointestinal tract (see Chapter 36).

Receptor tyrosine kinases such as RET dimerize as a consequence of ligand binding. Dimerization then leads to autophosphorylation of the receptor, and the phosphorylated receptor can bind or phosphorylate, or both, other molecules in a signaling cascade.[64] The RET protein, like other receptor tyrosine kinases, has extracellular, transmembrane, and intracellular (tyrosine kinase) domains (Fig. 35–3). The papillary cancer–specific *RET* rearrangements described to date involve a chromosomal break that fuses the intracellular tyrosine kinase domain–encoding portion of the *RET* gene to one of several alternative partners.[60] The *RET* fusion partner gene segment provides a new promoter that is constitutively active in thyroid cells and encodes a new in-frame N-terminus for the oncoprotein (see Fig. 35–3).

Three major classes of *RET* fusion oncogenes are called *RET-PTC1*, *RET-PTC2*, and *RET-PTC3;* the corresponding fusion partner genes are *H4*, *R1α*, and *ELE1*.[60] The N-termini of these fusion oncoproteins allow dimerization and activation of the RET tyrosine kinase, bypassing the usual requirement for ligand binding.

The specificity of these *RET* fusion oncogenes for papillary-type thyroid cancer is not well understood. It appears that only this thyroid cell type tends to produce such fusions or that only this cell has the molecular machinery that can respond to this form of RET kinase activation. Perhaps development of a papillary cancer may be an inevitable response to the occurrence of the *RET* rearrangement early in the life of a thyroidal neoplasm.

Finally, the *RET* proto-oncogene and its fusion partners, especially *ELE1*, may be highly susceptible to breakage and fusion as a consequence of ionizing radiation. More than 60% of papillary cancers that have developed in young people exposed to the nuclear fallout from the Chernobyl reactor contain *RET-PTC* fusion oncogenes.[65, 66] The spatial contiguity of RET and its rearrangement partners in the interphase thyroid cell nucleus may provide a structural basis for the occurrence of such rearrangements by enabling a single radiation particle track to cause a double-stranded DNA break that is misrepaired.[66]

GERM LINE MUTATIONS PREDISPOSING TO ENDOCRINE NEOPLASIA: EXAMPLES

Patients in whom a particular tumor develops on the basis of a strong inherited predisposition typically constitute only a minority of patients with that tumor. Nonetheless, the lessons learned from identifying the molecular basis of inherited tumor predisposition are important, both clinically and from a fundamental biologic perspective. In addition, some genes in which germ line mutations cause rare genetic syndromes have subsequently been found to be somatically mutated in the more common, sporadic occurrences of the same tumors.

Germ line mutations that predispose to neoplasia can occur in either proto-oncogenes or tumor suppressor genes; in other words, mutations that cause inherited tumor syndromes can be of either the gain-of-function or the loss-of-function type. However, most germ line mutations identified to date are inactivating mutations, thus identifying the affected genes as tumor suppressors by definition. A few genes responsible for heritable endocrine neoplasia syndromes have been discovered, and others are still being sought.

RET Mutations in Multiple Endocrine Neoplasia Type 2

Multiple endocrine neoplasia type 2 (MEN 2) is a collection of three syndromes:

- MEN 2A
- Familial medullary thyroid cancer
- MEN 2B

These syndromes are detailed in Chapter 36.

All are autosomal dominant syndromes in which the most consistent feature is predisposition to medullary thyroid cancer. Genetic linkage analysis demonstrated that the *MEN 2* gene or genes must lie near the centromere on chromosome 10, and an evaluation of candidate genes known to map to this region led to the identification of germ line *RET* point mutations that co-segregated with the disease.[67] The existence of de novo *RET* mutations in patients with an MEN 2 phenotype, but a negative family history and the demonstration that the

Table 36–1. Features of Multiple Endocrine Neoplasia Type 1 with Estimated Average Penetrance (in parentheses) among Adults

Endocrine Features	Nonendocrine Features
Parathyroid adenoma (95%)	Facial angiofibroma (85%)
Enteropancreatic	Collagenoma (70%)
Gastrinoma (40%)*	Lipoma (30%)
Insulinoma (10%)	Leiomyoma (5%)
Nonfunctioning,† including *pancreatic polypeptide-oma*‡ (20%)	Ependymoma (<1%)
Other: *glucagonoma*, *VIPoma*, *somatostatinoma*, etc. (each <2%)	
Foregut carcinoid	
Thymic carcinoid nonfunctioning (2%)	
Bronchial carcinoid nonfunctioning (4%)	
Gastric enterochromaffin-like tumor nonfunctioning (10%)	
Anterior pituitary	
Prolactinoma (25%)	
Other: nonfunctioning (10%), growth hormone + prolactin, growth hormone (both 5%), ACTH (2%), thyrotropin (rare)	
Adrenal	
Cortex	
Nonfunctioning (30%)	
Functioning or cancer (2%)	
Medulla: pheochromocytoma (<1%)	

*Italics indicate tumor type with substantial (>20% of cases) malignant potential.
†Many "nonfunctioning" MEN1 tumors synthesize a peptide hormone or other factors (such as small amine) but do not oversecrete enough to produce a hormonal expression.
‡Omits nearly 100% prevalence of nonfunctioning and clinically silent tumors, some of which are detected incidental to enteropancreatic surgery in MEN1.
ACTH, adrenocorticotropic hormone; VIP, vasoactive intestinal peptide.

Hyperparathyroidism in Multiple Endocrine Neoplasia Type 1

MEN1 is uncommon with a population prevalence of about 1 in 30,000 and accounts for only about 1% to 3% of cases of primary hyperparathyroidism.[18] Hyperparathyroidism is the most common hormonal manifestation of MEN1 (Table 36–1).[6, 12, 14, 18–22] Prospective tumor surveillance in members of MEN1 families has shown hyperparathyroidism as early as age 8 years[12, 14, 23–27]; by age 40 years, about 95% of MEN1 carriers have been hypercalcemic.[12, 20, 19]

Expressions of Hyperparathyroidism

Hyperparathyroidism in MEN1 is most frequently asymptomatic; expressions include hypercalcemia, urolithiasis, parathyroid hormone (PTH)–induced bone abnormalities, musculoskeletal complaints, weakness, and alterations of mental status. These features are similar to those associated with other forms of hyperparathyroidism (see Chapter 26).

Hyperparathyroidism in MEN1 differs in some ways from that caused by a sporadic adenoma. The first way is a difference in epidemiology. Hyperparathyroidism in MEN1 has an earlier age of onset (typically 25 years versus 55 years)[20, 21] (Fig. 36–1) and lack of gender imbalance (1:1 versus 3:1 female/male ratio). Earlier onset implies that it can last longer. In particular, bone undermineralization among women with MEN1–related hyperparathyroidism seems increased by their 20s and 30s.[28] Second is a different parathyroid pathology; enlargement, albeit highly asymmetric, of multiple parathyroid glands* is usually present at the time of parathyroid exploration in MEN1 (Fig. 36–2).[29, 30] Third, the distributions of outcomes of parathyroid surgery differ. The presence of multiglandular disease and the need to examine each gland during a surgical procedure inevitably result in a higher postoperative rate of hypoparathyroidism and a lower rate of euparathyroidism.[29, 31] Successful subtotal parathyroidectomy is also followed within 10 years by recurrent hyperparathyroidism in half of MEN1 cases.[29, 31] In fact, true recurrent hyperparathyroidism in sporadic hyperparathyroidism is unusual, and recurrence should suggest the possibility of MEN1. True recurrent hyperparathyroidism, as with other tumor recurrences in MEN1, could arise theoretically from a small remnant of tumor tissue or from new mutation (second hit) in residual normal tissue. Fourth, hyperparathyroidism in MEN1 almost never progresses to parathyroid cancer, despite the fact that hyperparathyroidism occurs earlier in MEN1 than in sporadic cases.[32]E

There are several characteristics of hyperfunctioning parathyroid cells in MEN1 that may have mechanistic implications. First, most or all parathyroid glands have been overgrown by one or a few neoplastic clones by the time of surgery in MEN1 (Fig. 36–3, *top*).[33] Second, a circulating growth factor is specific to the plasma of MEN1 cases and mitogenic toward normal parathyroid cells in vitro (see later).[34] Third, a phenomenon observed in sporadic parathyroid adenomas, a rightward shift in the set-point for calcium suppression of PTH secretion, occurs to a lesser extent in MEN1 parathyroid tumors[35] (see Chapter 26). This set-point abnormality may be caused by secondary decrease in the amount of the calcium-sensing receptor on the parathyroid cell surface.[36]

**Parathyroid hyperplasia* is a term that has long-standing histologic usage. It is sometimes applied in a mechanistic meaning to all states with multiple parathyroid tumors. Because the multiple parathyroid tumors, particularly in MEN1, are all or mostly monoclonal or oligoclonal,[33] terminology and histologic features of hyperplasia cause confusion about etiology. MEN1 hyperparathyroidism is best considered mechanistically as multigland hyperparathyroidism or multiple adenomas, not hyperplasia.

Hyperparathyroidism Management

Decision for Surgery

Surgery is the treatment of choice for hyperparathyroidism in MEN1, although the timing and the type of operation remain controversial. Parathyroid surgery is definitely indicated in a MEN1 patient with an elevated PTH and other moderately advanced features, such as an albumin-adjusted serum calcium level higher than 3.0 mmol/L (12.0 mg/dL), kidney stones, or PTH-induced bone disease.

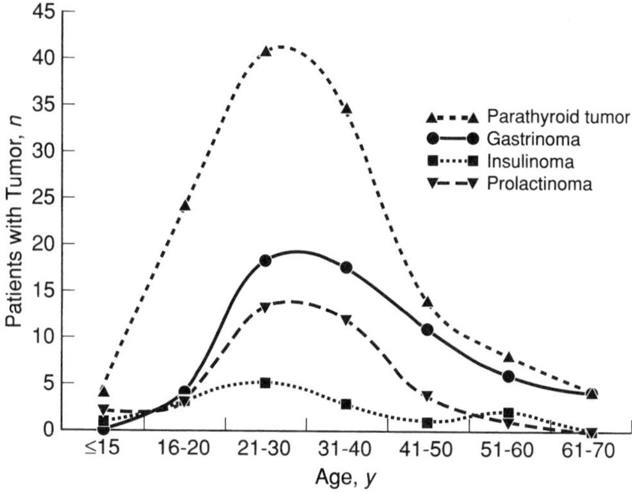

Figure 36–1. Age at onset for endocrine tumor expressions in multiple endocrine neoplasia type 1 (MEN1). Data from retrospective analysis of multiple tumor expressions in 130 inpatients with MEN1 during 15 years. Age of tumor onset was defined as the earlier of age at first symptom and age at first abnormal test result. (Modified from Marx S, Spiegel AM, Skarulis MC, et al. Multiple endocrine neoplasia type 1: clinical and genetic topics. Ann Intern Med 1998; 129:484–494.)

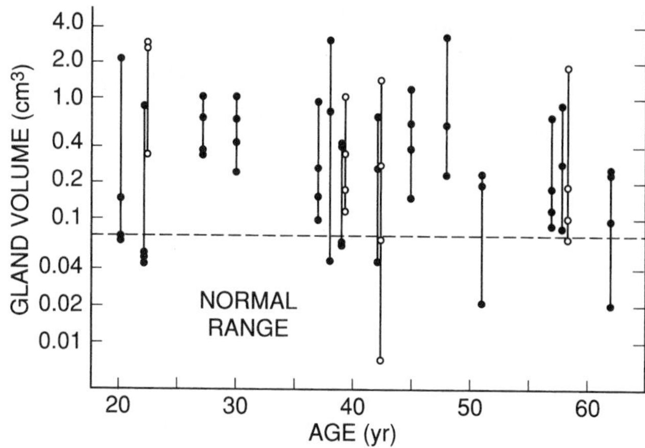

Figure 36–2. Parathyroid gland sizes at initial parathyroidectomy for 18 cases with familial multiple endocrine neoplasia type 1. Volumes of all glands at one operation are connected by a *vertical line. Dashed horizontal line* is upper limit of normal gland volume) 0.075 cm^3, equivalent to 75 mg mass). (Modified from Marx SJ, Menczel J, Campbell G, et al. Heterogeneous size of the parathyroid glands in familial multiple endocrine neoplasia type 1. Clin Endocrinol (Oxf) 1991; 35: 521–526.)

Prospective surveillance for hyperparathyroidism in MEN1 families has led to systematic identification of members with minimal elevations of serum calcium and PTH concentration. The optimal management of such patients is not clear. We favor a strategy of delaying parathyroid surgery for more advanced indications because parathyroidectomy has a lower likelihood of benefit in MEN1 than in adenoma (see later).[29] Delayed treatment is coupled with periodic assessment of serum indices, bone density, and urine calcium.

Early parathyroid surgery in MEN1 has been advocated by some on the basis of the philosophy that hyperparathyroidism should always be treated as early as possible or the speculation that normalization of the serum calcium concentration may lead to a reduction of gastrin secretion and, possibly, lowered pancreatic islet cell growth or transformation, or both.[18] Although parathyroidectomy can decrease gastrin secretion by gastrinoma in MEN1 (Fig. 36–4), there is no evidence that this intervention prevents or slows gastrin-cell transformation.[37] For this reason and because medical control of gastric acid oversecretion is excellent, the coexistence of a gastrinoma is not a sufficient indication for parathyroidectomy in MEN1, except in the rare case in which medical control of Zollinger-Ellison syndrome (ZES) is difficult.

Preoperative and Intraoperative Assessment of Tumors

Preoperative noninvasive imaging (ultrasonography or Tc99m-sestamibi, or both) for parathyroid surgery is being performed with increasing frequency.[38, 39] The major justification for the added costs of these procedures in sporadic hyperparathyroidism is to perform a unilateral or even more limited neck exploration, thereby reducing operative morbidity, time, and cost.[40] In MEN1 the likely presence of multiple parathyroid tumors makes it necessary to perform an exploration of four or more glands at initial surgery, thereby eliminating one major rationale for preoperative imaging procedures.[18] A much stronger case can be made for the use of these and other invasive procedures (ultrasound-guided fine-needle aspiration for PTH assay, selective arteriography, and selective venous sampling for PTH, when indicated) in MEN1 patients undergoing reoperation.[41, 42]

Several intraoperative tools can increase the likelihood of successful parathyroid surgery. Rapid "on-line" assay of PTH can be done at 5-minute intervals with a turnaround time of 10 minutes for each result.[43–45] A PTH fall of 50% or more from baseline predicts that no hyperfunctioning parathyroid tissue remains (Fig. 36–5). Sensitive ultrasound transducers routinely image parathyroid tumors intraoperatively in difficult locations, such as within the thyroid gland and within scar from prior surgery.[38] Availability of intraoperative PTH assay and ultrasonography may be useful as a backup option at initial parathyroid surgery, particularly in any patient expected to have multiple parathyroid tumors (as in MEN1). These tests are even more likely to be helpful during parathyroid reoperations in MEN1, as the number and locations of tumors during a second operative procedure are particularly hard to predict.

Surgical Objectives

The standard surgical approach for initial parathyroidectomy in MEN1 has been removal of 3.5 glands and conservation of approximately 50 mg of the most normal-appearing gland, attached to its vascular pedicle. Because eventual parathyroid reoperation in MEN1 is likely, the recording of careful operative notes and diagrams and the marking of remaining tissue with nonresorbable materials enhance the likelihood of success in subsequent operations.

An alternative is attempted complete removal of parathyroid tissue from the neck and immediate transplantation of small fragments to pockets in the nondominant forearm (Fig. 36–6).[46] Use of this strategy is dependent on the likelihood of achieving a high rate of graft success. This technique does not prevent recurrent hyperparathyroidism but may simplify its management. For example, a PTH concentration in the venous effluent of the graft greater than in the effluent from the contralateral arm confirms graft function (this does not exclude other parathyroid tissue in the neck or chest). Similarly, if peripheral PTH falls by more than 50% within minutes after inflation of a blood pressure cuff to occlude venous return from the graft, the graft is implicated as the main source of

Malignant Melanoma

This has occurred in at least seven MEN1 cases, but direct involvement of the *MEN1* gene has not been tested.[203]

Leiomyoma (of Esophagus, Lung, Rectum, or Uterus)

This has been reported in several MEN1 cases.[6, 19, 204, 205] Analyses of 11q13 LOH established that esophageal and uterine leiomyoma are specific to MEN1 cases.[206] Similar *MEN1* inactivation was not implicated in sporadic uterine leiomyoma.[206]

Varying Penetrance of Tumors by Tissue or by Age

MEN1 is perhaps the most heterogeneous of all multiple neoplasia syndromes.[207] The many tumors of MEN1 have a wide range of penetrance (see Table 36–1). If the organ is paired and the penetrance is high, the tumors are generally bilateral (i.e., parathyroid); if the tumor is rare in MEN1, its random occurrence is generally unilateral even in a paired organ (i.e., pheochromocytoma). Naturally, the apparent penetrance of any tumor type is heavily dependent upon the scrutiny that the organ is given. Thus, the frequent facial angiofibromas of MEN1 were not recognized until 1997.[199] When symptoms alone are the main basis for disease recognition, the first feature of MEN1 in adolescents is not hyperparathyroidism but rather prolactinoma or insulinoma.[208]

For each tumor type, penetrance necessarily increases with age (see Fig. 36–1). Overall, the penetrance for MEN1 (usually parathyroid) reaches nearly 100% by age 50,[20] but occasional obligate *MEN1* mutation carriers have not shown any tumor beyond age 70.[202] Earliest penetrance and earliest preventable morbidity must be evaluated in decisions about when to begin carrier ascertainment for tumors in a likely carrier. The earliest ages for identification of specific tumor expression in MEN1 have been as follows: prolactinoma at age 5,[161] insulinoma at age 6,[209] hyperparathyroidism at age 8,[20] and gastrinoma at age 12 (R. Jensen, personal communication). The information about morbidity for most of these cases is incomplete; thus, more information is needed before it is possible to make consensus recommendations regarding the correct age at which to begin tumor surveillance and possibly intervention.

Phenotypes or Varying Tumor Penetrance by Family

Clustering of clinical subvariants of MEN1, similar to that seen for MEN2 (see later in chapter), has been evaluated. Preliminary analyses in small MEN1 families suggested clusters of ACTH-producing pituitary tumors,[207] insulinomas[210, 211] carcinoids,[182] and aggressive gastrinomas.[184] Identification of a specific mutation that correlates with a specific clinical variant in multiple kindreds would be most meaningful. Although subsequent analysis has failed to identify such a relationship (see later), increasing the likelihood of random clustering in most of these families, it is important to continue evaluating such subvariants because some may be united by an as yet undiscovered molecular basis.

Prolactinoma Variant of MEN1

This is defined in a family with high penetrance for hyperparathyroidism and prolactinoma but low penetrance for gastrinoma (typically 90%, 50%, and 5%, respectively among adults). Four such families have been reported, each with eight or more affected members.[212–217] The largest family has over 100 affected members[214]; because their ancestors colonized the Burin Peninsula of Newfoundland, Canada, their trait has been termed $MEN1_{Burin}$.[213] Several smaller families seem similar.[178] Foregut carcinoid tumors were prominent in $MEN1_{Burin}$.[215] It has been argued that the prolactinoma variant is not a genuine MEN1 phenotype because prolactinoma has shown different penetrances among branches of one other large MEN1 family.[218]

Hyperparathyroidism Variant

Hyperparathyroidism is the most common clinical feature of MEN1 and occurs at a relatively young age. It would therefore not be surprising to identify isolated hyperparathyroidism in small families with early or occult MEN1, particularly those with a disproportionate number of young members. Larger families (four, five, or more affected members) have been identified with familial isolated hyperparathyroidism (FIH) and an identifiable *MEN1* mutation but still could represent a random part of the normal spectrum of MEN1 expression.[219] Eventually, most would probably develop other clinical features of MEN1.[220] Two FIH families with *MEN1* mutation have been particularly large, with 8 and 13 hyperparathyroid members, raising the likelihood that, in some families, isolated hyperparathyroidism may exist and continue as the only manifestation of *MEN1* mutation.[219, 221, 222] *MEN1* mutation is rare in families with FIH.[223]

Phenocopies and Differential Diagnoses of Multiple Endocrine Neoplasia Type 1

When MEN1 occurs in its typical forms, it is easily diagnosed. Presentation as a single sporadic tumor, as FIH, or as familial isolated pituitary tumor (see earlier) not only is rare but also presents the clinician with a difficult diagnostic challenge.

Sporadic Tumor or Tumors

MEN1 can occur without a recognized or even recognizable family history of MEN1. When sporadic cases present with two or more typical tumors, some cases meet the definition criteria for MEN1[17]; for others the suspicion of MEN1 is high. The prevalence of *MEN1* mutation is 10% to 90%, depending on the specific tumors (see later). When the sporadic case presents with tumor in only one tissue, the suspicion and the true frequency of *MEN1* mutation are low. The frequency of occult MEN1 with sporadic tumor can be estimated as follows: hyperparathyroidism (2%),[18, 224] gastrinoma (5%),[65] prolactinoma (5%).[155–157] Factors that increase the likelihood of MEN1 in these settings are earlier onset and tumor multiplicity in the same organ.

Familial Isolated Hyperparathyroidism

When hyperparathyroidism is familial and isolated, the main possibilities include occult MEN1 (see earlier), familial hypocalciuric hypercalcemia (FHH), hyperparathyroidism–jaw tumor syndrome (HPT-JT), MEN2A, and so-called true FIH[223] (see Chapter 26). FHH, with a frequency similar to that of MEN1, is an autosomal dominant disorder characterized by lifelong hypercalcemia with normal urine calcium excretion.[225, 226] PTH levels and parathyroid gland mass are normal or minimally increased.[227, 228] After subtotal parathyroidectomy, the residual parathyroid tissue directs persistent hypercalcemia after subtotal parathyroidectomy. The parathyroid dysfunction is not neoplastic but polyclonal.[229] A remarkably high rate of persistence after subtotal parathyroidectomy and a low morbidity without surgery justify efforts to avoid parathyroid surgery in FHH. Useful diagnostic features of FHH are the low ratio of renal calcium clearance to creatinine clearance (in the presence of hypercalcemia) and the onset of hypercalcemia in relatives typically before age 1 year. Two thirds of FHH index cases have an inactivating mutation of the calcium-sensing receptor gene (*CASR*)[35] Most of the rest are believed to have an undetected mutation of *CASR*, suggested by genetic linkage to chromosome 3q; occasional families have the FHH syndrome with mutation in unknown genes at 19p or 19q.[230, 231] One family with a missense mutation of *CASR* had features intermediate between FHH and typical hyperparathyroidism.[232]

HPT-JT is a syndrome of hyperparathyroidism, jaw tumors, and renal lesions.[233] Transmission is autosomal dominant, and it is caused only by the as yet unidentified *HRPT2* gene at 1q24-1q32.[234, 235] The commonest and sometimes the only feature is hyperparathyroidism.[236] The hyperparathyroidism typically involves one parathyroid gland at a time and there is a uniquely high malignant potential in the parathyroid tumor; 15% of reported cases have had parathyroid cancer.[223, 237] The associated jaw tumors are ossifying or cementifying fibromas.[234] Unlike the jaw tumors of hyperparathyroidism, they are not influenced by the hyperparathyroid status. The associated renal lesions are multiple renal cysts, hamartomas, or Wilms' tumor.[235] An international consortium is working to identify this gene.[238] Occult MEN2A, theoretically another cause of FIH, has not been identified in the form of FIH.[239, 240]

Many small kindreds with two or three affected members receive a diagnosis of FIH.[223, 241, 242] For years FIH was not pursued as a syndrome because of bland features and the belief that most kindreds had occult MEN1. A detailed analysis of many kindreds with FIH found occult MEN1, FHH, or HPT-JT in the minority.[223] Whether the remaining individuals have true FIH or some other genetic form of hyperparathyroidism will become clear only with long-term follow-up or when robust deoxyribonucleic acid (DNA) tests become available for all of the genes for FHH (at least three genes), HPT-JT, and other hereditary forms of hyperparathyroidism.

Familial Isolated Pituitary Tumor

Familial isolated tumor of the anterior pituitary has been recognized in several small and few large families.[243, 244, 645–653] The tumors are usually somatotropinomas, occasionally prolactinomas. In theory, familial isolated tumor of the anterior pituitary could be an expression of occult MEN1. To date, however, no family with familial isolated somatotropinoma has had a *MEN1* mutation (see later). It is more likely that most of these families harbor mutations of another unknown gene or genes.

The *MEN1* Gene: Normal or Mutated

The Normal *MEN1* Gene and Normal Menin

Larsson and colleagues[245] showed in 1988 that the *MEN1* gene mapped to chromosome 11q13 and that it was probably a tumor suppressor gene (see the following).[246, 247] However, almost a full decade passed before the *MEN1* gene was identified by positional cloning.[247b] This strategy involved a progressive narrowing of the candidate gene interval,[248] cloning all the DNA in the narrowed interval,[249] and identifying all or most genes therein.[249] The final step required sequence analysis of each of these genes in a panel of DNA from familial MEN1 index cases, a systematic process that led to the identification of the one gene that carried the defining mutations.[245, 250, 251]

The *MEN1* gene is 10 kilobases (kb) in size and encodes transcripts of 2.7 and 3.1 kb.[252] The transcripts are expressed in all or most tissues and with little cell cycle dependence.[253] They encode a 610-amino-acid protein termed menin. Rat, mouse, zebra fish, snail, *Drosophila*, and human menins are highly homologous.[254]

Menin has two nuclear localization signals near the carboxyl terminus that are likely to be responsible for its predominantly nuclear compartmentalization.[253] The first interacting protein partner identified for menin was selectively junD but not other members of the activator protein-1 (AP1) transcription factor family including fos, fra, or other jun proteins.[255, 256] The menin-junD interaction may confer upon junD unique effects by which junD differs from other members of the AP1 transcription family. For example, junD has several actions opposite to those of C-jun, and in the absence of menin binding to it, junD behaves more like C-jun.[257] The importance of the menin-junD interaction for the development of MEN1 is unclear. Homozygous knockout of junD in the mouse resulted in no identifiable abnormality of tissues involved in MEN1.[258] Other studies have identified SMAD3, PEM, NM23, nuclear factor κB, and several other proteins that potentially interact with menin. Each interaction has unknown importance.[259]

Tumorigenesis: Sequential Two-Step Inactivation of the *MEN1* Gene

The first DNA-based discoveries in MEN1 suggested that the *MEN1* gene was a tumor suppressor[245–247] (see Chapter 35), observations supported by subsequent studies (see later). Complete inactivation of a gene's function requires, in addition to the inherited or somatically acquired first hit (inactivating mutation), a second hit at the same genetic locus that finishes the inactivation of both copies of the *MEN1* gene. Inactivation of the second allele can be by mutation or other (epigenetic) means such as promoter methylation, though the latter has not been found for MEN1.[284] A two-hit model for tumorigenesis was developed by Alfred Knudson[246, 247] to account for epidemiologic observations in retinoblastoma: that, in comparison with sporadic cases, some hereditary tumors occurred earlier and in multiple sites. This can now be generalized to say that, in a hereditary tumor, the germ line mutation is obligatorily present in every cell. Thus, the earliest step seen in sporadic tumorigenesis caused by the *MEN1* gene is bypassed. Multiple independent cells in susceptible organs are thus primed for somatic mutations at the second and still normal copy to cause early and multiple tumors. This model can be extended to stepwise tumorigenesis by an oncogene such as *RET* (see later).

Somatic Point Mutations (First Hits) of the MEN1 *Gene in Sporadic Tumors*

MEN1 is one of the most frequently mutated genes in sporadic endocrine tumors. The frequency of *MEN1* mutation is 10% to 20% in parathyroid adenomas,[260–263] 25% in gastrinomas,[264–266] 10% to 20% in insulinomas,[264, 267] 50% in VIPomas,[264, 267] and 25% to 35% in bronchial carcinoids.[264, 268] Other sporadic endocrine tumors show a lower frequency of *MEN1* somatic mutation: 0% to 5% in anterior pituitary tumor,[269–273] 0% in thyroid tumor,[197] 0% in benign or malignant adrenocortical neoplasm,[274, 275] 0% in uremic secondary hyperparathyroidism,[274, 277] and 0% in parathyroid cancer.[278] Sporadic nonendocrine tumors have undergone little evaluation; the *MEN1* mutation frequency was 2/19 in angiofibromas,[279] 1/6 in lipomas,[280] 0% in lung cancer other than carcinoid,[281] 1% in malignant melanoma,[203, 282] and 0% in leukemia.[283]

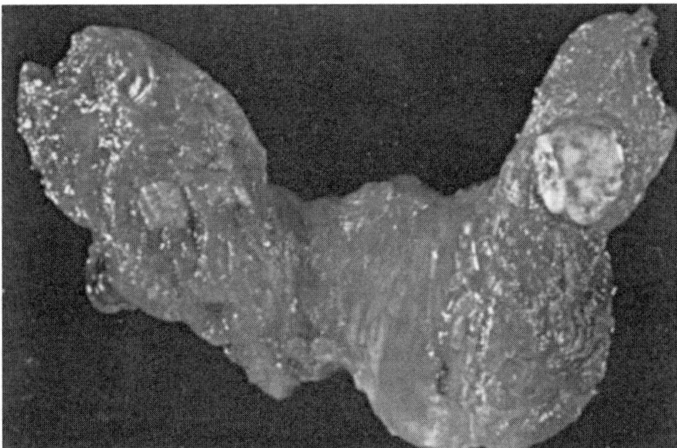

Figure 36–10. Bilateral medullary thyroid carcinoma in multiple endocrine neoplasia type 2A. Large bilateral foci of medullary thyroid carcinoma are located in each lobe of the thyroid gland.

as appropriate, a sequence of confirmation, exclusion of false-positives, a decision whether to proceed with staging or surgery or both, and finally preoperative and intraoperative tumor imaging tests (see Fig. 36–9). The specific details differ for each tumor type.

MULTIPLE ENDOCRINE NEOPLASIA TYPE 2

Multiple Endocrine Neoplasia Type 2A

In 1959, John Sipple was asked to see a hypertensive patient who subsequently died. At autopsy Sipple "was amazed when [he] saw large, bilateral pheochromocytomas and a 2-cm pale tan mass in each lobe of the thyroid gland and nodular enlargement of the only parathyroid gland [they] could find."[328] He reported this case and reviewed five others from the literature[5]; subsequently, the familial nature of the syndrome[7, 329] and the recognition of the thyroid tumor as medullary thyroid carcinoma were clarified by others.[330] Williams[331] reasoned that because MTC was a malignancy of the C cells it might produce calcitonin, a concept that led to the use of serum calcitonin measurements for early diagnosis of MTC and of MEN2.[8, 10, 332, 333]

The clinical syndrome of MEN2A, as described by Sipple[5] and others,[7] consists of bilateral and multicentric MTC, unilateral or bilateral pheochromocytoma, and, less commonly, parathyroid hyperplasia or adenomas. In the decade after Sipple's description, patients with this syndrome frequently presented with manifestations of a pheochromocytoma, a thyroid nodule, hypercalcemia, or some combination of the three. Such clinical presentations are still observed, but MEN2 syndrome identification and routine carrier ascertainment in affected families now make early thyroid C-cell hyperplasia or microscopic MTC without metastasis the most common initial presentation.[11, 13, 16, 334–343] Pheochromocytomas are subsequently identified in about half of patients, and parathyroid abnormalities occur in 10% to 35%.[7, 8, 239, 344, 345]

A feature of MEN2 that differs from MEN1 is clear progression of histologic changes from normal to hyperplasia to adenoma (pheochromocytoma or parathyroid adenoma) or carcinoma (MTC). The development of hyperplasia is probably a multicentric process, with each focus of tumor derived from a single clone. This point has been proved for only one manifestation of the syndrome (MTC)[346] but is likely to be true for other tumors as well.[347] The heterozygous activating mutations of the *RET* proto-oncogene may be the stimulus for hyperplasia, whereas additional mutational events appear to be required for progression of this process (to be discussed later).

Medullary Thyroid Carcinoma in Multiple Endocrine Neoplasia Type 2

Evolution of C-Cell Abnormalities

MTC in all variants of MEN2 is a multicentric neoplasm of the parafollicular or C cell of the thyroid gland (Fig. 36–10). The earliest demonstrable abnormality in the thyroid gland of individuals with this syndrome is hyperplasia of C cells,[348, 349] followed by progression to nodular hyperplasia, microscopic MTC, and finally frank MTC (Fig. 36–11). These changes are multicentric, with the frequent occurrence of more than one type of histologic lesion in one or both lobes of the thyroid.[350] The time required for progression through these several histo-

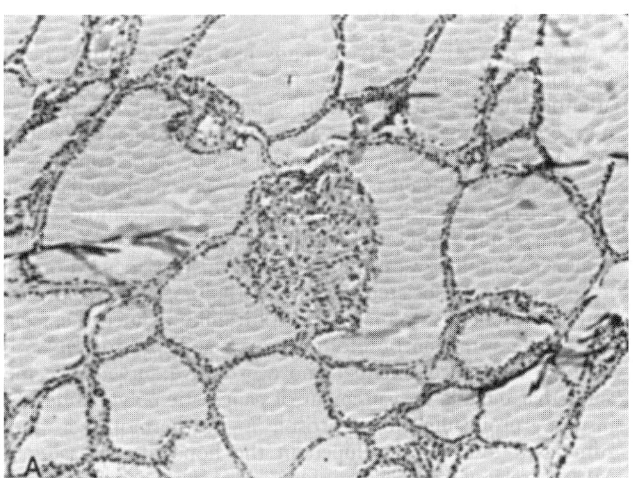

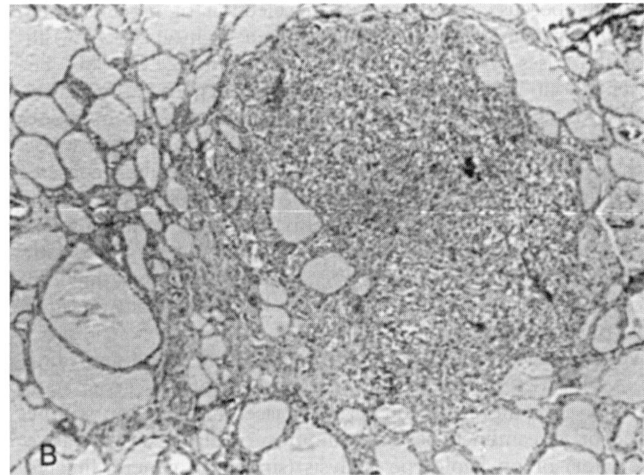

Figure 36–11. Progression of histologic changes from C-cell hyperplasia to medullary thyroid carcinoma. These sections were taken from a single thyroid lobe of a patient with hereditary medullary thyroid carcinoma and demonstrate the multicentric nature of this tumor. *A*, Nodular hyperplasia with containment of C cells within a thyroid follicle. Magnification ×250. *B*, Microscopic medullary thyroid carcinoma that is locally invasive. Magnification ×100.

logic stages is not known, but such changes have been noted as early as 3 years of age in MEN2A and during the first month of life in MEN2B.[350–352] It is also not known at which earliest histologic stage metastasis occurs, but local lymph node metastasis is common when the tumor diameter is larger than 1 cm,[8, 9, 338, 340] whereas lymph node metastasis is rare in a case with only C-cell hyperplasia.[10, 11, 13, 353–355] Occasionally, foci of MTC occur in extrathyroidal locations such as the thymus gland. Whether these lesions are primary or metastatic has not been determined with certainty.

Tumor Markers Associated with Medullary Thyroid Carcinoma

Proteins expressed by the normal C cell and by MTC include calcitonin, calcitonin gene–related peptide,[356] somatostatin,[357] dihydroxyphenylalanine decarboxylase,[358] and chromogranin-A.[359] Proteins that are not normally expressed in the C cell but that are expressed by MTC include pro-opiomelanocortin, thyrotropin-releasing hormone,[360] gastrin-releasing peptide,[361] VIP, neurotensin, substance P, carcinoembryonic antigen, histaminase,[362] and others.[363] The only reported clinical syndrome associated with ectopic hormone production is the ectopic ACTH syndrome in fewer than 5% of patients with extensive MTC (see Chapter 40). It is presumed that the diarrhea associated with advanced MTC is caused by a secretory product of the transformed C cell, although the specific causative agent has not been identified. With the exception of calcitonin and carcinoembryonic antigen, these markers are not generally used for recognition of a tumor in MEN2 and are rarely used for monitoring a tumor.

Treatment of Medullary Thyroid Carcinoma

Total thyroidectomy is mandatory for prevention or cure of hereditary MTC, although protocols for intervention are specific to each MEN2 variant. Abnormalities of the C cell in MEN2 are almost always bilateral and multicentric,[364] and even if C cells remaining after surgery are not malignant, transformation may occur later, suggesting that the posterior capsule of the thyroid gland should be removed. The probability of metastasis to central or other neck lymph nodes is high, approaching 75% in some series for even small intrathyroidal tumors.[365] Surgical removal of all central lymph nodes and selective removal of the lateral lymph nodes of the neck can result in cure of the disease, even in the presence of nodal metastasis.[8, 16, 333, 341, 366] Studies to exclude hyperparathyroidism and pheochromocytoma are mandatory; pheochromocytomas should be removed before thyroid surgery.

Younger individuals diagnosed by *RET* mutation analysis as described subsequently should have a total thyroidectomy.[13, 367, 368] C-cell hyperplasia and microscopic MTC (see Fig. 36–11) without metastatic disease are the most common histologic findings in these patients, although minimal or no abnormalities of C cells have been identified in some younger gene carriers.[353–355] A case can be made for a central node dissection even in early disease because of the finding of metastasis in young children,[352] although a more extensive lymph node dissection is generally not recommended.[354, 367] Children with MEN2B may have earlier metastasis, and consideration should be given to more extensive lymph node dissection. Surgical management for children identified by DNA testing is discussed in a subsequent section.

Monitoring after Surgery for Medullary Thyroid Carcinoma

At 3 to 6 months following thyroidectomy, patients should be reevaluated by measurement of serum calcitonin and an ultrasound examination of the neck. Earlier measurement of serum calcitonin is discouraged because serum calcitonin values may remain elevated for 3 to 6 months after thyroid surgery and become normal at a later time.[11, 16] The elevated calcitonin values are presumed to be related to the generalized rise in serum calcitonin that occurs during inflammation or sepsis.[369–371] Equally important, the fact that calcitonin gene expression can be activated in inflamed or infected tissue unrelated to the C cell suggests that one should be careful about overinterpreting the significance of a minimal or transient rise in the serum calcitonin value. Stimuli as nonspecific as exercise can cause a serum calcitonin rise.[372]

It may be useful to measure calcitonin after calcium or pentagastrin stimulation at 6 to 12 months if basal serum calcitonin values are undetectable. In general, it is useful to perform this procedure only if it would direct a specific clinical action (discussed in the next paragraph). Serial measurement of the serum calcitonin or carcinoembryonic antigen is a useful indicator of long-term disease progression and helps define the aggressiveness of MTC in a patient with metastatic disease. This type of information may be useful in making decisions regarding intervention with chemotherapy or reoperation. Calcitonin is a secretory peptide, and there is considerable variability of the serum concentration. Serum calcitonin values may vary by as much as 50% or more from measurement to measurement without evidence of progression of disease. However, a plot of values over months or years is useful to establish a trend of disease activity.

Management of Locally Metastatic Medullary Thyroid Carcinoma

Reoperation for persistent MTC was attempted with initially poor results.[366, 373] However, improvement of surgical techniques led to the normalization of serum calcitonin values in approximately one third of reoperated patients.[374] This experience has led others to examine the usefulness of reoperation, and a larger experience suggests that approximately 15% to 20% of carefully selected patients (patients with no evidence of pulmonary, hepatic, or bone metastasis) have normal or nondetectable calcitonin values after reoperation.[374–378]

A major question confronting the physician contemplating reoperation is whether the tumor is located in the neck or whether distant metastases are present. Techniques that have been used with variable success for localizing the tumor include scanning with thallium[379] and metaiodobenzylguanidine,[380–382] octreotide scanning,[383] and venous catheterization for measurement of calcitonin in blood from selectively catheterized veins.[384]

Several lines of evidence suggest that nondetectable basal and calcium- or pentagastrin-stimulated calcitonin after surgery is likely to be indicative of a cure. These include promising results after the short-term follow-up (5 to 10 years) of reoperated patients[374, 376, 385] and the generally favorable long-term outcome in patients with MTC and local nodal metastasis who had nondetectable calcitonin values after primary surgery.[16, 339, 373] Whether a 20% cure rate justifies the extensive repeat operative procedure is unclear, but the generally poor outcomes of reoperative strategies suggested by earlier reports[340, 386] should be reconsidered in light of this newer experience. One concern related to reoperation is a higher incidence of hypoparathyroidism.[378]

Pheochromocytoma in Multiple Endocrine Neoplasia Type 2

Evolution of Pheochromocytoma

Adrenal chromaffin tissue in patients with MEN2A undergoes the same type of histologic progression as observed for

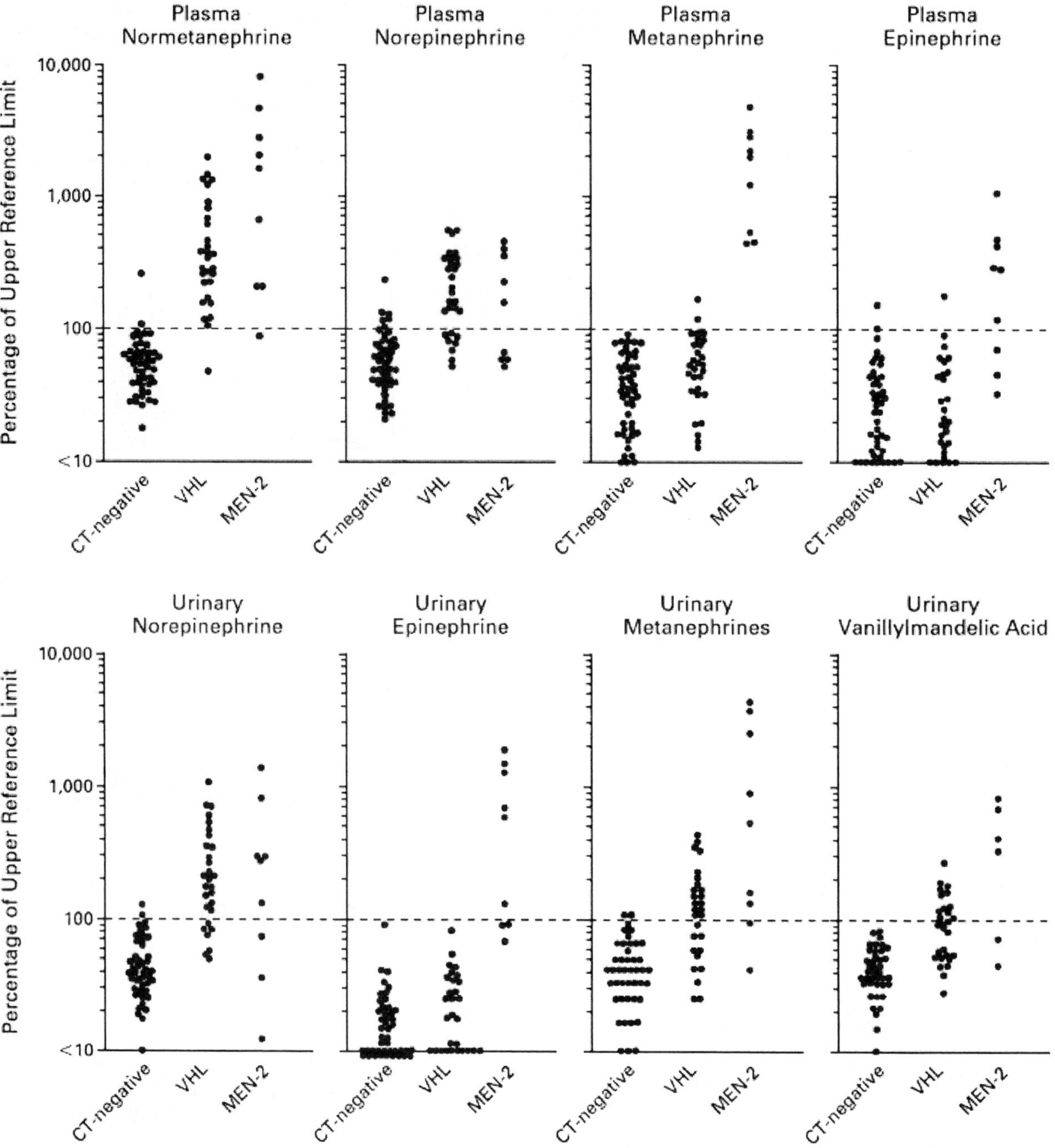

Figure 36–13 *Continued. Panel B,* Plasma concentrations of normetanephrine, norepinephrine, metanephrine, and epinephrine *(top)* and urinary excretion of norepinephrine, epinephrine, metanephrines, and vanillylmandelic acid *(bottom)*. The values are expressed as percentages of the upper reference limit for each test. Data on individual patients are shown for three groups of patients with von Hippel–Lindau (VHL) disease and MEN2 as follows: patients with VHL disease or MEN2 in whom a pheochromocytoma was ruled out on the basis of normal computed tomography (CT-negative), patients with VHL disease who had histologically verified pheochromocytomas (VHL), and patients with MEN2 who had histologically verified pheochromocytomas (MEN2). The values for patients with pheochromocytoma were determined when the tumors were first identified by CT. The dotted *horizontal line* represents the upper reference limit for each test. The scales are logarithmic. (*A,* From Gagel RF, Tashjian AH Jr, Cummings T, et al. The clinical outcome of prospective calcitonin-based surveillance for multiple endocrine neoplasia type 2A: an 18-year experience. N Engl J Med 1988; 318:478–484. *B,* Data from Eisenhofer G, Lenders JWM, Linehan WM, et al. Plasma normetanephrine and metanephrine for detecting pheochromocytoma in von Hippel–Lindau disease and multiple endocrine neoplasia type 2. N Engl J Med 1999; 340:1872–1879.)

Unilateral Pheochromocytoma

Unilateral pheochromocytomas may be identified by the development of adrenergic symptoms, abnormal urine or plasma catecholamines, or by an imaging procedure. The unilateral adrenal nodule in MEN2A or 2B is most commonly a pheochromocytoma, although metastatic MTC or benign adrenal cortical nodules have occasionally been identified. It is difficult and time consuming to differentiate between pheochromocytoma, metastatic MTC, or a benign cortical nodule in this situation. If catecholamines or metanephrine measurements are abnormal, it is appropriate to perform adrenal surgery. Computed tomography-guided fine-needle aspiration or selective adrenal vein sampling is generally discouraged.

Two different approaches have been employed to treat unilateral pheochromocytomas. The first is unilateral laparoscopic adrenalectomy. Reports of several deaths caused by adrenocortical insufficiency over the past decade[413, 414] raise the distinct possibility that, at present, corticoid deficiency is a greater threat to life in MEN2 than a pheochromocytoma and, therefore, the contralateral normal adrenal should remain untouched if radiographically normal. A second approach, developed to maintain adrenocortical function, is cortical sparing adrenalectomy. This is an old technique that has gained increasing favor as the risks of death from adrenocortical insufficiency associated with bilateral adrenalectomy have become apparent. This approach has been applied to small groups of patients with MEN2–related pheochromocytomas with retention of adrenal function in approximately 80% of treated patients.[397, 415–418]

Resection of an intra-adrenal pheochromocytoma with retention of cortical tissue raises the inevitable possibility of late recurrence of pheochromocytoma caused by adrenal chromaffin tissue at the corticomedullary interface, which develops into a tumor at a later time in approximately 20% of cases.[397] If retention of adrenocortical function is considered essential (e.g., for employment purposes),[416] consideration should be given to performance of a cortical sparing adrenalectomy on the first identified pheochromocytoma, thereby providing an opportunity for a successful procedure on the contralateral adrenal gland if the first procedure fails. It is also difficult to know whether the first procedure is successful without detailed studies of corticoid secretory function that involve venous catheterization with selective sampling.[419] Cortical sparing adrenalectomy is generally performed through a flank incision; although it is technically feasible to perform this procedure by a laparoscopic approach, a successful example after this approach has not been described.

Bilateral Pheochromocytoma

Bilateral pheochromocytomas eventually develop in approximately one half of MEN2A or MEN2B gene carriers, although there has been a change in the clinical presentation. Twenty-five years ago, pheochromocytomas were generally detected at a much later stage in the clinical course of the disease and, therefore, a higher percentage of patients had bilateral pheochromocytomas at presentation. Measurement of catecholamines and metanephrines, now routinely employed, has led to routine identification of pheochromocytoma at an earlier stage, yielding a higher percentage of unilateral pheochromocytomas at initial presentation. Of those who initially present with a unilateral pheochromocytoma, 50% have a pheochromocytoma develop in the contralateral adrenal gland over a period of 8 to 10 years.[16] Thus, the mode of clinical evolution has changed, but eventually approximately one half of MEN2A or 2B patients experience pheochromocytoma.

The management for patients with bilateral pheochromocytomas follows a paradigm similar to that described for a unilateral pheochromocytoma. Because bilateral tumors are more likely to produce catecholaminergic signs and symptoms, adrenergic antagonists and inhibition of catecholamine synthesis with α-methyltyrosine become doubly important (see Chapter 15). Bilateral laparoscopic adrenalectomy[420–423] or cortical sparing adrenalectomy[397] should be performed. In patients with very large pheochromocytomas, laparoscopic adrenalectomy may not be possible, necessitating bilateral flank approaches or the less preferred anterior abdominal approach.

Hyperparathyroidism

Reports from the 1960s and early 1970s described hyperparathyroidism in 10% to 35% of individuals with MEN2A.[7, 8, 239, 240, 366, 413] These reports described the presence of either parathyroid hyperplasia or multiple parathyroid adenomas in association with hypercalcemia, urolithiasis, or osteitis fibrosa cystica. A careful review of the histology of these tumors has demonstrated occasional adenomatous formation with a background of parathyroid hyperplasia,[424] a finding that is analogous to that observed for C-cell hyperplasia in the thyroid gland and chromaffin cell hyperplasia in the adrenal medulla.

Simultaneous hyperparathyroidism is almost never seen in patients thyroidectomized for early C-cell abnormalities, although histologic findings consistent with parathyroid hyperplasia have been observed.[16] Partly for this reason most surgeons attempt to preserve parathyroid tissue, particularly in children who have a prophylactic total thyroidectomy. Whether patients who have had a prophylactic thyroidectomy for MTC eventually experience hyperparathyroidism is unknown. Surgical management of hyperparathyroidism is similar to that described for MEN1, although recurrent hyperparathyroidism is a less common occurrence in MEN2.

One concern related to thyroid surgery is the potential for development of hypoparathyroidism after aggressive thyroidectomy. A careful review of most series documents an incidence of hypoparathyroidism that is comparable to or higher than that for other thyroid surgical indications. To address this issue, some surgeons routinely perform a total thyroidectomy and removal and reimplantation of parathyroid tissue into the nondominant arm.[354, 425]

Variants of Multiple Endocrine Neoplasia Type 2A

A number of MEN2A variants have been described (Table 36–3). The most common is familial medullary thyroid carcinoma (FMTC) without pheochromocytoma or parathyroid disease.[426] Kindreds with this syndrome account for approximately 10% to 15% of all those with hereditary MTC. Familial MTC

Table 36–3. Multiple Endocrine Neoplasia Type 2

Multiple endocrine neoplasia type 2A (MEN2A)
Medullary thyroid carcinoma (100%)
Pheochromocytoma (50%)
Parathyroid neoplasia (10%–35%)
Variants of MEN2A
MEN2A with cutaneous lichen amyloidosis (MEN2A/CLA)
MEN2A or FMTC with Hirschsprung's disease
Familial medullary thyroid carcinoma (FMTC)
Multiple endocrine neoplasia type 2B (MEN2B)
Medullary thyroid carcinoma (100%)
Pheochromocytoma (50%)
Absence of parathyroid disease
Marfanoid habitus (>95%)
Intestinal ganglioneuromatosis and mucosal neuromas (>98%)

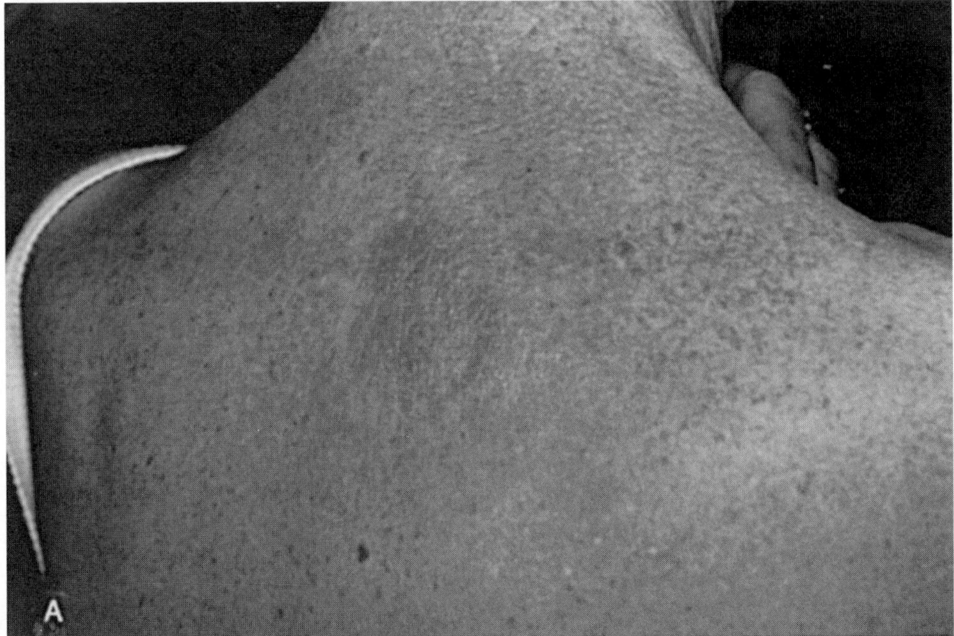

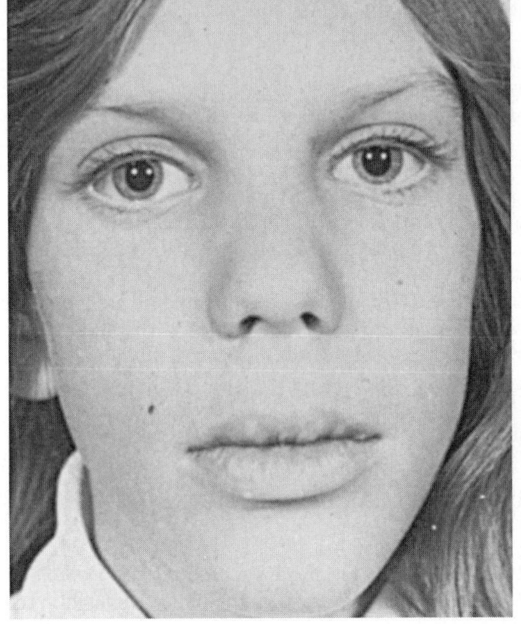

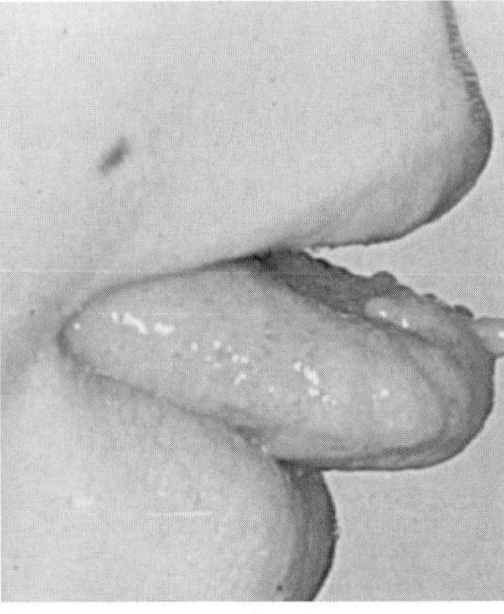

Figure 36–14. Cutaneous and oral manifestations in multiple endocrine neoplasia type 2 (MEN2) variants. *A*, The characteristic clinical picture of cutaneous lichen amyloidosis associated with MEN2A. The pruritic skin lesion may cover a small area or the entire right or left upper back, as shown in this patient. *B* and *C*, Patient with MEN2B demonstrating thick bumpy lips and eversion of upper eyelids *(B)* and neuromas on anterior third of tongue *(C)*. (*A*, From Gagel RF, Levy ML, Donovan DT, et al. Multiple endocrine neoplasia type 2A associated with cutaneous lichen amyloidosis. Ann Intern Med 1989; 111:802–806; *B* and *C*, from Brown RS, Colle E, Tashjian AH Jr. The syndrome of multiple mucosal neuromas and medullary thyroid carcinoma in childhood. Importance of recognition of the phenotype for the early detection of malignancy. J Pediatr 1975; 86:77–83.)

is most likely to be confused with sporadic MTC because of the absence of dramatic symptomatology associated with pheochromocytomas that is found in MEN2A. Because the penetrance of pheochromocytoma in MEN2A is much lower than that for MTC, it is possible to designate small kindreds with MEN2A incorrectly as having FMTC. The concern, of course, is that there will be a failure to screen for and diagnose pheochromocytomas in such kindreds.

At least 15 families have been identified with the MEN2A/cutaneous lichen amyloidosis variant.[427, 428] In these families, affected individuals had a pruritic skin lesion over the scapular region of the upper back consisting of multiple infiltrated papules overlying a well-demarcated plaque (Fig. 36–14*A*). The histology is that of cutaneous lichen amyloidosis (deposition of amyloid at the juncture of the epidermis and dermis) in patients with the fully formed skin lesion. Immunohistochemical staining of the amyloid for keratin but not calcitonin was observed, which indicates that the amyloid is probably of dermal origin and not the result of deposition of calcitonin gene products from the thyroid carcinoma.[427] In most patients, intense pruritus precedes the development of the skin lesion by 3 to 5 years, suggesting that the primary defect may be a sensory abnormality in the C6-T6 dermatomes leading to chronic irritation and friction amyloidosis.[429, 430] In support of this hypothesis is the fact that there is RET expression in the normal dorsal root ganglion, the site at which the sensory nerve cells for this region are located.[431] Neurologic and electromyographic abnormalities have been observed in some of these patients.[432]

A third variant is MEN2A associated with Hirschsprung disease,[433] which can be differentiated by rectal biopsy from the ganglioneuromatosis identified in MEN2B. Although this variant was considered uncommon a decade ago, the increasing focus on the role of the *RET* proto-oncogene in the development of the enteric nervous system has led to more frequent identification of this variant.[434–442]

Multiple Endocrine Neoplasia Type 2B

The association of MTC and pheochromocytoma with multiple mucosal neuromas is termed MEN2B (formerly MEN3).[331, 443] The hallmark of this syndrome is the presence of characteristic mucosal neuromas on the distal portion of the tongue (Fig. 36–14*B* and *C*), on the lips and subconjunctival areas, and throughout the gastrointestinal tract.[443–445] Thickened corneal nerves may be identified by slit lamp examination, and enlarged nerves are frequently noted during neck or abdominal surgery. Ganglioneuromatosis of the gastrointestinal tract can cause obstruction, dilation of the colon, or a colic-like childhood syndrome with associated diarrhea[446, 447] and may be the first clinical manifestation of MEN2B. Other features associated with this syndrome include a marfanoid habitus, pectus excavatum, slipped femoral epiphysis, and long, thin extremities.[443–445]

The mucosal neuroma phenotype is associated, in all reported cases, with bilateral and multicentric C-cell hyperplasia or MTC, or both. The MTC in this syndrome is more aggressive than that in MEN2A. Metastatic C-cell disease can occur in children younger than 1 year of age,[13, 351, 448–451] and there is a shorter average survival time in patients with metastatic disease.[452] However, the presence of multigenerational families and a more extensive compilation of outcomes suggest that long-term survival is more common than indicated by earlier reports.[453, 454] MEN2B is transmitted as an autosomal dominant trait,[455–457] but a large percentage of cases appear to represent new mutations.[458] Unilateral or bilateral pheochromocytoma occurs in approximately half of the individuals with this disorder,[455–457, 459] occurs at similar ages,[391] and is histologically similar to that seen in MEN2A.

The identification of the mucosal neuroma phenotype in a child should alert the physician to the diagnosis of MTC. It is important to confirm the diagnosis of MEN2B by DNA testing (discussed later) because there are rare examples of mucosal neuromas without other features of MEN2B or a *RET* mutation.[460–462] In most cases, a *RET* mutation is identified; in those who do not have a codon 918, 883, or 922 mutation, calcitonin testing would be appropriate. In children with MEN2B, total thyroidectomy should be performed during the first month of life. It is not known whether such treatment is curative because experience is limited. The expressivity of the mucosal neuroma phenotype may be less than 100%. A case report in which a mother and one child had mucosal neuromas and MTC and a second child had MTC but no evidence of the mucosal neuroma syndrome suggests this possibility.[463] Therefore, all children born to a parent expressing the phenotype, whether or not clinical evidence of ganglioneuromatosis is present, should have carrier analysis for MEN2B as discussed subsequently. Hyperparathyroidism is rare in MEN2B.[455]

RET Proto-oncogene: Normal or Mutated

Linkage analysis led to the mapping of all variants of MEN2 to proximal chromosome 10,[464–469] and in 1993 mutations of the *RET* proto-oncogene were identified in MEN2A and FMTC.[470, 471] Subsequent workers confirmed these observations[437] and identified point mutations of the *RET* proto-oncogene in MEN2B,[458, 472, 473] MEN2A/Hirschsprung disease variant,[440, 474, 475] MEN2A/cutaneous lichen amyloidosis,[437, 476] and Hirschsprung disease (Table 36–4).[477–479] Later reports identified somatic (present only in the tumor) *RET* proto-oncogene point mutations in at least 25% of sporadic MTCs (Table 36–4 and Fig. 36–15).[475, 480–482]

To understand better how and why small DNA changes within the ret tyrosine kinase receptor cause the unique clinical syndromes associated with MEN2, it is important to review current understanding of the ret receptor complex and the expression of its components and gain insight into its physiologic function. A brief synopsis is presented next.

The Discovery of *RET* and Elucidation of Its Transforming Effects

The *RET* proto-oncogene was discovered in 1985 by Takahashi and colleagues[483] as a result of a chance rearrangement of this gene during DNA extraction. This rearranged form was shown to cause transformation (RET = *re*arranged during *t*ransfection). The *RET* gene has 21 exons covering more than 60 kb of genomic DNA. It encodes a tyrosine kinase receptor composed of a large extracellular domain, a single transmembrane region, and an intracellular tyrosine kinase domain.[484] The extracellular domain includes a cadherin ligand–binding site that may be important for cell-cell signaling and a cysteine-rich extracellular region that is important for receptor dimerization. A number of variants of ret with different molecular weights have been identified, most of which result from alternative RNA processing events.

The *RET* gene was first shown to be a naturally occurring oncogene with the discovery of the papillary thyroid carcinoma oncogene (*RET-PTC* oncogene) 5 years later.[485–487] More than eight different rearrangements (three account for most of the identified forms) have been identified in 25% to 35% of papillary thyroid carcinomas.[488–490] The rearrangements permanently fuse two different genes, appear to result from physical adjacency of *RET* and other genes,[491] and appear to be triggered randomly by insults such as radiation.[492] The net effect of these rearrangements is that the tyrosine kinase of RET is expressed in a cell type (the thyroid follicular cell) that does not normally express this gene. These rearrangements involve two different genes and differ substantially from the single nucleotide changes most frequently associated with MEN2, discussed later. These gene rearrangements lead to expression of a structurally normal RET kinase domain fused to one of several proteins expressed in thyroid follicular cells. Other than a few reports of rearrangement of *RET* in lymphoma and Hürthle cell neoplasms,[493] activated forms of the *RET* gene are frequently involved only in the pathogenesis of two malignant neoplasms, papillary thyroid carcinoma and the several neoplasms found in MEN2.[490]

Normal Physiologic Functions of RET Protein

RET and a second extracellular protein, GFRα-1, together form a receptor for glial cell–derived neurotrophic factor (GDNF), a secretory peptide. A fascinating series of experiments led investigators to piece together the components of this signaling system.[488, 490] Investigators seeking to understand the roles of RET and GDNF created transgenic knockout mouse models for these two genes and independently discovered a nearly identical phenotype in both.[494–498] In a parallel search for a GDNF receptor, a 468-amino-acid protein that bound GDNF was isolated from an embryonic rat midbrain complementary DNA library.[499] This protein was designated GDNFRα-1/GDNF receptor α, now GFRα-1. GFRα-1 is a glycosyl-phosphatidylinositol–linked cell-surface protein that lacks cytoplasmic and transmembrane domains. It is expressed in GDNF-responsive cells and binds GDNF with high affin-

Table 36–4. Germline Mutations of the *RET* Proto-oncogene in Multiple Endocrine Neoplasia Type 2*

Affected Codon	Exon	Amino Acid Change Normal→Mutant	Nucleotide Change Normal→Mutant	Clinical Syndrome	Percentage of All MEN2 Mutations
609	10	Cys→Arg	TGC→CGC	MEN2A/FMTC	0–1
		Cys→Tyr	TGC→TAC†		
611	10	Cys→Tyr	TGC→TAC	MEN2A/FMTC	2–3
		Cys→Trp	TGC→TGG	FMTC	
		Cys→Gly	TGC→GGC		
618	10	Cys→Ser	TGC→AGC‡	MEN2A/FMTC	3–5
		Cys→Gly	TGC→GGC		
		Cys→Arg	TGC→CGC		
		Cys→Phe	TGC→TTC		
		Cys→Ser	TGC→TCC		
		Cys→Tyr	TGC→TAC		
		Cys→End	TGC→TGA		
620	10	Cys→Arg	TGC→CGC§	MEN2A/FMTC	6–8
		Cys→Tyr	TGC→TAC‖		
		Cys→Phe	TGC→TTC		
		Cys→Ser	TGC→TCC		
		Cys→Gly	TGC→GGC		
630	11	Cys→Phe	TGC→TTC	FMTC	<0.1
634	11	Cys→Ser	TGC→AGC	MEN2A¶	80–90
		Cys→Gly	TGC→GGC		
		Cys→Arg	TGC→CGC		
		Cys→Tyr	TGC→TAC		
		Cys→Phe	TGC→TTC		
		Cys→Ser	TGC→TCC		
		Cys→Trp	TGC→TGG		
768	13	Glu→Asp	GAG→GAC	FMTC	0–1
790	13	Leu→Phe	TTG→TTT	MEN2A/FMTC	<0.1
791	13	Tyr→Phe	TAT→TTT	FMTC	<0.1
804	14	Val→Met	GTG→ATG	FMTC	0–1
		Val→Leu	GTG→TTG		
883	15	Ala→Phe	GCT→TTT	MEN2B	—
891	15	Ser→Ala	TCG→GCG	FMTC	0–1
918	16	Met→Thr	ATG→ACG	MEN2B	10–20

*This table describes *RET* mutations identified in most germline carriers of MEN2. A more complete listing of rare mutations can be found in the Human Gene Mutation Database (http://archive.uwcm.ac.uk/uwcm/mg/ns/1/120346.html#ref35) and Online Mendelian Inheritance in Man (http://www.ncbi.nlm.nih.gov/htbin-post/Omim/dispmin?164761). In addition, there are rare mutations that have been identified in individual patients or in sporadic tumors. In some cases the physical location of these rare coding changes adjacent to a sequence known to be mutated gives credibility to the role of the mutant sequence; in others the relevance is unclear. Further clarification of their relevance awaits examination of their transforming abilities or additional genotype-phenotype correlation.

†, §Mutations of these two codons have been reported in Hirschsprung disease.

†, ‡, ‖Reported cases of MEN2A/Hirschsprung disease variants have these mutations.

¶A codon 634 cys→arg (TGC→CGC) mutation accounts for approximately 50% of all mutations associated with MEN2A.

FMTC, familial medullary thyroid carcinoma; MEN2A, multiple endocrine neoplasia type 2A.

ity.[499] GFRα-1 is required for GDNF to bind and activate the RET receptor, forming a multisubunit receptor system in which GFRα-1 is a ligand-binding component and RET is the signaling component (Fig. 36–16).[500, 501] Subsequent experiments showed that targeted disruption of GFRα-1 produced the same phenotype as disruption of RET or GDNF.[502] During the past 5 years, a family of GFR proteins (GFRα-2, GFRα-3) and GDNF-related ligands (artemin, persephin, and neurturin) has been identified. Each of these is likely to have an important developmental role, but there is currently no evidence for their involvement in MEN2.

One important and well-defined function of the RET receptor complex is to direct normal migration of several cell types during embryologic development. The targeting occurs through an interaction of the RET receptor system (RET and GFRα-1) with GDNF. RET is expressed in several tissues of neural crest derivation including C cells of the thyroid gland,[503] adrenal medulla,[504] and parasympathetic, sympathetic, and enteric ganglia.[505, 506] It is also expressed in parathyroid cells derived from the branchial arches[507] and in the ureteric bud.[508] The most well-characterized description of the role played by the RET/GFRα-1/GDNF receptor system is in the developing kidney. Normally, the developing ureteric bud invades the mesonephros, developing into the kidney collecting system by branching during growth into the kidney. RET and GFRα-1 are expressed in the ureteric bud; GDNF is expressed in the mesonephros. Targeted disruption of any of the *RET*, GFRα-1, or GDNF genes in mice causes renal agenesis. In the case of the GDNF knockout, the knockout phenotype can be rescued by implantation of pellets containing GDNF into the developing kidneys.[509] Thus, it appears that GDNF expression in the mesoderm entices the RET/GFRα-1–expressing neurons to grow into the developing kidney.

There is a similar relationship in the gastrointestinal tract. RET/GFRα-1–expressing neurons from the neural crest migrate into the developing gastrointestinal tract, presumably enticed by GDNF-expressing cells.[509] Predictably, disruption of any component of this system leads to a disordered migration of neurons into the gastrointestinal tract and a Hirschsprung-like phenotype. These observations are clinically relevant to both the development of mucosal neuromas (derived from the enteric nervous system) in MEN2B and disordered neural ganglia found in Hirschsprung disease. The *RET* mutations found in MEN2B are activating,[473, 510] whereas about 50% of hereditary Hirschsprung disease is attributable to inactivating mutations of *RET*.[511] There is an unresolved and interesting

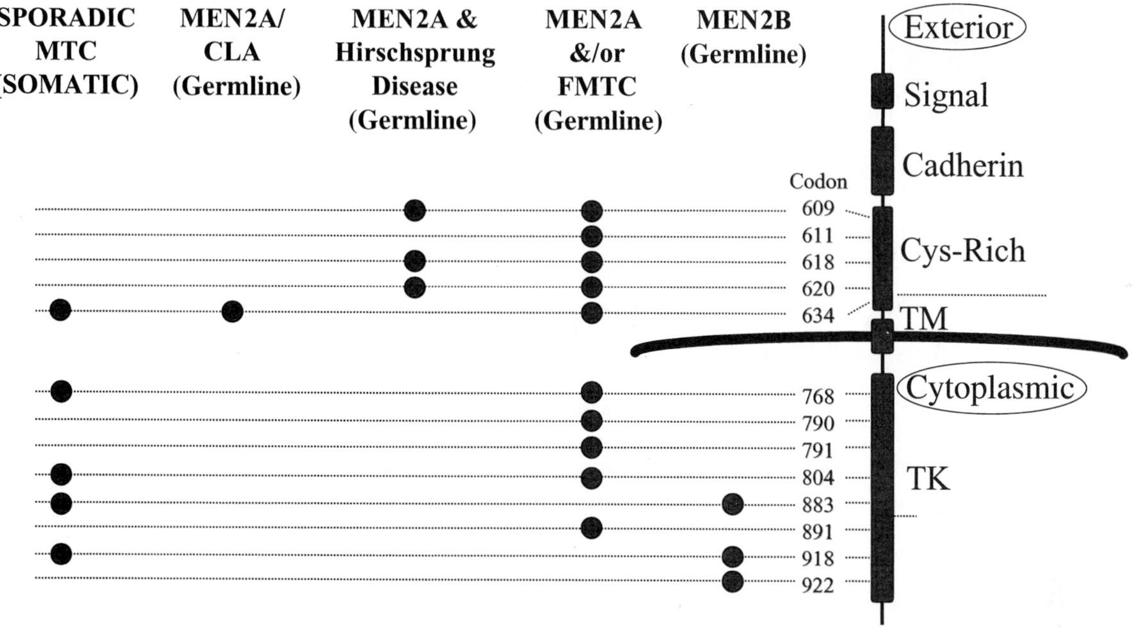

Figure 36–15. Molecular abnormalities of the *RET* proto-oncogene in multiple endocrine neoplasia type 2 (MEN2). Mutations of the *RET* proto-oncogene have been identified in MEN2A, familial medullary thyroid carcinoma (FMTC), MEN2A associated with Hirschsprung disease, MEN2A associated with cutaneous lichen amyloidosis (CLA), and as somatic mutations in sporadic MTC. Two regions of the RET tyrosine kinase are affected. The first is a cysteine-rich extracellular domain (Cys-Rich) important for dimerization of the ret receptor (codons 609, 611, 618, 620, 634). Mutations of individual cysteines at these codons cause RET dimerization, activation, autophosphorylation, and transformation. Mutations of the second region, the intracellular tyrosine kinase (TK) domain involving codons 768, 790, 791, 804, 883, 891, 918, and 922, cause activation, autophosphorylation, and transformation. A role for the cadherin-like region (Cadherin) has not been defined, although it may be involved in an interaction with the glial cell line–derived neurotrophic factor receptor. The most common germ line mutation is a codon 634 mutation that converts a cysteine to an arginine and accounts for 50% or more of all MEN2 mutations. Somatic mutations of codons 768, 804, and 918 have been identified as somatic mutations in sporadic MTC. Codon 768 and 804 mutations are rare; a somatic codon 918 mutation is identified in approximately 25% of sporadic MTCs. (TM, transmembrane domain.)

paradox of hereditary Hirschsprung disease arising from either activating or inactivating mutation of *RET*.

Mutations of the *RET* Proto-oncogene: Correlations with Multiple Endocrine Neoplasia Type 2 Variant or with Tumor Phenotype

RET can undergo gain of function by two types of mutation. The first, discussed two sections earlier, is a rearrangement in which genomic DNA from the *RET* kinase region is fused to a promoter sequence of another gene, creating the *RET-PIC* oncogene. The mutations of *RET* found in MEN2 are missense (amino acid or codon change) mutations. *RET* missense mutations in MEN2 fall into two broad categories: those that affect a group of highly conserved extracellular cysteine residues and a second group of intracellular mutations.

Germ Line RET *Mutations*

The most common mutations in MEN2 affect codons 609, 611, 618, 620, 630, and 634, all encoding extracellular cysteine residues (see Fig. 36–15).[437, 470, 471, 512] Mutations at codon 634 account for more than 80% of mutations in MEN2, and a single coding change, cysteine to arginine at codon 634, is found in approximately 50% of cases.[437] In contrast to MEN1, in which there is no relationship between a specific mutation and clinical phenotype, in MEN2 there is a high degree of correlation. Kindreds with any substitution at codon 634 invariably have MEN2A or one of its variants (Table 36–3), and all reported patients with the MEN2A/cutaneous lichen amyloidosis variant have a mutation at the same codon. Mutations of codons 609, 618, and 620 have been identified in the MEN2A/Hirschsprung variant of MEN2.[435, 475] Other less common extracellular mutations are listed in Table 36–4.

Mutations of the intracellular domain of RET predominantly affect codons 768, 790, 791, 804, 883, 891, 918, and 922. Most cases of MEN2B have a codon 918 mutation, although there are rare examples of codon 883 and 922 mutations. Codon 883, 918, and 922 mutations account for approximately 5% of all mutations in hereditary MTC. The other intracellular domain mutations (codons 768, 790, 791, 804, and 891) are uncommon and account for 2% to 3% of all mutations.[513] They are, however, important because mutations at these codons are most commonly associated with FMTC and are the most likely to be confused with sporadic MTC.

Familial MTC has been identified in kindreds with codon

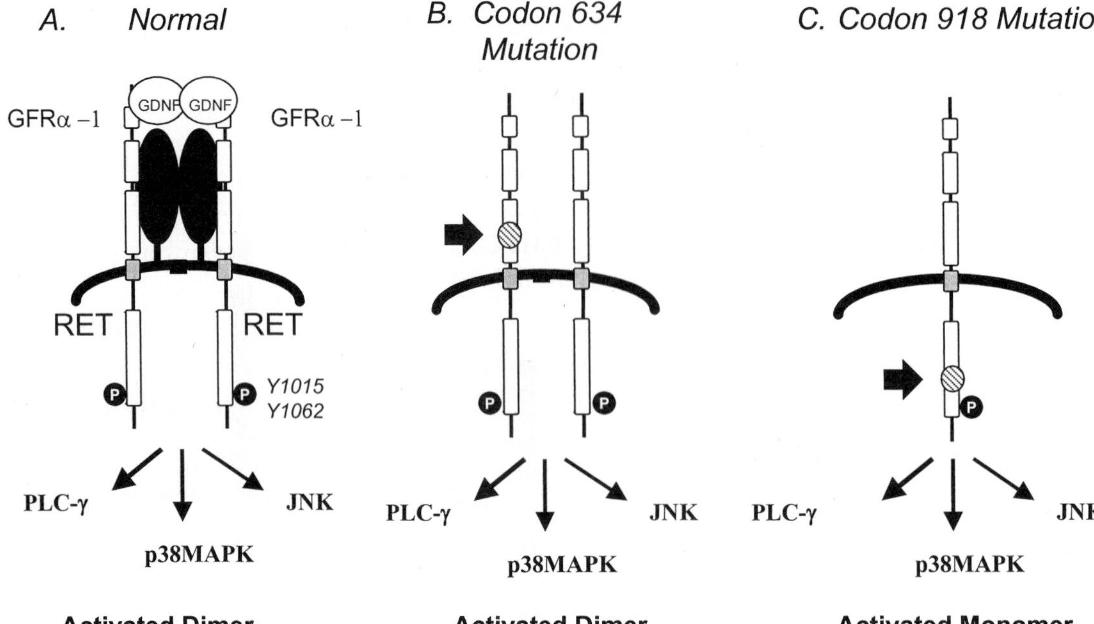

Figure 36–16. The RET tyrosine kinase and glial cell line–derived neurotrophic factor receptor signaling system. *A*, The RET receptor is a tyrosine kinase receptor that couples with the glial cell line–derived neurotrophic factor receptor (GFRα-1) to form a receptor for glial cell line–derived neurotrophic factor (GDNF). In the absence of GDNF, RET and GFRα-1 exist in an undimerized form. Addition of ligand results in activation of the receptor system, autophosphorylation (P), and activation of downstream signaling pathways (phospholipase Cγ [PLCγ], p38MAPK, and JNK pathways). *B*, Mutations of the extracellular cysteine-rich domain (codon 634) cause dimerization, autophosphorylation of the RET receptor complex, and activation of downstream signaling pathways. *C*, Mutations of the intracellular tyrosine kinase (codon 918) cause autophosphorylation and activation of the kinase domain in the absence of dimerization. (MAPK, mitogen-activated protein kinase; JNK, c-Jun N-terminal terminal.)

609, 611, 618, 620, 768, V804M, and 891 mutations,[471, 514–520] making the genotype-phenotype correlation for this clinical syndrome the least specific of the MEN2 variants. Indeed, there is overlap between FMTC and MEN2A for codon 609, 611, 618, and 620 mutations. In a large French series, 60% of 148 patients with FMTC in 47 kindreds had intracellular non-cysteine mutations (codons 768, 790, 804, 891); the remaining 40% had extracellular cysteine mutations at codons 611, 618, and 620.[513] One experimentally based hypothesis to explain this overlap is that mutations of codons 609, 611, 618, 620, 768, 804, and 891, relative to codon 634 or 918 mutations, have a lower in vitro transforming efficiency.[521] Because MTC is most commonly the earliest manifestation of MEN2A, it is possible that kindreds with these *RET* mutations would develop other manifestations of MEN2A if they lived long enough. Alternatively, other potential explanations such as small population-based polymorphisms of the *RET* gene or GFRα-1 or GDNF causing differential activity of this receptor system could be invoked.

The *RET* genotype-phenotype correlation is remarkable. Not only is it possible to predict the clinical phenotype with reasonable certainty (see Fig. 36–15), it is also possible to predict, albeit with considerably less certainty, the aggressiveness of MTC associated with a particular germ line mutation. There is an evolving literature attempting to correlate the clinical aggressiveness of MTC with in vitro studies of transforming efficiency.[521, 522] Although it is possible to make broad correlations, they are at present imperfect in most respects. However, within a given family specific mutations appear to behave in a more predictable manner. For example, in some kindreds with intracellular domain mutations with FMTC, there has never been a death caused by MTC, although the same mutations in other kindreds can be associated with more aggressive disease. These findings suggest that genetic differences of the *RET* gene or other components of the RET signaling system (GDNF, GFRα-1, or downstream effectors in the kinase signaling cascade) may modify the impact of a particular mutation. Clearly, there is more to learn.

Germ line mutations of the *RET* proto-oncogene have also been identified in Hirschsprung disease. Most of these are inactivating mutations,[477–479, 523, 524] although the association of Hirschsprung disease alone, or the MEN2A/Hirschsprung disease variant, with apparent activating mutations at codons 609, 618, and 620 (see Table 36–4) suggests that disordered expression can also lead to this phenotype.[479]

Sporadic (Nonhereditary) RET *Mutations*

Somatic mutation of the *MEN1* gene contributes to the causation of certain sporadic tumors, with a spectrum similar to that of the tumors seen in MEN1. A similar phenomenon is seen for somatic *RET* mutations in sporadic MTC and, to a much lesser extent, pheochromocytoma. Twenty-five percent of sporadic MTCs have a *somatic RET* mutation (60 of 236 cases).[473, 515, 525–537] The most common is a somatic codon 918 mutation identical to that found in the germ line in MEN2B, but other codons (609, 611, 618, 620, 631, 634, 768, 804, 883, and 891) are also mutated somatically. The presence of a codon 918 somatic mutation in an MTC is associated with a greater frequency of distant metastasis[481] and shorter survival.[533] In this respect, the behavior of the sporadic tumor with a somatic mutation parallels the aggressive behavior of MTC in the context of MEN2B caused by a germ line codon 918 mutation.[17]

Somatic RET mutations are considerably less common in sporadic pheochromocytomas than in sporadic MTC. Somatic *RET* mutations were identified in 2 of 35,[538] 2 to 4 of 48,[539] and 0 of 17[540] sporadic pheochromocytomas, for a total of 4 to

6 of 100 (4% to 6%). These results indicate that somatic *RET* mutation is an infrequent cause of sporadic pheochromocytoma. Similarly, in the only study to examine for the presence of somatic *RET* mutations in sporadic parathyroid tumors, none of 35 tumors examined had codon 609, 611, 618, 620, 630, 634, or 918 mutations, making it unlikely that somatic *RET* mutations play any significant role in sporadic hyperparathyroidism.[507]

RET-PTC mutations in papillary thyroid cancer and in a few other neoplasms have already been described. These too are somatic *RET* mutations, but they have no counterpart in the form of *RET* germ line mutations.

Tumorigenesis: Mechanism of *RET*-Induced Transformation

The *RET* gene is normally expressed in the several cell types involved in MEN2, including the C cell, the parathyroid cell, and the adrenal medullary cell. Studies demonstrating tumorigenic mechanisms were performed in an in vitro transformation assay (the NIH3T3 cell culture system), utilizing a cell type that does not usually express RET (hence only the mutant RET was expressed) and is readily transformed. These studies, from several different laboratories,[541–543] provide evidence for two different mechanisms of transformation.

The first mechanism is applicable to extracellular cysteine mutations (prototype was mutant codon 634). The cysteine-rich region has been shown to be important for normal RET receptor dimerization. Homozygous expression of a mutant RET receptor in NIH3T3 cells resulted in dimerization in the absence of either ligand or GFRα-1 and activation of downstream signaling pathways.[541, 542] There is evidence that GDNF is not required for activation of the dimerized ret and, indeed, does not further activate the tyrosine kinase.[544] A second mechanism has been demonstrated for a mutation of the tyrosine kinase domain at codon 918. This mutation causes autophosphorylation of the kinase domain and phosphorylation of downstream substrates (in the absence of RET dimerization or interaction with either GFRα-1 or GDNF). It has been shown experimentally that GDNF can further activate RET kinase in the presence of a codon 918 mutation.[544]

Activation of RET by GDNF or by intragenic activating mutations leads to autophosphorylation of the tyrosine at codons 1015 and 1062 (see Fig. 36–16).[545] There is considerable evidence that autophosphorylation of tyrosine 1062 is required for activation of downstream effector pathways and transformation.[546–548]

A third mechanism results from the gene termed *RET-PTC;* this is *RET* fused to regulatory elements of one of a small number of other genes, most commonly in the thyroid follicular cell (see earlier). These rearrangements drive RET expression in a cell type that does not normally express this gene and promote dimerization.

Tumorigenesis: Steps Distal to Ret

At least three different pathways, JNK,[549] p38MAPK,[550] and phospholipase C gamma,[488, 551] are activated through shc-grb2-src proteins linked to ret.[552, 553] There is also evidence that nuclear factor κB is activated by mutant *RET* and is dependent upon activation of raf and MEKK1.[554] It appears that additional genetic events are involved in the development or progression of the transformed phenotype. Multiple studies have demonstrated a consistent LOH of chromosome 1p, 3p, and 22q in MEN2–related MTC[555–557] and pheochromocytoma.[555–560]

Loss of the normal *RET* allele or amplification of the mutant *RET* allele is found in a significant number of MEN2 tumors.[561, 562] These studies demonstrate somatic amplification of the mutant *RET* allele by at least two different mechanisms: trisomy of chromosome 10 (Fig. 36–17) and duplication of the mutant *RET* allele.[562, 563] Alternatively, in a small percentage of tumors there is loss of the normal *RET* allele. These mutational rearrangements are formally analogous to the second hit at a tumor suppressor gene (see earlier). They help explain why germ line gain-of-function tumorigenesis as in MEN2 shares major properties with germ line loss-of-function tumorigenesis as in MEN1; specifically, both processes have early onset and tumor multiplicity.

It is hypothesized that the effect of amplification of the mutant *RET* allele or loss of the normal copy results in predominant expression of a mutant RET receptor, a model analogous to that demonstrated for *KRAS*[564] and *MET*.[565] In these examples, the normal oncogene moderates the impact of the mutant version. Several mechanisms could be envisioned to explain this mechanism for RET that are directly related to dimerization of the receptor, interaction of the receptor variants with GDNF or linker molecules, or differential activation of downstream mediators by the two different variants. None of these has been proved. This mechanism of unbalanced *RET* expression was not identified earlier, presumably because LOH of chromosome 10, in fact, occurs in only a small percentage of tumors.[566, 567]

Testing for Carrier State and for Tumor Emergence in Multiple Endocrine Neoplasia Type 2

The identification of *RET* proto-oncogene mutations causing MEN2 and FMTC has simplified carrier ascertainment and MTC surveillance in families with identifiable mutations (see Table 36–4).[353–355] Several different analytic techniques have been applied to the identification of mutations,[568] although direct DNA sequencing remains the most widely used. These analytic tests are readily available throughout North America and Europe at modest cost from several commercial sources.* Almost 10 years have passed since the discovery of *RET* mutations in MEN2, and it is now clear that DNA-based diagnosis will replace measurement of calcitonin after pentagastrin or calcium stimulation for carrier ascertainment.[353–355, 568–570] During this period, additional mutations have been described with some regularity and there are now few kindreds with hereditary MTC that do not have an identifiable mutation. In the rare kindred in which a mutation is not identified, continued calcitonin stimulation testing with calcium or pentagastrin (pentagastrin is not currently available in the United States but is available in other countries) is required.

Calcitonin Measurement for Carrier Ascertainment and for Tumor Surveillance

The pentagastrin test is performed by measuring the serum calcitonin level before and 2, 5, and 10 minutes after the intravenous injection of pentagastrin (0.5 μg/kg body weight).[10, 571] Administration of calcium immediately before the pentagastrin injection enhances the sensitivity of the test.[10] A short calcium infusion (15 minutes) can also be used to stimulate calcitonin release.[572] Calcium is the only potent calcitonin secretagogue currently available in the United States.

A positive test is one in which either the basal serum calcitonin concentration is elevated and is further increased by the administration of pentagastrin or calcium or one in which the basal value is normal but increases into the abnormal range

*A listing of available commercial testing sources is available through a Web site: http://www.genetests.org.

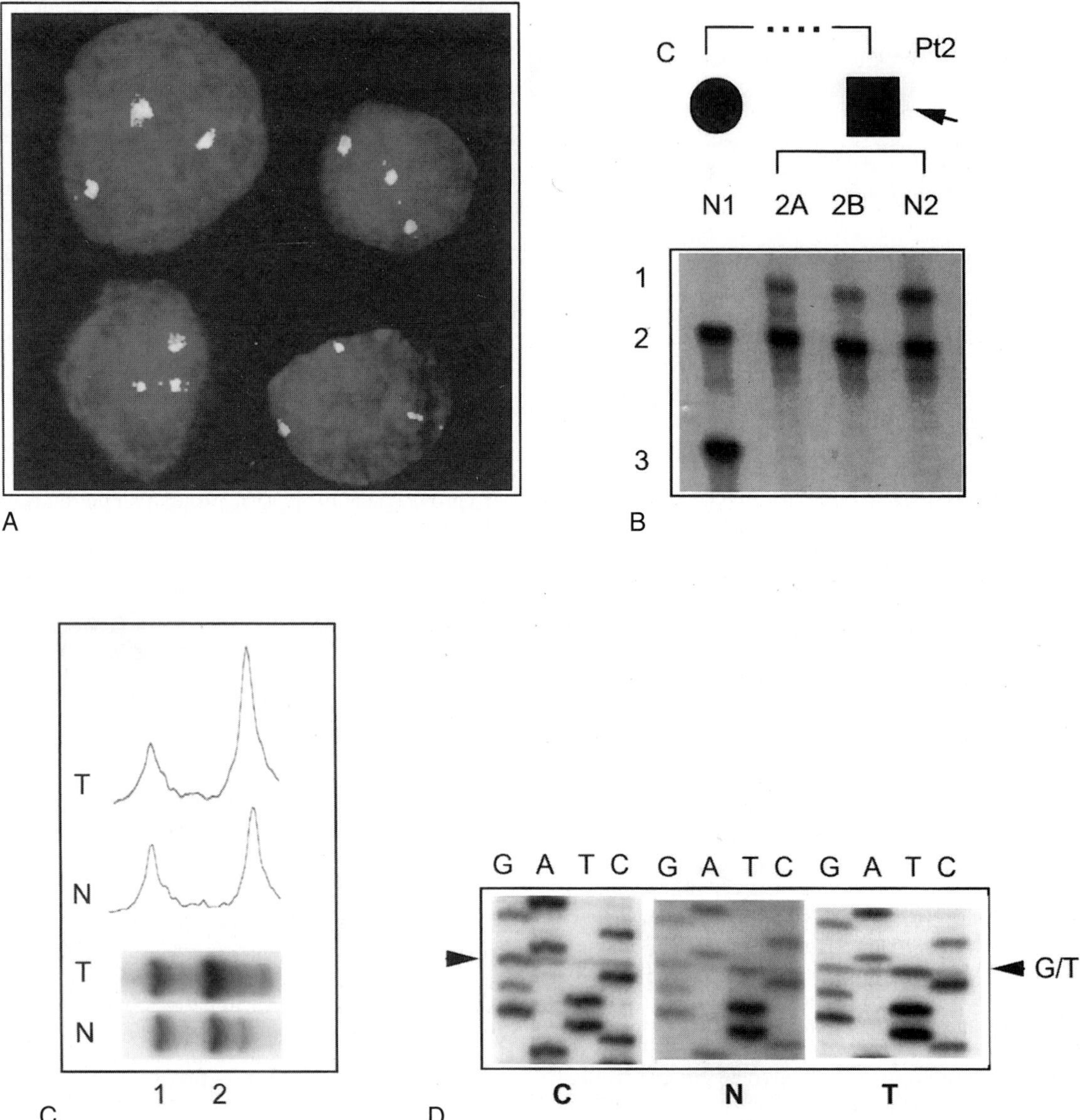

Figure 36–17. Trisomy 10 with nonrandom duplication of the mutant *RET* allele in pheochromocytoma associated with multiple endocrine neoplasia type 2 (MEN2). *A*, Representative interphase fluorescence in situ hybridization analysis of tumor touch preparation from patient 2 (tumor 2A). Three copies of chromosome 10 are shown using a centromeric satellite probe (fluorescein isothiocyanate, green signal) specific for chromosome 10. *B*, Combined pedigree and tumor allelic analysis of patient 2 (Pt2). *Arrow*, patient 2. *Filled symbols*, individuals with MEN2. Genotypes are shown for the chromosome 10 microsatellite marker *D10S1239* linked to the *RET* locus. Allele 2 of *D10S1239* is coinherited with the disease in this patient's family. In patient 2, allele 2 shows greater intensity in lanes 2A and 2B (tumors) than allele 1, representing the wild-type allele, as compared with lane N2 (blood DNA). Lane N1 (blood DNA) shows equal intensities of mutant and wild-type allele in the patient's affected cousin (C). *C*, Representative results of microsatellite and phosphorimage analyses. After polymerase chain reaction amplification using marker *D10S1239*, quantitative measurement of allelic intensity was performed using phosphorimage analysis. In tumor tissue (T), allele 2 is more intense than allele 1. Phosphorimage densitometry shows a 2:1 imbalance between the two alleles in the tumor (T) compared with the normal tissue (N). *D*, Representative results of sequencing analysis of *RET* in tumor 3A. Blood DNA from an unaffected healthy individual (C, *left*) shows the wild-type *RET* sequence (codon 631 GAC). Blood DNA from patient 3 (N, *middle*) shows the germ line mutation (G/T). Tumor DNA (T, *right*) shows a higher intensity of the mutant nucleotide (T) compared with the wild type. (From Huang SC, Koch CA, Vortmeyer AO, et al. Duplication of the mutant *RET* allele in trisomy 10 or loss of the wild-type allele in multiple endocrine neoplasia type 2–associated pheochromocytomas. Cancer Res 2000; 60:6223–6226.) (See also Color Plate.)

after the administration of pentagastrin or calcium. It is important that the samples be analyzed with the most sensitive assay available and with proper control samples; it is now possible to measure normal serum calcitonin levels (0.15 to 3 pmol/L [0.5 to 10 pg/mL]) routinely,[573–576] thereby making it possible to separate normal subjects from most with early C-cell hyperplasia. Criteria that are useful for separation of normal from abnormal kindred members include a parent known to be affected and a consistently abnormal test result (two or more nonconsecutive test results that are abnormal).[11, 16]

It is important to point out, however, that there is considerable overlap between the normal range of serum calcitonin after a provocative test and that observed in patients with early abnormalities of the C cell, a finding that was not fully recognized until *RET* mutation testing became available in 1993. In nearly every large kindred in which calcitonin abnormalities were used to determine carrier status, there are examples of false-positive calcitonin tests that in some kindreds approached 15% of the total number of carriers. In retrospect, the use of calcitonin testing was less of a "gold standard" than thought at the time.

The clinician confronted with the necessity to continue calcitonin testing in a kindred with no identifiable *RET* mutation should keep this experience in mind when assessing minor calcitonin abnormalities in such kindreds. Despite this caveat, it has been the authors' experience that when an abnormal calcitonin test result has been identified, pressure builds to consider total thyroidectomy. A discussion with the family of the risks (hypoparathyroidism, need for continued thyroid supplementation, and recurrent laryngeal nerve damage) and a firm plan of continued testing at 6- to 12-month intervals often allay parental concern or provide a more balanced viewpoint. It is clear from the 25-year experience with provocative calcitonin testing that there is progression of calcitonin abnormalities over a several year period in carriers, adding certainty to the diagnosis. Whether a deferral of decision to operate increases the risk of metastatic disease is unknown, although long-term experience with children with codon 634 mutations indicates that 85% to 90% remain disease-free 25 years after total thyroidectomy, performed at an average age of 13 years.[16]

An elevation of the basal serum calcitonin level with no further increase after a provocative test can be difficult to interpret. Such a test result can be seen in association with C-cell abnormalities, but this type of result is most likely to be caused by a nonspecific or false-positive increase of the serum calcitonin concentration[16, 577] or by production of calcitonin by a tumor other than MTC (lung carcinoma, hepatoma, pheochromocytoma, pancreatic islet cell tumor, or benign liver disease). Separation of a false-positive test result from a true elevation of the serum calcitonin concentration can be achieved by a radioimmunoassay using a different polyclonal antiserum or a two-site immunoradiometric assay.[575, 576] Establishment of ectopic production of calcitonin by a tumor other than MTC can be more difficult because calcitonin release is frequently enhanced by calcium or pentagastrin[578]; however, such tumors frequently produce a high-molecular-weight form of unprocessed procalcitonin, a finding that may be helpful in selected cases.[579]

Method of *RET* Sequence Testing in DNA

DNA diagnostic techniques currently in use to identify MEN2 gene carriers are based on the use of polymerase chain reaction techniques to amplify selected portions of the *RET* proto-oncogene known to be mutated in MEN2. All laboratories analyze for mutations in exons 10, 11, and 16 (codons 609, 611, 618, 620, 630, 634, and 918), those most commonly found in MEN2. If a mutation is not identified in one of these codons, some but not all laboratories analyze for mutations in exons 13, 14, and 15 (codons 768, 790, 791, 804, 883, and 891). If a mutation is not identified in exon 10, 11, or 16, it is important to identify a laboratory that will examine the other exons before concluding that no mutation is present. This is particularly true for kindreds with FMTC, a disproportionate number of which have an exon 13, 14, or 15 mutation.[513] Although there is a potential for several types of errors in mutational analysis,[355, 580] a repeated analysis of each positive or negative test result in a separate testing facility with an independently obtained DNA sample provides nearly 100% certainty that an individual test result is accurate. About 10 years of experience with this type of testing[17] has provided insight into its usefulness in various clinical settings.

Germ Line *RET* Mutation: Three Categories of Risk

There is now consensus that all patients with a *RET* mutation should be offered a total thyroidectomy. In the almost 10 years since the identification of these mutations, greater awareness of the relationship between mutation at a specific *RET* codon and the clinical aggressiveness of the MTC has developed. Although imperfect in many respects, a consensus has developed within the field that these difference should be considered in the decision-making process regarding early thyroidectomy. The consensus guidelines have divided hereditary MTC into three different risk categories.[17]

Category 1. Highest risk: In the highest risk category are those with MEN2B and a codon 883, 918, or 922 *RET* mutation. In these children MTC with metastasis may occur during the first year of life,[351, 448–451] prompting a recommendation for total thyroidectomy and central lymph node dissection in such children during the first 6 months of life and preferably during the first month. During this procedure, other level II to V lymph nodes should be sampled with performance of more extensive lymph node dissection if metastatic disease is identified.

Category 2. High risk: Cases with *RET* mutations of codons 609, 611, 618, 620, or 634 are classified as having high risk. They should have a total thyroidectomy, including removal of the posterior capsule, before the age of 5 years. This recommendation is based on the finding of microscopic MTC in two children with a codon 634 mutation at age 2 years[581, 582] and nodal metastasis in children at age 5[352, 450] and 6[583] years. There is less consensus regarding the need for central node dissection, although a majority of surgeons perform this dissection during the primary surgery so that they do not need to reoperate in the central compartment in the event that primary surgery is not curative.[17, 354, 377]

Category 3. Intermediate risk: Cases with codon 768, 790, 791, 804, or 891 mutations are classified as having intermediate risk. The biologic behavior and clinical aggressiveness of MTC in patients with such mutations vary, but the MTC tends to be less aggressive. Lymph node metastasis and death have been identified with all these mutations except codon 791. There is no consensus regarding the age of total thyroidectomy in such children. Two approaches are used. Some classify these patients with the high-risk category and perform a total thyroidectomy by the age of 5 years. Some recommend thyroidectomy by the age of 10 years. Others observe cases with these mutations with periodic provocative tests for calcitonin and perform a total thyroidectomy when calcitonin levels become clearly abnormal. There is consensus, however, that these patients should be followed up especially carefully if an early thyroidectomy is not performed. There are large kindreds with some of these mutations in which there has never been a death caused by MTC, making it difficult to convince family members that early thyroidectomy is indicated.

Multiple Endocrine Neoplasia Type 2 Kindred with Known *RET* Mutation

A normal *RET* analysis in a kindred with a known *RET* mutation excludes the carrier state with nearly 100% certainty. An individual with two independently obtained negative DNA test results in the context of a family with an identified missense mutation can be excluded from further carrier ascertainment. Pentagastrin testing in this situation adds almost nothing to the diagnostic accuracy and may actually confuse the clinical assessment because of a high incidence of false-positive results.[355]

Occult Phenotypes. Should *RET* Germ Line be Tested in a Case with an Apparently Sporadic Tumor in the Spectrum of Multiple Endocrine Neoplasia Type 2?

Germ Line Mutations in Sporadic Medullary Thyroid Carcinoma

A compilation of over 200 patients with apparent sporadic MTC who were examined for *germ line RET* mutations (codons 609, 611, 618, 620, 630, and in some cases 768) has identified mutations in approximately 6% of the total (this contrasts with data to be presented subsequently showing that approximately 25% of sporadic MTCs have a *somatic RET* mutation without a corresponding germ line abnormality).[475, 527, 537, 584] Subsequent investigation of the individuals in these studies with germ line *RET* mutations has demonstrated that the majority were members of previously unidentified kindreds or descendants of gene carriers who were separated from their families without knowledge of MEN2 in the family. There have been at least eight examples of de novo germ line mutations in which the affected individual carries a *RET* proto-oncogene mutation but neither parent is affected.[475, 537, 585, 586] In four of these cases in which it was tested and in most new MEN2B probands,[458] the newly mutated allele is derived from the unaffected father, suggesting acquisition of the mutation during spermatogenesis.

The finding that 6% of patients with apparent sporadic MTC carry germ line *RET* mutations suggests that all patients with MTC should have a *RET* germ line analysis performed. This is especially important because identification of one hereditary case may have a multiplier effect, leading to the diagnosis of unsuspected cases in the family and effective early treatment.[475] Negative family history, although useful, clearly does not exclude hereditary disease. A second reason for performing a *RET* germ line analysis is to reassure the patient and family members that there is no hereditary component. If the *RET* analysis is negative, hereditary disease can be excluded with greater than 99% certainty.[475] Most families of patients with sporadic MTC are assured by a less than 1% probability of hereditary disease; for those who want hereditary MTC excluded with 100% certainty, continued provocative calcitonin testing in relatives is required.

Germ Line Mutations in Sporadic Pheochromocytoma

The situation is less clear for apparently sporadic pheochromocytoma. Three genetic syndromes—MEN2, VHL, and hereditary pheochromocytoma or paraganglioma syndrome—can present as a sporadic pheochromocytoma. This presentation is unlikely for type 1 neurofibromatosis. Estimates of frequency of heredity for pheochromocytoma in the general population have ranged from 9%[333] to as high as 23%[587] in some series. It is important to recognize that these estimates came from tertiary care centers and in one, located in southwest Germany, there is a high incidence of VHL (84% of those with apparent sporadic pheochromocytomas found to have hereditary disease had VHL and with likely descent from one ancestor), raising the question of whether these percentages are relevant to the general population.[587]

Estimates based on genetic testing of *RET* in three other studies were that 2 of 230 patients (<1%) with apparently sporadic pheochromocytoma had a *germ line* mutation.[538, 539, 588] The low frequency is not surprising because pheochromocytomas in MEN2 are most commonly found with codon 634 RET mutations. The 50% penetrance of pheochromocytomas in these families makes it likely that the hereditary nature of these tumors can be identified by a careful family history. Germ line mutation of GDNF has been identified in 1 of 50 sporadic pheochromocytomas.[589, 590] The significance of this single mutation is unclear. Similarly, germ line VHL mutations in apparent sporadic pheochromocytoma are uncommon, being found in only 9 of 173 sporadic pheochromocytomas (5.2%) in four series.[540, 588, 591, 592] Finally, there are at least four different familial pheochromocytoma-paraganglionoma syndromes that have been mapped (PGL1, PGL2, PGL3, and familial pheochromocytoma-paraganglioma syndrome). Mutations of components of the succinate dehydrogenase complex gene, putative tumor suppressor genes because each of the mutations appears to be inactivating, have been identified in three of the four variants.[593–595, 654–656] There is currently no information regarding the frequency of these mutations.

The decision to pursue *RET* and *VHL* germ line testing in patients with apparent sporadic pheochromocytoma is somewhat more complicated than testing for MTC. There are several arguments for testing. When the incidences of *RET* and *VHL* mutations are combined (~6%), they approximate the incidence observed for germ line *RET* mutations in apparent sporadic MTC. In addition, the argument can be advanced that identification of hereditary pheochromocytoma prevents sudden death or significant morbidity related to pheochromocytoma or, in the case of MEN2A, results in earlier identification of MTC in other affected family members. The arguments against testing include the low frequency of mutations (particularly for *RET*), the necessity to test for both MEN2A and VHL (and possibly familial pheochromocytoma-paraganglionoma syndrome) leading to a substantial expenditure, and the fact that most hereditary pheochromocytoma comes to attention because of its distinctive clinical features before serious morbidity. A pragmatic approach is to apply criteria similar to those outlined for carrier ascertainment in MEN1. The information is useful, helps families to address health problems, provides reassurance if the test is negative, and leads to appropriate screening when a mutation is identified. It is, however, not absolutely necessary because no specific clinical action other than screening for pheochromocytoma or other neoplastic components of VHL or MEN2 is based on the test result.

Periodic Tumor Surveillance in a Known Carrier. Should Evaluation for Tumors Other than Medullary Thyroid Carcinoma Be Performed in Kindreds with Familial Medullary Thyroid Carcinoma?

Mutations at codons 768, 791, V804M, and 891 have been associated exclusively with FMTC; nonetheless, it would be prudent to consider a screening urine catecholamines or metanephrine test for pheochromocytoma at the time of diagnosis and perhaps at 5-year intervals. Codon 609, 611, 618, 620, or 630 mutations have been associated with either FMTC or MEN2A. Unless there is a several generation pattern of FMTC in more than 10 affected family members, it would be prudent to screen every 1 to 3 years for pheochromocytoma. The molecular basis for the phenotypic variability (FMTC or MEN2A) with codon 609, 611, 618, 620, or 630 mutations is unknown at present, although an answer may be found in the population-based polymorphisms discussed earlier in this chapter.

Management of an Established Multiple Endocrine Neoplasia Type 2 Kindred

Counseling

Family education is an important component in the management of MEN2. Although a physician's legal responsibility may end after immediate family members have been notified of the genetic nature of the disease, it is prudent to encourage patients to make even family members at distant risk aware of the nature of the disease. The fact that the disease appears to be benign in one generation should not deter carrier ascertainment and tumor surveillance efforts because the disease may assume a more virulent expression in a subsequent generation.[596] This notification can be done by giving pamphlets describing the syndrome to immediate family members for distribution to more distant relatives (available at www.endocrine.mdacc.tmc.edu).

Prospects for Surgical Cure of Medullary Thyroid Carcinoma in Multiple Endocrine Neoplasia Type 2

Widespread prospective carrier ascertainment and tumor surveillance have had an impact on the natural history of the syndrome. The age at carrier ascertainment has progressively fallen from a mean of 33 years when prospective carrier ascertainment through tumor surveillance first began in 1969 to a mean below 13 years in 1988.[597, 598] The current mean age with widespread DNA testing is likely to be below the age of 5 years. Testing for *RET* mutations now makes it possible to identify carrier status at birth or in utero.

Whether prospective DNA-based ascertainment and early thyroidectomy are curative for the thyroid neoplasm is less clear. Follow-up data from several groups indicate that approximately 85% to 90% but not 100% of kindred members who were thyroidectomized for early disease on the basis of pentagastrin testing have normal or nondetectable calcitonin values at mean follow-up periods ranging from 1 to 15 years.[13, 16, 339] It can be anticipated that earlier DNA-based ascertainment and treatment are likely to improve the outcome in gene carriers. None of the cases of MEN2A or FMTC identified by DNA-based carrier ascertainment and operated before the age of 5 years have had identifiable metastasis,[353–355, 582, 583, 599–604] although there was considerable variability in these small series in the numbers of nodes sampled.

The identification of MTC (without nodal metastasis) in a significant number of children with MEN2A between the ages of 2 and 5 years[581, 582] suggests that a child younger than 5 years with metastatic disease may be identified. There are insufficient data regarding the impact of a specific mutation on the presence or absence of metastasis in younger children, although several groups are now combining information from national databases, making it possible that such data will be available in the next few years. In summary, early carrier ascertainment and treatment by total thyroidectomy at an early age appear to identify and treat patients before there is identifiable lymph node metastasis. Thus, it is possible that death from hereditary MTC will be largely eliminated by this early intervention, making it the first example of successful use of genetic ascertainment to eliminate death from malignancy. However, it will be many years before the impact of this earlier intervention on cure of MTC will be demonstrated.

MULTIPLE ENDOCRINE NEOPLASIA OF MIXED TYPE

Overlap Syndromes

Overlap syndromes in single patients include gastrinoma in a MEN2 patient,[605] adenomatous polyposis coli with MEN1 or MEN2B,[606, 607] posterior pituitary tumor and MEN1,[608] prolactinoma in a patient with MEN2A,[609] and pheochromocytomas in MEN1 (see earlier). There is a single case report of an ovarian strumal carcinoid tumor, a variant of an ovarian teratoma, in a patient with MEN2A. The tumor was composed of neuroendocrine cells with thyroid-like follicles that stained positive for thyroglobulin.[610]

Most cases of overlap of MEN1 and MEN2 were published before the era of discovery of syndrome-causing genes. Currently, most can be understood as follows:

1. Unusual expressions of a syndrome. Thus, VHL can cause pheochromocytoma and islet tumor (see later), neurofibromatosis type 1 (NF1) can cause pheochromocytoma and duodenal somatostatinoma (see later), and MEN1 can cause pheochromocytoma with any other feature of MEN1 (see before).
2. Coexistence of two rare disorders.
3. Rare syndromes that have not yet been characterized sufficiently.
4. Few cases of unexplained overlap. In this regard, a mouse model (see earlier) has many features of both MEN1 and MEN2, suggesting a single pathway to both syndromes or an overlap.[302]

Familial Occurrence of Two or More Endocrine Neoplastic Disorders

MEN1 and MEN2 are the only multiple neoplasia syndromes in which the two most prominent features are hormone-secreting tumors. In other MEN syndromes, nonhormonal tumors are more urgent. For example, the McCune-Albright syndrome (which is not hereditary) features fibrous dysplasia of bone and café-au-lait spots of skin (Chapter 27) and VHL syndrome features papillary renal cancer and central nervous system hemangioblastomas.

Von Hippel–Lindau Syndrome

VHL syndrome is an autosomal dominant neoplastic syndrome characterized by hemangioblastomas of the central nervous system, retinal angiomas, renal cell carcinomas, visceral cysts, pheochromocytoma, and islet cell tumors.[611, 612] More than 90% of gene carriers express one or more of the manifestations of this disorder by the age of 60 years. Over 70% of gene carriers have one or more central nervous system tumors.[613] Of particular relevance to endocrinologists is the observation that 25% to 35% of these patients have unilateral or bilateral pheochromocytomas and 15% to 20% have islet cell tumors.[62, 611, 614] Although the islet cell tumors may immunostain weakly for insulin, they virtually never hypersecrete it.[62]

The *VHL* gene was mapped to chromosome 3p25.3[615] and identified by positional cloning.[616] This gene is a tumor suppressor gene, implying that loss of function or inactivating mutations of both alleles or copies of this gene are associated with tumor formation. Studies have described an inhibitory effect of the *VHL*-encoded protein on transcription elongation through its binding to an elongin B/C complex. Mutation of the *VHL* gene, particularly in the region of codons 150 to 170, interferes with this interaction, resulting in an accelerated rate of transcription elongation.[617–619] Another mechanism may explain many of the properties of the *VHL* protein and disease. The action of the VHL protein to facilitate the proteasome-mediated degradation of the hypoxia-inducible factor 1 (HIF-1) protein and other proteins may prove central to many manifestations of *VHL* gene alteration.[620] Mutation of codon 238 was identified in over 40% of VHL families with pheochromocytoma, suggesting that families with a mutation in this codon should be surveyed routinely for pheochromocytoma.[621] As with other recessive oncogenes such as *MEN1*, *p53*, *BRCA1*, or retinoblastoma gene, a large number of inactivating mutations have been described for *VHL*.

Clinical management for patients with VHL syndrome is often complicated by the presence of renal or central nervous system tumors. Pheochromocytomas or islet cell tumors associated with hypertension, cardiac arrhythmias, hypoglycemia, watery diarrhea, carcinoid, or a glucagonoma-like picture should be surgically excised. Judgment is required in the management of other malignant features associated with VHL. For example, a less aggressive approach to the management of pheochromocytoma or islet cell tumor may be indicated in a patient with VHL and a renal cell carcinoma with metastasis. An adrenal cortical sparing operation may be appropriate for pheochromocytoma in such a patient.[397, 416]

The association of pheochromocytoma and islet cell tumors can occur in familial[622–624] or nonfamilial[625–628] patterns. There is little information about the molecular genetics of these rare disorders, although it is possible that abnormalities of the *VHL* gene may be involved.

Neurofibromatosis Type 1

The main features of NF1 are neurofibromas and dermal café-au-lait spots. NF1 has been associated with a variety of endocrine neoplasms including pheochromocytoma,[629] hyperparathyroidism,[630] somatostatin-producing carcinoid tumors of the duodenal wall,[631–633] MTC,[634] and hypothalamic or optic nerve tumors that cause precocious puberty.[635] The causative gene for NF1 encodes a res guanosine triphosphatase (GTPase)–activating protein (GAP) of 2818 amino acids, named neurofibromin, which accelerates GTP hydrolysis on p21 res. Loss of the GTPase-activating function of neurofibromin (through mutation or allelic loss) leads to p21 *ras* activation.[636] More specific evidence for a role of this protein in endocrine tumors is shown by allelic loss of this gene in NF1-associated[637] or sporadic[638] pheochromocytomas. Targeted disruption of the mouse *NF1* gene resulted in sympathetic ganglia hyperplasia, providing additional evidence for a potential role of this gene in the genesis of endocrine tumors derived from neural crest tissue.[639]

Carney's Complex

Carney's complex comprises myxomas of the heart, skin, and breast; spotty skin pigmentation; testicular, adrenal cortical, and growth hormone–secreting pituitary tumors; and peripheral nerve schwannomas.[640–642] Linkage analysis has identified a locus at 2p in half of the families and another locus at 17q in most others.[643] The gene at 17q has been identified as encoding the regulatory subunit (type IA) of protein kinase A (*PRKA1A*), and it has tumor suppressor properties.[644] The activating *GNAS1* mutations in McCune-Albright syndrome and the inactivating *PRKA1A* mutations in Carney's complex are likely to cause tumors in selected tissues with a similar tissue spectrum by raising cyclic adenosine monophosphate.

Confusion and Contrasts between Multiple Endocrine Neoplasia Type 1 and Type 2

There is occasional confusion between MEN1 and MEN2, particularly among patients, paramedical personnel, and nonspecialists. The main source of confusion is the similar syndrome names. Several other similarities are recognized (see the introduction). In fact, the differences are more important than the similarities. MEN2 includes a cancer that can be prevented or cured by timely surgery. MEN1 also causes cancers, but these mostly cannot be prevented or cured. The principal tumors differ between MEN1 and MEN2, as do surveillance protocols and treatments. Gene testing in MEN2 should be started extremely early and management should be dependent on the phenotype or genotype. Gene testing in MEN1 has debatable indications for early usage and no genotype-phenotype correlation. Mutations of *RET* cause tumors in MEN2 by gain of function, whereas *MEN1* does this by loss of function. As a result, the oncogenic *RET* mutations are confined to selected loci of the gene and are thus easier to identify than those in the *MEN1* gene.

References

1. Erdheim J. Zur normalen und pathologischen Histologie der Glandula Thyreoidea, Parathyreoidea und Hypophysis. Beitr Pathol Anat 1903; 33:158–236.
2. Underdahl LO, Woolner LB, Black BM. Multiple endocrine adenomas: report of 8 cases in which the parathyroids, pituitary and pancreatic islets were involved. J Clin Endocrinol 1953; 13:20–47.
3. Moldawer MP, Nardi GL, Raker JW. Concomitance of multiple adenomas of parathyroids and pancreatic islets with tumor of pituitary: syndrome with familial incidence. Am J Med Sci 1954; 228:190–206.
4. Wermer P. Genetic aspects of adenomatosis of endocrine glands. Am J Med 1954; 16:363–371.
5. Sipple JH. The association of pheochromocytoma with carcinoma of the thyroid gland. Am J Med 1961; 31:163–166.
6. Ballard HS, Frame B, Hartsock RJ. Familial multiple endocrine adenoma-peptic ulcer complex. Medicine (Baltimore) 1964; 43: 481–516.
7. Steiner AL, Goodman AD, Powers SR. Study of a kindred with pheochromocytoma, medullary carcinoma, hyperparathyroidism and Cushing's disease: multiple endocrine neoplasia, type 2. Medicine (Baltimore) 1968; 47:371–409.
8. Melvin KEW, Tashjian AH Jr, Miller HH. Studies in familial (medullary) thyroid carcinoma. Recent Prog Horm Res 1972; 28: 399–470.
9. Chong GC, Beahrs OH, Sizemore GW, et al. Medullary carcinoma of the thyroid gland. Cancer 1975; 35:695–704.
10. Wells SA Jr, Ontjes DA, Cooper CW, et al. The early diagnosis of medullary carcinoma of the thyroid gland in patients with multiple endocrine neoplasia type II. Ann Surg 1975; 182:362–370.
11. Graze K, Spiler IJ, Tashjian AH Jr, et al. Natural history of familial medullary thyroid carcinoma: effect of a program for early diagnosis. N Engl J Med 1978; 299:980–985.
12. Marx SJ, Vinik AI, Santen RJ, et al. Multiple endocrine neoplasia type I: assessment of laboratory tests to screen for the gene in a large kindred. Medicine (Baltimore) 1986; 65:226–241.
13. Telander RL, Zimmerman D, van Heerden JA, et al. Results of early thyroidectomy for medullary thyroid carcinoma in children with multiple endocrine neoplasia type 2. J Pediatr Surg 1986; 21:1190–1194.
14. Benson L, Ljunghall S, Akerstrom G, et al. Hyperparathyroidism presenting as the first lesion in multiple endocrine neoplasia type 1. Am J Med 1987; 82:731–737.
15. Norton JA, Cornelius MJ, Doppman JL, et al. Effect of parathy-

roidectomy in patients with hyperparathyroidism, Zollinger-Ellison syndrome, and multiple endocrine neoplasia type I: a prospective study. Surgery 1987; 102:958–966.
16. Gagel RF, Tashjian AH Jr, Cummings T, et al. The clinical outcome of prospective screening for multiple endocrine neoplasia type 2a: an 18-year experience. N Engl J Med 1988; 318:478–484.
17. Brandi ML, Gagel RF, Angeli A, et al. Guidelines for diagnosis and therapy of MEN type 1 and type 2. J Clin Endocrinol Metab 2001; 86:5658–5671.
18. Marx S. Multiple endocrine neoplasia type 1. In Bilezekian JP, Marcus R, Levine MA (eds). The Parathyroids: Basic and Clinical Concepts, 2nd ed. San Diego, Academic Press, 2001, pp 535–584.
19. Eberle F, Grun R. Multiple endocrine neoplasia, type I (MEN I). Ergeb Inn Med Kinderheilkd 1981; 46:76–149.
20. Trump D, Farren B, Wooding C, et al. Clinical studies of multiple endocrine neoplasia type 1 (MEN1). Q J Med 1996; 89:653–669.
21. Marx S, Spiegel AM, Skarulis MC, et al. Multiple endocrine neoplasia type 1: clinical and genetic topics. Ann Intern Med 1998; 129:484–494.
22. Lamers CB, Froeling PG. Clinical significance of hyperparathyroidism in familial multiple endocrine adenomatosis type I (MEA I). Am J Med 1979; 66:422–424.
23. Jackson CE, Boonstra CE. The relationship of hereditary hyperparathyroidism to endocrine adenomatosis. Am J Med 1967; 43:727–734.
24. Johnson GJ, Summerskill WH, Anderson VE, et al. Clinical and genetic investigation of a large kindred with multiple endocrine adenomatosis. N Engl J Med 1967; 277:1379–1385.
25. Craven DE, Goodman D, Carter JH. Familial multiple endocrine adenomatosis: multiple endocrine neoplasia, type I. Arch Intern Med 1972; 129:567–569.
26. Snyder N III, Scurry MT, Deiss WP. Five families with multiple endocrine adenomatosis. Ann Intern Med 1972; 76:53–58.
27. Jung RT, Grant AM, Davie M, et al. Multiple endocrine adenomatosis (type I) and familial hyperparathyroidism. Postgrad Med 1978; 54:92–94.
28. Burgess JR, David R, Greenaway TM, et al. Osteoporosis in multiple endocrine neoplasia type 1: severity, clinical significance, relationship to primary hyperparathyroidism, and response to parathyroidectomy. Arch Surg 1999; 134:1119–1123.
29. Rizzoli R, Green J III, Marx SJ. Primary hyperparathyroidism in familial multiple endocrine neoplasia type I: long-term follow-up of serum calcium levels after parathyroidectomy. Am J Med 1985; 78:467–474.
30. Marx SJ, Menczel J, Campbell G, et al. Heterogeneous size of the parathyroid glands in familial multiple endocrine neoplasia type 1. Clin Endocrinol (Oxf) 1991; 35:521–526.
31. Hellman P, Skogseid B, Oberg K, et al. Primary and reoperative parathyroid operations in hyperparathyroidism of multiple endocrine neoplasia type 1. Surgery 1998; 124:993–999.
32. Sato M, Miyauchi A, Namihira H, et al. A newly recognized germline mutation of *MEN1* gene identified in a patient with parathyroid adenoma and carcinoma. Endocrine 2000; 12:223–226.
33. Friedman E, Sakaguchi K, Bale AE, et al. Clonality of parathyroid tumors in familial multiple endocrine neoplasia type 1. N Engl J Med 1989; 321:213–218.
34. Brandi ML, Aurbach GD, Fitzpatrick LA, et al. Parathyroid mitogenic activity in plasma from patients with familial multiple endocrine neoplasia type 1. N Engl J Med 1986; 314:1287–1293.
35. Brown EM, Pollak M, Hebert SC. The extracellular calcium-sensing receptor: its role in health and disease. Annu Rev Med 1998; 49:15–29.
36. Kifor O, Moore FD Jr, Wang P, et al. Reduced immunostaining for the extracellular Ca^{2+}-sensing receptor in primary and uremic secondary hyperparathyroidism. J Clin Endocrinol Metab 1996; 81:1598–1606.
37. Jensen RT. Management of the Zollinger-Ellison syndrome in patients with multiple endocrine neoplasia type 1. J Intern Med 1998; 243:477–488.
38. Shawker TH, Avila N, Premkumar A, et al. Ultrasound evaluation of primary hyperparathyroidism. Ultrasound Q 2000; 16:73–87.
39. Pattou F, Torres G, Mondragon-Sanchez A, et al. Correlation of parathyroid scanning and anatomy in 261 unselected patients with sporadic primary hyperparathyroidism. Surgery 1999; 126:1123–1131.
40. Norman J, Chheda H, Farrell C. Minimally invasive parathyroidectomy for primary hyperparathyroidism: decreasing operative time and potential complications while improving cosmetic results. Am Surg 1998; 64:391–395; discussion 395–396.
41. Thompson GB, Grant CS, Perrier ND, et al. Reoperative parathyroid surgery in the era of sestamibi scanning and intraoperative parathyroid hormone monitoring. Arch Surg 1999; 134:699–704; discussion 704–705.
42. Jaskowiak N, Norton JA, Alexander HR, et al. A prospective trial evaluating a standard approach to reoperation for missed parathyroid adenoma. Ann Surg 1996; 224:308–320; discussion 320–321.
43. Irvin GL 3rd, Molinari AS, Figueroa C, et al. Improved success rate in reoperative parathyroidectomy with intraoperative PTH assay. Ann Surg 1999; 229:874–878; discussion 878–879.
44. Tonelli F, Spini S, Tommasi M. Intraoperative PTH measurement in patients with MEN1 syndrome and hyperparathyroidism. World J Surg 1999; 24:556–563.
45. Libutti SK, Alexander HR, Bartlett DL, et al. Kinetic analysis of the rapid intraoperative parathyroid hormone assay in patients during operation for hyperparathyroidism. Surgery 1999; 126:1145–1150; discussion 1150–1151.
46. Feldman AL, Sharaf RN, Skarulis MC, et al. Results of heterotopic parathyroid autotransplantation: a 13-year experience. Surgery 1999; 126:1042–1048.
47. Majewski JT, Wilson SD. The MEA-I syndrome: an all or none phenomenon. Surgery 1979; 86:475–484.
48. Skogseid B, Oberg K, Eriksson B, et al. Surgery for asymptomatic pancreatic lesion in multiple endocrine neoplasia type I. World J Surg 1996; 20:872–876; discussion 877.
49. Wilkinson S, Teh BT, Davey KR, et al. Cause of death in multiple endocrine neoplasia type 1. Arch Surg 1993; 128:683–690.
50. Doherty GM, Olson JA, Frisella MM, et al. Lethality of multiple endocrine neoplasia type I. World J Surg 1998; 22:581–586; discussion 586–587.
51. Yu F, Venzon DJ, Serrano J, et al. Prospective study of the clinical course, prognostic factors, causes of death, and survival in patients with long-standing Zollinger-Ellison syndrome. J Clin Oncol 1999; 17:615–630.
52. Kloppel G, Willemer S, Stamm B, et al. Pancreatic lesions and hormonal profile of pancreatic tumors in multiple endocrine neoplasia type I: an immunocytochemical study of nine patients. Cancer 1986; 57:1824–1832.
53. Le Bodic MF, Heymann MF, Lecomte M, et al. Immunohistochemical study of 100 pancreatic tumors in 28 patients with multiple endocrine neoplasia, type I. Am J Surg Pathol 1996; 20:1378–1384.
54. Pipeleers-Marichal M, Somers G, Willems G, et al. Gastrinomas in the duodenums of patients with multiple endocrine neoplasia type 1 and the Zollinger-Ellison syndrome. N Engl J Med 1990; 322:723–727.
55. Vance JE, Stoll RW, Kitabchi AE, et al. Familial nesidioblastosis as the predominant manifestation of multiple endocrine adenomatosis. Am J Med 1972; 52:211–227.
56. Ariel I, Kerem E, Schwartz-Arad D, et al. Nesidiodysplasia: a histologic entity? Hum Pathol 1988; 19:1215–1218.
57. Lubensky IA, Debelenko LV, Zhuang Z, et al. Allelic deletions on chromosome 11q13 in multiple tumors from individual MEN1 patients. Cancer Res 1996; 56:5272–5278.
58. Debelenko LV, Zhuang Z, Emmert-Buck MR, et al. Allelic deletions on chromosome 11q13 in multiple endocrine neoplasia type 1–associated and sporadic gastrinomas and pancreatic endocrine tumors. Cancer Res 1997; 57:2238–2243.
59. Crabtree JS, Scacheri PC, Ward JM, et al. A mouse model of multiple endocrine neoplasia, type 1, develops multiple endocrine tumors. Proc Natl Acad Sci USA 2001; 98:1118–1123.
60. Tragl K-H, Mayr WR. Familial islet-cell adenomatosis. Lancet 1977; 2:426–428.
61. Maioli M, Ciccarese M, Pacifico A, et al. Familial insulinoma: description of two cases. Acta Diabetol 1992; 29:38–40.
62. Lubensky IA, Pack S, Ault D, et al. Multiple neuroendocrine

tumors of the pancreas in von Hippel–Lindau disease patients: histopathological and molecular genetic analysis. Am J Pathol 1998; 153:223–231.

63. Bardram L, Stage JG. Frequency of endocrine disorders in patients with the Zollinger-Ellison syndrome. Scand J Gastroenterol 1985; 20:233–238.
64. Farley DR, van Heerden JA, Grant CS, et al. The Zollinger-Ellison syndrome: a collective surgical experience. Ann Surg 1992; 215:561–569; discussion 569–570.
65. Serrano J, Gobel SU, Heppner C, et al. Occurrence of multiple endocrine neoplasia type 1 (*MEN1*) gene mutations in Zollinger-Ellison syndrome (ZES) (abstract). Gastroenterology 1998; 114: G2022.
66. Waxman I, Gardner JD, Jensen RT, et al. Peptic ulcer perforation as the presentation of Zollinger-Ellison syndrome. Dig Dis Sci 1991; 36:19–24.
67. Metz DC, Jensen RT, Bale AE, et al. Multiple endocrine neoplasia type 1: clinical features and management. In Bilezekian JP, Levine MA, Marx SJ (eds). The Parathyroids, 1st ed. New York, Raven Press, 1994, pp 591–646.
68. Benya RV, Metz DC, Hijazi YJ, et al. Fine needle aspiration cytology of submucosal nodules in patients with Zollinger-Ellison syndrome. Am J Gastroenterol 1993; 88:258–265.
69. Roy PK, Venzon DJ, Shojamanesh H, et al. Zollinger-Ellison syndrome: clinical presentation in 261 patients. Medicine (Baltimore) 2000; 79:379–411.
70. Norton JA, Fraker DL, Alexander HR, et al. Surgery to cure the Zollinger-Ellison syndrome. N Engl J Med 1999; 341:635–644.
71. Gibril F, Venzon DJ, Ojeaburu JV, et al. Prospective study of the natural history of gastrinoma in patients with MEN1: definition of an aggressive and a nonaggressive form. J Clin Endocrinol Metab 2001; 86:5282–5293.
72. Ruszniewski P, Podevin P, Cadiot G, et al. Clinical, anatomical, and evolutive features of patients with the Zollinger-Ellison syndrome combined with type I multiple endocrine neoplasia. Pancreas 1993; 8:295–304.
73. Stadil F, Bardram L, Gustafsen J, et al. Surgical treatment of the Zollinger-Ellison syndrome. World J Surg 1993; 17:463–467.
74. Thompson NW. Current concepts in the surgical management of multiple endocrine neoplasia type 1 pancreatic-duodenal disease: results in the treatment of 40 patients with Zollinger-Ellison syndrome, hypoglycaemia or both. J Intern Med 1998; 243:495–500.
75. Frucht H, Maton PN, Jensen RT. Use of omeprazole in patients with Zollinger-Ellison syndrome. Dig Dis Sci 1991; 36:394–404.
76. Maton PN. Omeprazole. N Engl J Med 1991; 324:965–975.
77. Maton PN. Review article: the management of Zollinger-Ellison syndrome. Aliment Pharmacol Ther 1993; 7:467–475.
78. Jensen RT. Gastrinoma as a model for prolonged hypergastrinemia. In Walsh JH (ed). Gastrin. New York, Raven Press, 1993, pp 373–393.
79. Solcia E, Capella C, Fiocca R, et al. Gastric argyrophil carcinoidosis in patients with Zollinger-Ellison syndrome due to type 1 multiple endocrine neoplasia: a newly recognized association. Am J Surg Pathol 1990; 14:503–513.
80. Maton PN, Lack EE, Collen MJ, et al. The effect of Zollinger-Ellison syndrome and omeprazole therapy on gastric oxyntic endocrine cells. Gastroenterology 1990; 99:943–950.
81. Cadiot G, Lehy T, Ruszniewski P, et al. Gastric endocrine cell evolution in patients with Zollinger-Ellison syndrome: influence of gastrinoma growth and long-term omeprazole treatment. Dig Dis Sci 1993; 38:1307–1317.
82. Gyr KE, Whitehouse I, Beglinger C, et al. Human pharmacological effects of SMS 201-995 on gastric secretion. Scand J Gastroenterol Suppl 1986; 119:96–102.
83. Kvols LK, Buck M, Moertel CG. Treatment of metastatic islet cell carcinoma with a somatostatin analogue (SMS 201-995). Ann Intern Med 1987; 107:162–168.
84. Shojamanesh H, Gibril F, Louie A, et al. Prospective study of the antitumor efficacy of long-term octreotide treatment in patients with progressive metastatic gastrinoma. Cancer Res 2002; 94: 331–343.
85. Tomassetti P, Migliori M, Caletti GC, et al. Treatment of type II gastric carcinoid tumors with somatostatin analogues. N Engl J Med 2000; 343:551–554.
86. Wells SA Jr. Surgery for the Zollinger-Ellison syndrome. N Engl J Med 1999; 341:689–690.
87. Service FJ, McMahon MM, O'Brien PC, et al. Functioning insulinoma—incidence, recurrence, and long-term survival of patients: a 60-year study. Mayo Clin Proc 1991; 66:711–719.
88. Proye C, Malvaux P, Pattou F, et al. Noninvasive imaging of insulinomas and gastrinomas with endoscopic ultrasonography and somatostatin receptor scintigraphy. Surgery 1998; 124:1134–1143; discussion 1143–1144.
89. Grant CS, van Heerden J, Charboneau JW, et al. Insulinoma: the value of intraoperative ultrasonography. Arch Surg 1988; 123: 843–848.
90. Norton JA. Intra-operative procedures to localize endocrine tumours of the pancreas and duodenum. Ital J Gastroenterol Hepatol 1999; 31(suppl 2):S195–S197.
91. Boukhman MP, Karam JM, Shaver J, et al. Localization of insulinomas. Arch Surg 1999; 134:818–822; discussion 822–823.
92. Doppman JL, Chang R, Fraker DL, et al. Localization of insulinomas to regions of the pancreas by intra-arterial stimulation with calcium. Ann Intern Med 1995; 123:269–273.
93. Proye C, Pattou F, Carnaille B, et al. Intraoperative insulin measurement during surgical management of insulinomas. World J Surg 1998; 22:1218–1224.
94. Stefanini P, Carboni M, Patrassi N, et al. The surgical treatment of occult insulinomas: a review of the problem. Br J Surg 1974; 61:1–4.
95. Stefanini P, Carboni M, Patrassi N, et al. Beta-islet cell tumors of the pancreas: results of a study on 1,067 cases. Surgery 1974; 75:597–609.
96. Goode PN, Farndon JR, Anderson J, et al. Diazoxide in the management of patients with insulinoma. World J Surg 1986; 10: 586–592.
97. Lamberts SW, Pieters GF, Metselaar HJ, et al. Development of resistance to a long-acting somatostatin analogue during treatment of two patients with metastatic endocrine pancreatic tumours. Acta Endocrinol (Copenh) 1988; 119:561–566.
98. Leichter SB. Clinical and metabolic aspects of glucagonoma. Medicine (Baltimore) 1980; 59:100–113.
99. Guillausseau PJ, Guillausseau C, Villet R, et al. [Glucagonomas: clinical, biological, anatomopathological and therapeutic aspects (general review of 130 cases)]. Gastroenterol Clin Biol 1982; 6: 1029–1041.
100. Boden G. Glucagonomas and insulinomas. Gastroenterol Clin North Am 1989; 18:831–845.
101. Montenegro RF, Samaan NA. Glucagonoma tumors and syndrome. Curr Probl Cancer 1981; 6:1–54.
102. Gorden P, Comi RJ, Maton PN, et al. NIH conference. Somatostatin and somatostatin analogue (SMS 201-995) in treatment of hormone-secreting tumors of the pituitary and gastrointestinal tract and non-neoplastic diseases of the gut. Ann Intern Med 1989; 110:35–50.
103. Altimari AF, Bhoopalam N, O'Dorsio T, et al. Use of a somatostatin analog (SMS 201-995) in the glucagonoma syndrome. Surgery 1986; 100:989–996.
104. Park SK, O'Dorisio MS, O'Dorisio TM. Vasoactive intestinal polypeptide–secreting tumours: biology and therapy. Baillieres Clin Gastroenterol 1996; 10:673–696.
105. Yamaguchi K, Abe K, Otsubo K, et al. The WDHA syndrome: clinical and laboratory data on 28 Japanese cases. Peptides 1984; 5:415–421.
106. Namihira Y, Achord JL, Subramony C. Multiple endocrine neoplasia, type 1, with pancreatic cholera. Am J Gastroenterol 1987; 82:794–797.
107. Lee CH, Ching KN, Lui WY, et al. Carcinoid tumor of the pancreas causing the diarrheogenic syndrome: report of a case combined with multiple endocrine neoplasia, type I. Surgery 1986; 99:123–129.
108. Hohmann EL, Levine L, Tashjian AH Jr. Vasoactive intestinal peptide stimulates bone resorption via a cyclic adenosine 3′,5′-monophosphate–dependent mechanism. Endocrinology 1983; 112:1233–1239.
109. Wu TJ, Lin CL, Taylor RL, et al. Increased parathyroid hormone–related peptide in patients with hypercalcemia associated with islet cell carcinoma. Mayo Clin Proc 1997; 72:1111–1115.
110. Thorner MO, Perryman RL, Cronin MJ, et al. Somatotroph hyperplasia: successful treatment of acromegaly by removal of a pancreatic islet tumor secreting a growth hormone–releasing factor. J Clin Invest 1982; 70:965–977.

111. Thorner MO, Frohman LA, Leong DA, et al. Extrahypothalamic growth-hormone-releasing factor (GRF) secretion is a rare cause of acromegaly: plasma GRF levels in 177 acromegalic patients. J Clin Endocrinol Metab 1984; 59:846–849.
112. Sano T, Yamasaki R, Saito H, et al. Growth hormone–releasing hormone (GHRH)–secreting pancreatic tumor in a patient with multiple endocrine neoplasia type I. Am J Surg Pathol 1987; 11: 810–819.
113. Asa SL, Singer W, Kovacs K, et al. Pancreatic endocrine tumour producing growth hormone–releasing hormone associated with multiple endocrine neoplasia type I syndrome. Acta Endocrinol (Copenh) 1987; 115:331–337.
114. Ramsay JA, Kovacs K, Asa SL, et al. Reversible sellar enlargement due to growth hormone–releasing hormone production by pancreatic endocrine tumors in a acromegalic patient with multiple endocrine neoplasia type I syndrome. Cancer 1988; 62:445–450.
115. Sano T, Asa SL, Kovacs K. Growth hormone–releasing hormone–producing tumors: clinical, biochemical, and morphological manifestations. Endocr Rev 1988; 9:357–373.
116. Liu SW, van de Velde CJ, Heslinga JM, et al. Acromegaly caused by growth hormone–relating hormone in a patient with multiple endocrine neoplasia type I. Jpn J Clin Oncol 1996; 26: 49–52.
117. Ezzat S, Asa SL, Stefaneanu L, et al. Somatotroph hyperplasia without pituitary adenoma associated with a long standing growth hormone–releasing hormone–producing bronchial carcinoid. J Clin Endocrinol Metab 1994; 78:555–560.
118. Pedrazzoli S, Pasquali C, Sperti C, et al. Clinically silent pancreatic "somatostatinoma" in MEN1 syndrome, and literature review. GI Cancer 1996; 1:191–206.
119. Fleury A, Flejou JF, Sauvanet A, et al. Calcitonin-secreting tumors of the pancreas: about six cases. Pancreas 1998; 16:545–550.
120. Skogseid B, Oberg K, Benson L, et al. A standardized meal stimulation test of the endocrine pancreas for early detection of pancreatic endocrine tumors in multiple endocrine neoplasia type 1 syndrome: five years experience. J Clin Endocrinol Metab 1987; 64:1233–1240.
121. Mutch MG, Frisella MM, DeBenedetti MK, et al. Pancreatic polypeptide is a useful plasma marker for radiographically evident pancreatic islet cell tumors in patients with multiple endocrine neoplasia type 1. Surgery 1997; 122:1012–1019; discussion 1019–1020.
122. Yim JH, Siegel BA, DeBenedetti MK, et al. Prospective study of the utility of somatostatin-receptor scintigraphy in the evaluation of patients with multiple endocrine neoplasia type 1. Surgery 1998; 124:1037–1042.
123. Skogseid B, Oberg K, Akerstrom G, et al. Limited tumor involvement found at multiple endocrine neoplasia type I pancreatic exploration: can it be predicted by preoperative tumor localization? World J Surg 1998; 22:673–677; discussion 667–668.
124. Pisegna JR, Doppman JL, Norton JA, et al. Prospective comparative study of ability of MR imaging and other imaging modalities to localize tumors in patients with Zollinger-Ellison syndrome. Dig Dis Sci 1993; 38:1318–1328.
125. Frilling A, Malago M, Martin H, et al. Use of somatostatin receptor scintigraphy to image extrahepatic metastases of neuroendocrine tumors. Surgery 1998; 124:1000–1004.
126. Cadiot G, Bonnaud G, Lebtahi R, et al. Usefulness of somatostatin receptor scintigraphy in the management of patients with Zollinger-Ellison syndrome. Groupe de Recherche et d'Etude du Syndrome de Zollinger-Ellison (GRESZE). Gut 1997; 41:107–114.
127. Doppman JL, Miller DL, Chang R, et al. Gastrinomas: localization by means of selective intraarterial injection of secretin. Radiology 1990; 174:25–29.
128. Alexander HR, Fraker DL, Norton JA, et al. Prospective study of somatostatin receptor scintigraphy and its effect on operative outcome in patients with Zollinger-Ellison syndrome. Ann Surg 1998; 228:228–238.
129. Legmann P, Vignaux O, Dousset B, et al. Pancreatic tumors: comparison of dual-phase helical CT and endoscopic sonography. AJR 1998; 170:1315–1322.
130. Sheridan MB, Ward J, Guthrie JA, et al. Dynamic contrast-enhanced MR imaging and dual-phase helical CT in the preoperative assessment of suspected pancreatic cancer: a comparative study with receiver operating characteristic analysis. AJR 1999; 173:583–590.
131. Ichikawa T, Peterson MS, Federle MP, et al. Islet cell tumor of the pancreas: biphasic CT versus MR imaging in tumor detection. Radiology 2000; 216:163–171.
132. Bansal R, Tierney W, Carpenter S, et al. Cost effectiveness of EUS for preoperative localization of pancreatic endocrine tumors. Gastrointest Endosc 1999; 49:19–25.
133. Suits J, Frazee R, Erickson RA. Endoscopic ultrasound and fine needle aspiration for the evaluation of pancreatic masses. Arch Surg 1999; 134:639–642; discussion 642–643.
134. Hiramoto JS, Feldstein VA, LaBerge JM, et al. Intraoperative ultrasound and preoperative localization detects all occult insulinomas. Arch Surg 2001; 136:1020–1025; discussion 1025–1026.
135. Granberg D, Stridsberg M, Seensalu R, et al. Plasma chromogranin A in patients with multiple endocrine neoplasia type 1. J Clin Endocrinol Metab 1999; 84:2712–2717.
136. Nobels FR, Kwekkeboom DJ, Coopmans W, et al. Chromogranin A as serum marker for neuroendocrine neoplasia: comparison with neuron-specific enolase and the alpha-subunit of glycoprotein hormones. J Clin Endocrinol Metab 1997; 82:2622–2628.
137. Goebel SU, Serrano J, Yu F, et al. Prospective study of the value of serum chromogranin A or serum gastrin levels in the assessment of the presence, extent, or growth of gastrinomas. Cancer 1999; 85:1470–1483.
138. Weber HC, Venzon DJ, Lin JT, et al. Determinants of metastatic rate and survival in patients with Zollinger-Ellison syndrome: a prospective long-term study. Gastroenterology 1995; 108:1637–1649.
139. Cadiot G, Vuagnat A, Doukhan I, et al. Prognostic factors in patients with Zollinger-Ellison syndrome and multiple endocrine neoplasia type 1. Groupe d'Etude des Néoplasies Endocriniennes Multiples (GENEM) and Groupe de Recherche et d'Etude du Syndrome de Zollinger-Ellison (GRESZE). Gastroenterology 1999; 116:286–293.
140. Lowney JK, Frisella MM, Lairmore TC, et al. Pancreatic islet cell tumor metastasis in multiple endocrine neoplasia type 1: correlation with primary tumor size. Surgery 1998; 124:1043–1048, discussion 1048–1049.
141. Wiedenmann B, Jensen RT, Mignon M, et al. Preoperative diagnosis and surgical management of neuroendocrine gastroenteropancreatic tumors: general recommendations by a consensus workshop. World J Surg 1998; 22:309–318.
142. Lairmore TC, Chen VY, DeBenedetti MK, et al. Duodenopancreatic resections in patients with multiple endocrine neoplasia type 1. Ann Surg 2000; 231:909–918.
143. Carty SE, Jensen RT, Norton JA. Prospective study of aggressive resection of metastatic pancreatic endocrine tumors. Surgery 1992; 112:1024–1031; discussion 1031–1032.
144. Kim YH, Ajani JA, Carrasco CH, et al. Selective hepatic arterial chemoembolization for liver metastases in patients with carcinoid tumor or islet cell carcinoma. Cancer Invest 1999; 17:474–478.
145. Ajani JA, Carrasco CH, Charnsangavej C, et al. Islet cell tumors metastatic to the liver: effective palliation by sequential hepatic artery embolization. Ann Intern Med 1988; 108:340–344.
146. Eriksson B, Oberg K, Alm G, et al. Treatment of malignant endocrine pancreatic tumours with human leucocyte interferon. Lancet 1986; 2:1307–1309.
147. Moertel CG, Lefkopoulo M, Lipsitz S, et al. Streptozocin-doxorubicin, streptozocin-fluorouracil or chlorozotocin in the treatment of advanced islet-cell carcinoma. N Engl J Med 1992; 326: 519–523.
148. Pisegna JR, Slimak GG, Doppman JL, et al. An evaluation of human recombinant alpha interferon in patients with metastatic gastrinoma. Gastroenterology 1993; 105:1179–1183.
149. Frank M, Klose KJ, Wied M, et al. Combination therapy with octreotide and alpha-interferon: effect on tumor growth in metastatic endocrine gastroenteropancreatic tumors. Am J Gastroenterol 1999; 94:1381–1387.
150. Tomassetti P, Migliori M, Corinaldesi R, et al. Treatment of gastroenteropancreatic neuroendocrine tumours with octreotide LAR. Aliment Pharmacol Ther 2000; 14:557–560.
151. Maton PN, Gardner JD, Jensen RT. Use of long-acting somatostatin analog SMS 201-995 in patients with pancreatic islet cell tumors. Dig Dis Sci 1989; 34:28S–39S.

152. Wymenga AN, Eriksson B, Salmela PI, et al. Efficacy and safety of prolonged-release lanreotide in patients with gastrointestinal neuroendocrine tumors and hormone-related symptoms. J Clin Oncol 1999; 17:1111.
153. di Bartolomeo M, Bajetta E, Buzzoni R, et al. Clinical efficacy of octreotide in the treatment of metastatic neuroendocrine tumors: a study by the Italian Trials in Medical Oncology Group. Cancer 1996; 77:402–408.
154. Verges B, Boureille F, Goudet P, et al. Pituitary disease in MEN type 1 (MEN1): data from the France-Belgium MEN1 multicenter study. J Clin Endocrinol Metab 2002; 87:457–465.
155. Andersen HO, Jorgensen PE, Bardram L, et al. Screening for multiple endocrine neoplasia type 1 in patients with recognized pituitary adenoma. Clin Endocrinol (Oxf) 1990; 33:771–775.
156. Corbetta S, Pizzocaro A, Peracchi M, et al. Multiple endocrine neoplasia type 1 in patients with recognized pituitary tumours of different types. Clin Endocrinol (Oxf) 1997; 47:507–512.
157. Tortosa F, Chico A, Rodriguez-Espinosa J, et al. Prevalence of MEN 1 in patients with prolactinoma. MEN1 Study Group of the Hospital de la Santa Creu i Sant Pau of Barcelona. Clin Endocrinol (Oxf) 1999; 50:272.
158. Wynne AG, Gharib H, Scheithauer BW, et al. Hyperthyroidism due to inappropriate secretion of thyrotropin in 10 patients. Am J Med 1992; 92:15–24.
159. Yoshimoto K, Saito S. [Clinical characteristics in multiple endocrine neoplasia type 1 in Japan: a review of 106 patients]. Nippon Naibunpi Gakkai Zasshi 1991; 67:764–774.
160. Carty SE, Helm AK, Amico JA, et al. The variable penetrance and spectrum of manifestations of multiple endocrine neoplasia type 1. Surgery 1998; 124:1106–1113; discussion 1113–1114.
161. Stratakis CA, Schussheim DH, Freedman SM, et al. Pituitary macroadenoma in a 5-year-old: an early expression of multiple endocrine neoplasia type 1. J Clin Endocrinol Metab 2000; 85: 4776–4780.
162. Sahdev A, Jager R. Bilateral pituitary adenomas occurring with multiple endocrine neoplasia type one. AJNR 2000; 21:1067–1069.
163. Weil RJ, Vortmeyer AO, Huang S, et al. 11q13 allelic loss in pituitary tumors in patients with multiple endocrine neoplasia syndrome type 1. Clin Cancer Res 1998; 4:1673–1678.
164. Scheithauer BW, Laws ERJ, Kovacs K, et al. Pituitary adenomas of the multiple endocrine neoplasia type I syndrome. Semin Diagn Pathol 1987; 4:205–211.
165. O'Brien T, O'Riordan DS, Gharib H, et al. Results of treatment of pituitary disease in multiple endocrine neoplasia, type I. Neurosurgery 1996; 39:273–278; discussion 278–279.
166. Weil C. The safety of bromocriptine in long-term use: a review of the literature. Curr Med Res Opin 1986; 10:25–51.
167. Fossati P, Dewailly D, Thomas DP, et al. Medical treatment of hyperprolactinemia. Horm Res 1985; 22:228–238.
168. Ferrari C, Crosignani PG. Medical treatment of hyperprolactinaemic disorders. Hum Reprod 1986; 1:507–514.
169. Bevan JS, Webster J, Burke CW, et al. Dopamine agonists and pituitary tumor shrinkage. Endocr Rev 1992; 13:220–240.
170. McCutcheon IE. Management of individual tumor syndromes: pituitary neoplasia. Endocrinol Metab Clin North Am 1994; 23: 37–51.
171. Thakker RV, Pook MA, Wooding C, et al. Association of somatotrophinomas with loss of alleles on chromosome 11 and with gsp mutations. J Clin Invest 1993; 91:2815–2821.
172. Oka H, Kameya T, Sato Y, et al. Significance of growth hormone–releasing hormone receptor mRNA in non-neoplastic pituitary and pituitary adenomas: a study by RT-PCR and in situ hybridization. J Neurooncol 1999; 41:197–204.
173. Ezzat S, Snyder PJ, Young WF, et al. Octreotide treatment of acromegaly: a randomized, multicenter study. Ann Intern Med 1992; 117:711–718.
174. Newman CB, Melmed S, Snyder PJ, et al. Safety and efficacy of long-term octreotide therapy of acromegaly: results of a multicenter trial in 103 patients—a clinical research center study. J Clin Endocrinol Metab 1995; 80:2768–2775.
175. Stewart PM. Current therapy for acromegaly. Trends Endocrinol Metab 2000; 11:128–132.
176. Skogseid B, Larsson C, Lindgren PG, et al. Clinical and genetic features of adrenocortical lesions in multiple endocrine neoplasia type 1. J Clin Endocrinol Metab 1992; 75:76–81.
177. Houdelette P, Chagnon A, Dumotier J, et al. [Malignant adrenocortical tumor as a part of Wermer's syndrome. Apropos of a case]. J Chir (Paris) 1989; 126:385–387.
178. Abe T, Yoshimoto K, Taniyama M, et al. An unusual kindred of the multiple endocrine neoplasia type 1 (MEN1) in Japanese. J Clin Endocrinol Metab 2000; 85:1327–1330.
179. Zahner J, Borchard F, Schmitz U, et al. [Thymus carcinoid in multiple endocrine neoplasms type I]. Dtsch Med Wochenschr 1994; 119:135–140.
180. Teh BT, McArdle J, Chan SP, et al. Clinicopathologic studies of thymic carcinoids in multiple endocrine neoplasia type 1. Medicine (Baltimore) 1997; 76:21–29.
181. Harpole DH Jr, Feldman JM, Buchanan S, et al. Bronchial carcinoid tumors: a retrospective analysis of 126 patients. Ann Thorac Surg 1992; 54:50–54; discussion 54–55.
182. Teh BT, Zedenius J, Kytola S, et al. Thymic carcinoids in multiple endocrine neoplasia type 1. Ann Surg 1998; 228:99–105.
183. Teh BT. Thymic carcinoids in multiple endocrine neoplasia type 1. J Intern Med 1998; 243:501–504.
184. Burgess JR, Greenaway TM, Parameswaran V, et al. Enteropancreatic malignancy associated with multiple endocrine neoplasia type 1: risk factors and pathogenesis. Cancer 1998; 83:428–434.
185. Chughtai TS, Morin JE, Sheiner NM, et al. Bronchial carcinoid: twenty years' experience defines a selective surgical approach. Surgery 1997; 122:801–808.
186. Gould PM, Bonner JA, Sawyer TE, et al. Bronchial carcinoid tumors: importance of prognostic factors that influence patterns of recurrence and overall survival. Radiology 1998; 208:181–185.
187. Musi M, Carbone RG, Bertocchi C, et al. Bronchial carcinoid tumours: a study on clinicopathological features and role of octreotide scintigraphy. Lung Cancer 1998; 22:97–102.
188. Bordi C, Falchetti A, Azzoni C, et al. Aggressive forms of gastric neuroendocrine tumors in multiple endocrine neoplasia type I. Am J Surg Pathol 1997; 21:1075–1082.
189. Anderson RE. A familial instance of appendiceal carcinoid. Am J Surg 1966; 111:738–740.
190. Moertel CG, Dockerty MB. Familial occurrence of metastasizing carcinoid tumors. Ann Intern Med 1973; 78:389–390.
191. Wale RJ, Williams JA, Beeley AH, et al. Familial occurrence in carcinoid tumours. Aust NZ J Surg 1983; 53:325–328.
192. Yeatman TJ, Sharp JV, Kimura AK. Can susceptibility to carcinoid tumors be inherited? Cancer 1989; 63:390–393.
193. Oliveira AM, Tazelaar HD, Wentzlaff KA, et al. Familial pulmonary carcinoid tumors. Cancer 2001; 91:2104–2109.
194. Babovic-Vuksanovic D, Constantinou CL, Rubin J, et al. Familial occurrence of carcinoid tumors and association with other malignant neoplasms. Cancer Epidemiol Biomarkers Prev 1999; 8:715–719.
195. Hemminki K, Li X. Familial carcinoid tumors and subsequent cancers: a nation-wide epidemiologic study from Sweden. Int J Cancer 2001; 94:444–448.
196. Cote GJ, Lee JE, Evans DB, et al. The spectrum of mutations in the MEN1 variant syndromes. Program of the Annual Meeting of the Endocrine Society 1998; 106.
197. Nord B, Larsson C, Wong FK, et al. Sporadic follicular thyroid tumors show loss of a 200-kb region in 11q13 without evidence for mutations in the MEN1 gene. Genes Chromosomes Cancer 1999; 26:35–39.
198. Reference deleted.
199. Darling TN, Skarulis MC, Steinberg SM, et al. Multiple facial angiofibromas and collagenomas in patients with multiple endocrine neoplasia type 1. Arch Dermatol 1997; 133:853–857.
200. Pack S, Turner ML, Zhuang Z, et al. Cutaneous tumors in patients with multiple endocrine neoplasia type 1 show allelic deletion of the *MEN1* gene. J Invest Dermatol 1998; 110:438–440.
201. Kato H, Uchimura I, Morohoshi M, et al. Multiple endocrine neoplasia type 1 associated with spinal ependymoma. Intern Med 1996; 35:285–289.
202. Giraud S, Choplin H, Teh BT, et al. A large multiple endocrine neoplasia type 1 family with clinical expression suggestive of anticipation. J Clin Endocrinol Metab 1997; 82:3487–3492.
203. Nord B, Platz A, Smoczynski K, et al. Malignant melanoma in patients with multiple endocrine neoplasia type 1 and involvement of the *MEN1* gene in sporadic melanoma. Int J Cancer 2000; 87:463–467.

204. Vortmeyer AO, Lubensky IA, Skarulis M, et al. Multiple endocrine neoplasia type 1: atypical presentation, clinical course, and genetic analysis of multiple tumors. Mod Pathol 1999; 12:919–924.
205. Dackiw AP, Cote GJ, Fleming JB, et al. Screening for *MEN1* mutations in patients with atypical endocrine neoplasia. Surgery 1999; 126:1097–1103; discussion 1103–1104.
206. McKeeby JL, Li X, Zhuang Z, et al. Multiple leiomyomas of the esophagus, lung, and uterus in multiple endocrine neoplasia type 1. Am J Pathol 2001; 159:1121–1127.
207. Fearon ER. Human cancer syndromes: clues to the origin and nature of cancer. Science 1997; 278:1043–1050.
208. Shepherd JJ. The natural history of multiple endocrine neoplasia type 1: highly uncommon or highly unrecognized? Arch Surg 1991; 126:935–952.
209. Giraud S, Zhang CX, Serova-Sinilnikova O, et al. Germ-line mutation analysis in patients with multiple endocrine neoplasia type 1 and related disorders. Am J Hum Genet 1998; 63:455–467.
210. Skogseid B, Eriksson B, Lundqvist G, et al. Multiple endocrine neoplasia type 1: a 10-year prospective screening study in four kindreds. J Clin Endocrinol Metab 1991; 73:281–287.
211. Gaitan D, Loosen PT, Orth DN. Two patients with Cushing's disease in a kindred with multiple endocrine neoplasia type I. J Clin Endocrinol Metab 1993; 76:1580–1582.
212. Marx SJ, Powell D, Shimkin PM, et al. Familial hyperparathyroidism. Ann Intern Med 1973; 78:371–377.
213. Farid NR, Buehler S, Russell NA, et al. Prolactinomas in familial multiple endocrine neoplasia syndrome type I: relationship to HLA and carcinoid tumors. Am J Med 1980; 69:874–880.
214. Green JS, Rigatto C, Parfrey PS, et al. MEN1 (Burin): update on a unique phenotypic variant (abstract). Am J Hum Genet 1999; 65(suppl):A128.
215. Hershon KS, Kelley WA, Shaw CM, et al. Prolactinomas as part of the multiple endocrine neoplastic syndrome type 1. Am J Med 1983; 74:713–720.
216. Heppner C, Agarwal SK, Kester MB, et al. Genotype-phenotype analysis in kindreds with familial multiple endocrine neoplasia type 1 (abstract). J Bone Miner Res 1997; 12(suppl 1):S107.
217. Waterlot C, Porchet N, Bauters C, et al. Type 1 multiple endocrine neoplasia (MEN1): contribution of genetic analysis to the screening and follow-up of a large French kindred. Clin Endocrinol (Oxf) 1999; 51:101–107.
218. Burgess JR, Shepherd JJ, Parameswaran V, et al. Prolactinomas in a large kindred with multiple endocrine neoplasia type 1: clinical features and inheritance pattern. J Clin Endocrinol Metab 1996; 81:1841–1845.
219. Kassem M, Kruse TA, Wong FK, et al. Familial isolated hyperparathyroidism as a variant of multiple endocrine neoplasia type 1 in a large Danish pedigree. J Clin Endocrinol Metab 2000; 85: 165–167.
220. Marx SJ, Spiegel AM, Levine MA, et al. Familial hypocalciuric hypercalcemia: the relation to primary parathyroid hyperplasia. N Engl J Med 1982; 307:416–426.
221. Kassem M, Zhang X, Brask S, et al. Familial isolated primary hyperparathyroidism. Clin Endocrinol (Oxf) 1994; 41:415–420.
222. Teh BT, Esapa CT, Houlston R, et al. A family with isolated hyperparathyroidism segregating a missense *MEN1* mutation and showing loss of the wild-type alleles in the parathyroid tumors. Am J Hum Genet 1998; 63:1544–1549.
223. Simonds WF, James-Newton LA, Agarwal SK, et al. Familial isolated hyperparathyroidism: clinical and genetic characteristics of 36 kindreds. Medicine (Baltimore) 2002; 81:1–26.
224. Uchino S, Noguchi S, Sato M, et al. Screening of the Men1 gene and discovery of germ-line and somatic mutations in apparently sporadic parathyroid tumors. Cancer Res 2000; 60:5553–5557.
225. Marx SJ, Attie MF, Levine MA, et al. The hypocalciuric or benign variant of familial hypercalcemia: clinical and biochemical features in fifteen kindreds. Medicine (Baltimore) 1981; 60:397–412.
226. Law WM Jr, Heath H III. Familial benign hypercalcemia (hypocalciuric hypercalcemia): clinical and pathogenetic studies in 21 families. Ann Intern Med 1985; 102:511–519.
227. Firek AF, Kao PC, Heath H 3rd. Plasma intact parathyroid hormone (PTH) and PTH-related peptide in familial benign hypercalcemia: greater responsiveness to endogenous PTH than in primary hyperparathyroidism. J Clin Endocrinol Metab 1991; 72: 541–546.
228. Thorgeirsson U, Costa J, Marx SJ. The parathyroid glands in familial hypocalciuric hypercalcemia. Hum Pathol 1981; 12:229–237.
229. Marx SJ. Clinical review 109: contrasting paradigms for hereditary hyperfunction of endocrine cells. J Clin Endocrinol Metab 1999; 84:3001–3009.
230. Heath H 3rd, Jackson CE, Otterud B, et al. Genetic linkage analysis in familial benign (hypocalciuric) hypercalcemia: evidence for locus heterogeneity. Am J Hum Genet 1993; 53:193–200.
231. Lloyd SE, Pannett AA, Dixon PH, et al. Localization of familial benign hypercalcemia, Oklahoma variant (FBHOk), to chromosome 19q13. Am J Hum Genet 1999; 64:189–195.
232. Carling T, Szabo E, Bai M, et al. Familial hypercalcemia and hypercalciuria caused by a novel mutation in the cytoplasmic tail of the calcium receptor. J Clin Endocrinol Metab 2000; 85:2042–2047.
233. Jackson CE, Norum RA, Boyd SB, et al. Hereditary hyperparathyroidism and multiple ossifying jaw fibromas: a clinically and genetically distinct syndrome. Surgery 1990; 108:1006–1012.
234. Szabo J, Heath B, Hill VM, et al. Hereditary hyperparathyroidism–jaw tumor syndrome: the endocrine tumor gene HRPT2 maps to chromosome 1q21-q31. Am J Hum Genet 1995; 56: 944–950.
235. Teh BT, Farnebo F, Kristoffersson U, et al. Autosomal dominant primary hyperparathyroidism and jaw tumor syndrome associated with renal hamartomas and cystic kidney disease: linkage to 1q21-q32 and loss of the wild type allele in renal hamartomas. J Clin Endocrinol Metab 1996; 81:4204–4211.
236. Teh BT, Farnebo F, Twigg S, et al. Familial isolated hyperparathyroidism maps to the hyperparathyroidism–jaw tumor locus in 1q21-q32 in a subset of families. J Clin Endocrinol Metab 1998; 83:2114–2120.
237. Streeten EA, Weinstein LS, Norton JA, et al. Studies in a kindred with parathyroid carcinoma. J Clin Endocrinol Metab 1992; 75:362–366.
238. Sood R, Bonner TI, Makalowska I, et al. Cloning and characterization of 13 novel transcripts and the human RGS8 gene from the 1q25 region encompassing the hereditary prostate cancer (HPC1) locus. Genomics 2001; 73:211–222.
239. Keiser HR, Beaven MA, Doppman J, et al. Sipple's syndrome: medullary thyroid carcinoma, pheochromocytoma, and parathyroid disease. Ann Intern Med 1973; 78:561–579.
240. Schuffenecker I, Virally-Monod M, Brohet R, et al. Risk and penetrance of primary hyperparathyroidism in multiple endocrine neoplasia type 2A families with mutations at codon 634 of the RET proto-oncogene. Groupe d'Etude des Tumeurs a Calcitonine. J Clin Endocrinol Metab 1998; 83:487–491.
241. Huang SM, Duh QY, Shaver J, et al. Familial hyperparathyroidism without multiple endocrine neoplasia. World J Surg 1997; 21:22–28; discussion 29.
242. Watanabe T, Tsukamoto F, Shimizu T, et al. Familial isolated hyperparathyroidism caused by single adenoma: a distinct entity different from multiple endocrine neoplasia. Endocr J 1998; 45: 637–646.
243. Berezin M, Karasik A. Familial prolactinoma. Clin Endocrinol (Oxf) 1995; 42:483–486.
244. Gadelha MR, Une KN, Rohde K, et al. Isolated familial somatotropinomas: establishment of linkage to chromosome 11q13.1-11q13.3 and evidence for a potential second locus at chromosome 2p16-12. J Clin Endocrinol Metab 2000; 85:707–714.
245. Larsson C, Skogseid B, Oberg K, et al. Multiple endocrine neoplasia type 1 gene maps to chromosome 11 and is lost in insulinoma. Nature 1988; 332:85–87.
246. Knudson AG Jr. Mutation and cancer: statistical study of retinoblastoma. Proc Natl Acad Sci USA 1971; 68:820–823.
247. Knudson AG. Hereditary cancer: two hits revisited. J Cancer Res Clin Oncol 1996; 122:135–140.
247b. Chandrasekharappa SC, Guru SC, Manickam P, et al. Positional cloning of the gene for multiple endocrine neoplasm type 1. Science 1997; 276:404–407.
248. Emmert-Buck MR, Lubensky IA, Dong Q, et al. Localization of the multiple endocrine neoplasia type I (MEN1) gene based on tumor loss of heterozygosity analysis. Cancer Res 1997; 57:1855–1858.

249. Guru SC, Agarwal SK, Manickam P, et al. A transcript map for the 2.8-Mb region containing the multiple endocrine neoplasia type 1 locus (letter). Genome Res 1997; 7:725–735.
250. Lemmens I, Van de Ven WJ, Kas K, et al. Identification of the multiple endocrine neoplasia type 1 (MEN1) gene. The European Consortium on MEN1. Hum Mol Genet 1997; 6:1177–1183.
251. Mayr B, Brabant G, von zur Muhlen A. Menin mutations in MEN1 patients (letter; comment). J Clin Endocrinol Metab 1998; 83:3004–3005.
252. Guru SC, Olufemi SE, Manickam P, et al. A 2.8-Mb clone contig of the multiple endocrine neoplasia type 1 (MEN1) region at 11q13. Genomics 1997; 42:436–445.
253. Guru SC, Goldsmith PK, Burns AL, et al. Menin, the product of the *MEN1* gene, is a nuclear protein. Proc Natl Acad Sci USA 1998; 95:1630–1634.
254. Manickam P, Vogel AM, Agarwal SK, et al. Isolation, characterization, expression and functional analysis of the zebrafish ortholog of MEN1. Mamm Genome 2000; 11:448–454.
255. Agarwal SK, Guru SC, Heppner C, et al. Menin interacts with the AP1 transcription factor JunD and represses JunD-activated transcription. Cell 1999; 96:143–152.
256. Gobl AE, Berg M, Lopez-Egido JR, et al. Menin represses JunD-activated transcription by a histone deacetylase-dependent mechanism. Biochim Biophys Acta 1999; 1447:51–56.
257. Knapp JI, Heppner C, Hickman AB, et al. Identification and characterization of JunD missense mutants that lack menin binding. Oncogene 2000; 19:4706–4712.
258. Thepot D, Weitzman JB, Barra J, et al. Targeted disruption of the murine *junD* gene results in multiple defects in male reproductive function. Development 2000; 127:143–153.
259. Kaji H, Canaff L, Lebrun JJ, et al. Inactivation of menin, a Smad3-interacting protein, blocks transforming growth factor type beta signaling. Proc Natl Acad Sci USA 2001; 98:3837–3842.
260. Heppner C, Kester MB, Agarwal SK, et al. Somatic mutation of the *MEN1* gene in parathyroid tumours. Nat Genet 1997; 16: 375–378.
261. Farnebo F, Teh BT, Kytola S, et al. Alterations of the *MEN1* gene in sporadic parathyroid tumors. J Clin Endocrinol Metab 1998; 83:2627–2630.
262. Carling T, Correa P, Hessman O, et al. Parathyroid *MEN1* gene mutations in relation to clinical characteristics of nonfamilial primary hyperparathyroidism. J Clin Endocrinol Metab 1998; 83: 2960–2963.
263. Farnebo F, Kytola S, Teh BT, et al. Alternative genetic pathways in parathyroid tumorigenesis. J Clin Endocrinol Metab 1999; 84: 3775–3780.
264. Zhuang Z, Vortmeyer AO, Pack S, et al. Somatic mutations of the *MEN1* tumor suppressor gene in sporadic gastrinomas and insulinomas. Cancer Res 1997; 57:4682–4686.
265. Wang EH, Ebrahimi SA, Wu AY, et al. Mutation of the MENIN gene in sporadic pancreatic endocrine tumors. Cancer Res 1998; 58:4417–4420.
266. Goebel SU, Heppner C, Burns AL, et al. Genotype/phenotype correlation of multiple endocrine neoplasia type 1 gene mutations in sporadic gastrinomas. J Clin Endocrinol Metab 2000; 85:116–123.
267. Gortz B, Roth J, Krahenmann A, et al. Mutations and allelic deletions of the *MEN1* gene are associated with a subset of sporadic endocrine pancreatic and neuroendocrine tumors and not restricted to foregut neoplasms. Am J Pathol 1999; 154:429–436.
268. Debelenko LV, Brambilla E, Agarwal SK, et al. Identification of *MEN1* gene mutations in sporadic carcinoid tumors of the lung. Hum Mol Genet 1997; 6:2285–2290.
269. Zhuang Z, Ezzat SZ, Vortmeyer AO, et al. Mutations of the *MEN1* tumor suppressor gene in pituitary tumors. Cancer Res 1997; 57:5446–5451.
270. Tanaka C, Kimura T, Yang P, et al. Analysis of loss of heterozygosity on chromosome 11 and infrequent inactivation of the *MEN1* gene in sporadic pituitary adenomas. J Clin Endocrinol Metab 1998; 83:2631–2634.
271. Prezant TR, Levine J, Melmed S. Molecular characterization of the men1 tumor suppressor gene in sporadic pituitary tumors. J Clin Endocrinol Metab 1998; 83:1388–1391.
272. Tanaka C, Yoshimoto K, Yamada S, et al. Absence of germ-line mutations of the multiple endocrine neoplasia type 1 (*MEN1*) gene in familial pituitary adenoma in contrast to MEN1 in Japanese. J Clin Endocrinol Metab 1998; 83:960–965.
273. Schmidt MC, Henke RT, Stangl AP, et al. Analysis of the *MEN1* gene in sporadic pituitary adenomas. J Pathol 1999; 188:168–173.
274. Gortz B, Roth J, Speel EJ, et al. *MEN1* gene mutation analysis of sporadic adrenocortical lesions. Int J Cancer 1999; 80:373–379.
275. Heppner C, Reincke M, Agarwal SK, et al. *MEN1* gene analysis in sporadic adrenocortical neoplasms. J Clin Endocrinol Metab 1999; 84:216–219.
276. Shan L, Nakamura Y, Murakami M, et al. Clonal emergence in uremic parathyroid hyperplasia is not related to *MEN1* gene abnormality. Jpn J Cancer Res 1999; 90:965–969.
277. Tahara H, Imanishi Y, Yamada T, et al. Rare somatic inactivation of the multiple endocrine neoplasia type 1 gene in secondary hyperparathyroidism of uremia. J Clin Endocrinol Metab 2000; 85:4113–4117.
278. Imanishi Y, Palanisamy N, Tahara H, et al. Molecular pathogenetic analysis of parathyroid carcinoma (abstract). J Bone Miner Res 1999; 14(suppl 1):S421.
279. Boni R, Vortmeyer AO, Pack S, et al. Somatic mutations of the *MEN1* tumor suppressor gene detected in sporadic angiofibromas (letter). J Invest Dermatol 1998; 111:539–540.
280. Vortmeyer AO, Boni R, Pak E, et al. Multiple endocrine neoplasia 1 gene alterations in MEN1-associated and sporadic lipomas (letter). J Natl Cancer Inst 1998; 90:398–399.
281. Debelenko LV, Swalwell JI, Kelley MJ, et al. *MEN1* gene mutation analysis of high-grade neuroendocrine lung carcinoma. Genes Chromosomes Cancer 2000; 28:58–65.
282. Boni R, Vortmeyer AO, Huang S, et al. Mutation analysis of the *MEN1* tumour suppressor gene in malignant melanoma. Melanoma Res 1999; 9:249–252.
283. Thieblemont C, Pack S, Sakai A, et al. Allelic loss of 11q13 as detected by MEN1-FISH is not associated with mutation of the *MEN1* gene in lymphoid neoplasms. Leukemia 1999; 13:85–91.
284. Herman JG, Latif F, Weng Y, et al. Silencing of the *VHL* tumor-suppressor gene by DNA methylation in renal carcinoma. Proc Natl Acad Sci USA 1994; 91:9700–9704.
285. Agarwal SK, Debelenko LV, Kester MB, et al. Analysis of recurrent germline mutations in the *MEN1* gene encountered in apparently unrelated families. Hum Mutat 1998; 12:75–82.
286. Kishi M, Tsukada T, Shimizu S, et al. A large germline deletion of the *MEN1* gene in a family with multiple endocrine neoplasia type 1. Jpn J Cancer Res 1998; 89:1–5.
287. Teh BT, Kytola S, Farnebo F, et al. Mutation analysis of the *MEN1* gene in multiple endocrine neoplasia type 1, familial acromegaly and familial isolated hyperparathyroidism. J Clin Endocrinol Metab 1998; 83:2621–2626.
288. Poncin J, Abs R, Velkeniers B, et al. Mutation analysis of the *MEN1* gene in Belgian patients with multiple endocrine neoplasia type 1 and related diseases. Hum Mutat 1999; 13:54–60.
289. Mutch MG, Dilley WG, Sanjurjo F, et al. Germline mutations in the multiple endocrine neoplasia type 1 gene: evidence for frequent splicing defects. Hum Mutat 1999; 13:175–185.
290. Mayer K, Ballhausen W, Rott HD. Mutation screening of the entire coding regions of the *TSC1* and the *TSC2* gene with the protein truncation test (PTT) identifies frequent splicing defects. Hum Mutat 1999; 14:401–411.
291. Olufemi SE, Green JS, Manickam P, et al. Common ancestral mutation in the *MEN1* gene is likely responsible for the prolactinoma variant of MEN1 (MEN1Burin) in four kindreds from Newfoundland. Hum Mutat 1998; 11:264–269.
292. Reference deleted.
293. Thakker RV, Bouloux P, Wooding C, et al. Association of parathyroid tumors in multiple endocrine neoplasia type 1 with loss of alleles on chromosome 11. N Engl J Med 1989; 321:218–224.
294. Debelenko LV, Emmert-Buck MR, Zhuang Z, et al. The multiple endocrine neoplasia type I gene locus is involved in the pathogenesis of type II gastric carcinoids. Gastroenterology 1997; 113:773–781.
295. Tahara H, Smith AP, Gaz RD, et al. Genomic localization of novel candidate tumor suppressor gene loci in human parathyroid adenomas. Cancer Res 1996; 56:599–605.

296. Arnold A, Brown MF, Urena P, et al. Monoclonality of parathyroid tumors in chronic renal failure and in primary parathyroid hyperplasia. J Clin Invest 1995; 95:2047–2053.
297. Falchetti A, Bale AE, Amorosi A, et al. Progression of uremic hyperparathyroidism involves allelic loss on chromosome 11. J Clin Endocrinol Metab 1993; 76:139–144.
298. Farnebo F, Farnebo LO, Nordenstrom J, et al. Allelic loss on chromosome 11 is uncommon in parathyroid glands of patients with hypercalcaemic secondary hyperparathyroidism. Eur J Surg 1997; 163:331–337.
299. Jakobovitz O, Nass D, DeMarco L, et al. Carcinoid tumors frequently display genetic abnormalities involving chromosome 11. J Clin Endocrinol Metab 1996; 81:3164–3167.
300. Williamson C, Pannett A, Pang JT, et al. Localisation of a tumour suppressor gene causing endocrine tumours to a four centimorgan region on chromosome 1 (abstract). Program of the Annual Meeting of the Endocrine Society 1996.
301. Kytola S, Makinen MJ, Kahkonen M, et al. Comparative genomic hybridization studies in tumours from a patient with multiple endocrine neoplasia type 1. Eur J Endocrinol 1998; 139: 202–206.
302. Franklin DS, Godfrey VL, O'Brien DA, et al. Functional collaboration between different cyclin-dependent kinase inhibitors suppresses tumor growth with distinct tissue specificity. Mol Cell Biol 2000; 20:6147–6158.
303. Pestell RG, Albanese C, Reutens AT, et al. The cyclins and cyclin-dependent kinase inhibitors in hormonal regulation of proliferation and differentiation. Endocr Rev 1999; 20:501–534.
304. Gustavson KH, Jansson R, Oberg K. Chromosomal breakage in multiple endocrine adenomatosis (types I and II). Clin Genet 1983; 23:143–149.
305. Benson L, Gustavson KH, Rastad J, et al. Cytogenetical investigations in patients with primary hyperparathyroidism and multiple endocrine neoplasia type 1. Hereditas 1988; 108:227–229.
306. Scappaticci S, Maraschio P, del Ciotto N, et al. Chromosome abnormalities in lymphocytes and fibroblasts of subjects with multiple endocrine neoplasia type 1. Cancer Genet Cytogenet 1991; 52:85–92.
307. Scappaticci S, Fossati GS, Valenti L, et al. A search for double minute chromosomes in cultured lymphocytes from different types of tumors. Cancer Genet Cytogenet 1995; 82:50–53.
308. Sakurai A, Katai M, Itakura Y, et al. Premature centromere division in patients with multiple endocrine neoplasia type 1. Cancer Genet Cytogenet 1999; 109:138–140.
309. Ikeo Y, Sakurai A, Suzuki R, et al. Proliferation-associated expression of the *MEN1* gene as revealed by in situ hybridization: possible role of the menin as a negative regulator of cell proliferation under DNA damage. Lab Invest 2000; 80:797–804.
310. Vortmeyer AO, Boni R, Pack SD, et al. Perivascular cells harboring multiple endocrine neoplasia type 1 alterations are neoplastic cells in angiofibromas. Cancer Res 1999; 59:274–278.
311. Deng G, Lu Y, Zlotnikov G, et al. Loss of heterozygosity in normal tissue adjacent to breast carcinomas. Science 1996; 274: 2057–2059.
312. Zimering MB, Katsumata N, Sato Y, et al. Increased basic fibroblast growth factor in plasma from multiple endocrine neoplasia type 1: relation to pituitary tumor. J Clin Endocrinol Metab 1993; 76:1182–1187.
313. Agarwal SK, Kester MB, Debelenko LV, et al. Germline mutations of the *MEN1* gene in familial multiple endocrine neoplasia type 1 and related states. Hum Mol Genet 1997; 6:1169–1175.
314. Larsson C, Calender A, Grimmond S, et al. Molecular tools for presymptomatic testing in multiple endocrine neoplasia type 1. J Intern Med 1995; 238:239–244.
315. Committee of Bioethics. American Academy of Pediatrics: Ethical issues with genetic testing in pediatrics. Pediatrics 2001; 107: 1451–1460.
316. Roijers JF, de Wit MJ, van der Luijt RB, et al. Criteria for mutation analysis in MEN1–suspected patients: MEN1 case-finding. Eur J Clin Invest 2000; 30:487–492.
317. Bassett JH, Forbes SA, Pannett AA, et al. Characterization of mutations in patients with multiple endocrine neoplasia type 1. Am J Hum Genet 1998; 62:232–244.
318. Hai N, Aoki N, Matsuda A, et al. Germline *MEN1* mutations in sixteen Japanese families with multiple endocrine neoplasia type 1 (MEN1). Eur J Endocrinol 1999; 141:475–480.
319. Morelli A, Falchetti A, Martineti V, et al. *MEN1* gene mutation analysis in Italian patients with multiple endocrine neoplasia type 1. Eur J Endocrinol 2000; 142:131–137.
320. Larsson C, Shepherd J, Nakamura Y, et al. Predictive testing for multiple endocrine neoplasia type 1 using DNA polymorphisms. J Clin Invest 1992; 89:1344–1349.
321. Courseaux A, Grosgeorge J, Gaudray P, et al. Definition of the minimal MEN1 candidate area based on a 5-Mb integrated map of proximal 11q13. The European Consortium on Men1, (GENEM 1; Groupe d'Etude des Néoplasies Endocriniennes Multiples de type 1). Genomics 1996; 37:354–365.
322. Stock JL, Warth MR, Teh BT, et al. A kindred with a variant of multiple endocrine neoplasia type 1 demonstrating frequent expression of pituitary tumors but not linked to the multiple endocrine neoplasia type 1 locus at chromosome region 11q13. J Clinical Endocrinol Metab 1997; 82:486–492.
323. Hai N, Aoki N, Shimatsu A, et al. Clinical features of multiple endocrine neoplasia type 1 (MEN1) phenocopy without germline *MEN1* gene mutations: analysis of 20 Japanese sporadic cases with MEN1. Clin Endocrinol (Oxf) 2000; 52:509–518.
324. Grayson RH, Halperin JM, Sharma V, et al. Changes in plasma prolactin and catecholamine metabolite levels following acute needle stick in children. Psychiatry Res 1997; 69:27–32.
325. Benya RV, Metz DC, Venzon DJ, et al. Zollinger-Ellison syndrome can be the initial endocrine manifestation in patients with multiple endocrine neoplasia-type I. Am J Med 1994; 97:436–444.
326. Burgess JR, Nord B, David R, et al. Phenotype and phenocopy: the relationship between genotype and clinical phenotype in a single large family with multiple endocrine neoplasia type 1 (MEN 1). Clin Endocrinol (Oxf) 2000; 53:205–211.
327. Oberg K, Skogseid B. The ultimate biochemical diagnosis of endocrine pancreatic tumours in MEN1. J Intern Med 1998; 243: 471–476.
328. Sipple JH. Multiple endocrine neoplasia type 2 syndromes: historical perspectives. Henry Ford Hosp Med J 1984; 32:219–221.
329. Cushman P Jr. Familial endocrine tumors: report of two unrelated kindred affected with pheochromocytomas, one also with multiple thyroid carcinomas. Am J Med 1962; 32:352–360.
330. Hazard JB, Hawk WA, Crile G Jr. Medullary (solid) carcinoma of the thyroid: a clinicopathologic entity. J Clin Endocrinol Metab 1959; 19:152–161.
331. Williams ED. A review of 17 cases of carcinoma of the thyroid and phaeochromocytoma. J Clin Pathol 1965; 18:288–292.
332. Melvin KEW, Miller HH, Tashjian AH Jr. Early diagnosis of medullary carcinoma of the thyroid gland by means of calcitonin assay. N Engl J Med 1971; 285:1115–1120.
333. Sizemore GW, Carney JA, Heath H III. Epidemiology of medullary carcinoma of the thyroid gland: a 5 year experience. Surg Clin North Am 1977; 57:633–645.
334. Gagel RF, Melvin KE, Tashjian AH Jr, et al. Natural history of the familial medullary thyroid carcinoma–pheochromocytoma syndrome and the identification of preneoplastic stages by screening studies: a five-year report. Trans Assoc Am Physicians 1975; 88:177–191.
335. Gagel RF, Costanza ME, DeLellis RA, et al. Streptozocin-treated Verner-Morrison syndrome: plasma vasoactive intestinal peptide and tumor responses. Arch Intern Med 1976; 136:1429–1435.
336. Block MA, Jackson CE, Tashjian AH Jr. Management of occult medullary thyroid carcinoma of thyroid: evidence only by serum calcitonin elevations after apparently adequate neck operation. Arch Surg 1978; 113:368–372.
337. Baylin SB. The multiple endocrine neoplasia syndromes: implications for the study of inherited tumors. Semin Oncol 1978; 5:35–45.
338. Sizemore GW, Heath H III, Carney JA. Multiple endocrine neoplasia type 2. Clin Endocrinol Metab 1980; 9:299–315.
339. Wells SA Jr, Baylin SB, Leight GS, et al. The importance of early diagnosis in patients with hereditary medullary thyroid carcinoma. Ann Surg 1982; 195:595–599.
340. Jackson CE, Talpos GB, Kambouris A, et al. The clinical course after definitive operation for medullary thyroid carcinoma. Surgery 1983; 94:995–1001.
341. Russell CF, Van Heerden JA, Sizemore GW, et al. The surgical management of medullary thyroid carcinoma. Ann Surg 1983; 197:42–48.

342. Gagel RF, Tashjian AH Jr, Cummings T, et al. Impact of prospective screening for multiple endocrine neoplasia type 2. Henry Ford Hosp Med J 1987; 35:94–98.
343. Jackson CE, Norum RA, Talpos GB, et al. Clinical value of calcitonin and carcinoembryonic antigen doubling times in medullary thyroid carcinoma. Henry Ford Hosp Med J 1987; 35:120–121.
344. Heath H III, Sizemore GW, Carney JA. Preoperative diagnosis of occult parathyroid hyperplasia by calcium infusion in patients with multiple endocrine neoplasia, type 2a. J Clin Endocrinol Metab 1976; 43:428–435.
345. Howe JR, Norton JA, Wells SA Jr. Prevalence of pheochromocytoma and hyperparathyroidism in multiple endocrine neoplasia type 2A: results of long-term follow-up. Surgery 1993; 114:1070–1077.
346. Baylin SB, Gann DS, Hsu SH. Clonal origin of inherited medullary thyroid carcinoma and pheochromocytoma. Science 1976; 193:321–323.
347. Arnold A, Staunton CE, Kim HG, et al. Monoclonality and abnormal parathyroid hormone genes in parathyroid adenomas. N Engl J Med 1988; 318:658–662.
348. Wolfe HJ, Melvin KEW, Cervi-Skinner SJ, et al. C-cell hyperplasia preceding medullary thyroid carcinoma. N Engl J Med 1973; 289:437–441.
349. DeLellis RA, Dayal Y, Tischler AS, et al. Multiple endocrine neoplasia (MEN) syndromes: cellular origins and interrelationships. Int Rev Exp Pathol 1986; 28:163–215.
350. Wolfe HJ, DeLellis RA. Familial medullary thyroid carcinoma and C-cell hyperplasia. Clin Endocrinol Metab 1981; 10:351–365.
351. Samaan NA, Draznin MB, Halpin RE, et al. Multiple endocrine syndrome type IIb in early childhood. Cancer 1991; 68:1832–1834.
352. Graham SM, Genel M, Touloukian RJ, et al. Provocative testing for occult medullary carcinoma of the thyroid: findings in seven children with multiple endocrine neoplasia type IIa. J Pediatr Surg 1987; 22:501–503.
353. Lips CJ, Landsvater RM, Hoppener JW, et al. Clinical screening as compared with DNA analysis in families with multiple endocrine neoplasia type 2A. N Engl J Med 1994; 331:828–835.
354. Wells SA Jr, Chi DD, Toshima K, et al. Predictive DNA testing and prophylactic thyroidectomy in patients at risk for multiple endocrine neoplasia type 2A. Ann Surg 1994; 220:237–247; discussion 247–250.
355. Gagel RF, Cote GJ, Martins Bugalho MJG, et al. Clinical use of molecular information in the management of multiple endocrine neoplasia type 2A. J Intern Med 1995; 238:333–341.
356. Cote GJ, Gould JA, Huang SC, et al. Studies of short-term secretion of peptides produced by alternative RNA processing. Mol Cell Endocrinol 1987; 53:211–219.
357. Gagel RF, Palmer WN, Leonhart K, et al. Somatostatin production by a human medullary thyroid carcinoma cell line. Endocrinology 1986; 118:1643–1651.
358. Atkins FL, Beaven MA, Keiser HR. Dopa decarboxylase in medullary carcinoma of the thyroid. N Engl J Med 1973; 289:545–548.
359. O'Connor DT, Deftos LJ. Secretion of chromogranin A by peptide-producing endocrine neoplasms. N Engl J Med 1986; 314:1145–1151.
360. Sevarino KA, Wu P, Jackson IMD, et al. Biosynthesis of thyrotropin releasing hormone by a rat medullary thyroid carcinoma cell line. J Biol Chem 1988; 263:620–623.
361. Yamaguchi K, Abe K, Adachi I, et al. Concomitant production of immunoreactive gastrin-releasing peptide and calcitonin in medullary carcinoma of the thyroid. Metabolism 1984; 33:724–727.
362. Baylin SB, Beaven MA, Buja LM, et al. Histaminase activity: a biochemical marker for medullary carcinoma of the thyroid. Am J Med 1972; 53:723–733.
363. Gagel R. Tumor markers of medullary thyroid carcinoma. In Fishman W (ed). Oncodevelopmental Markers: Biologic, Diagnostic and Monitoring Aspects. New York, Academic Press, 1983, pp 222–239.
364. Block MA, Jackson CE, Greenawald KA, et al. Clinical characteristics distinguishing hereditary from sporadic medullary thyroid carcinoma. Arch Surg 1980; 115:142–148.
365. Moley JF, DeBenedetti MK. Patterns of nodal metastases in palpable medullary thyroid carcinoma: recommendations for extent of node dissection. Ann Surg 1999; 229:880–887; discussion 887–888.
366. Cance WG, Wells SA Jr. Multiple endocrine neoplasia type IIa. Curr Probl Surg 1985; 22:1–56.
367. Leape LL, Miller HH, Graze K, et al. Total thyroidectomy for occult familial medullary carcinoma of the thyroid in children. J Pediatr Surg 1976; 11:831–837.
368. Block MA, Jackson CE, Tashjian AH Jr. Management of occult medullary thyroid carcinoma: evidenced only by serum calcitonin level elevations after apparently adequate neck operations. Arch Surg 1978; 113:368–372.
369. Becker KL, Walton-Moss BJ. Young woman with recurrent yeast infections. Lippincotts Prim Care Pract 2000; 4:125–131.
370. Muller B, Becker KL, Schachinger H, et al. Calcitonin precursors are reliable markers of sepsis in a medical intensive care unit. Crit Care Med 2000; 28:977–983.
371. Whang KT, Vath SD, Becker KL, et al. Procalcitonin and proinflammatory cytokine in interactions in sepsis. Shock 1999; 12:268–273.
372. Aloia JF, Rasulo P, Deftos LJ, et al. Exercise-induced hypercalcemia and the calciotropic hormones. J Lab Clin Med 1985; 106:229–232.
373. Samaan NA, Schultz PN, Hickey RC. Medullary thyroid carcinoma: prognosis of familial versus sporadic disease and the role of radiotherapy. J Clin Endocrinol Metab 1988; 67:801–805.
374. Tisell L, Hansson G, Jansson S, et al. Reoperation in the treatment of asymptomatic metastasizing medullary thyroid carcinoma. Surgery 1986; 99:60–66.
375. Moley JF, Dilley WG, DeBenedetti MK. Improved results of cervical reoperation for medullary thyroid carcinoma. Ann Surg 1997; 225:734–740; discussion 740–743.
376. Buhr HJ, Kallinowski F, Raue F, et al. Microsurgical neck dissection for metastasizing medullary thyroid carcinoma. Eur J Surg Oncol 1995; 21:195–197.
377. Evans DB, Fleming JB, Lee JE, et al. The surgical treatment of medullary thyroid carcinoma. Semin Surg Oncol 1999; 16:50–63.
378. Fleming JB, Lee JE, Bouvet M, et al. Surgical strategy for the treatment of medullary thyroid carcinoma. Ann Surg 1999; 230:697–707.
379. Talpos GB, Jackson CE, Froelich JW, et al. Localization of residual medullary thyroid cancer by thallium/technetium scintigraphy. Surgery 1985; 98:1189–1196.
380. Itoh H, Sugie K, Toyooka S, et al. Detection of metastatic medullary thyroid cancer with ^{131}I-MIBG scans in Sipple's syndrome. Eur J Nucl Med 1986; 11:502–504.
381. Baulieu JL, Guilloteau D, Delisle MJ, et al. Radioiodinated metaiodobenzylguanidine uptake in medullary thyroid cancer: a French cooperative study. Cancer 1987; 60:2189–2194.
382. Yobbagy JJ, Levatter R, Sisson JC, et al. Scintigraphic portrayal of the syndrome of multiple endocrine neoplasia type-2B. Clin Nucl Med 1988; 13:433–437.
383. Krenning EP, Kwekkeboom DJ, Bakker WH, et al. Somatostatin receptor scintigraphy with [^{111}In-DTPA-D-Phe^1]- and [^{123}I-Tyr^3]-octreotide: the Rotterdam experience with more than 1000 patients. Nucl Med 1993; 20:716–731.
384. Frank-Raue K, Raue F, Buhr HJ, et al. Localization of occult persisting medullary thyroid carcinoma before microsurgical reoperation: high sensitivity of selective venous catheterization. Thyroid 1992; 2:113–117.
385. Moley JF, Wells SA, Dilley WG, et al. Reoperation for recurrent or persistent medullary thyroid carcinoma. Surgery 1993; 114:1090–1096.
386. van Heerden JA, Grant CS, Gharib H, et al. Long-term course of patients with persistent hypercalcitoninemia after apparent curative primary surgery for medullary thyroid carcinoma. Ann Surg 1990; 212:395–400.
387. Carney JA, Sizemore GW, Tyce GM. Bilateral adrenal medullary hyperplasia in multiple endocrine neoplasia, type 2: the precursor of bilateral pheochromocytoma. Mayo Clin Proc 1975; 50:3–10.
388. Carney JA, Sizemore GW, Sheps SG. Adrenal medullary disease in multiple endocrine neoplasia, type 2: pheochromocytoma and its precursors. Am J Clin Pathol 1976; 66:279–290.
389. DeLellis RA, Wolfe HJ, Gagel RF, et al. Adrenal medullary hyperplasia: a morphometric analysis in patients with familial medullary thyroid carcinoma. Am J Pathol 1976; 83:177–196.

390. Webb TA, Sheps SG, Carney JA. Differences between sporadic pheochromocytoma and pheochromocytoma in multiple endocrine neoplasia, type 2. Am J Surg Pathol 1980; 4:121–126.
391. Carney JA, Sizemore GW, Hayles AB. Multiple endocrine neoplasia, type 2b. Pathobiol Annu 1978; 8:105–153.
392. Lips KJ, Van der Sluys Veer J, Struyvenberg A, et al. Bilateral occurrence of pheochromocytoma in patients with the multiple endocrine neoplasia syndrome type 2A (Sipple's syndrome). Am J Med 1981; 70:1051–1060.
393. Modigliani E, Vasen H, Raue K, et al. Pheochromocytoma in multiple endocrine neoplasia type 2: European study. J Int Med 1995; 238:363–367.
394. Sisson JC, Shapiro B, Beierwaltes WH. Scintigraphy with I-131 MIBG as an aid to the treatment of pheochromocytomas in patients with the multiple endocrine neoplasia type 2 syndromes. Henry Ford Hosp Med J 1984; 32:254–261.
395. Casanova S, Rosenberg-Bourgin M, Farkas D, et al. Phaeochromocytoma in multiple endocrine neoplasia type 2 A: survey of 100 cases. Clin Endocrinol (Oxf) 1993; 38:531–537.
396. Westfried M, Mandel D, Alderete MN, et al. Sipple's syndrome with a malignant pheochromocytoma presenting as a pericardial effusion. Cardiology 1978; 63:305–311.
397. Lee JE, Curley SA, Gagel RF, et al. Cortical-sparing adrenalectomy for patients with bilateral pheochromocytoma. Surgery 1996; 120:1064–1070; discussion 1070-1071.
398. Chevinsky AH, Minton JP, Falko JM. Metastatic pheochromocytoma associated with multiple endocrine neoplasia syndrome type II. Arch Surg 1990; 125:935–938.
399. Namba H, Kondo H, Yamashita S, et al. Multiple endocrine neoplasia type 2 with malignant pheochromocytoma: long term follow-up of a case by ^{131}I-meta-iodobenzylguanidine scintigraphy. Ann Nucl Med 1992; 6:111–115.
400. Hinze R, Machens A, Schneider U, et al. Simultaneously occurring liver metastases of pheochromocytoma and medullary thyroid carcinoma: a diagnostic pitfall with clinical implications for patients with multiple endocrine neoplasia type 2a. Pathol Res Pract 2000; 196:477–481.
401. Gentile S, Rainero I, Savi L, et al. Brain metastasis from pheochromocytoma in a patient with multiple endocrine neoplasia type 2A. Panminerva Med 2001; 43:305–306.
402. Scopsi L, Castellani MR, Gullo M, et al. Malignant pheochromocytoma in multiple endocrine neoplasia type 2B syndrome: case report and review of the literature. Tumori 1996; 82:480–484.
403. Chodankar CM, Abhyankar SC, Deodhar KP, et al. Sipple's syndrome (multiple endocrine neoplasia) in pregnancy: case report. Aust NZ J Obstet Gynaecol 1982; 22:243–244.
404. Moraca Kvapilova L, Op de Coul AA, Merkus JM. Cerebral haemorrhage in a pregnant woman with a multiple endocrine neoplasia syndrome (type 2A or Sipple's syndrome). Eur J Obstet Gynecol Reprod Biol 1985; 20:257–263.
405. Hamilton BP, Landsberg L, Levine RJ. Measurement of urinary epinephrine in screening for pheochromocytoma in multiple endocrine neoplasia type II. Am J Med 1978; 65:1027–1032.
406. Takai S, Miyauchi A, Matsumoto H, et al. Multiple endocrine neoplasia type 2 syndromes in Japan. Henry Ford Hosp Med J 1984; 32:246–250.
407. Eisenhofer G, Lenders JW, Linehan WM, et al. Plasma normetanephrine and metanephrine for detecting pheochromocytoma in von Hippel–Lindau disease and multiple endocrine neoplasia type 2. N Engl J Med 1999; 340:1872–1879.
408. Valk TW, Frager MS, Gross MD, et al. Spectrum of pheochromocytoma in multiple endocrine neoplasia: a scintigraphic portrayal using ^{131}I-metaiodobenzylguanidine. Ann Intern Med 1981; 94:762–767.
409. Tibblin S, Dymling JF, Ingemansson S, et al. Unilateral versus bilateral adrenalectomy in multiple endocrine neoplasia IIA. World J Surg 1983; 7:201–208.
410. Jansson S, Tisell LE, Fjalling M, et al. Early diagnosis of and surgical strategy for adrenal medullary disease in MEN II gene carriers. Surgery 1988; 103:11–18.
411. Lips CJ, Minder WH, Leo JR, et al. Evidence of multicentric origin of the multiple endocrine neoplasia syndrome type 2a (Sipple's syndrome) in a large family in the Netherlands: diagnostic and therapeutic implications. Am J Med 1978; 64:569–578.
412. van Heerden JA, Sizemore GW, Carney JA, et al. Surgical management of the adrenal glands in the multiple endocrine neoplasia type II syndrome. World J Surg 1984; 8:612–621.
413. Lairmore TC, Ball DW, Baylin SB, et al. Management of pheochromocytomas in patients with multiple endocrine neoplasia type 2 syndromes. Ann Surg 1993; 217:595–601; discussion 601–603.
414. Telenius-Berg M, Ponder MA, Berg B, et al. Quality of life after bilateral adrenalectomy in MEN2. Henry Ford Hosp Med J 1989; 37:160–163.
415. Irvin GL III, Fishman LM, Sher JA. Familial pheochromocytoma. Surgery 1983; 94:938–940.
416. van Heerden JA, Sizemore GW, Carney JA, et al. Bilateral subtotal adrenal resection for bilateral pheochromocytomas in multiple endocrine neoplasia, type IIa: a case report. Surgery 1985; 98: 363–366.
417. Hamberger B, Telenius BM, Cedermark B, et al. Subtotal adrenalectomy in multiple endocrine neoplasia type 2. Henry Ford Hosp Med J 1987; 35:127–128.
418. Albanese CT, Wiener ES. Routine total bilateral adrenalectomy is not warranted in childhood familial pheochromocytoma. J Pediatr Surg 1993; 28:1248–1251; discussion 1251–1252.
419. Evans DB, Lee JE, Merrell RC, et al. Adrenal medullary disease in multiple endocrine neoplasia type 2: appropriate management. Endocrinol Metab Clin North Am 1994; 23:167–176.
420. Nguyen L, Niccoli-Sire P, Caron P, et al. Pheochromocytoma in multiple endocrine neoplasia type 2: a prospective study. Eur J Endocrinol 2001; 144:37–44.
421. Brunt LM, Moley JF, Doherty GM, et al. Outcomes analysis in patients undergoing laparoscopic adrenalectomy for hormonally active adrenal tumors. Surgery 2001; 130:629–634; discussion 634-635.
422. Sprung J, O'Hara JF Jr, Gill IS, et al. Anesthetic aspects of laparoscopic and open adrenalectomy for pheochromocytoma. Urology 2000; 55:339–343.
423. Terachi T, Yoshida O, Matsuda T, et al. Complications of laparoscopic and retroperitoneoscopic adrenalectomies in 370 cases in Japan: a multi-institutional study. Biomed Pharmacother 2000; 54(suppl 1):211s-214s.
424. Carney JA, Roth SI, Heath H III, et al. The parathyroid glands in multiple endocrine neoplasia type 2b. Am J Pathol 1980; 99: 387–398.
425. Skinner MA, Norton JA, Moley JF, et al. Heterotopic autotransplantation of parathyroid tissue in children undergoing total thyroidectomy. J Pediatr Surg 1997; 32:510–513.
426. Farndon JR, Leight GS, Dilley WG, et al. Familial medullary thyroid carcinoma without associated endocrinopathies: a distinct clinical entity. Br J Surg 1986; 73:278–281.
427. Gagel RF, Levy ML, Donovan DT, et al. Multiple endocrine neoplasia type 2a associated with cutaneous lichen amyloidosis. Ann Intern Med 1989; 111:802–806.
428. Nunziata V, di Giovanni G, Lettera AM, et al. Cutaneous lichen amyloidosis associated with multiple endocrine neoplasia type 2A. Henry Ford Hosp J 1989; 37:144–146.
429. Chabre O, Labat F, Pinel N, et al. Cutaneous lesion associated with multiple endocrine neoplasia type 2A: lichen amyloidosis or notalgia paresthetica. Henry Ford Hosp J 1992; 40:245–248.
430. Wong C-K, Lin C-S. Friction amyloidosis. Int J Dermatol 1988; 27:302–307.
431. Durbec PL, Larsson-Blomberg LB, Schuchardt A, et al. Common origin and developmental dependence on c-ret of subsets of enteric and sympathetic neuroblasts. Development 1996; 122: 349–358.
432. Gagel RF. When "The 7-Year Itch" is indicative of an endocrine malignant condition. Endocr Pract 2002; 8:72–74.
433. Verdy MB, Cadotte M, Schurch W, et al. A French Canadian family with multiple endocrine neoplasia type 2 syndromes. Henry Ford Hosp Med J 1984; 32:251–253.
434. Blank RD, Sklar CA, Dimich AB, et al. Clinical presentations and *RET* protooncogene mutations in seven multiple endocrine neoplasia type 2 kindreds. Cancer 1996; 78:1996–2003.
435. Borst M, Peacock BA, Minth C, et al. Mutational analysis of Hirschsprung's disease associated with multiple endocrine neoplasia type 2A. Presented as abstract at the Fifth International Workshop on Multiple Endocrine Neoplasia, Stockholm, Sweden, 1994.
436. Decker RA, Peacock ML, Watson P. Hirschsprung disease in MEN2A: increased spectrum of RET exon 10 genotypes and strong genotype-phenotype correlation. Hum Mol Genet 1998; 7: 129–134.

437. Eng C, Clayton D, Schuffenecker I, et al. The relationship between specific *RET* proto-oncogene mutations and disease phenotype in multiple endocrine neoplasia type 2. International RET mutation consortium analysis. JAMA 1996; 276:1575–1579.
438. Inoue K, Shimotake T, Tokiwa K, et al. Mutational analysis of the *RET* proto-oncogene in a kindred with multiple endocrine neoplasia type 2A and Hirschsprung's disease. J Pediatr Surg 1999; 34:1552–1554.
439. Ito S, Iwashita T, Asai N, et al. Biological properties of Ret with cysteine mutations correlate with multiple endocrine neoplasia type 2A, familial medullary thyroid carcinoma, and Hirschsprung's disease phenotype. Cancer Res 1997; 57:2870–2872.
440. Lacroix A, Blanchard L, Villeneuve L, et al. Cosegregation of Hirschsprung's disease (HSCR) with chromosome 10 markers and a ret mutation in a French Canadian family with MEN 2A. Presented as abstract at the Fifth International Workshop on Multiple Endocrine Neoplasia, Stockholm, Sweden, 1994.
441. Peretz H, Luboshitsky R, Baron E, et al. Cys 618 Arg mutation in the *RET* proto-oncogene associated with familial medullary thyroid carcinoma and maternally transmitted Hirschsprung's disease suggesting a role for imprinting. Hum Mutat 1997; 10:155–159.
442. Sasaki Y, Shimotake T, Go S, et al. Total thyroidectomy for hereditary medullary thyroid carcinoma 12 years after correction of Hirschsprung's disease. Eur J Surg 2001; 167:467–469.
443. Williams ED, Pollock DJ. Multiple mucosal neuromata with endocrine tumours: a syndrome allied to von Recklinghausen's disease. J Pathol Bacteriol 1966; 91:71–80.
444. Rashid M, Khairi MR, Dexter RN, et al. Mucosal neuroma, pheochromocytoma and medullary thyroid carcinoma: multiple endocrine neoplasia type 3. Medicine (Baltimore) 1975; 54:89–112.
445. Carney JA, Sizemore GW, Hayles AB. C-cell disease of the thyroid gland in multiple endocrine neoplasia, type 2b. Cancer 1979; 44:2173–2183.
446. Carney JA, Go VL, Sizemore GW, et al. Alimentary-tract ganglioneuromatosis: a major component of the syndrome of multiple endocrine neoplasia, type 2b. N Engl J Med 1976; 295:1287–1291.
447. Khan AH, Desjardins JG, Youssef S, et al. Gastrointestinal manifestations of Sipple syndrome in children. J Pediatr Surg 1987; 22:719–723.
448. Stjernholm MR, Freudenbourg JC, Mooney HS, et al. Medullary carcinoma of the thyroid before age 2 years. J Clin Endocrinol Metab 1980; 51:252–253.
449. Kaufman FR, Roe TF, Isaacs H Jr, et al. Metastatic medullary thyroid carcinoma in young children with mucosal neuroma syndrome. Pediatrics 1982; 70:263–267.
450. Gill JR, Reyes-Mugica M, Iyengar S, et al. Early presentation of metastatic medullary carcinoma in multiple endocrine neoplasia, type IIA: implications for therapy. J Pediatr 1996; 129:459–464.
451. Smith VV, Eng C, Milla PJ. Intestinal ganglioneuromatosis and multiple endocrine neoplasia type 2B: implications for treatment. Gut 1999; 45:143–146.
452. Kakudo K, Carney JA, Sizemore GW. Medullary carcinoma of thyroid: biologic behavior of the sporadic and familial neoplasm. Cancer 1985; 55:2818–2821.
453. Sizemore GW, Carney JA, Gharib H, et al. Multiple endocrine neoplasia type 2B: eighteen-year follow-up of a four-generation family. Henry Ford Hosp J 1992; 40:236–244.
454. Vasen HFA, van der Feltz M, Raue F, et al. The natural course of multiple endocrine neoplasia type IIb: a study of 18 cases. Arch Intern Med 1992; 152:1250–1252.
455. Dyck PJ, Carney JA, Sizemore GW, et al. Multiple endocrine neoplasia, type 2b: phenotype recognition; neurological features and their pathological basis. Ann Neurol 1979; 6:302–314.
456. Aine E, Aine L, Huupponen T, et al. Visible corneal nerve fibers and neuromas of the conjunctiva: a syndrome of type-3 multiple endocrine adenomatosis in two generations. Graefes Arch Clin Exp Ophthalmol 1987; 225:213–216.
457. Hubner A, Holschneider AM. Multiple endocrine neoplasias in 3 generations. Langenbecks Arch Chir 1987; 372:747–750.
458. Carlson KM, Bracamontes J, Jackson CE, et al. Parent-of-origin effects in multiple endocrine neoplasia type 2B. Am J Hum Genet 1994; 55:1076–1082.
459. Norton JA, Froome LC, Farrell RE, et al. Multiple endocrine neoplasia type IIb: the most aggressive form of medullary thyroid carcinoma. Surg Clin North Am 1979; 59:109–118.
460. Pujol RM, Matias-Guiu X, Miralles J, et al. Multiple idiopathic mucosal neuromas: a minor form of multiple endocrine neoplasia type 2B or a new entity? J Am Acad Dermatol 1997; 37:349–352.
461. Gomez JM, Biarnes J, Volpini V, et al. Neuromas and prominent corneal nerves without MEN2B. Ann Endocrinol 1998; 59:492–494.
462. Valentines J, Marigo M, Quintana M, et al. Familial mucosal neuromatosis: a minor form of the MEN2b syndrome. J Fr Ophtalmol 1984; 7:479–484.
463. Sciubba JJ, D'Amico E, Attie JN. The occurrence of multiple endocrine neoplasia type IIb, in two children of an affected mother. J Oral Pathol 1987; 16:310–316.
464. Mathew CG, Chin KS, Easton DF, et al. A linked genetic marker for multiple endocrine neoplasia type 2A on chromosome 10. Nature 1987; 328:527–528.
465. Simpson NE, Kidd KK, Goodfellow PJ, et al. Assignment of multiple endocrine neoplasia type 2A to chromosome 10 by linkage. Nature 1987; 328:528–530.
466. Norum RA, Lafreniere RG, O'Neal LW, et al. Linkage of the multiple endocrine neoplasia type 2B gene (*MEN2B*) to chromosome 10 markers linked to *MEN2A*. Genomics 1990; 8:313–317.
467. Lairmore TC, Howe JR, Korte JA, et al. Familial medullary thyroid carcinoma and multiple endocrine neoplasia type 2B map to the same region of chromosome 10 as multiple endocrine neoplasia type 2A. Genomics 1991; 9:181–192.
468. Angrist M, Kauffman E, Slaugenhaupt SA, et al. A gene for Hirschsprung disease (megacolon) in the pericentromeric region of human chromosome 10. Nat Genet 1993; 4:351–356.
469. Lyonnet S, Bolino A, Pelet A, et al. A gene for Hirschsprung disease maps to the proximal long arm of chromosome 10. Nat Genet 1993; 4:346–350.
470. Mulligan LM, Kwok JB, Healey CS, et al. Germ-line mutations of the *RET* proto-oncogene in multiple endocrine neoplasia type 2A. Nature 1993; 363:458–460.
471. Donis-Keller H, Dou S, Chi D, et al. Mutations in the *RET* proto-oncogene are associated with MEN2A and FMTC. Hum Mol Genet 1993; 2:851–856.
472. Carlson KM, Dou S, Chi D, et al. Single missense mutation in the tyrosine kinase catalytic domain of the *RET* protooncogene is associated with multiple endocrine neoplasia type 2B. Proc Natl Acad Sci USA 1994; 91:1579–1583.
473. Hofstra RM, Landsvater RM, Ceccherini I, et al. A mutation in the *RET* proto-oncogene associated with multiple endocrine neoplasia type 2B and sporadic medullary thyroid carcinoma. Nature 1994; 367:375–376.
474. Borst MJ, Van Camp JM, Peacock ML, et al. Mutational analysis of multiple endocrine neoplasia type 2A associated with Hirschsprung's disease. Surgery 1995; 117:386–391.
475. Wohllk N, Cote GJ, Bugalho MMJ, et al. Relevance of *RET* proto-oncogene mutations in sporadic medullary thyroid carcinoma. J Clin Endocrinol Metab 1996; 81:3740–3745.
476. Ceccherini I, Romei C, Barone V, et al. Identification of the cys 634-to-tyr mutation of the *RET* proto-oncogene in a pedigree with multiple endocrine neoplasia type 2A and localized cutaneous lichen amyloidosis. J Endocr Invest 1994; 17:201–204.
477. Edery P, Lyonnet S, Mulligan LM, et al. Mutations of the *RET* proto-oncogene in Hirschsprung's disease. Nature 1994; 367:378–380.
478. Romeo G, Ronchetto P, Luo Y, et al. Point mutations affecting the tyrosine kinase domain of the *RET* proto-oncogene in Hirschsprung's disease. Nature 1994; 367:377–378.
479. Angrist M, Bolk S, Thiel B, et al. Mutation analysis of the RET receptor tyrosine kinase in Hirschsprung's disease. Hum Mol Genet 1995; 4:821–830.
480. Eng C, Mulligan LM, Smith DP, et al. Low frequency of germline mutations in the *RET* proto-oncogene in patients with apparently sporadic medullary thyroid carcinoma. Clin Endocrinol 1995; 43:123–127.
481. Zedenius J, Larsson C, Bergholm U, et al. Mutations of codon 918 in the *RET* proto-oncogene correlate to poor prognosis in sporadic medullary thyroid carcinomas. J Clin Endocrinol Metab 1995; 80:3088–3090.
482. Komminoth P, Kunz E, Hiort O, et al. Detection of *RET* proto-

oncogene point mutations in paraffin-embedded pheochromocytoma specimens by nonradioactive single-strand conformation polymorphism analysis and direct sequencing. Am J Pathol 1994; 145:922–929.
483. Takahashi M, Ritz J, Cooper GM. Activation of a novel human transforming gene, *ret*, by DNA rearrangement. Cell 1985; 42: 581–588.
484. Takahashi M, Buma Y, Iwamoto T, et al. Cloning and expression of the *ret* proto-oncogene encoding a tyrosine kinase with two potential transmembrane domains. Oncogene 1988; 3:571–578.
485. Donghi R, Sozzi G, Pierotti MA, et al. The oncogene associated with human papillary thyroid carcinoma (PTC) is assigned to chromosome 10 q11-q12 in the same region as multiple endocrine neoplasia type 2A (*MEN2A*). Oncogene 1989; 4:521–523.
486. Bongarzone I, Pierotti MA, Monzini N, et al. High frequency of activation of tyrosine kinase oncogenes in human papillary thyroid carcinoma. Oncogene 1989; 4:1457–1462.
487. Grieco M, Santoro M, Berlingieri MT, et al. *PTC* is a novel rearranged form of the *ret* proto-oncogene and is frequently detected in vivo in human thyroid papillary carcinomas. Cell 1990; 60:557–563.
488. Takahashi M. The GDNF/RET signaling pathway and human diseases. Cytokine Growth Factor Rev 2001; 12:361–373.
489. Vecchio G, Santoro M. Oncogenes and thyroid cancer. Clin Chem Lab Med 2000; 38:113–116.
490. Hoff AO, Cote GJ, Gagel RF. Multiple endocrine neoplasias. Annu Rev Physiol 2000; 62:377–411.
491. Nikiforova MN, Stringer JR, Blough R, et al. Proximity of chromosomal loci that participate in radiation-induced rearrangements in human cells. Science 2000; 290:138–141.
492. Nikiforov YE, Rowland JM, Bove KE, et al. Distinct pattern of *ret* oncogene rearrangements in morphological variants of radiation-induced and sporadic thyroid papillary carcinomas in children. Cancer Res 1997; 57:1690–1694.
493. Chiappetta G, Toti P, Cetta F, et al. The *RET/PTC* oncogene is frequently activated in oncocytic thyroid tumors (Hurthle cell adenomas and carcinomas), but not in oncocytic hyperplastic lesions. J Clin Endocrinol Metab 2002; 87:364–369.
494. Sanchez M, Silos-Santiago I, Frisen J, et al. Newborn mice lacking GDNF display renal agenesis and absence of enteric neurons, but no deficits in midbrain dopaminergic neurons. Nature 1996; 382:70–73.
495. Robbins J, Gulick J, Sanchez A, et al. Mouse embryonic stem cells express the cardiac myosin heavy chain genes during development in vitro. J Biol Chem 1990; 265:11905–11909.
496. Moore MW, Klein RD, Farinas I, et al. Renal and neuronal abnormalities in mice lacking GDNF. Nature 1996; 382:76–79.
497. Pichel JG, Shen L, Sheng HZ, et al. Defects in enteric innervation and kidney development in mice lacking GDNF. Nature 1996; 382:73–76.
498. Schuchardt A, D'Agati V, Larsson-Blomberg L, et al. Defects in the kidney and enteric nervous system of mice lacking the tyrosine kinase receptor Ret. Nature 1994; 367:380–383.
499. Jing S, Wen D, Yu Y, et al. GDNF-induced activation of the Ret protein tyrosine kinase is mediated by GDNFR-α, a novel receptor for GDNF. Cell 1996; 85:1113–1124.
500. Durbec P, Marcos-Gutierrez CV, Kilkenny C, et al. GDNF signalling through the ret receptor tyrosine kinase. Nature 1996; 381:789–793.
501. Treanor JJ, Goodman L, de Sauvage F, et al. Characterization of a multicomponent receptor for GDNF. Nature 1996; 382:80–83.
502. Cacalano G, Farinas I, Wang LC, et al. GFRalpha1 is an essential receptor component for GDNF in the developing nervous system and kidney. Neuron 1998; 21:53–62.
503. Santoro M, Rosati R, Grieco M, et al. The *ret* proto-oncogene is consistently expressed in human pheochromocytomas and thyroid medullary carcinomas. Oncogene 1990; 5:1595–1598.
504. Edstrom E, Frisk T, Farnebo F, et al. Expression analysis of RET and the GDNF/GFRalpha-1 and NTN/GFRalpha-2 ligand complexes in pheochromocytomas and paragangliomas. Int J Mol Med 2000; 6:469–474.
505. Pachnis V, Mankoo B, Costantini F. Expression of the c-*ret* proto-oncogene during mouse embryogenesis. Development 1993; 119:1005–1017.
506. Tsuzuki T, Takahashi M, Asai N, et al. Spatial and temporal expression of the *ret* proto-oncogene product in embryonic, infant and adult rat tissues. Oncogene 1995; 10:191–198.
507. Pausova Z, Soliman E, Amizuka N, et al. Role of the *RET* proto-oncogene in sporadic hyperparathyroidism and in hyperparathyroidism of multiple endocrine neoplasia type 2. J Clin Endocrinol Metab 1996; 81:2711–2718.
508. Attie-Bitach T, Abitbol M, Gerard M, et al. Expression of the *RET* proto-oncogene in human embryos. Am J Med Genet 1998; 80:481–486.
509. Pichel JG, Shen L, Sheng HZ, et al. Defects in enteric innervation and kidney development in mice lacking GDNF. Nature 1996; 382:73–76.
510. Carlson KM, Dou S, Chi D, et al. Single missense mutation in the tyrosine kinase catalytic domain of the *RET* protooncogene is associated with multiple endocrine neoplasia type 2B. Proc Natl Acad Sci USA 1994; 91:1579–1583.
511. Attie T, Pelet A, Edery P, et al. Diversity of *RET* proto-oncogene mutations in familial and sporadic Hirschsprung disease. Hum Mol Genet 1995; 4:1381–1386.
512. Mulligan LM, Eng C, Attie T, et al. Diverse phenotypes associated with exon 10 mutations of the *RET* proto-oncogene. Hum Mol Genet 1994; 3:2163–2167.
513. Niccoli-Sire P, Murat A, Rohmer V, et al. Familial medullary thyroid carcinoma with noncysteine ret mutations: phenotype-genotype relationship in a large series of patients. J Clin Endocrinol Metab 2001; 86:3746–3753.
514. Kitamura Y, Goodfellow PJ, Shimizu K, et al. Novel germline *RET* proto-oncogene mutations associated with medullary thyroid carcinoma (MTC): mutation analysis in Japanese patients with MTC. Oncogene 1997; 14:3103–3106.
515. Eng C, Smith DP, Mulligan LM, et al. A novel point mutation in the tyrosine kinase domain of the *RET* proto-oncogene in sporadic medullary thyroid carcinoma and in a family with FMTC. Oncogene 1995; 10:509–513.
516. Bolino A, Schuffenecker I, Luo Y, et al. *RET* mutations in exons 13 and 14 of FMTC patients. Oncogene 1995; 10:2415–2419.
517. Moers AM, Landsvater RM, Schaap C, et al. Familial medullary thyroid carcinoma: not a distinct entity? Genotype-phenotype correlation in a large family. Am J Med 1996; 101:635–641.
518. Berndt I, Reuter M, Saller B, et al. A new hot spot for mutations in the *ret* protooncogene causing familial medullary thyroid carcinoma and multiple endocrine neoplasia type 2A. J Clin Endocrinol Metab 1998; 83:770–774.
519. Hofstra RM, Fattoruso O, Quadro L, et al. A novel point mutation in the intracellular domain of the *ret* protooncogene in a family with medullary thyroid carcinoma. J Clin Endocrinol Metab 1997; 82:4176–4178.
520. Dang GT, Cote GJ, Schultz PN, et al. A codon 891 exon 15 *RET* proto-oncogene mutation in familial medullary thyroid carcinoma: a detection strategy. Mol Cell Probes 1999; 13:77–79.
521. Iwashita T, Kato M, Murakami H, et al. Biological and biochemical properties of Ret with kinase domain mutations identified in multiple endocrine neoplasia type 2B and familial medullary thyroid carcinoma. Oncogene 1999; 18:3919–3922.
522. Carlomagno F, Salvatore G, Cirafici AM, et al. The different *RET*-activating capability of mutations of cysteine 620 or cysteine 634 correlates with the multiple endocrine neoplasia type 2 disease phenotype. Cancer Res 1997; 57:391–395.
523. Edery P, Pelet A, Mulligan LM, et al. Long segment and short segment familial Hirschsprung's disease: variable clinical expression at the RET locus. J Med Genet 1994; 31:602–606.
524. Lyonnet S, Edery P, Mulligan LM, et al. [Mutations of *RET* proto-oncogene in Hirschsprung disease]. C R Acad Sci III 1994; 317:358–362.
525. Alemi M, Lucas SD, Sallstrom JF, et al. A complex nine base pair deletion in *RET* exon 11 common in sporadic medullary thyroid carcinoma. Oncogene 1997; 14:2041–2045.
526. Chiefari E, Russo D, Giuffrida D, et al. Analysis of *RET* proto-oncogene abnormalities in patients with MEN2A, MEN2B, familial or sporadic medullary thyroid carcinoma. J Endocrinol Invest 1998; 21:358–364.
527. Eng C, Mulligan LM, Smith DP, et al. Mutation of the *RET* protooncogene in sporadic medullary thyroid carcinoma. Genes Chromosomes Cancer 1995; 12:209–212.
528. Frilling A, Bockhorn M, Kalinin V, et al. [Somatic *ret* proto-oncogene mutations in sporadic C-cell carcinoma of the thyroid gland]. Chirurg 1997; 68:789–793.
529. Huang CN, Wu SL, Chang TC, et al. *RET* protooncogene mu-

tations in patients with apparently sporadic medullary thyroid carcinoma. J Formos Med Assoc 1998; 97:541–546.
530. Maeda S, Namba H, Takamura N, et al. A single missense mutation in codon 918 of the *RET* proto-oncogene in sporadic medullary thyroid carcinomas. Endocr J 1995; 42:245–250.
531. Marsh DJ, Learoyd DL, Andrew SD, et al. Somatic mutations in the *RET* proto-oncogene in sporadic medullary thyroid carcinoma. Clin Endocrinol 1996; 44:249–257.
532. Eng C, Mulligan L, Healey CS, et al. Heterogeneous mutations of the RET proto-oncogene in subpopulations of medullary thyroid carcinoma. Cancer Res 1996; 56:2167–2170.
533. Schilling T, Burck J, Sinn HP, et al. Prognostic value of codon 918 (ATG→ACG) RET proto-oncogene mutations in sporadic medullary thyroid carcinoma. Int J Cancer 2001; 95:62–66.
534. Scurini C, Quadro L, Fattoruso O, et al. Germline and somatic mutations of the *RET* proto-oncogene in apparently sporadic medullary thyroid carcinomas. Mol Cell Endocrinol 1998; 137: 51–57.
535. Takano T, Miyauchi A, Yoshida H, et al. Large-scale analysis of mutations in *RET* exon 16 in sporadic medullary thyroid carcinomas in Japan. Jpn J Cancer Res 2001; 92:645–648.
536. Uchino S, Noguchi S, Yamashita H, et al. Somatic mutations in *RET* exons 12 and 15 in sporadic medullary thyroid carcinomas: different spectrum of mutations in sporadic type from hereditary type. Jpn J Cancer Res 1999; 90:1231–1237.
537. Zedenius J, Wallin G, Hamberger B, et al. Somatic and MEN 2A de novo mutations identified in the *RET* proto-oncogene by screening of sporadic MTCs. Hum Mol Genet 1994; 3:1259–1262.
538. Rodien P, Jeunemaitre X, Dumont C, et al. Genetic alterations of the *RET* proto-oncogene in familial and sporadic pheochromocytomas. Horm Res 1997; 47:263–268.
539. Eng C, Crossey PA, Mulligan LM, et al. Mutations in the *RET* proto-oncogene and the von Hippel–Lindau disease tumour suppressor gene in sporadic and syndromic phaeochromocytomas. J Med Genet 1995; 32:934–937.
540. Bender BU, Gutsche M, Glasker S, et al. Differential genetic alterations in von Hippel–Lindau syndrome–associated and sporadic pheochromocytomas. J Clin Endocrinol Metab 2000; 85: 4568–4574.
541. Asai N, Iwashita T, Matsuyama M, et al. Mechanism of activation of the *ret* proto-oncogene by multiple endocrine neoplasia 2A mutations. Mol Cell Biol 1995; 15:1613–1619.
542. Santoro M, Carlomagno F, Romano A, et al. Activation of *RET* as a dominant transforming gene by germline mutations of MEN2A and MEN2B. Science 1995; 267:381–383.
543. Xing S, Smanik PA, Oglesbee MJ, et al. Characterization of *ret* oncogenic activation in MEN2 inherited cancer syndromes. Endocrinology 1996; 137:1512–1519.
544. Carlomagno F, Melillo RM, Visconti R, et al. Glial cell line–derived neurotrophic factor differentially stimulates ret mutants associated with the multiple endocrine neoplasia type 2 syndromes and Hirschsprung's disease. Endocrinology 1998; 139: 3613–3619.
545. Salvatore D, Barone MV, Salvatore G, et al. Tyrosines 1015 and 1062 are in vivo autophosphorylation sites in ret and ret-derived oncoproteins. J Clin Endocrinol Metab 2000; 85:3898–3907.
546. Ishiguro Y, Iwashita T, Murakami H, et al. The role of amino acids surrounding tyrosine 1062 in ret in specific binding of the shc phosphotyrosine-binding domain. Endocrinology 1999; 140: 3992–3998.
547. Asai N, Murakami H, Iwashita T, et al. A mutation at tyrosine 1062 in MEN2A-Ret and MEN2B-Ret impairs their transforming activity and association with shc adaptor proteins. J Biol Chem 1996; 271:17644–1769.
548. Hayashi Y, Iwashita T, Murakamai H, et al. Activation of BMK1 via tyrosine 1062 in RET by GDNF and MEN2A mutation. Biochem Biophys Res Commun 2001; 281:682–689.
549. Chiariello M, Visconti R, Carlomagno F, et al. Signalling of RET receptor tyrosine kinase through the C-Jun NH2-terminal protein kinases (JNKS): evidence for a divergence of the erks and jnks pathways induced by RET. Oncogene 1998; 16:2435–2445.
550. De Vita G, Melillo RM, Carlomagno F, et al. Tyrosine 1062 of RET-MEN2A mediates activation of Akt (protein kinase B) and mitogen-activated protein kinase pathways leading to PC12 cell survival. Cancer Res 2000; 60:3727–3731.
551. Hayashi H, Ichihara M, Iwashita T, et al. Characterization of intracellular signals via tyrosine 1062 in *RET* activated by glial cell line–derived neurotrophic factor. Oncogene 2000; 19:4469–4475.
552. Ohiwa M, Murakami H, Iwashita T, et al. Characterization of Ret-Shc-Grb2 complex induced by GDNF, MEN 2A, and MEN 2B mutations. Biochem Biophys Res Commun 1997; 237:747–751.
553. Melillo RM, Barone MV, Lupoli G, et al. Ret-mediated mitogenesis requires Src kinase activity. Cancer Res 1999; 59:1120–1126.
554. Ludwig L, Kessler H, Wagner M, et al. Nuclear factor-kappaB is constitutively active in C-cell carcinoma and required for *RET*-induced transformation. Cancer Res 2001; 61:4526–4535.
555. Khosla S, Patel VM, Hay ID, et al. Loss of heterozygosity suggests multiple genetic alterations in pheochromocytomas and medullary thyroid carcinomas. J Clin Invest 1991; 87:1691–1699.
556. Yang KP, Nguyen CV, Castillo SG, et al. Deletion mapping on the distal third region of chromosome 1p in multiple endocrine neoplasia type IIA. Anticancer Res 1990; 10:527–533.
557. Takai S, Tateishi H, Nishisho I, et al. Loss of genes on chromosome 22 in medullary thyroid carcinoma and pheochromocytoma. Jpn J Cancer Res 1987; 78:894–898.
558. Benn DE, Dwight T, Richardson AL, et al. Sporadic and familial pheochromocytomas are associated with loss of at least two discrete intervals on chromosome 1p. Cancer Res 2000; 60:7048–7051.
559. Moley JF, Brother MB, Fong CT, et al. Consistent association of 1p loss of heterozygosity with pheochromocytomas from patients with multiple endocrine neoplasia type 2 syndromes. Cancer Res 1992; 52:770–774.
560. Shin E, Fujita S, Takami K, et al. Deletion mapping of chromosome 1p and 22q in pheochromocytoma. Jpn J Cancer Res 1993; 84:402–408.
561. Uchino S, Noguchi S, Adachi M, et al. Novel point mutations and allele loss at the *RET* locus in sporadic medullary thyroid carcinomas. Jpn J Cancer Res 1998; 89:411–418.
562. Huang SC, Koch CA, Vortmeyer AO, et al. Duplication of the mutant RET allele in trisomy 10 or loss of the wild-type allele in multiple endocrine neoplasia type 2-associated pheochromocytomas. Cancer Res 2000; 60:6223–6226.
563. Koch CA, Huang SC, Moley JF, et al. Allelic imbalance of the mutant and wild-type RET allele in MEN 2A–associated medullary thyroid carcinoma. Oncogene 2001; 20:7809–7811.
564. Zhang Z, Wang Y, Vikis HG, et al. Wildtype Kras2 can inhibit lung carcinogenesis in mice. Nat Genet 2001; 29:25–33.
565. Zhuang Z, Park WS, Pack S, et al. Trisomy 7–harbouring nonrandom duplication of the mutant *MET* allele in hereditary papillary renal carcinomas. Nat Genet 1998; 20:66–69.
566. Okazaki M, Miya A, Tanaka N, et al. Allele loss on chromosome 10 and point mutation of *ras* oncogenes are infrequent in tumors of MEN 2A. Henry Ford Hosp Med J 1989; 37:112–115.
567. Landsvater RM, de Wit MJ, Zewald RA, et al. Somatic mutations of the *RET* proto-oncogene are not required for tumor development in multiple endocrine neoplasia type 2 (MEN 2) gene carriers. Cancer Res 1996; 56:4853–4855.
568. Cote GJ, Wohllk N, Evans D, et al. *RET* proto-oncogene mutations in multiple endocrine neoplasia type 2 and medullary thyroid carcinoma. Bailliere's Clin Endocrinol Metab 1995; 9:609–630.
569. Decker R, Borst M, Peacock M. Rapid screening for *ret* mutations in multiple endocrine neoplasia type 2 by denaturing gradient electrophoresis. Presented at the Fifth International Workshop on Multiple Endocrine Neoplasia, Stockholm, Sweden, July 1994.
570. Decker RA, Peacock ML, Borst MJ, et al. Progress in genetic screening of multiple endocrine neoplasia type 2A: is calcitonin testing obsolete? Surgery 1995; 118:257–264.
571. Wells SA Jr, Baylin SB, Linehan WM, et al. Provocative agents and the diagnosis of medullary carcinoma of the thyroid gland. Ann Surg 1978; 188:139–141.
572. Parthemore JG, Bronzert D, Roberts G, et al. A short calcium infusion in the diagnosis of medullary thyroid carcinoma. J Clin Endocrinol Metab 1974; 39:108–111.
573. Body JJ, Heath H III. Estimates of circulating monomeric calcitonin: physiological studies in normal and thyroidectomized man. J Clin Endocrinol Metab 1983; 57:897–903.
574. Catherwood BD, Deftos LJ. General principles, problems and

interpretation in the radioimmunoassay of calcitonin. Biomed Pharmacother 1984; 38:235–241.

575. Motte P, Vauzelle P, Gardet P, et al. Construction and clinical validation of a sensitive and specific assay for serum mature calcitonin using monoclonal anti-peptide antibodies. Clin Chim Acta 1988; 174:35–54.
576. Seth R, Motte P, Kehely A, et al. A sensitive and specific two-site enzyme-immunoassay for human calcitonin using monoclonal antibodies. J Endocrinol 1988; 119:351–357.
577. Body JJ, Heath HI. Nonspecific increases in plasma immunoreactive calcitonin in healthy individuals: discrimination from medullary thyroid carcinoma by a new extraction technique. Clin Chem 1984; 30:511–514.
578. Samaan NA, Castillo S, Schultz PN, et al. Serum calcitonin after pentagastrin stimulation in patients with bronchogenic and breast cancer compared to that in patients with medullary thyroid carcinoma. J Clin Endocrinol Metab 1980; 51:237–241.
579. Ghillani P, Motte P, Bohuon C, et al. Monoclonal antipeptide antibodies as tools to dissect closely related gene products: a model using peptides encoded by the calcitonin gene. J Immunol 1988; 141:3156–3163.
580. Wohllk N, Cote GJ, Evans D, et al. Application of genetic screening information to the management of medullary thyroid carcinoma and multiple endocrine neoplasia. Endocrine Metab Clin North Am 1996; 25:1–25.
581. Scopsi L, Sampietro G, Boracchi P, et al. Multivariate analysis of prognostic factors in sporadic medullary carcinoma of the thyroid: a retrospective study of 109 consecutive patients. Cancer 1996; 78:2173–2183.
582. van Heurn LW, Schaap C, Sie G, et al. Predictive DNA testing for multiple endocrine neoplasia 2: a therapeutic challenge of prophylactic thyroidectomy in very young children. J Pediatr Surg 1999; 34:568–571.
583. Arts CH, Bax NM, Jansen M, et al. [Prophylactic total thyroidectomy in childhood for multiple endocrine neoplasia type 2A: preliminary results]. Ned Tijdschr Geneeskd 1999; 143:98–104.
584. Komminoth P, Kunz EK, Matias-Guiu X, et al. Analysis of *RET* proto-oncogene point mutations distinguishes heritable from nonheritable medullary thyroid carcinomas. Cancer 1995; 76: 479–489.
585. Shirahama S, Ogura K, Takami H, et al. Mutational analysis of the *RET* proto-oncogene in 71 Japanese patients with medullary thyroid carcinoma. J Hum Genet 1998; 43:101–106.
586. Mulligan LM, Eng C, Healey CS, et al. A de novo mutation of the *RET* proto-oncogene in a patient with MEN2A. Hum Mol Genet 1994; 3:1007–1008.
587. Neuman HPH, Bausch B, McWhinney SR, et al. Germ-line mutations in nonsyndromic pheochromocytoma. N Engl J Med 2002; 346:1459–1466.
588. Brauch H, Hoeppner W, Jahnig H, et al. Sporadic pheochromocytomas are rarely associated with germline mutations in the *vhl* tumor suppressor gene or the ret protooncogene. J Clin Endocrinol Metab 1997; 82:4101–4104.
589. Woodward ER, Eng C, McMahon R, et al. Genetic predisposition to phaeochromocytoma: analysis of candidate genes *GDNF*, *RET* and *VHL*. Hum Mol Genet 1997; 6:1051–1056.
590. Dahia PL, Toledo SP, Mulligan LM, et al. Mutation analysis of glial cell line–derived neurotrophic factor (GDNF), a ligand for the RET/GDNF receptor alpha complex, in sporadic phaeochromocytomas. Cancer Res 1997; 57:310–313.
591. van der Harst E, de Krijger RR, Dinjens WN, et al. Germline mutations in the vhl gene in patients presenting with phaeochromocytomas. Int J Cancer 1998; 77:337–340.
592. Bar M, Friedman E, Jakobovitz O, et al. Sporadic phaeochromocytomas are rarely associated with germline mutations in the von Hippel–Lindau and *RET* genes. Clin Endocrinol (Oxf) 1997; 47: 707–712.
593. Astuti D, Douglas F, Lennard TW, et al. Germline *SDHD* mutation in familial phaeochromocytoma. Lancet 2001; 357:1181–1182.
594. Niemann S, Muller U. Mutations in *SDHC* cause autosomal dominant paraganglioma, type 3. Nat Genet 2000; 26:268–270.
595. Astuti D, Latif F, Dallol A, et al. Gene mutations in the succinate dehydrogenase subunit *SDHB* cause susceptibility to familial pheochromocytoma and to familial paraganglioma. Am J Hum Genet 2001; 69:49–54.
596. Ponder BA, Ponder MA, Coffey R, et al. Risk estimation and screening in families of patients with medullary thyroid carcinoma. Lancet 1988; 1:397–401.
597. Gagel RF, Jackson CE, Block MA, et al. Age-related probability of development of hereditary medullary thyroid carcinoma. J Pediatr 1982; 101:941–946.
598. Easton DF, Ponder MA, Cummings T, et al. The clinical and screening age-at-onset distribution for the MEN2 syndrome. Am J Hum Genet 1989; 44:208–215.
599. Machens A, Gimm O, Hinze R, et al. Genotype-phenotype correlations in hereditary medullary thyroid carcinoma: oncological features and biochemical properties. J Clin Endocrinol Metab 2001; 86:1104–1109.
600. Niccoli-Sire P, Murat A, Baudin E, et al. Early or prophylactic thyroidectomy in MEN2/FMTC gene carriers: results in 71 thyroidectomized patients. The French Calcitonin Tumours Study Group (GETC). Eur J Endocrinol 1999; 141:468–474.
601. Sanso G, Domene HM, Iorcansky S, et al. [Early diagnosis of multiple endocrine neoplasia type 2 (MEN2) by detection of mutated *RET* proto-oncogene carriers]. Medicina (B Aires) 1998; 58:179–184.
602. Lallier M, St-Vil D, Giroux M, et al. Prophylactic thyroidectomy for medullary thyroid carcinoma in gene carriers of MEN2 syndrome. J Pediatr Surg 1998; 33:846–848.
603. Dralle H, Gimm O, Simon D, et al. Prophylactic thyroidectomy in 75 children and adolescents with hereditary medullary thyroid carcinoma: German and Austrian experience. World J Surg 1998; 22:744–750; discussion 750–751.
604. Frank-Raue K, Hoppner W, Buhr H, et al. Results and follow-up in eleven MEN2A gene carriers after prophylactic thyroidectomy. Exp Clin Endocrinol Diabetes 1997; 105:76–78.
605. Cameron D, Spiro HM, Landsberg L. Zollinger-Ellison syndrome with multiple endocrine adenomatosis type II (letter). N Engl J Med 1978; 299:152–153.
606. Sakai Y, Koizumi K, Sugitani I, et al. Familial adenomatous polyposis associated with multiple endocrine neoplasia type 1–related tumors and thyroid carcinoma: a case report with clinicopathologic and molecular analyses. Am J Surg Pathol 2002; 26: 103–110.
607. Perkins JT, Blackstone MO, Riddell RH. Adenomatous polyposis coli and multiple endocrine neoplasia type 2b: a pathogenetic relationship. Cancer 1985; 55:375–381.
608. Tuch BE, Carter JN, Armellin GM, et al. The association of a tumour of the posterior pituitary gland with multiple endocrine neoplasia type 1. Aust NZ J Med 1982; 12:179–181.
609. Bertrand JH, Ritz P, Reznik Y, et al. Sipple's syndrome associated with a large prolactinoma. Clin Endocrinol (Oxf) 1987; 27: 607–614.
610. Tamsen A, Mazur MT. Ovarian strumal carcinoid in association with multiple endocrine neoplasia, type IIA. Arch Pathol Lab Med 1992; 116:200–203.
611. Binkovitz LA, Johnson CD, Stephens DH. Islet cell tumors in von Hippel–Lindau disease: increased prevalence and relationship to the multiple endocrine neoplasias. AJR 1990; 155:501–505.
612. Hough DM, Stephens DH, Johnson CD, et al. Pancreatic lesions in von Hippel–Lindau disease: prevalence, clinical significance, and CT findings. AJR 1994; 162:1091–1094.
613. Filling-Katz MR, Choyke PL, Oldfield E, et al. Central nervous system involvement in von Hippel–Lindau disease. Neurology 1991; 41:41–46.
614. Neumann HP, Dinkel E, Brambs H, et al. Pancreatic lesions in the von Hippel–Lindau syndrome. Gastroenterology 1991; 101: 465–471.
615. La Forgia S, Lasota J, Latif F, et al. Detailed genetic and physical map of the 3p chromosome region surrounding the familial renal cell carcinoma chromosome translocation, t(3;8)(p14.2; q24.1). Cancer Res 1993; 53:3118–3124.
616. Latif F, Tory K, Gnarra J, et al. Identification of the von Hippel–Lindau disease tumor suppressor gene. Science 1993; 260:1317–1320.
617. Aso T, Lane WS, Conaway JW, et al. Elongin (SIII): a multisubunit regulator of elongation by RNA polymerase II. Science 1995; 269:1439–1443.
618. Duan DR, Pause A, Burgess WH, et al. Inhibition of transcription elongation by the VHL tumor suppressor protein. Science 1995; 269:1402–1406.

619. Kibel A, Iliopoulos O, De Caprio JA, et al. Binding of the von Hippel–Lindau tumor suppressor protein to elongin B and C. Science 1995; 269:1444–1446.
620. Maxwell PH, Wiesener MS, Chang GW, et al. The tumour suppressor protein VHL targets hypoxia-inducible factors for oxygen-dependent proteolysis. Nature 1999; 399:271–275.
621. Chen F, Kishida T, Yao M, et al. Germline mutations in the von Hippel–Lindau disease tumor suppressor gene: correlations with phenotype. Hum Mutat 1995; 5:66–75.
622. Janson KL, Roberts JA, Varela M. Multiple endocrine adenomatosis: in support of the common origin theories. J Urol 1978; 119:161–165.
623. Hull MT, Warfel KA, Muller J, et al. Familial islet cell tumors in Von Hippel–Lindau's disease. Cancer 1979; 44:1523–1526.
624. Carney JA, Go VLW, Gordon H, et al. Familial pheochromocytoma and islet cell tumor of the pancreas. Am J Med 1980; 68: 515–521.
625. Mori Y, Kiyohara H, Miki T, et al. Pheochromocytoma with prominent calcification and associated pancreatic islet cell tumor. J Urol 1977; 118:843–844.
626. Probst A, Lotz M, Heitz P. Von Hippel–Lindau's disease, syringomyelia and multiple endocrine tumors: a complex neuroendocrinopathy. Virchows Arch A Pathol Anat Histol 1978; 378:265–272.
627. Nathan DM, Daniels GH, Ridgway EC. Gastrinoma and phaeochromocytoma: is there a mixed multiple endocrine adenoma syndrome? Acta Endocrinol (Copenh) 1980; 93:91–93.
628. Zeller JR, Kauffman HM, Komorowski RA, et al. Bilateral pheochromocytoma and islet cell adenoma of the pancreas. Arch Surg 1982; 117:827–830.
629. Cantor AM, Rigby CC, Beck PR, et al. Neurofibromatosis, phaeochromocytoma, and somatostatinoma. Br Med J 1982; 285: 1618–1619.
630. Chakrabarti S, Murugesan A, Arida EJ. The association of neurofibromatosis and hyperparathyroidism. Am J Surg 1979; 137:417–420.
631. Saurenmann P, Binswanger R, Maurer R, et al. [Somatostatin-producing endocrine pancreatic tumor in Recklinghausen's neurofibromatosis: case report and literature review]. Schweiz Med Wochenschr 1987; 117:1134–1139.
632. Chen CH, Lin JT, Lee WY, et al. Somatostatin-containing carcinoid tumor of the duodenum in neurofibromatosis: report of a case. J Formos Med Assoc 1993; 92:900–903.
633. van Basten JP, van Hoek B, de Bruine A, et al. Ampullary carcinoid and neurofibromatosis: case report and review of the literature. Neth J Med 1994; 44:202–206.
634. Hansen OP, Hansen M, Hansen HH, et al. Multiple endocrine adenomatosis of mixed type. Acta Med Scand 1976; 200:327–331.
635. Habiby R, Silverman B, Listernick R, et al. Precocious puberty in children with neurofibromatosis type 1. J Pediatr 1995; 126:364–367.
636. Nur EKMS, Varga M, Maruta H. The GTPase-activating NF1 fragment of 91 amino acids reverses v-Ha-Ras–induced malignant phenotype. J Biol Chem 1993; 268:22331–22337.
637. Gutmann DH, Cole JL, Stone WJ, et al. Loss of neurofibromin in adrenal gland tumors from patients with neurofibromatosis type I. Genes Chromosomes Cancer 1994; 10:55–58.
638. Gutmann DH, Geist RT, Rose K, et al. Loss of neurofibromatosis type I (NF1) gene expression in pheochromocytomas from patients without NF1. Genes Chromosomes Cancer 1995; 13: 104–109.
639. Brannan CI, Perkins AS, Vogel KS, et al. Targeted disruption of the neurofibromatosis type-1 gene leads to developmental abnormalities in heart and various neural crest–derived tissues. Genes Dev 1994; 8:1019–1029.
640. Carney JA, Gordon H, Carpenter PC, et al. The complex of myxomas, spotty pigmentation, and endocrine overactivity. Medicine (Baltimore) 1985; 64:270–283.
641. Carney JA. The Carney complex (myxomas, spotty pigmentation, endocrine overactivity, and schwannomas). Dermatol Clin 1995; 13:19–26.
642. Stratakis CA, Kirschner LS, Carney JA. Clinical and molecular features of the Carney complex: diagnostic criteria and recommendations for patient evaluation. J Clin Endocrinol Metab 2001; 86:4041–4046.
643. Stratakis CA. Genetics of Peutz-Jeghers syndrome, Carney complex and other familial lentiginoses. Horm Res 2000; 54:334–343.
644. Kirschner LS, Carney JA, Pack SD, et al. Mutations of the gene encoding the protein kinase A type I-alpha regulatory subunit in patients with the Carney complex. Nat Genet 2000; 26:89–92.
645. Abbassioun K, Fatourehchi V, Amirjamshidi A, et al. Familial acromegaly with pituitary adenoma: report of three affected siblings. J Neurosurg 1986; 64:510–512.
646. Benlian P, Giraud S, Lahlou N, et al. Familial acromegaly: a specific clinical entity—further evidence from the genetic study of a three-generation family. Eur J Endocrinol 1995; 133:451–456.
647. Himuro H, Kobayashi E, Kono H, et al. Familial occurrence of pituitary adenoma. No Shinkei Geka 1976; 4:371–377.
648. Kurisaka M, Takei Y, Tsubokawa T, et al. Growth hormone–secreting pituitary adenoma in uniovular twin brothers: case report. Neurosurgery 1981; 8:226–230.
649. Levin SR, Hofeldt FD, Becker N, et al. Hypersomatotropism and acanthosis nigricans in two brothers. Arch Intern Med 1974; 134: 365–367.
650. Matsuno A, Teramoto A, Yamada S, et al. Gigantism in sibling unrelated to multiple endocrine neoplasia: case report. Neurosurgery 1994; 35:952–955; discussion 955–956.
651. McCarthy MI, Noonan K, Wass JA, et al. Familial acromegaly: studies in three families. Clin Endocrinol (Oxf) 1990; 32:719–728.
652. Pestell RG, Alford FP, Best JD. Familial acromegaly. Acta Endocrinol (Copenh) 1989; 121:286–289.
653. Tamburrano G, Jaffrain-Rea ML, Grossi A, et al. Familial acromegaly: apropos of a case. Review of the literature. Ann Endocrinol (Paris) 1992; 53:201–207.
654. Gimenez-Roqueplo AP, Favier J, Rustin P, et al. The R22X mutation of the *SDHD* gene in hereditary paraganglioma abolishes the enzymatic activity of complex II in the mitochondrial respiratory chain and activates the hypoxia pathway. Am J Hum Genet 2001; 69:1186–1197.
655. Gimm O, Armanios M, Dziema H, et al. Somatic and occult germ-line mutations in *SDHD*, a mitochondrial complex II gene, in nonfamilial pheochromocytoma. Cancer Res 2000; 60:6822–6825.
656. Chew SL. Paraganglioma genes. Clin Endocrinol (Oxf) 2001; 54: 573–574.

37 The Immunoendocrinopathy Syndromes

George S. Eisenbarth and Peter A. Gottlieb

Geneticists, immunologists, and endocrinologists have generated a wealth of new information concerning the pathogenesis of the polyendocrine autoimmune syndromes and their component disorders.[1–3] In particular, the genetic loci underlying disease susceptibility and organ-specific autoantigens targeted by the immune system are being defined. Multiple distinct molecules are often the targets of autoimmunity for a single organ-specific autoimmune disorder, and in polyendocrine autoimmunity multiple molecules of multiple organs are usually targeted.

Autoantibodies highly specific for a given disorder are present before disease onset, such as anti-islet antibodies (GAD, islet cell antibody [ICA] 512 [IA-2], and insulin) in type 1 diabetes and 21-hydroxylase autoantibodies in Addison's disease. Each specific autoantibody reacts with only a single autoantigen, although autoantigens may be present in multiple tissues. For example, 17α-hydroxylase is present in both adrenal gland and gonads, and the coincidence of Graves' hyperthyroidism and Graves' ophthalmopathy implies a specific shared immune target. For the most part, however, the targets of autoantibodies appear to be unrelated except for their presence as differentiation antigens in specific cells and cellular sites.

In contrast, less is known concerning the specificity of pathogenic T cells. Given the observation that cross-reactive recognition by pathogenic T-cell clones may be determined by as few as four properly spaced amino acids of a nonapeptide[4] and the estimate that each T-cell receptor may react with a million different peptides, there is considerable potential for patterns of autoimmunity to be determined by cross-reactive T cells. One development has been the discovery within the thymus and other lymphoid tissues of what are termed peripheral antigen-expressing cells that express autoantigens such as insulin or glutamic acid decarboxylase (GAD65).[5, 6] Minute quantities of such molecules within the thymus can contribute to tolerance. Insulin messenger ribonucleic acid within the thymus is regulated by genetic polymorphisms of the insulin gene associated with diabetes risk.[5]

Two distinct autoimmune polyendocrine syndromes with characteristic groupings of manifestations are readily recognized (Table 37–1). *Autoimmune polyendocrine syndrome type I* (APS-I) is a rare disorder with autosomal recessive inheritance that has been shown to be caused by defects in the autoimmune regulator *(AIRE)* gene on chromosome 21.[7, 8] In contrast, the most common syndrome discussed in this chapter, *autoimmune polyendocrine syndrome type II* (APS-II), is less well defined, including overlapping groups of disorders. A unifying characteristic within APS-II is the strong association with polymorphic genes of the human leukocyte antigen (HLA) region located on the short arm of chromosome 6 (band 6p21.3). In addition to HLA, many other genetic loci are likely to contribute to susceptibility to APS-II.

APS-II has also been known by various other names: Schmidt's syndrome, polyglandular autoimmune disease, polyglandular failure syndrome, organ-specific autoimmune disease, and polyendocrinopathy diabetes. Such diverse names reflect the large number of studies and case reports of this syndrome and its historical importance. Studies of patients with APS-II were instrumental in the identification of the autoimmune basis of several diseases and the development of autoantibody assays (e.g., type 1 diabetes and cytoplasmic ICAs). Each of the preceding names has some shortcomings, such as failure to include the fact that both hyperfunction and hypofunction of endocrine glands can occur or failure to recognize that nonendocrine disorders such as pernicious anemia and celiac disease are a part of the syndrome.

Some authors have even broken APS-II into a third grouping called *APS-III* on the basis of the presence (APS-II) or absence (APS-III), for example, of autoimmune thyroid disease and type 1 diabetes without Addison's disease. Subdividing APS-II on the basis of specific groups of component diseases appears to add little information in terms of predicting future disorders likely to develop in affected individuals or disorders likely to be present among their relatives. Therefore, in this chapter we distinguish between APS-I and APS-II. The spectrum of disorders that may be present in these syndromes is listed in Table 37–1, and the major differences between the two syndromes are highlighted in Table 37–2.

AUTOIMMUNITY PRIMER

Major determinants of autoimmune endocrine disease are T lymphocytes and autoantibodies produced by B lymphocytes.

Table 37–1. Component Disorders of the Autoimmune Polyendocrine Syndromes*

Type I	Type II
Endocrine	
Addison's disease[13, 70, 79, 122]	**Addison's disease**[13, 79, 123–126]
Hypoparathyroidism[13, 70]	"Geriatric" hypoparathyroidism[23, 127]
Primary hypogonadism[70, 122, 128, 129]	Primary hypogonadism[129–131]
Type 1 diabetes[13, 70]	**Type 1 diabetes**[124, 125, 132, 133]
Hypothyroidism[13, 70]	**Hypothyroidism**[40, 123, 134, 135]
	Graves' disease[40]
	Hypophysitis[136–142]
Gastrointestinal	
Mucocutaneous candidiasis[13, 70]	
Chronic active hepatitis[13, 70]	
Malabsorption[13, 70, 74, 143, 144]	Celiac disease[17, 145–147]
Oral squamous cell carcinoma[70]	
Dermatologic	
Mucocutaneous candidiasis[13, 70]	
Alopecia[13, 70, 148, 149]	Alopecia[150]
Vitiligo[13, 70, 151]	Vitiligo[152]
Nail dystrophy[70]	
	Dermatitis herpetiformis[147]
Hematologic	
Pernicious anemia[70]	Pernicious anemia[153]
	Idiopathic thrombocytopenic purpura[154, 155]
Pure red cell hypoplasia[156, 157]	
Neurologic	
Myopathy[158]	Myasthenia gravis[159, 160]
	Stiff-man syndrome[161]
	Parkinson's disease[162]
Other Manifestations	
Dental enamel hypoplasia[70, 72, 163]	Immunoglobulin A deficiency[164, 165]
Keratopathy[166]	Serositis[167]
Tympanic membrane calcification[71]	Goodpasture's syndrome[168]
Vascular calcification[169]	Idiopathic heart block[170]
Asplenism[73]	

*The most common features are shown in bold type.

Table 37–2. Contrasting Features of the Polyendocrine Syndromes

Type I	Type II
Autosomal recessive inheritance (only siblings affected)	Polygenic inheritance (multiple generations may be affected)
No +HLA association (linked to chromosome 21q22.3)[87]	HLA-DR3 and HLA-DR4 associated
Equal sex incidence	Female preponderance
Onset in infancy or youth	Peak incidence ages 20 to 60 years
Mucocutaneous candidiasis	No mucocutaneous candidiasis
Destructive hypoparathyroidism	Hypoparathyroidism rare (antibody mediated)[23]
Type 1 diabetes mellitus rare in children (but lifetime frequency ~18%[70])	Type 1 diabetes mellitus common

HLA, human leukocyte antigen.

These two arms of the immune system differ fundamentally in their recognition of target antigens. Autoantibodies react with intact molecules (including both soluble and cell-surface molecules) and usually interact with conformational determinants of the autoantigen.

In contrast, T lymphocytes recognize peptide fragments of autoantigens, often 8 to 12 amino acids in length. Furthermore, T cells can recognize peptides only if they are presented on the surface of another cell by major histocompatibility molecules, also known as HLAs. $CD4^+$ (helper) T cells react with peptides that are derived from the extracellular fluid and bound by class II histocompatibility molecules (HLA-DP, HLA-DQ, or HLA-DR in humans). Effective presentation requires specialized antigen-presenting cells (APCs) such as macrophages, dendritic cells, and B lymphocytes. Helper T cells secrete various lymphokines, leading to an immune response to the antigen. $CD8^+$ (cytotoxic) T cells react with peptides bound by class I histocompatibility molecules (HLA-A, HLA-B, and HLA-C). *Class I* molecules are present on the surface of nearly all nucleated cells. The antigen peptide in this case is derived from within the presenting cell. Recognition of antigen of viral origin typically leads to the release of cytotoxic chemicals that kill the infected cell.

However, the simple expression of histocompatibility molecules and recognition of antigen by a T cell are not sufficient for T-cell activation. The interaction of major histocompatibility complex (MHC), peptide, and T-cell receptor (called *signal one*) is critical to the activation process, and other molecules help to define the nature of the immune response (signal two). Co-stimulatory molecules are required for T-cell activation. For example, the cell-surface molecule B7 engages the CD28 receptor on the T cell and amplifies signal one, which leads to T-cell activation.

Cytotoxic T lymphocyte–associated antigen (CTLA)-4 is a similar receptor but one for which engagement appears to down-regulate T cells.[9] Co-stimulatory signaling includes both cell surface–bound receptors on APCs and secreted substances called cytokines, such as interferon γ and interleukin-4 (IL-4), which can modify the type of immune response elicited to the same antigen. In the absence of co-stimulatory molecules, engagement of a T-cell receptor leads to inactivation rather than stimulation. Co-stimulatory molecules are expressed or secreted primarily by professional APCs. The hypothesis that expression by endocrine cells of class II molecules is the cause rather than the consequence of autoimmunity (cytokine-induced) has largely been abandoned as the preceding pathway for T-cell stimulation has been unraveled.

The crystal structure of histocompatibility molecules has been elucidated, and these molecules resemble a "hot dog bun" with the antigenic peptide (the hot dog) bound in the groove of the histocompatibility molecule (the bun). Histocompatibility molecules are extremely polymorphic, with different amino acids lining the peptide-binding groove. These variable amino acids determine which peptides are bound and presented to T lymphocytes.

Molecular HLA typing has revealed many subtypes of the older serologically defined alleles, and the unique genetic sequence encoding each polymorphic chain of the histocompatibility molecules is now given a unique identifying number. Thus, for the DQ molecule, which is the histocompatibility molecule most strongly associated with endocrine autoimmunity, a number is given for each alpha and beta chain. Examples are DQA1*0501 for the alpha chain and DQB1*0201 for the beta chain of the DQ molecule commonly encoded on DR3 (DRB1*0301) haplotypes. This DQ molecule (also termed DQ2) is strongly associated with type 1A diabetes, Addison's disease, Graves' disease, and celiac disease.[10] Each allele with its amino acid sequence is inherited in mendelian fashion.

On activation, $CD8^+$ T cells can directly lyse cells. $CD4^+$ cells are also capable (without $CD8^+$ T cells) of destroying target cells. $CD4^+$ T cells apparently kill through indirect pathways that include the induction of macrophages to produce cytokines and free radicals. $CD4^+$ T lymphocytes are also essential for activation and maturation of B lymphocytes, which produce autoantibodies.

As a simplification, there are two major pathways of $CD4^+$ T-cell activation, with subsets of helper T cells, termed T_H1 and T_H2. T_H1 cells produce proinflammatory cytokines such as interferon γ, IL-2, and tumor necrosis factor α. T_H2 cells produce lymphokines that suppress T_H1 cells and favor antibody production (e.g., IL-4, IL-5, IL-10, transforming growth factor β). Thus, depending on the context of T-cell stimulation, T-cell activation may actually down-regulate rather than promote autoimmunity. The T_H2 pathway is probably important for the induction of mucosal tolerance from either the oral or nasal route and may be initiated by other forms of antigen vaccination such as the use of altered peptide ligands that can suppress autoimmunity. Such types of therapy are being studied for the prevention and reversal of several autoimmune disorders, including type 1A diabetes, multiple sclerosis, and uveitis.

The natural history of autoimmune disorders can be divided into a series of stages beginning with genetic susceptibility, followed by triggering of autoimmunity (e.g., dietary gliadin exposure in celiac disease), active autoimmunity preceding clinical manifestations (e.g., progressive glandular destruction), and finally overt disease. An etiologic classification of autoimmunity based on initiating factors can be developed, illustrating the many ways autoimmunity, even to a single organ, can be initiated (Table 37–3). For example, myasthenia gravis has a drug-induced form (penicillamine), an oncogenic form (thymoma-associated), and the most common idiopathic form.

AUTOIMMUNE POLYENDOCRINE SYNDROME TYPE II

Clinical Definition

APS-II is the more common of the immunoendocrinopathy syndromes. It occurs more often in females than in males, frequently has its onset in adulthood, and exhibits familial aggregation. APS-II is usually defined by the occurrence in the same individual of two or more of the following: primary adrenal insufficiency (Addison's disease) (Fig. 37–1), Graves' disease, autoimmune thyroiditis, type 1A diabetes mellitus, primary hypogonadism, myasthenia gravis, or celiac disease. Vitiligo, alopecia, serositis, and pernicious anemia also occur with increased frequency in individuals with this syndrome and their family members.

The diagnosis of APS-II can be confirmed when one of the component disorders is present; an associated disorder occurs more commonly than in the general population. Furthermore, circulating organ-specific autoantibodies are often present even in the absence of overt clinical disease. In our assessment of APS-II families with Addison's disease, we have noted that up to 15% of relatives have 21-hydroxylase autoantibodies (Addison's disease), anti-islet autoantibodies, or transglutaminase (TG) autoantibodies (celiac disease). In a study of 10 families with APS-II, one in seven relatives had unsuspected illness, most commonly autoimmune thyroid disease.[11] The initial lesion and precipitating events that result in the syndrome are unknown, but immunogenetic and immunologic similarities are present with regard to both the time course and the pathogenesis of each of the component disorders.

The chronic development of organ-specific autoimmunity necessitates endocrinologic evaluation over time of patients with the syndrome and of their families. In a family in which the syndrome has been documented, relatives should be advised of the early symptoms and signs of the principal component diseases. A list is available at www.barbaradaviscenter.org. Relatives of patients with multiple disorders should have a medical history, physical examination, and screening every 3 to 5 years with measurement of anti-islet autoantibodies, a sensitive thyrotropin assay, measurement of serum vitamin B_{12} levels, and, if there are any symptoms or signs or 21-hydroxylase autoantibodies[12] that suggest adrenal insufficiency are present, annual assay of basal corticotropin and corticotropin-stimulated cortisol levels.

Among 224 patients with Addison's disease and APS-II reported by Neufeld and colleagues,[13] type 1 diabetes (52%) and autoimmune thyroid disease (69%) were the most common coexisting conditions. Other components were less common, including vitiligo (5%) and gonadal failure (4%). $CD8^+$, $CTLA^+$, intercellular adhesion molecule–positive ($ICAM^+$), and $HLA\text{-}DR^+$ cells representing activated cytotoxic T cells have been found at the sites of disappearing melanocytes, suggesting their involvement in the process of destruction that leads to loss of pigmentation in vitiligo lesions.[14] One target antigen for the antibody response noted in this disorder is tyrosinase.[15] Other reports have questioned whether this is the correct or dominant antigen and suggested that a protein comigrating with tyrosinase is the antigen of interest.[16]

Among patients with type 1A diabetes, thyroid autoimmunity and celiac disease coexist with sufficient frequency to justify screening. Thyroid peroxidase autoantibodies are present in 10% of children with type 1 diabetes,[17] and this frequency increases with age. However, thyroid autoantibodies are common without progression to overt disease in the absence of subclinical elevations of thyrotropin. Thus, annual screening of patients with type 1 diabetes with determination of thyrotropin levels is recommended as a cost-effective approach.

Previous reports have suggested that 2% to 3% of patients with type 1 diabetes have celiac disease.[18] With the identification of tissue transglutaminase (tTG) as the major endomysial autoantigen of celiac disease, radioimmunoassays were developed and demonstrated that 10% to 12% of patients with type 1 diabetes have tTG autoantibodies.[19] The prevalence of TG autoantibodies was higher in diabetic patients with HLA-DQ2; one third of DQ2-homozygous subjects were found to express anti-TG antibody. Seventy percent of those with high-titer antibody who underwent biopsy were subsequently found to have disease.[20] Therefore, screening with anti-TG antibody can be carried out; if the results are positive, small bowel biopsy to document celiac disease is warranted, with institution of a gluten-free diet if the disease is present. Many individuals have asymptomatic celiac disease that may nevertheless be associated with osteopenia[21] and impaired growth.[18] Untreated, symptomatic celiac disease is also associated with an increased risk of gastrointestinal malignancy, especially lymphoma.[22]

Hypoparathyroidism frequently occurs in APS-I but is rare in APS-II. If hypocalcemia occurs in a patient with the type II syndrome, celiac disease may be a more likely diagnosis than primary hypoparathyroidism. Nevertheless, we have described several elderly patients with APS-II who had a distinct form of hypoparathyroidism that, on the basis of a small series of patients, may be termed *geriatric hypoparathyroidism*.[23] These pa-

Table 37–3. An "Etiologic" Classification of Autoimmunity

Category	Example	Autoimmune Disease	HLA Association
Oncogenic	Ovarian carcinoma	Cerebellar degeneration[172]	
Drug-induced	Methimazole	Insulin autoimmune syndrome[173]	DR4 (DRB1*0405)
	Penicillamine	Myasthenia gravis[174]	DR7 (DQA1*0201, DQB1*0201)
Diet-induced	Gluten	Celiac disease[28]	DR3 or DR5/DR7 in *trans* (DQA1*0501, DQB1*0201)
Infectious	Group B streptococci	Rheumatic heart disease[175]	
	Congenital rubella	Increased frequency of type 1 diabetes mellitus[109]	DR3 (DQA1*0501, DQB1*0201)/DR4 (DQA1*0301, DQB1*0302)
Cytokine-induced	Interferon α	Thyroiditis[176]	
Unknown		Type 1 diabetes mellitus[177]	DR3 (DQA1*0501, DQB1*0201)/DR4 (DQA1*0301, DQB1*0302)
		Addison's disease[13]	DR3 (DQA1*0501, DQB1*0201)/DR4 (0404) (DQA1*0301, DQB1*0302)
		Multiple sclerosis[178]	DR2 (DQA1*0102, DQB1*0602)
		Stiff-man syndrome[179]	DR3 (DQB1*0201)

Adapted from Eisenbarth G, Bellgrau D. Autoimmunity. Sci Med 1994; 1:38–47.

tients form a distinct group because they have antibodies to the surface of parathyroid cells capable of suppressing parathyroid function and have a self-limited course of antibody presence and hypoparathyroidism.

Immunogenetics

Although there is familial aggregation of APS-II and its component disorders, there is no clearly discernible pattern of inheritance. Susceptibility is probably determined by multiple genetic loci (with HLA having the strongest effect) interacting with environmental factors. In the case of celiac disease, a dietary precipitating antigen (gliadin) has been identified. For type 1 diabetes, the concordance of identical twins is approximately 50%,[24] suggesting a possible role for environmental or other nongenetic factors, such as somatic mutation or the random rearrangement of T-cell receptors that occurs during the development of the immune system. We found that diabetes developed in identical twins much more often if it arose in the proband before 25 years of age[24] but that initially discordant twins can become diabetic even after a prolonged period of discordance.[24] Furthermore, approximately 40% of long-term discordant twins (>7 years) have persistent autoantibodies or loss of first-phase insulin release, or both. Identical twins may also be discordant for Addison's disease as well as type 1 diabetes.

Many of the disorders of APS-II are associated with an HLA extended haplotype formed by HLA-A1, B8, DR3, DQA1*0501, DQB1*0201[25] and HLA-DR4, DQA1*0301, DQB1*0302.[26] These include Graves' disease, atrophic thyroiditis, type 1A diabetes (also DR4-associated), Addison's disease (also DR4-associated), myasthenia gravis, and celiac disease.[10, 13, 27, 28] Figure 37–2 illustrates a family in which seven members have type 1 diabetes and three have Addison's dis-

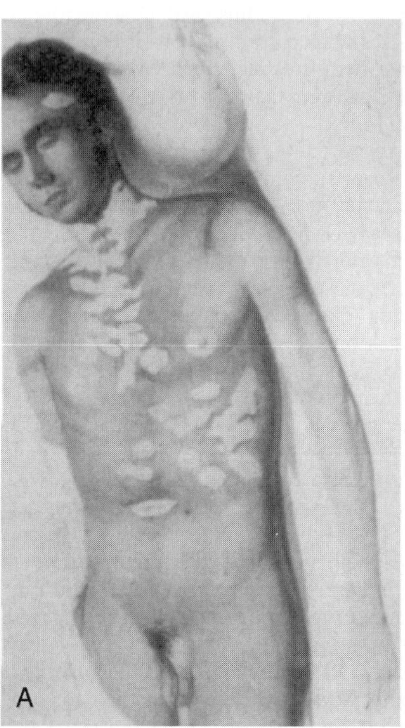

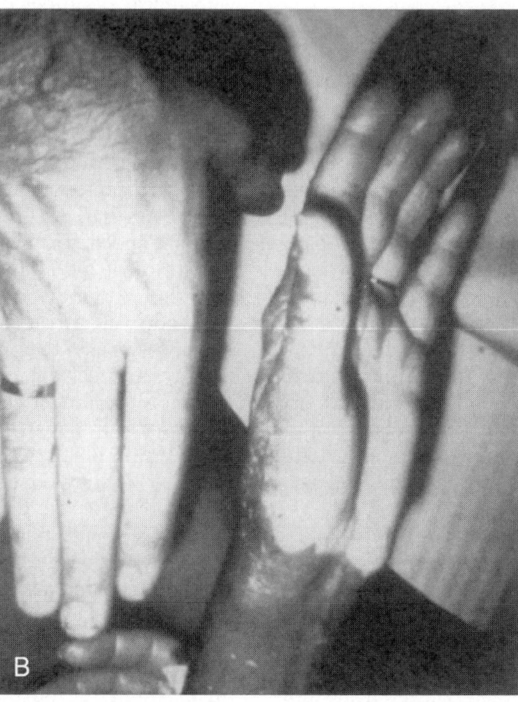

Figure 37–1. Reproduction of a plate from Addison's initial description of primary adrenal insufficiency (Addison's disease) *(A)* and hand of a patient with vitiligo and hyperpigmentation of Addison's disease *(B)*. (*A*, From Addison T. On the Constitutional and Local Effects of Disease of the Supra-renal Capsules. London, Samuel Highley, 1855, plate XI; *B*, courtesy of F. Neelon.)

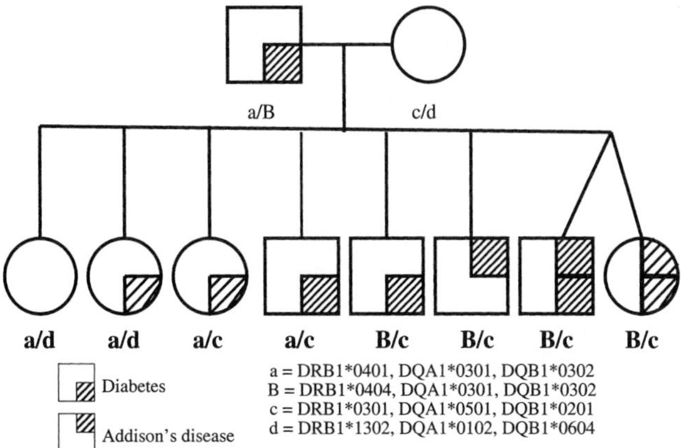

Figure 37–2. Autoimmune polyendocrine syndrome type II family with Addison's disease and type 1 diabetes.

ease. The HLA alleles help to explain the high frequency of autoimmunity in this family. The father is homozygous for the high-risk DR4, DQA1*0301, DQB1*0302 haplotype, and thus all of his offspring inherited this allele. The mother is heterozygous for the high-risk DR3 haplotype that was inherited by six of her eight children.

For some disorders, the complete HLA haplotype is associated with disease; for celiac disease, the most specific association is with the two chains of the DQ molecule. Celiac disease occurs primarily in individuals expressing DQA1*0501, DQB1*0201, either in *cis* (with both of these alleles from the preceding extended DR3 haplotype on the same chromosome) or in *trans* (with DR5 with DQA1*0501, DQB1*0301 from a DR5 haplotype on one chromosome 6 and DQA1*0201, DQB1*0201 from DR7 on the other chromosome 6). There are more than 100 genes within the MHC on the short arm of chromosome 6, including genes that influence the processing and transport of antigenic peptides. For celiac disease, it appears that the HLA contribution to disease may be limited to the DQ molecule (DQA1*0501, DQB1*0201). In contrast, for type 1A diabetes and several other component disorders of APS-II, HLA alleles of genes such as *A2*, *A24*,[29, 30] *DP2002*,[31] and *DQ* may contribute to susceptibility.[32] The MHC class I chain–related *(MIC-A)* gene encodes an unusual class I molecule in the MHC. A specific allele of the *MIC-A* gene, 5.1, is strongly associated with Addison's disease.[33]

Whereas some HLA alleles increase disease risk, others are associated with protection from disease. For example, the DQ alleles DQA1*0102, DQB1*0602 (usually associated with DR2) confer strong protection from type 1A diabetes in a dominant fashion[34] but confer susceptibility to another autoimmune disorder, multiple sclerosis. Furthermore, this protection appears to be organ specific because no protection from Addison's disease is afforded by DQB1*0602.

For both type 1A diabetes and Addison's disease in APS-II, the highest risk is conferred by heterozygosity for the DR3 (DQA1*0501, DQB1*0201) and DR4 (DQA1*0301, DQB1*0302) haplotypes.[27] The DRB1*0404 subtype is found more frequently in those with familial Addison's disease and so is consistent with APS-II.[26] Approximately 2% to 3% of the United States population carries the high-risk DR3-DR4 combination, compared with about 35% of individuals who have type 1A diabetes and about 60% of patients in the United States with Addison's disease.

Given the hypothesis that HLA molecules may predominantly determine the tissue targeting of autoimmunity (although other genetic loci may predispose to autoimmunity in general), there has been an intensive effort to identify non-HLA loci. Unlike the situation in APS-I (see later), multiple genetic loci are probably involved in APS-II. For type 1A diabetes, polymorphisms of the insulin gene region contribute to disease susceptibility.[35] There is some evidence of linkage to several loci, including insulin-dependent diabetes mellitus 17 *(IDDM17)*, which was found on chromosome 10 and conferred a 40% risk for diabetes in combination with HLA genes in the Bedouin Arab family in which it was identified.[36] Other loci have been described, including a locus on chromosome 6 (6q) termed *IDDM15* that has been confirmed in several studies. Analysis of mutations of the *AIRE* gene (see later) indicates that it does not play a role in APS-II or sporadic Addison's disease, with 1 of 90 (1.1%) patients with Addison's disease (non–APS-I) and 1 of 576 (0.2%) control subjects having *AIRE* mutations.[37] The G allele at the CTLA-4 A/G polymorphism was associated with Addison's disease,[37] especially in patients with APS-II and in those with Graves' disease.[38, 39]

Several disorders of the polyendocrine autoimmune syndrome are not associated with DR3.[40, 41] These disorders include pernicious anemia, goitrous thyroiditis, and vitiligo. Vitiligo is a classic component of the syndrome and was included in Addison's original description (see Fig. 37–1). These relatively common disorders may have more than one pathogenic mechanism, one of which is associated with polyendocrine autoimmunity. For example, a polymorphism—106–base pair (bp) allele: $(AT)_n$ repeat in exon 3—of CTLA-4 was associated with vitiligo only in patients who had an autoimmune disease.[42]

Organ-Specific Autoantibodies

Improved assays for several organ-specific autoantibodies have been developed with the cloning of specific autoantigens and the development of assays that use recombinant antigens. These radioimmunoassays are superior to assays based on immunofluorescence with tissue sections, such as ICA testing. The most notable finding is the identification of a large number of different autoantigens that are targeted even in single autoimmune disorders. Most of the endocrine autoantigens are hormones (such as insulin) or enzymes associated with differentiated endocrine function: thyroid peroxidase in thyroiditis; glutamic acid decarboxylase,[43] carboxypeptidase H,[28] and ICA512/IA-2[44] in type 1 diabetes; 17α-hydroxylase[12] and 21-hydroxylase in Addison's disease (Fig. 37–3)[45, 46]; and the parietal cell enzyme H^+/K^+-adenosine triphosphatase in pernicious anemia.[47]

In type 1 diabetes, the four most informative assays currently available determine autoantibodies that react with insulin, GAD65 (glutamic acid decarboxylase), ICA512/IA-2, and ICA512β/IA-2β.[44] In a similar manner, a radioassay format for the detection of autoantibodies that react with the enzyme 21-hydroxylase in Addison's disease has been developed and provides excellent disease specificity and sensitivity.[26, 48–50] Adrenal autoantibodies reacting with recombinant 21-hydroxylase[45, 51] usually precede the development of Addison's disease.[52] However, as with thyroid autoantibodies, there may be individuals who present with antibodies but have normal production of cortisol in response to adrenocorticotropic hormone (ACTH). Continued rescreening every year initially and then biyearly is indicated in this situation.

In contrast to the autoimmune polyendocrine disorders with T cell–mediated glandular destruction, autoantibodies may also be pathogenic. A hallmark of pathogenic autoantibodies is the existence of a neonatal form of the disorder, secondary to transplacental passage of the autoantibody. Examples include neonatal Graves' disease (anti–thyrotropin receptor autoantibodies) and neonatal myasthenia gravis (anti–acetyl choline receptor autoantibodies).[53]

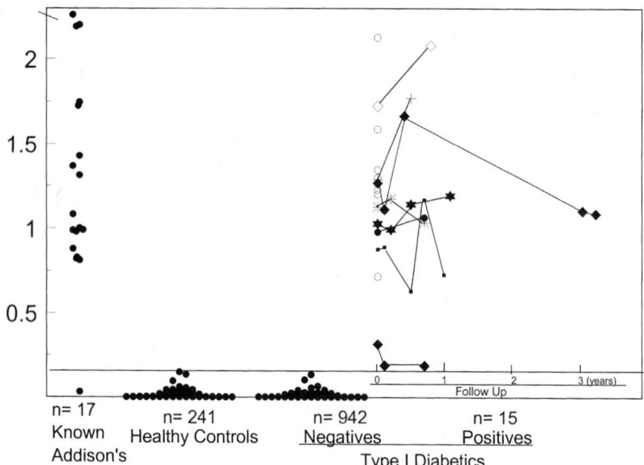

Figure 37–3. 21-Hydroxylase autoantibodies of patients with known Addison's disease, normal control subjects, and patients with type 1 diabetes mellitus. Data for the 15 patients with type 1 diabetes discovered to be 21-hydroxylase positive on screening are plotted on the *right*; where multiple different serum samples are available for an individual, values for each individual are connected by *lines*. (From Yu L, Brewer KW, Gates S, et al. DRB1*04 and DQ alleles: expression of 21-hydroxylase autoantibodies and risk of progression to Addison's disease. J Clin Endocrinol Metab 1999; 84:328–335.)

Therapy

Treatment of the individual diseases of the polyendocrine autoimmune syndrome is discussed in other chapters. Therapeutic considerations related specifically to APS-II include the following:

1. Many of the component disorders of the syndrome have a long prodromal phase and are associated with the expression of autoantibodies before overt disease. The manner in which the disorders develop allows the consideration of disease prediction and of clinical trials for prevention. This is particularly important for type 1A diabetes but is also likely to apply to Addison's disease, hypogonadism, and Graves' disease.
   a. Because of the autoimmune nature of these disorders, several studies have evaluated immunosuppressive drugs. Such studies have contributed to our understanding of autoimmunity, and drugs such as cyclosporine have preserved some residual insulin secretion. However, the nephrotoxicity and potential for oncogenicity of cyclosporine have precluded its more generalized use. Newer immunosuppressive agents (mycophenolate mofetil or sirolimus) and biologics such as anti–IL-2 receptor (daclizumab) or "nonmitogenic" CD3 antibodies, for example, hOKT3(ala-ala), may be more effective and have a better safety profile, and these are currently in clinical trials in patients with new-onset diabetes. With further research, immunomodulatory therapies have been developed that are remarkably effective in preventing type 1A diabetes of the BioBreeding (BB) rat and nonobese diabetic (NOD) mouse models of type 1A diabetes.
   b. There are also relatively benign therapies, such as administration of high doses of the vitamin nicotinamide or administration of immune adjuvants that appear to interfere with selected effector pathogenic mechanisms. Small trials of bacille Calmette-Guérin (BCG) vaccine[54, 55] and nicotinamide[56] treatment suggest that these agents have little if any effect in humans, but large randomized trials of nicotinamide are under way in Europe that should define its potential within the next 2 years.
   c. Mucosal administration of antigens is frequently associated with bystander immunosuppression, in which T cells specific to the antigen are apparently induced to produce suppressive T_H2-like or T_H3-like cytokines (e.g., IL-4, IL-10, and transforming growth factor β).[57] In addition, subcutaneous administration of insulin prevents diabetes and insulitis in animal models, and subcutaneous administration of insulin peptides in adjuvants can prevent diabetes but not insulitis. When such animal trials were extended to humans, oral insulin at diabetes onset had no effect[58] but a small pilot trial[59] suggested that a combination of daily subcutaneous insulin and intermittent intravenous insulin may delay the development of type 1A diabetes in humans. A large National Institutes of Health trial, the Diabetes Prevention Trial–Type I (DPT-I), is under way in the United States to test this hypothesis directly. DPT-I has two arms: (1) intravenous-subcutaneous for those at high risk and (2) oral insulin for those at moderate risk. Subcutaneous insulin injection did not slow progression to diabetes, and results of the oral trial should be known by 2003.
   d. Hashizume and co-workers[60] reported a lower relapse rate in women with Graves' disease who were given thyroxine at 100 μg daily than in those who did not receive thyroxine. Takasu and colleagues[61] reported that autoimmune thyroiditis may be reversible with the disappearance of autoantibodies and maintenance of a euthyroid state in a minority of patients after the cessation of thyroxine therapy. However, subsequent trials have not confirmed such protection, suggesting that other factors may influence the occurrence of disease (iodine intake, for example). In the BB rat model, the administration of thyroxine resulted in a reduced frequency of appearance of lymphocytic thyroiditis.[62] In preclinical Addison's disease, a short course of glucocorticoids appeared to suppress the expression of adrenal autoantibodies and prevent progressive adrenal destruction.[63]
   e. De Bellis and co-workers[63] screened patients with organ-specific autoimmune disorders and found that 0.9% were positive for adrenal autoantibodies. Three patients with high-titer adrenal autoantibodies and an impaired cortisol response to ACTH experienced remission and had negative results on assay for adrenal autoantibodies when treated with corticosteroids for Grave's ophthalmopathy (Fig. 37–4). In contrast, in 11 other patients with high-titer adrenal autoantibodies, the antibodies persisted and various abnormalities developed, including elevated plasma renin activity, impaired cortisol response to ACTH, elevated ACTH, and overt Addison's disease. Feedback inhibition of endocrine gland function may decrease the exposure of autoantigens to the immune system or decrease the susceptibility of the targeted tissue to immune attack. This preliminary observation requires direct testing in a larger population and in randomized fashion.
2. Thyroxine therapy can precipitate a life-threatening addisonian crisis in a patient with untreated adrenal insufficiency and hypothyroidism. Thus, it is necessary to evaluate adrenal function in all hypothyroid patients in whom the syndrome is suspected before the institution of such therapy.
3. A decreasing insulin requirement in a patient with insulin-dependent diabetes mellitus can be one of the earliest indications of adrenal insufficiency, occurring before the

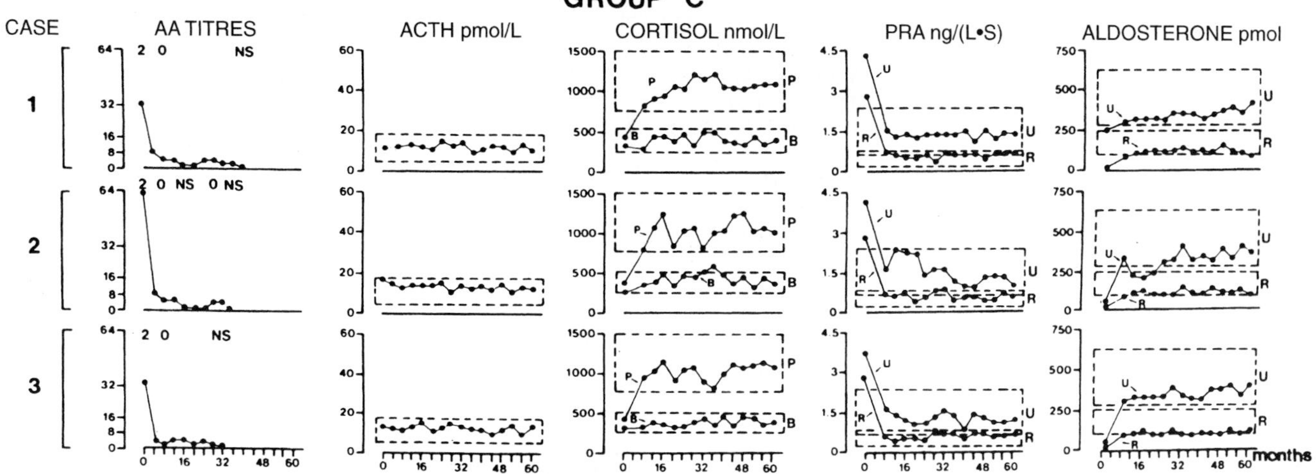

Figure 37–4. Adrenal antibody (AA) titers and levels of adrenocorticotropic hormone (ACTH), cortisol, plasma renin activity (PRA), and aldosterone in three anti–adrenal autoantibody–positive patients treated for 6 months with glucocorticoids for concomitant Graves' ophthalmopathy. (From De Bellis A, Bizzaro A, Rossi R, et al. Remission of subclinical adrenocortical failure in subjects with adrenal autoantibodies. J Clin Endocrinol Metab 1993; 76:1002–1007.)

development of hyperpigmentation or electrolyte abnormalities.

4. In patients with both adrenal insufficiency and primary hypothyroidism, thyroid function may improve after glucocorticoid replacement.[64]
5. Addisonian crisis that responds to mineralocorticoid therapy can occur in patients receiving high-dose glucocorticoids for inflammatory disease.[65]
6. Immunologic therapies, especially in patients with an autoimmune disease, may induce autoimmunity. A remarkable example is the treatment of patients with multiple sclerosis with an anti-CD52 monoclonal antibody. One third of 27 patients given the monoclonal developed anti–thyrotropin receptor autoantibodies and hyperthyroidism.[66] Interferon α therapy for hepatitis has been associated with thyroid autoimmunity[67] and potentially type 1 diabetes.[68]

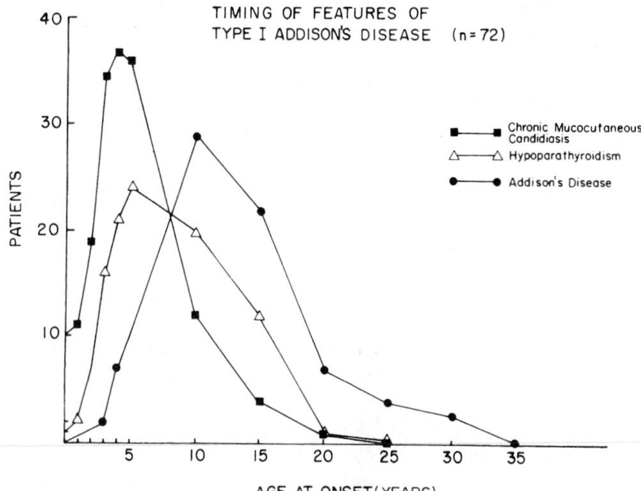

Figure 37–5. Age at onset of mucocutaneous candidiasis, hypoparathyroidism, and adrenal insufficiency in patients with autoimmune polyendocrine syndrome type I. (From Neufeld M, Maclaren NK, Blizzard RM. Two types of autoimmune Addison's disease associated with different polyglandular autoimmune [PGA] syndromes. Medicine [Baltimore] 1981; 60:355–362.)

AUTOIMMUNE POLYENDOCRINE SYNDROME TYPE I

Clinical Features

APS-I, also known as *autoimmune polyendocrinopathy–candidiasis–ectodermal dystrophy* (APECED), is characterized by the classic triad of mucocutaneous candidiasis, autoimmune hypoparathyroidism, and Addison's disease, although the presence of all three is not needed to make the diagnosis and various other manifestations may be present (see Table 37–1). The association of mucocutaneous candidiasis with glandular failure was recognized by Thorpe and Handley in 1929.[69] More than 140 patients have since been reported, including two large series from Finland[70, 71] and the United States.[13]

APS-I is characteristically recognized in early childhood, whereas APS-II has its peak incidence in middle age. Chronic mucocutaneous candidiasis is often the first manifestation, followed by hypoparathyroidism and Addison's disease (Fig. 37–5), but new components can develop at any age.[13, 70] Decades may elapse between the diagnosis of one disorder and the onset of another in the same individual. Consequently, lifelong follow-up is important to allow the early detection of additional components.

In a series of 68 Finnish patients described by Ahonen and co-workers,[70] all had chronic candidiasis at some time, 79% had hypoparathyroidism, 72% had Addison's disease, and 51% had all three of these classical components. Gonadal failure (60% in women, 14% in men) and hypoplasia of the dental enamel (77%) were also frequent findings. Other manifestations that occurred less frequently included alopecia (29%), vitiligo (13%), intestinal malabsorption (18%), type 1 diabetes (18%), pernicious anemia (13%), chronic active hepatitis (12%), and hypothyroidism (4%).[71] The onset of chronic active hepatitis suggested by hepatomegaly, jaundice, or elevated liver

Table 37–4. Mutations of the *AIRE* (Autoimmune Regulator) Gene

Population	Exon 8 13-bp deletion (1094–1106)	R257X	R139X	Other
Britain (n = 12)				
APS-I	71% (17/24)	4% (1/24)		21% (5/24)
Normal population	0.2% (1/576)			
United States (*n* = 16)[8, 180]	50% (16/32)	16% (5/32?)		(?11/32)
Sardinia (*n* = 10)[181]				
APS-I	5% (1/20)		90% (18/20)	5%
Normal population			1.7%	
Northern Italy (*n* = 9)[182]	27% (5/18)	56% (10/18)		17%

APS-I, autoimmune polyendocrine syndrome type I.

enzymes is a serious complication requiring therapy. The presence of chronic candidiasis suggests that a defect in T-cell function may underlie the development of multiple autoimmune disorders in this syndrome. Recurrent candidiasis commonly affects the mouth and nails and, less frequently, the skin and esophagus.[70]

Other infections do not occur with such increased frequency. Ectodermal dystrophy is another non-autoimmune part of the syndrome (manifested by pitted nails, keratopathy, and enamel hypoplasia) and cannot be attributed to hypoparathyroidism. Enamel hypoplasia may precede the onset of hypoparathyroidism and, despite adequate replacement therapy, may also affect teeth forming after the onset of hypoparathyroidism.[72] Friedman and colleagues[73] reported the frequent occurrence of asplenism and cholelithiasis as additional features of APS-I. Malabsorption with steatorrhea is of uncertain origin, is usually intermittent, and may be exacerbated by hypocalcemia. Bereket and associates[74] reported a case with patchy intestinal lymphangiectasia discovered by endoscopically directed biopsy. Pancreatic insufficiency has been treated with cyclosporine.[75]

Antiparathyroid and antiadrenal antibodies have been reported.[76] Cross-reactive autoantibodies may play a role in the multiorgan involvement of these disorders, as noted in several case reports. A target antigen for the autoantibodies found in autoimmune hypoparathyroidism was described by Li and colleagues,[77] who showed that 56% of 25 patients, 17 with APS-1, reacted to the extracellular domain of a membrane-associated antigen of 120 to 140 kd, which was identified as the calcium-sensing receptor. Whereas 21-hydroxylase appears to be the major autoantigen in isolated Addison's disease and in Addison's disease associated with APS-II, autoantibodies against 17α-hydroxylase and P450 side-chain cleavage enzyme (CYP11A1) have also been reported in Addison's disease associated with APS-I.[78–80]

Other autoantibodies that may be involved in other components of this disorder have been reported. These include antibodies to tryptophan hydroxylase in intestinal disease, tyrosine hydroxylase in alopecia areata, and L-amino acid decarboxylase in hepatitis and vitiligo, and phenylalanine hydroxylase[80, 81] and antibodies reacting with hair follicles.[82]

As with APS-II, Tuomi and co-workers[83] originally observed that many more patients (41%) express anti-GAD65 autoantibodies than become diabetic. Among patients with APS-I in this study in whom diabetes developed, GAD autoantibodies could be detected up to 8 years before the onset of overt diabetes. They subsequently noted that many of the antibody-negative patients can demonstrate T-cell responses to GAD65. Nearly 76% of all tested subjects showed either autoantibody or T-cell responses to GAD65 but only 18% had diabetes (8 of 44 subjects[84]), again suggesting that reactivity to this single autoantigen has low predictive value.

Genetics

APS-I is unique among autoimmune endocrine disorders, in that it is not associated with high-risk class II HLA alleles, although the protective allele DQB1*0602 may protect against type 1 diabetes but not Addison's disease.[13, 83] Addison's disease in APS-II is strongly associated with HLA-DR3 and HLA-DR4. APS-I shows an autosomal recessive pattern of inheritance, with a 25% recurrence risk for siblings of affected individuals.[85] The disorder has a high prevalence in Finland and in consanguineous Iranian Jewish families.[86]

The etiologic gene was localized to the short arm of chromosome 21 (near markers D21s49 and D21s171 on 21p22.3) by Aaltonen and co-workers[87] and identified as *AIRE*. The gene encodes a putative deoxyribonucleic acid (DNA)-binding protein of unknown function expressed in the thymus and in lymphoid and other tissues.[7, 88, 89] Multiple mutations are causative, and the frequency of specific mutations varies in different populations (Table 37–4). For example, in Sardinia, a deletion of amino acid 257 is present in 90% of mutated alleles. A 136-bp deletion in exon 8 is present in 71% of British alleles and 56% of alleles in the United States. Analysis of haplotypes indicates that this deletion has arisen on multiple occasions.

Therapy

Note the following principles:

1. The treatment of adrenal insufficiency and hypoparathyroidism is the same as that discussed in Chapters 14 and 26, respectively, with the caveat that malabsorption may complicate treatment.
2. The therapy for mucocutaneous candidiasis has been improved with orally active antifungal drugs such as fluconazole[90] and ketoconazole.[91] Infection often recurs when the drug is discontinued or when the dosage is decreased. Patients must be monitored carefully because ketoconazole may inhibit adrenal and gonadal steroid synthesis and may precipitate adrenal failure. It is also associated with transient elevation of liver enzyme levels and, occasionally, hepatitis. Fluconazole is associated with a lower frequency of hepatitis and does not inhibit steroidogenesis when given in the recommended doses.[90]
3. Screening to allow the early detection of new disorders before overt symptoms and signs develop is recommended, including autoantibody studies, electrolytes, calcium and phosphorus levels, thyroid and liver function tests, blood smear, and plasma vitamin B_{12} levels. Patients at risk for adrenal failure can be screened by measurement of basal ACTH and supine plasma renin activity (PRA) levels,[92] followed by dynamic testing as appropriate. Evaluation for asplenism[73] with

abdominal ultrasonography and blood smear examination for Howell-Jolly bodies is warranted, with pneumococcal vaccination and appropriate antibiotic coverage for affected patients.

4. Hypocalcemia has been associated with the intermittent steatorrhea characteristic of APS-I, and therapies that restore calcium levels have been beneficial. Treatment includes magnesium replacement for hypomagnesemia. Nevertheless, in individual patients, specific etiologic factors have been implicated, including pancreatic insufficiency, *Giardia lamblia* infection, and lymphangiectasia, and individualized therapy is required for these potentially diverse causes.

5. There are case reports of severely affected patients who have benefited from immunosuppressive therapy. For example, Ward and colleagues[93] treated a 13-year-old patient who had keratoconjunctivitis, hepatitis, and severe pancreatic insufficiency. Treatment with cyclosporine was associated with normalization of stool fat (from 31.5 g/day to 2.5 g/day).

OTHER POLYENDOCRINE DEFICIENCY AUTOIMMUNE SYNDROMES

Anti–Insulin Receptor Antibodies

In this rarely reported disorder (~25 patients), also known as *type B insulin resistance* and acanthosis nigricans, insulin resistance is due to the presence of anti–insulin receptor antibodies.[94] Approximately one third of patients with these antibodies have an associated autoimmune illness such as systemic lupus erythematosus (SLE) or Sjögren's syndrome. Arthralgia, vitiligo, alopecia, and secondary amenorrhea have also been reported. One patient had a daughter with hyperthyroidism and a granddaughter with SLE. Autoimmune thyroid disease has been described in two such patients, one with hypothyroidism and the other with antithyroid antibodies. Antinuclear antibodies and an elevated erythrocyte sedimentation rate, hyperglobulinemia, leukopenia, and hypocomplementemia are common.[95]

The major clinical manifestations are related to the anti–insulin receptor antibodies. Severe insulin resistance is profound, and up to 175,000 U of insulin given intravenously per day may be ineffective in lowering the elevated glucose level. Despite hyperglycemia and marked insulin resistance, ketoacidosis is uncommon. The course of the diabetes is variable, and several patients have had spontaneous remissions. Other patients have had severe hypoglycemia (perhaps related to the insulin-like effects of anti-insulin receptor antibodies demonstrable in vitro).[95] The acanthosis nigricans, which is due to hypertrophy and folding of otherwise histologically normal skin, appears to be related to the insulin-resistant state. Other forms of marked insulin resistance in the absence of antireceptor antibodies are also associated with acanthosis nigricans.

POEMS Syndrome

The components of the multisystem disorder *POEMS* (*p*lasma cell dyscrasia with polyneuropathy, *o*rganomegaly, *e*ndocrinopathy, *M* protein, and *s*kin changes or Crow-Fukase syndrome) consist of diabetes mellitus (50% of patients), primary gonadal failure (70% of patients), plasma cell dyscrasia, sclerotic bone lesions, and neuropathy.[96–101] Patients usually present with severe progressive sensorimotor polyneuropathy, hepatosplenomegaly, lymphadenopathy, and hyperpigmentation. On evaluation, they are found to have plasma cell dyscrasia and sclerotic bone lesions.

POEMS is assumed to be secondary to circulating immunoglobulins, but binding of antibody directly to involved tissues has not been demonstrated. There is evidence implicating cytokines such as IL-1β, IL-6, and tumor necrosis factor α in addition to the M protein in the pathogenesis of this disorder. Several studies have also demonstrated that elevated levels of vascular endothelial growth factor (VEGF) correlate with the disease state and that treatment with immunosuppressive agents reduced both symptoms of the disease and levels of VEGF, suggesting that this growth factor may play a role in the disease.[102, 103] A therapeutic trial of an anti-VEGF antibody would provide more definitive evidence for this hypothesis. The diabetes mellitus responds to small subcutaneous doses of insulin. The hypogonadism is associated with elevated plasma levels of follicle-stimulating hormone and luteinizing hormone. Temporary resolution of disease, including a return of the blood glucose level to normal, may occur after radiotherapy for localized plasma cell lesions of bone.

Kearns-Sayre Syndrome

The rare Kearns-Sayre syndrome, also known as oculocraniosomatic disease or oculocraniosomatic neuromuscular disease with ragged red fibers, is characterized by myopathic abnormalities leading to ophthalmoplegia and progressive weakness in association with several endocrine abnormalities, including hypoparathyroidism, primary gonadal failure, diabetes mellitus, and hypopituitarism.[104] Crystalline mitochondrial inclusions are found in muscle biopsy specimens, and such inclusions have also been observed in the cerebellum. The relationship between the mitochondrial disorders and endocrinologic abnormalities is not known. Other abnormalities include retinitis pigmentosa and heart block.

Antiparathyroid antibodies have not been described; however, antibodies to the anterior pituitary gland and striated muscle have been found, and the disease may have autoimmune components.

Thymic Tumors

The thymus has a central role in the ontogeny of cell-mediated immunity. DiGeorge described congenital aplasia of the thymus and parathyroid glands, both of which are derived from the third and fourth pharyngeal pouches. Affected infants present with tetany secondary to hypocalcemia, severe infections with markedly suppressed T-cell immunity, and normal humoral immunity.

The thymus is a complex tissue with a specialized endocrine epithelium that synthesizes a variety of biologically active peptides involved in the control of T-cell maturation. This epithelium is derived from the neural crest and contains complex gangliosides that react with monoclonal antibody (A2B5) and tetanus toxin in a manner similar to that of pancreatic islets. The role of these biologically active peptides of the thymus has not been defined, but they may be trophic factors in T-cell activation and increase in situations of primary failure of T-cell activation, just as the levels of trophic hormones increase in primary endocrine failure.

The illnesses associated with thymomas are similar to those in APS-II,[105] although the frequency of specific disorders is different. In one review of patients with thymoma, myasthenia gravis occurred in 44% of the patients, red blood cell aplasia in approximately 20%, hypoglobulinemia in 6%, autoimmune thyroid disease in 2%, and adrenal insufficiency in 1 of 423 patients. The frequency of autoimmune thyroid disease reported in patients with thymoma is probably an underestimate, given the frequency of unsuspected thyroid disease in patients with myasthenia gravis. Mucocutaneous candidiasis in adults is also associated with thymomas. In most patients, the thymomas are malignant, although temporary remissions of the autoimmune disease can occur with resection of the tumor.

Trisomy 21

Down syndrome, or trisomy 21, is associated with the development of insulin-dependent diabetes mellitus and thyroiditis. We have observed one patient with a partial distal translocation "leading" to trisomy 21 and "associated" with adrenal insufficiency, celiac disease, hypothyroidism, and insulin-dependent diabetes. Patients with trisomy 21 also have T-cell abnormalities, including increased Ia-positive T cells and a premature increase in the 3G5 age-related T-cell subset.[106] It is not known whether the observed chromosomal abnormality influences the development of autoimmunity or whether part of the susceptibility to autoimmunity is associated with chromosomal disorders.[107] Organ-specific autoimmunity also occurs with gonadal dysgenesis.[108]

Congenital Rubella

Patients with congenital rubella have an almost 20% risk of acquiring diabetes mellitus and a higher than normal risk of acquiring thyroiditis and hypothyroidism.[109, 110] Those at highest risk for diabetes express diabetes-associated HLA-DR3 and HLA-DR4 alleles.[111] Rubella appears to be associated with diabetes primarily after fetal infection, and it is not known whether the virus increases the probability of subsequent autoimmunity because it has permanent effects on the developing immune system.[112]

Organ-specific autoimmunity is readily induced in animal models by perturbations of neonatal immune function (neonatal thymectomy, neonatal cyclosporine administration[113]). Congenital diabetes, although rare, may occur as illustrated by a case report describing lymphocytic infiltration of the pancreas with CD45RO$^+$ memory phenotype cells and the presence of autoantibodies to GAD and insulin in a child born with congenital diabetes and without serologic evidence of viral infection.[114]

Wolfram Syndrome

Wolfram syndrome is a rare autosomal recessive disease that is also called DIDMOAD, which stands for *d*iabetes *i*nsipidus, *d*iabetes *m*ellitus, progressive bilateral *o*ptic *a*trophy, and sensorineural *d*eafness. In addition, neurologic and psychiatric disturbances are prominent in most patients and may cause severe disability.

Linkage analysis of several families with this disorder has identified a locus of chromosome 4 that was highly associated with the disease.[115] Segregation analysis of the mutations found in familial and sporadic cases of Wolfram syndrome led to the identification of wolframin, or WFS1, a 100-kd transmembrane protein encoded by a gene located at 4p16.1.[116] The disease has been mapped to a locus on the short arm of chromosome 4.[115] Atrophic changes in the brain have been found with magnetic resonance imaging.[117]

Wolfram syndrome appears to be a slowly progressive neurodegenerative process, and there is also (non-autoimmune) selective destruction of the pancreatic beta cells. This association may be related to the many molecules and metabolic pathways shared by islets and neurons. Diabetes mellitus with an onset in childhood is usually the first manifestation. Diabetes mellitus and optic atrophy are present in all reported cases, but expression of the other features is variable. Linkage to other loci in addition to *WFS1* may explain the variability in phenotype seen in this disorder. In one case report, two related children with Wolfram syndrome had megaloblastic and sideroblastic anemia that responded to treatment with thiamine. Furthermore, thiamine treatment was associated with a marked decrease in insulin requirements.[118]

X-Linked Syndrome of Polyendocrinopathy, Immune Dysfunction, and Diarrhea (XPID)

XPID was first described in 1982 and was noted to be an X-linked immunodeficiency syndrome characterized by autoimmune enteropathy, polyendocrinopathy, atopic dermatitis, and fatal infections.[119] Activated T cells can be found in the circulation and in the infiltrates along affected gut tissue. Linkage analysis demonstrated that a 17-cM stretch of the X chromosome is associated with XPID; this site is distinct from the adjacent site, which is associated with the similar Wiskott-Aldrich syndrome.[120] The syndrome consists of loss of pancreatic islets (diabetes mellitus), infection, severe enteropathy, thrombocytopenia and anemia, endocrinopathy and eczema, and growth retardation, and is often fatal in infancy. It differs from Wiskott-Aldrich syndrome in that activated CD4$^+$ T cells are found. Characteristics of the scurfy mouse (gene *sf*) bear a number of similarities to this syndrome, and abnormalities in the *sf* gene lead to abnormalities in the amount and function of scurfin, a DNA-binding protein. Wildin and colleagues studied four individuals with XPID for abnormalities in the *sf* gene and found that each had either nonconservative substitutions or deletion or insertion mutations that could affect function of this protein.[121] This study indicates that this disorder is tied to abnormalities in the *sf* gene.

SUMMARY

The most basic pathogenic lesion of the polyendocrine autoimmune syndromes is an inherited tendency to target self-molecules immunologically. The disease associations and the inheritance pattern make it possible to detect additional components of these syndromes in patients before the appearance of serious manifestations and to make the diagnosis in some first-degree relatives with unrecognized disease. Detection and diagnosis can now be facilitated by autoantibody assays with excellent sensitivity and specificity.

References

1. Schatz WA, Winter WE. Autoimmune polyendocrine syndrome Type II. Endocrinol Metab Clin North Am 2002; 31:339–352.
2. Perheentupa J. APS-I/APECED: The clinical disease and therapy. Endocrinol Metab Clin North Am 2002; 31:339–352.
3. Betterle C, Volpato M, Greggio AN, Presotto F. Type 2 polyglandular autoimmune disease (Schmidt's syndrome). J Pediatr Endocrinol Metab 1996; 9:113–123.
4. Wucherpfennig KW, Strominger JL. Molecular mimicry in T cell–mediated autoimmunity: viral peptides activate human T cell clones specific for myelin basic protein. Cell 1995; 80:695–705.
5. Pugliese A, Zeller M, Fernandez A, et al. The insulin gene is transcribed in the human thymus and transcription levels correlate with allelic variation at the INS VNTR-IDDM2 susceptibility locus for type I diabetes. Nat Genet 1997; 15:293–297.
6. Hanahan D. Peripheral-antigen–expressing cells in thymic medulla: factors in self-tolerance and autoimmunity. Curr Opin Immunol 1998; 10:656–662.
7. Aaltonen J, Björses P, Perheentupa J, et al. An autoimmune disease, APECED, caused by mutations in a novel gene featuring two PHD-type zinc-finger domains. Nat Genet 1997; 17:399–403.
8. Heino M, Scott HS, Chen Q, et al. Mutation analyses of North American APS-1 patients. Hum Mutat 1999; 13:69–74.
9. Luhder F, Chambers C, Allison JP, et al. Pinpointing when T

cell costimulatory receptor CTLA-4 must be engaged to dampen diabetogenic T cells. Proc Natl Acad Sci USA 2000; 97:12204–12209.

10. Badenhoop K, Walfish PG, Rau H, et al. Susceptibility and resistance alleles of human leukocyte antigen (HLA) DQA1 and HLA DQB1 are shared in endocrine autoimmune disease. J Clin Endocrinol Metab 1995; 80:2112–2117.
11. Eisenbarth GS, Wilson PW, Ward F, et al. The polyglandular failure syndrome: disease inheritance, HLA-type and immune function. Ann Intern Med 1979; 91:528–533.
12. de Carmo S, Kater CE, Dib SA, et al. Autoantibodies against recombinant human steroidogenic enzymes 21-hydroxylase, side-chain cleavage and 17α-hydroxylase in Addison's disease and autoimmune polyendocrine syndrome type III. Eur J Endocrinol 2000; 142:187–194.
13. Neufeld M, Maclaren NK, Blizzard RM. Two types of autoimmune Addison's disease associated with different polyglandular autoimmune (PGA) syndromes. Medicine (Baltimore) 1981; 60:355–362.
14. van den Wijngaard R, Wankowicz-Kalinska A, Le Poole C, et al. Local immune response in skin of generalized vitiligo patients: destruction of melanocytes is associated with the prominent presence of CLA^+ T cells at the perilesional site. Lab Invest 2000; 80:1299–1309.
15. Song Y-H, Connor E, Li Y, et al. The role of tyrosinase in autoimmune vitiligo. Lancet 1994; 344:1049–1052.
16. Xie Z, Chen D, Jiao D, Bystryn JC. Vitiligo antibodies are not directed to tyrosinase. Arch Dermatol 1999; 135:417–422.
17. Verge CF, Howard NJ, Rowley MJ, et al. Anti–glutamate decarboxylase and other antibodies at the onset of childhood IDDM: a population-based study. Diabetologia 1994; 37:1113–1120.
18. Barera G, Bianchi C, Calisti L, et al. Screening of diabetic children for coeliac disease with antigliadin antibodies and HLA typing. Arch Dis Child 1991; 66:491–494.
19. Bao F, Yu L, Babu S, et al. One third of HLA DQ2 homozygous patients with type 1 diabetes express celiac disease associated transglutaminase autoantibodies. J Autoimmun 1999; 13:143–148.
20. Hoffenberg EJ, Bao F, Eisenbarth GS, et al. Transglutaminase antibodies in children with a genetic risk for celiac disease. J Pediatr 2000; 137:356–360.
21. Mora S, Weber G, Barera G, et al. Effect of gluten-free diet on bone mineral content in growing patients with celiac disease. Am J Clin Nutr 1993; 57:224–228.
22. Holmes GKT, Prior P, Lane MR, et al. Malignancy in coeliac disease: effect of a gluten free diet. Gut 1989; 30:333–338.
23. Posillico JT, Wortsman J, Srikanta S, et al. Parathyroid cell surface autoantibodies that inhibit parathyroid hormone secretion from dispersed human parathyroid cells. Bone Miner Res 1986; 1:475–483.
24. Redondo MJ, Yu L, Hawa M, et al. Heterogeneity of type 1 diabetes: analysis of monozygotic twins in Great Britain and the United States. Diabetologia 2001; 44:354–362.
25. Huang W, Connor E, Rosa TD, et al. Although DR3-DQB1*0201 may be associated with multiple component diseases of the autoimmune polyglandular syndromes, the human leukocyte antigen DR4-DQB1*0302 haplotype is implicated only in beta-cell autoimmunity. J Clin Endocrinol Metab 1996; 81:2559–2563.
26. Yu L, Brewer KW, Gates S, et al. DRB1*04 and DQ alleles: expression of 21-hydroxylase autoantibodies and risk of progression to Addison's disease. J Clin Endocrinol Metab 1999; 84:328–335.
27. Thomson G, Robinson WP, Kuhner MK, et al. Genetic heterogeneity, modes of inheritance, and risk estimates for a joint study of Caucasians with insulin-dependent diabetes mellitus. Am J Hum Genet 1988; 43:799–816.
28. Bao F, Rewers M, Scott F, Eisenbarth GS. Celiac disease. In Eisenbarth GS (ed). Endocrine and Organ Specific Autoimmunity. Austin, Tex, RG Landes Company, 1999, pp 85–96.
29. Nakanishi K, Kobayashi T, Murase T, et al. Association of HLA-A24 with complete β-cell destruction in IDDM. Diabetes 1993; 42:1086–1098.
30. Yamamoto AM, Deschamps I, Garchon HJ, et al. Young age and HLA markers enhance the risk of progression to type 1 diabetes in antibody-positive siblings of diabetic children. J Autoimmun 1998; 11:643–650.
31. Elbein SC, Hoffman MD, Mayorga RA, et al. Do non–insulin dependent diabetes mellitus (NIDDM) and insulin-dependent diabetes mellitus (IDDM) share genetic susceptibility loci? An analysis of putative IDDM susceptibility regions in familial NIDDM. Metabolism 1997; 46:48–52.
32. Van der Auwera B, Van Waeyenberge C, Schuit F, et al. DRB1*0403 protects against IDDM in Caucasians with the high-risk heterozygous DQA1*0301-DQB1*0302/DQA1*501-DQB1*0201 genotype. Diabetes 1995; 44:527–530.
33. Gambelunghe G, Falorni A, Ghaderi M, et al. Microsatellite polymorphism of the MHC class I chain-related (MIC-A and MIC-B) genes marks the risk for autoimmune Addison's disease. J Clin Endocrinol Metab 1999; 84:3701–3707.
34. Baisch JM, Weeks T, Giles R, et al. Analysis of HLA-DQ genotypes and susceptibility in insulin-dependent diabetes mellitus. N Engl J Med 1990; 322:1836–1841.
35. Bennett ST, Lucassen AM, Gough SCL, et al. Susceptibility to human type I diabetes at IDDM2 is determined by tandem repeat variation at the insulin gene minisatellite locus. Nat Genet 1995; 9:284–292.
36. Verge CF, Vardi P, Babu S, et al. Evidence for oligogenic inheritance of type 1A diabetes in a large Bedouin Arab family. J Clin Invest 1998; 102:1569–1575.
37. Vaidya B, Imrie H, Geatch DR, et al. Association analysis of the cytotoxic T lymphocyte antigen-4 *(CTLA-4)* and autoimmune regulator-1 *(AIRE-1)* genes in sporadic autoimmune Addison's disease. J Clin Endocrinol Metab 2000; 85:688–691.
38. Heward JM, Allahabadia A, Armitage M, et al. The development of Graves' disease and the *CTLA-4* gene on chromosome 2q33. J Clin Endocrinol Metab 1999; 84:2398–2401.
39. Gough SC. The genetics of Graves' disease. Endocrinol Metab Clin North Am 2000; 29:255–266.
40. Santamaria P, Barbosa JJ, Lindstrom AL, et al. HLA-DQB1–associated susceptibility that distinguishes Hashimoto's thyroiditis from Graves' disease in type I diabetic patients. J Clin Endocrinol Metab 1994; 78:878–883.
41. Inoue D, Sato K, Sugawa H, et al. Apparent genetic difference between hypothyroid patients with blocking-type thyrotropin receptor antibody and those without, as shown by restriction fragment length polymorphism analyses of HLA-DP loci. J Clin Endocrinol Metab 1993; 77:606–610.
42. Kemp EH, Ajjan RA, Waterman EA, et al. Analysis of a microsatellite polymorphism of the cytotoxic T-lymphocyte antigen-4 gene in patients with vitiligo. Br J Dermatol 1999; 140:73–78.
43. Baekkeskov S, Aanstoot H-J, Christgau S, et al. Identification of the 64K autoantigen in insulin-dependent diabetes as the GABA-synthesizing enzyme glutamic acid decarboxylase [erratum in Nature 1990; 347:782]. Nature 1990; 347:151–156.
44. Kawasaki E, Gill RG, Eisenbarth GS. Type I diabetes mellitus. In Eisenbarth GS (ed). Endocrine and Organ Specific Autoimmunity. Austin, Tex, RG Landes Company, 1999, pp 149–182.
45. Bednarek J, Furmaniak J, Wedlock N, et al. Steroid 21-hydroxylase is a major autoantigen involved in adult onset autoimmune Addison's disease. FEBS Lett 1992; 309:51–55.
46. Baumann-Antczak A, Wedlock N, Bednarek J, et al. Autoimmune Addison's disease and 21-hydroxylase. Lancet 1992; 340:429–430.
47. Karlsson FA, Burman P, Loof L, Mardh S. Major parietal cell antigen in autoimmune gastritis and pernicious anemia is the acid producing H^+,K^+-adenosine triphosphatase of the stomach. J Clin Invest 1988; 81:475–479.
48. Falorni A, Nikoshkov A, Laureti S, et al. High diagnostic accuracy for idiopathic Addison's disease with a sensitive radiobinding assay for autoantibodies against recombinant human 21-hydroxylase. J Clin Endocrinol Metab 1995; 80:2752–2755.
49. Laureti S, Aubourg P, Calcinaro F, et al. Etiological diagnosis of primary adrenal insufficiency using an original flowchart of immune and biochemical markers. J Clin Endocrinol Metab 1998; 89:3163–3168.
50. Betterle C, Volpato M, Pedini B, et al. Adrenal-cortex autoantibodies and steroid-producing cells autoantibodies in patients with Addison's disease: comparison of immunofluorescence and immunoprecipitation assays. J Clin Endocrinol Metab 1999; 84:618–622.
51. Winqvist O, Karlsson FA, Kampe O. 21-Hydroxylase, a major autoantigen in idiopathic Addison's disease. Lancet 1992; 339:1559–1562.

52. Betterle C, Zanette F, Zanchetta R, et al. Complement-fixing adrenal autoantibodies as a marker for predicting onset of idiopathic Addison's disease. Lancet 1983; 1:1238–1241.
53. Drachman DB. Myasthenia gravis. N Engl J Med 1995; 330: 1797–1810.
54. Pozzilli P. BCG vaccine in insulin-dependent diabetes mellitus. IMDIAB Group. Lancet 1997; 349:1520–1521.
55. Allen HF, Klingensmith GJ, Jensen P, et al. Effect of BCG vaccination on new-onset insulin-dependent diabetes mellitus: a randomized clinical study. Diabetes Care 1998; 22:1703–1707.
56. Lampeter EF, Klinghammer A, Scherbaum WA, et al. The Deutsche Nicotinamide Intervention Study: an attempt to prevent type 1 diabetes. DENIS Group. Diabetes 1998; 47:980–984.
57. Schloot N, Eisenbarth GS. Isohormonal therapy of endocrine autoimmunity. Immunol Today 1995; 16:289–294.
58. Pozzilli P, Pitocco D, Visalli N, et al. No effect of oral insulin on residual beta-cell function in recent-onset type I diabetes (the IMDIAB VII). IMDIAB Group. Diabetologia 2000; 43:1000–1004.
59. Keller RJ, Eisenbarth GS, Jackson RA. Insulin prophylaxis in individuals at high risk of type I diabetes. Lancet 1993; 341:927–928.
60. Hashizume K, Ichikawa K, Nishi Y, et al. Effect of administration of thyroxine on the risk of postpartum recurrence of hyperthyroid Graves' disease. J Clin Endocrinol Metab 1992; 75:6–10.
61. Takasu N, Yamada T, Takasu M, et al. Disappearance of thyrotropin-blocking antibodies and spontaneous recovery from hypothyroidism in autoimmune thyroiditis. N Engl J Med 1992; 326: 513–518.
62. Banovac K, Ghandur-Mnaymeh L, Zakarija M, et al. The effect of thyroxine on spontaneous thyroiditis in BB/W rats. Int Arch Allergy Immunol 1988; 87:301–305.
63. De Bellis A, Bizzarro A, Rossi R, et al. Remission of subclinical adrenocortical failure in subjects with adrenal autoantibodies. J Clin Endocrinol Metab 1993; 76:1002–1007.
64. Petersen HD, Bergman M. Cortisone-induced remission of hypothyroidism in Schmidt's syndrome. Acta Med Scand 1980; 208: 125–127.
65. Jacobs TP, Whitlock RT, Edsall J, Holub DA. Addisonian crisis while taking high-dose glucocorticoids: an unusual presentation of primary adrenal failure in two patients with underlying inflammatory diseases. JAMA 1988; 260:2082–2084.
66. Coles AJ, Wing M, Smith S, et al. Pulsed monoclonal antibody treatment and autoimmune thyroid disease in multiple sclerosis. Lancet 1999; 354:1691–1695.
67. Gisslinger H, Gilly B, Woloszczuk W, et al. Thyroid autoimmunity and hypothyroidism during long-term treatment with recombinant interferon-alpha. Clin Exp Immunol 1992; 90:363–367.
68. Murakami M, Iriuchijima T, Mori M. Diabetes mellitus and interferon-α therapy. Ann Intern Med 1995; 123:318.
69. Thorpe ES, Handley HE. Chronic tetany and chronic mycelial stomatitis in a child aged four-and-one-half years. Am J Dis Child 1929; 38:328–338.
70. Ahonen P, Myllarniemi S, Sipila I, Perheentupa J. Clinical variation of autoimmune polyendocrinopathy–candidiasis–ectodermal dystrophy (APECED) in a series of 68 patients. N Engl J Med 1990; 322:1829–1836.
71. Perheentupa J, Miettinen A. Autoimmune polyendocrinopathy–candidiasis–ectodermal dystrophy. In Eisenbarth GS (ed). Endocrine and Organ Specific Autoimmunity. Austin, Tex, RG Landes Company, 1999, pp 19–40.
72. Walls AWG, Soames JV. Dental manifestations of autoimmune hypoparathyroidism. Oral Surg Oral Med Oral Pathol 1993; 75: 452–454.
73. Friedman TC, Thomas PM, Fleisher TA, et al. Frequent occurrence of asplenism and cholelithiasis in patients with autoimmune polyglandular disease type I. Am J Med 1991; 91:625–630.
74. Bereket A, Lowenheim M, Blethen SL, et al. Intestinal lymphangiectasia in a patient with autoimmune polyglandular disease type I and steatorrhea. J Clin Endocrinol Metab 1995; 80:933–955.
75. Friend PJ, Hale G, Chatenoud L, et al. Phase I study of an engineered aglycosylated humanized CD3 antibody in renal transplant rejection. Transplantation 1999; 68:1632–1637.
76. Blizzard RM, Chee D, Davis W. The incidence of parathyroid and other antibodies in the sera of patients with idiopathic hypoparathyroidism. Clin Exp Immunol 1966; 1:119–128.
77. Li Y, Song Y-H, Rais N, et al. Autoantibodies to the extracellular domain of the calcium sensing receptor in patients with acquired hypoparathyroidism. J Clin Invest 1996; 97:910–914.
78. Krohn K, Uibo R, Aavik E, et al. Identification by molecular cloning of an autoantigen associated with Addison's disease as steroid 17α-hydroxylase. Lancet 1992; 339:770–773.
79. Uibo R, Aavik E, Peterson P, et al. Autoantibodies to cytochrome P450 enzymes P450scc, P450c17, and P450c21 in autoimmune polyglandular disease types I and II and in isolated Addison's disease. J Clin Endocrinol Metab 1994; 78:323–328.
80. Ekwall O, Hedstrand H, Haavik J, et al. Pteridin-dependent hydroxylases as autoantigens in autoimmune polyendocrine syndrome type I. J Clin Endocrinol Metab 2000; 85:2944–2950.
81. Husebye ES, Boe AS, Rorsman F, et al. Inhibition of a aromatic L-amino acid decarboxylase activity by human autoantibodies. Clin Exp Immunol 2000; 120:420–423.
82. Hedstrand H, Perheentupa J, Ekwall O, et al. Antibodies against hair follicles are associated with alopecia totalis in autoimmune polyendocrine syndrome type I. J Invest Dermatol 1999; 113: 1054–1058.
83. Tuomi T, Björses P, Falorni A, et al. Antibodies to glutamic acid decarboxylase and insulin-dependent diabetes in patients with autoimmune polyendocrine syndrome type I. J Clin Endocrinol Metab 1996; 81:1488–1494.
84. Klemetti P, Bjorses P, Tuomi T, et al. Autoimmunity to glutamic acid decarboxylase in patients with autoimmune polyendocrinopathy–candidiasis–ectodermal dystrophy (APECED). Clin Exp Immunol 2000; 119:419–425.
85. Ahonen P. Autoimmune polyendocrinopathy–candidosis–ectodermal dystrophy (APECED): autosomal recessive inheritance. Clin Genet 1985; 27:535–542.
86. Zlotogora J, Shapiro MS. Polyglandular autoimmune syndrome type I among Iranian Jews. J Med Genet 1992; 29:824–826.
87. Aaltonen J, Björses P, Sandkuijl L, et al. An autosomal locus causing autoimmune disease: autoimmune polyglandular disease type I assigned to chromosome 21. Nat Genet 1994; 8:83–87.
88. Heino M, Peterson P, Kudoh J, et al. Autoimmune regulator is expressed in the cells regulating immune tolerance in thymus medulla. Biochem Biophys Res Commun 1999; 257:821–825.
89. Bjorses P, Aaltonen J, Horelli-Kuitunen N, et al. Gene defect behind APECED: a new clue to autoimmunity. Hum Mol Genet 1998; 7:1547–1553.
90. Como JA, Dismukes WE. Oral azole drugs as systemic antifungal therapy. N Engl J Med 1994; 330:263–272.
91. Ahonen P, Myllarniemi S, Kahanpaa A, Perheentupa J. Ketoconazole is effective against the chronic mucocutaneous candidosis of autoimmune polyendocrinopathy–candidosis–ectodermal dystrophy (APECED). Acta Med Scand 1986; 220:333–339.
92. Ketchum CH, Riley WJ, Maclaren NK. Adrenal dysfunction in asymptomatic patients with adrenocortical autoantibodies. J Clin Endocrinol Metab 1984; 58:1166–1170.
93. Ward L, Paquette J, Seidman E, et al. Severe autoimmune polyendocrinopathy–candidiasis–ectodermal dystrophy in an adolescent girl with a novel *AIRE* mutation: response to immunosuppressive therapy. J Clin Endocrinol Metab 1999; 84:844–852.
94. Kahn CR, Flier JS, Bar RS, et al. The syndromes of insulin resistance and acanthosis nigricans: insulin-receptor disorders in man. N Engl J Med 1976; 294:739–745.
95. Flier JS, Bar RS, Muggeo M, et al. The evolving clinical course of patients with insulin receptor autoantibodies: spontaneous remission or receptor proliferation with hypoglycemia. J Clin Endocrinol Metab 1978; 47:985–995.
96. Bardwick PA, Zvaifler NJ, Gill GN, et al. Plasma cell dyscrasia with polyneuropathy, organomegaly, endocrinopathy, M protein, and skin changes: the POEMS syndrome. Medicine (Baltimore) 1980; 59:311–322.
97. Amiel LL, Machover D, Droz JP. Dyscrasie plasmocytaire avec artériopathie, polyneuropathie, syndrome endocrinien. Ann Med Interne (Paris) 1975; 126:745–749.
98. Imawari M, Akatsuka N, Ishibashi M, et al. Syndrome of plasma cell dyscrasia, polyneuropathy, and endocrine disturbances. Ann Intern Med 1974; 81:490–493.
99. Iwashita H, Ohnishi A, Asada M, et al. Polyneuropathy, skin hyperpigmentation, edema, and hypertrichosis in localized osteosclerotic myeloma. Neurology 1977; 27:675–681.
100. Meshkinpour H, Myung CG, Kramer LS. A unique multisys-

temic syndrome of unknown origin. Arch Intern Med 1977; 137: 1719–1721.
101. Saihan EM, Burton JL, Heaton KW. A new syndrome with pigmentation, scleroderma, gynaecomastia, Raynaud's phenomenon and peripheral neuropathy. Br J Dermatol 1978; 99:437–440.
102. Soubrier M, Dubost JJ, Serre AF, et al. Growth factors in POEMS syndrome: evidence for a marked increase in circulating vascular endothelial growth factor. Arthritis Rheum 1997; 40: 786–787.
103. Watanabe O, Maruyama I, Arimura K, et al. Overproduction of vascular endothelial growth factor/vascular permeability factor is causative in Crow-Fukase (POEMS) syndrome. Muscle Nerve 1998; 21:1390–1397.
104. Harvey JN, Barnett D. Endocrine dysfunction in Kearns-Sayre syndrome. Clin Endocrinol 1992; 37:97–104.
105. Combs RM. Malignant thymoma, hyperthyroidism and immune disorder. South Med J 1968; 61:337–341.
106. Rabinowe SL, Rubin IL, George KL, et al. Trisomy 21 (Down's syndrome): autoimmunity, aging and monoclonal-antibody defined T-cell abnormalities. J Autoimmun 1989; 2:25–30.
107. Fialkow PJ, Thuline HC, Hecht F, Bryant J. Familial predisposition to thyroid disease in Down's syndrome: controlled immunoclinical studies. Am J Hum Genet 1971; 23:67–86.
108. Fleming S, Cowell C, Bailey J, Burrow GN. Hashimoto's disease in Turner's syndrome. Clin Invest Med 1988; 11:243–246.
109. Menser MA, Forrest JM, Bransby RD. Rubella infection and diabetes mellitus. Lancet 1978; 1:57–60.
110. Clarke WL, Shaver KA, Bright GM, et al. Autoimmunity in congenital rubella syndrome. J Pediatr 1984; 104:370–373.
111. Rubinstein P, Walker ME, Fedun B, et al. The HLA system in congenital rubella patients with and without diabetes. Diabetes 1982; 31:1088–1091.
112. Rabinowe SL, George KL, Loughlin R, et al. Congenital rubella: monoclonal antibody–defined T cell abnormalities in young adults. Am J Med 1986; 81:779–782.
113. Sakaguchi N, Sakaguchi S. Causes and mechanism of autoimmune disease: cyclosporin A as a probe for the investigation. J Invest Dermatol 1992; 98:70S–76S.
114. Cilio CM, Bosco A, Moretti C, et al. Congenital autoimmune diabetes mellitus (letter). N Engl J Med 2000; 342:1529–1531.
115. Polymeropoulos MH, Swift RG, Swift M. Linkage of the gene for Wolfram syndrome to markers on the short arm of chromosome 4. Nat Genet 1994; 8:95–97.
116. Strom TM, Hortnagel K, Hofmann S, et al. Diabetes insipidus, diabetes mellitus, optic atrophy and deafness (DIDMOAD) caused by mutations in a novel gene (wolframin) coding for a predicted transmembrane protein. Hum Mol Genet 1998; 7: 2021–2028.
117. Rando TA, Horton JC, Layzer RB. Wolfram syndrome: evidence of a diffuse neurodegenerative disease by magnetic resonance imaging. Neurology 1992; 42:1220–1224.
118. Borgna-Pignatti C, Marradi P, Pinelli L, et al. Thiamine-responsive anemia in DIDMOAD syndrome. J Pediatr 1989; 114:405–410.
119. Powell BR, Buist NR, Stenzel P. An X-linked syndrome of diarrhea, polyendocrinopathy, and fatal infection in infancy. J Pediatr 1982; 100:731–737.
120. Bennett CL, Yoshioka R, Kiyosawa H, et al. X-linked syndrome of polyendocrinopathy, immune dysfunction, and diarrhea maps to Xp11.23-Xq13.3. Am J Hum Genet 2000; 66:461–468.
121. Wildin RS, Ramsdell F, Peake J, et al. Mutations in the novel forkhead/winged-helix protein scurfin cause neonatal diabetes, enteropathy, thrombocytopenia, and endocrinopathy syndrome, the human equivalent of the scurfy mouse (abstract). Am J Hum Genet 2000; 67:41.
122. Ahonen P, Miettinen A, Perheentupa J. Adrenal and steroidal cell antibodies in patients with autoimmune polyglandular disease type I and risk of adrenocortical and ovarian failure. J Clin Endocrinol Metab 1987; 64:494–500.
123. Schmidt MB. Eine biglandulare Erkrankung (Nebennieren und Schilddruse) bei Morbus Addisonii. Verh Dtsch Ges Pathol 1926; 21:212–221.
124. Irvine WJ. Autoimmunity in endocrine disease. Recent Prog Horm Res 1980; 36:509–527.
125. Nerup J. Addison's disease—clinical studies: a report of 108 cases. Acta Endocrinol 1974; 76:127–141.
126. Zelissen PM, Bast EJEG, Croughs RJM. Associated autoimmunity in Addison's disease. J Autoimmun 1995; 8:121–130.
127. McElduff A, Lackmann M, Wilkinson M. Antiidiotypic PTH antibodies as a cause of elevated immunoreactive parathyroid hormone in idiopathic hypoparathyroidism, a second case: another manifestation of autoimmune endocrine disease? Calcif Tissue Int 1992; 51:121–126.
128. Tsatsoulis A, Shalet SM. Antisperm antibodies in the polyglandular autoimmune (PGA) syndrome type I: response to cyclical steroid therapy. Clin Endocrinol (Oxf) 1991; 35:299–303.
129. Smith BR, Furmaniak J. Adrenal and gonadal autoimmune diseases (editorial). J Clin Endocrinol Metab 1995; 80:1502–1505.
130. Irvine WJ, Chand MMM, Scarth L, et al. Immunological aspects of premature ovarian failure associated with idiopathic Addison's disease. Lancet 1968; 2:883–887.
131. Turkington RW, Lebovitz HE. Extra-adrenal endocrine deficiencies in Addison's disease. Am J Med 1967; 43:499–507.
132. Bosi E, Becker F, Bonifacio E, et al. Progression to type I diabetes in autoimmune endocrine patients with islet cell antibodies. Diabetes 1991; 40:977–984.
133. Landin-Olsson M, Karlsson FA, Lernmark Å Sundkvist G. Islet cell and thyrogastric antibodies in 633 consecutive 15- to 34-yr-old patients in the diabetes incidence study in Sweden. Diabetes 1992; 41:1022–1027.
134. Riley WJ, Maclaren NK, Lezotte DC, et al. Thyroid autoimmunity in insulin-dependent diabetes mellitus: the case for routine screening. J Pediatr 1981; 99:350–354.
135. Alvarez-Marfany M, Roman SH, Drexler AJ, et al. Long-term prospective study of postpartum thyroid dysfunction in women with insulin dependent diabetes mellitus. J Clin Endocrinol Metab 1994; 79:10–16.
136. Barkan AL, Kelch RP, Marshall JC. Isolated gonadotrope failure in the polyglandular autoimmune syndrome. N Engl J Med 1985; 312:1535–1540.
137. Kojima I, Nejima I, Ogata E. Isolated adrenocorticotropin deficiency associated with polyglandular failure. J Clin Endocrinol Metab 1982; 54:182–186.
138. Goudie RB, Pinkerton PH. Anterior hypophysitis and Hashimoto's disease in a young woman. J Pathol Bacteriol 1957; 83: 584–585.
139. Bevan JS, Othman S, Lazarus JH, et al. Reversible adrenocorticotropin deficiency due to probable autoimmune hypophysitis in a woman with postpartum thyroiditis. J Clin Endocrinol Metab 1992; 74:548–552.
140. Ozawa Y, Shishiba Y. Recovery from lymphocytic hypophysitis associated with painless thyroiditis: clinical implications of circulating antipituitary antibodies. Acta Endocrinol 1993; 128:493–498.
141. Paja M, Estrada J, Ojeda A, et al. Lymphocytic hypophysitis causing hypopituitarism and diabetes insipidus, and associated with autoimmune thyroiditis, in a non-pregnant woman. Postgrad Med J 1994; 70:220–224.
142. Thodou E, Asa SL, Kontogeorgos G, et al. Clinical case seminar: lymphocytic hypophysitis—clinicopathological findings. J Clin Endocrinol Metab 1995; 80:2302–2311.
143. Heubi JE, Partin JC, Schubert WK. Hypocalcemia and steatorrhea: clues to etiology. Dig Dis Sci 1983; 28:124–128.
144. Scire G, Magliocca FM, Cianfarani S, et al. Autoimmune polyendocrine candidiasis syndrome with associated chronic diarrhea caused by intestinal infection and pancreas insufficiency (letter). J Pediatr Gastroenterol Nutr 1991; 13:224–227.
145. Thain ME, Hamilton JR, Ehrlich RM. Coexistence of diabetes mellitus and celiac disease. J Pediatr 1974; 85:527–529.
146. Savilahti E, Simell O, Koskimies S, et al. Celiac disease in insulin-dependent diabetes mellitus. J Pediatr 1986; 108:690–693.
147. Reunala T, Salmi J, Karvonen J. Dermatitis herpetiformis and celiac disease associated with Addison's disease. Arch Dermatol 1987; 123:930–932.
148. Garty BZ, Kauli R. Alopecia universalis in autoimmune polyglandular syndrome type I. West J Med 1990; 152:76–77.
149. Stankler L, Bewsher PD. Chronic mucocutaneous candidiasis, endocrine deficiency and alopecia areata. Br J Dermatol 1972; 86: 238–245.
150. Eisenbarth GS, Wilson P, Ward F, Lebovitz HE. HLA type and occurrence of disease in familial polyglandular failure. N Engl J Med 1978; 298:92–94.

151. Betterle C, Caretto A, Pedini B, et al. Complement-fixing activity to melanin-producing cells preceding the onset of vitiligo in a patient with type I polyglandular failure. Arch Dermatol 1995; 128:123–124.
152. Peserico A, Rigon F, Semsenzato G, et al. Vitiligo and polyglandular autoimmune disease with autoantibodies to melanin-producing cells: a new syndrome? Arch Dermatol 1981; 117:751–752.
153. Riley WJ, Toskes PP, Maclaren NK, Silverstein JH. Predictive value of gastric parietal cell autoantibodies as a marker for gastric and hematologic abnormalities associated with insulin-dependent diabetes. Diabetes 1982; 31:1051–1055.
154. Candrina R, Giustina A. Development of type II autoimmune polyglandular syndrome in a patient with idiopathic thrombocytopenic purpura. Isr J Med Sci 1988; 24:57–58.
155. Segal BM, Weintraub MI. Hashimoto's thyroiditis, myasthenia gravis, idiopathic thrombocytopenic purpura. Ann Intern Med 1976; 85:761–763.
156. Hara T, Mizuno Y, Nagata M, et al. Human gamma delta T-cell receptor–positive cell-mediated inhibition of erythropoiesis in vitro in a patient with type I autoimmune polyglandular syndrome and pure red blood cell aplasia. Blood 1990; 75:941–950.
157. Mandel M, Etzioni A, Theodor R, Passwell JH. Pure red cell hypoplasia associated with polyglandular autoimmune syndrome type I. Isr J Med Sci 1989; 25:138–141.
158. Segawa F, Yamada H, Tomi H, et al. A case of autoimmune polyglandular deficiency associated with progressive myopathy [in Japanese]. Rinsho Shinkeigaku 1992; 32:501–505.
159. Bosch EP, Reith PE, Granner DK. Myasthenia gravis and Schmidt syndrome. Neurology 1994; 27:1179–1180.
160. Kane CA, Weed L. Myasthenia gravis associated with adrenocortical insufficiency. N Engl J Med 1950; 243:939–944.
161. Solimena M, Folli F, Denis-Donini S, et al. Autoantibodies to glutamic acid decarboxylase in a patient with stiff-man syndrome, epilepsy, and type I diabetes mellitus. N Engl J Med 1988; 318: 1012–1020.
162. Rabinowe SL. Immunology of diabetic and polyglandular neuropathy. Diabetes Metab Rev 1990; 6:169–188.
163. Porter SR, Haria S, Scully C, Richards A. Chronic candidiasis, enamel hypoplasia, and pigmentary anomalies. Oral Surg Oral Med Oral Pathol 1992; 74:312–314.
164. Smith WI, Rabin BS, Huellmantel A, et al. Immunopathology of juvenile-onset diabetes mellitus. I. IgA deficiency and juvenile diabetes. Diabetes 1978; 27:1092–1097.
165. Torrelo A, España A, Balsa J, Ledo A. Vitiligo and polyglandular autoimmune syndrome with selective IgA deficiency. Int J Dermatol 1992; 31:343–344.
166. Gass JD. The syndrome of keratoconjunctivitis, superficial moniliasis, idiopathic hypoparathyroidism and Addison's disease. Am J Ophthalmol 1962; 54:660–674.
167. Tucker WS Jr, Niblack GD, McLean RH, et al. Serositis with autoimmune endocrinopathy: clinical and immunogenetic features. Medicine (Baltimore) 1987; 66:138–147.
168. Moss M, Neff TA, Colby TV, et al. Diffuse alveolar hemorrhage due to antibasement membrane antibody disease appearing with a polyglandular autoimmune syndrome. Chest 1994; 105:296–298.
169. Shikata A, Sugimoto T, Kosaka K, et al. Thoracic aortic calcification in 3 children with candidiasis-endocrinopathy syndrome. Pediatr Radiol 1993; 23:100–103.
170. Fairfax AJ, Leatham A. Idiopathic heart block: association with vitiligo, thyroid disease, pernicious anemia, and diabetes mellitus. Br Med J 1975; 4:322–324.
171. Eisenbarth G, Bellgrau D. Autoimmunity. Sci Med 1994; 1:38–47.
172. Hetzel DJ, Stanhope R, O'Neill BP, Lennon VA. Gynecologic cancer in patients with subacute cerebellar degeneration predicted by anti–Purkinje cell antibodies and limited in metastatic volume. Mayo Clin Proc 1990; 65:1558–1563.
173. Uchigata Y, Kuwata S, Tsushima T, et al. Patients with Graves' disease who developed insulin autoimmune syndrome (Hirata disease) possess HLA-Bw62/Cw4/DR4 carrying DRB1*0406. J Clin Endocrinol Metab 1993; 77:249–254.
174. Garlepp MI, Dawkins RL, Christiansen FT. HLA antigens and acetylcholine receptor antibodies in penicillamine induced myasthenia gravis. Br Med J (Clin Res Ed) 1983; 286:1442–1443.
175. Yoshinaga M, Figueroa F, Wahid MR, et al. Antigenic specificity of lymphocytes isolated from valvular specimens of rheumatic fever patients. J Autoimmun 1995; 8:601–613.
176. Imagawa A, Itoh N, Hanafusa T, et al. Autoimmune endocrine disease induced by recombinant interferon-α therapy for chronic active type C hepatitis. J Clin Endocrinol Metab 1995; 80:922–926.
177. Nepom GT. Immunogenetics and IDDM. Diabetes Rev 1993; 1: 93–103.
178. Steinman L. Autoimmune disease. Sci Am 1993; 269(3):106–114.
179. Pugliese A, Solimena M, Awdeh ZL, et al. Association of HLA-DQB1*0201 with stiff-man syndrome. J Clin Endocrinol Metab 1993; 77:1550–1553.
180. Wang CY, Davoodi-Semiromi A, Huang W, et al. Characterization of mutations in patients with autoimmune polyglandular syndrome type 1 (APS1). Hum Genet 1998; 103:681–685.
181. Rosatelli MC, Meloni A, Devoto M, et al. A common mutation in Sardinian autoimmune polyendocrinopathy-candidiasis–ectodermal dystrophy patients. Hum Genet 1998; 103:428–434.
182. Scott HS, Heino M, Peterson P, et al. Common mutations in autoimmune polyendocrinopathy–candidiasis–ectodermal dystrophy patients of different origins. Mol Endocrinol 1998; 12:1112–1119.

38 Gastrointestinal Hormones and Gut Endocrine Tumors

Robin P. Boushey and Daniel J. Drucker

Endocrine tumors originating from islet, or *enteroendocrine*, cells may present with unique clinical symptoms that reflect the biologic actions of secreted peptide hormones. In this chapter, we discuss how endocrine cell lineages develop during organogenesis in the endocrine pancreas and intestine and review the biologic actions of peptide hormones produced in pancreatic and intestinal endocrine cells and enteric nerves. Although numerous physiologic actions of these peptides are still poorly understood and under active investigation, excessive production of one or more of these peptides frequently accounts for the clinical symptoms attributable to endocrine tumors arising from the gastrointestinal tract and pancreas.

ENDOCRINE CELL DEVELOPMENT IN THE PANCREAS

The endocrine and exocrine pancreas develop from the primitive foregut endoderm. Pancreatic morphogenesis is a complex process that begins with the evagination of the embryonic foregut into ventral and dorsal buds at 28 days' gestation in humans and at *embryonic day* (ED) 8 in mice.[1] Rotation of the stomach and duodenum during development results in simultaneous rotation of the ventral bud that undergoes fusion with the dorsal bud to give rise to the primitive pancreas. The ventral bud develops into the posterior portion of the pancreatic head, including the uncinate process, while the remaining pancreas derives from the dorsal bud. In mice, a complex tree-like, epithelial-lined ductal system develops within the pancreatic diverticula with glucagon immunoreactive cells detected as early as ED 9.5, followed by detection of cells containing insulin at ED 10.5. Stem cells that give rise to both terminally differentiated endocrine and exocrine acinar cells are thought to reside within the ductal epithelium.

In humans, islet formation begins at *gestational week* (GW) 12 with the aggregation of polyclonal endocrine cells. Between GWs 13 and 16, small aggregates of endocrine cells arise from the pancreatic duct and develop their own blood supply. At GWs 17 to 20, fewer islets are observed in contact with the ducts, and a mantle of non-beta endocrine cells forms around the beta cells. Between GWs 21 and 26, a continual increase in the proportion of islet tissue and in the average size of the islets is observed with occasional non-beta cells in the center of the islet, a morphologic appearance that is characteristic of the postnatal islet.

At birth, the endocrine pancreas accounts for 1% to 2% of the entire pancreatic cell mass. The neuroendocrine marker nestin appears to be expressed on islet and ductal cells that exhibit properties consistent with human islet stem cells in vitro.[2]

Although genetic studies in mice have yielded valuable insights into the ontogeny of islet development, the relative order of appearance of unique populations of hormone-producing islet endocrine cells differs in humans and mice. Somatostatin- and pancreatic polypeptide (PP)-positive cells are detected at GW 7 in the human pancreas scattered among ductal cells. One week later, glucagon cells appear, and by

Table 38–1. Effects of Disrupting Genes on Pancreatic Endocrine Cell Development

Gene	Phenotype in Homozygous (−/−) Mutant Mice
Hes-1	Increased glucagon-positive alpha cells, pancreatic hypoplasia
Hlxb-9	Dorsal lobe agenesis, small islets, reduced beta cells
Isl-1	Loss of differentiated islet cells
Nkx2.2	Absent mature beta cells, reduced alpha and pancreatic polypeptide cells
Nkx6.1	Reduced beta cell precursors
NeuroD	Reduced beta cells, arrested islet morphogenesis
ngn3	Absent islet cells and defective enteroendocrine cell formation
Pax4	Absent islet beta and delta cells
Pax6	Absent islet alpha cells
Pdx-1	Pancreatic agenesis

GW 9 to 10, insulin-producing cells are detectable. In mice, both insulin- and glucagon-expressing cells are first detected between ED 9.5 and 10.5, whereas somatostatin and PP are expressed later, by ED 15.5. Although cells coexpressing insulin and glucagon are detected during early islet development, cell lineage studies employing specific transgenes that mark or ablate islet cell precursors suggest that the alpha and beta cell lineages arise independently during ontogeny in the mouse.[3, 4] Peptide YY (PYY) co-localizes with each of the four main islet hormones in the developing pancreas.[5] However genetic evidence for an essential role of a PYY-producing precursor cell in pancreatic endocrine development has not yet been forthcoming.

Delineation of the genetic determinants that regulate the developmental formation and organization of pancreatic endocrine cell populations has been facilitated by studies of mice with disruption of candidate regulatory genes, principally islet transcription factors (Table 38–1). The homeobox transcription factor *Pdx-1* is required for insulin gene transcription in the adult beta cell and for developmental formation of the entire pancreas. Mice homozygous for a null mutation in *Pdx-1* fail to develop a pancreas,[6, 7] whereas restricted inactivation of *Pdx-1* in the murine beta cell produces insulin deficiency and diabetes mellitus.[8] Similarly, pancreatic agenesis has also been reported in human subjects homozygous for a loss of function *Pdx-1* mutation,[9] whereas subjects heterozygous for *Pdx-1* develop a form of maturity-onset diabetes mellitus of the young *(MODY4)*.

Targeted disruption of the LIM domain *Isl-1* gene in mice results in abnormal development of the dorsal pancreatic mesenchyme and abnormal differentiation of islet cells,[10] whereas a heterozygous human *ISL-1* mutation has been reported in a single patient with type 2 diabetes mellitus. Although mutations in the *Pax4* and *Pax6* genes produce profound abnormalities in developmental formation of murine pancreatic endocrine cells,[11] islet function has not been extensively studied in human subjects with *PAX* mutations. Nevertheless, binding sites for the MODY genes *Pdx-1*, *HNF1α*, and *HNF4α* have been identified in the *Pax4* promoter, suggesting that MODY genes may be upstream regulators of genes critical for islet cell formation and islet function in the pancreas.[12]

Genes encoding members of the notch receptor family, their ligands, and downstream targets are essential for developmental formation of the endocrine pancreas (see Table 38–1). Targeted inactivation of genes in the notch signaling pathway markedly perturbs the normal development and differentiation of pancreatic endocrine cells.[13] Mice lacking neurogenin 3 *(ngn3)*, a basic helix-loop-helix (bHLH) transcription factor, fail to develop pancreatic endocrine cells and die of diabetes mellitus postnatally, whereas overexpression of *ngn3* produces accelerated differentiation of pancreatic endocrine cells. These findings, taken together with the loss of *Isl-1*, *Pax4*, *Pax6*, and *NeuroD* expression in *ngn3* −/− mice, implicate *ngn3* as a key upstream regulator of pancreatic endocrine cell development.[14–16]

Research into the identification of upstream control mechanisms and downstream targets that promote islet cell formation, growth, and differentiation is likely to proceed rapidly in the next few years, providing scientists and clinicians with an enhanced understanding of the genetic determinants regulating the growth of normal and neoplastic endocrine cells. A summary of genetic mutations associated with abnormal formation of pancreatic endocrine cells is provided in Table 38–1.

ENDOCRINE CELL DEVELOPMENT IN THE INTESTINE

Stem cells associated with the intestinal epithelium differentiate into four different cell lineages: (1) enterocytes, (2) Paneth cells, (3) goblet cells, and (4) enteroendocrine cells.

The enteroendocrine cell population comprises less than 1% of all intestinal epithelial cells but represents the largest mass of endocrine cells in the body. Compared with studies of pancreatic endocrine cell development, much less is known about the molecular control of enteroendocrine cell formation and differentiation.

Numerous enteroendocrine cell types have been identified that can be classified according to morphologic criteria and expression of one or more secretory products.[17, 18] In the stomach, gastrin cells first appear in the duodenum, followed by their localization to the antrum and pylorus in adult gastric mucosa. In the small bowel, a secretin precursor cell appears important for enteroendocrine cell lineage formation.[19] In the murine colon, PYY is the first detectable hormone marking appearance of enteroendocrine cells[20] and is coexpressed in most endocrine cells in the large intestine as they first differentiate.

The notch signaling pathway is essential for developmental formation of enteroendocrine cells. Activation of notch results in increased expression of the bHLH transcriptional repressor *Hes1* that functionally antagonizes bHLH genes that regulate cellular differentiation. Mice deficient in *Hes1* demonstrate premature cellular differentiation and severe pancreatic hypoplasia due to depletion of pancreatic epithelial precursors.[21] These mice also demonstrate excessive differentiation of multiple endocrine cell types in the developing stomach and gut, suggesting that *Hes1* is a negative regulator of endodermal endocrine differentiation. Both *Notch1* and *ngn3* act upstream of BETA2/NeuroD, a bHLH protein important for differentiation of endocrine cells in both the pancreas and intestine[22] (Table 38–2).

Mice homozygous for a null mutation in the *Pdx-1* gene demonstrate poorly differentiated duodenal intestinal epithelium with absence of Brunner's glands and a deficiency of gastrin cells in the stomach. Just distal to the abnormal epithelium, a reduction in the number of enteroendocrine cells is observed. In contrast, expression of *Pdx-1* in gut epithelial cells redirects cell lineage toward an enteroendocrine phenotype.[23] Inactivation of BETA2/NeuroD in mice results in absence of secretin-producing and cholecystokinin (CCK)-producing enteroendocrine cells.[22] The complexity of lineage relationships between gut endocrine cell populations is further illustrated by studies in mice with targeted ablation of secretin-producing cells. These mice exhibit nearly complete elimination of enter-

Table 38–2. Effects of Disrupting Genes on Enteroendocrine Cell Development

Gene	Phenotype in Homozygous (−/−) Mutant Mice
Hes-1	Enhanced numbers of enteroendocrine cells
NeuroD	Absent secretin and CCK lineages
Pax4	Reduced endocrine cell lineages in duodenum and stomach
Pax6	Reduced number of GIP-positive K cells, antral gastrin and somatostatin cells, and L cells
Pdx-1	Reduced enteroendocrine cells in stomach and duodenum
Ihh	Reduced enteroendocrine cells in duodenum

CCK, cholecystokinin; GIP, gastric inhibitory polypeptide.

oendocrine cell populations producing CCK and PYY/glucagon and a reduction in cells producing gastric inhibitory polypeptide (GIP), somatostatin, and serotonin.[19]

Members of the *Pax* gene family are also essential for the formation of enteroendocrine cells (see Table 38–2). Targeted disruption of *Pax4* markedly reduces the number of murine duodenal cells immunopositive for serotonin, secretin, GIP, PYY, and CCK and decreases the number of somatostatin- and serotonin-positive cells in the stomach. Complete disruption of the *Pax6* locus more selectively reduces the number of duodenal cells expressing GIP and CCK[24] and decreases the number of gastrin-immunopositive and somatostatin-immunopositive cells in the stomach, whereas SEY^{Neu} mice that express a dominant negative mutant *Pax6* allele demonstrate markedly reduced levels of proglucagon messenger RNA (mRNA) transcripts in both the small and large intestine, with almost complete depletion of enteroendocrine cells exhibiting glucagon-like peptide 1 (GLP-1) and GLP-2 immunoreactivity (Fig. 38–1) (see also Color Plate).[25]

At present, the classification of enteroendocrine cells is based principally on the phenotype ascribed to the production of one or more peptide hormones. Nevertheless, it seems likely that additional enteroendocrine cell subpopulations will be described in different regions of the gut that exhibit considerable biologic complexity beyond that which is currently appreciated.

PANCREATIC AND GUT HORMONES (Table 38–3)

Amylin

Amylin, also known as *islet amyloid–associated peptide*, is a 37–amino acid hormone produced in islet beta cells and in scattered endocrine cells in the stomach and in the proximal small intestine. Exogenous administration of amylin inhibits gastric emptying and glucagon secretion in rodents and humans. Excess amylin secretion and deposition in the endocrine pancreas have been implicated as a potential pathogenic feature in some subjects with type 2 diabetes mellitus. Amylin exerts its physiologic actions through interaction with the calcitonin receptor in the presence of a receptor activity–modifying protein (RAMP). Mice deficient in amylin display modest perturbations in islet function and enhanced glucose clearance following glucose challenge.

The role of gut-derived amylin in human physiology has not been clearly established. Although amylin expression has been detected in both pancreatic and gut endocrine tumors, a specific syndrome attributable to amylin overexpression has not been delineated.

Calcitonin Gene-Related Peptide

Calcitonin gene-related peptide (CGRP) is a member of a larger family of peptides that includes calcitonin, amylin, and adrenomedullin. In humans, distinct genes *CALC-A* and *CALC-B* encode for both calcitonin and CGRP and give rise to two 37–amino acid C-terminal amidated neuropeptides, designated *α-CGRP* and *β-CGRP*. These neuropeptides share considerable amino acid sequence homology differing by only three amino acids in humans. α-CGRP is expressed predominantly in primary afferent sensory neurons arising from the spinal cord, whereas β-CGRP is expressed in enteric neurons.[26] Two calcitonin/CGRP seven-transmembrane domain G-protein coupled receptors[27] both interact with a family of RAMPs; coexpression of calcitonin receptor-like receptor with RAMP1 results in ligand specificity for CGRP, whereas expression of the same receptor with RAMP2 results in specificity for adrenomedullin.[28]

CGRP immunoreactivity has been localized to enteroendocrine cells of the human rectum and to endocrine cells and neurons in the small intestine. Intestinal CGRP is released in response to glucose and by gastric acid secretion. CGRP produces marked vasodilation in the stomach, splanchnic, and peripheral circulation through stimulating nitric oxide (NO) release. CGRP also inhibits gastric acid and pancreatic exocrine secretion likely through stimulating somatostatin release. Although focal CGRP positivity has been detected in some human carcinoid and pancreatic endocrine tumors (PETs), its usefulness as a tumor marker has not been firmly established.

Cholecystokinin

Cholecystokinin (CCK) was first characterized as a factor that stimulates gallbladder contraction. The CCK gene is expressed in "open-type" enteroendocrine I cells in the proximal

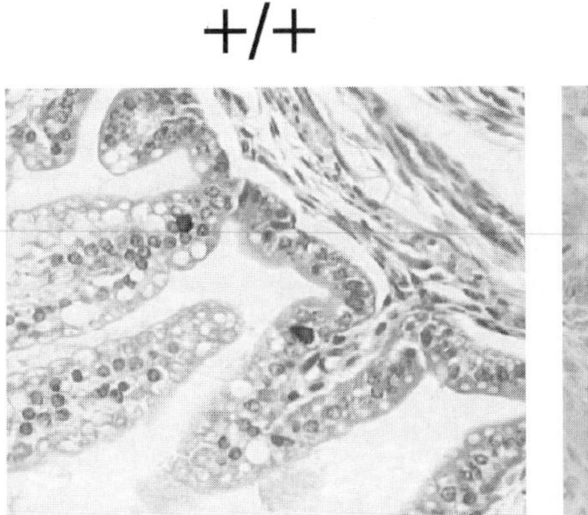

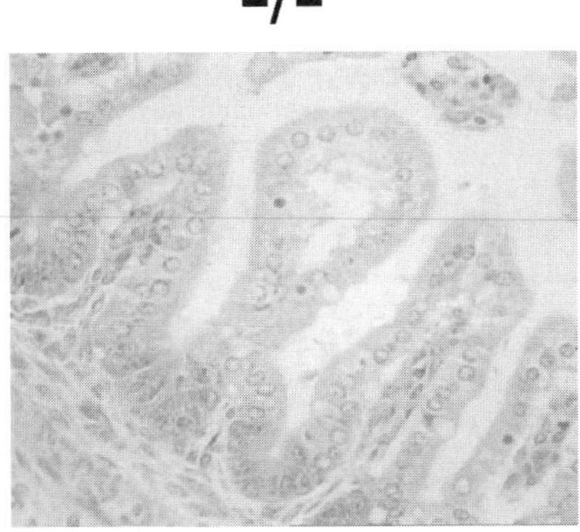

Figure 38–1. Essential requirement for *Pax6* for glucagon-positive enteroendocrine cell formation in the murine intestine. *Pax6* SEY^{NEU} mutant mice (−/−) exhibit markedly reduced numbers of glucagon-immunopositive cells in the small and large intestine. (See also Color Plate.)

Table 38–3. Summary of Gastrointestinal-Derived Hormones

Hormone	Cell/Tissue of Origin	Related Peptides	Actions	Secretory Stimuli
Amylin	Pancreatic B cell, endocrine cells of stomach and small intestine	Calcitonin, calcitonin gene-related peptide, adrenomedulin	1. Inhibits gastric emptying 2. Inhibits arginine-stimulated and postprandial glucagon secretion 3. Inhibits insulin secretion 4. Satiety factor	1. Co-secreted with insulin in response to oral nutrient ingestion
Calcitonin gene-related peptide (CGRP)	α-CGRP is expressed predominantly in afferent sensory nerves from the spinal cord; β-CGRP is expressed in enteric neurons and enteroendocrine cells of the rectum	Calcitonin, amylin, adrenomedulin	1. Produces marked vasodilatation in the splanchnic and peripheral circulation by stimulating nitric oxide release 2. Inhibits gastric acid and pancreatic exocrine secretion 3. Induces intestinal smooth muscle relaxation	1. Glucose and gastric acid secretion
Cholecystokinin (CCK)	Enteroendocrine I cells and enteric nerves, central nervous system, pituitary corticotrophs, C cells of the thyroid, adrenal medulla, and the acrosome of developing and mature spermatozoa		1. Inhibits proximal gastric motility while increasing antral and pyloric contractions 2. Regulates meal-stimulated pancreatic enzyme secretion and gallbladder contraction 3. Trophic effects on pancreatic acini in rats 4. Postprandial satiety 5. In the brain, CCK affects memory, sleep, sexual behavior, and anxiety	1. Oral nutrient ingestion 2. Several intestine-derived hormones, including GRP and bombesin 3. Activation of β-adrenergic receptors
Galanin	Central and peripheral nervous systems, pituitary, neural structures of the gut, pancreas, thyroid, and adrenal gland		1. In the brain, regulation of food intake, memory and cognition, and antinociception 2. Inhibits pancreatic exocrine secretion and intestinal ion transport 3. Induces both contraction and relaxation of intestinal smooth muscle, depending on the species examined 4. Delays gastric emptying and prolongs colonic transit times 5. Inhibits the secretion of insulin, PYY, gastrin, somatostatin, enteroglucagon, neurotensin, and pancreatic polypeptide	1. Intestinal distention 2. Chemical stimulation of the intestinal mucosa 3. Electrical stimulation of periarterial nerves 4. Extrinsic sympathetic neurons
Gastric inhibitory polypeptide/ glucose-dependent insulinotropic polypeptide (GIP)	Neuroendocrine K cells in the duodenum and proximal jejunum		1. Inhibits gastric acid secretion and gastrointestinal motility 2. Increases insulin release and regulates glucose and lipid metabolism 3. Exerts anabolic actions in bone	1. Oral nutrient ingestion, especially long-chain fatty acids
Gastrin	Predominantly enteroendocrine G cells of the stomach and duodenal bulb; central and peripheral nervous systems, pituitary, adrenal gland, genital tract, respiratory tract, fetal pancreas		1. Induces gastric acid secretion 2. Amidated gastrins are trophic to the oxyntic mucosa of the stomach 3. Progastrin and glycine-extended gastrin induce colonic epithelial proliferation	1. Luminal contents, especially partially digested aromatic amino acids, small peptides, calcium, coffee, and ethanol 2. Humoral and neural influences, including the vagus nerve, β-adrenergic and γ-aminobutyric acid neurons, and gastrin-releasing peptide 3. Somatostatin inhibits secretion

Table 38–3. Summary of Gastrointestinal-Derived Hormones *Continued*

Hormone	Cell/Tissue of Origin	Related Peptides	Actions	Secretory Stimuli
Gastrin-releasing peptide (GRP) and related peptides	Central nervous system, enteric nervous system; reproductive tract, and lung, where it acts as a neurotransmitter; GRP neurons also distributed throughout the human pancreas	Bombesin, neuromedin B, neuromedin C	1. Stimulates smooth muscle contraction in the stomach, intestine, and gallbladder 2. Stimulates the release of CCK, gastrin, GIP, glucagon, GLP-1, GLP-2, motilin, PP, PYY, and somatostatin 3. Stimulates gastric acid secretion via direct effect on G cells 4. In the brain, regulates appetite, memory, thermogenesis, and cardiac function 5. Stimulates pancreatic growth 6. In the lung, growth factor for both normal and neoplastic tissue	1. Cholinergic stimulation
Ghrelin	Central nervous system, stomach, small intestine, and colon	Motilin	1. Stimulates growth hormone release 2. Stimulates gastric kinetic activity 3. Orexigenic activity 4. Stimulates energy production and signals hypothalamic regulatory nuclei that control energy homeostasis	1. Fasting
Glucagon	Pancreatic A cell, central nervous system		1. Primary counterregulatory mechanism to restore plasma glucose levels in the setting of hypoglycemia by increasing gluconeogenesis, glycogenolysis, and protein-lipid flux in both the liver and periphery 2. Gastrointestinal smooth muscle relaxation	1. Neural and humoral factors released in response to hypoglycemia
Glucagon-like peptide 1 (GLP-1)	Enteroendocrine L cells located in the ileum and colon, central nervous system		1. Enhances glucose disposal following nutrient ingestion by inhibiting gastric emptying, stimulating insulin secretion, and inhibiting glucagon secretion 2. Inhibits food intake 3. Stimulates pancreatic islet neogenesis and proliferation 4. Inhibits sham feeding–induced gastric acid secretion	1. Oral nutrient ingestion, especially carbohydrates and fat-rich meals 2. Vagus nerve, GRP, and GIP 3. Acetylcholine and neuromedin C 4. Somatostatin inhibits secretion
Glucagon-like peptide-2 (GLP-2)	As described above for GLP-1		1. Induces small intestinal and colonic mucosal growth by stimulating crypt cell proliferation and inhibiting apoptosis 2. Inhibits centrally induced antral motility and meal-stimulated gastric acid secretion 3. Enhances intestinal epithelial barrier function 4. Stimulates intestinal hexose transport 5. Inhibits short-term control of food intake	As described above for GLP-1

Table continued on following page

Table 38–3. Summary of Gastrointestinal-Derived Hormones *Continued*

Hormone	Cell/Tissue of Origin	Related Peptides	Actions	Secretory Stimuli
Motilin	Brain, bronchoepithelial cells, and enteroendocrine M cells located in the duodenum and proximal jejunum	Ghrelin	1. Induces phase III contractions in the stomach 2. Stimulates gastric and pancreatic enzyme secretion 3. Induces contraction of the gallbladder, sphincter of Oddi, and lower esophageal sphincter	1. Duodenal alkalinization, sham feeding, gastric distention; opioid agonists promote secretion 2. Unlike most gastrointestinal hormones, secretion is suppressed in the presence of duodenal nutrients
Neuropeptide Y (NPY)	Central and peripheral nervous systems, pancreatic islet cells	PYY and PP	1. Potent stimulator of oral nutrient intake 2. Inhibits glucose-stimulated insulin secretion 3. Reduces gastrointestinal fluid and electrolyte secretion 4. Inhibits gastric and small intestinal motility 5. Induces marked vasoconstriction of the splanchnic circulation	1. Oral nutrient ingestion 2. Activation of the sympathetic nervous system
Neurotensin (NT)	N cells located in the small intestinal mucosa, especially the ileum; central and peripheral nervous systems, including the enteric nervous system; heart, adrenal gland, pancreas, and respiratory tract	Neuromedin N, xenin, and xenopsin	1. Stimulates growth of the colonic epithelium 2. Inhibits postprandial gastric acid secretion and pancreatic exocrine secretion 3. Stimulates colonic motility but inhibits gastric and small intestinal motility 4. Facilitates fatty acid uptake in the proximal small intestine and induces histamine release from mast cells 5. Trophic in some pancreatic and colon cancer cell lines in vitro 6. In the brain, neuromodulator of dopamine transmission and anterior pituitary hormone secretion, hypothermia, analgesic effects; reduces food intake	1. Luminal nutrients, especially lipids, but not amino acids or carbohydrates 2. GRP and bombesin 3. Somatostatin inhibits secretion
Pancreatic polypeptide (PP)	Major site of expression is pancreatic endocrine cells located in periphery of islets in pancreatic head and uncinate process	NPY and PYY	1. Reduces CCK-induced gastric acid secretion 2. Increases intestinal transit times by reducing gastric emptying and upper intestinal motility 3. Inhibits postprandial exocrine pancreas secretion via a vagal-dependent pathway	1. Stimulated by nutrients, hormones, neurotransmitters, gastric distention, insulin-induced hypoglycemia, and direct vagal nerve stimulation 2. Hyperglycemia, bombesin, and somatostatin inhibit secretion
Peptide YY (PYY)	Enteroendocrine cells, developing endocrine pancreas, subpopulation of pancreatic A cells in mature islets	NPY and PP	1. Enterogastrone inhibits both gastric acid secretion and gastric motility 2. Increases intestinal transit time by reducing intestinal motility 3. Inhibits pancreatic exocrine secretion 4. Role as an intestinal epithelial growth factor remains controversial 5. Peripheral vasoconstriction and reduced mesenteric and pancreatic vascular blood flow	1. Following oral nutrient ingestion, early secretion is mediated by the vagus nerve and hormonal influences; subsequently, secretion occurs as a result of direct L-cell stimulation 2. Bile acids and fatty acids 3. Amino acids administered intracolonically

Table 38–3. Summary of Gastrointestinal-Derived Hormones *Continued*

Hormone	Cell/Tissue of Origin	Related Peptides	Actions	Secretory Stimuli
Pituitary adenylate cyclase–activating peptide (PACAP)	Brain, respiratory tract, and enteric nervous system	Vasoactive intestinal peptide (VIP), peptide histidine isoleucine (PHI), and peptide histidine methionine (PHM)	1. Stimulates histamine release from the stomach 2. Increases the secretion of pancreatic fluid, protein, and bicarbonate 3. Stimulates insulin and catecholamine release 4. Neural regulation of gastric acid secretion	1. Activation of the central nervous system
Secretin	Central nervous system, fetal endocrine pancreas, and enteroendocrine S cells located in the duodenum and proximal jejunum		1. Principal hormonal stimulant of pancreatic and biliary bicarbonate and water secretion 2. Regulates pancreatic enzyme secretion 3. Stimulates gastric secretion of pepsinogen 4. Inhibits lower esophageal sphincter tone, postprandial gastric emptying, gastrin release, and gastric acid secretion	1. Gastric acid, bile salts, and luminal nutrients, especially fatty acids, peptides, and ethanol 2. Somatostatin inhibits secretion
Somatostatin	Central nervous system, pancreatic D cells, enteroendocrine D cells		1. Inhibits secretion of islet hormones, including insulin, glucagon, and PP 2. Inhibits the secretion of gut peptides, including gastrin, secretin, VIP, CCK, GLP-1, and GLP-2 3. Inhibits pancreatic exocrine secretion 4. Acts in a paracrine manner on G cells, enterochromaffin-like cells, and parietal cells to inhibit gastric acid secretion 5. Reduces splanchnic blood flow, intestinal motility, and carbohydrate absorption while increasing water and electrolyte absorption	1. Luminal nutrients 2. Gastrin, CCK, bombesin, GLP-1, and GIP 3. Neural influences, including PACAP, VIP, and β-adrenergic agonists stimulate while acetylcholine inhibits secretion
Tachykinins	Throughout the central and peripheral nervous systems, including the respiratory tract, skin, sensory organs, and the urogenital tract; In the gastrointestinal tract, neurons localized in the submucous and myenteric plexuses, extrinsic sensory fibers, and enterochromaffin cells in the gut epithelium	Substance P, neurokinin A, and neurokinin B	1. Regulate vasomotor and gastrointestinal smooth muscle contractility 2. Chemotaxis and activation of immune cells, mucus secretion, water absorption and secretion 3. Role in visceral inflammation, hyperreflexia, and hyperalgesia	1. Direct and/or indirect activation of neurons
Thyrotropin-releasing hormone (TRH)	Central and enteric nervous system, colon, G cells of the stomach, pancreatic islet beta cells		1. Suppresses pentagastrin-stimulated gastric acid secretion 2. Chronic administration induces pancreatic hyperplasia and inhibits amylase release 3. Attenuates CCK-induced gallbladder smooth muscle contraction 4. Inhibits cholesterol synthesis within the intestinal mucosa	1. In the stomach, histamine and serotonin stimulate and endogenous opioids inhibit secretion

Table continued on following page

Table 38–3. Summary of Gastrointestinal-Derived Hormones *Continued*

Hormone	Cell/Tissue of Origin	Related Peptides	Actions	Secretory Stimuli
Vasoactive intestinal peptide (VIP)	Widely expressed in the central and peripheral nervous system (including the enteric nervous system)	PACAP, PHI and PHM	1. Induces relaxation of vascular and nonvascular smooth muscle 2. Mediates relaxation of the lower esophageal sphincter, sphincter of Oddi, and anal sphincter 3. Regulates relaxation-associated gut contraction and may be involved with reflex vasodilation in the small intestine 4. Inhibits gastric acid secretion 5. Stimulates biliary water, bicarbonate, pancreatic enzyme, and intestinal chloride secretion 6. Some evidence suggesting a role in regulating pancreatic release of insulin and glucagon	1. Mechanical stimulation 2. Activation of the central and peripheral nervous systems

small intestine (Table 38–4) and in nerve fibers branching to the gastric and colonic myenteric plexus and submucosal plexus where CCK acts as a neurotransmitter. CCK-immunoreactive peptides are found in the cerebral cortex and limbic system and in pituitary corticotrophs, C cells of the thyroid, adrenal medulla, and the acrosome of the developing and mature spermatozoa. The *CCK* gene encodes a 94–amino acid prohormone that is post-translationally processed in a tissue-specific fashion into multiple molecular forms of CCK-83, -58, -39, -33, -22, -8, and -5, all sharing a common C-terminus. The major active form, CCK-8, is an octapeptide containing a sulfated tyrosine residue and an amidated C-terminal phenylalanine residue, whereas CCK-33 appears to be the predominant circular form in human plasma.[29]

CCK binds with high affinity to the CCK-A receptor, a seven-transmembrane domain G-protein–coupled receptor expressed in pancreatic acinar cells, gallbladder, smooth muscle, chief and D cells of the gastric mucosa, and the central and peripheral nervous systems. In the stomach, CCK inhibits proximal gastric motility while increasing the force of antral and pyloric contractions.[30] CCK also regulates meal-stimulated pancreatic enzyme secretion and gallbladder contraction.

CCK exhibits trophic effects on pancreatic acini in rats.[31] Experimental manipulations that increase levels of circulating CCK, such as treatment with soybean trypsin inhibitor, or long-term pancreatobiliary diversion result in pancreatic growth and premalignant changes.[31] Elevated circulating levels of CCK also enhanced the development of preneoplastic acinar lesions induced by azaserine, a pancreatic carcinogen in rats. In contrast, the Otsuka Long-Evans Tokushima Fatty (OLETF) rat fails to express a functional CCK-A receptor and demonstrates reduced pancreatic size.[32]

Exogenous administration of CCK decreases the size of spontaneously ingested meals, whereas CCK-A receptor antagonists increase appetite. A human subject with polyglandular syndrome type I exhibited severe diarrhea and malabsorption in association with reduced numbers of enteroendocrine cells and CCK deficiency.[33] Thus, CCK secretion in response to oral nutrient ingestion likely regulates nutrient absorption and postprandial satiety. Nevertheless, CCK receptors do not appear essential for weight regulation in vivo because mice with targeted disruption of the CCK-A and CCK-B receptors exhibit normal food intake and weight gain well into adult life.[34]

Table 38–4. Location of Enteroendocrine Cells and Their Associated Peptide Hormones in the Gastrointestinal Tract

Hormones	Enteroendocrine Cell	Location
Somatostatin	D	Stomach, duodenum, small intestine, colon
Gastrin, TRH	G	Stomach and duodenum
CCK	I	Duodenum and jejunum
GIP	K	Duodenum and proximal jejunum
GLP-1, GLP-2, PYY	L	Ileum, colon, and rectum
Motilin	M	Duodenum and proximal jejunum
Neurotensin	N	Small intestine, especially ileum
Secretin	S	Duodenum and proximal jejunum

CCK, cholecystokinin; GIP, gastric inhibitory polypeptide; GLP-1, -2, glucagon-like peptide 1, 2; PYY, peptide YY; TRH, thyrotropin-releasing hormone.

Galanin

Galanin was initially isolated from porcine intestine as a 29–amino acid C-terminally amidated neuropeptide. In humans, two molecular forms of galanin exist that are 19 and 30 amino acids in length. Galanin is expressed in the central and peripheral nervous systems and pituitary gland and in neural structures of the gut, pancreas, thyroid, and adrenal gland. In the intestine, galanin immunoreactivity is detected predominantly within enteric neurons located in the myenteric and submucosal plexuses that innervate the mucosa and the circular and longitudinal smooth muscle layer. Galanin is released by enteric neurons in response to intestinal distention, chemical stimulation of the mucosa, electrical stimulation of periarterial nerves, and extrinsic sympathetic neurons.

At least three different galanin receptor subtypes have been identified—GalR1, GalR2, and GalR3. These subtypes are widely expressed in gastric and intestinal smooth muscle cells, pancreas, and the central nervous system.[35] The actions of galanin include regulation of food intake, memory and cognition, antinociception, and modulation of multiple neuroendocrine systems in the pituitary, pancreas, and gut. The importance of galanin for pituitary lactotroph biology is exemplified by studies of galanin knockout mice that exhibit normal growth rates but reduced levels of prolactin and complete failure of lactation.[36]

Although galanin can inhibit GIP-induced and GLP-1–induced proinsulin gene transcription and insulin secretion, infusion of galanin in humans has no effect on levels of plasma insulin.[37] Galanin also inhibits both pancreatic exocrine secretion and intestinal ion transport and induces the contraction and relaxation of intestinal smooth muscle. In humans, intravenous administration of galanin delays gastric emptying and prolongs colonic transit times. Although galanin expression has been detected in hypothalamic, pituitary, and adrenal tumors, galanin immunopositivity in pancreatic or gut endocrine tumor cells is rare.

Gastric Inhibitory Polypeptide

Also known as *glucose-dependent insulinotropic polypeptide*, GIP is a 42–amino acid peptide secreted by enteroendocrine K cells located in the duodenum and proximal jejunum. GIP levels rise immediately following nutrient ingestion, leading to modest inhibitory effects on gastric acid secretion and gastrointestinal motility.

The precise role of GIP as an enterogastrone remains controversial because supraphysiologic concentrations of GIP are required to inhibit both gastric acid secretion and gastric emptying in humans. The actions of GIP on the pancreatic beta cell are primarily those of an incretin, a gut-derived peptide that stimulates insulin secretion in the setting of raised plasma glucose levels following oral nutrient ingestion.[38] GIP receptor knockout mice are viable but exhibit impaired oral glucose tolerance and enhanced susceptibility to diabetes mellitus following high-fat feeding.[39] Although GIP-secreting endocrine tumors are rare, gut-derived GIP may contribute to the development of food-induced Cushing's syndrome in a subset of patients with adrenal adenomas that express the GIP receptor.[40]

Gastrin

A single mRNA transcript encodes a pre-progastrin precursor of 101 amino acids that undergoes post-translational processing into multiple biologically active molecular forms of circulating gastrin, including G34, G17, and G14. Gastrin is produced predominantly in G cells located in the gastric antrum and duodenal bulb; however, gastrin immunoreactivity has also been detected in the central and peripheral nervous systems, pituitary, adrenal gland, genital tract, and respiratory tract and in tumors.[41] The fetal endocrine pancreas produces large amounts of amidated gastrin, suggesting a possible role of gastrin in pancreatic development. However, gastrin-deficient mice do not demonstrate overt abnormalities in pancreatic islet morphology.[42] A possible role for gastrin in human islet biology derives from studies of the CCK-2 receptor on pancreatic A cells, which secrete glucagon in response to gastrin in vitro.[43]

G cells are open-type endocrine cells subject to regulation by luminal contents in addition to humoral and neural influences. The effects of gastrin on acid secretion are mediated by the fully processed amidated forms of gastrin (G17 and G34) at the CCK-2 receptor (formerly known as the CCK-B/gastrin receptor) located on the enterochromaffin-like (ECL) cells of the oxyntic mucosa.[44] Gastrin stimulates histamine synthesis and release from ECL cells, which then induce acid secretion by binding to the histamine 2 (H_2) receptor located on the basolateral aspect of the parietal cell. Gastrin also stimulates acid secretion from parietal cells via the CCK-2 receptor.

The physiologic roles of progastrin and glycine-extended gastrin (G-Gly) are less completely defined but may involve regulation of the growth and differentiation of the gastrointestinal tract. Amidated gastrin is trophic to the oxyntic mucosa of the stomach, where it stimulates proliferation of gastric stem cells and ECL cells, resulting in increased parietal and ECL mass. G-Gly exerts trophic effects on the colonic mucosa. Transgenic mice expressing progastrin[45] or G-Gly[46] exhibit increased colonic proliferation and mucosal thickness and are more prone to formation of aberrant crypt foci following treatment with azoxymethane,[47] whereas inactivation of the gastrin gene results in reduced basal rates of colonic proliferation.[42]

Gastrin has been reported to induce proliferation of colon cancer cell lines expressing the CCK-2 receptor; however, most colon cancers and normal colonic epithelium do not normally express the CCK-2 receptor. A truncated gastrin-binding receptor has been described in some colon cancer cell lines,[48] and a constitutively active CCK-2 receptor mutant that confers ligand-independent growth to transfected cells has been identified in human colorectal cancers.[49] The trophic effects of gastrin have led to studies of gastrin-neutralizing antisera for the potential treatment of intestinal neoplasia.[50]

Gastrin-Releasing Peptide and Related Peptides

The *bombesin* family of peptides was originally isolated from frog skin[51] and includes bombesin, gastrin-releasing peptide (GRP—the mammalian homologue of bombesin), neuromedin B (NMB), and neuromedin C (NMC). Gastrin-releasing peptide is a 27–amino acid peptide, whereas both NMB and NMC are decapeptides. These peptides share an identical C-terminal α-amidated heptapeptide sequence that is essential for biologic activity. GRP is expressed in the central, peripheral, and enteric nervous systems, reproductive tract, and lung, where it acts as a neurotransmitter.[52] NMB is expressed predominantly in the brain and gastrointestinal tract. Within the intestine, GRP and NMB are localized to neurons in the submucosal and myenteric plexuses of the stomach, small intestine, and colon. GRP-containing neurons are also distributed throughout the human pancreas. Bombesin and GRP stimulate smooth muscle cell contraction in the stomach, intestine, and gallbladder. GRP stimulates the release of CCK, gastrin, GIP, glucagon, GLP-1 and GLP-2, motilin, PP, PYY, and somatostatin in some, but not all, species.

Three GRP receptor subtypes have been cloned that are seven-transmembrane domain G-protein–coupled receptors that bind bombesin-like peptides, including a GRP-preferring subtype (expressed throughout the intestine), NMB-preferring subtype (expressed in the esophageal and intestinal muscularis), and a third subtype, designated *bombesin receptor subtype 3*, which preferentially binds GRP over NMB and is expressed in testes and small cell lung cancer. GRP regulates appetite, memory, and thermoregulation and suppresses appetite following intracerebroventricular or systemic administration.[53] GRP stimulates pancreatic growth in part via a CCK-dependent mechanism. The expression of GRP in human tumors with neuroendocrine properties such as small cell carcinoma and medullary thyroid carcinoma, taken together with its autocrine and endocrine effects on cell growth, suggests that GRP may contribute to regulation of tumor cell growth.[54–57]

Ghrelin

Ghrelin, a motilin-related peptide, is a 28–amino acid growth hormone–releasing factor originally purified from rat stomach[58] that stimulates growth hormone release via the growth hormone secretagogue receptor (GHS-R). Fasting increases gastric ghrelin gene expression, and ghrelin exhibits gastric prokinetic activity and orexigenic activity following both intracerebroventricular and peripheral administration via the ghrelin receptor expressed in hypothalamic nuclei. Ghrelin expression is also induced by stressors, and ghrelin may play a role in the anxiogenic stress response in a corticotropin-releasing hormone (CRH)-dependent manner in mice.[59]

The majority of rat and human gut endocrine cells that express ghrelin are localized to the stomach, with a small number of ghrelin-positive cells identified in the small and large intestine. GHS-R is also expressed in the gut; however, the function of the intestinal ghrelin/GHS-R axis remains poorly understood. Circulating levels of ghrelin in human subjects increase and fall before and after food ingestion,[60] consistent with a role for ghrelin in appetite regulation.

Glucagon, Glucagon-like Peptide 1, and Glucagon-like Peptide 2

The proglucagon gene is expressed in the pancreatic A cell, intestinal L cell, and specialized regions of the brain, primarily neurons in the brain stem and, to a lesser extent, hypothalamus. In mammals, a single proglucagon precursor is differentially processed to yield multiple proglucagon-derived peptides (PGDPs), including glucagon in the islet A cell, and glicentin, oxyntomodulin, glucagon-like peptide 1 (GLP-1), GLP-2, and several spacer or intervening peptides in the gut enteroendocrine L cell.[61]

Pancreatic glucagon is a 29–amino acid peptide that regulates plasma glucose levels via effects on gluconeogenesis and glycogenolysis. Increased glucagon secretion functions as the primary counterregulatory mechanism to restore normal levels of plasma glucose in the setting of hypoglycemia. In contrast, GLP-1 secreted from the gut endocrine cell enhances glucose disposal following nutrient ingestion by inhibition of gastric emptying, stimulation of insulin secretion, and inhibition of glucagon secretion.[61] GLP-1 also inhibits food intake and stimulates pancreatic islet neogenesis and proliferation, biologic actions that facilitate long-term control of nutrient homeostasis.

GLP-2 is a 33–amino acid peptide that is co-secreted with GLP-1, oxyntomodulin, and glicentin from enteroendocrine cells in a nutrient-dependent manner. GLP-2 inhibits both centrally induced antral motility and meal-stimulated gastric acid secretion. GLP-2 exhibits trophic actions in the small intestine and colon via stimulation of crypt cell proliferation and reduction of apoptosis within the crypt and villus compartments.[62] GLP-2 also exerts actions independent of intestinal growth, including enhancement of intestinal epithelial barrier function and stimulation of intestinal hexose transport.[63] The beneficial therapeutic actions of GLP-2 in experimental models of intestinal injury and in human subjects with short bowel syndrome suggest that GLP-2 may be useful for preventing injury and enhancing repair and regeneration in the gastrointestinal epithelium.[61]

Although the actions of GLP-1 and GLP-2 are transduced via distinct GLP-1 and GLP-2 receptors, both GLP-1 and GLP-2 are rapidly inactivated by the same enzyme, dipeptidyl peptidase IV (DP-IV).[64] The GLP-1 receptor is widely expressed in GLP-1 target tissues, and disruption of the GLP-1 receptor in mice produces mild glucose intolerance and beta-cell dysfunction.[65] The GLP-2 receptor is expressed in subsets of enteroendocrine cells[66]; hence, many of the gastrointestinal actions of GLP-2 are likely indirect and mediated via enteroendocrine-derived factors. The coexpression of the GLP-2 receptor in minor subsets of distinct enteroendocrine subpopulations in the stomach and small and large intestine further illustrates the phenotypic complexity in defining subsets of functionally unique enteroendocrine cells (Fig. 38–2) (see also Color Plate). The GLP-2 receptor is also expressed in the central nervous system,[66] where both GLP-1 and GLP-2 regulate the short-term control of food intake.[67]

In contrast with the biologic actions of GLP-1 and GLP-2, those of glicentin and oxyntomodulin are less well established. Glicentin appears trophic for the gut mucosal epithelium, whereas oxyntomodulin inhibits food intake and pentagastrin-stimulated gastric acid secretion both in vitro and in vivo. Although distinct G protein–coupled receptors (GPCRs) for

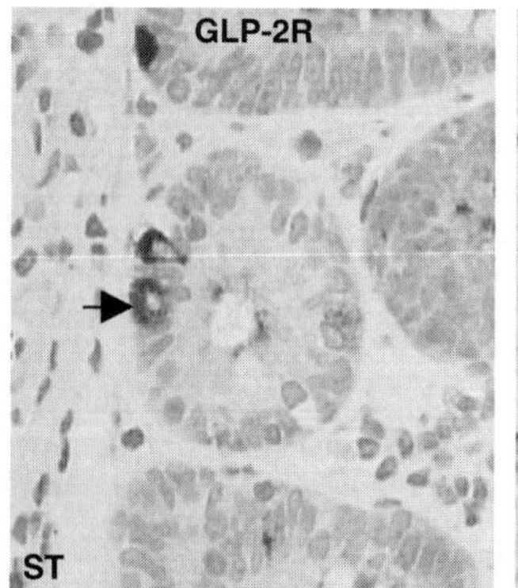

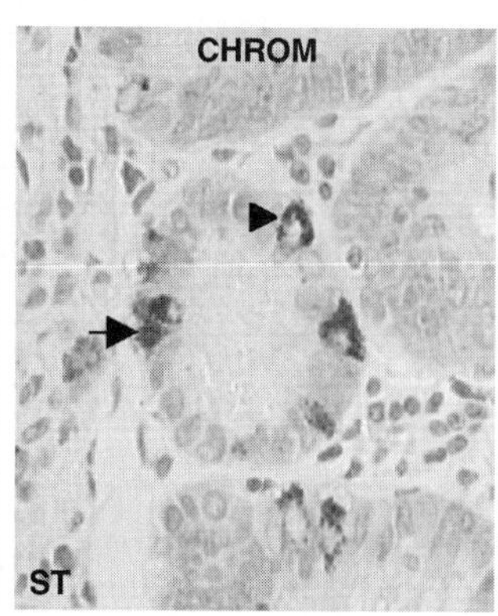

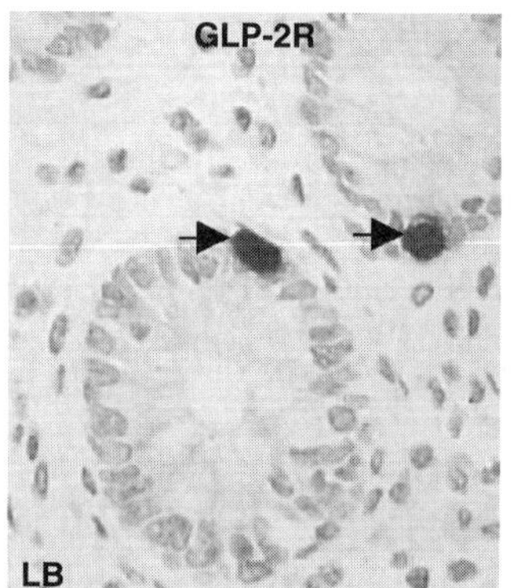

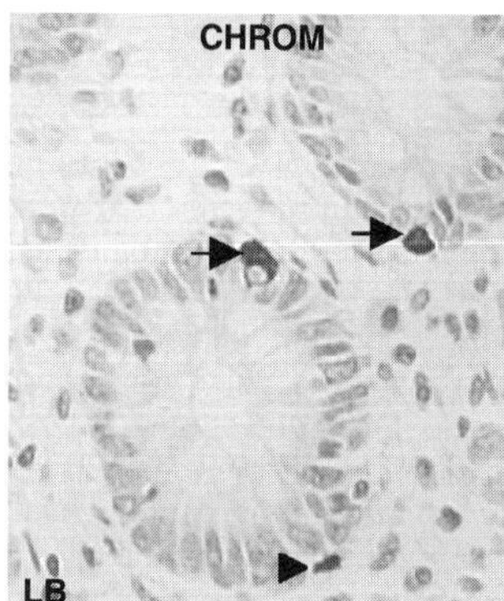

Figure 38–2. Glucagon-like peptide II receptor (GLP-2R) expression in subsets of endocrine cells in the human stomach (ST) and large bowel (LB). Most cells exhibiting positivity with antisera against the human GLP-2R also exhibited immunopositivity for an endocrine marker such as chromogranin (CHROM). In contrast, most endocrine cells in the stomach and both small and large intestine did not express the GLP-2R. *Arrows* denote cells positive for both the GLP-2R and chromogranin, and *arrowheads* denote cells positive for the GLP-2R or chromogranin. (From Yusta B, Huang L, Munroe D, et al. Endocrine localization of GLP-2 expression in humans and rodents. Gastroenterology 2000; 119:744–755.) (See also Color Plate.)

glucagon, GLP-1, and GLP-2 have been characterized, separate receptors that mediate the actions of glicentin and oxyntomodulin have not yet been identified.

Motilin

Motilin is a 22–amino acid peptide originally isolated from porcine intestine. Motilin immunoreactivity has been detected in open-type enteroendocrine epithelial M cells located predominantly in the duodenum and proximal jejunum. Secretion of motilin occurs in a cyclical manner during the interdigestive state between meals. The presence of nutrients in the duodenum suppresses the endogenous release of motilin in both dogs and humans.[68] Duodenal alkalinization, sham feeding, gastric distention, and administration of opioid agonists promote motilin secretion. A putative motilin receptor has been cloned that exhibits 52% amino acid identity with the human receptor for growth hormone secretagogues. The motilin receptor is expressed in multiple regions of the gastrointestinal tract, predominantly in smooth muscle and enteric neurons, and also recognizes the macrolide antibiotic erythromycin.[69]

Motilin induces phase 3 contractions in the stomach, an effect that can be abolished by food ingestion, duodenal acidification, somatostatin, pentagastrin, and CCK.[70] Atropine and 5-hydroxytryptamine antagonists also abolish phase 3 contractions, emphasizing the importance of the cholinergic and serotoninergic neuronal pathways. Motilin stimulates gastric and pancreatic enzyme secretion and induces contraction of the gallbladder, sphincter of Oddi, and lower esophageal sphincter.

Neuropeptide Y

Neuropeptide Y (NPY) is primarily synthesized and secreted by neurons in the central and peripheral nervous systems. In the brain, NPY is expressed not only in the hypothalamus, where it exhibits extremely potent effects on nutrient intake, but also in the cortex, hippocampus, basal forebrain striation, limbic structures, amygdala, and brain stem. In the peripheral nervous system, expression occurs predominantly in sympathetic neurons and in the myenteric and submucous plexuses of the enteric nervous system.

NPY and vasoactive intestinal peptide (VIP) are often coexpressed in enteric neurons. NPY is synthesized in and released from pancreatic islet cells and inhibits glucose-stimulated insulin secretion via the Y1 receptor. Elevated circulating NPY levels are observed following sympathetic nervous system activation and in patients with pancreatic endocrine tumors, carcinoid tumors, and neurogenic tumors, including neuroblastomas and pheochromocytomas.[71]

NPY exerts its actions via several receptor subtypes, including the Y1 and Y2 receptors that bind NPY and PYY with similar affinities and the Y3 receptor that exhibits a preference for NPY over PYY.[72] NPY and PYY are targets for N-terminal degradation by the enzyme DP-IV, leading to the generation of NPY (3-36) and PYY (3–36), peptides that exhibit preferential binding to the Y2 receptor.[64] In the gastrointestinal tract, NPY reduces fluid and electrolyte secretion and inhibits both gastric and small intestinal motility.[73] Intravascular administration of NPY is associated with marked vasoconstriction of the splanchnic circulation, an effect that is not altered by α-adrenergic or β-adrenergic blockade.

Neurotensin

Neurotensin (NT) is a 13–amino acid peptide originally detected in bovine hypothalamus. NT-related peptides include neuromedin N, a 6–amino acid NT-like peptide co-encoded in proneurotensin, as well as xenin, and xenopsin. In the gastrointestinal tract, NT processing favors the generation of NT in N cells of the ileum and in enteric neurons. NT is also produced in the central and peripheral nervous systems, heart, adrenal gland, pancreas, and respiratory tract. NT secretion is stimulated by luminal nutrients, especially lipids, but not amino acids or carbohydrates. GRP also stimulates NT release, whereas somatostatin exerts an inhibitory effect.

At least three different NT receptor/binding proteins (NTS-1 to NTS-3) have been identified. NTS-1 and NTS-2 belong to the GPCR family, whereas NTS-3 represents a structurally unrelated protein with NT-binding properties.[74] NTS-1 is expressed in both the brain and intestine, whereas NTS-2 and NTS-3 are expressed exclusively in the brain.

NT administration to rats augments the adaptive response to small bowel resection in the intestinal remnant,[75] and NT stimulates growth of the colonic epithelium in vivo.[76] NT also inhibits postprandial gastric acid secretion and pancreatic exocrine secretion, stimulates colonic motility, and inhibits gastric and small intestinal motility.[77] NT facilitates fatty acid uptake in the proximal small intestine and induces histamine release from mast cells. NT receptor expression has been detected in a subset of human colon and pancreatic ductal cancers, and NT is trophic for some pancreatic and colon cancer cells in vitro.

Pancreatic Polypeptide

Pancreatic polypeptide (PP) was isolated from chicken pancreatic extracts as a by-product of insulin purification. The majority of PP is expressed in pancreatic endocrine cells located predominantly in the periphery of islets in the pancreatic head and uncinate process. Elevated plasma levels of PP have been detected in patients with gastrointestinal endocrine tumors; hence, PP may be used as a tumor marker in appropriate clinical scenarios. Nutrients, hormones, neurotransmitters, gastric distention, insulin-induced hypoglycemia, and direct vagal nerve stimulation regulate PP secretion, whereas hyperglycemia, bombesin, and somatostatin inhibit PP secretion.[78]

The actions of PP are mediated by the Y4 receptor, a GPCR coupled to the inhibition of cyclic adenosine monophosphate accumulation.[79] The human Y4 receptor is expressed in the stomach, small intestine, colon, pancreas, prostate, and enteric nervous system and in select central nervous system neurons. Exogenous administration of PP reduces CCK-induced gastric acid secretion and increases intestinal transit times by reducing gastric emptying and upper intestinal motility. PP also inhibits postprandial exocrine pancreas secretion via a vagal-dependent pathway. Transgenic mice that overexpress PP exhibit reduced weight gain and rate of gastric emptying and decreased fat mass.[80] The biologic actions of PP in the gastrointestinal tract and pancreas are in part centrally mediated, because intracisternal injections of PP cause an increase in gastric acid secretion and gastric motility and a reduction in pancreatic secretion.

Peptide YY

Peptide YY (PYY), together with NPY, and PP are members of the PP family.[81] These peptides consist of 36 amino acids, contain several tyrosine residues, and share considerable amino acid identity with amidated C-terminal ends. Although these peptides likely share a common ancestry, they exhibit unique actions and patterns of tissue-specific expression, with PYY and PP acting as hormones, whereas NPY acts primarily as a neurotransmitter.

PYY is expressed in the fetal and adult gastrointestinal tract in enteroendocrine cells. Distinct enteroendocrine subpopulations have been identified that express PYY alone, or both PYY and GLP-1, in the ileum, colon, and rectum.[82] Immunoreactive PYY has also been detected in the developing endocrine pancreas and in a subpopulation of glucagon-producing A cells in mature islets.[5] PYY is secreted as a 36–amino acid peptide and circulates as two molecular forms: PYY (1-36) and an N-terminally truncated form, PYY (3-36). Luminal nutrients, CCK, GRP, and vagal tone regulate PYY secretion.

PYY exerts its actions in part through the NPY Y1 and Y2 receptors and a separate PYY receptor.[83] Whereas PYY (1-36) binds both Y1 and Y2 receptors, PYY (3-36) is selective for the Y2 receptor. PYY demonstrates inhibitory effects on gastrointestinal secretion, motility, and blood flow. In the stomach, PYY functions as an enterogastrone, inhibiting both gastric acid secretion and gastric emptying. PYY also increases intestinal transit times by inhibiting small and large intestinal motility. The role of PYY as an intestinal epithelial growth factor remains unclear because some, but not all, studies demonstrate an intestinotrophic effect of PYY in rodents.[84] In the pancreas, both PYY (1-36) and PYY (3-36) inhibit pancreatic exocrine secretion.

Pituitary Adenylate Cyclase–Activating Peptide

Pituitary adenylate cyclase–activating peptide (PACAP), VIP, and GRF are structurally related members of the glucagon/secretin superfamily.[85] PACAP-immunoreactive nerve fibers are distributed along the gastrointestinal tract from the esophagus to the colon. Both PACAP-38 and PACAP-27 are detected in many tissues, with PACAP-38 generally the predominant peptide. PACAP stimulates histamine release from the stomach; increases the secretion of pancreatic fluid, protein, and bicarbonate; and stimulates insulin secretion and catecholamine release. PACAP signaling in gastric ECL cells may also constitute an important component of the neural regulation of gastric acid secretion.

Three PACAP receptors—*PAC1*, *VPAC1*, and *VPAC2*—have been cloned and bind PACAP and VIP with varying affinities. Consistent with the putative importance of PACAP for islet function, PAC1 receptor knockout mice exhibit defective glucose-stimulated insulin secretion.[86]

Secretin

Secretin is a 27–amino acid peptide synthesized predominantly in the brain and gastrointestinal tract. In the gut, secretin is produced by the enteroendocrine S cell in the duodenum and proximal jejunum. Gastric acid, bile salts, and luminal nutrients stimulate, and somatostatin inhibits, the release of secretin.[87] Secretin stimulates pancreatic and biliary bicarbonate and water secretion and may regulate pancreatic enzyme secretion. Secretin also stimulates the gastric secretion of pepsinogen and inhibits lower esophageal sphincter tone, postprandial gastric emptying, gastrin release, and gastric acid secretion.

Although secretin is expressed in the fetal endocrine pancreas, its function in islet biology remains uncertain. To date, only a single secretin receptor has been isolated and characterized. Secretin has been proposed as a treatment for autism; however, clinical trial results examining this issue have not been consistently positive.[88]

Somatostatin

Somatostatin, originally isolated as a hypothalamic growth hormone release–inhibiting factor, is also expressed in the intestine and pancreas. Post-translational processing of prosomatostatin results in the generation of SS-14 and SS-28, biologically active peptides corresponding to the C-terminal 14 and 28 amino acids of prosomatostatin. SS-28 is the predominant molecular form liberated by enteroendocrine D cells, whereas SS-14 is the predominant species liberated by D cells in the stomach and pancreas.

Five somatostatin receptor subtypes (SST-1 to SST-5) have been identified that are expressed in a tissue-specific manner.[89] Somatostatin's actions are generally inhibitory; that is, somatostatin inhibits the secretion of growth hormone and thyrotropin in the pituitary, and insulin, glucagon, and PP in the endocrine pancreas.[90] In the gastrointestinal tract, somatostatin inhibits the secretion of a broad range of gut peptides. Somatostatin inhibits pancreatic exocrine secretion and also acts in a paracrine manner on G cells, ECL cells, and parietal cells to inhibit gastric acid secretion.[91]

The inhibitory properties of somatostatin make it suitable for the treatment of conditions characterized by excess hormone secretion.[92] Although the circulating half-life of native somatostatin is short, longer-acting synthetic somatostatin analogues such as octreotide and lanreotide are useful in the treatment of neuroendocrine tumors, acromegaly, and portal hypertension.[93, 94] Both octreotide and lanreotide are octapeptides that bind the SST-2 and SST-5 somatostatin receptor subtypes, receptors commonly expressed in neuroendocrine tumors. Somatostatin analogues are also employed for the treatment of portal hypertension and gastrointestinal bleeding. Tumor-associated somatostatin receptor expression forms the basis for the radiolabeled octreotide scan, a test that appears useful for the detection of a broad spectrum of human neoplasms.[95] Somatostatin-deficient mice exhibit normal growth but defects in sexually dimorphic hepatic gene expression.[96]

Tachykinins

The family of tachykinins includes substance P (SP), neurokinin-A (NKA), and neurokinin-B (NKB), all of which share a common C-terminal pentapeptide sequence essential for biologic action. Two genes encode the tachykinins: a pre-protachykinin-A gene that encodes SP and NKA and a preprotachykinin-B gene that encodes NKB. Tachykinins are synthesized within neurons localized to the submucous and myenteric plexuses,[97] extrinsic sensory fibers, and in enterochromaffin cells in the gut epithelium.[98] Tachykinins are also widely distributed throughout the central and peripheral nervous systems, the respiratory tract, skin, sensory organs, and the urogenital tract.

Four different tachykinin receptors *(NK1* to *NK4)* have been cloned and bind tachykinin peptides with different affinities. NK1 receptors preferentially bind SP, NK2 preferentially binds NKA, and both NK3 and NK4 preferentially bind NKB.[99]

The tachykinins regulate vasomotor and gastrointestinal motor activity.[100] The ability of tachykinins to induce vasodilatation or vasoconstriction appears to be specific to the species and to the vascular bed. Tachykinins exhibit both direct and indirect effects on intestinal smooth muscle contractile activity.

Activation of NK1 receptors on the interstitial cells of Cajal and NK2 receptors on intestinal smooth muscle cells directly promotes peristalsis, whereas activation of NK3 receptors on enteric neurons exerts a prokinetic effect that is indirectly mediated through cholinergic stimulation of enteric smooth muscle cells. The NK1 and NK3 receptors can exhibit inhibitory effects on intestinal motility by inducing the release of inhibitory molecules such as NO and VIP from inhibitory neurons. NK2 receptors can also inhibit intestinal motility by either stimulation of sympathetic ganglia or activation of nonadrenergic inhibitory mechanisms. NK2 receptor antagonists reduce or prevent trinitrobenzene sulfonic acid–induced weight loss and intestinal injury,[101] whereas an NK1 receptor antagonist exhibits protective effects in acetic acid–induced colitis.[102]

Tachykinins are commonly produced by gut carcinoids and

may be responsible for mediating some of the clinical manifestations associated with these tumors.

Thyrotropin-Releasing Hormone

Originally isolated as a hypothalamic regulatory peptide, thyrotropin-releasing hormone (TRH) is expressed throughout the gastrointestinal tract, including the stomach, colon, and pancreas.[103] In the pancreas, TRH is most abundantly expressed during perinatal development. Pre-pro-TRH is synthesized by islet beta cells, G cells in the stomach, and neurons comprising the myenteric plexus of the esophagus, stomach, and intestine. In the stomach, histamine and serotonin stimulate, and endogenous opioids inhibit, TRH release.

TRH acts via two related GPCRs: TRH receptor 1 (TRHR1) and TRH receptor 2 (TRHR2).[104] TRH suppresses pentagastrin-stimulated gastric acid secretion, and chronic administration of TRH induces pancreatic hyperplasia and inhibits amylase release. TRH also attenuates CCK-induced gallbladder smooth muscle contraction and inhibits cholesterol synthesis within the intestinal mucosa.

Vasoactive Intestinal Peptide

Vasoactive intestinal peptide (VIP) is a 28–amino acid member of a peptide superfamily that includes PACAP, peptide histidine isoleucine, and peptide histidine methionine, all neurotransmitters and neuromodulators of the enteric nervous system. The VIP gene is widely expressed in the central and peripheral nervous systems. Receptors for VIP and PACAP belong to the same family of GPCRs.[105] The PAC1 receptor binds both PACAP (1-27) and PACAP (1-38) with the same affinity but is unable to bind VIP, whereas the VPAC1 and VPAC2 receptors recognize both VIP and PACAP.[85]

In the digestive tract, VIP functions as an inhibitory neurotransmitter that induces relaxation of vascular and nonvascular smooth muscle. VIP mediates the relaxation of the lower esophageal sphincter, the sphincter of Oddi, and the anal sphincter. VIP also regulates relaxation associated with gut contraction and may be involved in reflex vasodilatation in the small intestine, in part through a NO-dependent mechanism. In humans, VIP and PACAP may be co-localized to some neuronal subpopulations and are co-released as neurotransmitters leading to NO regeneration.[106] VIP inhibits gastric acid secretion but stimulates biliary water and bicarbonate, pancreatic enzyme, and intestinal chloride secretion. VIP may also regulate pancreatic release of both insulin and glucagon and exerts either trophic or growth inhibitory effects on both normal and neoplastic cells.[107]

Miscellaneous Gut Endocrine Peptides

In addition to the several peptide hormones outlined earlier and summarized in Table 38–3, several other gut endocrine peptides exist. Chromogranins and secretogranins are a family of secretory proteins that are found in secretory vesicles of both endocrine cells and neurons. Chromogranin-A (CgA) is a protein belonging to this family of peptides and is secreted into the circulation by several neuroendocrine tumors, especially small gastrinomas and pheochromocytomas.[108] A direct correlation exists between circulating levels of CgA and tumor burden, making this a well-suited marker for assessing treatment response. In addition, opioid peptides regulate intestinal motility and gastric acid secretion and inhibit secretion.[109] Neuromedin U is a neurotransmitter that is expressed in the enteric nervous system, where it regulates intestinal motility and ion secretion.[110]

A number of hormones are secreted by the gastrointestinal tract directly into the lumen, where they modulate secretion and the release of other hormones. Guanylin and uroguanylin stimulate water, bicarbonate, and chloride secretion by the intestine while inhibiting sodium reabsorption.[111] Other luminally secreted peptides include sorbin (a 153–amino acid peptide involved with monitoring fluid and sodium fluxes in the duodenum)[112] and monitor peptide (a 61–amino acid peptide that stimulates CCK release).[113]

PANCREATIC AND GUT ENDOCRINE TUMORS

Understanding the ontogeny of pancreatic and gut endocrine cell development provides some insight into the molecular pathophysiology of pancreatic endocrine tumors. Although gastrin is not normally produced in human adult islets of Langerhans, the finding of gastrinomas arising from the adult endocrine pancreas may reflect the dedifferentiation of neoplastic endocrine tumor cells that recapitulates, in part, patterns of islet gene expression observed during embryonic development. Similarly, the observation that pancreatic and gut endocrine tumors are frequently plurihormonal is consistent with studies demonstrating co-localization of peptide hormones in both fetal and adult endocrine cells in the pancreas and gut.

Pancreatic endocrine tumors may present in isolation or as part of a genetic syndrome such as multiple endocrine neoplasia type 1 (MEN-1), or the phakomatoses such as von Hippel–Lindau disease, von Recklinghausen's disease (neurofibromatosis type 1), and tuberous sclerosis. Defects in distinct tumor suppressor genes account for the phenotypic manifestations and development of tumors in these syndromes (Table 38–5). Loss of heterozygosity at 10q has been detected in several sporadic pancreatic endocrine tumors, with cellular rather than nuclear localization of PTEN (phosphatase and tensin homologue deleted on chromosome 10) detected in a substantial proportion of malignant pancreatic endocrine tumors.[114] Similarly, loss of heterozygosity at the 11q13 *MEN1* locus has also been detected in a few sporadic pancreatic endocrine tumors.

Genetic mutations in the *menin* gene give rise to the MEN-1 syndrome associated with an increased incidence of endocrine tumors in many organs, including the pancreas and gut carcinoids in the stomach.[115] The *MEN1* gene encodes a 610–amino acid nuclear protein that interacts with the *N*-terminus of the *JunD* transcription factor, presumably resulting in derepressed cell growth. About 10% of all *MEN1* germline mutations arise de novo. The current usefulness of genetic testing for all patients with suspected MEN-1 syndrome remains un-

Table 38–5. Genetic Diseases Associated with the Development of Pancreatic or Gut Endocrine Tumors

Gene	Disease	Phenotype
menin	MEN-1	Parathyroid, pituitary, and pancreatic endocrine tumors
VHL	von Hippel–Lindau disease	Pancreatic endocrine tumors, hemangiomas, and multiple neoplasms
NF-1	Neurofibromatosis	Neurofibromas, pheochromocytomas
TSC1/2	Tuberous sclerosis	Pancreatic endocrine tumors, hamartomas

MEN-1, multiple endocrine neoplasia type 1.

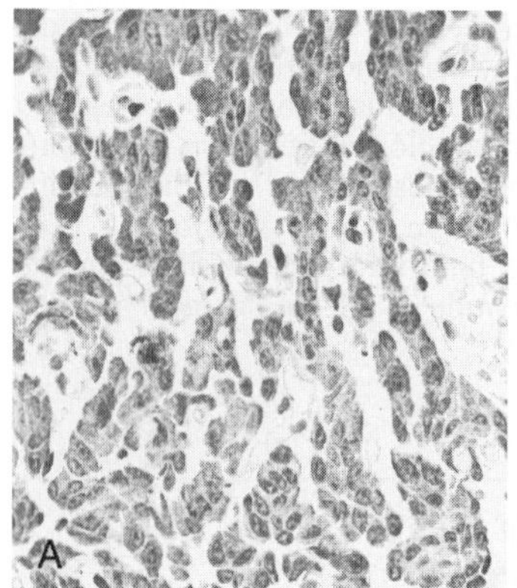

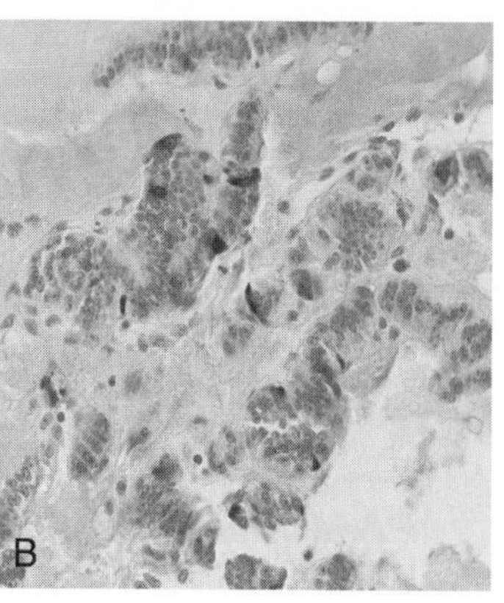

Figure 38–3. Clinically "nonfunctioning" tumors are often found to express one or more peptide hormones after immunocytochemical analyses. The photomicrographs represent histologic sections from the identical nonfunctioning human pancreatic endocrine tumor that exhibit immunopositivity for glucagon (*A*) and pancreatic polypeptide (*B*). (Courtesy of Dr. G. Rindi, Brescia, Italy.) (See also Color Plate.)

clear owing to the large number of heterogeneous mutations identified in the *menin* gene. Potentially affected family members may find utility in ruling out the diagnosis with genetic testing, thereby precluding years of biochemical testing and imaging studies.

A search for clinical manifestations of diseases associated with these genetic syndromes is an important component in the initial diagnosis and ongoing management of patients with pancreatic endocrine tumors. More careful clinical phenotype-genotype analyses have ascertained that facial angiofibromas, collagenomas, lipomas, leiomyomas, and adrenocortical tumors all may be seen with increased frequency in patients with MEN-1.[116] Moreover, somatic mutations of the *menin* gene have been described in isolated cases of gastrinomas, insulinomas, and gut endocrine tumors.[116]

The secretion of one or more peptide hormones resulting in the production of symptoms attributable to hormone excess, such as hypoglycemia, gastric ulceration, or profuse watery diarrhea in patients with insulinoma, gastrinoma, or VIPoma, respectively, clearly facilitates the diagnosis of a hormone-secreting endocrine tumor. In some instances, pancreatic or gut endocrine tumors may not be associated with clinically or biochemically detectable hormone excess, and the development of a recognizable syndrome and analysis of the tumor may fail to reveal evidence for peptide hormone biosynthesis.

Nonfunctioning pancreatic endocrine tumors are more common, often larger, and more frequently malignant at the time of diagnosis. The term nonfunctioning may be a misnomer, because these tumors may produce peptide hormones (Fig. 38–3) (see also Color Plate) whose biologic actions are less clinically apparent. In some instances, tumor-associated defects in post-translational processing may preclude the efficient synthesis and secretion of peptide hormones. Factors affecting prognosis include the presence of liver metastases, incomplete resection of the primary tumor, and poorly differentiated tumor cells.[117]

The use of somatostatin receptor scintigraphy (SRS) and measurement of gene products commonly expressed in endocrine cells such as chromogranin, PP, neuron-specific enolase, or glycoprotein hormone subunits may be useful as an adjunct for monitoring the tumor response to therapy.[118] The widespread expression of receptors for somatostatin and multiple peptide hormone GPCRs has stimulated efforts directed at developing novel radiolabeled peptide ligands for the localization and treatment of both endocrine and nonendocrine neoplasms.[119]

Despite the large number and complexity of endocrine cell populations in the human small bowel, gut endocrine tumors, including ileal carcinoids, are comparatively rare. Similarly, although human colon cancer remains a major cause of cancer-associated morbidity and mortality, peptide hormone–secreting carcinoid tumors arising from the colon are comparatively much less common compared with colonic adenocarcinomas. The molecular basis for the infrequent malignant transformation of human gut endocrine cells remains incompletely understood. Mutations in the *regIα* gene have been identified in a subset of patients with ECL tumors and associated hypergastrinemia; however, the contribution of this genetic mutation to transformation of ECL cells remains unclear.[120] The clinical presentation, diagnosis, and treatment of several more common pancreatic and gut endocrine tumors are reviewed later, and both medical and surgical perspectives to treatment have been reviewed.[121, 122]

Gastrinoma (Zollinger-Ellison Syndrome)

In 1955, Zollinger and Ellison described two patients with intractable peptic ulcer disease and pancreatic islet cell tumors.[123] Subsequent studies demonstrated elevated levels of circulating gastrin associated with gastric acid hypersecretion in patients with Zollinger-Ellison syndrome (ZES).

Although the gastrin gene is not normally expressed in the adult pancreas, gastrinomas commonly arise from within the pancreas and present as endocrine carcinomas, solitary adenomas, microadenomas, or endocrine cell hyperplasia. Gastrinomas and insulinomas represent the two most common pancreatic endocrine tumors. A smaller proportion of gastrin-secreting tumors (20% to 40%) arise from the duodenum. Most (75%) gastrinomas occur sporadically, whereas approximately 25% are associated with MEN-1 syndrome. MEN-1–related patients tend to exhibit a younger age of onset at the time of diagnosis.[124] Sporadic tumors are most often solitary and malignant, whereas MEN-1–associated tumors are usually multiple but may be more localized at the time of diagnosis. It is estimated that 50% to 60% of gastrinomas are malignant, based on the presence of metastases at the time of diagnosis, perhaps due in part to the long delay between the initial clinical presentation and the diagnosis of ZES. Nevertheless, gastrin-secreting tumors are often slow growing and associated with prolonged survival, despite complications arising from intestinal ulceration.

Clinical manifestations of gastrinomas are usually related to excessive gastric acid secretion resulting in severe refractory peptic ulceration complicated by hemorrhage, perforation, and stricture. Many patients report symptoms for 5 to 6 years before the diagnosis of ZES is established. Abdominal pain, diarrhea, and heartburn are common presenting symptoms, with diarrhea and pain observed in more than 70% of patients with ZES.[124] The diarrhea results in part from fat malabsorption due to pancreatic lipase degradation by excess gastric acid. Small-bowel inflammation and impaired nutrient absorption may also arise from excess gastric acid. Antisecretory therapy

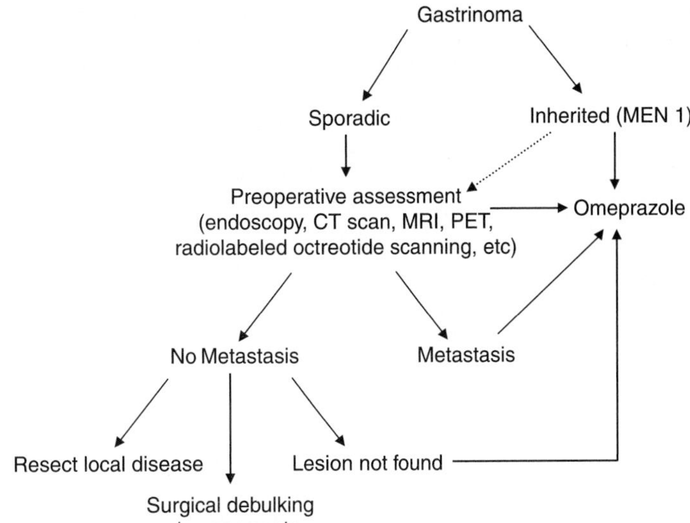

Figure 38–4. Treatment algorithm for the management of a patient with gastrinoma. The *dotted line* indicates that in some circumstances, patients with familial gastrinoma may also be candidates for surgical resection if disease is highly limited. MEN 1, multiple endocrine neoplasia type 1; CT, computed tomography; MRI, magnetic resonance imaging; PET, positron emission tomography.

usually abolishes the diarrhea and diminishes many clinical features of ZES.

The diagnosis of gastrinoma is based on the detection of elevated fasting circulating gastrin levels (>200 pg/mL) and gastric acid hypersecretion (basal acid output > 15 mEq/hour with an intact stomach or > 5 mEq/hour after ulcer surgery) in patients off all acid antisecretory medication (14 days for H^+,K^+-ATPase inhibitors and 3 days for H_2-receptor antagonists).[124, 125] Although many patients with ZES have serum gastrin values that exceed 500 pg/mL, a secretin stimulation test may be performed when the serum gastrin levels are in the range of 200 to 500 pg/mL to confirm the diagnosis. Provocative testing requires overnight fasting and the intravenous administration of secretin (2-unit/kg bolus), followed by serial measurement of circulating gastrin levels at 2, 5, 10, 15, and 20 minutes. A rise in the serum gastrin level of more than 200 pg/mL within 15 minutes or a doubling of the fasting gastrin levels strongly suggests the presence of a gastrinoma.

Provocative testing may be useful in distinguishing gastrinomas from other causes of ulcerogenic hypergastrinemia, such as gastric outlet obstruction, retained antrum after a Billroth II gastrectomy, antral G-cell hyperplasia, and *Helicobacter pylori* infection, that demonstrate a flat gastrin response to secretin. Nevertheless, difficulty in obtaining clinical supplies of secretin may preclude the routine use of the secretin test. More than 90% of patients exhibit prominent gastric folds at the time of endoscopy, consistent with the trophic effect of gastrin on the stomach mucosa.[124] Serum calcium and PTH, along with baseline pituitary function and imaging studies, should also be considered to rule out the presence of MEN-1 syndrome.[126]

Localization of small primary tumors or endocrine hyperplasia can be difficult. Conventional endoscopy or an upper gastrointestinal series can occasionally be used to directly visualize duodenal lesions; however, tumors are often confined to the submucosa, making detection and biopsy challenging. Radiolabeled octreotide scanning can be useful for detecting the primary tumor and metastases.[127] Magnetic resonance imaging (MRI) or computed tomography (CT) scans can also be informative; however, the primary tumor may not be detected with these modalities alone. Endoscopic ultrasonography has been used for tumor localization with increasing success,[128] and, less commonly, angiography with selective venous sampling may be helpful in localizing occult tumors. Primary tumors may also be localized to lymph nodes, and ectopic gastrinomas in sites such as the ovary have also been reported.

Initial treatment of patients with gastrinoma is directed at pharmacologic reduction of gastric acid secretion. Although H_2 blockers have been used with some success, H^+,K^+-ATPase inhibitors such as omeprazole have become the drug of choice owing to their longer duration of action.[129] Doses should be titrated to keep the H^+ ion output to less than 10 mEq/hour (5 mEq/hour in patients with previous acid-reducing surgery) for the hour prior to receiving the next dose of the drug.

As outlined in Figure 38–4, in the absence of unresectable disease all patients with sporadic gastrinoma should undergo surgical exploration with the intent of curative surgical resection. Exploration should include a combination of duodenal palpation, endoscopic transillumination, intraoperative ultrasonography, and duodenotomy.[130] In as many as 20% of patients undergoing surgical exploration, the primary tumor remains undetected at laparotomy despite meticulous exploration of the abdominal cavity. Total gastrectomy should be performed only under rare circumstances in patients with severe ulcer disease refractory to medical therapy in which the primary tumor cannot be resected. Surgery is generally not indicated in patients with gastrinoma and MEN-1 syndrome because these individuals often have multiple, small pancreatic tumors that are not all amenable to surgical resection.

Glucagonoma

Most glucagonomas are pancreatic in origin. Approximately 80% of tumors occur sporadically, with the remainder associated with MEN-1 syndrome. Most glucagonomas (~75%) are malignant and have metastasized by the time of diagnosis.

The clinical presentation reflects the various actions of the PGDPs and may vary depending on the profile of PGDPs liberated due to tumor-specific differences in the post-translational processing of proglucagon. A hallmark of this syndrome is necrolytic migratory erythema, a skin rash that usually begins in the groin and perineum as a raised, erythematous patch with occasional bullae that may also involve the lower extremities and perioral area.[131] The exact etiology of the skin rash remains unknown, and elevated plasma glucagon levels, as well as deficiencies of zinc, amino acids, and fatty acids may represent contributing factors.

Patients with glucagonomas may exhibit weight loss, abdominal pain, diabetes mellitus, stomatitis, glossitis, cheilitis, nail dystrophy, thromboembolic events, anemia, hypoaminoacidemia, and neuropsychiatric symptoms.[132] The triad of hyperglucagonemia, necrolytic migratory erythema, and a pancreatic tumor is seen in a minority of cases. Intestinal obstructive symptoms and increased intestinal transit times have also been reported and may reflect tumor-specific liberation of GLP-1 and GLP-2, peptides with antimotility and intestinotrophic properties, respectively.

The diagnosis may be confirmed by the presence of significantly elevated levels of plasma glucagon in association with a pancreatic mass. Extremely high levels of glucagon are more often seen with the classic glucagonoma syndrome, whereas more modest elevations of glucagon are detected in the setting of plurihormonal tumors.[133] In contrast with insulinomas, glucagonomas are often large and more easily localized with imaging modalities. SRS is effective in detecting metastatic disease that most commonly involves the liver, lymph nodes, adrenal glands, or vertebrae.

Therapy with a somatostatin analogue may be useful in the setting of metastatic disease by reducing levels of circulating glucagon via the SST2 receptor, improving the skin rash, and promoting weight gain.[92, 134] The skin rash may also respond to selective nutrient supplementation. Although somatostatin analogues may reduce glucagon secretion and tumor-associated symptoms, effects on tumor growth are often modest. Patients with nonresectable or recurrent disease can be treated with chemotherapeutic agents such as streptozotocin and dacarbazine or interferon or with the selective use of arterial embolization.

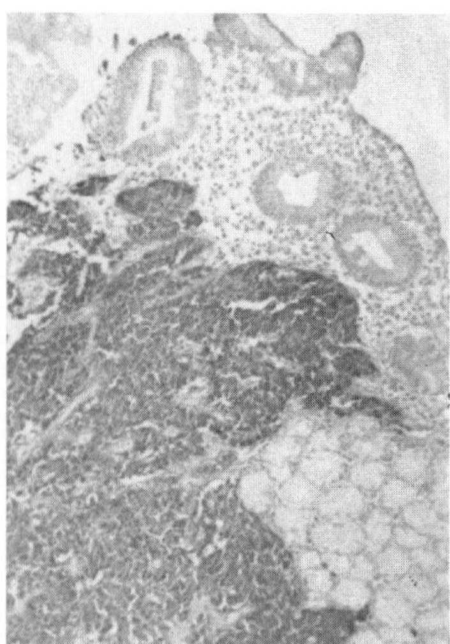

Figure 38–5. Somatostatin immunoreactivity in a human duodenal D cell tumor. The low-power micrograph illustrates the diffuse somatostatin immunoreactivity. Brunner's glands and the partly eroded mucosa are seen in the lower and upper right areas, respectively, in relation to the immunopositive endocrine tumor. (See also Color Plate.)

Somatostatinoma

Somatostatinomas are extremely rare tumors that arise in the pancreas and the duodenum. Most clinical symptoms observed in the originally described somatostatinoma syndrome reflect the inhibitory properties of somatostatin on most digestive organs.[135] A classic triad involving mild diabetes mellitus, steatorrhea, and cholelithiasis is observed in a few patients due to reduced insulin secretion, reduced biliary and pancreatic secretions, and inhibition of gallbladder motility. More prominent symptoms seen with duodenal tumors may include weight loss, postprandial fullness and abdominal pain, cholelithiasis, anemia, and hypochlorhydria.[136] Many patients do not present with the classic triad and exhibit only nonspecific symptoms. As a result, somatostatinomas are frequently malignant with extensive metastasis to the liver by the time of diagnosis.

Duodenal tumors are more frequently seen in association with neurofibromatosis type 1 or, less commonly, von Hippel–Lindau disease, and therefore may be associated with pheochromocytomas. Most duodenal tumors are not associated with symptoms of classic somatostatinoma syndrome and may present with local obstruction and abdominal pain. Pancreatic tumors usually occur sporadically or as part of MEN-1 syndrome and are most commonly located in the head of the pancreas.

The diagnosis is confirmed by the presence of markedly elevated levels of plasma somatostatin. CT scan and both conventional and endoscopic ultrasonography may localize the duodenal tumors (Fig. 38–5) (see also Color Plate). In the small proportion of patients with localized disease, surgical resection can be curative. Patients with incurable or recurrent disease can be treated with the chemotherapeutic agents streptozotocin and dacarbazine.

Vasoactive Intestinal Peptide–Secreting Tumors

The VIPoma syndrome is also known as *pancreatic cholera*, *Verner-Morrison syndrome*, or WDHA (*w*atery *d*iarrhea, *h*ypokalemia, and *a*chlorhydria) syndrome. Approximately 90% of individuals present with a pancreatic endocrine tumor that secretes VIP and often prostaglandins. The remaining tumors are extrapancreatic, usually involving the sympathetic chain or adrenal medulla. VIPomas may present as sporadic tumors or as part of MEN-1 syndrome.

Clinical manifestations include intermittent, severe watery diarrhea that contains large quantities of potassium, bicarbonate, and chloride.[137] As a result, patients may exhibit signs and symptoms of hypokalemia, metabolic acidosis, and dehydration. Hypotension can occur due to dehydration and the vasodilator effects of VIP. Diarrhea is secretory and does not respond to antidiarrheal medications. Gastric analysis usually reveals hypochlorhydria or achlorhydria, although an appropriate increase in acid secretion is observed in response to a pentagastrin challenge. Glucose intolerance may be present due to hypokalemia and altered insulin sensitivity. Cutaneous flushing of the head and trunk may be observed in 15% of patients, usually during a bout of diarrhea, and may be associated with a patchy erythematous rash.

The diagnosis of VIPoma may be challenging due to the intermittent nature of the symptoms. A history of severe recurrent, severe diarrhea, together with elevated fasting levels of plasma VIP (>200 pg/mL), should prompt a search for a pancreatic tumor. Increased circulating levels of peptide histidine methionine, PP, NT, and prostaglandins have also been detected in patients with VIP-producing tumors. VIPomas can be localized by ultrasonography, CT scan, and SRS imaging, and exploratory laparotomy with intraoperative ultrasonography may also be used to identify the tumor.

Initial treatment of patients with VIPoma syndrome involves aggressive fluid and electrolyte replacement. Somatostatin analogues may be used preoperatively to control the diarrhea by both lowering circulating VIP and directly inhibiting intestinal secretion.[138] Definitive treatment requires surgical resection of the tumor, commonly located in the body or tail of the pancreas. Although tumors are usually solitary, 60% are malignant at the time of diagnosis, with 75% metastasizing to the liver and regional lymph nodes, and, less commonly, to the lungs, mediastinum, stomach, and kidney.

If a pancreatic tumor cannot be identified, exploration of the retroperitoneum that includes the adrenal glands and sympathetic chains is indicated. If no pancreatic tumor is identified, some patients may elect to be closely monitored, whereas others may opt for a 80% distal pancreatectomy. This latter strategy may be beneficial for the 10% to 20% of symptomatic patients with diffuse islet cell hyperplasia. In patients with inoperable or metastatic tumor, a combination of 5-fluorouracil and streptozotocin may be effective.

Miscellaneous Gut Hormone–Producing Tumors

Although rare, pancreatic endocrine tumors may secrete PTH, growth hormone–releasing hormone, and adrenocorticotropic hormone, leading to the development of hypercalcemia, acromegaly, and Cushing's syndrome, respectively. A large number of peptide hormones may be produced by pancreatic endocrine tumor cells, including PYY, calcitonin, NT, melanocyte-stimulating hormone, corticotropin-releasing hormone, NPY, NMB, CGRP, GRP, and motilin. In some cases, the hormone precursors may be produced, but the correctly processed intact hormone may not be secreted by the tumor. Accordingly, excessive production of many of these hormones may not always be associated with characteristic signs and symptoms. Similarly, carcinoid tumors of the gastrointestinal tract often exhibit immunopositivity for multiple peptide hormones in the absence of a recognizable clinical syndrome.

SUMMARY

A large number of peptides are synthesized in and secreted by endocrine cells of the pancreas and gastrointestinal tract. Many of these peptides circulate as hormones, but they also function as paracrine modulators or neurotransmitters not only in the gut but in the central and peripheral nervous systems. Although some biologic actions for many of these peptides have been delineated, it seems likely that new peptides, receptors, and novel biologic functions will continue to be discovered, which may provide new opportunities for understanding the pathophysiology, diagnosis, and treatment of endocrine disease.

References

1. Peters J, Jurgensen A, Kloppel G. Ontogeny, differentiation and growth of the endocrine pancreas. Virchows Arch 2000; 436:527–538.
2. Zulewski H, Abraham EJ, Gerlach MJ, et al. Multipotential nestin-positive stem cells isolated from adult pancreatic islets differentiate ex vivo into pancreatic endocrine, exocrine, and hepatic phenotypes. Diabetes 2001; 50:521–533.
3. Herrera PL, Huarte J, Zufferey R, et al. Ablation of islet endocrine cells by targeted expression of hormone-promoter–driven toxigenes. Proc Natl Acad Sci U S A 1994; 91:12999–13003.
4. Herrera PL. Adult insulin- and glucagon-producing cells differentiate from two independent cell lineages. Development 2000; 127:2317–2322.
5. Upchurch BH, Apone GW, Leiter AB. Expression of peptide YY in all four islet cell types in the developing mouse pancreas suggests a common peptide YY–producing progenitor. Development 1994; 120:245–252.
6. Jonsson J, Carlsson L, Edlund T, Edlund H. Insulin-promoter-factor 1 is required for pancreas development in mice. Nature 1994; 371:606–609.
7. Offield MF, Jetton TL, Labosky PA, et al. *PDX-1* is required for pancreatic outgrowth and differentiation of the rostral duodenum. Development 1996; 122:983–995.
8. Ahlgren U, Jonsson J, Jonsson L, et al. β-Cell–specific inactivation of the mouse *Ipf1/Pdx1* gene results in loss of the β-cell phenotype and maturity-onset diabetes. Genes Dev 1998; 12: 1763–1768.
9. Stoffers DA, Zinkin NT, Stanojevic V, et al. Pancreatic agenesis attributable to a single nucleotide deletion in the human *IPF1* gene coding sequence. Nat Genet 1997; 15:106–110.
10. Ahlgren U, Pfaff SL, Jessell TM, et al. Independent requirement for *ISL1* in formation of pancreatic mesenchyme and islet cells. Nature 1997; 385:257–260.
11. Dohrmann C, Gruss P, Lemaire L. *Pax* genes and the differentiation of hormone-producing endocrine cells in the pancreas. Mech Dev 2000; 92:47–54.
12. Smith SB, Watada H, Scheel DW, et al. Autoregulation and maturity-onset diabetes of the young transcription factors control the human *PAX4* promoter. J Biol Chem 2000; 275:36910–36919.
13. Edlund H. Pancreas: how to get there from the gut? Curr Opin Cell Biol 1999; 11:663–668.
14. Apelqvist A, Li H, Sommer L, et al. Notch signalling controls pancreatic cell differentiation. Nature 1999; 400:877–881.
15. Gradwohl G, Dierich A, LeMeur M, et al. Neurogenin3 is required for the development of the four endocrine cell lineages of the pancreas. Proc Natl Acad Sci U S A 2000; 97:1607–1611.
16. Jensen J, Heller RS, Funder-Nielsen T, et al. Independent development of pancreatic alpha- and beta-cells from neurogenin3-expressing precursors: a role for the notch pathway in repression of premature differentiation. Diabetes 2000; 49:163–176.
17. Cheng H, Leblond CP. Origin, differentiation, and renewal of the four main epithelial cell types in the mouse small intestine. Am J Anat 1974; 141:537–562.
18. Sjolund K, Sanden G, Hakanson R, et al. Endocrine cells in human intestine: an immunocytochemical study. Gastroenterology 1983; 85:1120–1130.
19. Rindi G, Ratineau C, Ronco A, et al. Targeted ablation of secretin-producing cells in transgenic mice reveals a common differentiation pathway with multiple enteroendocrine cell lineages in the small intestine. Development 1999; 126:4149–4156.
20. Upchurch BH, Fung BP, Rindi G, et al. Peptide YY expression is an early event in colonic endocrine cell differentiation: evidence from normal and transgenic mice. Development 1996; 122:1157–1163.
21. Jensen J, Pedersen EE, Galante P, et al. Control of endodermal endocrine development by *Hes-1*. Nat Genet 2000; 24:36–44.
22. Naya FJ, Huang H, Qiu Y, et al. Diabetes, defective pancreatic morphogenesis, and abnormal enteroendocrine differentiation in *BETA2/NeuroD*-deficient mice. Genes Dev 1997; 11:2323–2334.
23. Yamada S, Kojima H, Fujimiya M, et al. Differentiation of immature enterocytes into enteroendocrine cells by *Pdx1* overexpression. Am J Physiol Gastrointest Liver Physiol 2001; 281: G229–G236.
24. Larsson LI, St-Onge L, Hougaard DM, et al. *Pax4* and *6* regulate gastrointestinal endocrine cell development. Mech Dev 1998; 79:153–159.
25. Hill MF, Asa SL, Drucker DJ. Essential requirement for *Pax6* in control of enteroendocrine proglucagon gene transcription. Mol Endocrinol 1999; 13:1474–1486.
26. Mulderry PK, Ghatei MA, Spokes RA, et al. Differential expression of alpha-CGRP and beta-CGRP by primary sensory neurons and enteric autonomic neurons of the rat. Neuroscience 1988; 25: 195–205.
27. Wimalawansa SJ. Calcitonin gene-related peptide and its receptors: molecular genetics, physiology, pathophysiology, and therapeutic potentials. Endocr Rev 1996; 17:533–585.
28. McLatchie LM, Fraser NJ, Main MJ, et al. RAMPs regulate the transport and ligand specificity of the calcitonin receptor-like receptor. Nature 1998; 393:333–339.
29. Rehfeld JF, Sun G, Christensen T, et al. The predominant cholecystokinin in human plasma and intestine is cholecystokinin-33. J Clin Endocrinol Metab 2001; 86:251–258.
30. Crawley JN, Corwin RL. Biological actions of cholecystokinin. Peptides 1994; 15:731–755.
31. Povoski SP, Zhou W, Longnecker DS, et al. Stimulation of growth of azaserine-induced putative preneoplastic lesions in rat pancreas is mediated specifically by way of cholecystokinin-A receptors. Cancer Res 1993; 53(17):3925–3929.
32. Moran TH, Katz LF, Plata-Salaman CR, et al. Disordered food intake and obesity in rats lacking cholecystokinin A receptors. Am J Physiol 1998; 274:R618–R625.

33. Hogenauer C, Meyer RL, Netto GJ, et al. Malabsorption due to cholecystokinin deficiency in a patient with autoimmune polyglandular syndrome type I. N Engl J Med 2001; 344:270–274.
34. Kopin AS, Mathes WF, McBride EW, et al. The cholecystokinin A receptor mediates inhibition of food intake yet is not essential for the maintenance of body weight. J Clin Invest 1999; 103: 383–391.
35. Branchek TA, Smith KE, Gerald C, et al. Galanin receptor subtypes. Trends Pharmacol Sci 2000; 21:109–117.
36. Wynick D, Small CJ, Bacon A, et al. Galanin regulates prolactin release and lactotroph proliferation. Proc Natl Acad Sci U S A 1998; 95:12671–12676.
37. McDonald TJ, Tu E, Brenner S, et al. Canine, human, and rat plasma insulin responses to galanin administration: species response differences. Am J Physiol 1994; 266:E612–E617.
38. Habener JF. The incretin concept and its relevance to diabetes. Endocrinol Clin North Am 1993; 22:775–794.
39. Miyawaki K, Yamada Y, Yano H, et al. Glucose intolerance caused by a defect in the entero-insular axis: a study in gastric inhibitory polypeptide receptor knockout mice. Proc Natl Acad Sci U S A 1999; 96:14843–14847.
40. Lacroix A, Ndiaye N, Tremblay J, et al. Ectopic and abnormal hormone receptors in adrenal Cushing's syndrome. Endocr Rev 2001; 22:75–110.
41. Dockray GJ. Topical review: gastrin and gastric epithelial physiology. J Physiol (Lond) 1999; 518:315–324.
42. Koh TJ, Goldenring JR, Ito S, et al. Gastrin deficiency results in altered gastric differentiation and decreased colonic proliferation in mice. Gastroenterology 1997; 113:1015–1025.
43. Saillan-Barreau C, Dufresne M, Clerc P, et al. Evidence for a functional role of the cholecystokinin-B/gastrin receptor in the human fetal and adult pancreas. Diabetes 1999; 48:2015–2021.
44. Koh TJ, Chen D. Gastrin as a growth factor in the gastrointestinal tract. Regul Pept 2000; 93:37–44.
45. Wang TC, Koh TJ, Varro A, et al. Processing and proliferative effects of human progastrin in transgenic mice. J Clin Invest 1996; 98:1918–1929.
46. Koh TJ, Dockray GJ, Varro A, et al. Overexpression of glycine-extended gastrin in transgenic mice results in increased colonic proliferation. J Clin Invest 1999; 103:1119–1126.
47. Singh P, Velasco M, Given R, et al. Mice overexpressing progastrin are predisposed for developing aberrant colonic crypt foci in response to AOM. Am J Physiol Gastrointest Liver Physiol 2000; 278:G390–G399.
48. McWilliams DF, Watson SA, Crosbee DM, et al. Coexpression of gastrin and gastrin receptors (CCK-B and delta CCK-B) in gastrointestinal tumour cell lines. Gut 1998; 42:795–798.
49. Hellmich MR, Rui XL, Hellmich HL, et al. Human colorectal cancers express a constitutively active cholecystokinin-B/Gastrin receptor that stimulates cell growth. J Biol Chem 2000; 275: 32122–32128.
50. Watson SA, Morris TM, Varro A, et al. A comparison of the therapeutic effectiveness of gastrin neutralisation in two human gastric cancer models: relation to endocrine and autocrine/paracrine gastrin-mediated growth. Gut 1999; 45:812–817.
51. Anastasi A, Erspamer V, Bucci M. Isolation and structure of bombesin and alytesin, two analogous active peptides from the skin of the European amphibians Bombina and Alytes. Experientia 1971; 27:166–167.
52. Ghatei MA, Bloom SR, Langevin H, et al. Regional distribution of bombesin and seven other regulatory peptides in the human brain. Brain Res 1984; 293:101–109.
53. Merali Z, McIntosh J, Anisman H. Role of bombesin-related peptides in the control of food intake. Neuropeptides 1999; 33: 376–386.
54. Guo YS, Townsend CM Jr. Roles of gastrointestinal hormones in pancreatic cancer. J Hepatobiliary Pancreat Surg 2000; 7:276–285.
55. Ferris HA, Carroll RE, Lorimer DL, et al. Location and characterization of the human GRP receptor expressed by gastrointestinal epithelial cells. Peptides 1997; 18:663–672.
56. Wang QJ, Knezetic JA, Schally AV, et al. Bombesin may stimulate proliferation of human pancreatic cancer cells through an autocrine pathway. Int J Cancer 1996; 68:528–534.
57. Saurin JC, Rouault JP, Abello J, et al. High gastrin-releasing peptide receptor mRNA level is related to tumour dedifferentiation and lymphatic vessel invasion in human colon cancer. Eur J Cancer 1999; 35:125–132.
58. Kojima M, Hosoda H, Date Y, et al. Ghrelin is a growth hormone–releasing acylated peptide from stomach. Nature 1999; 402:656–660.
59. Asakawa A, Inui A, Kaga T, et al. A role of ghrelin in neuroendocrine and behavioral responses to stress in mice. Neuroendocrinology 2001; 74:143–147.
60. Cummings DE, Purnell JQ, Frayo RS, et al. A preprandial rise in plasma ghrelin levels suggests a role in meal initiation in humans. Diabetes 2001; 50:1714–1719.
61. Drucker DJ. Minireview: the glucagon-like peptides. Endocrinology 2001; 142:521–527.
62. Drucker DJ, Ehrlich P, Asa SL, et al. Induction of intestinal epithelial proliferation by glucagon-like peptide-2. Proc Natl Acad Sci U S A 1996; 93:7911–7916.
63. Drucker DJ. Glucagon-like peptide 2. J Clin Endocrinol Metab 2001; 86:1759–1764.
64. Mentlein R. Dipeptidyl-peptidase IV (CD26)—role in the inactivation of regulatory peptides. Regul Pept 1999; 85:9–24.
65. Scrocchi LA, Brown TJ, MacLusky N, et al. Glucose intolerance but normal satiety in mice with a null mutation in the glucagon-like peptide receptor gene. Nature Med 1996; 2:1254–1258.
66. Yusta B, Huang L, Munroe D, et al. Enteroendocrine localization of GLP-2 receptor expression in humans and rodents. Gastroenterology 2000; 119:744–755.
67. Lovshin J, Estall J, Yusta B, et al. Glucagon-like peptide-2 action in the murine central nervous system is enhanced by elimination of GLP-1 receptor signaling. J Biol Chem 2001; 276:21489–21499.
68. Dawson J, Bryant MG, Bloom SR, et al. Gastrointestinal regulatory peptide storage granule abnormalities in jejunal mucosal diseases. Gut 1984; 25:636–643.
69. Feighner SD, Tan CP, McKee KK, et al. Receptor for motilin identified in the human gastrointestinal system. Science 1999; 284:2184–2188.
70. Itoh Z. Motilin and clinical application. Peptides 1997; 18:593–608.
71. Allen JM, Yeats JC, Causon R, et al. Neuropeptide Y and its flanking peptide in human endocrine tumors and plasma. J Clin Endocrinol Metab 1987; 64:1199–1204.
72. Michel MC, Beck-Sickinger A, Cox H, et al. XVI. International Union of Pharmacology recommendations for the nomenclature of neuropeptide Y, peptide YY, and pancreatic polypeptide receptors. Pharmacol Rev 1998; 50:143–150.
73. Sheikh SP. Neuropeptide Y and peptide YY: major modulators of gastrointestinal blood flow and function. Am J Physiol 1991; 261: G701–G715.
74. Vincent JP, Mazella J, Kitabgi P. Neurotensin and neurotensin receptors. Trends Pharmacol Sci 1999; 20:302–309.
75. Izukura M, Evers BM, Parekh D, et al. Neurotensin augments intestinal regeneration after small bowel resection in rats. Ann Surg 1992; 215:520–527.
76. Evers BM, Izukura M, Chung DH, et al. Neurotensin stimulates growth of colonic mucosa in young and aged rats. Gastroenterology 1992; 103:86–91.
77. Tyler-McMahon BM, Boules M, Richelson E. Neurotensin: peptide for the next millennium. Regul Pept 2000; 93:125–136.
78. Ahren B, Veith RC, Paquette TL, et al. Sympathetic nerve stimulation versus pancreatic norepinephrine infusion in the dog: II. Effects on basal release of somatostatin and pancreatic polypeptide. Endocrinology 1987; 121:332–339.
79. Lundell I, Blomqvist AG, Berglund MM, et al. Cloning of a human receptor of the NPY receptor family with high affinity for pancreatic polypeptide and peptide YY. J Biol Chem 1995; 270: 29123–29128.
80. Ueno N, Inui A, Iwamoto M, et al. Decreased food intake and body weight in pancreatic polypeptide–overexpressing mice. Gastroenterology 1999; 117:1427–1432.
81. Larhammar D. Evolution of neuropeptide Y, peptide YY, and pancreatic polypeptide. Regul Pept 1996; 62:1–11.
82. Ali-Rachedi A, Varndell IM, Adrian TE, et al. Peptide YY (PYY) immunoreactivity is co-stored with glucagon-related immunoreactants in endocrine cells of the gut and pancreas. Histochem J 1984; 80:487–491.

83. Jackerott M, Larsson LI. Immunocytochemical localization of the *NPY/PYY Y1* receptor in enteric neurons, endothelial cells, and endocrine-like cells of the rat intestinal tract. J Histochem Cytochem 1997; 45:1643–1650.
84. Guan D, Rivard N, Morisset J, et al. Effects of peptide YY on the growth of the pancreas and intestine. Endocrinology 1993; 132:219–223.
85. Vaudry D, Gonzalez BJ, Basille M, et al. Pituitary adenylate cyclase–activating polypeptide and its receptors: from structure to functions. Pharmacol Rev 2000; 52:269–324.
86. Jamen F, Persson K, Bertrand G, et al. PAC1 receptor–deficient mice display impaired insulinotropic response to glucose and reduced glucose tolerance. J Clin Invest 2000; 105:1307–1315.
87. Schaffalitzky de Muckadell OB, Fahrenkrug J. Secretion pattern of secretin in man: regulation by gastric acid. Gut 1978; 19:812–818.
88. Sandler AD, Sutton KA, DeWeese J, et al. Lack of benefit of a single dose of synthetic human secretin in the treatment of autism and pervasive developmental disorder. N Engl J Med 1999; 341:1801–1806.
89. Patel YC, Greenwood MT, Panetta R, et al. The somatostatin receptor family. Life Sci 1995; 57:1249–1265.
90. Mandarino L, Stenner D, Blanchard W, et al. Selective effects of somatostatin-14, -25, and -28 on in vitro insulin and glucagon secretion. Nature 1981; 291:76–77.
91. de Lecea L, Criado JR, Prospero-Garcia O, et al. A cortical neuropeptide with neuronal depressant and sleep-modulating properties. Nature 1996; 381:242–245.
92. Kahn CR, Bhathena SJ, Recant L, et al. Use of somatostatin and somatostatin analogs in a patient with a glucagonoma. J Clin Endocrinol Metab 1984; 53:543–549.
93. Lamberts SW, van der Lely AJ, de Herder WW, et al. Octreotide. N Engl J Med 1996; 334:246–254.
94. Arnold R, Simon B, Wied M. Treatment of neuroendocrine GEP tumours with somatostatin analogues: a review. Digestion 2000; 62:84–91.
95. Kaltsas G, Korbonits M, Heintz E, et al. Comparison of somatostatin analog and meta-iodobenzylguanidine radionuclides in the diagnosis and localization of advanced neuroendocrine tumors. J Clin Endocrinol Metab 2001; 86:895–902.
96. Low MJ, Otero-Corchon V, Parlow AF, et al. Somatostatin is required for masculinization of growth hormone–regulated hepatic gene expression but not of somatic growth. J Clin Invest 2001; 107:1571–1580.
97. Holzer P, Holzer-Petsche U. Tachykinins in the gut. I: Expression, release, and motor function. Pharmacol Ther 1997; 73:173–217.
98. Simon C, Portalier P, Chamoin MC, et al. Substance P–like immunoreactivity release from enterochromaffin cells of rat caecum mucosa: inhibition by serotonin and calcium-free medium. Neurochem Int 1992; 20:529–536.
99. Donaldson LF, Haskell CA, Hanley MR. Functional characterization by heterologous expression of a novel cloned tachykinin peptide receptor. Biochem J 1996; 320:1–5.
100. Lecci A, Giuliani S, Tramontana M, et al. Peripheral actions of tachykinins. Neuropeptides 2000; 34:303–313.
101. Mazelin L, Theodorou V, More J, et al. Comparative effects of nonpeptide tachykinin receptor antagonists on experimental gut inflammation in rats and guinea-pigs. Life Sci 1998; 63:293–304.
102. Cutrufo C, Evangelista S, Cirillo R, et al. Effect of MEN 11467, a new tachykinin NK1 receptor antagonist, in acute rectocolitis induced by acetic acid in guinea pigs. Eur J Pharmacol 1999; 374:277–283.
103. Leppaluoto J, Vuolteenaho O, Koivusalo F. Thyrotropin-releasing factor: radioimmunoassay and distribution in biological fluids and tissues. Med Biol 1981; 59:85–91.
104. O'Dowd BF, Lee DK, Huang W, et al. TRH-R2 exhibits similar binding and acute signaling but distinct regulation and anatomic distribution compared with TRH-R1. Mol Endocrinol 2000; 14: 183–193.
105. Ulrich CD II, Holtmann M, Miller LJ. Secretin and vasoactive intestinal peptide receptors: members of a unique family of G protein–coupled receptors. Gastroenterology 1998; 114:382–397.
106. Grider JR, Murthy KS, Jin JG, et al. Stimulation of nitric oxide from muscle cells by VIP: prejunctional enhancement of VIP release. Am J Physiol 1992; 262:G774–G778.
107. Waschek JA. Vasoactive intestinal peptide: an important trophic factor and developmental regulator? Dev Neurosci 1995; 17:1–7.
108. Helman LJ, Gazdar AF, Park J-G, et al. Chromogranin-A expression in normal and malignant human tissues. J Clin Invest 1988; 82:686–690.
109. Corazziari E. Role of opioid ligands in the irritable bowel syndrome. Can J Gastroenterol 1999; 13(Suppl A):71A–75A.
110. Nandha K, Bloom SR. Neuromedin U—an overview. Biomed Res 1993; 14(Suppl 3):71–76.
111. Semrad CE. Guanylin: where it's at! Why's it there? Gastroenterology 1997; 113:1036–1038.
112. Charpin G, Chikh-Issa AR, Guignard H, et al. Effect of sorbin on duodenal absorption of water and electrolytes in the rat. Gastroenterology 1992; 103:1568–1573.
113. Miyasaka K, Funakoshi A. Luminal feedback regulation, monitor peptide, CCK-releasing peptide, and CCK receptors. Pancreas 1998; 16:277–283.
114. Perren A, Komminoth P, Saremaslani P, et al. Mutation and expression analyses reveal differential subcellular compartmentalization of PTEN in endocrine pancreatic tumors compared to normal islet cells. Am J Pathol 2000; 157:1097–1103.
115. Chandrasekharappa SC, Guru SC, Manickam P, et al. Positional cloning of the gene for multiple endocrine neoplasia-type 1. Science 1997; 276:404–407.
116. Schussheim DH, Skarulis MC, Agarwal SK, et al. Multiple endocrine neoplasia type 1: new clinical and basic findings. Trends Endocrinol Metab 2001; 12:173–178.
117. Madeira I, Terris B, Voss M, et al. Prognostic factors in patients with endocrine tumours of the duodenopancreatic area. Gut 1998; 43:422–427.
118. Eriksson B, Oberg K, Stridsberg M. Tumor markers in neuroendocrine tumors. Digestion 2000; 62:33–38.
119. Heppeler A, Froidevaux S, Eberle AN, et al. Receptor targeting for tumor localisation and therapy with radiopeptides. Curr Med Chem 2000; 7:971–994.
120. Higham AD, Bishop LA, Dimaline R, et al. Mutations of RegI-alpha are associated with enterochromaffin-like cell tumor development in patients with hypergastrinemia. Gastroenterology 1999; 116:1310–1318.
121. Brentjens R, Saltz L. Islet cell tumors of the pancreas: the medical oncologist's perspective. Surg Clin North Am 2001; 81:527–542.
122. Azimuddin K, Chamberlain RS. The surgical management of pancreatic neuroendocrine tumors. Surg Clin North Am 2001; 81:511–525.
123. Zollinger RM, Ellison EH. Primary peptide ulcerations of the jejunum associated with islet cell tumors of the pancreas. Ann Surg 1955; 142:709–728.
124. Roy PK, Venzon DJ, Shojamanesh H, et al. Zollinger-Ellison syndrome: clinical presentation in 261 patients. Medicine (Baltimore) 2000; 79:379–411.
125. Mozell E, Stenzel P, Woltering EA, et al. Functional endocrine tumors of the pancreas: clinical presentation, diagnosis, and treatment. Curr Probl Surg 1990; 27:301–386.
126. Jensen RT. Management of the Zollinger-Ellison syndrome in patients with multiple endocrine neoplasia type 1. J Intern Med 1998; 243:477–488.
127. Meko JB, Doherty GM, Siegel BA, et al. Evaluation of somatostatin-receptor scintigraphy for detecting neuroendocrine tumors. Surgery 1996; 120:975–983; discussion 983–974.
128. Anderson MA, Carpenter S, Thompson NW, et al. Endoscopic ultrasound is highly accurate and directs management in patients with neuroendocrine tumors of the pancreas. Am J Gastroenterol 2000; 95:2271–2277.
129. McArthur KE, Collen MJ, Maton PN, et al. Omeprazole: effective, convenient therapy for Zollinger-Ellison syndrome. Gastroenterology 1985; 88:939–944.
130. Meko JB, Norton JA. Management of patients with Zollinger-Ellison syndrome. Annu Rev Med 1995; 46:395–411.
131. Sweet RD. A dermatosis specifically associated with a tumour of pancreatic alpha cells. Br J Dermatol 1974; 90:301–308.
132. Bloom SR, Polak JM. Glucagonoma syndrome. Am J Med 1987; 82:25–36.
133. Wermers RA, Fatourechi V, Kvols LK. Clinical spectrum of hyperglucagonemia associated with malignant neuroendocrine tumors. Mayo Clin Proc 1996; 71:1030–1038.

134. Benali N, Ferjoux G, Puente E, et al. Somatostatin receptors. Digestion 2000; 62:27–32.
135. Krejs GJ, Orci L, Conlon JM, et al. Somatostatinoma syndrome: biochemical, morphologic, and clinical features. N Engl J Med 1979; 301:285–292.
136. Tanaka S, Yamasaki S, Matsushita H, et al. Duodenal somatostatinoma: a case report and review of 31 cases with special reference to the relationship between tumor size and metastasis. Pathol Int 2000; 50:146–152.
137. Bloom SR, Polak JM, Pearce AGE. Vasoactive intestinal peptide and watery diarrhoea syndrome. Lancet 1973; 2:14–16.
138. Jensen RT. Overview of chronic diarrhea caused by functional neuroendocrine neoplasms. Semin Gastrointest Dis 1999; 10: 156–172.

39 Endocrine-Responsive Cancer

Richard Santen

BREAST CANCER

Etiology

A variety of data suggest that estrogens directly cause or contribute to the development of breast cancer.[1] Administration of exogenous estrogens to various animal species results in breast cancer. Spontaneous development of breast cancer in aging rats can be prevented by oophorectomy or administration of aromatase inhibitors to block estrogen production.[2, 3] Oophorectomy before age 35 years in women lowered the risk of breast cancer by 75% over a 25-year period.[4] Administration of antiestrogens caused a 50% reduction in breast cancers diagnosed in women at high risk for development of breast cancer.[5] These observations and other data have led to the classification of estrogen as a carcinogen.[5a]

Sources of Estrogen

The breast derives estradiol from three separate sources: the ovary, extraglandular tissues, and the breast itself. First, direct glandular secretion by the ovary results in delivery of estradiol to the breast through an endocrine mechanism in premenopausal women. Second, after the menopause, extraglandular production of estrogen from ovarian and adrenal androgens provides the second source of estradiol.[6] Third, the breast itself can synthesize estradiol through aromatization of androgens to estrogens or cleavage of estrone sulfate to estrone by the enzyme sulfatase.[7–10] Estradiol acts through paracrine, autocrine, and intracrine mechanisms on cells in the breast.[11] Several factors regulate in situ estradiol synthesis but the most important is the degree of obesity, which increases the amount of aromatase in breast and, consequently, estradiol production.[6, 12]

Estrogen-Induced Carcinogenesis

Mutations of key genes involved in cell proliferation, deoxyribonucleic acid (DNA) repair, or apoptosis must accumulate to produce cancer.[13–22] It is likely that mitogenic as well as mutagenic effects of estradiol act in concert to initiate and promote the development of breast cancer (Fig. 39–1).[23, 24] As a rule, the frequency of mutations increases in parallel with the number of mitotic divisions in a proliferating tissue. Accordingly, estrogens may *initiate* mutations leading to neoplastic transformation by increasing the rate of cell proliferation. As cells divide more rapidly, less time is available for DNA repair. Estrogens also enhance tumor *promotion* by increasing the rate of cell division with propagation of the mutations already present.

Metabolites of estradiol may be directly mutagenic through a pathway involving the 1B1 cytochrome P450 enzyme.[25–28] This catalyzes conversion of estradiol to the catechol-estrogen 4-hydroxyestradiol, which is then further metabolized to 3,4-estradiol-quinone.[29–33] This highly reactive species binds covalently to guanine or adenine molecules in the DNA helix, which activates a glycosidase and results in depurination. Error-prone or replicative repair of the depurinated site leads to point mutations.[15] Recent studies directly demonstrated estradiol-guanine conjugates in benign and malignant human breast

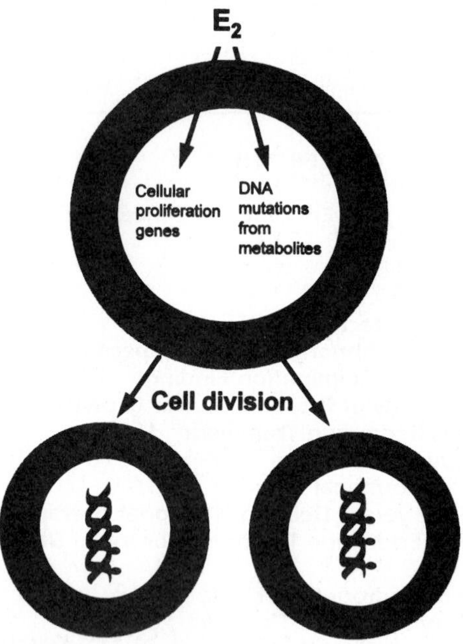

Figure 39–1. Diagrammatic representation of mechanisms by which estradiol causes breast cancer. By binding to its receptor and stimulating genes involved in cell proliferation, estradiol (E_2) increases the rate of cell division. The chances of error during deoxyribonucleic acid (DNA) replication increase as the number of dividing cells is enhanced. The number of mutations increases, and cancer ultimately develops. This mechanism can be called the *cell proliferation mechanism of cancer* (see Preston-Martin et al, 1993[24]). Increasing data suggest that metabolites of estradiol are directly genotoxic and result in deletions of DNA segments and point mutations (see Jefcoate et al, 2000[28]; Yager and Liehr, 1996[29]; and Cavalieri et al, 2000[468]). These two mechanisms may act in an additive or synergistic fashion to cause breast cancer. (From Santen RJ. Symposium overview. J Natl Cancer Inst Monogr 2000; 27:15–16.)

tissue, establishing the activity of the genotoxic pathway in women.[33] Support for the quinone-depurination hypothesis derives from correlative studies relating mutations of key enzymes in this pathway to breast cancer risk.[34–36] In addition, studies have directly demonstrated the mutagenic potential of estradiol in an in vitro assay as well as the transforming effect of estradiol on benign breast cells.[37–39]

Estradiol is not the sole factor mediating the development of breast cancer. A number of specific genetic mutations are associated with a high incidence of breast cancer.[40–42] Studies in twins suggest that approximately 27% of breast cancers arise because of genetic factors.[42, 43] The most common mutations involve the *BRCA1* and *BRCA2* genes and cause approximately 5% of breast cancer cases.[44–47] Rarer genetic syndromes include mutations of the *p53* gene in the Li-Fraumeni syndrome,[48] impaired cell cycle check point surveillance in the ataxia-telangiectasia syndrome,[49] mutations in the *PTEN* gene in the Cowden syndrome,[50] the *MLH1* and *MSH2* genes in the Muir-Torre syndrome,[51] and an *STK11* mutation in the Peutz-Jeghers syndrome.[52]

Dietary and environmental factors play a key role in breast cancer etiology and contribute to the fourfold difference in incidence between Japan, with a rate of 23 women per 100,000 per year, and the United States, at 90 per 100,000 per year.[53, 54] Epidemiologic observations suggest a role for a high-fat diet and resultant obesity in the genesis of breast cancer. In Japan, the rate of breast cancer peaks at the age of menopause; in the United States, however, the incidence continues to increase until age 90 years. The difference in postmenopausal patterns may result from the increase in obesity and associated aromatase increments in women in the United States compared with those in Japan. This differential postmenopausal rate does not appear to be genetic because Japanese women who move to the United States experience an increased rate of breast cancer that later approaches that of American women.[55]

Hormonal Risk Factors for Breast Cancer

Most risk factors for breast cancer are related to the duration or intensity of a woman's exposure to endogenous or exogenous estrogens (Fig. 39–2). Early menarche or late

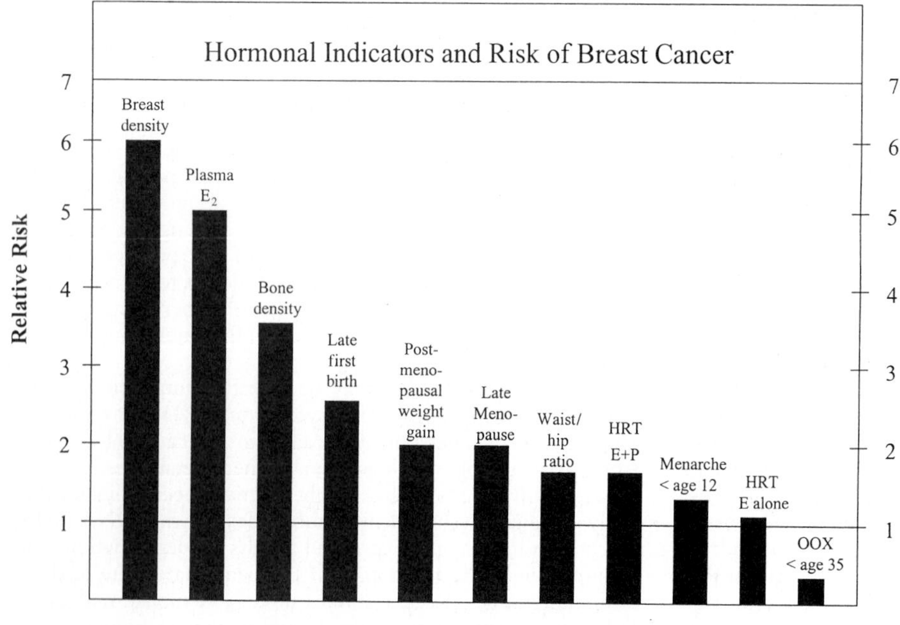

Figure 39–2. Relative risk of breast cancer as a function of several factors related to long-term exposure to estradiol (see Zhang et al, 1997[67]; Boyd et al, 1995[469]; Cauley et al, 1996[470]; Hulka, 1997[471]; Huang et al, 1997[472]; and Mouridsen, 2001[473]). E, estrogen; E_2, estradiol; HRT, hormone replacement therapy; OOX, oophorectomy; P, progesterone.

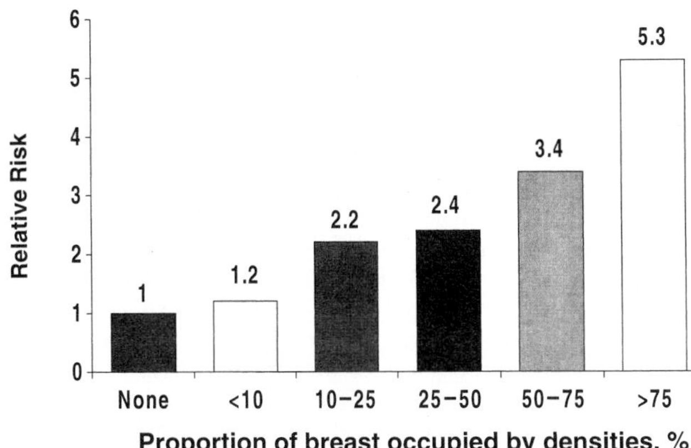

Figure 39–3. Relative risk of breast cancer as a function of the degree of mammographic density (From Boyd NF, Byng JW, Jong RA, et al. Quantitative classification of mammographic densities and breast cancer risk: results from the Canadian National Breast Screening Study. J Natl Cancer Inst 1995; 87:670–675.[469] Reprinted with permission of the publisher.)

menopause, or both increase breast cancer risk.[56, 57] Elevations in circulating estradiol levels predict the risk for development of breast cancer over the ensuing years in postmenopausal women.[58, 58a] An estradiol level in the top quintile is associated with an increase in the relative risk of breast cancer by fivefold.[59–65] Putative markers of long-term estrogen exposure such as bone density are also predictive. Women in the top quartile of bone density[56, 57, 66–68] have a threefold increase in risk of breast cancer.

Late first birth increases the risk 2.8-fold and is believed to be related to the lack of the differentiating effect of pregnancy on the type of breast lobule present.[69] Gain of at least 20 kg as an adult increases breast cancer risk twofold, probably as a result of increasing aromatase activity and estrogen production by adipose tissue.[70] Increased waist-hip ratio is associated with a similar increase in risk.[71] Several but not all studies suggest that alcohol intake can increase the risk of breast cancer,[72] perhaps by decreasing the clearance of estradiol.[73] Increased exposure to estradiol in utero, as shown by twin studies, may increase the risk of breast cancer by as much as twofold.[74] Early pregnancy and prolonged duration of breast-feeding diminish the risk.[57] More dramatic is the 75% reduction in risk caused by bilateral oophorectomy before age 35 years.[4, 75]

Mammographic density represents the most powerful risk factor for breast cancer. Increased breast density probably reflects either an increase in exposure to estrogen or sensitivity to it.[76–78] Exogenous estrogens increase[77, 79–81] and antiestrogens reduce breast density.[82] Because of these effects, hormone replacement therapy (HRT) alters the sensitivity and specificity associated with interpreting mammograms.[83, 84] The increase in breast cancer risk from the lowest to the highest breast density category is on the order of sixfold, depending on the age of the patient (Fig. 39–3), with a greater relative risk seen in older women.

Exogenous Estrogens and Breast Cancer Risk

In premenopausal women, use of oral contraceptives for 10 or more years increases the relative risk of breast cancer by approximately 10%.[85–87] However, this increase in relative risk affects few women because the age-related incidence of breast cancer is quite low in women taking oral contraceptives. Controversy surrounds the concept that HRT in postmenopausal women increases the risk of breast cancer. More than 50 observational studies have examined this question but have reported conflicting results.[88] However, a key study clarified the factors responsible for the different conclusions in the various reports. A meta-analysis from the Collaborative Group on Hormonal Factors in Breast Cancer[88] examined data for 52,705 women with breast cancer and 108,411 without. Five objective factors that confounded the interpretation of prior studies were identified.

1. The relative risk of breast cancer associated with estrogen replacement therapy is small, and large studies are required to minimize type I and type II statistical errors.
2. The risk of breast cancer appears to increase linearly with duration of HRT use. Accordingly, comparisons of "ever users" with "never users" are invalid because the duration of estrogen use is not considered.
3. The increased risk of breast cancer associated with estrogens appears to dissipate within 4 years of cessation of therapy. Therefore, only women using estrogen within 4 years of the study might be found to be at increased risk.
4. Breast cancer risk diminishes over a 4-year period after the menopause, presumably reflecting decreased estrogen levels. As a result, analyses of observational studies need to match users and nonusers according to time after menopause.
5. The increased risk of breast cancer appears to be limited to nonobese women (i.e., body mass index [BMI] < 25 kg/m^2). Inclusion of a large proportion of obese women in a single study might obscure an association between estrogen use and breast cancer risk.

Taking into account these five factors, the meta-analysis concluded that the relative risk of breast cancer increases linearly by 2.3% per year of HRT for up to 25 years.[88] Both the slope of the risk-time analysis (*P* value) and the overall risk of breast cancer among estrogen users (*P* value) were highly statistically significant. This study detected no increased risk associated with HRT use in obese women (i.e., BMI > 25 kg/m^2). A hypothetical explanation for the differences between obese and thin women involves the degree of in situ estrogen production. Obese women may have an increase in breast tissue estrogen as a result of increased aromatase activity, whereas lean women have lower levels. Exogenous estrogen might then produce a greater percentage increase in estrogen levels in thin than in obese women.

Data suggest that addition of a progestin to an estrogen replacement therapy regimen enhances the risk of breast cancer to a greater extent than estrogen alone (Fig. 39–4*A* and *B*).[89–91a] The physiologic basis for this conclusion rests on data indicating that progestins are mitogenic to breast tissue in contrast to their antimitogenic effects on the uterus.[92, 93] Although data from cell cultures or animal studies are not conclusive, the weight of evidence from patients suggests that progestins are mitogenic in breast.

Mammographic studies demonstrate that breast density in women taking an estrogen-progestin combination is greater than breast density in those taking estrogen alone.[77] Histologic examination demonstrated increased cell proliferation and percentage of the breast containing glandular tissue as a function of duration of progestin usage.[92] Increased proliferation would be expected to increase both *initiation* and *promotion* of breast cancer in a manner similar to that for estrogens.

A number of observational studies have suggested an increase in breast cancer risk in women receiving an estrogen-progestin combination, but these were not considered conclusive.[89–95] Recent results from a large, prospective, randomized, placebo-controlled trial in postmenopausal women now provide compelling evidence for this effect. Nearly 16,000 postmenopausal women with an average age of 63 enrolled in the

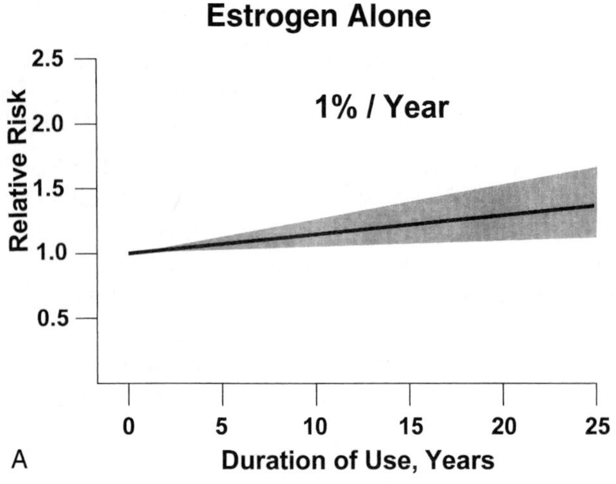

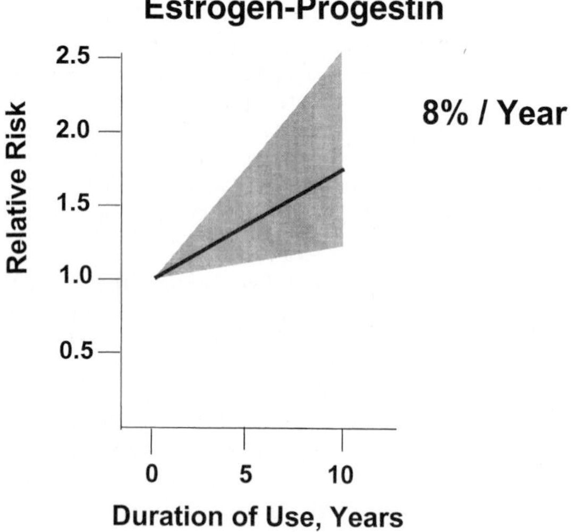

Figure 39–4. *A*, Increase in relative risk of breast cancer in women taking estrogen alone as hormone replacement therapy (HRT). *Solid line* represents the mean increase in relative risk over time. *Shaded area* represents the 95% confidence limits of that risk. *B*, Increase in relative risk of breast cancer in women taking estrogen plus a progestin as HRT. *Solid line* represents the mean increase in relative risk over time. *Shaded area* represents the 95% confidence limits of that risk. (From Santen RJ, Pinkerton J, McCartney C, et al. Risk of breast cancer with progestins in combination with estrogen as hormone replacement therapy. J Clin Endocrinol Metab 2001; 86:16–23.)

Women's Health Initiative study and received either placebo or conjugated estrogens plus medroxyprogesterone-acetate for 5 years on average. The study was terminated early because of an increased incidence of breast cancer in the HRT group with a relative risk of 1.26 and 95% confidence interval of 1.00 to 1.59. The absolute excess of cases was small, with only 8 more invasive breast cancers per 10,000 person-years in the HRT group. Nonetheless, these data confirm the prior observational studies and indicate a relative risk increase of 5.5% per year in those receiving HRT. This is similar to the 8% per year increase reported in the observational studies (Fig. 39–4). At the present time it is not known whether the type or dose of progestin can alter breast cancer risk. Various observational studies have examined differences between combined continuous and sequential regimens and various types of progestins but data are insufficient to make definitive conclusions. It has been suggested that certain types of progestin may exert no effects on breast cancer risk, but this requires further study. With respect to estrogen alone and breast cancer, another Women's Health Initiative study is currently comparing placebo with estrogen alone in women who had previously undergone a total abdominal hysterectomy. This study continues and has not at this time shown a sufficient increase in breast cancer with estrogen alone to warrant terminating the study.

Review of the totality of basic and clinical data strongly supports an adverse effect of adding progestins to estrogens in women. Regarding the effects of estrogen alone on breast cancer risk, one must interpret the existing data cautiously because of the retrospective/observational nature of available studies. Definitive information will await prospective information from the Women's Health Initiative study that is comparing estrogen alone to placebo. In the meantime, it is considered prudent to advise patients about the worst case conclusion, that estrogen alone may increase their risk of breast cancer. Additional risks may also be imparted for ovarian and uterine cancer.

Relative, Absolute, and Attributable Risks

Epidemiologists use *relative risk analysis* as a tool that provides substantial power to determine statistical significance.[97] However, this term is misleading to patients because actual risk is quite small in magnitude. The lay press, patients, and many physicians confuse the terms relative, absolute, and attributable risk.

Relative risk is defined as the ratio of risk under one condition to risk under another condition and does not take into account the frequency of occurrence of that condition.

Absolute risk is determined by multiplying the underlying incidence rate in the group being considered by relative risk.

Table 39–1. Attributable Risks from Hormone Replacement Therapy

			Attributable Risk of Breast Cancer	
Hormone	**Age Initiated (yr)**	**Duration of Use (yr)**	**Per 100 Women**	**As Numeric Chance**
Estrogen alone	50	2	0.0101	1:9925
Estrogen-progestin	50	2	0.0806	1:1241
Estrogen alone	50	10	0.252	1:397
Estrogen-progestin	50	10	2.016	1:50
Estrogen alone	60	10	0.350	1:286
Estrogen-progestin	60	10	2.780	1:36

From Santen RJ, Pinkerton J, McCartney C, et al. Risk of breast cancer with progestins in combination with estrogen as hormone replacement therapy. J Clin Endocrinol Metab 2001; 86:16–23.

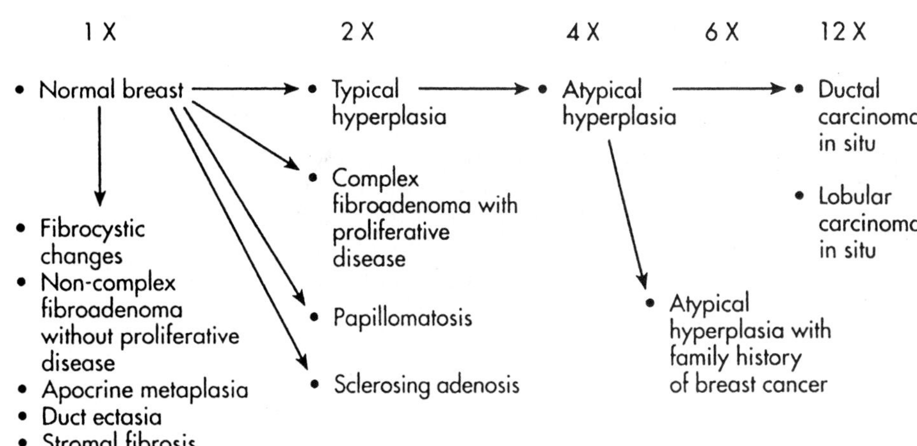

Figure 39–5. Relative risk of invasive breast cancer related to several benign breast lesions in women with long-term follow-up.

For example, the absolute risk of breast cancer development for an average 50-year-old woman in the United States is 2.52 per 100 women over a 10-year period. A 10% increase in relative risk resulting from estrogens alone would increase a woman's absolute risk of breast cancer to 2.77 per 100 women.

Attributable risk is defined as the number of women who would develop breast cancer that would not have occurred unless they had used estrogen replacement. Using the preceding example, the difference between breast cancer risk of 2.52 per 100 and 2.77 per 100 represents the increased risk *attributable* to estrogen or 0.252 per 100 women.

Attributable risks can be translated into the numeric odds of one's being adversely affected by estrogen (Table 39–1). For example, the chance of an estrogen-induced breast cancer in a 50-year-old woman receiving estrogen replacement therapy over 2 years is 1 in 9925; over 10 years, it would be 1 in 397. For a woman taking estrogen plus a progestin, the comparable odds are 1 in 1241 for 2 years of use and 1 in 50 for 10 years.

Benign Breast Disease and Risk of Breast Cancer

Benign breast lesions with an enhanced rate of proliferation or increased degree of atypical features predict an increased incidence of breast cancer over time (Fig. 39–5).[20–22, 98–109] Some of these lesions contain genetic mutations, and many lesions are analogous to adenomas because of clonal populations of mutated cells. Hyperplastic ductal lesions are often multicentric, suggesting that some type of underlying abnormality or *field defect* is present that predisposes to such lesions. The multifocal nature of the associated benign hyperplastic lesions is most apparent in breast tissue from women with cancer. Examination of tissue adjacent to an invasive breast cancer or in the contralateral breast reveals one or more additional hyperplastic lesions in approximately 40% of patients.[20]

The nature of the field defect has not been specifically identified, but hypothetically it may represent a single mutation of a gene controlling local estrogen production, cellular proliferation, DNA repair, metabolism of procarcinogens to carcinogens, or other cellular events. Preliminary data suggest progression from adenomas to frank neoplasms. Eighty percent to 90% of hyperplastic lesions contain DNA mutations similar to those in the contiguous tumors.[20] Extensive molecular genetic studies have now shown progression of abnormalities in the spectrum of breast lesions.

A major consideration for women who present with breast problems is whether they have a higher than normal risk of breast cancer. Certain breast lesions, such as fibrocystic changes, are associated with no increased risk of subsequent breast cancer (see Fig. 39–5), whereas other lesions, such as atypical ductal hyperplasia, involve an increased risk.[99, 100] The relative risk of development of invasive cancer is increased 10-fold to 12-fold when *ductal carcinoma in situ* (DCIS) and *lobular carcinoma in situ* (LCIS) are present.[110–114]

Estimating Breast Cancer Risk

To aid in assessment of breast cancer risk, a questionnaire developed by Gail and co-workers utilizes answers to seven questions to calculate the 5-year and lifetime risks of breast cancer.[115–117] This model has recognized deficiencies, in that it does not consider breast density, plasma estradiol levels, bone density, BMI, weight gain in adulthood, second-degree relatives with breast cancer, proliferative lesions of breast other than atypical ductal hyperplasia, alcohol intake, or birth control pill and HRT use.

Nonetheless, two major prospective studies validated the Gail model in a high-risk (National Surgical Adjuvant Breast and Bowel Project [NSABP] prevention study)[5] and in an average-risk population of women (the Nurses Health Study).[117] The ratio of observed to expected cancers with this tool is 1.03 (95% confidence limits of 0.88 to 1.21) in the high-risk patients and 0.94 (95% confidence interval [CI] 0.89 to 0.99) in average-risk women, and both are highly statistically significant. This risk tool, called the RISK DISK, is available from the National Cancer Institute. When second-degree relatives with breast cancer represent the major risk factor, the Claus model is a more valid risk assessment tool.[118, 118a]

Breast Cancer Risk and Clinical Decisions

Knowledge about underlying breast cancer risk influences advice given by health care providers and choices made by patients. Women known to be at high risk for breast cancer frequently choose a surrogate for estrogen (see later) to obtain its benefits while avoiding its risks. Those at low risk usually choose estrogen or an estrogen-progestin combination to relieve symptoms of estrogen deficiency or to prevent osteoporosis. Those at intermediate risk have several options, including use of a selective estrogen receptor modulator (SERM), other alternatives to estrogen, watchful waiting, or HRT.

As a working guide, we arbitrarily define risk categories on the basis of the Gail model:

- High risk, more than a 3% chance of breast cancer in 5 years

- Intermediate risk, 1.5% to 3% chance
- Low risk, less than 1.5%

Women classified as *high risk* include patients with a strong family history of breast cancer (particularly if associated with ovarian cancer), a prior history of atypical ductal hyperplasia or LCIS, and age older than 60 years when combined with early menarche, late menopause, or late first live birth. *Intermediate-risk* patients have some risk factors but not others. *Low-risk patients* are younger than 60 years, have a late onset of menarche, early menopause, early age of first live birth, and no family history of breast cancer or prior predisposing breast lesions.

Because no formal risk tool incorporates breast density, bone density, or plasma estradiol levels in its assessment, a physician must take these factors into account in advising patients.

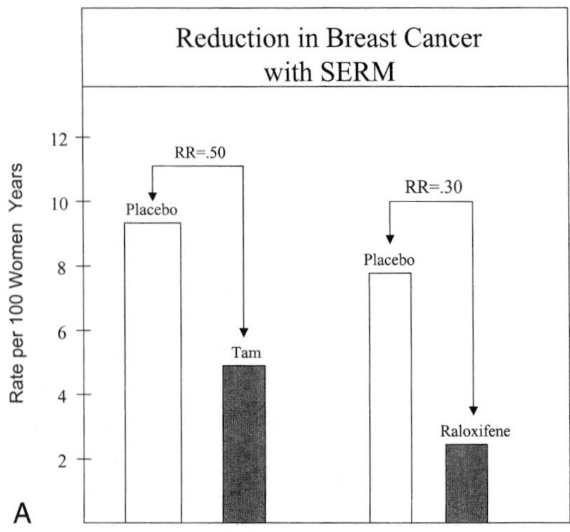

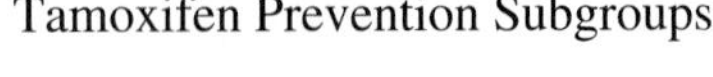

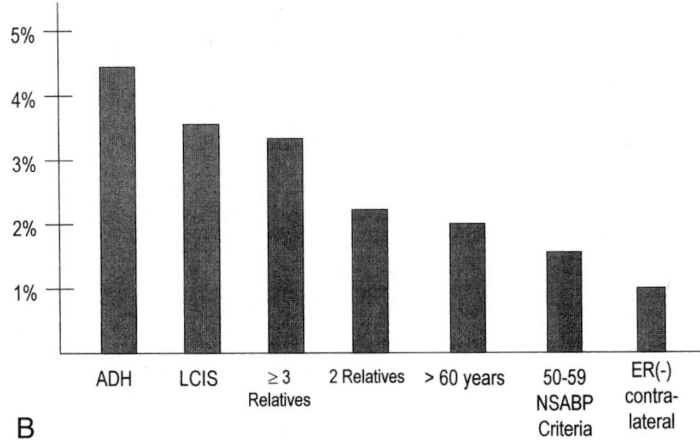

Figure 39–6. *A*, Reduction in risk of breast cancer in response to administration of tamoxifen (TAM) or raloxifene for a mean duration of 4 years (see Fisher et al, 1998[5]; and Cummings et al, 1999[122]). RR, relative risk; SERM, selective estrogen receptor modulator. *B*, Absolute benefit from tamoxifen expressed as percentage of women whose breast cancer was prevented as a function of the underlying risk factor present. ADH, atypical ductal hyperplasia; ER, estrogen receptor; LCIS, lobular carcinoma in situ; NSABP, National Surgical Adjuvant Breast Project.

Prevention of Breast Cancer

Depending on their risk category, women may wish to take tamoxifen or raloxifene to prevent breast cancer. Only the antiestrogen tamoxifen is approved for this use in the United States. Although evidence supporting antiestrogens for prevention is substantial, results from individual studies are conflicting. Five clinical trials provided data regarding the efficacy of antiestrogens for prevention of breast cancer.[5, 119–122]

The most definitive trial, the NSABP P-1 study, involved 13,388 women randomly assigned to receive either placebo or 20 mg of tamoxifen daily.[5] Eligibility for the study required an intermediate or high risk of breast cancer, defined in the study as a 1.67% or greater chance of development of a new breast cancer over a 5-year period. The rate of breast cancers was 9.4 per 1000 women-years in the placebo group versus 4.7 in the tamoxifen group, a relative risk reduction of 0.50 (Fig. 39–6*A*). Considered separately, the risk of invasive breast cancer was reduced by 49% and of noninvasive breast cancer by 50%. This effect occurred in women of all ages studied (younger than age 49, 50 to 59, 60 to 69, and older than 70 years) and in those with LCIS, atypical ductal hyperplasia, and a family history of breast cancer. The benefits of tamoxifen were related to the underlying risk of breast cancer and the specific risk factor present (Fig. 39–6*B*).

Two other published tamoxifen cancer prevention trials did not find a statistically significant reduction of breast cancer risk. Both studies were much smaller than the NSABP trial (2471 women in the United Kingdom study and 5408 women in the Italian study)[120, 121] and are considered flawed because of concomitant estrogen use (the United Kingdom study) or frequency of oophorectomy (the Italian study).[123]

A fourth trial (Multiple Outcomes of Raloxifene [MORE]) involved more than 7705 women taking the antiestrogen raloxifene or a placebo.[122] Although breast cancer incidence was only a secondary study end point, a highly significant 70% reduction in new breast cancers (relative risk 0.30) was observed after 48 months of raloxifene use (see Fig. 39–6). A fifth study examined the effect of tamoxifen on contralateral breast cancer in women with diagnosed DCIS and found a significant reduction.[119] Review of these prevention trials led a panel of experts commissioned by the American Society of Clinical Oncology (ASCO) to conclude that tamoxifen does reduce the incidence of newly diagnosed breast cancer in high-risk women.[124]

Tamoxifen in the breast cancer treatment setting is considered well tolerated and safe. However, for use in otherwise normal women, infrequent side effects and toxicity become more important. Up to 40% of women who start tamoxifen do not continue it because of perceived side effects, including depression and mood changes.[125, 126] Tamoxifen belongs to the class of agents called SERMs. Agents in this class exert antiestrogenic effects on tissues such as breast but estrogenic effects on other tissues such as uterus and liver. These various actions of the SERMs must be factored in when estimating risks and benefits in the setting of breast cancer prevention.

To compare risks and benefits in a meaningful way, the NSABP data are expressed as the number of women per 100 with a specific benefit or adverse event after 5 years of study. With respect to benefits, new invasive breast cancers were prevented in 1.7 of 100 women, noninvasive cancers in 0.67, and bone fractures in 0.50, for a total of 2.87 in 100 benefited after 5 years. Risks of tamoxifen are primarily related to its estrogenic effects on the uterus, a prothrombotic effect, and adverse effects on the lens of the eye. To estimate actual risks validly for a patient, one must correct for the underlying risks in the population under study. For that reason, analysis of adverse events includes determination of attributable risk[97] and involves subtracting the underlying rate from the total observed with tamoxifen. This analysis indicates an excess of 1.5 of 100 women who experienced cataracts, 0.69 with endometrial cancer (nearly exclusively in postmenopausal women), 0.27 with cerebrovascular accident (CVA), 0.25 with deep venous thrombosis (DVT), and 0.23 with pulmonary embolus, or a total of 2.94 per 100.[5] The new endometrial cancers were exclusively stage I and pulmonary emboli nonfatal. Neither risk nor benefit was observed regarding cardiovascular effects,[127] but the number of patients was not sufficient for statistical significance.

The increased incidence of uterine cancer in patients receiving tamoxifen presents a clinical management problem. Substantial study has been addressing how best to detect this cancer early.[128–130]

Transvaginal ultrasonography was initially proposed as a means of assessing both endometrial hyperplasia, as a precursor lesion, and early cancer. A prospective study demonstrated a mean increase in endometrial thickness from 3.5 ± 1.1 to 9.2 ± 5.1 mm in response to 5 years of tamoxifen. In 20% of women, endometrial thickness exceeded 10 mm or appeared suspicious for neoplasm. In this subset of women, biopsies revealed atrophy in 73%, polyps in 17%, and hyperplasia in 7.7% but endometrial cancer in only one patient.[129] The findings of this study and others[128–130] suggested that endometrial thickness does not usually indicate hyperplasia but, rather, the presence of edema and dilated myometrial glands.[129] It should be noted that nonprospective studies reported a higher prevalence of benign polyps (5% to 55%) and hyperplasia (8% to 16%),[131–134] but these are likely to be overestimates resulting from selection bias.

On the basis of these studies, recommendations for screening include a yearly gynecologic examination with reservation of endometrial sampling and ultrasonography for patients with signs of abnormal vaginal bleeding.[129, 130]

Guidelines for Breast Cancer Prevention

Premenopausal women with a 5-year risk of breast cancer greater than 1.67% are candidates for tamoxifen unless they are at increased risk for DVT or pulmonary emboli. Postmenopausal women are candidates for this approach if they no longer have a uterus and lack a predisposing risk for DVT or pulmonary emboli. The decision to take tamoxifen should be made by the patient in partnership with her health care provider and based on a full discussion of individual risks and benefits expressed in absolute and not relative terms.[124, 124a]

Critical Assessment of Breast Cancer Prevention Strategies

Estimates indicate that between 20 and 100 women (depending on underlying risk) must be treated to prevent one breast cancer. Clinical decisions depend on analysis of risk/benefit ratios and should be made after full discussion between health care provider and patient.[135] Regarding efficacy, available data demonstrate a reduction in newly diagnosed breast cancers. It is too early to assess overall survival. It is not known whether tamoxifen prevents breast cancer, cures some preexisting subclinical cancers, or delays the onset of small tumors. Mathematical modeling techniques suggest that the "preventive effects" are equally divided between blockade of growth of occult tumors and prevention of new ones.[136] Tumors whose growth was blocked by tamoxifen during 5 years of administration might be expected to regrow later. For this reason, data on overall survival (to be available from ongoing European studies) are critically important.[124]

Because reports indicate that both tamoxifen and raloxifene prevent breast cancer, it is expected that many women will ask their physicians about these two agents. The use of raloxifene exclusively for breast cancer prevention is not currently recommended. Although the MORE study demonstrated a reduction of breast cancers diagnosed in women taking raloxifene, breast cancer prevention was not a primary end point.[122, 137] The ongoing STAR (Study of Tamoxifen and Raloxifene) trial is currently testing the efficacy of tamoxifen versus raloxifene for breast cancer prevention.[138]

Future studies are needed that utilize additional factors to select women at higher risk for development of breast cancer. A study of raloxifene examined women with factors suggesting high long-term exposure to estrogen (i.e., increased bone mineral density, high BMI, and high plasma estradiol levels). Results indicated that raloxifene was more effective in preventing breast cancer in women with high, long-term estrogen exposure than in those with low exposure (94% versus 56% for BMD; 82% versus 64% for BMI; and 77% versus 55% for estradiol levels, $P < .005$).[139]

Treatment of Established Breast Cancers

In the year 2000, there were 184,000 new cases of breast cancer diagnosed in the United States and 41,000 deaths. The mechanisms whereby estradiol stimulates breast cancer growth are complex and involve direct regulation of genes involved in control of proliferation and apoptosis, induction of growth factors through secondary actions, and cross-talk between growth factor and estrogen pathways at both upstream and downstream levels.[14, 16, 17, 140–145] Nongenomic effects of estradiol on mitogenic pathways may also be involved.[146–147a] Treatment strategies utilize agents that abrogate the effects of estrogen on these pathways and thus inhibit growth and induce apoptosis.

Common approaches involve blockade of estrogen action with antiestrogens or estrogen synthesis with aromatase inhibitors or gonadotropin-releasing hormone (GnRH) superagonist analogues.[148] Patients who initially respond to hormonal therapy eventually have relapses. The biologic mechanisms for this phenomenon are not fully understood. A standard situation is that responders to the first-line treatment benefit from secondary and tertiary hormonal therapies upon relapse. The sequential responses to hormonal therapies suggest an adaptive process whereby tumors do not become totally resistant to hormonal therapy but develop a transitional state in which alternative means of blocking hormonal pathways cause tumor regression.[149]

Patients who have relapses after oophorectomy or tamoxifen treatment commonly respond secondarily to inhibitors of estrogen production (aromatase inhibitors) or, rarely, to the withdrawal of tamoxifen.[148] A hypothesis to explain this phenomenon is that these tumors become hypersensitive to lower amounts of circulating estrogen or to the estrogen agonist properties of tamoxifen.[150] Experimental support for this concept comes from observations in xenograft models and in vitro studies. Breast tumor xenografts adapt to long-term exposure to tamoxifen by responding to it as an estrogen rather than as an antiestrogen. Under these circumstances, the pure antiestrogen ICI 182,780 (fluvestrant [Faslodex]) caused tumor regression.[151] In an in vitro model system, long-term deprivation of estradiol rendered breast cancer cells hypersensitive to the proliferative effects of this sex steroid.[152] This adaptive process is associated with increments in mitogen-activated protein (MAP) kinase, an enzyme that stimulates cell proliferation.[150, 153] The hypersensitivity concept may explain secondary responses to aromatase inhibitors in patients who have relapses after oophorectomy or tamoxifen and secondary responses to the pure antiestrogen Faslodex.

Development of Hormonal Resistance

Women respond to each hormonal therapy on average for 12 to 18 months and then experience relapse.[148] At some time in their course, tumors become totally resistant to further hormonal therapy. Several explanations for development of resistance have been suggested, including[154–157]:

1. Changes in metabolism of tamoxifen with production of estrogenic metabolites.
2. Constitutive increase in growth factor production as a result of additional oncogene mutations.
3. Enhanced growth factor receptor functionality.
4. Down-regulation of transcriptional corepressors.
5. Outgrowth or selection of hormone-resistant clones of tumors cells.
6. Other adaptive mechanisms.

Prognostic Factors

Clinical decision making requires knowledge of the degree of aggressiveness and natural history of the diagnosed breast cancer. Numerous histologic types occur, and pathologic features provide information related to the prognosis. Much attention has been directed toward multivariate and neural network analysis to calculate the precise prognosis in individual women. In general, these methods have not been particularly useful in practical decision making and individual factors are used in treatment algorithms.[158–160]

Figure 39–7 illustrates the prognostic power of various biologic factors by comparing the effects of individual parameters on 5-year survival.[158–161] The most powerful prognostic parameters are related to tumor size, invasiveness, nodal status, histologic grade and type, and hormone and human epidermal growth factor receptor 2 (HER2)/neu receptor status (see Fig. 39–7). Other less useful prognostic characteristics include DNA labeling index (LI), percent S phase, percent PCNA or Ki67 positivity (markers of proliferation), degree of aneuploidy, and overexpression of certain oncogenes or coactivators (e.g., D1 cyclin, A1B1, MAP kinase, Ras, HER3 and HER4, heregulin, c-Src, and ODC [ornithine decarboxylase] levels).[141, 142, 144, 145, 162–164]

Finally, tumors diagnosed in postmenopausal women receiving HRT have a lower histologic grade and a 10% better prognosis than those in women not receiving HRT.[160, 165, 166]

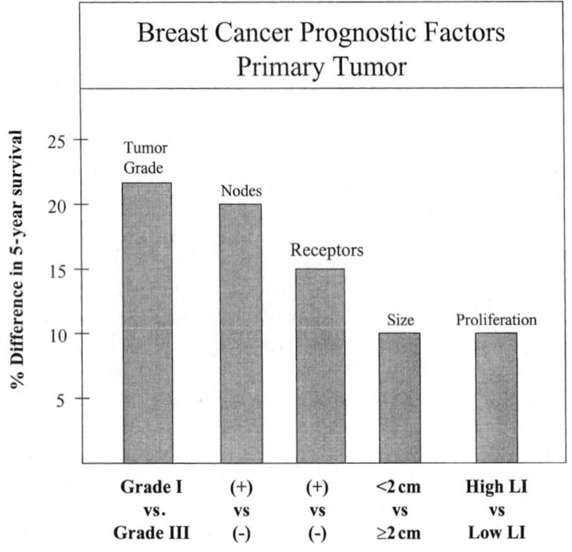

Figure 39–7. Prognostic value of several parameters related to patients with an initial diagnosis of breast cancer. All values are presented as the percent difference in survival at the 5-year interval. This method of presentation allows one to determine the increased number of women per 100 who will be alive at 5 years if they have a favorable prognostic factor compared with those with an unfavorable factor. LI, labeling index.

Predictive Factors

Certain other biologic parameters allow assessment of the potential effectiveness of certain therapies. Older age, long disease-free survival, high degree of tumor differentiation, and prior response to endocrine therapy predict a higher likelihood of responses to hormonal therapy.[148] The ability to measure receptors markedly improves the process of selection of patients for hormonal therapy. Absence of estrogen receptor (ER) in the tumor predicts that fewer than 5% to 10% of women will respond to hormonal therapy. If both ER and progesterone receptor (PR) are negative, an even lower percentage respond. Patients with both ER-positive and PR-positive tumors respond to hormonal therapy 50% to 75% of the time, whereas 30% to 50% of patients with ER-positive but PR-negative tumors are responsive.[148, 167] Preliminary but conflicting data suggest that patients with ER- and PR-positive tumors respond to hormonal therapy less frequently if HER2/neu is positive.[167–171]

Receptor measurements are commonly performed by immunocytochemical analysis, which correlates well with ligand-binding assays.[172] Immunocytochemical techniques measure only ER alpha and not ER beta, but 76% of ER alpha–positive tumors also contain ER beta (S. Fuqua, personal communication, 2001). Currently, it is not clear whether measurement of ER beta would provide important clinical information. Data suggest that certain tumors make ER beta variant proteins that can heterodimerize with full-length ER alpha or beta and exert dominant negative effects.[173] This concept suggests that further refinement of receptor assays may improve their predictive value.

Predictive parameters for chemotherapy are more limited. Measurement of HER2/neu content predicts responses to trastuzumab (Herceptin), an antibody directed against HER2/neu.[174] Preliminary data suggest that this also predicts which ER-positive patients will not respond to hormonal therapy.[167–171] A concept proposed many years ago was that ER-negative tumors responded better to chemotherapy than ER-positive tumors because of the more rapid proliferation rate of ER-negative tumors. Although originally controversial, meta-analyses now demonstrate the positive predictive value of a negative ER for chemotherapy.[175]

Hormonal Therapies for Breast Cancer: Mechanism of Action

Surgical Ablative Therapies

Historically, the initial approaches to hormonal therapy involved surgical removal of endocrine glands responsible for synthesis of estrogen or its precursors. In 1896, Beatson first demonstrated that oophorectomy caused regression of breast cancer in premenopausal women; comprehensive studies later documented responses in one third of patients.[148] The availability of glucocorticoid replacement therapy in the 1940s enabled the use of adrenalectomy or hypophysectomy. These maneuvers produced similar rates of response as a result of a reduction in estradiol levels and perhaps also of pituitary factors in the case of hypophysectomy. The development of medical means to block hormone synthesis or action has largely replaced adrenalectomy and hypophysectomy but surgical oophorectomy persists.[148]

Hormone Additive Therapies

Clinicians learned from empirical observations that high doses of estrogen, androgen, or progestins caused tumor regression.[148, 176] The mechanism whereby estrogens paradoxically inhibit tumor growth is unknown. This therapy is most effective in women who experienced menopause several years previously. A subsequent study suggested that high-dose estrogen might trigger a wave of apoptotic cell death in breast tumors as a mechanism of action.[177] With respect to androgens, a variety of observations suggest that an increased ratio of androgens to estrogens exerts an antagonistic effect on breast tissue. Progestins have glucocorticoid actions that suppress circulating estrogen levels and can also act through progestogenic mechanisms.[178]

Medical Ablative Therapies

Medical means of ablating hormone secretion or action avoid the need for major surgery and can effectively replicate the hormonal and clinical effects of these procedures. High doses of GnRH agonist analogues suppress ovarian function to the same extent as surgical oophorectomy.[179–182] Physiologically, the pituitary requires pulsatile exposure to GnRH to maintain gonadotropin secretion. GnRH agonists suppress luteinizing hormone (LH) and follicle-stimulating hormone by exposing the pituitary to a continuous GnRH stimulus that causes a paradoxical gonadotropin inhibition. Preparations lasting 3 to 4 months can be given by intramuscular injection. For the first several days after initiation of therapy, an increase in LH, follicle-stimulating hormone, and estradiol occurs, but thereafter these hormones fall to suppressed levels.[183]

Antiestrogens with Mixed Agonist-Antagonistic Actions

Blockade of estrogen action rather than synthesis provides an additional strategy. These agents, called antiestrogens, exert effects similar to those of surgical oophorectomy in premenopausal women and hypophysectomy or adrenalectomy in postmenopausal women. Tamoxifen, the initial antiestrogen of this type, was introduced for use in the United States in the mid-1970s.[148] Early clinical observations indicated that this drug has an antiestrogen effect on breast tissue but an estrogen agonist effect on uterus, vagina, bone, pituitary gland, and liver.[148]

Attempts to determine the divergent actions of tamoxifen led to an understanding of the complexity of ER-mediated transcriptional regulation and actions of the antiestrogens. Tamoxifen binds to both ER alpha and ER beta in the ligand binding domain (AF 2) of the receptor, which then facilitates the binding of the antiestrogen-ER complex to specific estrogen response elements on DNA.[157, 184–190] Conformational changes in the ER binding pocket at helix 12 induced by antiestrogens interfere with binding of coactivators to the ER but rather facilitate binding of corepressors to this area. The continued presence of corepressor in the complex is thought to explain the antiestrogenic properties of tamoxifen. The relative amounts of corepressor and coactivator in certain tissues and the presence of other unknown factors determine whether tamoxifen acts as an agonist or antagonist.[173] Additional estrogenic effects are mediated by nongenomic actions at the cell membrane as well as by protein-protein interactions with c-Jun, specificity protein 1 (SP-1), insulin-like growth factor receptor, phosphatidylinositol-3-kinase (PI-3-kinase), HER2/neu, c-Src, and potentially other factors.[189, 191, 192]

On the basis of the SERM concept, other agents have been introduced or are being developed to enhance breast antagonistic and bone agonistic properties.[193, 194] One of these, toremifene, is quite similar to tamoxifen although slightly less effective as an agonist to bone.[194] Raloxifene, however, appears not to stimulate the uterus or cause endometrial cancer and yet is an antiestrogen to breast. This agent is under trial as a breast cancer preventive drug but has not been extensively tested for treatment of breast cancer.[195–198] Preliminary results for other agents have been reported.[196–199]

Pure Antagonist Antiestrogens

Clinical and experimental data suggested that long-term exposure to tamoxifen might induce tumors to undergo adaptive mechanisms to cause the agonistic properties of this SERM to predominate. On the basis of these observations, antiestrogens were developed that were devoid of agonist properties. Faslodex, the prototype drug, increases the rate of degradation of the ER and also inhibits estradiol-mediated transcription by favoring binding of corepressors to the Faslodex-ER complex.[200–202]

Inhibitors of Estradiol Synthesis

Aromatase catalyzes the rate-limiting step in the conversion of androgens to estrogens.[203] Aromatase has been a key target for development of inhibitors over the past 25 years.[148] The first-generation inhibitor aminoglutethimide inhibited aromatase by 90% in postmenopausal women and was as effective as tamoxifen in causing breast tumor regressions.[204–206] However, it blocked cortisol production and induced significant side effects. The efficacy of aminoglutethimide in postmenopausal women served as an impetus to develop second-generation and third-generation inhibitors.[148, 204, 205]

Three third-generation agents (anastrozole, letrozole, and exemestane) are now approved drugs in the United States and Europe.[203, 207–222] These agents are 100-fold to 10,000-fold more potent than aminoglutethimide and are called selective aromatase inhibitors because they do not inhibit other enzymatic steps. The two major subclasses are nonsteroidal competitive inhibitors and steroidal enzyme inactivators.[203] The competitive inhibitors bind to the active site of the enzyme with high affinity and compete with substrate. Aromatase inactivators bind covalently to the enzyme and permanently destroy its activity. Theoretically, the inactivators could have advantages over the competitive aromatase inhibitors because inhibition might continue if one missed one or more doses of medication and the degree of blockade could theoretically be superior.

Both classes of drugs reduce aromatase to 1% to 10% of baseline activity,[223–228] substantially reduce plasma estradiol levels, and suppress tissue concentrations of this steroid in breast tumors (Fig. 39–8). The greater degree of suppression with the third-generation inhibitors may explain their enhanced efficacy in causing tumor regression compared with first-generation inhibitors.[229, 230] Because they lack estrogen agonistic properties, aromatase inhibitors do not increase the incidence of endometrial cancer, as occurs with tamoxifen. If they are used for long periods, one would expect acceleration of bone loss and perhaps cardiovascular disease as a result of total body aromatase inhibition. Studies evaluating these effects are ongoing. Preliminary data do not show adverse effects on lipid concentrations.[208]

Chemical Castration

Chemotherapeutic agents destroy granulosa cells in the ovary and result in transient or permanent amenorrhea in pre-

parameters with objective response rates of 30% versus 20%, clinical benefit of 49% versus 38%, and median time to treatment failure of 9 versus 5.8 months ($P < .0001$ by log rank test).[220]

Pooled data indicate that tamoxifen was associated with DVT and pulmonary emboli (7.6% versus 4.5%) significantly more frequently than anastrozole.[213] If one combines observations from all three trials, it appears that nausea, hot flashes, and gastrointestinal distress were comparable with either agent. A fourth but smaller study (238 patients) involving only ER-positive patients also demonstrated superiority of anastrozole over tamoxifen ($P = .05$).[221]

Taken together, these trials provide evidence that the third-generation aromatase inhibitors are superior in efficacy and toxicity to tamoxifen in the advanced disease setting. Letrozole and anastrozole have now been approved in the United States as first-line therapy for breast cancer. These three large aromatase inhibitor trials showed for the first time in a head-to-head randomized trial that one endocrine therapy is superior to another. Before these studies, it was thought that the available endocrine therapies produced similar rates of response and could be distinguished only on the basis of side effects and cost. Direct comparisons of letrozole and anastrozole are now needed to determine whether one agent is superior to the other. This is particularly important because hormonal data suggest that letrozole may be more potent as an aromatase inhibitor than anastrozole.[228a]

At present, the choice of aromatase inhibitors over tamoxifen as first-line therapy for advanced disease is warranted but based on incomplete data. Comparisons of tamoxifen with the first-generation aromatase inhibitor aminoglutethimide demonstrated equal efficacy but a different pattern of cross-resistance.[148] The aromatase inhibitors were efficacious if used after tamoxifen; in contrast, tamoxifen, when used after the aromatase inhibitors, appeared less effective. If this were true for the third-generation aromatase inhibitors, one might still wish to use tamoxifen as the first-line agent. However, preliminary data suggest that tamoxifen is effective after crossover from the aromatase inhibitor anastrozole.[209] In a crossover comparison, 51% of 98 patients experienced clinical benefit from tamoxifen when used as a second-line agent after initial use of letrozole. By comparison, second-line letrozole after initial tamoxifen produced clinical benefit in 66% of 61 patients.

The aromatase inactivator exemestane is currently being tested as a first-line agent for treatment of advanced breast cancer. Preliminary data for 122 patients showed 44.6% objective responses (complete response and partial response) with exemestane and 14.3% with tamoxifen.[252] Currently, exemestane is approved for clinical use in the United States as a second-line hormonal agent for treatment of breast cancer.[250, 251]

Hormone Additive Therapy

Androgens or estrogens are generally considered inferior to tamoxifen, aromatase inhibitors, and megestrol acetate. High-dose estrogen has been used sparingly since the advent of tamoxifen. However, a 20-year follow-up of a randomized comparison of tamoxifen with high-dose diethylstilbestrol (DES) reported a significant survival advantage in patients receiving the estrogen and lack of cross-resistance between these two therapeutic approaches. This surprising study suggests reconsideration of high-dose estrogen for selected patients.[253]

Surgical Oophorectomy

Although still used in both the adjuvant and advanced disease settings, surgical oophorectomy may be replaced by use of GnRH agonists. Laparoscopic oophorectomy, however, may make this a more attractive approach. Prophylactic oophorectomy represented the first adjuvant endocrine therapy for breast cancer. Although it was initially thought to be ineffective, meta-analyses demonstrate a clear benefit with a 6% absolute survival advantage at 15 years for patients younger than 50 years of age (Fig. 39–13).[254] Because the receptor status of the patients in these trials was unknown, a large fraction of receptor-negative patients were probably included. One would expect better results if only hormone receptor–positive patients were so treated.[254] In the advanced disease setting, surgical oophorectomy was clinically beneficial in approximately 50% of patients who were ER-positive or PR-positive, or both.[148]

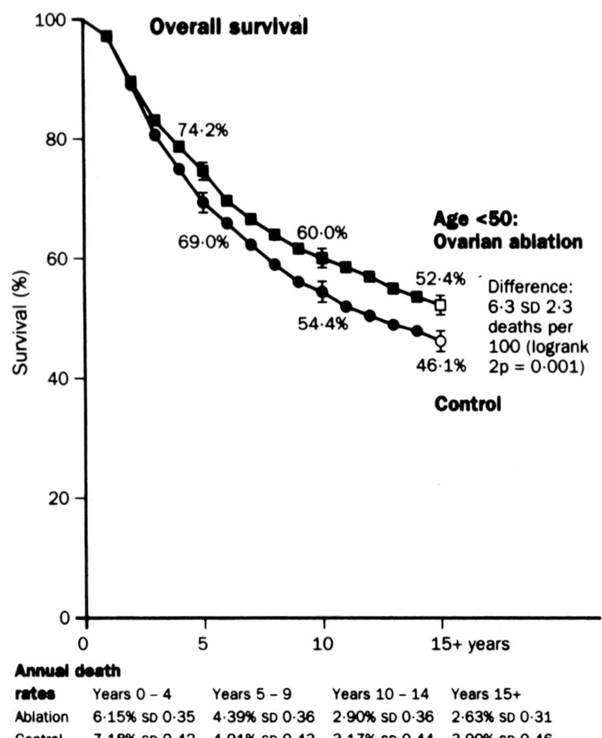

Figure 39–13. Survival data for patients undergoing a prophylactic oophorectomy in comparison with a group of women not receiving this therapy. (From Ovarian ablation in early breast cancer: overview of the randomized trials. Early Breast Cancer Trialists' Collaborative Group. Lancet 1996; 348:1189–1196. Reprinted with permission of the Lancet.)

Medical Oophorectomy

Emerging data support the use of medical oophorectomy in the adjuvant setting, and research emphasis focuses on this strategy. Demonstration of the effectiveness of prophylactic oophorectomy (see Fig. 39–13) was surprising to the medical community and led to reconsideration of this approach, although with use of GnRH agonists rather than surgery. The goal of these studies has been to determine the efficacy of medical oophorectomy in patients who are exclusively ER-positive. Two studies in the advanced setting indicated that the GnRH analogues produce clinical effects similar to those induced by surgical oophorectomy.[255, 256] Accordingly, one would expect similar effects in the adjuvant setting. Preliminary results from a four-arm trial suggested that this may be the case.[257] Benefit appeared to be greater in women younger than 45 years and with ER-positive tumors.

Further studies are required to determine whether the GnRH agonist approach is superior to the use of tamoxifen in this setting. Long-term studies have clearly shown the efficacy

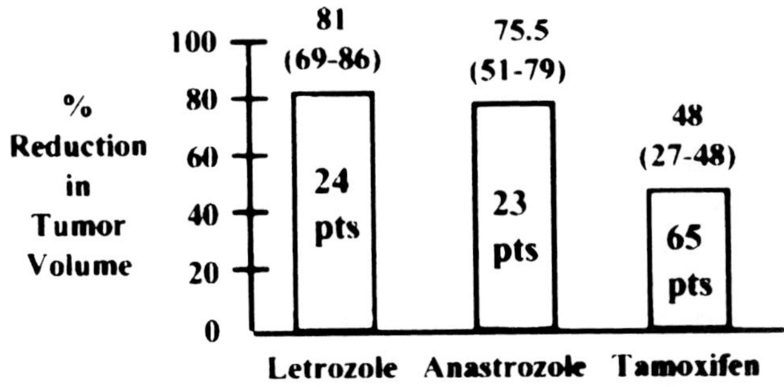

Figure 39–14. Percent reduction in tumor volume in response to either letrozole, anastrozole, or tamoxifen given for 3 months prior to the time of excisional surgery and used as neoadjuvant therapy. (From Dixon JM. Neoadjuvant endocrine therapy. In Miller WR, Santen RJ (eds). Aromatase Inhibition and Breast Cancer. New York, Marcel Dekker, 2001, p 109.)

of tamoxifen as adjuvant therapy.[175] Because four studies in the advanced disease setting suggested that tamoxifen is as effective as the GnRH agonists,[258] these analogues[259–261] may produce similar results in the adjuvant setting as well. Current studies are examining the use of GnRH agonists in comparison with chemotherapy in the adjuvant setting rather than with placebo (see "Chemical Castration"). Additional trials are needed to compare GnRH analogues with tamoxifen in this adjuvant setting.

Complete Estrogen Blockade

Medical oophorectomy alone has been compared with medical oophorectomy plus tamoxifen in the advanced disease setting. The rationale for the combined approach is to inhibit secretion of estradiol by the ovary and, at the same time, to block the action of residual estrogens of adrenal origin. This strategy, called complete estrogen blockade, appeared superior to tamoxifen alone in a single large trial and in a meta-analysis of four similar studies.[182, 256, 262] The combined approach resulted in more frequent objective responses as well as improved progression-free and overall survival. This strategy has not yet been studied in the adjuvant setting and particularly in comparison with chemotherapy. Because premenopausal women in the United States are usually treated first with adjuvant chemotherapy, the approach of complete estrogen blockade needs to be explored in this setting.[262, 262a]

Chemical Castration

Studies are ongoing to determine the mechanism of action of chemotherapy in premenopausal women. At least three possibilities exist: hormonal effects resulting from chemotherapeutic destruction of the ovary, direct cytotoxic effects on the tumor, or a combination of these two effects.

Eight trials have compared adjuvant chemotherapy with medical castration with and without tamoxifen in premenopausal women. The chemotherapy and hormonal therapies appeared to produce comparable antitumor effects.[257, 263–265, 269–271] However, trends suggest that chemotherapy is more effective than medical castration in ER-negative patients and that medical castration is superior in ER-positive patients.[271] These results suggest that at least part of the benefit of chemotherapy in premenopausal women results from chemical castration. These studies also provide further support for the benefit of medical oophorectomy in the adjuvant setting. The enhanced survival produced by chemotherapy compared with a placebo may be improved further by the effects of estradiol deprivation.

Further support for the medical castration hypothesis comes from studies showing that chemotherapy is less effective in patients without complete cessation of menses.[272, 273] Although effects of varying chemotherapeutic regimens on ovarian function differ, nearly 100% of women older than 40 years experience permanent amenorrhea after adjuvant chemotherapy (see Fig. 39–9).

From these data, it appears that comparisons of chemotherapy and endocrine therapy are not yet definitive. Further trials comparing medical oophorectomy alone with chemotherapy alone in receptor-positive, premenopausal patients are required. In the meantime, medical oophorectomy is a reasonable alternative to chemotherapy as adjuvant treatment for premenopausal women who are ER-positive or PR-positive, or both, and for various reasons are not candidates for chemotherapy.

Combination of Hormonal Therapy and Chemotherapy

On the basis of a meta-analysis, the combination of surgical or medical oophorectomy (GnRH agonists or tamoxifen) with chemotherapy provides additional benefit over chemotherapy alone in the adjuvant setting. The addition of the GnRH agonists might be particularly important for women younger than 40 years in whom estradiol remains in the premenopausal range after chemotherapy, as suggested by one trial.[232]

New Approaches to Adjuvant Endocrine Therapy

Aromatase inhibitors may provide a means to block estrogen effectively without the emergence of estrogen agonistic effects in the adjuvant setting. Detrimental effects on vaginal mucosa, bone density, and cholesterol levels could result from deprivation of estradiol.

A large ongoing trial is comparing tamoxifen alone, anastrozole alone, and the combination (Anastrazole and Tamoxifen Alone and in Combination [ATAC] trial). Preliminary data demonstrate statistically significant superiority of anastrozole with respect to recurrence-free survival and to number of new contralateral tumors.[232a] Subanalyses will compare potential detrimental effects on estrogen target organs such as bone, uterus, and liver. Other ongoing trials are examining sequential regimens with 2 to 5 years of tamoxifen and 2 to 5 years of an aromatase inhibitor with comparison of various inhibitors, dosages, and sequences. These results should be available in 3 to 5 years and should be helpful in suggesting optimal regimens.

Emerging Therapies

The concept of neoadjuvant chemotherapy has been adopted in clinical practice, and neoadjuvant hormonal therapy is now undergoing clinical trials. The rationale is to decrease tumor size before surgery to allow breast conservation. This type of therapy is selected for patients with tumors larger than 2 cm.

A nonrandomized trial demonstrated an 81% reduction in tumor volume with letrozole versus 75% with anastrozole and 48% with tamoxifen (Fig. 39–14).[274–276] A randomized trial involving 324 patients compared letrozole at 2.5 mg daily with tamoxifen at 20 mg daily in women with ER-positive tumors larger than 2 cm.[275] Letrozole resulted in a 55% rate of objective response (CR and PR) compared with 36% for tamoxifen ($P < .001$). Breast-conserving surgery was chosen by 45% of patients receiving letrozole and 35% receiving tamoxifen ($P < .001$). Approximately half of the patients experienced a sufficient reduction in size of the tumor to allow lumpectomy. Comparison of groups of patients treated conventionally and

Hormonal Treatment Sequence

Adjuvant Therapy	
Pre-menopausal	Post-menopausal
Chemotherapy + Antiestrogen	Antiestrogen with Consideration of chemotherapy

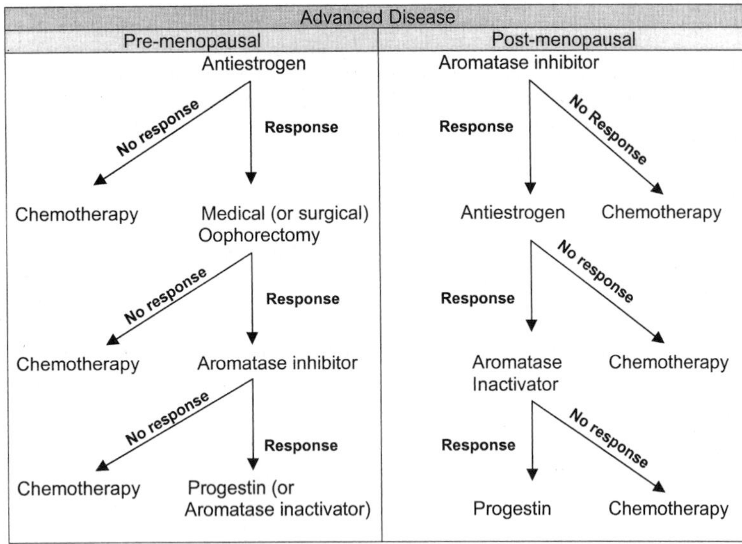

Figure 39–15. Decision-making algorithm for breast cancer. Top, Approach to adjuvant hormonal therapy in premenopausal and postmenopausal women. Bottom, Sequence of therapies for advanced disease in women still considered to have hormone-dependent breast cancer and with estrogen and/or progesterone receptor positive tumors (see text). (From Goss PE, Strasser K. Aromatase inhibitors I in the treatment and prevention of breast cancer. J Clin 2001; 19: 881–894.[280])

with neoadjuvant endocrine therapy is required before recommendations regarding this approach are warranted.

Recommended Approaches to Hormonal Treatment of Breast Cancer

Adjuvant Therapy

Premenopausal Women

Current opinion recommends chemotherapy for premenopausal women with ER-positive tumors and the addition of tamoxifen for 5 years (Fig. 39–15), a meta-analysis demonstrated statistically significant prolongation of survival with a combination of tamoxifen plus chemotherapy versus chemotherapy alone.[175] Medical oophorectomy with or without tamoxifen could be considered as an alternative for women adverse to chemotherapy.[182, 233, 256]

Postmenopausal Women

Tamoxifen is the preferred adjuvant therapy for postmenopausal women with tumors larger than 1 cm that are ER-positive or PR-positive, or both. For some women, chemotherapy in combination with or followed by tamoxifen may be chosen. In younger postmenopausal women with more aggressive tumors, chemotherapy may be preferred but clinical trial data regarding this are incomplete. Information obtained from meta-analyses suggests that the combination of chemotherapy and tamoxifen may be preferable to use of tamoxifen alone, and this approach is often chosen.[232] Early studies showed adverse drug-drug interactions between melphalan (L-Pam) and tamoxifen. However, this does not occur with CMF (cyclophosphamide [Cytoxan], methotrexate, fluorouracil) and CAF (Cytoxan, doxorubicin [Adriamycin], fluorouracil) regimens[277] and chemotherapy and tamoxifen can thus be given concomitantly.[175] The main consideration is whether the modest benefit accrued by adding chemotherapy is worth the additional toxicity encountered.

Small Tumors in Premenopausal and Postmenopausal Women

No randomized trial has examined the use of tamoxifen in women with tumors 1 cm or smaller in size. However, pooled data from four NSABP[278, 279] trials indicate a 4% absolute benefit in disease-free status and a 5% survival benefit for this group of women when given tamoxifen. Individual decisions are made on the basis of risk-benefit analysis, and not all women are offered this therapy.

Ductal Carcinoma in Situ

Adjuvant tamoxifen appears to provide benefit for women with noninvasive tumors (i.e., DCIS).[119] In a large NSABP clinical trial, 13% of women treated with lumpectomy, irradiation, and placebo experienced a new tumor event over 5 years. One third of these new events involved appearance of a contralateral breast cancer, one third a new ipsilateral tumor, and one third local recurrence of the original tumors. Tamoxifen reduced these events in absolute terms by 5% with equal benefit in reducing new contralateral, ipsilateral, and original tumor events. Risk-benefit analysis is also required to advise patients appropriately; benefit is not judged to outweigh risks in all patients.

Decision Making

(See Fig. 39–15.) An overview of these data suggests that all women with tumors that are ER-positive or PR-positive, or both, are potential candidates for tamoxifen as adjuvant therapy. In order to make a decision, one must determine whether the benefits of tamoxifen outweigh the risks in individual patients. From the NSABP prevention trial, the absolute risks of tamoxifen are known and include uterine cancer, cataracts,

DVT, pulmonary emboli, and cerebrovascular accident.[5] Presence of a uterus, a history of DVT or pulmonary embolus, or existing cataract would enhance these risks. Presence of larger or invasive tumors would enhance the absolute benefits of tamoxifen.

In general, most women with invasive tumors larger than 1 cm should be advised to take tamoxifen. Those with small or noninvasive tumors should be counseled on the basis of risk-benefit ratios. Those without a prior history of a thromboembolic event or cataract and with prior hysterectomy might be advised to take tamoxifen, particularly if they also have osteopenia. Raloxifene has not been used in the adjuvant setting and would not be advised for the patients discussed here.[124]

Treatment of Advanced Disease

The majority of women who have advanced disease had previously received tamoxifen as adjuvant therapy. Those experiencing tumor recurrence while receiving tamoxifen or within 1 year of its cessation are considered resistant to this antiestrogen. For them, other hormonal therapies are chosen. In the other group of women, tumors recur more than 1 year after cessation of tamoxifen, and these patients are candidates for an additional course of tamoxifen. An algorithm can then be used to choose hormonal therapy for women considered candidates for tamoxifen (see Fig. 39–15). For those resistant to tamoxifen, the next therapy in the sequential approach can be utilized.

Premenopausal Women

Aromatase inhibitors do not effectively inhibit ovarian estrogen production in premenopausal women, and tamoxifen (or toremifene) is usually considered first-line therapy for recurrent tumors. On the basis of current data, this might be combined with a GnRH analogue. If the initial therapy is tamoxifen alone, medical oophorectomy with use of a GnRH agonist analogue as second-line therapy would be recommended. Surgical oophorectomy can be substituted for the GnRH analogue.[182, 256] Aromatase inhibitors can be used if the GnRH analogue is continued. Megestrol acetate is then advised as additional therapy.

Postmenopausal Women

Data from trials comparing aromatase inhibitors with tamoxifen as first-line therapy for advanced disease suggest that aromatase inhibitors be considered the first choice of endocrine therapy.[217, 218, 220] Responders would be treated with tamoxifen as second-line therapy upon relapse, but nonresponders would be treated with chemotherapy.[280] Third-line therapy would utilize megestrol acetate and fourth-line therapy the aromatase inactivator exemestane. After this, high-dose estrogen or androgens might be chosen. If rapidly progressive disease develops at any time in this sequence, chemotherapy may be chosen instead of the next endocrine therapy.

Chemotherapy

The detailed management of breast diseases with chemotherapy has been addressed in the work of Ellis and colleagues.[167]

Long-Term Quality of Life in Breast Cancer Survivors

With earlier diagnosis of breast cancer, an increasing percentage of women survive breast cancer in the long term. Two thirds of these women are menopausal at the time of diagnosis, and half of the premenopausal women undergo permanent ovarian failure as a result of chemotherapy.[231] HRT is generally thought to be contraindicated in these women because estrogens may cause regrowth of residual tumor tissue after surgery or cause a second primary.[281, 282] Data from observational studies, however, do not provide evidence of a deleterious effect.[281] Study of the safety of HRT in this setting is currently undergoing testing in a moderately large group of women in the Habits trial (a large, multi-institutional Scandinavian and European trial coordinated by Dr. Lars Hølmberg, Uppsala University, Sweden).[283] Until the results are available, it is prudent to avoid estrogens in breast cancer survivors if alternatives to estrogen are effective.[282]

As reviewed previously, effective agents are available to substitute for estrogen,[284] including the following:

1. Bisphosphonates to prevent or treat osteoporosis.
2. Statins to prevent heart disease.
3. Selective serotonin reuptake inhibitors (SSRIs) to diminish the number and severity of hot flashes.
4. Low-dose vaginal estrogen for symptoms of urogenital atrophy.
5. SSRIs for depression thought to be related to estrogen deficiency.

Alternatives to HRT would not protect against Alzheimer's disease or improve cognitive function; however, the benefits of estrogen to protect against Alzheimer's disease have not been proven in randomized prospective studies and estrogens have not shown cognitive benefit in patients with Alzheimer's disease. Yet, estradiol does provide cognitive benefit in non-Alzheimer's patients.[285–287] Some women, then, might wish to consider the use of HRT to prevent Alzheimer's disease or improve cognitive function. If alternatives to estrogen are not satisfactory, women could receive HRT after a full discussion of the risks and benefits and with the informed consent of the patient.

Breast Cancer in Men

The incidence of breast cancer in men is 100-fold lower than in women with 1400 new cases in 2000 and 400 deaths. Risk factors include clinical disorders associated with reduced testosterone production or estrogen excess such as orchitis, undescended testes, testicular injury, Klinefelter's syndrome, chronic liver disease, and gynecomastia.[288] The breast cancer susceptibility genes *BRCA1* and *BRCA2* are also believed to increase the risk in men.[289] Breast cancer is suspected when a subareolar or upper outer quadrant, firm painless lesion is palpated. A diagnosis is then made by mammography and biopsy of the lesion. Most tumors are ER-positive, and patients are then treated by mastectomy and adjuvant tamoxifen. Later therapy may include aromatase inhibitors or progestins.[290]

ENDOMETRIAL CANCER

Etiology

Approximately 36,000 new cases of endometrial cancer occur annually in the United States, and 6500 die of this disease.[291] Risk factors are related to conditions causing overexposure to endogenous or exogenous estrogen. Enhanced tumor initiation and promotion mediated by the proliferative effects of estrogen occur as with breast cancer (see earlier). Progestins are antimitogenic to the endometrium, as opposed to breast tissue, and result in a decreased rate of cell proliferation. Thus, unopposed estrogen increases the risk of endometrial cancer and progestins reduce that risk.[292–295]

Continued stimulation of the endometrium without progestin-induced endometrial shedding causes an increase in the cell proliferation rate and a concomitant increase in genetic mutations. The mutations that are not repaired accumulate and ultimately result in neoplastic growth. With prolonged stimulation of the endometrial lining, typical hyperplasia occurs first, followed by atypical adenomatous hyperplasia, a premalignant lesion. It is thought that 30% of such lesions later progress to frank cancer.[296] Animal studies suggest that carcinogenic metabolites of estradiol may contribute to development of endometrial cancer in a fashion similar to that for breast cancer.[267, 297]

Several clinical states are characterized by increased estradiol production and anovulation, a state in which the proliferative effects of estrogen are not opposed by the antimitotic effects of progesterone. One of these involves *exogenous obesity*. As the number of adipocytes increases, the amount of aromatase enzyme increases proportionately.[6, 298] With a normal amount of androgenic substrate, estradiol production increases as a function of the amount of enzyme present and in proportion to the degree of obesity.

Polycystic ovarian syndrome is associated with increases in estrone levels and lack of cyclic increments in progesterone as a result of absence of the luteal phase of the cycle. The syndrome is associated with decreased sex steroid–binding globulin and, presumably, an increase in the free fraction of estradiol and an increased rate of conversion of androgens to estrogens (i.e., aromatase excess). Estrogen-producing ovarian and adrenal tumors are also conditions of unopposed estrogen and an increased incidence of endometrial cancer.[299] Other risk factors for endometrial cancer include nulliparity, late menopause, radiation to the pelvis, diabetes, hypertension, and estrogen-producing ovarian and adrenal tumors.[300, 301]

In postmenopausal women, HRT with estrogen, unopposed by a progestin, increases the relative risk of endometrial cancer by twofold to fourfold, depending on the duration of use.[292–295] This risk increases over time; the relative risk is 1.30 for 2 years of use of unopposed estrogen, 2.22 for 2 to 5 years, and 4.49 for 5 to 10 years.[292, 293, 295] Progestins reduce this risk by opposing the mitogenic effects of estrogen on the endometrium and reducing the proliferative stimulus.

Treatment

Three regimens of HRT have been used: combined continuous estrogen plus progestin, sequential addition of progestin for 10 or more days each month, and sequential addition for less than 10 days, usually 5 to 7 days. The combined continuous regimen reduces the risk of endometrial carcinoma substantially, if not completely.

Pike and colleagues[293] reported a relative risk of 1.07 (95% confidence limits 0.80 to 1.43) for combined continuous estrogen plus progesterone but a nonsignificant trend of increased risk for more than 5 years of use (relative risk 1.34, no confidence limits given). For sequential use of a progestin for 10 or more days each month and use for less than 5 years, there was no increase in endometrial cancer risk[293] (Pike and colleagues,[293] relative risk 1.07, 95% CI 0.82 to 1.41; Beresford and co-workers,[294] relative risk 0.7, 95% CI 0.4 to 1.4).[294] There is a trend, however, for an increase in endometrial cancer with longer term use of this continuous regimen. Beresford and co-workers[294] reported a relative risk of 2.7 (95% CI 1.2 to 6.0) for current users of this regimen for more than 5 years, whereas Pike's group[293] reported a relative risk of 1.09 (nonsignificant).

Caution should be advised concerning long-term use of such regimens. Sequential regimens in which a progestin is administered for less than 10 days are associated with an increase in risk of endometrial cancer. Pike and colleagues[293] reported an increase in relative risk of 1.87 per 5 years of use (95% CI 1.33 to 2.65), and Beresford and co-workers[294] reported a relative risk of 2.1 (0.9 to 4.7) for less than 5 years of use and 4.8 (95% CI 2.0 to 11.0) for more than 5 years of use. Taken together, these data suggest that progestins do not protect against estrogen-induced endometrial cancer unless taken continuously. In premenopausal women, oral contraceptives containing both estrogen and a progestin decrease the risk. Multiple pregnancies also increase the duration of exposure to large amounts of progesterone and decrease the risk of endometrial cancer.

Use of tamoxifen as adjuvant therapy for breast cancer or prevention is associated with an increased risk of endometrial cancer as well as hyperplasia and polyps (see earlier). It is interesting that raloxifene, another SERM, did not cause an increase in endometrial cancer in a large study monitoring this as a safety parameter.[122] Animal studies with raloxifene suggested that this SERM does not exert estrogen agonistic effects on the uterus, whereas tamoxifen does.[302]

Endocrinology of Endometrial Cancer

Most endometrial cancers contain appreciable levels of ER, whereas only differentiated ones generally have PRs.[303] Tumors resulting from estrogen replacement therapy are generally well differentiated, have ERs and PRs, and are of low grade and stage. The diagnosis is suspected when unexplained vaginal bleeding is detected. Instillation of saline into the uterine cavity followed by ultrasonography can reveal an area of focal thickening that is shown by biopsy to be cancer. An associated finding is generalized thickening of the endometrial stripe to greater than 6 mm as a sign of concomitant endometrial hyperplasia. Any unexplained vaginal bleeding in a postmenopausal women requires such evaluation to rule out endometrial cancer.

Treatment

Treatment requires initial hysterectomy and bilateral oophorectomy in all patients. Patients at risk for vaginal spread are pretreated with brachytherapy implants in the vagina. Those with a poor prognosis (~25% of patients) are treated postoperatively with brachytherapy implants or external beam radiotherapy.[301] Upon recurrence, high doses of systemic progestagens may be used. Response to therapy is independent of age, site of metastasis, or previous or concurrent therapy. Two large gynecologic oncology studies reported that objective responses to a progestin occurred in 24% to 25% of patients.[304, 305]

The exact mechanism of tumor regression is unknown but may involve the following:

1. Direct effects on tumor cells.
2. Stimulation of the inactivating 17β-hydroxysteroid dehydrogenase type I enzyme, which converts estradiol to estrone.
3. Inhibition of the production by the adrenal glands of androgenic estrogen precursors.
4. Down-regulation of estrogen receptors by progestagen.
5. Suppression of gonadotropin production in premenopausal women.

Experimental trials are ongoing to test the efficacy of aromatase inhibitors, antiestrogens, GnRH analogues, and combinations of these agents.[301] Various chemotherapeutic regimens are also available for such patients.

Hormone Replacement Therapy in Endometrial Cancer Survivors

Patients with an excellent prognosis and disease-free survival for at least 1 year can be treated with HRT to relieve menopausal symptoms.[306]

PROSTATE CANCER

Incidence

In the United States, 198,000 new cases of prostate cancer and 31,500 deaths were predicted in the year 2001.[291] Black men have an age-adjusted relative risk of 1.73 (95% CI 1.23 to 2.45) compared with white men. The mortality of black men is nearly twice that of white men.[307] Introduction of prostate-specific antigen (PSA) screening in the mid-1980s resulted in a tripling of prostate cancer detection rates between 1985 and 1997 from 96,000 per year to 334,500 per year.[308a, 308b] However, estimated case detection rates have gradually declined to 198,000 as the pool of previously undiagnosed patients has diminished. With the advent of PSA screening, 1 in 6.25 men will be diagnosed with prostate cancer during their lifetimes.[309] As a result of PSA screening, 75% of patients present with organ-confined disease compared with only 25% before PSA screening.

Etiology

Environment, Diet

Environmental and *dietary factors* play a major role in prostate cancer etiology, as evidenced by epidemiologic data. Global incidence figures vary widely from 1.08 per 100,000 per year in China to 190 per 100,000 per year in the United States. Dietary or environmental explanations for this wide variance are likely. Japanese men who move to the United States have rates of prostate cancer that ultimately approach those of United States citizens.[55] Differences in ingestion of high-fat diets, green tea, or soy products provide potential explanations for the divergent rates of prostate cancer among different populations.[55, 310–322] The incidence of premalignant prostate lesions and latent prostate cancer[323, 324] is the same in Japan and China as in the United States, whereas the rates of invasive cancer differ markedly.[325–329] The additional mutations or promotional factors necessary to convert latent to invasive cancer apparently occur less commonly in Japanese and Chinese men living in Asia. In contrast, the initial mutation or mutations leading to latent cancer occur at the same rate. This observation suggests that environmental or dietary factors may influence the later additional mutations or tumor promotion more specifically.

Hormonal and Genetic Factors

Hormonal factors and particularly circulating androgens probably play a role in the initiation and promotion of prostate cancer. Prostate cancer rarely develops in men surgically orchiectomized before the age of 30 years, although this has been difficult to document in the published literature (P. Gann, Fang-Liu Gu, Peking University, personal communications).[329a]

Genetic factors play an important role as well.[330–332] Twin studies suggest a genetic component in 44% of patients with prostate cancer.[42, 333] Men with prostate cancer report a family history of this tumor 3.1 to 4.3 times more commonly than healthy men. The relative risk of prostate cancer is increased approximately twofold in men with one first-degree relative with prostate cancer.[334] Specific genetic lesions resulting in prostate cancer are uncommon. The *BRCA2* gene probably accounts for a small percentage of prostate cancer cases. An increase in the number of glutamine repeats in the variable region of the androgen receptor from germ line cells occurs in 10% of patients with prostate cancer.[335, 336] Data from a Utah pedigree identified another high-risk gene on chromosome 17p called *ELAC2*.[337]

Ross and associates[338] suggested that the lower frequency of prostate cancer in Japanese and Chinese populations may be related to a lower level of 5α-reductase activity than in their white counterparts, perhaps on a genetic basis. This may lead to lower levels of dihydrotestosterone (DHT) in prostatic tissue and less androgen-induced proliferation. However, direct isotopic kinetic measurements of 5α-reductase activity in Chinese versus white men demonstrated no differences in the levels of this enzyme.[339]

Early Case Detection

Until the introduction of PSA measurements, digital rectal examination (DRE), followed by biopsy, represented the standard screening procedure. Currently, PSA measurements detect cancers at a time when most are not palpable by DRE. The principle behind PSA screening is that tumors release more PSA into the blood stream per gram of tissue than does tissue with benign prostatic hyperplasia or normal tissue.[340] PSA may be transiently increased by prostatitis, after endoscopic urethral manipulation, by prostatic biopsy, or to a lesser extent by ejaculation. Routine DRE has a minimal effect on PSA levels, but most physicians defer PSA testing until several days after this examination.[341–346]

The sensitivity of case detection with PSA is high but the specificity is low, and routine PSA screening has been controversial. In addition, there may be no advantage in detecting "latent" prostate cancers.[347] Attempts to increase specificity include use of age-related PSA normal ranges and PSA density (i.e., PSA divided by ultrasonographically determined prostate volume). Other methods to enhance specificity include PSA velocity (rate of increase in PSA over time), and percentage of free PSA.[348–354]

The free PSA measurement may provide the most useful information. A higher fraction of free PSA is present in men without prostate cancer.[341, 355–361] When free PSA was used in patients with borderline PSA values of 4.0 to 10.0 and a normal DRE, the rate of biopsy-proven prostate cancer increased from 8% to 20% to 56% with free PSA fractions of more than 25%, 15% to 20%, and 0% to 10%, respectively.

Various professional societies have provided guidelines for PSA screening, but no general agreement exists.[309] Randomized trials to determine whether screening improves survival are not yet conclusive,[362] although one study demonstrated benefit.[363] A commonsense approach suggests screening only when test results would dictate diagnostic and therapeutic decisions. The patient should understand the consequences of a positive result and be willing to proceed with further diagnostic and therapeutic measures if the PSA findings are positive.[364] Accordingly, patients selected for screening should be those for whom definitive treatment or hormonal manipulations, and not watchful waiting, would be the likely choice if cancer were detected.[364] On the basis of this reasoning, informed consent of the patient is required before embarking on screening with PSA.

Jewett Classification

STAGE A	STAGE B	STAGE C	STAGE D
A1 A2	B1 B2 B3	C	D

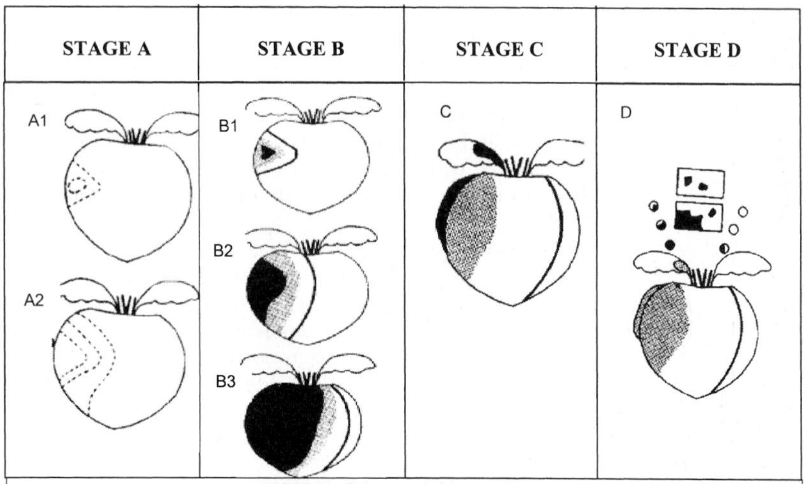

TNM Classification

T1 N0 M0	T2, N0 M0	T3, N0 M0	T2-4, Nx Mx
T1a – incidental tumor ≤ 5% T1b – incidental tumor > 5% T1c – identified by biopsy – PSA screening N0, M0	T2a – palpable or seen on TRUS – one lobe T2b – palpable or seen on TRUS – 2 lobes N0, M0	T3a – extracapsular Extension T3b – seminal vesicle involvement N0, M0	T4 – bladder neck, external sphincter, rectal levator muscles, or pelvic wall involvement N0 – no regional nodes or N1 – regional nodes M1 – nonregional nodes M1b – bone M1c – other sites

Figure 39–16. Two analogous systems for classification of prostate cancer. The Tumor-Node-Metastasis (TNM) system is generally used for a wide range of neoplasms; it involves an estimate of tumor size and presence of distant metastases or lymph nodes that contain tumor. The Jewett classification integrates these factors into stages A to D, which indicate progressively more severe disease. Both are used by various authors, and the parallels between the two systems are demonstrated here. PSA, prostate-specific antigen; TRUS, transrectal ultrasonography.

Evaluation of Abnormal Prostate-Specific Antigen or Digital Rectal Examination Findings

If the PSA is elevated to greater than 10 ng/mL or the DRE is abnormal, transrectal ultrasound–guided biopsy is indicated.[365–369] An algorithm for those with PSA values between 4 and 10 has been described.[370] Common practice involves obtaining biopsy specimens of ultrasound-detected hypoechoic lesions as well as "blind" biopsies.

Clinical staging of prostate cancer provides a means of determining the prognosis and is used for making treatment decisions. Two analogous systems have been used in the past (Fig. 39–16), but the Tumor-Node-Metastasis (TNM) classification is now preferred.

Endocrinology of Prostatic Cancer Growth

DHT, the 5α-reduced product of testosterone, binds to androgen receptors with 2.5-fold higher affinity than testosterone itself and serves as the major regulator of prostatic tumor growth. Direct effects of androgen, indirect effects induced by stimulation of growth factors, or a combination of these two mechanisms may mediate androgen-induced proliferation (Fig. 39–17).[371] Approximately 7000 μg of testosterone is secreted daily by the testes, of which 500 μg is converted into DHT in various peripheral tissues.[371] The adrenal gland provides an additional 5% of the androgen produced in adult men.[372] Testosterone as well as preandrogens such as androstenedione, dehydroepiandrosterone (DHEA or alternatively DHA), and DHEA sulfate (DHEAS) originate in the adrenal gland and are also converted in peripheral tissues into DHT. In addition to peripheral conversion, a large fraction of the DHT present in benign and malignant prostatic tissue is produced locally in the prostate gland from circulating precursors. Approximately 40% of prostatic DHT originates from steroids of adrenal origin.[373]

Prostate cancer cells contain androgen receptors that bind DHT and transmit proliferative signals in androgen-dependent prostate cancer.[374–378] As opposed to the use of receptor assays in breast cancer, measurement of the androgen receptor does not provide predictive information regarding hormone responsiveness. Mutations of the androgen receptor occur, but the frequency in primary prostate cancer is controversial.[379, 380] An early study found a 30% incidence of androgen receptor mutations in primary prostate cancers.[381] Others have found a much lower frequency ranging from 0% to 5%. All investigators found mutations in metastatic disease ranging from 21% to 50%.[380a] The frequency and type of mutation appear to be influenced by the selective pressure exerted by antiandrogens. For example, 5 of 16 men receiving flutamide had mutations compared with 1 of 17 not receiving flutamide.[380] Most of these cases involved a mutation at amino acid 877, the site involved in LnCAP cells (a type of prostate cancer cell model named for Ln [lymph node] Ca [carcinoma] P [prostate]), which allows flutamide to become an androgen agonist. This finding may explain the occurrence of flutamide withdrawal responses in men with prostatic cancer (see later).[382–385]

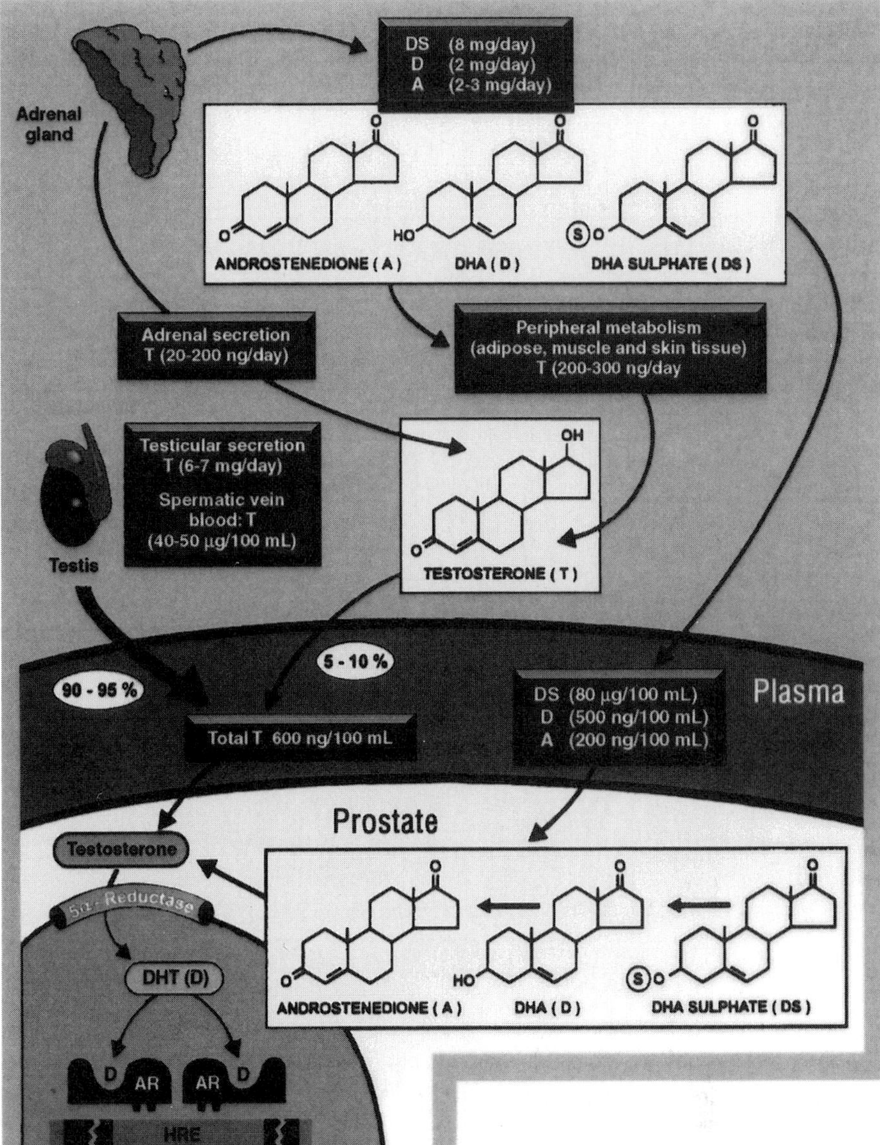

Figure 39–17. Diagrammatic representation of the endocrinology of prostate cancer growth. Androgens are directly secreted by the testis into the circulation, are synthesized in peripheral tissues from steroidal precursors, and are formed directly in the prostate gland. AR, androgen receptor; DHA, dehydroepiandrosterone; DHT, dihydrotestosterone; HRE, hormone response element. (From Denis LJ, Griffiths K. Endocrine treatment in prostate cancer. Semin Surg Oncol 2000; 18:52–54. Published with permission of Seminars in Surgical Oncology.)

Decisions Regarding Treatment

One of three strategies can be chosen for treatment of prostate cancer: watchful waiting, hormonal manipulation, or definitive (curative) therapy. The first decision after a diagnosis of prostate cancer is whether to recommend therapy or to advise watchful waiting. The underlying principle in decision making is that some prostate cancers are latent. The term *latent prostate cancer* has been applied to small lesions, generally smaller than 0.5 cm in volume, that do not progress and do not result in cause-specific death.[347]

In older men with other medical conditions, the risks of definitive therapy may outweigh the benefits, particularly if latent disease is present. Only a small percentage of men with limited disease die of prostate cancer each year after diagnosis (Fig. 39–18), and those with a limited expected life span because of other diseases may die with prostate cancer and not because of it. In general, watchful waiting is reserved for patients in older age groups (older than age 70 years) and those with a low stage and grade, localized disease, and a life expectancy of less than 10 years.[386] A reasonable working construct is that the younger and more healthy the patient, the more likely the benefit from definitive therapy. Prognostic factors that can be used to assess aggressiveness include tumor stage and tumor grade, as assessed by the Gleason score, and PSA.

Several competing approaches have been developed for definitive therapy. Radical prostatectomy with nerve sparing is one option. A risk stratification tool developed to assess the likelihood of recurrence after this procedure includes the initial PSA level and Gleason score. Low-risk patients (initial PSA < 10 and Gleason score equal to or less than 6) had a 5-year relapse-free survival of 81% versus 40% for high-risk patients (PSA > 10 and Gleason score greater than or equal to 7).[387] Conventional radiation, three-dimensional conformal radiation, or brachyradiation techniques provide other alternatives.[388–393] Patients are informed of the various treatment modalities, and a participatory decision is made on the basis of the best expected outcome. The younger and healthier the patient, the more reasonable is the recommendation of radical prostatectomy.

An experimental therapeutic option for locally advanced disease that avoids surgery and radiation involves monotherapy with an antiandrogen. The concept is that hormonal therapy shrinks the primary tumor and prevents metastatic spread. Pre-

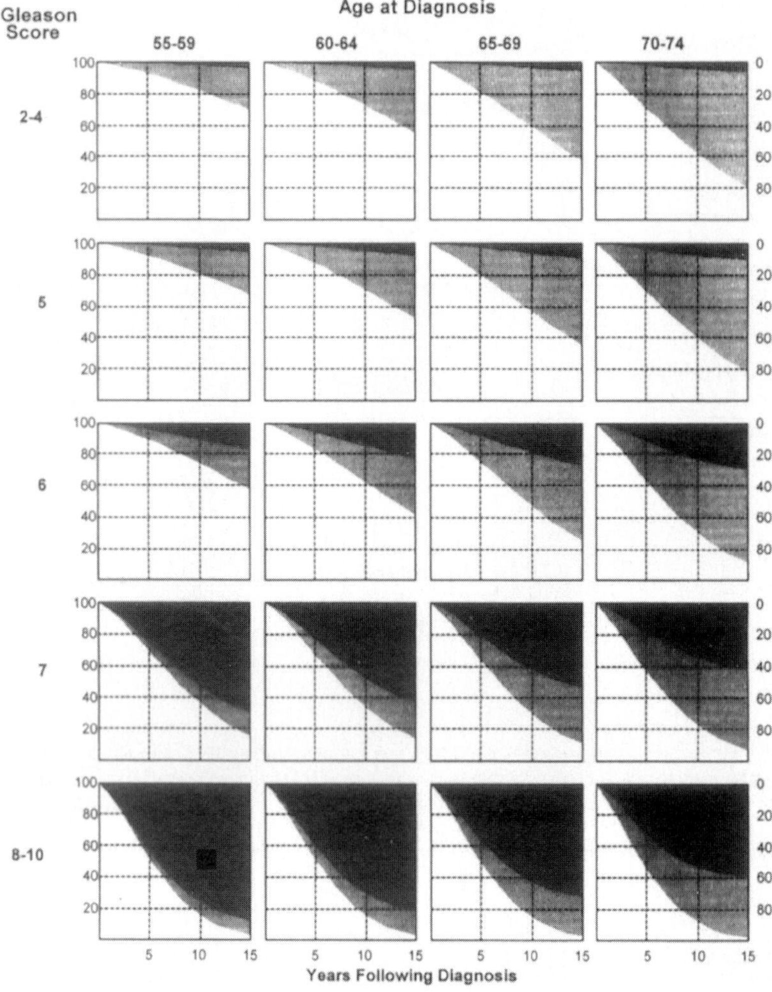

Figure 39–18. Illustration of death rates in men of various ages with prostate cancer. *Heavily shaded areas* represent death from all causes. *Lightly shaded areas* indicate prostate cancer–related death rates. (From Albertsen PC, Hanley JA, Gleason DF, Barry MJ. Competing risk analysis of men aged 55 to 74 years at diagnosis managed conservatively for clinically localized prostate cancer. JAMA 1998; 280:975. Reprinted with permission of the American Medical Association.)

liminary reports of three exploratory studies of antiandrogens in the setting of previously untreated locally advanced disease have appeared. These studies compare antiandrogens not with prostatectomy or radiation but with castration. Pooled mature data suggested no survival difference between bicalutamide at 150 mg daily and surgical castration in this setting.[394]

Another large study recruited 1453 men with confirmed metastatic disease or T3 to T4 disease with elevated PSA into two trials comparing castration with bicalutamide. Pooled data demonstrated decreased efficacy of bicalutamide with respect to survival (hazard ratio 1.3).

Taken together, these data suggest that bicalutamide is not as effective as castration.[395–397] Even though antiandrogen monotherapy is not as effective as castration, some men may choose this therapy in preference to watchful waiting.[394, 397a, 398]

Neoadjuvant Hormonal Therapy

Neoadjuvant therapy is defined as use of hormonal therapy before definitive treatment and involves (1) medical castration with GnRH analogues, (2) steroidal or nonsteroidal antiandrogens, or (3) a combination.

Radical Prostatectomy

Neoadjuvant strategies used for 3 to 6 months prior to radical prostatectomy resulted in an increase in organ-confined cancers and decrease in positive surgical margins.[399–404] However, no differences in PSA-detectable relapse rates have been observed in several trials. Data are not yet sufficiently mature to assess overall survival rates. However, the efficacy of this maneuver is still undetermined because longer follow-up is needed before definitive conclusions regarding overall survival can be reached.

Radiation Therapy

Radiation Therapy Oncology Group (RTOG) trial 86-10 examined the role of neoadjuvant endocrine therapy prior to radiation.[405] The incidence of local progression at 5 years was 46% for patients with T2 to T4 tumors receiving adjuvant hormonal therapy and 71% for those receiving radiation alone ($P = .001$), but no difference in overall survival was noted.

Adjuvant Hormonal Therapy

Therapy given with the initial definitive treatment and before evidence of recurrence is termed adjuvant hormonal treatment[406–408] (Fig. 39–19). Two large multicenter trials provided evidence of the efficacy of this approach. An RTOG study[409] involved patients with stage T3 and stage T4 disease given radiation therapy followed by medical castration with goserelin starting in the last week of radiation. Disease-free survival at 5 years was 60% for the goserelin arm and 44% for radiation alone ($P < .0001$). Only the subset of men with Gleason grade 8 to 10 tumors experienced a survival benefit from 55% to 66% ($P = .03$).

In a similar trial of the European Organization for Research and Treatment of Cancer (EORTC),[410] the 5-year disease-free survival was 85% in the adjuvant hormone–treated group (goserelin) versus 48% in the group given radiation alone (P = .001). Overall survival was 79% for the adjuvant hormonal group versus 62% for the radiation-alone group, and this difference was statistically significant (P = .001).

The majority of data favor the use of adjuvant hormonal therapy in patients undergoing radiation therapy as definitive treatment for prostate cancer.[411, 412] An analysis of pooled data from the RTOG neoadjuvant and adjuvant trials concluded that the key consideration may be the necessity for long-term rather than short-term hormonal therapy in either the neoadjuvant or adjuvant therapy approach.[412] In men receiving short-term hormonal therapy (goserelin and flutamide for 2 months before and 2 months after radiotherapy), statistically significant improvements were observed for two end points, distant metastasis–free and evaluable disease–free intervals, but not for overall survival. Only long-term adjuvant therapy improved overall survival and only in the subset of men with Gleason grade 7 to 10 tumors. These conclusions concerning long-term versus short-term adjuvant hormonal therapy were supported by a nonrandomized Canadian trial.[413]

In a large ongoing study, men are randomly assigned to placebo or 150 mg of bicalutamide daily after radical prostatectomy or radiotherapy or during watchful waiting. A total of 8055 patients have been entered. Bicalutamide significantly reduced the incidence of disease progression by 42% (hazard ratio 0.58, 95% CI 0.51 to 0.66, $P < .0001$). This encouraging result needs to be confirmed with respect to overall survival.[413a]

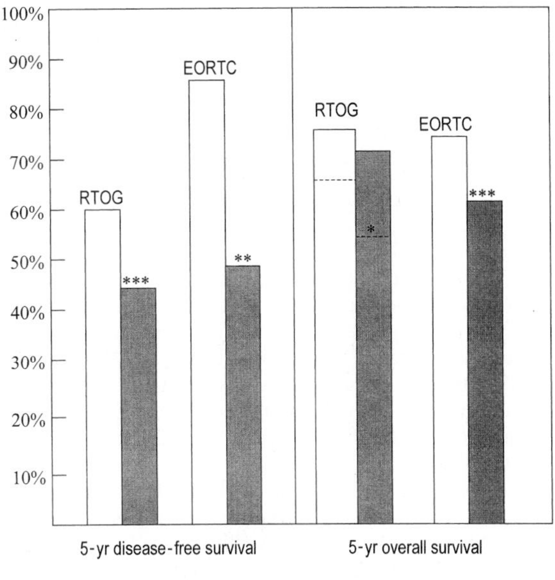

Figure 39–19. Two trials illustrate the benefit of adjuvant androgen deprivation therapy in patients with locally advanced disease treated with radiation therapy and either placebo *(open bars)* or medical orchiectomy with a gonadotropin-releasing hormone agonist analogue *(solid bars)*. EORTC, European Organization for Research and Treatment of Cancer; RTOG, Radiation Therapy Oncology Group.

Immediate versus Delayed Hormonal Therapy

Approximately 25% of men now present either with metastatic (M+ or stage D) disease or with local spread into lymph nodes (N+). Whether to initiate hormonal treatment immediately in these patients or to defer treatment until symptoms occur is a major question. Because cure with hormones is not possible, the two goals of treatment are to increase life expectancy and to relieve symptoms. If treatment is advocated for asymptomatic patients, it should improve their length of survival.

Rigorously controlled series from the Veterans Administration Cooperative Urological Research Group (VACURG) trials during the 1960s indicated no clear survival benefit from endocrine therapy in patients with stage C or D disease at the time of diagnosis.[414, 415] On the basis of these findings, standard practice usually involved withholding hormonal therapy until symptomatic metastatic (stage D) disease was present. However, two later studies provided evidence favoring therapy immediately upon detection of metastatic disease.

Messing and colleagues[416] studied men with prostate cancer found to have positive pelvic lymph nodes at the time of radical prostatectomy. They randomly assigned these men to an immediate therapy group (medical or surgical orchiectomy) or to a group observed until an indication occurred. Death from prostate cancer occurred in 3 of 47 men in the immediate treatment group and 16 of 51 in the deferred group ($P < .01$).[416]

In another study, 934 men with locally advanced prostate cancer or with asymptomatic metastatic disease were randomly assigned to immediate or deferred hormonal therapy. There were 203 deaths from prostate cancer in the immediate therapy arm and 257 in the deferred group (P = .02).[417] There were fewer cases of spinal cord compression (9 versus 23) and pathologic fracture (11 versus 21) in the immediate treatment group.[418, 419]

Other evidence of efficacy comes from nonrandomized studies from the Mayo Clinic that demonstrate a statistically significant survival advantage for early endocrine therapy (castration) in men with stage D1 (T0 to T3, N1 and N2, M0) disease.[420, 421] Seventy-three patients underwent either radical retropubic prostatectomy or radical prostatectomy plus orchiectomy. An advantage of immediate adjuvant therapy was demonstrated in that 5-year survival rates were 93% in the immediate orchiectomy group and 80% in the deferred orchiectomy group. In another study, a benefit was seen only in patients with diploid and not in those with tetraploid or aneuploid tumors.[422]

Finally, a subset analysis in the RTOG 85-31 study examined a group of 139 men with capsular penetration or seminal vesical involvement. Seventy-one men received radiation therapy plus luteinizing hormone-releasing hormone (LHRH) agonist therapy and 68 received radiation therapy alone. A statistically significant improvement in progression-free survival and freedom from biochemical relapse (i.e., PSA) was observed in the LHRH group. Overall survival was not statistically significantly different in this relatively small subset of men with follow-up for only a median of 5 years.[423]

Taken together, these data suggest, but do not prove, that immediate hormonal therapy may be efficacious for asymptomatic men presenting with lymph node spread.[423a] The data at present do not provide definitive evidence that early endocrine therapy is beneficial regarding survival of patients presenting with metastatic (M+) disease, but evidence from one study is suggestive.[382]

Men who experience a rising PSA (biochemical failure) after an initial fall to undetectable levels following radical prostatectomy may also benefit from hormonal therapy. Data indicate that a rapid rise in PSA suggests the presence of metastatic disease, whereas a slow rise suggests local recurrence.[424–426] In a single small study, 68% of men progressed to detectable clinical disease upon observation for a median of 19 months. With adjuvant hormonal therapy or radiotherapy, the rate of progression to clinically detectable disease decreased to 21%.[387] Use of the capromab pendetide (ProstaScint) radioisotopic scan has been advocated to identify patients with distant metastatic disease under these circumstances.[427–429] Such patients would not be considered candidates for salvage radiotherapy to the pelvis.

Choice of Endocrine Treatment for Initial Disease

Which endocrine therapy to use initially is a major question. Surgical orchiectomy produces a rapid decrease in serum androgen levels, does not require the patient's long-term compliance, and is effective in inducing tumor regression in nearly 90% of patients. The clinician can be assured that testicular androgens are completely suppressed. However, nearly 50% of men in the United States prefer medical castration[430] as a means to avoid surgery.

Highly potent agonist analogues of GnRH, called *superagonist analogues*, have been approved for use in prostate cancer and effectively produce a medical orchiectomy. These compounds paradoxically inhibit LH secretion by the pituitary gland and thereby suppress testicular testosterone production. Clinically, the GnRH agonists stimulate LH threefold to fourfold and testosterone twofold for 1 to 2 weeks from initiation of therapy.[431] Thereafter, LH is profoundly depressed and the plasma testosterone level falls from approximately 500 ng/dL to a castration level of 15 ng/dL. No escape from inhibition occurs for up to 2 years of continuous therapy.

The initial rise in testosterone causes a transient disease flare in 5% to 10% of patients. This flare produces an objective increase in tumor size in approximately 3% of patients and a subjective increase in bone pain in the remainder. Although tumor flare[432, 433] is usually transient, severe reactions with spinal cord compression or death have been observed in occasional patients. For this reason, it is necessary to administer an antiandrogen for the first month after starting GnRH agonist therapy.[434] GnRH antagonists are now in clinical trial as a means to abrogate this problem.[429]

The rationale for using GnRH agonists is to induce a medical castration selectively and without unwanted side effects. Testosterone and DHT levels in patients treated with GnRH agonists and with surgical orchiectomy fall to a similar extent.[431] Hormonal effects with the GnRH agonists are selective with no alterations of adrenal, thyroid, parathyroid, or pancreatic function. Objective regressions occur as frequently as with orchiectomy. The efficacy of medical castration is equal to that observed with surgical castration or use of DES.[435, 436]

Initially, a major problem with GnRH agonist therapy was the requirement for daily subcutaneous administration with the possibility of noncompliance with daily injections and incomplete androgen suppression.[435] Third-generation formulations are now available that allow injections at 3- or 4-month intervals. These biodegradable preparations appear highly effective and are well tolerated and acceptable to patients. The frequency of tumor regression or stabilization does not appear to differ in patients treated with orchiectomy or long-acting GnRH agonists.[436] Because some androgen-responsive cells remain in prostate tumors after relapse with the GnRH agonists, continued GnRH agonist treatment is advocated when disease relapse occurs and preferably for the remainder of the patient's life.

Monotherapy with antiandrogens provides an alternative to surgical or medical castration. These agents can be subclassified as steroidal and nonsteroidal antiandrogens. The nonsteroidal agents, flutamide and bicalutamide, bind to androgen receptors and block the cellular effects of circulating testosterone and DHT on cell proliferation. Interruption of the androgen negative feedback system results in reflex increments in serum LH, testosterone, and DHT levels. Studies with antiandrogens suggested that these agents preserve erectile function. More recent data suggest that only 20% maintain morning erections and sexual activity,[437] but this is still higher than after castration (18% reduction with bicalutamide versus 37% with castration).[438] Side effects include hot flashes and diarrhea, particularly with flutamide.[394] Long-term effects on bone density require more detailed study.

Randomized trials have compared antiandrogens as monotherapy with medical or surgical castration.[397, 439] Initial studies showed that 50 mg of bicalutamide is not as effective as orchiectomy.[397] Later studies compared 150 mg of bicalutamide with medical or surgical castration in patients with locally advanced (T1 to T4, N+, M0) and metastatic (T1 to T4, Nx, M0) disease. Bicalutamide was equivalent to medical or surgical castration for locally advanced[438] but not metastatic disease (hazard ratio for survival of 1.3).[398]

Another study examined whether 150 mg of bicalutamide was the equivalent of *maximal androgen blockade* (MAB) in the setting of locally advanced or M1 disease. In this study of Boccardo and colleagues,[395] bicalutamide was as effective as MAB for locally advanced (T1 to T4, N+, M0) disease but not for metastatic disease (M0). Taken together, these data suggest that antiandrogens as monotherapy may not block androgen effects as effectively as medical or surgical castration.

Administration of high-dose estrogen in the form of DES has been used as a treatment for prostate cancer since the 1940s. In the VACURG studies, 5 mg of DES decreased the rate of recurrence of prostate cancer but increased the cardiovascular death rate.[414, 415] After this observation, careful dose-response studies indicated that 3 mg of DES daily minimizes the risk of cardiovascular disease acceleration and maximizes the beneficial effects on prostate cancer. Gynecomastia and impotence are the major side effects.

Comparison of these monotherapies was the subject of a meta-analysis involving 10 separate trials. It was concluded by the Technology Evaluation Center, an agency of the Agency for Health Care Policy and Research,[440] that orchiectomy, GnRH agonist analogues, and DES produced equivalent survival in men and that no differences existed among the various GnRH analogues that are available.

Complete Androgen Blockade

A more comprehensive strategy for the endocrine treatment of prostate cancer has been proposed. The rationale for complete, or maximal, androgen blockade (CAB, complete androgen blockade; MAB, maximal androgen blockade) rests upon three considerations:

1. The adrenal glands contribute 5% of the total androgen pool.[372]
2. The concentrations of DHT in prostate cancer tissue of patients fall by only 50% to 80% after surgical orchiectomy[373] and DHT levels in that tissue after castration are still higher than in nonandrogen target tissues (Fig. 39–20).
3. In vitro systems demonstrate that some tumor cell clones are hypersensitive to the proliferative effects of androgen.[441]

On the basis of these considerations, inhibition of both testicular and adrenal androgens (MAB) might be more effective than inhibition of testicular androgens alone (testicular androgen suppression).

Thirty-six studies have examined the concept of MAB as initial endocrine therapy for advanced disease (stage D or Tx Nx M+ disease) in randomized trials, but the results and con-

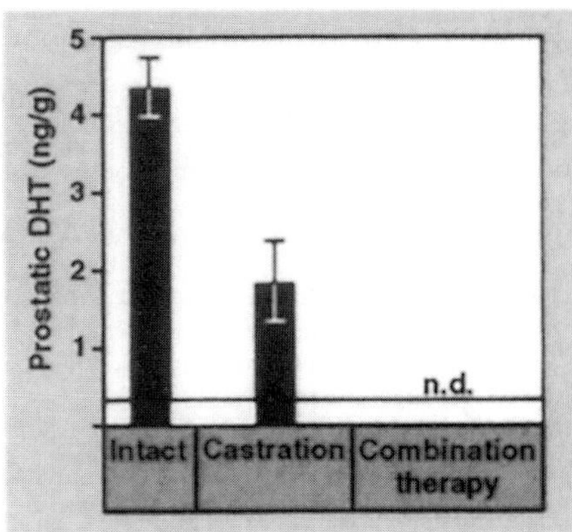

Figure 39–20. Prostate tissue levels of dihydrotestosterone (DHT) in the normal prostate gland and after surgical orchiectomy alone and in combination with suppression of adrenal androgens. n.d., nondetectable. (From Denis LJ, Griffiths K. Endocrine treatment in prostate cancer. Semin Surg Oncol 2000; 18:52–74. With permission of the publisher.)

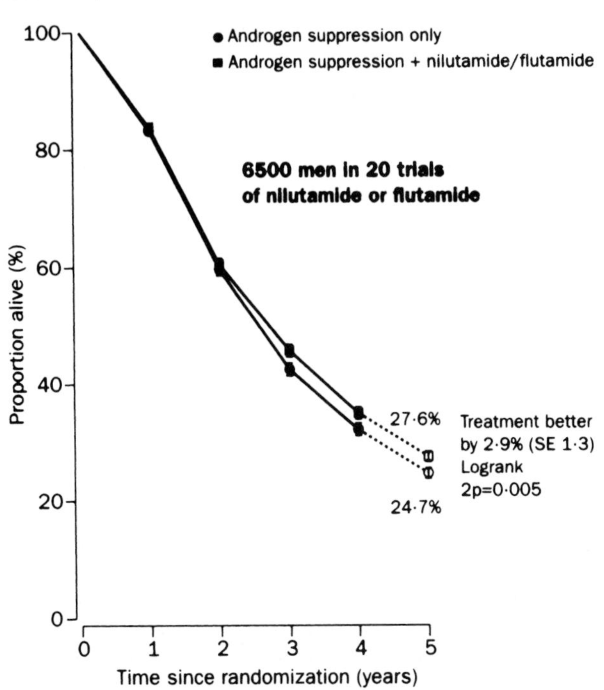

Figure 39–21. Results of complete versus partial androgen blockade in men with prostate cancer. Survival curves represent pooled data from a meta-analysis of multiple studies. (From Maximum androgen blockade in advanced prostate cancer: an overview of the randomised trials. Prostate Cancer Trialists' Collaborative Group. Lancet 2000; 355: 1491–1498. With permission of the publisher.)

clusions drawn from the studies are conflicting.[371, 442] However, a meta-analysis involving nearly 90% of men treated worldwide provided several definitive conclusions and reasons for discrepancies among prior results[443]:

1. MAB regimens using nonsteroidal antiandrogens provide a 2.9% improvement in overall survival from 24.7% to 27.6% at 5 years (Fig. 39–21). This difference is statistically significant ($P = .005$) but of marginal significance clinically.
2. MAB regimens using the steroidal antiandrogen cyproterone acetate produce adverse survival effects compared with testicular androgen suppression.
3. Analyses of studies of MAB that pool patients treated with either cyproterone acetate or nonsteroidal antiandrogens demonstrate no survival benefit produced by MAB over testicular androgen suppression.
4. Men with disease limited to the axial skeleton did not gain more benefit from MAB than those with metastases to the appendicular skeleton. A large prior study had reported this to be the case.[444]
5. Results were similar when subsets of men treated with surgical or medical castration or with flutamide or nilutamide were examined.

Past controversies about MAB can be explained by fact that some trials used cyproterone acetate, an antiandrogen that shortens survival in these patients.[443] Other trials did not use a short-term antiandrogen in the medical castration group, and the disease flare may have compromised overall efficacy. Finally, early trials used daily GnRH injections, which may not have induced effective medical castration because of the need for compliance with daily injections for 5 years.

It should be noted that no properly designed study has compared MAB with sequential androgen blockade (defined as initial castration followed by antiandrogen upon relapse). In the largest study of MAB,[445] the use of antiandrogen upon relapse in the placebo group was left to the investigator's discretion and only 50% of men in the placebo arm later took an antiandrogen. For this reason, there is no information about whether antiandrogen therapy given at the time of relapse after medical or surgical orchiectomy (i.e., sequential androgen blockade) is as effective as MAB. This is an important issue because flutamide given upon relapse after castration (sequential androgen blockade) resulted in objective benefit in 23% of patients.[446]

On the basis of the data presented and the additional considerations discussed, this author and others favor the sequential androgen blockade strategy and use of antiandrogens only after relapse from medical or surgical orchiectomy.[446a] However, if GnRH agonists are used to produce a medical orchiectomy, short-term use of an antiandrogen to prevent disease flare is necessary.[447, 448]

Secondary Hormonal Therapy

Men who experience cancer recurrence after medical or surgical orchiectomy are treated with secondary hormonal therapies. Before the use of PSA measurements, the clinician had to rely on bone radiographs and soft tissue changes to document responses and these were rarely observed. Consequently, the efficacy of secondary hormonal therapies was controversial. Clinicians have now accepted a 50% decline in PSA as reflecting an objective response to therapy.[449] Studies have shown that this PSA end point predicts a significantly prolonged median overall survival, objective progression-free survival, and time to pain progression.[450] Using PSA measurements, it is now possible to demonstrate the efficacy of a number of secondary hormonal therapies. Responses to antiandrogens, ketoconazole, flutamide, bicalutamide, aminoglutethimide, DES, and glucocorticoids alone range from 14% to 60% (Table 39–2). Head-to-head comparisons are unavailable for these agents, and relative efficacy cannot be compared.[383, 385, 451]

Antiandrogen Withdrawal Phenomena

Experimental studies with LnCAP cells in vitro detected a mutation in the androgen receptor in this cell line that caused it to respond to flutamide with increased proliferation.[452] As a result of this observation, clinical studies examined whether tumors in some patients might adapt to flutamide by develop-

Table 39–2. Prostate Cancer: Secondary Hormonal Therapies

Modality	Responders	Total Patients	Responses (%)	Clinical Setting	References
Flutamide	23	100	23	First relapse after medical or surgical orchiectomy	446
Prednisone	21	101	21	First relapse after medical or surgical orchiectomy	446
Flutamide withdrawal	29	138	21	Relapse after combined androgen blockade or flutamide monotherapy	385, 474
AG/HC	14	29	49	After antiandrogen withdrawal	475
HC	20	48	40	After antiandrogen withdrawal	385
Ketoconazole/HC	43	72	60	After antiandrogen withdrawal	385, 476
Megestrol acetate	17	119	14	After antiandrogen withdrawal	477
Diethylstilbestrol	71	243	29	After antiandrogen withdrawal	478

AG, aminoglutethimide; HC, hydrocortisone.

ing mutations, allowing flutamide to behave as an androgen agonist. In support of this possibility, approximately 40% of men receiving flutamide experienced tumor regression after withdrawal of flutamide (so-called withdrawal responses). These data suggest that a first step in patients receiving flutamide, either as part of a complete androgen blockade regimen or as secondary hormonal therapy, is to stop flutamide. These responses occur with bicalutamide as well but with lower frequency.[384, 453–458]

Other Secondary Hormonal Therapies

Prior to the PSA era, objective regression, stabilization, or symptomatic relief was reported with several agents. These included a high-dose formulation of DES called Stilphostrol[459, 460] and tamoxifen. A subsequent study using high-dose tamoxifen (160 mg/m^2 per day) observed only a 3.3% rate of objective response on the basis of PSA in heavily pretreated men with prostate cancer.[461] Each of these agents could be considered for patients who have slow relapses after castration.

Experimental Hormonal Approaches

Experimental data for Shionogi tumors in mice suggest that intermittent androgen withdrawal might control tumor growth and delay development of hormonal resistance. Several pilot reports suggest the feasibility of this approach,[462, 463] and observations are ongoing. This approach cannot be recommended until sufficient data are available to support its efficacy.[446a] Another approach undergoing extensive testing of efficacy is PS SPES, an herbal supplement.[463a]

Development of Androgen-Independent Tumor Growth

At some point in the patient's course, the tumor becomes refractory to hormonally based therapies. Current theory holds that tumors escape androgenic regulation of growth and co-opt mechanisms utilizing ligand-independent activation of androgen receptors, up-regulation of growth factor pathways, or a combination of these mechanisms.[371] Considerable experimental support for these concepts derives from the demonstration of increased activated MAP kinase activity (a protein that mediates mitogenesis) and enhanced phosphorylation of the androgen receptor, a marker of ligand-independent receptor activation.[464]

A major decision at the time of prostate cancer relapse after medical or surgical castration is whether to use hormonal therapy or chemotherapy. No diagnostic test is available to make the distinction between hormone dependence and independence. Men with a rapid downhill course with widespread systemic metastases should probably receive chemotherapy. Others have already been treated with all available options of endocrine therapy. Chemotherapy or combination chemohormonal therapy is chosen at that point. The choice of agents is beyond the scope of this chapter, and the interested reader is referred to the comprehensive treatise of Carroll and colleagues.[370]

Algorithm for Treatment of Prostate Cancer

To date, no standard approach to the treatment of prostate cancer has been universally accepted. To outline the options available, the algorithm in Figure 39–22 details decision branch points and currently accepted approaches with asterisks to indicate therapies that are controversial.

Initial Treatment of Nonmetastatic Prostate Cancer

No consensus exists regarding the selection of radical prostatectomy, radiation therapy, or watchful waiting. Patients with potentially curable, nonmetastatic (T1 to T3, N0, M0; stages A to C) prostate cancer are commonly treated by radical prostatectomy, radiation therapy, or watchful waiting.[370] Individual considerations, including age, risk factors for recurrence, and overall health of the patient, influence these decisions, which are often based on personal choices. In general, the younger and healthier the patient, the more likely is a choice of radical prostatectomy. The older and more debilitated the patient, the more likely is the choice of watchful waiting. Radiotherapy is often selected for patients falling at neither extreme.[465]

Patients with T1 to T3, N0, M0 (stages A to C) prostate cancer are commonly treated with radical prostatectomy. Neoadjuvant or adjuvant hormonal therapy is not usually recommended for these patients. Upon first recurrence, these men are then treated with either medical or surgical orchiectomy.

In men undergoing radiation as definitive treatment, adjuvant hormonal therapy appears to be warranted. Neoadjuvant therapy has not been adequately tested in a trial in which this step is added to long-term adjuvant therapy.[466] Nonetheless, neoadjuvant therapy would appear reasonable on the basis of the minimal additional toxicity and side effects associated with

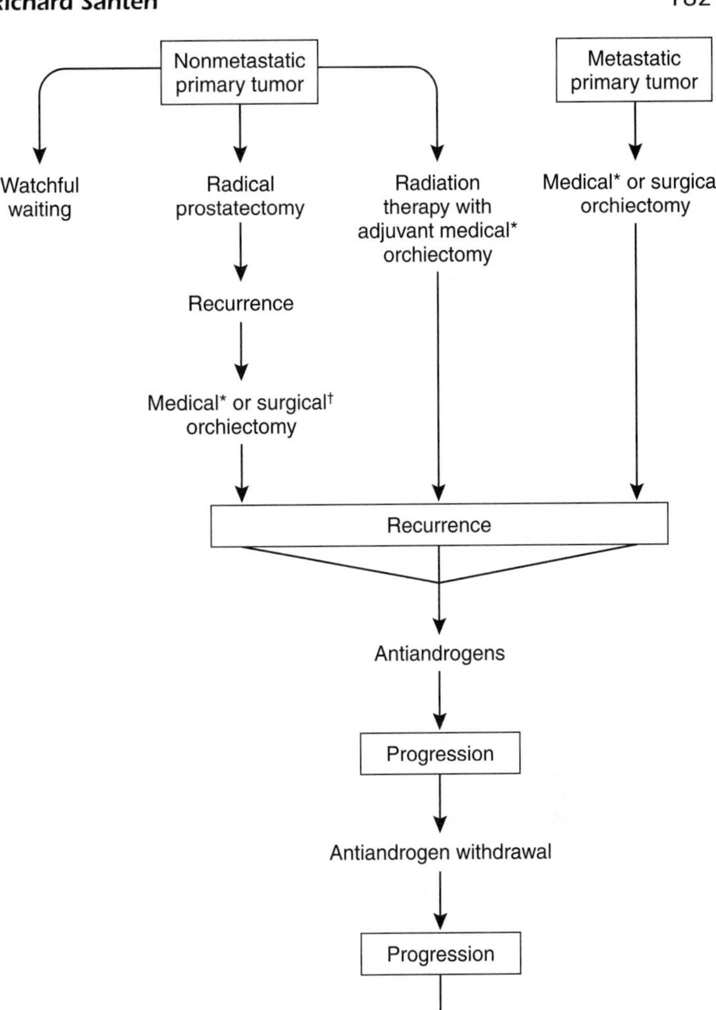

Figure 39–22. Algorithm of preferred treatment strategies for localized and advanced prostate cancer. Controversial therapies are represented by an asterisk or dagger.

this therapy for an additional 3 to 6 months before radiation therapy.

Watchful waiting is selected for men whose other illnesses would be expected to result in demise before death related to prostatic cancer.

Initial Therapy for Men with Metastatic Disease at Time of Diagnosis

Men with metastatic disease (T1 to T4, N+, or M+) at presentation are not treated definitively with radical prostatectomy or irradiation but are frequently offered hormonal therapy before the development of symptomatic disease. This decision is based on incomplete data suggesting superior efficacy of early rather than late hormonal therapy for locally advanced disease.[416] Randomized trials with a large number of patients are required before definitive advice can be given regarding management of PSA relapses.[467]

Which hormonal therapy to use is a matter of choice. A meta-analysis of 10 trials suggested that medical castration, surgical castration, and DES all have equal efficacy,[467] but individual trials indicated that antiandrogens are less effective. In this author's opinion, surgical orchiectomy appears preferable for the initial treatment of these patients. The operation is relatively minor and can be performed under local anesthesia, if desired. Rapid and complete cessation of testicular androgen secretion ensues, and the patient's compliance after surgery is not a factor. Unwarranted cardiovascular or other toxic side effects, such as those occurring with DES, are unknown. The incidence of impotence and loss of libido is the same as with other available therapies with the exception of the antiandrogens.

In practice, nearly half of patients in the United States prefer a form of medical castration for psychological or other reasons. The greater safety of the GnRH agonists favor their use over DES. To prevent tumor flare, antiandrogens should be used for at least 1 month during and after initiation of GnRH therapy. In the long term, MAB (maximal androgen blockade) is not recommended, according to the individual studies and meta-analysis already reviewed.[443, 446a] Some patients may choose to continue the antiandrogens in the long term to gain the slight (2.9%) maximal benefit from MAB. An antiandrogen or DES, 3 mg/day, can be chosen as an alternative but is not preferred.[467a]

At present, medical castration with GnRH agonists can be achieved with a 3- or 4-monthly injection that is well tolerated and should not be associated with cardiovascular complications. Cost (~$2700 for the 4-month injection) is the limiting factor. When concern about erectile dysfunction is a limiting factor, the persistence of libido and erectile function in a subset of patients treated with antiandrogens as primary therapy may be a decisive factor. Under these circumstances, some men may choose monotherapy with antiandrogens, even though this approach is not as effective as medical or surgical castration. This decision is related to quality of life, which is an increasingly important consideration in prostate cancer therapy.[362]

Disease Recurrence

Antiandrogen therapy provides a reasonable next option unless it has previously been given as part of an MAB regimen. Patients receiving an antiandrogen as part of a complete androgen blockade regimen are observed for an antiandrogen withdrawal response. Regarding the choice of antiandrogen, bicalutamide is preferred to flutamide because of its better side effect profile and potentially superior efficacy. Upon relapse, men are observed for an antiandrogen withdrawal response and treated further only when progressive disease is documented.

A variety of therapies are available for men experiencing relapse after antiandrogen withdrawal. One group[385] preferred ketoconazole and hydrocortisone because of their lack of toxicity and observed efficacy (i.e., 60% PSA response rate). The other agents listed in Table 39–2 can be used as alternatives or as third-line therapies. Further choices of chemotherapy alone or chemotherapy in combination with hormonal agents are a matter of individual preference.

References

1. Zumoff B. Does postmenopausal estrogen administration increase the risk of breast cancer? Contributions of animal, biochemical, and clinical investigative studies to a resolution of the controversy. Proc Soc Exp Biol Med 1998; 217:30–37.
2. Hollingsworth AB, Lerner MR, Lightfoot SA, et al. Prevention of DMBA-induced rat mammary carcinomas comparing leuprolide, oophorectomy, and tamoxifen. Breast Cancer Res Treat 1998; 47:63–70.
3. Gunson DE, Steele RE, Chau RY. Prevention of spontaneous tumours in female rats by fadrozole hydrochloride, an aromatase inhibitor. Br J Cancer 1995; 72:72–75.
4. Trichopoulos D, MacMahon B, Cole P. Menopause and breast cancer risk. J Natl Cancer Inst 1972; 48:605–613.
5. Fisher B, Costantino JP, Wickerham DL, et al. Tamoxifen for prevention of breast cancer: report of the National Surgical Adjuvant Breast and Bowel Project P-1 Study. J Natl Cancer Inst 1998; 90:1371–1388.

5a. IARC (International Agency for Research on Cancer) Monographs on the evaluation of carcinogenic risks to humans. Vol 72: Hormonal contraception and postmenopausal hormone therapy, 1999, Lyon, France, p 503.

6. Siiteri PK. Adipose tissue as a source of hormones. Am J Clin Nutr 1987; 45(1 Suppl):277–282.
7. Santner SJ, Pauley RJ, Tait L, et al. Aromatase activity and expression in breast cancer and benign breast tissue stromal cells. J Clin Endocrinol Metab 1997; 82:200–208.
8. Newman SP, Purohit A, Ghilchik MW, et al. Regulation of steroid sulphatase expression and activity in breast cancer. J Steroid Biochem Mol Biol 2000; 75:259–264.
9. Santen RJ, Martel J, Hoagland M, et al. Demonstration of aromatase activity and its regulation in breast tumor and benign breast fibroblasts. Breast Cancer Res Treat 1998; 49(Suppl 1): S93-S99.
10. Yue W, Santen RJ, Wang JP, et al. Aromatase within the breast. Endocr Relat Cancer 1999; 6:157–164.
11. Mor G, Yue W, Santen RJ, et al. Macrophages, estrogen and the microenvironment of breast cancer. J Steroid Biochem Mol Biol 1998; 67:403–411.
12. Zhao Y, Agarwal VR, Mendelson CR, et al. Transcriptional regulation of CYP19 gene (aromatase) expression in adipose stromal cells in primary culture. J Steroid Biochem Mol Biol 1997; 61: 203–210.
13. Amundadottir LT, Merlino G, Dickson RB. Transgenic mouse models of breast cancer. Breast Cancer Res Treat 1996; 39:119–135.
14. Rosfjord EC, Dickson RB. Growth factors, apoptosis, and survival of mammary epithelial cells. J Mammary Gland Biol Neoplasia 1999; 4:229–237.
15. Sekowski JW, Malkas LH, Schnaper L, et al. Human breast cancer cells contain an error-prone DNA replication apparatus. Cancer Res 1998; 58:3259–3263.
16. Reed JC. Balancing cell life and death: bax, apoptosis, and breast cancer. J Clin Invest 1996; 97:2403–2404.
17. Done SJ, Arneson NC, Ozcelik H, et al. p53 mutations in mammary ductal carcinoma in situ but not in epithelial hyperplasias. Cancer Res 1998; 58:785–789.
18. Elledge RM, Allred DC. Prognostic and predictive value of p53 and p21 in breast cancer. Breast Cancer Res Treat 1998; 52:79–98.
19. Yashima K, Milchgrub S, Gollahon LS, et al. Telomerase enzyme activity and RNA expression during the multistage pathogenesis of breast carcinoma. Clin Cancer Res 1998; 4:229–234.
20. Allred DC, Hilsenbeck SG. Biomarkers in benign breast disease: risk factors for breast cancer. J Natl Cancer Inst 1998; 90:1247–1248.
21. Nayar R, Zhuang Z, Merino MJ, et al. Loss of heterozygosity on chromosome 11q13 in lobular lesions of the breast using tissue microdissection and polymerase chain reaction. Hum Pathol 1997; 28:277–282.
22. Dillon EK, de Boer WB, Papadimitriou JM, et al. Microsatellite instability and loss of heterozygosity in mammary carcinoma and its probable precursors. Br J Cancer 1997; 76:156–162.
23. Preston-Martin S, Pike MC, Ross RK, et al. Increased cell division as a cause of human cancer. Cancer Res 1990; 50:7415–7421.
24. Preston-Martin S, Pike MC, Ross RK, et al. Epidemiologic evidence for the increased cell proliferation model of carcinogenesis. Environ Health Perspect 1993; 101(Suppl 5):137–138.
25. Spink DC, Spink BC, Cao JQ, et al. Differential expression of *CYP1A1* and *CYP1B1* in human breast epithelial cells and breast tumor cells. Carcinogenesis 1998; 19:291–298.
26. Cavalieri E, Frenkel K, Liehr JG, et al. Estrogens as endogenous genotoxic agents: DNA adducts and mutations. J Natl Cancer Inst Monogr 2000; (27):75–93.
27. Roy D, Liehr JG. Estrogen, DNA damage and mutations. Mutat Res 1999; 424:107–115.
28. Jefcoate CR, Liehr JG, Santen RJ, et al. Tissue-specific synthesis and oxidative metabolism of estrogens. J Natl Cancer Inst Monogr 2000; (27):95–112.
29. Yager JD, Liehr JG. Molecular mechanisms of estrogen carcinogenesis. Annu Rev Pharmacol Toxicol 1996; 36:203–232.
30. Liehr JG, Ricci MJ. 4-Hydroxylation of estrogens as marker of human mammary tumors. Proc Natl Acad Sci USA 1996; 93: 3294–3296.
31. Liehr JG. Dual role of oestrogens as hormones and pro-carcinogens: tumour initiation by metabolic activation of oestrogens. Eur J Cancer Prev 1997; 6:3–10.
32. Roy D, Liehr JG. Estrogen, DNA damage and mutations. Mutat Res 1999; 424:107–115.
33. Badawi AF, Devanesan PD, Edney JA, et al. Estrogen metabolites and conjugates: biomarkers of susceptibility to human breast cancer. Proc Am Assoc Cancer Res 2001; 42:664.
34. Spurdle AB, Hopper JL, Dite GS, et al. CYP17 promoter polymorphism and breast cancer in Australian women under age forty years. J Natl Cancer Inst 2000; 92:1674–1681.
35. Mitrunen K, Jourenkova N, Kataja V, et al. Polymorphic catechol-*O*-methyltransferase gene and breast cancer risk. Cancer Epidemiol Biomarkers Prev 2001; 10:635–640.
36. Thompson PA, Ambrosone C. Molecular epidemiology of genetic polymorphisms in estrogen metabolizing enzymes in human breast cancer. J Natl Cancer Inst Monogr 2000; (27):125–134.
37. Russo J, Hu YF, Tahin Q, et al. Carcinogenicity of estrogens in human breast epithelial cells. APMIS 2001; 109:39–52.
38. Kong LY, Szaniszlo P, Albrecht T, et al. Frequency and molecular analysis of *hprt* mutations induced by estradiol in Chinese hamster V79 cells. Int J Oncol 2000; 17:1141–1149.
39. Rajah TT, Pento JT. The mutagenic potential of antiestrogens at the *HPRT* locus in V79 cells. Res Commun Mol Pathol Pharmacol 1995; 89:85–92.
40. Armstrong K, Eisen A, Weber B. Assessing the risk of breast cancer. N Engl J Med 2000; 342:564–571.
41. Martin AM, Weber BL. Genetic and hormonal risk factors in breast cancer. J Natl Cancer Inst 2000; 92:1126–1135.

42. Lichtenstein P, Holm NV, Verkasalo PK, et al. Environmental and heritable factors in the causation of cancer: analyses of cohorts of twins from Sweden, Denmark, and Finland. N Engl J Med 2000; 343:78–85.
43. Tonin PN. Genes implicated in hereditary breast cancer syndromes. Semin Surg Oncol 2000; 18:281–286.
44. Welcsh PL, King MC. *BRCA1* and *BRCA2* and the genetics of breast and ovarian cancer. Hum Mol Genet 2001; 10:705–713.
45. Vahteristo P, Eerola H, Tamminen A, et al. A probability model for predicting *BRCA1* and *BRCA2* mutations in breast and breast-ovarian cancer families. Br J Cancer 2001; 84:704–708.
46. Orlando R III. Risk of breast cancer in carriers of *BRCA* gene mutations. N Engl J Med 1997; 337:787.
47. Taylor MR. Genetic testing for inherited breast and ovarian cancer syndromes: important concepts for the primary care physician. Postgrad Med J 2001; 77:11–15.
48. Malkin D, Li FP, Strong LC, et al. Germ line *p53* mutations in a familial syndrome of breast cancer, sarcomas, and other neoplasms. Science 1990; 250:1233–1238.
49. Lynch HT, Lynch J, Conway T, et al. Hereditary breast cancer and family cancer syndromes. World J Surg 1994; 18:21–31.
50. Celebi JT, Wanner M, Ping XL, et al. Association of splicing defects in PTEN leading to exon skipping or partial intron retention in Cowden syndrome. Hum Genet 2000; 107:234–238.
51. Propeck PA, Warner T, Scanlan KA. Sebaceous carcinoma of the breast in a patient with Muir-Torre syndrome. AJR 2000; 174: 541–542.
52. Chen J, Lindblom A. Germline mutation screening of the *STK11/LKB1* gene in familial breast cancer with LOH on 19p. Clin Genet 2000; 57:394–397.
53. Eide GE, Heuch I, Albrektsen G. Re: population attributable risk for breast cancer: diet, nutrition, and physical exercise. J Natl Cancer Inst 2000; 92:843–844.
54. Buell P. Changing incidence of breast cancer in Japanese-American women. J Natl Cancer Inst 1973; 51:1479–1483.
55. Shimizu H, Ross RK, Bernstein L, et al. Cancers of the prostate and breast among Japanese and white immigrants in Los Angeles County. Br J Cancer 1991; 63:963–966.
56. Clemons M, Goss P. Estrogen and the risk of breast cancer. N Engl J Med 2001; 344:276–285.
57. Hulka BS. Epidemiologic analysis of breast and gynecologic cancers. Prog Clin Biol Res 1997; 396:17–29.
58. Hankinson SE, Willett WC, Manson JE, et al. Plasma sex steroid hormone levels and risk of breast cancer in postmenopausal women. J Natl Cancer Inst 1998; 90:1292–1299.
59. Cummings SR, Duong T, Kenyon E, et al. Serum estradiol level and risk of breast cancer during treatment with raloxifene. JAMA 2002; 287:216–220.
60. Thomas HV, Key TJ, Allen DS, et al. A prospective study of endogenous serum hormone concentrations and breast cancer risk in post-menopausal women on the island of Guernsey. Br J Cancer 1997; 76:401–405.
61. Dorgan JF, Baer DJ, Albert PS, et al. Serum hormones and the alcohol–breast cancer association in postmenopausal women. J Natl Cancer Inst 2001; 93:710–715.
62. Dorgan JF, Longcope C, Stanczyk FZ, et al. Re: plasma sex steroid hormone levels and risk of breast cancer in postmenopausal women. J Natl Cancer Inst 1999; 91:380–381.
63. Dorgan JF, Longcope C, Stephenson HE Jr, et al. Relation of prediagnostic serum estrogen and androgen levels to breast cancer risk. Cancer Epidemiol Biomarkers Prev 1996; 5:533–539.
64. Toniolo PG, Levitz M, Zeleniuch-Jacquotte A, et al. A prospective study of endogenous estrogens and breast cancer in postmenopausal women. J Natl Cancer Inst 1995; 87:190–197.
65. Thomas HV Reeves GK, Key TJ. Endogenous estrogen and postmenopausal breast cancer: a quantitative review. Cancer Causes & Control 1997; 8:922–928.
66. Kuller LH, Cauley JA, Lucas L, et al. Sex steroid hormones, bone mineral density, and risk of breast cancer. Environ Health Perspect 1997; 105(Suppl 3):593–599.
67. Zhang Y, Kiel DP, Kreger BE, et al. Bone mass and the risk of breast cancer among postmenopausal women. N Engl J Med 1997; 336:611–617.
68. Leon DA, Carpenter LM, Broeders MJ, et al. Breast cancer in Swedish women before age 50: evidence of a dual effect of completed pregnancy. Cancer Causes Control 1995; 6:283–291.
69. Russo J, Hu YF, Yang X, et al. Developmental, cellular, and molecular basis of human breast cancer. J Natl Cancer Inst Monogr 2000; (27):17–37.
70. Huang Z, Hankinson SE, Colditz GA, et al. Dual effects of weight and weight gain on breast cancer risk. JAMA 1997; 278: 1407–1411.
71. Friedenreich CM. Review of anthropometric factors and breast cancer risk. Eur J Cancer Prev 2001; 10:15–32.
72. Smith-Warner SA, Spiegelman D, Yaun SS, et al. Alcohol and breast cancer in women: a pooled analysis of cohort studies. JAMA 1998; 279:535–540.
73. Ginsburg ES. Estrogen, alcohol and breast cancer risk. J Steroid Biochem Mol Biol 1999; 69:299–306.
74. Ekbom A, Hsieh CC, Lipworth L, et al. Intrauterine environment and breast cancer risk in women: a population-based study. J Natl Cancer Inst 1997; 89:71–76.
75. Feinleib M. Breast cancer and artificial menopause: a cohort study. J Natl Cancer Inst 1968; 41:315–329.
76. Byrne C, Schairer C, Wolfe J, et al. Mammographic features and breast cancer risk: effects with time, age, and menopause status. J Natl Cancer Inst 1995; 87:1622–1629.
77. Greendale GA, Reboussin BA, Sie A, et al. Effects of estrogen and estrogen-progestin on mammographic parenchymal density. Postmenopausal Estrogen/Progestin Interventions (PEPI) Investigators. Ann Intern Med 1999; 130:262–269.
78. Rutter CM, Mandelson MT, Laya MB, et al. Changes in breast density associated with initiation, discontinuation, and continuing use of hormone replacement therapy. JAMA 2001; 285:171–176.
79. Salminen TM, Saarenmaa IE, Heikkila MM, et al. Is a dense mammographic parenchymal pattern a contraindication to hormonal replacement therapy? Acta Oncol 2000; 39:969–972.
80. Bouras T, Southey MC, Venter DJ. Overexpression of the steroid receptor coactivator AIB1 in breast cancer correlates with the absence of estrogen and progesterone receptors and positivity for p53 and HER2/neu. Cancer Res 2001; 61:903–907.
81. Lundstrom E, Wilczek B, von Palffy Z, et al. Mammographic breast density during hormone replacement therapy: differences according to treatment. Am J Obstet Gynecol 1999; 181:348–352.
82. Son HJ, Oh KK. Significance of follow-up mammography in estimating the effect of tamoxifen in breast cancer patients who have undergone surgery. AJR 1999; 173:905–909.
83. Litherland JC, Evans AJ, Wilson AR. The effect of hormone replacement therapy on recall rate in the National Health Service Breast Screening Programme. Clin Radiol 1997; 52:276–279.
84. Kavanagh AM, Mitchell H, Giles GG. Hormone replacement therapy and accuracy of mammographic screening. Lancet 2000; 355:270–274.
85. Breast cancer and hormonal contraceptives: further results. Collaborative Group on Hormonal Factors in Breast Cancer. Contraception 1996; 54(3 Suppl):1S–106S.
86. Brinton LA, Brogan DR, Coates RJ, et al. Breast cancer risk among women under 55 years of age by joint effects of usage of oral contraceptives and hormone replacement therapy. Menopause 1998; 5:145–151.
87. Ursin G, Ross RK, Sullivan-Halley J, et al. Use of oral contraceptives and risk of breast cancer in young women. Breast Cancer Res Treat 1998; 50:175–184.
88. Breast cancer and hormone replacement therapy: collaborative reanalysis of data from 51 epidemiological studies of 52,705 women with breast cancer and 108,411 women without breast cancer. Collaborative Group on Hormonal Factors in Breast Cancer. Lancet 1997; 350:1047–1059.
89. Colditz G, Rosner B. Use of estrogen plus progestin is associated with greater increase in breast cancer risk than estrogen alone. Am J Epidemiol 1998; 147:S45.
90. Ross RK, Paganini-Hill A, Wan PC, et al. Effect of hormone replacement therapy on breast cancer risk: estrogen versus estrogen plus progestin. J Natl Cancer Inst 2000; 92:328–332.
91. Schairer C, Lubin J, Troisi R, et al. Menopausal estrogen and estrogen-progestin replacement therapy and breast cancer risk. JAMA 2000; 283:485–491.
91a. Chen CL, Weiss NS. Hormone replacement therapy in relation to breast cancer. JAMA 2002; 287:734–741.
92. Hofseth LJ, Raafat AM, Osuch JR, et al. Hormone replacement therapy with estrogen or estrogen plus medroxyprogesterone ace-

tate is associated with increased epithelial proliferation in the normal postmenopausal breast. J Clin Endocrinol Metab 1999; 84:4559–4565.
93. Santen RJ, Pinkerton J, McCartney C, et al. Risk of breast cancer with progestins in combination with estrogen as hormone replacement therapy. J Clin Endocrinol Metab 2001; 86:16–23.
94. Druckmann R. Mammary effects of progestins. J Womens Cancer 2000; 2:85–92.
95. Wiebe JP, Muzia D, Hu J, et al. The 4-pregnene and 5alpha-pregnane progesterone metabolites formed in nontumorous and tumorous breast tissue have opposite effects on breast cell proliferation and adhesion. Cancer Res 2000; 60:936–943.
95a. Writing group for the Women's Health Initiative Investigators. Risks and benefits of estrogen plus progestin in healthy postmenopausal women. Principal results from the Women's Health Initiative Randomized Controlled Trial. JAMA 2002; 288:321–333.
96. Rodriguez C, Patel AV, Calle EE, et al. Estrogen replacement therapy and ovarian cancer mortality in a large prospective study of US women. JAMA 1921; 285:1460–1465.
97. Santen RJ, Petroni GR. Relative versus attributable risk of breast cancer from estrogen replacement therapy. J Clin Endocrinol Metab 1999; 84:1875–1881.
98. Dupont WD, Page DL, Rogers LW, et al. Influence of exogenous estrogens, proliferative breast disease, and other variables on breast cancer risk. Cancer 1989; 63:948–957.
99. Dupont WD, Page DL. Risk factors for breast cancer in women with proliferative breast disease. N Engl J Med 1985; 312:146–151.
100. Page DL, Dupont WD, Rogers LW, et al. Atypical hyperplastic lesions of the female breast: a long-term follow-up study. Cancer 1985; 55:2698–2708.
101. Carter CL, Corle DK, Micozzi MS, et al. A prospective study of the development of breast cancer in 16,692 women with benign breast disease. Am J Epidemiol 1988; 128:467–477.
102. Marshall LM, Hunter DJ, Connolly JL, et al. Risk of breast cancer associated with atypical hyperplasia of lobular and ductal types. Cancer Epidemiol Biomarkers Prev 1997; 6:297–301.
103. O'Connell P, Pekkel V, Fuqua SA, et al. Analysis of loss of heterozygosity in 399 premalignant breast lesions at 15 genetic loci. J Natl Cancer Inst 1998; 90:697–703.
104. Rosenberg CL, Larson PS, Romo JD, et al. Microsatellite alterations indicating monoclonality in atypical hyperplasias associated with breast cancer. Hum Pathol 1997; 28:214–219.
105. Fisher ER, Costantino J, Fisher B, et al. Pathologic findings from the National Surgical Adjuvant Breast Project (NSABP) Protocol B-17: five-year observations concerning lobular carcinoma in situ. Cancer 1996; 78:1403–1416.
106. Visscher DW, Wallis TL, Crissman JD. Evaluation of chromosome aneuploidy in tissue sections of preinvasive breast carcinomas using interphase cytogenetics. Cancer 1996; 77:315–320.
107. Lundin C, Mertens F. Cytogenetics of benign breast lesions. Breast Cancer Res Treat 1998; 51:1–15.
108. Smith HS, Lu Y, Deng G, et al. Molecular aspects of early stages of breast cancer progression. J Cell Biochem Suppl 1993; 17G: 144–152.
109. Khan SA, Rogers MA, Obando JA, et al. Estrogen receptor expression of benign breast epithelium and its association with breast cancer. Cancer Res 1994; 54:993–997.
110. Bodian CA, Perzin KH, Lattes R. Lobular neoplasia: long term risk of breast cancer and relation to other factors. Cancer 1996; 78:1024–1034.
111. Morrow M, Schnitt SJ. Lobular carcinoma *in situ*. In Harris JR, Lippman M, Morrow M, Osborne CK. Diseases of the Breast. Philadelphia: Lippincott-Williams & Wilkins, 2001, pp 377–381.
112. Page DL, Dupont WD, Rogers LW, et al. Continued local recurrence of carcinoma 15–25 years after a diagnosis of low grade ductal carcinoma in situ of the breast treated only by biopsy. Cancer 1995; 76:1197–1200.
113. Wickerham DL. Ductal carcinoma-in-situ. J Clin Oncol 2001; 19:(Supply):100S.
114. Morrow M, Schnitt SJ, Harris JR. Ductal carcinoma in situ and microinvasive carcinoma. In Harris JR, Lippman M, Morrow M, Osborne CK. Diseases of the Breast. Philadelphia: Lippincott-Williams & Wilkins, 2000, pp 383–401.
115. Gail MH, Brinton LA, Byar DP, et al. Projecting individualized probabilities of developing breast cancer for white females who are being examined annually. J Natl Cancer Inst 1989; 81:1879–1886.
116. Gail MH, Costantino JP. Validating and improving models for projecting the absolute risk of breast cancer. J Natl Cancer Inst 2001; 93:334–335.
117. Rockhill B, Spiegelman D, Byrne C, et al. Validation of the Gail et al. model of breast cancer risk prediction and implications for chemoprevention. J Natl Cancer Inst 2001; 93:358–366.
118. McTiernan A, Kuniyuki A, Yasui Y, et al. Comparisons of two breast cancer risk estimates in women with a family history of breast cancer. Cancer Epidemiol Biomarkers Prev 2001; 10:333–338.
118a. Claus EB, Risch N, Thompson WD. Autosomal dominant inheritance of early-onset breast cancer. Implications for risk prediction. Cancer 1994; 73:643–651.
119. Fisher B, Dignam J, Wolmark N, et al. Tamoxifen in treatment of intraductal breast cancer: National Surgical Adjuvant Breast and Bowel Project B-24 randomised controlled trial. Lancet 1999; 353:1993–2000.
120. Veronesi U, Maisonneuve P, Costa A, et al. Prevention of breast cancer with tamoxifen: preliminary findings from the Italian randomised trial among hysterectomised women. Italian Tamoxifen Prevention Study. Lancet 1998; 352:93–97.
121. Powles T, Eeles R, Ashley S, et al. Interim analysis of the incidence of breast cancer in the Royal Marsden Hospital tamoxifen randomised chemoprevention trial. Lancet 1998; 352:98–101.
122. Cummings SR, Eckert S, Krueger KA, et al. The effect of raloxifene on risk of breast cancer in postmenopausal women: results from the MORE randomized trial. Multiple Outcomes of Raloxifene Evaluation. JAMA 1999; 281:2189–2197.
123. Pritchard KI. Is tamoxifen effective in prevention of breast cancer? Lancet 1998; 352:80–81.
124. Chlebowski RT, Collyar DE, Somerfield MR, et al. American Society of Clinical Oncology technology assessment on breast cancer risk reduction strategies: tamoxifen and raloxifene. J Clin Oncol 1999; 17:1939–1955.
124a. Gail MH, Costantino JP, Bryant J, et al. Weighing the risks and benefits of tamoxifen treatment for preventing breast cancer. J Natl Cancer Inst 1999; 91:1829–1846.
125. Thompson DS, Spanier CA, Vogel VG. The relationship between tamoxifen, estrogen, and depressive symptoms. Breast J 1999; 5:375–382.
126. Day R, Ganz PA, Costantino JP, et al. Health-related quality of life and tamoxifen in breast cancer prevention: a report from the National Surgical Adjuvant Breast and Bowel Project P-1 Study. J Clin Oncol 1999; 17:2659–2669.
127. Reis SE, Costantino JP, Wickerham DL, et al. Cardiovascular effects of tamoxifen in women with and without heart disease: breast cancer prevention trial. National Surgical Adjuvant Breast and Bowel Project Breast Cancer Prevention Trial Investigators. J Natl Cancer Inst 2001; 93:16–21.
128. Love CD, Muir BB, Scrimgeour JB, et al. Investigation of endometrial abnormalities in asymptomatic women treated with tamoxifen and an evaluation of the role of endometrial screening. J Clin Oncol 1999; 17:2050–2054.
129. Gerber B, Krause A, Muller H, et al. Effects of adjuvant tamoxifen on the endometrium in postmenopausal women with breast cancer: a prospective long-term study using transvaginal ultrasound. Proc Am Soc Clin Oncol 2000; 19:76a.
130. Barakat RR. Screening for endometrial cancer in the patient receiving tamoxifen for breast cancer. J Clin Oncol 1999; 17:1967–1968.
131. Timmerman D, Deprest J, Bourne T, et al. A randomized trial on the use of ultrasonography or office hysteroscopy for endometrial assessment in postmenopausal patients with breast cancer who were treated with tamoxifen. Am J Obstet Gynecol 1998; 179:62–70.
132. Tesoro MR, Borgida AF, MacLaurin NA, et al. Transvaginal endometrial sonography in postmenopausal women taking tamoxifen. Obstet Gynecol 1999; 93:363–366.
133. Mourits MJ, Van der Zee AG, Willemse PH, et al. Discrepancy between ultrasonography and hysteroscopy and histology of endometrium in postmenopausal breast cancer patients using tamoxifen. Gynecol Oncol 1999; 73:21–26.
134. Ozsener S, Ozaran A, Itil I, et al. Endometrial pathology of 104 postmenopausal breast cancer patients treated with tamoxifen. Eur J Gynaecol Oncol 1998; 19:580–583.

135. Gail MH, Costantino JP, Bryant J, et al. RESPONSE: re: weighing the risks and benefits of tamoxifen treatment for preventing breast cancer. J Natl Cancer Inst 2000; 92:758.
136. Radmacher MD, Simon R. Estimation of tamoxifen's efficacy for preventing the formation and growth of breast tumors. J Natl Cancer Inst 2000; 92:48–53.
137. Cauley JA, Norton L, Lippman ME, et al. Continued breast cancer risk reduction in postmenopausal women treated with raloxifene: 4-year results from the MORE trial. Multiple Outcomes of Raloxifene Evaluation. Breast Cancer Res Treat 2001; 65:125–134.
138. STAR: first-year recruitment efforts set brisk pace for future. CA Cancer J Clin 2000; 50:271–272.
139. Lippman ME, Krueger KA, Eckert S, et al. Indicators of lifetime estrogen exposure: effect on breast cancer incidence and interaction with raloxifene therapy in the multiple outcomes of raloxifene evaluation study participants. J Clin Oncol 2001; 19:3111–3116.
140. Padgett RW, Das P, Krishna S. TGF-beta signaling, Smads, and tumor suppressors. Bioessays 1998; 20:382–390.
141. Nass SJ, Dickson RB. Defining a role for c-Myc in breast tumorigenesis. Breast Cancer Res Treat 1997; 44:1–22.
142. Nass SJ, Dickson RB. Epidermal growth factor–dependent cell cycle progression is altered in mammary epithelial cells that overexpress c-myc. Clin Cancer Res 1998; 4:1813–1822.
143. Prall OW, Rogan EM, Sutherland RL. Estrogen regulation of cell cycle progression in breast cancer cells. J Steroid Biochem Mol Biol 1998; 65:169–174.
144. Barnes DM, Gillett CE. Cyclin D1 in breast cancer. Breast Cancer Res Treat 1998; 52:1–15.
145. Sgambato A, Zhang YJ, Ciaparrone M, et al. Overexpression of p27Kip1 inhibits the growth of both normal and transformed human mammary epithelial cells. Cancer Res 1998; 58:3448–3454.
146. Migliaccio A, Castoria G, Di Domenico M, et al. Steroid-induced androgen receptor–oestradiol receptor beta-Src complex triggers prostate cancer cell proliferation. EMBO J 2000; 19:5406–5417.
147. Castoria G, Barone MV, Di Domenico M, et al. Non-transcriptional action of oestradiol and progestin triggers DNA synthesis. EMBO J 1999; 18:2500–2510.
147a. Song RX, McPherson RA, Adam L. Linkage of rapid estrogen action to MAPK activation by ERalpha-Shc association and Shc pathway activation. Molec Endocrinol 2002; 16:116–127.
148. Santen RJ, Manni A, Harvey H, et al. Endocrine treatment of breast cancer in women. Endocr Rev 1990; 11:221–265.
149. Shim WS, Conaway M, Masamura S, et al. Estradiol hypersensitivity and mitogen-activated protein kinase expression in long-term estrogen deprived human breast cancer cells in vivo. Endocrinology 2000; 141:396–405.
150. Narod SA. Modifiers of risk of hereditary breast and ovarian cancer. Nature Rev 2002; 2:113–123.
151. Gottardis MM, Jiang SY, Jeng MH, et al. Inhibition of tamoxifen-stimulated growth of an MCF-7 tumor variant in athymic mice by novel steroidal antiestrogens. Cancer Res 1989; 49:4090–4093.
152. Fuqua SA, Wiltschke C, Zhang QX, et al. A hypersensitive estrogen receptor-alpha mutation in premalignant breast lesions. Cancer Res 2000; 60:4026–4029.
153. Coutts AS, Murphy LC. Elevated mitogen-activated protein kinase activity in estrogen-nonresponsive human breast cancer cells. Cancer Res 1998; 58:4071–4074.
154. Osborne CK, Coronado E, Allred DC, et al. Acquired tamoxifen resistance: correlation with reduced breast tumor levels of tamoxifen and isomerization of *trans*-4-hydroxytamoxifen. J Natl Cancer Inst 1991; 83:1477–1482.
155. Levenson AS, MacGregor Schafer JI, Bentrem DJ, et al. Control of the estrogen-like actions of the tamoxifen-estrogen receptor complex by the surface amino acid at position 351. J Steroid Biochem Molec Biol 2001; 76:61–70.
156. Van der FS, Brinkman A, Look MP, et al. Bcar1/p130Cas protein and primary breast cancer: prognosis and response to tamoxifen treatment. J Natl Cancer Inst 2000; 92:120–127.
157. Katzenellenbogen BS, Montano MM, Ekena K, et al. William L. McGuire Memorial Lecture. Antiestrogens: mechanisms of action and resistance in breast cancer. Breast Cancer Res Treat 1997; 44:23–38.
158. Hellman S, Harris JR. Natural history of breast cancer. In Harris JR, Lippman M, Morrow M, Osborne CK. Diseases of the Breast. Philadelphia: Lippincott-Williams & Wilkins, 2000, pp 407–424.
159. Schnitt SJ, Guidi AJ. Pathology of invasive breast cancer. In Harris JR, Lippman M, Morrow M, Osborne CK. Diseases of the Breast. Philadelphia: Lippincott-Williams & Wilkins, 2000, pp 425–470.
160. Clark GM. Prognostic and predictive factors. In Harris JR, Lippman M, Morrow M, Osborne CK. Diseases of the Breast. Philadelphia: Lippincott-Williams & Wilkins, 2000, pp 489–514.
161. Wenger CR, Clark GM. S-phase fraction and breast cancer: a decade of experience. Breast Cancer Res Treat 1998; 51:255–265.
162. Klijn JG, Berns PM, Schmitz PI, et al. The clinical significance of epidermal growth factor receptor (EGF-R) in human breast cancer: a review on 5232 patients. Endocr Rev 1992; 13:3–17.
163. Manni A, Mauger D, Gimotty P, et al. Prognostic influence on survival of increased ornithine decarboxylase activity in human breast cancer. Clin Cancer Res 1996; 2:1901–1906.
164. Hayes DF, Trock B, Harris AL. Assessing the clinical impact of prognostic factors: when is "statistically significant" clinically useful? Breast Cancer Res Treat 1998; 52:305–319.
165. Gapstur SM, Morrow M, Sellers TA. Hormone replacement therapy and risk of breast cancer with a favorable histology: results of the Iowa Women's Health Study. JAMA 1999; 281:2091–2097.
166. Clarke R, Leonessa F, Brunner WN, et al. In vitro models. In Harris JR, Lippman M, Morrow M, Osborne CK. Diseases of the Breast. Philadelphia: Lippincott-Williams & Wilkins, 2000, pp 335–354.
167. Ellis MJ, Hayes DF, Lippman M. Treatment of metastatic breast cancer. In Harris JR, Lippman M, Morrow M, Osborne CK. Diseases of the Breast. Philadelphia: Lippincott-Williams & Wilkins, 2000, pp 749–797.
168. Riou G, Mathieu MC, Barrois M, et al. c-*erbB-2* (*HER-2/neu*) gene amplification is a better indicator of poor prognosis than protein over-expression in operable breast-cancer patients. Int J Cancer 2001; 95:266–270.
169. Elledge RM, Green S, Ciocca D, et al. *HER-2* expression and response to tamoxifen in estrogen receptor–positive breast cancer: a Southwest Oncology Group Study. Clin Cancer Res 1998; 4:7–12.
170. Yamauchi H, O'Neill A, Gelman R, et al. Prediction of response to antiestrogen therapy in advanced breast cancer patients by pretreatment circulating levels of extracellular domain of the HER-2/c-neu protein. J Clin Oncol 1997; 15:2518–2525.
171. De Placido S, Carlomagno C, De Laurentiis M, et al. c-*erbB2* expression predicts tamoxifen efficacy in breast cancer patients. Breast Cancer Res Treat 1998; 52:55–64.
172. Elledge RM, Green S, Pugh R, et al. Estrogen receptor (ER) and progesterone receptor (PgR), by ligand-binding assay compared with ER, PgR and pS2, by immuno-histochemistry in predicting response to tamoxifen in metastatic breast cancer: a Southwest Oncology Group Study. Int J Cancer 2000; 89:111–117.
173. Pettersson K, Gustafsson JA. Role of estrogen receptor beta in estrogen action. Annu Rev Physiol 2001; 63:165–192.
174. Schnitt SJ. Breast cancer in the 21st century: neu opportunities and neu challenges. Mod Pathol 2001; 14:213–218.
175. Tamoxifen for early breast cancer: an overview of the randomised trials. Early Breast Cancer Trialists' Collaborative Group. Lancet 1998; 351:1451–1467.
176. Ingle JN, Ahmann DL, Green SJ, et al. Randomized clinical trial of diethylstilbestrol versus tamoxifen in postmenopausal women with advanced breast cancer. N Engl J Med 1981; 304:16–21.
177. Song RX, Mor G, Naftolin F, et al. Effect of long-term estrogen deprivation on apoptotic responses of breast cancer cells to 17beta-estradiol. J Natl Cancer Inst 2001; 93:1714–1723.
178. Lundgren S, Helle SI, Lonning PE. Profound suppression of plasma estrogens by megestrol acetate in postmenopausal breast cancer patients. Clin Cancer Res 1996; 2:1515–1521.
179. Jonat W, Kaufmann M, Blamey RW, et al. A randomised study to compare the effect of the luteinising hormone releasing hormone (LHRH) analogue goserelin with or without tamoxifen in pre- and perimenopausal patients with advanced breast cancer. Eur J Cancer 1995; 31A:137–142.

180. McInerney EM, Weis KE, Sun J, et al. Transcription activation by the human estrogen receptor subtype beta (ER beta) studied with ER beta and ER alpha receptor chimeras. Endocrinology 1998; 139:4513–4522.
181. Klijn JG, Beex LV, Mauriac L, et al. Combined treatment with buserelin and tamoxifen in premenopausal metastatic breast cancer: a randomized study. J Natl Cancer Inst 2000; 92:903–911.
182. Klijn JG, Duchateau L. Response: re: combined treatment with buserelin and tamoxifen in premenopausal metastatic breast cancer: a randomized study. J Natl Cancer Inst 2000; 92:2041–2042.
183. Santen RJ, Manni A, Harvey H. Gonadotropin releasing hormone (GnRH) analogs for the treatment of breast and prostatic carcinoma. Breast Cancer Res Treat 1986; 7:129–145.
184. Beato M, Sanchez-Pacheco A. Interaction of steroid hormone receptors with the transcription initiation complex. Endocr Rev 1996; 17:587–609.
185. Jackson TA, Richer JK, Bain DL, et al. The partial agonist activity of antagonist-occupied steroid receptors is controlled by a novel hinge domain-binding coactivator L7/SPA and the corepressors N-CoR or SMRT. Mol Endocrinol 1997; 11:693–705.
186. Shiau AK, Barstad D, Loria PM, et al. The structural basis of estrogen receptor/coactivator recognition and the antagonism of this interaction by tamoxifen. Cell 1998; 95:927–937.
187. Lavinsky RM, Jepsen K, Heinzel T, et al. Diverse signaling pathways modulate nuclear receptor recruitment of N-CoR and SMRT complexes. Proc Natl Acad Sci USA 1998; 95:2920–2925.
188. El Tanani MK, Green CD. Two separate mechanisms for ligand-independent activation of the estrogen receptor. Mol Endocrinol 1997; 11:928–937.
189. Paech K, Webb P, Kuiper GG, et al. Differential ligand activation of estrogen receptors ERalpha and ERbeta at AP1 sites. Science 1997; 277:1508–1510.
190. Horwitz KB, Jackson TA, Bain DL, et al. Nuclear receptor coactivators and corepressors. Mol Endocrinol 1996; 10:1167–1177.
191. Porter W, Saville B, Hoivik D, et al. Functional synergy between the transcription factor Sp1 and the estrogen receptor. Mol Endocrinol 1997; 11:1569–1580.
192. Filardo EJ, Quinn JA, Bland KI, et al. Estrogen-induced activation of Erk-1 and Erk-2 requires the G protein–coupled receptor homolog, GPR30, and occurs via *trans*-activation of the epidermal growth factor receptor through release of HB-EGF. Mol Endocrinol 2000; 14:1649–1660.
193. Lien EA, Lonning PE. Selective oestrogen receptor modifiers (SERMs) and breast cancer therapy. Cancer Treat Rev 2000; 26: 205–227.
194. Buzdar AU, Hortobagyi GN. Tamoxifen and toremifene in breast cancer: comparison of safety and efficacy. J Clin Oncol 1998; 16:348–353.
195. Gradishar W, Glusman J, Lu Y, et al. Effects of high dose raloxifene in selected patients with advanced breast carcinoma. Cancer 2000; 88:2047–2053.
196. Johnston SRD, Detre S, Riddler S, et al. SCH 57058 is a selective estrogen receptor modulator (SERM) without uterotrophic effects compared with either tamoxifen or raloxifene. Twenty-Third Annual San Antonio Breast Cancer Symposium, December 6–9, 2000, San Antonio, Texas. Breast Cancer Research and Treatment 2000; 64:51. Abstract #163.
197. Fabian C, Kimler B, Anderson J, et al. Phase I biomarker and toxicity evaluation of LY 353384 (a 3rd generation selective estrogen receptor modulator, SERM) in breast cancer. Proc Am Soc Clin Oncol 2000; 19:75a.
198. Couillard S, Gutman M, Roy J, et al. Comparison of the effects of EM-652.HCI (SCH-57068.HC1), tamoxifen, toremifene, droloxifene, idoxifene, GW-5638 and raloxifene on the growth of human ZR-75-1 breast tumors in nude mice. Proc Am Soc Clin Oncol 2000; 19:76a.
199. Martel C, Labrie F, Labrie C, et al. Effects of EM-652.HCI (SCH 57068.HCI), raloxifene and tamoxifen, administered alone or in combination, or rat endometrial epithelial height and vaginal weight. Proc Am Soc Clin Oncol 2000; 19:191a.
200. Howell A, Osborne CK, Morris C, et al. ICI 182,780 (Faslodex): development of a novel, "pure" antiestrogen. Cancer 2000; 89: 817–825.
201. Robertson JFR. A comparison of the single-dose pharmacokinetics of 'Faslodex' (fulvestrant) 250 mg when given as either a one × 5-ml intra-muscular (i.m.) injection or two × 2.5-ml injections in postmenopausal women with advanced breast cancer. Twenty-Third Annual San Antonio Breast Cancer Symposium, December 6–9, 2000, San Antonio, Texas. Abstracts Poster Session, 2000; 64:53. Abstract #172.
202. Osborne CK. A double-blind randomized trial comparing the efficacy and tolerability of Faslodex with Arimidex in postmenopausal women with advanced breast cancer. Twenty-Third Annual San Antonio Breast Cancer Symposium, December 6–9, 2000, San Antonio, Texas. Abstracts General Sessions 2000; 64: 27. Abstract #7.
203. Santen RJ, Harvey HA. Use of aromatase inhibitors in breast carcinoma. Endocr Relat Cancer 1999; 6:75–92.
204. Smith IE, Harris AL, Morgan M, et al. Tamoxifen versus aminoglutethimide in advanced breast carcinoma: a randomized cross-over trial. Br Med J Clin Res Ed 1981; 283:1432–1434.
205. Smith IE, Harris AL, Morgan M, et al. Tamoxifen versus aminoglutethimide versus combined tamoxifen and aminoglutethimide in the treatment of advanced breast carcinoma. Cancer Res 1982; 42(8 Suppl):3430s–3433s.
206. Gale KE, Andersen JW, Tormey DC, et al. Hormonal treatment for metastatic breast cancer: an Eastern Cooperative Oncology Group Phase III trial comparing aminoglutethimide to tamoxifen. Cancer 1994; 73:354–361.
207. Ingle JN, Suman VJ, Johnson PA, et al. Evaluation of tamoxifen plus letrozole with assessment of pharmacokinetic interaction in postmenopausal women with metastatic breast cancer. Clin Cancer Res 1999; 5:1642–1649.
208. Dewar J, Nabholtz J-M, Bonneterre J, et al. The effect of anastrozole on serum lipids: data from a randomized comparison of anastrozole vs. tamoxifen in postmenopausal women with advanced breast cancer. Twenty-Third Annual San Antonio Breast Cancer Symposium, December 6–9, 2000, San Antonio, Texas. Breast Cancer Research and Treatment 2000; 64:51. Abstract #164.
209. Thurlimann B, Robertson JFR, Bonneterre J, et al. Efficacy of tamoxifen following Arimidex as first-line treatment for advanced breast cancer in postmenopausal women. Twenty-Third Annual San Antonio Breast Cancer Symposium, December 6–9, 2000, San Antonio, Texas. Abstracts Poster Session 2000; 64:51. Abstract #162.
210. Bajetta E, Zilembo N, Dowsett M, et al. Double-blind, randomised, multicentre endocrine trial comparing two letrozole doses, in postmenopausal breast cancer patients. Eur J Cancer 1999; 35: 208–213.
211. Bajetta E, Zilembo N, Bichisao E, et al. Steroidal aromatase inhibitors in elderly patients. Crit Rev Oncol Hematol 2000; 33: 137–142.
212. Hamilton A, Piccart M. The third-generation non-steroidal aromatase inhibitors: a review of their clinical benefits in the second-line hormonal treatment of advanced breast cancer. Ann Oncol 1999; 10:377–384.
213. Buzdar A, Nabholtz J-M, Robertson J, et al. Anastrozole versus tamoxifen as first-line therapy for advanced breast cancer in postmenopausal women: combined analysis from two identically designed multicenter trials. Proc Am Soc Clin Oncol 2000; 19: 154a.
214. Buzdar A. An overview of the use of non-steroidal aromatase inhibitors in the treatment of breast cancer. Eur J Cancer 2000; 36(Suppl 4):82–84.
215. Buzdar AU. Critique of survival update analysis from two phase III anastrozole clinical trials. Ann Surg Oncol 1999; 6(8 Suppl): 8S–11S.
216. Jones S, Vogel C, Arkhipov A, et al. Multicenter, phase II trial of exemestane as third-line hormonal therapy of postmenopausal women with metastatic breast cancer. Aromasin Study Group. J Clin Oncol 1999; 17:3418–3425.
217. Bonneterre J, Thurlimann B, Robertson JF, et al. Anastrozole versus tamoxifen as first-line therapy for advanced breast cancer in 668 postmenopausal women: results of the tamoxifen or Arimidex randomized group efficacy and tolerability study. J Clin Oncol 2000; 18:3748–3757.
218. Nabholtz JM, Buzdar A, Pollak M, et al. Anastrozole is superior to tamoxifen as first-line therapy for advanced breast cancer in postmenopausal women: results of a North American multicenter randomized trial. J Clin Oncol 2000; 18:3758–3767.
219. Bisagni G, Cocconi G, Scaglione F, et al. Letrozole, a new oral

non-steroidal aromatase inhibitor in treating postmenopausal patients with advanced breast cancer: a pilot study. Ann Oncol 1996; 7:99–102.

220. Smith R, Sun Y, Garin A, et al. Femara showed significant improvement in efficacy over tamoxifen as first-line treatment in postmenopausal women with advanced breast cancer. Twenty-Third Annual San Antonio Breast Cancer Symposium, December 6–9, 2000, San Antonio, Texas. Breast Cancer Research and Treatment 2000; 64:27. Abstract #8.
221. Milla-Santos A, Milla L, Rallo L, et al. Anastrozole vs. tamoxifen in hormonodependent advanced breast cancer: a phase II randomized trial. Twenty-Third Annual San Antonio Breast Cancer Symposium, December 6–9, 2000, San Antonio, Texas. Breast Cancer Research and Treatment 2000; 64:54. Abstract #173.
222. Wischnewsky MB, Schmid P, Boehm R, et al. Letrozole and megestrol acetate in patients with advanced breast cancer resistant to tamoxifen. Twenty-Third Annual San Antonio Breast Cancer Symposium, December 6–9, 2000, San Antonio, Texas. Breast Cancer Research and Treatment 2000; 64:54. Abstract #174.
223. Dowsett M, Jones A, Johnston SR, et al. In vivo measurement of aromatase inhibition by letrozole (CGS 20267) in postmenopausal patients with breast cancer. Clin Cancer Res 1995; 1:1511–1515.
224. Geisler J, King N, Anker G, et al. In vivo inhibition of aromatization by exemestane, a novel irreversible aromatase inhibitor, in postmenopausal breast cancer patients. Clin Cancer Res 1998; 4: 2089–2093.
225. Geisler J, King N, Dowsett M, et al. Influence of anastrozole (Arimidex), a selective, non-steroidal aromatase inhibitor, on in vivo aromatisation and plasma oestrogen levels in postmenopausal women with breast cancer. Br J Cancer 1996; 74:1286–1291.
226. Jones AL, MacNeill F, Jacobs S, et al. The influence of intramuscular 4-hydroxyandrostenedione on peripheral aromatisation in breast cancer patients. Eur J Cancer 1992; 28A:1712–1716.
227. Lonning PE, Jacobs S, Jones A, et al. The influence of CGS 16949A on peripheral aromatisation in breast cancer patients. Br J Cancer 1991; 63:789–793.
228. MacNeill FA, Jones AL, Jacobs S, et al. The influence of aminoglutethimide and its analogue rogletimide on peripheral aromatisation in breast cancer. Br J Cancer 1992; 66:692–697.
228a. Geisler JH. Influence of letrozole and anastrozole on total body aromatization and plasma estrogen levels in postmenopausal breast cancer patients evaluated in a randomized, cross-over study. J Clin Oncol 2002; 20:751–757.
229. Gershanovich M, Chaudri HA, Campos D, et al. Letrozole, a new oral aromatase inhibitor: randomised trial comparing 2.5 mg daily, 0.5 mg daily and aminoglutethimide in postmenopausal women with advanced breast cancer. Letrozole International Trial Group (AR/BC3). Ann Oncol 1998; 9:639–645.
230. Goss PE. Pre-clinical and clinical review of vorozole, a new third generation aromatase inhibitor. Breast Cancer Res Treat 1998; 49(Suppl 1):559–565.
231. Goodwin PJ, Ennis M, Pritchard KI, et al. Risk of menopause during the first year after breast cancer diagnosis. J Clin Oncol 1999; 17:2365–2370.
232. Davidson N, O'Neill A, Vukov A, et al. Effect of chemohormonal therapy in premenopausal, node (+), receptor (+) breast cancer: an Eastern Cooperative Oncology Group phase III intergroup trial (E5188, INT-0101). Proc Am Soc Clin Oncol 1999; 18:67a. Abstract #249.
232a. Fisher MD, O'Shaughnessy J. Anastrozole may be superior to tamoxifen as adjuvant treatment for postmenopausal patients with breast cancer. Clinical Breast Cancer 2002; 4:269–271.
233. Henderson C. Expert perspectives: ovarian ablation comes around again. Breast Cancer Year Book Q 2000; 11:117–120.
234. Adjuvant tamoxifen in the management of operable breast cancer: the Scottish Trial. Report from the Breast Cancer Trials Committee, Scottish Cancer Trials Office (MRC), Edinburgh. Lancet 1987; 2:171–175.
235. Abe O. The role of chemoendocrine agents in postoperative adjuvant therapy for breast cancer: meta-analysis of the first collaborative studies of postoperative adjuvant chemoendocrine therapy for breast cancer (ACETBC). Breast Cancer 1994; P:P-9.
236. Carstensen J, Nordenskjold B, Rutqvist L, et al. Prolonged follow-up of the Swedish randomized trial of two versus five years of adjuvant tamoxifen for postmenopausal early stage breast cancer and relationships to hormone receptor and erbb2 levels. Proc Am Soc Clin Oncol 2000; 19:72a.
237. Cufer T. Adjuvant therapy of breast cancer: update. Ann Oncol 1999; 10(Suppl 6):129–137.
238. Delozier T, Switsers O, Genot JY, et al. Delayed adjuvant tamoxifen: ten-year results of a collaborative randomized controlled trial in early breast cancer (TAM-02 trial). Ann Oncol 2000; 11: 515–519.
239. Ferno M, Stal O, Baldetorp B, et al. Results of two or five years of adjuvant tamoxifen correlated to steroid receptor and S-phase levels. South Sweden Breast Cancer Group, and South-East Sweden Breast Cancer Group. Breast Cancer Res Treat 2000; 59:69–76.
240. Fisher B, Dignam J, Bryant J, et al. Five versus more than five years of tamoxifen therapy for breast cancer patients with negative lymph nodes and estrogen receptor–positive tumors. J Natl Cancer Inst 1996; 88:1529–1542.
241. Stewart HJ, Forrest AP, Everington D, et al. Randomised comparison of 5 years of adjuvant tamoxifen with continuous therapy for operable breast cancer. The Scottish Cancer Trials Breast Group. Br J Cancer 1996; 74:297–299.
242. Stewart HJ, Prescott RJ, Forrest APM. Scottish adjuvant tamoxifen trial: a randomized study updated to 15 years. J Natl Cancer Inst 1921; 93:456–462.
243. Santen RJ. Long-term tamoxifen therapy: can an antagonist become an agonist? J Clin Endocrinol Metab 1996; 81:2027–2029.
244. Howell A, Robertson JFR, Quaresma Albano J, et al. Comparison of efficacy and tolerability of fulvestrant with anastrozole in postmenopausal women with advanced breast cancer: preliminary results. Twenty-Third Annual San Antonio Breast Cancer Symposium, December 6–9, 2000, San Antonio, Texas. Breast Cancer Research and Treatment 2000; 64:27. Abstract #6.
245. Santen RJ, Harvey HA. Use of aromatase inhibitors in breast carcinoma. Endocr Relat Cancer 1999; 6:75–92.
246. Anker GB, Refsum H, Ueland PM, et al. Influence of aromatase inhibitors on plasma total homocysteine in postmenopausal breast cancer patients. Clin Chem 1999; 45:252–256.
247. Buzdar A, Jonat W, Howell A, et al. Anastrozole, a potent and selective aromatase inhibitor, versus megestrol acetate in postmenopausal women with advanced breast cancer: results of overview analysis of two phase III trials. Arimidex Study Group. J Clin Oncol 1996; 14:2000–2011.
248. Dombernowsky P, Smith I, Falkson G, et al. Letrozole, a new oral aromatase inhibitor for advanced breast cancer: double-blind randomized trial showing a dose effect and improved efficacy and tolerability compared with megestrol acetate. J Clin Oncol 1998; 16:453–461.
249. Dranitsaris G, Leung P, Mather J, et al. Cost-utility analysis of second-line hormonal therapy in advanced breast cancer: a comparison of two aromatase inhibitors to megestrol acetate. Anticancer Drugs 2000; 11:591–601.
250. Kaufmann M, Bajetta E, Dirix LY, et al. Exemestane improves survival compared with megoestrol acetate in postmenopausal patients with advanced breast cancer who have failed on tamoxifen: results of a double-blind randomised phase III trial. Eur J Cancer 2000; 36(Suppl 4):S86-S87.
251. Kaufmann M, Bajetta E, Dirix LY, et al. Exemestane is superior to megestrol acetate after tamoxifen failure in postmenopausal women with advanced breast cancer: results of a phase III randomized double-blind trial. The Exemestane Study Group. J Clin Oncol 2000; 18:1399–1411.
252. Paridaens R, Dirix L, Lohrisch C, et al. Promising activity and safety of exemestane as first-line hormonal therapy in metastatic breast cancer patients: final results of an EORTC randomised phase II trial. Twenty-Third Annual San Antonio Breast Cancer Symposium, December 6–9, 2000, San Antonio, Texas. Breast Cancer Research and Treatment 2000; 64:52. Abstract #167.
253. Peethambaram PP, Ingle JN, Suman VJ, et al. Randomized trial of diethylstilbestrol vs. tamoxifen in postmenopausal women with metastatic breast cancer: an updated analysis. Breast Cancer Res Treat 1999; 54:117–122.
254. Ovarian ablation in early breast cancer: overview of the randomised trials. Early Breast Cancer Trialists' Collaborative Group. Lancet 1996; 348:1189–1196.
255. Taylor CW, Green S, Dalton WS, et al. Multicenter randomized

clinical trial of goserelin versus surgical ovariectomy in premenopausal patients with receptor-positive metastatic breast cancer: an intergroup study. J Clin Oncol 1998; 16:994–999.

256. Boccardo F, Rubagotti A, Perrotta A, et al. Ovarian ablation versus goserelin with or without tamoxifen in pre-perimenopausal patients with advanced breast cancer: results of a multicentric Italian study. Ann Oncol 1994; 5:337–342.

257. Rutqvist LE. Zoladex and tamoxifen as adjuvant therapy in premenopausal breast cancer: a randomised trial by the Cancer Research Campaign (C.R.C.) Breast Cancer Trials Group, the Stockholm Breast Cancer Group and the Gruppo Interdisciplinare Valutazione Interventi in Oncologia (G.I.V.I.O). Proc Am Soc Clin Oncol 1999; 18:67A. Abstract #251.

258. Ingle JN, Krook JE, Green SJ, et al. Randomized trial of bilateral oophorectomy versus tamoxifen in premenopausal women with metastatic breast cancer. J Clin Oncol 1986; 4:178–185.

259. Buchanan RB, Blamey RW, Durrant KR, et al. A randomized comparison of tamoxifen with surgical oophorectomy in premenopausal patients with advanced breast cancer. J Clin Oncol 1986; 4:1326–1330.

260. Sawka CA, Pritchard KI, Shelley W, et al. A randomized crossover trial of tamoxifen versus ovarian ablation for metastatic breast cancer in premenopausal women: a report of the National Cancer Inst of Canada Clinical Trials Group (NCIC CTG) trial MA.1. Breast Cancer Res Treat 1997; 44:211–215.

261. Crump M, Sawka CA, DeBoer G, et al. An individual patient-based meta-analysis of tamoxifen versus ovarian ablation as first line endocrine therapy for premenopausal women with metastatic breast cancer. Breast Cancer Res Treat 1997; 44:201–210.

262. Klijn JG, Blamey RW, Boccardo F, et al. Combined tamoxifen and luteinizing hormone–releasing hormone (LHRH) agonist versus LHRH agonist alone in premenopausal advanced breast cancer: a meta-analysis of four randomized trials. J Clin Oncol 2001; 19:343–353.

262a. Michaud LB, Buzdar AU. Endocrine therapy of metastatic breast cancer. Seminars in Breast Disease 2000; 3:100–110.

263. Adjuvant ovarian ablation versus CMF chemotherapy in premenopausal women with pathological stage II breast carcinoma: the Scottish trial. Scottish Cancer Trials Breast Group and ICRF Breast Unit, Guy's Hospital, London. Lancet 1993; 341:1293–1298.

264. Ejlertsen B, Dombernowsky P, Mouridsen H, et al. Comparable effect of ovarian ablation (OA) and CMF chemotherapy in premenopausal hormone receptor positive breast cancer patients (PRP). Proc Am Soc Clin Oncol 1999; 18:66A. Abstract #248.

265. Jakesz R, Hausmaninger H, Samonigg H, et al. Comparison of adjuvant therapy with tamoxifen and goserelin vs. CMF in premenopausal stage I and II hormone-responsive breast cancer patients: four-year results of Austrian Breast Cancer Study Group (ABCSG) trial 5. Proc Am Soc Clin Oncol 1999; 18:67A. Abstract #250.

266. Mueck AO, Seeger H, Deuringer FU, et al. Effect of an estrogen/statin combination on biochemical markers of endothelial function in human coronary artery cell cultures. Menopause 2001; 8:216–221.

267. Liehr JG. Is estradiol a genotoxic mutagenic carcinogen? Endocr Rev 2000; 21:40–54.

268. Yager JD. Endogenous estrogens as carcinogens through metabolic activation. J Natl Cancer Inst Monogr 2000; (27):67–73.

269. Boccardo F, Rubagotti A, Amoroso D, et al. Cyclophosphamide, methotrexate, and fluorouracil versus tamoxifen plus ovarian suppression as adjuvant treatment of estrogen receptor–positive pre-/perimenopausal breast cancer patients: results of the Italian Breast Cancer Adjuvant Study Group 02 randomized trial. J Clin Oncol 2000; 18:2718–2727.

270. Roche HH, Kerbrat P, Bonneterre P, et al. Complete hormonal, blockade versus chemotherapy in premenopausal early-stage breast cancer patients with positive hormone-receptor and 1–3 node-positive tumor: results of the FASG 06 trial. American Society of Clinical Oncology 2000 Annual Meeting Summaries, 2000.

271. Jonat W. Zoladex vs. CMF as adjuvant therapy in pre/perimenopausal early (node positive) breast cancer: preliminary efficacy, QOL and BMD results from the ZEBRA study. Twenty-Third Annual San Antonio Breast Cancer Symposium, December 6–9, 2000, San Antonio, Texas. Breast Cancer Research and Treatment 2000; 64:29. Abstract #13.

272. Pagani O, O'Neill A, Castiglione M, et al. Prognostic impact of amenorrhoea after adjuvant chemotherapy in premenopausal breast cancer patients with axillary node involvement: results of the International Breast Cancer Study Group (IBCSG) Trial VI. Eur J Cancer 1998; 34:632–640.

273. Bianco AR, Del Mastro L, Gallo C, et al. Prognostic role of amenorrhea induced by adjuvant chemotherapy in premenopausal patients with early breast cancer. Br J Cancer 1991; 63:799–803.

274. Dixon JM, Renshaw L, Bellamy C, et al. The effects of neoadjuvant anastrozole (Arimidex) on tumor volume in postmenopausal women with breast cancer: a randomized, double-blind, single-center study. Clin Cancer Res 2000; 6:2229–2235.

275. Ellis MJ, Jaenicke F, Llombart-Cussac A, et al. A randomized double-blind multicenter study of pre-operative tamoxifen versus Femara for postmenopausal women with ER and/or PgR positive breast cancer ineligible for breast-conserving surgery: correlation of clinical response with tumor gene expression and proliferation. Twenty-Third Annual San Antonio Breast Cancer Symposium, December 6–9, 2000, San Antonio, Texas. Breast Cancer Research and Treatment 2000; 64:29. Abstract #14.

276. Dixon JM, Love CD, Renshaw L, et al. Lessons from the use of aromatase inhibitors in the neoadjuvant setting. Endocr Relat Cancer 1999; 6:227–230.

277. Albain K, Green S, Osborne CK, et al. Tamoxifen (T) versus cyclophosphamide, Adriamycin and 5-FU plus either concurrent or sequential T in postmenopausal, receptor(+), node(+) breast cancer: a Southwest Oncology Group phase III intergroup trial (SWOG-8814, INT-0100). Proc Am Soc Clin Oncol 1997; 16: 128a.

278. Fisher B, Dignam J, Tan-Chiu E, et al. Prognosis and treatment of patients with breast tumors of one centimeter or less and negative axillary lymph nodes. J Natl Cancer Inst 2001; 93:112–120.

279. Lippman ME, Hayes DF. Adjuvant therapy for all patients with breast cancer? J Natl Cancer Inst 2001; 93:80–82.

280. Goss PE, Strasser K. Aromatase inhibitors in the treatment and prevention of breast cancer. J Clin Oncol 2001; 19:881–894.

281. Santen R, Pritchard K, Burger H. The consensus conference on treatment of estrogen deficiency symptoms in women surviving breast cancer. Obstet Gynecol Surv 1998; 53(10 Suppl):S1-S83.

282. Treatment of estrogen deficiency symptoms in women surviving breast cancer. The Hormone Foundation, Canadian Breast Cancer Research Initiative, National Cancer Inst of Canada, Endocrine Society, and the University of Virginia Cancer Center and Woman's Place. J Clin Endocrinol Metab 1998; 83:1993–2000.

283. Vassilopoulou-Sellin R, Asmar L, Hortobagyi GN, et al. Estrogen replacement therapy after localized breast cancer: clinical outcome of 319 women followed prospectively. J Clin Oncol 1999; 17:1482–1487.

283a. Vassilopoulou-Sellin R. Estrogen replacement therapy and breast cancer. Seminars in Breast Disease 2000; 3:112–116.

284. Pinkerton JV, Santen R. Alternatives to the use of estrogen in postmenopausal women. Endocr Rev 1999; 20:308–320.

285. Mulnard RA, Cotman CW, Kawas C, et al. Estrogen replacement therapy for treatment of mild to moderate Alzheimer disease: a randomized controlled trial. Alzheimer's Disease Cooperative Study. JAMA 2000; 283:1007–1015.

286. Maki P, Zonderman A, Resnick S. Enhanced verbal memory in nondemented elderly women receiving hormone-replacement therapy. Am J Psychiatry 2001; 158:227–233.

287. LeBlanc ES, Janowsky J, Chan BK, et al. Hormone replacement therapy and cognition: systematic review and meta-analysis. JAMA 2001; 285:1489–1499.

288. Hsing AW, McLaughlin JK, Cocco P, et al. Risk factors for male breast cancer (United States). Cancer Causes Control 1998; 9: 269–275.

289. Liede A, Metcalfe K, Hanna D, et al. Evaluation of the needs of male carriers of mutations in *BRCA1* or *BRCA2* who have undergone genetic counseling. Am J Hum Genet 2000; 67:1494–1504.

290. Gradishar W. Male breast cancer. In Harris JR, Lippman M, Morrow M, Osborne CK. Diseases of the Breast. Philadelphia: Lippincott-Williams & Wilkins, 2000, pp 661–668.

291. Greenlee RT, Murray T, Bolden S, et al. Cancer statistics, 2000. CA Cancer J Clin 2000; 50:7–33.

292. Pike MC, Ross RK. Progestins and menopause: epidemiological studies of risks of endometrial and breast cancer. Steroids 2000; 65:659–664.

293. Pike MC, Peters RK, Cozen W, et al. Estrogen-progestin replacement therapy and endometrial cancer. J Natl Cancer Inst 1997; 89:1110–1116.
294. Beresford SA, Weiss NS, Voigt LF, et al. Risk of endometrial cancer in relation to use of oestrogen combined with cyclic progestagen therapy in postmenopausal women. Lancet 1997; 349: 458–461.
295. Brinton LA, Hoover RN. Estrogen replacement therapy and endometrial cancer risk: unresolved issues. The Endometrial Cancer Collaborative Group. Obstet Gynecol 1993; 81:265–271.
296. Kurman RJ, Kaminski PF, Norris HJ. The behavior of endometrial hyperplasia: a long-term study of "untreated" hyperplasia in 170 patients. Cancer 1985; 56:403–412.
297. Hajek RA, Robertson AD, Johnston DA, et al. During development, 17alpha-estradiol is a potent estrogen and carcinogen. Environ Health Perspect 1997; 105(Suppl 3):577–581.
298. Longcope C, Baker R, Johnston CC Jr. Androgen and estrogen metabolism: relationship to obesity. Metabolism 1986; 35:235–237.
299. Venkatesan AM, Dunaif A, Corbould A. Insulin resistance in polycystic ovary syndrome: progress and paradoxes. Recent Prog Horm Res 2001; 56:295–308.
300. Burke TW, Fowler WC Jr, Morrow CP. Clinical aspects of risk in women with endometrial carcinoma. J Cell Biochem Suppl 1995; 23:131–136.
301. Burke TW, Eifel PJ, Naftolin F. Cancer of the uterine body. In DeVita VT, Hellman S, Rosenberg SA. Cancer: Principles & Practice of Oncology. Philadelphia: Lippincott-Williams & Wilkins, 1993, pp 1573–1594.
302. Sato M, Bryant HU, Iversen P, et al. Advantages of raloxifene over alendronate or estrogen on nonreproductive and reproductive tissues in the long-term dosing of ovariectomized rats. J Pharmacol Exp Ther 1996; 279:298–305.
303. Ehrlich CE, Young PC, Stehman FB, et al. Steroid receptors and clinical outcome in patients with adenocarcinoma of the endometrium. Am J Obstet Gynecol 1988; 158:796–807.
304. Lentz SS, Brady MF, Major FJ, et al. High-dose megestrol acetate in advanced or recurrent endometrial carcinoma: a Gynecologic Oncology Group Study. J Clin Oncol 1996; 14:357–361.
305. Thigpen JT, Brady MF, Alvarez RD, et al. Oral medroxyprogesterone acetate in the treatment of advanced or recurrent endometrial carcinoma: a dose-response study by the Gynecologic Oncology Group. J Clin Oncol 1999; 17:1736–1744.
306. Burger CW, van Leeuwen FE, Scheele F, et al. Hormone replacement therapy in women treated for gynaecological malignancy. Maturitas 1999; 32:69–76.
307. Platz EA, Rimm EB, Willett WC, et al. Racial variation in prostate cancer incidence and in hormonal system markers among male health professionals. J Natl Cancer Inst 2000; 92: 2009–2017.
308. Potosky AL, Miller BA, Albertsen PC, et al. The role of increasing detection in the rising incidence of prostate cancer. JAMA 1995; 273:548–552.
308a. Silverberg E, Lubera J. Cancer statistics, 1987. Ca: a Cancer Journal for Clinicians 1987; 37:2–19.
308b. Parker SL, Tong T, Bolden S, et al. Cancer statistics, 1997. Ca: a Cancer Journal for Clinicians 1997; 47:5–27.
309. Barry MJ. Prostate-specific-antigen testing for early diagnosis of prostate cancer. N Engl J Med 2001; 344:1373–1377.
310. Hirayama T. Epidemiology of prostate cancer with special reference to the role of diet. Natl Cancer Inst Monogr 1979; (53): 149–155.
311. Gann PH, Hennekens CH, Sacks FM, et al. Prospective study of plasma fatty acids and risk of prostate cancer. J Natl Cancer Inst 1994; 86:281–286.
312. Giovannucci E, Rimm EB, Colditz GA, et al. A prospective study of dietary fat and risk of prostate cancer. J Natl Cancer Inst 1993; 85:1571–1579.
313. Hankin JH, Zhao LP, Wilkens LR, et al. Attributable risk of breast, prostate, and lung cancer in Hawaii due to saturated fat. Cancer Causes Control 1992; 3:17–23.
314. Fradet Y, Meyer F, Bairati I, et al. Dietary fat and prostate cancer progression and survival. Eur Urol 1999; 35:388–391.
315. Griffiths K, Morton MS, Denis L. Certain aspects of molecular endocrinology that relate to the influence of dietary factors on the pathogenesis of prostate cancer. Eur Urol 1999; 35:443–455.
316. Katiyar SK, Mukhtar H. Tea consumption and cancer. World Rev Nutr Diet 1996; 79:154–184.
317. Yang GY, Liao J, Kim K, et al. Inhibition of growth and induction of apoptosis in human cancer cell lines by tea polyphenols. Carcinogenesis 1998; 19:611–616.
318. Gupta S, Ahmad N, Mukhtar H. Prostate cancer chemoprevention by green tea. Semin Urol Oncol 1999; 17:70–76.
319. Chan JM, Stampfer MJ, Giovannucci EL. What causes prostate cancer? A brief summary of the epidemiology. Semin Cancer Biol 1998; 8:263–273.
320. Moyad MA, Brumfield SK, Pienta KJ. Vitamin E, alpha- and gamma-tocopherol, and prostate cancer. Semin Urol Oncol 1999; 17:85–90.
321. Clark LC, Dalkin B, Krongrad A, et al. Decreased incidence of prostate cancer with selenium supplementation: results of a double-blind cancer prevention trial. Br J Urol 1998; 81:730–734.
322. Yoshizawa K, Willett WC, Morris SJ, et al. Study of prediagnostic selenium level in toenails and the risk of advanced prostate cancer. J Natl Cancer Inst 1998; 90:1219–1224.
323. Yang CR, Ou YC, Ho HC, et al. Unsuspected prostate carcinoma and prostatic intraepithelial neoplasm in Taiwanese patients undergoing cystoprostatectomy. Mol Urol 1999; 3:33–39.
324. Shin M, Takayama H, Nonomura N, et al. Extent and zonal distribution of prostatic intraepithelial neoplasia in patients with prostatic carcinoma in Japan: analysis of whole-mounted prostatectomy specimens. Prostate 2000; 42:81–87.
325. Qian J, Wollan P, Bostwick DG. The extent and multicentricity of high-grade prostatic intraepithelial neoplasia in clinically localized prostatic adenocarcinoma. Hum Pathol 1997; 28:143–148.
326. Pienta KJ. The epidemiology of prostate cancer: clues for chemoprevention. In Vivo 1994; 8:419–422.
327. Muir CS, Nectoux J, Staszewski J. The epidemiology of prostatic cancer: geographical distribution and time-trends. Acta Oncol 1991; 30:133–140.
328. Meikle AW, Smith JA. Epidemiology of prostate cancer. Urol Clin North Am 1990; 17:709–718.
329. de la Torre M, Haggman M, Brandstedt S, et al. Prostatic intraepithelial neoplasia and invasive carcinoma in total prostatectomy specimens: distribution, volumes and DNA ploidy. Br J Urol 1993; 72:207–213.
329a. Ping WC, Fisher MD. The prostate in eunuchs. In EORTC Genitourinary Group Monograph 10-Urological Oncology: Reconstructive Surgery, Organ Conservation, and Restoration of Function 1991, pp 249–255.
330. Schuurman AG, Zeegers MP, Goldbohm RA, et al. A case-cohort study on prostate cancer risk in relation to family history of prostate cancer. Epidemiology 1999; 10:192–195.
331. McLellan DL, Norman RW. Hereditary aspects of prostate cancer. CMAJ 1995; 153:895–900.
332. McWhorter WP, Hernandez AD, Meikle AW, et al. A screening study of prostate cancer in high risk families. J Urol 1992; 148: 826–828.
333. Keetch DW, Rice JP, Suarez BK, et al. Familial aspects of prostate cancer: a case control study. J Urol 1995; 154:2100–2102.
334. Lightfoot N, Kreigr N, Sass-Kortsak A, et al. Prostate cancer risk: medical history, sexual, and hormonal factors. Ann Epidemiol 2000; 10:470.
335. Barrack ER. Androgen receptor mutations in prostate cancer. Mt Sinai J Med 1996; 63:403–412.
336. Hakimi JM, Schoenberg MP, Rondinelli RH, et al. Androgen receptor variants with short glutamine or glycine repeats may identify unique subpopulations of men with prostate cancer. Clin Cancer Res 1997; 3:1599–1608.
337. Tavtigian SV, Simard J, Teng DH, et al. A candidate prostate cancer susceptibility gene at chromosome 17p. Nat Genet 2001; 27:172–180.
338. Ross RK, Bernstein L, Lobo RA, et al. 5-alpha-reductase activity and risk of prostate cancer among Japanese and US white and black males. Lancet 1992; 339:887–889.
339. Santner SJ, Albertson B, Zhang GY, et al. Comparative rates of androgen production and metabolism in Caucasian and Chinese subjects. J Clin Endocrinol Metab 1998; 83:2104–2109.
340. Polascik TJ, Oesterling JE, Partin AW. Prostate-specific antigen: a decade of discovery—what we have learned and where we are going. J Urol 1999; 162:293–306.
341. Stenman UH, Leinonen J, Alfthan H, et al. A complex between

predicts metastatic versus local recurrence after definitive radiotherapy. Int J Radiat Oncol Biol Phys 1997; 38:941–947.
426. Patel A, Dorey F, Franklin J, et al. Recurrence patterns after radical retropubic prostatectomy: clinical usefulness of prostate-specific antigen doubling times and log slope prostate-specific antigen. J Urol 1997; 158:1441–1445.
427. Feneley MR, Chengazi VU, Kirby RS, et al. Prostatic radioimmunoscintigraphy: preliminary results using technetium-labelled monoclonal antibody, CYT-351. Br J Urol 1996; 77:373–381.
428. Kahn D, Williams RD, Haseman MK, et al. Radioimmunoscintigraphy with In-111–labeled capromab pendetide predicts prostate cancer response to salvage radiotherapy after failed radical prostatectomy. J Clin Oncol 1998; 16:284–289.
429. McCarthy JF, Catalona WJ, Hudson MA. Effect of radiation therapy on detectable serum prostate-specific antigen levels following radical prostatectomy: early versus delayed treatment. J Urol 1994; 151:1575–1578.
430. Cassileth BR, Soloway MS, Vogelzang NJ, et al. Patients' choice of treatment in stage D prostate cancer. Urology 1989; 33:57–62.
431. Warner B, Worgul TJ, Drago J, et al. Effect of very high dose D-leucine6-gonadotropin-releasing hormone proethylamide on the hypothalamic-pituitary testicular axis in patients with prostatic cancer. J Clin Invest 1983; 71:1842–1853.
432. Waxman J, Man A, Hendry WF, et al. Importance of early tumour exacerbation in patients treated with long acting analogues of gonadotrophin releasing hormone for advanced prostatic cancer. Br Med J Clin Res Ed 1985; 291:1387–1388.
433. Thompson IM, Zeidman EJ, Rodriguez FR. Sudden death due to disease flare with luteinizing hormone–releasing hormone agonist therapy for carcinoma of the prostate. J Urol 1990; 144:1479–1480.
434. Labrie F, Dupont A, Belanger A, et al. Flutamide eliminates the risk of disease flare in prostatic cancer patients treated with a luteinizing hormone–releasing hormone agonist. J Urol 1987; 138:804–806.
435. Leuprolide versus diethylstilbestrol for metastatic prostate cancer. The Leuprolide Study Group. N Engl J Med 1984; 311:1281–1286.
436. Soloway MS, Chodak G, Vogelzang NJ, et al. Zoladex versus orchiectomy in treatment of advanced prostate cancer: a randomized trial. Zoladex Prostate Study Group. Urology 1991; 37:46–51.
437. Schroder FH, Collette L, de Reijke TM, et al. Prostate cancer treated by anti-androgens: is sexual function preserved? Br J Cancer 2000; 82:283–290.
438. Iversen P, Tyrrell CJ, Kaisary AV, et al. Bicalutamide monotherapy compared with castration in patients with nonmetastatic locally advanced prostate cancer: 6.3 years of followup. J Urol 2000; 164:1579–1582.
439. Chang A, Yeap B, Davis T, et al. Double-blind, randomized study of primary hormonal treatment of stage D2 prostate carcinoma: flutamide versus diethylstilbestrol. J Clin Oncol 1996; 14: 2250–2257.
440. Relative Effectiveness and Cost-Effectiveness of Methods of Androgen Suppression in the Treatment of Advanced Prostatic Cancer. Summary, Evidence Report/Technology Assessment, 1999. AHCPR Publication No. 99-E011. http://www.ahrq.gov/clinic/prossamm.htm.
441. Labrie F, Veilleux R. A wide range of sensitivities to androgens develops in cloned Shionogi mouse mammary tumor cells. Prostate 1986; 8:293–300.
442. Caubet JF, Tosteson TD, Dong EW, et al. Maximum androgen blockade in advanced prostate cancer: a meta-analysis of published randomized controlled trials using nonsteroidal antiandrogens. Urology 1997; 49:71–78.
443. Maximum androgen blockade in advanced prostate cancer: an overview of the randomised trials. Prostate Cancer Trialists' Collaborative Group. Lancet 2000; 355:1491–1498.
444. Crawford ED, Eisenberger MA, McLeod DG, et al. A controlled trial of leuprolide with and without flutamide in prostatic carcinoma. N Engl J Med 1989; 321:419–424.
445. Eisenberger MA, Blumenstein BA, Crawford ED, et al. Bilateral orchiectomy with or without flutamide for metastatic prostate cancer. N Engl J Med 1998; 339:1036–1042.
446. Fossa SD, Slee PH, Brausi M, et al. Flutamide versus prednisone in patients with prostate cancer symptomatically progressing after androgen-ablative therapy: a phase III study of the European organization for research and treatment of cancer genitourinary group. J Clin Oncol 2000; 19:62–71.
446a. Carroll PR, Fair WR, Grossfeld GD, et al. Overview consensus statement. Urology 2001; 58(Suppl 4).
447. Schellhammer PF, Sharifi R, Block NL, et al. Clinical benefits of bicalutamide compared with flutamide in combined androgen blockade for patients with advanced prostatic carcinoma: final report of a double-blind, randomized, multicenter trial. Casodex Combination Study Group. Urology 1997; 50:330–336.
448. Sarosdy MF, Schellhammer PF, Sharifi R, et al. Comparison of goserelin and leuprolide in combined androgen blockade therapy. Urology 1998; 52:82–88.
449. Bubley GJ, Carducci M, Dahut W, et al. Eligibility and response guidelines for phase II clinical trials in androgen-independent prostate cancer: recommendations from the Prostate-Specific Antigen Working Group. J Clin Oncol 1999; 17:3461–3467.
450. Small EJ, McMillan A, Meyer M, et al. Serum prostate-specific antigen decline as a marker of clinical outcome in hormone-refractory prostate cancer patients: association with progression-free survival, pain end points, and survival. J Clin Oncol 2001; 19:1304–1311.
451. Scher HI, Liebertz C, Kelly WK, et al. Bicalutamide for advanced prostate cancer: the natural versus treated history of disease. J Clin Oncol 1997; 15:2928–2938.
452. Veldscholte J, Berrevoets CA, Ris-Stalpers C, et al. The androgen receptor in LNCaP cells contains a mutation in the ligand binding domain which affects steroid binding characteristics and response to antiandrogens. J Steroid Biochem Mol Biol 1992; 41: 665–669.
453. Scher HI, Zhang Z-F, Cohen L. Hormonally relapsed prostatic cancer: lessons from the flutamide withdrawal syndrome. Adv Urol 1995; 8:61.
454. Figg WD, Sartor O, Cooper MR, et al. Prostate-specific antigen decline following the discontinuation of flutamide in patients with stage D2 prostate cancer. Am J Med 1995; 98:412–414.
455. Herrada J, Dieringer P, Logothetis CJ. Characterization of patients with androgen-independent prostatic carcinoma whose serum prostate-specific antigen decreased following flutamide withdrawal. J Urol 1996; 155:620–623.
456. Nieh PT. Withdrawal phenomenon with the antiandrogen Casodex. J Urol 1995; 153:1070–1072.
457. Gomella LG, Ismail M, Nathan FE. Antiandrogen withdrawal syndrome with nilutamide. J Urol 1997; 157:1366.
458. Huan SD, Gerridzen RG, Yau JC, et al. Antiandrogen withdrawal syndrome with nilutamide. Urology 1997; 49:632–634.
459. Smith DC, Redman BG, Flaherty LE, et al. A phase II trial of oral diethylstilbestrol as a second-line hormonal agent in advanced prostate cancer. Urology 1998; 52:257–260.
460. Citrin DL, Kies MS, Wallemark CB, et al. A phase II study of high-dose estrogens (diethylstilbestrol diphosphate) in prostate cancer. Cancer 1985; 56:457–460.
461. Bergan RC, Reed E, Myers CE, et al. A phase II study of high-dose tamoxifen in patients with hormone-refractory prostate cancer. Clin Cancer Res 1999; 5:2366–2373.
462. Rambeaud J. Intermittent complete androgen blockade in metastatic prostate cancer. Eur Urol 1998; 35(Suppl S1):32–36.
463. Bruchovsky N, Klotz LH, Sadar M, et al. Intermittent androgen suppression for prostate cancer: Canadian Prospective Trial and related observations. Mol Urol 2000; 4:191–199.
463a. Chenn S. In vitro mechanism of PC SPES. Urology 2001; 58(Suppl 35).
464. Gioeli D, Mandell JW, Petroni GR, et al. Activation of mitogen-activated protein kinase associated with prostate cancer progression. Cancer Res 1999; 59:279–284.
465. Potosky AL, Legler J, Albertsen PC, et al. Health outcomes after prostatectomy or radiotherapy for prostate cancer: results from the Prostate Cancer Outcomes Study. J Natl Cancer Inst 2000; 92:1582–1592.
466. Bolla M. Adjuvant hormonal treatment with radiotherapy for locally advanced prostate cancer. Eur Urol 1999; 35(Suppl 1):23–25.
467. Aronson N, Seidenfeld J, Samson J, et al. Relative effectiveness and cost-effectiveness of methods of androgen suppression in the treatment of advanced prostatic cancer. Evidence Report/Tech-

nology Assessment No. 4. Blue Cross/Blue Shield Association Evidence-Based Practice Center. Rockville, Md: US Dept of Health and Human Services: Agency for Health Care Policy and Research, 1999.

467a. Malkowicz SB. The role of diethylstilbestrol in the treatment of prostate cancer. Urology 2001; 58(Suppl 13).

468. Cavalieri E, Frenkel K, Liehr JG, et al. Estrogens as endogenous genotoxic agents: DNA adducts and mutations. J Natl Cancer Inst Monographs 2000; (27):75–93.

469. Boyd NF, Byng JW, Jong RA, et al. Quantitative classification of mammographic densities and breast cancer risk: results from the Canadian National Breast Screening Study. J Natl Cancer Inst 1995; 87:670–675.

470. Cauley JA, Lucas FL, Kuller LH, et al. Bone mineral density and risk of breast cancer in older women: the study of osteoporotic fractures. Study of Osteoporotic Fractures Research Group. JAMA 1996; 276:1404–1408.

471. Hulka BS. Epidemiologic analysis of breast and gynecologic cancers. Prog Clin Biol Res 1997; 396:17–29.

472. Huang Z, Hankinson SE, Colditz GA, et al. Dual effects of weight and weight gain on breast cancer risk. JAMA 1997; 278: 1407–1411.

473. Mouridsen H, Gershanovich M, Sun Y, et al. Superior efficacy of letrozole versus tamoxifen as first-line therapy for postmenopausal women with advanced breast cancer: results of a phase III study of the International Letrozole Breast Cancer Group. J Clin Oncol 2001; 19:2596–2606.

474. Scher HI, Kelly WK. Flutamide withdrawal syndrome: its impact on clinical trials in hormone-refractory prostate cancer. J Clin Oncol 1993; 11:1566–1572.

475. Sartor O, Cooper M, Weinberger M, et al. Surprising activity of flutamide withdrawal, when combined with aminoglutethimide, in treatment of "hormone-refractory" prostate cancer. J Natl Cancer Inst 1994; 86:222–227.

476. Harris KA, Small EJ, Frohlich MW, et al. Prospective trial of low dose ketoconazole (LDK) in patients with androgen-independent prostate cancer. Proceedings of the Annual Meeting of the American Society of Clinical Oncology 2001; 20:2419 (Abstract).

477. Dawson NA, Small EJ, Winer EP, et al. Megestrol acetate in men with hormone-refractory prostate cancer: Prostate specific antigen response and anti-androgen withdrawal data: A Cancer and Leukemia Group B study. Proceedings of the Annual Meeting of the American Society of Clinical Oncology 1996; 15:241 (Abstract).

478. Shahidi M, Norman AR, Gadd J, et al. Prospective review of diethystilbestrol in advanced prostate cancer no longer responding to androgen suppression. Proceedings of the Annual Meeting of the American Society of Clinical Oncology 2001; 20:2455 (Abstract).

Cellular Basis of Ectopic Hormone Secretion

Why is the secretion of hormones by malignant neoplasms so commonplace? The simplest idea is that random sets of genes are "derepressed" in the cancer cell, including genes that code for hormones. For example, epigenetic phenomena such as demethylation of deoxyribonucleic acid (DNA) may derepress hormone genes.[16] However, the association of tumors and hormone secretion is nonrandom, with certain tumors (e.g., lung carcinoma) characteristically secreting certain hormones (e.g., corticotropin or vasopressin). Moreover, in a number of cases, the peptides that are secreted by tumors are the same peptides that are secreted by the normal cell of origin of the neoplasm. Derepression is again nonrandom and is a quantitative rather than a qualitative phenomenon.

The *dedifferentiation hypothesis* posits a retrograde movement of tumor cells along the pathway of differentiation, leading to the expression of fetal proteins (e.g., α-fetoprotein and carcinoembryonic antigen) or hormones that are normally formed in immature cells. This hypothesis would account for both the nonrandom nature of ectopic hormone secretion and the propensity for secretion of hormones that play a critical role in development, for example, IGF-II, PTHrP, and possibly GRP and other peptides of neuroendocrine cells. In addition, tumors frequently secrete other fetal proteins (carcinoembryonic antigen, α-fetoprotein). However, there is no compelling evidence for a generalized pattern of expression of primitive genes in tumor cells.

The *dysdifferentiation hypothesis* of Baylin and Mendelsohn[17] holds that epithelial malignancy is the result of clonal expansion of a particular cell type that occurs along a complex pathway of epithelial differentiation. This process may give rise to overexpression of a hormone because of (1) clonal expansion of a normally rare population of committed cells or (2) clonal expansion of a primitive cell type not normally present in the mature epithelium.

Because the defining characteristic of neoplastic cells is uncontrolled growth, it is worth considering the possible relationship of disordered growth and the secretion of hormones. In some instances, an oncogenic event might directly activate transcription of a hormone gene. One example of direct gene activation is the secretion of PTHrP in adult T-cell leukemia, with associated severe hypercalcemia.[18] The oncogenic event that gives rise to this form of leukemia involves integration of the human T-cell lymphotropic virus type I (HTLV-I), which can target the promoter of the PTHrP gene to induce its transcription using the *trans*-activating viral protein tax.[19–21] Loss of the tumor von Hippel–Lindau suppressor gene *VHL* is associated with the development of cerebellar hemangioblastoma and renal carcinoma. Evidence suggests that erythropoietin gene expression is directly up-regulated by this oncogenic event.[22–25]

Secretion of a hormone might stimulate the growth of tumor cells by an autocrine or a paracrine mechanism, so that hormone secretion may provide a growth advantage, leading to selective outgrowth of cells that secreted high levels of the hormone. One of the characteristic products of small cell lung carcinoma (SCLC) is GRP, the mammalian counterpart of the amphibian hormone bombesin. GRP fulfills criteria for being an autocrine growth factor in SCLC: (1) it is secreted by tumor cells and can stimulate replication of the cells via specific receptors, and (2) blockade of its action by neutralizing antibodies to GRP[26, 27] or peptide antagonists[28, 29] inhibits cell replication in vitro and tumor formation in vivo. β-Endorphin, one of the products of the pro-opiomelanocortin (*POMC*) gene, may also function as a growth factor in SCLC.[30]

Endothelin receptors are often coexpressed on tumor cells with endothelin-1, and endothelin-1 is reported to have paracrine effects on tumor cell growth.[31–34] Prolactin and its receptor are expressed by breast cancer cells, although rarely, if ever, at high enough levels to raise serum prolactin levels,[35–38] and an autocrine pathway has been described in which prolactin induces constitutive phosphorylation of *erbB-2* (Her/Neu), an oncogene that is important in growth of breast cancer.[39] Another ectopic hormone with growth factor activity is IGF-II, the factor that is believed to cause hypoglycemia in non–islet cell tumors.[8] However, there is no direct evidence for a role of IGF-II in the growth of these neoplasms.

Epigenetic events associated with tumorigenesis may activate the transcription of hormone genes. Altered methylation of CpG islands appears to play a role in the expression of PTHrP in renal carcinoma, with undermethylation of the PTHrP promoter in tumors that express the gene.[40] Evidence suggests that demethylation of the POMC promoter may also be involved in expression of corticotropin in neuroendocrine tumor cells.[41]

Thus, ectopic hormone production can be partly understood in the context of the determinants of tumor cell behavior generally. Nevertheless, why specific tumor types overexpress hormone genes and why overexpression occurs in some tumors of a given type (e.g., SCLC) and not others are questions that remain largely unanswered.

Neuroendocrine Cells and Hormone Secretion

Tumors that secrete corticotropin, vasopressin, calcitonin, gut peptides (GRP, somatostatin, vasoactive intestinal peptide [VIP]), and biogenic amines such as 5-hydroxytryptamine (5-HT) are characteristically of neuroendocrine cell origin. Neuroendocrine cells specialized for the production of peptide hormones and biogenic amines possess pathways for the rapid release of peptides or neurotransmitters in response to stimuli; such regulated pathways for protein secretion are distinct from the mechanism of constitutive secretion, which is ubiquitous in eukaryotic cells.

The most readily recognizable feature of the regulated pathway is the dense neurosecretory granule, which is designed for the secretion of peptides and amines.[42] The neurosecretory granule, which is involved in both the storage of hormones in concentrated form and the rapid release of these stores in response to stimulation, is recognizable histologically because it is electron dense and intensely argyrophilic, reflecting the dense, nearly crystalline packing of its contents.

The neurosecretory granule buds from the trans-Golgi network after it is packed with its peptide or neurotransmitter contents. Proteins on the surface of the neurosecretory granule, in the vesicular compartments from which the granule buds, and on the plasma membrane of neurosecretory cells collectively determine the properties of the regulated pathway of hormone secretion.[43] They are probably important in ectopic hormone secretion. In addition to stored hormones, the neuroendocrine granule contains one or more acidic proteins called *chromogranins*, which are released together with stored hormone and serve as additional neuroendocrine tumor markers, both in immunohistology and in the circulation.[44] The chromogranins are highly conserved in evolution and presumably play a role in the assembly, packing, or release of neurosecretory granules,[45–47] but this role has yet to be fully clarified.

The neurosecretory granules contain serine proteases called *prohormone convertases*, which process precursor proteins to their mature forms. The prohormone convertase family is widely distributed in evolution, and several members of the family, such as furin, are localized in the trans-Golgi network and process a wide variety of proteins in the constitutive pathway. The two members of the family that occur mainly in neurosecretory granules, PC2 (SPC2) and PC1/PC3 (SPC3), have acidic pH optima and are dependent on calcium, suiting them for the environment of the neurosecretory granule.[48, 48] Both enzymes cleave their substrate peptides on the carboxyl-terminal side of polybasic residues, but they have slightly different specificities, and their different distribution in the pituitary accounts for the differences in processing of POMC in the anterior and intermediate pituitary lobes.[48, 49]

The prohormone convertases are important for our understanding of ectopic hormone secretion. Their levels in tumor cells account for the efficiency of precursor processing to mature and biologically active versions of peptide hormones, thus determining whether a given tumor produces a clinical syndrome of hormone excess. Further, they determine the pattern of peptides produced (e.g., from the polyhormone precursor POMC) and thus the nature of the clinical syndrome.

Neuroendocrine cells are scattered through the bronchial mucosa of the developing and mature lung.[9, 10, 50] They occur singly and in distinct innervated corpuscles referred to as neuroepithelial bodies. Subpopulations of the cells contain the peptides calcitonin, GRP, vasopressin, and leu-enkephalin, and some may also contain somatostatin, motilin, or pancreatic polypeptide. Neuroendocrine (enterochromaffin) cells are also scattered through the gastrointestinal mucosa and are found in other organs, such as the ovaries and the prostate gland. Some years ago, Pearce suggested that neuroendocrine cells, which he called *APUD cells* (*a*mine *p*recursor *u*ptake and *d*ecarboxylation), although widely scattered in many tissues, have a common origin in the neural crest and represent a *diffuse neuroendocrine system*, a third branch of the nervous system.[51] Not all APUD cells are of neural crest origin, however; some arise from primitive endoderm.[52]

Neuroendocrine cells in the gut and lung are specified by a set of basic helix-loop-helix (bHLH) transcription factors that are involved in the determination of neuronal fate in mammals and *Drosophila.* Transient expression of the mouse achaete-scute homologue-1 (*mASH1*) is required for neurogenesis of autonomic and enteric neurons and adrenal chromaffin cells. Pulmonary neuroendocrine cells do not develop in mice deficient in mASH1[53] and forced expression of mASH1 induces metaplasia and cooperates with simian virus 40 (SV40) T antigen in tumorigenesis.[54] Neuroendocrine tumor cells such as SCLC cells express the human orthologue hASH1.[55–57]

Disruption of an inhibitory pathway may also lead to neuroendocrine cell expansion. *Drosophila* and vertebrate neurogenesis is characterized by lateral inhibition, a cell-cell interaction in which differentiating neuronal cells inhibit neuronal differentiation of their neighbors through actions of a transmembrane receptor, Notch, and the ligand Delta.[58] One of the chief targets of the inhibitory pathway is hairy-enhancer-of-split-1 (Hes-1), which inhibits the proneural genes neurogenin, neuroD, and ASH.[59, 60] Ablation of *Hes-1* leads to a marked increase in enteroendocrine cells,[59] and SCLC cells are characteristically deficient in Hes-1.[60] Collectively, these data delineate a pathway of origin of neuroendocrine tumor cells and identify transcription factors that may be directly involved in up-regulating expression in neuroendocrine cells. However, examples of direct regulation of hormonal expression by such genes have not yet been adduced.

Criteria for Diagnosis of Ectopic Hormone Secretion

Criteria for the diagnosis of ectopic hormone secretion, arranged in increasing order of stringency, are summarized in Table 40–3. The association of a clinical syndrome of hormone excess with a neoplasm provokes a search for inappropriate plasma or urinary hormone levels. In many cases, the clinician performs suppression tests because glandular hypersecretion of hormones is often suppressible whereas the secretion of hormones by neoplasms is typically autonomous and nonsuppressible. In the usual clinical circumstance, the last step is to exclude other possible causal mechanisms for hormone excess.

Table 40–3. Criteria for Diagnosis of Ectopic Hormone Secretion

Clinical criteria
1. A clinical syndrome of hormone excess is associated with a neoplasm.
2. Serum or urine levels of the hormone are inappropriately elevated.
3. The hormone level is nonsuppressible.
4. Other possible causal mechanisms are excluded.
5. The syndrome is reversed by resection of the tumor (rare).

Research criteria
1. The hormone can be detected in tumor tissue.
2. Messenger RNA for the hormone is present in tumor tissue.
3. The hormone is secreted from tumor cells in culture.
4. There is an arteriovenous gradient for the hormone across the tumor.

The coincidental occurrence of an endocrine tumor and a cancer is not uncommon; for example, primary hyperparathyroidism can be present in a patient who also has cancer and can be detected with relative ease using modern assays for PTH. Occasionally, the presence of an ectopic hormone syndrome can be confirmed by showing that resection of the tumor reverses the clinical syndrome. Because such syndromes are typically late manifestations of widespread neoplasms, these opportunities are sadly rare.

The remaining criteria for ectopic hormone secretion are useful mainly for research purposes. The detection of a hormone in tumor tissue by immunoassay methods provides evidence that the tumor is a site of its production, although caution must be exercised because of the possibility of false-positive reactions in immunohistochemistry and radioimmunoassay. An additional theoretical concern is that the tumor may accumulate hormone from the circulation; no examples of this phenomenon have been reported, however. Detection of mRNA for the hormone confirms that the tumor is indeed a site of synthesis of the peptide. For this evidence to be compelling, hormone mRNA should be detectable in solution hybridization or RNA blotting assays. The technique of reverse transcription and PCR is so sensitive that a signal can be obtained from samples containing only a few molecules of hormone mRNA, a level that may be insignificant. In addition, identification of hormone mRNA without hormone protein leaves open the possibility that the mRNA is not translated—for example, many normal tissues express a form of POMC mRNA that cannot be translated to protein.[61]

Demonstration of the presence of both hormone mRNA and protein provides strong evidence for synthesis in the tumor but does not directly establish that the hormone is secreted. The most rigorous criterion for ectopic hormone secretion is the demonstration of an arteriovenous gradient of the hormone across the tumor or of production and secretion of the hormone by tumor cells cultured in vitro. Unfortunately, selective catheterization to obtain a true arteriovenous gradient is often impossible, as many of the tumors are present in the pulmonary or splanchnic bed or are widely metastatic. Establishing tumor cells in culture provides an important research tool but requires an element of good fortune—many tumor cells, exuberant as their growth may be in the host, are difficult to propagate in cell culture.

MALIGNANCY-ASSOCIATED HYPERCALCEMIA

Clinical Features

Hypercalcemia is probably the most common endocrine complication of malignant tumors, occurring in as many as 5% of all cancers. The incidence of hypercalcemia in malignancy is 15 cases per 100,000 person-years, about one half the incidence of primary hyperparathyroidism,[62] and malignant tumors are the most common cause of hypercalcemia in hospitalized patients[63–65] (see Chapter 26).

Hypercalcemia in malignancy usually has a rapid onset and can cause confusion, stupor, nausea, vomiting, and dehydration. The offending neoplasm is almost always evident clinically, even when hypercalcemia is the initial manifestation. Thus, physical examination and a chest radiograph disclose the underlying tumor in about 98% of patients. Because hypercalcemia usually occurs in advanced malignancy, the prognosis is poor, with a median survival of only 4 to 8 weeks after the discovery of hypercalcemia.[66] Exceptions are breast carcinoma and multiple myeloma, in which successful treatment of the underlying malignancy may allow long survival of the hypercalcemic patient.

The frequency of individual tumors in patients with hypercalcemia is shown in Table 40–4. Lung carcinoma, breast carcinoma, and multiple myeloma account for more than 50% of all cases of malignancy-associated hypercalcemia. Lung carcinomas that produce hypercalcemia have squamous or large cell histology, whereas small cell carcinoma almost never causes hypercalcemia.[67] About two thirds of lung cancer patients have bone metastasis at the time when hypercalcemia develops. Among other solid tumors, the most common are squamous and renal carcinomas. Gastrointestinal tumors and prostate carcinoma are less common causes of hypercalcemia.

Hypercalcemia is uncommon in lymphomas and leukemia but occurs in two thirds of patients with adult T-cell leukemia syndrome, which is caused by the retrovirus HTLV-I.[18, 68, 69] Another rare variety of leukemia in which hypercalcemia is common is the M7 variant of acute myelogenous leukemia, megakaryocytic leukemia.[70, 71] Hypercalcemia is a common complication of multiple myeloma. Hypercalcemia in myeloma has been ascribed to a local osteolytic cause, but a substantial fraction of cases have increased PTHrP levels.[72–74] Pheochromocytomas may produce hypercalcemia by secretion of PTHrP.[75–77]

Table 40–4. Malignancy-Associated Hypercalcemia

Primary Site	No. (%) of Cases	Known Metastatic Disease (%)
Lung	111 (25.0)	62
Breast	87 (19.6)	92
Multiple myeloma	43 (9.7)	100
Head and neck	36 (8.1)	73
Renal and urinary tract	35 (7.9)	36
Esophagus	25 (5.6)	53
Female genitalia	24 (5.2)	81
Unknown primary	23 (5.2)	—
Lymphoma	14 (3.2)	91
Colon	8 (1.8)	—
Liver, biliary	7 (1.6)	—
Skin	6 (1.4)	—
Other	25 (5.6)	—
Total	444 (100)	

Data from references 63 to 65. Data on metastatic disease from references 64 and 65.

From Strewler GJ. Nonparathyroid hypercalcemia. Adv Intern Med 1987; 32: 235–258.

Laboratory Features

Overall, about 80% of cases, including most patients with solid tumors, have increased serum levels of PTHrP, which can be measured in two-site, amino-terminal or midregion assays (Fig. 40–1).[72, 78–84] Hypophosphatemia is common because of the phosphaturic effect of PTHrP. Although the combination of hypercalcemia and hypophosphatemia is consistent with the presence of primary hyperparathyroidism, the level of intact PTH is suppressed to less than 2 pmol/L (20 pg/mL) in patients with malignancy-associated hypercalcemia.[72, 85] The serum level of 1,25$(OH)_2D$ is also suppressed in hypercalcemic patients,[86, 87] except in lymphoma, in which 1,25$(OH)_2D$ levels are often high. Renal function may be impaired by hypercalcemia; the decreased glomerular filtration rate may lead to normalization of blood phosphate in patients with PTHrP-mediated hypercalcemia.

Pathogenesis

Hypercalcemia in malignancy is caused by excessive bone resorption. Multiple myeloma and some breast cancers induce hypercalcemia by local osteolytic mechanisms, but in most patients bone resorption is induced by humoral factors. The most common humoral factor is PTHrP, but 1,25$(OH)_2D$ is a hypercalcemic factor in lymphomas,[88–90] and in rare instances PTH is secreted ectopically by nonparathyroid tumors.[71, 91–93]

Parathyroid Hormone–Related Protein

PTHrP is related to PTH structurally (see Fig. 24–12) and shares a common receptor with PTH[11, 94, 95] (see Chapter 26 for a discussion of the chemistry of PTHrP). Because PTH and PTHrP share a receptor,[96, 97] their biologic actions are similar.[95] PTHrP produces hypercalcemia by increasing resorption of bone throughout the skeleton and by increasing the renal resorption of calcium and causes hypophosphatemia through a phosphaturic effect at the kidney.[94] The hypocalciuric effect of PTHrP probably plays a significant role in the pathogenesis of hypercalcemia,[98, 99] albeit secondary to the role of bone resorption. In some[100–102] but not all[87, 103] studies of bisphosphonate treatment of hypercalcemia, the effect of treatment was negatively correlated with the serum level of PTHrP, suggesting that increased renal calcium reabsorption may limit the response of some patients to treatment with inhibitors of bone resorption.

PTHrP functions in normal physiology as a tissue factor that regulates cellular proliferation and differentiation in fetal development and in tissues such as the breast, skin, and hair follicle in the adult[104] (see Chapter 26). Remarkably, PTHrP locally regulates development, in part acting via the same receptor that PTH uses systemically to regulate its target tissues, bone and kidney. However, when PTHrP is produced by a tumor of sufficient mass, it enters the systemic circulation, where it activates PTH-PTHrP receptors in bone and kidney and produces hypercalcemia.

PTHrP can either produce humoral hypercalcemia or cause local osteolytic hypercalcemia by direct activation of osteoclasts in the vicinity of bone metastases. In lung and renal carcinoma, PTHrP often acts as a humoral factor because hypercalcemia can occur without evidence of bone metastasis (see Table 40–1). Even when bone metastases are present, hypercalcemia is predominantly humoral because the serum calcium

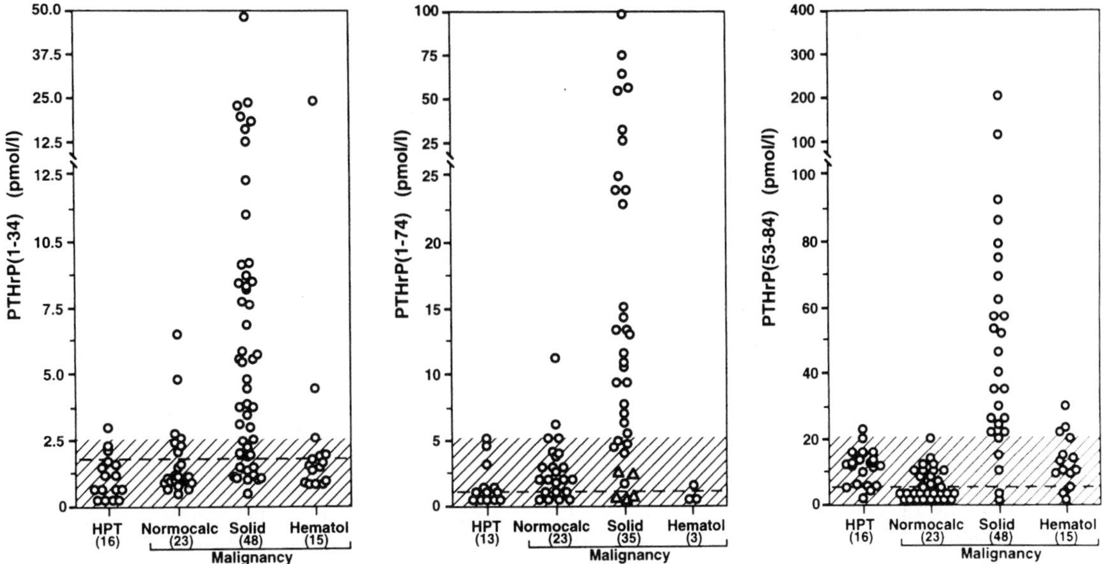

Figure 40–1. Plasma concentration of parathyroid hormone–related protein (PTHrP) in patients with hyperparathyroidism (HPT), normocalcemic patients with malignancy (Normocalc), and patients with hypercalcemia of malignancy caused by a solid tumor (Solid) or a hematologic malignancy (Hematol). Radioimmunoassay for amino-terminal PTHrP(1–34) *(left panel)*, an immunoradiometric assay for PTHrP(1–74) *(middle panel)*, and a radioimmunoassay for midregion PTHrP(53–84) *(right panel)*. The *hatched* area represents the normal ranges; the *dashed line* denotes the limits of detection; the numbers attached to each group indicate the number of patients. In the PTHrP(1–74) assay, the group Solid includes five patients classified as having local osteolytic type of hypercalcemia (Δ). Note the different scale of the y-axes. (Data from Budayr et al,[72] Burtis et al,[78] and Blind et al[81]; reprinted from Blind E, Nissenson RA, Strewler GJ. Parathyroid hormone–related protein. In Becker KL, Bremner WJ, Hung W, et al [eds]. Principles and Practice of Endocrinology and Metabolism, 2nd ed. Philadelphia, JB Lippincott, 1985.)

level correlates better with the level of PTHrP than with the number or size of bone metastases.

There is experimental evidence that PTHrP, when expressed in bone metastasis, can also be a local osteolytic factor. In an experimental model, transfection of PTHrP complementary DNA into breast carcinoma cells increased their propensity for bone metastasis, and bone metastasis induced local osteolysis without an increase in the circulating level of PTHrP.[105] This result is in agreement with the biology of human breast carcinoma, in which about 50% of hypercalcemic patients have extensive bone metastases without increased serum levels of PTHrP and are presumed to have local osteolytic hypercalcemia (see Table 40–4).[72, 78–81]

In humans, metastases of breast cancer to bone are immunohistochemically positive for PTHrP in 92% of cases, compared with 17% for nonosseous metastases.[106, 107] Tumor cells that secrete PTHrP have a selective advantage in bone, probably because they induce local resorption.[105] Moreover, transforming growth factor β (TGF-β) released from bone matrix as a result of bone resorption induces the expression of PTHrP, setting up a positive feedback loop to perpetuate the process.[108]

At least two aspects of the hypercalcemia syndrome associated with PTHrP are paradoxical. First, plasma levels of $1,25(OH)_2D$ tend to be low in malignancy,[86, 87] despite the acute effect of PTHrP to stimulate renal synthesis of $1,25(OH)_2D$.[109] This finding contrasts with normal to high levels of $1,25(OH)_2D$ in primary hyperparathyroidism.[86] This difference may be due to the capacity of hypercalcemia itself to suppress production of $1,25(OH)_2D$, tending to counteract the acute stimulatory effect of PTH or PTHrP. Thus, a continuous chronic infusion of PTH, in contrast to the effects of primary hyperparathyroidism, suppresses $1,25(OH)_2D$ levels, but clamping the serum calcium in the normal range prevents this suppression.[110] In the same vein, some patients with malignancy have a marked increase in $1,25(OH)_2D$ to supranormal levels when hypercalcemia is treated with bisphosphonates.[87] Perhaps the pattern of secretion of PTHrP (continuous?) or associated ancillary factors[111] increase the susceptibility of $1,25(OH)_2D$ synthesis to suppression by hypercalcemia.

A second paradox concerns bone turnover in the setting of high PTHrP levels. Despite avid bone resorption, bone formation is reduced in postmortem bone biopsy specimens from patients with malignancy and hypercalcemia.[112] This uncoupled state contrasts with primary hyperparathyroidism and most other resorptive states, which are characterized by coupled increases in bone formation, and also contrasts with the results of a PTHrP infusion.[113] It is possible that immobilization, inanition, illness, or other cytokines secreted by neoplasms depress osteoblastic activity.

Mechanisms involved in the activation of PTHrP gene expression in malignant tumors may include *trans*-activation by tumor-specific factors and differential methylation. The best example of *trans*-activation is adult T-cell leukemia, which is commonly characterized by PTHrP-dependent hypercalcemia.[18, 68, 69]

A specific *trans*-activating protein, called tax, in the genome of HTLV-I is capable of direct activation of PTHrP transcription, acting primarily at an Ets-1 site near the most downstream promoter.[19–21] The keratinocyte is a prominent site of normal PTHrP expression[114–116]; thus, secretion of PTHrP by squamous carcinomas can be regarded as eutopic. However, only a fraction of patients with squamous carcinomas have hypercalcemia. When PTHrP promoter constructs were fused to a reporter gene and transfected into squamous carcinoma cell lines, the relative level of expression of the reporter gene correlated with the intensity of endogenous PTHrP gene expression in the same cell lines,[117] suggesting that in this circumstance also, the expression of PTHrP is regulated in *trans* by a factor or factors that are differentially expressed in different squamous carcinomas.

PTHrP expression in human squamous carcinoma cells is repressed by mutant forms of the tumor suppressor gene p53.[118] Most squamous carcinomas express the PTHrP gene at some level,[119] but renal carcinomas are more sharply divided between PTHrP expressors and nonexpressors. The PTHrP gene is undermethylated in renal carcinomas that express PTHrP compared with those that do not.[40] This finding suggests that hypomethylation may be a mechanism by which the gene is expressed in some renal carcinomas.

1,25-Dihydroxyvitamin D

About 50% of lymphoma patients who become hypercalcemic have inappropriately high serum $1,25(OH)_2D$ levels.[88–90] In a few cases, lymph node tissue from such patients has been shown to produce $1,25(OH)_2D$ in vitro from 25-OHD.[120] Challenge of normocalcemic lymphoma patients with the precursor sterol 25-OHD resulted in increased serum $1,25(OH)_2D$ levels, increased serum calcium levels, and suppression of PTH.[120] This response is in marked contrast to that of normal individuals, who regulate the conversion of substrate to $1,25(OH)_2D$ tightly.

The enhanced responsiveness of normocalcemic lymphoma patients to vitamin D indicates that the fundamental abnormality in lymphoma, unregulated extrarenal production of $1,25(OH)_2D$, is more common than hypercalcemia. As would be expected from this interpretation, hypercalciuria is also more common than hypercalcemia in lymphoma patients[89] and presumably compensates at least in part for the inappropriate synthesis of $1,25(OH)_2D$. This syndrome resembles the hypercalcemia of sarcoidosis, which is also due to enhanced extrarenal production of $1,25(OH)_2D$.[121, 122] As in sarcoidosis, hypercalcemia in lymphoma is frequently responsive to administration of glucocorticoids. Hypercalcemia may not respond well to treatment with hydroxychloroquine.[123]

Parathyroid Hormone

Secretion of PTH from extraparathyroid tumors is extremely rare,[71, 91–93] although one case fulfilled the most rigorous criterion—demonstration of an arteriovenous gradient for PTH across the tumor.[124] Most nonparathyroid tumors that secrete PTH are neuroendocrine tumors, although one was an ovarian adenocarcinoma and one a hepatocellular carcinoma. The diagnosis should be considered in patients with malignant tumors (particularly small cell tumors), hypercalcemia, and elevated PTH levels. However, most patients with these findings have a malignant tumor with coincident primary hyperparathyroidism because this coincidence is more likely than the truly rare syndrome of ectopic PTH secretion. Consequently, exploration of the parathyroid glands may be indicated in patients who require treatment for hypercalcemia.

Local Osteolytic Hypercalcemia

Osteolytic lesions cause hypercalcemia by activation of osteoclasts and secretion of bone-resorbing cytokines. Cytokines with osteoclast-activating activity include interleukin-1, tumor necrosis factor α (TNF-α), interleukin-6, TGF-α, and PTHrP.[105, 125] As discussed earlier, PTHrP appears to be the local osteolytic factor that causes osteolytic hypercalcemia in breast carcinoma.[105–108]

The other classic example of local osteolytic hypercalcemia is multiple myeloma. Although at least one third of myeloma patients have hypercalcemia at some time during their disease, the offending cytokine has not been identified with certainty. Cultured human myeloma cell lines produce bone-resorbing factors that can be neutralized with antisera to interleukin-1β[126] or TNF-β (lymphotoxin),[127] but it is likely that other factors are responsible for the hypercalcemia.

A preliminary report suggested a strong association of hypercalcemia with secretion of the chemokine macrophage inflammatory protein 1.[128] It is clear that a fraction of hypercalcemic patients with multiple myeloma have high serum PTHrP levels and thus humoral rather than local osteolytic hypercalcemia.[72–74, 129] This finding raises the question of whether PTHrP, which may be expressed commonly in marrow myeloma cells,[130] is also a dominant local osteolytic factor in multiple myeloma and lymphoma.

Diagnosis

The diagnosis of malignancy-associated hypercalcemia is usually not difficult because the offending neoplasm is clinically evident. It is important to exclude intercurrent primary hyperparathyroidism by showing that the level of intact PTH is suppressed below 2 pmol/L (20 pg/mL). A low serum phosphorus level in conjunction with suppressed PTH levels suggests that the causative factor is PTHrP. Demonstration of elevated levels of PTHrP confirms the diagnosis in patients with solid tumors, but this is often unnecessary clinically. PTHrP is processed to amino-terminal, midregion, and carboxyl-terminal peptides,[11, 131] and similar assay performance has been achieved with assays of the amino terminus[72, 79] and midregion[81–83] and two-site immunoradiometric assays[78, 132, 133] (see Fig. 40–1). Two-site assays for PTHrP have become the standard.[72, 79, 80, 83, 84]

Treatment

The treatment of hypercalcemia is discussed in Chapter 26. The mainstays of therapy for tumor patients, in whom hypercalcemia is often acute and severe, are rehydration, institution of a saline diuresis, and institution of chronic treatment. In general, the treatment of choice is the second-generation bisphosphonate pamidronate, 60 to 90 mg by intravenous infusion. Patients with multiple myeloma or lymphoma often respond to glucocorticoid treatment.

SYNDROME OF INAPPROPRIATE VASOPRESSIN SECRETION

(See Chapter 9)

Clinical Features

The syndrome of inappropriate vasopressin secretion (commonly termed the syndrome of inappropriate antidiuretic hormone [SIADH]) is probably the second most common endocrine complication in cancer patients.[134–136] The secretion of vasopressin impairs the ability to dilute the urine, leading to a state of water intoxication with hypotonicity and hyponatremia. Patients with hyponatremia may be asymptomatic if the condition has developed gradually. Patients may experience weight gain because of water retention, but because the retained water is distributed among both extracellular and intracellular spaces, there is no edema. However, when the serum sodium level falls rapidly to below 120 mmol/L, somnolence, coma, and seizures can occur. Symptomatic hyponatremia carries a mortality rate of 10% to 15%, but this rate is higher when the serum sodium level is below 110 mmol/L.

By far, the most common tumor that causes SIADH is SCLC. SIADH occurs in 5% to 15% of patients with SCLC[135–139] and in fewer than 1% of patients with non–small cell lung cancer (non-SCLC).[140] Other neuroendocrine tumors, including carcinoids and small cell carcinomas of the prostate and cervix, can also cause SIADH. SIADH also occurs occasionally in a wide range of carcinomas, including as many as 2% of squamous carcinomas of the head and neck,[141] adenocarcinoma of the colon, Hodgkin's disease, non-Hodgkin's lymphomas, and several varieties of brain tumors.[135, 136] The finding of hyponatremia in cancer is nonspecific, and central secretion of vasopressin from various nonosmotic stimuli may be at fault in some of these patients, for example, patients with thoracic or intracranial tumors. However, vasopressin and associated neurophysins have been found in non-neuroendocrine tumor cells, and some epithelial tumors have the ability to secrete vasopressin.

Laboratory Features

The cardinal features of SIADH are hypotonicity with hyponatremia and an inappropriately concentrated urine. It is often unnecessary to measure serum osmolality directly in a hyponatremic patient because the effective serum osmolality—serum sodium (mmol/L) × 2 + glucose (mmol/L)—closely approximates direct measurements.[142] A urine osmolality greater than 50 to 60 mmol/L water is inappropriate in the setting of serum hypotonicity, which should inhibit the release of vasopressin and permit the excretion of a maximally dilute urine. The urine osmolality in SIADH is often higher than the serum osmolality, but that is not a necessary feature of the syndrome. If measured directly, vasopressin levels are inappropriately elevated, as are the levels of the associated neurophysins. However, it is rarely necessary to measure vasopressin. As discussed later, other causes of hypotonicity can generally be excluded with reasonable certainty by reliance on clinical and biochemical criteria.

Several other laboratory features of SIADH are helpful in diagnosis. The urinary sodium concentration is typically high, reflecting the natriuresis induced by expansion of extracellular fluid volume. However, the ability to conserve sodium in SIADH is usually unimpaired,[5] and the urinary sodium excretion can fall to low levels in the setting of reduced dietary sodium intakes. The blood urea nitrogen and serum uric acid levels are low,[143] again reflecting expanded extracellular fluid volumes and decreased tubular resorption of these solutes. Other electrolytes are diluted in proportion to the serum sodium, except for serum bicarbonate, which is normal.

Pathogenesis

Vasopressin is synthesized as a prohormone of 166 amino acids that is processed to produce three peptides: the mature octapeptide hormone, a midregion peptide of molecular weight 10,000 with vasopressin-binding activity called neurophysin II, and a C-terminal glycopeptide[144] (see Chapter 9). Vasopressin and its neurophysin are packaged together in neurosecretory granules, stored in nerve termini in the posterior pituitary, and released in response to hypotonicity or nonosmotic stimuli (baroreceptor stimulation, pain, nausea). Vasopressin is similarly processed in neuroendocrine tumor cells, but these cells frequently secrete not only vasopressin and neurophysin II but also vasopressin's sister peptide oxytocin together with its binding protein, neurophysin I.[145–147]

The molecular basis for inappropriate secretion of vasopressin from tumor cells is poorly understood. Immunoreactive vasopressin is identifiable in a portion of bronchial neuroendocrine cells, the presumed precursors of SCLC. Thus, like other hormonal products of neuroendocrine neoplasms, vasopressin may be regarded as secreted eutopically from neuroendocrine tumors. The usual coordinate expression of vasopressin and oxytocin precursors in tumor cells may be related to the physical linkage of the two genes, which are found within 12 kb of each other in the human genome with an inverted arrangement of the coding strands.[148] Either DNA rearrangements or *trans*-acting factors expressed in malignant tumors could simultaneously activate both promoters.

An E-box in the vasopressin promoter, a binding motif for bHLH transcription factors, is necessary for increased vasopressin gene expression in high-expressing SCLC cell lines.[149] This motif appears to bind the transcription factor USF (upstream transcription factor); a nearby sequence appears to interact and is a candidate for binding other bHLH factors. A neuron-specific silencer element has also been identified in the arginine vasopressin promoter.[150] Vasopressin receptors (V_{1A} and V_2 receptors) are present on SCLC cells,[151] and vasopressin can have paracrine effects on the growth of SCLC cells to promote their growth, but increased proliferation in response to vasopressin has not been observed.[152]

It is not known whether the secretion of neurohypophyseal peptides from tumor cells is under regulatory control. Four patterns of vasopressin release have been identified in SIADH.[153] Most commonly (37%), vasopressin levels fluctuate widely and independently of the serum osmolality. In a second group (33%), vasopressin is released in response to changes in osmolality, but the osmotic threshold for vasopressin release is decreased (reset osmostat). Other patients with SIADH manifest a constant leak of vasopressin or have no demonstrable abnormality in vasopressin secretion and could conceivably produce a different antidiuretic substance.

Patients with cancer and SIADH fall into all four categories. It is conceivable that those with a reset osmostat express both the vasopressin gene and an osmoreceptor in their tumors[154]; more likely, however, vasopressin is released centrally in these patients because of stimulation of baroreceptors in the pulmonary bed or periphery, invasion of the vagus nerve, or metastasis to regulatory centers, for example, the hypothalamus.

Expression and secretion of vasopressin are more common than hyponatremia in SCLC. More than 50% of SCLC patients have elevated plasma vasopressin levels,[155] and plasma levels of the neurophysins are increased in 44% to 65% of untreated patients with SCLC.[146, 147, 156, 157] Some tumors also express the gene for oxytocin,[145] but no clinical syndrome of inappropriate oxytocin release has been reported in tumor patients.

In patients with elevated vasopressin levels who do not have hyponatremia, abnormalities in water metabolism can be elicited by water loading, which discloses an impaired diuretic response in 47% of patients with limited SCLC and 86% of patients with extensive disease.[158] Patients with milder degrees of vasopressin excess probably compensate for reduced free water excretion by reducing fluid intake; only if free water intake exceeds the maximal excretion of free water does hyponatremia result. Thus, the development of hyponatremia is a function not only of the level of vasopressin but also of fluid intake. Although some tumors may secrete abnormally processed forms of vasopressin with reduced biologic activity, it is likely that compensatory mechanisms of this type account for the disparity in the frequency of biochemical and clinical abnormalities in SIADH.

When water is retained, extracellular and intracellular volumes are expanded. The expansion of extracellular fluid volume, probably by causing suppression of aldosterone and an increase in atrial natriuretic peptide (ANP),[159] induces the natriuresis that is characteristic of patients with SIADH who have an adequate intake of sodium. Plasma levels of ANP are normal or high in SIADH[159–161]; it is not clear whether high ANP levels are a compensatory response to extracellular fluid volume expansion or a consequence of release of ANP from the tumor. Many tumors that express the vasopressin gene also express the gene for ANP.[162–166] Restriction of sodium intake in patients with SIADH causes weight loss, however, and as the extracellular fluid volume returns to normal, natriuresis is reversed and sodium is conserved appropriately.[5] This suggests that the secretion of ANP is compensatory and that an ANP-induced natriuresis does not contribute significantly to the genesis of hyponatremia.

Acute water retention causes neurologic symptoms by rapidly increasing the intracellular volumes of brain cells and thus inducing cerebral edema. Chronic hyponatremia is probably less symptomatic because there is time for activation of compensatory volume-regulatory mechanisms in the central nervous system. Brain cells compensate for volume gain by activating ion transport processes that pump out intracellular potassium chloride (KCl) and sodium chloride (NaCl).[167, 168] This compensation has therapeutic importance because rapid correction of hyponatremia by infusion of hypertonic saline produces a transient hypertonic encephalopathy as water is drawn out of the already contracted intracellular space. This can cause permanent neurologic damage (e.g., central pontine myelinolysis) and death.

Diagnosis

The diagnosis of SIADH is usually made on clinical grounds. The first step is to establish that the urine is inappropriately concentrated in the presence of hypotonicity. In a hyponatremic patient, a urine osmolality higher than 50 to 60 mmol/L water is inappropriate, and many patients with SIADH have urine osmolalities higher than the plasma osmolality. Next, other causes of hypotonicity must be excluded. The differential diagnosis of hyponatremia includes states of true volume contraction; edematous states such as congestive heart failure and hepatic failure, in which the effective central plasma volume is diminished; adrenal insufficiency; hypothyroidism; drug effects; and SIADH (see Chapter 9).

Measurements of vasopressin are of little value in the differential diagnosis because vasopressin levels are increased in most hyponatremic states. True volume contraction and edematous states can usually be excluded on clinical grounds. It is appropriate to exclude adrenal insufficiency with a corticotropin stimulation test in patients with malignant tumors and SIADH, particularly because patients with bilateral adrenal metastases are at risk for adrenal insufficiency. Thyrotropin should be measured to exclude hypothyroidism. Among the drugs that stimulate the nonosmotic release of vasopressin are the cancer chemotherapeutic agents vincristine, vinblastine, and cyclophosphamide. Normovolemic patients without hormonal disorders or drug causes are presumed to have SIADH.

SIADH is a common cause of hyponatremia in hospitalized patients,[169, 170] but only a small minority of these patients develop the syndrome as the result of inappropriate secretion of vasopressin by a tumor. Furthermore, not all patients with cancer who meet the criteria for SIADH have ectopic secretion of vasopressin from a tumor. Not only are benign forms of SIADH more common, but the response of vasopressin to osmotic stimuli in some patients with malignant tumors[153] is consistent with eutopic secretion of the hormone from the pituitary.

The uncertainty regarding the etiology in an individual patient may be intellectually unsatisfying but is not of great practical importance. Patients with severe and symptomatic hyponatremia are more likely to have a true ectopic source of vasopressin. The treatment of hyponatremia in SIADH is similar regardless of the cause of the syndrome.

Treatment

Symptomatic hyponatremia in patients with a serum sodium level below 120 mmol/L requires immediate treatment (see Chapter 9). The therapeutic options include infusion or administration of hypertonic saline (3% or 5% saline) or of saline and furosemide.[171] The latter regimen has the advantage of not rapidly expanding extracellular fluid volume in an already volume-expanded patient. The goal of acute treatment is to raise the serum sodium level above 125 mmol/L. Such an increase takes the patient out of immediate danger, and further correction can be accomplished in a more leisurely fashion.

How rapidly the initial phase of correction should be carried out is controversial; one school argues for rapid correction in view of the high mortality of the untreated syndrome, and the other suggests that too rapid correction of hyponatremia can predispose to central pontine myelinolysis and other neurologic sequelae.[172] As discussed earlier, the risk of rapid correction probably has to do with brain shrinking in the presence of high concentrations of extracellular sodium and intracellular dehydration, which is exacerbated by prior loss of cell solute, the adaptive response of the central nervous system to hyponatremia (see Chapter 9). Under most circumstances, it seems best to correct hyponatremia at a rate of 0.5 mmol/L per hour until the serum sodium concentration reaches 120 to 125 mmol/L.

In asymptomatic patients or after acute correction of hyponatremia in symptomatic patients, the mainstay of chronic therapy is water restriction. Moderate fluid restriction may be reasonably well tolerated. The goal is to establish a fluid intake at which the intake of free water does not exceed the maximal free water clearance, which is determined by the circulating vasopressin level. If necessary, most patients can be maintained with severe restrictions to 800 to 1000 mL of fluid intake daily. At this level, the free water intake is actually negative because the patient is ingesting osmoles from food in excess of water. Therefore, even a patient who is obliged to excrete a concentrated urine and thus has negative free water excretion may be maintained in zero net water balance. However, severe fluid restrictions are onerous and difficult to maintain.

As an adjunct to water restriction, it can be beneficial to interfere with vasopressin action. The drug of choice for this purpose is demeclocycline, an antibiotic that blocks the action of vasopressin and produces nephrogenic diabetes insipidus. At a dose of 150 to 300 mg four times a day, demeclocycline has a reproducible effect on the urine-concentrating mechanism[173, 174] but up to 2 weeks may be necessary for the full effect. Side effects include photosensitive rashes and liver toxicity.

An alternative, fludrocortisone in doses of 0.1 to 0.3 mg/day, corrects hyponatremia partially but at the risk of causing edema and congestive heart failure. Lithium also produces nephrogenic diabetes insipidus, but its effects are less predictable than demeclocycline or fludrocortisone and the drug should be given only in refractory cases.[173] SCLC is now treated with aggressive combination chemotherapy, and SIADH often remits in responders to chemotherapy.[137]

ECTOPIC CORTICOTROPIN SYNDROME AND ECTOPIC SECRETION OF CORTICOTROPIN-RELEASING HORMONE

Clinical Features

The ectopic corticotropin syndrome accounts for 10% to 20% of cases of Cushing's syndrome.[175–177] Unlike Cushing's disease, with an 8:1 female preponderance, this syndrome is more common in men than in women. The typical presentation also differs; the onset is sudden, and progression is rapid. Patients complain of proximal myopathy and peripheral edema. Hypertension, hypokalemia, and severe glucose intolerance are often present. Hyperpigmentation may occur, but hirsutism is unusual. Other manifestations of cancer, such as anorexia, weight loss, and anemia, are common.

The somatic features of Cushing's syndrome are notably absent in the typical patient, perhaps because of the rapid evolution of the clinical picture. Patients with slowly growing carcinoid tumors of the bronchus or thymus have a more indolent disease and often present with the classic habitus of Cushing's syndrome—moon facies, centripetal obesity, proximal myopathy, polydipsia, and polyuria. Hyperpigmentation is common in these patients, as is hirsutism in women.

The tumors that produce the ectopic corticotropin syndrome are primarily of neuroendocrine cell origin. In published series, approximately 45% are SCLC, 15% are thymic carcinoids, 10% are bronchial carcinoids, 10% are islet cell tumors, 5% are other carcinoid tumors, 2% are pheochromocytomas, and 1% are ovarian adenocarcinomas. However, adenocarcinoma and squamous carcinoma are also occasionally associated with the syndrome. It appears that SCLC is greatly underrepresented in these referral series; it probably accounts for well over 50% of unselected cases.

Laboratory Features

Both the level of cortisol secretion and the level of corticotropin tend to be higher in ectopic than in pituitary Cushing's syndrome, although there is some overlap. In most ectopic cases, both cortisol and corticotropin levels are elevated to two to four times the normal morning values and the normal diurnal variation in their levels is lost. Urinary excretion of adrenal steroid metabolites is increased correspondingly. Two-site immunoradiometric assays, which are coming into common use for detection of corticotropin, give lower values for corticotropin in ectopic cases than older radioimmunoassays,[178] probably because they do not detect partially processed forms that are common in the ectopic syndrome.

Despite the abnormal processing of corticotropin by nonpituitary tumors, there is no other POMC peptide in serum whose presence is decisive in the diagnosis of the ectopic syndrome. More than one half of nonpituitary tumors that secrete corticotropin also secrete other peptides, including carcinoembryonic antigen, GRP, calcitonin, somatostatin, and corticotropin-releasing hormone (CRH), and the presence of these peptides is suggestive of the ectopic corticotropin syndrome.

Hypokalemia occurs in 80% to 100% of cases in various series, and potassium wasting is more severe than in pituitary Cushing's disease. The hypokalemia is probably explained by the mineralocorticoid effects of cortisol, which are more evident both because cortisol levels tend to be higher in ectopic than in pituitary Cushing's syndrome and because 11β-hydroxysteroid dehydrogenase activity appears for unknown reasons to be decreased in patients with ectopic corticotropin secretion.[179, 180] A deficiency of 11β-hydroxysteroid dehydrogenase activity impairs the inactivation of cortisol in the renal tubule, leading to increased exposure of mineralocorticoid receptors to cortisol. In disorders such as congenital deficiency of 11β-hydroxysteroid dehydrogenase and licorice intoxication, in which the activity of the enzyme is inhibited, normal levels of cortisol produce a state of pseudohyperaldosteronism.[181]

Pathogenesis

Although many nonpituitary tissues contain POMC mRNA, most are short transcripts (800 nucleotides) that are initiated by a downstream promoter at the third exon of the *POMC* gene and do not include coding sequences for the signal peptide that is necessary for direction of POMC into the secretory pathway.[61] Thus, nonpituitary POMC transcripts probably do not generate bioactive POMC products that can be secreted. In contrast, nonpituitary tumors that secrete corticotropin contain a 1150-nucleotide mRNA similar to the predominant pituitary species, and many nonpituitary tumors also contain 1350-nucleotide transcripts initiated from an upstream promoter that is largely quiescent in pituitary cells.[61, 182, 183]

Two regions of the POMC promoter contribute to activity in SCLC; the region that confers high POMC promoter activity on pituitary cells is not active.[184–186] One region binds the transcription factor E2F[186] in a methylation-sensitive fashion.[41] E2F is inactivated by the tumor suppressor gene Rb, which is inactive in 90% of cases of SCLC. Thus, both loss of Rb and differential methylation of the POMC promoter are potential mechanisms of POMC expression in SCLC.

Consistent with the nonsuppressibility of most nonpituitary tumors by glucocorticoids, the sensitivity of *POMC* gene expression to inhibition by glucocorticoids is reduced in SCLC cell lines. In some cell lines, glucocorticoid receptors are absent; in others, glucocorticoid receptor action appears to be defective.[183, 187, 188] Negative glucocorticoid regulatory elements are typically composite elements that require binding of regulatory factors in addition to the glucocorticoid receptor, leading to the possibility that such accessory factors may be abnormal in transformed cell lines. However, glucocorticoids also fail to stimulate transcription from classic glucocorticoid regulatory elements in SCLC cell lines, and this defect is overcome by overexpression of the wild-type glucocorticoid receptor.[183]

POMC processing in nonpituitary tumors is often incomplete, with the release into blood of POMC fragments with reduced biologic activity. These incompletely processed forms are larger than corticotropin by gel filtration and were first described in the serum of cancer patients with the ectopic corticotropin (ACTH) syndrome as *big ACTH*.[189] As noted earlier, some incompletely processed POMC peptides can be detected by radioimmunoassay techniques for corticotropin but not by two-site immunoradiometric assays.[178] In one study using a precursor-specific assay, the ratio of corticotropin precursors to corticotropin in plasma was 58:1 in the ectopic corticotropin syndrome and 5:1 in pituitary Cushing's disease.[190]

Unusual small peptides are also produced from POMC in nonpituitary tumors (Fig. 40–2). In anterior pituitary cortico-

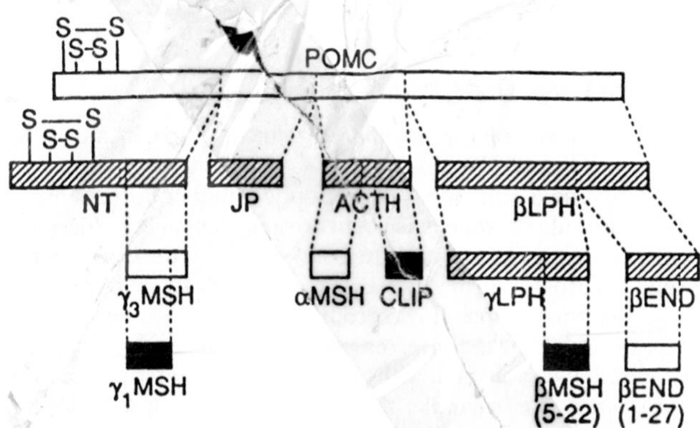

Figure 40–2. Processing of pro-opiomelanocortin (POMC) in normal pituitary (*hatched bars*), intermediate lobe (*open bars*), and nonpituitary neoplasms (*solid bars*). ACTH, adrenocorticotropic hormone (corticotropin); CLIP, corticotropin-like intermediate lobe peptide; END, endorphin; LPH, lipotropin; MSH, melanocyte-stimulating hormone. (Adapted from Schteingart DE. Ectopic secretion of peptides of the proopiomelanocortin family. Endocrinol Metab Clin North Am 1991; 20:453–471.)

trope cells, four of the six dibasic sites in POMC are cleaved by the prohormone convertase PC1/PC3,[191, 192] and the predominant products are six peptides:

- An NH_2-terminal peptide
- A joining peptide
- Corticotropin
- β-Lipotropin (β-LPH)
- Smaller amounts of γ-LPH and β-endorphin

Additional products that are detected routinely in extracts of nonpituitary tumors include the corticotropin-like intermediate lobe polypeptide (CLIP) and β-melanocyte–stimulating hormone (β-MSH) (5–22).[193] Both peptides are present in the intermediate lobe in the rodent pituitary gland, and their presence in nonpituitary tumors indicates that nonpituitary tumors contain the PC2 convertase,[194, 195] which is normally present in intermediate but not anterior pituitary cells.[194] These peptides are not secreted in large amounts and are not useful as tumor markers in blood, but the serum LPH/corticotropin ratio in the ectopic corticotropin syndrome is higher than in pituitary tumors,[196] possibly reflecting the increased PC2 activity in nonpituitary tumors.

Corticotropin-like activity can be identified in extracts of many non–SCLCs and in virtually all SCLCs,[197, 198] and at least one third of all SCLCs show POMC mRNA by in situ hybridization.[198] Yet only 1% to 3% of patients with SCLC have clinical evidence of corticotropin excess. Thus, the ectopic corticotropin syndrome is a good example of the principle that ectopic production of hormones is more common than clinical syndromes of hormone excess. Differences between tumors in *trans*-acting nuclear factors or epigenetic regulation of the POMC promoter by DNA methylation may account for differential expression of the POMC gene.[41, 186]

Patients with corticotropin-producing neoplasms are protected from the consequences of hormone excess by several mechanisms. Malignant tumors contain much smaller quantities of POMC mRNA and peptides than the pituitary and are thus inefficient in producing corticotropin. Tumor cells are much poorer in neurosecretory granules than pituitary corticotropes and are relatively deficient in the ability to process POMC efficiently and secrete the peptide products. Inefficient cleavage of POMC leads to incompletely processed forms of corticotropin with little biologic activity. Processing of POMC by tumors can also lead to production of biologically inactive products. For example, some tumors produce significant amounts of corticotropin but cleave it to the CLIP.[193]

Laboratory Diagnosis

The diagnosis of the ectopic corticotropin syndrome is described in Chapters 8 and 14.

The first step consists of determining whether cortisol excess is present and whether it is corticotropin-dependent. Increased basal cortisol secretion can often be shown by measurement of serum cortisol or urinary free cortisol, both of which are increased in the ectopic corticotropin syndrome. When the basal levels are not markedly increased, the presence of cortisol excess can be established with a low-dose dexamethasone suppression test, for example, the 1-mg overnight dexamethasone suppression test. The corticotropin dependence of cortisol excess can be established by measurement of corticotropin in the same sample in which cortisol is measured.

Corticotropin-dependent Cushing's syndrome results from either pituitary or ectopic secretion of corticotropin. In the classic form of the syndrome (e.g., corticotropin-secreting SCLC), secretion is nonsuppressible and there is little or no response of serum or urinary cortisol to the administration of high-dose dexamethasone, whereas the secretion of corticotropin by pituitary adenomas is dexamethasone-responsive. In a patient with a recognized malignancy and clinical features suggestive of the ectopic syndrome, the finding of nonsuppressible hypercortisolism usually suffices to make the diagnosis.

In occasional lung cancers and in about 50% of bronchial or thymic carcinoid tumors, the secretion of corticotropin can be suppressed with high-dose dexamethasone. This circumstance has been called the *occult ectopic corticotropin syndrome*[199] and presents a major diagnostic challenge because the clinical presentation and secretory dynamics may be identical to those of pituitary Cushing's syndrome and because neither these small tumors nor pituitary corticotroph adenomas may be evident on routine radiologic studies.

Although a number of noninvasive methods are used in this circumstance, none is definitive. Because nonpituitary tumors are not as well suppressed by glucocorticoids as corticotrope adenomas of the pituitary gland, it is useful to apply stringent criteria for glucocorticoid suppressibility, namely suppression of urinary free cortisol by more than 80% after administration of high-dose dexamethasone, which has a sensitivity of 81% and a specificity of 92% for pituitary Cushing's syndrome.[44] Stimulation with the ovine CRH test is valuable because nonpituitary tumors do not respond well to CRH. An increase in plasma corticotropin of 35% after administration of ovine CRH (1 μg/kg body weight) was reported to have a sensitivity of 93% and a specificity of 100% for the diagnosis of pituitary Cushing's syndrome.[200] Metyrapone testing in combination with high-dose dexamethasone may also improve diagnostic accuracy.[201]

The definitive study for distinguishing pituitary from nonpituitary forms of hypercortisolism is inferior *petrosal sinus sampling* with administration of ovine CRH.[202–204] The ratio of corticotropin in the inferior petrosal sinus to that in peripheral blood after administration of CRH is greater than 3 in patients with pituitary tumors and less than 2 in patients with corticotropin-secreting nonpituitary tumors. *Cavernous sinus sampling* has also been successful.[205] Localization of bronchial and thymic carcinoids may also be difficult. Thin-section computed tomography of the chest and scanning with labeled octreotide have sometimes been of use but have a high failure rate.[206]

Treatment

The management of Cushing's syndrome is discussed in Chapters 8 and 14.

When possible, the treatment of the ectopic corticotropin syndrome is surgical. With slow-growing carcinoid tumors of the bronchus, thymomas, or pheochromocytomas, surgical resection can be curative. If the tumor cannot be identified, it is necessary to block cortisol secretion with adrenolytic agents. Some patients ultimately require surgical adrenalectomy to control hypercortisolism.

Malignant nonpituitary neoplasms that secrete corticotropin are rarely amenable to resection because the tumor is usually advanced and inoperable by the time the clinical syndrome appears. With malignant neoplasms the aim is to palliate hypercortisolism by *medical adrenalectomy* using adrenolytic drugs, such as aminoglutethimide (250 mg three times a day) or metyrapone (250 to 500 mg three times a day).[207] Ketoconazole (200 to 400 mg twice a day) has also been useful for the treatment of ectopic corticotropin syndrome.[208, 209] A replacement dose of hydrocortisone should be administered with these drugs to avoid adrenal insufficiency. Some patients respond to the long-acting somatostatin agonist octreotide,[210] and the glucocorticoid antagonist mifepristone has also been used.[211]

Ectopic Secretion of Corticotropin-Releasing Hormone

Nonendocrine tumors rarely cause Cushing's syndrome by secretion of CRH.[175, 176, 212, 213] Patients have increased CRH levels in tumor tissue or in plasma and high plasma corticotropin levels. It is important to document that the site of corticotropin secretion is the pituitary gland because many nonendocrine tumors that secrete CRH also secrete corticotropin itself. Presumptive evidence of a pituitary source of corticotropin may come from demonstration that the gradient of corticotropin between the inferior petrosal sinus and peripheral blood is more than 3 : 1, from finding pituitary corticotropic hyperplasia in patients who underwent pituitary surgery for a presumed corticotropic adenoma, or from the failure to detect corticotropin in the nonendocrine tumor. When the nonendocrine tumor secretes both CRH and corticotropin, the true role of CRH in the clinical syndrome may be indeterminate.[175, 176]

Cushing's syndrome resulting from ectopic secretion of CRH does not have a distinctive presentation. In most cases, the hypercortisolism is unresponsive to dexamethasone suppression, but a normal response to high-dose dexamethasone has also been reported. The response to metyrapone is also variable. Tumors that secrete CRH include small cell carcinomas of the prostate and lung, medullary thyroid carcinoma, carcinoids, and a hypothalamic gangliocytoma. These neuroendocrine tumors are similar to the tumors that cause Cushing's syndrome by direct secretion of corticotropin.

The diagnosis of ectopic CRH secretion as the cause of Cushing's syndrome is usually made retrospectively. In view of the rarity of the disorder, it is probably inappropriate to measure CRH routinely in Cushing's syndrome. However, it may be worthwhile to determine the plasma CRH level when pituitary surgery has disclosed diffuse corticotropic hyperplasia in a patient with Cushing's syndrome.

HYPOGLYCEMIA WITH NON–ISLET CELL TUMORS

Clinical Features

Fasting hypoglycemia produced by non–islet cell tumors typically causes neuroglycopenic symptoms of obtundation, confusion, or behavioral aberrations, which may have been present for some time before the diagnosis is made.[8, 214–219] Non–islet cell tumors rarely secrete insulin, but a case of small cell cervical carcinoma with high levels of insulin, proinsulin, and C peptide has been reported; the tumor was found to contain insulin mRNA by in situ hybridization and immunoreactive insulin by immunohistochemical methods.[15]

Most extrapancreatic tumors that cause hypoglycemia do so by secreting IGF-II. The offending neoplasms are usually bulky, slow-growing mesenchymal tumors. Fibrosarcomas, rhabdomyosarcomas, leiomyosarcomas, mesotheliomas, and hemangiopericytomas account for more than 50% of cases. Hepatocellular carcinomas (hepatomas), carcinoid tumors, and adrenocortical carcinomas account for about 25% of cases, and the remainder are made up of various carcinomas, leukemias, and lymphomas. More than one third of the tumors are retroperitoneal, about one third are intra-abdominal, and the remainder are intrathoracic.

Pathogenesis

Fasting hypoglycemia produced by non–islet cell tumors results from increased peripheral utilization of glucose, primarily in skeletal muscle, coupled with decreased hepatic glucose output.[220–222] Lipolysis is inhibited, and free fatty acid levels are low. Although it had been suspected that bulky tumors themselves, sometimes weighing many kilograms, might metabolize enough glucose to exceed the capacity for hepatic glucose production, this phenomenon has not been documented. Despite insulin-like effects on glucose utilization, hepatic glucose production, and lipolysis, fasting insulin levels during hypoglycemia are appropriately suppressed. For this reason, it has appeared that an insulin-like factor is probably responsible for hypoglycemia.

Sera from patients with non–islet cell tumors contain elevated levels of an insulin-like activity by radioreceptor assay.[223] The level of IGF-II mRNA in non–islet cell tumors is often increased, even in patients with normal serum IGF-II levels.[224, 225] IGF-II levels are sometimes elevated during hypoglycemia but may be normal,[226–229] and the levels of IGF-I are typically suppressed.[228, 229] Although not all patients have high IGF-II levels, it appears that IGF-II is in fact the causative agent of hypoglycemia and can cause hypoglycemia at normal total serum levels as a consequence of altered processing and increased bioavailability.

Altered binding of IGF-II in the tumor-hypoglycemia syndrome increases its bioavailability to peripheral receptors. In normal serum, IGFs are bound largely in one of two complexes. Most IGF is normally bound to a heterotrimeric 150-kd complex consisting of the IGF, the binding protein IGFBP3, and an acid-labile glycoprotein. The large complex is retained in the circulation, and as a result the half-life of the IGF-II complex is relatively long, 12 to 15 hours. A minority of IGF circulates in a smaller 50-kd complex that contains mainly IGF and a different binding protein, IGFBP2. The small complex can cross capillaries and deliver IGF to tissue receptors, and IGF-II bound to this complex has a half-life of only about 30 minutes.[230] In sera from patients with non–islet cell tumors and hypoglycemia, the fraction of IGF-II bound to the small, bioavailable complex is increased, on average by threefold,[231–233] presumably increasing the access of IGF-II to the receptor, even in the setting of normal total IGF-II levels.

A substantial fraction of IGF-II in both tumors and sera is present in a high-molecular-weight form, *big IGF-II*,[225–227, 229] a partially processed form that contains a 21-amino-acid carboxyl-terminal extension from the E domain.[227] Big IGF-II was reported to lack O-linked glycosylation,[234] which may give it increased bioactivity,[235] but O-linked glycosylation was reported to be normal in another study.[236] Whether a decreased ability of big IGF-II to form a normal ternary complex contributes directly to its increased bioavailability remains to be determined.

Current concepts of the alteration in IGF-II binding are summarized in Figure 40–3.[8, 216] Oversecretion of big IGF-II suppresses the secretion of insulin, growth hormone (GH), and IGF-I.[237] In turn, suppression of GH and IGF-I down-regulates the synthesis of IGFBP3 and the acid-labile subunit, both of which are GH-dependent,[238] and up-regulates the synthesis of IGFBP2. Consistent with this proposal regarding the role of GH is the response of a patient to GH therapy.[239] Thus, IGF-II oversecretion leads to altered binding and increased bioactivity of IGF-II and can cause hypoglycemia even when total IGF-II levels are normal. The level of free IGF-II in serum is also increased.[240]

Laboratory Diagnosis

The fasting levels of insulin and C peptide are appropriately suppressed in samples obtained during hypoglycemia (insulin < 36 pmol/L [6 μU/mL], C peptide < 0.2 nmol/L [0.6 ng/

SYNDROMES CAUSED BY OTHER HORMONES

Erythropoietin and Erythrocytosis

Erythrocytosis occurs in 1% to 4% of renal carcinomas, 5% to 10% of hepatocellular carcinomas, and 10% to 20% of cerebellar hemangioblastomas. It has been observed in patients with uterine fibromyomas, adrenocortical carcinomas, or ovarian tumors.[274, 275] Renal and hepatocellular carcinomas account for 71% of cases; thus, erythrocytosis is most common in tumors arising from the tissues that normally secrete erythropoietin (the fetal liver and by the adult kidney).

The association of erythropoietin and vascular endothelial growth factor secretion from cerebellar hemangioblastoma and renal carcinoma raised the possibility that both of these hypoxia-responsive genes are specifically activated by loss of the von Hippel–Lindau tumor suppressor gene *VHL*.[22, 23] The VHL protein appears to stabilize mRNA for hypoxia-inducible proteins.[24] VHL-negative renal carcinomas display constitutively high levels of the hypoxia-inducible factor-1 (HIF-1), a heterodimeric member of the bHLH PAS family of transcription factors, composed of α and β subunits.[25] The action of the VHL protein to increase the proteasome-mediated degradation of the HIF-1α protein and other proteins may prove central to many manifestations of VHL gene alteration.[276]

The *VHL* gene also displays loss of heterozygosity in some hepatocellular carcinomas,[277] and tissue-specific inactivation of the *VHL* gene in hepatocytes gives rise to cavernous hemangioma of the liver and up-regulation of the erythropoietin gene.[278] It is thus likely that inactivation of *VHL* plays a central role in the induction of erythropoietin synthesis in each of the tumors classically associated with erythropoietin-dependent polycythemia, by either transcriptional or post-transcriptional mechanisms.

Early studies reported that erythropoietic bioactivity was frequently present in tumor extracts from polycythemic patients; erythropoietin mRNA has been demonstrated in extracts of renal carcinomas,[275] hepatocellular carcinoma,[279] and cerebellar hemangioblastoma.[22, 280] Erythrocytosis has been produced in nude mice by transplantation of erythropoietin-positive renal carcinoma cells and hepatocarcinoma cells.[281, 282] Some patients with tumors and erythrocytosis have increased serum erythropoietin levels.[275] However, in the best studied group, patients with hepatocellular carcinoma, it has been difficult to demonstrate a consistent relationship between the red blood cell mass and serum levels of erythropoietin.[283, 284] Increased serum levels of erythropoietin are common in patients with hepatocellular carcinoma; however, few of the patients with high erythropoietin levels have erythrocytosis, and some patients with erythrocytosis have normal levels of erythropoietin. Absence of erythrocytosis in the presence of high erythropoietin levels could reflect secretion of biologically inactive (e.g., precursor) forms of erythropoietin.

Calcitonin

Calcitonin is present in neuroendocrine cells of the normal bronchial epithelium[9, 10] and is frequently secreted by neuroendocrine tumors, including 18% to 60% of SCLCs.[285–289] Calcitonin is also secreted by other lung carcinomas, breast cancers, leukemias, and a broad spectrum of other neoplasms.[290] Estimates of the frequency of calcitonin secretion are lower in studies that rigorously control for assay artifacts,[287] but it is clear that some tumors express the gene for calcitonin/calcitonin gene–related peptide (CGRP) and secrete calcitonin in vitro.[291, 292]

Tumors frequently secrete large forms of calcitonin[287] and are less sensitive to stimulation than in patients with hypercalcitoninemia resulting from medullary thyroid carcinoma.[288, 293] CGRP, which is derived from alternative splicing of the calcitonin gene, is expressed in normal bronchial epithelium[10] and has been detected in tumor extracts and serum.[294] The levels of calcitonin in the sera of patients with lung carcinoma are lower than those in medullary thyroid carcinoma, and no clinical syndrome is associated with the secretion of calcitonin or CGRP.

Endothelin

The potent vasoconstrictor peptide endothelin is expressed in hepatocellular carcinoma,[295] breast carcinoma,[296] ovarian carcinoma,[32, 33] and prostate carcinoma.[34, 297–299] Endothelin receptors are often coexpressed on tumor cells, and endothelin-1 was reported to have paracrine effects on tumor cell growth.[31–34] Increased serum levels of endothelin-1 and a partially processed form of the peptide big endothelin-1 have been found in hepatocellular carcinoma.[295, 300] Arteriovenous differences, albeit small, have been found across the liver of patients with hepatocellular carcinoma.[295] No clinical manifestations of systemic secretion of endothelin have been reported, but endothelin-1 has been implicated as the factor causing the osteoblastic response to bone metastasis in breast carcinoma,[301] and a similar role was suggested in prostate carcinoma.[297, 299]

Vasoactive Intestinal Peptide

Inappropriate secretion of VIP produces pancreatic cholera, also known as the *WDHA syndrome* (watery diarrhea, hypokalemia, and achlorhydria) or *Verner-Morrison syndrome* (see Chapter 33). In addition to pancreatic islet cell tumors, other neuroendocrine tumors, including ganglioneuroma, ganglioneuroblastoma, neuroblastoma, pheochromocytoma, and medullary thyroid carcinoma, can produce the syndrome.[302] These tumors stain for VIP, and removal of the tumor causes return of peripheral VIP levels to normal and reverses the clinical syndrome. Increased VIP levels have also been reported in lung carcinoma[303] and in a neuroendocrine tumor of the kidney.[304] VIP is present in the central and peripheral nervous systems; thus, its production by neuroendocrine tumors may be regarded as eutopic rather than ectopic.

Other Gut Hormones

Somatostatin is frequently detectable in extracts of lung tumor[305, 306] and is secreted by cultured SCLC cells,[306] but elevated serum somatostatin concentrations are uncommon in lung cancer (see Chapter 35).[307, 308] Only one case of the *somatostatinoma syndrome* has been attributed to SCLC.[309] The *glucagonoma syndrome* occurred in a patient with a renal neuroendocrine tumor[310] and in a patient with a large cell lung carcinoma.[311]

GRP is often found in lung carcinomas,[305] cultured SCLC cells,[312, 313] and other tumors[314–316] but elevated serum levels are uncommon.[313, 317] Pro-GRP may be a better tumor marker.[318] The peptide is a mitogen for SCLC cells,[26, 319] and neutralizing studies with antibodies and antagonists[27–29, 320] suggested that it has an autocrine role as a growth factor. GRP was also reported to affect the motility of tumor cells.[316, 321] A variant form of the GRP receptor is expressed in human lung carcinoma cell lines.[322] GRP is expressed in neuroendocrine cells of bronchial mucosa,[9, 10] particularly at branch points,[323] and appears to have a developmental role in the regulation of branching morphogenesis of airways.[324, 325] Pancreatic polypeptide is occasionally detectable in the sera of patients with carcinoid tumors.[307, 326]

References

1. Brown WH. A case of pluriglandular syndrome: 'diabetes of bearded woman.' Lancet 1928; 2:1022.
2. Case Records of the Massachusetts General Hospital. Case 27461. N Engl J Med 1941; 225:789–791.
3. Plimpton CH, Gellhorn A. Hypercalcemia in malignant disease without evidence of bone destruction. Am J Med 1956; 21:750–759.
4. Connor TB, Thomas WC Jr. Etiology of hypercalcemia associated with lung carcinoma. J Clin Invest 1956; 35:697–701.
5. Schwartz WB, Bennett W, Curelop S, et al. A syndrome of renal sodium loss and hyponatremia probably resulting from inappropriate secretion of antidiuretic hormone. Am J Med 1957; 23: 529–542.
6. Meador CK, Liddle GW, Island DP, et al. Cause of Cushing's syndrome in patients with tumors arising from nonendocrine tissue. J Clin Endocrinol Metab 1962; 22:693–700.
7. Liddle GW, Nicholson WE, Island DP, et al. Clinical and laboratory studies of ectopic humoral syndromes. Recent Prog Horm Res 1969; 25:283–314.
8. Zapf J. Role of insulin-like growth factor (IGF) II and IGF binding proteins in extrapancreatic tumour hypoglycaemia. J Intern Med 1993; 234:543–552.
9. Cutz E, Chan W, Track N. Bombesin, calcitonin and leu-enkephalin immunoreactivity in endocrine cells of human lung. Experientia 1981; 37:765–767.
10. Gould V, Chan W, Lee I, et al. Immunohistochemical evaluation of neuroendocrine cells and neoplasms of the lung. Pathol Res Pract 1988; 183:200–213.
11. Broadus A, Stewart A. Parathyroid hormone–related protein: structure, processing, and physiological actions. In Bilezikian J, Levine M, Marcus R (eds). The Parathyroids. New York, Raven Press, 1994, pp 259–294.
12. Braunstein GD. Placental proteins as tumor markers. In Herberman R, Mercer DW (eds). Immunodiagnosis of Cancer, 2nd ed. New York, Marcel Dekker, 1991, pp 673–701.
13. Braunstein GD, Bridson WE, Glass A, et al. In vivo and in vitro production of human chorionic gonadotropin and alpha-fetoprotein by a virilizing hepatoblastoma. J Clin Endocrinol Metab 1972; 35:857–862.
14. Braunstein GD, Vaitukaitis JL, Carbone PP, et al. Ectopic production of human chorionic gonadotrophin by neoplasms. Ann Intern Med 1973; 78:39–45.
15. Seckl MJ, Mulholland PJ, Bishop AE, et al. Hypoglycemia due to an insulin-secreting small-cell carcinoma of the cervix. N Engl J Med 1999; 341:733–736.
16. Baylin SB, Herman JG, Graff JR, et al. Alterations in DNA methylation: a fundamental aspect of neoplasia. Adv Cancer Res 1998; 72:141–196.
17. Baylin SB, Mendelsohn G. Ectopic (inappropriate) hormone production by tumors: mechanisms involved and the biological and clinical implications. Endocr Rev 1980; 1:45–77.
18. Ikeda K, Ohno H, Hane M, et al. Development of a sensitive two-site immunoradiometric assay for parathyroid hormone–related peptide: evidence for elevated levels in plasma from patients with adult T-cell leukemia/lymphoma and B-cell lymphoma. J Clin Endocrinol Metab 1994; 79:1322–1327.
19. Dittmer J, Gitlin SD, Reid RL, et al. Transactivation of the P2 promoter of parathyroid hormone–related protein by human T-cell lymphotropic virus type I Tax1: evidence for the involvement of transcription factor Ets1. J Virol 1993; 67:6087–6095.
20. Dittmer J, Pise-Masison CA, Clemens KE, et al. Interaction of human T-cell lymphotropic virus type I Tax, Ets1, and Sp1 in transactivation of the PTHrP P2 promoter. J Biol Chem 1997; 272:4953–4958.
21. Dittmer J, Gegonne A, Gitlin SD, et al. Regulation of parathyroid hormone–related protein (PTHrP) gene expression. Sp1 binds through an inverted CACCC motif and regulates promoter activity in cooperation with Ets1. J Biol Chem 1994; 269:21428–21434.
22. Krieg M, Marti HH, Plate KH. Coexpression of erythropoietin and vascular endothelial growth factor in nervous system tumors associated with von Hippel–Lindau tumor suppressor gene loss of function. Blood 1998; 92:3388–3393.
23. Iliopoulos O, Levy AP, Jiang C, et al. Negative regulation of hypoxia-inducible genes by the von Hippel–Lindau protein. Proc Natl Acad Sci USA 1996; 93:10595–10599.
24. Lonergan KM, Iliopoulos O, Ohh M, et al. Regulation of hypoxia-inducible mRNAs by the von Hippel–Lindau tumor suppressor protein requires binding to complexes containing elongins B/C and Cul2. Mol Cell Biol 1998; 18:732–741.
25. Krieg M, Haas R, Brauch H, et al. Up-regulation of hypoxia-inducible factors HIF-1α and HIF-2α under normoxic conditions in renal carcinoma cells by von Hippel–Lindau tumor suppressor gene loss of function. Oncogene 2000; 19:5435–5443.
26. Cuttitta F, Desmond NC, Mulshine J, et al. Bombesin-like peptides can function as autocrine growth factors in human small-cell lung cancer. Nature 1985; 316:823–826.
27. Kelley MJ, Linnoila RI, Avis IL, et al. Antitumor activity of a monoclonal antibody directed against gastrin-releasing peptide in patients with small cell lung cancer. Chest 1997; 112:256–261.
28. Moody TW, Venugopal R, Zia F, et al. BW2258U89: a GRP receptor antagonist which inhibits small cell lung cancer growth. Life Sci 1995; 56:521–529.
29. Koppan M, Halmos G, Arencibia JM, et al. Bombesin/gastrin-releasing peptide antagonists RC-3095 and RC-3940-II inhibit tumor growth and decrease the levels and mRNA expression of epidermal growth factor receptors in H-69 small cell lung carcinoma. Cancer 1998; 83:1335–1343.
30. Melzig MF, Nulander I, Vlaskovska M, et al. β-Endorphin stimulates proliferation of small cell lung carcinoma cells in vitro via nonopioid binding sites. Exp Cell Res 1995; 219:471–476.
31. Shichiri M, Hirata Y, Nakajima T, et al. Endothelin-1 is an autocrine/paracrine growth factor for human cancer cell lines. J Clin Invest 1991; 87:1867–1871.
32. Bagnato A, Tecce R, Di Castro V, et al. Activation of mitogenic signaling by endothelin 1 in ovarian carcinoma cells. Cancer Res 1997; 57:1306–1311.
33. Bagnato A, Salani D, Di Castro V, et al. Expression of endothelin 1 and endothelin A receptor in ovarian carcinoma: evidence for an autocrine role in tumor growth. Cancer Res 1999; 59:720–727.
34. Nelson JB, Chan-Tack K, Hedican SP, et al. Endothelin-1 production and decreased endothelin B receptor expression in advanced prostate cancer. Cancer Res 1996; 56:663–668.
35. Fuh G, Wells JA. Prolactin receptor antagonists that inhibit the growth of breast cancer cell lines. J Biol Chem 1995; 270:13133–13137.
36. Reynolds C, Montone KT, Powell CM, et al. Expression of prolactin and its receptor in human breast carcinoma. Endocrinology 1997; 138:5555–5560.
37. Canbay E, Norman M, Kilic E, et al. Prolactin stimulates the JAK2 and focal adhesion kinase pathways in human breast carcinoma T47-D cells. Biochem J 1997; 324:231–236.
38. Clevenger CV, Chang WP, Ngo W, et al. Expression of prolactin and prolactin receptor in human breast carcinoma. Evidence for an autocrine/paracrine loop. Am J Pathol 1995; 146:695–705.
39. Yamauchi T, Yamauchi N, Ueki K, et al. Constitutive tyrosine phosphorylation of ErbB-2 via Jak2 by autocrine secretion of prolactin in human breast cancer. J Biol Chem 2000; 275:33937–33944.
40. Holt EH, Vasavada RC, Bander NH, et al. Region-specific methylation of the parathyroid hormone–related peptide gene determines its expression in human renal carcinoma cell lines. J Biol Chem 1993; 268:20639–20645.
41. Newell-Price J, King P, Clark AJ. The CpG island promoter of the human proopiomelanocortin gene is methylated in nonexpressing normal tissue and tumors and represses expression. Mol Endocrinol 2001; 15:338–348.
42. Kelly RB. Storage and release of neurotransmitters. Cell 1993; 72(Suppl):43–53.
43. Hannah MJ, Schmidt AA, Huttner WB. Synaptic vesicle biogenesis. Annu Rev Cell Dev Biol 1999; 15:733–798.
44. O'Connor DT, Wu H, Gill BM, et al. Hormone storage vesicle proteins. Transcriptional basis of the widespread neuroendocrine expression of chromogranin A, and evidence of its diverse biological actions, intracellular and extracellular. Ann NY Acad Sci 1994; 733:36–45.
45. Glombik MM, Kromer A, Salm T, et al. The disulfide-bonded loop of chromogranin B mediates membrane binding and directs sorting from the trans-Golgi network to secretory granules. EMBO J 1999; 18:1059–1070.

46. Mahata SK, Mahata M, Wakade AR, et al. Primary structure and function of the catecholamine release inhibitory peptide catestatin (chromogranin A(344–364)): identification of amino acid residues crucial for activity. Mol Endocrinol 2000; 14:1525–1535.
47. Parmer RJ, Mahata M, Gong Y, et al. Processing of chromogranin A by plasmin provides a novel mechanism for regulating catecholamine secretion. J Clin Invest 2000; 106:907–915.
48. Zhou A, Webb G, Zhu X, et al. Proteolytic processing in the secretory pathway. J Biol Chem 1999; 274:20745–20748.
49. Steiner DF. The proprotein convertases. Curr Opin Chem Biol 1998; 2:31–39.
50. Scheuermann DW, Adriaensen D, Timmermans JP, et al. Comparative histological overview of the chemical coding of the pulmonary neuroepithelial endocrine system in health and disease. Eur J Morphol 1992; 30:101–112.
51. Natori S, Huttner WB. Chromogranin B (secretogranin I) promotes sorting to the regulated secretory pathway of processing intermediates derived from a peptide hormone precursor. Proc Natl Acad Sci USA 1993; 9:4431–4436.
52. Le Douarin NM. On the origin of pancreatic endocrine cells. Cell 1988; 53:169–171.
53. Borges M, Linnoila RI, van de Velde HJ, et al. An achaete-scute homologue essential for neuroendocrine differentiation in the lung. Nature 1997; 386:852–855.
54. Linnoila RI, Zhao B, DeMayo JL, et al. Constitutive achaete-scute homologue-1 promotes airway dysplasia and lung neuroendocrine tumors in transgenic mice. Cancer Res 2000; 60:4005–4009.
55. Ball DW, Azzoli CG, Baylin SB, et al. Identification of a human achaete-scute homolog highly expressed in neuroendocrine tumors. Proc Natl Acad Sci USA 1993; 90:5648–5652.
56. Chen H, Biel MA, Borges MW, et al. Tissue-specific expression of human achaete-scute homologue-1 in neuroendocrine tumors: transcriptional regulation by dual inhibitory regions. Cell Growth Differ 1997; 8:677–686.
57. Soderholm H, Ortoft E, Johansson I, et al. Human achaete-scute homologue 1 (HASH-1) is downregulated in differentiating neuroblastoma cells. Biochem Biophys Res Commun 1999; 256:557–563.
58. Artavanis-Tsakonas S, Rand MD, Lake RJ. Notch signaling: cell fate control and signal integration in development. Science 1999; 284:770–776.
59. Jensen J, Pedersen EE, Galante P, et al. Control of endodermal endocrine development by Hes-1. Nat Genet 2000; 24:36–44.
60. Chen H, Thiagalingam A, Chopra H, et al. Conservation of the *Drosophila* lateral inhibition pathway in human lung cancer: a hairy-related protein (HES-1) directly represses achaete-scute homolog-1 expression. Proc Natl Acad Sci USA 1997; 94:5355–5360.
61. de Keyzer Y, Lenne F, Massias JF, et al. Pituitary-like proopiomelanocortin transcripts in human Leydig cell tumors. J Clin Invest 1990; 86:871–877.
62. Mundy GR, Cove DH, Fisken R. Primary hyperparathyroidism: changes in the pattern of clinical presentation. Lancet 1980; 1: 1317–1320.
63. Fisken RA, Heath DA, Bold AM. Hypercalcaemia: a hospital survey. Q J Med 1980; 49:405–418.
64. Fisken RA, Heath DA, Somers S. Hypercalcemia in hospital patients: clinical and diagnostic aspects. Lancet 1981; 1:202–207.
65. Singer FR, Sharp CF Jr, Rude RK. Pathogenesis of hypercalcemia of malignancy. Miner Electrolyte Metab 1979; 2:161–168.
66. Ralston SH, Gallacher SJ, Patel U, et al. Cancer-associated hypercalcemia: morbidity and mortality. Ann Intern Med 1990; 112: 499–504.
67. Bender RA, Hansen H. Hypercalcemia in bronchogenic carcinoma. Ann Intern Med 1974; 80:205–208.
68. Fukumoto S, Matsumoto T, Ikeda K, et al. Clinical evaluation of calcium metabolism in adult T-cell leukemia/lymphoma. Arch Intern Med 1988; 148:921–925.
69. Watanabe T, Yamaguchi K, Takatsuki K, et al. Constitutive expression of parathyroid hormone–related protein gene in human T cell leukemia virus type 1 (HTLV-1) carriers and adult T cell leukemia patients that can be trans-activated by HTLV-1 tax gene. J Exp Med 1990; 172:759–765.
70. Kumar S, Mow BM, Kaufmann SH. Hypercalcemia complicating leukemic transformation of agnogenic myeloid metaplasia-myelofibrosis. Mayo Clin Proc 1999; 74:1233–1237.
71. Wong KF, Chan JK, Ma SK, et al. Megakaryoblastic transformation of polycythemia vera associated with hypercalcemia. Am J Hematol 1993; 43:240–242.
72. Budayr AA, Nissenson RA, Klein RF, et al. Increased serum levels of a parathyroid hormone–like protein in malignancy-associated hypercalcemia. Ann Intern Med 1989; 111:807–812.
73. Firkin F, Seymour JF, Watson AM, et al. Parathyroid hormone–related protein in hypercalcaemia associated with haematological malignancy. Br J Haematol 1996; 94:486–492.
74. Firkin F, Schneider H, Grill V. Parathyroid hormone–related protein in hypercalcemia associated with hematological malignancy. Leuk Lymphoma 1998; 29:499–506.
75. Stewart AF, Hoecker JL, Mallette LE, et al. Hypercalcemia in pheochromocytoma. Ann Intern Med 1985; 102:776–777.
76. Kimura S, Nishimura Y, Yamaguchi K, et al. A case of pheochromocytoma producing parathyroid hormone–related protein and presenting with hypercalcemia. J Clin Endocrinol Metab 1990; 70:1559–1563.
77. Mune T, Katakami H, Kato Y, et al. Production and secretion of parathyroid hormone–related protein in pheochromocytoma: participation of an alpha-adrenergic mechanism. J Clin Endocrinol Metab 1993; 76:757–762.
78. Burtis WJ, Brady TG, Orloff JJ, et al. Immunochemical characterization of circulating parathyroid hormone–related protein in patients with humoral hypercalcemia of cancer. N Engl J Med 1990; 322:1106–1112.
79. Grill V, Hillary J, Ho PMW, et al. Parathyroid hormone–related protein: a possible endocrine function in lactation. Clin Endocrinol (Oxf) 1992; 37:405–410.
80. Ratcliffe WA, Norbury S, Stott RA, et al. Immunoreactivity of plasma parathyrin-related peptide: three region-specific radioimmunoassays and a two-site immunoradiometric assay compared. Clin Chem 1991; 37:1781–1787.
81. Blind E, Raue F, Gotzmann J, et al. Circulating levels of midregional parathyroid hormone–related protein in hypercalcaemia of malignancy. Clin Endocrinol (Oxf) 1992; 37:290–297.
82. Burtis WJ, Dann P, Gaich GA, et al. A high abundance midregion species of parathyroid hormone–related protein: immunological and chromatographic characterization in plasma. J Clin Endocrinol Metab 1994; 78:317–322.
83. Bucht E, Rong H, Pernow Y, et al. Parathyroid hormone–related protein in patients with primary breast cancer and eucalcemia. Cancer Res 1998; 58:4113–4116.
84. Wu TJ, Lin CL, Taylor RL, et al. Increased parathyroid hormone–related peptide in patients with hypercalcemia associated with islet cell carcinoma. Mayo Clin Proc 1997; 72:1111–1115.
85. Nussbaum SR, Zahradnik RJ, Lavigne JR, et al. Highly sensitive two-site immunoradiometric assay of parathyrin and its clinical utility in evaluating patients with hypercalcemia. Clin Chem 1987; 33:1364–1367.
86. Stewart AF, Horst R, Deftos LJ, et al. Biochemical evaluation of patients with cancer-associated hypercalcemia. N Engl J Med 1980; 303:1377–1383.
87. Budayr AA, Zysset E, Jenzer A, et al. Effects of treatment of malignancy-associated hypercalcemia on serum parathyroid hormone–related protein. J Bone Miner Res 1994; 9:521–526.
88. Adams JS, Fernandez M, Gacad MA, et al. Vitamin D metabolite–mediated hypercalcemia and hypercalciuria in patients with AIDS and non–AIDS-associated lymphoma. Blood 1989; 73:235–239.
89. Seymour JF, Gagel RF, Hagemeister FB, et al. Calcitriol production in hypercalcemic and normocalcemic patients with non-Hodgkin lymphoma. Ann Intern Med 1994; 121:633–640.
90. Seymour JF, Gagel RF. Calcitriol: the major humoral mediator of hypercalcemia in Hodgkin's disease and non-Hodgkin's lymphomas. Blood 1993; 82:1383–1394.
91. Strewler GJ, Budayr AA, Clark OH, et al. Production of parathyroid hormone by a malignant nonparathyroid tumor in a hypercalcemic patient. J Clin Endocrinol Metab 1993; 76:1373–1375.
92. Yoshimoto K, Yamasaki R, Sakai H, et al. Ectopic production of parathyroid hormone by small cell lung cancer in a patient with hypercalcemia. J Clin Endocrinol Metab 1989; 68:976–981.
93. Rizzoli R, Pache JC, Didierjean L, et al. A thymoma as a cause

of true ectopic hyperparathyroidism. J Clin Endocrinol Metab 1994; 79:912–915.
94. Strewler GJ, Nissenson RA. Hypercalcemia in malignancy. West J Med 1990; 153:635–640.
95. Orloff JJ, Reddy D, de Papp AE, et al. Parathyroid hormone-related protein as a prohormone: post-translational processing and receptor interactions. Endocr Rev 1994; 15:40–60.
96. Jüppner H, Abou-Samra AB, Uneno S, et al. The parathyroid hormone-like peptide associated with humoral hypercalcemia of malignancy and parathyroid hormone bind to the same receptor on the plasma membrane of ROS 17/2.8 cells. J Biol Chem 1988; 263:8557–8560.
97. Nissenson RA, Diep D, Strewler GJ. Synthetic peptides comprising the amino-terminal sequence of a parathyroid hormone-like protein from human malignancies: binding to parathyroid hormone receptors and activation of adenylate cyclase in bone cells and kidney. J Biol Chem 1988; 263:12866–12871.
98. Hirschel-Scholz S, Caverzasio J, Rizzoli R, et al. Normalization of hypercalcemia associated with a decrease in renal calcium. J Clin Invest 1986; 78:319–322.
99. Harinck HI, Bijvoet OL, Plantingh AS, et al. Role of bone and kidney in tumor-induced hypercalcemia and its treatment with bisphosphonate and sodium chloride. Am J Med 1987; 82:1133–1142.
100. Goodman EC, Iversen LL. Calcitonin gene-related peptide: novel neuropeptide. Life Sci 1986; 38:2169–2178.
101. Body JJ, Dumon JC, Thirion M, et al. Circulating PTHrP concentrations in tumor-induced hypercalcemia: influence on the response to bisphosphonate and changes after therapy. J Bone Miner Res 1993; 8:701–706.
102. Wimalawansa SJ. Significance of plasma PTHrP in patients with hypercalcemia of malignancy treated with bisphosphonate. Cancer 1994; 73:2223–2230.
103. Rizzoli R, Thiebaud D, Bundred N, et al. Serum parathyroid hormone-related protein levels and response to bisphosphonate treatment in hypercalcemia of malignancy. J Clin Endocrinol Metab 1999; 84:3545–3550.
104. Philbrick WM, Wysolmerski JJ, Galbraith S, et al. Defining the roles of parathyroid hormone-related protein in normal physiology. Physiol Rev 1996; 76:127–173.
105. Guise TA, Yin JJ, Taylor SD, et al. Evidence for a causal role of parathyroid hormone-related protein in the pathogenesis of human breast cancer-mediated osteolysis. J Clin Invest 1996; 98: 1544–1549.
106. Powell GJ, Southby J, Danks JA, et al. Localization of parathyroid hormone-related protein in breast cancer metastases: increased incidence in bone compared with other sites. Cancer Res 1991; 51:3059–3061.
107. Bundred NJ, Walker RA, Ratcliffe WA, et al. Parathyroid hormone related protein and skeletal morbidity in breast cancer. Eur J Cancer 1992; 28:690–692.
108. Yin JJ, Selander K, Chirgwin JM, et al. TGF-beta signaling blockade inhibits PTHrP secretion by breast cancer cells and bone metastases development. J Clin Invest 1999; 103:197–206.
109. Horiuchi N, Caulfield MP, Fisher JE, et al. Similarity of synthetic peptide from human tumor to parathyroid hormone in vivo and in vitro. Science 1987; 238:1566–1568.
110. Hulter HN, Halloran BP, Toto RD, et al. Long-term control of plasma calcitriol concentrations in dogs and humans. J Clin Invest 1985; 76:695–702.
111. Fukumoto S, Matsumoto T, Yamoto H, et al. Suppression of serum 1,25-dihydroxyvitamin D in humoral hypercalcemia of malignancy is caused by elaboration of a factor that inhibits renal 1,25-dihydroxyvitamin D_3 production. Endocrinology 1989; 124: 2057–2062.
112. Stewart AF, Vignery A, Silverglate A, et al. Quantitative bone histomorphometry in humoral hypercalcemia of malignancy. J Clin Endocrinol Metab 1982; 55:219–227.
113. Strewler GJ, Nissenson RA. Skeletal and renal actions of parathyroid hormone-related protein. In Bilezikian JP, Marcus R, Levine MA (eds). The Parathyroids: Basic and Clinical Concepts. New York, Raven Press, 1994, pp 311–320.
114. Merendino JJ Jr, Insogna KL, Milstone LM, et al. A parathyroid hormone-like protein from cultured human keratinocytes. Science 1986; 231:388–390.
115. Danks JA, Martin TJ, Moseley JM, et al. Do all epidermal keratinocytes contain parathyroid hormone related protein (PTHrP)? J Invest Dermatol 1991; 97:1086–1087.
116. Wysolmerski JJ, Broadus AE, Zhou J, et al. Overexpression of parathyroid hormone-related protein in the skin of transgenic mice interferes with hair follicle development. Proc Natl Acad Sci USA 1994; 91:1133–1137.
117. Wysolmerski JJ, Vasavada RC, Foley J, et al. Transactivation of the *PTHrP* gene in squamous carcinoma predicts the occurrence of hypercalcemia in athymic mice. Cancer Res 1996; 56:1043–1049.
118. Lafferty FW. Pseudohyperparathyroidism. Medicine (Baltimore) 1966; 45:247–260.
119. Danks JA, Ebeling PR, Hayman J, et al. Parathyroid hormone-related protein: immunohistochemical localization in cancers and in normal skin. J Bone Miner Res 1989; 4:273–278.
120. Davies M, Hayes ME, Yin JA, et al. Abnormal synthesis of 1,25-dihydroxyvitamin D in patients with malignant lymphoma. J Clin Endocrinol Metab 1994; 78:1202–1207.
121. Barbour GL, Coburn JW, Slatopolsky E, et al. Hypercalcemia in an anephric patient with sarcoidosis: evidence for extrarenal generation of 1,25-dihydroxyvitamin D. N Engl J Med 1981; 305: 440–443.
122. Stern PH, De Olazabal J, Bell NH. Evidence for abnormal regulation of circulating 1α,25-dihydroxyvitamin D in patients with sarcoidosis and normal calcium metabolism. J Clin Invest 1980; 66:852–855.
123. Adams JS, Kantorovich V. Inability of short-term, low-dose hydroxychloroquine to resolve vitamin D-mediated hypercalcemia in patients with B-cell lymphoma. J Clin Endocrinol Metab 1999; 84:799–801.
124. Nussbaum SR, Gaz RD, Arnold A. Hypercalcemia and ectopic secretion of parathyroid hormone by an ovarian carcinoma. N Engl J Med 1990; 323:1324–1328.
125. Mundy G. Hypercalcemic factors other than parathyroid hormone-related protein. Endocrinol Metab Clin North Am 1989; 18:795–805.
126. Kawano M, Yamamoto I, Iwato K, et al. Interkeukin-1 beta rather than lymphotoxin as the major bone resorbing activity in human multiple myeloma. Blood 1989; 73:1646–1649.
127. Garrett IR, Durie BGM, Nedwin GE, et al. Production of lymphotoxin, a bone-resorbing cytokine, by cultured human myeloma. N Engl J Med 1987; 317:526–532.
128. Han J-H, Choi SJ, Kurihara N, et al. Macrophage inflammatory protein-1α is an osteoclastogenic factor in myeloma that is independent of receptor activator of nuclear factor κB ligand. Blood 2001; 97:3349–3353.
129. Horiuchi T, Miyachi T, Arai T, et al. Raised plasma concentrations of parathyroid hormone related peptide in hypercalcemic multiple myeloma. Horm Metab Res 1997; 29:469–471.
130. Zeimer H, Firkin F, Grill V, et al. Assessment of cellular expression of parathyroid hormone-related protein mRNA and protein in multiple myeloma. J Pathol 2000; 192:336–341.
131. Wysolmerski JJ, Broadus AE. Hypercalcemia of malignancy—the central role of parathyroid hormone-related protein. Annu Rev Med 1994; 45:189–200.
132. Ratcliffe WA, Hutchesson AC, Bundred NJ, et al. Role of assays for parathyroid-hormone-related protein in investigation of hypercalcaemia. Lancet 1992; 339:164–167.
133. Pandian MR, Morgan CH, Carlton E, et al. Modified immunoradiometric assay of parathyroid hormone-related protein: clinical application in the differential diagnosis of hypercalcemia. Clin Chem 1992; 38:282–288.
134. Kovacs L, Robertson GL. Syndrome of inappropriate antidiuresis. Endocrinol Metab Clin North Am 1992; 21:859–875.
135. Moses AM, Scheinman SJ. Ectopic secretion of neurohypophyseal peptides in patients with malignancy. Endocrinol Metab Clin North Am 1991; 20:489–506.
136. Sorensen JB, Andersen MK, Hansen HH. Syndrome of inappropriate secretion of antidiuretic hormone (SIADH) in malignant disease. J Intern Med 1995; 238:97–110.
137. Hainsworth JD, Workman R, Greco FA. Management of the syndrome of inappropriate antidiuretic hormone secretion in small cell lung cancer. Cancer 1983; 51:161–165.
138. Passamonte PM. Hypouricemia, inappropriate secretion of antidi-

uretic hormone, and small cell carcinoma of the lung. Arch Intern Med 1984; 144:1569–1570.
139. List AF, Hainsworth JD, Davis BW, et al. The syndrome of inappropriate secretion of antidiuretic hormone (SIADH) in small-cell lung cancer. J Clin Oncol 1986; 4:1191–1198.
140. Rassam JW, Anderson G. Incidence of paramalignant disorders in bronchogenic carcinoma. Thorax 1975; 30:86–90.
141. Talmi YP, Hoffman HT, McCabe BF. Syndrome of inappropriate secretion of arginine vasopressin in patients with cancer of the head and neck. Ann Otol Rhinol Laryngol 1992; 101:946–949.
142. Gennari FJ. Current concepts: serum osmolality. Uses and limitations. N Engl J Med 1984; 310:102–105.
143. Beck LH. Hypouricemia in the syndrome of inappropriate secretion of antidiuretic hormone. N Engl J Med 1979; 301:528–530.
144. Gainer H, Wray S. Oxytocin and vasopressin: from genes to peptides. Ann NY Acad Sci 1992; 652:14–28.
145. North WG. Neuropeptide production by small cell carcinoma: vasopressin and oxytocin as plasma markers of disease. J Clin Endocrinol Metab 1991; 73:1316–1320.
146. North WG, Ware J, Maurer LH, et al. Neurophysins as tumor markers for small cell carcinoma of the lung: a cancer and Leukemia Group B evaluation. Cancer 1988; 62:1343–1347.
147. Legros JJ, Geenen V, Carvelli T, et al. Neurophysins as markers of vasopressin and oxytocin release. A study in carcinoma of the lung. Horm Res 1990; 34:151–155.
148. Sausville E, Carney D, Battey J. The human vasopressin gene is linked to the oxytocin gene and is selectively expressed in a cultured lung cancer cell line. J Biol Chem 1985; 260:10236–10241.
149. Coulson JM, Fiskerstrand CE, Woll PJ, et al. E-box motifs within the human vasopressin gene promoter contribute to a major enhancer in small-cell lung cancer. Biochem J 1999; 344: 961–970.
150. Coulson JM, Fiskerstrand CE, Woll PJ, et al. Arginine vasopressin promoter regulation is mediated by a neuron-restrictive silencer element in small cell lung cancer. Cancer Res 1999; 59: 5123–5127.
151. North WG, Fay MJ, Longo KA, et al. Expression of all known vasopressin receptor subtypes by small cell tumors implies a multifaceted role for this neuropeptide. Cancer Res 1998; 58:1866–1871.
152. Fay MJ, Friedmann AS, Yu XM, et al. Vasopressin and vasopressin-receptor immunoreactivity in small-cell lung carcinoma (SCCL) cell lines: disruption in the activation cascade of V1a-receptors in variant SCCL. Cancer Lett 1994; 82:167–174.
153. Zerbe R, Stropes L, Robertson G. Vasopressin function in the syndrome of inappropriate antidiuresis. Annu Rev Med 1980; 31: 315–327.
154. Kim JK, Summer SN, Wood WM, et al. Osmotic and non-osmotic regulation of arginine vasopressin (AVP) release, mRNA, and promoter activity in small cell lung carcinoma (SCLC) cells. Mol Cell Endocrinol 1996; 123:179–186.
155. North WG. Biosynthesis of vasopressin and neurophysins. In Gash DM, Boer GJ (eds). Vasopressin: Principles and Properties. New York, Plenum, 1987, p 175.
156. North WG, Maurer LH, Valtin H, et al. Human neurophysins as potential tumor markers for small cell carcinoma of the lung: application of specific radioimmunoassays. J Clin Endocrinol Metab 1980; 51:892–896.
157. Maurer LH, O'Donnell JF, Kennedy S, et al. Human neurophysins in carcinoma of the lung: relation to histology, disease stage, response rate, survival, and syndrome of inappropriate antidiuretic hormone secretion. Cancer Treat Rep 1983; 67:971–976.
158. Comis RL, Miller M, Ginsberg SJ. Abnormalities in water homeostasis in small cell anaplastic lung cancer. Cancer 1980; 45: 2414–2421.
159. Cogan E, Debieve MF, Pepersack T, et al. Natriuresis and atrial natriuretic factor secretion during inappropriate antidiuresis. Am J Med 1988; 84:409–418.
160. Kamoi K, Ebe T, Kobayashi O, et al. Atrial natriuretic peptide in patients with the syndrome of inappropriate antidiuretic hormone secretion and with diabetes insipidus. J Clin Endocrinol Metab 1990; 70:1385–1390.
161. Manoogian C, Pandian M, Ehrlich L, et al. Plasma atrial natriuretic hormone levels in patients with the syndrome of inappropriate antidiuretic hormone secretion. J Clin Endocrinol Metab 1988; 67:571–575.
162. Gross AJ, Steinberg SM, Reilly JG, et al. Atrial natriuretic factor and arginine vasopressin production in tumor cell lines from patients with lung cancer and their relationship to serum sodium. Cancer Res 1993; 53:67–74.
163. Bliss DP Jr, Battey JF, Linnoila RI, et al. Expression of the atrial natriuretic factor gene in small cell lung cancer tumors and tumor cell lines. J Natl Cancer Inst 1990; 82:305–310.
164. Yoshinaga K, Yamaguchi K, Abe K, et al. Production of immunoreactive atrial natriuretic polypeptide in neuroendocrine tumors. Cancer 1994; 73:1292–1296.
165. Campling BG, Sarda IR, Baer KA, et al. Secretion of atrial natriuretic peptide and vasopressin by small cell lung cancer. Cancer 1995; 75:2442–2451.
166. Johnson BE, Damodaran A, Rushin J, et al. Ectopic production and processing of atrial natriuretic peptide in a small cell lung carcinoma cell line and tumor from a patient with hyponatremia. Cancer 1997; 79:35–44.
167. Pollock AS, Arieff AI. Abnormalities of cell volume regulation and their functional consequences. Am J Physiol 1980; 239:F195–F205.
168. Grantham J, Linshaw M. The effect of hyponatremia on the regulation of intracellular volume and solute composition. Circ Res 1984; 54:483–491.
169. Anderson RJ, Chung HM, Kluge R, et al. Hyponatremia: a prospective analysis of its epidemiology and the pathogenetic role of vasopressin. Ann Intern Med 1985; 102:164–168.
170. Gross PA, Pehrisch H, Rascher W, et al. Pathogenesis of clinical hyponatremia: observations of vasopressin and fluid intake in 100 hyponatremic medical patients. Eur J Clin Invest 1987; 17:123–129.
171. Hantman D, Rossier B, Zohlman R, et al. Rapid correction of hyponatremia in the syndrome of inappropriate secretion of antidiuretic hormone. An alternative treatment to hypertonic saline. Ann Intern Med 1973; 78:870–875.
172. Arieff AI. Hyponatremia associated with permanent brain damage. Adv Intern Med 1987; 32:325–344.
173. Forrest JN Jr, Cox M, Hong C, et al. Superiority of demeclocycline over lithium in the treatment of chronic syndrome of inappropriate secretion of antidiuretic hormone. N Engl J Med 1978; 298:173–177.
174. De Troyer A. Demeclocycline. Treatment for syndrome of inappropriate antidiuretic hormone secretion. JAMA 1977; 237:2723–2726.
175. Wajchenberg BL, Mendonca BB, Liberman B, et al. Ectopic adrenocorticotropic hormone syndrome. Endocr Rev 1994; 15: 752–787.
176. Becker M, Aron DC. Ectopic ACTH syndrome and CRH-mediated Cushing's syndrome. Endocrinol Metab Clin North Am 1994; 23:585–606.
177. Magiakou MA, Mastorakos G, Oldfield EH, et al. Cushing's syndrome in children and adolescents. Presentation, diagnosis, and therapy. N Engl J Med 1994; 331:629–636.
178. Tabarin A, Corcuff J, Rashedi M, et al. Comparative value of plasma ACTH and beta-endorphin measurement with three different commercial kits for the etiological diagnosis of ACTH-dependent Cushing's syndrome. Acta Endocrinol (Copenh) 1992; 126:308–314.
179. Stewart PM, Walker BR, Holder G, et al. 11β-Hydroxysteroid dehydrogenase activity in Cushing's syndrome: explaining the mineralocorticoid excess state of the ectopic adrenocorticotropin syndrome. J Clin Endocrinol Metab 1995; 80:3617–3620.
180. Arteaga E, Fardella C, Campusano C, et al. Persistent hypokalemia after successful adrenalectomy in a patient with Cushing's syndrome due to ectopic ACTH secretion: possible role of 11β-hydroxysteroid dehydrogenase inhibition. J Endocrinol Invest 1999; 22:857–859.
181. Schambelan M, Slaton PE, Biglieri EG. Mineralocorticoid production in hyperadrenocorticism. Am J Med 1971; 51:299–303.
182. Chang AC, Israel A, Gazdar A, et al. Initiation of pro-opiomelanocortin mRNA from a normally quiescent promoter in a human small cell lung cancer cell line. Gene 1989; 84:115–126.
183. Ray DW, Littlewood AC, Clark AJ, et al. Human small cell lung

cancer cell lines expressing the proopiomelanocortin gene have aberrant glucocorticoid receptor function. J Clin Invest 1994; 93: 1625–1630.
184. Picon A, Bertagna X, de Keyzer Y. Analysis of proopiomelanocortin gene transcription mechanisms in bronchial tumour cells. Mol Cell Endocrinol 1999; 147:93–102.
185. Picon A, Leblond-Francillard M, Raffin-Sanson ML, et al. Functional analysis of the human pro-opiomelanocortin promoter in the small cell lung carcinoma cell line DMS-79. J Mol Endocrinol 1995; 15:187–194.
186. Picon A, Bertagna X, de Keyzer Y. Analysis of the human proopiomelanocortin gene promoter in a small cell lung carcinoma cell line reveals an unusual role for E2F transcription factors. Oncogene 1999; 18:2627–2633.
187. Ray DW, Davis JR, White A, et al. Glucocorticoid receptor structure and function in glucocorticoid-resistant small cell lung carcinoma cells. Cancer Res 1996; 56:3276–3280.
188. Parks LL, Turney MK, Detera-Wadleigh S, et al. An ACTH-producing small cell lung cancer expresses aberrant glucocorticoid receptor transcripts from a normal gene. Mol Cell Endocrinol 1998; 142:175–181.
189. Yalow RS, Berson SA. Size heterogeneity of immunoreactive human ACTH in plasma and in extracts of pituitary glands and ACTH-producing thymoma. Biochem Biophys Res Commun 1971; 44:439–445.
190. Ito H, Akiyama H, Shigeno C, et al. Hedgehog signaling molecules in bone marrow cells at the initial stage of fracture repair. Biochem Biophys Res Commun 1999; 262:443–451.
191. Rouille Y, Duguay SJ, Lund K, et al. Proteolytic processing mechanisms in the biosynthesis of neuroendocrine peptides: the subtilisin-like proprotein convertases. Front Neuroendocrinol 1995; 16:322–361.
192. Bertagna X. Proopiomelanocortin-derived peptides. Endocrinol Metab Clin North Am 1994; 23:467–485.
193. Vieau D, Massias JF, Girard F, et al. Corticotrophin-like intermediary lobe peptide as a marker of alternate pro-opiomelanocortin processing in ACTH-producing non-pituitary tumours. Clin Endocrinol (Oxf) 1989; 31:691–700.
194. Vieau D, Seidah NG, Mbikay M, et al. Expression of the prohormone convertase PC2 correlates with the presence of corticotropin-like intermediate lobe peptide in human adrenocorticotropin-secreting tumors. J Clin Endocrinol Metab 1994; 79:1503–1506.
195. Kimura N, Ishikawa T, Sasaki Y, et al. Expression of prohormone convertase, PC2, in adrenocorticotropin-producing thymic carcinoid with elevated plasma corticotropin-releasing hormone. J Clin Endocrinol 1996; 81:390–395.
196. Kuhn JM, Proeschel MF, Seurin DJ, et al. Comparative assessment of ACTH and lipotropin plasma levels in the diagnosis and follow-up of patients with Cushing's syndrome: a study of 210 cases. Am J Med 1989; 86:678–684.
197. Ratcliffe JG, Knight RA, Besser GM, et al. Tumor and plasma ACTH concentrations in patients with and without the ectopic ACTH syndrome. Clin Endocrinol (Oxf) 1972; 1:27–44.
198. Black M, Carey FA, Farquharson MA, et al. Expression of the pro-opiomelanocortin gene in lung neuroendocrine tumours: in situ hybridization and immunohistochemical studies. J Pathol 1993; 169:329–334.
199. Findling JW, Tyrrell JB. Occult ectopic secretion of corticotropin. Arch Intern Med 1986; 146:929–933.
200. Nieman LK, Oldfield EH, Wesley R, et al. A simplified morning ovine corticotropin-releasing hormone stimulation test for the differential diagnosis of adrenocorticotropin-dependent Cushing's syndrome. J Clin Endocrinol Metab 1993; 77:1308–1312.
201. Avgerinos PC, Yanovski JA, Oldfield EH, et al. The metyrapone and dexamethasone suppression tests for the differential diagnosis of the adrenocorticotropin-dependent Cushing syndrome: a comparison. Ann Intern Med 1994; 121:318–327.
202. Oldfield EH, Doppman JL, Nieman LK, et al. Petrosal sinus sampling with and without corticotropin-releasing hormone for the differential diagnosis of Cushing's syndrome. N Engl J Med 1991; 325:897–905.
203. Wiggam MI, Heaney AP, McIlrath EM, et al. Bilateral inferior petrosal sinus sampling in the differential diagnosis of adrenocorticotropin-dependent Cushing's syndrome: a comparison with other diagnostic tests. J Clin Endocrinol Metab 2000; 85:1525–1532.
204. Kaltsas GA, Giannulis MG, Newell-Price JD, et al. A critical analysis of the value of simultaneous inferior petrosal sinus sampling in Cushing's disease and the occult ectopic adrenocorticotropin syndrome. J Clin Endocrinol Metab 1999; 84:487–492.
205. Graham KE, Samuels MH, Nesbit GM, et al. Cavernous sinus sampling is highly accurate in distinguishing Cushing's disease from the ectopic adrenocorticotropin syndrome and in predicting intrapituitary tumor location. J Clin Endocrinol Metab 1999; 84: 1602–1610.
206. Tabarin A, Valli N, Chanson P, et al. Usefulness of somatostatin receptor scintigraphy in patients with occult ectopic adrenocorticotropin syndrome. J Clin Endocrinol Metab 1999; 84:1193–1202.
207. Miller JW, Crapo L. The medical treatment of Cushing's syndrome. Endocr Rev 1993; 14:443–458.
208. Sonino N, Boscaro M, Paoletta A, et al. Ketoconazole treatment in Cushing's syndrome: experience in 34 patients. Clin Endocrinol (Oxf) 1991; 35:347–352.
209. Sonino N. The use of ketoconazole as an inhibitor of steroid production. N Engl J Med 1987; 317:812–818.
210. Bertagna X, Favrod-Coune C, Escourolle H, et al. Suppression of ectopic adrenocorticotropin secretion by the long-acting somatostatin analog octreotide. J Clin Endocrinol Metab 1989; 68:988–991.
211. Sartor O, Cutler GB. Mifepristone-treatment of Cushing's syndrome. Clin Obstet Gynecol 1996; 39:506–510.
212. Carey RM, Varma SK, Drake CR Jr, et al. Ectopic secretion of corticotropin-releasing factor as a cause of Cushing's syndrome. N Engl J Med 1984; 311:13–20.
213. Auchus RJ, Mastorakos G, Friedman TC, et al. Corticotropin-releasing hormone production by small cell carcinoma in a patient with ACTH-dependent Cushing's syndrome. J Endocrinol Invest 1994; 17:447–452.
214. Service FJ. Hypoglycemic disorders. N Engl J Med 1995; 332: 1144–1152.
215. Daughaday WH. Hypoglycemia in patients with non–islet cell tumors. Endocrinol Metab Clin North Am 1989; 18:91–101.
216. Zapf J. Insulin-like growth factor binding proteins and tumor hypoglycemia. Trends Endocrinol Metab 1995; 6:37–42.
217. Koch CA, Rother KI, Roth J. Tumor hypoglycemia linked to IGF-II. In Rosenfeld RG, Roberts C Jr (eds). Contemporary Endocrinology: The IGF System. Totowa, NY, Humana Press, 1999, pp 675–698.
218. Marks V, Teale JD. Tumors producing hypoglycemia. In James V (ed). Hypoglycemia: Endocrine Related Cancer. 1998, pp 111–129.
219. Le Roith D. Tumor-induced hypoglycemia. N Engl J Med 1999; 341:757–758.
220. Moller N, Blum WF, Mengel A, et al. Basal and insulin stimulated substrate metabolism in tumour induced hypoglycaemia; evidence for increased muscle glucose uptake. Diabetologia 1991; 34:17–20.
221. Eastman RC, Carson RE, Orloff DG, et al. Glucose utilization in a patient with hepatoma and hypoglycemia Assessment by a positron emission tomography. J Clin Invest 1992; 89:1958–1963.
222. Chung J, Henry RR. Mechanisms of tumor-induced hypoglycemia with intraabdominal hemangiopericytoma. J Clin Endocrinol Metab 1996; 81:919–925.
223. Megyesi K, Kahn CR, Roth J, et al. Hypoglycemia in association with extrapancreatic tumors: demonstration of elevated plasma NSILA-s by a new radioreceptor assay. J Clin Endocrinol Metab 1974; 38:931–934.
224. Lowe WL Jr, Roberts CT Jr, LeRoith D, et al. Insulin-like growth factor-II in nonislet cell tumors associated with hypoglycemia: increased levels of messenger ribonucleic acid. J Clin Endocrinol Metab 1989; 69:1153–1159.
225. Shapiro ET, Bell GI, Polonsky KS, et al. Tumor hypoglycemia: relationship to high molecular weight insulin-like growth factor-II. J Clin Invest 1990; 85:1672–1679.
226. Daughaday WH, Emanuele MA, Brooks MH, et al. Synthesis and secretion of insulin-like growth factor II by a leiomyosarcoma with associated hypoglycemia. N Engl J Med 1988; 319: 1434–1440.
227. Daughaday WH, Trivedi B. Measurement of derivatives of proinsulin-like growth factor-II in serum by a radioimmunoassay

directed against the E-domain in normal subjects and patients with nonislet cell tumor hypoglycemia. J Clin Endocrinol Metab 1992; 75:110–115.
228. Wu JC, Daughaday WH, Lee SD, et al. Radioimmunoassay of serum IGF-I and IGF-II in patients with chronic liver diseases and hepatocellular carcinoma with or without hypoglycemia. J Lab Clin Med 1988; 112:589–594.
229. Hizuka N, Fukuda I, Takano K, et al. Serum insulin-like growth factor II in 44 patients with non–islet cell tumor hypoglycemia. Endocr J 1998; 45(Suppl):S61–S65.
230. Guler HP, Zapf J, Schmidt C, et al. Insulin-like growth factors I and II in healthy man: estimation of half-lives and production rates. Acta Endocrinol (Copenh) 1989; 121:753–758.
231. Zapf J, Futo E, Peter M, et al. Can 'big' insulin-like growth factor II in serum of tumor patients account for the development of extrapancreatic tumor hypoglycemia? J Clin Invest 1992; 90: 2574–2584.
232. Daughaday WH, Kapadia M. Significance of abnormal serum binding of insulin-like growth factor II in the development of hypoglycemia in patients with non–islet-cell tumors. Proc Natl Acad Sci USA 1989; 86:6778–6782.
233. Baxter RC, Daughaday WH. Impaired formation of the ternary insulin-like growth factor–binding protein complex in patients with hypoglycemia due to nonislet cell tumors. J Clin Endocrinol Metab 1991; 73:696–702.
234. Daughaday WH, Trivedi B, Baxter RC. Serum 'big insulin-like growth factor II' from patients with tumor hypoglycemia lacks normal E-domain O-linked glycosylation, a possible determinant of normal propeptide processing. Proc Natl Acad Sci USA 1993; 90:5823–5827.
235. Yang CQ, Zhan X, Hu X, et al. The expression and characterization of human recombinant proinsulin-like growth factor II and a mutant that is defective in the O-glycosylation of its E domain. Endocrinology 1996; 137:2766–2773.
236. Hizuka N, Fukuda I, Takano K, et al. Serum high molecular weight form of insulin-like growth factor II from patients with non–islet cell tumor hypoglycemia is O-glycosylated. J Clin Endocrinol Metab 1998; 83:2875–2877.
237. Ron D, Powers AC, Pandian MR, et al. Increased insulin-like growth factor II production and consequent suppression of growth hormone secretion: a dual mechanism for tumor-induced hypoglycemia. J Clin Endocrinol Metab 1989; 68:701–706.
238. Zapf J, Schmid C, Guler HP, et al. Regulation of binding proteins for insulin-like growth factors (IGF) in humans. Increased expression of IGF binding protein 2 during IGF I treatment of healthy adults and in patients with extrapancreatic tumor hypoglycemia. J Clin Invest 1990; 86:952–961.
239. Katz LE, Liu F, Baker B, et al. The effect of growth hormone treatment on the insulin-like growth factor axis in a child with nonislet cell tumor hypoglycemia. J Clin Endocrinol Metab 1996; 81:1141–1146.
240. Daughaday WH, Trevedi B, Baxter RC. Abnormal serum IGF-II transport in non–islet cell tumor hypoglycemia results from abnormalities of both IGF binding protein-3 and acid label subunit and leads to elevation of serum free IGF-II. Endocrine 1995; 3: 425–428.
241. Samaan NA, Pham FK, Sellin RV, et al. Successful treatment of hypoglycemia using glucagon in a patient with an extrapancreatic tumor. Ann Intern Med 1990; 113:404–406.
242. Hunter SJ, Daughaday WH, Callender ME, et al. A case of hepatoma associated with hypoglycaemia and overproduction of IGF-II (E-21): beneficial effects of treatment with growth hormone and intrahepatic Adriamycin. Clin Endocrinol (Oxf) 1994; 41:397–401.
243. Hoff AO, Vassilopoulou-Sellin R. The role of glucagon administration in the diagnosis and treatment of patients with tumor hypoglycemia. Cancer 1998; 82:1585–1592.
244. Faglia G, Arosio M, Bazzoni N. Ectopic acromegaly. Endocrinol Metab Clin North Am 1992; 21:575–595.
245. Melmed S. Extrapituitary acromegaly. Endocrinol Metab Clin North Am 1991; 20:507–518.
246. Melmed S, Ezrin C, Kovacs K, et al. Acromegaly due to secretion of growth hormone by an ectopic pancreatic islet-cell tumor. N Engl J Med 1985; 312:9–17.
247. Beuschlein F, Strasburger CJ, Siegerstetter V, et al. Acromegaly caused by secretion of growth hormone by a non-Hodgkin's lymphoma. N Engl J Med 2000; 342:1871–1876.
248. Guilemin R, Brazeau P, Bolhen P, et al. Growth hormone–releasing factor from a human pancreatic tumor that caused acromegaly. Science 1982; 218:585–587.
249. Rivier J, Spiess J, Thorner M, et al. Characterization of a growth hormone–releasing factor from a human pancreatic islet tumour. Nature 1982; 300:276–278.
250. Thorner MO, Frohman LA, Leong DA, et al. Extrahypothalamic growth-hormone–releasing factor (GRF) secretion is a rare cause of acromegaly: plasma GRF levels in 177 acromegalic patients. J Clin Endocrinol Metab 1984; 59:846–849.
251. Schopohl J, Losa M, Frey C, et al. Plasma growth hormone (GH)–releasing hormone levels in patients with lung carcinoma. Clin Endocrinol (Oxf) 1991; 34:463–467.
252. Moller DE, Moses AC, Jones K, et al. Octreotide suppresses both growth hormone (GH) and GH-releasing hormone (GHRH) in acromegaly due to ectopic GHRH secretion. J Clin Endocrinol Metab 1989; 68:499–504.
253. Drange MR, Melmed S. Long-acting lanreotide induces clinical and biochemical remission of acromegaly caused by disseminated growth hormone–releasing hormone–secreting carcinoid. J Clin Endocrinol Metab 1998; 83:3104–3109.
254. Ezzat S, Ezrin C, Yamashita S, et al. Recurrent acromegaly resulting from ectopic growth hormone gene expression by a metastatic pancreatic tumor. Cancer 1993; 71:66–70.
255. Weintraub BD, Rosen SW. Ectopic production of human chorionic somatomammotropin by nontrophoblastic cancers. J Clin Endocrinol Metab 1971; 32:94–101.
256. Rosen SW, Weintraub BD. Humours, tumors, and caveats. Ann Intern Med 1975; 82:274–276.
257. Sheth NA, Suraiya JN, Sheth AR, et al. Ectopic production of human placental lactogen by human breast tumors. Cancer 1977; 39:1693–1699.
258. Navarro C, Corretger JM, Sancho A, et al. Paraneoplastic precocious puberty: report of a new case with hepatoblastoma and review of the literature. Cancer 1985; 56:1725–1729.
259. Yokotani T, Koizumi T, Taniguchi R, et al. Expression of alpha and beta genes of human chorionic gonadotropin in lung cancer. Int J Cancer 1997; 71:539–544.
260. Kahn CR, Rosen SW, Weintraub BD, et al. Ectopic production of chorionic gonadotropin and its subunits by islet-cell tumors: a specific marker for malignancy. N Engl J Med 1977; 297:565–569.
261. Heitz PU, Kasper M, Kloppel G, et al. Glycoprotein-hormone alpha-chain production by pancreatic endocrine tumors: a specific marker for malignancy: immunocytochemical analysis of tumors of 155 patients. Cancer 1983; 51:277–282.
262. Blithe DL, Wehmann RE, Nisula BC. β-Core: chemical and clinical properties. Trends Endocrinol Metab 1990; 1:394–398.
263. Neven P, Iles RK, Lee CL, et al. Urinary chorionic gonadotropin subunits and beta-core in nonpregnant women: a study of benign and malignant gynecologic disorders. Cancer 1993; 71: 4124–4130.
264. Yoshimura M, Nishimura R, Murotani A, et al. Assessment of urinary beta-core fragment of human chorionic gonadotropin as a new tumor marker of lung cancer. Cancer 1994; 73:2745–2752.
265. Weidner N, Bar RS, Weiss D, et al. Neoplastic pathology of oncogenic osteomalacia/rickets. Cancer 1985; 55:1691–1705.
266. Schapira D, Ben Izhak O, Nachtigal A, et al. Tumor-induced osteomalacia. Semin Arthritis Rheum 1995; 25:35–46.
267. DiMeglio LA, White KE, Econs MJ. Disorders of phosphate metabolism. Endocrinol Metab Clin North Am 2000; 29:591–609.
268. Lyles KW, Berry WR, Haussler M, et al. Hypophosphatemic osteomalacia: association with prostatic carcinoma. Ann Intern Med 1980; 93:275–278.
269. Charhon SA, Chapuy MC, Delvin EE, et al. Histomorphometric analysis of sclerotic bone metastases from prostatic carcinoma special reference to osteomalacia. Cancer 1983; 51:918–924.
270. Cai Q, Hodgson SF, Kao PC, et al. Brief report: inhibition of renal phosphate transport by a tumor product in a patient with oncogenic osteomalacia. N Engl J Med 1994; 330:1645–1649.
271. White KE, Evans WE, O'Riordan JL, et al. Autosomal dominant hypophosphataemic rickets is associated with mutations in FGF23. Nat Genet 2000; 26:345–348.
272. White KE, Jonsson KB, Carn G, et al. The autosomal dominant hypophosphatemic rickets (*ADHR*) gene is a secreted polypeptide

overexpressed by tumors that cause phosphate wasting. J Clin Endocrinol Metab 2001; 86:497–500.
272a. Shimada T, Mizutani S, Muto T, et al. Cloning and characterization of FGF-23 as a causative factor of tumor-induced osteomalacia. Proc Natl Acad Sci USA 2001; 98(11):6500–6505.
273. Bowe AE, Finnegan R, Jan de Beur SM, et al. FGF-23 inhibits renal tubular phosphate transport and is a PHEX substrate. Biochem Biophys Res Commun 2001; 284(4):977–981.
274. Hammond D, Winnick S. Paraneoplastic erythrocytosis and ectopic erythropoietins. Ann NY Acad Sci 1974; 230:219–227.
275. Da Silva JL, Lacombe C, Bruneval P, et al. Tumor cells are the site of erythropoietin synthesis in human renal cancers associated with polycythemia. Blood 1990; 75:577–582.
276. Maxwell PH, Wiesener MS, Chang G-W, et al. The tumour suppressor protein VHL targets hypoxia-inducible factors for oxygen-dependent proteolysis. Nature 1999; 399:271–275.
277. Piao Z, Kim H, Jeon BK, et al. Relationship between loss of heterozygosity of tumor suppressor genes and histologic differentiation in hepatocellular carcinoma. Cancer 1997; 80:865–872.
278. Haase VH, Glickman JN, Socolovsky M, et al. Vascular tumors in livers with targeted inactivation of the von Hippel–Lindau tumor suppressor. Proc Natl Acad Sci USA 2001; 98:1583–1588.
279. Muta H, Funakoshi A, Baba T, et al. Gene expression of erythropoietin in hepatocellular carcinoma. Intern Med 1994; 33:427–431.
280. Trimble M, Caro J, Talalla A, et al. Secondary erythrocytosis due to a cerebellar hemangioblastoma: demonstration of erythropoietin mRNA in the tumor. Blood 1991; 78:599–601.
281. Shiramizu M, Katsuoka Y, Grodberg J, et al. Constitutive secretion of erythropoietin by human renal adenocarcinoma cells in vivo and in vitro. Exp Cell Res 1994; 215:249–256.
282. Horinouchi A, Miyamoto S, Sekiguchi M, et al. Erythropoietin mRNA in hepatocellular carcinomas and kidney in male B6C3F1 mice with secondary polycythemia. Toxicol Pathol 1998; 26:682–686.
283. Kew MC, Fisher JW. Serum erythropoietin concentrations in patients with hepatocellular carcinoma. Cancer 1986; 58:2485–2488.
284. Sawabe Y, Iida S, Tabata Y, et al. Serum erythropoietin measurements by a one-step sandwich enzyme linked immunosorbent assay in patients with hepatocellular carcinoma and liver cirrhosis. Jpn J Clin Oncol 1993; 23:273–277.
285. Coombes RC, Hillyard CJ, Greenberg PB, et al. Plasma immunoreactive calcitonin in patients with non-thyroid tumors. Lancet 1974; 1:1080–1082.
286. Silva O, Becker K, Primack A, et al. Increased calcitonin levels in bronchogenic cancer. Chest 1976; 69:495–501.
287. Roos BA, Lindall AW, Baylin SB, et al. Plasma immunoreactive calcitonin in lung cancer. J Clin Endocrinol Metab 1980; 50:659–666.
288. Samaan NA, Castillo S, Schultz PN, et al. Serum calcitonin after pentagastrin stimulation in patients with bronchogenic and breast cancer compared to that in patients with medullary thyroid carcinoma. J Clin Endocrinol Metab 1980; 51:237–241.
289. Sim SJ, Glassman AB, Ro JY, et al. Serum calcitonin in small cell carcinoma of the prostate. Ann Clin Lab Sci 1996; 26:487–495.
290. Foa P, Ortolani S, Pogliani EM, et al. Immunoreactive calcitonin: a tumor marker for myelogenous leukemias. Int J Biol Markers 1990; 5:27–30.
291. Zajac JD, Martin TJ, Hudson P, et al. Biosynthesis of calcitonin by human lung cancer cells. Endocrinology 1985; 116:749–754.
292. Symes AJ, Craig RK, Brickell PM. Loss of transcriptional repression contributes to the ectopic expression of the calcitonin/α-CGRP gene in a human lung carcinoma cell line. FEBS Lett 1992; 306:229–233.
293. Machens A, Haedecke J, Holzhausen HJ, et al. Differential diagnosis of calcitonin-secreting neuroendocrine carcinoma of the foregut by pentagastrin stimulation. Langenbecks Arch Surg 2000; 385:398–401.
294. Ghatei MA, Stratton MR, Allen JM, et al. Co-secretion of calcitonin gene–related peptide, gastrin-releasing peptide and ACTH by a carcinoid tumor metastasizing to the cerebellum. Postgrad Med J 1987; 63:123–130.
295. Ishibashi M, Fujita M, Nagai K, et al. Production and secretion of endothelin by hepatocellular carcinoma. J Clin Endocrinol Metab 1993; 76:378–383.
296. Alanen K, Deng DX, Chakrabarti S. Augmented expression of endothelin-1, endothelin-3 and the endothelin-B receptor in breast carcinoma. Histopathology 2000; 36:161–167.
297. Nelson JB, Hedican SP, George DJ, et al. Identification of endothelin-1 in the pathophysiology of metastatic adenocarcinoma of the prostate. Nat Med 1995; 1:944–949.
298. Nelson JB, Lee WH, Nguyen SH, et al. Methylation of the 5′ CpG island of the endothelin B receptor gene is common in human prostate cancer. Cancer Res 1997; 57:35–37.
299. Chiao JW, Moonga BS, Yang YM, et al. Endothelin-1 from prostate cancer cells is enhanced by bone contact which blocks osteoclastic bone resorption. Br J Cancer 2000; 83:360–365.
300. Nakamuta M, Ohashi M, Tabata S, et al. High plasma concentrations of endothelin-like immunoreactivities in patients with hepatocellular carcinoma. Am J Gastroenterol 1993; 88:248–252.
301. Yin JJ, Grubbs BG, Cui Y, et al. Endothelin A receptor blockade inhibits osteoblastic metastases. J Bone Miner Res 2001; 15(Suppl 1):S201.
302. Mendelsohn G, Eggleston JC, Olson JL, et al. Vasoactive intestinal peptide and its relationship to ganglion cell differentiation in neuroblastic tumors. Lab Invest 1979; 41:144–149.
303. Said SI, Faloona GR. Elevated plasma and tissue levels of vasoactive intestinal polypeptide in the watery-diarrhea syndrome due to pancreatic, bronchogenic and other tumors. N Engl J Med 1975; 293:155–160.
304. Hamilton I, Reis L, Bilimoria S, et al. A renal vipoma. Br Med J 1980; 281:1323–1324.
305. Wood SM, Wood JR, Ghatei MA, et al. Bombesin, somatostatin and neurotensin-like immunoreactivity in bronchial carcinoma. J Clin Endocrinol Metab 1981; 53:1310–1312.
306. Szabo M, Berelowitz M, Pettengill OS, et al. Ectopic production of somatostatin-like immuno- and bioactivity by cultured human pulmonary small cell carcinoma. J Clin Endocrinol Metab 1980; 51:978–987.
307. Noseda A, Peeters TL, Delhaye M, et al. Increased plasma motilin concentrations in small cell carcinoma of the lung. Thorax 1987; 42:784–789.
308. Penman E, Wass JA, Besser GM, et al. Somatostatin secretion by lung and thymic tumours. Clin Endocrinol (Oxf) 1980; 13:613–620.
309. Ghose RR, Gupta SK. Oat cell carcinoma of bronchus presenting with somatostatinoma syndrome. Thorax 1981; 36:550–551.
310. Gleeson MH, Bloom SR, Polak JM, et al. Endocrine tumour in kidney affecting small bowel structure, motility, and absorptive function. Gut 1971; 12:773–782.
311. Hunstein W, Trumper LH, Dummer R, et al. Glucagonoma syndrome and bronchial carcinoma. Ann Intern Med 1988; 109: 920–921.
312. Moody TW, Pert CB, Gazdar AF, et al. High levels of intracellular bombesin characterize human small-cell lung carcinoma. Science 1981; 214:1246–1248.
313. Sorenson GD, Bloom SR, Ghatei MA, et al. Bombesin production by human small cell carcinoma of the lung. Regul Pept 1982; 4:59–66.
314. Pansky A, De Weerth A, Fasler-Kan E, et al. Gastrin releasing peptide-preferring bombesin receptors mediate growth of human renal cell carcinoma. J Am Soc Nephrol 2000; 11:1409–1418.
315. Bartholdi MF, Wu JM, Pu H, et al. In situ hybridization for gastrin-releasing peptide receptor (GRP receptor) expression in prostatic carcinoma. Int J Cancer 1998; 79:82–90.
316. Saurin JC, Nemoz-Gaillard E, Sordat B, et al. Bombesin stimulates adhesion, spreading, lamellipodia formation, and proliferation in the human colon carcinoma Isreco1 cell line. Cancer Res 1999; 59:962–967.
317. Carney DN, Broder L, Edelstein M, et al. Experimental studies of the biology of human small cell lung cancer. Cancer Treat Rep 1983; 67:27–35.
318. Stieber P, Dienemann H, Schalhorn A, et al. Pro–gastrin-releasing peptide (ProGRP)—a useful marker in small cell lung carcinomas. Anticancer Res 1999; 19:2673–2678.
319. Weber S, Zuckerman JE, Bostwick DG, et al. Gastrin releasing peptide is a selective mitogen for small cell lung carcinoma in vitro. J Clin Invest 1985; 75:306–309.
320. Yang HK, Scott FM, Trepel JB, et al. Correlation of expression of bombesin-like peptides and receptors with growth inhibition by an anti-bombesin antibody in small-cell lung cancer cell lines. Lung Cancer 1998; 21:165–175.

321. Aprikian AG, Tremblay L, Han K, et al. Bombesin stimulates the motility of human prostate-carcinoma cells through tyrosine phosphorylation of focal adhesion kinase and of integrin-associated proteins. Int J Cancer 1997; 72:498–504.
322. Fathi Z, Corjay MH, Shipara H, et al. BRS-3: a novel bombesin receptor subtype selectively expressed in testis and lung carcinoma cells. J Biol Chem 1993; 268:5979–5984.
323. Cho T, Chan W, Cutz E. Distribution and frequency of neuroepithelial bodies in post-natal rabbit lung: quantitative study with monoclonal antibody against serotonin. Cell Tissue Res 1989; 255:353–362.
324. King KA, Torday JS, Sunday ME. Bombesin and [Leu^8]-phyllolitorin promote fetal mouse lung branching morphogenesis via a receptor-mediated mechanism. Proc Natl Acad Sci USA 1995; 92:4357–4361.
325. Li K, Nagalla SR, Spindel ER. A rhesus monkey model to characterize the role of gastrin-releasing peptide (GRP) in lung development. J Clin Invest 1994; 94:1605–1615.
326. Oberg K, Grimelius L, Lundqvist G, et al. Update on pancreatic polypeptide as a specific marker for endocrine tumours of the pancreas and gut. Acta Med Scand 1981; 210:145–152.

41 Carcinoid Tumors, Carcinoid Syndrome, and Related Disorders

Kjell Öberg

The first clinical and histopathologic description of carcinoid tumor was made by Otto Lubarsch in 1888.[1] He was impressed by the multicentric origin of carcinoid tumors of the gastrointestinal tract, their lack of gland formation, and their lack of similarity with the usual adenocarcinoma of the alimentary system.

The term *Karzinoide* was introduced in 1907 by the pathologist Oberndorffer[2] as a descriptive name for what he considered to be a "benign" type of neoplasm of the ileum, which could nevertheless behave like a carcinoma. It was subsequently generally accepted that the carcinoid tumor was a very-slow-growing and benign neoplasm with no potential for invasiveness and no tendency to give rise to metastases. This myth of benignity has survived to the present, even though in 1949 Pearson and Fitzgerald[3] described a large series of metastasizing carcinoid tumors.

Carcinoid tumors have subsequently been reported in a wide range of organs, but they most commonly involve the lungs and gastrointestinal tract. Carcinoid tumors of the thymus, ovaries, testes, heart, and middle ear have also been described. The clinically well-known *carcinoid syndrome* was described by Thorson and associates[4] in 1954; 1 year earlier, Lembeck[5] had extracted serotonin from a carcinoid tumor.

PHYLOGENESIS AND EMBRYOLOGY

Carcinoid tumors are derived from neuroendocrine cells, and Gosset and Masson[6] in 1914 were the first to point out the neuroendocrine properties of carcinoid tumors. Masson[7] later described the remarkable affinity for silver salts displayed by intracytoplasmic granules in tumor cells and noted that carcinoid tumors originate from enterochromaffin cells, the so-called Kulchitsky cells in the crypts of Lieberkühn in the intestinal epithelium. Furthermore, he suggested that the tumors were of endocrine origin (Fig. 41–1).

The mammalian gastrointestinal tract and pancreas contain a large number of endocrine cell types, which initially were thought to originate from the neuroectoderm. This observation gave rise to the *APUD concept* (*a*mine *p*recursor *u*ptake and *d*ecarboxylation) because of the ability of these cells to take up and decarboxylate amino acid precursors of biogenic amines such as serotonin and catecholamines.[8] It was later revised by others who postulated that these endocrine cells might also be derived from mesoderm and endoderm.[9] The neuronal phenotype is clearly seen when culturing carcinoid tumor cells in vitro. The enterochromaffin cells, from which many carcinoid tumors derive, have the property of producing and secreting amines (such as serotonin) and polypeptides (such as neurokinin-A and substance P).

Carcinoid tumors may also originate from other neuroendocrine cells, such as the enterochromaffin-like (ECL) cells of the gut and endocrine cells in the bronchi. The tumors derived from these cells are able to produce a wide range of hormones, such as gastrin, gastrin-releasing peptide (GRP), calcitonin, pancreatic polypeptide, adrenocorticotropic hormone (ACTH), corticotropin-releasing hormone (CRH), and growth hormone–releasing hormone (GHRH) as well as somatostatin, glucagon, and calcitonin gene–related peptide (CGRP).[10] A common secretory product from all types of carcinoid tumors is the glycoprotein chromogranin-A (CgA)—the most important general tumor marker in these patients (see later).

MOLECULAR GENETICS

Despite advances in the diagnosis, localization, and treatment of carcinoid tumors, no etiologic factor associated with the development of these tumors has been identified. Little is known about molecular genetic changes underlying tumorigenesis. Sporadic foregut carcinoids as well as the familial-type multiple endocrine neoplasia type 1 (MEN-1) frequently display allelic losses at chromosome 11q13, and somatic *MEN-1* gene mutations has been reported in one third of sporadic

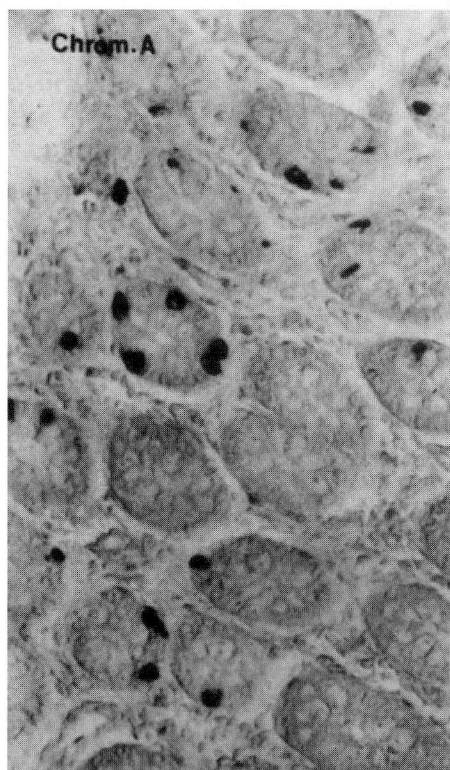

Figure 41-1. Normal human intestine stained with chromogranin A (Chrom. A) to delineate neuroendocrine cells. The cells are scattered in the intestinal mucosa.

foregut tumors.[11] In contrast with foregut carcinoids, molecular and cytogenetic data for midgut carcinoids are quite limited, and these tumors are not included in MEN-1 syndrome. Deletions of chromosomes 18q and 18p have been reported in 38% and 33%, respectively, of gastrointestinal carcinoids.[12]

In one recent publication, deletions on chromosome 18 were found in 88% of midgut carcinoid tumors but Smad 4/DPC4 locus was not deleted.[13] In addition to the consistent finding of deletions on chromosome 18, multiple deletions on other chromosomes (4, 5, 7, 9, 14, 20) were noticed in single tumors. The region telomeric to Smad 4/DPC 4/DCC loci must be further explored for possible losses of a tumor supressor gene in this area.

CLASSIFICATION

In 1963, Williams and Sandler reported a relationship between the embryonic origin of carcinoid tumors and the histologic, biochemical, and, to some extent, clinical features of the tumors.[14] Three distinct groups were formed (Table 41-1):

1. Foregut carcinoids (i.e., intrathoracic, gastric, and duodenal carcinoids).
2. Midgut carcinoids (carcinoids of the small intestine, appendix, and proximal colon).
3. Hindgut carcinoids (carcinoid tumors of the distal colon and rectum).

Although this original classification has been useful in the clinical assessment of patients with carcinoid tumors, it has demonstrated significant shortcomings. As a result, many investigators have adopted a new classification system that takes into account not only the site of origin but also variations in the histopathologic characteristics of carcinoid tumors.[15] In this revised system, typical tumors are classified as *well-differentiated* neuroendocrine tumors with their characteristic growth pattern (Fig. 41-2). These tumors are usually slow-growing, with low proliferation capacity (proliferation index <2%). They are usually confined to the mucosa and submucosa and are less than 1 to 2 cm in diameter. Tumors with increased nuclear atypia and high proliferation index (>10%) have been termed *atypical* or *anaplastic carcinoids* and have been subclassified to well-differentiated and poorly differentiated neuroendocrine carcinomas, depending on the growth pattern (Table 41-2).

The incidence of carcinoid tumors is similar in Western countries and is estimated to be 2.8 to 21 per 1 million people.[16-18] Because many carcinoid tumors are indolent, the true incidence may be higher. In particular, appendiceal carcinoids have not been included in many studies, but the high incidence of 21 per 1 million was found in an autopsy study when appendiceal carcinoids were included.[16] The incidence of patients with a carcinoid syndrome is about 0.5 per 100,000.[19] Data from the United States, based on results from the End Results Group and the Third National Cancer Survey, 1950 to 1969 and 1969 to 1971, respectively, found that the appendix

Table 41-1. Classification of Carcinoid Tumors

	Foregut	Midgut	Hindgut
Histopathology	Argyrophilic CgA-positive NSE-positive Synaptophysin-positive	Argentaffin-positive CgA-positive NSE-positive Synaptophysin-positive	Argyrophilic SVP-2-positive (CgA-positive NSE-positive) (Synaptophysin-positive)
Molecular Genetics	Chromosome 11q13 delection	Chromosome 18q, 18p deletion	Unknown
Secretory Products	CgA, 5-HT, 5-HTP, histamine, ACTH, GHRH, CGRP, somatostatin, AVP, glucagon, gastrin, NKA, substance-P, neurotensin, GRP	CgA, 5-HT, NKA, substance-P, prostaglandins E_1 and F_2, bradykinin	PP, PYY, somatostatin
Carcinoid Syndrome	Present (30%)	Present (70%)	Absent

ACTH, adrenocorticotropic hormone; AVP, arginine vasopressin; CgA, chromogranin-A, CGRP, calcitonin gene–related peptide; GHRH, growth hormone–releasing hormone; GRP, gastrin-releasing peptide; 5-HT, 5-hydroxytryptamine; 5-HTP, 5-hydroxytryptophan; NKA, neurokinin; NSE, neuron-specific enolase; PP, pancreatic peptide; PYY, peptide YY; SVP2, synaptic vesicle protein 2.

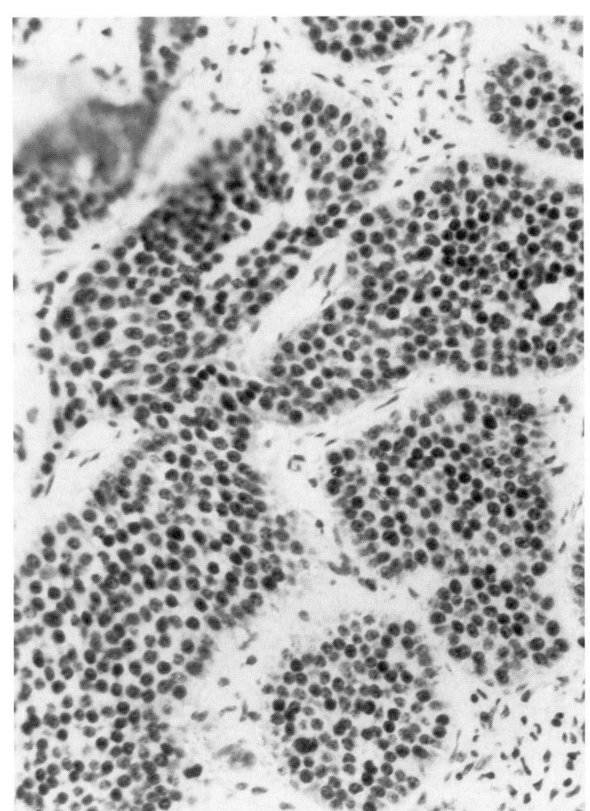

Figure 41–2. Histopathology of classic well-differentiated midgut carcinoid tumor.

was the most common site of carcinoid tumors, followed by the rectum, ileum, lungs, and bronchi.[20]

An analysis done in the Surveillance, Epidemiology, and End Results (SEER) program of the National Cancer Institute between 1973 and 1991 reported an increase in the proportion of pulmonary and gastric carcinoids and a decrease in the proportion of appendiceal carcinoids.[18]

BIOCHEMISTRY

The production of hormones appears to be a highly organized function of carcinoid cells. In 1953, Lembeck isolated serotonin from a carcinoid tumor; since then, the carcinoid syndrome has been related to serotonin overproduction.[5] The biosynthesis of serotonin and its metabolic degradation are outlined in Figure 41–3.

Carcinoid tumors of the midgut and foregut region with metastatic disease secrete serotonin and show elevated urinary excretion of 5-hydroxyindoleacetic acid (5-HIAA) in 76% and 30%, respectively.[21] Carcinoid tumors arising from the foregut, however, frequently have low levels of L-amino-acid decarboxylase, which converts 5-hydroxytryptophan (5-HTP) to serotonin. Thus, these tumors secrete primarily 5-HTP.[22, 23]

For many years, it was believed that the entire carcinoid syndrome could be explained by the secretion of these biologically active amines. However, further studies have indicated that serotonin is mainly involved in the pathogenesis of diarrhea and that other biologically active substances play a more important part in the carcinoid flush and bronchoconstriction.

Oates and associates[23] proposed that *kallikrein*, an enzyme found in carcinoid tumors, is released in association with flush and stimulates plasma kininogen to liberate lysyl-bradykinin and bradykinin. These are biologically active substances that cause vasodilation, hypotension, tachycardia, and edema.[24–26] Furthermore, prostaglandins (E_1, E_2, F_1, F_2) may also play a role in the carcinoid syndrome.[27] Gastric carcinoids as well as lung carcinoids have been found to contain and secrete histamine, which might be responsible for the characteristic bright red flush seen in these patients.[28–30] Metabolites of histamine are frequently present in high concentration in the urine from these patients. Dopamine and norepinephrine have also been found in carcinoid tumors.[31]

The occurrence of *substance-P* in carcinoid tumors was first demonstrated by Håkansson and co-workers in 1977.[32] Substance-P belongs to a family of polypeptides that share the same carboxyl terminus and are called *tachykinins* (Fig. 41–4). A number of tachykinin-related peptides have been isolated from carcinoid tumors, such as neurokinin-A, neuropeptide-K, and eledoisin. During stimulation of flush in patients with midgut carcinoids, multiple forms of tachykinins are released to the circulation (Fig. 41–5).[33–35]

Many different polypeptides (e.g., insulin, gastrin, somatostatin, S-100 protein, polypeptide YY, pancreatic polypeptide, human chorionic gonadotropin alpha subunit [hCG-α], motilin, calcitonin, vasoactive intestinal polypeptide [VIP], and endorphins) have been demonstrated in carcinoid tumors by immunohistochemical staining and sometimes in tumor extracts.[10] Ectopic ACTH or CRH production may be found in foregut carcinoids; in particular, patients with bronchial carcinoids seem susceptible to Cushing's syndrome.[36] Patients with carcinoid tumors of the foregut type might also present with acromegaly due to ectopic secretion of growth hormone–releasing hormone from the tumor.[37] Duodenal carcinoids as part of von Recklinghausen's disease can secrete somatostatin.[38]

The *chromogranin/secretogranin* family consists of CgA, CgB (sometimes called *secretogranin I*), secretogranin II (sometimes called *CgC*), and some other members. CgA was first isolated in 1965 as a water-soluble protein present in chromaffin cells from bovine adrenal medulla.[39] Its immunoreactivity has been found in all parts of the gastrointestinal tract and pancreas and has also been isolated from all endocrine glands.[40]

Table 41–2. Clinicopathologic Classification of Intestinal Endocrine Tumors

Well-differentiated endocrine tumor
Benign behavior: functioning or nonfunctioning, confined to mucosa-submucosa, nonangioinvasive
<1 or 2 cm* in diameter
Serotonin-producing tumor
Enteroglucagon-producing tumor
Uncertain behavior: functioning or nonfunctioning, confined to mucosa-submucosa, or angioinvasive
>1 or 2 cm† in diameter,
Serotonin-producing tumor
Enteroglucagon-producing tumor
Well-differentiated endocrine carcinoma
Low-grade malignant: deeply invasive (muscularis propria or beyond) or with metastases
Serotonin-producing carcinoma with or without carcinoid syndrome
Poorly differentiated endocrine carcinoma
High-grade malignant: small to intermediate cell carcinoma

*<1 cm for tumors of the small intestine; <2 cm for tumors of colon/rectum and appendix.

†>1 cm for tumors of the small intestine; >2 cm for tumors of colon/rectum and appendix.

Adapted from Solcia E, Rindi G, Paolotti D, et al. Clinico-pathological profile as a basis for classification of the endocrine tumors of the gastroentero-pancreatic tract. Ann Oncol 1999; 10(Suppl 2):S1–S7.

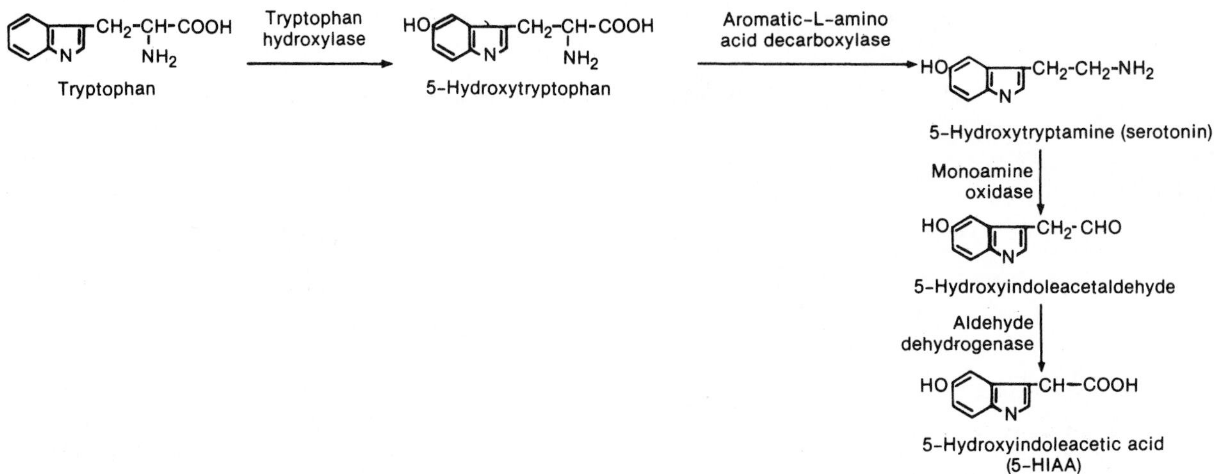

Figure 41–3. Biosynthesis and metabolism of 5-hydroxytryptamine (5-HT) (serotonin).

CgA is an acidic glycoprotein of 439 amino acids with a molecular weight of 48 kD. It can be spliced into smaller fragments at dibasic cleavage sites, generating multiple bioactive fragments such as vasostatins, chromostatin, and pancreastatin[40–44] (Fig. 41–6).

Amines and hormones are stored intracellularly in two types of vesicles: (1) large dense-core vesicles and (2) small synaptic-like vesicles. These vesicles are released on stimulation. Large dense-core vesicles contain the hormones and one or more members of the chromogranin/secretogranin family of proteins.[41, 45] Both amines and peptides are co-released (Fig. 41–7).

The physiologic function of CgA is not fully elucidated. Its ubiquitous presence in neuroendocrine tissues and its co-secretion with peptide hormones and amines indicate a storage role of the peptide within the secretory granule.[40, 41, 45] It also acts as a prohormone that can generate bioactive smaller fragments. CgA is an important tissue and serum marker for different types of carcinoid tumors, including those of the foregut, midgut, and hindgut (see Table 41–1 and later discussion).

CLINICAL PRESENTATION

The clinical presentation of carcinoid tumors depends on localization, hormone production, and extent of the disease. Usually, a lung carcinoid is diagnosed incidentally on routine pulmonary radiography, whereas a midgut carcinoid may be identified as a bowel obstruction or as a cause of abdominal discomfort or pain. Rectal carcinoids may cause bleeding or obstruction. However, lung carcinoids may also present clinically with Cushing's syndrome, due to secretion of CRH or ACTH, or with the carcinoid syndrome, due to production of serotonin, 5-HTP, or histamine.[46] A midgut carcinoid often presents with the carcinoid syndrome, due to production of serotonin and tachykinins.

The clinical manifestations at referral depend on the type of referral center. At our institution, which cares for patients with malignant tumors, 74% of the patients present with the carcinoid syndrome, 13% with abdominal pain, 12% with carcinoid heart disease, and 2% with bronchial constriction.[21] When unbiased material is analyzed, bowel obstruction is the most frequent problem leading to the diagnosis of ileal carcinoid tumor. The second most frequent symptom is abdominal pain. Flushing and diarrhea, which are components of the carcinoid syndrome, make up only the third most frequent presentations.[17, 47–49] Because many patients have vague symptoms, however, diagnosis of the tumor may be delayed by approximately 2 to 3 years.[19]

```
Substance P       Arg-Pro-Lys-Pro-Gln-Gln-Phe-Phe-Gly-Leu-Met-NH2
Neurokinin A              His-Lys-Thr-Asp-Ser-Phe-Val-Gly-Leu-Met-NH2
Neurokinin B                  Asp-Met-His-Asp-Phe-Val-Gly-Leu-Met-NH2
Eledoisin         Pyr-Pro-Ser-Lys-Asp-Ala-Phe-Ile-Gly-Leu-Met-NH2
Kassinin      Asp-Val-Pro-Lys-Ser-Asp-Glu-Phe-Val-Gly-Leu-Met-NH2
Physalemin        Pyr-Ala-Asp-Pro-Asn-Lys-Phe-Tyr-Gly-Leu-Met-NH2
Neuropeptide K    Arg-His-Lys-Thr-Asp-Ser-Phe-Val-Gly-Leu-Met-NH2
                 -Lys-His-Ser-Ile-Gln-Gly-His-Gly-Tyr-Leu-Ala-Lys
               Asp-Ala-Asp-Ser-Ser-Ile-Glu-Lys-Gln-Val-Ala-Leu-Leu
```

Figure 41–4. The tachykinin family of peptides shares the same carboxyl terminus. Neuropeptide-K is a prohormone containing neurokinin-A, which can be spliced off.

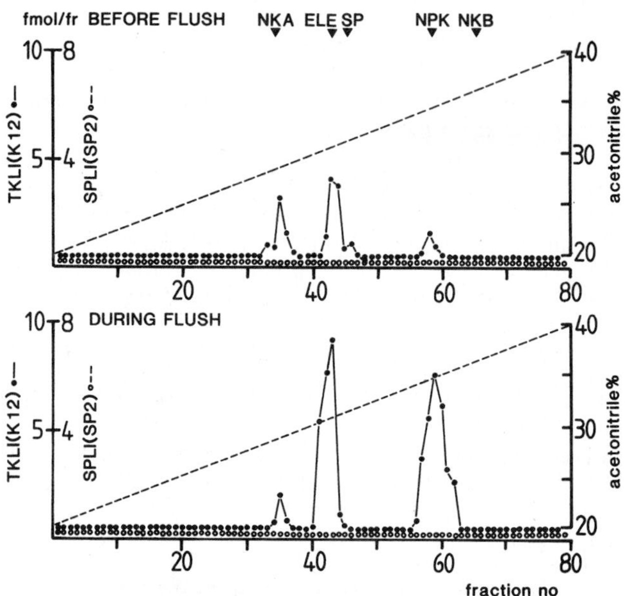

Figure 41–5. Chromatography samples of plasma from a patient with carcinoid before flush *(upper panel)* and during flush *(lower panel)*. Note the significant increase in eledoisin-like peptide as well as in neuropeptide-K.

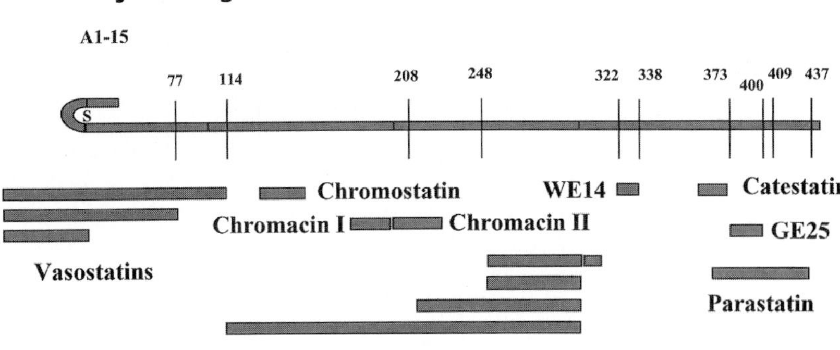

Figure 41–6. The glycoprotein chromogranin-A and related peptides.

The Carcinoid Syndrome

In 1954, Thorson and co-workers for the first time described the carcinoid syndrome as having the following features: malignant carcinoid of the small intestine with metastasis to the liver; valvular disease of the right side of the heart (pulmonary stenosis and tricuspidal insufficiency without septal defect); peripheral vasomotor symptoms; bronchial constriction; and an unusual type of cyanosis.[4] One year later, Dr. William Bean[50] gave this colorful description of the carcinoid syndrome:

> This witch's brew of unlikely signs and symptoms, intriguing to the most fastidious connoisseur of clinical esoterica—the skin underwent rapid and extreme changes—resembling in clinical miniature the fecal phantasmagoria of the aurora borealis.

The syndrome is thus well characterized and includes flushing, diarrhea, right-sided heart failure, and sometimes bronchial constriction and increased urinary levels of 5-HIAA.[51, 52] This is the classic carcinoid syndrome, but some patients may display only one or two of the features. Other symptoms related to the syndrome are weight loss, sweating, and pellagra-like skin lesions.

Development of the carcinoid syndrome is a function of tumor mass, extent and localization of metastases, and localization of the primary tumor. The syndrome is most common in tumors originating in the small intestine and proximal colon; 40% to 60% of patients with these tumors experience the syndrome.[21, 48, 51, 52] The disorders are less frequent in patients with bronchial carcinoids and do not occur in patients with rectal carcinoids.[46, 53, 54] The syndrome rarely occurs in patients with midgut carcinoids and a small tumor burden, such as only regional lymph node metastases.[49] Patients with the full syndrome usually have multiple liver metastases. The association with hepatic metastases is due to efficient inactivation by the liver of amines and peptides released into the portal circulation. The venous drainage of liver metastases is directly into the systemic circulation and bypasses hepatic inactivation.[55]

Other carcinoid tumors likely to be associated with the carcinoid syndrome in the absence of liver metastases are ovarian carcinoids and bronchial carcinoids, which release mediators directly into the systemic rather than the portal circulation. Retroperitoneal metastases from classic midgut carcinoid also release mediators directly into the circulation and might cause the carcinoid syndrome without any liver metastases.[51, 52]

Flushing

Four types of flushing have been described in the literature.[51, 52]

The first and most well-known type is the sudden, diffuse, erythematous flush, usually affecting the face, neck, and upper chest (i.e., the normal flushing area) (Fig. 41–8*A* and *B*) (see also Color Plate). This type of flush is commonly of short duration, lasting from 1 to 5 minutes, and is related to early-stage midgut carcinoids. Patients usually experience a sensation of warmth during flushing and sometimes heart palpitations. This type of flushing is reported in 20% to 70% of patients with midgut carcinoid at presentation of the disease.[19, 51, 52, 55]

The second type is the violaceous flush, which affects the same area of the body. It has roughly the same time course or sometimes lasts a little longer. Patients may also have facial telangiectasia. This flush is related to the later stages of midgut carcinoid (Fig. 41–9) (see also Color Plate) and is normally not felt by patients because they have become accustomed to the flushing reaction.

The third type is prolonged flushing that usually lasts a couple of hours but may last up to several days. This flush sometimes involves the whole body and is associated with profuse lacrimation, swelling of the salivary gland, hypotension, and facial edema (Fig. 41–10) (see also Color Plate). These symptoms are usually associated with malignant bronchial carcinoids.

The fourth type of flushing is a bright red, patchy flush, seen in patients with chronic atrophic gastritis and ECL-cell hyperplasia, or so-called ECL-oma (derived from ECL cells). This type of flushing is related to an increased release of histamine and histamine metabolites.

Flushes may be spontaneous or may be precipitated by (1) stress (physical and mental); (2) infection; (3) alcohol; (4) certain foods (spicy); or (5) drugs, such as by injections of catecholamines, calcium, or pentagastrin (see later). The pathophysiology of flushing in the carcinoid syndrome is not yet elucidated.[56–58] It was previously thought to be totally related to excess production of serotonin or serotonin metabolites.[57] However, several patients with high levels of plasma serotonin did not have any flushing, nor did a serotonin antagonist (e.g., methysergide, cyproheptadine, or ketanserin) have any effect on the flushing.[56, 59]

In a study from our own group in which we measured the release of tachykinins, neuropeptide-K, and substance-P during flushing provoked by pentagastrin or alcohol, a clear correlation was found between the onset and intensity of the flushing reaction and the release of tachykinins (see Fig. 41–5). Furthermore, when the release of tachykinins was blocked by prestimulatory administration of octreotide, little or no flushing was observed in the same patient (Fig. 41–11).[33–35] Other mediators of the flushing reaction may be kallikrein and bradykinins, which are released during provoked flushing.[24–26]

Histamine may be a mediator of the flushes seen both in lung carcinoids and in gastric carcinoids (ECL-omas).[28–30] Tachykinins, bradykinins, and histamines are well-known vasodilators, and somatostatin analogues may alleviate flushing by reducing circulating levels of these agents (see later).[33–35, 58–63] Furschgott and Zawadski have suggested that flushing is caused

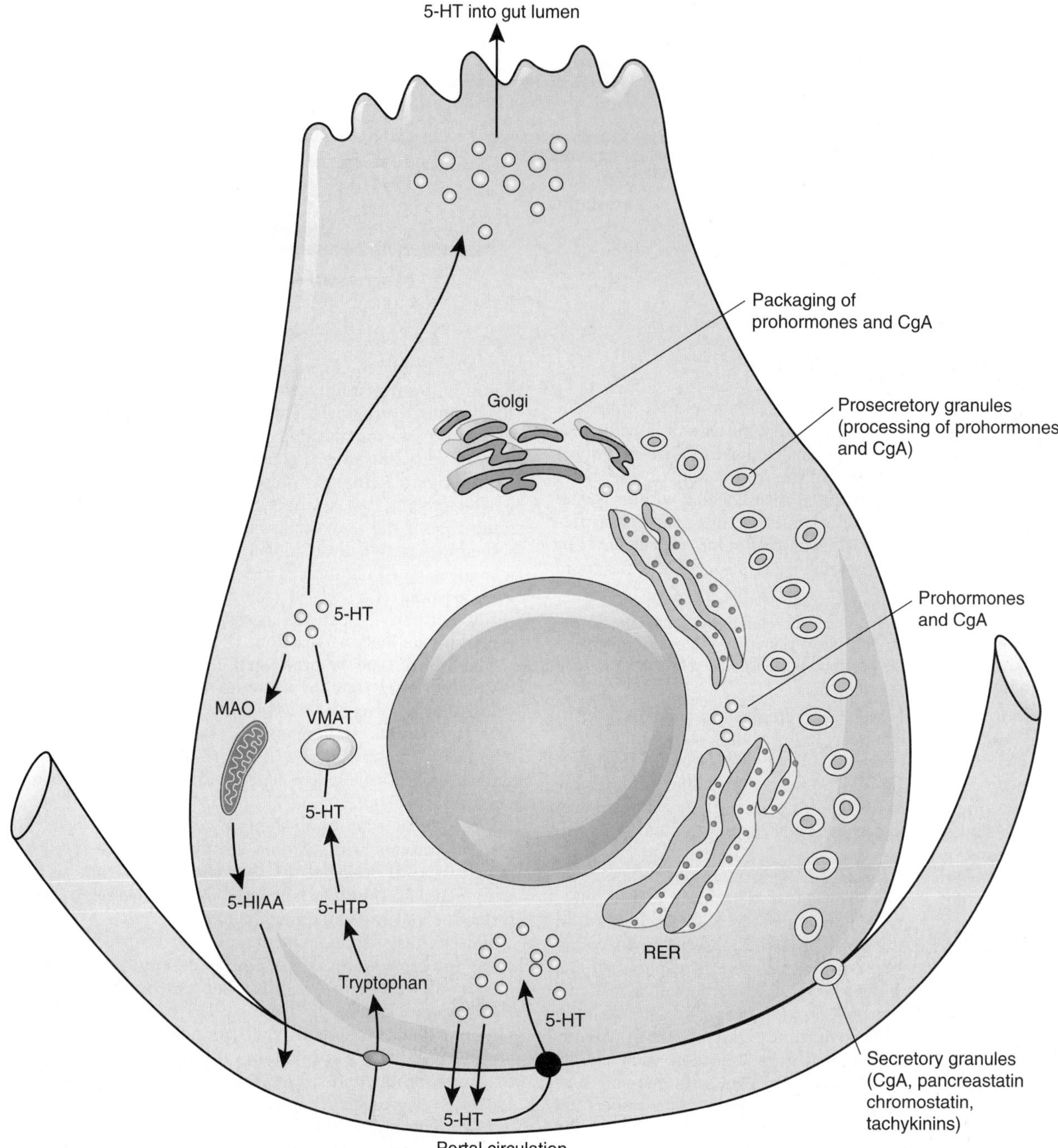

Figure 41–7. Schematic drawing of an enterochromaffin cell. The initial step in 5-hydroxytryptamine (5-HT) synthesis is carrier transport of the amino acid tryptophan from blood into the cell across the cell membrane. Intracellular tryptophan is first converted to 5-hydroxytryptophan (5-HTP), in turn converted to 5-HT and stored in secretory granules. The transport of 5-HT into granules requires vesicular membrane transporters (VMATs). Via the basal lateral membrane, 5-HT can be released into the circulation. There is also a membrane pump mechanism in the cell membrane responsible for amine reuptake. A minor part of 5-HT can also be released into the gut lumen. Monoamine oxidase (MAO) degrades 5-HT to 5-hydroxyindoleacetic acid (5-HIAA). Peptide prohormones are synthesized in the rough endoplasmic reticulum (RER) together with chromogranin-A (CgA) and other granula proteins. The products are transported to the Golgi apparatus (GA) for packaging into prosecretory granules. On stimulation, the secretory products are released from the granules by exocytosis.

by an indirect vasodilatation mediated by endothelium-derived relaxing factor (EDRF) or by nitric oxide released by 5-HTP during platelet activation.[64]

The facial flushing associated with carcinoid tumors should be distinguished from idiopathic flushing and menopausal "hot flashes." Patients with idiopathic flushes usually have a long history of flushing starting rather early in life and sometimes with a family history without occurrence of a tumor. Menopausal hot flashes usually involve the whole body and are accompanied by intense sweating. Postmenopausal women in whom a true carcinoid syndrome is developing can tell the difference between the two types of flushes.

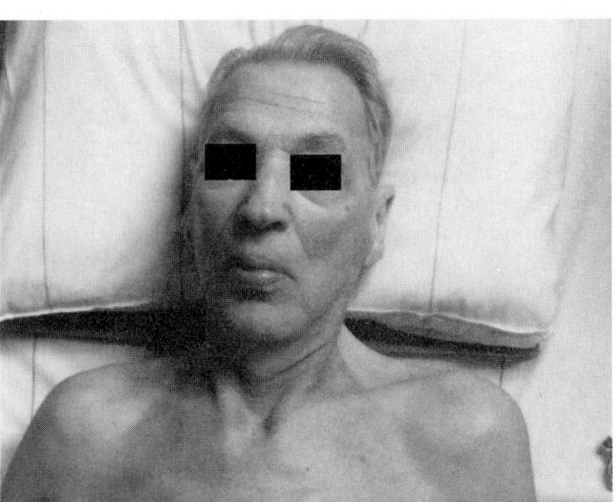

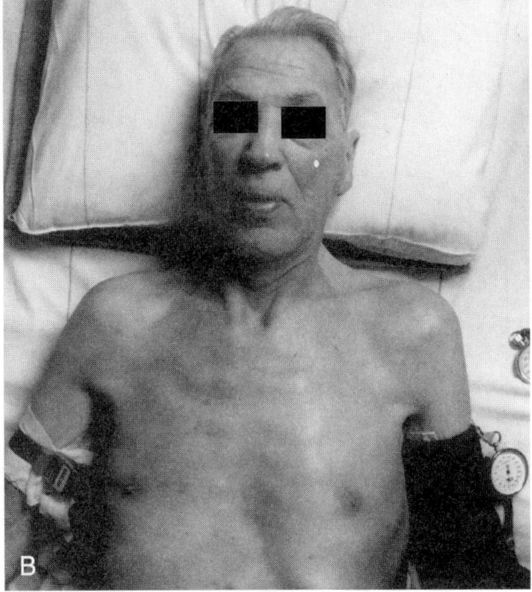

Figure 41–8. Carcinoid syndrome before and after provocation. *A*, Before flush provocation. *B*, Same patient after pentagastrin-stimulated flush. (See also Color Plate.)

Diarrhea

Diarrhea occurs in 30% to 80% of patients with the carcinoid syndrome.[19, 21, 51, 52] Its pathophysiology is poorly understood but is probably multifactorial. The diarrhea is frequently accompanied by abdominal cramping, and endocrine, paracrine, and mechanical factors contribute to this condition. A variety of tumor products, including serotonin, tachykinins, histamines, kallikrein, and prostaglandins, can stimulate peristalsis, electromechanical activity, and tone in the intestine.[58, 65–67] Secretory diarrhea may occur with fluid and electrolyte imbalance. Malabsorption may result from intestinal resections, lymph angiectasia, secondary to mesenteric fibrosis, bacterial overgrowth, and secondary to a tumor partially obstructing the small bowel or rapid intestinal transit. Increased secretion by the small bowel, malabsorption, or accelerated transit may overwhelm the normal storage and absorptive capacity of proximal colon and result in diarrhea, which may be aggravated if the reabsorbed function of the colon is impaired.

In a study of patients with elevated serotonin levels and the carcinoid syndrome, transit time in the small bowel and colon was significantly decreased in comparison with that of normal subjects.[68] The volume of the ascending colon was significantly

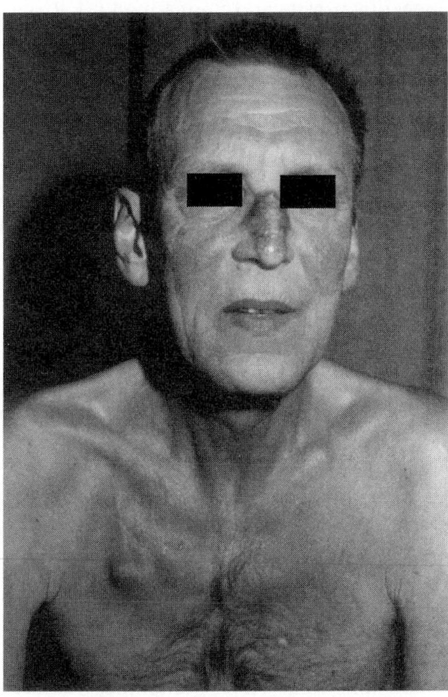

Figure 41–9. Long-lasting chronic flushing in a patient with long-standing carcinoid disease. Note the telangiectases. (See also Color Plate.)

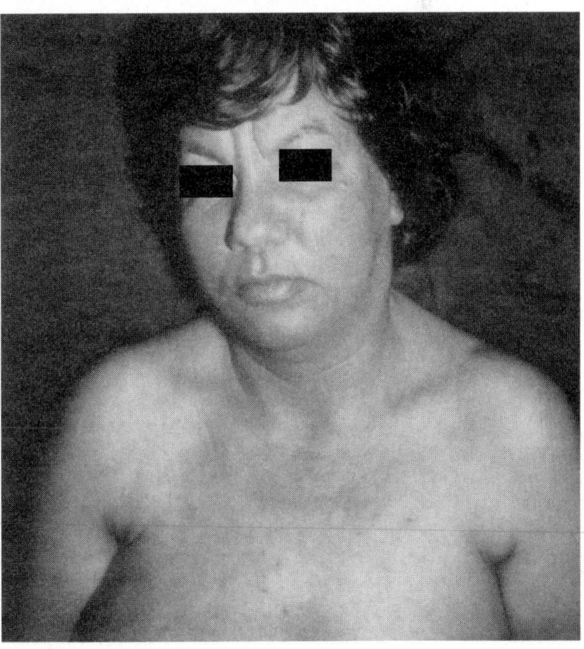

Figure 41–10. The patient has lung carcinoid and carcinoid syndrome with severe, long-standing flushing, lacrimation, and a swollen face. (See also Color Plate.)

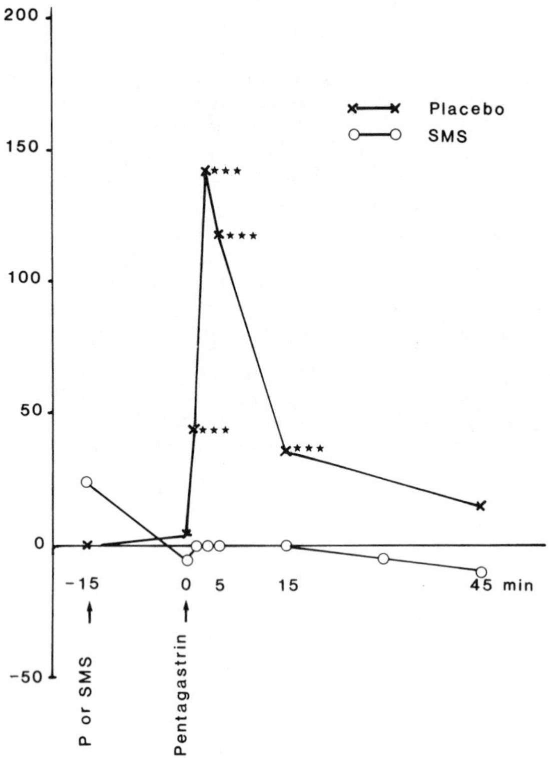

Figure 41–11. Tachykinin levels (TKLI) after stimulation with pentagastrin in patients with classic midgut carcinoids. Pretreatment for 15 minutes with somatostatin causes inhibition of tachykinin release and inhibition of the flush reaction (0–0). P, placebo.

smaller than in normal subjects, and the postprandial colonic tone was markedly increased. This indicates that in patients in whom the carcinoid syndrome is associated with diarrhea, major alterations in gut motor function occur that affect both the small intestine and the colon. Many patients with carcinoid tumors have undergone wide resection of the small intestine, and they may be affected by the symptoms of short-bowel syndrome.

Serotonin is thought to be responsible for the diarrhea in the carcinoid syndrome by its effects on gut motility and intestinal electrolyte and fluid secretion.[52, 65–67] Serotonin receptor antagonists, such as ondansetron and ketanserin, relieve the diarrhea to a certain degree.[65, 69–71]

Carcinoid Heart Disease

A unique endocrine effect of carcinoid tumors is the development of plaque-like thickenings of the endocardium of the heart, valve leaflets, atria, and ventricles in 10% to 20% of the patients.[72, 73] This fibrotic involvement causes stenosis and regurgitation of the blood flow. Findings of new collagen beneath the endothelium of the endocardium is almost pathognomonic for carcinoid heart disease.[72–74] The incidence of these lesions depends on the diagnostic methodology. Echocardiography can demonstrate early lesions in about 70% of patients with the carcinoid syndrome, whereas routine clinical examinations detect them in only 30% to 40%.[72, 73, 75] These figures have significantly dropped to 10% to 15%, probably because of earlier diagnosis and the use of biologic antitumor treatments such as somatostatin analogues and α-interferons. Both of these agents control the hormonal release and excess that might be involved in the fibrotic process.

In a study performed 15 years ago,[19] 40% of patients with carcinoid tumors died of cardiac complications related to the carcinoid disease. More recent data reveal that this complication is a rare event, and patients usually die of the effects of a progressive tumor.[21]

The precise mechanism behind the fibrosis in the right side of the heart has not been solved at the moment, but it occurs mainly in patients with liver metastases who usually also have the carcinoid syndrome.[72, 73] Substances inducing fibrosis are thought to be released directly into the right side of the heart and are then neutralized or degraded through the lung circulation because few patients present with similar lesions on the left side.[72, 73] However, patients with lung carcinoids occasionally display the same fibrotic changes on the left side. Histologically, the plaque-like thickenings in the endocardium consist of myofibroblasts and fibroblasts embedded in a stroma that is rich in mucopolysaccharides and collagen.[72]

We have previously shown that the transforming growth factor β (TGF-β) family of growth factors is up-regulated in carcinoid fibrous plaques on the right side of the heart.[76] The TGF-β family of growth factors is known to stimulate matrix formation and collagen deposition. The substances that induce TGF-β locally in the heart are not known, but serotonin, tachykinins, and insulin-like growth factor I (IGF-I) may be mediators.[72, 77]

A correlation has been found between circulating levels of serotonin and tachykinins and the degree and frequency of carcinoid heart lesion. The weight-reducing drugs fenfluramine and dexfenfluramine appear to interfere with normal serotonin metabolism and have been associated with valvular lesions identical to those seen in carcinoid heart disease.[78, 79] However, treatment resulting in decreased urinary 5-HIAA excretion does not result in regression of cardiac lesions.[80]

Another possible mediator might be IGF-I, which is released from carcinoid tumor cells. Treatment with somatostatin analogues, which down-regulate circulating IGF-I, has been able to prevent further development of carcinoid heart disease in two patients (data to be published).

Bronchial Constriction

A true asthma episode is a rare event in patients with the carcinoid syndrome.[19, 51, 52] The causative agents of bronchial constriction are not known, but both tachykinins and bradykinins have been suggested as mediators.[81, 82] These agents can constrict smooth muscles in the respiratory tract and may also cause local edema in the airways.

Other Manifestations of the Carcinoid Syndrome

Fibrotic complications other than heart lesions may be found in patients with carcinoid tumors. These include (1) intra-abdominal and retroperitoneal fibrosis, (2) occlusion of the mesenteric arteries and veins, (3) Peyronie's disease of the penis, and (4) carcinoid arthropathy.[51, 52]

Intra-abdominal fibrosis can lead to intestinal adhesions and bowel obstruction and is a more common cause of bowel obstruction than is the primary carcinoid tumor itself.[49, 83, 84] Retroperitoneal fibrosis can result in urethral obstruction that impairs kidney function, which sometimes requires treatment with urethral stents.

Narrowing and occlusion of arteries and veins by fibrosis are potentially life-threatening. Ischemic loops of the bowel may have to be removed, and this procedure ultimately causes short-bowel syndrome.[49, 84]

Other rare features of the syndrome are pellagra-like skin lesions with hyperkeratosis and pigmentation, myopathy, and sexual dysfunction.[52]

Carcinoid Crisis

Carcinoid crisis has become a rare event since the introduction of treatment with somatostatin analogues.[85] It might occur spontaneously or during induction of anesthesia, embolization procedures, chemotherapy, or infection. Carcinoid crisis is a clinical condition characterized by severe flushing, diarrhea, hypotension, hyperthermia, and tachycardia. Without treatment, patients might die during the crisis.[85–87]

Intravenous (IV) and/or subcutaneous somatostatin analogues are given before, during, and after surgery to prevent the development of carcinoid crisis.[85, 87–89] Patients with metastatic lung carcinoids are particularly difficult to treat during crisis. IV infusions of octreotide at doses of 50 to 100 μg/hour, supplemented with histamine H_1-receptor and H_2-receptor blockers and IV sodium chloride, are recommended.[90]

Other Clinical Manifestations of Carcinoid Tumors

Ectopic secretion of CRH and ACTH from pulmonary carcinoid tumors and thymic carcinoids accounts for 1% of all cases of Cushing's syndrome.[36, 91] Acromegaly due to ectopic secretion of GHRH has also been reported in foregut carcinoids.[37, 92] Gastric carcinoid tumors make up less than 1% of gastric neoplasms.[18] They can be separated into three distinct groups on the basis of both clinical and histologic characteristics and originate from gastric ECL cells[93]:

1. Those associated with chronic atrophic gastritis type A (80%) (type I).
2. Those associated with Zollinger-Ellison syndrome as part of MEN-1 syndrome (6%) (type II).
3. Sporadic gastric carcinoids (type III), which occur without hypergastrinemia and pursue a more malignant behavior, with 50% to 60% developing metastases.[93, 94]

About 80% of gastric carcinoids are associated with chronic atrophic gastritis type A, and more than 50% of patients with these carcinoids also have pernicious anemia. These tumors are more common in women than in men and are usually identified endoscopically during diagnostic evaluation for anemia or abdominal pain.[93, 95] They are often multifocal and localized in the gastric fundus area, and they are derived from ECL cells. Patients have hypochlorhydria and hypergastrinemia. Gastrin hypersecretion has been postulated to result in hyperplasia of the ECL cells, which might later develop into carcinoid tumors.[96, 97] Hyperplasia of ECL cells has been noticed in patients with long-standing proton-pump inhibitor therapy.[98, 99]

DIAGNOSIS

The diagnosis of a suspected carcinoid tumor must take into consideration tumor biology, histopathology, biochemistry, and localization. The diagnosis of a carcinoid may be suspected from clinical symptoms suggestive of the carcinoid syndrome or from the presence of other clinical symptoms, or it can be made in relatively asymptomatic patients from the histopathology at surgery or after liver biopsy for unknown hepatic lesions.

In one study involving 154 consecutive patients with gastrointestinal carcinoids found at surgery, 60% were asymptomatic.[100] In patients with symptomatic tumors, the time from onset of symptoms until diagnosis is frequently delayed, varying from 1 to 2 years.[17, 19] The current tumor biology program includes growth factors (platelet-derived growth factor, epidermal growth factor, IGF-I, TGF-β)[101, 103] and proliferation factors (measurements of the nuclear antigen Ki-67) as a proliferation index. Such index correlates with tumor aggressiveness and survival.[101, 102] Adhesion molecules such as CD-44, particularly exon-V6 and exon-V9, have been related to improved survival.[104] Determination of the expression of angiogenic factors basic fibroblast growth factor (b-FGF) and vascular endothelial growth factor (VEGF) should also be included in a tumor biology program. Somatostatin analogues are cornerstones in the treatment of the carcinoid syndrome; therefore, determination of the different subtypes of somatostatin receptors (sst-1 to sst-5) with specific antibodies is warranted.[105, 106]

The histopathologic diagnosis of carcinoids is based on immunohistochemistry using antibodies against CgA, synaptophysin, and neuron-specific enolase. These immunohistochemical stainings have replaced the old silver stainings, the so-called argyrophil stainings by Grimelius and Sevier-Munger. The argentaffin staining by Masson to demonstrate content of serotonin has also been replaced by immunocytochemistry with serotonin antibodies.[10] These neuroendocrine markers can be supplemented by specific immunocytochemistry to different hormones such as substance-P, gastrin, and ACTH.

Biochemical Diagnosis

In patients with flushing and other manifestations of the carcinoid syndrome, the diagnosis can be established by measuring the urinary excretion of 5-HIAA because levels are invariably elevated under these circumstances.[107] Patients with carcinoid tumors usually have urinary 5-HIAA levels of 100 to 3000 μmol/24 hours (15 to 60 mg/24 hours) (reference range <50 μmol/24 hours [10 mg/24 hours]). Assays for urinary 5-HIAA include high-pressure liquid chromatography (HPLC) with electrochemical detection and colorimetric and fluorescence methods.[108] Various foods and drugs can interfere with the measurement of urinary 5-HIAA, and patients should avoid these agents during the 24-hour sampling (Table 41–3).[109] Normally, two 24-hour urine collections are recommended. In a study of patients with malignant midgut carcinoid tumors, 60% to 73% presented with increased urinary 5-HIAA levels,[21, 51, 52] with a specificity of almost 100%.

Today measurement of urinary 5-HIAA for diagnosis of carcinoid tumor is the predominant biochemical analytic procedure. However, urinary and platelet measurement of serotonin itself may give additional information. In some studies, platelet serotonin levels were more sensitive than urinary 5-HIAA and urinary serotonin levels and were not affected by the patient's diet, as are 5-HIAA levels.

In a comparative study of 44 consecutive patients with carcinoid, the platelet serotonin, urinary 5-HIAA, and urinary serotonin levels were measured. In foregut carcinoids the sensitivities were 50%, 29%, and 55%, respectively. For midgut carcinoids, the sensitivities were 100%, 92%, and 82%, respectively, and for hindgut carcinoids, 20%, 0%, and 60%, respectively.[110]

Elevations of 5-HIAA can occur in malabsorption states and a number of other conditions. Foregut carcinoids tend to produce an atypical carcinoid syndrome with increased plasma 5-HTP, but not serotonin, because they lack the appropriate decarboxylase.[22, 31] That results in normal urinary 5-HIAA.

Table 41–3. Factors That Interfere with Determination of Urinary 5-HIAA

Factors That Produce False-Positive Results
Foods
Avocado
Banana
Chocolate
Coffee
Eggplant
Pecan
Pineapple
Plum
Tea
Walnuts
Drugs
Acetaminophen
Acetanilid
Caffeine
Fluorouracil
Guaifenesin
L-Dopa
Melphalan
Mephenesin
Methamphetamine
Methocarbamol
Methysergide maleate
Phenmetrazine
Reserpine
Salicylates
Factors That Cause False-Negative Results
Drugs
Corticotropin
p-Chlorophenylalanine
Chlorpromazine
Heparin
Imipramine
Isoniazid
Methenamine mandelate
Methyldopa
Monoamine oxidase inhibitors
Phenothiazine
Promethazine

However, some of the 5-HTP is decarboxylated in the intestine and other tissues, and many of these patients have slightly elevated U-5-HT or 5-HIAA levels.

Attempts have been made to identify more specific and sensitive serum markers for carcinoid that may allow earlier diagnosis. One such marker is CgA. It has been shown previously that CgA and CgB are more abundant than CgC in human neuroendocrine tissues.[40, 41, 111] In 44 patients with carcinoid tumors, CgA was increased in 99%, CgB in 88%, and CgC in only 6%[111] (Fig. 41–12). It has been proposed that CgA levels in plasma may reflect tumor size. In a study of 75 patients with midgut carcinoids and the carcinoid syndrome, CgA was elevated in 87% of carcinoid patients. Furthermore, a correlation between levels of plasma chromogranin and extent of disease was found ($P < .0001$).[21] In the same study, urinary 5-HIAA was elevated in 76% of midgut carcinoids, and there were no correlations with tumor size or extent of disease.

CgA is a more sensitive marker than urinary 5-HIAA in detection of carcinoid tumors, but because CgA is released and secreted from various types of neuroendocrine tumors, the specificity is lower.[111–114] Therefore, in a work-up of patients with the carcinoid syndrome, one should combine the determination of plasma CgA with urinary 5-HIAA or serotonin. Plasma neuron-specific enolase shows a lower sensitivity and specificity than does plasma CgA.[113] Serum hCG-α has been reported to be increased in 60% of patients with foregut carcinoid tumors and 50% of hindgut carcinoids but in only 11% of those patients with midgut carcinoids and the carcinoid syndrome. Plasma neuropeptide-K levels have been reported to be elevated in 46% of patients with midgut carcinoids, whereas only 9% of patients with foregut carcinoids displayed elevated levels.[112, 115] Plasma substance-P has a sensitivity of 32% and a specificity of 85%.[21, 33–35] Pancreatic polypeptide levels are also elevated in about one third of patients with midgut carcinoids and in as many with foregut carcinoids.[116, 117]

During therapy with somatostatin analogues, neither plasma CgA nor urinary 5-HIAA is a reliable marker of tumor size because somatostatin inhibits the synthesis and release of the hormones without changes in tumor size.

Localization Procedures

Numerous imaging techniques, including endoscopy, barium enema, chest radiography, ultrasonography, computed tomog-

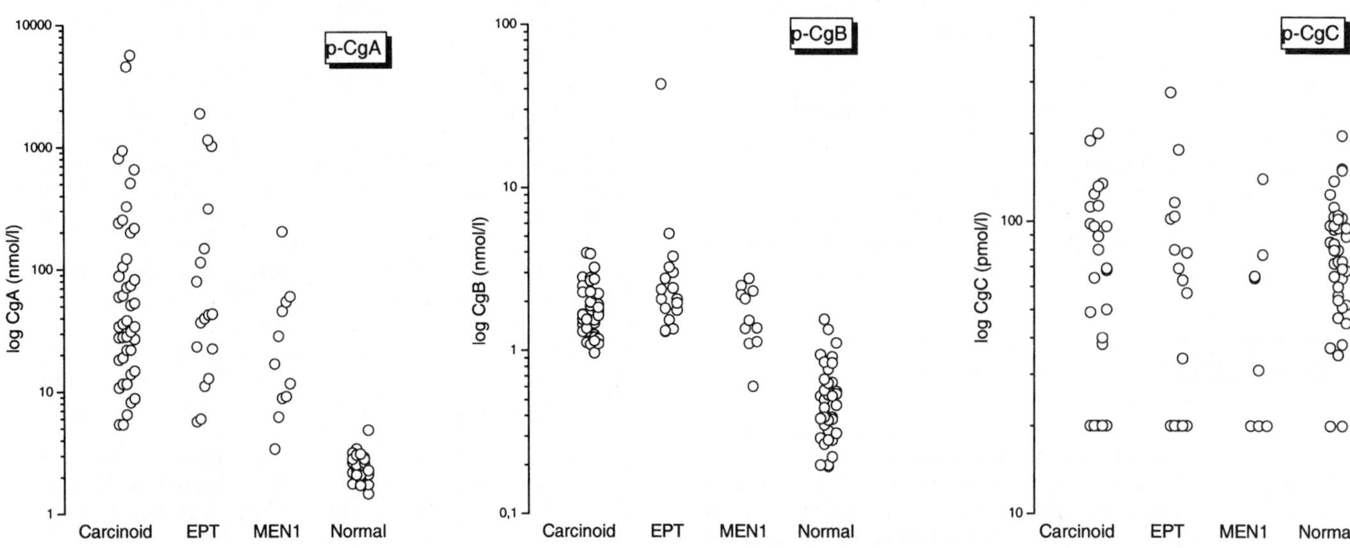

Figure 41–12. Plasma levels of chromogranin-A (CgA), CgB, and CgC in patients with various neuroendocrine tumors. EPTs, endocrine pancreatic tumors; MEN-1, multiple endocrine neoplasia type 1.

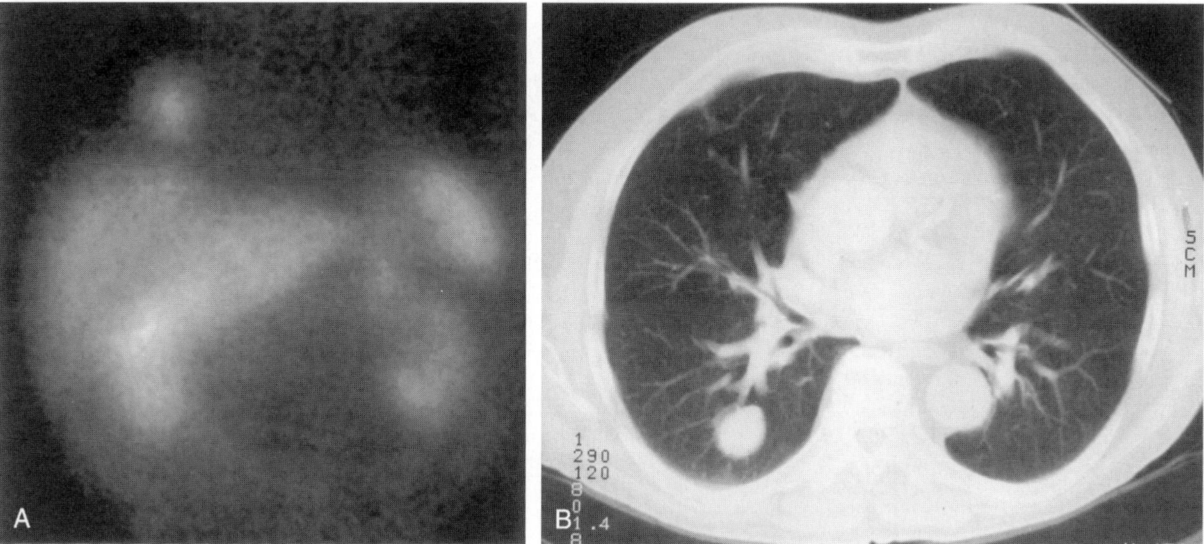

Figure 41–13. Bronchial carcinoid. *A*, Somatostatin-receptor scintigraphy in a patient with a bronchial carcinoid. (See also Color Plate.) *B*, CT scan in the same patient.

raphy (CT), magnetic resonance imaging (MRI), and angiography, have been used to determine the location of the primary tumor as well as the metastases in patients with carcinoid tumors. In more recent years, somatostatin-receptor scintigraphy (SRS) and iodinated meta-iodobenzylguanidine (^{131}I-MIBG) scanning have been used to localize and stage the disease.[118–121] Bronchial carcinoids are usually detected by chest radiography, CT, or, occasionally, by bronchoscopy.[122] The primary midgut tumor is usually small and difficult to localize with traditional diagnostic methods such as barium enema, CT scan, or MRI. Some of these tumors can be localized by angiography or SRS. Liver metastases are usually detected by CT or MRI. At present, CT or MRI and SRS are the primary diagnostic modalities for tumor staging (Fig. 41–13*A* and *B*) (see also Color Plate).

A more sensitive method is positron emission tomography (PET) using ^{11}C-5-HTP, the precursor of serotonin synthesis (Fig. 41–14) (see also Color Plate).[123, 124] This isotope is accumulated in carcinoid tumors, and with the recent development of PET cameras, tumors as small as 0.3 cm in diameter can be detected.[124] During treatment a close relationship has been found among changes in the PET scan, transport rate constant, and urinary 5-HIAA, suggesting that PET scanning may be useful in monitoring the results of therapy. PET scanning using fluorodeoxyglucose 18 (^{18}FDG) is not useful in detecting low-proliferating neuroendocrine tumors but can be beneficial in identifying poorly differentiated anaplastic tumors.

Carcinoid tumors contain high-affinity receptors for somatostatin in 80% to 100% of cases.[105, 106, 125] The receptors are present in both the primary tumor and metastases. Five subtypes of somatostatin receptors have been cloned (sst-1 to sst-5), and somatostatin receptor type 2 is the predominant subtype expressed in carcinoid tumors.

The most commonly available somatostatin analogue, *octreotide*, binds with high affinity to sst-2 and with lower affinity to sst-3 and sst-5.[126–128] SRS with ^{111}In-DTPA-Phe-octreotide has been reported with a sensitivity of 80% to 90% in patients with carcinoids.[128, 129] Many studies have demonstrated that SRS has greater sensitivity for localizing carcinoids compared with conventional imaging studies.[129, 131–134] False-positive scans can be encountered in patients with granulomas (e.g., sarcoidosis, tuberculosis), activated lymphocytes (lymphomas, chronic infection), thyroid diseases (goiter, thyroiditis), endocrine pancreatic tumors, and other endocrine tumors. Because of its high sensitivity and ability to image, whole-body SRS should be the initial imaging procedure to localize and establish the stage of the disease. Bone metastases, which are common in carcinoid tumors, are efficiently picked up by SRS, which is as sensitive as traditional bone scanning with technetium.[130, 132]

A diagnostic algorithm is outlined in Figure 41–15.

TREATMENT

Treatment of carcinoid tumors with the carcinoid syndrome requires a multimodal approach, including symptomatic control as well as tumor reduction. Most patients with the carcinoid

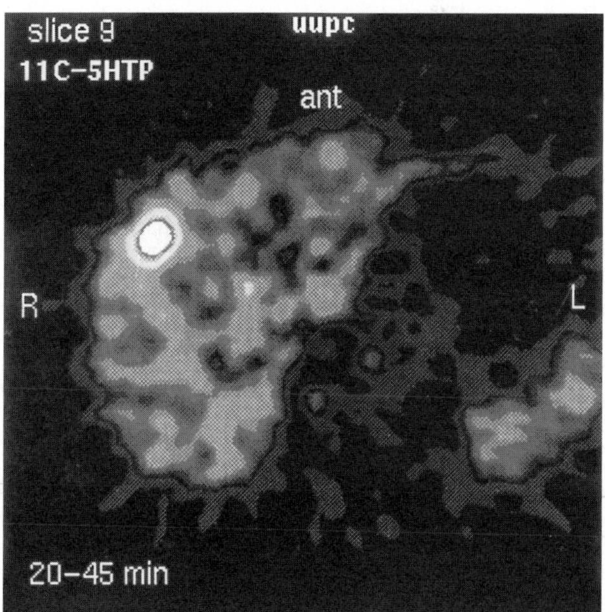

Figure 41–14. Positron emission tomography (PET) with ^{11}C-5-hydroxytryptophan. Note the metastasis in the liver. (See also Color Plate.)

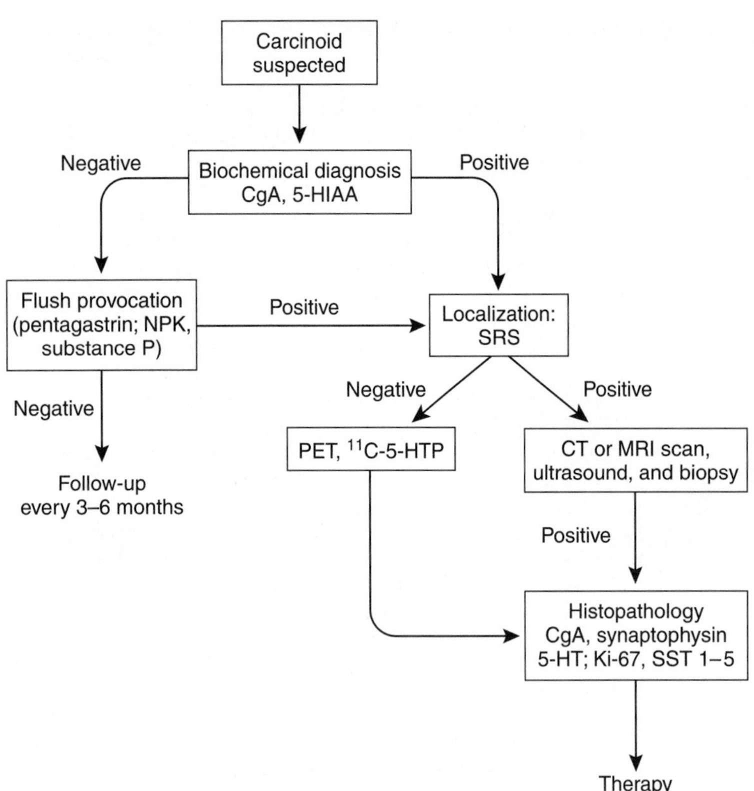

Figure 41–15. Diagnostic algorithm for patients with carcinoid tumor. CgA, chromogranin-A; ^{11}C-5-HTP, ^{11}C-5-hydroxytryptophan; 5-HIAA, 5-hydroxyindoleacetic acid; 5-HT, 5-hydroxytryptamine; NPK, neuropeptide-K; PET, positron emission tomography; SRS, somatostatin-receptor scintigraphy; sst 1–5, somatostatin-receptor subtypes 1–5.

syndrome have metastatic disease. The therapeutic goals are to ameliorate and improve clinical symptoms, abrogate the tumor growth, improve quality of life, and if possible, prolong overall survival.

Symptomatic control of the carcinoid syndrome includes lifestyle changes, dietary supplementation, and specific medical treatment that reduces the clinical symptoms related to the different components of the carcinoid syndrome. Avoiding stress, both psychological and physical, as well as substances such as alcohol, spicy food, and medication that precipitate a flushing reaction might be sufficient in early cases.[52]

Production of serotonin by the tumor consumes tryptophan. Normally, about 1% of the tryptophan is used for production of serotonin; in carcinoid tumors, however, as much as 60% of the available tryptophan may be consumed for the synthesis of serotonin, which can result in tryptophan and niacin deficiency. Therefore, supplemental niacin to prevent the development of pellagra has been recommended over the years. Because many patients have undergone resection of the terminal ileum, which may result in vitamin B_{12} and folic acid deficiency, vitamin B_{12} supplementation is needed in those patients.

Heart failure due to carcinoid heart disease may require diuretics or angiotensin-converting enzyme (ACE) inhibitors. A small number of patients need bronchodilators such as salbutamol, which interacts with β-adrenergic receptors and does not induce flushing. The diarrhea seen in the carcinoid syndrome might be controlled by loperamide or diphenoxylate.[135] If patients still have the carcinoid syndrome, they receive somatostatin analogue treatment, which has replaced most of the earlier types of serotonin and serotonin receptor inhibitors. Serotonin inhibitors (e.g., parachlorophenylalanine and α-methyldopa), which inhibit serotonin synthesis, and serotonin receptor antagonists (e.g., cyproheptadine, methysergide, and ketanserin) are not used routinely clinically.

These earlier treatments had limited efficacy in terms of inhibiting flushing and diarrhea and were accompanied by significant side effects. A combination of histamine H_1 and H_2-receptor antagonists is effective in the carcinoid syndrome that is caused by foregut carcinoids due to concomitant secretion of histamine and serotonin. Prednisolone in doses of 15 to 30 mg/day gives occasional relief in some cases with severe flushing and diarrhea.[135]

Somatostatin Analogues

Although natural somatostatin-14 reduces symptoms in patients with the carcinoid syndrome,[136] its use is limited by its short half-life (~2.5 minutes). During the last two decades, synthetic somatostatin analogues *(octapeptides)* have been developed for clinical use. Octreotide is the most commonly available drug; other analogues are lanreotide and vapreotide.[137–139]

The somatostatin analogues used in clinical practice (octreotide, lanreotide) (Fig. 41–16) both bind to receptors sst-1 and sst-5 and, with lower affinity, to sst-3. They exert their cellular action through interaction with specific cell and transmembrane receptors belonging to the superfamily of G protein–coupled membrane receptors. They inhibit adenylate cyclase activity, activate phosphotyrosine phosphatases (PTPs), and modulate mitogen-activated protein kinases (MAPKs).[126, 140–142] Receptor subtypes 2 and 5 modulate K^+ and Ca^{2+} fluxes in the cell.[140] Activation of all these pathways results in inhibition of known growth factor production and release as well as antiproliferative effects.[142–145]

Somatostatin receptor subtype 3 is known to mediate PTP-dependent apoptosis accompanied by activation of p53 and Bax.[146] Four of the five somatostatin receptor subtypes (sst-2 to sst-5) undergo rapid internalization after ligand binding, which has been explored by tumor-targeted radioactive somatostatin analogue therapy.[140, 142, 147]

An antiproliferative effect has been reported, probably through a combination of receptor subtype 2 and 5 activities, which inhibits MAPK and K^+ and Ca^{2+} fluxes leading to cell cycle arrest[143–145]; the precise antitumor mechanism, however, is not known.

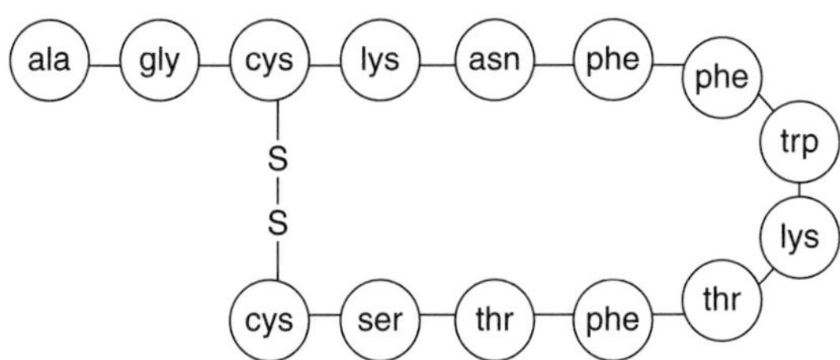

Human somatostatin

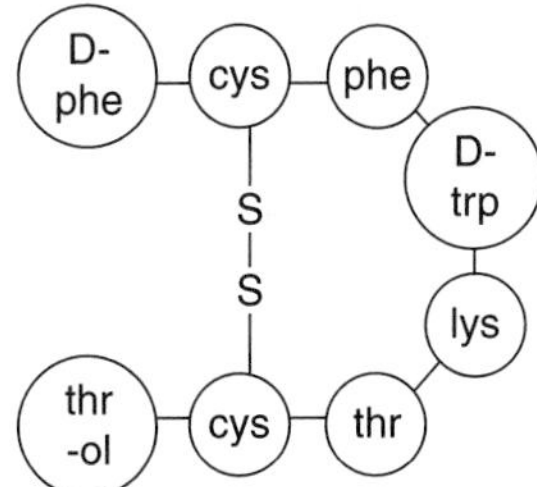

Octreotide acetate

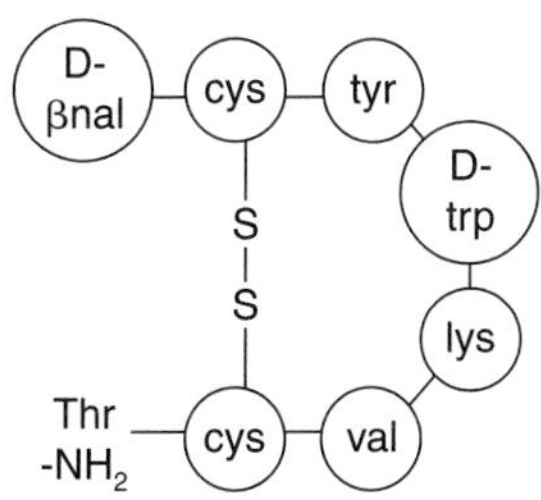

Lanreotide

Figure 41–16. Molecular structure of human somatostatin-14, octreotide acetate, and lanreotide.

It is now known that different subtypes of somatostatin receptors form heterodimers (sst-1 and sst-5) and heterodimers with dopamine receptor D2R. This cross-talk modulates the intracellular signal and gives a "fine tuning" of the mediated effects.[148]

All five subtypes of somatostatin receptors are expressed in carcinoid tumors; they are expressed in various combinations, although some tumors express all five subtypes.[140, 149–151] The receptors are expressed not only on tumor cells but also in peritumoral veins.[152] Antiangiogenesis might be another antitumor mechanism of somatostatin analogues.[153]

Subcutaneous administration of octreotide and lanreotide every 8 to 12 hours can control the clinical symptoms in about 60% to 70% of patients with the carcinoid syndrome; these agents are considered the drugs of choice.[154–159] Octreotide and lanreotide decrease serotonin and urinary 5-HIAA levels as well as plasma tachykinin and CgA levels. The recommended dose for octreotide is 100 μg two or three times a day, a standard treatment for controlling clinical symptoms.[158] However, some patients may require higher doses, up to a total of 3000 μg/day, to control the clinical symptoms and tumor growth, particularly during long-term therapy.

Tachyphylaxis (reduced sensitivity) to somatostatin analogues may develop during long-term therapy.[142] Long-acting, slow-release formulations of octreotide and lanreotide have been developed, and doses of 20 to 30 mg given once a month (octreotide) or every 2 weeks (lanreotide) control clinical symptoms and hormone levels in 50% to 60% of patients with the carcinoid syndrome.[160–162] The long-acting formulations of somatostatin analogues have clearly improved the quality of life of patients by reducing the number of injections and provide more stable control of clinical symptoms.[161]

High-dose therapy with lanreotide (12 mg/day) and octreotide (3 mg/day) has generated an increased number of significant tumor reductions (12% versus 5% for the standard dose).[163–166] Induction of apoptosis has been reported during high-dose therapy,[167] possibly mediated through activation of receptor subtype 3.

For patients at risk for carcinoid crisis, somatostatin analogue therapy is the treatment of choice. Carcinoid crisis is a life-threatening complication of the carcinoid syndrome and may occur spontaneously or may be associated with stress and anesthesia, chemotherapy, and infections (see earlier). Patients usually experience severe flushing, diarrhea, abdominal pain, and hypotension. Continuous infusion with somatostatin analogues, 50 to 100 μg/hour, is recommended and usually alters the life-threatening condition. It is also recommended that patients be given subcutaneous somatostatin analogues before surgery or before other stressful situations.

Side effects of somatostatin analogue therapy have been of a low-grade variety, occurring in 20% to 40% of patients. These include pain at the injection site, gas formation, diarrhea, and abdominal cramping. Significant long-term side effects include gallstone formation, "sludge" in the gallbladder, steatorrhea, deterioration of glucose tolerance, and hypocalcemia.[158, 160, 161] The incidence of gallstones in patients treated over the long term has varied from 5% to 70%, and the incidence of symptomatic gallstones requiring surgical treatment is less than 10%.[168]

Interferons

Interferon α—alone or in combination with somatostatin analogue—is effective in the treatment of the carcinoid syndrome. Symptomatic and biochemical control may be obtained in 40% to 50% of the patients with the recommended doses of 3 to 5 million units of recombinant interferon alfa-2a or alfa-2b three to five times per week subcutaneously.[169–175] Significant tumor reduction is reported in 10% to 20% of the patients.[169, 175]

Interferon α exerts a direct effect on the tumor cells by blocking cell division in the G1/S-phase, by inhibiting protein and hormone synthesis, and by reducing angiogenesis through inhibition of angiogenic factors b-FGF and VEGF. It has also an indirect effect through stimulation of the immune system, particularly T cells and natural killer cells.[176–179] Response to interferon α can be predicted by analyzing induction of 2′,5′-oligoadenylate synthetase or P68 (PKR) protein kinase, enzymes involved in cell cycle regulation and protein synthesis.[180, 181]

Treatment with interferon α induces an intratumoral fibrosis that is not picked up by regular CT scanning or ultrasonography; therefore, tumor size may remain unchanged.[182] The side effects of α-interferons are more pronounced than with somatostatin analogues and include chronic fatigue syndrome, anemia, leukopenia, and thrombocytopenia as well as the development of autoimmune reactions in 10% to 15% of the patients.[170, 183] Most of the side effects are dose-dependent and can be managed by individualizing the dose.

Patients with the carcinoid syndrome who have not responded to octreotide or interferon α alone may be given a combination of both agents. Such combinations have generated symptomatic control in 70% of patients and stabilization of tumor growth in 40% to 50% of patients.[184, 185] The combination also offers better tolerance of α-interferons when somato-

18. Modlin IM, Sandor A. An analysis of 8305 cases of carcinoid tumors. Cancer 1997; 79:813–829.
19. Norheim I, Oberg K, Theodorsson-Norheim E, et al. Malignant carcinoid tumors: an analysis of 103 patients with regard to tumor localization, hormone production, and survival. Ann Surg 1987; 206:215.
20. Godwin J. Carcinoid tumors: an analysis of 2837 cases of carcinoid Tumors. Cancer 1975; 36:560–569.
21. Tiensuu Janson E, Holmberg L, Stridsberg M, et al. Carcinoid tumors: an analysis of prognostic factors and survival in 301 patients from a referral center. Ann Oncol 1997; 8:685–690.
22. Sandler M, Scheuer PJ, Watt PJ. 5-Hydroxytryptophan-secreting bronchial carcinoid tumour. Lancet 1961; 2:1067–1069.
23. Oates JA, Sjoerdsma A. An unique syndrome associated with secretion of 5-hydroxytryptophan by metastatic gastric carcinoids. Am J Med 1962; 32:333–344.
24. Oates JA, Melmon KL, Sjoerdsma A. Release of a kinin peptide in the carcinoid syndrome. Lancet 1964; 1:514–517.
25. Lucas KJ, Feldman JM. Flushing in the carcinoid syndrome and plasma kallikrein. Cancer 1986; 58:2290–2293.
26. Gustafsen J, Boesby S, Nielsen F, et al. Bradykinin in carcinoid syndrome. Gut 1987; 28:1417–1419.
27. Metz SA, McRae JR, Robertson RP. Prostaglandins as mediators of paraneoplastic syndromes: review and update. Metabolism 1981; 30:299.
28. Roberts LJ II, Bloomgarden ZT, Marney SR Jr, et al. Histamine release from a gastric carcinoid: provocation by pentagastrin and inhibition by somatostatin. Gastroenterology 1983; 84:272–275.
29. Gilligan CJ, Lawton GP, Tang LH, et al. Gastric carcinoid tumors: the biology and therapy of an enigmatic and controversial lesion. Am J Gastroenterol 1995; 90:338–352.
30. Todd TR, Cooper JD, Weissberg D, et al. Bronchial carcinoid tumors: twenty years' experience. J Thorac Cardiovasc Surg 1980; 79:532–536.
31. Kema IP, deVries GE, Sloof MJH, et al. Serotonin, catecholamines, histamine, and their metabolites in urine, platelets, and tumor tissue of patients with carcinoid tumors. Clin Chem 1994; 40:86–95.
32. Håkansson R, Bergmark S, Brodin E, et al. Substance-P like immunoreactivity in intestinal carcinoid tumors. In von Euler US, Pernow B (eds). Substance-P. New York, Raven, 1977, pp 55–58.
33. Norheim I, Theodorsson-Norheim E, Brodin E, et al. Tachykinins in carcinoid tumors: use as a tumor marker and possible role in carcinoid flush. J Clin Endocrinol Metab 1986; 63:605–612.
34. Theodorsson-Norheim E, Norheim I, Öberg K, et al. Neuropeptide-K: a major tachykinin in plasma and tumor tissues from carcinoid patients. Biochem Biophys Res Comm 1985; 131:77–83.
35. Conlon JM, Deacon CF, Richter G, et al. Measurement and partial Characterization of the multiple forms of neurokinin A–like immunoreactivity in carcinoid tumors. Regul Pept 1986; 13: 183–196.
36. Becker M, Aron DC. Ectopic ACTH syndrome and CRH-mediated Cushing's syndrome. Endocrinol Metab Clin North Am 1994; 23:585.
37. Jensen RT, Norton JA. Endocrine neoplasms of the pancreas. In Yamada T, Alpers DH, Owyang C, et al (eds). Textbook of Gastroenterology. Philadelphia, JB Lippincott, 1998, p 2193.
38. Mao C, Shah A, Hanson DJ, et al. Von Recklinghausen's disease associated with duodenal somatostatinoma: contrast of duodenal versus pancreatic somatostatinoma. J Surg Oncol 1995; 59:67–73.
39. Banks P, Helle KB. The release of protein from stimulated adrenal medulla. Biochem J 1965; 97:40C–41C.
40. Fisher-Colbrie R. Chromogranins A, B, and C: widespread constituents of secretory vesicles. Ann NY Acad Sci 1987; 493:120–134.
41. Iacangelo AL, Eiden LE. Chromogranin A: current status as a precursor for bioactive peptides, a granulogenic/sorting factor in the regulated secretory pathway. Regul Pept 1995; 58:65–88.
42. Tatemoto K, Efendic S, Mutt V, et al. Pancreastatin, a novel pancreatic peptide that inhibits insulin secretion. Nature 1986; 324:476–478.
43. Angeletti RH, Mints L, Aber C, et al. Determination of residues in chromogranin A (16–40) required for inhibition of parathyroid secretion. Endocrinol 1996; 137:2918–2922.
44. Aardal S, Helle KB, Elsayed S, et al. Vasostatins comprising the *N*-terminal domain of chromogranin A, suppress tension in isolated human blood vessel segments. J Neuroendocrinol 1993; 5: 105–112.
45. Wiedenmann B, Huttner WB. Synaptophysin and chromogranins/secretogranins: widespread constituents of distinct types of neuro-endocrine vesicles and new tools in tumor diagnosis. Virchows Archiv B Cell Pathol 1989; 58:95–121.
46. Harpole DH Jr, Feldman JM, Buchanan S, et al. Bronchial carcinoid tumors: a retrospective analysis of 126 patients. Ann Thorac Surg 1992; 54:50–55.
47. Barcklay TH, Shapira DV. Malignant tumors of the small intestine. Cancer 1983; 51:878–881.
48. Moertel CG, Sauer WG, Dockerty MB, et al. Life history of the carcinoid tumor of the small intestine. Cancer 1961; 14:901–912.
49. Makridis C, Öberg K, Juhlin C, et al. Surgical treatment of midgut Carcinoid tumors. World J Surg 1990; 14:377–385.
50. Bean WB, Olch D, Weinberg HB. The syndrome of carcinoid and acquired valve lesions of the right side of the heart. Circulation 1955; 12:1–6.
51. Grahame-Smith DG. The carcinoid syndrome. Am J Cardiol 1968; 21:376.
52. Feldman JM. Carcinoid tumors and syndrome. Semin Oncol 1987; 14:237–246.
53. Smith RA. Bronchial carcinoid tumours. Thorax 1969; 24:43–50.
54. Caldarola VT, Jackman RJ, Moertel CG, et al. Carcinoid tumors of the rectum. Am J Surg 1964; 107:844–849.
55. Levin RJ, Elsas LJ, Duvall CP, et al. Malignant carcinoid tumors with and without flushing. JAMA 1963; 186:905–907.
56. Matuchansky C, Luanay JM. Serotonin, catecholamines, and spontaneous midgut carcinoid flush: plasma studies from flushing and nonflushing sites. Gastroenterology 1995; 108:743.
57. Robertson JIS, Peast WS, Andrews TM. The mechanism of facial flushes in the carcinoid syndrome. Q J Med 1962; 31:103–123.
58. Makridis C, Theodorsson E, Åkerström G, et al. Increased intestinal non-substance P tachykinin concentrations in malignant midgut carcinoid disease. J Gastroenterol Hepatol 1999; 14:500.
59. Creutzfeldt W, Stockmann F. Carcinoids and carcinoid syndrome. Am J Med 1987; 82:4.
60. Emson PC, Gilbert RF, Martensson H, et al. Elevated concentrations of substance P and 5-HT in plasma in patients with carcinoid tumors. Cancer 1984; 54:715–718.
61. Schaffalizky de Muckadell OB, Aggestrup P, Stentoft P. Flushing and plasma substance P concentration during infusion of synthetic substance P in normal man. Scand J Gastroenterol 1986; 21:498.
62. Frolich JC, Bloomgarden ZT, Oates JA, et al. The carcinoid flush: provocation by pentagastrin and inhibition by somatostatin. N Engl J Med 1978; 299:1055–1057.
63. Nawa H, Doteucki M, Iganok, et al. Substance-K: a novel mammalian tachykinin that differs from substance-P in its pharmacological profile. Life Sci 1984; 34:1153–1160.
64. Furschgott RF, Zawadski JU. The obligatory role of endothelial cells in the relaxation of arterial smooth muscle by acetylcholine. Nature 1980; 288:373–376.
65. Jensen RT. Overview of chronic diarrhea caused by functional neuroendocrine neoplasms. Semin Gastrointest Dis 1999; 10:156.
66. Donowitz M, Binder HJ. Jejunal fluid and electrolyte secretion in carcinoid syndrome. Am J Dig Dis 1975; 20:1115–1122.
67. Debonguie JC, Philips SF. Capacity of the human colon to absorb fluid. Gastroenterology 1978; 74:698–703.
68. Von der Otte MR, Camilieri M, Kvols LK, et al. Motor dysfunction of the small bowel and colon in patients with the carcinoid syndrome and diarrhea. N Engl J Med 1993; 329:1073–1078.
69. Wymenga AN, de Vries EG, Leijsma MK, et al. Effects of ondansetron on gastrointestinal symptoms in carcinoid syndrome. Eur J Cancer 1998; 34:1293.
70. Wilde MI, Markham A. Ondansetron: a review of its pharmacology and preliminary clinical findings in novel applications. Drugs 1996; 52:773.
71. Gustafsen J, Lindorf A, Raskev H, Boesby S. Ketanserin versus placebo in carcinoid syndrome: a clinical controlled trial. Scand J Gastroenterol 1986; 21:816.
72. Lundin L, Norheim I, Landelius J, et al. Carcinoid heart disease: relationship of circulating vasoactive substances to ultrasound-detectable cardiac abnormalities. Circulation 1988; 77:264–269.

73. Roberts WC, Sjoerdsma A. The cardiac disease associated with the carcinoid syndrome (carcinoid heart disease). Am J Med 1964; 36:5–34.
74. Ferrans VJ, Roberts WC. The carcinoid endocardial plaque: an ultrastructural study. Hum Pathol 1976; 7:387–409.
75. Lundin L, Landelius J, Andren B, et al. Transoesophageal echocardiography improves the diagnostic value of cardiac ultrasound in patients with carcinoid heart disease. Br Heart J 1990; 64:190–194.
76. Waltenberger J, Lundin L, Öberg K, et al. Involvement of transforming growth factor-β in the formation of fibrotic lesions in carcinoid heart disease. Am J Pathol 1993; 142:71–78.
77. Robiolo PA, Rigolin VH, Wilson JS, et al. Carcinoid heart disease: correlation of high serotonin levels with valvular abnormalities deleted by cardiac catheterization and echocardiography. Circulation 1995; 92:790–795.
78. Connoly HM, Crary JL, McGoon MD, et al. Valvular heart disease associated with fenfluramine-phentermine. N Engl J Med 1997; 337:581–588. (Erratum, N Engl J Med 1997; 337:1783.)
79. Khan MA, Herzog CA, St. Peter JV, et al. The prevalence of cardiac valvular insufficiency assessed by transthoracic echocardiography in obese patients treated with appetite-suppressant drugs. N Engl J Med 1998; 339:713–718.
80. Pellikka PA, Tajik AJ, Khandheria BK, et al. Carcinoid heart disease: clinical and echocardiographic spectrum in 74 patients. Circulation 1993; 87:1188–1196.
81. Hua XI, Lundberg JM, Theodorsson-Norheim E, et al. Comparison of cardiovascular and bronchoconstrictor effects of substance P, substance K, and other tachykinins. Naunyn Schmiedebergs Arch Pharmacol 1984; 328:196–201.
82. Gardner B, Dollinger M, Silen W, et al. Studies of the carcinoid syndrome: its relationship to serotonin, bradykinin, and histamine. Surgery 1967; 61:846–852.
83. Vinik AK, McLeod MK, Fig LM, et al. Clinical features, diagnosis, and localization of carcinoid tumors and their management. Gastroenterol Clin North Am 1989; 18:865–896.
84. Andaker L, Lamke LO, Smeds S. Follow-up of 102 patients operated on for gastrointestinal carcinoid. Acta Chir Scand 1985; 151:469.
85. Kvols LK, Martin JK, Mash HM, et al. Rapid reversal of carcinoid crisis with a somatostatin analogue (letter). N Engl J Med 1985; 313:1229–1230.
86. Vaughan DJ, Brunner MD. Anasthesia for patients with carcinoid syndrome. Int Anesthesiol Clin 1997; 35:129.
87. Veall GRQ, Peacock JE, Bax NDS, et al. Review of the anaesthetic management of 21 patients undergoing laparotomy for carcinoid syndrome. Br J Anaesth 1994; 72:335.
88. Harris AG, Redfern JS. Octreotide treatment of carcinoid syndrome: analysis of published dose-titration data. Aliment Pharmacol Ther 1995; 9:387.
89. Kvols LK. Therapy of the malignant carcinoid syndrome. Endocrinol Metab Clin North Am 1989; 18:557.
90. Roberts LJ, Marney SR Jr, Oates JA. Blockade of the flush associated with metastatic gastric carcinoid by combined histamine H_1 and H_2 receptor antagonists: evidence for an important role of H_2 receptors in human vasculature. N Engl J Med 1979; 300: 236–238.
91. Limper AH, Carpenter PC, Scheithauer B, et al. The Cushing syndrome induced by bronchial carcinoid tumors. Ann Intern Med 1992; 117:209–214.
92. Carroll DG, Delahunt JW, Teague CA, et al. Resolution of acromegaly after removal of a bronchial carcinoid shown to secrete growth hormone–releasing factor. Aust N Z J Med 1987; 17:63–67.
93. Rindi G, Bordi C, Rappel S, et al. Gastric carcinoids and neuroendocrine carcinoma pathogenesis, pathology, and behaviour. World J Surg 1996; 20:168.
94. Granberg D, Wilander E, Stridsberg M, et al. Clinical symptoms, hormone profiles, treatment, and prognosis in patients with gastric carcinoids. Gut 1998; 43:223.
95. Thomas RM, Baybick JH, Elsayed AM, et al. Gastric carcinoids: an immunohistochemical and clinicopathologic study of 104 patients. Cancer 1994; 73:2053–2058.
96. Sjoblom SM, Sipponen P, Karonen SL, et al. Mucosal argyrophil endocrine cells in pernicious anaemia and upper gastrointestinal carcinoid tumors. J Clin Pathol 1989; 42:371–377.
97. Solcia E, Fiocca R, Villani L, et al. Morphology and pathogenesis of endocrine hyperplasia, precarcinoid lesions, and carcinoids arising in chronic atrophic gastritis. Scand J Gastroenterol Suppl 1991; 180:146–159.
98. Havu N. Enterochromaffin-like cell carcinoids of gastric mucosa in rats after life-long inhibition of gastric secretion. Digestion 1986; 35(Suppl 1):42–55.
99. Rindi G, Luinetti O, Cornaggia M, et al. Three subtypes of gastric argyrophil carcinoid and the gastric neuroendocrine carcinoma: a clinicopathologic study. Gastroenterology 1993; 104: 994–1006.
100. Thompson GB, Van Heerden JA, Martin JK Jr, et al. Carcinoid tumors of the gastrointestinal tract: presentation management, and prognosis. Surgery 1985; 98:1054.
101. Chaudhry A, Oberg K, Wilander E, et al. A study of biological behaviour based on the expression of a proliferating antigen in neuroendocrine tumors of the digestive system. Tumour Biol 1992; 13:27.
102. von Herbay A, Sieg B, Shurmann G, et al. Proliferative activity of neuroendocrine tumours of the gastroenteropancreatic endocrine system: DNA flow cytometric and immunohistological investigations. Gut 1991; 32:949.
103. Chaudry A, Öberg K, Gobl A, et al. Expression of transforming growth factors β_1, β_2, β_3, in neuroendocrine of the digestive tract. Anticancer Res 1994; 14:2085–2092.
104. Granberg D, Wilander E, Öberg K, Skogseid B. Prognostic markers in patients in patients with typical bronchial carcinoid tumors. J Clin Endocrinol Metab 2000; 85:3425–3430.
105. Patel YC, Srikant CB. Somatostatin receptors. Trends Endocrinol Metab 1997; 8:398–405.
106. Schaer JC, Waser B, Mengod G, Reubi JC. Somatostatin receptor subtypes, sst_1, sst_2, sst_1, sst_5 expression in human pituitary, gastro-entero-pancreatic, and mammary tumors: comparison of mRNA analysis with receptor autoradiography. Int J Cancer 1997; 50:530–537.
107. Feldman JM. Urinary serotonin in the diagnosis of carcinoid tumors. Clin Chem 1986; 32:840.
108. Mailman RB, Kilts CD. Analytical considerations for quantitative determination of serotonin and its metabolically related products in biological matrices. Clin Chem 1985; 31:1849–1854.
109. Nuttall KL, Pingree SS. The incidence of elevations in urine 5-hydroxyindoleacetic acid. Am J Clin Nutr 1985; 42:639.
110. De Vries EGE, Kema IP, Slooff MJH, et al. Recent developments in diagnosis and treatment of metastatic carcinoid tumors. J Gastroenterol 1993; 28:87.
111. Stridsberg M, Öberg K, Li Q, et al. Measurements of chromogranin A, chromogranin B (secretogranin I), chromogranin C (secretogranin II), and pancreastatin in plasma and urine from patients with carcinoid tumors and endocrine pancreatic tumors. J Endocrinol 1995; 144:49–59.
112. Nobels FR, Kwekkeboom DJ, Coopmans W, et al. Chromogranin A as serum marker for neuroendocrine neoplasia: comparison with neuron-specific enolase and the alpha-subunit of glycoprotein hormones. J Clin Endocrinol Metab 1997; 82:2622.
113. Baudin E, Gigliotti A, Ducreux M, et al. Neuron-specific enolase and chromogranin A as markers of neuroendocrine tumours. Br J Cancer 1998; 78:1102.
114. Öberg K, Stridsberg M. Chromogranins as diagnostic and prognostic markers in neuroendocrine tumours. Adv Exp Med Biol 2000; 482:329–337.
115. Grossman M, Trautmann ME, Poertl S, et al. Alpha-subunit and human chorionic gonadotropin-β immunoreactivity in patients with malignant endocrine gastroentero-pancreatic tumours. Eur J Clin Invest 1994; 24:131.
116. Feldman JM, O'Dorisio TM. Role of neuropeptides and serotonin in the diagnosis of carcinoid tumors. Am J Med 1986; 81: 41.
117. Öberg K, Grimelius L, Lundquist G, et al. Update on pancreatic polypeptide as a specific marker for endocrine tumours of the pancreas and gut. Acta Medica Scand 1981; 210:145–152.
118. Mani S, Modlin IM, Ballantyne G, et al. Carcinoids of the rectum. J Am Coll Surg 1994; 179:231–248.
119. Krenning EP, Kwekkeboom DJ, Oei HY, et al. Somatostatin-receptor scintigraphy in gastroenteropancreatic tumors. Ann N Y Acad Sci 1994; 733:416.
120. Westlin JE, Janson ET, Arnberg H, et al. Somatostatin receptor